Selected Emergency Antidotes With Common Initial Doses[a]

Antidote	Indication and Dose	
N-Acetylcysteine	**Acetaminophen:** *Adults IV:* 150 mg/kg in 200 mL D_5W infused over 60 min followed by 50 mg/kg in 1,000 mL D_5W over 16 h. *Oral:* 140 mg/kg followed by 70 mg/kg every 4 h for 17 doses. **NOTE:** Special IV dilution required for children: www.acetadote.com/dosecalc.php.	
Atropine	**Cholinesterase inhibitors:** *Adults:* 1–2 mg (mild) or 3–5 mg (severe) IV, doubled every 3–5 min until bronchorrhea resolves. *Children:* 20 mcg/kg up to adult dose IV, doubled as for adults. Also for other cholinergics in similar dosing.	1503
L-Carnitine	**Valproic acid–induced hyperammonemia or valproic acid–induced elevated AST/ALT:** *Clinically ill:* 100 mg/kg (up to 6 g) infused IV over 30 min, followed by 15 mg/kg infused over 30 min every 6 h. *Clinically well:* 100 mg/kg/day given orally in divided dose every 8 h up to 3 g/day.	732
Deferoxamine	**Iron:** Begin continuous IV infusion at 5 mg/kg/h; titrate to 15 mg/kg/h as tolerated with a total dose of 6–8 g/for no more than 24 h	676
Digoxin-specific antibody fragments (Fab)	**Digoxin:** Known concentration: # of vials = Weight (kg) × Concentration (ng/mL)/100 rounded up to nearest vial. Empiric dosing: Acute: 10–20 vials. Chronic: *Adults:* 3–6 vials; *Children:* 1–2 vials. Usually given as IV infusion over 30 min. An IV bolus is acceptable for cardiac arrest. **NOTE:** For nondigoxin cardioactive steroids, use empiric dose.	977
Dimercaprol (BAL)	**Lead encephalopathy:** 75 mg/m² (~4 mg/kg) deep IM every 4 h. First dose to precede edetate calcium disodium ($CaNa_2EDTA$) by 4 h. Contraindicated if peanut allergy.	1251
Edetate calcium disodium ($CaNa_2EDTA$)	**Lead encephalopathy:** 1500 mg/m²/day (~50–75 mg/kg/day) as a continuous IV infusion (≤0.5% solution); maximum dose, 3 g/day; reduce dose if impaired kidney function. **NOTE:** Dimercaprol should be administered 4 h before starting this dose.	1315
Fomepizole	**Methanol or ethylene glycol:** 15 mg/kg diluted in 100 mL 0.9% NaCl or D_5W infused IV over 30 min; after 12 h, give next 4 doses at 10 mg/kg every 12 h; additional doses at 15 mg/kg every 12 h if needed. Adjust dose during hemodialysis.	1435
Glucagon	**β-Adrenergic antagonists or calcium channel blockers:** IV infusion over 3–10 min. *Adults and Children:* 50 mcg/kg. Repeat in 10 min for 1–2 doses as needed. Dose up to 10 mg are reasonable in an adult. Follow with a continuous infusion at 2–10 mg/h based on response. Emesis should be expected with higher doses and rates of administration.	941
Hydroxocobalamin	**Cyanide:** *Adults:* 5 g reconstituted with 200 mL 0.9% NaCl (invert for 60 sec) and infuse IV over 15 min. *Children:* 70 mg/kg up to 5 g. Repeat second dose as needed.	1694
Insulin (High-dose insulin {HDI}	**Calcium channel blockers or β-adrenergic antagonists:** 1 unit/kg IV bolus regular human insulin. Follow with infusion of 1 unit/kg/h. Use 10 units/mL insulin concentration. Titrate to 2 units/kg/h if no improvement in 15 min and titrate up to 10 units/kg/h as needed. If glucose <300 mg/dL, give 0.5 g/kg $D_{50}W$ bolus. Start 0.5 g/kg/h dextrose infusion. If glucose >300 mg/dL, hold glucose. Monitor glucose every 15–30 min until stable; then every 1–2 h. Maintain glucose 100–250 mg/dL. Monitor K^+ frequently to maintain K^+ in the "mildly hypokalemic" range (2.8–3.2 mEq/L).	953
Leucovorin (folinic acid)	**Methotrexate:** 100 mg/m² infused IV over 15–30 min every 3–6 h for several days or until serum methotrexate concentration $<0.01 \times 10^{-6}$ mol/L in the absence of bone marrow toxicity.	775
Lipid emulsion	**Cardiac arrest from lipid soluble xenobiotic (CCB, CA, local anesthetics):** Lipid emulsion 20% 1.5 mL/kg IV over 1 min. Follow with infusion at a rate of 0.25 mL/kg/min (15 mL/kg/h) over 30–60 min while continuing chest compressions. Repeat bolus for severe persistent symptoms.	1004
Methylene blue	**Methemoglobinemia:** 1 mg/kg (0.1 mL/kg) of 1% methylene blue IV over 5 min followed by a 30-mL fluid flush of 0.9% sodium chloride.	1713
Naloxone	**Opioid-induced respiratory depression:** *Adults:* 40–50 mcg (0.04–0.05 mg) IV titrated upward to reversal. Avoid opioid withdrawal and provide manual ventilation. *Children:* not receiving chronic opioids 0.1 mg/kg IV titrated as for adults.	538
Nitrites and sodium thiosulfate	**Cyanide:** *Adults:* (1) Sodium nitrite: 300 mg (10 mL of a 3% concentration) infused IV over 2–5 min. (2) Sodium thiosulfate: 12.5 g (50 mL of a 25% solution) infused IV over 10–30 min or as a bolus. *Children:* (1) Sodium nitrite: 6–8 mL/m² (0.2 mL/kg) of a 3% conc (maximum, 300 mg) infused IV over 2–5 min. (2) Sodium thiosulfate: 7 g/m² (0.5 g/kg) (maximum, 12.5 g) infused over 10–30 min or as a bolus. **NOTE:** In both adults and children, avoid sodium nitrite when carboxyhemoglobin is expected to be elevated.	1698
Octreotide	**Sulfonylurea-induced hypoglycemia:** *Adults:* 50 mcg SC every 6 h. *Children:* 1.25 mcg/kg (maximum, 50 mcg) SC every 6 h.	713
Physostigmine	**Anticholinergic syndrome:** IV infusion over 5 min. *Adults:* 1–2 mg. *Children:* 20 mcg/kg (maximum, 0.5 mg). Repeat the dose in 5–10 min if an adequate response is not achieved and cholinergic effects are not noted.	755
Pralidoxime	**Cholinesterase inhibitors:** *Adults:* 30 mg/kg (up to 2 g) over 15–30 min followed by a maintenance infusion of 8–10 mg/kg/h (up to 650 mg/h) for sickest patients. *Children:* 30 mg/kg (maximum, 2 g) infused IV over 15–30 min and then 10–20 mg/kg/h (maximum, 650 mg/h).	1508
Pyridoxine	**Isoniazid:** 1 g for each gram of isoniazid up to 70 mg/kg (maximum, 5 g) infused IV at 0.5 g/min until seizures stop, with the remainder infused IV over 4–6 h. Empiric dose: *Adults:* 5 g. *Children:* 70 mg/kg (maximum, 5 g) at specific dosing rate. Repeat dose 1–2 times if needed for the treatment of seizures or persistent depressed level of consciousness. Comparable therapy should be used following gyromitrin poisoning.	862
Succimer	**Lead poisoning:** *Adults and Children >5 years old:* 10 mg/kg orally every 8 h for 5 days followed by 10 mg/kg orally every 12 h for 14 days. *Children <5 years old:* 350 mg/m² orally as for adults.	1309

[a]Consult pages listed for complete information regarding dose, route, duration of therapy, adverse effects, safety issues, contraindications, and other considerations. For up-to-date information, contact your regional poison center at 800-222-1222 or a medical toxicologist.

CCB = calcium channel blocker; D_5W = dextrose 5% in water; $D_{50}W$ = dextrose 50% in water; IM = intramuscular; IV = intravenous; SC = subcutaneous; TCA, tricyclic antidepressant.

GOLDFRANK'S TOXICOLOGIC EMERGENCIES

EDITORS

First Edition
Lewis R. Goldfrank, MD, Robert Kirstein, MD

Second Edition
Lewis R. Goldfrank, MD, Neal E. Flomenbaum, MD, Neal A. Lewin, MD, Richard S. Weisman, PharmD

Third Edition
Lewis R. Goldfrank, MD, Neal E. Flomenbaum, MD, Neal A. Lewin, MD, Richard S. Weisman, PharmD, Mary Ann Howland, PharmD, Alan G. Kulberg, MD

Fourth Edition
Lewis R. Goldfrank, MD, Neal E. Flomenbaum, MD, Neal A. Lewin, MD, Richard S. Weisman, PharmD, Mary Ann Howland, PharmD

Fifth Edition
Lewis R. Goldfrank, MD, Neal E. Flomenbaum, MD, Neal A. Lewin, MD, Richard S. Weisman, PharmD, Mary Ann Howland, PharmD, Robert S. Hoffman, MD

Sixth Edition
Lewis R. Goldfrank, MD, Neal E. Flomenbaum, MD, Neal A. Lewin, MD, Richard S. Weisman, PharmD, Mary Ann Howland, PharmD, Robert S. Hoffman, MD

Seventh Edition
Lewis R. Goldfrank, MD, Neal E. Flomenbaum, MD, Neal A. Lewin, MD, Mary Ann Howland, PharmD, Robert S. Hoffman, MD, Lewis S. Nelson, MD

Eighth Edition
Neal E. Flomenbaum, MD, Lewis R. Goldfrank, MD, Robert S. Hoffman, MD, Mary Ann Howland, PharmD, Neal A. Lewin, MD, Lewis S. Nelson, MD

Ninth Edition
Lewis S. Nelson, MD, Neal A. Lewin, MD, Mary Ann Howland, PharmD, Robert S. Hoffman, MD, Lewis R. Goldfrank, MD, Neal E. Flomenbaum, MD

Tenth Edition
Robert S. Hoffman, MD, Mary Ann Howland, PharmD, Neal A. Lewin, MD, Lewis S. Nelson, MD, Lewis R. Goldfrank, MD, Neal E. Flomenbaum, MD (Editor Emeritus)

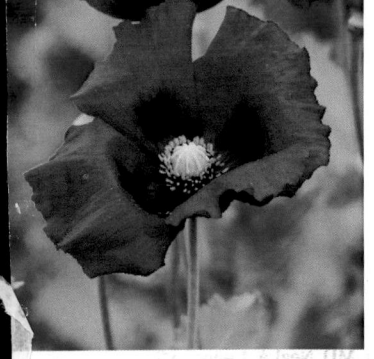

GOLDFRANK'S TOXICOLOGIC EMERGENCIES

Eleventh Edition

LEWIS S. NELSON, MD, FAACT, FACEP, FACMT, FAAEM, FASAM
Professor and Chair of Emergency Medicine
Department of Emergency Medicine
Director, Division of Medical Toxicology
Rutgers New Jersey Medical School
Chief of Service, Emergency Department
University Hospital of Newark
New Jersey Poison Information & Education System
Newark, New Jersey

MARY ANN HOWLAND, PharmD, DABAT, FAACT
Clinical Professor of Pharmacy
St. John's University College of Pharmacy and Health Sciences
Adjunct Professor of Emergency Medicine
Ronald O. Perelman Department of Emergency Medicine
New York University School of Medicine
Bellevue Hospital Center and New York University Langone Health
Senior Consultant in Residence
New York City Poison Control Center
New York, New York

NEAL A. LEWIN, MD, FACEP, FACMT, FACP
Druckenmiller Professor of Emergency Medicine and Medicine
Ronald O. Perelman Department of Emergency Medicine
New York University School of Medicine
Director, Didactic Education
Emergency Medicine Residency
Attending Physician, Emergency Medicine and Internal Medicine
Bellevue Hospital Center and New York University Langone Health
New York, New York

SILAS W. SMITH, MD, FACEP, FACMT
JoAnn G. and Kenneth Wellner Associate Professor of Emergency Medicine
Ronald O. Perelman Department of Emergency Medicine
New York University School of Medicine
Section Chief, Quality, Safety, and Practice Innovation
Attending Physician, Emergency Medicine
Bellevue Hospital Center and New York University Langone Health
New York, New York

LEWIS R. GOLDFRANK, MD, FAAEM, FAACT, FACEP, FACMT, FACP
Herbert W. Adams Professor of Emergency Medicine
Ronald O. Perelman Department of Emergency Medicine
New York University School of Medicine
Attending Physician, Emergency Medicine
Bellevue Hospital Center and New York University Langone Health
Medical Director, New York City Poison Control Center
New York, New York

ROBERT S. HOFFMAN, MD, FAACT, FACMT, FRCP Edin, FEAPCCT
Professor of Emergency Medicine and Medicine
Ronald O. Perelman Department of Emergency Medicine
New York University School of Medicine
Director, Division of Medical Toxicology
Attending Physician, Emergency Medicine
Bellevue Hospital Center and New York University Langone Health
New York, New York

Editor Emeritus

NEAL E. FLOMENBAUM, MD, FACP, FACEP
Professor of Clinical Medicine
Weill Cornell Medical College of Cornell University
Physician-in-Chief, Emergency Medical Services
Emergency Physician-in-Chief (1996-2016)
New York-Presbyterian Hospital
Weill Cornell Medical Center
New York, New York

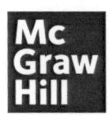
New York   Chicago   San Francisco   Athens   London   Madrid   Mexico City
Milan   New Delhi   Singapore   Sydney   Toronto

Goldfrank's Toxicologic Emergencies, Eleventh Edition

5 6 7 8 9   DUN   26 25 24 23

ISBN 978-1-259-85961-8
MHID 1-259-85961-4

NOTICE

Medicine is an ever-changing science. As new research and clinical experience broaden our knowledge, changes in treatment and drug therapy are required. The authors and the publisher of this work have checked with sources believed to be reliable in their efforts to provide information that is complete and generally in accord with the standards accepted at the time of publication. However, in view of the possibility of human error or changes in medical sciences, neither the authors nor the publisher nor any other party who has been involved in the preparation or publication of this work warrants that the information contained herein is in every respect accurate or complete, and they disclaim all responsibility for any errors or omissions or for the results obtained from use of the information contained in this work. Readers are encouraged to confirm the information contained herein with other sources. For example and in particular, readers are advised to check the product information sheet included in the package of each drug they plan to administer to be certain that the information contained in this work is accurate and that changes have not been made in the recommended dose or in the contraindications for administration. This recommendation is of particular importance in connection with new or infrequently used drugs.

This book was set in Kepler Std by Cenveo® Publisher Services.
The editors were Karen G. Edmonson and Robert Pancotti.
The production supervisor was Catherine H. Saggese.
Project management was provided by Revathi Viswanathan, Cenveo Publisher Services.
The text designer was Mary McKeon; the cover designer was W2 Design.
The main image on the cover is provided and used with permission and courtesy of Steven Foster. Mr. Foster is a photographer and medicinal plant specialist.

Library of Congress Cataloging-in-Publication Data

Names: Nelson, Lewis, 1963- editor.
Title: Goldfrank's toxicologic emergencies / [edited by] Lewis S. Nelson [and 6 others].
Other titles: Toxicologic emergencies
Description: Eleventh edition. | New York : McGraw-Hill Education, [2019] |
    Includes bibliographical references and index.
Identifiers: LCCN 2018003226| ISBN 9781259859618 (hardcover : alk. paper) |
    ISBN 1259859614 (hardcover : alk. paper)
Subjects: | MESH: Emergencies | Poisoning | Poisons | Case Reports
Classification: LCC RA1224.5 | NLM QV 600 | DDC 615.9/08—dc23
LC record available at https://lccn.loc.gov/2018003226

Neal E. Flomenbaum, MD, FACP, FACEP
Editor Emeritus

With the publication of the ninth edition of *Goldfrank's Toxicologic Emergencies*, Neal Flomenbaum informed us of his decision to step down as an editor in order to be able to devote more time to his growing interests in geriatric emergency medicine and prehospital care, while continuing to fulfill his clinical and administrative responsibilities as Chief of Emergency Medicine at New York Presbyterian Hospital-Weill Cornell Medical Center and as Medical Director of its extensive prehospital care system.

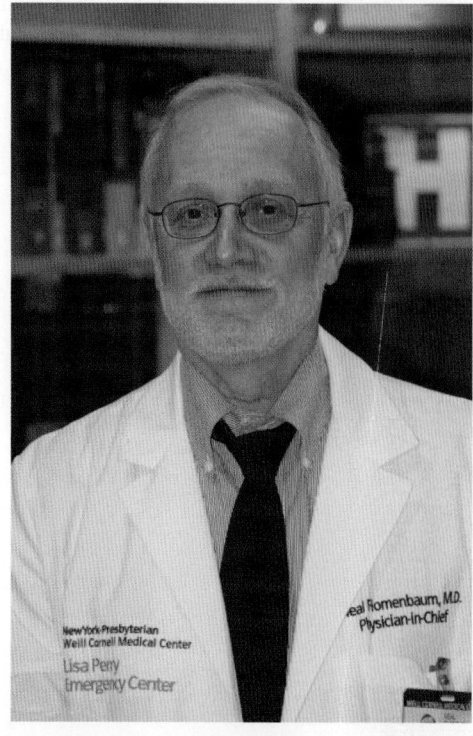

In 1979, Dr. Flomenbaum accepted an offer from Lewis Goldfrank to join him at New York University Bellevue Hospital as Associate Director of Emergency Services and Consultant (later, Chief Consultant) to the New York City Poison Control Center, and their subsequent collaborations resulted in many of the outstanding features of this textbook. Frequently, ideas and concepts Neal and Lewis developed for presenting clinical toxicology were recognized for their value to the textbook and then developed further by both, with considerable input and efforts by Neal Lewin, Richard Weisman, Mary Ann Howland, Robert Hoffman, and Lewis Nelson. Thus, an idea for a 1984 review article entitled "Newer Antidotes and Controversies in Antidotal Therapy," written to familiarize clinicians with the appropriate use of antidotes in patient management, became "Antidotes in Depth," a signature feature of this book.

Similarly, the idea for an organ system track in the NYU postgraduate toxicology courses that Neal and Lewis codirected in the early 1980s became "The Pathophysiologic Basis of Medical Toxicology: The Organ System Approach" in the textbook. This section, in turn, suggested another section entitled "The Biochemical and Molecular Basis of Medical Toxicology."

Additional ideas followed for making *Goldfrank's Toxicologic Emergencies* more accessible both as a teaching and a reference resource. A monthly case-based consultants' meeting at the New York City Poison Control Center was modeled after the successful format originated in the first edition of this book, and many of the cases discussed there were adapted for the text and related review books. Placing essential reference tables on the inside front and back covers of the textbook proved to be another useful feature, and Neal is particularly proud of the unique way the textbook acknowledges previous authors at the end of chapters. In addition to his ideas and his organizational and editorial contributions, Neal has written, coauthored, or contributed to dozens of chapters since 1982, including those on salicylates, rodenticides, and managing the acutely poisoned or overdosed patient.

In 1996, Neal Flomenbaum became the first Emergency Physician-in-Chief at New York Presbyterian Hospital/Weill Cornell Medical Center and built a multidisciplinary emergency department of over 50 attending emergency physicians, residents, nurses, nurse practitioners, physician assistants, paramedics, and EMTs. He created, developed, and supported traditional and nontraditional subspecialties and fellowships in pediatric emergency medicine, medical toxicology, prehospital care, global emergency medicine, geriatric emergency medicine, wilderness and environmental emergency medicine, and EM/critical care, each of which was heavily infused with the knowledge and information of age-specific poisonings, overdoses, adverse effects and drug interactions, polypharmacy, and environmental hazards found in these pages. Many of the faculty, in turn, have contributed to chapters in this textbook and peer-reviewed research papers in medial toxicology. These activities culminated in the establishment of an academic department of emergency medicine at Weill Cornell in early 2016. That same year, Neal received the Lifetime Achievement award from his alma mater, the Albert Einstein College of Medicine and, in 2015, the annual "Neal Flomenbaum, MD Prize for Excellence in Emergency Medicine" was established at Weill Cornell commencements.

Neal Flomenbaum first became interested in medical toxicology because of the clinical challenges it presented to emergency physicians, internists, and pediatricians, and he has remained focused on these clinical aspects. His creative energies, talents, and contributions to the second through ninth editions of this book have helped transform a case-based introduction to clinical toxicology into the 2000-page textbook it is today, and these contributions will remain an important part of future editions.

The cover image is the *Papaver somniferum* and is the source of opium. The plant is native to Southwestern Asia, but now grown around the globe. Its products have been used medicinally and recreationally for thousands of years. The beautiful flowers lose their petals with a resultant green capsule, which when lanced exudes the highly viscous opium. Opium contains numerous alkaloids of which morphine, codeine, papaverine, and thebaine are the most medically consequential. Morphine is an opioid agonist analgesic, which when diacetylated produces heroin. Naloxone, a pure opioid antagonist and derivative of thebaine, reverses most of the clinical effects of opioid agonists. Opioids in almost all forms are used with remarkable success for acute pain and conversely, misused and abused with tragic implications for patients, families, and society. The safe and appropriate use of the products and derivatives of *Papaver somniferum* will define much of the work of toxicologists in the twenty-first century.

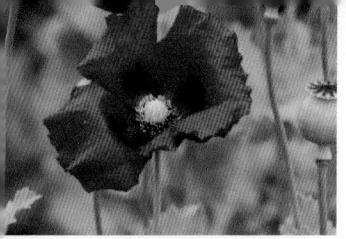

DEDICATION

To the staffs of our hospitals, emergency departments, intensive care units, and outpatient sites, who have worked with remarkable courage, concern, compassion, and understanding in treating the patients discussed in this text and many thousands more like them.

To the Emergency Medical Services personnel who have worked so faithfully and courageously to protect our patients' health and who have assisted us in understanding what happens in the home and the field.

To the staff of the New York City Poison Control Center, who have quietly and conscientiously integrated their skills with ours to serve these patients and prevent many patients from ever requiring a hospital visit.

To all the faculty, fellows, residents, nurses, nurse practitioners, physician assistants, and medical and pharmacy students who have studied toxicology with us, whose inquisitiveness has helped us continually strive to understand complex and evolving problems and develop methods to teach them to others. (Editors)

To my wife Laura for her unwavering support; to my children Daniel, Adina, and Benjamin for their fresh perspective, youthful insight, and appreciation of my passion; to my parents Myrna of blessed memory and Dr. Irwin Nelson for the foundation they provided; and to my family, friends, and colleagues who keep me focused on what is important in life. (L.N.)

To my husband Bob; to my children Robert, Marcy and Doug and my grandchildren Joey and Mackenzie; to my mother and to the loving memory of my father; and to family, friends, colleagues, and students for all their help and continuing inspiration. (M.A.H.)

To my wife Gail Miller; my sons Jesse Miller Lewin, MD and Justin Miller Lewin, MD and my daughters-in-law Alana Amarosa Lewin, MD and Alice Tang, MD; my granddaughter Isabelle Rose Lewin; and in memory of my parents. To all my patients, students, residents, fellows, and colleagues who constantly stimulate my being a perpetual student. (N.L.)

To my wife Helen, for her resolute support and understanding; to my children Addison and Alston, for their boundless enthusiasm and inquisitiveness; and to my parents. (S.W.S.)

To my children Rebecca and Ryan, Jennifer, Andrew and Joan, Michelle and James; to my grandchildren Benjamin, Adam, Sarah, Kay, Samantha, Herbert, Jonah, Susie, and Sasha, who have kept me acutely aware of the ready availability of possible poisons; and to my wife, partner, and best friend Susan (deceased) whose support was essential to help me in the development of the first ten editions and whose contributions continue to inspire me and will be found throughout the text. (L.G.)

To my wife Ali; my children Casey and Jesse; my parents; and my friends, family, and colleagues for their never-ending patience and forgiveness for the time I have spent away from them; to the many close colleagues and committee members who have helped me understand the fundamentals of evidence-based medicine and challenged me to be clear, precise, and definitive when making treatment recommendations. (R.S.H.)

To the memory of Louis R. Cantilena, MD, PhD. Lou was a wonderful collaborator, thoughtful intellectual, clinical pharmacologist and medical toxicologist who was a critical author for the previous five editions of our textbook. His warmth, enthusiasm and intellect will be missed.

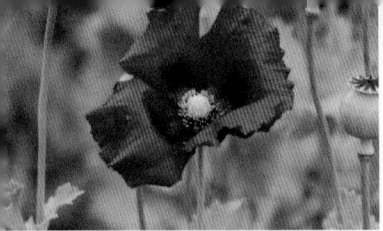

ANTIDOTES IN DEPTH

Editors: Mary Ann Howland and Silas W. Smith

Readers of previous editions of *Goldfrank's Toxicologic Emergencies* are undoubtedly aware that the editors have always felt that an emphasis on general management of patients who are poisoned or overdosed coupled with sound medical management is as important as the selection and use of a specific antidote. Nevertheless, there are some instances when nothing other than the timely use of a specific antidote is an essential lifesaving

intervention. For this reason, and also because the use of such strategies are often problematic, controversial, or unfamiliar to the practitioner as new therapeutic approaches continue to emerge and old standards are reevaluated, we have included a section (or sections) at the end of appropriate chapters in which an in-depth discussion of such material is relevant.

TABLE OF ANTIDOTES IN DEPTH

N-ACETYLCYSTEINE 492
Robert G. Hendrickson and Mary Ann Howland

ACTIVATED CHARCOAL 76
Silas W. Smith and Mary Ann Howland

ANTIVENOM FOR NORTH AMERICAN
VENOMOUS SNAKES (CROTALINE
AND ELAPID) 1627
Anthony F. Pizon and Anne-Michelle Ruha

ANTIVENOM: SCORPION.........................1563
Michael A. Darracq and Richard F. Clark

ANTIVENOM: SPIDER..............................1559
Michael A. Darracq and Richard F. Clark

ATROPINE..1503
Mary Ann Howland

BENZODIAZEPINES 1135
Fiona Garlich Horner, Robert S. Hoffman,
Lewis S. Nelson, and Mary Ann Howland

BOTULINUM ANTITOXIN..........................586
Silas W. Smith and Howard L. Geyer

CALCIUM 1403
Silas W. Smith and Mary Ann Howland

L-CARNITINE 732
Mary Ann Howland

DANTROLENE SODIUM 1029
Caitlin J. Guo and Kenneth M. Sutin

DEFEROXAMINE 676
Mary Ann Howland

DEXTROSE (D-GLUCOSE) 707
Vincent Nguyen and Larissa I. Velez

DIGOXIN-SPECIFIC ANTIBODY
FRAGMENTS 977
Silas W. Smith and Mary Ann Howland

DIMERCAPROL (BRITISH ANTI-LEWISITE
OR BAL) 1251
Mary Ann Howland

EDETATE CALCIUM DISODIUM
(CaNa$_2$EDTA) 1315
Mary Ann Howland

ETHANOL 1440
Mary Ann Howland

FLUMAZENIL 1094
Mary Ann Howland

FOLATES: LEUCOVORIN (FOLINIC ACID) AND
FOLIC ACID 775
Silas W. Smith and Mary Ann Howland

FOMEPIZOLE 1435
Mary Ann Howland

GLUCAGON 941
Mary Ann Howland and Silas W. Smith

GLUCARPIDASE (CARBOXYPEPTIDASE G$_2$) 782
Silas W. Smith

HIGH-DOSE INSULIN (HDI) 953
Samuel J. Stellpflug and William Kerns II

HYDROXOCOBALAMIN 1694
Mary Ann Howland

HYPERBARIC OXYGEN 1676
Stephen R. Thom

LIPID EMULSION....................................1004
Sophie Gosselin and Theodore C. Bania

MAGNESIUM 876
Silas W. Smith

METHYLENE BLUE 1713
Mary Ann Howland

NITRITES (AMYL AND SODIUM) AND
SODIUM THIOSULFATE.............................1698
Mary Ann Howland

OCTREOTIDE 713
Silas W. Smith and Mary Ann Howland

OPIOID ANTAGONISTS 538
Lewis S. Nelson and Mary Ann Howland

PENTETIC ACID OR PENTETATE (ZINC OR
CALCIUM) TRISODIUM (DTPA) 1779
Joseph G. Rella

PHYSOSTIGMINE SALICYLATE 755
Mary Ann Howland

POTASSIUM IODIDE 1775
Joseph G. Rella

PRALIDOXIME 1508
Mary Ann Howland

PROTAMINE 919
Mary Ann Howland

PROTHROMBIN COMPLEX CONCENTRATES
AND DIRECT ORAL ANTICOAGULANT
ANTIDOTES..908
Betty C. Chen and Mark K. Su

PRUSSIAN BLUE 1357
Robert S. Hoffman

PYRIDOXINE 862
Mary Ann Howland

SODIUM BICARBONATE 567
Paul M. Wax and Ashley Haynes

SUCCIMER (2,3-DIMERCAPTOSUCCINIC
ACID) AND DMPS (2,3-DIMERCAPTO-1-
PROPANESULFONIC ACID) 1309
Mary Ann Howland

THIAMINE HYDROCHLORIDE 1157
Robert S. Hoffman

URIDINE TRIACETATE..............................789
Silas W. Smith

VITAMIN K$_1$...915
Mary Ann Howland

WHOLE-BOWEL IRRIGATION AND OTHER
INTESTINAL EVACUANTS 83
Silas W. Smith and Mary Ann Howland

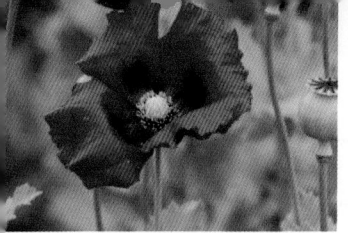

CONTENTS

Contributors .... *xiv*

Preface .... *xxv*

Acknowledgments .... *xxvi*

1. Historical Principles and Perspectives 1
   Paul M. Wax

2. Toxicologic Misfortunes and Catastrophes in History 16
   Paul M. Wax

PART A
THE GENERAL APPROACH TO THE PATIENT   27

CASE STUDY 1 27

3. Initial Evaluation of the Patient: Vital Signs and Toxic Syndromes ... 28
   Lewis S. Nelson, Mary Ann Howland, Neal A. Lewin, Silas W. Smith,
   Lewis R. Goldfrank, and Robert S. Hoffman

CASE STUDY 2 32

4. Principles of Managing the Acutely Poisoned or Overdosed Patient ... 33
   Lewis S. Nelson, Mary Ann Howland, Neal A. Lewin, Silas W. Smith,
   Lewis R. Goldfrank, and Robert S. Hoffman

SC1. PRINCIPLES OF ANTIDOTE STOCKING 42
   Silas W. Smith, Lewis R. Goldfrank, and Mary Ann Howland

5. Techniques Used to Prevent Gastrointestinal Absorption ... 48
   Lotte C. G. Hoegberg

SC2. DECONTAMINATION PRINCIPLES: PREVENTION OF DERMAL,
   OPHTHALMIC, AND INHALATIONAL ABSORPTION 71
   Scott Lucyk

A1. ACTIVATED CHARCOAL 76
   Silas W. Smith and Mary Ann Howland

A2. WHOLE-BOWEL IRRIGATION AND OTHER INTESTINAL EVACUANTS ... 83
   Silas W. Smith and Mary Ann Howland

6. Principles and Techniques Applied to Enhance Elimination ... 90
   David S. Goldfarb and Marc Ghannoum

7. Laboratory Principles 101
   Ami M. Grunbaum and Petrie M. Rainey

8. Principles of Diagnostic Imaging 114
   David T. Schwartz

9. Pharmacokinetic and Toxicokinetic Principles 140
   Mary Ann Howland

PART B
THE FUNDAMENTAL PRINCIPLES OF MEDICAL
TOXICOLOGY   155

SECTION I
BIOCHEMICAL AND MOLECULAR CONCEPTS

10. Chemical Principles 155
    Stephen J. Traub and Lewis S. Nelson

11. Biochemical and Metabolic Principles 167
    James D. Cao and Kurt C. Kleinschmidt

12. Fluid, Electrolyte, and Acid–Base Principles 189
    Alan N. Charney and Robert S. Hoffman

13. Neurotransmitters and Neuromodulators 203
    Steven C. Curry, Ayrn D. O'Connor, Kimberlie A. Graeme, and A. Min Kang

14. Withdrawal Principles 236
    Nicholas J. Connors and Richard J. Hamilton

SECTION II
PATHOPHYSIOLOGIC BASIS: ORGAN SYSTEMS

CASE STUDY 3 242

15. Cardiologic Principles I: Electrophysiologic and
    Electrocardiographic Principles 244
    Cathleen Clancy

16. Cardiologic Principles II: Hemodynamics 260
    Rachel S. Wightman and Robert A. Hessler

CASE STUDY 4 268

17. Dermatologic Principles 269
    Jesse M. Lewin, Neal A. Lewin, and Lewis S. Nelson

SC3. TRANSDERMAL TOXICOLOGY 284
    Lewis S. Nelson

18. Gastrointestinal Principles 287
    Matthew D. Zuckerman and Richard J. Church

19. Genitourinary Principles 297
    Jason Chu

20. Hematologic Principles 310
    Marco L. A. Sivilotti

21. Hepatic Principles 327
    Kathleen A. Delaney and Jakub Furmaga

CASE STUDY 5 339

22. Neurologic Principles 340
    Rama B. Rao

23. Oncologic Principles 349
    Richard Y. Wang

24. Ophthalmic Principles 356
    Adhi Sharma

25. Otolaryngologic Principles 363
    Mai Takematsu and William K. Chiang

26. Psychiatric Principles 373
    Andrea M. Kondracke, Justin M. Lewin, Cathy A. Kondas,
    and Erin A. Zerbo

SC4. PATIENT VIOLENCE 384
    Andrea M. Kondracke, Justin M. Lewin, Cathy A. Kondas,
    and Erin A. Zerbo

27. Renal Principles 389
    Marc Ghannoum and David S. Goldfarb

28. Respiratory Principles 399
    Andrew Stolbach and Robert S. Hoffman

29. Thermoregulatory Principles 411
    Susi U. Vassallo and Kathleen A. Delaney

SECTION III
SPECIAL POPULATIONS

30. Reproductive and Perinatal Principles 428
    Jeffrey S. Fine

31. Pediatric Principles 448
    Elizabeth Q. Hines and Jeffrey S. Fine

CASE STUDY 6 459

32. **Geriatric Principles** 460
     Michael E. Stern, Judith C. Ahronheim, and Mary Ann Howland

PART C
THE CLINICAL BASIS OF MEDICAL TOXICOLOGY   472

SECTION I

A. ANALGESICS AND ANTIINFLAMMATORY MEDICATIONS

33. **Acetaminophen** 472
     Robert G. Hendrickson and Nathanael J. McKeown

A3. *N*-ACETYLCYSTEINE 492
     Robert G. Hendrickson and Mary Ann Howland

34. **Colchicine, Podophyllin, and the Vinca Alkaloids** 501
     Cynthia D. Santos and Capt. Joshua G. Schier

35. **Nonsteroidal Antiinflammatory Drugs** 511
     William J. Holubek

36. **Opioids** 519
     Lewis S. Nelson and Dean Olsen

A4. OPIOID ANTAGONISTS 538
     Lewis S. Nelson and Mary Ann Howland

SC5. INTERNAL CONCEALMENT OF XENOBIOTICS 545
     Jane M. Prosser

SC6. PREVENTION, TREATMENT, AND HARM REDUCTION
     APPROACHES TO OPIOID OVERDOSES 551
     Daniel Schatz and Joshua D. Lee

37. **Salicylates** 555
     Daniel M. Lugassy

A5. SODIUM BICARBONATE 567
     Paul M. Wax and Ashley Haynes

B. FOOD, DIET, AND NUTRITION

38. **Botulism** 574
     Howard L. Geyer

A6. BOTULINUM ANTITOXIN 586
     Silas W. Smith and Howard L. Geyer

39. **Food Poisoning** 592
     Laura J. Fil and Michael G. Tunik

40. **Dieting Xenobiotics and Regimens** 606
     Jeanna M. Marraffa

41. **Athletic Performance Enhancers** 616
     Susi U. Vassallo

42. **Essential Oils** 627
     Lauren Kornreich Shawn

43. **Plant- and Animal-Derived Dietary Supplements** 638
     Lindsay M. Fox

44. **Vitamins** 654
     Beth Y. Ginsburg

45. **Iron** 669
     Jeanmarie Perrone

A7. DEFEROXAMINE 676
     Mary Ann Howland

C. PHARMACEUTICALS

46. **Pharmaceutical Additives** 681
     Sean P. Nordt and Lisa E. Vivero

47. **Antidiabetics and Hypoglycemics/Antiglycemics** 694
     George M. Bosse

A8. DEXTROSE (D-GLUCOSE) 707
     Vincent Nguyen and Larissa I. Velez

A9. OCTREOTIDE 713
     Silas W. Smith and Mary Ann Howland

48. **Antiepileptics** 719
     Suzanne Doyon

A10. L-CARNITINE 732
     Mary Ann Howland

CASE STUDY 7 736

49. **Antihistamines and Decongestants** 738
     Sophie Gosselin

A11. PHYSOSTIGMINE SALICYLATE 755
     Mary Ann Howland

50. **Chemotherapeutics** 759
     Richard Y. Wang

51. **Methotrexate, 5-Fluorouracil, and Capecitabine** 767
     Richard Y. Wang

A12. FOLATES: LEUCOVORIN (FOLINIC ACID) AND FOLIC ACID 775
     Silas W. Smith and Mary Ann Howland

A13. GLUCARPIDASE (CARBOXYPEPTIDASE G_2) 782
     Silas W. Smith

A14. URIDINE TRIACETATE 789
     Silas W. Smith

SC7. INTRATHECAL ADMINISTRATION OF XENOBIOTICS 793
     Rama B. Rao

SC8. EXTRAVASATION OF XENOBIOTICS 802
     Richard Y. Wang

52. **Antimigraine Medications** 805
     Jason Chu

53. **Thyroid and Antithyroid Medications** 812
     Nicole C. Bouchard

D. ANTIMICROBIALS

54. **Antibacterials, Antifungals, and Antivirals** 821
     Christine M. Stork

55. **Antimalarials** 836
     James David Barry

56. **Antituberculous Medications** 850
     Christina H. Hernon and Jeffrey T. Lai

A15. PYRIDOXINE 862
     Mary Ann Howland

E. CARDIOPULMONARY MEDICATIONS

57. **Antidysrhythmics** 865
     Maryann Mazer-Amirshahi and Lewis S. Nelson

A16. MAGNESIUM 876
     Silas W. Smith

58. **Antithrombotics** 883
     Betty C. Chen and Mark K. Su

A17. PROTHROMBIN COMPLEX CONCENTRATES AND DIRECT ORAL
     ANTICOAGULANT ANTIDOTES 908
     Betty C. Chen and Mark K. Su

A18. VITAMIN K_1 915
     Mary Ann Howland

A19. PROTAMINE 919
     Mary Ann Howland

CASE STUDY 8 924

59. **β-Adrenergic Antagonists** 926
     Jeffrey R. Brubacher

A20. GLUCAGON 941
     Mary Ann Howland and Silas W. Smith

60. Calcium Channel Blockers.........................945
David H. Jang

A21. HIGH-DOSE INSULIN 953
Samuel J. Stellpflug and William Kerns II

61. Miscellaneous Antihypertensives and Pharmacologically Related Agents 959
Hallam Melville Gugelmann and Francis Jerome DeRoos

62. Cardioactive Steroids 969
Jason B. Hack

A22. DIGOXIN-SPECIFIC ANTIBODY FRAGMENTS 977
Silas W. Smith and Mary Ann Howland

63. Methylxanthines and Selective β₂-Adrenergic Agonists.........985
Robert J. Hoffman

F. ANESTHETICS AND RELATED MEDICATIONS

64. Local Anesthetics 994
Matthew D. Sztajnkrycer

A23. LIPID EMULSION 1004
Sophie Gosselin and Theodore C. Bania

65. Inhalational Anesthetics 1011
Caitlin J. Guo and Brian S. Kaufman

66. Neuromuscular Blockers..........................1018
Caitlin J. Guo and Kenneth M. Sutin

A24. DANTROLENE SODIUM 1029
Caitlin J. Guo and Kenneth M. Sutin

G. PSYCHOTROPIC MEDICATIONS

67. Antipsychotics 1032
David N. Juurlink

68. Cyclic Antidepressants............................1044
Matthew Valento and Erica L. Liebelt

69. Serotonin Reuptake Inhibitors and Atypical Antidepressants.........1054
Christine M. Stork

70. Lithium 1065
Howard A. Greller

71. Monoamine Oxidase Inhibitors..................1075
Alex F. Manini

72. Sedative–Hypnotics................................1084
Payal Sud and David C. Lee

A25. FLUMAZENIL 1094
Mary Ann Howland

H. SUBSTANCES OF ABUSE

73. Amphetamines 1099
Meghan B. Spyres and David H. Jang

74. Cannabinoids......................................1111
Jeff M. Lapoint

75. Cocaine 1124
Craig G. Smollin and Robert S. Hoffman

A26. BENZODIAZEPINES................................1135
Fiona Garlich Horner, Robert S. Hoffman, Lewis S. Nelson, and Mary Ann Howland

76. Ethanol 1143
Luke Yip

A27. THIAMINE HYDROCHLORIDE....................1157
Robert S. Hoffman

77. Alcohol Withdrawal...............................1165
Jeffrey A. Gold and Lewis S. Nelson

78. Disulfiram and Disulfiramlike Reactions 1172
Amit K. Gupta

79. Hallucinogens......................................1178
Mark J. Neavyn and Jennifer L. Carey

80. γ-Hydroxybutyric Acid (γ-Hydroxybutyrate) 1188
Rachel Haroz and Brenna M. Farmer

81. Inhalants...1193
Heather Long

82. Nicotine..1203
Denise Fernández and Sari Soghoian

83. Phencyclidine and Ketamine 1210
Ruben E. Olmedo

I. METALS

CASE STUDY 9 1222

84. Aluminum 1223
Stephen A. Harding and Brenna M. Farmer

85. Antimony 1228
Asim F. Tarabar

86. Arsenic 1237
Stephen W. Munday

A28. DIMERCAPROL (BRITISH ANTI-LEWISITE OR BAL)....1251
Mary Ann Howland

87. Bismuth 1255
Rama B. Rao

88. Cadmium 1259
Stephen J. Traub and Robert S. Hoffman

89. Cesium 1264
Zhanna Livshits

90. Chromium 1268
Steven B. Bird

91. Cobalt 1273
Gar Ming Chan

92. Copper 1283
Lewis S. Nelson

93. Lead 1292
Diane P. Calello and Fred M. Henretig

A29. SUCCIMER (2,3-DIMERCAPTOSUCCINIC ACID) AND DMPS (2,3-DIMERCAPTO-1-PROPANESULFONIC ACID) 1309
Mary Ann Howland

A30. EDETATE CALCIUM DISODIUM (CaNa₂EDTA) 1315
Mary Ann Howland

94. Manganese...1319
Elizabeth Q. Hines and Sari Soghoian

95. Mercury..1324
Young-Jin Sue

96. Nickel 1333
John A. Curtis

97. Selenium...1339
Diane P. Calello

98. Silver...1344
Melisa W. Lai-Becker and Michele M. Burns

99. Thallium..1350
Maria Mercurio-Zappala and Robert S. Hoffman

A31. PRUSSIAN BLUE 1357
Robert S. Hoffman

100. Zinc 1362
Nima Majlesi

J. HOUSEHOLD PRODUCTS

101. Antiseptics, Disinfectants, and Sterilants 1368
Ashley Haynes and Paul M. Wax

102. Camphor and Moth Repellents 1380
Hong K. Kim

103. Caustics 1388
  Rachel S. Wightman and Jessica A. Fulton

104. Hydrofluoric Acid and Fluorides 1397
  Mark K. Su

A32. CALCIUM 1403
  Silas W. Smith and Mary Ann Howland

105. Hydrocarbons 1409
  Morgan A. A. Riggan and David D. Gummin

CASE STUDY 10 1420

106. Toxic Alcohols 1421
  Sage W. Wiener

A33. FOMEPIZOLE 1435
  Mary Ann Howland

A34. ETHANOL 1440
  Mary Ann Howland

SC9. DIETHYLENE GLYCOL 1444
  Capt. Joshua G. Schier

K. PESTICIDES

CASE STUDY 11 1450

107. Barium 1454
  Andrew H. Dawson

108. Fumigants 1457
  Shahin Shadnia and Kambiz Soltaninejad

109. Herbicides 1466
  Darren M. Roberts

110. Insecticides: Organic Phosphorous Compounds and Carbamates 1486
  Michael Eddleston

A35. ATROPINE 1503
  Mary Ann Howland

A36. PRALIDOXIME 1508
  Mary Ann Howland

111. Insecticides: Organic Chlorines, Pyrethrins/Pyrethroids, and Insect Repellents 1514
  Michael G. Holland

112. Phosphorus 1528
  Michael C. Beuhler

113. Sodium Monofluoroacetate and Fluoroacetamide 1533
  Fermin Barrueto Jr.

114. Strychnine 1536
  Yiu-Cheung Chan

L. NATURAL TOXINS AND ENVENOMATIONS

115. Arthropods 1540
  Daniel J. Repplinger and In-Hei Hahn

A37. ANTIVENOM: SPIDER 1559
  Michael A. Darracq and Richard F. Clark

A38. ANTIVENOM: SCORPION 1563
  Michael A. Darracq and Richard F. Clark

116. Marine Envenomations 1567
  Eike Blohm and D. Eric Brush

117. Mushrooms 1581
  Lewis R. Goldfrank

118. Plants 1597
  Lewis S. Nelson and Lewis R. Goldfrank

119. Native (US) Venomous Snakes and Lizards 1617
  Anne-Michelle Ruha and Anthony F. Pizon

A39. ANTIVENOM FOR NORTH AMERICAN VENOMOUS SNAKES (CROTALINE AND ELAPID) 1627
  Anthony F. Pizon and Anne-Michelle Ruha

SC10. EXOTIC NONNATIVE SNAKE ENVENOMATIONS 1633
  Keith J. Boesen, Kelly A. Green Boesen, Nicholas B. Hurst, and Farshad Mazda Shirazi

M. OCCUPATIONAL AND ENVIRONMENTAL TOXINS

CASE STUDY 12 1639

120. Smoke Inhalation 1640
  Nathan P. Charlton and Mark A. Kirk

CASE STUDY 13 1650

121. Simple Asphyxiants and Pulmonary Irritants 1651
  Lewis S. Nelson and Oladapo A. Odujebe

122. Carbon Monoxide 1663
  Christian Tomaszewski

A40. HYPERBARIC OXYGEN 1676
  Stephen R. Thom

123. Cyanide and Hydrogen Sulfide 1684
  Christopher P. Holstege and Mark A. Kirk

A41. HYDROXOCOBALAMIN 1694
  Mary Ann Howland

A42. NITRITES (AMYL AND SODIUM) AND SODIUM THIOSULFATE 1698
  Mary Ann Howland

124. Methemoglobin Inducers 1703
  Dennis P. Price

A43. METHYLENE BLUE 1713
  Mary Ann Howland

125. Nanotoxicology 1717
  Silas W. Smith

N. DISASTER PREPAREDNESS

126. Chemical Weapons 1741
  Jeffrey R. Suchard

127. Biological Weapons 1753
  Jeffrey R. Suchard

128. Radiation 1762
  Joseph G. Rella

A44. POTASSIUM IODIDE 1775
  Joseph G. Rella

A45. PENTETIC ACID OR PENTETATE (ZINC OR CALCIUM) TRISODIUM (DTPA) 1779
  Joseph G. Rella

PART D
POPULATION HEALTH

SECTION I

POISON CONTROL CENTERS, HEALTH SYSTEMS, AND EPIDEMIOLOGY

129. Poison Prevention and Education 1782
  Lauren Schwartz

130. Poison Control Centers and Poison Epidemiology 1789
  Mark K. Su and Robert S. Hoffman

131. Principles of Occupational Toxicology: Diagnosis and Control 1797
  Peter H. Wald

132. Hazardous Materials Incident Response 1806
  Brandy Ferguson and Bradley J. Kaufman

133. Risk Assessment and Risk Communication 1814
  Charles A. McKay

CASE STUDY 14 1820

134. Medication Safety and Adverse Drug Events 1822
  Brenna M. Farmer

135. **Drug Development, Adverse Drug Events, and Postmarketing Surveillance**.. 1833
Louis R. Cantilena

136. **International Perspectives on Medical Toxicology**........................ 1844
Sari Soghoian

137. **Principles of Epidemiology and Research Design**......................... 1852
Alex F. Manini

SECTION II

LEGAL ASPECTS OF TOXICOLOGY

138. **Risk Management and Legal Principles**... 1860
Barbara M. Kirrane

139. **Medicolegal Interpretive Toxicology** 1868
Robert A. Middleberg

SC11. **ASSESSMENT OF ETHANOL-INDUCED IMPAIRMENT** 1876
Robert B. Palmer

140. **Postmortem Toxicology**... 1884
Rama B. Rao and Mark A. Flomenbaum

SC12. **ORGAN PROCUREMENT FROM POISONED PATIENTS** 1892
Rama B. Rao

Index 1895

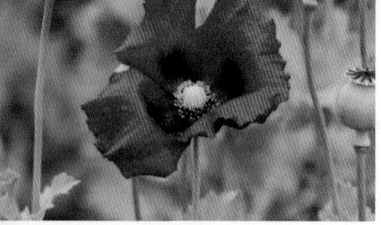

CONTRIBUTORS

Judith C. Ahronheim, MD
Clinical Professor of Medicine
New York Medical College
Valhalla, New York
Chapter 32, "Geriatric Principles"

Theodore C. Bania, MD, MS
Assistant Professor of Emergency Medicine
Director of Research and Toxicology
Mt. Sinai West and Mt. Sinai St. Luke's Hospitals
Department of Emergency Medicine
Associate Dean for Human Subject Research
Associate Director Program for the Protection
    of Human Subjects
Icahn School of Medicine at Mount Sinai
New York, New York
Antidotes in Depth: A23, "Lipid Emulsion"

Fermin Barrueto Jr., MD, MBA, FACEP
Volunteer Associate Professor of Emergency
    Medicine
University of Maryland School of Medicine
Baltimore, Maryland
Senior Vice President
Chief Medical Officer
University of Maryland Upper Chesapeake Health
Bel Air, Maryland
*Chapter 113, "Sodium Monofluoroacetate and
    Fluoroacetamide"*

James David Barry, MD
Clinical Professor of Emergency Medicine
University of California, Irvine School of Medicine
Irvine, California
Associate Director, Emergency Department
Long Beach VA Medical Center
Long Beach, California
Chapter 55, "Antimalarials"

Michael C. Beuhler, MD
Professor of Emergency Medicine
Carolinas HealthCare System
Medical Director, Carolinas Poison Center
Charlotte, North Carolina
Chapter 112, "Phosphorus"

Rana Biary, MD
Assistant Professor of Emergency Medicine
New York University School of Medicine
Program Director, Medical Toxicology Fellowship
Emergency Physician
Ronald O. Perelman Department of Emergency
    Medicine
Bellevue Hospital Center and NYU Langone
    Health
New York, New York
Case Studies

Steven B. Bird, MD
Professor of Emergency Medicine
University of Massachusetts Medical School
UMass Memorial Medical Center
Worcester, Massachusetts
Chapter 90, "Chromium"

Eike Blohm, MD
Assistant Professor of Surgery
Division of Emergency Medicine
Toxicology Consultant Northern New England
    Poison Center
University of Vermont Larner College of Medicine
University of Vermont Medical Center
Burlington, Vermont
Chapter 116, "Marine Envenomations"

Keith J. Boesen, PharmD, FAZPA
Instructor, University of Arizona College of
    Pharmacy
Director, Arizona Poison and Drug Information
    Center
Tucson, Arizona
*Special Considerations: SC10, "Exotic Nonnative
    Snake Envenomations"*

Kelly A. Green Boesen, PharmD
Clinical Pharmacist
Tucson, Arizona
*Special Considerations: SC10, "Exotic Nonnative
    Snake Envenomations"*

George M. Bosse, MD
Professor of Emergency Medicine
University of Louisville School of Medicine
Medical Director, Kentucky Poison Center
Louisville, Kentucky
*Chapter 47, "Antidiabetics and Hypoglycemics/
    Antiglycemics"*

Nicole C. Bouchard, MD, FACMT, FRCPC
Assistant Clinical Professor of Emergency
    Medicine
Donald and Barbara Zucker School of Medicine
    at Hofstra/Northwell
Emergency Physician
Lenox Health in Greenwich Village, Northwell
    Health
New York, New York
Chapter 53, "Thyroid and Antithyroid Medications"

Jeffrey R. Brubacher, MD, MSc, FRCPC
Associate Professor of Emergency Medicine
University of British Columbia
Emergency Physician
Vancouver General Hospital
Vancouver, British Columbia, Canada
Chapter 59, "β-Adrenergic Antagonists"

D. Eric Brush, MD, MHCM
Clinical Associate Professor of Emergency
    Medicine
University of Massachusetts Medical School
Division of Toxicology
Director of Clinical Operations
UMass Memorial Medical Center
Worcester, Massachusetts
Chapter 116, "Marine Envenomations"

Michele M. Burns, MD, MPH
Assistant Professor of Pediatrics and Emergency
    Medicine
Harvard Medical School
Director, Medical Toxicology Fellowship
Medical Director, Regional Center for Poison
    Control and Prevention
Attending Physician, Pediatric Emergency
    Medicine
Boston Children's Hospital
Boston, Massachusetts
Chapter 98, "Silver"

Diane P. Calello, MD
Associate Professor of Emergency Medicine
Rutgers New Jersey Medical School
Executive and Medical Director
New Jersey Poison Information and Education
    System
Newark, New Jersey
Chapter 93, "Lead"
Chapter 97, "Selenium"

Louis R. Cantilena, MD, PhD (Deceased)
Professor of Medicine and Pharmacology
Director, Division of Clinical Pharmacology and
    Medical Toxicology
Department of Medicine
Uniformed Services University
Bethesda, Maryland
*Chapter 135, "Drug Development, Adverse Drug
    Events, and Postmarketing Surveillance"*

James D. Cao, MD
Assistant Professor of Emergency Medicine
Division of Medical Toxicology
University of Texas Southwestern Medical School
Program Director, Medical Toxicology
University of Texas Southwestern Medical Center
Dallas, Texas
*Chapter 11, "Biochemical and Metabolic
    Principles"*

Jennifer L. Carey, MD
Assistant Professor of Emergency Medicine
Division of Medical Toxicology
University of Massachusetts Medical School
UMass Memorial Medical Center
Worcester, Massachusetts
Chapter 79, "Hallucinogens"

Gar Ming Chan, MD, FACEM
Emergency Medicine Specialist
Calvary Health Care, Lenah Valley
Tasmania, Australia
Chapter 91, "Cobalt"

Yiu-Cheung Chan, MD, MBBS, FRCS (Ed), FHKCEM, FHKAM
Consultant, Accident and Emergency Department,
United Christian Hospital
Hong Kong Poison Information Centre
Hong Kong SAR, China
Chapter 114, "Strychnine"

Nathan P. Charlton, MD
Associate Professor of Emergency Medicine
Program Director, Medical Toxicology
University of Virginia School of Medicine
Charlottesville, Virginia
Chapter 120, "Smoke Inhalation"

Alan N. Charney, MD
Professor of Medicine
New York University School of Medicine
New York, New York
Chapter 12, "Fluid, Electrolyte, and Acid–Base Principles"

Betty C. Chen, MD
Assistant Professor of Emergency Medicine
University of Washington School of Medicine
Harborview Medical Center
Toxicology Consultant, Washington Poison Center
Seattle, Washington
Chapter 58, "Antithrombotics"
Antidotes in Depth: A17, "Prothrombin Complex Concentrates and Direct Oral Anticoagulant Antidotes"

William K. Chiang, MD
Professor of Emergency Medicine
New York University School of Medicine
Emergency Physician
Ronald O. Perelman Department of Emergency Medicine
Bellevue Hospital Center and NYU Langone Health
New York, New York
Chapter 25, "Otolaryngologic Principles"

Jason Chu, MD
Associate Professor of Emergency Medicine
Icahn School of Medicine at Mount Sinai
Emergency Physician and Medical Toxicologist
Mt. Sinai West and Mt. Sinai St. Luke's Hospitals
New York, New York
Chapter 19, "Genitourinary Principles"
Chapter 52, "Antimigraine Medications"

Richard J. Church, MD, FACEP, FACMT
Associate Professor of Emergency Medicine and Medical Toxicology
Assistant Program Director, Emergency Medicine Residency
University of Massachusetts Medical School
UMass Memorial Medical Center
Worcester, Massachusetts
Chapter 18, "Gastrointestinal Principles"

Cathleen Clancy, MD
Associate Professor of Emergency Medicine
The George Washington University Medical Center
Emergency Physician
Walter Reed National Military Medical Center
Associate Medical Director
Program Director, Medical Toxicology Fellowship
National Capital Poison Center
Washington, District of Columbia
Chapter 15, "Cardiologic Principles I: Electrophysiologic and Electrocardiographic Principles"

Richard F. Clark, MD
Professor of Emergency Medicine
Director, Division of Medical Toxicology
University of California, San Diego
San Diego, California
Antidotes in Depth: A37, "Antivenom: Spider"
Antidotes in Depth: A38, "Antivenom: Scorpion"

Nicholas J. Connors, MD
Associate Professor of Emergency Medicine
Medical University of South Carolina
Charleston, South Carolina
Medical Toxicologist
Palmetto Poison Center
Columbia, South Carolina
Chapter 14, "Withdrawal Principles"

Steven C. Curry, MD
Professor of Medicine and Emergency Medicine
Division of Medical Toxicology and Precision Medicine
Division of Clinical Data Analytics and Decision Support
Center for Toxicology and Pharmacology Education and Research
University of Arizona College of Medicine—Phoenix
Banner—University Medical Center, Phoenix
Phoenix, Arizona
Chapter 13, "Neurotransmitters and Neuromodulators"

John A. Curtis, MD
Emergency Physician
Cheshire Medical Center-Dartmouth Hitchcock Keene
Keene, New Hampshire
Chapter 96, "Nickel"

Michael A. Darracq, MD, MPH
Associate Professor of Clinical Emergency Medicine
University of California, San Francisco (UCSF)-Fresno
Medical Education Program
Department of Emergency Medicine
Division of Medical Toxicology
Fresno, California
Antidotes in Depth: A37, "Antivenom: Spider"
Antidotes in Depth: A38, "Antivenom: Scorpion"

Andrew H. Dawson, MBBS, FRACP, FRCP, FCCP
Clinical Professor of Medicine, University of Sydney
Clinical Director, NSW Poisons Information Centre
Director, Clinical Toxicology
Royal Prince Alfred Hospital
Sydney, Australia
Chapter 107, "Barium"

Kathleen A. Delaney, MD, FACP, FACMT
Academic Chair of Emergency Medicine, Emeritus
John Peter Smith Health Science Center
Fort Worth, Texas
Chapter 21, "Hepatic Principles"
Chapter 29, "Thermoregulatory Principles"

Francis Jerome DeRoos, MD
Associate Professor of Emergency Medicine
Perelman School of Medicine at the University of Pennsylvania
Hospital of the University of Pennsylvania
Philadelphia, Pennsylvania
Chapter 61, "Miscellaneous Antihypertensives and Pharmacologically Related Agents"

Suzanne Doyon, MD, MPH, ACEP, FACMT, FASAM
Assistant Professor of Emergency Medicine
Medical Director, Connecticut Poison Control Center
University of Connecticut School of Medicine
Farmington, Connecticut
Chapter 48, "Antiepileptics"

Michael Eddleston, BM, ScD
Professor of Clinical Toxicology
University of Edinburgh
Consultant Clinical Toxicologist
Royal Infirmary of Edinburgh and National Poisons Information Service, Edinburgh
Edinburgh, United Kingdom
Chapter 110, "Insecticides: Organic Phosphorus Compounds and Carbamates"

Brenna M. Farmer, MD
Assistant Professor of Clinical Medicine
Weill Cornell Medical College of Cornell
    University
Emergency Physician
Assistant Program Director of Emergency
    Medicine
New York-Presbyterian Hospital
Director of Patient Safety
Weill Cornell Emergency Department
New York, New York
*Chapter 80, "γ-Hydroxybutyric Acid
    (γ-Hydroxybutyrate)"*
Chapter 84, "Aluminum"
*Chapter 134, "Medication Safety and Adverse Drug
    Events"*

Brandy Ferguson, MD
Assistant Professor of Emergency Medicine
New York University School of Medicine
Emergency Physician
Ronald O. Perelman Department of Emergency
    Medicine
Bellevue Hospital Center and NYU Langone
    Health
New York, New York
*Chapter 132, "Hazardous Materials Incident
    Response"*

Denise Fernández, MD
Assistant Professor of Emergency Medicine
Albert Einstein College of Medicine
Medical Toxicologist
Emergency Physician
Jacobi Medical Center/North Central Bronx
    Hospital
Bronx, New York
Chapter 82, "Nicotine"

Laura J. Fil, DO, MS
Adjunct Professor
Department of Primary Care
Touro College of Osteopathic Medicine
Middletown, New York
Emergency Physician
Department of Emergency Medicine
Vassar Brothers Medical Center
Poughkeepsie, New York
Chapter 39, "Food Poisoning"

Jeffrey S. Fine, MD
Associate Professor of Emergency Medicine and
    Pediatrics
New York University School of Medicine
Emergency Physician
Ronald O. Perelman Department of Emergency
    Medicine
Bellevue Hospital Center and NYU Langone
    Health
New York, New York
*Chapter 30, "Reproductive and Perinatal
    Principles"*
Chapter 31, "Pediatric Principles"

Mark A. Flomenbaum, MD, PhD
Chief Medical Examiner, State of Maine
Augusta, Maine
Chapter 140, "Postmortem Toxicology"

Lindsay M. Fox, MD
Assistant Professor of Emergency Medicine
Rutgers New Jersey Medical School
University Hospital
Toxicology Consultant, New Jersey Poison
    Information and Education System
Newark, New Jersey
*Chapter 43, "Plant- and Animal-Derived Dietary
    Supplements"*

Jessica A. Fulton, DO
Emergency Physician
Grandview Hospital
Sellersville, Pennsylvania
Chapter 103, "Caustics"

Jakub Furmaga, MD
Assistant Professor of Emergency Medicine
University of Texas Southwestern Medical School
Division of Medical Toxicology
University of Texas Southwestern Medical Center
Dallas, Texas
Chapter 21, "Hepatic Principles"

Howard L. Geyer, MD, PhD
Assistant Professor of Neurology
Director, Division of Movement Disorders
Montefiore Medical Center
Albert Einstein College of Medicine
Bronx, New York
Chapter 38, "Botulism"
Antidotes in Depth: A6, "Botulinum Antitoxin"

Marc Ghannoum, MD, MSc
Associate Professor of Medicine
University of Montreal
Nephrology and Internal Medicine
Verdun Hospital
Montreal, Québec, Canada
*Chapter 6, "Principles and Techniques Applied to
    Enhance Elimination"*
Chapter 27, "Renal Principles"

Beth Y. Ginsburg, MD
Assistant Professor of Emergency Medicine
Icahn School of Medicine at Mount Sinai
New York, New York
Emergency Physician
Elmhurst Hospital Center
Elmhurst, New York
Chapter 44, "Vitamins"

Jeffrey A. Gold, MD
Professor of Medicine
Chief, Division of Pulmonary and Critical Care
    (Interim)
Associate Director, Adult Cystic Fibrosis Center
Oregon Health and Science University
Portland, Oregon
Chapter 77, "Alcohol Withdrawal"

David S. Goldfarb, MD, FASN
Professor of Medicine and Physiology
New York University School of Medicine
Clinical Chief, Nephrology Division
NYU Langone Health
Chief, Nephrology Section
New York Harbor VA Healthcare System
Consultant, New York City Poison Control Center
New York, New York
*Chapter 6, "Principles and Techniques Applied to
    Enhance Elimination"*
Chapter 27, "Renal Principles"

**Lewis R. Goldfrank, MD, FAAEM, FAACT,
    FACEP, FACMT, FACP**
Herbert W. Adams Professor of Emergency
    Medicine
New York University School of Medicine
Emergency Physician
Ronald O. Perelman Department of Emergency
    Medicine
Bellevue Hospital Center and NYU Langone
    Health
Medical Director, New York City Poison Control
    Center
New York, New York
*Chapter 3, "Initial Evaluation of the Patient: Vital
    Signs and Toxic Syndromes"*
*Chapter 4, "Principles of Managing the Acutely
    Poisoned or Overdosed Patient"*
Chapter 117, "Mushrooms"
Chapter 118, "Plants"
*Special Considerations: SC1, "Principles of
    Antidote Stocking"*

**Sophie Gosselin, MD, CSPQ, FRCPC, FAACT,
    FACMT**
Associate Professor, Department of Medicine
    McGill University
Emergency Physician
McGill University Health Center & Hôpital
    Charles-Lemoyne
Montréal, Québec, Canada
Medical Toxicologist
Centre Antipoison du Québec
Québec City, Québec, Canada
Chapter 49, "Antihistamines and Decongestants"
Antidotes in Depth: A23, "Lipid Emulsion"

Kimberlie A. Graeme, MD
Clinical Associate Professor of Emergency
    Medicine
University of Arizona College of
    Medicine—Phoenix
Department of Medical Toxicology
Banner—University Medical Center Phoenix
Phoenix, Arizona
*Chapter 13, "Neurotransmitters and
    Neuromodulators"*

Howard A. Greller, MD, FACEP, FACMT
Department of Clinical Medicine,
    Affiliated Medical Professor
City University of New York School of Medicine
Director of Research and Medical Toxicology
SBH Health System Department of Emergency
    Medicine
St. Barnabas Hospital
Bronx, New York
Chapter 70, "Lithium"

Ami M. Grunbaum, MD, FRCPC
Adjunct Professor of Medicine
Medical Biochemist, MUHC and CISSS-Laval
McGill University
Montreal, Québec, Canada
Chapter 7, "Laboratory Principles"

Hallam Melville Gugelmann, MD, MPH
Assistant Clinical Professor
Division of Clinical Pharmacology and Medical
    Toxicology, Department of Medicine,
    University of California, San Francisco
Emergency Physician, CPMC St. Luke's Hospital
    Emergency Department
Assistant Medical Director, California Poison
    Control System-San Francisco Division
San Francisco, California
*Chapter 61, "Miscellaneous Antihypertensives and
    Pharmacologically Related Agents"*

David D. Gummin, MD, FAACT, FACEP, FACMT
Professor of Emergency Medicine, Pediatrics,
    Pharmacology and Toxicology
Section Chief, Medical Toxicology
Medical College of Wisconsin
Medical Director, Wisconsin Poison Center
Milwaukee, Wisconsin
Chapter 105, "Hydrocarbons"

Caitlin J. Guo, MD, MBA
Assistant Professor of Anesthesiology,
    Perioperative Care and Pain Medicine
New York University School of Medicine
Attending Physician
Bellevue Hospital Center and NYU Langone
    Health
New York, New York
Chapter 65, "Inhalational Anesthetics"
Chapter 66, "Neuromuscular Blockers"
Antidotes in Depth: A24, "Dantrolene Sodium"

Amit K. Gupta, MD
Assistant Professor of Emergency Medicine
Seton Hall Medical School
Assistant Residency Director, Department of
    Emergency Medicine
Hackensack University Medical Center
Hackensack, New Jersey
*Chapter 78, "Disulfiram and Disulfiramlike
    Reactions"*

Jason B. Hack, MD
Professor of Emergency Medicine
Program Director, Division of Medical Toxicology
The Warren Alpert Medical School of Brown
    University
Rhode Island Hospital
Providence, Rhode Island
Chapter 62, "Cardioactive Steroids"

In-Hei Hahn, MD, FACEP, FACMT
Expedition Medical Officer
Research Associate
Division of Paleontology
American Museum of Natural History
New York, New York
Chapter 115, "Arthropods"

**Richard J. Hamilton, MD, FAAEM, FACEP,
FACMT**
Professor and Chair of Emergency Medicine
Drexel University College of Medicine
Philadelphia, Pennsylvania
Chapter 14, "Withdrawal Principles"

Stephen A. Harding, MD
Assistant Professor of Emergency Medicine
Henry J. N. Taub Department of Emergency
    Medicine
Baylor College of Medicine
Houston, Texas
Chapter 84, "Aluminum"

Rachel Haroz, MD
Assistant Professor of Emergency Medicine
Cooper University Health Care
Camden, New Jersey
*Chapter 80, "γ-Hydroxybutyric Acid
    (γ-Hydroxybutyrate)"*

Ashley Haynes, MD, FACEP
Assistant Professor of Emergency Medicine
Division of Toxicology
University of Texas Southwestern Medical School
Attending Physician
Parkland Hospital
Clements University Hospital
Children's Medical Center
Dallas, Texas
*Chapter 101, "Antiseptics, Disinfectants, and
    Sterilants"*
Antidotes in Depth: A5, "Sodium Bicarbonate"

Robert G. Hendrickson, MD, FACMT, FAACT
Professor of Emergency Medicine
Program Director, Fellowship in Medical
    Toxicology
Associate Medical Director, Oregon Poison
    Center
Oregon Health and Science University
Portland, Oregon
Chapter 33, "Acetaminophen"
Antidotes in Depth: A3, "N-Acetylcysteine"

Fred M. Henretig, MD, FAAP, FACMT
Professor Emeritus of Pediatrics
Perelman School of Medicine, University of
    Pennsylvania
Senior Toxicologist, The Poison Control Center at
    the Children's Hospital of Philadelphia
Philadelphia, Pennsylvania
Chapter 93, "Lead"

Christina H. Hernon, MD
Lecturer in Emergency Medicine
Harvard Medical School
Department of Emergency Medicine
Division of Medical Toxicology
Cambridge Health Alliance
Cambridge, Massachusetts
Chapter 56, "Antituberculous Medications"

Robert A. Hessler, MD, PhD
Associate Professor of Emergency Medicine
New York University School of Medicine
Emergency Physician
Ronald O. Perelman Department of Emergency
    Medicine
Bellevue Hospital Center, NYU Langone Health
    and VA NY Harbor Healthcare System
New York, New York
*Chapter 16, "Cardiologic Principles II:
    Hemodynamics"*

Elizabeth Quaal Hines, MD
Clinical Assistant Professor of Pediatrics
Division of Pediatric Emergency Medicine
University of Maryland School of Medicine
Toxicology Consultant, Maryland Poison Center
Baltimore, Maryland
Chapter 31, "Pediatric Principles"
Chapter 94, "Manganese"

**Lotte C. G. Hoegberg, MS (Pharm), PhD,
FEAPCCT**
Pharmacist, Medical Toxicologist
The Danish Poisons Information Centre
Department of Anesthesia and Intensive Care
Copenhagen University Hospital Bispebjerg
Copenhagen, Denmark
*Chapter 5, "Techniques Used to Prevent
    Gastrointestinal Absorption"*

Robert J. Hoffman, MD, MS, FACMT, FACEP
Medical Director, Qatar Poison Center
Sidra Medicine
Doha, Qatar
*Chapter 63, "Methylxanthines and Selective
    β₂-Adrenergic Agonists"*

Robert S. Hoffman, MD, FAACT, FACMT, FRCP Edin, FEAPCCT
Professor of Emergency Medicine and Medicine
New York University School of Medicine
Director, Division of Medical Toxicology
Ronald O. Perelman Department of Emergency Medicine
Emergency Physician
Bellevue Hospital Center and NYU Langone Health
New York, New York
Chapter 3, "Initial Evaluation of the Patient: Vital Signs and Toxic Syndromes"
Chapter 4, "Principles of Managing the Acutely Poisoned or Overdosed Patient"
Chapter 12, "Fluid, Electrolyte, and Acid–Base Principles"
Chapter 28, "Respiratory Principles"
Chapter 75, "Cocaine"
Chapter 88, "Cadmium"
Chapter 99, "Thallium"
Chapter 130, "Poison Control Centers and Poison Epidemiology"
Antidotes in Depth: A26, "Benzodiazepines"
Antidotes in Depth: A27, "Thiamine Hydrochloride"
Antidotes in Depth: A31, "Prussian Blue"

Michael G. Holland, MD, FEAPCCT, FAACT, FACMT, FACOEM, FACEP
Clinical Professor of Emergency Medicine
SUNY Upstate Medical University
Syracuse, New York
Medical Toxicologist, Upstate New York Poison Center
Syracuse, New York
Director of Occupational Medicine, Glens Falls Hospital Center for Occupational Health
Glens Falls, New York
Senior Medical Toxicologist, Center for Toxicology and Environmental Health
North Little Rock, Arkansas
Chapter 111, "Insecticides: Organic Chlorines, Pyrethrins/Pyrethroids and Insect Repellents"

Christopher P. Holstege, MD
Professor of Emergency Medicine and Pediatrics
Chief, Division of Medical Toxicology
University of Virginia School of Medicine
Medical Director, Blue Ridge Poison Center
University of Virginia Health System
Charlottesville, Virginia
Chapter 123, "Cyanide and Hydrogen Sulfide"

William J. Holubek, MD, MPH, CPE, FACEP, FACMT
Vice President of Medical Affairs
WellStar Atlanta Medical Center
Atlanta, Georgia
Chapter 35, "Nonsteroidal Antiinflammatory Drugs"

Fiona Garlich Horner, MD
Clinical Assistant Professor of Emergency Medicine
Keck School of Medicine of the University of Southern California
Los Angeles, California
Antidotes in Depth: A26, "Benzodiazepines"

Mary Ann Howland, PharmD, DABAT, FAACT
Clinical Professor of Pharmacy
St. John's University College of Pharmacy and Health Sciences
Adjunct Professor of Emergency Medicine
New York University School of Medicine
Ronald O. Perelman Department of Emergency Medicine
Bellevue Hospital Center and NYU Langone Health
Senior Consultant in Residence
New York City Poison Control Center
New York, New York
Chapter 3, "Initial Evaluation of the Patient: Vital Signs and Toxic Syndromes"
Chapter 4, "Principles of Managing the Acutely Poisoned or Overdosed Patient"
Chapter 9, "Pharmacokinetic and Toxicokinetic Principles"
Chapter 32, "Geriatric Principles"
Antidotes in Depth: A1, "Activated Charcoal"
Antidotes in Depth: A2, "Whole-Bowel Irrigation and Other Intestinal Evacuants"
Antidotes in Depth: A3, "N-Acetylcysteine"
Antidotes in Depth: A4, "Opioid Antagonists"
Antidotes in Depth: A7, "Deferoxamine"
Antidotes in Depth: A9, "Octreotide"
Antidotes in Depth: A10, "L-Carnitine"
Antidotes in Depth: A11, "Physostigmine Salicylate"
Antidotes in Depth: A12, "Folates: Leucovorin (Folinic Acid) and Folic Acid"
Antidotes in Depth: A15, "Pyridoxine"
Antidotes in Depth: A18, "Vitamin K₁"
Antidotes in Depth: A19, "Protamine"
Antidotes in Depth: A20, "Glucagon"
Antidotes in Depth: A22, "Digoxin-Specific Antibody Fragments"
Antidotes in Depth: A25, "Flumazenil"
Antidotes in Depth: A26, "Benzodiazepines"
Antidotes in Depth: A28, "Dimercaprol (British Anti-Lewisite or BAL)"
Antidotes in Depth: A29, "Succimer (2,3-dimercaptosuccinic acid) and DMPS (2,3-dimercapto-1-propanesulfonic acid)"
Antidotes in Depth: A30, "Edetate Calcium Disodium (CaNa₂EDTA)"
Antidotes in Depth: A32, "Calcium"
Antidotes in Depth: A33, "Fomepizole"
Antidotes in Depth: A34, "Ethanol"
Antidotes in Depth: A35, "Atropine"
Antidotes in Depth: A36, "Pralidoxime"
Antidotes in Depth: A41, "Hydroxocobalamin"
Antidotes in Depth: A42, "Nitrites (Amyl and Sodium) and Sodium Thiosulfate"
Antidotes in Depth: A43, "Methylene Blue"
Special Considerations: SC1, "Principles of Antidote Stocking"

Nicholas B. Hurst, MD, MS, FAAEM
Assistant Professor of Emergency Medicine
Medical Toxicology Consultant
Arizona Poison and Drug Information Center
University of Arizona College of Medicine-Tucson
Tucson, Arizona
Special Considerations: SC10, "Exotic Nonnative Snake Envenomations"

David H. Jang, MD, MSc, FACMT
Assistant Professor of Emergency Medicine
Divisions of Medical Toxicology and Critical Care Medicine (ResCCU)
Perelman School of Medicine, University of Pennsylvania
Philadelphia, Pennsylvania
Chapter 60, "Calcium Channel Blockers"
Chapter 73, "Amphetamines"

David N. Juurlink, MD, PhD, FRCPC, FAACT, FACMT
Professor of Medicine, Pediatrics and Health Policy, Management and Evaluation
Director, Division of Clinical Pharmacology and Toxicology
University of Toronto
Senior Scientist, Institute for Clinical Evaluative Sciences
Medical Toxicologist, Ontario Poison Centre
Toronto, Ontario, Canada
Chapter 67, "Antipsychotics"

A. Min Kang, MD, MPhil, FAAP, FASAM
Assistant Professor of Child Health and Medicine
University of Arizona College of Medicine—Phoenix
Section Chief, Toxicology, Phoenix Children's Hospital
Medical Toxicologist, Banner—University Medical Center Phoenix
Associate Medical Director, Banner Poison and Drug Information Center
Phoenix, Arizona
Chapter 13, "Neurotransmitters and Neuromodulators"

Bradley J. Kaufman, MD, MPH, FACEP, FAEMS
Associate Professor of Emergency Medicine
Donald and Barbara Zucker School of Medicine at Hofstra/Northwell
Hempstead, New York
Emergency Physician
Long Island Jewish Medical Center
New Hyde Park, New York
First Deputy Medical Director
Fire Department of the City of New York
New York, New York
Chapter 132, "Hazardous Materials Incident Response"

Brian S. Kaufman, MD
Professor of Medicine, Anesthesiology, Neurology and Neurosurgery
New York University School of Medicine
NYU Langone Health
New York, New York
Chapter 65, "Inhalational Anesthetics"

William Kerns II, MD, FACEP, FACMT
Professor of Emergency Medicine and Medical
  Toxicology
Division of Medical Toxicology
Department of Emergency Medicine
Carolinas Medical Center
Charlotte, North Carolina
Antidotes in Depth: A21, "High-Dose Insulin (HDI)"

Hong K. Kim, MD, MPH
Assistant Professor of Emergency Medicine
University of Maryland School of Medicine
Baltimore, Maryland
Chapter 102, "Camphor and Moth Repellents"

Mark A. Kirk, MD
Associate Professor of Emergency Medicine
University of Virginia
Charlottesville, Virginia
Director, Chemical Defense
Countering Weapons of Mass Destruction
Department of Homeland Security
Washington, District of Columbia
Chapter 120, "Smoke Inhalation"
Chapter 123, "Cyanide and Hydrogen Sulfide"

Barbara M. Kirrane, MD, MPH
Medical Toxicology Consultant, Department of
  Emergency Medicine
Physician Advisor, Department of Case
  Management
Saint Barnabas Medical Center
Livingston, New Jersey
*Chapter 138, "Risk Management and Legal
  Principles"*

Kurt C. Kleinschmidt, MD, FACMT, DABAM
Professor of Emergency Medicine
Division Chief, Medical Toxicology
University of Texas Southwestern Medical School
Medical Director, Perinatal Intervention Program
Parkland Health and Hospital System
Dallas, Texas
*Chapter 11, "Biochemical and Metabolic
  Principles"*

Cathy A. Kondas, MD, MBS
Assistant Professor of Psychiatry
New York University School of Medicine
Attending Psychiatrist
Director, Women's Mental Health Fellowship
Associate Director, Consultation-Liaison
  Psychiatry
Bellevue Hospital Center
New York, New York
Chapter 26, "Psychiatric Principles"
Special Considerations: SC4, "Patient Violence"

Andrea Martinez Kondracke, MD
Assistant Professor of Psychiatry and Internal
  Medicine
New York University School of Medicine
Division Chief, Department of Medical Psychiatry
  and Consultation Liaison Psychiatry
Bellevue Hospital Center
New York, New York
Chapter 26, "Psychiatric Principles"
Special Considerations: SC4, "Patient Violence"

Jeffrey T. Lai, MD
Assistant Professor of Emergency Medicine
Department of Emergency Medicine
University of Massachusetts Medical School
UMass Memorial Medical Center
Worcester, Massachusetts
Chapter 56, "Antituberculous Medications"

Melisa W. Lai-Becker, MD, FACEP, FAAEM
Instructor in Emergency Medicine
Harvard Medical School
Chief, CHA Everett Hospital Emergency
  Department
Director, CHA Division of Medical Toxicology
Cambridge Health Alliance
Boston, Massachusetts
Chapter 98, "Silver"

Jeff M. Lapoint, DO
Director, Division of Medical Toxicology
Department of Emergency Medicine
Southern California Permanente Group
San Diego, California
Chapter 74, "Cannabinoids"

David C. Lee, MD
Professor of Emergency Medicine
Donald and Barbara Zucker School of Medicine
  at Hofstra/Northwell
Hempstead, New York
Chair, Department of Emergency Medicine
WellSpan York Hospital
York, Pennsylvania
Chapter 72, "Sedative-Hypnotics"

Joshua D. Lee, MD
Associate Professor of Population Health
New York University School of Medicine
New York, New York
*Special Considerations: SC6, "Prevention,
  Treatment, and Harm Reduction Approaches to
  Opioid Overdoses"*

Jesse M. Lewin, MD, FAAD
Mohs Micrographic and Dermatologic Surgery
Director of Dermatologic Surgery Education
Assistant Professor of Dermatology
Department of Dermatology
Columbia University Irving Medical Center
New York, New York
Chapter 17, "Dermatologic Principles"

Justin M. Lewin, MD
Assistant Professor of Psychiatry
New York University School of Medicine
Comprehensive Psychiatric Emergency Program
Consultation-Liaison Psychiatry
Bellevue Hospital Center
New York, New York
Chapter 26, "Psychiatric Principles"
Special Considerations: SC4, "Patient Violence"

Neal A. Lewin, MD, FACEP, FACMT, FACP
Druckenmiller Professor of Emergency Medicine
  and Professor of Medicine
New York University School of Medicine
Ronald O. Perelman Department of Emergency
  Medicine
Director, Didactic Education
Emergency Medicine Residency
Attending Physician, Emergency Medicine and
  Internal Medicine
Bellevue Hospital Center and NYU Langone
  Health
New York, New York
*Chapter 3, "Initial Evaluation of the Patient: Vital
  Signs and Toxic Syndromes"*
*Chapter 4, "Principles of Managing the Acutely
  Poisoned or Overdosed Patient"*
Chapter 17, "Dermatologic Principles"

Erica L. Liebelt, MD, FACMT
Clinical Professor of Pediatrics and Emergency
  Medicine
University of Washington School of Medicine
Medical/Executive Director
Washington Poison Center
Seattle, Washington
Chapter 68, "Cyclic Antidepressants"

Zhanna Livshits, MD
Assistant Professor of Medicine
Weill Cornell Medical College of Cornell
  University
Emergency Physician and Medical Toxicologist
New York Presbyterian Weill Cornell Medical
  Center
New York, New York
Chapter 89, "Cesium"

Heather Long, MD
Associate Professor of Emergency Medicine
Director, Medical Toxicology
Albany Medical Center
Albany, New York
Chapter 81, "Inhalants"

Scott Lucyk, MD, FRCPC
Clinical Assistant Professor of Emergency
  Medicine
Medical Toxicologist
Associate Medical Director, Poison and Drug
  Information Service (PADIS)
Program Director, Clinical Pharmacology and
  Toxicology
Alberta Health Services
Calgary, Alberta, Canada
*Special Considerations: SC2, "Decontamination
  Principles: Prevention of Dermal, Ophthalmic
  and Inhalational Absorption"*

Daniel M. Lugassy, MD
Assistant Professor of Emergency Medicine
Medical Director, New York Simulation Center for
the Health Sciences (NYSIM)
New York University School of Medicine
Division of Medical Toxicology
Ronald O. Perelman Department of Emergency
Medicine
Emergency Physician, Bellevue Hospital Center
and NYU Langone Health
Toxicology Consultant
New York City Poison Control Center
New York, New York
Chapter 37, "Salicylates"

Nima Majlesi, DO
Assistant Professor of Emergency Medicine
Donald and Barbara Zucker School of Medicine
at Hofstra/Northwell
Director of Medical Toxicology
Staten Island University Hospital
Staten Island, New York
Chapter 100, "Zinc"

Alex F. Manini, MD, MS, FACMT, FAACT
Professor of Emergency Medicine
Division of Medical Toxicology
Icahn School of Medicine at Mount Sinai
Elmhurst Hospital Center
New York, New York
Chapter 71, "Monoamine Oxidase Inhibitors"
*Chapter 137, "Principles of Epidemiology and
Research Design"*

Jeanna M. Marraffa, PharmD, DABAT, FAACT
Associate Professor of Emergency Medicine
Clinical Toxicologist
Assistant Clinical Director, Upstate New York
Poison Center
Upstate Medical University
Syracuse, New York
Chapter 40, "Dieting Xenobiotics and Regimens"

**Maryann Mazer-Amirshahi, PharmD,
MD, MPH**
Associate Professor of Emergency Medicine
Georgetown University School of Medicine
Emergency Physician,
Department of Emergency Medicine
MedStar Washington Hospital Center
Washington, District of Columbia
Chapter 57, "Antidysrhythmics"

Charles A. McKay, MD, FACMT, FACEP
Associate Clinical Professor of Emergency
Medicine
University of Connecticut School of Medicine
Consulting Toxicologist
Division of Medical Toxicology
Hartford Hospital and University of Connecticut
Health Center
Associate Medical Director
Connecticut Poison Control Center
Farmington, Connecticut
*Chapter 133, "Risk Assessment and Risk
Communication"*

Nathanael J. McKeown, DO, FACMT
Assistant Professor of Emergency Medicine
Oregon Health & Science University
Medical Toxicologist
Oregon Poison Center
Chief, Emergency Medicine Service
VA Portland Health Care System
Portland, Oregon
Chapter 33, "Acetaminophen"

Maria Mercurio-Zappala, RPh, MS
Assistant Professor of Emergency Medicine
New York University School of Medicine
Ronald O. Perelman Department of Emergency
Medicine
Associate Director
New York City Poison Control Center
New York, New York
Chapter 99, "Thallium"

**Robert A. Middleberg, PhD, F-ABFT,
DABCC(TC)**
Adjunct Assistant Professor of Pharmacology and
Experimental Therapeutics
Thomas Jefferson University
Philadelphia, Pennsylvania
Laboratory Director
NMS Labs
Willow Grove, Pennsylvania
Chapter 139, "Medicolegal Interpretive Toxicology"

Stephen W. Munday, MD, MPH, MS
Chair, Department of Occupational Medicine and
Chief Medical Toxicologist
Sharp Rees-Stealy Medical Group
San Diego, California
Chapter 86, "Arsenic"

Mark J. Neavyn, MD
Assistant Professor of Emergency Medicine
Program Director, Fellowship in Medical
Toxicology
University of Massachusetts Medical School
UMass Memorial Medical Center
Worcester, Massachusetts
Chapter 79, "Hallucinogens"

**Lewis S. Nelson, MD, FAACT, FACEP, FACMT,
FAAEM, FASAM**
Professor and Chair of Emergency Medicine
Director, Division of Medical Toxicology
Rutgers New Jersey Medical School
Chief of Service, Emergency Department
University Hospital of Newark
New Jersey Poison Information and Education
System
Newark, New Jersey
*Chapter 3, "Initial Evaluation of the Patient: Vital
Signs and Toxic Syndromes"*
*Chapter 4, "Principles of Managing the Acutely
Poisoned or Overdosed Patient"*
Chapter 10, "Chemical Principles"
Chapter 17, "Dermatologic Principles"
Chapter 36, "Opioids"
Chapter 57, "Antidysrhythmics"
Chapter 77, "Alcohol Withdrawal"
Chapter 92, "Copper"
Chapter 118, "Plants"
*Chapter 121, "Simple Asphyxiants and Pulmonary
Irritants"*
Antidotes in Depth: A4, "Opioid Antagonists"
Antidotes in Depth: A26, "Benzodiazepines"
*Special Considerations: SC3, "Transdermal
Toxicology"*

Vincent Nguyen, MD
Assistant Professor of Emergency Medicine
Medical Toxicologist
Albert Einstein College of Medicine
Jacobi Medical Center/North Central Bronx
Medical Center
The Bronx, New York
Antidotes in Depth: A8, "Dextrose (D-Glucose)"

**Sean Patrick Nordt, MD, PharmD, DABAT,
FAACT, FAAEM, FACMT**
Associate Dean, Academic Affairs
Gavin Herbert Endowed Professor of Pharmacy
Chief Medical Officer
Chapman University School of Pharmacy
Crean College of Health and Behavioral Sciences
Chapman University
Adjunct Associate Professor of Emergency
Medicine
Department of Emergency Medicine
University of California, Irvine
Irvine, California
Chapter 46, "Pharmaceutical Additives"

Ayrn D. O'Connor, MD
Associate Professor of Emergency Medicine
Program Director, Medical Toxicology Fellowship
University of Arizona College of Medicine
Phoenix
Department of Medical Toxicology
Banner—University Medical Center Phoenix
Phoenix, Arizona
*Chapter 13, "Neurotransmitters and
Neuromodulators"*

Ruben E. Olmedo, MD
Associate Clinical Professor of Emergency
    Medicine
Icahn School of Medicine at Mount Sinai
Director, Division of Toxicology
Mount Sinai Hospital
New York, New York
Chapter 83, "Phencyclidine and Ketamine"

Dean Olsen, DO
Assistant Professor of Emergency Medicine and
    Toxicology
NYIT College of Osteopathic Medicine
Old Westbury, New York
Director, Residency in Emergency Medicine
Nassau University Medical Center
East Meadow, New York
Chapter 36, "Opioids"

Robert B. Palmer, PhD, DABAT, FAACT
Assistant Clinical Professor of Emergency
    Medicine (Medical Toxicology)
University of Colorado School of Medicine
Attending Toxicologist
Medical Toxicology Fellowship Program
Rocky Mountain Poison and Drug Center
Denver, Colorado
*Special Considerations: SC11, "Assessment of
    Ethanol-Induced Impairment"*

Jeanmarie Perrone, MD, FACMT
Professor of Emergency Medicine
Director of Medical Toxicology
Perelman School of Medicine, University of
    Pennsylvania
Philadelphia, Pennsylvania
Chapter 45, "Iron"

Anthony F. Pizon, MD
Associate Professor of Emergency Medicine
University of Pittsburgh School of Medicine
Chief, Division of Medical Toxicology
University of Pittsburgh Medical Center
Pittsburgh, Pennsylvania
*Chapter 119, "Native (US) Venomous Snakes and
    Lizards"*
*Antidotes in Depth: A39, "Antivenom for North
    American Venomous Snakes (Crotaline and
    Elapid)"*

Dennis P. Price, MD
Assistant Professor of Emergency Medicine
New York University School of Medicine
Emergency Physician
Ronald O. Perelman Department of Emergency
    Medicine
Bellevue Hospital Center and NYU Langone
    Health
New York, New York
Chapter 124, "Methemoglobin Inducers"

Jane M. Prosser, MD
Medical Toxicologist
Emergency Physician
Department of Emergency Medicine
Kaiser Permanente Northern California
Kaiser Permanente
Vallejo, California
*Special Considerations: SC5, "Internal
    Concealment of Xenobiotics"*

Petrie M. Rainey, MD, PhD, FACMT
Professor Emeritus of Laboratory Medicine
University of Washington School of Medicine
University of Washington Medical Center
Seattle, Washington
Chapter 7, "Laboratory Principles"

Rama B. Rao, MD, FACMT
Associate Professor of Medicine
Weill Cornell Medical College of Cornell
    University
Chief, Division of Medical Toxicology
Emergency Physician
New York-Presbyterian Hospital
New York, New York
Chapter 22, "Neurologic Principles"
Chapter 87, "Bismuth"
Chapter 140, "Postmortem Toxicology"
*Special Considerations: SC7, "Intrathecal
    Administration of Xenobiotics"*
*Special Considerations: SC12, "Organ Procurement
    from Poisoned Patients"*

Joseph G. Rella, MD
Assistant Professor of Medicine
Weill Cornell Medical College of Cornell
    University
Emergency Physician
New York-Presbyterian Hospital
New York, New York
Chapter 128, "Radiation"
Antidotes in Depth: A44, "Potassium Iodide"
*Antidotes in Depth: A45, "Pentetic Acid or
    Pentetate (Zinc or Calcium) Trisodium
    (DTPA)"*

Daniel J. Repplinger, MD
Assistant Clinical Professor of Emergency
    Medicine
University of California, San Francisco
Zuckerberg San Francisco General Hospital
San Francisco, California
Chapter 115, "Arthropods"

Morgan A. A. Riggan, MD, FRCPC
Assistant Professor of Emergency Medicine
Western University
Emergency Physician
London Health Sciences Centre
London, Ontario, Canada
Medical Toxicologist
Poison and Drug Information Service (PADIS)
Alberta Health Services
Calgary, Alberta, Canada
Chapter 105, "Hydrocarbons"

Darren M. Roberts, MBBS, PhD, FRACP
Conjoint Associate Professor
University of New South Wales
Consultant Physician and Clinical Toxicologist
St. Vincent's Hospital and New South Wales
    Poisons Information Centre
Sydney, Australia
Chapter 109, "Herbicides"

Anne-Michelle Ruha, MD
Professor of Internal Medicine and Emergency
    Medicine
Departments of Internal Medicine and
    Emergency Medicine
University of Arizona College of
    Medicine—Phoenix
Department of Medical Toxicology
Banner—University Medical Center Phoenix
Phoenix, Arizona
*Chapter 119, "Native (US) Venomous Snakes and
    Lizards"*
*Antidotes in Depth: A39, "Antivenom for North
    American Venomous Snakes (Crotaline and Elapid)"*

Cynthia D. Santos, MD
Assistant Professor of Emergency Medicine
Emergency Physician
University Hospital of Newark
Rutgers New Jersey Medical School
Toxicology Consultant
New Jersey Poison Information and Education
    System
Newark, New Jersey
*Chapter 34, "Colchicine, Podophyllin, and the
    Vinca Alkaloids"*

Daniel Schatz, MD
Addiction Medicine Fellow
Department of Medicine
New York University School of Medicine
Bellevue Hospital Center
New York, New York
*Special Considerations: SC6, "Prevention,
    Treatment, and Harm Reduction Approaches to
    Opioid Overdoses"*

Capt. Joshua G. Schier, MD, MPH, USPHS
Lead, Environmental Toxicology Team
Centers for Disease Control and Prevention
Assistant Professor of Emergency Medicine
Emory University School of Medicine
Associate Director, Emory/CDC Medical
    Toxicology Fellowship
Consultant, Georgia Poison Center
Atlanta, Georgia
*Chapter 34, "Colchicine, Podophyllin, and the
    Vinca Alkaloids"*
Special Considerations: SC9, "Diethylene Glycol"

David T. Schwartz, MD
Associate Professor of Emergency Medicine
New York University School of Medicine
Emergency Physician
Ronald O. Perelman Department of Emergency
    Medicine
Bellevue Hospital Center and NYU Langone
    Health
New York, New York
Chapter 8, "Principles of Diagnostic Imaging"

Lauren Schwartz, MPH
Assistant Professor of Emergency Medicine
New York University School of Medicine
Ronald O. Perelman Department of Emergency
    Medicine
Director, Public Education
New York City Poison Control Center
New York, New York
Chapter 129, "Poison Prevention and Education"

Shahin Shadnia, MD, PhD, FACMT
Professor of Clinical Toxicology
Head of Clinical Toxicology Department
School of Medicine
Shahid Beheshti University of Medical Sciences
Chairman of Loghman Hakim Hospital Poison
    Center
Tehran, Iran
Chapter 108, "Fumigants"

Adhi Sharma, MD, FACMT, FACEP
Clinical Associate Professor of Emergency
    Medicine
Donald and Barbara Zucker School of Medicine
    at Hofstra/Northwell
Hempstead, New York
Senior Vice President, Medical Affairs
Chief Medical Officer
South Nassau Communities Hospital
Oceanside, New York
Chapter 24, "Ophthalmic Principles"

Lauren Kornreich Shawn, MD
Assistant Professor of Emergency Medicine
Icahn School of Medicine at Mount Sinai
Mount Sinai St. Luke's, Mount Sinai West
New York, New York
Chapter 42, "Essential Oils"

**Farshad Mazda Shirazi, MSc, MD, PhD, FACEP,
FACMT**
Associate Professor of Emergency Medicine,
    Pharmacology and Pharmacy Practice and
    Science
University of Arizona College of
    Medicine—Tucson
Program Director, Medical Toxicology
Medical Director, Arizona Poison and Drug
    Information Center
Tucson, Arizona
*Special Considerations: SC10, "Exotic Nonnative
    Snake Envenomations"*

**Marco L. A. Sivilotti, MD, MSc, FRCPC,
    FACMT, FAACT**
Professor of Emergency Medicine and of
    Biomedical and Molecular Sciences
Queen's University
Kingston, Ontario, Canada
Consultant, Ontario Poison Centre
Toronto, Ontario, Canada
Chapter 20, "Hematologic Principles"

Silas W. Smith, MD, FACEP, FACMT
JoAnn G. and Kenneth Wellner Associate
    Professor of Emergency Medicine
New York University School of Medicine
Section Chief, Quality, Safety, and Practice
    Innovation
Associate Program Director, Medical Toxicology
    Fellowship
Emergency Physician
Ronald O. Perelman Department of Emergency
    Medicine
Bellevue Hospital Center and NYU Langone
    Health
New York, New York
*Chapter 3, "Initial Evaluation of the Patient: Vital
    Signs and Toxic Syndromes"*
*Chapter 4, "Principles of Managing the Acutely
    Poisoned or Overdosed Patient"*
Chapter 125, "Nanotoxicology"
Antidotes in Depth: A1, "Activated Charcoal"
*Antidotes in Depth: A2, 'Whole-Bowel Irrigation
    and Other Intestinal Evacuants"*
Antidotes in Depth: A6, "Botulinum Antitoxin"
Antidotes in Depth: A9, "Octreotide"
*Antidotes in Depth: A12, "Folates: Leucovorin
    (Folinic Acid) and Folic Acid"*
*Antidotes in Depth: A13, "Glucarpidase
    (Carboxypeptidase G₂)"*
Antidotes in Depth: A14, "Uridine Triacetate"
Antidotes in Depth: A16, "Magnesium"
Antidotes in Depth: A20, "Glucagon"
*Antidotes in Depth: A22, "Digoxin-Specific
    Antibody Fragments"*
Antidotes in Depth: A32, "Calcium"
*Special Considerations: SC1, "Principles of
    Antidote Stocking"*

Craig G. Smollin, MD, FACMT
Associate Professor of Emergency Medicine
Program Director, Medical Toxicology
University of California, San Francisco
Medical Director, California Poison Control
    System–San Francisco Division
San Francisco, California
Chapter 75, "Cocaine"

Sari Soghoian, MD, MA
Associate Professor of Emergency Medicine
New York University School of Medicine
New York, New York
Clinical Coordinator, Korle Bu Teaching Hospital
Department of Emergency Medicine
Accra, Ghana
Chapter 82, "Nicotine"
Chapter 94, "Manganese"
*Chapter 136, "International Perspectives on
    Medical Toxicology"*

Kambiz Soltaninejad, PharmD, PhD
Associate Professor of Toxicology
Department of Forensic Toxicology
Legal Medicine Research Center
Legal Medicine Organization
Tehran, Iran
Chapter 108, "Fumigants"

Meghan B. Spyres, MD
Assistant Professor of Clinical Emergency
    Medicine
Division of Medical Toxicology
University of Southern California, Keck School of
    Medicine
Los Angeles, California
Chapter 73, "Amphetamines"

**Samuel J. Stellpflug, MD, FAACT, FACMT,
FACEP, FAAEM**
Associate Professor of Emergency Medicine
University of Minnesota Medical School
Minneapolis, Minnesota
Director, Clinical Toxicology
Regions Hospital
Saint Paul, Minnesota
Antidotes in Depth: A21, "High-Dose Insulin (HDI)"

Michael E. Stern, MD
Associate Professor of Clinical Medicine
Chief, Geriatric Emergency Medicine
New York Presbyterian Weill Cornell Medical
    Center, Cornell University
New York, New York
Chapter 32, "Geriatric Principles"

**Andrew Stolbach, MD, MPH, FAACT,
    FACEP, FACMT**
Associate Professor of Emergency Medicine
Johns Hopkins University School of Medicine
Toxicology Consultant
Maryland Poison Center
Baltimore, Maryland
Chapter 28, "Respiratory Principles"

**Christine M. Stork, BS, PharmD, DABAT,
    FAACT**
Professor of Emergency Medicine
Clinical Director, Upstate NY Poison Center
Upstate Medical University
Syracuse, New York
*Chapter 54, "Antibacterials, Antifungals, and
    Antivirals"*
*Chapter 69, "Serotonin Reuptake Inhibitors and
    Atypical Antidepressants"*

Mark K. Su, MD, MPH
Associate Professor of Emergency Medicine
New York University School of Medicine
Emergency Physician
Ronald O. Perelman Department of Emergency
    Medicine
Bellevue Hospital Center and NYU Langone
    Health
Director, New York City Poison Control Center
New York, New York
Chapter 58, "Antithrombotics"
Chapter 104, "Hydrofluoric Acid and Fluorides"
*Chapter 130, "Poison Control Centers and Poison
    Epidemiology"*
*Antidotes in Depth: A17, "Prothrombin Complex
    Concentrates and Direct Oral Anticoagulant
    Antidotes"*

Jeffrey R. Suchard, MD
Professor of Clinical Emergency Medicine and
    Pharmacology
University of California, Irvine School of Medicine
Irvine, California
Chapter 126, "Chemical Weapons"
Chapter 127, "Biological Weapons"

Payal Sud, MD, FACEP
Assistant Professor of Emergency Medicine
Donald and Barbara Zucker School of Medicine
    at Hofstra/Northwell
Hempstead, New York
Director of Performance Improvement
Department of Emergency Medicine
Long Island Jewish Medical Center
Assistant Program Director
Medical Toxicology Fellowship
Northwell Health
New Hyde Park, New York
Chapter 72, "Sedative-Hypnotics"

Young-Jin Sue, MD
Clinical Associate Professor of Pediatrics
Albert Einstein College of Medicine
Attending Physician, Pediatric Emergency
    Services
The Children's Hospital at Montefiore
Bronx, New York
Chapter 95, "Mercury"

Kenneth M. Sutin, MS, MD, FCCP, FCCM
Professor of Anesthesiology
New York University School of Medicine
Attending Physician, Department of
    Anesthesiology
Bellevue Hospital Center
New York, New York
Chapter 66, "Neuromuscular Blockers"
Antidotes in Depth: A24, "Dantrolene Sodium"

Matthew D. Sztajnkrycer, MD, PhD
Professor of Emergency Medicine
Mayo Clinic College of Medicine and Science
Staff Toxicologist
Minnesota Poison Control System
Rochester, Minnesota
Chapter 64, "Local Anesthetics"

Mai Takematsu, MD
Assistant Professor of Emergency Medicine
Albert Einstein College of Medicine
Director, Division of Medical Toxicology
Montefiore Medical Center
Bronx, New York
Chapter 25, "Otolaryngologic Principles"

Asim F. Tarabar, MD, MS
Assistant Professor of Emergency Medicine
Yale University School of Medicine
Director, Medical Toxicology
Yale New Haven Hospital
New Haven, Connecticut
Chapter 85, "Antimony"

Stephen R. Thom, MD, PhD
Professor of Emergency Medicine
Director of Research
University of Maryland School of Medicine
Baltimore, Maryland
Antidotes in Depth: A40, "Hyperbaric Oxygen"

**Christian Tomaszewski, MD, MS, MBA,
FACMT, FACEP**
Professor of Clinical Emergency Medicine
University of California, San Diego Health
Chief Medical Officer, El Centro Regional Medical
    Center
San Diego, California
Chapter 122, "Carbon Monoxide"

Stephen J. Traub, MD
Associate Professor of Emergency Medicine
Mayo Clinic College of Medicine and Science
Chairman, Department of Emergency Medicine
Mayo Clinic Arizona
Phoenix, Arizona
Chapter 10, "Chemical Principles"
Chapter 88, "Cadmium"

Michael G. Tunik, MD
Associate Professor of Emergency Medicine and
    Pediatrics
New York University School of Medicine
Director of Research, Division of Pediatric
    Emergency Medicine
Emergency Physician
Ronald O. Perelman Department of Emergency
    Medicine
Bellevue Hospital Center and NYU Langone
    Health
New York, New York
Chapter 39, "Food Poisoning"

Matthew Valento, MD
Assistant Professor of Emergency Medicine
Site Director for Medical Toxicology
University of Washington School of Medicine
Attending Physician
Harborview Medical Center
Seattle, Washington
Chapter 68, "Cyclic Antidepressants"

Susi U. Vassallo, MD
Professor of Emergency Medicine
New York University School of Medicine
Emergency Physician
Ronald O. Perelman Department of Emergency
    Medicine
Bellevue Hospital Center and NYU Langone
    Health
New York, New York
Chapter 29, "Thermoregulatory Principles"
Chapter 41, "Athletic Performance Enhancers"

Larissa I. Velez, MD, FACEP
Professor of Emergency Medicine
University of Texas Southwestern Medical School
Vice Chair of Education
Program Director of Emergency Medicine
Department of Emergency Medicine
University of Texas Southwestern Medical Center
Staff Toxicologist, North Texas Poison Center
Dallas, Texas
Antidotes in Depth: A8, "Dextrose (D-Glucose)"

Lisa E. Vivero, PharmD
Drug Information Specialist
Irvine, California
Chapter 46, "Pharmaceutical Additives"

Peter H. Wald, MD, MPH
Adjunct Professor of Public Health
San Antonio Regional Campus
University of Texas School of Public Health
Houston, Texas
Enterprise Medical Director, USAA
San Antonio, Texas
Houston, Texas
*Chapter 131, "Principles of Occupational
    Toxicology: Diagnosis and Control"*

Richard Y. Wang, DO
Senior Medical Officer
National Center for Environmental Health
Centers for Disease Control and Prevention
Atlanta, Georgia
Chapter 23, "Oncologic Principles"
Chapter 50, "Chemotherapeutics"
*Chapter 51, "Methotrexate, 5-Flourouracil, and
    Capecitabine"*
*Special Considerations: SC8, "Extravasation of
    Xenobiotics"*

Paul M. Wax, MD
Clinical Professor of Emergency Medicine
University of Texas Southwestern Medical School
Dallas, Texas
Executive Director
American College of Medical Toxicology
Phoenix, Arizona
Chapter 1, "Historical Principles and Perspectives"
*Chapter 2, "Toxicologic Misfortunes and
    Catastrophes in History"*
*Chapter 101, "Antiseptics, Disinfectants, and
    Sterilants"*
Antidotes in Depth: A5, "Sodium Bicarbonate"

Sage W. Wiener, MD
Assistant Professor of Emergency Medicine
SUNY Downstate Medical Center College of
    Medicine
Director of Medical Toxicology
SUNY Downstate Medical Center/Kings County
    Hospital
Brooklyn, New York
Chapter 106, "Toxic Alcohols"

Rachel S. Wightman, MD
Assistant Professor of Emergency Medicine
Division of Medical Toxicology
The Warren Alpert Medical School of Brown
    University
Rhode Island Hospital
Providence, Rhode Island
*Chapter 16, "Cardiologic Principles II:
    Hemodynamics"*
Chapter 103, "Caustics"

Luke Yip, MD
Consultant and Attending Staff Medical
   Toxicologist
Denver Health
Rocky Mountain Poison and Drug Center
Department of Medicine
Section of Medical Toxicology
Denver, Colorado
Senior Medical Toxicologist
Centers for Disease Control and Prevention
Office of Noncommunicable Diseases, Injury, and
   Environmental Health
National Center for Environmental Health/Agency
   for Toxic Substances and Disease Registry
Atlanta, Georgia
Chapter 76, "Ethanol"

Erin A. Zerbo, MD
Assistant Professor of Psychiatry
Associate Director, Medical Student Education in
   Psychiatry
Rutgers New Jersey Medical School
Newark, New Jersey
Chapter 26, "Psychiatric Principles"
Special Considerations: SC4, "Patient Violence"

Matthew D. Zuckerman, MD
Assistant Professor of Emergency Medicine/
   Medical Toxicology
University of Colorado School of Medicine
Denver, Colorado
Chapter 18, "Gastrointestinal Principles"

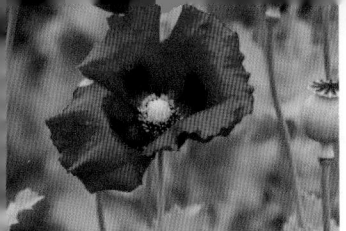

PREFACE

Goldfrank's Toxicologic Emergencies is a multiauthored text of approximately 2,000 pages prepared by using the educational and management principles we apply at the New York City Poison Control Center, New Jersey Poison Information & Education System, and at our clinical sites. In this eleventh edition of *Goldfrank's Toxicologic Emergencies*, we proudly offer readers an approach to medical toxicology using evidence-based principles viewed through the lens of an active bedside clinical practice.

Some would ask why create textbooks and e-books in an era when podcasts and blogs appear so successful. We still believe that the slow, thoughtful, rigorous investigation of all available information by a team of authors and editors required to create and revise this text is essential to analyze the complex problems that challenge our daily practices. Although in our field we have made great progress, the level of uncertainty remains substantial. We have attempted to integrate the collaborative wisdom of experts from diverse backgrounds in order to provide the information necessary to achieve excellence. We offer our readers the evidence, shared thoughts, and structured analysis necessary to arrive at a decision. Evidence is created not only with randomized clinical trials, observational studies, case control studies, and case reports, but also with the insights of six toxicologists who work together continuously, along with the gifted scholars we selected as authors. We have worked together defining and redefining the scope and context of chapters, Antidotes in Depth, and Special Considerations. We then shared our ideas with many respected local, national, and international toxicologists, thus creating new chapters that these toxicologists have revised by adding information and insight that has come to light since the publication of the tenth edition of the text. In this way, knowledge from their experience as toxicologists and related disciplines is merged with ours, allowing us to create chapters that represent our collective thoughts. This iterative process is continued until the authors and editors are satisfied that we have closely approximated the best strategy to evaluate and care for poisoned or overdosed patients. This is a fascinating process. In this edition, we have tried to enhance our rigor focusing on as precise an analysis of the literature as we can all do and an attempt to tell you as clearly as possible what we and our authors think and how we practice. Because we occasionally disagree, we then reread, research, look for special cases, and reflect on a final version with our authors.

In this edition, we have asked Rana Biary, MD to expand the concept of the patient narrative in the Case Studies section. These are the patients who challenge us to be vigilant as toxicologists. Such patients, whose signs and symptoms are related to the whole book or to several chapters, serve to return us to focus on the unknown, the differential diagnosis, and problem solving and include contextual cases representative of our work. Patients with a pesticide exposure, bradycardia, metabolic acidosis, medication error, seizures, coma or agitation, and hyperthermia are offered as examples for contemplation. We believe that analyzing the care of these complex, undifferentiated patients will help you as much as they have helped us and those who read the first edition of this book. These cases act as the building blocks for chapters in this edition and represent provocative introductions to several sections of this text. We have demonstrated our thought processes so that you can understand our approach to patient management. This classic Socratic development of knowledge and improvement of clinical decision making will improve problem solving, stimulate creative investigation, and enhance care. We hope to facilitate your participation in the intellectual processes that we believe to be essential in order to create a fine book for thoughtful readers who desire to render excellent attention to their patients. The cases serve as the transition between the patient and population as you diminish the gap between your roles as a medical or clinical toxicologist at the bedside and that of a toxicologist serving the needs of the community. Our hope is that these cases re-create the clinicians' thoughts prior to, during, and after care is initiated.

In this eleventh edition, Silas W. Smith, MD, became an editor reflecting his superior work on prior editions. We are sure that his knowledge and thoughtfulness will be appreciated by all.

The Editors

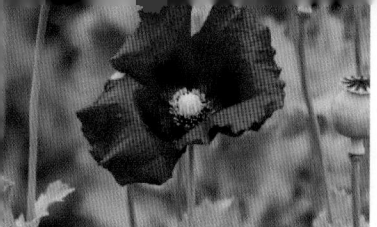

ACKNOWLEDGMENTS

We are grateful to Joan Demas, who worked extensively with the local, national, and international authors to ensure that their ideas were effectively expressed. She has assisted all of us in checking the facts, finding essential references, and improving the structure and function of our text, while dedicating her efforts to ensuring the precision and rigor of the text for her fifth consecutive edition. She has helped authors new and old achieve their commitment with the skill of an exceptional publishing professional. The authors' and editors' work is better because of her devotion to excellence, calm demeanor in the face of editorial chaos, and consistent presence throughout each stage of the production of this text. We are deeply appreciative of the wonderful effort she provides for our readers and colleagues.

The many letters and verbal communications we have received with the reviews of the previous editions of this book continue to improve our efforts. We are deeply indebted to our friends, associates, residents, fellows, and students, who stimulated us to begin this book with their questions and then faithfully criticized our answers.

We appreciate the assistance of Dorice Vieira, Associate Curator, Medical Library, and Clinical Outreach and Graduate Medical Education Librarian, in her commitment to helping us find essential information.

We thank the many volunteers, students, librarians, and particularly the St. John's University College of Pharmacy and Health Sciences students and drug information staff who provide us with vital technical assistance in our daily attempts to deal with toxicologic emergencies.

No words can adequately express our indebtedness to the many authors who worked on earlier editions of many of the chapters in this book. As different authors write and rewrite topics with each new edition, we recognize that without the foundational work of their predecessors this book would not be what it is today.

We appreciate the creative skills in design and scientific art that the McGraw-Hill team, led by Armen Ovsepyan, have added to the text. The devotion to the creation of high-quality art graphics and tables is greatly appreciated. The support for excellence in this edition was facilitated by the constant vigilance of our longstanding collaborator Senior Content Acquisitions Editor Karen Edmonson whose thoughtful, and cooperative spirit persists after all these years. Her intelligence and ever vigilant commitment to our efforts has been wonderful. We are pleased with the creative developmental editorial efforts of Robert Pancotti. The organized project management by Revathi Viswanathan has found errors hiding throughout our pages. Her carefully posed questions have facilitated the process of correcting the text. It has been a pleasure to have her assistance. We greatly appreciate the compulsion that Maria van Beuren has applied to make the index of this edition one of unique value. She demonstrated exceptional rigor with a twist of copy editing to find many unseen errors, saving the reader confusion and us embarrassment. We appreciate the work of Catherine Saggese in ensuring the quality of production in the finished work.

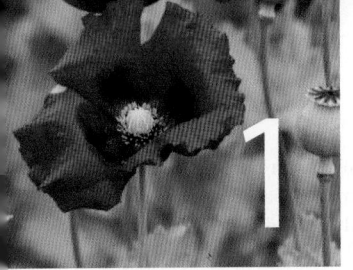

1 HISTORICAL PRINCIPLES AND PERSPECTIVES

Paul M. Wax

The term *poison* first appeared in the English literature around 1225 A.D. to describe a potion or draught that was prepared with deadly ingredients.[8,155] The history of poisons and poisoning, however, dates back thousands of years. Throughout the millennia, poisons have played an important role in human history—from political assassination in Roman times, to weapons of war, to contemporary environmental concerns, and to weapons of terrorism.

This chapter offers a perspective on the impact of poisons and poisoning on history. It also provides a historic overview of human understanding of poisons and the development of toxicology from antiquity to the present. The development of the modern poison control center, the genesis of the field of medical toxicology, and the increasing focus on medication errors are examined. Chapter 2 describes poison plagues and unintentional disasters throughout history and examines the societal consequences of these unfortunate events. An appreciation of past failures and mistakes in dealing with poisons and poisoning promotes a keener insight and a more critical evaluation of present-day toxicologic issues and helps in the assessment and management of future toxicologic problems.

POISONS, POISONERS, AND ANTIDOTES OF ANTIQUITY

The earliest poisons consisted of plant extracts, animal venoms, and minerals. They were used for hunting, waging war, and sanctioned and unsanctioned executions. The *Ebers Papyrus*, an ancient Egyptian text written circa 1500 B.C. that is considered to be among the earliest medical texts, describes many ancient poisons, including aconite, antimony, arsenic, cyanogenic glycosides, hemlock, lead, mandrake, opium, and wormwood.[102,155] These poisons were thought to have mystical properties, and their use was surrounded by superstition and intrigue. Some agents, such as the Calabar bean (*Physostigma venenosum*) containing physostigmine, were referred to as "ordeal poisons." Ingestion of these substances was believed to be lethal to the guilty and harmless to the innocent.[130] The "penalty of the peach" involved the administration of peach pits, which we now know contain the cyanide precursor amygdalin, as an ordeal poison. Magicians, sorcerers, and religious figures were the toxicologists of antiquity. The Sumerians, in circa 4500 B.C., were said to worship the deity Gula, who was known as the "mistress of charms and spells" and the "controller of noxious poisons" (Table 1–1).[155]

Arrow and Dart Poisons

The prehistoric Masai hunters of Kenya, who lived 18,000 years ago, used arrow and dart poisons to increase the lethality of their weapons.[20] One of these poisons appears to have consisted of extracts of *Strophanthus* species, an indigenous plant that contains strophanthin, a digitalislike substance.[102] Cave paintings of arrowheads and spearheads reveal that these weapons were crafted with small depressions at the end to hold the poison.[156] In fact, the term *toxicology* is derived from the Greek terms *toxikos* ("bow") and *toxikon* ("poison into which arrowheads are dipped").[6,156]

References to arrow poisons are cited in a number of other important literary works. The ancient Indian text *Rig Veda*, written in the 12th century B.C., refers to the use of *Aconitum* species for arrow poisons.[20] In the *Odyssey*, Homer (ca. 850 B.C.) wrote that Ulysses anointed his arrows with a variety of poisons, including extracts of *Helleborus orientalis* and snake venoms. The writings of Ovid (43 B.C.–18 A.D.), describe weapons poisoned with the blood of serpents.[164]

Classification of Poisons

The first attempts at poison identification and classification and the introduction of the first antidotes took place during Greek and Roman times.

An early categorization of poisons divided them into fast poisons, such as strychnine, and slow poisons, such as arsenic. In his treatise, *Materia Medica*, the Greek physician Dioscorides (40–80 A.D.) categorized poisons by their origin—animal, vegetable, or mineral.[156] This categorization remained the standard classification for the next 1,500 years.[156]

Animal Poisons

Animal poisons usually referred to the venom from poisonous animals. Although the venom from poisonous snakes has always been among the most commonly feared poisons, poisons from toads, salamanders, jellyfish, stingrays, and sea hares are often as lethal. Nicander of Colophon (204–135 B.C.), a

TABLE 1–1	Important Early People in the History of Toxicology	
Person	**Date**	**Importance**
Gula	ca. 4500 B.C.	First deity associated with poisons
Shen Nung	ca. 2000 B.C.	Chinese emperor who experimented with poisons and antidotes and wrote treatise on herbal medicine
Homer	ca. 850 B.C.	Wrote how Ulysses anointed arrows with the venom of serpents
Aristotle	384–322 B.C.	Described the preparation and use of arrow poisons
Theophrastus	ca. 370–286 B.C.	Referred to poisonous plants in *De Historia Plantarum*
Socrates	ca. 470–399 B.C.	Executed by poison hemlock
Nicander	204–135 B.C.	Wrote two poems, "Theriaca" and "Alexipharmaca," that are among the earliest works on poisons
King Mithridates VI	ca. 132–63 B.C.	Fanatical fear of poisons; developed mithridatum, one of the universal antidotes
Sulla	81 B.C.	Issued *Lex Cornelia*, the first antipoisoning law
Cleopatra	69–30 B.C.	Committed suicide with deliberate cobra envenomation
Andromachus	37–68 A.D.	Refined mithridatum; known as the Theriac of Andromachus
Dioscorides	40–80 A.D.	Wrote *Materia Medica*, which classified poisons by animal, vegetable, and mineral
Galen	ca. 129–200 A.D.	Prepared "nut theriac" for Roman emperors, a remedy against bites, stings, and poisons; wrote *De Antidotis I* and *II*, which provided recipes for different antidotes, including mithridatum and panacea
Ibn Wahshiya	9th century	Famed Arab toxicologist; wrote toxicology treatise *Book on Poisons*, combining contemporary science, magic, and astrology
Moses Maimonides	1135–1204	Wrote *Treatise on Poisons and Their Antidotes*
Petrus Abbonus	1250–1315	Wrote *De Venenis*, major work on poisoning

Greek poet and physician who is considered to be one of the earliest toxicologists, experimented with animal poisons on condemned criminals.[142] Nicander's poems *Theriaca* and *Alexipharmaca* are considered to be the earliest extant Greek toxicologic texts, describing the presentations and treatment of poisonings from animal xenobiotics.[155] A notable fatality from the effects of an animal xenobiotic was Cleopatra (69–30 B.C.), who reportedly committed suicide by deliberately falling on an asp.[76]

Vegetable Poisons

Theophrastus (ca. 370–286 B.C.) described vegetable poisons in his treatise *De Historia Plantarum*.[77] Notorious poisonous plants included *Aconitum* species (monkshood, aconite), *Conium maculatum* (poison hemlock), *Hyoscyamus niger* (henbane), *Mandragora officinarum* (mandrake), *Papaver somniferum* (opium poppy), and *Veratrum album* (hellebore). Aconite was among the most frequently encountered poisonous plants and was described as the "queen mother of poisons."[155] Hemlock was the official poison used by the Greeks and was used in the execution of Socrates (ca. 470–399 B.C.) and many others.[144] Poisonous plants used in India at this time included *Cannabis indica* (marijuana), *Croton tiglium* (croton oil), and *Strychnos nux vomica* (poison nut, strychnine).[77]

Mineral Poisons

The mineral poisons of antiquity consisted of the metals antimony, arsenic, lead, and mercury. Undoubtedly, the most famous of these was lead. Lead was discovered as early as 3500 B.C. Although controversy continues about whether an epidemic of lead poisoning among the Roman aristocracy contributed to the fall of the Roman Empire, lead was certainly used extensively during this period.[55,118] In addition to its considerable use in plumbing,[44] lead was also used in the production of food and drink containers.[62] It was common practice to add lead directly to wine or to intentionally prepare the wine in a lead kettle to improve its taste. Not surprisingly, chronic lead poisoning became widespread. Nicander described the first case of lead poisoning in the 2nd century B.C.[159] Dioscorides, writing in the 1st century A.D., noted that fortified wine was "most hurtful to the nerves."[159] Lead-induced gout ("saturnine gout") may have also been widespread among the Roman elite.[118]

Gases

Although not animal, vegetable, or mineral in origin, the toxic effects of gases were also appreciated during antiquity. In the 3rd century B.C., Aristotle commented that "coal fumes lead to a heavy head and death,"[74] and Cicero (106–43 B.C.) referred to the use of coal fumes in suicides and executions.

Poisoners of Antiquity

Given the increasing awareness of the toxic properties of some naturally occurring xenobiotics and the lack of analytical detection techniques, homicidal poisoning was common during Roman times. During this period, members of the aristocracy commonly used "tasters" to shield themselves from potential poisoners, a practice also in vogue during the reign of Louis XIV in 17th-century France.[164]

One of the most infamous poisoners of ancient Rome was Locusta, who was known to experiment on slaves with poisons that included aconite, arsenic, belladonna, henbane, and poisonous fungi. In 54 A.D., Nero's mother, Agrippina, hired Locusta to poison Emperor Claudius (Agrippina's husband and Nero's stepfather) as part of a scheme to make Nero emperor. As a result of these activities, Claudius, who was a great lover of mushrooms, died from *Amanita phalloides* poisoning,[18] and in the next year, Britannicus (Nero's stepbrother) also became one of Locusta's victims. In this case, Locusta managed to fool the taster by preparing unusually hot soup that required additional cooling after the soup had been officially tasted. At the time of cooling, the poison was surreptitiously slipped into the soup. Almost immediately after drinking the soup, Britannicus collapsed and died. The exact poison remains in doubt, although some authorities suggest that it was a cyanogenic glycoside.[147]

Early Quests for the Universal Antidote

The recognition, classification, and use of poisons in ancient Greece and Rome were accompanied by an intensive search for a universal antidote. In fact, many of the physicians of this period devoted significant parts of their careers to this endeavor.[155] Mystery and superstition surrounded the origins and sources of these proposed antidotes. One of the earliest specific references to a protective therapy can be found in Homer's *Odyssey*, when Ulysses is advised to protect himself by taking the antidote "moli." Recent speculation suggests that moli referred to *Galanthus nivalis*, which contains a cholinesterase inhibitor. Moli could have been used as an antidote against poisonous plants such as *Datura stramonium* (jimsonweed) that contain the anticholinergic alkaloids scopolamine, atropine, and hyoscyamine.[127]

Theriacs and the Mithridatum

The Greeks referred to the universal antidote as the *alexipharmaca* or *theriac*.[79,155] The term *alexipharmaca* was derived from the words *alexipharmakos* ("which keeps off poison") and *antipharmakon* ("antidote"). Over the years, *alexipharmaca* was increasingly used to refer to a method of treatment, such as the induction of emesis by using a feather. Theriac, which originally had referred to poisonous reptiles or wild beasts, was later used to refer to the antidotes. Consumption of the early theriacs (ca. 200 B.C.) was reputed to make people "poison proof" against bites of all venomous animals except the asp. Their ingredients included aniseed, anmi, apoponax, fennel, meru, parsley, and wild thyme.[155]

The quest for the universal antidote was epitomized by the work of King Mithridates VI of Pontus (135–63 B.C.).[75] After repeatedly being subjected to poisoning attempts by his enemies during his youth, Mithridates sought protection by the development of universal antidotes. To find the best antidote, he performed acute toxicity experiments on criminals and slaves. The theriac he concocted, known as the "mithridatum," contained a minimum of 36 ingredients and was thought to be protective against aconite, scorpions, sea slugs, spiders, vipers, and all other poisonous substances. Mithridates took his concoction every day. Ironically, when an old man, Mithridates attempted suicide by poison but supposedly was unsuccessful because he had become poison proof. Having failed at self-poisoning, Mithridates was compelled to have a soldier kill him with a sword. Galen described Mithridates' experiences in a series of three books: *De Antidotis I*, *De Antidotis II*, and *De Theriaca ad Pisonem*.[75,160]

The Theriac of Andromachus, also known as the "Venice treacle" or "galene," is probably the most well-known theriac.[64] According to Galen, this preparation, formulated during the 1st century A.D., was considered an improvement over the mithridatum.[146] It was prepared by Andromachus (37–68 A.D.), physician to Emperor Nero. Andromachus added to the mithridatum ingredients such as the flesh of vipers, squills, and generous amounts of opium.[167] Other ingredients were removed. Altogether, 73 ingredients were required. It was advocated to "counteract all poisons and bites of venomous animals," as well as a host of other medical problems, such as colic, dropsy, and jaundice, and it was used both therapeutically and prophylactically.[155,160] As evidence of its efficacy, Galen demonstrated that fowl receiving poison followed by theriac had a higher survival rate than fowl receiving poison alone.[155] It is likely, however, that the scientific rigor and methodology used differed from current scientific practice.

By the Middle Ages, the Theriac of Andromachus contained more than 100 ingredients. Its synthesis was quite elaborate; the initial phase of production lasted months followed by an aging process that lasted years, somewhat similar to that of vintage wine.[98] The final product was often more solid than liquid in consistency.

Other theriac preparations were named after famous physicians (Damocrates, Nicolaus, Amando, Arnauld, and Abano) who contributed additional ingredients to the original formulation. Over the centuries, certain localities were celebrated for their own peculiar brand of theriac. Notable centers of theriac production included Bologna, Cairo, Florence, Genoa, Istanbul, and Venice. At times, theriac production was accompanied by great fanfare. For example, in Bologna, the mixing of the theriac could take place only under the direction of the medical professors at the university.[155]

Whether these preparations were of actual benefit is uncertain. Some suggest that the theriac had an antiseptic effect on the gastrointestinal (GI) tract, but others state that the sole benefit of the theriac derived from its formulation with opium.[98] Theriacs remained in vogue throughout the Middle Ages and Renaissance, and it was not until 1745 that their efficacy was finally questioned by William Heberden in *Antitheriaka: An Essay on Mithridatum and Theriaca*.[75] Nonetheless, pharmacopeias in France, Spain, and Germany continued to list these preparations until the last quarter of the 19th century, and theriac was still available in Italy and Turkey in the early 20th century.[19,98]

Sacred Earth

Beginning in the 5th century B.C., an adsorbent agent called *terra sigillata* was promoted as a universal antidote. This xenobiotic, also known as the "sacred sealed earth," consisted of red clay that could be found on only one particular hill on the Greek island of Lemnos. Perhaps somewhat akin to the 20th-century "universal antidote," it was advocated as effective in counteracting all poisons.[155] With great ceremony, once per year, the terra sigillata was retrieved from this hill and prepared for subsequent use. According to Dioscorides, this clay was formulated with goat's blood to make it into a paste. At one time, it was included as part of the Theriac of Andromachus. Demand for terra sigillata continued into the 15th century. Similar antidotal clays were found in Italy, Malta, Silesia, and England.[155]

Charms

Charms, such as toadstones, snakestones, unicorn horns, and bezoar stones, were also promoted as universal antidotes. Toadstones, found in the heads of old toads, were reputed to have the capability to extract poison from the site of a venomous bite or sting. In addition, the toadstone was supposedly able to detect the mere presence of poison by producing a sensation of heat upon contact with a poisonous substance.[155]

Similarly, snakestones extracted from the heads of cobras (known as *piedras della cobra de Capelos*) were also reported to have magical qualities.[14] The 17th-century Italian philosopher Athanasius Kircher (1602–1680) became an enthusiastic supporter of snakestone therapy for the treatment of snakebite after conducting experiments, demonstrating the antidotal attributes of these charms "in front of amazed spectators." Kircher attributed the efficacy of the snakestone to the theory of "attraction of like substances." Francesco Redi (1626–1698), a court physician and contemporary of Kircher, debunked this quixotic approach. A harbinger of future experimental toxicologists, Redi was unwilling to accept isolated case reports and field demonstrations as proof of the utility of the snakestone. Using a considerably more rigorous approach, *provando et riprovando* (by testing and retesting), Redi assessed the antidotal efficacy of snakestone on different animal species and different xenobiotics and failed to confirm any benefit.[14]

Much lore has surrounded the antidotal effects of the mythical unicorn horn. Ctesias, writing in 390 B.C., was the first to chronicle the wonders of the unicorn horn, claiming that drinking water or wine from the "horn of the unicorn" would protect against poison.[155] The horns were usually narwhal tusks or rhinoceros horns, and during the Middle Ages, the unicorn horn may have been worth as much as 10 times the price of gold. Similar to the toadstone, the unicorn horn was used both to detect poisons and to neutralize them. Supposedly, a cup made of unicorn horn would sweat if a poisonous substance was placed in it.[96] To give further credence to its use, a 1593 study on dogs poisoned by arsenic reportedly showed that the horn was protective.[96]

Bezoar stones, also touted as universal antidotes, consisted of stomach or intestinal calculi formed by the deposition of calcium phosphate around a hair, fruit pit, or gallstone. They were removed from wild goats, cows, and apes and administered orally to humans. The Persian name for the bezoar stone was *pad zahr* ("expeller of poisons"); the ancient Hebrews referred to the bezoar stone as *bel Zaard* ("every cure for poisons"). Over the years, regional variations of bezoar stones were popularized, including an Asian variety from wild goat of Persia, an Occidental variety from llamas of Peru, and a European variety from chamois of the Swiss mountains.[50,155]

OPIUM, COCA, CANNABIS, AND HALLUCINOGENS IN ANTIQUITY

Although it was not until the mid-19th century that the true perils of opioid addiction were first recognized, juice from the *Papaver somniferum* was known for its medicinal value in Egypt at least as early as the writing of the *Ebers Papyrus* in 1500 B.C. Egyptian pharmacologists of that time reportedly recommended opium poppy extract as a pacifier for children who exhibited incessant crying.[141] In Ancient Greece, Dioscorides and Galen were early advocates of opium as a therapeutic xenobiotic. During this time, it was also used as a means of suicide. Mithridates' lack of success in his own attempted suicide by poisoning may have been the result of an opium tolerance that had developed from previous repetitive use.[141] One of the earliest descriptions of the abuse potential of opium is attributed to Epistratos (304–257 B.C.), who criticized the use of opium for earache because it "dulled the sight and is a narcotic."[141]

Cocaine use dates back to at least 300 B.C., when South American Indians reportedly chewed coca leaves during religious ceremonies.[112] Chewing coca to increase work efficacy and to elevate mood has remained commonplace in some South American societies for thousands of years. An Egyptian mummy from about 950 B.C. revealed significant amounts of cocaine in the stomach and liver, suggesting oral use of cocaine occurred during this time period.[116] Large amounts of tetrahydrocannabinol (THC) were also found in the lung and muscle of the same mummy. Another investigation of 11 Egyptian (1079 B.C.–395 A.D.) and 72 Peruvian (200–1500 A.D.) mummies found cocaine, thought to be indigenous only to South America, and hashish, thought to be indigenous only to Asia, in both groups.[126]

Cannabis use in China dates back even further, to around 2700 B.C., when it was known as the "liberator of sin."[112] In India and Iran, cannabis was used as early as 1000 B.C. as an xenobiotic known as *bhang*.[115] Other currently abused xenobiotics that were known to the ancients include cannabis, hallucinogenic mushrooms, nutmeg, and peyote. As early as 1300 B.C., Peruvian Indian tribal ceremonies included the use of mescaline-containing San Pedro cacti.[112] The hallucinogenic mushroom, *Amanita muscaria*, known as "fly agaric," was used as a ritual drug and may have been known in India as "soma" around 2000 B.C.

EARLY ATTEMPTS AT GASTROINTESTINAL DECONTAMINATION

Nicander's *Alexipharmaca* (*Antidotes for Poisons*) recommended induction of emesis by one of several methods: (a) ingesting warm linseed oil, (b) tickling the hypopharynx with a feather, or (c) "emptying the gullet with a small twisted and curved paper."[98] Nicander also advocated the use of suction to limit envenomation.[156] The Romans referred to the feather as the "vomiting feather" or "pinna." Most commonly, the feather was used after a hearty feast to avoid the GI discomfort associated with overeating. At times, the pinna was dipped into a nauseating mixture to increase its efficacy.[101]

TOXICOLOGY DURING THE MEDIEVAL AND RENAISSANCE PERIODS

After Galen (ca. A.D. 129–200), there is relatively little documented attention to the subject of poisons until the works of Ibn Wahshiya in the 9th century. Citing Greek, Persian, and Indian texts, Wahshiya's work, titled *Book of Poisons*, combined contemporary science, magic, and astrology during his discussion of poison mechanisms (as they were understood at that time), symptomatology, antidotes (including his own recommendation for a universal antidote), and prophylaxis. He categorized poisons as lethal by sight, smell, touch, and sound, as well as by drinking and eating. For victims of an aconite-containing dart arrow, Ibn Wahshiya recommended excision followed by cauterization and topical treatment with onion and salt.[93]

Another significant medieval contribution to toxicology can be found in Moses Maimonides' (1135–1204) *Treatise on Poisons and Their Antidotes* (1198). In part one of this treatise, Maimonides discussed the bites of snakes and mad dogs and the stings of bees, wasps, spiders, and scorpions.[139] He also discussed the use of cupping glasses for bites (a progenitor of the modern suctioning device) and was one of the first to differentiate the hematotoxic (hot) from the neurotoxic (cold) effects of poison. In part two, he discussed mineral and vegetable poisons and their antidotes. He described belladonna poisoning as causing a "redness and a sort of excitation."[139] He suggested that emesis should be induced by hot water, *Anethum graveolens* (dill), and oil, followed by fresh milk, butter, and honey. Although he rejected some of the popular treatments of the day, he advocated the use of the great theriac and the mithridatum as first- and second-line xenobiotics in the management of snakebite.[139]

On the subject of oleander poisoning, Petrus Abbonus (1250–1315) wrote that those who drink the juice, spines, or bark of oleander will develop anxiety, palpitations, and syncope.[22] He described the clinical presentation of opium overdose as someone who "will be dull, lazy, and sleepy, without feeling, and he will neither understand nor feel anything, and if he does not receive succor, he will die." Although this "succor" is not defined, he recommended that treatment of opium toxicity include drinking the strongest wine, rubbing the extremities with alkali and soap, and olfactory stimulation with pepper. To treat snakebite, Abbonus suggested the immediate application of a tourniquet, as well as oral suctioning of the bite wound, preferably performed by a servant. Interestingly, from a 21st-century perspective, Abbonus also suggested that St. John's wort had the magical power to free anything from poisons and attributed this virtue to the influence of the stars.[22]

The Scientists

Paracelsus' (1493–1541) study on the dose–response relationship is usually considered the beginning of the scientific approach to toxicology (Table 1–2). He was the first to emphasize the chemical nature of toxic xenobiotics.[123] Paracelsus stressed the need for proper observation and experimentation regarding the true response to xenobiotics. He underscored the need to differentiate between the therapeutic and toxic properties of chemicals when he stated in his *Third Defense*, "What is there that is not poison? All things are poison and nothing [is] without poison. Solely, the dose determines that a thing is not a poison."[43]

Although Paracelsus is the best known Renaissance toxicologist, Ambroise Pare (1510–1590) and William Piso (1611–1678) also contributed to the field. Pare argued against the use of the unicorn horn and bezoar stone.[100] He also wrote an early treatise on carbon monoxide poisoning. Piso is credited as one of the first to recognize the emetic properties of ipecacuanha.[136]

Medieval and Renaissance Poisoners

Along with these advances in toxicologic knowledge, the Renaissance is mainly remembered as the age of the poisoner, a time when the art of poisoning reached new heights (Table 1–3). In fact, poisoning was so rampant during this time that in 1531, King Henry VIII decreed that convicted poisoners should be boiled alive.[52] From the 15th to 17th centuries, schools of poisoning existed in Venice and Rome. In Venice, poisoning services were provided by a group called the Council of Ten, whose members were hired to perform murder by poison.[164]

Members of the infamous Borgia family were considered to be responsible for many poisonings during this period. They preferred to use a poison called "La Cantarella," a mixture of arsenic and phosphorus.[157] Rodrigo Borgia (1431–1503), who became Pope Alexander VI, and his son, Cesare Borgia, were reportedly responsible for the poisoning of cardinals and kings.

In the late 16th century, Catherine de Medici, wife of Henry II of France, introduced Italian poisoning techniques to France. She experimented on the poor, the sick, and the criminal. By analyzing the subsequent complaints of her victims, she is said to have learned the sites of action and times of onset, the clinical signs and symptoms, and the efficacies of poisons.[56] Murder by poison remained quite popular during the latter half of the 17th and the early part of the 18th centuries in Italy and France.

The Marchioness de Brinvilliers (1630–1676) tested her poison concoctions on hospitalized patients and on her servants and allegedly murdered her husband, father, and two siblings.[54,147] Among the favorite poisons of the Marchioness were arsenic, copper sulfate, corrosive sublimate (mercury bichloride), lead, and tartar emetic (antimony potassium tartrate).[157]

TABLE 1–2	Important People in the Later History of Toxicology	
Person	**Date**	**Importance**
Paracelsus	1493–1541	Introduced the dose–response concept to toxicology
Ambroise Pare	1510–1590	Argued against unicorn horns and bezoars as antidotes
William Piso	1611–1678	First to study emetic qualities of ipecacuanha
Bernardino Ramazzini	1633–1714	Father of occupational medicine; wrote *De Morbis Artificum Diatriba*
Richard Mead	1673–1754	Wrote English-language book about poisoning
Percivall Pott	1714–1788	Wrote the first description of occupational cancer, relating the chimney sweep occupation to scrotal cancer
Felice Fontana	1730–1805	First scientific study of venomous snakes
Philip Physick	1767–1837	Early advocate of orogastric lavage to remove poisons
Baron Guillaume Dupuytren	1777–1835	Early advocate of orogastric lavage to remove poisons
Francois Magendie	1783–1855	Discovered emetine and studied the mechanisms of cyanide and strychnine
Bonaventure Orfila	1787–1853	Father of modern toxicology; wrote *Traite des Poisons*; first to isolate arsenic from human organs
James Marsh	1794–1846	Developed reduction test for arsenic
Robert Christison	1797–1882	Wrote *Treatise on Poisons,* one of the most influential texts of the early 19th century
Grand Marshall Bertrand	1813	Demonstrated the efficacy of charcoal in arsenic ingestion
Claude Bernard	1813–1878	Studied the mechanisms of toxicity of carbon monoxide and curare
Edward Jukes	1820	Self-experimented with orogastric lavage apparatus known as Jukes syringe
Theodore Wormley	1826–1897	Wrote *Micro-Chemistry of Poisons,* the first American book devoted exclusively to toxicology
Pierre Touery	1831	Demonstrated the efficacy of charcoal in strychnine ingestion
Hugo Reinsch	1842–1884	Developed qualitative tests for arsenic and mercury
Alfred Garrod	1846	Conducted the first systematic study of charcoal in an animal model
Max Gutzeit	1847–1915	Developed method to quantitate small amounts of arsenic
Benjamin Howard Rand	1848	Conducted the first study of the efficacy of charcoal in humans
O.H. Costill	1848	Wrote the first book on symptoms and treatment of poisoning
Louis Lewin	1850–1929	Studied many toxins, including methanol, chloroform, snake venom, carbon monoxide, lead, opioids, and hallucinogenic plants
Rudolf Kobert	1854–1918	Studied digitalis and ergot alkaloids
Albert Niemann	1860	Isolated cocaine alkaloids
Alice Hamilton	1869–1970	Conducted landmark investigations associating worksite chemical hazards with disease; led reform movement to improve worker safety

TABLE 1–3	Notable Poisoners from Antiquity to the Present		
Poisoner	**Date**	**Victim(s)**	**Poison(s)**
Locusta	54–55 A.D.	Claudius and Britannicus	*Amanita phalloides*, cyanide
Cesare Borgia	1400s	Cardinals and kings	La Cantarella (arsenic and phosphorus)
Catherine de Medici	1519–1589	Poor, sick, criminals	Unknown
Hieronyma Spara	Died 1659	Taught women how to poison their husbands	Mana of St. Nicholas of Bari (arsenic trioxide)
Marchioness de Brinvilliers	Died 1676	Hospitalized patients, husband, father	Antimony, arsenic, copper, lead, mercury
Catherine Deshayes	Died 1680	>2,000 infants, many husbands	La poudre de succession (arsenic mixed with aconite, belladonna, and opium)
Madame Giulia Toffana	Died 1719	>600 people	Aqua toffana (arsenic trioxide)
Mary Blandy	1752	Father	Arsenic
Anna Maria Zwanizer	1807	Random people	Antimony, arsenic
Marie Lefarge	1839	Husband	Arsenic (first use of Marsh test)
John Tawell	1845	Mistress	Cyanide
William Palmer, MD	1855	Fellow gambler	Strychnine
Madeline Smith (acquitted)	1857	Lover	Arsenic
Edmond de la Pommerais, MD	1863	Patient and mistress	Digitalis
Edward William Pritchard, MD	1865	Wife and mother-in-law	Antimony
George Henry Lamson, MD	1881	Brother-in-law	Aconite
Adelaide Bartlett (acquitted)	1886	Husband	Chloroform
Florence Maybrick	1889	Husband	Arsenic
Thomas Neville Cream, MD	1891	Prostitutes	Strychnine
Johann Hoch	1892–1905	Serial wives	Arsenic
Cordelia Botkin	1898	Rival woman	Arsenic (in chocolate candy)
Roland Molineux	1898	Acquaintance	Cyanide of mercury
Hawley Harvey Crippen, MD	1910	Wife	Hyoscine
Frederick Henry Seddon	1911	Boarder	Arsenic (fly paper)
Henri Girard Landru	1912	Acquaintances	*Amanita phalloides*
Robert Armstrong	1921	Wife	Arsenic (weed killer)
Landru	1922	Many women	Cyanide
Suzanne Fazekas	1929	Supplied poison to 100 wives to kill husbands	Arsenic
Sadamichi Hirasawa	1948	Bank employees	Potassium cyanide
Christa Ambros Lehmann	1954	Friend, husband, father-in-law	E-605 (parathion)
Nannie Doss	1954	11 relatives, including five husbands	Arsenic
Carl Coppolino, MD	1965	Wife	Succinylcholine
Graham Frederick Young	1971	Stepmother, coworkers	Antimony, thallium
Judias V. Buenoano	1971	Husband, son	Arsenic
Ronald Clark O'Bryan	1974	Son and neighborhood children	Cyanide (in Halloween candy)
Governmental	1978	Georgi Markov, Bulgarian dissident	Ricin
Jim Jones	1978	>900 people in mass suicide	Cyanide
Harold Shipman, MD	1974–1998	>100 patients	Heroin
Unidentified	1982	Seven random people	Extra Strength Tylenol mixed with cyanide

(Continued)

TABLE 1–3	Notable Poisoners from Antiquity to the Present *(Continued)*		
Poisoner	**Date**	**Victim(s)**	**Poison(s)**
Donald Harvey	1983–1987	Patients	Arsenic
George Trepal	1988	Neighbors	Thallium
Michael Swango, MD	1980s–1990s	Hospitalized patients	Arsenic, potassium chloride, succinylcholine
Charles Cullen, RN	1990s–2003	Hospitalized patients	Digoxin
State sponsored	2004	Viktor Yushchenko, Ukrainian presidential candidate	Dioxin
State sponsored	2006	Alexander Litvinenko	Polonium-210
State sponsored	2017	Kim Jong-nam	VX

Catherine Deshayes (1640–1680), a fortuneteller and sorceress, was one of the last "poisoners for hire" and was implicated in countless poisonings, including the killing of more than 2,000 infants.[56] Better known as "La Voisine," she reportedly sold poisons to women wishing to rid themselves of their husbands. Her particular brand of poison was a concoction of aconite, arsenic, belladonna, and opium known as "la poudre de succession."[157] Ultimately, de Brinvilliers was beheaded, and Deshayes was burned alive for her crimes. In an attempt to curtail these rampant poisonings, Louis XIV issued a decree in 1662 banning the sale of arsenic, mercury, and other poisons to customers not known to apothecaries and requiring buyers to sign a register declaring the purpose for their purchase.[147]

A major center for poison practitioners was Naples, the home of the notorious Madame Giulia Toffana. She reportedly poisoned more than 600 people, preferring a particular solution of white arsenic (arsenic trioxide), better known as "aqua toffana," and dispensed under the guise of a cosmetic. Eventually convicted of poisoning, Madame Toffana was executed in 1719.[21]

EIGHTEENTH- AND NINETEENTH-CENTURY DEVELOPMENTS IN TOXICOLOGY

The development of toxicology as a distinct specialty began during the 18th and 19th centuries (Table 1–2).[125] The mythological and magical mystique of poisoners began to be gradually replaced by an increasingly rational, scientific, and experimental approach to these xenobiotics. Much of the poison lore that had survived for almost 2,000 years was finally debunked and discarded. The 18th-century Italian Felice Fontana was one of the first to usher in the modern age. He was an early experimental toxicologist who studied the venom of the European viper and wrote the classic text *Traite sur le Venin de la Vipere* in 1781.[82] Through his exacting experimental study on the effects of venom, Fontana brought a scientific insight to toxicology previously lacking and demonstrated that clinical symptoms resulted from the poison (venom) acting on specific target organs. During the 18th and 19th centuries, attention focused on the detection of poisons and the study of toxic effects of xenobiotics in animals.[117] Issues relating to adverse effects of industrialization and unintentional poisoning in the workplace and home environment were raised. Also during this time, early experience and experimentation with methods of GI decontamination took place.

Development of Analytical Toxicology and the Study of Poisons

The French physician Bonaventure Orfila (1787–1853) is often called the father of modern toxicology.[117] He emphasized toxicology as a distinct, scientific discipline, separate from clinical medicine and pharmacology.[11] He was also an early medicolegal expert who championed the use of chemical analysis and autopsy material as evidence to prove that a poisoning had occurred. His treatise *Traite des Poisons* (1814)[122] evolved over five editions and was regarded as the foundation of experimental and forensic toxicology.[163] This text classified poisons into six groups: acrids, astringents, corrosives, narcoticoacrids, septics and putrefiants, and stupefacients and narcotics.

A number of other landmark works on poisoning also appeared during this period. In 1829, Robert Christison (1797–1882), a professor of medical jurisprudence and Orfila's student, wrote *A Treatise on Poisons*.[32] This work simplified Orfila's poison classification schema by categorizing poisons into three groups: irritants, narcotics, and narcoticoacrids. Less concerned with jurisprudence than with clinical toxicology, O.H. Costill's *A Practical Treatise on Poisons*, published in 1848, was the first modern clinically oriented text to emphasize the symptoms and treatment of poisoning.[36] In 1867, Theodore Wormley (1826–1897) published the first American book written exclusively on poisons titled the *Micro-Chemistry of Poisons*.[48,166]

During this time, important breakthroughs in the chemical analysis of poisons resulted from the search for a more reliable assay for arsenic.[66,162] Arsenic was widely available and was the suspected cause of a large number of deaths. In one study, arsenic was used in 31% of 679 homicidal poisonings.[157] A reliable means of detecting arsenic was much needed by the courts.

Until the 19th century, poisoning was mainly diagnosed by its resultant symptoms rather than by analytic tests. The first use of a chemical test as evidence in a poisoning trial occurred in the 1752 trial of Mary Blandy, who was accused of poisoning her father with arsenic.[104] Although Blandy was convicted and hanged publicly, the test used in this case was not very sensitive and depended in part on eliciting a garlic odor upon heating the gruel that the accused had fed to her father.

During the 19th century, James Marsh (1794–1846), Hugo Reinsch (1842–1884), and Max Gutzeit (1847–1915) each worked on this problem. Assays bearing their names are important contributions to the early history of analytic toxicology.[105,117] The "Marsh test" to detect arsenic was first used in a criminal case in 1839 during the trial of Marie Lefarge, who was accused of using arsenic to murder her husband.[147] Orfila's trial testimony that the victim's viscera contained minute amounts of arsenic helped to convict the defendant, although subsequent debate suggested that contamination of the forensic specimen may have also played a role.

In a further attempt to curtail criminal poisoning by arsenic, the British Parliament passed the Arsenic Act in 1851. This bill, which was one of the first modern laws to regulate the sale of poisons, required that the retail sale of arsenic be restricted to chemists, druggists, and apothecaries and that a poison book be maintained to record all arsenic sales.[15]

Homicidal poisonings remained common during the 19th century and early 20th century. Infamous poisoners of that time included William Palmer, Edward Pritchard, Harvey Crippen, and Frederick Seddon.[157] Many of these poisoners were physicians who used their knowledge of medicine and toxicology in an attempt to solve their domestic and financial difficulties by committing the "perfect" murder. Some of the poisons used were aconitine (by Lamson, who was a classmate of Christison), *Amanita phalloides* (by Girard), arsenic (by Maybrick, Seddon, and others), antimony (by Pritchard), cyanide (by Molineux and Tawell), digitalis (by Pommerais), hyoscine (by Crippen), and strychnine (by Palmer and Cream) (Table 1–3).[24,91,155,157]

In the early 20th century, forensic investigation into suspicious deaths, including poisonings, was significantly advanced with the development of the medical examiner system replacing the much-flawed coroner system that was subject to widespread corruption. In 1918, the first centrally controlled medical examiner system was established in New York City. Alexander Gettler, considered the father of forensic toxicology in the United States, established a toxicology laboratory within the newly created New York City Medical Examiner's Office. Gettler pioneered new techniques for the detection of a variety of substances in biologic fluids, including carbon monoxide, chloroform, cyanide, and heavy metals.[49,117]

Systematic investigation into the underlying mechanisms of toxic substances also commenced during the 19th century. Francois Magendie (1783–1855) studied the mechanisms of toxicity and sites of action of cyanide, emetine, and strychnine.[47] Claude Bernard (1813–1878), a pioneering physiologist and a student of Magendie, made important contributions to the understanding of the toxicity of carbon monoxide and curare.[90] Rudolf Kobert (1854–1918) studied digitalis and ergot alkaloids and authored a textbook on toxicology for physicians and students.[87,120] Louis Lewin (1850–1929) was the first person to intensively study the differences between the pharmacologic and toxicologic actions of xenobiotics. Lewin studied chronic opium intoxication, as well as the toxicity of carbon monoxide, chloroform, lead, methanol, and snake venom. He also developed a classification system for psychoactive drugs, dividing them into euphorics, phantastics, inebriants, hypnotics, and excitants.[99]

The Origin of Occupational Toxicology

The origins of occupational toxicology can be traced to the early 18th century and to the contributions of Bernardino Ramazzini (1633–1714). Considered the father of occupational medicine, Ramazzini wrote *De Morbis Artificum Diatriba* (*Diseases of Workers*) in 1700, which was the first comprehensive text discussing the relationship between disease and workplace hazards.[53] Ramazzini's essential contribution to patient care is epitomized by the addition of a standard question to a patient's medical history: "What occupation does the patient follow?"[51] Altogether Ramazzini described diseases associated with 54 occupations, including hydrocarbon poisoning in painters, mercury poisoning in mirror makers, and pulmonary diseases in miners.

In 1775, Sir Percivall Pott proposed the first association between workplace exposure and cancer when he noticed a high incidence of scrotal cancer in English chimney sweeps. Pott's belief that the scrotal cancer was caused by prolonged exposure to tar and soot was confirmed by further investigation in the 1920s, indicating the carcinogenic nature of the polycyclic aromatic hydrocarbons contained in coal tar (including benzo[*a*]pyrene).[73]

Dr. Alice Hamilton (1869–1970) was another pioneer in occupational toxicology, whose rigorous scientific inquiry had a profound impact on linking chemical xenobiotics with human disease. A physician, scientist, humanitarian, and social reformer, Hamilton became the first female professor at Harvard University and conducted groundbreaking studies of many different occupational exposures and problems, including carbon monoxide poisoning in steelworkers, mercury poisoning in hatters, and wrist drop in lead workers. Hamilton's overriding concerns about these "dangerous trades" and her commitment to improving the health of workers led to extensive voluntary and regulatory reforms in the workplace.[60,65]

Advances in Gastrointestinal Decontamination

Using gastric lavage and charcoal to treat poisoned patients was introduced in the late 18th and early 19th century. A stomach pump was first designed by Munro Secundus in 1769 to administer neutralizing substances to sheep and cattle for the treatment of bloat.[25] The American surgeon Philip Physick (1768–1837) and the French surgeon Baron Guillaume Dupuytren (1777–1835) were two of the first physicians to advocate gastric lavage for the removal of poisons.[25] As early as 1805, Physick demonstrated the use of a "stomach tube" for this purpose. Using brandy and water as the irrigation fluid, he performed stomach washings in twins to wash out excessive doses of tincture of opium.[25] Dupuytren performed gastric emptying by first introducing warm water into the stomach via a large syringe attached to a long flexible sound and then withdrawing the "same water charged with

poison."[25] Edward Jukes, a British surgeon, was another early advocate of poison removal by gastric lavage. Jukes first experimented on animals, performing gastric lavage after the oral administration of tincture of opium. Attempting to gain human experience, he experimented on himself, by first ingesting 10 drams (600 g) of tincture of opium and then performing gastric lavage using a 25-inch-long, 0.5-inch-diameter tube, which became known as Jukes syringe.[111] Other than some nausea and a 3-hour sleep, he suffered no ill effects, and the experiment was deemed a success.

The principle of using charcoal to adsorb xenobiotics was first described by Scheele (1773) and Lowitz (1785), but the medicinal use of charcoal dates to ancient times.[35] The earliest reference to the medicinal uses of charcoal is found in Egyptian papyrus from about 1500 B.C.[35] The charcoal used during Greek and Roman times, referred to as "wood charcoal," was used to treat those with anthrax, chlorosis, epilepsy, and vertigo. By the late 18th century, topical application of charcoal was recommended for gangrenous skin ulcers, and internal use of a charcoal–water suspension was recommended for use as a mouthwash and in the treatment of bilious conditions.[35]

The first hint that charcoal might have a role in the treatment of poisoning came from a series of courageous self-experiments in France during the early 19th century. In 1813, the French chemist Bertrand publicly demonstrated the antidotal properties of charcoal by surviving a 5-g ingestion of arsenic trioxide that had been mixed with charcoal.[69] Eighteen years later, before the French Academy of Medicine, the pharmacist Touery survived an ingestion consisting of 10 times the lethal dose of strychnine mixed with 15 g of charcoal.[69] One of the first reports of charcoal used in a poisoned patient was in 1834 by the American Hort, who successfully treated a mercury bichloride–poisoned patient with large amounts of powdered charcoal.[3]

In the 1840s, Garrod performed the first controlled study of charcoal when he examined its utility on a variety of poisons in animal models.[69] Garrod used dogs, cats, guinea pigs, and rabbits to demonstrate the potential benefits of charcoal in the management of strychnine poisoning. He also emphasized the importance of early use of charcoal and the proper ratio of charcoal to poison. Other toxic substances, such as aconite, hemlock, mercury bichloride, and morphine, were also studied during this period. The first charcoal efficacy studies in humans were performed by the American physician B. Rand in 1848.[69]

But it was not until the early 20th century that an activation process was added to the manufacture of charcoal to increase its effectiveness. In 1900, the Russian Ostrejko demonstrated that treating charcoal with superheated steam significantly enhanced its adsorbing power.[35] Despite this improvement and the favorable reports mentioned, charcoal was only occasionally used in GI decontamination until the early 1960s, when Holt and Holz repopularized its use.[63]

The Increasing Recognition of the Perils of Drug Abuse
Opioids

Although the medical use of opium was promoted by Paracelsus in the 16th century, its popularity was given a significant boost when the distinguished British physician Thomas Sydenham (1624–1689) formulated laudanum, which was a tincture of opium containing cinnamon, cloves, saffron, and sherry. Sydenham also formulated a different opium concoction known as "syrup of poppies."[86] A third opium preparation called Dover's powder was designed by Sydenham's protégé, Thomas Dover; this preparation contained ipecac, licorice, opium, salt-peter, and tartaric acid.

John Jones, the author of the 18th-century text *The Mysteries of Opium Reveal'd*, was another enthusiastic advocate of its "medicinal" uses.[86] A well-known opium user himself, Jones provided one of the earliest descriptions of opioid addiction. He insisted that opium offered many benefits if the dose was moderate but that discontinuation or a decrease in dose, particularly after "leaving off after long and lavish use," would result in such symptoms as sweating, itching, diarrhea, and melancholy. His recommendation for the treatment of these withdrawal symptoms included decreasing the dose of opium by 1% each day until the drug was totally withdrawn. During this period, a number of English writers became well-known opium addicts including Elizabeth Barrett Browning, Samuel Taylor Coleridge, and Thomas De Quincey. De Quincey, author of *Confessions of an English Opium Eater*, was an early advocate of the recreational use of opioids. The famed Coleridge poem *Kubla Khan* referred to opium as the "milk of paradise," and De Quincey's *Confessions* suggested that opium held the "key to paradise." In many of these cases, the initiation of opium use for medical reasons led to recreational use, tolerance, and dependence.[86]

Although opium was first introduced to Asian societies by Arab physicians some time after the fall of the Roman Empire, the use of opium in Asian countries grew considerably during the 18th and 19th centuries. The growing dependence of China on opium was spurred on by the English desire to establish and profit from a flourishing drug trade.[141] Opium was grown in India and exported east. Despite Chinese protests and edicts against this practice, the importation of opium persisted throughout the 19th century, with the British going to war twice to maintain their right to sell opium. Not surprisingly, by the beginning of the 20th century, opium abuse in China was endemic.

In England, opium use continued to increase during the first half of the 19th century. During this period, opium was legal and freely available from the neighborhood grocer. To many, its use was considered no more problematic than alcohol use.[58] The Chinese usually self-administered opium by smoking, a custom that was brought to the United States by Chinese immigrants in the mid-19th century; the English use of opium was more often by ingestion, that is, "opium eating."

The liberal use of opioids as infant-soothing xenobiotics was one of the most unfortunate aspects of this period of unregulated opioid use.[87] Godfrey's Cordial, Mother's Friend, Mrs. Winslow's Soothing Syrup, and Quietness were among the most popular opioids for children.[94] They were advertised as producing a natural sleep and recommended for teething and bowel regulation, as well as for crying. Because of the wide availability of opioids during this period, the number of acute opioid overdoses in children was consequential and would remain problematic until these unsavory remedies were condemned and removed from the market.

With the discovery of morphine in 1805 and Alexander Wood's invention of the hypodermic syringe in 1853, parenteral administration of morphine became the preferred route of opioid administration for therapeutic use and abuse.[71] A legacy of the generous use of opium and morphine during the US Civil War was "soldiers' disease," referring to a rather large veteran population that returned from the war with a lingering opioid habit.[133] One hundred years later, opioid abuse and addiction would again become common among US military serving during the Vietnam War. Surveys indicated that as many as 20% of American soldiers in Vietnam were addicted to opioids during the war—in part because of their widespread availability and high purity there.[138]

Growing concerns about opioid abuse in England led to the passing of the Pharmacy Act of 1868, which restricted the sale of opium to registered chemists. But in 1898, the Bayer Pharmaceutical Company of Germany synthesized heroin from opium and also introduced aspirin in the late 1890s.[148] Although initially touted as a nonaddictive morphine substitute, problems with heroin use quickly became evident in the United States. Illicit heroin use reached epidemic proportions after World War II and again in the late 1960s.[72] Although heroin use appeared to have leveled off by the end of the 20th century, an epidemic of prescription opioid abuse followed by a resurgence in heroin use occurred during the first years of the 21st century.[85]

Cocaine

Ironically, during the later part of the 19th century, Sigmund Freud and Robert Christison, among others, promoted cocaine as a treatment for opioid addiction. After Albert Niemann's isolation of cocaine alkaloid from coca leaf in 1860, growing enthusiasm for cocaine as a panacea ensued.[80] Some of the most important medical figures of the time, including William Halsted, the famed Johns Hopkins surgeon, also extolled the virtues of cocaine use. Halsted championed the anesthetic properties of this drug, although his own use of cocaine and subsequent morphine use in an attempt to overcome his cocaine dependency would later take a considerable toll.[121] In 1884, Freud wrote *Uber Cocaine*,[27] advocating cocaine as a cure for opium and morphine addiction and as a treatment for fatigue and hysteria.

During the last third of the 19th century, cocaine was added to many popular nonprescription tonics. In 1863, Angelo Mariani, a Frenchman, introduced a new wine, "Vin Mariani," that consisted of a mixture of cocaine and wine (6 mg of cocaine alkaloid per ounce) and was sold as a digestive aid and restorative.[112] In direct competition with the French tonic was the American-made Coca-Cola, developed by J.S. Pemberton. It was originally formulated with coca and caffeine and marketed as a headache remedy and invigorator. With the public demand for cocaine increasing, patent medication manufacturers were adding cocaine to thousands of products. One such asthma remedy was "Dr. Tucker's Asthma Specific," which contained 420 mg of cocaine per ounce and was applied directly to the nasal mucosa.[80] By the end of the 19th century, the first American cocaine epidemic was underway.[114]

Similar to the medical and societal adversities associated with opioid use, the increasing use of cocaine led to a growing concern about comparable adverse effects. In 1886, the first reports of cocaine-related cardiac arrest and stroke were published.[134] Reports of cocaine habituation occurring in patients using cocaine to treat their underlying opioid addiction also began to appear. In 1902, a popular book, *Eight Years in Cocaine Hell*, described some of these problems. *Century Magazine* called cocaine "the most harmful of all habit-forming drugs," and a report in *The New York Times* stated that cocaine was destroying "its victims more swiftly and surely than opium."[42] In 1910, President William Taft proclaimed cocaine to be "public enemy number 1."

In an attempt to curb the increasing problems associated with drug abuse and addiction, the 1914 Harrison Narcotics Act mandated stringent control over the sale and distribution of narcotics (defined as opium, opium derivatives, and cocaine).[42] It was the first federal law in the United States to criminalize the nonmedical use of drugs. The bill required doctors, pharmacists, and others who prescribed narcotics to register and to pay a tax. A similar law, the Dangerous Drugs Act, was passed in the United Kingdom in 1920.[58] To help enforce these drug laws in the United States, the Narcotics Division of the Prohibition Unit of the Internal Revenue Service (a progenitor of the Drug Enforcement Agency) was established in 1920. In 1924, the Harrison Act was further strengthened with the passage of new legislation that banned the importation of opium for the purpose of manufacturing heroin, essentially outlawing the medicinal uses of heroin. With the legal venues to purchase these drugs now eliminated, users were forced to buy from illegal street dealers, creating a burgeoning black market that still exists today.

Sedative–Hypnotics

The introduction to medical practice of the anesthetics nitrous oxide, ether, and chloroform during the 19th century was accompanied by the recreational use of these anesthetics and the first reports of volatile substance abuse. Chloroform "jags," ether "frolics," and nitrous parties became a new type of entertainment. Humphry Davy was an early self-experimenter with the exhilarating effects associated with nitrous oxide inhalation. In certain Irish towns, especially where the temperance movement was strong, ether drinking became quite popular.[107] Horace Wells, the American dentist who introduced chloroform as an anesthetic, became dependent on this volatile solvent and later committed suicide.

Until the last half of the 19th century aconite, alcohol, hemlock, opium, and prussic acid (cyanide) were the primary xenobiotics used for sedation.[33] During the 1860s, new, more specific sedative–hypnotics, such as chloral hydrate and potassium bromide, were introduced into medical practice. In particular, chloral hydrate was hailed as a wonder drug that was relatively safe compared with opium and was recommended for insomnia, anxiety, and delirium tremens, as well as for scarlet fever, asthma, and cancer. But within a few years, problems with acute toxicity of chloral hydrate, as well as its potential to produce tolerance and physical dependence, became apparent.[33] Mixing chloral hydrate with ethanol, both of which inhibit each other's metabolism by competing with alcohol dehydrogenase, was noted to produce a rather powerful "knockout" combination that would become known as a "Mickey Finn," allegedly named after a Chicago saloon proprietor.[16] Abuse of chloral hydrate, as well as other new sedatives such as potassium bromide, would prove to be a harbinger of 20th-century sedative–hypnotic abuse.

Absinthe, an ethanol-containing beverage that was manufactured with an extract from wormwood (*Artemisia absinthium*), was very popular during the last half of the 19th century.[89] This emerald-colored, very bitter drink was memorialized in the paintings of Degas, Toulouse-Lautrec, and Van Gogh and was a staple of French society during this period.[12] α-Thujone, a psychoactive component of wormwood and a noncompetitive γ-aminobutyric acid type A (GABA$_A$ antagonist), is thought to be responsible for the pleasant feelings, hyperexcitability, and significant neurotoxicity associated with this drink.[68] Van Gogh's debilitating episodes of psychosis were likely exacerbated by absinthe drinking.[152] Because of the medical problems associated with its use, absinthe was banned throughout most of Europe by the early 20th century.

Hallucinogens

Native Americans used peyote in religious ceremonies since at least the 17th century. Hallucinogenic mushrooms, particularly *Psilocybe* mushrooms, were also used in the religious life of Native Americans. These were called "teonanacatl," which means "God's sacred mushrooms" or "God's flesh."[128] Interest in the recreational use of cannabis also accelerated during the 19th century after Napoleon's troops brought the drug back from Egypt, where its use among the lower classes was widespread. In 1843, several French Romantics, including Balzac, Baudelaire, Gautier, and Hugo, formed a hashish club called "Le Club des Hachichins" in the Parisian apartment of a young French painter. Fitz Hugh Ludlow's *The Hasheesh Eater*, published in 1857, was an early American text espousing the virtues of marijuana.[97]

A more recent event that had significant impact on modern-day hallucinogen use was the synthesis of lysergic acid diethylamide (LSD) by Albert Hofmann in 1938.[67] Working for Sandoz Pharmaceutical Company, Hofmann synthesized LSD while investigating the pharmacologic properties of ergot alkaloids. Subsequent self-experimentation by Hofmann led to the first description of its hallucinogenic effects and stimulated research into the therapeutic use of LSD. Hofmann is also credited with isolating psilocybin as the active ingredient in *Psilocybe mexicana* mushrooms in 1958.[112]

TWENTIETH- AND TWENTY-FIRST-CENTURY EVENTS
Early Regulatory Initiatives

The development of medical toxicology as a medical subspecialty and the important role of poison control centers began shortly after World War II. Before then, serious attention to the problem of household poisonings in the United States was limited to a few federal legislative antipoisoning initiatives (Table 1–4). The 1906 Pure Food and Drug Act was the first federal legislation that sought to protect the public from problematic and potentially unsafe drugs and food. The driving force behind this reform was Harvey Wiley, the chief chemist at the Department of Agriculture. Beginning in the 1880s, Wiley investigated the problems of contaminated food. In 1902, he organized the "poison squad," which consisted of a group of volunteers who did self-experiments with food preservatives.[4] Revelations from the "poison squad," as well as the publication of Upton Sinclair's muckraking novel *The Jungle*[146] in 1906, exposed unhygienic practices of the meatpacking industry and led to growing support for legislative intervention. Samuel Hopkins Adams' reports about the patent medicine industry revealed that some drug manufacturers added opioids to soothing syrups for infants and led to the call for reform.[135] Although the 1906 regulations were mostly concerned with protecting the public from adulterated food, regulations protecting against misbranded patent medications were also included.

The Federal Caustic Poison Act of 1927 was the first federal legislation to specifically address household poisoning. As early as 1859, bottles clearly demarcated "poison" were manufactured in response to a rash of unfortunate dispensing errors that occurred when oxalic acid was unintentionally substituted for a similarly appearing Epsom salts solution.[28] Before 1927, however, "poison" warning labels were not required on chemical containers, regardless of toxicity or availability. The 1927 Caustic Act was spearheaded by the efforts of Chevalier Jackson, an otolaryngologist, who showed that unintentional exposures to household caustics were an increasingly frequent cause of severe oropharyngeal and GI burns. Under this statute, for the first time, alkali- and acid-containing products had to clearly display a "poison" warning label.[78,154]

The most pivotal regulatory initiative in the United States before World War II—and perhaps the most significant American toxicologic regulation of the 20th century—was the Federal Food, Drug, and Cosmetic Act of 1938. Although the Food and Drug Administration (FDA) had been established in 1930 and legislation to strengthen the 1906 Pure Food and Drug Act was considered by Congress in 1933, the proposed revisions still had not been passed by 1938. Then the elixir of sulfanilamide tragedy in 1938 (Chap. 2) claimed the lives of 105 people who had ingested a prescribed liquid preparation of the antibiotic sulfanilamide inappropriately dissolved in diethylene glycol. This event finally provided the catalyst for legislative intervention.[109,161] Before the elixir disaster, proposed legislation called only for the banning of false and misleading drug labeling and for the outlawing of dangerous drugs without mandatory drug safety testing. After the tragedy, the proposal was strengthened to require assessment of drug safety before marketing, and the legislation was ultimately passed.

The Development of Poison Control Centers

World War II led to the rapid proliferation of new xenobiotics in the marketplace and in the household.[39] At the same time, suicide was recognized as a leading cause of death from these xenobiotics.[9] Both of these factors led the medical community to develop a response to the serious problems of unintentional and intentional poisonings. In Europe during the late 1940s, special toxicology wards were organized in Copenhagen and Budapest,[59] and a poison information service was begun in the Netherlands (Table 1–5).[158] A 1952 American Academy of Pediatrics study revealed that more than 50% of childhood "accidents" in the United States were the result of unintentional poisonings.[61] This study led Edward Press to open the first US poison control center in Chicago in 1953.[129] Press believed that it was extremely difficult for individual physicians to keep abreast of product information, toxicity, and treatment for the rapidly increasing number of potentially poisonous household products. His initial center was organized as a cooperative effort among the departments of pediatrics at several Chicago medical schools, with the goal of collecting and disseminating product information to inquiring physicians, mainly pediatricians.[132]

By 1957, 17 poison control centers were operating in the United States.[39] With the Chicago center serving as a model, these early centers responded to physician callers by providing ingredient and toxicity information about drug and household products and making treatment recommendations. Records were kept of the calls, and preventive strategies were introduced into the community. As more poison control centers opened, a second important function, providing information to calls from the general public, became increasingly common. The physician pioneers in poison prevention and poison treatment were predominantly pediatricians who focused on unintentional childhood ingestions.[137]

During these early years in the development of poison control centers, each center had to collect its own product information, which was a laborious and often redundant task.[38] In an effort to coordinate its operations and to avoid unnecessary duplication, Surgeon General James Goddard responded to the recommendation of the American Public Health Service and established the National Clearinghouse for Poison Control Centers in 1957.[106] This organization, placed under the Bureau of Product Safety of the Food and Drug Administration, disseminated 5-inch by 8-inch index cards containing poison information to each center to help standardize poison control center information resources. The Clearinghouse also collected and tabulated poison data from each of the centers.

Between 1953 and 1972, a rapid, uncoordinated proliferation of poison control centers occurred in the United States.[103] In 1962, there were 462 poison control centers. By 1970, this number had risen to 590,[95] and by 1978, there were 661 poison control centers in the United States, including 100 centers

TABLE 1–4	Protecting Our Health: Important US Regulatory Initiatives Pertaining to Xenobiotics	
Date	Federal Legislation	Intent
1906	Pure Food and Drug Act	Early regulatory initiative; prohibits interstate commerce of misbranded and adulterated foods and drugs.
1914	Harrison Narcotics Act	First federal law to criminalize the nonmedical use of drugs. Taxed and regulated distribution and sale of narcotics (opium, opium derivatives, and cocaine).
1927	Federal Caustic Poison Act	Mandated labeling of concentrated caustics.
1930	Food and Drug Administration (FDA)	Established successor to the Bureau of Chemistry; promulgation of food and drug regulations.
1937	Marijuana Tax Act	Applied controls to marijuana similar to those applied to narcotics.
1938	Federal Food, Drug, and Cosmetic Act	Required toxicity testing of pharmaceuticals before marketing.
1948	Federal Insecticide, Fungicide, and Rodenticide Act	Provided federal control for pesticide sale, distribution, and use.
1951	Durham-Humphrey Amendment	Restricted many therapeutic drugs to sale by prescription only.
1960	Federal Hazardous Substances Labeling Act	Mandated prominent labeling warnings on hazardous household chemical products.
1962	Kefauver-Harris Drug Amendments	Required drug manufacturers to demonstrate efficacy before marketing.
1963	Clean Air Act	Regulated air emissions by setting maximum pollutant standards.
1966	Child Protection Act	Banned hazardous toys when adequate label warnings could not be written.
1970	Comprehensive Drug Abuse and Control Act	Replaced and updated all previous laws concerning narcotics and other dangerous drugs.
1970	Environmental Protection Agency (EPA)	Established and enforced environmental protection standards.
1970	Occupational Safety and Health Act (OSHA)	Enacted to improve worker and workplace safety. Created National Institute for Occupational Safety and Health (NIOSH) as research institution for OSHA.
1970	Poison Prevention Packaging Act	Mandated child-resistant safety caps on certain pharmaceutical preparations to decrease unintentional childhood poisoning.
1972	Clean Water Act	Regulated discharge of pollutants into US waters.
1972	Consumer Product Safety Act	Established Consumer Product Safety Commission (CPSC) to reduce injuries and deaths from consumer products.
1972	Hazardous Material Transportation Act	Authorized the Department of Transportation to develop, promulgate, and enforce regulations for the safe transportation of hazardous materials.
1973	Drug Enforcement Administration (DEA)	Successor to the Bureau of Narcotics and Dangerous Drugs; charged with enforcing federal drug laws.
1973	Lead-based Paint Poison Prevention Act	Regulated the use of lead in residential paint. Lead in some paints was banned by Congress in 1978.
1974	Safe Drinking Water Act	Set safe standards for water purity.
1976	Resource Conservation and Recovery Act (RCRA)	Authorized EPA to control hazardous waste from the "cradle to grave," including the generation, transportation, treatment, storage, and disposal of hazardous waste.
1976	Toxic Substances Control Act	Emphasis on law enforcement. Authorized EPA to track 75,000 industrial chemicals produced or imported into the United States. Required testing of chemicals that pose environmental or human health risk.
1980	Comprehensive Environmental Response Compensation and Liability act (CERCLA)	Set controls for hazardous waste sites. Established trust fund (Superfund) to provide cleanup for these sites. Agency for Toxic Substances and Disease Registry (ATSDR) created.
1983	Federal Anti-Tampering Act	Response to cyanide laced Tylenol deaths. Outlawed tampering with packaged consumer products.
1986	Controlled Substance Analogue Enforcement Act	Instituted legal controls on analog (designer) drugs with chemical structures similar to controlled substances.
1986	Drug-Free Federal Workplace Program	Executive order mandating drug testing of federal employees in sensitive positions.
1986	Superfund Amendments and Reauthorization Act (SARA)	Amendment to CERCLA. Increased funding for the research and cleanup of hazardous waste (SARA) sites.
1988	Labeling of Hazardous Art Materials Act	Required review of all art materials to determine hazard potential and mandated warning labels for hazardous materials.
1994	Dietary Supplement Health and Education Act	Permitted dietary supplements including many herbal preparations to bypass FDA scrutiny.
1997	FDA Modernization Act	Accelerated FDA reviews, regulated advertising of unapproved uses of approved drugs.
2002	The Public Health Security and Bioterrorism Preparedness and Response Act	Tightened control on biologic agents and toxins; increased safety of the US food and drug supply and drinking water; and strengthened the Strategic National Stockpile.
2005	Combat Methamphetamine Epidemic Act	Part of the Patriot Act, this legislation restricted nonprescription sale of the methamphetamine precursor drugs ephedrine and pseudoephedrine used in the home production of methamphetamine.
2009	Family Smoking Prevention and Tobacco Control Act	Empowered FDA to set standards for tobacco products.
2016	Comprehensive Addiction and Recovery Act (CARA)	Federal response to prescription opioid and heroin epidemic providing for expansion of medication-assisted treatment with buprenorphine and methadone and expanded use of naloxone by first responders and community members.

TABLE 1–5	Milestones in the Development of Medical Toxicology in the United States
Year	Milestone
1952	American Academy of Pediatrics study shows that 51% of children's "accidents" are the result of the ingestion of potential poisons
1953	First US poison control center opens in Chicago
1957	National Clearinghouse for Poison Control Centers established
1958	American Association of Poison Control Centers (AAPCC) founded
1961	First Poison Prevention Week
1963	Initial call for development of regional Poison Control Centers (PCCs)
1964	Creation of European Association for PCCs
1968	American Academy of Clinical Toxicology (AACT) established
1972	Introduction of microfiche technology to poison information
1974	American Board of Medical Toxicology (ABMT) established
1978	AAPCC introduces standards of regional designation
1983	First examination given for Specialist in Poison Information (SPI)
1985	American Board of Applied Toxicology (ABAT) established
1992	Medical Toxicology recognized by American Board of Medical Specialties (ABMS)
1993	American College of Medical Toxicology established
1994	First ABMS examination in Medical Toxicology
2000	Accreditation Council for Graduate Medical Education (ACGME) approval of residency training programs in Medical Toxicology
2000	Poison Control Center Enhancement and Awareness Act
2004	Institute of Medicine (IOM) report on the future of poison control centers is released, calling for a greater integration between public health sector and poison control services

in the state of Illinois alone.[143] The nature of calls to centers changed as lay public–generated calls began to outnumber physician-generated calls. Recognizing the public relations value and strong popular support associated with poison control centers, some hospitals started poison control centers without adequately recognizing or providing for the associated responsibilities. Unfortunately, many of these centers offered no more than a part-time telephone service located in the back of the emergency department or pharmacy, staffed by poorly trained personnel.[143]

Despite the "growing pains" of these poison services during this period, many significant achievements were made. A dedicated group of physicians and other health care professionals began devoting an increasing proportion of their time to poison related matters. In 1958, the American Association of Poison Control Centers (AAPCC) was founded to promote closer cooperation between poison control centers, to establish uniform standards, and to develop educational programs for the general public and health care professionals.[61] Annual research meetings were held, and important legislative initiatives were stimulated by the organization.[106] Examples of such legislation include the Federal Hazardous Substances Labeling Act of 1960, which improved product labeling; the Child Protection Act of 1966, which extended labeling statutes to pesticides and other hazardous xenobiotics; and the Poison Prevention Packaging Act of 1970, which mandated safety packaging. In 1961, in an attempt to heighten public awareness of the dangers of unintentional poisoning, the third week of March was designated as the Annual National Poison Prevention Week.

Another organization that would become important, the American Academy of Clinical Toxicology (AACT), was founded in 1968 by a diverse group of toxicologists.[34] This group was "interested in applying principles of rational toxicology to patient treatment" and in improving the standards of care on a national basis.[140] The first modern textbooks of clinical toxicology began to appear in the mid-1950s with the publication of Dreisbach's *Handbook of Poisoning* (1955);[45] Gleason, Gosselin, and Hodge's *Clinical Toxicology of Commercial Products* (1957);[57] and Arena's *Poisoning* (1963).[10] Major advancements in the storage and retrieval of poison information were also instituted during these years. Information as noted earlier on consumer products initially appeared on index cards distributed regularly to poison control centers by the National Clearinghouse, and by 1978, more than 16,000 individual product cards had been issued.[143] The introduction of microfiche technology in 1972 enabled the storage of much larger amounts of data in much smaller spaces at the individual poison control centers. Toxifile and POISINDEX, two large drug and poison databases using microfiche technology, were introduced and gradually replaced the much more limited index card system.[143] During the 1980s, POISINDEX, which had become the standard database, was made more accessible by using CD-ROM technology. Sophisticated information about the most obscure xenobiotics was now instantaneously available by computer at every poison control center.

In 1978, the poison control center movement entered an important new stage in its development when the AAPCC introduced standards for regional poison control center designation.[103] By defining strict criteria, the AAPCC sought to improve poison control center operations significantly and to offer a national standard of service. These criteria included using poison specialists dedicated exclusively to operating the poison control center 24 hours per day and serving a catchment area of between 1 and 10 million people. Not surprisingly, this professionalization of the poison control center movement led to a rapid consolidation of services. An AAPCC credentialing examination for poison information specialists was inaugurated in 1983 to help ensure the quality and standards of poison control center staff.[7]

In 2000, the Poison Control Center Enhancement and Awareness Act was passed by Congress and signed into law by President Clinton. For the first time, federal funding became available to provide assistance for poison prevention and to stabilize the funding of regional poison control centers. This federal assistance permitted the establishment of a single nationwide toll-free phone number (800-222-1222) to access poison control centers. At present, 55 centers contribute data to a National Poison Database System (NPDS), which from 1983 to 2006 was known as Toxic Exposure Surveillance System (TESS). The Centers for Disease Control and Prevention (CDC) collaborates with the AAPCC to conduct real-time surveillance of these data to help facilitate the early detection of chemical exposures of public health importance.[165]

A poison control center movement has also grown and evolved in Europe over the past 35 years, but unlike the movement in the United States, it focused from the beginning on establishing strong centralized toxicology treatment centers.[131] In the late 1950s, Gaultier in Paris developed an inpatient unit dedicated to the care of poisoned patients.[59] In the United Kingdom, the National Poison Information Service developed at Guys Hospital in 1963 under Roy Goulding. Henry Matthew initiated a regional poisoning treatment center in Edinburgh about the same time.[131] In 1964, the European Association for Poison Control Centers was formed at Tours, France.[59]

The Rise of Environmental Toxicology and Further Regulatory Protection from Toxic Substances

The rise of the environmental movement during the 1960s can be traced, in part, to the publication of Rachel Carson's *Silent Spring* in 1962, which revealed the perils of an increasingly toxic environment.[29] The movement also benefited from the new awareness by those involved with the poison movement of the growing menace of xenobiotics in the home environment.[26] Battery casing fume poisoning, resulting from the burning of discarded lead battery cases, and acrodynia, resulting from exposure to a variety of mercury-containing products,[41] both demonstrated that young children are particularly vulnerable to low-dose exposures from certain xenobiotics. Worries about the persistence of pesticides in the ecosystem and the increasing number of chemicals introduced into the environment added to concerns of the environment as a potential source of illness, heralding a drive for additional regulatory protection.

Starting with the Clean Air Act in 1963, laws were passed to help reduce the toxic burden on our environment (Table 1–4). The establishment of the Environmental Protection Agency (EPA) in 1970 spearheaded this attempt at protecting our environment, and during the next 10 years, numerous protective regulations were introduced. Among the most important initiatives was the Occupational Safety and Health Act of 1970, which established the Occupational Safety and Health Administration (OSHA). This act mandates that employers provide safe work conditions for their employees. Specific exposure limits to toxic chemicals in the workplace were promulgated. The Consumer Product Safety Commission was created in 1972 to protect the public from consumer products that posed an unreasonable risk of illness or injury. Cancer-producing xenobiotics, such as asbestos, benzene, and vinyl chloride, were banned from consumer products as a result of these new regulations. Toxic waste disasters such as those at Love Canal, New York, and Times Beach, Missouri, led to the passing of the Comprehensive Environmental Response, Compensation, and Liability Act (CERCLA, also known as the Superfund) in 1980. This fund is designed to help pay for cleanup of hazardous substance releases posing a potential threat to public health. The Superfund legislation also led to the creation of the Agency for Toxic Substances and Disease Registry (ATSDR), a federal public health agency charged with determining the nature and extent of health problems at Superfund sites and advising the US EPA and state health and environmental agencies on the need for cleanup and other actions to protect the public's health. In 2003, the ATSDR became part of the National Center for Environmental Health of the CDC.

Medical Toxicology Comes of Age

Over the past 50 years, the primary specialties of medical toxicologists have changed. The development of emergency medicine and preventive medicine as medical specialties led to the training of more physicians with a dedicated interest in toxicology. By the early 1990s, emergency physicians accounted for more than half the number of practicing medical toxicologists. The increased diversity of medical toxicologists with primary training in emergency medicine, pediatrics, preventive medicine, or internal medicine has helped broaden the goals of poison control centers and medical toxicologists beyond the treatment of acute unintentional childhood ingestions. The scope of medical toxicology now includes a much wider array of toxic exposures, including acute and chronic, adult and pediatric, unintentional and intentional, and occupational and environmental exposures.

The development of medical toxicology as a medical subspecialty began in 1974, when the AACT created the American Board of Medical Toxicology (ABMT) to recognize physician practitioners of medical toxicology.[5] From 1974 to 1992, 209 physicians obtained board certification, and formal subspecialty recognition of medical toxicology by the American Board of Medical Specialties (ABMS) was granted in 1992. In that year, a conjoint subboard with representatives from the American Board of Emergency Medicine, American Board of Pediatrics, and American Board of Preventive Medicine was established, and the first ABMS-sanctioned examination in medical toxicology was offered in 1994. By 2016, a total of more than 600 physicians were board certified in medical toxicology. The American College of Medical Toxicology (ACMT) was founded in 1994 as a physician-based organization designed to advance clinical, educational, and research goals in medical toxicology. In 1999, the Accreditation Council of Graduate Medical Education (ACGME) in the United States formally recognized postgraduate education in medical toxicology, and by 2018, 27 fellowship training programs were approved. During the 1990s in the United States, some medical toxicologists began to work on establishing regional toxicology treatment centers. Adapting the European model, such toxicology treatment centers could serve as referral centers for patients requiring advanced toxicologic evaluation and treatment. Goals of such inpatient regional centers included enhancing care

of poisoned patients, strengthening toxicology training, and facilitating research. The evaluation of the clinical efficacy and fiscal viability of such programs is ongoing. More recently, an increasing number of medical toxicologists have expanded their practice into addiction medicine responding to the prescription opioid crisis.[88]

The professional maturation of advanced practice pharmacists and nurses with primary interests in clinical toxicology occurred over the past two decades. In 1985, the AACT established the American Board of Applied Toxicology (ABAT) to administer certifying examinations for nonphysician practitioners of medical toxicology who meet their rigorous standards.[4] By 2017, more than 115 toxicologists, who mostly held either a PharmD or a PhD in pharmacology or toxicology, were certified by this board.

Recent Poisonings and Poisoners
Although accounting for just a tiny fraction of all homicidal deaths (0.16% in the United States), notorious lethal poisonings continued throughout the 20th and 21st centuries (Table 1–3).[1]

In England, Graham Frederick Young developed a macabre fascination with poisons.[30] In 1971, at age 14 years, he killed his stepmother and other family members with arsenic and antimony. Sent away to a psychiatric hospital, he was released at age 24 years, when he was no longer considered to be a threat to society. Within months of his release, he again engaged in lethal poisonings, killing several of his coworkers with thallium. Ultimately, he died in prison in 1990.

In 1978, Georgi Markov, a Bulgarian defector living in London, developed multisystem failure and died 4 days after having been stabbed by an umbrella carried by an unknown assailant. The postmortem examination revealed a pinhead-sized metal sphere embedded in his thigh where he had been stabbed. Investigators hypothesized that this sphere had most likely carried a lethal dose of ricin into the victim.[37] This theory was greatly supported when ricin was isolated from the pellet of a second victim who was stabbed under similar circumstances.

In 1982, deliberate tampering with nonprescription Tylenol preparations with potassium cyanide caused seven deaths in Chicago.[46] Because of this tragedy, packaging of nonprescription medications was changed to decrease the possibility of future product tampering.[113] The perpetrator(s) were never apprehended, and other deaths from nonprescription product tampering were reported in 1991.[31]

In 1998, Judias Buenoano, known as the "black widow," was executed for murdering her husband with arsenic in 1971 to collect insurance money. She was the first woman executed in Florida in 150 years. The fatal poisoning had remained undetected until 1983, when Buenoano was accused of trying to murder her fiancé with arsenic and by car bombing. Exhumation of the husband's body, 12 years after he died, revealed substantial amounts of arsenic in the remains.[2]

Health care providers continue to be implicated in several poisoning homicides as well. An epidemic of mysterious cardiopulmonary arrests at the Ann Arbor Veterans Administration Hospital in Michigan in July and August 1975 was attributed to the homicidal use of pancuronium by two nurses.[153] Intentional digoxin poisoning by hospital personnel may have explained some of the increased number of deaths on a cardiology ward of a Toronto pediatric hospital in 1981, but the cause of the high mortality rate remained unclear.[23] In 2000, an English general practitioner Harold Shipman was convicted of murdering 15 female patients with heroin and may have murdered as many as 297 patients during his 24 year career. These recent revelations prompted calls for strengthening the death certification process, improving preservation of case records, and developing better procedures to monitor controlled drugs.[70]

Also in 2000, Michael Swango, an American physician, pleaded guilty to the charge of poisoning a number of patients under his care during his residency training. Succinylcholine, potassium chloride, and arsenic were used to kill his patients.[151] Attention to more careful physician credentialing and to maintenance of a national physician database arose from this case because the poisonings occurred at multiple hospitals across the country. Continuing concerns about health care providers acting as serial killers is highlighted by a recent case in New Jersey in which a nurse, Charles Cullen, was found responsible for killing patients with digoxin.[17]

By the end of the 20th century, 24 centuries after Socrates was executed by poison hemlock, the means of implementing capital punishment had come full circle. Government-sanctioned execution in the United States again favored the use of a "state" poison—this time, employing single drug and multiple drug protocols using sodium thiopental, pentobarbital, midazolam, hydromorphone, pancuronium, and potassium chloride.[81]

The use of a poison to achieve political ends has again resurfaced in several incidents from the former Soviet Union and its allies. In December 2004, it was announced that the Ukrainian presidential candidate Viktor Yushchenko was poisoned with 2,3,7,8-tetrachlorodibenzo-p-dioxin (TCDD), a potent dioxin.[149] The dramatic development of chloracne over the face of this public person during the previous several months suggested dioxin as a possibly culprit. Given the paucity of reports of acute dioxin poisoning, however, it was not until laboratory tests confirmed that Yushchenko's dioxin concentrations were more than 6,000 times normal that this diagnosis was confirmed. In another case, a former KGB agent and Russian dissident Alexander Litvinenko was murdered with polonium-210. Initially thought to be a possible case of heavy metal poisoning, Litvinenko developed acute radiation syndrome manifested by GI symptoms followed by alopecia and pancytopenia before he died.[108] In February 2017, the nerve agent VX was believed responsible for the death of the North Korean leader's elder brother Kim Jong-nam.[124]

Other Developments
Medical Errors
Beginning in the 1980s, several highly publicized medication errors received considerable public attention and provided a stimulus for the initiation of change in policies and systems. Ironically, all of the cases occurred at nationally preeminent university teaching hospitals. In 1984, 18-year-old Libby Zion died from severe hyperthermia soon after hospital admission. Although the cause of her death was likely multifactorial, drug–drug interactions and the failure to recognize and appropriately treat her agitated delirium also contributed to her death.[13] State and national guidelines for closer house staff supervision, improved working conditions, and a heightened awareness of consequential drug–drug interactions resulted from the medical, legislative, and legal issues of this case. In 1994, a prominent health journalist for the *Boston Globe*, Betsy Lehman, was the unfortunate victim of another preventable dosing error when she inadvertently received four times the dose of the chemotherapeutic cyclophosphamide as part of an experimental protocol.[83] Despite treatment at a world-renowned cancer center, multiple physicians, nurses, and pharmacists failed to notice this erroneous medication order. An overhaul of the medication-ordering system was implemented at that institution after this tragic event.

Another highly publicized death occurred in 1999, when 18-year-old Jesse Gelsinger died after enrolling in an experimental gene-therapy study. Gelsinger, who had ornithine transcarbamylase deficiency, died from multiorgan failure 4 days after receiving, by hepatic infusion, the first dose of an engineered adenovirus containing the normal gene. Although this unexpected death was not the direct result of a dosing or drug–drug interaction error, the FDA review concluded that major research violations had occurred, including failure to report adverse effects with this therapy in animals and earlier clinical trials and to properly obtain informed consent.[145] In 2001, Ellen Roche, a 24-year-old healthy volunteer in an asthma study at John Hopkins University, developed a progressive pulmonary illness and died 1 month after receiving 1 g of hexamethonium by inhalation as part of the study protocol.[150] Hexamethonium, a ganglionic blocker, was once used to treat hypertension but was removed from the market in 1972. The investigators were cited for failing to indicate on the consent form that hexamethonium was experimental and not FDA approved. Calls for additional safeguards to protect patients in research studies resulted from these cases.

In late 1999, the problems of medical errors finally received the high visibility and deserved attention in the United States with the publication and subsequent reaction to an Institute of Medicine (IOM) report suggesting that 44,000 to 98,000 fatalities each year were the result of medical errors.[84] Many of these errors were attributed to preventable medication errors. The IOM report focused on its findings that errors usually resulted from system faults and not solely from the carelessness of individuals.

Toxicology in the Twenty-First Century
As new challenges and opportunities arise in the 21st century, new toxicologic disciplines have emerged such as toxicogenomics, precision medicine, and nanotoxicology.[40,92,119] These nascent fields constitute the toxicologic responses to rapid advances in genetics and material sciences. Toxicogenomics combines toxicology with genomics dealing with how genes and proteins respond to toxic substances. The study of toxicogenomics attempts to better decipher the molecular events underlying toxicologic mechanisms, develop predictors of toxicity through the establishment of better molecular biomarkers, and better understand genetic susceptibilities that pertain to toxic substances such as unanticipated idiosyncratic drug reactions. Applying the principles of toxicogenomics has given birth to the field of precision medicine, also known as personalized medicine. Using such an approach drug therapy may be able to be individually tailored improving the prediction of drug efficacy and safety by accounting for genomic and metabolomics factors.[110]

Nanotoxicology refers to the toxicology of engineered tiny particles, usually smaller than 100 nm. Given the extremely small size of nanoparticles, typical barriers at portals of entry may not prevent absorption or may themselves be adversely affected by the nanoparticles. Ongoing studies focus on the translocation of these particles to sensitive target sites such as the central nervous system or bone marrow (Chap. 125).[119,168]

SUMMARY
- Since the dawn of recorded history, toxicology has impacted greatly on human events and our ecosystem.
- Over the millennia, although the important poisons of the day have changed to some degree, toxic xenobiotics continue to challenge our safety.
- The era of poisoners for hire may have long ago reached its pinnacle, but problems with drug abuse, intentional self-poisoning, and exposure to environmental chemicals continue to challenge us.
- Knowledge acquired by one generation is often forgotten or discarded inappropriately by the next generation, leading to a cyclical historic course.

REFERENCES
1. Adelson L. Homicidal poisoning. A dying modality of lethal violence? *Am J Forensic Med Pathol.* 1987;8:245-251.
2. Anderson C, McGehee S. *Bodies of Evidence: The True Story of Judias Buenoano: Florida's Serial Murderess.* New York, NY: St. Martin's; 1993.
3. Anderson H. Experimental studies on the pharmacology of activated charcoal. *Acta Pharmacol.* 1946;2:69-78.
4. Anonymous. American Board of Applied Toxicology. *AACTion.* 1992;1:3.
5. Anonymous. American Board of Medical Toxicology. *Vet Hum Toxicol.* 1987;29:510.
6. Anonymous. *American Heritage Dictionary.* 2nd college ed. Boston: Houghton Mifflin; 1991.
7. Anonymous. Certification examination for poison information specialists. *Vet Human Toxicol.* 1983;25:54-55.
8. Anonymous. *Oxford English Dictionary.* 3rd ed. Oxford: Oxford University Press; 2006. http://www.oed.com/view/Entry/146669?result=1&rskey=Elm5Hg&.
9. Anonymous. Suicide: a leading cause of death. *JAMA.* 1952;150:696-697.
10. Arena JM. *Poisoning: Chemistry, Symptoms, Treatments.* Springfield, IL: Charles C. Thomas; 1963.
11. Arena JM. The pediatrician's role in the poison control movement and poison prevention. *Am J Dis Child.* 1983;137:870-873.
12. Arnold WN. Vincent van Gogh and the thujone connection. *JAMA.* 1988;260: 3042-3044.
13. Asch DA, Parker RM. The Libby Zion case. One step forward or two steps backward? *N Engl J Med.* 1988;318:771-775.
14. Baldwin M. The snakestone experiments. An early modern medical debate. *Isis.* 1995;86:394-418.

15. Bartrip P. A "pennurth of arsenic for rat poison": the Arsenic Act, 1851 and the prevention of secret poisoning. *Med Hist.* 1992;36:53-69.

16. Baum CR. A century of Mickey Finn—but who was he? *J Toxicol Clin Toxicol.* 2000; 38:683.

17. Becker C. Killer credentials. In wake of nurse accused of killing patient, the health system wrestles with balancing shortage, ineffectual reference process. *Mod Health.* 2003;33:6-7, 1.

18. Benjamin DR. *Mushrooms: Poisons and Panaceas.* New York, NY: WH Freeman; 1995.

19. Berman A. The persistence of theriac in France. *Pharm Hist.* 1970;12:5-12.

20. Bisset NG. Arrow and dart poisons. *J Ethnopharmacol.* 1989;25:1-41.

21. Bond RT. *Handbook for Poisoners: A Collection of Great Poison Stories.* New York, NY: Collier Books; 1951.

22. Brown HM. De Venenis of Petrus Abbonus: a translation of the Latin. *Ann Med Hist.* 1924;6:25-53.

23. Buehler JW, et al. Unexplained deaths in a children's hospital. An epidemiologic assessment. *N Engl J Med.* 1985;313:211-216.

24. Burchell HB. Digitalis poisoning: historical and forensic aspects. *J Am Coll Cardiol.* 1983;1(2, pt 1):506-516.

25. Burke M. Gastric lavage and emesis in the treatment of ingested poisons: a review and a clinical study of lavage in ten adults. *Resuscitation.* 1972;1:91-105.

26. Burnham JC. How the discovery of accidental childhood poisoning contributed to the development of environmentalism in the United States. *Environ Hist Rev.* 1995;19:57-81.

27. Byck R, ed. *Cocaine Papers by Sigmund Freud (English Translation).* New York, NY: Stonehill Publishing; 1975:48-73.

28. Campbell WA. Oxalic acid, Epsom salt and the poison bottle. *Hum Toxicol.* 1982;1: 187-193.

29. Carson RL. *Silent Spring.* Boston: Houghton Mifflin; 1962.

30. Cavanagh JBJ. What have we learnt from Graham Frederick Young? Reflections on the mechanism of thallium neurotoxicity. *Neuropathol Appl Neurobiol.* 1991;17:3-9.

31. Centers for Disease Control (CDC). Cyanide poisonings associated with over-the-counter medication—Washington State, 1991. *MMWR Morb Mortal Wkly Rep.* 1991;40:242.

32. Christison R. *A Treatise on Poisons.* London: Adam Black; 1829.

33. Clarke MJ. Chloral hydrate: medicine and poison? *Pharm Hist.* 1988;18:2-4.

34. Comstock EG. Roots and circles in medical toxicology: a personal reminiscence. *J Toxicol Clin Toxicol.* 1998;36:401-407.

35. Cooney DO. *Activated Charcoal in Medical Applications.* 2nd ed. Taylor & Francis, Boca Boca Raton, FL: Taylor &Francis; 1995.

36. Costill OH. *A Practical Treatise on Poisons.* Philadelphia, PA: Grigg, Elliot; 1848.

37. Crompton R, Gall D. Georgi Markov—death in a pellet. *Med Leg J.* 1980;48:51-62.

38. Crotty J, Armstrong G. National Clearinghouse for Poison Control Centers. *Clin Toxicol.* 1978;12:303-307.

39. Crotty JJ, Verhulst HL. Organization and delivery of poison information in the United States. *Pediatr Clin North Am.* 1970;17:741-746.

40. Curtis JJ, et al. Nanotechnology and nanotoxicology: a primer for clinicians. *Toxicol Rev.* 2006;25:245-260.

41. Dally A. The rise and fall of pink disease. *Soc Hist Med.* 1997;10:291-304.

42. Das G. Cocaine abuse in North America: a milestone in history. *J Clin Pharmacol.* 1993;33:296-310.

43. Deichmann WB, et al. What is there that is not poison? A study of the Third Defense by Paracelsus. *Arch Toxicol.* 1986;58:207-213.

44. Delile H, et al. Lead in ancient Rome's city waters. *Proc Natl Acad Sci U S A.* 2014;111: 6594-6599.

45. Dreisbach RH. *Handbook of Poisoning: Diagnosis and Treatment.* Los Altos, CA: Lange; 1955.

46. Dunea G. Death over the counter. *Br Med J (Clin Res Ed).* 1983;286:211-212.

47. Earles MP. Early theories of mode of action of drugs and poisons. *Ann Sci.* 1961;17:97-110.

48. Eckert WG. Historical aspects of poisoning and toxicology. *Am J Forensic Med Pathol.* 1981;2:261-264.

49. Eckert WG. Medicolegal investigation in New York City. History and activities 1918-1978. *Am J Forensic Med Pathol.* 1983;4:33-54.

50. Elgood C. A treatise on the bezoar stone. *Ann Med Hist.* 1935;7:73-80.

51. Felton JS. The heritage of Bernardino Ramazzini. *Occup Med (Oxf).* 1997;47:167-179.

52. Ferner RE. *Forensic Pharmacology: Medicine, Mayhem, and Malpractice.* Oxford: Oxford University Press; 1996.

53. Franco G. Ramazzini and workers' health. *Lancet.* 1999;354:858-861.

54. Funck-Brentano F. *Princes and Poisoners: Studies of the Court of Louis XIV.* London: Duckworth & Co.; 1901.

55. Gaebel RE. Saturnine gout among Roman aristocrats. *N Engl J Med.* 1983;309:431.

56. Gallo MA. History and scope of toxicology. In: Klassen CD, ed. *Casarett and Doull's Toxicology: The Basic Science of Poisons.* 5th ed. New York, NY: McGraw-Hill; 1996:3-11.

57. Gleason MN, et al. *Clinical Toxicology of Commercial Products: Acute Poisoning (Home and Farm).* Baltimore, MD: Williams & Wilkins; 1957.

58. Golding AM. Two hundred years of drug abuse. *J R Soc Med.* 1993;86:282-286.

59. Govaerts M. Poison control in Europe. *Pediatr Clin North Am.* 1970;17:729-739.

60. Grant MP. *Alice Hamilton: Pioneer Doctor in Industrial Medicine.* London: Abelard-Schuman; 1967.

61. Grayson R. The poison control movement in the United States. *Indust Med Surg.* 1962;31:296-297.

62. Green DW. The saturnine curse: a history of lead poisoning. *South Med J.* 1985;78: 48-51.

63. Greensher J, et al. Ascendency of the black bottle (activated charcoal). *Pediatrics.* 1987;80:949-951.

64. Griffin JP. Venetian treacle and the foundation of medicines regulation. *Br J Clin Pharmacol.* 2004;58:317-325.

65. Hamilton A. Landmark article in occupational medicine. "Forty years in the poisonous trades." *Am J Indust Med.* 1985;7:3-18.

66. Hempel S. *The Inheritor's Powder: A Tale of Arsenic, Murder, and the New Forensic Science.* New York, NY: W.W. Norton & Company; 2013.

67. Hofmann A. How LSD originated. *J Psychedelic Drugs.* 1979;11:53-60.

68. Hold KM, et al. Alpha-thujone (the active component of absinthe): gamma-aminobutyric acid type A receptor modulation and metabolic detoxification. *Proc Natl Acad Sci U S A.* 2000;97:3826-3831.

69. Holt LE, Holz PH. The black bottle: a consideration of the role of charcoal in the treatment of poisoning in children. *J Pediatr.* 1963;63:306-314.

70. Horton R. The real lessons from Harold Frederick Shipman. *Lancet.* 2001;357:82-83.

71. Howard-Jones N. The origins of hypodermic medication. *Sci Am.* 1971;224:96-102.

72. Hughes PHP, Rieche OO. Heroin epidemics revisited. *Epidemiol Rev.* 1995;17:66-73.

73. Hunter D. *The Diseases of Occupations.* 6th ed. London: Hodder & Stoughton; 1978.

74. Jain KK. *Carbon Monoxide Poisoning.* St. Louis: Warren H. Green; 1990:3-5.

75. Jarcho S. Medical numismatic notes. VII. Mithridates IV. *Bull N Y Acad Med.* 1972;48:1059-1064.

76. Jarcho S. The correspondence of Morgagni and Lancisi on the death of Cleopatra. *Bull Hist Med.* 1969;43:299-325.

77. Jensen LB. *Poisoning Misadventures.* Springfield, IL: Charles C. Thomas; 1970.

78. Jones MM, Benrubi ID. A contentious history of consumer protection against dangerous household chemicals in the United States. *Am J Public Health.* 2013;103:801-812.

79. Karaberopoulos D, et al. The theriac in antiquity. *Lancet.* 2012;379:1942-1943.

80. Karch SB. The history of cocaine toxicity. *Hum Pathol.* 1989;20:1037-1039.

81. Kas K, et al. Lethal drugs in capital punishment in USA: history, present, and future perspectives. *Res Social Adm Pharm.* 2016;12:1026-1034.

82. Knoefel PK. Felice Fontana on poisons. *Clio Med.* 1980;15:35-66.

83. Knox RA. Doctor's orders killed cancer patient: Dana Farber admits drug overdose caused death of Globe columnist, damage to second woman. *Boston Globe.* March 23, 1995:1.

84. Kohn LT, et al. *To Err Is Human: Building a Safer Health System.* Washington, DC: National Academy of Science, Institute of Medicine; 2002.

85. Kolodny A, et al. The prescription opioid and heroin crisis: a public health approach to an epidemic of addiction. *Annu Rev Public Health.* 2015;36:559-574.

86. Kramer JC. Opium rampant: medical use, misuse and abuse in Britain and the West in the 17th and 18th centuries. *Br J Addict Alcohol Other Drugs.* 1979;74:377-389.

87. Kramer JC. The opiates: two centuries of scientific study. *J Psychedelic Drugs.* 1980;12:89-103.

88. Laes JR. The integration of medical toxicology and addiction medicine: a new era in patient care. *J Med Toxicol.* 2015;12:79-81.

89. Lanier D. *Absinthe: The Cocaine of the Nineteenth Century.* Jefferson, NC: McFarland; 1995.

90. Lee JA. Claude Bernard (1813-1878). *Anaesthesia.* 1978;33:741-747.

91. Lee MRM. Solanaceae III: henbane, hags and Hawley Harvey Crippen. *J R Coll Physicians Edinb.* 2006;36:366-373.

92. Lenfant C. Prospects of personalized medicine in cardiovascular diseases. *Metabolism.* 2013;62:S6-S10.

93. Levey M. Medieval Arabic toxicology: the book on poison of Ibn Wahshiya and its relation to early Indian and Greek texts. *Trans Am Philosph Soc.* 1966;56:5-130.

94. Lomax E. The uses and abuses of opiates in nineteenth-century England. *Bull Hist Med.* 1973;47:167-176.

95. Lovejoy FHJ, Alpert JJ. A future direction for poison centers. A critique. *Pediatr Clin North Am.* 1970;17:747-753.

96. Lucanie R. Unicorn horn and its use as a poison antidote. *Vet Hum Toxicol.* 1992;34:563.

97. Ludlow FH. *The Hasheesh Eater Microform: Being Passages from the Life of a Pythagorean.* New York, NY: Harper; 1857.

98. Lyon AS. *Medicine: An Illustrated History.* New York, NY: Abradale; 1978.

99. Macht DI. Louis Lewin: pharmacologist, toxicologist, medical historian. *Ann Med Hist.* 1931;3:179-194.

100. Magner LN. *A History of Medicine.* New York, NY: Marcel Dekker; 1992.

101. Major RH. History of the stomach tube. *Ann Med Hist.* 1934;6:500-509.

102. Mann RH. *Murder, Magic, and Medicine.* New York, NY: Oxford University Press; 1992.

103. Manoguerra AS, Temple AR. Observations on the current status of poison control centers in the United States. *Emerg Med Clin North Am.* 1984;2:185-197.

104. Mant AK. Forensic medicine in Great Britain. II. The origins of the British medicolegal system and some historic cases. *Am J Forensic Med Pathol.* 1987;8:354-361.

105. Marsh J. Account of a method of separating small quantities of arsenic from substances with which it may be mixed. *Edinb New Phil J.* 1836;21:229-236.

106. McIntire M. On the occasion of the twenty-fifth anniversary of the American Association of Poison Control Centers. *Vet Hum Toxicol.* 1983;25:35-37.

107. Mead GO. Ether drinking in Ireland. *JAMA.* 1891;16:391-392.

108. Miller CWC, et al. Murder by radiation poisoning: implications for public health. *J Environ Health.* 2012;74:8-13.

109. Modell W. Mass drug catastrophes and the roles of science and technology. *Science.* 1967;156:346-351.

110. Monte AA, et al. Improved drug therapy: triangulating phenomics with genomics and metabolomics. *Hum Genomics.* 2014;8:16.

111. Moore SW. A case of poisoning by laudanum, successfully treated by means of Juke's syringe. *NY Med Phys J.* 1825;4:91-92.

112. Moriarty KM, et al. Psychopharmacology. An historical perspective. *Psychiatr Clin North Am.* 1984;7:411-433.

113. Murphy DH. Cyanide-tainted Tylenol: what pharmacists can learn. *Am Pharm.* 1986;NS26:19-23.

114. Musto DF. America's first cocaine epidemic. *Wilson Q.* 1989;13:59-64.

115. Nahas GG. Hashish in Islam 9th to 18th century. *Bull N Y Acad Med.* 1982;58:814-831.

116. Nerlich AG, et al. Extensive pulmonary haemorrhage in an Egyptian mummy. *Virchows Arch.* 1995;427:423-429.

117. Niyogi SK. Historic development of forensic toxicology in America up to 1978. *Am J Forensic Med Pathol.* 1980;1:249-264.

118. Nriagu JO. Saturnine gout among Roman aristocrats. Did lead poisoning contribute to the fall of the Empire? *N Engl J Med.* 1983;308:660-663.

119. Oberdörster G, et al. Nanotoxicology: an emerging discipline evolving from studies of ultrafine particles. *Environ Health Perspect.* 2005;113:823.

120. Oehme FW. The development of toxicology as a veterinary discipline in the United States. *Clin Toxicol.* 1970;3:211-220.

121. Olch PD. William S. Halsted and local anesthesia: contributions and complications. *Anesthesiology.* 1975;42:479-486.

122. Orfila MP. *Traites Des Poisons.* Paris: Ches Crochard; 1814.

123. Pachter HM. *Paracelsus: Magic Into Science.* New York, NY: Collier; 1961.

124. Paddock RC, et al. In Kim Jong-Nam's death, North Korea lets loose a weapon of mass destruction. *The New York Times.* https://www.nytimes.com/2017/02/24/world/asia/north-korea-kim-jong-nam-vx-nerve-agent.html?_r=0

125. Pappas AA, et al. Toxicology: past, present, and future. *Ann Clin Lab Sci.* 1999;29: 253-262.

126. Parsche F, et al. Drugs in ancient populations. *Lancet.* 1993;341:503.

127. Plaitakis A, Duvoisin RC. Homer's moly identified as Galanthus nivalis L.: physiologic antidote to stramonium poisoning. *Clin Neuropharmacol.* 1983;6:1-5.

128. Pollack SH. The psilocybin mushroom pandemic. *J Psychedelic Drugs.* 1975;7:73-84.

129. Press E, Mellins RB. A poisoning control program. *Am J Public Health Nations Health.* 1954;44:1515-1525.

130. Proudfoot A. The early toxicology of physostigmine: a tale of beans, great men and egos. *Toxicol Rev.* 2006;25:99-138.

131. Proudfoot AT, et al. Clinical toxicology in Edinburgh, two centuries of progress. *Clin Toxicol (Phila).* 2013;51:509-514.

132. Proudfoot AT. Clinical toxicology—past, present and future. *Hum Toxicol.* 1988;7:481-487.

133. Quinones MA. Drug abuse during the Civil War (1861-1865). *Int J Addict.* 1975;10: 1007-1020.

134. Randall T. Cocaine deaths reported for century or more. *JAMA.* 1992;267:1045-1046.

135. Regier CC. The struggle for federal food and drugs legislation. *Law Contemp Prob.* 1933;1:3-15.

136. Reid DH. Treatment of the poisoned child. *Arch Dis Child.* 1970;45:428-433.

137. Robertson WO. National organizations and agencies in poison control programs: a commentary. *Clin Toxicol.* 1978;12:297-302.

138. Robins LN, et al. Narcotic use in southeast Asia and afterward. An interview study of 898 Vietnam returnees. *Arch Gen Psychiatry.* 1975;32:955-961.

139. Rosner F. Moses Maimonides' treatise on poisons. *JAMA.* 1968;205:914-916.

140. Rumack BH, et al. Regionalization of poison centers—a rational role model. *Clin Toxicol.* 1978;12:367-375.

141. Sapira JD. Speculations concerning opium abuse and world history. *Perspect Biol Med.* 1975;18:379-398.

142. Scarborough J. Nicander's toxicology II: spiders, scorpions, insects and myriapods. *Pharm Hist.* 1979;21:73-92.

143. Scherz RG, Robertson WO. The history of poison control centers in the United States. *Clin Toxicol.* 1978;12:291-296.

144. Scutchfield FD, Genovese EN. Terrible death of Socrates: some medical and classical reflections. *Pharos.* 1997;60:30-33.

145. Silberner J. A gene therapy death. *Hastings Cent Rep.* 2000;30:6.

146. Sinclair U. *The Jungle.* New York, NY: Doubleday; 1906.

147. Smith S. Poisons and poisoners through the ages. *Med Leg J.* 1952;20:153-167.

148. Sneader W. The discovery of heroin. *Lancet.* 1998;352:1697-1699.

149. Sorg O, et al. 2,3,7,8-tetrachlorodibenzo-p-dioxin (TCDD) poisoning in Victor Yushchenko: identification and measurement of TCDD metabolites. *Lancet.* 2009;374: 1179-1185.

150. Steinbrook R. Protecting research subjects—the crisis at Johns Hopkins. *N Engl J Med.* 2002;346:716-720.

151. Stewart JB. *Blind Eye: The Terrifying Story of a Doctor Who Got Away with Murder.* New York, NY: Touchstone; 1999.

152. Strang J, et al. Absinthe: what's your poison? Though absinthe is intriguing, it is alcohol in general we should worry about. *BMJ.* 1999;319:1590-1592.

153. Stross JK, et al. An epidemic of mysterious cardiopulmonary arrests. *N Engl J Med.* 1976;295:1107-1110.

154. Taylor HM. A preliminary survey of the effect which lye legislations had had on the incident of esophageal stricture. *Ann Otol Rhinol Laryngol.* 1935;44:1157-1158.

155. Thompson CJ. *Poison and Poisoners.* London: Harold Shaylor; 1931.

156. Timbrell JA. *Introduction to Toxicology.* London: Taylor & Francis; 1989.

157. Trestrail JH. *Criminal Poisoning: Investigational Guide for Law Enforcement, Toxicologists, Forensic Scientists, and Attorneys.* Totowa, NJ: Humana Press; 2000.

158. Vale JA, Meredith TJ. Poison information services. In: Vale JA, Meredith TJ, eds. *Poisoning, Diagnosis and Treatment.* London: Update Books; 1981:9-12.

159. Waldron HA. Lead poisoning in the ancient world. *Med Hist.* 1973;17:391-399.

160. Watson G. *Theriac and Mithridatum: A Study in Therapeutics.* London: Wellcome Historical Medical Library; 1966.

161. Wax PM. Elixirs, diluents, and the passage of the 1938 Federal Food, Drug and Cosmetic Act. *Ann Intern Med.* 1995;122:456-461.

162. Whorton JC. *The Arsenic Century: How Victorian Britain Was Poisoned at Home, Work and Play.* Oxford: Oxford University Press; 2010.

163. Witthaus RA, Becker TC. *Medical Jurisprudence: Forensic Medicine and Toxicology.* Vol 1. New York, NY: William Wood; 1894.

164. Witthaus RA. *Manual of Toxicology.* New York, NY: William Wood; 1911.

165. Wolkin AF, et al. Early detection of illness associated with poisonings of public health significance. *Ann Emerg Med.* 2006;47:170-176.

166. Wormley TG. *Micro-Chemistry of Poisons.* New York, NY: William Wood; 1869.

167. Wright-St Clair RE. Poison or medicine? *N Z Med J.* 1970;71:224-229.

168. Yildirimer L, et al. Toxicological considerations of clinically applicable nanoparticles. *Nano Today.* 2011;6:585-607.

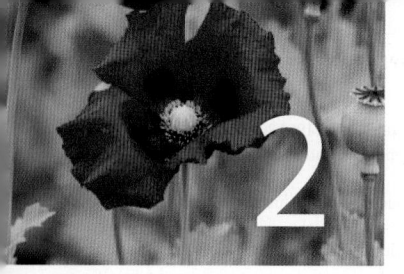

2 TOXICOLOGIC MISFORTUNES AND CATASTROPHES IN HISTORY

Paul M. Wax

Throughout history, mass poisonings have caused suffering and misfortune. From the ergot epidemics of the Middle Ages to contemporary industrial disasters, these mass events have had great political, economic, social, and environmental ramifications. Particularly within the past 100 years, as the number of toxins and potential toxins has risen dramatically, toxic disasters have become increasingly common events. The sites of some of these events—Bhopal (India), Chernobyl (Ukraine), Jonestown (Guyana), Love Canal (New York), Minamata Bay (Japan), Seveso (Italy), West Bengal (India)—have come to symbolize our increasing potential for environmental toxicity. Globalization has led to the proliferation and rapid distribution of toxic chemicals throughout the world. Many factories that store large amounts of potentially lethal chemicals are not secure. Given the increasing attention to terrorism preparedness, an appreciation of chemicals as agents of opportunity for terrorists has suddenly assumed great importance. This chapter provides an overview of some of the most consequential and historically important toxin-associated mass poisonings that represent human and environmental disasters.

GAS DISASTERS

Inhalation of toxic gases and oral ingestions resulting in food poisoning tend to subject the greatest number of people to adverse consequences of a toxic exposure. Toxic gas exposures may be the result of a natural disaster (volcanic eruption), industrial mishap (fire, chemical release), chemical warfare, or an intentional homicidal or genocidal endeavor (concentration camp gas chamber). Depending on the toxin, the clinical presentation may be acute, with a rapid onset of toxicity (cyanide), or subacute or chronic, with a gradual onset of toxicity (air pollution).

One of the earliest recorded toxic gas disasters resulted from the eruption of Mount Vesuvius near Pompeii, Italy, in 79 A.D. (Table 2–1). Poisonous gases generated from the volcanic activity reportedly killed thousands of people.[35] A more recent natural disaster occurred in 1986 in Cameroon, when excessive amounts of carbon dioxide spontaneously erupted from Lake Nyos, a volcanic crater lake.[19] Approximately 1,700 human and countless animal fatalities resulted from exposure to this asphyxiant.

A toxic gas leak at the Union Carbide pesticide plant in Bhopal, India, in 1984 resulted in one of the greatest civilian toxic disasters in modern history.[144] An unintended exothermic reaction at this carbaryl-producing plant caused the release of more than 24,000 kg of methyl isocyanate. This gas was quickly dispersed through the air over the densely populated area surrounding the factory where many of the workers lived, resulting in at least 2,500 deaths and 200,000 injuries.[88] The initial response to this disaster was greatly limited by a lack of pertinent information about the toxicity of this chemical as well as the poverty of the residents. A follow-up study 10 years later showed persistence of small-airway obstructive disease among survivors as well as chronic ophthalmic problems.[31] Calls for improvement in disaster preparedness and strengthened "right-to-know" laws regarding potential toxic exposures resulted from this tragedy.[50,144]

The release into the atmosphere of 26 tons of hydrofluoric acid at a petrochemical plant in Texas in October 1987 resulted in 939 people seeking medical attention at nearby hospitals. Ninety-four people were hospitalized, but there were no deaths.[154]

More than any other single toxin, carbon monoxide is involved in the largest number of toxic disasters. Catastrophic fires, such as the Cocoanut Grove Nightclub fire in 1943, have caused hundreds of deaths at a time, many of them from carbon monoxide poisoning.[37] A 1990 fire deliberately started at the Happy Land Social Club in the Bronx, New York, claimed 87 victims,

including a large number of nonburn deaths,[78] and the 2003 fire at the Station nightclub in West Warwick, Rhode Island, killed 98 people.[128] Carbon monoxide poisoning was a major determinant in many of these deaths, although hydrogen cyanide gas and simple asphyxiation may have also contributed to the overall mortality.

Another notable toxic gas disaster involving a fire occurred at the Cleveland Clinic in Cleveland, Ohio, in 1929, where a fire in the radiology department resulted in 125 deaths.[34] The burning of nitrocellulose radiographs produced nitrogen dioxide, cyanide, and carbon monoxide gases held responsible for many of the fatalities. In 2003, at least 243 people died and 10,000 became ill after a drilling well exploded in Xiaoyang, China, releasing hydrogen sulfide and natural gas into the air.[159] A toxic gas cloud covered 25 square kilometers. Ninety percent of the villagers who lived in the village adjoining the gas well died.

The release of a dioxin-containing chemical cloud into the atmosphere from an explosion at a hexachlorophene production factory in Seveso, Italy

TABLE 2–1	Gas Disasters		
Xenobiotic	**Location**	**Date**	**Significance**
Poisonous volcanic gases	Pompeii, Italy	79 A.D.	>2,000 deaths from eruption of Mt. Vesuvius
Smog (SO$_2$)	London, England	1873	268 deaths from bronchitis
NO$_2$, CO, CN	Cleveland Clinic, Cleveland, OH	1929	Fire in radiology department; 125 deaths
Smog (SO$_2$)	Meuse Valley, Belgium	1930	64 deaths
CO, CN	Cocoanut Grove Lounge, Boston, Mass	1942	498 deaths from fire
CO	Salerno, Italy	1944	>500 deaths on a train stalled in a tunnel
Smog (SO$_2$)	Donora, PA	1948	20 deaths; thousands ill
Smog (SO$_2$)	London, England	1952	4,000 deaths attributed to the fog and smog
Dioxin	Seveso, Italy	1976	Unintentional industrial release of dioxin into environment; chloracne
Methyl isocyanate	Bhopal, India	1984	>2,500 deaths; 200,000 injuries
Carbon dioxide	Cameroon, Africa	1986	>1,700 deaths from release of gas from Lake Nyos
Hydrofluoric acid	Texas City, TX	1987	Atmospheric release; 94 hospitalized
CO, CN	Happy Land Social Club, Bronx, NY	1990	87 deaths in fire from toxic smoke
Hydrogen sulfide	Xiaoyang, China	2003	243 deaths and 10,000 became ill from gas poisoning after a gas well exploded
CO, CN	West Warwick, RI	2003	98 deaths in fire

in 1976, resulted in one of the most serious exposures to dioxin (2,3,7,8-tetra-chlorodibenzo-*p*-dioxin {TCDD}).[49] The lethality of this xenobiotic in animals has caused considerable concern for acute and latent injury from human exposure. Although chloracne was the only significant clinical finding related to the dioxin exposure at 5-year follow-up[9] more recent data after 30 years suggest a positive correlation between TCDD serum concentration and cancer incidence.[147]

Air pollution is another source of toxic gases that causes significant disease and death. Complaints about smoky air date back to at least 1272, when King Edward I banned the burning of mineral coal.[142] By the 19th century, the era of rapid industrialization in England, winter "fogs" became increasingly problematic. An 1873 London fog was responsible for 268 deaths from bronchitis. Excessive smog (a portmanteau of smoke and fog) in the Meuse Valley of Belgium in 1930 and in Donora, Pennsylvania, in 1948, was also blamed for excess morbidity and mortality. In 1952, another dense sulfur dioxide–laden smog in London was responsible for 4,000 deaths.[74] Both the initiation of long-overdue air pollution reform in England and the passing of the 1956 Clean Air Act by Parliament resulted from this latter "fog."

WARFARE AND TERRORISM

Exposure to xenobiotics with the deliberate intent to inflict harm claimed an extraordinary number of victims during the 20th century (Table 2–2). During World War I, chlorine, phosgene, and the liquid vesicant mustard were used as battlefield weapons, with mustard causing approximately 80% of the chemical casualties.[130] Reportedly, 100,000 deaths and 1.2 million casualties were attributable to these chemical attacks.[37] The toxic exposures resulted in severe airway irritation, acute respiratory distress syndrome, hemorrhagic pneumonitis, skin blistering, and ophthalmic damage. Mustard was used again in the 1980s during the war between Iran and Iraq.

The Nazis used poisonous gases during World War II to commit genocide. Initially, the Nazis used carbon monoxide to kill. To expedite the killing process, Nazi scientists developed Zyklon-B gas (hydrogen cyanide gas). As many as 10,000 people per day were killed by the rapidly acting cyanide, and millions of deaths were attributable to the use of these gases.

Agent Orange was widely used as a defoliant during the Vietnam War. This herbicide consisted of a mixture of 2,4,5-trichlorophenoxy-acetic acid (2,4,5-T) and 2,4-dichlorophenoxyacetic acid (2,4-D), as well as small amounts of a contaminant, TCDD. Over the years, a large number of adverse health effects have been attributed to Agent Orange exposure. Although a 2002 Institute of Medicine study concluded that among Vietnam veterans, there was sufficient evidence to demonstrate an association between this herbicide exposure and chronic lymphocytic leukemia, soft tissue sarcomas, non-Hodgkin lymphomas, Hodgkin disease, and chloracne,[55] a 2015 critical review concluded that causation has yet to be established.[123]

Mass exposure to the very potent organic phosphorus compound sarin occurred in March 1995, when terrorists released this chemical weapon in three separate Tokyo subway lines.[104] Eleven people were killed, and 5,510 people sought emergency medical evaluation at more than 200 hospitals and clinics in the area.[131] This calamity introduced the spectra of terrorism to the modern emergency medical services system, resulting in a greater emphasis on hospital preparedness, including planning for the psychological consequences of such events. Sarin exposure also resulted in several deaths and hundreds of casualties in Matsumoto, Japan, in June 1994.[93,101] During the Syrian Civil War, sarin and chlorine were used on multiple occasions.[75]

After the terrorist attacks on New York City in September 11, 2001, that resulted in the collapse of World Trade Center, persistent cough and increased bronchial responsiveness were noted among 8% of New York City Fire Department workers who were exposed to large amounts of dust and other particulates during the clean-up.[110,111] This condition, known as World Trade Center cough syndrome, is characterized by upper airway (chronic rhinosinusitis) and lower airway findings (bronchitis, asthma, or both) as well as, at times, gastroesophageal reflux dysfunction. The risk of development of hyperreactivity and reactive airways dysfunction was clearly associated with the intensity of exposure.[16] A World Trade Center health registry was established to investigate and care for those exposed workers who may be at increased risk for development of cancer and other chronic diseases.[72,98] Registry data suggest that some workers appear to be at an increased risk for development of sarcoidosis[58] and persistent lower respiratory tract symptoms.[57]

The Russian military used a mysterious "gas" to incapacitate Chechen rebels at a Moscow theatre in 2002, resulting in the deaths of more than 120 hostages. One report suggested that the gas contained a mixture of the highly potent aerosolized fentanyl derivatives carfentanil and remifentanil.[115] Better preparation of the rescuers with suitable amounts of naloxone might have helped prevent some of these seemingly unanticipated casualties.[148]

Ricin was found in several government buildings, including a mail processing plant in Greenville, South Carolina, in 2003 and the Dirksen Senate Office Building in Washington, DC, in 2004. Although no cases of ricin-associated illness ensued, increased concern was generated because the method of delivery was thought to be the mail, and irradiation procedures designed to kill microbials such as anthrax would not inactivate chemical toxins such as ricin.[14,124]

TABLE 2–2	Warfare and Terrorism Disasters			
Toxin	*Location*	*Date*	*Significance*	
Chlorine, mustard gas, phosgene	Ypres, Belgium	1915–1918	100,000 dead and 1.2 million casualties from chemicals during World War I	
Cyanide, Carbon Monoxide	Europe	1939–1945	Millions murdered by Zyklon-B (HCN) gas	
Agent Orange	Vietnam	1960s	Contained dioxin; excess skin cancer	
Mustard gas	Iraq–Iran	1982	New cycle of war gas casualties	
Yet to be determined	Persian Gulf	1991	Gulf War syndrome	
Sarin	Matsumoto, Japan	1994	First terrorist attack in Japan using sarin	
Sarin	Tokyo, Japan	1995	Subway exposure; 5,510 people sought medical attention	
Dust and other particulates	New York, NY	2001	World Trade Center collapse from terrorist air strike	
Carfentanil & Remifentanil	Moscow, Russia	2002	Used by the Russian military to subdue terrorists in Moscow theater	
Ricin	Washington, DC	2004	Detected in Dirksen Senate Office Building; no illness reported	
Chlorine	Iraq	2007	Used against US troops and Iraqi civilians	
Sarin	Syria	2013, 2017	Used against Syrian civilians	

FOOD DISASTERS

Unintentional contamination of food and drink has led to numerous toxic disasters (Table 2–3). Ergot, produced by the fungus *Claviceps purpurea*, caused epidemic ergotism as the result of eating breads and cereals made from rye contaminated by *C. purpurea*. In some epidemics, convulsive manifestations predominated, and in others, gangrenous manifestations predominated.[90] Ergot-induced severe vasospasm was thought to be responsible for both presentations.[89,90] In 994 A.D., 40,000 people died in Aquitania, France, in one such epidemic.[70] Convulsive ergotism was initially described as a "fire which twisted the people," and the term "St. Anthony's fire" (*ignis sacer*) was used to refer to the excruciating burning pain experienced in the extremities that is an early manifestation of gangrenous ergotism. The events surrounding the Salem, Massachusetts, witchcraft trials have also been attributed to the ingestion of contaminated rye. The bizarre neuropsychiatric manifestations exhibited by some of the individuals associated with this event may have been caused by the hallucinogenic properties of ergotamine, a lysergic acid diethylamide (LSD) precursor.[23,84]

During the last half of the 20th century, unintentional mass poisoning from food and drink contaminated with toxic chemicals became all too common. One of the more unusual poisonings occurred in Turkey in 1956 when wheat seed intended for planting was treated with the fungicide hexachlorobenzene and then inadvertently used for human consumption. Approximately 4,000 cases of porphyria cutanea tarda were attributed to the ingestion of this toxic wheat seed.[125]

Another example of chemical food poisoning took place in Epping, England, in 1965. In this incident, a sack of flour became contaminated with methylenedianiline when the chemical unintentionally spilled onto the flour during transport to a bakery. Subsequent ingestion of bread baked with the contaminated flour produced hepatitis in 84 people. This outbreak of toxic hepatitis became known as Epping jaundice.[63]

The manufacture of polybrominated biphenyls (PBBs) in a factory that also produced food supplements for livestock resulted in the unintentional contamination of a large amount of livestock feed in Michigan in 1973.[24] Significant morbidity and mortality among the livestock population resulted, and increased human tissue concentrations of PBBs were reported,[155] although human toxicity seemed limited to vague constitutional symptoms and abnormal liver function test results.

The chemical contamination of rice oil in Japan in 1968 caused a syndrome called Yusho ("rice oil disease"). This occurred when heat-exchange fluid containing polychlorinated biphenyls (PCBs) and polychlorinated dibenzofurans (PCDFs) leaked from a heating pipe into the rice oil. More than 1,600 people developed chloracne, hyperpigmentation, an increased incidence of liver cancer, or adverse reproductive effects. In 1979 in Taiwan, 2,000 people developed similar clinical manifestations after ingesting another batch of PCB-contaminated rice oil. This latter epidemic was referred to as Yu-Cheng ("oil disease").[56] These polychlorinated chemicals are very biopersistent, with follow-up testing 40 years later demonstrating blood half-lives approaching infinity in some patients.[85]

In another oil contamination epidemic, consumption of illegally marketed cooking oil in Spain in 1981 was responsible for a mysterious poisoning epidemic that affected more than 19,000 people and resulted in at least 340 deaths. Exposed patients developed a multisystem disorder referred to as

TABLE 2–3	Food Disasters		
Xenobiotic	**Location**	**Date**	**Significance**
Ergot	Aquitania, France	994 A.D.	40,000 died in the epidemic
Ergot	Salem, MA	1692	Neuropsychiatric symptoms may be attributable to ergot
Lead	Devonshire, England	1700s	Colic from cider contaminated during production
Lead	Canada	1846	134 men died during the Franklin expedition, possibly because of contamination of food stored in lead cans
Cadmium	Japan	1939–1954	Itai-Itai ("ouch-ouch") disease
Hexachlorobenzene	Turkey	1956	4,000 cases of porphyria cutanea tarda
Methyl mercury	Minamata Bay, Japan	1950s	Consumption of organic mercury poisoned fish
Triorthocresyl phosphate	Meknes, Morocco	1959	Cooking oil adulterated with turbojet lubricant
Methylenedianiline	Epping, England	1965	Jaundice
Polychlorinated biphenyls	Japan	1968	Yusho ("rice oil disease")
Methyl mercury	Iraq	1971	>400 deaths from contaminated grain
Polybrominated biphenyls	Michigan	1973	97% of Michigan residents contaminated through food chain
Polychlorinated biphenyls	Taiwan	1979	Yu-Cheng ("oil disease")
Rapeseed oil (denatured)	Spain	1981	Toxic oil syndrome affected 19,000 people
Arsenic	Buenos Aires	1987	Malicious contamination of meat; 61 people underwent chelation
Arsenic	Bangladesh and West Bengal, India	1990s–present	Contaminated ground water; millions exposed; 100,000s with symptoms; greatest mass poisoning in history
Tetramine	China	2002	Snacks deliberately contaminated, resulting in 42 deaths and 300 people with symptoms
Arsenic	Maine	2003	Intentional contamination of coffee; one death and 16 cases of illness
Nicotine	Michigan	2003	Deliberate contamination of ground beef; 92 people became ill
Melamine	China	2008	50,000 hospitalized from tainted infant formula

toxic oil syndrome (or toxic epidemic syndrome), characterized by pneumonitis, eosinophilia, pulmonary hypertension, scleroderma-like features, and neuromuscular changes. Although this syndrome was associated with the consumption of rapeseed oil denatured with 2% aniline, the exact etiology was not definitively identified at the time. Subsequent investigations suggest that the fatty acid oleyl anilide may have been the putative xenobiotic.[59,60,108]

In 1999, an outbreak of health complaints related to consuming Coca-Cola occurred in Belgium, when 943 people, mostly children, complained of gastrointestinal (GI) symptoms, malaise, headaches, and palpitations after drinking Coca-Cola.[102] Many of those affected complained of an "off taste" or bad odor to the soft drink. In some of the Coca-Cola bottles, the carbon dioxide was contaminated with small amounts of carbonyl sulfide, which hydrolyzes to hydrogen sulfide, and may have been responsible for odor-triggered reactions. Mass psychogenic illness may have contributed to the large number of medical complaints because the concentrations of the carbonyl sulfide and hydrogen sulfide were very low and unlikely to cause systemic toxicity.[39]

Epidemics of heavy metal poisoning from contaminated food and drink have also occurred throughout history. Epidemic lead poisoning is associated with many different vehicles of transmission, including leaden bowls, kettles, and pipes. A famous 18th-century epidemic was known as the Devonshire colic. Although the exact etiology of this disorder was unknown for many years, later evidence suggested that the ingestion of lead-contaminated cider was responsible.[145]

Intentional chemical contamination of food may also occur. Multiple cases of metal poisoning occurred in Buenos Aires in 1987, when vandals broke into a butcher's shop and poured an unknown amount of a 45% sodium arsenite solution over 200 kg of partly minced meat.[117] The contaminated meat was purchased by 718 people. Of 307 meat purchasers who submitted to urine sampling, 49 had urine arsenic concentrations of 76 to 500 mcg/dL, and 12 had urine arsenic concentrations above 500 mcg/dL (normal urine arsenic concentration is <50–100 mcg/dL).

Cases of deliberate mass poisoning have heightened concerns about food safety and security. In China in 2002, a jealous food vendor adulterated fried dough sticks, sesame cakes, and rice prepared in a rival's snack bar by surreptitiously putting a large amount of tetramine (tetramethylene disulfotetramine) into the raw pastry material. More than 300 people who consumed these adulterated snacks became ill, and 42 died.[30] In Maine in 2003, a disillusioned parishioner contaminated the communal coffee pot at a church bake sale with arsenic. One victim died within 12 hours, and five others developed hypotension.[156] In 2003 in Michigan, 92 people became ill after ingesting contaminated ground beef deliberately contaminated with a nicotine pesticide by a supermarket employee.[6]

At the end of the 20th century and beginning of the 21st century, what may be the greatest mass poisoning in history occurred in Bangladesh and India's West Bengal State[33,95,112,135] (Chap. 86). In Bangladesh alone, 60 million people routinely drank arsenic-contaminated ground water, and at least 220,000 inhabitants of India's West Bengal were diagnosed with arsenic poisoning.[94] Symptoms reported include melanosis, depigmentation, hyperkeratosis, hepatomegaly, splenomegaly, squamous cell carcinoma, intraepidermal carcinoma, and gangrene.[33] In a country long plagued by dysentery, attempts to purify the water supply led to the drilling of millions of wells into the superficial water table. Unknown to the engineers, this water was naturally contaminated with arsenic, creating several thousand tube wells with extremely high concentrations of arsenic—up to 40 times the acceptable concentration. Although toxicity from arsenic-contaminated groundwater was previously reported from other areas of the world, including Argentina, China, Mexico, Taiwan (black foot disease), and Thailand, the number of people at risk in Bangladesh and West Bengal is by far the largest. A 2016 report suggests that 40 million people in Bangladesh may still be exposed to unsafe concentrations of arsenic in the water with tens of thousands of deaths per year attributed to arsenic exposure.[73]

Methyl mercury is responsible for several poisoning epidemics in the past half century. During the 1950s, a Japanese chemical factory that manufactured vinyl chloride and acetaldehyde routinely discharged mercury into Minamata Bay, resulting in contamination of the aquatic food chain. An epidemic of methyl mercury poisoning ensued as the local people ate the poisoned fish.[109,141] Chronic brain damage, tunnel vision, deafness, and severe congenital defects were associated with this mass poisoning.[109] Another mass epidemic of methyl mercury poisoning occurred in Iraq in 1971, when the local population consumed homemade bread prepared from wheat seed treated with a methyl mercury fungicide.[15] Six thousand hospital admissions and more than 400 deaths were associated with this mass poisoning. As was the case of the hexachlorobenzene exposure in Turkey 15 years previously, the treated grain, intended for use as seed, was instead utilized as food.

From 1939 to 1954, contamination of the local water supply with the wastewater runoff from a zinc–lead–cadmium mine in Japan was believed responsible for causing Itai-Itai ("ouch-ouch") disease, an unusual chronic syndrome manifested by extreme bone pain and osteomalacia. The local water was used for drinking and irrigation of the rice fields. Approximately 200 people who lived along the banks of the Jintsu River developed these peculiar symptoms, which were thought most likely to be caused by the cadmium.[2]

More than 50,000 infants were hospitalized in China in 2008 from the ill effects of melamine-contaminated powdered infant formulae.[54] Melamine (1,3,5-triazine–2,4,6-triamine) is a component in many adhesives, glues, plastics, and laminated products (eg, plywood, cleaners, cement, cleansers, fire-retardant paint). More than 20 Chinese companies produced the tainted formula. Analysis of these formulas found melamine concentrations as high as 2,500 ppm. Clinically, exposure to high doses of melamine has been associated with the development of nephrolithiasis, obstructive uropathy, and in some cases acute kidney failure.[146] Melamine contamination of pet food resulting in deaths in dogs and cats was previously reported.[22] The melamine disaster also demonstrates that globalization and international agribusiness may facilitate worldwide distribution of contaminated foodstuffs. After the initial reports of melamine contamination in China, investigation in the United States revealed that certain brands of cookies, biscuits, candies, and milk sold in this country were also tainted with melamine, some of which was traced to an origin in China.[54]

MEDICINAL DRUG DISASTERS

Illness and death as a consequence of therapeutic drug use occur as sporadic events, usually affecting individual patients, or as mass poisoning, affecting multiple (sometimes hundreds or thousands) patients. Sporadic single-patient medication-induced tragedies usually result from errors (Chaps. 1 and 135) or unforeseen idiosyncratic reactions. Mass therapeutic drug disasters have generally occurred secondary to poor safety testing, a lack of understanding of diluents and excipients, drug contamination, or problems with unanticipated drug–drug interactions or drug toxicity (Table 2–4).

In September and October 1937, more than 105 deaths were associated with the use of one of the early sulfa preparations—elixir of sulfanilamide-Massengill—that contained 72% diethylene glycol as the vehicle for drug delivery. Little was known about diethylene glycol toxicity at the time, and many cases of acute kidney failure and death occurred.[41] To avoid similar tragedies in the future, animal drug testing was mandated by the Food, Drug, and Cosmetic Act of 1938.[149] Unfortunately, diethylene glycol continues to be sporadically used in other countries as a medicinal diluent, resulting in deaths in South Africa (1969), India (1986), Nigeria (1990), Bangladesh (1990–1992), and Haiti (1995–1996).[150] In 1996 in Haiti, at least 88 Haitian children died (case fatality rate of 98% for those who remained in Haiti) after ingesting an acetaminophen (APAP) elixir formulated with diethylene glycol–contaminated glycerin.[103,122] In Panama in 2006, glycerin contaminated with diethylene glycol found in prescription liquid cough syrup resulted in at least 121 cases of poisoning and 78 deaths (case fatality rate, 65.5%).[18,114] Investigators of this last outbreak discovered that the contaminated glycerin was imported to Panama from China via a European broker, demonstrating that improprieties in pharmaceutical manufacturing may have worldwide implications. In Nigeria in 2009, a tainted teething formula was responsible for 84 deaths in children.[7] The pharmaceutical manufacturers intended to

TABLE 2–4	Medicinal Disasters		
Xenobiotic	*Location*	*Date*	*Significance*
Thallium	United States	1920s–1930s	Treatment of ringworm; 31 deaths
Diethylene glycol	United States	1937	Elixir of sulfanilamide; kidney failure
Thorotrast	United States	1930s–1950s	Hepatic angiosarcoma
Phenobarbital	United States	1940–1941	Contaminated sulfathiazole: 82 deaths
Diethylstilbestrol	United States, Europe	1940s–1970s	Vaginal adenocarcinomas in patients' daughters and urogenital abnormalities in sons
Stalinon	France	1954	Severe neurotoxicity from triethyltin
Clioquinol	Japan	1955–1970	Subacute myelooptic neuropathy; 10,000 symptomatic
Thalidomide	Europe	1960s	5,000 cases of phocomelia
Isoproterenol 30%	Great Britain	1961–1967	3,000 excess asthma deaths
Pentachlorophenol	United States	1967	Used in hospital laundry; nine neonates ill, two deaths
Benzyl alcohol	United States	1981	Neonatal gasping syndrome
Tylenol–cyanide	Chicago	1982	Tampering incident resulted in seven homicides
L-Tryptophan	United States	1989	Eosinophilia myalgia syndrome
Diethylene glycol	Haiti	1996	Contaminated acetaminophen elixir; kidney failure; >88 pediatric deaths
Diethylene glycol	Panama	2006	Contaminated cough preparation, causing 78 deaths
Diethylene glycol	Nigeria	2009	Contaminated teething formula, causing 84 deaths

purchase propylene glycol, a component of the teething formula, but had bought the diluent in a jerrycan instead of the original container, and the chemical contained diethylene glycol (Special Considerations: SC9).

A lesser known drug manufacturing event, also involving an early sulfa antimicrobial, occurred in 1940 to 1941, when at least 82 people died from the therapeutic use of sulfathiazole that was contaminated with phenobarbital (Luminal).[136] The responsible pharmaceutical company, Winthrop Chemical, produced both sulfathiazole and phenobarbital, and the contamination likely occurred during the tableting process because the tableting machines for the two medications were adjacent to each other and were used interchangeably. Each contaminated sulfathiazole tablet contained about 350 mg of phenobarbital (and no sulfathiazole), and the typical sulfathiazole dosing regimen was several tablets within the first few hours of therapy. Twenty-nine percent of the production lot was contaminated. Food and Drug Administration (FDA) intervention was required to assist with the recovery of the tablets, although 22,000 contaminated tablets were never found.[136]

In the early 1960s, one of the worst drug-related modern-day events occurred with the release of thalidomide as an antiemetic and sedative–hypnotic.[32] Its use as a sedative–hypnotic by pregnant women caused about 5,000 babies to be born with severe congenital limb anomalies.[90] This tragedy was largely confined to Europe, Australia, and Canada, where the drug was initially marketed. The United States was spared because of the length of time required for review and the rigorous scrutiny of new drug applications by the FDA.[86]

A major therapeutic drug event that did occur in the United States involved the recommended and subsequent widespread use of diethylstilbestrol (DES) for the treatment of threatened and habitual abortions. Despite the lack of convincing efficacy data, as many as 10 million Americans received DES during pregnancy or in utero during a 30-year period, until the drug was prohibited for use during pregnancy in 1971. Adverse health effects associated with DES use include increased risk for breast cancer in "DES mothers" and increased risk of a rare form of vaginal cancer, reproductive tract anomalies, and premature births in "DES daughters."[43,48]

Thorotrast (thorium dioxide 25%) is an intravenous radiologic contrast medium that was widely used between 1928 and 1955. Its use was associated with the delayed development of hepatic angiosarcomas, as well as skeletal sarcomas, leukemia, and "thorotrastomas" (malignancies at the site of extravasated thorotrast).[134,151]

The use of thallium to treat ringworm infections in the 1920s and 1930s also led to needless morbidity and mortality.[44] Understanding that thallium caused alopecia, dermatologists and other physicians prescribed thallium acetate, both as pills and as a topical ointment (Koremlu), to remove the infected hair. A 1934 study found 692 cases of thallium toxicity after oral and topical application and 31 deaths after oral use.[97] "Medicinal" thallium was subsequently removed from the market.

The "Stalinon affair" in France in 1954 involved the unintentional contamination of a proprietary oral medication that was marketed for the treatment of staphylococcal skin infections, osteomyelitis, and anthrax. Although it was supposed to contain diethyltin diiodide and linoleic acid, triethyltin, a potent neurotoxin and the most toxic of organotin compounds, and trimethyltin were present as impurities. Of the approximately 1,000 people who received this medication, 217 patients developed symptoms, and 102 patients died.[10,17]

An unusual syndrome, featuring a constellation of abdominal symptoms (pain and diarrhea) followed by neurologic symptoms (peripheral neuropathy and visual disturbances, including blindness) was experienced by approximately 10,000 Japanese people between 1955 and 1970, resulting in several hundred deaths.[66] This presentation, subsequently labeled subacute myelooptic neuropathy (SMON), was associated with the use of the GI disinfectant clioquinol, known in the West as Entero-Vioform and most often used for the prevention of travelers' diarrhea.[100] In Japan, this drug was referred to as "sei-cho-zai" ("active in normalizing intestinal function"). It was incorporated into more than 100 nonprescription medications and was used by millions of people, often for weeks or months. The exact mechanism of toxicity has not been determined, but recent investigators theorize that clioquinol may enhance the cellular uptake of certain metals, particularly zinc, and that the clioquinol–zinc chelate may act as a mitochondrial toxin, causing this syndrome.[13] New cases declined rapidly when clioquinol was banned in Japan.

In 1981, a number of premature neonates died with a "gasping syndrome," manifested by severe metabolic acidosis, respiratory depression with gasping, and encephalopathy.[42] Before the development of these findings, the infants had all received multiple injections of heparinized bacteriostatic sodium chloride solution (to flush their indwelling catheters) and bacteriostatic water (to mix medications), both of which contained 0.9% benzyl alcohol. Accumulation of large amounts of benzyl alcohol and its metabolite benzoic acid in the blood was thought to be responsible for this syndrome.[42]

In 1989 and 1990, eosinophilia-myalgia syndrome, a debilitating syndrome somewhat similar to toxic oil syndrome, developed in more than 1,500 people who had used the dietary supplement L-tryptophan.[143] These patients presented with disabling myalgias and eosinophilia, often accompanied by extremity edema, dyspnea, and arthralgias. Skin changes, neuropathy, and weight loss sometimes developed. Intensive investigation revealed that all affected patients had ingested L-tryptophan produced by a single manufacturer that had recently introduced a new process involving genetically altered bacteria to improve L-tryptophan production. A contaminant produced by this process probably was responsible for this syndrome.[20] The banning of L-tryptophan by the FDA set in motion the passage of the Dietary Supplement Health and Education Act of 1994. This legislation, which attempted to regulate an uncontrolled industry, facilitated industry marketing of dietary supplements bypassing FDA scrutiny. In 2001, the FDA loosened the restrictions on the marketing of tryptophan, which is now sold through some compounding pharmacies.

A number of pharmaceuticals previously approved by the FDA have been withdrawn from the market because of concerns about health risks.[158] Many more drugs have been given "black box warnings" by the FDA because of their propensity to cause serious or life-threatening adverse effects.[83] Some of the withdrawn drugs were responsible for causing serious drug–drug interactions (astemizole, cisapride, mibefradil, terfenadine).[96] Other drugs were withdrawn because of a propensity to cause hepatotoxicity (troglitazone), anaphylaxis (bromfenac sodium), valvular heart disease (fenfluramine, dexfenfluramine), rhabdomyolysis (cerivastatin), hemorrhagic stroke (phenylpropanolamine), and other adverse cardiac and neurologic effects (ephedra, rofecoxib). One of the more disconcerting drug problems to arise was the development of cardiac valvulopathy and pulmonary hypertension in patients taking the weight-loss drug combination fenfluramine and phentermine (fen-phen) or dexfenfluramine.[28,129] The histopathologic features observed with this condition were similar to the valvular lesions associated with ergotamine and carcinoid syndrome. Interestingly, appetite suppressant medications, as well as ergotamine and the carcinoid syndrome, all increase available serotonin.

ALCOHOL AND ILLICIT DRUG DISASTERS

Unintended toxic disasters have also involved the use of alcohol and other drugs of abuse (Table 2–5). Arsenical neuropathy developed in an estimated 40,000 people in France in 1828, when wine and bread were unintentionally contaminated by arsenious acid.[82] The use of arsenic-contaminated sugar in the production of beer in England in 1900 resulted in at least 6,000 cases of peripheral neuropathy and 70 deaths (Staffordshire beer epidemic).[5]

TABLE 2–5	Alcohol and Illicit Drug Disasters		
Xenobiotic	**Location**	**Date**	**Significance**
Arsenious acid	France	1828	40,000 cases of polyneuropathy from contaminated wine and bread
Arsenic	Staffordshire, England	1900	Contaminated sugar used in beer production
Triorthocresyl phosphate	United States	1930–1931	Ginger Jake paralysis
Methanol	Atlanta, GA	1951	Epidemic from ingesting bootleg whiskey
Cobalt	Quebec City, Canada and others	1960s	Beer cardiomyopathy
Methanol	Jackson, MI	1979	Occurred in a prison
MPTP	San Jose, CA	1982	Illicit meperidine manufacturing resulting in drug-induced parkinsonism
Heroin heated on aluminum foil	Netherlands	1982	Spongiform leukoencephalopathy
3-Methyl fentanyl	Pittsburgh, PA	1988	"China-white" epidemic
Methanol	Baroda, India	1989	Moonshine contamination; 100 deaths
Fentanyl	New York City	1990	"Tango and Cash" epidemic
Methanol	New Delhi, India	1991	Antidiarrheal medication contaminated with methanol; >200 deaths
Methanol	Cuttack, India	1992	Methanol-tainted liquor; 162 deaths
Scopolamine	US East Coast	1995–1996	325 cases of anticholinergic poisoning in heroin users
Methanol	Cambodia	1998	>60 deaths
Opioids	United States	1999–present	Epidemic of opioid fatalities from prescription opioids and heroin with >42,420 opioid deaths in 2016
Methanol	Nicaragua	2006	800 ill, 15 blind, 45 deaths
Methanol	India	2011	>143 deaths
Methanol	Czech Republic	2012	121 ill; 41 deaths
Methanol	Libya	2013	1066 ill; 101 deaths
Methanol	Kenya	2014	Two outbreaks: 341 ill and 100 deaths; 126 ill and 26 deaths
Fentanyl and analogs	United States	2015–present	Dramatic increase in opioid deaths from fentanyl and analogs such as carfentanil

MPTP = 1-methyl-4-phenyl-1,2,3,6-tetrahydropyridine.

During the early 20th century, particularly during Prohibition, the ethanolic extract of Jamaican ginger (sold as "the Jake") was a popular ethanol substitute in the southern and Midwestern United States.[91] It was sold legally because it was considered a medical supplement to treat headaches and aid digestion and was not subject to Prohibition. For years, the Jake was sold adulterated with castor oil, but in 1930, as the price of castor oil rose, the Jake was reformulated with an alternative adulterant, triorthocresyl phosphate (TOCP). Little was previously known about the toxicity of this compound, and TOCP proved to be a potent neurotoxin. From 1930 to 1931, at least 50,000 people who drank the Jake developed TOCP poisoning, manifested by upper and lower extremity weakness ("ginger Jake paralysis") and gait impairment ("Jake walk" or "Jake leg").[91] A quarter century later, in Morocco, the dilution of cooking oil with a turbojet lubricant containing TOCP caused an additional 10,000 cases of TOCP-induced paralysis.[132]

In the 1960s, cobalt was added to several brands of beer as a foam stabilizer. Certain local breweries in Quebec City, Canada; Minneapolis, Minnesota; Omaha, Nebraska; and Louvain, Belgium, added 0.5 to 5.5 ppm of cobalt to their beer. This resulted in epidemics of fulminant heart failure among heavy beer drinkers (named cobalt-beer cardiomyopathy).[1,92]

Epidemic methanol poisoning among those seeking ethanol and other inebriants is well described. In one such incident in Atlanta, Georgia, in 1951, the ingestion of methanol-contaminated bootleg whiskey caused 323 cases of methanol poisoning, including 41 deaths.[21] In another epidemic in 1979, 46 prisoners became ill after ingesting a methanol-containing diluent used in copy machines.[137]

In recent years, major mass methanol poisonings have continued to occur in developing countries, where store-bought alcohol is often prohibitively expensive. In Baroda, India, in 1989, at least 100 people died, and another 200 became ill after drinking a homemade liquor that was contaminated with methanol.[4] In New Delhi, India, in 1991, an inexpensive antidiarrheal medicine, advertised to contain large amounts of ethanol, was instead contaminated with methanol, causing more than 200 deaths.[27] The following year, in Cuttack, India, 162 people died, and an additional 448 were hospitalized after drinking methanol-tainted liquor.[11] A major epidemic of methanol poisoning occurred in 1998 in Cambodia, when rice wine was contaminated with methanol.[3] At least 60 deaths and 400 cases of illness were attributed to the methanol. In 2011 in Sangrampur, India, more than 143 died from drinking methanol-tainted bootleg alcohol.[77] A mass methanol poisoning in the Czech Republic in 2012 in 121 people resulted in a fatality rate of 34%.[160] Most recently in 2013 in Libya, more than 1,000 people were poisoned with methanol with a fatality rate of 10%, and in 2014 in Kenya, two outbreaks of methanol poisoning occurred among 341 and 126 people with fatality rates of 29% and 21% respectively.[118]

So-called designer drugs are responsible for several toxicologic disasters. In 1982, several injection drug users living in San Jose, California, who were attempting to use a meperidine analog, MPPP (1-methyl-4-phenyl-4-propionoxy-piperidine), developed a peculiar, irreversible neurologic disease closely resembling Parkinson disease.[68] Investigation revealed that these patients had unknowingly injected trace amounts of MPTP (1-methyl-4-phenyl-1,2,3,6-tetrahydropyridine), which was present as an inadvertent product of the clandestine MPPP synthesis. The subsequent metabolism of MPTP to MPP$^+$ resulted in a toxic compound that selectively destroyed cells in the substantia nigra, depleting dopamine stores or products and causing severe and irreversible parkinsonism. The vigorous pursuit of the cause of this disaster led to a better understanding of the pathophysiology of parkinsonism.

Another example of a "designer drug" poisoning occurred in the New York City metropolitan area in 1991, when a sudden epidemic of opioid overdoses occurred among heroin users who bought envelopes labeled "Tango and Cash."[38] Expecting to receive a new brand of heroin, the drug users instead purchased the much more potent fentanyl. Increased and unpredictable toxicity resulted from the inability of the dealer to adjust ("cut") the fentanyl dose properly. Some purchasers presumably received little or no fentanyl, but others received potentially lethal doses.

A similar epidemic involving 3-methylfentanyl occurred in 1988 in Pittsburgh, Pennsylvania.[80]

At least 325 cases of anticholinergic poisoning occurred among heroin users in New York City; Newark, New Jersey; Philadelphia, Pennsylvania; and Baltimore, Maryland, from 1995 to 1996.[8] The "street drug" used in these cases was adulterated with scopolamine. Whereas naloxone treatment was associated with increased agitation and hallucinations, physostigmine administration resulted in resolution of symptoms. Why the heroin was adulterated was unknown, although the use of an opiate–scopolamine mixture was reminiscent of the morphine–scopolamine combination therapy known as "twilight sleep" that was extensively used in obstetric anesthesia during the early 20th century.[106] Another unexpected complication of heroin use was observed in the Netherlands in the 1980s, when 47 heroin users developed mutism and spastic quadriparesis that was pathologically demonstrated to be spongiform leukoencephalopathy.[157] In these and subsequent cases in Europe and the United States, the users inhaled heroin vapors after the heroin powder had been heated on aluminum foil, a drug administration technique known as "chasing the dragon."[64,157] The exact toxic mechanism has not been elucidated.

Since 1999, an epidemic of opioid deaths has occurred in the United States. Described by the Centers for Disease Control and Prevention (CDC) as the worst drug overdose epidemic in US history,[62] from 1999 to 2014, the number of drug overdose deaths nearly tripled in the United States.[119] Drug overdose deaths now surpass the number of fatalities from motor vehicle collisions and are similar in number to the annual mortality at the height of the HIV/AIDS epidemic in the US. According to the CDC, in 2016, of the 63,632 drug overdose deaths in the United States, opioids were implicated in approximately 42,420 (66.4%) deaths.[119] This opioid overdose epidemic was fueled by an exponential increase in prescription opioid consumption, including a 500% increase in oxycodone consumption. Accompanying this epidemic has been a 900% increase in individuals seeking treatment for opioid use disorders.[62] What began as an epidemic of prescription opioid overdose deaths has now been associated with an epidemic of heroin overdose deaths as prescription opioid abusers switched to easier-to-obtain heroin as their opioid of choice. In 2015 and 2016, an increase in designer opioid overdose deaths emerged, including deaths attributed to fentanyl and fentanyl analogs such as carfentanil.[121,133]

OCCUPATION-RELATED CHEMICAL DISASTERS

Unfortunately, occupation-related toxic epidemics have become increasingly common (Table 2–6). Such poisoning syndromes tend to have an insidious onset and may not be recognized clinically until years after the exposure. A specific xenobiotic may cause myriad problems, among the most worrisome being the carcinogenic and mutagenic potentials.

Although the 18th-century observations of Ramazzini and Pott introduced the concept of certain diseases as a direct result of toxic exposures in the workplace, it was not until the height of the 19th-century industrial revolution that the problems associated with the increasingly hazardous workplace became apparent.[53] During the 1860s, a peculiar disorder, attributed to the effects of inhaling mercury vapor, was described among manufacturers of felt hats in New Jersey.[152] Mercury nitrate was used as an essential part of the felting process at the time. "Hatter's shakes" refers to the tremor that developed in an estimated 10% to 60% of hatters surveyed.[152] Extreme shyness, another manifestation of mercurialism, also developed in many hatters in later studies. Five percent of hatters during this period died from renal failure.

Other notable 19th-century and early 20th-century occupational tragedies included an increased incidence of mandibular necrosis (phossy jaw) among workers in the matchmaking industry who were exposed to white phosphorus,[51] an increased incidence of bladder tumors among synthetic dye makers who used β–naphthylamine,[45] and an increased incidence of aplastic anemia among artificial leather manufacturers who used benzene.[127] The epidemic of phossy jaw among matchmakers had a latency period of 5 years and a mortality rate of 20% and has been called the "greatest tragedy

TABLE 2–6	Occupational Disasters		
Xenobiotic	*Location*	*Date*	*Significance*
Polycyclic aromatic hydrocarbons	England	1700s	Scrotal cancer among chimney sweeps; first description of hydrocarbons occupational cancer
Mercury	New Jersey	Mid to late 1800s	Outbreak of mercurialism in hatters
White phosphorus	Europe	Mid to late 1800s	Phossy jaw in matchmakers
β-Naphthylamine	Worldwide	Early 1900s	Bladder cancer in dye makers
Benzene	Newark, NJ	1916–1928	Aplastic anemia among artificial leather manufacturers
Asbestos	Worldwide	20th century	Millions at risk for asbestos-related disease
Vinyl chloride	Louisville, KY	1960s–1970s	Hepatic angiosarcoma among plastics workers
Chlordecone	James River, VA	1973–1975	Neurologic abnormalities among insecticide workers
1,2-Dibromochloropropane	California	1974	Infertility among pesticide makers
Lead	Zamfara, Nigeria	2010	400 deaths in children exposed to lead from artisanal mining operation

in the whole story of occupational disease."[25] The problem continued in the United States until Congress passed the White Phosphorus Match Act in 1912, which established a prohibitive tax on white phosphorus matches.

Since antiquity, occupational lead poisoning has been a constant threat. Workplace exposure to lead was particularly problematic during the 19th century and early 20th century because of the large number of industries that relied heavily on lead. One of the most notorious of the "lead trades" was the actual production of white lead and lead oxides. Palsies, encephalopathy, and deaths from severe poisoning were reported.[47] Other occupations that resulted in dangerous lead exposures included pottery glazing, rubber manufacturing, pigment manufacturing, painting, printing, and plumbing.[79] Given the increasing awareness of harm suffered in the workplace, the British Factory and Workshop Act of 1895 required governmental notification of occupational diseases caused by lead, mercury, and phosphorus poisoning, as well as of occupational diseases caused by anthrax.[69]

In 2010, an outbreak of fatal lead poisoning in children who were environmentally exposed to lead from an artisanal gold mining operation in Zamfara, Nigeria, was reported.[46] Approximately 400 deaths from lead poisoning occurred over a 3-month period. As a result of this mass lead poisoning outbreak, 1,156 children underwent chelation therapy. Of 3,180 treatment courses administered, 36% commenced with venous blood lead concentrations greater than 80 mcg/dL, and 6% had concentrations greater than 120 mcg/dL.[140]

Exposures to asbestos during the 20th century have resulted in continuing extremely consequential occupational and environmental disasters.[29,99] Even though the first case of asbestosis was reported in 1907, asbestos was heavily used in the shipbuilding industries in the 1940s as an insulating and fireproofing material. Since the early 1940s, 8 to 11 million individuals were occupationally exposed to asbestos,[71] including 4.5 million individuals who worked in the shipyards. Asbestos-related diseases include mesothelioma, lung cancer, and pulmonary fibrosis (asbestosis). A threefold excess of cancer deaths, primarily of excess lung cancer deaths, has been observed in asbestos-exposed insulation workers.[126]

The manufacture and use of a variety of newly synthesized chemicals has also resulted in mass occupational poisonings. In Louisville, Kentucky, in 1974, an increased incidence of angiosarcoma of the liver was first noticed among polyvinyl chloride polymerization workers who were exposed to vinyl chloride monomer.[36] In 1975, chemical factory workers exposed to the organochlorine insecticide chlordecone (Kepone) experienced a high incidence of neurologic abnormalities, including tremor and chaotic eye movements.[138] An increased incidence of infertility among male Californian pesticide workers exposed to 1,2-dibromochloropropane (DBCP) was noted in 1977.[153]

RADIATION DISASTERS

A discussion of mass poisonings is incomplete without mention of the large number of radiation disasters that have characterized the 20th century (Table 2–7). The first significant mass exposure to radiation occurred among several thousand teenage girls and young women employed in the dial-painting industry.[26] These workers painted luminous numbers on watch and instrument dials with paint that contained radium. Exposure occurred by licking the paint brushes and inhaling radium-laden dust. Studies showed an increase in bone-related cancers, as well as aplastic anemia and leukemia, in exposed workers.[81,107]

At the time of the "watch" disaster, radium was also being sold as a nostrum touted to cure all sorts of ailments, including rheumatism, syphilis, multiple sclerosis, and sexual dysfunction. Referred to as "mild radium therapy" to differentiate it from the higher dose radium that was used in the treatment of cancer at that time, such particle-emitting isotopes were hailed as powerful natural elixirs that acted as metabolic catalysts to deliver direct energy transfusions.[76]

During the 1920s, dozens of patent medications containing small doses of radium were sold as radioactive tablets, liniments, or liquids. One of the most infamous preparations was Radithor. Each half-ounce bottle contained slightly more than one curie of radium (^{228}Ra and ^{226}Ra). This radioactive

TABLE 2–7	Radiation Disasters		
Xenobiotic	*Location*	*Date*	*Significance*
Radium	Orange, NJ	1910s–1920s	Increase in bone cancer in dial-painting workers
Radium	United States	1920s	"Radithor" (radioactive water) sold as radium-containing patent medication
Radiation	Hiroshima and Nagasaki, Japan	1945	First atomic bombs dropped at the end of World War II; clinical effects still evident today
Radiation	Chernobyl, Ukraine	1986	Unintentional radioactive release; acute radiation sickness
Cesium	Goiania, Brazil	1987	Acute radiation sickness and radiation burns
Cesium, iodine	Fukushima, Japan	2011	Unintentional radioactive release after earthquake and tsunami

water was sold all over the world "as harmless in every respect" and was heavily promoted as a sexual stimulant and aphrodisiac, taking on the glamour of a recreational drug for the wealthy.[76] More than 400,000 bottles were sold. The 1932 death of Eben Byers a Radithor connoisseur, from chronic radiation poisoning drew increased public and governmental scrutiny to this unregulated radium industry and helped end the era of radioactive patent medications.[76]

Concerns about the health effects of radiation have continued to escalate since the dawn of the nuclear age in 1945. Long-term follow-up studies 50 years after the atomic bombings at Hiroshima and Nagasaki demonstrate an increased incidence of leukemia, other cancers, radiation cataracts, hyperparathyroidism, delayed growth and development, and chromosomal anomalies in exposed individuals.[61]

The unintentional nuclear disaster at Chernobyl, Ukraine, in April 1986 again forced the world to confront the medical consequences of 20th-century scientific advances that created the atomic age.[40] The release of radioactive material resulted in 31 deaths and the hospitalization of more than 200 people for acute radiation sickness. By 2003, the predominant long-term effects of the event appeared to be childhood thyroid cancer and psychological consequences.[113] In some areas of heavy contamination, the increase in childhood thyroid cancer has increased 100-fold.[120]

Another serious radiation event occurred in Goiania, Brazil, in 1987 when an abandoned radiotherapy unit was opened in a junkyard and 244 people were exposed to cesium (^{137}Cs). Of those exposed, 104 showed evidence of internal contamination, 28 had local radiation injuries, and 8 developed acute radiation syndrome. There were at least 4 deaths.[105,116]

In September 1999, a nuclear event at a uranium-processing plant in Japan set off an uncontrolled chain reaction, exposing 49 people to radiation.[65] Radiation measured outside the facility reached 4,000 times the normal ambient level. Two workers died from the effects of the radiation.

A 9.0 magnitude earthquake and tsunami in Japan in March 2011 caused equipment failure at the Fukushima Daiichi nuclear plant resulted in a release of radioactive material into the atmosphere and seawater. Nearby foodstuff and drinking water was contaminated with cesium (^{137}Cs) and iodine (^{131}I).[139] Although there were no cases of acute radiation syndrome, significant psychological and social effects resulted from this incident.[87]

MASS SUICIDE BY POISON

Mass poisonings have also manifested themselves as events of mass suicide. In 1978 in Jonestown, Guyana, 911 members of the Peoples Temple died after drinking a beverage containing cyanide.[12] In 1997, phenobarbital and ethanol (sometimes assisted by physical asphyxiation) was the suicidal method favored by 39 members of the Heavens Gate cult in Rancho Santa Fe, California, a means of suicide recommended in the book *Final Exit*.[52] Apparently, the cult members committed suicide to shed their bodies in hopes of hopping aboard an alien spaceship they believed was in the wake of the Hale-Bopp comet.[67]

SUMMARY

- There are significant lessons to be learned from mass poisonings.
- An understanding of the pathogenesis of these mass poisonings pertaining to drug, food, and occupational safety is critically important to prevent future disasters.
- Such events make us aware that many of the toxic xenobiotics involved are potential agents of opportunity for terrorists and nonterrorists who seek to harm others.
- Given the practical and ethical limitations in studying the effects of many specific xenobiotics in humans, lessons from these unfortunate tragedies must be fully mastered and retained for future generations.

REFERENCES

1. Alexander CS. Cobalt-beer cardiomyopathy. A clinical and pathologic study of twenty-eight cases. *Am J Med.* 1972;53:395-417.
2. Anonymous. Cadmium pollution and Itai-itai disease. *Lancet.* 1971;1:382-383.
3. Anonymous. Cambodian mob kills two Vietnamese in poisoning hysteria. *Deutsche Presse-Agentur.* September 4, 1998.
4. Anonymous. Fatal moonshine in India. *Newsday.* March 6, 1989.
5. Anonymous. Final report of the Royal Commission on Arsenical Poisoning. *Lancet.* 1903;2:1674-1676.
6. Anonymous. Nicotine poisoning after ingestion of contaminated ground beef—Michigan, 2003. *MMWR Morb Mortal Wkly Rep.* 2003;52:413-416.
7. Anonymous. Nigeria: 12 held over tainted syrup. *The New York Times.* February 12, 2009.
8. Anonymous. Scopolamine poisoning among heroin users—New York City, Newark, Philadelphia, and Baltimore, 1995 and 1996. *MMWR Morb Mortal Wkly Rep.* 1996;45:457-460.
9. Anonymous. Seveso after five years. *Lancet.* 1981;2:731-732.
10. Anonymous. Stalinon: a therapeutic disaster. *Br Med J.* 1958;1:515.
11. Anonymous. Tainted liquor kills 162, sickens 228. *Los Angeles Times.* May 10, 1992.
12. Anonymous. The Guyana tragedy—an international forensic problem. *Forensic Sci Int.* 1979;13:167-172.
13. Arbiser JL, et al. Clioquinol-zinc chelate: a candidate causative agent of subacute myelo-optic neuropathy. *Mol Med.* 1998;4:665-670.
14. Audi J, et al. Ricin poisoning: a comprehensive review. *JAMA.* 2005;294:2342-2351.
15. Bakir F, et al. Methylmercury poisoning in Iraq. *Science.* 1973;181:230-241.
16. Banauch GI, et al. Persistent hyperreactivity and reactive airway dysfunction in firefighters at the World Trade Center. *Am J Respir Crit Care Med.* 2003;168:54-62.
17. Barnes JM, Stoner HB. The toxicology of tin compounds. *Pharmacol Rev.* 1959;11:211-232.
18. Barr DBD, et al. Identification and quantification of diethylene glycol in pharmaceuticals implicated in poisoning epidemics: an historical laboratory perspective. *J Anal Toxicol.* 2007;31:295-303.
19. Baxter PJ, et al. Lake Nyos disaster, Cameroon, 1986: the medical effects of large scale emission of carbon dioxide? *BMJ.* 1989;298:1437-1441.
20. Belongia EA, et al. An investigation of the cause of the eosinophilia-myalgia syndrome associated with tryptophan use. *N Engl J Med.* 1990;323:357-365.
21. Bennett IL, et al. Acute methyl alcohol poisoning: a review based on experiences in an outbreak of 323 cases. *Medicine.* 1953;32:431-463.
22. Brown CA, et al. Outbreaks of renal failure associated with melamine and cyanuric acid in dogs and cats in 2004 and 2007. *J Vet Diagn Invest.* 2007;19:525-531.
23. Caporael LR. Ergotism: the Satan loosed in Salem? *Science.* 1976;192:21-26.
24. Carter LJ. Michigan PBB incident: chemical mix-up leads to disaster. *Science.* 1976;192:240-243.
25. Cherniack MG. Diseases of unusual occupations: an historical perspective. *Occup Med.* 1992;7:369-384.
26. Clark C. *Radium Girls: Women and Industrial Health Reform, 1910-1935.* Chapel Hill: University of North Carolina Press; 1997.
27. Coll S. Tainted foods, medicine make mass poisoning rife in India: critics press for tougher inspections, more accurate labels. *Washington Post.* December 8, 1991:A36.
28. Connolly HM, et al. Valvular heart disease associated with fenfluramine-phentermine. *N Engl J Med.* 1997;337:581-588.
29. Corn JK, Starr J. Historical perspective on asbestos: policies and protective measures in World War II shipbuilding. *Am J Indust Med.* 1987;11:359-373.
30. Croddy E, Croddy E. Rat poison and food security in the People's Republic of China: focus on tetramethylene disulfotetramine (tetramine). *Arch Toxicol.* 2004;78:1-6.
31. Cullinan P, et al. Respiratory morbidity 10 years after the Union Carbide gas leak at Bhopal: a cross sectional survey. The International Medical Commission on Bhopal. *BMJ.* 1997;314:338-342.
32. Dally A. Thalidomide: was the tragedy preventable? *Lancet.* 1998;351:1197-1199.
33. Das D, et al. Arsenic in ground water in six districts of West Bengal, India: the biggest arsenic calamity in the world. Part 2. Arsenic concentration in drinking water, hair, nails, urine, skin-scale and liver tissue (biopsy) of the affected people. *Analyst.* 1995;120:917-924.
34. Easton WH. Smoke and fire gases. *Indust Med.* 1942;11:466-468.
35. Eckert WG. Mass deaths by gas or chemical poisoning. A historical perspective. *Am J Forens Med Path.* 1991;12:119-125.
36. Falk H, et al. Hepatic disease among workers at a vinyl chloride polymerization plant. *JAMA.* 1974;230:59-63.
37. Faxon NW, Churchill ED. The Cocoanut Grove disaster in Boston: a preliminary account. *JAMA.* 1942;120:1385-1388.
38. Fernando D. Fentanyl-laced heroin. *JAMA.* 1991;265:2962.
39. Gallay AA, et al. Belgian Coca-Cola-related outbreak: intoxication, mass sociogenic illness, or both? *Am J Epidemiol.* 2002;155:140-147.
40. Geiger HJ. The accident at Chernobyl and the medical response. *JAMA.* 1986;256:609-612.
41. Geiling E, Cannon PR. Pathologic effects of elixir of sulfanilamide (diethylene glycol) poisoning. *JAMA.* 1938;111:919-926.
42. Gershanik J, et al. The gasping syndrome and benzyl alcohol poisoning. *N Engl J Med.* 1982;307:1384-1388.
43. Giusti RM, et al. Diethylstilbestrol revisited: a review of the long-term health effects. *Ann Intern Med.* 1995;122:778-788.
44. Gleich M. Thallium acetate poisoning in the treatment of ringworm of the scalp: report of two cases. *JAMA.* 1931;97:851-851.
45. Goldblatt MW. Vesical tumours induced by chemical compounds. *Br J Indust Med.* 1949;6:65-81.

46. Greig J, et al. Association of blood lead level with neurological features in 972 children affected by an acute severe lead poisoning outbreak in Zamfara State, northern Nigeria. Chen A, ed. *PLoS ONE.* 2014;9:e93716-e93719.

47. Hamilton A. Landmark article in occupational medicine. "Forty years in the poisonous trades." *Am J Indust Med.* 1985;7:3-18.

48. Herbst AL, et al. Adenocarcinoma of the vagina. Association of maternal stilbestrol therapy with tumor appearance in young women. *N Engl J Med.* 1971;284:878-881.

49. Holmstedt B. Prolegomena to Seveso. Ecclesiastes I 18. *Arch Toxicol.* 1980;44:211-230.

50. Hood E. Lessons learned? Chemical plant safety since Bhopal. *Environ Health Perspect.* 2004;112:A352-A359.

51. Hughes JP, et al. Phosphorus necrosis of the jaw: a present day study. *Br J Indust Med.* 1962;19:83-99.

52. Humphry D. *Final Exit.* New York, NY: Dell; 1991.

53. Hunter D. *The Diseases of Occupations.* 6th ed. London: Hodder & Stoughton; 1978.

54. Ingelfinger JR. Melamine and the global implications of food contamination. *N Engl J Med.* 2008;359:2745-2748.

55. Institute of Medicine. *Veterans and Agent Orange: Update 2002.* Washington, DC: National Academies Press; 2002.

56. Jones GR. Polychlorinated biphenyls: where do we stand now? *Lancet.* 1989;2:791-794.

57. Jordan HT, et al. Risk factors for persistence of lower respiratory symptoms among community members exposed to the 2001 World Trade Center terrorist attacks. *Occup Environ Med.* 2017;74:449-455.

58. Jordan HT, et al. Sarcoidosis diagnosed after September 11, 2001, among adults exposed to the World Trade Center disaster. *J Occup Environ Med.* 2011;53:966-974.

59. Kilbourne EM, et al. Toxic oil syndrome: a current clinical and epidemiologic summary, including comparisons with the eosinophilia-myalgia syndrome. *J Am Coll Cardiol.* 1991;18:711-717.

60. Kilbourne EM, et al. Clinical epidemiology of toxic-oil syndrome. Manifestations of a new illness. *N Engl J Med.* 1983;309:1408-1414.

61. Kodama K, et al. A long-term cohort study of the atomic-bomb survivors. *J Epidemiol.* 1996;6(3 suppl):S95-S105.

62. Kolodny A, et al. The prescription opioid and heroin crisis: a public health approach to an epidemic of addiction. *Annu Rev Public Health.* 2015;36:559-574.

63. Kopelman H, et al. The Epping jaundice. *Br Med J.* 1966;5486:514-516.

64. Kriegstein AR, et al. Leukoencephalopathy and raised brain lactate from heroin vapor inhalation ("chasing the dragon"). *Neurology.* 1999;53:1765-1773.

65. Lamar J. Japan's worst nuclear accident leaves two fighting for life. *BMJ.* 1999;319:937.

66. Lambert ED. *Modern Medical Mistakes.* Bloomington, IN: Indiana University Press; 1978.

67. Lang J. Heavens's gate suicide still a mystery 1 year later. *Arizona Republic.* March 26, 1998:A11.

68. Langston JW, et al. Chronic Parkinsonism in humans due to a product of meperidine-analog synthesis. *Science.* 1983;219:979-980.

69. Lee WR. The history of the statutory control of mercury poisoning in Great Britain. *Br J Ind Med.* 1968;25:52-62.

70. Leschke E. *Clinical Toxicology: Modern Methods in the Diagnosis and Treatment of Poisoning.* Baltimore, MD: William Wood; 1934.

71. Levin SM, et al. Medical examination for asbestos-related disease. *Am J Indust Med.* 2000;37:6-22.

72. Li J, et al. Association between World Trade Center exposure and excess cancer risk. *JAMA.* 2012;308:2479-2488.

73. Loewenberg S. World Report in Bangladesh, arsenic poisoning is a neglected issue. *Lancet.* 2016;388:2336-2337.

74. Logan WPD. Mortality in the London fog incident, 1952. *Lancet.* 1953;1:336-338.

75. Loveluck L. Sarin was used in deadly Syria attack, chemical weapons watchdog confirms. *Washington Post.* April 19, 2017.

76. Macklis RM. Radithor and the era of mild radium therapy. *JAMA.* 1990;264:614-618.

77. Magnier M. Bootleg liquor laced with methanol kills 143people in India. *LA Times.* http://www.thestar.com/news/world/2011/12/15/bootleg_liquor_laced_with_methanol_kills_143_people_in_india.html. December 15, 2011.

78. Magnuson E. The devil made him do it. *Time.* April 1990:38.

79. Markowitz GG, Rosner DD. "Cater to the children": the role of the lead industry in a public health tragedy, 1900-1955. *Am J Public Health (N Y).* 2000;90:36-46.

80. Martin M, et al. China White epidemic: an eastern United States emergency department experience. *Ann Emerg Med.* 1991;20:158-164.

81. Martland HS. Occupational poisoning in manufacture of luminous watch dials. *JAMA.* 1929;92:466-473.

82. Massey EW, et al. Arsenic: homicidal intoxication. *South Med J.* 1984;77:848-851.

83. Matlock A, et al. A continuing black hole? The FDA boxed warning: an appeal to improve its clinical utility. *Clin Toxicol.* 2011;49:443-447.

84. Matossian MK. Ergot and the Salem witchcraft affair. *Am Sci.* 1982;70:355-357.

85. Matsumoto S. Unexpectedly long half-lives of blood 2,3,4,7,8-pentachlorodibenzofuran (PeCDF) levels in Yusho patients. *Environ Health.* 2015;14:1-6.

86. McFadyen RE. Thalidomide in America: a brush with tragedy. *Clio Med.* 1976;11:79-93.

87. Hasegawa A, et al. Health effects of radiation and other health problems in the aftermath of nuclear accidents, with an emphasis on Fukushima. *Lancet.* 2015;386:479-488.

88. Mehta PS, et al. Bhopal tragedy's health effects. A review of methyl isocyanate toxicity. *JAMA.* 1990;264:2781-2787.

89. Merhoff GC, Porter JM. Ergot intoxication: historical review and description of unusual clinical manifestations. *Ann Surg.* 1974;180:773-779.

90. Modell W. Mass drug catastrophes and the roles of science and technology. *Science.* 1967;156:346-351.

91. Morgan JP. The Jamaica ginger paralysis. *JAMA.* 1982;248:1864-1867.

92. Morin YL, et al. Quebec beer-drinkers' cardiomyopathy: forty-eight cases. *Can Med Assoc J.* 1967;97:881-883.

93. Morita H, et al. Sarin poisoning in Matsumoto, Japan. *Lancet.* 1995;346:290-293.

94. Mudur G. Arsenic poisons 220,000 in India. *BMJ.* 1996;313:9.

95. Mudur G. Half of Bangladesh population at risk of arsenic poisoning. *BMJ.* 2000;320:822.

96. Mullins ME, et al. Life-threatening interaction of mibefradil and beta-blockers with dihydropyridine calcium channel blockers. *JAMA.* 1998;280:157-158.

97. Munch JC. Human thallotoxicosis. *JAMA.* 1934;102:1929-1934.

98. Murphy J, et al. Measuring and maximizing coverage in the World Trade Center Health Registry. *Stat Med.* 2007;26:1688-1701.

99. Murray R. Asbestos: a chronology of its origins and health effects. *Br J Ind Med.* 1990;47:361-365.

100. Nakae K, et al. Relation between subacute myelo-optic neuropathy (S.M.O.N.) and clioquinol: nationwide survey. *Lancet.* 1973;1:171-173.

101. Nakajima T, et al. Epidemiological study of sarin poisoning in Matsumoto City, Japan. *J Epidemiol.* 1998;8:33-41.

102. Nemery B, et al. The Coca-Cola incident in Belgium, June 1999. *Food Chem Toxicol.* 2002;40:1657-1667.

103. O'Brien KLK, et al. Epidemic of pediatric deaths from acute renal failure caused by diethylene glycol poisoning. Acute Renal Failure Investigation Team. *JAMA.* 1998;279:1175-1180.

104. Okumura T, et al. Report on 640 victims of the Tokyo subway sarin attack. *Ann Emerg Med.* 1996;28:129-135.

105. Oliveira AR, et al. Medical and related aspects of the Goiania accident: an overview. *Health Phys.* 1991;60:17-24.

106. Pitcock CDC, Clark RBR. From Fanny to Fernand: the development of consumerism in pain control during the birth process. *Am J Obstet Gynecol.* 1992;167:581-587.

107. Polednak AP, Stehney AF. Mortality among women first employed before 1930 in the US radium dial-painting industry a group ascertained from employment lists. *Am J Epidemiol.* 1978;107:179-195.

108. Posada de la Paz M, et al. Toxic oil syndrome: the perspective after 20 years. *Epidemiol Rev.* 2001;23:231-247.

109. Powell PP. Minamata disease: a story of mercury's malevolence. *South Med J.* 1991;84:1352-1358.

110. Prezant DJ, et al. Cough and bronchial responsiveness in firefighters at the World Trade Center site. *N Engl J Med.* 2002;347:806-815.

111. Prezant DJ. World Trade Center cough syndrome and its treatment. *Lung.* 2008;186:94-102.

112. Rahman MM, et al. Chronic arsenic toxicity in Bangladesh and West Bengal, India—a review and commentary. *J Toxicol Clin Toxicol.* 2001;39:683-700.

113. Rahu M. Health effects of the Chernobyl accident: fears, rumours and the truth. *Eur J Cancer.* 2003;39:295-299.

114. Rentz ED, et al. Outbreak of acute renal failure in Panama in 2006: a case-control study. *Bull World Health Organ.* 2008;86:749-756.

115. Riches JR, et al. Analysis of clothing and urine from Moscow Theatre siege casualties reveals carfentanil and remifentanil use. *J Anal Toxicol.* 2012;36:647-656.

116. Roberts L. Radiation accident grips Goiania. *Science.* 1987;238:1028-1031.

117. Roses OE, et al. Mass poisoning by sodium arsenite. *J Toxicol Clin Toxicol.* 1991;29:209-213.

118. Rostrup M, et al. The methanol poisoning outbreaks in Libya 2013 and Kenya 2014. *PLoS ONE.* 2016;11:e0152676.

119. CDC. Wide-ranging online data for epidemiologic research (WONDER). Atlanta, GA: US Department of Health and Human Services, CDC, National Center for Health Statistics; 2016. https://wonder.cdc.gov.

120. Rytomaa T. Ten years after Chernobyl. *Ann Med.* 1996;28:83-87.

121. Sanburn J. Heroin is being laced with a terrifying new substance: what to know about carfentanil. *Time.* December 2016. http://time.com/4485792/heroin-carfentanil- drugs-ohio/.

122. Scalzo AJ. Diethylene glycol toxicity revisited: the 1996 Haitian epidemic. *J Toxicol Clin Toxicol.* 1996;34:513-516.

123. Madeen EP, et al. A critical review of the epidemiology of Agent Orange or 2,3,7,8-tetrachlorodibenzo-p-dioxin and lymphoid malignancies. *Ann Epidemiol.* 2015;25:275-292.e30.

124. Schier JG, et al. Public health investigation after the discovery of ricin in a South Carolina postal facility. *Am J Public Health (N Y).* 2007;97(suppl 1):S152-S157.

125. Schmid R. Cutaneous porphyria in Turkey. *N Engl J Med.* 1960;263:397-398.

126. Selikoff IJ, et al. Mortality experience of insulation workers in the United States and Canada, 1943-1976. *Ann N Y Acad Sci.* 1979;330:91-116.

127. Sharpe WD. Benzene, artificial leather and aplastic anemia: Newark, 1916-1928. *Bull N Y Acad Med.* 1993;69:47-60.

128. Sheridan RLR, et al. Case records of the Massachusetts General Hospital. Weekly clinicopathological exercises. Case 6-2004. A 35-year-old woman with extensive, deep burns from a nightclub fire. *N Engl J Med.* 2004;350:810-821.

129. Shively BK, et al. Prevalence and determinants of valvulopathy in patients treated with dexfenfluramine. *Circulation*. 1999;100:2161-2167.

130. Sidell FR, et al., eds. *Medical Aspects of Chemical and Biological Warfare*. Washington, DC: Office of the Surgeon General; 1997.

131. Sidell FR. Chemical agent terrorism. *Ann Emerg Med*. 1996;28:223-224.

132. Smith HV, Spalding J. Outbreak of paralysis in Morocco due to ortho-cresyl phosphate poisoning. *Lancet*. 1959;2:1019-1021.

133. Somerville NJ, et al. Characteristics of fentanyl overdose—Massachusetts, 2014-2016. *MMWR Morb Mortal Wkly Rep*. 2017;66:382-386.

134. Stover BJ. Effects of Thorotrast in humans. *Health Phys*. 1983;44(suppl 1):253-257.

135. Subramanian KS, Kosnett MJ. Human exposures to arsenic from consumption of well water in West Bengal, India. *Int J Occup Environ Health*. 1998;4:217-230.

136. Swann JP. The 1941 sulfathiazole disaster and the birth of good manufacturing practices. *PDA J Pharm Sci Technol*. 1999;53:148-153.

137. Swartz RD, et al. Epidemic methanol poisoning: clinical and biochemical analysis of a recent episode. *Medicine*. 1981;60:373-382.

138. Taylor JR, et al. Chlordecone intoxication in man. I. Clinical observations. *Neurology*. 1978;28:626-630.

139. Thielen H. The Fukushima Daiichi nuclear accident—an overview. *Health Phys*. 2012;103:169-174.

140. Thurtle N, et al. Description of 3,180 courses of chelation with dimercaptosuccinic acid in children ≤5 y with severe lead poisoning in Zamfara, Northern Nigeria: a retrospective analysis of programme data. Lanphear BP, ed. *PLoS Med*. 2014;11:e1001739-18.

141. Tsuchiya K. The discovery of the causal agent of Minamata disease. *Am J Indust Med*. 1992;21:275-280.

142. Urbinato D. London's historic pea-soupers. *EPA Journal*. 1994;20:1-3.

143. Varga J, et al. The cause and pathogenesis of the eosinophilia-myalgia syndrome. *Ann Intern Med*. 1992;116:140-147.

144. Varma DR, Guest I. The Bhopal accident and methyl isocyanate toxicity. *J Toxicol Environ Health*. 1993;40:513-529.

145. Waldron HA. The Devonshire colic. *J Hist Med Allied Sci*. 1970;25:383-413.

146. Wang P-X, et al. The clinical profile and prognosis of Chinese children with melamine-induced kidney disease: a systematic review and meta-analysis. *Biomed Res Int*. 2013; 2013:1-7.

147. Warner MM, et al. Dioxin exposure and cancer risk in the Seveso Women's Health Study. *Environ Health Perspect*. 2011;119:1700-1705.

148. Wax PM, et al. Unexpected "gas" casualties in Moscow: a medical toxicology perspective. *Ann Emerg Med*. 2003;41:700-705.

149. Wax PM. Elixirs, diluents, and the passage of the 1938 Federal Food, Drug and Cosmetic Act. *Ann Intern Med*. 1995;122:456-461.

150. Wax PM. It's happening again—another diethylene glycol mass poisoning. *J Toxicol Clin Toxicol*. 1996;34:517-520.

151. Weber E, et al. Abdominal pain: do not forget Thorotrast! *Postgrad Med J*. 1995;71: 367-368.

152. Wedeen RP. Were the hatters of New Jersey "mad"? *Am J Indust Med*. 1989;16:225-233.

153. Whorton D, et al. Infertility in male pesticide workers. *Lancet*. 1977;2:1259-1261.

154. Wing JS, et al. Acute health effects in a community after a release of hydrofluoric acid. *Arch Environ Health*. 1991;46:155-160.

155. Wolff MS, et al. Human tissue burdens of halogenated aromatic chemicals in Michigan. *JAMA*. 1982;247:2112-2116.

156. Wolkin AF, et al. Early detection of illness associated with poisonings of public health significance. *Ann Emerg Med*. 2006;47:170-176.

157. Wolters EC, et al. Leucoencephalopathy after inhaling "heroin" pyrolysate. *Lancet*. 1982;2:1233-1237.

158. Wysowski DK, Swartz L. Adverse drug event surveillance and drug withdrawals in the United States, 1969-2002: the importance of reporting suspected reactions. *Arch Intern Med*. 2005;165:1363-1369.

159. Yardley J. 40,000 Chinese evacuated from explosion "death zone." *New York Times*. December 27, 2003:A3.

160. Zakharov S, et al. Czech mass methanol outbreak 2012: epidemiology, challenges and clinical features. *Clin Toxicol*. 2014;52:1013-1024.

CASE STUDY 1

History Police were called to a public area where a young man was shirtless and acting bizarrely. It was a hot summer day with a temperature of 92°F (33°C) and a dew point of 75°F (24°C). The man, who appeared confused, was pacing and gesturing as if he was hallucinating. When the police approached him, he began to run away, but after a struggle, he was subdued. The paramedics were called because of his behavior. When they arrived, they found an agitated and confused man whose arms and legs were restrained and in a full-body bag. He was diaphoretic with 6 to 7 mm pupils, and he was breathing rapidly and had a pulse of 180 beats/min. Because of the restraints, no other vital signs were obtained, and the patient was transported to the emergency department (ED).

Physical Examination On arrival to the ED, a team of physicians, nurses, and hospital security personnel removed the patient from the body bag, restrained him, and transfered him to a hospital stretcher. An arm was held in place, and an intravenous (IV) line was administered. Blood was obtained for analysis, and midazolam (10 mg IV) was given. Within a few moments, the patient became calmer, and the following vital signs were obtained: blood pressure, 198/122 mm Hg; pulse, 188 beats/min; respiratory rate, 38 breaths/min; tympanic temperature, 104.6°F (40.3°C); oxygen saturation, 98% on room air; and glucose, 187 mg/dL. Physical examination revealed a diaphoretic young man who was mumbling incoherently and was hot to the touch. There were no signs of trauma, and his pupils were 7 mm and reactive to light. His chest was clear, and his heart rate was regular and tachycardic without extra sounds. His abdomen was soft and nontender with normal bowel sounds. A complete neurologic assessment could not be performed, as he was disoriented, distracted, and unable to follow commands. His pupils were reactive, and oculocephalic reflexes were present. Muscle tone was increased symmetrically, and reflexes were brisk, with three to four beats of clonus noted at both ankles. His toes were downgoing.

What Is the Toxicologic Differential Diagnosis? This patient presents with agitation, tachycardia, hypertension, hyperthermia, diaphoresis, mydriasis, and disorientation. Although this presentation is fairly characteristic of a sympathomimetic toxic syndrome (Chaps. 3, 73, and 75) additional considerations must include alcohol and sedative–hypnotic withdrawal (Chaps. 14 and 77), hallucinogens (Chap. 79), and phencyclidine (Chap. 83). These and other etiologies for the hyperthermia are listed in Table CS1–1.

Initial Management A rectal probe was inserted, and the patient's core temperature was noted to be 109.2°F (42.9°C). This single vital sign abnormality takes precedence over the others and requires emergent intervention, regardless of the etiology. An additional 5 mg of IV midazolam was administered (Antidotes in Depth: A26) to further control the agitation, and the patient was placed in an ice-water bath (Chap. 29). While in the bath, another 5 mg of midazolam was needed to control his behavior. One liter of 0.9 sodium chloride was infused through the peripheral IV line, and a Foley catheter was inserted, which drained a scant amount of dark yellow urine.

Within 15 minutes, the patient's core temperature fell to 101.4°F (38.6°C); he was removed from the ice bath, dried, and placed on a clean, dry stretcher. At that time, the following vital signs were obtained: blood pressure, 148/94 mm Hg; pulse, 120 beats/min; respiratory rate, 24 breaths/min; core temperature, 99.2°F (37.3°C); oxygen saturation, 96% on room air; and end-tidal carbon dioxide, 46 mm Hg.

What Clinical and Laboratory Analyses Can Help Exclude Life-Threatening Consequences of This Patient's Presentation? The consequences of hyperthermia include injury to many organ systems as outlined in Table CS1–2. An electrocardiogram (ECG) should be obtained because it can rapidly detect critical myocardial injury and life-threatening electrolyte abnormalities. A rapid assessment of electrolytes, kidney and liver function, coagulation status, acid–base balance, creatine kinase, troponin, and a urinalysis are all indicated. Severe abnormalities should be addressed as detected. In this case, although the urine dipstick showed the large presence of blood, no red blood cells were seen or microscopic analysis leading to a clinical suspicion of rhabdomyolysis. The patient was started on fluids at twice his maintenance requirement as well as a bicarbonate infusion (Antidotes in Depth: A5).

Further Diagnosis and Treatment The patient remained calm and began to answer questions a few hours later. The ECG showed sinus tachycardia with normal intervals and no pattern of injury. However, the laboratory results were remarkable for a creatinine of 3.4 mg/dL, a bicarbonate of 12 mEq/L, an anion gap of 30 mEq/L, and a creatine kinase of greater than 100,000 IU/L, compatible with an acute kidney injury to rhabdomyolysis. Although repeat electrolytes showed a rapid correction of the bicarbonate and anion gap, the creatinine continued to rise, and the creatine kinase remained greater than 100,000 IU/L. A nephrology consult was obtained because of the potential need for hemodialysis, but the patient continued to have an adequate urine output, and urine electrolytes demonstrated a retained ability to concentrate the urine.

The patient regained a normal mental status and related that the last thing he remembered was smoking crack cocaine. Over the course of one week, the creatine kinase fell, and the serum creatinine stabilized at 1.7 mg/dL. Referrals were made to an outpatient detoxification center and a primary physician, and the patient was discharged.

TABLE CS1–1	Xenobiotics, Potentiators and Interactions Associated with Life-Threatening Hyperthermia
• Alcohol withdrawal	• Oxidative phosphorylation uncouplers (dinitrophenol, salicylates)
• Anticholinergics (atropine, antihistamines)	
• Malignant hyperthermia	• Phencyclidine
• Monoamine oxidase inhibitor overdose	• Sedative–hypnotic withdrawal
• Neuroleptic malignant syndrome	• Serotonin toxicity
	• Sympathomimetics (cocaine, amphetamines)
	• Thyrotoxicosis factitia

TABLE CS1–2	Major Organ System Complications of Hyperthermia
Organ System	**Complication**
Brain	Cerebral edema
Lungs	Acute respiratory distress syndrome
Heart	Myocardial stunning, myocardial infarction, dysrhythmias
Gastrointestinal	Hepatic injury
Kidneys	Acute kidney injury
Hematological	Coagulopathy
Muscle	Rhabdomyolysis

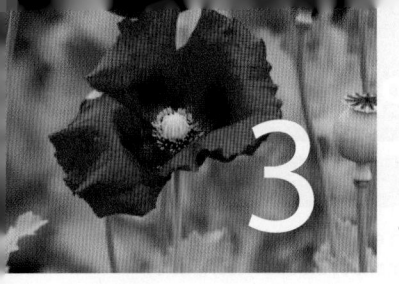

3 INITIAL EVALUATION OF THE PATIENT: VITAL SIGNS AND TOXIC SYNDROMES

Lewis S. Nelson, Mary Ann Howland, Neal A. Lewin, Silas W. Smith, Lewis R. Goldfrank, and Robert S. Hoffman

For more than 200 years, American health care providers have attempted to standardize their approach to the assessment of patients. At the New York Hospital in 1865, pulse rate, respiratory rate, and temperature were incorporated into the bedside chart and called "vital signs."[9] It was not until the early part of the 20th century, however, that blood pressure determination also became routine. Additional components of the present standard emergency assessment, such as oxygen saturation by pulse oximetry, capillary blood glucose, and pain severity, are sometimes considered vital signs. Although they are essential components of the clinical evaluation and are important considerations throughout this text, they are not discussed in this chapter. Similarly, invasive and noninvasive modalities for the bedside assessment of organ function, such as capnometry, focused ultrasonography, arterial Doppler analysis, arterial catheterization, and tissue oxygen saturation, are not discussed here but appear in relevant sections of this textbook.[1]

In the practice of medical toxicology, vital signs play an important role beyond assessing and monitoring the overall status of a patient, because they frequently provide valuable physiologic clues to the toxicologic etiology and severity of an illness. The vital signs also are a valuable parameter used to assess and monitor a patient's response to treatment and antidotal therapy.

Table 3–1 presents the normal vital signs for various age groups. However, this broad range of values considered normal should serve merely as a guide. Only a complete assessment of a patient can determine whether or not a particular vital sign is truly clinically normal in the particular clinical setting. This table of normal vital signs is useful in assessing children because normal values for children vary considerably with age, and knowing the range of normal variation is essential. Normal rectal temperature in adults is defined as 96.8° to 100.4°F (35°–38°C), and, although less reliable, a normal oral temperature is considered 95.0° to 99.6°F (36.4°–37.5°C).

The difficulty in defining what constitutes "normal" vital signs in an emergency setting is inadequately addressed and may prove to be an impossible undertaking. Published normal values likely have little relevance for an acutely ill or anxious patient in the emergency setting, yet that is precisely the environment in which abnormal vital signs must be identified and addressed. Even in nonemergent situations, "normalcy" of vital signs depends on the clinical condition of the patient. A sleeping or comatose patient may have physiologic bradycardia, although a slow heart rate is often appropriate for this low energy requiring state. For these reasons, descriptions of vital signs as "normal" or "stable" are too nonspecific to be meaningful and therefore should never be accepted as defining normalcy in an individual patient. Conversely, no patient should be considered too agitated, too young, or too gravely ill for the practitioner to obtain a complete set of vital signs; indeed, these patients urgently need a thorough evaluation that includes all of the vital signs. Also, the vital signs must be recorded as accurately as possible, first in the prehospital setting, again, with precision and accuracy, as soon as a patient arrives in the emergency department (ED), and continuously thereafter as clinically indicated to identify trends.

Many xenobiotics affect the autonomic nervous system, which in turn affects the vital signs via the sympathetic pathway, the parasympathetic pathway, or both. Meticulous attention to both the initial and repeated determinations of vital signs is of extreme importance in identifying a pattern of changes suggesting a particular xenobiotic or group of xenobiotics. The value of serial monitoring of the vital signs is demonstrated by the patient who presents with anticholinergic toxicity and receives the antidote, physostigmine. In this situation, it is important to recognize when tachycardia becomes bradycardia (eg, anticholinergic syndrome followed by physostigmine excess). Meticulous attention to these changes ensures that the therapeutic interventions should be modified or adjusted accordingly.

Similarly, a patient who has opioid-induced bradypnea (a decreased rate of breathing) will either normalize or develop tachypnea (an increased rate of breathing) after the administration of the opioid antagonist naloxone. The analysis becomes exceedingly complicated when that patient is potentially exposed to two or more xenobiotics, such as an opioid combined with cocaine. In this situation, the effects of cocaine become "unmasked" by the naloxone used to counteract the opioid, and the clinician must then differentiate naloxone-induced opioid withdrawal from cocaine toxicity. The assessment starts by analyzing diverse information, including vital signs, history, and physical examination.

Table 3–2 describes the most typical toxic syndromes. This table includes only vital signs that are thought to be characteristically abnormal or pathognomonic and directly related to the toxicologic effect of the xenobiotic. The primary purpose of the table, however, is to include many findings, in addition to the vital signs, that together constitute a toxic syndrome. Mofenson and Greensher[8] coined the term *toxidromes* from the words *toxic syndromes* to describe the groups of signs and symptoms that consistently result from particular toxins. These syndromes are usually best described by a combination of the vital signs and clinically apparent end-organ manifestations. The signs that prove most clinically useful are those involving the central nervous system (CNS; mental status), ophthalmic system (pupil size), gastrointestinal system (peristalsis), dermatologic system (skin dryness versus diaphoresis), mucous membranes (moistness versus dryness), and genitourinary system (urinary retention versus incontinence).

Table 3–2 includes some of the most important signs and symptoms and the xenobiotics most commonly responsible for these manifestations.

	Systolic BP (mm Hg)	Diastolic BP (mm Hg)	Pulse (beats/min)	Respirations (breaths/min)[b]
TABLE 3–1	**Normal Vital Signs by Age[a]**			
Age				
Adult	120	80	50–90	16–24
16 years	≤120	<80	80	16–30
12 years	119	76	85	16–30
10 years	115	74	90	16–30
6 years	107	69	100	20–30
4 years	104	65	110	20–30
4 months	90	50	145	30–35
2 months	85	50	145	30–35
Newborn	65	50	145	35–40

[a]The normal rectal temperature is defined as 96.8°F to 100.4°F (35°–38°C) for all ages. For children 1 year of age or younger, these values are the mean values for the 50th percentile. For older children, these values represent the 90th percentile at a specific age for the 50th percentile of weight in that age group.

These respiration values were determined in the emergency department and may be environment and situation dependent.

BP = blood pressure.

TABLE 3–2	Toxic Syndromes								
	Vital Signs								
Group	BP	P	R	T	Mental Status	Pupil Size	Peristalsis	Diaphoresis	Other
Anticholinergics	–/↑	↑	±	↑	Delirium	↑	↓	↓	Dry mucous membranes, flush, urinary retention
Cholinergics	±	±	±	–	Normal to depressed	±	↑	↑	Salivation, lacrimation, urination, diarrhea, bronchorrhea, fasciculations, paralysis
Ethanol or sedative–hypnotics	↓	↓	↓	–/↓	Depressed, agitated	±	↓	–	Hyporeflexia, ataxia
Opioids	↓	↓	↓	↓	Depressed	↓	↓	–	Hyporeflexia
Serotonin toxicity	↑	↑	–/↑	–/↑	Normal to agitated delirium	–/↑	↑	↑	Clonus, tremor, seizures
Sympathomimetics	↑	↑	↑	↑	Agitated	↑	–/↑	↑	Tremor, seizures diaphoresis
Withdrawal from ethanol or sedative–hypnotics	↑	↑	↑	↑	Agitated, disoriented hallucinations	↑	↑	↑	Tremor, seizures diaphoresis
Withdrawal from opioids	↑	↑	–	–	Normal, anxious	↑	↑	↑	Vomiting, rhinorrhea, piloerection, diarrhea, yawning

↑ = increases; ↓ = decreases; ± = variable; – = change unlikely; BP = blood pressure; P = pulse; R = respirations; T = temperature.

A detailed analysis of each sign, symptom, and toxic syndrome can be found in the pertinent chapters throughout the text. In this chapter, the most typical toxic syndromes are considered to enable the appropriate assessment and differential diagnosis of a poisoned patient.

In considering a toxic syndrome, the reader should always remember that the actual clinical manifestations of a poisoning are far more variable than the syndromes described in Table 3–2. The concept of the toxic syndrome is most useful when thinking about a clinical presentation and formulating a framework for assessment. Although some patients present in a "classic" fashion, others manifest partial toxic syndromes or formes frustes. These incomplete syndromes still provide at least a clue to the correct diagnosis. It is important to understand that incomplete or atypical presentations (particularly in the presence of multiple xenobiotics) do not necessarily imply less severe disease and, therefore, are comparably important to appreciate.

In some instances, an unexpected combination of findings is particularly helpful in identifying a xenobiotic or a combination of xenobiotics. For example, a dissociation between such typically paired changes as an increase in pulse with a decrease in blood pressure (cyclic antidepressants or phenothiazines) or the presentation of a decrease in pulse with an increase in blood pressure (ergot alkaloids) may be extremely helpful in diagnosing a toxic etiology. The use of these unexpected or atypical clinical findings is demonstrated in Chap. 16.

BLOOD PRESSURE

Xenobiotics cause hypotension by four major mechanisms: decreased peripheral vascular resistance, decreased myocardial contractility, dysrhythmias, and depletion of intravascular volume. Many xenobiotics initially cause orthostatic hypotension without marked supine hypotension, and any xenobiotic that affects autonomic control of the heart or peripheral capacitance vessels may lead to orthostatic hypotension (Table 3–3). Hypertension from xenobiotics is caused by CNS sympathetic overactivity, increased myocardial contractility, increased peripheral vascular resistance, or a combination thereof.

Blood pressure and pulse rate may vary significantly as a result of changes in receptor responsiveness, degree of physical fitness, and degree of vascular elasticity. Changing patterns of blood pressure often assist in the diagnostic evaluation: overdose with a monoamine oxidase inhibitor characteristically causes an initial normal blood pressure followed by hypertension, which in turn is followed abruptly by severe hypotension (Chap. 71).

PULSE RATE

Extremely useful clinical information can be obtained by evaluating the pulse rate (Table 3–4 and Chap. 16). Although the carotid artery is usually easily palpable, for reasons of both safety and reliability, the brachial artery is preferred in infants and the radial artery in adults older than 60 years. The normal heart rate for adults was defined by consensus studies suggesting that 95% of the population has bradycardia and tachycardia thresholds of 50 beats/min and 90 beats/min, making absolute definitions unrealistic, particularly in the ED.

TABLE 3–3	Common Xenobiotics That Affect the Blood Pressure[a]
Hypotension	Hypertension
α_1-Adrenergic antagonists	α_1-Adrenergic agonists
α_2-Adrenergic agonists (central)	α_2-Adrenergic agonists (central) (early)
β-Adrenergic antagonists	α_2-Adrenergic antagonists
β_2-Adrenergic agonists	Ergot alkaloids
Angiotensin-converting enzyme inhibitors	Ethanol and sedative-hypnotic withdrawal
Angiotensin receptor blockers	Lead (chronic)
Antidysrhythmics	Monoamine oxidase inhibitors (overdose early and drug–food interaction)
Calcium channel blockers	
Cyanide	Nicotine (early)
Cyclic antidepressants	Phencyclidine
Ethanol and other alcohols	Sympathomimetics
Iron	
Methylxanthines	
Nitrates and nitrites	
Nitroprusside	
Opioids	
Phenothiazines	
Phosphodiesterase-5 inhibitors	
Sedative–hypnotics	

[a]Chapter 16 lists additional xenobiotics that affect hemodynamic function.

TABLE 3–4   Common Xenobiotics That Affect the Pulse Rate[a]

Bradycardia	Tachycardia
α₂-Adrenergic agonists (central)	α₁-Adrenergic antagonists
β-Adrenergic antagonists	Anticholinergics
Baclofen	Antipsychotics
Calcium channel blockers	β-Adrenergic agonists
(nondihydropyridine)	Cyclic antidepressants
Carbamates	Disulfiram–ethanol interaction
Cardioactive steroids	Ethanol and sedative–hypnotic withdrawal
Ciguatoxin	Iron
Ergot alkaloids	Methylxanthines
γ-Hydroxybutyric acid	Phencyclidine
Opioids	Sympathomimetics
Organic phosphorus compounds	Thyroid hormone
Synthetic cannabinoids	Thiamine deficiency
	Yohimbine

[a]Chapter 16 lists additional xenobiotics that affect the heart rate.

Because pulse rate is the net result of a balance between sympathetic (adrenergic) and parasympathetic (muscarinic and nicotinic) tone, many xenobiotics that exert therapeutic or toxic effects or cause pain syndromes, hyperthermia, or volume depletion also affect the pulse rate. Whereas hypotension, such as that related to vasodilation or hypovolemia, generally leads to a reflex tachycardia, abrupt hypertension occasionally causes reflex bradycardia. Additionally, there is a direct correlation between pulse rate and temperature in that pulse rate increases approximately 8 beats/min for each 1.8°F (1°C) elevation in temperature.[7]

The inability to differentiate easily between sympathomimetic and anticholinergic xenobiotic effects by vital signs alone illustrates the principle that no single vital sign abnormality can definitively establish a toxicologic diagnosis. In trying to differentiate between a sympathomimetic and anticholinergic toxic syndrome, it should be understood that although tachycardia commonly results from both sympathomimetic and anticholinergic xenobiotics, when tachycardia is accompanied by diaphoresis or increased bowel sounds, sympathomimetic toxicity is suggested, but when tachycardia is accompanied by decreased sweating, absent bowel sounds, and urinary retention, anticholinergic toxicity is likely.

RESPIRATORY RATE

Establishment of an airway and evaluation of respiratory status are the initial priorities in patient stabilization. Although respirations are typically assessed initially for rate alone, careful observation of the depth and pattern is essential (Table 3–5) for establishing the etiology of a systemic illness or toxicity.[3] Unfortunately, very few investigators have actually measured

TABLE 3–5   Common Xenobiotics That Affect Respiration[a]

Bradypnea	Tachypnea
α₂-Adrenergic agonists (central)	Cyanide
Botulinum toxin	Dinitrophenol and congeners
Carbamates	Epinephrine
Elapidae venom	Ethylene glycol
Ethanol and other alcohols	Hydrogen sulfide
γ-Hydroxybutyric acid	Methanol
Magnesium	Methemoglobin producers
Neuromuscular blockers	Methylxanthines
Opioids	Nicotine (early)
Organic phosphorus compounds	Pulmonary irritants
Sedative–hypnotics	Salicylates
Tetanospasmin	Sympathomimetics
Tetrodotoxin	

[a]Chapter 28 lists additional xenobiotics affecting respiratory rate.

the respiratory rate in large populations of normal people, let alone in ED patients. Two papers investigating respiratory rates in ED patients differ substantially in their determinations of normal ranges from the remainder of the literature.[4,5] The combined results of these investigations suggest "normal" respiratory rates are 16 to 24 breaths/min in adults with more rapid rates that are inversely related to age in children.

Hyperventilation means an increase in minute ventilation above normal and it may result from tachypnea, hyperpnea or both. Tachypnea can also produce hypoventilation. When hyperventilation results solely or predominantly from hyperpnea, clinicians may miss this important finding entirely, instead erroneously describing such a hyperventilating patient as normally ventilating or even *hypoventilating* if bradypnea is also present. The ventilatory status of the patient must be viewed in the context of the patient's physiologic condition. Even in patients admitted to an intensive care unit and therefore with a high likeliness of illness, the sensitivity of clinical assessment on the ability to predict severe respiratory dysfunction was only 70%.[11]

Hyperventilation results from the direct effect of a CNS stimulant, such as salicylates, on the brainstem. However, salicylate poisoning characteristically produces hyperventilation by tachypnea, but it also produces hyperpnea with or without tachypnea. Metabolic acidosis, whether of a toxicologic etiology or not, typically results in an attempt by the patient to normalize her or his blood pH through hyperventilation. Pulmonary injury from any source, including aspiration of gastric contents, may lead to hypoxemia with a resultant tachypnea. Later, tachypnea may change to bradypnea, hypopnea (shallow breathing), or both. Bradypnea may occur when a CNS depressant acts on the brainstem. A progression from fast to slow breathing may also occur in a patient exposed to increasing concentrations of cyanide or carbon monoxide.

TEMPERATURE

Temperature evaluation and control are critical, yet our ability to recognize abnormal temperatures by clinical examination is limited.[6] However, temperature assessment can be done only if safe and reliable equipment is used. The risks of inaccuracy are substantial when an oral temperature is taken in a tachypneic patient, an axillary temperature or a temporal artery temperature is taken in any patient (especially those found outdoors), or a tympanic temperature is taken in a patient with cerumen impaction.[10] Obtaining rectal temperatures using a nonglass probe is essential for safe and accurate temperature determinations in agitated individuals and is considered the standard method of temperature determination in this textbook. Although concerns for infection control have limited the use of rectal temperatures, screening by other routes is acceptable, but rectal temperature assessments remain the most accurate.[10] Rectal temperatures should be obtained when the temperature obtained by another route is not consistent with the expected clinical findings.

The core temperature or deep internal temperature (T) is relatively stable (98.6° ± 1.08°F; 37° ± 0.6°C) under normal physiologic circumstances. Hypothermia (T <95.0°F; <35°C) and hyperthermia (T >100.4°F; >38°C) are common manifestations of toxicity. Severe or significant hypothermia and hyperthermia, unless immediately recognized and managed appropriately, may result in grave complications and inappropriate or inadequate resuscitative efforts. Life-threatening hyperthermia (T >106°F; >41.1°C) from any cause may lead to extensive rhabdomyolysis, myoglobinuric kidney failure, and direct liver and brain injury and must therefore be identified and corrected immediately.

Hyperthermia often results from a distinct neurologic response to a signal demanding thermal "upregulation." This signal can be from internal generation of heat beyond the capacity of the body to dissipate heat, such as occurs in association with agitation or mitochondrial uncoupling, or from an externally imposed physical or environmental factor, such as the environmental conditions causing heat stroke or the excessive swaddling in clothing causing hyperthermia in infants. Fever, or pyrexia, is hyperthermia caused by an elevation in the hypothalamic thermoregulatory setpoint.[2]

Regardless of etiology, core temperatures higher than 106°F (41.1°C) are extremely rare unless normal feedback mechanisms are overwhelmed.

TABLE 3–6	Common Xenobiotics that Affect Temperature[a]	
Hyperthermia	*Hypothermia*
Anticholinergics	α_2-Adrenergic agonists (central)
Chlorophenoxy herbicides	Anesthetics (general and intravenous)
Dinitrophenol and congeners	Cannabinoids
Malignant hyperthermia	Carbon monoxide
Monoamine oxidase inhibitors	Ethanol
Neuroleptic malignant syndrome	γ-Hydroxybutyric acid
Phencyclidine	Hypoglycemics
Salicylates	Opioids
Sedative–hypnotic or ethanol withdrawal	Sedative–hypnotics
Serotonin toxicity	(particularly barbiturates)
Sympathomimetics	Thiamine deficiency
Thyroid hormone	

[a]Chapter 29 lists additional xenobiotics that affect temperature.

Hyperthermia of this extreme nature is usually attributed to environmental heat stroke, extreme psychomotor agitation, or xenobiotic-related temperature disturbances such as malignant hyperthermia, serotonin toxicity, or the neuroleptic malignant syndrome. Numerous medications (anticholinergics, antiepileptics, antihistamines, antihypertensives, antipsychotics and diuretics) can also complicate or contribute to environmental hyperthermia. Xenobiotics, such as ethanol, CNS depressants, and general anesthetics, that render humans poikilothermic—in which body temperature approaches the ambient environmental temperature—present a particular risk. A hot environment, in combination with CNS alteration that precludes movement to a safe locale, requires external monitoring and interventions to address the significant patient temperature excursions that occur.

A common xenobiotic-related hyperthermia pattern that frequently occurs in the ED is the cooling that occurs after an acute temperature elevation resulting from psychomotor agitation or a grand mal seizure. Table 3–6 is a representative list of xenobiotics that affect body temperature. (Chap. 29 provides greater detail.)

Hypothermia is probably less of an immediate threat to life than hyperthermia, but it requires rapid appreciation, accurate diagnosis, and skilled management because it may suggest energy failure. Hypothermia impairs the metabolism of many xenobiotics, leading to unpredictable delayed and/or prolonged toxicologic effects when the patient is warmed. Many xenobiotics that lead to an alteration of mental status or poikilothermia place patients at great risk for becoming concerningly hypothermic from exposure to cold climates. Most important, a hypothermic patient should never be declared dead without both an extensive assessment and a full resuscitative effort of adequate duration, taking into consideration the difficulties in resuscitating cold but living patients. This is true whenever the body temperature remains less than 95.0°F (36°C) (Chap. 29).

SUMMARY

- Early, accurate determinations followed by serial monitoring of the vital signs are as essential in medical toxicology as in any other type of emergency or critical care medicine.
- Careful observation of the vital signs helps to determine appropriate therapeutic interventions and guide the clinician in making necessary adjustments to initial and subsequent therapeutic interventions.
- When pathognomonic clinical and laboratory findings are combined with accurate initial and sometimes changing vital signs, a toxic syndrome may become evident, which aids in both general supportive and specific antidotal treatment.
- Correct identification of toxic syndromes also guides further diagnostic testing.

Acknowledgment

Neal E. Flomenbaum contributed to this chapter in previous editions.

REFERENCES

1. Bartels K, et al. Blood pressure monitoring for the anesthesiologist: a practical review. *Anesth Analg.* 2016;122:1866-1879.
2. Childs C. Human brain temperature: regulation, measurement and relationship with cerebral trauma: Part 1. *Br J Neurosurg.* 2009;22:486-496.
3. Gravelyn TR, Weg JG. Respiratory Rate as an indicator of acute respiratory dysfunction. *JAMA.* 1980;244:1123-1125.
4. Hooker EA, et al. Respiratory rates in pediatric emergency patients. *J Emerg Med.* 1992;10:407-410.
5. Hooker EA, et al. Respiratory rates in emergency department patients. *J Emerg Med.* 1989;7:129-132.
6. Hung OL, et al. Evaluation of the physician's ability to recognize the presence or absence of anemia, fever, and jaundice. *Acad Emerg Med.* 2000;7:146-156.
7. Karjalainen J, Viitasalo M. Fever and cardiac rhythm. *Arch Intern Med.* 1986;146:1169-1171.
8. Mofenson HC, Greensher J. The unknown poison. *Pediatrics.* 1974;54:336-342.
9. Musher DM, et al. Edouard Seguin and the social power of thermometry. *N Engl J Med.* 1987;316:115-117.
10. Niven DJ, et al. Accuracy of peripheral thermometers for estimating temperature. *Ann Intern Med.* 2015;163:768-777.
11. Tulaimat A, et al. The validity and reliability of the clinical assessment of increased work of breathing in acutely ill patients. *J Crit Care.* 2016;34:111-115.

CASE STUDY 2

History A 22-year-old man was brought to the emergency department after being found unconscious at a movie theater. In the field, the paramedics inserted an intravenous (IV) line, performed a rapid reagent glucose test that was recorded as 88 mg/dL, and administered oxygen via nasal cannula at 4 L/min when his room air pulse oximetry was determined to be 91%. The patient had no medical records at the receiving hospital, and no useful information was found among his belongings.

Physical Examination On arrival at the ED, the patient was unconscious, with no response to physical stimuli. Vital signs were: blood pressure, 92/56 mm Hg; pulse, 52 beats/min; respiratory rate, 10 breaths/min; temperature, 97.4°F (36.3°C) {rectal}; and oxygen saturation, 98% on 4 L O_2/min. A repeat rapid reagent glucose was unchanged. Examination was notable for 2- to 3-mm pupils that responded to light, normal oculocephalic testing, nearly flaccid muscle tone, and downgoing toes bilaterally. His head was without signs of trauma, and his neck was supple. Examination of the chest revealed scattered coarse breath sounds and a regular heart rhythm with normal heart sounds and no murmurs. The abdomen was soft, bowel sounds were present, and no abnormalities were noted on the skin or extremities. When oxygen was removed, his saturation fell to 92%, and a continuous end-tidal CO_2 monitor measured 48 mm Hg.

Immediate Management Given the patient's hypoventilation and small pupils, graded doses of naloxone were given (0.04, 0.1, and 2 mg IV) without response (Antidotes in Depth: A4). On further examination, the patient's gag reflex was absent, prompting endotracheal intubation, which was performed without medications, and the patient was attached to a mechanical ventilator. A postintubation arterial blood gas, a complete blood count, electrolytes, and ethanol and acetaminophen (APAP) concentrations were obtained. Electrocardiography (ECG) showed sinus bradycardia with normal axis and intervals, and normal ST segments and

T-waves were observed. A total of 1 L of 0.9% sodium chloride was infused, and his blood pressure increased to 102/60 mm Hg, with no change in his pulse. A nasogastric tube was inserted through which 60 g of activated charcoal was instilled into the stomach.

What Is the Differential Diagnosis? This patient was comatose, with remarkable vital signs (hypotension, bradycardia, and hypoventilation) and remarkable physical findings (miosis, coma, flaccid muscles). The differential diagnosis is extensive and includes many xenobiotics from diverse chemical classes. The most common causes are listed in Table CS2–1. In many cases, it is not necessary to establish the correct diagnosis but rather to exclude diagnoses that require specialized care or are amenable to specific interventions.

What Clinical and Laboratory Analyses Help Exclude Life-Threatening Causes of This Patient's Presentation? Either a rapid reagent glucose determination should be obtained or hypertonic dextrose should be administered in every comatose patient (Chaps. 3 and 4 and Antidotes in Depth: A1 and A8). A normal blood glucose concentration or failure to respond to an appropriate dose of hypertonic dextrose essentially excludes persistent hypoglycemia. When hypoventilation is present, a graded trial of naloxone is indicated recognizing that patients who have overdosed on clonidine and similarly acting antihypertensives may respond

TABLE CS2–1	Common Causes of Coma with Limited Abnormalities in Vital Signs and the Physical Examination
Antidepressants	Ethanol and other toxic alcohols (early)
Antiepileptics	Gabapentin and pregabalin
Antipsychotics	γ-Hydroxybutyric acid
Baclofen	Inhalants
Clonidine and other centrally acting α-adrenergic agonists	Insulin secretagogues
	Sedative–hypnotics

(Antidotes in Depth: A4). A screening ECG is essential and may guide diagnosis and management (Chap. 15). Prolongation of the QRS complex occurs with some antidepressants, antipsychotics, and antiepileptics, and it may indicate the need to administer hypertonic sodium bicarbonate (Antidotes in Depth: A5). In addition, prolongation of the QT interval is commonly recognized with many antipsychotic and antidepressant overdoses (Chaps. 67 and 68). Although metabolic acidosis with an elevated anion gap is not typical of the xenobiotics listed, it might be indicative of a serious coingestant. Similarly, coma is not expected after a typical APAP overdose, but APAP is commonly ingested and coformulated with sedatives and opioids.

When a patient presents with coma, mildly abnormal vital signs, and flaccid muscles and if ECG results and glucose, oxygenation, anion gap, and APAP are normal or can be corrected, then the patient will likely do well with supportive care.

Further Diagnosis and Treatment The arterial blood gas and electrolytes showed no evidence of acidosis and a normal anion gap and a normal osmol gap. Other than bradycardia, the ECG was normal. The serum APAP concentration was 162 mcg/mL. Because the time of ingestion was unknown, N-acetylcysteine (NAC) was initiated (Antidotes in Depth: A3). After some time, a family member was contacted who disclosed that the patient had several previous suicide attempts and was known to be taking phenobarbital. A serum phenobarbital concentration was obtained on original blood in the laboratory and was reported to be 132 mcg/mL. A bicarbonate infusion was started to alkalinize the urine of the patient (Antidotes in Depth: A5). A 21-hour NAC regimen was completed at which time the patient's APAP was not detectable, and the aminotransferases were within normal limits. Over the next 48 hours, the patient regained consciousness and was extubated. A consultation with a psychiatrist determined the need for involuntary hospitalization, and the patient was transferred to the psychiatric service.

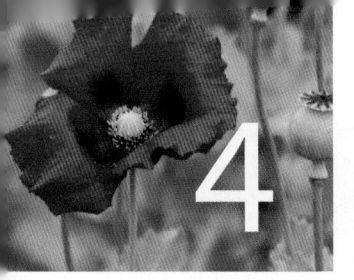

4 PRINCIPLES OF MANAGING THE ACUTELY POISONED OR OVERDOSED PATIENT

Lewis S. Nelson, Mary Ann Howland, Neal A. Lewin, Silas W. Smith, Lewis R. Goldfrank, and Robert S. Hoffman

OVERVIEW

For more than 5 decades, medical toxicologists and poison information specialists have used a clinical approach to poisoned or overdosed patients that emphasizes treating the patient rather than treating the poison.[3] Too often in the past, patients were initially ignored while attention was focused on the ingredients listed on the containers of the product(s) to which they presumably were exposed. Although astute clinicians must always be prepared to administer a specific antidote immediately in instances when nothing else will save a patient, such as with cyanide poisoning,[7] all poisoned or overdosed patients benefit from an organized, rapid clinical management plan (Fig. 4–1). However, clinicians should use caution when applying management advice from compendia and other non–toxicologic-specific sources because they may contain serious discrepancies with current standard expert advice.[2,10] Consultation with a poison control center or a medical or clinical toxicologist should be obtained if any questions or concerns arise about the management of a potentially poisoned or exposed patient.

Over the past 5 decades, some tenets and long-held beliefs regarding the initial therapeutic interventions in toxicologic management have been questioned and subjected to an "evidence-based" analysis. For example, in the mid-1970s, most medical toxicologists began to advocate a standardized approach to a comatose and possibly poisoned adult patient, typically calling for the intravenous (IV) administration of 50 mL of dextrose 50% in water ($D_{50}W$), 100 mg of thiamine, and 2 mg of naloxone along with 100% oxygen at high flow rates. The rationale for this approach was to compensate for the previously idiosyncratic style of management encountered in different health care settings. It was not unusual then to discover from a laboratory chemistry report more than 1 hour after a supposedly overdosed comatose patient had arrived in the emergency department (ED) that the patient had hypoglycemia—a critical delay in the management of unsuspected and consequently untreated hypoglycemic coma. Today, however, with the widespread availability of accurate rapid bedside testing for capillary blood glucose, pulse oximetry for oxygen saturation, and end-tidal CO_2 monitors coupled with a much greater appreciation by all physicians of what needs to be done for each suspected overdose patient, clinicians can safely provide a more rational, individualized approach to determine the need for, and in some instances more precise amounts of, dextrose, thiamine, naloxone, and oxygen.

A second major approach to providing more rational individualized early treatment for patients with toxicologic emergencies involves a closer examination of the actual risks and benefits of various gastrointestinal (GI) decontamination interventions. Appreciation of the potential for significant adverse effects associated with all types of GI decontamination interventions and recognition of the absence of clear evidence-based support of efficacy have led to abandoning of syrup of ipecac-induced emesis, an almost complete elimination of orogastric lavage, and a significant reduction in the routine use of activated charcoal. The value of whole-bowel irrigation (WBI) with polyethylene glycol electrolyte solution (PEG-ELS) appears to be much more specific and limited than originally thought, and some of the limitations and (uncommon) adverse effects of activated charcoal are now more widely recognized (Chap. 5). However, as with many issues in clinical medicine, properly selected procedures performed in properly selected patients can lead to an acceptable risk benefit profile, and blanket elimination of these GI decontamination procedures is not optimal and will lead to suboptimal care.

Similarly, interventions to eliminate absorbed xenobiotics from the body are now much more narrowly defined or, in some cases, have been abandoned. Multiple-dose activated charcoal (MDAC) is useful for select but not all xenobiotics. Ion trapping in the urine is only beneficial, achievable, and relatively safe when the urine can be maximally alkalinized after a significant salicylate or phenobarbital exposure (Antidotes in Depth: A5 and Table A5-1). Finally, the roles of hemodialysis, hemoperfusion, and other extracorporeal techniques are now much more specifically defined.[5] With the foregoing in mind, this chapter represents our current efforts to formulate a logical and effective approach to managing a patient with probable or actual toxic exposure.

The management of most patients with toxicologic clinical syndromes cannot be based on specific antidotal therapies but rather relies on the application of directed supportive or pharmacologic care. These forms of care include the extension of therapies from the management of related clinical syndromes caused by other xenobiotics or from other nontoxicologic etiologies. Examples include the use of vasopressors to manage hypotension from dihydropyridine calcium channel blockers and the use of anticonvulsant benzodiazepines to manage bupropion induced seizures. Table 4–1 provides a recommended stock list of antidotes and therapeutics for the treatment of poisoned or overdosed patients (Special Considerations: SC1). Consensus antidote stocking guidelines exist as well.[4]

MANAGING ACUTELY POISONED OR OVERDOSED PATIENTS

Rarely, if ever, are all of the circumstances involving a poisoned patient known. The history may be incomplete, unreliable, or unobtainable; multiple xenobiotics may be involved; and even when a xenobiotic etiology is identified, it may not be easy to determine whether the problem is an overdose, an allergic or idiosyncratic reaction, or a drug–drug interaction. Similarly, it is sometimes difficult or impossible to differentiate between the adverse effects of a correct dose of medication and the consequences of a deliberate or unintentional overdose. The patient's presenting signs and symptoms may force an intervention at a time when there is almost no information available about the etiology of the patient's condition (Table 4–2), and as a result, therapeutics must be thoughtfully chosen empirically to treat or diagnose a condition without exacerbating the situation. See Fig. 4-1 for an algorithmic approach to managing poisoned patients.

Initial Management of Patients with a Suspected Exposure

Similar to the management of any seriously compromised patient, the clinical approach to the patient potentially exposed to a xenobiotic begins with the recognition and treatment of life-threatening conditions, including airway compromise, breathing difficulties, and circulatory problems such as hemodynamic instability and serious dysrhythmias. After the "ABCs" (airway, breathing, and circulation) are addressed, the patient's level of consciousness should be assessed because it helps determine the techniques to be used for further management of the exposure.

Management of Patients with Altered Mental Status

Altered mental status (AMS) is defined as the deviation of a patient's sensorium from its baseline. Although it is commonly misconstrued as a depression in the patient's level of consciousness, a patient with agitation, delirium, psychosis, and other deviations from normal is also considered to have an AMS. The spectrum of deviation may range from hyperactive agitated

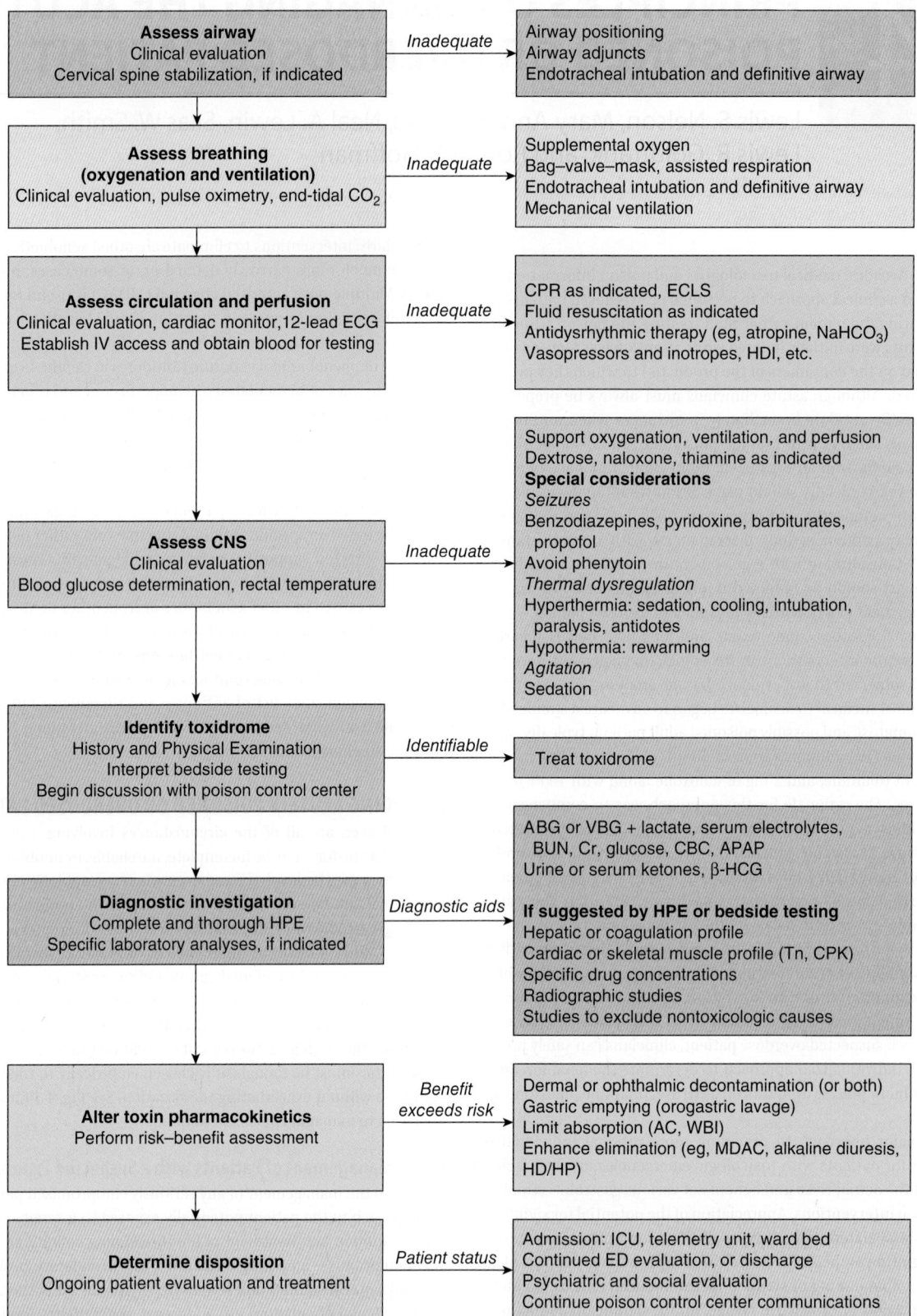

FIGURE 4–1. This algorithm is a basic guide to the management of poisoned patients. A more detailed description of the steps in management may be found in the accompanying text. This algorithm is only a guide to actual management, which must, of course, consider the patient's clinical status. ABG = arterial blood gas; AC = activated charcoal; APAP = acetaminophen; β-HCG = β-human chorionic gonadotropin; CBC = complete blood count; CNS = central nervous system; CPK = creatine phosphokinase; CPR = cardiopulmonary resuscitation; Cr, creatinine; ECG = electrocardiograph; ECLS = extracorporeal life support; HD = hemodialysis; HDI = high dose insulin; HP = hemoperfusion; ICU = intensive care unit; MDAC = multiple-dose activated charcoal; Tn = troponin; VBG = venous blood gas; WBI = whole-bowel irrigation.

TABLE 4–1   Antidotes and Therapeutics for the Treatment of Poisonings and Overdoses[a]

Therapeutics[b]	Indications	Therapeutics[b]	Indications
Acetylcysteine (p. 492)	Acetaminophen and other causes of hepatotoxicity	Hydroxocobalamin (p. 1694)	Cyanide
Activated charcoal (p. 76)	Adsorbent xenobiotics in the GI tract	Idarucizumab (p. 911)	Dabigatran
Antivenom (*Centruroides* spp) (p. 1563)	Scorpion envenomation	Insulin (p. 953)	β-Adrenergic antagonists, CCBs, hyperglycemia
Antivenom (*Crotalinae*) (p. 1627)	Crotaline snake envenomations	Iodide (SSKI) (p. 1775)	Radioactive iodine (I^{131})
Antivenom (*Micrurus fulvius*) (p. 1631)	Coral snake envenomations	Lipid emulsion (p. 1004)	Local anesthetics
Antivenom (*Latrodectus mactans*) (p. 1559)	Black widow spider envenomations	Magnesium sulfate injection (p. 876)	Cardioactive steroids, hydrofluoric acid, hypomagnesemia, ethanol withdrawal, torsade de pointes
Antivenom (*Synanceja* spp) (p. 1578)	Stonefish envenomation		
Atropine (p. 1503)	Bradydysrhythmias, cholinesterase inhibitors (organic phosphorus compounds, physostigmine) muscarinic mushrooms (*Clitocybe, Inocybe*) ingestions	Methylene blue (1% solution) (p. 1713)	Methemoglobinemia, ifosfamide, vasoplegic syndrome, shock
		Naloxone (p. 538)	Opioids, clonidine
		Norepinephrine (p. 950)	Hypotension
Benzodiazepines (p. 1135)	Seizures, agitation, stimulants, ethanol and sedative–hypnotic withdrawal, cocaine, chloroquine, organic phosphorus compounds	Octreotide (p. 713)	Insulin secretagogue induced hypoglycemia
		Oxygen (Hyperbaric) (p. 1676)	Carbon monoxide, cyanide, hydrogen sulfide
Botulinum antitoxin (Heptavalent) (p. 586)	Botulism	D-Penicillamine (p. 1215)	Copper
Calcium chloride, calcium gluconate (p. 1403)	Fluoride, hydrofluoric acid, ethylene glycol, CCBs, hypermagnesemia, β-adrenergic antagonists, hyperkalemia	Phenobarbital (p. 1087)	Seizures, agitation, stimulants, ethanol and sedative–hypnotic withdrawal
L-Carnitine (p. 732)	Valproic acid: hyperammonemia	Phentolamine (p. 1129)	Vasoconstriction: cocaine, MAOI interactions, epinephrine, and ergot alkaloids
Cyanide kit (nitrites, p. 1698; sodium thiosulfate, p. 1698)	Cyanide	Physostigmine (p. 755)	Anticholinergics
Cyproheptadine (p. 1001)	Serotonin toxicity	Polyethylene glycol electrolyte lavage solution (p. 83)	Decontamination
Dantrolene (p. 1029)	Malignant hyperthermia		
Deferoxamine (p. 676)	Iron, aluminum	Pralidoxime (p. 1508)	Acetylcholinesterase inhibitors (organic phosphorus compounds and carbamates)
Dextrose in water (50% adults; 20% pediatrics; 10% neonates) (p. 707)	Hypoglycemia	Protamine (p. 919)	Heparin anticoagulation
Digoxin-specific antibody fragments (p. 977)	Cardioactive steroids	Prussian blue (p. 1357)	Thallium, cesium
Dimercaprol (British anti-Lewisite [BAL]) (p. 1251)	Arsenic, mercury, gold, lead	Pyridoxine (vitamin B_6) (p. 862)	Isoniazid, ethylene glycol, gyromitrin-containing mushrooms
Diphenhydramine (p. 741)	Dystonic reactions, allergic reactions		
DTPA (p. 1779) calcium trisodium pentetate	Radioactive isotopes; americium, curium, plutonium	Sodium bicarbonate (p. 567)	Ethylene glycol, methanol, salicylates, cyclic antidepressants, methotrexate, phenobarbital, quinidine, chlorpropamide, class I antidysrhythmics, chlorophenoxy herbicides, sodium channel blockers
Edetate calcium disodium (calcium disodium versenate, $CaNa_2EDTA$) (p. 1315)	Lead, other selected metals		
Ethanol (p. 1440)	Ethylene glycol, methanol, diethylene glycol	Starch (p. 1371)	Iodine
Flumazenil (p. 1094)	Benzodiazepines	Succimer (p. 1309)	Lead, mercury, arsenic
Folinic acid (p. 775)	Methotrexate, methanol	Thiamine (vitamin B_1) (p. 1309)	Thiamine deficiency, ethylene glycol, chronic ethanol consumption ("alcoholism")
Fomepizole (p. 1435)	Ethylene glycol, methanol, diethylene glycol	Uridine triacetate (p. 789)	Fluorouracil, capecitabine
Glucagon (p. 941)	β-Adrenergic antagonists, CCBs		
Glucarpidase (p. 782)	Methotrexate	Vitamin K_1 (p. 915)	Warfarin or rodenticide anticoagulants

[a]Each emergency department should have the vast majority of these antidotes immediately available; some of these antidotes may be stored in the pharmacy, and others may be available from the Centers for Disease Control and Prevention, but the precise mechanism for locating each one must be known by each staff member (Special Considerations: SC1).

[b]A detailed analysis of each of these antidotes is found in the text in the Antidotes in Depth section on the page cited to the right of each antidote or therapeutic listed.

CCB = calcium channel blocker; DTPA = diethylenetriaminepentaacetic acid; EDTA = ethylenediamine tetraacetic acid; GI = gastrointestinal; MAOI = monoamine oxidase inhibitor; SSKI = saturated solution of potassium iodide.

TABLE 4–2	Clinical and Laboratory Findings in Poisoning and Overdose
Agitation	Anticholinergics,[a] hypoglycemia, phencyclidine, sympathomimetics,[b] synthetic cannabinoid receptor agonists, withdrawal from ethanol and sedative–hypnotics
Alopecia	Alkylating agents, radiation, selenium, thallium
Ataxia	Benzodiazepines, carbamazepine, carbon monoxide, ethanol, hypoglycemia, lithium, mercury, nitrous oxide, phenytoin
Blindness or decreased visual acuity	Caustics (direct), cisplatin, cocaine, ethambutol, lead, mercury, methanol, quinine, thallium
Blue skin	Amiodarone, FD&C #1 dye, methemoglobinemia, silver
Constipation	Anticholinergics,[a] botulism, lead, opioids, thallium (severe)
Deafness, tinnitus	Aminoglycosides, carbon disolfide, cisplatin, loop diuretics, macrolides, metals, quinine, quinolones, salicylates
Diaphoresis	Amphetamines, cholinergics,[c] hypoglycemia, opioid withdrawal, salicylates, serotonin toxicity, sympathomimetics,[b] withdrawal from ethanol and sedative–hypnotics
Diarrhea	Arsenic and other metals, boric acid (blue-green), botanical irritants, cathartics, cholinergics,[c] colchicine, iron, lithium, opioid withdrawal, radiation
Dysesthesias, paresthesias	Acrylamide, arsenic, ciguatera, cocaine, colchicine, thallium
Gum discoloration	Arsenic, bismuth, hypervitaminosis A, lead, mercury
Hallucinations	Anticholinergics,[a] dopamine agonists, ergot alkaloids, ethanol, ethanol and sedative–hypnotic withdrawal, LSD, phencyclidine, sympathomimetics,[b] tryptamines
Headache	Carbon monoxide, hypoglycemia, MAOI–food interaction (hypertensive crisis), serotonin toxicity
Metabolic acidosis (elevated anion gap)	Methanol, uremia, ketoacidosis (diabetic, starvation, alcoholic), paraldehyde, metformin, iron, isoniazid, lactic acidosis, cyanide, protease inhibitors, ethylene glycol, salicylates, toluene
Miosis	Cholinergics,[c] clonidine, opioids, phencyclidine, phenothiazines
Mydriasis	Anticholinergics,[a] botulism, opioid withdrawal, sympathomimetics[b]
Nystagmus	Barbiturates, carbamazepine, carbon monoxide, dextromethorphan, ethanol, lithium, MAOIs, phencyclidine, phenytoin, quinine, synthetic cannabinoid receptor agonists
Purpura	Anticoagulant rodenticides, corticosteroids, heparin, pit viper venom, quinine, salicylates, anticoagulants, levamisole
Radiopaque ingestions	Arsenic, halogenated hydrocarbons, iodinated compounds metals (eg, iron, lead), potassium compounds
Red skin	Anticholinergics,[a] boric acid, disulfiram, hydroxocobalamin, scombroid, vancomycin
Rhabdomyolysis	Carbon monoxide, doxylamine, HMG-CoA reductase inhibitors, sympathomimetics,[b] *Tricholoma equestre* mushrooms
Salivation	Arsenic, caustics, cholinergics,[c] clozapine, ketamine, mercury, phencyclidine, strychnine
Seizures	Bupropion, camphor, carbon monoxide, cyclic antidepressants, *Gyromitra* mushrooms, hypoglycemia, isoniazid, methylxanthines, ethanol and sedative–hypnotic withdrawal
Tremor	Antipsychotics, arsenic, carbon monoxide, cholinergics,[c] ethanol, lithium, mercury, methyl bromide, sympathomimetics,[b] thyroid hormones
Weakness	Botulism, diuretics, magnesium, paralytic shellfish, steroids, toluene
Yellow skin	APAP (late), pyrrolizidine alkaloids, β carotene, amatoxin mushrooms, dinitrophenol

[a]Anticholinergics, including antihistamines, atropine, cyclic antidepressants, and scopolamine.

[b]Sympathomimetics, including adrenergic agonists, amphetamines, cocaine, and ephedrine.

[c]Cholinergics, including muscarinic mushrooms; organic phosphorus compounds and carbamates, including select Alzheimer disease drugs and physostigmine; and pilocarpine and other direct-acting xenobiotics.

APAP = acetaminophen; HMG-CoA = 3-hydroxy-3-methyl-glutaryl-CoA); LSD = lysergic acid diethylamide; MAOI = monoamine oxidase inhibitor.

conditions typified by sympathomimetics such as cocaine or amphetamines to depressed levels of consciousness that typify opioid and sedative hypnotic exposures. "Awake" but "altered" conditions also include delirium or psychoses, such as those induced by lithium, salicylate, or antimuscarinic toxicity.

After airway patency is assured, an initial bedside assessment should be made regarding the adequacy of breathing. Although it is often not possible to assess the adequacy of the depth of ventilation, at least the rate and pattern of breathing should be determined. In this setting, any irregular or slow breathing pattern, particularly with an elevated end-tidal CO_2 measurement, should be considered a possible sign of the incipient apnea, requiring

ventilation using 100% oxygen by bag–valve–mask followed as soon as possible by endotracheal intubation and mechanical ventilation. Endotracheal intubation and mandatory ventilation is often indicated for patients with coma resulting from a toxic exposure to ensure and maintain control of the airway and to enable safe performance of procedures to prevent GI absorption or eliminate previously absorbed xenobiotic.

Although in many instances, the widespread availability of pulse oximetry to determine O_2 saturation and end-tidal CO_2 monitors have made arterial blood gas (ABG) analysis less of an immediate priority, these technical advances have not entirely eliminated the importance of blood gas analysis.

An ABG determination will more accurately define the adequacy not only of oxygenation (PO_2, O_2 saturation) and ventilation (PCO_2) but may also alert the physician to possible toxic-metabolic etiologies of coma characterized by acid–base disturbances (pH, PCO_2)[11] (Chap. 12). In addition, carboxyhemoglobin determinations are now available by point-of-care testing, and both carboxyhemoglobin and methemoglobin may be determined on either venous or arterial blood specimens (Chaps. 122 and 124). In every patient with an AMS, a bedside rapid glucose concentration should be obtained as soon as possible.

After the patient's respiratory status is assessed and managed appropriately, the strength, rate, and regularity of the pulse should be evaluated and the blood pressure and rectal temperature determined. Both an initial 12-lead electrocardiogram (ECG) and continuous rhythm monitoring are essential. Monitoring will alert the clinician to dysrhythmias that are related to toxic exposures either directly or indirectly via hypoxemia or electrolyte imbalance. For example, a 12-lead ECG demonstrating QRS widening and a right axis deviation might indicate a life-threatening exposure to a cyclic antidepressant or another xenobiotic with sodium channel–blocking properties. In these cases, the physician can anticipate such serious sequelae as ventricular tachydysrhythmias, seizures, and cardiac arrest and plan for both the early use of specific treatment (antidotes), such as IV sodium bicarbonate, and avoidance of medications, such as procainamide and other class IA and IC antidysrhythmics, that could exacerbate toxicity.

Extremes of core body temperature must be addressed early in the evaluation and treatment of a comatose patient. Life-threatening hyperthermia (temperature >106°F; >41.1°C) is usually appreciated when the patient is touched (although the widespread use of gloves as part of universal precautions has made this less apparent than previously). Individuals with severe hyperthermia, regardless of the etiology, should have their temperatures immediately reduced to about 101.5°F (38.7°C) by sedation if they are agitated or displaying muscle rigidity or by ice water immersion (Chap. 29). Hypothermia is probably easier to overlook than hyperthermia, especially in northern regions during the winter months, when most arriving patients feel cold to the touch. Early recognition of hypothermia, however, helps to avoid administering a variety of medications that are ineffective until the patient warms, at which point iatrogenic toxicity may result because of a sudden response to xenobiotics previously administered.

For a hypotensive patient with clear lungs and an unknown overdose, a fluid challenge with IV 0.9% sodium chloride or lactated Ringer solution should be administered. If the patient remains hypotensive or cannot tolerate fluids, an antidote, a vasopressor, or an inotrope is often indicated along with invasive monitoring.

At the time that the IV catheter is inserted, blood samples for glucose, electrolytes, blood urea nitrogen (BUN), a complete blood count (CBC), and any indicated toxicologic analyses should be obtained. A pregnancy test should be obtained in any woman of childbearing age. If the patient has an AMS, there may be a temptation to send blood and urine specimens to identify any central nervous system (CNS) depressants or so-called drugs of abuse in addition to other medications. But the indiscriminate ordering of these tests rarely provides clinically useful information.[1] For a potentially suicidal patient, an APAP concentration should be routinely requested along with tests affecting the management of any specific xenobiotic, such as carbon monoxide (CO), lithium, theophylline, iron, salicylates, and digoxin (or other cardioactive steroids), as suggested by the patient's history, physical examination, or bedside diagnostic tests. In many cases, the blood tests that are most useful in diagnosing toxicologic emergencies are not the toxicologic assays but rather the "nontoxicologic" routine metabolic profile tests such as CBC, BUN, glucose, electrolytes, liver function tests, and blood gas analysis.

Xenobiotic-related seizures are broadly divided into three categories: (1) those that respond to standard antiepileptic treatment (typically using a benzodiazepine); (2) those that either require specific antidotes to control seizure activity or that do not respond consistently to standard anticonvulsant treatment, such as isoniazid-induced seizures requiring pyridoxine administration; and (3) those that may appear to respond to initial treatment with cessation of tonic–clonic activity but that leave the patient exposed to the underlying, unidentified xenobiotic or to continued electrical seizure activity, as is the case with CO poisoning and hypoglycemia.

Within the first 5 minutes of managing a patient with an AMS, four therapeutic interventions should be administered if indicated and not contraindicated:

1. Supplemental oxygen to treat xenobiotic-induced hypoxia
2. Hypertonic dextrose: 0.5 to 1.0 g/kg of $D_{50}W$ for an adult or a more dilute dextrose solution ($D_{10}W$ or $D_{25}W$) for a child; the dextrose is administered as an IV bolus as specific or empiric therapy for hypoglycemia (Antidotes in Depth: A8)
3. Thiamine (100 mg IV for an adult; usually unnecessary for a child) to prevent Wernicke encephalopathy (Antidotes in Depth: A27)
4. Naloxone (0.04 mg IV with upward titration) for an adult or child with opioid-induced respiratory compromise (Antidotes in Depth: A4)

The clinician must be aware that hypoglycemia may be the sole or contributing cause of coma even when the patient manifests focal neurologic findings; therefore, dextrose administration should only be omitted when hypoglycemia can be definitely excluded by accurate rapid bedside testing. Also, while examining a patient for clues to the etiology of a presumably toxic-metabolic form of AMS, it is important to search for any indication that trauma caused, contributed to, or resulted from the patient's condition. Conversely, the possibility of a concomitant xenobiotic ingestion or toxic metabolic disorder in a patient with obvious head trauma should also be assessed.

The remainder of the physical examination should be performed rapidly but thoroughly. In addition to evaluating the patient's level of consciousness, the physician should note abnormal posturing (decorticate or decerebrate), abnormal or unilateral withdrawal responses, and pupil size and reactivity. Pinpoint pupils suggest exposure to opioids or organic phosphorus compounds, and widely dilated pupils suggest anticholinergic or sympathomimetic poisoning. The presence or absence of nystagmus, abnormal reflexes, and any other focal neurologic findings may provide important clues to a structural cause of AMS. For clinicians accustomed to applying the Glasgow Coma Scale (GCS) to all patients with AMS, assigning a score to the overdosed or poisoned patient may provide a useful measure for assessing changes in neurologic status. However, in this situation, the GCS should never be used for prognostic purposes because despite a low GCS score, complete recovery from properly managed toxic-metabolic coma is the rule rather than the exception (Chap. 22).

Characteristic breath or skin odors may identify the etiology of coma. The fruity odor of ketones on the breath suggests diabetic or alcoholic ketoacidosis but also the possible ingestion of acetone or isopropyl alcohol, which is metabolized to acetone. The pungent, minty odor of oil of wintergreen on the breath or skin suggests methyl salicylate poisoning. The odors of other substances such as cyanide ("bitter almonds"), hydrogen sulfide ("rotten eggs"), and organic phosphorus compounds ("garlic") are described in detail in Chap. 25 and summarized in Table 25–1.

Further Evaluation of All Patients with Suspected Xenobiotic Exposures

Auscultation of breath sounds, particularly after a fluid challenge, helps to diagnose pulmonary edema, acute respiratory distress syndrome, or aspiration pneumonitis. Coupled with an abnormal breath odor of hydrocarbons or organic phosphorus compounds, for example, crackles and rhonchi may point to a toxic pulmonary etiology instead of a cardiac etiology; this is important because the administration of certain cardioactive medications may be inappropriate or dangerous in the former circumstances.

Heart murmurs in an injection drug user, especially when accompanied by fever, suggest infectious endocarditis. Dysrhythmias suggest overdoses or inappropriate use of cardioactive xenobiotics, such as digoxin and other cardioactive steroids, β-adrenergic antagonists, calcium channel blockers, and cyclic antidepressants.

The abdominal examination often reveal signs of trauma or alcohol-related hepatic disease. The presence or absence of bowel sounds helps to exclude or to diagnose anticholinergic toxicity and is important in considering whether to manipulate the GI tract in an attempt to remove the toxin. A large palpable bladder often signal urinary retention as a further manifestation of anticholinergic toxicity.

Examination of the extremities will reveal clues to current or former drug use (track marks, skin-popping scars); metal poisoning (Mees lines, arsenical dermatitis); and the presence of cyanosis or edema suggesting preexisting cardiac, pulmonary, or kidney disease.

Repeated evaluation of the patient suspected of an overdose is essential for identifying new or developing findings or toxic syndromes and for early identification and treatment of a deteriorating condition. Until the patient is completely recovered or considered no longer at risk for the consequences of a xenobiotic exposure, frequent reassessment must be provided even as the procedures described later are carried out. Toxicologic etiologies of abnormal vital signs and physical findings are summarized in Tables 3–1 to 3–6. Toxic syndromes, sometimes called "toxidromes," are summarized in Table 3–1.

Typically, in the management of patients with toxicologic emergencies, there is both a necessity and an opportunity to obtain various diagnostic studies and ancillary tests interspersed with stabilizing the patient's condition, obtaining the history, and performing the physical examination. Chapters 7, 8, and 15 discuss the timing and indications for qualitative and quantitative diagnostic laboratory studies, diagnostic imaging procedures, and the use and interpretation of the ECG in evaluating and managing poisoned or overdosed patients, respectively.

The Role of Gastrointestinal Decontamination

A series of highly individualized treatment decisions regarding limiting the exposure to the xenobiotic follow the initial stabilization and assessment of the patient. As noted previously and as discussed in detail in Chap. 5, evacuation of the GI tract or administration of activated charcoal can no longer be considered standard or routine toxicologic care for most patients. Instead, the decision to perform GI decontamination should be based on the specifics of the ingestion, estimated quantity, formulation, and size of the pill or tablet, time since the exposure, concurrent ingestions, coexisting medical conditions, and age and size of the patient. The indications, contraindications, and procedures for performing orogastric lavage and for administering WBI, activated charcoal, MDAC, and cathartics are listed in Tables 5–1 to 5–7 and are discussed both in Chap. 5 and in the specific Antidotes in Depth sections immediately following Chap. 5.

Eliminating Absorbed Xenobiotics from the Body

After deciding whether or not an intervention to try to prevent absorption of a xenobiotic is indicated, the clinician must next assess the applicability of techniques available to eliminate xenobiotics already absorbed. Detailed discussions of the indications for and techniques of manipulating urinary pH (ion trapping), diuresis, hemodialysis, hemoperfusion, continuous renal replacement therapy, and exchange transfusion are found in Chap. 6. Briefly, patients who are likely to benefit from these procedures are those who have systemically absorbed xenobiotics amenable to one of these techniques and whose clinical conditions are both serious (or potentially serious) and unresponsive to supportive care or whose physiologic route of elimination (liver–feces, kidney–urine) is impaired.

Alkalinization of the urinary pH to enhance the renal excretion of acidic xenobiotics has only limited applicability. Commonly, sodium bicarbonate is used to alkalinize the urine (as well as the blood) and enhance salicylate elimination (other xenobiotics are discussed in Chap. 6), and sodium bicarbonate also prevents toxicity from methotrexate (Antidotes in Depth: A5). Acidifying the urine to hasten the elimination of alkaline substances is difficult to accomplish, of limited value, and possibly dangerous and therefore has no role in poisoning management. Forced diuresis also has no indication and may endanger the patient by causing pulmonary or cerebral edema.

If extracorporeal elimination is contemplated, hemodialysis is used for patients who overdose with salicylates, methanol, ethylene glycol, lithium, valproic acid, or xenobiotics that are either dialyzable or cause fluid and electrolyte abnormalities. Advances in hemodialysis technology allow the efficient removal of theophylline, phenobarbital, and carbamazepine and have replaced hemoperfusion, which is nearly unavailable in the US. Peritoneal dialysis is too ineffective to be of practical utility, and continuous renal replacement therapies are not as efficacious as hemodialysis or hemoperfusion, although they may play a role between multiple runs of dialysis or in hemodynamically compromised patients who cannot tolerate hemodialysis. In theory, both hemodialysis and hemoperfusion in series is useful for a very few life-threatening overdoses such as thallium or salicylates. Plasmapheresis and exchange transfusion are used to eliminate xenobiotics with large molecular weights that are not dialyzable (Chap. 10).

AVOIDING PITFALLS

The history alone is not a reliable indicator of which patients require naloxone, hypertonic dextrose, thiamine, and oxygen. Instead, the need for these therapies should be evaluated and performed if indicated (unless specifically contraindicated) only after a clinical assessment for all patients with AMS. The physical examination should be used to guide the use of naloxone. If dextrose or naloxone is indicated, sufficient amounts should be administered to exclude or treat hypoglycemia or opioid toxicity, respectively.

Attributing an AMS to alcohol because of an odor on a patient's breath is potentially misleading. Small amounts of alcohol or alcoholic beverage congeners generally produce the same breath odor as do intoxicating amounts. Conversely, even when an extremely high blood ethanol concentration is confirmed by laboratory analysis, it is dangerous to ignore other possible causes of an AMS. Because some individuals with chronic alcohol use disorder are alert with ethanol concentrations in excess of 500 mg/dL, a concentration that would result in coma and possibly apnea and death in a nontolerant person, finding a high ethanol concentration does not eliminate the need for further search into the cause of a depressed level of consciousness.

The metabolism of ethanol is fairly constant at 15 to 30 mg/dL/h. Therefore, as a general rule, regardless of the initial blood alcohol concentration, a presumably "inebriated" comatose patient who remains unarousable 3 to 4 hours after initial assessment should be considered to have an intracranial process, such as hemorrhage, or another comorbid medical condition, such as meningitis, as the etiology for the alteration in consciousness until proven otherwise. Careful neurologic evaluation of the completely undressed patient supplemented by a head computed tomography scan is frequently indicated in such cases. A lumbar puncture or additional laboratory testing should be performed based on the need to exclude CNS infection or toxic-metabolic etiologies, respectively. This is especially important in dealing with chronic or heavy users of ethanol given their predisposition to such injuries and diseases.

ADDITIONAL CONSIDERATIONS IN MANAGING PATIENTS WITH A NORMAL MENTAL STATUS

As in the case of patients with AMS, vital signs must be obtained and recorded. If the patient is alert, talking, and in no respiratory distress, all that remains to document are the respiratory rate and rhythm. Because the patient is alert, additional history should be obtained, keeping in mind that information regarding the number and types of xenobiotics ingested, time elapsed, prior vomiting, and other critical information may be unreliable.

Under certain circumstances, such as when the patient has an AMS or is at risk for self-harm, the history should be privately and independently obtained from a friend or relative after the patient has been initially stabilized. Recent emphasis on compliance with the federal Health Insurance Portability and Accountability Act (HIPAA) may inappropriately discourage clinicians from attempting to obtain information necessary to evaluate and treat patients. Obtaining such information from a friend or relative without unnecessarily giving that person information about the patient is the key to successfully helping such a patient without violating confidentiality.

Speaking to a friend or relative of the patient may provide an opportunity to learn useful and reliable information regarding the exposure, the patient's frame of mind, a history of previous exposures, and the type of support that is available if the patient is discharged from the ED. At times, it is essential to initially separate the patient from any relatives or friends to obtain greater cooperation from the patient and avoid violating confidentiality and because their anxiety may interfere with therapy. Even if the history obtained from a patient with an exposure proves to be unreliable, it may nevertheless provide clues to an overlooked possibility of a second exposure or reveal the patient's mental and emotional condition. As is often true of the history, physical examination, or laboratory assessment in other clinical situations, the information obtained often confirms but rarely excludes possible causes.

At this point in the management of a conscious patient, a focused physical examination should be performed, concentrating on the pulmonary, cardiac, and abdominal examinations. A neurologic survey should emphasize reflexes and any focal findings.

APPROACHING PATIENTS WITH INTENTIONAL EXPOSURES

Initial efforts at establishing rapport with the patient by indicating to the patient concern about the events that led to the ingestion and the availability of help after the xenobiotic is removed (if such procedures are planned) often facilitates management. If GI decontamination is deemed beneficial, the reason for and nature of the procedure should be clearly explained to the patient together with reassurance that after the procedure is completed, there will be ample time to discuss his or her concerns and provide additional care. These considerations are especially important in managing the patient with an intentional self-harm attempt who is often seeking psychiatric help or emotional support. In deciding on the value of performing GI decontamination, it is important to understand that a resistant patient may transform a procedure of limited benefit into one with serious risks.

SPECIAL CONSIDERATIONS FOR MANAGING PREGNANT PATIENTS

In general, a successful outcome for both the mother and fetus depends on optimum management of the mother, and proven effective treatment for a potentially serious toxic exposure to the mother should never be withheld based on theoretical concerns regarding the fetus (Chap. 30).

Physiologic Factors

A pregnant woman's total blood volume and cardiac output are elevated through the second trimester and into the later stages of the third trimester. This means that signs of hypoperfusion and hypotension manifest later than they would in a woman who is not pregnant, and when they do, uterine blood flow may already be compromised. For these reasons, the possibility of hypotension in a pregnant woman must be more aggressively sought and, if found, more rapidly treated. Maintaining the patient in the left-lateral decubitus position helps prevent supine hypotension resulting from impairment of systemic venous return by compression of the inferior vena cava. The left lateral decubitus position is also the preferred position for orogastric lavage if this procedure is deemed necessary.

Because the tidal volume is increased in pregnancy, the baseline PCO_2 will normally be lower by approximately 10 mm Hg. Appropriate adjustment for this effect should be made when interpreting blood gas results.

Use of Antidotes

Limited data are available on the use of antidotes in pregnancy. In general, antidotes should not be used if the indications for use are equivocal. On the other hand, antidotes should not be withheld if they have the potential to reduce potential morbidity and mortality. Risks and benefits of either decision must be assessed. For example, reversal of opioid-induced respiratory depression calls for the use of naloxone, but in an opioid-dependent woman, the naloxone can precipitate acute opioid withdrawal, including uterine contractions and possible induction of labor. Very slow, careful, IV titration starting with 0.04 mg of naloxone is indicated unless apnea is present or cessation of breathing appears imminent. In these instances, it is preferable

to either administer naloxone in higher doses (ie, 0.4–2.0 mg) or manually assist ventilation. A combination of transient assisted ventilation followed by small doses of naloxone optimizes the benefits of both techniques.

An APAP overdose is a serious maternal problem when it occurs at any stage of pregnancy, but the fetus is at greatest risk in the third trimester. Although APAP crosses the placenta easily, acetylcysteine (NAC) has somewhat diminished transplacental passage. During the third trimester, when both the mother and the fetus are at substantial risk from a significant APAP overdose with manifest hepatotoxicity, immediate delivery of a mature or viable fetus has to be considered.

In contrast to the situation with APAP, the fetal risk from iron poisoning is less than the maternal risk. Because deferoxamine is a large charged molecule with little transplacental transport, deferoxamine should never be withheld out of unwarranted concern for fetal toxicity when indicated to treat the mother.

Carbon monoxide poisoning is particularly threatening to fetal survival. The normal PO_2 of the fetal blood is approximately 15 to 20 mm Hg. Oxygen delivery to fetal tissues is impaired by the presence of carboxyhemoglobin, which shifts the oxyhemoglobin dissociation curve to the left, potentially compromising an already tenuous balance. For this reason, hyperbaric oxygen is recommended for much lower carboxyhemoglobin concentrations in a pregnant compared with a nonpregnant woman (Chap. 122 and Antidotes in Depth: A40). Early notification of the obstetrician and close cooperation among involved physicians are essential for the best results in all of these instances.

MANAGEMENT OF PATIENTS WITH CUTANEOUS EXPOSURE

The xenobiotics that people are commonly exposed to externally include household cleaning materials; organic phosphorus or carbamate mark in color so they can compare from crop dusting, gardening, or pest extermination; acids from leaking or exploding batteries; alkalis, such as lye; and lacrimators that are used in crowd control. In all of these cases, the principles of management are as follows:

1. Avoid secondary exposures by wearing protective (rubber or plastic) gowns, gloves, and shoe covers. Cases of serious secondary poisoning have occurred in emergency personnel after contact with xenobiotics such as organic phosphorus compounds on the victim's skin or clothing.
2. Remove the patient's clothing, place it in plastic bags, and then seal the bags.
3. Wash the patient with soap and copious amounts of water twice regardless of how much time has elapsed since the exposure.
4. Make no attempt to neutralize an acid with a base or a base with an acid. Further tissue damage may result from the heat generated by this exothermic reaction.
5. Avoid using any greases or creams because they will only keep the xenobiotic in close contact with the skin and ultimately make removal more difficult.

Chapter 17 discusses the principles of managing cutaneous exposures, and Special Considerations: SC2 discusses the principles of preventing dermal absorption.

MANAGEMENT OF PATIENTS WITH OPHTHALMIC EXPOSURES

Although the vast majority of toxicologic emergencies result from ingestion, injection, or inhalation, the eyes are occasionally the routes of systemic absorption or are the organs at risk from ophthalmic exposures. The eyes should be irrigated with the eyelids fully retracted for no less than 20 minutes. To facilitate irrigation, a drop of an anesthetic (proparacaine and tetracaine) in each eye should be used, and the eyelids should be kept open with an eyelid retractor. An adequate irrigation stream is obtained by running 1 L of 0.9% sodium chloride through regular IV tubing held a few inches from the eye or by using an irrigating lens. Checking the eyelid fornices with pH paper strips is important to ensure adequate irrigation; the pH should normally be 6.5 to 7.6 if accurately tested, although when using paper test strips, the measurement will often be near 8.0. Chapter 24 describes the management of toxic ophthalmic exposures in more detail, and Special Considerations: SC2 discusses the principles of preventing dermal absorption.

IDENTIFYING PATIENTS WITH NONTOXIC EXPOSURES

Many exposures, whether caused by the nature or quantity of the xenobiotic or the clinical circumstances, are reliably predictable to be nonconsequential. More than 40% of exposures reported to poison control centers annually are nontoxic or minimally toxic. In this patient population, there are considerable risks of needlessly subjecting a patient to potential harm through unnecessarily aggressive treatment. For example, GI decontamination techniques or antidotes that are indicated for patients with serious exposures carry risks that are only acceptable if there is potential to offset the risk with clinical benefit. The following general guidelines for considering an exposure nontoxic or minimally toxic will assist clinical decision making:[6,8,9]

1. Identification of the product and its ingredients is possible.
2. None of the US Consumer Product Safety Commission's "signal words" (CAUTION, WARNING, or DANGER) appear on the product label.
3. The route of exposure is known.
4. A reliable approximation of the maximum exposure quantity is able to be made.
5. Based on the available medical literature and clinical experience, the potential effects related to the exposure are expected to be benign or at worst self-limited and not likely to require the patient to access health care.
6. The patient is asymptomatic or has developed the maximal expected self-limited toxicity.
7. Adequate time has occurred to assess the potential for the development of toxicity.

For any patient in whom there is a question about the nature of the exposure, it is not appropriate to consider that exposure nontoxic. All such patients, and all patients for whom the health care provider is unsure of the risks associated with a given exposure, should be referred either to the regional poison control center or health care facility for further evaluation.

DISPOSITION OF PATIENTS

Determining the appropriate transition of care may occur once or several times during the management of a poisoned patient. The poison control center must determine the need for direct medical care in a hospital or whether the patient has had a nontoxic exposure (discussed earlier) and can be managed at home. In the ED, many patients are discharged after their evaluation and treatment and after psychiatric and social services evaluations are obtained as needed. Among clinically ill poisoned patients, the decision is generally simplified based on the relative abilities of the various units within the medical facility. Critical care units expend the highest level of resources to assure both intensive monitoring and the provision of timely care and are necessary for patients who are currently ill or currently stable but likely to decompensate. See Table 4–3 for a description of patients best suited for critical care unit admission. General hospital beds, often called medical/surgical beds, provide only intermittent nursing and medical care and are sufficient for patients unlikely to undergo abrupt concerning changes in the clinical status but who nonetheless need clinical monitoring. The capabilities of medical/surgical beds vary widely by hospital. Stepdown or intermediate care units and telemetry units bridge the divide between these two extremes of care, and variably provide enhanced technological support and monitoring and higher nurse-to-patient ratios. Determining the optimal disposition for a poisoned patient requires an evaluation of the nature of the exposure, the patient, and the capabilities of the community and the institution. Most often such decisions are made conservatively and cautiously, given the unpredictable nature of human poisoning.

ENSURING AN OPTIMAL OUTCOME

The best way to ensure an optimal outcome for the patient with a suspected toxic exposure is to apply the principles of basic and advanced life support in conjunction with a planned and stepwise approach. Always bear in mind that a toxicologic etiology or co-etiology for any abnormal conditions

TABLE 4-3	Define the Indications for Intensive Care Unit Admission	
Patient Characteristics	*Xenobiotic Characteristics*	*Capabilities of the Inpatient or Observation Unit*

Does the patient have any signs of serious end-organ toxicity? Are the end-organ effects progressing? Are laboratory data suggestive of serious toxicity? Is the patient a high risk for complications requiring ICU intervention?
    Seizures
    Unresponsive to verbal stimuli
    Level of consciousness impaired to the point of potential airway compromise
    PCO_2 >45 mm Hg
    Systolic blood pressure <80 mm Hg (in an adult)
    Cardiac dysrhythmias (ventricular dysrhythmias, high-grade conduction abnormalities)
    Abnormal ECG complexes and intervals (QRS duration ≥0.10 seconds; QT prolongation)
    Refractory or recurrent hypoglycemia
Is the patient at high risk for complications such as aspiration pneumonitis, anoxic brain injury, rhabdomyolysis, or compartment syndrome?
Does the patient have preexisting medical conditions that could predispose to complications?
    Alcohol or drug dependence
    Liver disease
    Acute kidney injury or chronic kidney disease
    Heart disease
    Pregnancy: Is the xenobiotic or the antidote teratogenic?
Is the patient suicidal?
	Are there known serious sequelae (eg, cyclic antidepressants, CCBs)?
	Can the patient deteriorate rapidly from its toxic effects?
	Is the onset of toxicity likely to be delayed (eg, sustained-release preparation, slowed GI motility, or delayed toxic effects)?
	Does the xenobiotic have effects that will require cardiac monitoring?
	Is the amount ingested a potentially serious or potentially lethal dose?
	Are xenobiotic concentrations rising?
	Is the required or planned therapy unconventional (eg, large doses of atropine for treating overdoses of organic phosphorus compounds; or high dose insulin for CCB overdose)?
	Does the therapy have potentially serious adverse effects?
	Is there insufficient literature to describe the potential human toxic effects?
	Are potentially serious coingestants likely (must take into account the reliability of the history)?
		Does the admitting health care team appreciate the potential seriousness of a toxicologic emergency?
		Is the nursing staff:
		    Familiar with this toxicologic emergency?
		    Familiar with the potential for serious complications?
		Is the staffing adequate to monitor the patient?
		    What is the ratio of nurses to patients?
		    Are time-consuming nursing activities required and realistic?
		Can a safe environment be provided for a suicidal patient?
		    Can a patient have suicide precautions and monitoring with a medical floor bed?
		    Can a one-to-one observer be present in the room with the patient?
		    Can the patient be restrained or sedated?

CCB = calcium channel blocker; ECG = electrocardiogram; GI = gastrointestinal; ICU = intensive care unit.

necessitates modifying whatever standard approach is brought to the bedside of a severely ill patient. For example, it is extremely important to recognize that xenobiotic-induced dysrhythmias and cardiac instability require alterations in standard protocols that assume a primary cardiac or nontoxicologic etiology (Chaps. 15 and 16).

Involvement of the expertise of a poison control center, a medical toxicologist, or a clinical toxicologist can help direct both diagnosis and management strategies to improve the efficiency and outcome of the patient.

Typically, only some of the xenobiotics to which a patient is exposed will ever be confirmed by laboratory analysis. The thoughtful combination of stabilization, general management principles, and both empiric and specific treatment when indicated will result in successful outcomes in the majority of patients with actual or suspected exposures.

SUMMARY

- Patients with a suspected overdose or poisoning and an AMS present some of the most complex initial challenges.
- Pregnant patients with possible xenobiotic exposures raise additional management issues, as do those with toxic cutaneous or ophthalmic exposures.
- Among the most frequent toxicologic emergencies that clinicians must address is a patient with a suspected toxic exposure to an unidentified xenobiotic (medication or substance), sometimes referred to as an unknown overdose.

- Consider self-harm, the use of illicit drugs, and those who are unknowingly exposed to xenobiotics as having the potential for serious adverse consequences because of the limited accurate historical information that can be obtained.

REFERENCES

1. Broderick KB, et al. Emergency physician practices and requirements regarding the medical screening examination of psychiatric patients. *Acad Emerg Med.* 2002;9:88-92.
2. Brubacher JR, et al. Salty broth for salicylate poisoning? Adequacy of overdose management advice in the 2001 *CMAJ.* 2002;167:992-996.
3. Clemmesen C, Nilsson E. Therapeutic trends in the treatment of barbiturate poisoning. The Scandinavian method. *Clin Pharmacol Ther.* 1961;2:220-229.
4. Dart RC, et al. Expert consensus guidelines for stocking of antidotes in hospitals that provide emergency care. *Ann Emerg Med.* 2009;54:386-394.e1.
5. Ghannoum M, Gosselin S. Enhanced poison elimination in critical care. *Adv Chronic Kidney Dis.* 2013;20:94-101.
6. McGuigan MA, Guideline Consensus Panel. Guideline for the out-of-hospital management of human exposures to minimally toxic substances. *J Toxicol Clin Toxicol.* 2003;41:907-917.
7. Mitchell LJ, et al. "Do you know where your cyanide kit is?": A study of perceived and actual antidote availability to emergency departments in the South West of England. *Emerg Med J.* 2012;30:43-48.
8. Mofenson HC, Greensher J. The nontoxic ingestion. *Pediatr Clin North Am.* 1970;17: 583-590.
9. Mofenson HC, Greensher J. The unknown poison. *Pediatrics.* 1974;54:336-342.
10. Mullen WH, et al. Incorrect overdose management advice in the Physicians' Desk Reference. *Ann Emerg Med.* 1997;29:255-261.
11. Sheta MA, et al. Physiological approach to assessment of acid-base disturbances. *N Engl J Med.* 2015;372:194-195.

PRINCIPLES OF ANTIDOTE STOCKING

Silas W. Smith, Lewis R. Goldfrank, and Mary Ann Howland

Most patients with xenobiotic exposures do well with supportive care and close attention to vital physiology. However, one of the fundamental principles of managing an acutely poisoned patient is appropriate and timely antidotal administration when indicated. According to the last available US Poison Control Center data, a therapeutic intervention which includes specific antidotes was used in 18.5% of all poisoning exposures (Chap. 130).[16,41]

Sufficient antidote stocking is a best practice; failure to do so presents a clear and present danger to patient safety. Death and serious harm resulted from the delay to administer appropriate antidotes, reversal agents, and rescue agents.[28] Many poisonings are acute unanticipated emergencies, which would presumably invoke the protections of the Emergency Medical Treatment and Labor Act of 1986, which mandates public access to emergency services regardless of ability to pay. The Joint Commission (TJC) is the accrediting body for hospitals. The Joint Commission's elements of performance require that "emergency medications and their associated supplies are readily available," as well as written criteria determining which medications are available for dispensing or administering to patients.[55,56] The Joint Commission also recognizes the difficulties presented by medication shortages and requires staff communication, written medication substitution protocols approved by leadership and the medical staff, and review of the impact of substitutions (eg, medication errors and adverse drug events).[57] It is an Institute for Safe Medication Practices best practice to "ensure all appropriate antidotes, reversal agents, and rescue agents are readily available."[28] The World Health Organization devotes an entire section to antidotes and other substances used in poisonings that are considered of paramount importance in its model list of essential medicines.[65] Because many antidotes are used in practice to reverse potential medication errors, overdoses, or adverse clinical conditions, the Department of Veterans Affairs (VA) National Center for Patient Safety considers it mandatory that reversal agents such as flumazenil, naloxone, protamine, and others are available in the clinical setting.[60] Antidotes are a fundamental aspect of response (as medical countermeasures) to chemical, biological, and radiologic terrorism. As such, provisioning and antidotal administration are Critical Target Capabilities in the US National Preparedness Guidelines.[59] These national Preparedness Measures include quarterly updates to the federal government on the status of critical items; memoranda of understanding to determine collective inventory accessibility and to ramp up manufacturing capability; and maintenance by pharmaceutical manufacturers and distributors of increased inventory amounts of critical items.[59] Many professional organizations such as the American Heart Association, American Hospital Association, American Medical Association, American College of Medical Toxicology, and American Academy of Clinical Toxicology consider drug and antidote shortages a significant threat to public health and patient outcomes.[5,6,8,9]

LOCAL AVAILABILITY

Decades of research have consistently documented inadequate stocking of antidotes, which are required at critical instances. In 1986, the lack of any antidotal capacity within a 50-mile radius to treat a case of pyrinuron (Vacor) overdose was reported, with ultimate patient mortality.[26] A 1996 study of Colorado, Montana, and Nevada pharmacies found that only 1 of 108 (0.9%) responding hospitals had adequate supplies of eight antidotes (Crotalidae antivenin, cyanide kit, deferoxamine, digoxin immune Fab, ethanol, naloxone, pralidoxime chloride, and pyridoxine).[17] A 1997 survey of

Massachusetts hospitals found that only 8 of 82 hospitals (9.8%) stocked all of 14 common antidotes.[64] A 1999 study determined that no Alabama hospital had adequate supplies of all nine essential antidotes (digoxin-specific antibody fragments [DSFab], pyridoxine, ethanol, pralidoxime, Crotalidae antivenin, deferoxamine, cyanide antidote, naloxone, and fomepizole).[53] In 1999, a tertiary care New Mexico hospital was unable to adequately respond to three separate poisoning episodes (ethylene glycol, organic phosphorus compounds, and rattlesnake envenomation).[47] Rural hospitals are even more likely to lack antidotes.[15,16,22] To complicate medication management, multiple antidotes, such as bromocriptine, carnitine, cyproheptadine, glucagon, octreotide, and high-dose insulin, are not specifically labeled for use as such or are used at different dosages than that of the labeled indication.

With its small vial size, pyridoxine was particularly problematic in the past. Only half of the hospitals with pediatric emergency medicine (EM) fellowships and only two-thirds of hospitals with EM residencies had adequate pyridoxine stores, and of those that did, more than 70% of the time it was stored away from the emergency department (ED) in the hospital's pharmacy.[49] One isoniazid overdose case depleted the intravenous pyridoxine supply for a significant region of a state (Nebraska).[40] A similar isoniazid overdose case left a patient continually seizing because of an inadequate supply at a treating hospital and three of four surrounding hospitals.[38] In one study of 21 patients, 85% of patients failed to receive adequate initial intravenous pyridoxine because of inadequate hospital stocking, with resultant severe toxicity to one patient until antidote procurement.[13]

Antidotes specific to known chemical disaster scenarios are equally poorly accessible. Evaluations of a US city's preparedness in 1996 and 2000 determined that only 4.8% of local hospitals had sufficient atropine and pralidoxime to address a nerve agent incident, and none had sufficient cyanide antidotal capacity.[31] In a survey of Philadelphia hospitals in 2002, 87% of ED directors did not believe or did not know if adequate antidote stores for nerve agent and cyanide poisoning were available onsite.[23] This antidotal preparedness gap had not narrowed by 2013, when a report of US hospitals determined that only 16% of emergency care hospitals had sufficient cyanide antidote to treat just two 100-kg patients.[21]

The failure to adequately stock antidotes is also well described internationally. In a survey of Quebec hospital pharmacies, the number of adequately stocked antidotes ranged from 0 to 9 (of 13) and was correlated with N-acetylcysteine and naloxone utilization, annual ED visits, and weekend pharmacy coverage, suggesting that smaller hospitals were poorly positioned to adequately care for poisoned patients.[12] Ontario hospitals were no better; only 1 of 179 hospitals (0.6%) stocked adequate amounts of 10 basic antidotes, and more than half were stocked less than 50% of the time.[29] A 2003 study of British Columbia hospitals found zero hospitals with adequate stocking of 14 antidotes, with poor availability of DSFab, glucagon, pyridoxine, and antivenom.[22] In follow-up in 2005, only 51% to 70% had adequate folic acid, glucagon, methylene blue, atropine, pralidoxime, leucovorin, pyridoxine, and deferoxamine; fewer than 50% had adequate DSFab; and only 7 (8.9%) hospitals sufficiently stocked 21 essential antidotes.[63] Similar deficiencies in antidote stocking are reported in Greece,[48] Lebanon,[34] Malaysia,[2] Spain,[45] sub-Saharan Africa,[52] and Taiwan.[46] Hospitals in the United Kingdom generally had access to N-acetylcysteine, activated charcoal, dantrolene, desferrioxamine, naloxone, flumazenil, and vitamin K but lacked cyanide antidotes, cyproheptadine, ethanol, fomepizole, pralidoxime, succimer, and viper antivenom.[54] Antidote stocking in New Zealand was generally robust, with only very rarely used antidotes being unavailable (eg, Prussian blue).[1]

NATIONAL AVAILABILITY

National shortages can impede institutional attempts to obtain and sustain necessary antidotes. The underlying causes of antidote shortages are complex and include a constricted supplier and manufacturer pool, supply chain disruptions, manufacturing delays, demand issues, economic factors, legal decisions, and the unintended consequences of well-intentioned regulatory approaches (eg, regulatory inspections and the Food and Drug Administration {FDA} Unapproved Drugs Initiative).[24,37,58] Novel regulatory requirements present a particular threat to antidotes that are not specifically labeled for toxicologic use or are used at different dosages than the FDA-approved labeling. The 2011 American Hospital Association survey on drug shortages reported that 99.5% of hospitals reported experiencing one or more drug shortage in the previous 6 months, 82% of hospitals had to delay patient treatment as a result of a drug shortage, and hospitals rarely or never received advance notice of drug shortages and were not informed of the cause or the expected duration of the shortage.[7] To address this crisis, the 2012 Food and Drug Administration Safety and Innovation Act[11] required manufacturers to notify the Secretary of Health and Human Services of significant medications disruptions, required the development and implementation of a plan to prevent and mitigate drug shortages, and required the Comptroller General of the United States to conduct a study to examine the reasons for drug shortages and formulate recommendations on remediation.[5] Tragically, US national drug shortages continue to number in the hundreds of medications.[10] Certain shortages do challenge credulity. Salt, sugar, and baking soda do not suffer from a lack of raw materials or natural abundance, but 0.9% saline, dextrose, and sodium bicarbonate for parenteral administration are intermittently difficult to obtain.[10] Other specific antidote shortages have included atropine, benzodiazepines, black widow spider (*Latrodectus mactans*) antivenin, CaNa$_2$EDTA, dexrazoxane, digoxin immune Fab, epinephrine, ethanol, lipid emulsion (20%), leucovorin, methylene blue, *N*-acetylcysteine, naloxone, North American coral snake (*Micrurus fulvius*) antivenin, octreotide, and vitamin K.[5] In one study, 141 of 1,751 (8.1%) drug shortages were products used to treat poisoned patients.[37] Associated medications for critical care such as inotropes, analgesics, induction agents and paralytics for intubation, and sedatives for mechanical ventilation have not been spared.[10,36,62] This pervasive systemic failure to provide basic medications undermines adequate "modern" health care. Internationally, entire countries have reported a substantial rise in hard endpoints such as mortality because of an inability to obtain of antidotes. For example, death rates rose threefold when digoxin immune Fab stocks were exhausted in Sri Lanka.[18]

The use of substitute or atypical medications can engender side effects or toxicity that would require alternative antidotes. One study of directors of pharmacy found multiple adverse events associated with drug shortages, including omission, wrong dose dispensing and administration, wrong drug dispensing and administration, treatment delays, and requirements for increased patient monitoring.[39] Most patients want to be informed of drug shortages and the side effects of substitutes, and drug shortages lead to patient complaints.[27,39] Antidote shortages are particularly vexing because of a relatively narrow number of agents "in class," or appropriate to the poisoning. In many situations, suitable alternatives either do not exist or create new benefit–side effect conundrums. For example, sodium acetate substitution for sodium bicarbonate is limited by ceilings in acute dosing

and the side effects of myocardial depression, hypotension, hypopnea, and hypoxemia.[43,44]

COST

Cost can present a significant barrier to antidote acquisition, particularly for those that are infrequently used. The reasons for this are complex and include market exclusivity, generic availability, development costs, and "what the market will bear."[32] However, even simple antidotes that are years since introduction are associated with massive cost increases. Without significant new research, the original cyanide antidote kit, containing amyl nitrite, sodium nitrite, and sodium thiosulfate, was rebranded and released as "new" Nithiodote without amyl nitrite, with subsequent market exclusivity and elimination of generic competition.[19] In one of the most egregious examples, Valeant Pharmaceuticals raised the price of CaNa$_2$EDTA from $950 to $26,927 within a year.[50] Similar massive increases in the cost of vital drugs such as epinephrine and naloxone are described.[20] In a broader analysis, the average wholesale price of 15 of 33 antidotes had a greater than 50% price increase, and 8 of 33 had greater than $1,000 increase from 2010 to 2015.[25] Similar marked cost increases are detailed in in the position statements of toxicologic organizations.[4] Even in the hospital setting, where providers and patients are typically insulated from cost, massive price increases (sometimes upwards of 70 times) have led to medication abandonment and presumably alternative medication use.[33] Shortages themselves exacerbate cost pressures, as pharmacy directors reported a 300% to 500% markup on medications on shortage lists.[14] Although factors other than cost such as frequency of use, shelf life, and outdated product returns or recycling factor into decision making, hospital emphasis on cost alone might cause EDs to forgo the most appropriate antidote.[51] To address these costs and provide economies of scale, standardized, regional antidote collections with online administration guidelines have demonstrated success in providing antidote coverage.[42]

RECOMMENDATIONS

Because the needs of each hospital are different, a hazard vulnerability assessment approach is recommended.[16] Conclusions on necessary antidotes could be similarly derived from a quality and safety framework provided by the analogous VA National Center for Patient Safety's Safety Assessment Code (SAC) Matrix.[61] This would include evaluating which pharmaceutical products are used as therapeutics, hospital catchment area (ie, nearby industries, indigenous creatures and plants, agricultural operations, and military or government facilities), referral patterns and mutual aid agreements, local use history or experience, anticipated volume of use, and anticipated time to restocking or resupply of antidote.[16] This need to understand the local ecology extends to specific clinical practice areas as well. For example, oncologic centers should address their need for leucovorin, glucarpidase, and uridine triacetate. This review should also include addressing access to specialty antidotes for other oncologic conditions, such as extravasation, that are not typically included on antidote lists, for example, dexrazoxane and sodium thiosulfate for extravasation, amifostine for radiotherapy and cisplatin bladder toxicity, mesna for cyclophosphamide and ifosfamide bladder toxicity, and colony-stimulating and growth factors (eg, darbepoetin alfa, erythropoietin, granulocyte colony-stimulating factor, granulocyte-macrophage colony-stimulating factor, oprelvekin, and palifermin).

Table SC1–1 summarizes our recommendations for the availability and storage of necessary antidotes. To achieve these goals of adequate stockings, several strategies are provided in Table SC2–2.

TABLE SC1–1   Antidote Stocking: Indications, Availability, and Storage[16,35,65]

Antidote (Generic Name)	Indications	Recommended Stocking Level (24 h)	Storage Information	Immediately Available	Available <60 min
Acetylcysteine IV (N-Acetylcysteine)	APAP and other causes of hepatotoxicity	20% IV solution 6 × 30 mL	Store unopened vials at 20°C–25°C (68°F–77°F). Do not use previously opened vials.	N	Y
Acetylcysteine, oral	APAP toxicity	20% oral solution 7 × 30 mL + 7 × 10 mL	Use diluted preparation within 1 h.	N	Y
Activated charcoal	Xenobiotic adsorption	4 bottles, 50 g each 2 bottles, 25 g each	Store in closed container at room temperature away from heat, direct light, and moisture.	Y	Y
Antivenom (Centruroides)	Scorpion envenomation	3 vials or local zoo access	Store at room temperature (up to 25°C [77°F]). Brief temperature excursions are permitted up to 40°C (104°F). DO NOT FREEZE.	N	Y
Antivenom (Crotalidae)	Crotalinae snake envenomation	12–18 vials or zoo	Store at 2°C–8°C (36°F–46°F). Do not freeze. The product must be used within 4 h after reconstitution.	N	Y
Antivenom (Elapidae)	Coral snake envenomation	Local zoo access		N	Y
Antivenom (Latrodectus mactans)	Black widow spider envenomation	Local zoo access		N	N
Atropine	Bradydysrhythmias, cholinesterase inhibitor toxicity	165 mg (available in 0.4 mg/mL, 1 mg/mL solution for injection and a variety of concentrations as auto-injectors and prefilled syringes)	Protect from light and store in airtight containers.	Y	Y
Benztropine	Acute dystonia	3 × 2 mL, 1 mg/mL	Store at room temperature away from moisture and heat.	Y	Y
Botulinum antitoxin	Botulism	CDC or Health Department		N	N
Calcium disodium EDTA	Lead	2 × 5 mL, 200 mg/mL	Store at 15°C–30°C (59°F–86°F).	N	N
Calcium chloride/gluconate	Oxalates, fluoride, hydrofluoric acid, ethylene glycol, calcium channel blockers, β-adrenergic antagonist, hypermagnesemia, hypocalcemia	Ca gluconate 4.65 mEq (1 g)/10 mL—30 vials (preferred) $CaCl_2$ 13.6 mEq (1 g)/10 mL—10 vials	Store at 15°C–30°C (59°F–86°F).	Y	Y
Calcium trisodium pentetate (calcium DTPA)	Internal contamination with radioactive plutonium, americium, curium	200 mg/mL 5 mL × 1	Store at 15°C–30°C (59°F–86°F).	N	N
Cyproheptadine	Serotonin toxicity	36 mg (4 mg tablets or 2 mg/5 mL syrup)	Store at 15°C–30°C (59°F–86°F) in a well-closed container.	N	N
Coagulation factor Xa (recombinant), inactivated-zhzo	Rivaroxaban or apixaban reversal	18 × 100 mg vials	Store at 2°C-8°C (36°F-46°F). Do not freeze.	Y	Y
Dantrolene	Malignant hyperthermia	50 × 20 mg vials or Ryanodex 4 × 250 mg vials	Avoid excessive heat over 40°C (104°F).	Y	Y
Deferoxamine mesylate	Iron	12 × 500 mg vials	Do not store above 25°C (77°F).	N	Y
Dextrose ($D_{50}W$)	Hypoglycemia	10 × 50 mL (25 g)	Store at 15°C–30°C (59°F–86°F).	Y	Y
Digoxin-specific antibody fragments	Cardioactive steroids	15 vials	Refrigerate at 2°C–8°C (36°F–46°F). After reconstitution, store at 2°C–8°C (36°F–46°F) for up to 4 h.	Y	Y
Dimercaprol	Arsenic, lead, mercury	8 × 3 mL, 100 mg/mL	Store at 20°C–25°C (68°F–77°F).	N	Y
Diphenhydramine	Acute dystonia, histamine receptor blockade	10 × 1 mL, 50 mg/mL	Control room temperature at 15°C–30°C (59°F–86°F). Avoid freezing and light.	Y	Y
Ethanol, oral	Methanol, ethylene glycol, diethylene glycol	1 bottle of 40%/16 oz	Store at room temperature.	N	Y
Flumazenil	Benzodiazepines	6 × 10 mL, 0.1 mg/mL	Store at 15°C–30°C (59°F–86°F).	Y	Y

(Continued)

TABLE SC1–1   Antidote Stocking: Indications, Availability, and Storage[16,35,65] (Continued)

Antidote (Generic Name)	Indications	Recommended Stocking Level (24 h)	Storage Information	Immediately Available	Available <60 min
Fomepizole	Ethylene glycol, methanol, diethylene glycol	4 × 1.5 mL, 1 g/mL	Store at controlled room temperature, 20°C–25° C (68°F–77°F).	N	Y
Glucagon	β-Adrenergic antagonists, calcium channel blockers	100 × 1 mg	Store at 15°C–30°C (59°F–86°F). Use immediately after reconstituted. Discard extra.	Y	Y
Glucarpidase	Methotrexate	5 × 1,000 units/vial	Store at 36°F–46°F (2°C–°C). Do not freeze.	N	N
Hydroxocobalamin	Cyanide	2 × 5 g	Lyophilized form: Store at 15°F–30°F. Cyanokit may be exposed during short periods of temperature variations of usual transport. Reconstituted solution: Store up to 6 h at temperature not exceeding 104°F (40°C). Do not freeze. Discard any unused portion after 6 h.	Y	Y
Idarucizumab	Dabigatran	2 × 50 mL, 2.5 g/50 mL	Store in the refrigerator at 2°C–8°C (36°F–46°F). Do not freeze. Do not shake. Before use, the unopened vial may be kept at room temperature 25°C (77°F) for up to 48 h, if stored in the original package, to protect from light or up to 6 h when exposed to light.	Y	Y
Insulin, regular	Calcium channel blockers, β-adrenergic antagonists	20 × 10 mL 100 units/mL	Store unopened containers in refrigerator at 2°C–8°C (36°F–46°F). Do not freeze. Vial in use may be stored under refrigeration or at room temperature; store below 30°C (86°F) away from direct heat or light.	Y	Y
Leucovorin calcium/folinic acid	Methotrexate, methanol	2 × 50 mL, 10 mg/mL	Store at 2°C–8°C. Refrigerate; do not freeze. Protect from light.	N	Y
L-carnitine	Valproic acid	15 × 5 mL, 1 g/5 mL	Store vials at 25°C. Discard unused portion of an opened vial.	N	Y
Lipid emulsion	Local anesthetics	1 × 1,000 mL 20% + 1 × 250 mL 20%	Store below 25°C; do not freeze. Emulsions that have been frozen should be discarded.	Y	Y
Methylene blue	Methemoglobinemia	6 × 10 mL, 10 mg/mL	Store at 20°–25°C (68°–77°F).	Y	Y
Naloxone	Opioids	10 × 1 mL, 0.4 mg/mL 30 × 2 mL, 1 mg/mL	Store at 20°–25°C (68°–77°F); protect from light.	Y	Y
Octreotide	Sulfonylureas	5 × 1 mL, 50 mcg/mL	Store in refrigerator at 2°C–8 °C for prolonged storage. Protect from light. At 20°C–30°C or 70°F–86°F), it is stable for 14 days if protected from light.	N	Y
Physostigmine	Anticholinergics	4 × 2 mL, 1 mg/mL	Store unopened vial at 15°C–30°C.	Y	Y
Phytonadione/vitamin K₁	Warfarin, rodenticide toxicity	10 × 1 mL, 10 mg/mL; 20 × 5 mg tablets	Store in the tight, light-resistant, original container at 15°C–30°C.Protect from light.	Y	Y
Polyethylene glycol electrolyte lavage solution	Gastrointestinal decontamination	10 L	Store in sealed container at 59°–86°F. When reconstituted, keep solution refrigerated. Use within 48 h. Discard unused portion.	Y	Y
Potassium iodide	Radioactive iodine	1 × 30 mL, 65 mg/mL (use with accompanying dropper)	Store at 25°C (77°F). Excursions permitted to 15°C–30°C (59°–86°F). Keep container tightly closed. Keep in carton protected from light.	N	Y
Pralidoxime	Cholinesterase inhibitor (organic phosphorus compounds, carbamates)	18 × 1-g vials	Store at controlled room temperature 20°C–25° C (68°F–77° F).	N	Y

(Continued)

TABLE SC1–1   Antidote Stocking: Indications, Availability, and Storage[16,35,65]   (Continued)

Antidote (Generic Name)	Indications	Recommended Stocking Level (24 h)	Storage Information	Immediately Available	Available <60 min
Protamine	Heparin	4 × 25 mL, 10 mg/mL 4 vials 50 mg/5 mL	Store at 15°C–30°C. Do not freeze.	Y	Y
Prothrombin complex concentrate (three-factor) Prothrombin complex concentrate (four-factor) and vitamin K₁	Vitamin K antagonist–induced anticoagulation; coagulopathy from other direct oral anticoagulants	5 × 1,000 units	Store at 2–25°C (36–77°F) (this includes room temperature); not to exceed 25°C (77°F). Do not freeze.	Y	Y
Prussian blue	Thallium, cesium	18 g (36 caps)	Store in the dark at 25°C (77°F), excursions permitted to 15°C–30°C (59°F–86°F).	N	N
Pyridoxine	Ethylene glycol, isoniazid, *Gyromitrin* mushroom toxicity	15 g 150 × 1 mL, 100 mg/mL	Store at room temperature away from moisture and heat.	Y	Y
Sodium bicarbonate	Cyclic antidepressants, salicylates, metabolic acidosis	10 vials or syringes (~50 mEq/50 mL)	Store at 15°C–30°C; freezing should be avoided.	Y	Y
Sodium nitrite Sodium thiosulfate Hydroxocobalamin preferred	Cyanide	2 × 10 mL, 30 mg/mL 2 × 50 mL, 250 mg/mL	Protect from direct light. Do not freeze. Store at controlled room temperature between 20°C and 25°C (68°F–77°F); excursions permitted to 15°C–30°C (59°F–86°F).	Y	Y
Succimer	Arsenic, lead, mercury	30 × 100 mg capsules	Store between 15°C and 25°C and avoid excessive heat.	N	Y
Sugammadex	Reversal of neuromuscular blockade induced by rocuronium and vecuronium	4 × 5 mL, 100 mg/mL	Store at 25°C (77°F); excursions permitted to 15°C to 30°C (59°F to 86°F)	Y	Y
Thiamine	Thiamine deficiency, Wernicke-Korsakoff syndrome, ethylene glycol	8 × 2 mL, 100 mg/mL	Store in tight, light-resistant containers at a temperature <40°C, preferably between 15°C and 30°C.	Y	Y
Uridine triacetate	5-Fluorouracil, capecitabine	4 × 10-g packets	Store at USP-controlled room temperature, 25°C (77°F); excursions permitted to 15°C–30°C (59°F–86°F).	N	N

APAP = acetaminophen; CDC = Centers for Disease Control and Prevention; DTPA = diethylenetriaminepentaacetic acid; EDTA = ethylenediaminetetraacetic acid; IV = intravenous; N = no; USP = United States Pharmacopeia; Y = yes.

TABLE SC1–2   Strategies to Address Antidote Stocking and Administration

Conduct a risk assessment (hazard vulnerability assessment or safety assessment) for antidotes.

Establish dedicated spaces within emergency departments, critical care areas, and the main pharmacy for antidote stocking.

Ensure close contact and communication with regional poison control centers that may be able to assist with antidote procurement (ie, Antivenom Index), guide appropriate antidote dosing and substitution, and assist in managing poisoned patients.

Establish a systematic mechanism for evaluating antidotal stocks, dating procedures, and resupply.

Establish surveillance mechanisms and written policies and procedures for potential antidote and medication shortages.

Establish local and regional strategies for antidote sharing and distribution.

Establish local and regional strategies for patient transfer to sites with toxicologic expertise.

Coordinate with prehospital and EMS providers antidote administration and transport guidelines (eg, atropine, hydroxocobalamin, naloxone, pralidoxime, sodium nitrite, sodium thiosulfate).

Coordinate, align, and integrate antidote stocking and policies with hospital, local, and regional disaster plans (eg, atropine, botulism antitoxin, calcium trisodium pentetate, hydroxocobalamin, potassium iodide, pralidoxime, Prussian blue, sodium nitrite, sodium thiosulfate).

Establish written policies and procedures for unfamiliar antidotes.

Establish written policies and procedures to anticipate emergent requests for formulary additions for antidotal substitutions.

Establish and implement an approved medication substitution protocol, to include staff communication and education.

Monitor the effects of medication substitution.

EMS = emergency medical services.
Recommendations are derived from references 3, 5, 30, 56.

REFERENCES

1. Abbott V, et al. Access in New Zealand to antidotes for accidental and intentional drug poisonings. *J Prim Health Care.* 2012;4:100-105.

2. Al-Sohaim SI, et al. Evaluate the impact of hospital types on the availability of antidotes for the management of acute toxic exposures and poisonings in Malaysia. *Hum Exp Toxicol.* 2012;31:274-281.

3. American College of Medical Toxicology. Institutions housing venomous animals. *J Med Toxicol.* 2015;11:155-156.

4. American College of Medical Toxicology. ACMT position statement: addressing the rising cost of prescription antidotes. *J Med Toxicol.* 2017, Nov 28. [Epub ahead of print.]

5. American College of Medical Toxicology, American Academy of Clinical Toxicology. Antidote shortages in the USA: impact and response. *J Med Toxicol.* 2015;11:144-146.

6. American Heart Association Inc. Our policy positions. access to care—other policy statements. Cardiovascular Drug Shortages. 2017. http://www.heart.org/HEARTORG/Advocate/Our-Policy-Positions_UCM_450349_Article.jsp - .WfbHNRQwcdq. Accessed October 30, 2017.

7. American Hospital Association. AHA survey on drug shortages: American Hospital Association. 2011. http://www.aha.org/content/11/drugshortagesurvey.pdf. Accessed October 30, 2017.

8. American Hospital Association. Small volume parenteral medication shortages: strategies for conservation. 2017. http://www.aha.org/advocacy-issues/tools-resources/advisory/2017/171025-quality-advisory-medication-shortages.pdf. Accessed October 30, 2017.

9. American Medical Association. Drug Shortages. 2017. https://www.ama-assn.org/delivering-care/drug-shortages. Accessed October 30, 2017.

10. American Society of Health-System Pharmacists. Drug shortages list. Current drug shortage bulletins: American Society of Health-System Pharmacists. 2017. http://www.ashp.org/menu/DrugShortages/CurrentShortages.aspx. Accessed October 29, 2017.

11. Anonymous. Food and Drug Administration Safety and Innovation Act (FDASIA). Public Law 112-144, 126 Stat. 993. http://wwwgovtrackus/congress/bills/112/s3187/text. Accessed 14 August 2012.

12. Bailey B, Bussieres JF. Antidote availability in Quebec hospital pharmacies: impact of N-acetylcysteine and naloxone consumption. *Can J Clin Pharmacol.* 2000;7:198-204.

13. Burda AM, et al. Inadequate pyridoxine stock and its effect on patient outcome. *Am J Ther.* 2007;14:262-264.

14. Caulder CR, et al. Impact of drug shortages on health system pharmacies in the southeastern united states. *Hosp Pharm.* 2015;50:279-286.

15. Chyka PA, Conner HG. Availability of antidotes in rural and urban hospitals in Tennessee. *Am J Hosp Pharm.* 1994;51:1346-1348.

16. Dart RC, et al. Expert consensus guidelines for stocking of antidotes in hospitals that provide emergency care. *Ann Emerg Med.* 2018;71:314-325.e1.

17. Dart RC, et al. Insufficient stocking of poisoning antidotes in hospital pharmacies. *JAMA.* 1996;276:1508-1510.

18. Eddleston M, et al. Deaths due to absence of an affordable antitoxin for plant poisoning. *Lancet.* 2003;362:1041-1044.

19. Food and Drug Administration. Sodium nitrite injection and sodium thiosulfate injection drug products labeled for the treatment of cyanide poisoning: enforcement action dates. *Fed Reg.* 2012;77:71006-1008.

20. Gabrielli A, et al. The tragedy of the commons—drug shortages and our patients' health. *Am J Med.* 2016 Oct 28. pii: S0002-9343(31013-0. [Epub ahead of print].

21. Gasco L, et al. Insufficient stocking of cyanide antidotes in US hospitals that provide emergency care. *J Pharmacol Pharmacother.* 2013;4:95-102.

22. Gorman SK, et al. Antidote stocking in British Columbia hospitals. *CJEM.* 2003;5:12-17.

23. Greenberg MI, et al. Emergency department preparedness for the evaluation and treatment of victims of biological or chemical terrorist attack. *J Emerg Med.* 2002;22:273-278.

24. Gupta R, et al. The FDA Unapproved Drugs Initiative: an observational study of the consequences for drug prices and shortages in the United States. *J Manag Care Spec Pharm.* 2017;23:1066-1076.

25. Heindel GA, et al. Rising cost of antidotes in the U.S.: cost comparison from 2010 to 2015. *Clin Toxicol (Phila).* 2017;55:360-363.

26. Howland MA, et al. Nonavailability of poison antidotes. *N Engl J Med.* 1986;314:927-928.

27. Hsia IK, et al. Survey of the National Drug Shortage Effect on Anesthesia and Patient Safety: a patient perspective. *Anesth Analg.* 2015;121:502-506.

28. Institute for Safe Medication Practices. 2016-2017 targeted medication safety best practices for hospitals. Horsham, PA Institute for Safe Medication Practices. 2017. https://www.ismp.org/tools/bestpractices/TMSBP-for-Hospitals.pdf. Accessed October 28, 2017.

29. Juurlink DN, et al. Availability of antidotes at acute care hospitals in Ontario. *CMAJ.* 2001;165:27-30.

30. Kearney TE. New Antidotes for Poisoning and Overdose Kearney TE. Therapeutic Drugs and Antidotes. In: Eds. Olson KR, Anderson IB, Benowitz NL, et al. Poisoning and Drug Overdose, 7th ed. McGraw-Hill Education, New York, NY, 2018. https://accessmedicine.mhmedical.com/content.aspx?bookid=2284&sectionid=177338518 Last accessed July 25, 2018..

31. Keim ME, et al. Lack of hospital preparedness for chemical terrorism in a major US city: 1996-2000. *Prehosp Disaster Med.* 2003;18:193-199.

32. Kesselheim AS, et al. The high cost of prescription drugs in the United States: origins and prospects for reform. *JAMA.* 2016;316:858-871.

33. Khot UN, et al. Nitroprusside and isoproterenol use after major price increases. *N Engl J Med.* 2017;377:594-595.

34. Mansour A, et al. National study on the adequacy of antidotes stocking in Lebanese hospitals providing emergency care. *BMC Pharmacol Toxicol.* 2016;17:51.

35. Marraffa JM, et al. Antidotes for toxicological emergencies: a practical review. *Am J Health Syst Pharm.* 2012;69:199-212.

36. Mazer-Amirshahi M, et al. U.S. drug shortages for medications used in adult critical care (2001-2016). *J Crit Care.* 2017;41:283-288.

37. Mazer-Amirshahi M, et al. Drug shortages: implications for medical toxicology. *Clin Toxicol (Phila).* 2015;53:519-524.

38. McFee RB, et al. Understocking antidotes for common toxicologic emergencies: a neglected public health problem. *Adv Stud Med.* 2005;5:262-263.

39. McLaughlin M, et al. Effects on patient care caused by drug shortages: a survey. *J Manag Care Pharm.* 2013;19:783-788.

40. Morrow LE, et al. Acute isoniazid toxicity and the need for adequate pyridoxine supplies. *Pharmacotherapy.* 2006;26:1529-1532.

41. Mowry JB, et al. 2015 Annual report of the American Association of Poison Control Centers' National Poison Data System (NPDS): 33rd annual report. *Clin Toxicol (Phila).* 2016;54:924-1109.

42. Murphy NG, et al. A system-wide solution to antidote stocking in emergency departments: the Nova Scotia antidote program. *CJEM.* 2017, Sep 20:1-10. [Epub ahead of print].

43. Neavyn MJ, et al. Sodium acetate as a replacement for sodium bicarbonate in medical toxicology: a review. *J Med Toxicol.* 2013;9:250-254.

44. New York State Poison Centers. *Alternatives for Sodium Bicarbonate Shortage.* New York, NY: New York State Poison Centers; 2017.

45. Nogue S, et al. Antidotes: availability, use and cost in hospital and extra-hospital emergency services of Catalonia (Spain). *Arch Toxicol Suppl.* 1997;19:299-304.

46. Ong HC, et al. Inadequate stocking of antidotes in Taiwan: is it a serious problem? *J Toxicol Clin Toxicol.* 2000;38:21-28.

47. Pettit HE, et al. Toxicology cart for stocking sufficient supplies of poisoning antidotes. *Am J Health Syst Pharm.* 1999;56:2537-2539.

48. Plataki M, et al. Availability of antidotes in hospital pharmacies in Greece. *Vet Hum Toxicol.* 2001;43:103-105.

49. Santucci KA, et al. Acute isoniazid exposures and antidote availability. *Pediatr Emerg Care.* 1999;15:99-101.

50. Silverman E. Doctors have toxic reaction to Valent pricing for a lead poisoning drug. Boston, MA: STAT. 2016. https://www.statnews.com/pharmalot/2016/10/11/valeant-drug-prices-lead-poisoning/. Accessed October 30, 2017.

51. Sivilotti ML, et al. Can emergency departments not afford to carry essential antidotes? *CJEM.* 2002;4:23-33.

52. Stock RP, et al. Bringing antivenoms to sub-saharan Africa. *Nat Biotechnol.* 2007;25:173-177.

53. Teresi WM, King WD. Survey of the stocking of poison antidotes in Alabama hospitals. *South Med J.* 1999;92:1151-1156.

54. Thanacoody RH, et al. National audit of antidote stocking in acute hospitals in the UK. *Emerg Med J.* 2013;30:393-396.

55. The Joint Commission. Revisions to the medication management standards regarding sample medications: The Joint Commission. 2013. http://www.jointcommission.org/assets/1/6/samplemedications_hap.pdf. Accessed October 28, 2017.

56. The Joint Commission. Standards FAQ details. Emergency cart—medication security. 2017. https://www.jointcommission.org/standards_information/jcfaqdetails.aspx?StandardsFAQId=1378. Accessed October 28, 2017.

57. The Joint Commission. Medication management (MM) (critical access hospitals/critical access hospitals). Medication selection and procurement—managing medication shortages. What are The Joint Commission requirements for managing medication shortages? 2017. https://www.jointcommission.org/standards_information/jcfaqdetails.aspx?StandardsFAQId=1530&StandardsFAQChapterId=27&ProgramId=0&ChapterId=0&IsFeatured=False&IsNew=False&Keyword=. Accessed October 28, 2017.

58. US Food and Drug Administration. Executive summary: a review of FDA's approach to medical product shortages. Silver Spring, MD: US Department of Health & Human Services. 2011. https://www.fda.gov/aboutfda/reportsmanualsforms/reports/ucm277744.htm. Accessed October 30, 2017.

59. US Department of Homeland Security. Target capabilities list. A companion to the National Preparedness Guidelines. 2007. http://wwwfemagov/pdf/government/training/tclpdf. Accessed August 14, 2012.

60. US Department of Veterans Affairs. VA National Center for Patient Safety: Patient Safety Assessment Tool (PSAT) [software tool]. Washington DC: US Department of Veterans Affairs. 2017. https://www.patientsafety.va.gov/professionals/onthejob/assessment.asp. Accessed October 29, 2017.

61. VA National Center for Patient Safety: Safety Assessment Code (SAC) Matrix. Washington DC: US Department of Veterans Affairs. 2017. https://www.patientsafety.va.gov/professionals/publications/matrix.asp. Accessed October 30, 2017.

62. Vail E, et al. Association between US norepinephrine shortage and mortality among patients with septic shock. *JAMA.* 2017;317:1433-1442.

63. Wiens MO, et al. Adequacy of antidote stocking in British Columbia hospitals: the 2005 Antidote Stocking Study. *CJEM.* 2006;8:409-416.

64. Woolf AD, Chrisanthus K. On-site availability of selected antidotes: results of a survey of Massachusetts hospitals. *Am J Emerg Med.* 1997;15:62-66.

65. World Health Organization. WHO model list of essential medicines, 20th list. Geneva, Switzerland: World Health Organization. 2017. http://www.who.int/entity/medicines/publications/essentialmedicines/20th_EML2017_FINAL_amendedAug2017.pdf?ua=1. Accessed October 28, 2017.

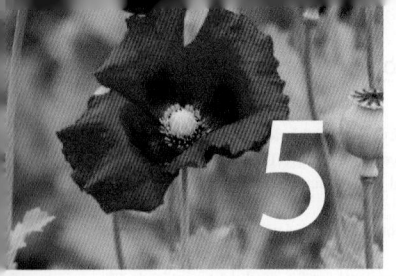

5 TECHNIQUES USED TO PREVENT GASTROINTESTINAL ABSORPTION

Lotte C. G. Hoegberg

Gastrointestinal (GI) decontamination is a highly controversial issue in medical toxicology. It can play an essential role in the initial phase of management of orally poisoned patients and frequently is the only treatment available other than routine supportive care. Unfortunately, as is true in most areas of medical toxicology, rigorous studies that demonstrate the effects of GI decontamination on clinically meaningful endpoints are difficult to find. The heterogeneity of poisoned patients demands that very large randomized studies be performed because patients who present to an emergency department (ED) typically have both unreliable histories and low-risk exposures (Chaps. 4 and 130). These factors, as well as other significant sources of bias, are often hidden in inclusion and exclusion criteria of even the best available studies. Numerous determinants contribute to the difficulties in designing and completing studies that provide sound evidence for or against a particular therapeutic option. Incontrovertible endpoints, such as complication-specific mortality, also demand exceptionally large studies because the overall morbidity and mortality of poisoned patients are quite low (Chap. 130). Whereas other endpoints, such as the length of stay in the hospital or intensive care unit (ICU), change in xenobiotic concentration, the rate of secondary complications, such as seizures or QT interval prolongation, and the need for specific treatments requiring expensive antidotes, must all be considered, these surrogate markers are not adequately rigorous and are inadequately precise measures of morbidity. In the science of decontamination investigators are also faced with the dilemma that randomizing half of a group of potentially ill patients to no decontamination is a significant ethical concern. Acetaminophen is often used both as the xenobiotic of choice in volunteer studies[64,124,141,237,373] and in the evaluation of actually poisoned patients.[78] However, despite its widespread use as a model, the applicability of the management approach for APAP poisoning to other ingestions is limited. It is our recommendation that decontamination should rarely be omitted unless a minimally toxic exposure has occurred.

As might be suspected, no available study provides adequate guidance for the management of a patient who has definitely ingested an unknown xenobiotic at an unknown time. Fortunately, in most cases, there is some component of the history or clinical presentation, such as vital signs, physical examination, or focused diagnostic studies such as an electrocardiogram (ECG) and anion gap, that offers insight into the nature of the ingested xenobiotic (Chap. 3).

For many, the ongoing controversy or debate on GI decontamination culminated in 1997 with the publication of the position statements on activated charcoal (AC), orogastric lavage, syrup of ipecac–induced emesis, and whole-bowel irrigation (WBI) from the American Academy of Clinical Toxicology (AACT) and the European Association of Poisons Centres and Clinical Toxicologists (EAPCCT),[66,186,331,351,352] and evolved toward sequentially lesser aggressive approaches after subsequent revisions.[33,67,186,332,334, 353] Contrary to initial expectations of some, these excellent reviews failed to end the debate; they simply highlighted many shortcomings and ambiguities within the field. A 2000 study concluded that despite having the evidence reviewed and consensus recommendations made, poison specialists at North American poison control centers still offered a wide variety of recommendations for GI decontamination.[173] The study evaluated decontamination options for a theoretical patient with a serious potentially life-threatening overdose of enteric-coated aspirin. The recommendations made were often inconsistent with the published position statements and in some cases were dangerous. Even toxicologists who made substantial contributions to the development of these consensus statements disagreed

on certain aspects of the treatment but to a lesser extent. In a similar study, when an interactive questionnaire was sent to 11 European poison control centers, significant differences in the protocols for the recommended method of GI decontamination, timing, and intervention doses were found.[122] Subsequently published locally adjusted recommendations for specific xenobiotics such as APAP indicate a shift away from the position statements.[61,151] Although the revisions include some new evidence, these differences suggest that there is still inadequate evidence available to produce a proper evidence-based answer for many of the clinical decisions we face. In most of the clinical studies that provide evidence to form the basis for the consensus statements and subsequent works, the proportion of patients with life-threatening ingestions is very small, the exclusion criteria were too broad, or the health care delivery model was too limited to provide widespread applicability to currently poisoned patients. Similarly, there are few or no studies for most drugs with modified release kinetics or altered kinetics in overdose; for the never-ending flood of newly marketed pharmaceuticals; and for patients with mixed overdoses, extremes of age, or significant end-organ dysfunction. Thus, clinicians must often make decisions based on a theoretical approach emphasizing an understanding of basic principles rather than evidence with a substantial level of uncertainty.

The reported trends in the use of GI decontamination demonstrate a continued decline in the United States (Chap. 130). The frequency of AC use declined from 4.6% of all exposures in 2006 to 1.97% in 2015, and a similar decline was observed in the frequency of orogastric lavage (4.2% in 2006 to 0.08% in 2015) and WBI (0.11% in 2006 to 0.08% in 2015) (Chap. 130). The decline in the use of GI decontamination likely results from an epidemiologic shift in the developed countries away from overdoses of more difficult to treat or more lethal xenobiotics, such as salicylates, theophylline, barbiturates, and tricyclic antidepressants, toward benzodiazepines, prescription opioids, serotonergic reuptake inhibitors, and APAP, with a natural resultant decrease in morbidity and mortality or the availability of an excellent antidote. Although true for the developed countries, studies in developing countries indicate a different pattern of poisonings, with patients ingesting xenobiotics such as organic phosphorus compounds and other pesticides and herbicides with a more lethal toxicologic profile.[46,92,93]

Similar to the overall trend in decontamination, the use of orogastric lavage is continually declining (Chap. 130).[196] The frequency of orogastric lavage varies from lowest frequency (percent of lavage compared with total decontaminations using AC, orogastric lavage, and WBI) in North America (0.08%, US) (Chap. 130) and Scandinavia (7.9%–9%; Denmark and Norway),[207,367] in Mediterranean countries and Russia (30%–33%; Spain, Palestine, and Russia),[14,184,197,304] to the highest frequency in Asia and South American countries, India (34%–50%),[35,159,203,240] Nepal (43%),[47] and Bolivia (96%).[105] As noted earlier, the frequency tends to correlate with the type of xenobiotic ingested, with highest frequency of lavage in regions where insecticides such as organic phosphorus compounds and carbamates are more commonly ingested.[35,47,105,159] Additionally, the use of decontamination seems to correlate inversely with availability of costly antidotes and ICUs. Numbers available on cause of death in the different regions of the world are estimates at best because data gaps are common because of the limited functionality of existing death-registration systems.[368]

This chapter does not discuss details with regard to the risk assessment and general principles of managing acutely poisoned or overdosed patients;

these issues are discussed in Chap. 4. Rather, the focus is on when to do GI decontamination and what to do, that is, determining which decontamination technique or combination of techniques is preferred after an indication for GI decontamination is established. The literature published since the previous edition of this book is emphasized, existing evidence is summarized, and areas necessitating further investigation are identified. Detailed discussions of AC and WBI are found in the corresponding Antidotes in Depth sections, Activated Charcoal (Antidotes in Depth: A1) and Whole-Bowel Irrigation and Other Intestinal Evacuants (Antidotes in Depth: A2). In addition, when the ingested xenobiotic is known, readers should also refer to the decontamination sections found in Chap. 132 and Special Considerations SC2, which offer insight into xenobiotic-specific issues that may alter decontamination strategies.

The efficacy of techniques used to prevent absorption of xenobiotics from the GI tract depend on one simple concept: At the time of the intervention, there must be enough xenobiotic in the GI tract to alter the patient's outcome if absorbed. Although this is a very simple requirement, in reality, it is almost never known, but rather is inferred from the history, particular formulation of the xenobiotic, and clinical findings. Because the concept of time is so critical to an understanding of the role of GI decontamination, this will be discussed before the individual techniques are described.

TIME

The most common route of exposure in poisoning in the United States continues to be ingestion (Chap. 130). Similar information on routes of exposure cannot be extracted from the data available from other parts of the world.[104,368] After ingestion, rates of absorption of pharmaceuticals are based on pharmacokinetic studies that are typically performed on fasting healthy human volunteers given a minimal number of pills with a small amount of liquid. In contrast, most overdose patients take large numbers of pills with some liquid or food. Gastric emptying time is prolonged by the presence of food or other solids compared with liquid.[300] Whereas gastric emptying of liquids begins instantly in an exponential fashion, for solids, a linear emptying phase begins after a lag phase.[50,183]

The short (1-hour) time frame when it is theoretically possible to obtain a clinical beneficial effect from GI decontamination that was initially recommended in the position statements[33,67,353] or clinical studies[72] is now being challenged,[171,205,230,266,285] and guidelines for certain xenobiotics such as APAP reinforce the acceptability of delayed GI decontamination especially in the setting of massive single dose ingestions (>30 g) or modified release preparation ingestions.[61,62]

Case reports and clinical practice demonstrate that poisoned patients still have xenobiotics in their stomachs as residuals or pharmacobezoars, from hours up to several days after ingestion and even on autopsy.[88,101,180,205,267,285] Details of a selection of these reports are summarized in Table 5–1.

In a prospective study of 85 poisoned patients, markedly prolonged gastric emptying half-lives and gastric hypomotility were demonstrated using gastric scintigraphy (Table 5–1).[1] The authors speculated that stress in an overdosed patient might be part of the etiology of the hypomotility observed and that the management of patients should not be based on the assumption that GI motility is normal.

The most meaningful study was a systematic attempt to evaluate the residual contents of the stomach using upper GI endoscopy in 167 adult patients presenting to an ED after an oral drug overdose.[230] The results demonstrate that residual gastric contents were found in 60% of the patients presenting more than 1 hour after the tablet ingestion and was classified as either tablet or soluble.[230] In fact, many patients had significant material remaining in the stomach hours later (Table 5–1).

Finally, in a review of 1,038 autopsies, 92 (9%) showed tablet or capsule residues in the GI tract. Although the time from ingestion to death could not be determined, data showed several cases in which it was estimated that death occurred more than 1 hour after ingestion[205] (Table 5–1).

Collectively, these data challenge both the position statement recommendations[33,67] and the general practice because they evaluate the

patient's actual phase of gastric emptying before the initiation of GI decontamination rather than studying the retrieval efficiency. The results emphasize the impact of well-validated imaging studies attempting to confirm the presence of medication (tablets or capsules) or liquid contents in the stomach of overdosed patients that support existing case reports and case series.[179,180,229,231,252,285,326,374]

Although the ability of xenobiotics to be removed by orogastric lavage is variable and unknown, the ability to prevent absorption by adsorption of the xenobiotic to AC is likely also beneficial far later than the time frame that is widely promoted.[230] The time before maximum absorption is reached depends on several factors. These include but are not limited to, patient-specific variables such as gut perfusion, the nature of the xenobiotic (medication, plant, or mushroom materials, chemical, etc.) physical characteristic (physical state, formulation, solubility, ionization, etc.), ingested amount, and presence of other material or coingestants in the GI tract. Further special considerations should be taken into account regarding medications. The estimated time to maximum absorption depends on the pharmaceutical preparation (liquid or solid preparation, dissolution of solid preparations, immediate- versus extended-release tablets or capsules), the nature of the active pharmaceutical ingredient (leading to increased or reduced gastric emptying), and the volume or amount of ingested xenobiotics.

Absorption from solid preparations is generally slower than liquid preparations, as a disintegration step precedes the xenobiotic dissolution that is required to be ready for absorption. In addition, extended-release tablets and capsules are designed to disintegrate or release drug more slowly than their immediate-release counterparts. These effects cause both a delayed onset of symptoms and prolonged toxicity in overdoses compared with therapeutic use. Usual treatment nomograms calculated for immediate release formulations of some xenobiotics such as APAP, are not appropriate for controlled-release formulations because the absorption phase is prolonged, and the time to maximum plasma concentration is correspondingly prolonged.[299] Furthermore, the maximum blood concentrations obtained after the ingestion of a specific dose of an extended-release formulation will most probably not rise as high as for the same dose of an immediate-release preparation.

The formulation of the extended-release tablet is critical to the risk of development of a pharmacobezoar.[285,286] Many different extended-release drug delivery systems are available.[250] They include hydrophilic matrix systems, in which the polymeric coating swells in contact with an aqueous medium to form a gel layer on the surface of the tablet (Fig. 5–1), which tends to cause tablet adherence in aqueous acidic media (Fig. 5–2).[286] This adherence is also recognized in case reports associated with the formation of pharmacobezoars.[24,285,312] The active xenobiotic is ultimately released by dissolution, diffusion, or erosion.[209,250]

Extended-release preparations or xenobiotics known to slow gastric transit time were the predominantly retained xenobiotics in the retrospective review of autopsy reports.[205] Gastroscopy revealed pharmacobezoar formations in approximately 50% of the cases after ingestion of quetiapine extended-release tablets.[285] The formation of pharmacobezoars necessitates treatment recommendations based on nonexistent toxicologic data, and recommendations for the management of immediate-release pharmaceuticals are without utility.[61,151,299] The release of xenobiotic(s) retained within the pharmacobezoar is slower compared with the release from individual tablets because the surface-to-volume ratio is lower, thereby reducing the rate of dissolution.[19,145,286] The time to appearance of symptoms in the patient is expected to be both delayed and prolonged and the maximum serum concentration possibly lower, but as long as the xenobiotic(s) remains in the pharmacobezoar, continuous release will occur. There are no specific rules that adequately predict when pharmacobezoars form or in which patients they form, and after they have formed, pharmacobezoars are difficult to identify.[320] Evidence of continuing absorption should raise suspicion for pharmacobezoar formation. The most effective methods of GI dissolution of pharmacobezoars are yet to be explored.[39,320]

TABLE 5–1	Evidence to Suggest a Utility of Gastrointestinal Decontamination Beyond 1 Hour Postingestion				
Author	**Citation**	**Study Method**	**Outcome Measure**	**Main Result**	**Comments**
Volunteer Data					
Christophersen et al. 2002	64	RCT, cross-over study ($n = 12$); APAP 50 mg/kg, either given alone (control) or with AC 50 g at 1 or 2 h.	PK parameters for APAP: AUC_{0-inf}, C_{max}, t_{max}, and $t_{1/2}$ calculated to evaluate the effects of AC on APAP absorption.	AC at 1 h reduced APAP AUC by 66% at 1 h compared with control; AC at 2 h reduced APAP AUC by 22.7% compared with control.	AC was effective in reducing the systemic absorption of APAP when administered both 1 and 2 h after ingestion.
Green et al. 2001	124	RCT, crossover study ($n = 10$); compared four groups given 4 g of APAP either alone (control) or with AC 50 g at 1, 2, or 3 h postdose.	PKs were calculated to evaluate the effects of AC on APAP absorption.	Only the 1-h group was significantly different from control, showing a 30.3% in AUC.	Benefits from AC administered 1 h after APAP; AC at 2 or 3 h had no significant effect.
Ollier et al. 2017	257	RCT, crossover study ($n = 12$); compared 4 groups given 40 mg of rivaroxaban either administered alone (control) or with AC 50 g at 2, 5, or 8 h postdose.	PKs were calculated to evaluate if AC interfered with rivaroxaban absorption. Estimated PKs were further investigated at 14, 20, and 26 h by nonlinear mixed-effect PK modeling.	AC at 2, 5, and 8 h significantly reduced rivaroxaban AUC by 43%, 31%, and 29%, respectively. Modeling at 14, 20, and 26 h showed reductions in AUC of 23%, 16%, and 10%, respectively.	Benefits of AC up to 8 h and possibly beyond likely secondary to the prolonged absorption profile of rivaroxaban, incomplete initial dissolution, and possible enteroenteric recycling.
Sato et al. 2003	303	RCT ($n = 46$); APAP 2 g in 13; 3 g in 33 volunteers. After 3 h, half of the participants received 75 g of AC.	Serum APAP concentrations at 4 and 7 h after the administration were compared.	APAP concentrations in the AC group were reduced by 23% at 4 h and by 62% at 7 h compared with control.	Benefits of AC administered 3 h after APAP.
Wang et al. 2014	366	RCT, crossover study ($n = 18$); compared three groups given 20 mg of apixaban either alone (control) or with AC 50 g at 2 or 6 h postdose.	PKs were calculated to evaluate the effect of AC on apixaban absorption.	AC at 2 and 6 h significantly decreased apixaban AUC by 50% and 28%, respectively, and decreased elimination half-life to 5.3 h and 4.9 h, respectively, compared with control. There was no effect of AC on C_{max} or t_{max}.	Benefits of AC up to 6 h. The reduced exposure in apixaban from AC dosing appeared by a combination of decreased bioavailability and increased elimination in the GI tract by interruption of its enteroenteric recirculation.
Yeates et al. 2000	373	RCT, crossover study ($n = 10$); compared four groups given 3 g of APAP either alone (control) or with AC 50 g at 1, 2, or 4 h postdose.	PKs were calculated to evaluate the effects of AC on APAP absorption.	AC at 1 and 2 h significantly reduced APAP AUC by 56% and 22%, respectively. At 4 h, the reduction of 8% was not significant.	Benefits of AC up to 2 h after APAP.
Actual Overdose Data					
Adams et al. 2004	1	Prospective cohort of poisoned patients who underwent gastric scintigraphy shortly after presentation and again at follow-up.	Gastric emptying half-time was compared in 104 patients at initial presentation and again in 85 at follow-up.	APAP, APAP–opioid combinations, CAs, and carbamazepine but not phenytoin had prolonged gastric emptying half-times that were significantly shorter on followup. For all patients combined, the mean gastric emptying half-time was 99.5 min on presentation vs 40 min at follow up ($P <0.0001$).	For many xenobiotics, the presence of an overdose itself decreases gastric motility and increases the likelihood of having material present in the stomach for a longer period of time. For the entire group, >50% of gastric contents present at presentation was still in the stomach 1.5 h later.
Chiew et al. 2017	62	Combined prospective observational study (two PCC) and retrospectively (three clinical toxicology unit databases) of APAP overdoses ≥40 g ingested over ≤8 h.	Acute liver injury, liver transplant, and death. APAP concentration at 4–16 h postingestion relative to 4-h standard nomogram line.	Of 200 cases, 14% developed hepatotoxicity, one liver transplant and one non-APAP–related death; AC was dosed to 25% at median of 2 h postingestion. AC within 4 h of ingestion reduced the APAP ratio and rates of hepatotoxicity compared with no AC. The APAP ratio was ≥2 in 40%, and 22% received an increased dose of acetylcysteine (200 mg/kg/16 h) in the first 21 h, significantly reducing the risk of hepatotoxicity.	AC dosed within 4 h of APAP ingestion significantly reduced APAP concentrations and risk of hepatotoxicity.
Cooper et al. 2015	80	Population PK study of sertraline overdose using data collected prospectively from 28 patients overdosed with sertraline; median dose, 1,550 mg.	PK parameters, including $t_{1/2}$, C_{max}, t_{max}, and AUC.	AC significantly increased sertraline clearance by an estimated factor of 1.9. AC significantly reduced $t_{1/2}$ and AUC of sertraline if dosed up to 4 h after drug ingestion.	PK benefits of AC up to 4 h after sertraline ingestion compared with no AC.

(Continued)

TABLE 5–1	Evidence to Suggest a Utility of Gastrointestinal Decontamination Beyond 1 Hour Postingestion (*Continued*)				
Author	*Citation*	*Study Method*	*Outcome Measure*	*Main Result*	*Comments*
Friberg et al. 2005	112	Population PK study of data from 63 citalopram overdose events in 53 patients; median dose, 270 mg. PK parameters were elicited from 14 studies on therapeutic citalopram dosing.	Comparison of AC given between 0.5 and 4 h overdose.	AC increased clearance by 72% and decreased bioavailability by 22%. In most patients, the AC was dosed more than 1 h after ingestion. Only 1 patient received AC within 1 h, 9 received AC within 1–2 h, and 7 patients received AC within 2–4 h.	Benefits of AC on clearance and relative fraction absorbed up to 4 h after citalopram ingestion.
Isbister et al. 2007	163	Prospective study describing quetiapine PK in overdose using Bayesian population PK analysis in 54 overdose events; median dose, 2,700 mg.	Comparison of AC given between 0.5 and 6 h.	PK estimated AC to reduce absorbed quetiapine fraction by 35%.	AC leads to a pronounced decrease in the relative fraction of quetiapine absorbed even when given after 1 h.
Livshits et al. 2015	205	Retrospective review of autopsy reports; cause of death was determined as *intoxication* or *overdose*. Decedents of all ages with solid drug ingestions.	Assessment of unabsorbed drug present in the GI tract and to analyze pharmacologic characteristics of retained drugs when present.	92 of 1038 autopsies had solid drug material in the GI tract; in 98%, the material was either modified-release preparations or drugs known to slow GI transit; most common were opioids and anticholinergics.	Unabsorbed drug can be found in the GI tract for a substantial time after oral drug ingestion of either modified-release preparations or substances known to slow GI tract motility.
Miyauchi et al. 2015	230	Cohort data from 167 overdoses prospectively collected. Endoscopy was performed on admission. Patients were classified into three groups; tablet/food phase, soluble/fluid phase, and reticular/empty phase.	The groups were compared with respect to time elapsed since ingestion and numbers and variety of orally overdosed drugs.	In the tablet/food group, 12 of 73 patients (16%) presented within 1 h, and 3 patients presented >12 h since ingestion. In the soluble/fluid phase group, 9 of 50 patients (18%) presented within 1 h, and 2 patients presented >12 h. In the reticular/empty phase group, 28 of 44 patients presented 1–6 h, 3 <1 h, and 13 >6 h since ingestion.	>60% of patients had substantial gastric contents >1 h after ingestion, and materials were found in 17% >4 h after ingestion.
Papazoglu et al. 2015	267	Case report in a 65-year-old patient.	Serum APAP concentration.	A combination of APAP–opioid ingestion a second APAP peak after completing 21 h of NAC. 9 h after finishing NAC, removal of the NG tube showed solid fragments in the tube lumen; continued absorption was confirmed by a serum APAP concentration.	Prolongation of NAC infusion beyond the standard protocol was necessary to prevent the development of hepatocellular damage.
Rauber-Lüthy et al. 2013	285	Case series of overdose patients undergoing gastroscopy (*n* = 9). Ingested quetiapine doses were 6–24.4 g.	Gastroscopy findings in quetiapine extended-release tablet poisonings.	The time from ingestion to gastroscopy was known in 7 cases (2.25–13 h). In all patients, gastroscopic removal of a pharmacobezoar was performed.	Tablets present in the stomach many hours postingestion.

AC = activated charcoal; APAP = acetaminophen; AUC = area under the concentration vs time curve; C_{max} = maximal concentration; GI = gastrointestinal; inf = infinity; NAC = *N*-acetylcysteine; NG = nasogastric; PCC = Poison Control Center; PK = pharmacokinetics; RCT = randomized controlled trial; $t_{1/2}$ = terminal elimination half-life; t_{max} = time to maximal concentration; TCA = tricyclic antidepressant.

OROGASTRIC LAVAGE

The principal theory governing orogastric lavage for gastric emptying is very simple: if a portion of a xenobiotic with substantial toxic potential is removed before absorption, toxicity should be either prevented or diminished. The relevant amount of xenobiotic that needs to be removed to obtain a beneficial treatment effect varies depending on the xenobiotic, the amount ingested, the overall health of the patient, and the shape of the dose–response curve for the individual xenobiotic. One group of authors defined

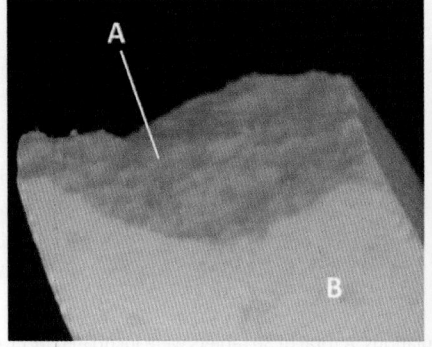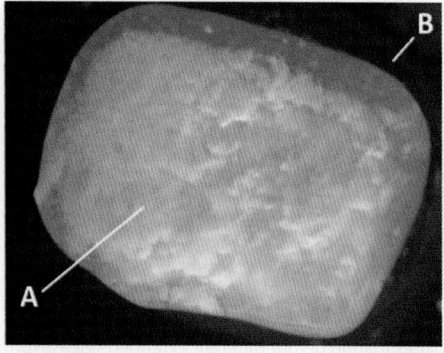

FIGURE 5-1. Acetaminophen 500-mg extended-release tablet microscopy. The tablet cut was in halves and showed as the dry tablet at the left and after incubation in 1 L of simulated gastric fluid for 4 hours at 37°C.[286] **A,** Tablet core. **B,** Hydrogel polymer coating material (*left*) forming the swelled gel-layer (*right*) surface of the tablet. (*Used with permission from Lotte C. G. Hoegberg as supervisor, mentor and collaborator with Refsgaard F, Petersen SH. In Vitro Investigation of Potential Pharmacobezoar Formation and Their Dissolution of Extended Release Tablets [master's thesis]. Copenhagen: Section of Toxicology, Department of Pharmacy, School of Pharmaceutical Sciences, Faculty of Health Sciences, University of Copenhagen; 2016.*)

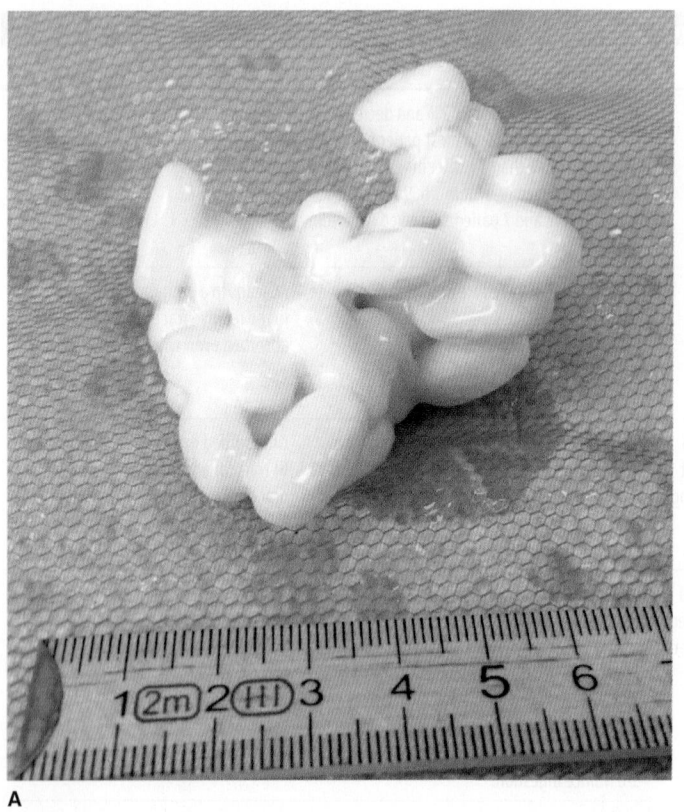

A

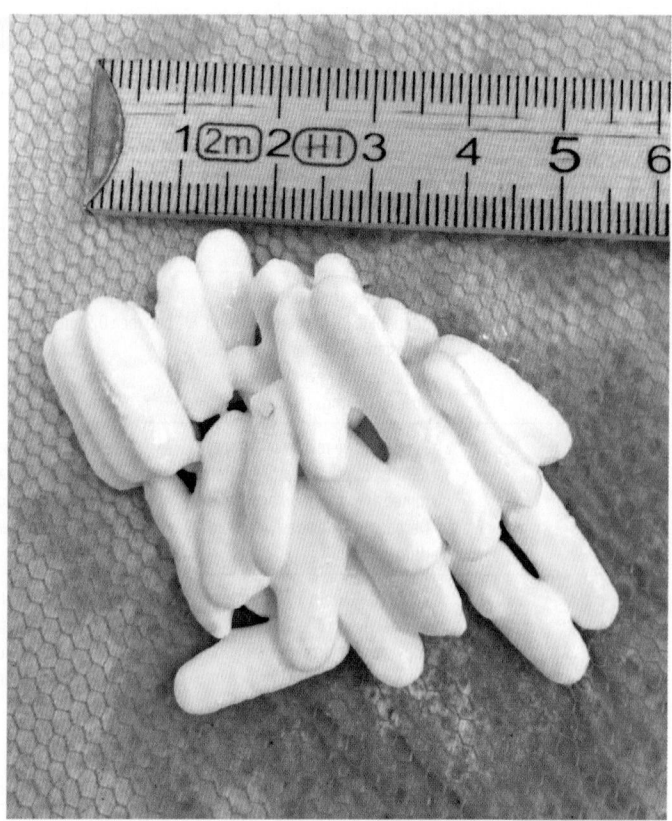

B

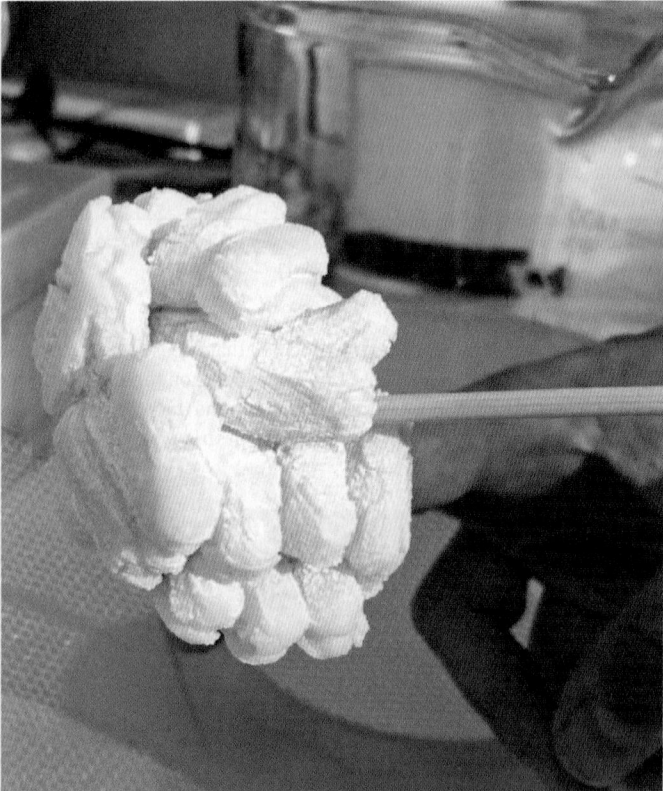

C

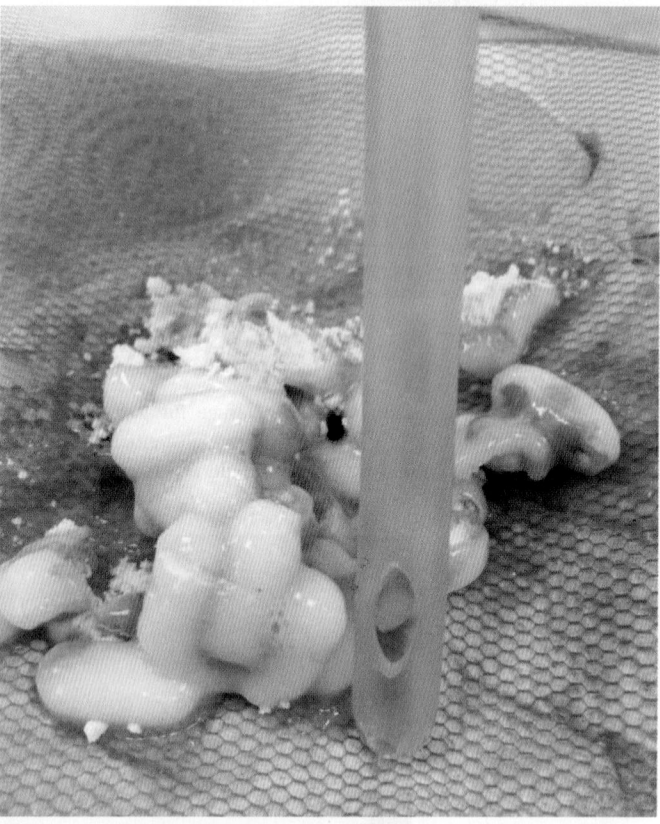

D

FIGURE 5-2. Pharmacobezoar formation of four different extended-release formulations. A total of 30 tablets were incubated in 1 L of simulated gastric fluid (Ph.Eur., omitting pepsin) for up to 48 hours at 37°C.[286] **A,** Acetaminophen extended release, 500 mg, 4 hours. **B,** Acetaminophen combined immediate and extended release, 665 mg, 4 hours. **C,** Verapamil extended release, 240 mg, 48 hours. **D,** Quetiapine extended release, 50 mg, 4 hours, and orogastric tube size 30 Fr. (*Used with permission from Lotte C. G. Hoegberg as supervisor, mentor and collaborator with Refsgaard F, Petersen SH. In Vitro Investigation of Potential Pharmacobezoar Formation and Their Dissolution of Extended Release Tablets [master's thesis]. Copenhagen: Section of Toxicology, Department of Pharmacy, School of Pharmaceutical Sciences, Faculty of Health Sciences, University of Copenhagen; 2016.*)

the efficacy of orogastric lavage by the number of therapeutic doses recovered, with more than two or more than 10 therapeutic doses representing possible and definite clinical benefit, respectively. In 76 patients poisoned by sedative–hypnotics, they reported that 10 therapeutic doses were recovered in 6.6% of the patients lavaged, and two therapeutic doses were recovered in 15.8% of the cases.[73] This approach is emphasized to highlight the confusion, given that knowing the amount recovered fails to expand understanding without knowing either the dose ingested or the dose remaining.

Even though the benefit of orogastric lavage is questionable, many publications demonstrate that there is a continued frequent or routine use of orogastric lavage, without reflection on the clinical effect obtained or fragments or volume of the xenobiotic retrieved.[3,15,39,56,68,102,119,132,133,154,160,175,187,204,211,228,236,238,280,283,296,315,318,327,370,374] Only a few authors report that actual fragments or specific volumes were retrieved during the procedure.[28,29,117,179,227,269,301,315,369] This lack of precision supports the concept that routine use of orogastric lavage should be avoided.

More than a quarter of a century ago, several important clinical trials attempted to define the role of gastric emptying in poisoned patients[10,43,72,155,188,226,279,350] (Table 5–2). Although all of these studies were limited because of the inclusion of a large number of low-risk patients, numerous restrictive exclusion criteria, and methodologic biases, they clearly demonstrated that many patients can be successfully managed without orogastric lavage. From 1995 until the present, few additional studies were published, and the series of updated position papers in 2004 and 2013 and reviews further emphasized the limited need for gastric emptying in poisoned patients.[11,33,36,41,184,185,353,375] No new clear evidence to support the clinical effectiveness of orogastric lavage is available,[40,43,60,64,72,95,103,126,127,159,188,226,279,329,330,350] and studies and reports describe a modest, varied, and unreliable effect.[89,110,125,127,157,184,193,195,200,210,295,371] The difficulties involved with attempting to evacuate ingested fragments were described in the 1970s, and a possible benefit from multiple orogastric lavage procedures was suggested.[157,316] Orogastric lavage using potassium permanganate lavage solutions or vegetable oils that were theoretically effective at protecting against the xenobiotic by change of oil–water equilibrium or chemical reaction were tried and abandoned because of variably poor efficacy.[4,215,223]

The ability to visualize fragments before determination of the need for GI decontamination has revitalized interest in selected use of orogastric lavage, and studies and case reports evaluate the amount of xenobiotic in the stomach before the initiation of orogastric lavage. Gastric tablet fragments are identified by endoscopy[229-231] using ultrathin esophagogastroduodenoscopy to confirm gastric presence of the ingested xenobiotic and thereby not only determine whether a potential benefit from orogastric lavage is present but also guide the actual orogastric lavage procedure. In two cases of potentially severe poisonings, direct visualization allowed observation of the effectiveness of orogastric lavage and aided clinicians in evacuating tobacco extract and the cyclic antidepressant amitriptyline.[229,231,251,252] Similarly, abdominal computed tomography was used to identify tablets, capsules, or liquid corresponding to the ingested xenobiotic up to 5 hours after the ingestion.[2,179,180,374] Unfortunately, transabdominal ultrasonography was neither able to determine the presence nor absence of tablets in simulated overdose studies, and both sensitivity and specificity were poor, leading the authors to conclude that ultrasonography is not a useful screening tool for the detection of gastric tablets and tablet residues.[252,326]

The clinical parameters listed in Table 5–3 help to identify individuals for whom orogastric lavage is usually not indicated based on a risk-to-benefit analysis. In contrast, for a small subset of patients (Table 5–3), gastric emptying is still recommended. A thorough understanding of this risk analysis is essential when deciding whether orogastric lavage is appropriate for a patient who has ingested a xenobiotic.

Time is an important consideration because for orogastric lavage to be beneficial, a consequential amount of xenobiotic must still be present in the stomach. Demographic studies have found that very few poisoned patients arrive at the ED within 1 to 2 hours after ingestion. In most studies, the average time from ingestion to presentation is approximately 3 to

4 hours, with significant variations.[174,185,188,230,335] This delay diminishes the likelihood of recovering a large percentage of the xenobiotic from the stomach to reduce a grave or possible lethal amount to a survivable amount except in those who have taken a massive amount. Many authors have adopted the consensus approach that orogastric lavage should not be considered unless a patient has ingested an amount of a xenobiotic with the potential to be severely harmful to organs or life threatening and when the procedure can be undertaken within 60 minutes of ingestion.[89,289] As discussed earlier and shown in Table 5–1, there is growing evidence to support the delayed persistence of significant amounts of drug in the stomach of selected overdose patients, thereby invalidating any concept of a hard stop occurring 60 minutes postingestion.

Assessment of whether or not orogastric lavage is appropriate for a patient must include an evaluation for potential contraindications (Table 5–4). Regardless of the severity of the ingestion and other contributing factors, such as time, there must be no contraindication to orogastric lavage procedures. Because the demonstrable benefit of orogastric lavage after ingestion of an unidentified xenobiotic is marginal at best, even relative contraindications usually dictate that the procedure should not be attempted. However, the clinical benefit could be significant if the ingested dose places the patient on the steep portion of the dose–response curve (Chap. 9). Under these circumstances, a small reduction in dose available for absorption would translate into a significant reduction in the potential for toxicity.

It is important to highlight the differences between volunteer studies using therapeutic doses of drugs and actual patients with clinically significant overdoses. The most important aspect of this comparison is a bias against gastric emptying and toward a benefit with AC. The drugs used in volunteer studies are typically well adsorbed by AC, and the doses of AC are significantly in excess of the AC–drug ratios that can be achieved in clinically significant overdoses. Larger overdoses, as might occur in patients with clinically important ingestions, are likely to saturate AC. An additional bias is introduced against gastric emptying in volunteer studies because the small amounts of any study xenobiotic used are unlikely to alter gastric motility, and thus the xenobiotics are more likely to pass through the pylorus before orogastric lavage is performed. A synthesis of available data can be used to develop indications for orogastric lavage (Table 5–4). Use of combination therapies with administration of AC after orogastric lavage was described by several,[6,7,14,37,47,100,108,166,169,197,224,226,272,287,343,354] but the procedure was not more effective than AC alone,[41,64,193-195] and it is unclear whether the outcome was due to orogastric lavage, other treatments, or their combination, and the procedure sometimes resulted in increased xenobiotic concentration and worsened clinical outcome.[14] In some cases, orogastric lavage delays AC administration further, and it is reasonable to eliminate orogastric lavage and only administer AC in cases when the benefits of orogastric lavage are estimated to be minimal to initiate the fastest decontamination procedure.

The procedure should always be performed by trained health care professionals and in health care settings. When deciding whether to actually perform orogastric lavage for a poisoned patient, these indications, contraindications, and potential adverse effects must be considered. Table 5–5 summarizes our recommended technique of orogastric lavage.

The tube size used for the procedure must be considered before initiation of the procedure if orogastric lavage is to be of value. Only gastric contents able to pass through the tube will be removed by the procedure (eg, liquid is able to pass through a small size tube, but a large tube might be necessary for tablets). If the ingested tablets are of known origin, it can be determined whether the tablets or capsules are able to pass through the tube at all in addition to difficulty of a pharmacobezoar that is unable to pass through any orogastric lavage tubes (Fig. 5–2).[19,88,145,210,285,286,311,312]

The volume of fluid used during orogastric lavage is not reported in most cases. Reported volumes vary from a few deciliters to 1 to 5 L[51,194,216,219,364] and up to 40 L,[202] or cycles of 250 mL until clear return fluid,[188] 200 to 400 mL cycles after aspiration of gastric content,[73] 400 to more than 1,000 mL each cycle,[94] or 8 mL/kg repeated five times.[120] Others are nonspecific, such as "one or more liters" or "lavage until the fluid was clear," in both children[44] and

TABLE 5–2	Summary of Studies Evaluating the Effect of Gastric Lavage on the Absorption of Diverse Xenobiotics				
Author	**Citation**	**Study Method**	**Outcome Measure**	**Main Result**	**Comments**
Volunteer Studies					
Christophersen et al. 2002	64	RCT; efficacy of AC and GL + AC 1 h compared with control (no AC) after a 50-mg/kg APAP dose ($n = 12$).	PK parameters for APAP: AUC_{0h-inf}, C_{max}, t_{max}, and $t_{1/2}$.	AC reduced APAP absorption by 66%, GL + AC reduced by 48.2% with controls; no significant difference between AC and GL+AC.	Combination treatment with GL + AC is not better in reducing APAP absorption compared with AC alone.
Grierson et al. 2000	127	RCT; crossover; two sessions ($n = 10$). Effect of GL to reduce absorption of liquids; 4 g of APAP, no GL vs GL (minimum 5× 200-mL cycles) after 1 h after ingestion.	PK parameters for APAP: AUC_{0-8h}, C_{max}, C_{4h}, and t_{max}.	No difference in C_{max} or t_{max}; reduction after GL in C_{4h} and AUC APAP absorption reduced by 20% (high SD).	Does not support of GL because clinical benefit was deemed unlikely, and other more effective treatments are available for APAP poisonings.
Lapatto-Reiniluoto et al. 2000	195	RCT; three sessions ($n = 9$); 25 g of AC vs GL (10 × 200 mL) at 30 min after 150 mg of moclobemide, 10 mg of temazepam, and 80 mg of verapamil.	PK variables AUC_{0-24h}, C_{max}, t_{max}, $t_{1/2}$ of moclobemide, temazepam, and verapamil compared with control.	AC – AUC_{0-24h} reduction: moclobemide, 55%; temazepam, 45%; verapamil, NS. C_{max} reduction: moclobemide, 40%; temazepam, 29%; verapamil, 16%. GL – AUC_{0-24h} reduction: moclobemide, 44%; temazepam, NA; verapamil, NS. C_{max} reduction: NS for all drugs.	GL was less effective in reducing absorption of moclobemide, temazepam, and verapamil.
Actual Overdose Data: Case Reports (Examples), Case Series, Cohort, Retrospective					
Comstock et al. 1981	73	Efficacy of GL (200- to 400-mL cycles) in 76 patients with sedative–hypnotic drug ingestions determined as recovered therapeutic doses. An efficacious lavage is suggested to be defined as recovery of at least either 2 or 10 therapeutic doses.	Drug concentrations in GL fluid and blood; time since ingestion when this could be determined.	Two or more therapeutic doses were recovered from 15.8% of the lavage samples, and 10 or more therapeutic doses were recovered from 6.6%. Poorest recoveries were obtained in patients lavaged more than 2 h after ingestion.	The majority of the patients did not benefit from GL.
Donkor et al. 2016	89	Retrospective review of 923 PCC records; Determine case type, location, and complications of GL cases.	Mortality, details of the xenobiotic ingestion (substance(s), time, dose), clinical effects, needs for care, decontamination method, GL outcome.	381 single and 540 multiple-xenobiotic ingestions: Non-TCA psychotropics, BZDs, and APAP were most common; 5 deaths; in 58% of cases GL was performed by PCC recommendation, in 42% without recommendation; complications reported in 20 cases; xenobiotic fragments were retrieved in 27%.	Inappropriate used of GL frequent; questionable effect beyond 1 h.
Leao et al. 2015	200	Retrospective data, 2012, carbamate or OP poisoning ($n = 70$; 77% carbamates, 23% OPs).	Clinical characteristics and treatment patterns (atropine, GL, AC), length of stay.	OP poisonings were more severe, with 68.75% of patients presenting moderate to severe toxicity. Atropine and AC significantly reduced signs and symptoms; GL was not effective.	GL contraindicated in acute toxicity from carbamates or OPs.
Magdalan et al. 2013	210	Case report; 42-year-old patient; clomipramine extended-release tablets, unknown dose, 14 h before. Treatment included GL and then 50 g AC every 4 h.	CA level on admission, 1,955 ng/mL; postmortem blood clomipramine, 1,729 ng/mL and nor-clomipramine, 431 ng/mL, myocardium clomipramine, 14,420 ng/g, nor-clomipramine, 35,930 ng/g.	Died; prolonged toxicity related to a large gastric pharmacobezoar.	GL revealed no tablets in lavage fluids.
Woo et al. 2013	371	Case report; 57-year-old patient; dabigatran 11.25 g, alprazolam unknown dose, 1 h before. Treatment included GL and then AC.	Blood dabigatran, 970 ng/mL; thrombin clotting times measured above the testable limits (>120 s) until 52 h postarrival.	Nontraditional intervention using GL in addition to AC in a coagulopathic patient.	The direct impact and efficacy of including GL was unclear.
Controlled Studies in Patients					
Bosse et al. 1995	43	RCT; prospective evaluation in 51 patients with TCA poisoning. Compared 50 g of AC, saline GL + 50 g AC, and 25 g AC + GL + 25 g AC. GL used 2 L or more as needed to produce a clear effluent.	Mortality; duration of hospital stay, ICU stay, mechanical ventilation, cardiotoxic symptoms and their duration (tachycardia, hypotension, wide QRS complex, ventricular dysrhythmias).	No deaths were reported. No statistically significant differences in clinical outcomes were shown between groups.	The clinical outcomes were similar using all three decontamination methods.

(Continued)

TABLE 5–2	Summary of Studies Evaluating the Effect of Gastric Lavage on the Absorption of Diverse Xenobiotics (*Continued*)				
Author	**Citation**	**Study Method**	**Outcome Measure**	**Main Result**	**Comments**
Comstock et al. 1982	72	Prospective evaluation in 339 patients with acute oral overdose of efficacy of AC after GL. All received GL, and 131 were randomly chosen also to receive AC.	Blood drug concentrations were continuously monitored to determine continued absorption after GI decontamination procedure.	The trend suggested that continued absorption was less frequent in the AC group. Ingestion time >1 h.	No clear additional benefit from AC.
Indira et al. 2013	159	Prospective evaluation in 176 patients with OP poisoning. Identified clinical profile of intermediate syndrome influencing the clinical course. All received GL and AC. Compared early (<1 h) vs late (>1 h) GL and single GL vs two GLs.	Mortality; vital signs; atropinization; pulse oximetry; cholinergic signs; specific treatment, including number of performed GL and antidote pralidoxime in OP poisonings.	Mortality rate was 28.4% (n = 50), all secondary to respiratory failure. Mortality with single vs double GL was 23 vs 25 (P = 0.99); 80 received single GL, 87 two GLs. Mortality with early vs late GL 12 vs 36 (P = 0.5), 48 received GL <1 h, 119 >1 h; 9 patients did not receive GL; 31 had intermediate syndrome.	No significant protection by early GL. No difference between early vs late GL. More than one GL procedure was protective against intermediate syndrome but not final outcome. Intermediate syndrome: Strongly associated with mortality; lower in multiple GL group; no association with GL timing.
Krayeva et al. 2013	184	Prospective prehospital study on poisoning epidemiology, treatment, and complications from treatment (n = 2,536).	Mortality, xenobiotic, clinical findings, treatment.	Overall mortality rate, 1.5%; mortality in +GL/+intubated 2.5%, in +GL/-intubation 2%, in -GL/- intubation 0%; Prehospital GL in 34% (n = 852) (20% <1 h, 61% <2 h), all performed in the patients' homes.	High prevalence of GL differing from recommended treatment practice; GL performed by tradition after corrosive substance ingestions. Nonrandomized, so outcome differences unclear.
Kulig et al. 1985	188	RCT; prospective evaluation in 592 overdose patients of the clinical outcome of AC (oral in alert patients or by NG tube in obtunded pts) compared with GL + AC.	Severity based on clinical course by symptoms (mild, moderate, severe) continuously the first 6 h.	GL within 1 h in obtunded pts improved clinical outcome; no difference between other groups.	Management without gastric emptying preferable in many patients; GE should not be standard care; benefit questionable effect of GL if initiated >1 h. Exclusion criteria biased against a benefit of GL.
Merigian et al. 1990	226	Prospective evaluation of GE (ipecac or GL) + AC or AC in the self-poisoned patient. AC was dosed in asymptomatic patients (n = 451), GE + AC was dosed in symptomatic patients (n = 357); 4-h observation. Sustained-release products and mushrooms were excluded because of potential late (>4 h) onset of symptoms.	Vital signs, supportive therapy, intubation, deterioration, duration of intubation, clinical disposition, disposition time, and total time in the ED.	No clinical deterioration occurred in the asymptomatic patients treated without GE. AC did not alter outcome measures in asymptomatic patients. GL was associated with a higher prevalence of ICU admissions and aspiration pneumonia. The data support the management of selected acute overdose patients without GE and failed to show a benefit from AC in asymptomatic overdose patients.	No additional benefits from GL. Increased prevalence of side effects and ICU care from GL. Large proportion of low-risk cases and extensive exclusion criteria biased against a benefit of GL and drove the negative outcome.
Pond et al. 1995	279	RCT; prospective evaluation in 876 overdose patients of the efficacy and safety of AC (oral or by NG tube in obtunded patients) compared with GL + AC.	Clinical course by symptoms (mild, moderate, severe) assessed every 1–2 h the first 6 h; length of hospital stay; complications.	Authors report no difference between groups after discounting positive cases.	No benefit of GL before AC. Exclusion criteria biased against a benefit of GL.
Saetta et al. 1991	295	RCT; prospective evaluation of gastric emptying procedures' (GL or ipecac) ability to force gastric contents into the small bowel using barium-impregnated polythene pellets (n = 60).	Abdominal radiograph after pellet ingestion and GL (n = 20) using 3.5–6 L of fluid.	51.8% pellets retained after GL of which 33.3% in the small intestine. Significantly fewer pellets (16.3%) had passed into the small intestine in the control group (n = 20).	GL was inefficient and forced gastric content into the small intestine. Time from xenobiotic ingestion to pellet ingestion was unknown.
Underhill et al. 1990	350	RCT; prospective evaluation in 60 patients; APAP >5 g ingestion within 4 h; compared efficacy of GL and AC.	Percentage change between first and last APAP plasma concentrations.	Mean percentage falls in APAP concentrations were 39.3% for GL and 52.2% for AC.	AC was more effective in limiting APAP absorption compared with GL.

AC = activated charcoal; APAP = acetaminophen; AUC = area under the concentration vs time curve; BZD = benzodiazepine; C_{max} = maximal concentration; CA = cyclic antidepressant; GE = gastric emptying; GI = gastrointestinal; GL = orogastric lavage; h = hour; ICU = intensive care unit; NAC = N-acetylcysteine; NG = nasogastric; NS = not significant; OP = organic phosphorus compound; PCC = Poison Control Center; PK = pharmacokinetics; RCT = randomized controlled trial; SD = standard deviation; $t_{1/2}$ = terminal elimination half-life; t_{max} = time to maximal concentration.

TABLE 5–3	Risk Assessment: When to Consider Orogastric Lavage
Orogastric Lavage Is Usually Not Indicated[a]	**Orogastric Lavage Is Indicated**[b]
The xenobiotic has limited toxicity at almost any dose.	The ingested xenobiotic is known to produce life-threatening toxicity *or* the patient has obvious signs or symptoms of life-threatening toxicity and
Although the xenobiotic ingested is potentially toxic, the dose ingested is likely less than that expected to produce significant illness.	■ There is reason to believe that, given the time of ingestion, a significant amount of the ingested xenobiotic is still present in the stomach *or*
The ingested xenobiotic is well adsorbed by AC, and the amount ingested is not expected to exceed the adsorptive capacity of AC.	■ The ingested xenobiotic is not adsorbed by AC or AC is unavailable *or*
Significant spontaneous emesis has already occurred.	■ Although the ingested xenobiotic is adsorbed by AC, the amount ingested exceeds the AC–xenobiotic ratio of 10:1 even when using a dose of AC that is twice the standard dose recommended *and*
The patient presents many hours postingestion and has minimal signs or symptoms of poisoning.	
The ingested xenobiotic has a highly efficient antidote (eg, APAP and *N*-acetylcysteine).	■ The patient has not had spontaneous emesis *or*
The procedure cannot be accomplished appropriately or safely (wrong tube size, lack of provider skill, anticipated extant esophageal or gastric injury, etc.)	■ No highly effective specific antidote exists or alternative therapies (eg, hemodialysis) pose a significant risk to the patient.

[a]Patients who fulfill some of these criteria can be decontaminated safely with activated charcoal alone or in many cases require no decontamination at all. [b]Patients who fulfill these criteria should undergo orogastric lavage *if* there are no contraindications or other compelling time-dependent interventions. For individuals who meet some of these criteria but who are judged not to be candidates for orogastric lavage, single- or multiple-dose activated charcoal or whole-bowel irrigation (or both) should be used.

AC = activated charcoal; APAP = acetaminophen.

adults. Simple tube aspiration of gastric contents not followed by a formal lavage procedure is reported by some to be more effective.[70,219,226] No recent literature distinguishes aspiration and lavage as different procedures, and we consider the aspiration as an initial part of the full procedure. The specific fluid volume needed for the procedure to be optimal has not been formally studied, and severe adverse effects caused by the use of excessive volumes are described.[94] A review of controlled clinical trials of orogastric lavage in acute organic phosphorus compound poisoning concluded that excessive volumes of fluid or repetitive use of orogastric lavage were unlikely to increase the yield compared with that of a single aspiration while avoiding the risk of electrolyte disturbances.[202] Our general recommendation of volume is included in Table 5–5.

TABLE 5–4	Orogastric Lavage: Indications and Contraindications	
Indications	**Contraindications**	
The patient meets some of the criteria for orogastric lavage (Table 5–3).	The patient does not meet any of the criteria for orogastric lavage (Table 5–3).	
	The patient has lost or will likely lose his or her airway protective reflexes without being intubated. (After intubation, orogastric lavage can be performed if otherwise indicated).	
The benefits of orogastric lavage outweigh the risks.	Ingestion of a xenobiotic with a high aspiration potential (eg, a hydrocarbon) in the absence of endotracheal intubation.	
	Ingestion of an alkaline caustic.	
	Ingestion of a foreign body (eg, a drug packet).	
	The patient is at risk of hemorrhage or gastrointestinal perforation because of underlying pathology, recent surgery, or another medical condition that could be further compromised by the use of orogastric lavage.	
	Ingestion of a xenobiotic in a form known to be too large to fit into the lumen of the lavage tube (eg, many modified-release preparations).	

TABLE 5–5	Technique for Performing Orogastric Lavage
Select the correct tube size	
Adults and adolescents: 36–40 Fr	
Children: 22–28 Fr	
Procedure	

1. If there is potential for airway compromise, endotracheal intubation should precede orogastric lavage.
2. The patient should be kept in the left lateral decubitus position if possible. Because the pylorus points upward in this orientation, this positioning theoretically helps prevent the xenobiotic from advancing through the pylorus during the procedure.
3. Before insertion, the proper length of tubing to be passed should be measured and marked on the tube. The length should allow the most proximal tube opening to be passed beyond the lower esophageal sphincter.
4. After the tube is inserted, it is essential to confirm that the distal end of the tube is in the stomach by withdrawal of material; injecting air; or if unable to clinically confirm placement, use radiographic confirmation.
5. Any material present in the stomach should be withdrawn.
6. In adults, 250-mL aliquots of a room temperature 0.9% saline lavage solution is instilled via a funnel or lavage syringe. In children, aliquots should be 10–15 mL/kg to a maximum of 250 mL.
7. Orogastric lavage should continue for at least several liters in an adult and for at least 0.5 to 1.0 L in a child or until a colorless particulate matter returns and the effluent lavage solution is clear.
8. After orogastric lavage, the same tube should be used to instill AC if indicated.
9. The tube should be withdrawn/removed.

Adverse effects of orogastric lavage include injury to the esophagus and stomach,[22,51,83,128,172,188,216,219,248,265,364] vomiting, bloody fluid return, and seizures,[89] as well as significant decreases in serum calcium,[120] ionized calcium,[120] and magnesium;[120] severe hypernatremia;[232] and leukocytosis.[166] Hypernatremia resulted from a lavage performed with 12 L of hypertonic saline.[232] An observational case series studying 14 consecutive orogastric lavages performed in a resource-poor location found three deaths directly related to the procedure, all of which seemed to result from inadequate airway protection.[94] These cases, as well as other well-known complications such as respiratory events, including the need for mechanical ventilation,[167] hypoxemia,[167] ECG changes,[336] respiratory failure,[365] and a higher frequency of aspiration pneumonitis,[33,44,167,219,226,323,352,353,365] demonstrate that orogastric lavage is associated with risk and should only be performed based on the rigorous indications for gastric emptying listed in Tables 5–3 and 5–4.

ACTIVATED CHARCOAL

Activated charcoal is an effective method for reducing the absorption of many xenobiotics.[5,11,21,27,115,129,165,176,244,257,259,366] For certain xenobiotics, it also enhances elimination through interruption of either the enterohepatic or enteroenteric cycle.[74,257,366] Its superb adsorptive properties theoretically make it the single most useful management strategy for diverse patients with acute oral overdoses.[16-18,41,64,74,75,118,142,152,273,274]

Mechanism

The entire effect of AC takes place in the GI tract. Oral AC is not absorbed through the wall of the GI tract but rather passes straight through the gut unchanged. To be adsorbed to AC, the xenobiotic must be dissolved in the GI liquid phase and be in physical contact with the AC. The possible sites of adsorption are demonstrated in Fig. 5–3. The surface (internal and external) of AC is specifically manufactured to chemically adsorb certain xenobiotics. Activated charcoal forms an equilibrium between free xenobiotic and xenobiotic that is adsorbed to it through relatively weak intermolecular forces.

$$\text{Free xenobiotic} + \text{AC} \Leftrightarrow \text{Xenobiotic–AC complex}$$

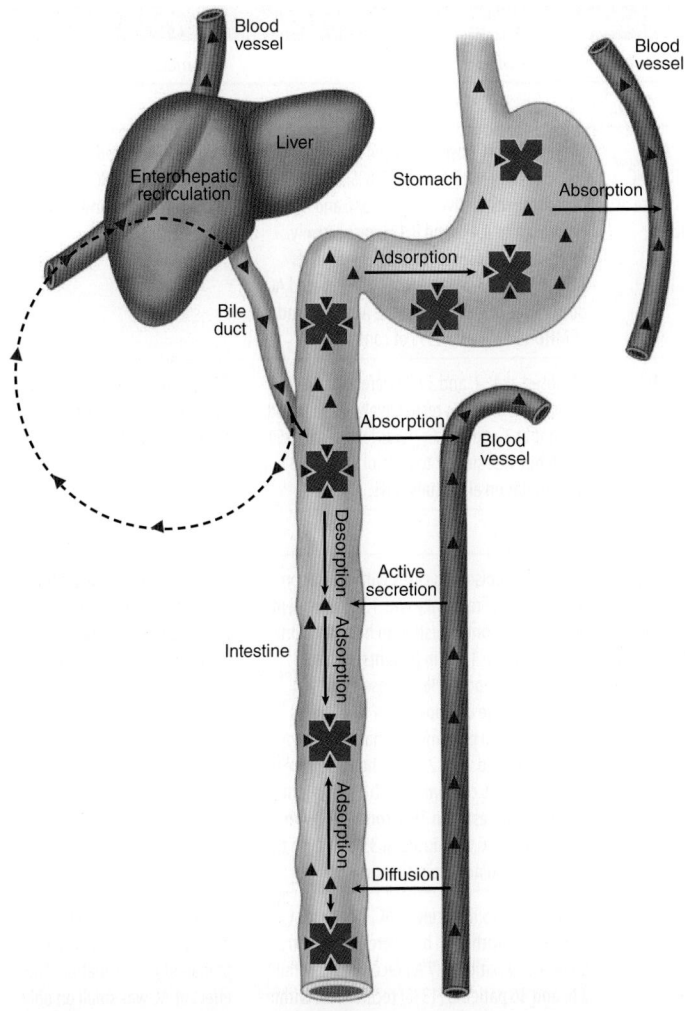

FIGURE 5-3. Mechanism of xenobiotic (▼) removal by AC in the luminal space of the gastrointestinal tract. The position of systemic xenobiotic absorption depends on the physical chemical characteristics of the xenobiotic and takes place from stomach, intestine, or both. Xenobiotic reentry into the luminal space can take place by enterohepatic recirculation and enteroenteric recirculation by active secretion and passive diffusion. Excess and continued supply of activated charcoal facilitates adsorption of recycled xenobiotic and favors continued active and passive diffusion of xenobiotic to the luminal space and adsorption of xenobiotic.

Desorption of the adsorbed xenobiotic occurs, but if sufficient AC is present (see dosing listed later), the equilibrium will be shifted toward the xenobiotic–AC complex. The effect is a low free xenobiotic concentration in the GI liquid phase and reduced xenobiotic absorption.[74,107]

Efficacy

However, as is true for the other methods of GI decontamination, there is a lack of sound evidence of its benefits as defined by clinically meaningful endpoints. This opinion is reflected both in the consensus statements and reviews and in the overall poison control center trend toward not performing decontamination (Chap. 130).[11,67,165,225] The consensus opinion concluded that *a single dose of activated charcoal should not be administered routinely in the management of poisoned patients and, based on volunteer studies, the effectiveness of activated charcoal decreased with time, providing the greatest benefit in severely poisoned patients if dosed within 1 hour of ingestion.* There was no evidence that the administration of a single dose of AC improved clinical outcome. These opinions are unfortunately biased by the fact that most "routinely" poisoned patients have low-risk exposures and do well with minimal interventions. Additionally, it is generally accepted that unless either airway protective reflexes are intact (and expected to remain so) or the patient's

airway has been protected, the administration of AC is contraindicated.[67] Despite little scientific basis or support from clinical trials, less severely poisoned patients might theoretically benefit from AC in terms of reduced need for life support, monitoring, and antidotes,[165] and many reports of poisoned cases include AC as part of treatment to reduce the clinical effect of xenobiotics of various origin—medications,[62,87,91,132,153,217,253,298,309,319,345] plants,[49,198,262,327,337] mushrooms,[113,123,182,260,359] pesticides,[187,200,235,282,369] and other chemicals.[135,377]

Theoretically, early administration of AC to a patient presenting with a significant oral overdose of a potentially toxic xenobiotic would lower systemic exposure to that xenobiotic and thus be of benefit to the patient.[80,257,366] The precise definition of "early" is yet to be defined, as discussed in the section about time. Some studies failed to show benefit from the use of AC beyond a 1-hour limit.[124,138,373] Although these data do not support the administration of AC as a GI decontamination strategy more than 1 hour after an overdose, the applicability of these results to actual overdosed patients is not adequately evaluated.

However, a range of reports show significant effect if dosing is delayed up to 4 hours after the xenobiotic ingestion.[91,112,161,162,165,171,237,322] In fact, studies suggest efficacy up to 6 hours after ingestion for some xenobiotics.[171,353] A meta-analysis was performed to evaluate the effect of AC on xenobiotic absorption during the first 6 hours after ingestion. Data were obtained from 64 controlled studies in which AC was compared with placebo up to 6 hours after drug ingestion in volunteers. Activated charcoal was most effective when administered immediately after xenobiotic ingestion. However, even with a delay of 4 hours after ingestion, 25% of the participants achieved at least a 32% reduction in absorption.[171] The theoretical intuitive result has been difficult to demonstrate using clinically relevant endpoints in large unselected populations of poisoned patients, again most likely as a result of the inclusion of large numbers of minimally exposed low-risk individuals. Several randomized controlled trials failed to show a benefit of AC over either emesis or no therapy at all. Most suffer from inclusion of a large number of low-risk patients and selection biases from extensive exclusion criteria.[79,96,290] Data are summarized in Table 5–6. Furthermore, in an article on compliance related to AC nested within one randomized, controlled trial, it is stated that a large number of patients included in the trial had undergone gastric emptying in some form before being transferred from peripheral hospitals.[233]

Evaluations of the efficacy of AC are often performed by comparisons of pharmacokinetic parameters, such as area under the blood xenobiotic concentration–time curve (AUC), maximum blood concentration of the xenobiotic (C_{max}), time to maximum blood concentration (T_{max}), and elimination half-life ($t_{1/2}$) (Chap. 9). More novel approaches include population pharmacokinetics.[64,80,112,162,257,303,366,373] Studies are summarized in Tables 5–1, 5–2, and 5–6.

Further increased effect of AC in reducing APAP absorption was observed in the presence of concomitant anticholinergic activity,[125] an observation relevant to consider in polydrug ingestions.

Thus, it should be clear that the use of a 1-hour time frame should serve as a guideline rather than an absolute endpoint. It is only logical that if an intervention is effective at 59 minutes, it will also be beneficial at 61 minutes. Although it is logical that efficacy decreases as time from ingestion increases, in certain cases, some benefit will be derived many hours after ingestion. Because after massive life-threatening ingestions, the absorption of xenobiotics is prolonged, there is no exact time limit for AC use.[243] As discussed earlier, good data from patients with actual ingestions demonstrate that a significant amount of xenobiotic is found in the stomach beyond this arbitrary 1-hour time frame. It is therefore recommended to administer AC to *prevent absorption* in poisoned patients even when they present late to medical care if there is a potential for clinically significant ongoing absorption. Additional benefits on enhanced elimination are discussed next.

Prehospital Use

One of the first controlled trials of GI decontamination noted that many patients present hours after oral overdose, with children presenting earlier than adults (mean, 68 minutes versus 3.3 hours).[188] Over a 6-month

TABLE 5–6	Summary of Studies Evaluating the Effect of Activated Charcoal on the Absorption of Diverse Xenobiotics				
Author	Citation	Study Method	Outcome Measure	Main Result	Comments
Volunteer Data					
Keranen et al. 2010	176	RCT; crossover; three sessions, ($n =$ 12) LTG 100 mg and OXC 600 mg were given orally, each to six subjects. Control = no AC vs either 50 g of AC once at 30 min or repeated 20 g AC doses 6–72 h after LTG and 12–48 h after OXC.	PK variables AUC_{0h-inf}, AUC_{6h-inf}, C_{max}, t_{max}, $t_{1/2}$, Ke of LTG, OXC, and the active metabolite of oxcarbazepine (MHD).	Single-dose AC dose decreased AUC_{0-inf} of LTG, OXC, and MHD to 58%, 2.8%, and 4.2% of control, respectively. T_{max} of OXC and MHD decreased to 4.4% and 8.1%, respectively. Repeated AC doses after LTG decreased its AUC_{6h-inf} to 39% and $t\frac{1}{2}$ to 44%. Repeated AC doses after OXC decreased the $AUC_{12h-inf}$ and $t\frac{1}{2}$ of MHD to 46% and 45% of control.	AC greatly reduced GI absorption of LTG and OXC, and it accelerated the elimination of LTG and MHD.
Mullins et al. 2009	237	RCT; crossover; four sessions ($n = 9$). Effect of delayed AC on a simulated overdose of 5 g of APAP + 0.5 mg/kg of oxycodone. No AC vs 50 g of AC was dosed at 1, 2, or 3 h after ingestion.	PK parameters for APAP: AUC_{0-8h}, C_{max}, t_{max}, and $t_{1/2}$.	AC dosed at 1, 2, and 3 h lowered the AUC by 43%, 24%, and 8%, respectively. This was significant at 1 and 2 h. C_{max} was lowered by 25% at 1 h but was similar to control at 2 and 3 h. $t_{1/2}$ was similar on all 4 study days.	AC was more beneficial if dosed early. Effect demonstrable up to 2 h.
Actual Overdose Data: Case Reports, Case Series, and Cohort Studies					
Isbister et al. 2004	161	Retrospective cohort of unselected population of overdose patients; characterization of aspiration pneumonitis frequency, outcomes, and factors that predispose to aspiration pneumonitis.	Poisoned patients with aspiration pneumonitis. Length of stay (in hours), GCS score (15 or <15), spontaneous emesis, treatment with AC, alcohol, and other coingestions.	71 of 4,562 poisoning cases with aspiration pneumonitis. Frequency was 1.0% in patients whose time from ingestion to hospital admission was <4 h; 1.9% in patients admitted 4–24 h after, and 4.4% in those admitted >24 h after the overdose. 62% of patients with aspiration pneumonitis had a GCS score of <15, compared with 23% without. Seizure was present in 16% compared with 2% without. TCA was coingested in 19% compared with 7% without. AC was dosed in 33% of both the aspiration and nonaspiration groups.	AC was not an independent risk factor for aspiration pneumonitis. Spontaneous vomiting, xenobiotic, and seizures are potential risk factors.
Isbister et al. 2009	162	Retrospective cohort of 176 patients on 286 occasions with quetiapine overdose; median dose was 2 g; evaluation of whether AC improves outcomes or shortens treatment requirement.	Measured intubation, duration of ventilation, and cardiac monitoring.	42 patients (15%) received AC, 4 patients (1%) received AC within 1 h but were excluded from analysis, 19 patients (7%) received AC within 2 h, and 36 patients (13%) received AC within 4 h. Single-dose AC within 2 h reduced the probability of intubation from 10% to 7% for 2-g ingestions only. AC between 2 and 4 h did not reduce the probability of intubation. The median duration of ventilation was not affected by AC. Abnormal QT intervals occurred in 8.4%, all with HR >100 beats/min.	Quetiapine dose and AC dosing (<2 h) influenced the probability of intubation. The effect of AC was small on only if given within 2 h.
Spiller et al. 2006	322	Nonrandomized prospective, multicenter, observational case series. Efficacy of AC in addition to standard NAC when AC given >4 h after APAP overdose. 145 patients included; 58 (40%) received NAC only, and 87 (60%) received NAC and AC.	Serum aminotransferase (ALT, AST).	23 patients had elevations of AST or ALT >1,000 IU/L, of which 21 patients received NAC only (38% of total NAC only group) and 2 patients received NAC and AC (2% of total NAC+AC group).	AC in addition to standard NAC was associated with a reduced incidence of liver injury from APAP.
Controlled Studies					
Cooper et al. 2005	79	RCT of overdosed patients presenting to one urban hospital. Excluding transfers, late presenters (>12 h), xenobiotics not adsorbed by AC, administration of AC contraindicated, and very serious ingestions. Patients were randomized to either AC or no decontamination. ($n = 327$ adults).	Primary outcome: length of stay (the time of presentation until the patient was declared medically fit for discharge); secondary outcomes: need for ventilation, vomiting after admission, occurrence of aspiration, or death.	The study excluded seven severely poisoned patients who all arrived within 1 h of ingestion; the majority of the patients in the trial (nearly 60%) arrived within 2 h postingestion. No difference in clinical endpoints. The most common xenobiotics ingested were APAP, benzodiazepines, and newer antidepressants, all of which have low case-fatality rates.	There was no benefit of AC compared with no treatment in a general population with low risk ingestions after severely poisoned patients are excluded.

(Continued)

TABLE 5–6		Summary of Studies Evaluating the Effect of Activated Charcoal on the Absorption of Diverse Xenobiotics *(Continued)*			
Author	*Citation*	*Study Method*	*Outcome Measure*	*Main Result*	*Comments*
de Silva et al. 2003	85	RCT (*n* = 401); all with yellow oleander poisoning. All received one dose of AC and were then randomly assigned either 50 g of AC every 6 h for 3 days or sterile water.	Primary outcome: mortality; secondary outcomes: life-threatening cardiac dysrhythmias, dose of atropine used, need for cardiac pacing, admission to ICU, and length of stay. Analysis was by intention to treat.	201 patients received MDAC; 200 received water. Lower mortality rate reported in the MDAC group (5 {2.5%} vs 16 {8%}), and differences favored MDAC for all secondary endpoints, except length of stay.	MDAC reduced the number of deaths and life-threatening cardiac dysrhythmias after yellow oleander poisoning. This was a unique study in that all patients ingested life-threatening toxins. The number needed to treat to save a life was 18.
Duffull and Isbister, 2013	91	Prospectively collected APAP patients. Two groups: presenting early (4–7 h) and presenting late (7–16 h) (*n* = 1,303 patients with 1,571 admissions).	Primary outcome: reported APAP dose predictive of the need for NAC; measures included time from APAP ingestion, timed APAP concentrations (4 and 16 h), ALT >1,000 U/L (hepatotoxicity), AC, and NAC.	Patients presenting late were more likely to have hepatotoxicity (5.5% vs. 0.4%; *P* <0.0001), have a toxic APAP concentration (34% vs 18%; *P* <0.0001), and receive NAC (48% vs 23%; *P* <0.0001). The probability of requiring NAC if AC was not administered was 5% at 6–9 g of APAP, increasing to 90% at 48–50 g of APAP. AC reduced the probability of needing NAC, up to 14% at 28 g APAP and <10% at APAP doses <19 g or >37 g.	Benefits of AC if dosed up to 3 h postingestion.
Eddleston et al. 2008	96	RCT (*n* = 4,629 acute self-poisoned patients) in a developing nation. Primary toxins were pesticides and yellow oleander seeds. Patients were randomized to no AC, single-dose AC, or MDAC.	Death.	No difference in mortality rates between groups. Many patients had GL before randomization; Audit of AC dosing shows limited compliance. Authors claim that logistic regression analysis found no influence of GL on their results.	MDAC did not reduce the number of deaths. The health care setting and xenobiotics were different from developed nations. The first 1,904 control patients received GL, as was the case for all patients presenting within 2 h of ingestion of substantial amounts of pesticides or potentially toxic xenobiotics.
Kulig et al. 1985	188	RCT, prospectively collected overdose patients (*n* = 592); efficacy in altering clinical outcome of AC (oral in alert patients or by NG tube in obtunded pts) compared with GL + AC.	Severity based on clinical course by symptoms (mild, moderate, severe) continuously the first 6 h.	GL within 1 h in obtunded patients improved clinical outcome; there was no difference between other groups.	Management without gastric emptying is preferable in many patients; GE should not be standard care; benefit of GL in sickest subset with in the first hour; questionable effect of GL if initiated >1 h. Exclusion criteria were biased toward an AC effect.
Merigian and Blaho, 2002	225	RCT (*n* = 1,479 adults); self-poisoning in a single hospital. Determine the effects of AC. Patients either received 50 g of AC or supportive care only.	Outcomes: clinical deterioration, length of stay in the ED or hospital, and complication rate.	The findings were no significant differences between groups when comparing the length of intubation time, length of hospital stay, and complication rates associated with the overdose. The AC group reported a higher incidence of vomiting and longer length of ED stay.	AC provided no additional benefit to supportive care alone and did not improve clinical outcome. AC was associated with a higher incidence of vomiting and a longer length of ED stay. Overall, most ingestions were benign and most serious xenobiotics as well as those not adsorbed to AC were excluded.
Roberts et al. 2006	290	RCT; acute self-poisoned patients (subgroup of Eddleston 2008 above who ingested yellow oleander seeds. (*n* = 104).	Plasma clearance of the yellow oleander cardenolides.	Both AC and MDAC significantly increased the plasma clearance of cardenolides. There was no difference between groups in mortality, but given the absolute numbers of two to three deaths per group, this could be related to a lack of power in the study design.	A favorable influence of AC was shown on the PK profile of ingested yellow oleander cardenolides.

AC = activated charcoal; ALT = alanine transaminase; APAP = acetaminophen; AST = aspartate transaminase; AUC = area under the concentration versus time curve; C_{max} = maximal concentration; ED = emergency department; GCS = Glasgow Coma Scale; GL = gastric lavage; h = hours; HR = heart rate; inf = infinity; Ke = rate constant of elimination; LTG = lamotrigine; MDAC = multiple-dose activated charcoal; NAC = N-acetylcysteine; OXC = oxcarbazepine; PK = pharmacokinetics; RCT = randomized controlled trial; $t_{1/2}$ = terminal elimination half-life; t_{max} = time to maximal concentration; TCA = tricyclic antidepressant.

period, another study of 63 patients who had taken potentially serious overdoses demonstrated a median time of arrival to a health care facility of 136 minutes after the overdose. Only 15 patients presented within 1 hour, and only 4 of 10 patients who qualified actually received AC within 1 hour. The results demonstrate not only the difficulty in clinically assessing patients before 1 hour but also the difficulty in adhering to the principle of treating patients with AC when they arrive within a few hours of ingestion unless AC could be safely administered to appropriate patients in the prehospital setting.[174] Enhanced communication between a poison control center and both emergency medical services and an ED was able to decrease the time to administration of AC.[348,349]

Prehospital use of AC has not gained wide acceptance because of unfounded concerns that it would not be administered properly by the untrained lay public and that many children would refuse to drink the charcoal slurry. In fact, an 18-month consecutive case series demonstrated that AC could be administered successfully in the home when given by the lay public. Home use of AC significantly reduced the time to AC administration after xenobiotic ingestion from a mean of 73 ± 18.1 minutes for ED treatment to a mean of 38 ± 18.3 minutes for home treatment.[321] Additionally, prehospital AC did not markedly delay transport or arrival of overdose patients into the ED and was generally safe in 441 cases collected retrospectively in which prehospital AC was given. The average elapsed time between xenobiotic ingestion and AC was 49.8 minutes (range, 7–199 minutes). Activated charcoal was administered more than 1 hour (22%) and more than 2 hours (3%) after the xenobiotic ingestion. Complications included emesis in 6.6% of the patients, as well as hypotension, hypoxia, and declining mental status, but authors attributed these events to the xenobiotic ingested rather than the AC itself.[362]

A prospective follow-up study evaluated adherence to a protocol of administering AC in the prehospital setting. Activated charcoal was indicated in 722 of 2,047 patients. Of these patients, 555 actually received AC at a mean of 88 minutes after ingestion; 72 patients refused to drink the AC, and no adverse effects were noted.[9]

However, many authorities recommend that AC should neither be a standard nor be administered at home and that administration should only be carried out by health professionals (Chap. 4).[13,65,214,221,307,308] However, we recommend that prehospital AC be used in rural and remote areas if the transport time to health care facilities exceeds the time frame of possible beneficial effect of AC, and its administration is expected to reduce the risk of appearance of life-threatening symptoms but only after consultation with a knowledgeable health care professional.

Dosing

The optimal dose of oral AC has never been fully established. Since the initiation of its clinical use as a GI decontaminant, various factors are recommended for determining the optimal dose of AC. Two factors commonly discussed are the patient's weight and the quantity of the xenobiotic ingested. The problems in using the quantity of the xenobiotic as a basis for AC dosing are that the amount is usually unknown, and there is an implication that nothing else in the GI tract will occupy binding sites on AC. Additionally, the xenobiotic is often unknown, and xenobiotics vary enormously in their toxicities, rate of absorption, and the clinical effects they produce such as respiratory depression, convulsions, and effect on gastric emptying rate. Some xenobiotics are well adsorbed to AC, but others are not.[74] Because of variables such as the physical properties of the formulation ingested (liquid, solid, or sustained-release tablet), the volume and pH of gastric and intestinal fluids, and the presence of other xenobiotics adsorbed by AC,[16-18,25,140,144,201,254,256] the optimal dose cannot be known with certainty in any given patient.

Information concerning the maximum adsorptive capacity of AC for the particular xenobiotic ingested permits a theoretical calculation of an adequate dose,[8,16,23,26,59,75,245,246,254,255,291,292,294,314,340,346] assuming that the amount of xenobiotic ingested is known. However, clinicians must remain cognizant of the risk of approaching or exceeding the adsorptive capacity of the standard dose of approximately 1 g/kg of body weight of AC.[8,26,53,144,156,242,294,358]

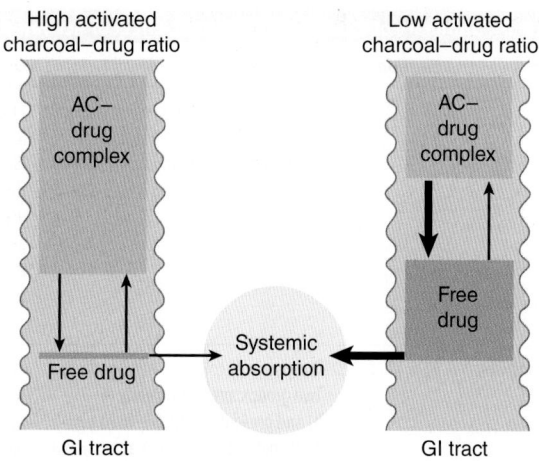

FIGURE 5-4. The effect of high and low ratios of AC to xenobiotic in the gastrointestinal (GI) tract. The reduced systemic absorption achieved when the AC–xenobiotic ratio is high (*left*) is compared with the increased systemic absorption at a low activated charcoal–xenobiotic ratio (*right*).

Thus, the idea that a fixed ratio of AC to xenobiotic is appropriate for all xenobiotics is clearly inappropriate. It is possible, however, to develop a logical approach to dosing based on available data. The effect of the ratio of AC to xenobiotic is such that theoretically increasing the ratio enhances the completeness of adsorption corresponding to a higher percentage of adsorption and total amount of adsorbed xenobiotic (Fig. 5–4).[243] A meta-analysis demonstrated an increasing effect of AC with increasing AC–xenobiotic dose, up to a 40:1 ratio.[171] The optimal AC dose is theoretically the minimum dose that completely adsorbs the ingested xenobiotic and, if relevant, that maximizes enhanced elimination. The results of in vitro studies show that the ideal AC–xenobiotic ratio varies widely, but a common recommendation is to deliver an AC–xenobiotic ratio of 10:1, or 50 to 100 g of AC to adult patients, whichever is greater. From a theoretical perspective, this amount will adsorb 5 to 10 g of a xenobiotic, which should be adequate for most poisonings.[16,17,67,74,255] In human volunteers, the APAP clearance was increased with increasing doses of AC.[130] Fixed doses of 50, 25, or 5 g of AC were administered 1 hour after 50 mg/kg of APAP was given. The apparent half-life of APAP was significantly reduced from 2.5 hours for the 5-g AC dose to 1.9 hours and 1.6 hours for the 25- and 50-g doses, respectively.[130] The effect of larger doses of AC adsorbing larger amounts of xenobiotics was supported by the meta-analysis mentioned earlier.[171] Based on available data from in vivo and in vitro studies, we recommend the dosing regimen for activated charcoal is 50 to 100 g in adults (1 g/kg of body weight) and 0.5 to 1.0 g/kg of body weight in children.[67,74] These recommendations are generally based more on AC tolerance than on efficacy. When calculation of a 10:1 ratio exceeds these recommendations and the ingestion is potentially severely toxic, either orogastric lavage should be performed expeditiously before dosing of AC or multiple-dose AC (MDAC) therapy should be administered.

For example, consider a patient who intentionally overdosed by ingesting 30 (0.25-mg) digoxin tablets (total dose, 7.5 mg). Achieving a 10:1 ratio is quite easy, and a standard dose of 1 g/kg might exceed a 10,000:1 ratio. In comparison, consider a patient who intentionally ingests 30 (325-mg) aspirin tablets (total dose, 9.75 g). In this case, obtaining a 10:1 AC–xenobiotic ratio is more difficult and is even less likely if a patient ingests 60 or 100 of the aspirin tablets. Poisoning with a combination of xenobiotics sometimes approaches or exceeds the maximum adsorptive capacity for the standard dose of AC, and increasing the dose to reach a higher AC–xenobiotic ratio will be necessary in patients with severe poisonings from multiple xenobiotics.[144]

Methods to Increase the Palatability of Activated Charcoal

Activated charcoal has a pronounced gritty texture, and it immediately sticks in the throat because it adheres to the mucosal surfaces and begins to cake.[74] In addition, the black appearance and insipid taste of AC make it less attractive.

There have been numerous attempts at making AC more appealing by providing flavors, including jam,[84] chocolate syrup,[218,241] cherry extract or syrup,[131,263,372] cookies,[181] juice,[263] sorbitol,[76,81,220] saccharin,[76,77] strawberry flavor,[261] orange or peppermint oil,[74] melted milk chocolate,[97,98] chocolate milk,[58,131,263] soda,[58,131,263,284] yogurt,[143] and ice cream.[59,141,333] The general recommendation, however, remains that AC should be mixed with water.[13,170] Because AC adsorbs the flavoring agents, the palatable taste from added flavors often disappears within minutes after mixing.[74,76,77,84] However, in cases in which the AC does not completely adsorb the flavoring agents, they provided a pleasant taste without significantly reducing the adsorptive properties of the AC.[74,76,77,141,143]

Effect on Oral Therapeutics

The nonspecific nature and high adsorptive capacity of AC raise concerns about the simultaneous use of orally administered therapeutics. It would be expected that therapeutics administered shortly before or simultaneously with AC would be extensively adsorbed, greatly reducing therapeutic efficacy. Restored utility of a therapeutic would be complex and depend on all of the factors that influence the efficacy of AC. Additional concerns arise regarding the administration of oral maintenance medications. For example, AC will likely alter the kinetics of the new oral anticoagulants (dabigatran, apixaban, and rivaroxaban).[257,310,366] The issue is described to a limited extent and not in the context of poisoning.[281,324]

Contraindications and Complications

Few clinically significant adverse effects are associated with the use of AC for poisoned patients.[74,281] Adverse GI effects are most commonly described, but the frequency varies,[48,281,297] and it might be difficult to differentiate from adverse effects resulting from the ingested xenobiotic.[191,303] In a study of 24 volunteers, mild adverse effects such as abdominal fullness or constipation (46%) and nausea (17%) were common.[303] In a randomized clinical trial, vomiting was not more frequent in patients treated with AC than those who did not receive AC.[79] Similarly, although vomiting was observed in 22% of patients in a randomized controlled trial of 1,103 patients with intentional poisoning; a nonsignificant difference in incidence was reported between patients who had or had not received GI emptying procedures.[233] A prospective cohort study estimating the incidence of vomiting subsequent to the therapeutic administration of AC in poisoned children younger than 18 years of age showed that one of five of these children vomited. Children with previous vomiting or nasogastric tube administration were at highest risk.[264] This incidence of vomiting appears to be greater when AC was administered with sorbitol[351] and after rapid ingestion of larger doses.[243] Although the coingestion of ethanol theoretically increases the risk of vomiting, ethanol does not interfere with the adsorptive capacity of AC in vivo.[142]

Pulmonary aspiration of gastric contents containing AC and inadvertent direct instillation of AC into the lungs from a misplaced nasogastric tube are rare but severe events[79,86,111,121,136,313,360] that might lead to airway obstruction, bronchospasm, hypoxemia, aspiration, permanent lung injury, and even death.[249,259,360] Administration of AC to intubated patients is associated with a low incidence of aspiration pneumonia.[234] In fact, pulmonary complications associated with AC aspiration appear to be primarily related to the aspiration of acidic gastric contents and not directly related to aspiration of AC.[277,293] A retrospective study found that only 1.6% of unselected overdose patients aspirated and that administration of AC was not an associated risk factor.[161] Pulmonary aspiration in overdose patients who have received AC is more easily recognized and thus documented because AC is a very identifiable marker.

Although relatively few reports of clinically significant emesis and pulmonary aspiration resulting from the administration of AC exist, the severity of these complications is clear. Consequently, it is important to evaluate whether AC therapy is likely to be beneficial based on the indications and contraindications listed in Table 5-7. This is especially true in small children, in whom the risks of nasogastric tube use often outweigh the benefits of AC.

TABLE 5–7	Single-Dose Activated Charcoal Therapy: Indications and Contraindications	
Indications	**Contraindications**
The patient does not meet criteria for orogastric lavage (Table 5–1) or orogastric lavage is likely to be harmful.	Activated charcoal is known not to adsorb a clinically meaningful amount of the ingested xenobiotic.
The patient has ingested a potentially toxic amount of a xenobiotic that is well adsorbed by AC.	Airway protective reflexes are absent or expected to be lost, and the patient is not intubated.
The ingestion occurred within a time frame amenable to adsorption by AC or clinical factors are present that suggest that not all of the xenobiotic has already been systemically absorbed.	Gastrointestinal perforation is likely, as in cases of caustic ingestions.
Patients who have potentially life-threatening toxicity regardless of the time since ingestion as long as no absolute contraindications exist.	Therapy will likely increase the risk and severity of aspiration, such as in the presence of hydrocarbons with a high aspiration potential.
	Endoscopy will be an essential diagnostic modality (caustics).

MULTIPLE-DOSE ACTIVATED CHARCOAL

Multiple-dose AC is defined as at least two sequential doses of AC.[351] In many cases, the actual number of doses administered is substantially greater. This technique serves two purposes: (1) to prevent ongoing absorption of a xenobiotic that persists in the GI tract (such as modified-release preparation) and (2) to enhance elimination in the postabsorptive phase by either disrupting enterohepatic recirculation or enteroenteric recirculation ("gut dialysis").

The 1999 position statement of the AACT and the EAPCCT concluded that based on clinical studies, MDAC should be considered only if a patient has ingested a potentially life-threatening amount of carbamazepine, dapsone, phenobarbital, quinine, or theophylline. Although data have confirmed enhanced elimination of these drugs, no controlled studies have demonstrated clinical benefit after their ingestion. Volunteer studies demonstrate that MDAC increases the elimination of amitriptyline, dextropropoxyphene, digitoxin, digoxin, disopyramide, nadolol, phenylbutazone, phenytoin, piroxicam, and sotalol, but the position statement concluded that there are insufficient clinical data to support or exclude the use of MDAC in these patients.[351] A possibly beneficial effect of MDAC was shown in poisonings including *Amanita phalloides* and other *Amanita* spp,[57,118,168,276] amiodarone,[328] carbamazepine,[38,354] digoxin,[192,278] dosulepin,[222] duloxetine,[100] diquat,[344] *Gymnopilus penetrans*,[239] lamotrigine,[100] phenobarbital,[69] phenytoin,[54] quetiapine,[38] theophylline,[55] valproic acid,[356] verapamil,[305] and vinorelbine.[376] Furthermore, MDAC is recommended in severe poisonings, such as colchicine[42] and quinine.[166]

Although technically correct, the preceding statements suffer from a lack of high-quality evidence. Because the clinical studies used to formulate this opinion all lack sufficient numbers of significantly poisoned patients, they induce a bias against any benefit of MDAC. Additionally, none of the studies included a detailed analysis of sustained- or extended-release formulations, which are currently widely used. Finally, it is noteworthy that the definition of "life threatening" is highly subjective. Endpoints such as decreased morbidity or rigorously determined lengths of stay should be considered essential in any study design. Three studies with these clinical endpoints were previously discussed.[130] Unfortunately, their results were discordant, highlighting the difficulties within this field of study.[45,85,96] However one study is unique in that all 401 patients ingested life-threatening doses of yellow oleander seeds. The patients arrived within 24 hours of ingestion, all received 50 g of AC on arrival, and they were then randomly assigned either 50 g of AC every 6 hours (MDAC) for 3 days or sterile water. Death was the primary outcome, and secondary outcomes included life-threatening cardiac dysrhythmias, dose of atropine used, need for antidigoxin Fab fragments, need for cardiac pacing, admission to the ICU, and length of stay. Analysis was by intention to treat. A total of 201 patients received MDAC; 200 received water. The mortality rate was lower in the MDAC group (5 {2.5%} versus 16 {8%}), and differences favored MDAC for all secondary outcomes, except length of stay. MDAC reduced the number of deaths and life-threatening cardiac dysrhythmias after yellow oleander poisoning. Furthermore, antidigoxin antibody Fab fragments was needed in seven patients in the placebo group, but none in the MDAC group needed the antidote.[85]

Dosing

Various MDAC regimens were evaluated to optimize the efficacy of AC.[158,176] Reduced xenobiotic absorption and enhanced elimination were demonstrated compared with either single-dose AC or control without AC.[176] The effect of MDAC on elimination was studied in volunteers who were given lamotrigine and oxcarbazepine in therapeutic doses.[176] The MDAC dose regimen was 25 g of AC at 6, 12, 24, 36, 48, and 72 hours after a 100-mg lamotrigine dose or 20 g of AC at 12, 24, 36, and 48 hours after a 300-mg oxcarbazepine dose. Both AC regimens significantly reduced the total systemic xenobiotic load compared with control participants with reductions of 51% for lamotrigine and 41% for 10-hydroxy-carbazepine. The elimination half-life for both xenobiotics was significantly shortened with MDAC: 11 ± 3.5 hours (MDAC) versus 25 ± 4.3 hours (control) for lamotrigine and 9.0 ± 1.5 (MDAC) versus 20 ± 12 hours (control) for 10-hydroxy-carbazepine.[176]

Intravenous administration of a xenobiotic is an ideal method to evaluate the ability of different MDAC dose regimens to enhance elimination of a xenobiotic in the postabsorptive phase. A total dose of 150 g of oral AC, given as a loading dose of 50 g and the remaining 100 g divided in 12.5 g every hour, 25.0 g every 2 hours, or 50.0 g every 4 hours during a total time of 8 hours was equally effective in reducing the mean area under the concentration versus time curve (AUC) in volunteers receiving 8 mg/kg of aminophylline intravenously over a period of 60 minutes.[158] In a similar study, the AUC and $t_{1/2}$ of aminophylline were reduced by 46% and 49%, respectively, by MDAC using a dosing regimen of 40-g loading dose and then five 20-g doses divided over 12 hours.[34]

Contraindications and Complications

Similar to single-dose AC, MDAC can produce emesis, with subsequent pulmonary aspiration of gastric contents containing AC. It is intuitive that these risks are greater with MDAC than with single-dose therapy. One retrospective study attempted to determine the frequency of complications associated with the use of MDAC.[90] The authors identified nearly 900 patients who had received MDAC and found that only 0.6% of patients had clinically significant pulmonary aspiration. Although no patients developed GI obstruction, 9% had hypernatremia or hypermagnesemia without any clinical consequences noted. The authors did not specify whether the multiple-dose regimens administered included the use of cathartics, but the profile of the adverse reactions suggests that these electrolyte abnormalities were probably associated with cathartic use. Despite the obvious limitations, this study demonstrates a reasonably low rate of complications associated with MDAC.

Table 5–8 summarizes the indications and contraindications for MDAC therapy. Table 5–9 lists our recommended dosing regimens. Because the optimal doses and intervals for MDAC are not established, recommendations are based more on amounts that can be tolerated than on amounts that might be considered pharmacologically appropriate. Larger doses and shorter intervals should be used for patients with more severe toxicity. It is reasonable to base endpoints either on the patient's clinical condition or on xenobiotic concentrations when they are easily measured.

Further clinical and toxicokinetic studies concerning MDAC are needed to establish an optimal dosing regimen and to confirm an effect on relevant endpoints. From available data discussed earlier, the dosing and most appropriate dosing intervals should be evaluated in each individual overdose case including compliance and clinical challenges from complications (eg, emesis and vomiting). Readers are referred to Antidotes in Depth: A1 for a more detailed discussion of single-dose AC and MDAC therapy.

TABLE 5–8	Multiple-Dose Activated Charcoal Therapy: Indications and Contraindications	
Indications		**Contraindications**
Ingestion of a life-threatening amount of *Amanita* spp., amiodarone, amitriptyline, carbamazepine, colchicine, dextropropoxyphene, digitoxin, digoxin, disopyramide, dosulepin, duloxetine, diquat, *Gymnopilus penetrans*, lamotrigine, nadolol, phenobarbital, phenylbutazone, phenytoin, piroxicam, quetiapine, quinine, sotalol, theophylline, valproic acid, verapamil, or vinorelbine.		Any contraindication to single-dose activated charcoal. The presence of an ileus or other causes of diminished peristalsis.
Ingestion of a life-threatening amount of a xenobiotic that undergoes enterohepatic or enteroenteric recirculation and that is adsorbed to activated charcoal.		
Ingestion of a significant amount of any slowly released xenobiotic or of a xenobiotic known to form concretions or bezoars.		

WHOLE-BOWEL IRRIGATION

Whole-bowel irrigation represents a method of purging the GI tract in an attempt to expeditiously achieve gut clearance and prevent further absorption of xenobiotics. This is achieved through the oral or nasogastric administration of large amounts of an osmotically balanced polyethylene glycol electrolyte lavage solution (PEG-ELS). WBI was subjected to a thorough literature review, which was published as a revised position statement in 2015.[334] No new evidence was available that required a major revision of the conclusions of the 2004 position statement.[332] The position statement was unable to establish a clear set of evidence-based indications for the use of WBI because no clinical outcome studies have ever been performed. When experimental, theoretical, and anecdotal human experience is considered, the use of WBI with PEG-ELS is reasonable for patients with potentially toxic ingestions of modified release pharmaceuticals and substantial amounts of metals. Other indications include the ingestion of large amounts of a xenobiotic with a slow absorptive phase in which morbidity is expected to be high, the ingested xenobiotic is not adsorbed by AC, and other methods of GI

TABLE 5–9	Technique of Administering Multiple-Dose Activated Charcoal Therapy
Initial dose orally or via orogastric or nasogastric tube:	
Adults and children: 1 g/kg of body weight or a 10:1 ratio of activated charcoal to xenobiotic, whichever is greater. After massive ingestions, 2 g/kg of body weight is reasonable if such a large dose can be tolerated.	
Repeat doses orally or via orogastric or nasogastric tube:	
Adults and children: 0.5 g/kg of body weight every 4–6 h for 12–24 h in accordance with the dose and dosage form of xenobiotic ingested (larger doses or shorter dosing intervals are reasonable in high-risk cases).	

Procedure

1. Add eight parts of water to the selected amount of powdered form. All formulations, including prepacked slurries, should be shaken well for at least 1 min to form a transiently stable suspension before the patient drinks or has it instilled via orogastric or nasogastric tube.

2. A cathartic can be added to AC *for the first dose only* when indicated. Cathartics should not be administered routinely and never be repeated with subsequent doses of activated charcoal.

3. If the patient vomits the dose of activated charcoal, it should be repeated. Smaller, more frequent doses or continuous nasogastric administration is better tolerated. Administration of an antiemetic is recommended.

4. If a nasogastric or orogastric tube is used for MDAC administration, time should be allowed for the last dose to pass through the stomach before the tube is removed. Suctioning the tube itself before removal will theoretically lessen the risk of subsequent activated charcoal aspiration.

MDAC = multiple-dose activated charcoal.

decontamination are unlikely to be either safe or beneficial.[334] The removal of packets of xenobiotics from body packers can be considered a unique indication for WBI (Special Considerations: SC5).[31,341]

Whole-bowel irrigation cannot be applied safely if the GI tract is not intact; there is an adynamic or obstructive ileus; in the presence of significant GI hemorrhage; or in patients with inadequate airway protection, uncontrolled vomiting, or hemodynamic instability that compromises GI function or integrity.[82,332] Compliance is often an issue because 1 to 2 L/h of PEG-ELS is required for rapid bowel cleansing in adults. These large volumes are facilitated when the solution is administered via a nasogastric tube.[206] Additionally, in vitro, the combination of WBI and AC decreases the adsorptive capacity of AC or increases the desorption of xenobiotic from AC,[23,148,212] especially when the WBI solution is premixed with AC.[212,334] When AC is necessary, it is reasonable to administer it immediately after the WBI procedure rather than simultaneously.

Results from volunteer studies often offer extreme variability in results,[189,190,193,208] and significant variations are noted when individual subjects are simultaneously given three different modified-release xenobiotics.[193] In one study, nine volunteers took sustained-release preparations of 200 mg of carbamazepine, 200 mg of theophylline, and 120 mg of verapamil, and 1 hour after ingestion, they were assigned to 25 g of AC followed by WBI, 1 L/h PEG-ELS, 25 g of AC, or water (200 mL). When the combination therapy was compared with AC alone, it was not more efficient at reducing pharmacokinetic parameters such as AUC (0–24 hours) and C_{max} for carbamazepine and theophylline, but for verapamil, the combination therapy was more effective than AC alone.[193] Similarly, in a volunteer study in which WBI was initiated 30 minutes after sustained-release APAP (75 mg/kg) ingestion, it did not significantly reduce the AUC compared with control.[208] In this study, a gelatin capsule containing 24 radiopaque polyvinyl chloride markers measuring 1 by 4.5 mm, which was given simultaneously with APAP, reached the colon more rapidly and in a "collected cluster" on the day of WBI administration compared with the control when the 24 markers were spread throughout the GI tract.

In both of these studies, therapeutic or nontoxic doses of pharmaceuticals were used as marker xenobiotics. In actual overdoses, the pharmacokinetic properties of pharmaceuticals and the effects of decontamination likely differ substantially. As mentioned earlier, study designs using AC and small doses of xenobiotics tend to bias the study toward a benefit of AC. In an overdose scenario, when the adsorptive capacity of AC is exceeded, it is intuitive that the benefits of other modalities would be more evident.

Pharmacokinetic and pharmacodynamic evaluation in venlafaxine-overdosed patients showed that compared with AC alone, combination therapy of WBI and AC decreased venlafaxine bioavailability (29% reduction), increased venlafaxine clearance (35% increase), lowered venlafaxine peak concentrations[190] and resulted in a decreased probability of venlafaxine induced seizures (odds ratio, 0.25 for the combination therapy versus 0.48 for AC alone).[189]

A small, retrospective, descriptive case series of 16 body packers treated with WBI supports the safety of WBI for body packers. Although the complication rate was reported as 12.5% (two of 16), these complications were not serious. One case of mild cocaine toxicity resulted from leakage, and one heroin body packer had to undergo surgery because of retained packages. There was no correlation between the dose of PEG-ELS, drug type, or packet quantity and length of hospital stay. Because there was no control group, it is not possible to evaluate whether WBI influenced any clinical outcome.[106] A variety of treatments were used to enhance GI clearance rates of cocaine packets in 61 verified body packers who were judged not to be able to clear the packets from their gut. In 33% of the procedures, PEG-ELS was used, and the dosage regimen of 1.5 L/h of PEG-ELS was continued until all packets had passed, with no limit on the total volume given.[31]

Whole-bowel irrigation is acceptable to treat overdoses in pregnant women and children. Two such cases involved iron overdoses in women during the second and third trimesters of pregnancy; both women were treated successfully without complications.[347,355] Pediatric case reports

TABLE 5–10	Whole-Bowel Irrigation: Indications and Contraindications
Indications	**Contraindications**
Potentially toxic ingestions of sustained-release and modified release drugs.	Airway protective reflexes are absent or expected to become so in a patient who is not intubated.
Ingestion of a toxic amount of a xenobiotic that is not adsorbed to AC when other methods of GI decontamination are not possible or not efficacious.	The GI tract is not intact. There are signs of ileus, obstruction, significant GI hemorrhage, or hemodynamic instability that might compromise GI motility.
Removal of illicit drug packets from body packers.	Persistent vomiting.
	Signs of leakage from cocaine packets (indication for surgical removal).

GI = gastrointestinal.

Reproduced with permission from Shargel L, Yu A: Applied Biopharmaceutics and Pharmacokinetics, 3rd ed. Norwalk, CT: Appleton & Lange; 1993.

describe combined WBI with succimer therapy[71] and eventually colonoscopic removal of ingested lead pellets.[71,137] Abdominal radiographs showed two small lead pellets, which WBI failed to remove, therefore requiring endoscopic removal.[71] Seven days of WBI, however, was ineffective in the removal of approximately 800 ingested lead pellets, which necessitated removal by colonoscopy.[137] Several reports support the use of WBI in children, including an intentional ingestion of mercury,[302] two pediatric body packers,[342] and a 16 month-old boy who had ingested a significant amount of iron.[361] In the latter case, despite WBI, the iron bezoar was not removed, treatment was eventually stopped, and the bezoar was expelled after a normal diet was resumed.[361]

The current evidence for the clinical efficacy of WBI is divergent, depending on the xenobiotic and its formulation. Additional case reports and series demonstrate the overall safety of WBI as well as some beneficial effects on secondary endpoints, but the benefits remain generally theoretical. The safety of using PEG-ELS was investigated with regard to its impact on the dissolution time of tablets. Although a hastened dissolution of immediate release APAP was shown in one study, no accelerated dissolution was observed from a variety of extended-release morphine formulations.[139,251]

The indications for WBI with PEG-ELS are patients with potentially toxic ingestions of modified-release pharmaceuticals, xenobiotic ingestions with slow absorptive phases when morbidity is expected to be high, and foreign body ingestions. The combination of WBI and AC is reasonable when adsorption of the ingested xenobiotic to AC is expected to be high. Other uses of WBI remain theoretical because the only support for the efficacy comes from surrogate markers and anecdotal experience. Table 5–10 summarizes the indications and contraindications for WBI.

CATHARTICS

At present, there is no indication for the routine use of cathartics as a method of either limiting absorption or enhancing elimination. It is reasonable to administer a single dose as an adjunct to AC therapy when there are no contraindications and constipation or an increased GI transit time is expected. Multiple-dose cathartics should never be used, and magnesium- and phosphate-containing cathartics should be avoided in patients with kidney disease (Antidotes in Depth: A2).

SURGERY AND ENDOSCOPY

Surgery and endoscopy are occasionally indicated for decontamination of poisoned patients. As might be expected, no controlled studies have been conducted, and potential indications are based largely on case reports and case series. A prospective, uncontrolled series of 50 patients with cocaine packet ingestion was published more than 30 years ago.[52] The patients were conservatively managed and only underwent surgery if there were signs of leakage or mechanical bowel obstruction. Bowel obstruction occurred in three patients, who promptly underwent successful emergency laparotomy; another six patients chose elective surgery. The authors concluded that body packers should be treated conservatively and only operated on for xenobiotic leakage or bowel obstruction.[52] A similar study performed a 16-year retrospective analysis of all body packers treated in a single center.[306] Of the 2,880 body packers who were identified, 63 (2.2%) developed symptoms of severe cocaine toxicity after rupture of a package, 43 of the 63 symptomatic patients (68%) died before surgery could be initiated, and the 20 (32%) who underwent emergency laparotomy to remove the drug packets survived. Another report described two body packers who successfully underwent surgery to remove drug packets. In one case, the indications were rupture and signs of cocaine toxicity. In the other case, the indication for surgery was bowel obstruction.[258] Because most packages do not spontaneously rupture, mechanical obstruction is probably the most common reason for surgical removal of ingested drug packets.[341] Leakage from heroin-containing packages should be managed by naloxone infusion, but the lack of antidote when cocaine packages rupture necessitates surgery (Special Considerations: SC5).[341]

Over the years, case reports, presented mixed results for the endoscopic removal of drug packets, pharmacobezoars, or foreign material from the stomach.[31,63,88,150,178,210,247,312,317,325,341] At present, this method is not routinely recommended for the removal of drug packets because of the concern regarding packet rupture. The procedure is reasonable for removal of a compact pharmacobezoar containing a xenobiotic causing severe and continued poisoning.[150,210,247,312] Emergency GI endoscopy was performed in a patient with a case of Portland cement ingestion. Within 40 minutes of ingestion, the patient vomited grayish material. Gray material was found by endoscopy in the esophagus and gastric fundus, portions of which had become solid masses. Most materials were carefully washed out with suction, and the solid masses were removed with a retrieval net. Gastric lavage was deemed contraindicated because of the risk of esophageal perforation from caustic injury and tracheal aspiration of the stomach contents.[178]

A tablet conglomerate of 43 etilefrin hydrochloride 430-mg tablets in the stomach, which could neither be effectively treated with AC nor by orogastric lavage, was fragmented endoscopically. Removal of the tablet fragments led to the elimination of the residual tablets, and symptoms of toxicity resolved rapidly.[312] Under exceptional circumstances, there is certainly a precedent for attempting this procedure in a highly controlled setting such as an ICU or operating room.

In rare cases of massive iron overdoses when emesis, orogastric lavage, and gastroscopy failed or were estimated to result in an insufficient treatment outcome, gastrotomy was performed. The significant clinical improvement and postoperative recovery indicated that surgery in these particular cases was the correct approach.[109,134,271] In a case of zinc toxicity resulting from massive chronic coin ingestion, laparotomy and gastrotomy proved essential to remove the more than 270 coins ingested (Chap. 100).[268]

OTHER ADJUNCTIVE METHODS USED FOR GASTROINTESTINAL DECONTAMINATION

Other xenobiotics, such as cholecystokinin, were studied as adjuncts to standard measures for GI decontamination.[99,146] Pharmaceuticals that either speed up GI passage or slow down gastric emptying were administered in an attempt to minimize the absorption of a xenobiotic. In all cases, the results were negligible, and the potential risks of administering additional pharmacologically active xenobiotics to an already poisoned patient seem to outweigh any benefit.[12,363] Interventions that reduce the absorption of xenobiotics from the GI tract other than AC were also studied, including sodium polystyrene sulfonate for lithium[32,116,208,212,213,289,339] or thallium overdose.[149] Human studies showed minimal decreased absorption and increased clearance of lithium when sodium polystyrene sulfonate was administered, and it is therefore not routinely recommended.[116,289] Similarly, case reports describe the use of the lipid-lowering resins cholestyramine and colestipol to interrupt the enterohepatic circulation of digoxin, digitoxin, and chlordane to increase elimination.[30,114,177,275] With the increased use of AC and availability of digoxin-specific Fab fragments, indications for lipid-lowering resins for cardioactive steroid ingestions seem obsolete. Studies on clay products in

vitro have demonstrated a lower efficacy compared with AC and AC–kaolin products in the adsorption of *Nerium oleander* cardioactive steroids.[338]

POST–BARIATRIC SURGERY PATIENTS

Patients who have undergone bariatric surgery represent a subgroup of patients who need special caution before GI decontamination procedures can be initiated. Bariatric surgery procedures differ, but they all alter the gastric anatomy and reduce the gastric volume significantly. Limited data are available in the literature, and a single report demonstrated that orogastric lavage was impossible because of resistance in the midesophagus. An 8-cm gastric pouch and a gastrojejunal anastomosis was shown on abdominal radiography, and instillation of AC–sorbitol via the gastric tube resulted in prompt oropharyngeal reflux.[288] Two retrospective case series discuss considerations in GI decontamination procedures in this subgroup of poisoned patients.[199,270] A retrospective poison control center study in 19 cases reported very poor results from orogastric lavage in four patients, with minor gastric bleeding caused by the procedure in one of the patients. No apparent complications were reported from AC dosing that was given in several instances (the specific number was not reported). Whole-bowel irrigation was used in two cases.[270] The use of GI decontamination procedures in a post–bariatric surgery population was retrospectively described in 527 cases. Activated charcoal was used in 14% of cases, MDAC in less than 1%, orogastric lavage in 2%, and WBI in less than 1%. Adverse effects for the procedures included nausea in 12%, vomiting in 9%, and hematemesis in less than 1%. Death unrelated to the toxic exposure was reported in 1%.[199]

Unfortunately, no studies investigated the optimal GI decontamination procedure in this subgroup of patients, and until studies are available, caution is required. Orogastric lavage is not indicated in a patient who has undergone bariatric surgery because the placement of a gastric tube possesses a risk of perforation injuries because of the altered gastric anatomy. The reduced gastric volume makes it impossible for the patient to hold more than an estimated volume of 100 mL of fluid at the time. Dosing of AC is possible but should be divided into smaller portions using a maximum volume of 100 mL. WBI is reasonable after ingestion of large amounts of slow-release formulations.

GENERAL GUIDANCE

Only a few studies provide guidance based on meaningful clinical endpoints for GI decontamination. Pharmacokinetic and pharmacodynamic parameters were introduced and systematically evaluated in human overdoses,[162-164,189,190,357] of the increasingly popular pharmaceuticals known to cause central nervous system and cardiac toxicity: venlafaxine, citalopram, escitalopram, and quetiapine. Cohort studies[162-164,189,190] evaluated the effect of GI decontamination with the aim to predict cardiotoxicity and the effects of the GI decontamination method chosen in real-life situations that are often inconsistent with the recommendations of the position papers.[33,66,185,332,334,351,353] In a cohort of 436 venlafaxine overdoses, AC increased venlafaxine clearance and decreased the probability of seizures.[189,190] Similarly, 77 patients with escitalopram overdoses were used to develop a pharmacokinetic–pharmacodynamic model that predicted the probability of having abnormal QT interval as a surrogate for torsade de pointes.[357] In this model, AC decreased the bioavailability by 31% and reduced the relative risk reduction of prolonged QT interval by 35% after the ingestion of 200 mg of escitalopram or more.[357] The interruption of the enteroenteric recirculation of therapeutic doses of rivaroxaban and apixaban showed an effect of AC 6 hours after a therapeutic dose and pharmacokinetic modeling suggested effects from AC more than 8 hours after rivaroxaban dosing.[257,366]

The trends in GI decontamination have dramatically shifted toward less intervention over the years. In 2015, of the 2,168,371 human exposure reported to the American Association of Poison Control Centers (Chap. 130), it is remarkable that only 41,598 patients were given single-dose AC, 1,114 were given MDAC, 1,745 underwent lavage, and 1,683 received WBI. At the same time, the more serious exposures (major, moderate, and death) increased and the less serious exposures (no effect, minor effect, not followed (nontoxic), decreased; Chap. 130). Similar trends in GI decontamination are reported elsewhere with no apparent worsening of outcome.[20] These trends in practice reflect the overall combined philosophy of the position statements, which are applicable to the vast majority of poisoned patients. They highlight the benign nature, in the developed world, of many exposures and the benefits of good supportive care in the typical patient for whom the interventions of GI decontamination represent more risk than benefit. In contrast, the survey mentioned at the beginning of this chapter regarding recommendations for a theoretical patient with a serious enteric-coated aspirin overdose reveals less consensus in that 36 different courses of action were proposed for the same patient—a situation in which nonintervention would likely be of greater risk to the patient than decontamination. Most of the poison control centers and toxicologists did, however, recommend at least one dose of AC.[173] This distinction serves as a reminder that the existing studies and consensus statements cannot be applied to all cases and that a lack of data produces significant uncertainty in choices for GI decontamination in either atypical or severely poisoned patients.[147]

It is essential to note that only one study has ever demonstrated a survival advantage for any form of GI decontamination of poisoned patients.[85] Its unique design, involving a cohort of patients with life-threatening toxicity, forces a reassessment of all previous and subsequent literature and confirms that the principles of decontamination are sound. It also suggests that the failure of most studies to demonstrate a benefit results not from a failure of the techniques used but from applying decontamination techniques to subsets of patients who were likely to have good outcomes regardless of intervention. By consulting experts within clinical and medical toxicology, treating clinicians will be assisted in the risk assessment and evaluation of poisoned patients, and guidelines for specific management can be provided, thereby initially obtaining correct and goal-directed treatment.

SUMMARY

- The approach to GI decontamination must be individualized. No decontamination method is completely free of risks. The indications and contraindications for GI decontamination must be well defined for each patient, and the method of choice must depend largely on what was ingested, how much was ingested, who ingested it, and when it was ingested.

- Evidence points away from the routine GI decontamination of most patients presenting to an ED with an oral pharmaceutical drug overdose.

- A single dose of AC alone will be sufficient in moderate-risk patients, and only in a small subset of exceptionally high-risk patients will the benefit of orogastric lavage outweigh the risks.

- Orogastric lavage as a single intervention is reserved for cases in which the ingested xenobiotic is not adsorbed by AC and there is reason to believe that the ingested xenobiotic is both life threatening *and* remains in the stomach.

- Multiple-dose activated charcoal and WBI have narrowly defined indications, which will likely change as more investigators address poisoned patients.

- The absolute time frame for when GI decontamination is indicated depends on many factors, such as the rate of gastric emptying, the rate of release of the xenobiotic from modified-release pharmaceuticals, the rate of xenobiotic absorption, and the possibility of enterohepatic and enteroenteric recirculation. The commonly stated short time frame of up to 1 hour postingestion for intervention is an artificially constructed framework that limits the potential benefits of GI decontamination and places many seriously poisoned patients at substantial risk of unnecessary morbidity and mortality.

REFERENCES

1. Adams BK, et al. Prolonged gastric emptying half-time and gastric hypomotility after drug overdose. *Am J Emerg Med*. 2004;22:548-554.

2. Adler P, et al. Hypothermia: an unusual indication for gastric lavage. *J. Emerg Med*. 2011;40:176-178.

3. Aghabiklooei A, et al. Acute colchicine overdose: report of three cases. *Reumatismo*. 2014;65:307-311.

4. Agrawal VK, et al. Aluminum phosphide poisoning: possible role of supportive measures in the absence of specific antidote. *Indian J Crit Care Med*. 2015;19:109-112.

5. Ahishali E, et al. Approach to mushroom intoxication and treatment: can we decrease mortality? *Clin Res Hepatol Gastroenterol*. 2012;36:139-145.

6. Aksakal E, et al. Prolonged QT interval after fexofenadine overdose in the presence of hypokalemia and hypocalcaemia. *Hong Kong J Emerg Med*. 2010;17:75-78.

7. Akyildiz BN, et al. Cyanide poisoning caused by ingestion of apricot seeds. *Ann Trop Paediatr*. 2010;30:39-43.

8. al-Shareef AH, et al. Drug adsorption to charcoals and anionic binding resins. *Hum Exp Toxicol*. 1990;9:95-97.

9. Alaspaa AO, et al. Out-of-hospital administration of activated charcoal by emergency medical services. *Ann Emerg Med*. 2005;45:207-212.

10. Albertson TE, et al. Superiority of activated charcoal alone compared with ipecac and activated charcoal in the treatment of acute toxic ingestions. *Ann Emerg Med*. 1989;18:56-59.

11. Albertson TE, et al. Gastrointestinal decontamination in the acutely poisoned patient. *Int J Emerg Med*. 2011;4:65.

12. Amato CS, et al. Evaluation of promotility agents to limit the gut bioavailability of extended-release acetaminophen. *J Toxicol Clin Toxicol*. 2004;42:73-77.

13. American Academy of Pediatrics Committee on Injury, Violence, and Poison Prevention. Poison treatment in the home. American Academy of Pediatrics Committee on Injury, Violence, and Poison Prevention. *Pediatrics*. 2003;112:1182-1185.

14. Amigo M, et al. [Efficacy and safety of gut decontamination in patients with acute therapeutic drug overdose]. *Med Clin (Barc)*. 2004;122:487-492.

15. Aminiahidashti H, et al. Conservative care in successful treatment of abamectin poisoning. *Toxicol Int*. 2014;21:322-324.

16. Andersen AH. Experimental studies on the pharmacology of activated charcoal. I; adsorption power of charcoal in aqueous solutions. *Acta Pharmacol Toxicol (Copenh)*. 1946;2:69-78.

17. Andersen AH. Experimental studies on the pharmacology of activated charcoal. II; the effect of pH on the adsorption by charcoal from aqueous solutions. *Acta Pharmacol Toxicol (Copenh)*. 1947;3:199-218.

18. Andersen AH. Experimental studies on the pharmacology of activated charcoal. III; adsorption power of charcoal in aqueous solutions. *Acta Pharmacol Toxicol (Copenh)*. 1948;4:275-284.

19. Annas A, et al. Disintegration and possible bezoar formation of large sized extended release tablets—an in vitro study. *Clin Toxicol*. 2017;55:371-544.

20. Ardagh M, et al. Limiting the use of gastrointestinal decontamination does not worsen the outcome from deliberate self-poisoning. *N Z Med J*. 2001;114:423-425.

21. Arroyo AM, Kao LW. Calcium channel blocker toxicity. *Pediatr Emerg Care*. 2009;25: 532-538; quiz 539-540.

22. Askenasi R, et al. Esophageal perforation: an unusual complication of gastric lavage. *Ann Emerg Med*. 1984;13:146.

23. Atta-Politou J, et al. An in vitro evaluation of fluoxetine adsorption by activated charcoal and desorption upon addition of polyethylene glycol-electrolyte lavage solution. *J Toxicol Clin Toxicol*. 1998;36:117-124.

24. Attou R, Reper P. Slow-release clomipramine acute poisoning with radio-opaque gastric bezoar. *Intensive Care Med*. 2013;39:1320.

25. Bailey DN, Briggs JR. The effect of ethanol and pH on the adsorption of drugs from simulated gastric fluid onto activated charcoal. *Ther Drug Monit*. 2003;25:310-313.

26. Bainbridge CA, et al. In vitro adsorption of acetaminophen onto activated charcoal. *J Pharm Sci*. 1977;66:480-483.

27. Bandara V, et al. A review of the natural history, toxinology, diagnosis and clinical management of Nerium oleander (common oleander) and Thevetia peruviana (yellow oleander) poisoning. *Toxicon*. 2010;56:273-281.

28. Barton CA, et al. Successful treatment of a massive metoprolol overdose using intravenous lipid emulsion and hyperinsulinemia/euglycemia therapy. *Pharmacotherapy*. 2015;35:e56-60.

29. Bartos M, Knudsen K. Use of intravenous lipid emulsion in the resuscitation of a patient with cardiovascular collapse after a severe overdose of quetiapine. *Clin Toxicol (Phila)*. 2013;51:501-504.

30. Bazzano G, Bazzano GS. Digitalis intoxication. Treatment with a new steroid-binding resin. *JAMA*. 1972;220:828-830.

31. Beckley I, et al. Clinical management of cocaine body packers: the Hillingdon experience. *Can J Surg*. 2009;52:417-421.

32. Belanger DR, et al. Effect of sodium polystyrene sulfonate on lithium bioavailability. *Ann Emerg Med*. 1992;21:1312-1315.

33. Benson BE, et al. Position paper update: gastric lavage for gastrointestinal decontamination. *Clin Toxicol (Phila)*. 2013;51:140-146.

34. Berlinger WG, et al. Enhancement of theophylline clearance by oral activated charcoal. *Clin Pharmacol Ther*. 1983;33:351-354.

35. Bhat NK, et al. Profile of poisoning in children and adolescents at a North Indian tertiary care centre. *J Indian Acad Clin J Med*. 2012;13:37-42.

36. Bhoelan BS, et al. Barium toxicity and the role of the potassium inward rectifier current. *Clin Toxicol (Phila)*. 2014;52:584-593.

37. Bianchi Stefano SB, et al. An epidemiological analysis of poisonings in the Italian region of Emilia Romagna from 2005 to 2009. *Eur J Hosp Pharm*. 2012;19:222-223.

38. Bogevig S, Petersen TS. Lack of symptoms following a large combined carbamazepine and quetiapine overdose: the role of enzyme induction by carbamazepine. *Clin Toxicol*. 2016;54:418.

39. Bologa C, et al. Lipid emulsion therapy in cardiodepressive syndrome after diltiazem overdose—case report. *Am J Emerg Med*. 2013;31:1154.e1153-1154.

40. Bond GR. Home syrup of ipecac use does not reduce emergency department use or improve outcome. *Pediatrics*. 2003;112:1061-1064.

41. Bond GR. The role of activated charcoal and gastric emptying in gastrointestinal decontamination: a state-of-the-art review. *Ann Emerg Med*. 2002;39:273-286.

42. Bora KM, et al. Colchicine kinetics in non-fatal overdose. *Clin Toxicol*. 2009;47:763-764.

43. Bosse GM, et al. Comparison of three methods of gut decontamination in tricyclic antidepressant overdose. *J. Emerg Med*. 1995;13:203-209.

44. Boxer L, et al. Comparison of ipecac-induced emesis with gastric lavage in the treatment of acute salicylate ingestion. *J Pediatr*. 1969;74:800-803.

45. Brahmi N, et al. Influence of activated charcoal on the pharmacokinetics and the clinical features of carbamazepine poisoning. *Am J Emerg Med*. 2006;24:440-443.

46. Buckley NA, et al. Overcoming apathy in research on organophosphate poisoning. *BMJ*. 2004;329:1231-1233.

47. Budhathoki S, et al. Clinical profile and outcome of children presenting with poisoning or intoxication: a hospital based study. *Nepal Med Coll J*. 2009;11:170-175.

48. Burillo Putze G, et al. [Adverse events caused by activated charcoal in an emergency services survey]. *An Sist Sanit Navar*. 2015;38:203-211.

49. Calpin P, Daniels F. Heart-block smoothie. *Irish J Med Sci*. 2015;1:S338.

50. Camilleri M, et al. Relation between antral motility and gastric emptying of solids and liquids in humans. *Am J Physiol*. 1985;249(5 Pt 1):G580-585.

51. Caravati EM, et al. Esophageal laceration and charcoal mediastinum complicating gastric lavage. *J. Emerg Med*. 2001;20:273-276.

52. Caruana DS, et al. Cocaine-packet ingestion. Diagnosis, management, and natural history. *Ann Intern Med*. 1984;100:73-74.

53. Cassidy SL, et al. In vitro drug adsorption to charcoal, silicas, acrylate copolymer and silicone oil with charcoal and with acrylate copolymer. *Hum Exp Toxicol*. 1997;16:25-27.

54. Chan BSH, et al. Use of multi-dose activated charcoal in phenytoin toxicity secondary to genetic polymorphism. *Clin Toxicol*. 2015;53:131-133.

55. Chan TYK, et al. Overdose of methyldopa, indapamide and theophylline resulting in prolonged hypotension, marked diuresis and hypokalaemia in an elderly patient. *Pharmacoepidemiol Drug Saf*. 2009;18:977-979.

56. Chaouali N, et al. [Acute poisoning with anticholinesterase carbamate pesticides: methomyl-lannate(R)]. *Ann Biol Clin (Paris)*. 2014;72:723-729.

57. Chen WC, et al. A rare case of amatoxin poisoning in the state of Texas. *Case Rep Gastroenterol*. 2012;6:350-357.

58. Cheng A, Ratnapalan S. Improving the palatability of activated charcoal in pediatric patients. *Pediatr Emerg Care*. 2007;23:384-386.

59. Cheng M, Robertson WO. Charcoal "flavored" ice cream. *Vet Hum Toxicol*. 1989;31:332.

60. Cherukuri H, et al. Demographics, clinical characteristics and management of herbicide poisoning in tertiary care hospital. *Toxicol Int*. 2014;21:209-213.

61. Chiew AL, et al. Summary statement: new guidelines for the management of paracetamol poisoning in Australia and New Zealand. *Med J Aust*. 2015;203:215-218.

62. Chiew AL, et al. Massive paracetamol overdose: an observational study of the effect of activated charcoal and increased acetylcysteine dose (ATOM-2). *Clin Toxicol*. 2017;55:1055-1065.

63. Choudhary AM, et al. Endoscopic removal of a cocaine packet from the stomach. *J Clin Gastroenterol*. 1998;27:155-156.

64. Christophersen AB, et al. Activated charcoal alone or after gastric lavage: a simulated large paracetamol intoxication. *Br J Clin Pharmacol*. 2002;53:312-317.

65. Chyka PA, et al. Dextromethorphan poisoning: an evidence-based consensus guideline for out-of-hospital management. *Clin Toxicol (Phila)*. 2007;45:662-677.

66. Chyka PA, Seger D. Position statement: single-dose activated charcoal. American Academy of Clinical Toxicology; European Association of Poisons Centres and Clinical Toxicologists. *J Toxicol Clin Toxicol*. 1997;35:721-741.

67. Chyka PA, et al. Position paper: single-dose activated charcoal. *Clin Toxicol (Phila)*. 2005;43:61-87.

68. Cibickova L, et al. Multi-drug intoxication fatality involving atorvastatin: a case report. *Forensic Sci Int*. 2015;257:e26-31.

69. Ciszowski K, et al. Phenobarbital poisoning: the old problem anew—two case reports with toxicokinetics. *Clin Toxicol*. 2009;47:482.

70. Clemmesen C, Nilsson E. Therapeutic trends in the treatment of barbiturate poisoning. The Scandinavian method. *Clin Pharmacol Ther*. 1961;2:220-229.

71. Clifton JC, 2nd, et al. Acute pediatric lead poisoning: combined whole bowel irrigation, succimer therapy, and endoscopic removal of ingested lead pellets. *Pediatr Emerg Care*. 2002;18:200-202.

72. Comstock EG, et al. Assessment of the efficacy of activated charcoal following gastric lavage in acute drug emergencies. *J Toxicol Clin Toxicol*. 1982;19:149-165.

73. Comstock EG, et al. Studies on the efficacy of gastric lavage as practiced in a large metropolitan hospital. *Clin Toxicol*. 1981;18:581-597.

74. Cooney DO. *Activated Charcoal in Medical Applications*. New York: Marcel Dekker; 1995.

75. Cooney DO. In vitro adsorption of phenobarbital, chlorpheniramine maleate, and theophylline by four commercially available activated charcoal suspensions. *J Toxicol Clin Toxicol*. 1995;33:213-217.

76. Cooney DO. Palatability of sucrose-, sorbitol-, and saccharin-sweetened activated charcoal formulations. *Am J Hosp Pharm*. 1980;37:237-239.

77. Cooney DO. Saccharin sodium as a potential sweetener for antidotal charcoal. *Am J Hosp Pharm*. 1977;34:1342-1344.

78. Cooper GM, Buckley NA. Activated charcoal RCT. *Am J Ther*. 2003;10:235-236.

79. Cooper GM, et al. A randomized clinical trial of activated charcoal for the routine management of oral drug overdose. *QJM*. 2005;98:655-660.

80. Cooper JM, et al. The pharmacokinetics of sertraline in overdose and the effect of activated charcoal. *Br J Clin Pharmacol*. 2015;79:307-315.

81. Cordonnier JA, et al. In vitro adsorption of tilidine HCl by activated charcoal. *J Toxicol Clin Toxicol*. 1986;24:503-517.

82. Cumpston KL, et al. Whole bowel irrigation and the hemodynamically unstable calcium channel blocker overdose: primum non nocere. *J Emerg Med*. 2010;38:171-174.

83. Cuperus BK, et al. [Diagnostic image (65). Unintentional biopsies of the gastric mucosa, obtained by withdrawal of a stomach tube]. *Ned Tijdschr Geneeskd*. 2001;145:2271.

84. De Neve R. Antidotal efficacy of activated charcoal in presence of jam, starch and milk. *Am J Hosp Pharm*. 1976;33:965-966.

85. de Silva HA, et al. Multiple-dose activated charcoal for treatment of yellow oleander poisoning: a single-blind, randomised, placebo-controlled trial. *Lancet*. 2003;361:1935-1938.

86. De Weerdt A, et al. Rapid-onset adult respiratory distress syndrome after activated charcoal aspiration. A pitch-black tale of a potential to kill. *Am J Respir Crit Care Med*. 2015;191:344-345.

87. Dinesh Kumar R, et al. Case report—acetaminophen poisoning. *Res J Pharm Biol Chem Sci*. 2015;6:4-7.

88. Djogovic D, et al. Gastric bezoar following venlafaxine overdose. *Clin Toxicol (Phila)*. 2007;45:735.

89. Donkor J, et al. Analysis of gastric lavage reported to a statewide poison control system. *J Emerg Med*. 2016;51:394-400.

90. Dorrington CL, Johnson DW, Brant R; Multiple Dose Activated Charcoal Complication Study Group. The frequency of complications associated with the use of multiple-dose activated charcoal. *Ann Emerg Med*. 2003;41:370-377.

91. Duffull SB, Isbister GK. Predicting the requirement for N-acetylcysteine in paracetamol poisoning from reported dose. *Clin Toxicol (Phila)*. 2013;51:772-776.

92. Eddleston M. Patterns and problems of deliberate self-poisoning in the developing world. *QJM*. 2000;93:715-731.

93. Eddleston M, Chowdhury FR. Pharmacological treatment of organophosphorus insecticide poisoning: the old and the (possible) new. *Br J Clin Pharmacol*. 2016;81:462-470.

94. Eddleston M, et al. The hazards of gastric lavage for intentional self-poisoning in a resource poor location. *Clin Toxicol (Phila)*. 2007;45:136-143.

95. Eddleston M, et al. Does gastric lavage really push poisons beyond the pylorus? A systematic review of the evidence. *Ann Emerg Med*. 2003;42:359-364.

96. Eddleston M, et al. Multiple-dose activated charcoal in acute self-poisoning: a randomised controlled trial. *Lancet*. 2008;371:579-587.

97. Eisen TF, et al. The adsorption of salicylates by a milk chocolate-charcoal mixture. *Ann Emerg Med*. 1991;20:143-146.

98. Eisen TF, et al. The palatability of a new milk chocolate-charcoal mixture in children. *Vet Hum Toxicol*. 1988;30:351-352.

99. el-Bahie N, et al. The effect of activated charcoal and hyoscine butylbromide alone and in combination on the absorption of mefenamic acid. *Br J Clin Pharmacol*. 1985;19:836-838.

100. Eleftheriou G, et al. Ischemic colitis following duloxetine and lamotrigine poisoning: is there a relationship? *Clin Toxicol*. 2010;48:282.

101. England G, et al. Forensic features of pharmacobezoars. *J Forensic Sci*. 2015;60:341-345.

102. Erden A, et al. Colchicine intoxication: a report of two suicide cases. *Ther Clin Risk Manag*. 2013;9:505-509.

103. Erenler AK, et al. Investigation of toxic effects of mushroom poisoning on the cardiovascular system. *Basic Clin Pharmacol Toxicol*. 2016;119:317-321.

104. EUROSTAT. Accidents and injuries statistics, 2016. http://ec.europa.eu/eurostat/statistics-explained/index.php/Accidents_and_injuries_statistics.

105. Exner CJ, Ayala GU. Organophosphate and carbamate intoxication in La Paz, Bolivia. *J Emerg Med*. 2009;36:348-352.

106. Farmer JW, Chan SB. Whole body irrigation for contraband bodypackers. *J Clin Gastroenterol*. 2003;37:147-150.

107. Filippone GA, et al. Reversible Adsorption desorption of aspirin from activated charcoal. *Arch Intern Med*. 1987;147:1390-1392.

108. Finkelstein Y, et al. Colchicine poisoning: the dark side of an ancient drug. *Clin Toxicol*. 2010;48:407-414.

109. Foxford R, Goldfrank L. Gastrotomy—a surgical approach to iron overdose. *Ann Emerg Med*. 1985;14:1223-1226.

110. Franchitto N, et al. Self-intoxication with baclofen in alcohol-dependent patients with co-existing psychiatric illness: an emergency department case series. *Alcohol Alcohol*. 2014;49:79-83.

111. Francis RCE, et al. Acute respiratory failure after aspiration of activated charcoal with recurrent deposition and release from an intrapulmonary cavern. *Intensive Care Med.* 2009;35:360-363.

112. Friberg LE, et al. The population pharmacokinetics of citalopram after deliberate self-poisoning: a Bayesian approach. *J Pharmacokinet Pharmacodyn.* 2005;32:571-605.

113. Garcia J, et al. Co-ingestion of amatoxins and isoxazoles-containing mushrooms and successful treatment: a case report. *Toxicon.* 2015;103:55-59.

114. Garrettson LK, et al. Subacute chlordane poisoning. *J Toxicol Clin Toxicol.* 1984;22:565-571.

115. Gawarammana IB, Buckley NA. Medical management of paraquat ingestion. *Br J Clin Pharmacol.* 2011;72:745-757.

116. Ghannoum M, et al. Successful treatment of lithium toxicity with sodium polystyrene sulfonate: a retrospective cohort study. *Clin Toxicol (Phila).* 2010;48:34-41.

117. Giampreti A, et al. Recurrent tonic-clonic seizures and coma due to ingestion of Type I pyrethroids in a 19-month-old patient. *Clin Toxicol (Phila).* 2013;51:497-500.

118. Giannini L, et al. Amatoxin poisoning: a 15-year retrospective analysis and follow-up evaluation of 105 patients. *Clin Toxicol (Phila).* 2007;45:539-542.

119. Gibiino S, et al. Coma after quetiapine fumarate intentional overdose in a 71-year-old man: a case report. *Drug Saf Case Rep.* 2015;2:3.

120. Gokel Y, et al. Gastric lavage with normal saline: effects on serum electrolytes. *Bratisl Lek Listy.* 2010;111:216-218.

121. Golej J, et al. Severe respiratory failure following charcoal application in a toddler. *Resuscitation.* 2001;49:315-318.

122. Good AM, et al. Differences in treatment advice for common poisons by poisons centres—an international comparison. *Clin Toxicol (Phila).* 2007;45:234-239.

123. Grabhorn E, et al. Successful outcome of severe Amanita phalloides poisoning in children. *Pediatr Transplant.* 2013;17:550-555.

124. Green R, et al. How long after drug ingestion is activated charcoal still effective? *J Toxicol Clin Toxicol.* 2001;39:601-605.

125. Green R, et al. Effect of anticholinergic drugs on the efficacy of activated charcoal. *J Toxicol Clin Toxicol.* 2004;42:267-272.

126. Gregoriano C, et al. Acute thiopurine overdose: analysis of reports to a National Poison Centre 1995-2013. *PLoS One.* 2014;9:e86390.

127. Grierson R, et al. Gastric lavage for liquid poisons. *Ann Emerg Med.* 2000;35:435-439.

128. Griffiths EA, et al. Thirty-four cases of esophageal perforation: the experience of a district general hospital in the UK. *Dis Esophagus.* 2009;22:616-625.

129. Gude AB, Hoegberg LC. Techniques used to prevent gastrointestinal absorption. In: Nelson LS, Lewin NA, Howland MA, et al, eds. *Goldfrank's Toxicologic Emergencies.* 9th ed. New York, NY: McGraw-Hill Medical; 2011:90-103.

130. Gude AB, et al. Dose-dependent adsorptive capacity of activated charcoal for gastrointestinal decontamination of a simulated paracetamol overdose in human volunteers. *Basic Clin Pharmacol Toxicol.* 2010;106:406-410.

131. Guenther Skokan E, et al. Taste test: children rate flavoring agents used with activated charcoal. *Arch Pediatr Adolesc Med.* 2001;155:683-686.

132. Gulec H, et al. Seizure due to multiple drugs intoxication: a case report. *Braz J Anesthesiol.* 2016;66:651-653.

133. Gumber MR, et al. Successful treatment of severe iron intoxication with gastrointestinal decontamination, deferoxamine, and hemodialysis. *Ren Fail.* 2013;35:729-731.

134. Haider F, et al. Emergency laparoscopic-assisted gastrotomy for the treatment of an iron bezoar. *J Laparoendosc Adv Surg Tech A.* 2009;19(suppl 1):S141-S143.

135. Halprashanth DS, et al. Camphor poisoning in adult an unusual cause of seizure. *Ann Indian Acad Neurol.* 2014;17:S241-S242.

136. Harris CR, Filandrinos D. Accidental administration of activated charcoal into the lung: aspiration by proxy. *Ann Emerg Med.* 1993;22:1470-1473.

137. Hays H, et al. 800 Pebbles in a stream: whole bowel irrigation and colonoscopy for staggered lead shot ingestion. *Clin Toxicol.* 2012;50:661-662.

138. Hendrix L, et al. Deliberate self-poisoning: characteristics of patients and impact on the emergency department of a large university hospital. *Emerg Med J.* 2013;30:e9.

139. Hodgman M, et al. The influence of polyethylene glycol solution on the dissolution rate of sustained release morphine. *J Med Toxicol.* 2016;12:391-395.

140. Hoegberg LC, et al. Effect of ethanol and pH on the adsorption of acetaminophen (paracetamol) to high surface activated charcoal, in vitro studies. *J Toxicol Clin Toxicol.* 2002;40:59-67.

141. Hoegberg LC, et al. The effect of food and ice cream on the adsorption capacity of paracetamol to high surface activated charcoal: in vitro studies. *Pharmacol Toxicol.* 2003;93:233-237.

142. Hoegberg LC, et al. The effect of ethanol on paracetamol absorption and activated charcoal efficacy, in a simulated human paracetamol overdose. *Clin Toxicol.* 2012;50:276.

143. Hoegberg LC, et al. Comparison of the adsorption capacities of an activated-charcoal—yogurt mixture versus activated-charcoal—water slurry in vivo and in vitro. *Clin Toxicol (Phila).* 2005;43:269-275.

144. Hoegberg LCG, et al. Combined paracetamol and amitriptyline adsorption to activated charcoal. *Clin Toxicol.* 2010;48:898-903.

145. Hoegberg LCG, et al. Potential pharmacobezoar formation of extended-release tablets and their dissolution—an in vitro study. *Clin Toxicol.* 2017;55:371-544.

146. Hofbauer RD, Holger JS. The use of cholecystokinin as an adjunctive treatment for toxin ingestion. *J Toxicol Clin Toxicol.* 2004;42:61-66.

147. Hoffman RS. Does consensus equal correctness? *J Toxicol Clin Toxicol.* 2000;38:689-690.

148. Hoffman RS, et al. Theophylline desorption from activated charcoal caused by whole bowel irrigation solution. *J Toxicol Clin Toxicol.* 1991;29:191-201.

149. Hoffman RS, et al. Comparative efficacy of thallium adsorption by activated charcoal, prussian blue, and sodium polystyrene sulfonate. *J Toxicol Clin Toxicol.* 1999;37:833-837.

150. Hojer J, Personne M. Endoscopic removal of slow release clomipramine bezoars in two cases of acute poisoning. *Clin Toxicol (Phila).* 2008;46:317-319.

151. Hojer J, et al. Overdose of modified-release paracetamol calls for changed treatment routines. New guidelines from the Swedish Poisons Information Centre. *Lakartidningen.* 2016;113:D93C.

152. Holt LM, Holz PH. The black bottle. A consideration of the role of charcoal in the treatment of poisoning in children. *J Pediatr.* 1963;63:306-314.

153. Hondebrink L, et al. Prospective follow-up study on potential toxic methylphenidate exposures. *Clin Toxicol.* 2013;51:298-299.

154. Hsieh YW, et al. Paraquat poisoning in pediatric patients. *Pediatr Emerg Care.* 2013;29:487-491.

155. Hulten BA, et al. Activated charcoal in tricyclic antidepressant poisoning. *Hum Toxicol.* 1988;7:307-310.

156. Hussain K, et al. Adsorption of paracetamol on activated charcoal in the presence of dextropropoxyphene hydrochloride, N-acetylcysteine and sorbitol. *Lat Am J Pharm.* 2010;29:883-888.

157. Iliev YT, et al. Acute poisoning with dapsone and olanzapine: severe methemoglobinemia and coma with a favourable outcome. *Folia Med (Plovdiv).* 2015;57:122-126.

158. Ilkhanipour K, et al. The comparative efficacy of various multiple-dose activated charcoal regimens. *Am J Emerg Med.* 1992;10:298-300.

159. Indira M, et al. Incidence, predictors, and outcome of intermediate syndrome in cholinergic insecticide poisoning: a prospective observational cohort study. *Clin Toxicol (Phila).* 2013;51:838-845.

160. Inoue Y, et al. Factors associated with severe effects following acute glufosinate poisoning. *Clin Toxicol (Phila).* 2013;51:846-849.

161. Isbister GK, et al. Aspiration pneumonitis in an overdose population: frequency, predictors, and outcomes. *Crit Care Med.* 2004;32:88-93.

162. Isbister GK, Duffull SB. Quetiapine overdose: predicting intubation, duration of ventilation, cardiac monitoring and the effect of activated charcoal. *Int Clin Psychopharmacol.* 2009;24:174-180.

163. Isbister GK, et al. Pharmacokinetics of quetiapine in overdose and the effect of activated charcoal. *Clin Pharmacol Ther.* 2007;81:821-827.

164. Isbister GK, et al. Activated charcoal decreases the risk of QT prolongation after citalopram overdose. *Ann Emerg Med.* 2007;50:593-600, 600 e591-546.

165. Isbister GK, Kumar VV. Indications for single-dose activated charcoal administration in acute overdose. *Curr Opin Crit Care.* 2011;17:351-357.

166. Jaeger A. Quinine and chloroquine. *Medicine.* 2012;40:154-155.

167. Jayashree M, et al. Predictors of outcome in children with hydrocarbon poisoning receiving intensive care. *Indian Pediatr.* 2006;43:715-719.

168. Jiranantakan T, et al. Acute pancreatitis in Amanita phalloides poisoning. *Clin Toxicol.* 2009;47:730-731.

169. John S, et al. A unique presentation of massive quetiapine overdose: prolonged anticholinergic delirium and acute reversal with physostigmine. *Crit Care Med.* 2010;38:A258.

170. Jones A, Dargan P. *Churchill's Pocketbook of Toxicology.* London: Churchill Livingstone; 2001.

171. Jurgens G, et al. The effect of activated charcoal on drug exposure in healthy volunteers: a meta-analysis. *Clin Pharmaol Ther.* 2009;85:501-505.

172. Justiniani FR, et al. Charcoal-containing empyema complicating treatment for overdose. *Chest.* 1985;87:404-405.

173. Juurlink DN, McGuigan MA. Gastrointestinal decontamination for enteric-coated aspirin overdose: what to do depends on who you ask. *J Toxicol Clin Toxicol.* 2000;38:465-470.

174. Karim A, et al. How feasible is it to conform to the European guidelines on administration of activated charcoal within one hour of an overdose? *Emerg Med J.* 2001;18:390-392.

175. Katabami K, et al. Severe methemoglobinemia due to sodium nitrite poisoning. *Case Rep Emerg Med.* 2016;2016:9013816.

176. Keranen T, et al. Effects of charcoal on the absorption and elimination of the antiepileptic drugs lamotrigine and oxcarbazepine. *Arzneimittelforschung.* 2010;60:421-426.

177. Kilgore TL, Lehmann CR. Treatment of digoxin intoxication with colestipol. *South Med J.* 1982;75:1259-1260.

178. Kim KH, et al. Ingestion of Portland cement. *J Emerg Med.* 2015;49:e19-21.

179. Kimura Y, et al. Efficacy of abdominal computed tomography and nasogastric tube in acute poisoning patients. *Am J Emerg Med.* 2008;26:738.e733-735.

180. Kimura Y, et al. A patient with numerous tablets remaining in the stomach even 5 hours after ingestion. *Am J Emerg Med.* 2008;26:118 e111-112.

181. Klein-Schwartz W, et al. Drug adsorption efficacy and palatability of a novel charcoal cookie formulation. *Pharmacotherapy.* 2010;30:888-894.

182. Koksal O, et al. A 4 year retrospective analysis of our patients with mushroom poisoning. *Hong Kong J Emerg Med.* 2013;20:105-110.

183. Kong F, Singh RP. Disintegration of solid foods in human stomach. *J Food Sci.* 2008;73:R67-80.

184. Krayeva YV, et al. Pre-hospital management and outcome of acute poisonings by ambulances in Yekaterinburg, Russia. *Clin Toxicol (Phila).* 2013;51:752-760.

185. Krenzelok EP, et al. Position paper: ipecac syrup. *J Toxicol Clin Toxicol.* 2004;42:133-143.

186. Krenzelok EP, et al. Position statement: ipecac syrup. American Academy of Clinical Toxicology; European Association of Poisons Centres and Clinical Toxicologists. *J Toxicol Clin Toxicol.* 1997;35:699-709.

187. Ku JE, et al. A case of survival after chlorfenapyr intoxication with acute pancreatitis. *Clin Exp Emerg Med.* 2015;2:63-66.

188. Kulig K, et al. Management of acutely poisoned patients without gastric emptying. *Ann Emerg Med.* 1985;14:562-567.

189. Kumar VV, et al. The effect of decontamination procedures on the pharmacodynamics of venlafaxine in overdose. *Br J Clin Pharmacol.* 2011;72:125-132.

190. Kumar VV, et al. The effect of decontamination procedures on the pharmacokinetics of venlafaxine in overdose. *Clin Pharmacol Ther.* 2009;86:403-410.

191. Kyan R, et al. Severe accidental colchicine poisoning by the autumn crocus: a case of successful treatment. *J Acute Med.* 2015;5:103-106.

192. Lalonde RL, et al. Acceleration of digoxin clearance by activated charcoal. *Clin Pharmacol Ther.* 1985;37:367-371.

193. Lapatto-Reiniluoto O, et al. Activated charcoal alone and followed by whole-bowel irrigation in preventing the absorption of sustained-release drugs. *Clin Pharmacol Ther.* 2001;70:255-260.

194. Lapatto-Reiniluoto O, et al. Effect of activated charcoal alone or given after gastric lavage in reducing the absorption of diazepam, ibuprofen and citalopram. *Br J Clin Pharmacol.* 1999;48:148-153.

195. Lapatto-Reiniluoto O, et al. Efficacy of activated charcoal versus gastric lavage half an hour after ingestion of moclobemide, temazepam, and verapamil. *Eur J Clin Pharmacol.* 2000;56:285-288.

196. Larkin GL, Claassen C. Trends in emergency department use of gastric lavage for poisoning events in the United States, 1993-2003. *Clin Toxicol (Phila).* 2007;45:164-168.

197. Larrode I, et al. Drug poisoning: a reason for care in a hospital emergencies unit. *Eur J Hospital Pharm.* 2012;19:119-120.

198. Larsson S, et al. Poisoning with Cicuta virosa in Sweden. *Clin Toxicol.* 2015;53:345.

199. Layton GM, et al. Gastrointestinal decontamination considerations in weight loss surgery patients. *Clin Toxicol.* 2015;53:702.

200. Leao SC, et al. Management of exogenous intoxication by carbamates and organophosphates at an emergency unit. *Rev Assoc Med Bras (1992).* 2015;61:440-445.

201. Levy G, Houston JB. Effect of activated charcoal on acetaminophen absorption. *Pediatrics.* 1976;58:432-435.

202. Li Y, et al. Systematic review of controlled clinical trials of gastric lavage in acute organophosphorus pesticide poisoning. *Clin Toxicol (Phila).* 2009;47:179-192.

203. Liu Y, et al. The mastery of antidotes: a survey of antidote knowledge and availability among emergency physicians in registered hospitals in China. *Hum Exp Toxicol.* 2016;35:462-471.

204. Liu Z, et al. Acute self-induced poisoning with sodium ferrocyanide and methanol treated with plasmapheresis and continuous renal replacement therapy successfully: a case report. *Medicine (Baltimore).* 2015;94:e890.

205. Livshits Z, et al. Retained drugs in the gastrointestinal tracts of deceased victims of oral drug overdose. *Clin Toxicol.* 2015;53:113-118.

206. Lo JCY, et al. A retrospective review of whole bowel irrigation in pediatric patients. *Clin Toxicol.* 2012;50:414-417.

207. Lund C, et al. A one-year observational study of all hospitalized acute poisonings in Oslo: complications, treatment and sequelae. *Scand J Trauma Resusc Emerg Med.* 2012;20:49.

208. Ly BT, et al. Effect of whole bowel irrigation on the pharmacokinetics of an acetaminophen formulation and progression of radiopaque markers through the gastrointestinal tract. *Ann Emerg Med.* 2004;43:189-195.

209. Maderuelo C, et al. Critical factors in the release of drugs from sustained release hydrophilic matrices. *J Control Release.* 2011;154:2-19.

210. Magdalan J, et al. Suicidal overdose with relapsing clomipramine concentrations due to a large gastric pharmacobezoar. *Forensic Sci Int.* 2013;229:e19-22.

211. Mahendrakar K, et al. Glyphosate surfactant herbicide poisoning and management. *Indian J Crit Care Med.* 2014;18:328-330.

212. Makosiej FJ, et al. An in vitro evaluation of cocaine hydrochloride adsorption by activated charcoal and desorption upon addition of polyethylene glycol electrolyte lavage solution. *J Toxicol Clin Toxicol.* 1993;31:381-395.

213. Manoguerra AS, Cobaugh DJ; Guidelines for the Management of Poisoning Consensus Panel. Guideline on the use of ipecac syrup in the out-of-hospital management of ingested poisons. *Clin Toxicol (Phila).* 2005;43:1-10.

214. Manoguerra AS, et al. Valproic acid poisoning: an evidence-based consensus guideline for out-of-hospital management. *Clin Toxicol (Phila).* 2008;46:661-676.

215. Marashi SM, et al. Hydroxyethyl starch could save a patient with acute aluminum phosphide poisoning. *Acta Med Iran.* 2016;54:475-478.

216. Mariani PJ, Pook N. Gastrointestinal tract perforation with charcoal peritoneum complicating orogastric intubation and lavage. *Ann Emerg Med.* 1993;22:606-609.

217. Masi L, et al. Conservative management of intentional massive dabigatran overdose. *Italian J Med.* 2015;9:66.

218. Mathur LK, et al. Activated charcoal-carboxymethylcellulose gel formulation as an antidotal agent for orally ingested aspirin. *Am J Hosp Pharm.* 1976;33:717-719.

219. Matthew H, et al. Gastric aspiration and lavage in acute poisoning. *Br Med J.* 1966;1:1333-1337.

220. Mayersohn M, et al. Evaluation of a charcoal-sorbitol mixture as an antidote for oral aspirin overdose. *Clin Toxicol.* 1977;11:561-567.

221. McGregor T, et al. Evaluation and management of common childhood poisonings. *Am Fam Physician.* 2009;79:397-403.

222. Meert A, et al. Brugada-like ECG pattern induced by tricyclic antidepressants. *Eur J Emerg Med.* 2010;17:325-327.

223. Mehrpour O, et al. Successful treatment of cardiogenic shock with an intraaortic balloon pump following aluminium phosphide poisoning. *Arh Hig Rada Toksikol.* 2014;65:121-126.

224. Mehrpour O, et al. A systematic review of aluminium phosphide poisoning. *Arh Hig Rada Toksikol.* 2012;63:61-73.

225. Merigian KS, Blaho KE. Single-dose oral activated charcoal in the treatment of the self-poisoned patient: a prospective, randomized, controlled trial. *Am J Ther.* 2002;9:301-308.

226. Merigian KS, et al. Prospective evaluation of gastric emptying in the self-poisoned patient. *Am J Emerg Med.* 1990;8:479-483.

227. Mikaszewska-Sokolewicz MA, et al. Coma in the course of severe poisoning after consumption of red fly agaric (Amanita muscaria). *Acta Biochim Pol.* 2016;63:181-182.

228. Miranda Arto P, et al. [Acute poisoning in patients over 65 years of age]. *An Sist Sanit Navar.* 2014;37:99-108.

229. Miyauchi M, et al. Gastric lavage guided by ultrathin transnasal esophagogastroduodenoscopy in a life-threatening case of tobacco extract poisoning: a case report. *J Nippon Med Sch.* 2013;80:307-311.

230. Miyauchi M, et al. Evaluation of residual toxic substances in the stomach using upper gastrointestinal endoscopy for management of patients with oral drug overdose on admission: a prospective, observational study. *Medicine (Baltimore).* 2015;94:e463.

231. Miyauchi M, et al. Successful retrieval using ultrathin transnasal esophagogastroduodenoscopy of a significant amount of residual tricyclic antidepressant following serious toxicity: a case report. *Int J Emerg Med.* 2013;6:39.

232. Mofredi A, et al. Severe hypernatremia secondary to gastric lavage. *Ann Fr Anesth Reanim.* 2000;19:219-220.

233. Mohamed F, et al. Compliance for single and multiple dose regimens of superactivated charcoal: a prospective study of patients in a clinical trial. *Clin Toxicol (Phila).* 2007;45:132-135.

234. Moll J, et al. Incidence of aspiration pneumonia in intubated patients receiving activated charcoal. *J. Emerg Med.* 1999;17:279-283.

235. Moon J, et al. An exploratory study; the therapeutic effects of premixed activated charcoal-sorbitol administration in patients poisoned with organophosphate pesticide. *Clin Toxicol (Phila).* 2015;53:119-126.

236. Moon JM, Chun BJ. Clinical characteristics of patients after dicamba herbicide ingestion. *Clin Toxicol (Phila).* 2014;52:48-53.

237. Mullins M, et al. Effect of delayed activated charcoal on acetaminophen concentration after simulated overdose of oxycodone and acetaminophen. *Clin Toxicol (Phila).* 2009;47:112-115.

238. Mumoli N, et al. Conservative management of intentional massive dabigatran overdose. *J Am Geriatr Soc.* 2015;63:2205-2207.

239. Murray M, et al. Delayed-onset gastrointestinal symptoms after gymnopilus penetrans ingestion: a case report. *Clin Toxicol.* 2015;53:754-755.

240. Naderi S, et al. The use of gastric lavage in India. *Acad Emerg Med.* 2011;1(suppl):S132.

241. Navarro RP, et al. Relative efficacy and palatability of three activated charcoal mixtures. *Vet Hum Toxicol.* 1980;22:6-9.

242. Neijzen R, et al. Activated charcoal for GHB intoxication: an in vitro study. *Eur J Pharm Sci.* 2012;47:801-803.

243. Neuvonen PJ. Clinical pharmacokinetics of oral activated charcoal in acute intoxications. *Clin Pharmacokinet.* 1982;7:465-489.

244. Neuvonen PJ. Towards safer and more predictable drug treatment—reflections from studies of the first BCPT prize awardee. *Basic Clin Pharmacol Toxicol.* 2012;110:207-218.

245. Neuvonen PJ, et al. Capacity of two forms of activated charcoal to adsorb nefopam in vitro and to reduce its toxicity in vivo. *J Toxicol Clin Toxicol.* 1983;21:333-342.

246. Neuvonen PJ, et al. Effect of ethanol and pH on the adsorption of drugs to activated charcoal: studies in vitro and in man. *Acta Pharmacol Toxicol (Copenh).* 1984;54:1-7.

247. Ng HW, et al. Endoscopic removal of iron bezoar following acute overdose. *Clin Toxicol (Phila).* 2008;46:913-915.

248. Nithin MD, et al. Iatrogenic perforation of stomach—a case report. *Kathmandu Univ Med J.* 2015;13:175-177.

249. Nobre LF, et al. Pulmonary instillation of activated charcoal: early findings on computed tomography. *Ann Thorac Surg.* 2011;91:642-643.

250. Nokhodchi A, et al. The role of oral controlled release matrix tablets in drug delivery systems. *Bioimpacts.* 2012;2:175-187.

251. Nordt SP, Clark RF. "Go lytely" dissolves more quickly. *Clin Toxicol.* 2009;47:717-718.

252. Nordt SP, et al. Ultrasound visualization of ingested tablets: a pilot study. *Pharmacotherapy.* 2011;31:273-276.

253. O'Connell CW, et al. A retrospective analysis of phenytoin toxicity. *Clin Toxicol.* 2014;52:776-777.

254. Olkkola KT. Does ethanol modify antidotal efficacy of oral activated charcoal studies in vitro and in experimental animals. *J Toxicol Clin Toxicol.* 1984;22:425-432.

255. Olkkola KT. Effect of charcoal-drug ratio on antidotal efficacy of oral activated charcoal in man. *Br J Clin Pharmacol.* 1985;19:767-773.

256. Olkkola KT, Neuvonen PJ. Effect of gastric pH on antidotal efficacy of activated charcoal in man. *Int J Clin Pharmacol Ther Toxicol.* 1984;22:565-569.

257. Ollier E, et al. Effect of activated charcoal on rivaroxaban complex absorption. *Clin Pharmacokinet.* 2017;56:793-801.

258. Olmedo R, et al. Is surgical decontamination definitive treatment of "body-packers"? *Am J Emerg Med.* 2001;19:593-596.

259. Olson KR. Activated charcoal for acute poisoning: one toxicologist's journey. *J Med Toxicol.* 2010;6:190-198.

260. Olsson EK, Petersson E. Amatoxin poisoning during pregnancy: a case report and review of the literature. *Clin Toxicol.* 2016;54:504.

261. Oppenheim RC. Strawberry-flavoured activated charcoal. *Med J Aust.* 1980;1:39.

262. Ostapenko YN, et al. Fatal colchicine poisoning after accidental ingestion of autumn crocus (*Colchicum autumnale*). *Clin Toxicol.* 2016;54:503.

263. Osterhoudt KC, et al. Activated charcoal administration in a pediatric emergency department. *Pediatr Emerg Care.* 2004;20:493-498.

264. Osterhoudt KC, et al. Risk factors for emesis after therapeutic use of activated charcoal in acutely poisoned children. *Pediatrics.* 2004;113:806-810.

265. Padmanabhan K, et al. Acute mediastinal widening following endotracheal intubation and gastric lavage. Esophageal perforation, with mediastinal abscess. *West J Med.* 1991;155:419-420.

266. Palmer RB, Aks SE. Retained pill fragments at autopsy: time to rethink gastric decontamination? *Clin Toxicol (Phila).* 2015;53:82-84.

267. Papazoglu C, et al. Acetaminophen overdose associated with double serum concentration peaks. *J Community Hosp Intern Med Perspect.* 2015;5:29589.

268. Pawa S, et al. Zinc toxicity from massive and prolonged coin ingestion in an adult. *Am J Med Sci.* 2008;336:430-433.

269. Peetermans M, et al. Idarucizumab for dabigatran overdose. *Clin Toxicol (Phila).* 2016;54:644-646.

270. Personne M, Westberg US. Gastric decontamination in poisoned patients operated for bariatric surgery. *Clin Toxicol.* 2014;52:412.

271. Peterson CD, Fifield GC. Emergency gastrotomy for acute iron poisoning. *Ann Emerg Med.* 1980;9:262-264.

272. Petronijevic Z, et al. Combined extracorporal methods in mushroom poisoning treatment. *Int J Artific Organs.* 2010;33:453.

273. Picchioni AL. Activated charcoal as an antidote for poisons. *Am J Hosp Pharm.* 1967;24:38-39.

274. Picchioni AL. Management of acute poisonings with activated charcoal. *Am J Hosp Pharm.* 1971;28:62-64.

275. Pieroni RE, Fisher JG. Use of cholestyramine resin in digitoxin toxicity. *JAMA.* 1981;245:1939-1940.

276. Pold K, et al. Poisoning by *Amanita phalloides.* *Clin Toxicol.* 2010;48:312.

277. Pollack MM, et al. Aspiration of activated charcoal and gastric contents. *Ann Emerg Med.* 1981;10:528-529.

278. Ponampalam R. Effectiveness of multiple-dose activated charcoal in digoxin overdose: a case report. *Toxicol Lett.* 2015;(suppl 1):S141.

279. Pond SM, et al. Gastric emptying in acute overdose: a prospective randomised controlled trial. *Med J Aust.* 1995;163:345-349.

280. Purg D, et al. Low-dose intravenous lipid emulsion for the treatment of severe quetiapine and citalopram poisoning. *Arh Hig Rada Toksikol.* 2016;67:164-166.

281. Qureshi Z, Eddleston M. Adverse effects of activated charcoal used for the treatment of poisoning. *Adverse Drug React Bull.* 2011;1023-1026.

282. Rahmani A, et al. Medical management and outcome of paraquat poisoning in Ahvaz, Iran: a hospital-based study. *Asia Pac J Med Toxicol.* 2015;4:74-78.

283. Rakotomavo F, et al. *Datura stramonium* intoxication in two children. *Pediatr Int.* 2014;56:e14-16.

284. Rangan C, et al. Treatment of acetaminophen ingestion with a superactivated charcoal-cola mixture. *Ann Emerg Med.* 2001;37:55-58.

285. Rauber-Lüthy C, et al. Gastric pharmacobezoars in quetiapine extended-release overdose: a case series. *Clin Toxicol (Phila).* 2013;51:937-940.

286. Refsgaard F, Petersen SH. *In Vitro Investigation of Potential Pharmacobezoar Formation and Their Dissolution of Extended Release Tablets* [master's thesis]. Copenhagen: Section of Toxicology, Department of Pharmacy, School of Pharmaceutical Sciences, Faculty of Health Sciences, University of Copenhagen; 2016.

287. Ricci G, et al. A bittersweet symphony. *Clin Toxicol.* 2010;48:310-311.

288. Rinder HM, et al. Impact of unusual gastrointestinal problems on the treatment of tricyclic antidepressant overdose. *Ann Emerg Med.* 1988;17:1079-1081.

289. Roberge RJ, et al. Use of sodium polystyrene sulfonate in a lithium overdose. *Ann Emerg Med.* 1993;22:1911-1915.

290. Roberts DM, et al. Pharmacokinetics of digoxin cross-reacting substances in patients with acute yellow Oleander (*Thevetia peruviana*) poisoning, including the effect of activated charcoal. *Ther Drug Monit.* 2006;28:784-792.

291. Roivas L, Neuvonen PJ. Drug adsorption onto activated charcoal as a means of formulation. *Methods Find Exp Clin Pharmacol.* 1994;16:367-372.

292. Roivas L, et al. The bioavailability of two beta-blockers preadsorbed onto charcoal. *Methods Find Exp Clin Pharmacol.* 1994;16:125-132.

293. Roy TM, et al. Pulmonary complications after tricyclic antidepressant overdose. *Chest.* 1989;96:852-856.

294. Rybolt TR, et al. In vitro coadsorption of acetaminophen and N-acetylcysteine onto activated carbon powder. *J Pharm Sci.* 1986;75:904-906.

295. Saetta JP, et al. Gastric emptying procedures in the self-poisoned patient: are we forcing gastric content beyond the pylorus? *J R Soc Med.* 1991;84:274-276.

296. Sagah GA, et al. Evaluation of potential oxidative stress in Egyptian patients with acute zinc phosphide poisoning and the role of vitamin C. *Int J Health Sci (Qassim).* 2015;9:375-385.

297. Sahlner Y, et al. The frequency of intestinal obstruction associated with the use of activated charcoal in multiple doses. *Eur Surg Res.* 2013;50:103.

298. Sajkov D, Gallus A. Accidental rivaroxaban overdose in a patient with pulmonary embolism: some lessons for managing new oral anticoagulants. *Clin Med Insights Case Rep.* 2015;8:57-59.

299. Salmonson H, et al. The standard treatment protocol is inadequate following overdose of extended release paracetamol: a pharmacokinetic and clinical analysis of 53 cases. *Clin Toxicol.* 2016;54:424.

300. Sanaka M, et al. Gastric emptying of liquids is delayed by co-ingesting solids: a study using salivary paracetamol concentrations. *J Gastroenterol.* 2002;37:785-790.

301. Santana NO, Gois AF. Rhabdomyolysis as a manifestation of clomipramine poisoning. *Sao Paulo Med J.* 2013;131:432-435.

302. Satar S, et al. Intoxication with 100 grams of mercury: a case report and importance of supportive therapy. *Eur J Emerg Med.* 2001;8:245-248.

303. Sato RL, et al. Efficacy of superactivated charcoal administered late (3 hours) after acetaminophen overdose. *Am J Emerg Med.* 2003;21:189-191.

304. Sawalha AF, et al. Pesticide poisoning in Palestine: a retrospective analysis of calls received by Poison Control and Drug Information Center from 2006-2010. *Int J Risk Saf Med.* 2012;24:171-177.

305. Sawatzki M, et al. Seizure and non-cardiogenic pulmonary edema after intoxication. *Internist.* 2010;51:528-532.

306. Schaper A, et al. [Cocaine-body-packing. Infrequent indication for laparotomy]. *Chirurg.* 2003;74:626-631.

307. Scharman EJ, et al. Methylphenidate poisoning: an evidence-based consensus guideline for out-of-hospital management. *Clin Toxicol (Phila).* 2007;45:737-752.

308. Scharman EJ, et al. Diphenhydramine and dimenhydrinate poisoning: an evidence-based consensus guideline for out-of-hospital management. *Clin Toxicol (Phila).* 2006;44:205-223.

309. Schrettl V, et al. A case of mono-intoxication with duloxetine: clinical presentation and serum concentrations. *Clin Toxicol.* 2016;54:488.

310. Schulman S, Crowther MA. How I treat with anticoagulants in 2012: new and old anticoagulants, and when and how to switch. *Blood.* 2012;119:3016-3023.

311. Schwartz HS. Acute meprobamate poisoning with gastrotomy and removal of a drug-containing mass. *N Engl J Med.* 1976;295:1177-1178.

312. Schwerk C, et al. Etilefrinhydrochloride tablet ingestion: successful therapy by endoscopic removal of tablet conglomerate. *Klin Padiatr.* 2009;221:93-96.

313. Seger D. Single-dose activated charcoal—backup and reassess. *J Toxicol Clin Toxicol.* 2004;42:101-110.

314. Sellers EM, et al. Comparative drug adsorption by activated charcoal. *J Pharm Sci.* 1977;66:1640-1641.

315. Shang AD, Lu YQ. A case report of severe paraquat poisoning in an HIV-positive patient: an unexpected outcome and inspiration. *Medicine (Baltimore).* 2015;94:e587.

316. Sharman JR, et al. Drug overdoses: is one stomach washing enough? *N Z Med J.* 1975;81:195-197.

317. Sherman A, Zingler BM. Successful endoscopic retrieval of a cocaine packet from the stomach. *Gastrointest Endosc.* 1990;36:152-154.

318. Shirota T, et al. Successful living donor liver transplantation for acute liver failure after acetylsalicylic acid overdose. *Clin J Gastroenterol.* 2015;8:97-102.

319. Shively RM, et al. Salicylate poisoning: risk factors for severe outcome. *Clin Toxicol.* 2016;54:426.

320. Simpson SE. Pharmacobezoars described and demystified. *Clin Toxicol.* 2011;49:72-89.

321. Spiller HA, Rodgers GC Jr. Evaluation of administration of activated charcoal in the home. *Pediatrics.* 2001;108:E100.

322. Spiller HA, et al. Efficacy of activated charcoal administered more than four hours after acetaminophen overdose. *Emerg Med J. Emerg Med.* 2006;30:1-5.

323. Spray SB, et al. Aspiration pneumonia; incidence of aspiration with endotracheal tubes. *Am J Surg.* 1976;131:701-703.

324. Strobel J, et al. Charcoal intake and oral anticoagulation. *J Travel Med.* 2010;17:287-288.

325. Suarez CA, et al. Cocaine-codom ingestion. Surgical treatment. *JAMA.* 1977;238:1391-1392.

326. Sullivan SMD, et al. Accuracy of trans-abdominal ultrasound in a simulated massive acute overdose[white star]. *Am J Emerg Med.* 2016;34:1455-1457.

327. Tak S, et al. Aconite poisoning with arrhythmia and shock. *Indian Heart J.* 2016;68(suppl 2):S207-S209.

328. Takei T, et al. Acute amiodarone poisoning occurring twice in the same subject. *Clin Toxicol (Phila).* 2011;49:944-945.

329. Teece S, Crawford I. Best evidence topic report. Gastric lavage in aspirin and non-steroidal anti-inflammatory drug overdose. *Emerg Med J.* 2004;21:591-592.

330. Teece S, Hogg K. Best evidence topic reports. Gastric lavage in paracetamol poisoning. *Emerg Med J.* 2004;21:75-76.

331. Tenenbein M. Position statement: whole bowel irrigation. American Academy of Clinical Toxicology; European Association of Poisons Centres and Clinical Toxicologists. *J Toxicol Clin Toxicol.* 1997;35:753-762.

332. Tenenbein M, Lheureux P. Position paper: whole bowel irrigation. *J Toxicol Clin Toxicol*. 2004;42:843-854.

333. Teubner DJO. Absence of ice-cream interference with the adsorption of paracetamol onto activated charcoal. *Emerg Med*. 2000;12:326-328.

334. Thanacoody R, et al. Position paper update: whole bowel irrigation for gastrointestinal decontamination of overdose patients. *Clin Toxicol (Phila)*. 2015;53:5-12.

335. Thomas SH, et al. Presentation of poisoned patients to accident and emergency departments in the north of England. *Hum Exp Toxicol*. 1996;15:466-470.

336. Thompson AM, et al. Changes in cardiorespiratory function during gastric lavage for drug overdose. *Hum Toxicol*. 1987;6:215-218.

337. Thornton SL, et al. Castor bean seed ingestions: a state-wide poison control system's experience. *Clin Toxicol (Phila)*. 2014;52:265-268.

338. Tiwary AK, et al. In vitro study of the effectiveness of three commercial adsorbents for binding oleander toxins. *Clin Toxicol*. 2009;47:213-218.

339. Tomaszewski C, et al. Lithium absorption prevented by sodium polystyrene sulfonate in volunteers. *Ann Emerg Med*. 1992;21:1308-1311.

340. Tomaszewski C, et al. Cocaine adsorption to activated charcoal in vitro. *Emerg Med J. Emerg Med*. 1992;10:59-62.

341. Traub SJ, et al. Body packing—the internal concealment of illicit drugs. *N Engl J Med*. 2003;349:2519-2526.

342. Traub SJ, et al. Pediatric "body packing." *Arch Pediatr Adolesc Med*. 2003;157:174-177.

343. Tsai TY, et al. Suicide victim of paraquat poisoning make suitable corneal donor. *Hum Exp Toxicol*. 2011;30:71-73.

344. Tsamadou A, et al. Intentional ingestion of diquat: a case report with fatal outcome. *Clin Toxicol*. 2009;47:508.

345. Tsay ME, et al. Toxicity and clinical outcomes of paliperidone exposures reported to U.S. Poison Centers. *Clin Toxicol (Phila)*. 2014;52:207-213.

346. Tsitoura A, et al. In vitro adsorption study of fluoxetine onto activated charcoal at gastric and intestinal pH using high performance liquid chromatography with fluorescence detector. *J Toxicol Clin Toxicol*. 1997;35:269-276.

347. Turk J, et al. Successful therapy of iron intoxication in pregnancy with intravenous deferoxamine and whole bowel irrigation. *Vet Hum Toxicol*. 1993;35:441-444.

348. Tuuri RE, et al. Does emergency medical services transport for pediatric ingestion decrease time to activated charcoal? *Prehosp Emerg Care*. 2009;13:295-303.

349. Tuuri RE, et al. Does prearrival communication from a poison center to an emergency department decrease time to activated charcoal for pediatric poisoning? *Pediatr Emerg Care*. 2011;27:1045-1051.

350. Underhill TJ, et al. A comparison of the efficacy of gastric lavage, ipecacuanha and activated charcoal in the emergency management of paracetamol overdose. *Arch Emerg Med*. 1990;7:148-154.

351. Vale A, et al. Position statement and practice guidelines on the use of multi-dose activated charcoal in the treatment of acute poisoning. American Academy of Clinical Toxicology; European Association of Poisons Centres and Clinical Toxicologists. *J Toxicol Clin Toxicol*. 1999;37:731-751.

352. Vale JA. Position statement: gastric lavage. American Academy of Clinical Toxicology; European Association of Poisons Centres and Clinical Toxicologists. *J Toxicol Clin Toxicol*. 1997;35:711-719.

353. Vale JA, Kulig K; American Academy of Clinical Toxicology; European Association of Poisons Centres and Clinical Toxicologists. Position paper: gastric lavage. *J Toxicol Clin Toxicol*. 2004;42:933-943.

354. Valette E, et al. Case report: management of a severe carbamazepine intoxication. *Fundam Clin Pharmacol*. 2012;26:68.

355. Van Ameyde KJ, Tenenbein M. Whole bowel irrigation during pregnancy. *Am J Obstet Gynecol*. 1989;160:646-647.

356. van den Broek MP, et al. Severe valproic acid intoxication: case study on the unbound fraction and the applicability of extracorporeal elimination. *Eur J Emerg Med*. 2009;16:330-332.

357. van Gorp F, et al. Population pharmacokinetics and pharmacodynamics of escitalopram in overdose and the effect of activated charcoal. *Br J Clin Pharmacol*. 2012;73: 402-410.

358. van Ryn J, et al. Dabigatran etexilate—a novel, reversible, oral direct thrombin inhibitor: interpretation of coagulation assays and reversal of anticoagulant activity. *Thromb Haemost*. 2010;103:1116-1127.

359. Varvenne D, et al. Amatoxin-containing mushroom (*Lepiota brunneoincarnata*) familial poisoning. *Pediatr Emerg Care*. 2015;31:277-278.

360. Vasama J, et al. Fatal outcome after suicidal subcutaneous injection of E-cigarette liquid. *Clin Toxicol*. 2016;54:371-372.

361. Velez LI, et al. Iron bezoar retained in colon despite 3 days of whole bowel irrigation. *J Toxicol Clin Toxicol*. 2004;42:653-656.

362. Villarreal J, et al. A retrospective review of the prehospital use of activated charcoal. *Am J Emerg Med*. 2015;33:56-59.

363. Visser L, et al. Do not give paraffin to packers. *Lancet*. 1998;352:1352.

364. Wald P, et al. Esophageal tear following forceful removal of an impacted oral-gastric lavage tube. *Ann Emerg Med*. 1986;15:80-82.

365. Wang CY, et al. Early onset pneumonia in patients with cholinesterase inhibitor poisoning. *Respirology*. 2010;15:961-968.

366. Wang X, et al. Effect of activated charcoal on apixaban pharmacokinetics in healthy subjects. *Am J Cardiovasc Drugs*. 2014;14:147-154.

367. Westergaard B, et al. Adherence to international recommendations for gastric lavage in medical drug poisonings in Denmark 2007-2010. *Clin Toxicol*. 2012;50:129-135.

368. World Health Organization. *World Health Statistics*. Geneva: World Health Organization; 2016.

369. Wiles DA, et al. Massive lindane overdose with toxicokinetics analysis. *J Med Toxicol*. 2015;11:106-109.

370. Woo JH, Lim YS. Severe human poisoning with a flufenoxuron-containing insecticide: report of a case with transient myocardial dysfunction and review of the literature. *Clin Toxicol (Phila)*. 2015;53:569-572.

371. Woo JS, et al. Positive outcome after intentional overdose of dabigatran. *J Med Toxicol*. 2013;9:192-195.

372. Yancy RE, et al. In vitro and in vivo evaluation of the effect of cherry flavoring on the adsorptive capacity of activated charcoal for salicylic acid. *Vet Hum Toxicol*. 1977;19:163-165.

373. Yeates PJ, Thomas SH. Effectiveness of delayed activated charcoal administration in simulated paracetamol (acetaminophen) overdose. *Br J Clin Pharmacol*. 2000;49:11-14.

374. Yoshida S, et al. Much caution does no harm! Organophosphate poisoning often causes pancreatitis. *J Intensive Care*. 2015;3:21.

375. Zakharov S, et al. Non-fatal suicidal self-poisonings in children and adolescents over a 5-year period (2007-2011). *Basic Clin Pharmacol Toxicol*. 2013;112:425-430.

376. Zuccoli ML, et al. Unusual management of an inadvertent overdosage of vinorelbine in a child: a case report. *Clin Toxicol*. 2015;53:379-380.

377. Zuccoli ML, et al. Improper use of a medicine bottle to prepare an e-cigarette refill liquid. *Clin Toxicol*. 2016;54:389.

SC2

DECONTAMINATION PRINCIPLES: PREVENTION OF DERMAL, OPHTHALMIC, AND INHALATIONAL ABSORPTION

Scott Lucyk

Decontamination is a term that describes limiting or minimizing the exposure of a patient to a xenobiotic. This involves removal of a xenobiotic by physical means or by chemical neutralization before it can be systemically absorbed. Despite limited controlled studies assessing its efficacy, decontamination remains the mainstay of initial treatment for a patient exposed to a potentially harmful xenobiotic. Decontamination strategies in toxicology often refer to gastrointestinal (GI) techniques to minimize absorption or enhance elimination in orally poisoned patients (Chaps. 5 and 6). These same principles apply to other exposure routes where local or systemic absorption and toxicity occur, including dermal, ophthalmic, and pulmonary routes. An important point to note is that as opposed to GI decontamination, in which initial patient assessment and management always comes first, in the case of dermal and pulmonary contamination, in which there is risk for contamination and harm to health care personnel, the use of appropriate personal protective equipment (PPE) is paramount before initiation of patient decontamination. The benefits of decontamination to remove or neutralize a xenobiotic are severalfold and include (1) prevention of further absorption and toxicity in exposed patients, (2) prevention of secondary contamination of other staff or equipment, and (3) prevention of contamination of the health care facility and other patients.

An organized approach to decontamination is required following the release of hazardous materials. Unintentional release of hazardous materials occurs at industrial sites, chemical manufacturing plants, pipelines, and waste sites.[25] Also, the threat of terrorist attack using hazardous materials mandates that the health care community be prepared to effectively manage these situations in a safe and efficient manner that optimally treats patients while at the same time maintains the safety of the health care providers.

This Special Consideration focuses on situations that require health care facility–based dermal, ophthalmic, and pulmonary decontamination. The approach to the decontamination process is discussed, but the acute medical management of specific local and systemic toxicities is covered in other chapters. Dealing with mass casualty events and the incident command system, as well as prehospital decontamination are covered in detail elsewhere (Chap. 132). In addition, approaches to patient triage, runoff control, and isolation requirements are not covered here.

HAZARDOUS MATERIALS

Typically, decontamination efforts are initiated by first responders, including hazardous materials teams (HAZMAT), who respond to the site of initial xenobiotic release. However, in an instance when emergency medical services (EMS) is unable or uncertain how to decontaminate a patient or for patients who self-present to the hospital, it is prudent that health care providers are prepared to carry out effective decontamination. In fact, up to 80% of patients from a scene of xenobiotic release self-present to a hospital without undergoing any prior decontamination, mandating that hospital personnel have the appropriate knowledge and follow an organized approach to patient decontamination to ensure their personal safety and the safety of other health care providers and patients.[5,39,40] Close cooperation between the emergency department (ED) and prehospital providers, including HAZMAT teams responding to the initial site of exposure, help to

identify the xenobiotic involved and help to guide decontamination efforts. Appropriate communication with these teams before hospital arrival is paramount to ED preparations for a particular xenobiotic number of patients being brought by EMS, degree of prehospital decontamination, and associated injuries. Secondary contamination data from the Agency for Toxic Substances and Disease Registry (ATSDR) Hazardous Substances Emergency Events Surveillance system was studied. Between 1995 and 2001, six events involving 15 ED personnel, and from 2003 to 2006, 15 events involving at least 17 medical personnel were identified in which secondary contamination occurred.[20,21] After the Tokyo sarin subway attacks in 1995, many patients presented directly to a hospital as their first site of health care contact. Hospital-based decontamination attempts were not universal, with a limited number of patients receiving a change of clothes or shower, which resulted in approximately 23% of staff experiencing secondary contamination.[41]

A vast number of xenobiotics are involved in patient exposures, either from their deliberate use or from unintentional exposure. Identification of specific substances and their properties is helpful to determine specific toxic properties and the likelihood of systemic absorption. However, on initial hospital presentation, the exact xenobiotic or xenobiotics are often unknown, mandating that general safety and decontamination measures are promptly initiated to provide maximal safety to health care providers, with subsequent adjustments made as more product information becomes available.

In addition to concerns for toxicity related to hazardous materials, many of these exposures have nontoxicologic medical concerns that must be addressed simultaneously. Patients from industrial incidents often present with traumatic injuries or multiorgan dysfunction that require appropriate basic and advanced life support measures are instituted. Evaluation and support of patient airway, breathing, and circulation should ideally be done concomitantly with decontamination efforts, as long as health care providers are protected using appropriate PPE.

PERSONAL PROTECTIVE EQUIPMENT

As noted earlier, the most important aspects of managing patients contaminated with hazardous materials are to protect health care providers and to prevent worsening the situation by creating additional exposed individuals. There are several levels of PPE, classified according to the Environmental Protection Agency from level A to D, that provide varied levels of protection against exposure to gases, vapors, aerosols, liquids, and solids. The type of exposure dictates the level of PPE that is required for appropriate (Chap. 132).

DECONTAMINATION

Dermal Exposures

The majority of decontamination for patients presenting after hazardous materials exposures will involve dermal decontamination. Patients exposed to liquids, aerosols, or solids require dermal decontamination. Patients who do not pose a risk of secondary contamination to health care workers include those who have undergone appropriate prehospital decontamination and those exposed only to vapors or gases with no signs of skin or eye irritation and who do not have gross deposition of the material on their clothing or skin. These patients should proceed directly to the treatment area without further ED dermal decontamination.[4,16,22,24] However, gases or vapors condense on patient clothing, leading to secondary contamination from off-gassing if appropriate care is not taken in managing personal belongings (see later discussion). In addition, if a patient has ingested a chemical, vomitus poses a danger to health care providers through direct contact or off-gassing.[4] If able, patients should assist in their own decontamination efforts.

Methods of dermal decontamination include physical removal (clothing removal, removal of visible solid particles), adsorption (Fuller earth, activated charcoal, flour), dilution (flushing), or acts to neutralize the xenobiotic.[30]

Physical Removal

Before initiation of dermal decontamination, the most important step is to remove contaminated clothing, which removes from 75% to 90% of the contaminants.[13,22,26,39] Clothing should be cut off rather than pulled off because pulling off clothing will worsen contaminant exposure to the patient and health care staff.[22,39] Clothing and personal belongings should be double bagged in sealed plastic bags with the patient's information written on it.[3] Appropriate sealing is required to prevent evaporation or aerosolization of the xenobiotic.[4,30] Dermal decontamination also includes physical removal of the xenobiotic with forceps or gentle removal with brushing or use of a towel on the skin. Another method is to gently scrape the xenobiotic from the skin using a flat edge such as a tongue depressor.[24] Care must be taken to gently remove xenobiotics, as abrasive cleansers increase systemic absorption. Flushing the skin with copious amounts of water is also effective at physically removing xenobiotics.

A method of dry decontamination using activated charcoal, flour, or Fuller Earth is suggested by some groups to adsorb certain nerve agents and sulfur mustard, after which the adsorbed compound is gently brushed or wiped off with a towel.[22,24] The US military also uses a compound called M-291, a carbon-based adsorbent–polystyrene polymeric–ion exchange resin, for local, dermal decontamination.[22,24] Although dry decontamination is effective for localized exposures, it is unlikely to be useful in the hospital setting and therefore is not recommended because a lack of familiarity will lead to delays in initiating more effective decontamination strategies.

Dilution and Neutralization

Water only, soap and water, and 0.5% hypochlorite solutions are used to decontaminate skin after hazardous material exposures. The main factors determining usefulness of a hospital-based decontamination solution include safety (nontoxic and noncorrosive), availability, ease of use, affordability, and ease of disposal. The solution must also be nonirritating, rapid acting, and not produce toxic endproducts or enhance percutaneous absorption.[11,24] Regardless of the solution used to flush contaminated skin, the most important factor is that it must be done as soon as possible to minimize the inflammatory response and potential for local and systemic toxicity; after a xenobiotic is absorbed, topical decontamination is of limited utility.

Flushing contaminated skin with high volumes of low-pressure water will aid in physical removal and significant dilution of the xenobiotic. A military study showed that an oil-based xenobiotic was removed from 90% of subjects within 30 seconds and 100% of subjects at 90 seconds using a water only decontamination method.[36] Overall, showering with tepid water and liquid soap (mild, nonabrasive soap such as hand dishwashing soap) is the most effective, easiest, and most readily available method for removing hazardous materials from patients' hair and skin.[6,39] Use of alkaline soaps produces hydrolysis and neutralization of some xenobiotics; however, this contributes far less than the benefits of physical removal and dilution.[24] In addition, for patients exposed to non–water-soluble, oily, or adherent xenobiotics such as mustard or blister agents, addition of mild liquid soap and gentle scrubbing with a sponge or cloth helps to aid removal. Skin damage should be avoided to prevent further absorption of the xenobiotic. Patients should be scrubbed downward from head to toe with care taken to avoid contaminating unexposed areas.

Chemical alteration and deactivation, including hydrolysis and oxidative chlorination, were studied by the military in response to chemical weapons and suggest some benefit. However, these approaches do not have any significant role in the hospital setting because they require prolonged contact time to be effective.[22,32] Hydrolysis through the addition of acidic solutions is prohibitively slow, and alkaline solutions require a pH that would damage skin or mucosa (ie, pH 10–11).[24] Oxidative chlorination with the addition of dilute (0.5%) hypochlorite solution, although still recommended by the military and effective for decontaminating oxidizing mustard agents and some organic phosphorus compounds, is not acceptable for use on ophthalmic or mucosal surfaces, in open wounds, or exposed nerve tissue.[22,24] Both the difficulty in obtaining 0.5% hypochlorite solution and its propensity to worsen certain tissue injuries make its use impractical in the hospital setting.

There are no controlled studies to assess the optimal duration of showering or skin rinsing and no current consensus exists. Recommendations for duration of water-based decontamination range from 3 to 30 minutes.[4,7,12,39,48] It is reasonable to wash exposed areas with tepid water and liquid soap for 5 to 15 minutes, with an additional 10 to 15 minutes for contaminated open wounds.[7] The US military has several processes to assess efficacy of decontamination (eg, M8 paper, M9 tape, chemical agent monitor); however, these are not readily available or realistic for use in the hospital setting.[24]

Certain exposures benefit from a different decontamination strategy, and in certain instances, use of water may actually worsen toxicity. Exceptions to the water-first approach are solid alkali metals, including sodium, potassium, and lithium because water causes these metals to form their corresponding bases (sodium, potassium, or lithium hydroxide) and liberate a substantial amount of heat.[6] In addition, alkyl metals such as alkyl of aluminum, zinc, magnesium, or lithium cause similar reactions.[8] Radioactive compounds (cesium and rubidium) also react on contact with water.[27] Specific dusts (pure magnesium, white phosphorus, sulfur, strontium, titanium, uranium, yttrium, zinc, and zirconium) spontaneously ignite on contact with air. If these compounds are suspected on patient skin or clothing, residual metal should be removed with forceps and stored in mineral oil.[27] As mentioned previously, the identification is often delayed, and because the time to removal is paramount, when uncertain exposures are encountered, exposed patients should be immediately washed with copious amounts of soap and water.

Ophthalmic Exposures

There are more than 25,000 xenobiotics, including acids, bases, oxidizers, reducers, alkylators, chelators, and solvents, that cause chemical burns.[44] Acids and alkalis are the most commonly implicated xenobiotics in ophthalmic chemical exposures.[33,44] The severity of ophthalmic burns is determined by several factors, including solution concentration, pH, duration of exposure, extent of surface damaged, and degree of intraophthalmic penetration.[35,43] Liquid xenobiotics are most commonly implicated, but gases (eg, chlorine, ammonia, nerve agents) dissolve on the surface of the eye and be absorbed into the lacrimal fluid or diffuse through the lacrimal fluid (eg, mustard gas). Solids or powders also lead to ophthalmic injury if not removed promptly.

Decontamination

The single most important intervention after ophthalmic chemical injuries is immediate and copious irrigation because concentrated solutions penetrate the eye within seconds to minutes.[9,44] In one cohort of 101 patients with 131 burnt eyes, patients with delayed or no rinsing had a significant increase in number of operations required, worse visual outcomes, and increased length of stay in hospital compared with patients receiving immediate irrigation.[28,45] Contact lenses should be carefully removed to prevent any additional injury to the eye.[4] Often in industrial exposures, worksite safety precautions mandate that eyewash stations be readily available and that patients have initiated eye flushing before presentation to a health care facility. Some sites also have a portable eyewash station to be transported with the patient to hospital so that irrigation can be continued en route.

To adequately irrigate the eye and surrounding structures, the eye should be held open and continuously flushed. This process can be painful and irritating, so topical anesthetic should be applied before initiation. Solution can either be poured slowly into the eyes by gently pulling apart the patient's eyelids and tilting the head to the side or by using specially designed lenses that are placed beneath the eyelids to be in direct contact with the surface of the eye to enable direct flushing. The patient should be instructed to roll the eyeball to remove any particles retained beneath the eyelids.[9] The eyelids should be gently everted to assess for the presence of particulate debris that should be removed using a moist cotton tip. Irrigation should be continued for cycles of 10 to 15 minutes followed by pH rechecks (Chap. 24).[1,45] Ocular pH should be checked using litmus paper with a goal to continue irrigation until the pH is 7.5 to 8. Ophthalmic burns from strong or concentrated acids or alkalis require irrigation for at least 2 to 3 hours and immediate ophthalmologic consultation (Chap. 24).

Many different solutions and buffers were assessed in laboratory experiments while considering important ophthalmic properties, including osmolar regulation of tissues. Some experts caution that use of a low-osmolarity solution such as tap water will promote diffusion of the diluted xenobiotic into the deeper layers of the cornea and cause corneal edema.[44,45]

Overly complicated ocular decontamination protocols lead to physician uncertainty and delays in initiating treatment. Copious irrigation of the eye should be started promptly because time to irrigation is the most important factor. Any solution with a pH between 5 and 9 and temperature between 10° and 42°C is adequate for initial irrigation.[44] In residential exposures, prompt irrigation with any nontoxic liquid (eg, tap water) before and en route to a health care facility will significantly reduce injury. Although many different solutions and protocols have been studied, more evidence is required before these can be considered standard of care.

After appropriate irrigation has been effectively performed, a complete ophthalmologic assessment of consequential risk should be carried out, including visual acuity and intraocular pressure measurements for those with a toxic xenobiotic. Patients with ophthalmic exposure to chemicals should be assessed by an ophthalmologist because these patients are at risk for functional or anatomical loss of the eye, corneal ulceration, variations in ocular pressure, eyelid deformity and dysfunction, and tear abnormalities.[9] Decontamination attempts with copious flushing normalize the pH at the ophthalmic surface, however, the pH is not always reflective of the deeper structures of the globe, because xenobiotics will penetrate deeper into the eye.[44] Further treatments including cycloplegics, mydriatics, steroids, and topical antibiotics are beyond the scope of this chapter and should be discussed with an ophthalmologist (Chap. 24).

Inhalational Exposures

Internal decontamination of the pulmonary system is rarely required, specifically when an individual is exposed to a xenobiotic in which continued damage is expected and the xenobiotic is not able to rapidly diffuse from the pulmonary system. Removal of xenobiotics from the pulmonary tree requires use of bronchoalveolar lavage. The rare instances when this is required include removal of carbonaceous material after smoke inhalation and after exposure to large amounts of insoluble radioisotopes such as the alpha emitter plutonium.[47] Health care providers performing bronchoalveolar lavage should use appropriate PPE, as determined by the hospital Radiation Safety Officer. All lavage fluid should be collected and disposed of according to hospital policies.

SPECIFIC DECONTAMINATION EXAMPLES
Corrosives

A review of controlled clinical studies concluded that water was the best decontaminating solution for dermal corrosive exposures and that time to decontamination was the most important factor in limiting morbidity and improving outcomes.[6] Only four controlled clinical studies were published comparing early extensive water decontamination with none or lesser dilutional treatments in patients with corrosive dermal injury. One controlled

cohort study of 35 patients compared those treated with "immediate" water irrigation (within 10 minutes and continued for at least 15 minutes) with those receiving water irrigation after they arrived at hospital. Despite having mean total burn surface area twice as large (12% versus 6%), the immediate water irrigation group had significantly fewer burns that progressed to full thickness (12.5% versus 63%) and shorter mean hospital stays (7.7 days versus 20.5 days).[29] A follow-up study by the same group published 10 years of experience and included 83 patients (including the 35 patients from the previous study) treated with copious water irrigation within 3 minutes of exposure. These patients were less likely to progress to full-thickness burns (13.5% versus 60.8%) and had fewer delayed complications (5.4% versus 30.4%) and shorter lengths of hospital stay (6.2 versus 22 days) than those not decontaminated with water early.[38]

Other solutions were investigated for the purpose of "active rinsing." They are postulated to not only provide the irrigation benefits of water but also act to neutralize the offending xenobiotic. One decontamination solution investigated for use in chemical exposures and burns is an emergency aqueous rinsing solution that contains unspecified amphoteric salts.[18,33] In vitro studies suggest the emergency rinsing solution can neutralize alkaline or acidic substances without significant release of exothermic energy.[33] Animal studies suggest that an emergency rinsing solution helps to minimize ocular burns and is associated with improved wound healing and pain alleviation after dermal burns.[10,17] Use of an amphoteric, emergency rinsing solution was studied after implementation at three alumina refineries and included 180 patients with dermal alkali exposures, predominantly sodium hydroxide.[14,15] An emergency rinsing solution-first compared with water-first decontamination approach was associated with a not statistically significant difference in signs of chemical burns (47.1% versus 78.6% although when burns were present, patients treated with emergency rinsing solution had fewer blisters or severe signs compared with those who had water treatment (7.9% versus 23.8%; $P < 0.001$). A recent review of an emergency rinsing solution suggested it was a safe and effective method for improving healing time, healing sequelae, and pain management for chemical burns involving the skin and eyes of humans.[31] However, lack of treatment randomization, observer blinding, uncertain initial time to decontamination between the groups, and significant conflicts of interest limit the applicability of the studies. Further research and increased availability of amphoteric, emergency rinsing solutions are required before this can be recommended as a first-line therapy in preference to rapid and widely available water rinsing.

Hydrofluoric Acid

Hydrofluoric acid is a weak acid (pKa = 3.2) that can cause severe burns and life-threatening electrolyte abnormalities. Standard decontamination includes immediate and prolonged water rinsing of exposed areas followed closely by administration of calcium gluconate by one of several routes (Chap. 104). Dermal or ophthalmic exposures to hydrofluoric acid to the skin or eyes should be flushed with plain water or 0.9% saline for at least 20 minutes.[2] Another use of emergency aqueous rinsing solution containing unspecified amphoteric salts was advanced for decontaminating hydrofluoric acid and fluoride ions in an acidic environment. Such solutions provide the flushing effect of water but also act to chelate fluoride ions and neutralize acidic ions without creating a significant exothermic reaction.[33] Several case series involving workplace decontamination with an emergency rinsing solution claim minimization or avoidance of burn severity and minimal lost work time.[34,46] However, a study in rats with hydrofluoric acid exposure showed no difference between skin cleansing with an emergency rinsing solution versus water only in causing electrolyte abnormalities.[23] In fact, there was a trend toward milder hypocalcemia and hyperkalemia in rats decontaminated with 500 mL of water followed by a single application of 2.5% calcium gluconate gel compared with the emergency rinsing solution. Prior studies using the same skin cleansing technique showed that those treated with water and calcium gluconate gel had less severe burns compared with the emergency rinsing solution group.[19] Further research with amphoteric blends of emergency rinsing solutions is required before it can be recommended for treatment of hydrofluoric acid exposures.

Phenol

Phenol, also known as carbolic acid, is a colorless compound used in the production of many products, including phenolic resins, industrial coatings, dyes, perfumes, fungicides, plastics, explosives, and fertilizers. Concentrated phenol solutions cause severe chemical burns. Phenol is also used for chemical face peeling and is occasionally used in medicine in specific topical and oropharyngeal analgesics and ointments.[37] After exposure to concentrated solutions, skin will turn white initially followed by yellow-brown discoloration. Because toxicity is often significant, adequate dermal decontamination is vital. As in the case of all caustics, both the skin surface area exposed and the product concentration determine local and systemic toxicity. A porcine model assessed the optimal dermal decontamination strategy to minimize local damage based on histologic assessment and systemic absorption.[37] Histologic injury compared 10 different decontamination strategies, including water washes ranging from 1 to 30 minutes, alternating soap and water washes, and 15 minutes of alternating 1-minute water and 1-minute treatment washes. The treatment washes compared included polyethylene glycol (PEG) 400, PEG 400–industrial methylated spirits (IMS), PEG 400–ethanol, polyvinylpyrrolidone (PVP)–isopropyl alcohol (IPA), and IPA. The PEG 400 and IPA washes were more effective than the other treatments at reducing morphologic changes, including papillary dermal edema, pyknotic basal cells, and collagen necrosis.[37] In vitro studies using isolated perfused porcine skin flaps were then assessed and found that all three decontamination strategies studied (15 minutes of alternating water and PEG 400 washes, alternating water and IPA washes, or water-only washes) statistically reduced the amount of systemically absorbed phenol compared with controls but did not show significant differences between each of the treatment arms.[37] A swine study of phenol exposure found that decontamination for 15 minutes with either PEG 300–IMS or water shower found no significant differences in amount of phenol absorbed, as judged by plasma phenol concentrations.[42]

Given the inconclusive findings in prior studies, decontamination using inexpensive, readily available tepid water should be performed. Further studies on the safety and efficacy of using IPA and PEG–IMS are required before their use should be applied systematically to patients with phenol burns presenting to hospital.

Unknown Xenobiotics

Patients often present to health care facilities after exposure to an unknown xenobiotic. In these cases, patients should have clothing removed and affected areas washed with tepid water and liquid soap for 5 to 15 minutes, with an additional 10 to 15 minutes for contaminated open wounds. Ophthalmic exposures should have immediate water irrigation for cycles of 10 to 15 minutes followed by pH rechecks with goal pH of 7.5 to 8.

SUMMARY

- An organized approach to patient decontamination after hazardous materials exposure is paramount to ensure best patient outcomes, prevention of secondary contamination of health care providers, and optimal functioning of the health care facility.
- As opposed to GI decontamination, dermal decontamination must be performed concurrently with the initial evaluation.
- Many different products were evaluated for dermal and ophthalmic decontamination. At this time, there is insufficient evidence and availability to recommend use of one product over another. Use of tepid water is the most reasonable option for most exposures.
- Regardless of the solution used, the most important aspect is time to decontamination; after health care providers have donned appropriate PPE, prompt initiation of decontamination is vital.
- Removal of clothing and showering with soap and water to clean the skin and hair is the easiest, most efficacious way to minimize primary and secondary contamination.
- Pulmonary decontamination is rarely required for exposures causing contamination of the pulmonary tree when continued exposure is expected, such as with insoluble radioisotopes.

REFERENCES

1. Agency for Toxic Substances and Disease Registry (ATSDR). Medical Management Guidelines (MMG) for Acute Chemical Exposure. Toxic Substances Portal—Ammonia. October 21, 2014. https://www.atsdr.cdc.gov/MMG/MMG.asp?id=7&tid=2. Accessed January 31, 2017.
2. Agency for Toxic Substances and Disease Registry (ATSDR). Medical Management Guidelines (MMG) for Acute Chemical Exposure. Toxic Substances Portal—Hydrogen Fluoride (HF). October 21, 2014. https://www.atsdr.cdc.gov/mmg/mmg.asp?id=1142&tid=250. Accessed February 1, 2017.
3. Agency for Toxic Substances and Disease Registry (ATSDR). Medical Management Guidelines (MMG) for Acute Chemical Exposure. Toxic Substances Portal—Nerve Agents (GA, GB, GD, VX). October 21, 2014. http://www.atsdr.cdc.gov/mmg/mmg.asp?id=523&tid=93. Accessed August 1, 2016.
4. Agency for Toxic Substances and Disease Registry (ATSDR). Medical Management Guidelines (MMG) for Acute Chemical Exposure. Toxic Substances Portal—Unidentified Chemical. October 21, 2014). https://www.atsdr.cdc.gov/mmg/mmg.asp?id=1138&tid=243. Accessed November 15, 2016.
5. Auf der Heide E. The importance of evidence-based disaster planning. *Ann Emerg Med.* 2006;47:34-49.
6. Brent J. Water-based solutions are the best decontaminating fluids for dermal corrosive exposures: a mini review. *Clin Toxicol (Phila).* 2013;51:731-736.
7. Burgess JL, et al. Emergency department hazardous materials protocol for contaminated patients. *Ann Emerg Med.* 1999;34:205-212.
8. Burgher F, et al. Damaged skin. In: Maibach HI, Hall AH, eds. *Chemical Skin Injury: Mechanisms, Prevention, Decontamination, Treatment.* Springer-Verlag, Berlin; 2014:73-196.
9. Burns FR, Paterson CA. Prompt irrigation of chemical eye injuries may avert severe damage. *Occup Health Saf.* 1989;58:33-36.
10. Cavallini M, Casati A. A prospective, randomized, blind comparison between saline, calcium gluconate and Diphoterine for washing skin acid injuries in rats: effects on substance P and beta-endorphin release. *Eur J Anaesthesiol.* 2004;21:389-392.
11. Chan HP, et al. Skin decontamination: principles and perspectives. *Toxicol Ind Health.* 2013;29:955-968.
12. Cibulsky SM, et al. Patient decontamination in a mass chemical exposure incident: national planning guidance for communities. Security USDoH, Services USDoHaH/Division; (2014). https://www.dhs.gov/sites/default/files/publications/Patient Decon National Planning Guidance_Final_December 2014.pdf. Accessed April 1, 2017.
13. Cox RD. Decontamination and management of hazardous materials exposure victims in the emergency department. *Ann Emerg Med.* 1994;23:761-770.
14. Donoghue AM. Diphoterine for alkali chemical splashes to the skin at alumina refineries. *Int J Dermatol.* 2010;49:894-900.
15. Donoghue AM. Diphoterine(R) for alkali splashes to the skin. *Clin Toxicol (Phila).* 2014;52:148.
16. Georgopoulos PG, et al. Hospital response to chemical terrorism: personal protective equipment, training, and operations planning. *Am J Ind Med.* 2004;46:432-445.
17. Gerard M, et al. [Is there a delay in bathing the external eye in the treatment of ammonia eye burns? Comparison of two ophthalmic solutions: physiological serum and Diphoterine]. *J Fr Ophthalmol.* 2000;23:449-458.
18. Hall AH, et al. Safety of dermal Diphoterine application: an active decontamination solution for chemical splash injuries. *Cutan Ocul Toxicol.* 2009;28:149-156.
19. Hojer J, et al. Topical treatments for hydrofluoric acid burns: a blind controlled experimental study. *J Toxicol Clin Toxicol.* 2002;40:861-866.
20. Horton DK, et al. Secondary contamination of ED personnel from hazardous materials events, 1995-2001. *Am J Emerg Med.* 2003;21:199-204.
21. Horton DK, et al. Secondary contamination of medical personnel, equipment, and facilities resulting from hazardous materials events, 2003-2006. *Disaster Med Public Health Prep.* 2008;2:104-113.
22. Houston M, Hendrickson RG. Decontamination. *Crit Care Clin.* 2005;21:653-672, v.
23. Hulten P, et al. Hexafluorine vs. standard decontamination to reduce systemic toxicity after dermal exposure to hydrofluoric acid. *J Toxicol Clin Toxicol.* 2004;42:355-361.
24. Hurst CG. Decontamination. In: Sidell FR, Takafuji ET, Franz DR, eds. *Medical Aspects of Chemical and Biological Warfare.* Washington, DC: Office of the Surgeon General, TMM Publications; 1997:351-359.
25. Kirk MA, et al. Emergency department response to hazardous materials incidents. *Emerg Med Clin North Am.* 1994;12:461-481.
26. Koenig KL. Strip and shower: the duck and cover for the 21st century. *Ann Emerg Med.* 2003;42:391-394.
27. Koenig KL, et al. Health care facility-based decontamination of victims exposed to chemical, biological, and radiological materials. *Am J Emerg Med.* 2008;26:71-80.
28. Kuckelkorn R, et al. Poor prognosis of severe chemical and thermal eye burns: the need for adequate emergency care and primary prevention. *Int Arch Occup Environ Health.* 1995;67:281-284.
29. Leonard LG, et al. Chemical burns: effect of prompt first aid. *J Trauma.* 1982;22:420-423.
30. Levitin HW, et al. Decontamination of mass casualties—re-evaluating existing dogma. *Prehosp Disaster Med.* 2003;18:200-207.
31. Lynn DD, et al. The safety and efficacy of Diphoterine for ocular and cutaneous burns in humans. *Cutan Ocul Toxicol.* 2017;36:185-192.

32. Macintyre AG, et al. Weapons of mass destruction events with contaminated casualties: effective planning for health care facilities. *JAMA*. 2000;283:242-249.

33. Mathieu L, et al. Comparative evaluation of the active eye and skin chemical splash decontamination solutions Diphoterine and Hexafluorine with water and other rinsing solutions: effects on burn severity and healing. *J Chem Health Saf*. 2007;14:32-39.

34. Mathieu L, et al. Efficacy of Hexafluorine for emergent decontamination of hydrofluoric acid eye and skin splashes. *Vet Hum Toxicol*. 2001;43:263-265.

35. Merle H, et al. Alkali ocular burns in Martinique (French West Indies) Evaluation of the use of an amphoteric solution as the rinsing product. *Burns*. 2005;31:205-211.

36. Moffett PM, et al. Evaluation of time required for water-only decontamination of an oil-based agent. *Mil Med*. 2010;175:185-187.

37. Monteiro-Riviere NA, et al. Efficacy of topical phenol decontamination strategies on severity of acute phenol chemical burns and dermal absorption: in vitro and in vivo studies in pig skin. *Toxicol Ind Health*. 2001;17:95-104.

38. Moran KD, et al. Chemical burns. A ten-year experience. *Am Surg*. 1987;53:652-653.

39. Occupational Safety and Health Administration. *Best Practices for Hospital-Based First Receivers of Victims from Mass Casualty Incidents Involving the Release of Hazardous Substances*. Report No.: OSHA 3249-08N. Washington, DC: Occupational Safety and Health Administration; 2005.

40. Okumura T, et al. The Tokyo subway sarin attack: disaster management, Part 1: community emergency response. *Acad Emerg Med*. 1998;5:613-617.

41. Okumura T, et al. The Tokyo subway sarin attack: disaster management, Part 2: hospital response. *Acad Emerg Med*. 1998;5:618-624.

42. Pullin TG, et al. Decontamination of the skin of swine following phenol exposure: a comparison of the relative efficacy of water versus polyethylene glycol/industrial methylated spirits. *Toxicol Appl Pharmacol*. 1978;43:199-206.

43. Rozenbaum D, et al. Chemical burns of the eye with special reference to alkali burns. *Burns*. 1991;17:136-140.

44. Schrage NF. Rinsing therapy of eye burns. In: Schrage NF, Burgher F, Blomet J, et al, eds. *Chemical Ocular Burns: New Understanding and Treatments*. Springer-Verlag, Berlin; 2011:77-92.

45. Schrage NF, et al. Eye burns: an emergency and continuing problem. *Burns*. 2000;26:689-699.

46. Soderberg K, Kuusinen P, Mathieu L, et al. An improved method for emergent decontamination of ocular and dermal hydrofluoric acid splashes. *Vet Hum Toxicol*. 2004;46:216-218.

47. Sugarman SL, et al. The Radiation Emergency Assistance Center/Training Site: The Medical Aspects of Radiation Incidents. U.S. Department of Energy, Oak Ridge Associated Universities/Division. 2013. Accessed February 1, 2017.

48. U.S. Army Center for Health Promotion and Preventative Medicine. Personal Protective Equipment Guide for Military Medical Treatment Facility Personnel Handling Casualties from Weapons of Mass Destruction and Terrorism Events (Technical Guide 275). 2003. http://www.hsdl.org/?view&did=460845. Accessed January 15, 2017.

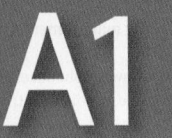

Antidotes in Depth

A1 ACTIVATED CHARCOAL

Silas W. Smith and Mary Ann Howland

INTRODUCTION

Activated charcoal (AC) is an excellent nonspecific adsorbent. Conclusions regarding the role of AC in poison management are achieved through the integration of pharmacologic data, controlled volunteer trials, studies in heterogeneous patients with overdose or poisoning, and clinical experience. Activated charcoal is provided to a patient after a risk-to-benefit assessment of the presumed ingested xenobiotic and patient-specific factors and circumstances. Benefits include preventing absorption or enhancing elimination by blocking enterohepatic or enteroenteric recirculation of a potentially toxic xenobiotic; risks include vomiting and subsequent aspiration pneumonitis. A detailed discussion of the merits of AC as a decontamination strategy is presented in Chap. 5.

HISTORY

Charcoal a fine, black, odorless powder, has been recognized for more than two centuries as an effective adsorbent of many substances. Organic chemist Scheele first used charcoal to absorb gases in 1773 and was followed in 1791 by Lowitz's use of charcoal with colored liquids.[6,89] Bertrand attributed his survival in 1811 from separate mercuric chloride and arsenic trioxide ingestions to their antecedent admixture with charcoal.[119] In 1830, the French pharmacist Touery demonstrated the powerful adsorbent qualities of charcoal by ingesting several lethal doses of strychnine mixed with charcoal in front of colleagues, suffering no ill effects.[6] An American physician, Holt, first used charcoal to "save" a patient from mercury bichloride poisoning in 1834.[6,89] However, it was not until the 1940s that Andersen began to systematically investigate the adsorbency of charcoal and unquestionably demonstrate that charcoal is an excellent, broad-spectrum gastrointestinal (GI) adsorbent.[6-8]

PHARMACOLOGY

Chemistry and Preparation

Activated charcoal is produced in a two-step process, beginning with the pyrolysis of various carbonaceous materials such as wood, coconut, petroleum, or peat to produce charcoal. This processing is followed by treatment at high temperatures (600°–900°C) with a variety of oxidizing (activating) agents such as steam, carbon dioxide, or acids to increase adsorptive capacity through formation of an internal maze of pores.[30,60,121] Typical AC surface areas average 800 to 1,200 m²/g.[117]

Mechanism of Action

The actual adsorption of a xenobiotic by AC relies on hydrogen bonding, ion-ion, dipole, and van der Waals forces, suggesting that most xenobiotics are best adsorbed by AC in their dissolved, nonionized form.[30,63,117,151]

Pharmacokinetics

Activated charcoal is pharmacologically inert and unabsorbed. Its GI transit time is influenced by the type and quantity and ingested xenobiotic, fasting and hydration status, perfusion, and the use of associated cathartics or evacuants, among other factors. The transit of AC is superimposed on a wide range of interindividual variation in gastric emptying and small bowel transit times, even in healthy volunteers.[62] In six volunteers acting as their own controls, AC alone or administered with sodium chloride, sodium sulfate, magnesium sulfate, or a proprietary cathartic "salt" (36.7% anhydrous

citric acid, 17.65% magnesium sulfate, and 45.6% sodium bicarbonate), the GI transit times to fecal evacuation ranged from 29.3 ± 1.2 hours to 17.3 ± 1.9 hours.[120] In 59 overdose patients compared with 104 overdose historical control participants who ingested acetaminophen (APAP), carbamazepine, cyclic antidepressants, opioid–APAP combinations, and phenytoin, the addition of 70% sorbitol solution to 25 to 50 g of AC decreased the median half-lives for gastric emptying (from 100 to 82 minutes), small intestinal transit (from 209 to 180 minutes), and orocecal transit (from 270 to 210 minutes).[1,2]

Pharmacodynamics

The adsorption rate to AC depends on external surface area, and the adsorptive capacity depends on the far larger internal surface area.[30,31,110] The adsorptive capacity is modified by altering the size of the pores. Current AC products have pore sizes that range from 10 to 1,000 angstroms (Å), with most of the internal surface area created by 10- to 20 Å-sized pores.[30,32] Most xenobiotics are of moderate molecular weight (100–800 Da) and adsorb well to pores in the range of 10 to 20 Å. Mesoporous charcoals with a pore size of 20 to 200 Å have a greater capacity to adsorb larger xenobiotics as well as those in their larger hydrated forms but are not available for clinical use.[86]

When the AC surface area is large, the adsorptive capacity is increased, but affinity is decreased because van der Waals forces and hydrophobic forces diminish.[151] According to the Henderson-Hasselbalch equation, weak bases are best adsorbed at basic pHs, and weak acids are best adsorbed at acidic pHs. For example, cocaine, a weak base, binds to AC with a maximum adsorptive capacity of 273 mg of cocaine per gram of AC at a pH of 7.0; this capacity is reduced to 212 mg of cocaine per gram of AC at a pH of 1.2.[85] Activated charcoal binds amitriptyline hydrochloride with adsorption capacities of 120 and 100 mg per gram of AC in simulated gastric and intestinal fluids, respectively.[150] The adsorption to AC of a weakly dissociated metallic salt such as mercuric chloride ($HgCl_2$) decreases with decreasing pH because the number of complex ions of the type $HgCl_3$ and $HgCl_4$ increases, and the number of electroneutral molecules ($HgCl_2$) is reduced.[7] Nonpolar, poorly water-soluble organic substances are more likely to be adsorbed from an aqueous solution than polar, water-soluble substances.[30] Among the organic molecules, aromatics are better adsorbed than aliphatics; molecules with branched chains are better adsorbed than those with straight chains; and molecules containing nitro groups are better adsorbed than those containing hydroxyl, amino, or sulfonic groups.[30]

Activated charcoal decreases the systemic absorption of most xenobiotics, including APAP, aspirin, barbiturates, cyclic antidepressants, phenytoin, theophylline, and other inorganic and organic materials.[49,106,123] Notable xenobiotics not amenable to AC are the alcohols, acids, alkalis, iron, lead, lithium, magnesium, potassium, and sodium salts.[53] Although the binding of AC to cyanide is less than 4%, the toxic dose is small, and 50 g of AC would theoretically be able to bind more than 10 lethal doses of potassium cyanide. Activated charcaol is capable of rapidly removing volatile anesthetic gases such as isoflurane, sevoflurane, and desflurane from anesthetic breathing circuits, which is potentially important in patients who are susceptible to or develop malignant hyperthermia.[14]

The efficacy of AC is directly related to the quantity administered. The effect of the AC to drug ratio on adsorption was demonstrated both in vitro and in vivo with para-aminosalicylate (PAS). In vitro, the fraction of unadsorbed PAS decreased from 55% to 3% as the AC-to-PAS ratio increased from 1:1 to 10:1 at a pH of 1.2.[114] This study provides the best scientific basis for the 10:1 AC-to-drug ratio dose typically recommended. In human volunteers, as the AC-to-PAS ratio increased from 2.5:1 to 50:1, the total 48-hour urinary excretion decreased from 37% to 4%.[114] Presumably, this occurred because more of the PAS was adsorbed by AC in the lumen of the GI tract rather than being absorbed systemically. These same studies demonstrate AC saturation at low ratios of AC to drug and argue for a 10:1 ratio of AC to xenobiotic. A meta-analysis of 64 controlled volunteer studies demonstrated that the percentage of reduction in drug exposure provided by AC followed a sigmoidal dose–response curve.[69] Activated charcoal to drug ratios of 1:1, 5:1, 10:1, 20:1, 25:1, and 50:1 reduced drug exposures by 9.0%, 30.2%, 44.6%, 58.9%, 62.9%, and 73.0%, respectively.[69] In a subsequent study of volunteers ingesting 50 mg/kg of APAP, reducing a 1-hour postingestion 50 g AC dose to 25 or 5 g caused the APAP area under the concentration versus time curve (AUC) to increase by 23.6% and 59.0%, respectively.[55]

In vitro studies demonstrate that adsorption begins within about 1 minute of AC administration but does not achieve equilibrium for 10 to 25 minutes.[31,106] The clinical efficacy of AC to prevent absorption is inversely related to the time elapsed after ingestion and depends largely on the rate of absorption of the xenobiotic. According to a meta-analysis of volunteer studies, the median reductions of drug exposure when AC was administered at 0 to 5 minutes, 30 minutes, 60 minutes, 120 minutes, 180 minutes, 240 minutes, and 360 minutes after ingestion were 88.4%, 48.5%, 38.4%, 24.4%, 13.6%, 27.4%, and 11%, respectively.[69] Early AC administration is more important with rapidly absorbed xenobiotics, in which AC functions to prevent xenobiotic absorption by achieving rapid adsorption in the GI tract. After a xenobiotic is systemically absorbed or parenterally administered, AC can enhance elimination through enterohepatic and enteroenteric recirculation as opposed to affecting absorption.

Desorption (drug dissociation from AC) can occur, especially weak acids, as the AC–drug complex transits the stomach and intestine and as the pH changes from acidic to basic.[50,113,147] Whereas strongly ionized and dissociated salts, such as sodium chloride and potassium chloride, are poorly adsorbed, nonionized or weakly dissociated salts, such as iodine and mercuric chloride, respectively, are adsorbed. Binding of γ-hydroxybutyrate (800 mg) to AC (10 g) decreased from 84.3% to 23.3% when exchanging simulated gastric for intestinal fluid.[105] Diminished AC adsorptive capacity in the intestinal lumen can also occur because of the rapid adsorption by AC of intestinal fatty acids, which rapidly cover the surface of carbon granules.[89] Desorption can lead to ongoing systemic xenobiotic absorption over days. In this case, the apparent elimination half-life of the xenobiotic increases, but peak concentrations remain unaffected.[111] The clinical effects of desorption can be minimized by providing sufficient AC to overcome the decreased affinity of the xenobiotic secondary to pH change, such as by using multiple-dose AC (MDAC).[73,96,109,124,140] Although ethanol and other solvents such as polyethylene glycol (PEG) are minimally adsorbed by AC, they can decrease AC adsorptive capacity for a coingested xenobiotic by competing for AC binding.[12,111,113,115]

Concomitant Administration of Activated Charcoal with Cathartics or Evacuants

Cathartics are often used with AC; however, evidence suggests that AC alone is comparably effective to AC plus a single dose of cathartic (sorbitol or magnesium citrate).[3,73,90,92,96,104,110,122] If a cathartic is used, it should be used only once. Repeated doses of magnesium-containing cathartics are associated with hypermagnesemia,[99,142] and repeated doses of any cathartic are associated with salt and water depletion, hypotension, and severe or fatal fluid and electrolyte derangements.[48] Activated charcoal with sorbitol is not recommended for children younger than 1 year of age.[121]

Whole-bowel irrigation (WBI) with PEG electrolyte lavage solution can significantly decrease the in vitro and in vivo adsorptive capacity of AC, depending on the individual xenobiotic, its formulation, and the GI location. For example, experiments demonstrate desorption of cocaine, fluoxetine,

salicylate, and theophylline from AC,[10,76,85] but chlorpromazine was not significantly affected by PEG at gastric pH.[11] A controlled crossover study compared the addition of a short course of WBI (1 L/h) with AC alone in nine healthy participants who were provided simultaneous carbamazepine (200 mg), theophylline (200 mg), and verapamil (120 mg).[80] Polyethylene glycol decreased AC's efficacy for carbamazepine and theophylline but was synergistic with AC for verapamil.[80] Whole-bowel irrigation did not improve upon AC's nonstatistically significant 11% decrease in absorption in volunteers ingesting 2.88 g of aspirin.[91] The most likely explanation is competition by PEG for the surface of the AC for solute adsorption. Activated charcoal and WBI interactions are further discussed in Antidotes in Depth: A2.

Related Formulations

Porous carbon microsphere compounds (eg, AST-120) are clinically used to adsorb endogenous enteric uremic toxins to mitigate glomerular hypertrophy, interstitial fibrosis, and progression of chronic kidney disease.[136,137,161]

ROLE OF ACTIVATED CHARCOAL IN GASTROINTESTINAL DECONTAMINATION

Single-Dose Activated Charcoal

It is difficult to assess the efficacy of single-dose AC (SDAC) in a prospective study involving consecutive adults receiving 50 g of AC for self-poisonings because of the exclusions of multiple xenobiotic and sustained-release products and because SDAC was used in combination with other forms of GI decontamination in all symptomatic patients.[97] Not surprisingly, a beneficial effect of SDAC on outcome measures could not be demonstrated in asymptomatic patients. Similarly, a study of routine SDAC administration after oral overdose consisting primarily of benzodiazepines, APAP, and selective serotonin reuptake inhibitors could not demonstrate differences in mortality, length of stay, vomiting, or intensive care admissions.[33] A prospective trial of 876 patients comparing SDAC alone with SDAC plus gastric emptying was unable to demonstrate a difference in outcomes, with the exception of patients presenting within 1 hour of ingestion, although this difference was not sustained after being adjusted for severity.[127] Subsequent studies touting the lack of benefit of AC are of limited value because of similar design flaws such as including irrelevant exposures or those to which AC would not adsorb or conflating AC administration outcomes with orogastric lavage.[118] When evaluating SDAC alone, a meta-analysis of 64 controlled volunteer studies found significant reductions in ingested xenobiotic amounts when SDAC was provided in appropriate quantity (eg, a 10:1 AC: xenobiotic ratio) and within 240 minutes of exposure.[69]

Research subsequent to this meta-analysis has sustained primarily pharmacokinetic advantage of SDAC, although some improvements in clinically important endpoints were demonstrated. A healthy volunteer study in 12 patients in which SDAC was provided 15 minutes after supratherapeutic APAP ingestions (60 mg/kg) reduced APAP absorption by a mean of 41%.[154] In nine human volunteers ingesting 5 g of APAP and 0.5 mg/kg of oxycodone, 50 g of SDAC at 1, 2, or 3 hours reduced the APAP AUC by 43%, 22%, and 15%, respectively.[103] In six volunteers, concentrations of lamotrigine (100 mg); oxcarbazepine (600 mg); and oxcarbazepine's active metabolite, 10,11-dihydro-10-hydroxy-carbamazepine were reduced by 42%, 97.2%, and 95.8%, respectively, by 50 g of AC provided 30 minutes after ingestion.[74]

In a pharmacokinetics and pharmacodynamics evaluation of escitalopram overdosed patients, SDAC reduced the absorbed fraction by 31% and reduced the risk of QT prolongation by approximately 35% for escitalopram doses above 200 mg.[152] In 319 patients with 436 venlafaxine overdoses, SDAC or SDAC with WBI significantly decreased the odds of seizure to 0.48 and 0.25, respectively, compared with no decontamination.[79] In 176 patients presenting with 286 separate quetiapine overdoses, SDAC administration within 2 hours reduced the probability of intubation by 7% for a 2-g ingestion and by 17% for a 10-g ingestion, although time to extubation was unaffected.[67] In pharmacokinetic modeling study of sertraline overdose that was limited by uncertainty in ingestion time and dose, SDAC decreased the AUC and decreased the maximum plasma concentration when administered between 1 and 4 hours after overdose.[34] Volunteer studies evaluated late AC administration in factor Xa inhibitor ingestions. Activated charcoal decreased ingested rivaroxaban AUCs by 43%, 31%, and 29% when administered 2 hours, 5 hours, and 8 hours postdose, respectively.[116] Similarly, for apixaban, which undergoes enteroenteric recirculation, AC decreased AUCs by 50% and 28%, when administered 2 hours and 6 hours postdose, respectively, as well as decreasing its apparent half-life from 13.4 hours to approximately 5 hours.[155] A retrospective observational study showed neither benefit nor harm of AC in organic phosphorus compounds or carbamate poisoning.[101] In light of further pharmacokinetic understanding and the potential for larger ingestions, more recent recommendations have relaxed the narrow AC administration "window" to support its utilization beyond 1 hour. This is true even in cases of ingestions for which an antidote exists, such as APAP.[20,25,118]

Multiple-Dose Activated Charcoal

Multiple-dose AC functions both to prevent the absorption of xenobiotics that are slowly absorbed from the GI tract and to enhance the elimination of suitable xenobiotics that have already been absorbed. Multiple-dose AC decreases xenobiotic absorption when large amounts of xenobiotics are ingested and dissolution is delayed (eg, masses, bezoars), when xenobiotic formulations exhibit a delayed or prolonged release phase (eg, enteric coated, extended release), when GI motility is impaired because of coingestants, or when reabsorption can be prevented (eg, enterohepatic circulation of active xenobiotic, active metabolites, or conjugated xenobiotic hydrolyzed by gut bacteria to active xenobiotic).

The ability of MDAC to enhance elimination after absorption had already occurred was first reported in 1982.[13] This report concluded that orally administered MDAC enhanced the total body clearance (nonrenal clearance) of six healthy volunteers given 2.85 mg/kg of body weight of intravenous (IV) phenobarbital.[13] The serum half-life of phenobarbital decreased from 110 ± 8 to 45 ± 6 hours. An editorial suggested that MDAC enhanced the diffusion of phenobarbital from the blood into the GI tract and trapped it there for later fecal excretion. In this manner, AC was said to perform as an "infinite sink," allowing for "gastrointestinal dialysis" to occur.[81] These findings were confirmed by studies in dogs and rats using IV aminophylline and shown to be independent of theophylline enterohepatic circulation.[39,78,94] Subsequent studies using MDAC with IV aminophylline further extended these results to humans.[64] Using an isolated perfused rat small intestine, the concept of GI dialysis[94] was elegantly demonstrated because AC dramatically affected the pharmacokinetics of theophylline and produced a constant intestinal clearance that approximated intestinal blood flow.[94] In 114 hemodialysis patients who received a mean AC daily dose of 3.19 ± 0.81 g/day in three divided doses, mean serum phosphate concentrations decreased by 2.60 ± 0.11 mg/dL, further supporting the concept of "GI dialysis."[156]

The toxicokinetic considerations underlying MDAC's ability to enhance elimination are similar to those involved in deciding whether hemodialysis would be appropriate for a given xenobiotic. Successful MDAC requires the xenobiotic to be in the blood compartment (low volume of distribution), have limited protein binding, and have prolonged endogenous clearance. Experimental evidence suggests a role for MDAC in the absence of available Prussian blue (Antidotes in Depth: A31) to treat thallium poisoning.[59] Although MDAC increases to varying degrees the elimination of amitriptyline,[61] cyclosporine,[61] carbamazepine,[15,17,157] dapsone,[108] digitoxin,[35,126] nadolol,[43] nortriptyline,[36] phenobarbital,[128] phenylbutazone,[107] propoxyphene,[71] quinine,[28] salicylate,[58,75] and theophylline,[14,84,146] its clinical utility remains to be defined.[28,72,145]

An analysis of 28 volunteer studies involving 17 xenobiotics was unable to correlate the physical chemical properties of a particular xenobiotic with MDAC's ability to decrease the plasma half-life of that xenobiotic.[22] Although the half-life was not thought to be the best marker of enhanced elimination, it was the only parameter consistently evaluated in these exceptionally diverse studies. The xenobiotics with the longest intrinsic plasma half-lives seemed to demonstrate the largest percent reduction in plasma half-life

when MDAC was used. A subsequent animal model with therapeutic doses of four simultaneously administered IV xenobiotics (APAP, digoxin, theophylline, and valproic acid) clarified the role of pharmacokinetics on MDAC's effectiveness.[27] Theophylline, APAP, and valproic acid all have small volumes of distribution. However, of the three, only valproic acid is highly protein bound at the doses used, which probably accounted for MDAC's inability to increase its clearance while increasing clearance of the three other xenobiotics. However, volunteer studies do not accurately reflect the overdose situation[95] in which saturation of plasma protein binding, saturation of first-pass metabolism, and acid–base disturbances may make more free xenobiotic available for an enteroenteric effect and therefore more amenable to MDAC use. The most rapid and dramatic effect of MDAC was on theophylline clearance. Large volumes of distribution alone do not necessarily exclude MDAC's benefit. Although digoxin has a large volume of distribution, it requires several hours to distribute from the blood to the tissues. Multiple-dose AC is beneficial as long as the digoxin remains in the blood compartment and distribution is incomplete.

In one case series of infants with aminophylline and theophylline overdoses, MDAC appeared to reduce theophylline half-lives (2–12 hours) compared with historical values.[138] Multiple-dose AC added as an adjunct to phototherapy in neonatal hyperbilirubinemia produced a significantly greater decline in bilirubin concentrations than in those receiving phototherapy alone.[5] In a randomized clinical study, patients with phenobarbital overdoses were given SDAC or MDAC.[128] Although the phenobarbital half-life was significantly decreased in the MDAC group (36 versus 93 hours), the length of intubation time required by each group did not differ from one another. This study was criticized for small size, unevenly matched groups, and focus on a single endpoint (extubation) potentially dependent on factors other than patient condition (eg, the time of day). In 15 adult patients with supratherapeutic phenytoin concentrations, MDAC reduced the time to phenytoin concentration less than 25 mg/L from 41.1 to 19.3 hours, although clinical endpoints were again unchanged.[141] Multiple-dose AC markedly decreased the apparent phenytoin half-lives in patients with prolonged half-lives because of CYP2C9 enzyme genetic polymorphisms.[23]

A compelling demonstration of MDAC's benefits in the overdose setting comes from a study performed in Sri Lanka in patients with severe cardiac toxicity caused by intentional overdose with yellow oleander seeds.[38] An initial AC dose of 50 g was administered to all patients, who were then randomized to 50 g of AC every 6 hours for 3 days or placebo. There were statistically fewer deaths and fewer life-threatening dysrhythmias in the MDAC group. Subsequent randomized, controlled trials further evaluated no AC, SDAC, and MDAC in self-poisoned patients. In 104 patients ingesting yellow oleander seeds in Sri Lanka, despite erratic and prolonged absorption, SDAC and MDAC significantly and equivalently reduced cardiac glycoside 24-hour mean residence time (which quantifies the time course of a xenobiotic through the body) from 11.21 ± 1.55 hours (no AC) to 10.36 ± 1.14 hours (SDAC) and 10.20 ± 0.99 hours (MDAC), respectively, and apparent terminal half-life from 62.9 hours (no AC) to 33.9 hours (SDAC) and 32.3 hours (MDAC), respectively.[131] Despite this, neither SDAC nor MDAC reduced the mortality rate among 4,629 randomized, poisoned patients.[44] However, in this study, about one-third of the patients had ingested yellow oleander seeds, slightly less than one-third ingested pesticides, and mechanical forced emesis or gastric lavage occurred in 54.0% and 7.5% of patients prerandomization.[44] It is unclear how these trials apply to management in developed countries, where the use of antidotes such as digoxin-specific antibody fragments for cardioactive steroid poisoning and atropine and pralidoxime for organic phosphorus pesticide poisoning routinely complement GI decontamination and the absorption kinetics of most prescription medications differ from the substances ingested in the trial.[68] A systematic review concluded that MDAC could enhance phenobarbital or primidone elimination in severe poisonings, although supportive care is the relevant clinical intervention.[130]

Ultimately, the decision to administer SDAC or MDAC should involve a patient-tailored, risk-to-benefit analysis. Potential adverse effects are weighed against the particular ingested xenobiotic, its quantity, and formulation; dose–response curve of the xenobiotic; the impact of SDAC or MDAC on this curve; the time since ingestion; coingestants; gastric motility and contents; available antidotes, therapies, and medical support; the severity of presentation; anticipated sequelae; patient cooperativity; and other patient-specific factors and comorbidities.[68,117,121,143]

ADVERSE EFFECTS AND SAFETY ISSUES

Contraindications to AC include presumed GI perforation or discontinuity or the need for endoscopic visualization (eg, in caustic ingestions). To prevent aspiration pneumonitis from oral AC administration, an airway assessment must occur, and potential airway compromise should be excluded. Subsequently, a risk-to-benefit assessment with regard to the need for airway protection and the need for AC should be made. Other considerations include a determination of adequate GI motility (appropriate bowel sounds to ensure peristalsis) and normal abdominal examination findings and absent distension or signs of an acute abdomen. With compromised bowel function, AC should be withheld or delayed until the stomach can be decompressed to decrease the risk of subsequent vomiting and aspiration.

Although the use of AC is relatively safe, emesis, which typically occurs after rapid administration; constipation; and diarrhea are frequently reported after AC administration.[110] Constipation and diarrhea are more likely to result from the ingestion itself than from the AC. However, black stools that are negative for occult blood, black tongues, and darkened mucous membranes are frequently observed. Serious adverse effects of AC include pulmonary aspiration of AC with or without gastric contents, leading to airway obstruction (potentially of rapid onset), acute respiratory distress syndrome, bronchiolitis obliterans, and death;[9,40,47,52,57,70,117,121,125,139] peritonitis from spillage of enteric contents, including AC, into the peritoneum after GI perforation;[88] and intestinal obstruction and pseudo-obstruction, especially after repeated AC doses in the presence of either dehydration or prior bowel adhesions.[19,54,83,98,158] Although a significant number of patients aspirate gastric contents before endotracheal intubation and AC administration,[100,132] the incidence of AC aspiration after endotracheal intubation varies from 4% to 25%, depending on the nature of the study. Another retrospective investigation demonstrated a 1.6% incidence of aspiration pneumonitis in unselected overdosed patients. Altered mental status, spontaneous emesis, and cyclic antidepressant overdose were associated risk factors; AC was not in itself a risk factor.[66] Because sorbitol is hepatically metabolized to fructose, the package insert warns against administration of AC with sorbitol to patients with a genetic intolerance to fructose.[121]

Adverse Effects of Multiple-Dose Activated Charcoal

Complications observed with SDAC increase with MDAC. Other adverse effects of MDAC include diarrhea when multiple sorbitol-containing AC preparations are used, constipation, vomiting with a subsequent risk of aspiration, intestinal ileus and obstruction, and a reduction of serum concentrations of therapeutically used xenobiotics.[42,98,117,125] One retrospective review of 834 poisoned patients uncontrolled for type of ingestion found that MDAC was associated with clinically significant pulmonary aspiration in 0.6%, GI obstruction in 0%, hypernatremia in 6.0%, and hypermagnesemia in 3.1%.[42] Administration of multiple sorbitol-containing AC preparations infrequently produces salt and water depletion, hypotension, and potentially fatal electrolyte derangements, especially in children.[48,102]

PREGNANCY AND LACTATION

The safety in pregnancy category for AC is undetermined. The benefit of preventing absorption with AC should outweigh the risk of administration to the pregnant patient. The underlying elevated prevalence of nausea and vomiting in pregnancy[77] might predispose pregnant patients to a potentially higher rate of vomiting, although this is speculative. Single-dose AC and MDAC have been safely administered to pregnant patients as part of poisoning management.[18,26,37,93,133] Murine and lapine studies have not demonstrated any teratogenic risk.[121] The lack of absorption of AC would not predispose it to breast milk excretion, although definitive safety in lactation has not been established.[121]

DOSING AND ADMINISTRATION

Single-dose AC should be administered when a xenobiotic is still expected to be available for adsorption in the GI tract and the benefit of preventing absorption outweighs the risk. The optimal SDAC dose is unknown.[28] However, most authorities recommend a minimum AC dose of 1 g/kg of body weight or a 10:1 ratio of AC to xenobiotic, up to an amount that can be tolerated by the patient and safely administered, which usually represents 50 to 100 g in adults. For some ingestions (eg, salicylate or APAP), a 10:1 ratio would be impracticable to achieve, although the 1-g/kg dose appears to be efficacious. This is supported by volunteer studies of supratherapeutic ingestions.[55,69] Activated charcoal that is not premixed is best administered as a slurry in a 1:8 ratio of AC to suitable liquid, such as water or cola.

Prehospital Administration

Prehospital AC administration by emergency medical personnel expedites the administration after overdose.[4,159] However, the implementation costs and potential adverse effects have to be weighed against the small number of patients who would actually benefit.[65] In a study simulating home administration in 50 young children, 86% readily drank the AC–water slurry, and 76% of them consumed 95% to 100% of the total dose.[21] Of seven children in a simulated home environment administered AC in regular cola, three drank 1 g/kg, two drank about half of this therapeutic dose, and the other two drank very little.[134] A prospective poison control center case series demonstrated successful home AC administration. In this series, the median age of the patients was 3 years, and the median AC dose ingested was 12 g.[144] However, other attempts at getting children to ingest AC were not as successful. Difficulty was noted in 70% of attempts to administer a standard AC dose to children in the home setting.[41] A review of AC in the home suggested variable success depending on the parent and child.[46] A retrospective review of poisoned children concluded that those who were preannounced to an emergency department by the poison control center received AC earlier (59 ± 34 minutes) than patients without a referral (71 ± 43 minutes).[148] One additional retrospective review determined that prehospital paramedic-administered AC did not increase EMS encounter duration.[153]

Hospital Administration

Administration in children is facilitated by offering an opaque, decorated, covered cup and a straw.[160] The black color and gritty nature of AC have led to the development of many formulations to improve palatability and patient acceptance. Bentonite, carboxymethyl cellulose, and starch[56,104,135] are used as thickening agents, and cherry syrup, chocolate syrup, sorbitol, sucrose, saccharin, and ice cream have been used as flavoring agents.[31,82,87,162] Most additives do not decrease the adsorptive capacity; however, improvements in palatability and acceptance have been minimal or nonexistent with all of these formulations.[30] Although a milk chocolate AC formulation evaluated by children was rated superior in palatability to standard AC preparations,[45] it was never marketed in the United States. A marketed cherry-flavored AC product was rated by adult volunteers as preferable over plain AC, and a statistically significant larger quantity of the flavored AC was ingested.[29] This difference was not maintained in adult overdosed patients; most patients consumed the entire bottle of AC independent of cherry flavoring. Cold cola was used to enhance palatability in volunteer children and adults. Children preferred regular cola over diet cola. Teenagers preferred the palatability of AC mixed with chocolate milk or cola over AC mixed with water, but this did not significantly improve ease of swallowing.[24] Adults rated cola–AC preferable to plain AC.[129,134] Other studies in adult overdosed patients compared different AC brands without additives or flavoring to determine the AC quantity typically ingested.[16,51] In one study, approximately half of the 50 g of AC offered was ingested, and 7% of the patients vomited.[16] In the other study, 60 g of AC as Liqui-Char (standard AC) or CharcoAid G (superactivated granulated AC) was offered, and approximately 95% of each formulation was consumed in 20 minutes. There was no difference in the amount consumed even though the palatability of the granular form of AC (CharcoAid G) was rated higher.[51]

Multiple-Dose Activated Charcoal Administration

An initial AC loading dose should be administered to adults and children in an attempt to achieve a AC-to-xenobiotic ratio of 10:1 or 1 g/kg of body weight (if the xenobiotic exposure amount is unknown). The correct AC dose and interval for multiple dosing, when it is indicated, is best tailored to the amount and dosage form of the xenobiotic ingested, the severity of the overdose, the potential lethality of the xenobiotic, and the patient's ability to tolerate AC. Benefit should always be weighed against risk. Doses of AC for multiple dosing have varied considerably in the past, ranging from 0.25 to 0.5 g/kg of body weight every 1 to 6 hours to 20 to 60 g for adults every 1, 2, 4, or 6 hours. Some evidence suggests that the total dose administered may be more important than the frequency of administration.[64,149] Continuous nasogastric administration of AC is reported, especially when vomiting is a problem, although the risk-to-benefit assessment would require consideration.[50,112,149] After the initial AC loading dose of 1 g/kg, subsequent doses of of 0.5 g/kg (~25–50 g in adults) every 4 to 6 hours for up to 12 to 24 hours is reasonable in most circumstances.

FORMULATION AND ACQUISITION

Activated charcoal is supplied in bottles or tubes as a ready-to-use aqueous suspension in multiple doses formulations (eg, suspensions of 15 g, 25 g, and 50 g of AC in 72 mL, 120 mL, and 240 mL at a fixed concentration of 208 mg/mL AC).[121] Some AC suspensions are also premixed with sorbitol (eg, 25 and 50 g AC with 48 or 96 g of sorbitol to yield 208 mg/mL of AC and 400 mg/mL of sorbitol).[121] When not premixed, it is recommended to create a slurry of AC in a 1:8 ratio of AC to suitable liquid (eg, water, cola).

SUMMARY

- Activated charcoal is an effective, nonspecific adsorbent.
- Absent contraindications, AC should be of benefit to a patient with a potentially life-threatening ingestion of a xenobiotic that is adsorbed by AC and is expected to be present in the GI tract at the time of administration. Activated charcoal does not adsorb alcohols, acids, alkalis, iron, lead, lithium, magnesium, potassium, or sodium salts.
- Multiple-dose AC is useful to prevent systemic absorption of xenobiotics with prolonged absorptive phases such as extended-release formulations or enteroenteric recirculation.
- In the postabsorptive phase, MDAC decreases the elimination half-lives of certain xenobiotics.
- Care must be taken to avoid pulmonary aspiration and intestinal obstruction when administering AC and MDAC.
- Home availability of AC should be encouraged in remote locations where prehospital care is not immediately available.

REFERENCES

1. Adams BK, et al. Prolonged gastric emptying half-time and gastric hypomotility after drug overdose. *Am J Emerg Med.* 2004;22:548-554.
2. Adams BK, et al. The effects of sorbitol on gastric emptying half-times and small intestinal transit after drug overdose. *Am J Emerg Med.* 2006;24:130-132.
3. Al-Shareef AH, et al. The effects of charcoal and sorbitol (alone and in combination) on plasma theophylline concentrations after a sustained-release formulation. *Hum Exp Toxicol.* 1990;9:179-182.
4. Allison TB, et al. Potential time savings by prehospital administration of activated charcoal. *Prehosp Emerg Care.* 1997;1:73-75.
5. Amitai Y, et al. Treatment of neonatal hyperbilirubinemia with repetitive oral activated charcoal as an adjunct to phototherapy. *J Perinat Med.* 1993;21:189-194.
6. Andersen AH. Experimental studies on the pharmacology of activated charcoal. I. Adsorption power of charcoal in aqueous solutions. *Acta Pharmacol Toxicol (Copenh).* 1946;2:69-78.
7. Andersen AH. Experimental studies on the pharmacology of activated charcoal. II. The effect of pH on the adsorption by charcoal from aqueous solutions. *Acta Pharmacol Toxicol (Copenh).* 1947;3:119-218.
8. Andersen AH. Experimental studies on the pharmacology of activated charcoal. III. Adsorption from gastro-intestinal contents. *Acta Pharmacol Toxicol (Copenh).* 1948;4:275-284.
9. Anderson IMWC. Syrup of ipecacuanha [letter]. *Br Med J.* 1987;294:578.
10. Atta-Politou J, et al. An in vitro evaluation of fluoxetine adsorption by activated charcoal and desorption upon addition of polyethylene glycol-electrolyte lavage solution. *J Toxicol Clin Toxicol.* 1998;36:117-124.
11. Atta-Politou J, et al. The effect of polyethylene glycol on the charcoal adsorption of chlorpromazine studied by ion selective electrode potentiometry. *J Toxicol Clin Toxicol.* 1996;34:307-316.
12. Bailey DN, Briggs JR. The effect of ethanol and pH on the adsorption of drugs from simulated gastric fluid onto activated charcoal. *Ther Drug Monit.* 2003;25:310-313.
13. Berg MJ, et al. Acceleration of the body clearance of phenobarbital by oral activated charcoal. *N Engl J Med.* 1982;307:642-644.
14. Berlinger WG, et al. Enhancement of theophylline clearance by oral activated charcoal. *Clin Pharmacol Ther.* 1983;33:351-354.
15. Boldy DA, et al. Activated charcoal for carbamazepine poisoning. *Lancet.* 1987;1:1027.
16. Boyd R, Hanson J. Prospective single blinded randomised controlled trial of two orally administered activated charcoal preparations. *J Accid Emerg Med.* 1999;16:24-25.
17. Brahmi N, et al. Prognostic value of human erythrocyte acetyl cholinesterase in acute organophosphate poisoning. *Am J Emerg Med.* 2006;24:822-827.
18. Brost BC, et al. Diphenhydramine overdose during pregnancy: lessons from the past. *Am J Obstet Gynecol.* 1996;175:1376-1377.
19. Brubacher JR, et al. Intestinal pseudo-obstruction (Ogilvie's syndrome) in theophylline overdose. *Vet Hum Toxicol.* 1996;38:368-370.
20. Buckley NA, et al. Treatments for paracetamol poisoning. *BMJ.* 2016;353:i2579.
21. Calvert WE, et al. Orally administered activated charcoal: acceptance by children. *JAMA.* 1971;215:641-641.
22. Campbell JW, Chyka PA. Physicochemical characteristics of drugs and response to repeat-dose activated charcoal. *Am J Emerg Med.* 1992;10:208-210.
23. Chan BS, et al. Use of multi-dose activated charcoal in phenytoin toxicity secondary to genetic polymorphism. *Clin Toxicol (Phila).* 2015;53:131-133.
24. Cheng A, Ratnapalan S. Improving the palatability of activated charcoal in pediatric patients. *Pediatr Emerg Care.* 2007;23:384-386.
25. Chiew AL, et al. Summary statement: new guidelines for the management of paracetamol poisoning in Australia and New Zealand. *Med J Aust.* 2015;203:215-218.
26. Chomchai C, Tiawilai A. Fetal poisoning after maternal paraquat ingestion during third trimester of pregnancy: case report and literature review. *J Med Toxicol.* 2007;3: 182-186.
27. Chyka PA, et al. Correlation of drug pharmacokinetics and effectiveness of multiple-dose activated charcoal therapy. *Ann Emerg Med.* 1995;25:356-362.
28. Chyka PA, et al. Position paper: single-dose activated charcoal. *Clin Toxicol (Phila).* 2005;43:61-87.
29. Cohen V, et al. Palatability of Insta-Char with cherry flavoring: a human volunteer study [abstract]. *J Toxicol Clin Toxicol.* 1996;34:635.
30. Cooney DO. Effect of type and amount of carboxymethylcellulose on in vitro salicylate adsorption by activated charcoal. *J Toxicol Clin Toxicol.* 1982;19:367-376.
31. Cooney DO. In vitro adsorption of phenobarbital, chlorpheniramine maleate, and theophylline by four commercially available activated charcoal suspensions. *J Toxicol Clin Toxicol.* 1995;33:213-217.
32. Cooney DO, Kane RP. "Superactive" charcoal adsorbs drugs as fast as standard antidotal charcoal. *Clin Toxicol.* 1980;16:123-125.
33. Cooper GM, et al. A randomized clinical trial of activated charcoal for the routine management of oral drug overdose. *QJM.* 2005;98:655-660.
34. Cooper JM, et al. The pharmacokinetics of sertraline in overdose and the effect of activated charcoal. *Br J Clin Pharmacol.* 2015;79:307-315.
35. Critchley JA, Critchley LA. Digoxin toxicity in chronic renal failure: treatment by multiple dose activated charcoal intestinal dialysis. *Hum Exp Toxicol.* 1997;16:733-735.
36. Crome P, et al. Effect of activated charcoal on absorption of nortriptyline. *Lancet.* 1977;2:1203-1205.
37. Crowell C, et al. Caring for the mother, concentrating on the fetus: intravenous *N*-acetylcysteine in pregnancy. *Am J Emerg Med.* 2008;26:735 e1-2.
38. de Silva HA, et al. Multiple-dose activated charcoal for treatment of yellow oleander poisoning: a single-blind, randomised, placebo-controlled trial. *Lancet.* 2003;361:1935-1938.
39. de Vries MH, et al. Pharmacokinetic modelling of the effect of activated charcoal on the intestinal secretion of theophylline, using the isolated vascularly perfused rat small intestine. *J Pharm Pharmacol.* 1989;41:528-533.
40. De Weerdt A, et al. Rapid-onset adult respiratory distress syndrome after activated charcoal aspiration. A pitch-black tale of a potential to kill. *Am J Respir Crit Care Med.* 2015;191:344-345.
41. Docksteder LL, et al. Home administration of activated charcoal: feasibility and acceptance [abstract]. *Vet Hum Toxicol.* 1986;28:471.
42. Dorrington CL, et al. The frequency of complications associated with the use of multiple-dose activated charcoal. *Ann Emerg Med.* 2003;41:370-377.
43. DuSoeuch P, et al. Reduction of nadolol plasma half-life by activated charcoal and antibiotics in man [letter]. *Clin Pharmacol Ther.* 1982;31:222.
44. Eddleston M, et al. Multiple-dose activated charcoal in acute self-poisoning: a randomised controlled trial. *Lancet.* 2008;371:579-587.
45. Eisen TF, et al. The adsorption of salicylates by a milk chocolate-charcoal mixture. *Ann Emerg Med.* 1991;20:143-146.
46. Eldridge DL, et al. Pediatric toxicology. *Emerg Med Clin North Am.* 2007;25:283-308; abstract vii-viii.
47. Elliott CG, et al. Charcoal lung. Bronchiolitis obliterans after aspiration of activated charcoal. *Chest.* 1989;96:672-674.

48. Farley TA. Severe hypernatremic dehydration after use of an activated charcoal-sorbitol suspension. *J Pediatr.* 1986;109:719-722.

49. Farrar HC, et al. Acute valproic acid intoxication: enhanced drug clearance with oral-activated charcoal. *Crit Care Med.* 1993;21:299-301.

50. Filippone GA, et al. Reversible adsorption (desorption) of aspirin from activated charcoal. *Arch Intern Med.* 1987;147:1390-1392.

51. Fischer TF, Singer AJ. Comparison of the palatabilities of standard and superactivated charcoal in toxic ingestions: a randomized trial. *Acad Emerg Med.* 1999;6:895-899.

52. Francis RC, et al. Acute respiratory failure after aspiration of activated charcoal with recurrent deposition and release from an intrapulmonary cavern. *Intensive Care Med.* 2009;35:360-363.

53. Gades NM, et al. Activated charcoal and the absorption of ferrous sulfate in rats. *Vet Hum Toxicol.* 2003;45:183-187.

54. Goulbourne KB, Cisek JE. Small-bowel obstruction secondary to activated charcoal and adhesions. *Ann Emerg Med.* 1994;24:108-110.

55. Gude AB, et al. Dose-dependent adsorptive capacity of activated charcoal for gastrointestinal decontamination of a simulated paracetamol overdose in human volunteers. *Basic Clin Pharmacol Toxicol.* 2010;106:406-410.

56. Gwilt PR, Perrier D. Influence of "thickening" agents on the antidotal efficacy of activated charcoal. *Clin Toxicol.* 1976;9:89-92.

57. Hack JB, et al. Images in emergency medicine. Activated charcoal aspiration. *Ann Emerg Med.* 2006;48:522.

58. Hillman RJ, Prescott LF. Treatment of salicylate poisoning with repeated oral charcoal. *Br Med J (Clin Res Ed).* 1985;291:1472-1472.

59. Hoffman RS, et al. Comparative efficacy of thallium adsorption by activated charcoal, Prussian blue, and sodium polystyrene sulfonate. *J Toxicol Clin Toxicol.* 1999;37:833-837.

60. Holt LE, Holz PH. The black bottle. A consideration of the role of charcoal in the treatment of poisoning in children. *J Pediatr.* 1963;63:306-314.

61. Honcharik N, Anthone S. Activated charcoal in acute cyclosporin overdose. *Lancet.* 1985;1:1051-1051.

62. Hung GU, et al. Development of a new method for small bowel transit study. *Ann Nucl Med.* 2006;20:387-392.

63. Ibezim EC, et al. In vitro adsorption of ciprofloxacin on activated charcoal and Talc. *Am J Ther.* 1999;6:199-201.

64. Ilkhanipour K, et al. The comparative efficacy of various multiple-dose activated charcoal regimens. *Am J Emerg Med.* 1992;10:298-300.

65. Isbister GK, et al. Feasibility of prehospital treatment with activated charcoal: who could we treat, who should we treat? *Emerg Med J.* 2003;20:375-378.

66. Isbister GK, et al. Aspiration pneumonitis in an overdose population: frequency, predictors, and outcomes. *Crit Care Med.* 2004;32:88-93.

67. Isbister GK, Duffull SB. Quetiapine overdose: predicting intubation, duration of ventilation, cardiac monitoring and the effect of activated charcoal. *Int Clin Psychopharmacol.* 2009;24:174-180.

68. Isbister GK, Kumar VV. Indications for single-dose activated charcoal administration in acute overdose. *Curr Opin Crit Care.* 2011;17:351-357.

69. Jurgens G, et al. The effect of activated charcoal on drug exposure in healthy volunteers: a meta-analysis. *Clin Pharmacol Ther.* 2009;85:501-505.

70. Justiniani FR, et al. Charcoal-containing empyema complicating treatment for overdose. *Chest.* 1985;87:404-405.

71. Karkkainen S, Neuvonen PJ. Effect of oral charcoal and urine pH on dextropropoxyphene pharmacokinetics. *Int J Clin Pharmacol Ther Toxicol.* 1985;23:219-225.

72. Karkkainen S, Neuvonen PJ. Pharmacokinetics of amitriptyline influenced by oral charcoal and urine pH. *Int J Clin Pharmacol Ther Toxicol.* 1986;24:326-332.

73. Keller RE, et al. Contribution of sorbitol combined with activated charcoal in prevention of salicylate absorption. *Ann Emerg Med.* 1990;19:654-656.

74. Keranen T, et al. Effects of charcoal on the absorption and elimination of the antiepileptic drugs lamotrigine and oxcarbazepine. *Arzneimittel-Forschung.* 2010;60:421-426.

75. Kirshenbaum LA, et al. Does multiple-dose charcoal therapy enhance salicylate excretion? *Arch Intern Med.* 1990;150:1281-1283.

76. Kirshenbaum LA, et al. Interaction between whole-bowel irrigation solution and activated charcoal: implications for the treatment of toxic ingestions. *Ann Emerg Med.* 1990;19:1129-1132.

77. Kramer J, et al. Nausea and vomiting of pregnancy: prevalence, severity and relation to psychosocial health. *MCN Am J Matern Child Nurs.* 2013;38:21-27.

78. Kulig KW, et al. Intravenous theophylline poisoning and multiple-dose charcoal in an animal model. *Ann Emerg Med.* 1987;16:842-846.

79. Kumar VV, et al. The effect of decontamination procedures on the pharmacodynamics of venlafaxine in overdose. *Br J Clin Pharmacol.* 2011;72:125-132.

80. Lapatto-Reiniluoto O, et al. Activated charcoal alone and followed by whole-bowel irrigation in preventing the absorption of sustained-release drugs. *Clin Pharmacol Ther.* 2001;70:255-260.

81. Levy G. Gastrointestinal clearance of drugs with activated charcoal. *N Engl J Med.* 1982;307:676-678.

82. Levy G, et al. Inhibition by ice cream of the antidotal efficacy of activated charcoal. *Am J Hosp Pharm.* 1975;32:289-291.

83. Longdon P, Henderson A. Intestinal pseudo-obstruction following the use of enteral charcoal and sorbitol and mechanical ventilation with papaveretum sedation for theophylline poisoning. *Drug Saf.* 1992;7:74-77.

84. Mahutte CK, et al. Increased serum theophylline clearance with orally administered activated charcoal. *Am Rev Respir Dis.* 1983;128:820-822.

85. Makosiej FJ, et al. An in vitro evaluation of cocaine hydrochloride adsorption by activated charcoal and desorption upon addition of polyethylene glycol electrolyte lavage solution. *J Toxicol Clin Toxicol.* 1993;31:381-395.

86. Malik DJ, et al. The characterization and development of microstructured carbons for the treatment of drug overdose [abstract]. *J Toxicol Clin Toxicol.* 2003;41:694.

87. Manes M, Mann JP. Easily swallowed formulations of antidote charcoals. *Clin Toxicol.* 1974;7:355-364.

88. Mariani PJ, Pook N. Gastrointestinal tract perforation with charcoal peritoneum complicating orogastric intubation and lavage. *Ann Emerg Med.* 1993;22:606-609.

89. Marketos SG, Androutsos G. Charcoal: from antiquity to artificial kidney. *J Nephrol.* 2004;17:453-456.

90. Mathur LK, et al. Activated charcoal-carboxymethylcellulose gel formulation as an antidotal agent for orally ingested aspirin. *Am J Hosp Pharm.* 1976;33:717-719.

91. Mayer AL, et al. Multiple-dose charcoal and whole-bowel irrigation do not increase clearance of absorbed salicylate. *Arch Intern Med.* 1992;152:393-396.

92. Mayersohn M, et al. Evaluation of a charcoal-sorbitol mixture as an antidote for oral aspirin overdose. *Clin Toxicol.* 1977;11:561-567.

93. McElhatton PR, et al. Paracetamol overdose in pregnancy analysis of the outcomes of 300 cases referred to the Teratology Information Service. *Reprod Toxicol.* 1997;11:85-94.

94. McKinnon RS, et al. Studies on the mechanisms of action of activated charcoal on theophylline pharmacokinetics. *J Pharm Pharmacol.* 1987;39:522-525.

95. McLuckie A, et al. Role of repeated doses of oral activated charcoal in the treatment of acute intoxications. *Anaesth Intensive Care.* 1990;18:375-384.

96. McNamara RM, et al. Sorbitol catharsis does not enhance efficacy of charcoal in a simulated acetaminophen overdose. *Ann Emerg Med.* 1988;17:243-246.

97. Merigian KS, et al. Prospective evaluation of gastric emptying in the self-poisoned patient. *Am J Emerg Med.* 1990;8:479-483.

98. Mezutani T, et al. Rectal ulcer with massive hemorrhage due to activated charcoal treatment in oral organophosphate poisoning. *Hum Exp Toxicol.* 1991;10:385-386.

99. Mofenson HC, Caraccio TR. Magnesium intoxication in a neonate from oral magnesium hydroxide laxative. *J Toxicol Clin Toxicol.* 1991;29:215-222.

100. Moll J, et al. Incidence of aspiration pneumonia in intubated patients receiving activated charcoal. *J Emerg Med.* 1999;17:279-283.

101. Moon J, et al. An exploratory study; the therapeutic effects of premixed activated charcoal-sorbitol administration in patients poisoned with organophosphate pesticide. *Clin Toxicol (Phila).* 2015;53:119-126.

102. Moore CM. Hypernatremia after the use of an activated charcoal-sorbitol suspension. *J Pediatr.* 1988;112:333.

103. Mullins M, et al. Effect of delayed activated charcoal on acetaminophen concentration after simulated overdose of oxycodone and acetaminophen. *Clin Toxicol (Phila).* 2009;47:112-115.

104. Navarro RP, et al. Relative efficacy and palatability of three activated charcoal mixtures. *Vet Hum Toxicol.* 1980;22:6-9.

105. Neijzen R, et al. Activated charcoal for GHB intoxication: an in vitro study. *Eur J Pharm Sci.* 2012;47:801-803.

106. Neuvonen PJ. Clinical pharmacokinetics of oral activated charcoal in acute intoxications. *Clin Pharmacokinet.* 1982;7:465-489.

107. Neuvonen PJ, Elonen E. Effect of activated charcoal on absorption and elimination of phenobarbitone, carbamazepine and phenylbutazone in man. *Eur J Clin Pharmacol.* 1980;17:51-57.

108. Neuvonen PJ, et al. Oral activated charcoal and dapsone elimination. *Clin Pharmacol Ther.* 1980;27:823-827.

109. Neuvonen PJ, Olkkola KT. Effect of purgatives on antidotal efficacy of oral activated charcoal. *Hum Toxicol.* 1986;5:255-263.

110. Neuvonen PJ, Olkkola KT. Oral activated charcoal in the treatment of intoxications. Role of single and repeated doses. *Med Toxicol Adverse Drug Exp.* 1988;3:33-58.

111. Neuvonen PJ, et al. Effect of ethanol and pH on the adsorption of drugs to activated charcoal: studies in vitro and in man. *Acta Pharmacol Toxicol (Copenh).* 1984;54:1-7.

112. Ohning BL, et al. Continuous nasogastric administration of activated charcoal for the treatment of theophylline intoxication. *Pediatr Pharmacol (New York).* 1986;5:241-245.

113. Olkkola KT. Does ethanol modify antidotal efficacy of oral activated charcoal studies in vitro and in experimental animals. *J Toxicol Clin Toxicol.* 1984;22:425-432.

114. Olkkola KT. Effect of charcoal-drug ratio on antidotal efficacy of oral activated charcoal in man. *Br J Clin Pharmacol.* 1985;19:767-773.

115. Olkkola KT, Neuvonen PJ. Do gastric contents modify antidotal efficacy of oral activated charcoal? *Br J Clin Pharmacol.* 1984;18:663-669.

116. Ollier E, et al. Effect of activated charcoal on rivaroxaban complex absorption. *Clin Pharmacokinet.* 2017;56:793-801.

117. Olson KR. Activated charcoal for acute poisoning: one toxicologist's journey. *J Med Toxicol.* 2010;6:190-198.

118. Orfanidou G, et al. Activated charcoal may not be necessary in all oral overdoses of medication. *Am J Emerg Med.* 2016;34:319-321.

119. Orfila MP (abridged and partially translated by Nancrede, JG). *Of Charcoal, Considered as an Antidote of Arsenic and Corrosive Sublimate. A General System of Toxicology: or, A Treatise on Poisons, found in the Mineral, Vegetable, and Animal Kingdoms, Considered*

in their Relations with Physiology, Pathology, and Medical Jurisprudence. Philadelphia, PA: M. Carey & Son; 1817.

120. Orisakwe OE, Ogbonna E. Effect of saline cathartics on gastrointestinal transit time of activated charcoal. *Hum Exp Toxicol.* 1993;12:403-405.

121. Paddock Laboratories LRLPC. ACTIDOSE-AQUA & ACTIDOSE® WITH SORBITOL. ACTIDOSE® WITH SORBITOL. ACTIDOSE®-AQUA. ACTIVATED CHARCOAL SUSPENSION [product label]. Minneapolis, MN: Paddock Laboratories, LLC; 2014.

122. Park GD, et al. Effect of the surface area of activated charcoal on theophylline clearance. *J Clin Pharmacol.* 1984;24:289-292.

123. Picchioni AL. Activated charcoal. A neglected antidote. *Pediatr Clin North Am.* 1970;17:535-543.

124. Picchioni AL, et al. Evaluation of activated charcoal-sorbitol suspension as an antidote. *J Toxicol Clin Toxicol.* 1982;19:433-444.

125. Pollack MM, et al. Aspiration of activated charcoal and gastric contents. *Ann Emerg Med.* 1981;10:528-529.

126. Pond S, et al. Treatment of digitoxin overdose with oral activated charcoal. *Lancet.* 1981;2:1177-1178.

127. Pond SM, et al. Gastric emptying in acute overdose: a prospective randomised controlled trial. *Med J Aust.* 1995;163:345-349.

128. Pond SM, et al. Randomized study of the treatment of phenobarbital overdose with repeated doses of activated charcoal. *JAMA.* 1984;251:3104-3108.

129. Rangan C, et al. Treatment of acetaminophen ingestion with a superactivated charcoal-cola mixture. *Ann Emerg Med.* 2001;37:55-58.

130. Roberts DM, Buckley NA. Enhanced elimination in acute barbiturate poisoning—a systematic review. *Clin Toxicol (Phila).* 2011;49:2-12.

131. Roberts DM, et al. Pharmacokinetics of digoxin cross-reacting substances in patients with acute yellow Oleander (*Thevetia peruviana*) poisoning, including the effect of activated charcoal. *Ther Drug Monit.* 2006;28:784-792.

132. Roy TM, et al. Pulmonary complications after tricyclic antidepressant overdose. *Chest.* 1989;96:852-856.

133. Saygan-Karamursel B, et al. Mega-dose carbamazepine complicating third trimester of pregnancy. *J Perinat Med.* 2005;33:72-75.

134. Scharman EJ, et al. Home administration of charcoal: can mothers administer a therapeutic dose? *J Emerg Med.* 2001;21:357-361.

135. Scholtz EC, et al. Evaluation of five activated charcoal formulations for inhibition of aspirin absorption and palatability in man. *Am J Hosp Pharm.* 1978;35:1355-1359.

136. Schulman G. A nexus of progression of chronic kidney disease: tryptophan, profibrotic cytokines, and charcoal. *J Ren Nutr.* 2012;22:107-113.

137. Schulman G, et al. Risk factors for progression of chronic kidney disease in the EPPIC trials and the effect of AST-120. *Clin Exp Nephrol.* 2017 Jul 24. doi: 10.1007/s10157-017-1447-0. [Epub ahead of print].

138. Shannon M, et al. Multiple dose activated charcoal for theophylline poisoning in young infants. *Pediatrics.* 1987;80:368-370.

139. Silberman H, et al. Activated charcoal aspiration. *N C Med J.* 1990;51:79-80.

140. Sketris IS, et al. Saline catharsis: effect on aspirin bioavailability in combination with activated charcoal. *J Clin Pharmacol.* 1982;22:59-64.

141. Skinner CG, et al. Randomized controlled study on the use of multiple-dose activated charcoal in patients with supratherapeutic phenytoin levels. *Clin Toxicol (Phila).* 2012;50:764-769.

142. Smilkstein MJ, et al. Severe hypermagnesemia due to multiple-dose cathartic therapy. *West J Med.* 1988;148:208-211.

143. Smith SW. Drugs and pharmaceuticals: management of intoxication and antidotes. *EXS.* 2010;100:397-460.

144. Spiller HA, Rodgers GC. Evaluation of administration of activated charcoal in the home. *Pediatrics.* 2001;108:E100.

145. Swartz CM, Sherman A. The treatment of tricyclic antidepressant overdose with repeated charcoal. *J Clin Psychopharmacol.* 1984;4:336-340.

146. True RJ, et al. Treatment of theophylline toxicity with oral activated charcoal. *Crit Care Med.* 1984;12:113-114.

147. Tsuchiya T, Levy G. Relationship between effect of activated charcoal on drug absorption in man and its drug adsorption characteristics in vitro. *J Pharm Sci.* 1972;61:586-589.

148. Tuuri RE, et al. Does prearrival communication from a poison center to an emergency department decrease time to activated charcoal for pediatric poisoning? *Pediatric Emerg Care.* 2011;27:1045-1051.

149. Vale JA, Proudfoot AT. How useful is activated charcoal? *BMJ.* 1993;306:78-79.

150. Valente Nabais JM, et al. Removal of amitriptyline from simulated gastric and intestinal fluids using activated carbons. *J Pharm Sci.* 2011;100:5096-5099.

151. Van de Graaff WB, et al. Adsorbent and cathartic inhibition of enteral drug absorption. *J Pharmacol Exp Ther.* 1982;221:656-663.

152. van Gorp F, et al. Population pharmacokinetics and pharmacodynamics of escitalopram in overdose and the effect of activated charcoal. *Br J Clin Pharmacol.* 2012;73:402-410.

153. Villarreal J, et al. A retrospective review of the prehospital use of activated charcoal. *Am J Emerg Med.* 2015;33:56-59.

154. Wananukul W, et al. Effect of activated charcoal in reducing paracetamol absorption at a supra-therapeutic dose. *J Med Assoc Thai.* 2010;93:1145-1149.

155. Wang X, et al. Effect of activated charcoal on apixaban pharmacokinetics in healthy subjects. *Am J Cardiovasc Drugs.* 2014;14:147-154.

156. Wang Z, et al. Oral activated charcoal suppresses hyperphosphatemia in hemodialysis patients. *Nephrology (Carlton).* 2012;17:616-620.

157. Wason S, et al. Carbamazepine overdose—the effects of multiple dose activated charcoal. *J Toxicol Clin Toxicol.* 1992;30:39-48.

158. Watson WA, et al. Gastrointestinal obstruction associated with multiple-dose activated charcoal. *J Emerg Med.* 1986;4:401-407.

159. Wax PM, Cobaugh DJ. Prehospital gastrointestinal decontamination of toxic ingestions: a missed opportunity. *Am J Emerg Med.* 1998;16:114-116.

160. West L. Innovative approaches to the administration of activated charcoal in pediatric toxic ingestions. *Pediatr Nurs.* 1997;23:616-619.

161. Yamaguchi J, et al. Effect of AST-120 in chronic kidney disease treatment: still a controversy? *Nephron.* 2017;135:201-206.

162. Yancy RE, et al. In vitro and in vivo evaluation of the effect of cherry flavoring on the adsorptive capacity of activated charcoal for salicylic acid. *Vet Hum Toxicol.* 1980;22:163-165.

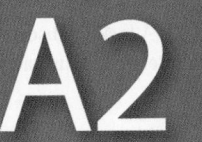

A2 WHOLE-BOWEL IRRIGATION AND OTHER INTESTINAL EVACUANTS

Silas W. Smith and Mary Ann Howland

INTRODUCTION

One approach to altering the pharmacokinetics of a xenobiotic is to administer a gastrointestinal (GI) evacuant. Selected patients benefit from minimizing systemic exposure by decreasing GI transit time and increasing rectal evacuation. The most effective process of evacuating the GI tract in poisoned patients is referred to as whole-bowel irrigation (WBI). Whole-bowel irrigation is typically accomplished using polyethylene glycol with a balanced electrolyte lavage solution (PEG-ELS). Unless stated otherwise, WBI will mean WBI with PEG-ELS. A detailed discussion of the merits of WBI in the context of various decontamination strategies is provided in Chap. 5.

HISTORY

In 1625 while endeavoring to recover from the febrile "Hungarian disease," Johann Glauber drank from a well from which he later isolated *sal mirabile*, now known as sodium sulfate, Na_2SO_4.[54] He advocated its use as a purgative and determined a synthetic production method.[54] In 1675, Nehemiah Grew first observed the presence of the eponymous purgative salt in the springs at Epsom, later determined to be magnesium sulfate.[125] Phosphate of soda, called "tasteless purging salt," was found in the urine by Hellot in 1737 and introduced into clinical practice as a purgative by George Pearson some 50 years later.[119] In 1882 and 1883, Hay reported a series of experiments that provided the foundational understanding of the mechanism of action of the saline cathartics. He identified the viscus as the main source of bowel fluid, which was secretory in nature, and established the dose–response principle of decreased time to stool as salt concentrations were increased.[50,51] Polyethylene glycol was initially introduced in 1957 as a nonabsorbable marker for the study of human fat, carbohydrate, and protein absorption.[20] Experimental studies of intestinal lavage in normal human subjects appeared in 1968.[89] In 1973, Hewitt and colleagues reported on WBI in clinical practice using their method of "whole-gut irrigation" with a solution of sodium chloride, potassium chloride, and sodium bicarbonate in distilled water to prepare the large bowel for surgery.[53] In 1976, WBI was used therapeutically for poisoning in a patient ingesting 300 lead air-gun pellets who was unresponsive to oral magnesium sulfate purgation.[159]

PHARMACOLOGY
Nomenclature

Xenobiotics that promote intestinal evacuation are referred to as laxatives, cathartics, purgatives, promotility agents, and evacuants. Depending on the dose, the same xenobiotic might accomplish some or all of these tasks, with differing side effect profiles. Laxatives promote a soft-formed or semifluid stool within 6 hours to 3 days. Cathartics promote a rapid, watery evacuation within 1 to 3 hours.[131] The term *purgative* relates the force associated with bowel evacuation. Evacuants are commonly used for preprocedural bowel cleansing, with an onset of action of as little as 30 to 60 minutes, but typically require 4 hours for a more complete effect. Promotility xenobiotics stimulate GI motor function via the enteric nervous system through a variety of acetylcholine, dopamine, guanylate cyclase-C, motilin, opioid, and serotonin receptor and intestinal chloride channel interactions.

Laxatives are further classified into categories of bulk-forming, softener or emollient, lubricant, stimulant or irritant, saline, hyperosmotic, and evacuant. Bulk-forming laxatives include high-fiber products such as methylcellulose, polycarbophil, and psyllium; softeners or emollients include docusate calcium. Mineral oil is the sole lubricant. These cathartics are not used therapeutically in medical toxicology because their onset of action is delayed. Stimulant or irritant laxatives include anthraquinones (sennosides, aloe, and casanthranol), diphenylmethane (bisacodyl), and castor oil. Saline (meaning salt) cathartics, which include magnesium citrate, magnesium hydroxide, magnesium sulfate, sodium phosphate, and sodium sulfate, are used infrequently. Hyperosmotic xenobiotics, generally nonabsorbable sugars and alcohols, including sorbitol and lactulose, are occasionally used in poisoned patients. The most common process of evacuating the intestinal tract in poisoned patients is WBI.

Chemistry and Preparation

Magnesium citrate and magnesium sulfate ("Epsom salt") are water-soluble salts of magnesium; magnesium hydroxide ("milk of magnesia") is insoluble.[64] Sodium sulfate is prepared either through purification of naturally occurring brine deposits or other manufacturing processes. Sodium phosphate is supplied as a combination of the monobasic monohydrate and dibasic anhydrous forms. D-Sorbitol, an isomer of mannitol, is a hexitol naturally occurring in many fruits and is produced commercially by the reduction of glucose. Lactulose is a water-soluble, synthetic disaccharide, 4-O-β-D-galactopyranosyl-D-fructofuranose. Sodium picosulfate is a monohydrate, disodium salt prodrug.

The addition reaction of ethylene oxide to an ethylene glycol equivalent polymerizes ethylene oxide into PEG. The "n" in the molecular structure of PEG, $H\text{-}(OCH_2CH_2)_n\text{-}OH$ refers to the average number of repeating oxyethylene groups.[69] The number after PEG represents its average molecular weight (MW). Also known as macrogol, PEG has numerous medicinal applications. It can be conjugated to pharmaceuticals to delay vascular clearance or preclude blood–brain barrier transit ("PEGylation"), serve as a solvent in oral liquids and soft capsules, function as a nonalcohol solubilizer and diluent for liquid oral-dose medications, provide a base for medical ointment and cosmetics, and act as a base liquid for producing vapor in electronic cigarettes.[1] Low-molecular-weight PEG (eg, 300 or 400 Da), because of its advantageous solvent properties, is used to decontaminate phenol burns, although animal studies demonstrated the equal efficacy of copious (ie, deluge) quantities of water.[59] Higher-molecular-weight variants are used to promote laxation. Although PEG's physical properties (eg, water solubility, hygroscopicity, vapor pressure, melting or freezing range, and viscosity) vary with MW and blending because of chain-length effects, the chemical properties are similar.[145] Polyethylene glycol 3350 used in pharmaceutical, personal care, and food applications is water soluble. It has a MW range of 3,015 to 3,685 Da, an average number of 75.7 repeating oxyethylene units, a pH of a 5% aqueous solution of 4.5 to 7.5 at 25°C, a density of 1.09 g/cm³ at 60°C, a melting or freezing range between 53° and 57°C, a water solubility of 67% by weight at 20°C, and a viscosity of 90.8 centistokes at 100°C.[144] Polyethylene glycol 3350 without electrolytes is sold for nonprescription use for short-term treatment of constipation. Whole-bowel irrigation used in poison management is typically accomplished using PEG 3350 added to a balanced electrolyte lavage solution (PEG-ELS), which contains an isotonic mixture of sodium sulfate, sodium bicarbonate, sodium chloride, and potassium chloride.[131]

Mechanisms of Action

The effects of saline cathartics are largely attributed to their relatively non-absorbable ions that establish an osmotic gradient and draw water into the gut.[116] The increased water leads to increased intestinal pressure and a subsequent increase in intestinal motility. Magnesium ions also lead to the release of cholecystokinin from the duodenal mucosa, which stimulates intestinal motor activity and alters fluid movement, contributing to catharsis.[19,131,138] A lack of endogenous hydrolytic enzymes allows sorbitol, lactulose, and sodium picosulfate to reach the colon unchanged. Colonic bacteria metabolize sorbitol into acetic and short-chain fatty acids and lactulose into lactic acid and small amounts of formic and acetic acids. This results in a slight acidification of colonic contents, an increase in osmotic pressure that draws water into the lumen, and stimulation of colonic propulsive motility.[131] Colonic bacteria hydrolyze sodium picosulfate, marketed in the United States for bowel preparation in combination with magnesium oxide and citric acid, which create magnesium citrate in solution, to active 4,4'-dihydroxydiphenyl-(2-pyridiyl) methane, a stimulant laxative.[4,72]

Long-chain PEGs (eg, MW ~3,350 Da) are nonabsorbable, isoosmotic, indigestible molecules that remain in the colon together with the water diluent, resulting in WBI primarily by the mechanical effect of large-volume lavage. As assessed in controlled clinical trials in patients undergoing colonoscopy, the added balanced electrolyte solution practically eliminates electrolyte abnormalities and helps preclude fluid shifts across the GI mucosa.[16,83] Sodium sulfate in many preparations reduces sodium absorption in the small intestine because of the absence of chloride, which is the accompanying anion necessary for active absorption against the electrochemical gradient.[94]

Promotility xenobiotics such as metoclopramide and erythromycin stimulate gut motor function. Metoclopramide mediates GI 5-hydroxy tryptamine ($5HT_4$) receptor agonist and dopamine (D_2) receptor antagonist activity, which both result in increased acetylcholine release and GI motility. Erythromycin stimulates gut motor function via direct stimulation of GI motilin receptors.[151] Prucalopride (approved outside of the United States) and tegaserod (withdrawn from the US market because of adverse cardiovascular effects but supplied in emergency situations) are selective, $5\text{-}HT_4$ receptor agonists. Tegaserod and WBI were combined together in an attempt to improve colonoscopy preparations but not in poisoned patients.[3] Lubiprostone activates chloride channel protein 2 to induce chloride secretion and to enhance the contraction of gastric and colonic musculature.[70] Lubiprostone is sometimes used with WBI to treat constipation but not in poisoned patients. Linaclotide and plecanatide are guanylate cyclase-C agonists that increase intracellular and extracellular cGMP concentrations to stimulate secretion of chloride and bicarbonate and water into the intestinal lumen primarily through activation of the cystic fibrosis transmembrane conductance regulator ion channel.[140] Use in poisoning is unstudied. Nonselective μ-opioid antagonists (naloxone and naltrexone), although primarily used to reverse central nervous system–associated effects, also mitigate acute and chronic opioid-associated constipation; they are used in combination with WBI in certain opioid poisonings (eg, enteral concealment of drug packets and transdermal fentanyl patch ingestion).[43,147] Use of peripherally acting μ-opioid antagonists (methylnaltrexone, naloxegol, and alvimopan) in poisoning is not yet reported.

Pharmacokinetics

Absorption of magnesium, phosphate, and other electrolytes contained in hypertonic products is well described.[34,110,116] In one prospective, nonrandomized study, 9 of 14 patients developed elevated magnesium concentrations (2.2–5.0 mEq/L) after multiple doses of magnesium-containing cathartics were administered for suspected drug overdose despite normal blood urea nitrogen and creatinine concentrations.[135] During the 24 hours after administration of oral sodium phosphate solution in seven healthy volunteers, serum phosphorus reached a mean peak concentration of 7.6 mg/dL (range, 3.6–12.4 mg/dL), and ionized calcium reached a mean nadir concentration of 4.6 mg/dL (range, 4.4–5.2 mg/dL).[34]

By virtue of its high osmotic nature, long-chain PEG is poorly absorbed, is retained in the lumen, and does not distribute. Polyethylene glycol is therefore eliminated unmetabolized in rectal effluent. A lack of absorption presents sorbitol, lactulose, and sodium picosulfate to endogenous bacteria for metabolism within the gut lumen.

Pharmacodynamics

Patients who ingested 45 mL of an aqueous sodium phosphate preparation taken the evening before and the morning of a procedure had stool production within 1.7 hours of the first dose and within 0.7 hours of the second dose, with a mean duration of activity of 4.6 and 2.9 hours, respectively, and termination of increased stool production within 4 to 5 hours.[85] In six volunteers, saline cathartics decreased activated charcoal (AC) mean GI transit time from 29.3 ± 1.2 hours to 24.4 ± 1.2 hours, 15.4 ± 3.0 hours, 17.3 ± 1.9 hours, and 17.5 ± 2.3 hours with sodium chloride, sodium sulfate, magnesium sulfate, and a proprietary cathartic "salt" (36.7% anhydrous citric acid, 17.65% magnesium sulfate, and 45.6% sodium bicarbonate), respectively.[117] When different cathartics were compared with respect to time to first stool and number of stools,[62,78,108,109,139] sorbitol produced 10 to 15 watery stools and the most abdominal cramping before catharsis. Sorbitol produced stools in the shortest amount of time, which also was associated with the highest incidence of nausea, vomiting, generated gas, and flatus.[71,74,111] In one systematic review, the mean transit times after administration of sorbitol, magnesium citrate, magnesium sulfate, and sodium sulfate were 0.9 to 8.5 hours, 3 to 14 hours, 9.3 hours, and 4.2 to 15.4 hours, respectively.[9] In comparison, the first bowel movement typically occurs relatively quickly after the initiation of WBI. Patients ingesting PEG-ELS (1.2–1.8 L/h until the rectal effluent was clear) completed their colonic preparation goals within 1.5 to 3 hours after averaging a total of 5.5 L per patient (range, 3–8 L).[46] As assessed by magnetic resonance imaging in 24 healthy volunteers, ingesting either a split dose (1 L the evening before and 1 L on the study day) or single dose (2 L) of WBI rapidly increased small bowel water content by fourfold over baseline, increased total colonic volume by $35 \pm 8\%$ (split dose) and $102 \pm 27\%$ (single dose), and dramatically increased the ascending colon motility index.[97]

ROLE OF GASTROINTESTINAL EVACUATION IN POISONING MANAGEMENT

Cathartics should not be used in the routine management of overdosed patients.[9] Intuitively, the advantages of cathartics appear to result from their ability to decrease the potential for constipation or obstruction from AC and hasten the delivery of AC to the small intestine. However, these theoretical advantages were never demonstrated clinically.

Studies demonstrate that when administered alone, cathartics such as sorbitol or sodium sulfate decrease peak or total absorption of some xenobiotics, but no study of cathartics alone has achieved pharmacokinetic results comparable to that of AC alone.[6,30,100,120,153] When comparing the efficacy of a single dose of AC alone with that of AC plus a single dose of cathartic, studies suggest the combination to be equal to,[6,105,114,134] slightly better than,[30,71] or even slightly worse than AC alone.[100,153] We currently advocate WBI to hasten the elimination of poorly absorbed xenobiotics or sustained-release medications before they can be absorbed. This approach is theoretically sound and does not produce the fluid and electrolyte complications associated with cathartics. Unfortunately, evidence of efficacy is limited to anecdotal case reports and volunteer studies.

Many studies of WBI demonstrate patient acceptance, effectiveness, and safety when used for bowel preparation, its labeled indication.[8,17,21,22,35,38,39,121,146,149] Animal models suggest that WBI enhances systemic clearance via GI dialysis, similar to multiple-dose AC (MDAC).[84] In actuality, low flow rates, the typical delay in administering WBI in actual clinical situations, and the inconvenience of this procedure make it highly unlikely that enhanced systemic clearance can be achieved in humans. In human volunteer studies, WBI was more effective than AC with sorbitol for enteric-coated acetylsalicylic acid (ASA) when administered 4 hours after ingestion,[74] decreased peak lithium concentrations, and lithium area under the plasma drug concentration versus time curve (AUC) compared with control participants;[136] decreased the bioavailability of two sustained-release medications;[26,81] and propelled radiopaque markers through the gut more efficiently than control participants.[91] In a retrospective analysis of 59 acute-on-chronic lithium overdoses, those decontaminated at an early stage with sodium polystyrene sulfonate, WBI, or both achieved statistically significant and clinically relevant decreases in peak serum lithium concentrations compared with those with delayed (>12 hours) or no decontamination (2.39 versus 4.08 mEq/L).[23] A retrospective chart review of 176 pediatric cases documented WBI use in 72 cases involving sustained- and delayed-release medications, such as nifedipine, bupropion, verapamil, diltiazem, and felodipine.[86] Abdominal radiographs were performed in 36 patients, of whom 16 had demonstrable radiopaque pills. Four of these individuals had repeat abdominal radiographs, all of which demonstrated a decrease in opacities.

As expected, WBI was inferior to AC with regard to prevention of absorption when administered after 650 mg of immediate-release aspirin.[124] Additionally, after the aspirin was absorbed, WBI was unable to enhance systemic clearance.[99] Likewise, only a small, statistically insignificant effect of WBI could be demonstrated on the absorption of extended-release acetaminophen (APAP) in a human volunteer study.[91] These findings highlight the limited utility of WBI to assist in the prevention of absorption of relatively rapidly absorbed xenobiotics. Reports suggest successful WBI use in the management of overdoses of iron,[40,68,96,141,142] sustained-release theophylline,[63] sustained-release verapamil,[24] modified-release fenfluramine,[107] zinc sulfate,[25] lead,[104,106,128,159] arsenic trioxide,[61] arsenic-containing herbicide,[82] mercuric oxide powder,[92] strontium,[73] potassium chloride capsules,[49,58] clonidine and fentanyl transdermal patches[43,60] and in body packers.[57,147] Whole-bowel irrigation for 5 hours after ingestion of 10 fluorescent coffee beans by each of seven volunteers removed an average of only four beans (range, 1–8).[126] Similar failures are reported with jequirity beans (Abrus precatorium),[25] iron,[29,154] and button batteries.[141] It can be argued that because of physical characteristics (eg, density, solubility, size, or pharmacobezoar formation), these cases might not be representative of xenobiotics amenable to WBI. The American Academy of Clinical Toxicology/European Association of Poisons Centres and Clinical Toxicologists (AACT/EAPCCT) 2015 WBI position paper recapitulates the 2004 guidelines that WBI "can be considered for potentially toxic ingestions of sustained-release or enteric-coated drugs, drugs not adsorbed by activated charcoal (eg, lithium, potassium, and iron) and for removal of illicit drugs in body 'packers' or 'stuffers,'" but there was no evidence to demonstrate improved outcomes.[143] Whole-bowel irrigation is recommended for evacuation of highly toxic xenobiotics with a slow absorption phase and not adsorbed to AC (eg iron, lead, lithium, potassium). When AC is expected to be of benefit, it is recommended that it be administered prior to WBI to achieve its greatest effect.

Internal Drug Concealment

The approach to patients with internal concealment and enteral transport of illicit substances (eg, cocaine, heroin, amphetamines, and hashish) is comprehensively reviewed in Special Considerations: SC5. In uncontrolled poison control center studies, these patients, along with incarcerated patients, had a higher utilization of WBI and presented a high risk for major adverse events, including death.[27] Close coordination with surgical services is advised because of the risks of obstruction, intestinal retention, or rupture. Because mineral oil rapidly degrades latex condoms,[156] its use in evacuating drug packets, which can be constructed in this fashion, risks fatal rupture[155] and is therefore contraindicated. In a retrospective descriptive case series of 16 body packers, management with WBI was successful in 14; a ruptured cocaine packet produced mild toxicity in 1 patient, and packets were retained in 1 heroin body packer.[42] In another retrospective analysis of 34 cocaine body stuffers who were asymptomatic on presentation, 14 received AC (2 left against medical advice before 24 hours), 1 received WBI alone, and 19 received AC plus WBI and remained asymptomatic and were discharged after 24 hours.[66] A review of 1,250 confirmed body packers found the success rate of WBI to be 98%.[95] All WBI-managed patients passed all of their packets within 5 days. WBI occasionally fails to evacuate all of the drug packets because of inadequate dosing, partial obstruction, or the nature of the procedure. In one case, prolonged WBI failed to clear packets from

a methamphetamine body stuffer who engaged in "parachuting (swallowing powdered or crushed drugs by rolling or folding in toilet paper or other paper)."[52] As a result of these failures, promotility xenobiotics were added to WBI and presumably successfully enhanced bowel evacuation in two body packers suspected of having ingested well-constructed drug packets.[148]

ADVERSE EFFECTS AND SAFETY ISSUES

Potential adverse effects associated with various cathartics and promotility xenobiotics include salt and water depletion, hypernatremia, hypermagnesemia, hyperphosphatemia, hypokalemia, and metabolic (contraction) alkalosis, absorption of magnesium or other absorbable electrolytes, activation of the renin–angiotensin–aldosterone system, phosphate-induced nephropathy, and colonic fermentation of digestible sugars.[28,44,133] Cathartic-induced rectal prolapse is reported in geriatric patients.[76] The use of repetitive doses of cathartics, either by design or unintentionally, has led to hypermagnesemia, altered mental status, and death.[65,110,135,158] Hypocalcemia, hyperphosphatemia, and hypokalemia have accompanied the use of hypertonic phosphate enemas and oral sodium phosphate despite adherence to recommended dosing.[36,44,48,88,98,122,137] Frail elderly patients, children, and those with decreased kidney function are most susceptible to adverse effects.[15,18] On January 8, 2014, the US Food and Drug Administration issued a safety warning that using more than one dose of nonprescription sodium phosphate–containing drugs in 24 hours to treat constipation risked rare but serious severe salt and water depletion, electrolyte abnormalities, acute kidney injury, dysrhythmias, and death.[5]

Softeners increase intestinal permeability and therefore increase the absorption of some xenobiotics.[13,131] Stimulant and irritant laxatives are rarely used today in medical toxicology because of their significant GI side effects, including abdominal discomfort, cramping, and tenesmus and with chronic administration, bowel habituation, and intestinal tissue damage.

Contraindications to WBI include prior, current, or anticipated diarrhea; salt and water depletion; significant GI anatomical or functional compromise such as colitis, hemorrhage, ileus, obstruction, perforation, or toxic megacolon; an unprotected or compromised airway; and hemodynamic instability.[10,141]

Multiple-dose AC regimens containing 70% sorbitol used to enhance elimination cause severe cathartic-related adverse effects (salt and water depletion)[7,41,87,101] The potential for sorbitol-related adverse events from the unintentional use of repetitive AC dosing was emphasized by a survey revealing that 16% of hospitals surveyed only stocked AC premixed with sorbitol.[157] The retention of sorbitol after repetitive doses in an aperistaltic gut can lead to significant morbidity from gas formation and abdominal distension as a result of the digestive action of gut bacteria.[87]

Adverse effects resulting from the use of WBI include vomiting, particularly after rapid administration, abdominal bloating, fullness, cramping, flatulence, and pruritus ani. In 176 pediatric cases detailed in the California Poison Control System electronic database, 16 vomited, and 1 experienced abdominal pain.[86] In an alternative administration strategy in which 46 children were provided 238 g of PEG 3350 mixed with 1.9 L of Gatorade, rates of nausea and vomiting, abdominal pain and cramping, and fatigue and weakness were 60%, 44%, and 40%, respectively.[2] Typically, patients need to remain near a commode for 4 to 6 hours to complete WBI therapy. Slow or low-volume administration of WBI results in sodium absorption. If a total of 500 mL of WBI was used instead of multiple liters, potentially 1.5 g of sodium can be absorbed.[37] This adverse effect is suggested to have resulted in the exacerbation of congestive heart failure in an unstable patient with cardiac and renal dysfunction.[47] An unusual complication of WBI is colonic perforation, which occurred in a patient with acute diverticulitis.[80] Other adverse effects noted by the manufacturer include isolated reports of upper GI bleeding from a Mallory-Weiss tear, esophageal perforation, aspiration pneumonitis after vomiting, and acute respiratory distress syndrome (ARDS). Rare cases of both hypo- and hypernatremia, leading to altered consciousness, seizures, cerebral edema, and death, are reported with PEG, alone or in combination with ELS.[14,112,127]

Unintentional administration of WBI by other than the enteral route has occurred. A 4-year-old child inadvertently received 390 mL of WBI intravenously with no obvious adverse result.[123] In contrast, ARDS developed in an 11-year-old child administered WBI through a nasogastric tube inadvertently inserted in the trachea.[113] In a similar case, an inappropriately used nasogastric tube was responsible for WBI aspiration in a 3-year-old boy, with resultant hypoxia and hemodynamic instability requiring endotracheal intubation.[45] An 8-year-old girl who developed emesis during nasogastric infusion of 1 L of WBI experienced gagging, coughing, emesis, and respiratory distress 2 hours after infusion; she progressed to ARDS and required intubation and ventilatory support for 2 days.[118] A report of 2 cases suggests that vomiting and aspiration are more frequent than previously recognized in hemodynamically unstable patients.[33] Presumably, a patient's hypotension results in GI hypoperfusion and ileus, which, with the continued administration of WBI in the presence of decreased GI motility, produces abdominal distension and vomiting.

For MiraLAX (electrolyte-free PEG 3350 powder) to be useful in WBI, it would need to be administered at a dose of 2 L/h (8 heaping teaspoons in 2 L of water/h) in adults. This is not recommended for WBI because it does not contain any added electrolytes and could result in an electrolyte imbalance and shifts. Use of sodium picosulfate with magnesium citrate was associated with a 65.2% adverse event rate (vomiting, abdominal pain, paresthesias, nausea, bloating, and thirst) in a study of 153 patients undergoing routine bowel preparation.[72]

XENOBIOTIC, ACTIVATED CHARCOAL, AND WHOLE-BOWEL IRRIGATION INTERACTIONS

Theoretically, WBI might worsen drug toxicity by facilitating drug dissolution because of the addition of the large volume of WBI, increasing drug solubility (lower molecular weight PEGs are used as pharmaceutical excipients and solvents), or through compromise of the adsorbent benefits of coadministered AC. In a simulated gastric fluid model containing 5 g of APAP, 0.5 L of WBI increased APAP concentrations at all time points and increased the $AUC_{0-90 min}$ from 315 mg-min/L to 6233 mg-min/L compared with 0.9% sodium chloride control.[115] Whole-bowel irrigation did not accelerate the release of extended-release morphine in a separate simulated gastric fluid model maintained in an acid pH.[55] In a prospective, randomized, crossover study of 10 volunteers administered 75 mg/kg of a bilayer, delayed-release APAP preparation, WBI initiated 30 minutes after ingestion resulted in a statistically insignificant decrease in the APAP AUC.[91]

Several in vitro studies with cocaine, chlorpromazine, fluoxetine, salicylate, and theophylline demonstrate that the addition of WBI to AC significantly decreases the adsorptive capacity of AC.[11,12,56,75,93] Some interactions were affected by pH and magnified by high ratios of WBI to AC.[12,75,93] The most likely explanation is competition with the AC surface for solute adsorption. Additionally, in an animal model, WBI appeared to have an adverse effect by washing the AC away from the sustained-release theophylline.[26] One controlled study evaluated the effect of WBI added to 25 g of AC in nine healthy human volunteers simultaneously ingesting 200 mg of carbamazepine, 200 mg of theophylline, and 120 mg of verapamil.[81] Compared with AC alone, WBI and AC significantly decreased verapamil peak concentration (C_{max}) and AUC but significantly increased carbamazepine C_{max} and AUC and nonsignificantly increased theophylline C_{max} and AUC. One case report documents rapid increases in carbamazepine concentrations temporally related to the initiation of WBI.[90] Although the patient received MDAC and hemoperfusion, xenobiotic concentrations were increasing 58 hours after ingestion. It is possible that WBI competed for carbamazepine binding to AC, displacing some drug and making it available for absorption. A similar rapidly increasing drug concentration occurred after the initiation of WBI in a patient with a reported 10-g phenytoin overdose.[32] In this case, AC was not given before the initiation of WBI. One possible explanation is that the massive dose of phenytoin prevented its own absorption by exceeding its solubility, but the administration of WBI provided sufficient diluent to allow phenytoin dissolution before GI emptying with subsequent absorption. One human study evaluated the influence of various decontamination strategies on the probability of seizures in 319 patients who overdosed on venlafaxine on 436 occasions.[79]

Whole-bowel irrigation added to AC alone in a mean ingestion of 2100 mg further reduced the odds ratio (OR) of a seizure to 0.25 (0.08–0.62) compared with an OR of 0.48 (0.25–0.89) with AC alone. Most of these patients ingested extended-release venlafaxine. These results demonstrate that combining AC and WBI provided a greater benefit than the sum of the independent effects of single-dose AC and WBI, and argued against adverse clinical effects caused by desorption in venlafaxine ingestion.[79] Problems with this study include assumptions on dose, weight, and time of ingestion, as well as all the limitations associated with nonrandomization of decontamination procedures.

PREGNANCY AND LACTATION

Commercial preparations of WBI are pregnancy category C.[21,22,129,130] Animal reproduction studies have not been conducted with Colyte, GoLYTELY, NuLYTELY, or TriLyte.[21,22,129,130] The underlying elevated prevalence of nausea and vomiting in pregnancy[77] might predispose pregnant patients to vomit more frequently, although this is speculative. Whole-bowel irrigation with large volumes of fluid was used successfully in pregnant women at 26 and 38 weeks of gestation.[150,152] The lack of absorption of WBI would not predispose it to excretion in breast milk, although definitive safety in lactation is not established.

DOSING AND ADMINISTRATION

The usual nonprescription daily dose for the short-term treatment (2 weeks) of occasional constipation is 17 g of PEG 3350 without electrolytes powder in 8 oz (240 mL) of water. The recommended dose of WBI is considerably larger: 0.5 L/h or 25 mL/kg/h for small children and 1.5 to 2.0 L/h or 20 to 30 mL/min for adolescents and adults. Whole-bowel irrigation solution is administered orally or through a nasogastric tube for 4 to 6 hours or until the rectal effluent becomes clear. If the xenobiotic being removed is radiopaque, a diagnostic imaging technique demonstrating the absence of the xenobiotic is a reasonable clinical endpoint (Special Considerations: SC5). An antiemetic such as metoclopramide or a 5-HT$_3$ serotonin antagonist is recommended for the treatment of nausea or vomiting. In carefully select patients, promotility agents serve as useful adjuncts.[148]

FORMULATION AND ACQUISITION

The original WBI solution was GoLYTELY manufactured by Braintree. This solution contained PEG with electrolytes and sodium sulfate as an added laxative. Colyte is manufactured by Schwartz Pharma and is similar to GoLYTELY. Braintree later introduced NuLYTELY, a PEG formulation with 52% less total salt than GoLYTELY without added sodium sulfate. These changes decreased the salty taste and the risk of fluid- or electrolyte-related complications.[102] Many products are available with flavors. The available WBI products are prepared by filling the container to the 4-L (or 1-gal) mark with water and shaking vigorously several times to ensure dissolution. Lukewarm water facilitates dissolution, but subsequent chilling improves palatability. Chilled solutions are not recommended for infants because of hypothermia risk. Products are stable with refrigeration for 48 hours after reconstitution. Available WBI products (eg, GoLYTELY, Colyte, NuLYTELY, TriLyte) differ slightly in their composition. All contain PEG 3350 with varying amounts of sodium chloride, potassium chloride, sodium sulfate, and sodium bicarbonate, which upon reconstitution yield the following concentrations: sodium, 65 to 125 mEq/L; potassium, 5 to 10 mEq/L; chloride, 35 to 53 mEq/L; bicarbonate, 17 to 20 mEq/L; and sulfate, 0 to 80 mEq/L.[21,22,129,130]

MiraLAX contains electrolyte-free PEG 3350 powder meant for oral administration after dissolution in water, juice, or soda. It is indicated for occasional constipation and not for poisoning management, with a recommended dose of 1 heaping teaspoon (17 g) in 8 oz (240 mL) of liquid per day. However, alternative WBI formulations using electrolyte-free PEG 3350 with Gatorade have been used clinically. One study of 139 patients comparing 4 L of PEG-ELS with electrolyte-free PEG combined with 1.9 L of Gatorade and found no differences in colonoscopy preparation scores, higher overall patient satisfaction scores with the Gatorade mixture, and fewer adverse effects (bloating and nausea).[103] In 46 children provided PEG 3350 mixed with 1.9 L of Gatorade over a few hours, 93.5% completed the regimen, and 77%

achieved effective colonic visualization.[2] In a retrospective evaluation of an endoscopic database analysis, patients undergoing bowel preparation using PEG 3350 without electrolytes (238 g of MiraLAX in 64 oz of Gatorade) and four 5-mg bisacodyl tablets were more likely to achieve an excellent or good bowel cleansing compared with patients receiving a GoLYTELY preparation (93.3% versus 89.3%), without any adverse events.[132] Coffee added to 1.5 L of PEG for bowel preparation improved perceived ease of drinking, taste, and preference.[67] Similarly, in a trial of 107 patients, admixing 2 L of PEG–ascorbic acid with orange juice significantly improved palatability and diminished nausea from 59.3%.to 26.4%.[31]

SUMMARY

- Cathartics are not considered part of routine management of poisoning and overdose in children or adults and should not be used as an AC substitute when xenobiotics known to be adsorbed to AC are involved.

- When MDAC is administered, if a cathartic is used, it should be provided only with the first dose of AC. Sufficient oral fluids should always accompany cathartic administration to avoid salt and water depletion and inspissation.

- Activated charcoal should be given first to patients for whom it is indicated, and if WBI is being performed in conjunction, a comparable dose of AC should be given after WBI to prevent or overcome the potential desorption and possible further systemic absorption of the xenobiotic.

- Unless contraindicated, WBI is recommended over repetitive-dose cathartics for evacuation of modified release or poorly soluble xenobiotics not adsorbed to AC.

- The precise role of WBI and the interactions between PEG-ELS and AC in overdosed patients remain incompletely defined. Absent controlled clinical studies to assess outcome, WBI is recommended for ingestions of xenobiotics not adsorbed by AC (eg, iron, lead, lithium); and foreign body ingestions, specifically drug packets in body packers, and xenobiotic ingestions with a slow absorptive phase and a high expectation of morbidity.

REFERENCES

1. Anonymous. Polyethylene glycol: a fly in the ointment? *Food Chem Toxicol.* 1983;21: 680-681.
2. Abbas MI, et al. Prospective evaluation of 1-day polyethylene glycol-3350 bowel preparation regimen in children. *J Pediatr Gastroenterol Nutr.* 2013;56:220-224.
3. Abdul-Baki H, et al. A randomized, controlled, double-blind trial of the adjunct use of tegaserod in whole-dose or split-dose polyethylene glycol electrolyte solution for colonoscopy preparation. *Gastrointest Endosc.* 2008;68:294-300; quiz 34, 36.
4. Adamcewicz M, et al. Mechanism of action and toxicities of purgatives used for colonoscopy preparation. *Expert Opin Drug Metab Toxicol.* 2011;7:89-101.
5. US Food and Drug Administration. FDA Drug Safety Communication: FDA warns of possible harm from exceeding recommended dose of over-the-counter sodium phosphate products to treat constipation. Silver Spring, MD: US Food and Drug Administration; 2014. https://www.fda.gov/Drugs/DrugSafety/ucm380757.htm. Accessed March 27, 2017.
6. Al-Shareef AH, et al. The effects of charcoal and sorbitol (alone and in combination) on plasma theophylline concentration after a sustained release formulation. *Hum Exp Toxicol.* 1990;9:179-182.
7. Allerton JP, Strom JA. Hypernatremia due to repeated doses of charcoal-sorbitol. *Am J Kidney Dis.* 1991;17:581-584.
8. Ambrose NS, et al. A physiological appraisal of polyethylene glycol and a balanced electrolyte solution as bowel preparation. *Br J Surg.* 1983;70:428-430.
9. American Academy of Clinical Toxicology and the European Association of Poison Centres and Clinical Toxicologists: position paper: cathartics. *J Toxicol Clin Toxicol.* 2004;42:243-253.
10. American Academy of Clinical Toxicology and the European Association of Poison Centres and Clinical Toxicologists: position paper: whole bowel irrigation. *J Toxicol Clin Toxicol.* 2004;42:843-854.
11. Atta-Politou J, et al. An in vitro evaluation of fluoxetine adsorption by activated charcoal and desorption upon addition of polyethylene glycol-electrolyte lavage solution. *J Toxicol Clin Toxicol.* 1998;36:117-124.
12. Atta-Politou J, et al. The effect of polyethylene glycol on the charcoal adsorption of chlorpromazine studied by ion selective electrode potentiometry. *J Toxicol Clin Toxicol.* 1996;34:307-316.
13. Aungst BJ. Intestinal permeation enhancers. *J Pharm Sci.* 2000;89:429-442.
14. Ayus JC, et al. Fatal dysnatraemia caused by elective colonoscopy. *BMJ.* 2003;326: 382-384.
15. Azzam I, et al. Life threatening hyperphosphataemia after administration of sodium phosphate in preparation for colonoscopy. *Postgrad Med J.* 2004;80:487-488.
16. Bae SE, et al. A comparison of 2 L of polyethylene glycol and 45 mL of sodium phosphate versus 4 L of polyethylene glycol for bowel cleansing: a prospective randomized trial. *Gut Liver.* 2013;7:423-429.
17. Beck DE, et al. Bowel cleansing with polyethylene glycol electrolyte lavage solution. *South Med J.* 1985;78:1414-1416.
18. Beloosesky Y, et al. Electrolyte disorders following oral sodium phosphate administration for bowel cleansing in elderly patients. *Arch Intern Med.* 2003;163:803-808.
19. Binder HJ. Pharmacology of laxatives. *Annu Rev Pharmacol Toxicol.* 1977;17:355-367.
20. Borgstrom B, et al. Studies of intestinal digestion and absorption in the human. *J Clin Invest.* 1957;36:1521-1536.
21. Braintree Laboratories. GoLYTELY(R). PEG-3350 and Electrolytes for Oral Solution [Prescribing Information]. Braintree, MA; Braintree Laboratories; 2000.
22. Braintree Laboratories. NuLYTELY(R) With Flavor Packs. PEG-3350, Sodium Chloride, Sodium Bicarbonate, and Potassium Chloride for Oral Solution [Prescribing Information]. Braintree, MA: Braintree Laboratories; 2008.
23. Bretaudeau Deguigne M, et al. Lithium poisoning: the value of early digestive tract decontamination. *Clin Toxicol.* 2013;51:243-248.
24. Buckley N, et al. Slow-release verapamil poisoning. Use of polyethylene glycol whole-bowel lavage and high-dose calcium. *Med J Aust.* 1993;158:202-204.
25. Burkhart KK, et al. Whole-bowel irrigation as treatment for zinc sulfate overdose. *Ann Emerg Med.* 1990;19:1167-1170.
26. Burkhart KK, et al. Whole-bowel irrigation as adjunctive treatment for sustained-release theophylline overdose. *Ann Emerg Med.* 1992;21:1316-1320.
27. Butterfield M, et al. Symptomatic exposures among California inmates 2011-2013. *J Med Toxicol.* 2015;11:309-316.
28. Carl DE, Sica DA. Acute phosphate nephropathy following colonoscopy preparation. *Am J Med Sci.* 2007;334:151-154.
29. Carlsson M, et al. Severe iron intoxication treated with exchange transfusion. *BMJ Case Rep.* 2009;93:321-322.
30. Chin L, et al. Saline cathartics and saline cathartics plus activated charcoal as antidotal treatments. *Clin Toxicol.* 1981;18:865-871.
31. Choi HS, et al. Orange juice intake reduces patient discomfort and is effective for bowel cleansing with polyethylene glycol during bowel preparation. *Dis Colon Rectum.* 2014;57:1220-1227.
32. Craig S. Phenytoin overdose complicated by prolonged intoxication and residual neurological deficits. *Emerg Med Australas.* 2004;16:361-365.
33. Cumpston KL, et al. Whole bowel irrigation and the hemodynamically unstable calcium channel blocker overdose: primum non nocere. *J Emerg Med.* 2010;38:171-174.
34. Curran MP, Plosker GL. Oral sodium phosphate solution: a review of its use as a colorectal cleanser. *Drugs.* 2004;64:1697-1714.
35. Davis GR, et al. Development of a lavage solution associated with minimal water and electrolyte absorption or secretion. *Gastroenterology.* 1980;78:991-995.
36. Davis RF, et al. Hypocalcemia, hyperphosphatemia, and dehydration following a single hypertonic phosphate enema. *J Pediatr.* 1977;90:484-485.
37. DiPalma J, et al. Braintree polyethylene glycol (PEG) laxative for ambulatory and long-term care facility constipation patients: report of randomized, cross-over trials. *Online J Dig Health.* 1999;1:1-10.
38. DiPalma JA, et al. Comparison of colon cleansing methods in preparation for colonoscopy. *Gastroenterology.* 1984;86:856-860.
39. Erstoff J, et al. A randomized blinded clinical trial of a rapid colonic lavage solution (GoLYTELY) compared with standard preparation for colonoscopy and barium enema. *Gastroenterology.* 1983;84:1512-1516.
40. Everson GW, et al. Use of whole bowel irrigation in an infant following iron overdose. *Am J Emerg Med.* 1991;9:366-369.
41. Farley TA. Severe hypernatremic dehydration after use of an activated charcoal-sorbitol suspension. *J Pediatr.* 1986;109:719-722.
42. Farmer JW, Chan SB. Whole body irrigation for contraband bodypackers. *J Clin Gastroenterol.* 2003;37:147-150.
43. Faust AC, et al. Management of an oral ingestion of transdermal fentanyl patches: a case report and literature review. *Case Rep Med.* 2011;2011:495938.
44. Forman J, et al. Hypokalemia after hypertonic phosphate enemas. *J Pediatr.* 1979;94:149-151.
45. Givens ML, Gabrysch J. Cardiotoxicity associated with accidental bupropion ingestion in a child. *Pediatr Emerg Care.* 2007;23:234-237.
46. Goldman J, Reichelderfer M. Evaluation of rapid colonoscopy preparation using a new gut lavage solution. *Gastrointest Endosc.* 1982;28:9-11.
47. Granberry MC, et al. Exacerbation of congestive heart failure after administration of polyethylene glycol-electrolyte lavage solution. *Ann Pharmacother.* 1995;29:1232-1235.
48. Grissinger M. Bowel preparations might pose problems in renal patients. *P&T.* 2002;27.
49. Gunja N. Decontamination and enhanced elimination in sustained-release potassium chloride poisoning. *Emerg Med Australas.* 2011;23:769-772.
50. Hay M. The action of saline cathartics. *J Anat Physiol.* 1882;16:243-282.
51. Hay M. The action of saline cathartics. *J Anat Physiol.* 1883;17:405-441.
52. Hendrickson RG, et al. "Parachuting" meth: a novel delivery method for methamphetamine and delayed-onset toxicity from "body stuffing." *Clin Toxicol.* 2006;44:379-382.

53. Hewitt J, et al. Whole-gut irrigation in preparation for large-bowel surgery. *Lancet.* 1973;2:337-340.

54. Hill JC. Johann Glauber's discovery of sodium sulfate—Sal Mirabile Glauberi. *J Chem Educ.* 1979;56:593.

55. Hodgman M, et al. The influence of polyethylene glycol solution on the dissolution rate of sustained release morphine. *J Med Toxicol.* 2016;12:391-395.

56. Hoffman RS, et al. Theophylline desorption from activated charcoal caused by whole-bowel irrigation. *Clin Toxicol.* 1991;29:191-202.

57. Hoffman RS, et al. Whole bowel irrigation and the cocaine body-packer: a new approach to a common problem. *Am J Emerg Med.* 1990;8:523-527.

58. Hojer J, Forsberg S. Successful whole bowel irrigation in self-poisoning with potassium capsules. *Clin Toxicol (Phila).* 2008;46:1102-1103.

59. Horch R, et al. Phenol burns and intoxications. *Burns.* 1994;20:45-50.

60. Horowitz R, et al. Accidental clonidine patch ingestion in a child. *Am J Ther.* 2005;12:272-274.

61. Isbister GK, et al. Arsenic trioxide poisoning: a description of two acute overdoses. *Hum Exp Toxicol.* 2004;23:359-364.

62. James LP, et al. A comparison of cathartics in pediatric ingestions. *Pediatrics.* 1995;96:235-238.

63. Janss GJ. Acute theophylline overdose treated with whole bowel irrigation. *S D J Med.* 1990;43:7-8.

64. Joint FAO/WHO Expert Committee on Food Additives. Magnesium sulfate. In: *Compendium of Food Additive Specifications.* FAO JECFA Monographs 4. Rome, Italy: FAO (Food and Agriculture Organization of the United Nations); 2007. ftp://ftp.fao.org/docrep/fao/010/a1447e/a1447e.pdf. Accessed July 13, 2013.

65. Jones J, et al. Cathartic-induced magnesium toxicity during overdose management. *Ann Emerg Med.* 1986;15:1214-1218.

66. June R, et al. Medical outcome of cocaine bodystuffers. *J Emerg Med.* 2000;18:221-224.

67. Jung SW, et al. Effect of coffee added to a polyethylene glycol plus ascorbic acid solution for bowel preparation prior to colonoscopy. *J Gastrointestin Liver Dis.* 2016;25:63-69.

68. Kaczorowski JM, Wax PM. Five days of whole-bowel irrigation in a case of pediatric iron ingestion. *Ann Emerg Med.* 1996;27:258-263.

69. Kahovec J, et al. Nomenclature of regular single-strand organic polymers (IUPAC Recommendations 2002). *Pure Appl Chem.* 2002;74:1921-1956.

70. Kapoor S. Lubiprostone: clinical applications beyond constipation. *World J Gastroenterol.* 2009;15:1147.

71. Keller RE, et al. Contribution of sorbitol combined with activated charcoal in prevention of salicylate absorption. *Ann Emerg Med.* 1990;19:654-656.

72. Kim HG, et al. Sodium picosulfate with magnesium citrate (SPMC) plus laxative is a good alternative to conventional large volume polyethylene glycol in bowel preparation: a multicenter randomized single-blinded trial. *Gut Liver.* 2015;9:494-501.

73. Kirrane BM, et al. Massive strontium ferrite ingestion without acute toxicity. *Basic Clin Pharmacol Toxicol.* 2006;99:358-359.

74. Kirshenbaum LA, et al. Whole-bowel irrigation versus activated charcoal in sorbitol for the ingestion of modified-release pharmaceuticals. *Clin Pharmacol Ther.* 1989;46:264-271.

75. Kirshenbaum LA, et al. Interaction between whole-bowel irrigation solution and activated charcoal: implications for the treatment of toxic ingestions. *Ann Emerg Med.* 1990;19:1129-1132.

76. Korkis AM, et al. Rectal prolapse after oral cathartics. *J Clin Gastroenterol.* 1992;14:339-341.

77. Kramer J, et al. Nausea and vomiting of pregnancy: prevalence, severity and relation to psychosocial health. *MCN Am J Matern Child Nurs.* 2013;38:21-27.

78. Krenzelok EP, et al. Gastrointestinal transit times of cathartics combined with charcoal. *Ann Emerg Med.* 1985;14:1152-1155.

79. Kumar VV, et al. The effect of decontamination procedures on the pharmacodynamics of venlafaxine in overdose. *Br J Clin Pharmacol.* 2011;72:125-132.

80. Langdon DE. Colonic perforation with volume laxatives. *Am J Gastroenterol.* 1996;91:622-623.

81. Lapatto-Reiniluoto O, et al. Activated charcoal alone and followed by whole-bowel irrigation in preventing the absorption of sustained-release drugs. *Clin Pharmacol Ther.* 2001;70:255-260.

82. Lee DC, et al. Whole-bowel irrigation as an adjunct in the treatment of radiopaque arsenic. *Am J Emerg Med.* 1995;13:244-245.

83. Lee KJ, et al. Electrolyte changes after bowel preparation for colonoscopy: a randomized controlled multicenter trial. *World J Gastroenterol.* 2015;21:3041-3048.

84. Lenz K, et al. Effect of gut lavage on phenobarbital elimination in rats. *J Toxicol Clin Toxicol.* 1983;20:147-157.

85. Linden TB, Waye JD. Sodium phosphate preparation for colonoscopy: onset and duration of bowel activity. *Gastrointest Endosc.* 1999;50:811-813.

86. Lo JC, et al. A retrospective review of whole bowel irrigation in pediatric patients. *Clin Toxicol (Phila).* 2012;50:414-417.

87. Longdon P, Henderson A. Intestinal pseudo-obstruction following the use of enteral charcoal and sorbitol and mechanical ventilation with papaveretum sedation for theophylline poisoning. *Drug Saf.* 1992;7:74-77.

88. Loughnan P, Mullins GC. Brain damage following a hypertonic phosphate enema. *Am J Dis Child.* 1977;131:1032.

89. Love AH, et al. Water and sodium absorption in the human intestine. *J Physiol.* 1968;195:133-140.

90. Lurie Y, et al. Limited efficacy of gastrointestinal decontamination in severe slow-release carbamazepine overdose. *Ann Pharmacother.* 2007;41:1539-1543.

91. Ly BT, et al. Effect of whole bowel irrigation on the pharmacokinetics of an acetaminophen formulation and progression of radiopaque markers through the gastrointestinal tract. *Ann Emerg Med.* 2004;43:189-195.

92. Ly BT, et al. Mercuric oxide poisoning treated with whole-bowel irrigation and chelation therapy. *Ann Emerg Med.* 2002;39:312-315.

93. Makosiej FJ, et al. An in vitro evaluation of cocaine hydrochloride adsorption by activated charcoal and desorption upon addition of polyethylene glycol electrolyte lavage solution. *J Toxicol Clin Toxicol.* 1993;31:381-395.

94. Mamula P, et al. Colonoscopy preparation. *Gastrointest Endosc.* 2009;69:1201-1209.

95. Mandava N, et al. Establishment of a definitive protocol for the diagnosis and management of body packers (drug mules). *Emerg Med J.* 2011;28:98-101.

96. Mann KV, et al. Management of acute iron overdose. *Clin Pharm.* 1989;8:428-440.

97. Marciani L, et al. Stimulation of colonic motility by oral PEG electrolyte bowel preparation assessed by MRI: comparison of split vs single dose. *Neurogastroenterol Motil.* 2014;26:1426-1436.

98. Martin RR, et al. Fatal poisoning from sodium phosphate enema. Case report and experimental study. *JAMA.* 1987;257:2190-2192.

99. Mayer AL, et al. Multiple-dose charcoal and whole-bowel irrigation do not increase clearance of absorbed salicylate. *Arch Intern Med.* 1992;152:393-396.

100. Mayershohn M, et al. Evaluation of a charcoal-sorbitol mixture as an antidote for oral aspirin overdose. *Clin Toxicol.* 1977;11:561-567.

101. McCord M. Toxicity of sorbitol-charcoal suspension. *J Pediatr.* 1987;110:307-308.

102. McKee K. A guide to colon preps. *Outpatient Surgery Magazine.* February 2002. http://wwwoutpatientsurgerynet/issues/2002/02/a-guide-to-colon-preps Accessed July 12, 2013.

103. McKenna T, et al. Colonoscopy preparation: polyethylene glycol with Gatorade is as safe and efficacious as four liters of polyethylene glycol with balanced electrolytes. *Dig Dis Sci.* 2012;57:3098-3105.

104. McKinney PE. Acute elevation of blood lead levels within hours of ingestion of large quantities of lead shot. *J Toxicol Clin Toxicol.* 2000;38:435-440.

105. McNamara RM, et al. Sorbitol catharsis does not enhance efficacy of charcoal in a simulated acetaminophen overdose. *Ann Emerg Med.* 1988;17:243-246.

106. McNutt TK, et al. Bite the bullet: lead poisoning after ingestion of 206 lead bullets. *Vet Hum Toxicol.* 2001;43:288-289.

107. Melandri R, et al. Whole bowel irrigation after delayed release fenfluramine overdose. *J Toxicol Clin Toxicol.* 1995;33:161-163.

108. Minocha A, et al. Effect of activated charcoal in 70% sorbitol in healthy individuals. *J Toxicol Clin Toxicol.* 1984;22:529-536.

109. Minocha A, et al. Dosage recommendations for activated charcoal-sorbitol treatment. *J Toxicol Clin Toxicol.* 1985;23:579-587.

110. Mofenson HC, Caraccio TR. Magnesium intoxication in a neonate from oral magnesium hydroxide laxative. *J Toxicol Clin Toxicol.* 1991;29:215-222.

111. Muller-Lissner SA. Adverse effects of laxatives: fact and fiction. *Pharmacology.* 1993;47(suppl 1):138-145.

112. Nagler J, et al. Severe hyponatremia and seizure following a polyethylene glycol-based bowel preparation for colonoscopy. *J Clin Gastroenterol.* 2006;40:558-559.

113. Narsinghani U, et al. Life-threatening respiratory failure following accidental infusion of polyethylene glycol electrolyte solution into the lung. *J Toxicol Clin Toxicol.* 2001;39:105-107.

114. Neuvonen PJ, Olkkola KT. Effect of purgatives on antidotal efficacy of oral activated charcoal. *Hum Toxicol.* 1986;5:255-263.

115. Nordt S, RF C. "Go Lytely" dissolves more quickly [abstract]. *Clin Toxicol.* 2009;47:717-718.

116. Nyberg C, et al. The safety of osmotically acting cathartics in colonic cleansing. *Nat Rev Gastroenterol Hepatol.* 2010;7:557-564.

117. Orisakwe OE, Ogbonna E. Effect of saline cathartics on gastrointestinal transit time of activated charcoal. *Hum Exp Toxicol.* 1993;12:403-405.

118. Paap CM, Ehrlich R. Acute pulmonary edema after polyethylene glycol intestinal lavage in a child. *Ann Pharmacother.* 1993;27:1044-1047.

119. Pereira J. 62. Sodea phosphas—phosphate of soda. In: *The Elements of Materia Medica and Therapeutics,* 4th ed., vol. 1. London: Wilson and Ogilvy. Printed for Longman, Brown, Green, and Longmans; 1854.

120. Picchioni AL, et al. Evaluation of activated charcoal-sorbitol suspension as an antidote. *J Toxicol Clin Toxicol.* 1982;19:433-444.

121. Postuma R. Whole bowel irrigation in pediatric patients. *J Pediatr Surg.* 1982;17:350-352.

122. Reedy JC, Zwiren GT. Enema-induced hypocalcemia and hyperphosphatemia leading to cardiac arrest during induction of anesthesia in an outpatient surgery center. *Anesthesiology.* 1983;59:578-579.

123. Rivera W, et al. Unintentional intravenous infusion of Golytely in a 4-year-old girl. *Ann Pharmacother.* 2004;38:1183-1185.

124. Rosenberg PJ, et al. Effect of whole-bowel irrigation on the antidotal efficacy of oral activated charcoal. *Ann Emerg Med.* 1988;17:681-683.

125. Sakula A. Doctor Nehemiah Grew (1641-1712) and the Epsom salts. *Clio Med.* 1984;19:1-21.

126. Scharman EJ, et al. Efficiency of whole bowel irrigation with and without metoclopramide pretreatment. *Am J Emerg Med.* 1994;12:302-305.

127. Schroppel B, et al. Hyponatremic encephalopathy after preparation for colonoscopy. *Gastrointest Endosc.* 2001;53:527-529.
128. Schwarz KA, Alsop JA. Pediatric ingestion of seven lead bullets successfully treated with outpatient whole bowel irrigation. *Clin Toxicol (Phila).* 2008;46:919.
129. Schwarz Pharma. Colyte(R) with Flavor Packs (PEG-3350 and Electrolytes) for Oral Solution [Prescribing Information]. Milwaukee, WI: Schwarz Pharma.
130. Schwarz Pharma. TriLyte® with flavor packs (PEG-3350, sodium chloride, sodium bicarbonate and potassium chloride). Milwaukee, WI: Schwarz Pharma.
131. Sharkey K, MacNaughton WK. Gastrointestinal Motility and Water Flux, Emesis, and Biliary and Pancreatic Disease. In: Brunton LL, Hilal-Dandan R, Knollmann BC, eds. *Gooodman & Gilman's The Pharmacological Basis of Therapeutics.* 3rd ed. New York, NY: McGraw-Hill; 2018.
132. Shieh FK, et al. MiraLAX-Gatorade bowel prep versus GoLytely before screening colonoscopy: an endoscopic database study in a community hospital. *J Clin Gastroenterol.* 2012;46:e96-e100.
133. Sica DA, et al. Acute phosphate nephropathy—an emerging issue. *Am J Gastroenterol.* 2007;102:1844-1847.
134. Sketris IS, et al. Saline catharsis: effect on aspirin bioavailability in combination with activated charcoal. *J Clin Pharmacol.* 1982;22:59-64.
135. Smilkstein MJ, et al. Magnesium levels after magnesium-containing cathartics. *J Toxicol Clin Toxicol.* 1988;26:51-65.
136. Smith SW, et al. Whole-bowel irrigation as a treatment for acute lithium overdose. *Ann Emerg Med.* 1991;20:536-539.
137. Sotos JF, et al. Hypocalcemic coma following two pediatric phosphate enemas. *Pediatrics.* 1977;60:305-307.
138. Stewart JJ. Effects of emetic and cathartic agents on the gastrointestinal tract and the treatment of toxic ingestion. *J Toxicol Clin Toxicol.* 1983;20:199-253.
139. Sue YJ, et al. Efficacy of magnesium citrate cathartic in pediatric toxic ingestions. *Ann Emerg Med.* 1994;24:709-712.
140. Synergy Pharmaceuticals. Trulance (plecanatide) tablets, for oral use [prescribing information]. New York, NY: Synergy Pharmaceuticals; 2017.
141. Tenenbein M. Whole bowel irrigation as a gastrointestinal decontamination procedure after acute poisoning. *Med Toxicol Adverse Drug Exp.* 1988;3:77-84.
142. Tennebein M, et al. Gastrotomy and whole bowel irrigation in iron poisoning. *Pediatr Emerg Care.* 1991;7:286-288.
143. Thanacoody R, et al. Position paper update: whole bowel irrigation for gastrointestinal decontamination of overdose patients. *Clin Toxicol (Phila).* 2015;53:5-12.
144. The Dow Chemical Company. Technical Data Sheet. CARBOWAX(TM) SENTRY(TM) Polyethylene Glycol (PEG) 3350. December 2011. http://msdssearch.dow.com/PublishedLiteratureDOWCOM/dh_0889/0901b8038088978a.pdf?filepath=polyglycols/pdfs/noreg/118-01815.pdf&fromPage=GetDoc. Accessed July 12, 2013.
145. The Dow Chemical Company. CARBOWAX(TM) SENTRY(TM) Polyethylene Glycols. Innovation, Performance, Flexibility and Compliance from the Global Leader in PEGs. 2011. http://www.dow.com/scripts/litorder.asp?filepath=polyglycols/pdfs/noreg/118-01790.pdf. Accessed July 12, 2013.
146. Thomas G, et al. Patient acceptance and effectiveness of a balanced lavage solution (Golytely) versus the standard preparation for colonoscopy. *Gastroenterology.* 1982;82:435-437.
147. Traub SJ, et al. Pediatric "body packing." *Arch Pediatr Adolesc Med.* 2003;157:174-177.
148. Traub SJ, et al. Use of pharmaceutical promotility agents in the treatment of body packers. *Am J Emerg Med.* 2003;21:511-512.
149. Tuggle DW, et al. The safety and cost-effectiveness of polyethylene glycol electrolyte solution bowel preparation in infants and children. *J Pediatr Surg.* 1987;22:513-515.
150. Turk J, et al. Successful therapy of iron intoxication in pregnancy with intravenous deferoxamine and whole bowel irrigation. *Vet Hum Toxicol.* 1993;35:441-444.
151. Utsunomiya S, et al. Critical residues in the transmembrane helical bundle domains of the human motilin receptor for erythromycin binding and activity. *Regul Pept.* 2013;180:17-25.
152. Van Ameyde KJ, Tenenbein M. Whole bowel irrigation during pregnancy. *Am J Obstet Gynecol.* 1989;160:646-647.
153. Van de Graaff WB, et al. Adsorbent and cathartic inhibition of enteral drug absorption. *J Pharmacol Exp Ther.* 1982;221:656-663.
154. Velez LI, et al. Iron bezoar retained in colon despite 3 days of whole bowel irrigation. *J Toxicol Clin Toxicol.* 2004;42:653-656.
155. Visser L, et al. Do not give paraffin to packers. *Lancet.* 1998;352:1352.
156. Voeller B, et al. Mineral oil lubricants cause rapid deterioration of latex condoms. *Contraception.* 1989;39:95-102.
157. Wax PM, et al. Prevalence of sorbitol in multiple-dose activated charcoal regimens in emergency departments. *Ann Emerg Med.* 1993;22:1807-1812.
158. Weng YM, et al. Hypermagnesemia in a constipated female. *J Emerg Med.* 2013;44:e57-60.
159. Woo P, et al. Whole-gut perfusion for therapeutic purgation. *Br Med J.* 1976;1:433-434.

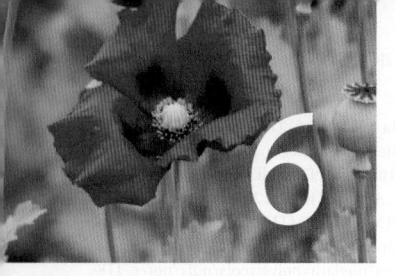

6 PRINCIPLES AND TECHNIQUES APPLIED TO ENHANCE ELIMINATION

David S. Goldfarb and Marc Ghannoum

Enhancing the elimination of a xenobiotic from a poisoned patient is a logical step after initial stabilization of the airway, breathing, and circulation; supportive measures; and techniques to inhibit absorption. Table 6–1 lists methods that might be used to enhance elimination. In this chapter, hemodialysis, hemoperfusion, and hemofiltration are considered *extracorporeal treatments* (ECTRs) because xenobiotic removal occurs in a blood circuit outside the body. Extracorporeal treatments are used infrequently because most poisonings are not amenable to removal by these methods. In addition, because these elimination techniques have associated adverse effects, costs, and complications, the risk-to-benefit analysis suggests they are only indicated in a relatively small proportion of patients and situations.

EPIDEMIOLOGY

Although undoubtedly an underestimate of true use, enhanced elimination techniques were performed relatively infrequently in the cohorts of millions of patients reported by the American Association of Poison Control Centers (AAPCC) National Poison Data System (NPDS) (Chap. 130). Alkalinization of the urine was reportedly used 11,651 times, multiple-dose activated charcoal (MDAC) 1,104 times, hemodialysis 2,663 times, and hemoperfusion 49 times. As in the past, there continue to be many instances of inappropriate use of ECTRs, such as in the treatment of overdoses of cyclic antidepressants (CAs).[35]

The AAPCC data reveal that there is a continued increase in the reported use of hemodialysis, paralleling a decline in reports of charcoal hemoperfusion (Chap. 130) (Table 6–2). Lithium and ethylene glycol were the most common xenobiotics for which hemodialysis was used between 1985 and 2014 (Fig. 6–1).[18] Possible reasons for the decline in use of charcoal and resin hemoperfusion are described in the section on hemoperfusion in this chapter. Peritoneal dialysis (PD), a slower modality that should have little or no role in any poisoning, is no longer reported separately. "Other extracorporeal procedures" in past AAPCC reports include continuous modalities (discussed later in the section Continuous Hemofiltration and Hemodiafiltration), plasmapheresis, and PD.

Very few prospective, randomized, controlled clinical trials have been conducted to determine which groups of patients actually benefit from enhanced elimination of various xenobiotics and which modalities are most efficacious. For most poisonings, it is unlikely that such studies will ever be performed, given the relative scarcity of appropriate cases of sufficient severity and because of the many variables that would hinder controlled comparisons. Thus, limited evidence deemed of high quality exists. We must therefore rely on an understanding of the principles of these methods to identify the individual patients for whom enhanced elimination is indicated. In particular, isolated case reports in which the kinetics are well described, including half-lives with and without enhanced elimination, clearance, and quantification of removal are very useful in establishing the efficacy of a method. Fortunately, in the absence of robust evidence, consensus-based recommendations have now been published and are being developed to guide clinical decisions. The American Academy of Clinical Toxicology (AACT) and the European Association of Poisons Centres and Clinical Toxicologists (EAPCCT) published joint position papers on urine alkalinization[50] and MDAC.[56] The Extracorporeal Treatments in Poisoning (EXTRIP) work group, a collaboration of experts from diverse specialties (clinical toxicology, nephrology, pharmacology, critical care, emergency medicine) representing more than 30 international societies, has published several recommendations regarding the indications for dialysis and other ECTRs for overdose[3,9,17,20,23,24,26,29,39,43,52,58] (see also http://extrip-workgroup.org).

GENERAL INDICATIONS FOR ENHANCED ELIMINATION

Enhanced elimination is generally indicated for several types of patients, with the preexisting condition that the responsible xenobiotic is removable.[22]

- *Patients who fail to respond adequately to comprehensive supportive care.* Such patients have evidence of poor prognostic factors such as intractable hypotension, heart failure, seizures, metabolic acidosis, or dysrhythmias. Hemodialysis is much better tolerated than in the past and offers potentially life-saving opportunities for patients with toxicity caused by theophylline, lithium, salicylates, or toxic alcohols, among others.
- *Patients in whom the normal route of elimination of the xenobiotic is impaired.* Such patients have kidney or hepatic dysfunction, either preexisting or caused by the overdose. For example, a patient with impaired kidney function is more likely to develop toxicity from a large lithium ingestion and require hemodialysis as treatment.
- *Patients in whom the amount of xenobiotic absorbed or its high concentration in serum indicates that serious morbidity or mortality is likely.* Such patients do not necessarily appear acutely ill on initial evaluation. Xenobiotics in this group include ethylene glycol, lithium, methanol, paraquat, salicylates, and theophylline.
- *Patients with concurrent disease or in an age group (very young or old) associated with increased risk of morbidity or mortality from the overdose.* Such patients are intolerant of prolonged coma, immobility, and hemodynamic instability. An example is a patient with both severe underlying respiratory disease and chronic salicylate poisoning.
- *Patients with concomitant electrolyte disorders that could be corrected with hemodialysis.* An example is the metabolic acidosis with elevated lactate associated with metformin toxicity discussed in the hemodialysis section of this chapter.

TABLE 6–1	Potential Methods of Enhancing Elimination of Xenobiotics
Occurring Inside the Body	**Occurring Outside the Body (Extracorporeal)**
Cerebrospinal fluid replacement	Exchange transfusion
Forced diuresis	Hemodialysis
Manipulation of urine pH	Hemofiltration and hemodiafiltration
Metal chelators	Hemoperfusion (charcoal, resin)
Multiple-dose activated charcoal	Liver support devices
Peritoneal dialysis	Plasmapheresis
Resins (Prussian blue, sodium polystyrene sulfonate, cholestyramine, colestipol)	

TABLE 6–2	Changes in AAPCC Annual Reported Use of Extracorporeal Therapies[a]						
	1986	1990	2001	2004	2007	2011	2015
Hemodialysis	297	584	1,280	1,726	2,106	2,323	2,663
Charcoal hemoperfusion	99	111	45	20	16	14	49
Resin	23	37	—	—	—	—	—
Peritoneal dialysis	62	27	—	—	—	—	—
Other extracorporeal: Such as CVVH and CVVHD	—	—	26	33	24	26	51

CVVH, continuous venovenous hemofiltration; CVVHD, continuous venovenous hemodialysis.
[a]Data from American Association of Poison Control Centers annual reports.

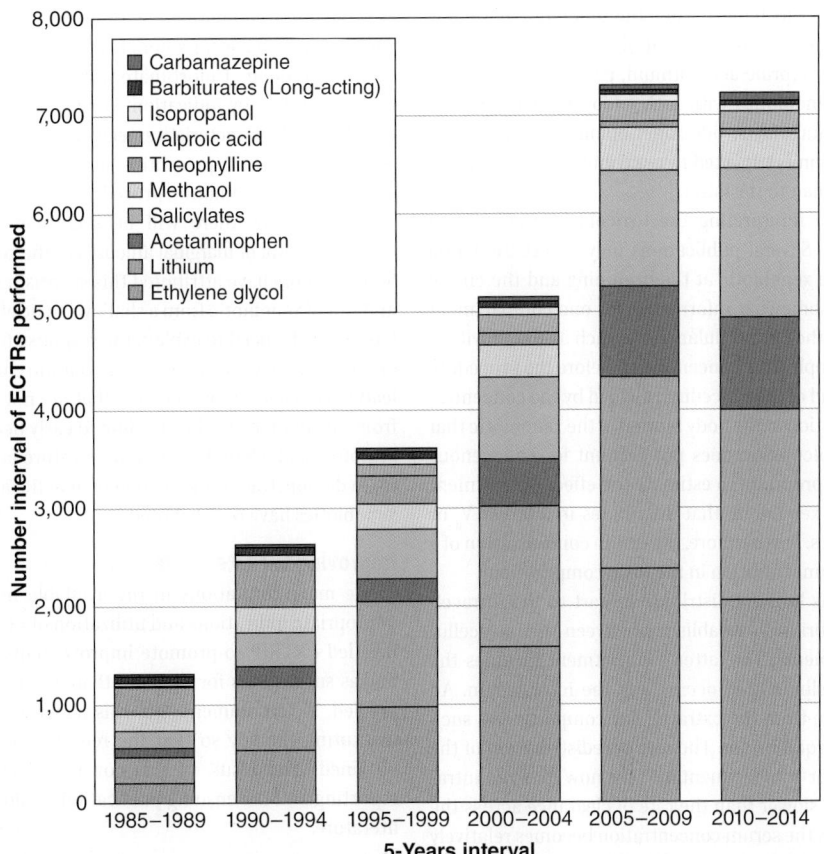

FIGURE 6–1. Xenobiotics that were most commonly reported by the AAPCC as treated with extracorporeal therapies per 5 year intervals. ECTR = extracorporeal treatment.

Ideally, these techniques are applied to poisonings for which studies suggest an improvement in outcome in treated patients compared with patients not treated with extracorporeal removal. As previously mentioned, these data are rarely available.[21]

The need for extracorporeal elimination is less clear for patients who are poisoned with xenobiotics that are known to be removed by an ECTR but that cause limited morbidity if supportive care is provided. Relatively high rates of endogenous clearance would also make extracorporeal elimination redundant. Examples of such xenobiotics include ethanol and some barbiturates; both are subject to substantial rates of hepatic metabolism, and neither would be expected to lead to significant morbidity after the affected patient has had endotracheal intubation and is mechanically ventilated. There may be instances of severe toxicity from these two xenobiotics for which enhanced elimination will reduce the length of intensive care unit (ICU) stays and the associated nosocomial risks; extracorporeal elimination would then be a reasonable option. Dialysis should be avoided if other more effective and less invasive modalities are available. For example, a patient with an acetaminophen (APAP) overdose should be initially treated with N-acetylcysteine instead of hemodialysis unless evidence of mitochondrial injury is apparent.[26]

CHARACTERISTICS OF XENOBIOTICS APPROPRIATE FOR EXTRACORPOREAL THERAPY

The appropriateness of any modality for increasing the elimination of a given xenobiotic depends on various properties of the molecules in question. Effective removal by the ECTR and other methods listed in Table 6–1 is limited by a number of factors, including a large volume of distribution (V_d), molecular and compartmental factors. The V_d relates to the concentration of the xenobiotic in the blood or serum as a proportion of the total body burden. The V_d can be envisioned as the apparent volume in which a known total dose of drug is distributed before metabolism and excretion occur:

$$V_d \text{ (L/kg)} \times \text{Patient weight (kg)} = \text{Dose (mg)}/\text{Concentration (mg/L)}$$

The larger the V_d, the less the xenobiotic is present in the blood compartment for elimination. A xenobiotic with a V_d below 1 L/kg is usually considered amenable to extracorporeal elimination. Methanol is an example of a xenobiotic with a small V_d, approximately equal to total body water (0.6 L/kg). A substantial fraction of a dose of methanol can be removed by hemodialysis. In addition to the alcohols, other xenobiotics with a relatively low V_d include phenobarbital, lithium, salicylates, valproic acid, bromide and fluoride ions, and theophylline. In contrast, lipid-soluble xenobiotics have large volumes of distribution (≥1 L/kg of body weight); an insignificant fraction of digoxin with a large V_d (5–12 L/kg of body weight) would be removed by hemodialysis. Other high V_d xenobiotics include many β-adrenergic antagonists (with the possible exception of atenolol), diazepam, organic phosphorus compounds, antipsychotics, quinidine, and the CAs.

Pharmacokinetics also influences the ability to enhance elimination of a xenobiotic. Kinetic parameters after an overdose often differ from those after therapeutic or experimental doses. For instance, carrier- or enzyme-mediated elimination processes may be overwhelmed by higher concentrations of the xenobiotic in question, making extracorporeal removal potentially more useful. Similarly, plasma protein- and tissue-binding sites may all be saturated at higher concentrations, making extracorporeal removal feasible in instances in which it would have no role in less significant overdoses. Examples include salicylates and valproic acid, which are poorly dialyzed at nontoxic concentrations because of high protein binding. However, at higher concentrations, protein-binding sites become saturated and lead to a higher proportion of the drug free in the serum, amenable to removal by hemodialysis at a clinically relevant rate. Estimated endogenous elimination rates of a xenobiotic should be derived by proper toxicokinetic models and not by pharmacokinetic data after therapeutic doses.

When assessing the efficacy of any technique of enhanced elimination, a generally accepted principle is that the intervention is worthwhile only if a large portion of total body drug burden can be eliminated or if total body clearance of the xenobiotic is increased by a factor of at least 2.[36]

This substantial increase is easier to achieve when the xenobiotic has a low endogenous clearance. Examples of xenobiotics with low endogenous clearances (<4 mL/min/kg) include valproic acid, lithium, paraquat, phenytoin, salicylate, and theophylline. Xenobiotics with high endogenous clearances include many β-adrenergic antagonists, lidocaine, opioids, nicotine, and CAs. Enhancement of elimination is expected to contribute more to overall clearance of the former group than to the latter.

There are many caveats in interpreting the toxicokinetic efficacy of any technique of elimination.[37] Several publications only report the blood or serum concentrations of the xenobiotic at the beginning and the end of the procedure; these data are somewhat informative for one-compartment xenobiotics that are limited to the extracellular space, such as theophylline. The difference between the theophylline concentration before the procedure and the concentration at the end of the procedure, divided by the concentration at the beginning, is the fraction of the body burden of the xenobiotic that is eliminated. However, this calculation does not account for endogenous clearance and would not be appropriate to estimate the effect of treatment on the total body burden of a xenobiotic that distributes in a larger V_d or with multicompartment kinetics. Furthermore, the serum concentration of a xenobiotic seldom reflects its concentration in the toxic compartment.

Certain xenobiotics, such as lithium, distribute in part to the intracellular compartment, and equilibrium is established between the intracellular and extracellular compartments. The latter compartment includes the blood from which xenobiotic elimination occurs and the interstitium. An increase in the elimination rate from the extracellular compartment, such as by hemodialysis, alters this equilibrium. The rate of redistribution of the xenobiotic from the intracellular compartment into the now dialyzed intravascular compartment is often slower than the rate of clearance across the dialysis membrane. In that case, the serum concentration becomes relatively low despite a substantial intracellular burden. This low serum concentration reduces the concentration gradient for diffusion from serum to dialysate so that dialysance (the dialysis clearance) is reduced. Thus, although serum concentrations decrease precipitously during the procedure, the total-body burden of the xenobiotic is not affected significantly if it does not move from cells to the dialyzable intravascular compartment. To fully appreciate the limitation of only observing serum concentration, the following example can be illustrated: a 60-kg patient ingests 100 (25-mg) amitriptyline tablets, a CA.[14] Because of significant lipophilicity, this class of xenobiotics has a high V_d. Assuming that the drug is fully absorbed, the 2,500 mg of amitriptyline distributes in an apparent volume of 40 L/kg of body weight to achieve a serum concentration of 1,000 ng/mL, a potentially toxic concentration. One might consider dialysis useful if the serum concentration of amitriptyline decreases from 1,000 ng/mL to 400 ng/mL during a 4-hour dialysis. If dialysis is performed with a blood flow rate of 350 mL/min (plasma flow rate of 200 mL/min, assuming a hematocrit of ~43%) and the extraction ratio is 100%, the clearance of drug is 200 mL/min or 200 mcg/min. In 4 hours (240 minutes) of treatment, only 48 mg (48,000 mcg), or less than 2% of the amount ingested, would be removed. The treatment would not affect toxicity despite decreasing serum concentrations.

When assessing overall efficacy, the evidence of enhanced elimination must be considered in the context of the clinical response. In some instances, observed improvement is not predicted by the kinetics of the parent xenobiotic and may not result from the intervention. For example, in severe cases of CA poisoning, unexpected improvement during hemoperfusion could be fortuitous because the toxicity is manifested early and ameliorates rapidly during the initial distribution phase.

Beginning a procedure during the initial distribution phase will likely increase the fraction of the drug burden that can be removed. Later, after the xenobiotic has distributed into fat, moved intracellularly, or has been bound by plasma or tissue proteins, administration of ECTR will have much lower clearance rates and benefits. Examples of xenobiotics that might be better removed soon after ingestion include paraquat and thallium.

The extent of xenobiotic removal by enhanced elimination is not necessarily correlated to clinical improvement. For example, no difference was observed between patients with lithium poisoning for whom hemodialysis was done and those for whom it was recommended by a poison control center but not done.[4] Unfortunately, this study was underpowered and limited by confounding by indication. Furthermore, although paraquat exhibits all the chemical characteristics necessary for high extracorporeal removal, the outcome of patients presenting late after paraquat ingestion remains dismal despite active elimination procedures.

Occasionally, there will be unanticipated evidence of improvement despite removal of marginal amounts of the xenobiotic and active metabolites. Some authors have attributed this surprising finding to removal of a critical amount of xenobiotic from a shallow "toxic effect" compartment. This theory has been advanced to explain the response to hemodialysis of patients overdosed with the CAs and the antipsychotic chlorprothixene. Such effects may lead to transient improvements that are not sustained as drug redistributes from one pool to another, leading to early benefit but eventual recurrence of symptoms. Much of the relevant literature fails to provide long-term follow-up to demonstrate prolongation of benefits after the ECTR is completed and xenobiotics have redistributed.

Improving the Literature

These many limitations in the available medical literature regarding the appropriate indications and utilization of ECTRs in the treatment of poisonings led EXTRIP to promote improvements in case reporting.[37] The paper makes suggestions for the data that should be obtained when the ECTR is applied. We recommend that this paper be reviewed when possible before instituting therapy so that the requisite and comprehensive data will be obtained. The result of this consideration will be more thorough case reporting and the ensuing publication of more thorough and useful medical literature.

TECHNIQUES TO ENHANCE REMOVAL OF XENOBIOTICS

Although the efficacy of, or need for, removal of many xenobiotics remains controversial, consensus regarding the indications for these procedures has developed. This consensus has led to consistent application of several techniques of enhanced elimination for some toxic exposures that occur relatively more frequently.

Multiple-Dose Activated Charcoal: "Gastrointestinal Dialysis"

Oral administration of multiple doses of activated charcoal increases elimination of some xenobiotics present in the blood. This modality is discussed in more detail in Antidotes in Depth: A1 and will not be discussed here.

Resins

Resins are sometimes used in poisoning management. They can reduce the bioavailability of ingested drugs and act as decontaminants, similarly to activated charcoal. In addition, however, they can promote elimination of certain xenobiotics by enhancing their back-diffusion from plasma to gut (gastrointestinal dialysis) and interrupt enterohepatic recirculation.

The most commonly used resins are sodium polystyrene sulfonate (Kayexalate), cholestyramine, and Prussian blue. Sodium polystyrene sulfonate is an ion exchanger that is used regularly for hyperkalemia in patients with chronic kidney disease. Limited data now exist on its potential use in lithium poisoning, although treatment results in hypokalemia.[19] Prussian blue is also an ion exchanger used for treatment of poisoning by cesium or thallium (Antidotes in Depth: A31). Cholestyramine, a bile acid sequestrant, binds several xenobiotics, including digoxin, ibuprofen, and mycophenolate mofetil, although its application in poisoning is doubtful (Chap. 62).

Forced Diuresis

Forced diuresis by volume expansion with isotonic sodium–containing solutions, such as 0.9% sodium chloride and Ringer's lactate (RL) solution with or without the addition of a diuretic, does increase renal clearance of some molecules. This therapy would theoretically be most useful for xenobiotics such as lithium for which the glomerular filtration rate (GFR), representing the volume of plasma filtered across the glomerular basement membrane per minute, is an important determinant of excretion. In people with normal extracellular fluid (ECF) volume, the increase in GFR and increase in xenobiotic renal elimination expected with plasma volume expansion is variable and unpredictable and not likely to be clinically significant. The effect is potentially more important in patients who have contraction of the ECF volume; loss of extracellular volume leads to a reduction of GFR partly as a result of decreased cardiac preload and cardiac output, which, in turn, reduces renal plasma flow. This circumstance is also accompanied by activation of angiotensin II, a small peptide that acts as a pressor and stimulates sodium reabsorption in the proximal tubule. Because small molecules such as lithium are both filtered at the glomerulus and reabsorbed by the proximal tubule, especially when volume depletion has occurred and angiotensin II has been activated, repletion of ECF volume with 0.9% sodium chloride will increase GFR and suppress proximal tubular sodium reabsorption. The result is an increase in excretion of low-molecular-weight xenobiotics such as lithium. After the ECF volume is restored, the continued infusion of 0.9% sodium chloride or RL will not enhance elimination of lithium to any major extent.

The major risk of excessive volume repletion is ECF volume overload, manifested by pulmonary and cerebral edema. This complication is particularly likely in patients with baseline chronic kidney disease such as is associated with long-standing lithium use. Other patients with acute kidney injury (AKI) not mediated by ECF volume depletion are also at risk. Knowing the result of past serum creatinine concentrations permits distinction between acute from chronic kidney disease in such cases. Administration of diuretics such as furosemide along with saline diminishes the risk of ECF volume overload but complicates the therapy, confuses the assessment of ECF volume, and increases the risk of metabolic alkalosis and hypokalemia. The unproven efficacy of enhanced diuresis in the management of *any* overdose has led most experts to abandon its use. On the other hand, the repletion of ECF volume when volume contraction is present, as determined by the history and physical examination, is, of course, appropriate. Saline diuresis may be used to treat toxin-induced hypercalcemia, which can result from excessive ingestion of calcium supplements or vitamin D ingestion.

Manipulations of Urinary pH

Many xenobiotics are weak acids or bases that are ionized in aqueous solution to an extent that depends on the pK_a of the xenobiotic and the pH of the solution. Knowing these variables, the Henderson-Hasselbalch equation (Chaps. 9 and 10) can be used to determine the relative proportions of the acids, bases, and buffer pairs. Whereas cell membranes are relatively impermeable to ionized, or polar molecules (eg, an unprotonated salicylate anion), nonionized, nonpolar forms (eg, the protonated, noncharged salicylic acid) cross more easily. As xenobiotics pass through the kidney, they may be filtered, secreted, and reabsorbed. If the urinary pH is manipulated to favor the formation of the ionized form in the tubular lumen, the xenobiotic is trapped in the tubular fluid and is not passively reabsorbed into the bloodstream. This is referred to as ion trapping. Hence, the rate and extent of its elimination can be increased. To make manipulation of urinary pH worthwhile, the renal excretion of the xenobiotic must be a major route of elimination. The 2004 position paper of the AACT and EAPCCT emphasizes that, as discussed earlier for extracorporeal therapies, enhanced removal does not necessarily translate into a clinical benefit with improved outcomes.[50]

Alkalinization of the urine to enhance elimination of weak acids has a role for salicylates, phenobarbital, chlorpropamide, formate, diflunisal, fluoride, methotrexate, and the herbicide 2,4-dichlorophenoxyacetic acid (2,4-D). These weak acids are ionized at alkaline urine pH, and tubular reabsorption is thereby greatly reduced. Alkalinization is achieved by the intravenous administration of sodium bicarbonate (1–2 mEq/kg rapid initial infusion with additional dosing) to increase urinary pH to 7 to 8. This degree of alkalinization will be difficult, if not impossible, if metabolic acidosis and acidemia are present, as often is the case in patients with salicylate poisoning. In this situation, bicarbonate (administered as the sodium salt, sodium bicarbonate) is consumed by titration of plasma protons before it

can appear in the urine. On the other hand, salicylate poisoning often causes respiratory alkalosis as well. In that case, when the PCO_2 is low, raising serum bicarbonate, equivalent to the induction of metabolic alkalosis, may lead to profound, life-threatening alkalemia. Finally, as for the case of 0.9% sodium chloride or RL, there is a risk of ECF volume overload with sodium bicarbonate administration. Modest reductions in GFR also reduce the likelihood of successful urinary alkalinization and increase the risk of pulmonary edema. Hypernatremia may also occur, especially if sodium bicarbonate is given as a hypertonic solution. Bicarbonaturia is also associated with urinary potassium losses, so the patient's serum potassium concentration should be monitored frequently and the appropriate dose of potassium administered as long as GFR is not impaired. A further complication of alkalemia is a decrease of ionized calcium, which becomes bound by albumin as protons are titrated off serum proteins; in this event, tetany, prolonged QT interval, and cardiac dysrhythmias are risks. If these complications can be identified and dealt with judiciously and safely, the renal clearance of salicylate increases fourfold as urine pH increases from 6.5 to 7.5 with alkalinization.[49] Increasing urine pH by decreasing proximal tubular bicarbonate reabsorption via administration of carbonic anhydrase inhibitors such as acetazolamide is not recommended. Although an alkaline urine pH will result and elimination of a xenobiotic enhanced, this is achieved at the expense of inducing a metabolic acidosis. In the case of salicylates, acidemia increases distribution into the central nervous system. The role of urinary alkalinization in the management of patients with salicylate poisoning is discussed further in Chap. 37.

Alkalinization is also used to increase the solubility of methotrexate and its metabolites and thereby prevents their precipitation in tubules when patients are given high-dose methotrexate.[8] Precipitation of sulfonamide antibiotics, resulting in crystalluria, kidney stones, or kidney failure, can be prevented by alkalinization. Administration of sodium bicarbonate, sodium chloride, or RL also protects the kidneys from the toxic effects of myoglobinuria in patients with extensive rhabdomyolysis. Acidification of the urine by systemic administration of HCl or NH_4Cl to enhance elimination of weak bases, such as phencyclidine or the amphetamines, is not useful and is potentially dangerous. The technique was abandoned because it does not significantly enhance removal of xenobiotics and is complicated by acidemia.

Peritoneal Dialysis

Peritoneal dialysis is a technique in which a solution is introduced into the abdomen via a catheter so that the patient's peritoneum can act as a membrane across which water, solutes, and xenobiotics are exchanged with the blood. Theoretically, PD enhances the elimination of water-soluble, low-molecular-weight, non–protein-bound xenobiotics with a low V_d. Clearance of xenobiotics by PD is related to the number of exchanges, the dwell time of dialysate, the surface area of the peritoneum, and the molecular weight of the compound. The highest clearances are achieved for xenobiotics with molecular weights below 500 Da. The efficacy of PD is markedly decreased when the patient is hypotensive.

Although PD is a relatively simple method to enhance xenobiotic elimination, it is too slow to be clinically useful.[46] Consequently, PD is not the ECTR of choice unless other more efficient techniques are unavailable. Besides exchange transfusion, it may be the only practical option in small children when experience with extracorporeal techniques in younger age groups is lacking or until a child can be transported to an appropriate center where hemodialysis can be performed.

Hemodialysis

Hemodialysis has been used for 100 years, ever since the discovery by John J. Abel and coworkers that dialysis could remove substantial amounts of salicylates from animals.[1] During conventional hemodialysis, blood and countercurrent dialysate are separated by a semipermeable membrane (*dialyzer*). Xenobiotics then diffuse across the membrane from blood into the dialysate down the concentration gradients (Fig. 6–2). Blood is pumped through one lumen of a temporary dialysis catheter, passed through the machine, and returned to the venous circulation through the second lumen.

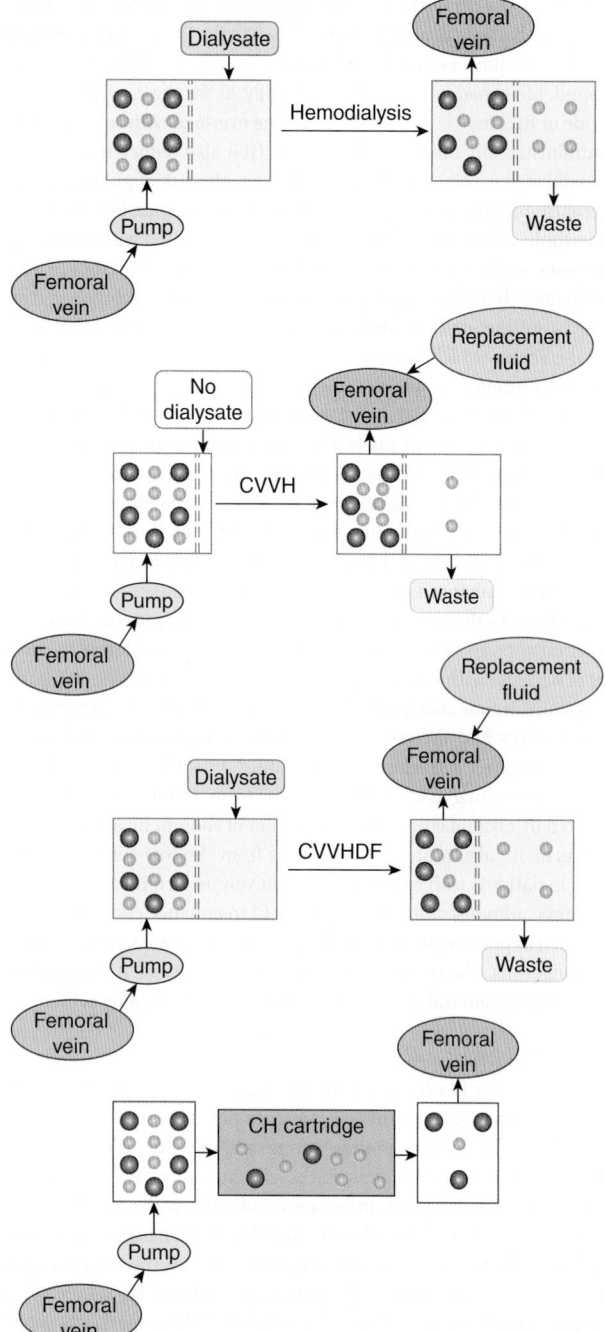

FIGURE 6–2. Comparative schematic layouts of hemodialysis (HD), continuous venovenous hemofiltration (CVVHDF), continuous venovenous hemofiltration with dialysis (CVVHD), and hemoperfusion (HP). *Red circles* are high molecular-weight (MW) xenobiotics, such as methotrexate, whose high MW makes them too large to be removed by HD. *Yellow circles* are low MW diffusible solutes such as urea or methanol. In dialysis, solute moves across a semipermeable membrane (*dashed lines*) from a solution in which it is present in a high concentration (blood) to one in which it is at a low concentration (dialysate). In CVVH and CVVHDF, plasma moves across a similar membrane in response to hydrostatic pressures; replacement fluid must be provided. The latter also uses a dialysate to augment clearance. The availability of blood pumps has made arteriovenous modalities nearly obsolete. Charcoal hemoperfusion (CH) requires movement of blood through a sorbent-containing cartridge and does not include dialysis or hemofiltration.

The utility of hemodialysis for the treatment of patients with toxicity caused by lithium, toxic alcohols, salicylates, or theophylline is unquestionable and is not dealt with here; each of these xenobiotics is described in detail in separate chapters that also review their toxicity and indications for

extracorporeal therapies. This section describes the hemodialysis procedure and its application in general.

Prompt consultation with a nephrologist is always indicated in the case of poisoning with a xenobiotic that might benefit from extracorporeal removal. Annual AAPCC data consistently suggest that some salicylate-related deaths, for example, could have been prevented if hemodialysis had been instituted earlier (Chap. 130).[12] To perform hemodialysis, a nephrologist must be available along with a nurse. The dialysis machine requires preparation, and a vascular access catheter must be inserted. A delay, ranging from one to several hours before hemodialysis can be instituted should be anticipated, particularly during hours when the hospital's dialysis unit, if there is one, is closed. If indicated, modalities of treatment such as fomepizole or ethanol for poisoning with toxic alcohols should be administered, and other modalities to enhance elimination, such as urinary alkalinization or oral MDAC, should be used when appropriate.

The technical details of performing hemodialysis for treatment of patients with poisonings do not differ markedly from those used in the treatment of patients with acute kidney failure. Several technologic advances have enabled improved xenobiotic clearance while limiting side effects and enabling better tolerance of dialysis.

Vascular access is obtained via a double-lumen catheter that is made of silicon, polyethylene, polyurethane, or polytetrafluoroethylene (Teflon). The catheter is usually inserted via the femoral, subclavian, or jugular vein. Whereas the subclavian and internal jugular veins have the added risk of pneumothorax and necessitate radiographic confirmation of catheter position, femoral catheters have increased blood recirculation (ie, lower efficacy of ~10%–15%).[38] Hemostasis after catheter removal is also more easily achieved at the femoral site. Bleeding or thrombosis at the site used for vascular access occur in approximately 5% to 10% of cases but can be minimized by ultrasonographic placement of the catheter and addressed by adequate postprocedure tamponade of the catheter site. Larger catheters now permit blood flow rates that can be as high as 450 to 500 mL/min, although 350 mL/min is sometimes the maximum rate achievable. Nosocomial bacteremia occurs when central catheters are indwelling but are exceedingly rare if they are in place for less than 3 days. This complication is therefore unusual in poisoning in which ECTRs are necessary for relatively short periods of time. Femoral venous lines should always be removed in patients who are mobile and out of bed.

Because modern dialysis membranes also have higher water permeability, computerized ultrafiltration control is necessary. These membranes, composed of polysulfone, polyamide, polyacrylonitrile, and other synthetic polymers, have better biocompatibility than older, cellulose-derived membranes. Better biocompatibility translates into lesser activation of inflammatory mediators and better dialytic tolerance. It is unlikely that better biocompatibility will affect outcomes for dialysis of poisoned patients who require only one or two treatments.

Dialysis membrane composition has also continually evolved. The hollow-fiber dialyzer, almost universally used today, is composed of thousands of blood-filled capillary tubes held together in a bundle and bathed in the machine-generated dialysate. Hemodialysis efficacy for poisonings with low-molecular-weight xenobiotics should improve with the use of larger membranes with larger clearances. "High-flux," synthetic dialyzers have larger pores and increased surface area that allow greater clearance of larger molecules. With the use of high-flux and high-efficiency dialyzers, small molecule clearance has more than doubled, but clearance of larger molecules, such as β_2-microglobulin (molecular weight, 11,800 Da) has increased by a factor of five compared with cellulose-based dialyzers. There are some instances in which high-flux dialyzers might be important in promoting clearance of larger molecules, such as vancomycin (molecular weight, 1,449 Da), which were not readily removed by conventional low-flux membranes.[10] However, the indications for performing hemodialysis to enhance removal of vancomycin and other xenobiotics with higher molecular weights have not been delineated. Nonetheless, a sound pharmacologic basis for the efficacy of dialysis must still be present; no amount of increased clearance will eliminate a xenobiotic with a large V_d or significant protein or tissue binding. However, it is important to consider that clearance rates for many xenobiotics reported in the literature of the 1970s and 1980s significantly underestimate currently achievable clearance rates.

To limit the risk of hemodynamic instability during hemodialysis, the blood lines and artificial kidney (the dialysis membrane) should be primed with an appropriate volume of fluid at the onset of the procedure. Furthermore, for many years, the source of base in dialysate has been sodium bicarbonate rather than sodium acetate; the latter caused hypotension and decreased cardiac output. Computerized machines allow fine control of ultrafiltration rates to limit volume losses; in the past, imprecise calculations and manipulations led to frequent episodes of hypotension. As a result of such innovations, treatment can be delivered in more instances than was previously possible. Hypotension still occurs in some in critically ill patients but can often be corrected with 0.9% sodium chloride, colloid, vasopressors, or inotropes.

Full anticoagulation with heparin is usually required to avoid clotting of the circuit. A typical adult heparin dose is 1,000 to 5,000 units as a bolus followed by 500 to 1,000 units hourly, but lower doses can also be given. Alternatively, in patients at high risk of bleeding (eg, methanol), periodic 0.9% sodium chloride flushes of the dialysis membrane often suffice.

In poisoned patients, hemodialysis is usually performed for 4 to 8 hours but needs to be prolonged in some cases if there is a large poison body burden, as is sometimes necessary for toxic alcohols. Some precautions are needed for the prescription of the dialysis parameters because poisoned patients have different characteristics than chronic kidney disease patients. In particular, serum potassium, phosphorus, and pH can be markedly different. Assuming that the patient's serum potassium concentration is normal, a standard bicarbonate-based dialysate with a potassium concentration of 3 or 4 mEq/L and a calcium concentration of 3 mEq/L, flowing at 600 to 800 mL/min, is indicated. If dialysis is performed in a dialysis unit, the dialysate is a mix of a concentrate with sodium bicarbonate and highly purified water, usually derived by reverse osmosis or deionization. Phosphate can be added to the dialysate bath if needed or administered intravenously if needed. Ultrafiltration is rarely required unless oliguric AKI associated with volume expansion is present. In rare circumstances, when the toxic burden of a xenobiotic is overwhelming, there have been reports of using two dialysis catheters and two independent dialysis circuits to provide maximal xenobiotic clearance.[13] Complications specifically related to the dialysis procedure are rare. Furthermore, centers administering dialysis treatments are increasingly common today, and costs of the procedure are on the decline. For these reasons, if dialysis appears required for survival of a poisoned patient, it should usually be attempted.

Table 6–3 lists the characteristics of xenobiotics that make them amenable to hemodialysis. These requirements greatly reduce the number of xenobiotics that can be expected to be cleared by dialysis. During hemodialysis, clearance of a xenobiotic (Cl_x) can be calculated by:

$$Cl_x = Q_p \times ER$$

where Q_p is the plasma flow rate and ER is the extraction ratio.

$$Q_p = Q_b \times (1 - Hct)$$

where Q_B is blood flow rate and Hct is hematocrit. The ER is a measure of the percentage of xenobiotic passing through the artificial kidney or charcoal hemoperfusion cartridge. This can be calculated as:

$$ER = \frac{C_{in} - C_{out}}{C_{in}} \times 100$$

where C_{in} is the concentration of the xenobiotic in blood entering the system and C_{out} is the concentration in blood leaving the system.
Thus:

$$Cl_X = [Q_p(C_{in} - C_{out})]/C_{in}$$

TABLE 6–3	Characteristics of Xenobiotics That Allow Clearance by Hemodialysis, Hemoperfusion, and Hemofiltration		
For All Three Techniques	**For Hemodialysis**	**For Hemoperfusion**	**For Hemofiltration**
Low V_d (<1 L/kg)	MW <5,000 Da	MW <50,000 Da	MW <40,000 Da
Single-compartment first-order kinetics	Low protein binding	Adsorption by activated charcoal	Low protein binding
Low endogenous clearance (<4 mL/min/kg)			

MW = molecular weight; V_d = volume of distribution.

With the current routine use of high flux membranes, hemodialysis appears, in some cases, as efficient as hemoperfusion to remove certain xenobiotics. Because valproic acid is increasingly prescribed for nonseizure disorders, the incidence of both intentional and unintentional overdoses of this drug will also increase. As discussed previously, valproic acid is largely protein bound at therapeutic serum concentrations. Toxic concentrations saturate protein-binding sites, leading to a higher proportion of unbound drug in the serum and a lower apparent V_d, thereby making the drug more dialyzable. Indeed, several case reports have demonstrated that the clearance of valproic acid with high-flux hemodialysis is at least equivalent to, if not greater than, that of charcoal hemoperfusion.[27,32] Although carbamazepine has a low molecular weight and a V_d that would allow for clearance by hemodialysis, its high protein binding and lack of water solubility are expected to impede the efficacy of hemodialysis. Nonetheless, current evidence shows that high-flux hemodialysis has comparable efficacy to charcoal hemoperfusion for carbamazepine toxicity.[47] Because of its potential efficacy and availability, lower cost, and preferable adverse event profile, high-flux hemodialysis should probably replace charcoal hemoperfusion as the treatment modality of choice when extracorporeal elimination is to be performed. As stated earlier, however, effective clearance is not necessarily a surrogate for improved outcomes.

In addition to removing xenobiotics, hemodialysis can correct acid–base and electrolyte abnormalities such as metabolic acidosis or alkalosis, hyperkalemia, and ECF volume overload. Consequently, hemodialysis is preferred, if not essential, for poisonings characterized by these disorders, especially when clearance rates resulting from hemoperfusion and hemodialysis are relatively similar. Examples include salicylate and toxic alcohol poisoning, which is often associated with metabolic acidosis. Valproic acid toxicity causes hyperammonemia, which is reduced by hemodialysis, possibly contributing to the benefit of the procedure.

A more controversial question is the role of dialysis in the treatment of metformin-associated lactic acidosis. Although debated, present evidence now suggests that metformin intoxication itself induces metabolic acidosis with elevated lactate concentration. Here, the small molecular weight and negligible plasma protein binding of metformin allow for adequate drug removal despite a relatively large V_d.[7] Endogenous renal elimination of metformin is quite high, and dialysis has therefore less impact on total metformin clearance in patients with intact kidney function. In addition, hemodialysis would rapidly correct acidosis via administration of sodium bicarbonate without the complication of volume overload. Clinical improvement with hemodialysis results as much or more from rapid correction of the acidosis as from removal of the drug.

An important unwanted effect of hemodialysis is the removal of therapeutic drugs and antidotes. Doses of these xenobiotics need to be increased during dialysis or administered immediately afterward. Examples include ethanol, fomepizole,[44] N-acetylcysteine,[16] many antibiotics, and water-soluble vitamins.

Hemoperfusion

During hemoperfusion, blood is pumped via a catheter through a cartridge containing a very large surface area of sorbent, either activated charcoal or a resin, on to which the xenobiotic can be directly adsorbed (Fig. 6–2). The activated charcoal sorbent is coated with a very thin layer of polymer membrane such as cellulose acetate (Adsorba; Gambro, Lakewood, CO), heparin-hydrogel, or polyHEMA.[15] The membrane prevents direct contact between blood and sorbent, improves biocompatibility, and helps prevent activated charcoal embolization.

Other adsorptive resins were used for hemoperfusion in the past, such as the synthetic Amberlite XAD-2 and XAD-4 and anion exchange resins such as Dow 1X-2. None of these columns is currently approved or available for use in the United States, but they remain available in other countries. The literature regarding their efficacy is scant and relatively anecdotal. Although in vitro evidence suggests that these resins may have greater adsorptive capacities than activated charcoal, there are few, if any, meaningful comparisons in a clinical setting.

The adsorptive capacity of the cartridge is reduced with use because of deposition of cellular debris and blood proteins and saturation of active sites by the xenobiotic in question. Hemoperfusion is usually performed for 4 to 6 hours at flow rates that can usually not exceed 350 mL/min because of the risk of hemolysis.[51] The technique can be used in adults or children.

The characteristics of xenobiotics that make them amenable to hemoperfusion (Table 6–3) differ slightly from those for hemodialysis in that hemoperfusion is not as limited by plasma protein binding, although this is less true with the advent of new dialysis membranes, which now permit removal of significant amounts of highly bound xenobiotics. Some xenobiotics are poorly adsorbed by activated charcoal, including the alcohols, lithium, and many metals (Antidotes in Depth: A1), making hemoperfusion inappropriate in their management.[15] Hemodialysis and hemoperfusion are sometimes combined to optimize clearance (Fig. 6–3), with greater removal rates than with either procedure alone, although it is unclear if this marginal benefit outweighs the cost and added complication rates of this combination.

Added to the questionable benefits of hemoperfusion, multiple limitations make their use less attractive compared with hemodialysis. A practical problem limiting the use of charcoal hemoperfusion is the availability of the cartridges. In a survey of New York City hospital dialysis units taking

911 calls, only 10 of 34 units had cartridges.[54] Saturation of the cartridge is apparent within 1 hour of use and markedly decreases absorptive capacity at 2 hours, but no such decreased performance is apparent with hemodialyzers. Compared with hemodialysis, patients must be anticoagulated with greater amounts of heparin. The cartridges are expensive (~$600 compared with the maximal cost for a high-flux dialysis membrane at less than $40), especially if cartridges are replaced regularly. Some have expiration dates, limiting their shelf life. Others have an indefinite shelf life but must be autoclaved before use, which will likely delay their use in an emergency. Complications of hemoperfusion are more common than with hemodialysis: thrombocytopenia, leukopenia, and hypocalcemia.[55] Finally, hemoperfusion cannot correct acid–base or electrolyte abnormalities and cannot provide ultrafiltration if volume overload occurs.

Although hemoperfusion has historically been considered the preferred method to enhance the elimination of carbamazepine, phenobarbital, phenytoin, and theophylline (Table 6–4), older comparisons of hemodialysis and hemoperfusion clearance rates are now obsolete. The most frequent indication for charcoal hemoperfusion in the past was theophylline toxicity, and theophylline is rarely used today in the treatment of obstructive lung disease and asthma and is consequently less often implicated in acute and chronic poisoning. In a review of the AAPCC annual data, theophylline was the most common xenobiotic for which hemoperfusion was reported from 1985 to 2000, but carbamazepine became the most frequent xenobiotic removed by hemoperfusion after 2001.[18,28] As in the case of hemodialysis, doses of drugs used therapeutically will need to be increased if they are removed by hemoperfusion.

Liver Support Devices

A newer concept for poisonings is that of liver support devices or liver dialysis. These procedures are currently available in the United States, mostly for the treatment of liver failure. Several techniques have been developed; the following three are the most common. (1) Single-pass albumin dialysis (SPAD) is similar to hemodialysis but has albumin added to the dialysate in counter-directional flow, which is then discarded after passing through a filter. (2) The Molecular Adsorbents Recirculation System (MARS) is identical to SPAD, but the albumin-enhanced dialysate (with the adsorbed xenobiotics) is itself recycled after going through another dialysis circuit and through both resin and activated charcoal cartridges. (3) The Prometheus system is a device that combines albumin adsorption with high-flux hemodialysis after selective filtration of the albumin fraction through a polysulfone filter. In all of these techniques, the dialysate bathing the fibers contains human serum albumin that binds the xenobiotic of interest. A steep concentration gradient from blood to dialysate is established so that even highly protein-bound xenobiotics can be removed from the plasma. The membrane is impermeable to albumin, which remains in the dialysate.

These extracorporeal devices are all able to remove protein-bound xenobiotics, but their use in poisoning remains limited to rare case reports. These devices are mostly used in patients with hepatic encephalopathy and liver failure and as a bridge to hepatic transplantation.[42] In toxicology, their use is mostly described in hepatic failure following toxicity of APAP or *Amanita* toxin exposure (Chap. 117). The reasons why the procedure might offer significant benefits are not completely understood, although it does remove both water-soluble and protein-bound compounds, such as bile salts and aromatic amino acids, to account for the therapeutic advantage in hepatic failure. Specific uses for liver support devices for elimination enhancement has been described in poisoning with phenytoin,[53] theophylline,[33] valproic acid,[11] and *Amanita* mushrooms.[31] Whether these relatively expensive (in excess of $10,000 per treatment), complicated, and nonspecific procedures would offer benefit in a handful of instances in which protein binding limits removal of xenobiotics is not known.

Hemofiltration

Hemofiltration is the movement of plasma across a semipermeable membrane in response to an active hydrostatic pressure by convection. In pure

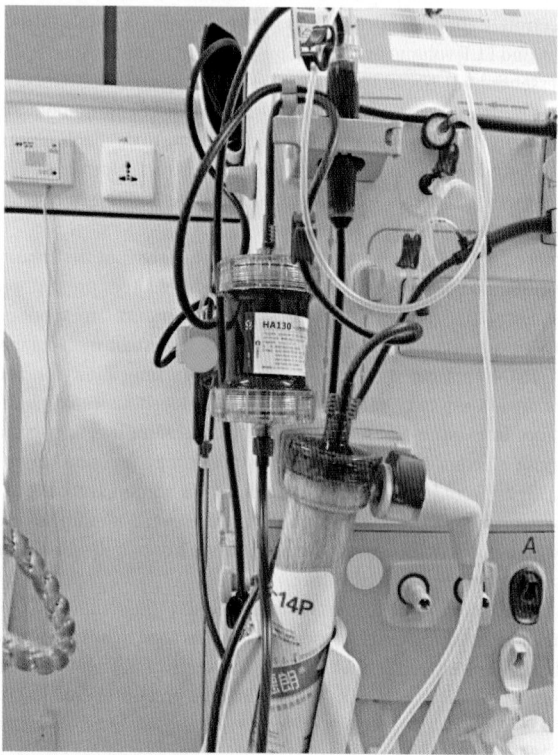

FIGURE 6–3. Example of a hemodialyzer (*orange circle*) used in series with a charcoal cartridge (*green circle*) for a paraquat poisoning.

TABLE 6–4   Properties of Xenobiotics Grouped by Benefit of Extracorporeal Techniques for Elimination

Xenobiotic	MW (Da)	Water Soluble	V_d (L/Kg)	Protein Binding (%)	Endogenous Clearance (mL/min/kg)	Comments
Clinically Beneficial						
Bromide	35	Yes	0.7	0	0.1	Falsely elevated chloride measurement
Caffeine	194	Yes	0.6	36	1.3	Hyperglycemia, hypokalemia, metabolic acidosis
Ethylene glycol	62	Yes	0.6	0	2.0	Oxaluria, kidney failure
Diethylene glycol	106	Yes	0.5	0	NA	Kidney failure
Isopropanol	60	Yes	0.6	0	1.2	No acidosis, ketosis and ketonuria
Lithium	7	Yes	0.8	0	0.4	Low anion gap, low Cl in kidney failure
Metformin	129	Yes	3–5	0	8	Very low Cl in kidney failure
Methanol	32	Yes	0.6	0	0.7	Risk of CNS hemorrhage
Propylene glycol	76	Yes	0.6	0	1.7	Lactic acidosis
Salicylate	138	Yes	0.2	50 (saturable)	0.9	Cl and protein binding ↓, with ↑ dose; HD also corrects electrolytes and acid–base disturbance
Theophylline	180	Yes	0.5	56	0.7	HP and HD can also be combined
Valproic acid	144	Yes	0.2	90 (saturable)	0.1	↑ Concentrations associated with ↓ % protein binding, HD also clears ammonia when elevated
Possibly Clinically Beneficial						
Acetaminophen	151	Yes	0.9	30	2.0	For coma and mitochondrial injury
Amatoxins	373–990	Yes	0.3	0	2.7–6.2	Possibly effective if performed within the first 24 h of exposure
Aminoglycosides	>500	Yes	0.3	1.5	<10	Cl ↓ with kidney failure
Atenolol	255	Yes	1.0	2.5	<5	Useful if Cl ↓ caused by kidney failure
Carbamazepine	236	No	1.4	74	1.3	Cl↑ in patients on long-term therapy
Disopyramide	340	No	0.6	1.2	1.6	Protein binding ↓ as concentration ↑
Fluoride	19	Yes	0.3	50	2.5	Hypocalcemia may be improved by HD
Methotrexate	454	Yes	0.6	50	1.5	Urine alkalinization is indicated, good antidote
Paraquat	186	Yes	1.0	6	24.0	Tight tissue binding precludes efficacy unless initiated early
Phenobarbital	232	No	0.5	24	0.1	Only for prolonged coma
Phenytoin	252	No	0.6	90	0.3	Cl ↓ as dose ↑; HD efficient

CL = clearance; CNS = central nervous system; HD = hemodialysis; HF = hemofiltration; HP = hemoperfusion; MW = molecular weight; NA = not available; V_d = volume of distribution.

hemofiltration, there is no dialysate solution on the other side of the dialysis membrane (Fig. 6–2). Molecules are transported across the membrane with plasma water, a mechanism known as *convective transport* or *bulk flow*. The ECF volume status of the patient determines whether replacement of all or some of the filtered plasma with physiologic electrolyte solution (RL or other commercially available preparations) is indicated. Although this technique can be done intermittently using a hemodialysis machine, it has been adapted for use in ICUs as a continuous form of treatment, particularly when removal of ECF is indicated. Hemofiltration is classically administered continuously for patients with AKI, although there is growing interest of this technique as a chronic treatment for patients with end-stage kidney disease. Compared with hemodialysis (diffusion), hemofiltration favors the elimination of larger xenobiotics (eg, myoglobin, molecular weight = 17,000 Da) but is slightly less performant for the removal of smaller molecules.[6] Because most xenobiotics of interest in toxicology are smaller than 1,000 Da, it is unclear if hemofiltration has any advantage over pure hemodialysis. Solute clearance can be significantly enhanced by combining both diffusion and convection, a technique known as *hemodiafiltration*. Table 6–3 summarizes the properties of xenobiotics that make them amenable to hemofiltration.

Continuous Techniques

Continuous techniques are referred to collectively as modalities of *continuous renal replacement therapy* (CRRT). The blood flow and effluent flow are lower than those administered during intermittent techniques, so the achievable xenobiotic clearance is lower. However, what they lack in removal rates is compensated by longer administration (they can be performed without interruption for several days).

For all of these procedures, the patient usually must be fully anticoagulated, with either heparin or with citrate. Continuous techniques include *continuous venovenous hemofiltration* (CVVH), *continuous venovenous hemodialysis* (CVVHD), and *continuous venovenous hemodiafiltration* (CVVHDF) (Fig. 6–2). These have largely replaced arteriovenous techniques, which did not require a blood pump but presented a high incidence of thrombotic and bleeding complications at the catheter site.

There are several possible advantages of continuous modalities; the major benefits are a slower fluid removal rate and solute flux, which are pertinent for acutely ill patients who are hemodynamically unstable, fluid overloaded, and oliguric. Another practical advantage of CRRT is that the procedure is usually done in ICUs by ICU nurses, and when available in such units, it might not require dialysis personnel. Familiarity of ICU staff with the procedure is critical to its availability when needed; it is most likely to be used effectively in hospitals with higher incidence rates of AKI. In clinical toxicology, CRRT is sometimes used after hemodialysis or hemoperfusion to further remove a xenobiotic, especially those that distribute slowly from tissue-binding sites or from the intracellular compartment.[41]

However, the rate of removal with this form of therapy is considerably inferior to that achieved by intermittent hemodialysis or hemoperfusion and so is not ideal for severely poisoned patients.[46] Patients who can tolerate slower clearance rates may not require this enhanced elimination therapy at all. It is true that a prolonged slower treatment can prevent a rebound of the xenobiotic's serum concentrations that commonly occurs after high-efficiency techniques. However, rebound occurs at the expense of diminishing xenobiotic concentration in the deeper and potentially toxic compartments, as has been shown nearly 50 years ago for lithium.[2] Rebound may therefore not be worrisome and may in fact be desirable while providing for an additional opportunity to remove more xenobiotic with hemodialysis. Rebound should be distinguished from increasing plasma values caused by ongoing intestinal absorption of the xenobiotic because these two entities do not carry the same prognostic relevance.

For these reasons, intermittent hemodialysis is preferable over CRRT for removal of xenobiotics.[25] Continuous modalities are best suited for hemodynamically unstable patients who require net ultrafiltration, although this situation is infrequent unless oliguric AKI is present. Of the guidelines published by EXTRIP to date, none has yet considered any CRRT technique superior to hemodialysis or the first choice of therapy when hemodialysis is available.

Plasmapheresis and Exchange Transfusion

Plasmapheresis and exchange transfusion are intended to eliminate xenobiotics that are either extremely large (>100,000 Da, typified by immunoglobulins) or extensively protein bound. The xenobiotic to be eliminated should also have limited endogenous metabolism to make pheresis or exchange worthwhile.[30] By removing plasma proteins, both techniques offer the consequent potential benefit of removal of protein-bound xenobiotics such as *Amanita* toxins, thyroxine, vincristine, monoclonal antibodies, or complexes of digoxin and antidigoxin antibodies. However, there is little evidence that either technique affects the clinical course and prognosis of a patient poisoned by any of these or other xenobiotics.

Pheresis is particularly expensive, and both pheresis and exchange transfusion expose the patient to the risks of infection with plasma- or blood-borne diseases. Replacement of the removed plasma during plasmapheresis can be accomplished with fresh-frozen plasma, albumin, or combinations of both. The former is associated with hypersensitivity reactions, such as fever, urticaria, wheezing, and hypotension.

A different setting in which exchange transfusion may be an appropriate technique is in the management of small infants or neonates in whom dialysis or hemoperfusion is often technically difficult or impossible, such as in the neonatal population. In premature neonates, a single volume exchange appeared to alleviate manifestations of aminophylline toxicity.[45] The therapy has been successfully used to treat other pediatric patients with poisonings, including severe salicylism.[40]

OTHER TECHNIQUES TO ENHANCE ELIMINATION

Further discussions of some of the techniques to enhance elimination that are not discussed here may be found in Special Considerations: SC7 (cerebrospinal fluid drainage and replacement), Antidotes in Depth: A22 (toxin-specific antibodies), and Chap. 93 (chelation). All of these techniques have

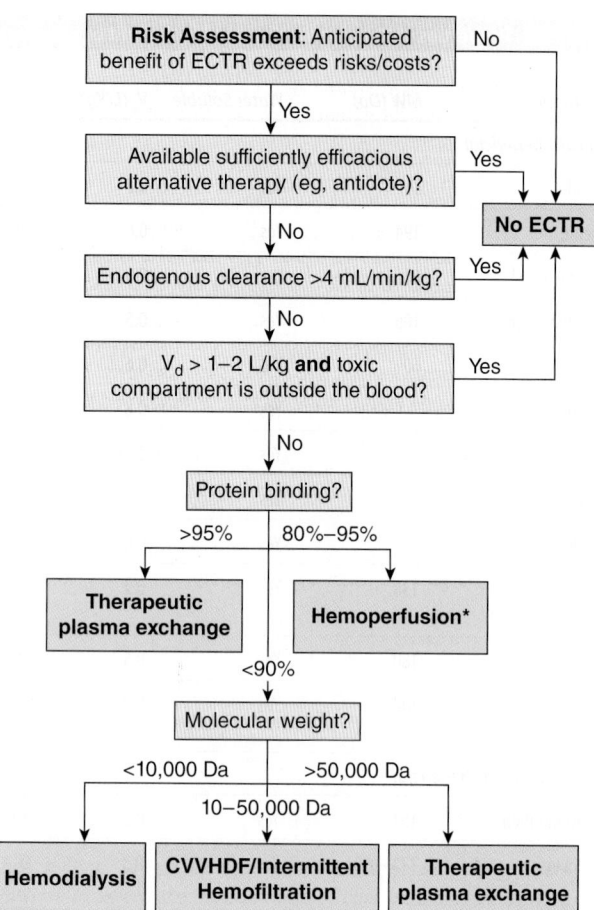

FIGURE 6–4. Clinical approach to consideration of using an extracorporeal treatment (ECTR) in poisoning situation. This assessment requires analysis of the patient's condition, the specific xenobiotic, alternative treatments, molecular and toxikinetic characteristics, and available modalities. * If the xenobiotic is adsorbed to activated charcoal, hemoperfusion is preferred, it not then evaluate based on molecular weight.

limited and very specific indications. A summarized approach to the use of ECTRs is shown in Fig. 6–4.

TOXICOLOGY OF HEMODIALYSIS

Unlike patients who receive acute hemodialysis once or twice in the management of poisoning, patients with chronic kidney failure are repeatedly exposed to large volumes of water derived from municipal reservoirs during the course of their hemodialysis treatments. If an "average" regimen consists of three treatments of 4 hours each week, with dialysate flows of 800 mL/min, patients will be exposed to nearly 600 L of water separated from them only by a semipermeable membrane designed to allow solute passage in either direction. Problems with dialysate generation therefore have the potential to be lethal to this population by exposing them to significant quantities of toxins. There are two potential sources of dialysate contamination: the municipal reservoirs and water treatment plants and the dialysis unit.[48]

Contamination of dialysate from the municipal water supply may occur as a result of xenobiotic runoff into reservoirs or as a result of inadvertent or intentional addition of a chemical by the municipality. Chlorine and chloramine are frequently added to municipal water supplies to control bacterial populations. However, chlorine may combine with nitrogenous compounds and form chloramine, which causes nausea, vomiting, methemoglobinemia, and hemolytic anemia.[57] Chloramine has been blamed for decreased bone marrow sensitivity to erythropoietin. Aluminum is present in some municipal water supplies, and before it was recognized as a problem, aluminum led to encephalopathy characterized by seizures, myoclonus, and dementia, as well as osteomalacia and microcytic anemia.

Water from the municipal supply may be treated with a variety of ways. It firsts enter the dialysis unit and is treated with a water softener to remove calcium and magnesium. It is then run through an activated charcoal bed to adsorb chloramine. The potential toxicity (hemolysis and death) from this compound has caused the Association for the Advancement of Medical Instrumentation (AAMI), which sets the standards for performance of dialysis, to mandate a redundancy in the carbon beds; when the active sites in one carbon bed are exhausted, a second will ensure that no toxicity will occur. Most commonly, water for dialysate is then generated by reverse osmosis, a process that requires that water, in response to applied hydrostatic pressure (and against the osmotic gradient), cross a membrane that is relatively impermeable to solutes, leaving them behind. Alternatively, but less commonly, water can also be purified using deionization, a technique that runs water over an exchange resin, releasing hydroxyl ions in exchange for charged species in the water.

Current requirements are that water be highly purified but not sterile, because bacteria cannot cross from the dialysate into the blood. However, small quantities of endotoxin (molecular weight, 5–15,000 Da) can cross, particularly in situations that include the use of high-flux membranes. Endotoxin is suspected of contributing to activation of circulating cytokines, malnutrition, fever, and other syndromes such as carpal tunnel syndrome, which are associated with chronic inflammation. Recommendations for the frequency of testing for endotoxin and the maximum amounts of endotoxin tolerated are established by the AAMI and are continually debated and continue to become more stringent. Water contamination should especially be suspected when multiple dialysis patients experience similar symptoms nearly simultaneously. General water chemistry and microbiology testing is mandated at regular intervals. Defects in any aspect of the hemodialysis apparatus with insufficient control and monitoring may lead to catastrophic outbreaks in dialysis units.[5] Similarly, nationwide aluminum contamination of dialysates for PD has been reported.[34]

SUMMARY

- Urinary alkalinization and many of the other techniques listed in Table 6–1 can be instituted quickly in the emergency department.
- The extracorporeal methods of xenobiotic removal, including hemodialysis, hemoperfusion, and continuous renal replacement therapies, all require consultation with a nephrologist, intensivist, or both.
- Timely use of these techniques requires mobilization of a competent team and preparation of the requisite equipment.
- Rapid identification of a toxic exposure for which these techniques are appropriate and the presence of more ominous prognostic features should lead to prompt notification of the appropriate consult services so that application of these techniques can proceed in an expeditious manner.
- The applicability of these techniques to new xenobiotics should be considered based on the principles discussed so that these and newer treatment modalities are not used indiscriminately.
- The literature regarding these techniques in general, and for the treatment of specific xenobiotic exposures in particular, should be read critically and with appropriate skepticism.

Acknowledgment
Daniel Matalon, MD, contributed to this chapter in previous editions.

REFERENCES

1. Abel JJ, et al. On the removal of diffusible substances from the circulating blood by dialysis. *Trans Assoc Am Physicians*. 1913;58:51-54.
2. Amdisen A, Skjoldborg H. Haemodialysis for lithium poisoning. *Lancet*. 1969;2(7613):213.
3. Anseeuw K, et al. Extracorporeal treatment in phenytoin poisoning: systematic review and recommendations from the EXTRIP (Extracorporeal Treatments in Poisoning) Workgroup. *Am J Kidney Dis*. 2016;67:187-197.
4. Bailey B, McGuigan M. Comparison of patients hemodialyzed for lithium poisoning and those for whom dialysis was recommended by PCC but not done: what lesson can we learn? *Clin Nephrol*. 2000;54:388-392.
5. Berend K, et al. Prosecution after an outbreak of subacute aluminum intoxication in a hemodialysis center. *Leg Med (Tokyo)*. 2004;6:1-10.
6. Bouchard J, et al. Principles and operational parameters to optimize poison removal with extracorporeal treatments. *Semin Dial*. 2014;27:371-380.
7. Calello DP, et al. Extracorporeal treatment for metformin poisoning: systematic review and recommendations from the Extracorporeal Treatments in Poisoning Workgroup. *Crit Care Med*. 2015;43:1716-1730.
8. Chan H, et al. Recovery from toxicity associated with high-dose methotrexate: prognostic factors. *Cancer Treat Rep*. 1977;61:797-804.
9. Decker BS, et al. Extracorporeal treatment for lithium poisoning: systematic review and recommendations from the EXTRIP Workgroup. *Clin J Am Soc Nephrol*. 2015;10:875-887.
10. Decker BS, et al. Vancomycin pharmacokinetics and pharmacodynamics during short daily hemodialysis. *Clin J Am Soc Nephrol*. 2010;5:1981-1987.
11. Dichtwald S, et al. Molecular adsorbent recycling system therapy in the treatment of acute valproic acid intoxication. *Isr Med Assoc J*. 2010;12:307-308.
12. Fertel BS, et al. The underutilization of hemodialysis in patients with salicylate poisoning. *Kidney Int*. 2009;75:1349-1353.
13. Friesecke S, et al. Combined renal replacement therapy for severe metformin-induced lactic acidosis. *Nephrol Dial Transplant*. 2006;21:2038-2039.
14. Garella S. Extracorporeal techniques in the treatment of exogenous intoxications. *Kidney Int*. 1988;33:735-754.
15. Ghannoum M, et al. Hemoperfusion for the treatment of poisoning: technology, determinants of poison clearance, and application in clinical practice. *Semin Dial*. 2014;27:350-361.
16. Ghannoum M, et al. Massive acetaminophen overdose: effect of hemodialysis on acetaminophen and acetylcysteine kinetics. *Clin Toxicol (Phila)*. 2016;54:519-522.
17. Ghannoum M, et al. Extracorporeal treatment for valproic acid poisoning: systematic review and recommendations from the EXTRIP workgroup. *Clin Toxicol (Phila)*. 2015;53:454-465.
18. Ghannoum M, et al. Practice trends in the use of extracorporeal treatments for poisoning in four countries. *Semin Dial*. 2016;29:71-80.
19. Ghannoum M, et al. Successful treatment of lithium toxicity with sodium polystyrene sulfonate: a retrospective cohort study. *Clin Toxicol (Phila)*. 2010;48:34-41.
20. Ghannoum M, et al. Extracorporeal treatment for thallium poisoning: recommendations from the EXTRIP Workgroup. *Clin J Am Soc Nephrol*. 2012;7:1682-1690.
21. Ghannoum M, et al. Blood purification in toxicology: nephrology's ugly duckling. *Adv Chronic Kidney Dis*. 2011;18:160-166.
22. Ghannoum M, et al. A stepwise approach for the management of poisoning with extracorporeal treatments. *Semin Dial*. 2014;27:362-370.
23. Ghannoum M, et al. Extracorporeal treatment for theophylline poisoning: systematic review and recommendations from the EXTRIP workgroup. *Clin Toxicol (Phila)*. 2015;53:215-229.
24. Ghannoum M, et al. Extracorporeal treatment for carbamazepine poisoning: systematic review and recommendations from the EXTRIP workgroup. *Clin Toxicol (Phila)*. 2014;52:993-1004.
25. Goodman JW, Goldfarb DS. The role of continuous renal replacement therapy in the treatment of poisoning. *Semin Dial*. 2006;19:402-407.
26. Gosselin S, et al. Extracorporeal treatment for acetaminophen poisoning: recommendations from the EXTRIP workgroup. *Clin Toxicol (Phila)*. 2014;52:856-867.
27. Hicks LK, McFarlane PA. Valproic acid overdose and haemodialysis. *Nephrol Dial Transplant*. 2001;16:1483-1486.
28. Holubek WJ, et al. Use of hemodialysis and hemoperfusion in poisoned patients. *Kidney Int*. 2008;74:1327-1334.
29. Juurlink DN, et al. Extracorporeal treatment for salicylate poisoning: systematic review and recommendations from the EXTRIP Workgroup. *Ann Emerg Med*. 2015;66:165-181.
30. Kale PB, et al. Evaluation of plasmapheresis in the treatment of an acute overdose of carbamazepine. *Ann Pharmacother*. 1993;27:866-870.
31. Kantola T, et al. Early molecular adsorbents recirculating system treatment of *Amanita* mushroom poisoning. *Ther Apher Dial*. 2009;13:399-403.
32. Kielstein JT, et al. Efficiency of high-flux hemodialysis in the treatment of valproic acid intoxication. *J Toxicol Clin Toxicol*. 2003;41:873-876.
33. Korsheed S, et al. Treatment of severe theophylline poisoning with the molecular adsorbent recirculating system (MARS). *Nephrol Dial Transplant*. 2007;22:969-970.
34. Lavergne V, et al. Risk factors and consequences of hyperaluminemia in a peritoneal dialysis cohort. *Perit Dial Int*. 2012;32:645-651.
35. Lavergne V, et al. Why are we still dialyzing overdoses to tricyclic antidepressants? A subanalysis of the NPDS database. *Semin Dial*. 2016;29:403-409.
36. Lavergne V, et al. The EXTRIP (Extracorporeal Treatments In Poisoning) workgroup: guideline methodology. *Clin Toxicol*. 2012;50:403-413.
37. Lavergne V, et al. Guidelines for reporting case studies on extracorporeal treatments in poisonings: methodology. *Semin Dial*. 2014;27:407-414.
38. Leblanc M, et al. Blood recirculation in temporary central catheters for acute hemodialysis. *Clin Nephrol*. 1996;45:315-319.
39. Mactier R, et al. Extracorporeal treatment for barbiturate poisoning: recommendations from the EXTRIP Workgroup. *Am J Kidney Dis*. 2014;64:347-358.
40. Manikian A, et al. Exchange transfusion in severe infant salicylism. *Vet Hum Toxicol*. 2002;44:224-227.

41. Meyer RJ, et al. Hemodialysis followed by continuous hemofiltration for treatment of lithium intoxication in children. *Am J Kidney Dis.* 2001;37:1044-1047.

42. Mitzner SR, et al. Extracorporeal detoxification using the molecular adsorbent recirculating system for critically ill patients with liver failure. *J Am Soc. Nephrol.* 2001;12(suppl 17): S75-S82.

43. Mowry JB, et al. Extracorporeal treatment for digoxin poisoning: systematic review and recommendations from the EXTRIP Workgroup. *Clin Toxicol (Phila).* 2016;54:103-114.

44. Mowry JB, et al. The effect of high flux hemodialysis on serum fomepizole concentrations. *Clin Toxicol (Phila).* 2005;43:774-775.

45. Osborn HH, et al. Theophylline toxicity in a premature neonate—elimination kinetics of exchange transfusion. *J Toxicol Clin Toxicol.* 1993;31(4):639-644.

46. Ouellet G, et al. Available extracorporeal treatments for poisoning: overview and limitations. *Semin Dial.* 2014;27:342-349.

47. Payette A, et al. Carbamazepine poisoning treated by multiple extracorporeal treatments. *Clin Nephrol.* 2015;83:184-188.

48. Pontoriero G, et al. The quality of dialysis water. *Nephrol Dial Transplant.* 2003;18(suppl 7): vii21-25; discussion vii56.

49. Proudfoot AT, et al. Does urine alkalinization increase salicylate elimination? If so, why? *Toxicol Rev.* 2003;22:129-136.

50. Proudfoot AT, et al. Position paper on urine alkalinization. *J Toxicol Clin Toxicol.* 2004;42:1-26.

51. Rahman MH, et al. Acute hemolysis with acute renal failure in a patient with valproic acid poisoning treated with charcoal hemoperfusion. *Hemodial Int.* 2006; 10:256-259.

52. Roberts DM, et al. Recommendations for the role of extracorporeal treatments in the management of acute methanol poisoning: a systematic review and consensus statement. *Crit Care Med.* 2015;43:461-472.

53. Sen S, et al. Treatment of phenytoin toxicity by the molecular adsorbents recirculating system (MARS). *Epilepsia.* 2003;44:265-267.

54. Shalkham AS, et al. The availability and use of charcoal hemoperfusion in the treatment of poisoned patients. *Am J Kidney Dis.* 2006;48:239-241.

55. Shannon MW. Comparative efficacy of hemodialysis and hemoperfusion in severe theophylline intoxication. *Acad Emerg Med.* 1997;4:674-678.

56. Vale J, et al. Position statement and practice guidelines on the use of multi-dose activated charcoal in the treatment of acute poisoning. American Academy of Clinical Toxicology; European Association of Poisons Centres and Clinical Toxicologists. *J Toxicol Clin Toxicol.* 1999;37:731-751.

57. Ward DM. Chloramine removal from water used in hemodialysis. *Adv Ren Replace Ther.* 1996;3:337-347.

58. Yates C, et al. Extracorporeal treatment for tricyclic antidepressant poisoning: recommendations from the EXTRIP Workgroup. *Semin Dial.* 2014;27:381-389.

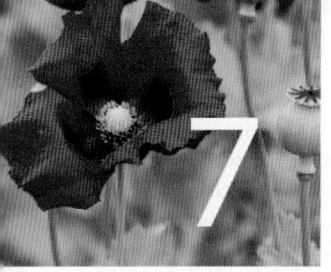

7 LABORATORY PRINCIPLES

Ami M. Grunbaum and Petrie M. Rainey

Clinical toxicology addresses the harm caused by acute and chronic exposures to excessive amounts of a xenobiotic. Detecting the presence or measuring the concentration of toxic xenobiotics is the primary activity of the analytical toxicology laboratory. Such testing is closely intertwined with therapeutic drug monitoring (TDM), in which drug concentrations are measured as an aid to optimizing drug dosing regimens. Another offshoot of laboratory toxicology that has become increasingly requested is testing for drugs of abuse.

The goal of the hospital toxicology laboratory is to provide clinically relevant test results to support the management of poisoned or intoxicated patients.

To be of optimal clinical value, the laboratory service requires both an appropriate test menu that meets quality criteria, as well as the ability to provide results within a clinically relevant time frame.

RECOMMENDATIONS FOR ROUTINELY AVAILABLE TOXICOLOGY TESTS

Despite a common focus, there is remarkable variability in the range of tests offered by clinical toxicologic laboratories. Test menus range from batched testing for routinely monitored drugs and common drugs of abuse to around-the-clock availability of a broad arsenal of assays with the potential to identify thousands of compounds. For most laboratories, it would be entirely impractical and inefficient to attempt to provide a full range of analyses in real-time because of cost constraints, staffing issues, and the required technical expertise.

Decisions on the test menu and turn-around times (TATs) to be offered should be made by the laboratory director in consultation with the medical toxicologists and other clinicians who will use the service. They should take into account regional patterns of the use of both licit and illicit xenobiotics and exposure to environmental xenobiotics as well as the available resources and competing priorities.

The essential questions that need to be addressed include:

1. Which tests should be available?
2. Do the assays require qualitative or quantitative results?
3. What specimen matrices will be tested (eg, blood, urine, other body fluid)?
4. When and how should the specimen be obtained?
5. What is the acceptable TAT?

From a consensus process that involved clinical biochemists, medical toxicologists, forensic toxicologists, and emergency physicians, the National Academy of Clinical Biochemists (NACB) recommended that hospital laboratories provide a two-tiered approach to toxicology testing.[27] In the United Kingdom, the National Poisons Information Service and the Association of Clinical Biochemists recommend a nearly identical list of tests, omitting the anticonvulsants.[21]

Tier 1 (Table 7–1) includes basic tests that should be offered locally because of their clinical relevance and the technical feasibility of rapid TATs. As with all laboratory tests, they should be selectively ordered based on the history, clinical presentation, and other relevant factors and not simply ordered as a general screening panel for all suspected cases of poisoning. The recommended TATs for most of the tests listed was 1 hour or less.

Unfortunately, on-site testing for the toxic alcohols is often difficult because of the complexity of their chromatography-based methodologies. As a compromise, a TAT of 2 to 4 hours was deemed acceptable. Another option is to calculate the serum osmolar gap (see later), which provides some important clinical information regarding the toxic alcohols.

TABLE 7–1 Tier-1 (Basic) Toxicology Assays	
Quantitative Serum Assays	**Qualitative Urine Assays**
Acetaminophen	Amphetamines
Alcohols (ethanol, methanol, ethylene glycol)	Barbiturates
Carbamazepine	Cocaine
Cooximetry (carboxyhemoglobin, methemoglobin, oxygen saturation)	Opiates
Digoxin	Phencyclidine
Iron (plus transferrin or iron-binding capacity)	Tricyclic antidepressants
Lithium	
Phenobarbital (if urine barbiturates positive)	
Phenytoin	
Salicylates	
Theophylline	
Valproic acid	

Data from Wu AH, McKay C, Broussard LA, et al: National academy of clinical biochemistry laboratory medicine practice guidelines: recommendations for the use of laboratory tests to support poisoned patients who present to the emergency department. Clin Chem. 2003 Mar;49(3):357-379.

Although the consensus for the menu of serum assays was generally excellent, there was less agreement as to the need for qualitative urine assays. This was largely a result of issues of poor sensitivity and specificity, poor correlation with clinical effects, and infrequent alteration of patient management. Although these were potential issues for all of the urine drug tests, they led to explicit omission of tests for tetrahydrocannabinol (THC) and benzodiazepines from the recommended list despite their widespread use. The results for THC have little value in managing patients with acute clinical concerns, and tests for benzodiazepines have an inadequate spectrum of detection. Testing for amphetamines, propoxyphene, and phencyclidine (PCP) is only recommended in areas where use is prevalent. It is also suggested that the diagnosis of tricyclic antidepressant (TCA) toxicity not be based solely on the results of a urine screening immunoassay because a number of other drugs cross-react. The significance of TCA results should always be correlated with electrocardiographic and clinical findings. The only urine test included in the United Kingdom guidelines was a spot test for paraquat.[21] Paraquat testing was omitted in the NACB guidelines because of a very low incidence of paraquat exposure in North America.[27]

The NACB guidelines also recommend additional tier 2 testing in selected patients whose clinical presentations are compatible with poisoning but remain undiagnosed and are not improving. In general, such testing should not be ordered until the patient is stabilized and input is obtained from a medical toxicologist or poison control center. This second level of testing may be provided directly by referral to a reference laboratory or a regional toxicology center. Such a system has the advantages of avoiding costly duplication of services and providing a pooled workload to enable the development of technical expertise for complex, low-volume methodologies.

Many physicians order a broad-spectrum toxicology panel, or a "tox screen" for a poisoned or overdosed patient if one is readily available, but only 7 % of clinical laboratories provide relatively comprehensive urine toxicology testing (as estimated from proficiency testing data).[6] Although broad-spectrum toxicology screens can identify many xenobiotics present in poisoned or overdosed patients, the results of broad-spectrum screens infrequently have altered management or outcomes.[4,14,15]

The extent to which the NACB recommendations are being followed may be estimated from the numbers of laboratories participating in various types of proficiency testing. Result summaries from the 2017 series of proficiency surveys administered by the College of American Pathologists suggest that among laboratories that offer routine clinical testing, only about 40% offer quantitative assays for lithium, phenobarbital and theophylline; 50% to 60% offer assays for acetaminophen (APAP), carbamazepine, carboxyhemoglobin, methemoglobin, ethanol, salicylates, and valproic acid; 60% to 70% offer digoxin, iron, and transferrin or iron-binding capacity; and 70% to 80% offer screening tests for drugs of abuse in urine.[6]

About 7% of laboratories participated in proficiency testing for a full range of toxicology services. These full-service laboratories typically offer quantitative assays for additional therapeutic drugs, particularly TCAs, as well as assays that are designated as broad-spectrum or comprehensive toxicology screens. About 7% of laboratories participated in proficiency testing for a full range of toxicology services. These full-service laboratories typically offer quantitative assays for additional therapeutic drugs, particularly TCAs, as well as assays that are designated as broad-spectrum or comprehensive toxicology screens. Only about 2% of laboratories offer testing for volatile alcohols other than ethanol; most of these also offer testing for ethylene glycol.[6]

Although relatively few laboratories offer a wide range of in-house testing, most laboratories offer a limited toxicology panel and send out specimens to reference laboratories that offer large toxicology menus. The TAT for such "send-out" tests ranges from a few hours to several days, depending on the proximity of the reference laboratory and the type of test requested.

Even in full-service toxicology laboratories, the test menus vary substantially from institution to institution. Larger laboratories typically offer one or more broad-spectrum test panels, often referred to as "tox screens." There is as much variety in the range of xenobiotics detected by various toxicologic screens as there is in the total menu of toxicologic tests. Routinely available tests are usually listed in a printed or online laboratory manual. Some laboratories with comprehensive services offer locally developed chromatographic assays for additional xenobiotics that are not listed. Testing that is sent to a reference laboratory is often not listed in the laboratory manual. The best way to determine if a particular xenobiotic can be detected or quantitated is to ask the director or supervisor of the toxicology or clinical chemistry section because laboratory clerical staff are likely only to be aware of tests listed in the manual.

USING THE TOXICOLOGY LABORATORY

There are many reasons for toxicologic testing. The most common function is to confirm or exclude suspected toxic exposures. A laboratory result provides a level of confidence not readily obtained otherwise and may avert other unproductive diagnostic investigations driven by the desire for completeness and medical certainty. Testing increased diagnostic certainty in more than half of cases,[1,15] and in some instances, a diagnosis is based primarily on the results of testing. This can be particularly important in poisonings or overdoses with xenobiotics having a delayed onset of clinical toxicity, such as APAP, or in patients exposed to multiple xenobiotics. In these instances, characteristic clinical findings typically have not developed at the time of presentation or are obscured or altered by the effects of coingestants.

Testing provides two key parameters that will have a major impact on the clinical course, namely, the xenobiotic involved and the intensity of the exposure. This information can assist in triage decisions and can facilitate management decisions, such as the use of specific antidotes or interventions to hasten elimination. Well-defined exposure information can also facilitate provision of optimum advice by poison control centers. Finally, positive findings for ethanol or drugs of abuse in trauma patients should serve as an indication for substance use intervention as well as a risk marker for the likelihood of future trauma.[15]

Laboratory support of a clinical diagnosis of poisoning provides important feedback, enabling the clinical team to confirm a suspected diagnosis. Another important benefit is reassurance that an unintentional ingestion did not result in absorption of a toxic amount of xenobiotic. This reassurance allows physicians to avoid spending excessive time with patients who are relatively stable. It also allows admissions and discharges to be made and interventions to be undertaken more confidently and efficiently than would be likely based solely on a clinical diagnosis. Testing is also indicated for medicolegal reasons to establish a diagnosis "beyond a reasonable doubt."

Unfortunately, clinicians are often unaware of the capabilities and limitations of their laboratory. A survey of emergency physicians found that more than 75% were not fully aware of the range of drugs detected and not detected by the toxicology screen of their laboratory. The majority believed that the screen was more comprehensive than it actually was.[12]

The key to optimal use of the toxicology laboratory is communication. This begins with learning the capabilities of the laboratory, including the xenobiotics on its menus, which can be quantitated and which merely detected, and the anticipated TATs. For screening assays, one should know which xenobiotics are routinely detected, which ones can be detected if specifically requested, and which ones cannot be detected even when present at concentrations that typically result in toxicity.

One should know the specimen type that is appropriate for the test requested. A general rule is that quantitative tests require serum (red stopper) or heparinized plasma (green stopper) but not ethylenediamine tetraacetic acid (EDTA) plasma (lavender stopper) or citrate plasma (light-blue stopper). Both EDTA and citrate bind divalent cations that serve as cofactors for enzymes used as reagents or labels in various assays. Additionally, liquid EDTA and citrate anticoagulants dilute the specimen. Serum or plasma separator tubes (gold or green stoppers with a separator gel at the bottom of the tube) are also acceptable, provided that prolonged gel contact before testing is avoided. Some hydrophobic drugs diffuse slowly into the gel, leading to falsely low results after several hours. A random, clean urine specimen is generally preferred for toxicology screens because the higher drug concentrations usually found in urine can compensate for the lower sensitivity of the broadly focused screening techniques. However, it should be emphasized that urine testing typically provides qualitative information and generally does not indicate the degree of clinical toxicity. The concentrations of xenobiotics and their metabolites are dramatically affected by the hydration status and underlying kidney function of the patient. A urine specimen of 20 mL is usually optimal. Requirements for all specimens vary from laboratory to laboratory.

When requesting a screening test, an important—and often overlooked—item of communication is specifying any xenobiotics of particular concern. This often enables faster results and a greater likelihood of detection. It is also important to provide sufficient clinical information, including the times and dates of suspected exposure and of specimen collection.

Most full-service toxicology laboratories welcome consultation on difficult cases or results that appear inconsistent with the clinical presentation. The laboratory will be familiar with the capabilities and limitations of their testing methods, as well as common sources of discrepant results. For example, they are aware of coadministered drugs or xenobiotics that interfere either positively or negatively with laboratory measurements.

METHODS USED IN THE TOXICOLOGY LABORATORY

Most tests in the toxicology laboratory are directed toward the identification or quantitation of xenobiotics. The primary techniques used include spot tests, spectrochemical tests, immunoassays, and chromatographic techniques. Mass spectrometry (MS) is also used, usually in conjunction with gas chromatography (GS) or liquid chromatography (LC). Table 7–2 compares the basic features of these methodologies. Other methodologies include ion-selective electrode measurements of lithium, atomic absorption spectroscopy or inductively coupled plasma mass spectroscopy for lithium and heavy metals, and anodic stripping methods for heavy metals. Many adjunctive tests, including glucose, creatinine, electrolytes, osmolality, metabolic products, and enzyme activities, are also useful in the management of poisoned or overdosed patients. The focus here is on the major methods used for directly measuring xenobiotics.

TABLE 7–2	Relative Comparison of Toxicology Methods					
Method	Sensitivity	Specificity	Quantitation	Analyte Range	Speed	Cost
Spot test	+	±	No	Few	Fast	$
Spectrochemical	+	+	Yes	Few	Medium	$
Immunoassay	++	++	Yes	Moderate	Variable	$$
TLC	+	++	No	Broad	Slow	$$
HPLC	++	++	Yes	Broad	Medium	$$
GC	++	++	Yes	Broad	Medium	$$
GC/MS	+++	+++	Yes	Broad	Slow	$$$
LC/MS/MS	+++	+++	Yes	Broad	Medium	$$$$

$ = very low cost; $$$$ = very high cost; GC = gas chromatography; GC/MS = gas chromatography/mass spectroscopy; HPLC = high-performance liquid chromatography; LC/MS/MS = liquid chromatography/tandem mass spectroscopy; TLC = thin-layer chromatography. Sensitivity and specificity - High (+++); Low (+).

Spot Tests

These are simple, noninstrumental, qualitative assays that rely on a rapid reaction between a xenobiotic and a chemical reagent to form a colored product. A classic example is the Trinder test for salicylates, in which salicylate is complexed with ferric ions to produce a violet-colored product.[2] Although once a mainstay of toxicologic testing, spot tests are rarely used today because of the significant variability in visual interpretation. However, the fundamental chemical reactions used in the tests are often used in modern quantitative methods.

Optical (Spectrophotometric) Tests

Spectrophotometry involves the measurement of light intensity at selected wavelengths. The method depends on the light-absorbing properties of a substance in solution. The intensity of transmitted light passing through the solution decreases in proportion to the concentration of the substance. The transmitted light is then measured and related to the concentration of the analyte.

Analytes that are intrinsically light absorbing are measured by *direct spectrometry*. An example of this is cooximetry for the measurement of hemoglobin and its variants in a whole blood sample. Because the absorbance of hemoglobin is altered by its oxidative state, measurements at multiple wavelengths are used to individually quantify the amounts of deoxyhemoglobin, oxyhemoglobin, carboxyhemoglobin, and methemoglobin. Classic pulse oximetry, which uses only two wavelengths, yields spurious results in the presence of significant amounts of methemoglobin or carboxyhemoglobin. Cooximetry is relatively free of interferences because the concentrations of the hemoglobins are so much higher than other substances in the blood. However, the presence of intensely colored substances such as methylene blue, hydroxocobalamin or unexpected hemoglobin species such as sulfhemoglobin cause spurious results or error flags.

Most analytes in physiologically relevant concentrations do not absorb enough light at a distinct wavelength or are not present at high enough concentrations to be measured by direct spectrometry. *Spectrochemical* methods use chemical reactions to produce intensely colored compounds that absorb light at specific wavelengths. The Trinder test described earlier is one early example. The difference between the spot test and the more advanced spectrochemical test versions is the degree of automation involved, and the spectrophotometer detector used to quantify the concentration of the colored product. The ultimate limitation of the Trinder test is its lack of specificity; a variety of both endogenous and exogenous compounds cross-react with the ferric reagents, yielding a large number of false positives.

Indirect spectrochemistry improves on the selectivity of the spectrochemical assays by increasing the selectivity of the reaction that generates the light-absorbing product. Enzymes that catalyze highly selective reactions are often used for this purpose. For example, many ethanol assays are based

on an indirect spectrochemical method that uses alcohol dehydrogenase to specifically catalyze the oxidation of ethanol to acetaldehyde with the concomitant reduction of the cofactor NAD^+ (oxidized nicotinamide adenine dinucleotide) into reduced NADH. The generation of NADH is spectrophotometrically monitored by the increase in absorbance at 340 nm. Reactions leading to the conversion of NAD^+ to NADH or vice versa are very common in the clinical laboratory.

In spectrochemical assays, light absorbance is measured after the completion of the reaction (endpoint method) or by making multiple measurements during the reaction to determine the rate of reaction (kinetic method). The initial rate of reaction is constant and proportional to the concentration of the analyte. Kinetic methods are typically faster and less sensitive to interference from other light-absorbing substances because their absorbance is constant and does not affect the measured rate. Kinetic methods are more complex and require precise timing.

Although enzymatic methods are more specific, they are not free of interferences from cross-reacting substrates. For example, some lactate assays use the enzyme lactate oxidase, which also accepts glycolic acid as a substrate. Consequently, patients who have high glycolate concentrations from metabolism of ingested ethylene glycol may have falsely elevated lactate measurements. Likewise, because endogenous lactate dehydrogenase can oxidize lactate to pyruvate with concomitant reduction of NAD^+ to NADH, patients with high serum lactate concentrations can convert NAD^+ to NADH via this pathway, leading to falsely increased results in assays based on NADH production.

Determination of Volatiles by Serum Osmol Gap

As mentioned earlier, because of their significant toxicity and the availability of an effective antidote such as fomepizole for methanol and ethylene glycol poisonings, their measurements are considered to be tier 1 tests. However, on-site availability is often limited. One possible alternative measure in such overdoses of toxic alcohols is the serum osmol gap, derived from the measured serum osmolality and calculated serum osmolarity:

$$\text{Osmol gap (mOsm/kg)} = \text{Measured serum osmolality} - \text{Calculated serum osmolarity}$$

where

$$\text{Calculated serum osmolarity} = 2 \times \text{Na (mmol/L)} + \text{Glucose (mg/dL)}/18 + \text{BUN (mg/dL)}/2.8$$

$$\text{or} = 2 \times \text{Na (mmol/L)} + \text{Glucose (mmol/L)} + \text{BUN (mmol/L)}$$

Normally, the osmol gap is less than -2 ± 6. Alcohols and acetone, when present at significant concentrations, increase the measured osmolality and would increase the osmol gap. An important caveat is that both measured osmolality and calculated osmolarity should be obtained from the same serum sample, and because of the volatile nature of these substances, the serum osmolality should be analyzed expeditiously by a freezing point depression osmometer. Furthermore, other substances that may be administered (eg, mannitol for osmotic diuresis or propylene glycol as a solvent for diazepam or phenytoin) also increase serum osmolality (Chap. 12).[2]

Immunoassays

The need to measure very low concentrations of an analyte with a high degree of specificity led to the development of immunoassays. The combination of high affinity and high selectivity makes antibodies excellent assay reagents. There are two common types of immunoassays: noncompetitive and competitive. In noncompetitive immunoassays, the analyte is sandwiched between two antibodies, each of which recognizes a different epitope on the analyte. In competitive immunoassays, analyte from the patient's specimen competes for a limited number of antibody binding sites with a known amount of a labeled version of the analyte provided in the reaction mixture. Because most xenobiotics are too small to have two distinct antibody binding sites, drug immunoassays are usually competitive.

Competitive immunoassays can either be heterogeneous or homogenous. An early example of the heterogeneous immunoassay was the radioimmunoassay (RIA). In this technique, the patient sample and radiolabeled antigen are added to a solution containing antibody fixed to a surface, such as the wall of a tube or beads, and compete for binding. A subsequent wash step removes any unbound radiolabel before the tube or beads are placed in a counter to measure the remaining radioactivity, which is inversely proportional to the amount of xenobiotic in the patient sample. Modern heterogeneous assays (Fig. 7–1) have largely replaced radioactive labels with fluorescent or luminescent moieties, often activated by an enzymatic reaction. The fixed surfaces have also been updated to microbeads with very large surface areas. These improvements have enabled methods with faster assay times than previously and higher sensitivities than attainable by homogenous assays.

Homogenous immunoassays are among the most widely used methods. In these techniques, the signal generated by the labeled moiety is modified by binding to the assay antibody. This negates the need to physically separate or wash out the unbound labels. Avoiding the separation step simplifies the methodology and facilitates automation. Commonly used homogenous techniques include the enzyme multiplied immunoassay technique (EMIT) and the cloned enzyme donor immunoassay (CEDIA).[2]

In the EMIT technique (Fig. 7–2), an enzyme-analyte conjugate is used as the label and competes with unlabeled substrate from the patient sample. If antibody binds to the labeled analyte, it blocks the active site and reduces the activity of the enzyme. Unlabeled substrate from the patient's specimen will displace the enzyme from the antibody and increase its activity in proportion to its concentration.

In the CEDIA technique, two complementary yet inactive fragments of a reporting enzyme are genetically engineered, in which one fragment is linked

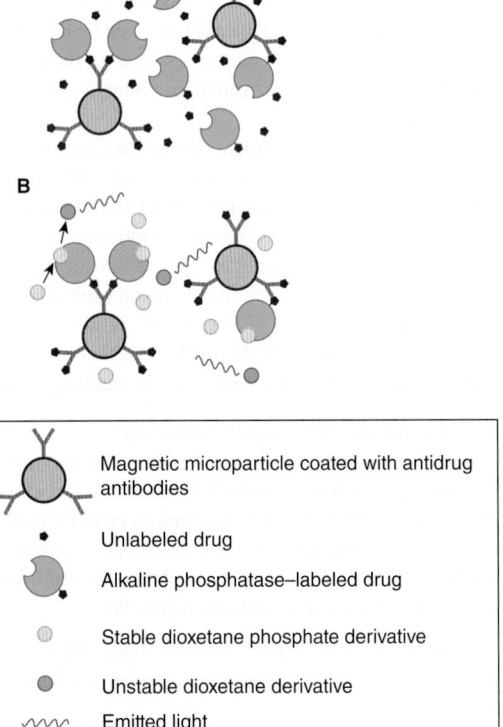

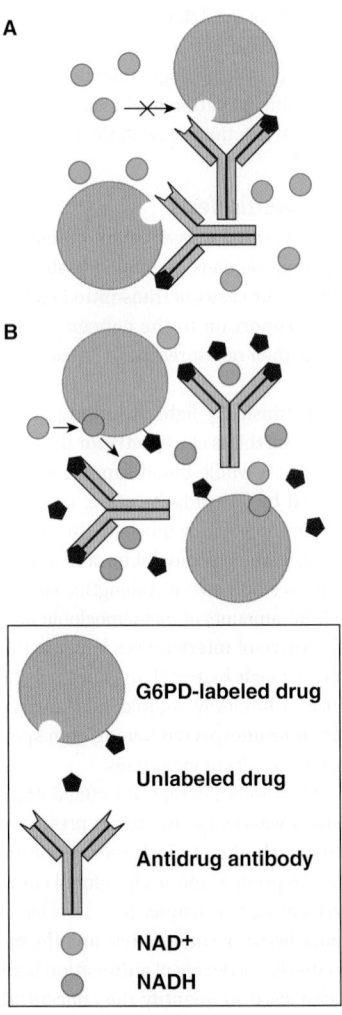

FIGURE 7–1. Magnetic microparticle chemiluminescent competitive immunoassay. (**A**) Unlabeled drug from the specimen competes with alkaline phosphatase–labeled drug for binding to antibody-coated magnetic microparticles. The microparticles are then held by a magnetic field while unbound material is washed away. (**B**) A dioxetane phosphate derivative is added and is dephosphorylated by microparticle-bound alkaline phosphatase to give an unstable dioxetane product that spontaneously decomposes with emission of light. The rate of light production is directly proportional to the amount of alkaline phosphatase bound to the microparticles and inversely proportional to the concentration of competing unlabeled drug from the specimen.

FIGURE 7–2. Enzyme multiplied immunoassay technique. The drug to be measured is labeled by being attached to the enzyme glucose-6-phosphate dehydrogenase (G6PD) near the active site. (**A**) Binding of the enzyme-labeled drug to the assay antibody blocks the active site, inhibiting conversion of NAD+ (oxidized form of nicotinamide adenine dinucleotide) to NADH (reduced form of nicotinamide adenine dinucleotide). (**B**) Unlabeled drug from the specimen can displace the drug–enzyme conjugate from the antibody, thereby unblocking the active site and increasing the rate of reaction.

to the target drug. These two fragments spontaneously reassemble into the active enzyme in solution. However, in the absence of substrate from patient's specimen, assay antibody will prevent formation of the active enzyme.

Both EMIT and CEDIA assays are used for quantitative TDM in blood and for qualitative screening of drugs of abuse in urine. Microparticle capture assays are a type of qualitative competitive immunoassay that have become very popular, especially for urine drug screening tests. The use of either colored latex or colloidal gold microparticles enables the result to be read visually as the presence or absence of a colored band, with no special instrumentation required. Competitive binding occurs as the assay mixture is drawn by capillary action through a porous membrane. This design feature is responsible for the alternate names of the technique: lateral flow immunoassay or immunochromatography.

The simplest microparticle capture design uses an antidrug antibody bound to colored microparticles and a capture zone consisting of immobilized drug (Fig. 7–3). If the specimen is xenobiotic free, the beads will bind to the immobilized analyte, forming a colored band. When the amount of xenobiotic in the patient specimen exceeds the detection limit, all of the antibody sites will be occupied by xenobiotic from the specimen, and no labeled antibody will be retained in the capture zone. The use of multiple antibodies and discrete capture zones with different immobilized analytes can allow several xenobiotics to be detected with a single device.

Although immunoassays have a high degree of sensitivity and selectivity, they are also subject to interferences and problems with cross-reactivity. Cross-reactivity refers to the ability of the assay antibody to bind to xenobiotics other than the target analyte. Xenobiotics with similar chemical structures may be efficiently bound, which can lead to falsely elevated results. In some situations, cross-reactivity can be beneficially exploited. For example, some immunoassays effectively detect classes of xenobiotics rather than one specific xenobiotic. Immunoassays for opioids use antibodies to morphine that cross-react to varying degrees with structurally related substances, including codeine, hydrocodone, and hydromorphone. Oxycodone typically has low cross-reactivity, and higher concentrations are required to give a positive result. The cross-reactivity of nonmorphine opiates varies with manufacturer. It is recommended that clinicians consult directly with their

laboratory for the relative sensitivities of the immunoassay used. Structurally unrelated synthetic opioids, such as meperidine and methadone, have little or no cross-reactivity and are not detected by opiate immunoassays. Immunoassays for the benzodiazepine class react with a wide variety of benzodiazepines but with varying degrees of sensitivity.[14,16] Because of the highly variable response of immunoassays to the various opiates and benzodiazepines, methods based on MS should be used for definitive results.

Cross-reactivity also leads to interferences between xenobiotics of similar structure. Assays for the TCA family have similar reactivity with amitriptyline, nortriptyline, imipramine, and desipramine and can be used to provide an estimate of the total concentration of any combination of these xenobiotics. However, a large number of other xenobiotics with tricyclic structures, including carbamazepine, many phenothiazines, and diphenhydramine, also cross-react and generate a signal, particularly at concentrations found in patients who are poisoned or overdosed.

Even when an antibody is selected to be specific to a single xenobiotic, it is common that metabolites of the target xenobiotic show some cross-reactivity. This cross-reactivity can lead to difficulties in interpretation because both active and inactive metabolites are measured, and not necessarily with similar sensitivities as the target xenobiotic.

Immunoassays are also subject to interference by xenobiotics that impair detection of the label. Elevated lactate concentrations often lead to spuriously increased xenobiotic concentrations in specimens tested by EMIT, as described earlier. Immunoassays that rely on enzyme labels are particularly sensitive to nonspecific interference because enzyme activity is highly dependent on reaction conditions. A number of substances that can inhibit the enzyme reaction in EMIT assays are used to adulterate urine submitted for drug abuse testing with the intent of producing false-negative results (see the later discussion of screening for drugs of abuse).

Chromatography

Essentially, chromatography is a separation method by which a complex mixture (eg, a biological fluid) is physically separated into its individual components. The fundamental principle of the methodology is the differential partitioning of a mixture between stationary and mobile phases. During the process, the mobile phase carries the mixture (sample) through a stationary phase. The different components of the sample will have differing affinities for the two phases and will spend more or less time interacting with the stationary phase and will elute at different rates. Under controlled separation conditions, the velocities of the different components in the sample are highly reproducible. A tremendous variety of xenobiotics can be identified based on their characteristic velocities, as measured by the time required to elute from the stationary phase (retention time, t_R).

To make clinical specimens compatible with the chromatographic separation requirements, the samples usually undergo an initial "clean-up" process to reduce their salt and protein content and to concentrate the analytes being measured for increased sensitivity. This process also enables an increased resolution of xenobiotics that would have otherwise migrated at similar rates and not been separately identifiable thereby increasing specificity.

Two common methods of clean-up or extraction include liquid–liquid extraction and solid-phase extraction (SPE).[2] The latter has become increasingly popular because it can be commercially prepared and purchased as single-use cartridges or multi-well plates, simplifying sample preparation and assisting automation. Solid-phase extraction is itself a modified chromatographic procedure in which a urine or serum patient specimen passes through a stationary phase that retains the analytes of interest. The retained xenobiotics are then selectively eluted with an organic solvent such as methanol.

Many analytes need to be chemically derivatized either before or after chromatographic separation to increase their ability to be detected. For example, to be detectable by a fluoroscopic detector, primary amines can be labeled with a fluorescamine tag.

There exist many different chromatographic modalities, including simple and inexpensive paper and thin-layer chromatography that are limited to

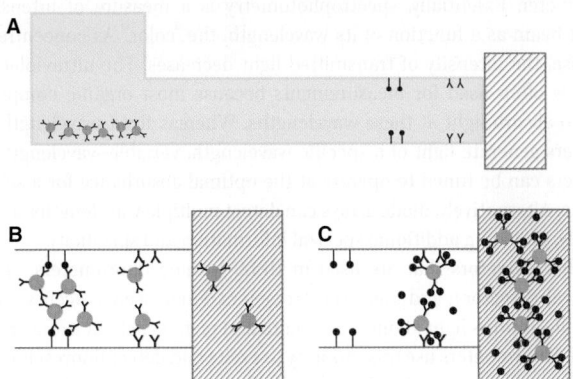

FIGURE 7–3. Microparticle capture immunoassay. (**A**) Diagram of a device before specimen addition. Colored microbeads (about the size of red blood cells) coated with antidrug antibodies (Y) are in the specimen well. At the far end of a porous strip are capture zones with immobilized drug molecules (•) and a control zone with antibodies recognizing the antibodies that coat the microbeads. (**B**) Adding the urine specimen suspends the microbeads, which are drawn by capillary action through the porous strip and into an absorbent reservoir (*hatched area*) at the far end of the strip. In the absence of drug in the urine, the antibodies will bind the beads to the capture zone containing the immobilized drug and form a colored band. Excess beads will be bound by antibody–antibody interactions in the control zone, forming a second colored band that verifies the integrity of the antibodies in the device. (**C**) If the urine contains the drug (•) in concentrations exceeding the detection limit, all of the antibodies on the microbeads will be occupied by drug from the specimen, and the microbeads will not be retained by the immobilized drug in the capture zone. No colored band will form. However, the beads will be bound and form a band in the control zone.

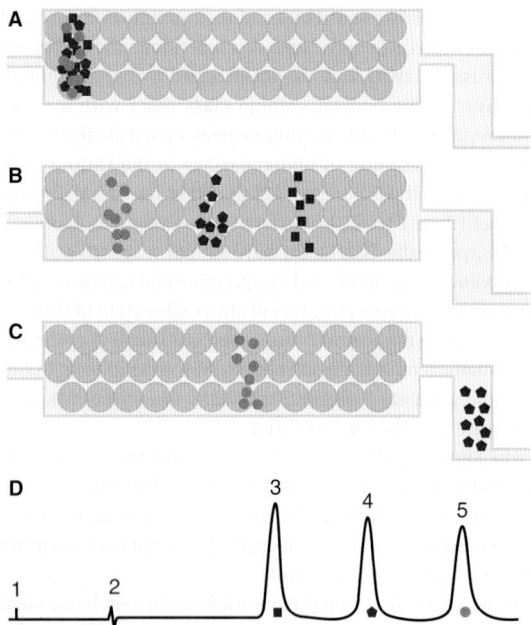

FIGURE 7–4. High-performance liquid chromatography (HPLC). HPLC is schematically shown. (**A**) A mixture of three compounds (■) (◉) (●) is injected into a column filled with a spherical reversed-phase packing. (**B**) The compounds move through the column at characteristic speeds. The most hydrophilic compound (■) moves most quickly, and the most hydrophobic compound (◉) moves most slowly. (**C**) The compound of intermediate polarity (●) has reached the detection cell, where it absorbs light directed through the cell and generates a signal proportional to its concentration. (**D**) Illustration of the HPLC tracing that might result: *1* indicates the time of injection. The artifact at *2* results when the injection solvent reaches the detector and indicates the retention time of a completely unretained compound. The peaks at *3, 4,* and *5* correspond to the separated compounds. For example, peak *4* might be amitriptyline, peak *3* might be the more polar metabolite, nortriptyline, and peak *5* could be the more hydrophobic internal standard *N*-ethylnortriptyline. Later-emerging peaks are typically wider and shorter because of more time for diffusive forces to spread out the molecules.

qualitative measures of analytes present in high concentrations. Liquid chromatography and GC are columnar techniques that require more technical expertise but permit identification and quantification of a large variety of xenobiotics with low limits of detection.

In **high-performance liquid chromatography (HPLC)**, a column is packed with solid particles that support a thin, liquid stationary phase. The mobile phase containing the specimen is pumped through under high pressure, and separation occurs between the two phases (Fig. 7–4). Smaller particles can be packed more densely, increasing the surface area of separation with improved column efficiency and resolution but at the expense of increased resistance to flow, requiring higher pumping pressures. Using high pressures with small particles, good separations can be achieved with relatively short assay times. Several different separation modalities are used in HPLC, including size exclusion, affinity, ion exchange, and partition separation. Xenobiotic assays most commonly use reverse-phase partitioning, in which separation occurs between a stationary nonpolar phase and a relatively polar mobile phase. Hydrophobic compounds are more strongly adsorbed by the stationary phase, and hydrophilic compounds tend to remain in the polar mobile phase. This results in the most hydrophilic xenobiotics eluting first followed by the progressively more hydrophobic xenobiotics. The most common reverse-phase columns use particles coated with octadecyl hydrocarbon chains and are referred to as C-18 columns.

In HPLC, the xenobiotics are detected after they exit the chromatographic column. The detector output is typically plotted as signal intensity versus time (Fig. 7–4D). Identification of the xenobiotics is made by their characteristic retention times and quantification is based on the area under the curve of the corresponding peak. To objectively validate the identity and

quantification of the xenobiotic, a structurally related calibrant (an "internal standard," shown as peak 5 in Fig. 7–4D) is added to the specimen in known concentrations.

The advantages of HPLC include the ability to separately identify and quantify multiple related xenobiotics and their metabolites (eg, opiates or benzodiazepines) in a single run of the same sample. By comparison, an immunoassay method would provide a single measurement that would either be unable to discriminate between related xenobiotics (lack of specificity) or be unable to identify them altogether (lack of sensitivity).

Disadvantages include relatively expensive instrumentation with complex specimen preparation that requires specialized expertise to design and execute.

Gas chromatography is similar in principle to HPLC but uses an inert carrier gas such as helium or nitrogen as the mobile phase pumped through a heated column to which the stationary phase is chemically bonded. The sample is heat vaporized and pumped through the column, and the xenobiotics are detected in the gas stream as they exit the column. The low flow resistance of gas allows very high flow rates and very long columns, enabling extremely high resolution in a short time. Analytes partition between the mobile gas phase and stationary phase based on their intrinsic volatility, which depends on temperature. Volatility can be optimized by adjusting the temperature of the system so that xenobiotics with a wide range of volatility can be analyzed in a single run.

Although the temperature-dependent partitioning and high flow rates of GC systems enable fast measurements and high resolution of multiple xenobiotics, the methodology is limited to analytes such as alcohols that are reasonably volatile at temperatures below 572°F (300°C) above which the stationary phase begins to break down. Another limitation is the limited column capacity, so that highly sensitive detectors are required to measure the small quantities that can be chromatographed.

By itself, chromatography is simply a separation method. It must be combined with a detection method to allow identification and, if desired, quantification of the separated substances. There exist a variety of different detectors, ranging from the extremely simple yet low sensitivity (visual) to the relatively complex with extremely low detection limits (mass spectrometers).

The most common detector used in HPLC assays remains the spectrophotometer. Essentially, spectrophotometry is a measure of intensity of a light beam as a function of its wavelength, the "color." As concentrations increase, the intensity of transmitted light decreases. The ultraviolet (UV) range is often used for measurements because most organic compounds tend to absorb light at these wavelengths. Whereas fixed-wavelength photometers generate light of a specific wavelength, variable-wavelength photometers can be tuned to operate at the optimal absorbance for a selected analyte. Alternatively, diode arrays can detect multiple wavelengths simultaneously, providing additional spectral information and specificity.

Other detectors that are used in HPLC include fluorometers, electrochemical detectors, and mass spectrometers. Fluorescence occurs when a molecule absorbs light at one wavelength and reemits light at a longer wavelength. Fluorometers use this property to excite and detect fluorescing xenobiotics. Analytes can either be naturally fluorescent or be derivatized with a fluorescent tag. Electrochemical detectors measure the electrical current produced by an electroactive analyte as it undergoes either reduction or oxidation at an electrode surface. These techniques (and MS, which is described later) are extremely sensitive and can detect picogram amounts of analytes.

The most common GC detector is the flame ionization detector (FID). As organic molecules emerge from the GC column, they are mixed with hydrogen and air and are burned by a flame. This creates charged combustion intermediates that can be measured as current. The amount of generated current is proportional to the mass of carbon burnt so that the FID is most sensitive to hydrocarbons, such as alcohols and other xenobiotics that are highly combustible. Nitrogen–phosphorus detectors are also widely used in xenobiotic analysis. In this modification of an FID, an alkali bead is heated above the flame. The presence of alkali atoms in the combusted xenobiotic generates enhanced electron emissions.

Mass Spectrometry

The chromatographic devices described earlier can detect broad ranges of xenobiotics but do not specifically identify them. The identity of the compounds detected must be inferred from the retention time. The mass spectrometer serves as a highly sensitive detector when paired with a chromatographic system and has the additional advantage of being able to definitively identify compounds by mass analysis. It is considered to be a "universal detector" because all compounds have mass and can, in theory, be detected.

Mass spectrometers determine the molecular weight of ions in vacuum. The basic design of the apparatus can be simplified into three components— the ion source in which the sample molecules are ionized; the mass analyzer in which the ions are separated according to their mass-to-charge (m/z) ratio; and the detector, which registers the signals. Important secondary components include a vacuum generator to avoid collisions between the ions generated and ambient air molecules and a computer for data analysis and recording.

Ion Source

A number of ionization techniques have been developed for MS. The most commonly used techniques for xenobiotic measurements include electron impact (EI) ionization in GC-coupled systems and electrospray ionization (ESI) in HPLC systems.

In EI, the gas phase analyte is introduced into the ionization chamber, where it is bombarded by a stream of electrons. Electron impact can dislodge an electron from the analyte, creating a positively charged ion and frequently imparting sufficient energy to the ion to break it into pieces. The ion fragments into which a molecule can break are characteristic properties of the xenobiotic, permitting its identification.

In ESI, an electrical charge is applied to the HPLC effluent entering the ionization chamber, producing a fine mist of charged droplets. As the solvent evaporates and the droplet size decreases, the surface charge increases. The repulsive force of like-charged particles causes further splitting into smaller droplets and eventual release of desolvated ions.[18]

A third MS ionization modality that has a limited role in toxicology is inductively coupled plasma (ICP). Whereas the EI and ESI are "soft" techniques, producing little fragmentation, ICP is the ultimate in "hard" ionization, in which samples are virtually completely atomized during ionization. Consequently, its primary use is for elemental analysis, as in the detection and measurement of trace metals and heavy metals in tissues and body fluids. It is an extremely sensitive technique, able to detect particles on the order of parts per trillion or lower. In ICP, a nebulized liquid sample is introduced into the ionization chamber, where it is injected into a hot argon plasma created by inductively coupling power into the plasma using a high-powered radiofrequency generator, reaching temperatures of approximately 10,000° K.

Mass Analyzer

Ionic species can be separated according to their m/z ratios by a variety of techniques, including ion traps, time-of flight instruments, and magnetic sector fields. Quadrupole mass spectrometers are the most common MS instruments found in clinical laboratories (Fig. 7–5).[18] This instrument consists of four parallel electrically conductive rods, which essentially function as a mass filter. Applying direct current (DC) and alternating current t (AC) in specific patterns creates an electromagnetic field through which only ions of a very narrow m/z range can pass to reach the detector. By rapidly and repeatedly scanning through many voltage settings, a range of m/z ions are sequentially allowed to reach the detector, generating a mass spectrum. The mass spectrum records the m/z ratios of the pieces produced by the ionic fragmentation of the parent ion, as well as their relative abundance. Fig. 7–6 shows the spectrum obtained from a gas chromatograph (GC-MS) at a time when the TMS derivative of the cocaine metabolite benzoylecgonine (TMS-BE) was emerging from the column. Because benzoylecgonine cannot be volatilized, it must be derivatized to be compatible with GC. The concentration of TMS-BE in the specimen is determined from the ratio of the peak height at m/z 240 to the height of a

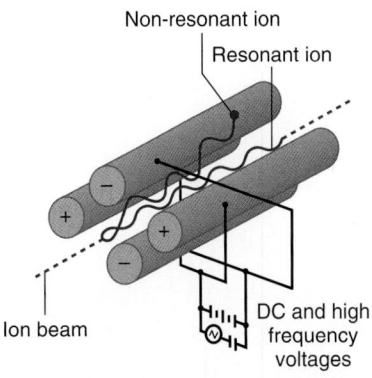

FIGURE 7–5. Principle of quadrupole analyzer. Four electrically conductive rods are arranged in parallel forming a channel through which the ion beam passes. By applying direct (DC) and alternating (AC) currents, an electromagnetic field is generated that permits only ions of a defined mass-to-charge (m/z) range to pass through to reach the mass detector while nonresonant ions are ejected radially. Modified after Manz A, Lossfidis D, Pamme N: Bioanalytical Chemistry. London: Imperial College Press; 2004. Chapter 4 Mass Spectrometry.

peak at m/z 243 that results from a corresponding fragment of the internal standard, TMS-BE labeled with three deuterium atoms (d3-TMS-BE). The specificity of the identification is verified by finding peaks at m/z 256 and m/z 361, with peak height ratios to the peak at m/z 240 comparable to the ratios seen with authentic TMS-BE. The detection at the correct retention time of a xenobiotic producing all three peaks in the correct ratios produces an extremely specific identification.

This *scanning mode* can be used for toxicologic screening because its permits identification of many different analytes in a single run. However, because a wide range of m/z need to be observed, the time spent on any specific value is limited, decreasing analytical sensitivity. Alternatively, when measuring for specific analytes, the analyzer can be set up in *selected ion monitoring (SIM) mode*. In this mode, the quadrupole mass filter is set to filter and detect only a few selected m/z. In the illustrated example of TMS-BE, the characteristic peaks at m/z 240, 256, and 361 are used, along with one or more of the corresponding peaks from the internal standard.

Tandem Mass Spectrometry

The high sensitivity and specificity afforded by chromatography/MS is being further improved by the related hybrid technique of liquid chromatography/tandem mass spectrometry (LC/MS/MS) (Fig. 7–7).[19] This technique is used in an increasing number of clinical toxicology laboratories for identification and quantification of suspected xenobiotics. In this setup, the effluent from a LC apparatus enters a soft ionization chamber (eg, ESI) that generates large, singly-charged ionic fragments that are directed into a series of three MS quadrupoles. The first quadrupole (Q1) selectively filters ions of specific m/z, called the "parent ion." The second quadrupole (Q2) is filled with inert gas and acts as a collision cell. As the filtered parent ions enter Q2 at high velocity, they collide with the gas molecules and are fragmented into smaller "daughter ions." These fragments are then introduced into the third quadrupole (Q3) for mass analysis. Characterizing the compounds by three physical properties (the parent and daughter ions masses, along with the chromatographic retention time) affords a high selectivity that dramatically reduces potential interferences.

Ion Detector

Because relatively few ions make it all the way through the mass spectrometer, the signals must be amplified in order to be measurable. Most MS detectors use electron multipliers for ion amplification and detection, in which ions impact a dynode, generating an electronic current that is amplified through a series of impacts on sequential dynodes before reaching the measuring anode.

A

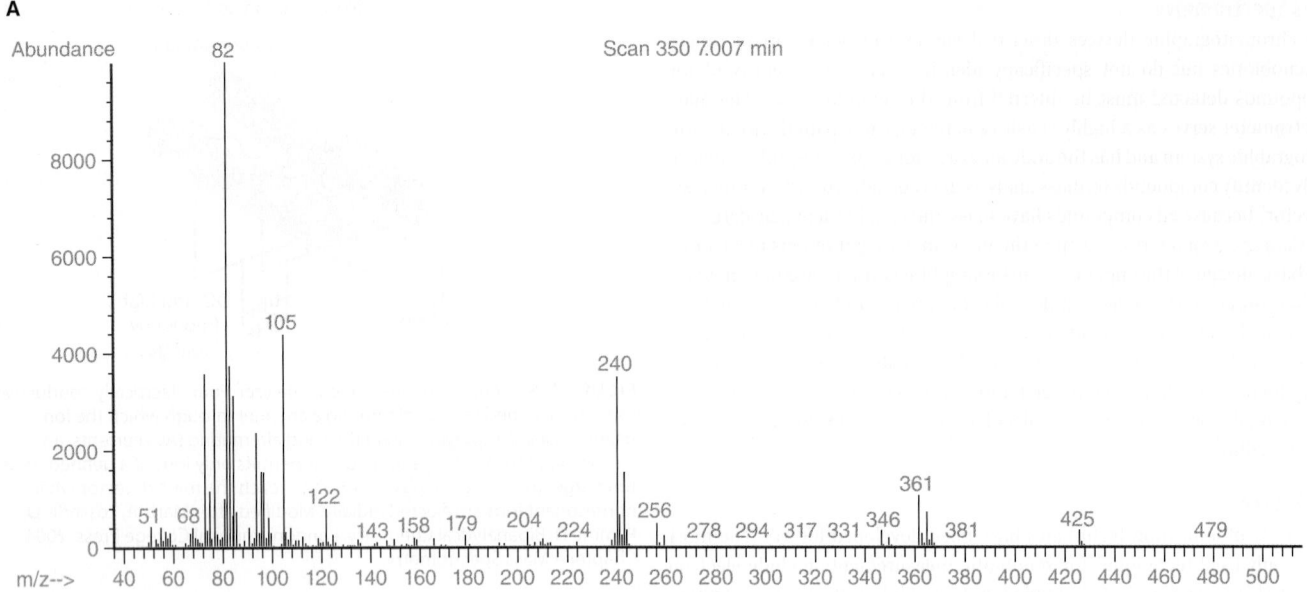

B

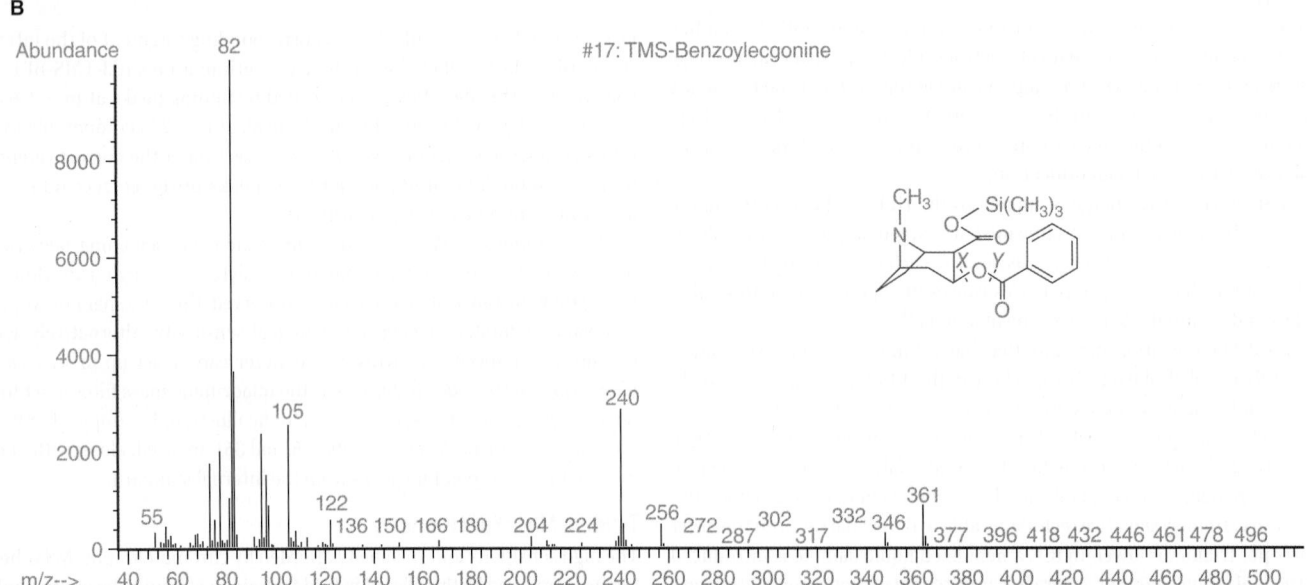

FIGURE 7-6. Mass spectrum of the trimethylsilyl derivative of benzoylecgonine (TMS-BE). (**A**) Mass spectrum of effluent from a gas chromatography (GC) column at the retention time of TMS-BE. The unfragmented parent ion of TMS-BE is at a mass-to-charge (m/z) ratio of 361. The two fragment peaks at m/z 243 and 259 result from fracture of the bonds at X and Y, respectively, in structure of TMS-BE (*inset* in **B**). Additional peaks at m/z 243, 259, and 361 are derived from trideuterated TMS-BZE (d3-TMS-BE) added as an internal standard. The mass spectrometer can identify and quantify TMS-BE and d3-TMS-BE independently of one another by measuring the heights of the peaks unique for each compound. The peak at m/z 425 is from a coeluting contaminant. (**B**) Mass spectrum of pure TMS-BE.

LABORATORY ERRORS

Laboratory testing is a complex process and, consequently, is prone to errors. But what are the sources of these errors? A more informative approach would be to break down the testing process into the preanalytical, analytical, and postanalytical phases. The preanalytical phase can be thought of as the test processing that takes place before the sample is placed on the analyzer, and the postanalytical phase involves the recording and transmission of test results.

Preanalytical errors include sample misidentification, inadequate tube filling, inappropriate containers, hemolysis, and delays in transport. A commonly cited source of analytical error is cross-reactivity with other compounds. Examples of postanalytical errors include erroneous transcription of test results and word misidentification.

With the advent of automation and test standardization, error rates decreased dramatically from approximately 160,000 errors per million tests in 1947 to 450 per million in 1997.[22] The majority (60%–70%) of modern laboratory errors occur in the preanalytical phase; approximately 10% to 15% of errors occur during the analytical phase and 15% to 20% in postanalysis.[22]

Errors, especially in the less automated preanalytical phase, can be minimized with appropriate procedures and training and good communication between the clinical and laboratory services. Analytical errors caused by cross-reactivity are typically methodology and test dependent and are described elsewhere in this chapter. A more detailed discussion of these sorts of errors is beyond the scope of this chapter. A good practical resource is the medical director of your local laboratory.

THERAPEUTIC DRUG MONITORING AND QUANTITATIVE DRUG MEASUREMENTS

Therapeutic drug monitoring (TDM) involves the quantification of drug concentrations in biological fluids (typically serum, plasma, or whole blood) to assess therapeutic compliance or efficacy or to elucidate the cause of

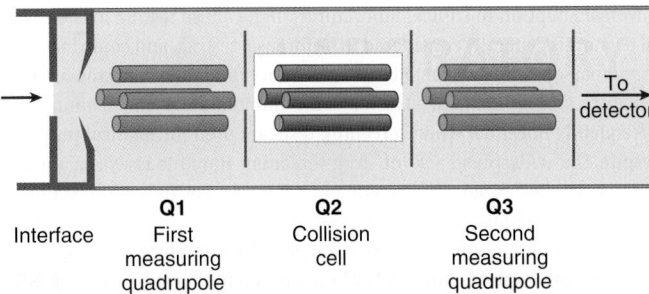

Q1
First
measuring
quadrupole

Q2
Collision
cell

Q3
Second
measuring
quadrupole

Interface

To
detector

FIGURE 7–7. Schematic of a tandem mass spectrometer. Effluent from an interfaced liquid chromatography (LC) system enters the ionization chamber where ion fragments are generated and directed into three successive quadrupoles (Q1, Q2, Q3). Q1 selectively filters ions of a specific mass-to-charge (m/z) (ie, "parent ions"). Q2 functions as a collision cell generating further ionic fragmentation. Q3 performs a second round of ion filtration before mass detection. By using a second round of ion fragmentation and filtering, higher selectivity and reduced interference are achieved. (*Data from Manz A, Lossfidis D, Pamme N: Bioanalytical Chemistry. London: Imperial College Press; 2004.*)

drug-induced toxicity. Therapeutic drug monitoring describes a patient's pharmacokinetic status at the moment of specimen collection. Pharmacokinetics is the relationship between the drug dose and the time course of drug absorption, distribution, metabolism, and elimination, which represent the effects of the body on the drug. Pharmacodynamics describes the effects of the drug on the body.

Drugs that are candidates for TDM share several characteristics:

1. Narrow therapeutic ranges.
2. Therapeutic effects and dose adjustments not readily assessed by clinical observation.
3. Unpredictable relationships between dose and clinical outcome. This is especially true during periods of physiological flux (eg, initiation of therapy acute illness, disease, puberty, pregnancy, aging, and polypharmacy).
4. Correlation between drug concentrations and their efficacy and toxicity
5. Drug toxicity leads to significant morbidity such as hospitalization, irreversible organ damage, and death.
6. Availability of appropriate analytic techniques.

When properly used to guide dosing adjustments, xenobiotic concentration measurements improve medical outcomes.[11] However, many therapeutic drug measurements are drawn at inappropriate times or are made without an appropriate therapeutic question in mind. An essential requirement for interpretation of xenobiotic concentrations is that the relationship between concentrations and effects must be known. Such knowledge is available for routinely monitored xenobiotics and is often encapsulated in published ranges of therapeutic and toxic concentrations. Concentrations designated as "toxic" are usually higher than the upper end of the therapeutic range and typically represent concentrations at which toxicity is acute and potentially serious (see back cover).

For most xenobiotics, the relationships between toxic concentrations and effects cannot be systematically studied in humans and consequently are often incompletely defined. These relationships are largely inferred from data provided in overdose case reports and case series. The measurement of xenobiotic concentrations in patients with poisonings or overdose cases in which concentration–effect relationships are not well defined contribute more to the management of future overdosed patients than to the management of the patient in whom the measurements were made.

For toxicologists, xenobiotic concentrations are especially useful in two ways. For xenobiotics, when toxicity is delayed or is clinically unapparent during the early phases of an overdose or poisoning, concentrations have substantial prognostic value and facilitate anticipatory management. These concentrations are also used to make decisions regarding the use of antidotes or of interventions to hasten drug elimination, such as hemodialysis.

Quantitative xenobiotic measurements are subject to various interferences, but these are less problematic than in qualitative assays. Signals generated by cross-reacting substances are generally weaker than those from the target analyte and are relatively unlikely to lead to a false diagnosis of toxicity, particularly if the target analyte is absent. Such cross-reactivity can be exploited in some instances to provide confirmatory evidence of a poison for which no specific assay is immediately available. For example, the immunoassay finding of apparent nontoxic concentrations of TCAs can help confirm a diphenhydramine overdose, and the finding of a measurable digoxin concentration in an unexposed patient suggests poisoning with other cardioactive steroids of plant or animal origin or endogenous production. Negative interferences are much less frequent. Interferences in chromatographic methods usually result from the presence of other compounds with migration rates similar to the target analyte. Because the migration rates are rarely exactly the same, the laboratory can often recognize the presence of the interference as an overlapping peak when both compounds are present. In such instances, the interference may impair accurate measurement of the xenobiotic concentration. When no target xenobiotic is present, misidentification of the interfering peak as the target becomes much more likely because a single peak is seen at approximately the expected position. Because interferences in chromatographic methods are generally unique to a specific method, information about these interferences should be obtained by asking the laboratory.

Xenobiotic measurements are unlike most other laboratory measurements in that the concentrations are highly dependent on the timing of the measurement. Knowledge of the pharmacokinetics of a xenobiotic can substantially enhance the ability to draw meaningful conclusions from a measured concentration. Some xenobiotics alter their pharmacokinetic behavior at very high concentrations. These changes in pharmacokinetics (called toxicokinetics) are often predictable from the mechanisms of drug clearance and the extent of binding to plasma proteins and to tissues (Chap. 9).

Knowledge of the relationship between xenobiotic concentrations and effects, or pharmacodynamics, is also important. Effects depend on local concentrations at the site of action, typically at cell membrane receptors, intracellular locations, or within deeper tissue compartments such as across the blood–brain barrier within the central nervous system. Serum or plasma concentrations can be correlated with effects only when these concentrations are in equilibrium with concentrations at the site of action. During the absorption and distribution phases, the concentration ratio will be higher than its equilibrium value, yet often the only xenobiotic concentration measured after an acute overdose is one obtained while absorption and distribution are still ongoing. This effect explains some observations of apparent poor correlation between measured concentrations and toxic effects.

Free Drug Monitoring

Drugs bind to serum proteins to various degrees. For example, whereas lithium is 0% protein bound, valproate and phenytoin are more than 90% protein bound at therapeutic concentrations. The major drug-binding proteins are albumin, α-1 acid glycoprotein, and the various lipoproteins.

For xenobiotics that bind significantly to plasma proteins, the concentration of xenobiotic that is not bound to proteins (the free-xenobiotic concentration) is in equilibrium with concentrations at the site of action. For most drugs at therapeutic concentrations, the free-drug concentration is an approximately constant percentage of the total drug concentration. The total concentration is what is usually measured in the laboratory. Under these conditions, the ratio of total concentration to active site concentration is approximately constant, and a reasonable correlation between total concentration and effects can be expected.

Although free-drug concentration can be estimated from total concentration in most cases, under certain pathological conditions, free-drug concentration may be significantly elevated even if the concentration of the total drug is within therapeutic range.

TABLE 7–3 Protein Binding Characteristics of Some Commonly Monitored Therapeutic Drugs[9]

Drug	Percent Protein Bound	Free-Drug Monitoring Candidate
Ethosuximide	0	No
Lithium	0	No
Procainamide	10–15	No
Digoxin	25	Yes
Theophylline	40	No
Phenobarbital	40	No
Lidocaine	60–80	Yes
Carbamazepine	80	Yes
Quinidine	80	Yes
Phenytoin	90	Yes
Valproate	90–95	Yes
Mycophenolate	92–98	Yes
Tacrolimus	97	Yes
Cyclosporine	98	Yes

These pathological conditions can include:

1. Uremia
2. Liver disease
3. Hypoalbuminemia
4. Polypharmacy, in which one strongly bound drug such salicylates can displace another phenytoin

In general, candidates for free drug monitoring are drugs that are greater than 80% protein bound. An exception is digoxin; although it is only 25% bound, after treatment with digoxin-specific antibody fragments, the free fraction is less than 1% of the total concentration.

The protein-binding characteristics of some commonly monitored therapeutic drugs are summarized in Table 7–3. In current clinical practice, free drug monitoring is best described for the classical anticonvulsants phenytoin, carbamazepine, and valproate.

The analytical considerations and limitations make the routine use of free drug monitoring prohibitive. To be able to quantify free drug, the analytical technique must first be able to isolate the unbound drug and then be sensitive enough to be able to measure the relatively low concentrations. The two most common separation techniques require either a prolonged separation time such as equilibrium dialysis or a series of manual steps that are difficult to automate in the modern clinical laboratory such as offline filtration and high-speed centrifugation. Because the concentrations of the free drugs are dramatically lower than the total drug, the analytical ranges and sensitivities of the measuring instruments are by necessity very different. It is recommended that clinicians contact their local clinical laboratory to find the specific tests (and TATs) that are available.

SCREENING FOR DRUGS OF ABUSE

Testing for drugs of abuse is a significant component of medical toxicology testing. These tests are widely used in the evaluation of potential poisonings and are assuming an increasing role in ensuring the appropriate use of analgesics.[8] Initial testing is usually done with a screening immunoassay. Although drug-screening immunoassays were initially developed for use in workplace drug-screening programs and are not always optimal for medical purposes, their wide availability, low cost, and ease of use led to their nearly universal adoption in clinical laboratories. Drug abuse testing for nonmedical reasons is generally considered to be forensic testing, and confirmation of immunoassay results is considered mandatory in such circumstances. Confirmatory testing compensates for some immunoassay shortcomings but is frequently not done when screening tests are used for medical purposes. Despite the widespread use of drug-screening immunoassays in medical practice, studies suggest that many physicians do not fully understand the capabilities and limitations of these tests.[23]

The most commonly tested-for xenobiotics are amphetamines, cannabinoids, cocaine, opioids, and PCP. These are often referred to as "the NIDA five" because they are the five drugs that were recommended in 1988 by the National Institute on Drug Abuse (NIDA) for drug screening of federal employees. The responsibility for recommendations for federal drug testing now lies with the Substance Abuse and Mental Health Services Administration (SAMHSA). Drug-screening immunoassays are also frequently done for oxycodone, methadone and benzodiazepines and less frequently for hydrocodone. Table 7–4 lists some of the general characteristics of these tests. Commercial urine immunoassays are also available for buprenorphine, lysergic acid diethylamide, methaqualone, methylenedioxymethamphetamine (MDMA), and hydrocodone. These screening immunoassays are available in a number of formats, which differ in performance. Almost all of them are designed to be used with urine specimens because these can be obtained noninvasively and generally have higher concentrations than serum, enhancing the sensitivity of the test.

The screening tests for cannabinoids and cocaine are directed toward metabolites rather than the parent compound. The parent xenobiotics, cocaine and THC, are both short lived and persist for no more than a few hours after use. The metabolites remain present for substantially longer periods of time. Detection of the metabolites increases the ability to detect any recent xenobiotic use. However, this limits the utility of the assays for determining whether a patient is currently under the influence of the drug. Because the metabolites are rapidly formed, a negative test result generally excludes toxicity, but a positive test result indicates only use in the recent past, not current toxicity.

The use of specific cutoff concentrations is nearly universal. Test results are considered positive only when the concentration of the xenobiotic in the specimen exceeds a predetermined threshold. This threshold should be set sufficiently high that false-positive results as a consequence of analytic variability or cross-reactivity are extremely infrequent. They should also be low enough to give consistent positive results in persons who are regularly using xenobiotics. Cutoff concentrations used vary with the xenobiotic or xenobiotic class under investigation. In some screening immunoassays, the laboratory has the option of selecting from several cutoff values.

The use of cutoff values sometimes creates confusion when a patient who is known to have recently used a xenobiotic has a negative result reported on a xenobiotic screen. In such instances, the drug is usually present but at a concentration below the cutoff value. A quantitative confirmatory test (see later) is usually able to demonstrate the presence of the drug or its metabolites under such circumstances. Another potential problem occurs when a patient's drug-screening test result is positive after previously having become negative. This is usually interpreted as indicating renewed drug use, but it may actually be due to variations in urine production. The rate of the urine flow may vary up to 100-fold, with a reflected change in the urine drug concentration. This effect is often exploited by individuals who drink large quantities of water before taking a urine drug test to increase urine flow and decrease urine drug concentrations. In contrast, a decrease in the rate of urine production could result in a positive test result after a negative one despite no new drug exposure. A similar effect is produced by changes in urine pH. Drugs containing a basic nitrogen (eg, amphetamine) demonstrate ionic trapping, with increasing concentrations as urine pH decreases. Similarly, excretion of an anionic drug such as salicylate increases with increasing urine pH.

Another widely used practice is the confirmation of positive screening results using an analytical methodology different from that used in the screen. The most common confirmatory methods are gas chromatography/mass

TABLE 7–4	Performance Characteristics of Common Urine Drug Screening Immunoassays[a]			
Drug/Class	Detection Limits (ng/mL)[b]	Confirmation Limits (ng/mL)[b]	Detection Interval[c]	Comments
Amphetamine/ methamphetamine	500	500	1–2 days (2–4 days)	Decongestants, ephedrine, L-methamphetamine, selegiline, and bupropion metabolites are reported to give false-positive test results with some assays; MDA, MDEA, and MDMA are variably detected.
Barbiturates	200		2–4 days	Phenobarbital detection interval is up to 4 weeks.
Benzodiazepines	100–300		1–30 days	Benzodiazepines vary in reactivity and potency. Hydrolysis of glucuronides increases sensitivity. False-positive test results are reported with oxaprozin.
Cannabinoids	50	15	1–3 days (1 month)	Screening assays detect inactive and active cannabinoids; confirmatory assay detects inactive metabolite THCA. Duration of positivity is highly dependent on screening assay detection limits.
Cocaine	150	100	2 days (1 wk)	Screening and confirmatory assays detect inactive metabolite BE. False-positive test results caused by cross-reactive compounds are unlikely.
Opiates			1–2 days (1 week)	Semisynthetic opioids derived from morphine show variable cross-reactivity. Fully synthetic opioids (eg, fentanyl, meperidine, methadone, tramadol) have minimal cross-reactivity. Quinolones are known to cross-react with some assays.
Codeine/morphine	2,000	2,000		
Hydrocodone/hydromorphone	300	100		
Oxycodone/oxymorphone	100	50		
6-Acetylmorphine	10	10		
Methadone	300		1–4 days	Doxylamine is reported to cross-react with some assays.
Phencyclidine	25	25	4–7 days (1 month)	Dextromethorphan, diphenhydramine, ketamine, and venlafaxine is reported to cross-react with some assays.

[a]Performance characteristics vary with manufacturer and may change over time. For the most accurate information, consult the package insert of the current lot or contact the manufacturer. [b]Substance Abuse and Mental Health Services Administration recommendations[10] are shown for amphetamines/methamphetamines, cannabinoids, cocaine, opiates, and phencyclidine immunoassays. Other commercial immunoassay cutoffs are also listed. Other cutoffs may be set by individual laboratories. [c]Values are after typical use; values in parentheses are after heavy or prolonged use.

BE = benzoylecgonine; MDA = methylenedioxyamphetamine; MDEA = methylenedioxyethylamphetamine; MDMA = methylenedioxymethamphetamine; THCA = tetrahydrocannabinolic acid.

spectrometry (GS/MS) and liquid chromatography/mass spectrometry (LC/MS). The high specificity afforded by the combination of the retention time and the mass spectrum makes false-positive results extremely unlikely. Chromatographic/MS methods also have greater sensitivity than the screening immunoassays, minimizing failed confirmations because of a drug concentration below the sensitivity of the confirmatory assay.

Immunoassay results are generally obtainable within 1 hour. Confirmatory testing usually requires at least several hours or longer for low-volume tests that are often batched and frequently have to be sent out to offsite laboratories. This creates a problem when confirmation of initial immunoassay results is required. Most laboratories provide a verbal report of a presumptive positive result to facilitate medical management but will not enter the result into a permanent record, such as the laboratory computer, until after confirmation is completed.

Confirmatory testing is less critical in an emergency department setting because a positive finding infrequently has consequences that extend beyond the medical management of the patient. An exception occurs when results of testing performed on motor vehicle crash victims are subsequently subpoenaed as evidence in legal proceedings. Confirmatory testing also becomes more important in drug abuse testing associated with chronic pain management programs, in which unexpected findings (whether positive or negative) may result in termination of care.

One workplace drug-screening practice that is not widely followed in medical toxicology is maintenance of a chain of custody. Employers generally insist on chain of custody for workplace testing because actions taken in response to a positive result are often contested in court. A chain of custody provides results that are readily defended in court. Laboratories providing testing for medical purposes rarely keep a chain of custody because it is quite expensive and does not benefit the patient. Additionally, the medical personnel responsible for obtaining the specimens are rarely trained in collection requirements for a chain of custody.

Another practice common in workplace testing but rare in medical laboratories is testing for specimen validity. It is common for individuals to try to "beat" obscure or falsify a workplace drug test through a variety of means, including diluting the specimen (either physiologically by water ingestion or by direct addition of water to the specimen), substituting "clean" urine obtained from another individual, or adding various substances that will either destroy drugs in the specimen or inactivate the enzymes or antibodies used in the screening immunoassays. Such substances include acids, bases, oxidizing agents (bleach, nitrite, peroxide, peroxidase, iodine, chromate), glutaraldehyde, pyridine, niacin, detergents, and soap. SAMHSA requires validity testing for all specimens in federal workplace testing, including measurement of urinary pH, specific gravity, and creatinine concentration, as well as tests for the presence of adulterants.[10] Dipsticks are available that detect the most common adulterants. However, manipulation or adulteration is rarely a problem in specimens obtained for emergency medical care, and most clinical laboratories do not provide validity testing.

A rapidly expanding epidemic of misuse of opioid analgesics and accompanying deaths caused by unintentional overdoses has led to the issuance of extensive recommendations, and often regulations, for managing chronic opioid therapy for noncancer pain. The use of periodic urine drug tests to monitor compliance with prescribed medications, as well as to detect use of illicit or unprescribed xenobiotics, is consistently a feature of such recommendations, although there is currently very little evidence that this practice reduces misuse or diversion of prescribed drugs or improves outcomes for patients.[5] There is evidence that the results of urine drug monitoring are inconsistent with the agreed-upon pain management plan in a very substantial fraction of patients so tested.[5]

The objectives of urine drug testing in chronic pain patients and abuse clinics are more complex in that negative results could signal misuse or diversion of a prescribed opioid, but positive results also indicate illicit xenobiotic use. In questionable cases, confirmatory testing by assays capable of distinguishing and quantitating prescription opiates and opioids, as well as key metabolites should be obtained. This done on specimens with a positive screening result to ensure that it is positive for the right reasons and for an unexpected negative result to address the possibility that the expected opioid or its metabolites are actually present but at concentrations too low to give a signal exceeding the cutoff value.

PERFORMANCE CHARACTERISTICS OF COMMON (URINE) DRUG SCREENING ASSAYS

There are problems with the performance characteristic summaries of all urine drug immunoassays (Table 7–4). Much of this confusion arises because there are multiple manufacturers of urine drug immunoassays. Each uses proprietary antibodies in a proprietary design and thus has unique performance characteristics, including differing reactivity with target drugs and cross-reactivity with interfering substances creating different false positives and false negatives. Reformulation of assays can remedy problems that previously existed, but this does not prevent older reports of false-positive results that are no longer valid from being cited repetitively in the current literature. For example, the interference of ibuprofen in a widely used assay for cannabinoids was corrected more than 20 years ago but continues to be cited in contemporary literature.[24] The best source of current information is the laboratory that is performing the testing or the assay manufacturer.

Immunoassays for opiates are directed toward morphine but have good cross-reactivity with many (but not all) structurally similar natural and semisynthetic opioids. The extent of cross-reactivity varies among manufacturers. For example, oxycodone exhibits approximately 30% cross-reactivity relative to morphine in a fluorescence polarization immunoassay but less than 5% cross-reactivity in a number of other screening assays.[16,26] A failure to appreciate the poor detection of oxycodone can create problems when opiate-screening immunoassays are used to confirm that patients receiving prescription oxycodone for chronic pain are indeed taking it rather than diverting it for illicit sale. If a low cross-reactivity assay is used, a patient taking oxycodone as prescribed might have a negative result, but another patient who is selling oxycodone and using the proceeds to buy heroin would have a positive result. To address this problem, assays specific for oxycodone were introduced. These assays are sensitive to therapeutic amounts of oxycodone but relatively insensitive to other opiates.

Synthetic opioids, such as dextromethorphan, fentanyl, meperidine, methadone, propoxyphene, and tramadol, have limited cross-reactivity with opiate immunoassays. Urine immunoassays specific for many of these compounds are available. Given the increasing importance of buprenorphine as maintenance therapy for opioid dependency, it is worth noting that the combination of high potency and low cross-reactivity means that buprenorphine will generally not be detected by opiate immunoassays. It was for this reason that immunoassays for specific detection of buprenorphine were developed.

A positive immunoassay result may reflect multiple contributions from various opiates and opiate metabolites. Concentrations of morphine glucuronide in the urine can up to 10-fold higher than the concentrations of unchanged morphine and can contribute substantially to positive results. A positive opiate result after the use of heroin (diacetylmorphine) is primarily a result of the morphine and morphine glucuronide that result from heroin metabolism. Distinguishing heroin from other opioids requires detection of 6-monoacetylmorphine, the heroin-specific metabolite.

The duration of positivity of an opiate immunoassay after last use depends on the identity and amount of the opiate used, the specific immunoassay, the cutoff value, and the pharmacokinetics of the individual. Currently, SAMHSA recommends a cutoff equivalent to 2,000 ng/mL of morphine for workplace screening because poppy seeds rarely produce transient positive results with the previously recommended cutoff of 300 ng/mL. However, most toxicology laboratories continue to use a 300-ng/mL cutoff.

Drug-screening assays for cocaine are actually assays for the cocaine metabolite benzoylecgonine, which is eliminated more slowly than cocaine. This extends the duration of positivity after last use from a few hours to 2 days and sometimes to 1 week or longer after significant or prolonged use.

Because the assay is directed toward a metabolite, positive results do not equate with toxicity but merely indicate recent exposure. The assay is highly specific for benzoylecgonine, and false-positive results due to an interfering substance are extremely uncommon.

Immunoassays for cannabinoids are also directed toward a metabolite, in this case tetrahydrocannabinoic acid (THC-COOH). These immunoassays exhibit cross-reactivity with other cannabinoids but little else. Because cannabinoids are structurally unique and occur only in plants of the genus *Cannabis*, false-positive results are uncommon. It is unusual, although possible, to become exposed to sufficient "secondhand" or sidestream marijuana smoke to develop a positive urine test result.[7] Legal hemp products include fiber, oil, and seedcake derived from *Cannabis* varieties with low concentrations of cannabinoids. Hemp food products contain insufficient amounts of THC to produce psychoactive effects and usually will not increase urinary cannabinoid concentrations above a 50-ng/mL screening threshold.[14,23]

Interpretation of a positive result for cannabinoids can be problematic. Urine is typically positive for up to 3 days after occasional recreational use. However, with significant or prolonged use, there is significant accumulation of cannabinoids in adipose tissue. These stored cannabinoids are slowly released into the bloodstream and produce positive findings for 1 month or more. Consequently, little can be concluded from a positive finding in terms of current clinical findings. Because positive results in the absence of toxicity are very common and because THC is rarely responsible for serious acute clinical manifestations, NACB guidelines recommend against its routine inclusion in drug screening for patients with acute symptoms.[27] Synthetic cannabinoids (found in products sold as "spice," "K2," and a variety of changing names) are generally not detected by cannabinoid assays, presumably because of a combination of very low concentrations in urine and limited cross-reactivity.

Amphetamine screening tests have the greatest problems with false-positive results. A number of structurally related xenobiotics have significant cross-reactivity, including bupropion metabolites[3] and nonprescription decongestants such as pseudoephedrine, as well as L-ephedrine, which is found in a variety of herbal preparations. Some nonprescription nasal inhalers contain L-methamphetamine, the less potent levorotary isomer of D-methamphetamine. It is particularly problematic because it not only cross-reacts in immunoassays but also cannot be distinguished from the D-isomer by MS.[13] This cross-reactivity is beneficial from the point of view of the medical toxicologist because all of these compounds similar produce toxicity. But it is problematic in drug abuse screening because of the widespread legitimate use of cold medications. Assays with greater selectivity for amphetamine or methamphetamine exist. Although these assays produce fewer false-positive results caused by decongestant cross-reactivity, they are also less sensitive for the detection of other abused amphetaminelike compounds, including methylenedioxyamphetamine (MDA), MDMA, and phentermine. Cross-reactivity patterns vary from assay to assay.[16] Literature produced by the manufacturer should be consulted for specific details. A number of designer phenethylamine derivatives (eg, those found in "bath salts") might be expected to cross-react in amphetamine assays because of structural similarity. However, they are typically much more potent than amphetamine or methamphetamine and do not achieve high enough concentrations to give a signal exceeding the cutoff.

Testing for benzodiazepines is complicated by the wide array of benzodiazepines that differ substantially in their potency, cross-reactivity, and half-lives. There are also substantial differences in the detection patterns of the various immunoassays.[14,16] This heterogeneity complicates the interpretation of benzodiazepine-screening assays. Screening results are typically positive in persons using low therapeutic doses of diazepam but negative after an overdose of a highly potent benzodiazepine such as clonazepam. To improve the scope of detection, some assays use antibodies to oxazepam, which is a metabolite of a number of different benzodiazepines. These assays have poor sensitivity to benzodiazepines that are not metabolized to oxazepam. False-negative results occur for benzodiazepines that are excreted in the urine almost entirely as glucuronides that have poor cross-reactivity with antibodies directed toward an unmodified benzodiazepine. This is one reason for the poor detectability of lorazepam in some screening assays. The latter situation has led to the recommendation that specimens be treated with β-glucuronidase before analysis.[20] Some assays now include β-glucuronidase in the reagent mixture or use antibodies directed toward glucuronidated metabolites. The frequency of false-negative results and the fact that benzodiazepines are relatively benign in overdose have led the NACB guidelines to withhold recommendation for routine screening of urine for benzodiazepines until these problems with the immunoassays are addressed.[27]

Barbiturates are comparable to benzodiazepines in their heterogeneity of potency, cross-reactivity, and half-lives, although the differences are less substantial. Specific assays for serum phenobarbital can often help to clarify the significance of a positive barbiturate screen.

Some PCP screening assays give positive results with dextromethorphan, ketamine, or diphenhydramine but only when these are used in amounts above usual therapeutic quantities. A positive result may serve as a clue to a possible overdose with any of these substances. Furthermore, much of the illicit PCP actually consists of a mixture of various congeners and byproducts of synthesis. The cross-reactivity of these xenobiotics with the assay varies significantly and may result in false-negative assay results in patients who use PCP.

SUMMARY

- Most hospital laboratories offer basic, clinically relevant tests that are needed on an urgent basis locally (tier 1 testing). Additional (tier 2) testing in selected patients who are not improving in whom unconfirmed poisoning is still suspected is typically referred out to reference toxicology laboratories.
- Although broad-spectrum toxicology screens can identify many drugs present in overdosed patients, the results of broad-spectrum screens infrequently have altered management outcomes.
- When requesting a screening test, an important and often overlooked item of communication is specifying any xenobiotics of particular concern.
- Xenobiotic concentrations are often useful to make decisions regarding the use of antidotes or if interventions to hasten drug elimination, such as hemodialysis, are indicated.
- Test errors can originate from the preanalytical, analytical, or postanalytical testing phases, with most occurring preanalytically. Adherence to procedure protocols and effective communication between personnel and services is key in reducing these errors.
- The predictive power of the result of a toxicology screen depends on a number of factors, including the likelihood of poisoning before receiving the test results (the prior probability or the prevalence), the range of xenobiotics effectively detected, and the frequency of false-positive test results.

FOR MORE INFORMATION

Additional information about clinical toxicology laboratories, including topics not covered in this chapter, may be found in contemporary textbooks.[2,17,25]

REFERENCES

1. Buck C, et al. Evaluation of rapid urine toxicological testing in patients with altered mental status in the emergency department [abstract]. *J Toxicol Clin Toxicol*. 1999;37:597-598.
2. Burtis C, et al, eds. *Tietz Textbook of Clinical Chemistry and Molecular Diagnostics*. 5th ed. St. Louis, MO: Elsevier; 2012.
3. Casey ER, et al. Frequency of false positive amphetamine screens due to bupropion using the Syva EMIT II immunoassay. *J Med Toxicol*. 2011;7:105-108.
4. Christian MR, et al. Do rapid comprehensive urine drug screens change clinical management in children? *Clin Toxicol (Phila)*. 2017;57:977-980.
5. Christo PJ, et al. Urine drug testing in chronic pain. *Pain Physician*. 2011;14:123-143.
6. College of American Pathologists Participant Summaries. *Chemistry/Therapeutic Drug Monitoring Survey Set C-C; Serum Alcohol/Volatiles Survey Set AL2-C; Blood Oximetry Survey Set SO-C; Toxicology Survey Set T-C; Urine Drug Testing (Screening) Set UDS6-B; Urine Toxicology Survey Set UT-C*. Northfield, IL: College of American Pathologists; 2017.
7. Cone EJ, et al. Passive inhalation of marijuana smoke: urinalysis and room air levels of delta-9-tetrahydrocannabinol. *J Anal Toxicol*. 1987;11:9-96.
8. Couto JE, et al. High rates of inappropriate drug use in the chronic pain population. *Popul Health Manag*. 2009;12:185-190.
9. Dasgupta A, ed. *Handbook of Drug Monitoring Methods: Therapeutics and Drugs of Abuse*. Totowa, NJ: Humana Press; 2008.
10. Department of Health and Human Services, Substance Abuse and Mental Health Services Administration. Mandatory guidelines and proposed revisions to mandatory guidelines for federal workplace drug testing programs. *Fed Reg*. 2015;80:28101-28151.
11. Destache CJ, et al. Does accepting pharmacokinetic recommendations impact hospitalization? A cost-benefit analysis. *Ther Drug Monit*. 1990;12:427-433.
12. Durback LF, et al. Emergency physicians' perceptions of drug screens at their own hospitals. *Vet Hum Toxicol*. 1998;40:234-237.
13. Franke JP, de Zeeuw RA. Solid-phase extraction procedures in systematic toxicological analysis. *J Chromatogr B*. 1998;713:51-59.
14. Gourlay DL, et al. *Urine Drug Testing in Clinical Practice*. 6th ed. https://www.remitigate.com/wp-content/uploads/2015/11/Urine-Drug-Testing-in-Clinical-Practice-Ed6_2015-08.pdf. Accessed March 29, 2018.
15. Hammett-Stabler CA, et al. Urine drug screening in the medical setting. *Clin Chim Acta*. 2002;315:125-135.
16. Magnani B. Concentrations of compounds that produce positive results. In: Shaw LM, Kwong TC, Rosano TG, et al, eds. *The Clinical Toxicology Laboratory: Contemporary Practice of Poisoning Evaluation*. Washington, DC: AACC Press; 2001:481-497.
17. Magnani B, et al, eds. *Clinical Toxicology Testing: A Guide for Laboratory Professionals*. Northfield, IL: CAP Press; 2012.
18. Manz A, et al. *Bioanalytical Chemistry*. London: Imperial College Press; 2004.
19. Maurer HH. Current role of liquid chromatography-mass spectrometry in clinical and forensic toxicology. *Anal Bioanal Chem*. 2007;388:1315-1325.
20. Meatherall R. Benzodiazepine screening using EMIT II and TDx: urine hydrolysis pretreatment required. *J Anal Toxicol*. 1994;18:385-390.
21. National Poisons Information Service, Association of Clinical Biochemists: Laboratory analyses for poisoned patients: joint position paper. *Ann Clin Biochem*. 2002;39:328-339.
22. Plebani M. The detection and prevention of errors in laboratory medicine. *Ann Clin Biochem*. 2010;47:101-110.
23. Reisfield GM, et al. Rational use and interpretation of urine drug testing in chronic opioid therapy. *Ann Clin Lab Sci*. 2007;4:301-314.
24. Reisfield GM, Bertholf RL. "Practical guide" to urine drug screening clarified. *Mayo Clin Proc*. 2008;83:848-849.
25. Shaw LM, et al, eds. *The Clinical Toxicology Laboratory: Contemporary Practice of Poisoning Evaluation*. Washington, DC: AACC Press; 2001.
26. Stull TM, et al. Variation in proficiency testing performance by testing site. *JAMA*. 1998;279:463-467.
27. Wu AH, et al. National Academy of Clinical Biochemistry laboratory medicine practice guidelines: recommendations for the use of laboratory tests to support poisoned patients who present to the emergency department. *Clin Chem*. 2003;49:357-379.

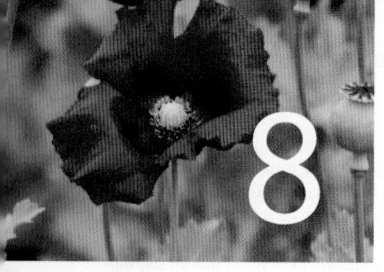

8 PRINCIPLES OF DIAGNOSTIC IMAGING

David T. Schwartz

Diagnostic imaging plays a significant role in the management of many patients with toxicologic emergencies. Radiography can confirm a diagnosis (eg, by visualizing the xenobiotic), assist in therapeutic interventions such as monitoring gastrointestinal (GI) decontamination, and detect complications of the xenobiotic exposure (Table 8–1).[219]

Conventional radiography is readily available in the emergency department (ED) and is the imaging modality most frequently used in acute patient management. Other imaging modalities are used in certain toxicologic emergencies, including computed tomography (CT); enteric and intravascular contrast studies; ultrasonography; transesophageal echocardiography (TEE); magnetic resonance imaging (MRI) and magnetic resonance angiography (MRA); and nuclear scintigraphy, including positron emission tomography (PET) and single-photon emission tomography (SPECT).

VISUALIZING THE XENOBIOTIC

A number of xenobiotics are radiopaque and can potentially be detected by conventional radiography. Radiography is most useful when a substance that is known to be radiopaque is ingested or injected. When the identity of the xenobiotic is unknown, the usefulness of radiography is very limited. When ingested, a radiopaque xenobiotic is often seen on an abdominal radiograph as described in detail in this chapter. Injected radiopaque xenobiotics are also visualized by radiography. If the toxic material itself is available for examination, it can be radiographed outside of the body to detect its radiopacity or any radiopaque contents (Fig. 102–2).[92]

RADIOPACITY

The radiopacity of a xenobiotic is determined by several factors. First, the intrinsic radiopacity of a substance depends on its physical density (g/cm³) and the atomic numbers of its constituent atoms. Biologic tissues are composed mostly of carbon, hydrogen, and oxygen and have an average atomic number of approximately 6. Substances that are more radiopaque than soft tissues include bone, which contains calcium (atomic number 20), radio-contrast agents containing iodine (atomic number 53) and barium (atomic number 56), iron (atomic number 26), and lead (atomic number 82). Some xenobiotics have constituent atoms of high atomic number, such as chlorine (atomic number 17), potassium (atomic number 19), and sulfur (atomic number 16) that contribute to their radiopacity.

The thickness of an object also affects its radiopacity. Small particles of a moderately radiopaque xenobiotic are often not visible on a radiograph. Finally, the radiographic appearance of the surrounding area also affects the detectability of an object. A moderately radiopaque tablet is easily seen against a uniform background, but in a patient, overlying bone or bowel gas often obscures the tablet.

ULTRASONOGRAPHY

Compared with conventional radiography, ultrasonography theoretically is a useful tool for detecting ingested xenobiotics because it depends on echogenicity rather than radiopacity for visualization.[40] Solid pills within the fluid-filled stomach infrequently have an appearance similar to gallstones within the gallbladder. In one in vitro study using a water-bath model, virtually all intact pills could be visualized.[8] The authors were also successful at detecting pills within the stomachs of human volunteers who ingested pills. Nonetheless, reliably finding pills scattered throughout the GI tract, which often contains air and feces that block the ultrasound beam, is a formidable task. In a well-controlled trial comparing participants who ingested 50 enteric-coated placebo tablets with control participants, ultrasonography of

the stomach had a sensitivity of only 62.5% at the time of ingestion and 20.8% after 1 hour and a specificity of 58.3% and 79%, respectively.[234] Ultrasonography, therefore, has limited clinical practicality and is therefore not routinely recommended.

INGESTION OF AN UNKNOWN XENOBIOTIC

Although a clinical policy issued by the American College of Emergency Physicians in 1995 suggested that an abdominal radiograph should be obtained in unresponsive overdosed patients in an attempt to identify the involved xenobiotic, the role of abdominal radiography in screening a patient who has ingested an unknown xenobiotic is questionable.[7] The number of potentially ingested xenobiotics that are radiopaque is limited. In addition, the radiographic appearance of an ingested xenobiotic is not sufficiently distinctive to determine its identity (Fig. 8–1).[1,248,266] However, when ingestion of a radiopaque xenobiotic such as ferrous sulfate tablets or another metal with a high atomic number is suspected, abdominal radiographs are helpful.[6] In addition, knowledge of potentially radiopaque xenobiotics is useful in suggesting diagnostic possibilities when a radiopaque xenobiotic is discovered on an abdominal radiograph that was obtained for reasons other than suspected xenobiotic ingestion, such as in a patient with abdominal pain (Fig. 8–2).[214,225]

Several investigators evaluated the radiopacity of various medications.[61,70,97,103,114,173,211,228,238] These investigators used an in vitro water-bath model to simulate the radiopacity of abdominal soft tissues.[211] The studies found that only a small number of medications exhibit some degree of radiopacity. A short list of the more consistently radiopaque xenobiotics is summarized in the mnemonic CHIPES—chloral hydrate, "heavy metals," iron, phenothiazines, and enteric-coated and sustained-release preparations.

The CHIPES mnemonic has several limitations.[211] It does not include all of the pills that are radiopaque in vitro such as acetazolamide and busulfan. Most radiopaque medications are only moderately radiopaque, and when ingested, they dissolve rapidly, becoming difficult or impossible to detect. "Psychotropic medications" include a wide variety of compounds of varying radiopacity.[173,211] For example, whereas trifluoperazine (containing fluorine; atomic number 9) is radiopaque in vitro, chlorpromazine (containing chlorine; atomic number 17) is not.[211] Sustained-release preparations and those with enteric coatings have variable composition and radiopacity. Pill formulations of fillers, binders, and coatings vary among manufacturers, and even a specific product can change depending on the date of manufacture. Furthermore, the insoluble matrix of some sustained-release preparations is radiopaque and when seen on a radiograph, these tablets once opened no longer contain active medication. Some sustained-release cardiac medications such as verapamil and nifedipine have inconsistent radiopacity.[140,227,240] Finally, this was a very old study, and many pills currently on the market have never been tested.

EXPOSURE TO A KNOWN XENOBIOTIC

When a xenobiotic that is known to be radiopaque is involved in an exposure, radiography plays an important role in patient care.[6] Radiography can confirm the diagnosis of a radiopaque xenobiotic exposure, quantify the approximate amount of xenobiotic involved, and monitor its removal from the body. Examples include ferrous sulfate, sustained-release potassium chloride,[123,232] and heavy metals.

Iron Tablet Ingestion

Adult-strength ferrous sulfate tablets are readily detected radiographically because they are highly radiopaque and disintegrate slowly when ingested.

TABLE 8–1	Xenobiotics with Diagnostic Imaging Findings	
Xenobiotic	Imaging Study[a]	Findings
Amiodarone	Chest	Phospholipidosis (interstitial and alveolar filling), pulmonary fibrosis
Asbestos	Chest	Interstitial fibrosis (asbestosis), calcified pleural plaques, mesothelioma
Beryllium	Chest	Acute: airspace filling; chronic: hilar adenopathy
Body packer	Abdominal	Ingested packets, ileus, bowel obstruction
	Enteric contrast or abdominal CT	Retained packets, bowel obstruction or perforation
	Ultrasonography	Ingested packets
Carbon monoxide	Head CT, MRI	Bilateral basal ganglion lucencies, white matter demyelinization
	SPECT, PET	Cerebral dysfunction
Caustic ingestion	Enteric contrast	Esophageal perforation or stricture
	CT	
Chemotherapeutics (busulfan, bleomycin)	Chest	Interstitial pneumonitis
Cholinergics	Chest	Diffuse airspace filling (bronchorrhea)
Cocaine	Chest, abdominal	Diffuse airspace filling, pneumomediastinum, pneumothorax, aortic dissection, perforation
	Noncontrast, head CT, MRI, TEE	SAH, intracerebral hemorrhage, infarction
	SPECT, PET	Cerebral dysfunction, dopamine receptor downregulation
Corticosteroids	Skeletal	Avascular necrosis (femoral head), osteoporosis
Ethanol	Chest	Dilated cardiomyopathy, aspiration pneumonitis, rib fractures
	Head CT, MRI	Cortical atrophy, cerebellar atrophy, SDH (head trauma)
	SPECT, PET	Cerebellar and cortical dysfunction
Fluorosis	Skeletal	Osteosclerosis, osteophytosis, ligament calcification
Hydrocarbons (low viscosity)	Chest	Aspiration pneumonitis
Inhaled allergens	Chest	Hypersensitivity pneumonitis
IDU injection drug use	Chest, skeletal, cranial CT	Septic emboli, pneumothorax, osteomyelitis (axial skeleton), AIDS-related infections
Iron	Abdominal	Radiopaque tablets
Irritant gases	Chest	Diffuse airspace filling thorax
Lead	Skeletal	Metaphyseal bands in children (proximal tibia, distal radius), bullets (dissolution near joints)
	Abdominal	Ingested leaded paint chips or other leaded compounds
Manganese	MRI brain	Basal ganglia and midbrain hyperintensity
Mercury (elemental)	Abdominal, skeletal, or chest	Ingested, injected, or embolic deposits
Metals (Pb, Hg, Tl, As)	Abdominal	Ingested xenobiotic
Nitrofurantoin	Chest	Hypersensitivity pneumonitis
Opioids	Chest	ARDS
	Abdominal	Ileus
Phenytoin	Chest, CT	Hilar lymphadenopathy, pseudolymphoma
Procainamide, isoniazid, hydralazine	Chest	Pleural and pericardial effusions (xenobiotic-induced lupus syndrome)
	Echocardiogram	Pericardial effusion
Salicylates	Chest	ARDS
Silica, coal dust	Chest	Interstitial fibrosis, hilar adenopathy (egg-shell calcification)
Thorium dioxide	Abdominal	Hepatic and splenic deposition

[a]Conventional radiography unless otherwise stated.

AIDS = acquired immune deficiency syndrome; ARDS = acute respiratory distress syndrome; CT = computed tomography; MRI = magnetic resonance imaging; PET = positron emission tomography; SAH = subarachnoid hemorrhage; SDH = subdural hematoma; SPECT = single-photon emission tomography; TEE = transesophageal echocardiography.

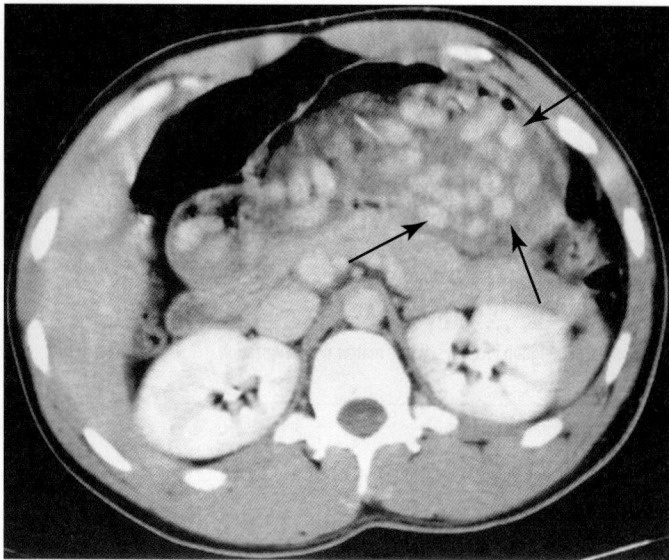

FIGURE 8–1. Ingestion of an unknown substance. A 46-year-old man presented to the emergency department with a depressed level of consciousness. Because he also complained of abdominal pain and mild diffuse abdominal tenderness, a computed tomography (CT) scan of the abdomen was obtained. The CT scan revealed innumerable tablet-shaped densities within the stomach (*arrows*). The CT finding was suspicious for an overdose of an unknown xenobiotic. Orogastric lavage was attempted, and the patient vomited a large amount of whole navy beans. Computed tomography is able to detect small, nearly isodense structures such as these that cannot be seen using conventional radiography. (*Used with permission from Dr. Earl J. Reisdorff, MD, Michigan State University, Lansing, MI.*)

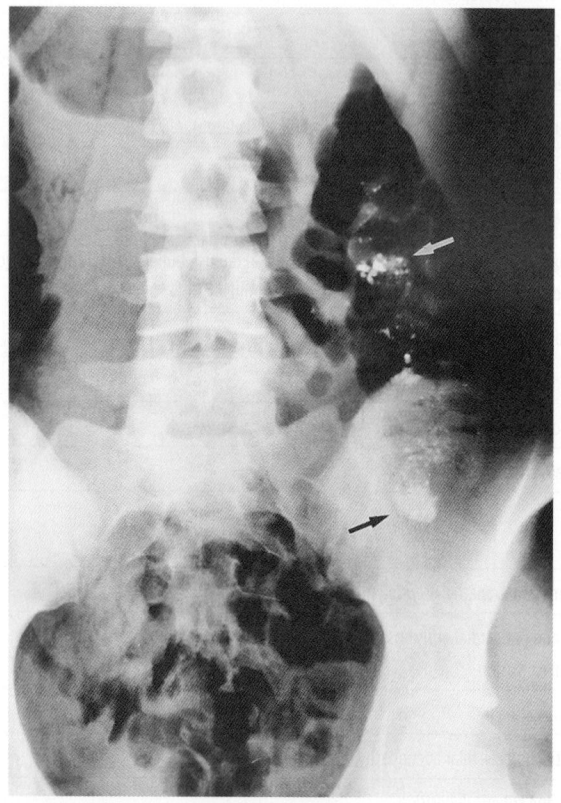

FIGURE 8–2. Detection of a radiopaque xenobiotic on an abdominal radiograph. An abdominal radiograph obtained on a patient with upper abdominal pain revealed radiopaque material throughout the intestinal tract (*arrows*). Further questioning of the patient revealed that he consumed bismuth subsalicylate (Pepto-Bismol) tablets to treat his peptic ulcer (bismuth; atomic number 83). The identification of radiopaque material does not allow determination of the nature of the substance.

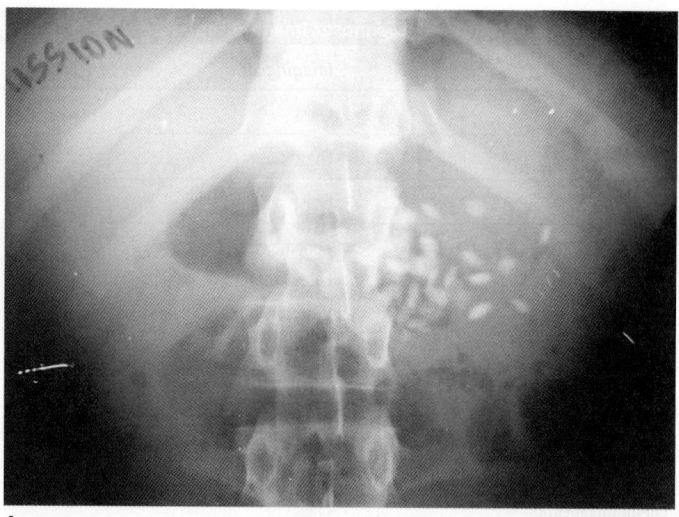

A

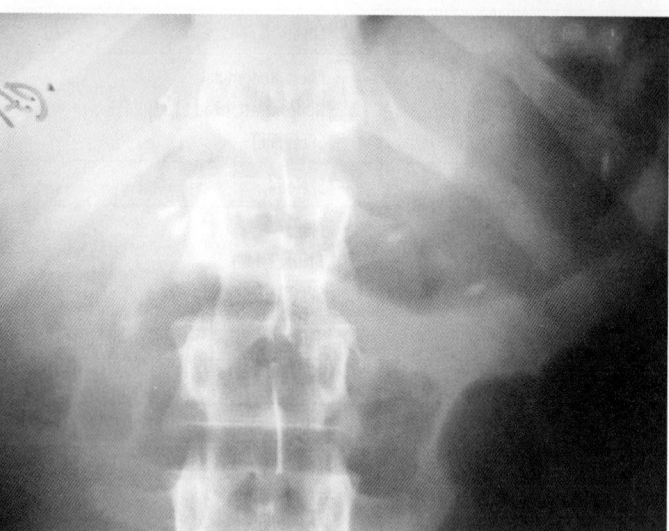

B

FIGURE 8–3. Iron tablet overdose. (**A**) Identification of the large amount of radiopaque tablets confirms the diagnosis in a patient with a suspected iron overdose and permits rough quantification of the amount ingested. (**B**) After emesis and whole-bowel irrigation, a second radiograph revealed some remaining tablets and indicated the need for further intestinal decontamination. (*Used with permission from the Fellowship in Medical Toxicology, NYU School of Medicine, New York City Poison Control Center.*)

Aside from confirming an iron tablet ingestion and quantifying the amount ingested, radiographs repeated after whole-bowel irrigation help to determine whether further GI decontamination is needed (Fig. 8–3).[60,74,118,123,172,178,181] Nonetheless, caution must be exercised in using radiography to exclude an iron ingestion. Some iron preparations are not radiographically detectable. Liquid, chewable, or encapsulated (Chap. 45) ("Spansule") iron preparations rapidly fragment and disperse after ingestion. Even when intact, these preparations are less radiopaque than ferrous sulfate tablets.[61]

Metals

Metals, such as arsenic, cesium, lead, manganese, mercury, potassium, and thallium, are often detected radiographically. Examples of metal exposure include leaded ceramic glaze (Fig. 8–4),[199] paint chips containing lead (Fig. 93–7),[131,158] mercuric oxide and elemental mercury (Fig. 95–1),[143] thallium salts (atomic number 81),[53,159] and zinc (atomic number 30).[28] Arsenic (Fig. 8–5) with a lower atomic number (atomic number 33) is also radiopaque.[93,136,246]

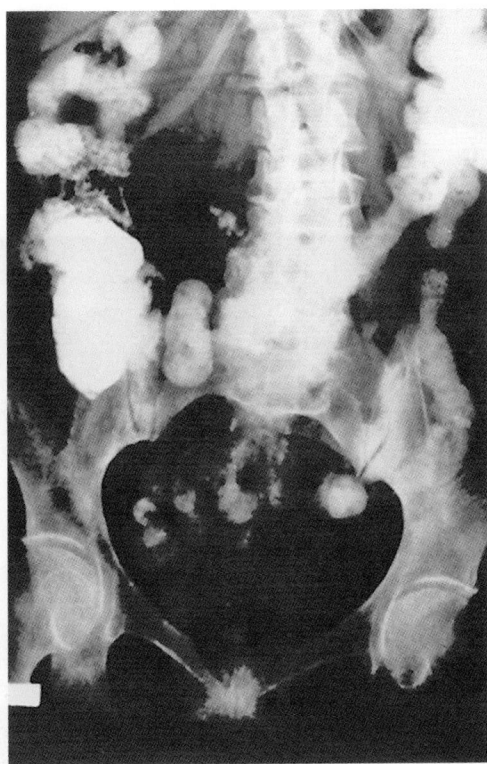

FIGURE 8–4. An abdominal radiograph of a patient who intentionally ingested ceramic glaze containing 40% lead. *(Used with permission from the Fellowship in Medical Toxicology, NYU School of Medicine, New York City Poison Control Center.)*

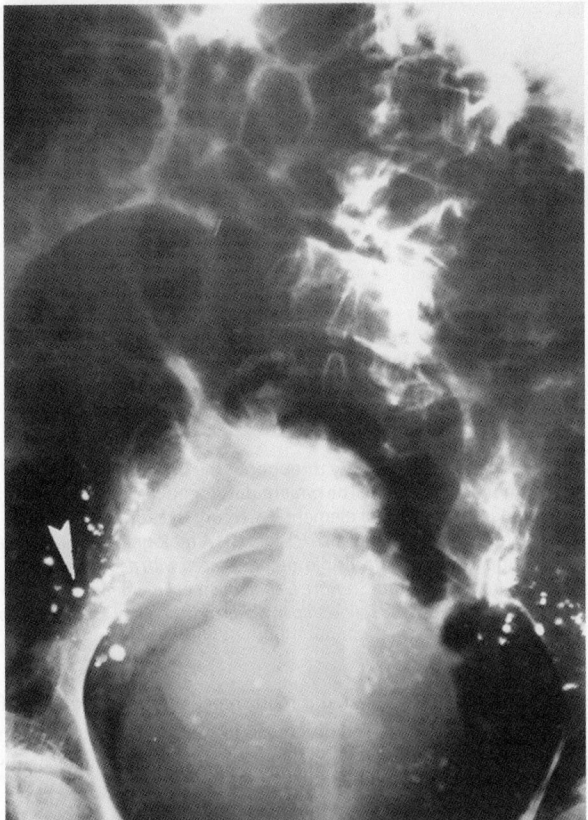

FIGURE 8–5. An abdominal radiograph in an elderly woman incidentally revealed radiopaque material in the pelvic region *(arrowhead)*. This was residual from gluteal injection of antisyphilis therapy she had received 35 to 40 years earlier. The injections may have contained an arsenical. *(Used with permission from Dr. Emil J. Balthazar, Department of Radiology, Bellevue Hospital Center.)*

Mercury

Unintentional ingestion of elemental mercury used to occur when a glass thermometer or a long intestinal tube with a mercury-containing balloon broke. Liquid elemental mercury is injected subcutaneously or intravenously. Radiographic studies assist débridement by detecting mercury that remains after the initial excision. Elemental mercury that is injected intravenously produces a dramatic radiographic picture of pulmonary embolization (Fig. 8–6).[32,47,148,169]

Lead

Ingested lead is detected only by abdominal radiography, such as in a child with lead poisoning who has ingested paint chips (Fig. 93–7). Metallic lead (eg, a bullet) that is embedded in soft tissues is not usually systemically absorbed. However, when the bullet is in contact with an acidic environment such as synovial fluid or cerebrospinal fluid (CSF), there significant absorption often occurs. Over many years, mechanical and chemical action within the joint causes the bullet to fragment and gradually dissolve.[52,54,62,231,236] Radiography confirms the source of lead poisoning by revealing metallic material in the joint or CSF (Fig. 8–7).

Xenobiotics in Containers

In some circumstances, ingested xenobiotics are seen even though they are of similar radiopacity to surrounding soft tissues. If a xenobiotic is ingested in a container, the container itself will be visible (Special Considerations: SC5).

Body Packers

"Body packers" are individuals who smuggle large quantities of illicit drugs across international borders in securely sealed packets.[4,18,20,31,43,65,69,111,129,146,157,184,220,223,243] The uniformly shaped, oblong packets are seen on abdominal radiographs either because there is a thin layer of air or metallic foil within the container wall or because the packets are outlined by bowel gas (Fig. 8–8). In some cases, a "rosette" representing the knot at the end of the packet is seen. Intraabdominal calcifications (pancreatic calcifications and bladder stones) have occasionally been misinterpreted as drug-containing packets.[244,261]

The sensitivity of abdominal radiography for such packets is high, in the range of 85% to 90%. The major role of radiography is as a rapid screening test to confirm the diagnosis in individuals suspected of smuggling drugs, such as persons being held by airport customs agents. However, because packets are occasionally not visualized and the rupture of even a single packet can be fatal, abdominal radiography should not be relied on to exclude the diagnosis of body packing.[204] Ultrasonography is used to rapidly detect packets, although it also should not be relied on to exclude such a life-threatening ingestion.[39,94,161] Computed tomography without oral contrast is more sensitive than radiography and ultrasonography (Figs. SC5-1 and SC5-2).[15,16,27,33,69,147,185,218,220] After intestinal decontamination, an upper GI series with oral contrast or CT without enteric contrast usually reveals any remaining packets (Fig. SC5–1).[96,107,152,174]

Body Stuffers

A "body stuffer" is an individual who, in an attempt to avoid imminent arrest, hurriedly ingests contraband in insecure packaging.[201] The risk of leakage from such haphazardly constructed containers is high. Unfortunately, radiographic studies cannot reliably confirm or exclude such ingestions.[226]

Occasionally, a radiograph will demonstrate the ingested container (Fig. 8–9). If the drug is in a glass or in a hard-plastic crack vial, the container is frequently seen.[106] If the body stuffer swallows soft plastic bags containing the drug, the containers are not usually visible. However, in three reported cases, "baggies" were visualized by abdominal CT.[44,57,99,101,125,186]

Halogenated Hydrocarbons

Some halogenated hydrocarbons are visualized radiographically.[38,45] Radiopacity is proportionate to the number of chlorine atoms. Both carbon tetrachloride (CCl_4) and chloroform ($CHCl_3$) are radiopaque. Because these liquids are immiscible in water, a triple layer is seen within the stomach on an upright abdominal radiograph—an uppermost air bubble, a middle

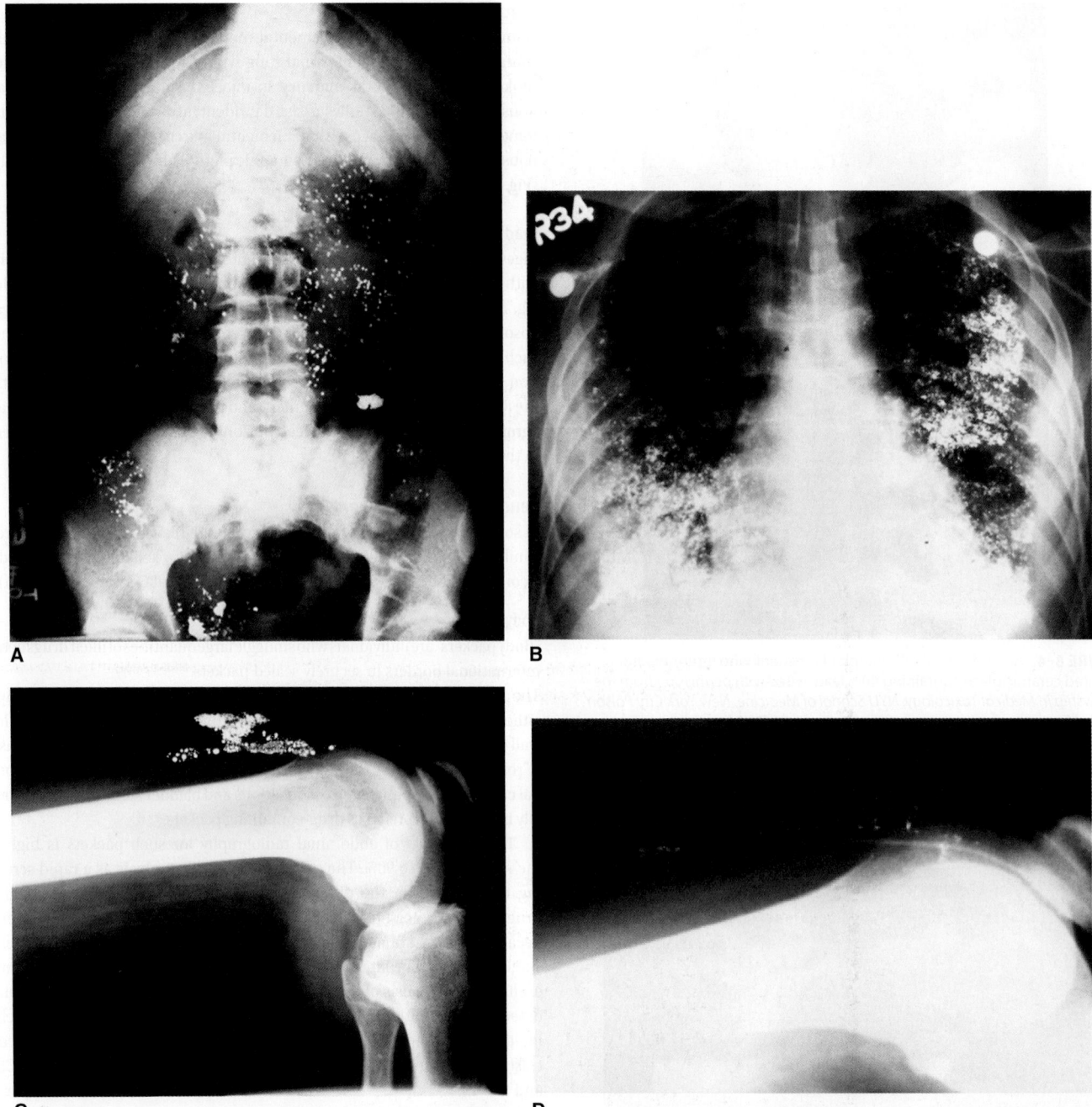

FIGURE 8–6. Elemental mercury exposures. (**A**) Unintentional rupture of a Cantor intestinal tube distributed mercury throughout the bowel. (**B**) The chest radiograph in a patient after intravenous injection of elemental mercury showing a metallic pulmonary embolism. The patient developed respiratory failure, pleural effusions, and uremia and died despite aggressive therapeutic interventions. (**C**) Subcutaneous injection of elemental mercury is readily detected radiographically. Because mercury is systemically absorbed from subcutaneous tissues, it must be removed by surgical excision. (**D**) A radiograph after surgical débridement reveals nearly complete removal of the mercury deposit. Surgical staples and a radiopaque drain are visible. *(Image A used with permission from Dr. Richard Lefleur, Department of Radiology, Bellevue Hospital Center; image B used with permission from Dr. N. John Stewart, Department of Emergency Medicine, Palmetto Health, University of South Carolina School of Medicine; and images C and D used with permission from the Fellowship in Medical Toxicology, NYU School of Medicine, New York City Poison Control Center.)*

radiopaque chlorinated hydrocarbon layer, and a lower gastric fluid layer. However, these ingestions are rare, and the quantity ingested is usually too small to show this effect. Other halogenated hydrocarbons such as methylene iodide are highly radiopaque.[259]

Moth Repellants

Some types of moth repellants (mothballs) can be visualized by radiography. Whereas relatively common and nontoxic paradichlorobenzene moth repellants (containing chlorine; atomic number 17) are moderately radiopaque, more toxic naphthalene moth repellants are faintly radiopaque.[233] If the patient is known to have ingested a moth repellant but the nature of the moth repellant is unknown, the difference in radiopacity helps determine the type. Radiographs of the moth repellant outside of the patient can distinguish these two types (Fig. 102–2).

Radiolucent Xenobiotics

A radiolucent xenobiotic is often visible because it is less radiopaque than surrounding soft tissues. Hydrocarbons such as gasoline are relatively radiolucent when embedded in soft tissues. The radiographic appearance resembles subcutaneous gas as seen in a necrotizing soft tissue infection (Fig. 8–10).[176]

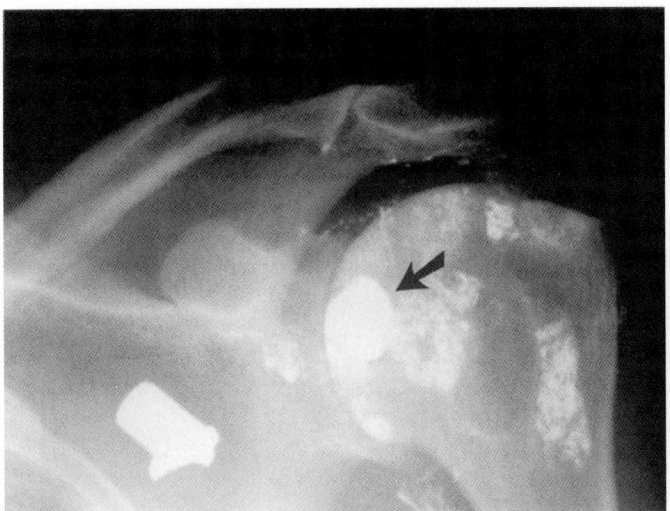

FIGURE 8–7. A "lead arthrogram" discovered many years after a bullet wound to the shoulder. At the time of the initial injury, the bullet was embedded in the articular surface of the humeral head (*arrow*). The portion of the bullet that protruded into the joint space was surgically removed, leaving a portion of the bullet exposed to the synovial space. A second bullet was embedded in the muscles of the scapula. Eight years after the injury, the patient presented with weakness and anemia. Extensive lead deposition throughout the synovium is seen. The blood lead concentration was 91 mcg/dL. (*Used with permission from the Fellowship in Medical Toxicology, NYU School of Medicine, New York City Poison Control Center.*)

EXTRAVASATION OF INTRAVENOUS CONTRAST MATERIAL

Extravasation of intravenous (IV) radiographic contrast material is a common occurrence. In most cases, the volume extravasated is small, and there are no clinical sequelae.[21,42,63,200] Rarely, a patient has an extravasation large enough to cause cutaneous necrosis and ulceration.

Recently, the incidence of sizable extravasations has increased because of the use of rapid-bolus automated power injectors for CT studies.[251] Fortunately, nonionic low-osmolality contrast solutions are currently nearly always used for these studies. These solutions are far less toxic to soft tissues than older ionic high-osmolality contrast materials.

The treatment of contrast extravasation has not been studied in a large series of human participants and is therefore controversial. Various strategies are proposed. The affected extremity should be elevated to promote drainage. Although topical application of heat causes vasodilation and could theoretically promote absorption of extravasated contrast material, the intermittent application of ice packs is recommended to lower the incidence of ulceration. Rarely, an extremely large volume of liquid is injected into the soft tissues, which requires surgical decompression when there are signs of a compartment syndrome. A radiograph of the extremity will demonstrate the extent of extravasation (Fig. 8–11).[42]

Precautions should be taken to prevent extravasation. A recently placed, well-running IV catheter should be used. The distal portions of the extremities (hands, wrist, and feet) should not be used as IV sites for injecting contrast. Patients who are more vulnerable to complications and those whose veins are more fragile, such as infants, debilitated patients, and those with an impaired ability to communicate, must be closely monitored to prevent or determine if extravasation occurs.

Summary

Obtaining an abdominal radiograph in an attempt to identify pills or other xenobiotics in a patient with an unknown ingestion is unlikely to be helpful and is, in general, not warranted. Radiography is most useful when the suspected xenobiotic is known to be radiopaque, as is the case with iron tablets and heavy metals. Radiography will demonstrate xenobiotic within the patient's abdomen; elsewhere in the patient's body; or, if the material is available, outside of the patient.

VISUALIZING THE EFFECTS OF A XENOBIOTIC ON THE BODY

The lungs, central nervous system (CNS), GI tract, and skeleton are the organ systems that are most amenable to diagnostic imaging. Disorders of the lungs and skeletal system are seen by plain radiography. For abdominal pathology, contrast studies and CT are more useful, although plain radiographs can diagnose intestinal obstruction, perforation, and radiopaque foreign bodies. Imaging of the CNS uses CT, MRI, and nuclear scintigraphy (PET and SPECT).[95]

Skeletal Changes Caused by Xenobiotics

A number of xenobiotics affect bone mineralization. Toxicologic effects on bone result in either increased or decreased density (Table 8–2). Some xenobiotics produce characteristic radiographic images, although exact diagnoses usually depend on correlation with the clinical scenario.[11,171] Furthermore, alterations in skeletal structure develop gradually and are usually not visible unless the exposure continues for at least 2 weeks.

Increase in Bone Density

Lead Poisoning. Skeletal radiography suggests the diagnosis of chronic lead poisoning in children even before the blood lead concentration is obtained. With lead poisoning, the metaphyseal regions of rapidly growing long bones develop transverse bands of increased density along the growth plate (Fig. 8–12).[25,189,191,209] Characteristic locations are the distal femur and proximal tibia. Flaring of the distal metaphysis also occurs. Such lead lines are also seen in the vertebral bodies and iliac crest. Detected in approximately 80% of children with a mean lead concentration of 49 ± 17 mcg/dL, lead lines usually occur in children between the ages of 2 and 9 years.[25] In most children, it takes several weeks for lead lines to appear, although in very young infants (2–4 months old), lead lines develop within days of exposure.[265] After exposure ceases, lead lines diminish and eventually disappear in some children.

Lead lines are caused by the toxic effect of lead on bone growth and do not represent deposition of lead in bone. Lead impedes resorption of calcified cartilage in the zone of provisional calcification adjacent to the growth plate. This is termed *chondrosclerosis*.[25,56] Other xenobiotics that cause metaphyseal bands are yellow phosphorus (Chap. 112), bismuth (Chap. 87), and vitamin D (Chap. 44).

Fluorosis. Fluoride poisoning causes a diffuse increase in bone mineralization. Endemic fluorosis occurs where drinking water contains very high concentrations of fluoride (≥2 or more parts per million), as an occupational exposure among aluminum workers handling cryolite (sodium–aluminum fluoride), or with excessive tea drinking. The skeletal changes associated with fluorosis are osteosclerosis (hyperostosis deformans), osteophytosis, and ligament calcification (Fig. 8–13). Fluorosis primarily affects the axial skeleton, especially the vertebral column and pelvis. Thickening of the vertebral column causes compression of the spinal cord and nerve roots. Without a history of fluoride exposure, the clinical and radiographic findings are mistaken for osteoblastic skeletal metastases. The diagnosis of fluorosis is confirmed by histologic examination of the bone and measurement of fluoride concentrations in the bone and urine (Figs. 81–1 and 81–2).[26,120,253]

Bisphosphonates. Bisphosphonates such as alendronate are commonly used to treat osteoporosis. They increase bone density by inhibiting osteoclast activity and decreasing bone resorption. However, by suppressing bone turnover and fracture healing, bisphosphonates are associated with accumulated microdamage to bone and skeletal weakening, which makes the bone vulnerable to fractures. Radiographically, there is thickening of the cortex of diaphyseal bone, typically the proximal femoral shaft. Such bone is associated with atypical proximal femoral shaft and subtrochanteric fractures after low-energy injuries such as a fall from standing. The fractures are transverse and have a characteristic "beaked" appearance caused by the cortical thickening (Fig. 8–14).[89,137,215-217,260]

Focal Loss of Bone Density

Skeletal disorders associated with focal diminished bone density (or mixed rarefaction and sclerosis) include osteonecrosis, osteomyelitis, and

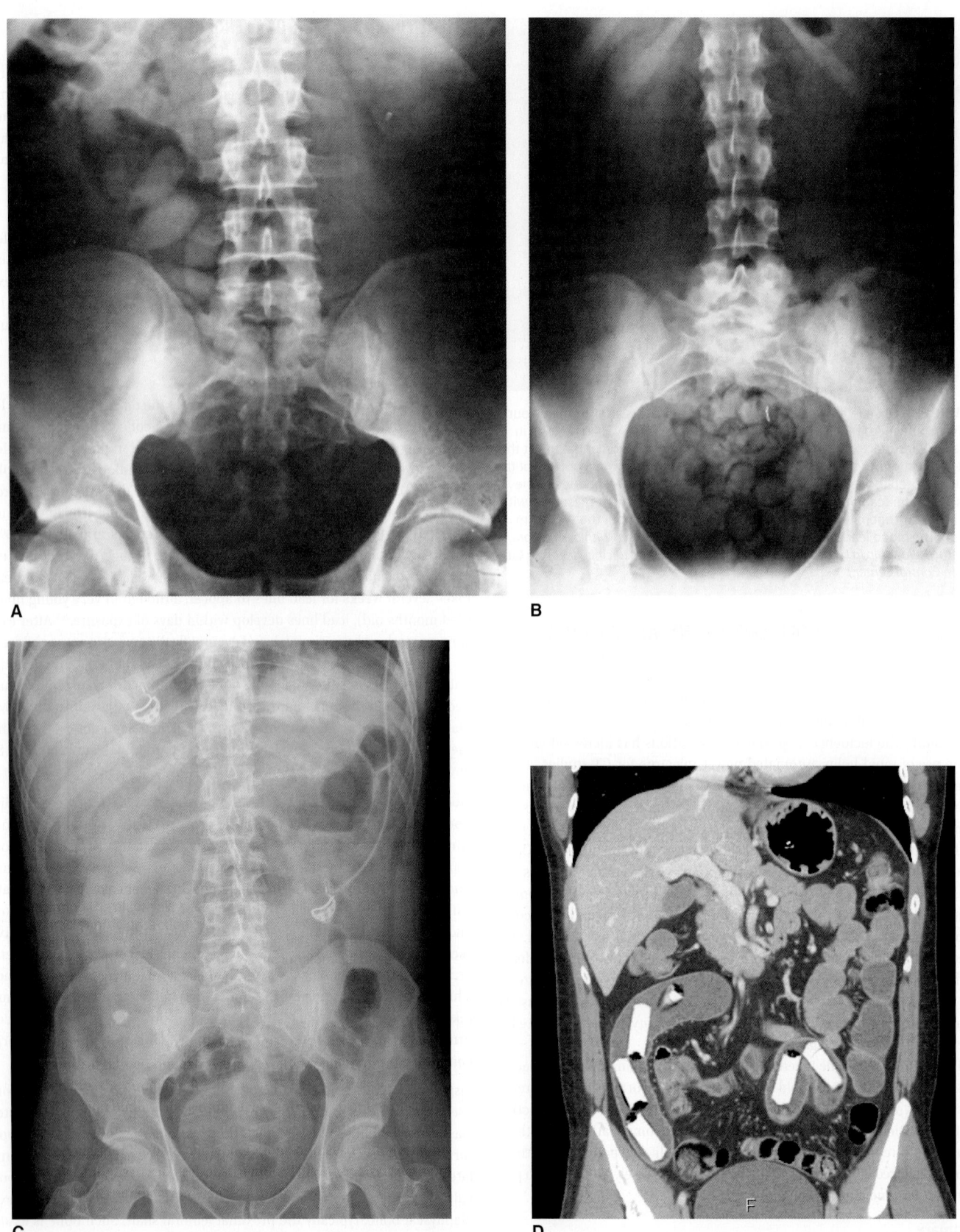

FIGURE 8–8. Three "body packers" showing the various appearances of drug packets. Drug smuggling is accomplished by packing the gastrointestinal tract with large numbers of manufactured, well-sealed containers. (**A**) Multiple oblong packages of uniform size and shape are seen throughout the bowel. (**B**) The packets are visible in this patient because they are surrounded by a thin layer of air within the wall of the packet. (**C** and **D**) Small bowel obstruction caused by drug packets in a man who developed abdominal pain and vomiting 1 day after arriving on a plane flight from Colombia. Computed tomography confirmed bowel obstruction, and the patient underwent laparotomy and removal of 15 packets through an enterotomy. *(Images A and B used with permission from Dr. Emil J. Balthazar, Department of Radiology, Bellevue Hospital Center. Images C and D used with permission from the Fellowship in Medical Toxicology, New York University School of Medicine, New York City Poison Center.)*

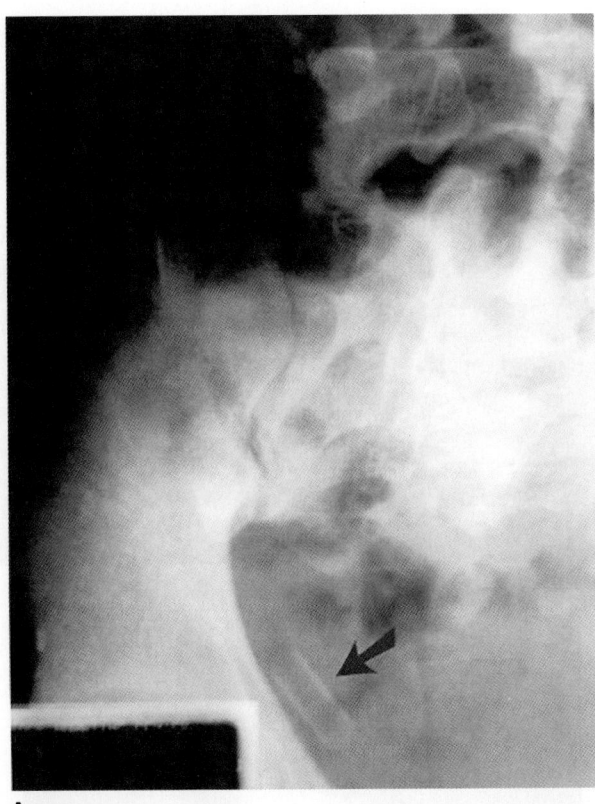
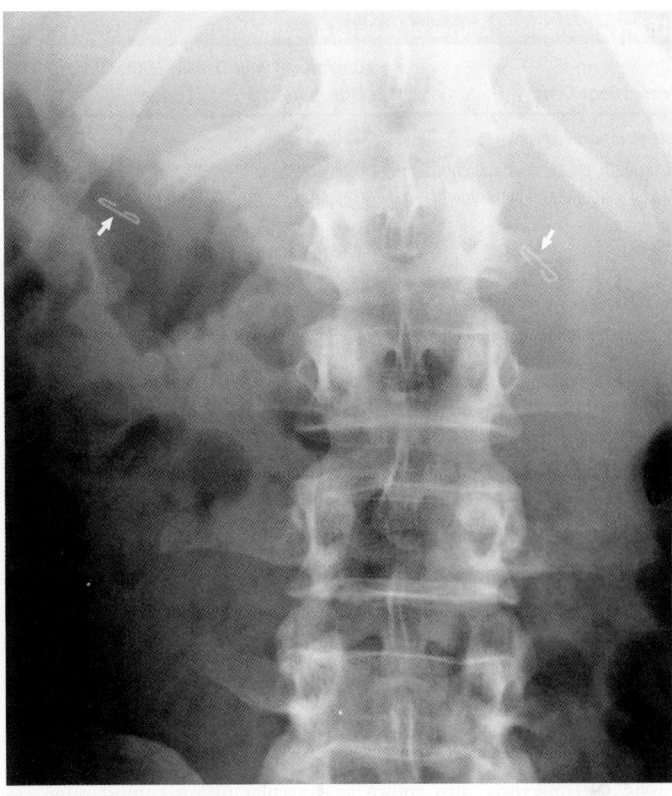

A

B

FIGURE 8-9. Two "body stuffers." Radiography infrequently helps with the diagnosis. (**A**) An ingested glass crack vial is seen in the distal bowel (*arrow*). The patient had ingested his contraband several hours earlier at the time of a police raid. Only the tubular-shaped container, and not the xenobiotic, is visible radiographically. The patient did not develop signs of cocaine toxicity during 24 hours of observation. (**B**) Another patient in police custody was brought to the emergency department for allegedly ingesting his drugs. The patient repeatedly denied this. The radiographs revealed "nonsurgical" staples in his abdomen (*arrows*). When questioned again, the patient admitted that he had swallowed several plastic bags that were stapled closed. (*Used with permission from the Fellowship in Medical Toxicology, NYU School of Medicine, New York City Poison Control Center.*)

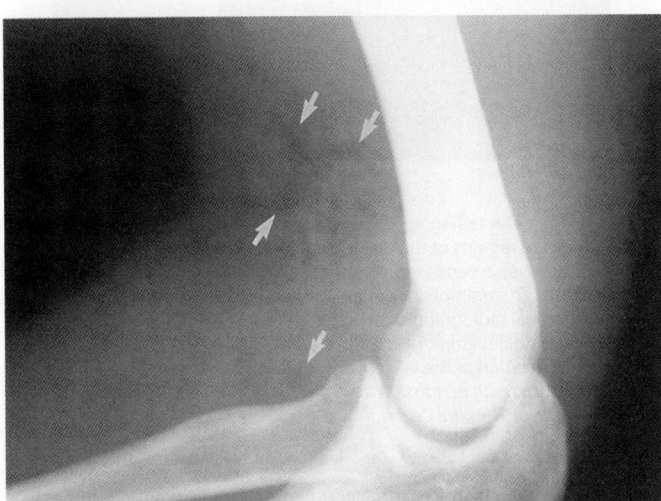

FIGURE 8-10. Subcutaneous injection of gasoline into the antecubital fossa. The radiolucent hydrocarbon mimics gas in the soft tissues that is seen with a necrotizing soft tissue infection such as necrotizing fasciitis or gas gangrene (*arrows*). (*Used with permission from the Fellowship in Medical Toxicology, NYU School of Medicine, New York City Poison Control Center.*)

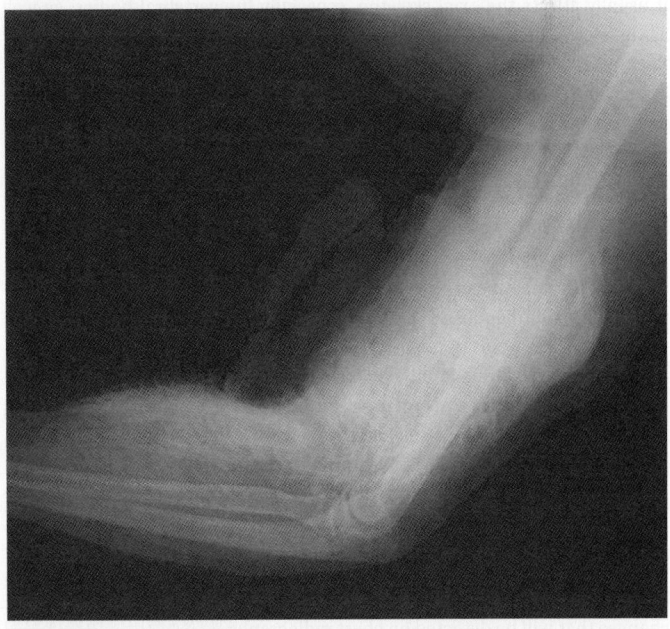

FIGURE 8-11. Extravasation of intravenous contrast into the soft tissues of the upper extremity that occurred during a computed tomography contrast bolus administered by a power injector. Despite the extensive extravasation, the patient was successfully managed with limb elevation and cool compresses. (*Used with permission from Mark Bernstein, MD, Department of Radiology, New York University School of Medicine.*)

TABLE 8–2   Xenobiotic Causes of Skeletal Abnormalities

Increased Bone Density	Diminished Bone Density (Either Diffuse Osteoporosis or Focal Lesions)
Metaphyseal bands (children) Lead, bismuth, phosphorus: chondrosclerosis caused by toxic effect on bone growth.	Corticosteroids: Osteoporosis: diffuse Osteonecrosis: focal avascular necrosis of the femoral head); loss of volume with both increased and decreased bone density Also occurs in alcoholism, bismuth arthropathy, Caisson disease (dysbarism), trauma
Diffuse increased bone density Fluorosis: osteosclerosis (hyperostosis deformans), osteophytosis, ligament calcification; usually involves the axial skeleton (vertebrae and pelvis) and can cause compression of the spinal cord and nerve roots Hypervitaminosis A (pediatric): cortical hyperostosis and subperiosteal new bone formation; diaphyses of long bones have an undulating appearance Hypervitaminosis D (pediatric): generalized osteosclerosis, cortical thickening, and metaphyseal bands	Hypervitaminosis D (adult): focal or generalized osteoporosis Injection drug use: osteomyelitis (focal lytic lesions) caused by septic emboli; usually affects vertebral bodies and sternomanubrial joint Vinyl chloride monomer: acroosteolysis (distal phalanges)

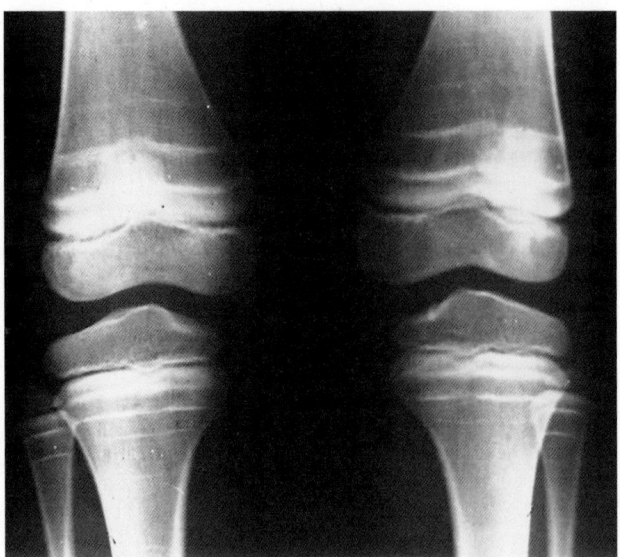

A

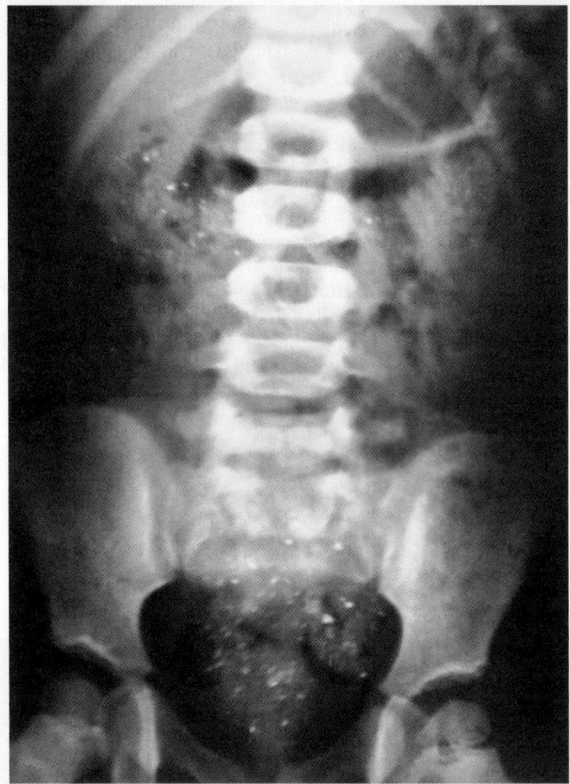

B

FIGURE 8–12. (**A**) A radiograph of the knees of a child with lead poisoning. The metaphyseal regions of the distal femur and proximal tibia have developed transverse bands representing bone growth abnormalities caused by lead toxicity. The multiplicity of lines implies repeated exposures to lead. (**B**) The abdominal radiograph of the child shows many radiopaque flakes of ingested leaded paint chips. Lead poisoning also caused abnormally increased cortical mineralization of the vertebral bodies, which gives them a boxlike appearance. *(Used with permission from Dr. Nancy Genieser, Department of Radiology, Bellevue Hospital Center.)*

osteolysis. Osteonecrosis, also known as avascular necrosis, most often affects the femoral head, humeral head, and proximal tibia.[149] There are many causes of osteonecrosis. Xenobiotic causes include long-term corticosteroid use and alcoholism. Radiographically, focal skeletal lucencies and sclerosis are seen, ultimately with loss of bone volume and collapse (Fig. 8–15A).

Acroosteolysis. Acroosteolysis is bone resorption of the distal phalanges and is associated with occupational exposure to vinyl chloride monomer. Protective measures have reduced its incidence since it was first described in the early 1960s.[192]

Osteomyelitis. Osteomyelitis is a serious complication of injection drug use. It usually affects the axial skeleton, especially the vertebral bodies, as well as the sternomanubrial and sternoclavicular joints (Figs. 8–15B and C).[90,95] Back pain or neck pain in injection drug users warrants careful consideration. Spinal epidural abscesses causing spinal cord compression accompany vertebral osteomyelitis. Radiographic findings are negative early in the disease course before skeletal changes are visible, and the diagnosis is confirmed by MRI or CT (Fig. 8–15D).

Soft Tissue Changes

Certain abnormalities in soft tissues, that occur predominantly as a consequence of infectious complications of injection drug use, are amenable to radiographic diagnosis.[90,95,116,239] In an injection drug user who presents with signs of local soft tissue infections, radiography is indicated to detect a retained metallic foreign body, such as a needle fragment, or subcutaneous gas, as is recognized in a necrotizing soft tissue infection such as necrotizing fasciitis. Computed tomography is more sensitive at detecting soft tissue gas than is conventional radiography. Computed tomography and ultrasonography also detect subcutaneous or deeper abscesses that require surgical or percutaneous drainage.

Pulmonary and Other Thoracic Problems

Many xenobiotics that affect intrathoracic organs produce pathologic changes that will be detected on chest radiographs.[10,30,58,76,105,144,165,195,203,230,262,263] The lungs are most often affected, resulting in dyspnea or cough, but the pleura, hila, heart, and great vessels are also involved. Patients with chest pain need to be evaluated for pneumothorax, pneumomediastinum, or aortic dissection. Patients with fever, with or without respiratory symptoms, can have focal infiltrates, pleural effusions, or hilar lymphadenopathy.

Chest radiographic findings suggest certain diseases, although the diagnosis ultimately depends on a thorough clinical history. When a specific xenobiotic exposure is known or suspected, the chest radiograph can confirm the diagnosis and help in assessment. If a history of xenobiotic exposure is not obtained, a patient with an abnormal chest radiograph can initially be misdiagnosed as having pneumonia or another disorder that is more

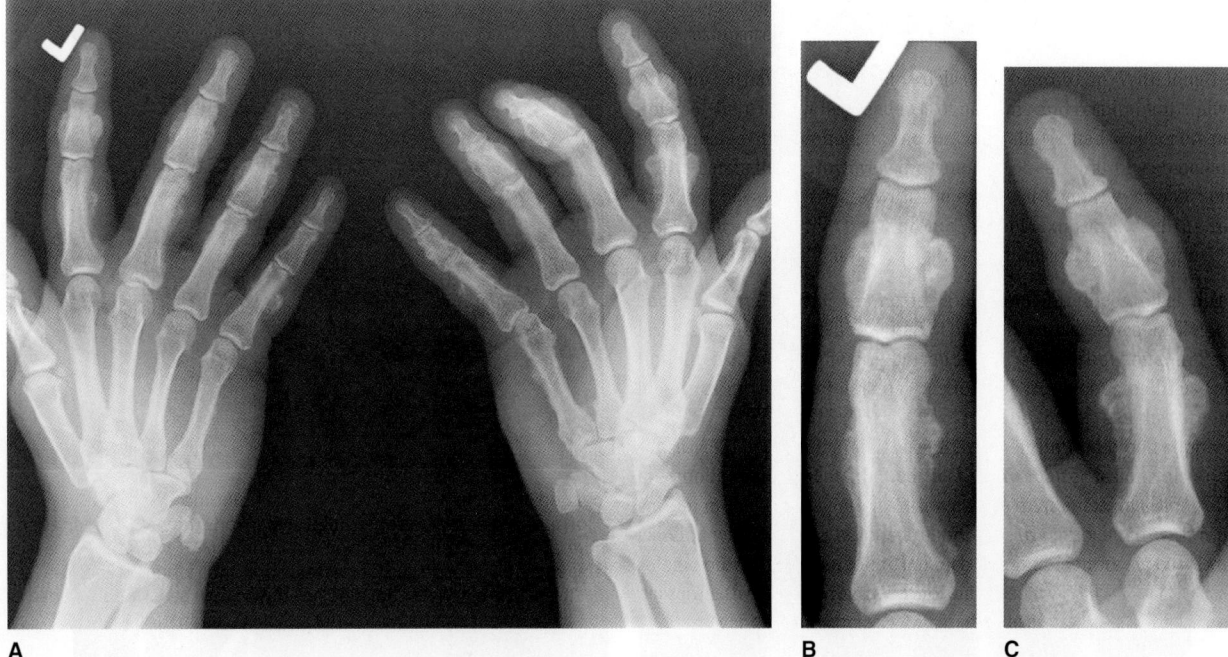

FIGURE 8-13. Skeletal fluorosis. A 28-year-old man developed progressive muscle and joint pain over 3 to 4 weeks particularly involving his hands with thickening of his fingers. The results of an evaluation for inflammatory rheumatologic disorders were negative. Radiographs of his hands showed exuberant periosteal new bone formation known as "periostitis deformans," which is characteristic of skeletal fluorosis. Further questioning revealed that the patient had been "huffing" the propellant of "Dust Off"; 225 cans were found at his residence. The propellant is difluoroethane (Freon 152a). The hydrocarbon is dehalogenated in the liver, and chronic exposure results in fluoride toxicity. *(Used with permission from Dr. Eric Lavonas, Rocky Mountain Poison and Drug Center, Denver Health and Hospital Authority, Denver, CO, and Dr. Shawn M. Varney, Department of Emergency Medicine, San Antonio Military Medical Center, TX.)*

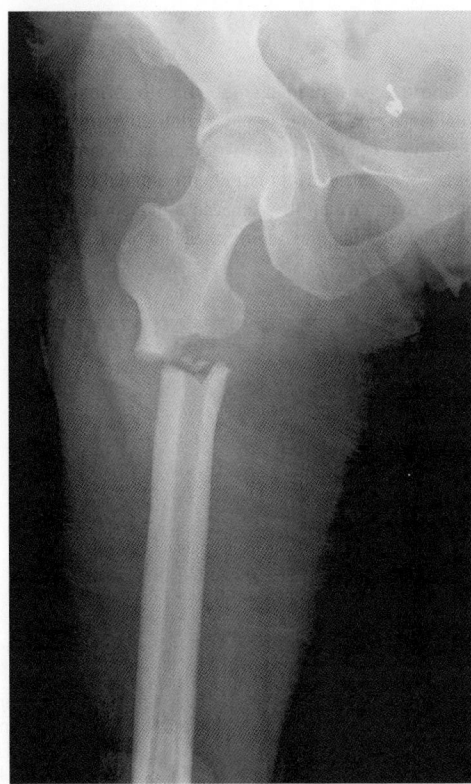

FIGURE 8-14. Bisphosphonate- (alendronate-) associated proximal femoral shaft fracture. A 61-year-old woman tripped on the sidewalk, falling on to her right side. She had been taking alendronate for 3 years for osteoporosis. There are diffuse cortical thickening of the femoral shaft and a transverse fracture in the subtrochanteric region with "beaking" of the fractured cortex on the medial side of the fracture. *(Used with permission from the Fellowship in Medical Toxicology, NYU School of Medicine, New York City Poison Control Center.)*

common than xenobiotic-mediated lung disease. Therefore, patients with chest radiographic abnormalities should be carefully questioned regarding possible xenobiotic exposures at work or at home, as well as the use of medications or other drugs.

Many pulmonary disorders are radiographically detectable because they result in fluid accumulation within the normally air-filled lung. Fluid accumulates within the alveolar spaces or interstitial tissues of the lung, producing the two major radiographic patterns of pulmonary disease, airspace filling and interstitial lung disease (Table 8–3). Most xenobiotics are widely distributed throughout the lungs and produce diffuse rather than focal radiographic abnormalities.

Diffuse Airspace Filling

Overdose with various xenobiotics, including salicylates, opioids, and paraquat, cause acute respiratory distress syndrome (ARDS) (formerly known as noncardiogenic pulmonary edema or acute lung injury) with or without diffuse alveolar damage and characterized by leaky capillaries (Fig. 8–16). There are, of course, many other causes of ARDS, including sepsis, anaphylaxis, and major trauma.[256] Other xenobiotic exposures that result in diffuse airspace filling include inhalation of irritant gases that are of low water solubility such as phosgene ($COCl_2$), nitrogen dioxide (silo filler's disease), chlorine, hydrogen sulfide, and sulfur dioxide (Chaps. 121 and 123).[122] Organic phosphorus compound poisoning causes cholinergic hyperstimulation, resulting in bronchorrhea (Chap. 110). Smoking "crack" cocaine is associated with diffuse alveolar hemorrhage (Chap. 75).[46,72,193]

Focal Airspace Filling

Focal infiltrates are usually caused by bacterial pneumonia, although aspiration of gastric contents also causes localized airspace disease.[235] Aspiration occurs during sedative–hypnotic or alcohol intoxication or during a seizure. During ingestion, low-viscosity hydrocarbons often enter the lungs while they are being swallowed (Figs. 8–17 and 105–1).[164] There is a typical delay in the development of radiographic abnormalities, and the chest radiograph abnormalities appear over the first 6 hours after the ingestion.[9] During

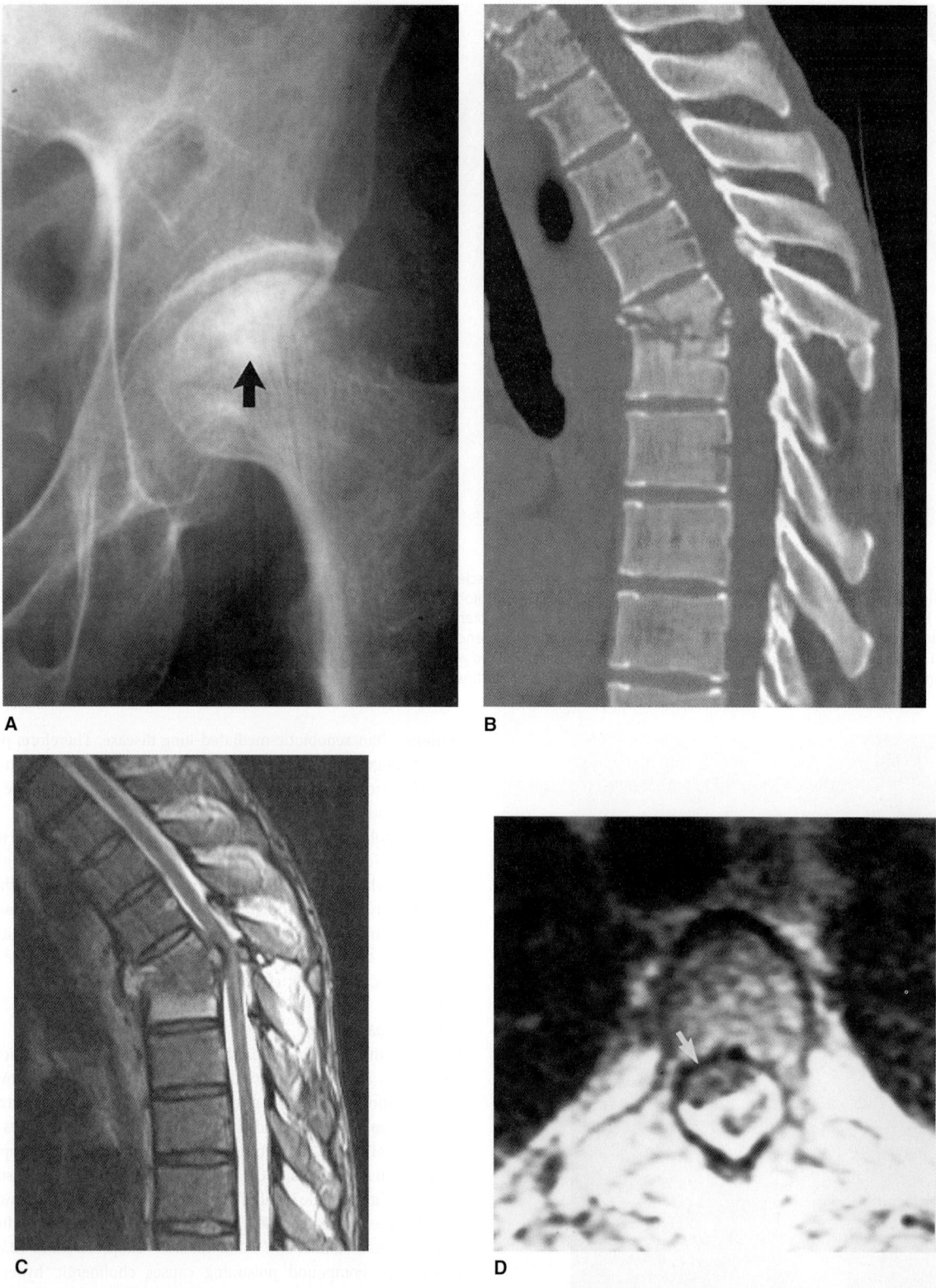

FIGURE 8–15. Focal loss of bone density and collapse: (**A**) Avascular necrosis causing collapse of the femoral head in a patient with long-standing steroid-dependent asthma (*arrow*). (**B** and **C**) Vertebral osteomyelitis in an injection drug user who presented with posterior thoracic pain for 2 weeks and then lower extremity weakness. As seen on computed tomography (CT), the infection begins in the intervertebral disk and then spreads to the adjacent vertebral bodies. Magnetic resonance image shows extension into the spinal canal causing spinal cord compression. (**D**) An injection drug user with thoracic back pain, leg weakness, and low-grade fever. Radiographic and CT findings of the spine were negative. Magnetic resonance image showing an epidural abscess (*arrow*) compressing the spinal cord. The cerebrospinal fluid in the compressed thecal sac is bright on this T2-weighted image. *(Reproduced with permission from Schwartz DT, Reisdorff EJ: Emergency Radiology. New York, NY: McGraw-Hill; 2000.)*

TABLE 8–3 Chest Radiographic Findings in Toxicologic Emergencies

Radiographic Finding	Responsible Xenobiotic	Disease Processes
Diffuse airspace filling	Opioids	ARDS
	Paraquat	
	Salicylates	
	Irritant gases: NO$_2$ (silo filler's disease), phosgene (COCl$_2$), Cl$_2$, H$_2$S	
	Organic phosphorus compounds, carbamates	Cholinergic stimulation (bronchorrhea)
	Alcoholic cardiomyopathy, cocaine, doxorubicin, cobalt	Congestive heart failure
Focal airspace filling	Low-viscosity hydrocarbons	Aspiration pneumonitis
	Gastric contents aspiration: CNS depressants, alcohol, seizures	
Multifocal airspace filling	Injection drug user	Septic emboli
Interstitial patterns	Inhaled organic allergens: farmer's lung, pigeon-breeder's lung	Hypersensitivity pneumonitis
Fine or coarse reticular or reticulonodular pattern	Nitrofurantoin, penicillamine	
Patchy airspace filling seen in some cases	Chemotherapeutics: bleomycin, busulfan, carmustine, cyclophosphamide, methotrexate	Cytotoxic lung damage
	Amiodarone	Phospholipidosis
	Talcosis (illicit drug contaminant)	Injected particulates
	Pneumoconiosis: asbestosis, berylliosis (chronic), coal dust, silicosis	Inhaled inorganic particulates

ARDS = acute respiratory distress syndrome; CNS = central nervous system.

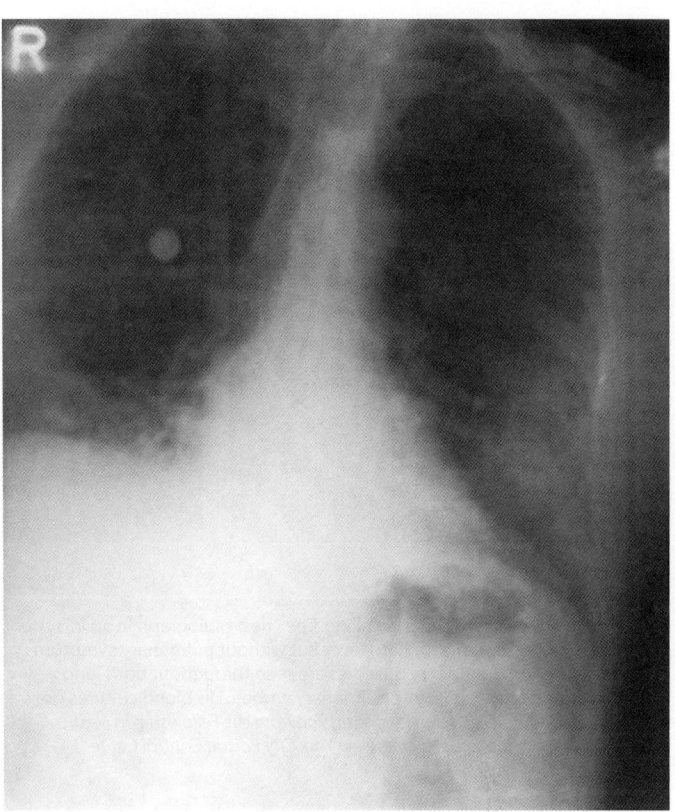

FIGURE 8–17. Focal airspace filling as a result of hydrocarbon aspiration. A 34-year-old man aspirated gasoline. The chest radiograph shows bilateral lower lobe infiltrates. *(Used with permission from the Fellowship in Medical Toxicology, NYU School of Medicine, New York City Poison Control Center.)*

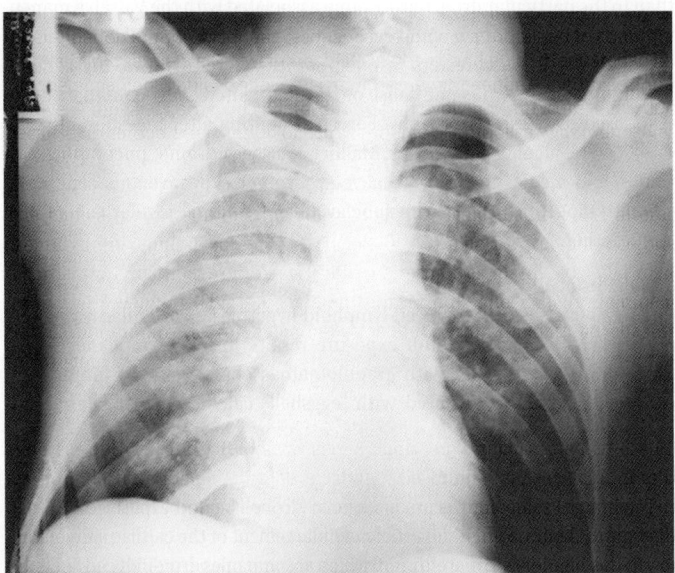

FIGURE 8–16. Diffuse airspace filling. The chest radiograph of a patient who had recently injected heroin intravenously presented with respiratory distress and acute respiratory distress syndrome. The heart size is normal.

aspiration, the most dependent portions of the lung are affected. When the patient is upright at the time of aspiration, the lower lung segments are involved. When the patient is supine, the posterior segments of the upper and lower lobes are affected.[75]

Multifocal Airspace Filling
Multifocal airspace filling occurs with septic pulmonary emboli, which is a complication of injection drug use and right-sided bacterial endocarditis. The foci of pulmonary infection often undergo necrosis and cavitation (Fig. 8–18).[91,95]

Interstitial Lung Diseases
Toxicologic causes of interstitial lung disease include hypersensitivity pneumonitis, use of medications with direct pulmonary toxicity, and inhalation or injection of inorganic particulates.[91] Interstitial lung diseases have acute, subacute, or chronic courses. On the chest radiograph, acute and subacute disorders cause a fine reticular or reticulonodular pattern (Fig. 8–19). Chronic interstitial disorders cause a coarse reticular "honeycomb" pattern.

Hypersensitivity Pneumonitis
Hypersensitivity pneumonitis is a delayed-type hypersensitivity reaction to an inhaled or ingested allergen.[49,113,195] Inhaled organic allergens such as those in moldy hay (farmer's lung) and bird droppings (pigeon breeder's lung) cause hypersensitivity pneumonitis in sensitized individuals. There are two clinical syndromes: an acute, recurrent illness and a chronic, progressive illness. The acute illness presents with fever and dyspnea. In these cases, the chest radiograph findings are normal or show fine interstitial or alveolar infiltrates. Chronic hypersensitivity pneumonitis causes progressive dyspnea, and the radiograph shows interstitial fibrosis.

The most common medication causing hypersensitivity pneumonitis is nitrofurantoin. Respiratory symptoms occur after taking the medication for

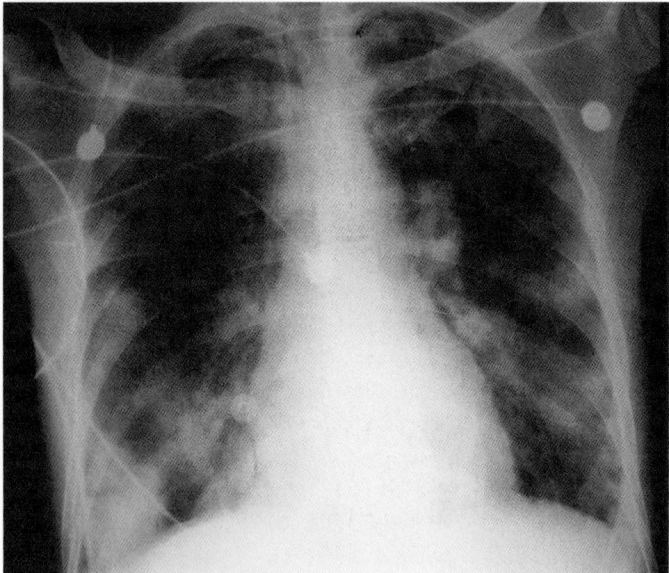

FIGURE 8–18. Multifocal airspace filling. The chest radiograph in an injection drug user who presented with high fever but without pulmonary symptoms. Multiple ill-defined pulmonary opacities are seen throughout both lungs, which are characteristic of septic pulmonary emboli. His blood cultures grew *Staphylococcus aureus*. (Used with permission from the Fellowship in Medical Toxicology, NYU School of Medicine, New York City Poison Control Center.)

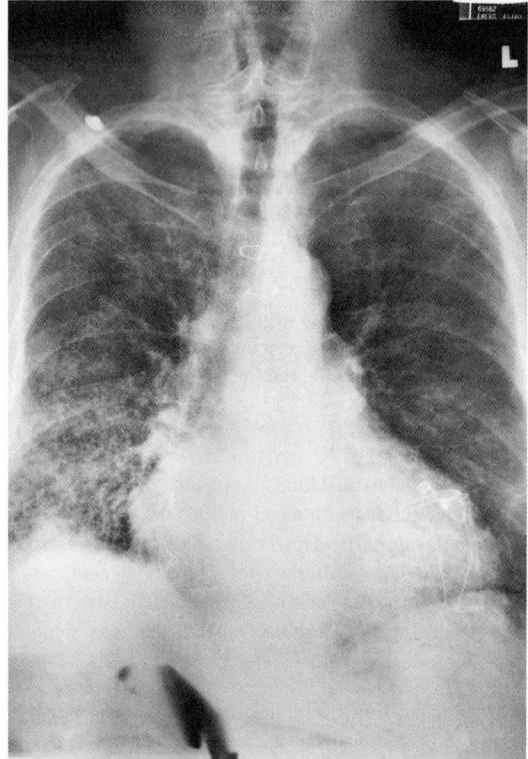

FIGURE 8–19. Reticular interstitial pattern. The chest radiograph of a patient with cardiac disease who presented to the emergency department with progressive dyspnea. The initial diagnostic impression was interstitial pulmonary edema. The patient was taking amiodarone for malignant ventricular dysrhythmias (note the implanted automatic defibrillator). The lack of response to diuretics and the high-resolution computed tomography pattern suggested that this was toxicity to amiodarone. The medication was stopped, and there was partial clearing over several weeks. (Used with permission from Dr. Georgeann McGuinness, Department of Radiology, New York University.)

1 to 2 weeks. Other medications that may cause hypersensitivity pneumonitis include sulfonamides and penicillins.

Chemotherapeutics

Various chemotherapeutics, such as bleomycin, busulfan, cyclophosphamide, and methotrexate, cause pulmonary injury by their direct cytotoxic effect on alveolar cells.[48,79] The radiographic pattern is usually interstitial (reticular or nodular) but also includes airspace filling or mixed patterns. The patient presents with dyspnea, fever, and pulmonary infiltrates that begin after several weeks of therapy. Other causes of these clinical and radiographic findings must be evaluated, including opportunistic infection, pulmonary carcinomatosis, pulmonary edema, and intraparenchymal hemorrhage. Symptoms usually resolve with discontinuation of the offending medication.

Amiodarone

Amiodarone toxicity causes phospholipid accumulation within alveolar cells and results in pulmonary fibrosis. An interstitial radiographic pattern is seen, although airspace filling also occur (Fig. 8–19) (Chap. 57).

Particulates

Inhaled inorganic particulates, such as asbestos, silica, and coal dust, cause pneumoconiosis. This is a chronic interstitial lung disease characterized by interstitial fibrosis and loss of lung volume.[2,198,258] Intravenous injection of illicit xenobiotics that have particulate contaminants, such as talc, causes a chronic interstitial lung disease known as talcosis.[2,64,255]

Pleural Disorders

Asbestos-related calcified pleural plaques develop many years after asbestos exposure (Fig. 8–20). These lesions do not cause clinical symptoms and have only a minor association with malignancy and interstitial lung disease. Asbestos-related pleural plaques should not be called *asbestosis* because that term refers specifically to the interstitial lung disease caused by asbestos. Pleural plaques must be distinguished from mesotheliomas, which are not calcified, enlarge at a rapid rate, and erode into nearby structures such as the ribs.

Pleural effusions occur with drug-induced systemic lupus erythematosus (SLE).[165] The medications most frequently implicated are procainamide, hydralazine, isoniazid, and methyldopa. The patient presents with fever as well as other symptoms of SLE.

Pneumothorax and pneumomediastinum are associated with illicit drug use. These complications are related to the route of administration rather than to the particular drug. Barotrauma associated with the Valsalva maneuver or intense inhalation with breath holding during the smoking of "crack" cocaine or marijuana results in pneumomediastinum (Fig. 8–21A).[24,59,91,177] Pneumomediastinum is one cause of cocaine-related chest pain that can be diagnosed by chest radiography. Forceful vomiting after ingestion of syrup of ipecac or alcohol produces a Mallory-Weiss syndrome, pneumomediastinum, and mediastinitis (Boerhaave syndrome).[264] Intravenous drug users who attempt to inject into the subclavian and internal jugular veins cause pneumothoraces.[55]

Lymphadenopathy

Phenytoin causes drug-induced lymphoid hyperplasia with hilar lymphadenopathy.[165] Chronic beryllium exposure results in hilar lymphadenopathy that mimics sarcoidosis, with granulomatous changes in the lung parenchyma. Silicosis is associated with "eggshell" calcification of hilar lymph nodes.

Cardiovascular Abnormalities

Dilated cardiomyopathy occurs in chronic alcoholism and exposure to cardiotoxic medications such as doxorubicin. Enlargement of the cardiac silhouette is also caused by a pericardial effusion, which accompanies drug-induced SLE. Aortic dissection is associated with use of cocaine and amphetamines.[80,91,134,180,190,194,221] The chest radiograph shows an enlarged or indistinct aortic knob and an enlarged ascending or descending aorta (Figs. 8–21B to D).

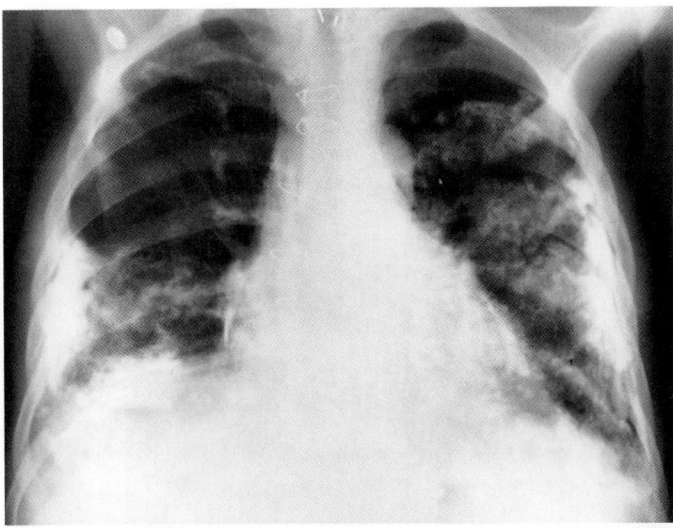

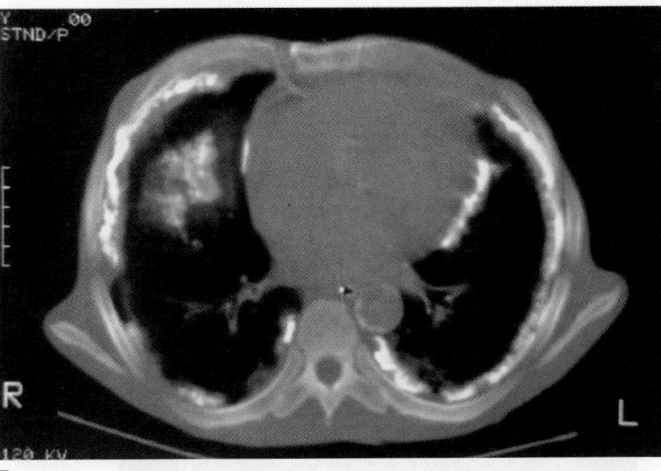

FIGURE 8–20. (**A**) Calcified plaques typical of asbestos exposure are seen on the pleural surfaces of the lungs, diaphragm, and heart. The patient was asymptomatic; this was an incidental radiographic finding. (**B**) The computed tomography (CT) scan demonstrates that the opacities seen on the chest radiograph do not involve the lung itself. A lower thoracic image shows calcified pleural plaques (the diaphragmatic plaque is seen on the *right*). The CT scan confirms that there is no interstitial lung disease ("asbestosis"). *(Used with permission from the Fellowship in Medical Toxicology, NYU School of Medicine, New York City Poison Control Center.)*

Abdominal Problems

Abdominal imaging modalities include conventional radiography, CT, GI contrast studies, and angiography.[82,222] Conventional radiography is limited in its ability to detect most intraabdominal pathology because most pathologic processes involve soft tissue structures that are not well seen. Plain radiography readily visualizes gas in the abdomen and is therefore useful to diagnose pneumoperitoneum (free intraperitoneal air) and bowel distension caused by mechanical obstruction or diminished gut motility (adynamic ileus). Other abnormal gas collections, such as intramural gas associated with intestinal infarction, are seen infrequently (Table 8–4).[88,141,151,162,225]

Pneumoperitoneum

Gastrointestinal perforation is diagnosed by the visualization of free intraperitoneal air under the diaphragm on an upright chest radiograph. Peptic ulcer perforation is associated with crack cocaine use.[3,36,127] Esophageal or gastric perforation (or tear) is a well reported complication of forceful emesis induced by syrup of ipecac or alcohol intoxication or attempted placement of a large-bore orogastric tube (Fig. 8–22).[264] Esophageal and gastric perforation

also occur after the ingestion of caustics such as iron, alkali, or acid.[121] Esophageal perforation causes pneumomediastinum and mediastinitis.

Obstruction and Ileus

Both mechanical bowel obstruction and adynamic ileus (diminished gut motility) cause bowel distension. With mechanical obstruction, there are a greater amount of intestinal distension proximal to the obstruction and a relative paucity of gas and intestinal collapse distal to the obstruction. In adynamic ileus, the bowel distension is relatively uniform throughout the entire intestinal tract. On the upright abdominal radiograph, both mechanical obstruction and adynamic ileus show air-fluid levels. In mechanical obstruction, air-fluid levels are seen at different heights and produce a "stepladder" appearance.

Mechanical bowel obstruction is caused by large intraluminal foreign bodies such as a body packer's packets or a medication bezoar.[77,238] Adynamic ileus results from the use of opioids, anticholinergics, and tricyclic antidepressants (Fig. 8–23).[18,82] Because adynamic ileus occurs in many diseases, the radiographic finding of an ileus is not helpful diagnostically. When the distinction between obstruction and adynamic ileus cannot be made based on the abdominal radiographs, abdominal CT can clarify the diagnosis.[160]

Mesenteric Ischemia

In most patients with intestinal ischemia, plain abdominal radiographs show only a nonspecific or adynamic ileus pattern. In a small proportion of patients with ischemic bowel (5%), intramural gas is seen.[18] Rarely, gas is also seen in the hepatic portal venous system. Computed tomography is better able to detect signs of mesenteric ischemia particularly bowel wall thickening (Fig. 8–24).[17]

Intestinal ischemia and infarction infrequently are caused by the use of cocaine; other sympathomimetics; and the ergot alkaloids, all of which induce mesenteric vasoconstriction.[95,130,154] Calcium channel blocker overdoses cause splanchnic vasodilation and hypotension that results in intestinal ischemia. Superior mesenteric vein thrombosis is caused by hypercoagulability associated with chronic oral contraceptive use.

Gastrointestinal Hemorrhage and Hepatotoxicity

Radiography is not usually helpful in the diagnosis of such common abdominal complications as GI hemorrhage and hepatotoxicity unless the bleeding is due to ingestion of ferrous sulfate tablets.

The now obsolete radiocontrast thorium dioxide (Thorotrast; thorium, atomic number 90) provides a unique example of pharmaceutical-induced hepatotoxicity. It was used as angiographic contrast until 1947, when it was found to cause hepatic malignancies. The radioactive isotope of thorium has a half-life of 400 years. It accumulates within the reticuloendothelial system and remains there for the life of the patient. It had a characteristic radiographic appearance, with multiple punctate opacities in the liver, spleen, and lymph nodes (Fig. 8–25). Patients who received thorium before its removal from the market still rarely present with hepatic malignancies.[22,247]

Contrast Esophagram and Upper Gastrointestinal Series

Ingestion of a caustic causes severe damage to the mucosal lining of the esophagus. This can be demonstrated by a contrast esophagram. However, in the acute setting, upper endoscopy should be performed rather than an esophagram because it provides more information about the extent of injury and prognosis. In addition, administration of barium will coat the mucosa, making endoscopy difficult. Computed tomography has been proposed as a noninvasive means to assess degree of esophageal injury and estimate the risk of later developing an esophageal stricture.[207] For later evaluation, a contrast esophagram identifies mucosal defects, scarring, and stricture formation (Figs. 8–26 and 103–4).[153,207]

The choice of radiographic contrast material (barium or water-soluble material) depends on the clinical situation. If the esophagus is severely strictured and there is a risk of aspiration, barium should be used because water-soluble contrast material is damaging to the pulmonary parenchyma. If, on the other hand, esophageal or gastric perforation is suspected, water-soluble

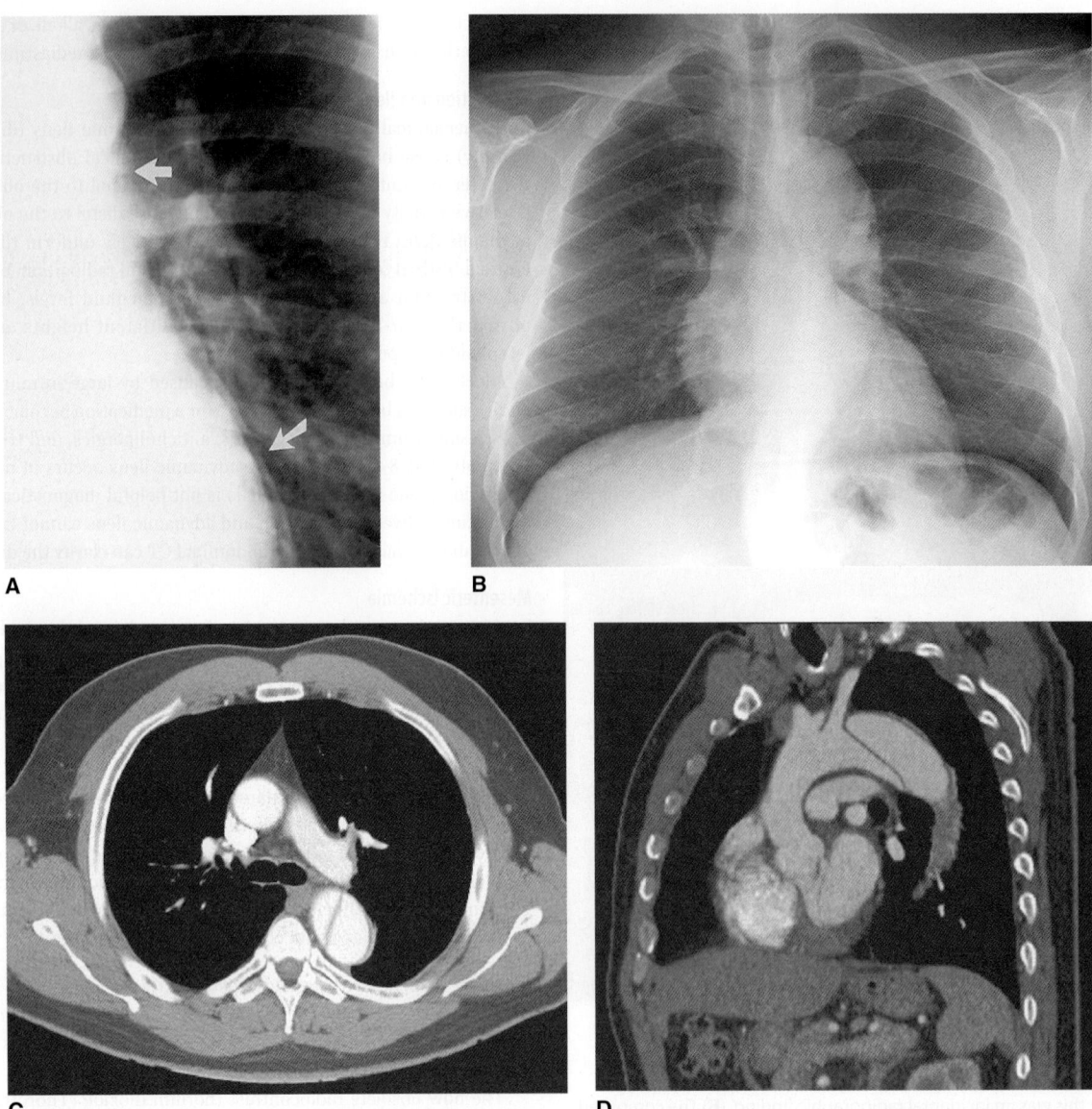

FIGURE 8–21. Two patients with chest pain after cocaine use. (**A**) Pneumomediastinum after forceful inhalation while smoking "crack" cocaine. A fine white line representing the pleura elevated from the mediastinal structures is seen (*arrows*). The patient's chest pain resolved during a 24-hour period of observation. (**B** to **D**) Thoracic aortic dissection after cocaine use. The patient presented with chest pain radiating to the back. He had a history of hypertension and was noncompliant with medications. Chest radiography shows an enlarged aorta caused by aortic wall weakening secondary to his long-standing hypertension. Computed tomography angiography shows the intraluminal dissection flap originating at the left subclavian artery and extending into the descending aorta. (*Used with permission from the Fellowship in Medical Toxicology, NYU School of Medicine, New York City Poison Control Center.*)

contrast is safer because extravasated barium is highly irritating to mediastinal and peritoneal tissues, but extravasated water-soluble contrast is gradually absorbed into the circulation.

Ingested foreign bodies cause esophageal and gastric outlet obstruction. Esophageal obstruction caused by a drug packet can be demonstrated by a contrast esophagram. Bezoars and concretions of ingested material in the stomach may cause gastric outlet obstruction. This is reported with potassium chloride tablets and enteric-coated aspirin.[12,224]

Abdominal Computed Tomography

CT provides great anatomic definition of intraabdominal organs and plays an important role in the diagnosis of a wide variety of abdominal disorders. In most cases, both oral and IV contrast are administered. Oral contrast delineates the intestinal lumen. Intravenous contrast is needed to reliably detect lesions in hepatic and splenic parenchyma, the kidneys, and the bowel wall.

Certain abdominal complications of poisonings are amenable to CT diagnosis. Intestinal ischemia causes bowel wall thickening; intramural hemorrhage; and at a later stage, intramural gas and hepatic portal venous gas (Fig. 8–24).[17] Hepatic portal venous gas is also seen after ingestion of high-concentration hydrogen peroxide (Fig. 8–27).[29,71,78,84,150,167,179,196] Splenic infarction and splenic and psoas abscesses are complications of IV drug use that are diagnosed on CT.[18] Radiopaque foreign substances such as intravenously injected elemental mercury may be detected and accurately localized by CT.[148] Ingested foreign bodies, such as a body packer's packets, are detected on noncontrast CT (Fig. 8–8D and Special Considerations: SC5–2 and 5–3).[16,99,101,147]

Vascular Lesions

Angiography detects such complications of injection drug use as venous thrombosis and arterial laceration causing pseudoaneurysm formation (Figs. 8–28 and 8–29). Intravenous injection of amphetamine, cocaine, or ergotamine causes necrotizing angiitis that is associated with microaneurysms, segmental stenosis, and arterial thrombosis. These lesions are seen in the kidneys, small bowel, liver, pancreas, and cerebral circulation (Fig. 8–30).[41,95]

TABLE 8–4 Plain Abdominal Radiography in Toxicologic Emergencies

Radiographic Finding	Xenobiotic
Pneumoperitoneum (hollow viscus perforation)	Caustics: iron, alkali, acids
	Cocaine
	GI decontamination (ipecac, lavage tube)
Mechanical obstruction (intraluminal foreign body)	Foreign-body ingestion
Intestinal	Body packer
Gastric outlet } Upper GI	Enteric-coated pills
Esophageal } series	Bezoar
Ileus (diminished gut motility)	Antimuscarinics
	Cyclic antidepressants
	Mesenteric ischemia caused by cocaine, oral contraceptives, cardioactive steroids
	Hypokalemia
	Hypomagnesemia
	Opioids
Intramural gas (intestinal infarction)	Calcium channel blockers
Bowel wall thickening	Cocaine
Hepatic portal venous gas	Ergot alkaloids
(CT is more sensitive)	Oral contraceptives
Foreign-body ingestion	Bismuth subsalicylate
	Body packers and stuffers
	Calcium carbonate
	Enteric-coated and sustained-release tablets
	Iron pills
	Metals (As, Cs, Hg, K, Pb, Tl)
	Pica (calcareous clay)
Nephrocalcinosis	Calcium
	Vitamin D

CT = computed tomography; GI = gastrointestinal.

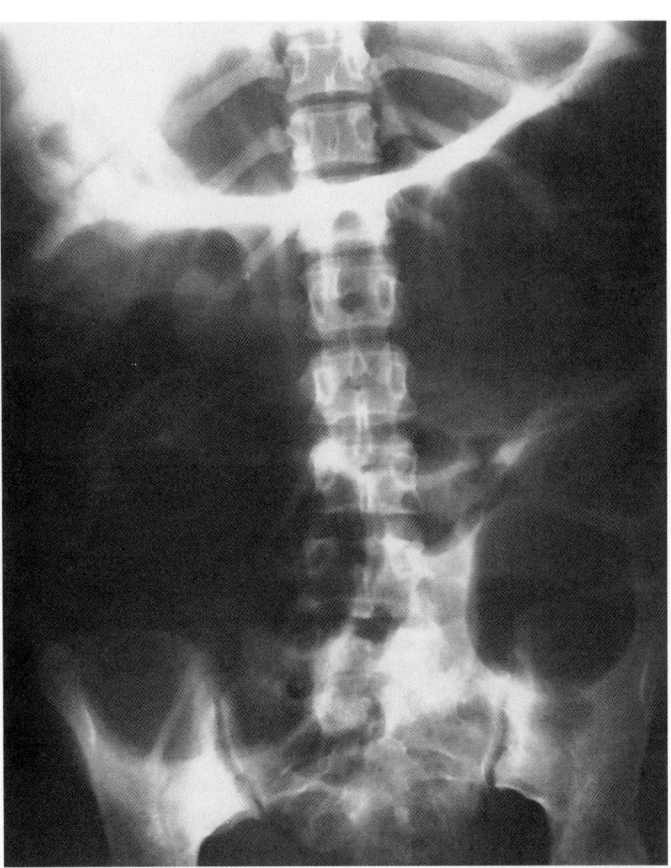

FIGURE 8–23. Methadone maintenance therapy causing marked abdominal distension. The radiograph reveals striking large bowel dilatation, termed *colonic ileus,* caused by chronic opioid use. A similar radiographic picture is seen with anticholinergic poisoning. A contrast enema can clarify the diagnosis. *(Used with permission from Dr. Emil J. Balthazar, Department of Radiology, Bellevue Hospital Center.)*

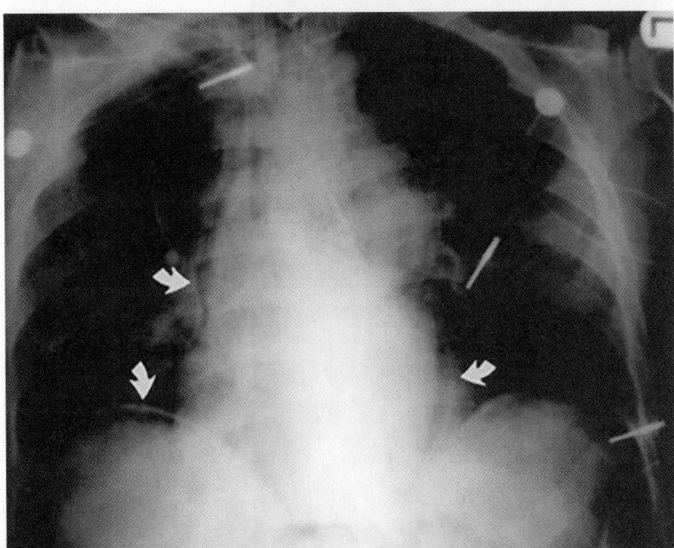

FIGURE 8–22. Gastrointestinal perforation after gastric lavage with a large-bore orogastric tube. The upright chest radiograph shows air under the right hemidiaphragm and pneumomediastinum *(arrows)*. An esophagram with water-soluble contrast did not demonstrate the perforation. Laparotomy revealed perforation of the anterior wall of the stomach. *(Used with permission from the Fellowship in Medical Toxicology, NYU School of Medicine, New York City Poison Control Center.)*

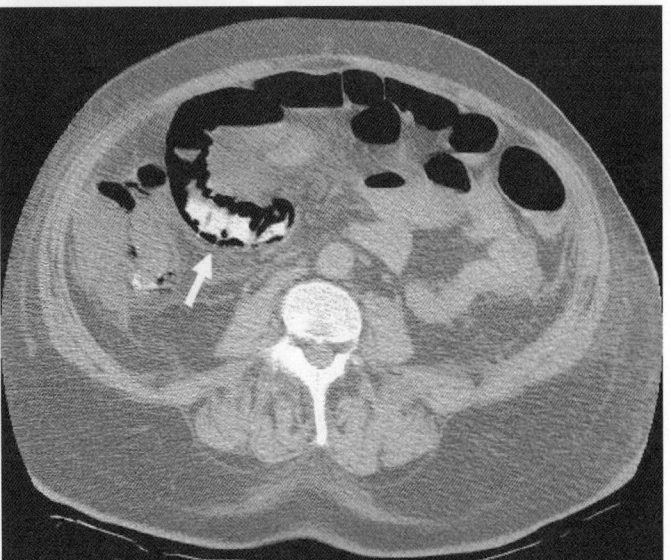

FIGURE 8–24. Bowel infarction in a 50-year-old man with an aspirin overdose. He presented with kidney failure, hypotension, and altered mental status. The next day after hemodialysis and hemofiltration, he developed abdominal distension and fever. Abdominal computed tomography showed extensive intramural gas *(arrow)* caused by bowel infarction, and the patient underwent surgical bowel resection. *(Used with permission from the Fellowship in Medical Toxicology, NYU School of Medicine, New York City Poison Control Center.)*

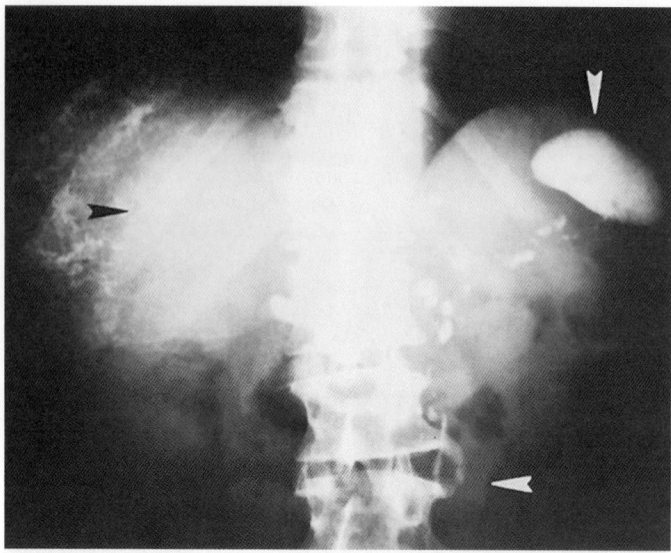

FIGURE 8–25. An abdominal radiograph of a patient who had received thorium dioxide (Thorotrast) for a radiocontrast study many years previously. The spleen (*vertical white arrowhead*), liver (*horizontal black arrowhead*), and lymph nodes (*horizontal white arrowhead*) are demarcated by thorium retained in the reticuloendothelial system. (*Used with permission from Dr. Emil J. Balthazar, Department of Radiology, Bellevue Hospital Center.*)

Complications include aneurysm rupture and visceral infarction. Renal lesions cause severe hypertension and acute kidney injury.[210]

Neurologic Problems

Diagnostic imaging studies have revolutionized the management of CNS disorders.[67,86] Both acute brain lesions and chronic degenerative changes are detected (Table 8–5).[139,237] Some xenobiotics have a direct toxic effect on the

CNS; others indirectly cause neurologic injury by causing hypoxia, hypotension, hypertension, cerebral vasoconstriction, head trauma, or infection.

Imaging Modalities

Computed tomography can directly visualize brain tissue and many intracranial lesions.[85] Computed tomography is the imaging study of choice in the emergency setting because it readily detects acute intracranial hemorrhage as well as parenchymal lesions that are causing mass effect. Computed tomography is fast, is widely available on an emergency basis, and can accommodate critical patient support and monitoring devices. Infusion of IV contrast further delineates intracerebral mass lesions such as tumors and abscesses.

Magnetic resonance imaging (MRI) has largely supplanted CT in nonemergency neurodiagnosis. It offers better anatomic discrimination of brain tissues and areas of cerebral edema and demyelinization. However, MRI is no better than CT in detecting acute blood collections or mass lesions. In the emergency setting, the disadvantages of MRI outweigh its strengths. Magnetic resonance imaging is often readily available on an emergency basis, but image acquisition time is long, and critical care supportive and monitoring devices are often incompatible with MR scanning machines.[142]

Nuclear scintigraphy that uses CT technology (SPECT and PET) is being used as a tool to elucidate functional characteristics of the CNS. Examples include both immediate and long-term effects of various xenobiotics on regional brain metabolism, blood flow, and neurotransmitter function.[73,135,182,250]

Emergency Cranial Computed Tomography Scanning

An emergency noncontrast CT scan is obtained to detect acute intracranial hemorrhage and focal brain lesions causing cerebral edema and mass effect. Patients with these lesions present with focal neurologic deficits, seizures, headache, or altered mental status. Toxicologic causes of intraparenchymal and subarachnoid hemorrhage include cocaine and other sympathomimetics (Fig. 8–31).[133,138] Cocaine-induced vasospasm causes ischemic infarction, although this is not well seen by CT until 6 to 24 or more hours after onset of

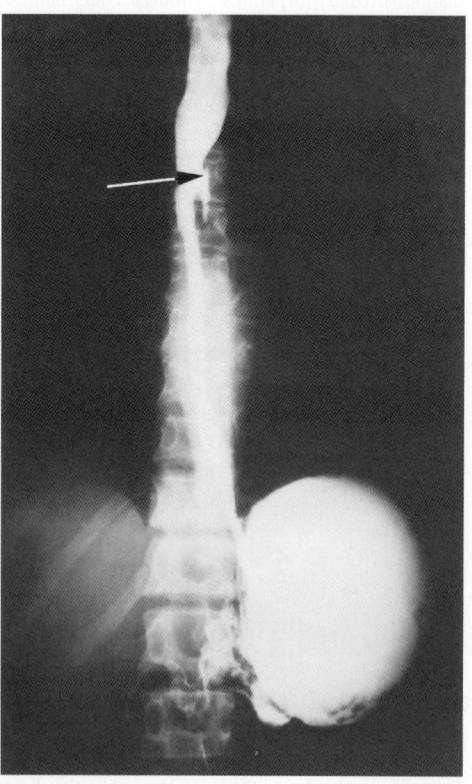
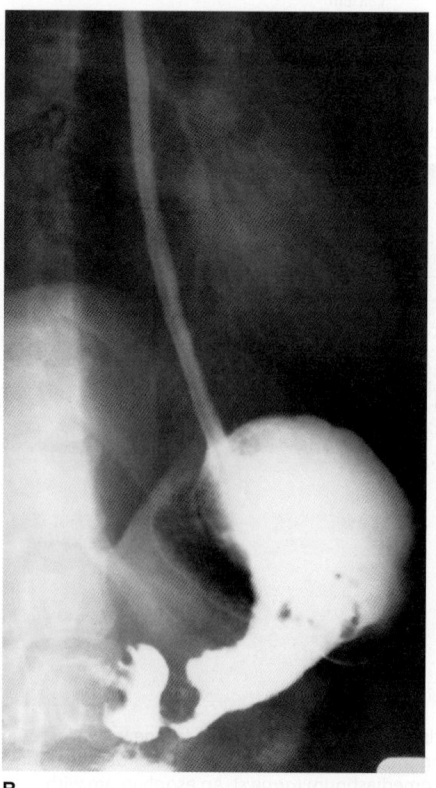

A   B

FIGURE 8–26. (**A**) A barium swallow performed several days after ingestion of liquid lye shows intramural dissection and extravasation of barium with early stricture formation. (**B**) At 3 weeks after ingestion, there are an absence of peristalsis, diffuse narrowing of the esophagus, and reduction in size of the fundus and antrum of the stomach as a result of scarring. (*Used with permission from Dr. Emil J. Balthazar, Department of Radiology, Bellevue Hospital Center.*)

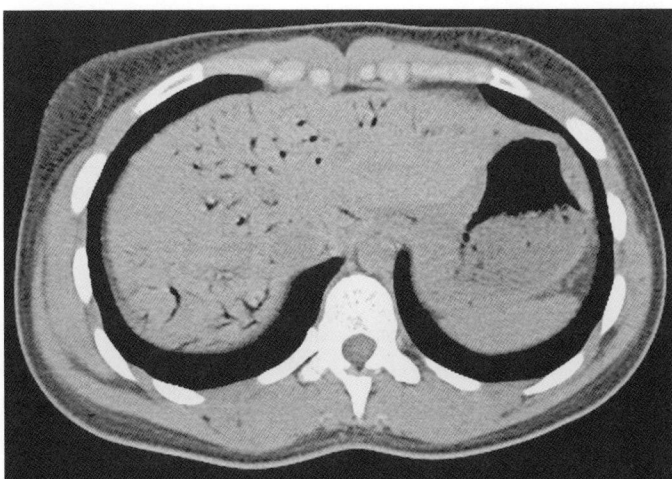

FIGURE 8–27. Abdominal computed tomography showing extensive hepatic portal venous gas in a woman who inadvertently ingested a small quantity of commercial concentration (35%) hydrogen peroxide. She also had gastric and esophageal erosions on endoscopy and was treated successfully with antacids and hyperbaric oxygen. *(Used with permission from the Fellowship in Medical Toxicology, NYU School of Medicine, New York City Poison Control Center.)*

the neurologic deficit (Fig. 8–32). Drug-induced CNS depression, most commonly ethanol intoxication, predisposes the patient to head trauma, which may result in a subdural hematoma or cerebral contusion (Fig. 8–33). Toxicologic causes of intracerebral mass lesions include septic emboli complicating injection drug use and HIV-associated CNS toxoplasmosis and lymphoma (Fig. 8–34).[23,90,95,175] On a contrast CT, such tumors and focal infections exhibit a pattern of "ring enhancement."

Xenobiotic-Mediated Neurodegenerative Disorders

A number of xenobiotics directly damage brain tissue, producing morphologic changes that may be detectable using CT and especially MRI. Such changes include generalized atrophy, focal areas of neuronal loss, demyelinization, and cerebral edema. Imaging abnormalities help establish a diagnosis or predict prognosis in a patient with neurologic dysfunction after a xenobiotic exposure. In some cases, the imaging abnormality will suggest a

toxicologic diagnosis in a patient with a neurologic disorder in whom a xenobiotic exposure was not suspected clinically.[5,14,67,117,124,183,237,257]

Atrophy. Ethanol is the most widely used neurotoxin. With long-term ethanol use, there is a widespread loss of neurons and resultant atrophy. In some individuals with alcoholism, the loss of brain tissue is especially prominent in the cerebellum. However, the amount of cerebral or cerebellar atrophy does not always correlate with the extent of cognitive impairment or gait disturbance.[51,81,100,102,126,252,254] Chronic solvent exposure, such as to toluene (occupational and illicit use), also causes diffuse cerebral atrophy.[109,202]

Focal Lesions. Carbon monoxide poisoning produces focal degenerative lesions in the brain. In about half of patients with severe neurologic dysfunction after carbon monoxide poisoning, CT scans show bilateral symmetric lucencies in the basal ganglia, particularly the globus pallidus (Figs. 8–35 and 122–1).[35,110,117,155,166,183,187,188,212,213,241,249] The basal ganglia are especially sensitive to hypoxic damage because of their limited blood supply and high metabolic requirements. Subcortical white matter lesions also occur after carbon monoxide poisoning. Although less frequent than lesions of the basal ganglia, white matter lesions are more clearly associated with a poor neurologic outcome. Magnetic resonance imaging is more sensitive than CT at detecting these white matter abnormalities.[35,67,119,188,241]

Basal ganglion lucencies, white matter lesions, and atrophy are caused by other xenobiotics such as methanol,[13,50,83,98,168,205] ethylene glycol, cyanide,[68,163] hydrogen sulfide, inorganic and organic mercury,[156,212] manganese,[14,229] heroin,[124,128] barbiturates, chemotherapeutics, solvents such as toluene,[67,109,202] and podophyllin.[34,170] Nontoxicologic disorders cause similar imaging abnormalities, including hypoxia, hypoglycemia, and infectious encephalitis.[98,104]

Focal lesions in the spinal cord are also caused by xenobiotic exposure, such as habitual use of nitrous oxide, and cause myelopathic symptoms. These lesions are visualized by MRI (Fig. 65–3).

Posterior Reversible Encephalopathy Syndrome. A wide range of medical conditions and medications cause symmetrical cortical and subcortical white matter changes that are reversible when the condition or xenobiotic is removed. This was formerly termed *reversible leukoencephalopathy syndrome*, but because the changes are not limited to the white matter and often involve the occipital lobes, it is now more commonly known as *posterior reversible encephalopathy syndrome*. However, this term too has been questioned because the changes are often more diffuse. These changes are most

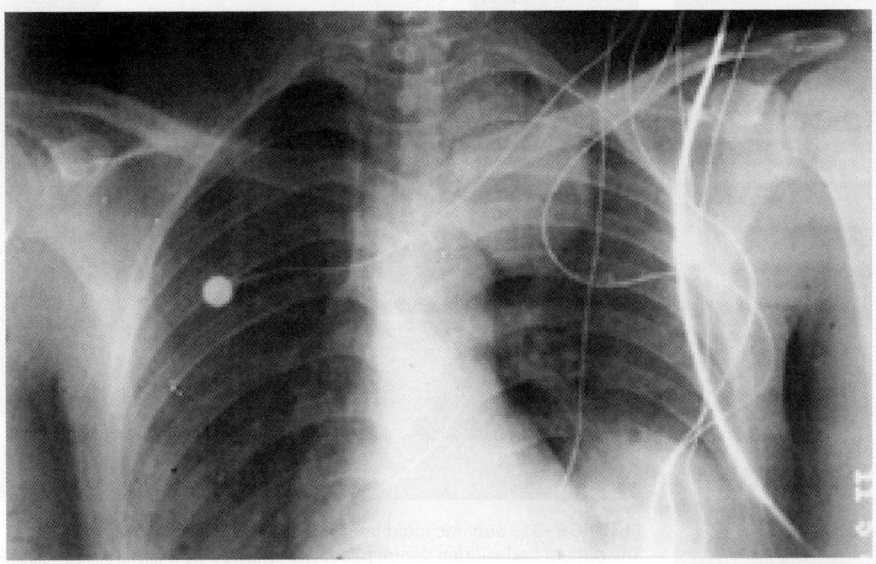
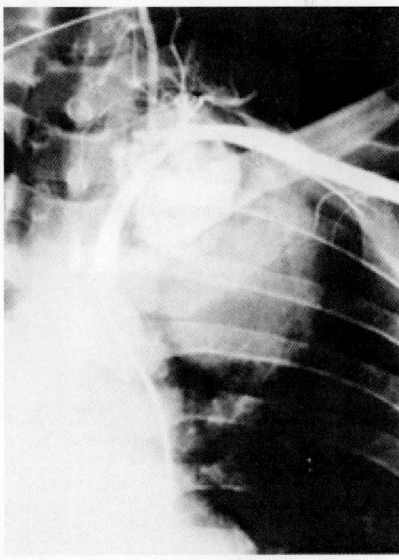

A   **B**

FIGURE 8–28. (**A**) Chest radiograph of a young drug user who used the supraclavicular approach for heroin injection. The large mass in the left chest was suspicious for a pseudoaneurysm. (**B**) An arch aortogram performed on the patient revealed a large pseudoaneurysm and hematoma subsequent to an arterial tear during attempted injection. Surgical repair was performed. *(Used with permission from Dr. Richard Lefleur, Department of Radiology, Bellevue Hospital.)*

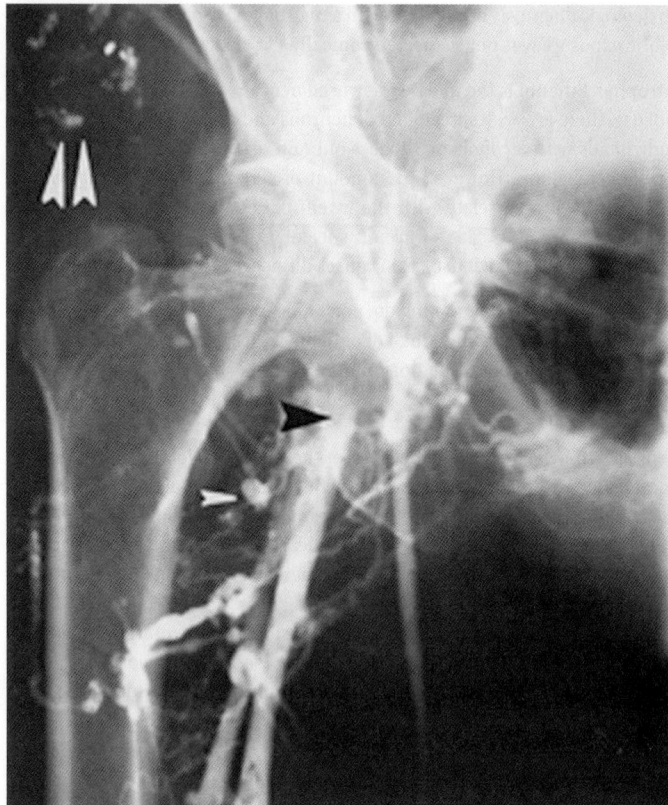

FIGURE 8–29. Venogram of a 50-year-old patient who routinely injected heroin into his groin. Occlusion of the femoral vein (*black arrowhead*) with diffuse aneurysmal dilatation (*small arrowhead*) and extensive collaterals are shown. Incidental radiopaque materials are noted in the right buttock (*double arrowheads*). By history, this represents either bismuth or arsenicals he received as antisyphilitic therapy. *(Used with permission from Dr. Richard Lefleur, Department of Radiology, Bellevue Hospital.)*

TABLE 8–5	Cranial Computed Tomography (Noncontrast) in Toxicologic Emergencies	
Computed Tomography Finding	Brain Lesion	Xenobiotic Etiology
Hemorrhage	Intraparenchymal hemorrhage	Sympathomimetics: cocaine ("crack"), amphetamine, phenylpropanolamine, phencyclidine, ephedrine, pseudoephedrine
	Subarachnoid hemorrhage	
		Mycotic aneurysm rupture (IDU)
	Subdural hematoma	Trauma secondary to ethanol, sedative–hypnotics, seizures
		Anticoagulants, NSAIDS, ASA
Brain lucencies	Basal ganglia focal necrosis (also sub-cortical white matter lucencies)	Carbon monoxide, cyanide, hydrogen sulfide, methanol, manganese
	Stroke: vasoconstriction	Sympathomimetics: cocaine ("crack"), amphetamine, phenylpropanolamine, phencyclidine; ephedrine, pseudoephedrine; ergotamine
	Mass lesion: tumor, abscess	Septic emboli, AIDS-related CNS toxoplasmosis or lymphoma
Loss of brain tissue	Atrophy: cerebral, cerebellar	Alcoholism, toluene

CNS = central nervous system; IDU = injection drug use; NSAIDs = nonsteroidal antiinflammatory drugs; ASA = Aspirin.

apparent on cranial MRI. The syndrome was initially described in association with hypertensive encephalopathy (malignant hypertension) and eclampsia, but it is associated with a variety of immunosuppressants and chemotherapeutics (cyclophosphamide, tacrolimus cisplatin, vincristine), as well as therapeutic monoclonal antibodies (bevacizumab, rituximab, adalimumab).

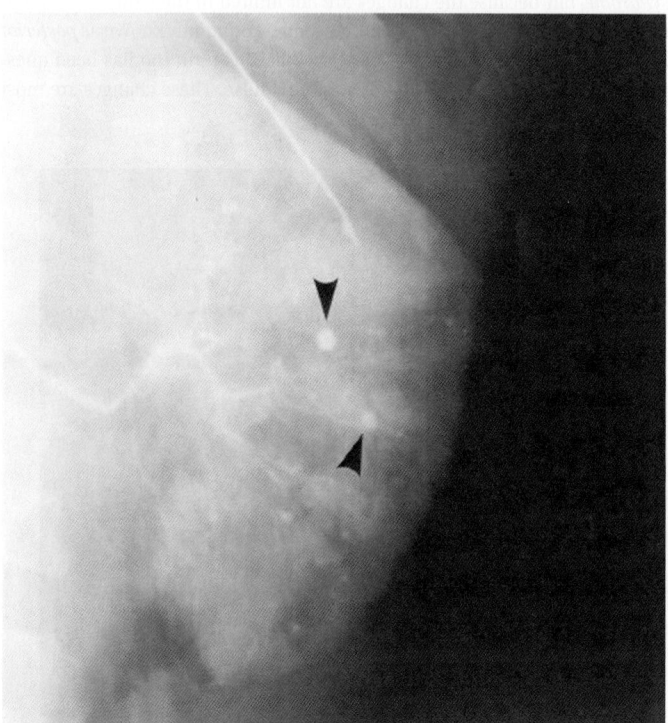

FIGURE 8–30. A selective renal angiogram in an injection methamphetamine user demonstrating multiple small and large aneurysms (*arrowheads*). *(Used with permission from Dr. Richard Lefleur, Department of Radiology, Bellevue Hospital.)*

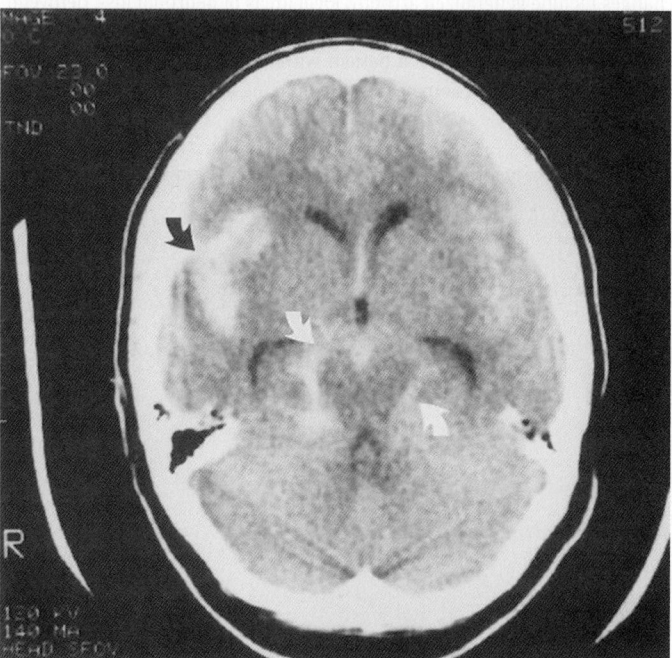

FIGURE 8–31. Subarachnoid hemorrhage after intravenous cocaine use. The patient had sudden severe headache followed by a generalized seizure. Extensive hemorrhage is seen surrounding the midbrain (*white arrows*) and in the right Sylvian fissure (*black arrow*). Angiography revealed an aneurysm at the origin of the right middle cerebral artery. *(Used with permission from The Fellowship in Medical Toxicology, New York University School of Medicine, New York City Poison Center.)*

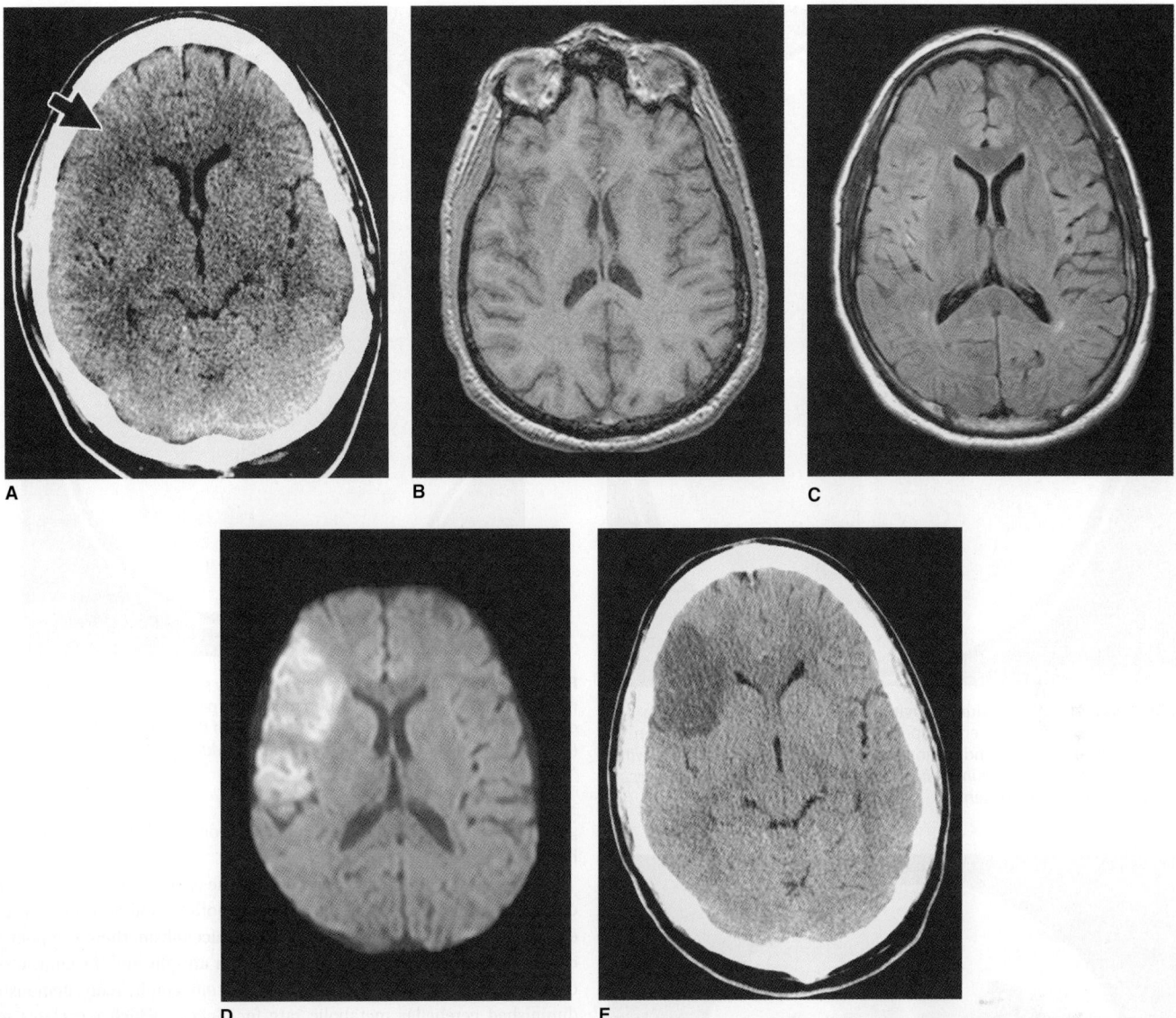

FIGURE 8–32. Acute stroke confirmed by diffusion-weighted magnetic resonance image (MRI). A 39-year-old man presented with left facial weakness that began 3 hours earlier after smoking crack cocaine. He also complained of left arm "tingling" but had normal examination findings. An emergency noncontrast computed tomography (CT) scan was obtained that was interpreted as normal (**A**), although in retrospect, there was subtle loss of the normal gray–white differentiation (*arrow*). Magnetic resonance imaging was obtained to confirm that the facial palsy was a stroke and not a peripheral seventh cranial nerve palsy. Standard MRI sequence (T1-weighted, T2-weighted, and fluid-attenuated inversion recovery) were normal in this early ischemic lesion (**B** and **C**). Diffusion-weighed imaging is able to show such early ischemic change—cytotoxic (intracellular) edema (**D**). The patient's facial paresis improved but did not entirely resolve. A repeat CT scan 2 days later showed an evolving (subacute) infarction with vasogenic edema (**E**). Infarction was presumably caused by vasospasm because no carotid artery lesion or cardiac source of embolism was found. *(Reproduced with permission from Schwartz DT: Emergency Radiology: Case Studies. New York, NY: McGraw-Hill; 2008.)*

The clinical manifestations include headache, visual disturbance, altered mental status, and seizures (Fig. 8–36).[19,112,132,206] These reversible cerebral disorders are distinct from irreversible white matter disease termed *toxic leukoencephalopathy*. This is associated with various cancer chemotherapeutics, carbon monoxide, toluene, methanol, and heroin inhalation ("chasing the dragon").[66,197,242]

Nuclear Scintigraphy

Whereas both CT and MRI display cerebral anatomy, nuclear medicine studies provide functional information about the brain. Nuclear scintigraphy uses radioactive isotopes that are bound to carrier molecules (ligands). The choice of ligand depends on the biologic function being studied. Brain cells take up the radiolabeled ligand in proportion to their physiologic activity or the regional blood flow. The radioactive emission from the isotope is detected by a scintigraphic camera, which produces an image showing the quantity and distribution of tracer. Better anatomic detail is provided by using CT

techniques to generate cross-sectional images. There are two such technologies: SPECT and PET. These imaging modalities are used in the research and clinical settings to study the neurologic effects of particular xenobiotics and the mechanisms of xenobiotic-induced neurologic dysfunction.

Single-photon emission computed tomography (SPECT) uses conventional isotopes such as technetium-99m and iodine-123.[135] These isotopes are bound to ligands that are taken up in the brain in proportion to regional blood flow, reflecting the local metabolic rate.

Position emission tomography (PET) uses radioactive isotopes of biologic elements such as carbon-11, oxygen-15, nitrogen-13, and fluoride-18 (a substitute for hydrogen).[182] These radioisotopes have very short half-lives so that PET scanning requires an onsite cyclotron to produce the isotope. The isotopes are incorporated into molecules such as glucose, oxygen, water, various neurotransmitters, and xenobiotics. Labeled glucose is taken up in proportion to the local metabolic rate for glucose. Uptake of labeled oxygen demonstrates the local metabolic rate for oxygen. Labeled neurotransmitters

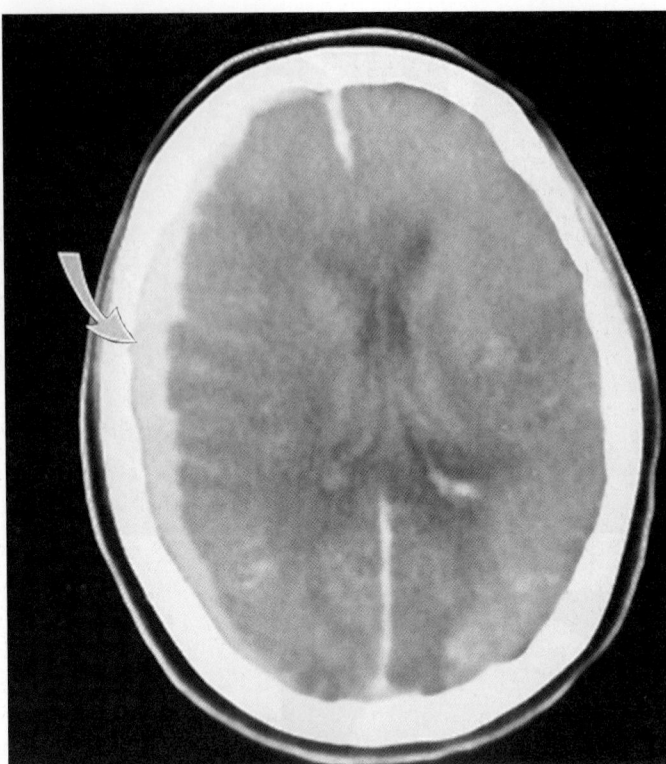

FIGURE 8-33. An acute subdural hematoma in a patient with alcoholism after an alcohol binge. A crescent-shaped blood collection is seen between the right cerebral convexity and the inner table of the skull *(arrow)*. *(Used with permission from the Fellowship in Medical Toxicology, NYU School of Medicine, New York City Poison Control Center.)*

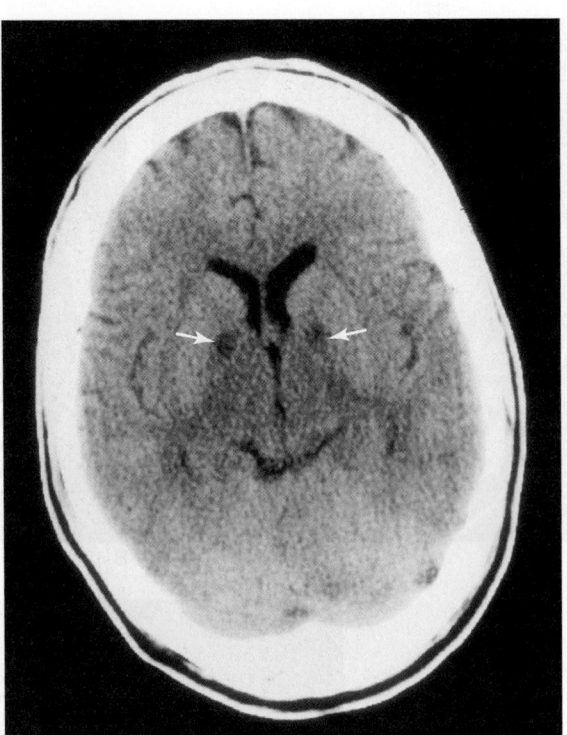

FIGURE 8-35. A head computed tomography scan of a patient with mental status changes after carbon monoxide poisoning. The scan shows characteristic bilateral symmetrical lucencies of the globus pallidus *(arrows)*. *(Used with permission from Dr. Paul Blackburn, Maricopa Medical Center, Arizona.)*

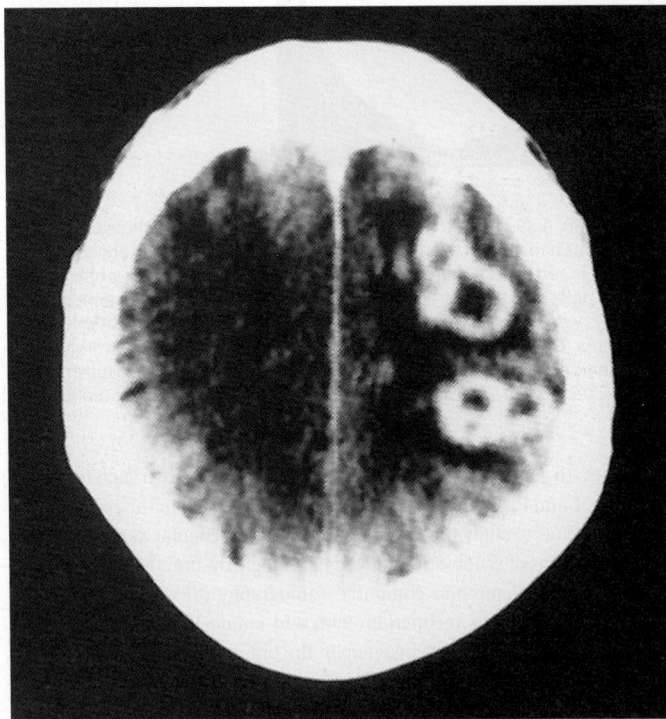

FIGURE 8-34. An injection drug user with ring-enhancing intracerebral lesions. The patient presented with fever and altered mental status. In this patient, the lesions represent multiple septic emboli complicating acute *Staphylococcus aureus* bacterial endocarditis. A similar ring-enhancing appearance is seen with lesions caused by toxoplasmosis or primary central nervous system lymphoma in patients with AIDS. This patient was HIV negative. *(Used with permission from the Fellowship in Medical Toxicology, NYU School of Medicine, New York City Poison Control Center.)*

generate images reflecting their concentration and distribution within the brain.

Both PET and SPECT are used to study the effects of various xenobiotics on cerebral function. For example, although both CT and MRI can detect cerebellar atrophy in individuals with chronic alcoholism, there is a poor correlation between the magnitude of cerebellar atrophy and the clinical signs of cerebellar dysfunction. Position emission tomography scans demonstrate diminished cerebellar metabolic rate for glucose, which correlates more accurately with the patient's clinical status.[87,252]

In patients with severe neurologic dysfunction after carbon monoxide poisoning, SPECT regional blood flow measurements show diffuse hypometabolism in the frontal cortex.[37] In one patient, severe perfusion abnormalities improved slightly over several months in proportion to the patient's gradual clinical improvement.[115,220] In another patient treated with hyperbaric oxygen, a SPECT scan revealed increased blood flow in the frontal lobes, although the blood flow still remained significantly diminished.[145]

In patients who chronically use cocaine, SPECT blood flow scintigraphy demonstrates focal cortical perfusion defects. The extent of these perfusion deficits correlates with the frequency of drug use. Focal perfusion defects probably represent local vasculitis or small areas of infarction.[108,245] Position emission tomography scanning has been used to demonstrate the effects of cocaine on cerebral blood flow and regional glucose metabolism. Position emission tomography neurotransmitter studies show promise in elucidating potential mechanisms of action of cocaine. Using radiolabeled dopamine analogs, downregulation of dopamine (D_2) receptors is noted after a cocaine binge. This finding is possibly associated with cocaine craving that occurs during cocaine withdrawal. Using ^{11}C-labeled cocaine, uptake of cocaine is demonstrated in the basal ganglia, a region rich in dopamine receptors.[250]

There are many advances in the use of these imaging modalities, and initial applications are being applied to patient care. These imaging modalities are capable of demonstrating abnormalities in many patients with xenobiotic exposures, although other patients with significant cerebral dysfunction have normal study findings.

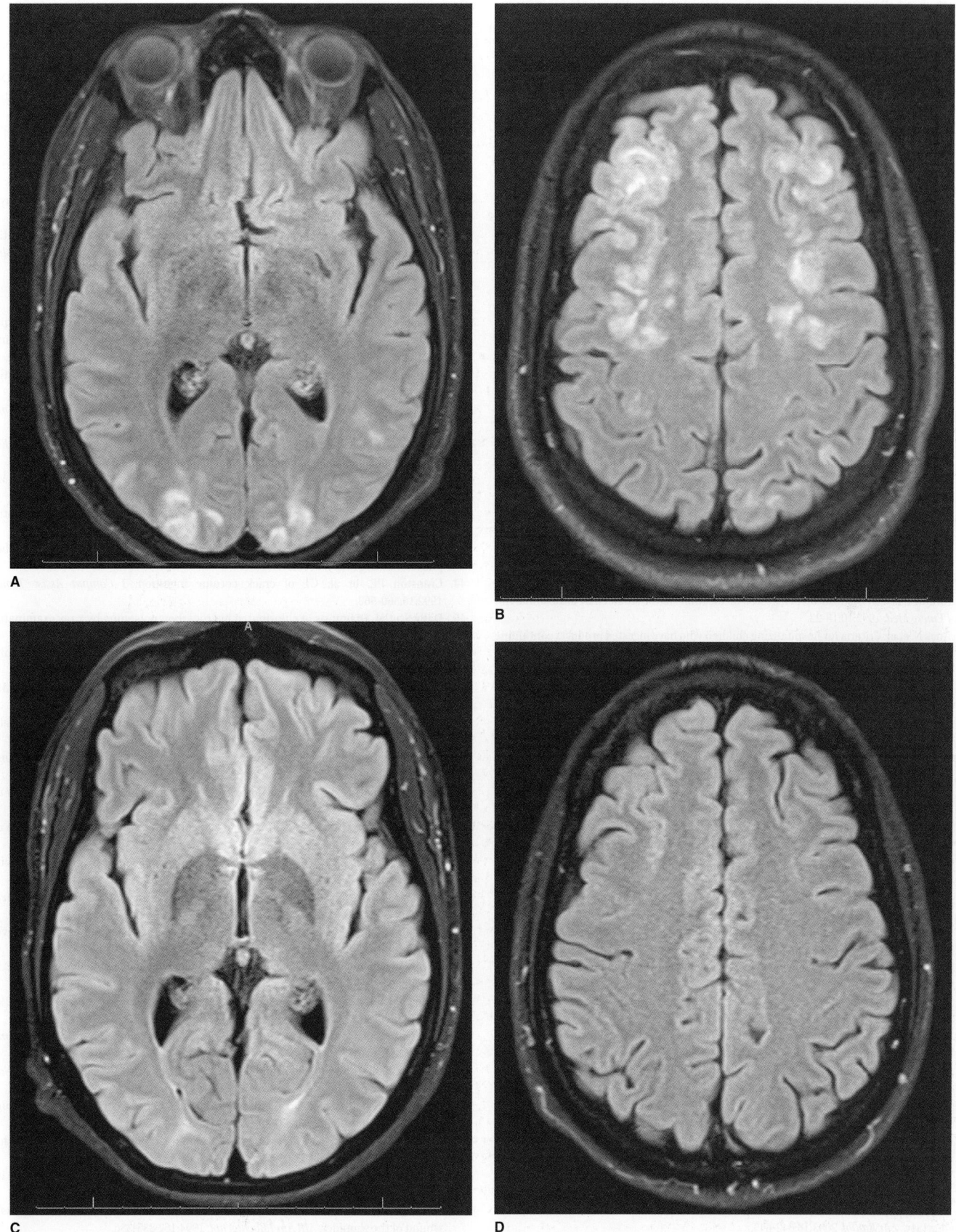

FIGURE 8–36. Posterior reversible encephalopathy syndrome (PRES) caused by cyclosporine. A 29-year-old man with severe aplastic anemia was treated with stem cell transplantation and cyclosporine to prevent subsequent graft versus host disease. The next day, he developed headache followed by a generalized tonic-clonic seizure with a prolonged postictal period. The head computed tomography scan was normal, and magnetic resonance imaging (MRI) revealed symmetric areas of fluid-attenuated inversion recovery hyperintensity involving the cortex and subcortical white matter of the occipital, frontal, and parietal lobes (**A** and **B**). Cyclosporine was stopped. The next day, he returned to his normal mental status. Follow-up MRI 1 week later revealed near-complete resolution (**C** and **D**). *(Used with permission from Dr. Alexander Baxter, Department of Radiology, New York University School of Medicine.)*

SUMMARY

This chapter has highlighted a variety of situations in which diagnostic imaging studies are useful in toxicologic emergencies.

- Imaging is an important tool in establishing a diagnosis, assisting in the treatment of patients, and detecting complications of a toxicologic emergency.
- The imaging modalities include plain radiography, CT, enteric and intravascular contrast studies, nuclear scintigraphy, and ultrasonography.
- Effective use of a diagnostic test requires a precise understanding of the clinical situations in which each test can be useful, knowledge of the capabilities and limitations of the tests, and how the results should be applied to the care of an individual patient.

REFERENCES

1. Adler P, et al. Hypothermia: an unusual indication for gastric lavage. *J Emerg Med.* 2011;40:176-178.
2. Akira M, et al. Inhalational talc pneumoconiosis: radiographic and CT findings in 14 patients. *AJR Am J Roentgenol.* 2007;188:326-333.
3. Albert P, Sadler MA. Duodenal perforation in a crack cocaine abuser. *Emerg Radiol.* 2000;7:248-249.
4. Algra PR, et al. Role of radiology in a national initiative to interdict drug smuggling: the Dutch experience. *AJR Am J Roentgenol.* 2007;189:331-336.
5. Alphs HH, et al. Findings on brain MRI from research studies of occupational exposure to known neurotoxicants. *AJR Am J Roentgenol.* 2006;187:1043-1047.
6. American College of Emergency Physicians. Clinical policy for the initial approach to patients presenting with acute toxic ingestion or dermal or inhalation exposure. *Ann Emerg Med.* 1999;33:735-761.
7. American College of Emergency Physicians. Clinical policy for the initial approach to patients presenting with acute toxic ingestion or dermal or inhalation exposure. American College of Emergency Physicians. *Ann Emerg Med.* 1995;25:570-585.
8. Amitai Y, et al. Visualization of ingested medications in the stomach by ultrasound. *Am J Emerg Med.* 1992;10:18-23.
9. Anas N, et al. Criteria for hospitalizing children who have ingested products containing hydrocarbons. *JAMA.* 1981;246:840-843.
10. Ansell G. The chest. In: Ansell G, ed. *Radiology of Adverse Reactions to Drugs and Toxic Hazards.* Rockville, MD: Aspen Systems; 1985:1-99.
11. Ansell G. Skeletal system and soft tissues. In: Ansell G, ed. *Radiology of Adverse Reactions to Drugs and Toxic Hazards.* Rockville, MD: Aspen Systems; 1985:254-326.
12. Antonescu CG, Barritt AS 3rd. Potassium chloride and gastric outlet obstruction. *Ann Intern Med.* 1989;111:855-856.
13. Aquilonius SM, et al. Cerebral computed tomography in methanol intoxication. *J Comput Assist Tomogr.* 1980;4:425-428.
14. Arjona A, et al. Diagnosis of chronic manganese intoxication by magnetic resonance imaging. *N Engl J Med.* 1997;336:964-965.
15. Asha SE, Cooke A. Sensitivity and specificity of emergency physicians and trainees for identifying internally concealed drug packages on abdominal computed tomography scan: do lung windows improve accuracy? *J Emerg Med.* 2015;49:268-273.
16. Asha SE, et al. Sensitivity and specificity of CT scanning for determining the number of internally concealed packages in "body-packers." *Emerg Med J.* 2014:1-5.
17. Balthazar EJ, et al. Computed tomography of intramural intestinal hemorrhage and bowel ischemia. *J Comput Assist Tomogr.* 1987;11:67-72.
18. Balthazar EJ, Lefleur R. Abdominal complications of drug addiction: radiologic features. *Semin Roentgenol.* 1983;18:213-220.
19. Bartynski WS. Posterior reversible encephalopathy syndrome, part 1: fundamental imaging and clinical features. *AJNR Am J Neuroradiol.* 2008;29:1036-1042.
20. Beerman R, et al. Radiographic evaluation of the cocaine smuggler. *Gastrointest Radiol.* 1986;11:351-354.
21. Bellin MF, et al. Contrast medium extravasation injury: guidelines for prevention and management. *Eur Radiol.* 2002;12:2807-2812.
22. Bensinger TA, et al. Thorotrast-induced reticuloendothelial blockade in man. Clinical equivalent of the experimental model associated with patent pneumococcal septicemia. *Am J Med.* 1971;51:663-668.
23. Berger JR, et al. The acquired immunodeficiency syndrome. In: Greenberg JO, Adams RD, eds. *Neuroimaging: A Companion to Adams and Victor's Principles of Neurology.* New York, NY: McGraw-Hill Health Professions Division; 1995:413-434.
24. Bernaerts A, et al. Pneumomediastinum and epidural pneumatosis after inhalation of "Ecstasy." *Eur Radiol.* 2003;13:642-643.
25. Blickman JG, et al. The radiologic "lead band" revisited. *AJR Am J Roentgenol.* 1986;146:245-247.
26. Bruns BR, Tytle T. Skeletal fluorosis. A report of two cases. *Orthopedics.* 1988; 11:1083-1087.
27. Bulakci M, et al. Comparison of diagnostic value of multidetector computed tomography and X-ray in the detection of body packing. *Eur J Radiol.* 2013;82: 1248-1254.
28. Burkhart KK, et al. Whole-bowel irrigation as treatment for zinc sulfate overdose. *Ann Emerg Med.* 1990;19:1167-1170.
29. Byrne B, et al. Hyperbaric oxygen therapy for systemic gas embolism after hydrogen peroxide ingestion. *J Emerg Med.* 2014;46:171-175.
30. Camus P, Rosenow EC 3rd. Iatrogenic lung disease. *Clin Chest Med.* 2004;25:XIII-XIX.
31. Caruana DS, et al. Cocaine-packet ingestion. Diagnosis, management, and natural history. *Ann Intern Med.* 1984;100:73-74.
32. Celli B, Khan MA. Mercury embolization of the lung. *N Engl J Med.* 1976;295: 883-885.
33. Cengel F, et al. The role of ultrasonography in the imaging of body packers comparison with CT: a prospective study. *Abdom Imaging.* 2015;40:2143-2151.
34. Chan YW. Magnetic resonance imaging in toxic encephalopathy due to podophyllin poisoning. *Neuroradiology.* 1991;33:372-373.
35. Chang KH, et al. Delayed encephalopathy after acute carbon monoxide intoxication: MR imaging features and distribution of cerebral white matter lesions. *Radiology.* 1992;184:117-122.
36. Cheng CL, Svesko V. Acute pyloric perforation after prolonged crack smoking. *Ann Emerg Med.* 1994;23:126-128.
37. Choi IS, et al. Evaluation of outcome of delayed neurologic sequelae after carbon monoxide poisoning by technetium-99m hexamethylpropylene amine oxime brain single photon emission computed tomography. *Eur Neurol.* 1995;35:137-142.
38. Choi SH, et al. Diagnostic radiopacity and hepatotoxicity following chloroform ingestion: a case report. *Emerg Med J.* 2006;23:394-395.
39. Chung C, Fung W. Detection of gastric drug packet by ultrasound scanning. *Eur J Emerg Med.* 2006;13:302-303.
40. Chung CH, Fung WT. Detection of gastric drug packet by ultrasound scanning. *Eur J Emerg Med.* 2006;13:302-303.
41. Citron BP, et al. Necrotizing angiitis associated with drug abuse. *N Engl J Med.* 1970;283:1003-1011.
42. Cohan RH, et al. Extravasation of radiographic contrast material: recognition, prevention, and treatment. *Radiology.* 1996;200:593-604.
43. Costello J, Townend W. Best evidence topic report. Abdominal radiography in "body packers." *Emerg Med J.* 2004;21:498.
44. Cranston PE, et al. CT of crack cocaine ingestion. *J Comput Assist Tomogr.* 1992;16:560-563.
45. Dally S, et al. Diagnosis of chlorinated hydrocarbon poisoning by x ray examination. *Br J Ind Med.* 1987;44:424-425.
46. de Almeida RR, et al. High-resolution computed tomographic findings of cocaine-induced pulmonary disease: a state of the art review. *Lung.* 2014;192:225-233.
47. de Souza AC, de Carvalho AM. Metallic mercury embolism to the hand. *N Engl J Med.* 2009;360:507.
48. Dee P, Armstrong P. Drug- and radiation-induced lung disease. In: Armstrong P, et al, eds. *Imaging of Diseases of the Chest.* 2nd ed. St. Louis, MO: Mosby; 1995:461-483.
49. Dee P, Armstrong P. Inhalational lung diseases. In: Armstrong P, et al, eds. *Imaging of Diseases of the Chest.* 2nd ed. St. Louis, MO: Mosby; 1995:426-460.
50. Degirmencia B, et al. Methanol intoxication: diffusion MR imaging findings. *Eur J Radiol Extra.* 2007;61:41-44.
51. Demaerel P, Van Paesschen W. Images in clinical medicine. Marchiafava-Bignami disease. *N Engl J Med.* 2004;351:e10.
52. DeMartini J, et al. Lead arthropathy and systemic lead poisoning from an intraarticular bullet. *AJR Am J Roentgenol.* 2001;176:1144.
53. Desenclos JC, et al. Thallium poisoning: an outbreak in Florida, 1988. *South Med J.* 1992;85:1203-1206.
54. Dillman RO, et al. Lead poisoning from a gunshot wound. Report of a case and review of the literature. *Am J Med.* 1979;66:509-514.
55. Douglass RE, Levison MA. Pneumothorax in drug abusers. An urban epidemic? *Am Surg.* 1986;52:377-380.
56. Edeiken J, et al. *Edeiken's Roentgen Diagnosis of Diseases of Bone.* 4th ed. 1990: 1401-1406.
57. Eng JG, et al. False-negative abdominal CT scan in a cocaine body stuffer. *Am J Emerg Med.* 1999;17:702-704.
58. Erasmus JJ, et al. High-resolution CT of drug-induced lung disease. *Radiol Clin North Am.* 2002;40:61-72.
59. Eurman DW, et al. Chest pain and dyspnea related to "crack" cocaine smoking: value of chest radiography. *Radiology.* 1989;172:459-462.
60. Everson GW, et al. Use of whole bowel irrigation in an infant following iron overdose. *Am J Emerg Med.* 1991;9:366-369.
61. Everson GW, et al. Effectiveness of abdominal radiographs in visualizing chewable iron supplements following overdose. *Am J Emerg Med.* 1989;7:459-463.
62. Farber JM, et al. Lead arthropathy and elevated serum levels of lead after a gunshot wound of the shoulder. *AJR Am J Roentgenol.* 1994;162:385-386.
63. Federle MP, et al. Frequency and effects of extravasation of ionic and nonionic CT contrast media during rapid bolus injection. *Radiology.* 1998;206:637-640.
64. Feigin DS. Talc: understanding its manifestations in the chest. *AJR Am J Roentgenol.* 1986;146:295-301.
65. Felson B, Spitz HB. Pelvic mass in a 12-year-old girl. *JAMA.* 1977;237:1255-1256.
66. Filley CM. Toluene abuse and white matter: a model of toxic leukoencephalopathy. *Psychiatr Clin North Am.* 2013;36:293-302.

67. Filley CM, Kleinschmidt-DeMasters BK. Toxic leukoencephalopathy. *N Engl J Med.* 2001;345:425-432.

68. Finelli PF. Case report. Changes in the basal ganglia following cyanide poisoning. *J Comput Assist Tomogr.* 1981;5:755-756.

69. Flach PM, et al. "Drug mules" as a radiological challenge: sensitivity and specificity in identifying internal cocaine in body packers, body pushers and body stuffers by computed tomography, plain radiography and Lodox. *Eur J Radiol.* 2012;81:2518-2526.

70. Florez MV, et al. The radiodensity of medications seen on x-ray films. *Mayo Clin Proc.* 1998;73:516-519.

71. Fok MC, et al. A naturopathic cause of portal venous gas embolism. Hydrogen peroxide ingestion causing significant portal venous gas and stomach wall thickening. *Gastroenterology.* 2013;144:509, 658-659.

72. Forrester JM, et al. Crack lung: an acute pulmonary syndrome with a spectrum of clinical and histopathologic findings. *Am Rev Respir Dis.* 1990;142:462-467.

73. Fowler JS, Volkow ND. PET imaging studies in drug abuse. *J Toxicol Clin Toxicol.* 1998;36:163-174.

74. Foxford R, Goldfrank L. Gastrotomy—a surgical approach to iron overdose. *Ann Emerg Med.* 1985;14:1223-1226.

75. Franquet T, et al. Aspiration diseases: findings, pitfalls, and differential diagnosis. *Radiographics.* 2000;20:673-685.

76. Fraser RO, et al. Drug- and poison-induced pulmonary disease. In: Fraser RG, Paré JAP, eds. *Diagnosis of Diseases of the Chest.* 3rd ed. Philadelphia, PA: WB Saunders; 1991:2417-2479.

77. Freed TA, et al. Case reports balloon obturation bowel obstruction: a hazard of drug smuggling. *AJR Am J Roentgenol.* 1976;127:1033-1034.

78. French LK, et al. Hydrogen peroxide ingestion associated with portal venous gas and treatment with hyperbaric oxygen: a case series and review of the literature. *Clin Toxicol (Phila).* 2010;48:533-538.

79. Fulkerson WJ, Gockerman JP. Pulmonary disease induced by drugs. In: Fishman AP, ed. *Pulmonary Diseases and Disorders.* 2nd ed. New York, NY: McGraw-Hill; 1988:793-811.

80. Gadaleta D, et al. Cocaine-induced acute aortic dissection. *Chest.* 1989;96:1203-1205.

81. Gallucci M, et al. MR imaging of white matter lesions in uncomplicated chronic alcoholism. *J Comput Assist Tomogr.* 1989;13:395-398.

82. Gatenby RA. The radiology of drug-induced disorders in the gastrointestinal tract. *Semin Roentgenol.* 1995;30:62-76.

83. Gaul HP, et al. MR findings in methanol intoxication. *Am J Neuroradiol.* 1995; 16:1783-1786.

84. Ghai S, O'Malley ME. Portal vein gas resulting from ingestion of hydrogen peroxide. *AJR Am J Roentgenol.* 2003;181:1719-1720.

85. Gibby WA, Zimmerman RA. X-ray computed tomography. In: Mazziotta JG, Gilman S, eds. *Clinical Brain Imaging: Principles and Applications.* Philadelphia, PA: FA Davis; 1992:3-34.

86. Gilman S. Advances in neurology (1). *N Engl J Med.* 1992;326:1608-1616.

87. Gilman S, et al. Cerebellar and frontal hypometabolism in alcoholic cerebellar degeneration studied with positron emission tomography. *Ann Neurol.* 1990;28:775-785.

88. Ginaldi S. Geophagia: an uncommon cause of acute abdomen. *Ann Emerg Med.* 1988;17:979-981.

89. Goh S-K, et al. Subtrochanteric insufficiency fractures in patients on alendronate therapy: a caution. *J Bone Joint Surg Br.* 2007;89-B:349-353.

90. Gordon RJ, FD. Bacterial infections in drug users. *N Engl J Med.* 2005;353:1945-1954.

91. Gotway MB, et al. Thoracic complications of illicit drug use: an organ system approach. *Radiographics.* 2002;22(Spec No):S119-S135.

92. Grabherr S, et al. Detection of smuggled cocaine in cargos by MDCT. *AJR Am J Roentgenol.* 2008;190:1390-1395.

93. Gray JR, et al. Acute arsenic toxicity—an opaque poison. *Can Assoc Radiol J.* 1989;40:226-227.

94. Greller HA, et al. Use of ultrasound in the detection of intestinal drug smuggling. *Eur Radiol.* 2005;15:193; author reply 194.

95. Hagan IG, Burney K. Radiology of recreational drug abuse. *Radiographics.* 2007;27:919-940.

96. Hahn IH, et al. Contrast CT scan fails to detect the last heroin packet. *J Emerg Med.* 2004;27:279-283.

97. Handy CA. Radiopacity of oral nonliquid medications. *Radiology.* 1971;98:525-533.

98. Hantson P, et al. Neurotoxicity to the basal ganglia shown by magnetic resonance imaging (MRI) following poisoning by methanol and other substances. *J Toxicol Clin Toxicol.* 1997;35:151-161.

99. Harchelroad F. Identification of orally ingested cocaine by CT scan. *Vet Hum Toxicol.* 1992;34:350.

100. Haubek A, Lee K. Computed tomography in alcoholic cerebellar atrophy. *Neuroradiology.* 1979;18:77-79.

101. Hibbard R, et al. Spiral CT imaging of ingested foreign bodies wrapped in plastic: a pilot study designed to mimic cocaine body stuffers [abstract]. *J Toxicol Clin Toxicol.* 1999;37:644.

102. Hillbom M, et al. The clinical versus radiological diagnosis of alcoholic cerebellar degeneration. *J Neurol Sci.* 1986;73:45-53.

103. Hinkel CL. The significance of opaque medications in the gastrointestinal tract, with special reference to enteric coated pills. *Am J Roentgenol Radium Ther Nucl Med.* 1951;65:575-581.

104. Ho VB, et al. Bilateral basal ganglia lesions: pediatric differential considerations. *Radiographics.* 1993;13:269-292.

105. Hoffman CK, Goodman PC. Pulmonary edema in cocaine smokers. *Radiology.* 1989;172:463-465.

106. Hoffman RS, et al. Prospective evaluation of "crack-vial" ingestions. *Vet Hum Toxicol.* 1990;32:164-167.

107. Hoffman RS, et al. Whole bowel irrigation and the cocaine body-packer: a new approach to a common problem. *Am J Emerg Med.* 1990;8:523-527.

108. Holman BL, et al. Regional cerebral blood flow improves with treatment in chronic cocaine polydrug users. *J Nucl Med.* 1993;34:723-727.

109. Hormes JT, et al. Neurologic sequelae of chronic solvent vapor abuse. *Neurology.* 1986;36:698-702.

110. Horowitz AL, et al. Carbon monoxide toxicity: MR imaging in the brain. *Radiology.* 1987;162:787-788.

111. Horrocks AW. Abdominal radiography in suspected "body packers." *Clin Radiol.* 1992;45:322-325.

112. How J, et al. Chemotherapy-associated posterior reversible encephalopathy syndrome: a case report and review of the literature. *Neurologist.* 2016;21:112-117.

113. Isabela C, et al. Hypersensitivity pneumonitis: spectrum of high-resolution CT and pathologic findings. *AJR Am J Roentgenol.* 2007;188:334-344.

114. Jaeger RW, et al. Radiopacity of drugs and plants in vivo-limited usefulness. *Vet Hum Toxicol.* 1981;23(suppl 1):2-4.

115. Jibiki I, et al. 123I-IMP brain SPECT imaging in a patient with the interval form of CO poisoning. *Eur Neurol.* 1991;31:149-151.

116. Johnston C, Keogan MT. Imaging features of soft-tissue infections and other complications in drug users after direct subcutaneous injection ("skin popping"). *AJR Am J Roentgenol.* 2004;182:1195-1202.

117. Jones JS, et al. Computed tomographic findings after acute carbon monoxide poisoning. *Am J Emerg Med.* 1994;12:448-451.

118. Kaczorowski JM, Wax PM. Five days of whole-bowel irrigation in a case of pediatric iron ingestion. *Ann Emerg Med.* 1996;27:258-263.

119. Kaineg B, Hudgins P. Wernicke's encephalopathy (images in clinical medicine). *N Engl J Med.* 2005;352:e18.

120. Kakumanu N, Rao SD. Skeletal fluorosis due to excessive tea drinking. *N Engl J Med.* 2013;368:1140-1140.

121. Kanne JP, et al. Delayed gastric perforation resulting from hydrochloric acid ingestion. *AJR Am J Roentgenol.* 2005;185:682-683.

122. Kanne JP, et al. Airway injury after acute chlorine exposure. *AJR Am J Roentgenol.* 2006;186:232-233.

123. Kazzi ZN, et al. Suicide attempt by multivitamin ingestion. *J Emerg Med.* 2011;40:328-329.

124. Keogh CF, et al. Neuroimaging features of heroin inhalation toxicity: "chasing the dragon." *AJR Am J Roentgenol.* 2003;180:847-850.

125. Keys N, et al. Cocaine body stuffers: a case series. *J Toxicol Clin Toxicol.* 1995;33:517.

126. Koller WC, et al. Cerebellar atrophy demonstrated by computed tomography. *Neurology.* 1981;31:405-412.

127. Kram HB, et al. Perforated ulcers related to smoking "crack" cocaine. *Am Surg.* 1992;58:293-294.

128. Kriegstein AR, et al. Heroin inhalation and progressive spongiform leukoencephalopathy. *N Engl J Med.* 1997;336:589-590.

129. Krishnan A, Brown R. Plain abdominal radiography in the diagnosis of the "body packer." *J Accid Emerg Med.* 1999;16:381.

130. Krupski WC, et al. Unusual causes of mesenteric ischemia. *Surg Clin North Am.* 1997;77:471-502.

131. Kulshrestha MK. Lead poisoning diagnosed by abdominal X-rays. *J Toxicol Clin Toxicol.* 1996;34:107-108.

132. Lamy C, et al. Posterior reversible encephalopathy syndrome. *Handb Clin Neurol.* 2014;121:1687-1701.

133. Landi JL, Spickler EM. Imaging of intracranial hemorrhage associated with drug abuse. *Neuroimag Clin North Am.* 1992;2:187-194.

134. Lange RA, Hillis LD. Cocaine associated cardiovascular events. *N Engl J Med.* 2001;345:351-358.

135. Lassen NA, Holm S. Single photon emission computerized tomography. In: Mazzotta JG, Gilman S, eds. *Clinical Brain Imaging: Principles and Applications.* Philadelphia, PA: FA Davis; 1992:108-134.

136. Lee DC, et al. Whole-bowel irrigation as an adjunct in the treatment of radiopaque arsenic. *Am J Emerg Med.* 1995;13:244-245.

137. Lenart BA, et al. Atypical fractures of the femoral diaphysis in postmenopausal women taking alendronate. *N Engl J Med.* 2008;358:1304-1306.

138. Levine SR, et al. Cerebrovascular complications of the use of the "crack" form of alkaloidal cocaine. *N Engl J Med.* 1990;323:699-704.

139. Lexa FJ. Drug-induced disorders of the central nervous system. *Semin Roentgenol.* 1995;30:7-17.

140. Linowiecki KA, et al. Radiopacity of modified release cardiac medications: a case report and in vitro analysis [abstract]. *Vet Hum Toxicol.* 1992;34:350.

141. Litovitz TL. Button battery ingestions. A review of 56 cases. *JAMA.* 1983; 249: 2495-2500.

142. Lufkin RB. Magnetic resonance imaging. In: Mazzotti JG, Gilman S, eds. *Clinical Brain Imaging: Principles and Applications.* Philadelphia, PA: FA Davis; 1992:36-69.

143. Ly BT, et al. Mercuric oxide poisoning treated with whole-bowel irrigation and chelation therapy. *Ann Emerg Med*. 2002;39:312-315.

144. Mabry B, et al. Patterns of heroin overdose-induced pulmonary edema. *Am J Emerg Med*. 2004;22:316.

145. Maeda Y, et al. Effect of therapy with oxygen under high pressure on regional cerebral blood flow in the interval form of carbon monoxide poisoning: observation from subtraction of technetium-99m HMPAO SPECT brain imaging. *Eur Neurol*. 1991;31:380-383.

146. Mahoney MS, Kahn M. A medical mystery. *N Engl J Med*. 1998;339:745.

147. Mandava N, et al. Establishment of a definitive protocol for the diagnosis and management of body packers (drug mules). *Emerg Med J*. 2011;28:98-101.

148. Maniatis V, et al. I.V. mercury self-injection: CT imaging. *AJR Am J Roentgenol*. 1997;169:1197-1198.

149. Mankin HJ. Nontraumatic necrosis of bone (osteonecrosis). *N Engl J Med*. 1992;326:1473-1479.

150. Manning EP, et al. Images in emergency medicine. Young woman with epigastric pain and vomiting. Ingestion of 35% hydrogen peroxide. *Ann Emerg Med*. 2014;64:330, 333.

151. Maravilla AM, Berk RN. The radiology corner. The radiographic diagnosis of pica. *Am J Gastroenterol*. 1978;70:94-99.

152. Marc B, et al. The cocaine body-packer syndrome: evaluation of a method of contrast study of the bowel. *J Forensic Sci*. 1990;35:345-355.

153. Martel W. Radiologic features of esophagogastritis secondary to extremely caustic agents. *Radiology*. 1972;103:31-36.

154. Martin TJ. Cocaine-induced mesenteric ischemia. *N C Med J*. 1991;52:429-430.

155. Martindale JL. Imaging abnormalities associated with carbon monoxide toxicity. *J Emerg Med*. 2013;44:1140-1141.

156. Matsumoto SC, et al. Minamata disease demonstrated by computed tomography. *Neuroradiology*. 1988;30:42-46.

157. McCarron MM, Wood JD. The cocaine 'body packer' syndrome. Diagnosis and treatment. *JAMA*. 1983;250:1417-1420.

158. McElvaine MD, et al. Prevalence of radiographic evidence of paint chip ingestion among children with moderate to severe lead poisoning, St Louis, Missouri, 1989 through 1990. *Pediatrics*. 1992;89(4 Pt 2):740-742.

159. Meggs WJ, et al. Thallium poisoning from maliciously contaminated food. *J Toxicol Clin Toxicol*. 1994;32:723-730.

160. Megibow AJ, et al. Bowel obstruction: evaluation with CT. *Radiology*. 1991;180:313-318.

161. Meijer R, Bots ML. Detection of intestinal drug containers by ultrasound scanning: an airport screening tool? *Eur Radiol*. 2003;13:1312-1315.

162. Mengel CE, Carter WA. Geophagia diagnosed by roentgenograms. *JAMA*. 1964;187:955-956.

163. Messing B, Storch B. Computer tomography and magnetic resonance imaging in cyanide poisoning. *Eur Arch Psychiatry Neurol Sci*. 1988;237:139-143.

164. Mi SY, et al. CT findings in hydrocarbon pneumonitis after diesel fuel siphonage. *AJR Am J Roentgenol*. 2009;193:1118-1121.

165. Miller WT Jr. Pleural and mediastinal disorders related to drug use. *Semin Roentgenol*. 1995;30:35-48.

166. Miura T, et al. CT of the brain in acute carbon monoxide intoxication: characteristic features and prognosis. *AJNR Am J Neuroradiol*. 1985;6:739-742.

167. Moon JM, et al. Hemorrhagic gastritis and gas emboli after ingesting 3% hydrogen peroxide. *J Emerg Med*. 2006;30:403-406.

168. Moral AR, et al. Putaminal necrosis after methanol intoxication. *Intensive Care Med*. 1997;23:234-235.

169. Naidich TP, et al. Metallic mercury emboli. *Am J Roentgenol Radium Ther Nucl Med*. 1973;117:886-891.

170. Nelson DL, et al. The CT and MRI features of acute toxic encephalopathies. *Am J Neuroradiol*. 1987;8:951.

171. Neustadter LM, Weiss M. Medication-induced changes of bone. *Semin Roentgenol*. 1995;30:88-95.

172. Ng RC, et al. Iron poisoning: assessment of radiography in diagnosis and management. *Clin Pediatr (Phila)*. 1979;18:614-616.

173. O'Brien RP, et al. Detectability of drug tablets and capsules by plain radiography. *Am J Emerg Med*. 1986;4:302-312.

174. Olmedo RE, et al. Limitations of whole bowel irrigation and laparotomy in a cocaine "body packer" [abstract]. *J Toxicol Clin Toxicol*. 1999;37:645.

175. Olsen WL, Cohen W. Neuroradiology of AIDS. In: Federle MP, Megibow AJ, Naidich DP, eds. *Radiology of Acquired Immune Deficiency Syndrome*. New York, NY: Raven Press; 1988:21-45.

176. Omori N, et al. Gas-producing cellulitis from injection of spot remover fluid (n-hexane). *J Emerg Med*. 2013;44:385-388.

177. Palat D, et al. Pneumomediastinum induced by inhalation of alkaloidal cocaine. *N Y State J Med*. 1988;88:438-439.

178. Palatnick W, Tenenbein M. Leukocytosis, hyperglycemia, vomiting, and positive X-rays are not indicators of severity of iron overdose in adults. *Am J Emerg Med*. 1996;14:454-455.

179. Papafragkou S, et al. Treatment of portal venous gas embolism with hyperbaric oxygen after accidental ingestion of hydrogen peroxide: a case report and review of the literature. *J Emerg Med*. 2012;43:e21-23.

180. Perron AD, Gibbs M. Thoracic aortic dissection secondary to crack cocaine ingestion. *Am J Emerg Med*. 1997;15:507-509.

181. Peterson CD, Field GC. Emergency gastrotomy for acute iron poisoning. *Ann Emerg Med*. 1980;9:262-264.

182. Phelps ME. Positron emission tomography. In: Mazzotta JG, Gilman S, eds. *Clinical Brain Imaging: Principles and Applications*. Philadelphia, PA: FA Davis, 1992:71-106.

183. Piatt JP, et al. Occult carbon monoxide poisoning in an infant. *Pediatr Emerg Care*. 1990;6:21-23.

184. Pidoto RR, et al. A new method of packaging cocaine for international traffic and implications for the management of cocaine body packers. *J Emerg Med*. 2002;23:149-153.

185. Poletti PA, et al. Screening of illegal intracorporeal containers ("body packing"): is abdominal radiography sufficiently accurate? A comparative study with low-dose CT. *Radiology*. 2012;265:772-779.

186. Pollack CV, Jr., et al. Two crack cocaine body stuffers. *Ann Emerg Med*. 1992;21:1370-1380.

187. Pracyk JB, et al. Brain computerized tomography after hyperbaric oxygen therapy for carbon monoxide poisoning. *Undersea Hyperb Med*. 1995;22:1-7.

188. Prockop LD, Naidu KA. Brain CT and MRI findings after carbon monoxide toxicity. *J Neuroimaging*. 1999;9:175-181.

189. Raber SA. The dense metaphyseal band sign. *Radiology*. 1999;211:773-774.

190. Rashid J, et al. Cocaine-induced aortic dissection. *Am Heart J*. 1996;132:1301-1304.

191. Resnick D. Heavy metal poisoning and deficiency. In: Resnick D, ed. *Diagnosis of Bone and Joint Disorders*. Philadelphia, PA: WB Saunders; 1995:3353-3364.

192. Resnick D, Niwayama G. Osteolysis and chondrolysis. In: Resnick D, ed. *Diagnosis of Bone and Joint Disorders*. Philadelphia, PA: WB Saunders; 1995:4467-4469.

193. Restrepo CS, et al. Pulmonary complications from cocaine and cocaine-based substances: imaging manifestations. *Radiographics*. 2007;27:941-956.

194. Restrepo CS, et al. Cardiovascular complications of cocaine: imaging findings. *Emerg Radiol*. 2009;16:11-19.

195. Richerson HB. Hypersensitivity pneumonitis (extrinsic allergic alveolitis). In: Fishman AP, ed. *Pulmonary Diseases and Disorders*. 2nd ed. New York, NY: McGraw-Hill; 1988:667-674.

196. Rider SP, et al. Cerebral air gas embolism from concentrated hydrogen peroxide ingestion. *Clin Toxicol (Phila)*. 2008;46:815-818.

197. Rimkus Cde M, et al. Toxic leukoencephalopathies, including drug, medication, environmental, and radiation-induced encephalopathic syndromes. *Semin Ultrasound CT MR*. 2014;35:97-117.

198. Roach HD, et al. Asbestos: when the dust settles an imaging review of asbestos-related disease. *Radiographics*. 2002;22(Spec No):S167-S184.

199. Roberge RJ, Martin TG. Whole bowel irrigation in an acute oral lead intoxication. *Am J Emerg Med*. 1992;10:577-583.

200. Roberts JR. Complications of radiographic contrast material. *Emerg Med News*. 2004:31-34.

201. Roberts JR, et al. The bodystuffer syndrome: a clandestine form of drug overdose. *Am J Emerg Med*. 1986;4:24-27.

202. Rosenberg NL, et al. Toluene abuse causes diffuse central nervous system white matter changes. *Ann Neurol*. 1988;23:611-614.

203. Rossi SE, et al. Pulmonary drug toxicity: radiologic and pathologic manifestations. *Radiographics*. 2000;20:1245-1259.

204. Rousset P, et al. Detection of residual packets in cocaine body packers: low accuracy of abdominal radiography: a prospective study. *Eur Radiol*. 2013;23:2146-2155.

205. Rubinstein D, et al. Methanol intoxication with putaminal and white matter necrosis: MR and CT findings. *AJNR Am J Neuroradiol*. 1995;16:1492-1494.

206. Rykken JB, McKinney AM. Posterior reversible encephalopathy syndrome. *Semin Ultrasound CT MR*. 2014;35:118-135.

207. Ryu HH, et al. Caustic injury: can CT grading system enable prediction of esophageal stricture? *Clin Toxicol (Phila)*. 2010;48:137-142.

209. Sachs HK. The evolution of the radiologic lead line. *Radiology*. 1981;139:81-85.

210. Saleem TM, et al. Renal infarction: a rare complication of cocaine abuse. *Am J Emerg Med*. 2001;19:528-529.

211. Savitt DL, et al. The radiopacity of ingested medications. *Ann Emerg Med*. 1987;16:331-339.

212. Sawada Y, et al. Correlation of pathological findings with computed tomographic findings after acute carbon monoxide poisoning. *N Engl J Med*. 1983;308:1296.

213. Sawada Y, et al. Computerised tomography as an indication of long-term outcome after acute carbon monoxide poisoning. *Lancet*. 1980;1:783-784.

214. Schabel SI, Rogers CI. Opaque artifacts in a health food faddist simulating ovarian neoplasm. *AJR Am J Roentgenol*. 1978;130:789-790.

215. Schilcher J, Aspenberg P. Atypical fracture of the femur in a patient using denosumab—a case report. *Acta Orthop*. 2014;85:6-7.

216. Schilcher J, et al. Risk of atypical femoral fracture during and after bisphosphonate use. *N Engl J Med*. 2014;371:974-976.

217. Schilcher J, et al. Bisphosphonate use and atypical fractures of the femoral shaft. *N Engl J Med*. 2011;364:1728-1737.

218. Schulz B, et al. Body packers on your examination table: how helpful are plain x-ray images? A definitive low-dose CT protocol as a diagnosis tool for body packers. *Clin Radiol*. 2014;69:e525-530.

219. Schwartz DT. Toxicologic emergencies. In: Schwartz DT, Reisdorff EJ, eds. *Emergency Radiology*. New York, NY: McGraw-Hill; 2000:627-648.

220. Sengupta A, Page P. Window manipulation in diagnosis of body packing using computed tomography. *Emerg Radiol.* 2008;15:203-205.
221. Shah R, et al. Cocaine-induced acute aortic dissection. *J Emerg Med.* 2015;49:e87-e89.
222. Shanbhogue AKP, et al. Spectrum of medication-induced complications in the abdomen: role of cross-sectional imaging. *AJR Am J Roentgenol.* 2011;197:286-294.
223. Sinner WN. The gastrointestinal tract as a vehicle for drug smuggling. *Gastrointest Radiol.* 1981;6:319-323.
224. Sogge MR, et al. Lavage to remove enteric-coated aspirin and gastric outlet obstruction. *Ann Intern Med.* 1977;87:721-722.
225. Spitzer A, et al. Radiopaque suppositories. *Radiology.* 1976;121:71-73.
226. Sporer KA, Firestone J. Clinical course of crack cocaine body stuffers. *Ann Emerg Med.* 1997;29:596-601.
227. Sporer KA, Manning JJ. Massive ingestion of sustained-release verapamil with a concretion and bowel infarction. *Ann Emerg Med.* 1993;22:603-605.
228. Staple TW, McAlister WH. Roentgenographic visualization of iron preparations in the gastrointestinal tract. *Radiology.* 1964;83:1051-1056.
229. Stepens A, et al. A parkinsonian syndrome in methcathinone users and the role of manganese. *N Engl J Med.* 2008;358:1009-1017.
230. Stern WZ, et al. The roentgen findings in acute heroin intoxication. *Am J Roentgenol Radium Ther Nucl Med.* 1968;103:522-532.
231. Stromberg BV. Symptomatic lead toxicity secondary to retained shotgun pellets: case report. *J Trauma.* 1990;30:356-357.
232. Su M, et al. Sustained-release potassium chloride overdose. *J Toxicol Clin Toxicol.* 2001;39:641-648.
233. Sue YJ, et al. Radiopacity of paradichlorobenzene-containing household products. *Vet Hum Toxicol.* 1992;34:350.
234. Sullivan S, et al. Accuracy of trans-abdominal ultrasound in a simulated massive acute overdose. *Am J Emerg Med.* 2016;34:1455-1457.
235. Swartz MN. Approach to the patient with pulmonary infections. In: Fishman AP, ed. *Pulmonary Diseases and Disorders.* 2nd ed. New York, NY: McGraw-Hill; 1988:1375-1750.
236. Switz DM, et al. Bullets, joints, and lead intoxication. A remarkable and instructive case. *Arch Intern Med.* 1976;136:939-941.
237. Tamrazi B, Almast J. Your brain on drugs: imaging of drug-related changes in the central nervous system. *Radiographics.* 2012;32:701-719.
238. Tatekawa Y, et al. Small bowel obstruction caused by a medication bezoar: report of a case. *Surg Today.* 1996;26:68-70.
239. Theodorou SJ, et al. Imaging findings of complications affecting the upper extremity in intravenous drug users. *Emerg Radiol.* 2008;15:227-239.
240. Tillman DJ, et al. Radiopacity study of extended-release formulations using digitalized radiography. *Am J Emerg Med.* 1994;12:310-314.
241. Tom T, et al. Neuroimaging characteristics in carbon monoxide toxicity. *J Neuroimaging.* 1996;6:161-166.
242. Tormoehlen LM. Toxic leukoencephalopathies. *Psychiatr Clin North Am.* 2013;36:277-292.
243. Traub SJ, et al. Body packing—the internal concealment of illicit drugs. *N Engl J Med.* 2003;349:2519-2526.
244. Traub SJ, et al. False-positive abdominal radiography in a body packer resulting from intraabdominal calcifications. *Am J Emerg Med.* 2003;21:607-608.
245. Tumeh SS, et al. Cerebral abnormalities in cocaine abusers: demonstration by SPECT perfusion brain scintigraphy. Work in progress. *Radiology.* 1990;176:821-824.
246. Vantroyen B, et al. Survival after a lethal dose of arsenic trioxide. *J Toxicol Clin Toxicol.* 2004;42:889-895.
247. Velasquez G, et al. Thorium dioxide: still around. *South Med J.* 1985;78:743-745.
248. Vernace MA, et al. Chronic salicylate toxicity due to consumption of over-the-counter bismuth subsalicylate. *Am J Med.* 1994;97:308-309.
249. Vieregge P, et al. Carbon monoxide poisoning: clinical, neurophysiological, and brain imaging observations in acute disease and follow-up. *J Neurol.* 1989;236:478-481.
250. Volkow ND, et al. Use of positron emission tomography to investigate cocaine. In: Nahas GG, Latour C, eds. *Physiopathology of Illicit Drugs: Cannabis, Cocaine, Opiates.* Pergamon Press, New York, NY. 1991:129-141.
251. Wang CL, et al. Frequency, management, and outcome of extravasation of nonionic iodinated contrast medium in 69,657 intravenous injections. *Radiology.* 2007;243:80-87.
252. Wang GJ, et al. Functional importance of ventricular enlargement and cortical atrophy in healthy subjects and alcoholics as assessed with PET, MR imaging, and neuropsychologic testing. *Radiology.* 1993;186:59-65.
253. Wang Y, et al. Endemic fluorosis of the skeleton: radiographic features in 127 patients. *AJR Am J Roentgenol.* 1994;162:93-98.
254. Warach SJ, Charness ME. Imaging the brain lesions of alcoholics. In: Greenberg JO, Adams RD, eds. *Neuroimaging: A Companion to Adams and Victor's Principles of Neurology.* New York, NY: McGraw-Hill Health Professions Division; 1995:503-515.
255. Ward S, et al. Talcosis associated with IV abuse of oral medications: CT findings. *AJR Am J Roentgenol.* 2000;174:789-793.
256. Ware LB, Matthay MA. The acute respiratory distress syndrome. *N Engl J Med.* 2000;342:1334-1349.
257. Weidauer S, et al. Wernicke encephalopathy: MR findings and clinical presentation. *Eur Radiol.* 2003;13:1001-1009.
258. Weill H, Jones RN. Occupational pulmonary diseases. In: Fishman AP, ed. *Pulmonary Diseases and Disorders.* 2nd ed. New York, NY: McGraw-Hill; 1988:1465-1474.
259. Weimerskirch PJ, et al. Methylene iodide poisoning. *Ann Emerg Med.* 1990;19:1171-1176.
260. Weinstein RS, et al. Giant osteoclast formation and long-term oral bisphosphonate therapy. *N Engl J Med.* 2009;360:53-62.
261. Wilgoren J. Misdiagnosis led to man's handcuffing, suit claims. *The New York Times.* December 6, 1998:62.
262. Williams MH. Pulmonary complications of drug abuse. In: Fishman AP, ed. *Pulmonary Diseases and Disorders.* 2nd ed. New York, NY: McGraw-Hill; 1988:819-860.
263. Wolff AJ, O'Donnell AE. Pulmonary effects of illicit drug use. *Clin Chest Med.* 2004;25:203-216.
264. Wolowodiuk OJ, et al. Pneumomediastinum and retropneumoperitoneum: an unusual complication of syrup-of-ipecac-induced emesis. *Ann Emerg Med.* 1984;13:1148-1151.
265. Woolf DA, et al. Lead lines in young infants with acute lead encephalopathy: a reliable diagnostic test. *J Trop Pediatr.* 1990;36:90-93.
266. Yanagawa Y, et al. Usefulness of computed tomography in the diagnosis of an overdose. *Acta Med Okayama.* 2011;65:33-39.

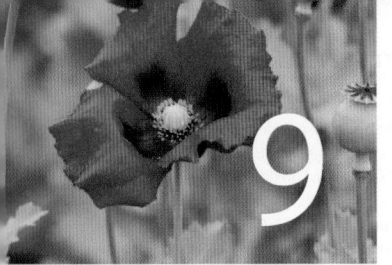

9 PHARMACOKINETIC AND TOXICOKINETIC PRINCIPLES

Mary Ann Howland

Pharmacokinetics is the study of the absorption, distribution, metabolism, and excretion of xenobiotics. Xenobiotics are substances that are foreign to the body and include natural or synthetic chemicals, drugs, pesticides, environmental agents, and industrial agents.[56] Mathematical models and equations are used to describe and to predict these phenomena. *Pharmacodynamics* is the term used to describe an investigation of the relationship of therapeutic xenobiotic concentration to its clinical effects. *Toxicokinetics*, which is analogous to pharmacokinetics, is the study of the absorption, distribution, metabolism, and excretion of a xenobiotic under circumstances that produce toxicity. *Toxicodynamics*, which is analogous to pharmacodynamics, is the study of the relationship of toxic xenobiotic concentrations to their clinical effects.

Overdoses challenge the mathematical precision of toxicokinetics and toxicodynamics because many of the variables, such as dose host variables, time of ingestion, and presence of vomiting, or diarrhea, that affect the result are often unknown. In contrast to the therapeutic setting, atypical solubility characteristics are noted, and saturation of enzymatic processes occurs. Intestinal or hepatic enzymatic saturation or alterations in transporters enhance absorption through a decrease in *first-pass effect* defined as metabolism before the xenobiotic reaches the systemic circulation.[5,85] Saturation of plasma protein binding results in the availability of more unbound xenobiotic in the plasma. Saturation of hepatic enzymes or saturation of active renal tubular secretion leads to prolonged elimination (metabolism and excretion). In addition, age, obesity, gender, pharmacogenetics and pharmacogenomics, chronopharmacokinetics (diurnal variations), and the effects of illness and impairment of hepatic and renal function, as well as cardiac output and splanchnic perfusion all further limit the ability to achieve precise analyses.[6,22,47,52,75,81] Furthermore, various treatments may alter one or more pharmacokinetic and toxicokinetic parameters. There are numerous approaches to recognizing these variables, such as obtaining historical information from the patient's family and friends, performing pill counts, procuring sequential serum concentrations during the phases of toxicity, and occasionally repeating a pharmacokinetic evaluation of that same xenobiotic during therapeutic dosing to obtain comparative data.

Although different, *plasma concentration* and *serum concentration* are terms often used interchangeably. When a reference or calculation is made with regard to a concentration in the body, it is actually a plasma concentration. When concentrations are measured in the laboratory, a serum concentration (clotted and centrifuged blood) is often determined. In reality, the laboratory measurements of most xenobiotics in serum or plasma are nearly equivalent. Frequently, this is not the case for whole-blood determination if the xenobiotic distributes into the erythrocyte, such as lead and most other heavy metals.

Despite all of the confounding and individual variability, toxicokinetic principles are nonetheless applied to facilitate our understanding and to make predictions. These principles are used to help evaluate whether a certain antidote or extracorporeal removal method is appropriate for use, when the serum concentration might be expected to decrease into the therapeutic range (if one exists), what dose might be considered potentially toxic, what the onset and duration of toxicity might be, and what the importance is of a serum concentration. While considering all of these factors, the clinical status of the patient is paramount, and mathematical formulas and equations can never substitute for a sound clinical assessment. This chapter explains the principles and presents the mathematics in a user-friendly fashion.[90]

ABSORPTION

Absorption is the process by which a xenobiotic enters the body. A xenobiotic must reach the bloodstream and then be distributed to the site or sites of action to cause a systemic effect. Both the rate (k_a) and extent (F) of absorption are measurable and important determinants of toxicity. The rate of absorption often predicts the onset of action and relies on dosage form, and the extent of absorption (*bioavailability*, or F) often predicts the intensity of the effect and depends in part on first-pass effects.[43,44] Fig. 9–1 depicts how changes in the rate of absorption may affect toxicity when the bioavailability is held constant versus how toxicity is increased as the bioavailability increases and the elimination rate constant (K_e) remains constant.

The route by which the xenobiotic enters the body significantly affects both the rate and extent of absorption. As an approximation, the rate of absorption proceeds in the following order from fastest to slowest: intravenous (IV), intraosseous, inhalation > sublingual > intramuscular, subcutaneous, intranasal, oral > cutaneous, rectal (may be unpredictable if bypasses first-pass elimination). After the oral intake of 200 mg (0.59 mmol) of cocaine hydrochloride, the onset of action is 20 minutes, with an average peak concentration of 200 ng/mL.[80] In marked contrast, smoking 200 mg (0.66 mmol) of alkaloidal cocaine (freebase) results in an onset of action of 8 seconds and a peak concentration of 640 ng/mL. When administered IV as 200 mg of

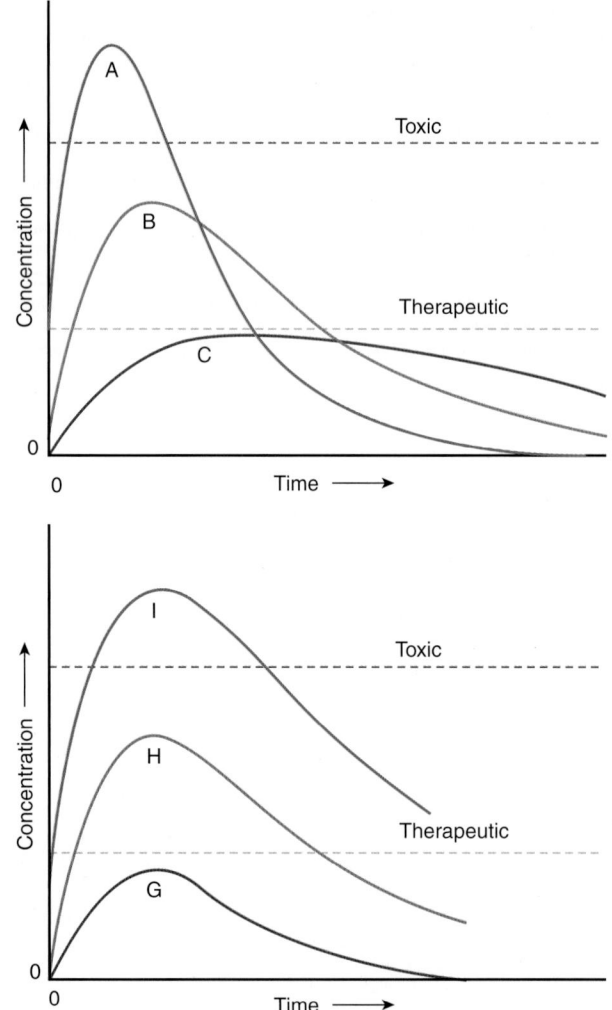

FIGURE 9–1. Effects of changes in k_a (rate of absorption) and F (bioavailability) on the blood concentration versus time graph and achieving a toxic threshold. In curves *A*, *B*, and *C*, F is constant as k_a decreases. In curves *G*, *H*, and *I*, toxicity increases as F increases from G to I while the K_e remains constant.[61]

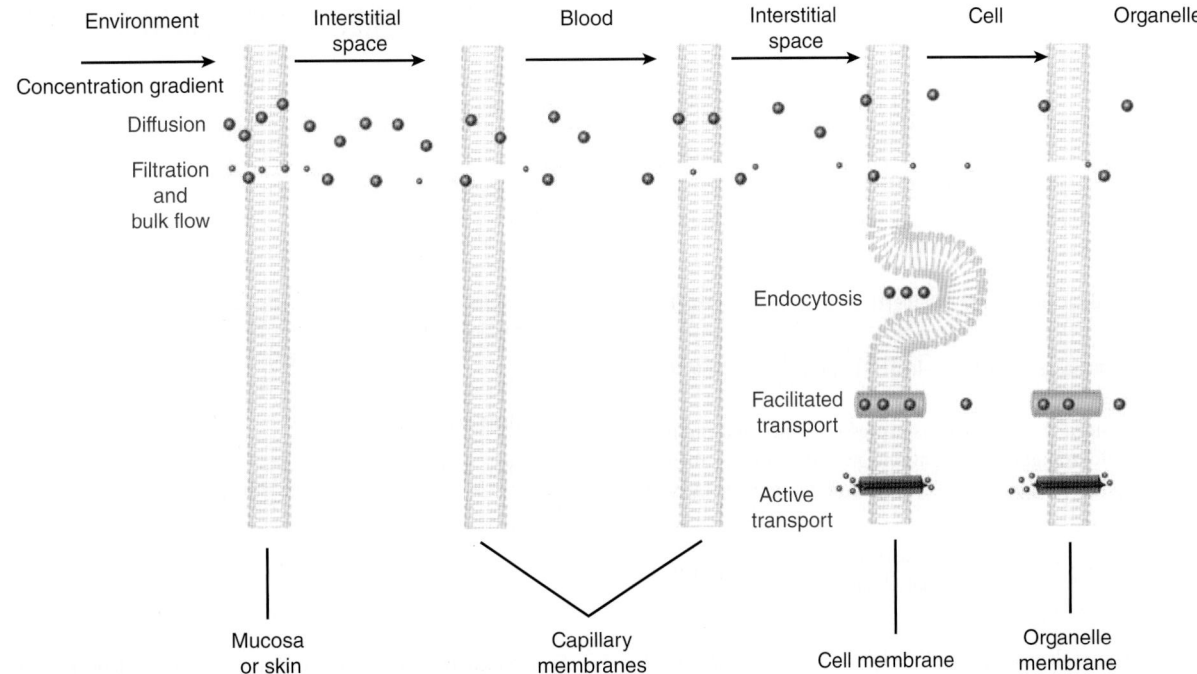

FIGURE 9–2. Illustration of the number of membranes encountered by a xenobiotic in the process of absorption and distribution and the transport mechanisms involved in the passage of xenobiotics across membranes. Examples include varying types of diffusion: nonpolar and uncharged (ethanol) and nonionized forms of weak acids (salicylic acid) and bases (amphetamines); endocytosis: Sabin polio virus vaccine; facilitated: 5-fluorouracil, lead, thallium; and active: thiamine and pyridoxine.

cocaine hydrochloride, the onset of action is 30 seconds and a peak concentration of 1,000 ng/mL.[80]

A xenobiotic must diffuse through a number of membranes before it reaches its site of action. Fig. 9–2 shows the number of membranes through which a xenobiotic typically diffuses. Membranes are predominantly composed of phospholipids and cholesterol in addition to other lipid compounds.[61] A phospholipid is composed of a polar head and a fatty acid tail, which are arranged in membranes so that the fatty acid tails are inside and the polar heads face outward in a mirror image.[65] Proteins are found on both sides of the membranes and often traverse the membrane.[61] Some of these proteins function as receptors and channels. Pores are found throughout the membranes. The principles relating to diffusion apply to absorption, distribution, certain aspects of elimination, and each mechanism that permits a xenobiotic to be transported through a membrane.

Transport through membranes occurs via (1) passive diffusion; (2) filtration or bulk flow, which is most important in renal and biliary secretion as the mechanism of transport associated with the movement of molecules with a molecular weight less than 100 Da, with water directly through aquapores; (3) carrier-mediated active and facilitated transports, which are saturable; and (4) rarely, endocytosis (Fig. 9–2). Most xenobiotics traverse membranes via simple passive diffusion. The rate of diffusion is determined by the Fick's law of diffusion:

$$\text{Rate of diffusion} = \frac{-dQ}{dt} = \frac{-DAK_{ow}(C_1 - C_2)}{h} \quad \text{(Eq. 9–1)}$$

where:

   D = diffusion coefficient
   A = surface area of the membrane
   h = membrane thickness
   K_{ow} = partition coefficient
   $C_1 - C_2$ = difference in concentrations of the xenobiotic on each side of the membrane

The driving force for passive diffusion is the difference between the concentrations of the xenobiotic on the opposing sides of the membrane. Each

xenobiotic has a constant D is derived when the difference in concentrations between the two sides of the membrane is one. The larger the surface area A, the higher the rate of diffusion. Most ingested xenobiotics are absorbed more rapidly in the small intestine than in the stomach because of the tremendous increase in surface area created by the presence of microvilli. The partition constant or ratio (previously called the coefficient) K_{ow} represents the lipid-to-water partitioning of the nonionized xenobiotic with pH adjustment to favor nonionized xenobiotic. To a substantial degree, the more lipid soluble a xenobiotic is, the more easily it crosses membranes. The logarithm of the K_{ow} is known as log P. Whereas log P represents the partitioning of the nonionized form, log D (logarithm of the distribution constant) represents the lipid-to-water partitioning of the sum of the nonionized plus ionized forms in the octanol and water phase and is pH dependent. Log D is most useful when measured at physiologic pH. Membrane thickness (h) is inversely proportional to the rate at which a xenobiotic diffuses through the membrane. Xenobiotics that are uncharged, nonpolar, of low molecular weight, and lipid soluble have the highest rates of passive diffusion.

The extent of ionization of weak electrolytes (weak acids and weak bases) affects their rate of passive diffusion. Nonpolar and uncharged molecules penetrate faster. The Henderson-Hasselbalch relationship is used to determine the degree of ionization. An acid (HA), by definition, gives up a proton, and a base (B) accepts a proton. Acids and bases can be nonionized (uncharged, molecular, free), positively charged (cationic), or negatively charged (anionic). Aspirin and phenobarbital are uncharged acids (RCOOH), and pseudoephedrine HCl is a cationic acid. Morphine, amphetamine, and amitriptyline are uncharged bases (RNH_2), and sodium valproate is an anionic base. The equilibrium dissociation constants K_a and K_b can then be described. $K_a \times K_b = K_w$, and K_w is the dissociation constant of water. Because these numbers are difficult to work with, they are transformed using logarithms. By Equations 9–2A and 9–2B:

For weak acids: $HA \underset{K_2}{\overset{K_1}{\rightleftharpoons}} H^+ + A^-$

$$K_a = \frac{[H^+][A^-]}{[HA]} \quad \text{(Eq. 9–2A)}$$

For weak bases: $BH^+ \underset{K_2}{\overset{K_1}{\rightleftarrows}} B + H^+$

$$K_b = \frac{[H^+][B]}{[BH^+]} \qquad \text{(Eq. 9–2B)}$$

$$B + H_2O \rightarrow BH^+ + OH^-$$

For a more facile mathematical utilization, the negative log of both sides is determined. The results are given in Equations 9–3A and 9–3B.

$$\text{For weak acids: } -\log K_a = -\log[H^+] - \log\frac{[A^-]}{[HA]} \qquad \text{(Eq. 9–3A)}$$

$$\text{For weak bases: } -\log K_b = -\log[H^+] - \log\frac{[B]}{[BA^+]} \qquad \text{(Eq. 9–3B)}$$

By definition, the negative log of $[H^+]$ is expressed as pH, and the negative log of K_a is pK_a. Rearranging the equations gives the familiar forms of the Henderson-Hasselbalch equations, as shown in Equations 9–4A, 9–4B, and 9–4C:

$$pH = pK_a + \log\frac{\text{Unprotonated species}}{\text{Protonated species}} \qquad \text{(Eq. 9–4A)}$$

$$\text{For weak acids: } pH = pK_a + \log\frac{[A^-]}{[HA]} \qquad \text{(Eq. 9–4B)}$$

$$\text{For weak bases: } pH = pK_b + \log\frac{[B]}{[BH^+]} \qquad \text{(Eq. 9–4C)}$$

Because uncharged molecules traverse membranes more rapidly, it is understood that weak acids cross membranes more rapidly in an acidic environment, and weak bases move more rapidly in a basic environment. When the pH equals the pK_a, half of the xenobiotic is charged (ionized), and half is uncharged (nonionized). An acid with a low pK_a is a strong acid, and a base with a low pK_a is a weak base. For an acid, a pH less than the pK_a favors the protonated or uncharged species facilitating membrane diffusion, and for a base, a pH greater than the pK_a achieves the same result. Table 9–1 lists the pH of selected body fluids, and Fig. 9–3 illustrates the extent of charged versus uncharged xenobiotic at different pH and pK_a and pK_b values.

Lipid solubility and ionization each have a distinct influence on absorption. Fig. 9–4 demonstrates these characteristics for three different xenobiotics. Although the three xenobiotics have similar pK_a and pK_b values, their different partition constants result in different degrees of absorption from the stomach.

TABLE 9–1	pH of Selected Body Fluids
Fluids	**pH**
Cerebrospinal	7.3
Gastric	1–3
Large intestine (adult stool)	>6
Ophthalmic (tears)	7–8
Plasma	7.4
Stool: Infants and children	7.2–12
Saliva	6.4–7.2
Small intestine: duodenum	5–6
Small intestine: ileum	8
Urine	4–8
Vaginal	3.8–4.5

Specialized transport mechanisms are either adenosine triphosphate (ATP) dependent to transport xenobiotics against a concentration gradient (ie, active transport) or ATP independent and lack the ability to transport against a concentration gradient (ie, facilitated transport). These transport mechanisms are of importance in numerous parts of the body, including the intestines, liver, lungs, kidneys, and biliary system. These same principles apply to a small number of lipid-insoluble molecules that resemble essential endogenous molecules.[34,71] For example, 5-fluorouracil resembles pyrimidine and is transported by the same system, and thallium and lead are actively absorbed by the endogenous transport mechanisms that absorb and transport potassium and calcium, respectively. Filtration is generally considered to be of limited importance in the absorption of most xenobiotics but is substantially more important with regard to renal and biliary elimination. Endocytosis, which describes the encircling of a xenobiotic by a cellular membrane, is responsible for the absorption of large macromolecules such as the oral Sabin polio vaccine.[71]

Gastrointestinal (GI) absorption is affected by xenobiotic-related characteristics, such as dosage form, degree of ionization, partition constant, and patient factors (eg, GI blood flow; GI motility; and the presence or absence of food, ethanol, or other interfering substances such as calcium) (Fig. 9–5).

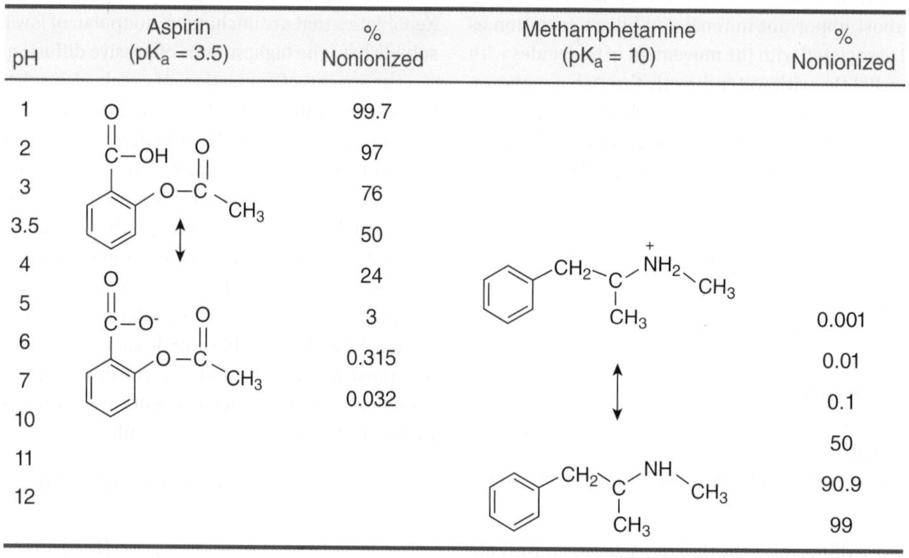

pH	Aspirin (pKa = 3.5)	% Nonionized	Methamphetamine (pKa = 10)	% Nonionized
1		99.7		
2		97		
3		76		
3.5		50		
4		24		
5		3		
6		0.315		0.001
7		0.032		0.01
10				0.1
11				50
12				90.9
				99

FIGURE 9–3. Effect of pH on the ionization of aspirin ($pK_a = 3.5$) and methamphetamine ($pK_a = 10$).

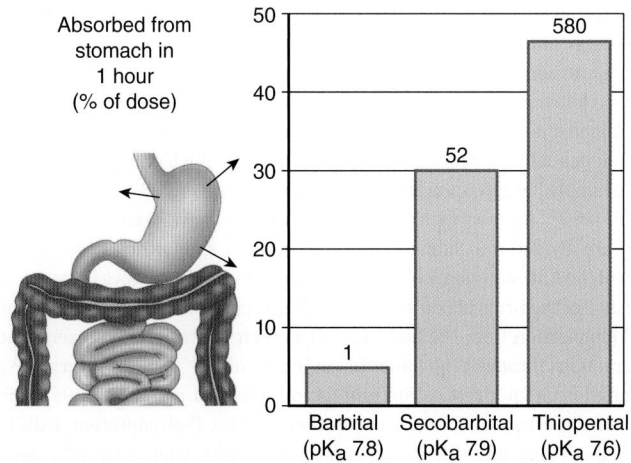

FIGURE 9–4. Influence of increasing lipid solubility on the amount of xenobiotic absorbed from the stomach for three xenobiotics with similar pK$_a$ values. The number above each column is the oil/water equilibrium partition coefficient. *(Reproduced with permission from Brody TM, Larner J, Minneman KP, et al: Human Pharmacology: Molecular to Clinical, 2nd ed. St. Louis, MO: Mosby; 1994.)*

TABLE 9–2	Xenobiotics That Form Concretions or Bezoars, Delay Gastric Emptying, or Result in Pylorospasm	
Anticholinergics		Iron
Barbiturates		Meprobamate
Bromides		Methaqualone
Carbamazepine		Opioids
Enteric-coated tablets		Phenytoin
Extended release (Acetaminophen, quetiapine)		Salicylates
Glutethimide		Verapamil

delayed-release preparations are enteric coated and specifically designed to bypass the stomach and to release drug in the small intestine. Other delayed-release formulations (eg, Verelan PM—verapamil) are designed to release the drug later but not specifically designed to bypass release in the stomach. Enteric-coated (acetylsalicylic acid, divalproex sodium—valproic acid) formulations resist disintegration and delay the time to onset of effect.[9] Dissolution is affected by ionization, solubility, and the partition coefficient. For example, only 1 g of aspirin is soluble in 100 mL of water at body temperature. In the overdose setting, the formation of poorly soluble or adherent masses such as concretions of foreign material termed *bezoars* significantly delay the time to onset of toxicity (Table 9–2).[7,14,35,37,67]

Most ingested xenobiotics are primarily absorbed in the small intestine as a result of the large surface area and extensive blood flow of the small intestines.[66] Critically ill patients who are hypotensive, have a reduced cardiac output, or are receiving vasopressors such as norepinephrine have a decreased perfusion of vital organs, including the GI tract, kidneys, and liver.[6] Not only is absorption delayed, but elimination is also diminished.[64] Total GI transit time ranges from 0.4 to 5 days, and small intestinal transit time is usually 3 to 4 hours. Extremely short GI transit times reduce absorption. This change in transit time is the unproven rationale for use of whole-bowel irrigation (WBI). Delays in emptying of the stomach impair absorption as a result of the delay in delivery to the small intestine. Delays in gastric emptying occur as a result of the presence of food, especially fatty meals; xenobiotics with anticholinergic, opioid, or antiserotonergic properties; ethanol; and any xenobiotic that results in pylorospasm (salicylates, iron).

Bioavailability is a measure of the amount of xenobiotic that reaches the systemic circulation unchanged (Equation 9–5).[45] The fractional absorption (F) of a xenobiotic is defined by the area under the plasma drug concentration versus time curve (AUC) of the designated route of absorption compared with the AUC of the IV route. The AUC for each route represents the amount absorbed.

$$F = \frac{(AUC)_{\text{route under study}}}{(AUC)_{IV}} \qquad \text{(Eq. 9–5)}$$

The formulation of a xenobiotic is extremely important in predicting GI absorption; for example, disintegration and dissolution must precede absorption. Disintegration is usually much more rapid than dissolution except for modified-release products. *Modified release* is a broad term that encompasses products that are delayed-release and extended-release formulations. These modified-release formulations are designed to release the xenobiotic over a prolonged period of time to attempt to produce the blood concentrations achieved with the use of a constant IV infusion. By definition, extended-release formulations decrease the frequency of drug administration by at least 50% compared with immediate-release formulations, and they include controlled-release, sustained-release, and prolonged-release formulations. These formulations minimize blood concentration fluctuations, reduce peak-related side effects, reduce dosing frequency, and improve patient compliance because fewer pills per day are needed. A variety of products use different pharmaceutical strategies, including dissolution control (encapsulation or matrix; Feosol—iron), diffusion control (membrane or matrix; Plendil ER—felodipine), erosion (Sinemet CR—levodopa carbidopa), osmotic pump systems (Procardia XL—nifedipine, Glucotrol XL—glipizide), and ion exchange resins (MS Contin suspension—morphine). Overdoses with modified-release formulations often result in a prolonged absorption phase, a delay to peak concentrations, and a prolonged duration of effect.[10] Some

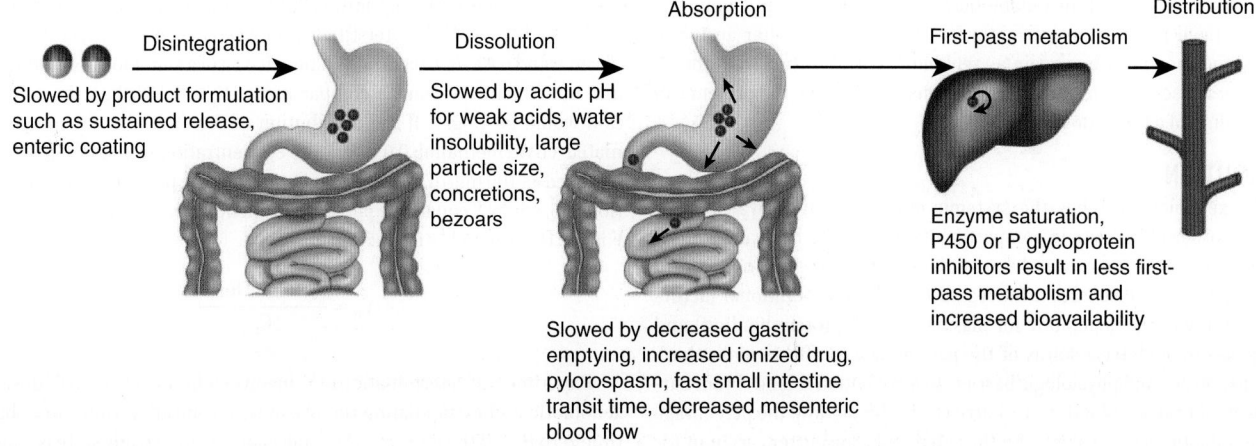

FIGURE 9–5. Determinants of absorption.

Gastric emptying and activated charcoal are used to decrease the bio-availability of ingested xenobiotics. The oral administration of certain chelators (deferoxamine, D-penicillamine) actually enhances the bioavailability of the complexed xenobiotic. The net effect of some chelators, such as succimer, is a reduction in body burden via enhanced urinary elimination even though GI absorption is enhanced.[38]

Presystemic metabolism may decrease or increase the bioavailability of a xenobiotic or a metabolite.[60] The GI tract contains microbial organisms (*Eggerthella lentum*) that can metabolize or degrade xenobiotics such as digoxin and oral contraceptives and enzymes, such as peptidases, that metabolize insulin.[61] However, in rare cases, GI hydrolysis can convert a xenobiotic into a toxic metabolite, as occurs when amygdalin is enzymatically hydrolyzed to produce cyanide, a metabolic step that does not occur when amygdalin is administered intravenously.[33] Xenobiotic metabolizing enzymes and influx and efflux transporters such as organic anion transporting polypeptides (OATPs) and P-glycoprotein (P-gp), respectively, also affect bioavailability. Xenobiotic-metabolizing enzymes are found in the lumen of the small intestine and can substantially decrease or increase the absorption of a xenobiotic.[51,82,89] Some of the xenobiotic that enters the cell is subsequently removed from the cell by the P-gp transporter and returned to the GI lumen, where it is reexposed to the metabolic enzymes.[51,82] Venous drainage from the stomach and intestines delivers orally (and intraperitoneally) administered xenobiotics to the liver via the portal vein and avoids direct delivery to the systemic circulation. This venous drainage allows hepatic metabolism to occur before the xenobiotic reaches the systemic circulation, and as previously mentioned, is referred to as the first-pass effect.[5,85] The hepatic extraction ratio is the percentage of xenobiotic metabolized in one pass of portal blood through the liver.[54] Xenobiotics that undergo significant first-pass metabolism (eg, propranolol, verapamil) are used at much lower IV doses than oral doses. Some drugs, such as lidocaine and nitroglycerin, are not administered by the oral route because of significant first-pass effect.[7] Instead, sublingual, transcutaneous (topical), and rectal administrations of drugs are used to bypass the portal circulation and avoid first-pass metabolism.

In the overdose setting, presystemic metabolism is often saturated, leading to an increased bioavailability of xenobiotics such as cyclic antidepressants, phenothiazines, opioids, and many β-adrenergic antagonists.[63] Hepatic metabolism usually transforms the xenobiotic into a less active metabolite but occasionally results in the formation of a more active or even toxic xenobiotic such as occurs with the transformation of parathion to paraoxon.[58] Biliary excretion into the small intestine usually occurs for these transformed xenobiotics of molecular weights greater than 350 Da and results in a xenobiotic appearing in the feces even though it had not was administered orally.[41,61,74] Hepatic conjugated metabolites such as glucuronides are hydrolyzed in the intestines to the parent form or to another active metabolite that can be reabsorbed by the enterohepatic circulation.[48,56,59,61] The enterohepatic circulation is responsible for what is termed a *double-peak phenomenon* after the administration of certain xenobiotics.[71] The double-peak phenomenon is characterized by a serum concentration that decreases (after an initial increase) and then increases again as xenobiotic is reabsorbed from the GI tract. Other causes include variability in stomach emptying, the presence of food, or failure of a tablet dosage form.[71]

DISTRIBUTION

After the xenobiotic reaches the systemic circulation, it is available for transport to peripheral tissue compartments and to the liver and kidney for elimination. Both the rate and extent of distribution depend on many of the same principles discussed with regard to diffusion. Additional factors include affinity of the xenobiotic for plasma (plasma protein binding) and tissue proteins, acid–base status of the patient (which affects ionization), drug transporters, and physiologic barriers to distribution (blood–brain barrier, placental transfer, blood–testis barrier).[29,42,65] Blood flow, the percentage of free xenobiotic in the plasma and the activity of transporters account for the initial phase of distribution, and xenobiotic affinities determine the final distribution pattern. Whereas the adrenal glands, kidneys, liver, heart, and

brain receive blood flow from 55 to 550 mL/min/100 g of tissue, the skin, muscle, connective tissue, and fat receive 1 to 5 mL/min/100 g of tissue.[69] Hypoperfusion of the various organs in the critically volume depleted ill and injured patients affects absorption, distribution, and elimination.[83]

Adenosine triphosphate-binding cassette (ABC) transporters are active ATP-dependent transmembrane protein carriers of which P-gp was the initial example.[12] P-glycoprotein (P-gp) is coded by the multiple drug resistance *MDRI* gene.[15] Approximately 50 ABC transporters have been identified, and they are divided into subfamilies based on their similarities. Several members of the ABC superfamily, including P-gp, are under extensive investigation because of their role in controlling xenobiotic entry into, distribution within, and elimination from the body as well as their contributions to xenobiotic interactions through P-gp inhibition or induction.[27,39,82] The discovery of P-gp resulted from an investigation into the reasons that certain tumors exhibit multidrug resistance to many chemotherapeutics. P-glycoprotein (ABCB1) as well as ABCC and ABCG2 are known to be efflux transporters located in the intestines, renal proximal tubules, hepatic bile canaliculi, placenta, and blood–brain barrier and are responsible for the intra- to extracellular transport of various xenobiotics.[21] Chemotherapy often induces P-gp expression, and extensive genetic polymorphism exists as in the case of CYPs.[15] First-generation transport inhibitors such as amiodarone, ketoconazole, quinidine, and verapamil are responsible for increasing body concentrations of P-gp substrates such as digoxin, the protease inhibitors, vinca alkaloids, and paclitaxel. St. John's wort is a transport inducer, and it lowers serum concentrations of these same xenobiotics. Second- and third-generation xenobiotics that will affect transport with a higher affinity and specificity are in development.[24,72] Many of the same xenobiotics that affect CYP3A4 also affect P-gp (Appendix Chap. 11: Cytochrome P450 Substrates Inhibitors and Inducers).

Other groups of transporters are found in the liver, kidneys, intestines, brain, and placenta that affect the absorption, distribution, and elimination of many xenobiotics and contribute to xenobiotic interactions. They include the organic anion transporters (OATs) and the organic cation transporters (OCTs).[24] For example, probenecid increases the serum concentrations of penicillin by inhibiting the OAT responsible for the active secretion of penicillin by the renal tubular cells, and cimetidine inhibits the OCT responsible for the renal elimination of procainamide and metformin. A variety of OAT inhibitors are being investigated to decrease the hepatic uptake of amatoxins[24] (Chap. 117).

Volume of distribution (V_d) is the proportionality term used to relate the dose of the xenobiotic that the individual receives with the resultant plasma concentration. Volume of distribution is an apparent or theoretical volume into which a xenobiotic distributes. It is a measure of how much xenobiotic is located inside versus outside of the plasma compartment after administration of a xenobiotic. Because only the plasma compartment is routinely assayed, the amount of xenobiotic that remains in the plasma can be used to calculate the movement out of the blood. In a 80-kg man, the total body water (TBW) is 60% of total body weight, or 48 L, with two-thirds (32 L) of the fluid accounted for by intracellular fluid. Of the 16 L of extracellular fluid, 13 L is considered interstitial or between the cells; 3.2 L, or 0.04 L/kg, is plasma; and 6.4 L, or 0.08 L/kg, is blood. If 48 g of a xenobiotic is administered and remains in the plasma compartment ($V_d = 0.04$ L/kg), the concentration would be 15 g/L. If the distribution of the 48 g of xenobiotic approximated TBW (methanol; 0.6 L/kg), the concentration would be 1 g/L (usually reported as 100 mg/dL). These calculations can be performed by using Equation 9–6, where S equals the percent pure xenobiotic if a salt form is used and F is the bioavailability or fraction absorbed.

$$V_d = \frac{S \times F \times Dose}{C_0} \qquad \text{(Eq. 9–6)}$$

Experimental determination of V_d involves administering an IV dose of the xenobiotic and extrapolating the plasma concentration time curve back to time zero (C_0). If the determination takes place after steady state is achieved, the volume of distribution is then referred to as the V_{dss}. For many xenobiotics, the V_d is known and readily available in the literature (Table 9–3). If the

TABLE 9–3 | Pharmacokinetic Characteristics of Xenobiotics Associated with Significant Morbidity and Mortality

	V_d (L/kg)	Protein Binding (%)	Renal Elimination (% Unchanged)	Hepatic Metabolism (CYP)	Active Metabolite	Enterohepatic Recirculation
Analgesics						
Acetaminophen	0.8–1	5–20	<5%	95% 5–10% (2E1)	N-acetyl-p-benzoquinoneimine	Yes
Aspirin	0.15–0.2	50–80 (salicylic acid) saturable	10 (pH dependent)	Majority	Salicylic acid	None
Methadone	3.59	71–87	5–10	Majority (2B6, 3A4); Minor (2C19, 2D6); N-demethylation	None	Yes
Morphine	1–6	35	<10		Morphine 6-glucuronide, morphine 3-glucuronide	Yes
Oxycodone	2.6	45	19	>64% (3A4, 2D6)	Oxymorphone Noroxycodone	No
Antidepressants						
Amitriptyline	18–22	96	18	Yes (2C9)	Nortriptyline (2D6)	Yes
Bupropion	20–47	84	2	Yes (2B6)	Hydroxybupropion	No
Citalopram	12	80	10	Yes (3A4, 2C19)	Desmethylcitalopram	Yes
Desipramine	33–42	92	0.3–2.6	Yes (2D6)	None	Yes
Doxepin	20 ± 8	80	<3	Yes (2D6, 2C19)	Desmethyldoxepin	Yes
Imipramine	15 ± 6	85	<5	Yes (2D6)	Desipramine	Yes
Lithium	0.3 initial 0.7–1 at SS	None	99	None	None	None
Cardiovascular						
Digoxin	5–7	20–25	50–80		Minor amount	Yes
Diltiazem	3–13	70–80	2–4	90% (3A4)	Yes, many	No
Nifedipine	0.8–1.4	92–98	?	98% (3A4)	None	No
Propranolol	4	90	>1	>95% (2D6, 1A2)	4-OH-propranolol	No
Verapamil	4	90	3–4%	97% (3A4, 1A2, 2C9)	Norverapamil	No
Stimulants and Drugs of Abuse						
Amphetamine	6.11 (in drug dependent) 3.5–4.6 (in naïve)	16	30–40 (pH dependent)	50%	Norephedrine, p-hydroxynorephedrine, 4-hydroxyamphetamine	No
Cocaine	1.96–2.7	8.7	9.5–20 (pH dependent)	5%–10%	Norcocaine, others	No
Heroin	25	40	Minor	Yes	Acetylmorphine, morphine	No
Methamphetamine	3.2–3.7	pH dependent			Amphetamine; p-hydroxymethamphetamine	No
Sedative–Hypnotics						
Alprazolam	1–2	80	100%	Yes (3A4)	4-hydroxyalprazolam, α-hydroxyalprazolam	No
Chloral hydrate	0.5–0.7	50–60	Minor	Alcohol dehydrogenase	Trichloroethanol	No
Phenobarbital	0.5–0.7	50–60	20–50 (pH dependent)	Yes (2C9, 2C19)	None	No
Quetiapine	10	83	0	Yes (3A4)	N-desalkylquetiapime	Yes
Alcohols						
Ethanol	0.5–0.6	None	Very little	95% alcohol dehydrogenase	Acetaldehyde	No

(Continued)

	V_d (L/kg)	Protein Binding (%)	Renal Elimination (% Unchanged)	Hepatic Metabolism (CYP)	Active Metabolite	Enterohepatic Recirculation
TABLE 9–3						

TABLE 9–3   Pharmacokinetic Characteristics of Xenobiotics Associated with Significant Morbidity and Mortality (Continued)

	V_d (L/kg)	Protein Binding (%)	Renal Elimination (% Unchanged)	Hepatic Metabolism (CYP)	Active Metabolite	Enterohepatic Recirculation
Ethylene glycol	0.6–0.8	None	20	Alcohol dehydrogenase	Oxalic and glycolic acids	No
Methanol	0.6–0.7	None	3–5	95% alcohol dehydrogenase	Formic acid	No
Miscellaneous						
Cyanide	0.4	60	0		Thiocyanate	None
Theophylline	0.5	50–60	7	90% (1A2, 2 E1 >3A4)	1,3-Dimethyluric acid; caffeine (in neonates)	
Organic Phosphorus Compounds						
Malathion	NA	None	?	CYP	Malaoxon	No
Chlorpyrifos	NA	None	?	Yes	3,5,6-Trichloro-2 pyridonol	No
Rodenticides						
Brodifacoum	0.985 (rats)	None		Yes	No	Yes
Strychnine	13	None	10–20 in 24 h	Yes	No	No

NA = not applicable; SS = steady state; V_d = volume of distribution.

peak plasma concentration and the V_d are known, then an approximation of total-body burden can be made ($Cp \times V_d/S \times F$ = Total-body burden) When the V_d and the dose ingested are known, a maximum predicted plasma concentration can be calculated after assuming all of the xenobiotic is absorbed and no elimination has occurred. This assumption usually overestimates the plasma concentration. Distribution is complex, and differential affinities for various storage sites in the body, such as plasma proteins, liver, kidney, fat, and bone, determine where a xenobiotic ultimately resides.

For the purposes of determining the utility of extracorporeal removal of a xenobiotic, a low V_d is often considered to be less than 1–2 L/kg. For some xenobiotics, such as digoxin (V_d = 5–7 L/kg) and the cyclic antidepressants (V_d = 10–20 L/kg), the V_d is much larger than the actual volume of the body. A large V_d indicates that the xenobiotic resides outside of the plasma compartment, but it is important to remember that it does not describe the actual site of distribution.

The site of accumulation of a xenobiotic is not necessarily the site of action or toxicity. If the site of accumulation is not a site of toxicity, then the storage depot is relatively inactive, and the accumulation at that site is theoretically protective.[65] Selective accumulation of xenobiotics occurs in certain areas of the body because of affinity for certain tissue-binding proteins. For example, the kidney contains metallothionein, which has a high affinity for metals such as cadmium, lead, and mercury.[29] The retina contains the pigment melanin, which binds and accumulates chlorpromazine, thioridazine, and chloroquine.[29] Other examples of xenobiotics accumulating at primary sites of toxicity are carbon monoxide binding to hemoglobin and myoglobin and paraquat distributing to type II alveolar cells in the lungs.[62] Dichlorodiphenyltrichloroethane (DDT), chlordane, and polychlorinated biphenyls are stored in fat and are mobilized should malnutrition develop.[86] Lead sequestered in bone[40] is not immediately toxic, but mobilization of bone through an increase in osteoclast activity[65] (hyperparathyroidism, pregnancy, immobilization) may liberate lead for distribution to sites of toxicity in the central nervous system (CNS) or blood.

Several plasma proteins bind xenobiotics and act as carriers and storage depots. The percentage of protein binding varies among xenobiotics, as do their affinities and potential for reversibility. After it is bound to a plasma protein, a xenobiotic with high binding affinity will remain largely confined to the plasma until elimination occurs. However, dissociation and reassociation may occur if another carrier is available with a higher binding affinity. Most plasma measurements of xenobiotic concentrations reflect total xenobiotic (bound plus unbound). Only the unbound xenobiotic is free to diffuse through membranes for distribution or for elimination. Albumin binds primarily to weakly acidic, poorly water-soluble xenobiotics, which include salicylates, phenytoin, and warfarin, as well as endogenous substances, including free fatty acids, cortisone, aldosterone, thyroxine, and unconjugated bilirubin.[69] α_1-Acid glycoprotein usually binds basic xenobiotics, including lidocaine, imipramine, and propranolol.[69] Transferrin, a β_1-globulin, transports iron, and ceruloplasmin carries copper.

Phenytoin is an example of a xenobiotic whose effects are significantly influenced by changes in concentration of plasma albumin because only free phenytoin is active. When albumin concentrations are in the normal range, approximately 90% of phenytoin is bound to albumin. As the albumin concentration decreases, more phenytoin is free for distribution, and a greater clinical response to the same serum phenytoin concentration is often observed. The free plasma phenytoin concentration can be calculated based on the albumin concentration. This achieves an appropriate interpretation (adjusted) of total phenytoin within the conventional therapeutic range of 10 to 20 mg/L of free plus bound phenytoin (Equation 9–7).

$$\text{Adjusted phenytoin concentration} = \frac{\text{Actual phenytoin concentration}}{0.25 \times [(\text{albumin}) + 0.1]} \quad \text{(Eq. 9–7)}$$

The clinical implications are that a malnourished or chronically ill patient with an albumin of 2 g/dL receiving phenytoin can manifest toxicity with a plasma phenytoin concentration of 14 mg/L. This measurement is total phenytoin (bound + unbound). Because the patient has a reduced albumin concentration, this actually represents a substantially higher proportion and absolute amount of active unbound phenytoin. Substitution into the above equation of 14 mg/L for actual plasma phenytoin concentration and 2 g/dL for albumin gives an adjusted plasma phenytoin concentration of 23.3 mg/L (therapeutic range, 10–20 mg/L).

Although drug interactions are often attributed to the displacement of xenobiotics from plasma protein binding, concurrent metabolic interactions are usually more consequential. Displacement transiently increases the amount of unbound, active drug. This results in an immediate increase in drug effect. This is usually followed by enhanced distribution of unbound drug out of the plasma compartment followed by elimination of unbound drug. Gradually, the unbound plasma concentration returns to predisplacement concentrations.[66]

Saturation of plasma proteins may occur in the therapeutic range for a drug such as valproic acid. Acute saturation of plasma protein binding after an overdose often leads to consequential adverse effects. Saturation of plasma protein binding with salicylates and iron after an overdose increase distribution to the CNS (salicylates) or to the liver, heart, and other tissues (iron), increasing toxicity.

Specific therapeutic interventions after an overdose are designed to alter xenobiotic distribution by inactivating or enhancing elimination to limit toxicity. These therapeutic interventions include manipulation of serum pH (tricyclic antidepressants, salicylates) or urine pH (salicylates), the use of chelators (lead), and the use of antibodies or antibody fragments (digoxin).

The V_d permits predictions about plasma concentrations and assists in defining whether an extracorporeal method of removal is beneficial for a particular toxin. If the V_d is large (>2 L/kg), it is unlikely that hemodialysis, hemoperfusion, or exchange transfusion would be effective because most of the xenobiotic is outside of the plasma compartment. Plasma protein binding also influences this decision. If the xenobiotic is more tightly bound to plasma proteins than to activated charcoal, then hemoperfusion is unlikely to be beneficial even if the V_d of the xenobiotic is small. In addition, high plasma protein binding limits the effectiveness of hemodialysis because only unbound xenobiotic will freely cross the dialysis membrane. However, in certain situations, although a xenobiotic such as valproic acid is highly protein bound at therapeutic concentrations, protein binding is saturated after an overdose, allowing free drug to be removed by extracorporeal methods.[77] Exchange transfusion can be effective for a xenobiotic with a small V_d and substantial plasma protein binding because both bound and free xenobiotic are removed simultaneously.

ELIMINATION

Removal of a parent xenobiotic from the body (elimination) begins as soon as the xenobiotic is delivered to clearance organs such as the liver, kidneys, and lungs. Elimination includes biotransformation and excretion. Elimination begins immediately but may not be the predominant kinetic process until absorption and distribution are substantially completed. The functional integrity of the cardiovascular, pulmonary, renal, and hepatic systems are major determinants of the efficiency of xenobiotic removal and of administered antidotes. Some xenobiotics themselves cause kidney or liver failure, subsequently compromising their own elimination. Other factors that influence elimination include older age, competition or inhibition of elimination processes by interacting xenobiotics, saturation of enzymatic processes, gender, pharmacogenetics and pharmacogenomics, obesity, and the physicochemical properties of the xenobiotic.[53]

Elimination can be accomplished by biotransformation to one or more metabolites or by excretion from the body of the parent xenobiotic. Excretion may occur via the kidneys, lungs, GI tract, and body secretions (sweat, tears, breast milk). Because of their water solubility, hydrophilic (polar) or charged xenobiotics and their metabolites are generally excreted via the kidney. The majority of xenobiotic metabolism occurs in the liver, but it also occurs in the blood, skin, GI tract, placenta, or kidneys. Lipophilic (uncharged or nonpolar) xenobiotics are usually metabolized in the liver to hydrophilic metabolites, which are then excreted by the kidneys.[30,58] These metabolites are generally inactive, but if active, they may contribute to toxicity. Examples of active metabolites include nortriptyline (derived from amitriptyline), normeperidine (derived from meperidine), hydroxybupropion (derived from bupropion), and desmethylcitalopram (derived from citalopram).

Metabolic reactions catalyzed by enzymes, categorized as either phase I or phase II, may result in pharmacologically active metabolites; frequently, the latter have toxicities that differ from those of the parent compounds. Phase I (asynthetic), or preparative metabolism, which may or may not precede phase II, is responsible for introducing polar groups onto nonpolar xenobiotics by oxidation (hydroxylation, dealkylation, deamination), reduction (alcohol dehydrogenase, azo reduction), and hydrolysis (ester hydrolysis).[28,56] Phase II, or synthetic reactions conjugate the polar group with a glucuronide, sulfate, acetate, methyl group, glutathione, or amino acids (eg, glycine, taurine, and glutamic acid), creating more polar metabolites.[18,28,56]

Comparatively, phase II reactions produce a much larger increase in hydrophilicity than phase I reactions. The enzymes involved in these reactions have low substrate specificity, and those in the liver are usually localized to either the endoplasmic reticulum (microsomes) or the soluble fraction of the cytoplasm (cytosol).[56] The location of the enzymes becomes important if they form reactive metabolites, which then concentrate at the sites of metabolism and cause toxicity. For example, acetaminophen (APAP) causes centrilobular necrosis because CYP2E1 that forms N-acetyl-p-benzoquinoneimine (NAPQI), the toxic metabolite, is located in their highest concentration in that zone of the liver.

The enzymes that metabolize the largest variety of xenobiotics are heme-containing proteins referred to as CYP monooxygenase enzymes.[34,56] This group of enzymes, formerly called the mixed function oxidase system, is found in abundance in the microsomal endoplasmic reticulum of the liver. These cytochrome P450 metabolizing enzymes (CYPs) primarily catalyze the oxidation of xenobiotics. Cytochrome P450 in a reduced state (Fe^{2+}) binds carbon monoxide. Its discovery and initial name resulted from spectral identification of the colored CO-bound cytochrome P450, which absorbs light maximally at 450 nm. The cytochrome P450 system is composed of many enzymes grouped according to their respective gene families and subfamilies, of which approximately 57 of these functional human genes have been sequenced. Members of a gene family have more than 40% similarity of their amino acid sequencing, and subfamilies have more than 55% similarity. For example, the *CYP2D6*1a* gene encodes wild-type protein (enzyme) CYP2D6, where 2 represents the family, D the subfamily and 6 the individual gene, and *1a the mutant allele; *CYP2D6*1* represents the most common or wild-type allele.

Toxicity may result from induction or inhibition of CYP enzymes by another xenobiotic, resulting in a consequential drug interaction (Chap. 11). Many of these interactions are predictable based on the known xenobiotic affinities and their capability to induce or inhibit the P450 system.[16,49,56,57,73] However, polymorphism (individual genetic expression of enzymes),[3] stereoisomer variability[84] (enantiomers with different potencies and isoenzyme affinities), and the capability to metabolize a xenobiotic by alternate pathways contribute to unexpected metabolic outcomes. The pharmaceutical industry is now using the concept of chiral switching (marketing a single enantiomer instead of the racemic mixture) to alter efficacy or side effect profiles. Enantiomers are named either according to the direction in which they rotate polarized light (*l* or – for levorotatory, and *d* or + for dextrorotatory) or according to the absolute spatial orientation of the groups at the chiral center (S or R). Chiral means "hand" in Greek, and the latter designations refer to either sinister (left-handed) or rectus (right-handed). There is no direct correlation between levorotatory or dextrorotatory and S and R, which indicates the direction polarized light is rotated by a solution of the xenobiotic.[78]

The percent of xenobiotic extracted from the blood during passage through the liver is termed the *hepatic extraction ratio*.[2,79] High extraction occurs when the liver can remove almost the entire drug (extraction ratio >0.7), and removal is based largely on hepatic blood flow. In this circumstance, the liver enzymes are so efficient that little xenobiotic passes through intact (Table 9–4, Equation 9–8).

TABLE 9–4	Hepatic Extraction of Xenobiotics	
High Liver Extraction (ER >0.7)	*Low Liver Extraction (ER <0.3)*
Cocaine	Acetaminophen
Desipramine	Carbamazepine
Lidocaine	Diazepam
Morphine	Phenobarbital
Nicotine	Salicylate
Nitroglycerin	Theophylline
Propranolol	Valproic acid
Verapamil	Warfarin

ER = extraction ratio.

$$Cl_H = Q \times ER, \text{ and if } ER \text{ approaches } 1, \text{ then } Cl_H = Q \qquad \text{(Eq. 9-8)}$$

where Cl_H = hepatic clearance

Q = blood flow

ER = extraction ratio = $(C_{in} - C_{out})/C_{in}$

C_{in} = xenobiotic concentration in fluid (blood or serum) entering the organ or device

C_{out} = xenobiotic concentration in fluid (blood or serum) leaving the organ or device

For oral drugs:

$$Cl_{oral} = f_u \times Cl_{int}$$
$$(f_u \times Cl_{int})$$

where f_u = fraction unbound

On the other hand, when the drug is poorly extracted by the liver (ER <0.3), it means that any change in protein binding or intrinsic metabolic activity will greatly influence hepatic clearance. In this case, the hepatic clearance is directly proportional to the unbound fraction (f_u) multiplied by intrinsic clearance (Cl_{int}) and hepatic blood flow has a limited impact.

The oral clearance of xenobiotics depends on their fraction unbound and the intrinsic ability of the liver to metabolize them.[79] High-extraction drugs have very low oral bioavailability. The fraction unbound times the intrinsic hepatic clearance is already more than liver blood flow, so the final clearance is dependent on liver blood flow. The fraction unbound times the intrinsic hepatic clearance for low extraction drugs is much lower than hepatic blood flow, so clearance is dependent on enzyme induction or inhibition and the amount of unbound xenobiotic.

Excretion is primarily accomplished by the kidneys, with biliary, pulmonary, and body fluid secretions contributing to lesser degrees. Urinary excretion occurs through glomerular filtration, tubular secretion, and passive tubular reabsorption. The glomerulus filters unbound xenobiotics of a particular size and shape in a manner that is not saturable (but is subject to renal blood flow and perfusion). Passive tubular reabsorption accounts for the reabsorption of uncharged, lipid-soluble xenobiotics and is therefore influenced by the pH of the urine and the pK_a of the xenobiotic. The principles of diffusion discussed earlier permit, for example, the ion trapping of salicylate ($pK_a = 3.0$) in the urine through urinary alkalinization. Tubular secretion is an active process carried out by drug transporters (OATs, OCTs) and subject to saturation and drug interactions (Table 9-5).

TABLE 9-5	Xenobiotics Secreted by Renal Tubules
Organic Anion Transport	**Organic Cation Transport**
ACEIs	Acetylcholine
Acetazolamide	Amiodarone
Acyclovir	Atropine
Bile salts	Cimetidine
Cephalosporins	Ciprofloxacin
Indomethacin	Digoxin
Hydrochlorothiazide	Diltiazem
Furosemide	Dopamine
Methotrexate	Epinephrine
Penicillin G	Metformin
Probenecid	Morphine
Prostaglandins	Neostigmine
Salicylates	Procainamide
	Quinidine
	Quinine
	Triamterene
	Trimethoprim
	Verapamil

ACEI = angiotensin-converting enzyme inhibitor.

The effects of obesity on elimination are intensely under study. Obesity is the accumulation of adipose tissue far in excess of what is considered normal for a person's age and gender. The National Institutes of Health defines obesity as a body mass index (BMI) greater than 30 and overweight as a BMI between 25 and 29.9. The BMI is calculated by dividing a person's weight in kilograms by the individual's height in meters squared (m^2). By this criterion, about one-third of the adult US population is obese. Obesity poses problems in determining the correct loading dose and maintenance dose for therapeutic xenobiotics and for the estimation of serum concentrations and elimination times in the overdose setting.[13,32,46,55] A number of formulas have been proposed to classify body size in addition to BMI, but none has been tested adequately in the obese population. Obese patients not only have an increase in adipose tissue but also an increase in lean body mass of 20% to 55%, which results in the alteration of the distribution of both lipophilic and hydrophilic xenobiotics. In general, the oral absorption of xenobiotics in obese patients does not appear to be affected, but subcutaneous and intramuscular absorption are affected.[91] A recent example of concern is whether an epinephrine autoinjector can achieve therapeutic plasma concentrations expeditiously.

Whereas distribution is often affected, the effect of obesity on hepatic metabolism requires additional study, although some studies suggest a nonlinear increase in clearance and differential effects depending on the CYP under study. The glomerular filtration rate increases in obesity but is not proportional to total body weight. For example, although aminoglycosides are hydrophilic, because of an increase in fat-free mass in obese patients, a dosing weight correction of 40% is used to calculate both the loading dose and the maintenance dose (Dosing body weight = 0.4 × {Actual body weight − Ideal body weight} + Ideal body weight). Preliminary studies with propofol, a very lipophilic drug, suggest that whereas induction doses correlate better with lean body weight, maintenance doses correlate better with actual body weight.[20,36] These equations are found in Table 9-6. One recent evaluation suggests using 40% of actual body weight instead of ideal body weight in the Cockcroft-Gault formula to estimate kidney function in obese patients.[87]

Now that bariatric surgery is more common, many pharmacokinetic issues arise in post–bariatric surgery patients.[1,4,23] Bariatric surgery works by increasing a patient's feeling of fullness by decreasing the size of the stomach (adjustable gastric banding, sleeve gastrectomy) or malabsorption in which the duodenum and parts of the jejunum are bypassed (Roux-en-Y gastric bypass {RYGB}). Absorption is particularly affected by gastric bypass. Calcium, vitamin D, iron, folate, vitamin B_{12}, and thiamine absorption is reduced and often needs supplementation. Modified-release xenobiotics are likely to have reduced absorption, but the onset of effect is quicker. First-pass metabolism is affected when a significant amount of the small intestine containing CYP3A4 is removed. Distribution and excretion are unlikely to be affected. Finally, after significant weight loss is achieved, the doses of medications often need to be reduced.

TABLE 9-6	Equations for Determining Body Size
$BMI = \dfrac{Weight\ (kg)}{Height\ (m^2)}$	
$BSA\ (m^2) = \dfrac{\sqrt{Height\ (cm) \times Weight\ (kg)}}{\sqrt{3600}}$	
IBW: Males (kg) = $50 + 2.3$ (Height >60 in)	
IBW: Females (kg) = $45.5 + 2.3$ (Height >60 in)	
$LBW: Males\ (kg) = \dfrac{9270 \times Weight\ (kg)}{6680 + \{(216 \times BMI\ (kg/m^2)\}}$	
$LBW: Females\ (kg) = \dfrac{9270 \times Weight\ (kg)}{8780 + \{(244 \times BMI\ (kg/m^2)\}}$	

BMI = body mass index; BSA = body surface area; IBW = ideal body weight; LBW = lean body weight.

CLASSICAL VERSUS PHYSIOLOGIC COMPARTMENT TOXICOKINETICS

Models exist to study and describe the movement of xenobiotics in the body with mathematical equations. Traditional compartmental models (one or two compartments) are data based and assume that changes in plasma concentrations represent proportional changes in tissue concentrations (Fig. 9–6).[54] Advances in computer technology facilitate the use of the classic concepts developed in the late 1930s.[76] Physiologic models describe the unique movement characteristics of xenobiotics based on known or theoretical biologic processes. This allows the prediction of tissue concentrations while incorporating the effects of changing physiologic parameters and affording better extrapolation from laboratory animals.[90] Unfortunately, physiologic modeling is still in its infancy, and the mathematical modeling it entails is often very complex.[25] The most common mathematical equations used are based on traditional compartmental modeling.

The one-compartment model is the simplest approach for analytic purposes and is applied to xenobiotics that enter and rapidly distribute throughout the body. This model assumes that changes in plasma concentrations will result in and reflect proportional changes in tissue concentrations. Many xenobiotics, such as digoxin, lithium, and lidocaine, do not instantaneously equilibrate with the tissues and are better described by a two-compartment model. In the two-compartment or more than two-compartment models, a xenobiotic is distributed instantaneously to highly perfused tissues (central compartment) and then is secondarily, and more slowly, distributed to a peripheral compartment. Elimination is assumed to take place from the central compartment.

If the rate of a reaction is directly proportional to the concentration of xenobiotic, it is termed *first order* or *linear* (Equation 9-9).

$$\text{Rate} \propto \text{concentration (C)} \qquad \text{(Eq. 9–9)}$$

Processes that are capacity limited or saturable are termed *nonlinear* (not proportional to the concentration of xenobiotic) and are described by the Michaelis-Menten equation, which is derived from enzyme kinetics. Calculus is used to derive the first-order equation.[90] Rate is directly proportional to concentration of xenobiotic, as in Equation 9–8.

Model 1. One-compartment open model, IV injection.

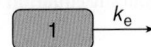

Model 2. One-compartment open model with first-order absorption.

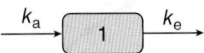

Model 3. Two-compartment open model, IV injection.

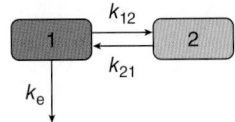

Model 4. Two-compartment open model with first-order absorption.

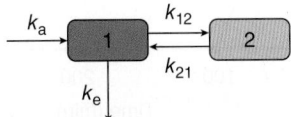

FIGURE 9–6. Various classical compartmental models. 1, plasma or central compartment; 2 = tissue compartment; IV = intravenous; k_a = absorption rate constant; k_e = elimination rate constants; k_{12} = rate constant into tissue from plasma; k_{21} = rate constant into plasma from tissue.

An infinitesimal change in concentration of a xenobiotic (dC) with respect to an infinitesimal change in time (dt) is directly proportional to the concentration (C) of the xenobiotic as in Equation 9–10:

$$\frac{d\text{C}}{dt} \propto \text{C} \qquad \text{(Eq. 9–10)}$$

The proportionality constant k is added to the right side of the expression to mathematically allow the introduction of an equality sign. The constant k represents all of the bodily factors, such as metabolism and excretion, that contribute to the determination of concentration (Equation 9–10).

$$\frac{d\text{C}}{dt} = k\text{C} \qquad \text{(Eq. 9–11)}$$

Introducing a negative sign to the left-hand side of the equation describes the "decay" or decreasing xenobiotic concentration (Equation 9–11).

$$-\frac{d\text{C}}{dt} = k\text{C} \qquad \text{(Eq. 9–12)}$$

This equation is impractical because of the difficulty of measuring infinitesimal changes in C or t. Therefore, the use of calculus allows the integration or summing of all of the changes from one concentration to another beginning at time zero and terminating at time t. This relationship is mathematically represented by the integration sign ($\int$). The sign $\int$ means to integrate the term from concentration at time zero (C_0) to concentration at a given time t (C_t). The second $\int$ means the same action with respect to time, where t_0 = zero. Before this application, the previous equation is first rearranged (Equation 9–13).

$$-\frac{d\text{C}}{\text{C}} = k\,dt$$
$$\int_{\text{C}_0}^{\text{C}_t} -\frac{d\text{C}}{\text{C}} = k\int_0^t dt \qquad \text{(Eq. 9–13)}$$

The integration of dC divided by C is the natural logarithm of C (ln C), and the integration of dt is t (Equation 9–14).

$$-\ln\text{C}\,\Big|_{\text{C}_0}^{\text{C}_t} = kt\,\Big|_{t_0}^{t} \qquad \text{(Eq. 9–14)}$$

The vertical straight lines proscribe the evaluation of the terms between those two limits. The following series of manipulations is then performed (Equation 9–15A–D).

$$-(\ln \text{C}_t - \ln \text{C}_0) = k(t - 0) \qquad \text{(Eq. 9–15A)}$$

$$-\ln \text{C}_t + \ln \text{C}_0 = kt \qquad \text{(Eq. 9–15B)}$$

$$-\ln \text{C}_t = -\ln \text{C}_0 + kt \qquad \text{(Eq. 9–15C)}$$

$-\ln \text{C}_t =$	$\ln \text{C}_0 -$	kt	
Can be measured	Can be selected	Constant	(Eq. 9–15D)

Equation 9–15D can be recognized as taking the form of an equation of a straight line (Equation 9–15), where the slope is equal to the negative rate constant k and the intercept is C_0.

$$y = b + mx \qquad \text{(Eq. 9–16)}$$

Instead of working with natural logarithms, an exponential form (the antilog) of Equation 9–15D may be used (Equation 9–17).

$$\text{C}_t = \text{C}_0 e^{-kt} \qquad \text{(Eq. 9–17)}$$

Graphing the (natural logarithm) of the concentration of the xenobiotic at various times for a first-order reaction is a straight line. Equation 9–17

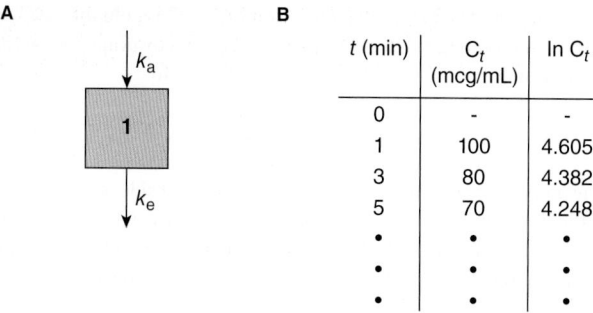

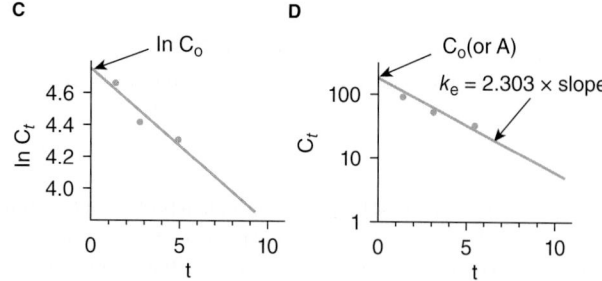

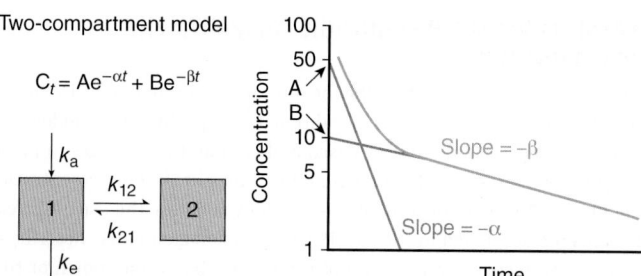

FIGURE 9–7. A one-compartment pharmacokinetic model demonstrating graphical illustration (**A**), hypothetical dataset (**B**), linear plot (**C**), and semilogarithmic plot (**D**).

FIGURE 9–8. Mathematical and graphical forms of a two-compartment classical pharmacokinetic model. k_a represents the absorption constant, k_e represents the elimination rate constant, α represents the distribution phase, and β represents the elimination phase.

describes the events when only one first-order process occurs. This is appropriate for a one-compartment model (Fig. 9–7).

In this model, regardless of the concentration of the xenobiotic, the rate (percentage) of decline is constant. The absolute amount of xenobiotic eliminated changes continuously while the percent eliminated remains constant. The rate constant k is reported in h^{-1}. A k_e of 0.10 h^{-1} means that the xenobiotic is being processed (eliminated) at a rate of 10% per hour. The rate constant k is often designated as k_e and referred to as the elimination rate constant. The time necessary for the xenobiotic concentration to be reduced by 50% is called the half-life. The half-life is determined by a rearrangement of Equation 9–15D whereby C_2 becomes C at time t_2 and C_1 becomes C at t_1 and by rearrangement giving Equation 9–18:

$$(t_1 - t_2) = \frac{(\ln C_1 - \ln C_2)}{k_e} \qquad \text{(Eq. 9–18)}$$

Substitution of 2 for C_1 and 1 for C_2 or 100 for C_1 and 50 for C_2 gives Equations 9–19A and 9–19B:

$$t_{1/2} = \frac{(\ln 2 - \ln 1)}{k_e} \qquad \text{(Eq. 9–19A)}$$

$$t_{1/2} = \frac{0.693}{k_e} \qquad \text{(Eq. 9–19B)}$$

The use of semilog paper facilitates graphing the first-order equation. If natural logs are used to calculate slope, then $k_e = -\text{slope}$, and if common logs are used to calculate slope, then $k_e = -2.303 \times \text{slope}$ (Fig. 9–7).

The mathematical modeling becomes more complex when more than one first-order process contributes to the overall elimination process. The equation that incorporates two first order rates is used for a two-compartment model and is Equation 9–20.

$$C_t = Ae^{-\alpha t} + Be^{-\beta t} \qquad \text{(Eq. 9–20)}$$

Fig. 9–8 demonstrates a two-compartment model where α often represents the distribution phase and β is the elimination phase.

The rate of reaction of a saturable process is not linear (ie, not proportional to the concentration of xenobiotic) when saturation occurs (Fig. 9–9). This model is best described by the Michaelis-Menten equation used in enzyme kinetics (Equation 9–20) in which v is the velocity or rate of the enzymatic reaction, C is the concentration of the xenobiotic, V_{max} is the maximum velocity of the reaction between the enzyme and the xenobiotic at high xenobiotic concentrations, and K_m is the substrate concentration at which the reaction rate is half of the V_{max}.[79]

$$v = \frac{V_{max} \times C}{K_m + C} \qquad \text{(Eq. 9–21)}$$

Application of this equation to toxicokinetics requires v to become the infinitesimal change in concentration of a xenobiotic (dC) with respect to an infinitesimal change in time (dt) as previously discussed (Equation 9–11). V_{max} and K_m both reflect the influences of diverse biologic processes. The Michaelis-Menten equation then becomes Equation 9–22, in which the negative sign again represents decay:

$$-\frac{dC}{dt} = \frac{V_{max} \times C}{K_m + C} \qquad \text{(Eq. 9–22)}$$

When the concentration of the xenobiotic is very low (C <<< K_m), it can be dropped from the bottom right of the equation because its contribution becomes negligible, and the resultant equation is described as a first-order

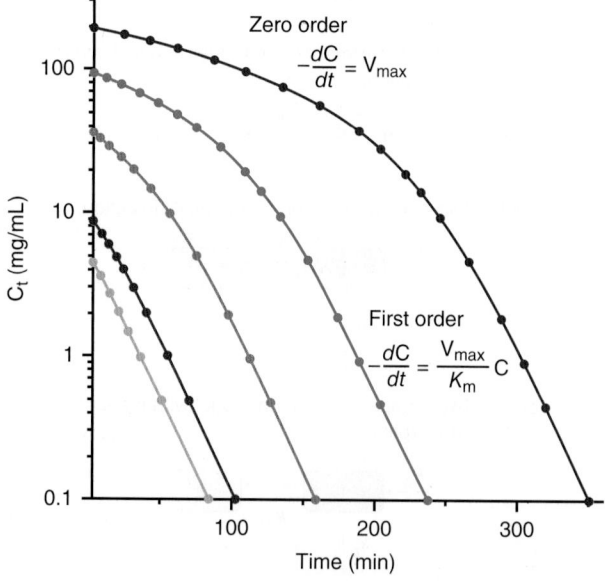

FIGURE 9–9. Concentration versus time curve for a xenobiotic showing nonlinear pharmacokinetics where concentrations below 10 mg/mL represent first-order elimination. C = concentration; K_m = affinity constant; V = velocity; V_{max}, maximum velocity.

process (Equations 9–23A and 9–23B). Conceptually, this is understandable because at a very low xenobiotic concentration, the process is not saturated.

$$-\frac{dC}{dt} = \frac{V_{max} \times C}{K_m} \qquad \text{(Eq. 9–23A)}$$

Because V_{max} divided by K_m is a constant, k, then:

$$-\frac{dC}{dt} = kC \qquad \text{(Eq. 9–23B)}$$

However, when the concentrations of the xenobiotic are extremely high and exceed the capacity of the system ($C >>> K_m$), the rate becomes fixed at a constant maximal rate (V_{max}) regardless of the exact concentration of the xenobiotic, termed a *zero-order reaction*. Tables 9–7A and 9–7B compare a first-order reaction with a zero-order reaction. In this example, zero order is faster, but if the fraction of xenobiotic eliminated in the first-order example were 0.4, then the amount of xenobiotic in the body would decrease below 100 before the xenobiotic in the zero-order example. It is inappropriate to perform half-life calculations on a xenobiotic displaying zero-order behavior because the metabolic rates are continuously changing. Sometimes the term *apparent half-life* is used if it is unclear if the xenobiotic is exhibiting zero-order or first-order pharmacokinetics. After an overdose, enzyme saturation is a common occurrence because the capacity of enzyme systems is overwhelmed.

CLEARANCE

Clearance (Cl) is the relationship between the rate of transfer or elimination of a xenobiotic from a reference fluid (usually plasma) to the plasma concentration (*Cp*) of the xenobiotic and is expressed in units of volume per unit time (milliliters per minute) (Equation 9–24).[31,54,68]

$$Cl = \frac{\text{Rate of elimination}}{Cp} \qquad \text{(Eq. 9–24)}$$

The determination of creatinine clearance is a well-known example of the concept of clearance. Creatinine clearance (Cl_{CR}) is determined by Equation 9–25:

$$Cl_{creatinine} = \frac{U \times V}{Cp} \qquad \text{(Eq. 9–25)}$$

in which *U* is the concentration of creatinine in urine (mg/mL), *V* is the volume flow of urine (mL/min), and *Cp* is the plasma concentration of creatinine (mg/mL) and the units for clearance are milliliters per minute. A creatinine clearance of 100 mL/min means that 100 mL of plasma is completely cleared of creatinine every minute. Clearance for a particular eliminating organ or for extracorporeal elimination is calculated with Equation 9–26:

TABLE 9–7A Illustration of 1,000 mg of a Xenobiotic in the Body after First-Order Elimination

Time After Administration (hour)	Amount in Body (mg)	Amount Eliminated over Preceding Hour (mg)	Fraction Eliminated over Preceding Hour
0	1,000	—	—
1	850	150	0.15
2	723	127	0.15
3	614	109	0.15
4	522	92	0.15
5	444	78	0.15
6	377	67	0.15

TABLE 9–7B Illustration of 1,000 mg of a Xenobiotic in the Body after Zero-Order Elimination

Time After Administration (hour)	Amount of Drug in Body (mg)	Amount of Drug Eliminated over Preceding Hour (mg)	Fraction of Drug Eliminated over Preceding Hour
0	1,000	—	—
1	850	150	0.15
2	700	150	0.18
3	550	150	0.21
4	400	150	0.27
5	250	150	0.38
6	100	150	0.60

$$Cl = Q_b \times (ER) = Q_b \times \frac{(C_{in} - C_{out})}{C_{in}} \qquad \text{(Eq. 9–26)}$$

Cl = clearance for the eliminating organ or extracorporeal device
Q_b = blood flow to the organ or device
ER = extraction ratio
C_{in} = xenobiotic concentration in fluid (blood or serum) entering the organ or device
C_{out} = xenobiotic concentration in fluid (blood or serum) leaving the organ or device

Clearance can be applied to any elimination process independent of the precise mechanisms (ie, first order, Michaelis-Menten) and represents the sum total of all of the rate constants for xenobiotic elimination. Total body clearance ($Cl_{total body}$) is the sum of the clearances of each of the individual eliminating processes, as seen in Equation 9–27:

$$Cl_{total body} = Cl_{renal} + Cl_{hepatic} + Cl_{chelation} + \cdots \qquad \text{(Eq. 9–27)}$$

For a first-order process (one-compartment model), clearance is given by Equation 9–28:

$$Cl = k_e V_d \qquad \text{(Eq. 9–28)}$$

Experimentally, the clearance can be derived by examining the IV dose of xenobiotic in relation to the AUC from time zero to time *t* (Equation 9–29). The AUC is calculated using the trapezoidal rule or through integral calculus (units, eg, {mg × hour}/mL) (Figs. 9–10 and 9–11).

$$Cl = \frac{Dose_{IV}}{AUC_{0-t}} \qquad \text{(Eq. 9–29)}$$

STEADY STATE

When exposure to a xenobiotic occurs at a fixed rate, the plasma concentration of the xenobiotic gradually achieves a plateau concentration at which the rate of absorption equals the rate of elimination and is termed *steady state* (Equations 9–30 and 9–31). The time to achieve 95% of steady-state concentration for a first-order process depends on the half-life and usually necessitates 5 half-lives; 10 half-lives are needed to achieve 99.9% of steady-state concentration. Similarly, after steady state is achieved, it would require 5 half-lives or 10 half-lives to remove 97% or 99.9% of the drug, respectively. The concentration achieved at steady state (Cpss) depends on the rate of exposure, the V_d, and the clearance (Cl).

$$\text{Rate of input} = (Dose \times S \times F/tau) \qquad \text{(Eq. 9–30)}$$

$$\text{Rate of elimination} = Cp \times Cl \qquad \text{(Eq. 9–31)}$$

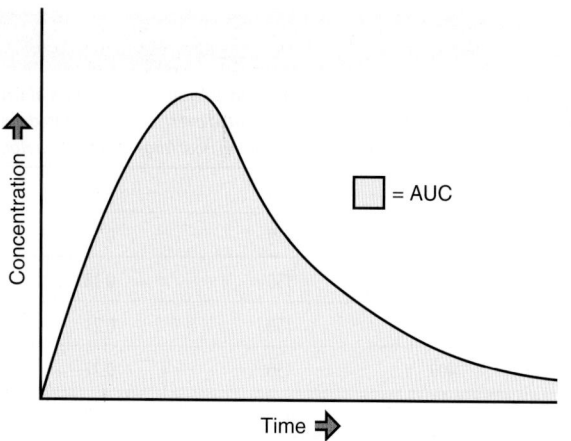

FIGURE 9–10. The area under the curve (AUC) profile obtained after extravascular administration of a xenobiotic.

At steady state, the rate of input is equal to the rate of elimination (Equations 32–35). Therefore, when the rate of input and the rate of elimination have remained constant for 4 to 5 half-lives:

$$[Dose \times S \times F/tau] = Cpss \times Cl \qquad (Eq.\ 9-32)$$

$$and\ Cpss = (Dose \times S \times F/tau) \qquad (Eq.\ 9-33)$$

$$Cl\ for\ first\text{-}order\ elimination\ Cl = keV_d \qquad (Eq.\ 9-34)$$

$$Therefore: Cpss = (Dose \times S \times F/tau)/(keV_d) \qquad (Eq.\ 9-35)$$

where S = fraction of administered salt or ester form of the drug that is active
F = bioavailability or the fraction of the administered dose that reaches the systemic circulation
tau = dosing interval

Iatrogenic toxicity occurs in the therapeutic setting when dosing decisions are based on serum concentrations determined before achieving a

steady state. This adverse event is particularly common when using xenobiotics with long half-lives such as digoxin[88] and phenytoin.

PEAK PLASMA CONCENTRATIONS

Peak plasma concentrations (C_{max}) of a xenobiotic occur at the time of peak absorption. At this point in time, the absorption rate is at least equal to the elimination rate. Thereafter, the elimination rate predominates, and plasma concentrations begin to decline. Whereas the C_{max} depends on the dose, the *rate of absorption* (k_a), and *the rate of* elimination (k_e), and the time to peak (t_{max}) are independent of dose and only depend on the k_a and k_e. For the same dose of xenobiotic, if the k_e remains constant and the rate of absorption decreases, then the t_{max} will occur later, and the C_{max} will be slightly lower (Table 9–8). Xenobiotics delivered with modified-release dosage forms or that form concretions have a decreased rate of absorption and will not achieve peak concentrations until many hours later than with an immediate-release preparation. The AUC will remain the same. However, if the k_a remains constant and the k_e is increased, then the t_{max} occurs sooner, the C_{max} decreases, and the AUC decreases (Table 9–8).[59] Values are based on a single oral dose (100 mg) that is 100% bioavailable (F = 1) and has an apparent V_d of 10 L. The drug follows a one-compartment open model. The AUC is calculated by the trapezoidal rule from 0 to 24 hours.

In the overdose setting, gastric emptying, single-dose activated charcoal, and WBI decrease k_a. Multiple-dose activated charcoal, manipulation of pH to promote ion trapping to facilitate elimination, and certain chelators (ie, succimer, deferoxamine) increase k_e and are likely to decrease C_{max}, t_{max}, and AUC.

INTERPRETATION OF SERUM CONCENTRATIONS

For serum concentrations to have significance, there must be an established relationship between effect and serum concentration. Many xenobiotics, such as valproic acid, digoxin, carbamazepine, lithium, and cyclosporine, have established therapeutic ranges. However, there are also many drugs (eg, diazepam, propranolol, verapamil) for which there is no established therapeutic range. Some xenobiotics (eg, physostigmine) exhibit hysteresis in which the effect increases as the serum concentration decreases. For many xenobiotics, very little information on toxicodynamics is available. Sequential serum concentrations are often collected for retrospective analysis in an attempt to correlate serum concentrations and toxicity. Tolerance to xenobiotics, such as

Compartment model

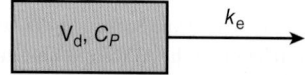

Static volume and first-order elimination are assumed. Plasma flow is not considered. $Cl_T = k_e V_d$.

Physiologic model

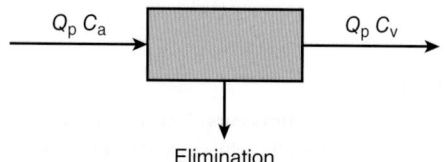

Clearance is the product of the plasma flow (Q_p) and the extraction ratio (ER). Thus, $Cl_T = Q_p\ ER$.

Model independent

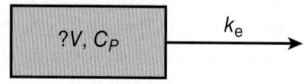

Volume and elimination rate constant not defined. $Cl_T = Dose \div [AUC]_0^\infty$.

FIGURE 9–11. General approaches to clearance.

Absorption Rate Constant k_a (h^{-1})	Elimination Rate Constant k_e (h^{-1})	t_{max} (h)	C_{max} (mcg/mL)	AUC (mcg.hr/mL)
0.1	0.2	6.93	2.50	50
0.2	0.1	6.93	5.00	100
0.3	0.1	5.49	5.77	100
0.4	0.1	4.62	6.26	100
0.5	0.1	4.02	6.69	100
0.6	0.1	3.58	6.69	100
0.3	0.1	5.49	5.77	100
0.3	0.2	4.05	4.44	50
0.3	0.3	3.33	3.68	33.3
0.3	0.4	2.88	3.16	25
0.3	0.5	2.55	2.79	20

TABLE 9–8 Pharmacokinetic Effects of the Absorption Rate Constant and Elimination Rate Constant

AUC = area under the (plasma drug concentration versus time) curve; C_{max} = peak xenobiotic concentration; t_{max} = time to peak plasma concentration.

Reproduced with permission from Shargel L, Yu A: Applied Biopharmaceutics and Pharmacokinetics, 3rd ed. Norwalk, CT: Appleton & Lange; 1993.

ethanol, also influences the interpretation of serum concentrations. Tolerance is an example of a pharmacodynamic or toxicodynamic effect as a result of cellular adaptation, and it occurs when larger doses of a xenobiotic are necessary to achieve the same clinical or pharmacologic result.

Other factors that influence the interpretation of serum concentrations include chronicity of dosing (a single dose versus multiple doses); whether absorption is still ongoing and therefore concentrations are still increasing; whether distribution is still ongoing and therefore concentrations are uninterpretable (Fig. 9–12); or whether the value is a peak, trough, or steady-state concentration. Collection of accurate data for analysis requires at least four data points during at least one elimination half-life. Clinical examples in which interpretation is dependent on the dosing pattern of a single dose versus multiple doses include digoxin, lithium, vancomycin, and APAP. Modified-release preparations and xenobiotics that delay gastric emptying or form concretions are expected to have prolonged absorptive phases and require serial serum concentrations to obtain a meaningful analysis of serum concentrations (Chap. 7). A combination of trough, peak, and minimum inhibitory concentrations is often consequential for monitoring antibiotics such as gentamicin.[11,50]

Pitfalls in interpretation arise when the units for a particular serum concentration are not obtained or are unfamiliar (eg, mmol/L) to the clinician.

The type of analysis generally applied clinically may not be appropriate to massive overdoses, and the laboratory may make errors in dilution, or errors can be inherent in the assay (Chap. 7). In these cases, the director of the laboratory should be consulted for advice with regard to the availability of a reference laboratory. The type of collection tube (eg, plasma or serum instead of whole blood for certain metals), the receptacle (metal free for certain metals, free of lithium heparin as the anticoagulant for serum lithium determinations), or the conditions during delivery of the sample result in inaccurate or inadequate information. When in doubt, the laboratory toxicologist or chemist should be called before sample collection. The laboratory usually measures total xenobiotic (free plus bound), and for xenobiotics that are highly plasma protein bound, reductions in albumin increase free concentrations and alter the interpretation of the reported concentration (Equation 9–7). Active metabolites may contribute to toxicity and are not measured.[44] During extracorporeal methods of elimination, ideal criteria for determining the amount removed require assay of the dialysate or activated charcoal cartridge or multiple simultaneous serum concentrations going into and out of the device along with timed urine concentrations and urine volume if renal elimination is significant rather than random serum concentrations (Chap. 6). Clearance calculations for drugs such as lithium that partition significantly into the red blood cells are more accurate when measurements are taken on whole blood.[17,26] The patient's weight and height and, when indicated, hemoglobin, creatinine, albumin, and other parameters to assess elimination pathways are helpful.

SUMMARY

- Pharmacokinetics and toxicokinetics are the study of the absorption, distribution, metabolism, and excretion of xenobiotics in the therapeutic and overdose settings, respectively (ie, what the body does to the xenobiotic).
- Pharmacokinetics and toxicokinetics can help predict the onset and duration of toxicity when serum concentrations are related to therapeutic and toxic effects.
- Pharmacodynamics and toxicodynamics are the study of the relationship of the xenobiotic concentration to clinical effect in the therapeutic and overdose settings, respectively (ie, what the xenobiotic does to the body).
- Interpretation of serum concentrations relies on many factors dependent on the xenobiotics (eg, dosage form, single versus multiple doses) and the patient (tolerance, genetic profile).

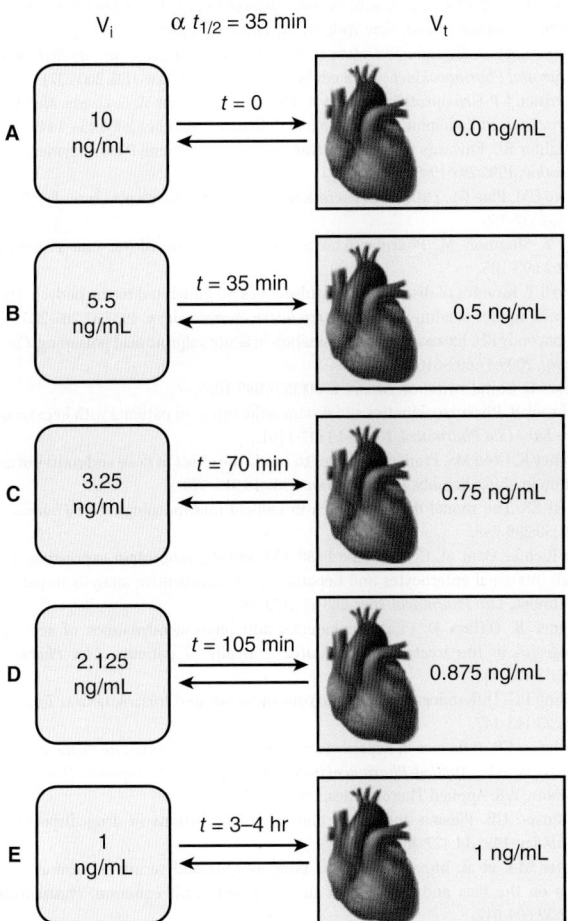

FIGURE 9–12. A theoretical two-compartment model for digoxin. Assume **A** to **E** represent the digoxin serum concentration equilibriums at different t (time) intervals between the plasma compartment and the tissue compartment. V_i (initial volume of distribution) is smaller than V_t (tissue volume of distribution). The myocardium sits in V_t. A is the time at which digoxin is administered. **E** represents distribution at 5 half-lives and it is assumed that the plasma and tissue compartments are now in equilibrium. The tissue compartments are extensive, and the graphic only represents the estimated cardiac fraction of the total distribution of this drug in the body.[78] *(Reproduced with permission from Winter ME. Basic Clinical Pharmacokinetics. 5th ed. Vancouver, WA: Applied Therapeutics; 2010.)*

REFERENCES

1. Azran C, et al. Oral drug therapy following bariatric surgery: an overview of fundamentals, literature and clinical recommendations. *Obesity Rev.* 2016;17:1050-1066.
2. Benet L, Zia-Amirhosseini P. Basic principles of pharmacokinetics *Toxicol Pathol.* 1995;23:115-123.
3. Bertilsson L. Geographical/interracial differences in polymorphic drug oxidation. *Clin Pharmacokinet.* 1995;29:192-209.
4. Bland C, et al. Long-term pharmacotherapy considerations in the bariatric surgery patient. *Am J Health-Sys Pharm.* 2016;73:1230-1242.
5. Blaschke TF, Rubin PC. Hepatic first-pass metabolism in liver disease. *Clin Pharmacokinet.* 1979;4:423-432.
6. Bodenham A, et al. The altered pharmacokinetics and pharmacodynamics of drugs commonly used in critically ill patients. *Clin Pharmacokinet.* 1988;14:347-373.
7. Bosse GM, Matyunas NJ. Delayed toxidromes. *J Emerg Med.* 1999;17:679-690.
8. Boyes RN, et al. Pharmacokinetics of lidocaine in man. *Clin Pharmacol Ther.* 1971;12:105-116.
9. Brubacher J, et al. Delayed toxicity following ingestion of enteric-coated divalproex sodium. *J Emerg Med.* 1999;3:463-467.
10. Buckley N, et al. Controlled-release drugs in overdose. *Drug Saf.* 1995;12:73-84.
11. Burgess D. Pharmacodynamic principles of antimicrobial therapy in the prevention of resistance. *Chest.* 1999;115(suppl):19S-23S.
12. Calcagno A, et al. ABC drug transporters as molecular targets for the prevention of multidrug resistance and drug-drug interactions. *Curr Drug Deliv.* 2007;4:324-333.
13. Casati A, Putzu M. Anesthesia in the obese patient: pharmacokinetic considerations. *J Clin Anesth.* 2005;17:134-145.
14. Chaikin P, Adir J. Unusual absorption profile of phenytoin in a massive overdose case. *J Clin Pharmacol.* 1987;27:70-73.
15. Chung FS, et al. Disrupting P-glycoprotein function in clinical settings: what can we learn from the fundamental aspects of this transporter? *Am J Cancer Res.* 2016;6:1583-1598.

16. Ciummo PE, Katz NL. Interactions and drug metabolizing enzymes. *Am Pharm.* 1995;9:41-51.

17. Clendenin N, et al. Potential pitfalls in the evaluation of the usefulness of hemodialysis for the removal of lithium. *J Toxicol Clin Toxicol.* 1982;19:341-352.

18. Dauterman WC. Metabolism of toxicants: phase II reactions. In: Hodgson E, Levi P, eds. *Introduction to Biochemical Toxicology.* Norwalk, CT: Appleton & Lange; 1994:113-132.

19. Dean B, et al. A study of iron complexation in a swine model. *Vet Hum Toxicol.* 1988;30:313-315.

20. De Baerdemaeker L, Margarson M. Best anaesthetic drug strategy for morbidly obese patients. *Curr Opin Anaesthesiol.* 2016;29:119-128.

21. de Boer AG, et al. The role of drug transporters at the blood–brain barrier. *Annu Rev Pharmacol Toxicol.* 2003;43:629-656.

22. DeGeorge JJ. Food and Drug Administration viewpoints on toxicokinetics: the view from review. *Toxicol Pathol.* 1995;23:220-225.

23. Edwards A, Ensom M. Pharmacokinetic effects of bariatric surgery. *Ann Pharmacother.* 2012;46:130-136.

24. Endres CJ, et al. The role of transporters in drug interactions. *Eur J Pharm Sci.* 2006;27:501-517.

25. Engasser JM, et al. Distribution, metabolism and elimination of phenobarbital in rats: physiologically based pharmacokinetic model. *J Pharm Sci.* 1981;70:1233-1238.

26. Ferron G, et al. Pharmacokinetics of lithium in plasma and red blood cells in acute and chronic intoxicated patients. *Int J Clin Pharmacol Ther.* 1995;33:351-355.

27. Fromm MF. Importance of P-glycoprotein at blood–tissue barriers. *Trends Pharmacol Sci.* 2004;25:423-429.

28. Gillette JR. Factors affecting drug metabolism. *Ann N Y Acad Sci.* 1971;179:43-66.

29. Gram TE. Drug absorption and distribution. In: Craig CR, Stitzel RE, eds. *Modern Pharmacology with Clinical Applications.* Boston: Little, Brown; 1997:13.

30. Guengerich FP, Liebler DC. Enzymatic activation of chemicals to toxic metabolites. *Crit Rev Toxicol.* 1985;14:259-307.

31. Gwilt PR. Pharmacokinetics. In: Craig CR, Stitzel RE, eds. *Modern Pharmacology with Clinical Applications.* Boston, MA: Little, Brown; 1997:49-58.

32. Han PY, et al. Dosing in obesity: a simple solution to a big problem. *Clin Pharmacol Ther.* 2007;82:505-508.

33. Hill HZ, et al. Blood cyanide levels in mice after administration of amygdalin. *Biopharm Drug Dispos.* 1980;1:211-220.

34. Hodgson E, Levi PE. Metabolism of toxicants phase I reactions. In: Hodgson E, Levi P, eds. *Introduction to Biochemical Toxicology.* Norwalk, CT: Appleton & Lange; 1994:75-111.

35. Iberti T, et al. Prolonged bromide intoxication resulting from a gastric bezoar. *Arch Intern Med.* 1984;144:402-403.

36. Ingrande J, Lemmens HJ. Dose adjustment of anaesthetics in the morbidly obese. *Br J Anaesth.* 2010;105(suppl 1):i16-23.

37. Jenis EH, et al. Acute meprobamate poisoning: a fatal case following a lucid interval. *JAMA.* 1969;207:361-365.

38. Kapoor SC, et al. Influence of 2,3-dimercaptosuccinic acid on gastrointestinal lead absorption and whole body lead retention. *Toxicol Appl Pharmacol.* 1989;97:525-529.

39. Kivisto KT, et al. Functional interaction of intestinal CYP3A4 and P-glycoprotein. *Fundam Clin Pharmacol.* 2004;8:621-626.

40. Klaassen CD, Shoeman DW. Biliary excretion of lead in rats, rabbits and dogs. *Toxicol Appl Pharmacol.* 1974;29:436-446.

41. Klaassen CD, Watkins JB. Mechanisms of bile formation, hepatic uptake, and biliary excretion. *Pharmacol Rev.* 1984;36:1-67.

42. Klotz U. Pathophysiological and disease-induced changes in drug distribution volume: pharmacokinetic implications. *Clin Pharmacokinet.* 1976;1:204-218.

43. Koch-Weser J. Bioavailability of drugs. Part I. *N Engl J Med.* 1974;291:233-237.

44. Koch-Weser J. Bioavailability of drugs. Part II. *N Engl J Med.* 1974;291:503-506.

45. Kwan KC. Oral bioavailability and first-pass effects. *Drug Metab Dispos.* 1997;25:1329-1336.

46. Lee J, et al. Pharmacokinetic changes in obesity. *Orthopedics.* 2006;29:984-988.

47. Lemmer B, Bruguerolle B. Chronopharmacokinetics, are they clinically relevant? *Clin Pharmacokinet.* 1994;26:419-427.

48. Levine WG. Biliary excretion of drugs and other xenobiotics. *Ann Rev Pharmacol Toxicol.* 1978;18:81-96.

49. Levy R, et al, eds. *Metabolic Drug Interactions.* Philadelphia, PA: Lippincott Williams & Wilkins; 2000.

50. Li R, et al. Achieving optimal outcome in the treatment of infections. *Clin Pharmacokinet.* 1999;37:1-16.

51. Lin JH, Yamazaki M. Role of P-glycoprotein in pharmacokinetics: clinical implications. *Clin Pharmacokinet.* 2003;42:59-98.

52. Marik P, Varon J. The obese patient in the ICU. *Chest.* 1998;113:492-498.

53. McCarthy J, Gram TE. Drug metabolism and disposition in pediatric and gerontological stages of life. In: Craig CR, Stitzel RE, eds. *Modern Pharmacology with Clinical Applications.* Boston: Little, Brown; 1997:43-48.

54. Medinsky MA, Klaassen CD. Toxicokinetics. In: Klaassen CD, ed. *Casarett & Doull's Toxicology: The Basic Science of Poisons.* 5th ed. New York, NY: McGraw-Hill; 1996:187-198.

55. Pai MP, Bearden DT. Antimicrobial dosing considerations in obese adult patients. *Pharmacotherapy.* 2007;27:1081-1091.

56. Parkinson A. Biotransformation of xenobiotics. In: Klaassen C, ed. *Casarett & Doull's Toxicology: The Basic Science of Poisons.* 5th ed. New York, NY: McGraw-Hill; 1996:113-186.

57. Pharmacist's Letter. Stockton, CA: Pharmacy Information Services, University of the Pacific; June 1985.

58. Pirmohamed M, et al. The role of active metabolites in drug toxicity. *Drug Saf.* 1994;11:114-144.

59. Plaa OL. The enterohepatic circulation. In: Gillette JR, Mitchell JR, eds. *Handbook of Experimental Pharmacology.* New York, NY: Springer; 1975:28,130-140, 480.

60. Pond SM, Tozer TN. First-pass elimination: basic concepts and clinical consequences. *Pharmacokinetics.* 1984;9:1-25.

61. Riviere JE. Absorption and distribution. In: Hodgson E, Levi P, eds. *Introduction to Biochemical Toxicology.* Norwalk, CT: Appleton & Lange; 1994:11-48.

62. Rose MS, et al. Paraquat accumulation: tissue and species specificity. *Biochem Pharmacol.* 1976;25:419-423.

63. Rosenberg J, et al. Pharmacokinetics of drug overdose. *Clin Pharmacokinet.* 1981;6:161-192.

64. Rowland M, Tozer TN. *Clinical Pharmacokinetics Concepts & Applications.* 2nd ed. Philadelphia, PA: Lea & Febiger; 1989.

65. Rozman KK, Klaassen CD. Absorption, distribution and excretion of toxicants. In: Klaassen CD, ed. *Casarett & Doull's Toxicology: The Basic Science of Poisons.* New York, NY: McGraw-Hill; 1996:91-112.

66. Sansom LN, Evans AM. What is the true clinical significance of plasma protein binding displacement interactions? *Drug Saf.* 1995;12:227-233.

67. Schwartz MD, Morgan BW. Massive verapamil pharmacobezoar resulting in esophageal perforation. *Int J Med Toxicol.* 2004;7:4.

68. Shargel L, et al. Drug elimination and clearance. In: *Applied Biopharmaceutics and Pharmacokinetics.* 5th ed. New York, NY: McGraw-Hill; 2005:131-160.

69. Shargel L, et al. Physiologic drug distribution and protein binding. In: *Applied Biopharmaceutics and Pharmacokinetics.* 5th ed. New York, NY: McGraw-Hill; 2005:251-301.

70. Shargel L, et al. Pharmacokinetics of oral absorption. In: *Applied Biopharmaceutics and Pharmacokinetics.* 5th ed. New York, NY: McGraw-Hill; 2005:161-184.

71. Shargel L, et al. Physiologic factors related to drug absorption. In: *Applied Biopharmaceutics and Pharmacokinetics.* 5th ed. New York, NY: McGraw-Hill; 2005:371-408.

72. Silverman J. P-Glycoprotein. In: Levy R, Thummel K, Trager W, et al, eds. *Metabolic Drug Interactions.* Philadelphia, PA: Lippincott Williams & Wilkins; 2000:135-144.

73. Slaughter RL, Edwards DJ. Recent advances: the cytochrome P450 enzymes. *Ann Pharmacother.* 1995;29:619-623.

74. Stowe CM, Plaa GL. Extrarenal excretion of drugs and chemicals. *Annu Rev Pharmacol.* 1968;8:337-356.

75. Sue Y, Shannon M. Pharmacokinetics of drugs in overdose. *Clin Pharmacokinet.* 1992;23:93-105.

76. Teorell T. Kinetics of distribution of substances administered to the body: I. The extravascular modes of administration. *Arch Int Pharmacodyn.* 1937;57:205-225.

77. Thanacoody RH. Extracorporeal elimination in acute valproic acid poisoning. *Clin Toxicol (Phila).* 2009;47:609-616.

78. Tucker G. Chiral switches. *Lancet.* 2000;355:1085-1087.

79. Verbeeck R. Pharmacokinetics and dosage adjustment in patients with hepatic dysfunction. *Eur J Clin Pharmacol.* 2008;64:1147-1161.

80. Verebey K, Gold MS. From coca leaves to crack: the effect of dose and routes of administration in abuse liability. *Psychiatr Ann.* 1988;18:513-520.

81. Vesell ES. The model drug approach in clinical pharmacology. *Clin Pharmacol Ther.* 1991;50:239-248.

82. von Richter O, et al. Cytochrome P450 3A4 and P-glycoprotein expression in human small intestinal enterocytes and hepatocytes: a comparative analysis in paired tissue specimens. *Clin Pharmacol Ther.* 2004;75:172-183.

83. Wagner B, O'Hara D. Pharmacokinetics and pharmacodynamics of sedatives and analgesics in the treatment of agitated critically ill patients. *Clin Pharmacokinet.* 1997;33:426-453.

84. Welling PG. Differences between pharmacokinetics and toxicokinetics. *Toxicol Pathol.* 1995;23:143-147.

85. Wilkinson GR. Influence of hepatic disease on pharmacokinetics. In: Evans WE, Schentag J, Justo W, eds. *Applied Pharmacokinetics: Principles of Therapeutic Drug Monitoring.* Spokane, WA: Applied Therapeutics; 1986:116-138.

86. Wilkinson GR. Plasma and tissue binding considerations in drug disposition. *Drug Metab Rev.* 1983;14:427-465.

87. Winter MA, et al. Impact of various body weights and serum creatinine concentrations on the bias and accuracy of the Cockcroft-Gault equation. *Pharmacotherapy.* 2012;32:604-612.

88. Winter ME. Digoxin. In: Koda-Kimble MA, Young LY, eds. *Basic Clinical Pharmacokinetics.* 3rd ed. Vancouver, WA: Applied Therapeutics; 1994:198-235.

89. Wu C, et al. Differentiation of absorption and first pass metabolism and hepatic metabolism in humans: studies with cyclosporine. *CP&T.* 1995;58:492-749.

90. Yang R, Andersen M. Pharmacokinetics. In: Hodgson E, Levi P, eds. *Introduction to Biochemical Toxicology.* Norwalk, CT: Appleton & Lange; 1994:49-73.

91. Zuckerman M, et al. A review of the toxicologic implications of obesity. *J Med Toxicol.* 2015;11:342-354.

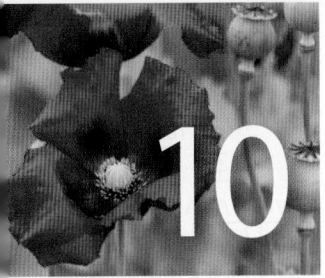

Section I Biochemical and Molecular Concepts

10 CHEMICAL PRINCIPLES

Stephen J. Traub and Lewis S. Nelson

Chemistry is the science of matter; it encompasses the structure, physical properties, and reactivities of atoms and their compounds. In many respects, toxicology is the science of the interactions of matter with living entities; chemistry and toxicology are therefore intimately linked. The study of the principles of inorganic, organic, and biologic chemistry offers important insight into the mechanisms and clinical manifestations of xenobiotics and poisoning.[5] This chapter reviews many of these tenets and provides relevance to the current practice of medical toxicology.

THE STRUCTURE OF MATTER
Basic Structure
Matter includes the substances of which everything is made. *Elements* are the foundation of matter, and all matter is made from one or more of the known elements. An *atom* is the smallest quantity of a given element that retains the properties of that element. Atoms consist of a nucleus, incorporating protons and neutrons, coupled with its orbiting electrons. The *atomic number* is the number of protons in the nucleus of an atom, and it is a whole number that is unique for each element. Thus, elements with 6 protons are always carbon, and all forms of carbon have exactly 6 protons. However, although the vast majority of carbon nuclei have 6 neutrons in addition to the protons, accounting for an *atomic mass* (protons plus neutrons) of 12 (^{12}C), a small proportion of naturally occurring carbon nuclei, called *isotopes*, have 8 neutrons and a mass number of 14 (^{14}C). This is the reason that the *atomic weight* of carbon displayed on the periodic table is 12.011, and not 12, as it actually represents the average atomic masses of all isotopes found in nature weighted by their frequency of occurrence. ^{14}C is also a *radioisotope*, which is an isotope with an unstable nucleus that emits radiation until it achieves a stable state (Chap. 128). The atomic weight, measured in grams per mole (g/mol), also indicates the molar mass of the element. That is, in one atomic weight of matter (12.011 g for carbon) there is one mole ($6.022140857 \times 10^{23}$) of atoms as defined by Avogadro's constant.

Elements combine chemically to form *compounds*, which generally have physical and chemical properties that differ from those of the constituent elements. The elements in a compound can be separated only by chemical means that destroy the original compound, as occurs during the burning (ie, oxidation) of a hydrocarbon, a process that releases the carbon principally as carbon dioxide and the hydrogen principally as water (H_2O). This important property differentiates compounds from *mixtures*. Mixtures are combinations of elements or compounds that can be separated by physical means, such as the distillation of petroleum into its hydrocarbon components or the evaporation of seawater to separate water from sodium chloride and other substances. With notable exceptions, such as the elemental forms of many metals or halogens (eg, Cl_2), most xenobiotics are compounds or mixtures.

Dmitri Mendeleev, a Russian chemist in the mid-19th century, recognized that when all of the known elements were arranged in order of atomic weight, certain patterns of reactivity became apparent. The result of his work was the Periodic Table of the Elements (Fig. 10–1), which, with some minor alterations, is still an essential tool today. All of the currently recognized elements are represented; those heavier than uranium do not occur in nature. Many of the symbols used to identify the elements refer to the Latin name of the element. For example, silver is Ag, for argentum, and mercury is Hg, for hydrargyrum, literally "silver water."

The periodicity of the table relates to the electrons that circle the nucleus in discrete orbitals. Although the details of quantum mechanics and electronic configuration are complex, it is important to review some aspects in order to predict chemical reactivity. Orbitals, or quantum shells, represent the energy levels in which electrons exist around the nucleus. The orbitals are identified by various schemes, but the maximum number of electrons each orbital can contain is calculated as $2x^2$, where x represents the numerical rank order of the orbital. Thus, the first orbital may contain 2 electrons, the second orbital may contain 8, the third may contain 18, and so on. However, the outermost shell (designated by s, p, d, f nomenclature) of each orbital may only contain up to 8 electrons. This is irrelevant through element 20, calcium, because there is no need to fill the third-level or d shells. Even though the third orbital may contain 18 electrons, once 8 are present the 4s electrons dip below the 3d electrons in energy and this shell begins to fill. This occurs at element 21, scandium, and accounts for its chemical properties and those of the other transition elements. Transition elements are chemically defined as elements that form at least one ion with a partially filled subshell of d electrons. The inert gas elements, which are also known as noble gases, have complete outermost orbitals, accounting for their lack of reactivity under standard conditions.

In general, only electrons in unfilled shells, or *valence shells*, are involved in chemical reactions. This property relates to the fact that the most stable form of an element occurs when the configuration of its valence shell resembles that of the nearest noble gas, found in group 18 on the periodic table. This state can be obtained through the gaining, losing, or sharing of electrons with other elements and is the basis for virtually all chemical reactions.

INORGANIC CHEMISTRY
The Periodic Table
Chemical Reactivity
Broadly, the periodic table is divided into metals and nonmetals. Metals, in their elemental form, are typically malleable solids that conduct electricity, whereas nonmetals are usually dull, fragile, nonconductive compounds (C, N, P, O, S, Se, and the halogens). Metals are found on the left side of the periodic table, and account for the majority of the elements, whereas nonmetals are on the right side. Separating the 2 groups are the metalloids, which fall on a jagged line starting with boron (B, Si, Ge, As, Sb, Te, At). Metalloids have chemical properties that are intermediate between the metals and the nonmetals. Each column of elements is termed a family or group, and each row is a period. Although the table is conceived and organized in periods, trends in the chemical reactivity, and therefore toxicity, typically exist within the groups.

In 1990, the International Union of Pure and Applied Chemistry (IUPAC) replaced the existing numbering schemes for the periodic table columns with a unified and simplified nomenclature. Using this format, which is included in this chapter, the groups are simply incrementally numbered from 1 to 18 from left to right.[2]

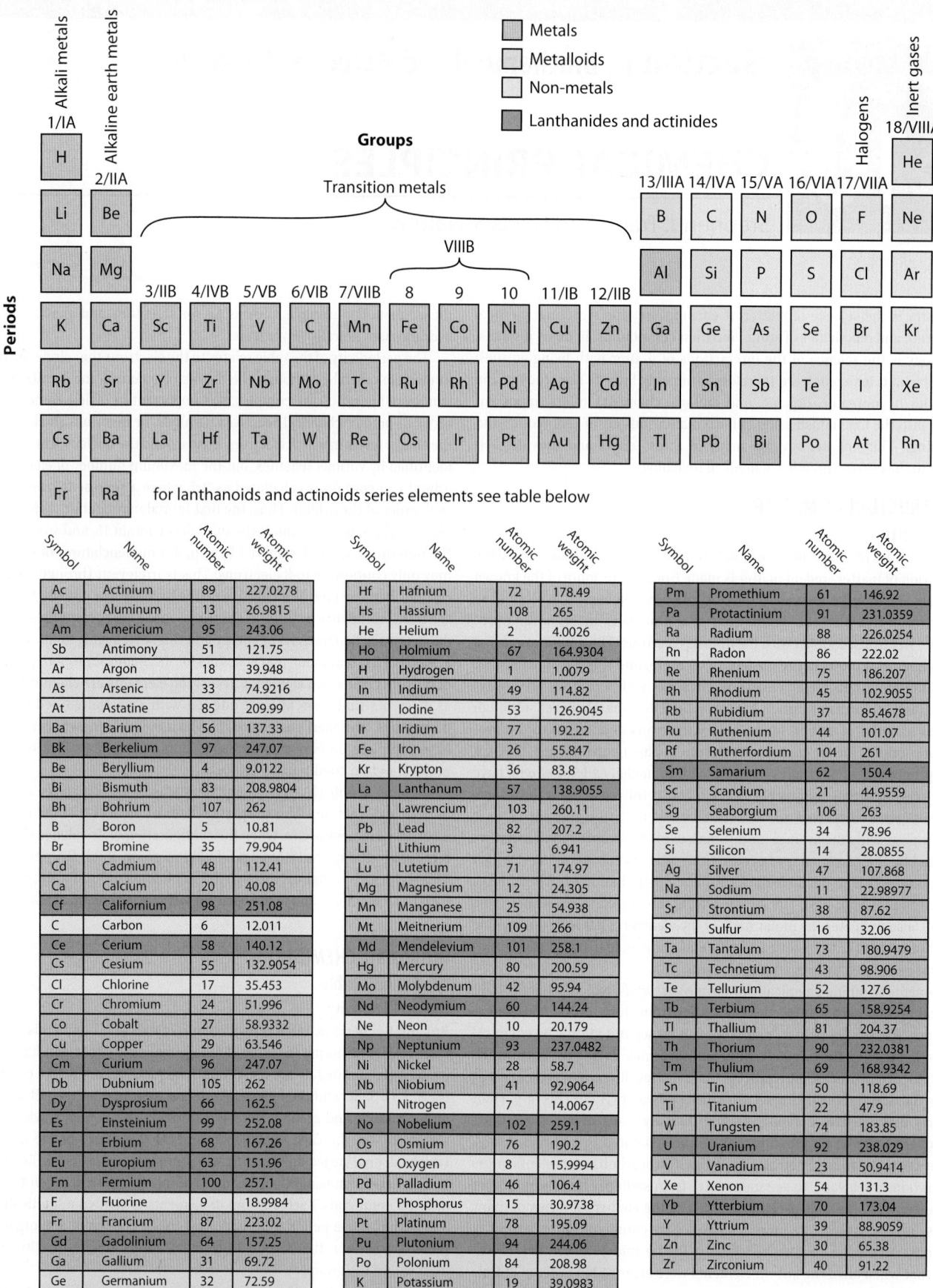

FIGURE 10–1. The Periodic Table of the Elements. Group numbering: 2 (Modern IUPAC) IIA (Classical).

The ability of any particular element to produce toxicologic effects relates directly to one or more of its many physicochemical properties. These properties will, to some extent, be predicted by their location on the periodic table. For example, arsenate will substitute for phosphate in the mitochondrial production of adenosine triphosphate (ATP), creating adenosine diphosphate monoarsenate (Chap. 11). Because this compound is unstable and not useful as an energy source, energy production by the cell fails; in this manner, arsenic interferes with oxidative phosphorylation. The existence of an interrelationship between Ca^{2+} and either Mg^{2+} or Ba^{2+} is predictable, although the actual effects are not. Under most circumstances, Mg^{2+} is a Ca^{2+} antagonist, and patients with hypermagnesemia present with neuromuscular weakness caused by the blockade of myocyte calcium channels. Alternatively, Ba^{2+} mimics Ca^{2+} and closes Ca^{2+}-dependent K^+ channels in myocytes, producing life-threatening hypokalemia. The physiologic relationships among the ions of lithium (Li^+), potassium (K^+), and sodium (Na^+) are also consistent with their chemical similarities (all alkali metals in Group IA). However, the clinical similarity between thallium (thallous) ion (Tl^+) and K^+ is not immediately predictable. Other than their monovalent nature (ie, 1+ charge), it is difficult to predict the substitution of Tl^+ (Group 13, Period 6) for K^+ (Group 1, Period 4) in membrane ion channel functions, until the similarity of their ionic radii is known (Tl^+, 1.47 Å; K^+, 1.33 Å).

An emerging physicochemical property of toxicological interest is particle size. The chemical and toxicologic properties of a given element or molecule change as the particle size is reduced. An entire field of nanotoxicology has emerged to study the adverse health effects of nanoparticles, which are ultrafinely divided particles, ranging from approximately 1 to 100 nm in diameter. Differences in absorption, biodistribution, and structure-activity effects, for example, enhance the toxicologic potential of otherwise nontoxic xenobiotics.[7]

Alkali and Alkaline Earth Metals
Alkali metals (Group 1, formerly Group IA: Li, Na, K, Rb, Cs, Fr) and hydrogen (not an alkali metal on Earth) have a single outer valence electron and lose this electron easily to form compounds with a valence of 1+. The alkaline earth metals (Group 2, formerly Group IIA: Be, Mg, Ca, Sr, Ba, Ra) are located between the alkali and rare earth (Group 3, formerly Group IIIB), readily lose 2 electrons, and form cations with a 2+ charge. In their metallic form, members of both of these groups react violently with water to liberate strongly basic solutions, accounting for the word alkali in their group names ($2Na^0 + 2H_2O \rightarrow 2NaOH + H_2$).

The soluble ionic forms of sodium, potassium, or calcium, which are critical to survival, also produce life-threatening symptoms following excessive intake (Chap. 12). Xenobiotics interfere with the physiologic role of these key electrolytes. Li^+ mimics K^+ after entering neurons through K^+ channels, and serves as an inadequate substrate for the repolarizing of Na^+,K^+-ATPase. Li^+ thus interferes with cellular K^+ homeostasis and alters neuronal repolarization, accounting for the neuroexcitability manifesting as tremor. Similarly, as noted previously, the molecular effects of Mg^{2+} and Ba^{2+} supplant those of Ca^{2+}.

More commonly, the consequential toxicities ascribed to alkali or alkaline earth salts relate to the anionic component. In the case of NaOH or $Ca(OH)_2$, it is the hydroxide anion, whereas with potassium cyanide (KCN) it is the cyanide (CN^-) anion. When the chemical reactivity of an ionic compound (including its cellular toxicity) can be ascribed solely to one of the ions, any other ion in the compound is referred to as a *spectator* ion.

Transition Metals
Unlike the alkali and alkaline earth metals, most other metallic elements are neither soluble nor reactive. This includes the transition metals (Groups 4-12; formerly Groups IB to VIIB, VIII, IB and IIB), a large group that contains several ubiquitous metals such as iron (Fe) and copper (Cu). These elements, in their metallic form, are widely used in both industrial and household applications because of their high tensile strength, density, and melting point, which is partly a result of their ability to delocalize the

electrons in the d orbital throughout the metallic lattice. Transition metals also form brightly colored salts that find widespread applications, including as pigments for paints or fireworks. The ionic forms of these elements are of greater toxicologic importance than their metallic/elemental forms. Chemically, transition elements form at least one ion with a partially filled subshell of d electrons. Because the transition metals have partially filled valence shells, they are capable of obtaining several, usually positive, oxidation states. This important mechanism explains the role of transition metals in oxidation/reduction (redox) reactions, generally as electron acceptors (see Reduction-Oxidation below). This reactivity is used by organisms in various physiologic, catalytic, and coordination roles, such as at the active sites of enzymes and in hemoglobin. As expected, the substantial reactivity of these transition metal elements is associated with cellular injury caused by several mechanisms, including the generation of reactive oxygen species (Fig. 10–2). Manganese ion, as an example, is implicated in free radical damage of the basal ganglia, causing parkinsonism.

Heavy Metals
Heavy metal is often loosely used to describe all metals of toxicologic significance, but in reality the term should be reserved to describe only those metals in the lower period of the periodic table, particularly those with atomic masses greater than 200 Da. The chemical properties and toxicologic predilection of these elements vary, but a unifying toxicologic mechanism is electrophilic interference with nucleophilic sulfhydryl-containing enzymes. Some of the heavy metals also participate in the generation of free radicals through Fenton chemistry (Fig. 10–2). The likely determinant of the specific toxicologic effects produced by each metal is the tropism for various physiologic systems, enzymes, or microenvironments; thus, lipophilicity, water solubility, ionic size, and other physicochemical parameters are undoubtedly critical. Also, because the chemistry of metals varies dramatically based on the chemical form (ie, organic, inorganic, or elemental), as well as the charge on the metal ion, prediction of the clinical effects of a particular metal is often difficult.

Mercury. Elemental mercury (Hg^0) is unique in that it is the only metal that exists in liquid form at room temperatures. As such, it is capable of creating semisolid solutions, or amalgams, with other metals. Although relatively innocuous if ingested as a liquid, elemental mercury is readily volatilized (as a result of its high vapor pressure), transforming it into a significant pulmonary mucosal irritant upon inhalation. Pulmonary exposure increases its systemic bioavailability. Elemental mercury undergoes biotransformation in the erythrocyte and brain to the mercuric (Hg^{2+}) form, which has a high affinity for sulfhydryl-containing molecules, such as proteins. This causes a depletion of glutathione in organs such as the kidney, and also initiates lipid peroxidation. The mercurous form (Hg^+) is considerably less toxic than the mercuric (Hg^{2+}) form, perhaps because of its reduced water solubility, which limits absorption. Organic mercurial compounds, such as methylmercury and dimethylmercury, are formed environmentally by anaerobic bacteria containing the methylating compound methylcobalamin, a vitamin B_{12} analog (Chap. 95).

$$H_2O_2 + Fe^{2+} \longrightarrow OH^- + OH\bullet + Fe^{3+}$$

Fenton

$$H_2O_2 + O_2^{\bar{\bullet}} \xrightarrow{Fe^{2+}/Fe^{3+}} O_2 + OH^- + OH\bullet$$

Haber-Weiss

FIGURE 10–2. The Fenton and Haber-Weiss reactions, which are the 2 most important mechanisms to generate hydroxyl radicals, are both mediated by transition metals. Typical transition metals include iron (Fe^{2+}, shown) or copper (Cu^+).

Thallium. Metallic thallium (Tl^0) is used in the production of electronic equipment, and is itself minimally toxic. Thallium ions, however, have physicochemical properties that closely mimic potassium ions, allowing them to participate in and often alter the myriad physiologic activities related to potassium. This property is exploited during a thallium-stress test to assess for myocardial ischemia or infarction; because ischemic myocardial cells lack adequate energy for normal Na^+,K^+-ATPase function, they cannot exchange sodium for potassium (or radioactive thallium administered during a stress test). This produces a "cold spot" in the ischemic areas on cardiac scintigraphy (Chap. 99).

Lead. Lead is not abundant in the Earth's crust (0.002%), but mining and industrial use make it a significant toxicologic concern. Lead exposure occurs during the smelting process or from one of its diverse commercial applications. Most of the useful lead compounds are inorganic plumbous (Pb^{2+}) salts, but plumbic (Pb^{4+}) compounds are also used. The Pb^{2+} compounds are typically ionizable, releasing Pb^{2+} when dissolved in a solvent, such as water. Lead ions are absorbed in place of Ca^{2+} ions by the gastrointestinal tract and replace Ca^{2+} in certain physiologic processes. This mechanism is implicated in the neurotoxic effect of lead ions. Lead compounds tend to be covalent compounds that do not ionize in water. Some Pb^{4+} compounds are oxidants. Although elemental lead is not itself toxic, it rapidly develops a coating of toxic lead oxide or lead carbonate on exposure to air or water (Chap. 93).

Metalloids

Although the metalloids (B, Si, Ge, As, Sb, Te, At) share many physical properties with metals, they differ in their propensity to form compounds with both metals and the nonmetals carbon, nitrogen, or oxygen. Metalloids are either oxidized or reduced in chemical reactions.

Arsenic. Toxicologically important inorganic arsenic compounds exist in either the pentavalent arsenite (As^{5+}) form or the trivalent arsenate (As^{3+}) form. The reduced water solubility of arsenate compounds (such as arsenic pentoxide) accounts for its limited clinical toxicity when compared to trivalent arsenic trioxide. The trivalent form of arsenic is primarily a nucleophilic toxin, binding sulfhydryl groups and interfering with enzymatic function (Chaps. 11 and 86).

Nonmetals

The nonmetals (C, N, P, O, S, Se, halogens) are highly electronegative and are toxic in either their compounded or their elemental form. The nonmetals with large electronegativity, such as O_2 or Cl_2, generally oxidize other elements in chemical reactions. Those with lesser electronegativity, such as C, behave as reducing agents.

Halogens. In their highly reactive elemental form, which is a covalent dimer of halogen atoms, the halogens (F, Cl, Br, I, At) carry the suffix *ine* (eg, Cl_2, chlorine). Halogens require the addition of one electron to complete their valence shell, and are strong oxidizing agents. Because they are highly electronegative, they readily form halides (eg, Cl^-, chloride) by abstracting electrons from less electronegative elements. Thus, the halogen ions, in their stable ionic form, generally carry a charge of –1. The halides, although much less reactive than their respective elemental forms, are reducing agents. The hydrogen halides (eg, HCl, hydrogen chloride) are gases under standard conditions, but they ionize when dissolved in aqueous solution to form hydrohalidic acids (eg, HCl, hydrochloric acid). All hydrogen halides except HF (hydrogen fluoride) ionize nearly completely in water to release H^+ and are considered *strong acids*. Because of its small ionic radius, lack of charge dispersion, and the intense electronegativity of the fluorine atom, HF ionizes poorly and is a *weak acid*. This specific property of HF has important toxicologic implications (Chap. 104).

Group 18 (formerly Group VIIIA): Inert Gases. Inert gases (He, Ne, Ar, Kr, Xe, Rn), also known as noble gases, maintain completed valence shells and are thus unreactive except under extreme experimental conditions. Despite their lack of chemical reactivity, the inert gases are toxicologically important as simple asphyxiants, causing hypoxia if they displace ambient oxygen from a confined space (Chap. 121). During high-concentration exposure, inert gases produce anesthesia, and xenon is used as an anesthetic agent. Radon, although chemically unreactive, is radioactive, and prolonged exposure is associated with the development of lung cancer.

Bonds

Electrons are not generally shared evenly between atoms when they form a compound unless the bond is between the same elements, as in Cl_2. When different elements are involved, one will exert a larger attraction for the shared electrons. The degree to which an element draws the shared electron is determined by the *electronegativity* of the element (Fig. 10–3). The electronegativity of each element was catalogued by Linus Pauling and relates to the ionic radius, or the distance between the orbiting electron and the nucleus, and the shielding effects of the inner electrons. Electronegativity rises toward the right of the periodic table, corresponding with the expected charge obtained on an element when it forms a bond. Fluorine has the highest electronegativity of all elements, which explains many of the toxicologic properties of fluorine.

Several types of bonds exist between elements when they form compounds. When one element gains valence electrons and another loses them, the resulting elements are charged and attract one another in an *ionic*, or *electrovalent*, bond. An example is sodium chloride (NaCl), or table salt, in which the electronegativity difference between the elements is 1.9, or greater than the electronegativity of the sodium (Fig. 10–3). Thus, the chloride wrests control of the electrons in this bond. In solid form, ionic compounds exist in a crystalline lattice, but when put into solution, as in water or in blood (serum), the elements separate and form charged particles, or *ions* (Na^+ and Cl^-). The ions are stable in solution because their valence shells contain 8 electrons and are complete. The properties of ions differ from both the original atom from which the ion is derived and the noble gas with which it shares electronic structure.

It is important to recognize that when a mole of a salt, such as NaCl (molecular weight 58.45 g/mol), is put in aqueous solution, 2 moles of particles result. This is because NaCl is essentially fully ionized in water; that is, it produces one mole of Na^+ (23 g/mol) and one mole of Cl^- (35.5 g/mol). For salts that do not ionize completely, less than the intrinsic number of moles are released and the actual quantity liberated can be predicted based on the defined solubility of the compound, or the solubility product constant (K_{sp}). For ions that carry more than a single charge, the term *equivalent* is often used to denote the number of moles of other particles to which one mole of the substance will bind. Thus, one equivalent of calcium ions will typically bind 2 moles (or equivalents) of chloride ions (which are monovalent) because calcium ions are divalent. Alternatively stated, a 10% calcium chloride ($CaCl_2$) aqueous solution contains approximately 1.4 mEq/mL or 0.7 mmol/mL of Ca^{2+}.

Compounds formed by 2 elements of similar electronegativity have little ionic character because there is little impetus for separation of charge.

1/IA			13/IIIA	14/IVA	15/VA	16/VIA	17/VIIA	18/VIIIA
H 2.20	2/IIA							He –
Li 0.98	Be 1.57		B 2.04	C 2.55	N 3.04	O 3.44	F 3.98	Ne –
Na 0.93	Mg 1.31		Al 1.61	Si 1.90	P 2.19	S 2.58	Cl 3.16	Ar –
K 0.82	Ca 1.00				As 3.18	Se 2.55	Br 2.96	Kr –

FIGURE 10–3. Electronegativity of the common elements. Note that the noble gases are not reactive and thus do not have electronegativity. The top row indicates modern IUPAC nomenclature/classical nomenclature.

Instead, these elements share pairs of valence electrons, a process known as *covalence*. The resultant molecule contains a *covalent bond*, which is typically very strong and generally requires a high-energy chemical reaction to disrupt it. There is wide variation in the extent to which the electrons are shared between the participants of a covalent bond, and the physicochemical and toxicologic properties of any particular molecule are in part determined by its nature. Sharing is rarely symmetric (as in oxygen {O_2} or chlorine {Cl_2}). When electrons are shared asymmetrically (localized to a greater degree around one of the component atoms), the bond is called *polar*. Importantly, however, the presence of polar bonds does not mean that the compound itself is polar. For example, methane contains a carbon atom that shares its valence electrons with 4 hydrogen atoms, in which there is a small charge separation between the elements (electronegativity {EN} difference = 0.40). Although each of the carbon hydrogen bonds is polar, however, the tetrahedral configuration of the molecule means that the asymmetries cancel each other out, resulting in no net polarity, rendering the compound *nonpolar*. The lack of polarity demonstrates that methane molecules have little affinity for other methane molecules and they are held together only by weak intermolecular bonds. This explains why methane is highly volatile and therefore exists as a gas under standard temperature and pressure.

Because the EN differences between hydrogen (EN = 2.20) and oxygen (EN = 3.44) are significant (EN difference = 1.24), the electrons in the hydrogen-oxygen bonds in water are drawn toward the oxygen atom, giving it a partial negative charge and the hydrogen a partial positive charge. Because H_2O is angular, not linear or symmetric, water is a polar molecule. Water molecules are held together by *hydrogen bonds*, which are bonds between electropositive hydrogen atoms and the strongly electronegative oxygen atoms. Hydrogen bonds are stronger than other intermolecular bonds (eg, *van der Waals forces*; see later). Hydrogen bonds have sufficient energy to open many ionic bonds and *solvate* ions (ie, cause ionic compounds to go into solution). In this process, the polar ends of the water molecule surround the charged particles of the dissolved salt. As one corollary, nonpolar molecules are relatively insoluble in polar compounds such as water, as there is little similarity between the nonpolar methane and the polar water molecules. As a second corollary, salts cannot be solvated by nonpolar compounds, and thus a salt, such as sodium chloride, has almost no solubility in a nonpolar solvent such as carbon tetrachloride.

Alternatively, the stability and irreversibility of the bond between an organic phosphorus compound and the cholinesterase enzyme are a result of covalent phosphorylation of an amino acid at the active site of the enzyme. The resulting bond is essentially irreversible in the absence of another chemical reaction (Fig. 110–3).

Compounds often share multiple pairs of electrons. For example, the 2 carbon atoms in acetylene (HC≡CH) share 3 pairs of electrons between them, and each shares one pair with a hydrogen. Carbon and nitrogen share 3 pairs of electrons in forming cyanide (C≡N⁻), making this bond very stable and accounting for the large number of xenobiotics capable of liberating cyanide. Complex ions are covalently bonded groups of elements that behave as a single element. For example, hydroxide (OH^-) and sulfate (SO_4^{2-}) form sodium salts as if they were simply the ion of a single element (such as chloride).

Noncovalent bonds, such as hydrogen or ionic bonds, are important in the interaction between ligands and receptors as well as between ion channels and enzymes. These are low-energy bonds and easily broken. Van der Waals forces, also known as London dispersion forces, are intermolecular forces that arise from induced dipoles as a consequence of nonuniform distribution of the molecular electron cloud. These forces become stronger as the atom (or molecule) becomes larger because of the increased polarizability of the larger, more dispersed electron clouds. This accounts for the fact that under standard temperature and pressure, fluorine and chlorine are gases, whereas bromine is a liquid, and iodine is a solid.

Reduction-Oxidation

Reduction-oxidation (*redox*) reactions involve the movement of electrons from one atom or molecule to another, and comprise 2 interdependent reactions (reduction and oxidation). *Reduction* is the gain of electrons by an atom that is thereby *reduced*. The electrons derive from a *reducing agent*, which in the process becomes *oxidized*. *Oxidation* is the loss of electrons from an atom, which is, accordingly, *oxidized*. An *oxidizing agent* accepts electrons and, in the process, is reduced. By definition, these chemical reactions involve a change in the valence of an atom. It is also important to note that acid-base and electrolyte chemical reactions involve electrical charge interactions but no change in valence of any of the involved components. The implications of redox chemistry for toxicology are significant. For example, the oxidation of ferrous (Fe^{2+}) to ferric (Fe^{3+}) iron within the hemoglobin molecule creates the dysfunctional methemoglobin molecule (Chap. 124).

The *oxidation state* of an atom or molecule plays an important role in its toxicity. Elemental lead and mercury are both intrinsically harmless metals, but when oxidized to their cationic forms produce devastating clinical effects. The metabolism of ethanol to acetaldehyde involves a change in the oxidation state of the molecule. In this case, an enzyme, alcohol dehydrogenase, oxidizes (ie, removes electrons from) the C-O bond and delivers the electrons to oxidized nicotinamide adenine dinucleotide (NAD^+), reducing it to NADH. As in this last example, *oxidation* is occasionally used to signify the gain of oxygen by a substance. That is, when elemental iron (Fe^0) undergoes rusting to iron oxide (Fe_2O_3), it is said to oxidize. The use of this term is consistent because in the process of oxidation, oxygen derives electrons from the atom with which it is reacting and combining.

Reactive Oxygen Species

Free radicals are reactive molecules that contain one or more unpaired electrons. They are typically neutral but also can be anionic or cationic. However, because certain toxicologically important reactive molecules, such as hydrogen peroxide (H_2O_2) and ozone (O_3), do not contain unpaired electrons, the term *reactive species* is preferred. The reactivity of these molecules directly relates to their attempts to fill their outermost orbitals by receiving an electron; the result is *oxidative stress* on the biologic system. Molecular oxygen is actually a diradical with 2 unpaired electrons in the outer orbitals. However, its reactivity is less than that of the other radicals because the unpaired electrons have parallel spins, so catalysts (ie, enzymes or metals) are typically involved in the use of oxygen in biologic processes.

Reactive species are continuously generated as a consequence of endogenous metabolism, and there is an efficient detoxification system for their control. However, under conditions of either excessive endogenous generation or exposure to exogenous reactive species, the physiologic defenses against these toxic products are overwhelmed. When this occurs, reactive species induce direct cellular damage and initiate a cascade of additional harmful oxidative reactions.[4]

Intracellular organelles, particularly the mitochondria, are damaged by various reactive species. This causes further injury to the cell as energy failure occurs. This initial damage is exacerbated by the activation of the host inflammatory response by chemokines that are released from cells in response to reactive species–induced damage. This inflammatory response aggravates cellular damage. The resultant membrane dysfunction or damage causes cellular apoptosis or necrosis.

The most important reactive oxygen species in medical toxicology are derived from oxygen, although those derived from nitrogen are also important. Table 10–1 lists some of the important reactive oxygen and nitrogen species.

The biradical nature of oxygen explains both the physiologic and toxicologic importance of oxygen in biologic systems. Physiologically, the majority of oxygen used by the body serves as the ultimate electron acceptor in the mitochondrial electron transport chain. In this situation, 4 electrons are added to each molecule of oxygen to form 2 water molecules ($O_2 + 4H^+ + 4e^- \rightarrow 2H_2O$).

Superoxide (O_2^-) is "mutated" from oxygen within neutrophil and macrophage lysosomes as part of the oxidative burst, which serves to help eliminate infectious agents and damaged cells. Superoxide is subsequently enzymatically converted, or "dismutated," into hydrogen peroxide by superoxide

TABLE 10–1	Structure of Important Reactive Species	
		Structure
Reactive Oxygen Species		
Free radicals		
Hydroxyl radical		OH•
Alkoxyl radical		RO•
Peroxyl radical		ROO•
Superoxide radical		$O_2^{\bar{}}$
Nonradicals		
Hydrogen peroxide		H_2O_2
Hypochlorous acid		HOCl
Singlet oxygen		[O] or $^1O_2$
Ozone		O_3
Reactive Nitrogen Species		
Free radicals		
Nitric oxide		NO•
Nitrogen dioxide		NO_2•
Nonradicals		
Peroxynitrite anion		$ONOO^-$
Nitronium cation		NO_2^+

dismutase (SOD). Hydrogen peroxide also can subsequently converted into hypochlorous acid by the enzymatic addition of chloride by myeloperoxidase. Both hydrogen peroxide and hypochlorite ion are more potent reactive oxygen species than superoxide. However, this lysosomal protective system is also responsible for tissue damage following poisoning as the innate inflammatory response attacks xenobiotic-damaged cells. Examples include acetaminophen (APAP)-induced hepatotoxicity (Chap. 33), carbon monoxide neurotoxicity (Chap. 122), and chlorine-induced pulmonary toxicity (Chap. 121), each of which is altered, at least in experimental systems, by the addition of scavengers of reactive species.

Although superoxide and hydrogen peroxide are reactive species, it is their conversion into the hydroxyl radical (OH·) that accounts for their most consequential effects. The hydroxyl radical is generated by the Fenton reaction (Fig. 10–2), in which hydrogen peroxide is decomposed in the presence of a transition metal.[3] This catalysis typically involves Fe^{2+}, Cu^+, Cd^{2+}, Cr^{5+}, Ni^{2+}, or Mn^{2+}. The Haber-Weiss reaction (Fig. 10–2), in which a transition metal catalyzes the combination of superoxide and hydrogen peroxide, is another important means of generating the hydroxyl radical. Alternatively, superoxide dismutase, within the erythrocyte, contains an ion of copper (Cu^{2+}) that participates in the catalytic reduction of superoxide to hydrogen peroxide and the subsequent detoxification of hydrogen peroxide by glutathione peroxidase or catalase.

Transition metal cations frequently bind to the cellular nucleus and locally generate reactive oxygen species, most importantly hydroxyl radicals. This results in DNA strand breaks and modification, accounting for the mutagenic effects of many transition metals. In addition to the important role that transition metal chemistry plays following iron or copper salt poisoning, the long-term consequences of chronic transition metal poisoning are exemplified by asbestos. The iron contained in asbestos serves as the source of the Fenton-generated hydroxyl radicals that are responsible for the pulmonary fibrosis and cancers associated with long-term exposure.

The most important toxicologic effects of reactive oxygen species occur on the cell membrane, and are caused by the initiation by hydroxyl radicals of the lipid peroxidative cascade. The alteration of these lipid membranes ultimately causes membrane destruction. Identification of released oxidative products such as malondialdehyde is a common method of assessing lipid peroxidation.

Under normal conditions, there is a delicate balance between the formation and immediate detoxification of reactive oxygen species. For example,

the conversion of the superoxide radical to hydrogen peroxide via SOD is rapidly followed by the transformation of hydrogen peroxide to water by glutathione peroxidase or catalase. The fact that transition metals exist in "free" form in only minute quantities in biologic systems minimizes the formation of hydroxyl radicals; that is, cells have developed extensive systems by which transition metal ions are sequestered and rendered harmless. Ferritin (binds iron), ceruloplasmin (binds copper), and metallothionein (binds cadmium) are all specialized proteins that safely sequester transition metal ions. Certain proteins and enzymes such as hemoglobin or SOD have critical biological functions associated with the transition metals at their active sites.

Detoxification of certain reactive species is difficult because of their extreme reactivity. Widespread antioxidant systems typically scavenge reactive species before tissue damage occurs. An example is glutathione, a reducing agent and nucleophile, which prevents both exogenous oxidants from producing hemolysis and the APAP metabolite N-acetyl-p-benzoquinoneimine (NAPQI) from damaging the hepatocyte (Chap. 33).

The key reactive nitrogen species is nitric oxide. At typical physiologic concentrations, this radical is responsible for vascular endothelial relaxation through stimulation of guanylate cyclase. However, during oxidative burst, high concentrations of nitric oxide are formed from L-arginine. At these concentrations, nitric oxide is directly damaging to tissue and also reacts with the superoxide radical to generate the peroxynitrite anion. This is particularly important because peroxynitrite spontaneously degrades to form the hydroxyl radical. Peroxynitrite ion is implicated in both the delayed neurologic effects of carbon monoxide poisoning and the hepatic injury from APAP.

Redox Cycling. Although transition metals are an important source of reactive species, certain xenobiotics are also capable of independently generating reactive species. Most do so through a process called *redox cycling*, in which a molecule accepts an electron from a reducing agent and subsequently transfers that electron to oxygen, generating the superoxide radical. At the same time, this second reaction regenerates the parent molecule, which itself can gain another electron and restart the process. The toxicity of paraquat (Chap. 109) is selectively localized to pulmonary endothelial cells. Its pulmonary toxicity results from redox cycling generation of reactive oxygen species (Fig. 109–3). A similar process, localized to the heart, occurs with anthracycline antineoplastics such as doxorubicin.

Acid-Base Chemistry

Water is *amphoter*ic, which means that it can function as either an acid or a base, much the same way as the bicarbonate ion (HCO_3^-). Because of the amphoteric nature of water, H^+, despite the nomenclature, does not ever actually exist in aqueous solution; rather, it is covalently bound to a molecule of water to form the hydronium ion (H_3O^+). However, the term H^+, or proton, is used for convenience.

Even in a neutral solution, a tiny proportion of water is always undergoing ionization to form both H^+ and OH^- in exactly equal amounts. By convention, however, it is the quantity of H^+ that is measured to determine the acidity or alkalinity of the solution. The units for this measurement are pH, which is $-\log[H^+]$. In a perfect system at equilibrium, the concentration of H^+ ions in water is precisely 0.0000001, or 10^{-7}, mol/L and that of OH^- is the same. The number of H^+ ions increases when an acid is added to the solution and falls when an alkali is added. The negative log of 10^{-7} is 7, and the pH of a neutral aqueous solution is thus 7. In actuality, the pH of water is approximately 6 because of dissolution of ambient carbon dioxide to form carbonic acid ($H_2O + CO_2 \rightarrow H_2CO_3$), which ionizes to form H^+ and bicarbonate (HCO_3^-).

There are many definitions of acid and base. The 3 commonly used definitions are those advanced by (1) Svante Arrhenius, (2) Brønsted and Lowry, and (3) Lewis. Because our focus is on physiologic systems, which are most commonly aqueous solutions, the original definition by the Swedish chemist Arrhenius is the most practical. In this view, an acid releases hydrogen ions, or protons (H^+), in water. Conversely, a base produces hydroxyl ions (OH^-) in water. Thus, hydrogen chloride (HCl), a neutral gas under standard conditions, dissolves in water to liberate H^+ and is therefore an acid.

For nonaqueous solutions, the Brønsted-Lowry definition is preferable. An acid, in this schema, is a substance that donates a proton and a base is one that accepts a proton. Thus, any molecule that has a hydrogen atom in the 1+ oxidation state is technically an acid, and any molecule with an unbound pair of valence electrons is a base. Because most of the acids or bases of toxicologic interest have ionizable protons or available electrons, respectively, the Brønsted-Lowry definition is most often considered when discussing acid-base chemistry (ie, $HA + H_2O \rightarrow H_3O^+ + A^-$; $B^- + H_2O \rightarrow HB + OH^-$). However, this is not a defining property of all acids or bases.

The Lewis classification offers the least-restrictive definition of such substances. A Lewis acid is an electron acceptor and a Lewis base is an electron donor.

Simplistically, acids are sour and turn litmus paper red; bases feel slippery (due to the dissolution of skin), are bitter, and turn litmus paper blue. Of note, the tasting and tactile assessment of substances to determine their acid-base status is not recommended.

Because acidity and alkalinity are determined by the number of available H^+ ions, it is useful to classify chemicals by their effect on the H^+ concentration. Strong acids ionize almost completely in aqueous solution, and very little of the parent compound remains. Thus, 0.001 (or 10^{-3}) mol of HCl, a strong acid, added to 1 L of water produces a solution with a pH of 3. Weak acids, on the other hand, reach an equilibrium between parent and ionized forms, and thus do not alter the pH to the same degree as a similar quantity of a strong acid. This chemical notation defines the strength or weakness of an acid and should not be confused with the concentration of the acid. Thus, the pH of a dilute strong acid solution is substantially less than that of a concentrated weak acid (Table 10–2).

The degree of ionization of an acid is determined by the pK_a, or the negative log of the *ionization constant*, which represents the pH at which an acid is half dissociated in solution. The same relationship applies to the pK_b of an

alkali, although pK_b is rarely used and the degree of ionization of bases is also expressed as pK_a (of note, $pK_a = 14 - pK_b$). The lower the pK_a, the stronger the acid; the higher the pK_a, the stronger the base. The pK of a strong acid is clinically irrelevant because it is nearly fully ionized under all but the most extremely acidic conditions. Importantly, knowledge of the pK_a does not itself denote the strength of an acid or an alkali. To some extent, this quality is predicted by its chemical structure or reactivity, or it can be obtained through direct measurement or from a reference source.

Because only uncharged compounds cross lipid membranes spontaneously, the pK_a has strong clinical relevance. Salicylic acid, a weak acid with a pK_a of 3, is nonionized in the stomach (pH = 2) and passive absorption occurs (Fig. 9–3). Because it is predominantly in the ionized form (ie, salicylate) in blood, which has a pH of 7.4, little of the ionized blood-borne salicylate passively enters the tissues. However, because in overdose the serum salicylate rises considerably, enough enters the tissue to result in clinical toxicity. Salicylate is the conjugate base of a weak acid (and thus itself a strong base). It diffuses into the mitochondrial intermembrane space (between the inner and outer mitochondrial membrane), where abundant protons exist that have been transported there via the electron transport chain of this organelle (Fig. 11–3). Because salicylate is a strong base, it protonates easily in this environment. In this nonionized form, some of the salicylic acid passes through the inner mitochondrial membrane, into the mitochondrial matrix, and again establish equilibrium by losing a proton. This is the uncoupling of oxidative phosphorylation, dispersing highly concentrated protons in the intermembrane space that are normally used to generate adenosine triphosphate (Chap. 11). Uncoupling contributes to a metabolic acidosis, which shifts the blood equilibrium of aspirin toward the nonionized, protonated form (salicylic acid), enabling it to cross the blood-brain barrier. Presumably, once in the brain, the salicylate uncouples the metabolic activity of neurons with the subsequent development of cerebral edema. Part of the treatment of patients with salicylate toxicity is interrupting the above chain of events with serum alkalinization (Chap. 37).

In a related manner, alkalinization of the patient's urine prevents reabsorption by ionization of the urinary salicylate. Salicylate anion excreted into acidic urine protonates, and the uncharged moiety then back-diffuses across the renal tubular epithelium and re-enter the body. Alkalinization of the urine "traps" salicylate in the deprotonated form, enhancing excretion. Conversely, because cyclic antidepressants are organic bases, alkalinization of the urine reduces their ionization and actually decreases the urinary elimination of the drug. However, in the management of cyclic antidepressant poisoning, because the other beneficial effects of sodium bicarbonate on the sodium channel outweigh the negative effect on drug elimination, serum alkalinization is recommended (Chap. 68).

ORGANIC CHEMISTRY

The study of carbon-based chemistry and the interaction of inorganic molecules with carbon-containing compounds is called *organic chemistry*, because the chemistry of living organisms is carbon based. *Biochemistry* (Chap. 11) is a subdivision of organic chemistry; it is the study of organic chemistry within biologic systems. This section reviews many of the salient points of organic chemistry, focusing on those with the most applicability to medicine and the study of toxicology: nomenclature, bonding, nucleophiles and electrophiles, stereochemistry, and functional groups.

Chemical Properties of Carbon

Carbon, atomic number 6, has a molecular weight of 12.011 g/mol. With few exceptions (notably cyanide ion and carbon monoxide), carbon forms 4 bonds in stable organic molecules. In organic compounds, carbon is commonly bonded to other carbon atoms, as well as to hydrogen, oxygen, nitrogen, or halides. Under certain circumstances, carbon is bonded to metals, as is the case with methylmercury.

Nomenclature

The most systematic method to name organic compounds is in accordance with standards adopted by the International Union of Pure and Applied

TABLE 10–2	pH of 0.10 *M* Solutions of Common Acids and Bases Represents the Strength of the Acid or Base
Acid/Base	**pH**
HCl (hydrochloric acid)	1.1
H_2SO_4 (sulfuric acid)	1.2
H_2SO_3 (sulfurous acid)	1.5
H_3PO_4 (phosphoric acid)	1.5
HF (hydrofluoric acid)	2.1
CH_3CO_2H (acetic acid)	2.9
H_2CO_3 (carbonic acid)	3.8
H_2S (hydrogen sulfide)	4.1
NH_4Cl (ammonium chloride)	4.6
HCN (hydrocyanic acid)	5.1
$NaHCO_3$ (sodium bicarbonate)	8.3
$NaCH_3CO_2$ (sodium acetate)	8.9
Na_2HPO_4 (sodium hydrogen phosphate)	9.3
Na_2SO_3 (sodium sulfite)	9.8
NaCN (sodium cyanide)	11.0
NH_4OH (ammonium hydroxide)	11.1
Na_2CO_3 (sodium carbonate)	11.6
Na_3PO_4 (sodium phosphate)	12.0
NaOH (sodium hydroxide)	13.0

Chemistry (IUPAC); these names are infrequently used, especially for larger molecules, and alternative names are common. The complete details of the IUPAC naming system are beyond the scope of this text and can be reviewed elsewhere (www.iupac.org), but a brief description of the fundamentals of this system is included here.

The carbon backbone of a molecule serves as the basis of its chemical name. Once the carbon backbone is identified and named, *substituents* (atoms or groups of atoms that substitute for hydrogen atoms) are identified, named, and numbered. The number refers to the carbon to which the substituent is attached. Some of the common substituents in organic chemistry are –OH (hydroxy), –NH$_2$ (amino), –Br (bromo), –Cl (chloro), and –F (fluoro). Substituents are then alphabetized and placed as prefixes to the carbon chain.

As an example, consider the molecule 2-bromo-2-chloro-1,1,1-trifluoroethane. The molecule has a 2-carbon backbone (ethane), 3 fluoride atoms on the first carbon, a bromine atom on the second carbon, and a chlorine atom on the second carbon (Fig. 10–4A). A basic understanding of a few simple rules of nomenclature thus allows one to quickly generate the molecular structure of a familiar compound, halothane.

Although the above-mentioned rules suffice to name simple structures, they are inadequate to describe many others, such as molecules with complex branching or ring structures. The IUPAC rules for naming compounds such as [1R-(exo,exo)]-3-(benzoyloxy)-8-methyl-8-azabicyclo[3,2,1]octane-2-carboxylic acid methyl ester, for example, are too complex to include here. Fortunately, many compounds with complex chemical names have simpler names for day-to-day use; as an example, this molecule is commonly referred to as cocaine (Fig. 10–4B).

Cocaine is an example of a *common* or *trivial* name: one without a systematic basis, but which is generally accepted as an alternative to (frequently unwieldy) proper chemical names. Common names often refer to the origin of the substance; for example, cocaine is derived from the coca leaf, and wood alcohol (methanol) can be prepared from wood. Alternatively, a common name frequently refers to the way in which a compound is used; for example, rubbing alcohol is a common name for isopropanol. Common names are often imprecise and generate some confusion, however, as evidenced by the fact that rubbing alcohol, when commercially marketed, is either ethanol or isopropanol.

An even less precise system of nomenclature is the use of *street* names. A street name is a slang term for a drug of abuse, such as "blow" (cocaine), "weed" (marijuana), or "smack" (heroin). The street name *ecstasy* refers to the stimulant 3,4-methylenedioxymethamphetamine (MDMA), which is most frequently consumed in pill form. It would stand to reason that *liquid ecstasy* might refer to a solution of MDMA, but street names are not necessarily logical. Instead, liquid ecstasy refers to the drug γ-hydroxybutyrate, a sedative-hypnotic with a completely different pharmacologic and toxicologic profile. Furthermore, there are no standards for the content of ecstasy, and many street pills contain other chemicals.

A final consideration must be given to *product names*. Product names are trade names under which a given compound might be marketed and are frequently different from both the chemical name and common name. Thus, the inhalational anesthetic in Fig. 10–4A with the chemical name 2-bromo-2-chloro-1,1,1-trifluoroethane has the common name halothane and the trade name Fluothane.

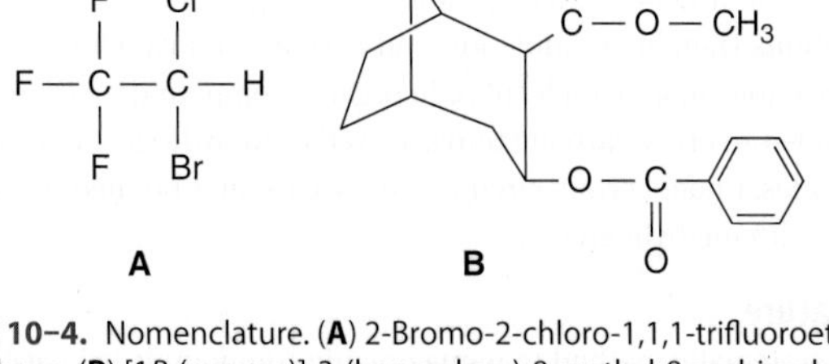

Bonding in Organic Chemistry

While much of the bonding in inorganic chemistry is ionic, the vast majority of bonding in organic molecules is *covalent*. Whereas electrons in ionic bonds are described as predominately "belonging" to one atom or another, electrons in covalent bonds are shared between 2 atoms; this type of bonding occurs when the difference in electronegativity between 2 atoms is insufficient for one atom to wrest control of an electron from another. Bonds are represented by lines between the atoms: one for a single bond, 2 for a double bond, and 3 for a triple bond.

Nucleophiles and Electrophiles

Many organic reactions of toxicologic importance are described as the reactions of *nucleophiles* with *electrophiles*. *Nucleophiles* (literally, nucleus-loving) are species with increased electron density, frequently in the form of a lone pair of electrons (as in the cases of cyanide ion and carbon monoxide). Nucleophiles, by virtue of their increased electron density, have an affinity for atoms or molecules that are electron deficient; such moieties are called *electrophiles* (literally, electron-loving). The electron deficiency of electrophiles is described as absolute or relative. Absolute electron deficiency occurs when an electrophile is charged, as is the case with cations such as Pb^{2+} and Hg^{2+}. Relative electron deficiency occurs when one atom or group of atoms shifts electrons away from a second atom, making the second atom relatively electron deficient. This is the case for the neurotoxin 2,5-hexanedione (Fig. 10–5); the electronegative oxygen of the carbon-oxygen double bond pulls electron density away from the second and fifth carbon atoms of this molecule, making these carbon atoms electrophilic.

The reaction of a nucleophile with an electrophile involves the movement of electrons, by forming or breaking bonds. This movement of electrons is frequently denoted by the use of curved arrows, which better demonstrates how the nucleophile and electrophile interact. The interaction of acetylcholinesterase with acetylcholine, organic phosphorus compounds, and pralidoxime hydrochloride provides an example of how the use of curved arrow notation leads to a better understanding of the reactions involved.

Under normal circumstances, the action of acetylcholine is terminated when the serine residue in the active site of acetylcholinesterase attacks this neurotransmitter, forming a transient serine-acetyl complex and liberating choline. This serine-acetyl complex is then rapidly hydrolyzed, producing an acetic acid molecule and regenerating the serine residue for another round of the reaction (Fig. 10–6A). In the presence of an organic phosphorus compound, however, this serine residue attacks the electrophilic phosphate atom, forming a stable serine-phosphate bond, which is not hydrolyzed (Fig. 10–6B). The enzyme, thus inactivated, can no longer break down acetylcholine, leading to an increase of this neurotransmitter in the synapse and possibly a cholinergic crisis.

The enzyme can be reactivated, however, by the use of another nucleophile. Pralidoxime hydrochloride (2-PAM) is referred to as a *site-directed nucleophile*. Because part of its chemical structure (the charged nitrogen atom) is similar to the choline portion of acetylcholine, this antidote is directed to the active site of acetylcholinesterase. Once in position, the nucleophilic oxime moiety (–NOH) that is remote from the positive charge of pralidoxime attacks the electrophilic phosphate moiety. This displaces the serine residue, regenerating the enzyme (Fig. 10–6C) (Chap. 110 and Antidotes in Depth: A36).

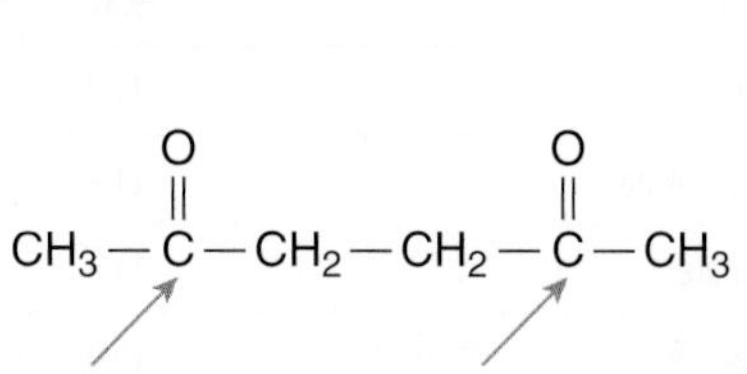

FIGURE 10–4. Nomenclature. (**A**) 2-Bromo-2-chloro-1,1,1-trifluoroethane, or halothane. (**B**) [1R-(exo,exo)]-3-(benzoyloxy)-8-methyl-8-azabicyclo[3,2,1]-octane-2-carboxylic acid methyl ester, or cocaine.

FIGURE 10–5. Chemical properties of 2,5-hexanedione. Arrows designate the electrophilic carbon atoms.

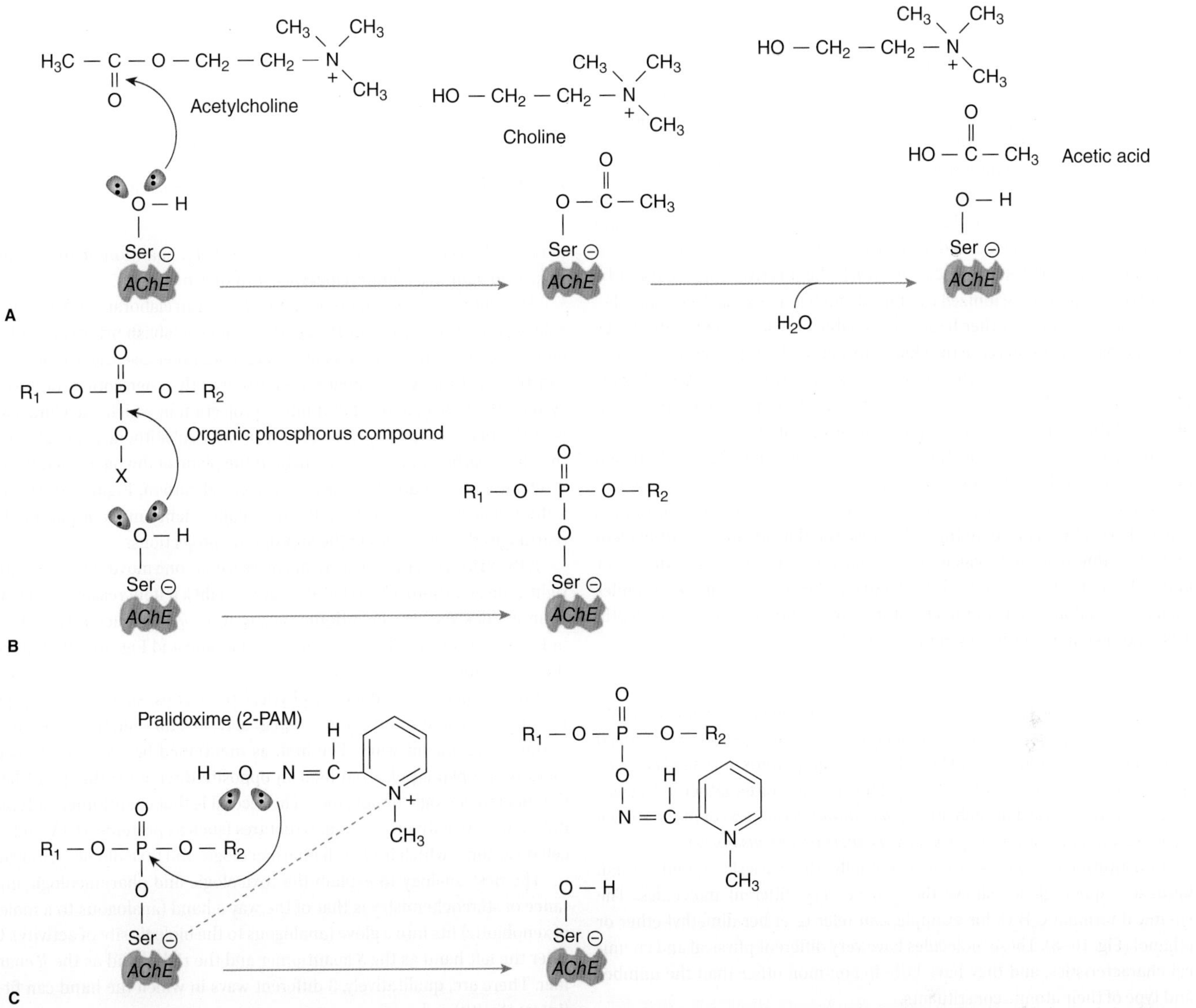

FIGURE 10–6. The reactions of acetylcholinesterase (AChE), organic phosphorus compounds, and pralidoxime hydrochloride (2-PAM). Curved arrows represent the movement of electrons as bonds are formed or broken. (**A**) Normal hydrolysis of acetylcholine by AChE. (**B**) Inactivation (phosphorylation) of AChE by organic phosphorus compound. (**C**) Reactivation by 2-PAM of functional AChE.

A second toxicologically important electrophile is NAPQI (Fig. 10–7). NAPQI is formed when the endogenous detoxification pathways of APAP metabolism (glucuronidation and sulfation) are overwhelmed (Chap. 33). As a result of the electron configuration of NAPQI, the carbon atoms adjacent to the *carbonyl carbon* (a carbon that is double bonded to an oxygen) are very electrophilic; the sulfur groups of cysteine residues of hepatocyte proteins react with NAPQI to form a characteristic *adduct* (formed when one compound is added to another), 3-(cystein-*S*-yl)APAP, in a multistep process. These adducts are released as hepatocytes die, and can be found in the blood of patients with APAP-related liver toxicity. Figure 10–7 diagrams the mechanism of the protein-NAPQI reaction (Chap. 33).

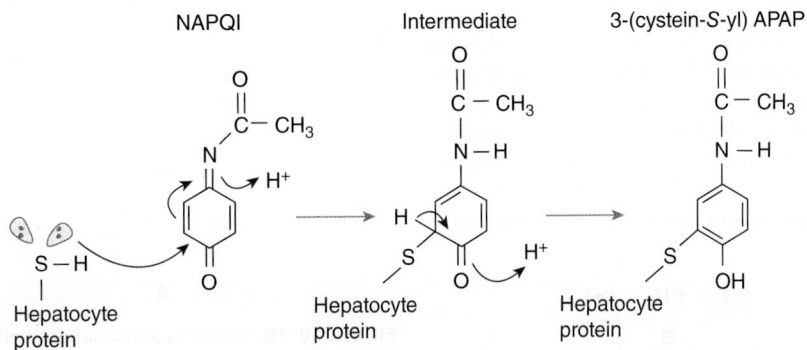

FIGURE 10–7. The reaction of cysteine residues on hepatocyte proteins with *N*-acetyl-*p*-benzoquinoneimine (NAPQI) to form the characteristic adducts 3-(cystein-*S*-yl) APAP.

Nucleophiles are often described by their strength, which by convention is related to the rate at which they react with a reference electrophile (CH_3I). Of more common use in pharmacology and toxicology, however, are the descriptive terms "hard" and "soft." Although imprecise, the designations hard and soft help to predict, qualitatively, how nucleophiles and electrophiles interact with one another.

Hard species have a charge (or partial charge) that is highly localized; that is, their charge-to-radius ratio is high. Hard nucleophiles are molecules in which the electron density or lone pair is tightly held; fluoride, a small atom that cannot spread its electron density over a large area, is an example. Similarly, hard electrophiles are species in which the positive charge cannot be spread over a large area; ionized calcium, a small ion, is a hard electrophile.

Soft species, on the other hand, are capable of delocalizing their charge over a larger area. In this case the charge-to-mass ratio is low, either because the atom is large or because the charge can be spread over a number of atoms within a given molecule. Sulfur is the prototypical example of a soft nucleophile, and the lead ion, Pb^{2+}, is a typical soft electrophile.

The utility of this classification lies in the observation that hard nucleophiles tend to react with hard electrophiles, and soft nucleophiles with soft electrophiles. For example, a principal toxicity of fluoride ion poisoning (Chap. 104) is hypocalcemia; this is because the fluoride ions (hard nucleophiles) readily react with calcium ions (hard electrophiles). On the other hand, the soft nucleophile lead is effectively chelated by soft electrophiles such as the sulfur atoms in the chelators dimercaprol (Antidotes in Depth: A28) and succimer (Antidotes in Depth: A29).[1]

Isomerism

*Isomer*ism describes the different ways in which molecules with the same chemical formula (ie, the same number and types of atoms) can be arranged to form different compounds. These different compounds are called *isomers*. Isomers always have the same chemical formula but differ either in the way that atoms are bonded to each other (*constitutional isomers*) or in the spatial arrangement of these atoms (*geometric isomers* or *stereoisomers*).

Constitutional isomers are conceptually the easiest to understand, because a quick glance shows them to be very different molecules. The chemical formula C_2H_6O, for example, can refer to either dimethyl ether or ethanol (Fig. 10–8). These molecules have very different physical and chemical characteristics, and they have little in common other than the number and type of their atomic constituents.

Stereoisomerism, also referred to as *geometric isomerism*, refers to the different ways in which atoms of a given molecule, with the same number and types of bonds, might be arranged. The most important type of stereoisomerism in pharmacology and toxicology is the stereochemistry around a *stereogenic* (sometimes called *chiral*) *carbon*.

Consider the 2 representations of halothane shown in Fig. 10–9. In this figure, the straight solid lines and the atoms to which they are bonded exist in the plane of the paper, the solid triangle and the atom to which it is bonded are coming out of the paper, and the dashed triangle and the atom to which it is bonded are receding into the paper. It is clear that, for the molecules in Figs. 10–9A and 10-9B, no amount of rotation or manipulation will make these molecules superimposable. They are, therefore, different compounds.

These molecules are *enantiomers* or *optical isomers*. They differ only in the way in which their atoms are bonded to a chiral carbon.[6] It is important to define the stereochemical configuration of these 2 molecules, which is done in one of 2 ways. In the first classification—the $d(+)/l(-)$ system—molecules are named empirically based on the direction in which they rotate plane-polarized light. Each enantiomer will rotate plane-polarized light in one direction; the enantiomer that rotates light clockwise (to the right) is referred to as

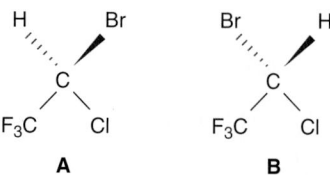

FIGURE 10–9. The graphic representation of the enantiomers of halothane.

$d(+)$, or *dextrorotatory*; the $l(-)$, or *levorotatory*, enantiomer rotates plane-polarized light in a counterclockwise fashion (to the left).

Alternatively, enantiomers are named using an elaborate and formal set of rules known as *Cahn-Ingold-Prelog*. These rules establish priority for substituents, based primarily on molecular weight, and then use the arrangement of substituents to assign a configuration. To correctly assign configuration in this system, the molecule is rotated into a projection in which the chiral carbon is in the plane of the page, the lowest priority substituent is directly behind the chiral carbon (and therefore behind the plane of the page), and the other 3 substituents are arranged around the chiral carbon. Figure 10–10 assigns Cahn-Ingold-Prelog priority to the halothane enantiomers of Fig. 10–9, and rearranges the molecules in the appropriate projections.

If the priority of the substituents increases as one moves clockwise (to the right), the enantiomer is R (Latin, *rectus* = right); if it increases as one moves counterclockwise, the enantiomer is S (Latin, *sinister* = left). Thus, the one in Fig. 10–10A is the R enantiomer of halothane and Fig. 10–10B represents the S enantiomer.

Enantiomers have identical physical properties, such as boiling point, melting point, and solubility in different solvents; they differ from each other in only 2 significant ways. The first, as mentioned before, is that enantiomers rotate plane-polarized light in opposite directions; this point has no practical toxicologic importance. The second is that enantiomers interact in different ways with other chiral structures (such as proteins, DNA, and other cell receptors), which is of both pharmacologic and toxicologic significance.[6]

The best analogy to explain the toxicologic and pharmacologic importance of stereochemistry is that of the way a hand (analogous to a molecule of xenobiotic) fits into a glove (analogous to the biologic site of activity). Consider the left hand as the S enantiomer and the right hand as the R enantiomer. There are, qualitatively, 3 different ways in which the hand can fit into (interact with) a glove.

First, if the glove is pliable and relatively fluid (such as a disposable latex glove), it can accept either the left hand or the right hand without difficulty;

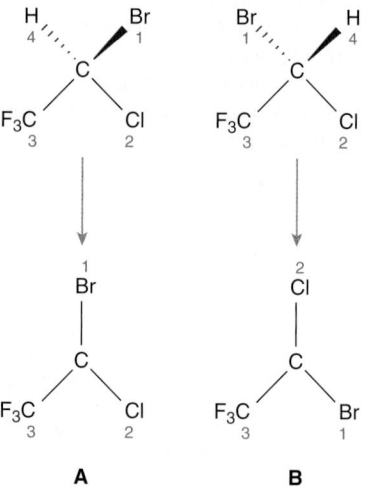

FIGURE 10–10. R and S enantiomers of halothane. (**A**) The substituents increase in a clockwise fashion, so the configuration is R. (**B**) The substituents increase in a counterclockwise fashion, so the configuration is S. In this projection, hydrogen atoms are directly behind the carbon atoms.

$$CH_3 - O - CH_3 \qquad CH_3 - CH_2 - OH$$

A   **B**

FIGURE 10–8. Two molecules with chemical formula C_2H_6O. (**A**) Dimethylether. (**B**) Ethanol (ethyl alcohol).

this is the case for halothane, whose *R* and *S* enantiomers interact with cell membranes rather than specific receptors and possess equal activity. Second, if a glove is constructed with greater (but imperfect) specificity, one hand will fit well and the other poorly; this is the case for many substances, such as epinephrine and norepinephrine, whose naturally occurring levorotatory enantiomers are 10-fold more potent than the synthetic dextrorotatory enantiomers. Finally, a glove can be made with exquisite precision, such that one hand fits perfectly, while the other hand does not fit at all. This is the case for physostigmine, in which the (–) enantiomer is biologically active whereas the (+) enantiomer is not.

Even the above analogy is oversimplified, however, as there are examples where one enantiomer of a drug is an agonist whereas the other enantiomer is an antagonist. Dobutamine, has one stereogenic carbon and thus 2 stereoisomers; at the α_1-adrenergic receptor, *l*-dobutamine is a potent agonist and *d*-dobutamine is a potent antagonist. Because dobutamine is marketed as a *racemic mixture* (a racemic mixture is a 1:1 mixture of enantiomers), however, these effects cancel each other out. Interestingly, at the β_1-adrenergic receptor, *d*- and *l*-dobutamine have unequal agonist effects, with *d*-dobutamine approximately 10 times more potent than *l*-dobutamine.

Functional Groups

There is perhaps no concept in organic chemistry as powerful as that of the *functional group*. Functional groups are atoms or groups of atoms that confer similar reactivity on a molecule; of less importance is the molecule to which it is attached. *Alcohols, carboxylic acids*, and *thiols* are functional groups; *hydrocarbons* are generally not considered functional groups per se, but rather are the structural backbone to which functional groups are attached. The functional groups discussed below are included to illustrate important principles, not because they represent an exhaustive list of important functional groups in toxicology.

Hydrocarbons, as their name implies, consist of only carbon and hydrogen. *Alkanes* are hydrocarbons that contain no multiple bonds; they are straight chain, usually designated by the prefix *n*- as in *n*-butane (Fig. 10–11A) or iso- if branched, as in isobutane (Fig. 10–11B). *Alkenes* contain carbon-carbon double bonds. *Alkynes*, which contain carbon-carbon triple bonds, are of limited toxicologic importance. Butane (found in lighter fluid) is an alkane, and gasoline is a mixture of alkanes.

Hydrocarbons are of toxicologic importance for 2 reasons. They are widely abused as inhalational drugs for their central nervous system (CNS) depressant effects, and cause profound toxicity when aspirated. Although these effects are physiologically disparate, they are readily understood in the context of the chemical characteristics of the hydrocarbon functional group.

Hydrocarbons do not contain *polar groups* (ie, groups that introduce full or partial charges into the molecule). As such, they interact readily with other nonpolar substances, such as lipids or lipophilic substances. Hydrocarbons readily interact with the myelin of the CNS, disrupting normal ion channel function and causing CNS depression. When aspirated, hydrocarbons interact with the fatty acid tail of surfactant, dissolving this protective substance and contributing to acute respiratory distress syndrome (Chap. 105).

Alcohols possess the hydroxyl (–OH) functional group, which adds polarity to the molecule and makes alcohols highly soluble in other polar substances, such as water. For example, ethane gas (CH_3CH_3) has negligible solubility in water, whereas ethanol (CH_3CH_2OH) is *miscible*, or infinitely soluble, in water. In biologic systems, alcohols are generally CNS depressants,

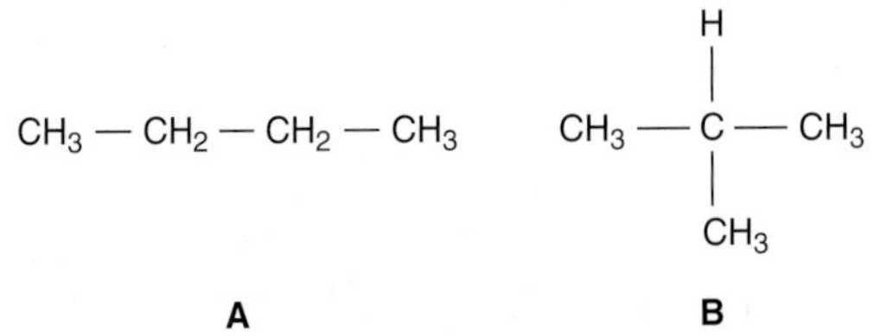

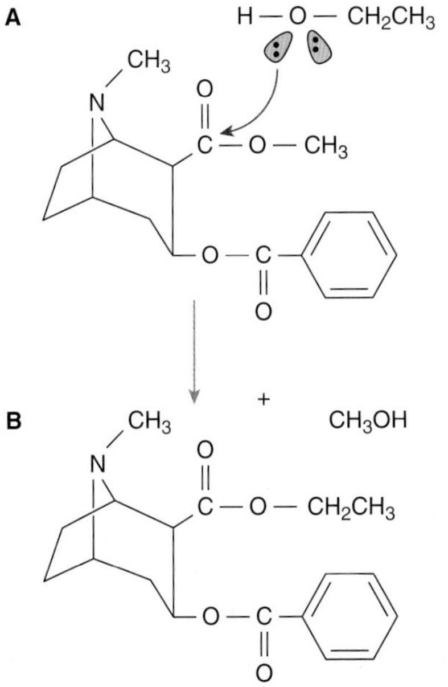

FIGURE 10–12. Transesterification reaction of cocaine with ethanol (**A**) to form cocaethylene and methanol (**B**).

but they can also act as nucleophiles. Ethanol reacts with cocaine to form cocaethylene, a longer-acting and more vasoactive substance than cocaine itself (Fig. 10–12) (Chap. 75).

Alcohols are categorized as primary, secondary, or tertiary, in which the reference carbon is bonded to 1, 2, or 3 carbons (respectively) in addition to the hydroxyl group. Methanol, in which the reference carbon is bonded to no other carbons, is not a primary alcohol per se but shares many of the reactivity patterns of primary alcohols. The difference between primary, secondary, and tertiary structures is important, because although the alcohol functional group imparts many qualities to the molecule, the degree of substitution can affect the chemical reactivity. Primary alcohols can undergo multistep oxidation to form carboxylic acids, whereas secondary alcohols generally undergo one-step metabolism to form ketones, and tertiary alcohols do not readily undergo oxidation. This is a point of significant toxicologic importance, and is discussed in more detail below.

Alcohols are named in several ways; the most common is to add *-ol* or *-yl alcohol* to the appropriate prefix. If the alcohol group is bonded to an interior carbon, the number to which the carbon is bonded precedes the suffix.

Carboxylic acids contain the functional group –COOH. As their name implies, they are (weakly) acidic, and the pK_a of carboxylic acids is generally 4 or 5, depending on the substitution of the molecule. Small-molecular-weight carboxylic acids are capable of producing an elevated anion gap metabolic acidosis, which is true whether the acids are endogenous or exogenous. Examples of endogenous acids are β-hydroxybutyric acid and lactic acid; examples of exogenous acids are formic acid (produced by the metabolism of methanol) and glycolic, glyoxylic, and oxalic acids (produced by the metabolism of ethylene glycol). Carboxylic acids are named by adding *-oic acid* to the appropriate prefix; the 4-carbon straight-chain carboxylic acid is thus butanoic acid.

Thiols contain a sulfur atom, which usually functions as a nucleophile. The sulfur atom of *N*-acetylcysteine regenerates glutathione reductase and also reacts directly with NAPQI to detoxify this electrophile. The sulfur atoms of many chelators, such as dimercaprol and succimer, are nucleophiles that are very effective at chelating electrophiles such as heavy metals. Thiols are generally named by adding the word *thiol* to the appropriate base. Thus, a 2-carbon thiol is ethane thiol.

As noted above, molecules with a given functional group often have more in common with molecules with the same functional group than they have in common with the molecules from which they were derived. The alkanes

FIGURE 10–11. Two isomers of the 4-carbon alkane, butane. (**A**) *n*-Butane. (**B**) Isobutane.

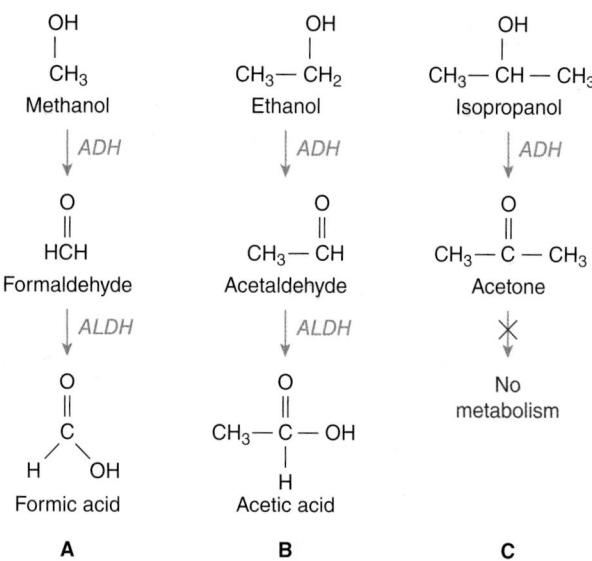

FIGURE 10–13. Oxidative metabolism of (**A**) methanol, (**B**) ethanol, and (**C**) isopropanol. Note that acetone does not undergo further oxidation in vivo. ADH = alcohol dehydrogenase; ALDH = aldehyde dehydrogenase.

methane, ethane, and propane are straight-chain hydrocarbons with similar properties. All are gases at room temperature, have almost no solubility in water, and have similar melting and boiling points. When these molecules are substituted with one or more hydroxide functional groups, they become alcohols: examples are methanol, ethanol, ethylene glycol (a *glycol* is a molecule that contains 2 alcohol functional groups), the primary alcohol 1-propanol, and the secondary alcohol 2-propanol (isopropanol). Each of these alcohols is a liquid at room temperature, and all are very soluble in water. All have boiling points that are markedly different from the alkane from which they were derived, and are very close to each other.

In addition to conferring different physical properties on the molecule, the addition of the alcohol functional group also confers different chemical properties and reactivities. For example, methane, ethane, and propane are virtually incapable of undergoing oxidation in biologic systems. The alcohols formed by the addition of one or more hydroxyl groups, however, are readily oxidized by alcohol dehydrogenase (Fig. 10–13).

As Fig. 10–13 indicates, the oxidation of the primary alcohols methanol and ethanol results in the formation of *aldehydes* (functional groups in which a carbon atom contains a double bond to oxygen and a single bond to hydrogen), whereas the oxidation of the secondary alcohol isopropanol results in the formation of a *ketone* (a functional group in which a carbon is double-bonded to an oxygen atom and single-bonded to 2 separate carbon atoms). Although both aldehydes and ketones contain the *carbonyl group* (a carbon-oxygen double bond), aldehydes and ketones are distinctly different functional groups, and they have different reactivity patterns. For instance, aldehydes can undergo enzymatic oxidation to carboxylic acids (Figs. 10–13A and 13B), whereas ketones cannot (Fig. 10–13C).

It is here that recognition of functional groups helps to understand the potential toxicity of an alcohol. Methanol, ethanol, and isopropanol are all alcohols; as such, their toxicity before metabolism is expected to be (and in fact is) quite similar to that of ethanol, producing CNS sedation. Because these toxins are primary and secondary alcohols, all can be metabolized to a carbonyl compound, either an aldehyde or a ketone. Here, however, the functional groups on the molecules have changed; whereas aldehydes can undergo metabolism to carboxylic acids (which can, in turn, cause an anion gap acidosis), ketones cannot. It is for this reason that methanol and ethylene glycol cause an anion gap acidosis whereas isopropanol does not (Chap. 106).

The concept of functional groups, however useful, has limitations. For example, although both formic acid and oxalic acid are organic acids, they cause different patterns of organ system toxicity. Formic acid is a mitochondrial toxin and exerts effects primarily in areas (such as the retina or basal ganglia) that poorly tolerate an interruption in the energy supplied by oxidative phosphorylation. Conversely, oxalic acid readily precipitates calcium and is toxic to renal tubular cells, which accounts for the nephrotoxicity that is characteristic of severe ethylene glycol poisoning. The concept of the functional group is thus an aid to understanding chemical reactivity, but not a substitute for a working knowledge of the toxicokinetic or toxicodynamic effects of xenobiotics in living systems.

SUMMARY

- Understanding key principles of inorganic and organic chemistry provide insight into the mechanisms by which xenobiotics function.
- The periodic table forms the basis for understanding inorganic chemistry and provides insight into the expected reactivity, and to a large extent the clinical effects, of an element.
- A growing understanding of how reactive species are formed and how they interfere with physiologic processes has led to new insights in the pathogenesis and treatment of toxin-mediated diseases.
- Changes in functional groups on organic molecules dramatically changes their chemical and toxicologic effects, and knowing the relevant general principles is essential to an understanding of biochemistry and pharmacology.

REFERENCES

1. Aaseth J, et al. Chelation in metal intoxication—Principles and paradigms. *J Trace Elem Med Biol.* 2015;31:260-266.
2. Fluck E. New notations in the periodic table. *Pure Appl Chem.* 1988;60:431-436.
3. Jomova K, Valko M. Advances in metal-induced oxidative stress and human disease. *Toxicology.* 2011;283:65-87.
4. Liochev SI. Reactive oxygen species and the free radical theory of aging. *Free Radical Biol Med.* 2013;60(C):1-4.
5. Manahan SE. *Fundamentals of Environmental and Toxicological Chemistry.* 4th ed. Boca Raton, FL: CRC Press; 2013.
6. Smith SW. Chiral toxicology: it's the same thing...only different. *Toxicol Sci.* 2009;110:4-30.
7. Winkler DA, et al. Applying quantitative structure–activity relationship approaches to nanotoxicology: Current status and future potential. *Toxicology.* 2013;313:15-23.

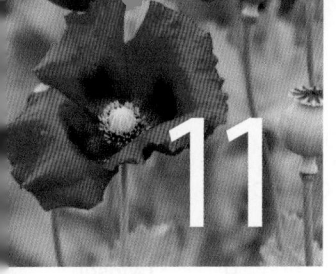

11 BIOCHEMICAL AND METABOLIC PRINCIPLES

James D. Cao and Kurt C. Kleinschmidt

Xenobiotics are compounds that are foreign to a living system. Toxic xenobiotics interfere with critical metabolic processes, cause structural damage to cells, or alter cellular genetic material. The specific biochemical sites of actions that disrupt metabolic processes are well characterized for many xenobiotics although mechanisms of cellular injury are not. This chapter reviews the biochemical principles that are relevant to an understanding of the biotransformation enzymes and their clinical implications and the damaging effects of toxic xenobiotics.

XENOBIOTIC CHARACTERISTICS AND TOXICITY

The capacity of a xenobiotic to produce injury is affected by many factors, including its absorption, distribution, elimination, genotypic/phenotypic states, synergistic/antagonistic coingestants, site of activation or detoxication, and site of action. This section focuses on how the route of exposure (absorption) and the ability to cross membranes in order to access particular organs (distribution) affect toxicity.

The route of exposure to a xenobiotic often confines damage primarily to one organ, for example, pulmonary injury that follows inhalation of an irritant gas or gastrointestinal (GI) injury that follows ingestion of a caustic. However, most xenobiotics have lipophilic properties that facilitate absorption across cell membranes of organs that are portals of entry into the body: the skin, GI tract, and lungs. Systemically circulating xenobiotics, such as cyanide or carbon monoxide, affect toxicity in multiple organs. The liver is particularly susceptible to xenobiotic-induced injury as it receives blood supply from both the portal venous system and from the hepatic artery containing xenobiotics absorbed from multiple sites of exposure.

Once systemically absorbed, various factors affect the distribution of a xenobiotic to a particular organ, including its molecular weight, protein binding, plasma pH/drug pKa, lipophilicity, in addition to the presence of membrane transporters, and physiologic barriers (Chap. 9). Restriction of distribution or preferential distribution into a target organ determines the ability of a xenobiotic to mediate tissue injury. For example, many potentially toxic xenobiotics fail to produce central nervous system (CNS) injury because they cannot cross the blood–brain barrier. The negligible CNS effects of the mercuric salts when compared with organic mercury compounds are related to their relative inability to penetrate the CNS. With respect to target organs, 2 potent biologic xenobiotics—ricin (from *Ricinus communis*) and α-amanitin (from *Amanita phalloides*)—block protein synthesis through the inhibition of RNA polymerase. However, they result in different clinical effects because they access different tissues. Ricin has a special binding protein that enables it to gain access to the endoplasmic reticulum in GI mucosal cells, where it inhibits cellular protein synthesis and causes severe diarrhea. α-Amanitin is transported into hepatocytes by bile salt transport systems, where inhibition of protein synthesis results in cell death. Finally, the electrical charge of a xenobiotic at tissue pH affects its ability to enter a cell. Unlike the ionized (charged) form of a xenobiotic, the un-ionized (uncharged) form is often lipophilic and passes through lipid cell membranes to enter the cells. The pK_a of an acidic xenobiotic ($HA \rightleftharpoons A^- + H^+$) is the pH at which 50% of the molecules are ionized (A^- form) and 50% is un-ionized (HA form). A xenobiotic with a low pK_a is more likely to be absorbed in an acidic environment in which the un-ionized form predominates. This conept is the basis for urine alkalinization and ion trapping in the management of salicylate toxicity (Chap. 37).

GENERAL ENZYME CONCEPTS

The capability to detoxify and eliminate both endogenous toxins and xenobiotics is crucial to the maintenance of physiologic homeostasis. A simple example is the detoxification of cyanide, a potent cellular poison that is

$$\begin{array}{c} NADH + H^+ \qquad NAD^+ \\ Drug\text{-}H + O_2 \xrightarrow[CYP]{} Drug\text{-}OH + H_2O \end{array}$$

FIGURE 11–1. A common oxidation reaction catalyzed by CYP enzymes: the hydroxylation of Drug-H to Drug-OH.

common in the environment and is also a product of normal metabolism. Mammals have evolved to have the enzyme rhodanese, which combines cyanide with thiosulfate to create the less toxic, renally excreted compound thiocyanate.[7]

The liver has the highest concentration of enzymes that metabolize xenobiotics. Enzymes found in the cytosol of hepatocytes that are specific for alcohols, aldehydes, esters, or amines act on many different substrates within these broad chemical classes. Enzymes that act on more lipophilic xenobiotics, including the cytochrome enzymes, are embedded in the lipid membranes of the cytosol-based endoplasmic reticulum. Cytochromes are a class of hemoprotein enzymes whose function is electron transfer, using a cyclical transfer of electrons between oxidized (Fe^{3+}) or reduced (Fe^{2+}) forms of iron. One type of cytochrome is cytochrome P450 (CYP) whose nomenclature derives from the spectrophotometric characteristics of its associated heme molecule. When bound to carbon monoxide, the maximal absorption spectrum of the reduced CYP (Fe^{2+}) enzyme occurs at 450 nm.[79] These CYP enzymes commonly split the 2 oxygen atoms of an oxygen molecule, incorporating one into the substrate and one into water and thus are called mixed-function oxidases or monooxygenases (Fig. 11–1). This differs from dioxygenases that incorporate both oxygen atoms into the substrate.[79,108]

Microsomes are the pieces of the endoplasmic reticulum that result when cells are disrupted. When cells are mechanically disrupted and centrifuged, these membrane-bound enzymes are found in the pellet, or microsomal fraction; hence, they are called *microsomal enzymes*. Enzymes located in the liquid matrix of cells are called *cytosolic enzymes* and are found in the supernatant when disrupted cells are centrifuged.[22]

BIOTRANSFORMATION OVERVIEW

The study of xenobiotic metabolism was established as a scientific discipline by the seminal publication of Williams in 1949.[120] Biotransformation is the physiochemical alteration of a xenobiotic, usually as a result of enzyme action. Most definitions also include that this action converts lipophilic substances into more polar, excretable substances.[70,108] Most xenobiotics undergo some biotransformation, the degree of which is affected by their chemical nature. The hydrophilic nature of ionized compounds such as carboxylic acids enables the kidneys to rapidly eliminate them. Very volatile compounds, such as enflurane, are expelled promptly via the lungs. Neither of these groups of xenobiotics undergo significant enzymatic metabolism.

Biotransformation usually results in "detoxification," a reduction in the toxicity, by the conversion to hydrophilic metabolites of the xenobiotic that can be renally eliminated.[70] However, this is not always the case. Many parent xenobiotics are inactive and must undergo "metabolic activation."[72] When metabolites are more toxic than the parent xenobiotic, biotransformation is said to have resulted in "toxification."[108] Biotransformation via acetylation or methylation enhances the lipophilicity of a xenobiotic. Biotransformation is accomplished by impressively few enzymes, reflecting broad substrate specificity. The predominant pathway for the biotransformation of an individual xenobiotic is determined by many factors, including the availability of cofactors, changes in the concentration of the enzyme caused by induction, and the presence of inhibitors. The predominant pathway is also affected by the rate of substrate metabolism, reflected by the K_m (Michaelis–Menten dissociation constant) of the biotransformation enzyme (Chap. 9).[108]

Biotransformation is often divided into phase I and phase II reactions, terminology first introduced in 1959.[120] Phase I reactions prepare lipophilic xenobiotics for the addition of functional groups or actually add the groups, converting them into more chemically reactive metabolites. This is usually followed by phase II synthetic reactions that conjugate the reactive products of phase I with other molecules that render them more water soluble, further detoxifying the xenobiotics and facilitating renal elimination. However, biotransformation often does not follow this stepwise process.[52] Some xenobiotics undergo only a phase I or a phase II reaction prior to elimination. Additionally, phase II reactions can precede phase I. While virtually all phase II synthesis reactions cause inactivation, a classic exception is fluoroacetate being metabolized to fluorocitrate, a potent inhibitor of the citric acid (tricarboxylic acid, or Krebs) cycle (Chap. 113).[90]

Biotransformed xenobiotics cannot be eliminated until they are moved back across cell membranes and out of the cells. Membrane transporters are proteins that move endobiotics/xenobiotics across the membranes without altering their chemical compositions Most membrane transporters are in the adenosine triphosphate binding cassette (ABC) family of transmembrane proteins that use energy from adenosine triphosphate (ATP) hydrolysis to move xenobiotics.[14,45,52] This family includes the P-glycoprotein family and the glutathione S-conjugate export pump.[103] The process of transport is sometimes termed a "phase III reaction." However, membrane transport does not always occur after phase I or II reactions, and some parent compounds, such as digoxin, are transported across membranes without any biotransformation at all.[25]

Phase I Biotransformation Reactions

Oxidation is the predominant phase I reaction, adding reactive functional groups suitable for synthetic conjugation during phase II. These groups include hydroxyl (–OH), sulfhydryl (–SH), amino (–NH$_2$), aldehyde (–CHO), or carboxyl (–COOH) moieties. Noncarbon elements such as nitrogen, sulfur, and phosphorus are also oxidized in phase I reactions. Other phase I reactions include hydrolysis (the splitting of a large molecule by the addition of water that is divided among the 2 products), hydration (incorporation of water into a complex molecule), hydroxylation (the attachment of –OH groups to carbon atoms), reduction, dehalogenation, dehydrogenation, and dealkylation.[70,108]

The CYP enzymes are the most numerous and important of the phase I enzymes. A common oxidation reaction catalyzed by CYP enzymes is illustrated by the hydroxylation of a xenobiotic R–H to R–OH (Fig. 11–1).[30] Membrane-bound flavin monooxygenase (FMO), a nicotinamide adenine dinucleotide phosphate (NADPH)-dependent oxidase located in the endoplasmic reticulum, is an important oxidizer of amines and other compounds containing nitrogen, sulfur, or phosphorus.[70]

The alcohol, aldehyde, and ketone oxidation systems use predominantly cytosolic enzymes that catalyze these reactions using nicotinamide adenine dinucleotide (NADH/NAD$^+$), but alcohol oxidation can also occur in microsomes via CYP enzymes and in peroxisomes via the enzyme catalase (Fig. 11–2).[65,108,123] Two classic phase I oxidation reactions are the metabolism of ethanol to acetaldehyde by alcohol dehydrogenase (ADH) followed by the metabolism of acetaldehyde to acetic acid by aldehyde dehydrogenase (ALDH). Alcohol dehydrogenase, which oxidizes many different alcohols, is found in the liver, lungs, kidneys, and gastric mucosa.[65] Variations in these enzymes have clinical implications. For example, young women have less ADH in their gastric mucosa than young men. This results in decreased first-pass metabolism of ethanol and increased ethanol absorption. Some populations, particularly Asians, are deficient in ALDH, resulting in increased acetaldehyde concentrations and symptoms (Chap. 78).[65]

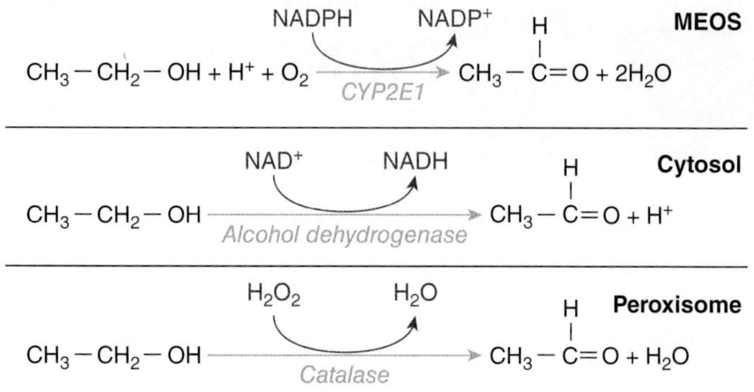

FIGURE 11–2. The conversion of ethanol to acetaldehyde by three pathways. In the microsomal ethanol oxidizing system (MEOS), CYP2E1 uses nicotinamide adenine dinucleotide phosphate (NADPH) and oxygen for the conversion. In the cytosol, alcohol dehydrogenase uses NAD$^+$. In peroxisomes, catalase uses H$_2$O$_2$. This illustrates how NAD$^+$ and NADPH can function in oxidation reactions in both their oxidized and reduced forms. Alcohol dehydrogenase has a low K_m for ethanol and is the predominant metabolic enzyme in moderate drinkers. *(Adapted with permission from Zakhari S: Overview: how is alcohol metabolized by the body? Alcohol Res Health 2006;29(4):245-254.)*

Oxidation Overview

Biotransformation often results in the oxidation or reduction of carbon. A substrate is oxidized when it transfers electrons to an electron-seeking (electrophilic or oxidizing) molecule, leading to reduction of the electrophilic molecule. These oxidation-reduction reactions are usually coupled to the cyclical oxidation and reduction of a cofactor, such as the pyridine nucleotides, NADH/NAD$^+$, or NADPH/NADP$^+$. The nucleotides alternate between their reduced (NADPH, NADH) and oxidized (NADP$^+$, NAD$^+$) forms. Because xenobiotic oxidation is the most common phase I reaction, the newly created reduced cofactors must have a place to unload their electrons; otherwise, biotransformation ends. The electron transport chain serves as the major electron recipient.

Electrons resulting from the catabolism of energy sources are extracted primarily by NAD$^+$, forming NADH. Within the mitochondria, NADH transports its electrons to the cytochrome-mediated electron transport chain. This results in the production of ATP, the reduction of molecular oxygen to water, and the regeneration of NAD$^+$—all parts critical to the maintenance of oxidative metabolism. Nicotinamide adenine dinucleotide phosphate, generated by the hexose monophosphate shunt, is used in the synthetic (anabolic) reactions of biosynthesis (especially fatty acid synthesis). Nicotinamide adenine dinucleotide phosphate is also the cofactor in the reduction of glutathione, a molecule vital to the protection of cells from oxidative damage.

Biotransformation often results in the oxidation or reduction of carbon. The oxidation state of a specific carbon atom is determined by counting the number of hydrogen and carbon atoms to which it is connected. The more reduced a carbon, the higher the number of connections. For example, the carbon in methanol (CH$_3$OH) has 3 carbon–hydrogen bonds and is more reduced than the carbon in formaldehyde (H$_2$C=O), which has two. Carbon–carbon double bonds count as only one connection.

Cytochrome Enzymes—An Overview

Cytochrome enzymes perform many functions. The biotransformation CYP enzymes are bound to the lipid membranes of the smooth endoplasmic reticulum. They execute 75% of all xenobiotic metabolism and most phase I oxidative biotransformations of xenobiotics.[39] A second role for CYP enzymes is synthetic: biotransforming endobiotics (chemicals endogenous to the body) to cholesterol, steroids, bile acids, fatty acids, prostaglandins, and other important lipids. Cytochromes also act within the mitochondrial electron transport chain.[41,78]

Although more than 6,000 CYP genes exist in nature, the human genome project determined that the number of human CYP genes was 57.[78] Cytochrome P450 enzymes are categorized according to the similarities of their amino acid sequences. They are in the same "family" if they are more than 40% comparable and same "subfamily" if they are more than 55% similar.[77] Families are designated by an Arabic numeral (n), subfamilies by a

TABLE 11–1	Characteristics of Different Cytochrome P450 Enzymes[26,33,123]						
CYP Enzyme	1A2	2B6	2C9	2C19	2D6	2E1	3A4
Percent of liver CYPs	4%–16%	2%–5%	5%–29%	1%–4%	1%–4%	6%–17%	15%–37%
Contribution to enterocyte CYPs	None	None	Minor	Minor	Minor	Minor	70%
Organs other than liver with enzyme	Lung	Kidney	Small intestine, nasal mucosa, heart	Small intestine, nasal mucosa, heart	Small intestine, kidney, lung, heart	Lung, small intestine, kidney	Much in small intestine; some in kidney, nasal mucosa, lung, stomach
Percent of metabolism of typically used pharmaceuticals	9%	7%	13%	7%	20%	3%	30%
Polymorphisms[a]	No	Yes	Yes	Yes	Yes	No	No
Allelic Frequency							
Decreased Activity							
African American		38%–62%	0%–3%	10%–17%	14%–30%		
Asian	—	14%–25%	2%–8%	25%–39%	47%–94%	—	—
Caucasian		23%–39%	16%–23%	6%–16%	31%–45%		
Increased Activity							
African American		0%–25%		15%–27%			
Asian	—	5%–15%	—	0%–2%	1%		
Caucasian		6%		21%–25%	1%–9%		
Ethiopian					30%		

[a] Polymorphism is a genetic change that exists in at least 1% of the human population. Interpersonal allelic variations exist even in those listed as "No" for polymorphism.

capital letter (X), and each individual enzyme by another numeral (m), resulting in the nomenclature CYPnXm for each enzyme. For example, CYP3A4 is enzyme number 4 of the CYP3A subfamily of the CYP3 family.[74] Genes coding for these enzymes contain sequence variations, designated by italicized style and an asterisk followed by an Arabic numeral (ie, *CYP2D6*4*), that lead to functional differences.[49,74] An allele is a form of a gene that often arises through mutation. If the same gene variation exists in greater than 1% of the human population, then the allele is termed a genetic polymorphism. Most xenobiotic metabolism is done by the CYP1, CYP2, and CYP3 families, with a small amount done by the CYP4 family.[13,117] Although 15 CYP enzymes metabolize xenobiotics,[86] nearly 90% is done by 6 CYP enzymes: 1A2, 2C9, 2C19, 2D6, 2E1, and 3A4 (Table 11–1).[78]

Most CYP enzymes are found in the liver, where they comprise 2% of the total microsomal protein.[86] High concentrations are also found in extrahepatic tissues, particularly the GI tract and kidney.[26,80] The lungs,[126] heart,[84] and brain[27] have the next highest amounts. Each tissue has a unique profile of CYP enzymes that determines its sensitivity to different xenobiotics.[26] The CYP enzymes in the enterocytes of the small intestine actually contribute significantly to "first-pass" metabolism of some xenobiotics.[56,78] Corrected for tissue mass, the CYP enzyme system in the kidneys is as active as that in the liver. The activity of the renal CYP enzymes is decreased in patients with chronic kidney disease, with relative sparing of CYPs 1A2, 2C19, and 2D6 compared with 3A4 and 2C9.[13]

Cytochrome P450 Enzyme Specificity for Substrates

In vitro models are used to define the specificities of CYP enzymes for their substrates and inhibitors. However, activity in a test tube does not always correlate with that in a cell. These models use substrate and inhibitor concentrations that are much higher than would be encountered in vivo, and the mathematical models that extrapolate to clinically relevant processes yield conflicting results. Discrepancies in reported substrates, inhibitors, and inducers of specific CYP enzymes results.[119]

Most CYP enzymes involved in xenobiotic biotransformation have broad substrate specificity and can metabolize many xenobiotics.[39] This is fortunate because the number of xenobiotic substrates likely already exceeds

200,000 and continues to grow.[64] Broad substrate specificity often results in multiple CYP enzymes being able to biotransform the same xenobiotic. This enables the ongoing biotransformation despite an inhibition or deficiency of an enzyme. When a substrate is biotransformed by more than one enzyme, the enzyme with the highest affinity for the substrate usually predominates at low substrate concentrations, whereas enzymes with lower affinity become important at high concentrations. This transition is usually concomitant with, but not dependent on, the saturation of the catalytic capacity of the primary enzyme as it reaches its maximum rate of activity.[39] The K_m, which is defined as the concentration of substrate that results in 50% of maximal enzyme activity, describes this property of enzymes. For example, ADH in the liver has a very low K_m for ethanol, making it the primary metabolic enzyme for ethanol when concentrations are low.[65] Ethanol is also biotransformed by the CYP2E1 enzyme, which has a high K_m for ethanol and only functions when ethanol concentrations are high. The CYP2E1 enzyme metabolizes little ethanol in moderate drinkers but accounts for significantly more biotransformation in alcoholics, as it is also inducible. As another example, diazepam is metabolized by both CYP2C19 and CYP3A4 enzymes. However, the affinity of CYP3A4 for diazepam is so low (ie, the K_m is high) that most diazepam is metabolized by CYP2C19.[44]

The substrate selectivity of some CYP enzymes is determined by molecular and physicochemical properties of the substrates. The CYP1A subfamily has greater specificity for planar polyaromatic substrates such as benzo[*a*]pyrene. The CYP2E enzyme subfamily targets low-molecular-weight hydrophilic xenobiotics, whereas the CYP3A4 enzyme has increased affinity for lipophilic compounds. Substrates of CYP2C9 are usually weakly acidic, whereas those of CYP2D6 are more basic.[64] High specificity also results from key structural considerations such as stereoselectivity. Some xenobiotics are racemic mixtures of 2 stereoisomers that are substrates for different CYP enzymes and have distinct affinities for the enzymes, resulting in different rates of metabolism. For example, *R*-warfarin is biotransformed by CYP3A4 and CYP1A2, whereas *S*-warfarin is metabolized by CYP2C9.[97]

The CYP enzymes that biotransform a specific xenobiotic cannot be predicted by its drug class. For example, the selective serotonin reuptake inhibitors (SSRIs) fluoxetine and paroxetine are both major substrates and potent inhibitors of CYP2D6, but sertraline is not extensively metabolized by this enzyme and exhibits minimal interaction with other antidepressants.[5] Most β-hydroxy-β-methylglutarylcoenzyme A (HMG-CoA) reductase inhibitors are metabolized by CYP3A4 (lovastatin, simvastatin, and atorvastatin); however, fluvastatin is metabolized by CYP2D6, and pravastatin undergoes virtually no CYP enzyme metabolism at all.[69] Among angiotensin-II receptor blockers, losartan and irbesartan are metabolized by CYP2C9, whereas valsartan, eprosartan, and candesartan are not substrates for any CYP enzyme. In addition, losartan is a prodrug whose active metabolite provides most of the pharmacologic activity, whereas irbesartan is the primary active compound. For these 2 drugs, the inhibition of CYP2C9 is predicted to have opposite effects.[31]

Cytochrome P450 and Drug–Drug/Drug–Xenobiotic Interactions

Adverse reactions to medications and drug–drug interactions are common causes of morbidity and mortality, the risk of which increases with the number of drugs taken (Chaps. 134 and 135). As many as 50% of adverse reactions are related to pharmacogenetic factors.[34] The most significant interactions are mediated by CYP enzymes.[78] The impacts of genetic polymorphism and enzyme induction or inhibition are addressed below.

The CYP enzymes are involved in many types of drug interactions. The ability of potential new drugs to induce or inhibit enzymes is an important consideration of industry. Drug development focuses on the potential of new xenobiotics to induce or inhibit other drugs or enzymes during the drug discovery phase. Various in vitro models enable this early determination.[66]

Many xenobiotics interact with the CYP enzymes. St. John's wort, an herb marketed as a natural antidepressant, induces multiple CYP enzymes, including 1A2, 2C9, and 3A4. The induction of CYP3A4 by St. John's wort is associated with a 57% decrease in effective serum concentrations of indinavir when given concomitantly.[88] Xenobiotics contained in grapefruit juice, such as naringin and furanocoumarins, are both substrates and inhibitors of CYP3A4. They inhibit the first-pass metabolism of CYP3A4 substrates by inhibiting CYP3A4 activity in both the GI tract and the liver.[21] Polycyclic hydrocarbons found in charbroiled meats and in cigarette smoke induce CYP1A2. Thus, for smokers who drink coffee, concentrations of caffeine, a CYP1A2 substrate, will increase following a permanent cessation of smoking.[30]

Genetic Polymorphism

The response to xenobiotics and to coadministration of inhibitory or inducing xenobiotics is highly variable. The translation of DNA sequences into proteins results in the phenotypic expression of the genes. When a genetic mutation occurs, the changed DNA may continue to exist, be eliminated, or propagate into a polymorphism. A polymorphism is a genetic change that exists in at least 1% of the human population.[34,74] A polymorphism in a biotransformation enzyme may change its rate of activity. The heterogeneity of CYP enzymes contributes to the differences in metabolic activity among patients.[34] Differences in biotransformation capacity that lead to toxicity, once thought to be "idiosyncratic" drug reactions, are likely caused by these inherited differences in the genetic complement of individuals.

An individual with 2 CYP alleles of "normal" catalytic speed is called extensive metabolizer, which usually represents a majority of the population. There are 3 major metabolizer phenotypes due to polymorphism: poor, intermediate, and ultrarapid. Poor and intermediate metabolizers have either loss-of-function variants or absent CYP alleles. Poor metabolizers have 2 inactive or absent alleles, whereas intermediate metabolizers will have either 2 reduced function alleles or one "normal" allele with one inactive or absent allele. On the other hand, an ultrarapid metabolizer will have either gain-of-function variants or gene duplication.[34,125] The *CYP2C19* and *CYP2D6* genes are highly polymorphic (Table 11–1). The *CYP2D6* gene, which has 157 alleles, is associated with both ultrarapid and poor metabolism.[49] The *CYP2C19* and *CYP2C9* genes are both associated with polymorphisms, resulting in poor metabolizers.[13,78]

The clinical implications of polymorphisms are vast. Prodrugs have limited activation in patients who are poor metabolizers. For example, clopidogrel mediates antiplatelet effects via an active thiol metabolite generated by CYP enzymes. Individuals with the loss-of-function *CYP2C19*2* allele have decreased generation of the active metabolite, decreased antiplatelet effects, and increased cardiovascular events while on clopidogrel.[55,99] Conversely, some ultrarapid metabolizers generate toxic concentrations of an active metabolic. Codeine (inactive) metabolizes to morphine (active) via CYP2D6. Ultrarapid metabolizers with CYP2D6 can have 2 to 13 copies of the gene leading to rapid conversion of codeine to morphine and as a consequence toxicity.[67] Finally, some active drugs with inactive metabolites fail to reach therapeutic concentrations in patients who are ultrarapid metabolizers.[34]

Polymorphisms exist for enzymes other than CYP enzymes. A classic example is the inheritance of rapid or slow "acetylator" phenotypes. Acetylation is important for the biotransformation of amines ($R–NH_2$) or hydrazines ($NH_2–NH_2$). Slow acetylators are at increased risk of toxicity associated with the slower biotransformation of certain nitrogen-containing xenobiotics such as isoniazid, procainamide, hydralazine, and sulfonamides.[101] Genetic polymorphism of UDP-glucuronosyl transferase 2B17 (UGT2B17) contributes to a bimodal distribution of urinary conjugated testosterone excretion. Since the testosterone isomer, epitestosterone, has little genetic variation and is not affected by testosterone metabolism, an elevated testosterone:epistestosterone (T:E) is indicative of the exogenous administration of testosterone.[115] The World Anti-Doping Agency sets the suspicious threshold ratio of T:E ratio at 4:1 in response to genetic variations.[95,121] Athletes with homozygote deletions of UGT2B17 have less conjugation of testosterone and have had false negative testing using the previous ratio of 6:1 (Chap. 41).[51]

Polymorphic genes that code for enzymes in important metabolic pathways affect the toxicity of a xenobiotic by altering the response to, or the disposition of, the xenobiotic. An example occurs in patients with glucose-6-phosphate dehydrogenase (G6PD) deficiency. Glucose-6-phosphate dehydrogenase is a critical enzyme in the hexose monophosphate shunt, a metabolic pathway located in the red blood cell (RBC) that produces NADPH, which is required to maintain RBC glutathione in a reduced state. In turn, reduced glutathione prevents hemolysis during oxidative stress.[15] In patients deficient in G6PD, oxidative stress produced by electrophilic xenobiotics results in hemolysis.

Induction of CYP Enzymes

Biotransformation by induced CYP enzymes results in either increased activity of prodrugs or enhanced elimination of drugs. Stopping an inducer results in the opposite effects. Either way, maintaining therapeutic concentrations of affected drugs is difficult, resulting in either toxic or subtherapeutic concentrations. Interestingly, not all CYP enzymes are inducible. The inducible enzymes include CYP1A, CYP2A, CYP2B, CYP2C, CYP2E, and CYP3A.[66]

Although varied mechanisms of induction exist, the most common and significant is nuclear receptor (NR)-mediated increase in gene transcription.[66] Nuclear receptors are the largest group of transcription factors (proteins) that switch genes on or off.[113] They regulate reproduction, growth, and biotransformation enzymes, including CYP enzymes.[109] Nuclear receptors exist mostly within the cytoplasm of cells. The CYP families 2 and 3 both have gene activation triggered through the NR pregnane X receptor (PXR) and the constitutive androstane receptor (CAR). The CYP1A subfamily uses the aryl hydrocarbon receptor (AhR) as its NR. Ligands, molecules that bind to and affect the reactivity of a central molecule, are typically small and lipophilic, enabling them to enter cells. Many xenobiotics are themselves ligands. Ligands bind the NRs, resulting in structural changes that enable the NR–ligand complexes to be translocated into the cell nucleus. Within the nucleus, NR–ligand complexes bind to proteins to create a heterodimer such as the retinoid X receptor (RXR) with either the PXR or the CAR. Similarly, the AhR interacts with the AhR nuclear translocator (Arnt) to create the nuclear heterodimer. This new heterodimer complex then interacts with specific response elements of DNA, initiating the transcription of a segment of DNA, and translation of its RNA resulting in the phenotypic expression of the respective CYP enzyme.

The ligand-binding domain of the PXR is very hydrophobic and flexible, enabling this pocket to bind many substrates of varied sizes and reflecting why the PXR is activated by a broad group of ligands.[85,109] For example, xenobiotic ligands that bind the NR PXR that targets the *CYP3A4* gene include rifampin, omeprazole, carbamazepine, and troleandomycin. Phenobarbital, a classic inducing xenobiotic, is a ligand that binds the CAR.[113] The induction of CYP1A subfamily enzymes is through the interaction with the NR AhR. Exogenous AhR ligands are hydrophobic, cyclic, planar molecules. Classic AhR ligands include polyaromatic hydrocarbons (PAHs) such as 2,3,7,8-tetrachlorodibenzo-*p*-dioxin and benzo[*a*]pyrene.[85]

Induction requires time to occur because it involves de novo synthesis of new proteins. Similarly, withdrawal of the inducer results in a slow return to the original enzyme concentration.[66] Polyaromatic hydrocarbons (PAHs) result in CYP1A subfamily induction within 3 to 6 hours with a maximum effect within 24 hours.[104] The inducer rifampin does not affect verapamil trough concentrations maximally until one week; followed by a 2-week return to baseline steady state after withdrawal of rifampin.[66] Xenobiotics with long half-lives require longer periods of time to reach steady-state concentrations that maximize induction. Phenobarbital and fluoxetine, which have long half-lives, fully manifest induction only after weeks of exposure. Conversely, xenobiotics with short half-lives, such as rifampin or venlafaxine reach maximum induction within days.[13]

Inconsistency in CYP induction exists in all organs and among individuals.[66,85] In an in vitro study of the effects of inducing xenobiotics on 60 livers, differences in enzyme induction ranged from 5-fold for CYP3A4 and CYP2C9 up to more than 50-fold for CYP2A6 and CYP2D6.[66] The inconsistency likely results from both polymorphisms and multiple environmental factors including diet, tobacco, and pollutants.[66] There is variation in the extent to which inducers generate new CYP enzymes. Identical dosing regimens with rifampin resulted in induction of in vivo hepatic CYP3A4 with up to 18-fold differences between subjects.[66] There is an inverse correlation of the degree of inducibility of an enzyme and the baseline enzyme concentration. Patients with a relatively low baseline concentration of a CYP enzyme will be more inducible than those with a high baseline concentration. Interestingly, the maximum concentrations of CYP enzymes seem to be quantitatively similar among individuals, suggesting a limit to which enzymes can be induced.[66]

Although the focus of this section is on CYP enzymes, it appears that most phases of xenobiotic metabolism are regulated by NRs.[11] Also, just as genetic polymorphisms exist for CYP enzymes, they exist for NRs including the AhR, the CAR, and the PXR. This results in varied sensitivities to the ligands that complex with the NRs, ultimately resulting in differences in CYP enzyme induction.[66,113]

Inhibition of CYP Enzymes

Inhibition of CYP enzymes result in either increased bioavailability of a drug or decreased bioactivation of a prodrug, and is the most common cause of harmful drug–drug interactions.[86] Severe inhibition of CYP enzymes by a coadministered xenobiotic resulted in the removal of many medications from the market, including terfenadine, mibefradil, bromfenac, astemizole, cisapride, cerivastatin, and nefazodone.[119] The appendix at the end of this chapter includes a comprehensive listing of CYP enzyme substrates, inhibitors, and inducers.

Inhibition mechanisms include irreversible (mechanism-based inhibition) and, the more common, reversible processes. The most common type of reversible inhibition is competitive, where the substrate and inhibitor both bind the active site of the enzyme.[86,119] Binding is weak and is formed and broken down easily, resulting in subsequent enzyme liberation. It occurs rapidly, usually beginning within hours.[13] Because the degree of inhibition varies with the concentration of the inhibitor, the time to reach the maximal effect correlates with the half-life of the xenobiotic in question.[13] A competitive inhibitor can be overcome by increasing the substrate concentration. Each substrate of a CYP enzyme is an inhibitor of the metabolism of all the other substrates of the same enzyme, thereby increasing their concentrations and half-lives. Reversible, noncompetitive inhibition occurs when an

inhibitor binds a location on an enzyme that is not the active site, resulting in a structural change that inhibits the active enzyme site. For example, noncompetitive inhibitors of CYP2C9 include nifedipine, tranylcypromine, and medroxyprogesterone.[100] Another reversible mechanism results from competition between one xenobiotic and a metabolite of a second xenobiotic at its CYP enzyme substrate binding site. For example, the metabolites of clarithromycin and erythromycin produced by CYP3A inhibit further CYP3A activity. The effect is reversible and usually increases with repeated dosing.[100] Some reversible inhibitors bind so tightly to the enzyme that they essentially function as irreversible inhibitors.[86]

Irreversible inhibitors have reactive groups that covalently, and thus permanently, bind the enzyme. They display time-dependent inhibition because the amount of active enzyme at a given concentration of irreversible inhibitor will be different depending on how long the inhibitor is preincubated with the enzyme. Because the enzyme will never be reactivated, inhibition lasts until new enzyme is synthesized.[86] One measure of inhibitor potency is the inhibitory concentration, K_i, the concentration of the inhibitor that produces 50% inhibition of the enzyme. The more potent the inhibitor, the lower the value.[104] Values below 1.0 μmol/L are regarded as potent.[82] The azole antifungals are very potent, with K_i values of 0.02 μmol/L.[104]

The impact of an inhibitor is also affected by the fraction of the substrate that is biotransformed by the inhibited, target enzyme. The inhibition of a CYP enzyme will have little impact if the enzyme only metabolizes a fraction of the affected xenobiotic.[82] Conversely, xenobiotics that are primarily metabolized by a single CYP enzyme are more susceptible to interactions.[86] Simvastatin is biotransformed primarily by CYP3A4. The potent and specific CYP3A inhibitor itraconazole prevents its metabolism, resulting in an increased risk of rhabdomyolysis.[1]

Specific CYP Enzymes
CYP1A1 and 1A2

Whereas 1A1 is located primarily in extrahepatic tissue, 1A2 is a hepatic enzyme and is involved in the metabolism of 10% to 15% of xenobiotics.[13,66] They both are very inducible by polycyclic aromatic hydrocarbons, including those in cigarette smoke and charred food. They bioactivate several procarcinogens, including benzo[*a*]pyrene.[57] Xenobiotics activated by the CYP1 enzyme family in the GI tract are linked to colon cancer.[78] A xenobiotic interaction through CYP1A2 involves the addition of ciprofloxacin, a moderate inhibitor of CYP1A2, to a patient using tizanidine for muscle spasms. Oral administration of tizanidine, an α_2 adrenergic agonist, yields low serum concentration because of extensive first-pass metabolism through CYP1A2. With concurrent ciprofloxacin dosing, serum tizanidine concentration increases significantly, and the interaction causes a clinically significant hypotension.[37]

CYP2B6

This enzyme metabolizes approximately 7% of xenobiotics with many overlapping substrates with other CYP enzymes, especially CYP3A4.[43,125] CYP2B6 comprises between 4% and 14% of total hepatic CYP enzymes and is polymorphic with 38 allele variations.[49,125] Cyclophosphamide and ifosfamide are commonly used nitrogen mustard class of chemotherapeutics that require bioactivation. Metabolism through CYP2B6 yields the therapeutic phosphamide mustard metabolite, whereas metabolism through CYP3A4 inactivates the compound. Preferential metabolism through the induction of CYP2B6 increases therapeutic efficacy of cyclophosphamide and ifosfamide.[43]

CYP2C9 and 2C19

The CYP2 enzyme family, with its 60 *CYP2C9* alleles and 35 *CYP2C19* alleles, is one of the most polymorphic of the CYP enzymes families (Table 11–1).[30,49,114] The CYP2C9 enzyme is the most abundant enzyme of the CYP2C enzyme subfamily, which, with CYP2C19, comprises approximately 10% to 20% of the CYP enzymes in the liver and is involved in 15% to 20% of all xenobiotic metabolism.[30,114] CYP2C9 biotransforms *S*-warfarin, the more active isomer of warfarin. Warfarin is one of the most commonly reported causes of adverse drug events. There is an association between slow metabolism and an increased risk of bleeding in patients taking warfarin.[16,97]

CYP2D6

This enzyme is of historical significance because the exploration of differences in pharmacokinetics among individuals taking the antihypertensive debrisoquine led to the discovery of CYP2D6 and marked the beginning of pharmacogenetics.[48] Debrisoquine through its effects on blood pressure acts as a probe molecule for enzymatic variations of CYP2D6. In fact, CYP2D6 is highly polymorphic with more than 109 allelic variants.[49] Twenty-five percent of pharmaceuticals, including 50% of the commonly used antipsychotics and antidepressants, are substrates for CYP2D6.[42,48,78,83] Because CYP2D6 is the only drug-metabolizing CYP enzyme that is noninducible, the polymorphisms are the primary reason for the substantial interindividual variation in enzyme activity.[50] CYP2D6 enzyme is strongly inhibited by common antidepressants such as bupropion, fluoxetine, and paroxetine. Between inhibitors and poor metabolizers, opioid substrates such as codeine, tramadol, and hydrocodone that are bioactivated through CYP2D6 have less clinical efficacy.[42] Ultrarapid metabolizers have higher incidences of postoperative and chemotherapy-induced vomiting when given ondansetron, a commonly used antiemetic metabolized by CYP2D6.[9]

CYP2E1

This enzyme comprises 7% of the total CYP enzyme content in the human liver.[79] It metabolizes small organic compounds, including ethanol, carbon tetrachloride, and halogenated anesthetics.[104] It also biotransforms low-molecular-weight xenobiotics, including benzene, acetone, and N-nitrosamines.[104] Some of its substrates are procarcinogens, which are bioactivated by CYP2E1.[78] The assessment for a relationship between CYP2E1 and cancer is intense because many of its substrates are environmental xenobiotics. The induction of CYP2E1 is associated with increased liver injury by reactive metabolites of carbon tetrachloride and vinyl chloride (Chap. 21).[36] During the metabolism of substrates that include carbon tetrachloride, ethanol, acetaminophen (APAP), aniline, and N-nitrosodimethylamine, CYP2E1 actively produces free radicals and other reactive metabolites associated with adduct formation and lipid peroxidation (Chaps. 9 and 33).[17] CYP2E1 is inhibited by acute elevations of ethanol, an effect illustrated by the acute administration of ethanol inhibiting the metabolism of APAP. The chronic ingestion of ethanol hastens its own metabolism through CYP2E1 induction.[36]

CYP3A4

CYP3A4 is the most abundant CYP in the human liver, comprising 40% to 55% of the mass of hepatic CYP enzymes.[13,30] The CYP3A4 enzyme is the most common one found in the intestinal mucosa and is responsible for much first-pass drug metabolism.[13] It is involved in the biotransformation of 50% to 60% of all pharmaceuticals.[79,127] It has broad substrate specificity because it accommodates large lipophilic substrates and can adopt multiple conformations. It can even simultaneously fit 2 relatively large compounds (ketoconazole, erythromycin) in its active site.[96]

Methadone, extensively metabolized by CYP3A4, is associated with many examples of adverse drug interactions.[54] Torsade de pointes due to the methadone dose–related prolongation of the QT_c interval is reported in patients who take methadone in addition to CYP3A4 inhibitors including ciprofloxacin,[75] itraconazole,[81] and the antiretrovirals atazanavir and ritonavir.[29] Ketoconazole inhibits CYP3A4, causing a 15- to 72-fold increase in serum concentrations of terfenadine, which also causes torsade de pointes.[78] Bioflavonoids in grapefruit juice decrease metabolism of some substrates by 5- to 12-fold.[13,78] The CYP3A4 enzyme does not exhibit significant genetic polymorphism; however, there are large interindividual variations in enzyme concentrations that can affect metabolic rates.[127]

Phase II Biotransformation Reactions

Phase II biotransformation reactions are synthetic, catalyzing the conjugation of products of phase I reactions or xenobiotics with endogenous molecules that are generally hydrophilic. Conjugation usually terminates the pharmacologic activity of xenobiotics and greatly increases their water solubility and excretability.[70,108,124] Conjugation occurs most commonly with glucuronic acid, sulfates, and glutathione. Less common phase II reactions include conjugation with amino acids such as glycine, glutamic acid, and taurine as well as acetylation and methylation.

Glucuronidation is the most common phase II synthesis reaction.[70] Glucuronyl-transferase has relatively low substrate affinity, but it has high capacity at higher substrate concentrations.[108] The glucuronic acid, donated by uridine diphosphate glucuronic acid, is conjugated with the nitrogen, sulfhydryl, hydroxyl, or carboxyl groups of substrates. Smaller conjugates usually undergo renal elimination, whereas larger ones undergo biliary elimination.[70] The process of glucuronidation is reversible via β-glucuronidases. Although the liver has an overall low concentration of β-glucuronidases, the gut flora have high β-glucuronidase activity. Cleavage of the glucuronide metabolite enhances the lipophilicity and thus reabsorption through intestinal walls. This process is termed enterohepatic circulation, which decreases elimination and prolong toxicity from xenobiotics such as carbamazepine and phenobarbital.[3,124] Multiple-dose activated charcoal provides therapeutic benefit to break enterohepatic circulation (Antidotes in Depth: A1).

Sulfation complements glucuronidation because it is a high-affinity but low-capacity reaction that occurs primarily in the cytosol. For example, the affinity of sulfate for phenol is very high (the K_m is low), so that when low doses of phenol are administered, the predominant excretion product is the sulfate ester. Because the capacity of this reaction is readily saturated, glucuronidation becomes the main method of detoxification when high doses of phenol are administered.[70,124] Sulfate conjugates are highly ionized and very water soluble.

Glutathione S-transferases are important because they catalyze the conjugation of the tripeptide glutathione (glycine-glutamate-cysteine, or GSH) with a diverse group of reactive, electrophilic metabolites of phase I CYP enzymes. The reactive compounds initiate an attack on the sulfur group of cysteine, resulting in conjugation with GSH that detoxifies the reactive metabolite. Of the 3 phase II reactions addressed, hepatic concentrations of glutathione by far account for the greatest amount of cofactors used. Although intracellular glutathione is difficult to deplete, when it does occur, severe hepatotoxicity often follows.[124] Some GSH conjugates are directly excreted. More commonly, the glycine and glutamate residues are cleaved and the remaining cysteine is acetylated to form a mercapturic acid conjugate that is readily excreted in the urine. A familiar example of this detoxification is the avid binding of N-acetyl-p-benzoquinoneimine (NAPQI), the toxic metabolite of APAP, by glutathione.[5,12]

As with the CYP enzymes, many phase II enzymes are inducible. For example, UDP-glucuronosyltransferase, which performs glucuronidation, is inducible via the PXR, CAR, and AhR nuclear receptors after binding with rifampin, phenobarbital, and PAHs, respectively. Its activity varies 6- to 15-fold in liver microsomes.[113] Similarly, UDP-glucuronosyltransferases are inhibited by xenobiotics such as amitriptyline, indinavir, phenylbutazone, and quinidine.[63,111] Inhibition of glucuronidation exacerbates hyperbilirubinemia in patients with underlying Gilbert syndrome (reduced UDP-glucuronosyltransferase activity on bilirubin).[111] Although inhibition of a high-capacity phase II metabolism step has theoretical implications and potential drug–drug interactions, the clinical implications are not well-studied.

Membrane Transporters

Although the focus on drug disposition has traditionally been on biotransformation, membrane transporter proteins greatly impact drug disposition.[45] Transporter proteins mediate the cellular uptake and efflux of endogenous compounds and xenobiotics.[128] Their baseline physiologic role is to transport sugars, lipids, amino acids, and hormones so as to regulate cellular solute and fluid balance. Biotransformation cannot occur unless xenobiotics are taken up into the cells via transport proteins. After xenobiotics have undergone phase I and II metabolism, the metabolites undergo transport protein mediated efflux from the cell, an action that has been called phase III metabolism.[52]

Xenobiotic absorption, compartmentalization, and elimination are facilitated or prevented by the transport proteins.[58] In the apical (luminal) membrane of the intestinal enterocytes, P-glycoprotein, part of the ABC family of transmembrane proteins, is important because it can actively extrude xenobiotics back into the intestinal lumen and effectively decreases absorption.[14] The degree of phenotypic expression of P-glycoprotein affects the bioavailability of many xenobiotics, including paclitaxel, digoxin, and protease inhibitors.[45] Transporter-mediated uptake of xenobiotics also occurs from the portal venous blood into the hepatocytes or from renal filtrate back into proximal tubular cells. α-Amanitin uses the sodium-dependent bile acid transporter, Na⁺-taurocholate cotransporting polypeptide, to enter hepatocytes, where it inhibits RNA-polymerase II and mediates cellular toxicity.[40] Alternatively, transport proteins decrease xenobiotic entry into specific cells or compartments. P-glycoprotein in endothelial cells of the blood–brain barrier prevent CNS entry of substrate xenobiotics. Finally, transport proteins mediate xenobiotic elimination via hepatocyte efflux transporters that move biotransformed xenobiotics into bile and via efflux from renal proximal tubular cells into urine.[14,45,128] Organs important for drug disposition have multiple transporters that have overlapping substrate capabilities, a redundancy that enhances protection.[45]

As with biotransformation enzymes and nuclear receptors, membrane transporters are also inhibited or induced. Digoxin, a high-affinity substrate for P-glycoprotein, has increased bioavailability when administered with P-glycoprotein inhibitors such as clarithromycin or atorvastatin.[45] Loperamide is a substrate for P-glycoprotein that limits its intestinal absorption

or CNS entry. Coadministration with quinidine, a P-glycoprotein inhibitor, or large dose ingestions (70–200 mg daily) that overwhelm the P-glycoprotein capacity result in increased opioid CNS effects of loperamide.[24,45] As with the biotransformation enzymes, polymorphisms exist for membrane transporters. However, the clinical significance of these is not clear.[19]

MECHANISMS OF CELLULAR INJURY

Ideally and commonly, potentially toxic metabolites produced by phase I reactions are detoxified during phase II reactions. However, detoxification does not always occur. This section reviews mechanisms of cellular injury related to xenobiotic biotransformation.

Synthesis of Toxins

Sometimes a xenobiotic is mistaken for an endogenous substrate by synthetic enzymes that biotransform it into an injurious compound. The incorporation of the rodenticide fluoroacetate into the citric acid cycle is an example of this mechanism of toxic injury (Fig. 11–3).[90] Another example is illustrated by analogs of purine or pyrimidine bases that are phosphorylated and inserted into growing DNA or RNA chains, resulting in mutations and disruption of cell division. This mechanism is used therapeutically with 5-fluorouracil (5-FU), an antitumor pyrimidine base analog. When phosphorylated to 5-fluoro-dUTP and incorporated into growing DNA chains, it causes structural instability of the cellular DNA and inhibits tumor growth.[94]

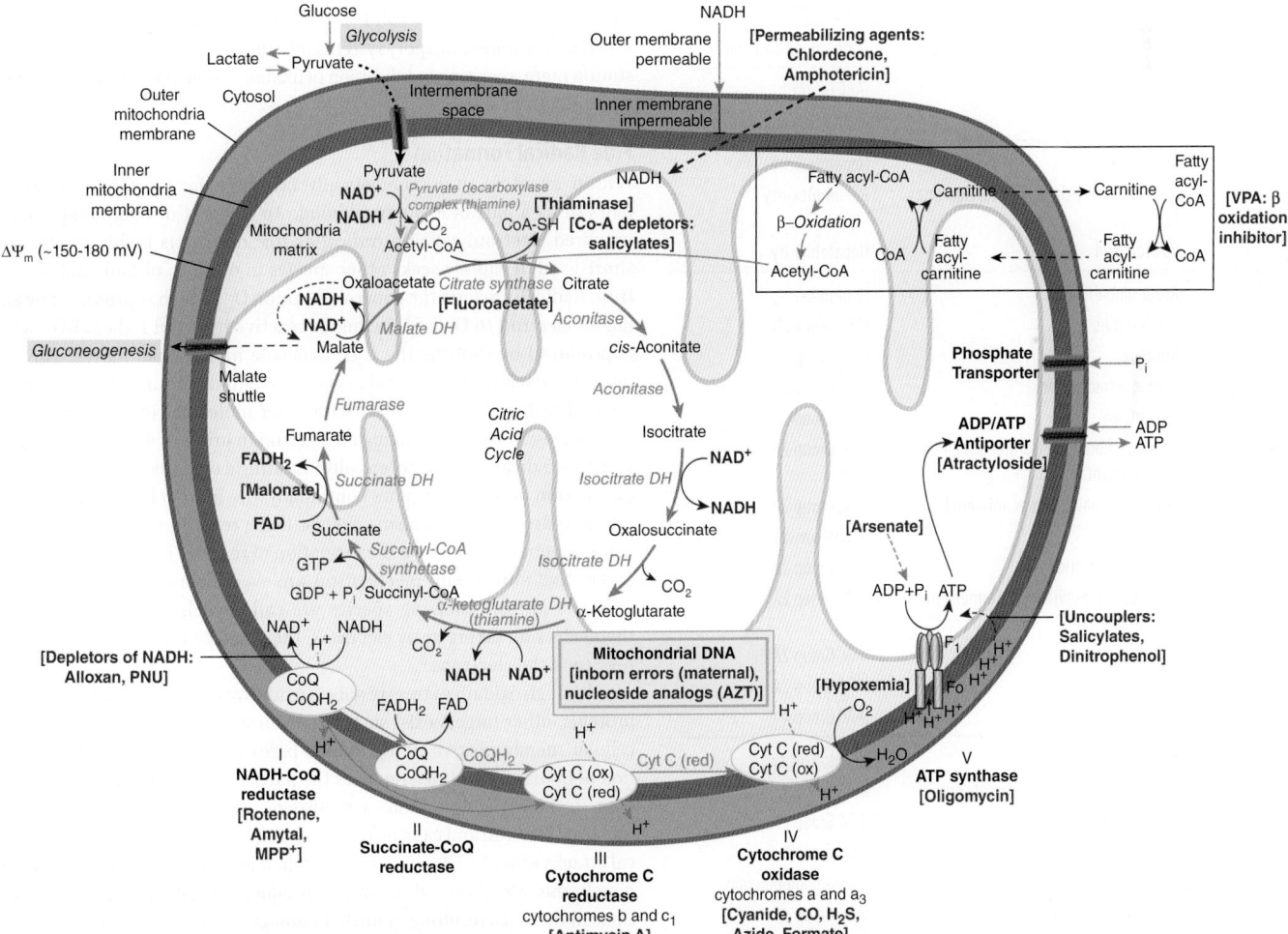

FIGURE 11–3. Pyruvate is converted to acetylcoenzyme A (acetyl-CoA), which enters the citric acid cycle as shown. Reducing equivalents, in the form of NADH and FADH, donate electrons to a chain of cytochromes beginning with NADH dehydrogenase. These reactions "couple" the energy released during electron transport to the production of ATP. Ultimately, electrons combine with oxygen to form water. The sites of action of xenobiotics that inhibit oxidative metabolism are shown. The sites where thiamine functions as a coenzyme are also illustrated.[87] $\Delta\Psi_m$ = mitochondrial membrane potential; DH = dehydrogenase. MPP⁺ =1-methyl-4-phenylpyridinium; PNU = N-3-pyridylmethyl-N-nitrophenyl urea; VPA = valproic acid.

Injury by Metabolites of Biotransformation

Many toxic products result from metabolic activation (Table 11–2).[53] The CYP enzymes most associated with bioactivation are 1A1, 1B1, 2A6, and 2E1, whereas 2C9 and 2D6 yield little toxic activation.[39]

Highly reactive metabolites exert damage at the site where they are synthesized; reacting too quickly with local molecules to be transported

TABLE 11–2	Examples of Xenobiotics Activated to Toxins by Human Cytochrome P450 Enzymes	
Enzyme	CYP Substrate	Toxicity
1A1	Benzo[a]pyrene (PAH)	IARC Group 1
1A2	Acetaminophen	Hepatotoxicity
	Aflatoxin B (Aspergillus mycotoxin)	IARC Group 1
	2-Naphthylamine (azo dye production)	IARC Group 1
	NNK (nitrosamine in tobacco)	IARC Group 1
	N-Nitrosodiethylamine (gas and lubricant additive, copolymer softener)	IARC Group 2A
2B6	Chrysene (PAH)	IARC Group 2B
	Cyclophosphamide	IARC Group 1
	Dapsone	Methemoglobinemia
2C8,9	Cyclophosphamide	IARC Group 1
	Phenytoin	IARC Group 2B
	Valproic acid	Hepatotoxicity
2C19	Dapsone	Methemoglobinemia
2D6	NNK	IARC Group 1
	Dapsone	Methemoglobinemia
2F1	Acetaminophen	Hepatotoxicity
	3-Methylindole (in perfumes, cigarettes for flavor)	Pneumotoxicity
	Valproic acid	Hepatotoxicity
2E1	Acetaminophen	Hepatotoxicity
	Acrylonitrile	IARC Group 2B
	Benzene	IARC Group 1
	Carbon tetrachloride	IARC Group 2B
	Chloroform	IARC Group 2B
	Ethylene dibromide (former gas additive and fumigant)	IARC Group 2A
	Ethyl carbamate (former antineoplastic)	IARC Group 2A
	Halothane	Hepatotoxicity
	Methylene chloride	IARC Group 2B
	N-Nitrosodimethylamine (formerly in rocket fuel)	IARC Group 2A
	Styrene	IARC Group 2A
	Trichloroethylene	IARC Group 2A
	Vinyl chloride	IARC Group 1
3A4	Acetaminophen	Hepatotoxicity
	Aflatoxin B₁ (Aspergillus mycotoxin)	IARC Group 1
	Chrysene (PAH)	IARC Group 2B
	Cyclophosphamide	IARC Group 1
	Dapsone	Methemoglobinemia
	1-Nitropyrene (PAH)	IARC Group 2B
	Senecionine (pyrrolizidine alkaloid)	Hepatotoxicity
	Sterigmatocystin (Aspergillus mycotoxin)	IARC Group 2B

Group 1 = known carcinogen; Group 2A = probable carcinogen; Group 2B = possible carcinogen; IARC = International Agency for Research on Cancer of the World Health Organization; NNK = nicotine-derived nitrosamine ketone; PAH = polycyclic aromatic hydrocarbon.

elsewhere. This commonly occurs in the liver, the major site of biotransformation of xenobiotics (Chap. 21).[38,102] However, metabolism in the lungs, skin, kidneys, GI tract, and nasal mucosa also create toxic metabolites that cause local injury.[12,61] Overdoses of APAP lead to excessive hepatic CYP2E1 production of the highly reactive, semiquinoneimine, electrophile NAPQI, which initiates a damaging covalent bond with hepatocytes (Chap. 33).[5] Acute renal tubular necrosis also occurs in patients with overdose of APAP, attributed to its biotransformation to NAPQI by prostaglandin H synthase within renal tubular cells.[28,118] Other toxic metabolites cause systemic toxicity. Dapsone (4,4'-diphenyldiaminosulfone) is a medication used in the treatment of *Pneumocystis jiroveci* pneumonia, malaria, and leprosy. Dapsone is metabolized primarily by CYP2C19 with contributions from CYP2B6, CYP2D6, and CYP3A4 to N-hydroxy metabolites such as dapsone hydroxylamine and monoacetyl hydroxylamine, which induce methemoglobinemia and cause hemolytic anemia.[6,33] These metabolites have a prolonged elimination half-life of approximately 30 hours and cause the well-described prolonged methemoglobinemia associated with dapsone.[6]

Monoamine oxidases (MAOs) are mitochondrial enzymes present in many tissues. They oxidize many amines, including dopamine, epinephrine, and serotonin, and xenobiotics such as primaquine and haloperidol. The metabolic activity of MAOs was responsible for the outbreak of parkinsonism associated with the use of methylphenyltetrahydropyridine (MPTP), an unintended by-product of attempts to synthesize a "designer" analog of meperidine, methylphenylpropionoxypiperidine (MPPP). After crossing the blood–brain barrier, MPTP is biotransformed by MAO in glial cells to methylphenyldihydropyridine (MPDP⁺), which is converted to the l-methyl-4-phenylpyridinium cation (MPP⁺). The MPP⁺ is subsequently taken up by specific dopamine transport systems into dopaminergic neurons in the substantia nigra, resulting in inhibition of oxidative phosphorylation and subsequent neuronal death.[35]

Free Radical Formation

Within an atom, it is energetically favorable for electrons to exist in pairs or as a part of a chemical bond. An element or compound with an unpaired electron, called a *radical* or *free radical*, is highly reactive and short-lived. It rapidly seeks other species in order to obtain another electron. Radicals include the superoxide anion $O_2^{\cdot-}$, which is produced by adding an electron to O_2, and the highly reactive hydroxyl radical HO•, which is produced by splitting the H_2O_2 molecule into 2 equal halves. The H_2O_2 molecule itself is reactive and is also associated with injury. The superoxide and hydroxyl radicals react with other molecules in order to stabilize themselves; however, by taking an electron in order to do so, they generate new free radical species, potentially initiating a chain reaction. Because the production of radicals occurs continually, the human body has developed effective defense mechanisms against these reactive molecules. However, some xenobiotics promote the formation of reactive oxidant species to the extent that antioxidant mechanisms are overwhelmed, a condition called *oxidative stress*. Oxidizing species are called such because, by reducing themselves by taking away electrons, they oxidize the species from which they took the electrons.[8]

Although oxidative stress results in oxidative damage to nucleic acids and proteins, other targets exist such as polyunsaturated fatty acids (PUFAs) in cellular membranes, resulting in lipid peroxidation (the oxidative destruction of lipids). This attack removes the particularly reactive hydrogen atom, with its lone electron, from a methylene carbon of a PUFA, leaving an unpaired electron and causing the formation of a lipid radical. This lipid radical attacks other PUFAs, initiating a chain reaction that destroys the cellular membrane. Membrane degradation products initiate inflammatory reactions in the cells, resulting in further damage.[8,102]

Molecular oxygen (O_2) has a lone pair of electrons in its orbit. Because oxygen is a relatively weak univalent electron acceptor (and most organic molecules are weak univalent electron donors), oxygen cannot efficiently oxidize amino acids and nucleic acids. However, the unpaired electrons of O_2 readily interact with the unpaired electrons of transition metals and

1. $O_2 + e^- \rightarrow O_2^{\bullet-}$

2. $O_2^{\bullet-} + 2H^+ + e^- \rightarrow H_2O_2$

3. $H_2O_2 \xrightarrow{Fe^{2+}} OH^- + OH\bullet$ (Fenton)

   $H_2O_2 + O_2^{\bullet-} \xrightarrow{Fe^{2+}} O_2 + OH^- + OH\bullet$ (Haber-Weiss)

FIGURE 11–4. Hydroxyl radical formation. (1) First is the addition of an electron to O_2 to create the superoxide ion. (2) Then the very reactive superoxide combines with hydrogen and another electron to produce hydrogen peroxide. (3) Finally, in the presence of a metal ion catalyst such as iron, hydrogen peroxide undergoes various reactions to produce the hydroxyl radical. The dot in these formulas represents an unpaired electron, the hallmark of a free radical.[47,70]

organic radicals. Metals frequently catalyze the creation of oxygen free radicals. Fig. 11–4 reflects the typical steps in the formation of a hydroxyl radical. The damaging effects of the free radicals are decreased by reaction with antioxidants such as ascorbate, tocopherols, and glutathione.[70] Deficiencies of antioxidants, especially glutathione, are associated with increased oxidative damage. Free radicals are also neutralized by several enzymes, including peroxidase, superoxide dismutase, and catalase.

The ethanol-inducible CYP2E1 enzyme produces significant amounts of superoxide and peroxide free radicals. In the presence of iron, these hydroxyl free radicals readily initiate lipid peroxidation. This was studied extensively in models of the metabolism of carbon tetrachloride, ethanol, and APAP.[23] The formation of free radicals is implicated in the pulmonary injury caused by paraquat, the myocardial injury caused by doxorubicin, and the hepatic injury caused by carbon tetrachloride.[73,91] Paraquat reacts with NADPH to form a pyridinyl free radical, which, in turn, reacts with oxygen to generate the superoxide anion radical. Doxorubicin is metabolized to a semiquinone free radical in the cardiac mitochondria, which, in the presence of oxygen, forms a superoxide anion radical that initiates myocardial lipid peroxidation.[73] Carbon tetrachloride (CCl_4) is metabolized to the trichloromethyl radical ($\bullet CCl_3$) that binds covalently to cellular macromolecules. In the presence of oxygen, this is converted to the trichloromethylperoxyl radical ($\bullet CCl_3O_2$) that can initiate lipid peroxidation (Fig. 11–5).[92] (Chap. 105 offers a more extensive discussion.)

CRITICAL BIOCHEMICAL PATHWAYS AND XENOBIOTICS THAT AFFECT THEM

Energy metabolism is the foundation of cellular function. It provides high-energy fuel, predominantly in the form of ATP, for all energy-dependent cellular processes such as synthesis, active transport, and maintenance of

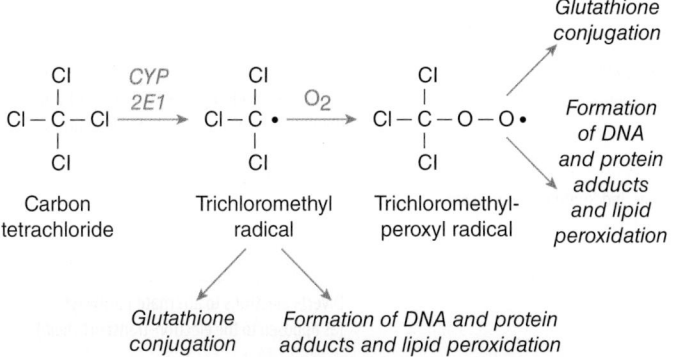

FIGURE 11–5. This is carbon tetrachloride metabolism by the hepatocyte. Under hypoxic conditions, the CCl_3 radical is the predominant species formed. At higher oxygen tensions, the CCl_3 radical is oxidized to the CCl_3OO^- radical, which is more readily detoxified by glutathione. Both free radicals bind to hepatocytes and cause cellular injury.

electrolyte balance and membrane integrity. Numerous pathways interconnect glycogen, fat, and protein reserves in many tissues that store and retrieve ATP and glucose. The brain and red blood cells (RBCs) are entirely dependent on glucose for energy production, although other tissues can also use ketone bodies and fatty acids to synthesize ATP. Rapid cell death occurs if the production or use of ATP is inhibited; thus, the goal of many metabolic processes is the production and mobilization of cellular energy.

Catabolic pathways, those that break down molecules into smaller units enabling the production of cellular energy, include glycolysis, the citric acid cycle, and oxidative phosphorylation via the electron transport chain. Glycolysis produces small amounts of ATP through the anaerobic metabolism of glucose. Pyruvate, the end product of glycolysis, yields far more ATP when it is converted to acetyl-coenzyme A (acetyl-CoA) and "processed" in the citric acid cycle (Fig. 11–3). Fat and protein yield their energy through their conversion to acetyl-CoA and other intermediates of the citric acid cycle. The citric acid cycle and oxidative phosphorylation, via the electron transport chain, result in most ATP synthesis. Oxidative phosphorylation disposes of electrons or "reducing equivalents" and converts their energy to ATP. A lack of oxygen stops the electron transport chain and ATP production. Oxidative metabolism is highly energy efficient, producing 36 moles of ATP for each mole of glucose metabolized, compared to the 2 moles of ATP produced by anaerobic glycolysis. The following sections review the basics of cellular energy metabolism and several important xenobiotics that affect these critical metabolic functions (Table 11–3).[30,59]

Glycolysis
Glycolysis is the first biochemical pathway in the metabolism of glucose. Other sugars enter this pathway after conversion to glycolytic intermediates (Fig. 11–6). The glycolytic process converts one molecule of glucose to 2 of pyruvate plus 2 molecules of ATP plus 2 molecules of NADH. Pyruvate may follow many paths. Under anaerobic conditions, the 2 pyruvate molecules produced from one glucose molecule are reduced by lactate dehydrogenase to 2 lactate molecules in an NADH-requiring step that regenerates NAD^+. Thus, anaerobic glycolysis yields 2 molecules of lactate plus 2 molecules of ATP. When NAD^+ and oxygen are available, pyruvate is transported from the cytosol into the mitochondria where it enters the citric acid cycle by being converted by pyruvate decarboxylase to acetyl-CoA (Fig. 11–3).[30,59] In energy-rich conditions, pyruvate is used for fatty acid synthesis, whereas in energy-poor situations, it is used for gluconeogenesis.

Arsenate (As^{5+}) affects the glycolytic step where 3-phosphoglyceraldehydedehydrogenase (3-PGA) catalyzes the oxidation of glyceraldehyde-3-phosphate to 1,3-diphosphoglycerate, a reaction that preserves a high-energy phosphate bond used to synthesize ATP in the next step of glycolysis (Fig. 11–6).[46] Arsenate acts as an analog of phosphate at this step, resulting in an unstable arsenate intermediate that is rapidly hydrolyzed to 3-phosphoglycerate. While glycolysis continues, there is the loss of ATP synthesis because 1,3 biphosphoglycerate is not made.[46]

Citric Acid Cycle
The citric acid cycle uses acetyl-CoA derived from glycolysis, fat, or protein to regenerate NADH from NAD^+. The cycle is a major source of electrons (in the form of NADH) and is critical to the aerobic production of ATP (Fig. 11–3). Each acetyl-CoA molecule that is oxidized within the citric acid cycle ultimately forms one molecule each of CO_2 and guanosine triphosphate (GTP), and more importantly, 3 molecules of NADH and one molecule of reduced flavin adenine dinucleotide ($FADH_2$). Both NADH and $FADH_2$ enter the electron transport chain to generate ATP via oxidative phosphorylation (details below). In addition, the citric acid cycle provides important intermediates for amino acid synthesis and for gluconeogenesis.[59]

Various xenobiotics inhibit the citric acid cycle. The rodenticides, sodium fluoroacetate and fluoroacetamide, are combined with coenzyme A, CoASH, to create fluoroacetyl CoA (FAcCoA). The FAcCoA substitutes for acetyl CoA, entering the citric acid cycle by condensation with oxaloacetate to form fluorocitrate. Fluorocitrate metabolism results in a metabolite that blocks

TABLE 11–3	Inhibitors of Glucose Metabolism and ATP Synthesis	
Step/Location	**Examples**	**Action**
Glycolysis	Iodoacetate (at GAPDH)	Inhibits NADH production
	NO⁺ (at GAPDH)	
	Arsenate, (As⁵⁺)	Bypasses ATP producing step
Gluconeogenesis	4-(Dimethylamino)phenol p-benzoquinone	Inhibits NADH production
	Hypoglycin A (ackee fruit)	
	Methylenecyclopropylacetic acid (lychee fruit)	
Fatty acid metabolism	Aflatoxin	Inhibits NADH production
	Amiodarone	
	Hypoglycin	
	Perhexiline	
	Protease inhibitors	
	Salicylates	
	Tetracycline	
	Valproic acid	
Citric acid cycle	Arsenite, (As³⁺)	Inhibits NADH production
	p-Benzoquinone	
	Fluoroacetate	
Electron-transport chain at complex I	MPP⁺	Inhibits electron transport
	Paraquat	
	Rotenone	
Electron-transport chain at complex III	Antimycin-A	Inhibits electron transport
	Funiculosin	
	Cations: Zn²⁺, Hg²⁺, Cu²⁺, and Cd²⁺	
	Substituted phenols (pentachlorophenol and dinitrophenol) (also uncouplers)	
Electron-transport chain at complex IV	Azide	Inhibits electron transport
	Carbon monoxide	
	Cyanide	
	Formate	
	Hydrogen sulfide	
	Nitric oxide	
	Phosphine	
	Protamine	
Electron-transport chain at ATP synthase	Arsenate, (As⁵⁺)	Inhibits ATP production
	Mycotoxins (numerous, including oligomycin)	
	Organic chlorines (DDT and chlordecone)	
	Organotins (cyhexatin)	
	Paraquat	
Mitochondria ADP/ATP antiporter	Atractyloside	Disrupts the movement of ADP into and ATP out of the mitochondria at the ADP/ATP antiporter
	DDT	
	Free fatty acids	
Mitochondria inner membrane	Substituted phenols (pentachlorophenol and dinitrophenol)	Uncouples oxidative phosphorylation by disrupting the proton gradient → stops proton flow at ATP synthase → stops ATP synthesis
	Lipophilic amines (amiodarone, perhexiline, buprenorphine)	
	Benzonitrile	
	Thiadiazol herbicides	
	NSAIDs with ionizable groups (salicylates, diclofenac, indomethacin, piroxicam)	
	Valinomycin	
	Chlordecone	
Mitochondria inner membrane	Doxorubicin	Diverts electrons to alternate pathways (as opposed to the electron-transport chain)
	MPP⁺	
	Naphthoquinones (menadione)	
	N-nitrosamines	
	Paraquat	

ADP = adenosine diphosphate; ATP = adenosine triphosphate; DDT = dichlorodiphenyltricholorethane; GAPDH = glyceraldehyde 3-phosphate dehydrogenase; MPP⁺ = 1-methyl-4-phenylpyridinium. NADH = Nicotinamide adenine dinucleoide; NSAIDs = nonsteroidal antiinflammatory drugs.

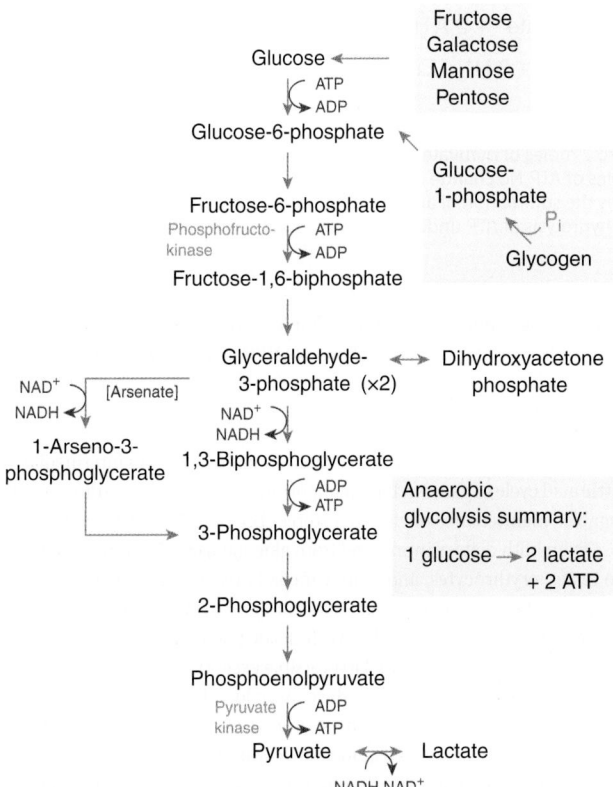

FIGURE 11–6. During glycolysis, the anaerobic metabolism of 1 mole of glucose to 2 moles of pyruvate results in the net production of 2 moles of ATP. Arsenate (As⁵⁺) results in the creation of an unstable intermediary that bypasses a step that typically creates one of those moles of ATP. Pyruvate kinase and phosphofructokinase, the enzymes whose activities are regulated by glucagon via cyclic adenosine monophosphate–dependent phosphokinase, are shown.

aconitase within the cycle, resulting in citrate accumulation and the termination of oxidative metabolism (Fig. 11–3) (Chap. 113).

Thiamine is an important cofactor for 2 citric acid cycle enzymes: the conversion of pyruvate to acetyl-CoA by pyruvate decarboxylase and for the conversion of α-ketoglutarate to succinyl-CoA by α-ketoglutarate dehydrogenase (Fig. 11–3).[30] The life-threatening effects of thiamine deficiency are likely related to impairment of these enzyme functions (Antidotes in Depth: A27). Chronic alcoholics have poor nutrition intake with impaired thiamine absorption. Thiamine deficiency damages cholinergic neurons in the basal forebrain leading to a syndrome of diencephalic amnesia and contributes to the pathophysiology of Wernicke encephalopathy and the Korsakoff psychosis. These cholinergic neurons have high energy demands and are more sensitive to inhibitions of glucose metabolism through thiamine-dependent enzymes.[76]

The Electron Transport Chain

The electron transport chain is the location where the "phosphorylation" of oxidative phosphorylation occurs. Oxidative phosphorylation is the creation of high-energy bonds by phosphorylation of adenosine diphosphate (ADP) to ATP, "coupled" to the transfer of electrons from reduced coenzymes to molecular oxygen via the electron transport chain. The success of aerobic metabolism requires the disposal of electrons within NADH and FADH₂, generated by oxidative metabolism within glycolysis and the citric acid cycle. The electron transport chain consists of a series of cytochrome–enzyme complexes within the inner mitochondrial membrane (Fig. 11–3). Within these complexes, NADH is split into NAD⁺ + H⁺ plus 2 electrons at complex I at the beginning of the chain whereas FADH₂ is split into FAD + 2H⁺ plus 2 electrons at complex II. These reactions have 2 results. First, the regenerated NAD⁺ and FAD are recycled back to the citric acid cycle, enabling oxidative metabolism to continue. Second, these actions provide the energy required to pump

protons (H⁺) from the mitochondrial matrix into the intermembrane space. This action causes the matrix to become relatively alkaline compared to the now acidified intermembrane space and the creation of a proton gradient across the inner mitochondrial membrane (mitochondrial membrane potential, $\Delta\psi_m \sim 150–180$ mV).[87] The final step in the electron flow of oxidative phosphorylation is the reduction of molecular oxygen to water by complex IV, cytochrome a-a₃ (Fig. 11–3).[30,59] This H⁺ gradient provides the energy needed to create the high-energy bonds of ATP at complex V (ATP synthase).

In total, aerobic glucose metabolism generates 36 moles of ATP. Glycolysis contributes 2 moles of ATP, 2 moles of NADH, and 2 moles of pyruvate. Pyruvate dehydrogenase converts pyruvate to acetyl-CoA while generating another 2 moles of NADH per mole of glucose. The citric acid cycle uses acetyl-CoA to generate 6 moles of NADH, 2 moles of FADH₂, and 2 mol of GTP per mole of glucose. Each mole of NADH via the electron transport chain produces 3 moles of ATP. Flavin adenine dinucleotide donates electrons later in the chain, so it only produces 2 moles of ATP. The entire process generates 2 moles of ATP, 10 moles of NADH (30 moles of ATP), and 2 moles of FADH₂ (4 moles of ATP) for a total of 36 moles of ATP and 2 moles of GTP per mole of glucose.

Mitochondria oxidize substrates, consume oxygen, produce CO_2, and make ATP. Xenobiotics that interrupt oxidative phosphorylation impair ATP production either by inhibiting specific electron chain complexes or by acting as "uncouplers." Both of these mechanisms result in rapid depletion of cellular energy stores, followed by failure of ATP-dependent active transport pumps, loss of essential electrolyte gradients, and increases in cell volume.[59]

Inhibitors of specific cytochromes block electron transport and cause an accumulation of reduced intermediates proximal to the site of inhibition. This stops the regeneration of oxidized substrates for the citric acid cycle, particularly NAD⁺ and FAD, further impairing oxidative metabolism. Cyanide, carbon monoxide, and hydrogen sulfide block the cytochrome a-a₃–mediated reduction of O_2 to H_2O. The very dramatic clinical effects of these exposures illustrate the importance of aerobic metabolism (Chap. 123). Other xenobiotics are less commonly associated with inhibition of the electron transport chain (Table 11–3).[110,116]

Severe metabolic acidosis is a clinical manifestation of xenobiotics that inhibit aerobic respiration. Lactate (the base form of lactic acid) accumulates during anaerobic respiration but is only a surrogate marker for metabolic acidosis associated with the impairment of oxidative metabolism.[60] The process of anaerobic glycolysis from glucose to pyruvate and subsequently to lactate is H⁺ neutral (Fig. 11–7, Equation 1). The H⁺ excess results from ATP hydrolysis by energy-requiring cellular processes. The hydrolysis of a high-energy bond in ATP yields ADP, phosphate, H⁺, and energy (Fig. 11–7, Equation 2). In total, 1 mole of glucose via anaerobic glycolysis yields 2 moles of lactate and 2 moles of H⁺ (Fig. 11–7, Equation 3). Therefore, the hydrolysis of ATP under anaerobic conditions contributes to metabolic acidosis rather than the dissociation of lactic acid to lactate.[68] Conversely during aerobic respiration and oxidative phosphorylation, the process of ATP generation via ATP synthase consumes the H⁺ gradient created by the electron transport chain and largely balances H⁺ production during ATP hydrolysis.

Xenobiotics that uncouple oxidative phosphorylation, like inhibitors of the electron transport chain, reduce ATP synthesis. However, with uncouplers, protons continue to be pumped into the intermembrane space, electrons continue to flow down the chain to reduce oxygen, and substrate consumption continues. Uncouplers dissipate the proton gradient across the mitochondrial inner membrane by allowing the protons to cross back into the mitochondrial matrix. Because it is the proton gradient that drives the production of ATP at complex V, ATP production is reduced. Thus, oxygen consumption is "uncoupled" from ATP production. The redox energy created by electron transport that cannot be coupled to ATP synthesis is released as heat. Various xenobiotics uncouple ATP synthesis (Table 11–3). A classic one is dinitrophenol, used as an herbicide and as a weight-loss product (Chap. 40). Xenobiotics that are capable of carrying hydrogen ions across membranes are generally lipophilic weak acids. These xenobiotics must have an acid-dissociable group to carry the proton and a bulky lipophilic group

$$\text{Equation 1. Glucose} + 2\ ADP^{3-} + 2\ Pi^{2-} \rightarrow 2\ Lactate^- + 2\ ATP^{4-} + 2\ H_2O$$

$$\text{Equation 2. } 2\ ATP^{4-} + 2\ H_2O \rightarrow 2\ ADP^{3-} + 2\ Pi^{2-} + 2\ H^+ + \text{Energy}$$

$$\text{Equation 3. Glucose} \rightarrow 2\ Lactate^- + 2\ H^+$$

FIGURE 11–7. Equation 1 describes anaerobic glycolysis. Glucose is initially converted to 2 moles of pyruvate via glycolysis and then under anaerobic conditions, pyruvate is converted to lactate. The net gain from these 2 processes is 2 moles of ATP. No change in H^+ concentration occurs. Equation 2 describes the hydrolysis of ATP, which yields both energy for cellular processes and H^+. Equation 3 is the summation of anaerobic glycolysis with ATP hydrolysis, which shows the conversion of 1 mole of glucose to 2 moles of lactate and 2 H^+. Therefore, the hydrolysis of ATP under anaerobic conditions contributes to metabolic acidosis rather than the dissociation of lactic acid to lactate. P: Inorganic phosphate.

to cross a membrane.[62] Dinitrophenol is able to carry its proton from the cytosol into the more alkaline mitochondrial matrix where it dissociates, acidifying the matrix and destroying the proton gradient across the inner mitochondrial membrane. Interestingly, the phenolate anion of dinitrophenol is relatively lipophilic and can cross back out to the cytosol where it gains a new proton and starts the process over again. Long-chain fatty acids uncouple oxidative phosphorylation by a similar mechanism.[62,116] Fatal exposures to dinitrophenol and to pentachlorophenol, a wood preservative, are associated with severe hyperthermia attributed to heat generation by uncoupled oxidative phosphorylation.[89] The hyperthermia and acidosis associated with severe salicylate poisoning are attributed to its uncoupling of oxidative phosphorylation.[107]

Hexose Monophosphate Shunt

The hexose monophosphate shunt provides the only source of cellular NADPH. Nicotinamide adenine dinucleotide phosphate is used in biosynthetic reactions, particularly fatty acid synthesis, and is an important source of reducing power for the maintenance of sulfhydryl groups that protect the cell from free radical injury.[10,47] As noted earlier, G6PD is a key enzyme in the pathway (Fig. 11–8). Reduced glutathione, which is quantitatively the most important antioxidant in cells, depends on the availability of NADPH. Red blood cells are especially vulnerable to deficiency of NADPH, which results in hemolysis during oxidative stress.

Another manifestation of oxidative stress in RBCs is the oxidation of the iron in hemoglobin from Fe^{2+} to Fe^{3+}, producing methemoglobin that occurs both spontaneously and as a response to xenobiotics such as nitrites and aminophenols. Because most reduction of methemoglobin is done by NADH-dependent methemoglobin reductase, which is not deficient in persons who lack G6PD, such persons do not develop methemoglobinemia under normal circumstances. However, when oxidative stress is severe

and methemoglobinemia develops, people who have G6PD deficiency have limited ability to use the alternative NADPH-dependent methemoglobin reductase (Chap. 124).[112]

Gluconeogenesis

Gluconeogenesis facilitates the conversion of amino acids and intermediates of the citric acid cycle to glucose. It is an important source of glucose during fasting and enables maintenance of glycogen stores. The brain is a major consumer of glucose from both dietary intake and from gluconeogenesis. Other tissues such as the testes, erythrocytes, and kidney medulla rely exclusively on glucose for energy production.[59] Gluconeogenesis occurs primarily in the liver but also in the kidney. Most of the steps in the synthesis of glucose from pyruvate are simply the reverse of glycolysis, with 3 irreversible exceptions: (1) the conversion of glucose-6-phosphate to glucose; (2) the conversion of fructose-1,6-diphosphate to fructose-6-phosphate; and (3) the synthesis of phosphoenolpyruvate from pyruvate. The synthesis of phosphoenolpyruvate from pyruvate is especially complex. Pyruvate is first converted to oxaloacetate within the mitochondria; then to malate, which is transported out of the mitochondria and converted in the cytosol back to oxaloacetate; and then to phosphoenolpyruvate (Fig. 11–9). Certain amino acids—notably alanine, glutamate, and aspartate—are readily converted to citric acid cycle intermediates and can be used in the synthesis of glucose through this cycle.[59] Glycerol, produced by the breakdown of triglycerides in adipose tissue, is another substrate for gluconeogenesis.

The regulation of gluconeogenesis is opposite to that of glycolysis, stimulated by glucagon and catecholamines but inhibited by insulin. Gluconeogenesis requires the cytosolic NAD^+ and mitochondrial NADH. It is impaired by processes that increase the cytosol-reducing potential as measured by the cytosol $NADH/NAD^+$ ratio (see discussion below).

A number of xenobiotics impair gluconeogenesis, resulting in hypoglycemia when glycogen stores are depleted (Table 11–3). Hypoglycin A, an unusual amino acid found in unripe ackee fruit that is the cause of Jamaican vomiting sickness, and its metabolite, methylenecyclopropylacetic acid (MCPA), found in lychee fruit, produce profound hypoglycemia.[98,105] Methylenecyclopropylacetic acid indirectly inhibits gluconeogenesis by blocking the oxidation of long-chain fatty acids, an important source of NADH in mitochondria. It also inhibits the metabolism of several glycogenic amino acids, including leucine, isoleucine, and tryptophan, and blocks their entrance into the citric acid cycle. Methylenecyclopropylacetic acid also prevents the transport of malate out of the mitochondria.[93,105,106] Hypoglycemia often occurs in fasting patients with elevated ethanol concentrations.[4,32,61] This is likely a result of the impairment of gluconeogenesis by the increased cytosolic $NADH:NAD^+$ ratio associated with the metabolism of ethanol. This inhibits the 2 cytosolic steps that require NAD^+—the conversions of lactate to pyruvate and of malate to oxaloacetate.[2,61]

Fatty Acid Metabolism

Fatty acid metabolism occurs primarily in hepatocytes. Fatty acids mobilized in adipose tissue enter hepatocytes by passive diffusion. Fatty acid synthesis is stimulated by insulin and inhibited by glucagon and epinephrine. Acetyl-CoA is the primary building block of free fatty acids (FFAs). In energy-depleted cells, fatty acids are combined with glycerol phosphate to form triacylglycerol (triglycerides), the first step in the synthesis of fat for storage. Hepatic triglycerides are bound to lipoprotein to form very-low-density lipoprotein and then transported and stored in adipocytes.

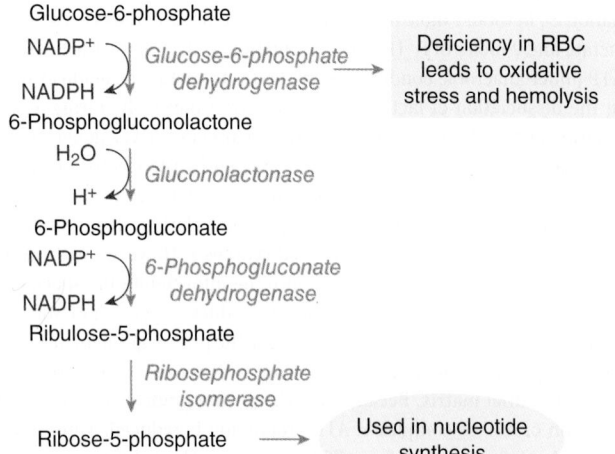

FIGURE 11–8. The oxidation reactions of the hexose monophosphate shunt are an important source of nicotinamide adenine dinucleotide phosphate (NADPH) for reductive biosynthesis and for protection of cells against oxidative stress. Deficiency of glucose-6-phosphate dehydrogenase, the first enzyme in the pathway, may result in red blood cell (RBC) hemolysis during oxidative stress.

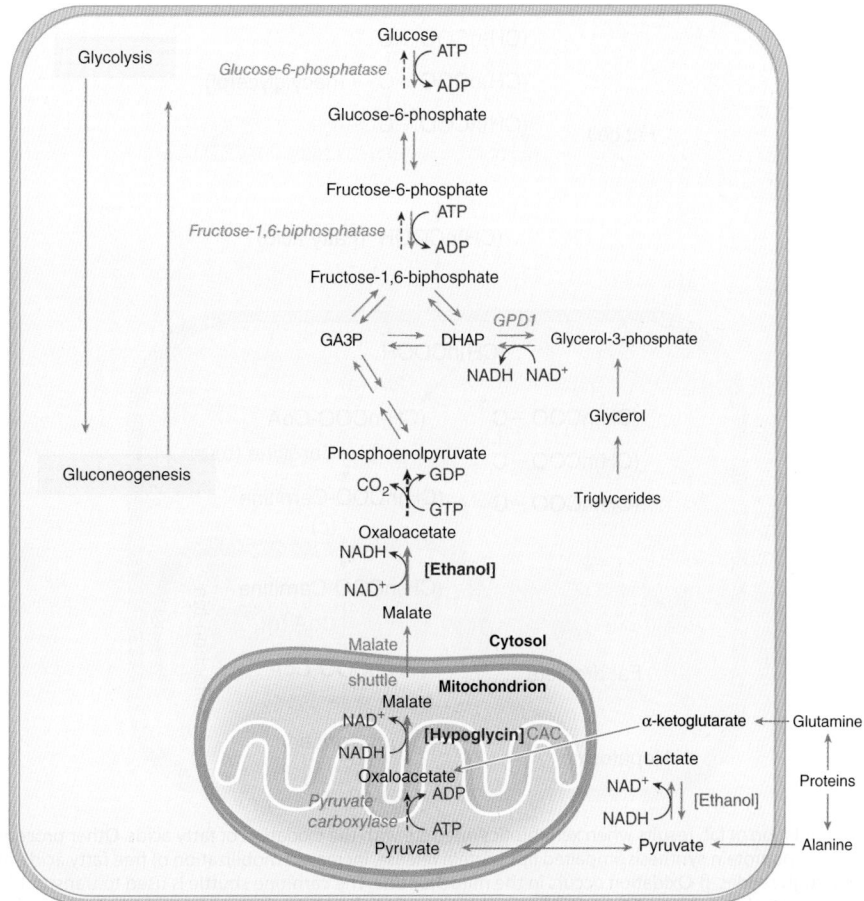

FIGURE 11–9. Gluconeogenesis reverses the steps of glycolysis, with the exception of the bypass of the 3 irreversible steps shown. The step from pyruvate to phosphoenolpyruvate involves both cytosolic and mitochondrial reactions that use ATP. Hypoglycin A inhibits the intramitochondrial conversion of oxaloacetate to malate by depleting NADH through interference with β-oxidation of fatty acids. Ethanol decreases cytosolic supplies of NAD$^+$. Alternative substrates for gluconeogenesis include glycerol from triglycerides and numerous amino acids. DHAP = dihydroxyacetone phosphate, GA3P = glyceraldehyde 3 phosphate, GPD1 = glycerol-3-phosphate dehydrogenase, CAC = citric acid cycle.

When hepatocytes are energy depleted, triglycerides are broken down to FFAs and glycerol. This process is suppressed by insulin but supported by glucagon or epinephrine. Free fatty acids undergo β-oxidation in the mitochondria, a process that breaks the FFA into acetyl-CoA molecules that can then enter the citric acid cycle. Free fatty acids require activation before transport into the mitochondria. This is accomplished by acyl-coenzyme A (acyl-CoA) synthetase, which adds a CoA group to the FFA in an energy-dependent synthetic reaction. These are transported into the mitochondria by a process that utilizes cyclical binding to carnitine, a "carnitine shuttle" (Fig. 11–3). Once inside the mitochondria, FFAs are converted to acetyl-CoA by β-oxidation, involving the sequential removal of 2-carbon fragments, each time acting at the second carbon (the β carbon) position of the fatty acid. Each 2-carbon mole removed from the FFA produces one NADH and one FADH$_2$, which are oxidized in the electron transport chain, and 1 mole of acetyl-CoA, which enters the citric acid cycle. This process produces 1.3 times more ATP per mole of carbon metabolized than does the oxidative metabolism of glucose or other carbohydrates.[59]

Many xenobiotics interrupt fatty acid metabolism at various steps, resulting in accumulation of triglycerides in the liver (Table 11–3; Fig. 11–10). The mechanisms of disruption of fatty acid metabolism are poorly defined.[18] Some xenobiotics, including ethanol, hypoglycin A, MCPA, and nucleoside analogs, inhibit β-oxidation, at least indirectly, through effects on NADH concentrations. Protease inhibitors are associated with a syndrome of peripheral fat wasting, central adiposity, hyperlipidemia, and insulin resistance.

The condition of alcoholic ketoacidosis is related in part to inhibition of gluconeogenesis in the alcoholic patient and in part to an exuberant response to nutritional needs by the fatty acid machinery. In a chronic alcohol-users,

decreased intake of carbohydrates and impaired thiamine absorption stimulates a starvation response with increases in serum glucagon, cortisol, growth hormone, and epinephrine concentrations, and decreases in serum insulin. With continued ethanol intake, the metabolism of ethanol via oxidation increases the NADH:NAD$^+$ ratio, which inhibits hepatic gluconeogenesis. When the need for carbohydrate is not met by gluconeogenesis, lipolysis, which is normally inhibited by insulin, is intensified and fatty acid mobilization progresses. The increased mitochondrial NADH:NAD$^+$ ratio favors the production of β-hydroxybutyrate over acetoacetate, its oxidized form. The administration of fluids, dextrose, and thiamine to the alcoholic patient leads to correction of this process (Chap. 76).[71]

Protein and Nitrogen Metabolism

Human nitrogen consumption occurs through dietary intake of free amino acids, polypeptides, and ammonia (via intestinal splitting of urea and amino acids). Amino acids are the basic building blocks of proteins and are built on a backbone of an amino group, a carboxylic acid group, and a middle α carbon attached to a variable group. The simplest amino acid is glycine, in which the variable group is a hydrogen. Of the 20 major amino acids involved in protein synthesis, 10 are considered essential and only available through dietary intake. The other amino acids can be synthesized by the body via other carbon- and nitrogen-containing molecules. As mentioned above, amino acids such as alanine, glutamate, and aspartate are available for use as citric acid cycle intermediates. Alanine is an important molecule for skeletal muscles for the elimination of nitrogen waste and for energy generation via the glucose-alanine cycle. Myocytes release alanine to the systemic circulation through which it goes to the liver. In the hepatocytes, alanine

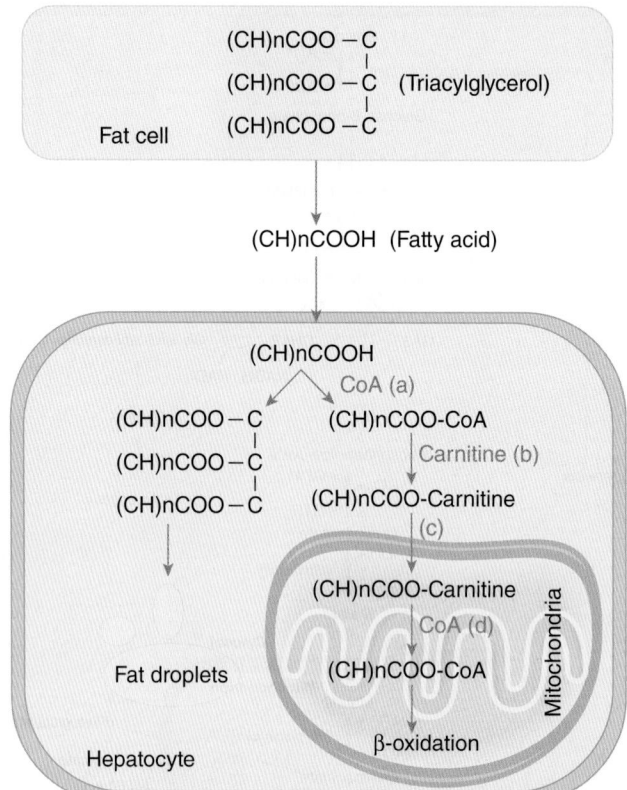

FIGURE 11–10. Steatosis, an accumulation of fat, results when xenobiotics interfere with the oxidation of fatty acids. Other processes that increase intracellular accumulation of fat include impaired lipoprotein synthesis, impaired lipoprotein release, increased mobilization of free fatty acids, increased uptake of circulating lipids, and increased production of triglycerides. β-Oxidation occurs in the mitochondria. The carnitine shuttle is used to transport long-chain fatty acids from the cellular cytosol across the mitochondrial membrane. The enzymes involved are (a) acyl-CoA synthetase, (b) carnitine palmitoyltransferase I, (c) carnitine acylcarnitine translocase, and (d) carnitine palmitoyltransferase II. Acyl-CoA is the intramitochondrial substrate for β-oxidation. Potential mechanisms of inhibition of β-oxidation include induction of carnitine deficiency, inhibition of the transferase or translocase, and increased NADH:NAD+ ratio via increased use of NAD+ or by inhibition of NADH use. The specific site of action is not defined for many toxins that cause steatosis.

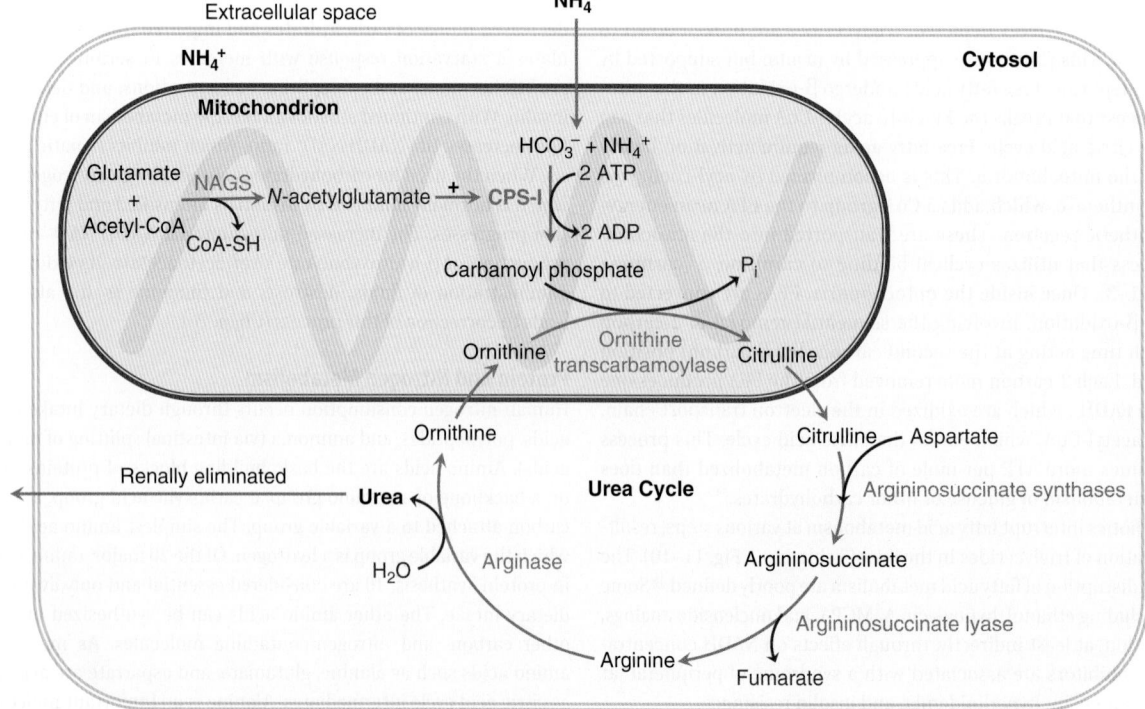

FIGURE 11–11. Hepatocytes extract circulating free ammonia and combine the ammonia with an amine group from aspartate to form urea, a water-soluble compound eliminated by the kidneys. Carbamoyl phosphate synthetase-1 (CPS-1) is the rate-limiting step of ammonia entry into the urea cycle. In turn, CPS-1 is positively regulated by the formation of N-acetylglutamate via N-acetylglutamate synthetase (NAGS).

TABLE 11–4	Xenobiotic Causes of Hyperammonemia

Anesthetics

Asparaginase

Carbamazepine

Ethylene glycol

5-Fluorouracil

Glycine

Hypoglycin A (ackee fruit)

Methanol

Methylenecyclopropylacetic acid (lychee fruit)

Pyrimethamine

Salicylates

Sulfadiazine

Topiramate

Valproic acid

Xenobiotics causing fulminant hepatic failure

converts to pyruvate via alanine transaminase (ALT), releasing its nitrogen group to glutamate. Pyruvate then undergoes gluconeogenesis, and glucose is released back to circulation for myocytes and other cells to use.[59]

Glutamine is the main storage molecule for total body nitrogen/ammonia. A single glutamine molecule contains 2 amino groups. The uptake of ammonia (NH_4^+) into glutamine protects the body from the neurotoxic and alkalemic effects of free ammonia. The removal of an ammonia yields glutamate (a neurotransmitter), and a removal of a second ammonia yields α-ketoglutarate (a citric acid cycle substrate). As free ammonia is released from glutamine, hepatocytes facilitate the removal of free ammonia from the body via generation of urea by the urea cycle (Fig. 11–11). The activation step of the urea cycle combines NH_4^+, bicarbonate, and 2 ATP molecules to create carbamoyl phosphate by carbamoyl phosphate synthetase-1 (CPS-1). This process requires an obligate cofactor of N-acetylglutamate, a product of glutamate and acetyl-CoA via N-acetylglutamate synthetase. Carbamoyl phosphate enters into the urea cycle through ornithine transcarbamylase (OTC), which catalyzes the addition of carbamoyl phosphate to ornithine to make citrulline. Citrulline is subsequently converted to arginosuccinate, arginine, and back to ornithine. The final step of arginine to ornithine by arginase releases urea. Urea is highly water soluble, and it is renally eliminated from the body.[59]

Inborn errors of metabolism involving the deficiencies of urea cycle enzymes lead to severe hyperammonemia and death if undiagnosed and/or untreated. X-linked OTC deficiency is the most common urea cycle disorder. Several xenobiotics can also induce secondary hyperammonemia by the inhibition of enzymes in the urea cycle (Table 11–4).[20] For example, valproic acid undergoes ω-oxidation to yield 2-propyl-4-pentenoate (4-en-VPA) and propionate in an overdose state or when secondary carnitine deficiencies prohibit adequate β-oxidation. Both 4-en-VPA and propionate decrease the generation of N-acetylglutamate, which effectively inhibits CPS-1 and subsequently the entire urea cycle. Hyperammonemia is a common clinical feature of valproic acid in overdose and occasionally in therapeutic use (Chap. 48).[122]

SUMMARY

- Biotransformation is a complex process, involving numerous enzyme systems, that usually detoxifies xenobiotics; however, "metabolic activation" occurs.
- Phase I reactions add functional groups to lipophilic xenobiotics to enhance their reactivity, preparing them for further detoxification by synthetic phase II reactions that enhance hydrophilicity and renal elimination.
- The phase I cytochrome P450 (CYP) enzymes biotransform most xenobiotics; CYP3A4 is the most abundant one, metabolizing 50% to 60% of all pharmaceuticals.

- Cytochrome P450 enzyme activity is quite variable because of genetic polymorphisms—genetic changes that exist in at least 1% of the human population. Enzyme activity also varies because of induction and inhibition.
- The most common method of induction is a nuclear receptor–mediated increase in gene transcription. Inhibition of CYP enzymes is the most common cause of harmful drug–drug interactions, the most common type being competitive, where the substrate and inhibitor both bind the active site of the enzyme.
- Xenobiotic disposition is also effected by membrane transporter (MT) proteins that mediate the cellular uptake and efflux of xenobiotics.
- P-glycoprotein is an MT protein that mediates the efflux of xenobiotics from the apical (luminal) membrane of intestinal enterocytes.

Acknowledgment
Kathleen A. Delaney, MD, contributed to this chapter in previous editions.

REFERENCES

1. Abernethy DR, Flockhart DA. Molecular basis of cardiovascular drug metabolism: implications for predicting clinically important drug interactions. *Circulation.* 2000;101:1749-1753.
2. Albert A. Fundamental aspects of selective toxicity. *Ann N Y Acad Sci.* 1965;123:5-18.
3. American Academy of Clinical Toxicology; European Association of Poisons Centres and Clinical Toxicologists Reference. Position statement and practice guidelines on the use of multi-dose activated charcoal in the treatment of acute poisoning. *J Toxicol Clin Toxicol.* 1999;37:731-751.
4. Arky RA, Freinkel N. Alcohol hypoglycemia. Effects of ethanol on plasma. 3. Glucose, ketones, and free fatty acids in "juvenile" diabetics: a model for "nonketotic diabetic acidosis"? *Arch Intern Med.* 1964;114:501-507.
5. Badr MZ, et al. Mechanism of hepatotoxicity to periportal regions of the liver lobule due to allyl alcohol: role of oxygen and lipid peroxidation. *J Pharmacol Exp Ther.* 1986;238:1138-1142.
6. Barclay JA, et al. Dapsone-induced methemoglobinemia: a primer for clinicians. *Ann Pharmacother.* 2011;45:1103-1115.
7. Baud FJ. Cyanide: critical issues in diagnosis and treatment. *Hum Exp Toxicol.* 2007;26:191-201.
8. Bayir H. Reactive oxygen species. *Crit Care Med.* 2005;33(12)(suppl):S498-S501.
9. Bell GC, et al. Clinical Pharmacogenetics Implementation Consortium (CPIC) guideline for CYP2D6 genotype and use of ondansetron and tropisetron. *Clin Pharmacol Ther.* 2017;102:213-218.
10. Beutler E. Glucose-6-phosphate dehydrogenase deficiency. *N Engl J Med.* 1991;324:169-174.
11. Bock KW, Kohle C. Coordinate regulation of drug metabolism by xenobiotic nuclear receptors: UGTs acting together with CYPs and glucuronide transporters. *Drug Metab Rev.* 2004;36:595-615.
12. Brittebo EB. Metabolism of xenobiotics in the nasal olfactory mucosa: implications for local toxicity. *Pharmacol Toxicol.* 1993;72(suppl) 3:50-52.
13. Brown C. Overview of drug interactions modulated by cytochrome P450. *US Pharmacists.* 2001;26:20-35.
14. Callaghan R, et al. P-Glycoprotein: so many ways to turn it on. *J Clin Pharmacol.* 2008;48:365-378.
15. Cappellini MD, Fiorelli G. Glucose-6-phosphate dehydrogenase deficiency. *Lancet.* 2008;371:64-74.
16. Carlquist JF, Anderson JL. Using pharmacogenetics in real time to guide warfarin initiation: a clinician update. *Circulation.* 2011;124:2554-2559.
17. Caro AA, Cederbaum AI. Oxidative stress, toxicology, and pharmacology of CYP2E1. *Annu Rev Pharmacol Toxicol.* 2004;44:27-42.
18. Carr A, et al. Pathogenesis of HIV-1-protease inhibitor-associated peripheral lipodystrophy, hyperlipidaemia, and insulin resistance. *Lancet.* 1998;351:1881-1883.
19. Chinn LW, Kroetz DL. ABCB1 pharmacogenetics: progress, pitfalls, and promise. *Clin Pharmacol Ther.* 2007;81:265-269.
20. Clay AS, Hainline BE. Hyperammonemia in the ICU. *Chest.* 2007;132:1368-1378.
21. Conney AH. Induction of drug-metabolizing enzymes: a path to the discovery of multiple cytochromes P450. *Annu Rev Pharmacol Toxicol.* 2003;43:1-30.
22. Cribb AE, et al. The endoplasmic reticulum in xenobiotic toxicity. *Drug Metab Rev.* 2005;37:405-442.
23. Dai Y, et al. Stable expression of human cytochrome P4502E1 in HepG2 cells: characterization of catalytic activities and production of reactive oxygen intermediates. *Biochemistry.* 1993;32:6928-6937.
24. Daniulaityte R, et al. "I just wanted to tell you that loperamide WILL WORK": a web-based study of extra-medical use of loperamide. *Drug Alcohol Depend.* 2013;130:241-244.
25. de Lannoy IA, Silverman M. The MDR1 gene product, P-glycoprotein, mediates the transport of the cardiac glycoside, digoxin. *Biochem Biophys Res Commun.* 1992;189:551-557.

26. Ding X, Kaminsky LS. Human extrahepatic cytochromes P450: function in xenobiotic metabolism and tissue-selective chemical toxicity in the respiratory and gastrointestinal tracts. *Annu Rev Pharmacol Toxicol.* 2003;43:149-173.

27. Dutheil F, et al. Xenobiotic metabolizing enzymes in the central nervous system: contribution of cytochrome P450 enzymes in normal and pathological human brain. *Biochimie.* 2008;90:426-436.

28. Eling TE, et al. Prostaglandin H synthase and xenobiotic oxidation. *Annu Rev Pharmacol Toxicol.* 1990;30:1-45.

29. Falconer M, et al. Methadone induced torsade de pointes in a patient receiving antiretroviral therapy. *Ir Med J.* 2007;100:631-632.

30. Farabee MJ. On-line biology book. http://www.emc.maricopa.edu/faculty/farabee/BIOBK/BioBookTOC.html. Published 2009. Accessed March 14, 2009.

31. Flockhart DA, Tanus-Santos JE. Implications of cytochrome P450 interactions when prescribing medication for hypertension. *Arch Intern Med.* 2002;162:405-412.

32. Freinkel N, et al. Alcohol hypoglycemia. I. Carbohydrate metabolism of patients with clinical alcohol hypoglycemia and the experimental reproduction of the syndrome with pure ethanol. *J Clin Invest.* 1963;42:1112-1133.

33. Ganesan S, et al. Cytochrome P450-dependent toxicity of dapsone in human erythrocytes. *J Appl Toxicol.* 2010;30:271-275.

34. Gardiner SJ, Begg EJ. Pharmacogenetics, drug-metabolizing enzymes, and clinical practice. *Pharmacol Rev.* 2006;58:521-590.

35. Gerlach M, et al. MPTP mechanisms of neurotoxicity and their implications for Parkinson's disease. *Eur J Pharmacol.* 1991;208:273-286.

36. Gonzalez FJ. The 2006 Bernard B. Brodie Award Lecture. CYP2E1. *Drug Metab Dispos.* 2007;35:1-8.

37. Granfors MT, et al. Ciprofloxacin greatly increases concentrations and hypotensive effect of tizanidine by inhibiting its cytochrome P450 1A2-mediated presystemic metabolism. *Clin Pharmacol Ther.* 2004;76:598-606.

38. Guengerich FP. Catalytic selectivity of human cytochrome P450 enzymes: relevance to drug metabolism and toxicity. *Toxicol Lett.* 1994;70:133-138.

39. Guengerich FP. Cytochrome p450 and chemical toxicology. *Chem Res Toxicol.* 2008;21:70-83.

40. Gundala S, et al. The hepatocellular bile acid transporter NTCP facilitates uptake of the lethal mushroom toxin alpha-amanitin. *Arch Toxicol.* 2004;78:68-73.

41. Handschin C, Meyer UA. Induction of drug metabolism: the role of nuclear receptors. *Pharmacol Rev.* 2003;55:649-673.

42. Haufroid V, Hantson P. CYP2D6 genetic polymorphisms and their relevance for poisoning due to amfetamines, opioid analgesics and antidepressants. *Clin Toxicol (Phila).* 2015;53:501-510.

43. Hedrich WD, et al. Insights into CYP2B6-mediated drug-drug interactions. *Acta Pharm Sin B.* 2016;6:413-425.

44. Hetu C, et al. Effect of chronic ethanol administration on bromobenzene liver toxicity in the rat. *Toxicol Appl Pharmacol.* 1983;67:166-177.

45. Ho RH, Kim RB. Transporters and drug therapy: implications for drug disposition and disease. *Clin Pharmacol Ther.* 2005;78:260-277.

46. Hughes MF. Arsenic toxicity and potential mechanisms of action. *Toxicol Lett.* 2002;133:1-16.

47. Imlay JA. Pathways of oxidative damage. *Annu Rev Microbiol.* 2003;57:395-418.

48. Ingelman-Sundberg M. Genetic polymorphisms of cytochrome P450 2D6 (CYP2D6): clinical consequences, evolutionary aspects and functional diversity. *Pharmacogenomics J.* 2005;5:6-13.

49. Ingelman-Sundberg M, et al. The Human Cytochrome P450 (CYP) Allele Nomenclature Database. http://www.cypalleles.ki.se/. Published 2015. Accessed February 23, 2017.

50. Ingelman-Sundberg M, et al. Influence of cytochrome P450 polymorphisms on drug therapies: pharmacogenetic, pharmacoepigenetic and clinical aspects. *Pharmacol Ther.* 2007;116:496-526.

51. Jakobsson J, et al. Large differences in testosterone excretion in Korean and Swedish men are strongly associated with a UDP-glucuronosyl transferase 2B17 polymorphism. *J Clin Endocrinol Metab.* 2006;91:687-693.

52. Josephy PD, et al. "Phase I and Phase II" drug metabolism: terminology that we should phase out? *Drug Metab Rev.* 2005;37:575-580.

53. Kalgutkar AS, et al. A comprehensive listing of bioactivation pathways of organic functional groups. *Curr Drug Metab.* 2005;6:161-225.

54. Kapur BM, et al. Methadone: a review of drug-drug and pathophysiological interactions. *Crit Rev Clin Lab Sci.* 2011;48:171-195.

55. Karazniewicz-Lada M, et al. The influence of genetic polymorphism of CYP2C19 isoenzyme on the pharmacokinetics of clopidogrel and its metabolites in patients with cardiovascular diseases. *J Clin Pharmacol.* 2014;54:874-880.

56. Kato M. Intestinal first-pass metabolism of CYP3A4 substrates. *Drug Metab Pharmacokinet.* 2008;23:87-94.

57. Kim D, Guengerich FP. Cytochrome P450 activation of arylamines and heterocyclic amines. *Annu Rev Pharmacol Toxicol.* 2005;45:27-49.

58. Kim RB. Drugs as *P*-glycoprotein substrates, inhibitors, and inducers. *Drug Metab Rev.* 2002;34:47-54.

59. King M. The Medical Biochemistry Page. http://themedicalbiochemistrypage.org/. Published 2017. Accessed January 20, 2017.

60. Kraut JA, Madias NE. Lactic acidosis. *N Engl J Med.* 2014;371:2309-2319.

61. Krishna DR, Klotz U. Extrahepatic metabolism of drugs in humans. *Clin Pharmacokinet.* 1994;26:144-160.

62. Labbe G, et al. Drug-induced liver injury through mitochondrial dysfunction: mechanisms and detection during preclinical safety studies. *Fundam Clin Pharmacol.* 2008;22:335-353.

63. Lankisch TO, et al. Gilbert's syndrome and hyperbilirubinemia in protease inhibitor therapy—an extended haplotype of genetic variants increases risk in indinavir treatment. *J Hepatol.* 2009;50:1010-1018.

64. Lewis DF. On the recognition of mammalian microsomal cytochrome P450 substrates and their characteristics: towards the prediction of human p450 substrate specificity and metabolism. *Biochem Pharmacol.* 2000;60:293-306.

65. Lieber CS. Metabolism of alcohol. *Clin Liver Dis.* 2005;9:1-35.

66. Lin JH. CYP induction-mediated drug interactions: in vitro assessment and clinical implications. *Pharm Res.* 2006;23:1089-1116.

67. Lundqvist E, et al. Genetic mechanisms for duplication and multiduplication of the human CYP2D6 gene and methods for detection of duplicated CYP2D6 genes. *Gene.* 1999;226:327-338.

68. Madias NE. Lactic acidosis. *Kidney Int.* 1986;29:752-774.

69. Maggo SD, et al. Clinical implications of pharmacogenetic variation on the effects of statins. *Drug Saf.* 2011;34:1-19.

70. Manahan SE. *Toxicological Chemistry and Biochemistry.* 3rd ed. Boca Raton, FL: Lewis; 2003.

71. McGuire LC, et al. Alcoholic ketoacidosis. *Emerg Med J.* 2006;23:417-420.

72. Miller EC, Miller JA. The presence and significance of bound amino azodyes in the livers or rats fed p-demethylaminoazobenzene. *Cancer Res.* 1947;7:468-480.

73. Myers CE, et al. Adriamycin: the role of lipid peroxidation in cardiac toxicity and tumor response. *Science.* 1977;197:165-167.

74. Nagata K, Yamazoe Y. Genetic polymorphism of human cytochrome p450 involved in drug metabolism. *Drug Metab Pharmacokinet.* 2002;17:167-189.

75. Nair MK, et al. Ciprofloxacin-induced torsades de pointes in a methadone-dependent patient. *Addiction.* 2008;103:2062-2064.

76. Nardone R, et al. Thiamine deficiency induced neurochemical, neuroanatomical, and neuropsychological alterations: a reappraisal. *ScientificWorldJournal.* 2013;2013:309143.

77. Nebert DW, et al. Human cytochromes P450 in health and disease. *Philos Trans R Soc Lond B Biol Sci.* 2013;368:20120431.

78. Nelson DR. The cytochrome p450 homepage. *Hum Genomics.* 2009;4:59-65.

79. Nelson DR, et al. Comparison of cytochrome P450 (CYP) genes from the mouse and human genomes, including nomenclature recommendations for genes, pseudogenes and alternative-splice variants. *Pharmacogenetics.* 2004;14:1-18.

80. Nolin TD. Altered nonrenal drug clearance in ESRD. *Curr Opin Nephrol Hypertens.* 2008;17:555-559.

81. NoorZurani MH, et al. Itraconazole-induced torsade de pointes in a patient receiving methadone substitution therapy. *Drug Alcohol Rev.* 2009;28:688-690.

82. Obach RS, et al. In vitro cytochrome P450 inhibition data and the prediction of drug-drug interactions: qualitative relationships, quantitative predictions, and the rank-order approach. *Clin Pharmacol Ther.* 2005;78:582-592.

83. Owen RP, et al. Cytochrome P450 2D6. *Pharmacogenet Genomics.* 2009;19:559-562.

84. Park BK. Cytochrome P450 enzymes in the heart. *Lancet.* 2000;355:945-946.

85. Pavek P, Dvorak Z. Xenobiotic-induced transcriptional regulation of xenobiotic metabolizing enzymes of the cytochrome P450 superfamily in human extrahepatic tissues. *Curr Drug Metab.* 2008;9:129-143.

86. Pelkonen O, et al. Inhibition and induction of human cytochrome P450 enzymes: current status. *Arch Toxicol.* 2008;82:667-715.

87. Perry SW, et al. Mitochondrial membrane potential probes and the proton gradient: a practical usage guide. *Biotechniques.* 2011;50:98-115.

88. Piscitelli SC, et al. Indinavir concentrations and St John's wort. *Lancet.* 2000;355:547-548.

89. Proudfoot AT. Pentachlorophenol poisoning. *Toxicol Rev.* 2003;22:3-11.

90. Proudfoot AT, et al. Sodium fluoroacetate poisoning. *Toxicol Rev.* 2006;25:213-219.

91. Rose MS, et al. Paraquat accumulation: tissue and species specificity. *Biochem Pharmacol.* 1976;25:419-423.

92. Rosen GM, Rauckman EJ. Carbon tetrachloride-induced lipid peroxidation: a spin trapping study. *Toxicol Lett.* 1982;10:337-344.

93. Ruderman N, et al. Relation of fatty acid oxidation tgluconeogenesis: effect of pentenoic acid. *Life Sci.* 1968;7:1083-1089.

94. Santi DV, et al. Mechanism of interaction of thymidylate synthetase with 5-fluorodeoxyuridylate. *Biochemistry.* 1974;13:471-481.

95. Saudan C, et al. Testosterone and doping control. *Br J Sports Med.* 2006;40 (suppl 1):i21-i24.

96. Schuster I, Bernhardt R. Inhibition of cytochromes p450: existing and new promising therapeutic targets. *Drug Metab Rev.* 2007;39:481-499.

97. Schwarz UI, Stein CM. Genetic determinants of dose and clinical outcomes in patients receiving oral anticoagulants. *Clin Pharmacol Ther.* 2006;80:7-12.

98. Shrivastava A, et al. Association of acute toxic encephalopathy with litchi consumption in an outbreak in Muzaffarpur, India, 2014: a case-control study. *Lancet Glob Health.* 2017;5:e458-e466.

99. Shuldiner AR, et al. Association of cytochrome P450 2C19 genotype with the antiplatelet effect and clinical efficacy of clopidogrel therapy. *JAMA.* 2009;302:849-857.

100. Si D, et al. Mechanism of CYP2C9 inhibition by flavones and flavonols. *Drug Metab Dispos.* 2009;37:629-634.

101. Sim E, et al. Arylamine *N*-acetyltransferases: structural and functional implications of polymorphisms. *Toxicology.* 2008;254:170-183.

102. Southorn PA, Powis G. Free radicals in medicine. I. Chemical nature and biologic reactions. *Mayo Clin Proc.* 1988;63:381-389.

103. Suzuki T, et al. The MRP family and anticancer drug metabolism. *Curr Drug Metab.* 2001;2:367-377.

104. Sweeney BP, Bromilow J. Liver enzyme induction and inhibition: implications for anaesthesia. *Anaesthesia.* 2006;61:159-177.

105. Tanaka K. On the mode of action of hypoglycin A. 3. Isolation and identification of *cis*-4-decene-1,10-dioic, *cis,cis*-4,7-decadiene-1,10-dioic, *cis*-4-octene-1,8-dioic, glutaric, and adipic acids, *N*-(methylenecyclopropyl)acetylglycine, and *N*-isovalerylglycine from urine of hypoglycin A-treated rats. *J Biol Chem.* 1972;247:7465-7478.

106. Tanaka K, et al. Jamaican vomiting sickness. Biochemical investigation of two cases. *N Engl J Med.* 1976;295:461-467.

107. Temple AR. Pathophysiology of aspirin overdosage toxicity, with implications for management. *Pediatrics.* 1978;62(5, pt 2, suppl):873-876.

108. Timbrell JA. *Principles of Biochemical Toxicology.* 4th ed. New York, NY: Informa Healthcare; 2009.

109. Timsit YE, Negishi M. CAR and PXR: the xenobiotic-sensing receptors. *Steroids.* 2007;72:231-246.

110. Toogood PL. Mitochondrial drugs. *Curr Opin Chem Biol.* 2008;12:457-463.

111. Uchaipichat V, et al. Selectivity of substrate (trifluoperazine) and inhibitor (amitriptyline, androsterone, canrenoic acid, hecogenin, phenylbutazone, quinidine, quinine, and sulfinpyrazone) "probes" for human udp-glucuronosyltransferases. *Drug Metab Dispos.* 2006;34:449-456.

112. Umbreit J. Methemoglobin—it's not just blue: a concise review. *Am J Hematol.* 2007;82:134-144.

113. Urquhart BL, et al. Nuclear receptors and the regulation of drug-metabolizing enzymes and drug transporters: implications for interindividual variability in response to drugs. *J Clin Pharmacol.* 2007;47:566-578.

114. Van Booven D, et al. Cytochrome P450 2C9-CYP2C9. *Pharmacogenet Genomics.* 2010;20:277-281.

115. van de Kerkhof DH, et al. Evaluation of testosterone/epitestosterone ratio influential factors as determined in doping analysis. *J Anal Toxicol.* 2000;24:102-115.

116. Wallace KB, Starkov AA. Mitochondrial targets of drug toxicity. *Annu Rev Pharmacol Toxicol.* 2000;40:353-388.

117. Waxman DJ. P450 gene induction by structurally diverse xenochemicals: central role of nuclear receptors CAR, PXR, and PPAR. *Arch Biochem Biophys.* 1999;369:11-23.

118. Whelton A. Renal and related cardiovascular effects of conventional and COX-2-specific NSAIDs and non-NSAID analgesics. *Am J Ther.* 2000;7:63-74.

119. Wienkers LC, Heath TG. Predicting in vivo drug interactions from in vitro drug discovery data. *Nat Rev Drug Discov.* 2005;4:825-833.

120. Williams RT. *Detoxication Mechanisms: The Metabolism of Drugs and Allied Organic Compounds.* London: Chapman & Hall Limited; 1959.

121. World Anti-Doping Agency. *Endogenous Anabolic Androgenic Steroids: Measurement and Reporting.* 2015.

122. Yamamoto Y, et al. Risk factors for hyperammonemia associated with valproic acid therapy in adult epilepsy patients. *Epilepsy Res.* 2012;101:202-209.

123. Zakhari S. Overview: how is alcohol metabolized by the body? *Alcohol Res Health.* 2006;29:245-254.

124. Zamek-Gliszczynski MJ, et al. Integration of hepatic drug transporters and phase II metabolizing enzymes: mechanisms of hepatic excretion of sulfate, glucuronide, and glutathione metabolites. *Eur J Pharm Sci.* 2006;27:447-486.

125. Zanger UM, Schwab M. Cytochrome P450 enzymes in drug metabolism: regulation of gene expression, enzyme activities, and impact of genetic variation. *Pharmacol Ther.* 2013;138:103-141.

126. Zhang JY, et al. Xenobiotic-metabolizing enzymes in human lung. *Curr Drug Metab.* 2006;7:939-948.

127. Zhou SF, et al. Clinically important drug interactions potentially involving mechanism-based inhibition of cytochrome P450 3A4 and the role of therapeutic drug monitoring. *Ther Drug Monit.* 2007;29:687-710.

128. Zolk O, Fromm MF. Transporter-mediated drug uptake and efflux: important determinants of adverse drug reactions. *Clin Pharmacol Ther.* 2011;89:798-805.

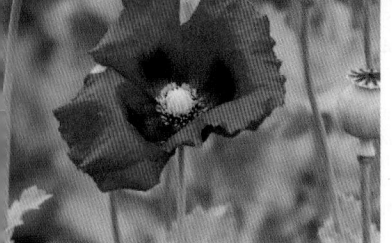

APPENDIX

Cytochrome P450 Substrates, Inhibitors, and Inducers[1-17]

	Substrates		Inhibitors		Inducers
1A2	**Analgesics** Acetaminophen Lidocaine Nabumetone Naproxen Ropivacaine Phenacetin **Antidepressants** Amitriptyline Clomipramine Duloxetine[b] Fluvoxamine Imipramine Mirtazapine **Antiemetics** Alosetron[b] Ondansetron Ramosetron[b] **Antipsychotics** Chlorpromazine Clozapine Haloperidol Olanzapine	**Cardiovascular** Ergotamines Frovatriptan Guanabenz Mexiletine Propafenone Propranolol Verapamil Zolmitriptan **Hormones** Estradiol Flutamide Melatonin[b] Ramelteon[b] Tasimelteon[b] **Others** Caffeine[b] Cyclobenzaprine Pirfenidone Riluzole Ropinirole Tacrine Theophylline[b] Tizanidine[b] Triamterene Warfarin-R	**Antibiotics (Fluoroquinolones)** Ciprofloxacin[d] Enoxacin[d] Norfloxacin **Antibiotics (Macrolides)** Clarithromycin Erythromycin Troleandomycin **Antidepressants** Duloxetine Fluvoxamine[d] **Antivirals** Acyclovir Efavirenz Peginterferon-α-2a	**Cardiovascular** Amiodarone Mexiletine Propafenone Ticlopidine Verapamil **NSAIDs** Rofecoxib Tolfenamic acid **Others** Allopurinol Cimetidine Disulfiram Famotidine Grapefruit juice Methoxsalen Oral contraceptives Zafirlukast[d]	**Antibiotics** Nafcillin Rifampin Primaquine **Antiepileptics** Carbamazepine Secobarbital Pentobarbital Phenobarbital Phenytoin **Antiretrovirals** Nelfinavir Ritonavir[a] **Proton Pump Inhibitors** Lansoprazole Omeprazole **Others** Antipyrine Coffee Cruciferous vegetables Insulin PCBs Polycyclic hydrocarbons (chargrilled meat, cigarette smoke) Sulfinpyrazone St. John's Wort Teriflunomide TCDD
2B6	**Analgesics** Aminopyrine Antipyrine Lidocaine Meperidine Methadone Tramadol **Antidepressants** Bupropion Selegiline Sertraline **Antiepileptics** Phenobarbital Phenytoin Propofol Valproic acid **Antimalarials** Artemether Artemisinin antimalarials **Antiretrovirals** Efavirenz Nevirapine	**Benzodiazepines** Diazepam Temazepam **Chemotherapeutics** Cyclophosphamide Ifosfamide **Insecticides** Chlorpyrifos DEET Endosulfan **Others** Coumarins Hexane Ketamine MDMA Mexiletine Nicotine **Testosterone**	**17-α-ethynylestradiol** Clopidogrel Clotrimazole Mifepristone (RU-486) Phencyclidine Sertraline Tenofovir ThioTEPA Ticlopidine Voriconazole		**Antibiotics** Artemisinin antimalarials Rifampin **Antiepileptics** Carbamazepine[e] Phenobarbital Phenytoin **Antiretrovirals** Efavirenz Nelfinavir Nevirapine Ritonavir **Others** Cyclophosphamide DEET Metamizole St. John's Wort Statins Vitamin D

(Continued)

Cytochrome P450 Substrates, Inhibitors, and Inducers[1-17] (*Continued*)

	Substrates		*Inhibitors*		*Inducers*
2C9	**Angiotensin II Receptor Blockers** Candesartan Irbesartan Losartan Valsartan **Antibiotics** Dapsone Sulfamethoxazole **Antidepressants** Amitriptyline Fluoxetine Sertraline **Antiepileptics** Phenobarbital Phenytoin[c] Valproic acid **Insulin Secretagogues** Chlorpropamide Glibenclamide Glimepiride Glipizide Glyburide Tolbutamide	**NSAIDs** Celecoxib[b] Diclofenac Flurbiprofen Ibuprofen Indomethacin Meloxicam Naproxen Piroxicam **Others** Cyclophosphamide Fluvastatin Rosiglitazone Rosuvastatin Tamoxifen Tetrahydrocannabinol Torsemide Voriconazole Warfarin-S[c] Zafirlukast	**Antibiotics (Macrolides)** Clarithromycin Erythromycin Troleandomycin **Antibiotics (Other)** Isoniazid[d] Metronidazole[d] Rifampin Sulfamethoxazole Trimethoprim **Antidepressants** Fluoxetine Fluvoxamine Paroxetine Sertraline **Antiepileptics** Felbamate Valproic acid	**Antifungals (Azoles)** Fluconazole[d] Itraconazole Ketoconazole Miconazole Sulphaphenazole Voriconazole **Antiretrovirals** Efavirenz Ritonavir[a] **HMG CoA Reductase Inhibitors** Fluvastatin Lovastatin **Others** Amiodarone Cimetidine Disulfiram Grapefruit juice	**Antibiotics** Rifampin Rifapentine **Antiepileptics** Amobarbital Carbamazepine Pentobarbital Phenobarbital Phenytoin Secobarbital **Antiretrovirals** Nelfinavir Nevirapine Ritonavir[a] **Steroids** Dexamethasone Prednisone **Others** Aminoglutethimide Antipyrine Aprepitant Avasimibe Bosentan Cigarette smoke Cyclophosphamide Enzalutamide Glutethimide Nifedipine St. John's Wort Statins
2C19	**Antidepressants** Amitriptyline Citalopram Clomipramine Desipramine Doxepin Escitalopram Fluoxetine Imipramine **Antiepileptics** Diazepam Hexobarbital Phenobarbital Phenytoin[b,c] **Cardiovascular** Labetalol Propranolol **Proton Pump Inhibitors** (Major for most) Esomeprazole Lansoprazole[b] Omeprazole[b] Pantoprazole Rabeprazole	**Others** Atomoxetine Carisoprodol Clopidogrel Cyclophosphamide Indomethacin Melatonin Meperidine Methadone Nelfinavir Olanzapine Progesterone Proguanil Ranitidine Voriconazole[b] Warfarin-R	**Antibiotics (Macrolides)** Clarithromycin Erythromycin Troleandomycin **Antibiotics (Others)** Chloramphenicol Isoniazid **Antidepressants** Citalopram Fluoxetine[d] Fluvoxamine[d] Moclobemide[d] Paroxetine Sertraline **Antiepileptics** Felbamate Oxcarbazepine Topiramate Valproic acid	**Antifungals** Fluconazole[d] Ketoconazole Voriconazole **Proton Pump Inhibitors** Esomeprazole Lansoprazole Omeprazole[d] Pantoprazole Rabeprazole **Others** Cimetidine Clopidogrel Grapefruit juice Indomethacin Oral contraceptives Ritonavir[a] Ticlopidine[d]	**Analgesics** Antipyrine Salicylates **Antibiotics** Artemisinin antimalarials Rifampin[e] Rifapentine **Antiepileptics** Carbamazepine Phenobarbital Phenytoin **Antiretrovirals** Efavirenz Nelfinavir Ritonavir[a,e] **Steroids** Dexamethasone Prednisone **Others** Enzalutamide St. John's Wort

(*Continued*)

Cytochrome P450 Substrates, Inhibitors, and Inducers[1-17] (Continued)

	Substrates		Inhibitors		Inducers
2D6	**Antidepressants (SSRIs)** Escitalopram Fluoxetine Fluvoxamine Paroxetine Sertraline **Antidepressants (Others)** (Major for most) Amitriptyline Clomipramine Desipramine[b] Doxepin Duloxetine Imipramine Maprotiline Mirtazapine Nortriptyline[b] Trimipramine Venlafaxine[b] **Antidysrhythmics** Encainide Flecainide Mexiletine Procainamide Quinidine **Antihistamines** Chlorpheniramine Desloratadine Diphenhydramine Loratadine **Antipsychotics** (Major for most) Aripiprazole Chlorpromazine Clozapine Fluphenazine Haloperidol Olanzapine Perphenazine[b] Promethazine Risperidone Thioridazine Zuclopenthixol	**β-Adrenergic Antagonists** Carvedilol Metoprolol Nebivolol[b] Pindolol Propafenone Propranolol Timolol **Opioids** Codeine Dextromethorphan[b] Hydrocodone Oxycodone Tramadol **Stimulants** Amphetamine Atomoxetine[b] MDMA **Others** Clomiphene Cyclobenzaprine Debrisoquine Donepezil Eliglustat[b] Galantamine Lidocaine Metoclopramide Ondansetron Sparteine Tamoxifen Tolterodine[b]	**Antidepressants** Bupropion[d] Citalopram Clomipramine Desvenlafaxine Doxepin Duloxetine Escitalopram Fluoxetine[d] Fluvoxamine Moclobemide Paroxetine[d] Sertraline **Antidysrhythmics** Amiodaron Flecainide Quinidine[d] **Antihistamines** Chlorpheniramine Cimetidine Diphenhydramine Hydroxyzine Ranitidine	**Antipsychotics** Aripiprazole Chlorpromazine Fluphenazine Haloperidol Perphenazine Promethazine Thioridazine **Antiretrovirals** Cobicistat Ritonavir[a] **Others** Abiraterone Celecoxib Chloramphenicol Chloroquine Cinacalcet Clobazam Cocaine Doxorubicin Labetalol Lorcaserin Methadone Mirabegron Terbinafine[d] Ticlopidine Vemurafenib	**No Clinically Significant Inducers of CYP2D6**
2E1	**Analgesics** Acetaminophen Salicylates **Inhaled Anesthetics** Enflurane Isoflurane Halothane Methoxyflurane Sevoflurane **Volatile Organic Compounds** Benzene Butadiene Dimethylformamide Ethyl carbamate Ethylene dibromide Methylene chloride *N*-Nitrosodimethylamine Styrene Tetrachloromethane (Carbon tetrachloride) Toluene Trichloroethylene Vinyl chloride	**Others** Acrylonitrile Aniline Chlorzoxazone Ethanol Isoniazid Ropivacaine Theophylline	Clomethiazole Diethyldithiocarbamate Disulfiram 4-Methylpyrazole Orphenadrine		Acetone ATRA Ethanol Isoniazid Smoking St. John's wort Styrene Toluene

Cytochrome P450 Substrates, Inhibitors, and Inducers[1-17] (Continued)

Substrates			Inhibitors		Inducers

3A4

Substrates

Analgesic (Non-opioid)
Acetaminophen
Antipyrine
Bupivacaine
Diclofenac
Lidocaine
Ropivacaine

Antibiotics
Clarithromycin
Dapsone
Erythromycin
Rifabutin
Telithromycin
Troleandomycin

Antidepressants
(Minor for most)
Amitriptyline
Buspirone[b]
Citalopram
Clomipramine
Escitalopram
Imipramine
Mirtazapine
Nefazodone
Sertraline
Trazodone
Venlafaxine

Antidysrhythmics
Amiodarone
Digitoxin
Disopyramide
Dronedarone
Quinidine[c]
Quinine

Antiemetics
Cisapride[c]
Granisetron
Ondansetron

Antifungals
Itraconazole
Ketoconazole
Voriconazole

Antihistamines
Astemizole[c]
Chlorpheniramine
Desloratadine
Ebastine[b]
Loratadine
Terfenadine[c]

Antipsychotics
(Minor for most)
Aripiprazole
Clozapine
Haloperidol
Lurasidone
Pimozide[c]
Quetiapine
Risperidone
Thioridazine
Ziprasidone

Antiretrovirals
Darunavir[b]
Indinavir
Maraviroc
Nelfinavir
Nevirapine
Ritonavir[a]
Saquinavir[b]
Tipranavir[b]

Hepatitis C Medications
Boceprevir
Telaprevir

Immune Modulators
Cyclosporine[c]
Everolimus[b]
Sirolimus[b,c]
Tacrolimus[b,c]
Tamoxifen

Opioids
Alfentanil[b,c]
Buprenorphine
Codeine
Dextromethorphan
Dextropropoxyphene
Fentanyl[c]
Hydromorphone
L-α-acetylmethadol
Loperamide
Meperidine
Methadone
Morphine
Oxycodone
Sufentanil
Tramadol

Proton Pump Inhibitors
(Minor for most)
Esomeprazole
Lansoprazole
Omeprazole
Pantoprazole
Rabeprazole

HMG CoA Reductase Inhibitors
Atorvastatin
Cerivastatin
Lovastatin[b]
Simvastatin[b]

Steroids and Hormones
Budesonide[b]
Cortisol
Dexamethasone
Estradiol
Flutamide
Fluticasone[b]
Hydrocortisone
Methylprednisolone
Prednisone
Progesterone
Testosterone

Inhibitors

Antibiotics (Macrolides)
Clarithromycin[d]
Erythromycin
Telithromycin[d]
Troleandomycin[d]

Antibiotics (Other)
Azithromycin
Chloramphenicol
Ciprofloxacin
Isoniazid
Norfloxacin

Antidepressants
Fluoxetine
Fluvoxamine
Nefazodone[d]
Norfluoxetine
Paroxetine
Sertraline

Antidysrhythmics
Amiodarone
Dronedarone
Quinine

Antifungals
Clotrimazole
Fluconazole
Itraconazole[d]
Ketoconazole[d]
Miconazole
Posaconazole[d]
Voriconazole[d]

Antihistamines
Cimetidine
Ranitidine

Antiretrovirals
Amprenavir
Atazanavir[d]
Cobicistat[d]
Danoprevir[d]
Elvitegravir[d]
Fosamprenavir
Indinavir[d]
Lopinavir[d]
Nelfinavir[d]
Paritaprevir[d]
Ritonavir[a,d]
Saquinavir[d]
Tipranavir[d]

Calcium Channel Blockers (CCBs)
Amlodipine
Diltiazem[b]
Nicardipine
Nifedipine
Verapamil

Cardiovascular (Not CBs)
Ergotamines
Ticagrelor

Chemotherapeutics
Crizotinib
Idelalisib[d]
Imatinib
Irinotecan

Hepatitis C Medications
Boceprevir[d]
Telaprevir[d]

Immune Modulators
Cyclosporine
Tacrolimus

Others
Aprepitant
Chlorzoxazone
Cilostazol
Cocaine
Conivaptan[d]
Ethinylestradiol
Felbamate
Fosaprepitant
Grapefruit Juice[d]
Istradefylline
Ivacaftor
Lomitapide
Mifepristone (RU-486)
Nicotine
Olanzapine
Propofol
Ranolazine
Tofisopam
Zileuton

Inducers

Antibiotics
Nafcillin
Rifabutin
Rifampin[e]
Rifapentine
Troleandomycin

Antiepileptics
Amobarbital
Carbamazepine[e]
Felbamate
Oxcarbazepine
Pentobarbital
Phenobarbital
Phetharbital
Phenytoin[e]
Rufinamide
Topiramate
Valproic acid

Antiretrovirals
Amprenavir
Efavirenz
Etravirine
Nelfinavir
Nevirapine
Ritonavir[a]
Tipranavir

Chemotherapeutics
Bexarotene
Enzalutamide[e]
Imatinib
Mitotane[e]
Vinblastine

Steroids
Dexamethasone
Methylprednisolone
Prednisolone
Prednisone

Others
Alitretinoin
Antipyrine
Aprepitant
Armodafinil
Artemisinin antimalarials
Avasimibe
Bosentan
Ethanol
Gingko biloba
Metamizole
Miconazole
Modafinil
Organochlorine compounds
Phenylbutazone
Pioglitazone
St. John's Wort[e]
Statins
Sulfinpyrazone
Troglitazone

Cytochrome P450 Substrates, Inhibitors, and Inducers[1-17] (Continued)

	Substrates		Inhibitors	Inducers
3A4	**Benzodiazepines** Alprazolam Clonazepam Diazepam Midazolam[b] Triazolam[b] **Calcium Channel Blockers (CCBs)** Amlodipine Diltiazem Felodipine[b] Nicardipine Nifedipine Nimodipine Nisoldipine[b] Nitrendipine Verapamil **Cardiovascular (Not CBs)** Ergotamines[c] Losartan Propranolol Ticagrelor **Chemotherapeutics** Cyclophosphamide Dasatinib Docetaxel Erlotinib Etoposide Gefitinib Ibrutinib[b] Ifosfamide Imatinib Irinotecan Teniposide Vincristine[b]	**Non-benzodiazepine Hypnotics (Z-Drugs)** Eszopiclone Zaleplon Zolpidem **PDE5 Inhibitors** Avanafil[b] Sildenafil[b] Tadalafil Vardenafil[b] **Others** Aflatoxin Aprepitant Carbamazepine Conivaptan[b] Cyclobenzaprine Darifenacin[b] Donepezil Eplerenone Glyburide Isotretinoin Lomitapide[b] Mifepristone (RU-486) Naloxegol[b] Pioglitazone Salmeterol Tetrahydrocannabinol Theophylline Tolvaptan Warfarin-R		

This table list is not complete and may reflect some variation in author opinions as to whether a xenobiotic is a substrate, inhibitor, or inducer.

[a]Ritonavir has paradoxical dose- and time-dependent inhibitory and induction effects.

[b]Substrate is sensitive; area under the concentration versus time curve (AUC) values have been shown to increase 5-fold or more when coadministered with a known CYP3A inhibitor.

[c]Substrate has a narrow therapeutic range, and safety concerns occur when coadministered with an inhibitor.

[d]A strong inhibitor (at least a 5-fold increase in AUC or greater than 80% decrease in clearance).

[e]A strong inducer (at least a 4-fold increase in enzyme activity).

ATRA = all-*trans*-retinoic acid; DMF = *N,N*-dimethylformamide; DEET = *N,N*-diethyl-meta-toluamide; MDMA = 3,4-methylenedioxymethamphetamine; NSAID = nonsteroidal antiinflammatory drug; PCB = polychlorinated biphenyl; PPI = proton pump inhibitor; SSRI = selective serotonin reuptake inhibitor; TCDD = 2,3,7,8-tetrachlorodibenzodioxin.

REFERENCES

1. Armstrong SC, Cozza KL. Antihistamines. *Psychosomatics.* 2003;44:430-434.
2. Bartra J, et al. Interactions of the H1 antihistamines. *J Investig Allergol Clin Immunol.* 2006;16(suppl 1):29-36.
3. Bertilsson L. Metabolism of antidepressant and neuroleptic drugs by cytochrome p450s: clinical and interethnic aspects. *Clin Pharmacol Ther.* 2007;82:606-609.
4. Bondy B, Spellmann I. Pharmacogenetics of antipsychotics: useful for the clinician? *Curr Opin Psychiatry.* 2007;20:126-130.
5. Caro AA, Cederbaum AI. Oxidative stress, toxicology, and pharmacology of CYP2E1. *Annu Rev Pharmacol Toxicol.* 2004;44:27-42.
6. Flockhart DA. Flockhart Table. 2016; http://medicine.iupui.edu/CLINPHARM/ddis/main-table. Accessed January 22, 2017.
7. Flockhart DA, Tanus-Santos JE. Implications of cytochrome P450 interactions when prescribing medication for hypertension. *Arch Intern Med.* 2002;162:405-412.
8. Hedrich WD, et al. Insights into CYP2B6-mediated drug-drug interactions. *Acta Pharm Sin B.* 2016;6:413-425.
9. Hukkanen J. Induction of cytochrome P450 enzymes: a view on human in vivo findings. *Expert Rev Clin Pharmacol.* 2012;5:569-585.
10. Nivoix Y, et al. The enzymatic basis of drug-drug interactions with systemic triazole antifungals. *Clin Pharmacokinet.* 2008;47:779-792.
11. Nowack R. Review article: cytochrome P450 enzyme, and transport protein mediated herb-drug interactions in renal transplant patients: grapefruit juice, St John's Wort—and beyond! *Nephrology (Carlton).* 2008;13:337-347.
12. Pai MP, et al. Antibiotic drug interactions. *Med Clin North Am.* 2006;90:1223-1255.
13. Pelkonen O, et al. Inhibition and induction of human cytochrome P450 enzymes: current status. *Arch Toxicol.* 2008;82:667-715.
14. Spriet I, et al. Mini-series: II. clinical aspects. clinically relevant CYP450-mediated drug interactions in the ICU. *Intensive Care Med.* 2009;35:603-612.
15. Sweeney BP, Bromilow J. Liver enzyme induction and inhibition: implications for anaesthesia. *Anaesthesia.* 2006;61:159-177.
16. US Food and Drug Administration. Drug Development and Drug Interactions: Table of Substrates, Inhibitors and Inducers. 2016. Accessed January 22, 2017.
17. Zanger UM, Schwab M. Cytochrome P450 enzymes in drug metabolism: regulation of gene expression, enzyme activities, and impact of genetic variation. *Pharmacol Ther.* 2013;138:103-141.

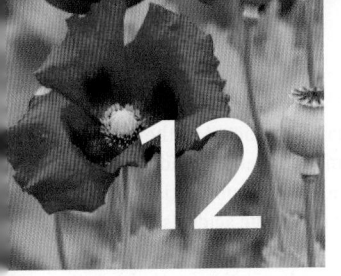

12 FLUID, ELECTROLYTE, AND ACID–BASE PRINCIPLES

Alan N. Charney and Robert S. Hoffman

A meaningful analysis of fluid, electrolyte, and acid–base abnormalities is dependent on the history and physical examination of each patient. Although a rigorous appraisal of laboratory parameters often yields the correct differential diagnosis, the clinical characteristics provide an understanding of the extracellular fluid volume (ECFV) and pathophysiology. Thus, the evaluation always begins with an overall assessment of the patient.

INITIAL PATIENT ASSESSMENT
History
The history should be directed toward clinical questions associated with fluid and electrolyte abnormalities. Xenobiotic exposure commonly results in fluid losses through the respiratory system (hyperpnea and tachypnea), gastrointestinal (GI) tract (vomiting and diarrhea), skin (diaphoresis), and kidneys (polyuria). Patients with ECFV depletion often complain of dizziness, thirst, and weakness. Usually the patients can identify the source of fluid loss.

A history of exposure to nonprescription and prescription medications, alternative or complementary therapies, and other xenobiotics can suggest the most likely electrolyte or acid–base abnormality. In addition, patient characteristics (race, gender, age), premorbid medical conditions, and the ambient temperature and humidity should always be considered.

Physical Examination
The vital signs are invariably affected by significant alterations in ECFV. Whereas hypotension and tachycardia often characterize life-threatening ECFV depletion, an increase of the heart rate and a narrowing of the pulse pressure are the earliest findings. Abnormalities are best recognized through an ongoing dynamic evaluation, realizing that the measurement of a single set of supine vital signs offers useful information only when markedly abnormal. Orthostatic pulse and blood pressure measurements provide a more meaningful determination of functional ECFV status (Chaps. 3 and 16).

The respiratory rate and pattern can give clues to the patient's metabolic status. In the absence of lung disease, hyperventilation (manifested by tachypnea, hyperpnea, or both) is often either caused by a primary respiratory stimulus (respiratory alkalosis) or is a response to the presence of metabolic acidosis. Although hypoventilation (bradypnea or hypopnea or both) is present in patients with metabolic alkalosis, it is rarely clinically significant except in the presence of chronic lung disease or in combination with respiratory depressant xenobiotics. More commonly, hypoventilation is caused by a primary depression of consciousness and respiration with resulting respiratory acidosis. Unless the clinical scenario (eg, nature of the poisoning, presence of renal or pulmonary disease, and findings on physical examination or laboratory testing) is classic, arterial or venous blood gas analysis is recommended to determine the acid–base disorder associated with a change in ventilation.

The skin should be evaluated for turgor, moisture, and the presence or absence of edema. The moisture of the mucous membranes can also provide valuable information. These are nonspecific parameters and often fail to correlate directly with the status of hydration. This dissociation is especially true with xenobiotic exposure because many xenobiotics alter skin and mucous membrane moisture without necessarily altering ECFV status. For example, antimuscarinics commonly result in dry mucous membranes and skin without producing ECFV depletion. Conversely, patients exposed to sympathomimetics such as cocaine or cholinergics such as organic phosphorus compounds have moist skin and mucous membranes even in the presence of significant fluid losses. This dissociation of ECFV and cutaneous characteristics reinforces the need to assess patients meticulously.

The physical findings associated with electrolyte abnormalities are generally nonspecific. Hyponatremia, hypernatremia, hypercalcemia, and hypermagnesemia all produce a depressed level of consciousness. Neuromuscular excitability such as tremor and hyperreflexia occurs with hypocalcemia, hypomagnesemia, hyponatremia, and hyperkalemia. Weakness results from both hyperkalemia and hypokalemia. Also, multiple, concurrent electrolyte disorders can produce confusing clinical presentations, or patients can appear normal. Diagnostic findings, such as Chvostek and Trousseau signs (primarily found in hypocalcemia), are useful in assessing patients with potential xenobiotic exposures.

Rapid Diagnostic Tools
The electrocardiogram (ECG) is a useful tool for screening several common electrolyte abnormalities (Chap. 15). It is easy to perform, rapid, inexpensive, and routinely available. Unfortunately, because poor sensitivity (0.43) and moderate specificity (0.86) were demonstrated when ECGs were used to diagnose hyperkalemia, in actuality the test is of limited diagnostic value.[151] However, the ECG is valuable for the evaluation of changes in serum potassium and calcium concentrations ($[K^+]$ and $[Ca^{2+}]$) in an individual patient.

Assessment of urine specific gravity by dipstick analysis provides valuable information about ECFV status. A high urine specific gravity (>1.015) signifies concentrated urine and is often associated with ECFV depletion. However, urine specific gravity is often similarly elevated in conditions of ECFV excess, such as congestive heart failure or third spacing. Similarly, patients with excess antidiuretic hormone (ADH) secretion (eg, due to methylenedioxymethamphetamine {MDMA} exposure) excrete concentrated urine (specific gravity >1.015) even in the presence of a normal or expanded ECFV. Furthermore, when renal impairment or diuretic use is the source of the volume loss, the specific gravity is usually approximately 1.010 (known as isosthenuria). Finally, patients with lithium-induced diabetes insipidus (DI) excrete dilute urine (specific gravity <1.010) despite ongoing water losses and contraction of the ECFV.

The urine dipstick is highly reliable and rapidly available for determining the presence of ketones, which are often associated with common causes of metabolic acidosis (eg, diabetic ketoacidosis, salicylate poisoning, alcoholic ketoacidosis). The urine ferric chloride test rapidly detects exposure to salicylates with a high sensitivity and specificity although it is rarely used today in locations where salicylate concentrations can be obtained rapidly (Chap. 37).

Laboratory Studies
A simultaneous determination of the venous serum electrolytes, blood urea nitrogen (BUN), glucose, and arterial or venous blood gases are adequate to determine the nature of the most common acid–base, fluid, and electrolyte abnormalities. More complex clinical problems require determinations of urine and serum osmolalities, urine electrolytes, serum ketones, serum lactate, and other tests. A systematic approach to common problems is discussed in the following sections.

ACID–BASE ABNORMALITIES
Definitions
The lack of a clear understanding and precise use of the terminology of acid–base disorders often leads to confusion and error. The following definitions provide the appropriate frame of reference for the remainder of the chapter and this textbook.

Whereas the terms *acidosis* and *alkalosis* refer to processes that tend to change pH in a given direction, *acidemia* and *alkalemia* only refer to the actual pH. By definition, a patient is said to have:

- A *metabolic acidosis* if the arterial pH is less than 7.40 and serum bicarbonate concentration ($[HCO_3^-]$) is less than 24 mEq/L. Because acidemia stimulates ventilation (respiratory compensation), metabolic acidosis is usually accompanied by a PCO_2 less than 40 mm Hg.
- A *metabolic alkalosis* if the arterial pH is greater than 7.40 and serum $[HCO_3^-]$ is greater than 24 mEq/L. Because alkalemia inhibits ventilation (respiratory compensation), metabolic alkalosis is usually accompanied by a PCO_2 greater than 40 mm Hg.
- A *respiratory acidosis* if the arterial pH is less than 7.40 and partial pressure of carbon dioxide (PCO_2) is greater than 40 mm Hg. Because an elevated PCO_2 stimulates renal acid excretion and the generation of HCO_3^- (renal compensation), respiratory acidosis is usually accompanied by a serum $[HCO_3^-]$ greater than 24 mEq/L.
- A *respiratory alkalosis* if the arterial pH is greater than 7.40 and PCO_2 is less than 40 mm Hg. Because a decreased PCO_2 lowers renal acid excretion and increases the excretion of HCO_3^- (renal compensation), respiratory alkalosis is usually accompanied by a serum $[HCO_3^-]$ less than 24 mEq/L.

It is important to note that under many circumstances, a venous pH permits an approximation of arterial pH. However, when rigorously compared, the arterial blood gas analysis outperforms the venous blood gas analysis especially when findings are subtle.[131] (See Chap. 28 for a further discussion of the relationship between arterial and venous pH.) Any combination of acidoses and alkaloses can be present in any one patient at any given time. The terms *acidemia* and *alkalemia* refer only to the resultant arterial pH of blood (acidemia referring to a pH <7.40 and alkalemia referring to a pH >7.40). These terms do not describe the processes that led to the alteration in pH. Thus, a patient with acidemia must have a primary metabolic or respiratory acidosis but potentially also has an alkalosis present at the same time. Clues to the presence of more than one acid–base abnormality include the clinical presentation, an apparent excess or insufficient "compensation" for the primary acid–base abnormality, a delta gap ratio {(Δ) anion gap/Δ$[HCO_3^-]$} that significantly deviates from one, or an electrolyte abnormality that is uncharacteristic of the primary acid–base disorder.

Determining the Primary Acid–Base Abnormality

It is helpful to begin by determining whether the patient has an acidosis or an alkalosis. This is followed by an assessment of the pH, PCO_2, and $[HCO_3^-]$. With these 3 parameters defined, the patient's primary acid–base disorder can be classified using the aforementioned definitions. Next it is important to determine whether the compensation of the primary acid–base disorder is appropriate. It is generally assumed that overcompensation cannot occur.[106] That is, if the primary process is metabolic acidosis, respiratory compensation tends to raise the pH toward normal but never to greater than 7.40. If the primary process is respiratory alkalosis, compensatory renal excretion of HCO_3^- tends to lower the pH toward normal but not to less than 7.40. The same is true for primary metabolic alkalosis and primary respiratory acidosis. As a rule, compensation for a primary acid–base disorder that appears inadequate or excessive is indicative of the presence of a second primary acid–base disorder.

Based on patient data, the Winters equation (Equation 12–1)[7] predicts the degree of the respiratory compensation (the decrease in PCO_2) in metabolic acidosis as follows:

$$PCO_2 = (1.5 \times [HCO_3^-]) + 8 \pm 2 \qquad \text{(Eq. 12–1)}$$

Thus, in a patient with an arterial $[HCO_3^-]$ of 12 mEq/L, the predicted PCO_2 is calculated as

$$(1.5 \times 12) + 8 \pm 2$$

or

$$26 \pm 2 \text{ mm Hg.}$$

If the actual PCO_2 is substantially lower than is predicted by the Winters equation, it can be concluded that both a primary metabolic acidosis and a primary respiratory alkalosis are present. If the PCO_2 is substantially higher than the predicted value, then both a primary metabolic acidosis and a primary respiratory acidosis are present.

An alternative to the Winters equation is the observation by Narins and Emmett that in compensated metabolic acidosis, the arterial PCO_2 is usually the same as the last 2 digits of the arterial pH.[106] For example, a pH of 7.26 predicts a PCO_2 of 26 mm Hg.

Guidelines are also available to predict the compensation for metabolic alkalosis,[64] respiratory acidosis, and respiratory alkalosis.[83] Patients with a metabolic alkalosis compensate by hypoventilating, resulting in an increase of their PCO_2 above 40 mm Hg. However, the concomitant development of hypoxemia limits this compensation so that respiratory compensation in the presence of a metabolic alkalosis usually results in a PCO_2 of 55 mm Hg or less. It is difficult to be more accurate about the expected respiratory compensation for a metabolic alkalosis, although the compensation, as in the case of metabolic acidosis, is nearly complete within hours of onset.

By contrast, the degree of compensation in primary respiratory disorders depends on the length of time the disorder has been present. In a matter of minutes, primary respiratory acidosis results in an increase in the serum $[HCO_3^-]$ of 0.1 times the increase in the PCO_2. This increase is a result of the production and dissociation of H_2CO_3. Over a period of days, respiratory acidosis causes the compensatory renal excretion of acid. This compensation increases the serum $[HCO_3^-]$ by 0.3 times the increase in PCO_2. Primary respiratory alkalosis acutely decreases the serum $[HCO_3^-]$ by 0.2 times the decrease in PCO_2. If a respiratory alkalosis persists for several days, renal compensation, by the urinary excretion of HCO_3^-, decreases the serum $[HCO_3^-]$ by 0.4 times the decrease in PCO_2.

Calculating the Anion Gap

The concept of the anion gap is said to have arisen from the "Gamblegram" originally described in 1939[51]; however, its use was not popularized until the determination of serum electrolytes became routinely available. The law of electroneutrality states that the net positive and negative charges of all fluids must be equal. Thus, all of the negative charges present in the serum must equal all of the positive charges, and the sum of the positive charges minus the sum of the negative charges must equal zero. The problem that immediately arose (and produced an "anion gap") was that all charged species in the serum are not routinely measured.

Normally present but not routinely measured cations include calcium and magnesium; normally present but not routinely measured anions include phosphate, sulfate, albumin, and organic anions (eg, lactate and pyruvate).[41] Whereas Na^+ and K^+ normally account for 95% of extracellular cations, Cl^- and HCO_3^- account for 85% of extracellular anions. Thus, because more cations than anions are among the electrolytes usually measured, subtracting the anions from the cations normally yields a positive number, known as the anion gap. The anion gap is therefore derived as shown in Equation 12–2:

$$[Na^+] + [K^+] + [\text{Unmeasured Cations } (U_c)] = [Cl^-] + [HCO_3^-] + [\text{Unmeasured Anions } (U_a)]$$
$$\text{Anion Gap} = [U_a] - [U_c]$$

or

$$\text{Anion Gap} = ([Na^+] + [K^+]) - ([Cl^-] + [HCO_3^-]) \qquad \text{(Eq. 12–2)}$$

Because the serum $[K^+]$ varies over a limited range of perhaps 1 to 2 mEq/L above and below normal and therefore rarely significantly alters the anion gap, it is often deleted from the equation for simplicity. Most prefer this approach, yielding Equation 12–3:

$$\text{Anion Gap} = ([Na^+]) - ([Cl^-] + [HCO_3^-]) \qquad \text{(Eq. 12–3)}$$

Using Equation 12–3, the normal anion gap was initially determined to be 12 ± 4 mEq/L.[41] However, because the normal serum $[Cl^-]$ is higher on

TABLE 12–1	Xenobiotic and Other Causes of a High Anion Gap
Increase in Unmeasured Anions	**Decrease in Unmeasured Cations**
Metabolic acidosis (Table 12–3)	Simultaneous hypomagnesemia, hypocalcemia, or hypokalemia
Therapy with sodium salts of unmeasured anions	
Sodium citrate	
Sodium lactate	
Sodium acetate	
Therapy with certain antibiotics	
Carbenicillin	
Sodium penicillin	
Alkalosis	

TABLE 12–3	Xenobiotic and Other Causes of a High Anion Gap Metabolic Acidosis
Carbon monoxide	Methanol
Cyanide	Paraldehyde
Ethylene glycol	Phenformin
Hydrogen sulfide	Propylene glycol
Isoniazid	Salicylates
Iron	Sulfur (inorganic)
Ketoacidoses (diabetic, alcoholic, and starvation)	Theophylline
Lactate	Toluene
Metformin	Uremia (acute or chronic kidney failure)

current laboratory instrumentation, the current range for a normal anion gap is 7 ± 4 mEq/L.[149]

A variety of pathologic conditions result in a rise or fall of the anion gap. High anion gaps result from increased presence of unmeasured anions or decreased presence of unmeasured cations (Table 12–1).[41,89] Conversely, a low anion gap results from an increase in unmeasured cations or a decrease in unmeasured anions (Table 12–2).[41,49,59,129]

Anion Gap Reliability

Several authors have discussed the usefulness of the anion gap determination.[21,50,72] When 57 hospitalized patients were studied to determine the cause of elevated anion gaps in patients whose anion gap was greater than 30 mEq/L, the cause was always a metabolic acidosis with elevations of lactate or ketones.[50] In patients with smaller elevations of the anion gap, the ability to define the cause of the elevation diminished; in only 14% of patients with anion gaps of 17 to 19 mEq/L could the cause be determined. Another study determined that although the anion gap is often used as a screening test for hyperlactatemia (as a sign of poor perfusion), only patients with the highest serum lactate concentrations had elevated anion gaps.[72] Finally, in a sample of 571 patients, those with greater elevations in anion gaps tended to have more severe illness. This logically correlated with higher admission rates, a greater percentage of admissions to intensive care units, and a higher mortality rate.[21] Thus, although the absence of an increased anion gap does not exclude significant illness, a very elevated anion gap can generally be attributed to a specific cause (typically a disorder that is associated with elevated lactate or ketones) and usually indicates a relatively severe illness.

Metabolic Acidosis

After the diagnosis of metabolic acidosis is established by finding an arterial pH less than 7.40, $[HCO_3^-] < 24$ mEq/L, and $PCO_2 < 40$ mm Hg, the serum anion gap should be analyzed. Indeed, the popularity of the anion gap is primarily based on its usefulness in categorizing metabolic acidosis as being of the high anion gap or normal anion gap type. This determination should be made after correcting the anion gap for the effect of hypoalbuminemia,

a common and important confounding factor in chronically ill patients. The anion gap decreases approximately 3 mEq/L per 1 g/dL decrease in the serum [albumin].[47] In general, the electrolyte abnormalities that frequently accompany metabolic acidosis usually have only small and insignificant effects on the anion gap.

It should be noted that although many clinicians rely on the mnemonics MUDPILES (M, methanol; U, uremia; D, diabetic ketoacidosis; P, paraldehyde; I, iron; L, lactic acidosis; E, ethylene glycol; and S, salicylates) or KULT (K, ketones; U, uremia; L, lactate; T, toxins), to help remember this differential diagnosis, these mnemonics include rarely used drugs (phenformin, paraldehyde) and omit important others (eg, metformin, cyanide).

A high anion gap metabolic acidosis results from the absorption or generation of an acid that dissociates into an anion other than Cl^- that has neither been excreted nor metabolized at the time the anion gap is determined. The retention of this "unmeasured" anion (eg, glycolate in ethylene glycol poisoning) increases the anion gap. By contrast, a normal anion gap metabolic acidosis results from the absorption or generation of an acid that dissociates into H^+ and Cl^-. In this case, the "measured" Cl^- is retained as HCO_3^-, is titrated, and its concentration reduced during the acidosis, and no increase in anion gap is produced. Normal anion gap acidosis, also referred to as hyperchloremic metabolic acidosis, is typically caused by intestinal or renal bicarbonate losses as in diarrhea or renal tubular acidosis, respectively. Other causes of high and normal anion gap metabolic acidoses are described elsewhere[3,4] and shown in Tables 12–3 and 12–4.

TABLE 12–4	Xenobiotic Causes of a Normal Anion Gap Metabolic Acidosis
Acetazolamide	
Acidifying agents	
Ammonium chloride	
Arginine hydrochloride	
Hydrochloric acid	
Lysine hydrochloride	
Calcineurin inhibitors (eg, tacrolimus, sirolimus)	
Cholestyramine	
Cleistanthus collinus (plant)	
Mafenide acetate (sulfamylon)	
Toluene	
Topiramate	

TABLE 12–2	Xenobiotic and Other Causes of a Low Anion Gap		
Increase in Unmeasured Cations	**Decrease in Unmeasured Anions**	**Overestimation of Chloride**
Hypercalcemia	Hypoalbuminemia	Bromism
Hypermagnesemia	Hemodilution	Iodism
Hyperkalemia		Nitrate excess
Lithium poisoning		
Multiple myeloma		

Narrowing the Differential Diagnosis of a High Anion Gap Metabolic Acidosis

The ability to diagnose the etiology of a high anion gap metabolic acidosis is an essential skill in clinical medicine. The following discussion provides a rapid and cost-effective approach to the problem. As always, the clinical history and physical examination provide essential clues to the diagnosis. For example, iron poisoning is virtually always associated with significant GI symptoms, the absence of which essentially excludes the diagnosis (Chap. 45). Furthermore, when iron overdose is suspected, an abdominal radiograph often shows the presence of iron-containing tablets. The acidosis associated with isoniazid (INH) toxicity results from seizures, the absence of which excludes INH as the cause of a metabolic acidosis (Chap. 56). Methanol poisoning is classically associated with visual complaints or abnormal finding on funduscopic examination (Chap. 106). Methyl salicylate has a characteristic wintergreen odor (Chap. 37). When these findings are absent, the laboratory analysis must be relied on, as follows:

1. *Begin with the serum electrolytes, BUN, creatinine, and glucose.* A rapid blood glucose reagent test should be performed to help confirm or exclude hyperglycemia. Although hyperglycemia should raise the possibility of diabetic ketoacidosis, the absence of an elevated serum glucose does not exclude the possibility of euglycemic diabetic ketoacidosis,[11,27,74] alcoholic or starvation ketoacidosis, which are often associated with normal or even low serum glucose concentrations. An elevated BUN and creatinine are essential to diagnose acute or chronic kidney failure.

2. *Proceed to the urinalysis.* If there is a suspicion of a high anion gap metabolic acidosis and only the arterial or venous blood gas analysis is completed, the evaluation can easily begin here while the electrolyte determinations are pending. A urine dipstick for glucose and ketones helps with the diagnosis of diabetic ketoacidosis and other ketoacidoses. However, the absence of urinary ketones does not exclude a diagnosis of alcoholic ketoacidosis[48] (Chap. 76), and ketones are often present in patients with severe salicylism (Chap. 37) and biguanide-associated metabolic acidosis (Chap. 47). If timed properly, the urine of a patient who has ingested fluorescein-containing antifreeze (ethylene glycol) fluoresces when exposed to a Wood lamp. Also, because ethylene glycol is metabolized to oxalate, calcium oxalate crystals are present in the urine of approximately half of poisoned patients. Although the presence of a fluorescent urine and calcium oxalate crystals are useful findings, their absence does not exclude ethylene glycol poisoning (Chap. 106). When clinically available, a urine ferric chloride test should be performed. Although highly sensitive and specific for the presence of salicylates, this test is not specific for the diagnosis of salicylism because small amounts of salicylate will be detected in the urine even days after its last use (Chap. 37). Thus, a serum salicylate concentration must be obtained to quantify the findings of a positive urine ferric chloride test result. A negative urine ferric chloride test result essentially excludes a diagnosis of salicylism.

3. A blood lactate concentration can be helpful. In theory, if the lactate (measured in mEq/L) can entirely account for the fall in serum $[HCO_3^-]$, the cause of the high anion gap can be attributed to lactic acidosis. In practicality we know that this unfortunately does not work largely because the volumes of distribution of bicarbonate and lactate are not identical, with the bicarbonate volume of distribution being very dependent on pH.[119] Another important example is that glycolate (a metabolite of ethylene glycol) can produce a false-positive elevation of the lactate concentration with many current laboratory techniques.[100,150]

When the above analysis of a high anion gap metabolic acidosis is nondiagnostic, the diagnosis is usually toxic alcohol ingestion, starvation, or alcoholic ketoacidosis (with minimal urine ketones), or a multifactorial process involving small amounts of lactate and other anions. One approach is to provide the patient with 1 to 2 hours of intravenous (IV) hydration, dextrose, and thiamine. If the acidosis improves, the etiology is either ketoacidosis or metabolic acidosis with hyperlacatemia. In the absence of improvement, a more detailed search for the toxic alcohols, involving measurement of either the osmol gap or actual methanol and ethylene glycol concentrations, should be initiated (discussed later).

The Δ Anion Gap-to-Δ[HCO₃⁻] Ratio

Many patients have mixed acid–base disorders such as metabolic acidosis and respiratory alkalosis. Depending on the relative effects of the acid–base disorders, the patient may have significant acidemia or alkalemia, minor alterations in pH, or even a normal pH. Although the clinical presentation, degree of compensation for the primary acid–base disorder, or the presence of unexpected electrolyte abnormalities suggest whether more than one primary acid–base disorder is present, comparing the Δ anion gap (ΔAG) with the $\Delta[HCO_3^-]$ provides additional information to help establish the correct diagnosis.

In a patient with a simple high anion gap metabolic acidosis, each 1 mEq/L decrease in the serum $[HCO_3^-]$ should (at least initially) be associated with a 1 mEq/L rise in the anion gap.[106] This occurs because the unmeasured anion is paired with the acid that is titrating the HCO_3^-. Any deviation from this direct relationship may be an indication of a mixed acid–base disorder.[60,106,111] Thus, the ratio of the change in the anion gap (ΔAG) to the deviation of the serum $[HCO_3^-]$ from normal (Equation 12–4) evolved:

$$\text{Anion gap ratio} = \Delta AG/\Delta[HCO_3^-] \qquad \text{(Eq. 12–4)}$$

A ratio close to one would suggest a pure high anion gap metabolic acidosis. When the ratio is greater than one, there is a relative increase in $[HCO_3^-]$ that can result only from a concomitant metabolic alkalosis or renal compensation such as renal generation of HCO_3^- for a respiratory acidosis. Alternatively, when the ratio is less than one, the additional presence of either hyperchloremic (normal anion gap) metabolic acidosis or compensated respiratory alkalosis is suggested. Although the usefulness of this relationship has been supported strongly by some authors,[109,111] others suggest that it is often flawed and frequently misleading.[34,125]

After reviewing the arguments, the statements of one author[34] are reasonable in concluding that "the exact relationship between the ΔAG and $\Delta[HCO_3^-]$ in a high anion gap metabolic acidosis is not readily predictable and deviation of the $\Delta AG/\Delta[HCO_3^-]$ ratio from unity does not necessarily imply the diagnosis of a second acid–base disorder." Regardless, very large deviations from a value of one usually are associated with the presence of a second primary acid–base disorder.

The Osmol Gap

The osmol gap, which is sometimes used to screen for toxic alcohol ingestion, is defined as the difference between the values for the measured serum osmolality and the calculated serum osmolarity. Osmolarity is a measure of the total number of particles in one liter of solution. Osmolality differs from osmolarity in that it represents the number of particles per kilogram of solution. Thus, osmolarity and osmolality represent molar and molal concentrations of solutes, respectively. In clinical medicine, osmolarity is usually calculated whereas osmolality is measured.

Calculating osmolarity requires a summing of the known particles in solution. Because molarity and milliequivalents are particle-based measurements, unlike weight or concentration, the known constituents of serum that are measured in the latter units (such as mg/dL) have to be converted to molar values. Assumptions are required based on the extent of dissociation of polar compounds (eg, NaCl), the water content of serum, and the contributions of various other solutes such as Ca^{2+} and Mg^{2+}. The nature and limitations of these assumptions are beyond the scope of this chapter. Readers are referred to several reviews for more details.[67,110] Many equations have been used and evaluated for calculating serum osmolarity. One investigation that used 13 different methods to evaluate sera from 715 hospitalized patients[36] concluded that Equation 12–5 provided the most accurate calculation:

$$1.86([Na^+] \text{ in mEq/L}) + ([Glucose] \text{ in mg/dL}/18)$$
$$+ ([BUN] \text{ in mg/dL}/2.8) \qquad \text{(Eq. 12–5)}$$

Obvious sources of potential error in this calculation include laboratory error in determining the measured parameters and the failure to account for a number of osmotically active particles.

The measurement of serum osmolality also has the potential for error stemming from the use of different laboratory technique.[40] It is essential to ensure that the freezing point depression technique or osmometry is used because when the boiling point elevation method is used, xenobiotics with low boiling points (ethanol, isopropanol, methanol) will not be detected.

Conceptual errors may also result. In methanol poisoning, the methanol molecule has osmotic activity that is measured but not calculated, and no increase in the anion gap is present until it is metabolized to formate. Although the metabolite also has osmotic activity, its activity is accounted for by Na^+ in the osmolarity calculation because it is largely dissociated, existing as Na^+ formate. Thus, shortly after a methanol ingestion, the patient will have an elevated osmol gap and a normal anion gap; later, the anion gap will increase, and the osmol gap will decrease (Fig. 106–4). This effect is highlighted by several case reports.[9,30]

Using Equation 12–5 to calculate osmolarity, it is often stated that the "normal" osmol gap is 10 ± 6 mOsm/L.[36] However, when more than 300 adult samples were studied with a more commonly used equation (Eq. 12–6),

$$2([Na^+] \text{ in mEq/L}) + ([Glucose] \text{ in mg/dL}/18)$$
$$+ ([BUN] \text{ in mg/dL}/2.8) \qquad \text{(Eq. 12–6)}$$

normal values for the osmol gap were -2 ± 6 mOsm/L.[67] Almost identical results are reported in children.[96]

The largest limitation of the osmol gap calculation is due to the documented large standard deviation around a small "normal" number.[36,67] An error of 1 mEq/L (<1.0%) in the determination of the serum $[Na^+]$ will result in an error of 2 mOsm/L in the calculation of the osmol gap. Considering this variability, the molecular weights (MWs) and relatively modest serum concentrations of the xenobiotics in question (eg, ethylene glycol; MW, 62 Da; at a concentration of 50 mg/dL theoretically contributes only 8.1 mOsm/L) and the predicted fall in the osmol gap as metabolism occurs, small or even negative osmol gaps can never be used to exclude toxic alcohol ingestion.[67] This overall concept is illustrated by an actual patient with an osmol gap of 7.2 mOsm (well within the normal range) who ultimately required hemodialysis for severe ethylene glycol poisoning.[138] An additional error may result when including ethanol in the determination of the osmol gap. When present, ethanol is osmotically active and should be included in the calculated osmolarity. In theory, because the MW of ethanol is 46 g/mol, dividing the serum ethanol concentration (in mg/dL) by 4.6 will yield the osmolar contribution in mmol/L. However, because the physical interaction of ethanol with water is complex, it is more scientifically accurate to divide by lower numbers as the ethanol concentration increases.[26,115] Therefore because the osmol gap is a screening tool, we suggest continuing to use the 4.6 divisor (or if in SI units using the unmodified molar concentration) in an attempt to reduce clinical false-negative test results.

Finally, although exceedingly large serum osmol gaps are suggestive of toxic alcohol ingestions, common conditions such as alcoholic ketoacidosis, metabolic acidosis with elevated lactate, kidney failure, and shock are all associated with elevated osmol gaps.[73,128,134] This may be surprising because lactate, acetoacetate, and β-hydroxybutyrate should not account for any increase in the osmol gap because they are charged (and accounted for in the osmolarity calculation). Apparently, these conditions are associated with the accumulation of small uncharged, unmeasured molecules in the serum.

Thus, although the negative and positive predictive values of the osmol gap are too poor to recommend this test to routinely screen for xenobiotic ingestion, the presence of very high osmol gaps (>50–70 mOsm/L) usually indicates a diagnosis of toxic alcohol ingestion (Chap. 106).

Differential Diagnosis of a Normal Anion Gap Metabolic Acidosis

Although the differential diagnosis of a normal anion gap metabolic acidosis is extensive (Table 12–4), most cases result from either urinary or GI HCO_3^- losses: renal tubular acidosis (RTA) or diarrhea, respectively. A number of

xenobiotics also cause this disorder, including toluene,[25] which also may cause a high anion gap metabolic acidosis. When the findings of the history and physical examination cannot be used to narrow the differential diagnosis, the use of a urinary anion gap is suggested.[15,120]

The urinary anion gap is calculated as shown in Equation 12–7:

$$([Na^+] + [K^+]) - [Cl^-] \qquad \text{(Eq. 12–7)}$$

The size of this gap is inversely related to the urinary ammonium (NH_4^+) excretion.[58] As NH_4^+ elimination increases, the urinary anion gap decreases and can actually become negative because NH_4^+ serves as an unmeasured urinary cation and is predominantly accompanied by Cl^-.

The normal anion gap metabolic acidosis associated with diarrhea results from HCO_3^- loss. During this process, the ability of the kidney to eliminate NH_4^+ is undisturbed; in fact, it increases as a normal response to the acidemia. Thus, with gastrointestinal HCO_3^- losses, the urinary anion gap should decrease and may become negative. By contrast, a patient with RTA has lost the ability to either reabsorb HCO_3^- (type 2 RTA) or increase NH_4^+ excretion in response to metabolic acidosis (types 1 and 4 RTA) and the urinary anion gap should become more positive. Indeed, when the urinary anion gap was calculated in patients with diarrhea or RTA, it was found that patients with diarrhea had a mean negative gap (-20 ± 5.7 mEq/L) compared with a positive gap (23 ± 4.1 mEq/L) in those with RTA.[58] Therefore, when evaluating the patient with a normal anion gap metabolic acidosis, the determination of a urinary anion gap is helpful to determine the source of the disorder when the history and physical examination are unclear.

Adverse Effects of Metabolic Acidosis

The acuity of onset and severity of metabolic acidosis determine the consequences of this disorder. Acute metabolic acidosis is usually characterized by obvious hyperventilation (caused by respiratory compensation). At arterial pH values less than 7.20, cardiac and central nervous system abnormalities are often present. These include decreases in blood pressure and cardiac output, cardiac dysrhythmias, and progressive obtundation.[3,4] Chronic metabolic acidosis is often not accompanied by overt clinical symptoms. The nonspecific symptoms of anorexia and fatigue are the most typical manifestations of chronic acidosis, and compensatory hyperventilation although present is often not evident. Because the consequences of even severe metabolic acidosis are nonspecific, the presence of metabolic acidosis is most often suggested by the history and physical examination and subsequently confirmed by laboratory testing.

Management Principles in Patients with Metabolic Acidosis

The treatment of metabolic acidosis depends on its severity and cause. In most cases of severe poisoning, with a serum $[HCO_3^-]$ concentration less than 8 mEq/L and an arterial pH value less than 7.20, we recommend treating with HCO_3^- to increase the pH to greater than 7.20, as described in detail elsewhere.[3,4] As an example, to raise the serum $[HCO_3^-]$ by 4 mEq/L in a 70-kg person with an apparent HCO_3^- distribution space of 50% of body weight, approximately 140 mEq must be administered. Unfortunately, because the apparent volume of distribution of HCO_3^- increases as the pH and serum $[HCO_3^-]$ fall, any given dose of exogenous HCO_3^- will have less of an effect on pH. When ECFV overload (caused by heart failure, kidney failure, or the sodium bicarbonate therapy itself) cannot be prevented or managed by administering loop diuretics, hemofiltration or hemodialysis will be necessary.

In patients with arterial pH values greater than 7.20, the cause of the acidosis should guide therapy. Metabolic acidosis primarily caused by the overproduction of acid, as in the case of ketoacidosis and toxic alcohol poisoning, requires very large quantities of HCO_3^- and typically does not respond well to sodium bicarbonate therapy. Treatment in these patients should be directed at the cause of acidosis (eg, insulin and IV fluids in diabetic ketoacidosis; fomepizole in methanol, ethylene glycol, and DEG poisonings (Antidotes in Depth: A33), fluids, dextrose, and thiamine in alcoholic ketoacidosis; fluid resuscitation, antibiotics, and vasopressors in sepsis-induced hyperlactatemia). Patients with metabolic acidosis primarily caused by insufficient excretion of acid (eg, acute or chronic kidney failure, RTA) should be treated with a low-protein diet (if feasible) and oral sodium bicarbonate or substances that generate HCO_3^- during metabolism. We recommended an oral sodium citrate solution such as Shohl solution, which yields 1 mEq base/mL. The goal of therapy is to increase the serum $[HCO_3^-]$ to 20 to 22 mEq/L and the pH to 7.30.

METABOLIC ALKALOSIS

Adverse Effects of Metabolic Alkalosis

Life-threatening metabolic alkalosis is rare but can result in tetany (from decreased ionized $[Ca^{2+}]$); weakness (from decreased serum $[K^+]$); or altered mental status leading to coma, seizures, and cardiac dysrhythmias. In addition, metabolic alkalosis shifts the oxyhemoglobin dissociation curve to the left, impairing tissue oxygenation (Chap. 28). The expected compensation for a metabolic alkalosis is hypoventilation and increased PCO_2. As discussed before, respiratory compensation is inadequate at best, invoking the teleological argument that hypoxia is more undesirable than alkalemia.[106] Several authors, however, have reported that severe hypoventilation and respiratory failure can occur in response to metabolic alkalosis, suggesting an actual, although uncommon, risk.[112]

Approach to the Patient with Metabolic Alkalosis

Metabolic alkalosis results from GI or urinary loss of acid, administration of exogenous base, or renal HCO_3^- retention (ie, impaired renal HCO_3^- excretion). Table 12-5 lists the causes of metabolic alkalosis. Compared with metabolic acidosis, metabolic alkalosis is less common and less frequently a consequence of xenobiotic exposure.

The etiologies of metabolic alkalosis are classically characterized from a therapeutic standpoint as chloride responsive or chloride resistant. Chloride-responsive etiologies such as diuretic use, vomiting, nasogastric suction, and Cl⁻ diarrhea are usually associated with a urinary $[Cl^-]$ <10 mEq/L.[64] Patients with these disorders respond rapidly to infusion of 0.9% NaCl solution when concomitant therapy addresses the underlying problem.[3,4] Chloride resistant disorders exemplified by hyperaldosteronism and severe K^+ depletion are characterized by urinary $[Cl^-]$ >10 mEq/L and tend to be resistant to 0.9% NaCl solution therapy.[53,64] Patients with these disorders often require K^+ repletion or drugs that reduce mineralocorticoid effects, such as spironolactone or eplerenone, before correction can occur.[53] When 0.9% NaCl solution repletion is ineffective or emergent correction of the alkalosis is required, some authors have suggested infusions of lysine or arginine HCl or dilute HCl.[3,4] However, this technique is rarely necessary and we do not routinely recommend it.

XENOBIOTIC-INDUCED AND OTHER ALTERATIONS OF WATER BALANCE

Significant fluid abnormalities commonly occur following xenobiotic exposure. Gastrointestinal losses in the form of vomiting, diarrhea, GI hemorrhage, and third spacing such as from GI burns result from a variety of xenobiotic toxicities and their management with emetics and cathartics. Renal fluid losses result from the ability of many xenobiotics to increase the glomerular filtration rate (inotropes), impair Na^+ reabsorption (diuretics), or increase urine volume in response to an obligate solute load (salicylates).

Fluid losses also occur through the skin as a result of sweating (sympathomimetics, cholinergics, and uncouplers of oxidative phosphorylation) or the lung as a result of increased minute ventilation (salicylates and sympathomimetics) or bronchorrhea (cholinergics). To the extent that these lost fluids contain Na^+, various signs, symptoms, and laboratory evidence of ECFV depletion develop.

The diagnosis and treatment of abnormal serum electrolyte concentrations are usually addressed after repletion of the ECFV deficit with isotonic, Na^+-containing fluids (eg, blood products, 0.9% NaCl solution, lactated Ringer solution). Other fluid balance issues are discussed in Chaps. 16 and 27 and other chapters relating to individual xenobiotics. This section focuses on body water balance (abnormalities of which manifest as hypernatremia and hyponatremia) and specifically on the toxicologically relevant syndromes of diabetes insipidus (DI) and the syndrome of inappropriate secretion of antidiuretic hormone (SIADH).

Sodium concentration in the extracellular space is intrinsically related to and directly reflects total body water balance. This occurs because the sodium cation is largely restricted to the extracellular space, and its serum concentration is primarily, if indirectly, controlled by factors that control water balance. Thus, both the serum $[Na^+]$ and plasma osmolality vary inversely with changes in the quantity of body water.

Plasma osmolality is maintained through a complex interaction between dietary water intake; the hypothalamus, pituitary gland, and kidney; and the effects of hormones such as arginine vasopressin (ADH) and adrenal mineralocorticoids.[17,20,108,146] Briefly, changes in osmolality are caused by changes in water intake and insensible (dermal, respiratory, and stool) and sensible (urinary, sweat) water losses. Urinary water losses are controlled by ADH. Increases in the osmolality of the extracellular fluid (ECF) stimulate anterior hypothalamic osmoreceptors, thereby stimulating thirst and ADH synthesis and release by the posterior pituitary gland. Arginine vasopressin release reaches its maximum concentration at a plasma osmolality of about 295 mOsm/kg. Arginine vasopressin is transported to the kidney via the bloodstream, where it stimulates the synthesis of cyclic adenosine monophosphate (cAMP). Cyclic adenosine monophosphate increases the water permeability of the distal convoluted tubule and collecting duct by stimulating the insertion of aquaporin (water) channels in the apical membrane, and thereby increasing water reabsorption and urine concentration, and minimizing urinary water losses. Conversely, as plasma osmolality falls, thirst and ADH release are diminished. This results in decreased renal cAMP generation, decreased water permeability of the distal convoluted tubule and collecting duct, and excretion of a relatively dilute urine that ultimately corrects the body water excess. Marked alterations in water intake combined with perturbations of these various processes often lead to hypernatremia or hyponatremia.

Hypernatremia

Table 12-6 summarizes the xenobiotics that cause hypernatremia. Hypernatremia occasionally results from the parenteral administration of sodium-containing drugs or rapid and excessive oral Na^+ intake.[1] Oral NaCl and oral sodium citrate were once used as emetics and antiemetics, respectively. As might be expected, they produced severe hypernatremia.[20] One case of unintentional fatal hypernatremia resulted from gargling with a supersaturated NaCl solution.[99] Similarly, massive ingestion of sodium hypochlorite bleach

TABLE 12-5	Xenobiotic and Other Causes of Metabolic Alkalosis		
Gastrointestinal Acid Loss	**Urinary Acid Loss**	**Base Administration**	**Renal Bicarbonate Retention**
Nasogastric suction (protracted)	Common	Acetate (dialysis or hyperalimentation)	Hypercapnia (chronic)
Vomiting	Diuretics	Bicarbonate	Hypochloremia
	Glucocorticoids	Carbonate (antacids)	Hypokalemia
	Rare	Citrate (posttransfusion)	Volume contraction
	Hypercalcemia	Milk alkali syndrome	
	Licorice (containing glycyrrhizic acid)		
	Magnesium deficiency		

TABLE 12–6 Xenobiotic Causes of Hypernatremia

Sodium Gain	Water Loss	Water Loss Due to Diabetes Insipidus
Antacids sodium bicarbonate	Cholestyramine	α-Adrenergic antagonists
Sodium salts (acetate, ascorbate, bicarbonate, chloride, citrate, hypochlorite, polystyrene sulfonate)	Diuretics	Amphotericin
	Lactulose	Antivirals: abacavir, adefovir, cidofovir, tenofovir
	Mannitol	Colchicine
Seawater	Povidone-iodine	Demeclocycline
	Sorbitol	Ethanol
	Urea	Foscarnet
		Glufosinate
		Ifosfamide
		Lithium
		Lobenzarit disodium
		Methoxyflurane
		Mesalazine
		Minocycline
		Opioid antagonists
		Propoxyphene
		Rifampin
		Streptozotocin
		Temozolomide
		V_2-receptor antagonists: conivaptan, tolvaptan
		Valproic acid

was associated with hypernatremia.[123] Unfortunately intentional salt poisoning is also reported.[37]

More commonly, hypernatremia results from relatively electrolyte-free (hypotonic) water losses due to xenobiotics or conditions that cause urinary, GI, and dermal fluid losses.[1] Indeed, all fluid losses from the body, except hemorrhage and those from fistulas, are hypotonic (and have the potential to cause hypernatremia). The lack of adequate fluid replacement is a key element in the development of hypernatremia because even the large fluid losses caused by DI or cholera-induced diarrhea will not cause hypernatremia if they are adequately replaced. Thus, in patients with hypernatremia caused by fluid losses, the reason why the losses were not replaced by the patient should always be sought.

Xenobiotics that produce significant diarrhea, such as lactulose, cause hypernatremia through unreplaced stool water losses. A similar pathogenesis accounts for the hypernatremia caused by the polyethylene-containing solution used for bowel preparation for colonoscopy.[13] Of particular concern is the use of cathartics in the management of poisonings, especially when fluid losses are not anticipated. For example, multiple doses of sorbitol reportedly produce severe hypernatremic dehydration and death in both children and adults.[23,44,55,147]

Significant water loss also occur through the skin. Although diffuse diaphoresis resulting from cocaine or organic phosphorus insecticide toxicity has the potential to produce hypernatremia, this rarely, if ever, occurs. However, application of a remedy containing hyperosmolar povidone–iodine to the skin of burned patients is reported to produce significant water losses and hypernatremia.[130]

Diagnosis and Treatment

The symptoms of significant hypernatremia consist largely of altered mental status ranging from confusion to coma, and neuromuscular weakness that occasionally results in respiratory paralysis. If hypernatremia is associated with Na^+ losses and marked ECFV depletion, cardiovascular symptoms, tachycardia, and orthostatic hypotension may be present. Treatment

consists of first replacing the Na^+ deficit if present (with isotonic fluids such as 0.9% NaCl solution), and then replacing the water deficit. The water deficit is estimated by assuming that the fractional increase in serum $[Na^+]$ is equal to the fractional decrease in total body water. Thus, a serum $[Na^+]$ that has increased by 10% (from 144 mEq/L to 158 mEq/L) indicates that the water deficit is 10% (3.6 L in a 60-kg person with 36 L of body water).

When hypernatremia develops over several hours, for example, as occurs after ingestion or administration of a sodium salt, rapid correction is indicated. However, when hypernatremia develops over several days or when the duration is unknown, slow correction of hypernatremia (over several days) is recommended.[1] The adaptation of brain cells to the water deficit (including the gain of intracellular solute including K^+, Na^+, inositol, glutamate, taurine, and creatine) makes cerebral edema a frequent complication of rapid water replacement. Although some sources suggest that 0.9% NaCl solution is an appropriate replacement fluid regardless of the magnitude of the water deficit, a more refined analysis emphasizes the use of hypotonic fluids to correct hypernatremia in the absence of a significant sodium deficit.[1]

Diabetes Insipidus

The greatest water losses and therefore the potentially most severe cases of hypernatremia occur during DI, which is always characterized by greater or lesser degrees of hypotonic polyuria. Diabetes insipidus is either characterized as neurogenic, resulting from failure to sense a rising osmolality or from a failure to release ADH, or nephrogenic, resulting from failure of the kidney to respond appropriately to ADH. Although there are many nontoxicologic causes of DI (eg, trauma, tumor, sarcoidosis, vascular, and congenital), xenobiotic-induced DI is also common and is mediated through either central or peripheral mechanisms.

Ethanol, opioid antagonists, and α-adrenergic agonists all suppress ADH release.[103,104] Lithium,[88,133] demeclocycline,[132] methoxyflurane,[83,92] propoxyphene, foscarnet,[107] mesalazine,[90] streptozotocin, amphotericin,[69] glufosinate,[141] lobenzarit,[124] rifampin,[116] temozolomide,[42] and colchicine[146] are associated with nephrogenic DI (Table 12–6). In addition, nephrogenic DI is reportedly caused by severe hypokalemia from diuretic use and hypercalcemia from vitamin D poisoning.[146] Of all of these xenobiotics, lithium has been the most extensively evaluated. Although polyuria is a common finding with lithium therapy (occurring in 20%–70% of patients on maintenance therapy), the exact incidence of DI and hypernatremia is unknown. Estimates range from 10% to 20% to as high as 80%.

Diagnosis

Patients with DI complain of polyuria and polydipsia. Urine volumes typically exceed 30 mL/kg/d[146] and can be as high as 9 L/d with nephrogenic DI[88] and 12 to 14 L/d with neurogenic (central) DI.[104] Nocturia, fatigue, and decreased work performance are often noted.[146] Neurogenic DI resulting from hypothalamic or pituitary damage is typically associated with other signs of neuroendocrine dysfunction.[104]

After polyuria is confirmed (eg, in adults, by measuring a urine output >200 mL over one hour), the urine osmolality or specific gravity should be measured. The diagnosis of DI is established by the occurrence of dilute urine (urine osmolality <300 mOsm/kg, urine specific gravity <1.010) in the presence of increased serum $[Na^+]$ and a serum osmolality greater than 295 mOsm/kg.[146] After this determination, a trial of desmopressin, an arginine vasopressin analog, helps to differentiate between neurogenic and nephrogenic DI. If the etiology of the DI is neurogenic, the patient will promptly respond to desmopressin with a decrease in urine output and increase in urine osmolality. In nephrogenic DI, desmopressin will have no significant effect.

Treatment

The initial approach to a hypernatremic patient with DI involves the repletion of the water deficit (as described earlier) and the restoration of electrolyte depletion, if necessary. If a reversible cause for the DI can be established, it should be corrected. Specifically, xenobiotics implicated as the cause of DI should be discontinued or their dose reduced. Patients with neurogenic DI should be maintained on either vasopressin or desmopressin. The latter is preferred because of the lack of vasopressor effects and ease of administration. In the past, patients were occasionally treated with oral medications known to produce SIADH (see later). Patients with nephrogenic DI can be treated with thiazide diuretics,[38] prostaglandin inhibitors,[33,86] or amiloride, all of which reduce the urine flow rate.[16]

Hyponatremia

Hyponatremia may be associated with a high, normal, or low serum osmolality. Some patients with myeloma or severe hyperlipidemia exhibit artifactual hyponatremia whenever the measurement technique requires dilution of the serum sample rather than direct measurement by a sodium electrode. These patients have a normal serum osmolality and no symptoms related to their artifactual hyponatremia, and they require no therapy for their "pseudohyponatremia."

Hyperglycemic patients develop hyponatremia because the increase in plasma osmolality caused by hyperglycemia results in a water shift from the intracellular to the extracellular space. The reduction in serum [Na+], which may cause symptoms, is approximately 1.6 mEq/L for every 100 mg/dL increase in serum glucose concentration above normal. The contribution of hyperglycemia to the hyponatremia should be calculated to determine if other causes of hyponatremia should also be sought. All other causes of hyponatremia are associated with a low plasma osmolality. In fact, in the absence of myeloma, hyperlipidemia, and hyperglycemia, the serum osmolality need not be measured in hyponatremic patients and should be assumed to be low.

Hyponatremia associated with a low plasma osmolality usually results from water intake in excess of the renal capacity to excrete it. When renal water excretion is normal, very large intake is required to cause hyponatremia. For example, large quantities of water are ingested over a short period of time by people with psychiatric or neurologic disorders such as psychogenic polydypsia.[57,121] Xenobiotic-induced water excess comparable to psychogenic polydypsia is quite uncommon. An example occurred during urologic procedures, such as transurethral resection of the prostate (TURP), in which large volumes of irrigation solution are required. Because the wounds were electrically cauterized, these fluids did not contain conductive electrolytes such as sodium. Sorbitol, dextrose, and mannitol were tried as irrigation solutions in an attempt to maintain a normal osmolality, but their optical characteristics were undesirable during the surgery. Thus, irrigation during TURP was performed with glycine-containing solutions. If a large volume of 1.5% glycine (osmolality, 220 mOsm/kg) is absorbed through the prostatic venous plexus, a rapid reduction in serum [Na+] results and will persist until the glycine is metabolized.[66,98] Symptoms in these patients are probably a result of several factors: hyponatremia, the glycine itself, and NH_3, a glycine metabolite. A similar complication is also described during hysteroscopy.[113]

Rarely, hyponatremia results from the loss of a body fluid with a [Na+] greater than the ECF [Na+] (of 145 mEq/L). This rarely occurs in patients with adrenal insufficiency through hypertonic urinary losses (although increased ADH secretion as a consequence of ECF sodium depletion is probably a more important mechanism; see later discussion). In burn patients, Na+ may be lost directly from the ECF. When treated with topical applications of silver nitrate cream, hyponatremia developed from the diffusion of sodium through permeable skin into the hypotonic dressing.[28] Ingestion of licorice that contains glycyrrhizic acid produces a syndrome of hyponatremia, hypokalemia, and hypertension that resembles mineralocorticoid excess. Although the exact mechanism of hyponatremia is debated, one report suggested that a glycyrrhizic acid–induced reduction in 11-β-hydroxysteroid dehydrogenase activity, an enzyme that metabolizes cortisol, could account for the findings.[43] Lithium, which is usually associated with DI and hypernatremia, is rarely reported to cause renal sodium wasting and hyponatremia that seems to be unrelated to ADH effects.[97]

Most cases of hyponatremia are caused by water intake in excess of a reduced renal excretory capacity. This reduction in urinary water excretion

may be physiologic (as during ECF sodium depletion) or pathologic (in association with kidney, heart, or liver failure).[2] Because these conditions are accompanied by alterations in renal sodium handling, signs and symptoms of ECFV depletion, such as postural hypotension, or ECFV excess, such as edema, usually accompany the hyponatremia. Other patients cannot excrete water normally because malignancy or various brain or pulmonary diseases cause ADH secretion.[2] In some cases, the tumors are associated with paraneoplastic disease and directly secrete ADH. Xenobiotics, such as diuretics, cause ECFV depletion, but most directly stimulate ADH secretion or augment the renal effects of ADH. Drugs such as the thiazide diuretics cause hyponatremia by several mechanisms, including interference with maximal urinary dilution, and by ADH-induced water retention in response to decreased ECFV.[2,46] Patients with excess secretion or action of ADH who have near-normal ECFV have the syndrome of inappropriate antidiuretic hormone (SIADH) secretion. Table 12–7 summarizes these and other causes of hyponatremia.

TABLE 12–7	Xenobiotic and Other Causes of Hyponatremia
Angiotensin-converting enzyme inhibitors	
Arginine	
Diuretics	
Glycine (transurethral prostatectomy syndrome)	
Licorice (containing glycyrrhizic acid)	
Lithium	
Nonsteroidal antiinflammatory drugs	
Primary polydipsia	
Silver	
Syndrome of inappropriate antidiuretic hormone secretion (SIADH)	
Amiloride	
Amiodarone	
Amitriptyline (and other cyclic antidepressants)	
Antipsychotics	
Atomoxetine	
Biguanides (metformin and phenformin)	
Bortezomib	
Carbamazepine (and oxcarbamazepine)	
Cisplatin (and other platinum chemotherapeutics)	
Clofibrate	
Cyclophosphamide	
Desmopressin (DDAVP)	
Diazoxide	
Duloxetine	
Eslicarbazepine	
Hallucinogenic amphetamines, MDMA (methylenedioxymethamphetamine), methylone, methcathinone	
Nicotine	
Opioids	
Oxytocin	
Pantoprazole	
Selective serotonin reuptake inhibitors	
Sibutramine	
Sulfonylureas	
Tramadol	
Tranylcypromine	
Trimethoprim	
Valproate	
Vasopressin	
Vincristine and vinblastine	
Vinorelbine	

Syndrome of Inappropriate Antidiuretic Hormone (SIADH)

The SIADH is characterized by hyponatremia and plasma hypotonicity in the absence of abnormalities of ECFV, or abnormal adrenal, thyroid, or kidney function. Early reviews claimed that SIADH was a disorder of volume overload based largely on evidence of weight gain.[103] The consistent absence of edema, however, and the fact that the decrease in serum [Na$^+$] cannot be accounted for by the fluid gain (weight gain) suggest that water retention is only part of the mechanism.[82] Urinary Na$^+$ loss and Na$^+$ redistribution from the extracellular to the intracellular space is apparently important as well.

There are many nontoxicologic etiologies of SIADH, most of which result from pulmonary or intracranial pathology. These causes include infections, malignancies, and surgery.[2,82,104] Table 12–7 summarizes xenobiotics and other causes known to produce SIADH. The antidiabetics, including both the sulfonylurea (eg, chlorpropamide) and biguanide (eg, metformin) classes, produce hyponatremia more commonly than other drugs.[102] Their actions are multifactorial and can include both the potentiation of endogenous ADH and the stimulation of ADH release.[102] Many psychiatric medications, including the selective serotonin reuptake inhibitors, cyclic antidepressants, and antipsychotics, are implicated in causing SIADH.[79,87,137,144] The effects of these drugs are mediated by the complex interactions between the dopaminergic and noradrenergic systems that control ADH release.[137] Additional evidence supports a role of serotonin in drug-induced SIADH. Serotonin (specifically 5-HT$_2$ or 5-HT$_{1C}$ agonism) directly stimulates ADH release[10] and water intake.[71] An important role of serotonin is supported by the occurrence of SIADH with MDMA use.[70]

Diagnosis

The clinical presentation of patients with hyponatremia depends on the cause, the absolute serum [Na$^+$], and the rate of decline in serum [Na$^+$]. Patients with associated ECFV excess or depletion present with evidence of altered ECFV, as well as signs and symptoms of the disease that caused the abnormality in ECFV, such as adrenal insufficiency or heart failure.[2] Rarely do these patients exhibit symptoms of hyponatremia and hyposmolality of body fluids per se. This is because of the moderate degree of hyponatremia (usually > 130 mEq/L) or the moderate rate of decline in [Na$^+$] or because the loss of Na$^+$ and water limits the development of cerebral edema.[85] It is important to note that patients with hyponatremia and a low plasma osmolality (excluding those with primary polydipsia) all have a urinary osmolality that is relatively high regardless of whether they have excess, diminished, or normal ECFV. Consequently, these disorders can only be differentiated by the history, physical examination, and other laboratory test results.

Patients with SIADH, if symptomatic, usually present with signs and symptoms of hyponatremia. As noted earlier, the clinical manifestations of hyponatremia are dependent on both the absolute serum [Na$^+$] and its rate of decline.[85,104] Whereas chronic slow depression of the [Na$^+$] is usually well tolerated, rapid decreases are associated with symptoms and sometimes catastrophic events. Symptoms include headache, nausea, vomiting, restlessness, disorientation, depression, apathy, irritability, lethargy, weakness, and muscle cramps. In more severe cases, respiratory depression, coma, and seizures develop.

The diagnosis of SIADH is based on establishing the presence of hyponatremia, a low serum osmolality, and impaired urinary dilution in the absence of edema, hypotension, hypovolemia, and kidney, adrenal, or thyroid dysfunction.[82] As discussed earlier, the presence of any of these clinical findings suggests that another cause of hyponatremia is present. A serum uric acid concentration is helpful in differentiating SIADH from other causes of hyponatremia. In the presence of hyponatremia and impaired urinary dilution, patients with SIADH have hypouricemia, whereas patients exhibiting ECFV excess or depletion characteristically have hyperuricemia.[31]

Treatment

Treatment of patients with demonstrable ECFV excess or depletion should be directed at the abnormal ECFV and its cause rather than the hyponatremia. In almost all cases, the hyponatremia will improve with correction of the ECFV.[2,85] In a similar way, correction of the serum glucose in hyperglycemic patients and the removal of glycine by hemodialysis in patients with the

TURP syndrome will correct the serum [Na$^+$]. The rate of correction of the serum [Na$^+$] in these patients is generally not of concern.

In patients with SIADH, treatment begins with fluid restriction. Because the goal of this therapy is to establish a negative fluid balance, careful attention to intake and output is required. If an offending xenobiotic is identified, it should be discontinued. Although most cases resolve in 1 to 2 weeks,[82,104] SIADH caused by chronic cerebral or pulmonary conditions or by malignancy often persists. If this occurs, therapy with demeclocycline, lithium, or tolvaptan is suggested because severe fluid restriction is often intolerable. Tolvaptan, an oral ADH antagonist with specificity for the V$_2$ receptor, is currently the recommended treatment for chronically hyponatremic patients in whom fluid restriction is unsuccessful because it is easier to titrate with fewer potential side effects than demeclocycline and lithium. In all asymptomatic or mildly symptomatic patients (usually patients with chronic hyponatremia of more than 2 days' duration), correction should proceed slowly and certainly at a rate less than 8.0 mEq/L during the first 24 hours and less than 16 mEq/L during the first 48 hours. This approach to correction is indicated because if hyponatremia resolution is faster than the reuptake of the solutes (K$^+$, Na$^+$, inositol, glutamate, taurine, and creatine) extruded from brain cells during the development of hyponatremia, brain shrinkage will occur with disruption of the blood–brain barrier. This effect is responsible for the osmotic demyelination syndrome (ODS). The ODS, which is associated with central pontine and extrapontine myelinolysis, often has a delayed onset of 2 to 6 days and causes irreversible brain damage and death in 50% and 15% of patients, respectively.[2,12,139] Risk factors for ODS, in addition to too rapid correction of chronic hyponatremia, include serum [Na$^+$] below 115 mEq/L and patients who are elderly, hypokalemic, alcoholic, or malnourished. In asymptomatic patients, as described earlier, water restriction is recommended and usually sufficient, but occasionally tolvaptan (an ADH V$_2$ receptor antagonist) is appropriate. When hyponatremia is associated with life-threatening clinical presentations, including respiratory depression, altered mental status, seizures, or coma, careful infusion of hypertonic 3% saline ([Na$^+$] = 513 mEq/L) (eg, 1–2 mL/kg/h), with or without furosemide, is indicated.[2,82] Alternatively, conivaptan (another ADH V$_2$ receptor antagonist) can be administered intravenously as an initial bolus of 20 mg followed by a continuous infusion of 40 mg/d for no more than 4 days.[62,65] In these symptomatic patients, the goal is to increase the serum [Na$^+$] 1 mEq/L/h (5–6 mEq/L over 6 hours) or until life-threatening symptoms resolve.[2,85] After this initial correction and improvement of symptoms, the serum [Na$^+$] should be increased at a rate less than 0.3 mEq/L/h, preferably by water restriction alone. Formulas are available to help calculate the rate of correction of hyponatremia.[2] Equation 12–8 is the equation we prefer.

When 1 L of fluid is infused:

$$\text{Change in serum [Na}^+] = \frac{\text{infusate [Na}^+] - \text{serum [Na}^+]}{\text{Total body water} + 1L} \quad \text{(Eq. 12–8)}$$

where the infusate [Na$^+$] in mEq/L equals:

3% sodium chloride	513
0.9% sodium chloride	154
Lactated Ringer solution	130
0.45% sodium chloride	77
0.33% sodium chloride	56

XENOBIOTIC-INDUCED ELECTROLYTE ABNORMALITIES
Potassium

Xenobiotic-induced alterations in serum [K$^+$] are potentially more serious than alterations in other electrolyte concentrations because of the critical role of potassium in a variety of homeostatic processes, most importantly, muscle strength and cardiac function. The total body potassium content of an average adult is about 54 mEq/kg, of which only 2% is located in the intravascular space. The large intracellular store of potassium is maintained by a variety of systems, the most important of which is membrane Na$^+$,K$^+$-adenosine triphosphatase (ATPase). The relationship between total body stores and serum [K⁺] is not linear, and small changes in the total body potassium often result in dramatic alterations in serum concentrations and, more importantly, in the ratio of extracellular to intracellular [K⁺].

People eating a Western diet ingest 50 to 150 mEq/d of potassium, approximately 90% of which is subsequently eliminated in the urine. The body has 2 major defenses against a potassium load: acutely, potassium is transferred into cells; chronically, potassium is excreted in the urine by decreased proximal tubular reabsorption and increased distal tubular secretion (to a maximum of 600–700 mEq/d).[22] After a meal, K⁺ transfers into the intracellular space through insulin and catecholamine-mediated uptake of potassium in liver and muscle cells.[122] Renal potassium excretion is primarily modulated by the renin–angiotensin–aldosterone system. In addition, the GI absorption of potassium decreases as the serum [K⁺] increases.

Hypokalemia results from decreased oral intake, GI losses caused by repeated vomiting or diarrhea, urinary losses through increased K⁺ secretion or decreased reabsorption, and processes that shift potassium into the intracellular compartment.[20,22,148] Table 12–8 summarizes the xenobiotics and other causes commonly associated with hypokalemia.

The neuromuscular manifestations of hypokalemia are reviewed elsewhere.[80] Patients with hypokalemia are often asymptomatic when the decrease in serum [K⁺] is mild (serum concentrations of 3.0–3.5 mEq/L). Occasionally, hypokalemia interferes with renal concentrating mechanisms, and polyuria is noted. More significant potassium deficits (serum concentrations of 2.0–3.0 mEq/L) cause generalized malaise and weakness. As the [K⁺] falls to less than 2 mEq/L, weakness becomes prominent, and areflexic paralysis and respiratory failure occur, often necessitating intubation and mechanical ventilation.[80] Rhabdomyolysis also occurs. These neuromuscular manifestations are so prominent that they are potentially erroneously attributed to a neuromuscular syndrome such as Guillain-Barré. Other clinical findings associated with hypokalemia include GI hypoperistalsis (ileus); manifestations of cardioactive steroid toxicity; worsening hyperglycemia in patients with diabetes; and the symptoms and signs of the metabolic abnormalities that often accompany hypokalemia, such as hyponatremia, metabolic acidosis, or alkalosis.[148]

Electrocardiographic changes also are common, even with mild potassium depletion, although the absence of ECG changes should never be used to exclude significant hypokalemia. Common ECG findings of hypokalemia include depression of the ST segment, decreased T-wave amplitude, and increased U-wave amplitude (Chap. 15). These findings may herald life-threatening rhythm disturbances, particularly polymorphic ventricular tachycardia.[148]

Treatment of hypokalemia involves discontinuing or removing the offending xenobiotic and correcting the potassium deficit. Potassium supplementation should be given, either orally or intravenously as acceptable. The choice of potassium salt should be based on the associated acid–base abnormality, if present. Thus, potassium chloride is preferred when metabolic alkalosis is present, and another salt of potassium (eg, potassium citrate or potassium bicarbonate) is preferable when metabolic acidosis is present.[148] Potassium phosphate should be used as part of the K⁺ supplement when hypophosphatemia is also present, as occurs in diabetic ketoacidosis, or when hyperchloremia is present. Hypomagnesemia, which either causes or accompanies hypokalemia (eg, in diuretic-induced hypokalemia), must be corrected because this abnormality often prevents successful potassium replacement.

The debate over the maximum safe infusion rate for IV potassium is summarized elsewhere.[84,148] Based on experience with more than 1300 infusions, one group concluded that under intensive care monitoring, IV administration of 20 mEq/h (by central or peripheral vein) is well tolerated. They also found that each 20 mEq of potassium administered resulted in an average increase in serum [K⁺] of 0.25 mEq/L. Under most circumstances we agree with these recommendations, but acknowledge that others have used significantly larger doses (up to 100 mEq/h) in unique life-threatening circumstances.[32]

Hyperkalemia results from decreased urinary elimination (renal insufficiency, potassium-sparing diuretics, hypoaldosteronism), increased intake (either orally or intravenously), or redistribution from tissue stores.[20,22] The last mechanism is of major toxicologic importance. Overdoses of both cardioactive steroids (Chap. 62) and β-adrenergic antagonists (Chap. 59) cause hyperkalemia by promoting net potassium release from intracellular reservoirs. Presumably because of other protective mechanisms, overdose with a β-adrenergic antagonist produces only a moderate rise in serum [K⁺] (usually to 5.0–5.5 mEq/L). By contrast, a similar rise in serum [K⁺] as a consequence of blockade of the Na⁺,K⁺-ATPase pump during acute cardioactive steroid toxicity may be lethal (Chap. 62). This suggests that hyperkalemia per se is not the cause of the lethality of cardioactive steroid toxicity. Thus, the focus of therapy should involve efforts to neutralize or eliminate the cardioactive steroid rather than reduce the serum [K⁺].[18] Table 12–8 lists xenobiotics and other causes of hyperkalemia.

After oral overdoses of potassium salts, patients usually complain of nausea and vomiting. Ileus, intestinal irritation, bleeding, and perforation reportedly complicate the clinical course.[126,127] In the absence of potassium ingestion, GI symptoms of hyperkalemia are usually very mild. Neuromuscular manifestations include weakness with an ascending flaccid paralysis and respiratory compromise, with intact sensation and cognition.[80,94,114] The similarity of these signs and symptoms to those associated with hypokalemia is striking, suggesting that hyperkalemia should only be diagnosed with certainty by laboratory measurement.

The cardiac manifestations of hyperkalemia are distinct, prominent, and life threatening. ECG patterns progress through characteristic changes.[127] Although the progression of ECG changes is reproducible, there is great individual variation with respect to the serum [K⁺] at which these ECG findings occur. Initially, the only ECG finding is the presence of tall, peaked

TABLE 12–8   Xenobiotic and Other Causes of Altered Serum Potassium

Hypokalemia	Hyperkalemia
β-Adrenergic agonists	α-Adrenergic agonists (phenylephrine)
Aminoglycosides	β-Adrenergic antagonists
Amphotericin	Aliskerin
Barium (soluble salts)	Amiloride
Bicarbonate	Angiotensin-converting enzyme inhibitors
Caffeine	Angiotensin receptor blockers
Carbonic anhydrase inhibitors	Arginine hydrochloride
Cathartics	Cardioactive steroids
Chloroquine	Cyclosporine
Cisplatin	Dabigatran
Dextrose	Drosperidone
Hydroxychloroquine	Fluoride
Infliximab	Glyphosate
Insulin	Heparin
Levetiracetam	Nicorandil
Licorice (containing glycyrrhizic acid)	Nonsteroidal antiinflammatory drugs
Loop diuretics	Penicillin (potassium)
Metabolic alkalosis	Pentamidine
Osmotic diuretics	Potassium salts
Quinine	Spironolactone
Salicylates	Succinylcholine
Sodium penicillin and its analogs	Tacrolimus
Sodium polystyrene sulfate	Triamterene
Sulfonylureas	Trimethoprim
Sympathomimetics	
Tenofovir	
Theophylline	
Thiazide diuretics	
Toluene	

T waves. As the serum [K⁺] concentration increases, the QRS complex tends to blend into the T waves, the P-wave amplitude decreases, and the PR interval becomes prolonged. Next, the P wave is lost, and ST-segment depression occurs. Finally, the distinction between the S and T waves becomes blurred, and the ECG takes on a sine wave configuration (Chap. 16). Hemodynamic instability and cardiac arrest can result. As the patient's serum [K⁺] falls with therapy, these ECG changes resolve in a reverse fashion.

The treatment of severe hyperkalemia focuses on methods to (1) reverse the ECG effects, (2) transfer K⁺ to the intracellular space, and (3) enhance K⁺ elimination. Pharmacologic interventions, extensively discussed elsewhere,[126] are summarized here. Calcium salts (eg, 10–20 mEq administered intravenously) (Antidotes in Depth: A29) work almost immediately to protect the myocardium against the effects of hyperkalemia, although it does not reduce the serum [K⁺]. However, a potentially life-threatening interaction occurs when the patient with cardioactive steroid toxicity is given calcium salts (Chap. 62).

The administration of insulin (and dextrose to prevent hypoglycemia unless hyperglycemia is present), sodium bicarbonate, or inhalation of a β-adrenergic agonist all stimulate potassium entry into cells.[8] They reduce the serum [K⁺] over approximately 30 minutes, but potassium begins to reenter the extracellular space over the next several hours. Caution is advised, when using insulin in patients with chronic kidney disease because hypoglycemia can be prolonged as a result reduced insulinase function. Cationic exchange resins, such as Na⁺ polystyrene sulfonate and patiromer, nonabsorbable polymers that binds potassium in exchange for calcium take longer to reduce the serum [K⁺] as they enhance GI potassium loss.[14,63,81] Hemodialysis or peritoneal dialysis are the most efficient means of rapidly reducing total body potassium stores, especially when significant renal impairment is present.

Calcium

Calcium is the most abundant mineral in the body, and 98% to 99% is located in bone. Approximately half of the remaining 1% to 2% of calcium in the body is bound to plasma proteins (mostly albumin), and most of the rest is complexed to various anions, with free, ionized calcium representing a very small fraction of extraosseous stores. The serum [Ca²⁺] is maintained through interactions between dietary intake and renal elimination, modulated by vitamin D activity, parathyroid hormone, and calcitonin. More extensive discussions of calcium physiology are found elsewhere.[6,105]

Xenobiotic-induced hypercalcemia is uncommon and usually caused by increased dietary calcium as a result of milk or antacid usage, calcium supplements, or a decrease in its renal excretion such as occurs with thiazide use.[6,20] Cholecalciferol, available as a rodenticide, can increase the serum [Ca²⁺] by increasing its release from bone, increasing GI absorption, and decreasing renal elimination. Vitamin D toxicity from excessive vitamin or milk intake also can cause hypercalcemia.[76] Table 12–9 lists other causes of hypercalcemia.

Symptoms of hypercalcemia consist of lethargy, muscle weakness, nausea, vomiting, and constipation. Life-threatening manifestations include complications from altered mental status such as aspiration pneumonia and cardiac dysrhythmias (Chap. 15). Treatment of clinically significant hypercalcemia focuses on removing the offending xenobiotic when possible, decreasing GI absorption by administering a binding agent, increasing distribution into bone with a bisphosphonate (onset 1–2 days), and enhancing renal excretion through forced diuresis with IV 0.9% NaCl solution and furosemide (onset 4–6 hours).[6,140] Hemodialysis is often required when significant renal impairment is present.

Xenobiotics more commonly cause hypocalcemia than hypercalcemia. Minor, usually clinically insignificant, decreases in serum [Ca²⁺] can occur in association with anticonvulsant and aminoglycoside therapy.[20] Severe, life-threatening hypocalcemia can occur, however, from ethylene glycol poisoning (Chap. 106) or as a manifestation of fluoride toxicity from either fluoride salts or hydrofluoric acid (Chap. 103).[39,142] Calcium complex formation with fluoride or oxalate ions is responsible for the rapid development of hypocalcemia

TABLE 12–9	Xenobiotic Causes of Altered Serum Calcium
Hypocalcemia	**Hypercalcemia**
Aminoglycosides	All-*trans*-retinoic acid (ATRA)
Bicarbonate	Aluminum
Bisphosphonates	Androgens
Calcitonin	Antacids (calcium containing)
Cinacalcet	Antacids (magnesium containing)
Citrate	Cholecalciferol and other vitamin D analogs
Denosumab	Lithium
Edetate disodium	Milk–alkali syndrome
Ethanol	Tamoxifen
Ethylene glycol	Thiazides
Fluoride	Vitamin A
Foscarnet	
Furosemide (and other loop diuretics)	
Mithramycin	
Neomycin	
Phenobarbital	
Phenytoin	
Phosphate	
Theophylline	
Valproate	

in these settings. Similar effects occur with excess phosphate[145] or citrate[93,143] intake. This mechanism (calcium complex formation) decreases the ionized [Ca²⁺] but may or may not reduce the measured total serum [Ca²⁺]. Other xenobiotics that produce hypocalcemia decrease absorption, enhance renal loss, or stimulate calcium entry into cells (Table 12–9).

Symptoms of hypocalcemia consist largely of neuromuscular findings, including paresthesias, cramps, carpopedal spasm, tetany, and seizures. Although ECG abnormalities are common (Chap. 15), life-threatening dysrhythmias are rare. Treatment strategies focus on calcium replacement. When hypomagnesemia or hyperphosphatemia is present, these abnormalities should be corrected, or calcium replacement will likely fail.

Magnesium

Magnesium is the fourth most abundant cation in the body (after Ca²⁺, Na⁺, and K⁺), with a normal total body store of about 2000 mEq in a 70-kg person.[117] Approximately 50% of magnesium is stored in bone, with most of the remainder distributed in the soft tissues. Because only approximately 1% to 2% of magnesium is located in the ECF, serum concentrations correlate poorly with total body stores.[118] Magnesium homeostasis is maintained through dietary intake and renal and GI excretion modulated by hormonal effects.[5]

Clinically significant hypermagnesemia is uncommon in the absence of kidney failure except when massive doses of magnesium salts overwhelm renal excretory mechanisms. This has been reported with inadvertent IV infusion,[19,24,68,101] urologic procedures involving irrigation with magnesium salts,[45,77] and ingestion of large quantities of magnesium-containing antacids[95] or cathartics.[52,56] Iatrogenic overdose was formerly of concern when magnesium-containing cathartics were routinely used in poison management.[54,78,135] In a series of poisoned patients, a single oral dose of a magnesium-containing cathartic (30 g of magnesium sulfate) failed to produce any demonstrable rise in serum [Mg²⁺].[136] However, patients who received 3 oral doses of magnesium sulfate over 8 hours had a significant increase in their serum [Mg²⁺].[136] Thus, the potential for iatrogenic toxicity exists, mandating cautious use of magnesium-containing cathartics, especially in patients with renal insufficiency. Table 12–10 lists xenobiotic causes of hypermagnesemia.

The symptoms of hypermagnesemia correlate with serum concentrations but depend somewhat on the rate of increase and host factors.

TABLE 12–10	Xenobiotic Causes of Altered Serum Magnesium
Hypomagnesemia	*Hypermagnesemia*
Aminoglycosides	Antacids (magnesium containing)
Amphotericin	Cathartics (magnesium containing)
Cetuximab	Lithium
Cisplatin	Magnesium salts
Citrate	
Cyclosporine	
DDT	
EGRF antibodies (panitumumab and cetuximab)	
Ethanol	
Fluoride	
Foscarnet	
Insulin	
Laxatives	
Levetiracetam	
Loop diuretics	
Methylxanthines	
Osmotic diuretics	
Phosphates	
Proton pump inhibitors	
Strychnine	
Tacrolimus	
Thiazides	

At serum $[Mg^{2+}]$ of about 3 to 10 mEq/L, patients feel weak, nauseated, flushed, and thirsty. Bradycardia, a widened QRS complex on ECG, hypotension, and decreased deep tendon reflexes are typically noted. As the $[Mg^{2+}]$ increases, hypoventilation, muscle paralysis, and ventricular dysrhythmias occur. Serum $[Mg^{2+}]$ greater than 10 mEq/L, especially those concentrations greater than 15 mEq/L, often cause death.

Hypermagnesemia is a life-threatening disorder. When significant neuromuscular or ECG manifestations are noted, administration of 5 to 20 mEq of Ca^{2+} should be administered by slow intravenous infusion to competitively antagonize the effects of the magnesium ion.[6,61] (Antidotes in Depth: A32) Further therapy should focus on enhancing renal excretion by administering fluids and loop diuretics such as furosemide.[61] In the presence of renal failure or inadequate renal excretion, hemodialysis will rapidly correct hypermagnesemia.

Xenobiotic-induced hypomagnesemia is common but rarely life threatening. Renal losses (caused by diuretics), GI losses (caused by ethanol), intracellular shifts caused by insulin[91] or β-adrenergic agonists, and complex formation (by fluoride or phosphate) are common.[5,6] Table 12–10 lists these and other xenobiotic causes of hypomagnesemia. Of note, many causes of hypomagnesemia also cause hypokalemia and hypocalcemia.[5] Therefore, when hypomagnesemia is suspected or discovered, the presence of other electrolyte abnormalities should be sought.

The symptoms of hypomagnesemia are lethargy, weakness, fatigue, neuromuscular excitation (tremor and hyperreflexia), nausea, and vomiting.[29,35] Dysrhythmias are reported, especially in patients treated with cardioactive steroids. Signs and symptoms consistent with hypocalcemia and hypokalemia also may be present.

Treatment involves removing the offending xenobiotic (if it can be identified) and restoring magnesium balance. Although either oral or parenteral supplementation is usually acceptable for mild hypomagnesemia, parenteral therapy is required when significant clinical manifestations are present. When oral therapy is indicated, a normal diet or magnesium oxide, magnesium chloride, or magnesium lactate in divided doses (magnesium 20–100 mEq/d) will often correct the hypomagnesemia.[5,6] When hypomagnesemia

is severe or symptomatic, and kidney function is normal, 16 mEq (2 g) of magnesium sulfate can be given intravenously over several minutes to a maximum of 1 mEq/kg of magnesium in a 24-hour period.[6,29,75] During any continuous magnesium infusion, frequent serum $[Mg^{2+}]$ determinations should be obtained and the presence of reflexes documented. If hyporeflexia occurs, the magnesium infusion should be discontinued and the patient assessed and treated for respiratory muscle weakness if present.

SUMMARY

- The management of poisoned patients must include an evaluation of their fluid, electrolyte, and acid–base status.
- Developing a stepwise approach to the evaluation of patients with a high anion gap metabolic acidosis is essential.
- The osmol gap can help confirm a suspicion of toxic alcohol poisoning but cannot exclude the diagnosis.
- Disorders of sodium (water) are common manifestations of xenobiotic exposure. Because fluid and electrolyte abnormalities result from both poisoning and the therapy of poisoned patients, reassessment and monitoring are essential to ensure a good clinical outcome.

REFERENCES

1. Adrogue HJ, Madias NE. Hypernatremia. *N Engl J Med.* 2000;342:1493-1499.
2. Adrogue HJ, Madias NE. Hyponatremia. *N Engl J Med.* 2000;342:1581-1589.
3. Adrogue HJ, Madias NE. Management of life-threatening acid-base disorders. First of two parts. *N Engl J Med.* 1998;338:26-34.
4. Adrogue HJ, Madias NE. Management of life-threatening acid-base disorders. Second of two parts. *N Engl J Med.* 1998;338:107-111.
5. Agus ZS. Hypomagnesemia. *J Am Soc Nephrol.* 1999;10:1616-1622.
6. Agus ZS, et al. Disorders of calcium and magnesium homeostasis. *Am J Med.* 1982;72:473-488.
7. Albert MS, et al. Quantitative displacement of acid-base equilibrium in metabolic acidosis. *Ann Intern Med.* 1967;66:312-322.
8. Allon M, et al. Nebulized albuterol for acute hyperkalemia in patients on hemodialysis. *Ann Intern Med.* 1989;110:426-429.
9. Ammar KA, Heckerling PS. Ethylene glycol poisoning with a normal anion gap caused by concurrent ethanol ingestion: importance of the osmolal gap. *Am J Kidney Dis.* 1996;27:130-133.
10. Anderson IK, et al. Central administration of 5-HT activates 5-HT1A receptors to cause sympathoexcitation and 5-HT2/5-HT1C receptors to release vasopressin in anaesthetized rats. *Br J Pharmacol.* 1992;107:1020-1028.
11. Andrews TJ, et al. Euglycemic diabetic ketoacidosis with elevated acetone in a patient taking a sodium-glucose cotransporter-2 (SGLT2) inhibitor. *J Emerg Med.* 2017;52:223-226.
12. Ayus JC, et al. Treatment of symptomatic hyponatremia and its relation to brain damage. A prospective study. *N Engl J Med.* 1987;317:1190-1195.
13. Ayus JC, et al. Fatal dysnatraemia caused by elective colonoscopy. *BMJ.* 2003;326:382-384.
14. Bakris GL, et al. Effect of patiromer on serum potassium level in patients with hyperkalemia and diabetic kidney disease: the AMETHYST-DN Randomized Clinical Trial. *JAMA.* 2015;314:151-161.
15. Batlle DC, et al. The use of the urinary anion gap in the diagnosis of hyperchloremic metabolic acidosis. *N Engl J Med.* 1988;318:594-599.
16. Batlle DC, et al. Amelioration of polyuria by amiloride in patients receiving long-term lithium therapy. *N Engl J Med.* 1985;312:408-414.
17. Berl T, et al. Clinical disorders of water metabolism. *Kidney Int.* 1976;10:117-132.
18. Bismuth C, et al. Hyperkalemia in acute digitalis poisoning: prognostic significance and therapeutic implications. *Clin Toxicol.* 1973;6:153-162.
19. Bourgeois FJ, et al. Profound hypotension complicating magnesium therapy. *Am J Obstet Gynecol.* 1986;154:919-920.
20. Brass EP, Thompson WL. Drug-induced electrolyte abnormalities. *Drugs.* 1982;24:207-228.
21. Brenner BE. Clinical significance of the elevated anion gap. *Am J Med.* 1985;79:289-296.
22. Brown RS. Extrarenal potassium homeostasis. *Kidney Int.* 1986;30:116-127.
23. Caldwell JW, et al. Hypernatremia associated with cathartics in overdose management. *West J Med.* 1987;147:593-596.
24. Cao Z, et al. Acute hypermagnesemia and respiratory arrest following infusion of MgSO4 for tocolysis. *Clin Chim Acta.* 1999;285:191-193.
25. Carlisle EJ, et al. Glue-sniffing and distal renal tubular acidosis: sticking to the facts. *Journal of the American Society of Nephrology: J Am Soc Nephrol.* 1991;1:1019-1027.
26. Carstairs SD, et al. Contribution of serum ethanol concentration to the osmol gap: a prospective volunteer study. *Clin Toxicol (Phila).* 2013;51:398-401.
27. Clement M, Senior P. Euglycemic diabetic ketoacidosis with canagliflozin: not-so-sweet but avoidable complication of sodium-glucose cotransporter-2 inhibitor use. *Can Fam Physician.* 2016;62:725-728.

28. Connelly DM. Silver nitrate. Ideal burn wound therapy? *N Y State J Med.* 1970;70:1642-1644.

29. Cronin RE, Knochel JP. Magnesium deficiency. *Adv Intern Med.* 1983;28:509-533.

30. Darchy B, et al. Delayed admission for ethylene glycol poisoning: lack of elevated serum osmol gap. *Intensive Care Med.* 1999;25:859-861.

31. Decaux G, et al. Uric acid, anion gap and urea concentration in the diagnostic approach to hyponatremia. *Clin Nephrol.* 1994;42:102-108.

32. DeFronzo RA, Bia M. Intravenous potassium chloride therapy. 1981;245:2446.

33. Delaney V, et al. Indomethacin in streptozocin-induced nephrogenic diabetes insipidus. *Am J Kidney Dis.* 1987;9:79-83.

34. DiNubile MJ. The increment in the anion gap: overextension of a concept? *Lancet.* 1988;2:951-953.

35. Dirks JH. The kidney and magnesium regulation. *Kidney Int.* 1983;23:771-777.

36. Dorwart WV, Chalmers L. Comparison of methods for calculating serum osmolality form chemical concentrations, and the prognostic value of such calculations. *Clin Chem.* 1975;21:190-194.

37. Dyer C. Mother found guilty in case of fabricated illness. *BMJ.* 2005;330:497.

38. Earley LE, Orloff J. The mechanism of antidiuresis associated with the administration of hydrochlorothiazide to patients with vasopressin-resistant diabetes insipidus. *J Clin Invest.* 1962;41:1988-1997.

39. Edelman P. Hydrofluoric acid burns. *Occup Med.* 1986;1:89-103.

40. Eisen TF, et al. Serum osmolality in alcohol ingestions: differences in availability among laboratories of teaching hospital, nonteaching hospital, and commercial facilities. *Am J Emerg Med.* 1989;7:256-259.

41. Emmett M, Narins RG. Clinical use of the anion gap. *Medicine (Baltimore).* 1977;56:38-54.

42. Faje AT, et al. Central diabetes insipidus: a previously unreported side effect of temozolomide. *J Clin Endocrinol Metab.* 2013;98:3926-3931.

43. Farese RV Jr, et al. Licorice-induced hypermineralocorticoidism. *N Engl J Med.* 1991;325:1223-1227.

44. Farley TA. Severe hypernatremic dehydration after use of an activated charcoal-sorbitol suspension. *J Pediatr.* 1986;109:719-722.

45. Fassler CA, et al. Magnesium toxicity as a cause of hypotension and hypoventilation. Occurrence in patients with normal renal function. *Arch Intern Med.* 1985;145:1604-1606.

46. Fichman MP, et al. Diuretic-induced hyponatremia. *Ann Intern Med.* 1971;75:853-863.

47. Figge J, et al. Anion gap and hypoalbuminemia. *Crit Care Med.* 1998;26:1807-1810.

48. Fulop M. Alcoholic ketoacidosis. *Endocrinol Metab Clin North Am.* 1993;22:209-219.

49. Gabow PA. Disorders associated with an altered anion gap. *Kidney Int.* 1985;27:472-483.

50. Gabow PA, et al. Diagnostic importance of an increased serum anion gap. *N Engl J Med.* 1980;303:854-858.

51. Gamble JL. *Chemical Anatomy, Physiology, and Pathology of Extracellular Fluids: A Lecture Series.* 6th ed. Cambridge, MA: Harvard University Press; 1960.

52. Garcia-Webb P, et al. Hypermagnesaemia and hypophosphataemia after ingestion of magnesium sulphate. *Br Med J (Clin Res Ed).* 1984;288:759.

53. Garella S, et al. Saline-resistant metabolic alkalosis or "chloride-wasting nephropathy." Report of four patients with severe potassium depletion. *Ann Intern Med.* 1970;73:31-38.

54. Garrelts JC, et al. Magnesium toxicity secondary to catharsis during management of theophylline poisoning. *Am J Emerg Med.* 1989;7:34-37.

55. Gazda-Smith E, Synhavsky A. Hypernatremia following treatment of theophylline toxicity with activated charcoal and sorbitol. *Arch Intern Med.* 1990;150:689, 692.

56. Gerard SK, et al. Extreme hypermagnesemia caused by an overdose of magnesium-containing cathartics. *Ann Emerg Med.* 1988;17:728-731.

57. Goldman MB, et al. Mechanisms of altered water metabolism in psychotic patients with polydipsia and hyponatremia. *N Engl J Med.* 1988;318:397-403.

58. Goldstein MB, et al. The urine anion gap: a clinically useful index of ammonium excretion. *Am J Med Sci.* 1986;292:198-202.

59. Goldstein RJ, et al. The myth of the low anion gap. *JAMA.* 1980;243:1737-1738.

60. Goodkin DA, et al. The role of the anion gap in detecting and managing mixed metabolic acid-base disorders. *Clin Endocrinol Metab.* 1984;13:333-349.

61. Graber TW, et al. Magnesium: physiology, clinical disorders, and therapy. *Ann Emerg Med.* 1981;10:49-57.

62. Greenberg A, Verbalis JG. Vasopressin receptor antagonists. *Kidney Int.* 2006;69:2124-2130.

63. Hagan AE, et al. Sodium polystyrene sulfonate for the treatment of acute hyperkalemia: a retrospective study. *Clin Nephrol.* 2016;85:38-43.

64. Harrington JT. Metabolic alkalosis. *Kidney Int.* 1984;26:88-97.

65. Hays RM. Vasopressin antagonists—progress and promise. *N Engl J Med.* 2006;355:2146-2148.

66. Hoekstra PT, et al. Transurethral prostatic resection syndrome—a new perspective: encephalopathy with associated hyperammonemia. *J Urol.* 1983;130:704-707.

67. Hoffman RS, et al. Osmol gaps revisited: normal values and limitations. *J Toxicol Clin Toxicol.* 1993;31:81-93.

68. Hoffman RS, et al. An "amp" by any other name: the hazards of intravenous magnesium dosing. *JAMA.* 1989;261:557.

69. Hohler T, et al. Indomethacin treatment in amphotericin B induced nephrogenic diabetes insipidus. *Clin Investig.* 1994;72:769-771.

70. Holden R, Jackson MA. Near-fatal hyponatraemic coma due to vasopressin over-secretion after "ecstasy" (3,4-MDMA). *Lancet.* 1996;347:1052.

71. Hubbard JI, et al. Subfornical organ lesions in rats abolish hyperdipsic effects of isoproterenol and serotonin. *Brain Res Bull.* 1989;23:41-45.

72. Iberti TJ, et al. Low sensitivity of the anion gap as a screen to detect hyperlactatemia in critically ill patients. *Crit Care Med.* 1990;18:275-277.

73. Inaba H, et al. Serum osmolality gap in postoperative patients in intensive care. *Lancet.* 1987;1:1331-1335.

74. Ireland JT, Thomson WS. Euglycemic diabetic ketoacidosis. *Br Med J.* 1973;3:107.

75. Iseri LT, et al. Magnesium deficiency and cardiac disorders. *Am J Med.* 1975;58:837-846.

76. Jacobus CH, et al. Hypervitaminosis D associated with drinking milk. *N Engl J Med.* 1992;326:1173-1177.

77. Jenny DB, et al. Hypermagnesemia following irrigation of renal pelvis. Cause of respiratory depression. *JAMA.* 1978;240:1378-1379.

78. Jones J, et al. Cathartic-induced magnesium toxicity during overdose management. *Ann Emerg Med.* 1986;15:1214-1218.

79. Kessler J, Samuels SC. Sertraline and hyponatremia. *N Engl J Med.* 1996;335:524.

80. Knochel JP. Neuromuscular manifestations of electrolyte disorders. *Am J Med.* 1982;72:521-535.

81. Kosiborod M, et al. Sodium zirconium cyclosilicate for urgent therapy of severe hyperkalemia. *N Engl J Med.* 2015;372:1577-1578.

82. Kovacs L, Robertson GL. Syndrome of inappropriate antidiuresis. *Endocrinol Metab Clin North Am.* 1992;21:859-875.

83. Krapf R, et al. Chronic respiratory alkalosis. The effect of sustained hyperventilation on renal regulation of acid-base equilibrium. *N Engl J Med.* 1991;324:1394-1401.

84. Kruse JA, Carlson RW. Rapid correction of hypokalemia using concentrated intravenous potassium chloride infusions. *Arch Intern Med.* 1990;150:613-617.

85. Lauriat SM, Berl T. The hyponatremic patient: practical focus on therapy. *J Am Soc Nephrol.* 1997;8:1599-1607.

86. Libber S, et al. Treatment of nephrogenic diabetes insipidus with prostaglandin synthesis inhibitors. *J Pediatr.* 1986;108:305-311.

87. Liu BA, et al. Hyponatremia and the syndrome of inappropriate secretion of antidiuretic hormone associated with the use of selective serotonin reuptake inhibitors: a review of spontaneous reports. *CMAJ.* 1996;155:519-527.

88. Lydiard RB, Gelenberg AJ. Hazards and adverse effects of lithium. *Annu Rev Med.* 1982;33:327-344.

89. Madias NE, et al. Increased anion gap in metabolic alkalosis: the role of plasma-protein equivalency. *N Engl J Med.* 1979;300:1421-1423.

90. Masson EA, Rhodes JM. Mesalazine associated nephrogenic diabetes insipidus presenting as weight loss. *Gut.* 1992;33:563-564.

91. Matsumura M, et al. Electrolyte disorders following massive insulin overdose in a patient with type 2 diabetes. *Intern Med.* 2000;39:55-57.

92. Mazze RI, et al. Methoxyflurane metabolism and renal dysfunction: clinical correlation in man. *Anesthesiology.* 1971;35:247-252.

93. McCarthy LJ, et al. Hypocalcemia secondary to citrate toxicity. *Ther Apher.* 1998;2:249.

94. McCarty M, et al. Hyperkalemic ascending paralysis. *Ann Emerg Med.* 1998;32:104-107.

95. McGuire JK, et al. Fatal hypermagnesemia in a child treated with megavitamin/megamineral therapy. *Pediatrics.* 2000;105:E18.

96. McQuillen KK, Anderson AC. Osmol gaps in the pediatric population. *Acad Emerg Med.* 1999;6:27-30.

97. Mercado R, Michelis MF. Severe sodium depletion syndrome during lithium carbonate therapy. *Arch Intern Med.* 1977;137:1731-1733.

98. Mizutani AR, et al. Visual disturbances, serum glycine levels and transurethral resection of the prostate. *J Urol.* 1990;144:697-699.

99. Moder KG, Hurley DL. Fatal hypernatremia from exogenous salt intake: report of a case and review of the literature. *Mayo Clin Proc.* 1990;65:1587-1594.

100. Morgan TJ, et al. Artifactual elevation of measured plasma L-lactate concentration in the presence of glycolate. *Crit Care Med.* 1999;27:2177-2179.

101. Morisaki H, et al. Hypermagnesemia-induced cardiopulmonary arrest before induction of anesthesia for emergency cesarean section. *J Clin Anesth.* 2000;12:224-226.

102. Moses AM, Miller M. Drug-induced dilutional hyponatremia. *N Engl J Med.* 1974;291:1234-1239.

103. Moses AM, et al. Pathophysiologic and pharmacologic alterations in the release and action of ADH. *Metabolism.* 1976;25:697-721.

104. Moses AM, Notman DD. Diabetes insipidus and syndrome of inappropriate antidiuretic hormone secretion (SIADH). *Adv Intern Med.* 1982;27:73-100.

105. Mundy GR. The hypercalcemia of malignancy. *Kidney Int.* 1987;31:142-155.

106. Narins RG, Emmett M. Simple and mixed acid-base disorders: a practical approach. *Medicine (Baltimore).* 1980;59:161-187.

107. Navarro JF, et al. Nephrogenic diabetes insipidus and renal tubular acidosis secondary to foscarnet therapy. *Am J Kidney Dis.* 1996;27:431-434.

108. Nielsen S, et al. Aquaporins in the kidney: from molecules to medicine. *Physiol Rev.* 2002;82:205-244.

109. Oster JR, et al. Use of the anion gap in clinical medicine. *South Med J.* 1988;81:229-237.

110. Osterloh JD, et al. Discrepancies in osmolal gaps and calculated alcohol concentrations. *Arch Pathol Lab Med.* 1996;120:637-641.

111. Perez GO, Oster JR. $\Delta AG/\Delta HCO_3$ in Evaluating Mixed Acid-Base Disorders: A Patient Management Problem. *South Med J.* 1986;79:882-886.

112. Perrone J, Hoffman RS. Compensatory hypoventilation in severe metabolic alkalosis. *Acad Emerg Med.* 1996;3:981-982.

113. Phillips DR, et al. Preventing hyponatremic encephalopathy: comparison of serum sodium and osmolality during operative hysteroscopy with 5.0% mannitol and 1.5% glycine distention media. *J Am Assoc Gynecol Laparosc.* 1997;4:567-576.
114. Ponce SP, et al. Drug-induced hyperkalemia. *Medicine (Baltimore).* 1985;64:357-370.
115. Purssell RA, et al. Derivation and validation of a formula to calculate the contribution of ethanol to the osmolal gap. *Ann Emerg Med.* 2001;38:653-659.
116. Quinn BP, Wall BM. Nephrogenic diabetes insipidus and tubulointerstitial nephritis during continuous therapy with rifampin. *Am J Kidney Dis.* 1989;14:217-220.
117. Randall RE Jr, et al. Hypermagnesemia in renal failure: etiology and toxic manifestations. *Ann Intern Med.* 1964;61:73-88.
118. Reinhart RA. Magnesium metabolism. A review with special reference to the relationship between intracellular content and serum levels. *Arch Intern Med.* 1988;148:2415-2420.
119. Repetto HA, Penna R. Apparent bicarbonate space in children. *ScientificWorldJournal.* 2006;6:148-153.
120. Richardson RM, Halperin ML. The urine pH: a potentially misleading diagnostic test in patients with hyperchloremic metabolic acidosis. *Am J Kidney Dis.* 1987;10:140-143.
121. Riggs AT, et al. A review of disorders of water homeostasis in psychiatric patients. *Psychosomatics.* 1991;32:133-148.
122. Rosa RM, et al. Adrenergic modulation of extrarenal potassium disposal. *N Engl J Med.* 1980;302:431-434.
123. Ross MP, Spiller HA. Fatal ingestion of sodium hypochlorite bleach with associated hypernatremia and hyperchloremic metabolic acidosis. *Vet Hum Toxicol.* 1999;41:82-86.
124. Sakane N, et al. Nephrogenic diabetes insipidus induced by lobenzarit disodium treatment in patients with rheumatoid arthritis. *Intern Med.* 1996;35:119-122.
125. Salem MM, Mujais SK. Gaps in the anion gap. *Arch Intern Med.* 1992;152:1625-1629.
126. Saxena K. Clinical features and management of poisoning due to potassium chloride. *Med Toxicol Adverse Drug Exp.* 1989;4:429-443.
127. Saxena K. Death from potassium chloride overdose. *Postgrad Med.* 1988;84:97-98, 101-102.
128. Schelling JR, et al. Increased osmolal gap in alcoholic ketoacidosis and lactic acidosis. *Ann Intern Med.* 1990;113:580-582.
129. Schnur MJ, et al. The anion gap in asymptomatic plasma cell dyscrasias. *Ann Intern Med.* 1977;86:304-305.
130. Scoggin C, et al. Hypernatraemia and acidosis in association with topical treatment of burns. *Lancet.* 1977;1:959.
131. Sheta MA, et al. Physiological approach to assessment of acid-base disturbances. *N Engl J Med.* 2015;372:194-195.
132. Singer I, Rotenberg D. Demeclocycline-induced nephrogenic diabetes insipidus. In-vivo and in-vitro studies. *Ann Intern Med.* 1973;79:679-683.
133. Singer I, Rotenberg D. Mechanisms of lithium action. *N Engl J Med.* 1973;289:254-260.
134. Sklar AH, Linas SL. The osmolal gap in renal failure. *Ann Intern Med.* 1983;98:481-482.
135. Smilkstein MJ, et al. Severe hypermagnesemia due to multiple-dose cathartic therapy. *West J Med.* 1988;148:208-211.
136. Smilkstein MJ, et al. Magnesium levels after magnesium-containing cathartics. *J Toxicol Clin Toxicol.* 1988;26:51-65.
137. Spigset O, Hedenmalm K. Hyponatraemia and the syndrome of inappropriate antidiuretic hormone secretion (SIADH) induced by psychotropic drugs. *Drug Saf.* 1995;12:209-225.
138. Steinhart B. Case report: severe ethylene glycol intoxication with normal osmolal gap—"a chilling thought." *J Emerg Med.* 1990;8:583-585.
139. Sterns RH, et al. Osmotic demyelination syndrome following correction of hyponatremia. *N Engl J Med.* 1986;314:1535-1542.
140. Suki WN, et al. Acute treatment of hypercalcemia with furosemide. *N Engl J Med.* 1970;283:836-840.
141. Takahashi H, et al. A case of transient diabetes insipidus associated with poisoning by a herbicide containing glufosinate. *J Toxicol Clin Toxicol.* 2000;38:153-156.
142. Tepperman PB. Fatality due to acute systemic fluoride poisoning following a hydrofluoric acid skin burn. *J Occup Med.* 1980;22:691-692.
143. Uhl L, et al. Unexpected citrate toxicity and severe hypocalcemia during apheresis. *Transfusion.* 1997;37:1063-1065.
144. Van Amelsvoort T, et al. Hyponatremia associated with carbamazepine and oxcarbazepine therapy: a review. *Epilepsia.* 1994;35:181-188.
145. Vincent JC, Sheikh A. Phosphate poisoning by ingestion of clothes washing liquid and fabric conditioner. *Anaesthesia.* 1998;53:1004-1006.
146. Vokes TJ, Robertson GL. Disorders of antidiuretic hormone. *Endocrinol Metab Clin North Am.* 1988;17:281-299.
147. Wax PM, et al. Prevalence of sorbitol in multiple-dose activated charcoal regimens in emergency departments. *Ann Emerg Med.* 1993;22:1807-1812.
148. Weiner ID, Wingo CS. Hypokalemia—consequences, causes, and correction. *J Am Soc Nephrol.* 1997;8:1179-1188.
149. Winter SD, et al. The fall of the serum anion gap. *Arch Intern Med.* 1990;150:311-313.
150. Woo MY, et al. Artifactual elevation of lactate in ethylene glycol poisoning. *J Emerg Med.* 2003;25:289-293.
151. Wrenn KD, et al. The ability of physicians to predict hyperkalemia from the ECG. *Ann Emerg Med.* 1991;20:1229-1232.

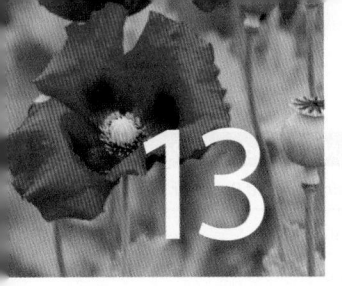

13 NEUROTRANSMITTERS AND NEUROMODULATORS

Steven C. Curry, Ayrn D. O'Connor, Kimberlie A. Graeme, and A. Min Kang

This chapter reviews the normal physiology of neurotransmission, the molecular action and biochemistry of several major neurotransmitters and their receptors, and the toxicologic mechanisms by which numerous xenobiotics act at the molecular level. Acetylcholine, norepinephrine, epinephrine, dopamine, serotonin, γ-aminobutyric acid (GABA), γ-hydroxybutyrate (GHB), glycine, glutamate, and adenosine are neurotransmitters and neuromodulators of toxicologic interest discussed herein.

When examining molecular actions of xenobiotics on neurotransmitter systems, it quickly becomes apparent that xenobiotics rarely possess single pharmacologic actions. As examples, doxepin, in part, antagonizes voltage-gated sodium channels, voltage-gated potassium channels, histaminic H_1 and H_2 receptors, α-adrenergic receptors, muscarinic acetylcholine receptors, dopamine D_2 receptors, and $GABA_A$ receptors; and inhibits norepinephrine, serotonin, and adenosine reuptake. Similarly, carbamazepine blocks voltage-gated sodium channels; inhibits the reuptake of norepinephrine, adenosine, and serotonin; antagonizes adenosine and muscarinic receptors; activates $GABA_B$ receptors; and binds to benzodiazepine-binding sites on mitochondria. For obvious reasons, then, this chapter cannot include every action of every xenobiotic on the nervous system. Nor is it meant to be a complete discussion of toxidromes produced by various xenobiotics, as these are discussed in specific chapters. Rather, this chapter provides a general and basic understanding of mechanisms of action of various xenobiotics affecting neurotransmitter function and receptors, especially in the central nervous system. With this focus, the clinical effects produced are more easily understood and predicted, and specific treatments can be rationally undertaken. Given the complexity of the nervous system and the numerous actions of a given xenobiotic, it is not always clear which neurotransmitter system is producing an observed effect. Therefore, specific xenobiotics are found in several sections. An attempt is made to note the major mechanism of action of a xenobiotic, although other actions are noted when possible.

NEURON PHYSIOLOGY AND NEUROTRANSMISSION

Membrane Potentials, Ion Channels, and Nerve Conduction

Membrane-bound sodium, potassium adenosine triphosphatase (ATPase) moves 3 sodium ions (Na^+) from inside the cell to the interstitial space while pumping 2 potassium ions (K^+) into the cell. Because the cell membrane is not freely permeable to large, negatively charged intracellular molecules, such as proteins, an equilibrium results in which the inside of the neuron is negative with respect to the outside. This typical neuronal resting membrane potential is –65 mV.

Sodium, calcium (Ca^{2+}), K^+, and chloride (Cl^-) ions move into and out of neurons through ion channels. When moving through ion channels, which are long polypeptides comprising several subunits that span the plasma membrane multiple times, ions always move passively down electrochemical gradients. Many different ion channels are structurally comparable, sharing similar amino acid sequences.[29] Channels for a specific ion also vary in structure, depending on the specific subunits that have combined to form the channel. Because of structural similarity of different channels, it is not surprising that many xenobiotics are able to bind to more than one type of ion channel.

More than 40 different ion channels have been described in various nerve terminals,[182] and it is estimated that a human being contains hundreds of different varieties of ion channels for Na^+, Cl^-, Ca^{2+}, and K^+. Most ion channels fall into 2 general classes: voltage-gated (voltage-dependent) ion channels and ligand-gated ion channels.[182] Voltage-gated channels open or close in response to changes in membrane potential. Ligand-gated channels open or close when a ligand (eg, neurotransmitter) binds to and changes the conformation of the channel.

A commonly accepted model describes voltage-gated Na^+ channels and some other voltage-gated ion channels in 3 possible states. Using Na^+ channels as an example, the Na^+ channel is closed at rest and impermeable to Na^+, preventing Na^+ from moving into the cell. When the channel undergoes activation, the channel opens, allowing Na^+ to move intracellularly, down its electrochemical gradient. The channel then undergoes a third conformational change by becoming inactivated, preventing further influx of Na^+. The term *recovery* describes the conversion of inactive channels back to the resting state, a process that requires repolarization of the cell membrane.

Depolarization of a neuron usually results from an initial inward flux of cations (Na^+ or Ca^{2+}), or prevention of K^+ efflux. The fall in membrane potential (movement toward 0 mV) results in further activation of these voltage-gated Na^+ channels, allowing yet a greater influx of cations. When the membrane potential falls to threshold, Na^+ channels are activated en masse, and there is a large influx of Na^+.

Depolarization of a segment of the neurolemma causes the adjacent neuronal membrane to reach threshold, resulting in the propagation of an action potential down the neuron. Sodium channel activation is quickly followed by inactivation, ending depolarization. Over the short term, repolarization of the neuron subsequently occurs mainly from efflux of K^+ and some influx of Cl^-.

Neurotransmitter Release

Neurotransmitters are chemicals that are released from nerve endings into the synapse, where they produce effects by binding to receptors on postsynaptic or presynaptic cell membranes. The receptors are also found on other neurons or effector organs such as smooth muscle. Concentrations of neurotransmitters in cytoplasm are kept low to prevent passive movement out of the nerve ending. To provide a source of neurotransmitters that is protected from cytoplasmic enzymatic degradation and that can rapidly be released, neurotransmitters are concentrated and stored within vesicles in the nerve terminal. As a wave of depolarization from Na^+ influx reaches the nerve ending, membrane depolarization opens voltage-gated Ca^{2+} channels, allowing Ca^{2+} to move rapidly into the cell. This influx of Ca^{2+} triggers exocytosis of vesicle contents into the synapse via the *snare* complex. The voltage-gated Ca^{2+} channels responsible for inward Ca^{2+} currents that trigger neurotransmitter release are members of the Ca_v2 subfamily (N, P/Q, and R subtypes).[188,233] Ziconotide, is a conotoxin derivative that is used for analgesia blocking N-type Ca^{2+} channels on nociceptive neurons in the dorsal root to prevent neurotransmitter release. Cardiovascular calcium channel blockers used in clinical practice do not block these subtypes of voltage-dependent Ca^{2+} channels, but block the L-subtype. However, L-subtype Ca^{2+} channels reside elsewhere on neurons.

Vesicle Transport of Neurotransmitters

The pH inside neurotransmitter vesicles is about 5.5, which is lower than that in the cytoplasm. A vacuolar ATPase in the vesicular membrane is responsible for movement of protons into the vesicular lumen at the expense of ATP hydrolysis. Vesicular uptake pumps (transporters) that move neurotransmitters or their precursors from the cytoplasm into the vesicle lumen, in turn, are powered by the electrochemical H^+ gradient. That is, the movement of an H^+ out of the vesicle into the cytoplasm is coupled to the movement of a neurotransmitter from the cytoplasm into the vesicle.

Various vesicular transporters for neurotransmitters have been sequenced to date. Vesicular GABA transporter (VGAT) (also known as VIAAT) transports GABA and glycine. Vesicular monamine transporter (VMAT2) transports all 3 monoamines, dopamine, norepinephrine, and serotonin (VMAT1 transports monoamines into non-neuronal vesicles). Vesicular acetylcholine transporter (VAChT) is responsible for acetylcholine (ACh) transport, and 3 vesicular glutamate transporter (VGluTs) (VGluT1-3) move glutamate into vesicles.

Neurotransmitters are confined within the vesicle, to a great extent, by ion trapping, as they are more ionized and less able to diffuse back out of the vesicle at the lower pH. Anything that causes a decrease in the pH gradient across the vesicle membrane results in the movement of neurotransmitters into the cytoplasm.[274] For example, amphetamine moves into vesicles, where it buffers protons, causing the movement of monoamine neurotransmitters out of vesicles, and raising cytoplasmic concentrations of neurotransmitters, and ultimately raising the synaptic monoamine concentrations.[274,275]

Neurotransmitter Reuptake

Although ACh is inactivated in the synapse by enzymatic degradation, other neurotransmitters have their synaptic effects terminated by active uptake into neurons or glial cells. These plasma membrane neurotransmitter transporters are distinct from those transporters responsible for movement of neurotransmitters into vesicles. Cell membrane transporters for different neurotransmitters are Na^+-dependent transport proteins, during which the uptake of neurotransmitters is accompanied by the movement of Na^+ across the synaptic membrane.[5] These uptake transporters are commonly known as either uptake or reuptake pumps; the term "reuptake" will be used in this chapter for purposes of consistency.

Neurotransmitter reuptake transporters are subdivided into 2 main families.[5] One family (SLC6) includes structurally similar uptake pumps for GABA, glycine, norepinephrine, dopamine, and serotonin. They generally comprise 600 to 700 amino acids and form loops spanning the plasma membrane 12 times. Four GABA reuptake transporters (GAT-1 through GAT-4) transport GABA into neurons and glial cells. Reuptake of dopamine, serotonin, and norepinephrine is achieved by DAT, SERT, and NET respectively. Glycine uptake into neurons and astrocytes is achieved by GLYT-1 and GLYT-2.

The second family (SLC1) comprises 5 glutamate reuptake transporters (excitatory amino acid transporters; EAATs), which appear to traverse the plasma membrane 10 times and move glutamate from the synapse into glial cells and neurons.

Several properties make transporter proteins of particular toxicologic significance. First, they are capable of moving neurotransmitters in either direction; when cytoplasmic neurotransmitter concentrations are significantly elevated, neurotransmitters are transported back into the synapse. Second, these transporters are not always completely specific. For instance, the uptake transporter for norepinephrine moves dopamine and other bioactive amines into the neuron. Third, a xenobiotic that acts at the level of the membrane transporter affects functions of several different neurotransmitters, depending on its specificity for a particular transporter. As an example, fluoxetine is fairly specific at inhibiting reuptake of serotonin, whereas cocaine inhibits the reuptake of serotonin, norepinephrine, and dopamine.

Neurotransmitter Receptors
Channel Receptors

The first general class of neurotransmitter receptors comprises ligand-gated ion channels (LGICs; channel receptors; ionotropic receptors), in which the receptor for the neurotransmitter is part of an ion channel. These channels comprise multiple subunits that combine in various combinations to create channels that vary in response to a given neurotransmitter or other agonist/antagonist. Ligand-gated ion channels for neurotransmitters discussed in this chapter are divided into 2 main groups, based on structure of subunits and assemblies. Most neurotransmitter LGICs are pentameric and display 4 transmembrane helices. Ligand-gated ion channels for glutamate, however, are tetrameric and comprise 3 transmembrane helices.[173]

By binding to its LGIC receptor, the neurotransmitter allosterically changes the configuration of the ion channel so that ions traverse the channel in greater quantities per unit time. As an example, the acetylcholine nicotinic ACh receptor at the neuromuscular junction is a ligand-gated Na^+ channel. When acetylcholine binds to the nicotinic receptor, the configuration of the channel changes, allowing Na^+ to move into the cell and trigger

TABLE 13–1	Types of Neurotransmitter and Neuromodulator Receptors
Ion Channel	*G Protein–Coupled Receptor*
ACh nicotinic	ACh muscarinic
$GABA_A$	Adenosine
Glycine (Inhibitory)	Dopamine
Glutamate AMPA	$GABA_B$
Glutamate NMDA	GHB
Glutamate kainate[a]	Glutamate metabotropic
$5-HT_3$	Norepinephrine
	$5-HT_{1,2,4-7}$

[a]There are data supporting a subset of glutamate kainate receptors coupled to G-proteins.
ACh = acetylcholine; AMPA = amino-3-hydroxy-5-methyl-4-isoxazole propionate;
GABA = γ-aminobutyric acid; 5-HT = 5-hydroxytryptamine (serotonin);
NMDA = N-methyl-D-aspartate; GHB = γ-hydroxybutyrate.

an action potential. The action potential then propagates down muscle via voltage-gated Na^+ channels. Table 13–1 lists other examples of channel receptors.

G Protein–Coupled Receptors

The second general class of neurotransmitter receptors are linked to G proteins, which are part of a superfamily of proteins with guanosine triphosphatase (GTPase) activity responsible for signal transduction across plasma membranes.[264] G proteins comprise 3 polypeptide subunits: α, β, and γ chains. These chains span the plasma membrane several times, and they associate with a separately transcribed neurotransmitter receptor that spans the cell membrane 7 times, with an external binding site for neurotransmitters. Some receptors (eg, $GABA_B$ receptor) coupled to G proteins are obligatory heterodimers comprising 2 separate proteins, both of which must be present for activity.

The α chain normally binds guanosine diphosphate (GDP) in the cytoplasm and is inactive. When a neurotransmitter binds to its receptor externally on the cell membrane, GDP dissociates from the α chain and guanosine triphosphate (GTP) binds in its place, activating the α subunit. The activated α subunit then dissociates from the receptor and from the β-γ chains. Both the activated α subunit and β-γ subunits modulate effectors in the plasma membrane.[264] The effector influenced by α or β-γ subunits is frequently an enzyme that the subunits stimulate or inhibit (eg, adenylate cyclase) or an ion channel that is opened or closed directly or through other chemical reactions (eg, channel phosphorylation).[48] Intrinsic GTPase activity in the α chain eventually converts the GTP to GDP, inactivating the α subunit and allowing it to reassociate with the β-γ chains and the neurotransmitter receptor, terminating the consequences of neurotransmitter binding.[264]

The type of the α chain that the G proteins contain determines the categorization. The 3 main families of G proteins coupled to neurotransmitter receptors are G_s (containing α_s), $G_{i/o}$ (containing α_i or α_o), and G_q (or $G_{q/11}$, containing α_q). G_s stimulates membrane-bound adenylate cyclase; activation of a neurotransmitter receptor coupled to G_s causes a rise in intracellular 3',5'-cyclic adenosine monophosphate (cAMP) concentration. Neurotransmitter receptors activating G_i may inhibit adenylate cyclase or modulate K^+ and Ca^{2+} channels. Receptors coupled to G_q act through membrane-bound phospholipase C to increase intracellular calcium concentrations. See Table 13–1 for a list of the neurotransmitter receptors coupled to G proteins. A given neurotransmitter can activate different classes of receptors (eg, ion-channel and G protein) or different types of receptors in the same class. For example, $GABA_A$ receptors are Cl^- channels, whereas $GABA_B$ receptors are coupled to G proteins. Dopamine D_1–like receptors (D_1 and D_5) are linked to G_s, whereas D_2-like receptors (D_2, D_3, and D_4) are most commonly linked to G_i or G_o.

Importantly, some single G protein–coupled receptors activate more than one type of G protein in the same cell, depending on various circumstances, including duration of receptor activation. Evidence continues to accumulate indicating that G protein–coupled receptors for the same or different neurotransmitters form both heterodimers and oligomers, resulting in yet more variation in response to neurotransmitter binding. Examples include combinations of various dopamine receptors, combinations of dopamine and 5-HT receptors, and combinations of dopamine and glutamate receptors.[189,191,245]

Receptor downregulation occurs at various levels. For example, prolonged receptor activation results in receptor phosphorylation by G protein kinases (GPKs), causing receptor binding to a member of the arrestin family of proteins. This, in turn, prevents further activation of the G protein by the receptor and eventually triggers receptor endocytosis.[7,150,259]

Neuronal Excitation and Inhibition

Excitatory neurotransmitters usually act postsynaptically by causing Na^+ or Ca^{2+} influx, or by preventing K^+ efflux, triggering depolarization and an action potential (Fig. 13–1). These effects usually are mediated by either ion channel or G protein–coupled receptors.

Postsynaptic inhibition results from actions on ion channel receptors or receptors coupled to G proteins (Fig. 13–1). Inhibition is usually accomplished by neuronal influx of Cl^- or efflux of K^+ to hyperpolarize the neuron and move membrane potential farther away from threshold, making it more difficult for a given stimulus to depolarize the membrane to threshold voltage.

Presynaptic inhibition, the prevention of neurotransmitter release, is usually mediated by receptors coupled to G proteins, but ligand-gated ion channels such as kainate glutamate receptors are found on neuronal terminals, as well. When a neurotransmitter released from a neuron binds to a receptor on that same neuron to limit further neurotransmitter release, the receptor is termed an *autoreceptor*.[252] Autoreceptors reside on dendrites, cell bodies, axons, and presynaptic terminals. Activation of autoreceptors on dendrites and cell bodies (somatodendritic autoreceptors) usually impairs neurotransmitter release by increasing K^+ efflux, thereby hyperpolarizing the neuron away from threshold (Fig. 13–2). However, activation of autoreceptors found on presynaptic terminals (terminal autoreceptors) usually limits

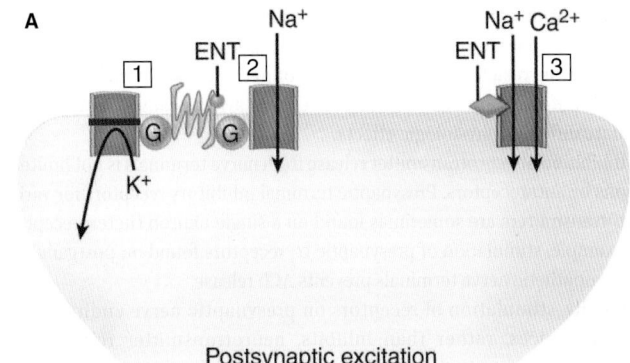

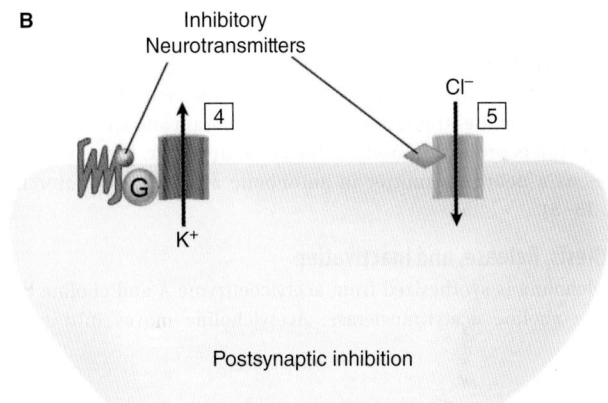

FIGURE 13–1. Common mechanisms of postsynaptic excitation and inhibition. (**A**) An excitatory neurotransmitter (ENT) binds to receptors linked to G proteins to prevent K^+ efflux [1] or to allow Na^+ influx [2], producing membrane depolarization. An ENT may bind to and activate a cation channel [3] to allow Na^+ and/or Ca^{2+} influx with resultant membrane depolarization. (**B**) An inhibitory neurotransmitter hyperpolarizes the membrane (makes membrane potential more negative) by binding to receptors linked to G proteins to enhance K^+ efflux [4], or to Cl^- channels to allow Cl^- influx [5]. Some Cl^- channels are regulated by G proteins as well. G = G protein.

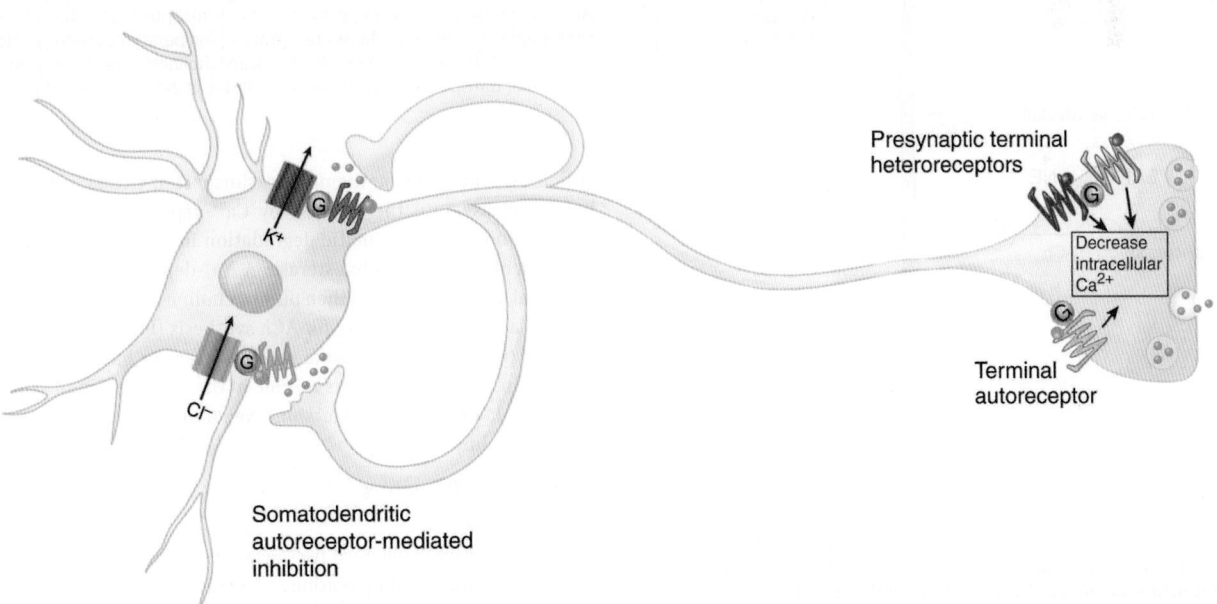

FIGURE 13–2. Common mechanisms of presynaptic inhibition (the inhibition of neurotransmitter {NT} release). A neuron releases NT (green dots), which returns to activate receptors on the cell body or dendrites (somatodendritic autoreceptors), or on the axonal terminal (terminal autoreceptors). Such activation limits further release of NT by completing a negative feedback loop. At somatodendritic autoreceptors, NT binding produces activation of G proteins, which promote either K^+ efflux or Cl^- influx; both processes hyperpolarize the neuron away from threshold. At terminal autoreceptors, NT binding activates G proteins, which, through various mechanisms, lower intracellular Ca^{2+} concentrations to prevent exocytosis of NT vesicles, despite depolarization. Presynaptic inhibitory receptors for other types of NTs (heteroreceptors) are also shown. Excitatory axonal terminal autoreceptors and heteroreceptors that serve to enhance neurotransmitter release are not illustrated. G = G protein.

increases in intracellular Ca^{2+} concentration by limiting Ca^{2+} influx or preventing Ca^{2+} release from intracellular stores, impairing exocytosis of neurotransmitter vesicles (Fig. 13–2). Types of neurotransmitter receptors that serve as autoreceptors also usually reside postsynaptically, where they may mediate different physiologic effects.

Inhibition of neurotransmitter release from nerve terminals is not limited to actions by autoreceptors. Presynaptic terminal inhibitory receptors for various neurotransmitters are sometimes found on a single neuron (heteroreceptors). For example, stimulation of presynaptic α_2 receptors found on postganglionic parasympathetic nerve terminals prevents ACh release.

Finally, stimulation of receptors on presynaptic nerve endings sometimes enhances, rather than inhibits, neurotransmitter release. Such receptors also are usually coupled to G proteins. For example, activation of β_2 receptors on adrenergic nerve terminals enhances norepinephrine release.

ACETYLCHOLINE

Acetylcholine (ACh) is a neurotransmitter of the central and peripheral nervous system. Centrally, it is found in both brain and spinal cord; cholinergic fibers project diffusely to the cerebral cortex. Peripherally, ACh serves as a neurotransmitter in autonomic and somatic motor fibers (Fig. 13–3).

Synthesis, Release, and Inactivation

Acetylcholine is synthesized from acetylcoenzyme A and choline by the enzyme choline acetyltransferase. Acetylcholine moves into synaptic

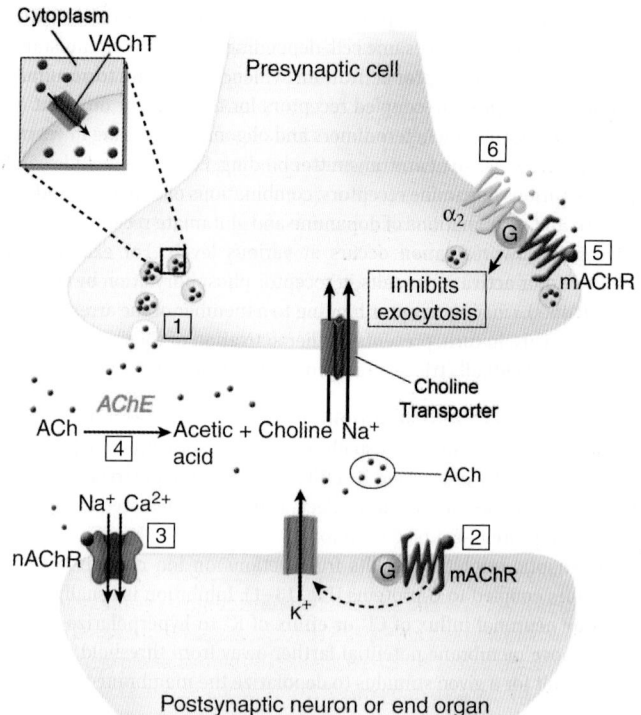

FIGURE 13–4. Cholinergic nerve ending. Activation of postsynaptic muscarinic receptors (mAChR) hyperpolarizes the postsynaptic membrane through G protein–mediated enhancement of K^+ efflux. Several subtypes of muscarinic receptors coupled to various G proteins exist—a muscarinic receptor coupled to a G protein that opens K^+ channels is shown only as an example [2]. Postsynaptic nicotinic receptor (nAChR) activation causes Na^+ influx and membrane depolarization [3]. Ca^{2+} influx appears to be the main cation involved with some neuronal nicotinic receptors. Presynaptic muscarinic and α_2-adrenergic receptor activation prevents ACh release through lowering of intracellular Ca^{2+} concentrations. The xenobiotics listed in Table 13–2 may act to enhance or prevent release of ACh [1]; activate or antagonize postsynaptic muscarinic (M) receptors [2]; activate or antagonize nicotinic (N) receptors [3]; inhibit acetylcholinesterase [4]; prevent ACh release by stimulating presynaptic muscarinic autoreceptors [5] or α_2-adrenergic heteroreceptors [6]; or enhance ACh release by antagonizing presynaptic autoreceptors [5] or by antagonizing presynaptic α_2-adrenergic heteroreceptors [6] (on parasympathetic postganglionic terminals). ACh = acetylcholine; AChE = acetylcholinesterase; G = G protein; VAChT = vesicular transporter for ACh. Norepinephrine is shown as light blue dots.

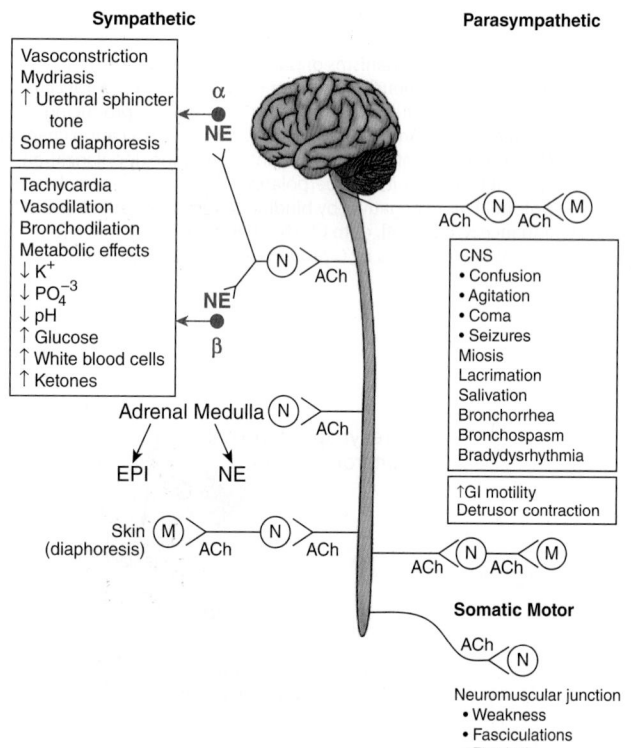

FIGURE 13–3. Diagram of the cholinergic nervous system, including adrenergic involvement in the autonomic nervous system. ACh binds to various nicotinic receptors (N) in CNS, in sympathetic and parasympathetic ganglia, and the adrenal glands. All nicotinic receptors shown are neuronal nicotinic receptors (neuronal nAChRs) except for those at skeletal muscle, which are neuromuscular junction nicotinic receptors (NMJ nAChRs). Acetylcholine (ACh) also binds to various subtypes of muscarinic (M) receptors in the CNS and on effector organs innervated by postsynaptic parasympathetic neurons and to most sweat glands. NE and/or EPI released in response to ACh stimulation of neuronal nAChRs activates α- and β-adrenergic receptors. ACh = acetylcholine; CNS = central nervous system; EPI = epinephrine; NE = norepinephrine.

vesicles via the vesicular membrane transporter, VAChT, where it is stored before release into the synapse by Ca^{2+}-dependent exocytosis. Acetylcholine undergoes enzymatic degradation in the synapse to choline and acetic acid by acetylcholinesterase. A Na^+-dependent transporter in the neuronal membrane (ChT) then pumps choline back into the cytoplasm to be used again as a substrate for ACh synthesis (Fig. 13–4). Pseudocholinesterase (also known as plasma cholinesterase or butyryl cholinesterase) is made in the liver and plays no role in the degradation of synaptic ACh. However, it does metabolize some xenobiotics, including cocaine and succinylcholine.

Acetylcholine Receptors

Nicotinic Receptors

After release from cholinergic nerve endings, ACh activates 2 main types of receptors: nicotinic and muscarinic.[151] Nicotinic receptors (nAChRs) reside in the CNS (mainly in spinal cord), on postganglionic autonomic neurons (both sympathetic and parasympathetic), in the adrenal medulla, and at skeletal neuromuscular junctions, where they mediate muscle contraction (Fig. 13–3).

Nicotinic receptors at neuromuscular junctions (NMJ nAChRs) are part of a Na^+ channel made from 5 protein subunits. Stimulation of these receptors by ACh results mainly in Na^+ influx, depolarization of the endplate, and triggering of an action potential that is propagated down the muscle by voltage-gated Na^+ channels.

Nicotinic receptors on central or peripheral neurons or in the adrenal gland are termed neuronal nAChRs. Neuronal nAChRs are also ion channels, although in some cases Ca^{2+} influx through the receptor may be more important than Na^+ influx. Neuronal nAChRs also comprise 5 subunits.

Muscarinic Receptors

Muscarinic receptors reside in the CNS (mainly in the brain), on end organs innervated by postganglionic parasympathetic nerve endings, and at most postganglionic sympathetically innervated sweat glands (Fig. 13–3). Five subtypes of muscarinic receptors, M_{1-5}, are recognized and linked to several G proteins. For example, in the heart, ACh released from the vagus nerve binds to M_2 receptors linked to G_i in pacemaker cells. G_i opens K^+ channels, allowing efflux of K^+ down its concentration gradient, which makes the inside of the cell more negative and more difficult to depolarize, slowing the heart rate. Different subtypes of muscarinic receptors also act as autoreceptors in various locations, M_1 being the most common.

Xenobiotics

Table 13–2 provides examples of xenobiotics that affect cholinergic neurotransmission.

TABLE 13–2   Examples of Xenobiotics Affecting Cholinergic Neurotransmission

Cholinomimetics	Cholinolytics
Cause ACh release	Direct nicotinic antagonists
α_2-Adrenergic receptor antagonists[a]	α-Bungarotoxin[c]
Aminopyridines	Nondepolarizing neuromuscular blockers
Black widow spider venom	Trimethaphan
Carbachol Guanidine	Indirect neuronal nicotinic antagonists
Anticholinesterases	Galantamine
Donepezil	Physostigmine
Edrophonium	Tacrine
N-Methylcarbamate compounds	Direct muscarinic antagonists
Organic phosphorus compounds	Antihistamines
Physostigmine	Atropine
Rivastigmine	Benztropine
Direct nicotinic agonists	Clozapine
Carbachol	Cyclic antidepressants
Coniine	Cyclobenzaprine
Cytisine	Disopyramide
Nicotine	Orphenadrine
Succinylcholine[b]	Phenothiazines
Varenicline	Procainamide
Indirect neuronal nicotinic agonists	Scopolamine
Chlorpromazine	Trihexyphenidyl
Ethanol	Inhibit ACh release
Ketamine	α_2-Adrenergic receptor agonists[d]
Local anesthetics	Botulinum toxins
Phencyclidine	Crotalinae venoms
Volatile anesthetics	Elapidae β-neurotoxins
Direct muscarinic agonists	Hypermagnesemia
Arecoline	
Bethanechol	
Carbachol	
Cevimeline	
Methacholine	
Muscarine	
Pilocarpine	

[a]Antagonism of α_2-adrenoceptors enhances ACh release from parasympathetic nerve endings.
[b]Depolarizing neuromuscular blockers. [c]α-Bungarotoxin exemplifies many elapid α-neurotoxins that produce paralysis and death from respiratory failure. [d]Stimulation of presynaptic α_2-adrenergic receptors on parasympathetic nerve endings prevents ACh release.
ACh = acetylcholine.

Modulators of Acetylcholine Release

Figure 13–4 illustrates sites of actions of numerous xenobiotics that influence the cholinergic nervous system. Botulinum toxins, some neurotoxins from pit vipers, and elapid β-neurotoxins prevent release of ACh from peripheral nerve endings.[101] This results in ptosis, other cranial nerve findings, weakness, and respiratory failure. Hypermagnesemia also inhibits ACh release, probably by inhibiting Ca^{2+} influx into the nerve endings.[151]

Guanidine, aminopyridines, and black widow spider venom enhance the release of ACh from nerve endings. Aminopyridines, in part, block voltage-gated K^+ channels to prevent K^+ efflux; the resultant action potential widening (delayed repolarization) causes prolongation of Ca^{2+}-channel activation, enhancing influx of Ca^{2+}, which promotes neurotransmitter release. Aminopyridines are used therapeutically in Lambert–Eaton syndrome, myasthenia gravis, multiple sclerosis, and experimentally in Ca^{2+}-channel channel blocker overdose.

Black widow spider venom causes ACh release by opening neuronal Ca^{2+}-channels with resultant muscle cramping and diaphoresis.[12]

Nicotinic Receptor Agonists and Antagonists

Xenobiotics that bind to and activate nicotinic receptors stimulate postganglionic sympathetic and parasympathetic neurons, skeletal muscle endplates, the adrenal medulla, and/or neurons within the CNS (Fig. 13–3). Prolonged depolarization at the receptor eventually causes diminution of responses to receptor occupancy.[214] For example, poisoning by nicotine, both a neuronal and NMJ nAChR agonist, produces hypertension, tachycardia, vomiting, diarrhea, muscle fasciculations, and convulsions, followed by hypotension, bradydysrhythmias, paralysis, and coma. Succinylcholine is a neuromuscular blocker that initially stimulates and then blocks muscular activity through prolonged depolarization of NMJ nAChRs.

Xenobiotics that block NMJ nAChRs without stimulation at skeletal neuromuscular junctions produce weakness and paralysis. Examples include tubocurarine and atracurium. α-Neurotoxins from elapids (eg, α-bungarotoxin) directly antagonize NMJ nAChRs, producing ptosis, weakness, and respiratory failure from paralysis.[296]

Peripheral neuronal nAChR blockade produces autonomic ganglionic blockade. Trimethaphan was used as a pharmacologic ganglionic blocker; however, it is not entirely specific for neuronal nAChRs. Occasionally, trimethaphan caused weakness and paralysis from NMJ nAChR blockade.

The functions of neuronal nAChRs are modulated by a variety of xenobiotics that do not bind to the ACh binding site, but bind instead to a number of distinct allosteric sites. For example, aside from their ability to inhibit acetylcholinesterase, physostigmine, tacrine, and galantamine bind to a noncompetitive allosteric activator site on neuronal nAChRs to enhance channel opening and ion conductance. Furthermore, a diverse range of xenobiotics, including chlorpromazine, phencyclidine, ketamine, local anesthetics, and ethanol bind to a noncompetitive negative allosteric site(s) on nAChRs to inhibit inward ion fluxes without directly affecting ACh binding. Some steroids desensitize neuronal nAChRs by binding to yet an additional allosteric site.[219]

Muscarinic Receptor Agonists and Antagonists

Peripheral muscarinic agonists produce bradycardia, miosis, salivation, lacrimation, vomiting, diarrhea, bronchospasm, bronchorrhea, and micturition. Central muscarinic agonists produce sedation, extrapyramidal dystonias, rigidity, coma, and convulsions. The anticholinergic toxidrome results from blockade of muscarinic receptors and is more appropriately referred to as an antimuscarinic toxidrome.[255] Central nervous system muscarinic blockade produces confusion, agitation, myoclonus, tremor, picking movements, abnormal speech, hallucinations, and coma. Peripheral antimuscarinic effects include mydriasis, anhidrosis, tachycardia, and urinary retention. Muscarinic antagonists number in the hundreds (Table 13–2 for common examples).

Acetylcholinesterase Inhibition

Xenobiotics inhibiting acetylcholinesterase (ie, anticholinesterase) raise ACh concentrations at both nicotinic and muscarinic receptors, producing a variety of CNS, sympathetic, parasympathetic, and skeletal muscle signs and symptoms.[50] Anticholinesterases include organic phosphorus compounds and *N*-methylcarbamates. Organic phosphorus compounds are usually encountered as insecticides, although topical medicinal organic phosphorus compounds are used for the treatment of glaucoma and lice. *N*-Methylcarbamates are found as insecticides and pharmaceuticals. Medicinal *N*-methylcarbamates include physostigmine, pyridostigmine, rivastigmine, and neostigmine. Edrophonium, galantamine, tacrine, donepezil, and metrifonate are non-carbamate, reversible anticholinesterases.

α₂-Adrenergic Receptor Agonists and Antagonists

Agonists and antagonists of α_2-adrenergic receptors are discussed in detail below. Briefly, stimulation of presynaptic α_2-adrenergic receptors on postganglionic parasympathetic nerve endings decreases ACh release. Conversely, presynaptic α_2 antagonism increases ACh release (Fig. 13–4).

NOREPINEPHRINE AND EPINEPHRINE

Norepinephrine (NE), epinephrine (EPI), dopamine (DA), and serotonin (5-hydroxytryptamine {5-HT}) are similar in many respects. Neurotransmitter synthesis, vesicle transport and storage, uptake, and degradation share many enzymes and structurally similar transport proteins. Cocaine, reserpine, amphetamine, and monoamine oxidase inhibitors (MAOIs) affect all four types of neurons. In addition, these xenobiotics produce several different effects in the same system. For example, in the noradrenergic neuron, amphetamines work mainly by causing the release of cytoplasmic NE, but they also inhibit NE reuptake, and their metabolites inhibit monoamine oxidase. Actions of xenobiotics that affect all bioactive amine neurotransmitters are described in the most detail for noradrenergic neurons. For the sake of brevity, similar mechanisms of action are simply noted in discussions of dopaminergic and serotonergic neurotransmission.

Norepinephrine is released from postganglionic sympathetic terminals (Fig. 13–3). The adrenal gland, acting as a modified sympathetic ganglion, releases EPI and lesser amounts of NE in response to stimulation of neuronal nAChRs. Epinephrine-containing neurons also reside in the brain stem.

The locus ceruleus is the main noradrenergic nucleus and resides in the floor of the fourth ventricle on each side of the pons. Axons radiate from this nucleus out to all layers of the cerebral cortex, to the cerebellum, and to other structures. Norepinephrine demonstrates both excitatory and inhibitory actions in the CNS. Norepinephrine released from locus ceruleus projections in the hippocampus increases cortical neuron activity through β-adrenergic receptor activation and G protein–mediated inhibition of K⁺ efflux. Norepinephrine released in outer cortical areas produces inhibitory effects mediated by α_2-adrenergic receptor activation. Consistent with this, NE demonstrates antiepileptic actions in animals. The antiepileptic action of carbamazepine may partly result from inhibition of NE uptake.[76] Despite antagonistic actions on different cortical neurons, electrical stimulation of the locus ceruleus produces widespread cortical activation and excitation. This overall effect explains a great deal of the hyperattentiveness and lack of fatigue that accompanies use of xenobiotics that mimic or increase noradrenergic activity in the brain. Neuronal firing in the locus ceruleus increases during waking and dramatically falls during sleep.

Synthesis, Release, and Reuptake

Figure 13–5 is a representation of a noradrenergic neuron. Tyrosine hydroxylase is the rate-limiting enzyme in NE synthesis and is sensitive to negative feedback by NE. This enzyme requires Fe^{2+} as a cofactor and exists as a homotetramer that is upregulated by chronic exposure to caffeine and nicotine. Under normal dietary conditions, tyrosine hydroxylase is completely saturated by tyrosine, and increasing dietary tyrosine does not appreciably increase dopa synthesis. Dopa undergoes decarboxylation by L-amino acid decarboxylase (DOPA decarboxylase) to DA. DOPA decarboxylase is not specific for DOPA. For example, it also catalyzes the formation of serotonin from 5-HT.

About one-half of cytoplasmic DA is actively pumped into vesicles by VMAT2. The remaining DA is quickly deaminated. In the vesicle, DA is converted to NE by dopamine-β-hydroxylase. Vesicles isolated from peripheral nerve endings contain DA, NE, dopamine-β-hydroxylase,

and ATP, and all of these substances are released into the synapse during Ca^{2+}-dependent exocytosis triggered by neuronal firing. In neurons containing EPI as a neurotransmitter, NE is released from vesicles into the cytoplasm, where it is converted to EPI by phenylethanolamine-*N*-methyl-transferase. Epinephrine is then transported back into vesicles before synaptic release.[151]

Norepinephrine is removed from the synapse, mainly by reuptake into the presynaptic neuron by the NE transporter (NET). Although this transporter has great affinity for NE, it also transports other amines, including DA, tyramine, MAOIs, and amphetamines. Once pumped back into the cytoplasm, NE is either transported back into vesicles for further storage and release, or quickly degraded by monoamine oxidase (MAO), an enzyme expressed on the outer mitochondrial membrane.

Monoamine oxidase (MAO) is present in all human tissues except red blood cells. It exists as 2 isoenzymes, MAO-A and MAO-B,[181] each with partially overlapping substrate affinities (Table 13–3). Neuronal MAO, bound to the outer mitochondrial membrane, oxidatively deaminates cytoplasmic amines, including neurotransmitters, to attenuate elevated cytoplasmic concentrations of bioactive amines. Hepatic and intestinal MAO prevents large quantities of dietary bioactive amines from entering the circulation and producing systemic effects.

Catechol-*O*-methyltransferase (COMT) mainly exists as a membrane-bound enzyme widely distributed throughout the body, including the central nervous system, which is responsible for metabolism of DA, L-dopa, NE, and EPI. It remains controversial as to whether enzymatic activity is focused on extracellular (synaptic) or cytoplasmic degradation of catecholamines. In extraneuronal tissue, COMT metabolizes catecholamines, including those that have entered the systemic circulation.

Adrenergic Receptors

The 2 main types of adrenergic receptors are α-adrenergic receptors and β-adrenergic receptors. All adrenergic receptors are coupled to G proteins.[222]

β-Adrenergic Receptors

β-Adrenergic receptors are divided into 3 major subtypes (β_1, β_2, and β_3), depending on their affinity for various agonists and antagonists.[257] β_1-adrenergic receptors and β_2-adrenergic receptors are linked to G_s, and their stimulation raises cAMP concentration and/or activates protein kinase A, which, in turn, produces several effects, including regulation of ion channels. At least some β_3-adrenergic receptors are coupled to $G_{i/o}$ proteins.

TABLE 13–3	Characteristics of Monoamine Oxidase (MAO) Isoenzymes	
	MAO Isoenzymes	
	MAO-A	**MAO-B**
Location		
Brain	+	+++
Intestines	+++	+
Liver	++	++
Platelets	+	++++
Placenta	++++	+
Substrates		
Norepinephrine	++++	+
Epinephrine	++	++
Dopamine	++	++
Serotonin	++++	+
Tyramine	++	++

Upregulation of β_3 receptors responsible for a negative inotropic effect in diseased myocardium appears to protect against adverse effects of chronic excessive catecholamine stimulation. β_3-receptor activation by nebivolol probably is responsible for nitric oxide production in some vascular beds.[88]

The β-adrenergic receptors are polymorphic, with genetic variation in humans.[41,121] Polymorphism influences response to medications, regulation of receptors, and clinical course of disease.[41,123,156] In general, peripheral β_1-adrenergic receptors are found mainly in the heart and in the juxtaglomerular apparatus. β_2-adrenergic receptors also reside in the heart as well as other organs where their activation mediates additional adrenergic effects such as bronchodilation and vasodilation.[123] Presynaptic β_2-adrenergic receptor activation causes release of NE from nerve endings (positive feedback). β_3-adrenergic receptors reside mainly in fat, but they also reside in skeletal muscle, gallbladder, and colon where they regulate metabolic processes. Polymorphism of β_3-adrenergic receptors is associated with clinical expressions of non–insulin-dependent diabetes and obesity.[41,273,298]

α-Adrenergic Receptors

α-Adrenergic receptors are linked to G proteins that inhibit adenylate cyclase to affect cAMP concentrations, affect ion channels, increase intracellular Ca^{2+} through inositol triphosphate and diacylglycerol production, or produce other actions.[222] These receptors are divided into 2 main types, α_1 and α_2, and at least 6 subtypes—α_{1A}, α_{1B}, α_{1D}, α_{2A}, α_{2B}, and α_{2C}.[68,110,257] Most α_1-adrenergic receptors are coupled to G_q, whereas most α_2-adrenergic receptors are coupled to $G_{i/o}$, although at least some α_{2A}-adrenergic receptors are coupled to G_s. The roles of α_2 receptor subtypes are not fully elucidated. Receptors of the α_{2A} type are the predominant form found in the CNS and are responsible mediating sedative, hypotensive and analgesic effects from α_2 agonists.[120,213]

In peripheral tissue, α_1-adrenergic receptors reside on the postsynaptic membrane in continuity with the synaptic cleft. Stimulation of these receptors on blood vessels results in vasoconstriction.

Central and peripheral α_2-adrenergic receptors are found at presynaptic and postganglionic sites. Presynaptic α_2-adrenergic receptor activation mediates negative feedback, limiting further release of NE (Fig. 13–5). Postganglionic parasympathetic neurons also contain presynaptic α_2-adrenergic receptors that, when stimulated, prevent release of ACh (Fig. 13–4).

Postsynaptic α_2-adrenergic receptors on vasculature also mediate vasoconstriction.[222] Initially, it was suggested that postsynaptic α_2-adrenergic receptors resided mainly outside of the synapse and mediated vasoconstrictive responses to circulating α-adrenergic agonists such as NE, whereas

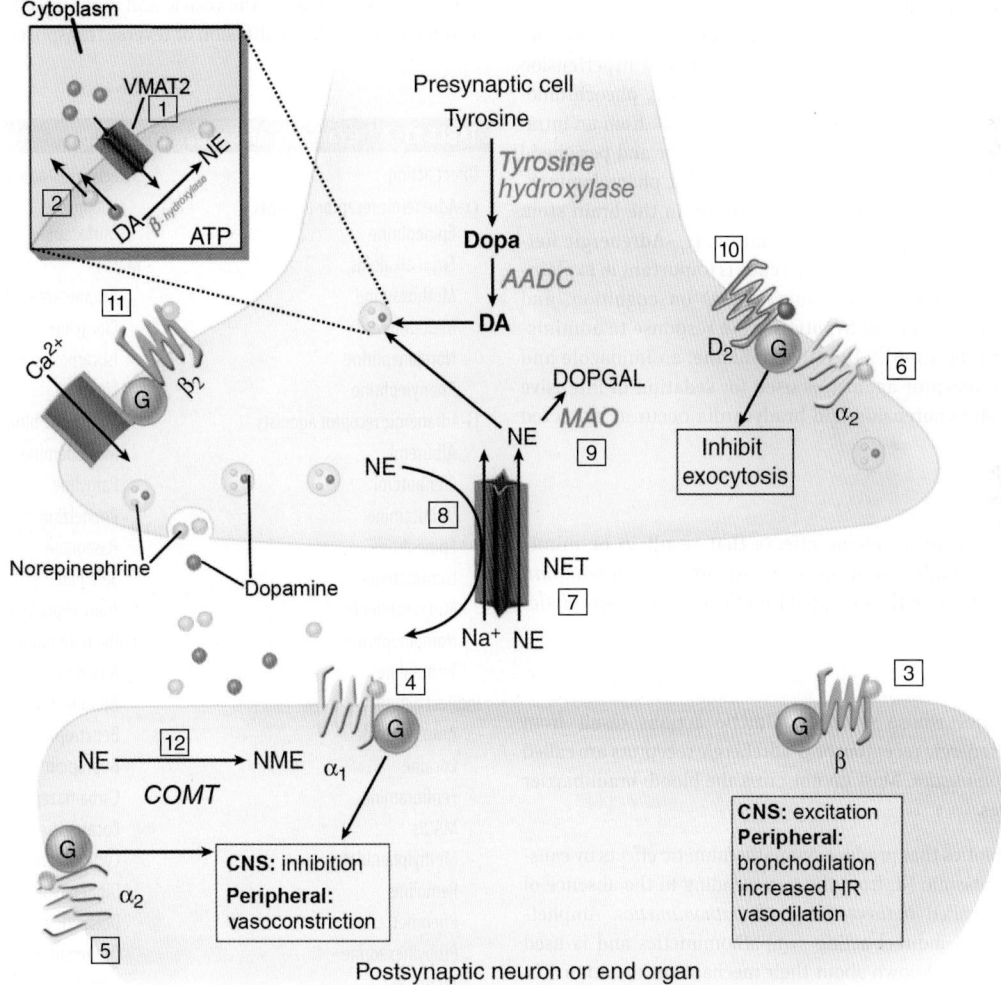

FIGURE 13–5. Noradrenergic nerve ending. The postsynaptic membrane may represent an end organ or another neuron in the CNS. Brief examples of effects resulting from postsynaptic receptor activation are shown. Xenobiotics in Tables 13–4 and 13–5 produce effects by inhibiting transport of dopamine (DA) or norepinephrine (NE) into vesicles through VMAT2 [1]; causing movement of NE and DA from vesicles into the cytoplasm [2]; activating or antagonizing postsynaptic α- and β-adrenergic receptors [3–5]; modulating NE release by activating or antagonizing presynaptic α_2-autoreceptors [6], dopamine$_2$ (D$_2$) heteroreceptors [10], or β_2-autoreceptors [11]; blocking reuptake of NE (NET inhibition) [7]; causing reverse transport of NE from the cytoplasm into the synapse via NET by raising cytoplasmic NE concentrations [8]; inhibiting monoamine oxidase (MAO) to prevent NE degradation [9]; or inhibiting COMT to prevent NE degradation [12]. Controversy exists as to whether COMT's enzymatic action mainly occurs in the synapse or intracellularly. AADC = aromatic L-amino acid decarboxylase; β-hydroxylase = dopamine-β-hydroxylase; COMT = catechol-O-methyltransferase; CNS = central nervous system; DOPGAL = 3,4-dihydroxyphenylglycoaldehyde; G = G protein; NET = membrane NE reuptake transporter; NME = normetanephrine; VMAT2 = vesicle uptake transporter for NE.

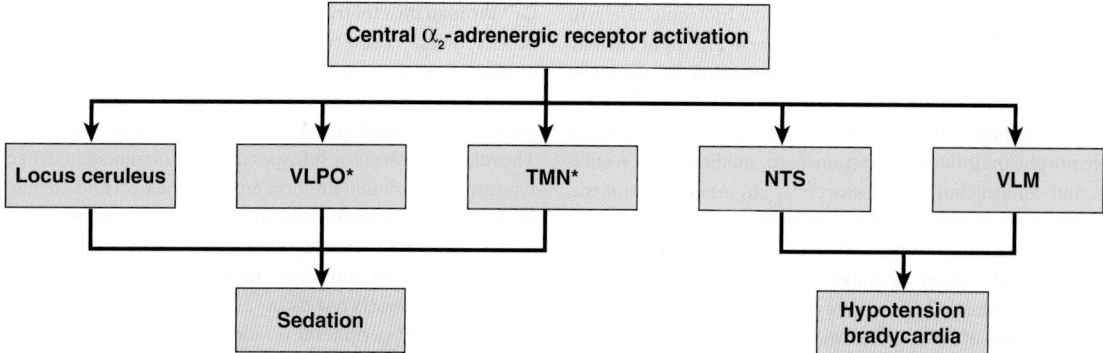

FIGURE 13–6. Central action of xenobiotics that activate α_2-adrenergic receptors. Activation of α_2-adrenergic receptors on noradrenergic neurons in the locus ceruleus produces sedation. Activation of receptors in the nucleus tractus solitarius (NTS) and ventrolateral medulla (VLM) contributes to hypotension and bradycardia. *In animal models, α_2-receptor activation of GABAergic neurons in the ventrolateral preoptic nucleus (VLPO) and of histaminergic neurons in the tuberomammillary nucleus (TMN) also contribute to sedation.

postsynaptic α_1-adrenergic receptors responded to NE released from nerve endings. However, in at least some tissues (eg, saphenous vein), NE released following nerve stimulation produces vasoconstriction through action at α_2-adrenergic receptors, making the previous differentiation not as distinct.[68,135] Because both α_1-adrenergic receptors and α_2-adrenergic receptors on non-cerebral vasculature mediate vasoconstriction, a patient with hypertension from high concentrations of circulating catecholamines (eg, pheochromocytoma or clonidine withdrawal) or from extravasation of NE from an intravenous line commonly requires both α_1-adrenergic receptor and peripheral α_2-adrenergic receptor blockade to vasodilate adequately (eg, phentolamine).

Activation of postsynaptic α_2-adrenergic receptors in the brain stem inhibits sympathetic output and produces sedation. α_{2A}-Adrenergic heteroreceptor activation on non-noradrenergic cells is important in explaining sedation, antinociception, hypothermia, effects on cognition, and centrally mediated bradycardia and hypotension in response to administration of α_2 agonists (Fig. 13–6).[93] Dexmedetomidine, an imidazole and potent α_{2A}-adrenergic receptor agonist, is used for sedation in intensive care patients, although hypotension and bradycardia occur as expected side effects.[27]

Xenobiotics

Xenobiotics producing pharmacologic effects that result in or mimic increased activity of the adrenergic nervous system are *sympathomimetics* (Table 13–4). Those with the opposite effect are *sympatholytics* (Table 13–5).

Sympathomimetics

Direct-Acting Xenobiotics whose sympathomimetic actions result from direct binding to α-adrenergic receptors or β-adrenergic receptors are called *direct-acting sympathomimetics*. Most do not cross the blood–brain barrier in significant quantities.

Indirect-Acting Xenobiotics that produce sympathomimetic effects by causing the release of cytoplasmic NE from the nerve ending in the absence of vesicle exocytosis are called *indirect-acting sympathomimetics*. Amphetamine is the prototype of indirect-acting sympathomimetics and is used for the discussion of what is known about their mechanisms of action.[45] In general, mechanisms of indirect release of NE by amphetamines, cocaine, phencyclidine, MAOIs, and mixed-acting xenobiotics noted in Table 13–4 are similar in that their actions depend on their ability to produce elevated cytoplasmic NE concentrations.

Amphetamine and structurally similar indirect-acting sympathomimetics move into the neuron mainly by the membrane transporter that transports NE into the neuron. Lipophilic indirect-acting sympathomimetics frequently move into the neuron by diffusion. From the cytoplasm, amphetamine is transported into neurotransmitter vesicles, where it buffers protons

to raise intravesicular pH. As noted earlier, much of the ability of the vesicle to concentrate NE (and other neurotransmitters) is a result of ion trapping of NE at the lower pH. The rise in intravesicular pH produced by amphetamine causes NE to leave the vesicle and move into the cytoplasm.[274,275] This movement results from diffusion or reverse transport of NE by VMAT2. In the

TABLE 13–4	Examples of Sympathomimetics
Direct acting	**Selective α_2-adrenergic receptor antagonists**
α-Adrenergic receptor agonists	Yohimbine
Epinephrine	Mirtazapine
Ergot alkaloids	**MAOIs**
Methoxamine	Amphetamine
Midodrine	Clorgyline
Norepinephrine	Isocarboxazid
Phenylephrine	Linezolid
β-Adrenergic receptor agonists	Methylene blue
Albuterol	Moclobemide
Clenbuterol	Pargyline
Dobutamine	Phenelzine
Epinephrine	Rasagiline
Isoproterenol	Selegiline
Metaproterenol	Tranylcypromine
Norepinephrine	**Inhibit norepinephrine reuptake**
Terbutaline	Amphetamine
Indirect acting	Atomoxetine
Amphetamine	Benztropine
Cocaine	Bupropion
Fenfluramine	Carbamazepine
MAOIs	Cocaine
Methylphenidate	Cyclic antidepressants
Pemoline	Diphenhydramine
Phenmetrazine	Duloxetine
Propylhexedrine	Orphenadrine
Tyramine	Pemoline
Mixed acting	Reboxetine
Dopamine	Tramadol
Ephedrine	Trihexyphenidyl
Mephentermine	Venlafaxine
Metaraminol	
Phenylpropanolamine	
Pseudoephedrine	

MAOI = monoamine oxidase inhibitor.

TABLE 13–5 Examples of Sympatholytics

α-Adrenergic receptor antagonists (non-selective or α₁)	α₂-Adrenergic receptor agonists[b]
Clozapine	α-Methyldopa[c]
Cyclic antidepressants	Apraclonidine
Doxazosin	Brimonidine
Ergot alkaloids	Clonidine
Olanzapine	Dexmedetomidine
Phenothiazines	Guanabenz
Phenoxybenzamine	Guanethidine
Phentolamine	Guanfacine
Prazosin	Moxonidine
Risperidone	Naphazoline
Terazosin	Oxymetazoline
Tolazoline	Rilmenidine
Trazodone	Tetrahydrozoline
Inhibit dopamine-β-hydroxylase	Tizanidine
Diethyldithiocarbamate	Xylazine
Disulfiram	Xylometazoline
MAOIs	Inhibitors of vesicle uptake
β-Adrenergic receptor antagonists[d]	Reserpine
Atenolol	Tetrabenazine
Esmolol	
Labetalol	
Nadolol	
Pindolol[a]	
Practolol[a]	
Propranolol	
Sotalol	

[a]Partial β-adrenergic receptor agonist. [b]Xenobiotics in these categories vary in their relative selectivity for α₂-adrenergic receptors or imidazoline-binding sites. [c]Metabolized to α-methylnorepinephrine, which activates α₂-adrenergic receptors. [d]Common examples.

MAOI = monoamine oxidase inhibitor.

cytoplasm, amphetamine also competes with NE and DA for transport into vesicles, which further contributes to elevated cytoplasmic NE concentrations. In the case of amphetamine, the rise in cytoplasmic concentrations of NE is further enhanced by the ability of amphetamine metabolites to inhibit MAO, which impairs NE degradation.

Every time the Na⁺-dependent uptake transporter, NET, moves a bioactive amine (eg, tyramine) into the neuron from which it is released, a binding site for NE on NET conceptually transiently faces inward and becomes available for reverse transport of NE out of the neuron. The normally low concentration of cytoplasmic NE prevents significant reverse transport. In the face of elevated cytoplasmic NE concentrations produced by indirect-acting sympathomimetics, NET moves NE out of the neuron and back into the synapse, where the neurotransmitter activates adrenergic receptors (indirect action). This process is sometimes referred to as facilitated exchange diffusion or displacement of NE from the nerve ending. Evidence supporting reverse transport produced by amphetamine is that inhibitors of the transporter (eg, tricyclic antidepressants) prevent amphetamine induced NE release.

While all indirect-acting sympathomimetics cause reverse NE transport by increasing cytoplasmic NE concentrations, those that move into the neuron by the membrane transporter (eg, amphetamines, MAOIs, DA, tyramine) further enhance reverse transport because their uptake causes more NE-binding sites on NET to face inward per unit time.

Although cocaine inhibits NET, it also causes some NE release. In fact, cocaine similarly lessens pH gradients across vesicle membranes to raise cytoplasmic concentrations of NE.[275] That cocaine produces less NE release than amphetamines is partly explained by cocaine induced inhibition of the

membrane transporter and possibly by the fact that cocaine does not move into the neuron by active uptake (ie, does not increase the number of NE-binding sites facing inward), but diffuses into the neuron. In fact, most of the severe sympathomimetic effects of cocaine appear to result from action on the brain rather than peripheral nerve endings.[284]

Phencyclidine (PCP) is a hallucinogen that possesses multiple pharmacologic actions. Like toxicity from many hallucinogens, PCP toxicity is accompanied by increased adrenergic activity, which results, in part, from PCP induced decreases in pH gradients across the vesicle membrane[275] and indirect release of NE. Like cocaine, PCP moves into the neuron by diffusion rather than uptake through the membrane transporter, at least partly explaining less PCP induced NE release than which contains typically occurs in amphetamine poisoning.

In addition to causing ACh release, black widow spider venom α-latrotoxin causes vesicle exocytosis of NE, producing hypertension and diaphoresis over the palms, soles, upper lip, and nose. All of the aforementioned indirectly acting sympathomimetics, except α-latrotoxin, enter the CNS.

Mixed-Acting Mixed-acting sympathomimetics act directly and indirectly. For example, ephedrine indirectly causes NE release and directly activates adrenergic receptors. Intravenously administered DA indirectly causes NE release, explaining most of its vasoconstricting activity, but also directly stimulates dopaminergic and β-adrenergic receptors. Direct α-agonism occurs at high doses. Except for DA, these xenobiotics cross the blood–brain barrier to produce central effects.

Reuptake Inhibitors Inhibitors of NE reuptake raise concentrations of NE in the synapse to produce excessive stimulation of adrenergic receptors.

There are 2 main means by which inhibitors of bioactive amine inhibit reuptake: competitive and noncompetitive. Noncompetitive inhibitors, such as cyclic antidepressants, carbamazepine, venlafaxine, methylphenidate, and cocaine, bind at or near the carrier site on NET to prevent NET from moving NE and similar xenobiotics into or out of the neuron. Various xenobiotics used for their antimuscarinic effects also block NET noncompetitively. These include atomoxetine, benztropine, diphenhydramine, trihexyphenidyl, and orphenadrine.[193]

The second mechanism, competitive inhibition of NET, characterizes most indirect-acting sympathomimetics, including amphetamine and structurally similar xenobiotics (eg, mixed-acting agents, MAOIs). These xenobiotics prevent NE reuptake by competing with synaptic NE for binding to the carrier site on NET, a mechanism by which they move into the neuron. In fact, an additional adrenergic action of amphetamines, mixed-acting xenobiotics, MAOIs, and tyramine is to raise synaptic NE concentrations by competing for uptake, thereby compounding their indirect or direct actions.

MAOIs Monoamine oxidase inhibitors (MAOIs) are transported by NET into the neuron, where in which they act through several mechanisms (Table 13–4).[3,181] Inhibition of MAO, their main pharmacologic effect, results in increased cytoplasmic concentrations of NE and some indirect release of neurotransmitter into the synapse. As a minor effect they also displace NE from vesicles by raising pH in a manner similar to amphetamines. These actions explain the initial sympathomimetic findings following MAOI overdose and also account for occasional and unpredictable adrenergic crises that occur despite dietary compliance.

Nonspecific MAOIs inhibit both enzymes of MAO, preventing intestinal and hepatic degradation of bioactive amines. A person taking such an MAOI who then is exposed to indirect-acting sympathomimetics (eg, tyramine in cheese, ephedrine, DA, amphetamines) has a much larger cytoplasmic concentration of NE to transport into the synapse and, therefore, develops central and peripheral sympathomimetic findings. Monoamine oxidase inhibitors (MAOIs) specific for the MAO-B enzyme are less likely to predispose to food or drug interactions by maintaining significant hepatic and intestinal MAO activity. Furthermore, reversible

MAO-A specific inhibitors are also less likely to provoke this reaction because their reversibility allows competition of exogenous amines with the inhibitor, resulting in its displacement from the enzyme and normal metabolism of the bioactive amines.[303] Isoenzyme specificity is lost as the dose of the MAOI is increased. In fact, selegiline, currently marketed as a selective MAO-B inhibitor, partially inhibits MAO-A activity at therapeutic doses. Rasagiline is a newer MAO-B inhibitor that has 100-fold greater affinity for MAO-B than MAO-A, but still loses specificity at supratherapeutic doses.[96,109] Monoamine oxidase inhibitors (MAOI) enzyme specificity is of lesser importance when indirect-acting xenobiotics are administered parenterally (eg, intravenous DA or amphetamines). Linezolid is an antibiotic that displays nonspecific MAO inhibition,[201] while methylene blue mainly inhibits MAO-A.[253]

Occasionally, patients suffering from refractory depression respond to a combination of MAOIs and tricyclic antidepressants. This combination therapy is usually unaccompanied by excessive adrenergic activity because the inhibition of the membrane uptake transporter by the tricyclic antidepressant attenuates excessive reverse transport of elevated cytoplasmic NE concentrations produced by MAOIs.

COMT Inhibitors Inhibitors of COMT are administered in the treatment of Parkinson disease to prevent the catabolism of concomitantly administered L-dopa. Entacapone only acts peripherally, whereas tolcapone also crosses the blood–brain barrier where it also prevents DA degradation as well.

α_2-Adrenergic Receptor Antagonists Yohimbine produces selective competitive antagonism of α_2-adrenergic receptors to produce a mixed clinical picture. Peripheral postsynaptic α_2 blockade produces vasodilation. Blockade of presynaptic α_2-adrenergic receptors on cholinergic nerve endings (Fig. 13–4) enhances ACh release, occasionally producing bronchospasm[146] and contributing to diaphoresis. Similar presynaptic actions on peripheral noradrenergic nerves enhance catecholamine release (Fig. 13–5). Antagonism of central α_2-adrenergic receptors in the locus ceruleus results in CNS stimulation, whereas blockade of postsynaptic α_2-adrenergic receptors in the nucleus tractus solitarius may enhance sympathetic output (Fig. 13–6). The final result includes hypertension, tachycardia, anxiety, fear, agitation, mania, mydriasis, diaphoresis, and bronchospasm.[158] Mirtazapine, an antidepressant, antagonizes central α_2-adrenergic receptors, which increases serotonin and NE release in the CNS.

Sympatholytics

Direct Antagonists Direct α-adrenergic receptor and β-adrenergic receptor antagonists are noted in Table 13–5. After overdose, β-adrenergic receptor selectivity is less significant. Some β-adrenergic receptor antagonists also are partial agonists.

Xenobiotics That Prevent Norepinephrine Release Xenobiotics that block the vesicle uptake transporter prevent the movement of NE into vesicles and deplete the nerve ending of this neurotransmitter, preventing NE release after depolarization. Reserpine and ketanserin inhibit both VMAT1 and VMAT2, whereas tetrabenazine only inhibits VMAT2. Like guanethidine, reserpine causes transient NE release with the initial dose or early in overdose. β-Adrenergic receptor antagonists block presynaptic β_2-adrenergic receptors to limit catecholamine release from nerve endings, although most of the antihypertensive action of β-adrenergic antagonists at therapeutic doses results from inhibition of renin release in the kidney.

α_2-Adrenergic Receptor Agonists Numerous imidazoline derivatives (eg, clonidine) and structurally similar xenobiotics used as centrally acting antihypertensives or long-acting topical vasoconstrictors act by activating α_2-adrenergic receptors. These xenobiotics also display various affinities for what are termed imidazoline-binding sites, apart from α_2-adrenergic receptors. Although imidazoline-binding sites are proposed and subdivided into I_1, I_2, and I_3,[73] and endogenous ligands for these binding sites are identified (eg, agmatine, imidazole acetic acid ribotide, harmane, other β-carbolines),[25,102,237] it must be recognized that the molecular structures

of imidazoline-binding sites have not been determined, nor have signaling pathways been characterized. As a result, major professional societies such as the International Union of Pharmacology Committee on Receptor Nomenclature and Drug Classification have not adopted the term imidazoline receptor.[154] The role of imidazoline-binding sites in mediating responses to xenobiotics remains controversial and ill-defined.

The ventromedial (depressor) and the rostral-ventrolateral (pressor) areas of the ventrolateral medulla (VLM) are responsible for the central regulation of cardiovascular tone and blood pressure. They receive afferent fibers from the carotid and aortic baroreceptors, which form the tractus solitarius via the nucleus tractus solitarius (NTS).[132]

Ingestions of xenobiotics that activate α_2-adrenergic receptors (Table 13–5) produce a mixed clinical picture. Peripheral postsynaptic α_2-adrenergic receptor stimulation produces vasoconstriction, pallor, and hypertension, often with reflex bradycardia (Fig. 13–5). Peripheral presynaptic α_2-adrenergic receptor stimulation prevents NE release (Fig. 13–5), reducing sympathetic activation. Central α_2-adrenergic receptor stimulation in the locus ceruleus accounts for CNS and respiratory depression (Fig. 13–6). Recently acquired knowledge about α_2-adrenergic receptor subtypes and their effects on non-adrenergic neurons makes analysis of their hypotensive and sedative effects complex. Recent animal evidence suggests that sedation is not entirely mediated by α_2-adrenergic receptor activation on noradrenergic neurons in the locus ceruleus.[93] Stimulation of postsynaptic α_{2A}-adrenergic receptors in the NTS in the VLM is thought to inhibit sympathetic output and enhance parasympathetic tone, explaining hypotension with bradycardia (Fig. 13–6).[132]

Dopamine-β-Hydroxylase Inhibition Inhibition of dopamine-β-hydroxylase, a copper-containing enzyme (Fig. 13–5), prevents the conversion of DA to NE, resulting in less NE release and less α- and β-adrenergic receptor stimulation. Disulfiram and diethyldithiocarbamate, copper chelators, produce such inhibition.[75] Because NE release mediates most of the ability of DA to cause vasoconstriction, NE is the vasopressor of choice in a hypotensive patient taking disulfiram. Monoamine oxidase inhibitors and α-methyldopa also inhibit dopamine-β-hydroxylase, although this is not their main mechanism of action.[181]

Dopamine is relatively contraindicated in hypotensive patients who have overdosed on MAOIs. First, DA acts indirectly, and its administration might produce excessive adrenergic activity and exaggerated rises in blood pressure. Second, even if an adrenergic storm does not occur, most of the α-mediated vasoconstriction of dopamine is secondary to NE release. In the presence of MAOIs, NE synthesis may be impaired from concomitant dopamine-β-hydroxylase inhibition, and DA might not reliably raise blood pressure if cytoplasmic and vesicular stores are depleted. In the presence of impaired NE release or α-adrenergic receptor blockade from any cause, unopposed dopamine-induced vasodilation from action on peripheral DA and β-adrenergic receptors paradoxically lowers blood pressure further. Norepinephrine and EPI are used to support blood pressure relatively safely in patients taking MAOIs because they have little or no indirect action and are metabolized by COMT when given intravenously.

DOPAMINE

Because DA is the direct precursor of NE, noradrenergic vesicles contain DA. The release of NE from peripheral sympathetic nerves, therefore, always results in release of some DA (Fig. 13–5), as does the release of NE and EPI from the adrenal gland, explaining most of DA in blood. In peripheral tissues, activation of DA receptors causes vasodilation of renal, mesenteric, and coronary vascular beds. Dopamine also stimulates β-adrenergic receptors and, at high doses, directly stimulates α-adrenergic receptors. When DA is administered intravenously, most vasoconstriction is caused by dopamine-induced NE release.

Dopamine accounts for about one-half of all catecholamines in the brain and is present in greater quantities than NE or 5-HT. By contrast to the diffuse projections of noradrenergic neurons, dopaminergic neurons and receptors are highly organized and concentrated in several areas, especially in the basal ganglia and limbic system.[144,254]

Excessive dopaminergic activity in the striatum and/or other areas from any cause (eg, increased release, impaired uptake, increased receptor sensitivity) produces acute choreoathetosis[136] and acute Gilles de la Tourette syndrome, with tics, spitting, and cursing. Excessive dopaminergic activity in the limbic system and frontal cortex, and perhaps in other areas, produces paranoia and psychosis. Dopaminergic activity in the nucleus accumbens is thought responsible for much of the drug craving and addictive behavior in patients abusing sympathomimetics, opioids, alcohol, and nicotine. Diminished dopaminergic tone (eg, impaired release, receptor blockade) in the striatum produces various extrapyramidal disorders such as acute dystonias and parkinsonism.[235,269,287]

Synthesis, Release, and Reuptake

The steps of DA synthesis and vesicle storage are the same as those for NE, except that DA is not converted to NE after transport into vesicles (Fig. 13–7). Dopamine is removed from the synapse via reuptake by DAT, the membrane-bound DA transporter. Dopamine transporter and NET exhibit 66% homology in their amino acid sequences. Like NET, DAT is not

completely specific for DA and transports amphetamines and other structurally similar sympathomimetics. Cytoplasmic DA has a fate similar to NE. It is pumped back into vesicles by VMAT2 (brain) and VMAT1 (neuroendocrine tissue, adrenal glands) or degraded by MAO and COMT.

Dopamine Receptors

All DA receptors are coupled to G proteins and are divided into 2 main groups. Dopamine D_1-like receptors (D_1 and D_5) are expressed as various subtypes and are linked to G_s to stimulate adenylate cyclase and to raise cAMP concentrations.[257] Dopamine (D_1) receptors are found in the nuclei of the basal ganglia and the cerebral cortex, and D_5 receptors are concentrated in the hippocampus and hypothalamus. Dopamine is 5 to 10 times more potent at D_5 receptors than it is at D_1 receptors.

Dopamine (D_2)-like receptors (D_2, D_3, D_4) most commonly are linked to $G_{i/o}$ to produce several actions, including inhibition of adenylate cyclase and the lowering of cAMP concentrations. Again, numerous subtypes of receptors exist (eg, D_{2s}, D_{2L}). Dopamine (D_2) receptors are concentrated in the basal ganglia and limbic system. Some D_2 receptors also reside on presynaptic membranes, where their activation limits neurotransmitter release, including the peripheral release of NE (Figs. 13–5 and 13–7). Dopamine (D_3)

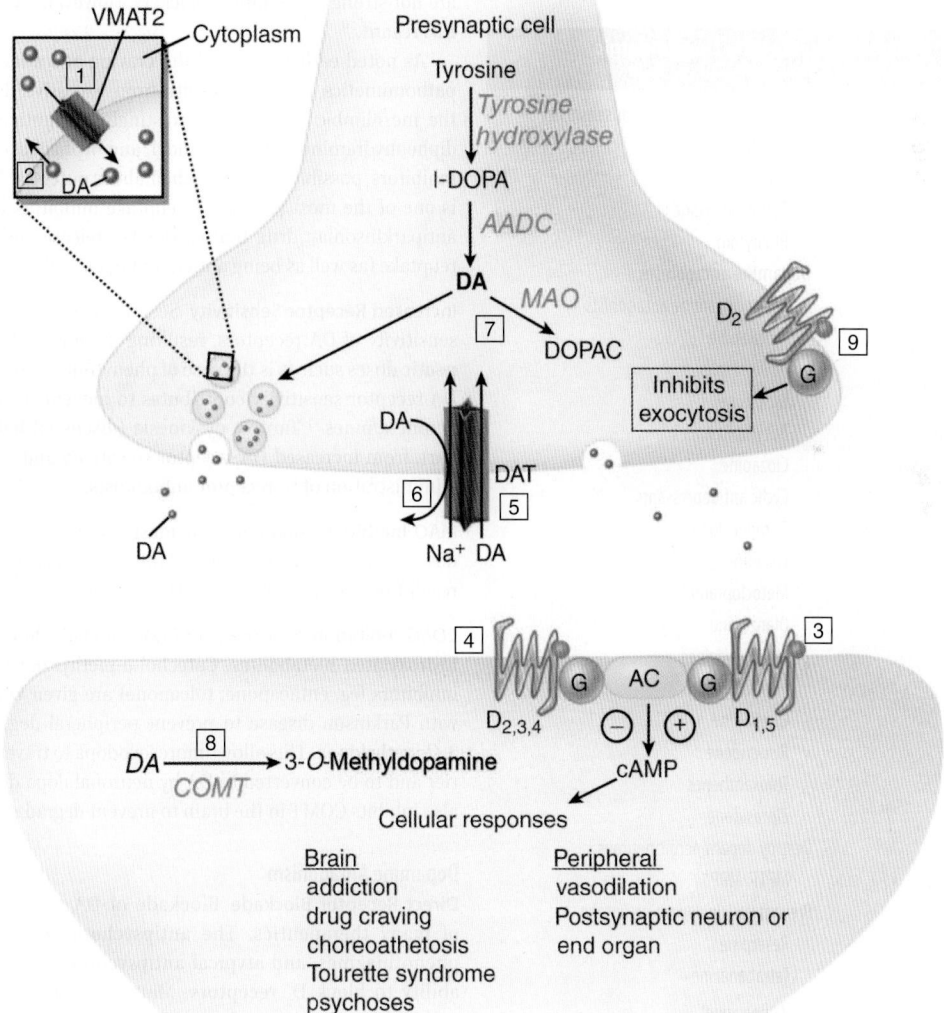

FIGURE 13–7. A dopaminergic nerve ending and postsynaptic membrane. Dopamine (DA) released from nerve endings binds to various postsynaptic DA receptors (D) on neurons or peripheral end organs. Stimulation of presynaptic D_2 receptors [9] lessens DA release. Xenobiotics in Table 13–6 have diverse activities including to inhibit vesicle uptake [1]; cause DA to leave the vesicle and move into the cytoplasm [2]; activate or antagonize DA receptors [3, 4, 9]; inhibit DAT to prevent DA reuptake [5]; cause reverse transport of cytoplasmic DA (via DAT) into the synapse by raising cytoplasmic DA concentrations [6]; prevent DA degradation by inhibiting monoamine oxidase (MAO) [7]; or prevent DA degradation by inhibiting catechol-O-methyltransferase (COMT) [8]. (Both DA and dopa are substrates for COMT.) Inhibition or stimulation of adenylate cyclase by DA receptors is shown for illustration, though other G protein–mediated effects can result. AADC = L-aromatic amino acid decarboxylase; DAT = membrane DA reuptake transporter; DOPAC = 3,4-dihydroxyphenylacetic acid; L-DOPA = VMAT2 = vesicle membrane uptake transporter.

receptors are concentrated in the hypothalamic and limbic nuclei, whereas D_4 receptors are concentrated in the frontal cortex and limbic nuclei (rather than basal ganglia nuclei). Most agonists bind to the D_3 receptors with higher affinity than to D_2 receptors, whereas most antagonists bind preferentially to D_2 receptors.[144,254] Most agonists and antagonists express a lower affinity for D_4 receptors than they express for D_2 receptors; a notable exception is clozapine.

Xenobiotics

Table 13–6 provides examples of xenobiotics that affect dopaminergic neurotransmission.

Dopamine Agonism

Indirect-Acting and Mixed-Acting Xenobiotics Most indirect-acting and mixed-acting sympathomimetics cause DA release. The mechanism of action is similar to that causing NE release. These xenobiotics diffuse into the neuron or undergo uptake by DAT before being transported into vesicles by VMAT2 where they buffer protons and displace DA into the cytoplasm for reverse transport by DAT into the synapse. Benztropine, diphenhydramine, trihexyphenidyl, and orphenadrine also cause DA release, perhaps contributing to their abuse potential, which is noted below.[193] Excessive dopaminergic

activity following therapeutic doses or overdoses of decongestants (eg, pseudoephedrine), amphetamines, methylphenidate, and pemoline can produce acute choreoathetosis and the Tourette Syndrome.[39,165] Ingestion of excessive doses of L-dopa (which is converted to DA) produces similar symptoms.

Direct Agonists Bromocriptine is an ergot derivative that directly activates DA receptors (mainly D_2-like). Toxic effects include those described above for indirect-acting xenobiotics. Apomorphine directly activates D_2 receptors. Such action at the chemoreceptor trigger zone (CTZ) produces vomiting, whereas agonism in the basal ganglia explains the use of apomorphine in the treatment of Parkinson disease. Fenoldopam is a D_1 receptor agonist that is used as a vasodilator in the treatment of hypertensive emergencies.

Dopamine (D_1-) and D_2-like receptor activation is the predominant mediator of locomotor effects from DA agonists. Activation of either D_1- or D_2-like receptors produces antiparkinsonian effects.[106,254] Cabergoline, ropinirole, and pramipexole are D_2-like receptor agonists used to treat Parkinson disease.[19,73,99]

Reuptake Inhibition Xenobiotics inhibiting DAT prevent DA reuptake and include cocaine, amphetamines, methylphenidate, and probably amantadine. Increased dopaminergic activity from cocaine toxicity produces choreoathetosis and Gilles de la Tourette syndrome. In general, antidepressants are not strong DA reuptake blockers. However, bupropion is more active in this regard.[247]

As noted earlier, much of the craving and addiction produced by sympathomimetics probably results from excessive dopaminergic activity in the mesolimbic system.[269] Interestingly, the anticholinergics benztropine, diphenhydramine, trihexyphenidyl, and orphenadrine are also DA reuptake inhibitors, possibly explaining their abuse potential.[193,265] In fact, benztropine is one of the most potent DA reuptake inhibitors known. Amantadine, an antiparkinsonian drug that causes DA release and some inhibition of DA reuptake (as well as being anticholinergic), is also abused.

Increased Receptor Sensitivity Several xenobiotics are thought to increase sensitivity of DA receptors, resulting in choreoathetosis, even with therapeutic doses such as is the case of phenytoin. Evidence exists that increased DA receptor sensitivity contributes to movement disorders resulting from amphetamines.[44] Tardive dyskinesia (discussed below) results, at least in part, from increased DA receptor sensitivity and occurs following chronic administration of D_2 receptor antagonists.

MAO Inhibition Monoamine oxidase inhibitors (MAOIs) inhibit the breakdown of cytoplasmic DA. Some of the food and drug interactions with MAOIs result from excessive release of DA from nerve endings.

COMT Inhibition Substrates of COMT include dopa, DA, NE, EPI, and their hydroxylated metabolites. Catechol-*o*-methyltransferase inhibitor (COMT) inhibitors (eg, entacapone, tolcapone) are given with levodopa to patients with Parkinson disease to prevent peripheral degradation of levodopa to 3-*O*-methyldopa. This allows more levodopa to traverse the blood–brain barrier and to be converted to DA by neuronal dopa decarboxylase. Tolcapone also inhibits COMT in the brain to prevent degradation of dopamine.[125]

Dopamine Antagonism

Direct Receptor Blockade Blockade of DA receptors is the specific aim of many therapeutics. The antipsychotic actions of butyrophenones, phenothiazines, and atypical antipsychotics mainly correlate with their ability to block D_2 receptors. Many phenothiazines block both D_1-like and D_2-like receptors, whereas haloperidol mainly blocks D_2-like receptors. Unfortunately, antipsychotics and metoclopramide also block DA receptors in the striatum, producing various extrapyramidal symptoms, including acute parkinsonism and dystonias.

Atypical antipsychotics produce fewer extrapyramidal effects and are thought to carry less risk of producing tardive dyskinesia.[241] The relative affinity of an antipsychotic for 5-HT_{2A} receptors over D_2 receptors has predictive value for atypical antipsychotics, with a lower risk of extrapyramidal

---

TABLE 13–6   Examples of Xenobiotics Affecting Dopaminergic Neurotransmission

Dopamine agonism	Increase dopamine receptor sensitivity
Direct stimulation of dopamine receptors	Amphetamine
Apomorphine	Antipsychotics
Bromocriptine	Metoclopramide
Cabergoline[a]	Phenytoin
L-Dopa[b]	**Dopamine antagonism**
Fenoldopam	Direct dopamine antagonists
Lisuride	Amoxapine
Pramipexole	Aripiprazole
Ropinirole	Buspirone
Inhibit dopamine metabolism	Butyrophenones
MAOIs	Clozapine
COMTIs	Cyclic antidepressants
Indirect acting	Domperidone
Amantadine	Loxapine
Amphetamine	Metoclopramide
Benztropine	Olanzapine
Diphenhydramine	Phenothiazines
MAOIs	Pimozide
Methylphenidate	Quetiapine
Pemoline	Risperidone
Trihexyphenidyl	Thioxanthenes
Inhibit dopamine reuptake	Ziprasidone
Amantadine	Destroy dopaminergic neurons
Amphetamine	MPTP/MPP$^+$
Benztropine	Prevent vesicle dopamine uptake
Bupropion	Reserpine
Cocaine	Tetrabenazine
Diphenhydramine	Valbenazine
Methylphenidate	
Orphenadrine	
Trihexyphenidyl	

[a]Associated with fibrotic valvulopathy due to 5-HT_{2B} agonism. [b]Metabolized to dopamine, which acts as an agonist.

COMTI = catechol-*o*-methyltransferase inhibitor; MAOI = monoamine oxidase inhibitor; MPTP = 1-methyl-4-phenyl-1,2,3,6-tetrahydropyridine; MPP$^+$ = 1-methyl-4-phenylpyridinium

symptoms.[228] These include clozapine, olanzapine, quetiapine, risperidone, and ziprasidone.

The ratio of muscarinic (M_1) blockade to D_2-receptor blockade is also important in limiting extrapyramidal symptoms. Antipsychotics exhibiting strong antimuscarinic effects (eg, olanzapine, clozapine, thioridazine) are also less likely to induce extrapyramidal symptoms.[241]

Buspirone, an anxiolytic, antagonizes D_2 receptors, which explains occasional extrapyramidal reactions. Various cyclic antidepressants, especially amoxapine, block D_2 receptors to some extent.

The chronic use of dopamine receptor antagonists causes upregulation of DA receptors. The continued use of or, especially, withdrawal of DA receptor antagonists (antipsychotics, metoclopramide, and occasionally antidepressants) results in excessive dopaminergic activity and tardive dyskinesia, characterized by choreiform movements typical of excessive dopaminergic influence in the striatum.

The blockade of DA receptors by numerous xenobiotics, including butyrophenones, phenothiazines, and metoclopramide, produces a poorly understood disorder called neuroleptic *malignant syndrome*. Neuroleptic malignant syndrome also rarely follows acute withdrawal of DA agonists (eg, stopping L-dopa, bromocriptine, or tolcapone). Neuroleptic malignant syndrome is characterized, in part, by mental status changes, autonomic instability, rigidity, and hyperthermia.

Indirect Antagonism

Reserpine and tetrabenazine inhibit VMAT to prevent transport of DA into storage vesicles and deplete nerve endings of DA. In fact, reserpine was used as an antipsychotic before the introduction of phenothiazines. 1-Methyl-4-phenyl-1,2,3,6-tetrahydropyridine (MPTP), a meperidine analog, undergoes activation by MAO-B, including that in glial cells, to a metabolite, 1-methyl-4-phenylpyridinium (MPP^+), that undergoes uptake by and causes death of dopaminergic neurons. Both MAOIs and inhibitors of DA transporters prevent MPTP-induced destruction of dopaminergic neurons.

SEROTONIN

Serotonin (5-hydroxytryptamine, 5-HT) is an indole alkylamine found throughout nature (animals, plants, venoms). The serotonergic system is extremely diverse, with 14 subtypes of receptors organized into 7 classes. All of the receptor classes are coupled to G proteins except for 5-HT_3, which is a ligand-gated ion channel.

In the CNS, several hundred thousand serotonergic neurons lie in or in juxtaposition to numerous midline nuclei in the brain stem (raphe nuclei), from which they project to virtually all areas of the brain and spinal cord. Serotonin is involved with mood, emotion, learning, memory, personality, affect, appetite, aggression, motor function, temperature regulation, sexual activity, pain perception, sleep induction, and other basic functions. Serotonin is not essential for any of these processes, but modulates their quality and extent. A number of psychiatric disorders, including depression, anxiety, obsessive-compulsive disorder, dementia, schizophrenia, and eating disorders, are linked to altered serotonin function. Consequently, modification of serotonergic neurotransmission is an integral part of the treatment plan for most of these conditions.[234] Serotonin is also the precursor for the pineal hormone, melatonin.

Despite the important role 5-HT plays in the CNS, less than 5% of the body's 5-HT is found within the CNS. The great majority of the body's 5-HT is located within enterochromaffin cells of the intestine, and a small amount is sequestered by platelets.[24] Peripherally, 5-HT is released by enterochromaffin cells in response to intestinal stimulation, which contributes to peristalsis and fluid secretion. Platelets take up 5-HT while passing through the enteric circulation. Serotonin is released from activated platelets to interact with other platelet membranes (promote aggregation) and with vascular smooth muscle.[24]

Experimentally, 5-HT exhibits diverse effects on the cardiovascular and peripheral nervous systems, although the importance of these actions remains uncertain in the normal physiologic state. Serotonin-induced vasoconstriction or vasodilation found in experimental studies involves multiple types of 5-HT receptors and, in turn, is influenced by multiple other factors. 5-HT_{1B} receptor agonists (eg, sumatriptan) produce coronary artery vasoconstriction in some patients as an adverse event.[202,289]

Centrally, it is particularly difficult to ascribe a specific symptom or physical finding to serotonergic neurons because of the diversity of their physiologic actions. However, 5-HT plays an important role in the action of many hallucinogenic or illusinogenic xenobiotics, which act as partial agonists at cortical 5-HT_2 receptors. Proserotonergic drugs are used to treat depression, whereas 5-HT receptor (5-HT_2) antagonists have greater importance in the management of schizophrenia.[89]

Generally, in areas where they overlap, 5-HT acts in opposition to DA. For example, 5-HT serves to increase prolactin, adrenocorticotropic hormone (ACTH), and growth hormone secretion, whereas DA decreases prolactin secretion. As another example, activation of basal ganglial 5-HT_{2A} receptors inhibits DA release.[89] However, well-known exceptions exist, such as cortical 5-HT_3 receptors[47] and 5-HT_{1A} receptors that are capable of promoting DA release under certain circumstances.[199]

Synthesis, Release, and Reuptake

Serotonin does not cross the blood–brain barrier but, rather, is synthesized from the amino acid L-tryptophan, which passes through the blood–brain barrier through a neutral amino acid transporter. Figure 13–8 illustrates 5-HT synthesis. Tryptophan-5-hydroxylase is the rate-limiting enzyme and converts L-tryptophan to 5-hydroxytryptophan (5-OHT) within the cytoplasm. Increasing tryptophan predictably increases 5-HT production. 5-Hydroxytryptophan (5-OHT) is then converted to 5-HT by L-amino acid decarboxylase (DOPA decarboxylase). 5-HT is transported into vesicles by VMAT2, where it is concentrated by ion trapping before release by Ca^{2+}-dependent exocytosis. In contrast to vesicles containing DA or NE, 5-HT vesicles contain almost no ATP. After release into the synapse, a transporter (SERT) in the neuronal membrane moves 5-HT back into the neuron, where it reenters vesicles or is degraded by MAO.[234]

Serotonin is preferentially metabolized by the MAO-A enzyme. Paradoxically, the serotonergic nerve terminal is almost devoid of MAO-A, but contains abundant amounts of MAO-B. It is hypothesized that the large amounts of MAO-B metabolize other xenobiotics that might inappropriately promote 5-HT release (eg, dopamine). However, the small amount of MAO-A found in serotonergic neurons provides adequate degradation of 5-HT.[196]

Serotonin Receptors

There are 7 major functioning receptor types (5-HT_1–5-HT_7), numerous subtypes, splice variants, and post-translational modifications that result in wide variation.

5-HT_1 Receptors

Five subtypes of 5-HT_1 receptors are known, encoded by the genes *HTR1A*, *HTR1B*, and *HTR1D* to *HTR1F* (1C was reclassified to 2C). These receptors are linked to G_i and inhibit adenylate cyclase, decreasing cAMP concentrations. Members of the 5-HT_1 receptor class express greatest affinity for 5-HT and are, thus, biologically active under normal physiologic conditions. 5-Hydroxytryptamine (5-HT_{1A}) receptors reside predominantly on raphe nuclei, where they act as somatodendritic autoreceptors.[145,186,210] Hippocampal 5-HT_{1A} receptors reside postsynaptically, where they also inhibit through similar mechanisms.[145]

Central 5-HT_{1B} and 5-HT_{1D} receptors primarily act as inhibitory terminal autoreceptors and heteroreceptors. They are found less commonly on postsynaptic membranes.[234] Originally 5-HT_{1B} receptors were not believed to exist in humans. However, most of the actions described in older literature regarding 5-HT_{1D} receptors are now attributed to 5-HT_{1B} receptors. Cranial blood vessels (eg, meninges) possess 5-HT_{1B} and 5-HT_{1D} receptors, whose activation produces vasoconstriction and decreased inflammation.[202,234] 5-Hydroxytryptamine (5-HT_{1B}) receptors are also found on smooth muscle cells in other

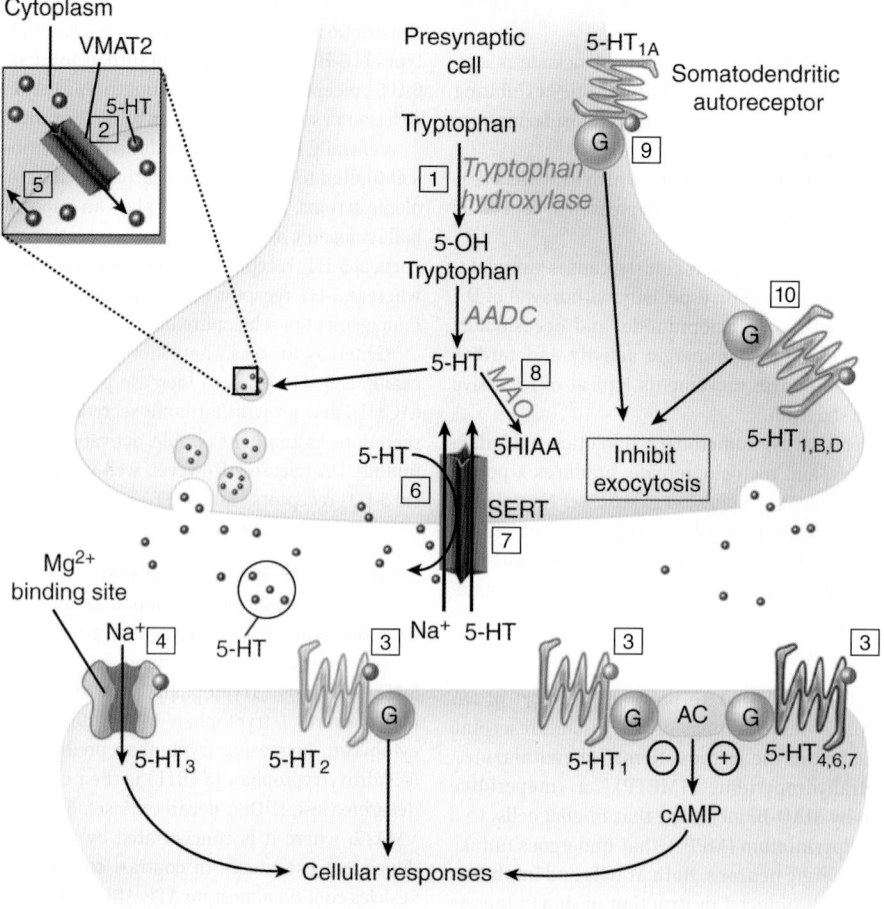

FIGURE 13–8. A serotonergic nerve ending and postsynaptic membrane. Tryptophan hydroxylase [1] converts tryptophan to 5-hydroxytryptophan (5-OHT). Aromatic L-amino acid decarboxylase (AADC) then metabolizes 5-OHT to serotonin (5-HT). Serotonin is concentrated within vesicles through uptake by VMAT2 before exocytosis [2]. After uptake into the neuron by SERT [7], 5-HT is transported back into vesicles or undergoes degradation by monoamine oxidase (MAO) to an intermediate compound, which is converted to 5-hydroxyindoleacetic acid (5-HIAA) [8]. $5-HT_{1,2,4,6,7}$ receptors [3,9,10] are coupled to G proteins, whereas $5-HT_3$ receptors [4] are ligand-gated cation channels that may conduct Na^+ and/or Ca^{2+} (only Na^+ is illustrated). $5-HT_3$ cation channels also appear to be blocked by Mg^{2+} until the cell is depolarized, allowing Mg^{2+} to dissociate—a mechanism similar to that found at NMDA glutamate receptors. In addition to residing on postsynaptic membranes, $5-HT_{1A}$, $5-HT_{1B}$, and $5-HT_{1D}$ receptors serve as presynaptic autoreceptors that, when stimulated, decrease further release of 5-HT [9,10]. Presynaptic $5-HT_{1A}$ receptors mainly serve as somatodendritic autoreceptors, whereas presynaptic $5-HT_{1B}$ and $5-HT_{1D}$ receptors serve as terminal autoreceptors. Xenobiotics in Table 13–7 act to enhance 5-HT synthesis [1]; inhibit VMAT2 to prevent vesicle uptake of 5-HT [2]; raise cytoplasmic concentrations of 5-HT, resulting in reverse transport of 5-HT into the synapse by SERT [6]; by displacing 5-HT from vesicles [5] or inhibiting MAO [8]; activate or antagonize 5-HT receptors [3,4,9,10]; or by inhibiting 5-HT reuptake [7]. G = G protein; SERT = membrane 5-HT uptake transporter; VMAT2 = vesicle membrane uptake transporter.

blood vessels, and this is a consideration when using $5-HT_{1B/1D}$ agonists for migraine.

5-Hydroxytryptamine ($5-HT_{1E}$) receptors are highly expressed in the frontal cortex, hippocampus, and the olfactory bulb.[137] The $5-HT_{1F}$ receptor is also found in brain and studies are under way to investigate its role in migraine using a new class of selective agonists.[239]

5-HT₂ Receptors

The 3 subtypes of $5-HT_2$ receptors are encoded by *HTR2A* to *HTR2C*. These receptors are coupled to G proteins, thus serving to decrease K^+ efflux and/or increase intracellular Ca^{2+} concentration by raising concentrations of inositol triphosphate and diacylglycerol.[234] The 3 subtypes of $5-HT_2$ receptors are so similar in characterization that investigational probes have great difficulty in distinguishing the subtypes. 5-Hydroxytryptamine ($5-HT_{2A}$) receptors are most concentrated in the cerebral cortex, where they serve as excitatory postsynaptic receptors. Their activation increases glutamate release from pyramidal cells, but also lead to release of GABA.[184] They also are a cellular receptor for JC virus, the cause of progressive multifocal leukoencephalopathy.[74]

Activation of $5-HT_{2A}$ receptors on platelets produces platelet aggregation. 5-Hydroxytryptamine ($5-HT_{2C}$) receptors (previously $5-HT_{1C}$) reside on the

choroid plexus, where they regulate cerebrospinal fluid production. Activation of $5-HT_{2B}$ receptors in the GI tract promotes gastric contraction.[234] At least some xenobiotics that activate $5-HT_{2B}$ receptors on cardiac valves cause a valvulopathy identical to that of carcinoid syndrome, though both sides of the heart commonly are involved following $5-HT_{2B}$ agonists, whereas carcinoid syndrome usually affects the right-sided valves.[38]

5-HT₃ Receptors

The $5-HT_3$ receptor is unique among the 5-HT receptor family members in being an ion channel, instead of being linked to a G protein. It belongs to the family of Cys-loop receptors and is a pentamer with the 5 subunits surrounding a central cation-selective pore, similar to the nicotinic acetylcholine receptor.[100] In humans, 5 different subunits are known, encoded by the genes *HTR3A* to *HTR3E*. Moreover, subunits have different splice isoforms and also have differential tissue expression. For example, while subunits HTR3A, B, and C are found in the brain, HTR3D subunits reside primarily in the GI tract, and HTR3E is found exclusively in the GI tract.[204] Functional homomeric receptors composed only of A subunits can form, but it appears receptors with other subunits require at least one A subunit.[168] Upon activation, postsynaptic receptors stimulate the neuron by opening the channel to cause depolarization through Na^+ and/or Ca^{2+} influx. In addition, these channels are normally blocked by Mg^{2+} in a voltage-dependent manner similar to glutamatergic NMDA receptors (see *Glutamate* later).

The chemoreceptor trigger zone (CTZ) has a large concentration of 5-HT$_3$ receptors, where their activation causes emesis. Consequently, 5-HT$_3$ receptor antagonists are used as antiemetics. These receptors also have a role in gut motility, and antagonists are finding use as treatment for diarrhea-predominant irritable bowel syndrome (IBS-D).

5-HT$_4$ Receptors

5-Hydroxytryptamine (5-HT$_4$) receptors (*HTR4*) have numerous splice variants and are found in the brain, intestines, and heart. They signal through G protein and G protein–independent pathways as well.[31] 5-Hydroxytryptamine (5-HT$_4$) receptors were investigated for effects on memory[134] and depression,[31] but their exact role in the brain is not yet clear. In the intestine, they are being investigated for constipation-predominant irritable bowel syndrome.[290]

5-HT$_5$ Receptors

The 5-HT$_{5A}$ receptor (*HTR5A*) is the only receptor from this subfamily found in humans and is limited to the brain,[236] particularly the cerebral cortex, hippocampus, and cerebellum.[218] The receptor is coupled to G$_i$ and inhibits both adenylate cyclase and ADP ribosyl cyclase, while stimulating a Ca^{2+}-dependent K$^+$ current.[206] Although there are hypotheses, the role of this receptor is unknown.[280]

5-HT$_6$ Receptors

5-Hydroxytryptamine (5-HT$_6$) receptors (*HTR6*) reside in several brain regions, especially in the caudate and putamen,[177] where their activation stimulates adenylate cyclase through coupling to G$_s$.[138] Although many antipsychotics antagonize these receptors,[30,138] and there are hypothesized effects on learning and memory,[134] their role remains unclear.

5-HT$_7$ Receptors

The 5-HT$_7$ receptor (*HTR7*) has several isoforms found in both brain and peripheral tissues, including liver, pancreas, spleen, and kidney.[18,104] The receptor is coupled to both G$_s$[18,246] and G$_{12}$.[143] One of the brain regions in which this receptor is found is the suprachiasmatic nucleus of the hypothalamus, where it appears to participate in regulating circadian rhythms, as agonists advance circadian rhythms in vitro[163] and in mice.[2] Other possible roles for this receptor, including neuroprotection against *N*-methyl-D-aspartate–induced toxicity and enhancement of morphine-induced antinociception, are also being investigated.[66] Additionally, some antipsychotics also antagonize this receptor.[30,281]

Xenobiotics

Table 13–7 provides examples of xenobiotics that affect serotonergic neurotransmission.

Serotonin Agonists

Orally ingested 5-HT is rapidly metabolized via intestinal and hepatic MAO. However, L-tryptophan, the amino acid precursor to 5-HT, is readily absorbed by the intestines. In fact, it was used as an unproven sleep aid until it was associated with the eosinophilia myalgia syndrome in 1990.[28] 5-Hydroxytryptophan (5-OHT), the immediate precursor to 5-HT, is available without a prescription. The anxiolytics, buspirone, gepirone, and ipsapirone act as partial agonists at somatodendritic and postsynaptic 5-HT$_{1A}$ receptors. Sumatriptan, an antimigraine medication, mainly activates 5-HT$_{1B}$ and 5-HT$_{1D}$ receptors.[202] The action of sumatriptan results from vasoconstriction of meningeal and other cranial, extracerebral vasculature; no impairment of cerebral blood flow follows its use. Other members of the triptan class include almotriptan, eletriptan, frovatriptan, naratriptan, rizatriptan, and zolmitriptan. Vilazodone is an antidepressant with both partial 5-HT$_{1A}$ receptor agonism and SERT inhibition.[62] Flibanserin, approved for hypoactive sexual desire disorder in women, is both a 5-HT$_{1A}$ agonist and 5-HT$_{2A}$ antagonist.[33]

Metoclopramide and tegaserod are prokinetic drugs that activate 5-HT$_4$ receptors to increase gut motility.[194] Because 5-HT$_4$ receptors are also found

TABLE 13–7	Examples of Xenobiotics Affecting Serotonergic Neurotransmission
Serotonin Agonism	Lamotrigine
Enhance 5-HT synthesis	Meperidine
L-Tryptophan	Nefazodone
5-Hydroxytryptophan	NSSRIs
Direct 5-HT agonists	SSRIs
Buspirone	Tramadol
Cisapride	Vilazodone
Ergots and indoles	Vortioxetine
Flibanserin	**Serotonin Antagonism**
Hallucinogenic substituted amphetamines	Direct 5-HT antagonists
mCPP	Agomelatine
Lisuride	Alosetron
Lurasidone	Aripiprazole
Mescaline	Clozapine
Metoclopramide	Cyclic antidepressants
Tegaserod	Cyproheptadine
Triptans	Ergots and indoles (eg, LSD)
Vilazodone	Flibanserin
Vortioxetine	Granisetron
Increase 5-HT release	Haloperidol
Amphetamine	Ketanserin
Cocaine	Lurasidone
Dexfenfluramine	Mescaline
Dextromethorphan	Methysergide
L-DOPA	Metoclopramide
Fenfluramine	Mirtazapine
MDMA	Nefazodone
Mirtazapine	Olanzapine
Reserpine (initial)	Ondansetron
Increase 5-HT tone by unknown mechanism	Paliperidone
Lithium	Palonosetron
Inhibit 5-HT breakdown	Phenothiazines
MAOIs	Phentolamine
Inhibit 5-HT reuptake	Propranolol
Amoxapine	Quetiapine
Amphetamines	Risperidone
Atomoxetine	Trazodone
Carbamazepine	Vortioxetine
Clomipramine[a]	Ziprasidone
Cocaine	Enhance 5-HT uptake
Cyclic antidepressants	Tianeptine
Dextromethorphan	Inhibit vesicle uptake
Duloxetine	Reserpine
	Ketanserin
	Tetrabenazine

[a]Clomipramine is the most potent 5-HT uptake inhibitor of the cyclic antidepressants.

5-HT, serotonin; LSD = lysergic acid diethylamide; MAOI = monoamine oxidase inhibitor; mCPP = *m*-chlorophenylpiperazine (metabolite of trazodone and nefazodone); MDMA = methylenedioxymethamphetamine.

SSRIs=selective serotonin reuptake inhibitors; NSSRIs=nonselective serotonin reuptake inhibitors

in the heart and urinary bladder detrusor muscle, 5-HT$_4$ agonists occasionally produce urinary incontinence and tachycardia.

Numerous indoles and phenylalkylamines, including ergot alkaloids, lysergic acid diethylamide (LSD), psilocybin, and mescaline, exhibit both agonistic and antagonistic properties at multiple 5-HT receptors. Their hallucinogenic/illusionogenic action is best explained by partial agonism at 5-HT$_{2A}$ receptors.[89] Some substituted amphetamines (eg, methylene-dioxymethamphetamine, XTC) directly stimulate 5-HT receptors.[275]

Cocaine and indirect-acting sympathomimetics, especially amphetamines, cause 5-HT release as previously described.[275] Centrally, DA undergoes uptake into serotonergic neurons to displace 5-HT from the neuron. Ingestion of L-dopa or other xenobiotics that increase synaptic DA concentrations can cause 5-HT release.[186]

Inhibitors of 5-HT reuptake include amphetamines, cocaine, various antidepressants, meperidine, tramadol, and dextromethorphan. Several antidepressants more specifically inhibit 5-HT reuptake. Examples of selective 5-HT reuptake inhibitors (SSRIs) include fluoxetine, sertraline, paroxetine, and citalopram. The use of SSRIs sometimes produces extrapyramidal side effects for reasons that remain unclear because of the numerous actions of 5-HT in the basal ganglia.[103] Vortioxetine is an SSRI that acts as a full agonist at the 5-HT$_{1A}$ and a partial agonist at the 5-HT$_{1B}$ receptors; conversely, it acts as an antagonist at 5-HT$_{1D}$, 5-HT$_3$, and 5-HT$_7$ receptors.[251] Two antiepileptics, carbamazepine and lamotrigine, inhibit 5-HT reuptake.[268] Again, reserpine and tetrabenazine prevent 5-HT uptake into vesicles.

Monoamine oxidase (MAO-A) accounts for most 5-HT degradation, and nonspecific MAOIs and MAO-A inhibitors (clorgyline, moclobemide) raise cytoplasmic 5-HT concentrations and, through indirect action, probably cause 5-HT release. Some medications (eg, methylene blue, procarbazine, linezolid) have the undesired side effect of causing MAO inhibition, which occasionally produces serotonin toxicity when combined with other serotonergic drugs.

Serotonin Antagonists

Trazodone and nefazodone act mainly as antagonists at 5-HT$_2$ receptors, but are also weak reuptake inhibitors. Both undergo metabolism to *m*-chlorophenylpiperazine (mCPP), which activates most 5-HT receptors, but is especially active at 5-HT$_{2C}$ receptors. Agomelatine is an antidepressant that antagonizes 5-HT$_{2C}$ receptors and stimulates melatonin MT$_1$ and MT$_2$ receptors.[71] Ketanserin and ritanserin specifically antagonize 5-HT$_{2C}$ receptors, while methysergide and cyproheptadine antagonize 5-HT$_1$ and 5-HT$_2$ receptors.[196]

Mirtazapine exhibits complex actions, including antagonism of 5-HT$_{2A}$, 5-HT$_{2C}$, and 5-HT$_3$ receptors.[92] It also indirectly increases 5-HT$_{1A}$ activity and enhances release of NE through antagonism of α_2-adrenergic receptors. Mirtazapine demonstrates potent antagonism of histaminic and muscarinic receptors.[92]

Most antipsychotics and cyclic antidepressants antagonize 5-HT$_{2A}$ and, to a lesser extent, 5-HT$_{2C}$ receptors. In fact, investigators are interested in developing antipsychotics similar to risperidone that possess potent antagonistic properties at 5-HT$_2$ receptors, without accompanying potent DA receptor antagonism, in order to limit extrapyramidal side effects. These investigations resulted in the introduction of olanzapine, sertindole, ziprasidone, zotepine, quetiapine, and amisulpride.[184]

5-Hydroxytryptamine (5-HT$_3$) receptor antagonists are commonly used as antiemetics. The first-generation 5-HT$_3$ receptor antagonists include ondansetron, granisetron, and dolasetron. Their antiemetic action is explained by several mechanisms, including antagonism of 5-HT$_3$ receptors in the CTZ and on visceral afferent neurons leading to the vomiting center in the medulla. Peripheral 5-HT$_3$ receptor antagonism in the gut prevents ACh release, decreasing gut motility. Alosetron was taken off the market because of ischemic colitis and severe constipation before being reintroduced with an indication for severe diarrhea-predominant irritable bowel syndrome (IBS-D) in women, only. Palonosetron is a second-generation receptor antagonist that causes receptor internalization and inhibits crosstalk with the neurokinin-1 receptor, making it effective for both acute and delayed phase chemotherapy-induced nausea and vomiting.[243] Metoclopramide antagonizes 5-HT$_3$ and D$_2$ receptors.

Tianeptine is an antidepressant with several pharmacologic effects, including enhancement of 5-HT reuptake, thus lowering synaptic 5-HT concentrations.[232]

Serotonin Toxicity

Serotonin toxicity (formerly called serotonin syndrome) represents an iatrogenic and largely idiosyncratic condition that is most commonly caused by the combination of 2 or more proserotonergic xenobiotics, although it can happen following single 5-HT agonists in overdose or at therapeutic dosages.[190] Animal models indicate that serotonin toxicity is prevented by the blockade of 5-HT$_{1A}$ receptors and 5-HT$_{2A}$ receptors.[111,196,199] Serotonin toxicity is characterized by alterations in mentation and cognition, autonomic nervous system dysfunction, and neuromuscular abnormalities. Symptoms include confusion, agitation, convulsions, coma, tachycardia, diaphoresis, hyperthermia, hypertension, shivering, myoclonus, tremor, hyperreflexia, and muscle rigidity (especially of legs).[190] Serotonin toxicity is often confused with neuroleptic malignant syndrome in its more severe presentation due to their similar manifestations. Serotonin toxicity usually responds to supportive care alone but temporally improves with 5-HT$_{1A}$ and 5-HT$_{2A}$ receptor antagonists such as cyproheptadine.[35,190] Serotonin toxicity results from xenobiotics that increase CNS 5-HT neurotransmission (Table 13–7). In addition, xenobiotics that act to increase CNS DA concentrations, such as levodopa and bromocriptine, have potential to precipitate serotonin toxicity by indirectly causing 5-HT release (Chap. 69).

γ-AMINOBUTYRIC ACID

γ-Aminobutyric acid (GABA) is one of 2 main inhibitory neurotransmitters of the central nervous system (glycine is discussed later). Xenobiotics that enhance GABA activity are generally used as antiepileptics, sedative-hypnotics, anxiolytics, and general anesthetics. Xenobiotics that antagonize GABA activity typically produce CNS excitation and convulsions. GABA is synthesized from glutamate, the brain's main excitatory neurotransmitter.

In general, GABA inhibition predominates in the brain. In the spinal cord, through monosynaptic and polysynaptic reflex pathways, GABA mediates a number of physiologically minor peripheral effects outside the CNS (eg, vasodilation, bladder relaxation). Spinal cord GABA is important in attenuating skeletal muscle reflex arcs.[175]

Synthesis, Release, and Reuptake

Figure 13–9 illustrates GABA synthesis. Glutamate is converted to GABA via glutamic acid decarboxylase (GAD), which requires pyridoxal phosphate (PLP) as a cofactor. Pyridoxal phosphate is synthesized from pyridoxine (vitamin B$_6$) by the enzyme pyridoxine kinase (PK).[187] VGAT, also known as VIAAT (vesicular inhibitory amino acid transporter), transports GABA into vesicles from where it is released through Ca^{2+}-dependent exocytosis into the synapse.[175] Reuptake of GABA from the synapse back into the presynaptic neurons is mediated by the Na$^+$-dependent transporter, GAT-1, whereas uptake into glial cells and possibly postsynaptic neurons is mediated by GAT-2, GAT-3, and GAT-4. Evidence also suggests that GABA is released into the synapse from cytoplasm by reverse transport under some conditions. In glial cells, cytoplasmic GABA can undergo degradation by GABA-transaminase (GABA-T) to succinic semialdehyde (SSA), part of which then undergoes oxidation to succinate. GABA-T also requires PLP as a cofactor.[209] The transamination of GABA to SSA by GABA-T results in the conversion of α-ketoglutarate to glutamate, which then moves back into neurons to be used for resynthesis of GABA.

GABA Receptors

There are 2 main types of GABA receptors (Table 13–8). GABA$_A$ receptors are members of pentameric ligand-gated ion channel family, along with nicotinic ACh, 5-HT$_3$, and inhibitory glycine receptors.[211] γ Aminobutyric acid (GABA$_A$) receptors are Cl$^-$ channels that mediate inhibition by allowing Cl$^-$ to move into and hyperpolarize the neuron. Most GABA$_A$ receptors are located postsynaptically and mediate fast or *phasic* inhibition. About 5% to 10% of GABA$_A$ receptors are located outside the synapse and are responsible for slower *tonic* current that is present at resting membrane potential.[102,164,195,250] Situated at various sites in relation to the GABA recognition site on the Cl$^-$ channel are sites for exogenous and endogenous modulators where numerous excitatory and depressant xenobiotics bind, and through

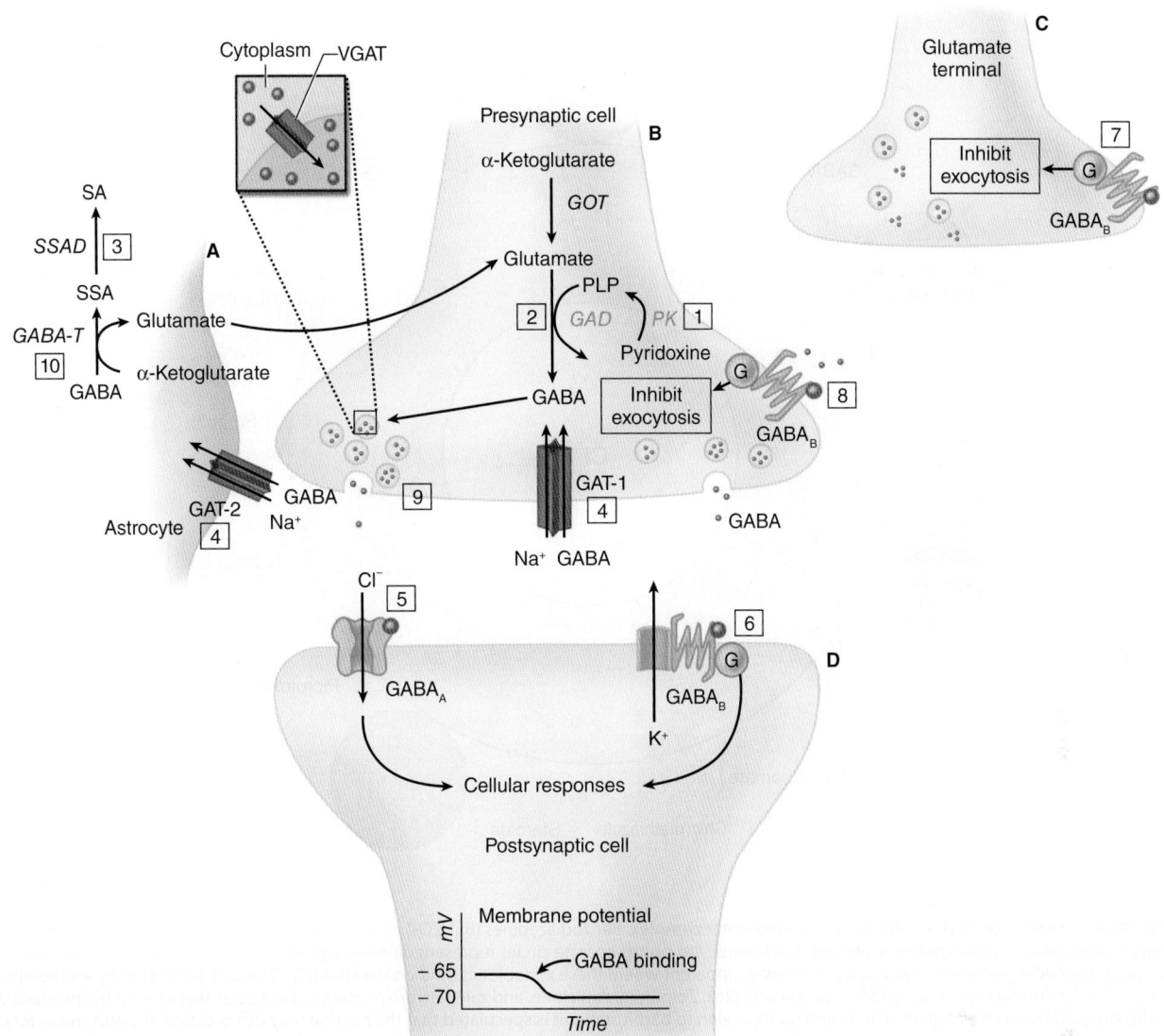

FIGURE 13–9. GABAergic neurotransmission. γ-aminobutyric acid (GABA) released from a presynaptic neuron (B) binds to postsynaptic GABA$_A$ or GABA$_B$ receptors to hyperpolarize and inhibit neuron D [5,6] or to presynaptic GABA$_B$ heteroreceptors on neuron C [7] to inhibit neurotransmitter release by blocking Ca^{2+} influx (an excitatory glutamatergic neuron is shown as an example). Stimulation of GABA$_B$ autoreceptors on neuron B [8] also reduces further release of GABA. Synaptic GABA undergoes reuptake into the presynaptic neuron by GAT-1, and uptake into glial cells and possibly postsynaptic neurons by GAT-2, GAT-3, and GAT-4 (GAT-2 is shown mediating uptake into glial cell A as an example.) Acute falls in pyridoxal phosphate (PLP) lead to impaired glutamic acid decarboxylase (GAD) activity and low GABA concentrations. Although GABA-transaminase (GABA-T) also requires PLP, acute falls in PLP do not affect this enzyme as dramatically because of tight PLP binding to the GABA-T complex. Xenobiotics in Table 13–9 act to impair PLP formation by inhibiting pyridoxine kinase (PK) [1]; to increase GABA concentrations by either stimulating GAD [2] or inhibiting SSAD [3]; to inhibit GABA reuptake [4]; to stimulate or block GABA receptors [5–8]; to cause GABA release [9]; or to inhibit GABA-T [10]. Glutamic-oxaloacetic transaminase (GOT), GABA-T, and SSAD are mitochondrial enzymes. G = G protein; GAT = membrane GABA reuptake transporter; SA = succinic acid; SSA = succinic semialdehyde; SSAD = SSA dehydrogenase; VGAT = vesicle membrane GABA uptake transporter; VGAT = Vesicular GABA transporter.

TABLE 13–8	GABA Receptors and Their Characteristics	
	GABA$_A$	GABA$_B$
Receptor	Cl$^-$ Channel	G Protein–Coupled
Baclofen agonism	Yes	No
Barbiturate agonism	No	Yes
Benzodiazepine agonism	Yes	No
Bicuculline antagonism	Yes	No
Picrotoxin antagonism	Yes	No

which GABA$_A$ receptor responsiveness is regulated under normal physiologic conditions (Fig. 13–10). The common denominator for modulation at the GABA$_A$ complex is an increase or decrease in inward Cl$^-$ current.

γ Aminobutyric acid (GABA$_A$) receptors exist as pentamers, composed of various subunits, and throughout the CNS there are regional variations in expressions of multiple subunit genes for GABA$_A$ complexes.[211] To date 19 subunits are identified (α$_1$-α$_6$, β$_1$-β$_3$, γ$_1$-γ$_3$, δ, ε, θ, π, ρ$_1$-ρ$_3$). γ Aminobutyric acid (GABA$_A$) receptors are composed most commonly of 2 α subunits, 2 β subunits, and either a γ or δ subunit. Multiple isoforms of subunits exist, but within a single receptor, the isoforms of individual subunits appear to be identical. Although the large numbers of isoforms and different combinations of subunits could theoretically produce more than 2,000 different GABA$_A$ Cl$^-$ channels, only a few dozen combinations exist naturally.[60,195] The

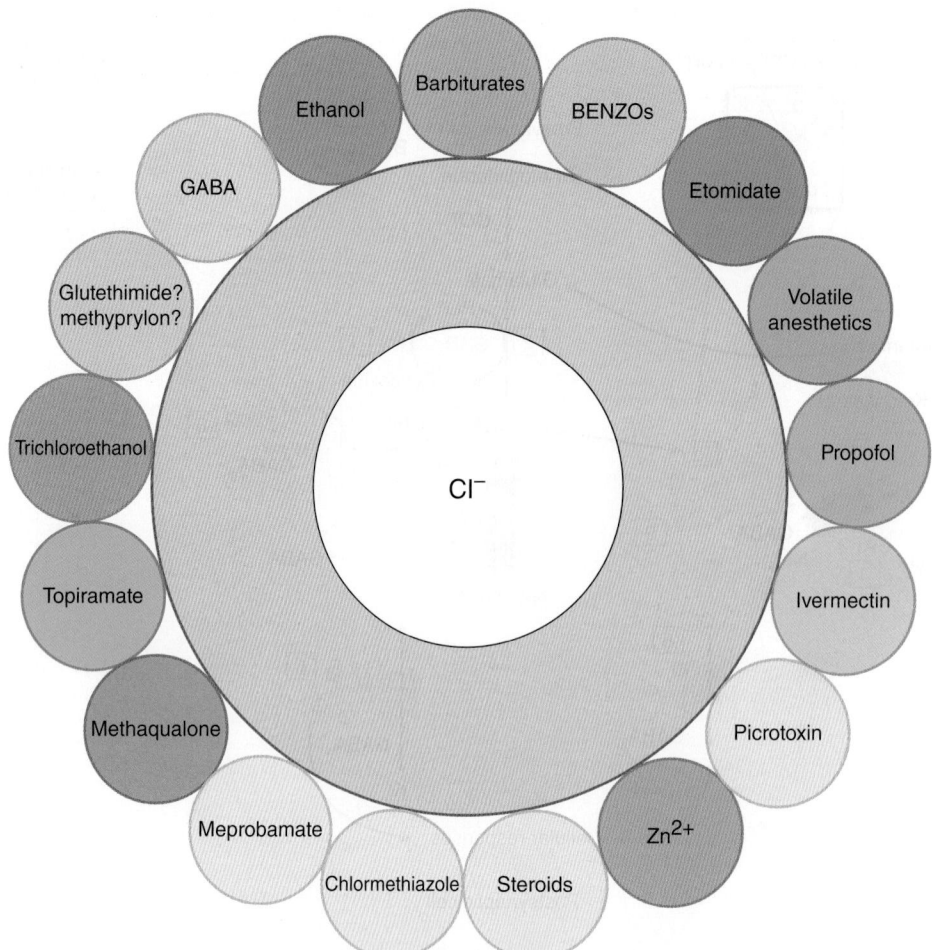

FIGURE 13–10. Representation of the GABA$_A$ Cl$^-$ channel receptor complex. Benzodiazepines (BENZOs), barbiturates, picrotoxin, steroids, and GABA (γ-aminobutyric acid) clearly bind to different sites on the channel. Although separate circles represent different agents capable of binding to and of modulating Cl$^-$ influx through the GABA$_A$ receptor complex, it is not always apparent where these xenobiotics bind on the channel. Chloral hydrate undergoes metabolism to trichloroethanol, which interacts with the GABA$_A$ receptor complex. Zolpidem, zopiclone, and zaleplon are nonbenzodiazepines that bind to the benzodiazepine site. Given the structural similarity of glutethimide and methyprylon to barbiturates, it is speculated that their action may be mediated at GABA$_A$ receptors.

most common is $\alpha_1\beta_2\gamma_2$.[19,263] Previously, GABA$_C$ receptors were classified as a separate type of GABA receptor, but are now classified as GABA$_A$ receptors comprising homo-oligomers and hetero-oligomers formed by ρ subunits (ρ$_1$ to ρ$_3$).

The second type of GABA receptor, GABA$_B$, is a G protein–coupled receptor found presynaptically, postsynaptically, and on extrasynaptic membranes.[211] GABA$_B$ receptors are obligate heterodimers formed by 2 subunits, GABA$_{B1}$ and GABA$_{B2}$. The GABA$_{B1}$ subunit exists as multiple isoforms, with GABA$_{B1a}$ and GABA$_{B1b}$ apparently the most relevant in human CNS.[129] γ Aminobutyric acid or other GABA$_B$ receptor ligands such as baclofen bind to the GABA$_{B1}$ subunit, whereas the GABA$_{B2}$ subunit couples the receptor with the effector G$_{i/o}$ protein.[23]

γ Aminobutyric acid (GABA$_B$) receptors are distributed both in the CNS and peripheral nervous system and mediate both presynaptic and postsynaptic inhibition.[34] Presynaptic inhibition results from preventing Ca^{2+} influx so as to impair exocytosis of neurotransmitter vesicles, including those containing glutamate. γ Aminobutyric acid (GABA$_B$) receptors are found in high density in the ventral tegmental area (VTA) of the midbrain at presynaptic DA and glutamatergic neurons, and animal studies show that their activation reduces DA release in regions crucial in reward pathways associated with addiction.[129,226]

Through presynaptic actions, GABA$_B$ receptors serve not only as heteroreceptors on glutamatergic and other nerve terminals but also as autoreceptors, where their activation in response to synaptic GABA provides feedback inhibition of further neurotransmitter release (Fig. 13–9).

Postsynaptic inhibition is mediated by increasing K$^+$ efflux through K$^+$ channels, resulting in hyperpolarization of the membrane away from threshold. In addition to their effects on ion channels, GABA$_B$ receptors inhibit adenylate cyclase via G$_{i/o}$ proteins and thus, the cAMP-protein kinase A pathway, which is necessary for phosphorylation and upregulation of glutamatergic NMDA receptors.[22]

Xenobiotics

Table 13–9 provides examples of xenobiotics that affect GABAergic neurotransmission.

Modulation of GABA Production and Degradation

Isoniazid (INH) and other hydrazines such as monomethylhydrazine lower CNS GABA concentrations by several mechanisms. Most important, they compete with pyridoxine for binding to PK, impairing PLP production.[187] Pyridoxal phosphate binding to the GAD complex is easily reversible.[209] The acute decrease in PLP concentration is rapidly accompanied by impaired GABA synthesis and a decrease in GABA concentration. Lack of normal GABA inhibition produces seizures typical of hydrazine toxicity. Although PLP is also required for GABA degradation by GABA-T, acute decreases in PLP do not affect this enzyme nearly as much, because PLP is more tightly bound to the GABA-T complex and remains associated with the enzyme.[209] To a lesser extent, isoniazid binds to the GAD-PLP complex to prevent GABA formation.

Large ingestions of *Ginkgo biloba* seeds produce recurrent seizures that may result from decreased GABA concentrations. Ginkgo seeds contain

TABLE 13–9	Examples of Xenobiotics Affecting GABAergic Neurotransmission

GABA Agonism	GABA Antagonism
Stimulate GAD	Direct GABA$_A$ antagonists
Valproate	Bicuculline
Direct GABA$_A$ agonists	Cephalosporins
Muscimol	Fluoroquinolones
Progabide[a]	Imipenem
Indirect GABA$_A$ agonists	Nalidixic acid
Barbiturates	Penicillins
Benzodiazepines	Indirect GABA$_A$ antagonists
Chloral hydrate	Aztreonam
Clomethiazole	Clozapine
Ethanol	Cyclic antidepressants
Etomidate	Flumazenil
Felbamate	Lindane
Ivermectin	MAOIs
Meprobamate	Maprotiline
Methaqualone	Organic chlorine insecticides
Propofol	Penicillins
Steroids	Pentylenetetrazol
Topiramate	Picrotoxin
Trichloroethanol	Inhibit GAD
Volatile anesthetics	Cyanide
Zaleplon	Domoic acid
Zolpidem	Hydrazines
Zopiclone	Isoniazid
Direct GABA$_B$ agonists	4-Methoxypyridoxine[d]
Baclofen	Direct GABA$_B$ antagonists
GHB	Phaclofen[b]
Phenibut	Saclofen[b]
Inhibit GABA-T	Inhibit PK
Vigabatrin	Hydrazines[c]
Inhibit GABA reuptake	Isoniazid[c]
Tiagabine	
Valproate	

[a]Directly activates GABA$_A$ and GABA$_B$ receptors as well as being metabolized to GABA. [b]Thought not to cross the blood–brain barrier in meaningful amounts. [c]Major site of action is PK inhibition, though some direct GAD inhibition occurs. [d]Found in *Gingko biloba*.

GABA = γ-aminobutyric acid; GABA-T = GABA transaminase; GAD = glutamic acid decarboxylase; GHB = γ-hydroxybutyric acid; PK = pyridoxine kinase; MAOI = monoamine oxidase inhibitor.

4-methoxypyridoxine, which acts as a competitive antagonist of pyridoxal kinase, thereby inhibiting glutamate decarboxylase and impairing GABA synthesis.[127,192]

Cyanide inhibits numerous enzymes besides cytochrome oxidase, including GAD. Domoic acid (see Glutamate later) inhibits GAD.[61]

In vitro studies demonstrate the ability of valproate to increase brain GABA concentrations, either by inhibition of succinic semialdehyde dehydrogenase or by activation of GAD.[124] Gabapentin may increase the rate of GABA synthesis in the brain by stimulating GAD, although the main mechanism of action of gabapentin is to bind to calcium channels.[279] Vigabatrin, an antiepileptic, acts by irreversibly inhibiting GABA-T.[271]

GABA$_A$ Agonism

Figure 13–10 schematically illustrates the GABA$_A$ receptor complex. In general, GABA$_A$ agonists cause CNS depression, ranging from mild sedation and nystagmus to ataxia, stupor, and coma. Many indirect agonists that bind to the GABA$_A$ complex have no activity in the absence of GABA. With some exceptions, their pharmacologic actions require the binding of GABA to its

receptor and do not result from a direct effect on Cl⁻ conductance exclusive of GABA binding. Many of these xenobiotics demonstrate additional actions that are not mediated through the GABA$_A$ complex.

Direct GABA Agonists The main direct GABA agonist of toxicologic interest is muscimol, found in some poisonous mushrooms. Muscimol binds at the GABA binding site on the GABA$_A$ complex to mimic the action of GABA.[212] Ibotenic acid, a direct glutamate agonist found in the same mushrooms, is decarboxylated to muscimol just as glutamate is decarboxylated to GABA.

Indirect GABA Agonists Benzodiazepines bind to GABA$_A$ complexes to increase the affinity of GABA for its receptor and to increase the frequency of Cl⁻ channel opening in response to GABA binding.[262] The benzodiazepine binding site on the GABA$_A$ receptor is located in a pocket between an α subunit and a γ$_2$ subunit.[291] Benzodiazepines also inhibit adenosine uptake apart from GABA$_A$ activity (see Adenosine later). The historical terms "benzodiazepine receptor" and "omega receptor" (for benzodiazepines) were abandoned, and benzodiazepine-binding sites on subtypes of GABA$_A$ receptors are categorized as high, intermediate, or low affinity benzodiazepine-binding sites, based on zolpidem binding.[249]

It follows that various isoforms of GABA$_A$ Cl⁻ channels differ in their affinity for different benzodiazepines. γ Aminobutyric acid (GABA$_A$) receptors containing γ$_2$ subunits are more sensitive to benzodiazepines than are GABA$_A$ receptors containing γ$_1$ and γ$_3$ subunits. Sensitivity and response to benzodiazepine binding is also highly dependent on the specific α subunit composition of the GABA$_A$ receptor. γ Aminobutyric acid (GABA$_A$) receptors containing an α$_4$ or α$_6$ subunit are completely insensitive to and will not bind benzodiazepines, whereas GABA$_A$ receptors containing α$_1$, α$_2$, α$_3$, or α$_5$ subunits are sensitive to benzodiazepine binding. This has important implications in that development of tolerance to ethanol confers cross-tolerance to benzodiazepines through a change in α subunits. In addition, specific subunits mediate different effects of benzodiazepines. For example, sedating and amnestic effects are mediated through binding to α$_1$ subunits, whereas anxiolytic and myorelaxant effects are mediated by binding to α$_2$ and α$_3$ subunits.[81]

Zolpidem, zaleplon, and zopiclone are non-benzodiazepines that act as agonists at the benzodiazepine binding site on the GABA$_A$ receptor. They exhibit a high selectivity for the α$_1$ subunit and low selectivity for α$_2$, α$_3$, and α$_5$ subunits.[266,291] Selective binding to α$_1$ subunits accounts for their relatively selective sedative properties at therapeutic doses and lack of anxiolysis, as compared to benzodiazepines.

Barbiturates bind to the GABA$_A$ complex to produce several effects.[140,262] All barbiturates enhance the action of GABA by producing more Cl⁻ influx for a given amount of GABA binding by increasing the duration of Cl⁻ channel opening. Whereas phenobarbital does not change the affinity of GABA or benzodiazepines for their binding sites, depressant barbiturates, such as pentobarbital, do increase GABA and benzodiazepine binding site affinities for their ligands, further enhancing inward Cl⁻ currents. At high concentrations, at least some barbiturates directly open Cl⁻ channels to cause Cl⁻ influx.[140] Phenobarbital can directly open the Cl⁻ channel at antiepileptic concentrations. In addition, barbiturates possess other actions that depress all excitable membranes, including cardiac and smooth muscle.

The intravenous anesthetics propofol and etomidate enhance inward GABA$_A$ Cl⁻ currents, and at high concentrations they directly open chloride channels in the absence of GABA.[15] The respiratory depressant and immobilizing effects of etomidate and propofol are mediated by β$_3$ subunits, whereas the sedative effects are mediated through agonism at β$_2$ subunits.[267,307] Volatile general anesthetics also directly activate GABA$_A$ Cl⁻ channels.

Some of the action of ethanol is mediated through binding to the GABA$_A$ complex. The degree to which ethanol enhances the effect of GABA on Cl⁻ influx depends on the GABA$_A$ receptor subunit composition. For example, receptors with an α$_4$ or α$_6$ subunit and a δ subunit respond to very low concentrations of ethanol.[276,294]

Methaqualone produces at least part of its pharmacologic effect through indirect GABA$_A$ activity. Little is known of the mechanisms of action of glutethimide and methyprylon. Their structural similarities to barbiturates suggest that they have activity at the $GABA_A$ receptor. Trichloroethanol, a metabolite of chloral hydrate, and clomethiazole interact at the $GABA_A$ complex in a manner similar to barbiturates, although it is not clear whether they are binding to an identical site on the Cl⁻ channel.[298] Ivermectin, an anthelmintic, activates $GABA_A$ Cl⁻ channels by increasing GABA binding. Meprobamate displays barbiturate like action at the $GABA_A$ receptor and, at high concentrations, is able to cause Cl⁻ influx in the absence of GABA.[240] High concentrations of felbamate also cause inward Cl⁻ currents in the presence of GABA, although this seems unimportant at therapeutic doses.[240] Part of the antiepileptic action of topiramate results from enhanced Cl⁻ influx through binding to $GABA_A$ receptors.[256]

Inhibition of GABA Reuptake Valproate and the antiepileptics guvacine and tiagabine work, in part, by inhibiting GABA reuptake. Although valproate is structurally similar to GABA, its inhibition of the GABA transporter does not appear to be competitive.[205]

$GABA_A$ Antagonism

Direct $GABA_A$ Antagonists Xenobiotics that act by any mechanism to decrease $GABA_A$ activity cause CNS excitation and convulsions by decreasing inhibitory inward Cl⁻ currents. Direct antagonists bind to the same site as GABA to prevent GABA binding, the prototype being bicuculline. Various antibiotics interact with the $GABA_A$ receptor to antagonize the action of GABA. In a dose-dependent manner, both imipenem and cephalosporins directly antagonize GABA binding and produce seizures at high doses or at therapeutic doses in susceptible individuals.[293] Evidence suggests that penicillin also directly antagonizes GABA binding. Electrophysiologic and radioligand-binding studies indicate that norfloxacin, ciprofloxacin, ofloxacin, and enoxacin interact with the GABA binding site to prevent GABA binding.[293] Theophylline and at least some nonsteroidal antiinflammatory drugs markedly enhance GABA antagonism by some fluoroquinolones in vitro.[293] Virol A, from *Cicuta virosa*, appears to directly antagonize binding of GABA to the $GABA_A$ receptor.[285]

Indirect $GABA_A$ Antagonists Penicillin is well known for producing convulsions at high doses (eg, >20 million units of penicillin per day with renal insufficiency), and both penicillin and aztreonam, a monobactam, block the Cl⁻ channel to prevent GABA-mediated inward Cl⁻ currents.[293]

Picrotoxin, from *Anamirta cocculus* (fish berries), is an equimolar mixture of picrotoxinin and picrotin and binds to the picrotoxin site of the $GABA_A$ receptor to block the Cl⁻ channel. Excessive doses produce CNS excitation and convulsions. Some organochlorine insecticides (eg, lindane) also inhibit the action of GABA by binding to what appears to be the picrotoxin site and cause convulsions.[167] Both α-thujone, the active component in wormwood oil, and cicutoxin from the water hemlock noncompetitively antagonize $GABA_A$ activity.[108,286] The explosive RDX (cyclotrimethylenetrinitramine) binds to the picrotoxin site to produce seizures.

Flumazenil competitively antagonizes benzodiazepines, zolpidem, zaleplon, and zopiclone at their binding sites to reverse their pharmacologic effects.[32,263] Paradoxically, large doses of flumazenil exhibit antiepileptic activity in animals. This is explained, at least in part, by the ability of flumazenil to inhibit adenosine reuptake.[227,272]

Cyclic antidepressants, including amoxapine and maprotiline, and at least 2 MAOIs (isocarboxazid and tranylcypromine) inhibit GABA-mediated Cl⁻ influx at $GABA_A$ receptors.[174,270] Their potency at inhibiting Cl⁻ influx correlates with the frequency of seizures that occur in patients taking therapeutic doses of these medications. Impaired $GABA_A$ activity is believed those to contributes to or is primarily responsible for seizures in those patients who overdose on these medications. Their exact binding on the $GABA_A$ receptor remains unknown, although some evidence suggests at least indirect activity at the picrotoxin-binding site.

Some subtypes of $GABA_A$ receptors are susceptible to inhibition by zinc ions.[262] What role this plays in normal physiology or toxicology is not established.

$GABA_A$ Withdrawal Acute withdrawal from all $GABA_A$ direct and indirect agonists clinically appears the same except for time course; the common denominator is impaired Cl⁻ influx. Withdrawal of all $GABA_A$ agonists causes tremor, hypertension, tachycardia, respiratory alkalosis, diaphoresis, agitation, hallucinations, and convulsions. When $GABA_A$ receptors are chronically exposed to an agonist, changes in gene expression of receptor subunits occur, which lessens Cl⁻ influx in response to GABA or drug binding, producing tolerance. Importantly, withdrawal of the agonist produces yet further changes in subunit expression. For example, benzodiazepine-insensitive $α_4$-subunit expression is increased following discontinuation of many GABA agonists, including benzodiazepines, zolpidem, zopiclone, zaleplon, neurosteroids, and ethanol. Expression of other subunits, including $α_1$, $γ_2$, $β_2$, and $β_1$, also change in response to exposure and/or withdrawal of $GABA_A$ agonists.[81] Alterations in $GABA_A$ receptor subunit composition following chronic exposure to and withdrawal of an agonist can, therefore, affect the ability to successfully treat withdrawal symptoms. Although any $GABA_A$ receptor agonist can be used to treat withdrawal from another, some xenobiotics work better than others in different clinical settings. For example, patients experiencing severe alcohol withdrawal have an increased proportion of $GABA_A$ receptors containing benzodiazepine-insensitive $α_4$ subunits, and contain fewer $GABA_A$ receptors with benzodiazepine-sensitive $α_1$ subunits.[42] Even extremely high doses of benzodiazepines in these patients often fail to effectively control severe alcohol withdrawal. A better treatment option in such a setting would be $GABA_A$ agonists such as propofol or phenobarbital that either act on a different site on the $GABA_A$ receptor or directly open the Cl⁻ channel.[15,42] Phenytoin and carbamazepine do not stop $GABA_A$ withdrawal seizures because their pharmacologic effects are independent of $GABA_A$ agonism.

$GABA_B$ Agonists The main $GABA_B$ receptor agonist of toxicologic significance is baclofen, which is used for treatment of spasticity and some types of neuropathic pain. Coma, hypothermia, hypotension, bradydysrhythmias, and seizures characterize its toxicity. The convulsions that occur in patients with baclofen overdose are proposed to result from disinhibition (inhibition of inhibitory neurons). Carbamazepine activates $GABA_B$ receptors, although this is not thought to explain most of its antiepileptic action. Some of the actions of γ-hydroxybutyrate following pharmacologic doses are mediated by activation of $GABA_B$ receptors. β-Phenyl-γ-amino butyric acid, or Phenibut, is structurally similar to baclofen and activates $GABA_B$ receptors.

$GABA_B$ Withdrawal Baclofen withdrawal is similar clinically to $GABA_A$ withdrawal. Hallucinations, agitation, tremor, increased sympathetic activity, and convulsions are the main characteristics. Withdrawal from chronic intrathecal baclofen administration is also accompanied by large swings in autonomic tone (hypotension, hypertension, tachycardia, bradycardia) and transient cardiomyopathy and shock. Reinstitution of oral baclofen therapy following oral withdrawal, or intrathecal baclofen following intrathecal withdrawal is the treatment of choice, when possible.[175]

γ-HYDROXYBUTYRATE

γ-Hydroxybutyrate (GHB, γ-hydroxybutyric acid) exists endogenously and is thought to affect sleep cycles, temperature regulation, cerebral glucose metabolism and blood flow, memory, and emotional control. Toxicologic interest stems from its use in supraphysiologic doses as a drug of abuse and as a treatment for narcolepsy.[26,78,153] γ-Hydroxybutyrate is rapidly absorbed and freely crosses the blood–brain barrier. Toxicity resulting from ingestion of GHB is explained by GHB receptor and $GABA_B$ receptor activation, comprising agitation, tremor, rapid onset of coma, vomiting, bradycardia, hypotension, hypotonia, and apnea that usually resolve within several hours. Although seizures are noted in experimental animals, it is debated whether GHB causes true convulsive activity in human beings. Human experiments with "therapeutic" doses of GHB do not demonstrate EEG changes consistent with seizure activity.[153] Interestingly, patients with the rare inborn error of metabolism, succinic semialdehyde dehydrogenase (SSAD) deficiency, have elevated GHB concentrations and experience seizures.[91] Valproate elevates endogenous GHB concentrations by inhibiting SSAD.

Controversy exists as to whether GHB should be considered a neurotransmitter or simply a neuromodulator, because it is unclear whether GHB is

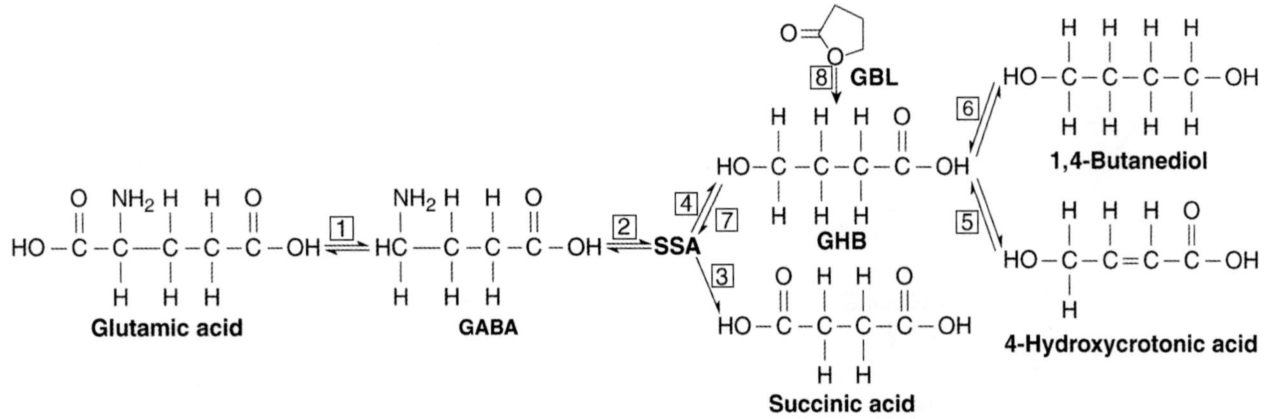

FIGURE 13–11. Potential pathways of γ-hydroxybutyrate (GHB) synthesis and degradation. GABA = γ-aminobutyric acid; GBL = γ-butyrolactone; SSA = succinic semialdehyde; [1] = glutamic acid decarboxylase; [2] = GABA-transaminase; [3] = succinic semialdehyde dehydrogenase; [4] = specific succinic semialdehyde reductase and/or nicotinamide adenine dinucleotide phosphate (NADPH)-dependent aldehyde reductase 2; [5] = mitochondrial β oxidation; [6] = alcohol dehydrogenase and aldehyde dehydrogenase; [7] = GHB dehydrogenase; [8] = γ-lactonase.

concentrated within vesicles for synaptic release. There is evidence supporting a sodium-dependent reuptake transporter for GHB. γ-Hydroxybutyrate (GHB) receptors or binding sites are heterogeneously distributed throughout the brain, with highest concentrations in the hippocampus, cortex, limbic areas, and thalamus, as well as in regions innervated by dopaminergic terminals and dopaminergic nuclei. γ-Hydroxybutyrate receptors exist on neurons, mainly at the synaptic level, but are absent from glial or peripheral cells. At least 2 general GHB receptors are thus far described, based on binding affinity for GHB and other ligands.

Several proposed pathways for endogenous GHB formation exist (Fig. 13–11).[26] Evidence exists for the metabolism of GHB back to GABA, although this appears minimal at physiologic GHB concentrations.[78] However, effects resulting from pharmacologic doses of GHB may result, in part, from secondary GABA formation.

Therapeutic doses of GHB inhibit DA release through activation of GABA$_B$ receptors[299] and GHB affects firing rates of DA neurons, and DA synthesis. Specific interactions between GHB and DA are not fully delineated. Although GHB suppresses signs of alcohol withdrawal, it is also addictive, and both tolerance and a withdrawal syndrome are described. Withdrawal is characterized, in part, by insomnia, cramps, paranoia, hallucinations, tremor, and anxiety.

GLYCINE

Glycine acts as an inhibitory neurotransmitter in the spinal cord, lower brain stem, and retina. In the CNS, serine is converted to glycine by serine hydroxymethyltransferase (SHMT). Some sources of serine include degradation of proteins and phospholipids through dietary intake and formation from 3-phosphoglycerate in a 3-step biosynthetic pathway. It is well established that both GABA and glycine are excitatory in the embryonic central nervous system prior to becoming the main inhibitory neurotransmitters of the mature CNS.[67,148,231]

Release and Reuptake

Glycine is transported into storage vesicles by VGAT (also known as VIAAT) and undergoes Ca^{2+}-dependent exocytosis upon neuronal depolarization (Fig. 13–12). Glycine is removed from the synapse through reuptake by a Na$^+$-dependent transporter into presynaptic neurons and into glial cells. Two glycine membrane transporters were cloned and share homology with GABA uptake transporters. Membrane glycine transporter (GLYT-1) is found both in astrocytes and neurons, whereas GLYT-2 is localized on axons and terminal boutons of neurons that contain vesicular glycine. Although both transporters are associated with glycinergic neurons in the brain stem and spinal cord, GLYT-1 is also found in the forebrain in regions devoid of glycinergic neurotransmission. At the latter location, GLYT-1 regulates extracellular glycine that is available for NMDA receptor activation, and

GLYT-1 inhibitors could then enhance NMDA responses (Table 13–11). Glycine transporters also function in reverse, moving glycine out of the cell.[9]

Glycine Receptors

The glycine receptor is a member of the Cys-loop family of ligand-gated ion channel receptors and is a Cl$^-$ channel that shares significant amino acid homology with the GABA$_A$ Cl$^-$ channel.[169] Glycine receptors are pentameric proteins made up of α and β subunits. To date, 4 isoforms of the α subunit and one isoform of the β subunit are described.[185] An anchoring protein, gephyrin, binds to the β subunit and allows for clustering of glycine receptors at postsynaptic membranes. Glycine receptor activation causes an inward Cl$^-$ current that hyperpolarizes the membrane. Presynaptic glycine receptors are identified that are also Cl$^-$ channels; the Cl$^-$ influx from their activation enhances release of several neurotransmitters. Glycine binding is also important for functioning of the NMDA receptor, as discussed later.

Xenobiotics

Table 13–10 provides examples of xenobiotics that affect inhibitory glycine Cl$^-$ channels. The amino acids β-alanine, taurine, and serine also activate glycinergic Cl$^-$ channels. Both ethanol and propofol potentiate glycine-mediated inward Cl$^-$ currents, just as they do at GABA$_A$ Cl$^-$ channels.[179,185] Volatile halogenated anesthetics, ivermectin, δ-9-tetrahydrocannabinol, and chlormethiazole also potentiate glycinergic transmission.[297] Clozapine inhibits glycine reuptake.[114]

Strychnine and tetanospasmin are the main xenobiotic affecting glycinergic transmission. Strychnine competitively inhibits glycine binding to its receptor, decreasing Cl$^-$ influx.[8,297] Antagonism of glycine produces increased muscle tone, rigidity, opisthotonus, trismus, rhabdomyolysis, and death from respiratory failure. Given the similarity in Cl$^-$ channels, it is not surprising that strychnine binds to the GABA$_A$ complex in vitro. However, the affinity of strychnine for this complex is less than that for glycine receptors, and most of its toxicologic action is a result of physiologic antagonism of glycine-induced inhibition.

Picrotoxin binds to the glycine receptor to impair Cl$^-$ influx.[170] Evidence exists for a direct antagonistic effect of picrotoxin at the glycine-binding site(s), in contrast to GABA$_A$ Cl$^-$ channels, where it acts at a site separate from where GABA binds. Ginkgolide X inhibits the glycine receptor by directly blocking the Cl$^-$ channel.[116] Tetanus toxin (tetanospasmin) produces rigidity and trismus by preventing glycine release from neuronal terminals in the spinal cord and brain stem.

GLUTAMATE

Glutamate is the main excitatory neurotransmitter in the CNS and the immediate precursor to the main inhibitory neurotransmitter, GABA. Balance between glutamatergic neuronal stimulation and GABAergic neuronal

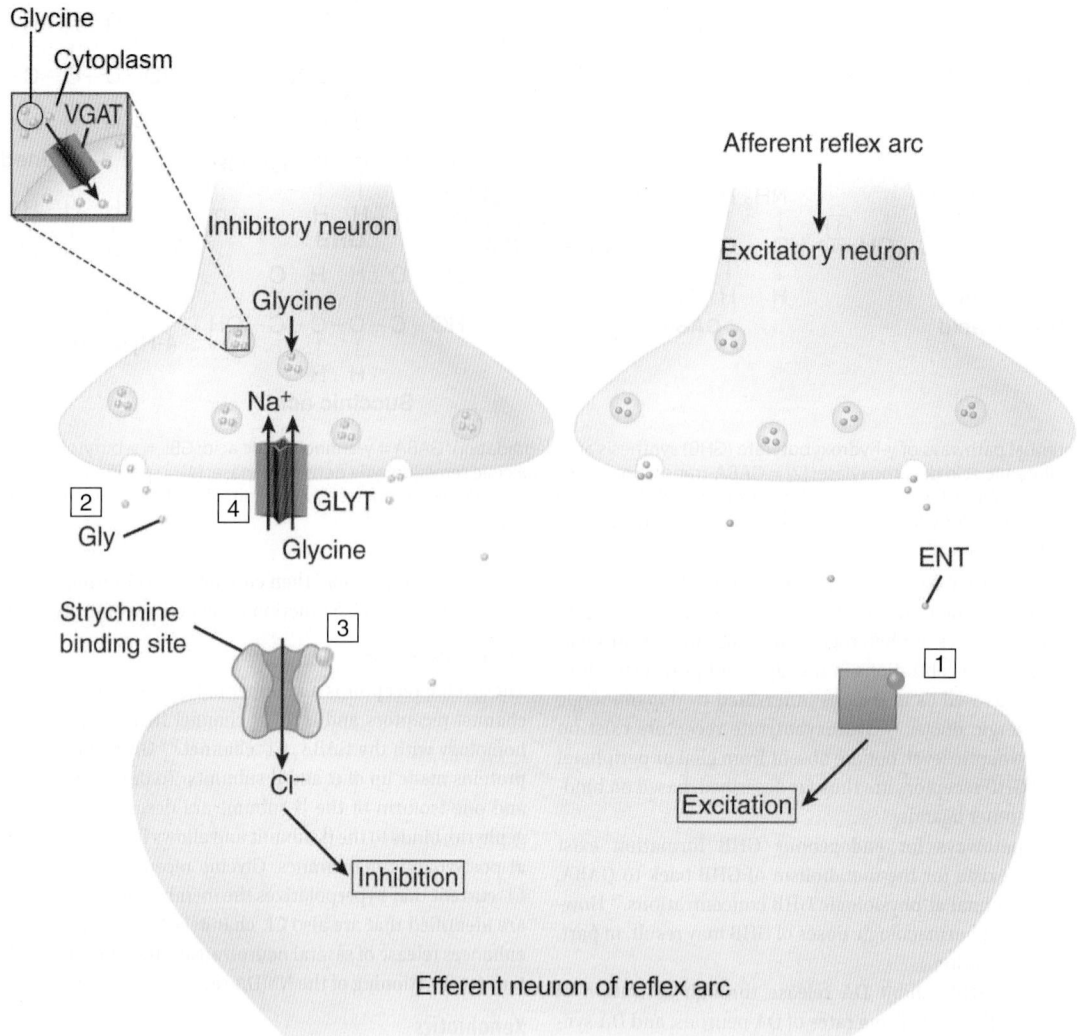

FIGURE 13–12. Inhibitory glycinergic neurotransmission. Glycine is concentrated within vesicles by uptake via VGAT, the vesicle membrane transporter. Signals from the afferent limb of a reflex arc (top right) cause the release of an excitatory neurotransmitter (ENT) that crosses the synapse to bind to a neuron in the efferent limb of the reflex arc [1]. To prevent excessive neuronal firing and motor activity, glycine (Gly) released from a glycinergic inhibitory neuron [2] binds to glycine Cl⁻ channel receptors [3] and causes inhibition by hyperpolarization through Cl⁻ influx. Synaptic glycine is transported back into the neuron by at least 2 subtypes of membrane glycine transporters, GLYT-1 and GLYT-2 [4]. Strychnine binds to the glycinergic Cl⁻ channel to decrease the binding of glycine, which prevents Cl⁻ influx. Although strychnine is shown to bind to a separate site from glycine, there is evidence that these sites may overlap. GLYT = glycine reuptake transporter.

inhibition is essential to maintain normal CNS function.[72,114,126,308] Glutamate is essential for memory, learning, perception, attention, locomotion, and neuropsychiatric well-being.[22,52,67,97] Although glutamate receptor stimulation is essential for normal brain activity, excessive endogenous or exogenous stimulation plays a significant role in mediating neuronal damage in acute, progressive, and chronic psychiatric and neurologic diseases, including trauma, ischemia, hypoglycemia, and status epilepticus.[22,180] A rise in synaptic glutamate concentrations after neurologic insult that induces further damage and apoptosis is termed glutamate-related excitotoxicity.[36,67,171,308] Conversely, glutamate antagonists demonstrate neuroprotective properties and antiepileptic activity in animal models of CNS injury. Unfortunately, clinical trials with currently available glutamate antagonists for treatment of patients with ischemic stroke and traumatic brain injury have proved disappointing.[36,67]

A number of psychiatric and neurologic disorders are associated with altered glutamatergic function, including schizophrenia, depression, anxiety, posttraumatic stress disorder, obsessive–compulsive disorder (OCD), substance use disorders and withdrawal, autism, intellectual disability, attention deficit hyperactivity disorder (ADHD), epilepsy, Alzheimer disease,

Parkinson disease, Huntington disease, amyotrophic lateral sclerosis (ALS) and neuropathic pain.[1,6,52,67,86,87,90,97,114,122,149,171,244]

Glutamatergic pathways intertwine with dopaminergic, serotonergic, and adenosinergic pathways, among others. For instance, illicit drug use may alter glutamatergic pathways, via interactive pathways involving dopaminergic neurons—heavy cannabis and cocaine users having decreased glutamate

TABLE 13–10	Examples of Xenobiotics Affecting Inhibitory Glycine Chloride Channels
Glycine Agonists	**Glycine Antagonists**
β-Alanine	Glycine reuptake inhibitor
Ethanol	Atropine
Halogenated anesthetics (volatile)	Clozapine
Ivermectin	Ginkgolide B
Propofol	Picrotoxin
Serine	Strychnine

in various brain areas.[43,53] It is thought that striatal dopamine modulates glutamate concentrations in the basal ganglia, and glutamate is involved in Parkinson disease with glutamatergic signals from the cortex interacting with the dopaminergic network of the substantia nigra; ionotropic glutamate receptors are being targeted to ameliorate the motor symptoms of Parkinson disease.[43,87,97] Although glutamate-modulating xenobiotics are being developed, with the hope of treating various neuropsychiatric illnesses, initial studies are disappointing.[97,112,292]

Synthesis, Release, and Reuptake

Glutamate does not cross the blood–brain barrier and must be synthesized from products of glucose metabolism or other precursors within the CNS. Glutamate primarily is synthesized from glutamine by the enzyme glutaminase located within the mitochondrial compartment.[82] Glutamate is stored within vesicles and then released into the synapse by Ca^{2+}-dependent exocytosis. Synaptic glutamate that is taken up by glial cells undergoes conversion back to glutamine by the enzyme glutamine synthase. Glial cells then release glutamine, which is taken up by neurons before conversion back to glutamate and subsequent transport into vesicles (Fig. 13–13).[36] Reverse transport of glutamate from the cytoplasm into the synapse by the membrane transporter occurs under some circumstances.[13] There are 5 different plasma membrane excitatory amino acid transporters (EAAT1-5) that differ in their predominant CNS locations. The EAATs play a role in controlling extracellular glutamate concentrations and cross-talk between synapses, making them important therapeutic targets.[36,215,308] Some EAATs function as chloride channels and function more as inhibitory glutamate receptors than as transporters. Interestingly, beta-lactam antibiotics, such as ceftriaxone, and orb weaver spider venom enhance EAAT2 transport activity.[308] Another membrane transporter is the glutamate-cystine exchanger (SLC7A11), by which uptake of cystine causes glutamate release.[308]

Glutamate Receptors

Once glutamate undergoes release into the synapse, it binds to one of 3 ionotropic receptors or 8 metabotropic receptors. The 3 ionotropic glutamate receptors are cation channels and named according to their affinity for specific agonists: kainate, AMPA (α-amino-3-hydroxy-5-methyl-4-isoxazole propionate), and NMDA (N-methyl-D-aspartate). All comprise 4 subunits, with associated modulatory sites that bind small ligands, termed allosteric modulators.[51,67,79,126,131,183,215,229,308] The NMDA and AMPA receptors compose the core of glutamatergic synapses and are responsible for fast excitatory glutamatergic activity, necessary for higher cognitive functions, such as memory and learning.[215] The NMDA receptors are critical for synaptic plasticity and play prominent roles in neurologic diseases.[215]

The 8 metabotropic receptors are linked to G proteins and produce actions that are slower, more diverse, and longer-lasting than those of inotropic receptors.[79,131] A single neuron may express numerous types of glutamate receptors. Every type of glutamate receptor has been identified on both presynaptic and postsynaptic membranes, but many are not active under normal physiologic conditions. This complexity offers protection against the devastating effects of uncontrolled excitatory neurotransmission.

Ionotropic Glutamate Receptors

Ionotropic cationic glutamate receptors share structural similarity, especially kainate and AMPA receptors. These receptors are homomeric or heteromeric tetramers with a central ion channel pore. The inward current carried through most ionotropic glutamate receptors results from Na^+ and/or Ca^{2+} influx.[126,183,282]

AMPA receptors are hetero- and homotetramers comprising GluA1–4 subunits and are the most common ionotropic glutamate receptors found in the brain. These receptors are responsible for most glutamatergic excitation, mainly through Na^+ influx under normal conditions.[46,126,200,217,282] Post-transcriptional modification or RNA editing of AMPA receptor subunits alters ion permeability and function. In adults, nearly all GluA2 subunits are edited, resulting in maintenance of Na^+ permeability, but loss of Ca^{2+}

permeability. In contrast, some unedited GluA2 subunits demonstrate Ca^{2+} and Zn^{2+} permeability.[67,126,183,200,223] These AMPA receptors permeable to Ca^{2+} are more prevalent in many neurologic diseases where they contribute to excitotoxicity.[126,183]

Kainate receptors are named for their affinity for kainate, found in red algae. These receptors comprise GluK1-5 subunits joined in homomeric and heteromeric tetramers.[57,119,126,242] Activation allows Na^+ influx, and lesser K^+ efflux, resulting in neuronal depolarization. Ribonucleic acid (RNA) editing of GluK1 and GluK2 subunits abolishes Ca^{2+} permeability while maintaining Na^+ conductance, but some subunits remain unedited and permeable to Ca^{2+}.[46,223] Recent studies indicate that some kainate receptors also signal through G proteins and are involved in long-term potentiation for learning and memory.[54,225]

N-methyl-D-aspartate (NMDA) receptors are heteromeric tetramers of subunits that may include GluN1, GluN2A-2D, and GluN3A-3B (7 isoforms), but most commonly comprise 2 GluN1 and 2 GluN2 subunits.[22,67,126,128,282,309] The principal endogenous agonists that bind to the GluN1 subunit are glycine and D-serine, whereas the principal endogenous agonist that binds to the GluN2 subunit is glutamate.[122] N-methyl-D-aspartate (NMDA) receptors reside near AMPA receptors, forming a functional synaptic unit at virtually all central synapses.[282] N-methyl-D-aspartate (NMDA) receptor activation allows for Ca^{2+} and Na^+ influx (and some K^+ efflux), resulting in neuronal depolarization and excitation (Fig. 13–14). The NMDA ion channel is normally blocked by Mg^{2+} in a voltage-dependent manner, preventing Ca^{2+} influx despite glutamate binding (Fig. 13–14).[114,128] For Ca^{2+} to flow through the channels, 3 conditions must be met: (1) the neuronal membrane must be depolarized by at least 20 to 30 mV through some other mechanism (eg, activation of an adjacent AMPA receptor) so that Mg^{2+} will leave the channel, (2) 2 molecules of glutamate must bind to the receptor, and (3) 2 molecules of glycine must bind to their binding sites on the receptor.[67,79,128,171] The amino acid D-serine may substitute for glycine at the glycine modulatory site.[17,22,126,215] Evidence suggests that D-serine is the primary co-agonist for synaptic, but not extra synaptic, NMDARs.[17] Thus, the NMDA receptor is both a ligand-gated and voltage-gated ion channel (Fig. 13–14).

Direct Ca^{2+} influx through both NMDA and Ca^{2+}-selective AMPA channel receptors contributes to excitotoxicity. Excessive stimulation of NMDA and AMPA receptors by glutamate released during times of ischemia, trauma, hypoglycemia, or convulsions triggers damaging rises in intracellular Ca^{2+} concentrations, activation of numerous enzymes, and free radical formation, all of which incite cell death.[180] Antagonists of NMDA Ca^{2+} channels are antiepileptic and neuroprotective. Zinc is packaged into synaptic vesicles in axons and is co-released with glutamate into the synaptic cleft during neuronal activity where it acts as a negative allosteric modulator of NMDA receptors.[282,309] Other endogenous substances, such as Mg^{2+}, protons, polyamines, neurosteroids, and fatty acids also modulate NMDA receptor activity.[122]

Metabotropic Glutamate Receptors

Metabotropic glutamate receptors (mGlus) are linked to various G proteins on post- and presynaptic membranes (Fig. 13–13). Eight different receptors (mGlu1-8) were isolated. In contrast to ionotropic glutamate receptors, metabotropic glutamate receptors either excite or inhibit at postsynaptic membranes, and mainly inhibit at presynaptic locations, regulating synaptic transmission and neuronal excitability.[215]

Metabotropic glutamate receptors are commonly subdivided into 3 main groups based on their sequence homology, intracellular signaling mechanisms, and response to specific experimental agonists.[258,277] As a general rule, group I receptors (mGlu1 [a,b,c,d] and mGlu5 [a,b]) reside postsynaptically; activation produces excitation through blockade of K^+ efflux or by activating phospholipase C, producing rises in intracellular Ca^{2+}, resulting in cell depolarization.[52,79,215,258,277] The mGlu5 receptors are physically coupled to NMDA receptors by scaffolding proteins and are functionally coupled to NMDA receptors by protein kinase C.[52,79,258,292] In animal experiments, agonists of group I receptors produce convulsions, while antagonists display antiepileptic action.[79,162,171,258] Negative allosteric modulators (NAMs)

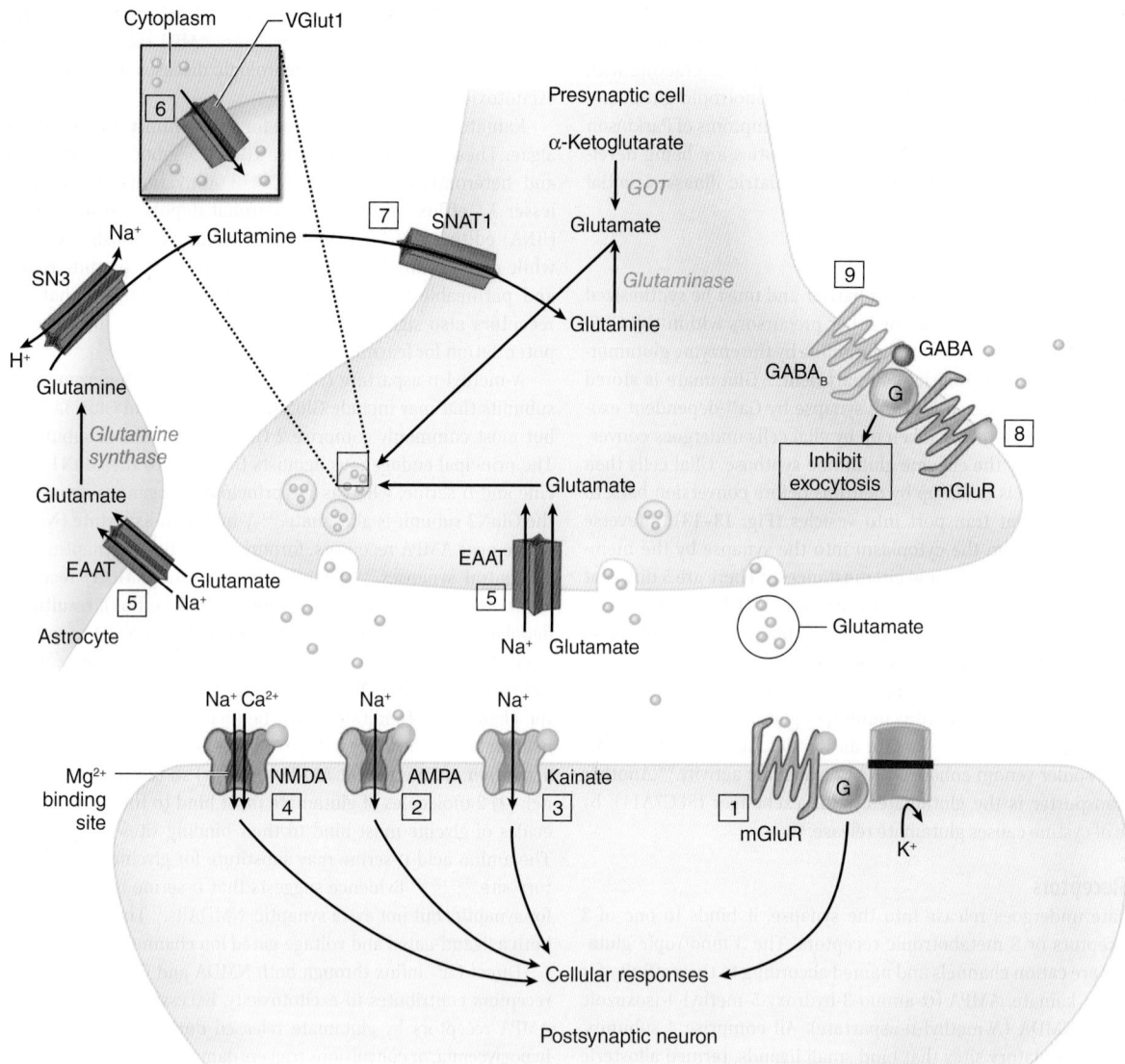

FIGURE 13–13. Glutamatergic neurotransmission. Aspartate aminotransferase (AST) converts α-ketoglutarate to glutamate in mitochondria. Glutamate also forms from glutamine via mitochondrial glutaminase. Glutamate is transported into vesicles [6] by VGlut1 (or possibly other subtypes) for exocytotic release into the synapse. Synaptic glutamate activates 4 main types of receptors. AMPA [2], kainate [3], and NMDA [4] receptors are cation channels. Membrane depolarization in response to their activation causes neuronal excitation through cation influx. All types of glutamate receptors have been found on pre- and postsynaptic membranes, including kainate receptors. However, ligand-gated ion channel glutamate receptors on the postsynaptic membrane only are illustrated in this figure. Metabotropic receptors (mGluR) [1,8] are coupled to G proteins and are expressed on pre- and postsynaptic membranes. In addition, some mGluRs reside outside of the synapse. Postsynaptic mGluR excitation in this example [1] results from preventing K^+ efflux, but other mechanisms of excitation exist. Presynaptic mGluRs act to inhibit [8] glutamate (and other neurotransmitter) release through modulating intracellular Ca^{2+} concentrations, as do presynaptic $GABA_B$ receptors in response to GABA binding [9]. Figure 13–14 provides a more detailed illustration of the NMDA receptor. Excessive influx of Ca^{2+} through NMDA receptors (and through some AMPA and kainate receptors) causes neuronal damage and cell death. A Mg^{2+} ion normally blocks the NMDA receptor channel to prevent Ca^{2+} influx despite glutamate binding. However, depolarization of the neuronal membrane by cation influx resulting from activation of any of the other receptor types causes Mg^{2+} to dissociate from the NMDA receptor and to allow potentially damaging inward Ca^{2+} currents in response to glutamate binding. Glutamate undergoes reuptake by neurons and glial cells by various subtypes of EAAT, the membrane-bound glutamate transporter [5]. In glial cells, glutamate is converted to glutamine by glutamine synthase, and glutamine is transported out of glial cells by the system N amino acid transporter (SN3). Glutamine then moves back into neurons through another amino acid transporter (SNAT1) [7] where it undergoes conversion back to glutamate. Various xenobiotics in Table 13–11 affect glutamatergic neurotransmission, in part, by stimulating or blocking the various glutamate receptors [1–4,8] or by preventing glutamate reuptake [5]. G = G protein.

for mGlu5 receptors are being investigated for the treatment of addiction, L-dopa–induced dyskinesia, depression, and OCD.

Group II (mGlu2, mGlu3) and Group III (mGlu4, mGlu6, mGlu7, mGlu8) metabotropic receptors most commonly serve as presynaptic autoreceptors and heteroreceptors and, when activated, inhibit adenylate cyclase activity.[52,79,215,229,245,277] This, in turn, prevents Ca^{2+} influx and inhibits release of neurotransmitters, including glutamate, GABA, DA, and adenosine. Group II presynaptic autoreceptors are believed to play an important role in decreasing further glutamate release during pathologic conditions, when extracellular concentrations of glutamate exceed

normal physiologic levels. They are positioned outside the synaptic active zone and, therefore, only become activated when glutamate spills out of the synapse.[229] Positive allosteric modulators of mGlu2 receptors are being investigated for the treatment of addiction relapse, depression, and schizophrenia. The mGlu7 receptor is positioned within the active zone of the synapse, but has a low affinity for glutamate, allowing for a continuous but mild inhibitory effect on glutamate release.[229,277] Agonists for mGlu7 receptors are being studied for analgesic effects.[261] Agonists of group II and III metabotropic receptors produce antiepileptic effects in animals.[178] Positive allosteric modulators of mGlu4 receptors are being

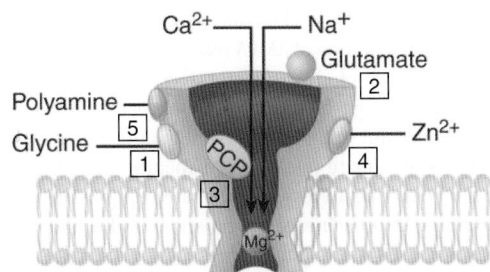

FIGURE 13–14. Representation of the NMDA glutamate receptor. The NMDA receptor is a voltage-gated and ligand-gated Ca^{2+} channel. Glutamate binds to its receptor on the channel [2] to open the Ca^{2+} channel and to allow Ca^{2+} and Na^+ influx and lesser amounts of K^+ efflux. Mg^{2+} normally blocks the Ca^{2+} channel, preventing cation influx in response to glutamate binding. Mg^{2+} leaves the channel when the membrane is depolarized by 20–30 mV. Glycine must also bind to its site on the NMDA receptor complex for successful glutamate agonism. Polyamines bind on the extracellular surface of the receptor [5]. Zn^{2+} binds [4] to inhibit Ca^{2+} influx. The phencyclidine (PCP) binding site [3] lies within the channel. Xenobiotics in Table 13–11 may antagonize glycine binding [1]; block the Ca^{2+} channel by binding to the PCP binding site [3]; bind to the polyamine binding site [5]; or directly stimulate the glutamate-binding site [2].

investigated for the treatment of Parkinson disease, anxiety, OCDs, and psychosis.

The glutamate-binding pocket is so well conserved among the metabotropic glutamate receptors that it is difficult to find subtype selective agonists or competitive antagonists. Therefore, drug development is now focused on negative and positive allosteric modulators (NAMs and PAMs).[245] Allosteric modulators bind to metabotropic glutamate receptors at a site distinct from the glutamate binding site and alter the functioning of the receptor in the presence of glutamate. The NAMs block activation of G proteins by the receptor, while PAMs facilitate the action of direct receptor agonists. Allosteric modulators are being developed to treat hyperlocomotion, psychosis, and schizophrenia.[52,79,245]

Xenobiotics

Table 13–11 provides examples of xenobiotics that affect glutamatergic neurotransmission.

Glutamate Agonism

Kainate is a strong neurotoxin that produces seizures through activation of kainate receptors.[57,95] Domoic acid, a kainate analog, produces amnestic shellfish poisoning, partly characterized by confusion, agitation, convulsions, memory disturbance, neuronal damage, and death.[95,105] The structural similarity between domoic acid and glutamate is thought to explain excessive activation of AMPA and kainate receptors with secondary NMDA receptor activation and resultant neuronal damage.[107] Domoic acid toxicity in birds is thought to have explained their attack on the city of Capitola, CA, in 1961, and may have partly inspired Hitchcock's creation of the movie, *The Birds*.[56] More recently, domoic acid toxicosis produced epidemics of bizarre behavior among coastal California sea lions.[95]

Investigators hypothesize that other naturally occurring glutamate receptor agonists produce additional neurologic diseases. The neurogenic form of lathyrism results from using chickling peas (*Lathyrus sativus*) as a food staple. Neurolathyrism was common in German concentration and prisoner of war camps during World War II and still occurs in some parts of the world. Chickling peas contain L-β-*N*-oxalyl-α,β-diaminopropionic acid (ODAP), previously known as β-*N*-oxalylamino-L-alanine (BOAA), an agonist of AMPA receptors.[142,288] Excitotoxicity with influx of Ca^{2+} likely contributes to motor neuron cell death in neurolathyrism.[288]

Endemic ALS–Parkinson disease in Guam is hypothesized to result from chronic toxicity by β-methylamino-L-alanine (BMAA), which is formed by cyanobacteria symbiotically residing within the roots of Cycads (*Cycas micronesica*). α-Amino-β-methylaminopropionic acid (BMAA) and its carbamate

TABLE 13–11	Examples of Xenobiotics That Affect Glutamatergic Neurotransmission	
Glutamate agonism		**AMPA receptor antagonists**
Direct glutamate receptor agonists		Perampanel
BMAA		Quinoxalinediones
Cinnabarinic acid		Talampanel
Domoic acid		Topiramate
Homoquinolinic acid		**NMDA receptor antagonists**
Ibotenic acid		Acamprosate
ODAP (previously BOAA)		Amantadine
Quisqualate (*Quisqualis indica*)		Atomoxetine
Willardine (*Acacia willardinia*)		Buprenorphine
Xanthurenic acid		Chlorpromazine
AMPA receptor modulators		Conatokins (*Conus* genus snails)
Aniracetam		Desipramine
BMAA		Dextromethorphan
Cyclothiazide		Dextrorphan
Dysiherbaine		Dimebon
Minocycline		Dizocilpine (MK801)
ODAP (previously BOAA)		Dynorpin peptides
Racetams		Esketamine
Thiazides		Ethanol[a]
Kainate receptor modulators		Ifenprodil
Concavanalin A		Ketamine
Domoic acid		Kynurenic acid
Dysiherbaine		Magnesium
Neodysiherbaine A		Memantine
NMDA receptor modulators		Meperidine
Aspartic acid		Methadone
Cannabidiol		Methoxetamine
N-Acetylcysteine		Neramexane
Nitric oxide		Orphenadrine
Piracetam		Pentamidine
Pregnenolone		Phencyclidine
Spermine		Promethazine
Glycine NMDA receptor agonists		Remacemide
Alanine		Selfotel
D-Cycloserine		Tramadol
Kynerenic acid		**NMDA glycine antagonists**
Milacemide		Felbamate
Rapastinel (Glyx-13)		Kynurenic acid
D- and L-serine**		Meprobamate
Glutamate uptake inhibitor		Xenon
Clozapine		**Kainate receptor antagonists**
Nitropropionic acid		Quinoxalinediones
Glycine reuptake inhibitor (GlyT1 antagonist)		Topiramate
Chlorpromazine		**Metabotropic negative allosteric**
Clozapine		**modulators (NAMs)**
Haloperidol		Dipraglurant
Sarcosine (*N*-methylglycine)		Fenobam
Thioridazine		Rufinamide
Polyamine agonists		**Polyamine antagonists**
Neomycin		Aptiganel
Glutamate antagonism		Arcaine
Prevent glutamate release		Argiotoxin (spider toxin)
Diazoxide		Diethylenetriamine
Felbamate		Eliprodil
Lamotrigine		Ifenprodil
Nimodipine		Joro spider toxins
Riluzole		Philanthotoxins (digger wasp)
Sulfasalazine		**Glutamate scavengers**
Increase glutamate reuptake		Oxaloacetate
Ceftriaxone		Pyruvate
Lithium		
Riluzole		

BMAA = α-amino-β-methylaminopropionic acid; ODAP = L-β-*N*-oxalyl-a,β-diaminopropionic acid; BOAA = β-*N*-oxalylamino-L-alanine; NMDA = *N*-methyl-D-aspartate; NAM = negative allosteric modulator; PAM = positive allosteric modulator.

[a]Ethanol is a noncompetitive antagonist of NMDA receptors, with sensitivity dependent upon the GluN2 subunit.

are structurally similar to glutamate,[37] and experiments demonstrate that prolonged exposure to BMAA produces Ca^{2+} influx into substantia nigra pars compacta dopaminergic neurons and excitotoxic effects through activation of metabotropic glutamate receptors (mGlu1), and to a lesser extent, AMPA receptors.[58] Consumption of raw *Cycas* seeds, or flour made from *Cycas*, or of animals that have eaten *Cycas*, results in an accumulation of protein-bound BMAA within brain tissues of humans that can be demonstrated at autopsy. However, autopsies of patients throughout the world with ALS, Alzheimer disease, and Parkinson disease, in absence of *Cycas* exposure, also demonstrate elevated brain BMAA concentrations, and cyanobacteria that produce BMAA are ubiquitous, making interpretation of BMAA's role in producing ALS–Parkinson disease difficult.

Ibotenic acid, from poisonous mushrooms, activates NMDA and some metabotropic glutamate receptors. It undergoes decarboxylation to muscimol, a direct agonist of $GABA_A$ receptors. Glufosinate is a tripeptide and glutamate analogue isolated from *Streptomyces* and utilized in herbicides. Glufosinate produces excitotoxicity in humans, manifesting as drowsiness, amnesia, confusion, coma, seizures or death, through activation of NMDA receptors.[176]

There is in vitro evidence that ketamine causes glutamate release from neuronal terminals. Ketamine and methoxetamine directly activate AMPA glutamate receptors, and this effect may explain their potential antidepressant action.[55,130,157,171,183,217] Despite memantine and ketamine both antagonizing NMDA receptors by occupying the ion channel, overlying the Mg^{2+} binding site, and occluding current flow, memantine has failed to show antidepressant action; this may be due to differences in downstream signaling and expression of key proteins.[122,130] Memantine and amantadine improve the motor effects of Parkinson disease when used in conjunction with levodopa.[87]

Because noncompetitive NMDA receptor antagonism reproduces many signs and symptoms of schizophrenia and autism, investigators are directing efforts at increasing activity at NMDA channels in an effort to treat these diseases,[149,260,305] and potentiating activity at the glycine-binding site should enhance NMDA receptor function. After crossing the blood–brain barrier, milacemide undergoes conversion to glycine, which is required for NMDA receptor activation.[260] D-Cycloserine also crosses the blood–brain barrier to stimulate glycine receptors on NMDA calcium channels.[128] D-Cycloserine significantly ameliorates social withdrawal and repetitive behaviors in patients with autism spectrum disorders.[149] Rapastinel (GLYX-13) is a NMDA receptor modulator with glycine-site partial agonist properties that produces antidepressant-like effects.[65,197] Sarcosine (*N*-methylglycine) is a glycine transporter-1 inhibitor, raising synaptic glycine concentrations near NMDA receptors.[115]

N-Acetylcysteine (NAC) modulates glutamate through the astrocytic antiporter cysteine/glutamate, resulting in stimulation of metabotropic glutamate receptors and activation of NMDA receptors. Also, NAC likely potentiates AMPA receptors. Some have suggested NAC as a treatment for Parkinson disease and for depressive symptoms of bipolar disease.[157] More recently, it was discovered that NAC activates mGlu2 receptors, and it is under evaluation for ethanol, cocaine, cannabis, and methamphetamine addiction treatment.[203]

L-Acetylcarnitine produces rapid, long-lasting antidepressantlike effects by up-regulating mGlu2 receptors and is utilized to treat persistent depressive disorders.[203] L-Acetylcarnitine is also being studied for the treatment of chronic pain.[207]

Aniracetam inhibits deactivation of AMPA receptors and is advocated as a nootropic agent for patients with dementia.[126,139] Minocycline and cyclothiazide attenuate receptor desensitization and demonstrate neuroprotective effects.[118,126,183]

Glutamate Antagonism

Prevention of Glutamate Release Riluzole is used to treat ALS and is being considered for neuroprotection in Parkinson disease and for treatment of depression. Overall, riluzole increases glutamine/glutamate ratios. It indirectly prevents release of glutamate by inhibiting voltage-dependent Na^+ channels and facilitates uptake of glutamate from the synapse by stimulating EAAT activity.[67,171,183] Riluzole also enhances AMPA trafficking, enhances membrane insertion of AMPA receptors, and promotes neurogenesis through stimulation of growth factors.[67,128,171] Lamotrigine diminishes glutamate release through blockade of voltage-gated Na^+ channels and increases AMPA receptor activity.[171] Felbamate antagonizes NMDA receptors and prevents glutamate release.[67] Gabapentin and pregabalin inhibit presynaptic Ca^{2+} channels to lessen glutamate release. The α_2-adrenergic agonists, clonidine, guanfacine, and tizanidine inhibit glutamate release. This action is proposed to explain their efficacy in the treatment of ADHD and the neuroprotective effects in animal models.[141,300] Tizanidine is used to treat stiff person syndrome.[306]

AMPA Receptor Antagonists Talampanel, a noncompetitive AMPA receptor antagonist, was investigated in the treatment of ALS and demonstrated antiepileptic properties.[183] Some wasp and spider venoms contain AMPA receptor antagonists.[183] Fluoxetine and desipramine inhibit Ca^{2+}-permeable AMPA receptors.[20,302]

NMDA Receptor Antagonists Phencyclidine, ketamine, and methoxetamine act as noncompetitive antagonists by binding within the ion channel (PCP-binding site) to block Ca^{2+} influx following glutamate binding (Fig. 13–14).[114,128] Tiletamine is an NMDA receptor antagonist utilized, in conjunction with the benzodiazepine zolazepam, in veterinary medicine as a tranquilizer. There are concerns of human misuse.[64]

Dextromethorphan and its metabolite, dextrorphan, exhibit antiepileptic activity and psychoactive effects in animals. Most of the actions of dextromethorphan are due to its metabolite, dextrorphan, which antagonizes the actions of glutamate at NMDA receptors by binding to the PCP binding site. Both compounds directly block N- and L-subtype voltage-dependent Ca^{2+} channels.[128,238]

Tramadol has multiple mechanisms of action as an analgesic, including a weak affinity for opioid receptors, inhibition of monoamine reuptake, and inhibition of glutamatergic activity at clinically relevant concentrations by an unknown mechanism.[98,117] Methadone, meperidine, and buprenorphine are opioid analgesics that antagonize NMDA receptors at therapeutic doses, and this mechanism of action may contribute to their analgesic effect.[63]

Dizocilpine (MK-801) antagonizes NMDA receptors by binding to the PCP binding site in the NMDA Ca^{2+} channel, producing adverse effects, similar to phencyclidine.[70] Amantadine, memantine, and orphenadrine act as low-affinity antagonists at the PCP site, but are not associated with psychotomimetic adverse effects from such action.[128] Memantine is a low-affinity NMDA receptor antagonist, which is approved for the treatment of Alzheimer disease, but was also recently utilized for the treatment of other neurologic and psychiatric disorders.[22,67,77,171,278,282] Ifenprodil is a GluN2B-subunit-selective antagonist of NMDA receptors that is advocated for neuroprotection in stroke patients.[208] Pentamidine antagonizes glutamate binding at NMDA channels.[70]

Ethanol noncompetitively antagonizes NMDA receptors, resulting in upregulation of this glutamatergic system.[282] Ethanol-tolerant individuals show marked reductions to subjective intoxicating effects of ketamine.[171] In some animal models of ethanol withdrawal seizures, NMDA receptor antagonists demonstrate better antiepileptic action than $GABA_A$ agonists.

Desipramine, atomoxetine, chlorpromazine, minocycline, and atomoxetine antagonize NMDA receptors.[20,166,244]

Glycine Antagonism The antiepileptic activity of felbamate results, in part, from antagonism of glycine at NMDA receptors.[221,301] Kynurenic acid, a metabolite of L-tryptophan, prevents NMDA activation through glycine antagonism. Meprobamate also antagonizes NMDA glutamate receptors by a yet-to-be-determined mechanism.[221] However, given the structural similarity to felbamate, meprobamate might antagonize the action of glycine.

Polyamine Antagonism Polyamines are GluN2B subunit allosteric modulators.[40] Ifenprodil and eliprodil antagonize the action of glutamate at NMDA channels by preventing polyamine binding.[94]

Glutamate Scavengers Glutamate scavengers are beneficial in nonhuman studies of traumatic brain injury, subarachnoid hemorrhage, epilepsy, glioma, and organic phosphorus–induced neuronal damage.[36] Oxaloacetate, pyruvate, glutamate-oxaloacetate transaminase, and glutamate-pyruvate transaminase reduce blood glutamate concentrations, and subsequently brain glutamate concentrations.[36] Other glutamate scavengers include estrogen, progesterone, beta-adrenergic activation, hypothermia, insulin, and glucagon.

Glutamate Receptor Antibodies Glutamate receptor antibodies (eg, anti-AMPA-GluR3, anti-NMDA-NR1, anti-NMDA-NR2A/B, anti-mGluR1, and anti-BluR5 antibodies) are associated with neurologic diseases (eg, epilepsy, encephalitis, neuropsychiatric systemic lupus erythematosus, schizophrenia), and some glutamate receptor antibodies, such as anti-NMDA-NR2A/B and GluR3B antibodies, activate glutamate receptors, resulting in excitotoxicity.[152,160] Perampanel is an antiepileptic that acts like talampanel.

ADENOSINE

Adenosine is an important modulator of brain activity and body physiology. Adenosine receptors are distributed throughout the body, emphasizing its pivotal role in neurotransmission and metabolic activity. The overall action of adenosine is to decrease oxygen requirements and to increase oxygen and substrate delivery.[83] In contrast to classical neurotransmitters that are secreted in discrete quanta upon stimulation of presynaptic neurons, adenosine is found in small concentrations in most extracellular fluids as a consequence of ATP metabolism. In fact, basal in vivo extracellular adenosine concentrations in the striatum are estimated to range from 40 to 460 nM (rat).[16] In the brain, adenosine primarily limits glutamate and ACh release, thereby preventing excessive postsynaptic neuronal stimulation.[161,283] Adenosine also counterbalances the effects of DA stimulation in the basal ganglia.[161,283]

Synthesis, Release, and Reuptake

Adenosine is commonly co-released with other neurotransmitters (eg, NE, ACh, glutamate) into the synapse before subsequent degradation by ectonucleotidases (Fig. 13–15). Intracellular adenosine concentrations increase rapidly during ischemia, hypoxia, or elevated metabolic activity (eg, seizures).[83,161] Synaptic adenosine then activates adenosine receptors on neuronal and non-neuronal tissue (eg, vasculature). The normal cellular preference is to convert adenosine back to ATP via adenosine kinase, but some adenosine also undergoes conversion to inosine by adenosine deaminase.[161] The actions of adenosine are terminated by reuptake into glial cells and neurons (Fig. 13–15).[161,283] Several members of a family of bidirectional equilibrative nucleoside transporters (ENTs) move adenosine down its concentration gradient.[14,295] Under normal conditions, transport is from the

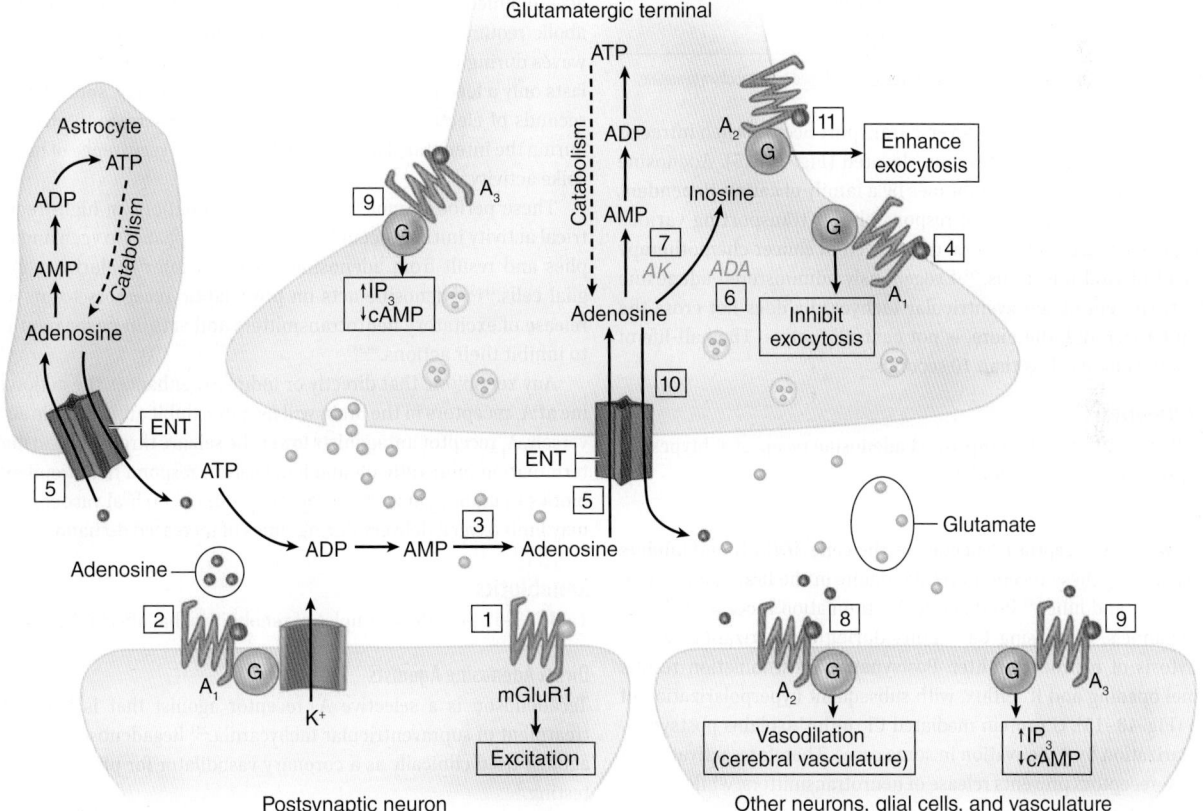

FIGURE 13–15. The role of adenosine in regulating excitatory neurotransmission, using glutamate as an example. In this example, glutamate excites a postsynaptic neuron by activating metabotropic glutamate receptors (mGluR1) [1]. ATP enters the synapse when glutamate is released. Adenosine formed from metabolism of ATP within the synapse [3] binds to postsynaptic A_1 receptors [2], which open K^+ channels to inhibit the neuron through hyperpolarization. Adenosine also activates presynaptic A_1 receptors [4] to lower intracellular Ca^{2+} concentrations, thereby impairing further glutamate release. Activation of presynaptic A_2 receptors has the opposite effect, enhancing glutamate exocytosis [11]. After uptake by ENT [5], adenosine is acted upon either by adenosine kinase (AK) [7] to form AMP, or by adenosine deaminase (ADA) [6] to form inosine. Adenosine also binds to neuronal postsynaptic A_2 receptors (especially in the striatum) and to vascular A_2 receptors to cause vasodilation [8]. A_3 receptors [9] are not activated by normal concentrations of adenosine. During times of excessive catabolism (eg, seizures, hypoglycemia, stroke) when intracellular adenosine concentrations rise markedly, adenosine moves into the synapse through reverse transport via ENT [5]. Resultant stimulation of A_1 and A_2 receptors results in inhibitory actions to decrease oxygen requirements and to increase substrate delivery through vasodilation as described above. However, the resultant stimulation of A_3 receptors [9] may contribute to neuronal damage and death. Not illustrated are cation-dependent adenosine transporters. Xenobiotics in Table 13–12 act to inhibit adenosine uptake [5]; to inhibit ADA [6]; to inhibit AK [7]; to increase adenosine release; and to antagonize A_1 [2,4] and A_2 [8,11] receptors. ADP = adenosine diphosphate; ATP = adenosine triphosphate; cAMP = cyclic adenosine monophosphate; ENT = equilibrative nucleoside transporter; G = G protein; IP_3 = inositol triphosphate.

TABLE 13–12   Examples of Xenobiotics Affecting Adenosine Receptors

Adenosine agonism	Inhibit adenosine deaminase
Direct nonselective agonists	Acadesine
Adenosine	Dipyridamole
ADAC (adenosine amine congener)	Pentostatin
Inosine	Inhibit adenosine kinase
Direct selective A_1 agonists	Acadesine
Tecadenoson	Increase adenosine release
Direct selective A_2 agonists	Opioids
Regadenoson	Inhibit xanthine oxidase
Inhibit reuptake	Allopurinol
Acadesine	Increase A_1 receptor activity
Acetate[a]	Isoflurane
Benzodiazepines	Sevoflurane
Calcium channel blockers	**Adenosine antagonism**
Carbamazepine	A_1 blockade
Cyclic antidepressants	Caffeine
Dipyridamole	Carbamazepine
Ethanol[a]	Theophylline
Indomethacin	A_2 blockade
Papaverine	Caffeine
	Theophylline
	A_{2A} blockade
	Istradefylline

[a]The inhibition of adenosine uptake by ethanol might, at least in part, be explained by metabolism to acetate.

synapse back into the neuron, but reverse transport occurs when intracellular adenosine concentrations become elevated (Fig. 13–15). Adenosine is also transported across cell membranes by a family of cation-dependent concentrative transporters that are responsible for transporting various nucleosides, nucleobases, and several drugs used in cancer chemotherapy and treatment of viral infections.[304] Exogenously administered adenosine used in the treatment of supraventricular tachycardia does not cross the blood–brain barrier and, therefore, is not centrally active. The half-life of adenosine in the blood is less than 10 seconds.

Adenosine Receptors

The purine P1 receptor family comprises 4 adenosine receptor subtypes, all linked to G proteins: A_1, A_{2A}, A_{2B}, and A_3.

A_1 Receptors

A single subtype of A_1 receptor is encoded by the gene *ADORA1* and inhibits adenylate cyclase.[155] These receptors reside mainly in the brain, but also in the heart, kidney, and lung.[248] Presynaptic A_1 stimulation modifies voltage-gated Ca^{2+}-channels, decreasing Ca^{2+} influx during depolarization, which limits exocytosis of neurotransmitter. Postsynaptic A_1 stimulation results in K^+ channel opening and K^+ efflux, with subsequent hyperpolarization of the neuron (Fig. 13–15). G protein mediated Cl^- influx explains postsynaptic hyperpolarization by A_1 activation in some cases. Therefore, activation of presynaptic A_1 receptors prevents release of neurotransmitters, while activation of postsynaptic receptors inhibits neuronal response.[161]

In the central and autonomic nervous systems, A_1 receptors serve as inhibitory modulators for numerous neurotransmitter systems; they are particularly prevalent in association with glutamatergic neurons in the CNS.[161] This receptor is prevalent throughout the central nervous system, with high concentrations in the cerebral cortex, hippocampus, cerebellum, thalamus, brain stem, and spinal cord. Agonism of A_1 receptors by adenosine produces sedation, neuroprotection, anxiolysis, temperature reduction, antiepileptic activity, and spinal analgesia.[84,283]

Peripheral A_1 receptor activation produces bronchoconstriction, decreased glomerular filtration, decreased heart rate, slowed atrioventricular conduction, and decreased atrial myocardial contractility.[84]

A mutation in *ADORA1* is suggested to cause a form of hereditary early-onset Parkinson disease and dementia.[113] Also, single-nucleotide polymorphisms in this gene are associated with aspirin-intolerant asthma in a South Korean sample of patients.[133]

A_2 Receptors

The 2 known types of A_2 receptors are encoded by *ADORA2A* and *ADORA2B*, and both stimulate adenylate cyclase.[172] In the CNS, A_{2A} receptors are colocalized with and inhibit D_2 receptors in the basal ganglia.[230,283]

Adenosine (A_{2B}) receptors are expressed diffusely throughout the brain, and are most commonly identified on glial cells. Adenosine (A_{2B}) receptors have low affinity for adenosine, and little is known of their physiologic role.[283] Both types of A_2 receptors cause vasodilation of most vascular beds, including the coronary circulation.[147]

A_3 Receptors

The A_3 receptor is encoded by *ADORA3* and inhibits adenylate cyclase.[248] It is expressed in many tissues, especially lung and liver,[248] but is also highly expressed in inflammatory cells where agonists are being investigated for treatment of conditions such as rheumatoid arthritis.[80]

Adenosine and Seizure Termination

In humans and in animal models of status epilepticus, including those from xenobiotics, there are 2 alternating phases of electrical activity noted on electroencephalography. Periods of high-frequency spike activity (ictal) are accompanied by marked increases in cerebral oxygen consumption and metabolic requirements and alternate with interictal periods of isolated spike waves during which metabolic demands are less. The high-frequency phase lasts only a few minutes before suddenly terminating, sometimes with a few seconds of electrocerebral silence. A gradual increase in electrical activity during the interictal phase eventually leads to a recurrence of high-frequency spike activity.[11]

These periodic, spontaneous self-terminations of high-frequency electrical activity initially occur before neurons exhaust oxygen and energy supplies and result from adenosine released from depolarizing neurons and glial cells.[11,69] Adenosine acts on presynaptic receptors to prevent further release of excitatory neurotransmitters and acts on postsynaptic receptors to inhibit their actions.[69,283]

Any xenobiotic that directly or indirectly enhances the action of adenosine at A_1 receptors in the brain will usually exhibit antiepileptic activity. Conversely, A_1 receptor antagonists lower the seizure threshold and make seizure termination more difficult and less likely to respond to antiepileptics. Xenobiotics that antagonize A_{2A} receptors produce cerebral vasoconstriction and may limit oxygen delivery during times of increased demand.[11]

Xenobiotics

Table 13–12 provides examples of xenobiotics that affect adenosine receptors.

Direct Adenosine Agonists

Tecadenoson is a selective A_1 receptor agonist that is being studied for treatment of supraventricular tachycardia.[224] Regadenoson is a selective A_{2A} agonist used clinically as a coronary vasodilator for pharmacological stress testing.[4]

Indirect Adenosine Agonists

Papaverine and dipyridamole inhibit adenosine reuptake.[84,85] Like other adenosine agonists, papaverine and dipyridamole demonstrate antiepileptic activity when injected into the CNS. Such actions are not achievable with safe systemic doses. Sevoflurane and isoflurane are 2 commonly used general anesthetic gases that activate adenosine receptors.[84]

In addition to their actions at $GABA_A$ receptors, benzodiazepines inhibit adenosine reuptake.[159] This might explain observations that methylxanthines, potent adenosine receptor antagonists, have reversed benzodiazepine-induced sedation in humans. The potencies of benzodiazepines as inhibitors of adenosine uptake show good correlation with clinical anxiolytic and anticonflict potencies, suggesting that such inhibition contributes to their action. The antiepileptic effect of large doses of flumazenil also results, at least in part, from inhibition of adenosine uptake. Carbamazepine inhibits adenosine reuptake, although this is not thought to account for most antiepileptic action.

Evidence suggests adenosine mediates many of the acute and chronic motor effects of ethanol on the brain. Ethanol, possibly through its metabolite, acetate, prevents adenosine reuptake to raise synaptic adenosine concentrations.[10] Excessive stimulation of several adenosine receptors in the cerebellum could explain much of the motor impairment from low ethanol concentrations. In fact, animals made tolerant to ethanol develop cross-tolerance to adenosine agonists. In mice, adenosine receptor agonists increase ethanol-induced incoordination whereas adenosine antagonists decrease this intoxicating response.[10]

There are numerous inhibitors of adenosine reuptake, including propentofylline, nimodipine, and other calcium channel blockers and cyclic antidepressants.[216,220] Adenosine (A_1) receptors located at the spinal cord are important modulators of pain transmission. Cyclic antidepressant-induced inhibition of adenosine uptake might explain some of their effectiveness in treating neuropathic pain.[85] The analgesic effectiveness of opioids is partially attributed to their ability to increase the release of adenosine within the spinal cord.[21,85]

Dipyridamole inhibits adenosine deaminase, raising adenosine concentrations. During times of elevated adenosine concentrations that occur with cardiac or cerebral ischemia, acadesine further enhances the beneficial actions of adenosine by 3 mechanisms: inhibition of adenosine kinase, inhibition of adenosine deaminase, and inhibition of adenosine reuptake.[198]

Adenosine Antagonists

The main adenosine antagonists of toxicologic concern are methylxanthines. Theophylline and caffeine are selective P1 antagonists, blocking both A_1 and A_2 receptors.[11,21] Human A_3 receptors demonstrate very low affinity for methylxanthines.[84]

Peripherally, methylxanthines cause excessive release of catecholamines from peripheral nerve endings (and probably the adrenal gland) by blocking presynaptic A_1 receptors. In turn, catecholamine-mediated responses are exaggerated by blockade of inhibitory postsynaptic A_1 receptors on end organs.[84]

Centrally, enhanced release and actions of excitatory neurotransmitters (eg, glutamate) explain methylxanthine-induced convulsions that are frequently refractory to antiepileptics. The reasons why theophylline convulsions carry such a high mortality stem from lack of A_1-mediated self-termination (continual high-frequency spike activity and large metabolic demands), compounded by vasoconstriction caused by blockade of vascular A_2 receptors.

Like phenytoin, the major antiepileptic effect of carbamazepine results from Na^+-channel blockade. Unlike phenytoin, carbamazepine antagonizes A_1 receptors.[49,59] This explains the higher frequency of seizures after carbamazepine overdose than after phenytoin overdose. The absence of A_2 blockade by carbamazepine theoretically allows for increases in cerebral blood flow to meet metabolic demands of the seizing brain.

Selective A_{2A} receptor antagonists are being studied in the treatment of Parkinson Disease. Istradefylline is used as an adjunct to decrease *OFF* time in patients being treated with levodopa.[230]

SUMMARY

- Neurotransmitter systems share common physiologic features, including neurotransmitter reuptake, vesicle membrane pumps, ion trapping of neurotransmitters within vesicles, calcium-dependent exocytosis, and receptors coupled to either G proteins or to ion channels.
- It is not surprising, then, that a single xenobiotic frequently produces effects on several different neurotransmitter systems. As the number of new xenobiotics encountered by man continues to grow, an understanding of their molecular actions in the nervous system helps to anticipate and better understand various pharmacologic and adverse effects resulting from therapeutic or toxic doses.

Acknowledgement

Anne-Michelle Ruha and Kirk Mills made significant contributions to this chapter in previous editions.

REFERENCES

1. Acher F, Goudet C. Therapeutic potential of group III metabotropic glutamate receptor ligands in pain. *Curr Opin Pharmacol.* 2015;20:64-72.
2. Adriani W, et al. Modulatory effects of two novel agonists for serotonin receptor 7 on emotion, motivation and circadian rhythm profiles in mice. *Neuropharmacology.* 2012;62:833-842.
3. Al-Nuaimi SK, et al. Monoamine oxidase inhibitors and neuroprotection: a review. *Am J Ther.* 2012;19:436-448.
4. Al Jaroudi W, Iskandrian AE. Regadenoson: a new myocardial stress agent. *J Am Coll Cardiol.* 2009;54:1123-1130.
5. Albers RW, Seigel GJ. Membrane transport. In: Seigel GJ, Agranoff BW, Albers RW, et al, eds. *Basic Neurochemistry.* 6th ed. Phildelphia, PA: Lippincott Williams & Wilkins; 1999:95-118.
6. Amalric M. Targeting metabotropic glutamate receptors (mGluRs) in Parkinson's disease. *Curr Opin Pharmacol.* 2015;20:29-34.
7. Andresen BT. A pharmacological primer of biased agonism. *Endocr Metab Immune Disord Drug Targets.* 2011;11:92-98.
8. Aprison MH, et al. Identification of a second glycine-like fragment on the strychnine molecule. *J Neurosci Res.* 1995;40:396-400.
9. Aragon C, Lopez-Corcuera B. Structure, function and regulation of glycine neurotransporters. *Eur J Pharmacol.* 2003;479:249-262.
10. Asatryan L, et al. Implication of the purinergic system in alcohol use disorders. *Alcohol Clin Exp Res.* 2011;35:584-594.
11. Avsar E, Empson RM. Adenosine acting via A1 receptors, controls the transition to status epilepticus-like behaviour in an in vitro model of epilepsy. *Neuropharmacology.* 2004;47:427-437.
12. Baba A, Cooper JR. The action of black widow spider venom on cholinergic mechanisms in synaptosomes. *J Neurochem.* 1980;34:1369-1379.
13. Bak LK, et al. The glutamate/GABA-glutamine cycle: aspects of transport, neurotransmitter homeostasis and ammonia transfer. *J Neurochem.* 2006;98:641-653.
14. Baldwin SA, et al. Functional characterization of novel human and mouse equilibrative nucleoside transporters (hENT3 and mENT3) located in intracellular membranes. *J Biol Chem.* 2005;280:15880-15887.
15. Bali M, Akabas MH. Defining the propofol binding site location on the $GABA_A$ receptor. *Mol Pharmacol.* 2004;65:68-76.
16. Ballarin M, et al. Extracellular levels of adenosine and its metabolites in the striatum of awake rats: inhibition of uptake and metabolism. *Acta Physiol Scand.* 1991;142:97-103.
17. Balu DT, Coyle JT. The NMDA receptor "glycine modulatory site" in schizophrenia: D-serine, glycine, and beyond. *Curr Opin Pharmacol.* 2015;20:109-115.
18. Bard JA, et al. Cloning of a novel human serotonin receptor (5-HT7) positively linked to adenylate cyclase. *J Biol Chem.* 1993;268:23422-23426.
19. Barnard EA, et al. International Union of Pharmacology. XV. Subtypes of gamma-aminobutyric acidA receptors: classification on the basis of subunit structure and receptor function. *Pharmacol Rev.* 1998;50:291-313.
20. Barygin OI, et al. Inhibition of the NMDA and AMPA receptor channels by antidepressants and antipsychotics. *Brain Res.* 2017;1660:58-66.
21. Benarroch EE. Adenosine and its receptors: multiple modulatory functions and potential therapeutic targets for neurologic disease. *Neurology.* 2008;70:231-236.
22. Benarroch EE. NMDA receptors: recent insights and clinical correlations. *Neurology.* 2011;76:1750-1757.
23. Benarroch EE. GABAB receptors: structure, functions, and clinical implications. *Neurology.* 2012;78:578-584.
24. Berger M, et al. The expanded biology of serotonin. *Annu Rev Med.* 2009;60:355-366.
25. Berkels R, et al. Agmatine signaling: odds and threads. *Cardiovasc Drug Rev.* 2004;22:7-16.
26. Bernasconi R, et al. Gamma-hydroxybutyric acid: an endogenous neuromodulator with abuse potential? *Trends Pharmacol Sci.* 1999;20:135-141.
27. Bhana N, et al. Dexmedetomidine. *Drugs.* 2000;59:263-268; discussion 269-270.
28. Blackburn WD Jr. Eosinophilia myalgia syndrome. *Semin Arthritis Rheum.* 1997;26:788-793.
29. Bloom FE. Neurotransmission and the central nervous system. In: Hardman JG, Limbird LE, Molinoff PB, Ruddon RW, Gilman AG, eds. *The Pharmacological Basis of Therapeutics.* 9th ed. New York, NY: McGraw-Hill; 1995:267-293.
30. Bobo WV. Asenapine, iloperidone and lurasidone: critical appraisal of the most recently approved pharmacotherapies for schizophrenia in adults. *Expert Rev Clin Pharmacol.* 2013;6:61-91.
31. Bockaert J, et al. 5-HT4 receptors, a place in the sun: act two. *Curr Opin Pharmacol.* 2011;11:87-93.
32. Bormann J. The "ABC" of GABA receptors. *Trends Pharmacol Sci.* 2000;21:16-19.
33. Borsini F, et al. Pharmacology of flibanserin. *CNS Drug Rev.* 2002;8:117-142.
34. Bowery NG, Enna SJ. Gamma-aminobutyric acid(B) receptors: first of the functional metabotropic heterodimers. *J Pharmacol Exp Ther.* 2000;292:2-7.

35. Boyer EW, Shannon M. The serotonin syndrome. *N Engl J Med.* 2005;352:1112-1120.

36. Boyko M, et al. Brain to blood glutamate scavenging as a novel therapeutic modality: a review. *J Neural Transm (Vienna).* 2014;121:971-979.

37. Bradley WG, Mash DC. Beyond Guam: the cyanobacteria/BMAA hypothesis of the cause of ALS and other neurodegenerative diseases. *Amyotroph Lateral Scler.* 2009;10(suppl 2):7-20.

38. Brea J, et al. Emerging opportunities and concerns for drug discovery at serotonin 5-HT2B receptors. *Curr Top Med Chem.* 2010;10:493-503.

39. Briscoe JG, et al. Pemoline-induced choreoathetosis and rhabdomyolysis. *Med Toxicol Adverse Drug Exp.* 1988;3:72-76.

40. Burnashev N, Szepetowski P. NMDA receptor subunit mutations in neurodevelopmental disorders. *Curr Opin Pharmacol.* 2015;20:73-82.

41. Buscher R, et al. Human adrenoceptor polymorphisms: evolving recognition of clinical importance. *Trends Pharmacol Sci.* 1999;20:94-99.

42. Cagetti E, et al. Withdrawal from chronic intermittent ethanol treatment changes subunit composition, reduces synaptic function, and decreases behavioral responses to positive allosteric modulators of GABAA receptors. *Mol Pharmacol.* 2003;63:53-64.

43. Caravaggio F, et al. The effect of striatal dopamine depletion on striatal and cortical glutamate: a mini-review. *Prog Neuropsychopharmacol Biol Psychiatry.* 2016;65:49-53.

44. Carpenter CL, et al. Dextromethorphan and dextrorphan as calcium channel antagonists. *Brain Res.* 1988;439:372-375.

45. Carvalho M, et al. Toxicity of amphetamines: an update. *Arch Toxicol.* 2012;86:1167-1231.

46. Catarzi D, et al. Competitive AMPA receptor antagonists. *Med Res Rev.* 2007;27:239-278.

47. Chameau P, van Hooft JA. Serotonin 5-HT(3) receptors in the central nervous system. *Cell Tissue Res.* 2006;326:573-581.

48. Clapham DE. Direct G protein activation of ion channels? *Annu Rev Neurosci.* 1994;17:441-464.

49. Clark M, Post RM. Carbamazepine, but not caffeine, is highly selective for adenosine A1 binding sites. *Eur J Pharmacol.* 1989;164:399-401.

50. Clark RF, Curry SC. Organophosphates and carbamates. In: Reisdorff E, Roberts MR, Wiegenstein JG, eds. *Pediatric Emergency Medicine.* Philadelphia, PA: Saunders; 1993:684-693.

51. Cleva RM, et al. mGluR5 positive allosteric modulation enhances extinction learning following cocaine self-administration. *Behav Neurosci.* 2011;125:10-19.

52. Cleva RM, Olive MF. Positive allosteric modulators of type 5 metabotropic glutamate receptors (mGluR5) and their therapeutic potential for the treatment of CNS disorders. *Molecules.* 2011;16:2097-2106.

53. Colizzi M, et al. Effect of cannabis on glutamate signalling in the brain: A systematic review of human and animal evidence. *Neurosci Biobehav Rev.* 2016;64:359-381.

54. Contractor A, et al. Kainate receptors coming of age: milestones of two decades of research. *Trends Neurosci.* 2011;34:154-163.

55. Coppola M, Mondola R. Methoxetamine: from drug of abuse to rapid-acting antidepressant. *Med Hypotheses.* 2012;79:504-507.

56. Costa LG, et al. Domoic acid as a developmental neurotoxin. *Neurotoxicology.* 2010;31:409-423.

57. Crepel V, Mulle C. Physiopathology of kainate receptors in epilepsy. *Curr Opin Pharmacol.* 2015;20:83-88.

58. Cucchiaroni ML, et al. Metabotropic glutamate receptor 1 mediates the electrophysiological and toxic actions of the cycad derivative beta-N-Methylamino-L-alanine on substantia nigra pars compacta DAergic neurons. *J Neurosci.* 2010;30:5176-5188.

59. Czuczwar SJ, et al. Differential effects of agents enhancing purinergic transmission upon the antielectroshock efficacy of carbamazepine, diphenylhydantoin, diazepam, phenobarbital, and valproate in mice. *J Neural Transm Gen Sect.* 1990;81:153-166.

60. Da Settimo F, et al. GABA A/Bz receptor subtypes as targets for selective drugs. *Curr Med Chem.* 2007;14:2680-2701.

61. Dakshinamurti K, et al. Domoic acid induced seizure activity in rats. *Neurosci Lett.* 1991;127:193-197.

62. Dawson LA, Watson JM. Vilazodone: a 5-HT1A receptor agonist/serotonin transporter inhibitor for the treatment of affective disorders. *CNS Neurosci Ther.* 2009;15:107-117.

63. De Kock MF, Lavand'homme PM. The clinical role of NMDA receptor antagonists for the treatment of postoperative pain. *Best Pract Res Clin Anaesthesiol.* 2007;21:85-98.

64. de la Pena JB, Cheong JH. The abuse liability of the NMDA receptor antagonist-benzodiazepine (tiletamine-zolazepam) combination: evidence from clinical case reports and preclinical studies. *Drug Test Anal.* 2016;8:760-767.

65. Dhir A. Investigational drugs for treating major depressive disorder. *Expert Opin Investig Drugs.* 2017;26:9-24.

66. Di Pilato P, et al. Selective agonists for serotonin 7 (5-HT7) receptor and their applications in preclinical models: an overview. *Rev Neurosci.* 2014;25:401-415.

67. Dobrek L, Thor P. Glutamate NMDA receptors in pathophysiology and pharmacotherapy of selected nervous system diseases. *Postepy Hig Med Dosw (Online).* 2011;65:338-346.

68. Docherty JR. Subtypes of functional alpha1- and alpha2-adrenoceptors. *Eur J Pharmacol.* 1998;361:1-15.

69. Dragunow M. Purinergic mechanisms in epilepsy. *Open Neurosci J.* 2010;4:31-34.

70. Dravid SM, et al. Subunit-specific mechanisms and proton sensitivity of NMDA receptor channel block. *J Physiol.* 2007;581:107-128.

71. Dubovsky SL, Warren C. Agomelatine, a melatonin agonist with antidepressant properties. *Expert Opin Investig Drugs.* 2009;18:1533-1540.

72. Duncan NW, et al. Associations of regional GABA and glutamate with intrinsic and extrinsic neural activity in humans—a review of multimodal imaging studies. *Neurosci Biobehav Rev.* 2014;47:36-52.

73. Eglen RM, et al. "Seeing through a glass darkly": casting light on imidazoline "I" sites. *Trends Pharmacol Sci.* 1998;19:381-390.

74. Elphick GF, et al. The human polyomavirus, JCV, uses serotonin receptors to infect cells. *Science.* 2004;306:1380-1383.

75. Eneanya DI, et al. The actions of metabolic fate of disulfiram. *Annu Rev Pharmacol Toxicol.* 1981;21:575-596.

76. Faingold CL, Browning RA. Mechanisms of anticonvulsant drug action. I. Drugs primarily used for generalized tonic-clonic and partial epilepsies. *Eur J Pediatr.* 1987;146:2-7.

77. Fakhri A, et al. Memantine Enhances the Effect of Olanzapine in Patients With Schizophrenia: A Randomized, Placebo-Controlled Study. *Acta Med Iran.* 2016;54:696-703.

78. Feigenbaum JJ, Howard SG. Gamma hydroxybutyrate is not a GABA agonist. *Prog Neurobiol.* 1996;50:1-7.

79. Field JR, et al. Targeting glutamate synapses in schizophrenia. *Trends Mol Med.* 2011;17:689-698.

80. Fishman P, Cohen S. The A3 adenosine receptor (A3AR): therapeutic target and predictive biological marker in rheumatoid arthritis. *Clin Rheumatol.* 2016;35:2359-2362.

81. Follesa P, et al. Changes in GABA(A) receptor gene expression induced by withdrawal of, but not by long-term exposure to, zaleplon or zolpidem. *Neuropharmacology.* 2002;42:191-198.

82. Foster AC, Kemp JA. Glutamate- and GABA-based CNS therapeutics. *Curr Opin Pharmacol.* 2006;6:7-17.

83. Fredholm BB. Adenosine receptors as drug targets. *Exp Cell Res.* 2010;316:1284-1288.

84. Fredholm BB, et al. International Union of Basic and Clinical Pharmacology. LXXXI. Nomenclature and classification of adenosine receptors—an update. *Pharmacol Rev.* 2011;63:1-34.

85. Fredholm BB, et al. Actions of adenosine at its receptors in the CNS: insights from knockouts and drugs. *Annu Rev Pharmacol Toxicol.* 2005;45:385-412.

86. Gandal MJ, et al. Mice with reduced NMDA receptor expression: more consistent with autism than schizophrenia? *Genes Brain Behav.* 2012;11:740-750.

87. Gardoni F, Di Luca M. Targeting glutamatergic synapses in Parkinson's disease. *Curr Opin Pharmacol.* 2015;20:24-28.

88. Gauthier C, et al. Beta-3 adrenoceptors as new therapeutic targets for cardiovascular pathologies. *Curr Heart Fail Rep.* 2011;8:184-192.

89. Geyer MA, Vollenweider FX. Serotonin research: contributions to understanding psychoses. *Trends Pharmacol Sci.* 2008;29:445-453.

90. Ghanizadeh A. Increased glutamate and homocysteine and decreased glutamine levels in autism: a review and strategies for future studies of amino acids in autism. *Dis Markers.* 2013;35:281-286.

91. Gibson KM, et al. 4-Hydroxybutyric acid and the clinical phenotype of succinic semialdehyde dehydrogenase deficiency, an inborn error of GABA metabolism. *Neuropediatrics.* 1998;29:14-22.

92. Gillman PK. A systematic review of the serotonergic effects of mirtazapine in humans: implications for its dual action status. *Hum Psychopharmacol.* 2006;21:117-125.

93. Gilsbach R, et al. Pre- versus postsynaptic signaling by alpha(2)-adrenoceptors. *Curr Top Membr.* 2011;67:139-160.

94. Gogas KR. Glutamate-based therapeutic approaches: NR2B receptor antagonists. *Curr Opin Pharmacol.* 2006;6:68-74.

95. Goldstein T, et al. Novel symptomatology and changing epidemiology of domoic acid toxicosis in California sea lions (*Zalophus californianus*): an increasing risk to marine mammal health. *Proc Biol Sci.* 2008;275:267-276.

96. Goren T, et al. Clinical pharmacology tyramine challenge study to determine the selectivity of the monoamine oxidase type B (MAO-B) inhibitor rasagiline. *J Clin Pharmacol.* 2010;50:1420-1428.

97. Grados MA, et al. A selective review of glutamate pharmacological therapy in obsessive-compulsive and related disorders. *Psychol Res Behav Manag.* 2015;8:115-131.

98. Hara K, et al. The effects of tramadol and its metabolite on glycine, gamma-aminobutyric acidA, and N-methyl-D-aspartate receptors expressed in Xenopus oocytes. *Anesth Analg.* 2005;100:1400-1405.

99. Hasler WL. Serotonin receptor physiology: relation to emesis. *Dig Dis Sci.* 1999;44:108S-113S.

100. Hassaine G, et al. X-ray structure of the mouse serotonin 5-HT3 receptor. *Nature.* 2014;512:276-281.

101. Hawgood B, Bon C. Snake venom presynaptic toxins. In: Tu AT, ed. *Reptile Venoms and Toxins: Handbook of Natural Toxins.* Vol 5. New York, NY: Marcel Dekker; 1991:3-52.

102. Head GA, Mayorov DN. Imidazoline receptors, novel agents and therapeutic potential. *Cardiovasc Hematol Agents Med Chem.* 2006;4:17-32.

103. Hedenmalm K, et al. Risk factors for extrapyramidal symptoms during treatment with selective serotonin reuptake inhibitors, including cytochrome P-450 enzyme, and serotonin and dopamine transporter and receptor polymorphisms. *J Clin Psychopharmacol.* 2006;26:192-197.

104. Heidmann DE, et al. Four 5-hydroxytryptamine7 (5-HT7) receptor isoforms in human and rat produced by alternative splicing: species differences due to altered intron-exon organization. *J Neurochem.* 1997;68:1372-1381.

105. Hesp BR, et al. Domoic acid preconditioning and seizure induction in young and aged rats. *Epilepsy Res.* 2007;76:103-112.

106. Hobson DE, et al. Ropinirole and pramipexole, the new agonists. *Can J Neurol Sci.* 1999;26(suppl 2):S27-S33.

107. Hogberg HT, Bal-Price AK. Domoic acid-induced neurotoxicity is mainly mediated by the AMPA/KA receptor: comparison between immature and mature primary cultures of neurons and glial cells from rat cerebellum. *J Toxicol.* 2011;2011:543512.

108. Hold KM, et al. Alpha-thujone (the active component of absinthe): gamma-aminobutyric acid type A receptor modulation and metabolic detoxification. *Proc Natl Acad Sci U S A.* 2000;97:3826-3831.

109. Hubalek F, et al. Inactivation of purified human recombinant monoamine oxidases A and B by rasagiline and its analogues. *J Med Chem.* 2004;47:1760-1766.

110. Insel PA. Seminars in medicine of the Beth Israel Hospital, Boston. Adrenergic receptors—evolving concepts and clinical implications. *N Engl J Med.* 1996;334:580-585.

111. Iqbal MM, et al. Overview of serotonin syndrome. *Ann Clin Psychiatry.* 2012;24:310-318.

112. Iwata Y, et al. Effects of glutamate positive modulators on cognitive deficits in schizophrenia: a systematic review and meta-analysis of double-blind randomized controlled trials. *Mol Psychiatry.* 2015;20:1151-1160.

113. Jaberi E, et al. Mutation in ADORA1 identified as likely cause of early-onset parkinsonism and cognitive dysfunction. *Mov Disord.* 2016;31:1004-1011.

114. Javitt DC. Glutamate as a therapeutic target in psychiatric disorders. *Mol Psychiatry.* 2004;9:984-997, 979.

115. Javitt DC. Glycine transport inhibitors in the treatment of schizophrenia. *Handb Exp Pharmacol.* 2012:367-399.

116. Jensen AA, et al. Ginkgolide X is a potent antagonist of anionic Cys-loop receptors with a unique selectivity profile at glycine receptors. *J Biol Chem.* 2010;285:10141-10153.

117. Jesse CR, Nogueira CW. Evidence for the involvement of glutamatergic and neurokinin 1 receptors in the antinociception elicited by tramadol in mice. *Pharmacology.* 2010;85:36-40.

118. Jin LJ, et al. The two different effects of the potential neuroprotective compound minocycline on AMPA-type glutamate receptors. *Pharmacology.* 2012;89:156-162.

119. Jin XT, Smith Y. Localization and functions of kainate receptors in the basal ganglia. *Adv Exp Med Biol.* 2011;717:27-37.

120. Jnoff E, et al. Discovery of selective alpha(2C) adrenergic receptor agonists. *ChemMedChem.* 2012;7:385-390.

121. Johnson JA, Liggett SB. Cardiovascular pharmacogenomics of adrenergic receptor signaling: clinical implications and future directions. *Clin Pharmacol Ther.* 2011;89:366-378.

122. Johnson JW, et al. Recent insights into the mode of action of memantine and ketamine. *Curr Opin Pharmacol.* 2015;20:54-63.

123. Johnson M. The beta-adrenoceptor. *Am J Respir Crit Care Med.* 1998;158:S146-S153.

124. Joy RM, Albertson TE. In vivo assessment of the importance of GABA in convulsant and anticonvulsant drug action. *Epilepsy Res Suppl.* 1992;8:63-75.

125. Kaakkola S. Clinical pharmacology, therapeutic use and potential of COMT inhibitors in Parkinson's disease. *Drugs.* 2000;59:1233-1250.

126. Kaczor AA, Matosiuk D. Molecular structure of ionotropic glutamate receptors. *Curr Med Chem.* 2010;17:2608-2635.

127. Kajiyama Y, et al. Ginkgo seed poisoning. *Pediatrics.* 2002;109:325-327.

128. Kalia LV, et al. NMDA receptors in clinical neurology: excitatory times ahead. *Lancet Neurol.* 2008;7:742-755.

129. Kasten CR, Boehm SL 2nd. Identifying the role of pre-and postsynaptic GABA(B) receptors in behavior. *Neurosci Biobehav Rev.* 2015;57:70-87.

130. Kavalali ET, Monteggia LM. How does ketamine elicit a rapid antidepressant response? *Curr Opin Pharmacol.* 2015;20:35-39.

131. Kew JN, Kemp JA. Ionotropic and metabotropic glutamate receptor structure and pharmacology. *Psychopharmacology (Berl).* 2005;179:4-29.

132. Khan ZP, et al. Alpha-2 and imidazoline receptor agonists. Their pharmacology and therapeutic role. *Anaesthesia.* 1999;54:146-165.

133. Kim S-H, et al. Adenosine deaminase and adenosine receptor polymorphisms in aspirin-intolerant asthma. *Respir Med.* 2009;103:356-363.

134. King MV, et al. A role for the 5-HT1A, 5-HT4 and 5-HT6 receptors in learning and memory. *Trends Pharmacol Sci.* 2008;29:482-492.

135. Kiowski W, et al. Alpha 2 adrenoceptor-mediated vasoconstriction of arteries. *Clin Pharmacol Ther.* 1983;34:565-569.

136. Klawans HL, Weiner WJ. The pharmacology of choreatic movement disorders. *Prog Neurobiol.* 1976;6:49-80.

137. Klein MT, et al. Toward selective drug development for the human 5-hydroxytryptamine 1E receptor: a comparison of 5-hydroxytryptamine 1E and 1F receptor structure-affinity relationships. *J Pharmacol Exp Ther.* 2011;337:860-867.

138. Kohen R, et al. Cloning, characterization, and chromosomal localization of a human 5-HT6 serotonin receptor. *J Neurochem.* 1996;66:47-56.

139. Koliaki CC, et al. Clinical efficacy of aniracetam, either as monotherapy or combined with cholinesterase inhibitors, in patients with cognitive impairment: a comparative open study. *CNS Neurosci Ther.* 2012;18:302-312.

140. Korpi ER, et al. GABA(A)-receptor subtypes: clinical efficacy and selectivity of benzodiazepine site ligands. *Ann Med.* 1997;29:275-282.

141. Koyuncuoglu H, et al. N-Methyl-D-aspartate antagonists, glutamate release inhibitors, 4-aminopyridine at neuromuscular transmission. *Pharmacol Res.* 1998;37:485-491.

142. Kuo YH, et al. Comparison of urinary amino acids and trace elements (copper, zinc and manganese) of recent neurolathyrism patients and healthy controls from Ethiopia. *Clin Biochem.* 2007;40:397-402.

143. Kvachnina E, et al. 5-HT7 receptor is coupled to G alpha subunits of heterotrimeric G12-protein to regulate gene transcription and neuronal morphology. *J Neurosci.* 2005;25:7821-7830.

144. Lachowicz JE, Sibley DR. Molecular characteristics of mammalian dopamine receptors. *Pharmacol Toxicol.* 1997;81:105-113.

145. Lacivita E, et al. The therapeutic potential of 5-HT1A receptors: a patent review. *Expert Opin Ther Pat.* 2012;22:887-902.

146. Landis E, Shore E. Yohimbine-induced bronchospasm. *Chest.* 1989;96:1424.

147. Layland J, et al. Adenosine: physiology, pharmacology, and clinical applications. *JACC Cardiovasc Interv.* 2014;7:581-591.

148. Le-Corronc H, et al. GABA(A) receptor and glycine receptor activation by paracrine/ autocrine release of endogenous agonists: more than a simple communication pathway. *Mol Neurobiol.* 2011;44:28-52.

149. Lee EJ, et al. NMDA receptor dysfunction in autism spectrum disorders. *Curr Opin Pharmacol.* 2015;20:8-13.

150. Lefkowitz RJ. Historical review: a brief history and personal retrospective of seven-transmembrane receptors. *Trends Pharmacol Sci.* 2004;25:413-422.

151. Lefkowitz RJ, et al. The autonomic and somatic motor nervous systems. In: Hardman JG, Limbird LE, Molinoff PB, et al, eds. *The Pharmacological Basis of Therapeutics.* 9th ed. Yew York, NY: McGraw-Hill; 1995:105-139.

152. Levite M. Glutamate receptor antibodies in neurological diseases: anti-AMPA-GluR3 antibodies, anti-NMDA-NR1 antibodies, anti-NMDA-NR2A/B antibodies, anti-mGluR1 antibodies or anti-mGluR5 antibodies are present in subpopulations of patients with either: epilepsy, encephalitis, cerebellar ataxia, systemic lupus erythematosus (SLE) and neuropsychiatric SLE, Sjogren's syndrome, schizophrenia, mania or stroke. These autoimmune anti-glutamate receptor antibodies can bind neurons in few brain regions, activate glutamate receptors, decrease glutamate receptor's expression, impair glutamate-induced signaling and function, activate blood brain barrier endothelial cells, kill neurons, damage the brain, induce behavioral/psychiatric/cognitive abnormalities and ataxia in animal models, and can be removed or silenced in some patients by immunotherapy. *J Neural Transm (Vienna).* 2014;121:1029-1075.

153. Li J, et al. A tale of novel intoxication: a review of the effects of gamma-hydroxybutyric acid with recommendations for management. *Ann Emerg Med.* 1998;31:729-736.

154. Li JX, Zhang Y. Imidazoline I2 receptors: target for new analgesics? *Eur J Pharmacol.* 2011;658:49-56.

155. Libert F, et al. The orphan receptor cDNA RDC7 encodes an A1 adenosine receptor. *EMBO J.* 1991;10:1677-1682.

156. Liggett SB. Molecular and genetic basis of beta2-adrenergic receptor function. *J Allergy Clin Immunol.* 1999;104:S42-46.

157. Linck VM, et al. AMPA glutamate receptors mediate the antidepressant-like effects of N-acetylcysteine in the mouse tail suspension test. *Behav Pharmacol.* 2012;23:171-177.

158. Linden CH, et al. Yohimbine: a new street drug. *Ann Emerg Med.* 1985;14:1002-1004.

159. Listos J, et al. Adenosine receptor antagonists intensify the benzodiazepine withdrawal signs in mice. *Pharmacol Rep.* 2006;58:643-651.

160. Liu Y, et al. GluR3B Ab's induced oligodendrocyte precursor cells excitotoxicity via mitochondrial dysfunction. *Brain Res Bull.* 2017;130:60-66.

161. Lopes LV, et al. Adenosine and related drugs in brain diseases: present and future in clinical trials. *Curr Top Med Chem.* 2011;11:1087-1101.

162. Loscher W, et al. mGlu1 and mGlu5 receptor antagonists lack anticonvulsant efficacy in rodent models of difficult-to-treat partial epilepsy. *Neuropharmacology.* 2006;50:1006-1015.

163. Lovenberg TW, et al. A novel adenylyl cyclase-activating serotonin receptor (5-HT7) implicated in the regulation of mammalian circadian rhythms. *Neuron.* 1993;11:449-458.

164. Lovinger DM, Homanics GE. Tonic for what ails us? high-affinity GABAA receptors and alcohol. *Alcohol.* 2007;41:139-143.

165. Lowe TL, et al. Stimulant medications precipitate Tourette's syndrome. *JAMA.* 1982;247:1168-1169.

166. Ludolph AG, et al. Atomoxetine acts as an NMDA receptor blocker in clinically relevant concentrations. *Br J Pharmacol.* 2010;160:283-291.

167. Lummis SC, et al. Blocking actions of heptachlor at an insect central nervous system GABA receptor. *Proc R Soc Lond B Biol Sci.* 1990;240:97-106.

168. Lummis SCR. 5-HT3 receptors. *J Biol Chem.* 2012;287:40239-40245.

169. Lynch JW. Glycine receptors. IUPHAR/BPS Guide to Pharmacology. http://www.guideto-pharmacology.org/GRAC/FamilyDisplayForward?familyId=73. Accessed February 14, 2017.

170. Lynch JW, et al. Mutations affecting the glycine receptor agonist transduction mechanism convert the competitive antagonist, picrotoxin, into an allosteric potentiator. *J Biol Chem.* 1995;270:13799-13806.

171. Machado-Vieira R, et al. Novel glutamatergic agents for major depressive disorder and bipolar disorder. *Pharmacol Biochem Behav.* 2012;100:678-687.

172. Maenhaut C, et al. RDC8 codes for an adenosine A2 receptor with physiological constitutive activity. *Biochem Biophys Res Commun.* 1990;173:1169-1178.

173. Maksay G. Ligand-gated pentameric ion channels, from binding to gating. *Curr Mol Pharmacol.* 2009;2:253-262.

174. Malatynska E, et al. Antidepressants and seizure-interactions at the GABA-receptor chloride-ionophore complex. *Life Sci.* 1988;43:303-307.

175. Malcangio M, Bowery NG. GABA and its receptors in the spinal cord. *Trends Pharmacol Sci.* 1996;17:457-462.

176. Mao YC, et al. Acute human glufosinate-containing herbicide poisoning. *Clin Toxicol (Phila).* 2012;50:396-402.
177. Marazziti D, et al. Distribution of serotonin receptor of type 6 (5-HT(6)) in human brain post-mortem. A pharmacology, autoradiography and immunohistochemistry study. *Neurochem Res.* 2012;37:920-927.
178. Marek GJ. Metabotropic glutamate 2/3 receptors as drug targets. *Curr Opin Pharmacol.* 2004;4:18-22.
179. Mascia MP, et al. A single amino acid determines differences in ethanol actions on strychnine-sensitive glycine receptors. *Mol Pharmacol.* 1996;50:402-406.
180. Matute C, et al. Glutamate-mediated glial injury: mechanisms and clinical importance. *Glia.* 2006;53:212-224.
181. McDaniel KD. Clinical pharmacology of monoamine oxidase inhibitors. *Clin Neuropharmacol.* 1986;9:207-234.
182. Meir A, et al. Ion channels in presynaptic nerve terminals and control of transmitter release. *Physiol Rev.* 1999;79:1019-1088.
183. Mellor IR. The AMPA receptor as a therapeutic target: current perspectives and emerging possibilities. *Future Med Chem.* 2010;2:877-891.
184. Meltzer HY, et al. Serotonin receptors as targets for drugs useful to treat psychosis and cognitive impairment in schizophrenia. *Curr Pharm Biotechnol.* 2012;13:1572-1586.
185. Mihic SJ. Acute effects of ethanol on GABA_A and glycine receptor function. *Neurochem Int.* 1999;35:115-123.
186. Millan MJ, et al. Signaling at G-protein-coupled serotonin receptors: recent advances and future research directions. *Trends Pharmacol Sci.* 2008;29:454-464.
187. Miller J, et al. Acute isoniazid poisoning in childhood. *Am J Dis Child.* 1980;134:290-292.
188. Miller RJ. Presynaptic receptors. *Annu Rev Pharmacol Toxicol.* 1998;38:201-227.
189. Milligan G. G protein-coupled receptor hetero-dimerization: contribution to pharmacology and function. *Br J Pharmacol.* 2009;158:5-14.
190. Mills KC. Serotonin syndrome. A clinical update. *Crit Care Clin.* 1997;13:763-783.
191. Missale C, et al. The neurobiology of dopamine receptors: evolution from the dual concept to heterodimer complexes. *J Recept Signal Transduct Res.* 2010;30:347-354.
192. Miwa H, et al. Generalized convulsions after consuming a large amount of gingko nuts. *Epilepsia.* 2001;42:280-281.
193. Modell JG, et al. Dopaminergic activity of the antimuscarinic antiparkinsonian agents. *J Clin Psychopharmacol.* 1989;9:347-351.
194. Modica MN, et al. Serotonin 5-HT3 and 5-HT4 ligands: an update of medicinal chemistry research in the last few years. *Curr Med Chem.* 2010;17:334-362.
195. Mody I, et al. A new meaning for "Gin & Tonic": tonic inhibition as the target for ethanol action in the brain. *Alcohol.* 2007;41:145-153.
196. Mohammad-Zadeh LF, et al. Serotonin: a review. *J Vet Pharmacol Ther.* 2008;31:187-199.
197. Moskal JR, et al. The Development of Rapastinel (Formerly GLYX-13); A Rapid Acting and Long Lasting Antidepressant. *Curr Neuropharmacol.* 2017;15:47-56.
198. Muller CE, Scior T. Adenosine receptors and their modulators. *Pharm Acta Helv.* 1993;68:77-111.
199. Muller CP, et al. Serotonin and psychostimulant addiction: focus on 5-HT1A-receptors. *Prog Neurobiol.* 2007;81:133-178.
200. Nakagawa T. The biochemistry, ultrastructure, and subunit assembly mechanism of AMPA receptors. *Mol Neurobiol.* 2010;42:161-184.
201. Narita M, et al. Linezolid-associated peripheral and optic neuropathy, lactic acidosis, and serotonin syndrome. *Pharmacotherapy.* 2007;27:1189-1197.
202. Newman CM, et al. Effects of sumatriptan and eletriptan on diseased epicardial coronary arteries. *Eur J Clin Pharmacol.* 2005;61:733-742.
203. Nicoletti F, et al. Metabotropic glutamate receptors as drug targets: what's new? *Curr Opin Pharmacol.* 2015;20:89-94.
204. Niesler B. 5-HT(3) receptors: potential of individual isoforms for personalised therapy. *Curr Opin Pharmacol.* 2011;11:81-86.
205. Nilsson M, et al. Transport of valproate and its effects on GABA uptake in astroglial primary culture. *Neurochem Res.* 1990;15:763-767.
206. Noda M, et al. Recombinant human serotonin 5A receptors stably expressed in C6 glioma cells couple to multiple signal transduction pathways. *J Neurochem.* 2003;84:222-232.
207. Notartomaso S, et al. Analgesia induced by the epigenetic drug, L-acetylcarnitine, outlasts the end of treatment in mouse models of chronic inflammatory and neuropathic pain. *Mol Pain.* 2017;13:1744806917697009.
208. Ogden KK, Traynelis SF. New advances in NMDA receptor pharmacology. *Trends Pharmacol Sci.* 2011;32:726-733.
209. Oja SS, Kontro P. Neurochemical aspects of amino acid transmitters and modulators. *Med Biol.* 1987;65:143-152.
210. Olivier B, van Oorschot R. 5-HT1B receptors and aggression: a review. *Eur J Pharmacol.* 2005;526:207-217.
211. Olsen R, et al. GABA receptors. IUPHAR/BPS Guide to PHARMACOLOGY. http://www.guidetopharmacology.org/GRAC/FamilyDisplayForward?familyId=72. Accessed February 14, 2017.
212. Olsen RW. The GABA postsynaptic membrane receptor-ionophore complex. Site of action of convulsant and anticonvulsant drugs. *Mol Cell Biochem.* 1981;39:261-279.
213. Ostopovici-Halip L, et al. Structural determinants of the alpha2 adrenoceptor subtype selectivity. *J Mol Graph Model.* 2011;29:1030-1038.
214. Palmer T. Agents acting at the neuromuscular junction and autonomic ganglia. In: Hardman JG, Limbird LE, Molinoff PB, et al, eds: *The Pharmacological Basis of Therapeutics.* 9th ed. New York, NY: McGraw-Hill; 1995:177-197.
215. Paoletti P, Pin JP. Editorial overview: neurosciences: targeting glutamatergic signaling in CNS diseases: new hopes? *Curr Opin Pharmacol* 2015;20:iv-vi.
216. Parkinson FE, et al. Propentofylline: a nucleoside transport inhibitor with neuroprotective effects in cerebral ischemia. *Gen Pharmacol.* 1994;25:1053-1058.
217. Partin KM. AMPA receptor potentiators: from drug design to cognitive enhancement. *Curr Opin Pharmacol.* 2015;20:46-53.
218. Pasqualetti M, et al. Distribution of the 5-HT5A serotonin receptor mRNA in the human brain. *Brain Res Mol Brain Res* 1998;56:1-8.
219. Paterson D, Nordberg A. Neuronal nicotinic receptors in the human brain. *Prog Neurobiol.* 2000;61:75-111.
220. Pelleg A, Porter RS. The pharmacology of adenosine. *Pharmacotherapy.* 1990;10:157-174.
221. Pellock JM, et al. Felbamate: consensus of current clinical experience. *Epilepsy Res.* 2006;71:89-101.
222. Perez D, et al. Adrenoceptors. IUPHAR/BPS Guide to PHARMACOLOGY. http://www.guidetopharmacology.org/GRAC/FamilyDisplayForward?familyId=4. Accessed March 27, 2017.
223. Perrais D, et al. Gating and permeation of kainate receptors: differences unveiled. *Trends Pharmacol Sci.* 2010;31:516-522.
224. Peterman C, Sanoski CA. Tecadenoson: a novel, selective A1 adenosine receptor agonist. *Cardiol Rev.* 2005;13:315-321.
225. Petrovic MM, et al. Metabotropic action of postsynaptic kainate receptors triggers hippocampal long-term potentiation. *Nat Neurosci.* 2017;20:529-539.
226. Phillips TJ, Reed C. Targeting GABAB receptors for anti-abuse drug discovery. *Expert Opin Drug Discov.* 2014;9:1307-1317.
227. Phillis JW, O'Regan MH. The role of adenosine in the central actions of the benzodiazepines. *Prog Neuropsychopharmacol Biol Psychiatry.* 1988;12:389-404.
228. Pin JP, Bockaert J. Get receptive to metabotropic glutamate receptors. *Curr Opin Neurobiol.* 1995;5:342-349.
229. Pinheiro PS, Mulle C. Presynaptic glutamate receptors: physiological functions and mechanisms of action. *Nat Rev Neurosci.* 2008;9:423-436.
230. Pinna A. Adenosine A2A Receptor antagonists in Parkinson's disease: progress in clinical trials from the newly approved istradefylline to drugs in early development and those already discontinued. *CNS Drugs.* 2014;28:455-474.
231. Planells-Cases R, Jentsch TJ. Chloride channelopathies. *Biochim Biophys Acta.* 2009;1792:173-189.
232. Proenca P, et al. Fatal intoxication with tianeptine (Stablon). *Forensic Sci Int.* 2007;170:200-203.
233. Pucilowski O. Psychopharmacological properties of calcium channel inhibitors. *Psychopharmacology (Berl).* 1992;109:12-29.
234. Pytliak M, et al. Serotonin receptors—from molecular biology to clinical applications. *Physiol Res.* 2011;60:15-25.
235. Redgrave P, et al. Is the short-latency dopamine response too short to signal reward error? *Trends Neurosci.* 1999;22:146-151.
236. Rees S, et al. Cloning and characterisation of the human 5-HT5A serotonin receptor. *FEBS Lett.* 1994;355:242-246.
237. Reis DJ, Regunathan S. Is agmatine a novel neurotransmitter in brain? *Trends Pharmacol Sci.* 2000;21:187-193.
238. Reissig CJ, et al. High doses of dextromethorphan, an NMDA antagonist, produce effects similar to classic hallucinogens. *Psychopharmacology (Berl).* 2012;223:1-15.
239. Reuter U, et al. The pharmacological profile and clinical prospects of the oral 5-HT1F receptor agonist lasmiditan in the acute treatment of migraine. *Ther Adv Neurol Disord.* 2015;8:46-54.
240. Rho JM, et al. Barbiturate-like actions of the propanediol dicarbamates felbamate and meprobamate. *J Pharmacol Exp Ther.* 1997;280:1383-1391.
241. Richelson E. Receptor pharmacology of neuroleptics: relation to clinical effects. *J Clin Psychiatry.* 1999;60(suppl 10):5-14.
242. Rodriguez-Moreno A, Sihra TS. Metabotropic actions of kainate receptors in the CNS. *J Neurochem.* 2007;103:2121-2135.
243. Rojas C, Slusher BS. Pharmacological mechanisms of 5-HT3 and tachykinin NK1 receptor antagonism to prevent chemotherapy-induced nausea and vomiting. *Eur J Pharmacol.* 2012;684:1-7.
244. Rojas DC. The role of glutamate and its receptors in autism and the use of glutamate receptor antagonists in treatment. *J Neural Transm (Vienna).* 2014;121:891-905.
245. Rondard P, et al. The complexity of their activation mechanism opens new possibilities for the modulation of mGlu and GABAB class C G protein-coupled receptors. *Neuropharmacology.* 2011;60:82-92.
246. Ruat M, et al. Molecular cloning, characterization, and localization of a high-affinity serotonin receptor (5-HT7) activating cAMP formation. *Proc Natl Acad Sci U S A.* 1993;90:8547-8551.
247. Rudorfer MV, Potter WZ. Antidepressants. A comparative review of the clinical pharmacology and therapeutic use of the "newer" versus the "older" drugs. *Drugs.* 1989;37:713-738.
248. Salvatore CA, et al. Molecular cloning and characterization of the human A3 adenosine receptor. *Proc Natl Acad Sci U S A.* 1993;90:10365-10369.

249. Sankar R. GABA(A) receptor physiology and its relationship to the mechanism of action of the 1,5-benzodiazepine clobazam. *CNS Drugs.* 2012;26:229-244.

250. Santhakumar V, et al. Ethanol acts directly on extrasynaptic subtypes of GABAA receptors to increase tonic inhibition. *Alcohol.* 2007;41:211-221; erratum in *Alcohol.* 2007;41:461.

251. Schatzberg AF, et al. An overview of vortioxetine. *J Clin Psychiatry.* 2014;75:1411-1418.

252. Scholz KP. Introductory perspective. In: Dunwiddie TV, Lovinger DM, eds. *Presynaptic Receptors in the Mammalian Brain.* Boston, MA: Birkhauser; 1993:1-11.

253. Schwiebert C, et al. Small doses of methylene blue, previously considered safe, can precipitate serotonin toxicity. *Anaesthesia.* 2009;64:924.

254. Sealfon SC. Dopamine receptors and locomotor responses: molecular aspects. *Ann Neurol.* 2000;47:S12-S19; discussion S19-S21.

255. Selden BS, Curry SC. Anticholinergics. In: Reisdorff E, Roberts MR, Wiegenstein JG, eds. *Pediatric Emergency Medicine.* Philadelphia, PA: Saunders; 1993:693-700.

256. Shank RP, et al. An overview of the preclinical aspects of topiramate: pharmacology, pharmacokinetics, and mechanism of action. *Epilepsia.* 2000;41(suppl 1):S3-S9.

257. Sharman JL, et al. IUPHAR-DB. New receptors and tools for easy searching and visualization of pharmacological data. Nucleic Acids Res. 2011;39:D534-D538.

258. Sheffler DJ, et al. Allosteric modulation of metabotropic glutamate receptors. *Adv Pharmacol.* 2011;62:37-77.

259. Shenoy SK, Lefkowitz RJ. Beta-Arrestin-mediated receptor trafficking and signal transduction. *Trends Pharmacol Sci.* 2011;32:521-533.

260. Shim SS, et al. Potentiation of the NMDA receptor in the treatment of schizophrenia: focused on the glycine site. *Eur Arch Psychiatry Clin Neurosci.* 2008;258:16-27.

261. Shivaprakash G, et al. Can metabotropic glutamate receptor 7 (mGluR 7) be a novel target for analgesia? *J Clin Diagn Res.* 2014;8:HC16-HC18.

262. Sieghart W. Structure and pharmacology of gamma-aminobutyric acidA receptor subtypes. *Pharmacol Rev.* 1995;47:181-234.

263. Sigel E, Buhr A. The benzodiazepine binding site of GABAA receptors. *Trends Pharmacol Sci.* 1997;18:425-429.

264. Simonds WF. G protein-regulated signaling dysfunction in human disease. *J Investig Med.* 2003;51:194-214.

265. Smith JM. Abuse of the antiparkinson drugs: a review of the literature. *J Clin Psychiatry.* 1980;41:351-354.

266. Smith TA. Type A gamma-aminobutyric acid (GABAA) receptor subunits and benzodiazepine binding: significance to clinical syndromes and their treatment. *Br J Biomed Sci.* 2001;58:111-121.

267. Solt K, Forman SA. Correlating the clinical actions and molecular mechanisms of general anesthetics. *Curr Opin Anaesthesiol.* 2007;20:300-306.

268. Southam E, et al. Lamotrigine inhibits monoamine uptake in vitro and modulates 5-hydroxytryptamine uptake in rats. *Eur J Pharmacol.* 1998;358:19-24.

269. Spanagel R, Weiss F. The dopamine hypothesis of reward: past and current status. *Trends Neurosci.* 1999;22:521-527.

270. Squires RF, Saederup E. Antidepressants and metabolites that block GABAA receptors coupled to 35S-t-butylbicyclophosphorothionate binding sites in rat brain. *Brain Res.* 1988;441:15-22.

271. Stahl SM. Anticonvulsants as anxiolytics, part 1: tiagabine and other anticonvulsants with actions on GABA. *J Clin Psychiatry.* 2004;65:291-292.

272. Stone TW. Actions of the benzodiazepines and the benzodiazepine antagonist flumazenil may involve adenosine. *J Neurol Sci.* 1999;163:199-201.

273. Strosberg AD. Association of beta 3-adrenoceptor polymorphism with obesity and diabetes: current status. *Trends Pharmacol Sci.* 1997;18:449-454.

274. Sulzer D, et al. Amphetamine and other weak bases act to promote reverse transport of dopamine in ventral midbrain neurons. *J Neurochem.* 1993;60:527-535.

275. Sulzer D, Rayport S. Amphetamine and other psychostimulants reduce pH gradients in midbrain dopaminergic neurons and chromaffin granules: a mechanism of action. *Neuron.* 1990;5:797-808.

276. Sundstrom-Poromaa I, et al. Hormonally regulated alpha(4)beta(2)delta GABA(A) receptors are a target for alcohol. *Nat Neurosci.* 2002;5:721-722.

277. Swanson CJ, et al. Metabotropic glutamate receptors as novel targets for anxiety and stress disorders. *Nat Rev Drug Discov.* 2005;4:131-144.

278. Szakacs R, et al. The "blue" side of glutamatergic neurotransmission: NMDA receptor antagonists as possible novel therapeutics for major depression. *Neuropsychopharmacol Hung.* 2012;14:29-40.

279. Taylor CP. Mechanisms of new antiepileptic drugs. In: Delgado-Escueta AV, Jasper HH, Herbert H, eds. *Jasper's Basic Mechanisms of the Epilepsies.* 3rd ed. Philadelphia, PA: Lippincott Williams & Wilkins; 1999:1018.

280. Thomas DR. 5-HT5A receptors as a therapeutic target. *Pharmacol Ther.* 2006;111:707-714.

281. Thomas DR, et al. Functional characterisation of the human cloned 5-HT7 receptor (long form); antagonist profile of SB-258719. *Br J Pharmacol.* 1998;124:1300-1306.

282. Traynelis SF, et al. Glutamate receptor ion channels: structure, regulation, and function. *Pharmacol Rev.* 2010;62:405-496.

283. Trincavelli ML, et al. Adenosine receptors: what we know and what we are learning. *Curr Top Med Chem.* 2010;10:860-877.

284. Tuncel M, et al. Mechanism of the blood pressure—raising effect of cocaine in humans. *Circulation.* 2002;105:1054-1059.

285. Uwai K, et al. Exploring the structural basis of neurotoxicity in C(17)-polyacetylenes isolated from water hemlock. *J Med Chem.* 2000;43:4508-4515.

286. Uwai K, et al. Virol A, a toxic trans-polyacetylenic alcohol of Cicuta virosa, selectively inhibits the GABA-induced Cl(−) current in acutely dissociated rat hippocampal CA1 neurons. *Brain Res.* 2001;889:174-180.

287. Vallone D, et al. Structure and function of dopamine receptors. *Neurosci Biobehav Rev.* 2000;24:125-132.

288. Van Moorhem M, et al. L-Beta-N-oxalyl-alpha,beta-diaminopropionic acid toxicity in motor neurons. *Neuroreport.* 2011;22:131-135.

289. Villalon CM, Centurion D. Cardiovascular responses produced by 5-hydroxytriptamine: a pharmacological update on the receptors/mechanisms involved and therapeutic implications. *Naunyn Schmiedebergs Arch Pharmacol.* 2007;376:45-63.

290. Wadhwa A, et al. New and investigational agents for irritable bowel syndrome. *Curr Gastroenterol Rep.* 2015;17:1-11.

291. Wafford KA, et al. Differentiating the role of gamma-aminobutyric acid type A (GABAA) receptor subtypes. *Biochem Soc Trans.* 2004;32:553-556.

292. Walker AG, Conn PJ. Group I and group II metabotropic glutamate receptor allosteric modulators as novel potential antipsychotics. *Curr Opin Pharmacol.* 2015;20:40-45.

293. Wallace KL. Antibiotic-induced convulsions. *Crit Care Clin.* 1997;13:741-762.

294. Wallner M, et al. Ethanol enhances alpha 4 beta 3 delta and alpha 6 beta 3 delta gamma-aminobutyric acid type A receptors at low concentrations known to affect humans. *Proc Natl Acad Sci U S A.* 2003;100:15218-15223.

295. Ward JL, et al. Kinetic and pharmacological properties of cloned human equilibrative nucleoside transporters, ENT1 and ENT2, stably expressed in nucleoside transporter-deficient PK15 cells. Ent2 exhibits a low affinity for guanosine and cytidine but a high affinity for inosine. *J Biol Chem.* 2000;275:8375-8381.

296. Watt G, et al. Positive response to edrophonium in patients with neurotoxic envenoming by cobras (*Naja naja philippinensis*). A placebo-controlled study. *N Engl J Med.* 1986;315:1444-1448.

297. Webb TI, Lynch JW. Molecular pharmacology of the glycine receptor chloride channel. *Curr Pharm Des.* 2007;13:2350-2367.

298. Whiting PJ, et al. Structure and pharmacology of vertebrate GABAA receptor subtypes. *Int Rev Neurobiol.* 1995;38:95-138.

299. Wong CG, et al. From the street to the brain: neurobiology of the recreational drug gamma-hydroxybutyric acid. *Trends Pharmacol Sci.* 2004;25:29-34.

300. Woo JH, et al. Effects of clonidine on the activity of the rat glutamate transporter EAAT3 expressed in Xenopus oocytes. *Korean J Anesthesiol.* 2012;62:266-271.

301. Yang J, et al. Felbamate but not phenytoin or gabapentin reduces glutamate release by blocking presynaptic NMDA receptors in the entorhinal cortex. *Epilepsy Res.* 2007;77:157-164.

302. Yi ES, et al. Chronic stress-induced dendritic reorganization and abundance of synaptosomal PKA-dependent CP-AMPA receptor in the basolateral amygdala in a mouse model of depression. *Biochem Biophys Res Commun.* 2017.

303. Youdim MB, et al. The therapeutic potential of monoamine oxidase inhibitors. *Nat Rev Neurosci.* 2006;7:295-309.

304. Young James D. The SLC28 (CNT) and SLC29 (ENT) nucleoside transporter families: a 30-year collaborative odyssey. *Biochem Soc Trans.* 2016;44:869-876.

305. Yuen EY, et al. The novel antipsychotic drug lurasidone enhances N-methyl-D-aspartate receptor-mediated synaptic responses. *Mol Pharmacol.* 2012;81:113-119.

306. Zdziarski P. A case of stiff person syndrome: immunomodulatory effect of benzodiazepines: successful rituximab and tizanidine therapy. *Medicine (Baltimore).* 2015;94:e954.

307. Zeller A, et al. Identification of a molecular target mediating the general anesthetic actions of pentobarbital. *Mol Pharmacol.* 2007;71:852-859.

308. Zhou Y, Danbolt NC. Glutamate as a neurotransmitter in the healthy brain. *J Neural Transm (Vienna).* 2014;121:799-817.

309. Zhu S, Paoletti P. Allosteric modulators of NMDA receptors: multiple sites and mechanisms. *Curr Opin Pharmacol.* 2015;20:14-23.

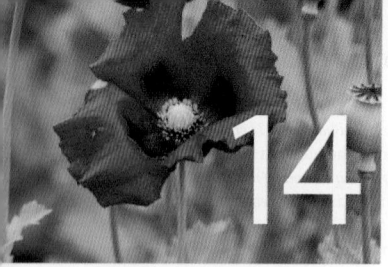

14 WITHDRAWAL PRINCIPLES

Nicholas J. Connors and Richard J. Hamilton

In the central nervous system (CNS), excitatory neurons fire regularly, and inhibitory neurons inhibit the transmission of these impulses. Whenever action is required, the inhibitory tone diminishes, permitting the excitatory nerve impulses to travel to their end organs. Thus, all action in human neurophysiology can be considered to result from disinhibition.

Tonic inhibition (sustained, as opposed to phasic or transient inhibition) triggered by the constant presence of a xenobiotic produces an adaptive change in the affected neuron such that the constant presence of that xenobiotic is required to prevent dysfunction. A withdrawal syndrome occurs when the constant presence of this xenobiotic is removed or reduced and the adaptive changes persist. Withdrawal is a dysfunctional condition in which tonic inhibitory neurotransmission is significantly reduced, essentially producing excitation (Fig. 14–1). Every withdrawal syndrome has 2 characteristics: (1) a preexisting compensatory physiologic adaptation to the continuous presence of a xenobiotic and (2) decreasing concentrations of that xenobiotic below some threshold necessary to prevent physiologic derangement. In contrast, simple tolerance to a xenobiotic is characterized by a shift in the dose–response curve to the right; that is, greater amounts of a xenobiotic are required to achieve a given effect. Physiologic dependence, commonly referred to as dependence, occurs when the absence of the xenobiotic leads to the development of a specific withdrawal syndrome. Dependence needs to be distinguished from addiction, which is compulsive drug-seeking behavior. The *Diagnostic and Statistical Manual of Mental Disorders, Fifth Edition* (DSM-5), uses the term *substance use* to combine the DSM-IV disorders of substance abuse and substance dependence.[1]

Withdrawal is manifested by either of the following: (1) a characteristic withdrawal syndrome for the xenobiotic, or (2) the same (or a closely related) xenobiotic is taken to relieve withdrawal symptoms. Note that either criterion fulfills this definition. Logically, all syndromes meet the first criterion, so it is the presence of the second criterion that is critical to understanding physiology and therapy.

For the purposes of defining a unifying pathophysiologic pattern of withdrawal syndromes, this chapter considers syndromes in which both features are present. An analysis from this perspective distinguishes xenobiotics that affect the inhibitory neuronal pathways from those that affect the excitatory neuronal pathways, such as cocaine. According to this definition, cocaine does not produce a withdrawal syndrome but rather a posttoxicity syndrome that often results in lethargy, hypersomnolence, movement disorders, and irritability. Although referred to as withdrawal, this syndrome does not meet the definition for a withdrawal syndrome because the same (or a closely related) xenobiotic is not taken to relieve or avoid withdrawal symptoms. This posttoxicity syndrome, the so-called "crack crash" or "washed-out syndrome," is caused by prolonged use of cocaine, and patients ultimately return to their premorbid function without intervention. This distinction is

Quantity	Ethanol status	Neuronal effect		Clinical effect
	Naïve-sober	Baseline inhibition	Baseline excitation	Baseline normal
	Naïve	Enhanced inhibition	Blocked excitation	Intoxication, sedation
	Tolerant	Downregulated, receptor shift → Desensitized inhibition	Upregulated, receptor multiplication → Controlled excitation	New baseline "normal"
	Abstinent	Loss of inhibition	Uncontrolled excitation	Withdrawal, autonomic instability

= GABA receptor with α_1 subunit

= GABA receptor with α_4 subunit

= NMDA receptor

= Ethanol

FIGURE 14–1. Ethanol intoxication, tolerance, and withdrawal. Ethanol consumption in an ethanol-naïve person produces intoxication and sedation by simultaneous agonism at the γ-aminobutyric acid (GABA) receptor–chloride channel complex and antagonism at the N-methyl-D-aspartate (NMDA) receptor. Continuous ethanol consumption leads to the development of tolerance through changes in both the GABA receptor–chloride channel complex (a subunit shift from α_1 to α_4, resulting in reduced sensitivity to the sedating effects of ethanol) and the NMDA subtype of glutamate receptor (upregulation in number, resulting in enhanced wakefulness). There is conceptually a concentration at which the tolerant patient may appear clinically normal despite having an elevated blood ethanol concentration. Tolerant patients who are abstinent lose the tonic effects of ethanol on these receptors, resulting in withdrawal.

important for toxicologists, because (1) withdrawal syndromes that demonstrate both features of the *DSM-5* criteria are treated with reinstatement and gradual withdrawal of a xenobiotic that has an effect on the receptor and (2) withdrawal syndromes that do not demonstrate the second feature require only supportive care and resolve spontaneously. The term "drug discontinuation syndrome" is used instead of withdrawal, for example, with serotonin reuptake inhibitors to describe the symptoms that result when a drug used therapeutically is discontinued, but this is in fact a withdrawal syndrome. Addiction and dependence are terms often used in the context of the psychosocial aspects of xenobiotic use and are meant to convey the continued use of a xenobiotic despite adverse consequences.

Finally, withdrawal syndromes are best described and treated according to the class of receptors primarily affected because this concept also organizes the approach to patient care. For each receptor and its agonists, research has identified genomic and nongenomic effects that produce neuroadaptation and withdrawal syndromes. Six mechanisms appear to be involved: (1) epigenetic mechanisms via micro-RNA (miRNA) and messenger RNA (mRNA) expression, DNA methylation, and histone modification; (2) second-messenger effects via protein kinases, cyclic adenosine monophosphate (cAMP),[44,48] or calcium ions; (3) receptor endocytosis; (4) expression of various receptor and neurotransmitter transporter subtypes depending on location within the synapse (synaptic localization); (5) intracellular signaling via effects on other receptors; and (6) neurosteroid modulation. Some or all of these mechanisms are demonstrated in each of the known withdrawal syndromes.[52,53] These mechanisms develop in a surprisingly rapid fashion and modify the receptor and its function in such complex ways as to depend on the continued presence of the xenobiotic to prevent dysfunction.[50,59,72,80,81]

GABA$_A$ RECEPTORS (BARBITURATES, BENZODIAZEPINES, ETHANOL, VOLATILE SOLVENTS)

γ-Aminobutyric acid type A (GABA$_A$) receptors are part of a superfamily of ligand-gated ion channels, including nicotinic acetylcholine receptors and glycine receptors, which exist as pentamers arranged around a central ion channel. When activated, they hyperpolarize the postsynaptic neuron by facilitating an inward chloride current (without a G protein messenger), decreasing the likelihood of the neuron firing an action potential. γ-Aminobutyric acid type A (GABA$_A$) receptors have separate binding sites for GABA, barbiturates, benzodiazepines, loreclezole, and picrotoxin (Chap. 13).[65] Barbiturates and benzodiazepines bind to separate receptor sites and enhance the affinity for GABA$_A$ at its receptor site.

The GABA receptor is a pentamer composed of 2 α subunits, 2 β subunits, and 1 additional subunit, most commonly γ, which is a key element in the benzodiazepine-binding site. Each receptor has 2 GABA-binding sites that are located in a homologous position to the benzodiazepine site between the α and β subunits. Although the mechanism is unclear, benzodiazepines have no direct functional effect without the presence of GABA. Conversely, certain barbiturates in a dose-dependent manner and propofol can directly increase the duration of channel opening, thereby producing a net increase in current flow without GABA binding. This process has therapeutic implications and explains why high-dose barbiturates are nearly universally successful in stopping status epilepticus and treating severe withdrawal.

This prototypical pentameric GABA$_A$ receptor assembly is derived from permutations and combinations of 2, 3, 4, or even 5 different protein subunits. The subtypes of GABA receptors can even vary on the same cell. In fact, GABA receptors are heterogeneous receptors with different subunits and distinct regional distribution. Although the preponderance of subtypes $\alpha_1\beta_2\gamma_2$, $\alpha_2\beta_3\gamma_2$, and $\alpha_3\beta_3\gamma_2$ accounts for 75% of GABA receptors, there are at least 16 other significant subtypes.[81] The recognition of additional subunits of GABA$_A$ receptors facilitated the development of targeted pharmaceuticals, such as zolpidem.[10]

Previously, ethanol was thought to have GABA receptor activity, although a clearly identified binding site was not evident. Traditional explanations for this effect included (1) enhanced membrane fluidity and allosteric potentiation (so-called cross-coupling) of the 5 proteins that construct the GABA$_A$

receptor; (2) interaction with a portion of the receptor; and/or (3) enhanced GABA release. Research with chimeric reconstruction of GABA$_A$ and *N*-methyl-D-aspartate (NMDA) channels demonstrates highly specific binding sites for high doses of ethanol that enhance GABA$_A$ and inhibit NMDA receptor-mediated glutamate neurotransmission. However, research has not clarified whether ethanol at low concentrations is a direct agonist of GABA$_A$ receptors or a potentiator of GABA$_A$ receptor binding.[66]

There are 6 mechanisms of adaptation to chronic ethanol exposure making it the prototypical xenobiotic for the study of neuroadaptation and withdrawal.[25,52,58] These 6 mechanisms appear to apply to benzodiazepines as well.[4,66] The 6 mechanisms are (1) altered GABA$_A$ receptor gene expression via alterations in miRNA, mRNA, and protein concentrations of GABA$_A$ receptor subunits in numerous regions of the brain (genomic mechanisms); (2) posttranslational modification through phosphorylation of receptor subunits with protein kinase C (second-messenger effects); (3) subcellular localization by an increased internalization of GABA$_A$ receptor α_1-subunit receptors (receptor endocytosis); (4) modification of GABA and NMDA receptor subtypes with differing affinities for agonists to the synaptic or nonsynaptic sites (synaptic localization) reducing the sensitivity of the receptor; (5) regulation via intracellular signaling by the NMDA, acetylcholine, serotonin, and β-adrenergic receptors; and (6) neurosteroidal modulation of GABA receptor sensitivity and expression.[20,21,44,54] Furthermore, changes in GABA$_A$ subunit composition and function are evident within one hour of administration of a single exposure to ethanol in animals.[57]

Intracellular signaling via the NMDA subtype of the glutamate receptor appears to explain the "kindling" hypothesis, in which successive withdrawal events become progressively more severe.[17,58] The activity of excitatory neurotransmission increases the more it fires, a phenomenon known as *long-term potentiation*, and is the result of increased activity of mRNA and receptor protein expression, a genomic effect of intracellular signaling.[77] As NMDA and other glutamatergic receptors (kainite and α-amino-3-hydroxy-5-methyl-4-isoxazoleproprionic acid {AMPA}) increase in number and function (upregulation) and GABA$_A$ receptor activity diminishes, withdrawal becomes more severe.[42,58,75] The dizocilpine (MK-801)-binding site of the NMDA receptor appears to be the major contributor, and this effect is recognized in neurons that express both NMDA and GABA$_A$ receptors.[5] When the concentration of ethanol or any xenobiotic with GABA agonist activity is diminished, inhibitory control of excitatory neurotransmission, such as that mediated by the now upregulated NMDA receptors, is lost.[59] Additionally, increased presynaptic glutamate release is noted in withdrawal.[27] These effects result in the clinical syndrome of withdrawal: CNS excitation (tremor, hallucinations, seizures) and autonomic stimulation (tachycardia, hypertension, hyperthermia, diaphoresis) (Chap. 77).[72]

Volatile solvents, such as gasoline, diethyl ether, and toluene, are widely abused xenobiotics whose effects also appear to be mediated by the GABA receptor (Chap. 81).[70,74] These solvents produce CNS inhibition and anesthesia at escalating doses via the GABA$_A$ receptor in a fashion similar to that of ethanol.[16,47,83]

In addition to GABA receptor/neurotransmitter effects, other neurotransmitters are important in the development of ethanol tolerance and withdrawal. These include an NMDA receptor subunit and anchoring protein, the dynorphin/kappa opioid receptor, the 5-HT$_{2C}$ serotonergic receptors, serum nerve growth protein, and brain voltage-gated calcium channels.[34,60] Ethanol use is also associated with increased expression of pronociceptin and increased activity in the dynorphin/kappa opioid receptor system causing an altered affective condition.[22,31] Symptoms of ethanol withdrawal correlate with increased synthesis of mRNA for the nociceptin/orphanin FQ (N/OFQ)-opioid peptide receptor, which are involved in CNS stress-regulatory systems.[11] Once withdrawal has started, increases are noted in serum nerve growth protein, which is theorized to counteract excitatory states, and decreases in methylation of the gene coding for its transcription.[43] Finally, electrical current through brain voltage-gated calcium channels is increased in those chronically exposed to ethanol, and increased Ca^{2+} conduction may play a role in ethanol withdrawal seizures.[62]

GABA$_B$ RECEPTORS (GHB AND BACLOFEN)

GABA$_B$ agonists such as γ-hydroxybutyric (GHB) acid, γ-hydroxybutyrate (GHB) precursors and analogs, and baclofen have similar clinical characteristics with regard to adaptation and withdrawal.[84] The GABA$_B$ receptor is a heterodimer of the GABA$_{B1}$ and GABA$_{B2}$ receptors. Unlike GABA$_A$, the GABA$_B$ receptor couples to various effector systems through a signal-transducing G protein.[24,84] GABA$_B$ receptors mediate presynaptic inhibition (by preventing Ca^{2+} influx) and postsynaptic inhibition (by increasing K$^+$ efflux). The postsynaptic receptors appear to have an inhibitory effect similar to that of the GABA$_A$ receptors, though the mechanism differs. The presynaptic receptors provide feedback inhibition of GABA release.

γ-Hydroxybutyric acid is a naturally occurring inhibitory neurotransmitter with its own distinct receptor (Chap. 80).[7] Physiologic concentrations of GHB activate at least 2 subtypes of a distinct GHB receptor (antagonist-sensitive and antagonist-insensitive). However, at supraphysiologic concentrations, such as those that occur after overdose and abuse, GHB binds directly to the GABA$_B$ receptor and is metabolized to GABA (which then activates the GABA$_B$ receptor). The GHB withdrawal syndrome clinically resembles the withdrawal syndrome from ethanol and benzodiazepines and can be severe. In most cases, distinctive clinical features of GHB withdrawal are relatively mild with brief autonomic instability and the persistence of psychotic symptoms.[79]

Baclofen is also a GABA$_B$ agonist. The presynaptic and postsynaptic inhibitory properties of baclofen allow it, paradoxically, to cause seizures associated with both acute overdose because of decreased release of presynaptic GABA via autoreceptor stimulation and withdrawal. Withdrawal is probably a result of the loss of the chronic inhibitory effect of baclofen on postsynaptic GABA$_B$ receptors. Discontinuation of baclofen produces hyperactivity of neuronal Ca^{2+} channels (N, P/Q type),[32] leading to seizures, hypertension, hallucinations, psychosis, and coma. However, many of these manifestations do not differ clinically from the withdrawal symptoms of GABA$_A$ agonists.

Typically, the development of a baclofen withdrawal occurs 24 to 48 hours after discontinuation or a reduction in the dose of baclofen. Case reports highlight the development of seizures, hallucinations, psychosis, dyskinesias, and visual disturbances. Additionally, the intrathecal baclofen pump is an effective replacement for oral dosing, but severe withdrawal can occur when the pump malfunctions or becomes disconnected.[12] Reinstatement of the prior baclofen-dosing schedule appears to resolve these symptoms within 24 to 48 hours. Benzodiazepines and GABA$_A$ agonists are the appropriate treatment for seizures induced by baclofen withdrawal.[73]

OPIOID RECEPTORS (OPIOIDS)

Similar to the behavior of ethanol and GABA$_A$ receptors, opioid binding to the opioid receptors results in a series of genomic and nongenomic neuroadaptations, especially via second-messenger effects. When opioids bind to opioid receptors, they alleviate pain by activating G$_s$ proteins and stimulating K$^+$ efflux currents hyperpolarizing the cell and inhibiting these neurons. Opioid receptors are also linked to the G$_{i/o}$ proteins that dissociate into the Gα and Gβγ subunits and go on to other intracellular effects such as inhibition of adenylate cyclase through the Gα subunit and inactivation of the inward Ca^{2+} current via the βγ subunit, thus suppressing the intrinsic excitability of a neuron by limiting its ability to depolarize (Chap. 36).[14,30,78] This inhibition permits the downstream disinhibition of dopaminergic neurons.[19] After chronic stimulation of opioid receptors, there is uncoupling of the receptor to the G$_{i/o}$ proteins, and coupling to the G$_z$ protein that upregulates the adenylate cyclase/cAMP pathway and results in multiple effects such as hyperalgesia.[69,78]

Chronic use of all xenobiotics with opioid-receptor affinity results in a decreased efficacy of the receptor to open potassium channels by genomic mechanisms and second-messenger effects. Following chronic opioid use, the expression of adenylate cyclase increases through activation of the transcription factor known as cAMP response element-binding protein (CREB) (Fig. 14–2).[41,63] This results in upregulation of cAMP-mediated responses like the inward Na$^+$ channels responsible for intrinsic excitability.

The net effect is that only higher concentrations of opioids result in analgesia and other opioid effects. In the dependent patient, when opioid concentrations drop, inward Na$^+$ flux occurs unchecked, and the patient experiences the opioid withdrawal syndrome. The clinical findings associated with this syndrome are largely a result of uninhibited activity at the locus ceruleus, mediated by orexin agonism at orexin receptors, thus decreasing the inhibitory activity of GABAergic neurons.[3,35,50,63] Chronic opioid use results in decreased expression of the excitatory amino acid transporter 3 (EAAT3), which prevents glutamate reuptake from the synapse and causes postsynaptic neuroexcitation.[39] Further, in the nucleus accumbens, opioid withdrawal causes activation of the NMDA receptor, increasing receptor phosphorylation and is associated with increased cell surface expression of excitatory NMDA receptors.[6] Additionally, there seems to be a role for peroxisome proliferator-activated receptor gamma (PPAR-γ) in the development of tolerance as PPAR-γ agonists decrease opioid tolerance and attenuate withdrawal through inhibition of cellular antiinflammatory effects.[26,38] Tolerance to

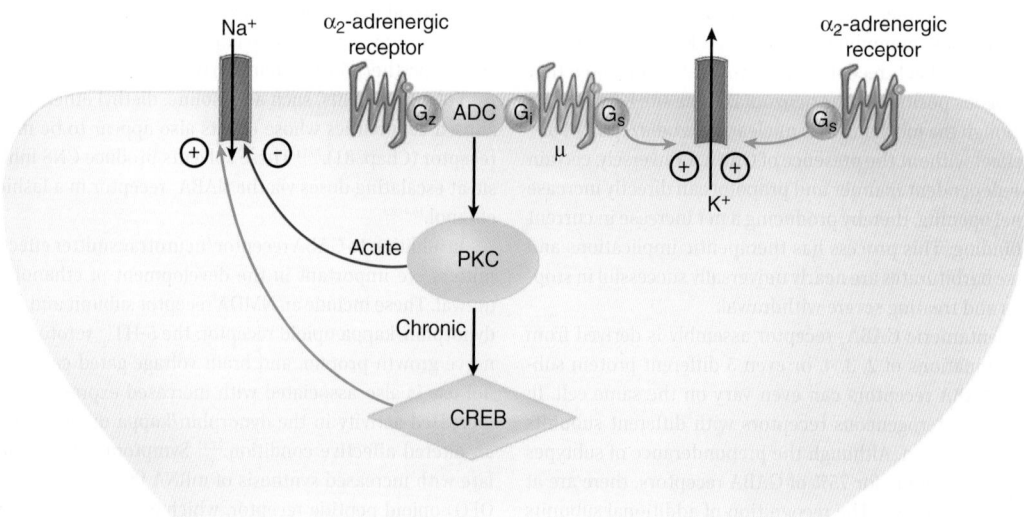

FIGURE 14–2. Immediate and long-term effects of opioids. The immediate effects of both opioids and α$_2$-adrenergic agonists are to increase inhibition through enhanced potassium efflux and inhibited sodium influx. Long-term effects alter gene expression to enhance sodium influx and restore homeostasis. CREB = cAMP response element-binding protein; ADC = adenylate cyclase; PKC = protein kinase C. (〰) = α$_2$-adrenergic receptor; (〰) = μ opioid receptor.

opioids is also mediated through histone acetylation by 2 enzymes, histone acetyltransferase (associated with the development of tolerance) and histone deacetylase (mediates the resolution of tolerance back to normal homeostasis).[56] Opioid tolerance and naloxone-precipitated withdrawal can be demonstrated in humans naïve to opioids after just 1 or 2 doses of morphine 15 mg/70 kg.[13]

Functional MRI data in humans with precipitated opioid withdrawal show increased neuronal activity in the caudate, pregenual cingulate, orbitofrontal gyrus, middle orbital gyrus, and putamen, areas associated with reward processing. There is decreased activity in networks involved in sensorimotor integration including bilateral precentral and postcentral gyri.[28] After precipitated opioid withdrawal, histone acetylation and increased expression of genes associated with neuronal plasticity are noted.[29]

In addition, opioid receptors and central α_2-adrenergic receptors both exert an analogous effect on the potassium channel in the locus ceruleus. Clonidine binds to the central α_2-adrenergic receptor and stimulates potassium efflux, as do opioids, and produces similar clinical findings, which explains why clonidine has efficacy in treating certain aspects of the opioid withdrawal syndrome (cross tolerance). In addition, the antagonistic effect of naloxone at the opioid receptor seems to partially reverse the effect of clonidine on this shared potassium efflux channel.

Rapid and ultrarapid opioid detoxification are forms of intentional iatrogenic withdrawal that use opioid antagonists to accelerate a return to premorbid receptor physiology. In theory, although not necessarily in practice, inducing opioid withdrawal under general anesthesia with high-dose opioid antagonists permits the transition from drug dependency to naltrexone maintenance without enduring an intense withdrawal syndrome (Chap. 36).[36,40,49]

α_2-ADRENERGIC RECEPTORS (CLONIDINE)

In a manner related to their role in treating opioid withdrawal, prolonged exposure to clonidine and related medications is associated with a withdrawal syndrome. α_2-Adrenergic receptors are located in the central and peripheral nervous systems. Clonidine is a central and peripheral α_2-adrenergic agonist. Stimulation of central presynaptic α_2-adrenergic receptors inhibits sympathomimetic output and results in bradycardia and hypotension. Within 24 hours after the discontinuation of chronic clonidine use, norepinephrine concentrations rise as a result of enhanced efferent sympathetic activity. This increase results in hypertension, tachycardia, anxiety, diaphoresis, and hallucinations.

Dexmedetomidine is widely used as a sedative in the intensive care unit. Like clonidine it is a central and peripheral presynaptic α_2-adrenergic agonist, but dexmedetomidine has greater specificity for the α_2-adrenergic receptor and hence stronger sedative properties. It cannot be given in bolus doses because it causes hypertension by stimulating peripheral α_2 receptors on vascular smooth muscle (much like the initial phase of a clonidine overdose) (Chap. 61).[51] Dexmedetomidine is occasionally used as an adjunct to treat ethanol, benzodiazepine, and opioid withdrawal and is reported to cause less respiratory depression than benzodiazepines but more bradycardia.[68] Importantly, dexmedetomidine has a withdrawal syndrome exactly like that of clonidine, including hypertension, tachycardia, and agitation. In fact, clonidine is reportedly used to treat this withdrawal successfully.[71,82]

ADENOSINE (A) RECEPTORS (CAFFEINE)

The release of most neurotransmitters is accompanied by the passive release of adenosine as a by-product of adenosine triphosphate (ATP) breakdown. The released adenosine binds to postsynaptic A_1 receptors where it typically has inhibitory effects on the postsynaptic neuron. It also binds to presynaptic A_1 autoreceptors to limit further release of neurotransmitters. A_2 receptors are found on the cerebral vasculature and peripheral vasculature where stimulation promotes vasodilation. Caffeine and other methylxanthines, such as theophylline, antagonize the inhibitory effect of adenosine, primarily on postsynaptic A_1 receptors. As a result, acute use results in increases in heart rate, ventilation, gastrointestinal motility, gastric acid secretion, and motor activity. Chronic caffeine use results in tolerance and the above symptoms diminish. Caffeine use upregulates A_1 receptors by a variety of mechanisms, including increases in receptor number, increases in receptor affinity, enhancement of receptor coupling to the G protein, and increases in G protein–stimulated adenyl cyclase. An animal study demonstrates that the adenosine receptor has a 3-fold increase in affinity for adenosine at the height of withdrawal symptoms. This model suggests that long-term caffeine administration results in an increase in receptor affinity for adenosine, thus restoring a state of physiologic balance (normal motor inhibitory tone). When caffeine concentrations are reduced below the concentration necessary to maintain this physiologic balance, the enhanced receptor affinity results in a strong adenosine effect and clinical symptoms of withdrawal: headache (cerebral vasodilation), fatigue, and hypersomnia (motor inhibition).

ACETYLCHOLINE RECEPTORS (NICOTINE)

The neuronal nicotinic acetylcholine receptors are pentamers made up of α and β subunits located in the autonomic ganglia, adrenal medulla, CNS, spinal cord, neuromuscular junction, and carotid and aortic bodies. Nicotinic receptors are upregulated in the brain in the setting of chronic nicotine exposure.[61] Nicotinic receptors are fast-response calcium channels that are not coupled to G proteins, distinguishing them from muscarinic receptors, but rather open voltage-gated calcium channels and thereby increasing intracellular calcium concentrations. Activation of calcium/calmodulin-dependent protein kinase II (CaMKII) causes downstream effects, partly through activation of GTPase proteins, and cause the release of GABA, glutamate, and dopamine. CaMKII is upregulated in chronically exposed neurons and synthesis decreases significantly in withdrawal.[45] GTPase activity is mediated by the upregulation of prenyltransferase enzyme systems in chronic nicotine exposure.[76] Nicotinic acetylcholine receptors have both excitatory and inhibitory effects. In the habenulo-interpeduncular pathway, specific nicotinic receptor subtypes ($\alpha5$ and $\beta4$) are concentrated and are associated with aversive effects of nicotine withdrawal. Of note, animal knockouts for $\alpha2$, $\alpha5$, and $\beta4$ display no somatic signs of withdrawal.[8,33] Physical signs of withdrawal in animals are also reduced by blocking $\alpha3\beta4$ receptor subunits.[46] Additionally, severe withdrawal occurs in people with variants of the gene encoding for the $\alpha4$ subunit, making it significantly more sensitive to acetylcholine. Varencycline, a treatment for nicotine abuse, is a partial agonist at $\alpha4\beta2$ nicotinic receptors.[55] As in other withdrawal syndromes, changes brought on by chronic use of nicotinic agonists, such as nicotine in cigarettes, appear to be related to selective upregulation of cAMP.[18,80] Decreased concentrations of synaptic glutamate are associated with the nicotine withdrawal syndrome.[23] Additionally, withdrawal is potentiated by increased concentrations of corticotropin-releasing factor and expression of mRNA for the receptor CRF1R.[15]

CANNABINOID RECEPTORS

Chronic use of cannabinoid receptor agonists causes dependence, and abrupt cessation results in a drug discontinuation syndrome (not withdrawal) that includes anxiety, irritability, abdominal pain, and insomnia. Δ^9-Tetrahydrocannabinol is an agonist at 2 G-protein coupled receptors, CB_1 and CB_2.[37] Agonism of the CB_1 receptor results in its downregulation whereas discontinuation of cannabinoids results in increased gene expression.[9]

SEROTONIN REUPTAKE INHIBITOR DISCONTINUATION SYNDROME

As mentioned above, *drug discontinuation syndrome* is a term used to describe the withdrawal syndrome associated with the therapeutic use of serotonin reuptake inhibitors. It meets the definition of withdrawal syndromes in that symptoms begin when xenobiotic concentrations diminish, and the syndrome abates when the xenobiotic is reintroduced.[64] Headache, nausea, fatigue, dizziness, and dysphoria are commonly described symptoms, with tremor, increased reflexes and muscle tone, tachypnea, and irritability noted in newborns.[2] The condition appears to be uncomfortable but not life threatening, rapidly resolves with reinstatement of a xenobiotic of the same class, and slowly resolves when the medication is discontinued after a more gradual taper (Chap. 69).[67]

SUMMARY

- Withdrawal occurs when a xenobiotic that has produced neuronal adaptive changes is removed.
- The treatment of a withdrawal or a discontinuation syndrome generally involves reintroduction of the xenobiotic from which the patient is withdrawing.
- In some situations, cross-tolerant xenobiotics (those with activity at the same receptor) are administered to treat withdrawal. Examples include the use of benzodiazepines and barbiturates to treat ethanol withdrawal or clonidine for opioid withdrawal.

REFERENCES

1. American Psychiatric Association. *Diagnostic and Statistical Manual of Mental Disorders.* 5th ed. Washington, DC: American Psychiatric Association; 2013.
2. Abdy NA, Gerhart K. Duloxetine withdrawal syndrome in a newborn. *Clin Pediatr (Phila).* 2013;52:976-977.
3. Ahmadi-Soleimani SM, et al. Orexin type 1 receptor antagonism in Lateral Paragiganto-cellularis nucleus attenuates naloxone precipitated morphine withdrawal symptoms in rats. *Neurosci Lett.* 2014;558:62-66.
4. Allison C, Pratt JA, Neuroadaptive processes in GABAergic and glutamatergic systems in benzodiazepine dependence. *Pharmacol Ther.* 2003;98:171-195.
5. Almiron RS, et al. MK-801 prevents the increased NMDA-NR1 and NR2B subunits mRNA expression observed in the hippocampus of rats tolerant to diazepam. *Brain Res.* 2004;1008:54-60.
6. Anderson EM, et al. Phosphorylation of the N-methyl-D-aspartate receptor is increased in the nucleus accumbens during both acute and extended morphine withdrawal. *J Pharmacol Exp Ther.* 2015;355:496-505.
7. Andriamampandry C, et al. Cloning and characterization of a rat brain receptor that binds the endogenous neuromodulator gamma-hydroxybutyrate (GHB). *FASEB J.* 2003;17:1691-1693.
8. Antolin-Fontes B, et al. The habenulo-interpeduncular pathway in nicotine aversion and withdrawal. *Neuropharmacology.* 2015;96(pt B):213-222.
9. Aracil-Fernandez A, et al. Pregabalin and topiramate regulate behavioural and brain gene transcription changes induced by spontaneous cannabinoid withdrawal in mice. *Addict Biol.* 2013;18:252-262.
10. Atack JR. Anxioselective compounds acting at the GABA(A) receptor benzodiazepine binding site. *Curr Drug Targets CNS Neurol Disord.* 2003;2:213-232.
11. Aujla H, et al. Modification of anxiety-like behaviors by nociceptin/orphanin FQ (N/OFQ) and time-dependent changes in N/OFQ-NOP gene expression following ethanol withdrawal. *Addict Biol.* 2013;18:467-479.
12. Awuor SO, et al. Intrathecal baclofen withdrawal: a rare cause of reversible cardiomyopathy. *Acute Card Care.* 2016;18:13-17.
13. Azolosa JL, et al. Opioid physical dependence development: effects of single versus repeated morphine pretreatments and of subjects' opioid exposure history. *Psychopharmacology (Berl).* 1994;114:71-80.
14. Bagley EE. Opioid and GABAB receptors differentially couple to an adenylyl cyclase/protein kinase A downstream effector after chronic morphine treatment. *Front Pharmacol.* 2014;5:148.
15. Baiamonte BA, et al. Nicotine dependence produces hyperalgesia: role of corticotropin-releasing factor-1 receptors (CRF1Rs) in the central amygdala (CeA). *Neuropharmacology.* 2014;77:217-223.
16. Bale AS, et al. Alterations in glutamatergic and gabaergic ion channel activity in hippocampal neurons following exposure to the abused inhalant toluene. *Neuroscience.* 2005;130:197-206.
17. Ballenger JC, Post RM. Kindling as a model for alcohol withdrawal syndromes. *Br J Psychiatry.* 1978;133:1-14.
18. Barik J, Wonnacott S. Molecular and cellular mechanisms of action of nicotine in the CNS. *Handb Exp Pharmacol.* 2009:173-207.
19. Barrot M. Ineffective VTA disinhibition in protracted opiate withdrawal. *Trends Neurosci.* 2015;38:672-673.
20. Beckley EH, et al. Decreased anticonvulsant efficacy of allopregnanolone during ethanol withdrawal in female Withdrawal Seizure-Prone vs. Withdrawal Seizure-Resistant mice. *Neuropharmacology.* 2008;54:365-374.
21. Bekdash RA, Harrison NL. Downregulation of Gabra4 expression during alcohol withdrawal is mediated by specific microRNAs in cultured mouse cortical neurons. *Brain Behav.* 2015;5:e00355.
22. Berger AL, et al. Affective cue-induced escalation of alcohol self-administration and increased 22-kHz ultrasonic vocalizations during alcohol withdrawal: role of kappa-opioid receptors. *Neuropsychopharmacology.* 2013;38:647-654.
23. Bowers MS, et al. N-Acetylcysteine decreased nicotine reward-like properties and withdrawal in mice. *Psychopharmacology (Berl).* 2016;233:995-1003.
24. Bowery NG, et al. International Union of Pharmacology. XXXIII. Mammalian gamma-aminobutyric acid(B) receptors: structure and function. *Pharmacol Rev.* 2002;54:247-264.
25. Cagetti E, et al. Withdrawal from chronic intermittent ethanol treatment changes subunit composition, reduces synaptic function, and decreases behavioral responses to positive allosteric modulators of GABAA receptors. *Mol Pharmacol.* 2003;63:53-64.
26. Charkhpour M, et al. Duloxetine attenuated morphine withdrawal syndrome in the rat. *Drug Res (Stuttg).* 2014;64:393-398.
27. Christian DT, et al. Thalamic glutamatergic afferents into the rat basolateral amygdala exhibit increased presynaptic glutamate function following withdrawal from chronic intermittent ethanol. *Neuropharmacology.* 2013;65:134-142.
28. Chu LF, et al. Acute opioid withdrawal is associated with increased neural activity in reward-processing centers in healthy men: a functional magnetic resonance imaging study. *Drug Alcohol Depend.* 2015;153:314-322.
29. Ciccarelli A, et al. Morphine withdrawal produces ERK-dependent and ERK-independent epigenetic marks in neurons of the nucleus accumbens and lateral septum. *Neuropharmacology.* 2013;70:168-179.
30. Connor M, et al. β-Arrestin-2 knockout prevents development of cellular mu-opioid receptor tolerance but does not affect opioid-withdrawal-related adaptations in single PAG neurons. *Br J Pharmacol.* 2015;172:492-500.
31. D'Addario C, et al. Different alcohol exposures induce selective alterations on the expression of dynorphin and nociceptin systems related genes in rat brain. *Addict Biol.* 2013;18:425-433.
32. Dang K, et al. Interaction of gamma-aminobutyric acid receptor type B receptors and calcium channels in nociceptive transmission studied in the mouse hemisected spinal cord in vitro: withdrawal symptoms related to baclofen treatment. *Neurosci Lett.* 2004;361:72-75.
33. Dani JA, De Biasi M. Mesolimbic dopamine and habenulo-interpeduncular pathways in nicotine withdrawal. *Cold Spring Harb Perspect Med.* 2013;3:a012138.
34. Daut RA, et al. Tolerance to ethanol intoxication after chronic ethanol: role of GluN2A and PSD-95. *Addict Biol.* 2015;20:259-262.
35. Davoudi M, et al. The blockade of GABAA receptors attenuates the inhibitory effect of orexin type 1 receptors antagonist on morphine withdrawal syndrome in rats. *Neurosci Lett.* 2016;617:201-206.
36. Dijkstra BA, et al. Does naltrexone affect craving in abstinent opioid-dependent patients? *Addict Biol.* 2007;12:176-182.
37. Gamage TF, et al. Differential effects of endocannabinoid catabolic inhibitors on morphine withdrawal in mice. *Drug Alcohol Depend.* 2015;146:7-16.
38. Ghavimi H, et al. Acute administration of pioglitazone attenuates morphine withdrawal syndrome in rat: a novel role of pioglitazone. *Drug Res (Stuttg).* 2015;65:113-118.
39. Guo M, et al. Chronic exposure to morphine decreases the expression of EAAT3 via opioid receptors in hippocampal neurons. *Brain Res.* 2015;1628(pt A):40-49.
40. Hamilton RJ, et al. Complications of ultrarapid opioid detoxification with subcutaneous naltrexone pellets. *Acad Emerg Med.* 2002;9:63-68.
41. Han MH, et al. Role of cAMP response element-binding protein in the rat locus ceruleus: regulation of neuronal activity and opiate withdrawal behaviors. *J Neurosci.* 2006;26:4624-4629.
42. Haugbol SR, et al. Upregulation of glutamate receptor subtypes during alcohol withdrawal in rats. *Alcohol Alcohol.* 2005;40:89-95.
43. Heberlein A, et al. Epigenetic down regulation of nerve growth factor during alcohol withdrawal. *Addict Biol.* 2013;18:508-510.
44. Hu Y, et al. Surface expression of GABA_A receptors is transcriptionally controlled by the interplay of cAMP-response element-binding protein and its binding partner inducible cAMP early repressor. *J Biol Chem.* 2008;283:9328-9340.
45. Jackson KJ, Imad Damaj M. Beta_2-containing nicotinic acetylcholine receptors mediate calcium/calmodulin-dependent protein kinase-II and synapsin I protein levels in the nucleus accumbens after nicotine withdrawal in mice. *Eur J Pharmacol.* 2013;701:1-6.
46. Jackson KJ, et al. The alpha3beta4* nicotinic acetylcholine receptor subtype mediates nicotine reward and physical nicotine withdrawal signs independently of the alpha5 subunit in the mouse. *Neuropharmacology.* 2013;70:228-235.
47. Jenkins A, et al. General anesthetics have additive actions on three ligand gated ion channels. *Anesth Analg.* 2008;107:486-493.
48. Johnston CA, Watts VJ. Sensitization of adenylate cyclase: a general mechanism of neuroadaptation to persistent activation of Galpha(i/o)-coupled receptors? *Life Sci.* 2003;73:2913-2925.
49. Kirchmayer U, et al. Naltrexone maintenance treatment for opioid dependence. *Cochrane Database Syst Rev.* 2000:CD001333.
50. Koch T, et al. Receptor endocytosis counteracts the development of opioid tolerance. *Mol Pharmacol.* 2005;67:280-287.
51. Kukoyi A, et al. Two cases of acute dexmedetomidine withdrawal syndrome following prolonged infusion in the intensive care unit: report of cases and review of the literature. *Hum Exp Toxicol.* 2013;32:107-110.
52. Kumar S, et al. Ethanol regulation of gamma-aminobutyric acid A receptors: genomic and nongenomic mechanisms. *Pharmacol Ther.* 2004;101:211-226.
53. Kumar S, et al. The role of GABA(A) receptors in the acute and chronic effects of ethanol: a decade of progress. *Psychopharmacology (Berl).* 2009;205:529-564.
54. Lack AK, et al. Chronic ethanol and withdrawal differentially modulate pre- and post-synaptic function at glutamatergic synapses in rat basolateral amygdala. *J Neurophysiol.* 2007;98:3185-3196.
55. Lazary J, et al. Massive withdrawal symptoms and affective vulnerability are associated with variants of the CHRNA4 gene in a subgroup of smokers. *PLoS One.* 2014;9:e87141.
56. Liang DY, et al. Epigenetic regulation of opioid-induced hyperalgesia, dependence, and tolerance in mice. *J Pain.* 2013;14:36-47.

57. Liang J, et al. Mechanisms of reversible GABAA receptor plasticity after ethanol intoxication. *J Neurosci*. 2007;27:12367-12377.

58. Little HJ, et al. Alcohol withdrawal and conditioning. *Alcohol Clin Exp Res*. 2005;29:453-464.

59. Malcolm RJ. GABA systems, benzodiazepines, and substance dependence. *J Clin Psychiatry*. 2003;64(suppl 3):36-40.

60. Marcinkiewcz CA, et al. Ethanol induced adaptations in 5-HT2c receptor signaling in the bed nucleus of the stria terminalis: implications for anxiety during ethanol withdrawal. *Neuropharmacology*. 2015;89:157-167.

61. McLaughlin I, et al. Nicotine withdrawal. *Curr Top Behav Neurosci*. 2015;24:99-123.

62. N'Gouemo P. Altered voltage-gated calcium channels in rat inferior colliculus neurons contribute to alcohol withdrawal seizures. *Eur Neuropsychopharmacol*. 2015;25:1342-1352.

63. Nestler EJ. Molecular mechanisms of drug addiction. *Neuropharmacology*. 2004; 47(suppl 1):24-32.

64. Nielsen M, et al. What is the difference between dependence and withdrawal reactions? A comparison of benzodiazepines and selective serotonin re-uptake inhibitors. *Addiction*. 2012;107:900-908.

65. Nutt DJ, Malizia AL. New insights into the role of the GABA(A)-benzodiazepine receptor in psychiatric disorder. *Br J Psychiatry*. 2001;179:390-396.

66. Pericic D, et al. Prolonged exposure to gamma-aminobutyric acid up-regulates stably expressed recombinant alpha 1 beta 2 gamma 2s GABAA receptors. *Eur J Pharmacol*. 2003;482:117-125.

67. Precourt A, et al. Multiple complications and withdrawal syndrome associated with quetiapine/venlafaxine intoxication. *Ann Pharmacother*. 2005;39:153-156.

68. Rayner SG, et al. Dexmedetomidine as adjunct treatment for severe alcohol withdrawal in the ICU. *Ann Intensive Care*. 2012;2:12.

69. Rehni AK, Singh TG. Pharmacological modulation of geranylgeranyltransferase and farnesyltransferase attenuates opioid withdrawal in vivo and in vitro. *Neuropharmacology*. 2013;71:19-26.

70. Riegel AC, et al. Toluene-induced locomotor activity is blocked by 6-hydroxydopamine lesions of the nucleus accumbens and the mGluR2/3 agonist LY379268. *Neuropsychopharmacology*. 2003;28:1440-1447.

71. Riker RR, et al. Dexmedetomidine vs midazolam for sedation of critically ill patients: a randomized trial. *JAMA*. 2009;301:489-499.

72. Sanna E, et al. Changes in GABA(A) receptor gene expression associated with selective alterations in receptor function and pharmacology after ethanol withdrawal. *J Neurosci*. 2003;23:11711-11724.

73. Schep LJ, et al. The clinical toxicology of gamma-hydroxybutyrate, gamma-butyrolactone and 1,4-butanediol. *Clin Toxicol (Phila)*. 2012;50:458-470.

74. Shah R, et al. Phenomenology of gasoline intoxication and withdrawal symptoms among adolescents in India: a case series. *Am J Addict* 1999;8:254-257.

75. Sheela Rani CS, Ticku MK. Comparison of chronic ethanol and chronic intermittent ethanol treatments on the expression of GABA(A) and NMDA receptor subunits. *Alcohol* 2006;38:89-97.

76. Singh TG, et al. Pharmacological modulation of farnesyltransferase subtype I attenuates mecamylamine-precipitated nicotine withdrawal syndrome in mice. *Behav Pharmacol*. 2013;24:668-677.

77. Smith SS, et al. Neurosteroid regulation of GABA(A) receptors: focus on the alpha4 and delta subunits. *Pharmacol Ther*. 2007;116:58-76.

78. Spahn V, et al. Opioid withdrawal increases transient receptor potential vanilloid 1 activity in a protein kinase A-dependent manner. *Pain*. 2013;154:598-608.

79. Tarabar AF, Nelson LS. The gamma-hydroxybutyrate withdrawal syndrome. *Toxicol Rev*. 2004;23:45-49.

80. Tzavara ET, et al. Nicotine withdrawal syndrome: behavioural distress and selective up-regulation of the cyclic AMP pathway in the amygdala. *Eur J Neurosci*. 2002;16:149-153.

81. Wafford KA. GABAA receptor subtypes: any clues to the mechanism of benzodiazepine dependence? *Curr Opin Pharmacol*. 2005;5:47-52.

82. Weber MD, et al. Acute discontinuation syndrome from dexmedetomidine after protracted use in a pediatric patient. *Paediatr Anaesth*. 2008;18:87-88.

83. Williams JM, et al. Effects of repeated inhalation of toluene on ionotropic GABA A and glutamate receptor subunit levels in rat brain. *Neurochem Int*. 2005;46:1-10.

84. Wong CG, et al. From the street to the brain: neurobiology of the recreational drug gamma-hydroxybutyric acid. *Trends Pharmacol Sci*. 2004;25:29-34.

CASE STUDY 3

History A 54-year-old man presented to the emergency department (ED) complaining that he was weak, dizzy, and felt as if he was about to pass out. His past medical history was significant for opioid dependence. Three hours earlier he saw an alternative medical provider and was given a natural remedy to help him "detoxify." Prior to this therapy, he was receiving daily methadone, but transitioned to hydrocodone in preparation for treatment. He denied nausea, vomiting, diarrhea, lacrimation, or other symptoms consistent with opioid withdrawal. In triage, his pulse was 35 beats/min, so the patient was immediately triaged to the critical care area.

Physical Examination On arrival to the critical care area he was awake but complaining of weakness. Vital signs were: blood pressure, 128/62 mm Hg; pulse, 35 beats/min; respiratory rate, 14 breaths/min; rectal temperature, 98.4°F (36.9°C); oxygen saturation, 98% on room air; and glucose, 110 mg/dL. A general physical examination was unremarkable and specifically noted the absence of mydriasis, piloerection, rhinorrhea, or lacrimation.

Initial Management The patient was immediately attached to continuous cardiac monitoring and an electrocardiogram (ECG) was obtained (**Fig. CS3–1**), which

was notable for sinus bradycardia with a QT interval of approximately 600 ms and an abnormally shaped T wave. An intravenous catheter (IV) was inserted and blood was sent for a complete blood count and electrolytes.

Suddenly, the patient lost consciousness and became pulseless. A rhythm strip captured the event (**Fig. CS3–2**), which was torsade de pointes (TdP) (Chap. 15). The event self-terminated, and the patient awoke, but syncope recurred 5 minutes later. Although he spontaneously recovered again, at this time he was administered 2 g of magnesium sulfate intravenously over several minutes followed by a continuous magnesium infusion at 1 g/h. His cardiac rhythm was converted to a normal sinus rhythm, and he was transferred to the cardiac intensive care unit (CCU), where a temporary transvenous pacemaker was inserted.

What Is the Differential Diagnosis? In addition to congenital and acquired intrinsic cardiac conditions and electrolyte abnormalities (Chap. 12), numerous xenobiotics from diverse chemical classes are associated with QT interval prolongation and the risk of TdP. These xenobiotics, which typically share an ability to block myocardial potassium channels (Chap. 15), can be found throughout this textbook. Common classes of xenobiotics that are associated with QT interval prolongation, and some

specific examples, are listed in **Table CS3–1**. Readers are referred to www.crediblemeds.com, a comprehensive website that risk stratifies a myriad of pharmaceuticals. It is noteworthy that many nonpharmaceutical xenobiotics also are listed in the table and textbook.

What Rapid Clinical and Laboratory Analyses Can Help Determine the Etiology and Guide Therapy for This Patient's Presentation? Because the differential diagnosis is so extensive, broad laboratory testing is not advocated to determine the etiology in patients with unclear causes for QT interval prolongation. Instead, efforts should be directed at a thorough history, because the cause may then become evident. Patients should have routine electrolytes measured, because hypokalemia, hypocalcemia, and hypomagnesemia can all either be the primary cause of QT interval prolongation or be contributory when another primary etiology exists. Because these electrolyte abnormalities can be rapidly corrected in most circumstances, they represent easy and important interventions. When acute overdose is suspected, gastrointestinal decontamination can help limit drug absorption or enhance elimination (Chap. 5 and Antidotes in Depth: A1, A2).

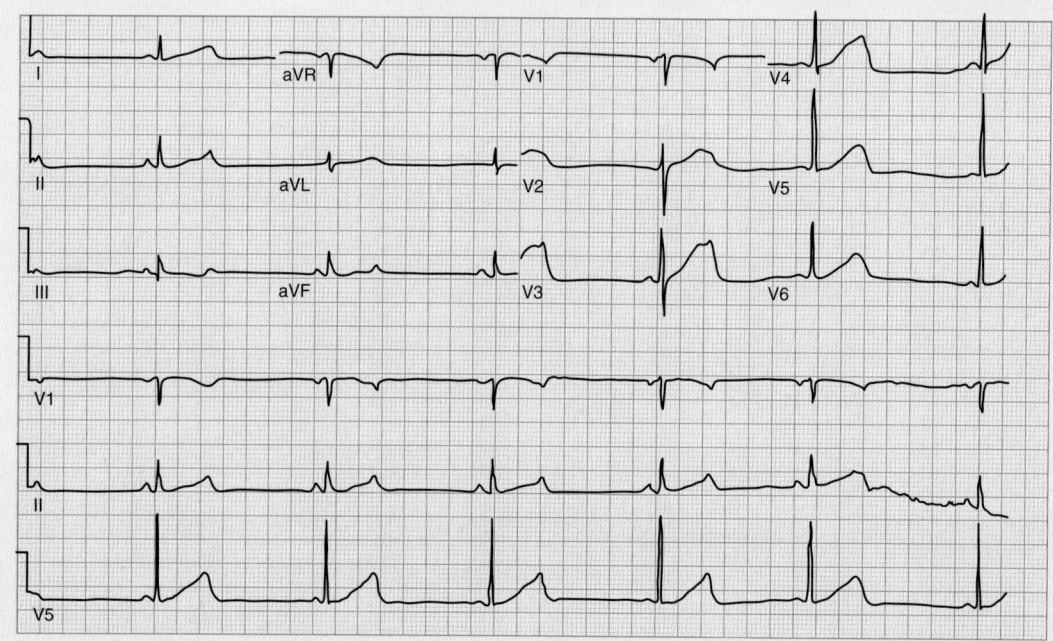

FIGURE CS3–1. Initial electrocardiograph demonstrating sinus bradycardia at a heart rate of 35 beats/min with a normal axis, normal PR interval of 120 ms, a normal QRS duration of 80 ms, and prolonged QT interval at nearly 600 ms with an abnormal T-wave morphology. (*Used with permission from The Fellowship in Medical Toxicology, New York University School of Medicine, New York City Poison Center.*)

CASE STUDY 3 (CONTINUED)

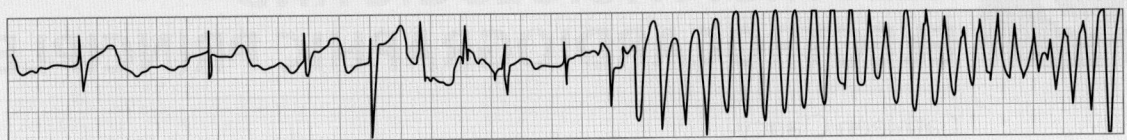

FIGURE CS3–2. Electrocardiograph associated with loss of consciousness demonstrating the transition from bradycardia to ventricular ectopy followed by an episode of torsade de pointes. *(Used with permission from The Fellowship in Medical Toxicology, New York University School of Medicine, New York City Poison Center.)*

TABLE CS3–1	Xenobiotics Associated With QT Interval Prolongation and Torsade de Pointes
Class	**Specific Examples**
β-Adrenergic antagonists	Sotalol
Antibiotics	Macrolides and fluoroquinolones
Antidysrhythmics	(Class IA, IC, and III)
Antiepileptics	Carbamazepine
Antimalarials	Chloroquine, mefloquine, halofantrine
Antipsychotics	Phenothiazines
Caustics	Hydrofluoric acid
Cyclic antidepressants	Most
Drugs of abuse	Cocaine
Herbals	Ibogaine
Metals	Arsenic, barium, cesium
Opioids	Methadone
Pesticides	Organic phosphorus compounds
Serotonin reuptake inhibitors	Citalopram

Further Diagnosis and Treatment

Laboratory evaluation demonstrated normal concentrations of magnesium whereas his calcium and potassium were low. The patient stated that he had received ibogaine therapy to treat his opioid dependence, which is associated with both bradycardia and QT interval prolongation. While in the CCU, he had several episodes of ventricular ectopy but no recurrent TdP. His hypokalemia was corrected with supplemental potassium chloride, stress echocardiogram showed no signs of structural heart disease. Several days later he was discharged with a normal heart rate and a minimally prolonged mild QT interval 470 ms.

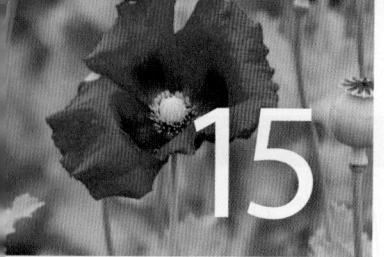

15 CARDIOLOGIC PRINCIPLES I: ELECTROPHYSIOLOGIC AND ELECTROCARDIOGRAPHIC PRINCIPLES

Cathleen Clancy

ELECTROPHYSIOLOGIC PRINCIPLES

The clinical tool most commonly used to assess cardiac function is the surface electrocardiogram (ECG). The ECG records the sum of the electrical changes occurring within the myocardium. The electrophysiologic basis of cardiac function and the ECG are complex and are subject to alteration by numerous xenobiotics. Ion currents flowing through various ion channels are responsible for cardiac function. Electrophysiologic studies identify the functional types of membrane receptors and ion channels. Molecular genetic studies identify the gene coding for the key cardiac ion channels and elucidate the structural and physiologic relationships that lead to the toxic effects of many xenobiotics. These channels are critical for maintenance of the intracellular ion concentrations necessary for action potential development, impulse conduction throughout the heart, and myocyte contraction. This chapter will first review the individual ion channels and their currents, and then summarize their contribution and effects on the ECG.

ION CHANNELS OF THE MYOCARDIAL CELL MEMBRANE

Sodium Channels

The voltage-sensitive sodium channels are responsible for the initiation of depolarization of the myocardial membrane. All currently identified voltage-sensitive channels, including the sodium and calcium channels, have structures similar to the potassium channel assembly. The sodium channel gene encodes a single protein that contains 4 functional domains (D I to D IV). Each of these domains has the 6 membrane-spanning regions characteristic of the voltage-gated potassium channel and is structurally similar to the α subunit of the potassium channel. The single, large α subunit of the sodium channel assembles with regulatory β subunits to form the functional unit of the sodium channel (Fig. 15–1A). The best characterized of the sodium channels, the *SCN5A* gene–encoded α channel, is inactivated by xenobiotic interactions between the D III and the D IV domains to physically block the inner mouth of the sodium channel pore.[29] Seven specific receptor sites are

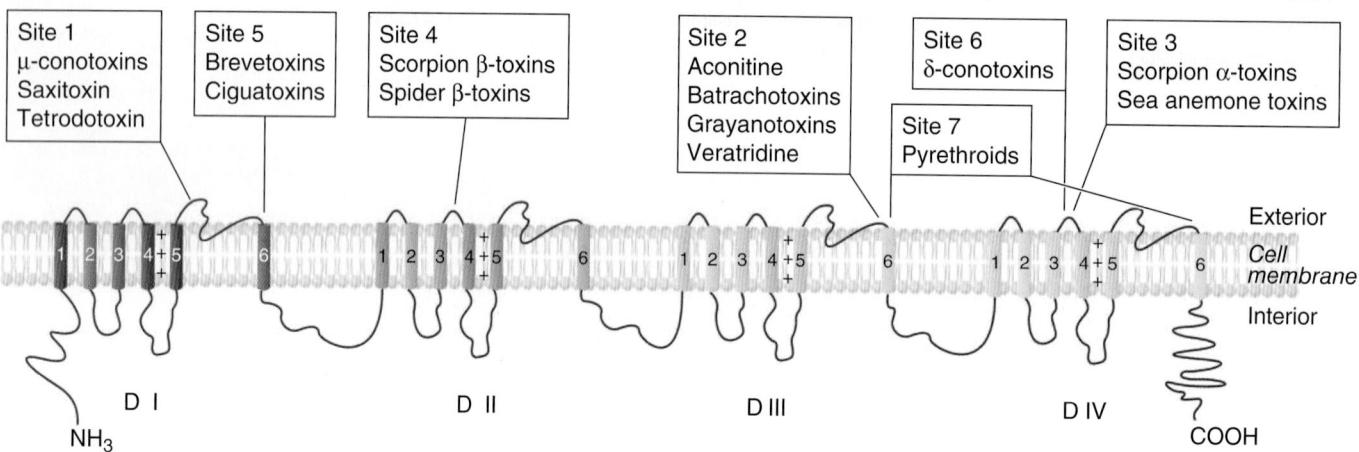

A

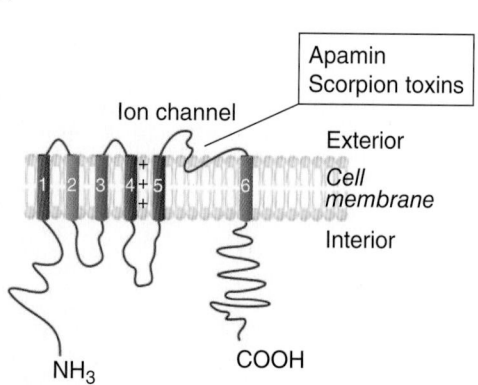

B

FIGURE 15–1. Structure of the sodium and potassium channels. (**A**) The structure of the α subunit of the sodium channel. The protein molecule has 4 functional domains (D I–D IV) each analogous to one of the potassium channel α subunits. One of these molecules assembles with β subunits to form the membrane sodium channel. Sites 1–7 are shown with individual toxins known to bind at these sites. (**B**) The structure of the α-subunit of the voltage-gated potassium channel. The protein molecule has 6 membrane-spanning regions (1–6); the voltage-sensitive region is at 4 and the actual ion channel is located between regions 5 and 6, similar to the α sodium channel. Four of these α-subunits assemble with 4 β subunits to form the potassium channel complex.

currently identified on the α subunit, with different xenobiotics binding at the specific sites: tetrodotoxin, saxitoxin, μ-conotoxin (site 1); aconitine, batrachotoxin, grayanotoxin, veratridine (site 2); α scorpion toxins, sea anemone toxins (site 3); β scorpion toxins, Chinese bird spider toxin (site 4); brevetoxins, ciguatoxins (site 5); δ-conotoxins (site 6); pyrethroids (site 7), and local anesthetics and related antidysrhythmics and antiepileptics binding at overlapping receptor sites.[14,57,61,71]

Potassium Channels

Ion channels that change their conductance of current with changes in the transmembrane voltage potential are called *rectifying channels*. The voltage-sensitive potassium channels are categorized based on their speed of activation and their voltage response. They include the "delayed rectifier" potassium currents, particularly the I_{Kr} (rapidly activating) and the I_{Ks} (slowly activating) channels.[43] Potassium channels form large multimolecular complexes with regulatory kinases, phosphatases, anchoring proteins, accessory subunits, and with each other.

The various voltage-gated potassium channels share an underlying structural similarity. The α subunit is a protein molecule with 6 membrane-spanning α-helical regions, 1 to 6 (Fig. 15–1B). The pore domain is located between the regions five and six of the α subunit. Region 4 is the voltage sensor region.[53,64] Apamin, found in apitoxin obtained from bee venom, is a potent blocker of a specific subset of Ca^{2+}-activated K^+ channels conferring atrial antidysrhythmic effects. The scorpion toxins scyllatoxin and tamapin block similar K^+ channels although they are structurally dissimilar.[57] There are more than 70 genes encoding K^+ channels in the human genome.[3] Human Ether-à-go-go Related Gene (hERG) encodes the α subunit that assembles with β subunit proteins to form the I_{Kr} potassium channel. The C-terminus region of the α subunit encoded by hERG has a cyclic nucleotide binding domain and an N-terminus region similar to domains involved in signal transduction in cells.[64]

Many xenobiotics interact with the hERG-encoded subunit of the potassium channel to reduce the current through the I_{Kr} channel and prolong the action potential duration. The hERG α subunit of the channel is particularly susceptible to xenobiotic-induced interactions because of 2 important differences from the other channels. First, region 6 of the hERG channel has aromatic side chains on the inner cavity pore that can bind to aromatic xenobiotics, for example, cisapride, haloperidol, and terfenadine.[55] Additionally, the inner cavity and entrance of the hERG channel is larger than the other voltage-gated potassium channels. This larger pore can accommodate larger xenobiotics that get trapped within the pore when the channel closes.[52,53,64]

Calcium Channels

Calcium channel conductivity across the myocardial cell membrane is critical for the maintenance of the appropriate duration of cell membrane depolarization and for initiation of cellular contraction. The best characterized of the calcium channels are the slow (L-type), the fast (T-type), and the ryanodine receptor calcium channel. They are more prominently involved in cardiac contractility and discussed in Chapter 16.

ION CHANNELS AND MYOCARDIAL CELL ACTION POTENTIAL

An understanding of the basic electrophysiology of the myocardial cell is essential to understand the toxicity of xenobiotics and to plan appropriate therapy. Figure 15–2A shows the typical action potential of myocardial cell depolarization, the electrolyte fluxes responsible for the action potential, and the resulting ECG complex (Fig. 15–2B). The action potentials of the contractile and the conductive cells are also shown.

The action potential is divided into 5 phases: phase 0, depolarization; phase 1, overshoot; phase 2, plateau; phase 3, repolarization; and phase 4, resting. Phase 0 begins when the cell is excited either by a stimulus from an adjoining cell or by spontaneous depolarization of a pacemaker cell. The stimulus causes selective voltage-gated fast sodium channels (I_{Na+}) to open, resulting in rapid depolarization of the membrane. At the end of phase 0, the

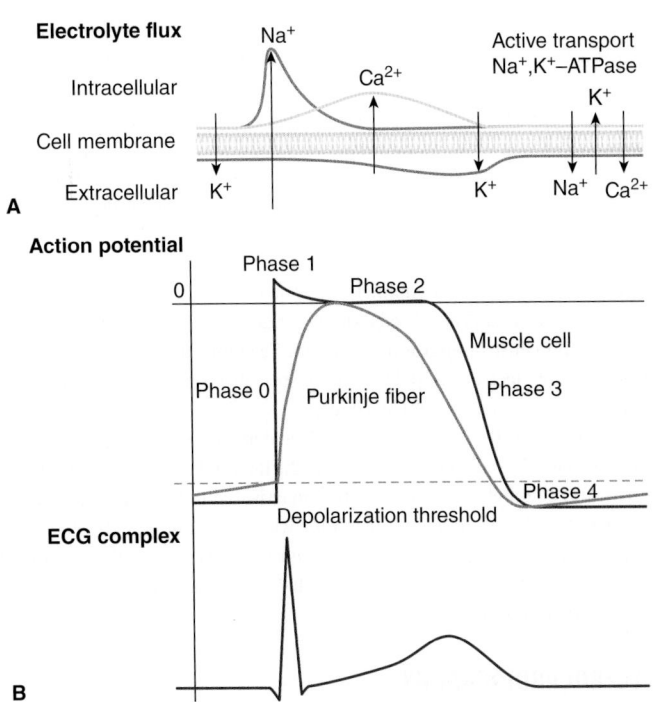

FIGURE 15–2. Relationship of electrolyte movement across the cell membrane (**A**) to the action potential and the surface ECG recording (**B**) over a single cardiac cycle.

voltage-sensitive sodium channels close and a transient outward potassium current (I_{To}) occurs, resulting in a partial repolarization of the membrane—this constitutes phase 1.

During phase 2 (plateau phase), the inward depolarizing calcium currents are largely balanced by the outward repolarizing potassium currents. Voltage-sensitive calcium channels that open allow Ca^{2+} movement down the 5,000–10,000-fold concentration gradient into the cell. These channels are categorized based on their conductance (fast or slow) and their sensitivity to voltage changes.[57] The calcium currents (mostly the "long-lasting" current) gradually decrease as the channels inactivate. Simultaneously, the outward potassium "delayed rectifier" currents, particularly the I_{Ks} (slowly activating) current increases, terminating the plateau phase of the action potential and initiating cellular repolarization (phase 3). Other, smaller, outward potassium currents (not shown in Fig. 15–2A) play a lesser role in the duration of the action potential and development of phase 3, including I_{Kur} (ultrarapid), I_{Kr} (rapidly activating), I_{K-Ach} (acetylcholine-dependent), and I_{K-ATP} (adenosine triphosphate–dependent) currents.

In phase 3, the rapid repolarization phase, the cell membrane repolarizes as a result of the voltage-gated currents, the delayed rectifier currents (I_{Kr}, I_{Ks}), and to a lesser extent the other K^+ currents, the Na^+,Ca^{2+} exchanger current, and the sodium/potassium pump (active transport via Na^+,K^+-ATPase.

Phase 4 is the resting state for much of the myocardium, except the pacemaker cells, and it corresponds to diastole in the cardiac cycle. During phases 3 and 4, active transport of Na^+, K^+, and Ca^{2+} against their electrochemical gradients returns the myocyte to its baseline resting state. The transmembrane electrochemical gradient is maintained during the resting state by a Ca^{2+},Na^+ exchange mechanism and by ATP-dependent pumps in the membrane that together move Ca^{2+} out of the cells.[57]

In the pacemaker cells during phase 4 of the action potential, gradual electrical depolarization of the membrane occurs due to potassium currents called the I_{kf} for "funny" or the I_{Kh} for "hyperpolarization-activated" current.[6,16] The membrane potential gradually increases in these pacemaker cells until the threshold potential is reached, the fast inward sodium channels open, and the I_{Na} current initiates the next phase 0. This electrical impulse is then propagated via the His-Purkinje conducting system of the heart.

In addition to its role in myocardial contractility, Ca^{2+} influx is also important in pacemaker function. Although spontaneous pacemaker cell depolarization has traditionally been ascribed to inward cation current through "pacemaker channels,"[16] more recent research suggests that it is actually driven by rhythmic release of calcium from the sarcoplasmic reticulum.[36,37] Regardless, Ca^{2+} flux plays an important role in the spontaneous depolarization (phase 4) of the action potential in the sinoatrial (SA) node.[38] The rate of pacemaker cell depolarization is enhanced by β-adrenergic stimulation through phosphorylation of proteins on the sarcoplasmic reticulum and by a phosphorylation-independent action of cAMP at the pacemaker channels.[42] Depolarization of cells in the SA node spreads to surrounding atrial cells where it triggers the opening of fast sodium channels and causes impulse propagation. Calcium flux also allows normal propagation of electrical impulses via the specialized myocardial conduction tissues in the atrioventricular (AV) node.

During phases 0 to 2, the cell cannot be depolarized again with another stimulus; the cell is absolutely *refractory*. During the latter half of phase 3, as the calcium channels recover from their inactivated to their resting state, an electrical stimulus of sufficient magnitude will cause another depolarization; the cell is said to be *relatively refractory*. During phase 4, the cell is no longer refractory and any appropriate stimulus that reaches the threshold level will cause depolarization.

ELECTROCARDIOGRAPHY

The ECG measures the sum of all electrical activity in the heart. It is used extensively in medicine and its interpretation is widely understood by physicians of nearly all disciplines. It is an invaluable diagnostic tool for patients with cardiovascular complaints. However, it is also a valuable source of information in poisoned patients and has the potential to enhance and direct their care. Although it seems obvious that an ECG would be required following exposure to a medication used for cardiovascular indications, many medications with no overt cardiovascular effects at therapeutic doses are cardiotoxic in overdose, for example loperamide. Furthermore, in patients with unknown exposures, the ECG can suggest specific xenobiotics or demonstrate electrolyte abnormalities, long before blood is drawn. For example, oropharyngeal or dermal burns in a patient whose ECG has evidence of hyperkalemia or hypocalcemia suggests exposure to hydrofluoric acid (Chap. 104).[69] Alternatively, a patient manifesting signs of the opioid toxidrome with runs of torsade de pointes might have ingested methadone (Chap. 36).[21] QT interval prolongation is a clue to the etiology of an overdose with an atypical antipsychotic such as quetiapine (Chap. 67). The ECG is used to predict complications of poisoning, such as seizures following a cyclic antidepressant overdose (Chap. 68). Therefore, an ECG should be examined early in the initial evaluation of most poisoned patients.

History of the ECG

In the 1900s, Willem Einthoven graphically displayed the electrical activity of the heart and named the different waves—P, QRS, and T. He called this tracing an "elektrokardiogramme," and was awarded a Nobel Prize in 1924 for his efforts. The acronym *EKG*, still employed by some authors, was derived from Einthoven's spelling. The acronym *ECG*, which is consistent with our current spelling of electrocardiogram, is used throughout this text.

Since this initial description, both the normal electrophysiology of the heart and the pharmacologic effects of various xenobiotics on the ECG have been described. Despite the large number, diversity, and complexity of the various cardiac toxins, there are a limited number of electrocardiographic manifestations.

Basic Electrophysiology of an ECG

Simplistically, a positive or upward deflection on the oscilloscope is generated when an electrical force moves toward an electrical sensor or electrode, and a downward deflection occurs if the force moves away. An ECG represents the sum of movement of all electrical forces in the heart in relation to the surface electrode, and the height above baseline represents the magnitude of the force (Fig. 15–2B). Only during depolarization or repolarization

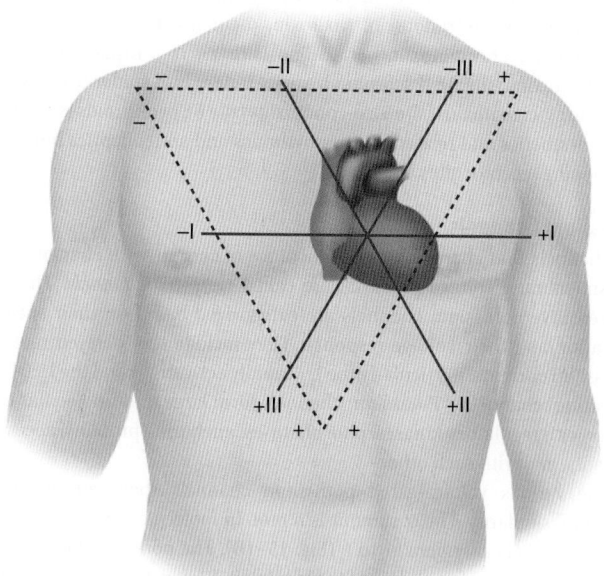

FIGURE 15–3. The hexaxial reference system derived from the Einthoven equilateral triangle defining the electrical potential vectors of electrocardiography. The relationships of the original 3 limb leads are illustrated. The equiangular (60°) Einthoven triangle formed by leads I, II, and III is shown (*dotted lines*), with positive and negative poles of each of the leads indicated. Leads I, II, and III are also presented as a triaxial reference system that intersects in the center of the ventricles.

does the ECG tracing leave the isoelectric baseline, because it is only during these periods that measurable net currents are flowing in the heart. During the other periods, mechanical effects are occurring in the myocardium, but large amounts of current are not flowing.

Leads

Although the reading from a single ECG lead can provide valuable information, to visualize the heart in a nearly 3-dimensional perspective, multiple leads must be assessed simultaneously. Given the cylindrical nature of both the heart and thorax, at any given moment some of these leads will record positive voltage and others negative. The lead placement that was described and refined by Einthoven forms the basis for the bipolar or limb leads, described as I, II, and III (Fig. 15–3). The Einthoven triangle is an equilateral triangle formed by the sum of these leads. Unipolar limb leads and precordial leads were subsequently added to the standard ECG. Unipolar leads were created when the limb leads were connected to a common point where the sum of the potentials from leads I, II, and III was zero. The currently used unipolar augmented (a) leads (aV_R, aV_L, and aV_F) are based on these unipolar leads (Fig. 15–4). The voltage potential of these unipolar, "augmented leads" is small; thus, it is amplified by incorporating the voltage change of the other 2 augmented leads. Together, leads I, II, III, aV_R, aV_L, and aV_F form the hexaxial reference system that is used to calculate the electrical axis of the heart in the frontal plane. The precordial leads, called V_1 through V_6, are also unipolar measurements of the change in electric potential measured from a central point to the sixth anterior and left lateral chest positions (Fig. 15–5). If V_2 is placed over the right ventricle, part of the initial positive ventricular deflection (QRS complex) reflects right ventricular activation, with electrical forces moving toward the electrode. The majority of the subsequent terminal negative deflection reflects activation of other muscle tissue (septum, left ventricular wall) when the electrical forces are moving away from the electrode. Recordings from each of these 12 leads (I, II, III, aV_R, aV_L, aV_F, V_{1-6}) evaluate the heart from 2 different planes in 12 different positions, yielding a 3-dimensional electrical "picture" of the heart, with respect aV_R, aV_L, aV_F, to time and voltage.

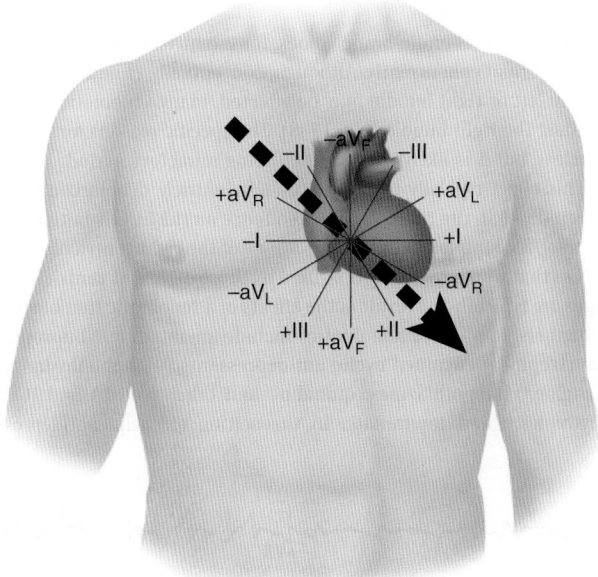

FIGURE 15–4. The hexaxial reference system derived from the Einthoven equilateral triangle defining the electrical potential vectors of electrocardiography showing the relationship between cardiac anatomy and electrocardiographic leads.

A continuous cardiac monitor often relies on recordings from one of 2 bipolar leads: a modified left chest lead (MCL$_1$) or a lead II. The recording from an MCL$_1$, in which the positive electrode is in the V$_1$ position, is similar in appearance to a V$_1$ recording on a 12-lead ECG. This lead visualizes ventricular activity well; however, lead II shows atrial activity (ie, the P wave) much more clearly. Right ventricular precordial leads (V$_1$, V$_{3-6}$R) are sensitive and specific for determining the presence of right ventricular myocardial infarctions, although specific applications to poisoning are not reported.

Various Intervals and Waves

The ECG tracing has specific nomenclature to define the characteristic patterns. Waves refer to positive or negative deflections from baseline, such as the P,

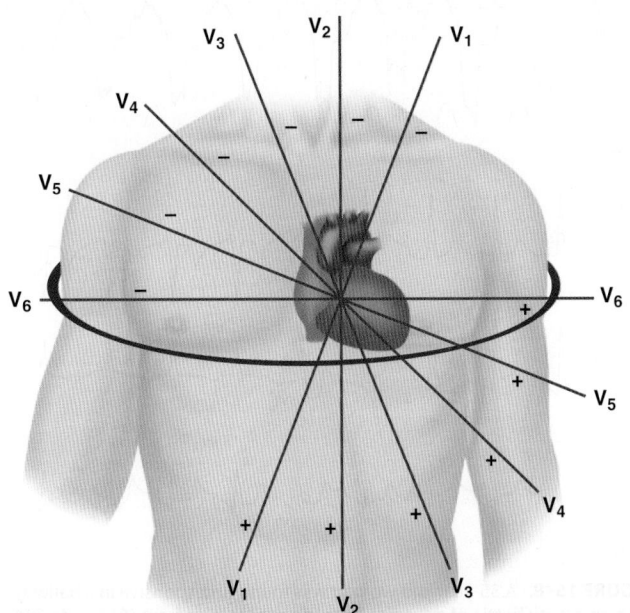

FIGURE 15–5. Visualized as a cross-section, each of the chest lead is oriented through the atrioventricular (AV) node and exits through the patient's back, which is negative.

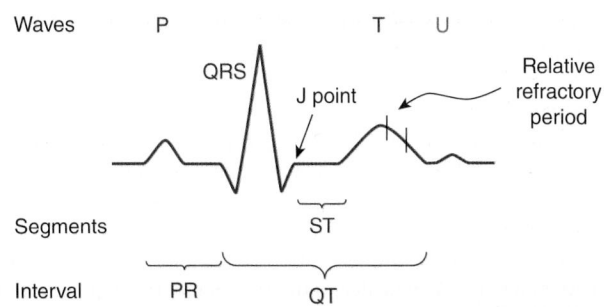

FIGURE 15–6. The normal ECG. The U wave is the small, positive deflection following the T wave. P wave, PR interval, atrial depolarization; QRS complex, ventricular depolarization; ST segment, T wave, QT interval, and U wave, and ventricular repolarization demonstrate the normal ECG.

T, or U waves. A segment is defined as the distance between 2 waves, such as the ST segment, and an interval measures the duration of a wave plus a segment, such as QT or PR interval. Complexes are a group of waves without intervals or segments between them (QRS complex). Electrophysiologically, the P wave and PR interval on the ECG tracing represent the depolarization of the atria. The QRS complex represents the depolarization of the ventricles. The plateau is depicted by the ST segment and repolarization is visualized as the T wave and the QT interval (QT). The U wave, when present, generally represents an afterdepolarization (Fig. 15–6).

The P Wave

The P wave is the initial deflection on the ECG that occurs with the initiation of each new cardiac cycle.

Electrophysiology

The early, middle, and late portions of the P wave are represented sequentially by the electrical potential initiated by the sinus node. The impulse is propagated directly through the right atrial muscle, producing contraction. The impulse is also propagated by specialized conduction tissue across the interatrial septum, to produce contraction of the left atrium. Additionally, internodal pathways rapidly conduct the impulse to the AV node. The electrical excitation of the sinus node differs from that of the ventricular myocardium in that current is mediated primarily by Ca^{2+} influx via slow T-type calcium channels, following hyperpolarization by the I$_{kf}$, mixed sodium-potassium current (f for "funny"). The "funny" current is also called the I$_{Kh}$ (h for "hyperpolarization-activated"). The vagus nerve and β-adrenergic stimulation also affect conduction across nodal tissues.[6]

Abnormal P Wave

Clinically, abnormalities of the P wave occur with xenobiotics that depress automaticity of the sinus node, causing sinus arrest and nodal or ventricular escape rhythms (β-adrenergic antagonists, calcium channel blockers). The P wave is absent in rhythms with sinus arrest, such as occurs with xenobiotics that increase vagal tone such as cardioactive steroids and cholinergics. A notched P wave suggests delayed conduction across the atrial septum and is characteristic of quinidine poisoning or atrial enlargement (Fig. 15–7). P waves

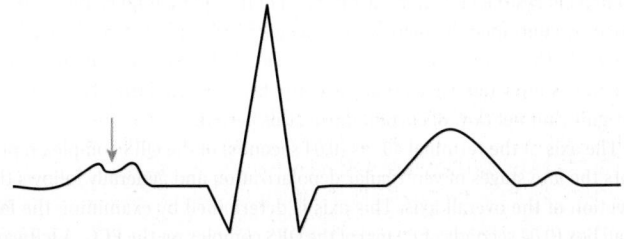

FIGURE 15–7. A notched P wave (arrow) suggests delayed conduction across the atrial septum and is characteristic of quinidine poisoning.

decrease in amplitude as hyperkalemia becomes more severe until they become indistinguishable from the baseline (Chap. 12).

PR Interval

The PR interval is measured from the beginning of the P wave to the beginning of the QRS complex (normal is 120–200 milliseconds {ms}).

Electrophysiology

Despite rapid conduction by specialized conduction tissue from the SA to the AV node, the AV node delays transmission of the impulse into the ventricles, ostensibly to allow for complete atrial emptying. Thus, the PR interval represents the interval between the onset of atrial depolarization and the onset of ventricular depolarization. Children usually have more rapid conduction and a shortened PR interval, and older adults generally have a prolonged PR interval. The segment between the end of the P wave and the beginning of the QRS complex (the PQ segment) reflects atrial contraction and is usually isoelectric. Atrial repolarization coincides with the Q wave, but the ECG evidence, or atrial T waves, are obscured by the QRS complex.

Abnormal PR Interval

Xenobiotics that decrease interatrial or AV nodal conduction cause marked prolongation of the PR segment until such conduction completely ceases. At this point, the P wave no longer relates to the QRS complex; this is AV dissociation, or complete heart block. Some xenobiotics suppress AV nodal conduction by blocking calcium channels in nodal cells, as does magnesium, β-adrenergic antagonists, or muscarinics through enhanced vagal tone. Although the therapeutic concentrations of digoxin, as well as early cardio-active steroid poisoning, cause PR prolongation through vagal tone, direct electrophysiologic effects account for the bradycardia of poisoning (Chap. 62 and Antidotes in Depth: A22).

QRS Complex

The QRS complex is the second and typically largest deflection on the ECG. The normal QRS duration in adults varies between 60 and 100 ms. A QRS duration that is prolonged from the patient's baseline in the setting of poisoning indicates toxicity even if the QRS is within the normal range. The normal QRS complex axis in the frontal plane lies between −30° and 90°, although most individuals have an axis between 30° and 75°. This axis will vary with the weight and age of the patient. Alterations in myocardial function will also alter the electrical axis of the heart.

Electrophysiology

The QRS complex reflects the electrical forces generated by ventricular depolarization mediated primarily by Na^+ influx into the myocardial cells. Although under normal conditions both ventricles depolarize nearly simultaneously, the greater mass of the left ventricle causes it to contribute the majority of the electrical forces. The QRS complex is primarily positive in leads I and aV_L on the surface ECG recording because under normal conditions the depolarization vector is directed at 60° and is thus moving toward these leads.

The simultaneous and rapid depolarization of the ventricles results in a very short period of electrical activity recorded on the electrocardiogram. Mechanical systole lasts well past the end of the QRS complex and is maintained by continued depolarization during the plateau phase of the action potential. The return to, and maintenance of, the baseline, or isoelectric potential, simply represents that the entire heart is depolarized and there is no significant net flow of current during this period.

The axis of the terminal 40 ms (0.04 seconds) of the QRS complex represents the late stages of ventricular depolarization and generally follows the direction of the overall axis. This axis is determined by examining the last small box (0.04 seconds or 40 ms) of the QRS complex on the ECG. A leftward shift of the terminal 40 ms axis of the QRS complex correlates with toxicity from xenobiotics with Na^+-channel–blocking effects (Chap. 68).

Abnormal QRS Complex

In the presence of a bundle-branch block, the 2 ventricles depolarize sequentially rather than concurrently. Although, conceptually, conduction through either the left or right bundle may be affected, many xenobiotics preferentially affect the right bundle (Fig. 15–8). The specific reasons for this effect are unclear, but it is likely related to differing refractory periods of the tissues. This effect typically results in the left ventricle depolarizing slightly more rapidly than the right. The consequence on the ECG is both a widening of the QRS complex and the appearance of the right ventricular electrical forces that were previously obscured by those of the left ventricle. These changes are typically the result of the effects of a xenobiotic that blocks fast Na^+ channels. Implicated xenobiotics include amantadine,[56] buproprion,[22] carbamazepine,[30] cocaine,[1] cyclic antidepressants,[11,12] diphenhydramine,[58] lamotrigine,[45] phenothiazines, quinidine and other type IA and IC antidysrhythmics,[17] and topiramate. In the setting of cyclic antidepressant

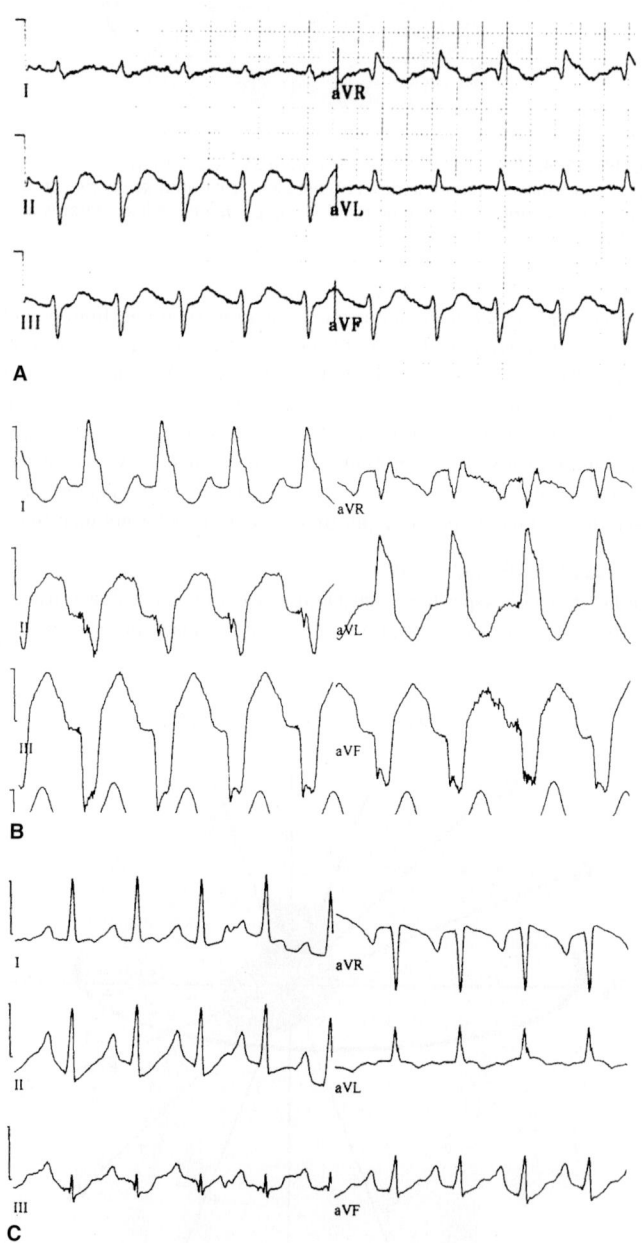

FIGURE 15–8. A 35-year-old woman was found unresponsive in a hallway with an empty bottle of doxepin. Note the progression from (**A**) a wide QRS interval (108 ms, axis +10); to (**B**) at >35 min: a right bundle branch block (RBBB) with an axis of −50 and a rightward shift of the terminal 40 ms of the QRS axis; and (**C**) in the next hour, marked improvement occurred after infusion of hypertonic sodium bicarbonate.

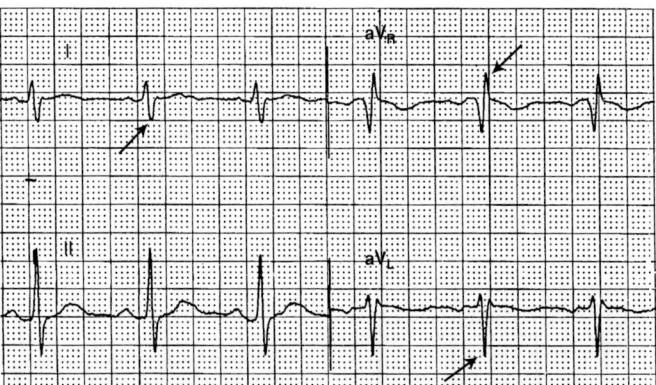

FIGURE 15–9. ECG of a patient with a tricyclic antidepressant overdose. The arrows highlight prominent S wave in leads I and aV_L, and the R wave in aV_R demonstrates the terminal 40-ms rightward axis shift. *(Used with permission from the Fellowship in Medical Toxicology, New York University School of Medicine, New York City Poison Center.)*

poisoning, a prolonged QRS duration has both prognostic and therapeutic value (Chap. 68).[8,12,25] In one prospective analysis of ECGs in cyclic antidepressant poisoned patients, the maximal limb lead QRS duration was prognostic of seizures (0% if <100 ms; 30% if greater) and ventricular dysrhythmias (0% if <160 ms; 50% if greater).[12]

The terminal 40-ms axis of the QRS complex also contains information regarding the likelihood, but not the extent, of poisoning by Na^+ channel blockers. In a patient poisoned by a Na^+ channel blocker, the terminal portion of the QRS has a rightward deviation greater than 120°. The common abnormalities include an R wave (positive deflection) in lead aV_R and an S wave (negative deflection) in leads I and aV_L.[33] The combination of a rightward axis shift in the terminal 40 ms of the QRS complex (Fig. 15–9) with a prolonged QT interval and a sinus tachycardia is highly specific and sensitive for cyclic antidepressant poisoning.[44] Another study suggests that although ECG changes, like a prolonged QRS duration, are better at predicting severe outcomes than the cyclic antidepressant concentration, neither is very accurate.[8] One retrospective study suggests that an absolute height of the terminal portion of aV_R that is greater than 3 mm predicted seizures or dysrhythmias in cyclic antidepressant–poisoned patients.[32] However, in infants younger than 6 months, a rightward deviation of the terminal 40-ms QRS axis is physiologic and not predictive of cyclic antidepressant toxicity.[11]

An apparent increase in QRS complex duration and morphology, which is an elevation or distortion of the J point called a J wave or an Osborn wave (Fig. 29–3) is a common finding in patients with hypothermia.[47,65] Hypermagnesemia is also associated with prolongation of the QRS complex duration. A slight narrowing of the QRS complex may occur with hypomagnesemia. Significant hyperkalemia also causes prolongation and distortion of the QRS complex.

ST Segment

The ST segment is defined as the distance between the end of the QRS complex and the beginning of the T wave.

Electrophysiology

The ST segment reflects the period of time between depolarization and the start of repolarization, or the plateau phase of the action potential. During this period, no major currents flow within the myocardium, which explains why under normal circumstances the ST segment is isoelectric. Although both the degree of displacement from the baseline and the length of this segment are important, the ST segment duration is usually measured by its effects on the QT interval duration (see "QT Interval").

Abnormal ST Segment

Displacement of the ST segment from its baseline typically characterizes myocardial ischemia or infarction (Fig. 15–10). The subsequent appearance of a Q wave is diagnostic of myocardial infarction. The ECG patterns of these

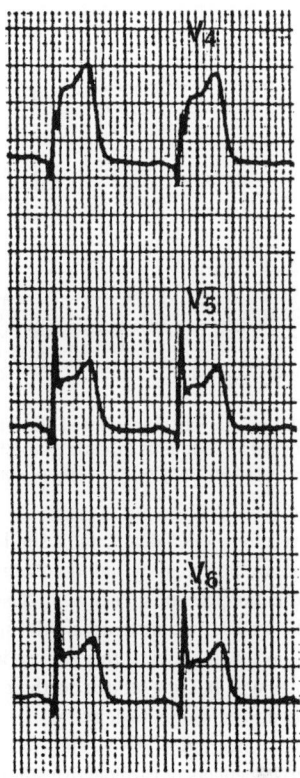

FIGURE 15–10. Leads V_4 to V_6 suggestive of a lateral ST elevation myocardial infarction (STEMI) are shown from the ECG of a 27-year-old man with substernal chest pain after using crack cocaine. *(Used with permission from The Fellowship in Medical Toxicology, New York University School of Medicine, New York City Poison Center.)*

entities reflect the different underlying electrophysiologic states of the heart. Ischemic regions are highly unstable and produce currents of injury because of inadequate repolarization, which is related to lack of energy substrate to power the Na^+,K^+-ATPase pump. Myocardial infarction represents the loss of electrical activity from the necrotic, inactive ventricular tissue, allowing the contralateral ventricular forces to be predominant on the ECG. Patients who are poisoned by xenobiotics that cause vasoconstriction, such as cocaine (Chap. 75), other α-adrenergic agonists, or the ergot alkaloids, are particularly prone to develop focal myocardial ischemia and infarction. The specific ECG manifestations help to identify the region of injury and are correlated with an arterial flow pattern: inferior (leads II, III, aV_F; right coronary artery); anterior (leads I, aV_L; left anterior descending artery); or lateral (leads aV_L, V_{5-6}; circumflex branch). However, any poisoning that results in profound hypotension or hypoxia also results in ECG changes of ischemia and injury. In these patients, the injury is more global, involving more than one arterial distribution. Diffuse myocardial damage may not be identifiable on the ECG because of global, symmetric electrical abnormalities. Under these circumstances, the diagnosis is established by other noninvasive testing, such as by echocardiogram or by finding elevated concentrations of serum markers for myocardial injury such as troponin.

Many young, healthy patients have ST segment abnormalities that mimic those of myocardial infarction. The most common normal variant is termed "early repolarization" or "J point elevation," and is identified as diffusely elevated, upwardly concave ST segments, located in the precordial leads and typically with corresponding T waves of large amplitude (Fig. 15–11).[13] The J point is located at the beginning of the ST segment just after the QRS complex. Because this ECG variant is common in patients with cocaine-associated chest pain (Chap. 75),[24] its recognition is critical to instituting appropriate therapy.

The Brugada electrocardiographic pattern (Fig. 15–12) is characterized by terminal positivity of the QRS complex and ST segment elevation in the right precordial leads. The Brugada pattern is found in some patients with mutations of the gene that codes for the α subunit of the sodium channel.

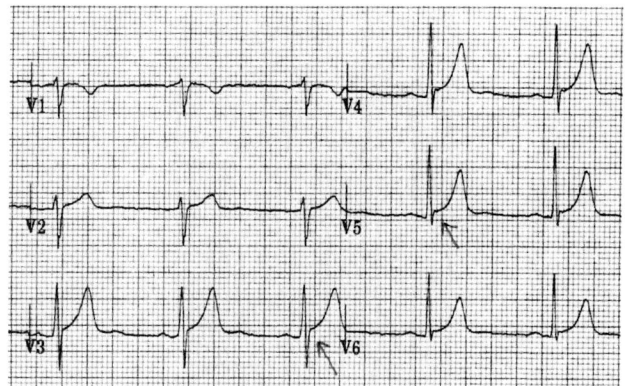

FIGURE 15–11. Healthy 34-year-old man whose ECG demonstrates diffusely elevated, upwardly concave ST segments in leads V3 to V5, and T waves of large amplitude suggestive of an "early repolarization" abnormality (J point).

These patients are at risk for sudden death, and a similar ECG pattern often occurs in patients who are poisoned by sodium-channel–blocking xenobiotics, including cyclic antidepressants, cocaine,[23] class IA (procainamide) antidysrhythmics and class IC (flecainide, encainide) antidysrhythmics.[34] In cyclic antidepressant–poisoned patients, this pattern is associated with an increased risk of hypotension, but not sudden death or dysrhythmias.[10] This pattern is also associated with lithium toxicity.[70]

Sagging ST segments, inverted T waves, and normal or shortened QT intervals are characteristic effects of cardioactive steroids, such as digoxin. These repolarization abnormalities are sometimes identified by their similar appearance to "Salvador Dali's mustache" (Fig. 15–13). As a group, these findings, along with PR prolongation, are commonly described as the "digitalis effect." They are found in patients with therapeutic digoxin concentrations and in patients with cardioactive steroid poisoning. As the serum concentration or, more precisely, the tissue concentration increases, clinical and electrocardiographic manifestations of toxicity will appear, which include profound bradycardia, AV nodal blockade, or ventricular dysrhythmias.

Changes in the ST segment duration are frequently caused by abnormalities in the serum Ca^{2+} concentration. Hypercalcemia causes shortening of the ST segment through enhanced Ca^{2+} influx during the plateau phase of the cardiac cycle, speeding the onset of repolarization. For practical purposes, this effect is more commonly identified by shortening of the QT duration (Fig. 15–14). In patients with hypercalcemia, the morphology and duration of the QRS complex and T and P waves remain unchanged. Xenobiotic-induced hypercalcemia results from exposure to antacids (ie, milk alkali syndrome), diuretics (eg, hydrochlorothiazide), cholecalciferol (vitamin D), vitamin A, and other retinoids. Hypocalcemia causes prolongation of the ST segment and QT interval.

T Wave

The T wave is the third deflection that occurs on the ECG.

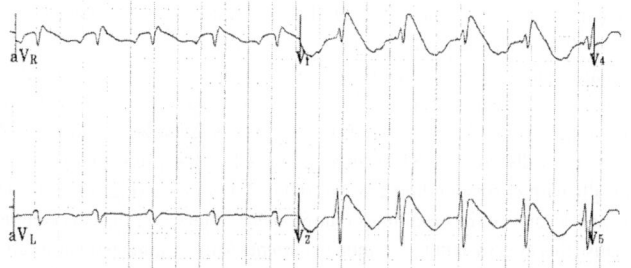

FIGURE 15–12. The Brugada pattern is characterized by terminal positivity of the QRS complex and ST segment elevation in the right precordial leads and is a similar ECG pattern to that noted in patients poisoned by sodium channel blocking xenobiotics such as cyclic antidepressants.[4] *(Used with permission from Vikhyat Bebarta, MD.)*

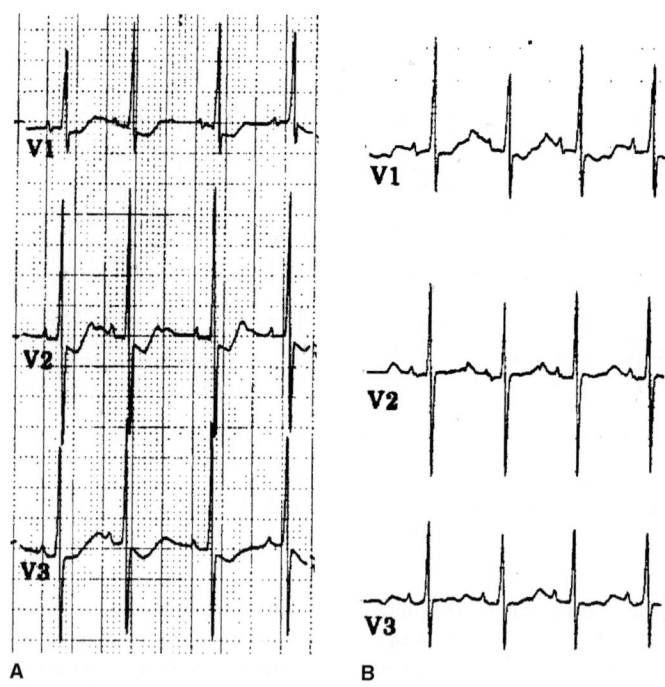

FIGURE 15–13. Two-day-old boy erroneously given 50 mcg/kg of digoxin initially presented with heart rate 60 beats/min, given Digibind. (**A**) ECG from hospital day 2, before digoxin-specific Fab, and shows "digitalis effect" of the ST segment in leads V1 to V3 (digoxin concentration 4 ng/mL). (**B**) This finding resolves after the child was switched to amiodarone; notice the QT interval prolongation.

Electrophysiology

The T wave represents ventricular repolarization, during which time current is again flowing, although at a cellular level in the opposite direction from that during depolarization. Cardiac repolarization on the larger level generally follows the same pattern as depolarization and thus the deflection is usually in the same direction as the QRS complex. During repolarization, the intracellular potential of the cardiac myocyte becomes more negative as a

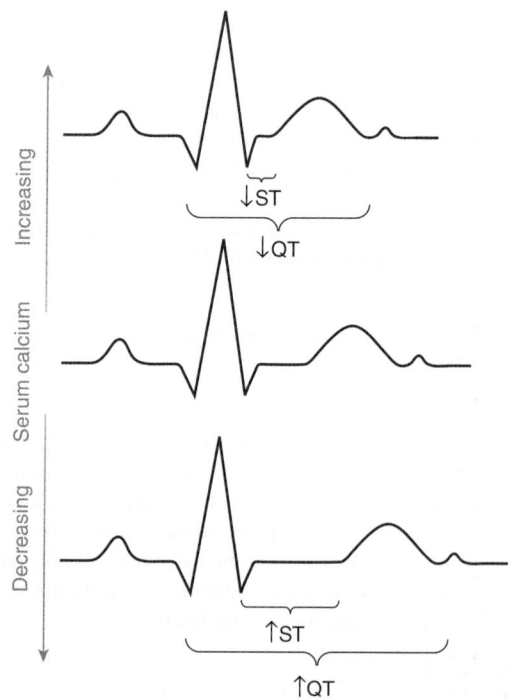

FIGURE 15–14. Electrocardiographic findings associated with changes in serum calcium concentration.

result of a net loss of positive charge because of the increasing outward flow of potassium ions. As repolarization progresses, the voltage-dependent ion channels "reset" themselves as the intracellular potential falls past their set points. Thus, the initial part of the T wave represents the absolute refractory period of the heart, because at this time there are an insufficient number of reset voltage-dependent calcium channels to allow an impulse to cause a contraction. The latter part of the T wave represents the relative refractory period of the heart, during which time a sufficient number of these calcium channels are available to open with an aberrant depolarization and initiate a contraction.

Abnormal T Wave

Isolated peaked T waves are usually evidence of early hyperkalemia.[39] Hyperkalemia initially causes tall, tented T waves with normal QRS and QT intervals, and a normal P wave (Fig. 15–15A). As the serum potassium concentration acutely rises to 6.5 to 8 mEq/L, the P wave diminishes in amplitude and the PR and QRS intervals prolong. Progressive widening of the QRS complex causes it to merge with the ST segment and T wave, forming a "sine wave" (Fig. 15-15B). ECG manifestations of hyperkalemia occur following chronic exposure to numerous xenobiotics, including potassium-sparing diuretics, angiotensin-converting enzyme inhibitors, angiotensin receptor blockers, or potassium supplements (Chap. 12). Fluoride, arsine, and cardioactive steroid poisoning can cause acute hyperkalemia, but the latter rarely produces hyperkalemic ECG changes. Peaked T waves also occur following myocardial ischemia and are often confused with early repolarization effects (ST segment). Consequently, the ability to properly identify electrolyte abnormalities by electrocardiography is often limited.

Hypokalemia typically reduces the amplitude of the T wave and, ultimately, causes the appearance of prominent U waves (Fig. 15–15A). Its effects on the ECG are manifestations of altered myocardial repolarization. Lithium similarly affects myocardial ion fluxes and causes reversible changes on the ECG that may mimic mild hypokalemia, although documentation of low cellular potassium concentrations is lacking.[59,68] Patients chronically poisoned with lithium have more T-wave abnormalities (typically flattening) than do those who are poisoned acutely, but these abnormalities are rarely of clinical significance.[60]

QT Interval

The QT interval is measured from the beginning of the QRS complex to the end of the T wave. The QT interval normally varies because of biologic diurnal effects and autonomic tone, age, gender, technical issues with the environment or with processing and acquiring the ECG, and observer variability.[2,40,41,49] The bipolar limb lead with the largest T wave should therefore be used for this measurement.

The QT interval is normally prolonged at slower heart rates and shortens as the heart rate increases. This is especially important since many of the xenobiotics that affect the QT interval also affect the heart rate. As the normal QT also varies with the heart rate, numerous formulas and tables are available to obtain the corrected QT, known as the QTc. Using the QTc allows the determination of the appropriateness of the QT independent of the heart rate.

With a rate of 50 to 90 beats/min, the commonly used Bazett formula ($QTc\ ms = QT\ (ms)/\sqrt{RR\ interval\ (seconds)}$) is adequate for determining a rate-corrected QT interval (QTc). If the RR interval is calculated as 60 beats/min, 99% of men have a QTc <450 ms and 99% of women have a QTc < 460 ms.[42] A QTc interval >500 ms weakly correlates with an increased risk of developing ventricular dysrhythmias. However, at higher heart rates, a normal patient will have an inaccurately calculated "prolonged" QTc interval using the Bazett formula. Studies suggest that medications such as bupropion prolong the QT interval when the "increase" in the QTc may be only a result of the increased heart rate.[26] A variety of formulas and corrections are proposed to attempt to identify normal QT intervals on ECGs at higher heart rates,[7,35] including the Fridericia formula ($QTc = QT/\sqrt[3]{RR\ interval\ (seconds)}$) and the Framingham linear regression analysis ($QT_{LC} = QT + 0.154\ (1 - RR)$).[54] Which

correction formula is optimal remains unknown, and the FDA requests that "presentation of data with a Fridericia correction is likely to be appropriate in most situations, but other methods could be more appropriate" when performing a "thorough QT study" for any drug with prodysrhythmic potential. A QT nomogram that plots QT interval duration versus heart rate may better predict the risk for lethal dysrhythmia.[15] The conventional use of QTc as a marker for dysrhythmia risk has a high false positive rate. The greatest discrepancy occurs during slow heart rates, 30 to 60 beats/min, when patients are at the highest risk for torsade de pointes. The nomogram that plots absolute QT interval duration versus heart rate is more sensitive. It is important to consider the known risk of the xenobiotic involved and whether the patient has an underlying abnormal QT interval (Fig. 15-16).[15,66] There is also evidence that the normal QT interval is shortened in adolescent males and varies substantially by age and gender.[49]

With slow heart rates, a prominent U wave can obscure the terminal portion of the T wave, and with fast heart rates the subsequent P wave can obscure the terminal portion of the T wave. In these patients, estimate the QTc by following the downslope of the T wave.

QT interval measurements from the computerized ECG algorithms are less accurate than careful manual determinations of the interval. In August 2000, a panel of experts convened to address these issues and suggested that the QT interval should be measured manually in one of the limb leads that best shows the end T wave; the QT interval should be measured and averaged over 3 to 5 beats; and large U waves should be included in the QT interval measurement if they merge into the T wave and obscure the end of the T wave.[5] However, a subsequent study of 334 health care professionals found that only 60% of the physicians were able to correctly measure a sample QT interval on the survey, although nearly all indicated correctly that the measurement should be from the beginning of the QRS to the end of the T wave.[31]

Electrophysiology

The QT represents the entire duration of ventricular systole and thus is composed of several electrophysiologic periods. Prolongation of the QT interval generally corresponds to a lengthening of the duration of phase 2 or 3 of the action potential. Although as noted above, depolarization abnormalities can affect the QT. These are uncommon, and the plateau phase and repolarization are primarily reflected by the QT. Variations in the speed of the paper,[19] T wave morphology, irregular baseline, and the presence of U waves makes this determination difficult.[5]

Abnormal QT Interval

A prolonged QT reflects more time that the heart is "vulnerable" to the initiation of ventricular dysrhythmias (Table 15–1, Fig. 15–17). This occurs because although some myocardial fibers are refractory during this time period, others are not (ie, relative refractory period). Early afterdepolarizations (EADs) occur in patients with a prolonged repolarization time (Table 15–2). An EAD occurs when a myocardial cell spontaneously depolarizes before its repolarization is complete (Fig. 15–18). If this depolarization is of sufficient magnitude, it captures and initiates a premature ventricular contraction, which itself initiates ventricular tachycardia, ventricular fibrillation, or torsade de pointes. There are 2 types of EADs based on whether they occur during phase 2 (type 1) or phase 3 (type 2) of the cardiac action potential. Early afterdepolarizations are primarily due to reactivation of the voltage-gated L-type calcium channels. The importance of a pathologic rise in the late Na^+ channel current (I_{Na-L}) in the genesis of EADs was studied using a sea anemone toxin (ATX II). ATX II specifically blocks I_{Na-L} with minimal effects on other ion currents, resulting in decreased EADs.[28] Early afterdepolarizations are also suppressed by magnesium.[9]

Xenobiotics that cause Na^+ channel blockade (Chaps. 64 and 68), prolong the QT duration by slowing cellular depolarization during phase 0. Thus, the QT duration lengthens because of a prolongation of the QRS complex duration, and the ST segment duration remains near normal. Xenobiotics that cause potassium channel blockade similarly prolong the QT, but through

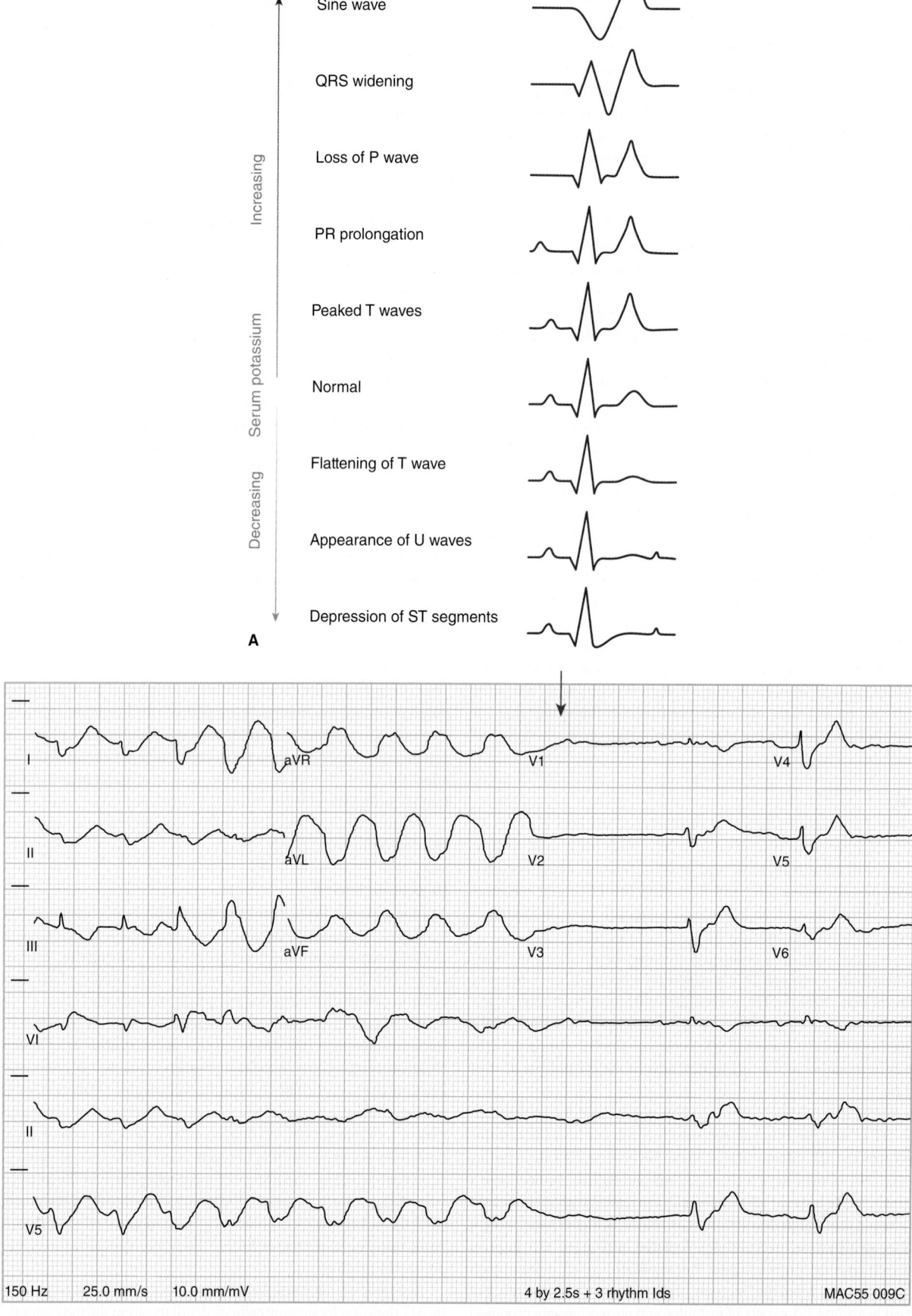

FIGURE 15–15 (**A**) Electrocardiographic manifestations associated with changes in serum potassium concentration. (**B**) A 45-year-old woman with chronic renal failure presents with a K⁺ of 7.2 mEq/L. This ECG reveals the sine-wave associated with severe hyperkalemia. Following treatment (↓) with calcium gluconate, her rhythm improved. *(Used with permission from Diane Sauter, MD, Washington Hospital Center.)*

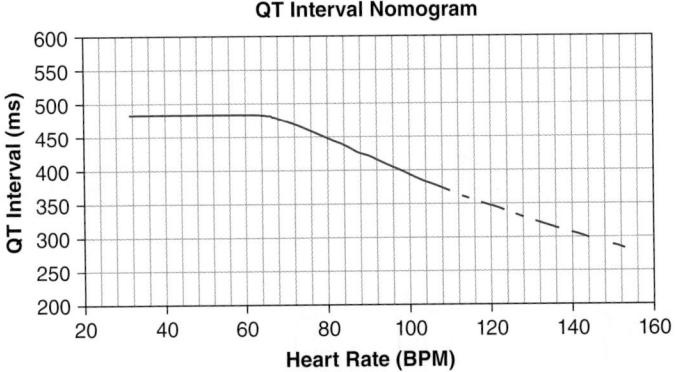

FIGURE 15–16. QT Interval Nomogram.[15] Solid line (_____) indicates heart rates that are not tachycardic. Dashed line (_ _ _ _) is extrapolated to allow assessment of faster heart rates. The QT nomogram is a plot of the QT interval versus the heart rate. A QT heart rate pair plotted above the line is associated with an increased risk of torsade de pointes. *(Reproduced with permission from Chan A, Isbister GK, Kirkpatrick CM, Dufful SB. Drug-induced QT prolongation and torsades de pointes: evaluation of a QT nomogram. QJM 2007 Oct;100(10):609-615.)*

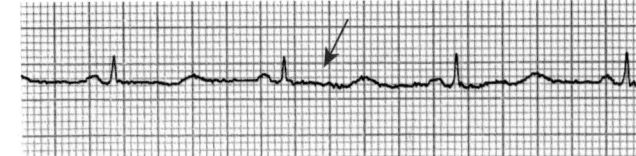

FIGURE 15–17. A 33-year-old woman who ingested excessive methadone along with ethanol 3 hours before admission. Her ECG shows a sinus bradycardia and QT prolongation (✓) of 500 ms.

prolongation of the plateau and repolarization phases. This specifically prolongs the ST segment duration. Although at a cellular level these xenobiotics are antidysrhythmic, the multicellular effects are prodysrhythmic. The highly selective serotonin reuptake inhibitors citalopram/escitalopram cause QT prolongation due to the potassium and calcium channel–blocking effects of the metabolite didesmethyl-citalopram. In a large retrospective cohort study, users of both typical antipsychotics (thioridazine and haloperidol) and atypical antipsychotics (clozapine, quetiapine, olanzapine, risperidone) had a risk of sudden cardiac death that was twice that of nonusers of antipsychotics. Xenobiotic-induced QT prolongation and the subsequent risk of dysrhythmias is the postulated etiology.[50] Loperamide has recently been recognized as a cause of QT prolongation and life-threatening ventricular tachycardia via inhibition of cardiac hERG channels.[18,63]

Hypocalcemia of sufficient severity produces a prolonged QT interval and is caused by a number of xenobiotics, including fluoride, calcitonin, phosphates, and mithramycin (Table 12–9). Hypokalemia alone does not usually prolong the QT. Arsenic poisoning cause prolongation of the QT and results in torsade de pointes. The mechanism is unknown, although increases in cardiac Ca^{2+} currents and reduction in surface expression of the cardiac potassium channel hERG are postulated.[20]

QT Dispersion

The QT interval varies in duration from lead to lead, reflecting a dispersion or variability in regional myocardial repolarization. Both QT and QTc dispersion can be calculated. The normal QT and QTc interval dispersions are 30 to 50 ms and 40 to 60 ms, respectively. The conduction characteristics vary regionally throughout the heart. For example, the subendocardial cells have a longer action potential duration than do epicardial cells; this is called dispersion of repolarization and is normal. This is important to allow the heart to contract and relax in an appropriate manner even though the impulse takes time to travel through the full thickness of the myocardial wall, from endocardium to epicardium. The subpopulations of the various ion channels (primarily potassium channels in the setting of repolarization) differ in character and density and account for this variation.[43] Ischemia and xenobiotics preferentially affect certain layers of the myocardium and alter—generally increasing—the regional heterogeneity of repolarization. M cells, located in the mid-myocardium, are very sensitive to the effects of xenobiotics that increase the repolarization heterogeneity.[27] This is reflected on the ECG as an increase in QT dispersion and a prolongation of the vulnerable period. This prolonged vulnerable phase is associated with occurrences of ventricular dysrhythmias. A measured QT dispersion greater than 80 ms after myocardial infarction was associated with ventricular tachycardia with a sensitivity rate of 73% and a specificity rate of 86%.[48] This heterogeneity is also correlated with both the efficacy and prodysrhythmic potential of therapy.[62] However, the overall assessment of QT dispersion (from a standard 12-lead ECG) has not gained popularity as a useful clinical tool.

U Wave

The U wave is a small deflection that occurs after the T wave and usually with a similar orientation. Distinguishing a U wave from a notched T wave is difficult. The apices of a notched T wave are usually <150 ms apart, and the peaks of a TU complex are >150 ms apart.

TABLE 15–1	Common Xenobiotic Causes of Prolonged QT[a]

Antidysrhythmics
    Classes IA, IC, and III antidysrhythmics
Antifungals: fluconazole, itraconazole, ketoconazole
Antihistamines: diphenhydramine
Antimicrobials: amantadine, chloroquine, fluoroquinolones, macrolides, pentamidine
Antiretrovirals: efavirenz, ritonavir-boosted saquinavir
Electrolyte disturbances
    Hypocalcemia: fluoride, oxalate (eg, ethylene glycol)
    Hypokalemia: barium soluble
    Hypomagnesemia: cathartics, diuretics
Other: arsenic trioxide, cocaine, foscarnet, hydroxychloroquine, loperamide, methadone, ondansetron, organic phosphorus compounds, tacrolimus
Psychotropics: atypical antipsychotics, citalopram, cyclic cardidepressants, droperidol, escitalopram, haloperidol, pimozide, phenothiazines, quetiapine, venlafaxine, ziprasidone

[a]Additional information can be found at www.crediblemeds.org, hosted by the Arizona CERT.

TABLE 15–2	Electrophysiologic Basis for Delayed Afterdepolarization and Early Afterdepolarization		
	Phase of Action Potential Affected by Depolarization	**Clinical Effect**	**Mechanism**
Delayed afterdepolarization	Phase 4	Cardioactive steroid–induced dysrhythmias	↑ Intracellular Ca^{2+} → Activation of a nonselective cation channel or Na^+,Ca^{2+} exchanger → Transient inward current carried mostly by Na^+ ions
Early afterdepolarization	Phase 2	↑ Repolarization time	Multifactorial (K^+, Na^+-K^+, Ca^{2+},Na^+ currents)
	Phase 3	Long QT syndrome (hereditary and acquired)	
		Drug-induced torsade de pointes, ventricular tachycardia	

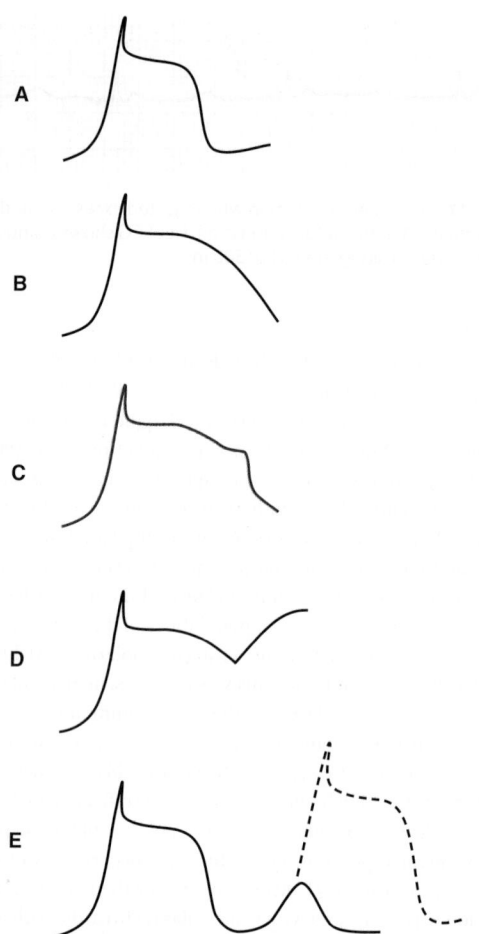

FIGURE 15–18. Afterdepolarization. (**A**) The normal action potential. (**B**) Prolonged duration action potential. (**C**) Prolonged duration action potential with an early after depolarization (EAD) occurring during the downslope of phase 3 of the action potential. (**D**) Early afterdepolarization that reaches the depolarization threshold and initiates another depolarization, or a triggered beat. (**E**) Delayed afterdepolarization, which occurs after repolarization is complete.

Electrophysiology

U waves occur when there is fluctuation in the membrane potential following myocardial repolarization. Prominent U waves are generally representative of an underlying electrophysiologic abnormality, although they may be physiologic. Physiologic U waves are caused by repolarization of the Purkinje fibers, or they correspond to late repolarization of myocardial cells in the midmyocardium, and are implicated in the initiation of cardiac dysrhythmias.[5]

Abnormal U Wave

Abnormal U waves are typically caused by spontaneous afterdepolarization of membrane potential that occurs in situations where repolarization is prolonged (Fig. 15–18). An EAD occurs in situations where the prolonged repolarization period allows calcium channels (which are both time and voltage dependent) to close and spontaneously reopen because they may close at a membrane potential that is above their threshold potential for opening. M cells in the mid-myocardium are particularly sensitive to xenobiotics causing prolonged repolarization and EADs. In this situation, the opening of the calcium channels produces a slight membrane depolarization identified as a U wave (Fig. 15-19). A delayed afterdepolarization (DAD) occurs during phase 4 of the action potential when the myocyte is overloaded with Ca^{2+}, as in the setting of cardioactive steroid toxicity. The excess intracellular Ca^{2+} can trigger the ryanodine receptors on the myocyte sarcoplasmic reticulum to release Ca^{2+}, causing slight depolarization that is erroneously recognized

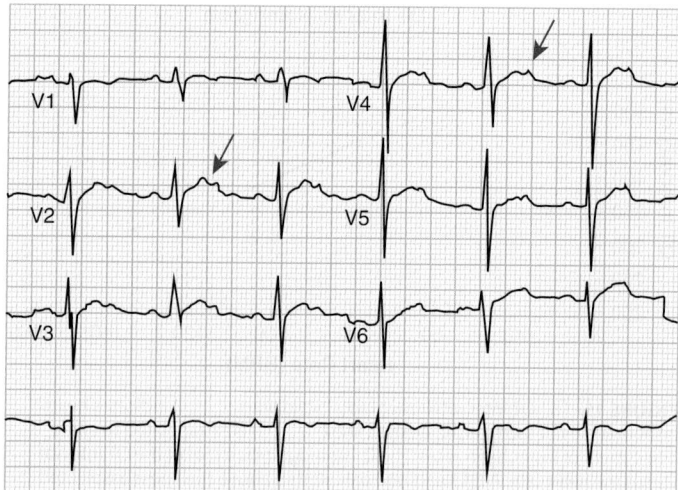

FIGURE 15–19. A 20-year-old man with a loperamide overdose. ECG shows QT prolongation (420 ms) and possible U waves with T wave notching. (✓) *(Used with permission from Thomas Oliver MD, Walter Reed National Military Medical Center Endocrinology.)*

as a U wave. If the afterdepolarization is of sufficient magnitude to reach the threshold, the cell can depolarize and initiate a premature ventricular contraction. Transient U-wave inversion can also be caused by myocardial ischemia or left ventricular overload as occurs in systemic hypertension.

Abnormal QU Interval

The QU interval is the distance between the end of the Q wave and the end of the U wave. Differentiation between the QU and the QT intervals is difficult if the T and U waves are superimposed (Fig. 15-19). When hypomagnesemia coexists with hypokalemia, as is usually the case, QU prolongation and torsade de pointes can occur.

CARDIAC DYSRHYTHMIAS AND CONDUCTION ABNORMALITIES

Xenobiotics produce adverse effects on the electrical activity of the heart, often by acting directly on the myocardial cells. Because metabolic abnormalities (especially acidemia, hypotension, hypoxia, and electrolyte abnormalities) further exacerbate the toxicity, or can actually be the sole cause of the cardiovascular abnormalities, correction of metabolic abnormalities must be a high priority in the treatment of patients with cardiovascular manifestations of poisoning. The terminal phase of any serious poisoning includes nonspecific hemodynamic abnormalities and cardiac dysrhythmias. However, many xenobiotics directly or indirectly affect cardiac rhythm or conduction, often through effects on the cardiac ion channels.

The distinction between xenobiotics that cause a rapid rate and those that cause a slow rate on the ECG is somewhat artificial, because many can do both. For example, patients poisoned by cyclic antidepressants almost always develop sinus tachycardia, but most who die will have a wide complex bradycardia immediately prior to death. In either case, abnormalities in the pattern or rate on the ECG can provide the clinician with immediate information about a patient's cardiovascular status. ECG disturbances in many poisoned patients are categorized in more than one manner (abnormal pattern, fast rate, slow rate). In any case, when ECG abnormalities are detected, appropriate interpretation, evaluation, and therapy must be rapidly performed.

Xenobiotics that directly cause dysrhythmias or cardiac conduction abnormalities usually affect the myocardial cell membrane. Other xenobiotics that modify ion channels alter the transmembrane potentials within myocytes and may result in the spontaneous generation of an abnormal rhythm.

Mechanisms of Dysrhythmia Initiation and Propagation

Dysrhythmias are related to one or more of 3 mechanisms: abnormal spontaneous depolarization (enhanced automaticity), afterdepolarization

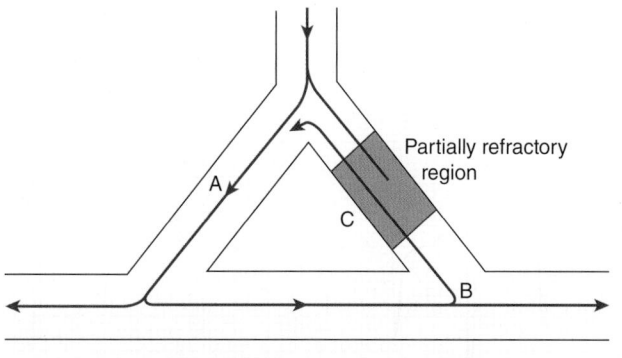

FIGURE 15–20. Mechanism of reentrant dysrhythmias. An impulse traveling down a conduction pathway reaches a branch point with one branch refractory (**C**). The impulse is conducted down branch **A** and spreads through the myocardium eventually to reach **B**, the distal end of the originally refractory branch. However, branch **C** is no longer refractory, and the impulse is conducted retrograde up through branch **C**, again to be conducted down branch **A**. The myocardium is depolarized during each loop around the circuit as the impulse spreads from the distal end of branch **A** to the rest of the heart.

(triggered automaticity), and reentry.[43] In normal myocardium, spontaneous, phase 4 depolarization occurs most rapidly in the sinus node, the normal pacemaker for the heart. Speeding or slowing the rate of phase 4 depolarization of the pacemaker cell results in sinus tachycardia or sinus bradycardia, respectively. However, xenobiotics can also speed the depolarization of other myocardial cells with pacemaker potential allowing them to overtake the sinus node as the primary pacemaker. This mechanism, called increased automaticity, accounts for many of the dysrhythmias that occur with cardioactive steroid and β-adrenergic agonist poisoning.

Afterdepolarizations, mentioned above, typically occur during phase 3 or 4 of the action potential and may reach the threshold potential, causing the fast Na+ channels to open and initiate an action potential. EADs account for the "trigger beats" that initiate episodes of ventricular tachycardia, commonly torsade de pointes (TdP), when the action potential is prolonged, as discussed below. DADs are typically associated with cardioactive steroid toxicity[43] and excessive sympathetic stimulation.

Most afterdepolarizations do not propagate rapidly throughout the myocardium and do not generate ectopic beats. However, because the normal dispersion of repolarization is increased by certain xenobiotics, ectopic beats (eg, atrial premature contraction or ventricular premature contraction) may propagate abnormally within the myocardium. Ectopy is the ECG manifestation of myocardial depolarization initiated from a site other than the sinus node. Ectopy may be lifesaving under circumstances in which the atrial rhythm cannot be conducted to the ventricles (ie, "escape rhythm"), as during high-degree AV blockade induced by cardioactive steroids (Chap. 62). Alternatively, ectopy may lead to dramatic alterations in the physiologic function of the heart or deteriorate into lethal ventricular dysrhythmias.

Occasionally, because of the altered regional repolarization (ie, increased dispersion of repolarization), an impulse reaches a branch point with a partial block (ie, relatively refractory) to conduction in one of the branches (Fig. 15–20). The impulse is carried through only one of the branches and then spreads through the myocardial cells. After a short delay, the impulse reaches the distal end of the previously blocked pathway. By this time, the region is no longer refractory and conducts the impulse in a retrograde fashion. The impulse continues in a continuous loop circuit, depolarizing the heart with each passage; this process is called reentry. Reentrant mechanisms appear to be responsible for the majority of the malignant tachydysrhythmias attributable to poisoning.

Tachydysrhythmias

Both supraventricular and ventricular tachydysrhythmias occur in poisoned patients (Table 15–3). Sinus tachycardia is the most common rhythm disturbance that occurs in poisoned patients. Parasympatholytic xenobiotics, such

TABLE 15–3	Xenobiotics Causing Ventricular and Supraventricular Tachydysrhythmias

Amantadine
Anticholinergics
Antidysrhythmics: classes IA, IC, and III (Table 57–1)
Antihistamines
Antipsychotics
Botanicals (Diverse) (Chap. 118)
Carbamazepine
Cardioactive steroids
Chloroquine and quinine
Cyclic antidepressants
Cyclobenzaprine
Hydrocarbons and solvents
   Halogenated hydrocarbons
   Inhalational anesthetics
Jellyfish venom
Metal salts
   Arsenic
   Lithium
   Magnesium
   Potassium
Pentamidine
Phenothiazines
Phosphodiesterase inhibitors (eg, methylxanthines)
Sedative-hypnotics
   Chloral hydrate
   Ethanol ("holiday heart")
Sympathomimetics (eg, cocaine)
Thyroid hormone

as atropine, raise the heart rate to its innate rate by eliminating the inhibitory tonic vagal influence. However, more rapid rates require direct myocardial stimulatory effects, generally mediated by β-adrenergic agonism. For example, catecholamine excess, as occurs in patients with cocaine use, psychomotor agitation, or fever, may cause sinus tachycardia with rates faster than 150 beats/min. Ventricular dysrhythmias frequently accompany hypotension, hypoxia, acidemia, electrolyte abnormalities, and other metabolic derangements that are present in poisoned patients or are a direct effect of the xenobiotic.

The intrinsic pacemaker cells of the heart undergo spontaneous depolarization and reach threshold at a predictable rate. Under normal circumstances, the sinus node is the most rapidly firing pacemaker cell of the heart; and as a result it controls the heart rate. Other potential pacemakers exist in the heart, but their rate of spontaneous depolarization is considerably slower than that of the sinus node. Thus, they are reset during depolarization of the myocardium and they never spontaneously reach threshold. Xenobiotics, such as sympathomimetics, which speed the rate of rise of phase 4, or diastolic depolarization, speed the rate of firing of the pacemaker cells. As long as the sinus node is preferentially affected, it maintains the pacemaker activity of the heart. If the firing rate of another intrinsic pacemaker exceeds that of the sinus node, ectopic rhythms develop.

Certain xenobiotics are highly associated with ventricular tachydysrhythmias following poisoning. Those that increase the adrenergic tone on the heart, either directly, or indirectly, cause ventricular dysrhythmias. Whether a result of excessive circulating catecholamines observed with cocaine and sympathomimetics, myocardial sensitization secondary to halogenated hydrocarbons or thyroid hormone, or increased second messenger activity secondary to methylxanthines, the extreme inotropic and chronotropic effects cause dysrhythmias. Altered repolarization, increased intracellular

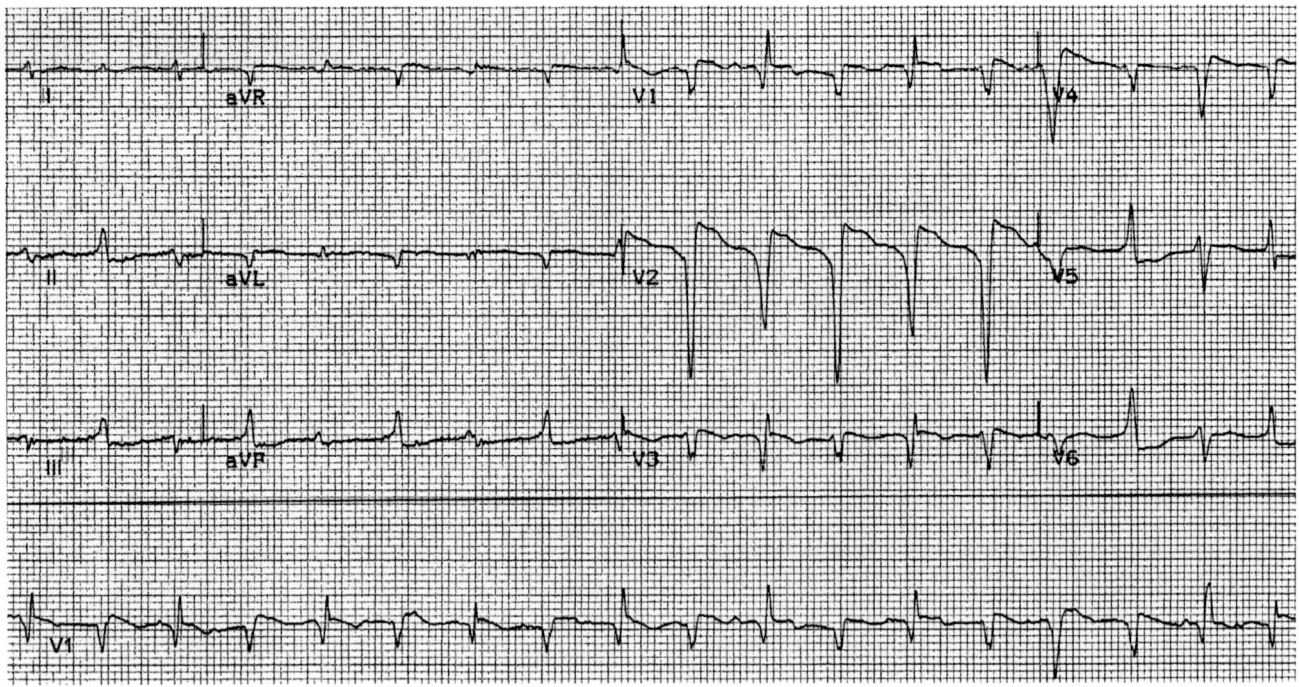

FIGURE 15–21. Digoxin-induced bidirectional ventricular tachycardia. The ECG demonstrates the alternating QRS axis characteristic of bidirectional ventricular tachycardia and is nearly pathognomonic for cardioactive steroid poisoning. The 89-year-old patient's serum digoxin concentration was 4.0 ng/mL. *(Used with permission from Ruben Olmedo, MD, Mount Sinai School of Medicine.)*

Ca^{2+} concentrations, or myocardial ischemia often cause dysrhythmias. Additionally, xenobiotics that produce focal myocardial ischemia, such as cocaine, ephedrine, or ergots often lead to malignant ventricular dysrhythmias. Finally, an uncommon cause of xenobiotic-induced ventricular dysrhythmias is persistent activation of sodium channels, such as following aconitine poisoning. Although not all prolonged QRS complex tachydysrhythmias are ventricular in origin, making this assumption is generally considered to be prudent. For example, in a patient poisoned with cyclic antidepressants or cocaine, the differentiation of aberrantly conducted sinus tachycardia (common) from ventricular tachycardia (rare) is important, but difficult. Although guidelines for determining the origin of a wide complex tachydysrhythmia exist, they are imperfect, difficult to apply, and unstudied in poisoned patients.[4,67]

Bidirectional ventricular tachycardia is associated with severe cardioactive steroid toxicity and results from alterations of intraventricular conduction, junctional tachycardia with aberrant intraventricular conduction, or, on rare occasions, alternating ventricular pacemakers (Fig. 15–21). Aconitine, usually obtained from traditional Chinese or other alternative therapies that contain plants of the *Aconitum* spp. (such as *Aconitum napellus* {monkshood}), cause bidirectional ventricular tachycardia (Chaps. 43 and 118).

Tachydysrhythmia Associated With a Prolonged QT Interval: Torsade de Pointes

Xenobiotics that alter myocardial repolarization and prolong the QT interval predispose to the development of afterdepolarization-induced contractions during the relative refractory period (R on T phenomena), which initiates ventricular tachycardia. If torsade de pointes (TdP) is noted, this is undoubtedly the mechanism, and the QT interval should be carefully assessed and appropriate treatment initiated (Fig. 15–22).

Ventricular tachycardia, including TdP, is usually a reentrant-type rhythm. The presence of a prolonged QT interval on the ECG indicates the possible existence of conditions within the myocardium that favor occurrence of reentry dysrhythmias, as discussed above. The long action potential duration resulting from prolongation in the duration of phase 2 or 3 increases the occurrence of EADs. These, in combination with an increased dispersion of repolarization, increase the risk for reentrant dysrhythmias, particularly TdP.

Many xenobiotics interact with cardiac membrane ion channels and increase the risk of TdP. Most of these xenobiotics interact with the hERG-encoded subunit of the potassium channel to reduce the current through the I_{Kr} channel and prolong the action potential duration. The hERG subunit of the channel is particularly susceptible to xenobiotic interactions because of the larger inner cavity with aromatic-binding domains.[51,512] Acquired QT interval prolongation and TdP from xenobiotics occur most often with class IA and IC antidysrhythmics, the cyclic antidepressants, and the antipsychotics. Although class IC antidysrhythmics (such as encainide and flecainide) cause greater QT interval prolongation, class IA antidysrhythmics (such as quinidine and procainamide) are responsible for more reported cases. This is probably a result of the relatively infrequent use of the class IC antidysrhythmics, due paradoxically, to concerns about the higher risk of prodysrhythmic effects. Class IB antidysrhythmics, such as lidocaine, have no significant effect on potassium channels and the QT interval, and do not cause TdP. Acquired QT interval prolongation and TdP also commonly result from metabolic and electrolyte abnormalities, particularly hypocalcemia, hypomagnesemia, and hypokalemia (Chaps. 12 and 57).

Bradydysrhythmias

Bradycardia, heart block, and asystole are the terminal events following fatal ingestions of many xenobiotics, but some xenobiotics tend to cause sinus bradycardia (Table 16–2) and conduction abnormalities (Table 15–4) early in the course of toxicity. Sinus bradycardia with an otherwise normal electrocardiogram is characteristic of xenobiotics that reduce central nervous system outflow (Chap. 16). Xenobiotics that cause CNS sedation, such as the sedative-hypnotics, most opioids, and α_2-adrenergic receptor agonist ("centrally acting") antihypertensives, and imidazolines will usually decrease sympathetic outflow to the heart and produce a heart rate in the range of 40 to 60 beats/min. Xenobiotics that directly affect ion flux across myocardial cell membranes cause abnormalities in AV nodal conduction. β-adrenergic antagonists, calcium channel blockers, and cardioactive steroids (Chaps. 59, 60, and 62) are the leading causes of sinus bradycardia and conduction disturbances. Indirect metabolic effects are also contributory, such as severe hyperkalemia (which may accompany any acidosis), causing a wide complex, sinusoidal bradycardic rhythm.

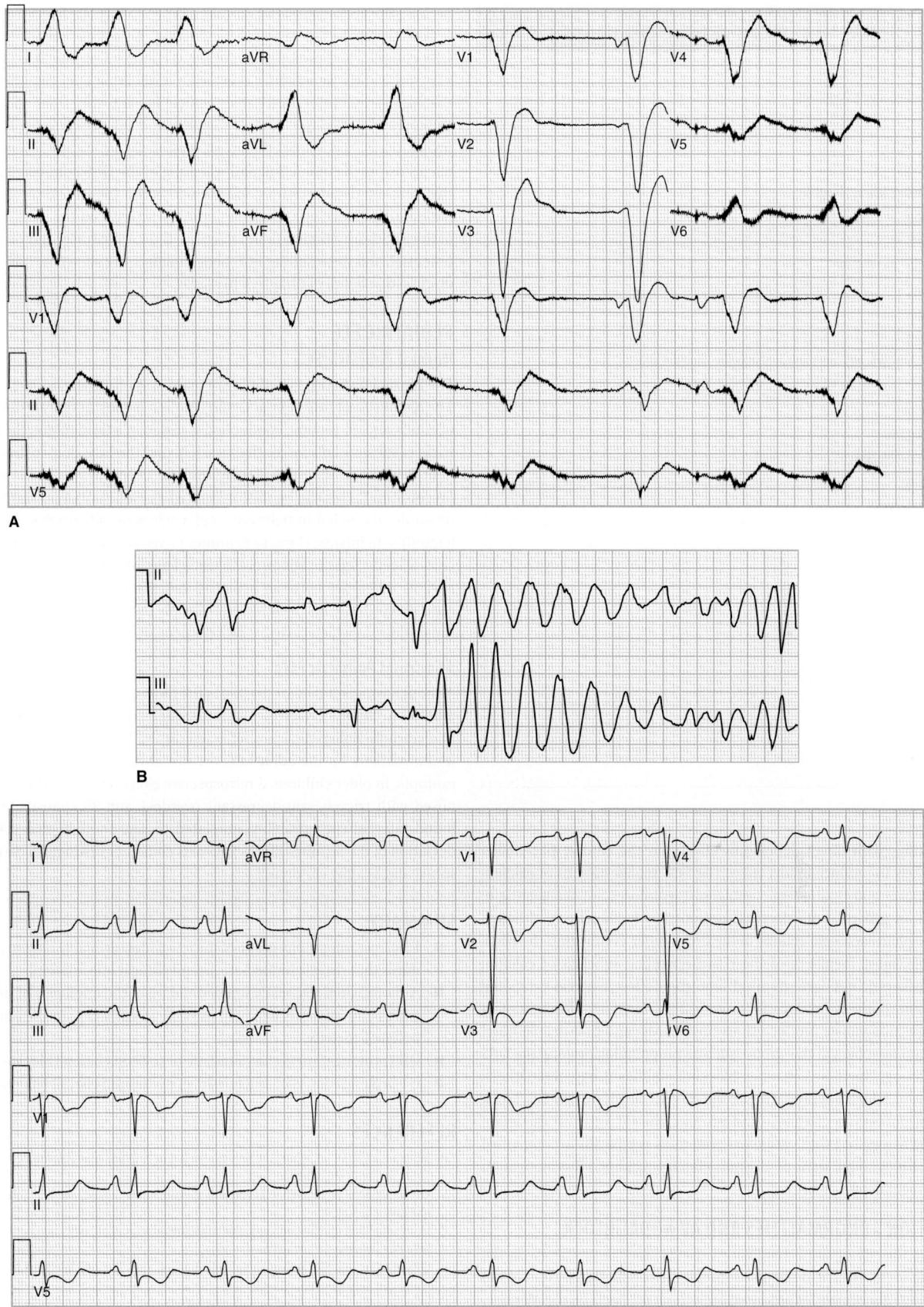

FIGURE 15–22. **(A)** This is the initial electrocardiograph of a 25-year-old woman who presented after a syncopal event. She was taking loperamide in addition to her chronic medications, quetiapine and escitalopram. Initial treatment included amiodarone and magnesium. She had recurrent episodes of wide complex tachycardia for 6 days. Her loperamide concentration was 130 ng/mL, and the metabolite desmethylloperamide was 500 ng/mL. **(B)** the rhythm strip from her cardiac monitor on the day of admission showed a wide complex dysrhythmia and torsade de pointes **(C)**. Two days later, she had a persistent long QT interval (QT/QTc: 600/584 ms). *(Used with permission from Jeanmarie Perrone, MD, University of Pennsylvania School of Medicine.)*

TABLE 15–4 Xenobiotics Causing Conduction Abnormalities and/or Heart Block

α_1- and α_2-adrenergic agonists
β_1- and β_2-adrenergic antagonists
Amantadine
Anesthetics (local)
Antidepressants
Antidysrhythmics (classes I and III)
Antihistamines
Antimicrobials
  Chloroquine and quinine
  Macrolides
  Quinolones
Antipsychotics
  Atypical antipsychotics (quetiapine, olanzapine, risperidone)
  Droperidol
  Haloperidol
  Phenothiazines
Calcium channel blockers
Carbamazepine
Cardioactive steroids
Cholinergics
Cocaine
Cyclic antidepressants
Cyclobenzaprine
Electrolytes
  Potassium
  Magnesium (hyper- and hypo-)
Metal salts
  Arsenic
Methadone
Pentamidine

Xenobiotics with direct depressant effects on the cardiac pacemaker are most likely to produce bradycardia. The ECG manifestations of calcium channel blocker and β-adrenergic antagonist overdoses are challenging to distinguish. In general, both decrease dromotropy (conduction), although the specific pharmacologic actions of the drugs differ even within the class. For example, most members of the dihydropyridine subclass of calcium channel blockers do not have any antidromotropic effect, whereas verapamil and diltiazem routinely produce PR prolongation. Similarly, although most β-adrenergic antagonists produce sinus bradycardia and first-degree heart block, certain members of this group, such as propranolol, prolong the QRS complex through their Na$^+$ channel–blocking abilities (Chap. 59). Others, such as sotalol, which has properties of the class III antidysrhythmics, block myocardial potassium channels and prolong the QT interval duration. Bradycardia associated with cardioactive steroids is typically accompanied by electrocardiographic signs of "digitalis effect," including PR prolongation and ST segment depression (Chap. 62).

CONDUCTION ABNORMALITIES AND AV NODAL BLOCK

The cardiac toxicity of some xenobiotics results from their effects on the propagation of the electrical impulse through the conduction system of the heart. The ECG abnormalities produced are a result of effects on the AV node, producing first-, second-, or third-degree (complete) heart block, or on the His-Purkinje system, producing intraventricular conduction delays such as bundle-branch blocks. The effects of xenobiotics on myocardial conduction are often mediated through interactions with the sodium or potassium membrane channels. For example, xenobiotics that affect the fast inward I_{Na} currents (such as the type I antidysrhythmics and cyclic antidepressants)

prolong the action potential duration, slow ventricular myocyte depolarization, and slow intraventricular conduction. This produces widening of the QRS complex and prolongation of the QT interval on the ECG. Table 15–4 lists some of the xenobiotics that cause conduction abnormalities. Many of the antidysrhythmics derive their clinical benefit from their ability to alter sodium and potassium channel function and slow conduction through the myocardium. Xenobiotics that depress phase 0 (the inward I_{Na} currents) produce slowing of conduction and widening of the QRS complex. Xenobiotics that prolong depolarization and repolarization (phase 2 or 3 of the action potential) produce prolongation of the QT interval on the ECG. The classes of the antidysrhythmics, their effects on the ion channels and on the action potential, and the resulting ECG abnormalities, are shown in Table 57–1 and discussed in detail in Chapters 16 and 57.

PEDIATRIC ECG

Normal Pediatric ECG

The normal pediatric ECG differs in many ways from the normal adult ECG. The resting heart rate of infants and children is substantially faster than that of adults and, in general, conduction is faster. In a term infant, the right ventricle is substantially larger than the left, and the ECG demonstrates prominent R waves in the right precordium and deep S waves in the left lateral precordium.[46] This can be misinterpreted as cyclic antidepressant toxicity.[11] An adult ratio of left to right ventricular size is usually reached by the age of 6 months. In infants, Q waves commonly exist in the inferior and lateral precordial leads, but are abnormal in leads I and aV$_L$. The T waves are the most notable difference between pediatric and adult ECGs. The T waves in the right precordial leads in children are deeply inverted until 7 years and sometimes older, in which case it is called a persistent juvenile T-wave pattern.

Abnormal Pediatric ECG

Although congenital heart disease is the most common cause of ECG abnormalities in children, electrolyte disorders and xenobiotics also cause changes in electrophysiology that are reflected on the ECG. Abnormalities that are useful markers on the adult ECG are not always as useful in children. For example, in older children, a retrospective chart review of 37 children diagnosed with tricyclic antidepressant overdose and 35 controls (<11 years) found interpatient variability, unrelated to age, so great that a rightward deviation of the terminal 40-ms QRS axis could not distinguish between poisoned and healthy children.[11]

SUMMARY

- Electrocardiography is one of the few widely available diagnostic procedures that reveals immediate, useful clinical information.
- A thorough mechanistic understanding of the etiologies of the various waves and intervals will help provide an early clue to the etiology of a patient's toxicity.
- QRS prolongation is characteristic of sodium channel blockade.
- QT prolongation is characteristic of potassium channel blockade.

REFERENCES

1. Afonso L, et al. Crack whips the heart: a review of the cardiovascular toxicity of cocaine. *Am J Cardiol.* 2007;100:1040-1043.
2. Al-Khatib SM, et al. What clinicians should know about the QT interval. *JAMA.* 2003;289:2120-2127.
3. Alexander SP, et al. The concise guide to pharmacology 2015/16: voltage-gated ion channels. *Br J Pharmacol.* 2015;172:5904-5941.
4. Alzand BS, Crijns HJ. Diagnostic criteria of broad QRS complex tachycardia: decades of evolution. *Europace.* 2011;13:465-472.
5. Anderson ME, et al. Cardiac repolarization: current knowledge, critical gaps, and new approaches to drug development and patient management. *Am Heart J.* 2002;144:769-781.
6. Antzelevitch C, Burashnikov A. Overview of basic mechanisms of cardiac arrhythmia. *Card Electrophysiol Clin.* 2011;3:23-45.
7. Aytemir K, et al. Comparison of formulae for heart rate correction of QT interval in exercise electrocardiograms. *Pacing Clin Electrophysiol.* 1999;22:1397-1401.
8. Bailey B, et al. A meta-analysis of prognostic indicators to predict seizures, arrhythmias or death after tricyclic antidepressant overdose. *J Toxicol Clin Toxicol.* 2004;42:877-888.

9. Bailie DS, et al. Magnesium suppression of early afterdepolarizations and ventricular tachyarrhythmias induced by cesium in dogs. *Circulation.* 1988;77:1395-1402.
10. Bebarta VS, et al. Incidence of Brugada electrocardiographic pattern and outcomes of these patients after intentional tricyclic antidepressant ingestion. *Am J Cardiol.* 2007;100:656-660.
11. Berkovitch M, et al. Assessment of the terminal 40-millisecond QRS vector in children with a history of tricyclic antidepressant ingestion. *Pediatr Emerg Care.* 1995;11:75-77.
12. Boehnert MT, Lovejoy FH Jr. Value of the QRS duration versus the serum drug level in predicting seizures and ventricular arrhythmias after an acute overdose of tricyclic antidepressants. *N Engl J Med.* 1985;313:474-479.
13. Brady WJ. Benign early repolarization: electrocardiographic manifestations and differentiation from other ST segment elevation syndromes. *Am J Emerg Med.* 1998;16:592-597.
14. Catterall WA, et al. International Union of Pharmacology. XLVII. Nomenclature and structure-function relationships of voltage-gated sodium channels. *Pharmacol Rev.* 2005;57:397-409.
15. Chan A, et al. Drug-induced QT prolongation and torsades de pointes: evaluation of a QT nomogram. *Q J Med.* 2007;100:609-615.
16. DiFrancesco D, Borer JS. The funny current: cellular basis for the control of heart rate. *Drugs.* 2007;67(suppl 2):15-24.
17. Ducroq J, et al. Action potential experiments complete hERG assay and QT-interval measurements in cardiac preclinical studies. *J Pharmacol Toxicol Methods.* 2007;56:159-170.
18. Eggleston W, et al. Loperamide abuse associated with cardiac dysrhythmia and death. *Ann Emerg Med.* 2017;69:83-86.
19. Faber TS, et al. Impact of electrocardiogram recording format on QT interval measurement and QT dispersion assessment. *Pacing Clin Electrophysiol.* 2001;24:1739-1747.
20. Ficker E, et al. Mechanisms of arsenic-induced prolongation of cardiac repolarization. *Mol Pharmacol.* 2004;66:33-44.
21. Food and Drug Administration. Methadone hydrochloride (marketed as Dolophine) information: Death, narcotic overdose, and serious cardiac arrhythmias. [FDA Alert]. http://www.fda.gov/Drugs/DrugSafety/PostmarketDrugSafetyInformationforPatientsandProviders/ucm142827.htm. Accessed March 14, 2017.
22. Franco F. Wide complex tachycardia after bupropion overdose. *Am J Emerg Med.* 2015;33:1540.e3-1540.e5.
23. Hoffman RS. Treatment of patients with cocaine-induced arrhythmias: bringing the bench to the bedside. *Br J Clin Pharmacol.* 2010;69:448-457.
24. Hollander JE, et al. "Abnormal" electrocardiograms in patients with cocaine-associated chest pain are due to "normal" variants. *J Emerg Med.* 1994;12:199-205.
25. Hulten BA, et al. Predicting severity of tricyclic antidepressant overdose. *J Toxicol Clin Toxicol.* 1992;30:161-170.
26. Isbister GK, Balit CR. Bupropion overdose: QTc prolongation and its clinical significance. *Ann Pharmacother.* 2003;37:999-1002.
27. Kao LW, Furbee RB. Drug-induced Q-T prolongation. *Med Clin North Am.* 2005;89:1125-1144.
28. Karagueuzian HS, et al. Enhanced late Na and Ca currents as effective antiarrhythmic drug targets. *Front Pharmacol.* 2017;8:36.
29. Keating MT, Sanguinetti MC. Molecular and cellular mechanisms of cardiac arrhythmias. *Cell.* 2001;104:569-580.
30. Kenneback G, et al. Electrophysiologic effects and clinical hazards of carbamazepine treatment for neurologic disorders in patients with abnormalities of the cardiac conduction system. *Am Heart J.* 1991;121:1421-1429.
31. LaPointe NM, et al. Knowledge deficits related to the QT interval could affect patient safety. *Ann Noninvasive Electrocardiol.* 2003;8:157-160.
32. Liebelt EL, et al. ECG lead aVR versus QRS interval in predicting seizures and arrhythmias in acute tricyclic antidepressant toxicity. *Ann Emerg Med.* 1995;26:195-201.
33. Liebelt EL, et al. Serial electrocardiogram changes in acute tricyclic antidepressant overdoses. *Crit Care Med.* 1997;25:1721-1726.
34. Littmann L, et al. Brugada syndrome and "Brugada sign": clinical spectrum with a guide for the clinician. *Am Heart J.* 2003;145:768-778.
35. Malik M, et al. Differences between study-specific and subject-specific heart rate corrections of the QT interval in investigations of drug induced QTc prolongation. *Pacing Clin Electrophysiol.* 2004;27:791-800.
36. Maltsev VA, Lakatta EG. Normal heart rhythm is initiated and regulated by an intracellular calcium clock within pacemaker cells. *Heart Lung Circ.* 2007;16:335-348.
37. Maltsev VA, et al. The emergence of a general theory of the initiation and strength of the heartbeat. *J Pharmacol Sci.* 2006;100:338-369.
38. Mangoni ME, Nargeot J. Genesis and regulation of the heart automaticity. *Physiol Rev.* 2008;88:919-982.
39. Mattu A, et al. Electrocardiographic manifestations of hyperkalemia. *Am J Emerg Med.* 2000;18:721-729.
40. Molnar J, et al. Diurnal pattern of QTc interval: how long is prolonged? Possible relation to circadian triggers of cardiovascular events. *J Am Coll Cardiol.* 1996;27:76-83.
41. Morganroth J, et al. Variability of the QT measurement in healthy men, with implications for selection of an abnormal QT value to predict drug toxicity and proarrhythmia. *Am J Cardiol.* 1991;67:774-776.
42. Moss AJ. Long QT syndrome. *JAMA.* 2003;289:2041-2044.
43. Nelson LS. Toxicologic myocardial sensitization. *J Toxicol Clin Toxicol.* 2002;40:867-879.
44. Niemann JT, et al. Electrocardiographic criteria for tricyclic antidepressant cardiotoxicity. *Am J Cardiol.* 1986;57:1154-1159.
45. Nogar JN, et al. Severe sodium channel blockade and cardiovascular collapse due to a massive lamotrigine overdose. *Clin Toxicol.* 2011;49:854-857.
46. O'Connor M, et al. The pediatric electrocardiogram, part I: age-related interpretation. *Am J Emerg Med.* 2008;26:506-512.
47. Osborn JJ. Experimental hypothermia: respiratory and blood pH changes in relation to cardiac function. *Am J Physiol.* 1953;175:389-398.
48. Puljevic D, et al. QT dispersion, daily variations, QT interval adaptation and late potentials as risk markers for ventricular tachycardia. *Eur Heart J.* 1997;18:1343-1349.
49. Rautaharju PM, et al. New age- and sex-specific criteria for QT prolongation based on rate correction formulas that minimize bias at the upper normal limits. *Int J Cardiol.* 2014;174:535-540. Erratum in: *Int J Cardiol.* 2015;178:299.
50. Ray WA, et al. Atypical antipsychotic drugs and the risk of sudden cardiac death. *N Engl J Med.* 2009;360:225-235.
51. Roden DM. Role of the electrocardiogram in determining electrophysiologic end points of drug therapy. *Am J Cardiol.* 1988;62:34H-38H.
52. Roden DM. Drug-induced prolongation of the QT interval. *N Engl J Med.* 2004;350:1013-1022.
53. Roden DM, et al. Cardiac ion channels. *Annu Rev Physiol.* 2002;64:431-475.
54. Sagie A, et al. An improved method for adjusting the QT interval for heart rate (the Framingham Heart Study). *Am J Cardiol.* 1992;70:797-801.
55. Saxena P, et al. New potential binding determinant for hERG channel inhibitors. *Sci Rep.* 2016;6:24182.
56. Schwartz M, et al. Cardiotoxicity after massive amantadine overdose. *J Med Toxicol.* 2008;4:173-179.
57. Schmitt N, et al. Cardiac potassium channel subtypes: new roles in repolarization and arrhythmia. *Physiol Rev.* 2014;94:609-653.
58. Sharma AN, et al. Diphenhydramine-induced wide complex dysrhythmia responds to treatment with sodium bicarbonate. *Am J Emerg Med.* 2003;21:212-215.
59. Singer I, Rotenberg D. Mechanisms of lithium action. *N Engl J Med.* 1973;289:254-260.
60. Singh D, et al. Electrocardiac effects associated with lithium toxicity in children: an illustrative case and review of the pathophysiology. *Cardiol Young.* 2016;26:221-229.
61. Stevens M, et al. Neurotoxins and their binding areas on voltage-gated sodium channels. *Front Pharmacol.* 2011;2:71.
62. Stone PH. Ranolazine: new paradigm for management of myocardial ischemia, myocardial dysfunction, and arrhythmias. *Cardiol Clin.* 2008;26:603-614.
63. Upadhyay A, et al. Loperamide induced life threatening ventricular arrhythmia. *Case Rep Cardiol.* 2016;2016:5040176.
64. Vandenberg JI, et al. hERG K+ channels: structure, function, and clinical significance. *Physiol Rev.* 2012;92:1393-1478.
65. Vassallo SU, et al. A prospective evaluation of the electrocardiographic manifestations of hypothermia. *Acad Emerg Med.* 1999;6:1121-1126.
66. Waring S, Graham A, Gray J, et al. Evaluation of a QT nomogram for risk assessment after antidepressant overdose. *Br J Clin Pharmacol.* 2010;70:881-885.
67. Wellens HJ. Electrophysiology: ventricular tachycardia: diagnosis of broad QRS complex tachycardia. *Heart.* 2001;86:579-585.
68. Woods JW, et al. Perturbation of sodium-lithium countertransport in red cells. *N Engl J Med.* 1983;308:1258-1261.
69. Wrenn KD, et al. The ability of physicians to predict electrolyte deficiency from the ECG. *Ann Emerg Med.* 1990;19:580-583.
70. Wright D, Salehian O. Brugada-type electrocardiographic changes induced by long-term lithium use. *Circulation.* 2010;122:e418-e419.
71. Zhang F, et al. Shellfish toxins targeting voltage-gated sodium channels. *Mar Drugs.* 2013;11:4698-4723.

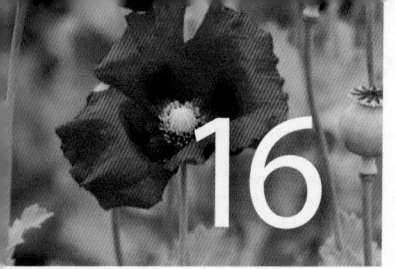

16 CARDIOLOGIC PRINCIPLES II: HEMODYNAMICS

Rachel S. Wightman and Robert A. Hessler

Adequate tissue perfusion depends on maintenance of volume status, vascular resistance, cardiac contractility, and cardiac rhythm. All of these components of the hemodynamic system are vulnerable to the effects of xenobiotics. Cardiovascular toxicity is manifested by the development of hemodynamic instability, heart failure, cardiac conduction abnormalities, or dysrhythmias. The presence of a specific pattern of cardiovascular anomalies (toxicologic syndrome or "toxidrome") often suggests a particular class or type of xenobiotic.

In addition, an alteration in hemodynamic functioning is frequently the indirect result of metabolic abnormalities. Poisoning with a xenobiotic often leads to development of acid–base disturbances, hypoxia, or electrolyte abnormalities with secondary hemodynamic changes. In these patients, supportive care with ventilation, oxygenation, and fluid and electrolyte repletion can dramatically improve the cardiovascular status.

PHYSIOLOGY OF THE CARDIOVASCULAR SYSTEM

Maintaining cardiac contractility, heart rate and rhythm, and vascular resistance requires complex modulation of the cardiac and vascular systems. Xenobiotics cause hemodynamic abnormalities as a result of direct effects on the myocardial cells, the cardiac conduction system, or on the arteriolar smooth muscle cells. These effects are frequently mediated by interactions with cellular ion channels or cell membrane neurohormonal receptors. These complex cellular systems provide multiple sites for xenobiotics to demonstrate their toxicologic effects. Xenobiotics and xenobiotic metabolites interact with the cellular receptors, intracellular signal mechanisms, effector enzymes, or intracellular organelles.

Toxic effects of xenobiotics can be due to direct poisoning from excessive amounts of a xenobiotic that follow an overdose. Slower accumulation of the xenobiotic or active metabolites (due to alterations in metabolism) also leads to adverse effects. Additionally, the toxic effects of a xenobiotic can be altered by the characteristics of the host subject. Underlying medical conditions, presence of other xenobiotics, electrolyte abnormalities, concurrent acid–base, and hydration status contribute to the potential adverse hemodynamic effects of a xenobiotic. Even with a small concentration of a xenobiotic, hemodynamic toxicity may occur due entirely to underlying genetic differences in the cellular receptors or the intracellular signal transducers in the particular patient.

This complex interaction between the xenobiotic and patient's physiology and genetic diversity is exemplified by the Brugada syndrome. This congenital cardiac channelopathy (Chaps. 15 and 57) predisposes to sudden cardiac death due to polymorphic ventricular tachycardia or ventricular fibrillation. Brugada syndrome is characterized by an atypical right bundle branch pattern with a characteristic cove-shaped ST segment elevation in leads V1 to V3 of the electrocardiogram (ECG) in the absence or structural heart disease, ischemia, or electrolyte disturbances).[10,83] This typical type 1 Brugada ECG pattern is shown in Fig. 15-12. However, this distinctive ECG pattern can be covert[30] and only unmasked by sleep, fever, bradycardia, or by xenobiotics such as vagotonic medications or class I antidysrhythmics (sodium channel blockers).[4,59] The reason for this variable and dynamic response to xenobiotics is the heterogeneous genetic basis of the disorder. Mutations in each of 10 different genes have been linked to the Brugada syndrome; more than 300 different mutations have been identified in the *SCN5A* gene alone which encodes the α subunit of the cardiac sodium channel. Brugada syndrome is also associated with mutations in other cardiac ion channels and with mutations of the glycerol-3-phosphate 1-like (GDP1L) gene, which interacts with the cardiac sodium channel subunits at the cell membrane.[5] The complexity

of the potential xenobiotic interactions and variable potential for toxicity has lead to the establishment of a Web page (www.brugadadrugs.org) to provide up-to-date classification of xenobiotics into those to avoid, those to preferably avoid, and those to potentially use for treatment.[11,59]

AUTONOMIC NERVOUS SYSTEM AND HEMODYNAMICS

In addition to the voltage-dependent ion channels, the cell membrane contains channels that open in response to receptor binding of neurotransmitters or neurohormones.[60,61] The hemodynamic effects of many xenobiotics are mediated by interactions with membrane receptors and by changes in the autonomic nervous system. The autonomic nervous system is functionally divided into the sympathetic (ie, adrenergic) and parasympathetic (ie, cholinergic) systems. The 2 systems, which share certain common features, function semi-independently of each other. The sympathetic nervous system is primarily responsible for the maintenance of arteriolar tone and cardiac inotropy and chronotropy through the release of norepinephrine and epinephrine. The parasympathetic nervous system opposes the sympathetic nervous system and reduces overall cardiovascular response such as through vagal nerve innervation of the heart, resulting in reduced heart rate. Through complex feedback, the 2 systems provide the balance needed for existence under changing external conditions.

Adrenergic Receptors

Cellular Physiology of Adrenergic Receptors

The effects of adrenergic xenobiotics on the cell are primarily mediated through a secondary messenger system of cyclic adenosine monophosphate (cAMP). The intracellular cAMP concentration is regulated by the membrane interaction of 3 components: the adrenergic receptor, a G-protein complex, and adenylate cyclase, the (enzyme that synthesizes cAMP in the cell.)[13,27,76,77] These receptors are described in detail in Chapter 13.

The G proteins serve as "signal transducers" between the receptor molecule in the cell membrane and the effector enzyme, adenylate cyclase, in the cytosol. The G proteins consist of 3 subunits: α, β, and γ.[17,54,55] The α subunit of a G protein complex binds to the adrenergic receptor in the cell membrane and to the adenylate cyclase enzyme. The G protein complex exists in several isomeric forms, depending on their interactions with adenylate cyclase. These forms, G_s, G_i, and G_q, have different functions in the regulation of cellular activity. The G_s protein complexes contain α_s subunits that stimulate adenylate cyclase when "activated" by adrenergic receptor interaction. These G_s complexes are primarily responsible for the stimulatory activity of β-adrenergic agonist agents. β_1- and β_2-adrenergic receptors interact primarily with β_s subunits in stimulatory G_s protein complexes. The α_i subunits of G_s proteins inhibit the activity of adenylate cyclase. Some β_2-adrenergic receptors and the α_2-adrenergic receptors interact with inhibitory G_i proteins to decrease the activity of adenylate cyclase. A third form, G_q, interacts with the α_1-adrenergic receptors but does not interact directly with adenylate cyclase. Instead, the G_q interacts with phospholipase C to mediate the cell response to α_1-adrenergic stimulation.

The G protein complex is composed of the cellular receptor and the 3 subunits, α, β, and γ, which are involved in the cellular response to catecholamines. In the absence of a catecholamine at the receptor site, the receptor protein is bound to the β and β-γ–dimer of the G protein, and guanosine diphosphate (GDP) is bound to the α subunit. Catecholamine binding to the receptor causes a conformational change in the α subunit; GDP dissociates and guanosine triphosphate (GTP) binds to the α subunit. The α subunit (with GTP bound) then dissociates from the receptor and from

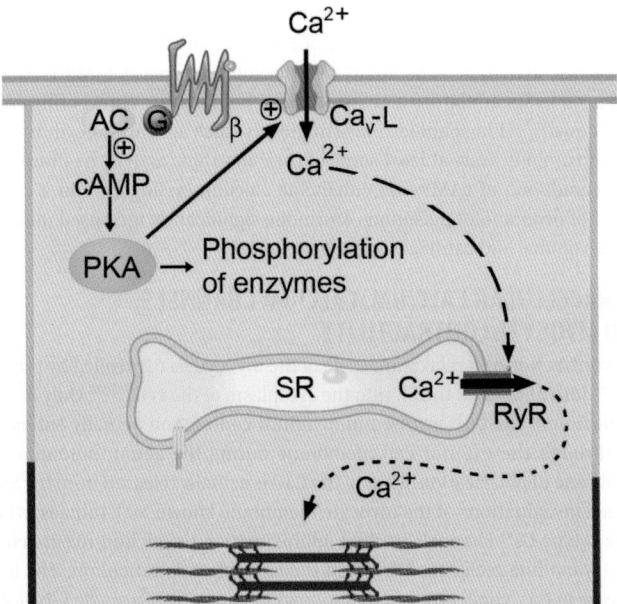

FIGURE 16–1. Binding of the β-adrenergic agonist to the β receptor of a myocardial cell causes the G$_s$ protein to activate AC to produce cAMP. The cAMP interacts with and activates PKA. Subsequent phosphorylation by PKA changes the activity of multiple other various cellular proteins, including phospholamban, calcium channels, and troponin, all of which increase the activity of the myocardial cell. Refer to the text for more details. AC = adenylate cyclase; cAMP = cyclic adenosine monophosphate; Ca$_v$-L = L-type voltage-dependent calcium channel; PKA = protein kinase A; RyR = ryanodine receptor; SR = sarcoplasmic reticulum.

the β-γ–dimer. This "activated" α subunit then interacts with adenylate cyclase or other effector enzymes. Interaction of the α$_s$ subunit with adenylate cyclase increases the activity of the enzyme, resulting in a rapid increase in the intracellular cAMP (Fig. 16–1).[13,17,45,54]

Cyclic AMP acts as a secondary messenger in the cell. Cyclic AMP interacts with protein kinase A (PKA) and other cAMP-dependent protein kinases to increase their protein phosphorylating activity.[44] In the absence of cAMP, PKA is a tetramer of 2 regulatory and 2 catalytic subunits. Cyclic AMP binds to the regulatory subunits to release the active enzymatic units from the tetramer (Fig. 16–1). The activated protein kinases then transfer phosphate groups from ATP to serine (as well as to threonine and tyrosine amino acid groups) on enzymes that are involved in intracellular regulation and activities. Phosphorylation increases or decreases the activity of specific enzymes, and specific protein kinases are highly selective in the proteins that they phosphorylate.[73,74]

Protein kinase A phosphorylates a variety of cellular proteins involved in Ca^{2+} regulation, including the voltage-sensitive Ca^{2+} channel, phospholamban, and troponin,[31,32,72] which are involved in the regulation and control of cellular muscle fiber contraction. Phosphorylation of the L-type calcium channel increases the entry of Ca^{2+} ions into the cell during membrane depolarization.[58] Phosphorylation of phospholamban decreases its ability to inhibit the calcium ATPase pump on the sarcoplasmic reticulum (SR). Decreased inhibition of the calcium ATPase pump on the SR increases the efficiency of Ca^{2+} storage in the SR, which enhances both the cellular contractility as the Ca^{2+} is released into the cell cytosol and the relaxation of muscle fibers as the Ca^{2+} is pumped back into the SR.[58]

Physiologic Effects of Adrenergic Receptor Subclasses

The existence of 2 types of adrenergic receptors, α and β, was first proposed in 1948 to explain both the excitatory and the inhibitory effects of catecholamines on different smooth muscle tissue.[1] The α receptor was subsequently subdivided into α$_1$ and α$_2$ when norepinephrine and other α-adrenergic agonists were found to inhibit the release of additional norepinephrine from neurons into the synapse. The α$_1$-adrenergic receptors are located on postsynaptic cells outside the central nervous system, primarily on blood vessels, and mediate arteriolar constriction. The "autoregulatory" α$_2$-adrenergic receptors are primarily located on the presynaptic neuronal membrane and, when stimulated, decrease release of additional norepinephrine into the synapse. Additionally, some α$_2$-adrenergic receptors are also found on the postsynaptic membrane in the central nervous system. Activation of these postsynaptic α$_2$-receptors in the cardiovascular control center in the medulla and elsewhere in the central nervous system decreases sympathetic outflow from the brain. Thus, α$_2$-adrenergic agonists generally decrease peripheral vascular resistance, decrease heart rate, and decrease blood pressure. The α$_1$- and α$_2$-adrenergic receptors also interact with circulating catecholamines and other sympathomimetics. The effects of sympathomimetics vary in the different organ systems as a result of differences in the adrenergic receptors and in the cellular responses to the receptor interactions.

The β-adrenergic receptors are subclassified into 3 subtypes: β$_1$, β$_2$, and β$_3$ (Table 16–1). The most prevalent β-adrenergic subtype in the heart is β$_1$ (80%), although β$_2$ (20%) and β$_3$ (few) receptors are also present.[9,20,26,60] Stimulation of the β$_1$-adrenergic receptors increases heart rate, contractility, conduction velocity, and automaticity. The β$_2$-adrenergic receptors primarily cause relaxation of smooth muscle with resulting bronchodilation and arteriolar dilation. The β$_3$ receptors are located primarily on adipocytes, where they play a role in lipolysis and thermogenesis.[14] With normal aging and in the setting of heart failure, a decline in β-adrenergic responsiveness referred to as "β-adrenergic desensitization" occurs. This process is believed to be due to a decrease in β$_1$-adrenergic receptor density in cardiac myocytes, alterations in signaling of G-proteins and kinase activity, and an increase in baseline circulating plasma norepinephrine and epinephrine levels.[22,81]

The β$_1$- and β$_2$-receptors interact with G$_s$ proteins and stimulate the adenylate cyclase enzyme. Differences in the resultant clinical effects are primarily related to the location and number of the different receptors in different tissues and to differences in the specificity of the tissue protein kinases activated by cAMP. Stimulation of the β$_1$-adrenergic receptor results in increased heart rate and increased contractility. β$_2$-Adrenergic receptor stimulation causes relaxation, as opposed to contraction, of smooth muscle. Because both β-adrenergic receptor subtypes interact with stimulatory G$_s$ proteins, their clinical effects would appear to be paradoxical. However, there are 2 primary reasons for their different effects when G$_s$ complexes are stimulated by β$_1$- or β$_2$-adrenergic agonists. First, PKA is

TABLE 16–1	Types and Function of the β-Adrenergic Receptors	
TYPE	**Location**	**Function**
β$_1$	Heart	Increase rate
		Increase inotropy
		Increase sinoatrial and atrioventricular node conduction
	Kidney	Increase renin
	Eye	Increase aqueous humor
	Adipose tissue	Increase lipolysis
β$_2$	Heart	Increase rate
		Increase inotropy
	Liver	Increase glycogenolysis
		Increase gluconeogenesis
	Skeletal muscle	Increase glycogenolysis
	Smooth muscle (bronchi, arterioles, gastrointestinal tract, uterus)	Relaxation
β$_3$	Adipose tissue	Increase lipolysis and thermogenesis
	Bladder	Increases relaxation
	Heart	Decrease inotropy

not a single enzyme, but a group of related enzymes variably expressed in different tissues.[8,35,56] The actions and the substrates of the varied protein kinase enzymes differs between β_1- and β_2-adrenergic responsive tissues. Second, whereas β_1-adrenergic stimulation results in cAMP-mediated effects throughout the cytoplasm, β_2-adrenergic stimulation is compartmentalized within the cell. The effect of β_2-adrenergic stimulation of G_s-type receptors is primarily localized phosphorylation of the L-type calcium channels, increasing their activity.[16,39,84,85] Additionally, some β_2-adrenergic receptors are also coupled to G_i-type receptors that inhibit adenylate cyclase and prevent the diffuse cytoplasmic increases in cAMP.[69,70,85] Also, β_2-adrenergic receptor stimulation does not result in phosphorylation of phospholamban[42] or troponins.[16]

The α_2-adrenergic receptor interacts with a G_i protein that has an inhibitory interaction with adenylate cyclase. Binding of α_2-adrenergic agonists to the receptor inhibits (not stimulates) adenylate cyclase and decreases intracellular cAMP.

The α_1-adrenergic receptors also are associated with G proteins. However, rather than being associated with G_s proteins and adenylate cyclase, the α_1-adrenergic receptors are associated with G_q proteins that are linked to phospholipase C.[75] Agonist binding to the receptor activates the hydrolysis of phosphatidyl inositol 4,5-bisphosphate (PIP$_2$) to 1,2-diacylglycerol (DAG) and inositol triphosphate (IP$_3$).[29] The IP$_3$ acts as an intracellular messenger, binds to receptors on the SR, and initiates the release of calcium ion.[6] 1,2-Diacylglycerol activates protein kinase C, which phosphorylates slow Ca^{2+} channels and other intracellular proteins, and increases the influx of Ca^{2+} ion into the cell (Fig. 16–2).[62,68,87]

Many xenobiotics interact with G-protein membrane receptors and alter the intracellular cAMP or Ca^{2+} concentration. β-Adrenergic antagonist overdose results in decreased stimulation of adenylate cyclase by G_s proteins, decreased production of cAMP, decreased activation of the cAMP-dependent kinases, and decreased Ca^{2+} release (Chap. 59). Similarly, by different mechanisms, Ca^{2+} channel blocker overdose results in decreased cytoplasmic [Ca^{2+}] concentration (Chap. 60).

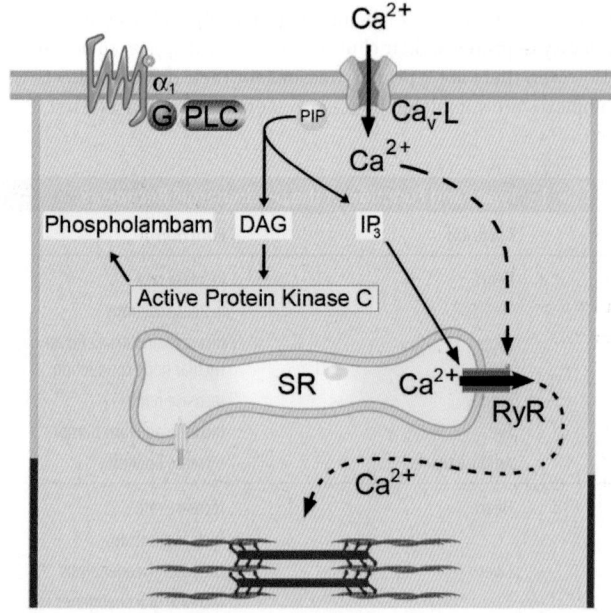

FIGURE 16–2. Binding of the α-adrenergic agonist to the α_1-adrenergic receptor causes the Gq protein to activate PLC. PLC catalyzes the hydrolysis of PIP to produce DAG and IP$_3$. IP$_3$ interacts with the RyR on the sarcoplasmic reticulum to enhance release of Ca^{2+} from this cellular store. The Ca^{2+} and DAG activate protein kinase C, which phosphorylates and changes the activity of various cellular proteins, including phospholamban. Refer to the text for more details. Ca$_v$-L = L-type voltage-dependent Ca^{2+} channel; DAG = 1,2-diacylglycerol; IP$_3$ = inositol triphosphate PIP = 4,5-bisphosphate; PLC = phospholipase C; RyR = ryanodine receptor.

Glucagon receptors, which resemble β-adrenergic receptors, are coupled to the same G_s proteins as β-adrenergic receptors and thus stimulate adenylate cyclase activity.[28,86] The ability of glucagon to increase cAMP is further enhanced by its inhibitory activity on phosphodiesterase (preventing cAMP breakdown).[21,51] Phosphodiesterase inhibitors, such as amrinone, milrinone, and enoximone, exert at least some of their inotropic activity by preventing the degradation of cAMP and enhancing calcium cycling.[46,79,82] In a canine model of propranolol poisoning, amrinone significantly increased inotropy, stroke volume, and cardiac output.[46]

INTRACELLULAR CALCIUM, CALCIUM CHANNELS, AND MYOCYTE CONTRACTILITY

The contraction and relaxation cycle of the myocyte is controlled by the flux of Ca^{2+} into and out of the SR into the cytoplasm of the cell.[18,43,63] Only a small proportion of the Ca^{2+} involved in myofibril contraction actually enters the cell through the exterior cell membrane during the action potential and membrane depolarization. Most of the Ca^{2+} is actually released from the SR of the cell invaginations of the myocyte membrane known as T-tubules, which place L-type Ca^{2+} channels in close approximation to calcium-release channels (ryanodine receptors {RyR}) on the sarcoplasmic reticulum. The local increase in Ca^{2+} concentration that follows the opening of a single L-type calcium channel triggers the opening of the associated RyR channels, resulting in a large release of Ca^{2+} from the SR.[15] Myocytes contain tens of thousands of *couplons*, clusters of L-type calcium channels and RyR channels. The Ca^{2+} released from one couplon is not sufficient to trigger firing of neighboring couplons. Therefore, myocyte contraction requires synchronized release of Ca^{2+} from numerous couplons throughout the myocyte. The cell membrane depolarization synchronizes opening of L-type channels and subsequent Ca^{2+} release from the sarcoplasmic reticulum.[19,58] This phenomenon of Ca^{2+}-induced Ca^{2+} release results in a rapid increase in the intracellular [Ca^{2+}] and initiates a rapid myosin and actin interaction.[18]

At the conclusion of cellular contraction, SR-associated Ca^{2+}-adenosine triphosphatase (ATPase) pumps return the cytosolic Ca^{2+}-ATPase into the SR. This SR-associated Ca^{2+}-ATPase pump is regulated by phospholamban, a cellular protein. When phospholamban is bound to the Ca^{2+}-ATPase pump, the activity of the pump is decreased and less Ca^{2+}-ATPase is stored in the SR. Phosphorylation of phospholamban decreases its affinity for binding to the Ca^{2+}-ATPase pump. Dissociation of the phosphorylated phospholamban increases the activity of the Ca^{2+}-ATPase pump. β-Adrenergic stimulation increases protein kinase activity and leads to phosphorylation of phospholamban, dissociation of the phosphorylated phospholamban from the pump, and an increase in the total SR Ca^{2+} stores.[24,25] The increased activity of the SR associated Ca^{2+}-ATPase pump enhances the contractility and increases the rate of relaxation of the myocytes.

Cellular contraction occurs when myosin filaments interact with the actin-tropomyosin helix. A complex of troponins T, I, and C binds to the actin helix near the myosin-binding site and act as regulators of the interaction. Troponin T binds the regulatory complex to the actin helix, troponin I prevents myosin from accessing its binding site on the actin helix, and troponin C acts as a Ca^{2+} trigger to initiate contraction. When the intracellular [Ca^{2+}] increases, 4 molecules of Ca^{2+} bind to troponin C and a conformational shift occurs in the troponin complex. Troponin I shifts away and the myosin-binding site is exposed. Myosin then binds to the exposed site and myofibril contraction occurs (Fig. 16–3).[36,37,64,65]

Calcium transport through the cellular membrane ion channels is critical for normal cardiac muscle function and contractility and for maintenance of vascular smooth muscle tone. The physiologic response to Ca^{2+} channel blockers and to xenobiotics that interact with the α- or β-adrenergic receptors is mediated through changes in the intracellular Ca^{2+} concentration. Calcium channel blockers in current clinical use primarily block the L-type Ca^{2+} channel, although their specificity differs for the Ca^{2+} channels on the vascular smooth muscle cells versus on the myocardial cells. Dihydropyridine Ca^{2+} channel blockers preferentially act on peripheral vascular smooth muscle cells, whereas non-dihydropyridine Ca^{2+} channel blockers exert

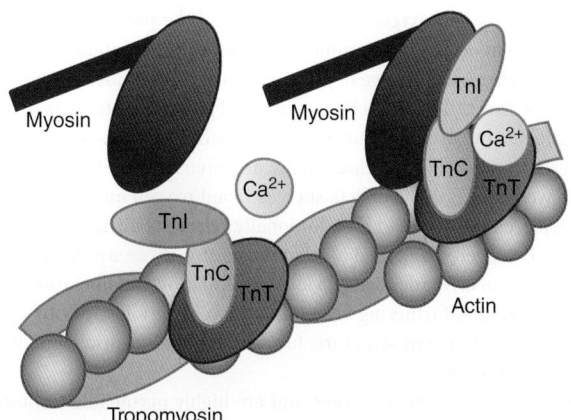

FIGURE 16–3. Troponin regulation of actin and myosin interaction. On the left, TnI blocks the binding site for myosin on the tropomyosin–actin helix. On the right, Ca^{2+} binding to TnC causes a conformational shift in the troponin molecules, and myosin binds to the actin helix and initiates myofibril contraction. TnC = troponin C; TnI = troponin I; TnT = troponin T.

TABLE 16–2	Common Xenobiotics Causing Bradycardia
α_1-Adrenergic agonists (reflex bradycardia)	Cholinergics
Phenylephrine	Carbamates or organic phosphorus
Phenylpropanolamine	compounds
α_2-Adrenergic agonists (centrally acting)	Edrophonium
Clonidine	Neostigmine
Imidazolines	Physostigmine
Methyldopa	Opioids
β-Adrenergic antagonists	Sedative hypnotics
Antidysrhythmics	Sodium channel openers
Amiodarone	Aconitine
Sotalol	Ciguatoxin
Calcium channel blockers	Grayanotoxin
Cardioactive steroids	Veratridine
	Synthetic cannabinoids

stronger central effects. This results in variable effects of the different Ca^{2+} channel blockers on the vascular tone and peripheral vascular resistance, and on the contractility and electrical activity of the myocardial cells.

Patients poisoned by Ca^{2+} channel blockers have less Ca^{2+} entry into the cell during cardiac membrane depolarization. Administration of exogenous Ca^{2+} increases the concentration gradient across the cell membrane, enhances flow through available Ca^{2+} channels, and restores the triggered response of the RyR-2 channels to release Ca^{2+} from the sarcoplasmic reticulum (Antidotes in Depth: A32). Because β-adrenergic antagonists have negative effects on Ca^{2+} handling by the SR, similar effects occur in the myocyte affected by β-adrenergic antagonists.

In the vascular smooth muscle, the cytosolic $[Ca^{2+}]$ maintains the basal contraction of the vascular muscle. Any decrease of Ca^{2+} influx results in relaxation and arterial vasodilation.[55] Any influx of Ca^{2+} binds calmodulin, and the resulting complex stimulates myosin light-chain kinase activity.[47] The myosin light-chain kinase phosphorylates myosin. The phosphorylated myosin has increased activity for binding to actin, which causes contraction (Fig. 60–1).[7,37]

CARDIOVASCULAR EFFECTS OF XENOBIOTICS

Certain xenobiotics produce adverse effects on the cardiovascular system by acting on the myocardial cells or the autonomic nervous system to directly affect the heart rate, blood pressure, or cardiac contractility. Because metabolic abnormalities (especially acidemia, hypotension, hypoxia, and electrolyte abnormalities) can further exacerbate toxicity, or can be the sole cause of the cardiovascular abnormalities, correction of metabolic abnormalities must be a high priority in the treatment of patients with cardiovascular manifestations of poisoning. The terminal phase of any serious poisoning includes nonspecific hemodynamic abnormalities and cardiac dysrhythmias.

Heart Rate Abnormalities

Xenobiotics that directly cause dysrhythmias or cardiac conduction abnormalities usually affect the myocardial cell membrane. These abnormal rhythms, cardiac conduction abnormalities, and heart blocks are discussed in Chap. 15.

Bradycardia

Sinus bradycardia is probably the most common xenobiotic-induced bradycardia. Xenobiotics (Table 16–2) produce bradycardia through different mechanisms. The xenobiotic influences the central or peripheral nervous systems affecting rhythm generation or conduction in the heart. Most xenobiotics that cause central nervous system depression, such as the sedative-hypnotics, opioids, and α_2-adrenergic receptor agonist ("centrally acting") antihypertensives, usually decrease sympathetic outflow to the heart and

produce sinus bradycardia in the range of 40 to 60 beats/min. Digoxin, certain cholinergics, and α_1 agonists produce bradycardia and heart block through the enhancement of vagal tone. Sodium channel activators, such as aconitine, cause bradycardia due to intracellular Na^+ overload with a resultant alteration in Ca^{2+} handling. The most profound bradycardia results from overdoses of xenobiotics that have direct depressant effects on the cardiac pacemakers.[71] The inability to propagate an impulse within the cardiac conducting system produces bradycardia or even asystole. Examples of xenobiotics that produce pacemaker or conduction effects include Ca^{2+} channel blockers and β-adrenergic antagonists.

Bradycardia, heart block, and asystole frequently are terminal events in patients with massive overdose of many noncardiotoxic xenobiotics. These dysrhythmias occur as a result of direct effects on the myocardium or of indirect metabolic effects. For example, severe hyperkalemia or metabolic acidosis results in a wide complex, sinusoidal bradycardic rhythm.

Tachycardia

Sinus tachycardia is the most common xenobiotic induced tachycardia. Parasympatholytic drugs, such as atropine, raise the heart rate by elimination of the inhibitory vagal influence. However, more rapid rates result from direct myocardial stimulatory effects, generally mediated by β-adrenergic agonism. For example, catecholamine excess (eg, cocaine, psychomotor agitation, methylxanthines, sedative-hypnotic withdrawal) causes sinus tachycardia with rates faster than 150 beats/min. Tachycardia is also an indirect effect in response to hypotension, hypoxia, acidemia, fever, electrolyte abnormalities, and other metabolic derangements that present in poisoned patients (Table 16–3).

Decreased Cardiac Contractility and Congestive Heart Failure

Xenobiotics reduce cardiac contractility, with a resulting decrease in cardiac ejection fraction and cardiac output, a decrease in blood pressure, and development of congestive heart failure (CHF). Cardiogenic pulmonary edema generally occurs as a result of the direct negative effects of the xenobiotic on the contractility, or inotropy, of the heart, or through increases in the preload or afterload. Acute cardiogenic pulmonary edema, resulting from impaired left heart filling, which often results from decreased cardiac output, occurs in patients poisoned by a nondihydropyridine calcium channel blocker or β-adrenergic receptor antagonist. Other xenobiotics that exert direct depressant effects on cardiac contractility, generally through sodium channel blockade, include antihistamines, phenothiazines, antidysrhythmics, and local anesthetics. By slowing intraventricular conduction these xenobiotics reduce the ability of the heart to contract efficiently. Pulmonary edema can result from the fluid overload accompanying infusion of large quantities of sodium-containing xenobiotics (eg, sodium penicillin), the renal effects of medications such as nonsteroidal antiinflammatory drugs, or as a late consequence of xenobiotics that cause kidney failure (Chap. 27).

TABLE 16–3	Common Xenobiotics Causing Sinus Tachycardia and/or Tachydysrhythmias
Amantadine	Pentamidine
Antidysrhythmics	Phenothiazines
Anticholinergics	Phosphodiesterase inhibitors
Antihistamines	Amrinone
Botanicals and plants (Chaps. 43 and 118)	Methylxanthines
Bupropion	Sedative–hypnotics
Carbamazepine	Chloral hydrate
Cardioactive steroids	Ethanol
Chloroquine and quinine	Sympathomimetics
Cyclic antidepressants	Amphetamines
Cyclobenzaprine	Catecholamines
Hydrocarbons and solvents	Cocaine
Halogenated hydrocarbons	Thyroid hormone preparations
Inhalational anesthetics	
Jellyfish venom (*Chironex fleckeri*)	
Loperamide	
Metal salts	
Arsenic	
Iron	
Lithium	
Magnesium	
Potassium	

Xenobiotics can cause cardiomyopathy through chronic toxic effects directly on the myocardium or indirectly through effects on blood pressure or cardiac vasculature (Table 16–4). In most cases, the exact mechanism of toxicity is not known. However, free radical generation, nitric oxide formation, acetaldehyde production, myocardial ischemia, mechanical overload, nutritional deficiency, and persistent tachycardia are each implicated in the cellular toxicity of the various xenobiotics and development of cardiomyopathy.[23,38,57,67,80]

Blood Pressure Abnormalities

Blood pressure is dependent upon cardiac and vascular function. (The blood pressure is directly related to the heart rate (HR), the stroke volume (SV), and the systemic vascular resistance (SVR): Blood pressure = HR × SV × SVR.) The systolic component of the blood pressure measurement is a reflection of the inotropic state of the myocardium, whereas the diastolic component reflects the vascular tone. Blood pressure is also expressed as the mean arterial pressure (MAP) during a single cardiac cycle. Because at normal heart rates the duration of diastole is approximately twice that of systole, the MAP is calculated as ($\{(2 \times \text{diastolic}) + (\text{systolic})\}/3$).

Systemic vascular resistance depends on vascular tone, vessel diameter, and flow properties of blood. Arteries are twice the thickness of veins and thus a higher resistance to flow and the ability to handle higher shear stress. The viscoelastic properties of large arteries dampen the pulsatile pressure and flow from cardiac output, which enables the microvasculature to steadily

TABLE 16–4	Xenobiotics Associated with Cardiomyopathy	
Amphetamines		Clozapine
Anabolic steroids		Cobalt
Anthracyclines (e.g. dactinomycin, doxorubicin)		Cocaine
Antimony		Ethanol
Catecholamines		HMG-CoA reductase inhibitors
Checkpoint inhibitors		Phenylpropanolamine, Zidovudine

HMG-CoA = β-hydroxy-β-methylglutarylcoenzyme A.

deliver nutrients and oxygen to tissues. Most of the pressure change in the vascular system occurs in precapillary arterioles. To maintain blood flow to vital organs over a wide range of pressures, the smooth muscle tone of these arterioles is directly linked to changes in blood pressure. Arteriolar resistance is also affected by vasoactive humoral and tissues factors such as bradykinin, vasopressin, circulating catecholamines, angiotensin II, and natriuretic peptides as well as metabolic effects such as blood oxygen and carbon dioxide content, pH, osmolarity, and K^+. Additionally, release of nitric oxide and prostaglandin I_2 triggered by metabolic factors and/or shear stress on the endothelial surface of arterioles leads to local vasodilation and liberation of nitric oxide downstream, furthering vessel dilatation. Arterioles vary by territory and, given their different structure, function and react variably in different locations in the body.[34]

Capillaries have very thin walls and are highly permeable to fluid. The low capillary pressure is important for maintenance of tissue fluid balance and nutrient and oxygen delivery to cells. The hydrostatic pressure within the early capillary section drives diffusion and filtration across the capillary beds, which is counterbalanced by the oncotic pressure. In the setting of circulatory shock, increased release of catecholamines causes reduced microvascular perfusion to nonessential organ systems in an attempt to maintain perfusion to vital organs. Tissue hypoxia and release of inflammatory mediators increase vascular permeability and ultimately decrease venous return and cardiac output. When blood pressure falls below the limits of autoregulation, cardiovascular instability occurs, leading first to decreased oxygen delivery and, if left uncorrected, to activation of an inflammatory cascade leading to cellular apoptosis and organ failure.[2,34,66]

Hypertension Caused by Xenobiotics

Hypertension can be the result of an increase in either inotropy or vascular resistance or both. For example, stimulation of the α_1-adrenergic receptor causes hypertension through vasoconstriction, and stimulation of the β_1-adrenergic receptor causes hypertension through enhanced myocardial contractility (Table 16–5).

The hemodynamic results of a xenobiotic overdose depend on the specific xenobiotic ingested and the relative action on the various types of receptors. This suggests that, among β-adrenergic agonists, only those with a predominant β_1-adrenergic effect cause hypertension. Nonselective β-adrenergic agonists (those that agonize at both β_1 and β_2) produce β_1-mediated systolic hypertension (through inotropic effects) with β_2-mediated vascular vasodilation and diastolic hypotension. This results in a widened pulse pressure, which is the numerical difference between the systolic and diastolic pressures. Exposure to selective β_2-adrenergic agonists such as albuterol result in tachycardia and enhanced inotropy with a widened pulse pressure in a manner analogous to nonselective β-adrenergic agonists. The resulting blood pressure depends on the relative physiologic balance between inotropy and vasodilation.

Xenobiotics that interact only with the α_1-adrenergic receptor (such as phenylephrine) cause vasoconstriction and hypertension. Baroreceptors detect the increased blood pressure and signal the parasympathetic nervous system neurons of the vagus nerve to fire and slow the heart rate. In the absence of β-adrenergic stimulation, a "reflex" bradycardia results. Norepinephrine is an α_1-adrenergic agonist with additional β-adrenergic activity. Profound hypertension is the primary hemodynamic toxic effect due to the activity of norepinephrine as both a positive inotrope (β_1) and a vasoconstrictor (α_1). Reflex bradycardia does not occur as a result of stimulation of the cardiac β_1-adrenergic receptors.

Hypotension Caused by Xenobiotics

Typically, hypotension in adults is arbitrarily defined as a systolic blood pressure of less than 90 mm Hg or a MAP of less than 70 mm Hg. However, this is not an adequate clinical parameter. Young children and adults with a small body habitus often have a normal systolic pressure less than 90 mm Hg (Chap. 3). Patients with hypothermia have decreased metabolic demands, and a lower blood pressure is often "normal" for these patients. Most importantly, patients with long-standing hypertension often have inadequate tissue

TABLE 16–5	Xenobiotics That Commonly Cause Hypertension
Hypertensive Effects Mediated by α-Adrenergic Receptor Interaction	**Hypertensive Effects Not Mediated by α-Adrenergic Receptor Interaction**
Direct α-adrenergic receptor agonists	β-Adrenergic receptor agonists[b]
Clonidine[a]	Nonselective
Epinephrine	Isoproterenol
Ergotamines	Cholinergics[a]
Methoxamine	Corticosteroids
Norepinephrine	Nicotine[a]
Phenylephrine	Thromboxane A$_2$
Tetrahydrozoline	Vasopressin
Indirect-acting agonists	
Amphetamines	
Cocaine	
Dexfenfluramine	
Monoamine oxidase inhibitors	
Phencyclidine	
Yohimbine	
Direct- and indirect-acting agonists	
Dopamine	
Ephedrine	
Metaraminol	
Naphazoline	
Oxymetazoline	
Phenylpropanolamine	
Pseudoephedrine	

[a]These cause transient hypertension followed by hypotension.
[b]These cause hypotension.

TABLE 16–6	Heart Rate and ECG Abnormalities of Xenobiotics That Commonly Cause Hypotension		
		Characteristic ECG Abnormalities	
Heart Rate	**Sinus Rhythm**	**Heart Block or Prolonged Intervals**	**Dysrhythmia**
Bradycardia	α$_2$-Adrenergic agonists	β-Adrenergic antagonists	Cardioactive steroids
	Opioids	Calcium channel blockers	Plant toxins
	Sedative-hypnotics	Cholinergics	Aconitine
		Cardioactive steroids	Grayanotoxin
		Magnesium (severe)	Veratridine
		Methadone	Propafenone
		Propafenone	Propoxyphene
		Sotalol	Sotalol
Tachycardia	Amphetamines	Anticholinergics	Anticholinergics
	Angiotensin-converting enzyme inhibitors	Antidysrhythmics	Antidysrhythmics
	Anticholinergics	Antihistamines	Antihistamines
	Arterial vasodilators	Arsenic	Arsenic
	Bupropion	Bupropion	Chloral hydrate
	Cocaine	Cocaine	Cocaine
	Disulfiram	Cyclic antidepressants	Cyclic antidepressants
	Diuretics	Phenothiazines	Loperamide
	Iron	Quinine/chloroquine	Methylxanthines
	Yohimbine		Noncyclic antidepressants
			Phenothiazines
			Sympathomimetics

perfusion even with a MAP of more than 70 mm Hg. The cerebral arterioles normally constrict or dilate to maintain a relatively constant cerebrovascular blood flow despite changes in the peripheral blood pressure. Chronically hypertensive patients lose this autoregulatory response as a consequence of atherosclerotic disease, arteriolar hypertrophy, or arteriolar smooth muscle constriction. These narrowed arterioles typically require a higher peripheral blood pressure to properly perfuse the brain.

Clinically, hypotension is defined as blood pressure that is inadequate to perfuse tissues. The clinical assessment of tissue perfusion is based on the vital signs, skin color, capillary refill, mental status, urine output and concentration, and acid–base balance (eg, serum lactate concentration). However, if a xenobiotic directly affects one or more of these parameters, the clinical assessment of volume and hemodynamic status may be difficult.

Poor tissue perfusion results from hypovolemia, decreased peripheral vascular resistance, myocardial depression, or a dysrhythmia that reduces cardiac output. A single xenobiotic can exert several effects on the hemodynamic system, such as diltiazem, a calcium channel blocker that causes negative inotropy and vasodilation. Appropriate treatment of the hypotension requires an understanding of the pathophysiologic consequences of the xenobiotic and the resultant hemodynamic derangement (Table 16–6).

Hypotension in a poisoned patient also results from intravascular volume depletion. Intravascular volume decreases as a result of gastrointestinal, urinary, or insensible losses; or fluid may redistribute from the intravascular space into the intracellular, interstitial, pleural, or peritoneal spaces. Xenobiotics cause significant intravascular volume depletion through all of these mechanisms.

Hypotension is also caused by xenobiotics that affect venous tone. These xenobiotics increase venous capacitance, decrease the central venous pressure, and result in relative hypovolemia. The effects are mediated via central effects on the sympathetic nervous system or direct effects on the peripheral vasculature. Sedative hypnotics and central α$_2$-adrenergic agonists

(eg, clonidine) decrease the central sympathetic outflow and result in hypotension. Other xenobiotics directly block peripheral α$_1$-adrenergic receptors or stimulate β$_2$-adrenergic receptors on the blood vessels to produce vascular smooth muscle relaxation, venodilation, and hypotension. A large number of xenobiotics are reported to cause hypotension; however, the hypotension often is not a direct action of the xenobiotic. Rather, the cause of hypotension is coexisting hypoxia, acidemia, anaphylaxis, volume depletion, or dysrhythmias.

Identification of the specific xenobiotic causing hypotension requires the integration of a detailed history, complete physical examination, and laboratory studies. Often the identification of the specific xenobiotic responsible for hypotension is based on other physical findings associated with the xenobiotic or recognition of a specific toxic syndrome.

ASSESSMENT OF HEMODYNAMIC STATUS IN THE POISONED PATIENT

Assessment of volume status can be particularly difficult in the poisoned patient because of functional alterations in the patient's autonomic nervous system and the pharmacologic effects of the xenobiotic. For example, the usual signs of salt and water depletion, such as dry mucous membranes, dry skin, low blood pressure, tachycardia, narrowed pulse pressure, altered sensorium, and decreased urine output, can be mimicked by a number of xenobiotics, including cyclic antidepressants. Additionally, hypovolemic patients present with diaphoresis, flushed skin, hypertension, bradycardia, or increased urine output following exposure to a cholinergic xenobiotic such as an organic phosphorus compound.

The most accurate immediate assessment of volume status in a patient is the demonstration of increased cardiac output after a fluid challenge. If concern about providing a fluid bolus exists, providers can perform the passive leg-raising test to functionally give the patient a fluid bolus to assess the adequacy of fluid resuscitation without adding to whole-body volume status. The test is performed by having the patient sit upright in a semi-recumbent position at about 45 degrees. The head is then lowered to the recumbent position and the legs are raised to about 45 degrees. This transiently increases the circulatory volume by approximately 130 to 300 mL, and it results in changes in the arterial pressure and heart rate.[33,53] Several studies demonstrate that this simple maneuver is a good predictor of hemodynamic response to a fluid bolus especially in intensive care patients.[12,40,41,47,49,50,52,78]

Other modes of hemodynamic monitoring have been proposed, including CVP, ultrasonography of the inferior vena (IVC), neck vein distension, and orthostatic vital sign monitoring. However, none of these modes have proven to be reliable or accurate markers of volume status and should not be relied upon when managing a critically ill poisoned patient. The only truly reliable means to assess the volume status of a patient and how a patient will respond to fluid is a trial bolus.

Lactate is a widely accepted diagnostic and prognostic marker of shock in medical and surgical patients due to trauma, sepsis, and cardiogenic shock. In circulatory failure, lactate is elevated as a result of a combination of increased production from tissue hypoxia, increased glucose metabolism/metabolic demands, and/or decreased clearance.[3] In a retrospective case–control study serum lactate concentration had excellent prognostic utility to predict drug-overdose fatality.[48] However lactate as a marker of adequate microcirculatory perfusion and overall hemodynamic status is nonspecific. Elevated lactate can occur due to factors outside hemodynamics including seizure (eg, methylxanthine or cocaine toxicity), mitochondrial DNA changes (eg, nucleoside inhibitors), increased production (eg, propylene glycol), or decreased clearance (eg, metformin).

If hypoperfusion and hypotension do not resolve after initial fluid resuscitation, an echocardiogram to assess cardiac output is a useful adjunct to guide further management. For example, a patient with a decreased ejection fraction and normal volume status, which occurs in a β-adrenergic antagonist overdose, can benefit from an inotrope such as dobutamine, whereas an α₁-adrenergic agonist such as phenylephrine is indicated for a patient with hypotension despite good cardiac contractility and adequate fluid resuscitation. Definitive care of the poisoned patient with hemodynamic compromise or a dysrhythmia begins with the recognition that a possible xenobiotic ingestion occurred. Infections, cardiovascular disease, and other metabolic disorders must always be considered; however, the toxic effects of xenobiotics must be included in the differential diagnosis. A variety of clinical clues, when present, should heighten the clinician's suspicion that a xenobiotic effect is responsible for the hemodynamic or dysrhythmic problem (Table 16–7).

TABLE 16–7   Clues That an Unanticipated Xenobiotic Might Be Causing Hemodynamic Compromise or Dysrhythmia

History
Concomitant seizure
Gastrointestinal disturbances (colicky pain, nausea, vomiting, diarrhea)
Prior ingestion of medications (consider possibility that the container is mislabeled or misidentified)
Depression (even if patient denies ingestion)
Suspected myocardial ischemia in patient < 35 years old
Treatment with any cardiac medications (especially antidysrhythmics or cardioactive steroids)
History of psychiatric illness, asthma, or hypertension
History of drug use or abuse

Physical Examination and Vital Signs
Heart rate
 Sinus tachycardia with rate > 130 beats/min
 Sinus tachycardia without apparent identified cause
 Sinus bradycardia
Respiratory rate
 Any unexplained depression or elevation in rate
Temperature
 Hyperthermia especially if > 106°F (> 41.1°C)
 Hypothermia if < 86°F (< 30°C)
Dissociation between typically paired changes, for example:
 Hypotension and bradycardia (tachycardia expected)
 Fever and dry skin (diaphoresis expected)
 Hypertension and tachycardia (reflex bradycardia anticipated)
 Depressed mental status and tachypnea (decreased respirations common)
Relatively rapid changes in vital signs
Initial hypertension becomes hypotension
Increasing sinus tachycardia or hypertension

General
Alteration in consciousness, such as depressed mental status, confusion, or agitation
Findings usually not associated with cardiovascular diseases
Ataxia, bullae, dry mucous membranes, lacrimation, miosis or mydriasis, nystagmus, unusual odor, flushed skin, salivation, tinnitus, tremor, visual disturbances
Findings consistent with a toxic syndrome
 Especially findings consistent with anticholinergics, sympathomimetics, or sedative hypnotics

Laboratory Tests
Any unexpected or unexplained laboratory result, especially:
 Metabolic acidosis
 Respiratory alkalosis
 Electrolyte abnormalities

SUMMARY

- Xenobiotics interact with the heart or blood vessels to produce hypotension or hypertension, congestive heart failure, dysrhythmias (including bradycardias and tachycardias), or cardiac conduction delays.
- These toxic effects often occur through interactions with specific receptors or with the ion channels in the cell membrane.
- Disruption of the normal cellular regulation of metabolic processes or of the cellular ionic status leads to the cardiovascular and hemodynamic compromise.
- The occurrence of these abnormalities, individually or in combination, might suggest a particular xenobiotic or class of xenobiotics as etiologic (toxic syndrome) and might dictate initial treatment.
- By understanding both the pharmacology of the xenobiotic and the physiology of the heart vasculature autonomic nervous system appropriately tailored treatment can be delivered.

REFERENCES

1. Ahlquist RP. A study of the adrenotropic receptors. *Am J Physiol.* 1948;153:586-600.
2. Aya HD, et al. From cardiac output to blood flow auto-regulation in shock. *Anaesthesiol Intensive Ther.* 2015;47 Spec No:s56-s62.
3. Bakker J. Lactate levels and hemodynamic coherence in acute circulatory failure. *Best Pract Res Clin Anaesthesiol.* 2016;30:523-530.
4. Baranchuk A, et al. Brugada phenocopy: new terminology and proposed classification. *Ann Noninvasive Electrocardiol.* 2012;17:299-314.
5. Berne P, Brugada J. Brugada syndrome 2012. *Circ J.* 2012;76:1563-1571.
6. Berridge MJ. Inositol trisphosphate and calcium signalling. *Nature.* 1993;361:315-325.
7. Berridge MJ. Smooth muscle cell calcium activation mechanisms. *J Physiol.* 2008;586:5047-5061.
8. Blackshear PJ, et al. Protein kinases 1988: a current perspective. *FASEB J.* 1988;2:2957-2969.
9. Brodde OE. The functional importance of beta 1 and beta 2 adrenoceptors in the human heart. *Am J Cardiol.* 1988;62:24C-29C.
10. Brugada P, Brugada J. Right bundle branch block, persistent ST segment elevation and sudden cardiac death: a distinct clinical and electrocardiographic syndrome. A multicenter report. *J Am Coll Cardiol.* 1992;20:1391-1396.
11. BrugadaDrugs.org. Safe drug use and the Brugada syndrome. http://www.brugadadrugs.org/. Accessed June 1, 2017.
12. Carsetti A, et al. Fluid bolus therapy: monitoring and predicting fluid responsiveness. *Curr Opin Crit Care.* 2015;21:388-394.

13. Casey PJ, Gilman AG. G protein involvement in receptor-effector coupling. *J Biol Chem.* 1988;263:2577-2580.

14. Celi FS. Brown adipose tissue—when it pays to be inefficient. *N Engl J Med.* 2009;360:1553-1556.

15. Chakraborti S, et al. Calcium signaling phenomena in heart diseases: a perspective. *Mol Cell Biochem.* 2007;298:1-40.

16. Chen-Izu Y, et al. G(i)-dependent localization of beta(2)-adrenergic receptor signaling to L-type Ca(2+) channels. *Biophys J.* 2000;79:2547-2556.

17. Clapham DE, Neer EJ. G protein beta gamma subunits. *Annu Rev Pharmacol Toxicol.* 1997;37:167-203.

18. Dibb KM, et al. Analysis of cellular calcium fluxes in cardiac muscle to understand calcium homeostasis in the heart. *Cell Calcium.* 2007;42:503-512.

19. Eisner DA, et al. Integrative analysis of calcium cycling in cardiac muscle. *Circ Res.* 2000;87:1087-1094.

20. Enocksson S, et al. Demonstration of an in vivo functional beta 3-adrenoceptor in man. *J Clin Invest.* 1995;95:2239-2245.

21. Fant JS, et al. The use of glucagon in nifedipine poisoning complicated by clonidine ingestion. *Pediatr Emerg Care.* 1997;13:417-419.

22. Ferrara N, et al. beta-adrenergic receptor responsiveness in aging heart and clinical implications. *Front Physiol.* 2014;4:396.

23. Figueredo VM. Chemical cardiomyopathies: the negative effects of medications and nonprescribed drugs on the heart. *Am J Med.* 2011;124:480-488.

24. Frank K, Kranias EG. Phospholamban and cardiac contractility. *Ann Med.* 2000; 32:572-578.

25. Frank KF, et al. Sarcoplasmic reticulum Ca^{2+}-ATPase modulates cardiac contraction and relaxation. *Cardiovasc Res.* 2003;57:20-27.

26. Gauthier C, et al. Functional beta3-adrenoceptor in the human heart. *J Clin Invest.* 1996;98:556-562.

27. Gilman AG. The Albert Lasker Medical Awards. G proteins and regulation of adenylyl cyclase. *JAMA.* 1989;262:1819-1825.

28. Glick G, et al. Glucagon. Its enhancement of cardiac performance in the cat and dog and persistence of its inotropic action despite beta-receptor blockade with propranolol. *Circ Res.* 1968;22:789-799.

29. Graham RM, et al. Alpha 1-adrenergic receptor subtypes. Molecular structure, function, and signaling. *Circ Res.* 1996;78:737-749.

30. Gussak I, et al. The Brugada syndrome: clinical, electrophysiologic and genetic aspects. *J Am Coll Cardiol.* 1999;33:5-15.

31. Hartzell HC, et al. Effects of protein phosphatase and kinase inhibitors on the cardiac L-type Ca current suggest two sites are phosphorylated by protein kinase A and another protein kinase. *J Gen Physiol.* 1995;106:393-414.

32. Hirayama Y, Hartzell HC. Effects of protein phosphatase and kinase inhibitors on Ca^{2+} and Cl- currents in guinea pig ventricular myocytes. *Mol Pharmacol.* 1997;52:725-734.

33. Jabot J, et al. Passive leg raising for predicting fluid responsiveness: importance of the postural change. *Intensive Care Med.* 2009;35:85-90.

34. Jacob M, et al. Regulation of blood flow and volume exchange across the microcirculation. *Crit Care.* 2016;20:319.

35. Jaken S. Protein kinase C isozymes and substrates. *Curr Opin Cell Biol.* 1996;8:168-173.

36. Katz AM. A growth of ideas: role of calcium as activator of cardiac contraction. *Cardiovasc Res.* 2001;52:8-13.

37. Katz AM, Lorell BH. Regulation of cardiac contraction and relaxation. *Circulation.* 2000;102(suppl 4):IV69-IV74.

38. Keefe DL. Trastuzumab-associated cardiotoxicity. *Cancer.* 2002;95:1592-1600.

39. Kuschel M, et al. G(i) protein-mediated functional compartmentalization of cardiac beta(2)-adrenergic signaling. *J Biol Chem.* 1999;274:22048-22052.

40. Lafanechère A, et al. Changes in aortic blood flow induced by passive leg raising predict fluid responsiveness in critically ill patients. *Crit Care Lond Engl.* 2006;10:R132.

41. Lamia B, et al. Echocardiographic prediction of volume responsiveness in critically ill patients with spontaneously breathing activity. *Intensive Care Med.* 2007;33:1125-1132.

42. Lee J. Glucagon use in symptomatic beta blocker overdose. *Emerg Med J EMJ.* 2004;21:755.

43. Lennon NJ, Ohlendieck K. Impaired Ca^{2+}-sequestration in dilated cardiomyopathy (review). *Int J Mol Med.* 2001;7:131-141.

44. Levitzki A, et al. The signal transduction between beta-receptors and adenylyl cyclase. *Life Sci.* 1993;52:2093-2100.

45. Limbird LE. Receptors linked to inhibition of adenylate cyclase: additional signaling mechanisms. *FASEB J.* 1988;2:2686-2695.

46. Love JN, et al. A comparison of amrinone and glucagon therapy for cardiovascular depression associated with propranolol toxicity in a canine model. *J Toxicol Clin Toxicol.* 1992;30:399-412.

47. Lukito V, et al. The role of passive leg raising to predict fluid responsiveness in pediatric intensive care unit patients. *Pediatr Crit Care Med.* 2012;13:e155-e160.

48. Manini AF, et al. Utility of serum lactate to predict drug-overdose fatality. *Clin Toxicol Phila.* 2010;48:730-736.

49. Marik PE, et al. Does central venous pressure predict fluid responsiveness? A systematic review of the literature and the tale of seven mares. *Chest.* 2008;134:172-178.

50. Marik PE, et al. The use of bioreactance and carotid Doppler to determine volume responsiveness and blood flow redistribution following passive leg raising in hemodynamically unstable patients. *Chest.* 2013;143:364-370.

51. Méry PF, et al. Glucagon stimulates the cardiac Ca^{2+} current by activation of adenylyl cyclase and inhibition of phosphodiesterase. *Nature.* 1990;345:158-161.

52. Monnet X, et al. Prediction of fluid responsiveness by a continuous non-invasive assessment of arterial pressure in critically ill patients: comparison with four other dynamic indices. *Br J Anaesth.* 2012;109:330-338.

53. Monnet X, Teboul J-L. Passive leg raising. *Intensive Care Med.* 2008;34:659-663.

54. Neer EJ. Heterotrimeric G proteins: organizers of transmembrane signals. *Cell.* 1995; 80:249-257.

55. Neer EJ, Clapham DE. Roles of G protein subunits in transmembrane signalling. *Nature.* 1988;333:129-134.

56. Paakkari P, et al. Evidence for differential opioid mu 1- and mu 2-receptor-mediated regulation of heart rate in the conscious rat. *Neuropharmacology.* 1992;31:777-782.

57. Packer M. Cobalt cardiomyopathy: a critical reappraisal in light of a recent resurgence. *Circ Heart Fail.* 2016;9:e003604.

58. Petrovic MM, et al. Ryanodine receptors, voltage-gated calcium channels and their relationship with protein kinase A in the myocardium. *Physiol Res.* 2008;57:141-149.

59. Postema PG, et al. Drugs and Brugada syndrome patients: review of the literature, recommendations, and an up-to-date website (www.brugadadrugs.org). *Heart Rhythm.* 2009;6:1335-1341.

60. Rasmussen H. The calcium messenger system (1). *N Engl J Med.* 1986;314:1094-1101.

61. Rasmussen H, et al. Calcium ion as intracellular messenger and cellular toxin. *Environ Health Perspect.* 1990;84:17-25.

62. Reuter H. Calcium channel modulation by beta-adrenergic neurotransmitters in the heart. *Experientia.* 1987;43:1173-1175.

63. Roden DM, et al. Cardiac ion channels. *Annu Rev Physiol.* 2002;64:431-475.

64. Rüegg JC. Cardiac contractility: how calcium activates the myofilaments. *Naturwissenschaften.* 1998;85:575-582.

65. Rüegg JC. Pharmacological calcium sensitivity modulation of cardiac myofilaments. *Adv Exp Med Biol.* 2003;538:403-410; discussion 410.

66. Secomb TW. Hemodynamics. *Compr Physiol.* 2016;6:975-1003.

67. Shah S, Nohria A. Advanced heart failure due to cancer therapy. *Curr Cardiol Rep.* 2015;17:16.

68. Sperelakis N, et al. Regulation of slow calcium channels of myocardial cells and vascular smooth muscle cells by cyclic nucleotides and phosphorylation. *Mol Cell Biochem.* 1994;140:103-117.

69. Steinberg SF. The cellular actions of beta-adrenergic receptor agonists: looking beyond cAMP. *Circ Res.* 2000;87:1079-1082.

70. Steinberg SF. The molecular basis for distinct beta-adrenergic receptor subtype actions in cardiomyocytes. *Circ Res.* 1999;85:1101-1111.

71. Stinson J, et al. Ventricular asystole and overdose with atenolol. *BMJ.* 1992;305:693.

72. Sulakhe PV, Vo XT. Regulation of phospholamban and troponin-I phosphorylation in the intact rat cardiomyocytes by adrenergic and cholinergic stimuli: roles of cyclic nucleotides, calcium, protein kinases and phosphatases and depolarization. *Mol Cell Biochem.* 1995;149-150:103-126.

73. Sunahara RK, et al. Exchange of substrate and inhibitor specificities between adenylyl and guanylyl cyclases. *J Biol Chem.* 1998;273:16332-16338.

74. Sunahara RK, et al. Complexity and diversity of mammalian adenylyl cyclases. *Annu Rev Pharmacol Toxicol.* 1996;36:461-480.

75. Talosi L, Kranias EG. Effect of alpha-adrenergic stimulation on activation of protein kinase C and phosphorylation of proteins in intact rabbit hearts. *Circ Res.* 1992; 70:670-678.

76. Tang WJ, Gilman AG. Type-specific regulation of adenylyl cyclase by G protein beta gamma subunits. *Science.* 1991;254:1500-1503.

77. Taussig R, et al. Distinct patterns of bidirectional regulation of mammalian adenylyl cyclases. *J Biol Chem.* 1994;269:6093-6100.

78. Teboul J-L, Monnet X. Prediction of volume responsiveness in critically ill patients with spontaneous breathing activity. *Curr Opin Crit Care.* 2008;14:334-339.

79. Travill CM, et al. The inotropic and hemodynamic effects of intravenous milrinone when reflex adrenergic stimulation is suppressed by beta-adrenergic blockade. *Clin Ther.* 1994;16:783-792.

80. Von Hoff DD, et al. Risk factors for doxorubicin-induced congestive heart failure. *Ann Intern Med.* 1979;91:710-717.

81. Wallukat G. The beta-adrenergic receptors. *Herz.* 2002;27:683-690.

82. Whitehurst VE, et al. Reversal of propranolol blockade of adrenergic receptors and related toxicity with drugs that increase cyclic AMP. *Proc Soc Exp Biol Med.* 1999; 221:382-385.

83. Wilde AAM, et al. Proposed diagnostic criteria for the Brugada syndrome: consensus report. *Circulation.* 2002;106:2514-2519.

84. Xiao RP. Cell logic for dual coupling of a single class of receptors to G(s) and G(i) proteins. *Circ Res.* 2000;87:635-637.

85. Xiao RP, et al. Recent advances in cardiac beta(2)-adrenergic signal transduction. *Circ Res.* 1999;85:1092-1100.

86. Yagami T. Differential coupling of glucagon and beta-adrenergic receptors with the small and large forms of the stimulatory G protein. *Mol Pharmacol.* 1995;48: 849-854.

87. Zaugg M, Schaub MC. Cellular mechanisms in sympatho-modulation of the heart. *Br J Anaesth.* 2004;93:34-52.

CASE STUDY 4

History A 32-year-old woman with no significant past medical history presented to the emergency department with a 2-day history of a painless, rapidly expanding lesion on her back. She reported subjective fever and malaise. She first noticed the lesion 2 days prior but did not recall any trauma or other inciting factors. The woman denied headache, shortness of breath, chest pain, nausea, vomiting, diarrhea or dysuria. She was not taking any medications, she drank alcohol socially, and she denied injection drug use. She worked as an accountant in New York City and traveled frequently to a vacation home in Montauk, Long Island.

Physical Examination On presentation to the emergency department, the patient was well appearing and in no apparent distress. Vital signs were: blood pressure, 102/52 mm Hg; pulse, 92 beats/min; respiratory rate, 16 breaths/min; tympanic temperature, 98.7°F (37.1°C); and oxygen saturation, 100% on room air. A complete physical examination was within normal limits, except for her skin examination. This was notable for a solitary 9-cm annular plaque on the upper back with central hemorrhagic crust overlying a 5-cm violaceous plaque surrounded by a ring of erythema with a dermatonecrotic lesion (**Fig. CS4–1**). The lesion was only mildly tender to palpation, and there was no underlying fluctuance.

Initial Management A more detailed history failed to reveal any clues. The woman specifically denied knowledge of tick or spider bites, and she neither worked, lived, nor vacationed in an area known to be inhabited by brown recluse spiders. However, she frequented an area of Long Island where ticks are endemic. An intravenous line was inserted and a complete blood count, basic metabolic panel, and liver function tests were sent; all were within normal limits. The patient was started on vancomycin to provide methicillin-susceptible *Staphylococcus aureus* as well as methicillin-resistant *S. aureus* coverage for a presumed bacterial infection or necrotizing soft tissue infection.

What Is the Differential Diagnosis? The only remarkable finding in this patient is the 2-day-old skin lesion, associated with subjective fever and malaise. The differential diagnosis includes infectious diseases such as cellulitis or a bacterially superinfected cyst or arthropod bite, sporotrichosis, Lyme disease, and anthrax (Chap. 127); drug reactions such as a fixed-drug eruption, or given the necrotic appearance of the lesion, necrosis due to warfarin or heparin therapy (Chaps. 17 and 58); and necrotic spider bites (Chap. 115).

Cases such as these require an immediate assessment for potential public health implications. Once a diagnosis of cutaneous anthrax is considered, the possibility of malicious exposure mandates a coordinated effort to establish a definitive diagnosis. It is important to recall that one of the cases of cutaneous anthrax that occurred following the malicious letters in New York in 2001 involved the case of a small child who was initially diagnosed with brown recluse spider envenomation. Additionally, although spider envenomation may occur outside of regions considered to be endemic as movement of spiders in suitcases, packages, or vehicles may occasionally occur, a new pattern of envenomation may represent a local infestation or the expansion of an endemic area resulting from climate changes. All of these scenarios may require public health interventions.

What Clinical and Laboratory Analyses Help Exclude Life-Threatening Causes of This Patient's Presentation? A dermatology consult was called, and a biopsy was taken for histologic evaluation of a permanent section as well as Gram stain. An acid-fast bacillus stain was also done on the tissue for mycobacterial infection and was negative. Extensive laboratory testing was ordered to help exclude uncommon etiologies for the skin lesion. The biopsy demonstrated epidermal necrosis and dermal abscess, which are nonspecific findings. A wound Gram stain and culture failed to show white blood cells or microorganisms.

Further Diagnosis and Treatment Serologic studies including a Lyme Western blot, Rocky Mountain spotted fever antibodies, and *Francisella tularensis* were all negative. The vancomycin was stopped, and the woman was discharged on a 21-day course of oral doxycycline for presumed Lyme disease given the history and morphology of the lesion. The lesion began to regress on oral doxycycline. Although a final diagnosis was never established, the working diagnosis was that of either Lyme disease or a necrotic spider envenomation, and the patient's Lyme Western blot was to be repeated in 3 to 4 weeks in order to further clarify between the two leading diagnoses: Lyme disease or necrotic spider envenomation.

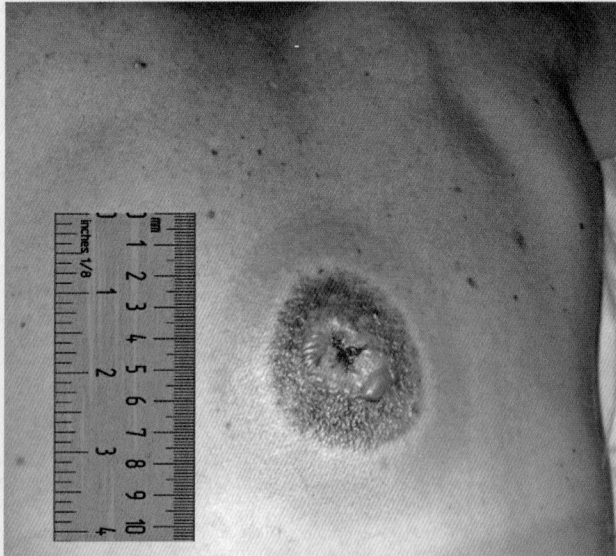

Figure CS4–1. The lesion on the woman's back, reproduced with her permission.

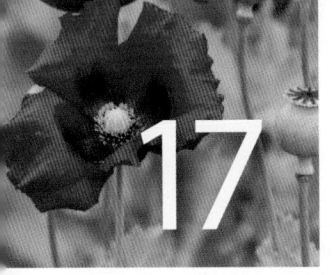

17 DERMATOLOGIC PRINCIPLES

Jesse M. Lewin, Neal A. Lewin, and Lewis S. Nelson

INTRODUCTION

Dermatology is a specialty in which visual inspection allows for rapid diagnosis. A brief physical examination prior to a lengthy history is valuable because some of the classic skin diseases with obvious morphologies allow a "doorway diagnosis" to be established. The tools the physician needs are readily available: magnifying glass, glass slide (for diascopy to determine if a lesion is blanchable), adequate lighting, a flashlight, alcohol pad to remove scale or makeup, scalpel, and at times a Wood lamp. Universal precautions should always be used.

The ability to describe lesions accurately is an important skill, as is the ability to recognize specific patterns. These abilities aid clinicians in their approach to the patient with a cutaneous eruption both in developing a differential diagnosis and while communicating with other physicians. The classic dermatologic lesions are defined in Table 17–1.

The skin shields the internal organs from harmful xenobiotics in the environment and maintains internal organ integrity. The adult skin covers an average surface area of 2 m². Despite its outwardly simple structure and function, the skin is extraordinarily complex. The skin is affected by xenobiotic exposures that occur through many routes. Dermal exposures themselves are important as they account for approximately 7% of all human exposures reported to the American Association of Poison Control Centers (Chap. 130). The clinician must obtain essential information as to the dose, timing, route, and location of exposure. Knowledge of the physical and chemical properties of the xenobiotic can be used to make relevant predictions of adverse cutaneous reactions and whether the response will be local or systemic. The location of xenobiotic exposure determines the histologic morphology, the severity of the reaction pattern, and the overall clinical findings. It should be noted, however, that different xenobiotics produce clinically similar skin changes and conversely that an individual xenobiotic produces diverse cutaneous lesions.

SKIN ANATOMY AND PHYSIOLOGY

The skin has 3 main components that interconnect anatomically and interact functionally: the epidermis, the dermis, and the subcutis or hypodermis (Fig. 17–1). Some experts further categorize the components of the skin into 3 reactive units: The superficial reactive unit, which is composed of the epidermis, the dermal–epidermal junction, and the superficial or papillary dermis with its vascular system; the dermal reactive unit, which is composed of the reticular layer of the dermis and the dermal microvascular plexus; and the subcutaneous reactive unit, which consists of fat lobules and septae.[38] The primary physiologic role of the epidermis, the outermost layer of the skin, is to serve as a barrier, maintain fluid balance, and prevent infection. The degree of barrier function of the epidermis varies with the thickness of the epidermis, which ranges from 1.5 mm on the palms and soles to 0.1 mm on the eyelids. The epidermis is composed of 4 layers: the horny layer (stratum corneum), the granular layer (stratum granulosum), the spinous layer (stratum spinosum), and the basal layer (stratum germinativum), which overlies the basement membrane zone (Fig. 17–1). The keratinocyte, or squamous cell, which is an ectodermal derivative, comprises the majority of cells in the epidermis.

The stratum corneum, a semipermeable surface composed of differentiated keratinocytes, is predominantly responsible for the physical barrier function of the skin. Disruption or abnormal formation of the stratum corneum leads to inadequate function of this barrier, whether by disorders of proliferation or desquamation. For example, accelerated cornification leads to retained nuclei in the stratum corneum (parakeratosis) causing gaps in the stratum corneum, as in psoriasis, which impedes barrier function.[38] Alternatively, in some forms of ichthyosis there is decreased desquamation leading to epidermal retention that influences the barrier function of the stratum corneum.[4] Barrier function is also partly maintained by the upper spinous and granular layers. In this layer, there are Odland bodies, also known as membrane-coating granules, lamellar granules, and keratinosomes. The contents of these organelles provide a barrier to water loss while mediating stratum corneum cell cohesion.[19] The stratum corneum is covered by a surface film composed of sebum emulsified with sweat and breakdown products of keratinocytes.[33] This surface film functions as an external barrier to protect from the entry of bacteria, viruses, and fungi. The role of the surface film, however, is limited with regard to percutaneous absorption. The major barrier molecules to percutaneous absorption in the skin are lipids called ceramides.[33] Diseases characterized by dry skin, such as atopic dermatitis and psoriasis, are in part caused by decreased concentrations of ceramide in the stratum corneum, which allows increased xenobiotic penetration because of barrier degradation.[33] Similarly, hydrocarbon solvents, including alcohols, or detergents, commonly produce a "defatting dermatitis" by keratolysis or the dissolution of these surface lipids.

The cells of the basal layer control the renewal of the epidermis. The basal layer contains stem cells and transient amplifying cells, which are the proliferative cells resulting in new epidermal formation that occurs approximately every 28 days.[38] As the basal cells migrate toward the skin surface they flatten, lose their nuclei, develop keratohyalin granules, and eventually develop into keratinocytes of the stratum corneum. The basal layer of the epidermis is just above the basement membrane zone and is also populated by melanocytes and Langerhans cells in addition to basal keratinocytes. Melanocytes

TABLE 17–1	Dermatologic Diagnostic Descriptions of Lesions of the Skin
Primary Cutaneous Lesions	**Secondary Cutaneous Lesions**
Comedone: open and closed dilated pores (blackheads and whiteheads, respectively)	**Erosion:** a loss of the epidermis up to the full thickness of the epidermis but not through the basement membrane
Macule: a circumscribed flat variation of color that is brown, blue, yellow, red, or hyper- or hypopigmented, <1 cm	**Ulcer:** a loss of full-thickness epidermis and papillary dermis, reticular dermis, or subcutis
Patch: a circumscribed flat variation of color that is brown, blue, yellow, red, or hyper- or hypopigmented, >1 cm	**Lichenification:** thickening of the epidermis and accentuation of natural skin lines
Papule: a circumscribed elevation of <1 cm in diameter	**Atrophy:** thinning of the epidermis
Plaque: a circumscribed elevation of >1 cm in diameter	**Scale:** flaking caused by accumulation of stratum corneum (hyperkeratosis) or delayed desquamation
Nodule: a circumscribed elevation often >2 cm in diameter, involves the dermis and at times subcutis	**Scar:** a thickened, often discolored surface
Pustule: a circumscribed collection of purulent fluid that varies in size	
Tumor: an elevation of >0.5 cm in diameter	
Vesicle: a circumscribed collection of clear fluid <1 cm in diameter	
Bulla: a circumscribed collection of clear fluid >1 cm in diameter	
Wheal: a firm edematous plaque resulting from infiltration of the dermis with fluid	

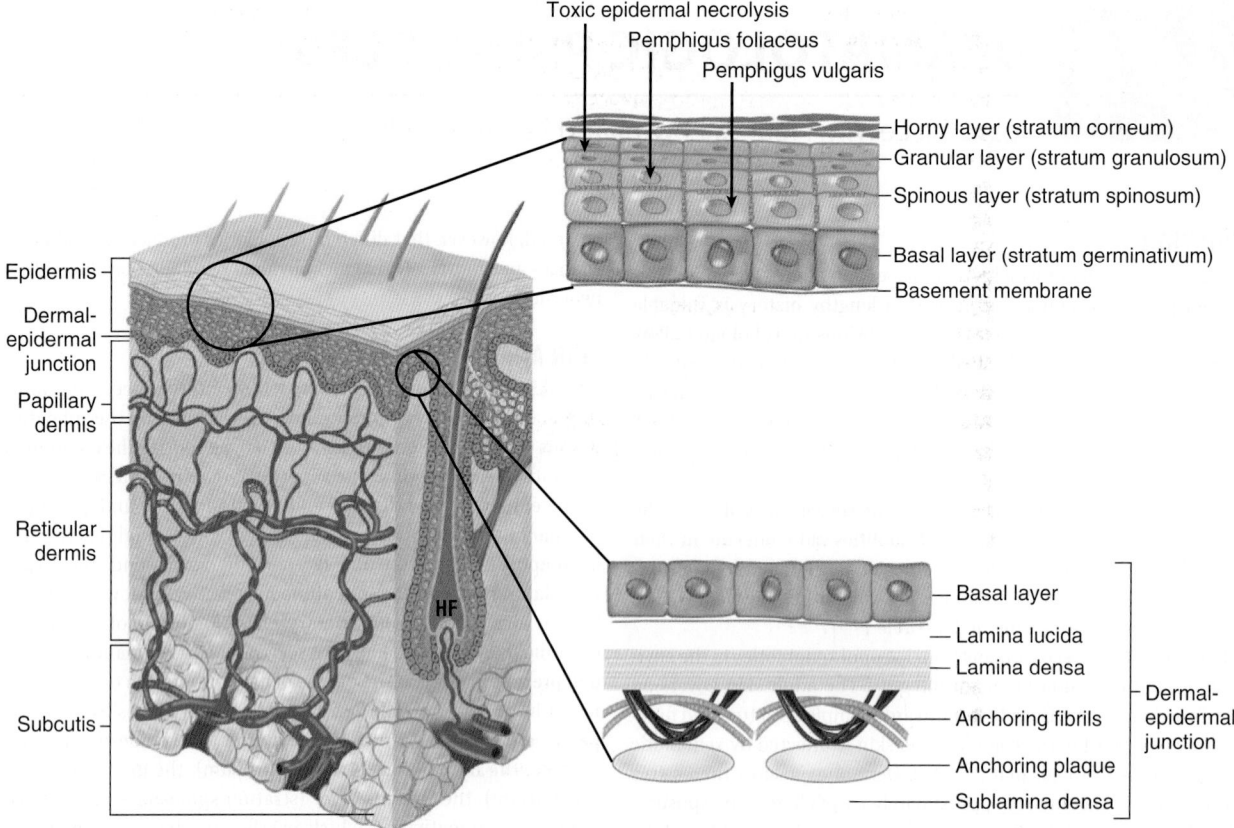

FIGURE 17–1. Skin histology and pathology. Intraepidermal cleavage sites in various xenobiotic-induced blistering diseases. In pemphigus foliaceus, the cleavage is below or within the granular layer, whereas in pemphigus vulgaris, it is suprabasilar. This accounts for the differing types of blisters found in the 2 diseases. HF = hair follicle.

contain melanin, which is the major chromophore in the skin that protects the skin from ultraviolet radiation. Melanocytes are primarily responsible for producing skin pigmentation. Langerhans cells are bone marrow–derived dendritic cells with a primary role in immunosurveillance. These cells function in the recognition, uptake, processing, and presentation of antigens to previously sensitized T lymphocytes. In addition, Langerhans cells also carry antigens via dermal lymphatics to regional lymph nodes.

The basement membrane zone (BMZ) consists of 3 layers—the lamina lucida, the lamina densa, and the sublamina densa (which is composed of anchoring fibrils) — and separates the epidermis from the dermis (Fig. 17–1). It provides a site of attachment for basal keratinocytes and permits epidermal–dermal interaction. The BMZ is also of clinical significance as it is the target of genetic defects and autoimmune attack, leading to a variety of inherited and acquired cutaneous diseases.

The dermal–epidermal junction (DEJ) provides resistance against trauma, gives support to the overlying structures, organizes the cytoskeleton in the basal cells, and serves as a semipermeable barrier. The dermis, below the DEJ, contains the adnexal structures, blood vessels, and nerves. It is arranged into 2 major regions, the upper papillary dermis and the deeper reticular dermis. The dermis provides structural integrity and contains many important appendageal structures. The structural support is provided by both collagen and elastin fibers embedded in glycosaminoglycans, such as chondroitin A and hyaluronic acid. Collagen accounts for 70% of the dry weight of the skin, whereas elastic fibers comprise 1% to 2% of the skin's dry weight. Several important cells, including fibroblasts, macrophages, and mast cells, are residents of the dermis, each with their own unique function. Traversing the dermis are venules, capillaries, arterioles, nerves, and glandular structures.

The arteriovenous framework of the skin is derived from a deep plexus of perforating vessels within the skeletal muscle and subcutaneous fat. From this deep plexus, smaller arterioles transverse upward to the junction of

the reticular and papillary dermis, where they form the superficial plexus. Capillary venules form superficial vascular loops that ascend into and descend from the dermal papillae (Fig. 17–1). The communicating blood vessels provide channels through which xenobiotics exposed on the skin surface can be transported internally. This circulatory network provides nutrition for the tissue and is involved in temperature and blood pressure regulation, wound repair, and numerous immunologic events.[12] Parallel to the vasculature are cutaneous nerves, which serve the dual function of receiving sensory input and carrying sympathetically mediated autonomic stimuli that induce piloerection and sweating.[22]

The apocrine glands consist of secretory coils and intradermal ducts ending in the follicular canal. The secretory coil is located in the subcutis and consists of a large lumen surrounded by columnar to cuboidal cells with eosinophilic cytoplasm.[22] Apocrine glands, which are concentrated in select areas of the body such as the axillae, eyelids, external auditory meatus, areolae, and anogenital region, produce secretions that are rendered odoriferous by cutaneous bacterial flora.

The eccrine glands, in contrast, produce an isotonic to hypotonic secretion that is modified by the ducts and emerges on the skin surface as sweat. The eccrine unit consists of a secretory gland as well as intradermal and intraepidermal ducts. The coiled secretory gland is located in the area of the deep dermis and subcutis. These glands are innervated by postganglionic sympathetic fibers that use acetylcholine neurotransmission, explaining the clinical effects of anticholinergic xenobiotics. Xenobiotics that are concentrated in the sweat increase the intensity of the local skin reactions. Certain chemotherapeutics, such as cytarabine or bleomycin, directly damage the eccrine sweat glands, resulting in neutrophilic eccrine hidradenitis.[65]

Sebaceous glands also reside in the dermis. They produce an oily, lipid-rich secretion that functions as an emollient for the hair and skin, and can be a reservoir of noxious environmental xenobiotics. Pilosebaceous follicles, which are present all over the body, consist of a hair shaft, hair follicle,

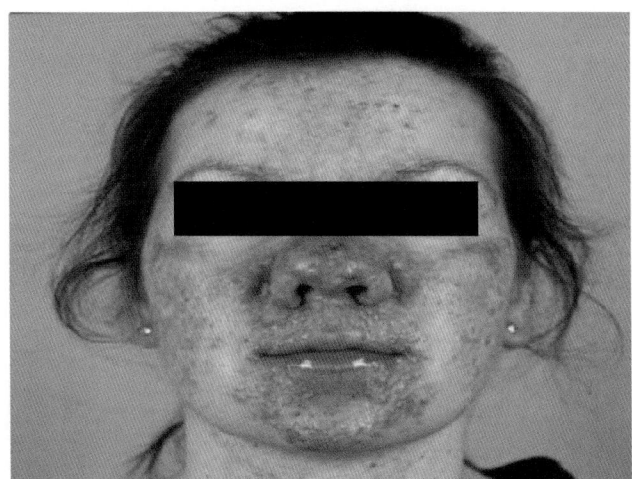

FIGURE 17–2. Chloracne due to dioxin intoxication. Comedones and papulopustular lesions, nodules, and cyst have led to a gross deformity of the nose. *(Used with permission from Dr. Alexandra Geusau.)*

sebaceous gland, sensory end organ, and erector pili. Certain halogenated aromatic chemicals, such as polychlorinated biphenyls (PCBs), dioxin, and 2,4-dichlorophenoxyacetic acid, are excreted in the sebum and cause hyperkeratosis of the follicular canal. This produces the syndrome, chloracne, which appears clinically like severe acne vulgaris but predominates in the malar, retroauricular, and mandibular regions of the head and neck and typically develops after several weeks of exposure (Fig. 17–2). Similar syndromes result from exposure to brominated and iodinated compounds, and are known as bromoderma and ioderma, respectively.[70]

The subcutis serves to insulate, cushion, and allow for mobility of the overlying skin structures. Adipocytes represent the majority of cells found in this layer. Leptin, an adipose-derived hormone responsible for feedback of appetite and satiety signaling, is synthesized and regulates fat mass (adiposity) in this layer.

The hair follicle is divided into 3 portions, the hair bulb, infundibulum, and isthmus.[57] The deepest portion of the hair follicle contains the bulb with matrix cells. The matrix cells are highly mitotically active and often are the target of cytotoxic xenobiotics. The rate of growth and the type of hair are unique for different body sites. Hair growth proceeds through 3 distinct phases: the active prolonged growth phase (anagen phase) during which matrix cell mitotic activity is high; a short involutional phase (catagen phase), and a resting phase (telogen phase). The length of the anagen phase determines the final length of the hair and varies depending on site of the body. For example, hair on the scalp has the longest anagen phase ranging from 2 to 8 years with hair growth at a rate of 0.37 to 0.44 mm/day.[38] Understanding the phases of hair growth is important because hair growth can be used to identify clues regarding the timing of exposure and the mechanism of action of a particular xenobiotic.

The nail plate, which is often considered analogous to the hair, is also a continuously growing structure. Fingernails grow at average of 2 to 3 mm per month and toenails grow approximately 1 mm per month. The mitotically active cells of the nail matrix that produce the nail plate are subject to both traumatic and xenobiotic injury, which in turn affects the appearance and growth of the nail plate. Because nail growth is relatively stable, location of an abnormality in the plate can predict the timing of exposure, such as Mees lines (transverse white lines).

TOPICAL TOXICITY
Transdermal Xenobiotic Absorption
Although there is no active cutaneous uptake mechanism for xenobiotics, many undergo percutaneous absorption by passive diffusion. Lipid solubility, concentration gradient, molecular weight, and certain specific skin characteristics are important determinants of dermal absorption.[23,24,50,54] Absorption is determined to a great extent by the lipid solubility of the specific xenobiotic.[15,39] The pharmacokinetic profile of transdermally administered xenobiotics is markedly different than by the enteral or other parenteral routes.[17] As with any other routes of administration, adverse effects are caused by excessive absorption following application or even with therapeutic use of a transdermal patch. Other xenobiotics, topically applied without a specific delivery device, including podophyllin, camphor, phenol, organic phosphorus compounds, ethanol, organochlorines, nitrates, and hexachlorophene, can lead to systemic morbidity and mortality (Special Considerations: SC3).

Direct Dermal Toxicity
Exposure to any of a myriad of industrial and environmental xenobiotics results in dermal "burns." Although the majority of these xenobiotics injure the skin through chemical reactivity rather than thermal damage, the clinical appearances of the two are often identical. Injurious xenobiotics act as oxidizing or reducing agents, corrosives, protoplasmic poisons, desiccants, or vesicants. Often an injury initially appears to be mild or superficial with minimal erythema, blanching, or discoloration of the skin. Over the subsequent 24 to 36 hours, the injury progresses to extensive necrosis of the skin and subcutaneous tissue.

Both inorganic and organic acids are capable of penetrating and damaging the epidermis via protein denaturation and cytotoxicity; however, organic acids tend to be less irritating. The damaged tissue coagulates and forms a thick eschar, which limits the spread of the xenobiotic. The histopathologic finding following acid injury is termed coagulative necrosis.[10] Inorganic acids that are frequently used in industry include hydrochloric and sulfuric acids which lead to the severe injury. The weakly acidic hydrofluoric (HF) acid, is used for the etching of glass, metal and stone. Hydrofluoric acid, because of its limited dissociation constant, is able to penetrate intact skin with subsequent penetration into deeper tissues. The fluoride ion is extremely cytotoxic, causing severe tissue damage, including bone destruction, by interfering with cellular enzymes. Severe pain is due to the capacity of fluoride ions to bind tissue calcium, thus affecting nerve conduction.[61] Once in the dermis, the proton (H$^+$) and fluoride ions (F$^-$) cause both acid-induced tissue necrosis and fluoride-induced toxicity (Chap. 104).[5]

Alkali exposures characteristically produce a liquefactive necrosis, which allows continued penetration of the corrosive. Consequently, cutaneous and subcutaneous injury following alkali exposure is typically more severe than after an acid exposure, with the exception of hydrofluoric acid. With alkali burns there are generally no vesicles, but rather necrotic skin due to the disruption of barrier lipids, including denaturation of proteins with subsequent fatty acid saponification. Common strong alkalis include sodium, ammonium, and potassium hydroxide; sodium and potassium carbonate; and calcium oxide. These are used primarily in the manufacture of bleaches, dyes, vitamins, pulp, paper, plastics, and soaps, and detergents. Alkali burns from wet cement, which has an initial pH of 10 to 12 that rises to 12 to 14 as the cement sets,[37] result from the liberation of calcium hydroxide.

Thermal damage also results from xenobiotic exposure. For example, the exothermic reaction generated by the wetting of elemental phosphorus or sodium results in a thermal burn.[18] In these circumstances, the products of reactivity, phosphoric acid and sodium hydroxide, respectively, produce secondary chemical injury. Alternatively, skin exposure to a rapidly expanding gas, such as nitrous oxide from a whipped cream cartridge or compressed liquefied nitrogen, or to frozen substances, such as dry ice (CO_2), produce a freezing injury, or frostbite. Dermatologists routinely use liquid nitrogen to induce a cold injury that destroys precancerous lesions such as actinic keratoses.

Hydrocarbon-based solvents are liquids that are capable of dissolving non–water-soluble solutes.[10] Although the most prominent effect is dermatitis due to loss of ceramides from the stratum corneum of the epidermis, prolonged exposure results in deeper dermal injury.

PRINCIPLES OF DERMAL DECONTAMINATION

On contact with xenobiotics, the skin should be thoroughly cleansed to prevent direct effects and systemic absorption. In general, water in copious amounts is the decontaminant of choice for skin irrigation. Soap should be used when adherent xenobiotics are involved. Following exposures to airborne xenobiotics, the mouth, nasal cavities, eyes, and ear canals should be irrigated with appropriate solutions such as water or a 0.9% NaCl solution. For nonambulatory patients, the decontamination process is conducted using special collection stretchers if available.[9]

There are a few situations in which water should not be used for skin decontamination. These situations include contamination with the reactive metallic forms of the alkali metals, sodium, potassium, lithium, cesium, and rubidium, which react with water to form strong bases. The dusts of pure magnesium, sulfur, strontium, titanium, uranium, yttrium, zinc, and zirconium will ignite or explode on contact with water. Following exposure to these metals, any residual metal should be removed mechanically with forceps, gauze, or towels and stored in mineral oil. Phenol, a colorless xenobiotic used in the manufacturing of plastics, paints, rubber, adhesives, and soap, has a tendency to thicken and become difficult to remove following exposure to water. Suggestions for phenol decontamination include alternating washing with water and polyethylene glycol (PEG 400) or 70% isopropanol for 1 minute each for a total of 15 minutes.[40] Our conclusions are that inexpensive readily available tepid water should be utilized (Special Considerations: SC2). Calcium oxide (quicklime) thickens and forms $Ca(OH)_2$ following exposure to water, which releases heat and causes cutaneous ulcerations, suggesting that mechanical removal as above is advised.

DERMATOLOGIC SIGNS OF SYSTEMIC DISEASES

Cyanosis

Normal cutaneous and mucosal pigmentation is caused by several factors, one of which is the visualization of the capillary beds through the translucent epidermis and dermis. Cyanosis manifests as a blue or violaceous appearance of the skin, mucous membranes, and nailbeds. It occurs when excessive concentrations of reduced hemoglobin (>5 g/dL) are present, as in hypoxia or polycythemia, or when oxidation of the iron moiety of heme to the ferric state (Fe^{3+}) forms methemoglobin, which is deeply pigmented (Chap. 124). The presence of the more deeply colored hemoglobin moiety within the dermis results in cyanosis that is most pronounced on areas of thin skin such as the mucous membranes or underneath fingernails. In the differential diagnosis of skin discoloration is pseudochromhidrosis, also termed extrinsic apocrine chromhidrosis. The discoloration is a product of staining of the sweat by chromogenic bacteria including *Corynebacterium*, *Malassezia furfur*, and *Bacillus* spp; the latter 2 species have been known to cause blue discoloration of the skin. Several cases of blue pseudochromhidrosis due to topiramate are reported in the literature, and diagnosis is established by the ability of the clinician to wipe off the discoloration with a damp cotton swab (Fig. 17–3).[11]

Xanthoderma

Xanthoderma is a yellow to yellow-orange macular discoloration of skin.[26] Xanthoderma is caused by xenobiotics such as carotenoids, which deposit in the stratum corneum, and causes carotenoderma. Carotenoids are lipid soluble and consist of α-carotene, β-carotene, β-cryptoxanthin, lycopene, lutein, and zeaxanthan, and serve as precursors of vitamin A (retinol). The carotenoids are excreted via sweat, sebum, urine, and GI secretions. Jaundice is typically a sign of hepatocellular failure or hemolysis and is caused by hyperbilirubinemia, either conjugated or unconjugated, deposits in the subcutaneous fat. Jaundice due to hyperbilirubinemia is often accompanied by other cutaneous stigmata including spider angiomas, telangiectasias, palmar erythema, and dilated superficial abdominal veins (caput medusae). True hyperbilirubinemia is differentiated from hypercarotenemia by the presence of scleral icterus in patients with hyperbilirubinemia. In addition, the cutaneous discoloration seen in hypercarotenemia can be removed by wiping the skin with an alcohol swab. Hypercarotenemia is reported among

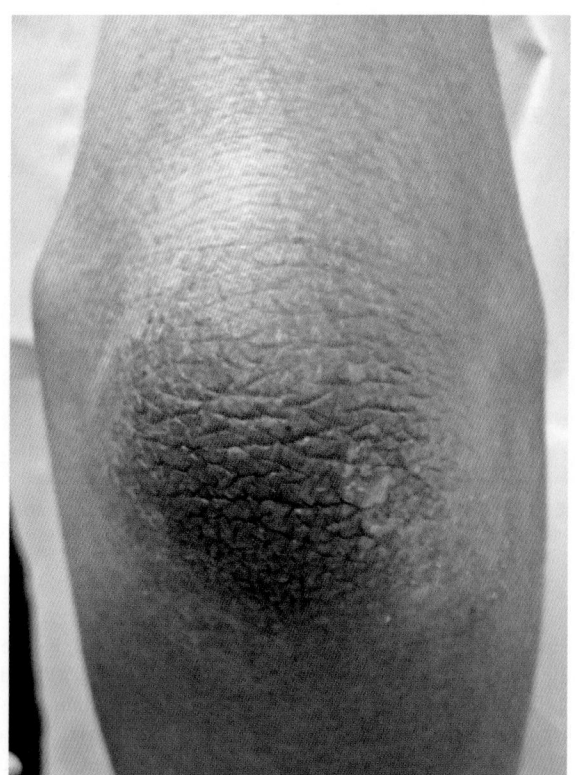

FIGURE 17–3. Pseudochromhidrosis. Blue discoloration on the elbow in a 28-year-old woman as a result of topiramate treatment for epilepsy. This entity is postulated to be a result of a decrease in sweat gland activity and a change in the skin's pH induced by topiramate, leading to the growth of chromogenic bacteria. *(Reproduced with permission from Castela E, Thomas P, Bronsard V, et al. Blue pseudochromhidrosis secondary to topiramate treatment. Acta Derm Venereol. 2009;89(5):538-539.)*

people who take carotene nutrient supplements (Fig. 17–4).[59] Lycopenemia, an entity similar to carotenemia, is caused by the excessive consumption of tomatoes, which contain lycopene. Additionally, topical exposure to dinitrophenol, picric acid, or stains from cigarette use produces localized yellow discoloration of the skin.

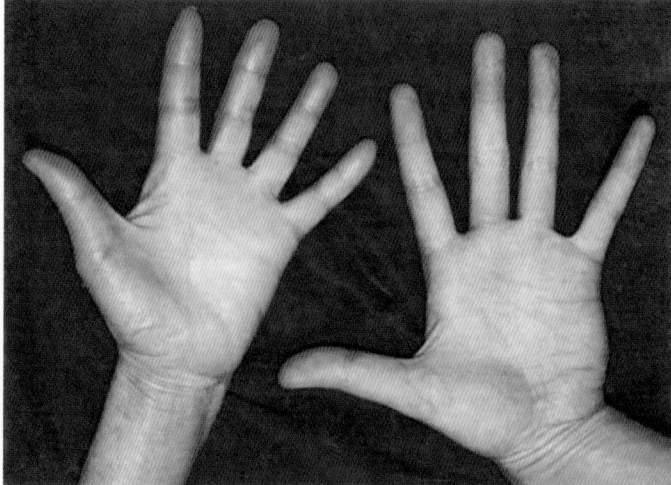

FIGURE 17–4. Carotenemia. Yellow-orange discoloration on the palm (left) as compared with that of a normal control (right). In the presence of excessive blood carotene concentrations, this yellow component is increased, and is most conspicuously accentuated where the skin is thick on the palms and soles. *(Reproduced with permission from Takita Y, Ichimiya M, Hamamoto Y, et al. A case of carotenemia associated with ingestion of nutrient supplements. J Dermatol. 2006 Feb;33(2):132-134.)*

Pruritus

Pruritus is the poorly localized, unpleasant sensation that elicits a desire to scratch. The biologic purpose of pruritus is to provoke the removal of a pruritogen, a response likely to have originated when most pruritogens were parasites. Pruritus is a common manifestation of urticarial reactions, but at times it is of nonimmunologic origin. Pruritus is the most common dermatologic symptom and can arise from a primary dermatologic condition or is a symptom of an underlying systemic disease in an estimated 10% to 50% of patients.[29] Pruritus is also caused by topical exposure to the urticating hairs of Tarantula spiders, spines of the stinging nettle plant (*Urtica* spp), or via stimulation of substance P by capsaicin.[25] Virtually any xenobiotic can cause a cutaneous reaction that can be associated with pruritus, whether by inducing hepatotoxicity, cholestasis, phototoxicity, or histamine release (ie, neurologically mediated). Xenobiotics commonly implicated in neurally mediated itch include tramadol, codeine, cocaine, morphine, butorphanol, and methamphetamine.[29]

Flushing

Vasodilation of the dermal arterioles leads to flushing, or transient reddening of the skin, commonly of the face, neck, and chest. Flushing occurs following autonomically mediated vasodilation, as occurs with stress, anger, or exposure to heat, or it can be induced by vasoactive xenobiotics. Xenobiotics that cause histamine release through a type I hypersensitivity reaction are the most frequent cause of xenobiotic-induced flush. Histamine poisoning produces flushing from the consumption of scombrotoxic fish (Chap. 39). Flushing after the consumption of ethanol is common in patients of Asian and Inuit descent and is similar to the reaction following ethanol consumption in patients exposed to disulfiram or similar xenobiotics (Chap. 78). The inability to efficiently metabolize acetaldehyde, the initial metabolite of ethanol, results in the characteristic syndrome of vomiting, headache, and flushing. Niacin causes flushing through an arachidonic acid–mediated pathway that is generally prevented by aspirin.[7,66] Vancomycin, if too rapidly infused, causes a transient bright red flushing, mediated by histamine and at times can be accompanied by hypotension. This reaction typically occurs during and immediately after the infusion, and is termed "red man syndrome." Idiopathic flushing is managed with nonselective beta-adrenergic antagonists (nadolol, propranolol) or clonidine, while anxiolytics are beneficial if emotional distress or anxiety is determined to be causative. Other nontoxicologic causes of flushing including carcinoid syndrome, pheochromocytoma, mastocytosis, anaphylaxis, medullary carcinoma of the thyroid, pancreatic cancer, menopausal flushing, and renal carcinoma, are in the differential diagnosis of the flushed patient.[28]

Sweating

Xenobiotic-induced diaphoresis is either part of a physiologic response to heat generation or is pharmacologically mediated following parasympathetic or sympathomimetic xenobiotic use. Because the postsynaptic receptor on the eccrine glands is muscarinic, most muscarinic agonists stimulate sweat production. Sweating occurs following exposure to cholinesterase inhibitors, such as organic phosphorus compounds, but also occurs with direct-acting muscarinic agonists such as pilocarpine. Alternatively, antimuscarinics, such as belladonna alkaloids or antihistamines, reduce sweating and produce dry skin. Certain xenobiotics have proven useful for the treatment of hyperhidrosis including the anticholinergics glycopyrrolate, propantheline bromide, and botulinum toxin. Botulinum toxin-A derived from *Clostridium botulinum*, which is FDA approved for the treatment of primary focal axillary hyperhidrosis, temporarily chemodenervates eccrine sweat glands at the neuroglandular junction via inhibition of presynaptic acetylcholine release.[1]

Xenobiotic-Induced Dyspigmentation

Cutaneous pigmentary changes can result from the deposition of xenobiotics that are ingested and carried to the skin by the blood or that permeate the skin from topical applications. Many heavy metals are associated with dyspigmentation. Argyria, a slate-colored discoloration of the skin resulting from the systemic deposition of silver particles in the skin after excessive ingestion of colloidal silver, can be localized or widespread. The discoloration tends to be most prominent in areas exposed to sunlight, probably because silver

stimulates melanocyte proliferation. Histologically, fine black granules are found in the basement membrane zone of the sweat glands, blood vessel walls, the dermoepidermal junction, and along the erector pili muscles (Chap. 98). Gold, which was historically used parenterally in the treatment of rheumatoid arthritis, caused a blue or slate-gray pigmentation, often periorbitally, known as chrysiasis. The pigmentation is also accentuated in sun-exposed areas but, unlike argyria, sun-protected areas do not histologically demonstrate gold. Also, melanin is not increased in the areas of hyperpigmentation. The hyperpigmentation is probably caused by the gold itself, but the cause of its distribution pattern remains unknown. Histologically, the gold is found within lysosomes of dermal macrophages and distributed in a perivascular and perieccrine pattern in the dermis. Bismuth produces a characteristic oral finding of the metallic deposition in the gums and tongue known as bismuth lines, as well as a blue-gray discoloration of the face, neck, and dorsal hands. Chronic arsenic exposure occurs following exposure to pesticides or contaminated well-water, which can cause cutaneous hyperpigmentation with a bronze hue, with areas of scattered hypopigmentation occurring between 1 and 20 years following exposure. Lead also deposits in the gums, causing the characteristic "lead lines," which are the result of subepithelial deposition of lead granules. Intramuscular injection of iron stains the skin, resulting in pigmentation similar to that seen in tattoos, and iron storage disorders, known as hemochromatosis, and results in a bronze appearance of the skin.[21]

Medications are also often implicated in dyspigmentation. The tetracycline-class antibiotic minocycline is a highly lipid-soluble, yellow crystalline xenobiotic that turns black with oxidation. Minocycline-induced discoloration of the skin is at times accompanied by darkening of the nails, sclerae, oral mucosa, thyroid, bones, and teeth. Hyperpigmentation from minocycline is divided into 3 types depending on the color, anatomic distribution, and whether iron- or melanin-containing granules are found within the skin. Other medications associated with hyperpigmentation include amiodarone, zidovudine, bleomycin, and other chemotherapeutics, antimalarials, and psychotropics (chlorpromazine, thioridazine, imipramine, desipramine, amitriptyline).[30] Although not true dyspigmentation, as noted above topiramate is linked to blue pseudochromhidrosis.[11]

XENOBIOTIC-INDUCED CUTANEOUS REACTIONS (DRUG REACTIONS)

The skin is one of the most common targets for adverse drug reactions.[3] Drug eruptions occur in approximately 2% to 5% of inpatients and in greater than 1% of outpatients. Several cutaneous reaction patterns account for the majority of clinical presentations of xenobiotic-induced dermatotoxicity (Table 17–2). The following drug reactions will be discussed in detail: urticaria, erythema multiforme, Steven-Johnson syndrome and toxic epidermal necrolysis, fixed eruptions, and drug-induced hypersensitivity syndrome (formerly called "DRESS" syndrome).

Urticarial Drug Reactions

Urticarial drug reactions are characterized by transient, pruritic, edematous, pink papules, or wheals that arise in the dermis, which blanch on palpation and are frequently associated with central clearing. At times, the urticarial lesions are targetoid and mimic erythema multiforme. Approximately 40% of patients with urticaria experience angioedema and anaphylactoid reactions as well.[2] The reaction pattern is representative of a type I, or IgE-dependent, immune reaction and commonly occurs as part of clinical anaphylaxis or anaphylactoid (non–IgE-mediated) reactions. Widespread urticaria occurs following systemic absorption of an allergen or following a minimal localized exposure in patients highly sensitized to the allergen. Regardless of whether the eruption is localized or widespread, it occurs as a result of immunologic recognition of a putative antigen by IgE antibodies, thus triggering the immediate degranulation of mast cells, which are distributed along the dermal blood vessels and nerves. The release of histamine, complements C3a and C5a, and other vasoactive mediators results in extravasation of fluid from dermal capillaries as their endothelial cells contract. This produces the characteristic urticarial lesions described above. Activation of the nearby sensory neurons produces pruritus.

TABLE 17–2	Xenobiotics Commonly Associated with Various Cutaneous Reaction Patterns			
Acneiform	Cimetidine	Oral contraceptives	Hydrochlorothiazide	Minocycline
ACTH	Codeine	D-Penicillamine	Hematoporphyrin (Porphyria)	NSAIDs
Amoxapine	Gold	Salicylates	Levofloxacin	Oral contraceptives
Androgens	Ethinyl estradiol	**Hair Loss**	NSAIDS	Penicillamine
Azathioprine	Furosemide	**Telogen Effluvium**	Oxybenzone	Penicillin
Bromides	Ketoconazole	β-Adrenergic antagonists	Piroxicam	Phenytoin
Corticosteroids	NSAIDs	(eg, timolol, propranolol)	Psoralen	Propylthiouracil
Dantrolene	Nitrogen mustard	Albendazole	Sulfanilamide	Quinolones
Halogenated hydrocarbons	Phenolphthalein	Anticoagulants (heparin, warfarin)	Tetracyclines	Serum (antithymocyte globulin)
Iodides	Phenothiazines	Antiepileptics (phenytoin, valproic	Tolbutamide	Sulfonamides
Isoniazid	Thiazides	acid, carbamazepine)	**Phototoxic Dermatitis**	**Vesiculobullous**
Lithium	**Erythroderma**	Antithyroid (propylthiouracil,	Celery	Amoxapine
Oral contraceptives	Allopurinol	methimazole)	Dispense blue 35	Barbiturates
Phenytoin	Antimicrobials (aminopenicillins,	Heavy metals	Eosin	Captopril
Allergic Contact Dermatitis	sulfonamides, vancomycin)	Interferon-α	Fig	Carbon monoxide
Bacitracin	Antiepileptics	Oral contraceptives	Fragrance materials	Chemotherapeutics
Balsam of Peru	Antimuscarinics	(discontinuation)	Lime	Dipyridamole
Benzocaine	Boric acid	Vitamin A excess	Parsnip	Furosemide
Carba mix	Calcium channel blockers	**Anagen Effluvium**	Tar	Griseofulvin
Catechol	Cimetidine	Alkylating agents: cyclophosphamide,	**Toxic Epidermal Necrolysis**	Penicillamine
Cobalt	Dapsone	ifosfamide, mechlorethamine	Allopurinol	Penicillin
Diazolidinyl urea	Gold	Anthracyclines: daunorubicin,	L-Asparaginase	Rifampin
Ethylenediamine dihydrochloride	Lithium	doxorubicin, idarubicin	Amoxapine	Sulfonamides
Formaldehyde	Niacin	Arsenic	Mithramycin	**Xanthoderma**
Fragrance mix	Quinidine	Bismuth	Nitrofurantoin	**Generalized**
Imidazolidinyl urea	Scombroid	Chemotherapeutics (taxanes:	NSAIDs	Carotenoderma
Lanolin	**Fixed Drug Eruptions**	paclitaxel, docetaxel,	Penicillin	Canthaxanthin (tanning pills)
Methylchloroisothiazolinone or	Acetaminophen	topoisomerase-1 inhibitors:	Phenytoin	Dipyridamole (yellow compound)
methylisothiazolinone	Allopurinol	topotecan, irinotecan, etoposide,	Prazosin	Hepatic jaundice (acetaminophen,
Neomycin sulfate	Barbiturates	vincristine, vinblastine, busulfan,	Pyrimethamine-sulfadoxine	isoniazid)
Nickel	Captopril	actinomycin D, gemcitabine)	Streptomycin	Hemolytic jaundice
p-tert-Butylphenol formaldehyde	Carbamazepine	Gold	Sulfonamides	Quinacrine
resin	Chloral hydrate	Thallium	Sulfasalazine	**Localized**
p-Phenylenediamine	Chlordiazepoxide	**Maculopapular or**	Trimethoprim–sulfamethoxazole	Dihydroxyacetone (spray tanning)
Quaternium-15	Chlorpromazine	**Exanthematous Drug Eruptions**	**Vasculitis**	Picric acid
Rosin (colophony)	Erythromycin	Antimicrobials (cephalosporins,	Allopurinol	Methylenedianiline
Sesquiterpene lactones	Fiorinal	sulfonamides and aminopenicillins)	Bortezomib	Phenol, topical
Thimerosal	Gold	Antiepileptics	Cephalosporins (commonly	**Nail Changes: Beau Lines and**
Urushiol	Griseofulvin	**Photosensitivity Reactions**	cefaclor)	**Mees Lines (Leukonychia)**
Erythema Multiforme	Lithium	Amiodarone	Cimetidine	Arsenic
Allopurinol	Phenolphthalein	Benoxaprofen	G-CSF	Cyclophosphamide
Antiepileptics (phenytoin,	Metronidazole	Chlorpromazine	Gold	Doxorubicin
carbamazepine)	Minocycline	Ciprofloxacin	Hydralazine	Hydroxyurea
Antimicrobial (sulfonamides,	Naproxen	Dacarbazine	Levamisole	Paclitaxel
aminopenicillins)	NSAIDs	5-Fluorouracil	Methotrexate	Thallium
Barbiturates		Furosemide		
		Griseofulvin		

ACTH = adrenocorticotrophic hormone; G-CSF = granulocyte colony–stimulating factor; NSAIDs = nonsteroidal antiinflammatory drugs.

Nonimmunologically mediated mast cell degranulation producing an identical urticarial syndrome also occurs following exposure to any xenobiotic.[14]

Erythema Multiforme

Historically, it was believed that erythema multiforme existed on a spectrum with Stevens-Johnson syndrome (SJS) and toxic epidermal necrolysis (TEN) given overlapping clinical features and morphology. However, these entities were reclassified on the basis that most cases of erythema multiforme are believed to be triggered by viral infection (herpes simplex virus most

commonly) and most cases of SJS/TEN are triggered by xenobiotics.[51] Erythema multiforme is an acute self-limited disease characterized by target-shaped, erythematous macules and patches on the palms and soles, as well as the trunk and extremities (Fig. 17–5). The Nikolsky sign, defined as sloughing of the epidermis when direct pressure is exerted on the skin, is absent. Mucosal involvement is absent or mild in erythema multiforme minor and severe in erythema multiforme major. While less common than viral-induced erythema multiforme, xenobiotics such as sulfonamides, phenytoin, antihistamines, many antibiotics, rosewood, and urushiol also elicit erythema multiforme.

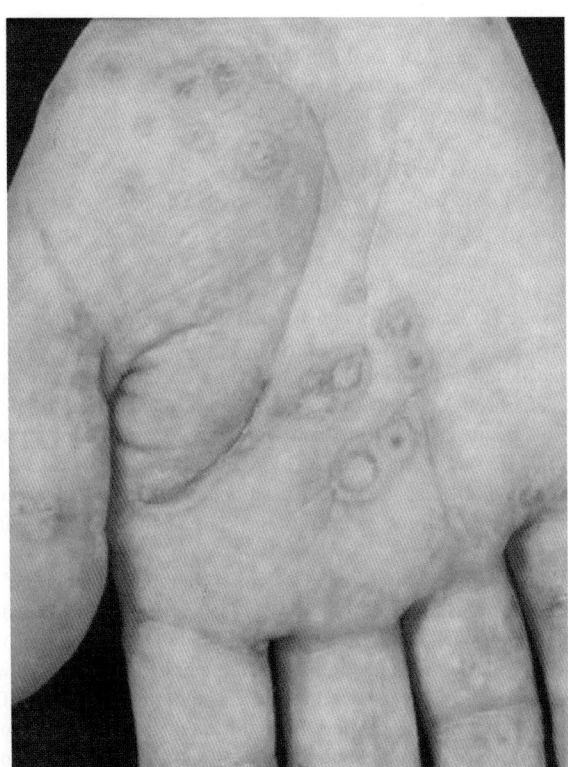

FIGURE 17–5. Erythema multiforme. Typical targetoid macules on the palm. *(Reproduced with permission from Wolff K, Goldsmith LA, Katz SI, et al. Fitzpatrick's Dermatology in General Medicine, 7th ed. New York, NY: McGraw-Hill; 2008.)*

Differentiating erythema multiforme from SJS/TEN, which can also present with targetoid lesions, can be difficult, especially in the case of bullous erythema multiforme. A skin biopsy revealing partial or full-thickness epidermal necrosis would favor a diagnosis of SJS/TEN rather than erythema multiforme.

Stevens-Johnson Syndrome and Toxic Epidermal Necrolysis

Toxic epidermal necrolysis (TEN) and Stevens-Johnson syndrome (SJS) (Fig. 17–6) are considered to be related disorders that belong to a spectrum of increasingly severe skin eruptions.[45] Stevens-Johnson syndrome is defined by lesser than 10% body surface area epidermal detachment, SJS-TEN overlap 10% to 30% involvement, and TEN greater than 30% epidermal sloughing. Although on a spectrum, SJS has a mortality rate of 5%, which is far lower than the approximate 25% to 50% mortality rate for patients with TEN.[49,52] However, a more recent series of 40 patients with TEN cared for at academic burn units revealed a 10% mortality rate.[35] Toxic epidermal necrolysis is a rare, life-threatening dermatologic emergency whose incidence is estimated at 0.4 to 1.2 cases per 1 million persons. More than 220 xenobiotics are causally implicated in 80% to 95% of the TEN cases. The largest study examining medication triggers of TEN divided these medications into long-term (used for months to years) and short-term. Short-term xenobiotics most commonly implicated in the development of TEN included trimethoprim-sulfamethoxazole and other sulfonamide antibiotics, followed by cephalosporins, quinolones, and aminopenicillins.[53] With chronic medication use, the increased risk largely occurred during the first 2 months of treatment and was greatest for carbamazepine, phenobarbital, phenytoin, valproic acid, the oxicam NSAIDs, allopurinol, and corticosteroids.

Classically, the eruption of TEN is painful and occurs within 1 to 3 weeks after the exposure to the implicated xenobiotic(s). The eruption is preceded by malaise, headache, abrupt onset of fever, myalgia, arthralgia, nausea, vomiting, diarrhea, chest pain, or cough. One to 3 days later, signs begin in the mucous membranes including the eyes, mouth, nose, and genitals in 90% of cases.[49] A macular erythema then develops that subsequently becomes raised and morbilliform on the face, neck, and central trunk and finally the extremities. Individual lesions can appear targetoid because of their dusky centers and progress to bullae in the following 3 to 5 days involving the entire thickness of the epidermis. This necrosis and sloughing can also lead to loss of the fingernails. A Nikolsky sign, or sloughing of the epidermis with gentle manual pressure, is suggestive of TEN but not pathognomonic. A Nikolsky sign occurs in a variety of other dermatoses, including pemphigus vulgaris. If the diagnosis is suspected, a punch biopsy should be performed for immediate frozen section and the suspected triggering xenobiotic discontinued immediately. The histopathology typically shows partial- or full-thickness epidermal necrosis, with subepidermal bullae with a sparse infiltrate, and vacuolization with numerous dyskeratotic keratinocytes along the dermoepidermal junction adjacent to the necrotic epidermis.

The incidence of TEN is higher in patients with advanced HIV disease.[45,62] There is general agreement that the keratinocyte cell death in TEN is the result of apoptosis, which is suggested based on electronic microscopic studies with DNA fragmentation analysis.[45] Cytotoxic T lymphocytes are the main effector cells and experimental evidence points to involvement of the Fas-ligand (FasL) and perforin/granzyme pathways.

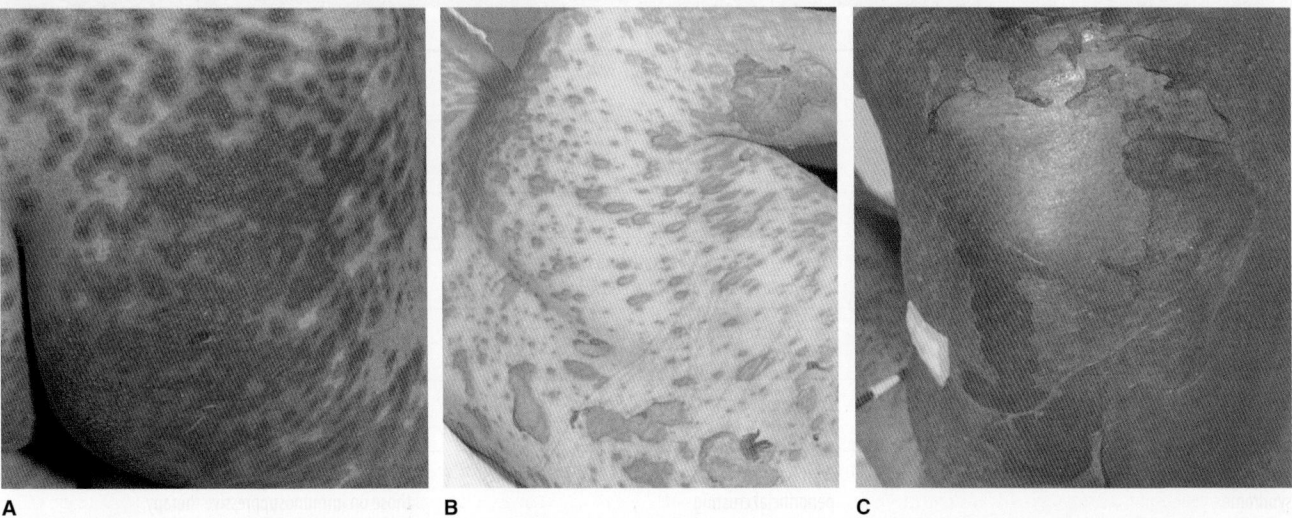

A   B   C

FIGURE 17–6. Toxic epidermal necrolysis. (**A**) Early eruption. Erythematous dusky red macules (flat atypical target lesions) that progressively coalesce and show epidermal detachment. (**B**) Advanced eruption. Blisters and epidermal detachment have led to large confluent erosions. (**C**) Full-blown epidermal necrolysis characterized by large erosive areas reminiscent of scalding. *(Reproduced with permission from Wolff K, Goldsmith LA, Katz SI, et al. Fitzpatrick's Dermatology in General Medicine, 7th ed. New York, NY: McGraw-Hill, 2008.)*

There are several theories as to the pathogenesis of SJS/TEN. These include that a xenobiotic could induce upregulation of Fas Ligand leading to a death receptor–mediated apoptotic pathway. A xenobiotic might interact with MHC class I–expressing cells and cause drug-specific CD8+ cytotoxic T lymphocytes to accumulate within epidermal blisters, releasing perforin and granzyme B that kills keratinocytes. Finally it has been proposed that the xenobiotic triggers the activation of CD8+ T lymphocytes, NK cells and NKT cells to secrete granulysin, with keratinocyte death not requiring cell contact.[44] Serum Fas ligand concentrations are elevated up to 4 days prior to mucosal involvement in patients with SJS/TEN and have the potential to be useful clinically as an early predictor of these severe dermatologic diseases.[43] Serum granulysin, a proinflammatory cytolytic enzyme released by CD8+ T lymphocytes found in the blisters of TEN was demonstrated to be a potential early predictive marker of SJS/TEN.[20] A rapid immunochromatographic test that detects elevated serum granulysin (>10 ng/mL) in 15 minutes demonstrates promise in a small study in which its sensitivity was noted to be 80% and specificity 95.8% for differentiating SJS/TEN from ordinary exanthematous drug eruptions.[20] However, this test is not yet commercially available.

Because immediate removal of the inciting xenobiotic is critical to survival, patients with TEN related to a xenobiotic with a long half-life have a poorer prognosis, and these patients should be transferred to a burn or other specialized center for sterile wound care. Risk factors for mortality include older patient age, higher total surface area of involvement, and more pre-existing comorbidities.[35] In a recent study, only serum bicarbonate less than 20 mmol/L was found to portend hospital mortality in patients with TEN.[68] Porcine xenografts or human skin allografts including amniotic membrane transplantation are used and are widely accepted therapy.[48] A meta-analysis of 17 studies revealed a trend toward improved mortality with high-dose IVIG in adults and good prognosis in children; however, there is insufficient evidence to support a clinical benefit.[27] Patients with TEN develop metabolic abnormalities, sepsis, multiorgan failure, pulmonary emboli, and gastrointestinal hemorrhages and should be closely monitored. The major microbes leading to sepsis are *Staphylococcus aureus* and *Pseudomonas aeruginosa*. In a patient with SJS/TEN with ophthalmic involvement, early ophthalmologic consultation is necessary because blindness is a potential complication.

Mimickers of TEN include SJS, staphylococcal scalded skin syndrome, severe exanthematous drug eruptions, erythema multiforme-major, linear IgA dermatosis, paraneoplastic pemphigus, acute graft versus host disease, drug-induced pemphigoid and pemphigus vulgaris, and acute generalized exanthematous pustulosis. Discussion of some of these entities is beyond the scope of this chapter (Table 17–3).

Bullous Reactions (Blistering Reactions)

In addition to SJS and TEN, other bullous cutaneous reactions include drug-induced pseudoporphyria, fixed drug eruption, acute generalized exanthematous pustulosis, phototoxic drug eruptions, and drug-induced autoimmune blistering diseases. Xenobiotic-related cutaneous blistering reactions are clinically indistinguishable from autoimmune blistering diseases such as pemphigus vulgaris or bullous pemphigoid (Fig. 17–7). Certain topically applied xenobiotics such as the vesicant cantharidin derived from "blister beetles" in the Coleoptera order and Meloidae family are used in the treatment of molluscum and viral warts. In high concentrations, xenobiotics lead to necrosis of both skin and mucous membranes. Other systemic xenobiotics cause a similar reaction pattern mediated by the production of antibody directed against the cells at the dermal–epidermal junction (Table 17–3).

A number of medications, many of which contain a "thiol group" such as penicillamine and captopril, induce either pemphigus resembling pemphigus foliaceus, a superficial blistering disorder in which the blister is at the level of the stratum granulosum, or pemphigus vulgaris, in which blistering occurs above the basal layer of the epidermis (Fig. 17–1). Other xenobiotics, such as furosemide, penicillin, and sulfasalazine produce tense bullae that resemble bullous pemphigoid. Direct immunofluorescence studies demonstrate epidermal intracellular immunoglobulin deposits at the dermal–epidermal junction. The offending xenobiotic should be discontinued and the patient should be referred to a dermatologist to determine treatment. The reaction may persist for up to 6 months after the offending xenobiotic is withdrawn.

Fixed Drug Eruptions

Fixed drug eruption is another bullous drug eruption and is characterized by well-circumscribed erythematous to dusky violaceous patches which with central bullae or erosions and develops 1 to 2 weeks after first exposure to the drug. This reaction pattern is so named because re-exposures to the xenobiotic cause lesions in the same area, typically within 24 hours of exposure (Fig. 17–8). Typical locations include acral extremities, genitals,

TABLE 17–3	Differential Diagnosis of Xenobiotic-Induced Blistering (Vesiculobullous) Disorders				
Disease	**Fever**	**Mucositis**	**Morphology**	**Onset**	**Miscellaneous**
Acute graft-versus-host disease	Yes	Present	Morbilliform rash, bullae and erosions	Acute	Closely resembles toxic epidermal necrolysis
Acute generalized exanthematous pustulosis	Yes	Rare	Superficial pustules	Acute	Self-limiting on discontinuation of drug
Linear IgA bullous dermatosis	No	Rare	Tense, subepidermal bullae	Acute	Vancomycin is most commonly implicated
Pemphigus	No	Usually absent	Erosions, crusts, patchy erythema (resembles pemphigus foliaceous)	Gradual	Commonly caused by penicillamine and other "thiol" drugs; often resolves after the inciting xenobiotic is discontinued
Pemphigoid	No	Rare	Tense bullae (sometimes hemorrhagic)	Acute	Diuretics a common cause, especially furosemide, spironolactone; often pruritic
Paraneoplastic pemphigus	No	Present (usually severe)	Polymorphous skin lesions, flaccid bullae	Gradual	Resistant to treatment; associated with malignancy, especially lymphoma
Staphylococcal scalded skin syndrome	Yes	Absent	Erythema, skin tenderness, periorificial crusting	Acute	Affects children younger than 5 years, adults on dialysis, and those on immunosuppressive therapy
Xenobiotic-triggered Pemphigus	No	Present	Mucosal erosions, flaccid bullae	Gradual	Caused by "nonthiol" xenobiotics which are more likely to persist after discontinuation of xenobiotic; may require long-term immunosuppressive therapy

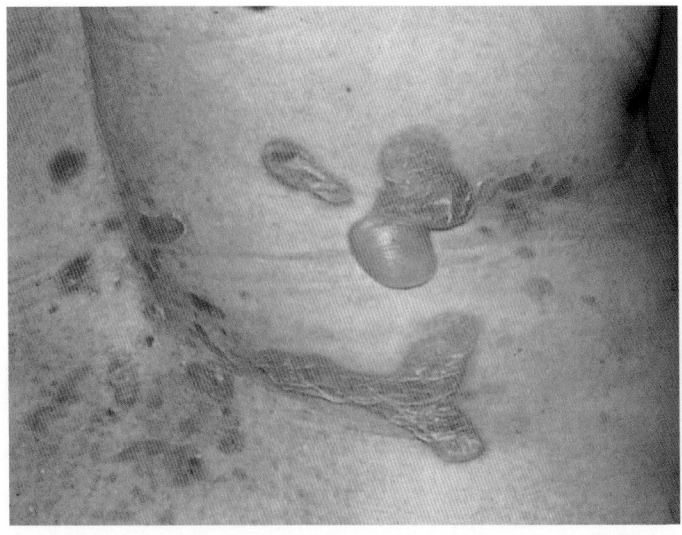

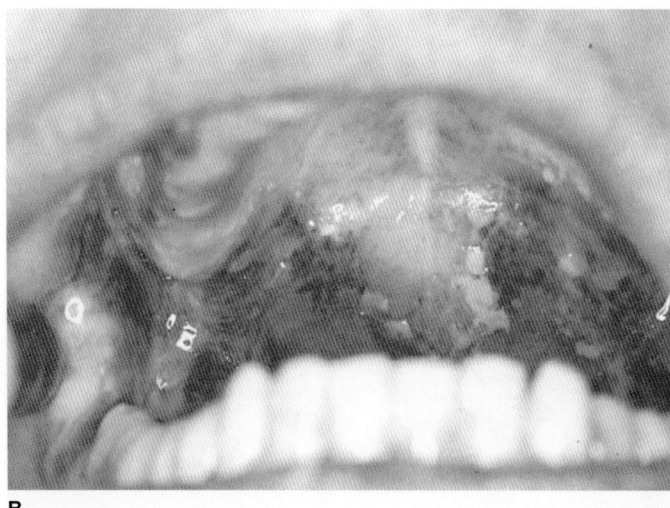

A   **B**

FIGURE 17–7. Pemphigus vulgaris. (**A**) Flaccid blisters. (**B**) Oral erosions. *(Part **A**, Used with permission from Lawrence Lieblich, MD. Part **B**, Reproduced with permission from Wolff K, Goldsmith LA, Katz SI, et al. Fitzpatrick's Dermatology in General Medicine, 7th ed. New York, NY: McGraw-Hill; 2008.)*

and intertriginous sites, and this process is confused with TEN if widely confluent as in a "generalized fixed drug eruption." This reaction pattern is generally not life threatening and heals with residual postinflammatory hyperpigmentation. Bullous fixed-drug reactions result from exposure to diverse xenobiotics such as angiotensin-converting enzyme inhibitors and a multitude of antibiotics. As mentioned above, EM can have a bullous variant that can also be confused with SJS/TEN.

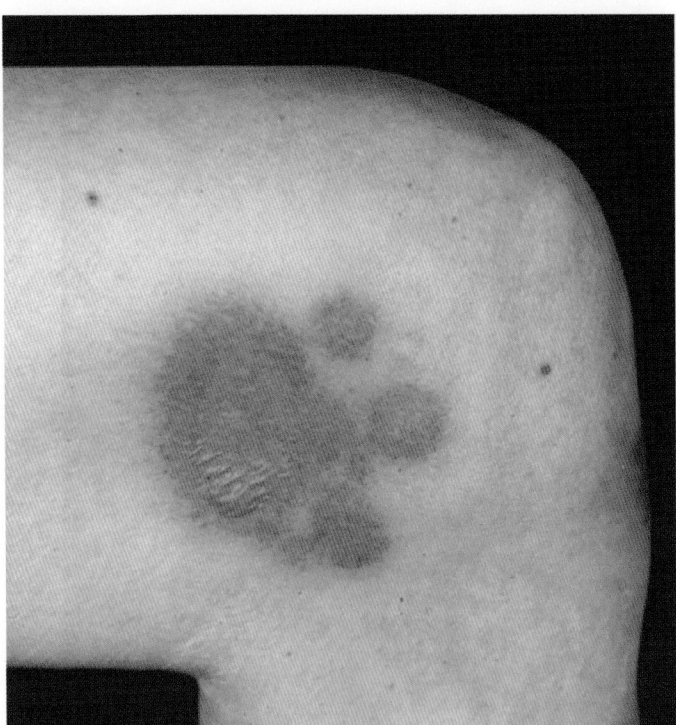

FIGURE 17–8. Fixed drug eruption due to tetracycline. A well-defined plaque on the knee, merging with 3 satellite lesions. The large plaque exhibits epidermal wrinkling, a sign of incipient blister formation. This was the second such episode after ingestion of a tetracycline. No other lesions were present. *(Reproduced with permission from Wolff K, Goldsmith LA, Katz SI, et al. Fitzpatrick's Dermatology in General Medicine, 7th ed. New York, NY: McGraw-Hill; 2008.)*

Coma Bullae

"Coma bullae" are tense bullae on normal-appearing skin that occur within 48 to 72 hours in comatose patients with sedative–hypnotic overdoses, particularly phenobarbital, or carbon monoxide, poisoning. They also occur in patients in coma from infectious, neurologic, or metabolic causes. Although these blisters are thought to result predominantly from pressure-induced epidermal necrosis, they occasionally occur in non–pressure-dependent areas, suggesting a systemic mechanism. Histologically, an intraepidermal or subepidermal blister is observed. There is accompanying eccrine duct and gland necrosis.

Drug-Induced Hypersensitivity Syndrome

The skin is linked with systemic immunologic diseases such that an alteration in the metabolism of certain xenobiotics leads to a hypersensitivity syndrome. The drug-induced hypersensitivity syndrome, formerly called Drug Reaction with Eosinophilia and Systemic Symptoms (DRESS), can be severe and potentially life threatening. The hypersensitivity syndrome is characterized by the triad of fever, skin eruption, and internal organ involvement.[32] The frequency is estimated between 1 in 1,000 to 1 in 10,000 with antiepileptic or sulfonamide antibiotic exposures and usually presents within 2 to 6 weeks of the initial exposure. For antiepileptics, the inability to detoxify arene oxide metabolites is suggested to be a key factor; once a patient has a documented drug-induced hypersensitivity syndrome to one antiepileptic, it is important to note that cross-reactivity between phenytoin, carbamazepine, and phenobarbital is well documented, both in vivo and in vitro.[47] In the case of sulfonamides, acetylator phenotype and lymphocytes' susceptibility to the metabolite hydroxylamine are risk factors for developing drug hypersensitivity syndrome. Further support for the role of genetic predisposition comes from data in Northern European populations in which the presence of the HLA-A*3101 allele significantly increases the risk of developing carbamazepine-induced hypersensitivity syndrome.[34] Fever and a cutaneous eruption are the most common symptoms. Accompanying malaise, pharyngitis, and cervical lymphadenopathy are frequently present. Atypical lymphocytes and eosinophilia occur initially. The exanthem is initially generalized and morbilliform, and conjunctivitis and angioedema occur (Fig. 17–9). Later the eruption becomes edematous, and facial edema, which is often present, is a hallmark of this syndrome. One-half of patients with drug induced hypersensitivity syndrome will have hepatitis, interstitial nephritis, vasculitis, CNS manifestations (including encephalitis, aseptic meningitis), interstitial pneumonitis, acute respiratory distress

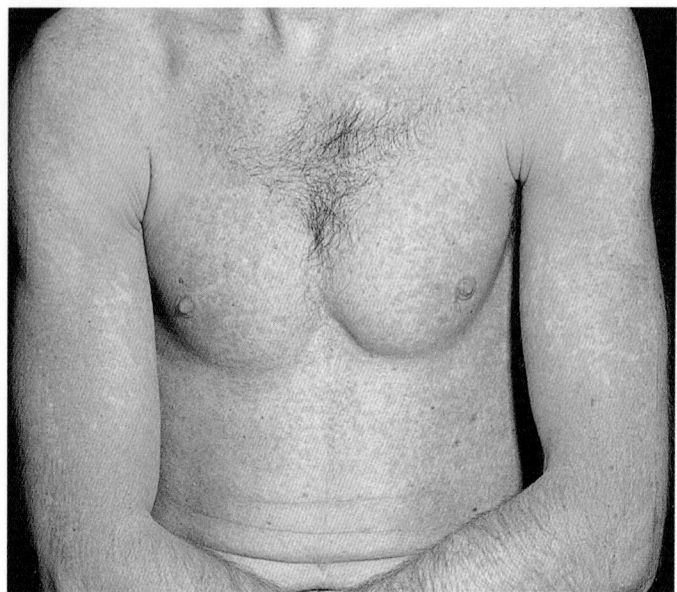

FIGURE 17–9. A patient with a hypersensitivity syndrome associated with phenytoin. He has a symmetric, bright red, and exanthematous eruption, confluent in some sites. The patient had associated lymphadenopathy. *(Reproduced with permission from Wolff K, Johnson RA. Fitzpatrick's Color Atlas and Synopsis of Clinical Dermatology, 6th ed. New York, NY: McGraw-Hill; 2009.)*

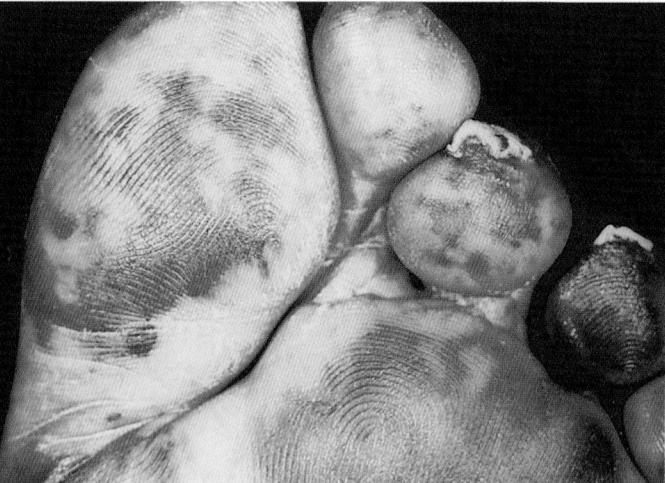

FIGURE 17–10. Leukocytoclastic vasculitis in a patient with mixed cryoglobulinemia manifested as palpable purpura and acrocyanosis. Patient with tuberculosis, positive antinuclear antibody, and hepatitis. *(Reproduced with permission from Wolff K, Goldsmith LA, Katz SI, et al. Fitzpatrick's Dermatology in General Medicine, 7th ed. New York, NY: McGraw-Hill; 2008.)*

syndrome, and autoimmune hypothyroidism. Hepatic involvement can be fulminant and is the most common cause of deaths associated with this syndrome. Colitis with bloody diarrhea and abdominal pain are associated. In addition to the aromatic antiepileptics (phenobarbital, carbamazepine, and phenytoin), lamotrigine, allopurinol, sulfonamide antibiotics, dapsone and the protease inhibitor abacavir are implicated. Early withdrawal of the offending xenobiotic is crucial and treatment is generally supportive.[42,67] If cardiac or pulmonary involvement is present, systemic corticosteroids should be initiated. However, their benefit on outcome has not been demonstrated, and relapse may occur during tapering, necessitating long-term (several month) courses of therapy. The authors recommend that patients with drug-induced hypersensitivity syndrome be managed in conjunction with a dermatologist and that adequate follow-up is ensured.

Erythroderma

Erythroderma, also known as exfoliative dermatitis, is defined as a generalized redness and scaling of the skin. However, it does not represent one disease entity, but rather it is a severe clinical presentation of a variety of skin diseases including psoriasis, atopic dermatitis, drug reactions, or cutaneous T-cell lymphoma (CTCL). At times, the underlying etiology of erythroderma is never discovered and this is termed "idiopathic erythroderma." The importance of this presentation is its association with systemic complications such as hypothermia, peripheral edema, and loss of fluid, electrolytes and albumin with subsequent tachycardia and cardiac failure. Many xenobiotics produce erythroderma (Table 17–2). Boric acid, when ingested, can cause systemic toxicity in addition to a bright red eruption ("lobster skin"), followed usually within 1 to 3 days by a generalized exfoliation.[55]

Vasculitis

Xenobiotic-induced vasculitis (Fig. 17–10) comprises 10% to 15% of secondary cutaneous vasculitis. It generally occurs from 7 to 21 days after initial exposure to the xenobiotic or 3 days after rechallenge and is considered to be a secondary cause of cutaneous small vessel vasculitis (typically involving dermal postcapillary venules). Many xenobiotics are implicated as triggers of cutaneous vasculitis (Table 17–2).[60] Cutaneous vasculitis is characterized by purpuric, nonblanching macules that usually become raised and palpable. The purpura tends to occur predominantly on gravity-dependent areas, including the lower extremities, particularly the feet, ankles, and buttocks (Fig. 17–11). Sometimes the reaction pattern has edematous purpuric wheals (urticarial vasculitis), hemorrhagic bullae, or ulcerations. Histologic examination of affected skin shows a leukocytoclastic vasculitis, which is characterized by fibrin deposition in the vessel walls. There is a perivascular infiltrate with intact and fragmented neutrophils that appear as black dots, known as "nuclear dust" and extravasated red blood cells. Vasculitis can be limited to the skin, or can involve other organ systems, particularly the kidneys, joints, liver, lungs, and brain.

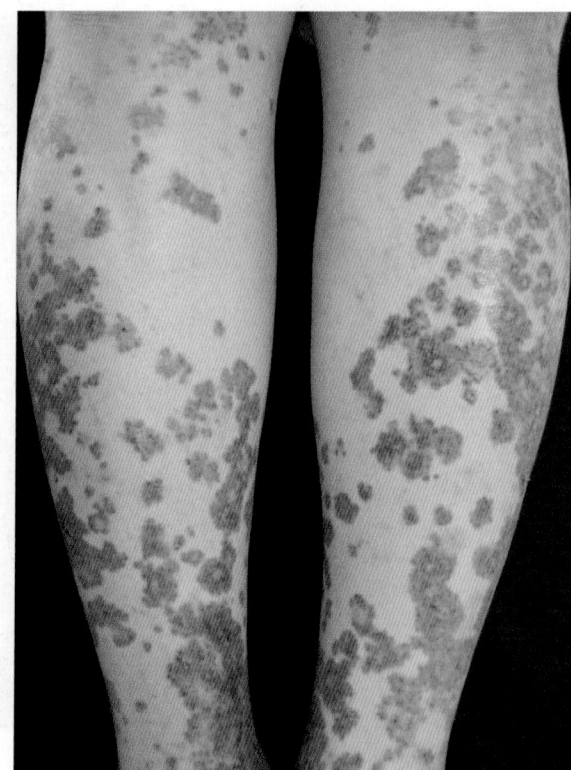

FIGURE 17–11. Purpura. Nonblanching red erythematous papules and plaques (palpable purpura) on the legs, representing leukocytoclastic vasculitis. *(Reproduced with permission from Wolff K, Goldsmith LA, Katz SI, et al. Fitzpatrick's Dermatology in General Medicine, 7th ed. New York, NY: McGraw-Hill; 2008.)*

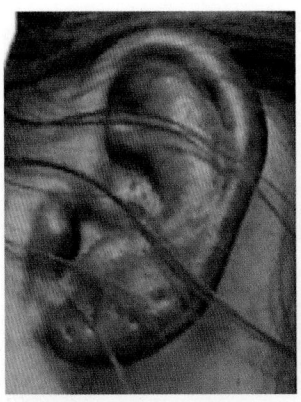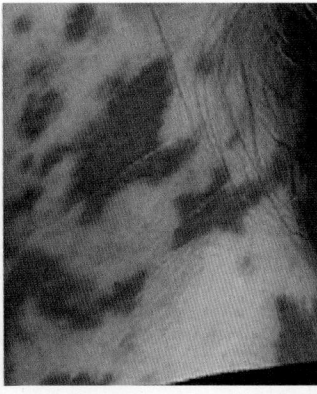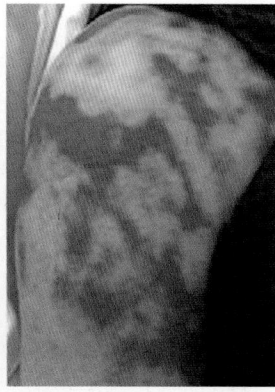

FIGURE 17–12. Levamisole-induced purpura: violaceous patches on the ear, neck, and thigh of 46-year-old woman exposed to levamisole-adulterated cocaine. *(Reproduced with permission from Chung C, Tumeh PC, Birnbaum R, et al. Characteristic purpura of the ears, vasculitis, and neutropenia—a potential public health epidemic associated with levamisole-adulterated cocaine. J Am Acad Dermatol. 2011 Oct;65(4):722-725.)*

The purpura results from the deposition of circulating immune complexes, which form as a result of hypersensitivity to a xenobiotic. Treatment consists of withdrawing the putative xenobiotic and initiating systemic corticosteroid therapy if systemic involvement is present. A syndrome of vasculitis, neutropenia, and retiform purpura occurs as a result of levamisole-adulterated cocaine (Fig. 17–12).[13] The earlobe is a common site of purpuric lesions from levamisole, and it was estimated that up to 70% of the cocaine sold in some areas during an epidemic in the United States contained levamisole.[6,63,64]

Purpura

Purpura is the multifocal extravasation of blood into the skin or mucous membranes (Fig. 17–12). Ecchymoses, therefore, are considered to be purpuric lesions. Chemotherapeutics that either diffusely suppress the bone marrow or specifically depress platelet counts below 30,000/mm³, predispose to purpuric macules. Xenobiotics that interfere with platelet aggregation, such as aspirin, clopidogrel, ticlopidine, valproic acid, and thrombolytics, cause purpura. Anticoagulants, such as heparin and warfarin, may also result in purpura (Chaps. 20 and 58).

Anticoagulant-Induced Skin Necrosis

Skin necrosis from warfarin, low-molecular-weight heparin, or unfractionated heparin usually begins 3 to 5 days after the initiation of treatment, which corresponds with the expected early decline of protein C function with warfarin (Fig. 17–13). The estimated risk is one in 10,000 persons. It is 4 times higher in women, especially if obese, with peaks in sixth to seventh decades of life. The necrosis is secondary to thrombus formation in vessels of the dermis and subcutaneous fat. Heparin-induced cutaneous necrosis results from antibodies that bind to complexes of heparin and platelet factor 4 and induce platelet aggregation and consumption. This causes bullae, ecchymosis, ulcers, and massive subcutaneous necrosis, usually in areas of abundant subcutaneous fat, such as the breasts, buttocks, abdomen, thighs, and calves. Heparin-induced necrosis is associated with protein C or S deficiency, anticardiolipin antibody syndrome, as well as factor V Leiden mutations.[46]

Contact Dermatitis

When a xenobiotic comes in contact with the skin, it can result in either an allergic contact dermatitis (20% of cases) or more commonly an irritant contact dermatitis (80% of cases). Contact dermatitis is characterized by inflammation of the skin with spongiosis (intercellular edema) of the epidermis that results from the interaction of a xenobiotic with the skin. Well-demarcated erythematous vesicular or scaly patches or plaques, and at times bullae, are noted on areas in direct contact with the xenobiotic, whereas the remaining areas are spared.

Allergic contact dermatitis fits into the classic delayed hypersensitivity, or type IV, immunologic reaction. The development of this reaction requires prior sensitization to an allergen, which, in most cases, acts as a hapten by binding with an endogenous molecule that is then presented to an appropriate immunologic T cell. Upon reexposure, the hapten diffuses to the Langerhans cell, is chemically altered, bound to an HLA-DR, and the complex is expressed on the Langerhans cell surface. This complex interacts with primed T cells either in the skin or lymph nodes, causing the Langerhans cells to make interleukin-1 and the activated T cells to make interleukin-2 and interferon. This subsequently activates the keratinocytes to produce cytokines and eicosanoids that activate mast cells and macrophages, leading to an inflammatory response (Fig. 17–14).[31]

Many allergens are associated with contact dermatitis (Table 17–2). Among the most common plant-derived sensitizers are urushiol (*Toxicodendron* species), sesquiterpene lactone (ragweed), and tuliposide A (tulip bulbs). Metals, particularly nickel, are commonly implicated in contact dermatitis and should be considered in patients with erythematous, vesicular, or scaly patches or plaques around the umbilicus from nickel buttons on pants, and on the ear lobes from earrings. Several industrial chemicals, such as the thiurams (rubber) and urea formaldehyde resins (plastics), account for the majority of occupational contact dermatitis. Medications, particularly topical

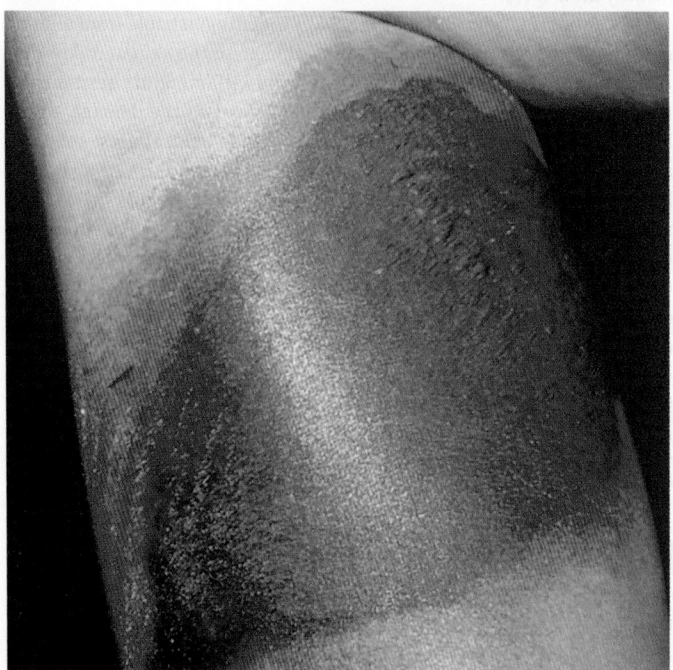

FIGURE 17–13. Skin necrosis in a patient after 4 days of warfarin therapy. *(Reproduced with permission from Wolff K, Goldsmith LA, Katz SI, et al. Fitzpatrick's Dermatology in General Medicine, 7th ed. New York, NY: McGraw-Hill; 2008.)*

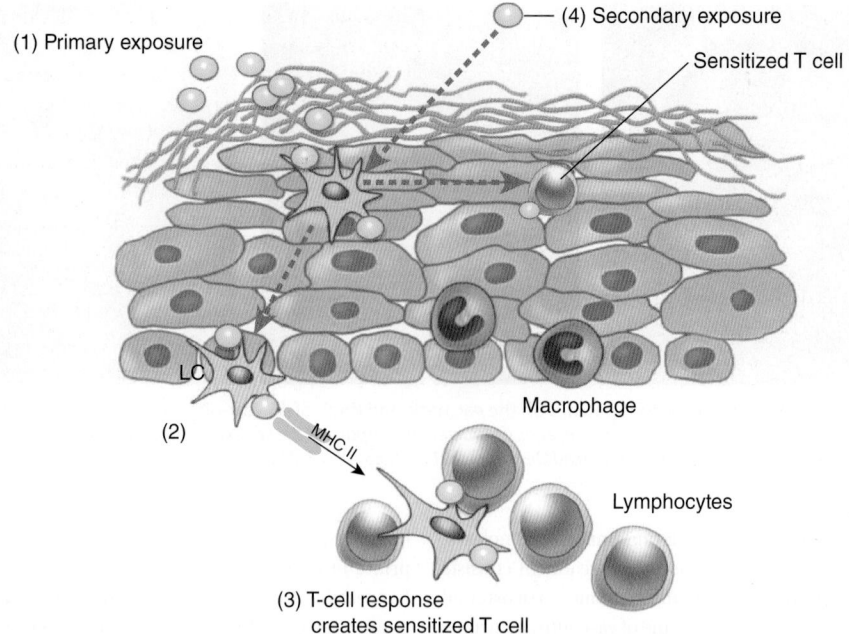

FIGURE 17–14. Contact dermatitis. **(1)** Causative xenobiotic, typically a hapten of <500 Da, diffuses through stratum corneum and binds to receptor on Langerhans cell (LC). **(2)** The antigen is processed with major histocompatibility complex II (MHC II) receptor site, presented to T-helper lymphocytes, and carried through the lymphatics to regional lymph nodes. (3) There it undergoes the sensitization phase by producing memory, effector, and suppressor T-lymphocytes. (4) On reexposure to the same, or to a cross-reactive antigen, the LC presents the antigen to T-lymphocytes (▬ ▬ ▬►), which are now sensitized. This initiates an inflammatory process that appears as indurated, scaly patches.

medications such as neomycin, commonly cause contact dermatitis. Another important allergen is paraphenylenediamine, a black dye in permanent and semipermanent hair coloring, leather, fur, textiles, industrial rubber products, and black henna tattoos. According to the North American Contact Dermatitis Group, the frequency of sensitization has been found to be 5%.[69] The management of contact dermatitis varies based on the severity of the reaction, ranging from treatment with topical steroids to oral cyclosporine (Table 17–4). A thorough history in addition to patch testing (the gold standard) will often identify the culprit.

Irritant dermatitis, although clinically indistinguishable from allergic contact dermatitis, results from direct damage to the skin and does not require prior antigen sensitization. Still, the inflammatory response to the initial mild insult is the cause of the majority of the damage. Xenobiotics that cause an irritant dermatitis include acids, bases, solvents, and detergents, many of which, in their concentrated form or after prolonged exposure, can cause direct cellular injury. The specific site of damage varies with the chemical nature of the xenobiotic. Many xenobiotics affect the lipid membrane of the keratinocyte, whereas others diffuse through the membrane, injuring the lysosomes, mitochondria, or nuclear components. When the cell membrane is injured, phospholipases are activated and affect the release of arachidonic acid and the synthesis of eicosanoids. The second-messenger system is then activated, leading to the expression of genes and the synthesis of various cell surface molecules and cytokines. Interleukin-1 is secreted, which can activate T cells directly and indirectly by stimulation of granulocyte-macrophage

colony–stimulating factor production. The treatment is similar to allergic contact dermatitis (Table 17–4).

Photosensitivity Reactions

Photosensitivity is caused by topical or systemic xenobiotics. Nonionizing radiation, particularly to ultraviolet A (UVA) (320–400 nm) and less often to ultraviolet B (UVB) (280–320 nm), are the wavelengths that commonly cause photosensitivity. There are generally 2 types of xenobiotic-related photosensitivity: phototoxic and photoallergic.[41] Phototoxic reactions occur within 24 hours of the first exposure, usually within hours, and are dose-related. These reactions result from direct tissue injury caused by ultraviolet-induced activation of a phototoxic xenobiotic. The clinical findings include erythema, edema, and vesicles in a light-exposed distribution, and resemble a severe sunburn that lasts days to weeks, with patients complaining of burning and stinging (Fig. 17–15). A subtype of phototoxic reaction is phytophotodermatitis, in which linear streaks of erythema occur due to skin contact with furocoumarins from plants followed by exposure to sunlight (Table 17–2). Photoallergic reactions occur less commonly, occur following even small exposures, and resemble allergic contact dermatitis with lichenoid papules or an eczematous dermatitis on exposed areas and is often pruritic. These are type IV hypersensitivity reactions that develop in response to a xenobiotic that has been altered by absorption of nonionizing radiation, acting as a hapten and eliciting an immune response on first exposure. Only on recurrent exposure do the lesions develop. Studies indicate that benzophenone-3 (oxybenzone), often found in sunscreen, is the most common cause of photoallergic dermatitis.[8,16] Other common photoallergens include xenobiotics such as promethazine, NSAIDs, fragrances, and antibiotics. Photoallergic reactions can be diagnosed by the use of photopatch tests. Both phototoxic and photoallergic reactions are managed with symptomatic treatment, including topical or, if needed, systemic corticosteroids. Identification and avoidance of the triggering xenobiotic are crucial in addition to avoidance of sun exposure and wearing a broad-spectrum sunscreen (SPF 30 or above) that blocks both UVA and UVB preferably without para-aminobenzoic acid (PABA) and oxybenzone. Para-amino benzoic acid is a sensitizer for many patients and is rarely included in current sunscreen products.

TABLE 17–4	Overview of Treatment of Acute Contact Dermatitis
Identification of contactant and future avoidance (consider patch testing to identify culprit)	
Emollients for lichenified lesions	
Topical or oral corticosteroids to treat dermatitis (may take 6 weeks of treatment)	
Topical calcineurin inhibitors (tacrolimus or pimecrolimus)	
Cyclosporine (oral)	
Phototherapy: narrow-band UVB	

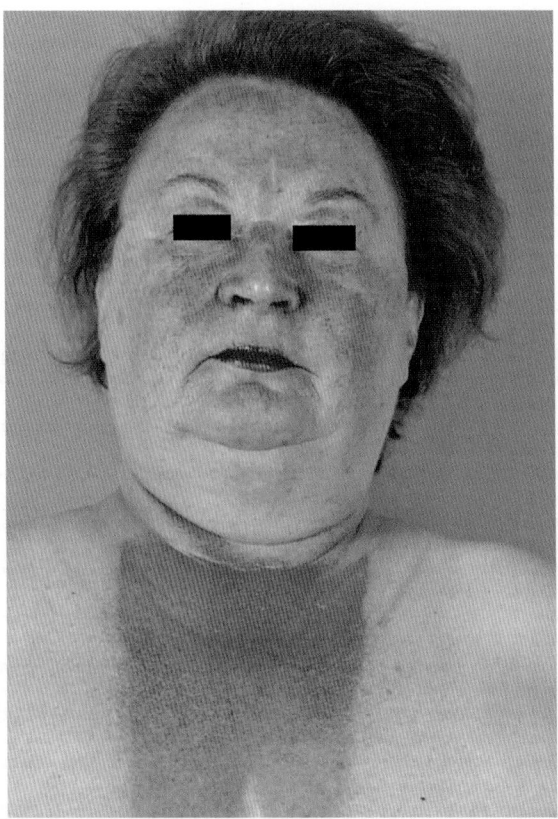

FIGURE 17–15. Phototoxicity associated with a cyclic antidepressant. Note erythema and edema on sun-exposed areas and sparing of sun-protected chest and shaded upper lip and neck. *(Reproduced with permission from Wolff K, Goldsmith LA, Katz SI, et al. Fitzpatrick's Dermatology in General Medicine, 7th ed. New York, NY: McGraw-Hill; 2008. Photo contributor: Dr. Adrian Tanew.)*

Scleroderma-Like Reactions

A number of environmental xenobiotics are associated with localized or diffuse scleroderma-like reactions. Scleroderma refers to a tightened indurated surface change of the skin that typically occurs on the face, hands, forearms, and trunk and is 3 times more common in women. This can be accompanied by facial telangiectasias and Raynaud syndrome. Raynaud syndrome consists of skin color changes of white, blue, and red accompanied by intense pain with exposure to cold, and can cause acral ulcerations, if untreated. The fibrotic process usually does not remit with removal of the external stimulus, and specific autoantibodies are absent. The association of scleroderma-like reactions with polyvinyl chloride manufacture is likely related to exposure to vinyl chloride monomers. Similar reports of this syndrome are associated with exposure to trichloroethylene and perchlorethylene, which are structurally similar to vinyl chloride. Epoxy resins, silica, and organic solvents are implicated as environmental causes. Bleomycin, carbidopa, pentazocine, and taxanes are also causative.

In Spain, patients exposed to imported rapeseed oil mixed with an aniline additive and colorant developed widespread cutaneous sclerosis. This became known as the "toxic oil syndrome." A similar syndrome following ingestion of contaminated L-tryptophan as a dietary supplement used as a sleeping aid resulted in the eosinophilia myalgia syndrome, which is characterized by myalgia, edema, arthralgias, alopecia, urticaria, mucinous yellow papules, and erythematous plaques.[56]

HAIR LOSS

Xenobiotics have the potential to cause distinctive patterns of hair loss (Table 17–2). Anagen effluvium, or hair loss during the anagen stage of the growth cycle, is caused by interruption of the rapidly dividing cells of the hair matrix, producing rapid hair loss within 2 to 4 weeks. Telogen

effluvium, or toxicity during the resting stage of the cycle, typically produces hair loss 2 to 4 months later and occurs as a side effect of a xenobiotic or in the setting of systemic disease or altered physiologic states (eg, postpartum). Anagen toxicity is commonly associated with xenobiotic exposures such as doxorubicin, cyclophosphamide, vincristine, and thallium.[58] Many chemotherapeutics reduce the mitotic activity of the rapidly dividing hair matrix cells, leading to the formation of a thin, easily breakable shaft. Thallium, classically associated with hair loss, causes alopecia by 2 mechanisms. Thallium distributes intracellularly, like potassium, altering potassium-mediated processes and thereby disrupting protein synthesis. By binding sulfhydryl groups, thallium also inhibits the normal incorporation of cysteine into keratin. Thallium toxicity results in alopecia 1 to 4 weeks after exposure. Within 4 days of exposure, a hair mount observed using light microscopy will demonstrate tapered or bayonet anagen hair with a characteristic bandlike black pigmentation at the base. Seeing this anagen effect can reveal the timing of exposure. Soluble barium salts, such as barium sulfide, are applied topically as a depilatory to produce localized hair loss. The mechanism of hair loss is undefined.

NAILS

The nail consists of a horny layer: the "nail plate" and 4 specialized epithelia—proximal nail fold, nail matrix, nail bed, and hyponychium. The nail matrix consists of keratinocytes, melanocytes, Langerhans cells, and Merkel cells.

Nail hyperpigmentation occurs for unclear reasons, but can be caused by focal stimulation of melanocytes in the nail matrix leading to melanonychia. The pigment deposition can be longitudinal, diffuse, or perilunar in orientation and typically develops several weeks after chemotherapy.[58] Dark-skinned patients are more commonly affected because of a higher concentration of melanocytes. Cyclophosphamide, doxorubicin, hydroxyurea, zidovudine, and bleomycin are among the most common xenobiotics that cause melanonychia, and the pigmentation generally resolves with cessation of therapy. When approaching a patient with a single streak of longitudinal melanonychia, it is crucial to include nail melanoma in the differential diagnosis, particularly if the band is greater than 3 mm in breadth and/or evolving.

Nail findings serve as important clues to xenobiotic exposures that occurred in the recent past. Matrix keratinization in a programmed and scheduled pattern leads to the formation of the nail plate. Certain changes

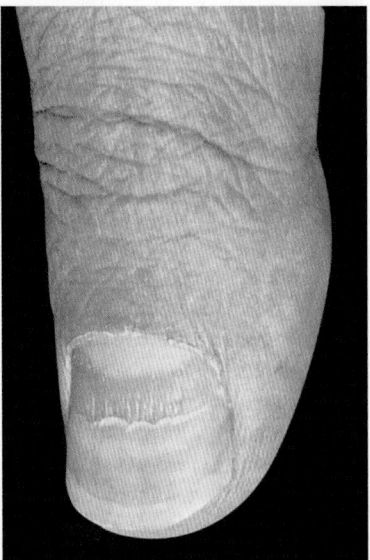

FIGURE 17–16. Presence of proximal indented Beau line and distal band of leukonychia due to cyclophosphamide 3 months after bone marrow transplantation. *(Reproduced with permission from Wolff K, Goldsmith LA, Katz SI, et al. Fitzpatrick's Dermatology in General Medicine, 7th ed. New York, NY: McGraw-Hill; 2008.)*

in nails, such as Mees lines and Beau lines, result from a temporary arrest of the proximal nail matrix proliferation. These lines can be used to predict the timing of a toxic exposure because of the reliability of rate of growth of the fingernails at approximately 2 to 3 mm per month. Mees lines, first described in 1919 in the setting of arsenic poisoning, can be used to approximate the date of the insult by the position of growth of the Mees line a patterned leukonychia (not indentation) causing transverse white lines.[36] Multiple Mees lines suggests multiple exposures over time. Arsenic, thallium, doxorubicin, vincristine, cyclophosphamide, methotrexate, and 5-fluorouracil cause Mees lines, but Mees lines can develop after any period of critical illness such as sepsis or trauma. Beau lines are transverse grooves or indentations more often in the central portion of the nail plate, most commonly caused by trauma (eg, manicures) or dermatologic disease affecting the proximal nail fold. Beau lines present on multiple digits, especially at the same level on each nail, indicate a systemic illness or xenobiotic exposure (Fig. 17–16).

SUMMARY

- The integument is constantly exposed to both topical and systemic xenobiotics, and these exposures result in reactive dermatoses.
- Prompt examination of the entire skin, hair, and nails provide invaluable clues about the route and nature of the offending xenobiotic.
- A careful history, clinical examination, and consultation with a dermatologist and biopsy when indicated can aid in identifying the etiology and nature of the reaction and lead to prompt treatment.
- Medication or drug reactions range from ordinary exanthematous reactions to potentially life-threatening drug-induced hypersensitivity reactions and SJS/TEN; these entities can be distinguished with a careful history, physical examination, and precise drug-exposure timeline.

Acknowledgment

Dr. Dina Began contributed to this chapter in previous editions.

REFERENCES

1. Allergan. Botox medication guide. FDA. http://www.fda.gov/downloads/drugs/drug-safety/ucm176360.pdf. Published 2016.
2. Amar SM, Dreskin SC. Urticaria. *Prim Care.* 2008;35:141-157.
3. Arndt KA, Jick H. Rates of cutaneous reactions to drugs. A report from the Boston Collaborative Drug Surveillance Program. *JAMA.* 1976;235:918-923.
4. Bastuji-Garin S, et al. Clinical classification of cases of toxic epidermal necrolysis, Stevens-Johnson syndrome, and erythema multiforme. *Arch Dermatol.* 1993;129:92-96.
5. Bertolini JC. Hydrofluoric acid: a review of toxicity. *J Emerg Med.* 1992;10:163-168.
6. Bradford M, et al. Bilateral necrosis of earlobes and cheeks: another complication of cocaine contaminated with levamisole. *Ann Intern Med.* 2010;152:758-759.
7. Brown BG. Expert commentary: niacin safety. *Am J Cardiol.* 2007;99:34.
8. Bryden AM, et al. Photopatch testing of 1155 patients: results of the U.K. multicentre photopatch study group. *Br J Dermatol.* 2006;155:737-747.
9. Burgess JL, et al. Emergency department hazardous materials protocol for contaminated patients. *Ann Emerg Med.* 1999;34:205-212.
10. Cartotto RC, et al. Chemical burns. *Can J Surg.* 1996;39:205-211.
11. Castela E, et al. Blue pseudochromhidrosis secondary to topiramate treatment. *Acta Derm Venereol.* 2009;89:538-539.
12. Chu D. *Development and Structure of Skin: Fitzpatrick's Dermatology in General Medicine.* 8th ed. New York, NY: McGraw-Hill; 2012.
13. Chung C, et al. Characteristic purpura of the ears, vasculitis, and neutropenia—a potential public health epidemic associated with levamisole-adulterated cocaine. *J Am Acad Dermatol.* 2011;65:722-725.
14. Clark S, Camargo CA. Epidemiology of anaphylaxis. *Immunol Allergy Clin North Am.* 2007;27:145-163.
15. Czerwinski SE, et al. Effect of octanol:water partition coefficients of organophosphorus compounds on biodistribution and percutaneous toxicity. *J Biochem Mol Toxicol.* 2006;20:241-246.
16. Darvay A, et al. Photoallergic contact dermatitis is uncommon. *Br J Dermatol.* 2001;145:597-601.
17. Duragesic [package insert]. Titusville, NJ: Janssen Pharmaceuticals, Inc; 2008.
18. Edlich RF, et al. Modern concepts of treatment and prevention of chemical injuries. *J Long Term Eff Med Implants.* 2005;15:303-318.
19. Fartasch M, Diepgen TL. The barrier function in atopic dry skin. Disturbance of membrane-coating granule exocytosis and formation of epidermal lipids? *Acta Derm Venereol Suppl (Stockh).* 1992;176:26-31.
20. Fujita Y, et al. Rapid immunochromatographic test for serum granulysin is useful for the prediction of Stevens-Johnson syndrome and toxic epidermal necrolysis. *J Am Acad Dermatol.* 2011;65:65-68.
21. Granstein RD, Sober AJ. Drug- and heavy metal–induced hyperpigmentation. *J Am Acad Dermatol.* 1981;5:1-18.
22. Groscurth P. Anatomy of sweat glands. *Curr Probl Dermatol.* 2002;30:1-9.
23. Guy RH, Hadgraft J. Physicochemical aspects of percutaneous penetration and its enhancement. *Pharm Res.* 1988;5:753-758.
24. Hadgraft J, Lane ME. Skin permeation: the years of enlightenment. *Int J Pharm.* 2005;305:2-12.
25. Harvell J, et al. Contact urticaria and its mechanisms. *Food Chem Toxicol.* 1994;32:103-112.
26. Haught JM, et al. Xanthoderma: a clinical review. *J Am Acad Dermatol.* 2007;57:1051-1058.
27. Huang YC, et al. The efficacy of intravenous immunoglobulin for the treatment of toxic epidermal necrolysis: a systematic review and meta-analysis. *Br J Dermatol.* 2012;167:424-432.
28. Izikson L, et al. The flushing patient: differential diagnosis, workup, and treatment. *J Am Acad Dermatol.* 2006;55:193-208.
29. Bernhard JD. *Itch: Mechanisms and Management of Pruritus.* New York, NY: McGraw-Hill; 1994.
30. Kang S, et al. Pigmentary disorders from exogenous causes. In: Levine N, ed. *Pigmentation and Pigmentary Disorders.* Boca Raton, FL: CRC Press; 1993.
31. Kligman AM. The spectrum of contact urticaria. Wheals, erythema, and pruritus. *Dermatol Clin.* 1990;8:57-60.
32. Knowles SR, Shear NH. Recognition and management of severe cutaneous drug reactions. *Dermatol Clin.* 2007;25:245-253.
33. Lebwohl M, Herrmann LG. Impaired skin barrier function in dermatologic disease and repair with moisturization. *Cutis.* 2005;76:7-12.
34. McCormack M, et al. HLA-A*3101 and carbamazepine-induced hypersensitivity reactions in Europeans. *N Engl J Med.* 2011;364:1134-1143.
35. McCullough M, et al. Steven Johnson syndrome and toxic epidermal necrolysis in a burn unit: a 15-year experience. *Burns.* 2017;43:200-205.
36. Mee R. Een verschijnsel bij polyneuritis arsenicosa. *Ned Tijdsch Geneeskd.* 1919;1:391-396.
37. Mehta RK, et al. Cement dermatitis and chemical burns. *Clin Exp Dermatol.* 2002;27:347-348.
38. Mihm MC, et al. Basic pathologic reactions of the skin. In: Fitzpatrick TB, Wolff K, eds. *Fitzpatrick's Dermatology in General Medicine.* 8th ed. New York: McGraw-Hill Medical; 2012.
39. Milewski M, Stinchcomb AL. Estimation of maximum transdermal flux of non-ionized xenobiotics from basic physicochemical determinants. *Mol Pharmacol.* 2012;9:2111-2120.
40. Monteiro-Riviere NA, et al. Efficacy of topical phenol decontamination strategies on severity of acute phenol chemical burns and dermal absorption: in vitro and in vivo studies in pig skin. *Toxicol Ind Health.* 2001;17:95-104.
41. Morison WL. Clinical practice. Photosensitivity. *N Engl J Med.* 2004;350:1111-1117.
42. Morkunas AR, Miller MB. Anticonvulsant hypersensitivity syndrome. *Crit Care Clin.* 1997;13:727-739.
43. Murata J, et al. Increased soluble Fas ligand levels in patients with Stevens-Johnson syndrome and toxic epidermal necrolysis preceding skin detachment. *J Allergy Clin Immunol.* 2008;122:992-1000.
44. Nickoloff BJ. Saving the skin from drug-induced detachment. *Nat Med.* 2008;14:1311-1313.
45. Pereira FA, et al. Toxic epidermal necrolysis. *J Am Acad Dermatol.* 2007;56:181-200.
46. Peterson CE, Kwaan HC. Current concepts of warfarin therapy. *Arch Intern Med.* 1986;146:581-584.
47. Pirmohamed M, et al. Carbamazepine-hypersensitivity: assessment of clinical and in vitro chemical cross-reactivity with phenytoin and oxcarbazepine. *Br J Clin Pharmacol.* 1991;32:741-749.
48. Prasad JK, et al. Use of amnion for the treatment of Stevens-Johnson syndrome. *J Trauma.* 1986;26:945-946.
49. Revuz J, et al. Toxic epidermal necrolysis. Clinical findings and prognosis factors in 87 patients. *Arch Dermatol.* 1987;123:1160-1165.
50. Riviere JE, Brooks JD. Prediction of dermal absorption from complex chemical mixtures: incorporation of vehicle effects and interactions into a QSPR framework. *SAR QSAR Environ Res.* 2007;18:31-44.
51. Roujeau JC. Stevens-Johnson syndrome and toxic epidermal necrolysis are severity variants of the same disease which differs from erythema multiforme. *J Dermatol.* 1997;24:726-729.
52. Roujeau JC, et al. Toxic epidermal necrolysis (Lyell syndrome). Incidence and drug etiology in France, 1981-1985. *Arch Dermatol.* 1990;126:37-42.
53. Roujeau JC, et al. Medication use and the risk of Stevens-Johnson syndrome or toxic epidermal necrolysis. *N Engl J Med.* 1995;333:1600-1607.
54. Scheindlin S. Transdermal drug delivery: past, present, future. *Mol Interv.* 2004;4:308-312.
55. Schillinger BM, et al. Boric acid poisoning. *J Am Acad Dermatol.* 1982;7:667-673.
56. Silver RM, et al. Scleroderma, fasciitis, and eosinophilia associated with the ingestion of tryptophan. *N Engl J Med.* 1990;322:874-881.

57. Stenn KS, Paus R. Controls of hair follicle cycling. *Physiol Rev.* 2001;81:449-494.

58. Susser WS, et al. Mucocutaneous reactions to chemotherapy. *J Am Acad Dermatol.* 1999;40:367-398.

59. Takita Y, et al. A case of carotenemia associated with ingestion of nutrient supplements. *J Dermatol.* 2006;33:132-134.

60. ten Holder SM, et al. Cutaneous and systemic manifestations of drug-induced vasculitis. *Ann Pharmacother.* 2002;36:130-147.

61. Vance MV. Hydrofluoric acid burns. In: Adams RM, ed. *Occupational Skin Disease.* 3rd ed. Philadelphia, PA: WB Saunders; 1999.

62. Viard I, et al. Inhibition of toxic epidermal necrolysis by blockade of CD95 with human intravenous immunoglobulin. *Science.* 1998;282:490-493.

63. Waller JM, et al. Cocaine-associated retiform purpura and neutropenia: is levamisole the culprit? *J Am Acad Dermatol.* 2010;63:530-535.

64. Walsh NM, et al. Cocaine-related retiform purpura: evidence to incriminate the adulterant, levamisole. *J Cutan Pathol.* 2010;37:1212-1219.

65. Wenzel FG, Horn TD. Nonneoplastic disorders of the eccrine glands. *J Am Acad Dermatol.* 1998;38:1-17; quiz 18-20.

66. Wilkin JK. The red face: flushing disorders. *Clin Dermatol.* 1993;11:211-223.

67. Wolverton SE. Update on cutaneous drug reactions. *Adv Dermatol.* 1997;13:65-84.

68. Yeong EK, et al. Serum bicarbonate as a marker to predict mortality in toxic epidermal necrolysis. *J Intensive Care Med.* 2011;26:250-254.

69. Zug KA, et al. Patch-test results of the North American Contact Dermatitis Group 2005-2006. *Dermatitis.* 2009;20:149-160.

70. Zugerman C. Chloracne. Clinical manifestations and etiology. *Dermatol Clin.* 1990;8:209-213.

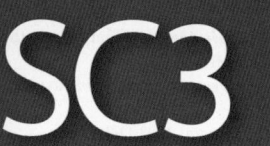
Lewis S. Nelson

HISTORY AND CURRENT USE

Applying a xenobiotic to the skin to treat a systemic medical condition is not new. Ointments and other salves have been applied topically for thousands of years for the treatment of local and systemic diseases. During World War I, dynamite workers used nitroglycerin applied to their hatbands to prevent angina when they were away from work and no longer exposed to organic nitrates.[36] Mustard seed plaster for chest congestion, releasing allyl isothiocyanate, and topical elemental mercurials for syphilis are other examples of such use in the beginning of the 20th century.[28] Over the past 30 years, an increasing number of medications have been formulated in transdermal delivery systems, or patches, to allow for systemic delivery of a xenobiotic. The first commercially available patch delivered scopolamine for motion sickness (1979), which was followed by nitroglycerin for chronic angina (1981) and then fentanyl for chronic pain management (1990). In the United States, the nicotine patch remains the most widely used transdermal patch, because of both the significant need for smoking cessation and its nonprescription availability. Certain medicinal xenobiotics, such as testosterone, can be administered without a patch, as a spray or gel.[22] Further, xenobiotics are absorbed transdermally, as occurs with nicotine following direct exposure to moist tobacco leaf in patients with "green tobacco sickness" or following direct contact with organic phosphorus compound spraying.[3]

The skin is the largest organ in the body, although it is not widely used as a route for intentional xenobiotic delivery. However, there are several benefits of transdermal delivery of xenobiotics. This route provides a non-invasive means to discretely administer xenobiotics. Patches result in steady plasma concentrations that reduce side effects, particularly for xenobiotics with short half-lives. Although metabolism occurs in the skin, metabolism does not appear to be highly consequential for the majority of currently used transdermal xenobiotics.[18] The patches are designed to be left in place for long periods of time, which improves compliance. Importantly, the avoidance of first-pass metabolism permits an effective means of delivery for poorly orally bioavailable xenobiotics. However, because absorption through the skin following simple application is passive, there is a large degree of variability among both patients and xenobiotics. Newer nanocarriers and minimally invasive technologies, as discussed below, attempt to overcome this limitation.[11,16]

This chapter does not cover xenobiotics applied to the skin to produce an effect locally. These xenobiotics are available in patch formulation (eg, lidocaine and capsaicin) or as a directly applied preparation, such as a variety of antibiotics or acne creams (eg, tretinoin). Locally acting formulations (eg, lidocaine) typically provide only trivial amounts of systemic xenobiotic;[6] for example, with tretinoin, despite devastating fetal complications when taken orally, these same effects do not occur when applied topically.[20] Some xenobiotics, such as capsaicin, have both local (for postherpetic neuralgia) and systemic (for cannabinoid hyperemesis syndrome) effects.[7,31]

TRANSDERMAL ADMINISTRATION PHARMACOLOGY
Passive Administration
The same hydrophobic property that allows the skin to prevent water loss hinders the ability to administer a water-soluble xenobiotic transdermally. In order to reach the systemic circulation, a xenobiotic applied to the stratum corneum (horny layer) (Fig. 17–1) must initially pass through about a dozen layers of keratinized epidermal cells and then into the dermis. This

keratinaceous horny layer is highly impervious to water movement because of the presence of ceramides, fatty acids, and other lipids.[5] This property maintains the ability of the skin to lose excess water in dry environments. Burn victims lose the capacity to regulate water loss through injury to the keratinaceous layer. In order for a xenobiotic to partition into the stratum corneum, it must be sufficiently lipid soluble. However, this same xenobiotic must subsequently partition out from the stratum corneum into the aqueous underlying tissue, and this requires sufficient hydrophilicity.[25] The ability to partition into these various phases (lipid and water) is described by the octanol–water partition coefficient. These vary widely among xenobiotics. For example, this coefficient for fentanyl (717) and nicotine (15) suggests sufficient ability to cross the stratum corneum, whereas morphine (0.7) cannot pass through this outer layer.

Fick's first law describes xenobiotic permeation across the stratum corneum. In this model, steady-state flux (J) is related to the diffusion coefficient (D) of the xenobiotic based on the thickness of the stratum corneum (h), the partition coefficient (P) between the stratum corneum and the xenobiotic in its vehicle, and the xenobiotic concentration (C) that is applied, which is assumed to be constant. This equation demonstrates the influence of solubility and partition coefficient of a xenobiotic on diffusion across the stratum corneum (Equation 9–1). Molecules showing intermediate partition coefficients have adequate solubility within the lipid domains of the stratum corneum to permit diffusion through this domain while still having sufficient hydrophilic nature to allow partitioning into the lower layers (stratum granulosum, stratum spinosum, and the stratum germinativum) of the epidermis.

Permeation enhancers improve absorption by solubilizing the xenobiotic or altering the characteristics of the stratum corneum, effectively increasing the lipid solubility of the xenobiotic.[19,32] Enhancers include solvents such as ethanol, fatty acids, fatty esters, and surfactants that serve as vehicles to improve the solubility of a xenobiotic in the lipids of the stratum corneum layer.[19] An alternative means of enhancing lipophilicity is the addition of organic functional groups to create a prodrug that is cleaved once absorbed.[29] This is similar to the significantly enhanced neurotoxicity of dimethylmercury compared to methylmercury when applied to the skin.[24] Additionally, the use of nanoparticles enhances xenobiotic solubility and surface contact area.[33]

Few xenobiotics have the essential molecular requirements to be systemically delivered by the transdermal route. The upper limit of the molecular weight of an acceptable drug is 500 Da (fentanyl is 337 Da), and the medication must be sufficiently potent to exert the desired effect at concentrations that can reliably be obtained. Although only small quantities, typically less than 2 mg daily are delivered, the largest nicotine patch delivers 21 mg daily.

As suggested by Fick's law, the ability to cross the dermis is related to the concentration gradient provided by the transdermal patch. To allow sufficient delivery, a large amount of xenobiotic is contained in the apparatus to maintain the concentration gradient over time. For example, the 50-mcg/hr fentanyl patch (which delivers 1.2 mg daily) contains 8.4 mg (8,400 mcg) of fentanyl in the patch.[13,36] This excess amount of drug minimizes the fluctuations in delivery over time as the concentration gradient naturally falls during movement of xenobiotic from the patch to the skin. Upon completion of the 3-day use of a fentanyl patch, the amount of fentanyl remaining in a patch ranged from 28% to 85%; at the end of use, 27% to 74% of the contents of a nicotine patch remained.[21,28] Furthermore, in order to prevent rapid movement into the skin, and also maintain a functional concentration gradient, a rate-controlling membrane is present that allows the passage of a measured amount of drug per area of skin contact surface.

Applying xenobiotic to broken skin or tissue lacking a stratum corneum, such as mucosa, results in a substantial increase in absorption, which is greater than 5- or greater than 30-fold, respectively, for fentanyl.[12,22] For example, application of salicylic acid for a treatment of hyperkeratinization disorders causes salicylate poisoning.[1,32] Because the pharmacokinetics of transmucosal delivery tend to be more predictable than by the transdermal route, certain formulations such as fentanyl citrate (Actiq, Subsys, Fentora) or nicotine (Nicorette gum) are administered transmucosally. However, the greater penetrability accounts for the toxicity associated with improper application to a mucosal surface, which lacks a stratum corneum.[5,26] A small amount of xenobiotic also enters the body by way of the skin appendages, such as the sweat glands or hair follicles.[5,25]

Properties of the skin that account for pharmacokinetic variability include hydration status and temperature. Absorption varies based on the site of application on the body and on both the thickness of the stratum corneum and the blood flow.[2,29,30] Although the average skin thickness of the human body is 40 μm, it ranges between 20 and 80 μm as a result of many factors including body location, race, age, and sex. As an example, in skin samples from 8 individuals, there was more than a 50% difference in the permeability of fentanyl.[17] Because the stratum corneum thickness is most relevant to diffusion rates, those areas that have similar thickness, such as the chest, extremities, and abdomen, provide the most consistent delivery and are generally used as sites for transdermal patch application.[30,33] Intertriginous areas, where skin contacts other skin (axillae, groin, inframammary, and intergluteal) allow greater absorption because of enhanced contact surface, temperature, and moisture.

Active Administration

As described earlier, passive administration requires the optimization of formulation- or xenobiotic-carrying vehicle to increase skin permeability. However currently used absorption enhancers do not greatly improve the permeation of xenobiotics with molecular weights greater than 500 Da.[27] In contrast, active methods, normally involving physical or mechanical methods of enhancing delivery are generally superior. The delivery of xenobiotics of differing lipophilicity and molecular weight including proteins, peptides, vaccines, and oligonucleotides are improved by active energy-requiring techniques such as electroporation, iontophoresis, and ultrasonography (Tables SC3–1 and SC3–2).[11,37]

Patch Technology

In most current patches, the drug to be delivered is also incorporated into the adhesive layer to reduce the delay to drug absorption. Multiple layers of

TABLE SC3–1   Examples of Xenobiotics Available in Patch Formulations
Buprenorphine
Clonidine
Estradiol
Estradiol/levonorgestrel
Fentanyl
Granisetron
Methylphenidate
Nicotine
Nitroglycerin
Norelgestromin/ethinyl estradiol
Oxybutynin
Rivastigmine
Rotigotine
Scopolamine
Selegiline
Testosterone

TABLE SC3–2   Description of Advanced Transdermal Drug Delivery Systems
Electroporation: uses high-voltage microsecond duration electrical pulses to create transient pores within the skin (for larger molecules such as peptides).
Iontophoresis: uses electrodes to pass a small current through a xenobiotic (pilocarpine for sweat testing for cystic fibrosis and for lidocaine).
Microneedle based devices: approximately 10–100 μm in length, and are generally arranged in arrays on patch devices. Each microneedle is coated in the xenobiotic to be delivered, and the small size avoids the production of pain.
Needleless injection: compressed air is used to force xenobiotics across the skin surface, and may deliver local anesthetics prior to intravenous line placement.
Ultrasound: low frequency ultrasound to promote transcutaneous delivery, also called sonophoresis.

adhesive are often separated by membranes that serve to regulate the release. To allow a longer duration of drug delivery, a reservoir is often added. This compartment contains the medication in solution or suspension, and a rate-regulating membrane ensures that the release follows zero-order kinetics to avoid fluctuations in concentration. Increasing the surface area of contact by enlarging the patch proportionally increases the amount of xenobiotic delivered. The membrane itself is not altered. Removal of the rate-regulating membrane, however, results in rapid absorption of toxic quantities of xenobiotic.[8]

The initial fentanyl patch used a reservoir that contained a large quantity of xenobiotic. This reservoir was at risk for access inadvertently by a child chewing the patch or intentionally by a person seeking to abuse the liquid contents.[23] Cutting the reservoir patch dispersed the fentanyl and would result in either overdose or loss of analgesia. Patch construction defects also occurred that potentially allowed leakage.[14] Alternatively, by incorporating the xenobiotic into a fabric mesh, the matrix patch eliminated the reservoir and reduced the risk for abuse. The matrix patch could be safely cut to change the dosage delivered, based on surface contact area, without risking spillage of any liquid content. The clinical pharmacology of the matrix fentanyl patch is similar to that of the reservoir patch.[9]

Pharmacokinetics

The initial detection of xenobiotic in the serum following transdermal application is not surprisingly delayed compared to other routes of administration. The delay is dependent on the properties of the xenobiotic, the skin, and the environment. Highly lipophilic xenobiotics form a depot in the subcutaneous tissue as the xenobiotic slowly dissolves in the aqueous tissue for diffusion to allow vascular uptake. Highly hydrophilic xenobiotics slowly penetrate the lipid layers of the epidermis, which is why ionic (salt) forms of drugs are administered by a subcutaneous or intramuscular route. For example, fentanyl concentrations will not be detected in the serum for 1 to 2 hours after placement of a patch, and the peak concentration is typically achieved in a day or longer.[13] For this reason the use of a fentanyl patch is not indicated for the treatment of acute pain, particularly postoperative pain.[23] Because the natural history of acute pain is to rapidly improve over several days, during which time the fentanyl concentrations continue to rise, the risk of toxicity also rises.[34] However, in patients with chronic pain, this pharmacokinetic profile will be beneficial, as long as opioids are indicated and safe use is monitored. Furthermore, as noted, permeation enhancers will commonly alter the xenobiotic or the skin sufficiently to alter the absorption kinetics.[19]

The pharmacokinetic profiles of serial doses of patches is based on removal of the patch after the specified time period, and application of a new patch at a different location.[23] This is important to allow a new subcutaneous depot to form while the existing depot from the initial patch is absorbed. If applied to the same location, rather than initiating absorption from a new site, the dose in the adhesive will combine with the existing depot and alter the clinical pharmacokinetics.

Washing the skin or removing the patch will not result in a rapid fall in serum concentrations or a reduction in clinical effect.[13] Rather, the concentration and clinical effects will resolve over several hours because of the persistence of the dermal depot, which is not removed by cleansing.[23] For example, the apparent half-life of fentanyl following removal of a fentanyl patch is approximately 18 hours.[13] Therefore, simple removal of a fentanyl patch will not be sufficient treatment of a patient with respiratory depression, and respiratory support or naloxone should be used.

ADVERSE EFFECTS

Because transdermal administration places the xenobiotic in close contact with the environment, there is substantial risk of variation in absorption as a result of changes in ambient conditions. For example, patches exposed to heat, from heating blankets or saunas, can release drug at a rate greater than expected under conventional ambient conditions.[4] Patches are periodically damaged, either during the manufacturing process or subsequently following application which alters their release profile, resulting in toxicity.[14] Certain patches, such as those with a metal backing, will frequently become exceedingly hot during exposure to magnetic resonance imaging studies and result in burns.

Despite these techniques to enhance xenobiotic delivery, transdermal systems require that large amounts of xenobiotic be present externally to maximize the transcutaneous gradient. Much of the xenobiotic typically remains in the patch when it is removed following its intended course of therapy,[21] raising concerns for safe disposal, especially for children[35] and abuse potential among others.[15]

Perhaps the most insidious adverse effects are related to their complicated pharmacokinetics. Because many prescribers are unfamiliar with the dosing and initiation of therapy with transdermal products, those xenobiotics with consequential adverse effects in overdose, such as fentanyl, are commonly linked to poor outcomes even with intended therapeutic use.[10,23]

SUMMARY

- A limited number of xenobiotics have the appropriate chemical properties, such as lipophilicity and potency, to permit transdermal absorption.
- Transdermal delivery of a xenobiotic has certain therapeutic advantages over other routes, such as bypassing first-pass hepatic metabolism and providing a discrete administration.
- The pharmacokinetics of transdermal xenobiotic delivery are unique; they are distinctly different than other routes. Absorption is typically slower but more prolonged, which is potentially beneficial in situations in which long-term, round-the-clock dosing is required.
- Because of the atypical pharmacokinetics, both the onset and offset of the clinical effects are slow and relatively unpredictable. The development of toxicity, in particular, is often insidious.

REFERENCES

1. Akhavan A, Bershad S. Topical acne drugs: review of clinical properties, systemic exposure, and safety. *Am J Clin Dermatol.* 2003;4:473-492.
2. Andrews SN, et al. Transdermal delivery of molecules is limited by full epidermis, not just stratum corneum. *Pharm Res.* 2013;30:1099-1109.
3. Arcury TA, et al. Green tobacco sickness and skin integrity among migrant Latino farmworkers. *Am J Ind Med.* 2008;51:195-203.
4. Ashburn MA, et al. The pharmacokinetics of transdermal fentanyl delivered with and without controlled heat. *J Pain.* 2003;4:291-297.
5. Benson HAE. Transdermal drug delivery: penetration enhancement techniques. *Curr Drug Deliv.* 2005;2:23-33.
6. Campbell BJ, et al. Systemic absorption of topical lidocaine in normal volunteers, patients with post-herpetic neuralgia, and patients with acute herpes zoster. *J Pharm Sci.* 2002;91:1343-1350.
7. Derry S, et al. Topical capsaicin (high concentration) for chronic neuropathic pain in adults. Derry S, ed. *Cochrane Database Syst Rev.* 2017;1:CD007393.
8. Fiset P, et al. Biopharmaceutics of a new transdermal fentanyl device. *Anesthesiology.* 1995;83:459-469.
9. Freynhagen R, et al. Switching from reservoir to matrix systems for the transdermal delivery of fentanyl: a prospective, multicenter pilot study in outpatients with chronic pain. *J Pain Symptom Manage.* 2005;30:289-297.
10. Gill JR, et al. Reliability of postmortem fentanyl concentrations in determining the cause of death. *J Med Toxicol.* 2013;9:34-41.
11. Gratieri T, et al. Next generation intra- and transdermal therapeutic systems: using non- and minimally-invasive technologies to increase drug delivery into and across the skin. *Eur J Pharm Sci.* 2013;50:609-622.
12. Gupta SK, et al. System functionality and physicochemical model of fentanyl transdermal system. *J Pain Symptom Manage.* 1992;7(suppl):S17-S26.
13. Janssen Pharmaceuticals. *Duragesic (Fentanyl Transdermal System) Prescribing Information.* Titusville, NJ; 2012:1-11.
14. Janssen Pharmaceuticals. *Urgent Class 1 Drug Recall Notification.* Titusville, NJ; 2004:1-2. https://www.fda.gov/downloads/Safety/MedWatch/UCM166412.pdf.
15. Jumbelic MI. Deaths with transdermal fentanyl patches. *Am J Forensic Med Pathol.* 2010;31:18-21.
16. Kurmi BD, et al. Transdermal drug delivery: opportunities and challenges for controlled delivery of therapeutic agents using nanocarriers. *Curr Drug Metab.* 2017;18:1-1.
17. Larsen RH, et al. Dermal penetration of fentanyl: inter- and intraindividual variations. *Pharmacol Toxicol.* 2003;93:244-248.
18. Li J, et al. The application of skin metabolomics in the context of transdermal drug delivery. *Pharmacol Rep.* 2016;69:252-259.
19. Lopes LB, et al. Chemical penetration enhancers. *Ther Deliv.* 2015;6:1053-1061.
20. Loureiro KD, et al. Minor malformations characteristic of the retinoic acid embryopathy and other birth outcomes in children of women exposed to topical tretinoin during early pregnancy. *Am J Med Genet A.* 2005;136:117-121.
21. Marquardt KA, et al. Fentanyl remaining in a transdermal system following three days of continuous use. *Ann Pharmacother.* 1995;29:969-971.
22. Martinez-Pajares et al. Peripheral precocious puberty due to inadvertent exposure to testosterone: case report and review of the literature. *J Pediatr Endocrinol Metab.* 2012;25:1007-1012.
23. Nelson L, Schwaner R. Transdermal fentanyl: pharmacology and toxicology. *J Med Toxicol.* 2009;5:230-241.
24. Nierenberg DW, et al. Delayed cerebellar disease and death after accidental exposure to dimethylmercury. *N Engl J Med.* 1998;338:1672-1676.
25. Prausnitz MR, et al. Current status and future potential of transdermal drug delivery. *Nat Rev Drug Discov.* 2004;3:115-124.
26. Prosser JM, et al. Complications of oral exposure to fentanyl transdermal delivery system patches. *J Med Toxicol.* 2010;6:443-447.
27. Ruan R, et al. Recent advances in peptides for enhancing transdermal macromolecular drug delivery. *Ther Deliv.* 2016;7:89-100.
28. Scheindlin S. Transdermal drug delivery: past, present, future. *Mol Interv.* 2004;4:308-312.
29. Sloan KB, et al. Dermal and transdermal delivery: prodrugs. *Ther Deliv.* 2011;2:83-105.
30. Solassol I, et al. Inter- and intraindividual variabilities in pharmacokinetics of fentanyl after repeated 72-hour transdermal applications in cancer pain patients. *Ther Drug Monit.* 2005;27:491-498.
31. Sorensen CJ, et al. Cannabinoid hyperemesis syndrome: diagnosis, pathophysiology, and treatment—a systematic review. *J Med Toxicol.* 2017;13:71-87.
32. Tiwary AK, et al. Innovations in transdermal drug delivery: formulations and techniques. *Recent Pat Drug Deliv Formul.* 2007;1:23-36.
33. Valenzuela P, Simon JA. Nanoparticle delivery for transdermal HRT. *Nanomedicine (Lond).* 2012;8(suppl 1):S83-S89.
34. van Bastelaere M, et al. Postoperative analgesia and plasma levels after transdermal fentanyl for orthopedic surgery: double-blind comparison with placebo. *J Clin Anesth.* 1995;7:26-30.
35. Wain AA, Martin J. Can transdermal nicotine patch cause acute intoxication in a child? A case report and review of literature. *Ulster Med J.* 2004;73:65-66.
36. Warren JV. Monday morning sudden death. *Trans Am Clin Climatol Assoc.* 1988;99:10-16.
37. Watkinson AC, et al. Future of the transdermal drug delivery market—have we barely touched the surface? *Expert Opin Drug Deliv.* 2016;13:523-532.

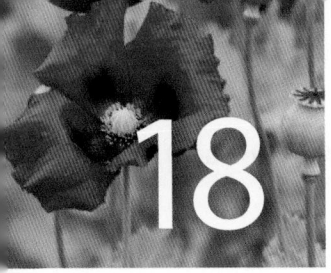

18 GASTROINTESTINAL PRINCIPLES

Matthew D. Zuckerman and Richard J. Church

Humans are in constant contact with xenobiotics. In addition to its critical role in absorbing nutrients, the gastrointestinal (GI) tract forms the initial functional barrier between ingested material and the body. An understanding of the structure, physiology, and innervation of the GI tract is critical to the toxicologic concepts of absorption, motility, and toxic insult. This chapter discusses the normal role of the GI tract and its relationship to toxicology. Anatomic, pathologic, and microbiologic principles are discussed, including the role of the GI tract in the metabolism of xenobiotics. Types of GI pathologies and their clinical manifestations are discussed, with examples when appropriate.

STRUCTURE AND INNERVATION OF THE GASTROINTESTINAL TRACT

The luminal GI tract is divided into 5 distinct structures: oral cavity and hypopharynx, esophagus, stomach, small intestine, and colon (Fig. 18–1). These environments differ in luminal pH, epithelial cell receptor types, and endogenous flora. The transitional areas between these distinct organs have specialized epithelia and muscular sphincters with specific functions and vulnerabilities. Knowing the anatomy of these transition zones is particularly important for the localization and management of foreign bodies. The functions of the pancreas and liver are closely integrated with those of the luminal organs. The pancreas is discussed here; the liver and its metabolic functions are discussed in Chaps. 11 and 21.

The visceral structures of the GI tract are composed of several layers, including the epithelium, lamina propria, submucosa, muscularis layers, and serosa (the last of which is only present in intraperitoneal organs). As the transition is made throughout the GI tract, differences in luminal pH, epithelial cell receptors, muscularity, and endogenous flora are encountered, affecting the absorption and metabolism of individual xenobiotics.

The epithelium, the innermost layer of the GI tract, is the most specialized cell type in the intestine and is composed of epithelial, endocrine, and receptor cells. The basal surface of epithelial cells faces the lamina propria, and the apical surface faces the lumen. They are further specialized for specific functions of secretion or absorption. Additionally, the epithelial cells form part of the mucosal immune defense, where they detect the presence of microbial pathogens and downregulate the immune system in the presence of nonpathogenic or probiotic microbes. The major barrier to penetration of xenobiotics and microbes is the GI epithelium, a single-cell-thick membrane. The cell membrane is a semipermeable lipid bilayer that contains aqueous pores through which certain materials pass, depending on size and molecular structure. The membrane is not continuous because it consists of individual epithelial cells; however, these cells are joined to each other by structures known as tight junctions. The tight junctions have a gap of about 8 Å, which allows passage only of water, ions, and low-molecular-weight substances.

The muscle layer found beneath the lamina propria is made up of the muscularis mucosa, the circular muscles, and the longitudinal muscles. Contraction of the muscularis mucosa causes a change in the surface area of the gut lumen that alters secretion or absorption of nutrients. Whereas depolarization of circular muscle leads to contraction of a ring of smooth muscle and a decrease in the diameter of that segment of the GI tract, depolarization of longitudinal muscle leads to contraction in the longitudinal direction and a decrease in the length of that segment. The function of the muscle layers is integrated with the enteric nervous system to provide for a coordinated movement of luminal contents through the GI tract to maximize absorption and maintain the gastrointestinal microbiota. This integration facilitates the flow of chyme (undigested food) via a coordinated sequence of muscular contractions and relaxations, leading to segmentation of luminal contents, peristaltic movements, and unidirectional flow through the intestine.

The GI tract is innervated by the autonomic nervous system via both extrinsic and intrinsic pathways (Fig. 18–2). The extrinsic innervation permits communication among the brain, spinal cord, and chemoreceptors and mechanoreceptors located in the gut. Parasympathetic stimulation in the extrinsic pathway tends to be excitatory ("rest and digest") and is carried via the vagus, splanchnic, and pelvic nerves to the myenteric and submucosal plexuses. In contrast, increased sympathetic tone ("fight or flight") inhibits digestive and peristaltic activity via fibers that originate in the thoracolumbar cord and terminate in the myenteric and submucosal plexuses. The intrinsic innervation of the GI tract, or enteric nervous system, constitutes a reflex arc that modulates both peristalsis (via the myenteric plexus) and secretion (via the submucosal plexus) in response to parasympathetic and sympathetic tone.

THE IMMUNE SYSTEM AND MICROBIOLOGY OF THE GASTROINTESTINAL TRACT

An elaborate mucosal immune system has evolved to protect the GI tract from pathogens and modulate functional gastrointestinal diseases.[35,44] Mucosal immunity consists of an afferent limb, which recognizes a pathogen and induces the proliferation and differentiation of immunocompetent cells, and an efferent limb, which coordinates and affects the immune response. The afferent system includes the lymphoid follicles and specialized M-cells found therein that promote transit of antigens to antigen-presenting cells.[37] Once sensitized, immune cells undergo a complicated process of clonal expansion and differentiation, which occurs in mucosal and mesenteric lymphoid follicles, and in extraintestinal sites. Immunocompetent cells then return to the intestine and other mucous membranes and are scattered diffusely within the epithelial and lamina propria compartments.

The normal endogenous flora in the GI tract includes more than 400 species of bacteria along with a small number of fungi and viruses. The intestinal mucosa is normally colonized by large numbers of nonpathogenic anaerobic strains of *Bacteroides* spp, *Eubacterium* spp, *Clostridium* spp, as well as aerobic strains of *Escherichia coli*, *Proteus* spp, *Enterobacter* spp, *Serratia* spp, *Lactobacillus* spp, *and Klebsiella* spp.[19] The concentration of luminal bacteria varies by site, from lowest in the proximal small intestine to highest in the large intestine. En masse, these bacteria are more metabolically active than the liver. Endogenous bacteria occupy unique niches related to host physiology, environmental pressures, and microbial interactions, which result in long-term stability. Following a course of ciprofloxacin, the gut microbiome of healthy volunteers demonstrated a marked shift and loss of biodiversity within days, but began to return to the initial state within a week of cessation.[13] Indeed, the cumulative total of microbial species in the enteric system (or enterotype) is remarkably consistent across countries and continents.[3]

The endogenous flora has multiple metabolic functions. A primary function in the colon is the salvage of malabsorbed carbohydrates by fermentation and production of short-chain fatty acids, a preferred substrate for colonic epithelial cells. This increased metabolic efficiency is best demonstrated when mice grown in germ-free conditions require a higher caloric intake to maintain weight.[48] This has led to some conjecture about the link between human flora and obesity.[16]

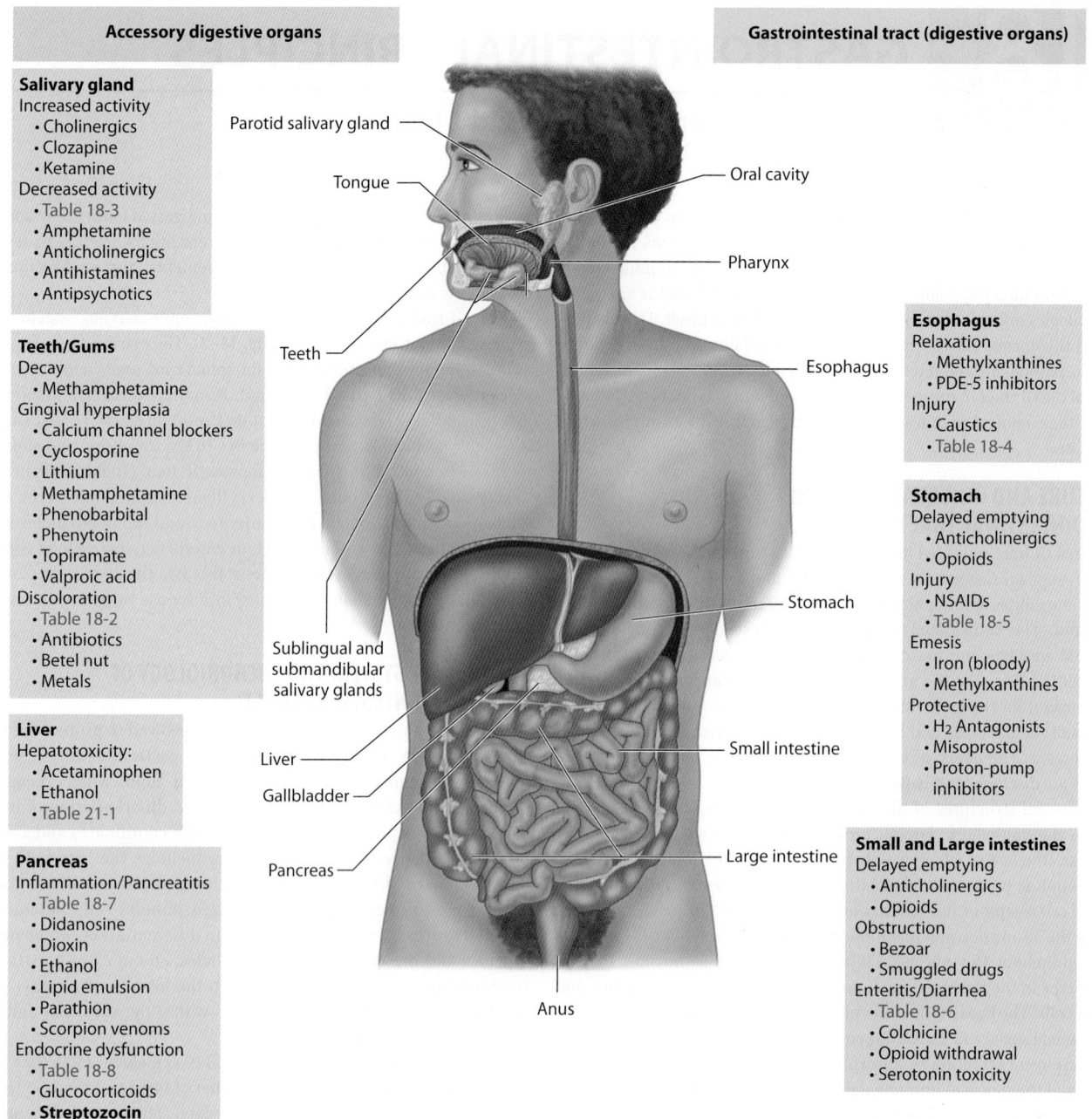

Accessory digestive organs

Salivary gland
Increased activity
• Cholinergics
• Clozapine
• Ketamine
Decreased activity
• Table 18-3
• Amphetamine
• Anticholinergics
• Antihistamines
• Antipsychotics

Teeth/Gums
Decay
• Methamphetamine
Gingival hyperplasia
• Calcium channel blockers
• Cyclosporine
• Lithium
• Methamphetamine
• Phenobarbital
• Phenytoin
• Topiramate
• Valproic acid
Discoloration
• Table 18-2
• Antibiotics
• Betel nut
• Metals

Liver
Hepatotoxicity:
• Acetaminophen
• Ethanol
• Table 21-1

Pancreas
Inflammation/Pancreatitis
• Table 18-7
• Didanosine
• Dioxin
• Ethanol
• Lipid emulsion
• Parathion
• Scorpion venoms
Endocrine dysfunction
• Table 18-8
• Glucocorticoids
• **Streptozocin**

Parotid salivary gland
Tongue
Teeth
Sublingual and submandibular salivary glands
Liver
Gallbladder
Pancreas
Anus

Gastrointestinal tract (digestive organs)

Oral cavity
Pharynx
Esophagus
Stomach
Small intestine
Large intestine

Esophagus
Relaxation
• Methylxanthines
• PDE-5 inhibitors
Injury
• Caustics
• Table 18-4

Stomach
Delayed emptying
• Anticholinergics
• Opioids
Injury
• NSAIDs
• Table 18-5
Emesis
• Iron (bloody)
• Methylxanthines
Protective
• H_2 Antagonists
• Misoprostol
• Proton-pump inhibitors

Small and Large intestines
Delayed emptying
• Anticholinergics
• Opioids
Obstruction
• Bezoar
• Smuggled drugs
Enteritis/Diarrhea
• Table 18-6
• Colchicine
• Opioid withdrawal
• Serotonin toxicity

FIGURE 18–1. Anatomy of the gastrointestinal system. (*Modified with permission from Mescher AL: Junqueira's Basic Histology, 13th ed. New York, NY: McGraw-Hill; 2013.*)

Bacterial metabolism significantly affects the disposition of enteral compounds.[23] For example, the bacterial metabolism of digoxin contributes to its steady-state concentrations, and antibiotic treatment reduces or eradicate the intestinal flora, predisposing to digoxin toxicity.[10] Bacterial contribution to vitamin K metabolism is also demonstrated, necessitating dose adjustments of warfarin during and after antibiotic therapy. The metabolic activity of intra-luminal bacteria is exploited in some treatment strategies. For example, sulfasalazine, used in the treatment of ulcerative colitis, is created through the linkage of 5-aminosalicylic acid to sulfapyridine. The azo bonds of the nonabsorbable sulfasalazine are broken by bacterial azoreductases, permitting the absorption of active metabolites in the colon at the site of inflammation.[41]

The normal flora of the gut consists of probiotics—live, nonpathogenic bacteria and fungi that are also used as prophylactic or therapeutic xenobiotics. These bacteria compete for and displace pathogenic bacteria, directly modulate intestinal immune function, and exert a trophic effect on the GI tract. They appear to serve to decrease traveler's diarrhea, suppress antibiotic-induced diarrhea, and reduce inflammation in ileal pouches after colectomy in patients with ulcerative colitis.[17,20,22]

REGULATORY SUBSTANCES OF THE GASTROINTESTINAL TRACT

There are 3 groups of regulatory peptide hormones that act on target cells within the GI tract. These are released from endocrine cells in the GI mucosa into the portal circulation and enter the systemic circulation to affect target cells. Gastrin, cholecystokinin (CCK), secretin, and glucose-dependent insulinotropic polypeptide (GIP; formerly gastric inhibitory peptide) are considered the primary GI hormones. Somatostatin and histamine comprise the paracrines, hormones that are released from endocrine cells and diffuse over short distances to act on target cells located in the GI tract. Vasoactive intestinal peptide (VIP), gastrin-releasing peptide (GRP), and enkephalins make up the last group known as neurocrines—substances that are synthesized in neurons of the GI tract, move by axonal transport down the axon, and are then released by action potentials in the nerves. The effects of these regulators are summarized in Table 18–1.[7]

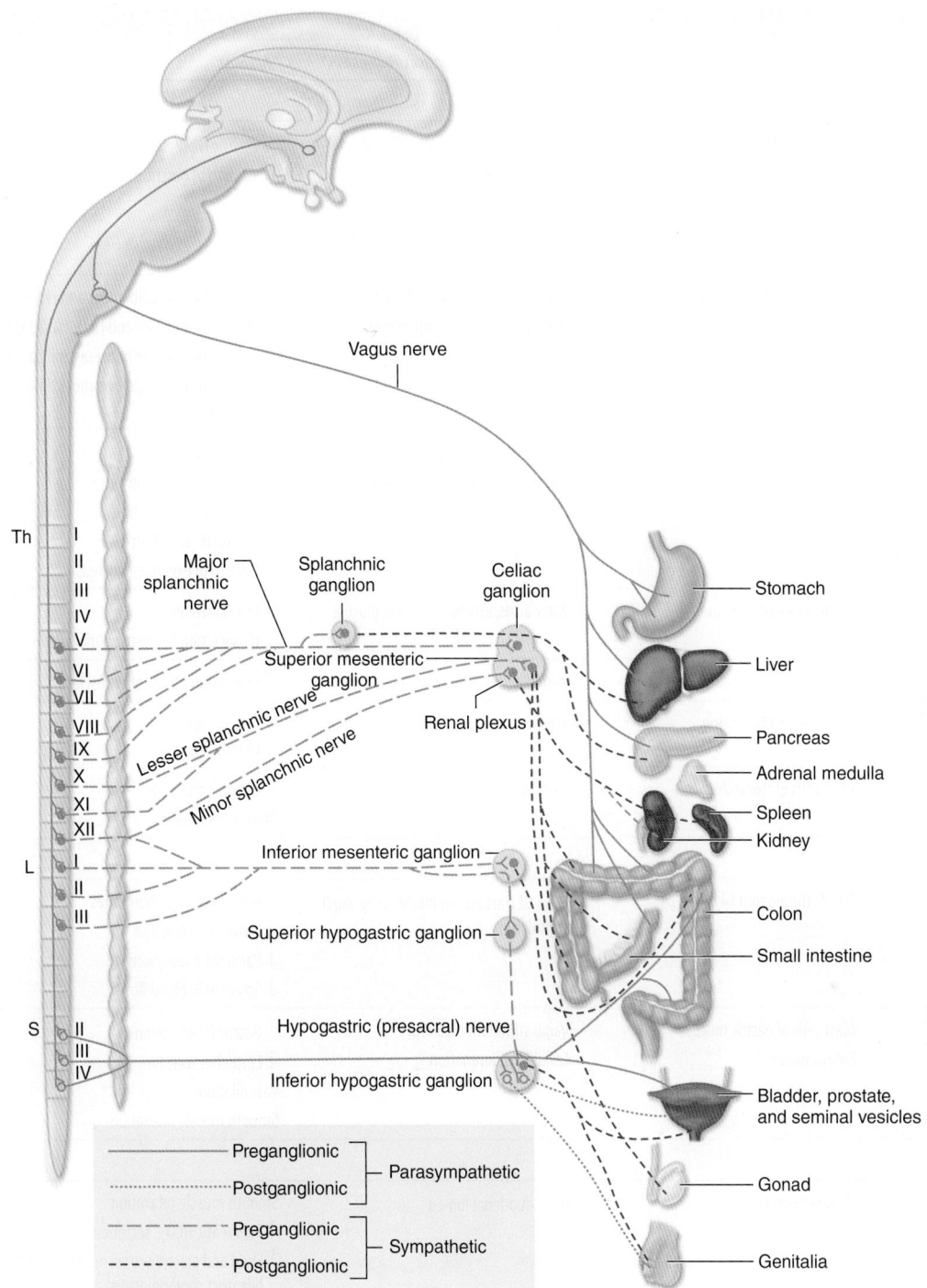

FIGURE 18–2. Innervation of the gastrointestinal system. *(Adapted with permission from McAninch JW, Lue TF, Smith DR: Smith and Tanagho's General Urology, 18th ed. New York, NY: McGraw-Hill Professional; 2013.)*

Xenobiotic effects on GI regulation have intended and unintended consequences. Somatostatins reduce splanchnic blood flow and portal blood pressure, leading to their use as therapeutics for bleeding esophageal varices. Erythromycin agonizes motilin receptors, leading to increased GI propulsion, cramping, and diarrhea.

ANATOMIC AND PHYSIOLOGIC PRINCIPLES

Oropharynx and Hypopharynx

The main functions of the mouth and oropharynx are chewing, lubrication of food with saliva, and swallowing. Saliva initiates digestion of starch by α-amylase (ptyalin), triglyceride digestion by lingual lipase, lubrication of

ingested food by mucus, and protection of the mouth and esophagus by dilution and buffering of ingested foods.

Saliva production is unique in that it is increased by both parasympathetic and sympathetic activity. Parasympathetic stimulation, via cranial nerves VII and IX, acts on muscarinic cholinergic receptors on acinar and ductal cells, increasing saliva production via vasodilation and increasing transport processes. Parasympathetic pathways are stimulated by food in the mouth, smells, conditioned reflexes, and nausea, and are inhibited by sleep, dehydration, and fear. Sympathetic stimulation originates from preganglionic nerves in the thoracic segments T1 to T3. When β-adrenergic receptors are triggered by norepinephrine, production of saliva increases but at a rate less than that

TABLE 18–1 Regulatory Substances of the GI Tract

Substance	Site of Secretion or Release	Stimulus for Secretion/Release	Actions
Endocrines			
Gastrin	G cells of gastric antrum	Small peptides and amino acids Stomach distention Vagal stimulation (via GRP) Inhibited by H^+ in stomach (negative feedback)	↑ Gastric H^+ secretion ↑ Growth of gastric mucosa
Cholecystokinin	I cells of duodenum and jejunum	Small peptides and amino acids Fatty acids and monoglycerides	↑ Contraction of gallbladder and relaxation of sphincter of Oddi ↑ Pancreatic enzyme and HCO_3^- secretion ↑ Growth of exocrine pancreas and gallbladder ↓ Gastric emptying (allows more time for digestion and absorption)
Secretin	S cells of duodenum	H^+ in duodenal lumen Fatty acids in duodenal lumen	↓ Small intestinal H^+ ↑ Pancreatic HCO_3^- secretion ↑ Biliary HCO_3^- secretion ↓ Gastric H^+ secretion ↑ Growth of exocrine pancreas
GIP	K cells of small intestine	Fatty acids, amino acids, oral glucose	↑ Insulin release ↓ H^+ secretion by gastric parietal cells
Motilin	Epithelial cells of duodenum	Periodic (not responsive to food)	↑ Propulsion of smooth muscle
Glucagonlike peptide 1	L cells of small intestine	Meal intake	↑ Insulin secretion ↓ GI motility
Ghrelin	P/D1 cells of stomach	Fasting	↑ Gastric emptying Stimulates feeding
Paracrines			
Somatostatin	D cells throughout GI tract	H^+ in GI tract lumen Inhibited by vagal stimulation	↓ Release of all GI hormones ↓ Gastric H^+ secretion ↓ Pancreatic secretions ↓ Splanchnic blood flow
Histamine	Mast cells of gastric mucosa	Vagal stimulation gastrin	↑ Gastric H^+ secretion
Nitric oxide	Enteric nerves	Cellular inflammation	↑ Epithelial secretion Vasodilation Smooth muscle relaxation
Neurocrines			
VIP	GI tract neurons	H^+ in duodenal lumen	Smooth muscle relaxation ↑ Pancreatic HCO_3^- secretion ↑ Fluid and electrolyte secretion from intestinal epithelium and bile duct cholangiocytes ↓ Gastric H^+ secretion
Gastrin-releasing peptide	Vagus nerves that innervate G cells	Vagal stimulation	↑ Gastrin release from G cells
Enkephalins (met-enkephalin, leu-enkephalin)	GI tract mucosa and smooth muscle neurons		↑ Contraction of GI smooth muscle ↓ Intestinal secretion of fluid and electrolytes

GIP = glucose-dependent insulinotropic polypeptide (*formerly* gastric inhibitory peptide); GRP = gastrin-releasing peptide; VIP = vasoactive intestinal peptide. G, I, S, K, L D cells are typical cells of a part of the intestine producing an endocrine substance: e.g. G cells of the antrum produce gastrin.

of parasympathetic stimulation.[11] It is theorized that the hypersalivation, or sialorrhea, associated with clozapine is related to agonism of parasympathetic muscarinic receptors or antagonism of adrenergic α receptors (resulting in unopposed β-adrenergic receptor–mediated vasodilation).[6] Conversely, dysfunction of saliva production, via the anticholinergic side effects of other antipsychotics, leads to dry mouth, or xerostomia.

Esophagus

The esophagus is a distensible muscular tube that extends from the epiglottis to the gastroesophageal junction. The lumen of the esophagus narrows at several points along its course, first at the cricopharyngeus muscle, then midway down alongside the aortic arch, and then distally where it crosses the diaphragm. The upper esophageal sphincter (UES) and lower esophageal sphincter (LES) are physiologic high-pressure regions that remain closed except during swallowing. Although the LES is a functional segment without anatomic features, the UES is marked by the presence of striated muscle.

The wall of the esophagus reflects the general structural organization of the GI tract noted previously, consisting of mucosa, submucosa, muscularis propria, and adventitia. The mucosal layer has 3 components. The nonkeratinizing stratified squamous epithelial layer faces the lumen; provides protection for underlying tissue; and houses several specialized cell types such as melanocytes, endocrine cells, dendritic cells, and lymphocytes. The lamina propria is the nonepithelialized portion of the mucosa, and the muscularis mucosa, a layer of longitudinally oriented smooth muscle bundles, is the third component.

The submucosa consists of loose connective tissue, and submucosal glands secrete a mucin-containing fluid via squamous epithelium–lined ducts, which facilitates lubrication of the esophageal lumen. The muscularis propria consists of an inner circular and outer longitudinal coat of smooth muscle; this layer also contains striated muscle fibers in the proximal esophagus that are responsible for voluntary swallowing.

The esophagus has no serosal lining. Only small segments of the intraabdominal esophagus are covered by adventitia, a sheathlike structure that also surrounds the adjacent great vessels, tracheobronchial tree, and other structures of the mediastinum.

The esophagus provides a conduit for food and fluids from the pharynx to the stomach, and the sphincters generally prevent reflux of gastric contents into the esophagus. Normal transit of food involves coordinated motor activity, including a wave of peristaltic contraction, relaxation of the LES (facilitated by nitric oxide and VIP), and subsequent closure of the LES (facilitated by several hormones and neurotransmitters such as gastrin, acetylcholine, serotonin, and motilin). Xenobiotics alter muscle tone in various segments of the esophagus, altering function. Caffeine is associated with relaxation of the LES and decreased peristalsis, increasing incidence of acid reflux.[34] Calcium channel blockers, nitroglycerin, β-adrenergic antagonists and phosphodiesterase inhibitors all relax esophageal smooth muscle, decreasing the pathologically elevated esophageal tone common to patients with achalasia.[9] Because of the rapid transit time of swallowed substances xenobiotics through this portion of the GI tract, digestion does not take place, and passive diffusion of xenobiotics from the food into the bloodstream is prevented.[11,59]

Stomach

The stomach is a saccular organ covered entirely by peritoneum that has a capacity greater than 3 L. The stomach is divided into 5 anatomic regions: the cardia, fundus, corpus or body, antrum, and pyloric sphincter. The gastric wall consists of mucosa, submucosa, muscularis propria, and serosa. The interior surface of the stomach is marked by coarse rugae, or longitudinal folds. The mucosa is composed of a superficial epithelial cell compartment and a deep glandular compartment. The mucous glands of the cardia, fundus, and body secrete mucus and pepsinogen. Oxyntic, or acid-forming, glands located in the fundus and body contain parietal, chief, and endocrine cells. The parietal cells contain vesicles that house hydrochloric acid–secreting proton pumps and secrete intrinsic factor, a substance necessary for the ileal absorption of vitamin B_{12}. Chief cells secrete the proteolytic proenzyme pepsinogen, which is cleaved to its active form, pepsin, upon exposure to the low luminal gastric pH of 3 to 4. Pepsin is subsequently inactivated in the duodenum when the pH increases to 6.0. The endocrine, or enterochromaffinlike (ECL), cells found in the mucosa of the body of the stomach produce histamine, which increases acid production and decreases gastric pH by stimulating H_2 receptors on the parietal cells. Somatostatin and endothelin, both modulators of acid production, are also produced in ECL cells (Fig. 49–4).

Hydrochloric acid is secreted when cephalic, gastric, and intestinal signals converge on the gastric parietal cells to activate proton pumps and release hydrochloric acid in an ATP-dependent process. During the cephalic phase, or the preparatory phase of the brain for eating and digestion,

acetylcholine is released from vagal afferents in response to sight, smell, taste, and chewing. Acetylcholine stimulates the parietal cells via muscarinic receptors, resulting in an increase in cytosolic calcium and activation of the proton pump. Antral G cells of the stomach, produce and release gastrin in response to luminal amino acids and peptides. Gastrin activates receptors within parietal cells, leading to a similar increase in cytosolic calcium. Additionally, gastrin and vagal afferents induce the release of histamine from ECL cells, which stimulates parietal cell H_2 receptors. Lastly, the intestinal phase is initiated when food containing digested protein enters the proximal small intestine and involves gastrin and several other polypeptides in the secretion of hydrochloric acid from the stomach[59] (Fig. 18–3).

The gastric mucosa is protected from gastric acidic secretions by several mechanisms, including a thin layer of surface mucus and channels that allow acid- and pepsin-containing fluids to exit glands without contact with the surface epithelium. Additionally, surface epithelium secretes bicarbonate, raising the pH at the cell surface. Prostaglandins produced in the mucosal cells stimulate production of bicarbonate and mucus, and inhibit parietal cell production of acid; prostaglandin inhibition by nonsteroidal antiinflammatory drugs (NSAIDs) plays an important role in the pathogenesis of peptic ulcer disease (PUD).[59]

In the stomach, ingested products are ground to particle sizes of less than 0.2 mm, which are then further processed and digested in preparation for absorption of nutrients in the small intestine. Many xenobiotics are weak acids that are no longer ionized in the acidic environment of the stomach, facilitating absorption through the lipid bilayer in the stomach. Other factors that affect xenobiotic absorption include particle size, transit time, and type of drug delivery system. Different drug formulations, such as time release, enteric coating, slowly dissolving matrices, dissolution control via osmotic pumps, ion exchange resins, and pH-sensitive mechanisms, affect bioavailability and the site of maximal release within the GI tract.

The time required for gastric emptying is determined by the complex interplay of innervation, muscle action, underlying illness, and xenobiotic exposure. Digestion and absorption are time-dependent processes, and optimal absorption requires adjustment of the luminal environment through secretion of ions and water, to accommodate meals that vary considerably in nutrient composition, water content, and density. Osmoreceptors and chemoreceptors in the GI tract adjust the digestive and absorptive processes by regulating transit and secretion using a variety of neurocrine, paracrine, and endocrine mechanisms. Interference with this integrated response either leads to stasis and bacterial overgrowth or to rapid transit with decreased absorption and development of diarrhea. Many mediators affect motility, including common neurotransmitters, such as acetylcholine and norepinephrine; hormones; cytokines; and inflammatory compounds. In general, whereas parasympathetic impulses promote motility, sympathetic stimulation inhibits motility. Other neurotransmitters, such as serotonin, promote transit, but dopamine and enkephalins slow motility. Some xenobiotics, such as opioids and diphenhydramine, delay gastric emptying, but other xenobiotics, such as metoclopramide, enhance gastric emptying. Our understanding of the complex neuroendocrine gastric axis continues to evolve in attempts to explain relatively new phenomenon, such as the cannabinoid hyperemesis syndrome, which appears to be caused by cannabinoid receptors in the brain or gut.[52]

Small and Large Intestines

In an average adult, the small intestine is approximately 6 m in length and begins retroperitoneally as the duodenum, becoming intraperitoneal at the jejunum and ileum. The boundary between the small intestine and large intestine is the ileocecal valve, and the large intestine typically measures 1.5 m in an adult. The large intestine (or colon) is further divided into cecal, ascending, transverse, descending, and sigmoid segments. The sigmoid colon is continuous with the rectum and terminates at the anus. Whereas anterograde and retrograde peristalsis occurs in the small intestine, anterograde peristalsis predominates in the large intestine. This movement allows for mixing of food, maximizes contact with the mucosa, and is mediated by

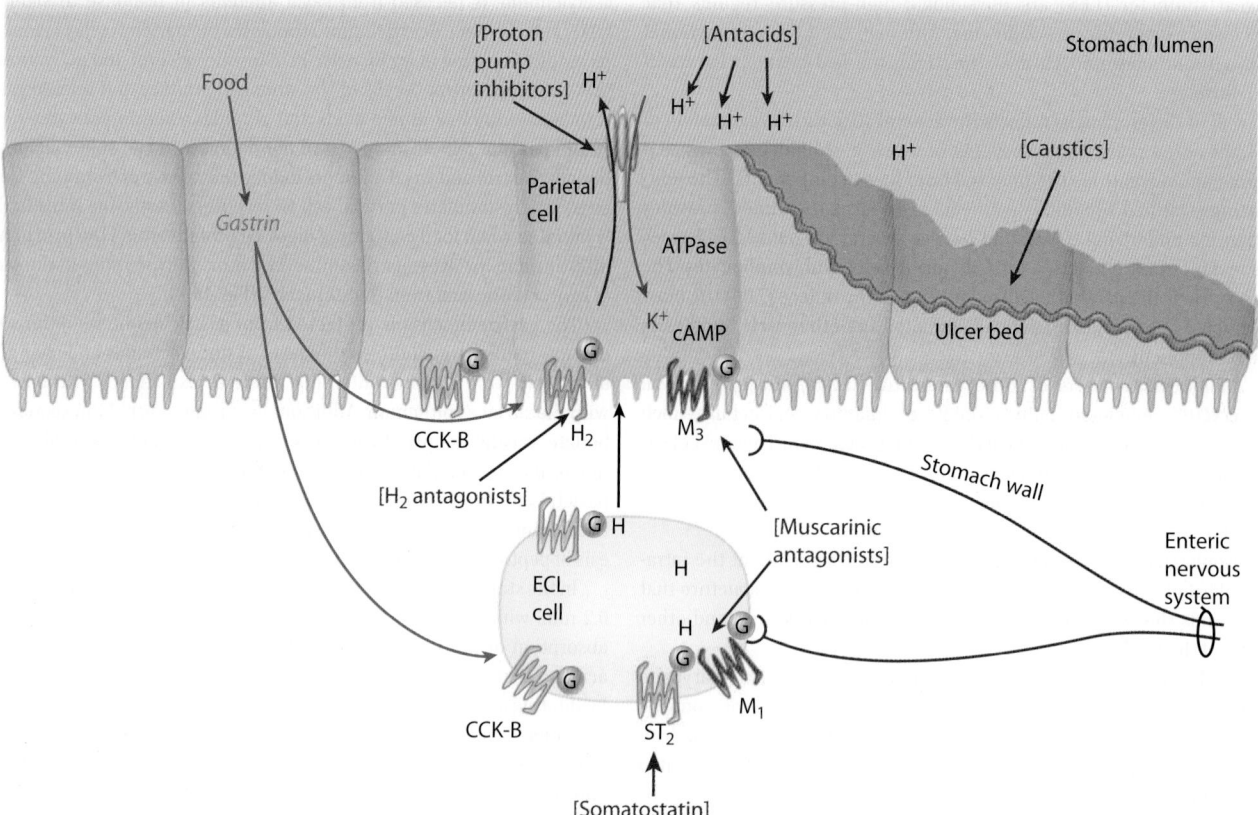

FIGURE 18–3. Effects of various xenobiotics on the gastrointestinal tract. CCK-B = cholecystokinin receptor B; ECL cell = enterochromaffinlike cell; H = histamine; H_2 = histamine-2 (H_2) receptor; M_1, M_3 = muscarinic receptors; ST_2 = somatostatin-2 receptor.

both the extrinsic and intrinsic nervous systems. The remarkable absorptive capacity of the small intestine is made possible by innumerable villi of the intestinal wall, which extend into the lumen and increase absorptive area. The epithelial border of the small intestine also contains mucin-secreting goblet cells, endocrine cells, and specialized absorptive cells; functionally, these cells create an ideal environment for nutrient absorption. The mucosa of the large intestine is devoid of villi. The large intestine functions primarily to absorb electrolytes and water, secrete potassium, salvage any remaining nutrients, and store and release waste. Intestinal epithelial cells also metabolize xenobiotics, a function typically attributed to the liver (see below).

Regeneration of injured or senescent intestinal epithelial cells begins in the crypts, with differentiation occurring as these cells migrate toward the intestinal lumen. This process occurs rapidly, with turnover of the small intestinal epithelium occurring every 4 to 6 days and large intestinal epithelium turnover occurring every 3 to 8 days. This rapid regeneration leaves the intestinal epithelium vulnerable to processes that interfere with cell replication (eg, radiation, chemotherapy). Sloughing of GI epithelium, typically manifested by hemorrhagic enteritis, is a valuable marker for xenobiotic insults that lead to mitotic arrest.

Pancreas

The pancreas is a retroperitoneal organ that serves both exocrine and endocrine functions. The exocrine portion of the gland produces digestive enzymes and occupies more than 80% to 85% of the mass of the pancreas. The exocrine pancreas is composed of acinar cells, specialized epithelial cells housing zymogen granules that release digestive enzymes and proenzymes into the duodenum. Columnar epithelial cells produce mucin, and ductal cuboidal epithelial cells secrete a bicarbonate-rich fluid that neutralizes gastric acids. The pancreas secretes 2 to 2.5 L/day of this mixed solution. Typically, the digestive enzymes are released as proenzymes, such as trypsinogen, chymotrypsinogen, and procarboxypeptidase, which are activated on contact with the higher pH of the duodenum; this process

usually helps to prevent autodigestion of the pancreas itself. Enzymes on the brush border of the duodenum, including enteropeptidase, cleave proenzymes to their active forms. Only pancreatic amylase and lipase are secreted in their active forms.

Secretion of pancreatic enzymes is regulated by multiple factors, the most important of which are cholecystokinin and secretin, both produced in the duodenum. Cholecystokinin is released from the duodenum in response to fatty acids and the products of protein catabolism such as peptides and amino acids. Cholecystokinin stimulates acinar cells to release digestive enzymes and proenzymes. Secretin is released by the duodenum in the presence of the decrease in pH caused by gastric acids and luminal fatty acids. Secretin triggers ductal cells to secrete bicarbonate and water. Acetylcholine also plays a role in the regulation of pancreatic exocrine function by stimulating digestive enzyme secretion from the acinus and potentiating the effects of secretin. Vagal reflexes increase acetylcholinergic tone in the setting of decreased pH, protein breakdown products, and fatty acids in the duodenal lumen.

The endocrine portion of the pancreas is composed of approximately one million clusters of cells known as the islets of Langerhans that secrete insulin, glucagon, and somatostatin. Other products of the endocrine pancreas include serotonin and VIP. Injury to the endocrine pancreas or alteration of physiologic functions often results in impaired glucose homeostasis, diabetes, and exocrine insufficiencies.[21,46] Calcium channel blockers interfere with Ca^{2+}-dependent insulin release, resulting in hyperglycemia. Sulfonylureas close ATP-sensitive K^+-channels, stimulating insulin release.

XENOBIOTIC METABOLISM

Although the liver is usually identified as the site of xenobiotic metabolism, a significant amount of CYP and other metabolic enzymes are found in the luminal GI tract, contributing to hydroxylation, sulfation, acetylation, and glucuronidation. In descending order, CYP3A, CYP2C9, and CYP2C19 are the most abundant CYP families in the small intestine.[39] Biotransformation, especially reduction and hydrolysis, is also a property of luminal bacteria.

Gut microbiomes can alter the metabolism of dozens of pharmaceuticals, in many cases changing their efficacy and side effect profiles.[53] First-pass metabolism by the intestine affects the amount of orally administered xenobiotic that enters hepatic portal circulation and, therefore, contributes greatly to the first-pass effect, or presystemic disposition.

One of the most well-described families of export proteins, P-glycoprotein (P-gp), is found in the mucosa of the small and large intestines, hepatocytes, adrenal cortex, renal tubules, and capillary cells lining the blood–brain barrier.[62] The P-gps are susceptible to induction and inhibition in a manner similar to hepatic cytochrome oxidase enzymes. Many of the inhibitors of CYP3A have inhibitory effects on P-gps. Inhibitors of P-gps raise serum concentrations of a xenobiotic, and inducers of P-gps have the potential to prevent therapeutic drug concentrations from ever reaching the target cell. The P-gp system is important in drug interactions and drug resistance (Chap. 9). Novel nanocarrier drug delivery systems containing both substrates and inhibitors of P-gps mitigate some of these effects.[47]

Postoperative Effects on the Gastrointestinal Tract

Anatomic and functional changes after bariatric surgery and bowel resection have important effects on drug bioavailability and toxicity. The common Roux-en-Y gastric bypass surgery, which diverts gastric contents into the distal small bowel, increases bioavailability by bypassing intestinal CYP3A and decreases bioavailability by bypassing the proximal jejunum as an area of drug absorption.[15] Alterations in stomach and bowel pH after surgery affect absorption of ionized drugs. Disruption of the enterohepatic recirculation enhances elimination of xenobiotics such as digoxin.[61] Many xenobiotics, such as ethanol, oral morphine, and caffeine, achieve maximum serum concentrations faster because of rapid transit. However, studies evaluating serum concentrations of known CYP substrates (caffeine [CYP1A2], tolbutamide [CYP2C9], omeprazole [CYP219], and midazolam [CYP3A]) in patients with gastric bypass surgery have not found any clinically significant changes in drug metabolism.[55] Because specific data are limited, current recommendations for dosing in postoperative patients are based on extrapolating from a xenobiotic site of absorption and kinetics and a particular patient's functional GI anatomy.

PATHOLOGIC CONDITIONS OF THE GASTROINTESTINAL TRACT

Oral Pathology

Discoloration of the teeth is reported with a number of medications, most notably tetracyclines (Table 18–2). Gingival hyperplasia, overgrowth of the gums around the teeth, is an uncommon adverse effect from chronic use of several xenobiotics. Some medications implicated in causing gingival hyperplasia include calcium channel blockers, cyclosporine, lithium, phenobarbital, phenytoin, topiramate, and valproic acid.[1] Xerostomia, or pathologic dryness of the mouth, is an uncomfortable effect of many xenobiotics that lead to increased dental decay. The list of xenobiotics that cause xerostomia

TABLE 18–2	Xenobiotics Causing Discoloration of the Teeth and Gums
Betel nut	Red
Cadmium	Yellow
Chlorhexidine oral rinse	Brown
Ciprofloxacin	Green
Doxycycline	Yellow
Fluoride	White flecking
Lead	Blue line
Quinine	Blue-gray or blue-black
Silver	Brown-gray to blue-gray
Tetracycline	Yellow to brown-gray

TABLE 18–3	Xenobiotics That Commonly Cause Xerostomia
α_1-Adrenergic antagonists	
α_2-Adrenergic agonists	
Amphetamines	
Anticholinergics	
Antidepressants (cyclic antidepressants, maprotiline)	
Antipsychotics	
H_1 antagonists	
Protease inhibitors	

is extensive, but the most common classes of xenobiotics causing xerostomia are listed in Table 18–3.[1] Chronic methamphetamine use is linked to characteristic oral pathology known as "meth mouth." This condition, which is common in both inhalational and intravenous users, is characterized by extensive and severe tooth decay and is linked to poor hygiene, bruxism, and xerostomia associated with methamphetamine use.[12] Notably, a case report involved a similar pattern of tooth decay in a heavy user of cocaine, heroin, and marijuana (not methamphetamine), thought to be related to sugary foods, lack of oral hygiene, and xerostomia.[28]

Esophagitis and Dysphagia

Xenobiotic-induced esophageal injury includes esophagitis (including pill esophagitis), ulceration, erosion, impacted pill fragments, perforation, and stricture.[27] The most common presenting complaint is a foreign body sensation in the throat.[26] Xenobiotics commonly implicated in esophagitis and esophageal ulcerations are listed in Table 18–4. Patients with preexisting esophageal motility disorders are at higher risk of esophageal pathology. Additionally, xenobiotics with a gelatin matrix, rapid dissolvability, and large size predispose to esophageal injury. Although most symptoms resolve with withdrawal of the offending xenobiotics, patients with persistent or severe odynophagia should be evaluated with endoscopy to identify pathology and prevent perforation caused by retained pills.

Webs, Strictures, and Esophageal Malignancy

Caustic injury is one of the most common causes of esophageal strictures and malignancies (Chap. 103). Some authors also postulate the role of pill esophagitis in the evolution of esophageal strictures.[8] As many as 4% of patients with esophageal cancer report a history of caustic injury, and patients with a prior history of caustic ingestion have more than a 1,000-fold higher risk of developing an esophageal malignancy than the general population.[29] Other xenobiotics known to cause esophageal strictures include aluminum phosphide and ionizing radiation.[54]

Gastritis and Peptic Ulcer Disease

Gastritis, or inflammation of the gastric mucosa, and PUD are commonly related to xenobiotic exposure (Table 18–5). Symptoms of gastritis and PUD include epigastric pain, nausea, and vomiting as well as hematemesis and melena. The primary distinction between gastritis and PUD is appearance at endoscopy: whereas gastritis is characterized by diffuse inflammation

TABLE 18–4	Xenobiotics Implicated in Esophagitis and Esophageal Ulcerations
Antipsychotics	
Bisphosphonates	
Chemotherapeutics	
Nonsteroidal antiinflammatory drugs	
Potassium salts	
Quinine	
Radiation (ionizing)	
Salicylates	
Tetracycline	

TABLE 18–5	Xenobiotics Commonly Implicated in Gastritis and Peptic Ulcer Disease

Corticosteroids
Ethanol
Nicotine
Nonsteroidal antiinflammatory drugs
Radiation (ionizing)
Salicylates

TABLE 18–6	Xenobiotic-Induced Enteritis	
Mechanism	**Xenobiotic**
Mechanical irritation	Aloe
	Bacterial food poisoning
	Laxatives
	Mushrooms (GI irritant group)
Cholinergic stimulation	Carbamates
	Neostigmine, physostigmine, pyridostigmine
	Mushrooms (muscarine containing)
	Nicotine
	Organic phosphorus compounds
Inhibitors of mucosal regeneration (hemorrhagic enteritis)	Arsenic
	Chemotherapeutics
	Colchicine
	Iron
	Mercuric salts
	Monochloroacetic acid
	Podophyllin
	Pokeweed (*Phytolacca americana*)
	Radiation (ionizing)
Mitochondrial poison	Thallium

of the gastric mucosa, an ulcer is a discrete lesion of the mucosa. Nonsteroidal antiinflammatory drugs remain an important part of the pathogenesis of gastritis and PUD by interfering with prostaglandin synthesis and subsequently impairing the integrity of the gastric mucosal barrier to acid. Cyclooxygenase-2 (COX-2) selective inhibitors promised to decrease the incidence of gastric pathology caused by chronic NSAID use; however, unexpected cardiovascular side effects limited their utility. New xenobiotics are focusing on inhibition of other inflammatory mediators that have been previously overlooked, and coadministration of protective xenobiotics. 5-Lipoxygenase (5-LOX) inhibitors reduce production of proinflammatory leukotrienes, and when coadministered with COX inhibitors, they decrease gastric toxicity. Other reformulated NSAIDs are designed to release molecules of NO and H_2S, which help maintain gastric mucosal integrity. These next generation of drugs may preserve systemic antiinflammatory effects while enhancing the gastric safety profile.[42]

Long-term treatment of PUD with antacids, H_2 antagonists, or proton pump inhibitors leads to hypochlorhydria or achlorhydria, the reduction or absence of gastric acid, respectively. By increasing the pH of the stomach, these conditions increase risk of bacterial overgrowth (*C. difficile*), atrophic gastritis, osteoporosis, hip fracture (via impaired calcium absorption), *Salmonella* and *Vibrio cholerae* infection, gastric carcinoma and impaired magnesium absorption.[60]

Enteritis and Diarrhea
The symptoms of GI distress are nonspecifically associated with xenobiotic exposure. However, certain xenobiotics that increase peristalsis or impair fluid absorption result in significant diarrhea. Opioid withdrawal, colchicine overdose, and serotonin toxicity are important toxidromes that often feature diarrhea as a prominent symptom. The rapid turnover of the GI mucosa makes it uniquely susceptible to xenobiotics that cause cell death and mitotic arrest. Hemorrhagic enteritis, manifested by hematochezia, is a characteristic finding of certain exposures (Table 18–6).

Bezoars
The term *bezoar* refers to a concretion formed anywhere in the alimentary system and is a rare complication of overdose. The risk of bezoar formation is increased in cases of massive pill ingestion and varies according to tablet size, adhesiveness, and liquid viscosity.[51] Comorbid illnesses or toxicities that delay gastric emptying and bowel transit time increase the risk of bezoar formation. Effects from bezoars range from mechanical obstruction to severe local irritation (and stricture formation) to continuous delayed absorption of xenobiotics and resulting toxicity. Suspicion for bezoar formation is raised in patients after ingestion who develop signs of obstruction (vomiting, abdominal pain, constipation) and in patients with delayed or prolonged toxicity (eg, rising serum iron concentrations 8 hours following ingestion) after overdose.[51] Depending on the nature of the bezoar, the diagnosis will be achieved by plain radiography; however, in some instances, computed tomography (CT) with oral contrast increases sensitivity. Recent studies have had limited success with ultrasonography as a diagnostic adjuvant, although this requires further study. Ultimately, a high suspicion of bezoar with negative radiographic evaluation findings should prompt consideration of direct visualization with endoscopy and colonoscopy or exploratory surgery. Bezoars frequently require surgical intervention, and several cases report dramatic recovery after removal.

Pancreatitis
Pancreatitis is an acute inflammatory process that results in autolysis of the pancreas from digestive enzymes. Cases range from mild to severe, with an overall mortality rate of 5%.[18] The most common causes of pancreatitis are alcohol abuse and gall bladder disease; however, nonalcoholic xenobiotic-induced pancreatitis accounts for 0.1% to 2% of cases of acute pancreatitis.[5] Populations at higher risk of xenobiotic-induced pancreatitis include children, women, elderly adults, and patients with HIV and inflammatory bowel disease.[5] Acute pancreatitis is defined as having 2 of the following 3 criteria: (1) abdominal pain consistent with acute pancreatitis, (2) serum amylase or lipase greater than 3 times the upper limit of normal (although amylase, which is also released by salivary glands, is less specific and often unnecessary), and (3) characteristic findings of acute pancreatitis on CT scan.[57] The diagnosis of xenobiotic-induced pancreatitis can be impossible to confirm because no diagnostic test or pattern of injury distinguishes xenobiotic-induced pancreatitis from other etiologies. However, the symptoms and laboratory abnormalities associated with xenobiotic-induced pancreatitis tend to resolve shortly after withdrawal of the offending xenobiotic; again, this is often challenging to differentiate from the natural course of mild to moderate disease. It is unclear whether rechallenge with an offending xenobiotic will cause pancreatitis again; however, any xenobiotic suspected of causing pancreatitis should be withheld unless the benefits outweigh this risk. The management of xenobiotic-induced pancreatitis does not differ from other causes and hinges on volume resuscitation, bowel rest, and careful monitoring.

Numerous xenobiotics are associated with pancreatitis, each with varying levels of quality and quantity of evidence; representative xenobiotics are listed in Table 18–7.[4,24] The pathogenic mechanism varies among xenobiotics. The nucleoside reverse transcriptase inhibitor didanosine and dioxin promote pancreatitis as a result of mitochondrial injury.[38,45,49] Cholinergic xenobiotics, such as parathion and certain scorpion venoms, result in pancreatitis caused by overstimulation.[30,43] Vasospasm and ischemia are also a purported mechanism, as in cases of pancreatitis secondary to ergot alkaloids.[14]

The endocrine functions of the pancreas are also susceptible to injury from pancreatitis or toxic insult. Typically, this results from injury to pancreatic β cells leading to impaired glucose homeostasis, similar to diabetes.

TABLE 18–7 Xenobiotics Commonly Associated with Pancreatitis

Alcohols: ethanol, methanol

Analgesics: acetaminophen, NSAIDs, codeine

Antibiotics: isoniazid, metronidazole, sulfonamides, tetracycline

Antiepileptics: valproic acid, carbamazepine

Antiretrovirals: didanosine, nelfinavir

Cardiovascular: ACE inhibitors and ARBs, methyldopa

Dioxin

Diuretics: loop diuretics

HMG-CoA reductase inhibitors

Hormones: corticosteroids, estrogens

Hypoglycemics: DPP-4 inhibitors

Immunosuppressants: azathioprine, corticosteroids, mesalamine

Pesticides: organic phosphorus compounds

Venoms: *Buthus quinquestriatus, Tityus discrepans*

ACE = angiotensin-converting enzyme; ARB = angiotensin II receptor blocker; DPP-4 = dipeptidyl peptidase-4 inhibitors; NSAIDs = nonsteroidal antiinflammatory drugs.

Streptozotocin is notable for its toxicity to pancreatic β cells and ability to induce diabetes in animal models. In one study of patients after episodes of alcoholic pancreatitis, more than one third developed impaired glucose tolerance.[46] There are rare xenobiotics that cause damage to α cells in animal models; however, they do not consistently cause hypoglycemia (Table 18–8).

Constipation

Decreased stooling (fewer than 3 bowel movements a week) associated with abdominal pain is a major source of morbidity for patients taking opioids and other drugs that slow gastric emptying and decrease gut motility. In its most extreme form, severe constipation is associated with bowel obstruction and perforation. The bowel function index, a simple 3-item assessment, is useful for assessing opioid induced constipation (OIC).[2] Novel therapeutics for OIC include peripherally acting μ-opioid receptor antagonists (PAMORAs) such as prolonged-release naloxone, methylnaltrexone, and naloxegol. Additional therapies aimed at altering fluid secretion include lubiprostone and linaclotide.[36] As OIC affects up to 40% of patients on long-term opioids, this is an active area of drug development.

FOREIGN BODIES

The esophagus is the most common site of impaction from symptomatic foreign bodies. They tend to be found just proximal to a pathologic esophageal narrowing or in one of 3 anatomic places: at the cervical esophagus near the cricopharyngeus muscle, at the level of the aortic arch, or just above the gastroesophageal junction. The likelihood that a foreign object will lodge in the esophagus is related to its size and shape. The major complications of foreign bodies in the esophagus include pain, bleeding, obstruction, or perforation, which sometimes lead to subsequent mediastinitis or fistula.

TABLE 18–8 Xenobiotics Associated with Endocrine Pancreatic Dysfunction

α Cells of the pancreas	
Cobalt salts	Decamethylene diguanidine

β Cells of the pancreas	
Alloxan	Glucocorticoids
Androgens	Growth hormone
Cyclizine	Pentamidine
Cyproheptadine	Somatostatin
Diazoxide	Streptozocin
Epinephrine	Sulfonamides
Glucagon	Vacor

They are often managed conservatively up to 12 hours after ingestion of the esophageal foreign body. If serial radiographs demonstrate no movement after 12 hours, endoscopic retrieval or surgery should be considered because the risk of perforation increases after that time; some authors extend this observation period to 24 hours.[25] Ingestion of button batteries proves an important exception to this rule. Esophageal button batteries can cause significant mucosal injury in 2 to 4 hours, with perforation in as little as 6 hours.[33] Proposed mechanisms for the rapid development of esophageal injury include alkaline burn, local current, and pressure necrosis (Chap. 103). Most recently, almost all button battery ingestions associated with serious or fatal outcomes were 20-mm lithium batteries, dangerous for their large size and higher voltage.[32,33,50] Of note, lithium batteries do not contain an alkali solution, lending support to the concept that electrical current results in morbidity rather than leakage of caustic battery contents. All suspected esophageal button batteries should therefore undergo immediate endoscopic removal within 2 hours; success rates with this modality are reported as excellent. Button batteries that are in the stomach or beyond should be allowed to pass spontaneously in asymptomatic patients. Some authors suggest removal of button batteries from the stomach to prevent injury.[40] Early research on specialized battery coatings to reduce mucosal injury during ingestion is promising.[31]

Foreign bodies are also commonly found in the stomach. Many small foreign bodies pass through the stomach and the remainder of the GI tract without difficulty. Objects greater than 5 cm in length or 2 cm in diameter are frequently unable to traverse the duodenum and require endoscopic or surgical removal. Foreign bodies beyond the duodenum usually do not require any intervention except observation; however, some objects become lodged at the ileocecal valve. Serial examinations and radiographs are used for asymptomatic patients; however, increasing abdominal pain or tenderness mandates further imaging and surgical consultation. Recent increase in pediatric ingestion of strong, small magnets present an exception to these recommendations. Multiple magnets attract across bowel walls, preventing transit and leading to intestinal perforation. Ingestion of a single magnet does not increase morbidity and should be managed as a benign foreign body above, but the ingestion of multiple magnets should be managed aggressively with surgical consultation for removal.[56] Body packers represent an unusual exception to these rules. Patients who are discovered to be internally concealing large quantities of illicit drugs frequently require whole-bowel irrigation to facilitate transit of colonic packets and even emergency laparotomy for obstruction or suspected packet rupture in cases of cocaine or methamphetamine smuggling[58] (Special Considerations: SC5).

SUMMARY

- The GI tract is vulnerable to a wide variety of pathogenic organisms.
- The GI tract modulates absorption and metabolism of xenobiotics.
- Normal GI tract function is dependent on the presence of metabolically active endogenous flora.
- The GI tract involves a complex interplay of regulatory hormones.
- As function follows structure, effects of various xenobiotics are often related to the specific parts of the GI tract that are affected.

Acknowledgment

Kavita Babu, MD; Neal E. Flomenbaum, MD; Donald P. Kotler, MD; and Martin Jay Smilkstein, contributed to this chapter in previous editions.

REFERENCES

1. Abdollahi M, et al. Current opinion on drug-induced oral reactions: a comprehensive review. *J Contemp Dent Pract.* 2008;9:1-15.
2. Argoff CE, et al. Consensus recommendations on initiating prescription therapies for opioid-induced constipation. *Pain Med.* 2015;16:2324-2337.
3. Arumugam M, et al. Enterotypes of the human gut microbiome. *Nature.* 2011;473:174-180.
4. Badalov N, et al. Drug-induced acute pancreatitis: an evidence-based review. *Clin Gastroenterol Hepatol.* 2007;5:648-661; quiz 644.
5. Balani AR, Grendell JH. Drug-induced pancreatitis: incidence, management and prevention. *Drug Saf.* 2008;31:823-837.

6. Bird AM, et al. Current treatment strategies for clozapine-induced sialorrhea. *Ann Pharmacother.* 2011;45:667-675.

7. Bohorquez DV, Liddle RA. Gastrointestinal hormones and neurotransmitters. In: Sleisenger MH, Feldman M, Friedman LS, et al, eds. *Sleisenger and Fordtran's Gastrointestinal and Liver Disease: Pathophysiology, Diagnosis, Management.* 10th ed. Philadelphia, PA: Saunders/Elsevier; 2015: 36-56.

8. Bonavina L, et al. Drug-induced esophageal strictures. *Ann Surg.* 1987;206:173-183.

9. Bortolotti M, et al. Effects of sildenafil on esophageal motility of patients with idiopathic achalasia. *Gastroenterology.* 2000;118:253-257.

10. Constantine PA. Antibiotic therapy and serum digoxin toxicity. *Am Fam Physician.* 1998;57:1239-1240.

11. Costanzo LS. *Physiology.* 6th ed. ed. Philadelphia, PA: Elsevier; 2018.

12. Curtis EK. Meth mouth: a review of methamphetamine abuse and its oral manifestations. *Gen Dent.* 2006;54:125-129; quiz 130.

13. Dethlefsen L, Relman DA. Incomplete recovery and individualized responses of the human distal gut microbiota to repeated antibiotic perturbation. *Proc Natl Acad Sci U S A.* 2011;108(suppl 1):4554-4561.

14. Deviere J, et al. Ischemic pancreatitis and hepatitis secondary to ergotamine poisoning. *J Clin Gastroenterol.* 1987;9:350-352.

15. Edwards A, Ensom MHH. Pharmacokinetic effects of bariatric surgery. *Ann Pharmacother.* 2012;46:130-136.

16. Festi D, et al. Gut microbiota and metabolic syndrome. *World J Gastroenterol.* 2014;20:16079-16094.

17. Gionchetti P, et al. Prophylaxis of pouchitis onset with probiotic therapy: a double-blind, placebo-controlled trial. *Gastroenterology.* 2003;124:1202-1209.

18. Granger J, Remick D. Acute pancreatitis: models, markers, and mediators. *Shock.* 2005;24(suppl 1):45-51.

19. Guarner F, Malagelada JR. Gut flora in health and disease. *Lancet.* 2003;361:512-519.

20. Hempel S, et al. Probiotics for the prevention and treatment of antibiotic-associated diarrhea: a systematic review and meta-analysis. *JAMA.* 2012;307:1959-1969.

21. Ho TW, et al. Change of both endocrine and exocrine insufficiencies after acute pancreatitis in non-diabetic patients: a nationwide population-based study. *Medicine (Baltimore).* 2015;94:e1123.

22. Johnston BC, et al. Probiotics for the prevention of pediatric antibiotic-associated diarrhea. *Cochrane Database Syst Rev.* 2011:CD004827.

23. Jourova L, et al. Human gut microbiota plays a role in the metabolism of drugs. *Biomed Pap Med Fac Univ Palacky Olomouc Czech Repub.* 2016;160:317-326.

24. Kale-Pradhan PB, Wilhelm SM. Pancreatitis. In: Tisdale JE, Miller DA, eds. *Drug-Induced Diseases: Prevention, Detection, and Management.* 2nd ed. Bethesda, MD: American Society of Health-System Pharmacists; 2010: 800-818.

25. Kay M, Wyllie R. Pediatric foreign bodies and their management. *Curr Gastroenterol Rep.* 2005;7:212-218.

26. Kikendall JW. Pill esophagitis. *J Clin Gastroenterol.* 1999;28:298-305.

27. Kim SH, et al. Clinical and endoscopic characteristics of drug-induced esophagitis. *World J Gastroenterol.* 2014;20:10994-10999.

28. Ko BE. "Meth Mouth" in a non-methamphetamine user. *J Mich Dent Assoc.* 2015;97:62-64.

29. Kochhar R, et al. Corrosive induced carcinoma of esophagus: report of three patients and review of literature. *J Gastroenterol Hepatol.* 2006;21:777-780.

30. Lankisch PG, et al. Painless acute pancreatitis subsequent to anticholinesterase insecticide (parathion) intoxication. *Am J Gastroenterol.* 1990;85:872-875.

31. Laulicht B, et al. Simple battery armor to protect against gastrointestinal injury from accidental ingestion. *Proc Natl Acad Sci U S A.* 2014;111:16490-16495.

32. Litovitz T, et al. Preventing battery ingestions: an analysis of 8648 cases. *Pediatrics.* 2010;125:1178-1183.

33. Litovitz T, et al. Emerging battery-ingestion hazard: clinical implications. *Pediatrics.* 2010;125:1168-1177.

34. Lohsiriwat S, et al. Effect of caffeine on lower esophageal sphincter pressure in Thai healthy volunteers. *Dis Esophagus.* 2006;19:183-188.

35. MacDonald TT, et al. Regulation of homeostasis and inflammation in the intestine. *Gastroenterology.* 2011;140:1768-1775.

36. Nelson AD, Camilleri M. Opioid-induced constipation: advances and clinical guidance. *Ther Adv Chronic Dis.* 2016;7:121-134.

37. Neutra MR. M cells in antigen sampling in mucosal tissues. *Curr Top Microbiol Immunol.* 1999;236:17-32.

38. Nyska A, et al. Exocrine pancreatic pathology in female Harlan Sprague-Dawley rats after chronic treatment with 2,3,7,8-tetrachlorodibenzo-*p*-dioxin and dioxin-like compounds. *Environ Health Perspect.* 2004;112:903-909.

39. Paine MF, et al. The human intestinal cytochrome P450 "pie." *Drug Metab Dispos.* 2006;34:880-886.

40. Patoulias I, et al. Multiple gastric erosion early after a 3 V lithium battery (CR2025) ingestion in an 18-month-old male patient: consideration about the proper time of intervention. *Case Rep Pediatr.* 2016;2016:3965393.

41. Peppercorn MA. Sulfasalazine. Pharmacology, clinical use, toxicity, and related new drug development. *Ann Intern Med.* 1984;101:377-386.

42. Pereira-Leite C, et al. Nonsteroidal anti-inflammatory therapy: a journey toward safety. *Med Res Rev.* 2017;37:802-859.

43. Possani LD, et al. Discharge effect on pancreatic exocrine secretion produced by toxins purified from *Tityus serrulatus* scorpion venom. *J Biol Chem.* 1991;266:3178-3185.

44. Powell N, et al. The mucosal immune system: master regulator of bidirectional gut-brain communications. *Nat Rev Gastroenterol Hepatol.* 2017;14:143-159.

45. Rozman K, et al. Histopathology of interscapular brown adipose tissue, thyroid, and pancreas in 2,3,7,8-tetrachlorodibenzo-*p*-dioxin (TCDD)-treated rats. *Toxicol Appl Pharmacol.* 1986;82:551-559.

46. Sand J, Nordback I. Acute pancreatitis: risk of recurrence and late consequences of the disease. *Nat Rev Gastroenterol Hepatol.* 2009;6:470-477.

47. Saneja A, et al. Co-formulation of *P*-glycoprotein substrate and inhibitor in nanocarriers: an emerging strategy for cancer chemotherapy. *Curr Cancer Drug Targets.* 2014;14:419-433.

48. Scarpellini E, et al. Gut microbiota and obesity. *Intern Emerg Med.* 2010;5(suppl 1): S53-S56.

49. Seidlin M, et al. Pancreatitis and pancreatic dysfunction in patients taking dideoxyinosine. *AIDS.* 1992;6:831-835.

50. Sharpe SJ, et al. Pediatric battery-related emergency department visits in the United States, 1990-2009. *Pediatrics.* 2012;129:1111-1117.

51. Simpson SE. Pharmacobezoars described and demystified. *Clin Toxicol (Phila).* 2011;49:72-89.

52. Sorensen CJ, et al. Cannabinoid hyperemesis syndrome: diagnosis, pathophysiology, and treatment—a systematic review. *J Med Toxicol.* 2017;13:71-87.

53. Spanogiannopoulos P, et al. The microbial pharmacists within us: a metagenomic view of xenobiotic metabolism. *Nat Rev Micro* 2016;14:273-287.

54. Talukdar R, et al. Aluminium phosphide-induced esophageal stricture. *Indian J Gastroenterol.* 2006;25:98-99.

55. Tandra S, et al. Effect of Roux-en-Y gastric bypass surgery on the metabolism of the orally administered medications. Paper presented at: Digestive Disease Week; May 7-11, 2011; Chicago, IL.

56. Tavarez MM, et al. Prevalence, clinical features and management of pediatric magnetic foreign body ingestions. *J Emerg Med.* 2013;44:261-268.

57. Tenner S, et al. American College of Gastroenterology guideline: management of acute pancreatitis. *Am J Gastroenterol.* 2013;108:1400-1415; 1416.

58. Traub SJ, et al. Body packing—the internal concealment of illicit drugs. *N Engl J Med.* 2003;349:2519-2526.

59. Robbins SL, et al, eds. *Robbins and Cotran: Pathologic Basis of Disease.* 8th ed. Philadelphia, PA: Saunders/Elsevier; 2010.

60. Vakil N. Prescribing proton pump inhibitors: is it time to pause and rethink? *Drugs.* 2012;72:437-445.

61. Ward N. The impact of intestinal failure on oral drug absorption: a review. *J Gastrointest Surg.* 2010;14:1045-1051.

62. Yu DK. The contribution of *P*-glycoprotein to pharmacokinetic drug-drug interactions. *J Clin Pharmacol.* 1999;39:1203-1211.

19 GENITOURINARY PRINCIPLES

Jason Chu

The genitourinary system encompasses 2 major organ systems, the reproductive and the urinary systems. Successful reproduction requires interaction between 2 sexually mature individuals. Xenobiotic exposures to either individual can have an adverse impact on fertility, which is the successful production of children, and fecundity, which is an individual's or a couple's capacity to produce children. The role of occupational and environmental exposures in the development of infertility is difficult to define.[12,42,88] Well-designed and conclusive epidemiologic studies are lacking because of the following factors: laboratory tests used to evaluate fertility are relatively unreliable, clinical endpoints are unclear, xenobiotic exposure is difficult to monitor, and indicators of biologic effects are imprecise. Although the negative impact of xenobiotics on fertility is often ignored, infertility evaluations are incomplete without a thorough xenobiotic exposure and occupational history. Differences in the toxicity of xenobiotics in individuals are sex related, age related, or both. Xenobiotic-related, primary infertility is the result of effects on the hypothalamic–pituitary–gonadal axis or a direct toxic effect on the gonads.[76] Fertility is also affected by exposures that cause abnormal sexual performance. Table 19–1 lists xenobiotics associated with infertility.

Aphrodisiacs are used to heighten sexual desire and to counteract sexual dysfunction. Humans have long sought the perfect aphrodisiac. However, of those tried, their effectiveness is variable, and toxic consequences occur commonly. Particularly popular are the various treatments for male sexual dysfunction, or erectile dysfunction.

Although many people search for a cure for impotence or infertility, others explore xenobiotics that can be used as abortifacients. Routes of administration used include oral, parenteral, and intravaginal, with an end result of pregnancy termination. However, many of these xenobiotics produce systemic toxic effects on the mother and a nonaborted fetus.

This chapter examines these issues, as well as the impact of xenobiotics on the urinary system, specifically, urinary retention and incontinence, and abnormalities detected in urine specimens. Renal (Chap. 27), reproductive (Chap. 31), and oncologic (Chap. 23) principles are discussed elsewhere in this text.

MALE FERTILITY

Male fertility is dependent on a normal reproductive system and normal sexual function. The male reproductive system is composed of the central nervous system (CNS) endocrine organs and the male gonads. The hypothalamus and the anterior pituitary gland form the CNS portion of the male reproductive system. Both organs begin low-level hormone secretion as early as in utero gestation. At puberty, the hypothalamus begins pulsatile secretion of gonadotropin-releasing hormone (GnRH). This stimulates the anterior pituitary gland to release follicle-stimulating hormone (FSH) and luteinizing hormone (LH) in a similarly pulsatile fashion. The hormones exert their effects on the male target organs, inducing spermatogenesis and secondary body sexual characteristics.

Disruption of the normal function of any part of the system affects fertility. A number of xenobiotics adversely affect the male reproductive system and sexual function as shown in Fig. 19–1.

Spermatogenesis

Central to the male reproductive system is the process of spermatogenesis, which occurs in the testes. The bulk of the testes consist of seminiferous tubules with germinal spermatogonia and Sertoli cells. The remainder of the gonadal tissue is interstitium with blood vessels, lymphatics, supporting

TABLE 19–1	Xenobiotics Associated with Infertility
Men	
Xenobiotic	*Effects*
Anabolic steroids	↓ LH, oligospermia
Androgens	↓ Testosterone production
Benzene	Chromosomal aberrations in sperm
Carbon disulfide	↓ FSH, ↓ LH, ↓ spermatogenesis
Chemotherapeutics	Gonadal toxicity
Chlorambucil	Oligospermia
Combination chemotherapy (CVP, MOPP, MVPP)	Oligospermia
Cyclophosphamide	Oligospermia
Methotrexate	Oligospermia
Chlordecone	Asthenospermia, oligospermia
Cimetidine	Oligospermia
Dibromochloropropane	Azoospermia, oligospermia
Diethylstilbestrol	Testicular hypoplasia
Ethanol	↓ Testosterone production, Leydig cell damage, asthenospermia, oligospermia, teratospermia
Ethylene oxide	Asthenospermia (in monkeys), oligospermia
Glycol ethers 2-Ethoxyethanol 2-Methoxyethanol	Azoospermia, oligospermia, testicular atrophy
Lead	↓ Spermatogenesis, asthenospermia, teratospermia
Nitrofurantoin	↓ Spermatogenesis
Opioids	↓ LH, ↓ testosterone
PCBs	↓ Sperm motility
Radiation (ionizing)	↓ Spermatogenesis
Styrene	Oligospermia
Sulfasalazine	↓ Spermatogenesis
Tobacco	↓ Testosterone
Women	
Xenobiotic	*Effects*
Chemotherapeutics	Gonadal toxicity
Cyclophosphamide	Ovarian failure
Busulphan	Amenorrhea
Combination chemotherapy	Amenorrhea
Diethylstilbestrol	Spontaneous abortions
Ethylene oxide	Spontaneous abortions
Lead	Spontaneous abortions, still births
Oral contraceptives	Affect hypothalamic–pituitary axis, end-organ resistance to hormones, amenorrhea
Thyroid hormone	↓ Ovulation

CVP = cyclophosphamide, vincristine, and prednisone; DBCP = dibromochloropropane; FSH = follicle-stimulating hormone; LH = luteinizing hormone; PCB = polychlorinated biphenyl.

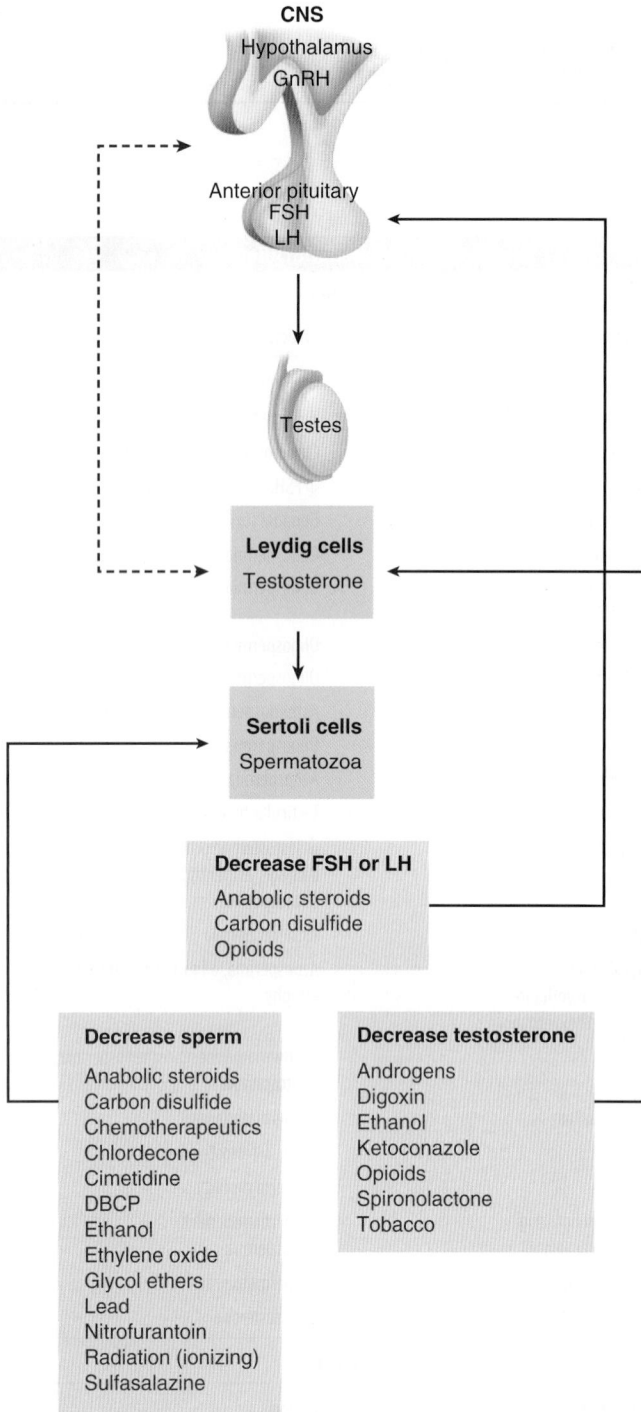

FIGURE 19–1. Schematic of the male reproductive axis and sites of xenobiotic effects. CNS = central nervous system; DBCP = dibromochloropropane; FSH = follicle-stimulating hormone; GnRH = gonadotropin-releasing hormone; LH = luteinizing hormone.

cells, and Leydig cells. Spermatogenesis begins with the maturation and differentiation of the germinal spermatogonia. The process is controlled by the secretion of GnRH from the hypothalamus, which in turn stimulates the pituitary to release FSH and LH. Follicle-stimulating hormone stimulates the development of Sertoli cells in the testes, which are responsible for the maturation of spermatids to spermatozoa. Luteinizing hormone promotes production of testosterone by Leydig cells. Testosterone concentrations must be maintained to ensure the formation of spermatids.[21] Both FSH and testosterone are required for initiation of spermatogenesis, but testosterone alone is sufficient to maintain the process.

Testicular Xenobiotics

Xenobiotics can affect any part of the male reproductive tract, but invariably, the end result is decreased sperm production defined as oligospermia, or absent sperm production, azoospermia. In contrast to oogenesis in women, spermatogenesis is an ongoing process throughout life that is inhibited by decreases in FSH or LH or by Sertoli cell toxicity. Spermatogenic capacity is evaluated by semen analysis, including sperm count, motility, sperm morphology, and penetrating ability. Normal sperm count is greater than 40 million sperm/mL semen, and a count less than 20 million/mL is indicative of infertility.[21] Decreased motility (asthenospermia) less than 40% of normal or abnormal morphology (teratospermia) of greater than 40% of the total number of sperm also indicates infertility.[21,102]

Physiology of Erection

The penis is composed of 2 corpus cavernosa and a central corpus spongiosum. The internal pudendal arteries supply blood to the penis via 4 branches. Blood outflow is via multiple emissary veins draining into the dorsal vein of the penis and plexus of Santorini. Within the penis, the corpora cavernosa share vascular supply and drainage because of extensive arteriolar, arteriovenous, and sinusoidal anastomoses.[121] Erection occurs when penile blood flow is greater than 20 to 50 mL/min, and tumescence is maintained with flow rates of 12 mL/min. The tunica albuginea limits the absolute size of erection.

In the flaccid state, sympathetic efferent nerves maintain arteriole constriction primarily through norepinephrine-induced α-adrenergic agonism. Whereas α-adrenergic receptor agonism in the erectile tissues decreases cyclic adenosine monophosphate (cAMP) to produce flaccidity, α-adrenergic antagonism can result in pathologic erection (priapism) as a consequence of parasympathetic dominance.[121] Other endogenous vasoconstrictors, such as endothelin, prostaglandin $F_{2\alpha}$ ($PGF_{2\alpha}$), and thromboxane A_2, play a role in maintaining corpus cavernosal smooth muscle tone in contraction, which results in a flaccid state.[83]

Normal penile erection is a result of both neural and vascular effects. Psychogenic neural stimulation arising from the cerebral cortex inhibits norepinephrine release from thoracolumbar sympathetic pathways, stimulates nitric oxide (NO) and acetylcholine release from sacral parasympathetic tracts, and stimulates acetylcholine release from somatic pathways.[83] Reflex stimulation also occurs from the sacral spinal cord. The pudendal nerves supply the afferent limb and the nervi erigentes (pelvic splanchnic nerves) supply the efferent limb of the reflex arc.

The central impulses stimulate various neurotransmitters to be released by peripheral nerves in the penis. Nonadrenergic–noncholinergic nerves and endothelial cells produce NO, which is the principal neurotransmitter mediating erection.[85] Nitric oxide activates guanylate conversion of guanosine triphosphate (GTP) to cyclic guanosine monophosphate (cGMP). Increasing concentrations of cGMP act as a second messenger, mediating arteriolar and trabecular smooth muscle relaxation to enable increased cavernosal blood flow and penile erection.[83] Both cGMP and cAMP pathways mediate smooth muscle relaxation. Cholinergic nerves release acetylcholine, which stimulates endothelial cells via M_3 receptors to produce NO and prostaglandin E_2 (PGE_2). Prostaglandin E_2 and nerves containing vasoactive intestinal peptide (VIP) and calcitonin gene-related peptide (CGRP) increase cellular cAMP to potentiate smooth muscle relaxation.

Penile corpus cavernosal smooth muscle relaxation allows increased blood flow into the corpus cavernosal sinusoids. Expansion of the sinusoids compresses the venous outflow and enables penile erection (Fig. 19–2).

Male Sexual Dysfunction

The sexual response cycle is divided in 4 stages—sexual desire or libido, sexual arousal of the genitalia, orgasm, and resolution.[99] Dopamine, melanocortin, testosterone, and estrogen facilitate libido. Libido is decreased by xenobiotics that either block central dopaminergic or adrenergic pathways while xenobiotics that increase dopamine improve sexual function.

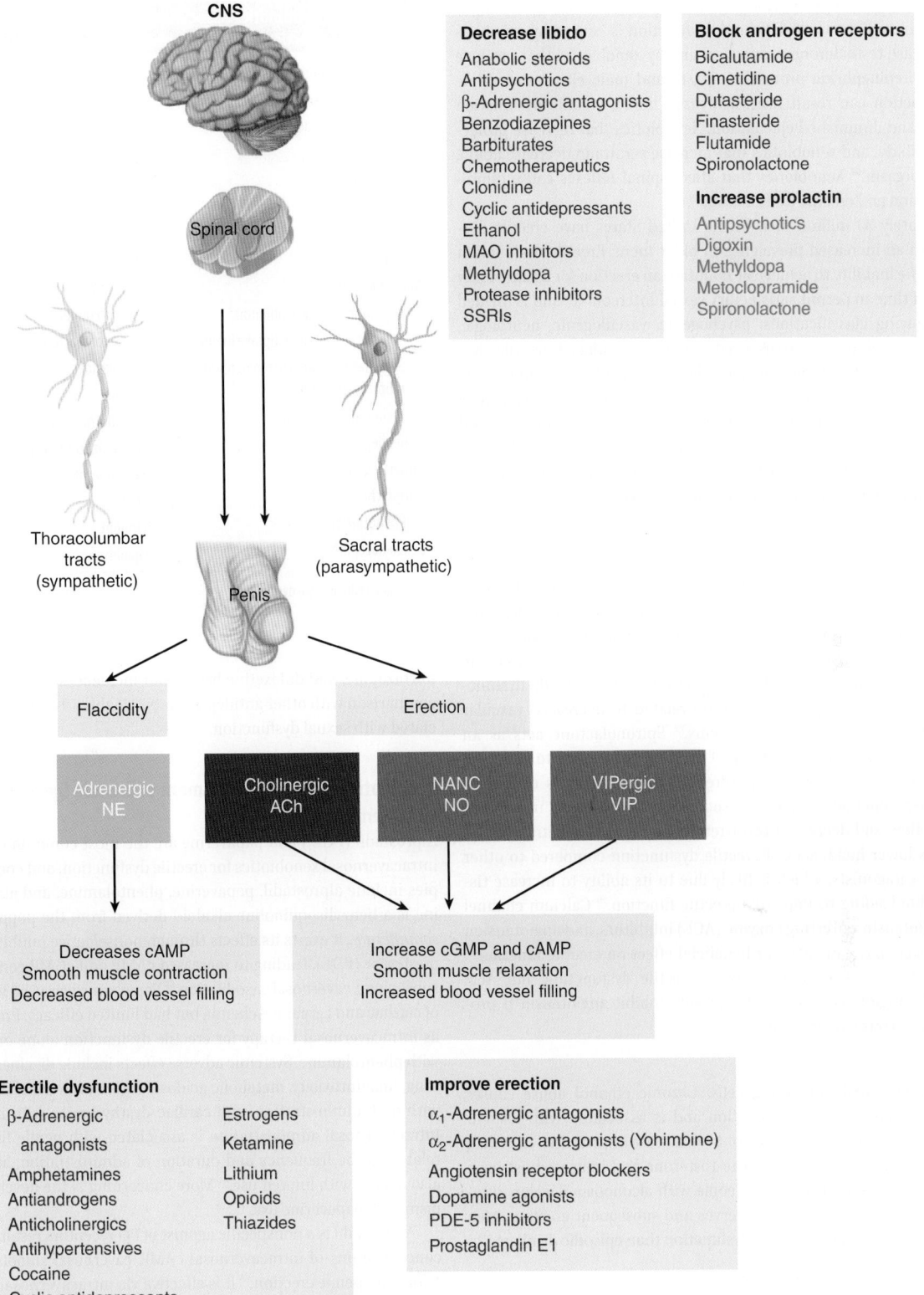

FIGURE 19–2. Schematic of erection and xenobiotics that cause sexual dysfunction. ACh = acetylcholine; cAMP = cyclic adenosine monophosphate; cGMP = cyclic guanosine monophosphate; MAOI = monoamine oxidase inhibitor; NANC = nonadrenergic-noncholinergic; NE = norepinephrine; NO = nitric oxide; PDE = phosphodiesterase; VIP = vasoactive intestinal peptide; SSRI = selective serotonin reuptake inhibitor.

Acetylcholine, NO, norepinephrine, melanocortin, testosterone, estrogen and dopamine mediate arousal. Sexual dysfunction is caused by xenobiotics that decrease testosterone production and by xenobiotics that produce dysphoria. Norepinephrine promotes orgasm and male ejaculation. Male sexual dysfunction can result from decreased libido, erectile dysfunction (impotence), and diminished ejaculation. Xenobiotics that increase prolactin decrease libido, and xenobiotics that increase serotonin decrease libido, arousal and orgasm.[64] Xenobiotics that affect spinal reflexes cause diminished ejaculation and erectile dysfunction.[119]

Approximately 30 million men in the United States have erectile dysfunction, with an increased prevalence in older men.[5] Erectile dysfunction is defined as the inability to achieve or maintain an erection for a sufficiently long period of time to permit satisfactory sexual intercourse[5] and is divided into the following classifications: psychogenic, vasculogenic, neurologic, endocrinologic, and xenobiotic-induced. Xenobiotic-induced erectile dysfunction is associated with the following classes of xenobiotics: antidepressants, antipsychotics, centrally and peripherally acting antihypertensives, CNS depressants, anticholinergics, exogenous hormones, antibiotics, and chemotherapeutics.[71,101,119] Treatment of this disorder is varied based on the etiology and includes vacuum-constriction devices, penile prostheses, vascular surgery, and medications that can be administered via the intracavernosal, transdermal, and oral routes.

Antihypertensives

Erectile dysfunction is reported as an adverse effect with many antihypertensives, and is caused, in part, by a decrease in hypogastric artery pressure, which impairs blood flow to the pelvis.[119] Centrally acting α_2-adrenergic agonists treat hypertension by inhibiting sympathetic outflow from the brain but this in turn causes male sexual dysfunction.[89] Erectile dysfunction associated with thiazide diuretics are related to decreased vascular resistance, diverting blood from the penis.[22] Spironolactone acts as an antiandrogen by inhibiting the binding of dihydrotestosterone to its receptors. Impotence related to use of β-adrenergic antagonists is caused by unopposed α-adrenergic–mediated vasoconstriction resulting in reduced penile blood flow and decreased testosterone and FSH concentrations.[30,37] Nebivolol has lower incidences of erectile dysfunction compared to other β-adrenergic antagonists, which is likely due to its ability to increase tissue nitric oxide leading to improved erectile function.[20] Calcium channel blockers, angiotensin-coverting enzyme (ACE) inhibitors, and angiotension receptor blockers have a neutral or beneficial effect on erectile function.[30] Angiotensin II vasoconstriction leads to erectile dysfunction, but ACE inhibitors and angiotension receptor blockers inhibit angiotensin II production in the corpus cavernosum.[14]

Ethanol

Ethanol is directly toxic to Leydig cells. Chronic ethanol abuse causes decreased libido and erectile dysfunction and is associated with testicular atrophy. In people with alcoholism, liver disease contributes to sexual dysfunction resulting from decreased testosterone and increased estrogen production or decreased breakdown. People with alcoholism develop autonomic neuropathies affecting penile nerves and subsequent erection. Men who drink heavily have more erectile dysfunction than episodic drinkers.[118]

Antidepressants and Antipsychotics

Individuals who take psychoactive medications therapeutically have varying degrees of sexual dysfunction related to their underlying disease and their medications. Antidepressant and antipsychotic inhibition of male sexual function is multifactorial and includes serotonin effects on $5HT_2$ receptors, anticholinergic, antihistaminergic, α-adrenergic receptor antagonism, dopamine blockage, and increased prolactin.[63,64] Monoamine oxidase inhibitors (MAOIs), cyclic antidepressants (CAs), antipsychotics, and selective serotonin reuptake inhibitors (SSRIs) are associated with decreased libido and erectile dysfunction in men.[34] Thioridazine is associated with significantly lower LH and testosterone concentrations in men in comparison with other antipsychotics.[21] Antidepressants such as bupropion, nefazodone,

TABLE 19–2	Xenobiotics Associated with Sexual Dysfunction (Particularly Diminished Libido and Erectile Dysfunction)
α_1-Adrenergic antagonists	Chemotherapeutics
α_2-Adrenergic agonists	Alkylating agents
β-Adrenergic antagonists[a]	Cytarabine
Amphetamines	Methotrexate
Anabolic steroids	Vinca alkaloids
Antiandrogens[a]	Cimetidine
Flutamide	Cocaine
Anticholinergics[a]	Digoxin
Antidepressants	Diuretics
Monamine oxidase inhibitors[a]	Loop diuretics
Selective serotonin reuptake inhibitors	Spironolactone
Selective serotonin/norepinephrine reuptake inhibitors	Thiazides
Cyclic antidepressants	Ethanol
Antiepileptics	Gonadotropin-releasing hormone agonists[a]
Antiestrogens	Hormonal contraceptives
Antipsychotics	Ketoconazole
Phenothiazines	Lead
Benzodiazepines	Lithium
	Opioids

[a]Associated with erectile dysfunction.

mirtazapine, and duloxetine have lower incidences of sexual dysfunction in comparison with other antidepressants.[103] Table 19–2 lists xenobiotics associated with sexual dysfunction.

Xenobiotics Used in the Treatment of Erectile Dysfunction
Intracavernosal and Intraurethral

Alprostadil (PGE_1) and papaverine are the most commonly used individual intracavernosal xenobiotics for erectile dysfunction, and combination therapies include alprostadil, papaverine, phentolamine, and atropine. Papaverine is a benzylisoquinoline alkaloid derived from the poppy plant *Papaver somniferum*. It exerts its effects through nonselective inhibition of phosphodiesterase (PDE), leading to increased cAMP and cGMP concentrations and subsequent cavernosal vasodilation.[55] Papaverine was used for the treatment of cardiac and cerebral ischemia but had limited efficacy. Presently, it is used as intracavernosal therapy for erectile dysfunction alone or in conjunction with phentolamine. Systemic adverse effects include dizziness, nausea, vomiting, hepatotoxicity, metabolic acidosis with elevated lactate concentration with oral administration, and cardiac dysrhythmias with intravenous use. Intracavernosal administration is associated with penile fibrosis, which is related to the frequency and duration of administration, although fibrosis also occurs with limited use.[65] More concerning is the development of priapism with papaverine use.

Alprostadil is a nonspecific agonist of PG receptors resulting in increased concentrations of intracavernosal cAMP, cavernosal smooth muscle relaxation, and penile erection.[55] It is effective via intracavernosal administration as monotherapy. Other preparations include an intraurethral preparation, which is less effective, and a topical gel formulation.[52] Penile fibrosis occurs, but the incidence is lower compared with papaverine. Other adverse effects include penile pain, secondary to its effects as a nonspecific PG receptor agonist, and priapism.

Phentolamine is a competitive α-adrenergic antagonist at both α_1 and α_2 receptors in cavernosal smooth muscle. Although this increases arterial blood flow and produces erection, it is not effective as a sole therapeutic.[55] It is usually combined with papaverine, alprostadil, or atropine as 2, 3 or 4 xenobiotic mixtures. Penile fibrosis, prolonged erection, and priapism are also more common with these xenobiotic combinations.[55]

Oral

Since the development of the PDE-5 inhibitors, oral therapy has replaced intracavernosal injections as the mainstay for treatment of erectile dysfunction. Sildenafil was the first drug developed followed by vardenafil, tadalafil, and avanafil in the United States and lodenafil, mirodenafil, and udenafil in other parts of the world. These medications share a mechanism of action but differ in their pharmacokinetics. Phosphodiesterase-5 inhibitors increase NO-induced cGMP concentrations by preventing PDE breakdown of cGMP, enhancing NO-induced vasodilation to promote penile vascular relaxation and erection.[18]

Sildenafil and vardenafil have similar times to peak concentration, ranging from 30 minutes to 2 hours. Avanafil has a shorter time to peak concentration (30–45 minutes) and tadalafil has a longer time to peak concentration (30 minutes to 6 hours).[62] The PDE-5 inhibitors have large volumes of distribution ranging from 63 L for tadalfil up to 208 L for vardenafil.[62] Elimination half-life is similar for avanafil, sildenafil, and vardenafil (4–5 hours), and tadalafil is longest at 17.5 hours.[62] Serum concentrations of sildenafil and vardenafil are increased in patients older than 65 years, hepatic dysfunction (Child Pugh A and B), severe kidney disease (creatinine clearance <30 mL/min).[28] Age, hepatic dysfunction, and kidney disease do not affect serum concentrations of avanafil or tadalfil.[62] Phosphodiesterase-5 inhibitors are metabolized primarily by the CYP3A4 pathway, with some minor metabolic activity via the CYP2C pathway for sildenafil, tadalafil, and vardenafil.[62] Strong CYP3A4 inhibitors like erythromycin, ketoconazole, cimetidine, protease inhibitors (indinavir, ritonavir, saquinavir), and grapefruit juice will increase PDE-5 inhibitor concentrations.[54] Inducers of CYP3A4 like rifampin, phenobarbital, phenytoin, and carbamazepine can decrease PDE-5 inhibitor concentrations.[79]

The most common adverse effects of the PDE-5 inhibitors are headache, flushing, dyspepsia, and rhinitis, which are related to PDE-1 inhibitory effects in the brain, myocardium, and vascular smooth muscle.[79] Blurred vision, increased light perception, and transient blue-green tinged vision are also reported and are related to the weak PDE-6 inhibition of sildenafil in the retina.[51] Vardenafil and tadalafil are associated with infrequent abnormal vision, including blurred and abnormal color vision.[53] Back pain and myalgia with PDE-5 inhibitor use is postulated to be from PDE-11 inhibition.[79]

More serious adverse effects of PDE-5 inhibitors include myocardial infarction, when used alone or with nitrates; subaortic obstruction; stroke; transient ischemic attack; priapism; and hearing loss.[10,43,58,78,104,110] Phosphodiesterase-5 inhibitors are associated with adverse bleeding events, including epistaxis, variceal bleeding, intracranial hemorrhages, and aortic dissection. The FDA updated the labeling of the PDE-5 inhibitors, warning of possible vision loss after reported cases of nonarteritic ischemic optic neuropathy associated with PDE-5 inhibitor use.[6,16,43]

When taken alone, the vasodilatory effects of PDE-5 inhibitors cause a modest decrease in systemic blood pressure. However, because of their mechanism of action via cGMP inhibition and vascular vasodilation, PDE-5 inhibitors can have synergistic interactions with the vasodilatory effects of nitrates, resulting in profound hypotension.[18,59] A study of healthy male volunteers taking sildenafil demonstrated significantly less tolerance to a nitroglycerin infusion in comparison with those who took placebo.[116] Because of this interaction, patients with acute myocardial ischemic syndromes using PDE-5 inhibitors should avoid taking organic nitrates as well.[28] α_1-Adrenergic antagonists are also contraindicated with concomitant PDE-5 inhibitor use because of increased hypotensive effects.[59] Hypotension occurred in patients using vardenafil in combination with terazosin and tamsulosin[59] and in patients using tadalafil with doxazosin.[60] However, patients using tadalafil with tamsulosin did not develop hypotension.[60]

Sublingual apomorphine effects erection through activation of central dopaminergic pathways, most likely D_2 receptors in the paraventricular nucleus of the hypothalamus.[56] It reaches maximum serum concentrations within 40 to 60 minutes after sublingual administration and is metabolized hepatically with a half-life of 2 to 3 hours.[9] Common adverse effects are nausea, vomiting, headache, dizziness, and syncope. Unlike the PDE-5 inhibitors, apomorphine is not associated with hypotension when used with antihypertensives, such as nitrates.

PRIAPISM

Priapism is defined as prolonged involuntary erection unassociated with sexual stimulation. Subtypes of priapism are ischemic (characterized by low cavernosal blood flow), nonischemic (characterized by increased arterial flow), and stuttering (recurrent ischemic priapism).[82] It most commonly occurs during the third and fourth decades of life and is caused by inflow of blood to the penis in excess of outflow. The corpora cavernosa become firm and the corpus spongiosum flaccid. Intracavernosal pressures exceed arterial systolic pressure, resulting in cell death. Priapism occurs from an imbalance in neural stimuli, interference with venous outflow or as a result of xenobiotic-induced inhibition of penile detumescence. α-Adrenergic antagonists prevent constriction of blood vessels supplying erectile tissue, resulting in priapism.[82] One in 10,000 patients taking trazodone develops priapism, which is thought to be related to its α-adrenergic antagonist effects.[98] Xenobiotics associated with priapism are listed in Table 19–3.

The goal in the treatment of priapism is detumescence with retention of potency. Initial therapy includes sedation with benzodiazepines, analgesia with opioids, ice packs, treatment of underlying systemic diseases such as sickle cell disease, and early urologic consultation. In ischemic priapism, aspiration with or without 9% NaCl solution irrigation of the corpora cavernosa is effective in 24% to 36% of cases, and adding intracavernosal injection of sympathomimetic agents increases priapism resolution to 43% to 81%.[82] The American Urology Association guidelines recommend phenylephrine (100–500 mcg/mL solution) injection into the corpora cavernosa at a dosage of 0.5 to 1 mL every 3 to 5 minutes up to 1 hour.[82] Oral xenobiotics are not recommended for ischemic priapism but oral terbutaline (5–10 mg) was

TABLE 19–3	Xenobiotics Associated with Priapism
Alprostadil	Cantharidin
Androgens	*Carukia barnesi* (Irukandji syndrome)
Anticoagulants	Cocaine
Direct oral acting anticoagulants	Hydroxyzine
Heparin	Intravenous lipid emulsion (parenteral nutrition)
Low-molecular-weight heparins	
Warfarin	Lithium
Antidepressants	Marijuana
Bupropion	Methylphenidate
Phenelzine	Oxcarbazepine
SSRIs	Papaverine
Trazodone	Phosphodiesterase-5 inhibitors
Antihypertensives	Propofol
α-Adrenergic antagonists	Scorpion envenomation
Guanethidine	Spider envenomation
Hydralazine	*Latrodectus mactans* (black widow)
Labetalol	*Phoneutria nigriventer* (Brazilian wandering spider)
Phentolamine	
Antipsychotics	Testosterone
Aripiprazole	Yohimbine
Butyrophenones	
Clozapine	
Olanzapine	
Phenothiazines	
Quetiapine	
Risperidone	
Ziprasidone	

SSRI = selective serotonin reuptake inhibitor.

effective for PGE_1-induced prolonged erections.[70,82,95] Intracavernosal methylene blue has been used successfully as an alternative to intracavernosal sympathomimetics.[74] If the above measures fail, an operative venous shunt placement is often required.[23]

FEMALE FERTILITY

The female reproductive system consists of the female gonadal organs and the respective hormonal system (Fig. 19–3). Fertility encompasses the reproductive system, the process of oocyte fertilization, and gestation. Female infertility results from changes in hormone concentrations, direct toxicity to the ovum, interference with the transport of the ovum, or inhibition of implantation of the ovum in the uterus. Women usually notice reproductive abnormalities more quickly than men because menses are affected, although infertility does occur while normal menses persists. Evaluation of female fertility is more difficult because of the complexity of the systems involved and the inaccessibility of the female germ cell. Investigations involve study of the anatomy and hormonal concentrations. The following is a discussion of oogenesis, xenobiotics that disrupt oogenesis, and xenobiotics that affect early embryo gestation.

Oogenesis

In contrast to men, women have a limited number of reproductive cells (ovarian follicles). Follicles are most numerous while a fetus is in utero, with the number decreasing to approximately 2 million at birth. By the time a woman reaches puberty, the majority of follicles have degenerated, leaving 300,000 to 400,000 ova, of which approximately 400 will eventually produce mature ova during a woman's reproductive years. In contrast, men produce millions of spermatozoa each day. The process of oogenesis requires secretion of GnRH from the hypothalamus, resulting in production of LH and FSH from the pituitary, which are required for ovarian follicle maturation.[21] Follicle-stimulating hormone induces early maturation by stimulating granulosa and thecal cell proliferation and estrogen production. Luteinizing hormone is required for ovulation and for the formation of the corpus luteum. The corpus luteum continues estrogen production and produces progesterone, which stimulates the uterus to develop an endometrium receptive to any fertilized ovum. Successful ovulation requires not only hormone secretion but also appropriate cyclic secretion.

Female Sexual Dysfunction

The National Health and Social Life Survey found that 43% of women in the United States (in comparison with 31% of men) reported having sexual dysfunction.[66] In 2013, the *Diagnostic and Statistical Manual of Mental Disorders*, fifth edition, categorized female sexual dysfunction into female orgasmic disorder, female sexual interest/arousal disorder, which includes the previously termed hypoactive sexual desire disorder, and genito-pelvic pain/penetration disorder.[2] The organic etiologies of female sexual dysfunction parallel those of male sexual and erectile dysfunction: vascular, neurologic, muscular, psychogenic, endocrinologic, and xenobiotic-induced causes.[15] Medications implicated in female sexual dysfunction are similar to those associated with male sexual dysfunction, with antihypertensives, antidepressants, especially SSRIs, and antipsychotics as the most frequent causes.[44]

Treatments for xenobiotic-induced female sexual dysfunction include decreasing medication dosages, switching to alternate medications with less adverse effects on sexual function such as bupropion and nefazodone, temporary cessation of the medication (drug holiday), or adding another medication to stimulate sexual function. Bupropion alone was as effective as fluoxetine for the treatment of depression but with less sexual dysfunction,[36] and when used in conjunction with SSRIs, bupropion improved sexual function compared with SSRIs alone.[26,33] Sildenafil was successful for treating spinal cord–induced[108] and antidepressant-induced sexual dysfunction,[87] but larger trials had mixed results with sildenafil for sexual arousal disorder.[13,25] Sublingual apomorphine improved sexual function in women with hypoactive sexual disorder.[24]

Flibanserin is the only FDA-approved medication for generalized hypoactive sexual desire disorder (HSDD) in premenopausal women but the mechanism of action is unknown. It is a $5HT_{1A}$ receptor agonist and $5HT_{2A}$ receptor antagonist with weaker antagonism of $5HT_{2B}$, $5HT_{2C}$, and dopamine D4 receptors.[109] Flibanserin has a 33% bioavailability, mean time to maximum concentration of 0.75 hours, 98% protein binding, mean terminal half-life of 11 hours, and is hepatically metabolized by CYP3A4 and CYP2C19.[97] In animal studies, flibanserin decreased CNS serotonin and increased dopamine and norepinephrine concentrations.[40] Common adverse effects are dizziness, somnolence, nausea, fatigue, insomnia, and dry mouth; serious adverse effects are CNS depression, hypotension, and syncope.[97] Flibanserin is contraindicated with concomitant alcohol usage, hepatic dysfunction, and CYP3A4 inhibitors.[97]

Other pharmacotherapies for female sexual dysfunction are estrogen and androgen supplementation. Estrogen replacement therapy is available in oral, dermal, vaginal ring, and topical cream formulations alone or in combination with progesterone.[115] Estrogen therapy is associated with a higher incidence of coronary disease, breast cancer, stroke, and venous thromboembolism. Androgen therapy includes testosterone, formulated as a transdermal patch or spray; methyltestosterone; micronized testosterone; and dehydroepiandrosterone.[7] Adverse effects are hirsutism, acne, weight gain, increased cholesterol concentrations and virilization.[7]

ABORTIFACIENTS

An abortifacient is defined as a xenobiotic that affects early embryonic gestation to induce abortion. Xenobiotics act by flushing the zygote from the fallopian tube, blocking the uterine horn inhibiting implantation, inducing fetal resorption, or producing oxytocin-like activity that results in uterine irritation and contraction. Abortifacients also indirectly affect pregnancy by altering hormonal concentrations through placental inhibition of human chorionic gonadotropin or progesterone production or through interference with progesterone receptors. Emergency contraceptive medications to prevent pregnancy include levonorgestrel as the most common single hormonal medication, ulipristal, and the combining oral hormonal contraceptive pills.[35] In early pregnancy, medications used for medical termination of pregnancy include mifepristone, methotrexate, prostaglandins (commonly misoprostol), or combinations of mifepristone or methotrexate with prostaglandins.[61]

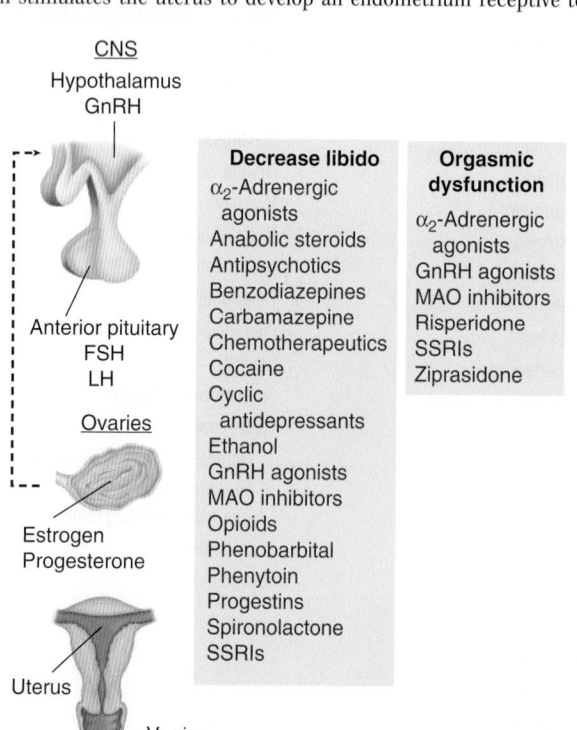

FIGURE 19–3. Schematic of female reproductive axis and sites of xenobiotic action. CNS = central nervous system; FSH = follicle-stimulating hormone; GnRH = gonadotropin-releasing hormone; LH = luteinizing hormone; MAO = monoamine oxidase; SSRI = selective serotonin reuptake inhibitor.

The toxic effects of abortifacients are varied. Many produce GI effects such as abdominal pain, nausea, and vomiting. Abdominal pain is related to the oxytocic uterine effects associated with misoprostol and mifepristone, cytotoxic effects on the GI mucosa associated with methotrexate, leading to stomatitis and ulcers or hepatoxicity associated with pennyroyal oil.[29] Mifepristone inhibits implantation or has abortive effects that cause severe vaginal bleeding. Other toxic effects are not necessarily related to their abortive mechanisms but due to the specific xenobiotic. Plant-derived abortifacients such as *Aristolochia* cause nephrotoxicity; dong quai causes photosensitivity; blue cohosh causes seizure; and quinine causes cardiac dysrhythmias.[86] Congenital abnormalities of the scalp and skull defects, cranial nerve palsies, and limb defects such as talipes equinovarus are also reported with misoprostol use that did not terminate pregnancy (Table 19–4).[29]

TABLE 19–4	Xenobiotics Used as Abortifacients		
Source	Common Name	Xenobiotic	Miscellaneous/Toxicity
Inhibit Implantation			
Abrus precatorius	Jequirity pea	Abrin	GI necrosis and multisystem organ failure
Acanthospermum hispidum	Bristly starbur	*Acanthospermum hispidum*	Impairs implantation
Aristolochia spp	Birthwort	Aristolochic acid	Nephrotoxicity
Momordica charantia	Bitter melon	α-Momorchin	Inhibits protein synthesis, ↓HCG, ↓progestera
Cajanus cajan	Pigeon pea	*Cajanus cajan*	Preimplantation effects
Hormonal therapy	—	Levonorgestrel, Yuzpe regimen: estradiol–levonorgestrel	Nausea, vomiting, abdominal pain, vaginal bleeding
Lagenaria breviflora	Wild colocynth	*Lagenaria breviflora*	Preimplantation effects
Juniperus sabina	Savin	Oil of savin	Hepatotoxicity in mice
Ricinus communis	Castor	Ricin	GI necrosis and multisystem organ failure
Ruta graveolens	Rue	Chalepesin	Hepatotoxicity, nephrotoxicity, photodermatitis
Selective progesterone receptor modulator	—	Mifepristone, ulipristal	Nausea, vomiting, abdominal pain, vaginal bleeding
Abortive			
Angelica sinensis	Dong quai	Furanocoumarin, phytoestrogen	Anticoagulant effects, gynecomastia, fetal demise
Daphne genkwa	Lilac daphne	Yuanhuacine	
Digoxin (intrafetal)			Fetal demise
Lysol disinfectant	—		Death after intrauterine administration
Mentha pulegium	Pennyroyal	Pulegone	Hepatotoxicity
Methotrexate	—		Cytotoxic effects
Mifepristone	—		Nausea, vomiting, abdominal pain, vaginal bleeding
Momordica charantia	Bitter melon	α-Momorchin	Inhibits protein synthesis ↓HCG, ↓progestera
Moringa oleifera	Horseradish tree	*Moringa oleifera*	100% abortifacient in rats
Podophyllum peltatum	Mayapple	Podophyllin	Nausea, vomiting, diarrhea
Ranunculus spp	Buttercup	Devil's claw	Hepatotoxicity
Trichosanthes kirilowii	Snake gourd	Trichosanthin (compound Q)	Inhibits protein synthesis, ↓ HCG, ↓ progesterone
Oxytocic			
Aristolochia spp	Birthwort	Aristolochic acid	Nephrotoxicity
Caulophyllum thalictroides	Blue cohosh	Methylcytosine	Salivation, nausea, vomiting
Cimicifuga racemosa	Black cohosh	Unknown	Nausea, vomiting, headache, rare hepatotoxicity
Cinchona spp	Quinine bark	Quinine	Nausea, vomiting, tinnitus
Claviceps purpurea	Ergot	Ergotamines	Vasospasm
Lagenaria breviflora Robert	Wild colocynth	*Lagenaria breviflora* Robert	Inhibits implantation, oxytocic
Misoprostol		Prostaglandin E analogue	Teratogenicity, vascular abnormalities
Ulipristal		Progesterone agonist/antagonist	Headache, nausea, abdominal pain

HCG = human chorionic gonadotropin; GI = Gastrointestinal.

In a US poison control center study, 5 of 43 pregnant women who intentionally overdosed used known abortifacients, including quinine, misoprostol, methylergonovine, and oral contraceptives. Four of these patients developed vaginal bleeding and cramping, but no short-term (1–3 days) fetal demise was reported.[94] The use of abortifacients is more common in underdeveloped countries and in people without access to safer methods for termination or prevention of pregnancy.

TOXICITY OF APHRODISIACS

Aphrodisiacs heighten sexual desire, pleasure, or performance and include xenobiotics from the plant, animal, and mineral kingdoms.[38] The search for an effective aphrodisiac has continued for thousands of years. Ancient fertility cults used *Datura*, belladonna, and henbane as aphrodisiacs. Mandrake was used in medieval Europe, and yohimbine was used by African cultures to enhance sexual performance. Yohimbine, an indole alkylamine alkaloid from the West African yohimbe tree (*Corynanthe yohimbe*), is an α_2-adrenergic antagonist with cholinergic activity and structurally similar to reserpine. It is rapidly absorbed, with peak serum concentrations within 45 to 60 minutes, elimination half-life of 36 minutes, and clearance by hepatic metabolism primarily.[90] Maximum pharmacologic effects occur 1 to 2 hours after ingestion, and effects persist for 3 to 4 hours.[69] Adverse effects include anxiety, headache, confusion, seizures, coma, tachycardia, hypertension, QRS interval widening, and priapism.[49] It is reasonable to administer activated charcoal to symptomatic patients. Clonidine is a reasonable treatment for the central and peripheral effects of yohimbine.[27] Arterial vasodilators and calcium channel blockers are not routinely recommended, and β-adrenergic antagonists are not recommended at this time. Benzodiazepines are reasonable to administer for agitation and seizures related to yohimbine.[27,49]

A small sampling of other xenobiotics used as aphrodisiacs include oysters, live beetles, vitamin E, ginseng, saffron, herba epimedii (horny goat weed), *Lepidium meyenii* (maca) and *Eurycoma longifolia* Jack (tongkat ali).[100,106] Most published studies evaluating aphrodisiacs were conducted in animals, and little information is available in humans. Toxicity occurs from either the aphrodisiac or adulterants[11] (Table 19–5).

TABLE 19–5 Xenobiotics Used as Aphrodisiacs

Xenobiotic	Toxicity
Oral	
Cantharidin	Vesicant actions—GI mucositis and hemorrhage, hematuria
Cathinone (hagigat)	Hypertension, tachycardia
Dapsone	Methemoglobinemia, hemolysis
Ginseng	GI distress impotence, vaginal bleeding
Lead	Anemia, abdominal pain
Mandragora officinarum (mandrake)	Anticholinergic
Myristica fragrans (nutmeg)	Hallucinogen, GI upset
Tribulus terrestris (Puncturevine)	Gynecomastia, seizures
Yohimbine	Paresthesias, hypertension
Topical	
Cantharidin	Vesicant actions—GI mucositis and hemorrhage, hematuria
Bufotoxin	Nausea, vomiting, dysrhythmias, death
Inhalation	
Alkyl nitrites (amyl, butyl, isobutyl nitrites)	Hemolytic anemia, methemoglobinemia, orthostasis

GI = Gastrointestinal.

Dopamine, NO, oxytocin, and ACTH facilitate sexual behavior. Dopamine stimulates the forebrain and midbrain and leads to an increase in sexual response and arousal. In animals, dopamine agonists, such as apomorphine and quinpirole, have proerectile effects through stimulation of dopamine pathways, increasing NO in the paraventricular nucleus in the hypothalamus, and releasing oxytocin.[83] Other preparations tested for the treatment of impotence include bromocriptine,[1,17] nitroglycerin,[84] zinc,[8] oxytocin,[68] and LH.[67] Endogenous opioids, GABA, and norepinephrine are associated with decreased sexual behavior. Serotonin is generally inhibitory to sexual function, but the effects are dependent on the receptor subclass. Whereas 5-HT_{1A} receptor stimulation inhibits erection but facilitates ejaculation in rats, 5-HT_{2C} receptors facilitate male sexual behavior.[83] Various serotonergic drugs, including trazodone, nefazodone, bupropion, and clomipramine, are reported to improve sexual dysfunction.[98,120]

URINARY SYSTEM

The urinary system is composed of the kidneys, ureters, bladder, and urethra (Chap. 27). Many xenobiotics are concentrated by the kidneys and eliminated in the urine. The following discusses the effect of xenobiotics on the bladder and urine.

Bladder Anatomy and Physiology

The bladder is a hollow, muscular reservoir composed of 2 parts—the body and the neck—and normally stores up to 350 to 450 mL of urine in adults. A smooth muscle, the detrusor muscle, makes up the bulk of the body and contracts during urination. Urine from the ureters enters the bladder at the uppermost part of the trigone, an area in the posterior wall of the bladder, and leaves via the neck and the posterior urethra. Surrounding the neck and posterior urethra is smooth muscle interlaced with elastic tissue to form the internal sphincter. Sympathetic innervation from the lumbar spinal cord to the internal sphincter maintains smooth muscle contraction. Distal to the internal sphincter is an area with voluntary skeletal muscle that forms the external sphincter and is innervated by somatic pudendal nerves.

The nerve supply and neurophysiology of urination involve interplay among lumbar sympathetic nerves, sacral parasympathetic nerves, and sacral somatic nerves. Figure 19–4 illustrates the physiology of micturition. With bladder filling, norepinephrine is released by sympathetic postganglionic fibers. α-Adrenergic receptors predominate in the internal sphincter and the bladder neck, and β-adrenergic receptors supply the detrusor wall of the bladder. Stimulation of α-adrenergic receptors results in internal sphincter contraction and increased bladder outlet resistance, and stimulation of β-adrenergic receptors leads to detrusor relaxation and bladder filling.[113] In micturition, parasympathetic pre- and postganglionic fibers release acetylcholine to M_2 and M_3 muscarinic receptors in the detrusor muscle. Stimulation of M_3 receptors is responsible for detrusor muscle contraction and bladder emptying.[26] Conversely, anticholinergics prevent bladder emptying and result in urinary retention.[31,46]

Urinary Abnormalities

Urinary incontinence is common in elderly. As age increases, bladder size decreases, resulting in more frequent emptying. Early detrusor contraction, even with low bladder volumes, occurs more commonly in elderly adults, causing a sense of urgency. There are many etiologies for urinary incontinence, including various xenobiotic exposures (Fig. 19–5). General or regional anesthesia, bladder instrumentation, and medications produce bladder atony, leading to incontinence.[31] Functional incontinence also result from the use of medications, such as sedative–hypnotics and opioids, that causes impaired cognition or decreased mobility.[31] Xenobiotics used in the treatment of urinary incontinence include anticholinergics (darifenacin, fesoterodine, oxybutynin, solifenacin, tolterodine, trospium), α_1-adrenergic antagonists, PDE_5 inhibitors, β_3-adrenergic antagonists (mirabegron), duloxetine, imipramine, and botulinum toxin A.[3,32] Urinary retention

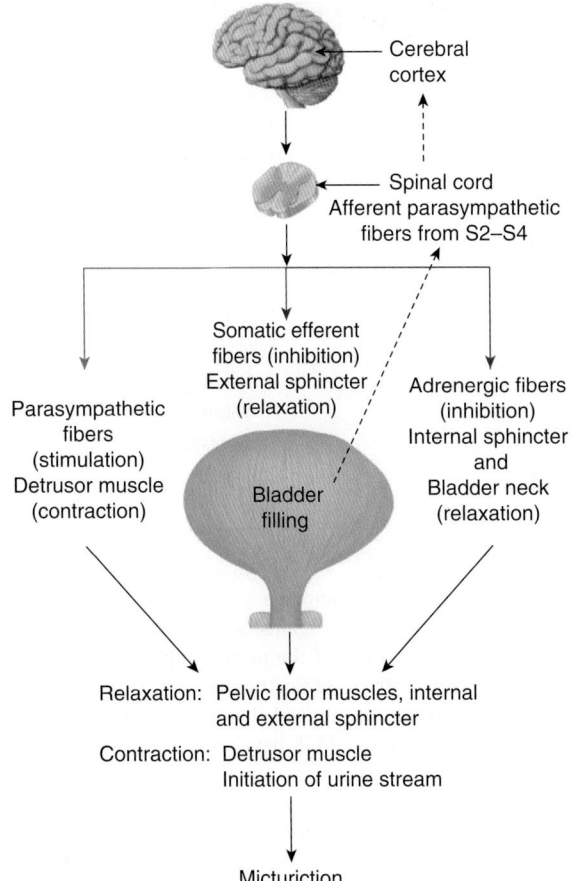

FIGURE 19–4. Schematic description of the physiology of micturition. (The dotted lines show the efferent pathway.)

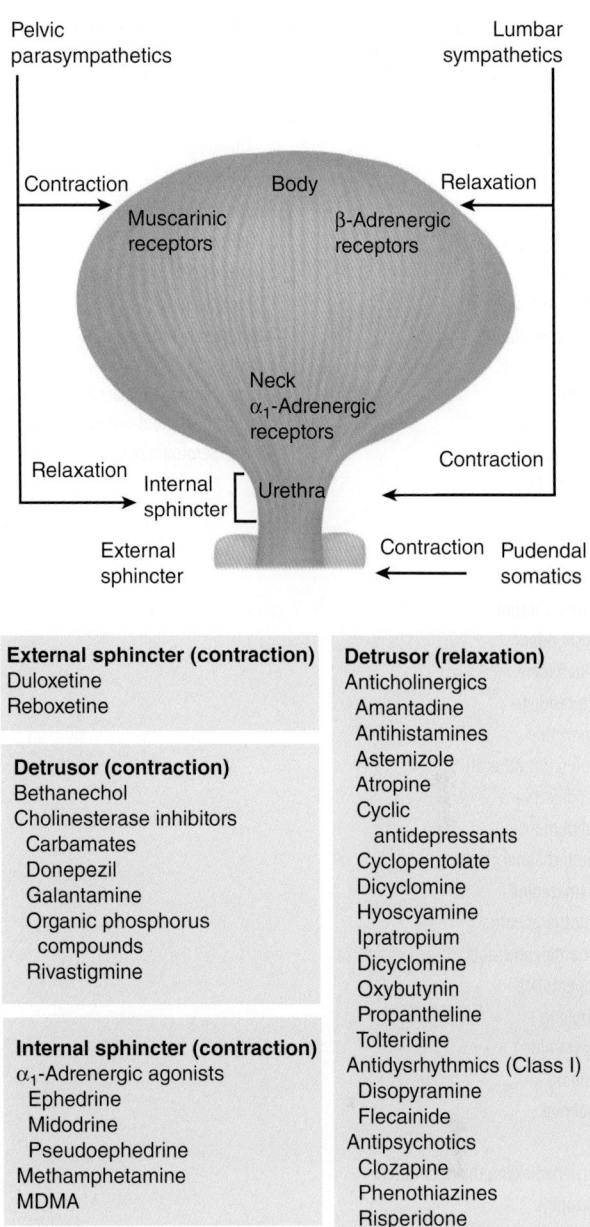

External sphincter (contraction)	Detrusor (relaxation)
Duloxetine	Anticholinergics
Reboxetine	Amantadine
	Antihistamines
Detrusor (contraction)	Astemizole
Bethanechol	Atropine
Cholinesterase inhibitors	Cyclic
Carbamates	antidepressants
Donepezil	Cyclopentolate
Galantamine	Dicyclomine
Organic phosphorus	Hyoscyamine
compounds	Ipratropium
Rivastigmine	Dicyclomine
	Oxybutynin
	Propantheline
Internal sphincter (contraction)	Tolteridine
α_1-Adrenergic agonists	Antidysrhythmics (Class I)
Ephedrine	Disopyramine
Midodrine	Flecainide
Pseudoephedrine	Antipsychotics
Methamphetamine	Clozapine
MDMA	Phenothiazines
	Risperidone
	Ziprasidone
Internal sphincter (relaxation)	α_1-Adrenergic
α-Adrenergic antagonists	antagonists
Doxazosin	Botulinum toxin
Phentolamine	Calcium channel
Prazonsin	blocker
Terazosin	Flunarizine
Antipsychotics	
Clozapine	
Thioridazine	

FIGURE 19–5. Graphic of the bladder and sites of xenobiotic effects. MDMA = 3,4-methylenedioxy-*N*-methylamphetamine.

is obstructive, neurogenic, psychogenic, or pharmacologic in origin. Medications associated with urinary retention include sympathomimetics, anticholinergics, antidysrhythmics (quinidine, procainamide, disopyramide), antidepressants, antipsychotics, hormones (progesterone, estrogen, testosterone), and muscle relaxants.[31,46] In men older than 50 years, benign prostatic hyperplasia is the most common cause of bladder outlet obstruction, leading to decreased urinary output and urinary retention. Treatment of benign prostatic hyperplasia consists of 5α-reductase inhibitors and α-adrenergic antagonists. 5α-Reductase inhibitors (finasteride, dutasteride) block the conversion of testosterone to dihydrotestosterone and thereby decrease prostate volume.[77] α_1-Adrenergic antagonists (doxazosin, terazosin, alfuzosin, tamsulosin) decrease urethral α-adrenergic contraction.[47] Table 19–6 lists xenobiotics associated with urinary retention increased urinary frequency and incontinence which may be due to overflow.

ABNORMALITIES IN URINALYSIS

Abnormalities of the urinalysis are often useful in identifying xenobiotic exposures. Crystalluria is a common finding and while normal, the presence of crystals may aid in diagnosis. Crystal formation is dependent on supersaturation of the urine and changes in the urine temperature or pH. The most common crystals are calcium oxalate, uric acid, and phosphate. However, crystals of various xenobiotics alone or in combination with other crystals are seen in ingestions.[39] The urinalysis in patients who ingest ethylene glycol reveals calcium oxalate or hippurate crystals in 45% to 63% of cases.[19,57] Calcium oxalate crystals are monohydrates (prism or needlelike) or dihydrates (envelope shaped). Hippurate crystals are needle shaped.[91] Birefringent single or conglomerates of hexagonal crystals are noted after massive primidone

poisoning and result from precipitation of primidone in the urine.[112] Crystalluria occurs with therapeutic doses of salicylate, phenacetin, sulfonamide, and quinolones. Oral sodium phosphate preparations for bowel cleansing have caused calcium phosphate calcifications leading to acute phosphate nephropathy.[72] After large exposures, crystals are also seen with, methotrexate, amoxicillin, cephalexin, ampicillin, and indinavir (Table 19–7).

Urine color is dependent on several factors, including pH, concentration, natural pigments, and length of time exposed to air. Normal urine

TABLE 19–6	Examples of Xenobiotics That Cause Urinary Retention, Frequent Urination and Incontinence
Retention	**Incontinence**
α_1-Adrenergic agonists	α_1-Adrenergic antagonists
Amantadine	Antipsychotics
Antihistamines	Clozapine
Anticholinergics	Chlorpromazine
Atropine	Haloperidol
Dicyclomine	Thioridazine
Glycopyrrolate	Cholinesterase inhibitors
Hyoscyamine	Diuretics
Ipratropium	Estrogen hormone replacement therapy
Oxybutynin	Naloxone (for opioid-induced retention)
Tiotropium	Selective serotonin reuptake inhibitors
Tolterodine	
Antipsychotics	
Aripiprazole	
Olanzapine	
Phenothiazines	
Risperidone	
Quetiapine	
Ziprasidone	
Atomoxetine	
Baclofen (intrathecal)	
Benzodiazepines	
Botulinum toxin	
Calcium channel blockers	
Carbamazepine	
Chemotherapeutics	
Cyclic antidepressants	
Cyclopentolate	
Dantrolene	
Disopyramide	
Flecainide	
Imiquimod	
Kava	
Methylenedioxymethamphetamine	
Mirtazapine	
Nonsteroidal antiinflammatory drugs	
Opioids	
Selective serotonin reuptake inhibitors	
Duloxetine	
Escitalopram	
Fluoxetine	
Fluvoxamine	
Milnacipran	
Reboxetine	
Theophylline	
Vincristine	

TABLE 19–7	Xenobiotics That Cause Crystalluria
Ampicillin	Nitrofurantoin
Amoxicillin	Orlistat
Antivirals	Primidone
Acyclovir	Protease inhibitors
Ganciclovir	Atazanavir
Valacyclovir	Indinavir
Ascorbic acid	Quinolones
Cephalexin	Salicylates
Ethylene glycol	Sodium phosphate
Felbamate	Sulfonamides
Flucytosine	Sulfadiazine
Foscarnet	Sulfamethoxazole
Melamine	Thiabendazole
Methotrexate	Triamterene
	Xylitol

added sodium fluorescein to examine physicians' ability to detect urinary fluorescence with a Wood lamp against a fluorometer. The fluorometer reported fluorescence in 100% of the urine samples, but the physicians reported fluorescence in 70% to 80% of the samples.[92] Urinary fluorescence, even when present, is not recommended as the sole means to establish a diagnosis at this time. Table 19–8 lists other causes of colored urine (Chap. 106).

There are multiple causes of hematuria[73] (Table 19–9). It can occur with xenobiotic-induced interstitial nephritis, a condition distinguished by fever, rash, eosinophilia, eosinophiluria, azotemia, and oliguria.[41] Hemorrhagic cystitis is a more frequent cause of hematuria and is associated with a number of xenobiotics. The clinical presentation of hemorrhagic cystitis includes hematuria, dysuria, and urinary frequency. Criteria for diagnosis of hemorrhagic cystitis include a history of gross hematuria, laboratory findings, of microscopic hematuria (>3 red blood cells/high-power field), platelet count above 50,000/mm³, and a negative urine culture result.[96] When in doubt, the diagnosis is confirmed by cystoscopy, which reveals an inflamed, hyperemic, and sometimes ulcerated bladder mucosa.

Cyclophosphamide-related hemorrhagic cystitis was first described in 1959 and is the best-documented type of xenobiotic-induced hemorrhagic cystitis.[81] As many as 40% to 60% of patients receiving cyclophosphamide develop hemorrhagic cystitis.[117] Acrolein, the causative xenobiotic, is a metabolite of cyclophosphamide that damages the urothelium when excreted (Chap. 50).[111] Cyclophosphamide and ifosfamide-induced hemorrhagic cystitis is reduced with mesna therapy.[4]

An outbreak of hemorrhagic cystitis occurred in workers in a packaging plant after exposure to chlordimeform, a formamidine insecticide used to control mites and insects on cotton. Nine workers developed abdominal pain, dysuria, urgency, and hematuria, with biopsy-proven hemorrhagic cystitis.[45] Eight young adults developed painful hematuria after consuming "bootleg" methaqualone. The cause was orthotoluidine, a compound used in the synthesis of methaqualone, and the findings occurred within 6 hours of ingestion.[50] Chronic ketamine and methoxetamine abuse is associated with the development of hemorrhagic ulcerative cystitis[105] (Fig. 83–2). Rare cases of hemorrhagic cystitis are also described with ticarcillin, nafcillin, penicillin G, carbenicillin, piperacillin, isoniazid, indomethacin, tiaprofenic acid, and busulphan.[48,75,80,107]

Treatment for hemorrhagic cystitis includes bladder irrigation with saline, alum, prostaglandins, silver nitrate, formalin, and phenol. Systemic therapy include estrogens, vasopressin, aminocaproic acid, and hyperbaric oxygen.[117] These therapies have inherent adverse effects as well. Aluminum toxicity was reported with alum bladder irrigation for hemorrhagic cystitis in patients with kidney failure.[93]

specimens should be clear and yellow in coloration. Whereas dilute urine secondary to diuretic use, diabetes mellitus, diabetes insipidus, or adequate hydration appears colorless, concentrated urine is usually orange. Fluorescein, present in some antifreeze products, is detected by illumination of the urine with a Wood lamp, although this diagnostic test has poor sensitivity and specificity for antifreeze exposure.[114] One study used urine samples from a group of unpoisoned children and 3 urine samples with

TABLE 19–8	Common Causes of Colored Urine

Milky white
- Chyle
- Lipids
- Pyuria
- Propofol

Reddish-brown
- Anthraquinone
- Bilirubin
- Chloroquine
- Ibuprofen
- Levodopa
- Methyldopa
- Metronidazole
- Nitrofurantoin
- Phenacetin
- Phenazopyridine
- Phenothiazines
- Phenytoin
- Porphyrins
- Trinitrophenol

Reddish-orange
- Aminopyrine
- Aniline dyes
- Antipyrine
- Chlorzoxazone
- Doxorubicin
- Ibuprofen
- Idarubicin
- Mannose
- Phenacetin
- Phenazopyridine
- Phenothiazines
- Phenytoin
- Rifampin
- Salicylazosulfapyridine
- Sulfasalazine
- Warfarin

Red
- Anthraquinones
- Beets
- Blackberries
- Deferoxamine
- Eosin
- Erythrocytes
- Hemoglobin
- Hydroxocobalamin
- Myoglobin
- Porphyrins
- Rhubarb

Yellow-brown
- Aloe
- Anthraquinones
- Chloroquine

- Fava beans
- Nitrofurantoin
- Primaquine
- Rhubarb
- Sulfamethoxazole

Yellow
- Fluorescein
- Phenacetin
- Quinacrine
- Riboflavin
- Santonin

Yellow-orange
- Aminopyrine
- Anisindione
- Carrots
- Sulfasalazine
- Vitamin A
- Warfarin

Black
- Alcaptonuria
- Homogentisic acid
- Melanin
- p-Hydroxyphenylpyruvic acid

Brown-black
- Carbidopa/levodopa
- Cascara
- Iron
- Methyldopa
- Phenylhydrazine
- Senna

Green or greenish-blue
- Amitriptyline
- Anthraquinones
- Biliverdin
- Cimetidine
- Chlorophyll breath mints
- Flavin derivatives
- Flutamide
- Food dye and Color Blue No. 1
- Indicans
- Indigo blue
- Indomethacin
- Magnesium salicylate
- Methocarbamol
- Methylene blue
- Metoclopramide
- Mitoxantrone
- Phenol
- Promethazine
- Propofol
- Thymol
- Triamterene
- Zaleplon

TABLE 19–9	Xenobiotics That Cause Hematuria

- Acyclovir
- Amitraz
- Anticoagulants
- Baclofen
- BCG (intravesicular)
- Cantharidin
- Cefaclor
- Chemotherapeutics
- Cyclophosphamide ifosfamide
- Chlordimeform
- Ciprofloxacin
- Clozapine
- Colchicine
- Crotaline envenomation
- Danazol
- Fibrinolytics
- Isoniazid

- Ketamine
- Mesalamine
- Nonsteroidal antiinflammatory drugs
- Orthotoluidine
- Penicillamine
- Penicillins
- Pentamidine
- Protease inhibitors
- Radiation
- Salicylates
- Solvents
  - Cyclohexane
  - Toluene
  - Xylene
- Statins

BCG = Bacillus Calmette-Guerin.

SUMMARY

- Xenobiotics decrease fertility and fecundity by decreasing FSH and LH centrally or altering sperm production in men and altering ovarian function in women.
- Xenobiotics that increase CNS serotonin or prolactin or decrease CNS urinary frequency dopamine cause sexual dysfunction by decreasing libido in men and women.
- Therapies for erectile dysfunction increase local nitric oxide production via cyclic AMP and cyclic GMP to increase penile blood flow but can result in priapism.
- Abortifacients usually prevent embryo implantation or induce uterine contractions leading to increased vaginal bleeding and abdominal pain.
- Xenobiotics alter bladder function to cause urinary retention or incontinence (at times due to overflow) as well as change the characteristics of urine in terms of color, hematuria, or crystal formation.

REFERENCES

1. Ambrosi B, et al. Study of the effects of bromocriptine on sexual impotence. *Clin Endocrinol (Oxf)*. 1977;7:417-421.
2. American Psychiatric Association. *Diagnostic and Statistical Manual of Mental Disorders*. 5th ed. Arlington, VA: American Psychiatric Association; 2013.
3. Andersson KE. The use of pharmacotherapy for male patients with urgency and stress incontinence. *Curr Opin Urol*. 2014;24:571-577.
4. Andriole GL, et al. The efficacy of mesna (2-mercaptoethane sodium sulfonate) as a uroprotectant in patients with hemorrhagic cystitis receiving further oxazaphosphorine chemotherapy. *J Clin Oncol*. 1987;5:799-803.
5. Anonymous. NIH Consensus Conference. Impotence. NIH Consensus Development Panel on Impotence. *JAMA*. 1993;270:83-90.
6. Anonymous. FDA updates labeling for erectile dysfunction drugs. *FDA Consum*. 2005;39:3.
7. Anonymous. ACOG Practice Bulletin No. 119: Female sexual dysfunction. *Obstet Gynecol*. 2011;117:996-1007.
8. Antoniou LD, et al. Reversal of uraemic impotence by zinc. *Lancet*. 1977;2:895-898.
9. Argiolas A, Hedlund H. The pharmacology and clinical pharmacokinetics of apomorphine SL. *BJU Int*. 2001;88(suppl 3):18-21.
10. Arora RR, et al. Acute myocardial infarction after the use of sildenafil. *N Engl J Med*. 1999;341:700.
11. Balayssac S, et al. Analysis of herbal dietary supplements for sexual performance enhancement: first characterization of propoxyphenyl-thiohydroxyhomosildenafil and identification of sildenafil, thiosildenafil, phentolamine and tetrahydropalmatine as adulterants. *J Pharm Biomed Anal*. 2012;63:135-150.
12. Baranski B. Effects of the workplace on fertility and related reproductive outcomes. *Environ Health Perspect*. 1993;101(suppl 2):81-90.

13. Basson R, et al. Efficacy and safety of sildenafil citrate in women with sexual dysfunction associated with female sexual arousal disorder. *J Womens Health Gend Based Med.* 2002;11:367-377.

14. Becker AJ, et al. Plasma levels of angiotensin II during different penile conditions in the cavernous and systemic blood of healthy men and patients with erectile dysfunction. *Urology.* 2001;58:805-810.

15. Berman JR. Physiology of female sexual function and dysfunction. *Int J Impot Res.* 2005;17(suppl 1):S44-S51.

16. Bollinger K, Lee MS. Recurrent visual field defect and ischemic optic neuropathy associated with tadalafil rechallenge. *Arch Ophthalmol.* 2005;123:400-401.

17. Bommer J, et al. Improved sexual function in male haemodialysis patients on bromocriptine. *Lancet.* 1979;2:496-497.

18. Boolell M, et al. Sildenafil: an orally active type 5 cyclic GMP-specific phosphodiesterase inhibitor for the treatment of penile erectile dysfunction. *Int J Impot Res.* 1996;8:47-52.

19. Brent J, et al. Fomepizole for the treatment of ethylene glycol poisoning. Methylpyrazole for Toxic Alcohols Study Group. *N Engl J Med.* 1999;340:832-838.

20. Brixius K, et al. Nitric oxide, erectile dysfunction and beta-blocker treatment (MR NOED study): benefit of nebivolol versus metoprolol in hypertensive men. *Clin Exp Pharmacol Physiol.* 2007;34:327-331.

21. Buchanan JF, Davis LJ. Drug-induced infertility. *Drug Intell Clin Pharm.* 1984;18:122-132.

22. Buffum J. Pharmacosexology update: prescription drugs and sexual function. *J Psychoactive Drugs.* 1986;18:97-106.

23. Burnett AL, Bivalacqua TJ. Priapism: new concepts in medical and surgical management. *Urol Clin North Am.* 2011;38:185-194.

24. Caruso S, et al. Placebo-controlled study on efficacy and safety of daily apomorphine SL intake in premenopausal women affected by hypoactive sexual desire disorder and sexual arousal disorder. *Urology.* 2004;63:955-959.

25. Caruso S, et al. Premenopausal women affected by sexual arousal disorder treated with sildenafil: a double-blind, cross-over, placebo-controlled study. *BJOG.* 2001;108:623-628.

26. Chapple CR, et al. Muscarinic receptor subtypes and management of the overactive bladder. *Urology.* 2002;60:82-88; discussion 88-89.

27. Charney DS, et al. Yohimbine induced anxiety and increased noradrenergic function in humans: effects of diazepam and clonidine. *Life Sci.* 1983;33:19-29.

28. Cheitlin MD, et al. ACC/AHA expert consensus document. Use of sildenafil (Viagra) in patients with cardiovascular disease. American College of Cardiology/American Heart Association. *J Am Coll Cardiol.* 1999;33:273-282.

29. Christin-Maitre S, et al. Medical termination of pregnancy. *N Engl J Med.* 2000;342:946-956.

30. Chrysant SG. Antihypertensive therapy causes erectile dysfunction. *Curr Opin Cardiol.* 2015;30:383-390.

31. Chutka DS, et al. Urinary incontinence in the elderly population. *Mayo Clin Proc.* 1996;71:93-101.

32. Cipullo LM, et al. Pharmacological treatment of urinary incontinence. *Female Pelvic Med Reconstr Surg.* 2014;20:185-202.

33. Clayton AH, et al. A placebo-controlled trial of bupropion SR as an antidote for selective serotonin reuptake inhibitor-induced sexual dysfunction. *J Clin Psychiatry* 2004;65:62-67.

34. Clayton DO, Shen WW. Psychotropic drug-induced sexual function disorders: diagnosis, incidence and management. *Drug Saf.* 1998;19:299-312.

35. Cleland K, et al. Emergency contraception review: evidence-based recommendations for clinicians. *Clin Obstet Gynecol.* 2014;57:741-750.

36. Coleman CC, et al. A placebo-controlled comparison of the effects on sexual functioning of bupropion sustained release and fluoxetine. *Clin Ther.* 2001;23:1040-1058.

37. Cordero A, et al. Erectile dysfunction in high-risk hypertensive patients treated with beta-blockade agents. *Cardiovasc Ther.* 2010;28:15-22.

38. Czajka P, et al. Case report: accidental aphrodisiac ingestion. *J Tenn Med Assoc.* 1978;71:747, 750.

39. Daudon P, Frochot V. Crystalluria. *Clin Chem Lab Med.* 2015;53(suppl 2):s1479-s1487.

40. Dhanuka I, Simon JA. Flibanserin for the treatment of hypoactive sexual desire disorder in premenopausal women. *Expert Opin Pharmacother.* 2015;16:2523-2529.

41. Ditlove J, et al. Methicillin nephritis. *Medicine (Baltimore).* 1977;56:483-491.

42. Dlugosz L, Bracken MB. Reproductive effects of caffeine: a review and theoretical analysis. *Epidemiol Rev.* 1992;14:83-100.

43. Egan R, Pomeranz H. Sildenafil (Viagra) associated anterior ischemic optic neuropathy. *Arch Ophthalmol.* 2000;118:291-292.

44. Finger WW, et al. Medications that may contribute to sexual disorders. A guide to assessment and treatment in family practice. *J Fam Pract.* 1997;44:33-43.

45. Folland DS, et al. Acute hemorrhagic cystitis. Industrial exposure to the pesticide chlordimeform. *JAMA.* 1978;239:1052-1055.

46. Fontanarosa PB, Roush WR. Acute urinary retention. *Emerg Med Clin North Am.* 1988;6:419-437.

47. Furuya S, et al. Alpha-adrenergic activity and urethral pressure in prostatic zone in benign prostatic hypertrophy. *J Urol.* 1982;128:836-839.

48. Ghose K. Cystitis and nonsteroidal antiinflammatory drugs: an incidental association or an adverse effect? *N Z Med J.* 1993;106:501-503.

49. Giampreti A, et al. Acute neurotoxicity after yohimbine ingestion by a body builder. *Clin Toxicol (Phila).* 2009;47:827-829.

50. Goldfarb M, Finelli R. Necrotizing cystitis. Secondary to "bootleg" methaqualone. *Urology.* 1974;3:54-55.

51. Goldstein I, et al. Oral sildenafil in the treatment of erectile dysfunction. Sildenafil Study Group. *N Engl J Med.* 1998;338:1397-1404.

52. Goldstein I, et al. A double-blind, placebo-controlled, efficacy and safety study of topical gel formulation of 1% alprostadil (Topiglan) for the in-office treatment of erectile dysfunction. *Urology.* 2001;57:301-305.

53. Goldstein I, et al. Vardenafil, a new phosphodiesterase type 5 inhibitor, in the treatment of erectile dysfunction in men with diabetes: a multicenter double-blind placebo-controlled fixed-dose study. *Diabetes Care.* 2003;26:777-783.

54. Gupta M, et al. The clinical pharmacokinetics of phosphodiesterase-5 inhibitors for erectile dysfunction. *J Clin Pharmacol.* 2005;45:987-1003.

55. Hatzimouratidis K, et al. Pharmacotherapy for erectile dysfunction: recommendations from the fourth International Consultation for Sexual Medicine (ICSM 2015). *J Sex Med.* 2016;13:465-488.

56. Heaton JP. Central neuropharmacological agents and mechanisms in erectile dysfunction: the role of dopamine. *Neurosci Biobehav Rev.* 2000;24:561-569.

57. Jacobsen D, et al. Urinary calcium oxalate monohydrate crystals in ethylene glycol poisoning. *Scand J Clin Lab Invest.* 1982;42:231-234.

58. Kassim AA, et al. Acute priapism associated with the use of sildenafil in a patient with sickle cell trait. *Blood.* 2000;95:1878-1879.

59. Kloner RA. Novel phosphodiesterase type 5 inhibitors: assessing hemodynamic effects and safety parameters. *Clin Cardiol.* 2004;27:I20-I25.

60. Kloner RA, et al. Interaction between the phosphodiesterase 5 inhibitor, tadalafil and 2 alpha-blockers, doxazosin and tamsulosin in healthy normotensive men. *J Urol.* 2004;172:1935-1940.

61. Kulier R, et al. Medical methods for first trimester abortion. *Cochrane Database Syst Rev.* 2011:CD002855.

62. Kyle JA, et al. Avanafil for erectile dysfunction. *Ann Pharmacother.* 2013;47:1312-1320.

63. La Torre A, et al. Sexual dysfunction related to psychotropic drugs: a critical review part II: antipsychotics. *Pharmacopsychiatry.* 2013;46:201-208.

64. La Torre A, et al. Sexual dysfunction related to psychotropic drugs: a critical review—part I: antidepressants. *Pharmacopsychiatry.* 2013;46:191-199.

65. Lakin MM, et al. Intracavernous injection therapy: analysis of results and complications. *J Urol.* 1990;143:1138-1141.

66. Laumann EO, et al. Sexual dysfunction in the United States: prevalence and predictors. *JAMA.* 1999;281:537-544.

67. Levitt NS, et al. Synthetic luteinizing hormone-releasing hormone in impotent male diabetics. *S Afr Med J.* 1980;57:701-704.

68. Lidberg L, Sternthal V. A new approach to the hormonal treatment of impotentia erectionis. *Pharmakopsychiatr Neuropsychopharmakol.* 1977;10:21-25.

69. Linden CH, et al. Yohimbine: a new street drug. *Ann Emerg Med.* 1985;14:1002-1004.

70. Lowe FC, Jarow JP. Placebo-controlled study of oral terbutaline and pseudoephedrine in management of prostaglandin E1-induced prolonged erections. *Urology.* 1993;42:51-53; discussion 53-54.

71. Lue TF. Erectile dysfunction. *N Engl J Med.* 2000;342:1802-1813.

72. Markowitz GS, et al. Acute phosphate nephropathy following oral sodium phosphate bowel purgative: an underrecognized cause of chronic renal failure. *J Am Soc Nephrol.* 2005;16:3389-3396.

73. Marks LB, et al. The response of the urinary bladder, urethra, and ureter to radiation and chemotherapy. *Int J Radiat Oncol Biol Phys.* 1995;31:1257-1280.

74. Martinez Portillo F, et al. Methylene blue as a successful treatment alternative for pharmacologically induced priapism. *Eur Urol.* 2001;39:20-23.

75. Marx CM, Alpert SE. Ticarcillin-induced cystitis. Cross-reactivity with related penicillins. *Am J Dis Child.* 1984;138:670-672.

76. Mattison DR, et al. Reproductive toxicity: male and female reproductive systems as targets for chemical injury. *Med Clin North Am.* 1990;74:391-411.

77. McConnell JD. Benign prostatic hyperplasia. Hormonal treatment. *Urol Clin North Am.* 1995;22:387-400.

78. McGwin G Jr. Phosphodiesterase type 5 inhibitor use and hearing impairment. *Arch Otolaryngol Head Neck Surg.* 2010;136:488-492.

79. Mehrotra N, et al. The role of pharmacokinetics and pharmacodynamics in phosphodiesterase-5 inhibitor therapy. *Int J Impot Res.* 2007;19:253-264.

80. Millard RJ. Busulphan haemorrhagic cystitis. *Br J Urol.* 1978;50:210.

81. Miller LJ, et al. Treatment of cyclophosphamide-induced hemorrhagic cystitis with prostaglandins. *Ann Pharmacother.* 1994;28:590-594.

82. Montague DK, et al. American Urological Association guideline on the management of priapism. *J Urol.* 2003;170:1318-1324.

83. Moreland RB, et al. The biochemical and neurologic basis for the treatment of male erectile dysfunction. *J Pharmacol Exp Ther.* 2001;296:225-234.

84. Mudd JW. Impotence responsive to glyceryl trinitrate. *Am J Psychiatry.* 1977;134:922-925.

85. Musicki B, Burnett AL. eNOS function and dysfunction in the penis. *Exp Biol Med (Maywood).* 2006;231:154-165.

86. Netland KE, Martinez J. Abortifacients: toxidromes, ancient to modern—a case series and review of the literature. *Acad Emerg Med.* 2000;7:824-829.

87. Nurnberg HG, et al. Sildenafil for women patients with antidepressant-induced sexual dysfunction. *Psychiatr Serv.* 1999;50:1076-1078.

88. Olsen J. Is human fecundity declining—and does occupational exposures play a role in such a decline if it exists? *Scand J Work Environ Health.* 1994;20 Spec No:72-77.

89. Oster JR, Epstein M. Use of centrally acting sympatholytic agents in the management of hypertension. *Arch Intern Med.* 1991;151:1638-1644.

90. Owen JA, et al. The pharmacokinetics of yohimbine in man. *Eur J Clin Pharmacol.* 1987;32:577-582.

91. Parry MF, Wallach R. Ethylene glycol poisoning. *Am J Med.* 1974;57:143-150.

92. Parsa T, et al. The usefulness of urine fluorescence for suspected antifreeze ingestion in children. *Am J Emerg Med.* 2005;23:787-792.

93. Perazella M, Brown E. Acute aluminum toxicity and alum bladder irrigation in patients with renal failure. *Am J Kidney Dis.* 1993;21:44-46.

94. Perrone J, Hoffman RS. Toxic ingestions in pregnancy: abortifacient use in a case series of pregnant overdose patients. *Acad Emerg Med.* 1997;4:206-209.

95. Priyadarshi S. Oral terbutaline in the management of pharmacologically induced prolonged erection. *Int J Impot Res.* 2004;16:424-426.

96. Relling MV, Schunk JE. Drug-induced hemorrhagic cystitis. *Clin Pharm.* 1986;5:590-597.

97. Robinson K, et al. First pharmacological therapy for hypoactive sexual desire disorder in premenopausal women: flibanserin. *Ann Pharmacother.* 2016;50:125-132.

98. Rosen RC, Ashton AK. Prosexual drugs: empirical status of the "new aphrodisiacs." *Arch Sex Behav.* 1993;22:521-543.

99. Rosen RC, et al. Effects of SSRIs on sexual function: a critical review. *J Clin Psychopharmacol.* 1999;19:67-85.

100. Sandroni P. Aphrodisiacs past and present: a historical review. *Clin Auton Res.* 2001;11:303-307.

101. Schlegel PN, et al. Antibiotics: potential hazards to male fertility. *Fertil Steril.* 1991;55:235-242.

102. Schrag SD, Dixon RL. Occupational exposures associated with male reproductive dysfunction. *Annu Rev Pharmacol Toxicol.* 1985;25:567-592.

103. Segraves RT. Sexual dysfunction associated with antidepressant therapy. *Urol Clin North Am.* 2007;34:575-579, vii.

104. Shah PK. Sildenafil in the treatment of erectile dysfunction. *N Engl J Med.* 1998;339:699; author reply 701-702.

105. Shahani R, et al. Ketamine-associated ulcerative cystitis: a new clinical entity. *Urology.* 2007;69:810-812.

106. Shamloul R. Natural aphrodisiacs. *J Sex Med.* 2010;7:39-49.

107. Shieh CC, et al. Late onset hemorrhagic cystitis after allogeneic bone marrow transplantation. *Taiwan Yi Xue Hui Za Zhi.* 1989;88:508-511.

108. Sipski ML, et al. Sildenafil effects on sexual and cardiovascular responses in women with spinal cord injury. *Urology.* 2000;55:812-815.

109. Stahl SM, et al. Multifunctional pharmacology of flibanserin: possible mechanism of therapeutic action in hypoactive sexual desire disorder. *J Sex Med.* 2011;8:15-27.

110. Stauffer JC, et al. Subaortic obstruction after sildenafil in a patient with hypertrophic cardiomyopathy. *N Engl J Med.* 1999;341:700-701.

111. Stillwell TJ, Benson RC Jr. Cyclophosphamide-induced hemorrhagic cystitis. A review of 100 patients. *Cancer.* 1988;61:451-457.

112. van Heijst AN, et al. Coma and crystalluria: a massive primidone intoxication treated with haemoperfusion. *J Toxicol Clin Toxicol.* 1983;20:307-318.

113. Verhamme KM, et al. Drug-induced urinary retention: incidence, management and prevention. *Drug Saf.* 2008;31:373-388.

114. Wallace KL, et al. Diagnostic use of physicians' detection of urine fluorescence in a simulated ingestion of sodium fluorescein-containing antifreeze. *Ann Emerg Med.* 2001;38:49-54.

115. Walsh KE, Berman JR. Sexual dysfunction in the older woman: an overview of the current understanding and management. *Drugs Aging.* 2004;21:655-675.

116. Webb DJ, et al. Sildenafil citrate and blood-pressure-lowering drugs: results of drug interaction studies with an organic nitrate and a calcium antagonist. *Am J Cardiol.* 1999;83:21C-28C.

117. West NJ. Prevention and treatment of hemorrhagic cystitis. *Pharmacotherapy.* 1997;17:696-706.

118. Wetterling T, et al. Drinking pattern and alcohol-related medical disorders. *Alcohol Alcohol.* 1999;34:330-336.

119. Wilson B. The effect of drugs on male sexual function and fertility. *Nurse Pract.* 1991;16:12-17, 21-24.

120. Woodrum ST, Brown CS. Management of SSRI-induced sexual dysfunction. *Ann Pharmacother.* 1998;32:1209-1215.

121. Yealy DM, Hogya PT. Priapism. *Emerg Med Clin North Am.* 1988;6:509-520.

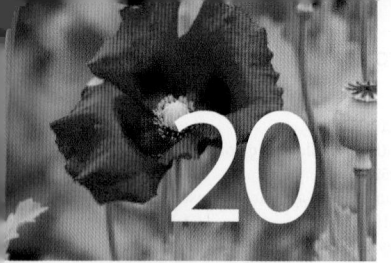

20 HEMATOLOGIC PRINCIPLES

Marco L. A. Sivilotti

Blood is rightfully considered the vital fluid, because every organ system depends on the normal function of blood. Blood delivers oxygen and other essential substances throughout the body, removes waste products of metabolism, transports hormones from their origin to site of action, signals and defends against threatened infection, promotes healing via the inflammatory response, and maintains the vascular integrity of the circulatory system through the clotting cascade. It also serves as the central compartment in classical pharmacokinetics and thereby comes into direct contact with virtually every systemic xenobiotic that acts on the organism.[92] The ease and frequency with which blood is assayed, its central role in functions vital to the organism, and the ability to analyze its characteristics, at first by light microscopy and more recently with molecular techniques, have enabled a detailed understanding of blood that continues to advance the frontiers of molecular medicine.

In addition to transporting xenobiotics throughout the body, blood and the blood-forming organs can at times be directly affected by these same xenobiotics. For example, decreased blood cell production, increased blood cell destruction, alteration of hemoglobin, and impairment of coagulation can all result from exposure to xenobiotics. The response in many cases depends on the nature and quantity of the xenobiotic as well as the capacity of the system to defend against the insult. In other cases, no clear and predictable dose–response relationship can be determined, especially when the interaction involves the immune system. These latter reactions are often termed idiosyncratic, reflecting an incomplete understanding of their causative mechanism. In general, such reactions can often be reclassified when advancing knowledge identifies the characteristics that render the individual vulnerable.

HEMATOPOIESIS

Hematopoiesis is the development of the cellular elements of blood. The majority of the cells of the blood system are classified as either lymphoid (B, T, and natural killer lymphocytes) or myeloid (erythrocytes, megakaryocytes, granulocytes, and monocytes). All of these cells originate from a small common pool of totipotent cells called *hematopoietic stem cells*. Indeed, the study of this process and its regulation has provided fundamental insight into embryogenesis, stem cell pluripotency, and complex cell-to-cell signaling and interaction.

Bone Marrow

Marrow spaces within bone begin to form in humans at about the fifth fetal month and become the sole site of granulocyte and megakaryocyte proliferation. Erythropoiesis moves from the liver to the marrow by the end of the last trimester. At birth, all marrow contributes to blood cell formation and is red, containing very few fat cells. By adulthood, the same volume of hematopoietic marrow is normally restricted to the sternum, ribs, pelvis, upper sacrum, proximal femora and humeri, skull, vertebrae, clavicles, and scapulae. Extramedullary hematopoiesis in the liver and spleen reemerges as a compensatory mechanism only under severe stimulation.

Progenitor cells must interact with a supportive microenvironment to sustain hematopoiesis. The hematopoietic stroma consists of macrophages, fibroblasts, adipocytes, and endothelial cells. The extracellular matrix is produced by the stromal cells and is composed of various fibrous proteins, glycoproteins, and proteoglycans, such as collagen, fibronectin, laminin, hemonectin, and thrombospondin. Hematopoietic progenitor cells have receptors to particular matrix molecules. The extracellular matrix provides a structural network to which the progenitors are anchored. As the cells approach maturity, they lose their surface receptors, allowing them to leave the hematopoietic space and enter the venous sinuses. Blood cell release depends on a pressure gradient that drives proliferating, mature cells through endothelial cells lining the sinusoidal spaces.[34] This pressure is contained by the surrounding rigid bone cortex and increases under the influence of erythropoietin and granulocyte colony-stimulating factor.

Stem Cells

A stem cell is capable of self-renewal, as well as differentiation into a specific cell type. The pluripotent hematopoietic stem cells can therefore continuously replicate while awaiting the appropriate signal to differentiate into either a myeloid or a lymphoid stem cell (Fig. 20–1). Stem cells represent only 1 in 100,000 of the nucleated cells of the bone marrow, and most of these stem cells are usually quiescent. Nevertheless, these relatively few cells are directly responsible for the estimated 200 billion red cells, 150 billion platelets, and 100 billion leukocytes produced each day.[34] In response to hemolysis or infection, substantially larger numbers of blood cells are produced.[73] Multiple steps are involved in the commitment of less-differentiated cells to more mature cell lines. The final steps in the maturation of erythrocytes alone, for example, involve extensive remodeling, the restructuring of cellular membranes, the accumulation of hemoglobin, and the loss of nuclei and organelles.

Multipotent mesenchymal stem cells capable of differentiating into other tissue lines, including hepatic, renal, muscle, and perhaps neuronal, are also found in the bone marrow.[41] Furthermore, tissue-specific stem cells capable of self-renewal reside in numerous other organs and to play a fundamental role in repair and regeneration.[21] A variety of strategies have likely evolved to protect the stem cell from injury due to xenobiotics and radiation, and a better understanding of these effects promises to improve our understanding of toxicity and treatment. The hematopoietic stem cell has provided fundamental insights into regenerative biology, and it remains a focus of intense research given the profound implications for organ homeostasis, tissue repair, and gene therapy.[59,62]

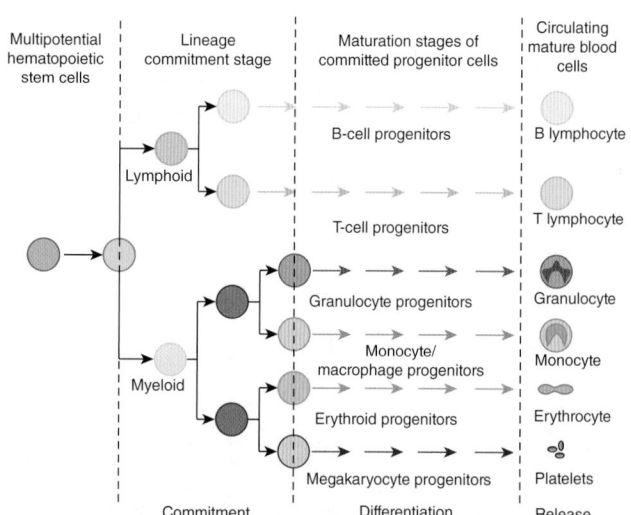

FIGURE 20–1. Principles of hematopoiesis. Commitment refers to the apparent inability of progenitor cells to generate hematopoietic stem cells. Following differentiation, the various mature blood cells are released into the circulation.

Cytokines

Cytokines are soluble mediators secreted by cells for cell-to-cell communication. Initially termed growth factors, it is now recognized that not all cytokines are growth factors. Cytokines promote or inhibit the differentiation, proliferation, and trafficking of blood cells and their precursors. Importantly, they can also inhibit apoptosis, and their absence therefore results in the self-destruction of unwanted cells. They include growth factors or colony-stimulating factors (CSFs), interleukins, monokines, interferons, and chemokines. At baseline, these act in concert to maintain normal blood counts. In response to antigens or other stimuli, cytokines are released to combat perceived infection. Recombinant cytokines are being used therapeutically in immunocompromised patients, transplant recipients, and those with hepatitis C, anemia, multiple sclerosis, and cancer. They are also being used in clinical toxicology, for example, for the treatment of leukocytopenia that results from colchicine and podophyllum toxicity.[29,44]

The growth factors are glycoproteins necessary for the differentiation and maturation of individual or multiple cell lines. They fall into 2 families based on their target receptors. The ligands of the cytokine receptor family include growth hormone, interleukin-2 (IL-2), macrophage colony-stimulating factor–1 (CSF-1), granulocyte-macrophage colony–stimulating factor (GM-CSF), γ-interferon, and granulocyte colony–stimulating factor (G-CSF), to name a few. The second group, the tyrosine kinase family, includes Kit ligand and insulinlike growth factor-1 receptor (IGF-1R), a member of the insulin family.

Cell Surface Antigens

Using monoclonal antibody technology, cell-surface antigens are used to characterize cell types. The cluster designation (CD) nomenclature was introduced by immunologists to ensure a common language when confronted with multiple antibodies to the same leukocyte cell-surface molecule, and hundreds of such unique molecules have been classified.[110] For example, the CD34 antigen is a 115-kilodalton (kDa) highly glycosylated transmembrane protein that is selectively expressed by primitive multipotent hematopoietic stem cells shortly after activation, but is absent from mature T and B lymphocytes.[64] Advances in genomics and proteomics now complement the immunologic designation, but the ability to subtype blood cells phenotypically has transformed the approach to the leukemias, autoimmune disease, transplantation medicine, and thromboembolic disease.

The human leukocyte antigen (HLA) system denotes the major histocompatibility complex in humans, a group of genes involved in antigen presentation to T lymphocytes, the complement system, cancer surveillance, and autoimmune disease. The rich variation in HLA genes, with more than 100 known alleles at 6 loci, may reflect selective evolutionary pressure to deter individuals with similar HLA from mating. Such sexual selection enhancing diversity would protect a population from coevolving pathogens that attempted to mimic a specific human epitope and avoid immune attack. Indeed, humans appear to be able to distinguish and preferentially choose partners with HLA alleles different from their own using smell, promoting heterozygous diversity.[68] Exposure to blood transfusions, pregnancy, and organ grafts can generate antibodies against non-self HLAs.

APLASTIC ANEMIA

Aplastic anemia is characterized by pancytopenia on peripheral smear, a hypocellular marrow, and delayed plasma iron clearance. Severe aplastic anemia denotes a granulocyte count of less than 500 cells/mm³, a platelet count of less than 20,000/mm³, and a reticulocyte count of less than 1% after correction for anemia. Following acute insult and depletion of extracirculatory reserves, cell line counts fall at a rate inversely proportional to their life span: granulocytes (circulating half-life 6–12 hours) disappear within days, platelets (life span of 7–10 days) decline by half in about one week, while erythrocytes (normal life span 120 days) decline over weeks in the absence of bleeding or hemolysis. Approximately 1,000 new cases of aplastic anemia are diagnosed yearly in the United States. The incidence is 2 to 3 times higher in Asia, perhaps because of a combination of genetic, environmental, and

TABLE 20–1	Selected Xenobiotics Associated with Aplastic Anemia
Analgesics	Antirheumatics
Acetaminophen	Gold salts
Diclofenac	Methotrexate
Dipyrone	D-Penicillamine
Indomethacin	Antithyroids
Phenylbutazone	Propylthiouracil
Salicylates	Chemotherapeutics[a]
Antidysrhythmics	Adriamycin[a]
Tocainide	Antimetabolites
Antiepileptics	Colchicine
Carbamazepine	Daunorubicin[a]
Felbamate	Mustards
Levetiracetam	Vinblastine
Antihistamines	Vincristine
Cimetidine	Diuretics
Antimicrobials	Acetazolamide
Albendazole	Metolazone
Chloramphenicol	Occupational
Mefloquine	Arsenic[a]
Penicillin	Benzene[a]
Zidovudine	Cadmium
Antiplatelets	Pesticides
Ticlopidine	Radiation[a]
Antipsychotics	
Chlorpromazine	
Clozapine	

[a]Denotes xenobiotics that predictably result in bone marrow aplasia following a sufficiently large exposure.

infectious factors.[108] Aplastic anemia may be inborn (as in Fanconi anemia) or acquired. A variety of xenobiotics such as benzene, pesticides, and chloramphenicol are associated with acquired aplastic anemia (Table 20–1),[20,109] but causality is uncertain given uncertain case ascertainment and other biases. Epidemiologic studies demonstrate that specific causes are identified in relatively few cases.[52]

Generally speaking, the majority of cases of so-called idiosyncratic aplastic anemia are caused by autoimmune attack on CD34+ hematopoietic stem cells. Following an exposure to an inciting antigen, cytotoxic T cells secrete interferon-γ and tumor necrosis factor α, which destroy progenitor cells, eventually depleting mature leukocytes, erythrocytes, and platelets in circulation.[109] As with other autoimmune diseases, certain HLA patterns are associated with a genetic predisposition for the condition, namely the HLA DR2. Clozapine-induced agranulocytosis is associated with the HLA B38, DR4, and DQ3 haplotypes.[74] Immunosuppressive therapy or allogenic stem cell transplantation allows recovery of hematopoiesis, and survival is now expected.[108]

It is important to distinguish immunologic xenobiotic-induced aplastic anemia from the direct myelotoxic effects of radiation and chemotherapy. Following exposure to ionizing radiation, a pancytopenia ensues as a result of injury to stem and progenitor cells. Although atom bomb survivors rarely developed aplastic anemia,[49] fractionated whole body radiation of at least 10 Gy is used to intentionally destroy bone marrow stem cells prior to hematopoietic stem cell transplantation. Cancer chemotherapy is often dosed to the endpoint of reversible hematopoietic toxicity. Vacuolated pronormoblasts are found in the bone marrow when aplasia is due to a myelotoxic drug, and treatment consists primarily of stopping the offending xenobiotic while supporting cell lines and preventing infection and bleeding. Other nonimmunologic mechanisms of aplasia are identified in specific cases. For example, the severe pancytopenia that occasionally occurs following 5-fluorouracil therapy is caused by a deficiency of dihydropyrimidine dehydrogenase present in 3% to 5% of whites.[104]

THE ERYTHRON

The erythron is often considered to be a single yet dispersed tissue, defined as the entire mass of erythroid cells from the first committed progenitor cell to the mature circulating erythrocyte (red blood cell). This functional definition emphasizes the integrated regulation of the erythron, both in health and disease. The primary function of the erythron is to transport molecular oxygen throughout the organism. To accomplish this, adequate numbers of circulating erythrocytes (nearly half of the blood by volume) must be maintained. These erythrocytes must be able to preserve their structure and flexibility to circuit repeatedly through the microcirculation and to resist oxidant stress accumulated during their life span.[84] The erythrocyte also plays a key role in modulating vascular tone. Interactions between oxyhemoglobin and nitric oxide help match vasomotor tone to local tissue oxygen demands.[30,39,43,67,91]

Homeostasis of erythron proliferation is primarily maintained by the equilibrium between stimulation via the hormone erythropoietin and apoptosis controlled by 2 receptors, Fas and FasL, expressed on the membranes of erythroid precursors. At the other extreme, erythrocytes are culled from the circulation at the end of their life span primarily by the action of the spleen. With age, erythrocytes become less able to negotiate the narrow red pulp passages in the spleen and are phagocytosed by macrophages. By filtering out these senescent cells, the spleen minimizes entrapment in the microvasculature of other organs and prevents spillage of intracellular contents including hemoglobin into the intravascular circulation.

Erythropoietin

Erythropoietin (EPO) is a glycoprotein hormone of molecular weight 34,000 Da that is produced in the epithelial cells lining the peritubular capillaries of the kidney. Anemia and hypoxemia stimulate its synthesis. Erythropoietin receptors are found in human erythroid cells, megakaryocytes, and fetal liver. Erythropoietin promotes erythroid differentiation, the mobilization of marrow progenitor cells, and the premature release of marrow reticulocytes. The cell most sensitive to EPO is a cell between the erythroid colony–forming unit (CFU-E) and the proerythroblast. The absence of EPO results in DNA cleavage and erythroid cell death.

The Mature Erythrocyte

The mature erythrocyte is a highly specialized cell, designed primarily for oxygen transport. Accordingly, it is densely packed with hemoglobin, which constitutes approximately 90% of the dry weight of the erythrocyte. During maturation, the erythrocyte loses its nucleus, mitochondria, and other organelles, rendering it incapable of synthesizing new protein, replicating, or using the oxygen being transported for oxidative phosphorylation. Its metabolic repertoire is severely limited and largely restricted to a few pathways (described below under Metabolism). In general, the enzymatic pathways are those required for optimizing oxygen and carbon dioxide exchange, transiting the microcirculation while maintaining cellular integrity and flexibility, and resisting oxidant stress on the iron and protein of the cell. The characteristic biconcave discocyte shape is dynamically maintained, increasing membrane surface-to-cell volume. This shape decreases intracellular diffusion distances to the cell membrane and allows plastic deformation when squeezing through the microcirculation. The shape is the net sum of elastic and electrostatic forces within the membrane, surface tension, and osmotic and hydrostatic pressures. The cell membrane contains globular proteins suspended within the phospholipid bilayer. The major blood group antigens are carried on membrane ceramide glycolipids and proteins, particularly glycophorin A and the Rh proteins. Membrane proteins generally serve to maintain the structure of the cell, to transport ions and other substances across the membrane, or to catalyze a limited number of specific chemical reactions for the cell.

Structural Proteins

The cell membrane is coupled to, and interacts dynamically with, the cytoskeleton, allowing changes in cell shape such as tank treading or rotation of the membrane relative to the cytoplasm. This cytoskeleton consists of a hexagonal lattice of proteins, especially spectrin, actin, and protein 4.1, which interact with ankyrin and band 3 in the membrane to provide a strong but flexible structure to the membrane. Other essential structural proteins include tropomyosin, tropomodulin, and adducin. The absence or abnormalities of these proteins results in abnormal erythrocyte shapes such as spherocytes and elliptocytes.

Transport Proteins

Many specialized transport proteins are embedded in the erythrocyte membrane. These include anion and cation transporters, glucose and urea transporters, and water channels. The erythrocyte membrane is relatively impermeable to ion flux. Band 3 anion-exchange protein plays an important role in the chloride–bicarbonate exchanges that occur as the erythrocyte moves between the lung and tissues. Glucose, the sole source of energy of the erythrocyte, crosses the membrane by facilitated diffusion mediated by a transmembrane glucose transporter. Sodium-potassium adenosine triphosphatase (Na^+,K^+,ATPase) maintains the primary cation gradient by pumping sodium out of the erythrocyte in exchange for potassium.

Membrane-Associated Enzymes

At least 50 membrane-bound or membrane-associated enzymes are known to exist in the human erythrocyte. Acetylcholinesterase is an externally oriented enzyme whose role in the function of the erythrocyte remains obscure. Its function is inhibited by certain xenobiotics, most notably the organic phosphorus compounds, and it is conveniently assayed as a marker for such exposures (Chap. 110).

Metabolism

Lacking mitochondria and the ability to generate adenosine triphosphate (ATP) using molecular oxygen, the mature erythrocyte has a severely limited repertoire of intermediary metabolism compared to most mammalian cells. Having lost its nucleus, ribosomes, and translational apparatus, new enzymes cannot be synthesized and existing enzymes decline in function over the lifetime of the cell. Fortunately, the metabolic demands of the erythrocyte are usually modest, but under conditions of stress that capacity can be overwhelmed, especially among senescent cells. The greatest expenditure of energy under physiologic conditions is for the maintenance of transmembrane gradients and for the contraction of cytoskeletal elements. However, oxidant stress can put severe strain on the metabolic reserves of the erythrocyte, and lead ultimately to the premature destruction of the cell, a process termed hemolysis.

Figure 20–2 illustrates the main metabolic pathways and their purpose. Embden-Meyerhof glycolysis is the only source of ATP for the erythrocyte and consumes approximately 90% of the glucose imported by the cell. The reduced nicotinamide adenine dinucleotide (NADH) generated during glycolysis, which would ordinarily be used for oxidative phosphorylation in cells containing mitochondria, is directed toward the reduction of either methemoglobin to hemoglobin by cytochrome b5 reductase, or of pyruvate to lactate. Both pyruvate and lactate are exported from the cell. In response to anemia, altitude, or changes in cellular pH, glycolysis is diverted into the Rapoport-Luebering shunt, generating 2,3-bisphosphoglycerate (2,3-BPG, formerly known as 2,3-diphosphoglycerate or 2,3-DPG) in lieu of ATP. 2,3-bisphosphoglycerate binds to deoxyhemoglobin to modulate oxygen affinity and to allow unloading of oxygen at the capillaries, thereby increasing oxygen delivery considerably. Reduced levels of 2,3-BPG in stored blood result in impaired oxygen delivery following massive transfusion.[101]

As an alternative to glycolysis, glucose is diverted to the hexose monophosphate shunt during times of oxidant stress. This pathway results in the generation of reduced nicotinamide adenine dinucleotide phosphate (NADPH), which the erythrocyte uses to maintain reduced glutathione. Reduced glutathione, in turn, inactivates oxidants and protects the sulfhydryl groups of hemoglobin and other proteins. The initial, rate-limiting step of this pathway is controlled by glucose-6-phosphate dehydrogenase (G6PD). Accordingly, cells deficient in this enzyme are less able to maintain reduced glutathione, and are vulnerable to irreversible damage under oxidant stress.

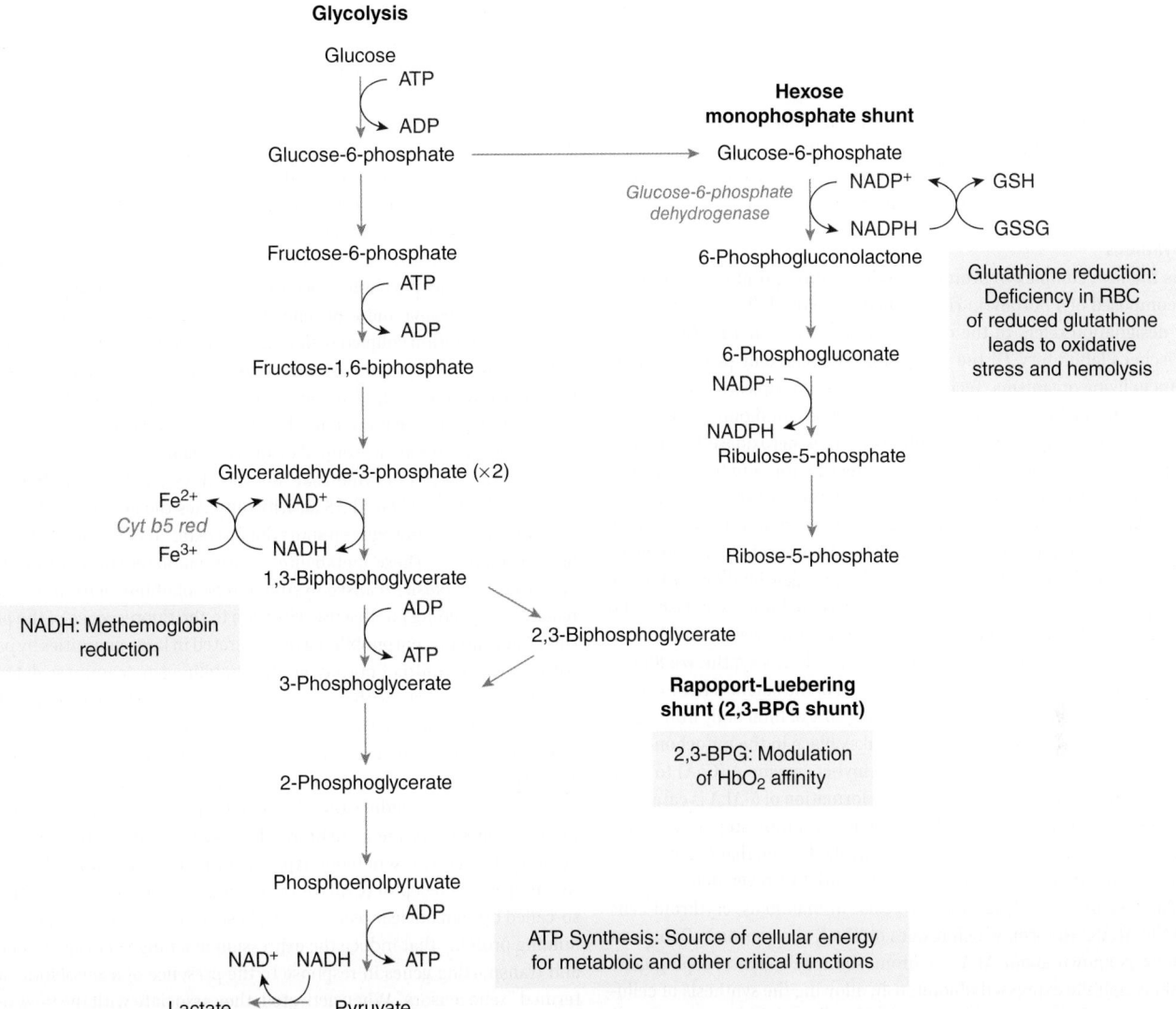

FIGURE 20–2. Metabolic pathways of the erythrocyte. The main metabolic pathways available to the mature erythrocyte are shown (rectangles). Glucose is imported into the cell, while pyruvate, lactate, and oxidized glutathione (GSSG) are exported. 2,3-BPG = 2,3-bisphosphoglycerate; ADP = adenosine diphosphate; ATP = adenosine triphosphate; cyt b5 red = cytochrome b5 reductase; G6PD = glucose-6-phosphate dehydrogenase; GSH = reduced glutathione; Hb = hemoglobin; NADH = reduced form of nicotinamide adenine dinucleotide (NAD+); NADPH = reduced form of nicotinamide adenine dinucleotide phosphate (NADP+); RBC = red blood cell (erythrocyte).

The consequences of this deficiency are discussed in greater detail below under Glucose-6-Phosphate Dehydrogenase Deficiencies.

The erythrocyte also contains enzymes to synthesize glutathione (γ-glutamyl-cysteine synthetase and glutathione synthetase), to convert CO_2 to bicarbonate ion (carbonic anhydrase I), to remove pyrimidines resulting from the degradation of RNA (pyrimidine 5′-nucleotidase), to protect against free radicals (catalase, superoxide dismutase, glutathione peroxidase), and to conjugate glutathione to electrophiles (ρ-glutathione-*S*-transferase).

Hemoglobin

Hemoglobin, the major constituent of the cytoplasm of the erythrocyte, is a conjugated protein with a molecular weight of 64,500 Da. To put things in perspective, the typical adult man has approximately 75 mL/kg of blood containing 15 g/100 mL of hemoglobin, or nearly 1 kg of hemoglobin. His 0.3-kg heart must pump this entire mass of hemoglobin every minute at rest, which is a substantial work expenditure. One molecule is composed of 4 protein (globin) chains, each attached to a prosthetic group called heme. Heme contains an iron molecule complexed at the center of a porphyrin ring. The globin chains are held together by noncovalent electrostatic attraction into a tetrahedral array. Hemoglobin is so efficient at binding and carrying

oxygen that it enables blood to transport nearly 100 times as much oxygen as could be carried by plasma alone (Chap. 28). In addition, the capacity of hemoglobin to modulate oxygen binding under different conditions allows adaptation to a wide variety of environments and demands. Three complex and integrated pathways are required for the formation of hemoglobin: globin synthesis, protoporphyrin synthesis, and iron metabolism.

Globin Synthesis

The protein chains of hemoglobin are produced with information from 2 different genetic loci. The α-globin gene cluster spans 30 kb on the short arm of chromosome 16, and codes for 2 identical adult α-chain genes, as well as the ζ-chain, an embryonic globulin. The β cluster is 50 kb on chromosome 11, and codes for the 2 adult globins β and δ, as well as 2 nearly identical γ chains expressed in the fetus and an embryonic globulin ε. The expression of genes in each family changes during embryonic, fetal, neonatal, and adult development. Until 8 weeks of intrauterine life, ε, ζ, γ, and α chains are produced and assembled in various combinations in yolk sac–derived erythrocytes. With the shift in erythropoiesis from yolk sac to fetal liver and spleen, embryonic hemoglobin disappears, and the α and γ globin chains are paired into fetal hemoglobin (HbF = $\alpha_2\gamma_2$). Erythrocytes containing HbF have a higher

O_2 affinity than those containing adult hemoglobin, which is important for oxygen transfer across the placenta into the relatively hypoxic uterine environment. Beginning shortly before birth, expression at the β cluster shifts to the β and δ globins. The predominant adult hemoglobin is termed hemoglobin A ($\alpha_2\beta_2$), whereas approximately 2.5% of normal adult hemoglobin is in the form of hemoglobin A_2 ($\alpha_2\delta_2$). The thalassemias, a group of inherited disorders, result from defective synthesis of one or more of the globin chains. Clinically this results in a hypochromic, microcytic anemia.

Heme Synthesis

Heme is the iron complex of protoporphyrin IX. Protoporphyrin IX is a tetramer composed of 4 porphyrin rings joined in a closed, flat-ring structure. The IX designation refers to the order in which it was first synthesized in Hans Fischer's laboratory. Of the 15 possible isomers, only protoporphyrin IX occurs in living organisms. Technically, only iron complexes with the iron in the Fe^{2+} state can be called heme, but the term is commonly used to refer to the prosthetic group of metalloproteins such as peroxidase (ferric) and cytochrome c (both ferric and ferrous), whether the iron is in the Fe^{2+} or Fe^{3+} state. The terms "hemiglobin" and "ferrihemoglobin" are synonymous with methemoglobin but rarely used. All animal cells can synthesize heme, with the notable exception of mature erythrocytes. Hemoproteins are involved in a multitude of biologic functions, including oxygen binding (hemoglobin, myoglobin), oxygen metabolism (oxidases, peroxidases, catalases, and hydroxylases), and electron transport (cytochromes), as well as metabolism of xenobiotics (cytochrome P450 family). Erythroid cells synthesize 85% of total body heme, with the liver synthesizing most of the balance. Hemoglobin is the most abundant hemoprotein, containing 70% of total body iron.

The first step in the synthesis of heme takes place in the mitochondrion and is the condensation of glycine and succinyl-coenzyme A (CoA) to form 5-aminolevulinic acid (ALA) (Fig. 20–3). The formation of 5-ALA is catalyzed by aminolevulinic acid synthase (ALAS), the rate-limiting step of the pathway. The rate of heme synthesis is closely controlled, given that free intracellular heme is toxic and that this first step is essentially irreversible.

Of the 2 isoforms of ALAS known to exist in mammals, erythroid cells express the ALAS2 isoform, which resides on the X chromosome. Comparatively more is known about ALAS1 (chromosome 3), a housekeeping gene with a short half-life expressed ubiquitously, allowing the synthesis of cellular and mitochondrial hemoproteins. Aminolevulinic acid synthase (ALAS1) activity is induced by many factors, which can increase its expression by 2 orders of magnitude. Moreover, it is strongly inhibited by heme in a classical negative feedback fashion. Aminolevulinic acid synthase (ALAS2) is constitutively expressed at very high concentrations in erythroid precursors, allowing sustained synthesis of heme during erythropoiesis. Pyridoxal phosphate (active vitamin B_6) serves as a cofactor to both isoforms of ALAS. The clinical consequences of pyridoxine deficiency include a hypochromic, microcytic anemia, iron overload, and neurologic impairment.

The next step in the synthesis of hemoglobin is the formation of the monopyrrole porphobilinogen via the condensation of 2 molecules of ALA.

The subsequent steps in heme synthesis involve the condensation of 4 molecules of porphobilinogen into a flat ring, which is transported back into the mitochondrion by an unknown mechanism. The final step is the insertion of iron into protoporphyrin IX, a reaction that is catalyzed by ferrochelatase (also known as heme synthase) to form heme.

Understanding this carefully regulated synthetic pathway is relevant to understanding the laboratory evidence of lead toxicity (Chap. 93), and predicting the response of porphyric patients to a range of xenobiotics. Most steps in the heme biosynthetic pathway are inhibited by lead. ALA dehydratase is the most sensitive, followed by ferrochelatase, coproporphyrinogen oxidase, and porphobilinogen deaminase. As a consequence, ALA is increased in plasma and especially urine. With increasing exposure, ferrochelatase inhibition coupled with iron deficiency causes zinc protoporphyrin to accumulate in erythrocytes, which can easily be detected by fluorescence. Coproporphyrinogen III also appears in the urine. Historically, these effects have served as the basis for a number of tests of lead exposure.

The porphyrias are a group of disorders resulting from an inherited deficiency of any given enzyme that follows ALAS on the heme biosynthetic pathway. As such, when ALAS activity outpaces the activity of the deficient enzyme, the rate-limiting step shifts downstream, and intermediate metabolites accumulate. These metabolites cause characteristic neuropsychiatric symptoms and palsies (caused by ALA and porphobilinogen), and cutaneous reactions, including photosensitivity (due to the fluorescence of the porphyrins). For example, porphobilinogen is excreted in large quantities by patients with acute intermittent porphyria (porphobilinogen deaminase deficiency), and the urine darkens with exposure to air and light due to oxidation to porphobilin and to nonenzymatic assembly into porphyrin rings. A variety of xenobiotics precipitate crises in susceptible individuals, by inducing ALAS1 and overloading the deficient enzyme.[100] The molecular mechanisms that allow xenobiotics to induce the ALAS1 gene closely resemble those accounting for induction of the cytochrome P450 (CYP) genes, which also require heme synthesis. The xenobiotic typically interacts with either the constitutive androstane receptor (CAR) or the pregnane X receptor (PXR), the 2 main so-called orphan nuclear receptors.[107] These transcriptional factors are DNA-binding proteins that induce the expression of a range of drug metabolizing and transporting genes in response to the presence of a xenobiotic and are termed "xenosensors." When activated, they associate with the 9-*cis* retinoic acid xenobiotic receptor (RXR), and then attach to enhancer sequences near the apoCYP or ALAS1 genes to enhance transcription.[81] The multifunctional inducers capable of activating a wide range of hepatic enzymes are therefore extremely porphyrogenic and include phenobarbital, phenytoin, carbamazepine, and primidone. Furthermore, because CYP 3A4 and 2C9 represent nearly half of the hepatic CYP pool, inducers of these isoforms also stimulate heme synthesis and induce porphyric crises. Examples include the anticonvulsants; nifedipine; sulfamethoxazole; rifampicin; ketoconazole; and the reproductive steroids progesterone, medroxyprogesterone, and testosterone. Glucocorticoids, on the other hand, despite binding to PXR, suppress ALAS1 induction and translation, and they are not porphyrogenic.[100]

Iron Metabolism

At equilibrium, approximately 1 to 2 mg of iron is absorbed from the diet, and a similar amount is shed from the intestinal epithelium each day. Unless appropriately chelated, free iron not bound by transport or storage proteins can generate harmful oxygen free radicals that damage cellular structures and metabolism (Chaps. 10 and 45). For this reason, serum iron circulates bound to a transfer protein, transferrin, and is stored in the tissues using ferritin (Fig. 20–4). Whereas each molecule of transferrin can bind 2 iron atoms, ferritin has a large internal cavity, approximately 80 Å in diameter, that can hold up to 4500 iron atoms per molecule. The amount of iron transported through plasma depends on total-body iron stores and the rate of erythropoiesis. Only about one-third of the iron-binding sites of circulating transferrin are normally saturated, as demonstrated by the usual serum iron content of 60 to 170 mcg/dL (10–30 μmol/L) as compared to the total iron-binding capacity of 280 to 390 mcg/dL (50–70 μmol/L).

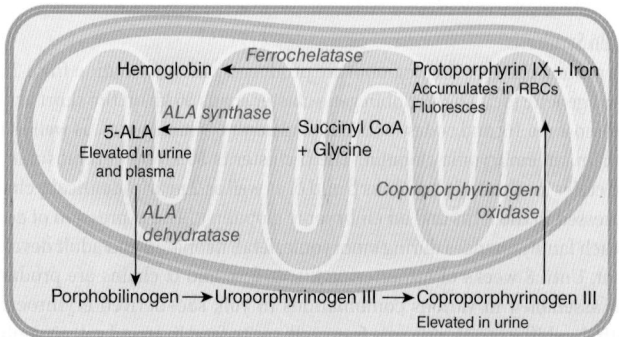

FIGURE 20–3. The heme synthesis pathway. The enzymatic steps inhibited by lead are marked in red. 5-ALA = 5-aminolevulinic acid; RBCs = red blood cells.

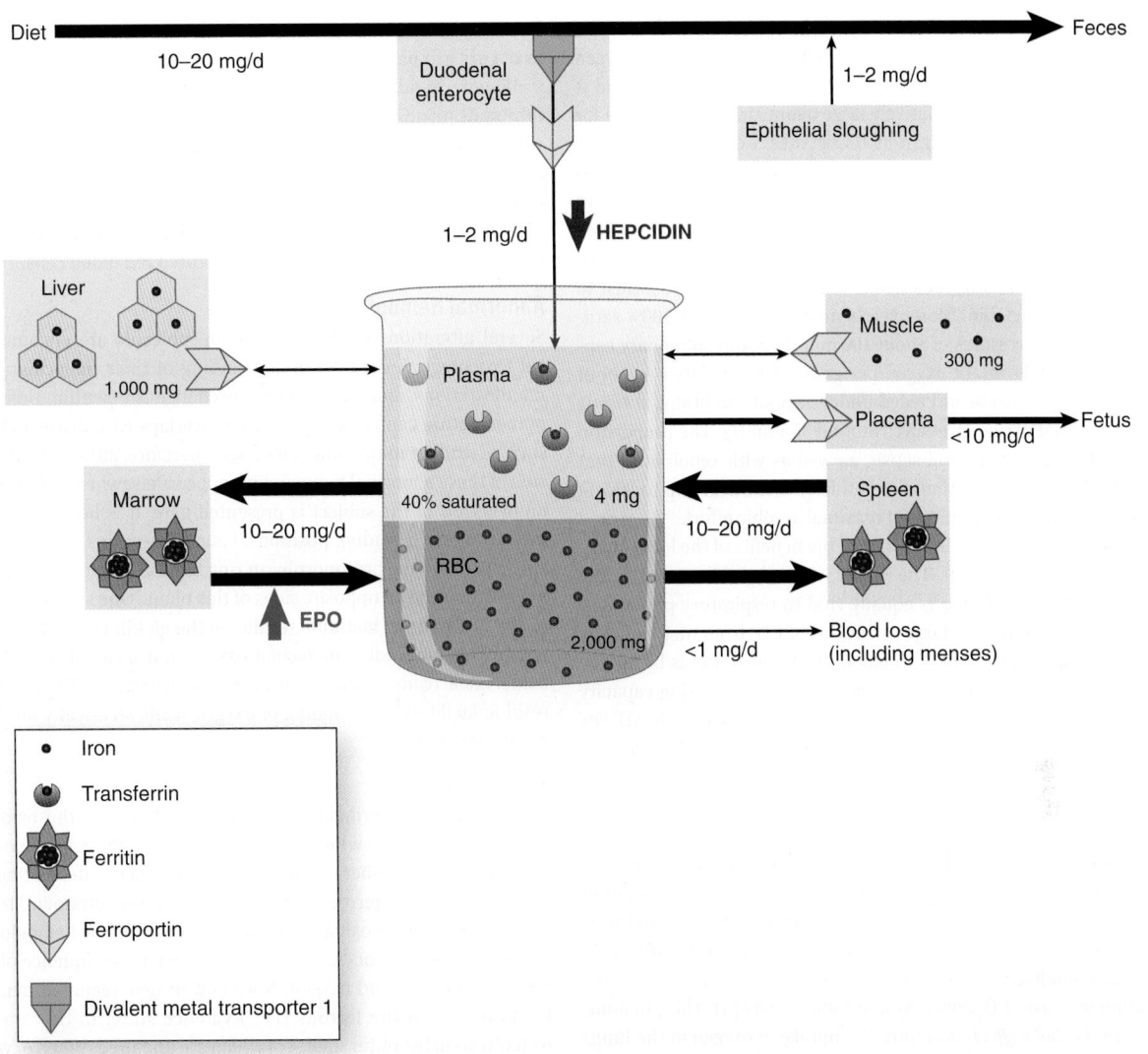

FIGURE 20–4. The iron cycle. The flow of iron is indicated by arrows, and average daily rates of flux are shown for an adult. Absorption at the duodenal enterocyte is tightly controlled, because there are few physiologic processes to regulate losses (other than pregnancy and menstruation). Atomic iron is absorbed via the divalent metal transporter 1, and heme-bound iron via heme carrier protein 1. Hepcidin is an important circulating peptide inhibitor of ferroportin, thereby limiting absorption when stores are adequate. Iron content (either atomic or heme bound) of specific organs or compartments is shown in milligrams. The largest stores of atomic iron are contained by ferritin, mostly in liver and spleen macrophages, and erythrocyte precursors in the marrow. Only a relatively small amount circulates in the plasma bound to transferrin, which is usually only partially saturated. EPO = erythropoietin; RBC = red blood cell.

Only transferrin can directly supply iron for hemoglobin synthesis. The iron–transferrin complex binds to transferrin receptors on the surface of developing erythroid cells in bone marrow. Iron in the erythroid cell is used for hemoglobin synthesis or is stored in ferritin.

The absorption of nonheme, free ferrous iron from the diet occurs via the divalent metal transporter 1 of the duodenal enterocyte, which then passes it into the circulation via ferroportin. Iron then circulates in the ferric form bound to transferrin.[46] Dietary iron complexed with heme can also be absorbed via the heme carrier protein-1, which transports either iron or zinc protoporphyrin into the enterocyte.[61] The iron may then be freed by microsomal heme oxygenase and follow the transport of atomic iron, or perhaps heme itself can be transferred to the circulation via specific export proteins and circulate bound to its carrier protein, hemopexin.[5]

When the erythrocyte is removed from the circulation by splenic macrophages, heme is degraded by heme oxygenase to carbon monoxide and biliverdin, and the iron extracted. Some iron remains in macrophages in the form of ferritin or hemosiderin. Most is delivered again by ferroportin back to the plasma and bound to transferrin.

Iron homeostasis is largely regulated at the level of absorption, with little physiologic control over its rate of loss. Excess absorption relative to body stores is the hallmark of hereditary hemochromatosis. The iron regulatory hormone hepcidin produced by the liver plays a central role in iron control, including the anemia of chronic disease caused by inflammatory signals.[46] Hepcidin is a 25–amino acid peptide that senses iron stores and controls the ferroportin-mediated release of iron from enterocytes, macrophages, and hepatocytes. The liver is an important reservoir of iron because it can store considerable amounts of iron taken from portal blood and release it when needed.

Oxygen–Carbon Dioxide Exchange

The evolutionary transition of organisms from anaerobic to aerobic life allowed the liberation of 18 times more energy from glucose. Vertebrates developed 2 important systems to overcome the relatively small quantities of oxygen dissolved in aqueous solutions under atmospheric conditions: the circulatory system and hemoglobin. The circulatory system allows delivery of oxygen and removal of carbon dioxide throughout the organism. Hemoglobin plays an essential role in the transport and exchange of both gases. Moreover, the interactions between these gases and hemoglobin are directly linked in a remarkable story of molecular evolution. Understanding this interplay allowed early insight into protein conformation and the importance of allosteric interactions between molecules.

The binding of each oxygen molecule to atomic iron in any of the 4 heme molecules results in conformational changes that affect binding of oxygen at the remaining sites. This phenomenon is known as *cooperativity*, and it is necessary for the transport of relatively large quantities of oxygen and for the unloading of most of this oxygen at tissue sites. Cooperativity results from the intramolecular interactions of the tetrameric hemoglobin, and is expressed in the sigmoidal shape of the oxyhemoglobin dissociation curve (Fig. 28–2). Conversely, the monomeric myoglobin has a hyperbolic oxygen binding curve. The partial pressure of oxygen at which 50% of the oxygen-binding sites of hemoglobin are occupied is about 26 mm Hg, in contrast to about 1 mm Hg for myoglobin. Moreover, hemoglobin is nearly 100% saturated at partial oxygen pressures of about 100 mm Hg in the pulmonary capillaries, transporting 1.34 mL of oxygen per gram of hemoglobin A. About one-third of this oxygen can be unloaded under normal conditions at tissue capillaries with partial oxygen pressures around 35 mm Hg. The proportion unloaded rises during exercise and sepsis, as well as with xenobiotics that uncouple oxidative phosphorylation. Elite athletes can extract up to 80% of the available oxygen under conditions of maximal aerobic effort.

The oxygen reserve, however, is only one of the benefits of the large quantity of hemoglobin in circulation. The ability of hemoglobin to buffer the acid equivalent of CO_2 in solution is equally vital to respiratory physiology, because it allows the removal of large quantities of CO_2 from metabolically active tissues with minimal changes in blood pH. Hemoglobin is by far the largest buffer in circulation, accounting for 7 times the buffering capacity of the serum proteins combined (28 versus 4 mEq H^+/L of whole blood). For every 1 mole of oxygen unloaded in the tissue, about 0.5 mole of H^+ is loaded onto hemoglobin.

The linked interaction between oxygen and carbon dioxide transport can be first considered from the perspective of oxygen binding to hemoglobin. The affinity of oxygen for hemoglobin is directly affected by pH, which is a function of the CO_2 content of the blood. The oxyhemoglobin dissociation curve shifts to the left in lungs, where the level of carbon dioxide, and thus carbonic acid, are kept relatively low as a result of ventilation, an effect that promotes oxygen binding. The curve shifts to the right in tissues where cellular respiration increases CO_2 concentrations and lowers pH. This phenomenon, known as the *Bohr effect*, promotes the uptake of oxygen in the lungs and the release of oxygen at tissue sites.

From the perspective of carbon dioxide transport, hemoglobin also plays an essential albeit indirect role. Carbon dioxide dissolves into plasma, and is slowly hydrated to carbonic acid, which dissociates to H^+ and HCO_3^- (pK_a 6.35). The speed of the hydration reaction is accelerated from about 40 seconds to 10 ms by the abundant enzyme carbonic anhydrase located within the erythrocyte. Most carbon dioxide collected at the tissues diffuses into erythrocytes, where it becomes H^+ and HCO_3^-. This HCO_3^- is then rapidly transported back to the serum in exchange for chloride ion via the band 3 anion exchange transporter located in the erythrocyte membrane, thereby shifting serum Cl^- into the erythrocyte (the *chloride shift*). The hydrogen ion is accepted by hemoglobin, largely at the imidazole ring of histidine residues, which have a pK_a of about 7.0. A small amount of CO_2 reacts directly with the amino terminal of the globin chains to form carbamino residues ($HbNHCOO^-$). Thus, most of the transported carbon dioxide is transformed by the erythrocyte into bicarbonate ion that is returned to the serum and hydrogen ion that is buffered by hemoglobin. Each liter of venous blood typically carries 0.8 mEq dissolved CO_2 + 16 mEq HCO_3^- in the plasma, and 0.4 mEq dissolved CO_2 + 4.6 mEq HCO_3^- + 1.2 mEq $HbNHCOO^-$ in the erythrocyte (a total of 23 mEq CO_2, equivalent to 510 mL CO_2/L blood). Although two-thirds of the total CO_2 content is ultimately carried in the plasma, nearly all of the bicarbonate is generated within erythrocytes. In the capillaries of the lungs, the reverse reactions occur to eliminate CO_2. Because deoxyhemoglobin is better able to buffer hydrogen ions, the release of oxygen from hemoglobin at the tissues facilitates the uptake of carbon dioxide into venous blood. This effect is known as the *Haldane effect*. In fact, 1 L of venous blood at 70% oxygen saturation can transport an additional 20 mL of CO_2 compared to arterial blood, which is nearly 100% saturated. Both the Bohr and Haldane effects

have important consequences at the extremes of acid–base perturbations, as occurs in a number of poisonings that interfere with oxygen metabolism.

Finally, in addition to inactivating nitric oxide, hemoglobin also reversibly binds nitric oxide as *S*-nitrosohemoglobin, thereby playing an important role in the regulation of microvascular circulation and oxygen delivery. The ability of hemoglobin to vasodilate the surrounding microvasculature in response to oxygen desaturation using nitric oxide provides new insight into oxygen delivery and may be pivotal in such disorders as septic shock, pulmonary hypertension, and senescence of stored red blood cells.[94]

Abnormal Hemoglobins

Several alterations of the hemoglobin molecule are encountered in clinical toxicology. A detailed understanding of their molecular basis, clinical manifestations, and effects on gas exchange is essential. Unfortunately, the nomenclature can be ambiguous and overlaps with distinct clinical entities such as oxidant injury and hemolysis. Therefore, although a detailed discussion of these abnormal hemoglobins appears elsewhere (Chaps. 122 and 124), an overview of the subject is presented here. It is helpful to recall that the iron atom has 6 binding positions. Four of these positions are attached in a single plane to the protoporphyrin ring to form heme. The remaining 2 binding positions lie on opposite sides of this plane. One site is ordinarily bonded to the F8 proximal histidine residue of the globin chain. The remaining site is available for binding molecular oxygen, but it can also bind carbon monoxide, nitric oxide, cyanide, a hydroxide ion, or water. The E7 distal histidine residue facilitates the binding of oxygen while stearically hindering carbon monoxide binding.

Methemoglobin

Methemoglobin (ferrihemoglobin or hemiglobin) is the oxidized form of deoxyhemoglobin in which at least one heme iron is in the oxidized (Fe^{3+}) valence state. A number of valency hybrids can occur, depending on the number of ferric versus ferrous heme units within the tetramer. Methemoglobin therefore represents oxidation (loss of electrons) of the hemoglobin molecule at the iron atom. It occurs spontaneously as a consequence of interactions between the iron and oxygen. Normally, in deoxygenated hemoglobin, the heme iron is in the ferrous (Fe^{2+}) valence state. In this state, there are 6 electrons in the outer shell, 4 of which are unpaired. When oxygen is bound, one of these electrons is partially transferred to it and the iron is reversibly oxidized. When oxygen is released, the electron is usually transferred back to heme iron, yielding the normal reduced state. Sometimes, the electron remains with the oxygen yielding a superoxide anion radical $O_2^{\bullet-}$ rather than molecular oxygen. In this case, heme iron is left in the Fe^{3+}, or oxidized, state and is unable to release another electron to bind oxygen. This oxidation is primarily reversed via the action of cytochrome b5 reductase, also known as NADH methemoglobin reductase, which uses the electron carrier NADH generated by glycolysis (Chap. 11). Minor pathways are also involved in methemoglobin reduction, including NADPH methemoglobin reductase, which normally reduces only approximately 5% of the methemoglobin, and vitamin C, a nonenzymatic reducing agent. The activity of NADPH methemoglobin reductase is significantly accelerated by the presence of the electron donor methylene blue (Antidotes in Depth: A43 and Chap. 124) or riboflavin. Equilibrium is maintained with methemoglobin concentrations of ~1% of total hemoglobin. Many xenobiotics increase the rate of methemoglobin formation by as much as 1,000-fold. Nitrites, nitrates, chlorates, and quinones are capable of directly oxidizing hemoglobin.[19] Certain individuals are especially vulnerable resulting from deficient methemoglobin reduction.[28] The fetus and neonate are more susceptible to methemoglobinemia than the adult, because HbF is more susceptible to oxidation of the heme iron than adult hemoglobin. The newborn also has a limited capacity to reduce methemoglobin, because adult concentrations of cytochrome b5 reductase are only achieved at about 6 months of age.

Carboxyhemoglobin

Carbon monoxide (CO) can reversibly bind to heme iron in lieu of molecular oxygen. The affinity of CO for hemoglobin is 200–300 times that of oxygen, despite the stearic hindrance of the E7 distal histidine. The presence of CO thereby precludes the binding of oxygen. In addition, CO binding within any one heme subunit degrades the cooperative binding of oxygen at the remaining heme groups of the same hemoglobin molecule. The oxyhemoglobin dissociation curve is therefore shifted to the left, reflecting the fact that oxygen is more tightly bound by hemoglobin and less able to be unloaded to the tissues. In addition, CO binds to the heme group of myoglobin and the cytochromes, interfering with cellular respiration and exacerbating the hypoxia (Chap. 122).[42]

Sulfhemoglobin

Sulfhemoglobin is a bright green molecule in which the hydrosulfide anion HS⁻ irreversibly binds to ferrous hemoglobin. The sulfur atom is probably attached to a β carbon in the porphyrin ring and not at the normal oxygen-binding site.[70] It has a spectrophotometric absorption band at approximately 618 nm,[16] is ineffective in oxygen transport, and clinically produces a condition that resembles cyanosis. The oxygen affinity of sulfhemoglobin is approximately 100 times less than that of oxyhemoglobin, shifting the oxyhemoglobin dissociation curve to the right, in favor of oxygen unbinding. Thus, the symptoms of hypoxia are not as severe with sulfhemoglobinemia as with carboxy- or methemoglobinemia.[77]

Oxidation of the Globin Chain

Oxidation can also occur at the amino acid side chains of the globin protein. In particular, sulfhydryl groups can oxidize to form disulfide links between cysteine residues, which leads to the unfolding of the protein chain, exposure of other side chains, and further oxidation. When these disulfide links join adjacent hemoglobin molecules, they cause the precipitation of the concentrated hemoglobin molecules out of solution. Covalent links can also form between hemoglobin and other cytoskeletal and membrane proteins.[25] Eventually, aggregates of denatured and insoluble protein are visible on light microscopy as Heinz bodies. The distortion of the cellular architecture and the loss of fluidity in particular signal reticuloendothelial macrophages to excise sections of erythrocyte membrane ("bite cells") or to remove the entire erythrocyte from the circulation (see below). To guard against these oxidation reactions, the erythrocyte maintains a pool of reduced glutathione via the actions of the NADPH generated in the hexose monophosphate shunt (assuming adequate G6PD activity to initiate this pathway). This glutathione transfers electrons to break open disulfide links and to preserve sulfhydryl groups in their reduced state.

Hemolysis

Hemolysis is merely the acceleration of the normal process by which senescent or compromised erythrocytes are removed from the circulation.[95] The normal life span of a circulating erythrocyte is approximately 120 days, and any reduction in this life span represents some degree of hemolysis. If sufficiently rapid, hemolysis can overwhelm the regenerative capacity of the erythron, resulting in anemia. Intravascular hemolysis occurs when the rate of hemolysis exceeds the capacity of the reticuloendothelial macrophages to remove damaged erythrocytes, and free hemoglobin and other intracellular contents of the erythrocyte appear in the circulation.

Reticulocytosis, polychromasia, unconjugated (indirect) hyperbilirubinemia, increased serum lactate dehydrogenase, and decreased serum haptoglobin are characteristic of hemolysis. A normal or elevated RBC distribution width (RDW) and thrombocytosis are usually present. The presence of spherocytes on peripheral blood smear suggests an autoimmune or hereditary process and can be pursued with a Coombs' test. Schistocytes suggest thrombotic thrombocytopenic purpura (TTP) or hemolytic uremic syndrome, disseminated intravascular coagulation, or valvular hemolysis. Thrombotic thrombocytopenic purpura and hemolytic uremic syndrome are characterized by a microangiopathic anemia, thrombocytopenia, and normal coagulation parameters (unlike disseminated intravascular coagulation). Thrombotic thrombocytopenic purpura is discussed under platelet disorders below. Hemoglobinemia, hemoglobinuria, and hemosiderinuria occur with intravascular hemolysis. Specialized tests to measure hemolysis

TABLE 20–2	Representative Xenobiotics Causing Acquired Hemolysis
Immune-mediated	
Type I: IgG against drug tightly bound to red cell	
High-dose penicillin	
Type II: Complement activated by antibodies against drug-membrane complex	
Cefotaxime, cefotetan, ceftriaxone, quinidine, stibophen	
Type III: True autoimmune response to red cell membrane	
Chlorpromazine, cladribine, cyclosporine, fludarabine, levodopa, methyldopa, procainamide	
Nonimmune-mediated	
Oxidants	
Aniline	
Benzocaine	
Chlorates	
Dapsone	
Hydrogen peroxide	
Hydroxylamine	
Methylene blue	
Naphthalene	
Nitrites	
Nitrofurantoin	
Oxygen	
Phenacetin	
Phenazopyridine	
Phenol	
Platinoids	
Sulfonamides	
Nonoxidants	
Arsine (AsH₃)	
Copper	
Lead	
Pyrogallic acid	
Stibine (SbH₃)	
Hypophosphatemia	
Microangiopathic (eg, ticlopidine, clopidogrel, prasugrel, cyclosporine, tacrolimus, mitomycin, gemcitabine)	
Osmotic agents (eg, water)	
Venoms (snake, spider)	

detect shortened erythrocyte survival, increased endogenous carbon monoxide generation from heme oxygenase, and increased fecal urobilinogen.

Table 20–2 presents a classification of acquired causes of hemolysis relevant to toxicology. Oxidant injury following xenobiotic exposure is one of the triggers of hemolysis, as it causes irreversible changes in the erythrocyte. Erythrocytes deficient in G6PD by virtue of cell age or enzyme mutations are particularly vulnerable to hemolysis following oxidant stress due to limited capacity to generate NADPH and reduced glutathione.[95] The immune-mediated hemolytic anemias occur when ingested xenobiotics trigger an antigen antibody reaction. In general, these molecules are too small to be sensitizing agents, but antigenicity is acquired after binding to carrier proteins in blood. The particulars of the xenobiotic-carrier immune activation sequence form the basis for the classification of this group of hemolytic anemias.[9]

Nonimmune-Mediated Causes of Xenobiotic-Induced Hemolysis

A number of xenobiotics or their reactive metabolites cause hemolysis via oxidant injury. A Heinz-body hemolytic anemia results, which typically resolves within a few weeks of drug discontinuation. Some xenobiotics cause hemolysis in the absence of overt oxidant injury (Table 20–2). Copper sulfate hemolysis is described in Chap. 92, whereas the delayed hemolysis following exposure to arsine or stibine is described here.

Arsine (AsH_3) is a colorless, odorless, nonirritating gas that is 2.5 times denser than air (Chap. 86). Clinical signs and symptoms appear after a latent period of up to 24 hours after exposure to concentrations above 30 ppm and may include headache, malaise, dyspnea, abdominal pain with nausea and vomiting, hepatomegaly, hemolysis with hemoglobinuric acute kidney injury, and death.[23,35,54,58,80] The mechanism of hemolysis is believed to involve the fixation of arsine by sulfhydryl groups of hemoglobin and other essential proteins.[40,106] Interestingly, hemolysis is prevented in vitro by conversion to carboxy- or methemoglobin.[45] Impairment of membrane proteins, including $Na^+,K^+,ATPase$, is another potential mechanism for arsine-induced hemolysis.[83] Chronic exposure to low levels of arsine can produce clinically significant disease.[23] Stibine (SbH_3), an antimony derivative, likely causes hemolysis via similar mechanisms (Chap. 85).

Glucose-6-Phosphate Dehydrogenase Deficiencies

Glucose-6-phosphate dehydrogenase deficiencies (G6PD) is the enzyme that catalyzes the first step of the hexose monophosphate shunt: the conversion of glucose-6-phosphate to phosphogluconolactone (Fig. 11–8). In the process, $NADP^+$ is reduced to NADPH, which the erythrocyte uses to maintain a supply of reduced glutathione and to defend against oxidation. It follows that erythrocytes deficient in G6PD activity are less able to resist oxidant attack and, in particular, to maintain sulfhydryl groups of hemoglobin in their reduced state, resulting in hemolysis. It is important to recognize that the term G6PD deficiency encompasses a wide range of differences in enzyme activities among individuals. These differences result from decreased enzyme synthesis, altered catalytic activity, or reduced stability of the enzyme. Approximately 7.5% of the world population is affected to some degree, with more than 400 variants having been identified. Most cases involve relatively mild deficiency and minimal morbidity. Ethnic populations from tropical and subtropical countries (the so-called malaria belt) have a much higher prevalence of G6PD deficiency, possibly because that phenotype protects against malaria.[72]

The gene that encodes for G6PD resides near the end of the long arm of the X-chromosome. Most mutations consist of a single amino acid substitution, as complete absence of this enzyme is lethal. Although men hemizygous for a deficient gene are more severely affected, women randomly inactivate one X-chromosome during cellular differentiation (the Lyon hypothesis). Thus, women carriers heterozygous for a deficient G6PD gene have a mosaic of erythrocytes, some proportion of which expresses the deficient gene during maturation. Accordingly, approximately 10% of carrier women are nearly as severely affected as males hemizygous for the same deficient gene. Because of the high gene frequency in certain ethnic groups, another approximately 10% of women are homozygous for the deficient gene.

Normal G6PD has a half-life of about 60 days. Because the erythrocyte cannot synthesize new protein, the activity of G6PD normally declines by approximately 75% over its 120-day life span. Consequently, even in unaffected individuals, susceptibility to oxidant stress varies based on the age mix of circulating erythrocytes. In all cases, older erythrocytes are less likely to recover following exposure to an oxidant and will hemolyze first. Moreover, after an episode of hemolysis following acute exposure to an oxidant stress, the higher G6PD activity of surviving erythrocytes will confer some resistance against further hemolysis in most individuals with relatively mild deficiency, even if the offending xenobiotic is continued. For this reason, phenotypic testing for G6PD deficiency is best done 2 to 3 months after a hemolytic crisis, which is when the reticulocyte count has usually normalized.

The World Health Organization classification of G6PD is based on the degree of enzyme deficiency and severity of hemolysis.[18] Both class I and class II patients are severely deficient, with less than 10% of normal G6PD activity. Class I individuals are prone to chronic hemolytic anemia, whereas class II patients experience intermittent hemolytic crises. Class III patients have only moderate (10%–60%) enzyme deficiency, and experience self-limiting hemolysis in response to certain xenobiotics and infections.

TABLE 20–3	Selected Xenobiotics That Cause Hemolysis in Patients with G6PD Deficiency	
Alkyl nitrites	Phenylhydrazine
Doxorubicin	Primaquine
Furazolidone	Sulfacetamide
Methylene blue	Sulfamethoxazole
Nalidixic acid	Sulfanilamide
Naphthalene	Sulfapyridine
Nitrofurantoin	Toluidine blue
Phenazopyridine	Trinitrotoluene

Data from Beutler E: Glucose-6-phosphate dehydrogenase deficiency. *N Engl J Med.* 1991;324:169–174 and Beutler E: G6PD deficiency. *Blood.* 1994;84:3613–3636.

Approximately 11% of African Americans have a class III deficiency, traditionally termed type A⁻, and experience a decline of no more than 30% of the red blood cell mass during any single hemolytic episode. Another 20% of African Americans have type A⁺ G6PD enzyme, which is functionally normal, and therefore of no consequence despite a one-base substitution compared to wild-type B. The Mediterranean type found in Sardinia, Corsica, Greece, the Middle East, and India is a class II deficiency, and hemolysis either occurs spontaneously or in response to ingestion of oxidants, such as the β-glycosides found in fava (*Vicia fava*) beans.

The most common clinical presentation of previously unrecognized G6PD deficiency is the acute hemolytic crisis. Typically, hemolysis begins 1 to 4 days following the exposure to an offending xenobiotic or infection (Table 20–3). Jaundice, pallor, and dark urine occur accompanied by abdominal and back pain. A decrease in the concentration of hemoglobin occurs. The peripheral smear demonstrates cell fragments and cells that have had Heinz bodies excised. Bone marrow stimulation results in a reticulocytosis by day 5 and an increased erythrocyte mass. In general, a normal bone marrow can compensate for ongoing hemolysis and can return the hemoglobin concentration to normal. Most crises are self-limiting because of the higher G6PD activity of younger erythrocytes. Historically, the anemia observed when primaquine was administered to type A⁻ military recruits for malaria prophylaxis resolved within 3 to 6 weeks in most cases.[17] Some xenobiotics, including APAP, vitamin C, and sulfisoxazole, are safe at therapeutic doses but can cause hemolysis in G6PD-deficient patients following overdose.

Other presentations of more severe variants of G6PD include neonatal jaundice and kernicterus, chronic hemolysis with splenomegaly and black pigment gallstones, megaloblastic crisis caused by folate deficiency, and aplastic crisis after parvovirus B19 infection.

Megaloblastic Anemia

Vitamin B_{12} and folate are essential for one-carbon metabolism in mammals. One-carbon fragments are necessary for the biosynthesis of thymidine, purines, serotonin, and methionine; the methylation of DNA, histones, and other proteins; and the complete catabolism of branched-chain fatty acids and histidine. Unable to synthesize vitamin B_{12} or folate, mammals are dependent on dietary sources and microorganisms for these cofactors. The hematologic manifestation of vitamin B_{12} or folate deficiency is a characteristic panmyelosis termed *megaloblastic anemia*. The hallmark nuclear-cytoplasmic asynchrony is due to disrupted DNA synthesis, halted interphase and ineffective erythropoiesis.[82] The hyperplastic bone marrow contains precursor cells with abnormal nuclei filled with incompletely condensed chromatin. Among circulating blood cells, macrocytic anemia (macro-ovalocytes) without reticulocytosis is followed by the appearance of granulocytes with an abnormally large, distorted nucleus (hypersegmented neutrophils with 6 or more lobes). Lymphocytes and platelets appear normal but are functionally impaired.

In addition to dietary deficiencies, which have become less common, macrocytic anemia with or without megaloblastosis in adults is usually caused by chronic ethanol abuse, chemotherapeutics, or antiretrovirals, especially when mean corpuscular volumes are only moderately elevated (100–120 fL).[90] The folate antagonists aminopterin, methotrexate, hydantoins, pyrimethamine, proguanil, sulfasalazine, trimethoprim sulfamethoxazole, and valproate can interfere with DNA synthesis. Ethanol affects folate metabolism and transport. A functional vitamin B_{12} deficiency is induced by chronic exposure to nitrous oxide, biguanides, colchicine, neomycin, and the proton pump inhibitors. Purine analogs (eg, azathioprine, 6-mercaptopurine, 6-thioguanine, acyclovir) and pyrimidine analogs (eg, 5-fluorouracil, floxuridine, 5-azacitidine, and zidovudine) also disrupt nucleic acid synthesis. Hydroxyurea and cytarabine, which inhibit ribonucleotide reductase, also delay nuclear maturation and function and frequently cause megaloblastosis.

Pure Red Cell Aplasia

Pure red cell aplasia is an uncommon condition in which erythrocyte precursors are absent from an otherwise normal bone marrow. It results in a normocytic anemia with inappropriately low reticulocyte count. The other blood cell lines are unaffected, unlike aplastic anemia. Pharmaceuticals cause fewer than 5% of cases of this uncommon condition, having been implicated in fewer than 100 human reports.[99] Only phenytoin, azathioprine, and isoniazid meet criteria for definite causality; chlorpropamide and valproic acid can be considered only as possible causes.[99] Most other xenobiotics are cited only in single case reports, and drug rechallenge was not used, making the association uncertain.

In part because of its rarity, a cluster of 13 cases in France of pure red cell aplasia in hemodialysis patients receiving subcutaneous recombinant EPO ultimately led to an international effort by researchers, regulatory authorities, and industry to identify the etiology.[12,26] To reduce theoretical concerns regarding transmission of variant Creutzfeldt-Jakob disease, human serum albumin was replaced with polysorbate 80 as the stabilizer in a formulation used in Europe and Canada. It is suspected that this change allowed rubber to leach from the uncoated stopper of prefilled syringes, triggering an immune response against both recombinant and endogenous EPO in some patients.[66] This episode not only serves as a recent example of successful pharmacovigilance for rare adverse drug effects but has also influenced safety assessments for an emerging class of biological therapies that include simple peptides, monoclonal antibodies, and recombinant DNA proteins.[14,66]

Erythrocytosis

Erythrocytosis denotes an increase in the red cell mass, either in absolute terms or relative to a reduced plasma volume. An increasingly recognized cause of drug-induced absolute erythrocytosis is the abuse of recombinant human EPO by athletes to enhance aerobic capacity (Chap. 41). Autologous blood transfusions (doping) are also used in this population, and both can cause dangerous increases in blood viscosity. Cobalt was once considered for the treatment of chronic anemia[32] because of its ability to cause a secondary erythrocytosis (Chap. 91). The mechanism is hypothesized to involve impaired degradation of the transcription factor hypoxia-inducible factor 1α, thereby prolonging EPO transcription. This effect is more pronounced in high-altitude dwellers, in whom elevated serum EPO concentrations persist despite hematocrits in excess of 75%, and chronic mountain sickness is associated with increased serum cobalt concentrations.[53]

THE LEUKON

The leukon represents all leukocytes (white blood cells), including precursor cells, cells in the circulation, and the large number of extravascular cells. It includes the granulocytes (neutrophils, eosinophils, and basophils), lymphocytes, and monocytes. Neutrophils (polymorphonuclear leukocytes) are highly specialized mediators of the inflammatory response, and are a primary focus of concern regarding hematologic toxicity of xenobiotics. B and T lymphocytes are involved in antibody production and cell-mediated immunity. Monocytes migrate out of the vascular compartment to become tissue macrophages and to regulate immune system function.

Immunity is generally divided into the *innate* and the *adaptive* responses. *Innate immunity* is an immediate but less specific defense that is highly conserved in evolutionary terms. It is centered on the neutrophil response, and it involves monocytes and macrophages as well as complement, cytokines, and acute phase proteins. The innate system responds primarily to extracellular pathogens, especially bacteria, by recognizing structures commonly found on pathogens, namely lipopolysaccharide (Gram-negative cell walls), lipoteichoic acid (Gram positive), and mannans (yeast). *Adaptive immunity* is demonstrated only in higher animals and is an antigen-specific response via T and B lymphocytes after antigen presentation and recognition. Although this reaction is more specific, it requires several days to develop, unless that antigen has previously triggered a response (so-called immune memory). This response can also at times be directed against self-antigens, resulting in autoimmune disorders.

The recruitment and activation of neutrophils provide the primary defense against the invasion of bacterial and fungal pathogens. They emerge from the bone marrow with the biochemical and metabolic machinery needed for the efficient killing of microorganisms. Activated macrophages release G-CSF and GM-CSF, which stimulate myeloid differentiation and are recognized on blood testing as the classic neutrophil leukocytosis. Neutrophils are activated when circulating cells detect chemokines released from sites of inflammation. On activation, they undergo conformational and biochemical changes that transform them into powerful host defenders. These changes allow rolling along the endothelial lining of postcapillary venules, migration toward the site of inflammation, adherence to the endothelium, migration through the endothelium to tissue sites, ingestion, killing, and digestion of invading organisms.

Neutrophils migrate to sites of infection along gradients of chemoattractant mediators. An acute inflammatory stimulus leads to the accumulation of neutrophils along the endothelium of postcapillary venules. The major molecules involved in this process are adhesion molecules, chemoattractants, and chemokines. Loose adhesions between neutrophils and endothelium are made and broken, resulting in the slow movement of leukocytes along endothelium and a more intense exposure of neutrophils to activating factors. Chemotaxis requires responses involving actin polymerization–depolymerization adhesion events mediated by integrins and involving microfilament–membrane interactions. All leukocytes including lymphocytes localize infection using these same mediators. Colchicine depolymerizes microfilaments, causing the dissolution of the fibrillar microtubules in granulocytes and other motile cells, impairing this response.

Opsonized particles, immune complexes, and chemotactic factors activate neutrophils in tissues by binding to cell surface receptors. The neutrophil makes tight contact with its target, and the plasma membrane surrounds the organism completely enclosing it. Two mechanisms are then responsible for the destruction of the organism: the oxygen-dependent respiratory burst, and the oxygen-independent response involving cationic enzymes found in cytoplasmic granules. The respiratory burst is caused by an NADPH oxidase complex that assembles at the phagosomal membrane. Electrons are transferred from cytoplasmic NADPH to oxygen on the phagosomal side of the membrane, generating superoxide, hydrogen peroxide, hydroxyl radical, singlet oxygen, hypochlorous acid, chloramines, nitric oxide, and peroxynitrite. Cytoplasmic granules within the neutrophil fuse with the phagosome and empty their contents into it. The components of these granules include myeloperoxidase (MPO), elastase, lipases, metalloproteinases, and a pool of CD11b/CD18 proteins required for adhesion and migration. Finally, the phagocytized organism is digested and eliminated by the neutrophil. Overstimulation of this complex and highly regulated but somewhat nonspecific system can at times become deleterious, as is postulated to occur with reperfusion injury or carbon monoxide poisoning, to cite 2 examples.[98] Vasculitis and the systemic inflammatory response syndrome are further examples of excessive activation of the innate response.

Neutropenia and Agranulocytosis

Neutropenia is a reduction in circulating neutrophils at least 2 standard deviations below the norm, but the threshold of 1500/mm³ (1.5×10^9/L) is often used instead.[48] Severe neutropenia is termed *agranulocytosis* and is generally defined to be an absolute neutrophil count of less than $500/mm^3$ (0.5×10^9/L). Neutropenia results from decreased production, increased destruction, or retention of neutrophils in the various storage pools. Their high rate of turnover renders neutrophils vulnerable to any xenobiotic that inhibits cellular reproduction. As such, the various antineoplastics including antimetabolites, alkylating agents, and antimitotics will predictably cause neutropenia. This predictable, dose-dependent reaction represents an important dose-limiting adverse effect of therapy. On the other hand, a number of xenobiotics are implicated in idiosyncratic neutropenia.[3,4] The parent drug or a metabolite usually acts as a hapten to trigger antineutrophil antibodies. Table 20–4 provides an abbreviated list.[2,79,97] Cocaine users are at very high risk for agranulocytosis because of the common contamination of this drug with levamisole (Chaps. 17 and 75).[22]

Eosinophilia

Eosinophils are primarily responsible for protecting against parasitic infection. Allergic reactions and malignancies such as lymphoma are also common causes of eosinophilia, especially where nematode infection is rare.[88] Eosinophils bind to antigen-specific IgE and discharge their large granules, which contain major basic protein, peroxidase, and eosinophil-derived neurotoxin, onto the surface of the antibody-coated organism. Two unusual toxicologic outbreaks were characterized by eosinophilia, acute cough, fever, and pulmonary infiltrates, followed by severe myalgia, neuropathy, and eosinophilia. The first outbreak, called the toxic oil syndrome, took place in central Spain in 1981, when industrial-use rapeseed oil denatured with 2% aniline was fraudulently sold as olive oil by door-to-door salesmen.[37] The precise causative agent remains uncertain but may include fatty acid esters of 3-(N-phenylamino)-1,2-propanediol.[37] The second outbreak, called the eosinophilia-myalgia syndrome, occurred during 1988 and 1989 in users of L-tryptophan supplements traced back to a single wholesaler in Japan.[6] The causative contaminant has not been identified but is believed to have been present in only trace quantities in the L-tryptophan purified from

TABLE 20–4	Selected Causes of Idiosyncratic Drug-Induced Agranulocytosis	
Antiepileptics		Antipsychotics
Carbamazepine		Clozapine[a]
Phenytoin		Phenothiazines
Antiinflammatories		Antithyroid agents
Aminopyrine		Methimazole[a]
Ibuprofen		Propylthiouracil[a]
Indomethacin		Cardiovascular
Phenylbutazone		Hydralazine
Antimicrobials		Lidocaine
β-Lactams, including penicillin G[a]		Procainamide[a]
Cephalosporins		Quinidine
Chloramphenicol		Ticlopidine[a]
Dapsone[a]		Vesnarinone
Ganciclovir		Diuretics
Isoniazid		Acetazolamide
Rifampicin		Hydrochlorothiazide
Sulfonamides		Hypoglycemics
Vancomycin		Chlorpropamide
Antirheumatics		Tolbutamide
Gold salts		Sedative–hypnotics
Levamisole[a]		Barbiturates
Penicillamine		Flurazepam
Sulfasalazine[a]		Other
		Deferiprone

[a]Denotes at least 10 cases reported.[2]

microbial culture. Both syndromes appear to be mediated by immunologic mechanisms.

Leukemia

The leukemias represent the malignant, unregulated proliferation of hematopoietic cells. Although monoclonal in origin, they affect all cell lines derived from the progenitor cell. Acute myeloid leukemia (AML) and the myelodysplastic syndromes are the most common leukemias associated with xenobiotics. The long-recognized association between AML and occupational benzene exposure, radiation, or treatment with alkylating antineoplastics has helped to advance understanding of the molecular mechanisms underlying leukemogenesis.[15] The necessary events are believed to involve several sequential genetic and epigenetic alterations, as evidenced by a distinct pattern of chromosomal deletions preceding the development of AML.[50,51] Other recognized xenobiotics that cause leukemia include topoisomerase II inhibitors, 1,3-butanediol, styrol, ethylene oxide, and vinyl chloride.[55,78] In many cases, the latency period between exposure and illness is prolonged. For example, leukemia linked to benzene is preceded by several months of anemia, neutropenia, and thrombocytopenia.

HEMOSTASIS

In the absence of pathology, blood remains in a fluid form with cells in suspension. Injury triggers coagulation and thrombosis. The resulting clot formation, retraction, and dissolution involve an interaction between the vessel endothelium, soluble constituents of the coagulation system, and proteins located on and within platelets. Platelets respond to signals within their immediate environment and from injured components of the distant microcirculation. A dynamic balance must be maintained between coagulation and fibrinolysis to maintain the integrity of the circulatory system (Fig. 20–5).

Coagulation

Two basic pathways termed *intrinsic* and *extrinsic* are involved in the initiation of coagulation. The more important extrinsic, or tissue factor, pathway is activated when blood is exposed to tissue factor (also known as thromboplastin) which is normally expressed on subendothelial cells and fibroblasts not in direct contact with blood. Tissue factor activates factor VII and together form the extrinsic tenase complex activating both factors X and IX. The intrinsic, or contact activation, pathway also activates factor IX, which forms the intrinsic tenase (i.e., "ten"-ase) complex with factor VIIIa. Both extrinsic and intrinsic tenase with calcium activate factor X, which binds to factor Va on the surface of activated platelets, forming the prothrombinase complex. The prothrombinase complex activates prothrombin, which results in the generation of thrombin activity. Thrombin activates platelets, promotes its own generation by activation of factors V, VIII, and XI, and converts fibrinogen to fibrin (Chap. 58).[47]

Laboratory Tests of Coagulation

An understanding of several widely available coagulation tests is important to achieve the correct interpretation of the effects of xenobiotics on hemostasis, whether for therapeutic drug monitoring or following overdose. Four studies—prothrombin time (PT, or international normalized ratio[96]), partial thromboplastin time (PTT), thrombin time, and fibrinogen-concentration—are particularly important in the classification of coagulation disorders.

The PT assesses the extrinsic coagulation pathway and is calculated by adding standardized thromboplastin reagent (phospholipid and tissue factor) to a sample of the patient's citrated plasma (the citrate removes calcium to prevent clotting). Calcium is then introduced, and the time to clotting measured. With the exception of factor X, the PT is unaffected by the presence or absence of factors VIII to XIII, platelets, prekallikrein, and high-molecular-weight kininogen (HMWK). An individual's PT was formerly expressed as a ratio (PT observed to PT control). Because this ratio is directly affected by both laboratory methodology and the source of the thromboplastin reagent used, the generated results suffered from significant variability between laboratories and countries. Thus, the INR was developed in an attempt to limit this variability. The INR is calculated by

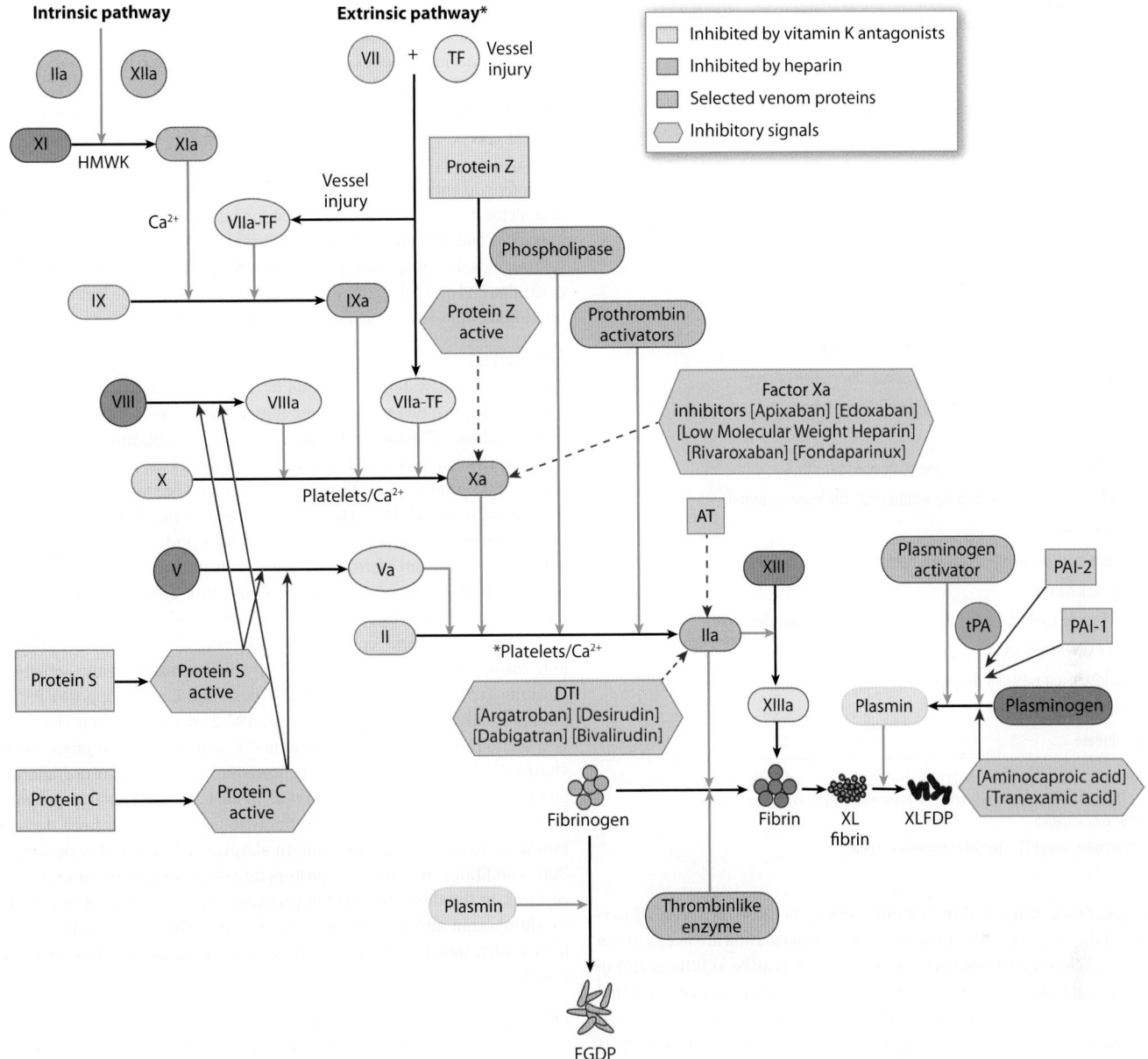

FIGURE 20–5. A schematic overview of the coagulation, platelet activation, and fibrinolytic pathways indicating where phospholipids on the platelet surface interact with the coagulation pathway intermediates. Arrows are not shown from platelets to phospholipids involved in the tissue factor VIIa and the factor IX to VIIIa interactions to avoid confusion. Interactions of selected venom proteins are indicated in the purple boxes. The diagram is not complete with reference to the multiple sites of interaction of the serine protease inhibitors (SERPINs) to avoid overcrowding. Solid red lines indicate inhibition of a reaction effect. Black arrows refer to chemical conversion of coagulation factors. Green arrows represent activation of the chemical conversion pathway. Dashed red lines indicate inhibition of a specific clotting factor. *Refer to Figs. 58–4 and 58–5 for the platelet activation pathway. DTI = direct thrombin inhibitor; FDP = fibrin degradation products; FGDP = fibrinogen degradation product; HMWK = high-molecular-weight kininogen; TF = tissue factor; t-PA = tissue plasminogen activator; XL = cross-linked.

raising the PT ratio to an exponent known as the International Sensitivity Index (ISI), that is, (PT ratio)[ISI]. The ISI is calibrated against an international standard to measure responsiveness of the particular thromboplastin to the effects of warfarin.

Although the use of the INR does not completely eliminate variability, it improves warfarin dosing and comparison with international norms. It should be noted that the ISI, and thus the INR, are designed for greater consistency in measuring coagulation changes due to warfarin, but are often more variable than the PT ratio for patients with other coagulation defects.[87] Specifically, replacing the PT with the INR for prognosis in the setting of fulminant hepatic failure, as occurs following APAP overdose, is controversial.[24] In these patients, the INR is more variable between laboratories, and the use of a substantially different ISI may be warranted.[11]

The PTT tests both the intrinsic and common coagulation pathway. It is measured by adding calcium and an activator (kaolin, silica, or celite)

to citrated plasma and the time to clotting observed. Some tests also use phospholipids in the reagent to activate the remaining coagulation factors, thereby giving rise to the term *activated partial thromboplastin time* (aPTT). Because the PTT and aPTT are essentially interchangeable, the term PTT is used hereafter to represent the concept. The PTT is not affected by alterations in factors VII, XIII, or platelets.

The thrombin time (or thrombin clotting time), determined by adding exogenous thrombin to citrated plasma, evaluates the ability to convert fibrinogen to fibrin, and is thus unaffected by abnormalities of factors II, V, VII to XIII, platelets, prekallikrein, or HMWK. Finally, either a fibrinogen concentration or a determination of fibrin degradation products will help distinguish between problems with clot formation and consumptive coagulopathy (disseminated intravascular coagulation). An evaluation of the combination of normal and abnormal results of these tests usually determines a patient's clotting abnormality (Table 20–5).

TABLE 20–5 Evaluation of Abnormal Coagulation Times

PT prolonged, PTT normal
Deficiency of factor VII
Warfarin therapy and other vitamin K antagonists (early)
Vitamin K deficiency (mild)
Liver disease (mild)

PT normal, PTT prolonged, bleeding
Deficiencies of factors VIII, IX, XI
von Willebrand disease

PT normal, PTT prolonged, no bleeding
Deficiencies of factor XII, prekallikrein
High-molecular-weight kininogen inhibitor syndrome

PT and PTT prolonged, thrombin time normal, fibrinogen normal
Deficiencies of factors II, V, IX; vitamin K deficiency (severe)
Warfarin therapy (late)
Factor Xa inhibitor therapy (eg, rivaroxaban, apixaban)[a,b]

PT and PTT prolonged, thrombin time abnormal, fibrinogen normal
Heparin therapy[a]
Direct thrombin inhibitor therapy (eg, dabigatran)[c]
Dysfibrinogenemia

PT and PTT prolonged, thrombin time abnormal, fibrinogen abnormal
Crotaline envenomation
Disseminated intravascular coagulation
Fibrinolytic therapy
Liver disease

[a]PTT insensitive to low-molecular-weight heparin effects and less sensitive than PT to factor Xa inhibitor therapy. [b]Normal PT does not exclude effect. [c]Prolongation of PTT is not linearly correlated with dabigatran concentration.

PT = prothrombin time; PTT = partial thromboplastin time.

Inhibitors are diagnosed by "mixing studies," because only a small percentage of the coagulation factors present in normal plasma are necessary to have normal clotting studies. Factor activity in blood can be as little as 25% of normal without affecting the PT or PTT. Thus, the presence of an abnormal PT or PTT that will not correct despite the addition of an equal volume of normal plasma demonstrates the presence of an inhibitor of coagulation as opposed to a factor deficiency. Heparin-induced anticoagulation results in an elevated PTT that does not correct when mixing studies are performed. More sophisticated studies are used to identify specific coagulation factor deficiencies.

Xenobiotic-Induced Defects in Coagulation

A rapidly increasing number of xenobiotics are in therapeutic use to antagonize coagulation (Chap. 58). The recognition of a hemorrhagic disease in cattle in the 1920s and the isolation of the causative agent dicoumarol from spoiled sweet clover in the 1940s resulted in the development of the warfarin-type anticoagulants. This group of anticoagulants indirectly inhibits hepatic synthesis of coagulation factors II, VII, IX, X, and proteins C, S, and Z by inhibiting the reductase that is responsible for the regeneration of vitamin K quinone from vitamin K epoxide. Because warfarin is widely prescribed and has a narrow therapeutic index, efforts to improve our understanding of the pharmacology of warfarin are advancing the fields of pharmacogenomics and drug interactions.[105]

Heparin is a highly sulfated glycosaminoglycan that is normally present in tissues. Commercial unfractionated heparin is either bovine or porcine in origin and consists of a mixture of polysaccharides with molecular weights ranging from 4,000 to 30,000 Da. The anticoagulant activity of heparin is through its catalytic activation of antithrombin III, a suicide inhibitor of the serine proteases thrombin and factors IXa, Xa, XIa, and XIIa.[71]

The low-molecular-weight heparins (LMWHs) have a mean molecular weight of 4,000–6,000 Da.[47] Their subcutaneous bioavailability, more predictable pharmacokinetics, lower protein binding, and longer half-life make them more convenient than unfractionated heparin.[71]

Heparinoids are glycosaminoglycans not derived from heparin with anticoagulant effects. This class includes dermatan sulfate and danaparoid sodium. Fondaparinux is a synthetic pentasaccharide that also inhibits factor Xa by binding to antithrombin III and therefore acts upstream of thrombin. Other oral factor Xa inhibitors are approved for human use, including rivaroxaban, apixaban, and edoxaban. Several direct thrombin inhibitors are also in clinical use, including parenterally administered lepirudin, argatroban, bivalirudin, desirudin, and oral dabigatran. These xenobiotics prolong the INR, aPTT, thrombin clotting time, and whole-blood activated clotting time.

Fibrinolysis

The coagulation system is opposed by 3 major inhibitory systems. Components of the fibrinolytic system circulate as zymogens, activators, inhibitors, and cofactors.[33] Plasminogen can be activated to plasmin by an intrinsic pathway involving factor XII, prekallikrein, and HMWK. This produces the degradation products and fibrin monomers that are found in disseminated intravascular coagulation. The extrinsic pathway involves the release of tissue plasminogen activator (t-PA) from tissues and urokinase plasminogen activator (u-PA) from secretions.[33] Once activated, plasmin degrades fibrinogen, fibrin, and coagulation factors V and VIII. The degradation of cross-linked fibrin strands results in the formation of D-dimers.

Several inhibitors oppose the fibrinolytic system, including α_2-antiplasmin, α_2-macroglobulin, both of which oppose plasmin activity, and plasminogen activator inhibitor (PAI) types 1 and 2, which oppose t-PA. Plasminogen activator inhibitor (PAI-1) and PAI-2 are opposed by activated protein C and protein S. Activated protein C is activated by thrombin. Another vitamin K–dependent glycoprotein, protein Z, accelerates the degradation of factor Xa. Congenital deficiencies of proteins C, S, and Z result in pathologic venous thrombosis. Decreased fibrinolytic activity results from decreased synthesis, release of t-PA, or from an elevation of the PAI-1 concentration. Both conditions are observed postoperatively, with the use of oral contraceptives, in the third trimester of pregnancy, and in obesity. The activity of α_2-antiplasmin and α_2-macroglobulin are increased in pulmonary fibrosis, malignancy, infection, and myocardial infarction, and in thromboembolic disease.[33]

Xenobiotic-Induced Defects in Fibrinolysis

Table 20–6 lists xenobiotics associated with an acquired defect of fibrinolysis. The chemotherapeutics result in a reduction in serine-protease inhibitors such as antithrombin. L-Asparaginase is associated with a reduction in

TABLE 20–6 Selected Xenobiotics and Endogenous Factors, Cytokines, and Hormones That Impair Fibrinolysis

Antifibrinolytics
ε-Aminocaproic acid
Aprotinin
Desmopressin
Tranexamic acid
Chemotherapeutics
Anthracyclines
L-Asparaginase
Methotrexate
Mithramycin
Coagulation factors
Cytokines
Erythropoietin
Thrombopoietin
Hormones, including conjugated estrogens

circulating t-PA concentrations. Methotrexate damages vascular endothelium, which triggers thrombosis (Chap. 51).[33] Hemostatic xenobiotics used therapeutically include the synthetic lysine derivatives aminocaproic acid and tranexamic acid, which bind reversibly to plasminogen; the bovine protease inhibitor aprotinin, which inhibits kallikrein; the vasopressin analog desmopressin, which increases plasma concentrations of factor VIII and vWF; and conjugated estrogens, which normalize bleeding times in uremia.[65]

PLATELETS

In the resting state, platelets maintain a discoid shape. The platelet membrane is a typical trilaminal membrane with glycoproteins, glycolipids, and cholesterol embedded in a phospholipid bilayer. The plasma membrane is in direct continuity with a series of channels, the surface-connected canalicular system (SCCS), which is sometimes referred to as the open canalicular system. The SCCS provides a route of entry and exit for various molecules, a storage pool for platelet glycoproteins, and an internal reservoir of membrane that is recruited to increase platelet surface area. This facilitates platelet spreading and pseudopod formation during the process of cell adhesion.

The glycocalyx, or outer coat, is heavily invested with glycoproteins that serve as receptors for a wide variety of stimuli. The β_1-integrin family includes receptors that mediate interactions between cells and mediators in the extracellular matrix, including collagen, laminin, and fibronectin. The β_2-integrin receptors are present in inflammatory cells and platelets and are important in immune activation. The β_3-integrin receptors (also known as cytoadhesins) include the glycoprotein (GP) IIb-IIIa fibrinogen receptor, as well as vitronectin.[47] Vitronectin has binding sites for other integrins, collagen, heparin, and components of complement. All of the integrins are active in the process of platelet adhesion to surfaces. Platelet aggregation is mediated by the GP IIb-IIIa receptors.[47]

The submembrane region contains actin filaments that stabilize the platelets' discoid shape and are involved in the formation and stabilization of pseudopods. They also generate the force needed for the movement of receptor–ligand complexes from the outer plasma membrane to the SCCS. These mobile receptors are important in the spreading of platelets on surfaces, and for binding fibrin strands and other platelets. Platelet cytoplasm contains 3 types of membrane-bound secretory granules.[47] The α granules contain β-thromboglobulin, which mediates inflammation, binds and inactivates heparin, and blocks the endothelial release of prostacyclin. In addition, platelet factor-4, which inactivates heparin, and fibrinogen are contained within the α granules. Dense granules store adenine nucleotides, serotonin, and calcium, which are secreted during the release reaction. Platelet lysosomes contain hydrolytic enzymes. Stimulation by platelet agonists causes the granules to fuse with the channels of the SCCS, driving the contents out of the platelets and into the surrounding media.

Platelet Adhesion

On the vessel wall, collagen, von Willebrand factor (vWF), and fibronectin are the adhesive proteins that play the most prominent role in the adhesion of platelets to vascular subendothelium. On the exposure of collagen (eg, following a laceration or the rupture of an atherosclerotic plaque), platelet adhesion is triggered. Under conditions of high shear (flowing blood), platelet adhesion is mediated by the binding of GP Ib-V-IX receptors on platelet membranes to vWF in the vascular subendothelium.[47] Following adherence of platelets to subendothelial vWF, a conformational change in GP IIb-IIIa on platelet membrane occurs, activating this receptor complex to ligate vWF and fibrinogen. The result is the amplification of platelet adhesion and aggregation. An important interaction occurs between thrombosis and inflammation. Platelet-activating factor is synthesized and coexpressed with P-selectin on the surface of the endothelium in response to mediators such as histamine or thrombin. Platelet-activating factor interacts with a receptor on the surface of neutrophils that activates the CD11/CD18 adhesion complex, and results in adhesion of neutrophils to endothelium and to platelets. This results in the synthesis of leukotrienes and other mediators of inflammation.

Platelet Activation

Thrombin, collagen, and epinephrine can activate platelets. In response to thrombin, granules fuse with each other and with elements of the SCCS to form secretory vesicles. These vesicles are believed to fuse with the surface membrane, releasing their contents into the surrounding medium. The membranes of the secretory granules become incorporated into the platelet surface membrane.

Platelet Aggregation

Following activation, GP IIb-IIIa is expressed in active form on the platelet surface, serving as the final common pathway for platelet aggregation regardless of the inciting stimulus. This receptor binds exogenous calcium and fibrinogen. GP IIb-IIIa ligates fibrinogen along with fibronectin, vitronectin, and vWF, resulting in the binding of platelets to other platelets, and ultimately the formation of the platelet plug. Collagen-induced platelet aggregation is mediated by adenosine diphosphate (ADP) and thromboxane A_2. Adenosine diphosphate binds to the metabotropic purine receptors $P2Y_1$ and $P2Y_{12}$, leading to transient and sustained aggregation, respectively.[36] Thromboxane A_2 is formed from arachidonic acid by the action of cyclooxygenase-1. It is a potent vasoconstrictor and inducer of platelet aggregation and release reactions.[47] Platelets participate in triggering the coagulation cascade by binding coagulation factors II, VII, IX, and X to membrane phospholipid, a calcium-dependent process.

Antiplatelet Xenobiotics
Aspirin
Aspirin inhibits prostaglandin H synthase (cyclooxygenase[27]) by irreversibly acetylating a serine residue at the active site of the enzyme. Aspirin inhibition of the COX-1 isoform of this enzyme is 100 to 150 times more potent than its inhibition of the COX-2 isoform. The inhibition of COX-1 results in the irreversible inhibition of thromboxane A_2 formation. Because platelets are activated by other mechanisms including thrombin, thrombosis can develop despite aspirin therapy (Chap. 37).[93]

Selective COX-2 Inhibitors
Platelets express primarily COX-1 and use it to produce mostly thromboxane A_2, which leads to platelet aggregation and vasoconstriction. Endothelial cells express COX-2 and use it to produce prostaglandin I_2, an inhibitor of platelet aggregation and a vasodilator. Whereas aspirin and traditional (nonselective) nonsteroidal antiinflammatory drugs inhibit the production of thromboxane A_2 and prostaglandin I_2 at both sites, the selective COX-2 inhibitors do not affect platelet-derived thromboxane A_2, perhaps accounting for the increase in cardiovascular events associated with long-term use of some of these xenobiotics.[27,102]

Glycoprotein IIb-IIIa Antagonists
The GP IIb-IIIa antagonist abciximab is a chimeric human-murine monoclonal antibody that binds the GP IIb-IIIa receptor of platelets and megakaryocytes. Two synthetic ligand-mimetic antagonists have also been developed: eptifibatide and tirofiban. These parenteral antagonists are used primarily in patients undergoing percutaneous coronary interventions.[47] By blocking the fibrogen-binding site of IIb-IIIa, platelet aggregation is reversed regardless of the inciting activation. Reversible thrombocytopenia occurs within hours of initiation of these xenobiotics.[89]

ADP Receptor Inhibitors
The thienopyridines clopidogrel, ticlopidine, and prasugrel antagonize platelet aggregation by irreversible inhibition of ADP binding to the $P2Y_{12}$ receptor. All 3 prodrugs are associated with TTP, as well as neutropenia and aplastic anemia.[13,75,76] The purine analogs ticagrelor and cangrelor are direct-acting, reversible allosteric antagonists that bind to a different site on the $P2Y_{12}$ receptor.

Dipyridamole
The pyrimidopyrimidine derivative dipyridamole inhibits cyclic nucleotide phosphodiesterase in platelets, resulting in the accumulation of cyclic

adenosine monophosphate and perhaps cyclic guanine monophosphate. It also inhibits cellular reuptake of adenosine, blocks thromboxane synthase, and inhibits the thromboxane receptor.

Xenobiotic-Induced Thrombocytopenia

Multiple xenobiotics are reported to cause thrombocytopenia, either via the formation of drug-dependent antiplatelet antibodies or as thrombocytopenic purpura (TTP). Drug-induced platelet antibodies are estimated to occur in 1 in 100,000 drug exposures. Reversible drug binding to platelet epitopes, such as GP Ib-V-IX, GP IIb-IIIa, and platelet–endothelial cell adhesion molecule-1, leads to a structural change that forms or exposes a neoepitope target for antibody formation. The presence of the drug is required for antibody binding and increased platelet destruction, but there is no covalent bond (as occurs in the hapten model of penicillin binding to the erythrocyte membrane).

Thrombocytopenia also occurs as a result of spurious clumping, pregnancy, hypersplenism with cirrhosis, idiopathic thrombocytopenic purpura, heparin-induced thrombocytopenia (Chap. 58), bone marrow toxicity, and TTP. After excluding these conditions and nontherapeutic exposures, a systematic literature search updated annually lists more than 1,000 cases reported in English involving more than 150 xenobiotics. Table 20–7 lists the xenobiotics appearing in multiple cases, satisfying criteria for probable to definite causality including drug rechallenge. Nevertheless, a common clinical problem is to distinguish drug-induced thrombocytopenia from idiopathic thrombocytopenic purpura in a patient on multiple medications who develops thrombocytopenia. In the absence of validated laboratory assays for drug-dependent platelet antibodies other than heparin, diagnosis still depends on the clinical course following drug discontinuation and perhaps rechallenge. Large databases provide some guidance regarding past reported experience.[38,63,85] Severe (<20,000 platelets/mm³) or acute transient thrombocytopenia are more likely to be drug-induced.[10]

In patients administered the sensitizing xenobiotic de novo, 5 to 7 days are typically required for the development of the immune response. During rechallenge, thrombocytopenia can develop within 12 hours.[10] Interestingly, the unique ability of GP IIb/IIIa inhibitors such as abciximab to cause thrombocytopenia within hours of first use suggests the presence of preformed antibodies directed against platelet epitopes, perhaps accounting for ex vivo clumping of platelets observed in approximately one of 500 normal

patients.[86] Clinically, fever, chills, pruritus, and lethargy occur. The onset of life-threatening bleeding may be abrupt. Hemorrhagic vesicles develop in the oral mucosa. Laboratory investigations will demonstrate an absence of platelets on peripheral smear, prolongation of the bleeding time, deficient clot retraction, and an abnormal prothrombin consumption test. Bone marrow aspiration will demonstrate normal or increased numbers of megakaryocytes and immature forms. Treatment includes the transfusion of blood products, glucocorticoids, and the withdrawal of the offending xenobiotic.[10]

Thrombotic Thrombocytopenic Purpura

Thrombocytopenic purpura is characterized by the triad of microangiopathic hemolytic anemia, severe thrombocytopenia, and fluctuating neurologic abnormalities.[69] Fever and acute kidney injury are also common, although overt kidney failure is rare. The hallmark is the presence of platelet aggregates throughout the microvasculature, without fibrin clot, unlike the fibrin-rich thrombi that occur in disseminated intravascular coagulation or the hemolytic uremic syndrome. In the acquired form, drug-induced autoantibodies inactivate a circulating zinc metalloprotease ADAMTS13, thereby blocking its ability to depolymerize large multimers of vWF and leading to platelet clumping.[7,8,13,60,103] Plasma exchange with fresh-frozen plasma replenishes ADAMTS13 and removes the inhibitory antibodies. Prior to understanding of the molecular mechanism, other causes of microvascular hemolysis with thrombocytopenia were often confused with TTP. These causes included hemolytic uremic syndrome due to shiga toxin, the HELLP syndrome of pregnancy, Rocky Mountain spotted fever, and paroxysmal nocturnal hemoglobinuria. Also included were cases secondary to xenobiotics such as cyclosporine, cocaine, gemcitabine, mitomycin C, and cisplatin, in which ADAMTS13 antibodies are not present.[31,103]

Heparin-Induced Thrombocytopenia

An immune response to both unfractionated and low-molecular-weight heparin, manifested clinically by the development of thrombocytopenia and, at times, venous thrombosis, is now recognized to result from IgG antibodies against platelet factor-4, a heparin-binding chemokine.[1] The diagnosis is confirmed by testing for these antibodies. The heparin–platelet factor-4 antibody complex results in the release of procoagulant microparticles which release tissue factor, provide an anionic phospholipid membrane surface on which clotting cascade complexes assemble, and can lead to paradoxical thrombosis, which can be limb- or life-threatening (Chap. 58).[56,57]

SUMMARY

- The mechanisms of toxic injury to the blood are extremely varied, reflecting the complexity of this vital fluid.
- Virtually all xenobiotics come into contact with blood, and have the potential to disrupt its essential functions of oxygen transport, gas exchange, signaling, host defense, and hemostasis.
- Xenobiotics directly injure mature cells, or prohibit their development by injuring the stem cell pool.
- Oxygen transport is disrupted in several distinct ways, including oxidation of the heme iron, protein globin chain disruption, and shift of the oxygen-hemoglobin dissociation curve and hemolysis.
- A common theme in hematologic toxicity is the perturbation of homeostatic equilibria that exist between cell proliferation and apoptosis, between immune activation and suppression, or between thrombophilia and thrombolysis.

TABLE 20–7	Selected Xenobiotics Causing Thrombocytopenia as a Result of Antiplatelet Antibodies[a]
Abciximab	Indinavir
Acetaminophen	Levamisole
Aminoglutethimide	Linezolid
Aminosalicylic acid	Meclofenamic acid
Amiodarone	Nalidixic acid
Amphotericin B	Orbofiban
Carbamazepine	Oxprenolol
Cimetidine	Phenytoin
Danazol	Piperacillin
Diclofenac	Procainamide
Digoxin	Quinidine
Dipyridamole	Quinine
Eptifibatide	Rifampin
Famotidine	Tirofiban
Furosemide	Trimethoprim-sulfamethoxazole
Gold salts	Valproate
Heparin	Vancomycin
Imipenem-cilastatin	

[a]Xenobiotics reported in at least 2 cases to have definitely caused immune thrombocytopenia or in at least 5 cases to have probably caused immune thrombocytopenia following therapeutic use.

Data from Li X, Swisher KK, Vesely SK, et al. Drug-induced thrombocytopenia: an updated systematic review. *Drug Safety.* 2007;30:185–186 and http://www.ouhsc.edu/platelets.

REFERENCES

1. Alberio L. Heparin-induced thrombocytopenia: some working hypotheses on pathogenesis, diagnostic strategies and treatment. *Curr Opin Hematol.* 2008;15:456-464.
2. Andersohn F, et al. Systematic review: agranulocytosis induced by nonchemotherapy drugs. *Ann Intern Med.* 2007;146:657-665.
3. Andres E, Maloisel F. Idiosyncratic drug-induced agranulocytosis or acute neutropenia. *Curr Opin Hematol.* 2008;15:15-21.
4. Andres E, et al. Life-threatening idiosyncratic drug-induced agranulocytosis in elderly patients. *Drugs Aging.* 2004;21:427-435.
5. Andrews NC. Understanding heme transport. *N Engl J Med.* 2005;353:2508-2509.

6. Armstrong C, et al. Eosinophilia-myalgia syndrome: selective cognitive impairment, longitudinal effects, and neuroimaging findings. *J Neurol Neurosurg Psychiatry.* 1997;63:633-641.

7. Aster RH. Drug-induced immune thrombocytopenia: an overview of pathogenesis. *Semin Hematol.* 1999;36(suppl 1):2-6.

8. Aster RH. Thrombotic thrombocytopenic purpura (TTP)—an enigmatic disease finally resolved? *Trends Mol Med.* 2002;8:1-3.

9. Aster RH. Drug-induced immune cytopenias. *Toxicology.* 2005;209:149-153.

10. Aster RH, Bougie DW. Drug-induced immune thrombocytopenia. *N Engl J Med.* 2007;357:580-587.

11. Bellest L, et al. A modified international normalized ratio as an effective way of prothrombin time standardization in hepatology. *Hepatology.* 2007;46:528-534.

12. Bennett CL, et al. Pure red-cell aplasia and epoetin therapy. *N Engl J Med.* 2004; 351:1403-1408.

13. Bennett CL, et al. Thrombotic thrombocytopenic purpura associated with clopidogrel. *N Engl J Med.* 2000;342:1773-1777.

14. Bennett CL, et al. Long-term outcome of individuals with pure red cell aplasia and antierythropoietin antibodies in patients treated with recombinant epoetin: a follow-up report from the Research on Adverse Drug Events and Reports (RADAR) Project. *Blood.* 2005;106:3343-3347.

15. Bergsagel DE, et al. Benzene and multiple myeloma: appraisal of the scientific evidence. *Blood.* 1999;94:1174-1182.

16. Berzofsky JA, et al. Sulfheme proteins. I. Optical and magnetic properties of sulfmyoglobin and its derivatives. *J Biol Chem.* 1971;246:3367-3377.

17. Beutler E, et al. The hemolytic effect of primaquine. IV. The relationship of cell age to hemolysis. *J Lab Clin Med.* 1954;44:439-442.

18. Beutler E, Vulliamy TJ. Hematologically important mutations: glucose-6-phosphate dehydrogenase. *Blood Cells Mol Dis.* 2002;28:93-103.

19. Bradberry SM. Occupational methaemoglobinaemia. Mechanisms of production, features, diagnosis and management including the use of methylene blue. *Toxicol Rev.* 2003;22:13-27.

20. Brodsky RA. Biology and management of acquired severe aplastic anemia. *Curr Opin Oncol.* 1998;10:95-99.

21. Bryder D, et al. Hematopoietic stem cells: the paradigmatic tissue-specific stem cell. *Am J Pathol.* 2006;169:338-346.

22. Buchanan JA, Lavonas EJ. Agranulocytosis and other consequences due to use of illicit cocaine contaminated with levamisole [review]. *Curr Opin Hematol.* 2012;19:27-31.

23. Bulmer FMR, et al. Chronic arsine poisoning among workers employed in the cyanide extraction of gold: a report of fourteen cases. *J Ind Hygiene Tox.* 1940;22:111-124.

24. Caldwell S, Shah N. The prothrombin time-derived international normalized ratio: great for Warfarin, fair for prognosis and bad for liver-bleeding risk. *Liver Int.* 2008;28:1325-1327.

25. Cappellini MD, et al. Metabolic indicators of oxidative stress correlate with haemichrome attachment to membrane, band 3 aggregation and erythrophagocytosis in beta-thalassaemia intermedia. *Br J Haematol.* 1999;104:504-512.

26. Casadevall N, et al. Pure red-cell aplasia and antierythropoietin antibodies in patients treated with recombinant erythropoietin. *N Engl J Med.* 2002;346:469-475.

27. Clark DW, et al. Do some inhibitors of COX-2 increase the risk of thromboembolic events? Linking pharmacology with pharmacoepidemiology. *Drug Saf.* 2004;27:427-456.

28. Coleman MD, Coleman NA. Drug-induced methaemoglobinaemia. Treatment issues. *Drug Saf.* 1996;14:394-405.

29. Critchley JA, et al. Granulocyte-colony stimulating factor in the treatment of colchicine poisoning. *Hum Exp Toxicol.* 1997;16:229-232.

30. Datta B, et al. Red blood cell nitric oxide as an endocrine vasoregulator: a potential role in congestive heart failure. *Circulation.* 2004;109:1339-1342.

31. Dlott JS, et al. Drug-induced thrombotic thrombocytopenic purpura/hemolytic uremic syndrome: a concise review. *Ther Apher Dial.* 2004;8:102-111.

32. Edwards MS, Curtis JR. Use of cobaltous chloride in anaemia of maintenance hemodialysis patients. *Lancet.* 1971;2:582-583.

33. Fareed J, et al. Acquired defects of fibrinolysis associated with thrombosis. *Semin Thromb Hemost.* 1999;25:367-374.

34. Fliedner TM, et al. Structure and function of bone marrow hemopoiesis: mechanisms of response to ionizing radiation exposure [review]. *Cancer Biother Radiopharm.* 2002;17:405-426.

35. Fowler BA, Weissberg JB. Arsine poisoning. *N Engl J Med.* 1974;291:1171-1174.

36. Gachet C. ADP receptors of platelets and their inhibition. *Thromb Haemost.* 2001;86:222-232.

37. Gelpi E, et al. The Spanish toxic oil syndrome 20 years after its onset: a multidisciplinary review of scientific knowledge. *Environ Health Perspect.* 2002;110:457-464.

38. George JN, et al. Drug-induced thrombocytopenia: a systematic review of published case reports. *Ann Intern Med.* 1998;129:886-890.

39. Gow AJ, et al. The oxyhemoglobin reaction of nitric oxide. *Proc Natl Acad Sci U S A.* 1999;96:9027-9032.

40. Graham AF, et al. The action of arsine on blood: observations on the nature of the fixed arsenic. *Biochem J.* 1946;40:256-260.

41. Gregory CA, et al. Non-hematopoietic bone marrow stem cells: molecular control of expansion and differentiation. *Exp Cell Res.* 2005;306:330-335.

42. Haab P. The effect of carbon monoxide on respiration. *Experientia.* 1990;46:1202-1203.

43. Hare JM. Nitroso-redox balance in the cardiovascular system. *N Engl J Med.* 2004;351:2112-2114.

44. Harris R, et al. Colchicine-induced bone marrow suppression: treatment with granulocyte colony-stimulating factor. *J Emerg Med.* 2000;18:435-440.

45. Hatlelid KM, et al. Reactions of arsine with hemoglobin. *J Toxicol Environ Health.* 1996;47:145-157.

46. Hentze MW, et al. Balancing acts: molecular control of mammalian iron metabolism. *Cell.* 2004;117:285-297.

47. Hirsh J, Weitz I. Thrombosis and anticoagulation. *Semin Hematol.* 1999;36:118-132.

48. Hsieh MM, et al. Prevalence of neutropenia in the U.S. population: age, sex, smoking status, and ethnic differences. *Ann Intern Med.* 2007;146:486-492.

49. Ichimaru M, et al. Incidence of aplastic anemia in A-bomb survivors. Hiroshima and Nagasaki, 1946-1967. *Radiat Res.* 1972;49:461-472.

50. Irons RD. Molecular models of benzene leukemogenesis. *J Toxicol Environ Health A.* 2000;61:391-397.

51. Irons RD, Stillman WS. The process of leukemogenesis. *Environ Health Perspect.* 1996;104(suppl 6):1239-1246.

52. Issaragrisil S, et al. The epidemiology of aplastic anemia in Thailand. *Blood.* 2006;107:1299-1307.

53. Jefferson JA, et al. Excessive erythrocytosis, chronic mountain sickness, and serum cobalt levels. *Lancet.* 2002;359:407-408.

54. Jenkins GC, et al. Arsine poisoning: massive haemolysis with minimal impairment of renal function. *Br Med J.* 1965;5453:78-80.

55. Karp JE, Smith MA. The molecular pathogenesis of treatment-induced (secondary) leukemias: foundations for treatment and prevention. *Semin Oncol.* 1997;24:103-113.

56. Kelton JG, et al. Nonheparin anticoagulants for heparin-induced thrombocytopenia. *N Engl J Med.* 2013;368:737-744.

57. Kelton JG, Warkentin TE. Heparin-induced thrombocytopenia: a historical perspective. *Blood.* 2008;112:2607-2616.

58. Kleinfeld MJ. Arsine poisoning. *J Occup Med.* 1980;22:820-821.

59. Korbling M, Estrov Z. Adult stem cells for tissue repair—a new therapeutic concept? *N Engl J Med.* 2003;349:570-582.

60. Kremer Hovinga JA, et al. Thrombotic thrombocytopenic purpura. *Nat Rev Dis Primers.* 2017;3:17020.

61. Latunde-Dada GO, et al. Recent advances in mammalian haem transport. *Trends Biochem Sci.* 2006;31:182-188.

62. Lennard AL, Jackson GH. Stem cell transplantation. *BMJ.* 2000;321:433-437. Erratum in *BMJ.* 2000;321:1331.

63. Li X, et al. Drug-induced thrombocytopenia: an updated systematic review, 2006. *Drug Saf.* 2007;30:185-186.

64. Majeti R, et al. Identification of a hierarchy of multipotent hematopoietic progenitors in human cord blood. *Cell Stem Cell.* 2007;1:635-645.

65. Mannucci PM. Hemostatic drugs. *N Engl J Med.* 1998;339:245-253.

66. McKoy JM, et al. Epoetin-associated pure red cell aplasia: past, present, and future considerations. *Transfusion.* 2008;48:1754-1762.

67. McMahon TJ, et al. Nitric oxide in the human respiratory cycle. *Nat Med.* 2002;8:711-717.

68. Milinski M, et al. Major histocompatibility complex peptide ligands as olfactory cues in human body odour assessment. *Proc R Soc London Ser B Biol Sci.* 2013;280:20122889. Erratum in *Proc Biol Sci.* 2013;280:20130381.

69. Moake JL. Thrombotic microangiopathies. *N Engl J Med.* 2002;347:589-600.

70. Morell DB, Chang Y. The structure of the chromophore of sulphmyoglobin. *Biochim Biophys Acta.* 1967;136:121-130.

71. Mousa SA. Comparative efficacy of different low-molecular-weight heparins (LMWHs) and drug interactions with LMWH: interactions for management of vascular disorders. *Semin Thromb Hemost.* 2000;26(suppl 1):1-46.

72. Nagel RL, Roth EF Jr. Malaria and red cell genetic defects. *Blood.* 1989;74:1213-1221.

73. Nardi NB, Alfonso ZZC. The hematopoietic stroma. *Braz J Med Biol Res.* 1999;32:601-609.

74. Nimer SD, et al. An increased HLA DTR2 frequency is seen in aplastic anemia patients. *Blood.* 1994;84:923-927.

75. Paradiso-Hardy FL, et al. Hematologic dyscrasia associated with ticlopidine therapy: evidence for causality. *CMAJ.* 2000;163:1441-1448.

76. Paradiso-Hardy FL, et al. Thrombotic thrombocytopenic purpura associated with clopidogrel: further evaluation. *Can J Cardiol.* 2002;18:771-773.

77. Park CM, Nagel RL. Sulfhemoglobinemia: clinical and molecular aspects. *N Engl J Med.* 1984;310:1579-1584.

78. Pedersen-Bjergaard J. Insights into leukemogenesis from therapy-related leukemia. *N Engl J Med.* 2005;352:1591-1594.

79. Piga A, et al. Deferiprone: new insight. *Ann N Y Acad Sci. Ann N Y Acad Sci.* 2005;1054:169-174.

80. Pinto SS. Arsine poisoning: evaluation of the acute phase. *J Occup Med.* 1976;18:633-635.

81. Podvinec M, et al. Identification of the xenosensors regulating human 5-aminolevulinate synthase. *Proc Natl Acad Sci U S A.* 2004;101:9127-9132.

82. Provan D, Weatherall D. Red cells II: acquired anaemias and polycythaemia. *Lancet.* 2000;355:1260-1268.

83. Rael LT, et al. The effects of sulfur, thiol, and thiol inhibitor compounds on arsine-induced toxicity in the human erythrocyte membrane. *Toxicol Sci.* 2000;55:468-477.

84. Reiter CD, et al. Cell-free hemoglobin limits nitric oxide bioavailability in sickle-cell disease. *Nat Med.* 2002;8:1383-1389.

85. Rizvi MA, et al. Drug-induced thrombocytopenia: an updated systematic review. *Ann Intern Med.* 2001;134:346.

86. Rizvi MA, et al. Drug-induced thrombocytopenia. *Curr Opin Hematol.* 1999;6:349-353.

87. Robert A, Chazouilleres O. Prothrombin time in liver failure: time, ratio, activity percentage, or international normalized ratio? *Hepatology.* 1996;24:1392-1394.

88. Rothenberg ME. Eosinophilia. *N Engl J Med.* 1998;338:1592-1600.

89. Said SM, et al. Glycoprotein IIb/IIIa inhibitor-induced thrombocytopenia: diagnosis and treatment. *Clin Res Cardiol.* 2007;96:61-69.

90. Savage DG, et al. Etiology and diagnostic evaluation of macrocytosis. *Am J Med Sci.* 2000;319:343-352.

91. Schechter AN, Gladwin MT. Hemoglobin and the paracrine and endocrine functions of nitric oxide. *N Engl J Med.* 2003;348:1483-1485.

92. Schrijvers D. Role of red blood cells in pharmacokinetics of chemotherapeutic agents. *Clin Pharmacokinet.* 2003;42:779-791.

93. Schror K. Aspirin and platelets: the antiplatelet action of aspirin and its role in thrombosis and treatment prophylaxis. *Semin Thromb Hemost.* 1997;23:349-356.

94. Singel DJ, Stamler JS. Chemical physiology of blood flow regulation by red blood cells: the role of nitric oxide and *S*-nitrosohemoglobin. *Annu Rev Physiol.* 2005;67:99-145.

95. Sivilotti MLA. Oxidant stress and hemolysis of the human erythrocyte. *Toxicol Rev.* 2004;23:169-188.

96. Smith RE. The INR: a perspective. *Semin Thromb Hemost.* 1997;23:547-549.

97. Stock W, Hoffman R. White blood cells 1: non-malignant disorders. *Lancet.* 2000;355:1351-1357.

98. Thom SR. Leukocytes in carbon monoxide-mediated brain oxidative injury. *Toxicol Applied Pharmacol.* 1993;123:234-247.

99. Thompson DF, Gales MA. Drug-induced pure red cell aplasia. *Pharmacotherapy.* 1996;16:1002-1008.

100. Thunell S, et al. Guide to drug porphyrogenicity prediction and drug prescription in the acute porphyrias. *Br J Clin Pharmacol.* 2007;64:668-679.

101. Tinmouth A, Chin-Yee I. The clinical consequences of the red cell storage lesion. *Transfus Med Rev.* 2001;15:91-107.

102. Topol EJ. Arthritis medicines and cardiovascular events—"house of coxibs." *JAMA.* 2005;293:366-368.

103. Tsai HM. Current concepts in thrombotic thrombocytopenic purpura. *Annu Rev Med.* 2006;57:419-436.

104. Vandendries ER, Drews RE. Drug-associated disease: hematologic dysfunction. *Crit Care Clin.* 2006;22:347-355, viii.

105. Wang L, et al. Genomics and drug response. *N Engl J Med.* 2011;364:1144-1153.

106. Winski SL, et al. Sequence of toxic events in arsine-induced hemolysis in vitro: implications for the mechanism of toxicity in human erythrocytes. *Fundam Appl Toxicol.* 1997;38:123-128.

107. Xie W, et al. Orphan nuclear receptor-mediated xenobiotic regulation in drug metabolism. *Drug Discov Today.* 2004;9:442-449.

108. Young NS, Kaufman DW. The epidemiology of acquired aplastic anemia. *Haematologica.* 2008;93:489-492.

109. Young NS, et al. Aplastic anemia. *Curr Opin Hematol.* 2008;15:162-168.

110. Zola H, et al. CD molecules 2005: human cell differentiation molecules. *Blood.* 2005;106:3123-3126.

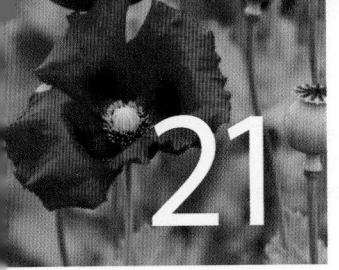

21 HEPATIC PRINCIPLES

Kathleen A. Delaney and Jakub Furmaga

The liver plays an essential role in metabolic homeostasis. Hepatic functions include the synthesis, storage, and breakdown of glycogen. In addition, the liver is important in the metabolism of lipids; the synthesis of albumin, clotting factors, and other important proteins; the synthesis of the bile acids necessary for absorption of lipids and lipid-soluble vitamins; and the metabolism of cholesterol. Hepatocytes facilitate the excretion of metals, most importantly iron, copper, zinc, manganese, mercury, and aluminum, as well as the detoxification of products of metabolism, such as bilirubin and ammonia.[27,59] Generalized disruption of these important functions results in manifestations of liver failure: hyperbilirubinemia, coagulopathy, hypoalbuminemia, hyperammonemia, and hypoglycemia. Disturbances of more specific functions result in accumulation of lipids, metals, and bilirubin, and the development of lipid-soluble vitamin deficiencies.[125]

The liver is also the primary site of biotransformation and detoxification of xenobiotics. The interposition of the liver between the gastrointestinal tract and systemic circulation makes it the first-pass recipient of ingested xenobiotics. The liver receives blood from the systemic circulation and participates in the detoxification and elimination of xenobiotics that reach the bloodstream through other routes, such as inhalation or cutaneous absorption.[112,125]

Many xenobiotics are lipophilic and inert, requiring chemical modification followed by conjugation to make them sufficiently water-soluble to be eliminated. The liver is the primary organ responsible for this biotransformation, and contains the highest concentration of cytochrome P450 (CYP) enzymes involved in the first stage of detoxification for many lipophilic xenobiotics (Chap. 11). Although many of the xenobiotics that are detoxified in the liver are subsequently excreted in the urine, the biliary tract provides an additional route for their elimination.[43] Although cytochrome P450 phase I activation of xenobiotics usually leads to detoxification, in some cases it can produce xenobiotics with increased toxicity and hepatocyte injury at the site of synthesis.[112]

MORPHOLOGY AND FUNCTION OF THE LIVER

Two pathologic concepts are used to describe the appearance and function of the liver: a structural one represented by the hepatic lobule, and a functional one represented by the acinus. The basic structural unit of the liver as characterized by light microscopy is the hepatic lobule, a hexagon with the hepatic vein at the center and the portal triads at the angles. The portal triad consists of the portal vein, the common bile duct, and the hepatic artery. Cords of hepatocytes are oriented radially around the central hepatic vein, forming sinusoids. In contrast, the acinus, or "metabolic lobule" is the functional unit of the liver. Located between 2 central hepatic veins, it is bisected by terminal branches of the hepatic artery and portal vein that extend from the bases of the acini toward hepatic venules at the apices. The acinus is subdivided into 3 metabolically distinct zones: Zone 1 lies near the portal triad, zone 3 lies near the central hepatic vein, and zone 2 is the intermediate area.[125] Figure 21–1 illustrates the relationship of the structural and functional concepts of the liver.

Approximately 75% of the blood supply to the liver is derived from the portal vein, which drains the gastrointestinal tract, spleen, and pancreas. This blood is enriched with nutrients and other absorbed xenobiotics and is poor in oxygen. The remainder of the hepatic blood flow comes from the hepatic artery, which delivers well-oxygenated blood from the systemic circulation. Blood from the hepatic artery and portal vein mixes in the sinusoids, coming in close contact with cords of hepatocytes before it exits through small fenestrations in the wall of the vein.[137] Oxygen content diminishes severalfold as blood flows from the portal area to the central hepatic vein.[53]

There are 6 types of cells in the liver. Hepatocytes and bile duct epithelia make up the parenchyma. Cells found near the sinusoids include endothelial cells, fixed macrophages (Kupffer cells), hepatic stellate cells (so-called Ito cells), and a large population of lymphocytes that roam the sinusoids. The sinusoidal lining formed by endothelial cells is thin and fenestrated, allowing transfer of fluid, chylomicrons, and proteins across the space of Disse, an extrasinusoidal space filled with microvilli.[137] Kupffer cells remove particles and cell debris that include bacteria and endotoxins from the portal circulation. They also clear many biologically active substances from the systemic circulation.[12] When immunologically activated by xenobiotics, Kupffer cells contribute to the generation of oxygen free radicals[110] and also participate in the production of autoimmune injury to hepatocytes, including activation of hepatic stellate cells.[58,110] Hepatic stellate cells are primary sites for the storage of fat and vitamin A.[36,45] In a quiescent state, they spread out between the sinusoidal endothelium and hepatic parenchymal cells. Filled with microtubules and microfilaments, they project cytoplasmic extensions that contact several cell types.[36,45] Activated stellate cells produce collagen, proteoglycans, and adhesive glycoproteins, which are crucial to the development of hepatic fibrosis.[34] The liver lymphocyte population is enriched with natural killer (NK) or pit cells, which play a key role in host defense by actively lysing tumor cells and virally infected cells[18,35] (Fig. 21–2). Evidence from animal models suggests that NK cells selectively kill activated stellate cells, inhibiting the development of liver fibrosis.[34,35]

Bile acids, organic anions, bilirubin, phospholipids, xenobiotics, and other molecules excreted in bile are actively transported across the hepatocyte plasma membrane into the bile canaliculi at sites that have specificity for acids, bases, and neutral xenobiotics.[94] Tight junctions separate the contents of the bile canaliculi from the sinusoids and hepatocytes, maintaining a rigid and functionally necessary compartmentalization. Bile acids use 3 active transport systems: a sodium-dependent bile salt transporter in the sinusoidal membrane, an adenosine triphosphate (ATP)-dependent bile salt carrier in the canalicular membrane, and a canalicular membrane transport site driven by the membrane proton gradient.[94] Xenobiotics bound to glucuronide are substrates for the bile acid transport systems and are actively secreted into bile. Xenobiotics with molecular weights greater than 500 Da are also preferentially secreted into bile. Like the transport and concentration of constituents from the sinusoids and hepatocytes, the flow of bile through the canaliculi is also an active process facilitated by ATP-dependent contractions of actin filaments that encircle the canaliculi.[94,129]

The enterohepatic recirculation of bile acids and certain vitamins plays a crucial role in their conservation. Unfortunately, this recirculation also impedes the fecal elimination of some xenobiotics by reabsorbing and returning them back into the systemic circulation, prolonging their apparent half-lives and toxicity. Xenobiotics that have low molecular weights and are not ionized at intestinal pH (ie, methylmercury, phencyclidine, and nortriptyline) are most likely to be reabsorbed.[109]

TYPES OF HEPATIC INJURY

Owing to its location at the end of the portal system and its substantial complement of biotransformation enzymes, the liver is especially vulnerable to toxic injury. The pathologic spectrum of liver injury includes combinations of hepatocellular necrosis with focal or generalized lysis of hepatocytes and elevations of aspartate aminotransferase (AST) and alanine aminotransferase (ALT); hepatitis associated with inflammatory cellular infiltrates and varied elevations of hepatocellular enzymes; cholestasis with pruritus, jaundice, and insignificant elevations of hepatocellular enzymes; steatosis

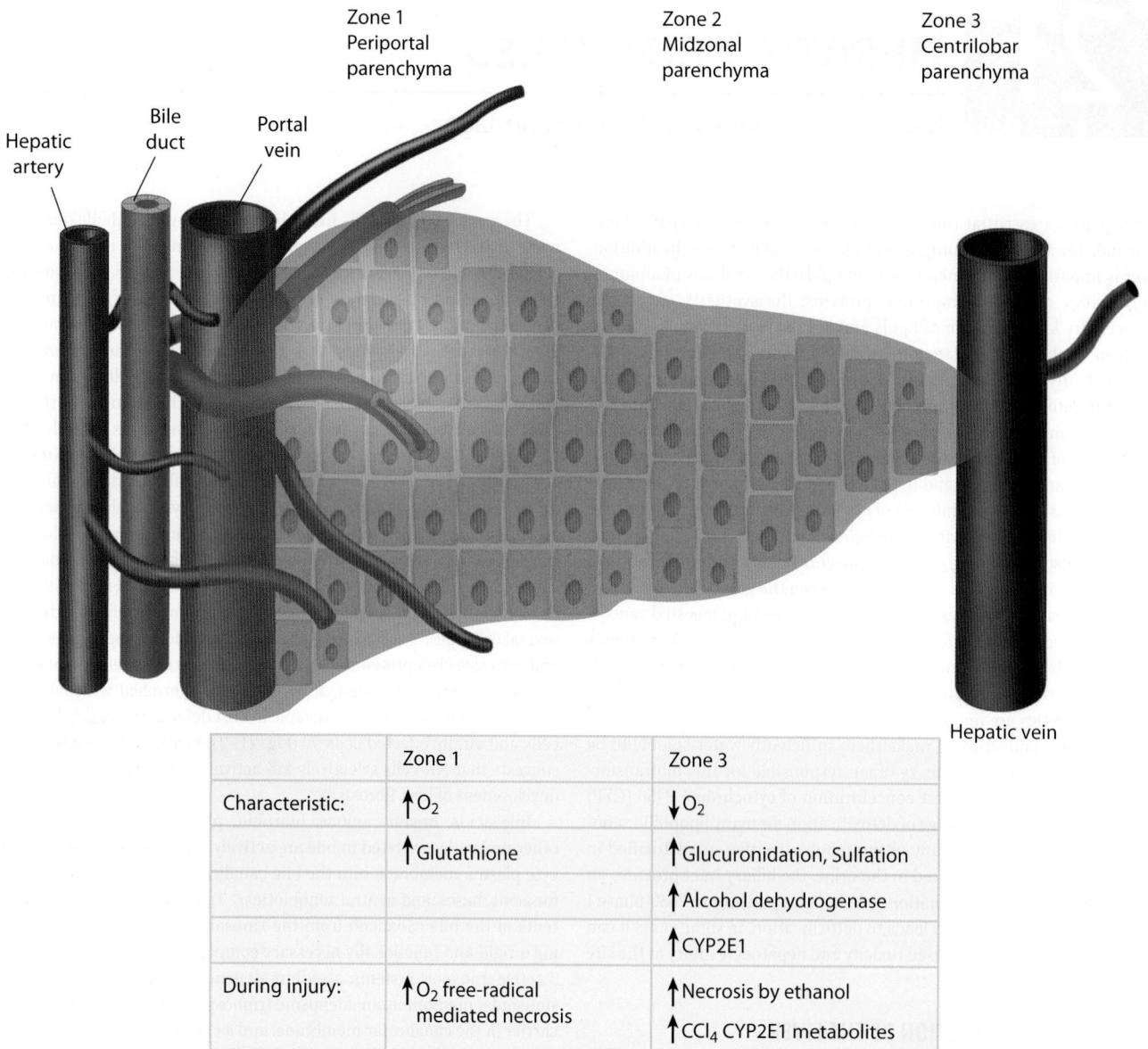

FIGURE 21–1. The acinus is defined by 3 functional zones. Specific contributions of each zone to the biotransformation of xenobiotics reflect various metabolic factors that include differences in oxygen content of blood as it flows from the oxygen-rich portal area to the central hepatic vein, differences in glutathione content, different capacities for glucuronidation and sulfation, and variations in content of metabolic enzymes such as CYP2E1. The hepatic lobule (not shown) is a structural concept, a hexagon with the central vein at the center surrounded by six portal areas that contain branches of the hepatic artery, bile duct, and portal vein. Injury to hepatocytes that is confined to zone 3 is called "centrilobular" because in the structure of the lobule, zone 3 encircles the central vein, which is the center of the hepatic lobule.

caused by intracellular deposits of fat; apoptosis, the formation of shrunken, nonfunctioning, eosinophilic bodies; and fibrosis.[125]

FACTORS THAT AFFECT THE ANATOMIC LOCALIZATION OF HEPATIC INJURY

Hepatocellular necrosis that occurs near the portal vein is called *periportal*, or *zone 1* necrosis. The term *centrilobular* or *zone 3* necrosis refers to injury that surrounds the central hepatic vein. Figure 21–3 shows centrilobular necrosis caused by exposure to acetaminophen. Metabolic characteristics of the zones of the acinus have important relevance to the anatomic distribution of toxic liver injury. Because of its location in the periportal area, zone 1 has a 2-fold higher oxygen content than zone 3. Hepatic injury that results from the metabolic production of oxygen free radicals predominates in zone 1. Allyl alcohol, an industrial chemical that is metabolized to a highly reactive aldehyde, is associated with oxygen-dependent lipid peroxidation injury to hepatocytes in zone 1.[3] The tendency for centrilobular or zone 3

accumulation of fat in patients with alcoholic steatosis is attributed to the effect of relative hypoxia in the central vein area on the oxidation potential of the hepatocyte.[6] The availability of substrates for detoxification and the localization of enzymes involved in biotransformation also affect the site of injury. Zone 1 has a higher concentration of glutathione, whereas zone 3 has a greater capacity for glucuronidation and sulfation.[130] Zone 3 has higher concentrations of alcohol dehydrogenase, which leads to increased production of its toxic metabolite acetaldehyde at centrilobular sites.[26,78] Zone 3 also has high concentrations of CYP2E1, which converts many xenobiotics including acetaminophen (APAP), nitrosamines, benzene, and carbon tetrachloride (CCl_4) to reactive intermediates that cause centrilobular injury. Although CCl_4 is metabolized to a highly reactive oxygen free radical in zone 1, it primarily injures zone 3 for the following reasons: CCl_4 is metabolized by CYP2E1 in zone 3 to a trichloromethyl free radical ($\cdot CCl_3$) that forms covalent bonds with cellular proteins, causes lipid peroxidation, or spontaneously reacts with oxygen to form the more highly reactive trichloromethyl peroxy

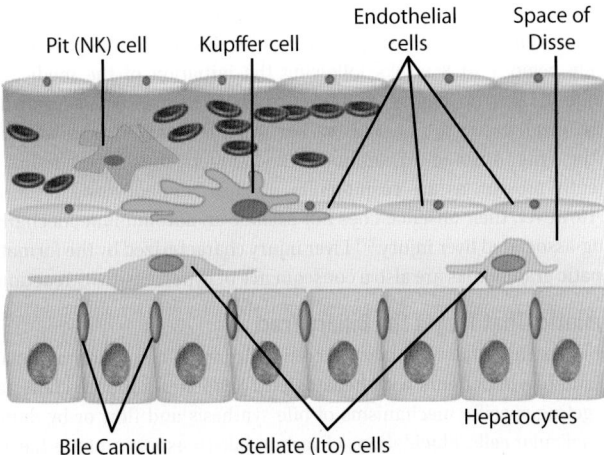

FIGURE 21–2. Blood flowing through the hepatic sinusoids is separated from hepatocytes by fenestrated endothelium that allows passage of many substances across the space of Disse. This figure shows 6 types of cells found in the liver and their localization in relation to the sinusoid. Stellate cells are fat storage cells that promote fibrosis when activated.[34] Kupffer cells are fixed macrophages that participate in immune surveillance and are a source of free radicals when activated. Natural killer (NK) cells are lymphocytes that float freely in the sinusoids, scavenging tumor and virus-infected cells.[18] Hepatocytes and bile epithelial cells form the hepatic parenchyma.

radical ($CCl_3OO\cdot$).[9,73] Higher oxygen tension in zone 1 fosters the formation of $CCl_3OO\cdot$, which is rapidly detoxified by glutathione. Because the less reactive $\cdot CCl_3$ that predominates in zone 3 is not readily detoxified by glutathione, zone 3 incurs the greater amount of injury. Hyperbaric oxygen increases the oxygen tension throughout the liver and decreases liver injury caused by CCl_4, possibly by increasing the formation of $CCl_3OO\cdot$ in zone 3, which is then efficiently detoxified by glutathione.[14] The observed effects of isoniazid (an inhibitor of CYP2E1) and chronic ethanol intake (an inducer of the CYP2E1) on injury in cell cultures from periportal and centrilobular areas exposed to CCl_4 support the association of CCl_4 injury with the localization of CYP2E1 activity. Acute exposure to isoniazid significantly decreases the injury associated with exposure of zone 3 cells to CCl_4, whereas chronic treatment with ethanol significantly enhances injury.[73]

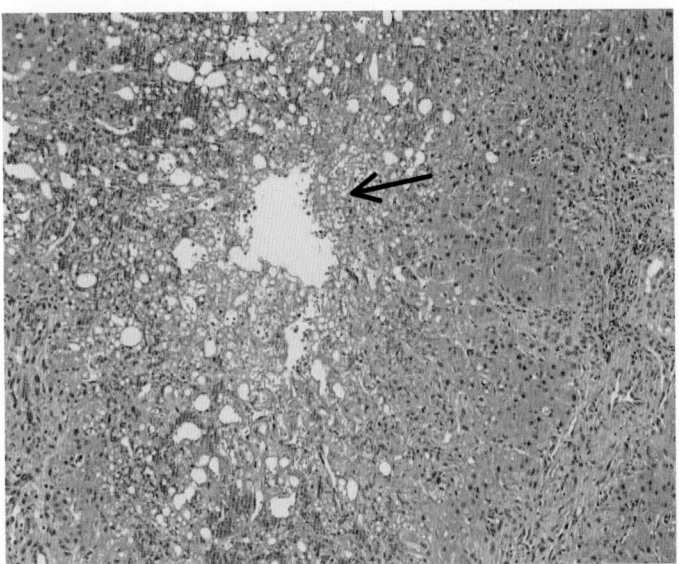

FIGURE 21–3. Biopsy showing centrilobular necrosis of a liver in a patient with acetaminophen toxicity. The arrow points to the necrotic area with cells without nuclei. There is also the presence of polymorphonuclear leukocyte infiltration in the periphery. (*Used with permission from Daniel Mais, MD, Professor of Pathology, University of Texas Health Science Center at San Antonio.*)

FACTORS THAT AFFECT THE DEVELOPMENT OF HEPATOTOXICITY

Xenobiotics that produce liver damage in all humans in a predictable and dose-dependent manner are called *intrinsic* hepatotoxins. They include APAP, CCl_4, and yellow phosphorus, to name a few. Those that cause liver damage in a small number of individuals and whose effect is not apparently predictable or dose dependent are called *idiosyncratic* hepatotoxins.[38]

Prediction of Drug-Induced Liver Injury

Drug-induced liver injury (DILI) refers to the production of liver injury by pharmaceuticals. It is the most common cause of acute liver failure in the United States, and is the most frequent adverse event responsible for the termination of clinical trials of new drugs, as well as postmarketing withdrawals of approved drugs.[98] LiverTox (https://livertox.nih.gov) is an up-to-date informational website about the incidence, diagnosis, and management of xenobiotic-associated liver injury.[8]

Prediction of DILI in any individual patient based on clinical trials is difficult because the incidence is rare. Drug-induced liver injury depends largely on factors that affect host susceptibility. These include age, gender, diet, underlying diseases, and concurrent exposure to other xenobiotics.[98] Genetic factors are increasingly elucidated. Many enzymes involved in biotransformation show genetic polymorphism. Inherited variations in CYP enzymes affect susceptibility to DILI.[2] For example, perhexiline, an antianginal marketed in Europe in the 1980s, caused severe liver injury and peripheral neuropathy in persons with an inability to metabolize debrisoquine.[118] The congenital disorder that results in Gilbert syndrome is characterized by decreased glucuronyltransferase. These patients demonstrate decreased glucuronidation and increased bioactivation of APAP during chronic therapeutic dosing, suggesting an increased risk of hepatic injury following ingestion of APAP.[23] Gastrointestinal toxicity due to irinotecan, an antineoplastic used in the treatment of colon cancer, is associated with deficiency of glucuronyltransferase.[87]

Studies that compare the genomes of patients who develop hypersensitivity reactions to various drugs with those who do not show significant associations with human leukocyte antigen (HLA) alleles.[41] Hypersensitivity reactions to abacavir are significantly associated with HLA-B*5701, such that the Food and Drug Administration now recommends HLA screening prior to the initiation of abacivir.[81] Human leukocyte antigen-B*5701 is also associated with cholestatic DILI in patients taking flucloxacillin, an antibiotic marketed in Europe.[21] Similarly, HLA-B27 predisposes to the development of agranulocytosis in levamisole-adulterated crack-cocaine exposure.[15] Severe hypersensitivity reactions to carbamazepine are associated with the HLA allele HLA-A*3101.[82] Specific HLA phenotypes are implicated in the development of cholestatic liver injury in patients exposed to amoxicillin-clavulanate.[76] Drug-induced liver injury in the form of elevation of the ALT occurred in 15% of patients exposed to the first-generation direct thrombin inhibitor ximelagatran, with some developing clinically significant hepatitis. This was associated with 2 specific HLA phenotypes-DRB1*07 and DQA1*02.[57]

Effects of Xenobiotics on Enzyme Function

Some xenobiotic combinations increase the possibility of hepatotoxic reactions because one xenobiotic alters the metabolism of the other, leading to the production of toxic metabolites. This is the case with combinations of rifampin and isoniazid,[132] amoxicillin and clavulanic acid,[24] and trimethoprim and sulfamethoxazole.[19] Changes in the activities of biotransformation enzymes that result in increased formation of hepatotoxic metabolites suggest increased susceptibility to hepatic injury. For example, chronic ethanol exposure causes proliferation of the smooth endoplasmic reticulum in the centrilobular areas resulting in increased CYP2E1 activity.[75] When bromobenzene, a xenobiotic whose metabolism and hepatotoxicity are similar to that of APAP (the toxic metabolite 3,4-epoxide is formed via CYP2E pathway), was administered to rats chronically exposed to ethanol, it caused a more rapid onset of hepatotoxicity compared to the controls. In addition, the dose of bromobenzene required for hepatic injury was not altered by immediate pretreatment with ethanol.[47] This means that hepatic toxicity caused by solvents such as CCl_4, dimethylformamide, and bromobenzene is likely exacerbated by chronic exposure to ethanol.[73,102]

Availability of Substrates

The availability of substrates for detoxification significantly affects both the likelihood and the localization of hepatic injury. The metabolism of APAP illustrates the effect of glutathione concentration on the delicate balance between detoxification and the production of injurious metabolites. In healthy adults taking therapeutic amounts of APAP, approximately 90% of hepatic metabolism results in formation of the glucuronide or sulfate metabolites. Most of the remainder undergoes oxidative metabolism to the toxic electrophile *N*-acetyl-*p*-benzoquinone imine (NAPQI) and is rapidly detoxified by conjugation with glutathione.[111] Glutathione is depleted during the course of metabolism of APAP by otherwise normal livers, but it is also decreased by inadequate nutrition or liver disease.[111] Excessive amounts of APAP result in increased synthesis of NAPQI, which, in the absence of glutathione, reacts avidly with hepatocellular macromolecules. The cellular concentration of glutathione correlates inversely with the demonstrable covalent binding of NAPQI to liver cells.[16] Centrilobular (zone 3) necrosis predominates in APAP-induced hepatic injury, likely related both to the centrilobular localization of CYP2E1 and to the relatively low glutathione concentrations in zone 3 compared to the periportal areas (zone 1).[48]

MECHANISMS OF HEPATIC INJURY

There are several mechanisms of xenobiotic-induced hepatotoxicity.

Immune-Mediated Liver Injury

Immune-mediated liver injury is an idiosyncratic and host-dependent hypersensitivity response xenobiotic exposure.[7] Damage to the hepatocytes is mediated by complement- or antibody-directed lysis, by specific cell-mediated cytotoxicity, or by an inflammatory response stimulated by immune complexes and complement.[123] The antibody or cell-mediated response is precipitated by a covalently bound xenobiotic-cell protein adduct that acts as a hapten. The resultant inflammatory response provokes secondary cytokine release that promotes further cell injury by neutrophils.[43] Subsequent apoptosis appears to be partly mediated by tumor necrosis factor (TNF).[123] Immune-mediated toxic hepatitis is differentiated from liver injury caused by other autoimmune disorders by the absence of self-perpetuation; that is, there is a need for continuous exposure to the xenobiotic to perpetuate the injury.[7] It is also less likely to recur following withdrawal of immune suppression therapy.[7]

Hypersensitivity reactions result in hepatitis, cholestasis, and mixed disorders. It is not clear whether all the autoantibodies stimulated by the xenobiotic–protein adducts are the actual mediators of cell injury.[7] In cases where the metabolite is highly unstable, an electrophilic attack is directed against the CYP enzyme at the site of formation of the metabolite.[74] The most severe form of idiosyncratic halothane liver injury is manifested as fulminant hepatic necrosis associated with the formation of adducts of its trifluoroacetyl chloride (TFA) metabolite with numerous hepatoproteins including CYP2E1 and pyruvate dehydrogenase.[28,55] Autoantibodies specifically directed against CYP enzymes are also demonstrated for dihydralazine[10] and phenytoin.[68]

Cell-mediated autoimmune mechanisms are also implicated in the idiosyncratic type of halothane hepatitis, and are now recognized in an increasing number of experimental xenobiotic-mediated liver injury models.[63] Polymorphonucleocyte (PMN) activation and infiltration appear to be an important factor in the production of cholangitis in a rat model of α-naphthyl-isothiocyanate (ANIT) liver injury. α-Naphthyl-isothiocyanate stimulates the release of cytotoxic lysosomal enzymes and oxygen free radicals by activated PMNs.[86] Antibodies directed against circulating neutrophils decrease the extent of liver damage caused by ANIT.[20] Natural Killer (NK) T cells are ubiquitous in the liver, and also serve an important role in the cell-mediated autoimmune liver injury.[35]

Drugs most commonly involved in autoimmune injury are nitrofurantoin and minocycline.[7] Drugs with hypersensitivity reactions that typically present with hepatitis include halothane,[63] trimethoprim-sulfamethoxazole,[80] antiepileptics,[139] and allopurinol.[122] Drugs associated with hypersensitivity that typically present with cholestatic signs include chlorpromazine, erythromycin estolate, penicillins, rifampin, and sulfonamides.[94] Signs of injury typically begin 1 to 8 weeks following the initiation of the medication, although it takes as long as 20 weeks for drugs such as isoniazid or dantrolene. In all cases, the onset is earlier when the patient is rechallenged with the drug. Antinuclear antibodies and smooth muscle antibodies are frequently present, as are eosinophilia, atypical lymphocytosis, fever, and rash. However, their absence does not exclude an autoimmune mechanism of drug-associated liver injury.[7,74] Liver injury characterized by the formation of hepatic granulomas are also a consequence of hypersensitivity reactions.[67]

Xenobiotics That Target the Biliary Tract

Xenobiotics that undergo biliary excretion are most commonly associated with jaundice in patients with hepatotoxicity. Xenobiotics induce cholestasis by targeting specific mechanisms of bile synthesis and flow or by damaging canalicular cells. Elucidations of various bile transport proteins have led to better understanding of mechanisms of cholestasis in toxic liver injury.[94] Cholestasis occurs with or without associated hepatitis. The development of jaundice following hepatic necrosis is a manifestation of general failure of liver function. More discrete mechanisms that result in intrahepatic cholestasis include (a) impairment of the integrity of tight membrane junctions that functionally isolate the canaliculus from the hepatocyte and sinusoids, (b) failure of transport of bile components across the hepatocytes, (c) blockade of specific membrane active transport sites, (d) decreased membrane fluidity resulting in altered transport, and (e) decreased canalicular contractility resulting in decreased bile flow.[11,61,94,115] Xenobiotics that specifically target bile canaliculi can lead to irreversible injury, the so-called vanishing bile duct syndrome.[127] Estrogens cause intrahepatic cholestasis by altering the composition of the lipid membrane and inhibiting the rate of secretion of bile into the canaliculi.[115] Rifampin impedes the uptake of bilirubin into hepatocytes. Methyltestosterone and C-17 alkylated anabolic steroids impair the secretion of bilirubin into canaliculi.[70] Cyclosporine inhibits sodium-dependent uptake of bile salts across the sinusoidal membrane and blocks ATP-dependent bile salt transport across the canalicular membrane.[11] Floxacillin causes cholestasis with minimal inflammation or evidence of hepatocellular injury.[131] Exposure of rats to ANIT causes a specific injury localized to the tight junctions that separate the hepatocytes from the canaliculi. This results in reflux of bile constituents into the sinusoidal spaces and increased access of sinusoidal molecules to the biliary tree.[138]

Mitochondrial Injury

Direct mitochondrial injury impairs cellular respiration and is associated with fat accumulation, diminution of ATP production, and metabolic acidosis with elevated lactate.[64] This involves attacks by xenobiotics on structural components of the mitochondria such as DNA, respiratory chain enzymes, and membranes. Nucleoside analogs that inhibit viral reverse transcriptase also inhibit mitochondrial DNA synthesis, leading to depletion of mitochondria.[17]

Other Targets

Stimulation of Kupffer cells enhances hepatic injury. When immunologically activated by xenobiotics, Kupffer cells contribute to the generation of oxygen free radicals and participate in the production of autoimmune injury to hepatocytes, including activation of hepatic stellate cells.[110] Activated stellate cells produce collagen, proteoglycans, and adhesive glycoproteins, which are crucial to the development of hepatic fibrosis.[34] Hepatic veno-occlusive disease is caused by xenobiotics that injure the endothelium of terminal hepatic venules, resulting in intimal thickening, edema, and non-thrombotic obstruction.[62]

MORPHOLOGIC MANIFESTATIONS OF TOXIC HEPATIC INJURY

The liver responds to injury in a limited number of ways. Cells may swell and accumulate fat or biliary material. They may necrose and lyse or undergo the slower process of apoptosis, forming shrunken, nonfunctioning, eosinophilic bodies. Necrosis can be focal or bridging, linking the periportal or centrilobular areas; zonal or panacinar; or it can be massive.[43] An autoimmune type of injury is characterized by hepatitis with a prominent plasma cell infiltrate.[7] Injury to the bile ducts results in cholestasis. Xenobiotics that target canalicular transport proteins can cause cholestasis in the absence of injury to hepatocytes.[94] Direct mitochondrial injury impairs cellular respiration and is associated with fat accumulation, diminution of ATP production, and metabolic acidosis.[95] Injuries to the intima of postsinusoidal veins cause obstruction to venous flow.[140] Table 21–1 lists characteristic morphologies of hepatic injury and associated xenobiotics.

Acute Hepatocellular Necrosis

Numerous xenobiotics are associated with hepatocellular necrosis (Table 21–1). Acetaminophen is a common cause, as are herbal remedies that contain hepatotoxins, whose risks are increasingly recognized.[29] Many halogenated hydrocarbons including carbon tetrachloride,[14] bromobenzene,[47] hydrochlorofluorocarbons,[49] halothane,[63] and antituberculous medications[113] also produce hepatocellular necrosis. A study of more than 11,000 patients exposed to isoniazid during preventive treatment showed that the risk of hepatocellular necrosis was low, occurring in 0.1% of those starting treatment, and in 0.15% of those completing treatment.[92] Risk factors for the development of hepatotoxicity from isoniazid exposure are female sex, increasing age, coadministration with rifampin, and alcoholism (Chap. 56).[144] The thiazolidinedione antidiabetics pioglitazone, rosiglitazone, and troglitazone are associated with acute hepatocellular necrosis.[33,39] Occupational exposure to solvents including dimethylformamide and CCl_4 causes dose-related hepatocellular necrosis.[102]

Acute necrosis of a hepatocyte disrupts all aspects of its function. Because there is a great deal of functional reserve in the liver, hepatic function is usually preserved despite the development of focal necrosis. However, extensive necrosis results in functional liver failure. The processes that lead to cell necrosis are not well known. Cell lysis is preceded by the formation of blebs in the lipid membrane and leakage of cytosolic enzymes, primarily aminotransferases and lactate dehydrogenase. Coalescence of blebs leads to rupture of the cellular membrane and acute irreversible cell death, with disintegration of the nucleus and termination of all cellular function. Prior to membrane rupture, this injury is reversible by membrane repair processes.[86] The release of intracellular constituents attracts circulating leukocytes and results in an inflammatory response in the hepatic parenchyma. A proposed mechanism of rapid injury to the cell membrane is the initiation of a cascading lipid peroxidation reaction following attack by a free radical. The CYP2E1 enzyme has a significant potential to produce oxygen free radicals, as do activated PMNs and Kupffer cells.[34] Oxidant stress is an important cause of liver injury during the metabolism of ethanol by CYP2E1. This results in cell death and the stimulation of stellate cells, which promotes fibrosis.[26] In addition to peroxidation of membrane lipids, the oxidation of proteins, phospholipid fatty acyl side chains, and nucleosides appear to be widespread. Mitochondrial injury and resultant ATP depletion can also be associated with necrosis.[54] Xenobiotics known to cause mitochondrial injury include antiretroviral drugs that inhibit the replication of mitochondrial DNA,[121] tetracycline,[116] valproic acid,[141] hypoglycin, margosa oil, and cereulide.[114]

Steatosis

Steatosis is the abnormal accumulation of fat in hepatocytes. It reflects abnormal cellular metabolism in conditions that include responses to xenobiotics. Cell injury depends on the severity of the underlying metabolic disturbance. Steatosis per se is normally well tolerated and reversible in many cases, although approximately one-third of patients with nonalcoholic steatosis develop steatohepatitis.[30] Nonalcoholic steatosis associated with obesity, insulin resistance, and the metabolic syndrome accounts for many cases of cryptogenic cirrhosis.[30] The β-oxidation of fatty acids depends on a steady synthesis of cellular energy in the form of ATP and takes place in the mitochondria. Mechanisms of impaired β-oxidation of fatty acids include direct inhibition or sequestration of critical cofactors such as coenzyme-A and L-carnitine.[64]

TABLE 21–1	Morphology of Liver Injury by Selected Xenobiotics	
Acute Hepatocellular Necrosis	**Microvesicular Steatosis**	**Venoocclusive Disease**
Acetaminophen	Aflatoxin	Cyclophosphamide
Allopurinol	Cereulide	Oxaliplatin
Amatoxin	Cocaine	Pyrrolizidine alkaloids
Arsenic	Dimethylformamide	
Beryllium	Fialuridine	**Peliosis Hepatis**
Carbamazepine	Hypoglycin	Androgenic hormones
Carbon tetrachloride	Jin bu huan	Contraceptive steroids
Chaparral leaf	Margosa oil	Thiopurine-derived
Chlordecone (less severe)	Nucleoside analogs (antiretrovirals)	chemotherapeutics
Clove oil	Tetracycline	Thorium dioxide
Cocaine	Valproic acid	
Cotrimoxazole		**Cholestasis**
Dimethylformamide	**Steatohepatitis**	Allopurinol
Ethanol	Amiodarone	Amoxicillin/clavulanic acid
Ferrous sulfate	Dimethylformamide	Anabolic steroids
Germander	Irinotecan	Androgenic steroids
Glue thistle	Perhexiline	Chaparral leaf
Halothane	Sodium azide	Chlorpromazine
Hydralazine		Chlorpropamide
Iron	**Granulomatous Hepatitis**	Clarithromycin
Isoniazid	Allopurinol	Cyclosporine
Ketoconazole	Beryllium	Erythromycin estolate
Methylenedioxymethamphetamine (MDMA)	BCG therapy for cancer	Estrogens
Methotrexate	Carbamazepine	Hydralazine
Methyldopa	Cephalexin	Methylenedianiline
Monoamine oxidase inhibitors	Chlorpromazine	Nimesulide
Nitrofurantoin	Chlorpropamide	Nitrofurantoin
Pennyroyal	Copper salts	Oral contraceptives
Phenytoin	Dapsone	Piroxicam
Phosphorus (yellow)	Diazepam	Rifampin
Pioglitazone	Diclofenac	Tetracycline
Procainamide	Dicloxacillin	Trimethoprim-sulfamethoxazole
Propylthiouracil	Diltiazem	
Quinine	Gold	**Autoimmune Hepatitis**
Rosiglitazone	Halothane	ACEIs
Sulfonamides	Hydralazine	Clometacin
Tetrachloroethane	Interferon	Dantrolene
Tetrachloroethylene	Isoniazid	Diclofenac
Tetracycline	Mesalamine	Methotrexate
Trinitrotoluene	Methyldopa	Methyldopa
Troglitazone	Metolazone	Minocycline
Valproic acid	Nitrofurantoin	Nafcillin
Vinyl chloride	Oxacillin	Nitrofurantoin
	Penicillins	Propylthiouracil
Neoplasms	Phenylbutazone	Sulfonamides
Anabolic steroids	Phenytoin	Tamoxifen
Androgenic hormones	Procainamide	Tegafur
Arsenic	Procarbazine	Trazodone
Copper salts	Quinidine	Uracil
Contraceptive steroids	Quinine	
Thorium dioxide	Salicylates	**Fibrosis and Cirrhosis**
Vinyl chloride	Sulfonamides	Ethanol
	Sulfonylureas	Methotrexate
Macrovesicular Steatosis		Vitamin A
Chlorinated hydrocarbons	**Bile Duct Damage**	
Ethanol	Amoxicillin	
5-Fluorouracil	Carbamazepine	
Gold	α-Naphthyl-isothiocyanate	
Steroids	Nitrofurantoin	
Total parenteral nutrition	Oral contraceptives	

ACEIs = angiotensin-converting enzyme inhibitors.

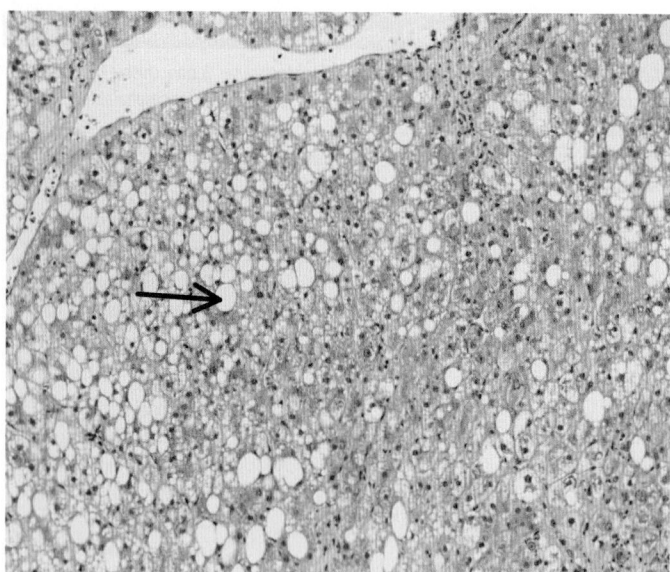

FIGURE 21–4. Biopsy showing macrovesicular steatosis in the liver of a patient with methotrexate toxicity. The arrow points to accumulated intracellular fat where the nucleus is pushed to the periphery by the accumulated fat. *(Used with permission from Daniel Mais, MD, Professor of Pathology, University of Texas Health Science Center at San Antonio.)*

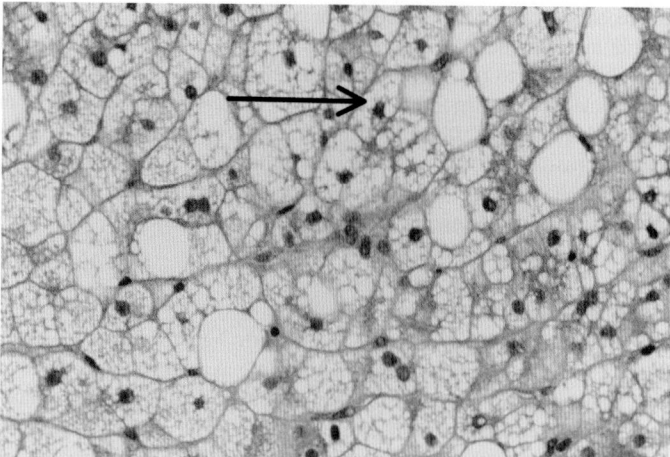

FIGURE 21–5. Biopsy showing microvesicular steatosis in the liver of a patient with valproate toxicity. The arrow demonstrated presence of centrally located nucleus despite fat accumulation. *(Used with permission from Daniel Mais, MD, Professor of Pathology, University of Texas Health Science Center at San Antonio.)*

Intracellular fat accumulation occurs as a result of any one or more of the following mechanisms: impaired synthesis of lipoproteins, increased mobilization of peripheral adipose stores, increased uptake of circulating lipids, increased triglyceride production, decreased binding of triglycerides to lipoprotein, and decreased release of very-low-density lipoproteins from the hepatocytes.[64,72] There are 2 light microscopic manifestations of steatosis: *macrovesicular* steatosis, in which the nucleus is displaced by large droplets of intracellular fat, and *microvesicular* steatosis, which is characterized by tiny cytoplasmic fat droplets that do not displace the nucleus. Xenobiotics associated with macrovesicular steatosis include ethanol and amiodarone. Ethanol increases the uptake of fatty acids into hepatocytes and decreases lipoprotein secretion. In addition, the increased ratio of the reduced form of nicotinamide adenine dinucleotide (NADH) to the oxidized form of nicotinamide adenine dinucleotide (NAD⁺), associated with hepatic metabolism of ethanol, decreases oxidation of fatty acids and promotes fatty acid synthesis.[72] An early pathologic lesion that occurs in alcoholic liver disease is reversible macrovesicular steatosis. Steatohepatitis is a more virulent form, characterized by swelling of the hepatocytes and apoptosis that may progress to cirrhosis.[69] Mallory bodies, eosinophilic cytoplasmic deposits of keratin filaments in degenerating hepatocytes, are also common microscopic findings in alcoholic liver disease.[77] Amiodarone hepatic toxicity resembles that of alcoholic hepatitis, with steatosis, Mallory bodies, and potential for progression to cirrhosis.[66] Lamellated intralysosomal phospholipid inclusion bodies are specific for amiodarone toxicity.[105] Figure 21–4 shows macrovesicular steatosis with Mallory bodies caused by methotrexate.

Steatosis Associated With Mitochondrial Dysfunction
Microvesicular steatosis is caused by severe impairment of β-oxidation of fatty acids. Valproic acid causes mild elevations of aminotransferases in approximately 11% of patients, usually during the first few months of therapy. The earliest pathologic lesion that signals progression of liver injury is microvesicular steatosis, which occurs in the absence of necrosis. An association between deficiency of carnitine, microsteatosis, and the development of hyperammonemia is observed in children treated with valproic acid.[71] A small percentage of patients progress to fulminant hepatic failure characterized by centrilobular necrosis.[141] The incidence of fatal hepatocellular injury is highest in children, approaching 1 in 800 children younger than 2 years of age.[99]

Microvesicular steatosis is described in patients taking antiretrovirals such as zidovudine, zalcitabine, and didanosine.[22] In all cases, metabolic acidosis with elevated lactate is a prominent biochemical feature.[22] The nucleoside analog fialuridine caused severe hepatotoxicity during a study of its use in the treatment of chronic hepatitis B infection. Microscopic examinations of liver specimens in these cases showed marked accumulation of fat with minimal necrosis or structural injury. Severe metabolic acidosis and failure of hepatic synthetic function suggested failure of cellular energy production. Mitochondria examined under the electron microscope are demonstrably abnormal.[84] Figure 21–5 demonstrates microvesicular steatosis in a patient with valproate hepatotoxicity. High doses of tetracycline produce microvesicular steatosis associated with moderate elevations of aminotransferases, markedly prolonged prothrombin time (PT), and progression to fulminant hepatic failure.[116] Microvesicular steatosis attributed to failure of mitochondrial energy production was reported in a fatal case of *Bacillus cereus* food poisoning, where high concentration of the bacterial emetic toxin cereulide was found in the bile and liver. In this case, microvesicular steatosis was associated with extensive hepatocellular necrosis.[79] Other xenobiotics that cause mitochondrial failure are hypoglycin, the cause of Jamaican vomiting sickness, aflatoxin, and margosa oil.[114] Steatosis is also observed following exposure to the industrial solvent dimethylformamide. Liver biopsies in patients with acute illness show focal hepatocellular necrosis and microvesicular steatosis. More prolonged, less symptomatic exposures result in significant macrovesicular steatosis with mild aminotransferase elevations.[101]

Venoocclusive Disease
Hepatic venoocclusive disease is caused by xenobiotics that injure the endothelium of terminal hepatic venules, resulting in intimal thickening, edema, and nonthrombotic obstruction. Central and sublobular hepatic veins become edematous and fibrosed. There is intense sinusoidal dilation in the centrilobular areas that is associated with liver cell atrophy and necrosis.[136] The gross pathologic appearance is that of a "nutmeg" liver.[62] Massive hepatic congestion and ascites ensue.[104] Hepatic venoocclusive disease is rapidly fatal in 15% to 20% of cases. It is associated with exposure to pyrrolizidine alkaloids found in many plant species including *Symphytum* (comfrey tea),[140] *Heliotrope*, *Senecio*, and *Crotalaria*.[62] It has occurred in epidemic proportions, in South Africa after the ingestion of flour contaminated with ragwort (*Senecio*), in Jamaica after the ingestion of "bush teas" (*Crotalaria* spp), and in India and Afghanistan when food was contaminated with *Heliotropium lasiocarpine* and *Crotalaria*.[13,88] A rapidly progressive form is also reported in bone marrow transplant patients following high-dose treatment with cyclophosphamide.[83]

Chronic Hepatitis

A form of toxic hepatitis that clinically resembles autoimmune hepatitis occurs with the chronic administration of xenobiotics such as nitrofurantoin, propylthiouracil, and diclofenac.[56,103,117] Many cases are associated with positive antinuclear antibody (ANA), smooth muscle antibody (SMA), and hyperglobulinemia. Jaundice is prominent and hepatocellular enzymes are elevated 5- to 60-fold. Liver biopsy commonly reveals intrahepatic cholestasis, as well as centrilobular inflammation.[7]

Granulomatous hepatitis is characterized by infiltration of the hepatic parenchyma with caseating granulomata. At least 60 xenobiotics are associated with this disorder. Fever and systemic symptoms are common, and 25% of patients have splenomegaly. Liver enzyme abnormalities are mixed, reflecting variable degrees of cholestasis and hepatocellular injury. Eosinophilia occurs in 30% as an extrahepatic manifestation of drug hypersensitivity. Continued exposure results in a more severe form of liver disease. Small vessel vasculitis, which involves the skin, lungs, and kidney, is a disturbing sign associated with increased mortality.[67,85,142] Table 21–1 lists a number of the xenobiotics that are implicated in this disorder.

Cirrhosis

Cirrhosis is caused by progressive fibrosis and scarring of the liver, which results in irreversible hepatic dysfunction and portal hypertension. This causes shunting of blood away from hepatocytes and subsequent hepatocellular dysfunction. Activated stellate cells produce collagen, proteoglycans, and adhesive glycoproteins, which are deposited in the space of Disse and are crucial to the development of hepatic fibrosis.[34] The development of fibrosis requires inflammation. Reactive oxygen species derived from lipid peroxidation, reduced NADPH, and apoptotic cells are important inflammatory stimuli that activate stellate cells.[34] In alcoholic cirrhosis, acetaldehyde and tumor necrosis factor provide a cytokine-mediated inflammatory stimulus.[6] Chronic ingestion of excessive amounts of vitamin A (25,000 units/day for 6 years or 100,000 units/day for 2.5 years) results in cirrhosis. An increase in the fat content of the sinusoidal stellate cells with increasing degrees of collagen formation are characteristic lesions that occur early in vitamin A toxicity (Chap. 44). Portal hypertension can be early and striking.[37] Like vitamin A, methyldopa and methotrexate also cause a slow progressive development of cirrhosis, with few clinical symptoms.[65,134] Methotrexate-induced hepatic fibrosis is dose dependent. Risk factors include associated ethanol intake and preexisting liver disease. Reduced dosing has largely eliminated the risk of the development of cirrhosis in patients receiving methotrexate.[134]

Hepatic Tumors

There is persuasive evidence that the use of oral contraceptive steroids increases the risk of hepatic adenomas.[1] Oral contraceptives also increase the overall risk of hepatocellular carcinoma; however, the number of cases associated with estrogen therapy is low.[51] Anabolic steroids are rarely associated with the development of both benign and malignant hepatic tumors.[120] Angiosarcoma is strongly associated with exposure to vinyl chloride, in addition to arsenic, thorium dioxide, and androgenic hormones.[50,97]

Hepatic Injury Associated With Plants and Herbs

In addition to the venoocclusive disease associated with pyrrolizidine alkaloids described above, herbal remedies are recognized as a cause of acute hepatocellular injury. Numerous plants or plant products are known or suspected to cause hepatic injury (Chaps. 43 and 118).[29]

CLINICAL PRESENTATION OF TOXIC LIVER INJURY

Clinical presentations range from indolent, often asymptomatic progression of impairment of hepatic function to rapid development of hepatic failure. Jaundice and pruritus are due to increased concentrations of bile acids and bilirubin in the blood. Failure of hepatocellular synthetic function results in bleeding due to coagulopathy and edema due to hypoalbuminemia. Encephalopathy is due to hypoglycemia, impaired neurotransmission, or accumulation of toxic products of metabolism such as ammonia. Fever occurs with autoimmune-mediated liver injury. Impaired hepatic blood flow results in

familiar manifestations of portal hypertension such as caput medusa, splenomegaly, ascites, and varices. Spider angiomata and gynecomastia also occur as a result of altered estrogen metabolism.[125]

Acute Liver Failure

Acute liver failure is defined as a rapid onset of liver injury progressing over 2 to 3 weeks that results in altered mental status, vasodilation, kidney and pulmonary failure, frequent infection, and a poor outcome without transplantation.[40] Complications from acute liver failure include encephalopathy, cerebral edema, coagulopathy, acute kidney injury, hypoglycemia, hypotension, acute respiratory distress syndrome, sepsis, and death. The encephalopathy associated with chronic liver disease should be considered separately from the rapidly progressive disorder of acute liver failure.[32] In some cases, patients progress from health to death in as little as 2 to 10 days.[32,67,91,106] Table 21–2 emphasizes the clinical progression of encephalopathy as acute liver failure develops. The prognosis of acute liver failure is related to the time that passes between the onset of jaundice and the onset of encephalopathy. Perhaps surprisingly, a better prognosis is associated with shorter (2–4 weeks) jaundice-to-encephalopathy intervals.[106,107] Most cases are caused by xenobiotics or viral hepatitis. Acute liver failure is usually associated with extensive necrosis.[46] Some xenobiotics that are associated with acute liver failure are listed in Table 21–1.

Hepatic Encephalopathy

Hepatic encephalopathy (HE) is a complex disorder that affects both cognitive and neuromuscular functions of the central nervous system. Cognitive changes range from barely discernible impairment evident only on psychometric testing to confusion, stupor and coma. Neuromuscular signs include slowed motor responses, asterixis, myoclonus, and rigidity.[108] Hepatic encephalopathy is potentially fully reversible, even in cases of deep coma.[31] Table 21–2 lists the clinical stages of acute HE. Ammonia concentrations are elevated in 60% to 80% of patients with HE.[108] The finding that ammonia is not elevated in many cases suggests that there are other etiologies and that HE is multifactorial.[107] Disruption of central neurotransmitter regulation including dopamine receptor binding may contribute.[133] There is evidence that liver failure is associated with the accumulation of substances that stimulate central benzodiazepine receptors, leading to enhancement of γ-aminobutyric acid transmission.[135] Other xenobiotics such as mercaptans, phenol, and manganese also play a role.[108] Inflammation and infection is also proposed as an important precipitant. Ammonia is produced in the colon by bacterial breakdown of ingested proteins, and is then transported to the liver via the portal circulation where it is detoxified to glutamine and urea by urea

TABLE 21–2	Stages of Hepatic Encephalopathy	
Clinical Stage	*Mental Status*	*Neuromotor Function*
Subclinical	Normal physical examination	Subtle impairment of neuromuscular function → driving or work injury hazard
I	Euphoric, irritable, depressed, fluctuating mild confusion, poor attention, sleep disturbance	Poor coordination; asterixis alone
II	Impaired memory, cognition, or simple mathematical tasks	Slurred speech, tremor, ataxia
III	Difficult to arouse, persistent confusion, incoherent	Hyperactive reflexes, clonus, nystagmus
IV	Coma; may respond to noxious stimuli	Decerebrate posturing; Cheyne-Stokes respirations; pupils are reactive and the oculocephalic reflex is intact; signs of ↑ intracranial pressure

cycle enzymes.[96] In the presence of liver failure, ammonia accumulates and is shunted into the systemic circulation, where it then crosses the blood–brain barrier. In the brain, the astrocytic glutamine synthetase converts glutamate and ammonia into glutamine, which acts as an osmolyte and increases cerebral volume.[135] Ammonia itself also acts as a neurotoxin, resulting in decreased excitatory neurotransmission.[135] Other processes that raise central nervous system ammonia concentrations include infection, hypokalemia, alkalemia, increased muscle wasting, volume depletion, azotemia, and gastrointestinal bleeding.[108] Alkalemia and hypokalemia facilitate conversion of NH_4^+ to NH_3, which moves more easily across the bowel wall and the blood–brain barrier. Acidification of the bowel by bacterial breakdown of lactulose creates a hostile environment for ammonia-producing bacteria and constructs a gradient that favors entrapment of ammonia in the bowel.[96] In a study of lactulose alone versus placebo, over a 14-month period 19.6% of patients on lactulose had recurrent HE, compared with 48.6% of patients on placebo.[119] A nonabsorbed broad-spectrum antibiotic rifaximin decreases the recurrence of HE in cirrhotic patients, presumably by decreasing the numbers of urease-containing colonic bacteria that produce ammonia.[4]

Flumazenil is proposed by some authors to treat HE. Studies evaluating flumazenil's effectiveness show short-term improvement but no change in patient recovery or survival.[135] Concordantly, benzodiazepines can make HE worse and should be avoided.

EVALUATION OF THE PATIENT WITH LIVER DISEASE

History is critical in establishing the etiologic diagnosis of the patient with liver disease. Medication history should include careful investigation of nonprescription xenobiotics, especially APAP and any alternative or complementary therapies including herbal and vitamin products. Nearly any chronically used medications should be suspect. An occupational history may indicate exposure to vinyl chloride (plastics industry), dimethylformamide (leather industry), or other industrial solvents. Table 21–3 lists occupational exposures that result in liver injury. Ethanol abuse is a common cause of acute hepatitis and the most common cause of cirrhosis in the United States.[6] A history of male homosexual contacts, health care occupation, or injection drug use indicates the possibility of hepatitis B or C infection. Recent travel

to a developing country suggests the possibility of hepatitis A and other viruses and parasites. In patients with significant pain, a diagnosis of cholelithiasis or cholecystitis should be evaluated.

Biochemical Patterns of Liver Injury

There are 2 basic biochemical patterns associated with xenobiotic-induced liver injury. The hepatocellular pattern is characterized by elevation of liver aminotransferases due to the destruction of hepatocytes by apoptosis or necrosis.[90] The cholestatic pattern is characterized by elevations of the serum alkaline phosphatase, concentration and conjugated bilirubin, and usually results from injury or functional impairment of the bile ductules.[42] Processes associated with intrahepatic cholestasis in the absence of hepatitis do not always lead to significant aminotransferase elevation.[89]

Aminotransferases

Laboratory tests are helpful, and certain patterns suggest specific etiologies (Table 21–4). Elevation of hepatocellular enzymes, especially the AST and ALT, indicates hepatocellular injury, and within a given clinical context, has useful diagnostic significance. Aminotransferases often are increased up to 500 times normal when hepatic necrosis is extensive, such as in severe acute viral or toxic hepatitis.[143] The degree of elevation does not always reflect the severity of injury because concentrations decline as liver failure progresses. Only moderately elevated, or occasionally normal, aminotransferase concentrations occur in some patients with hepatic failure caused by mitochondrial failure, cirrhosis, or venoocclusive disease.[84,141] Aminotransferase concentrations can be normal or only slightly elevated in processes associated with intrahepatic cholestasis in the absence of hepatitis.[89] In alcoholic liver disease, in contrast to other forms of hepatitis, the AST concentration is typically 2 to 3 times greater than the ALT. Elevation of either of these enzymes greater than 300 IU/L is inconsistent with injury caused by ethanol.[77] The measurement of γ-glutamyl transpeptidase (GGTP) is not very useful because it is present throughout the liver and its elevation is often nonspecific.[124]

Alkaline Phosphatase

In patients with cholestasis, bile acids stimulate the synthesis of alkaline phosphatase by hepatocytes and biliary epithelium in response to a number of pathologic processes in the liver. Elevations of the alkaline phosphatase as great as 10-fold can occur with infiltrative liver diseases, but are most commonly associated with extrahepatic obstruction.[124] Although the alkaline phosphatase can be normal or only minimally elevated in hepatocellular injury, it is unusual for obstruction to occur without some elevation of the alkaline phosphatase.

Bilirubin

Elevation of conjugated (direct) bilirubin implies impairment of secretion into bile, whereas elevation of unconjugated (indirect) bilirubin implies impairment of conjugation. Unconjugated hyperbilirubinemia also occurs during hemolysis and in rare disorders of hepatic conjugation such as Gilbert or Crigler-Najjar syndromes. Except in cases of pure unconjugated hyperbilirubinemia, the fractionation of bilirubin in the case of hepatobiliary disorders does not have any important diagnostic utility, and it will not distinguish patients with parenchymal disorders of the liver from intrinsic or extrinsic cholestasis. The presence of bilirubin in the urine implies elevation of conjugated (direct) bilirubin, which is water soluble and filtered by the glomerulus, obviating the need for laboratory fractionation.[125]

Urobilinogen is produced by the bacterial metabolism of bilirubin in the bowel lumen. It is absorbed and excreted in the urine. Its presence in the urine indicates the normal excretion of bilirubin in bile, while its absence is associated with complete biliary obstruction. As a result of more modern methods of detection of complete obstruction of the biliary tract, this test is mainly of historical interest.

Serum Albumin

Quantitatively, albumin is the most important protein that is made in the liver. With a half-life as great as 20 days, the albumin is usually normal in the previously healthy patient with acute liver injury. In the absence of disorders

TABLE 21–3	Occupational Exposures Associated With Liver Injury
Xenobiotic	**Type of Injury**
Arsenic	Cirrhosis, angiosarcoma
Beryllium	Granulomatous hepatitis
Carbon tetrachloride	Acute hepatocellular necrosis
Chlordecone	Minor hepatocellular necrosis
Copper salts	Granulomatous hepatitis, angiosarcoma
Dimethylformamide	Steatohepatitis
Methylenedianiline	Acute hepatocellular cholestasis
Phosphorus	Acute hepatocellular necrosis
Sodium azide	Steatohepatitis
Tetrachloroethane	Acute, subacute hepatocellular necrosis
Tetrachloroethylene	Acute hepatocellular necrosis
Toluene	Hepatocellular steatosis (minor)
Trichloroethane	Hepatocellular steatosis (minor)
Trinitrotoluene	Acute hepatocellular necrosis
Vinyl chloride	Acute hepatocellular necrosis, fibrosis, angiosarcoma
Xylene	Steatosis, hepatocellular vacuolation

TABLE 21–4 Laboratory Used to Evaluate Liver Function

Disorder	Alkaline Phosphatase	AST, ALT	Albumin	Prothrombin Time	Bilirubin	Ammonia	Anion Gap
Cholelithiasis	↑	N or ↑	N	N	N or ↑	N	N
Cholestasis	↑↑	N or ↑	N	N	↑	N	N
Chronic hepatitis	N or ↑	↑	N or ↓	N	N or ↑	N or ↑	N
Cirrhosis	N or ↑	↑	↓	N or ↑	N or ↑	N or ↑	N
Hepatocellular necrosis, acute focal (hepatitis)	N or ↑	↑↑↑	N	N or ↑	↑↑	N	N
Hepatocellular necrosis, acute massive	N or ↑	↑↑↑	N	↑↑	↑↑↑	↑↑	↑
Infiltrative disease, chronic (tumor, fatty liver)	↑↑↑	↑	N	N	N	N	N
Mitochondrial failure (acute)	N or ↑	N or ↑	N	↑↑	↑	↑↑	↑↑↑

↑ = increase; ↓ = decrease; N = normal; AST = aspartate aminotransferase; ALT = alanine aminotransferase.

that affect albumin, such as nephrotic syndrome, protein-losing enteropathy, or starvation, a low serum albumin concentration is a useful marker for the severity of chronic liver disease.[125]

Serum Prealbumin

Prealbumin is the earliest laboratory indicator of protein malnutrition, and is considered the best way to assess the severity of illness in both the critically ill and the chronically ill. Because albumin has a relatively large body pool, a half-life of 20 days, and its serum concentrations are affected by the patient's hydration status and kidney function, it is not as sensitive as prealbumin in identifying changes in nutrition. Because prealbumin has one of the highest essential-to-nonessential amino acid ratios in the body, it a great marker for protein synthesis.[5]

Coagulation Factors

Impairment of coagulation is a marker of the severity of hepatic dysfunction in both acute and chronic liver disease. Elevation of the PT in acute hepatitis is associated with a higher risk of hepatic failure.[44] Unlike the case with serum albumin, the onset of coagulopathy as a consequence of impaired synthesis of coagulation factors produced in the liver is rapid. Acute changes in coagulation reflect the concentration of factor VII, which has the shortest half-life.[52] The extrinsic coagulation pathway, as measured by the PT, is affected by reductions in factors VII, IX, and X. In addition to failure of hepatic synthesis, inadequate concentrations of factors II, VII, IX, and X can also result from ingestion of warfarin anticoagulants or malabsorption of vitamin K (Chap. 58).

Because different thromboplastin reagents give different PT values on the same sample, the international normalized ratio (INR) was developed to normalize PT measurements in patients treated with warfarin, allowing comparisons of therapeutic outcomes across different care settings and across the literature. The INR uses the International Sensitivity Index (ISI) that is derived from a cohort of patients on stable anticoagulant therapy. It normalizes the responsiveness of a given thromboplastin reagent in comparison to a WHO reference standard that is assigned a value of 1.0.[60] There is little controversy regarding the value of the INR in comparison with the PT ratio for measuring the extent of warfarin-induced anticoagulation. In patients with liver disease, use of the INR implies a normalized correlation that does not exist and is therefore potentially misleading. Because factor deficiencies in patients with liver disease are different from those in patients on warfarin, there is considerable controversy regarding which measurement is best for patients with liver disease.[25,60] Although comparison of factor concentrations in warfarin-treated patients with those with liver disease showed no difference in factor VII, there are significant differences in factors II, V, X, and fibrinogen. Comparison of the PT with INR in the evaluation of test results with 3 different thromboplastin reagents showed consistency among the control groups of warfarin-treated patients,

but no consistency among PT or INR measurements using the same thromboplastin reagents in patients with liver disease.[60] Because of a failure to demonstrate an advantage, liver specialists have supported the continued use of the PT to describe the degree of liver injury, lacking the availability of a single reliable standard that would help predict operative risk.[25] The implication for toxicologists is that caution should be exercised in relying too heavily on published INR values that purportedly predict the severity of illness in patients with acute liver failure.

A thoughtful review of bleeding risk due to coagulopathy in chronic liver disease discussed the balance of procoagulation forces (elevated factor VIII concentrations, elevated von Willebrand factor, decreased protein C and antithrombin) and anticoagulation forces (decreased fibrinogen and other clotting factors, high tissue plasminogen activator, low platelet count). The balance is simply characterized as a seesaw effect between stimulation of thrombin generation by factor VIII and the suppression of thrombin generation by protein C. This fragile balance between procoagulation and anticoagulation can be tipped by events such as acute kidney injury or infection. It is not effectively characterized by the INR or the PT. The review proposed that the standard belief that patients with liver failure are "auto-anticoagulated" and not at risk of venous or arterial thrombosis is erroneous. Neither the PT nor the INR predict bleeding risk in the cirrhotic patient, and other investigations are proposed to help identify bleeding risk and prevent or manage thrombotic events in cirrhotic patients.[128]

Ammonia

Severe generalized impairment of hepatic function leads to a rise in the serum ammonia concentration as a result of impairment of hepatic detoxification of ammonia produced during catabolism of proteins.[4] Urease-containing bacteria within the bowel, especially *Klebsiella* and *Proteus* species, are the most prominent producers of ammonia.[107] Some patients treated with valproic acid develop alterations in mental status associated with elevated ammonia concentrations in the absence of other laboratory indicators of hepatic injury.[100] Hyperammonemia in patients on valproic acid is also commonly asymptomatic.[126] This has been attributed to selective impairment of urea cycle enzymes ornithine transcarbamylase or carbamyl phosphate synthetase by pentanoic acid metabolites (Chap. 48).

Other Laboratory Tests

Serologic studies for the presence of markers of hepatitis A, B, and C should be obtained routinely in patients with hepatitis. In the patient with severe liver injury, hypoglycemia is a major concern because of impairment of glycogen storage and gluconeogenesis. Hyperglycemia also occurs as a result of the inability of the liver to handle a large glucose load. The arterial or venous blood gas commonly shows a respiratory alkalosis. Severe metabolic acidosis with elevated lactate occurs in patients with hepatic failure caused by mitochondrial injury. Measurement of serum lactate concentration is useful in identifying the cause of acidosis in a patient with suspected toxic liver injury.

Computed tomography and magnetic resonance imaging scans are useful tests for evaluation of parenchymal disease of the liver. An ultrasonographic examination reliably demonstrates dilation of the extrahepatic bile ducts. Liver biopsy is helpful but is not specifically diagnostic of xenobiotic-induced hepatic injury.

MANAGEMENT

In many patients, toxic liver injury resolves with simple withdrawal of the offending xenobiotic. In patients with severe injury, significant improvement in survival is associated with good supportive care in an intensive care environment. Transplantation is lifesaving for critically ill patients with acute liver failure. Early referral to a transplant center is indicated for patients with evidence of severe or rapidly progressive toxic injury.[93] For discussion of indications for the use of *N*-acetylcysteine and discussion of indications for hepatic transplantation see Chap. 33.

SUMMARY

- The primary role of the liver in the biotransformation of xenobiotics results in an increased risk of hepatotoxicity. Xenobiotic-induced liver injury is either dose-dependent and predictable or idiosyncratic and unpredictable.
- Predictability is evolving with the science of genome analysis. Injury that is apparently idiosyncratic is affected by host characteristics that include genetic makeup, concomitant or previous exposure to xenobiotics, and the underlying condition of the liver. The ability to predict this susceptibility is increasing.
- The pathologic spectrum of liver injury includes combinations of hepatocellular necrosis, hepatitis, cholestasis, steatosis, apoptosis, and fibrosis.
- Mechanisms of hepatic injury include cell-mediated immune mechanisms that result in inflammation and fibrosis; antibody-mediated immune mechanisms that attack various hepatocyte targets, including critical cellular enzymes; lipid peroxidation initiated by free radicals; and mitochondrial injury.

Acknowledgment
Charles Maltz, MD, PhD, and Todd Bania, MD, contributed to this chapter in previous editions.

REFERENCES

1. Agrawal S, et al. Management of hepatocellular adenoma: recent advances. *Clin Gastroenterol Hepatol.* 2015;13:1221-1230.
2. Ahmad J, Odin JA. Epidemiology and genetic risk factors of drug hepatotoxicity. *Clin Liver Dis.* 2017;21:55-72.
3. Badr MZ, et al. Mechanism of hepatotoxicity to periportal regions of the liver lobule due to allyl alcohol: role of oxygen and lipid peroxidation. *J Pharmacol Exp Ther.* 1986;238:1138-1142.
4. Bass NM, et al. Rifaximin treatment in hepatic encephalopathy. *N Engl J Med.* 2010;362:1071-1081.
5. Beck FK, Rosenthal TC. Prealbumin: a marker for nutritional evaluation. *Am Fam Physician.* 2002;65:1575-1578.
6. Beier JI, et al. Advances in alcoholic liver disease. *Curr Gastroenterol Rep.* 2011;13:56-64.
7. Bjornsson E, et al. Drug-induced autoimmune hepatitis: clinical characteristics and prognosis. *Hepatology.* 2010;51:2040-2048.
8. Björnsson ES. Hepatotoxicity by drugs: the most common implicated agents. *Int J Mol Sci.* 2016;17:224.
9. Boll M, et al. Mechanism of carbon tetrachloride-induced hepatotoxicity. Hepatocellular damage by reactive carbon tetrachloride metabolites. *Z Naturforsch C.* 2001;56:649-659.
10. Bourdi M, et al. Anti-liver microsomes autoantibodies and dihydralazine-induced hepatitis: specificity of autoantibodies and inductive capacity of the drug. *Mol Pharmacol.* 1992;42:280-285.
11. Böhme M, et al. Cholestasis caused by inhibition of the adenosine triphosphate-dependent bile salt transport in rat liver. *Gastroenterology.* 1994;107:255-265.
12. Bradfield JW. Control of spillover: the importance of Kupffer-cell function in clinical medicine. *Lancet.* 1974;304:883-886.
13. Bras G, et al. Veno-occlusive disease of liver with nonportal type of cirrhosis, occurring in Jamaica. *AMA Arch Pathol.* 1954;57:285-300.
14. Burk RF, et al. Hyperbaric oxygen protection against carbon tetrachloride hepatotoxicity in the rat. Association with altered metabolism. *Gastroenterology.* 1986;90:812-818.
15. Buxton JA, et al. Genetic determinants of cocaine-associated agranulocytosis. *BMC Res Notes.* 2015;8:240.
16. Corcoran GB, et al. Effects of *N*-acetylcysteine on acetaminophen covalent binding and hepatic necrosis in mice. *J Pharmacol Exp Ther.* 1985;232:864-872.
17. Côté HCF, et al. Changes in mitochondrial DNA as a marker of nucleoside toxicity in HIV-infected patients. *N Engl J Med.* 2002;346:811-820.
18. Crispe IN. The liver as a lymphoid organ. *Annu Rev Immunol.* 2009;27:147-163.
19. Cudmore J, et al. Methotrexate and trimethoprim-sulfamethoxazole: toxicity from this combination continues to occur. *Can Fam Physician.* 2014;60:53-56.
20. Dahm LJ, et al. An antibody to neutrophils attenuates alpha-naphthylisothiocyanate-induced liver injury. *J Pharmacol Exp Ther.* 1991;256:412-420.
21. Daly AK, et al. HLA-B*5701 genotype is a major determinant of drug-induced liver injury due to flucloxacillin. *Nat Genet.* 2009;41:816-819.
22. Day L, et al. Mitochondrial injury in the pathogenesis of antiretroviral-induced hepatic steatosis and lactic acidemia. *Mitochondrion.* 2004;4:95-109.
23. De Morais SM, et al. Decreased glucuronidation and increased bioactivation of acetaminophen in Gilbert's syndrome. *Gastroenterology.* 1992;102:577-586.
24. deLemos AS, et al. Amoxicillin-clavulanate-induced liver injury. *Dig Dis Sci.* 2016;61:2406-2416.
25. Denson KW, et al. Validity of the INR system for patients with liver impairment. *Thromb Haemost.* 1995;73:162.
26. Dey A, Cederbaum AI. Alcohol and oxidative liver injury. *Hepatology.* 2006;43(suppl 1):S63-S74.
27. Dutczak WJ, et al. Biliary-hepatic recycling of a xenobiotic: gallbladder absorption of methyl mercury. *Am J Physiol.* 1991;260(6, pt 1):G873-G880.
28. Eliasson E, Kenna JG. Cytochrome P450 2E1 is a cell surface autoantigen in halothane hepatitis. *Mol Pharmacol.* 1996;50:573-582.
29. Estes JD, et al. High prevalence of potentially hepatotoxic herbal supplement use in patients with fulminant hepatic failure. *Arch Surg.* 2003;138:852-858.
30. Farrell GC, Larter CZ. Nonalcoholic fatty liver disease: from steatosis to cirrhosis. *Hepatology.* 2006;43(suppl 1):S99-S112.
31. Ferenci P, et al. Hepatic encephalopathy—definition, nomenclature, diagnosis, and quantification: final report of the working party at the 11th World Congresses of Gastroenterology, Vienna, 1998. *Hepatology.* 2002;35:716-721.
32. Ferenci P. Brain dysfunction in fulminant hepatic failure. *J Hepatol.* 1994;21:487-490.
33. Floyd JS, et al. Case series of liver failure associated with rosiglitazone and pioglitazone. *Pharmacoepidemiol Drug Saf.* 2009;18:1238-1243.
34. Friedman SL. Mechanisms of hepatic fibrogenesis. *Gastroenterology.* 2008;134:1655-1669.
35. Gao B, Radaeva S. Natural killer and natural killer T cells in liver fibrosis. *Biochim Biophys Acta.* 2013;1832:1061-1069.
36. Geerts A. History, heterogeneity, developmental biology, and functions of quiescent hepatic stellate cells. *Semin Liver Dis.* 2001;21:311-335.
37. Geubel AP, et al. Liver damage caused by therapeutic vitamin A administration: estimate of dose-related toxicity in 41 cases. *Gastroenterology.* 1991;100:1701-1709.
38. Ghabril M, et al. Drug-induced liver injury: a clinical update. *Curr Opin Gastroenterol.* 2010;26:222-226.
39. Gitlin N, et al. Two cases of severe clinical and histologic hepatotoxicity associated with troglitazone. *Ann Intern Med.* 1998;129:36-38.
40. Gotthardt D, et al. Fulminant hepatic failure: etiology and indications for liver transplantation. *Nephrol Dial Transplant.* 2007;22(suppl 8):viii5-viii8.
41. Grant LM, Rockey DC. Drug-induced liver injury. *Curr Opin Gastroenterol.* 2012;28:198-202.
42. Grattagliano I, et al. Biochemical mechanisms in drug-induced liver injury: certainties and doubts. *World J Gastroenterol.* 2009;15:4865-4876.
43. Gunawan BK, Kaplowitz N. Mechanisms of drug-induced liver disease. *Clin Liver Dis.* 2007;11:459-475.
44. Harrison PM, et al. Serial prothrombin time as prognostic indicator in paracetamol induced fulminant hepatic failure. *BMJ.* 1990;301:964-966.
45. Hautekeete ML, Geerts A. The hepatic stellate (Ito) cell: its role in human liver disease. *Virchows Arch.* 1997;430:195-207.
46. He Y, et al. Mechanisms of fibrosis in acute liver failure. *Liver Int.* 2015;35:1877-1885.
47. Hétu C, et al. Effect of chronic ethanol administration on bromobenzene liver toxicity in the rat. *Toxicol Appl Pharmacol.* 1983;67:166-177.
48. Hinson JA, et al. Mechanisms of acetaminophen-induced liver necrosis. *Handb Exp Pharmacol.* 2010;196:369-405.
49. Hoet P, et al. Epidemic of liver disease caused by hydrochlorofluorocarbons used as ozone-sparing substitutes of chlorofluorocarbons. *Lancet.* 1997;350:556-559.
50. Huang N-C, et al. Arsenic, vinyl chloride, viral hepatitis, and hepatic angiosarcoma: a hospital-based study and review of literature in Taiwan. *BMC Gastroenterol.* 2011;11:142.
51. Ishak KG. Hepatic lesions caused by anabolic and contraceptive steroids. *Semin Liver Dis.* 1981;1:116-128.

52. Johnston M, et al. Reliability of the international normalized ratio for monitoring the induction phase of warfarin: comparison with the prothrombin time ratio. *J Lab Clin Med.* 1996;128:214-217.

53. Jungermann K, Kietzmann T. Oxygen: modulator of metabolic zonation and disease of the liver. *Hepatology.* 2000;31:255-260.

54. Kaplowitz N. Drug-induced liver injury. *Clin Infect Dis.* 2004;38(suppl 2):S44-S48.

55. Kenna JG. Immunoallergic drug-induced hepatitis: lessons from halothane. *J Hepatol.* 1997;26(suppl 1):5-12.

56. Kim BH, et al. The incidence and clinical characteristics of symptomatic propylthiouracil-induced hepatic injury in patients with hyperthyroidism: a single-center retrospective study. *Am J Gastroenterol.* 2001;96:165-169.

57. Kindmark A, et al. Genome-wide pharmacogenetic investigation of a hepatic adverse event without clinical signs of immunopathology suggests an underlying immune pathogenesis. *Pharmacogenomics J.* 2008;8:186-195.

58. Kita H, et al. The lymphoid liver: considerations on pathways to autoimmune injury. *Gastroenterology.* 2001;120:1485-1501.

59. Klaassen CD. Biliary excretion of metals. *Drug Metab Rev.* 2008;5:165-196.

60. Kovacs MJ, et al. Assessment of the validity of the INR system for patients with liver impairment. *Thromb Haemost.* 1994;71:727-730.

61. Krell H, et al. Drug-induced intrahepatic cholestasis: characterization of different pathomechanisms. *Arch Toxicol.* 1987;60:124-130.

62. Kumana CR, et al. Herbal tea induced hepatic veno-occlusive disease: quantification of toxic alkaloid exposure in adults. *Gut.* 1985;26:101-104.

63. Kurth MJ, et al. Halothane-induced hepatitis: paradigm or paradox for drug-induced liver injury. *Hepatology.* 2014;60:1473-1475.

64. Labbe G, et al. Drug-induced liver injury through mitochondrial dysfunction: mechanisms and detection during preclinical safety studies. *Fundam Clin Pharmacol.* 2008; 22:335-353.

65. Lee WM, Denton WT. Chronic hepatitis and indolent cirrhosis due to methyldopa: the bottom of the iceberg? *J S C Med Assoc.* 1989;85:75-79.

66. Lee WM. Drug-induced hepatotoxicity. *N Engl J Med.* 1995;333:1118-1127.

67. Lee WM. Drug-induced hepatotoxicity. *N Engl J Med.* 2003;349:474-485.

68. Leeder JS, et al. Non-monooxygenase cytochromes P450 as potential human autoantigens in anticonvulsant hypersensitivity reactions. *Pharmacogenetics.* 1998;8:211-225.

69. Lefkowitch JH. Morphology of alcoholic liver disease. *Clin Liver Dis.* 2005;9:37-53.

70. Lewis JH. Drug-induced liver disease. *Med Clin North Am.* 2000;84:1275-1311.

71. Lheureux PER, Hantson P. Carnitine in the treatment of valproic acid-induced toxicity. *Clin Toxicol (Phila).* 2009;47:101-111.

72. Lieber CS. Alcohol and the liver: 1994 update. *Gastroenterology.* 1994;106:1085-1105.

73. Lindros KO, et al. Role of ethanol-inducible cytochrome P-450 IIE1 in carbon tetrachloride-induced damage to centrilobular hepatocytes from ethanol-treated rats. *Hepatology.* 1990;12:1092-1097.

74. Liu Z-X, Kaplowitz N. Immune-mediated drug-induced liver disease. *Clin Liver Dis.* 2002;6:755-774.

75. Lu Y, Cederbaum AI. CYP2E1 and oxidative liver injury by alcohol. *Free Radic Biol Med.* 2008;44:723-738.

76. Lucena MI, et al. Susceptibility to amoxicillin-clavulanate-induced liver injury is influenced by multiple HLA class I and II alleles. *Gastroenterology.* 2011;141:338-347.

77. Lucey MR, et al. Alcoholic hepatitis. *N Engl J Med.* 2009;360:2758-2769.

78. Maddrey WC. Alcohol-induced liver disease. *Clin Liver Dis.* 2000;4:116-130.

79. Mahler H, et al. Fulminant liver failure in association with the emetic toxin of *Bacillus cereus.* *N Engl J Med.* 1997;336:1142-1148.

80. Mainra RR, Card SE. Trimethoprim-sulfamethoxazole-associated hepatotoxicity—part of a hypersensitivity syndrome. *Can J Clin Pharmacol.* 2003;10:175-178.

81. Mallal S, et al. HLA-B*5701 screening for hypersensitivity to abacavir. *N Engl J Med.* 2008;358:568-579.

82. McCormack M, et al. HLA-A*3101 and carbamazepine-induced hypersensitivity reactions in Europeans. *N Engl J Med.* 2011;364:1134-1143.

83. McDonald GB, et al. Veno-occlusive disease of the liver and multiorgan failure after bone marrow transplantation: a cohort study of 355 patients. *Ann Intern Med.* 1993; 118:255-267.

84. McKenzie R, et al. Hepatic failure and lactic acidosis due to fialuridine (FIAU), an investigational nucleoside analogue for chronic hepatitis B. *N Engl J Med.* 1995;333:1099-1105.

85. McMaster KR, Hennigar GR. Drug-induced granulomatous hepatitis. *Lab Invest.* 1981;44:61-73.

86. Mehendale HM, et al. Novel mechanisms in chemically induced hepatotoxicity. *FASEB J.* 1994;8:1285-1295.

87. Mehra R, et al. Severe irinotecan-induced toxicities in a patient with uridine diphosphate glucuronosyltransferase 1A1 polymorphism. *Clin Colorectal Cancer.* 2005;5:61-64.

88. Mohabbat O, et al. An outbreak of hepatic veno-occlusive disease in North-Western Afghanistan. *Lancet.* 1976;308:269-271.

89. Nair SS, et al. Trimethoprim-sulfamethoxazole-induced intrahepatic cholestasis. *Ann Intern Med.* 1980;92:511-512.

90. Navarro VJ, Senior JR. Drug-related hepatotoxicity. *N Engl J Med.* 2006;354:731-739.

91. Nicolas F, et al. Fulminant hepatic failure in poisoning due to ingestion of T 61, a veterinary euthanasia drug. *Crit Care Med.* 1990;18:573-575.

92. Nolan CM, et al. Hepatotoxicity associated with isoniazid preventive therapy: a 7-year survey from a public health tuberculosis clinic. *JAMA.* 1999;281:1014-1018.

93. O'Grady J. Timing and benefit of liver transplantation in acute liver failure. *J Hepatol.* 2014;60:663-670.

94. Padda MS, et al. Drug-induced cholestasis. *Hepatology.* 2011;53:1377-1387.

95. Pessayre D, et al. Central role of mitochondria in drug-induced liver injury. *Drug Metab Rev.* 2012;44:34-87.

96. Petersen KU. Rifaximin und polyethylene glycol as treatment modalities in hepatic encephalopathy. *J Med Drug Rev.* 2012;2:5-12.

97. Ramachandran R, Kakar S. Histological patterns in drug-induced liver disease. *J Clin Pathol.* 2009;62:481-492.

98. Raschi E, De Ponti F. Drug-induced liver injury: towards early prediction and risk stratification. *World J Hepatol.* 2017;9:30-37.

99. Raskind JY, El-Chaar GM. The role of carnitine supplementation during valproic acid therapy. *Ann Pharmacother.* 2000;34:630-638.

100. Rawat S, et al. Valproic acid and secondary hyperammonemia. *Neurology.* 1981; 31:1173-1173.

101. Redlich CA, et al. Liver disease associated with occupational exposure to the solvent dimethylformamide. *Ann Intern Med.* 1988;108:680-686.

102. Redlich CA, et al. Clinical and pathological characteristics of hepatotoxicity associated with occupational exposure to dimethylformamide. *Gastroenterology.* 1990;99:748-757.

103. Reinhart HH, et al. Combined nitrofurantoin toxicity to liver and lung. *Gastroenterology.* 1992;102:1396-1399.

104. Ridker PM, et al. Hepatic venoocclusive disease associated with the consumption of pyrrolizidine-containing dietary supplements. *Gastroenterology.* 1985;88:1050-1054.

105. Rigas B, et al. Amiodarone hepatotoxicity. A clinicopathologic study of five patients. *Ann Intern Med.* 1986;104:348-351.

106. Riordan SM, Williams R. Fulminant hepatic failure. *Clin Liver Dis.* 2000;4:25-45.

107. Riordan SM, Williams R. Gut flora and hepatic encephalopathy in patients with cirrhosis. *N Engl J Med.* 2010;362:1140-1142.

108. Riordan SM, Williams R. Treatment of hepatic encephalopathy. *N Engl J Med.* 1997; 337:473-479.

109. Roberts MS, et al. Enterohepatic circulation: physiological, pharmacokinetic and clinical implications. *Clin Pharmacokinet.* 2002;41:751-790.

110. Roberts RA, et al. Role of the Kupffer cell in mediating hepatic toxicity and carcinogenesis. *Toxicol Sci.* 2007;96:2-15.

111. Rumack BH, Bateman DN. Acetaminophen and acetylcysteine dose and duration: past, present and future. *Clin Toxicol (Phila).* 2012;50:91-98.

112. Russmann S, et al. Current concepts of mechanisms in drug-induced hepatotoxicity. *Curr Med Chem.* 2009;16:3041-3053.

113. Saukkonen JJ, et al. An official ATS statement: hepatotoxicity of antituberculosis therapy. *Am J Respir Crit Care Med.* 2006;174:935-952.

114. Schafer DF, Sorrell MF. Power failure, liver failure. *N Engl J Med.* 1997;336:1173-1174.

115. Schreiber AJ, Simon FR. Estrogen-induced cholestasis: clues to pathogenesis and treatment. *Hepatology.* 1983;3:607-613.

116. Schultz JC, et al. Fatal liver disease after intravenous administration of tetracycline in high dosage. *N Engl J Med.* 1963;269:999-1004.

117. Scully LJ, et al. Diclofenac induced hepatitis. 3 cases with features of autoimmune chronic active hepatitis. *Dig Dis Sci.* 1993;38:744-751.

118. Shah RR, et al. Impaired oxidation of debrisoquine in patients with perhexiline neuropathy. *Br Med J (Clin Res Ed).* 1982;284:295-299.

119. Sharma BC, et al. Secondary prophylaxis of hepatic encephalopathy: an open-label randomized controlled trial of lactulose versus placebo. *Gastroenterology.* 2009; 137:885-891.

120. Solbach P, et al. Testosterone-receptor positive hepatocellular carcinoma in a 29-year old bodybuilder with a history of anabolic androgenic steroid abuse: a case report. *BMC Gastroenterol.* 2015;15:60.

121. Soriano V, et al. Antiretroviral drugs and liver injury. *AIDS.* 2008;22:1-13.

122. Stamp LK, et al. Allopurinol hypersensitivity: investigating the cause and minimizing the risk. *Nat Rev Rheumatol.* 2016;12:235-242.

123. Stine JG, Chalasani NP. Drug hepatotoxicity: environmental factors. *Clin Liver Dis.* 2017;21:103-113.

124. Thapa BR, Walia A. Liver function tests and their interpretation. *Indian J Pediatr.* 2007;74:663-671.

125. Theise ND. Liver, gallbladder, and biliary tract. In: Kamur V, Abbas AK, Aster JC, et al., eds. *Robbins Basic Pathology.* 9th ed. Philadelphia, PA: Elsevier Saunders; 2013:603-644.

126. Thomas KL, et al. Valproic acid-induced hyperammonemia and minimal hepatic encephalopathy prevalence among psychiatric inpatients. *Ann Clin Psychiatry.* 2016; 28:37-42.

127. Trauner M, et al. Molecular pathogenesis of cholestasis. *N Engl J Med.* 1998;339: 1217-1227.

128. Tripodi A, Mannucci PM. The coagulopathy of chronic liver disease. *N Engl J Med.* 2011;365:147-156.

129. Tsukada N, Phillips MJ. Bile canalicular contraction is coincident with reorganization of pericanalicular filaments and co-localization of actin and myosin-II. *J Histochem Cytochem.* 1993;41:353-363.

130. Tsutsumi M, et al. The intralobular distribution of ethanol-inducible P450IIE1 in rat and human liver. *Hepatology.* 1989;10:437-446.

131. Victorino RM, et al. Floxacillin-induced cholestatic hepatitis with evidence of lymphocyte sensitization. *Arch Intern Med.* 1987;147:987-989.

132. Wang P, et al. Isoniazid metabolism and hepatotoxicity. *Acta Pharmaceutica Sinica B.* 2016;6:384-392.

133. Watanabe Y, et al. Selective alterations of brain dopamine D2 receptor binding in cirrhotic patients: results of a 11C-N-methylspiperone PET study. *Metab Brain Dis.* 2008; 23:265-274.

134. Whiting-O'Keefe QE, et al. Methotrexate and histologic hepatic abnormalities: a meta-analysis. *Am J Med.* 1991;90:711-716.

135. Wijdicks EFM. Hepatic Encephalopathy. *N Engl J Med.* 2016;375:1660-1670.

136. Williams DE, et al. Bioactivation and detoxication of the pyrrolizidine alkaloid senecionine by cytochrome P-450 enzymes in rat liver. *Drug Metab Dispos.* 1989;17:387-392.

137. Wisse E, et al. The liver sieve: considerations concerning the structure and function of endothelial fenestrae, the sinusoidal wall and the space of Disse. *Hepatology.* 1985; 5:683-692.

138. Woolley J, et al. Reflux of biliary components into blood in experimental intrahepatic cholestasis induced in rats by treatment with alpha-naphthylisothiocyanate. *Clin Chim Acta.* 1979;92:381-386.

139. Ye YM, et al. Hypersensitivity to antiepileptic drugs. *Immunol Allergy Clin North Am.* 2014;34:633-643.

140. Yeong ML, et al. Hepatic veno-occlusive disease associated with comfrey ingestion. *J Gastroenterol Hepatol.* 1990;5:211-214.

141. Zimmerman HJ, Ishak KG. Valproate-induced hepatic injury: analyses of 23 fatal cases. *Hepatology.* 1982;2:591-597.

142. Zimmerman HJ, Lewis JH. Chemical- and toxin-induced hepatotoxicity. *Gastroenterol Clin North Am.* 1995;24:1027-1045.

143. Zimmerman HJ, Maddrey WC. Acetaminophen (paracetamol) hepatotoxicity with regular intake of alcohol: analysis of instances of therapeutic misadventure. *Hepatology.* 1995;22:767-773.

144. American Thoracic Society, CDC, and Infectious Diseases Society of America. Treatment of tuberculosis. *MMWR Morb Mortal Wkly Rep.* 2003;52:1-72.

History Parents called 911 because they found their 5-year-old girl at home unresponsive. Shortly before emergency medical services (EMS) arrived, the girl had a witnessed self-limited convulsion that the parents described as the sudden onset of unresponsiveness with repetitive shaking and urinary incontinence. When EMS arrived, she was no longer shaking but could not be awoken. The paramedics recorded a respiratory rate of 30 breaths/min with a pulse of 150 beats/min and a point-of-care glucose of 122 mg/dL. They administered oxygen via nasal cannula and transported her to the emergency department (ED).

On arrival at the hospital, the parents reported that the child had no significant past medical history, had a pediatrician, was current with all vaccinations, and was not taking any prescription medications. Although she had a mild cough and nasal congestion, she was able to attend kindergarten the previous day. As further history was being obtained, the child began to shake repetitively once again.

Physical Examination The child was attached to continuous cardiac monitoring, and repeat vital signs were as follows: blood pressure, 108/80 mm Hg; pulse, 155 beats/min; respiratory rate, 32 breaths/min; rectal temperature, 99.4°F (37.4°C); oxygen saturation, 100% on a 100% nonrebreather face mask; and glucose, 143 mg/dL. Physical examination revealed a normal head without signs of trauma, pupils that were 4 to 5 mm and reactive, a clear chest, normal heart sounds, a soft abdomen with normal bowel sounds, and skin that was without rashes or other abnormalities. The child was still not verbal but appeared to localize pain and moved all extremities, and she had normal muscle tone.

Immediate Management The child was given an intramuscular injection of lorazepam (2 mg; 0.1 mg/kg for an estimated weight of 20 kg) while an intravenous (IV) line was being inserted. Within a few moments, the shaking stopped. Blood samples were sent for a complete blood count and electrolytes and an electrocardiogram (ECG) were ordered. The patient began to seize again, for which IV lorazepam (2 mg) was given with nearly an immediate response. Repeat vital signs and physical examination were essentially unchanged.

What Is the Differential Diagnosis? In addition to idiopathic epilepsy, trauma, infections, and structural brain lesions, seizures can result from both exposure to countless xenobiotics as well as withdrawal. In most instances, seizures are usually single and either self-limited or respond easily to an appropriate dose of a benzodiazepine. This child had three seizures in a brief period of time without regaining consciousness, which meets one of the criteria for status epilepticus. Although seizures are common, status epilepticus is rare, thereby narrowing the differential diagnosis to xenobiotics found in Table CS5–1.

Several features distinguish toxic–metabolic seizures from idiopathic epilepsy. With few exceptions, toxic–metabolic seizures often fail to respond to phenytoin. Phenytoin either has no efficacy or is actually detrimental in diverse or toxic–metabolic-induced convulsions associated with alcohol withdrawal, theophylline, cyclic antidepressants, antiepileptics, and cocaine. Conceptually, phenytoin fails because its ability to prevent secondary generalization of a focal seizure in idiopathic epilepsy is lost in toxic–metabolic etiologies where many areas of the brain are likely reaching the convulsive threshold simultaneously. Thus, when a toxic–metabolic cause is suspected, typically a barbiturate or propofol is added when benzodiazepines fail. In some cases, such as isoniazid, a specific antidote may be necessary (Antidotes in Depth: A15), and in others, such as theophylline, hemodialysis is often indicated (Chap. 6). Finally, it is important to recognize that the cessation of motor activity with toxic–metabolic seizures may be insufficient to prevent serious complications. For example, although it is common that patients with hypoglycemia, hyponatremia, or carbon monoxide poisoning can have their seizures terminated with benzodiazepines, the failure to correct these underlying issues will likely prevent complete neurologic recovery. The reader is referred to Antidotes in Depth: A26 for information regarding the choice, dose, and route of commonly used benzodiazepines.

What Clinical and Laboratory Analyses Can Help Exclude Life-Threatening Causes of This Patient's Presentation? Many rapidly reversible causes of seizures are assessed by the history and physical examination. Signs and symptoms of trauma, infection, and structural brain injury are often immediately evident. Bedside techniques can assess hypoxia, hypercarbia, and hypoglycemia, and a venous blood gas can confirm or exclude hyponatremia. An ECG provides rapid confirmation of sodium channel blockade, which is frequently associated with the risk of convulsions (Chaps. 15, 68). Potassium channel blockade can produce torsade de pointes (Chaps. 15, 67), which causes syncope that can be confused with convulsions in unmonitored patients. Vomiting would be commonly expected following overdose, especially with isoniazid (Chap. 56) and theophylline (Chap. 63). In some patients, computed tomography (CT) of the head, lumbar puncture, and empiric antimicrobials are indicated.

Further Diagnosis and Treatment Because of the child's continued depressed mental status, a clinical decision was made to protect her airway. During preparation for intubation, a unique "chemical" odor was noted in the oropharynx. When the parents were questioned, they confirmed that they recently bought camphor (Chap. 102) for use in a vaporizer in an attempt to help relieve the symptoms of an upper respiratory tract infection. The child had likely eaten some camphor, based on the odor and the recent purchase by the parents. Intubation was not performed when this history was obtained, because the girl's mental status appeared to be improving. A head CT scan was obtained without contrast and was interpreted as normal. Over the next day, the girl awakened and was neurologically normal. She was discharged after her parents were counseled about the safe storage of chemicals and medications.

TABLE CS5–1	Xenobiotics or Conditions Commonly Associated With Status Epilepticus
Bupropion	Insulin and insulin secretagogues
Camphor	
Carbon monoxide	Isoniazid
Chloroquine	Theophylline
Diphenhydramine	Cage convulsants
Hyponatremia	

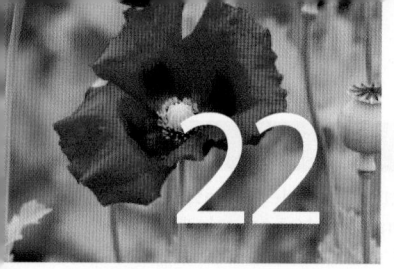

22 NEUROLOGIC PRINCIPLES

Rama B. Rao

INTRODUCTION

The central nervous system (CNS) coordinates responses to the fluctuating metabolic requirements of the body and modulates behavior, memory, and higher levels of thinking. These functions require diverse cells: astrocytes, neurons, ependymal cells, and vascular endothelial cells. Disruption or death of any one cell type can cause critical changes in the function or viability of another. This cellular interdependence, along with the high metabolic demands of the CNS, makes neurons especially vulnerable to injury from both endogenous neurotoxins and xenobiotics. Endogenous neurotoxins, such as the metals iron, copper, and manganese, are substances that are critical to CNS function but are harmful when their penetration into the CNS is poorly controlled.

The understanding of the normal chemical and molecular functions of the CNS is limited at best. Interestingly, cellular mechanisms are sometimes revealed by investigating xenobiotic-induced neuronal injuries.[39,69] For example, the pathophysiology of Parkinson disease, which affects movement and motor tone, was elucidated by the inadvertent exposure of individuals to 1-methyl-4-phenyl-1,2,3,6-tetrahydropyridine (MPTP), a by product of synthesis of a meperidine analog. The mechanisms of axonal transport were elucidated by investigations of the effects of acrylamide exposures in human and animal models.[59] The neurodegenerative changes of amyotrophic lateral sclerosis have a promising xenobiotic model in β-methylamino-L-alanine (BMAA), a neurotoxin found in the cyanobacteria associated with cycad plants ingested by the Chamorro people of Guam (Chap. 13).

There are few minimally invasive methods available to investigate xenobiotic-induced CNS injury. Biomarkers are usually nonspecific and not readily available. Xenobiotic concentrations of blood and urine rarely reflect tissue concentrations of the CNS.[61] Cerebrospinal fluid (CSF) is useful in excluding CNS injury from infection, hemorrhage, and inflammatory processes, but is, with few exceptions, poorly reflective of the etiology of neuronal injuries.[93] Similarly, electroencephalograms and electromyelograms are useful in only a few types of xenobiotic exposures, and neuroimaging, while progressively evolving,[55] is a poor substitute for neuroanatomical evaluations that are usually available only on autopsy. Much of the current study to elucidate the mechanisms of CNS injury uses animal models, cultured astrocytes, and other tissue, or postmortem investigations. Less commonly, occupational evaluations, such as the enzyme activity of cholinesterases, are used in pesticide-exposed workers.

This chapter reviews some basic anatomic and physiologic principles of the nervous system and the common mechanisms by which xenobiotics exploit the functional and protective components of the CNS, with a few relevant examples. The multiple factors determining the clinical expression of neurotoxicity are reviewed.

CELLS OF THE NERVOUS SYSTEM: AN OVERVIEW

Neurons

Neurons are the major pathway of cellular communication in the CNS. Having one of the highest metabolic rates in the body, these cells are especially sensitive to changes in the microenvironment and are dependent on astrocytes, choroidal epithelium, and capillary endothelium to confer protection and deliver glucose and other sources of energy.

Although each neuron is capable of receiving information through different neurotransmitters and receptor subtypes at the dendrite, neurons typically produce and release a single type of neurotransmitter at the axonal terminal. This specificity allows for cellular classification of neurons based on the neurotransmitter released, for example, serotonergic, cholinergic, and dopaminergic neurons (Chap. 13). Other substances such as adenosine are produced and released that are less specific to the neuron type.

The anatomic structure of neurons facilitates their function. Dendrites located on the cell body are lined with receptors that bind neurotransmitters and affect cellular changes via several mechanisms. The soma, or cell body, is responsible for coordination and production of multiple proteins required to carry out normal physiological functions. This synthesis occurs at a rate several times greater than that in the liver or kidney. These proteins, organelles, and substrates must then be transported across long distances to the terminal axon. This energy-dependent function is supported by a cytoskeleton composed of neurofilaments, microfilaments, microtubules, and complex transport proteins. Fast anterograde transport of membrane-bound organelles occurs through *kinesin*, a transport protein, at a rate of 200 to 400 mm/d. Channel proteins, synaptic vesicles, mitochondria, Na^+,K^+-ATPase, glycolipids, and other substances are transported by kinesin. Slow anterograde transport also occurs, but at a substantially slower rate (0.5–4 mm/d). The retrograde transport protein, *dynein*, is produced in the soma and delivered to the nerve terminal for the movement of larger vesicles and reusable proteins back to the cell body.

In the CNS, groups of neurons are organized into complex functional pathways, with a single class of neurons regulating different functions and clinical effects depending on the brain region. As an example, dopaminergic neurons regulate cravings, movement, and resting muscle tone, each of which is determined not only by dopaminergic neurons and receptor subtype, but the location in the cortex or basal ganglia (Chap. 13).

Neurons must be able to respond to changes in the local environment and alter the expression of different receptors in response to signaling from neurotrophic factors, variations in metabolic requirements, and xenobiotic interactions. This "neuroplasticity" accounts for the diversity of clinical responses to xenobiotics that induce tolerance such as ethanol (Chap. 14).

Glial Cells

Glial cells are composed of *astrocytes*, *oligodendrocytes*, *Schwann cells*, and *microglia*. These cells serve to support the neurons both structurally and functionally.

Astrocytes comprise between 25% and 50% of the brain volume.[1,3,4,12] In addition to the anatomic contribution to the blood–brain barrier (BBB), astrocytes play a critical role in maintaining neuronal function.[1,2,96] They contribute to 3 major areas: homeostasis of the extraneuronal environment, provision of energy substrates, and limitation of oxidative stress. In addition, astrocytes contribute to the "plasticity" of cells and receptor expression in the CNS (see later discussion).

In order for cells of all types to function in the CNS, membrane potentials must be adequately maintained. Astrocytes contribute to this by closely regulating the extracellular pH, water, and, like brain capillaries, the extracellular potassium concentration. Metallothioneins, which control the entry of metals necessary for CNS function, are produced by astrocytes.[29,96] Astrocytes also release energy substrates such as lactate, citrate, alanine, glutathione, and α-ketoglutarate for utilization by neurons.[12]

Astrocytes metabolize glutamate, the main excitatory amino acid (EAA) neurotransmitter in the CNS, as well as ammonia. These cells also produce superoxide dismutase and glutathione peroxidase to reduce free radical propagation. Glutathione, the major antioxidant for the brain, is predominantly located in the astrocytes. It is released into the extracellular space or cleaved for neuronal uptake and intracellular reformulation.[12]

Through the release of complex trophic factors, astrocytes control the expression of endothelial transporters of the BBB and the production of tight junctions in both the blood CSF barrier and BBB. Angiogenesis is similarly astrocyte regulated, as is detection of neuronal injury, immune mediation, and neurotransmitter production. The growth of neurites, the branches of neuronal cell bodies that eventually become dendrites or axons, is similarly modulated by astrocytes.

Oligodendrocytes are a type of glial cell that provide anatomical support, protective insulation, and facilitate rapid neuronal depolarization by the production of myelin. Myelin is the primary constituent of white matter in the CNS. The production of myelin in the peripheral nervous system (PNS) is performed by the Schwann cells. Although oligodendrocytes support several axons, each Schwann cell is anatomically dedicated to a single axon.

Finally, microglial cells modulate immune response, inflammation, and tissue repair from a variety of CNS injuries. Like neurons, microglia are dependent on signaling from astrocytes.

MECHANISMS OF NEUROPROTECTION

The nervous system has multiple protective mechanisms. Xenobiotics are prevented from accessing the CNS by the blood–brain and blood–CSF barriers. For xenobiotics that enter the CNS, there are multiple cellular specializations to limit oxidant stress as reviewed below.

Blood–Brain Barrier

The BBB confers an anatomic and functional barrier to xenobiotic entry into the CNS. Brain capillaries are surrounded by the foot processes of adjacent astrocytes. The potential spaces between endothelial cells are limited by tight junctions, or zonulae occludentes, which are between 50 and 100 times tighter than those found on peripheral capillaries.[1,2,4,53,64] This anatomic barrier prevents movement of substances between cells, also known as the paracellular aqueous pathway, due to osmotic and oncotic forces.[1,2,4,53,64]

Transendothelial movement of critical substrates and, potentially, xenobiotics occurs through 3 major mechanisms: diffusion, transport proteins, and endocytosis.[1,4] These routes allow carefully controlled entry of critical substrates and cofactors while limiting the potential for injury from either endogenous or exogenous neurotoxins.

Lipophilic substances can move directly across the luminal and abluminal endothelial membranes abutting the CNS. Other substances enter the endothelium through bidirectional transport proteins on the luminal surface. Some of these proteins are specific, such as the glucose transporter 1 (GLUT1) protein for uptake of glucose. Other less specific large neutral amino acid transporters can move amino acids and xenobiotics such as baclofen, intracellularly. These transporters also line the abluminal surface of the endothelial cell for movement of substrates and xenobiotics into the CNS. The third line of entry for larger proteins is via endocytosis. This is adsorptive, or mediated through specific receptors such as those for insulin or transferrin.[1,3,4,53,64,96]

Endothelial cells have other protective properties, including intracellular enzymes, to metabolize xenobiotics and efflux proteins to transport certain xenobiotics back into the capillary lumen. These efflux proteins include energy-dependent P-glycoproteins that are ATP-binding cassette transporters and are sometimes referred to as multidrug-resistant (MDR) proteins (Chap. 9). Several hydrophobic xenobiotics are prevented from accumulating in the CNS through these transporters, including vinca alkaloids, digoxin, cyclosporine A, and protease inhibitors. Nonsedating antihistamines and loperamide have limited sedative properties due, in part, to efflux through P-glycoproteins.[26,77] Another type of saturable transporter, known as organic acid transport (OAT) protein, facilitates the efflux of hydrophilic xenobiotics such as valproic acid or baclofen. The expression of each of these transporters is upregulated under certain conditions such as intermittent disruptions in the BBB from seizures. This expression upregulation is theorized to account for the resistance of anticonvulsant medications in patients with epilepsy. Comprehensive lists of xenobiotics that are substrates for these transporters are available elsewhere.[2,53,54]

Blood–Cerebrospinal Fluid Barrier

The ventricles of the brain are lined by the epithelial cells of the choroid plexus. These cells also have tight junctions but not as extensive as those of the BBB. They are, however, rich in glutathione peroxidase and other xenobiotic-metabolizing enzymes in concentrations approximating those of the liver. Similar to brain capillary cells, the choroid plexus contains efflux transporters for organic anions and cations, as well as MDR efflux proteins (P-glycoproteins) to limit entry of xenobiotics into the CSF.[1,4,53,96]

NEUROTOXIC PRINICPLES

Excitotoxicity

Neuronal function is strictly dependent on aerobic metabolism. When energy expenditure exceeds production, cellular dysfunction and ultimately cell death, or apoptosis, results. The specific cascade of molecular events relating to this process is termed *excitotoxicity*.[11,74]

The initial event is traced to an oxidant stress and excessive stimulation of *N*-methyl-D-aspartate (NMDA) receptors by glutamate, an EAA neurotransmitter. An influx of intracellular calcium changes membrane potentials across the cellular and mitochondrial membranes. The mitochondria become progressively more inefficient at ATP production and handling the resulting reactive oxygen species. As membrane damage is propagated, calcium further depolarizes the mitochondria, activating a permeability transition pore across the mitochondrial membrane. Gradients are further disrupted, precipitating more injury, energy failure, and ultimately cell death.

Excitotoxicity is considered a common mechanism of cell death due to xenobiotic, ischemic, traumatic, infectious, neoplastic, or neurodegenerative injury. It is the subject of study for many therapeutic interventions in CNS injury.

Determinants of Neurotoxicity

The clinical expression of neurotoxicity is related to many factors. These include the chemical properties of the xenobiotic, the dose and route of administration, xenobiotic interactions, and underlying patient characteristics including age, gender, and comorbid conditions.

Chemical Properties of Xenobiotics

One of the most important determinants of neurotoxicity is the ability of a xenobiotic to penetrate the BBB. Water-soluble molecules larger than 200 to 400 M_r (molecular weight ratio, or mass of a molecule relative to the mass of an atom) are unable to bypass the tight junctions.[4] Lipid-soluble xenobiotics (those with a high octanol/water partition coefficient) are more likely to passively penetrate the capillary endothelium, and potentially the BBB, whereas those with a low partition coefficient typically require energy-dependent facilitated transport.[64] Xenobiotics that are substrates for capillary endothelial efflux mechanisms will have limited penetration regardless of the coefficient.[1,4,53,64]

Route of Administration

The route of xenobiotic administration is also consequential. Although most xenobiotics gain access to the nervous system through the circulatory system, aerosolized solvents and heavy metals in industrial and occupational exposures gain CNS access through inhalation, traveling via olfactory and circulatory routes. Alternatively, some substances move from the PNS via retrograde axonal transport to the CNS. Naturally occurring proteins such as tetanospasmin, as well as rabies, polio, and herpes virus use this mechanism to access the PNS and CNS.[14,17,48] The toxalbumins ricin and abrin as well as bismuth salts also use this mechanism to a limited extent.[87,94] This understanding can prove beneficial from a therapeutic perspective. For example, in one small experimental series of patients experiencing severe pain, doxorubicin was injected into the involved peripheral nerves. Therapeutically, a chemical ganglionectomy occurred through retrograde "suicide" transport of doxorubicin, which provided substantial relief for these patients.[51]

Some xenobiotics are delivered directly into the CSF (intrathecally), the consequences of which are variable (Special Considerations: SC7).

Xenobiotic Interactions

Coadministration of xenobiotics can precipitate neurotoxicity by several mechanisms.[46] Extraaxially (outside of the CNS), xenobiotic interactions that result in an increase of the blood concentration of one or both can overwhelm the protective mechanisms of the BBB.[21] Similar effects can occur in the PNS, where elevated blood concentrations can enhance clinical effects resulting in peripheral neuropathies.[96]

Some xenobiotic interactions are synergistic, acting on the same neuroreceptor. Benzodiazepines and ethanol, for example, both stimulate the γ-aminobutyric acid type A (GABA$_A$) receptor. The excessive neuroinhibition results in enhanced sedation and even respiratory depression when these xenobiotics are administered simultaneously.

In some circumstances, xenobiotic interactions result in excessive neurotransmitter availability.[10] This neurotransmitter excess is demonstrated in patients with serotonin toxicity, which results from the coadministration of a monoamine oxidase inhibitor and a serotonin reuptake inhibitor or other serotonergics as an example (Chap. 69).

Access to the CNS can be altered by one of the xenobiotics, allowing the other to bypass the BBB. For example, mannitol causes transient opening of the BBB; as a result, therapeutic use of mannitol is under investigation for the delivery of chemotherapeutics that might otherwise be unable to access the nervous system.[54] Similarly, some xenobiotics, such as verapamil, cyclosporine, and probenecid, are blockers of capillary endothelium efflux.[4,96] These theoretically limit efflux of other substrates of P-glycoprotein or OAT. Loperamide penetration into the CNS is limited by P-glycoprotein. In healthy volunteers the coadministration of quinidine—another P-glycoprotein substrate—with loperamide results in respiratory depression suggestive of increased CNS penetration.[77] The clinical utility of employing such efflux blockers is under investigation as was done in a study in which primates received intrathecal methotrexate. The CSF clearance of methotrexate was reduced in animals administered intrathecal probenecid.[13,78]

Patient Characteristics

Patient-specific variables also affect the ability of a xenobiotic to penetrate the BBB and/or the clinical effects of a given exposure. For example, age of the patient at the time of exposure is critical, especially in the fetus and neonates.[80] The structural and enzymatic development of the BBB is incomplete, and synaptogenesis, or formation of intercellular relationships, is especially sensitive to impaired protein synthesis or other excitotoxic events. This is demonstrated classically by maternal exposure to methylmercury. The mother can be minimally affected, but the developing fetus suffers profound neurological and developmental consequences (Chaps. 30 and 95).

In neonates, immature liver function can lead to the accumulation of circulating bilirubin. Because of incomplete formation of the BBB, the bilirubin accesses the CNS and produces a form of encephalopathy known as *kernicterus*.

Elderly patients are also susceptible to neurotoxins as a result of relatively impaired circulation or age-related changes in mitochondrial function that predispose to excitotoxicity.[83] Xenobiotic-induced Parkinsonism, or the unmasking of subclinical idiopathic Parkinson disease occurs more readily than in younger patients. Animal models also suggest age-related sensitivity, with one study noting increased manganese toxicity with advanced age.[37]

Gender is contributory to the expression of xenobiotic induced neurologic injury. In animal models, the presence of estrogen-related and progesterone-related compounds are neuroprotective for some xenobiotic injuries.[65,72] In humans, women are more susceptible to some movement disorders such as xenobiotic-induced parkinsonism and tardive dyskinesia, whereas dystonias and bruxism are more prevalent in young men.[75] The etiologies of these gender-related differences are incompletely understood.

Neurologic Comorbidities

Conditions affecting the integrity of the BBB affect CNS penetration of xenobiotics and endogenous neurotoxins. For example, glutamate concentrations are normally higher in the circulatory system than the CNS.[58] Patients with trauma, ischemia, or lupus vasculitis[3] can experience neuropsychiatric disorders as a result of increased penetration of glutamate or sensitivity to additional xenobiotics. Similarly, inflammation associated with meningitis and encephalitis causes openings in the BBB, which is exploited therapeutically. Intravenous penicillin achieves a higher CSF concentration in animals with meningitis than in those without meningitis.[79]

In some patients, previously undiagnosed diseases become evident on exposure to xenobiotics. This is especially true in patients with peripheral neuropathies. For example, patients being treated with therapeutic doses of vincristine suffered a severe polyneuropathy due to unmasking of a previously undiagnosed Charcot-Marie-Tooth disease.[10,23] Similarly, patients with diabetes mellitus, the commonest cause of peripheral neuropathy, or human immunodeficiency virus disease have exacerbation of symptoms in the presence of antiretrovirals.[25,73] Patients with myasthenia gravis have exacerbation of weakness with aminoglycoside administration, which affects transmission at the neuromuscular junction (NMJ).[95]

Chronic exposures to some neuroinhibitory xenobiotics such as ethanol alter neuronal receptor expression and upregulate or increase the amount of receptors for EAAs. In addition to receptor augmentation, neurotransmitter concentrations of the excitatory neurotransmitters glutamate and aspartate are increased, as is homocysteine. These changes induce a tolerance to neuroinhibitory xenobiotics acting on the same receptor, and patients require escalating doses to achieve the same clinical effect. In such patients, cessation of ethanol intake results in a relative deficiency of exogenous inhibitory tone. The patient experiences neuroexcitability and the clinical syndrome of withdrawal[18,19] (Chap. 14).

Adequate nutritional status is important for the maintenance of normal neurologic function. The BBB is inadequately maintained in patients with malnutrition. Deficiencies of metal cofactors such as manganese, copper, zinc, and iron affect neurological function. In some cases, the deficiencies enhance absorption of other xenobiotics. For example, iron deficiency enhances lead and manganese absorption in the gastrointestinal tract, which can ultimately overwhelm neuroprotective mechanisms. Vitamins serve as enzymatic cofactors in modulating the production of glutamate, homocysteine, and other amino acids. Specific vitamin deficiencies precipitate neurologic syndromes such as Wernicke encephalopathy in thiamine-depleted patients (Antidotes in Depth: A27 and Chap. 44). The toxicity of xenobiotics is also enhanced. For example, a relative pyridoxine deficiency in patients with acute isoniazid overdose result in seizures as a result of a relative excess of EAAs (Antidotes in Depth: A15 and Chap. 56). Glucose is a critical energy substrate that causes profound neurologic impairment when delivery is inadequate (Antidotes in Depth: A8 and Chap. 47).

Interestingly, certain conditions such as temperature sometimes affect the toxicity of xenobiotics. For example, cooling limits the impedance of acetylcholine neurotransmission caused by botulinum toxin.[42]

Extraaxial Organ Dysfunction

Kidney failure impairs metabolism or elimination of xenobiotics or endogenous substances such as uremic toxins rendering them more available to the CNS. Hyperglycemia in patients with diabetes mellitus increases formation of CNS reactive oxygen species. Similarly, some patients with liver failure have elevations in CNS manganese resulting in Parkinsonism.[52,81]

Hepatic encephalopathy illustrates the concept of excitotoxicity from endogenous neurotoxins. Hyperammonemia increases oxidative stress and free radical formation in astrocytes. Ammonia potentially decreases critical metabolic enzymes such as catalases, superoxide dismutase, and glutathione peroxidase. Nitric oxide (NO) production is increased as a result of elevations in NO synthetase. Under these conditions, astrocytes upregulate the expression of the peripheral benzodiazepine receptor (PBR) on the outer mitochondrial membrane. The PBR modulates the production of neurosteroids and, in turn, the GABA$_A$ receptor. Continued CNS exposure to ammonia and other endogenous solutes propagates this oxidative and nitrosative stress to the mitochondrial membrane, potentially opening the mitochondrial permeability transition pore. Osmotic swelling of the mitochondrial membrane followed by excitotoxicity results in cerebral edema and hepatic encephalopathy.[65–67]

SPECIFIC MECHANISMS OF NEUROTOXICTY

Alteration of Endogenous Neurotransmission

Xenobiotics induce neurotoxicity by triggering changes in neurotransmission in either the CNS or PNS. In some cases, xenobiotics enhance neurotransmission through a specific receptor subtype. This enhanced transmission occurs through inhibition of presynaptic metabolism (monoamine oxidase inhibitors), stimulation of neurotransmitter release (amphetamines), impairment of neurotransmitter reuptake (cocaine), or inhibition of synaptic degradation (acetylcholinesterase inhibitors).

Alternatively, synaptic neurotransmission can be impaired.[82] Xenobiotics can inhibit the presynaptic release of neurotransmitters (botulinum toxin), block receptors (antimuscarinics), or alter membrane potentials at the postsynaptic membrane (tetrodotoxin).[33,34] Patients present with a clinical syndrome of toxicity associated with altered neurotransmission of the specific receptor (Chap. 3).

Direct Receptor Interaction

Some xenobiotics are able to directly stimulate receptors. Both kainate and α-amino-3-hydroxy-5-methyl-4-isoxazole propionate (AMPA) are subclasses of the glutamate receptor, which are targeted by some naturally occurring xenobiotics.[43] An example is β-N-oxalylamino-L-alanine (BOAA) found in the grass pea, *Lathyrus sativus*. β-N-Oxalyl-amino-L-alanine stimulates the AMPA receptor and inhibits specific mitochondrial enzymes, resulting in the spastic paraparesis of lathyrism.[70] Domoic acid stimulates the kainate receptor and causes the neuroexcitation associated with neurotoxic shellfish poisoning (Chap. 39). Direct inhibition is also possible, as exemplified by phencyclidine, an NMDA receptor antagonist.

Enzyme and Transporter Exploitation

The classic example of xenobiotics that exploit endogenous enzymes and/or transporters is MPTP.[39] Once MPTP crosses the BBB, it is converted by monoamine oxidase to the neurotoxic compound 1-methyl-4-phenylpyridine ion in astrocytes. 1-Methyl-4-phenylpyridine ion (MPP+) is taken up by dopamine transporters into the neurons of the substantia nigra pars compacta. It inhibits complex I of the mitochondrial electron transport chain resulting in dopaminergic excitotoxicity and the clinical syndrome similar to Parkinson disease (see below and Chap. 36).

Altered Conduction Along Membranes: Demyelinating Neurotoxins

Aside from xenobiotics that affect neurotransmission at the postsynaptic membrane, some affect the production or maintenance of myelin by oligodendrocytes and Schwann cells.[24,35,38,49] In the CNS, these are often associated with white matter abnormalities and a leukoencephalopathy.[35] Xenobiotics such as hexachlorophene, arsenic, inhibitors of tumor necrosis factor α, neural tissue–derived rabies vaccine, and inhaling some forms of volatilized heroin ("chasing the dragon") are associated with a demyelinating neurotoxicity.[24] In the PNS, suramin and tacrolimus are associated with peripheral demyelination.[47] Nitrous oxide affects the CNS and can also cause axonal degeneration in the PNS.[92]

Inhibition of Intracellular Functions

Some xenobiotics are nonspecific inhibitors of cellular function.[30] For example, the neurotoxicity of carbon monoxide (CO) or cyanide that can appear as a diffuse impairment of neuropsychiatric dysfunction or, depending on the dose and specific vulnerabilities of an exposed patient, be more focal. Some patients surviving acute CO exposure experience delayed neurologic sequelae that includes a diffuse impairment of neuropsychiatric function, or more focally, present with a xenobiotic-induced Parkinson syndrome (see below and Chap. 122). Patients ingesting inadequately prepared cassava are exposed to excessive linamarins that can result in spastic paralysis, visual disturbances, and somatosensory abnormalities.[88]

Chemotherapeutics affect the production of critical proteins required for cellular maintenance. These can be very specific such as the ability of vincristine and colchicine to impair cytoskeletal transport in the peripheral nervous system (Chap. 34).

CLINICALLY RELEVANT XENOBIOTIC-MEDIATED CONDITIONS

Alterations in Consciousness

The toxicologic differential diagnosis of xenobiotics that induce alterations in mental status or consciousness is expansive. These xenobiotics are broadly divided into those that produce some form of neuroexcitation and those that produce neuroinhibition. Although some xenobiotics such as phencyclidine have elements of both depending on dose, this categorization facilitates a general clinical understanding of neurotoxic alterations in mental status.

Xenobiotics resulting in neuroexcitation enhance neurotransmission of EAAs, or diminish inhibitory input from GABAergic neurons. The clinical presentation of the patient varies; some patients are alert and confused, or suffering from an agitated delirium, hallucinations, or a seizure.

Neuroinhibitory xenobiotics typically enhance GABA-mediated neurotransmission. These patients often are somnolent or in deep coma. Benzodiazepines hyperpolarize cells by increasing inward movement of Cl⁻ ions through the chloride channel of the GABA$_A$ receptor. This hyperpolarization limits subsequent neurotransmission (Chap. 13). Less commonly, neuroinhibition is a result of diminution of EAA. Patients presenting the day after binging on cocaine are often sleepy but arousable and oriented in what is termed cocaine "washout," theoretically related to depletion of EAA and dopamine. Xenobiotics that cause diffuse cortical dysfunction through impairment in the delivery or utilization of oxygen or glucose also present with depressed or altered consciousness.

Clinical evaluation of patients with altered consciousness includes obtaining complete history, including medications, comorbid conditions, occupation, and suicidal intent when relevant or available. Patients should have a complete physical examination, with particular attention paid to vital sign abnormalities or findings that indicate a toxic syndrome. Assessment and correction of hypoxia or hypoglycemia should be performed. An electrocardiogram is useful in some circumstances (Chap. 15).

Xenobiotic-Induced Seizures

Seizures are the most extreme form of neuroexcitation. As with alterations of consciousness, this can be due to enhanced EAA neurotransmission (domoic acid, sympathomimetics) or inhibition of GABAergic tone (isoniazid). Unlike in traumatic or idiopathic seizure disorders with an identifiable seizure focus, the initiation and propagation of xenobiotic-induced seizures is diffuse. It is for this reason that most non–sedative–hypnotic antiepileptics such as phenytoin are ineffective in terminating xenobiotic-induced seizures.

Seizures can be idiosyncratic as described with tramadol and bupropion, or they can be concentration-dependent events as described with theophylline and isoniazid toxicity. Alternatively, seizures can be a result of withdrawal from GABAergic substances.

Status epilepticus is variably defined but involves 2 or more seizures without a lucid interval, or continuous seizure activity for greater than 5 minutes.[60] True xenobiotic induced status epilepticus is rare. Cicutoxin, the toxin in water hemlock, *Cicuta maculata*, is a potent inhibitor of GABA$_A$ neurotransmission and can cause status epilepticus.

Theophylline toxicity precipitates seizures and status epilepticus through a different mechanism. Normally, endogenous termination of seizures is mediated through presynaptic release of adenosine during the release of the primary neurotransmitter at the terminal axon. Adenosine functions as a feedback inhibitor of the presynaptic neuron, disrupting propagation of excitatory neurotransmission. Theophylline is an adenosine antagonist. Adenosine administration is not a useful therapy for theophylline-induced seizures as adenosine is unable to cross the BBB. Generally high-dose sedative–hypnotics, affecting GABA$_A$ receptors, are required for seizure control.

TABLE 22–1	Xenobiotics That Commonly Induce Seizures		
Concentration Related	**Idiosyncratic**	**Withdrawal Related**	**Tonic-Clonic Seizurelike**
Antihistamines	Bupropion[a]	Baclofen	Strychnine
Baclofen	Carbamazepine	Barbiturates	Tetanospasmin
Camphor[a]	Ergotamines	Benzodiazepines	
Carbon monoxide	GHB	Ethanol	
Chloroquine[a]	Mefenamic acid	GHB	
Cicutoxin[a]	Tramadol		
Cyanide			
Diphenhydramine[a]			
Domoic acid			
Isoniazid[a]			
Hypoglycemics			
Gyromitrin[a]			
Lidocaine			
Meperidine metabolites			
Organic chlorines			
Organic phosphorus compounds			
Propoxyphene metabolites			
Strychnine			
Sympathomimetics			
Tetramethylene disulfotetramine (TETS)[a]			
Thallium			
Theophylline[a]			
Zinc phosphide			

[a]While therapeutic concentrations are associated with seizures idiosyncratically, high concentrations are associated with status epilepticus.

CNS = central nervous system; GHB = γ-hydroxybutyric acid.

TABLE 22–2	Xenobiotics Commonly Inducing Mood[a] and Neuropsychiatric Disorders	
Mania	**Depression[a]**	**Psychosis**
Acyclovir	β-Adrenergic antagonists	Amantadine
Amantadine	Amiodarone α	Glucocorticosteroids
Caffeine	Interferon	Sympathomimetics
Chloroquine	Isoretinoic acid	
Clarithromycin	Ribavirin	
CNS stimulants		
Corticosteroids		
Dextromethorphan		
Dehydroepiandrosterone		
L-Dopa		
Efavirenz		
Fenfluramine		
Fluoroquinolones		
Gabapentin		
Ginseng		
Ifosfamide		
Interferon-α		
Isoniazid		
Mefloquine		
Phentermine		
Phenylpropanolamine		
Pseudoephedrine		
Quetiapine		
St. John's wort		
Sympathomimetics		
Testosterone		
Tramadol		

[a]In some patients, antidepressants increase the risk of suicide by converting a vegetative depression to active depression.

CNS = central nervous system.

Some clinical conditions appear to be centrally mediated tonic–clonic movements but are due to glycine inhibition in the spinal cord. Glycine is the major inhibitory neurotransmitter of motor neurons of the spinal cord. Under normal conditions, glycine contributes to termination of reflex arcs. Glycine inhibition results in myoclonus, hyperreflexia, and opisthotonos, often without alteration in consciousness. Presynaptic glycine release inhibition is caused by tetanospasmin, the major neurotoxin from *Clostridium tetani*. Postsynaptic glycine inhibition is caused by strychnine, the toxin in *Strychnos nux-vomica*. Patients with exposures to tetanospasmin or strychnine are often treated in quiet environments where the stimuli to initiate hyperreflexia are minimized (Chap. 114 and Table 22–1).

Xenobiotic-Induced Mood Disorders

Certain xenobiotics are inconsistently associated with alterations in mood.[5,20] What predisposes individuals to xenobiotic-induced mood alterations is unclear. In some circumstances, patients with previously undiagnosed bipolar disorder are given a xenobiotic that unmasks their disease. Interestingly, antibiotic-induced mania is found in some patients without a previous psychiatric history. The symptoms of mania are usually evident within the first week of therapy and, unlike the mania of purely psychiatric origin, readily abate within 48 to 72 hours of the last antibiotic dose. Some patients with clarithromycin-induced mania have documented recurrence on rechallenge.[5] In general, xenobiotic-induced manias are idiopathic and very rare. More common are either psychosis from chronic CNS stimulant use or depression from ethanol or the xenobiotics listed in Table 22–2.

Disorders of Movement and Tone
Central Nervous System–Mediated Disorders

Most movement disorders, including akathisia, bradykinesia, tics, chorea, and dystonias, are mediated by the complex dopaminergic pathways of the basal ganglia. Different dopamine receptor subtypes are modulated by serotonergic, GABAergic, glutaminergic, and cholinergic neurons (Chap. 13).

Chorea rarely occurs in carbamazepine overdose, therapeutic oral contraceptive use,[32] and after cocaine use when the stimulant effects have subsided.[75]

Dopamine receptor antagonists precipitate acute dystonic reactions. The D_2 receptor antagonists, in conjunction with alterations in muscarinic cholinergic tone, are usually implicated. Animal models suggest possible mediation through σ receptors, the craniofacial distribution of which corresponds to the common clinical manifestations of acute dystonias.[50]

Diffusely increased motor tone occurs with glycine antagonists such as tetanospasmin and strychnine, and in adrenergic excess clinical conditions such as acute toxicity with sympathomimetics or withdrawal from sedative–hypnotics. The rare complication of bone fractures associated with severe muscle spasm and myoclonus is reported with chronic bismuth toxicity and inadvertent intrathecal administration of hyperosmolar contrast dye (Chap. 87 and Special Considerations: SC7).

Other centrally mediated disorders of tone include serotonin toxicity and neuroleptic malignant syndrome (NMS). Both of these potentially life-threatening disorders consist of altered consciousness, hyperthermia, rigidity, and autonomic instability. Neuroleptic malignant syndrome occurs in patients taking dopamine receptor antagonists such as antipsychotics or in those with idiopathic Parkinson disease who abruptly stop their dopamine agonist therapy. Dopamine receptor agonists such as bromocriptine or restoration of antiparkinson medications are used therapeutically in these circumstances (Chap. 67). The diagnosis and management of serotonin toxicity is reviewed in Chap. 69.

Parkinsonism

Xenobiotic-induced parkinsonism is a syndrome of unstable posture, rigidity, gait disturbance, loss of facial expression, hypokinesis, and variable presence of tremor.[8] The common neuroanatomic target involves the dopaminergic neurons of the basal ganglia, specifically the substantia nigra.[27,89] In some circumstances, the toxicity is transient and the mechanism inadequately understood.

TABLE 22–3	Xenobiotics Associated with Parkinsonism
Reversible[a]	**Irreversible**
Antipsychotics	Carbon disulfide
Calcium channel blockers	Carbon monoxide
Chemotherapeutics	Copper
Cyclosporine	Cyanide
Dopaminergic agonists (withdrawal)	Heroin
Kava kava	Hydrogen sulfide
Progesterone	Manganese
Valproate	MPTP
Trazodone	

[a]Although patients typically improve with removal of xenobiotic, sometimes persistent administration of dopaminergic therapy is required.

MPTP = 1-methyl-4-phenyl-1,2,3,6-tetrahydropyridine.

Some xenobiotics such as carbon monoxide and heroin produce tissue hypoxia and ischemia in the basal ganglia that occasionally results in xenobiotic-induced Parkinson syndrome.

Other xenobiotics such as MPTP, carbon disulfide, manganese, and the endogenous neurotoxin copper in patients with Wilson disease produce predictable mitochondrial impairment of the basal ganglia neurons. Viscose rayon workers exposed to carbon disulfide present with a Parkinson syndrome refractory to L-dopa administration[44,45] (see Enzyme and Transporter Exploitation earlier).

Manganese is a critical substrate for production and metabolism of several neurotransmitters including glutamate. Excessive manganese interferes with normal uptake of glutamate and is critical to the function of superoxide dismutase and glutamine synthetase.[31,36] In patients with liver failure, or who accumulate manganese from occupational exposure, reversal or treatment of liver disease, or removal from exposure can result in resolution of parkinsonism.[37,81]

A review of patients who intravenously injected illicit methcathinone described a Parkinson syndrome thought to be secondary to contamination with manganese from a precursor, potassium permanganate, which is used in methcathinone production. Unlike patients with idiopathic parkinsonism, these patients did not suffer from a resting tremor, and they had a specific gait abnormality in which they walked on the balls of their feet.[86] Like those with occupational manganese exposures and normal liver function, these patients did not respond to L-dopa (Table 22–3).

Tremors

Tremors are be observed with adrenergic excess, with specific xenobiotics such as lithium, or as a result of sedative–hypnotic withdrawal. These are well reviewed elsewhere.[63]

The Neuromuscular Junction

Flaccid paralysis usually occurs as a result of impaired transmission at the NMJ[15,16,82] or from xenobiotics causing demyelination.[56] Mechanisms of NMJ transmission impairment include impeded propagation of the action potential on the terminal neuron, impaired or excessive release of acetylcholine, depression of motor end-plate potential with failure of depolarization or recovery, or impedance of myofibril excitation[56,82] (Chap. 66).

Xenobiotics can enhance transmission at the NMJ. Latrotoxin, the toxic compound in the black widow spider (*Latrodectus* spp) venom causes enhanced release of acetylcholine at the NMJ with severe, painful muscle contractions. Some types of snake and scorpion venoms act similarly, as do carbamates and organic phosphorus compounds (Chap. 119).

NEUROPATHIES AND MYOPATHIES

Cranial Nerves

Xenobiotics are a relatively rare cause of cranial nerve impairment. Some neuropathies are a result of direct delivery of the xenobiotic to the affected cranial nerve. For example, some patients can have optic nerve impairment from intraorbital installation of silicone oil[7] or inadvertent deep space

injection of a local anesthetic during dental anesthesia with a resultant abducens palsy.[62] In some cases, a xenobiotic, methanol, is converted into a toxic substance such as formic acid in the retina.

The NMJ of the cranial nerves (CNs) is sensitive to disruptions in neurotransmission. When xenobiotics affect the occulomotor nerves (CNs III, IV, VI), patients describe diplopia or have gaze palsies on examination. Botulinum toxin, diethylene glycol toxicity, elapid snake venom, and the cranial neuropathy associated with the organic phosphorus compounds–induced intermediate syndrome are some examples.

Absence of glucose or thiamine results in ophthalmoplegia. In most cases, however, the mechanisms underlying the cranial neuropathy are poorly understood, such as is the case with antineoplastics. Some patients who survive ethylene glycol poisoning experience transient ophthalmoplegia days after the initial exposure.[57,84] Transient ataxia and ophthalmoplegia are described in a Nigerian population consuming the larvae of the moth *Anaphe venata* as a source of dietary protein. The larvae contain thiaminase, rendering patients acutely thiamine deficient[6] (Table 22–4 and Chap. 24).

Peripheral Nerves

Complaints of pain, paresthesias, numbness, or weakness of extremities are clinically termed *neuropathies*. The mechanisms of evolution are variable. Common to most xenobiotic-induced neuropathies is early symmetrical involvement of the lower extremities. This is due in part to the patient's rapid recognition of impairment during an attempt to ambulate. Additionally, the axons serving the lower extremities are longer. Maintenance and transportation of substrates is more energy dependent and sensitive to xenobiotic-induced disruptions.

In some cases, the anatomic structure of the nerve is maintained, but the xenobiotic affects neurotransmission. This can be due to direct impairment of specific enzymes at the NMJ, such as cholinesterase inhibitors.[28] Tri-*ortho*-cresyl phosphate (TOCP) is an inhibitor of neuropathic target esterase. Contamination of food and the alcoholic beverage "Ginger Jake" with TOCP resulted in irreversible lower extremity paralysis in several epidemic exposures during Prohibition.[71,91] Indirectly, the extracellular environment is altered as in the case of hypermagnesemia or hypokalemia, which is induced by multiple xenobiotics (Chap. 12). Ciguatoxin, a sodium channel opener, affects neurotransmission, causing paresthesias and the unusual symptom of temperature reversal in which the perception of temperature is opposite to the stimulus.

Xenobiotics such as amiodarone and tacrolimus induce peripheral demyelination. Patients present with weakness and flaccidity. Nitrous oxide impairs the production of *S*-adenosyl methionine essential to the production of myelin and is additive to the nitrous oxide disruptions of vitamin B_{12}, which further impair axonal function. Patients with chronic nitrous oxide misuse often have proprioceptive loss as a result.[92]

Other xenobiotics affect the structure or intracellular function of the peripheral nerves. Those that induce death of the cell body are termed *neuronopathies* and, at onset, are clinically indistinguishable from those that affect the axon, or *axonopathies*.

Peripheral nerve cell death is usually linked to injury at the spinal cord as was described above by the doxorubicin injection of the peripheral nerves.[51] Pyridoxine overdose is another cause of neuronopathy. However, neuronopathies are an unusual mechanism of peripheral nerve toxicity.

Unlike neuronopathies, axonopathies are potentially reversible and are the most common mechanism of xenobiotic-induced peripheral neuropathy. Xenobiotic-induced axonal injuries to the peripheral nerves are usually diffuse and bilateral, with preservation of the proximal cell body. These often target the cytoskeleton and impair the capacity for the microtubule system to deliver functional substrates.[22,41] Patients with occupational exposure to 2,5-hexanedione, a diketone metabolite of *n*-hexane present in certain glues, suffer from a sensorimotor axonopathy due to cross-linking of neurofilaments and impaired substrate transport.[68] Progressive neuropathy often occurs long after the initial exposure. Vincristine similarly affects axonal transport. Acrylamide impairs fast anterograde and retrograde transport in animal models, suggesting effects on both kinesin and dynein.

TABLE 22–4	Cranial Neuropathies		
Cranial Nerve	**Signs**	**Symptoms/Signs**	**Xenobiotics**[a]
I[b]		Failure to detect odor	Hydrogen sulfide: olfactory fatigue
II	Pupil unresponsive to light	Blindness	Amiodarone, ammonia, cisplatin, clioquinol, deferoxamine, DEG, dimethyl mercury, holocyclotoxin, interferon α, methanol, methotrexate, methyl iodide, oxaliplatin, quinine, solvents
III	Paralysis: ptosis, mydriasis: unresponsive or sluggish to light, motor impairment extraocular muscles, adduction	Photophobia	Amiodarone, antimuscarinics, botulinum toxin, DEG, holocyclotoxin, hypoglycemics, interferon α, methyl iodide, paralytics, thallium, venoms (Elapidae, scorpion)
	Stimulation: miosis	Dim vision	Cholinergic muscarinics
IV	Paralysis of the superior oblique muscle of eye with weakness of downward gaze, slight upward gaze of affected eye	Vertical and torsional diplopia that worsens on adduction and improves with tilt of head	Barbiturates, botulinum toxin, DEG, holocyclotoxin, thallium, venoms
V	Diminished facial sensation, weakness in chewing and swallowing	Paresthesias face, weakness in chewing	Botulinum toxin, ethylene glycol, holocyclotoxin, oxaliplatin, vincristine
	Excessive contraction	Trismus	Tetanospasmin and strychnine[c]
VI	Failure to abduct eye on lateral gaze	Diplopia	Botulinum toxin, DEG, holocyclotoxin, intrathecal water-soluble contrast agents, lithium, local anesthetics, MDMA, nitroglycerin, ornithine aminotransferase deficiency, oxaliplatin, thallium, thiamine deficiency, venom (elapid), vitamin A
VII[b]	Weakness of facial muscles, impaired expression	Facial droop, impaired taste	Botulinum toxin, DEG, ethylene glycol, holocyclotoxin
VIII[b]	Impaired hearing on auditory testing, nystagmus	Alterations in hearing, potential alterations in balance	Aminoglycosides, cisplatin, DEG, ethylene glycol, loop diuretics, oxalosis, quinine, salicylates, solvents
IX[d]	Decreased gag reflex	Impaired taste	Anesthetics (oral), botulinum toxin, cholinergic compounds, ethylene glycol, stibanate[d]
X[d,e]	Paralysis: Decreased gag reflex	Choking, change in voice	Botulinum toxin, ethylene glycol, stibanate[d]
	Stimulation: autonomic instability	Bradycardia, bronchorrhea	Cholinergics
	GI stimulation	bronchospasm, diarrhea, vomiting	
XI[d]	Weakness shoulder shrug	Weakness neck/shoulders	Botulinum toxin, cholinergic compounds,[d] paralytics
XII[d]	Impaired speech, tongue deviation	Dysarthria	Botulinum toxin, cholinergic compounds[d]

[a]Lists are not intended to be exclusive or exhaustive. [b]See also Chap. 25. [c]Tetanus causes indirect effects on masseter muscles; see section on xenobiotic-induced seizures or Chap. 114. [d]Weakness of cranial nerves IX–XII is often referred to as bulbar palsy and can be seen in the intermediate syndrome after acute organic phosphorus compound poisoning. This syndrome is often accompanied by paralysis of extraocular muscles (Chap. 110). [e]See Chap. 3.

DEG = diethylene glycol; MDMA = methylenedioxymethamphetamine.

Nucleoside reverse transcriptase inhibitors cause peripheral neuropathy by decreasing the production of mitochondrial DNA.

Myopathies

Some patients experience local muscle damage as a result of direct injury from extravasation of tissue toxic substances or enzymatic degradation associated with crotalid snake envenomations.

Most xenobiotic-induced muscle injuries or myopathies are more diffuse.[40,76,84,90] 3-Hydroxy-3-methylglutaryl–coenzyme A (HMG Co-A) reductase inhibitors infrequently cause myalgias, cramping, myositis, or rhabdomyolysis. The incidence appears to be higher in patients taking other medications that share the same liver metabolic enzymes. The mechanism underlying the myopathy is likely related to impaired cholesterol synthesis in myocytes or diminished production of regulatory proteins such as ubiquinone and GTP-binding proteins required for mitochondrial function.

Another myopathy that presents predominantly with weakness is the acute quadriplegic myopathy of intensive care patients. This syndrome was originally described in ventilated patients with asthma who received glucocorticoids and nondepolarizing neuromuscular blockers, but is also reported in other critically ill patients[9] (Chap. 66). The mechanisms underlying quadriplegic myopathy, eosinophilia myalgia syndrome, and toxic oil syndrome are poorly described. Xenobiotics associated with muscle injury are found in Table 22–5.

TABLE 22–5	Xenobiotics Associated with Muscle Toxicity*
ε-Aminocaproic acid	Niacin
Amiodarone	Organic phosphorus compounds
Chloroquine	D-Penicillamine
Cimetidine	Phencyclidine
Clofibrate	Procainamide
Clostridium toxins	Propylthiouracil
Cocaine	Rifampin
Colchicine	Snake venoms
Cyclosporine	Succinylcholine
Doxylamine	Sulfonamides
Ethanol	Syrup of ipecac
Ethchlorvynol	Toxic oil syndrome
Glucocorticosteroids	*Tricholoma equestre* (mushroom)
Heroin	L-Tryptophan
HMG-CoA reductase inhibitors	Vincristine
Hydroxychloroquine	Zidovudine
Loxosceles spp venom	

*Toxicity with adrenergics cause indirect rhabdomyolysis due to neurobehavioral muscular exertion and tonic contracture. Similarly xenobiotics which cause status epilepticus, as well as xenobiotics that precipitate NMS or serotonin toxicity also result in indirect rhabdomyolysis.

SUMMARY

- The central nervous system has unique anatomic and transporter mechanisms to limit xenobiotic penetration.
- Disruption of these protections can result in neurotoxicity.
- The chemical properties of the xenobiotic and the characteristic of the patient exposed affect the clinical expression of neurotoxicity.
- The peripheral nervous system is similarly vulnerable to toxicity and the patterns of injury are reflected in the clinical presentation.

Acknowledgment

E. John Gallagher, MD, contributed to this chapter in previous editions.

REFERENCES

1. Abbott NJ. Astrocyte-endothelial interactions and blood-brain barrier permeability. *J Anat.* 2002;200:629-638.
2. Abbott NJ. Inflammatory mediators and modulation of blood-brain barrier permeability. *Cell Mol Neurobiol.* 2000;20:131-147.
3. Abbott NJ, et al. The blood-brain barrier in systemic lupus erythematosus. *Lupus.* 2003;12:908-915.
4. Abbott NJ, Romero IA. Transporting therapeutics across the blood-brain barrier. *Mol Med Today.* 1996;2:106-113.
5. Abouesh A, et al. Antimicrobial-induced mania (antibiomania): a review of spontaneous reports. *J Clin Psychopharmacol.* 2002;22:71-81.
6. Adelmolekun B, Ibikunle FR. Investigation of an epidemic of seasonal ataxia in Ikare, Western Nigeria. *Acta Neurol Scand.* 1994;90:309-311.
7. Agrawal R, et al. Silicone oil-associated optic nerve degeneration. *Am J Ophthalmol.* 2002;133:429-430.
8. Anonymous. Parkinsonian syndrome and calcium channel blockers. *Prescrire Int.* 2003;12:62.
9. Argov Z. Drug-induced myopathies. *Curr Opin Neurol.* 2000;13:541-545.
10. Ariffin H, et al. Severe vincristine neurotoxicity with concomitant use of itraconazole. *J Paediatr Child Health.* 2003;39:638-639.
11. Arundine M, Tymianski M. Molecular mechanisms of calcium-dependent neurodegeneration in excitotoxicity. *Cell Calcium.* 2003;34:325-337.
12. Aschner M, et al. Astrocyte modulation of neurotoxic injury. *Brain Pathol.* 2002;12:475-481.
13. Balis FM, et al. Methotrexate distribution within the subarachnoid space after intraventricular and intravenous administration. *Cancer Chemother Pharmacol.* 2000;45:259-264.
14. Bearer EL, et al. Squid axoplasm supports the retrograde axonal transport of herpes simplex virus. *Biol Bull.* 1999;197:257-258.
15. Ben-Ami M, et al. The combination of magnesium sulphate and nifedipine: a cause of neuromuscular blockade. *Br J Obstet Gynaecol.* 1994;101:262-263.
16. Best JA, et al. Neuromuscular blockade after clindamycin administration: a case report. *J Oral Maxillofac Surg.* 1999;57:600-603.
17. Bhatia R, et al. Tetanus. *Neurol India.* 2002;50:398-407.
18. Bleich S, et al. Plasma homocysteine is a predictor of alcohol withdrawal seizures. *Neuroreport.* 2000;11:2749-2752.
19. Bleich S, et al. Homocysteine as a neurotoxin in chronic alcoholism. *Prog Neuropsychopharmacol Biol Psychiatry.* 2004;28:453-464.
20. Boffi BV, Klerman GL. Manic psychosis associated with appetite suppressant medication, phenylpropanolamine. *J Clin Psychopharmacol.* 1989;9:308-309.
21. Burneo JG, et al. Neurotoxicity following addition of intravenous valproate to lamotrigine therapy. *Neurology.* 2003;60:1991-1992.
22. Chang MH, et al. Reversible myeloneuropathy resulting from podophyllin intoxication: an electrophysiological follow up. *J Neurol Neurosurg Psychiatry.* 1992;55:235-236.
23. Chauvenet AR, et al. Vincristine-induced neuropathy as the initial presentation of Charcot-Marie-Tooth disease in acute lymphoblastic leukemia: a Pediatric Oncology Group study. *J Pediatr Hematol Oncol.* 2003;25:316-320.
24. Chen CY, et al. Heroin-induced spongiform leukoencephalopathy: value of diffusion MR imaging. *J Comput Assist Tomogr.* 2000;24:735-737.
25. Cherry CL, et al. Nucleoside analogues and neuropathy in the era of HAART. *J Clin Virol.* 2003;26:195-207.
26. Chishty M, et al. Affinity for the *P*-glycoprotein efflux pump at the blood-brain barrier may explain the lack of CNS side-effects of modern antihistamines. *J Drug Target.* 2001;9:223-228.
27. Chuang C, et al. Chemotherapy-induced parkinsonism responsive to levodopa: an underrecognized entity. *Mov Disord.* 2003;18:328-331.
28. Chuang CC, et al. Delayed neuropathy and myelopathy after organophosphate intoxication. *N Engl J Med.* 2002;347:1119-1121.
29. Chung RS, West AK. A role for extracellular metallothioneins in CNS injury and repair. *Neuroscience.* 2004;123:595-599.
30. Cliff J, et al. Association of high cyanide and low sulphur intake in cassava-induced spastic paraparesis. *Lancet.* 1985;2:1211-1213.
31. Dobson AW, et al. Manganese neurotoxicity. *Ann N Y Acad Sci.* 2004;1012:115-128.
32. Driesen JJ, Wolters EC. Bilateral ballism induced by oral contraceptives. A case report. *J Neurol.* 1986;233:379.
33. Dutta D, et al. Angiotensin converting enzyme inhibitor induced hyperkalaemic paralysis. *Postgrad Med J.* 2001;77:114-115.
34. Elinav E, Chajek-Shaul T. Licorice consumption causing severe hypokalemic paralysis. *Mayo Clin Proc.* 2003;78:767-768.
35. Ellis WG, et al. Leukoencephalopathy in patients treated with amphotericin B methyl ester. *J Infect Dis.* 1982;146:125-137.
36. Erikson KM, Aschner M. Manganese neurotoxicity and glutamate-GABA interaction. *Neurochem Int.* 2003;43:475-480.
37. Erikson KM, et al. Airborne manganese exposure differentially affects end points of oxidative stress in an age- and sex-dependent manner. *Biol Trace Elem Res.* 2004;100:49-62.
38. Freimer ML, et al. Chronic demyelinating polyneuropathy associated with eosinophilia-myalgia syndrome. *J Neurol Neurosurg Psychiatry.* 1992;55:352-358.
39. Fukuda T. Neurotoxicity of MPTP. *Neuropathology.* 2001;21:323-332.
40. George KK, Pourmand R. Toxic myopathies. *Neurol Clin.* 1997;15:711-730.
41. Graham DG. Neurotoxicants and the cytoskeleton. *Curr Opin Neurol.* 1999;12:733-737.
42. Grattan-Smith PJ, et al. Clinical and neurophysiological features of tick paralysis. *Brain.* 1997;120:1975-1987.
43. Hampson DR, Manalo JL. The activation of glutamate receptors by kainic acid and domoic acid. *Nat Toxins.* 1998;6:153-158.
44. Huang CC, et al. Clinical course in patients with chronic carbon disulfide polyneuropathy. *Clin Neurol Neurosurg.* 2002;104:115-120.
45. Huang CC, et al. Dopamine transporter binding study in differentiating carbon disulfide induced parkinsonism from idiopathic parkinsonism. *Neurotoxicology.* 2004;25:341-347.
46. Israel ZH, et al. Multifocal demyelinative leukoencephalopathy associated with 5-fluorouracil and levamisole. *Acta Oncol.* 2000;39:117-120.
47. Iwata K, et al. Neurologic problems associated with chronic nitrous oxide abuse in a non-healthcare worker. *Am J Med Sci.* 2001;322:173-174.
48. Jackson AC. Rabies virus infection: an update. *J Neurovirol.* 2003;9:253-258.
49. Jarosz JM, et al. Cyclosporine-related reversible posterior leukoencephalopathy: MRI. *Neuroradiology.* 1997;39:711-715.
50. Jeanjean AP, et al. Neuroleptic binding to sigma receptors: possible involvement in neuroleptic-induced acute dystonia. *Biol Psychiatry.* 1997;41:1010-1019.
51. Kato S, et al. Retrograde adriamycin sensory ganglionectomy: novel approach for the treatment of intractable pain. *Stereotact Funct Neurosurg.* 1990;54-55:86-89.
52. Klos KJ, et al. Neurologic spectrum of chronic liver failure and basal ganglia T1 hyperintensity on magnetic resonance imaging. *Arch Neurol.* 2005;62:1385-1390.
53. Kroll RA, Neuwelt EA. Outwitting the blood-brain barrier for therapeutic purposes: osmotic opening and other means. *Neurosurgery.* 1998;42:1083-1099.
54. Kroll RA, et al. Improving drug delivery to intracerebral tumor and surrounding brain in a rodent model: a comparison of osmotic versus bradykinin modification of the blood-brain and/or blood-tumor barriers. *Neurosurgery.* 1998;43:879-886.
55. Lang CJ. The use of neuroimaging techniques for clinical detection of neurotoxicity: a review. *Neurotoxicology.* 2000;21:847-855.
56. Levin KH. Variants and mimics of Guillain Barre syndrome. *Neurologist.* 2004;10:61-74.
57. Lewis LD, et al. Delayed sequelae after acute overdoses or poisonings: cranial neuropathy related to ethylene glycol ingestion. *Clin Pharmacol Ther.* 1997;61:692-699.
58. Lo EH, et al. Drug delivery to damaged brain. *Brain Res Brain Res Rev.* 2001;38:140-148.
59. LoPachin RM. The changing view of acrylamide neurotoxicity. *Neurotoxicology.* 2004;25:617-630.
60. Lowenstein DH, Bleck T, Macdonald RL. It's time to revise the definition of status epilepticus. *Epilepsia.* 1999;40:120-122.
61. Manzo L, et al. Assessing effects of neurotoxic pollutants by biochemical markers. *Environ Res.* 2001;85:31-36.
62. Marinho RO. Abducent nerve palsy following dental local analgesia. *Br Dent J.* 1995;179:69-70.
63. Morgan JC, Sethi KD. Drug-induced tremors. *Lancet Neurol.* 2005;4:866-876.
64. Neuwelt EA. Mechanisms of disease: the blood-brain barrier. *Neurosurgery.* 2004;54:131-140.
65. Nilsen J, Diaz Brinton R. Mechanism of estrogen-mediated neuroprotection: regulation of mitochondrial calcium and Bcl-2 expression. *Proc Natl Acad Sci U S A.* 2003;100:2842-2847.
66. Norenberg MD. Oxidative and nitrosative stress in ammonia neurotoxicity [comment]. *Hepatology.* 2003;37:245-248.
67. Norenberg MD, Jayakumar AR, Rama Rao KV. Oxidative stress in the pathogenesis of hepatic encephalopathy. *Metab Brain Dis.* 2004;19:313-329.
68. Oge AM, et al. Peripheral and central conduction in n-hexane polyneuropathy. *Muscle Nerve.* 1994;17:1416-1430.
69. Orth M, Tabrizi SJ. Models of Parkinson's disease. *Mov Disord.* 2003;18:729-737.
70. Pai KS, Ravindranath V. L-BOAA induces selective inhibition of brain mitochondrial enzyme, NADH-dehydrogenase. *Brain Res.* 1993;621:215-221.
71. Parascandola J. The Public Health Service and Jamaica ginger paralysis in the 1930s. *Public Health Rep.* 1995;110:361-363.
72. Picazo O, et al. Neuroprotective and neurotoxic effects of estrogens. *Brain Res.* 2003;990:20-27.
73. Pourmand R. Diabetic neuropathy. *Neurol Clin.* 1997;15:569-576.

74. Reynolds IJ. Mitochondrial membrane potential and the permeability transition in excitotoxicity. *Ann N Y Acad Sci.* 1999;893:33-41.

75. Rodnitzky RL. Drug-induced movement disorders in children. *Semin Pediatr Neurol.* 2003;10:80-87.

76. Rosenson RS. Current overview of statin-induced myopathy. *Am J Med.* 2004;116:408-416.

77. Sadeque AJ, et al. Increased drug delivery to the brain by P-glycoprotein inhibition. *Clin Pharmacol Ther.* 2000;68:231-237.

78. Salzer W, et al. Effect of probenecid on ventricular cerebrospinal fluid methotrexate pharmacokinetics after intralumbar administration in nonhuman primates. *Cancer Chemother Pharmacol.* 2001;48:235-240.

79. Sande MA, et al. Factors influencing the penetration of antimicrobial agents into the cerebrospinal fluid of experimental animals. *Scand J Infect Dis Suppl.* 1978;14:160-163.

80. Saunders NR, et al. Barriers in the immature brain. *Cell Mol Neurobiol.* 2000;20:29-40.

81. Schaumberg HH, et al. Occupational manganese neurotoxicity provoked by hepatitis C. *Neurology.* 2006;67:322-323.

82. Senanayake N, Roman GC. Disorders of neuromuscular transmission due to natural environmental toxins. *J Neurol Sci.* 1992;107:1-13.

83. Shigenaga MK, et al. Oxidative damage and mitochondrial decay in aging. *Proc Natl Acad Sci U S A.* 1994;91:10771-10778.

84. Sieb JP, Gillessen T. Iatrogenic and toxic myopathies. *Muscle Nerve.* 2003;27:142-156.

85. Spillane L, et al. Multiple cranial nerve deficits after ethylene glycol poisoning. *Ann Emerg Med.* 1991;20:208-210.

86. Stepens A, et al. A Parkinsonian syndrome in methcathione users and the role of manganese. *N Engl J Med.* 2008;358:1009-1017.

87. Stoltenberg M, et al. Retrograde axonal transport of bismuth: an autometallographic study. *Acta Neuropathol.* 2001;101:123-128.

88. Teive HA, et al. Parkinsonian syndrome induced by amlodipine: case report. *Mov Disord.* 2002;17:833-835.

89. Thompson PD, et al. Statin-associated myopathy. *JAMA.* 2003;289:1681-1690.

90. Tosi L, et al. October 1942: a strange epidemic paralysis in Saval, Verona, Italy. Revision and diagnosis 50 years later of tri-*ortho*-cresyl phosphate poisoning. *J Neurol Neurosurg Psychiatry.* 1994;57:810-813.

91. Tshala-Katumbay DD, et al. Cyanide and the human brain: perspective from a model of food (cassava) poisoning. *Ann N Y Acad Sci. Ann N Y Acad Sci.* 2016;1378:50-57.

92. Waclawik AJ, et al. Myeloneuropathy from nitrous oxide abuse: unusually high methylmalonic acid and homocysteine levels. *WMJ.* 2003;102:43-45.

93. Wagner AK, et al. Relationships between cerebrospinal fluid markers of excitotoxicity, ischemia, and oxidative damage after severe TBI: the impact of gender, age, and hypothermia. *J Neurotrauma.* 2004;21:125-136.

94. Wiley RG, et al. Suicide transport: destruction of neurons by retrograde transport of ricin, abrin, and modeccin. *Science.* 1982;216:889-890.

95. Yamada S, et al. Effects of aminoglycoside antibiotics on the neuromuscular junction: part I. *Int J Clin Pharmacol Ther Toxicol.* 1986;24:130-138.

96. Zheng W, et al. Brain barrier systems: a new frontier in metal neurotoxicological research. *Toxicol Appl Pharmacol.* 2003;192:1-11.

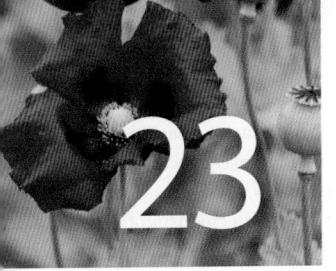

23 ONCOLOGIC PRINCIPLES

Richard Y. Wang

In 2012, there were 1.5 million persons with newly diagnosed invasive cancer in the United States.[41] Among patients receiving chemotherapy for their disease, some will seek further care at an emergency department and require inpatient hospitalization for effects related to their treatment.[10,35,38] In a prospective analysis of cancer registry data, 8.7% (179/2068) of patients receiving chemotherapy were admitted to the hospital for chemotherapy-related effects.[14] Fever, neutropenia, and severe gastroenteritis are common reasons for inpatient care among patients receiving chemotherapy.[14,21,35]

The chemotherapeutics employed in curative and palliative regimens in many cases preclude cell division via a variety of mechanisms. Chemotherapeutics have also found expanded use in a variety of rheumatologic, dermatologic, and autoimmune disorders. Clinicians caring for patients affected by chemotherapeutics should understand the expected cellular responses from an initial and long-term exposure perspective. Chemotherapeutics cause damage primarily to deoxyribonucleic acid (DNA). This chapter will provide the reader with a focused review of cellular growth and proliferation, DNA damage from chemotherapeutics, the response of the cell to DNA damage, and the response of the tissues commonly affected by chemotherapeutics. This information will enhance the clinician's management of patients affected by chemotherapeutics. New cancer therapies, such as targeted therapeutics and immunotherapies, are available for clinical use, and these therapies are discussed elsewhere (Chap. 50).[23]

CELL GROWTH AND PROLIFERATION

Cell Cycle

Cell activities are growth, metabolism, proliferation, apoptosis, and senescence. The cell cycle is the classic paradigm that depicts cell proliferation in sequential steps that are represented by phases, and it is coordinated by the cell-cycle control system (Fig. 23–1).[47] The phases are G_0 (resting phase), G_1, S (synthesis), G_2, and M (mitosis). Stem cells tend to reside at G_0. When cells are stimulated by a mitotic stimulant, such as a growth factor, they leave the resting phase and enter the cell cycle. G_1-, S-, and G_2-phases are known as the *interphase* of the cell cycle, and they encompass cell growth and DNA replication. G_1 and G_2 are growth or *gap phases*, and they allow for growth and regulatory processes that aid in the transition from the S-phase to the M-phase. The G_1-phase is the most variable in duration among cell types, and it controls or determines the length of the cell cycle. A typical cell cycle takes about 24 hours, and mitosis takes about 20 to 60 minutes.[15] The replication of DNA occurs in the S-phase, and mitosis and cytokinesis occur in the M-phase. The G_2-phase likely serves to prevent the unintended consequence of a cell undergoing separation with an incomplete copy of the DNA. The fidelity of cellular duplication is ensured by checkpoints located throughout the cell cycle.

DNA Replication

The process for DNA replication begins in the G_1-phase, occurs in the S-phase, and ends in the G_2-phase. There are several steps in the process, including identification of the origins for replication, incorporation of protein complexes at these origins, DNA unwinding, DNA elongation, and DNA termination. The cell enters mitosis at the completion of DNA replication.

In the G_1-phase, the replication origins on the DNA are identified and the pre-replication complex (pre-RC) is formed. This complex consists of the origin recognition complex, MCM (mini-microsomal maintenance) (inactive helicase), CDT1, and CDC6, which facilitates the loading of MCM into the pre-RC. In the transition from the G_1-phase to the S-phase, the pre-IC is

formed and it activates helicase (via the CDC45-MCM-GINS {CMG} helicase complex), which begins DNA replication in the S-phase.

In the S-phase, DNA unwinds using the CMG helicase complex, elongates, and undergoes synthesis. The replisome accomplishes these steps during DNA replication, which includes assembly of supporting proteins, unwinding, polymerization, synthesis of RNA primers, and coordination of the polymerization between the leading and lagging strands of DNA.

The replisome is comprised of DNA polymerase, helicase, single-strand DNA binding protein, trimetric clamp processivity factor (enables DNA polymerase to synthesize a continuous strand of DNA on a template DNA without frequent dissociation), pentameric clamp loader complex, and primase. In addition, the replisome contains a translesion DNA polymerase, which allows the cell to bypass extensively damaged DNA and continue with DNA replication.

In general, the replication process proceeds in the following manner: DNA unwinds, forms replication forks, strands are stabilized by single-strand-binding proteins to prevent coiling, tension on the DNA helix in front of the replication fork is relaxed by topoisomerases I and II, and the ATR-ATRIP complex (ataxia telangiectasia mutated and Rad3-related-ATR-interacting protein) limits excessive firing or activation of origin complexes during the S-phase. Deoxyribonucleic acid elongation uses various DNA polymerases (ie, alpha, delta, and epsilon) in the synthesis of DNA. RNA primase forms a RNA primer

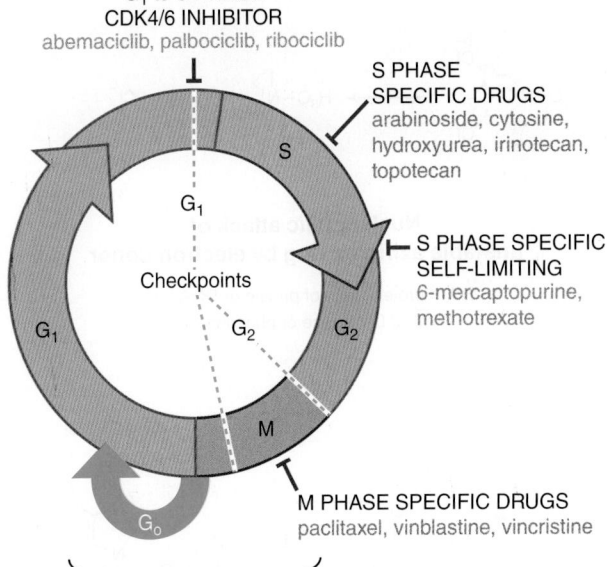

FIGURE 23–1. Cell cycle specificity of chemotherapeutics: selected class of cell cycle phase–specific chemotherapeutics and their sites of action in the cell cycle. Arrows represent the progression of the cell cycle by phases, G_0 (resting), G_1 (gap1), G_2 (gap2), M (mitosis), and S (DNA synthesis). The colors of each chemotherapeutic is matched with its cell cycle of activity. *(Reproduced with permission from Brunton LL, Hilal-Dandan R, Knollmann BC. Goodman & Gilman's: The Pharmacological Basis of Therapeutics, 13th ed. New York: NY: McGraw Hill Education; 2018.)*

that is used by DNA polymerase to synthesize a complementary chain to the template DNA chain in a 5′ to 3′ direction. In the leading strand, DNA is synthesized in a continuous manner as it follows behind the CMG helicase complex. In contrast to the leading strand, the lagging strand DNA is synthesized in fragments that are later joined to form a continuous strand. Deoxyribonucleic acid polymerase removes RNA primers and replaces the segments with deoxyribonucleotides. Deoxyribonucleic acid ligase joins remaining gaps between fragments. When DNA replication is complete, the cell will enter G_2/M-phase.

CELL INJURY AND DNA DAMAGE

Cellular injuries caused by chemotherapeutics are typically from a stress that impairs a DNA function, such as replication. Cells undergoing proliferation that are injured by stress to DNA will halt the cell cycle by activating a checkpoint, and it will attempt to repair the injury. If the repair is unsuccessful or there is a significant injury, the cell will undergo apoptosis or senescence. Stress may also be indirect, such as impairment of the spindle fibers during mitosis. When stress causes a structural change to DNA, such as a break in the strand of DNA or the presence of a bulky adduct, the result is considered a damaged DNA.[43] Structural damage to DNA can be repaired; however, errors in the repair can lead to mutations. Mutation is a heritable change in the encoded nucleotide sequence of the DNA. Cells with mutations and a slow replication tend to accumulate over time, and they will develop into tumors that occur at an increased age of the host organism. Cells with mutations and a fast replication tend to develop into tumors at an early age.

Some chemotherapeutics cause DNA damage by forming bulky adducts, such as by alkylation or intrastrand crosslinks. For example, cisplatin causes DNA crosslinks (approximately 90% intrastrand and <5% interstrand); and nitrogen mustard, nitrosoureas, and triazenes cause alkyl-DNA adducts (Fig. 23–2).[6] At very high doses, chemotherapeutics can cause additional

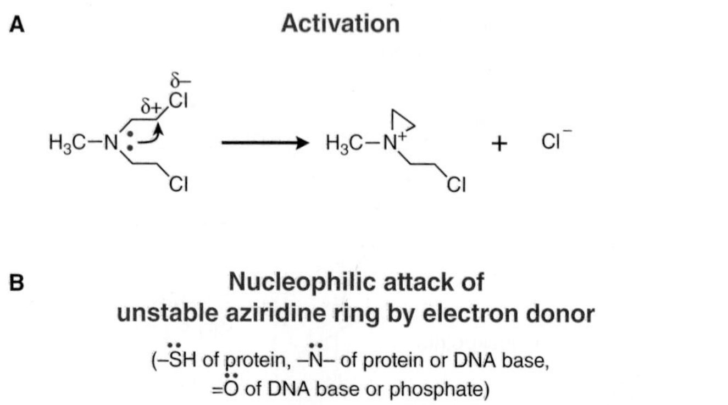

toxicities (Chaps. 50 and 51). Some chemotherapeutics act at specific phases in the cell cycle and they are known as cell cycle phase–specific chemotherapeutics. For example, vincristine acts specifically during the M-phase, and cytarabine acts during the S-phase based on the mechanism of action (Fig. 23–1). These chemotherapeutics will not affect cells in the G_0-phase. However, cell cycle phase–nonspecific chemotherapeutics, like alkylating agents, affect cells at all phases of the cell cycle.

Cell senescence is considered a protective outcome because it arrests DNA-damaged cells, and it is a process of aging. The factors determining cell senescence are the cell type, type of damage, and severity of damage. Although the specific initiators of senescence are unknown, these items likely involve dysfunctional telomeres, damaged DNA, dysfunctional chromatin, oncogenes, and other types of stresses to the cell. The pathways involved with senescence are p53 (primary) and p16-pRB (retinoblastoma protein) (secondary).

CHECKPOINTS THAT REGULATE DNA REPLICATION

Checkpoints work with the phases of the cell cycle to regulate cellular duplication so the process is accomplished in a correct manner. For example, cells with damaged DNA will not proceed in the cell cycle because this type of damage will lead to a cell with unstable genetic material during mitosis. Notable checkpoints are located at G_1/S, the S-phase, the G_2/M boundary, and the M-phase.[51] The checkpoint at G_1/S is the major one in humans. In the G-phase, DNA replication checkpoints arrest cell cycle progression and inhibit firing of late replication origins in response to stressors. The checkpoint in the S-phase slows down DNA replication and cell cycle progression when the DNA replication fork stalls. A stalled fork can result from an obstacle such as an adduct, a lack of substrates (eg, nucleotide), or an inactive enzyme.[28] The checkpoint at G_2/M is considered important for determining cell survival or death because many cells are observed to be halted at the G_2-phase. In the M-phase, a cell with damaged DNA can undergo apoptosis (initiated by spindle assembly checkpoint {SAC}), undergo endoreplication (ie, DNA replication but no cell division), or return to mitosis.[9] Cells with endoreplication will survive, but they cannot proliferate.

Cyclin-dependent kinases (Cdks) are a family of serine/threonine protein kinases that are responsible for the phosphorylation of specific proteins and the binding of inhibitory proteins in the cell cycle.[7,40] Cyclin-dependent kinases are activated by rising concentrations of specific cyclins and Cdk-activating kinases, and inhibited by other proteins and protein kinases. For example, in the G_1-phase, mitotic stimulants, such as growth factors, activate the complex cyclin D-Cdk4 by increasing cyclin D by gene expression, which binds to Cdk4. This complex activates the transcription factor E2F, which is important for entering the cell cycle. E2F promotes the expression of genes responsible for DNA synthesis and the production of cyclins E and A, which are needed for the G_1/S transition and the S-phase, respectively.

Cyclin E complexes with Cdk2, which activates the inhibitory pRb that regulates EF2 to ensure the expression of genes specific to G_1/S at the proper time in the cell cycle. Cyclin A complexes with Cdk2, which is involved with chromosome condensation and the firing of replication origins. In the M-phase, the increased concentration of cyclin A–Cdk complex, decreased concentrations of the protein kinases Wee1 and Myt1, and the increased concentration of the phosphatase Cdc25 activates the cyclin B–Cdk1 complex, which is necessary for the early stages of mitosis leading to metaphase and the activation of the anaphase-promoting complex (APC). The APC is a protease complex that degrades the remaining cyclins in the S- and M-phases, and it signifies the transition from metaphase to anaphase and the beginning of the exit from mitosis. When the cell leaves the M-phase and enters the G_1-phase, the Cdk concentration is kept low by decreased gene expression of cyclin and increased cyclin degradation. The cell cycle is activated by increasing the concentration of cyclin D at this phase.

A cascading event of inhibitory proteins and protein complexes halt the cell cycle by inhibiting Cdk activity in the G_1-phase when there is DNA damage. For example, when ATM kinase detects a DNA double-strand break (DSB) it rapidly halts the cell cycle by inhibiting the activation of

FIGURE 23–2. Mechanism of action of alkylating agents of mechlorethamine, a prototypic nitrogen mustard. (**A**) Activation reaction. (**B**) Alkylation of N7 of guanine. With bifunctional drugs such as nitrogen mustards, the second 2-chloroethyl side chain can undergo a similar activation crosslink of 2 nucleic acid chains or a nucleic acid to a protein. (*Modified with permission from Rollins DE, Blumenthal DK. Workbook and Casebook for Goodman and Gilman's The Pharmacological Basis of Therapeutics. New York: NY: McGraw-Hill Education; 2018.*)

Cdk2–cyclin through Chk2 and Cdc2. A later process that causes a prolonged cell arrest follows the rapid response and it involves p53. Ataxia telangiectasia mutated kinase activates p53, which causes p21 to bind and inactivate Cdk2–cyclin. When there is a stalled replication fork in the S-phase, ATR can activate p53 and p21 to halt the cell cycle. The cell cycle will restart after the DNA damage is repaired. If the damage cannot be repaired, p53 can remove the cell through apoptosis. The INK4 proteins (p15, p16, 18, and p19) inhibit the binding of Cdk4 and Cdk6 to cyclin D and the activation of cyclin D–Cdk, which halts the cell cycle at the beginning of the G_1-phase.

The SAC consists of several proteins that monitor the alignment of the spindle at the metaphase plate, the attachment of the chromosomes to the spindles through the kinetochore, and the binding of the kinetochore to spindle fibers at opposite poles.[7] If there is an irregularity in the centromere–kinetochore–microtubule interface or the tension among these structures, the SAC will inhibit the onset of anaphase by blocking the activation of APC, which is needed to activate the protease separase. Separase cleaves the protein complex that holds the sister chromatids together and this step initiates the separation of the sister chromatids during early anaphase. An irregularity in the spindle assembly results in chromosomal instability and abnormal chromosomes, such as aneuploidy. Microtubule inhibitors (eg, vinca alkaloids) prevent the proper assembly of the kinetochore microtubules and will activate the SAC.[48]

DNA REPAIR MECHANISMS

The DNA damage response (DDR) detects and repairs lesions in the DNA, and coordinates these activities with the cell cycle. The mechanism of the repair for lesions in the DNA depends on the type of the lesion and the location of the lesion in the cell cycle. When there is a lesion to a nucleotide or a single-strand break, the nuclear excision repair (NER) or the base excision repair (BER) mechanism is used to correct the lesion. When there is a double-strand break, the nonhomologous end joining (NHEJ) or the homologous recombination (HR) is used to correct the damage. Interstrand crosslinks in the DNA (caused by nitrogen mustards and cisplatin) are significant to the survival of the cell because these lesions cannot be easily repaired.[6,29] However, intrastrand crosslinks in the DNA can continue on in the cell cycle after the lesion is addressed by the NER.[18]

The DNA repair systems for interstrand crosslinks involve the NER and translesional synthesis (TLS) when the cell is in the G_0- or G_1-phase, and HR when the cell is in the S-phase. The TLS allows DNA replication to proceed when there is extensive DNA damage by using a low-fidelity translesion polymerase. The cell's capacity to repair the DNA also determines the repair mechanism. For example, a cell with a damaged DNA and with a mutation at p53 will bypass apoptosis and end up in the M-phase.[13,34]

DNA Double-Strand Break

When a DNA double-strand break is recognized, the MRN complex (Mre11-Rad50-Nbs1) and Ku proteins secure the ends and initiate a kinase-dependent pathway that halts the cell cycle. The process starts with the ATM (ataxia telangiectasia mutated) kinase, which activates cellular processes responsible for cell cycle arrest. The ATM kinase initially forms the ATR complex (ataxia telangiectasia mutated and Rad3-related), which activates Chk1 and Chk2. The latter items inhibit the activation of Cdks by inhibiting CDC25 phosphatase. The inhibition of Cdk1 and Cdk2 halts the cell cycle, prevents the entry of the cell into the S-phase, arrests progression in the S-phase, and arrests progression in the G_2/M-phase. When the cyclin concentration is high, such as in the S- or G_2-phase, the MRN complex resects the damaged ends, which will allow an ATR-mediated response and repair by using HR. When the cyclin concentration is low, such as in the G_1-phase, the MRN complex activates the ATM, which will repair the break by using NHEJ.

Nonhomologous end joining is a sequence-independent process, occurs in the G_1-phase, and is prone to errors because a template is not used in the repair process. The NHEJ process involves binding the DNA strands, processing the adjoining ends, and repairing the break. The proteins involved with the repair are DNA ligase IV, XRCC4 (x-ray repair cross complementing group 4),

DNA-dependent protein kinase catalytic subunit (DNA-PKcs), Ku proteins (Ku70-80), and nucleases (eg, Artemis).[33] The broken strands are initially bound by Ku proteins and DNA-PKcs, the ends are processed by DNA polymerase or Artemis, and finally the ends are joined by XRCC4 /DNA ligase IV complex.[33] X-ray repair cross complementing group 4 is the regulatory unit for DNA ligase IV, and its phosphorylation appears to inhibit the repair of DNA DSBs during mitosis.[44] The NHEJ repair typically results in the loss of a few nucleotides in the sequence and a small mutation. Small mutations accumulate over time from repairs by NHEJ.

Homologous recombination is a process that occurs during the S- or G_2-phase and it is usually activated by a stalled or broken replication fork. This process requires a template, usually a sister chromatid or a homologous chromosome, to repair the damaged strand, and it is less prone for errors than NHEJ.[15] The typical repair process for a DSB involves the following: resect the ends to form overhanging segments, identify homologous sequence in the complimentary strand-by-strand exchange, fill in the gap sequence, and ligate the remaining ends.

When DNA damage is detected by the DDR during mitosis, such as a result of a checkpoint failure or a chromosomal breakage during cytokinesis, the location of the damaged sites are retained, but the ability of DDR to halt the cell cycle is inactivated. The reason for inactivating DNA repair during mitosis appears to be the cell's lack of ability to distinguish damaged DNA strands form undamaged DNA ends containing telomeres. If the repair process were to continue, cells can repair and fuse DNA ends containing telomeres (ie, anaphase bridges), which will form abnormal chromosomes, such as aneuploidy.[32] Thus, when damaged DNA is identified, the broken strands are bound by the MRN complex. The damaged DNA will be repaired when the cell leaves mitosis and enters interphase.[12] Deoxyribonucleic acid with minor damage is repaired in the G_1-phase, and those with complicated damage are repaired later in the S-phase. However, DNA with significant damage affecting the centromere or defects in chromosomal alignment will activate the SAC and result in mitotic arrest and cell death or mutagenesis through mitotic slippage.[15] The SAC uses cyclin B1 to halt mitosis for a prolonged period that allows for cell death by a caspase-dependent pathway. When cyclin B1 concentrations fall before cell death occurs, there is "mitotic slippage" and a mutagenic cell exits from mitosis.

DNA Single-Strand Breaks and Nucleotide Lesions

Single-strand breaks and lesions in nucleotides are quickly (in minutes) repaired by using NER, BER, or the mismatch repair system (during replication).[3,22] In addition, there are specialized repair proteins for specific lesions in a nucleotide (eg, methylation by alkylating agents). Some examples of this direct reversal of a lesion in a nucleotide are the methylated adducts of O6-methylguanine, 1-methyladenine, and 3-methylcytosine.

Base excision repair occurs throughout the cell cycle and it removes small non–helix distorting nucleotide lesions from the DNA. Typical lesions amenable to BER are those that result from oxidation, deamination, or alkylation by methylation. The general steps in the repair process are recognition, excision of the base, end processing to remove the sugar phosphate backbone, gap filling, and ligation. Deoxyribonucleic acid polymerases use the other strand as a template to fill in the gap, and the ligation is accomplished by DNA ligases.

Nuclear excision repair removes bulky lesions that distort the helix, such as adducts with a large chemical. The general steps in this process are recognition, incision and end processing, gap filling, and ligation. Nucleases and helicases are used to remove the lesion in NER. The nucleotide is removed by sequential action of 5′ and 3′ endonucleases followed by polymerase to fill in the remaining gap. The gap filling is accomplished by DNA polymerases and the ligation is accomplished by DNA ligases.

INJURY TO CELL LINES FROM SELECTED TISSUES

Chemotherapeutics are toxic to cells, and the tissues commonly affected are those with a high turnover of cells. These cells are the hematopoietic cells, intestinal epithelium, epidermis and hair follicles, and sperm.[25] The following discussion will focus on the cell lines of the hematologic system and intestinal epithelium. The significance of the biology of stem cells for this discussion is it is a site of toxicity for chemotherapeutics, the toxicity to the cell line is typically not immediately apparent, and the effect to the cell line has long-term consequences.[24]

The duration of progression from a stem cell to a mature cell is clinically important because this timeline will contribute to the time of appearance of toxicity from the chemotherapeutic from the time of exposure. For example, tissue toxicity will not be immediately apparent when a chemotherapeutic is administered because mature cells maintain the functioning during their survival. However, toxicity will manifest as the mature cells die and they are not replaced over time because of toxicity to the stem cells. The time between the appearance of toxicity to the cell line and the onset of toxicity to the stem cell is known as the latency period for chemotherapeutics that are toxic to the mitotic cell. The duration of the latency period also depends on the physiological rate of loss (ie, life span) of the mature cells. The duration of recovery from toxicity depends on the dose and rate of administration of a chemotherapeutic because these factors will determine the extent of injury to stem and progenitor cells.

In addition, the chemotherapeutic's site of action in the cell cycle can predict the time of onset and duration of toxicity. For the hematopoietic system, cell cycle phase–specific chemotherapeutics (eg, antimetabolites, vinca alkaloids) cause early onset and recovery of myelosuppression.[16] Cell cycle phase–nonspecific chemotherapeutics result in intermediate to late onset and recovery of myelosuppression. However, nitrogen mustards tend to cause late onset and recovery of myelosuppression because they affect the primitive stem cells.

Stem Cells

The common features of stem cells are self-renewal and differentiation into specialized cell types, compartmentalization in the body, and existence in a micro-environment known as a niche. The niche consists of many elements, including stem cells, extracellular matrix providing structural support to the cells, and soluble factors, such as growth factors. The niche provides a supportive environment for the survival and self-renewal of the stem cell. In addition, this environment permits the transmission of feedback information that direct behaviors of the stem cell, including entry into the cell cycle, cell fate (resting, self-renewal, differentiation, and apoptosis), and cell motility.[46]

The fate of the stem cells is regulated by extrinsic and intrinsic factors. These factors determine the number of stem cells in the niche by adjusting the stem cell's type of cell division (symmetrical versus asymmetrical), cell cycle, fate, and motility.[8] The survival of a stem cell is mostly determined by extrinsic factors. The general order of differentiation by cell type in a cell lineage is stem cell, progenitor cell, and mature or specialized cell. A stem cell tends to stay in the Go-phase and a progenitor cell is continuously active in the cell cycle.

Hematopoietic Cells

In humans, hematopoiesis predominately occurs in the bone marrow. The majority of cells in the bone marrow transitions from the long bones in the child to the ribs, sternum, and vertebrae in the adult. The hematopoietic system consists of the red blood cells, white blood cells, and platelets. The mature forms of these cells reside in the peripheral compartment and are primarily formed in the central compartment or bone marrow. Stem cells are found in decreasing order at the following locations in the body: the bone marrow, spleen, and the peripheral compartment. A small percentage (10%) of hematopoietic stem cells exists as progenitor or multipotent stem cells in the vasculature.

The progression of the cellular lineage for hematopoietic cells is long-term hematopoietic stem cells (HSC), short-term HSCs (for 8–10 weeks), oligopotent (multi-) progenitor cells (lymphoid and myeloid), committed (limited) progenitor cells for colony forming unit (CFU)–erythroid, CFU–megakaryocyte, and CFU–granulocyte–monocyte, and mature cells (Fig. 23–3). Unlike stem cells, which have high renewal potential and low proliferative rate, committed progenitor cells have a high proliferative rate, which makes them vulnerable to toxicity from chemotherapeutics. The sparing of stem cells from toxicity permits the hematopoietic system to recover from chemotherapy. When stem cells are destroyed, the recovery period for the hematopoietic system is prolonged (ie, several weeks). In addition, age, the cumulative effect of recent chemotherapy, and concurrent infections delay the recovery of the hematopoietic system. Aging alters or decreases the ability of HSCs to respond to stress. The reasons for the former item are an accumulation of damaged DNA, a trend away from self-renewing HSCs, a preference toward myeloid instead of lymphoid lineage, and an increased amount of adipocytes in the niche.[26]

The red blood cell lasts for about 120 days in the peripheral compartment before splenic sequestration. It takes about 7 days before an immature red blood cell is released into the peripheral compartment. Although alkylating agents and antimetabolites can cause aplastic anemia, new-onset anemia occurring post-chemotherapy requires an immediate assessment for acute

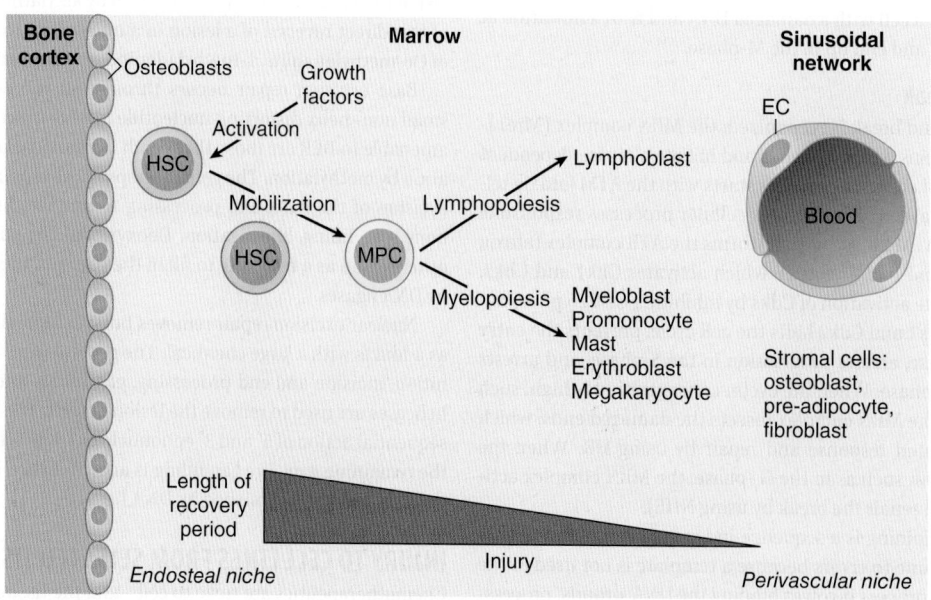

FIGURE 23–3. A schematic of the hematopoietic stem cell niche in the bone marrow. EC = endothelial cell; HSC = hematopoietic stem cell; MPC = multiprogenitor cell.

blood loss and is not directly attributed to the chemotherapeutic. The longevity of the white blood cell in the peripheral compartment is shorter than it is for the red blood cell, and it varies depending on the maturity and location of the cell. For example, the survival times in the circulation (and other compartments) for mature neutrophils is 12 hours (3 days for those residing in tissues), mature granulocytes is 7 to 24 hours (10–14 days when progenitor cells are committed to mature granulocytes in the bone marrow). The anticipated milestones for white blood cells in response to a chemotherapy schedule of every 3 to 4 weeks is, the nadir will appear at about 10 to 14 days, recovery will begin at 14 days, and full recovery will be at 21 days. Although mature lymphocytes survive for about 6 to 24 hours, lymphopenia is not directly attributed to toxicity from chemotherapy. If lymphopenia occurs soon after chemotherapy, other causes should be initially suspected, such as ionized radiation therapy. Platelets survive for about 10 days in the circulation, and the nadir occurs from 10 to 14 days from the start of chemotherapy. The completion of recovery is expected at about 3 weeks for platelets.

The primary compartment of the HSCs is the bone marrow for the postnatal human. Within the bone marrow, there are 2 niches that are important to HSCs. The endosteal niche (located at the space between the trabecular bone and the bone marrow) consists of quiescent HSCs (long term) (Fig. 23–3). The perivascular niche (located near to the sinusoidal endothelium) consists of actively cycling HSCs (short term). The role of the quiescent HSC is to maintain itself for self-renewal by preventing exhaustion. The roles of the actively cycling HSCs are differentiation and response to stressors, such as ionizing radiation and chemotherapeutics.[39] Hematopoietic stem cells balance the roles of these 2 niches to address the need of the situation.

The niche consists of HSCs, stromal cells, soluble factors, and the extracellular matrix environment. The stromal cells are fibroblasts, preadipocytes, and osteoblasts. The environmental matrix consists of fibronectin, proteoglycan, and hyaluronic acid. Soluble factors are cytokines (eg, IL-3 and IL-6), growth factors, transcription factors, and surface molecules (eg, CD44) produced by the stromal cells.[11] The anaerobic environment of the bone marrow favors glycolysis, which is consistent with the G_0-phase of the quiescent HSCs. When HSCs undergo differentiation, their metabolism converts to oxidative phosphorylation.[31]

The vascular supplies are arterioles for the endosteum and a sinusoidal network for the perivascular space. Following ionizing radiation injury, HSCs repopulate at the endosteum before the perivascular space because the sinusoid is more sensitive to this type of insult than the arteriole.[2] The HSC niche is regulated by sympathetic innervation, circadian rhythm, hormones, and hypoxia.[4] Hormones that affect HSC directly or indirectly through the niche are parathyroid hormone, estrogen, and prostaglandin E_2.[17] A disruption of the adrenergic innervation can impair HSC recovery from chemotherapy.[2]

HSC Response to Stress

Following an injury to the hematopoietic system, the initial response is myelosuppression. Bone marrow failure occurs when actively cycling cells in the marrow are severely injured. Significant injury to HSCs results in long-term consequences to the HSC, including a decrease in the reserve of HSCs or impaired self-renewal. Some potential consequences of a decreased reserve in HSC are hypoplastic anemia, myelodysplastic syndrome, and a diminished response to stress.[39] Hematopoietic stem cells can be injured by a quantitative reduction in HSCs, a qualitative alteration in the replicative function of HSCs, or a damage to the niche, such as the stromal cells.[39] For example, busulfan decreases the reserve of HSCs by inducing senescence.[27] Patients with a decreased reserve in HSCs typically recover with an unremarkable peripheral blood count during nonstressed conditions, but have an inadequate hematopoietic response to a stress that will occur in the future.

The toxicity of a chemotherapeutic on hematopoietic cells is demonstrated by the time of onset of the decline in the cell line, the time to recovery of the cell line, and the occurrence of residual or long-term effects to the cell line. The hematopoietic cells decline in the following order based on survival of the mature cell—granulocytes (48 hours), platelets (10–12 days), and

erythrocytes (120 days). In practice, the decline in granulocytes is usually evident at 1 to 2 weeks after the exposure to a chemotherapeutic because there are residual cells in peripheral tissue compartments.

Prolonged granulocytopenia (ie, neutropenia) results from direct damage to hematopoietic stem or progenitor cells, premature exhaustion of the reserve of HSCs (eg, repeated cycling), premature senescence, and damage to the niche architecture (eg, sinusoidal network by ionizing radiation) or stromal cells. For example, the nitrosourea BCNU (carmustine) damages the CFU-fibroblast, the alkyl sulfonate busulfan induces senescence in the HSC,[27] and cisplatin diminishes the reserve of the stem cell.[24,30] The nitrogen mustard analogue cyclophosphamide causes prolonged granulocytopenia at high and repeated doses.[45] Unlike the previously mentioned cell cycle phase–nonspecific agents, the cell cycle phase–specific agents such as cytosine arabinoside (ara-C, cytarabine) and 5-fluorouracil (5FU) do not cause prolonged myelosuppression.

There are a limited number of options for the medical treatment of hematopoietic injury: transfusion, growth factors, and bone marrow transplantation. The thresholds for the initiation of these therapies are determined by clinical practice.

Intestinal Epithelial Cells

Epithelial cells in the gastrointestinal tract develop from stem cells that are primarily located in the gastric glands and intestinal crypts, which serve as the niche. The cells in the small and large intestines are the predominate stem cells for the gastrointestinal epithelium. The stem cells for the large intestine are located at the ascending and descending portions of the colon. Intestinal stem cells (ISCs) develop from mesenchymal cells in the lamina propria, and they are supported by nutrients and soluble factors in the niche (Fig. 23–4). The hierarchical progression of intestinal epithelial cells is stem cell, progenitor cell (ie, transit-amplifying cell), and differentiated or mature cell. Mature cells are classified by their function (goblet cell, enterocyte, enteroendocrine cell, tuft cell, and Paneth cell) in the intestine. The mature cell is mitotically inactive, not renewed, and eventually sloughed off from the villi and into the gut lumen.

The intestinal epithelial cells are replaced daily because they undergo a high turnover rate. Differentiated epithelial cells migrate up the villi and are sloughed off after 3 to 5 days.[1] In contrast, the Paneth cell is located at the base of the crypt, and they turn over every 3 to 6 weeks. The amount of time it takes for the intestinal epithelium to become denuded following an injury depends on several factors, including the cell cycle time for the cell type (amount of time for one cell division), the number of cell divisions in the transit populations (from stem cell to mature cell), and the transit time for the postmitotic cell to migrate from the crypt to the villi.

The cell cycle times for the intestinal epithelium by section in humans are approximately 30 hours for the ileum, colon and rectum.[37] For comparison, the intestinal cell cycle times by section in mice are small to large bowel (11–26 hours), and in rats are small to large bowel (10–52 hours). The short cell cycle time for the ileum is reflected in the difference in the percentage of cells in mitosis for the total cell population among these sections in the intestine—ileum (53%), colon (25%), and rectum (16%).[36] The progenitor cell divides every 12 to 18 hours, and it undergoes 4 to 6 divisions before becoming a differentiated cell type.[20] An active stem cell (crypt base columnar cell) routinely enters into the cell cycle, but it occurs at a rate slower than the progenitor cell.[20] In a rodent model, it took about 3.2 days for the intestinal epithelium to become denuded following an exposure to ionizing radiation.[37]

Intestinal stem cells exist as 2 populations that function as active stem cells (crypt base columnar, CBC {leucine-rich repeat containing G protein–coupled receptor 5}) and quiescent stem cells (+4 stem cells) in the niche (Fig. 23–4).[1] The +4 stem cells are located at the fourth to fifth cell layer above the base of the crypt,[20] and they will undergo proliferation and differentiation when the active stem cells are damaged from an injury, such as an exposure to ionizing radiation or a chemotherapeutic. The CBC cells are located with the Paneth cells at the base of the crypt.

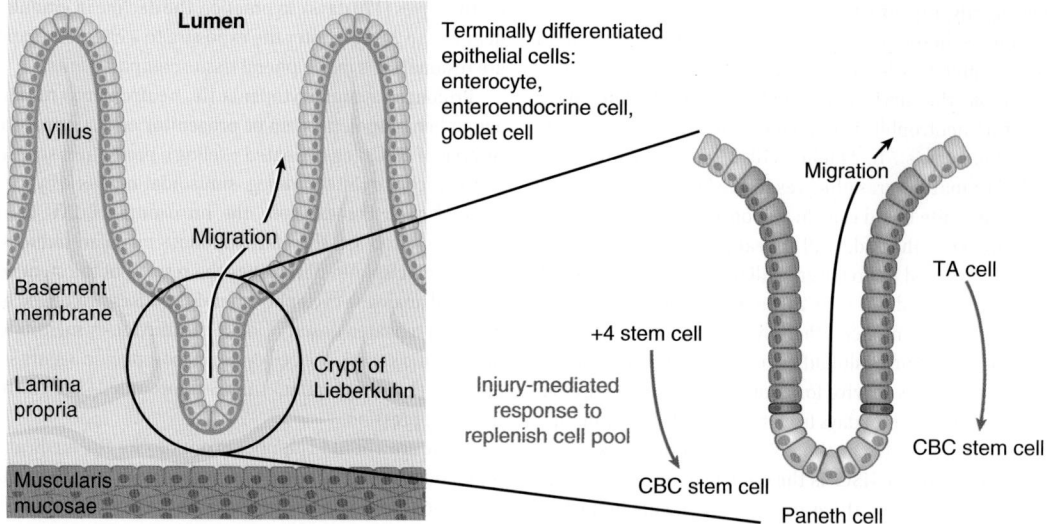

FIGURE 23–4. A schematic of the intestinal stem cell niche in the small intestine. +4 stem cells = quiescent stem cells; CBC = crypt base columnar; TA cell = transit-amplifying cell.

The CBC cells tend to replicate by symmetrical division, producing a pair of stem cells or transit-amplifying (progenitor) cells, to maintain epithelial homeostasis.[1]

There are several signaling pathways involved with the homeostasis of ISCs. One is the Wnt signaling pathway, and it acts on primarily stem cells to produce progenitor cells by activating the cell cycle. In addition, the pathway promotes the regulation of epithelial cell development along the lineage. Wnt appears to accomplish the former activities by stabilizing beta-catenin, which targets genes (CCND1 for cyclin D1 and MYC for c-MYC) that produce proteins involved with the regulation of the cell cycle. The Wnt/beta-catenin pathway appears to be involved with the regeneration of ISC following methotrexate treatment.[42]

There is a decreasing gradient for the Wnt signaling pathway as cells migrate from the crypt to the villi. The BMP signaling pathway serves as a negative regulator of cell proliferation in the crypt, and its gradient increases along the crypt–villi axis. The Notch signaling pathway promotes the maturation of progenitor cells to differentiated secretory cells.

ISC Response to Stress

Crypt base columnar cells and transit-amplifying cells are sensitive to ionizing radiation and chemotherapeutics and undergo apoptosis when exposed.[19,20,49,50] Although all chemotherapeutics used in a mouse model resulted in death of cells in the crypt, the level of injury in the crypt varied depending on exposure. For example, cell cycle phase–nonspecific chemotherapeutics (nitrosourea, nitrogen mustard analogues, anthracycline) affected cells at position +4 to 11 from the base of the crypt, and cell cycle phase–specific agents (antifolate, Vinca alkaloid, and antipyrimidine) affected cells from +8 to 11 in the crypt.[20] When CBC cells are injured, +4 stem cells and early transit-amplifying cells with regenerative capacity work to replenish the cell pool in the crypt.[1,5]

SUMMARY

- Chemotherapeutics cause various types of injuries to the cell. These injuries predominantly affect the DNA and they lead to damages of the DNA.
- Deoxyribonucleic acid damages result in cell death or senescence, tissue injury, and toxicity in the patient affected by these chemotherapeutics.
- The understanding of the mechanisms of these injuries and the responses of the cell and tissue to these injuries will enhance the clinician's management of the immediate and long-term consequences in patients affected by these chemotherapeutics.

Disclaimer

The findings and conclusions in this chapter are those of the author and do not necessarily represent the official position of the Centers for Disease Control and Prevention.

REFERENCES

1. Barker N. Adult intestinal stem cells: critical drivers of epithelial homeostasis and regeneration. *Nat Rev Mol Cell Biol.* 2014;15:19-33.
2. Boulais PE, Frenette PS. Making sense of hematopoietic stem cell niches. *Blood.* 2015; 125:2621-2629.
3. Caldecott KW. Single-strand break repair and genetic disease. *Nat Rev Genet.* 2008; 9:619-631.
4. Calvi LM, Link DC. Cellular complexity of the bone marrow hematopoietic stem cell niche. *Calcif Tissue Int.* 2014;94:112-124.
5. Carulli AJ, et al. Unraveling intestinal stem cell behavior with models of crypt dynamics. *Integr Biol (Camb).* 2014;6:243-257.
6. Deans AJ, West SC. DNA interstrand crosslink repair and cancer. *Nat Rev Cancer.* 2011; 11:467-480.
7. Elledge SJ. Cell cycle checkpoints: preventing an identity crisis. *Science.* 1996; 274:1664-1672.
8. Ema H, Suda T. Two anatomically distinct niches regulate stem cell activity. *Blood.* 2012;120:2174-2181.
9. Erenpreisa J, Cragg MS. Mitotic death: a mechanism of survival? A review. *Cancer Cell Int.* 2001;1:1.
10. Fitch K, Pyenson B. *Cancer Patients Receiving Chemotherapy: Opportunities for Better Management.* New York, NY: Millman, Inc; 2010.
11. Fukushima N, Ohkawa H. Hematopoietic stem cells and microenvironment: the proliferation and differentiation of stromal cells. *Crit Rev Oncol Hematol.* 1995;20:255-270.
12. Giunta S, et al. DNA damage signaling in response to double-strand breaks during mitosis. *J Cell Biol.* 2010;190:197-207.
13. Hanel W, Moll UM. Links between mutant p53 and genomic instability. *J Cell Biochem.* 2012;113:433-439.
14. Hassett MJ, et al. Chemotherapy-related hospitalization among community cancer center patients. *Oncologist.* 2011;16:378-387.
15. Heijink AM, et al. The DNA damage response during mitosis. *Mutat Res.* 2013;750:45-55.
16. Hoagland HC. Hematologic complications of cancer chemotherapy. *Semin Oncol.* 1982; 9:95-102.
17. Hoffman CM, Calvi LM. Minireview: complexity of hematopoietic stem cell regulation in the bone marrow microenvironment. *Mol Endocrinol.* 2014;28:1592-1601.
18. Huang Y, Li L. DNA crosslinking damage and cancer—a tale of friend and foe. *Transl Cancer Res.* 2013;2:144-154.
19. Ijiri K, Potten CS. Response of intestinal cells of differing topographical and hierarchical status to ten cytotoxic drugs and five sources of radiation. *Br J Cancer.* 1983;47:175-185.
20. Ijiri K, Potten CS. Further studies on the response of intestinal crypt cells of different hierarchical status to eighteen different cytotoxic agents. *Br J Cancer.* 1987;55:113-123.
21. Krzyzanowska MK, et al. Development of a patient registry to evaluate hospital admissions related to chemotherapy toxicity in a community cancer center. *J Oncol Pract.* 2005;1:15-19.
22. Li GM. Mechanisms and functions of DNA mismatch repair. *Cell Res.* 2008;18:85-98.

23. Luke JJ, et al. Targeted agents and immunotherapies: optimizing outcomes in melanoma. *Nat Rev Clin Oncol.* 2017;14:463-482.

24. Mauch P, et al. Hematopoietic stem cell compartment: acute and late effects of radiation therapy and chemotherapy. *Int J Radiat Oncol Biol Phys.* 1995;31:1319-1339.

25. Meistrich ML. Effects of chemotherapy and radiotherapy on spermatogenesis in humans. *Fertil Steril.* 2013;100:1180-1186.

26. Mendelson A, Frenette PS. Hematopoietic stem cell niche maintenance during homeostasis and regeneration. *Nat Med.* 2014;20:833-846.

27. Meng A, et al. Ionizing radiation and busulfan induce premature senescence in murine bone marrow hematopoietic cells. *Cancer Res.* 2003;63:5414-5419.

28. Mirkin EV, Mirkin SM. Replication fork stalling at natural impediments. *Microbiol Mol Biol Rev.* 2007;71:13-35.

29. Muniandy PA, et al. DNA interstrand crosslink repair in mammalian cells: step by step. *Crit Rev Biochem Mol Biol.* 2010;45:23-49.

30. Nikkels PG, et al. Long-term effects of cytostatic agents on the hemopoietic stroma: a comparison of four different assays. *Leuk Res.* 1987;11:817-825.

31. Oburoglu L, et al. Metabolic regulation of hematopoietic stem cell commitment and erythroid differentiation. *Curr Opin Hematol.* 2016;23:198-205.

32. Orthwein A, et al. Mitosis inhibits DNA double-strand break repair to guard against telomere fusions. *Science.* 2014;344:189-193.

33. Pastwa E, Blasiak J. Non-homologous DNA end joining. *Acta Biochim Pol.* 2003;50:891-908.

34. Pfeifer GP, et al. Tobacco smoke carcinogens, DNA damage and p53 mutations in smoking-associated cancers. *Oncogene.* 2002;21:7435-7451.

35. Pittman NM, et al. Emergency room visits and hospital admission rates after curative chemotherapy for breast cancer. *J Oncol Pract.* 2015;11:120-125.

36. Potten CS. The significance of spontaneous and induced apoptosis in the gastrointestinal tract of mice. *Cancer Metastasis Rev.* 1992;11:179-195.

37. Potten CS, Hendry JH. *Cytotoxic Insult to tissue: Effects on Cell Lineages.* Edinburgh, UK: Churchill Livingstone; 1983.

38. Sadik M, et al. Attributes of cancer patients admitted to the emergency department in one year. *World J Emerg Med.* 2014;5:85-90.

39. Shao L, et al. Hematopoietic stem cell injury induced by ionizing radiation. *Antioxid Redox Signal.* 2014;20:1447-1462.

40. Sherr CJ. The Pezcoller lecture: cancer cell cycles revisited. *Cancer Res.* 2000; 60:3689-3695.

41. Singh SD, et al. Surveillance for cancer incidence and mortality—United States, 2012. *MMWR Morb Mortal Wkly Rep.* 2016;63:17-58.

42. Sukhotnik I, et al. The role of Wnt/beta-catenin signaling in enterocyte turnover during methotrexate-induced intestinal mucositis in a rat. *PLoS One.* 2014;9:e110675.

43. Swenberg JA, et al. Biomarkers in toxicology and risk assessment: informing critical dose-response relationships. *Chem Res Toxicol.* 2008;21:253-265.

44. Terasawa M, et al. Canonical non-homologous end joining in mitosis induces genome instability and is suppressed by M-phase-specific phosphorylation of XRCC4. *PLoS Genet.* 2014;10:e1004563.

45. Testa NG, et al. Long-term bone marrow damage in experimental systems and in patients after radiation or chemotherapy. *Anticancer Res.* 1985;5:101-110.

46. Wagers AJ, et al. Cell fate determination from stem cells. *Gene Ther.* 2002;9:606-612.

47. Wong WM, Wright NA. Cell proliferation in gastrointestinal mucosa. *J Clin Pathol.* 1999;52:321-333.

48. Yamada HY, Gorbsky GJ. Spindle checkpoint function and cellular sensitivity to antimitotic drugs. *Mol Cancer Ther.* 2006;5:2963-2969.

49. Yu J. Intestinal stem cell injury and protection during cancer therapy. *Transl Cancer Res.* 2013;2:384-396.

50. Zhan Y, et al. beta-Arrestin1 inhibits chemotherapy-induced intestinal stem cell apoptosis and mucositis. *Cell Death Dis.* 2016;7:e2229.

51. Zhang H. DNA replication damage from environmental carcinogens. In: *SpringerBriefs in Biochemistry and Molecular Biology.* Dordrecht: Springer; 2015. http://BN7ZQ5YK2C.search.serialssolutions.com/?V=1.0&L=BN7ZQ5YK2C&S=JCs&C=TC0001500637&T=marc&tab=BOOKS.

24 OPHTHALMIC PRINCIPLES

Adhi Sharma

Although it is arguable that the eyes are the mirror to the soul, it is certain that the eyes reveal a great deal of information with regard to toxicology. In addition to exhibiting findings of systemic toxicity, they are also subject to the direct effects of xenobiotics and serve as a portal of entry for systemic absorption. An understanding of ophthalmic principles will allow the clinician to make timely and more accurate diagnoses that can be sight-saving or lifesaving and is essential to efficient, organized patient care.

OPHTHALMIC EXAMINATION

As a matter of convention, the routine eye examination is performed in the following sequence: visual acuity, pupillary response, extraocular muscle function, funduscopy, and, when indicated, a slit-lamp examination. Examination of the pupillary size and response to light can help determine the presence of a toxic syndrome. For example, opioids and cholinergics produce miosis, whereas anticholinergics and sympathomimetics produce mydriasis. Assessment of the extraocular muscles often reveals xenobiotic-induced nystagmus or cranial nerve abnormalities. Funduscopy typically reveals pink discs characteristic of poisoning by methanol or carbon monoxide. The slit-lamp examination allows for evaluation of toxic exposure to the lids, lacrimal systems, conjunctiva, sclera, cornea, and anterior chamber. However, before considering specific xenobiotic exposures in detail, it is important to review the anatomy and physiology of the visual pathways and how alteration of the normal physiology and anatomy correlate with clinical signs and symptoms.

OPHTHALMIC ANATOMY AND PHYSIOLOGY

The eye is a spherical structure referred to as a globe. The globe is divided into anterior and posterior structures (Fig. 24–1). The most anterior structures are the cornea, conjunctiva, and sclera. Posterior to the cornea are the iris, the lens, and the ciliary body. The space between the cornea and the iris is the anterior chamber, and the space between the iris and the retina is the posterior chamber. The anterior chamber contains *aqueous humor*, which is produced by the ciliary processes; this fluid nourishes the cornea, iris, and lens. The iris, the ciliary processes, and the choroid compose the uvea. The posterior chamber is filled with a transparent gelatinous mass termed the *vitreous humor*. The vitreous humor is an important body fluid in forensic toxicology as it is less susceptible to postmortem redistribution (Chaps. 139 and 140). The fundus is the most posterior structure and includes the retina, retinal vessels, and the head of the optic nerve or disc.

Visual Acuity and Color Perception

Normal vision is dependent on light transmission through the globe reaching intact posterior neural elements. As such, appropriate light transmission requires a clear cornea, clear aqueous humor, proper pupil size, an unclouded lens, and clear vitreous. The posterior neural elements include the retina, optic nerve, and the optic cortex; in turn, all of these structures require intact blood circulation for proper function. Decreased acuity results from abnormalities anywhere in the visual system that affect either light transmission or the neural elements.[4,12,22] Corneal injury or edema results in blurring of vision, characteristically described as "halos" around lights. Toxicologic causes of corneal abnormalities include direct exposure to chemicals, failure of corneal protective reflexes because of local anesthetic effects or a profoundly decreased level of consciousness, and incomplete eyelid closure during coma. Mydriasis (Table 24–1) interferes with the pupillary constriction necessary for accommodation, thereby resulting in decreased acuity for near objects. Lens clouding or cataract formation causes blurred vision and decreased light perception, as does blood

(hyphema), pus (hypopyon), or other deposits in the aqueous humor or vitreous humor (vitreous hemorrhage). Many xenobiotic-induced lens abnormalities are caused by chronic systemic exposures (Table 24–2).[17,22,30] Even if light reaches the retina without distortion, ischemia or injury to any neural element from the retina to the optic cortex will result in abnormal reception or transmission. Direct, acute, visual neurotoxic injury is rare and is caused almost exclusively by methanol or quinine.[17,43] Indirect injury following xenobiotic-induced central nervous system (CNS) ischemia or hypoxia is far more common. Alterations in color perception generally result from abnormalities in retinal or optic nerve function. Color–vision abnormalities are attributed to numerous xenobiotics, but most are caused by chronic xenobiotic exposure and rarely are features of acute toxicity.[17,22]

Cornea
Amiodarone
Caustics (acid, alkali, hydrofluoric acid)
Cocaine
Deferoxamine
Irritants (capsaicin, phenol, hydrogen sulfide)
Metal ions of (Cu, Au, Hg, Ag)

Lens
Amiodarone
Busulfan
Chlorpromazine
Corticosteroids
Iron

Iris
Bisphosphonates
Rifabutin
Sulfonamides

Optic nerve
Amiodarone
Disulfram
Ethambutol
Isoniazid
Lead
Linezolid
Thallium
Toluene

Retina
Cardioactive
 steroids
Cocaine
Deferoxamine
Methanol (formate)
Phosphodiesterase-5
 inhibitors
Quinine
Thallium

Visual cortex
Cisplatin
Cocaine
Cyclosporine
Hypoxic injury
 (CO, CN, H$_2$S)
Mercury
Vasoconstrictors
 (sympathomimetics,
 ergot alkaloids)

FIGURE 24–1. The major xenobiotics that cause ophthalmic toxicity and their areas of ophthalmic injury.

TABLE 24–1	Classic Ophthalmic Findings Caused by Acute Xenobiotic Exposures

Disconjugate gaze
Botulism
Elapid envenomation
Neuromuscular blockers
Paralytic shellfish poisoning
Secondary to decreased level of consciousness
Tetrodotoxin
Thiamine deficiency

Funduscopic abnormalities
Carbon monoxide (red)
Cocaine (vasoconstriction)
Cyanide (retinal vein arterialization)
Ergot alkaloids (vasoconstriction; disc pallor)
Injection drug use (attenuation or loss of small vessels due to emboli)
Methanol (disc and retinal pallor or hyperemia)
Methemoglobin (cyanosis)

Miosis
Cholinesterase inhibitors (carbamates, organic phosphorus compounds)
Coma from sedative–hypnotics (barbiturates, benzodiazepines, ethanol)
Decreased sympathetic tone (clonidine, opioids, valproic acid)
Increased cholinergic tone (pilocarpine, nicotine)

Mydriasis
Decreased cholinergic tone (antihistamines, atropine, cyclic antidepressants)
Increased sympathetic tone (cocaine, sedative-hypnotic withdrawal, lysergic acid diethylamide, monoamine oxidase inhibitors)
Nicotine

Nystagmus
Carbamazepine
Dextromethorphan
Ethanol
Ketamine and methoxetamine
Lithium
Monoamine oxidase inhibitors (oscillopsia or ping-pong nystagmus)
Phencyclidine (usually rotary nystagmus)
Phenytoin
Sedative–hypnotics
Scorpion venom
Thiamine deficiency

Opsoclonus
Diphenhydramine
Monoamine oxidase inhibitors
Scorpion venom
Serotonin toxicity

Papilledema
Amiodarone
Lead
Phenytoin
Vitamin A

TABLE 24–2	Examples of Ophthalmic Abnormalities Caused by Chronic Systemic Xenobiotic Exposures[a]

Alteration of color vision
Alkylamines (dimethylamine) (glaucopsia)
Ethyl chloride
Digoxin
Ethambutol
Sildenafil citrate (cyanopsia)
Styrene (color blindness)

Cataracts
Busulfan[c]
Corticosteroids[b]
Deferoxamine
Dinitrophenol (internal use)[d]
Trinitrotoluene[d]

Corneal deposits
Amiodarone[b]
Chloroquine
Chlorpromazine
Copper[d]
Gold
Mercury[d]
Retinoids
Silver (argyria)[d]
Vitamin D

Corneal/conjunctival inflammation
Cytosine arabinoside (Ara-C)
Isotretinoin[b]
Mercury (acrodynia)
Practolol[c]

Cortical blindness and reversible posterior leukoencephalopathy
Cisplatin
Cyclosporine
Glycine
Interleukin[c]
Methylmercury compounds[d]
Monoclonal antibodies (mabs)
Tacrolimus

Lens deposits
Amiodarone[b]
Chlorpromazine
Copper[d]
Iron
Mercury[d]
Silver[d]

Macular edema
Atorvastatin
Sildenafil
Thiazolidinediones

Myopia[c]
Acetazolamide
Diuretics (chlorthalidone, thiazides, spironolactone)
Retinoids
Sulfonamides
Topiramate

Retinal injury
Carbon disulfide[d]
Carmustine[c]
Chloramphenicol[c]
Chloroquine
Cinchona alkaloids (quinine)
Deferoxamine[c]
Ethambutol
Methanol
Thallium
Vigabatrin
Vincristine[c]

Retrobulbar and optic neuropathy
Carbon disulfide[d]
Chloramphenicol[d]
Dinitrobenzene[d]
Dinitrochlorobenzene[d]
Dinitrotoluene[d]
Disulfiram
Ethambutol[b]
Ethyl chloride
Isoniazid[c]
Lead[c]
Sildenafil (rare)
Thallium
Vincristine[c]

Uveitis
Bisphosphonates
Pamidronate
Rifabutin
Sulfonamides

[a]This list includes only selected examples and is not intended to be comprehensive. [b]Particularly important example. [c]Reported, but extremely rare from this exposure. [d]Mostly of historical interest; associated with patterns of use that are no longer common.

Pupil Size and Reactivity

Generally, pupils are round and symmetric with an average diameter of 3 to 4 mm under typical light conditions. Physiologic anisocoria (unequal pupils) is a normal variant and is defined as a difference in pupil size of 1 mm or less. However, in the absence of a history of physiologic anisocoria, any asymmetry in pupil size should be considered an abnormal finding. Pupils react directly and consensually to light intensity by either constricting or dilating. Constriction is also a component of the near reflex (accommodation) that occurs when the eye focuses on near objects. The iris controls pupil size through a balance of cholinergic innervation of the sphincter (constrictor) muscle by cranial nerve III and sympathetic innervation of the radial (dilator) muscle.[12]

Pupillary dilation (mydriasis) results from increased sympathetic stimulation of the radial muscle by endogenous catecholamines, or from the use of cocaine, amphetamines, and other sympathomimetics and ophthalmic instillation of sympathomimetics such as phenylephrine. Mydriasis also results from inhibition of muscarinic cholinergic-mediated innervation of the sphincter secondary to systemic or ophthalmic exposure to anticholinergics (Chap. 49). Because pupillary constriction in response to light is a major determinant of normal pupil size, blindness from ocular, retinal, or optic nerve disorders also leads to mydriasis as exemplified by methanol and quinine toxicity. As such, the reactivity of mydriatic pupils to light varies with the etiology of the mydriasis.[22] Although often difficult to appreciate, constriction to light is often elicited after sympathomimetic exposures because constrictor function is preserved, whereas this is often not the case when mydriasis results from anticholinergic excess since constrictor function is potently antagonized. Light reactivity is absent in complete blindness but is preserved if light perception persists.

Miosis results from either increased cholinergic stimulation such as opioids, pilocarpine, and cholinesterase inhibitors, such as organic phosphorus compounds, or inhibition of sympathetic dilation caused by clonidine. Miosis was the most common finding in victims of the Tokyo subway sarin attack of 1995 and was used to distinguish between mild and moderate exposure.[36]

There are conflicting reports regarding the pupillary reactions to many xenobiotics. Depending on the stage and severity of toxicity, the presence of coingestants or coexistent hypoxemia, and numerous other factors, many individual xenobiotics such as clonidine, nicotine, phencyclidine, and barbiturates cause mydriasis, miosis, or hippus, which is defined as a spasmodic and rhythmic, but regular, alteration between miosis and mydriasis.[22,31] For some xenobiotics, the pupillary examination provides consistent information (Table 24–1), but many factors are involved, and the significance of the pupil size and reactivity must always be considered in the context of the remainder of the patient evaluation.

Extraocular Movement, Diplopia, and Nystagmus
Maintenance of normal eye position and movement requires a coordinated function of a complex circuit involving bilateral frontal and occipital cortices, multiple brain stem nuclei, cranial nerves, and extraocular muscles.[2,12] Because of the many elements necessary for normal function, abnormalities of eye movement result from several causes and are extremely common.[22] Probably the most common abnormality is reversible nystagmus or rhythmic oscillations of the globes (Table 24–1). Nystagmus is divided into 2 types: jerk nystagmus, which has a slow phase and a fast phase, and pendular nystagmus, which has rhythmic oscillation. Either type can be torsional (rotatory) or in a horizontal or vertical direction. Xenobiotic-induced nystagmus takes many forms but is most commonly jerk nystagmus, as opposed to pendular. The nystagmus may be evident at rest but is accentuated by visual pursuit and extreme lateral gaze. Although nystagmus with extreme lateral gaze is a normal finding, it extinguishes within 2 to 5 beats; if nystagmus persists, it is evidence of underlying pathology. Vertical nystagmus in other settings is usually associated with a structural lesion of the CNS. However, xenobiotic-induced vertical nystagmus occurs with phencyclidine, ketamine, dextromethorphan, or phenytoin toxicity. Loss of conjugate gaze commonly results from CNS depression of any etiology, typically after sedative–hypnotic or ethanol poisoning. Except after extremely rare exposures to neurotoxins (Table 24–1), diplopia without a decreased level of consciousness should not be attributed to an acute toxicologic etiology. In addition to the transient effects of some xenobiotics, thallium, carbon disulfide, and carbon monoxide cause sustained gaze disorders as a consequence of residual cranial nerve and CNS injury.[22] Nystagmus and ophthalmoplegia caused by thiamine deficiency (Wernicke encephalopathy) usually improves after therapy, but on occasion the nystagmus completely resolves.[46]

DIRECT OPHTHALMIC TOXINS
Chemical Ophthalmic Injury
Chemical injury to the eye from a number of xenobiotics occurs in both residential and industrial settings, and also results from warfare or acts of terrorism. A recent study demonstrated that over a 4-year period there were more

than 144,000 ophthalmic burns recorded in emergency departments in the United States.[23] Although injuries were more common in men than women, children aged 1 to 2 years had the highest incidence of injury. Alkaline injuries resulted in more severe injuries than acids, and were more common.[23] Vision loss is associated with an increased risk for subsequent serious injuries, and will have long-lasting impact on general health.[29]

Caustics
The initial approach to all patients with ophthalmic caustic exposures should be immediate decontamination by irrigating with copious amounts of fluids.[9,47] Water, 0.9% sodium chloride solution, lactated Ringer solution, and balanced salt solution (BSS) are all appropriate choices. In theory, BSS is ideal, because it is both isotonic and buffered to physiologic pH. Lactated Ringer solution (pH 6–7.5) and 0.9% sodium chloride solution (pH 4.5–7) are also isotonic and therefore theoretically preferable to water.[24] The use of an ophthalmic anesthetic is usually required to perform irrigation properly. Irrigation is intended to accomplish at least 4 objectives: immediate dilution of the offending xenobiotic; removal of the xenobiotic; removal of any foreign body; and, in some cases, normalization of anterior chamber pH. Because delays of even seconds can dramatically affect outcome,[22] there is no justification for waiting for any specific solution if water is the first available therapy or in obtaining visual acuity prior to treatment. Irrigation must include the external and internal palpebral surfaces, as well as the cornea and bulbar conjunctiva and its recesses. Effective irrigation includes lid retraction and eversion or use of a scleral shell or other irrigating device. After irrigation, visual acuity testing, inspection of the eye, and slit-lamp examination should be performed. The immediacy with which an ophthalmologic consultation must be obtained will depend on the degree of injury.

Sulfur Mustard
This alkylating agent reacts with ophthalmic tissues, resulting in early and late toxic effects. Of note, there is a latency of 30 minutes to 8 hours, during which time victims will be relatively asymptomatic. Initial effects include pain, foreign body sensation (grittiness), lacrimation, photophobia, blepharospasm, corneal ulceration, and blindness.[26] Generally, injury is limited to the anterior chamber. More than 90% of exposed victims will experience late complications associated with conjunctival sensitivity to irritants, with resultant recurrent blepharoconjunctivitis. Fewer than 1% of severely toxic victims will suffer delayed keratopathy, resulting in thinning, neovascularization, and epithelial defects of the cornea.[26]

Management is directed at removal from the exposure and aggressive decontamination of the skin and eyes. Any of the irrigation solutions mentioned above will suffice. The goal is to provide irrigation as soon as possible; to this end, even tap water is an acceptable solution. Animal studies suggest that topical nonsteroidal antiinflammatory drugs (NSAIDs) drugs are helpful; as such, a short course of ophthalmic corticosteroids is reasonable.[5] Ophthalmic corticosteroid treatment should be used in consultation with an ophthalmologist. Late complications are best managed by an ophthalmologist.

Exposure-Specific Irrigating Solutions
Despite theoretical concern, there is probably no toxic exposure for which standard aqueous solutions are contraindicated. Of greatest concern are xenobiotics such as white or yellow phosphorus, metallic sodium, metallic potassium, and calcium oxide (cement) that typically react in the presence of water, leading to an exothermic or mechanical injury, or resulting in the generation of sodium hydroxide, potassium hydroxide, and calcium hydroxide.[22] Although not well studied, irrigation with large amounts of water probably dissipates the heat of the initial hydration reaction with conjunctival moisture more than it initiates a thermochemical reaction. In addition to removing the offending material, irrigation serves to dilute and remove the alkaline byproducts formed by reaction with conjunctival water. Table 24–3 summarizes recommended irrigation solutions for various xenobiotics.

The use of special irrigating solutions for more uncommon exposures, including hydrofluoric acid and phenols, is also debated. Animal models of

TABLE 24–3	Recommended Irrigation Solutions for Various Xenobiotics	
Xenobiotic	Irrigation Solution	Duration of Irrigation[a]
Capsaicin (pepper spray)	NS, LR, BSS	15–20 minutes
Caustics (acids/alkalis)	NS, LR, BSS	1–2 hours
Cyanoacrylate adhesives	Typically none needed	N/A
Hydrofluoric acid	NS	1–2 hours[a]
Phenol	NS, LR, BSS	15–20 minutes

[a]Duration of irrigation should be determined by other endpoints, including symptoms or conjunctival pH.
BSS = balanced saline solution (pH ~7.4); LR = lactated Ringer solution (pH 6.0–7.5); NS = 0.9% sodium chloride (pH ~5.5).

alkaline xenobiotics and nitrogen mustard injuries suggest that irrigation with amphoteric or buffered solutions rapidly restores anterior chamber pH.[20,41] Some authors have gone further to conclude that 0.9% sodium chloride solution should be avoided as an irrigation solution.[38] Use of these specialized irrigating solutions is beneficial for cutaneous burns;[14] however, the majority of the published human ophthalmic data are case reports. These solutions are probably best suited for first aid treatment at worksite eyewash stations and are neither practical nor proven for prolonged irrigation.

Hydrofluoric Acid

For hydrofluoric acid exposures (Chap. 104), experimental irrigation with calcium salt solutions was too irritating to the eye, but isotonic magnesium chloride solutions appear effective and not irritating, and are the preferred irrigant if available.[32,33] However, from a practical standpoint, 0.9% sodium chloride solution remains readily available, well studied, and effective. In one animal model, it was suggested that irrigation beyond the initial liter yielded worse outcomes; however, this was not demonstrated in humans.[32]

Phenol

For dermal exposure, topical low-molecular-weight polyethylene glycol (PEG) solutions are effective for treatment of experimental skin exposure; for eyes, copious water irrigation appears to be as effective as PEG.[7] There is, however, a report of superior efficacy of PEG-400 over water in treatment of actual phenol eye burns.[28] Although PEG-400 should be readily available at worksites where phenols are used, it is not a realistic option in the emergency department, and there should be no hesitation to use water, 0.9% sodium chloride solution, lactated Ringer solution, or BSS as lavage solutions.

Cyanoacrylate Adhesives

Ophthalmic exposures to cyanoacrylate adhesives such as Dermabond® and Krazy Glue® occasionally result in rapid adherence between the upper and lower eyelids that typically persists for days. Classically, such occurrences are associated with corneal abrasions,[13] but are otherwise relatively harmless. In fact, cyanoacrylate is used for the treatment of corneal perforations.[49] Solvents such as acetone or ethanol, which are often effective treatment for dermal-to-dermal adhesions caused by cyanoacrylates, should never be used in or around the eyes because they can result in a severe keratitis. Expectant management is the safest approach, because spontaneous rejection of the glue will occur over time. Application of gauze pads coated with antibiotic ophthalmic ointment will hasten recovery.[27] A thorough eye examination should be performed once the eyelids can be fully opened.

Other xenobiotic-specific treatments have been tried experimentally or clinically,[24] but none should be considered prior to, or instead of, copious irrigation. Most are not advocated, and consideration of such therapies should be vanishingly rare.

Duration of Irrigation

To accomplish the desired goals of irrigation, the appropriate duration varies with the exposure. Most solvents, for example, do not penetrate deeper than the superficial cornea, and 10–20 minutes of irrigation is generally sufficient.[22] After exposure to acids or alkalis, normalization of the conjunctival

pH is often suggested as a useful endpoint. Testing of pH should be done in every case of acid or alkali exposure, but the limitations of testing must be understood. When measured by sensitive experimental methods, normal pH of the conjunctival surface is 6.5 to 7.6.[1] This is highly method dependent, however, and normal values in the literature range from 5.2 to 8.6.[10] When measured by touching pH-sensitive paper to the moist surface of the conjunctival cul-de-sac, normal pH is most often near 8.[3] Therefore, after irrigation following alkali burns, pH should not be expected to reach 7 and is more likely to stabilize near 8.[22] In this setting, lower pH values likely indicate the pH of the irrigation solution rather than of the ophthalmic surface. Waiting for an interval of several minutes between irrigation and pH testing allows washout of any residual irrigant.[11] Choice of testing paper is important, because some are intended for use at extremes of pH and lack sensitivity in the clinically useful range.

Despite these limitations, a logical role for pH assessment is appropriate. A minimum of 500 to 1,000 mL of irrigant should be used for each affected eye before any assessment of pH, and after a waiting period (7–10 minutes), the pH of the lower fornix conjunctiva should be checked. Thereafter, cycles of 10 to 15 minutes of irrigation followed by rechecks should be continued until the pH is 7.5 to 8. This is certainly adequate for exposures to weak acids, which do not penetrate well, and for alkaline exposures where the pH is less than 12.

For strong or concentrated acid or alkali exposures, normal surface pH is not an adequate endpoint. After these burns, irrigation should be continued for at least 1 to 2 hours, regardless of surface pH, in an attempt to correct anterior chamber pH.[22,39,47] In addition, immediate ophthalmologic consultation is mandatory. Following this lengthy irrigation, it is important to verify that conjunctival pH has normalized. If not, irrigation must be continued, sometimes for 24 to 48 hours.

Others

Most solvents cause immediate pain and superficial injury because of dissolution of corneal epithelial lipid membranes but do not penetrate or react significantly with deeper tissue.[22] Consequently, even when the epithelial defect is large or complete, the limited depth of injury allows for rapid regeneration of normal epithelium. Detergents and surfactants cause variable injury, ranging from minor irritation from soaps to extensive injury from cationic detergents such as concentrated benzalkonium chloride.[22] Ophthalmic exposure to A-200 Pyrinate pediculicide shampoo causes typical detergent–surfactant injury, leading to extensive loss of corneal epithelium but with normal underlying stroma; therefore, complete healing occurs within days. Lacrimators (tear gases), such as chloroacetophenone, stimulate corneal nerve endings and cause pain, burning, and tearing, but produce no structural injury at low concentrations. At high concentrations, these xenobiotics typically produce significant corneal injury.

Pepper spray, often used for self-protection by civilians or to defuse a potentially violent event by law enforcement, contains the active ingredient oleoresin capsicum (OC). Oleoresin capsicum results in rapid depolarization of nociceptors containing substance P, resulting in immediate pain, blepharospasm, tearing, and blurred vision. In general, ophthalmic injury is uncommon, although corneal erosions are reported.[22] The solvent used for the spray is typically more injurious to the eye than the OC itself. Although most sprays use a water-based or oil-based solvent, some use alcohol, which can result in significant corneal damage.[50] Management of pepper spray exposure consists of rapid irrigation and pain control. Corneal erosions (epithelium intact) are often treated with artificial tears and antistaphylococcal antibiotics are recommended for corneal abrasions (epithelial defects). Specific information on numerous other xenobiotics is readily available.[22]

General Measures

There is a wide array of options for adjunctive therapy of chemical burns of the eye. In all cases in which serious injury is evident, the treatment plan must include consultation with an ophthalmologist. Generally, patients ophthalmic topical antibiotics providing antistaphylococcal and antipseudomonal coverage are recommended for corneal injuries. Cycloplegics not only reduce pain from ciliary spasm, but also decrease the likelihood of posterior synechiae (scar) formation. Topical nonsteroidal antiinflammatory drugs and systemic analgesics also improve patient comfort. Dispensing topical ophthalmic anesthetics is rarely recommended, because repeated use leads to further corneal disruption both by direct chemical effects and by eliminating corneal protective reflex sensation.

DISPOSITION

Disposition of patients with chemical burns of the cornea is frequently challenging. Patients with extensive burns to other parts of the body necessitate evaluation for transfer to a burn center. Grading the degree of injury in patients with isolated ophthalmic injury will guide disposition. The most commonly used grading system is the Roper-Hall modification of the Ballen classification system. Injury is graded on a 4-tier scale. Patients with mild conjunctival injection with corneal epithelial loss and minimal corneal haziness are classified as grades 1 and 2 (mild to moderate). These patients can be safely discharged from the emergency department with ophthalmology follow-up within 24 to 48 hours. Patients with severe corneal haziness or opacification with significant limbal ischemia (lack of blood vessels outside the periphery of the cornea) are classified as grade 3 or 4 (moderate to severe) and will benefit from immediate consultation with an ophthalmologist and consultation with a burn unit is advisable.

SYSTEMIC ABSORPTION AND TOXICITY FROM OPHTHALMIC EXPOSURES

Systemic absorption from ophthalmic exposure causes serious toxicity, morbidity, and even mortality.[15,25] Although the patterns of toxicity are characteristic of the xenobiotics involved, delays in recognition occur as a result of a failure to appreciate the eye as a significant route of absorption. Although transcorneal diffusion of xenobiotics is limited, there is substantial nasal mucosal absorption after nasolacrimal drainage, and absorption via conjunctival capillaries and lymphatics, which is markedly increased during conjunctival inflammation. Unlike the gastrointestinal route of absorption, there is no significant first-pass hepatic removal after ophthalmic absorption; consequently, bioavailability is much greater.[21,25,42] If nasolacrimal outflow is normal, up to 80% of instilled drug is absorbed systemically.[15] Unfortunately, by the time toxicity is apparent, there is no role for ophthalmic decontamination to prevent further absorption. After instillation of eye drops, absorption is generally complete within 7 minutes.

Children are at greatest risk, possibly because of the higher relative drug dose they experience when systemic absorption does occur.[15,37,42] Diligent attempts to comply with prescribed dosing in a struggling, crying infant often results in excessive dosing. As eye drop size (40–50 μL) exceeds ophthalmic cul-de-sac capacity (30 μL), overflow often occurs and is assumed to represent a failed instillation, which leads to unnecessary reinstillation. Also, as doses of ophthalmic medications are typically not adjusted based on patient weight, the consequences of equivalent degrees of systemic absorption are much greater for an infant than for an adult. Toxicity from eye drops is also a problem among the immunocompromised, probably because of the combination of greater use of potentially toxic ophthalmic medications and the presence of comorbid conditions.

Prevention of systemic toxicity from topical ophthalmic medications requires recognition of the risk, a careful history, use of the lowest effective concentration and dose, and patient education including proper administration instructions. To minimize inadvertent absorption, no more than one drop of any eye drop solution should be instilled at one time in the superolateral corner of the eye while using gentle finger compression of the medial canthus to limit nasolacrimal drainage.[15,25]

Mydriatics

Mydriatics are used almost exclusively to dilate the pupils prior to diagnostic evaluation of the eyes. This common practice is not generally considered to be potentially dangerous; however, the risks are substantial if the precautions

outlined are not considered. Anticholinergic poisoning is reported following ophthalmic use of atropine, cyclopentolate, or scopolamine eye drops, especially in infants.

The use of the α-adrenergic agonist phenylephrine eye drops in a 10% solution led to severe hypertension, subarachnoid hemorrhage, ventricular dysrhythmias, and myocardial infarction.[17] Fortunately, these effects are rare if the 2.5% ophthalmic phenylephrine is used. Mydriatics also risk precipitating acute angle closure glaucoma in susceptible individuals.

Miotics and Other Antiglaucoma Drugs

Miosis is induced by the cholinesterase inhibitor echothiophate (sometimes used to treat glaucoma or accommodative esotropia; a type of eye-turn related to extraocular muscle weakness). Echothiophate also exacerbates asthma, Parkinsonism, and cardiac disease, and prolongs the metabolism of certain medications such as succinylcholine.[25] Miosis is also produced by use of direct cholinergic agonists, such as pilocarpine. Although absorption is limited, nausea and abdominal cramps are reported at recommended doses. After excessive dosing, salivation, diaphoresis, bradycardia, and hypotension are all described.

β-Adrenergic antagonists, such as timolol, levobunolol, metipranolol, carteolol, and betaxolol, are used to lower intraocular pressure but infrequently cause a variety of adverse effects, including bradycardia, hypotension, myocardial infarction, syncope, transient ischemic attacks, congestive heart failure, exacerbation of asthma, and respiratory arrest. Timolol exacerbats weakness in patients with myasthenia gravis and is implicated in both causing and masking the signs and symptoms of hypoglycemia in diabetics.[44,45] Nonspecific complaints of anorexia, anxiety, depression, fatigue, hallucinations, headache, and nausea are also described after the use of timolol eye drops. Despite the cardioselectivity of betaxolol, respiratory effects occur.[15]

Dipivefrin, an esterified epinephrine derivative sometimes used to treat glaucoma, has caused systemic adrenergic effects, although less frequently than those caused by epinephrine. Ophthalmic formulations of highly selective α$_2$-adrenergic agonists, brimonidine and apraclonidine, were introduced to treat glaucoma.[15,48] Apraclonidine is expected to have a lower potential for toxicity because of limited CNS penetration. Systemic absorption of brimonidine eye drops in a child led to bradycardia, hypotension, and a decreased level of consciousness, similar to the central effects of other α$_2$-adrenoceptor agonists such as clonidine,[6] apparently mediated through both α$_2$-adrenoceptors and imidazoline receptors (Chap. 61).[8]

Antimicrobials

Life-threatening reactions to ophthalmic antimicrobials are unusual. Aplastic anemia occurred after prolonged use of chloramphenicol eye preparations,[16] and Stevens-Johnson syndrome was reported after short-term use of ophthalmic sulfacetamide in a patient with a history of allergy to sulfa drugs.[21]

TOXICITY TO OPHTHALMIC STRUCTURES FROM NONOPHTHALMIC EXPOSURES

Ophthalmic toxicity from systemic xenobiotics is almost always the result of chronic exposure, and the manifestations develop over a prolonged period of time. Thousands of xenobiotics are implicated, affecting every element of the visual system from the cornea to the optic cortex. Thorough discussion of this topic is beyond the scope of this text, but Table 24–2 lists examples of causative xenobiotics.[17,22] Many topical and systemic medications are associated with inflammation of the eye, such as the development of anterior or posterior uveitis (inflammation of the iris, ciliary process, or choroid membrane).[18] Unlike many other ophthalmic abnormalities caused by xenobiotics, uveitis should prompt immediate ophthalmologic consultation. Because in many cases the etiology is related to commonly prescribed medications, adverse drug effects should always be considered when patients present with visual abnormalities or unusual ophthalmic findings.

In the setting of emergency care, xenobiotic-induced disturbances of normal vision from systemic exposures take many forms. Impaired near-vision

TABLE 24–4 Common Xenobiotics Reported to Cause Visual Loss After Acute Exposures

Direct Causes	Indirect Causes[b]
Caustics	Cisplatin
Mercuric chloride[a]	Combined endocrine xenobiotics (thyrotropin-releasing hormone with gonadotropin-releasing hormone and glucagon)
Methanol	
Lead[a]	Embolization of foreign material (intravenous injection)
Quinine	Reversible posterior leukoencephalopathy
	Vasoactive xenobiotics
	Amphetamines
	Cocaine
	Ergot alkaloids
	Hypotension (eg, calcium channel blockers), diazoxide

[a]Distinctly rare with poisoning. [b]Distinctly rare with use of these xenobiotics; visual loss often instantaneous, secondary to sudden hypotension, vascular spasm, or embolization.

from mydriasis, and diplopia or nystagmus from interference with normal control of extraocular movements, are examples of common, usually harmless visual effects. Serious effects generally result from injury or dysfunction of the neural elements from the retina to the cortex. Such toxicity can be either direct (neurotoxic) or indirect (hypoxia, ischemia). Many xenobiotics historically reported to cause acute visual loss directly are no longer available.[22] Methanol and quinine are currently the most important xenobiotics that cause direct visual toxicity after acute oral poisoning. Many xenobiotics capable of causing vasospasm, hypotension, or embolization also cause acute visual loss (Table 24–4).[43] Blindness and other visual defects are described following recovery from severe toxicity with barbiturates and other sedative–hypnotics, opioids, carbon monoxide, and many others.[22]

OPHTHALMIC COMPLICATIONS OF ILLICIT DRUG USE
In addition to the well-known ophthalmic pupillary signs of opioid, cocaine, amphetamine, and phencyclidine toxicity, a number of complications result from short-term or long-term use of these xenobiotics.[34] Quinine amblyopia (Chap. 55) caused by intravenous use of quinine-adulterated heroin is one of many ophthalmic complications caused by injection of contaminants. Talc contaminants result in talc retinopathy, which was first described after prolonged intravenous use of adulterated methylphenidate,[19] but was also noted after intravenous use of heroin, methadone,[35] codeine, meperidine, and pentazocine. Talc retinopathy develops only after extensive intravenous drug use. In one study of intravenous methadone abusers, only patients who had injected more than 9,000 tablets developed this complication.[35] Infectious complications, such as fungal (Candida, Aspergillus) or bacterial (Staphylococcus spp, Bacillus cereus) endophthalmitis, are well known as both direct effects of intravenous drug use and secondary complications of acquired immunodeficiency syndrome (AIDS). In addition to AIDS-related ophthalmic infections such as cytomegalovirus, cryptococcus, toxoplasmosis retinitis, and choroidal Mycobacterium avium-intracellulare complex (MAC), other disorders include retinal cotton-wool spots, conjunctival Kaposi sarcoma, and ophthalmic motility disorders caused by infectious or neoplastic meningitis. Corneal defects are reported after smoking cocaine alkaloid ("crack eye").[40] Cocaine that is either volatilized or inadvertently introduced by direct contact probably results in corneal anesthesia and loss of corneal protective reflex sensation. Minor trauma, such as eye rubbing, then leads to corneal epithelial defects. In addition, there appears to be an increased incidence of infectious keratitis and corneal ulceration in these patients. The ability of local anesthetics to interfere with corneal epithelial adhesion may also play a role.

SUMMARY
■ Systemic and local toxicologic emergencies often have manifestations in the ophthalmic system.

■ Although the obvious physical injuries are apparent to the clinician, the subtler clues to toxicologic mechanisms that involve the ophthalmic and neurologic systems are made only by a meticulous examination of the eye.

■ Direct ophthalmic toxins should be washed out immediately without delays for determining visual acuity or locating toxin-specific irrigation solutions.

■ After initial management it is recommended that patients with moderate–severe injury be promptly referred to an ophthalmologist for further evaluation.

Acknowledgment
Martin J. Smilkstein, MD, and Frederick W. Fraunfelder, MD, contributed to this chapter in previous editions.

REFERENCES
1. Abelson MB, et al. Normal human tear pH by direct measurement. *Arch Ophthalmol.* 1981;99:301.
2. Adams RD, Victor M. *Disorders of Ocular Movement and Pupillary Function.* New York, NY: McGraw-Hill; 1993.
3. Adler IN, et al. The effects of pH on contact lens wearing. *Optom Assoc.* 1968;39:1000-1001.
4. Albert DM, et al, eds. *Principles and Practice of Ophthalmology.* Philadelphia, PA: Saunders; 2000.
5. Amir A, et al. Beneficial effects of topical anti-inflammatory drugs against sulfur mustard-induced ocular lesions in rabbits. *J Appl Toxicol* 2000;20(suppl):S109-S114.
6. Berlin RJ, et al. Ophthalmic drops causing coma in an infant. *J Pediatr.* 2001;138:441-443.
7. Brown VKH, et al. Decontamination procedures for skin exposed to phenolic substances. *Arch Environ Health.* 1975;30:1-6.
8. Burke J, et al. Adrenergic and imidazoline receptor-mediated responses to UK-14 (brimonidine) in rabbits and monkeys. A species difference. *Ann N Y Acad Sci.* 1995;763:304-318.
9. Burns FR, Paterson CA. Prompt irrigation of chemical eye injuries may avert severe damage. *Occup Health Saf.* 1989;58:33-36.
10. Carney LG, Hill RM. Human tear pH: diurnal variations. *Arch Ophthalmol.* 1976;94:821-824.
11. Chen FS, Maurice DM. The pH in the precorneal tear film and under a contact lens measured with a fluorescent probe. *Exp Eye Res.* 1990;50:251-259.
12. Davson H. *Physiology of the Eye.* London: Macmillan; 1990.
13. Dean BS, Krenzelok EP. Cyanoacrylates and corneal abrasions. *J Toxicol Clin Toxicol.* 1989;27:169-172.
14. Donoghue AM. Diphoterine for alkali chemical splashes to the skin at alumina refineries. *Int J Dermatol.* 2010;49:894-900.
15. Flach AJ. Systemic toxicity associated with topical ophthalmic medications. *J Fla Med Assoc.* 1994;81:256-260.
16. Fraunfelder FT, et al. Fatal aplastic anemia following topical administration of ophthalmic chloramphenicol. *Am J Ophthalmol.* 1982;93:356-360.
17. Fraunfelder FT, et al. *Clinical Ocular Toxicology: Drugs, Chemicals, and Herbs.* Philadelphia, PA: Elsevier Saunders; 2008.
18. Fraunfelder FW, Rosenbaum JT. Drug-induced uveitis incidence, prevention and treatment. *Drug Saf.* 1997;17:197-207.
19. Friberg TR, et al. Talc emboli and macular ischemia in intravenous drug abuse. *Arch Ophthalmol.* 1979;97:1089-1091.
20. Goldich Y, et al. Use of amphoteric rinsing solution for treatment of ocular tissues exposed to nitrogen mustard. *Acta Ophthalmol.* 2013;91:e35-e40.
21. Gottschalk HR, Orville J. Stone Stevens-Johnson syndrome from ophthalmic sulfonamides. *Arch Dermatol.* 1976;112:513-514.
22. Grant WM, Schuman JS. *Toxicology of the Eye.* Springfield, IL: C. Thomas; 1993.
23. Haring RS, et al. Epidemiologic trends of chemical ocular burns in the United States. *JAMA Ophthalmol.* 2016;134:1119-1124.
24. Herr RD, et al. Clinical comparison of ocular irrigation fluids following chemical injury. *Am J Emerg Med.* 1991;9:228-231.
25. Hugues FC, Jeunne C. Le Systemic and local tolerability of ophthalmic drug formulations. An update. *Drug Saf.* 1993;8:365-380.
26. Javadi MA, et al. Chronic and delayed-onset mustard gas keratitis: report of 48 patients and review of literature. *Ophthalmology.* 2005;112:617-625.
27. Kimbrough RL, et al. Conservative management of cyanoacrylate ankyloblepharon: a case report. *Ophthalmic Surg.* 1986;17:176-177.
28. Lang K. Treatment of phenol burns of the eye with polyethyleneglycol-400 [in German]. *Z Arztl Fortbild (Jena).* 1969;63:705-708.
29. Lee DJ, et al. Visual acuity impairment and mortality in US adults. *Arch Ophthalmol.* 2002;120:1544-1550.
30. Mattox C. *Table of toxicology.* In: Albert DM, Jakobiec FA, eds. Principles and Practice of Ophthalmology. 2nd ed. Philadelphia: WB Saunders; 2000:496-507.
31. McCarron MM, et al. Acute phencyclidine toxicity: incidence of clinical findings in 1,000 cases. *Ann Emerg Med.* 1981;10:237-242.

32. McCulley JP. Ocular hydrofluoric acid burns: animal model, mechanism of injury and therapy. *Trans Am Ophthalmol Soc.* 1990;88:649-684.

33. McCulley JP, et al. Hydrofluoric acid burns of the eye. *Med.* 1983;25:447-450.

34. McLane NJ, Carroll DM. Ocular manifestations of drug abuse. *Surv Ophthalmol.* 1986;30:298-311.

35. Murphy SB, et al. Talc retinopathy. *Can J Ophthalmol.* 1977;95:861-868.

36. Okumura T, et al. Report on 640 victims of the Tokyo subway sarin attack. *Ann Emerg Med.* 1996;28:129-135.

37. Palmer EA. How safe are ocular drugs in pediatrics? *Ophthalmology.* 1986;93:1038-1040.

38. Rihawi S, et al. Rinsing with isotonic saline solution for eye burns should be avoided. *Burns.* 2008;34:1027-1032.

39. Saari KM, et al. Management of chemical eye injuries with prolonged irrigation. *Acta Ophthalmol Suppl.* 1984;161:52-59.

40. Sachs R, et al. Corneal complications associated with the use of crack cocaine. *Ophthalmology.* 1993;100:181-191.

41. Schrage NF, et al. Use of an amphoteric lavage solution for emergency treatment of eye burns. First animal type experimental clinical considerations. *Burns.* 2002;28:782-786.

42. Shell JW. Pharmacokinetics of topically applied ophthalmic drugs. *Surv Ophthalmol.* 1982;26:207-217.

43. Smilkstein MJ, et al. Acute toxic blindness: unrecognized quinine poisoning. *Ann Emerg Med.* 1987;16:98-101.

44. Velde TM, Kaiser FE. Ophthalmic timolol treatment causing altered hypoglycemic response in a diabetic patient. *Arch Intern Med.* 1983;143:1627.

45. Verkijk A. Worsening of myasthenia gravis with timolol maleate eye-drops. *Ann Neurol.* 1985;17:211-212.

46. Victor M, Adams RD. The effect of alcohol on the nervous system. *Res Publ Assoc Res Nerv Ment Dis.* 1953;32:526-573.

47. Wagoner MD. Chemical injuries of the eye: current concepts in pathophysiology and therapy. *Surv Ophthalmol.* 1997;41:275-312.

48. Walters TR. Development and use of brimonidine in treating acute and chronic elevations of intraocular pressure: a review of safety, efficacy, dose response, and dosing studies. *Surv Ophthalmol.* 1996;41(suppl):S19-S26.

49. Webster RG, et al. The use of adhesive for the closure of corneal perforations: report of two cases. *Arch Ophthalmol.* 1968;80:705-709.

50. Zollman TM, et al. Clinical effects of oleoresin capsicum (pepper spray) on the human cornea and conjunctiva. *Ophthalmology.* 2000;107:2186-2189.

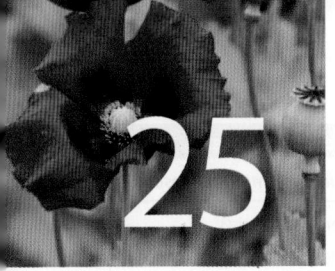

25 OTOLARYNGOLOGIC PRINCIPLES

Mai Takematsu and William K. Chiang

Many xenobiotics adversely affect the senses of olfaction, gustation, and cochlear–vestibular functions. Although these toxic effects are not life-threatening they are frequently distressful to patients. Furthermore, because of the dearth of access to standardized diagnostic techniques and normal parameters, such adverse effects are sometimes overlooked or dismissed by health care providers, despite significant patient distress and dysfunction. This is particularly true for disorders of olfaction and gustation. This chapter reviews the anatomy and physiology of these senses, describes the effects of xenobiotics on these senses, and examines the significant diagnostic information these senses contribute to identifying the presence of xenobiotics. Understanding the effects of xenobiotics on these senses allows for early detection, removal, and prevention of future events. In occupational settings, understanding these principles help prevent permanent and life-threatening injuries.

OLFACTION

Anatomy and Physiology

Olfactory receptors are bipolar neurons located in the superior nasal turbinates and the adjacent septum. There are 10 to 20 million receptor cells per nasal chamber, and the receptor portion of the cell undergoes continuous renewal from the olfactory epithelium.[122,127] Renewed olfactory receptors regenerate neural connections to the olfactory bulb. These olfactory receptor neurons are distinctive in their ability to regenerate.[26] The axons of these cells form small bundles that traverse the fenestrations of the cribriform plate of the ethmoid bone to the dura. Within the dura, these bundles form connections with the olfactory bulb from which neural projections then connect to the olfactory cortex. There are extensive interconnections to other parts of the brain, such as the hippocampus, thalamus, hypothalamus, and frontal lobe, suggesting effects on other biologic functions.[122] Although primary odor detection is a function of the olfactory nerve (CN I), some irritant odors, such as ammonia and acetone, are transmitted through the trigeminal nerve (CN V) and its receptors.[48,164]

The actual olfactory receptor sites are guanine nucleotide protein (G protein)-coupled receptors (GPCRs) similar to the taste receptors of the mouth and the photoreceptors of the retina. The receptor is a single-polypeptide chain consisting of approximately 350 amino acids, which folds back and forth onto itself to traverse the cellular membrane 7 times. The outer end of the polypeptide contains an amine group (N-terminal), and the cytosolic end contains a carboxyl group (C-terminal). The transmembranous portions determine the receptor shape and characteristics of the binding site. When a molecule binds to a specific receptor site, the resultant conformational change leads to the activation of the G protein system and calcium and/or sodium channel activation and neurotransmission.[86]

Smelling is an extremely sensitive mechanism of detecting xenobiotics. Olfactory receptors detect the presence of a few molecules of certain xenobiotics with a sensitivity that is superior to some of the most sophisticated laboratory detection instruments, even though human smell is several orders of magnitude less perceptive than other mammals.[78]

Clinical Use of Odor Recognition

The sense of smell is extremely useful as a toxicologic warning system. Human olfaction is a variable trait.[5,137,202] For example, 40% to 45% of people have specific anosmia (inability or loss of smell) for the bitter almond odor of cyanide.[49,101,137] There are limited data on the inheritance characteristics or genetic basis of these specific forms of anosmia. Although some studies suggest that the ability to detect the odor of cyanide is a sex-linked

recessive trait,[68] other studies yield conflicting results.[5,20,103] Women have a greater ability to detect androsterone, which is prominent in human underarm secretion.[78] Human olfaction usually can distinguish a mixture of no more than 4 xenobiotics;[107] therefore, specific odors are frequently masked by other stimuli.

Olfactory fatigue is the process of olfactory adaptation following exposure to a stimulus for a variable period of time. This leads to a temporal diminution of the smell. Unfortunately, this adaptation provides a false sense of security during continued exposure to a xenobiotic. For example, hydrogen sulfide, which inhibits cytochrome oxidase, is readily detectable as distinct and offensive at the very low concentration of 0.025 ppm. At a higher and potentially toxic concentration of 50 ppm, the odor is less offensive, and extinguishes recognition after 2 to 15 minutes of exposure.[8,177] At even higher concentrations when toxicity is likely, the onset of olfactory fatigue is even more rapid. The combination of the rapid onset of olfactory fatigue and systemic toxicity at high concentrations of hydrogen sulfide exposure contributes to numerous fatalities (Chap. 123).[1,27,185]

In industrial settings, it is important to be aware of impaired olfactory function in any worker who may be exposed to chemical vapors or gases.[84,177] Such workers are at increased risk for toxic injury. The National Institute for Occupational Safety and Health (NIOSH) requires that an individual using an air-purifying respirator be capable of detecting the odor of a xenobiotic at concentrations below those producing toxicity.[6,177] Sensory perception at this concentration ensures that the individual can detect filter cartridge "breakthrough" or failure at a safe concentration.[177] The odor safety factor refers to the ratio of the time-weighted average (TWA) threshold limit value (TLV) to the odor threshold for a given xenobiotic. A xenobiotic with a high odor safety factor is detectable despite prolonged exposure.[6] Nontoxic xenobiotics with a very high odor safety factor, such as ethyl mercaptan, are added to xenobiotics that are odorless with lower safety factors so that olfactory detection is predictable. This enhanced sensory awareness is the basis for the addition of mercaptans to the odorless natural gases used in the home so as to limit the potential for unrecognized hazardous exposure.

The recognition of odors was traditionally considered an important diagnostic skill in clinical medicine. Some diseases are diagnosed accurately by recognizable associated odors of various affected parts of the body such as the breath, sweat, urine, and wounds: diabetic ketoacidosis as a characteristically fruity odor of the breath; diphtheria as sweet; scurvy as putrid; typhoid fever as fresh-baked brown bread; and scrofula as stale beer.[42] Odors are also described for disorders of amino acid and fatty acid metabolism, such as phenylketonuria, maple syrup urine disease, hypermethioninemia, and isovaleric acidemia.[42]

The recognition of odors continues to be an important diagnostic skill for the rapid detection of some xenobiotics (Table 25–1). To increase awareness of odors of toxic xenobiotics, a "sniffing bar" of commonly available odors may be prepared.[73] Nontoxic xenobiotics that simulate the odors of toxic xenobiotics are placed in test tubes, numbered, and inserted in a test tube rack for circulation among staff. The sniffing bar, brief descriptions of clinical presentations, and a table of diagnostic odors (Table 25–1) is used to teach the recognition of odors in medical toxicology.[73]

Classification of Olfactory Impairment

There are different types of olfactory dysfunction. *Anosmia*, the inability to detect odors, and *hyposmia*, a decrease in the perception of certain odors, are the most common forms of olfactory impairment. The etiology of olfactory impairment is classified as conductive, from anatomic obstruction of inspired air, or perceptive, from dysfunction of the olfactory receptors or

TABLE 25–1	Odors Suggestive of a Xenobiotic
Odor	**Xenobiotic**
Bitter almond	Cyanide
Carrots	Cicutoxin (water hemlock)
Disinfectants	Creosote, phenol
Eggs (rotten)	Carbon disulfide, disulfiram, hydrogen sulfide, mercaptans, *N*-acetylcysteine
Fish or raw liver (musty)	Aluminum phosphide, zinc phosphide
Fruity	Nitrites (amyl, butyl)
Garlic	Arsenic, dimethyl sulfoxide, organic phosphorus compounds, phosphorus, selenium, tellurium, thallium
Hay	Phosgene
Mothballs	Camphor, naphthalene, *p*-dichlorobenzene
Pepper	*O*-Chlorobenzylidene malononitrile
Rope (burnt)	Marijuana, opium
Shoe polish	Nitrobenzene
Sweet fruity	Acetone, chloral hydrate, chloroform, ethanol, isopropanol, lacquer, methylbromide, paraldehyde, trichloroethane
Tobacco	Nicotine
Vinegar	Acetic acid
Violets	Turpentine (metabolites excreted in urine)
Wintergreen	Methyl salicylate

TABLE 25–2	Xenobiotics Responsible for Disorders of Smell	
Hyposmia/Anosmia		**Dysosmia/Cacosmia/Phantosmia**
Acrylic acid		β-Adrenergic antagonists
Antihyperlipidemics: cholestyramine, clofibrate, gemfibrozil, HMG-CoA reductase inhibitors		Amebicides/antihelminthics: metronidazole
		Anesthetics, local
Cadmium		Anticonvulsants: carbamazepine, phenytoin
Chlorhexidine		Antihistamines
Cocaine		Antihypertensives: angiotensin-converting enzyme inhibitors, diazoxide
Formaldehyde		Antimicrobials
Gentamicin nose drops		Antiinflammatory
Hydrocyanic acid		Antirheumatics: allopurinol, colchicine, gold, D-penicillamine
Hydrocarbons (volatile)		
Hydrogen sulfide		Antiparkinsonians: levodopa, bromocriptine
Methylbromide		Antithyroid drugs: methimazole, methylthiouracil, propylthiouracil
Nutritional		Calcium channel blockers
Vitamin B$_{12}$ deficiency		Dimethylsulfoxide
Zinc deficiency		Ethacrynic acid
Pentamidine		Insecticides
Sulfur dioxide		Lithium
		Nicotine
		Nonsteroidal antiinflammatory drugs
		Opioids
		Sympathomimetics
		Toothpastes
		Vitamin D

Anosmia = the loss of smell; cacosmia = sensation of a foul smell; dysosmia = a distorted perception of smell; hyposmia = a decreased perception of smell; phantosmia = sensation of smell without stimulus.

signal transmission. Most conductive olfactory dysfunction results in hyposmia, because the obstruction is usually incomplete.[122,161]

The most common causes of anosmia and hyposmia are viral infections, trauma, xenobiotics, tumors, and congenital and psychiatric disorders (Table 25–2).[48,147,153,161] Viral infections impair olfaction either by obstructing nasal airflow or by causing damage to the olfactory epithelium.[87] Trauma to the head or nose can shear fragile olfactory nerves crossing the cribriform plate.[164,187]

Chronic exposures to numerous xenobiotics are associated with olfactory dysfunction (Table 25–2). The most commonly cited toxic mechanism is perceptive olfactory dysfunction. This is a result of a direct injury, or of a structural alteration of the receptor or its components such as G proteins, adenylate cyclase, or receptor kinase.[85,86] Anosmia or hyposmia from hydrocarbons, formaldehyde, cadmium, and chemotherapeutics such as cytarabine results from direct effects on the receptor sites.[52,86,91] Local effects on the epithelium and the receptors from antibiotic nose drops leads to temporary anosmia and hyposmia.[97,201] Inhaled corticosteroids have local effects on the epithelium, as well as direct effects on both G proteins and adenylate cyclase.[88] Cocaine insufflation causes direct local effects such as nasal septum perforations, as well as effects on receptor functions.[74,76] Because of the limited local effects of most xenobiotics and the regenerative ability of the olfactory receptor neurons, most xenobiotic-induced olfactory dysfunction is reversible.

Many individuals determined to have anosmia actually have congenital anosmia for select molecules, such as hydrogen cyanide, *n*-butyl mercaptan, trimethylamine, and isovaleric acid.[7,48] Some extreme forms of congenital anosmia are associated with other abnormalities, such as Kallmann syndrome, a hereditary form of anosmia associated with hypogonadotropic hypogonadism in which agenesis of the olfactory bulbs and incomplete development of the hypothalamus are responsible for the anosmia.[48,164]

Dysosmia or *parosmia* is the distorted perception of smell (Table 25–2). Subclassifications of dysosmia include the perception of foul smell or *cacosmia*, or *phantosmia* the sensation of smell without a stimulus, or such as the sensation of the smell of a burnt or metallic material, *torqosmia*.[161] The etiologies are classified as peripheral or central. Peripheral etiologies include abnormalities of the nose, sinuses, and upper respiratory tract. Central etiologies are related to disorders such as Addison disease, hypothyroidism, temporal lobe epilepsy, psychosis, or pregnancy.[48,122,162] How these conditions actually alter the perception of smell is unclear. A number of xenobiotics with similar effects are listed in Table 25–2. Bromocriptine alters dopaminergic transmission and inhibits adenylate cyclase. Levodopa affects the dopaminergic transmission and also chelates zinc, which is important in the maintenance of normal receptor functions.[86,88]

Evaluation of Olfactory Impairment

General evaluation of olfactory function includes a detailed history, focusing on types, duration, and progression of symptoms, recent illnesses, head and nose trauma, sinus diseases, family history, occupational history, exposures hobbies, and xenobiotic exposures.[44,77] A physical examination with a detailed examination of the nasopharynx and sinuses is performed to assess the potential for inflammation or structural abnormality. A simple set of olfactory stimulants, such as ground coffee, almond extract, peppermint extract, and musk, is recommended to test each nostril individually with the patient's eyes closed.[77,164] Standardized smell tests such as the University of Pennsylvania Smell Identification Test (UPSIT) and the Connecticut Chemosensory Clinical Research Center (CCCRC) tests are commercially available, and a composite score based on a panel of tests determines the degree of olfactory dysfunction.[114] Pungent odors or stimulation associated with ammonia, capsaicin, acetone, and menthol are dependent on the trigeminal nerve (CN V) olfactory function, which is mainly responsible for tactile pressure, pain, and temperature sensation in the mouth and nasal cavity. A patient who has olfactory nerve damage should be able to detect these substances; conversely, a person with hysteria may deny detection of these substances that should physiologically be recognized.[77,164,201] If a xenobiotic-mediated mechanism is suspected, the offending xenobiotic should be discontinued. Coronal computed tomography of the sinuses and nose or magnetic resonance imaging of the brain should be obtained if structural abnormalities are suspected.[164,201] Gas chromatographic analysis of the urine is useful in patients with fish odor syndrome associated with trimethylaminuria.[108,174] Complicated cases and patients with significant impairment should be referred to an otolaryngologist or neurologist.

GUSTATION
Anatomy and Physiology
Taste, the sensory interpretation of oral materials, is determined by taste buds on the tongue, palate, throat, and upper third of the esophagus. The cells in the taste buds have a life span of 10 days and are constantly renewed.[11,164] The taste buds on the anterior two-thirds of the tongue and the palate are innervated by the facial nerve (CN VII), those on the posterior one-third of the tongue by the glossopharyngeal nerve (CN IX), and those on the laryngeal and epiglottal regions by the vagus nerve (CN X). The signals are sent to the solitary nucleus in the brain stem, where they are processed and distributed to various regions of the brain. There are at least 14 known chemical taste receptors responsible for the 5 primary taste sensations—sweet, sour, bitter, umami (savory), and salty: 2 sodium receptor types; 2 potassium receptor types; one chloride receptor; one adenosine receptor; 2 inosine receptors; 2 sweet receptor types; 2 bitter receptor types; one glutamate receptor; and one hydrogen ion receptor.[79] One substrate will typically activate multiple taste receptors; the combined effects of these stimulated receptors determine the taste of the substance.[66]

The structure of the taste receptors is similar to that of the olfactory receptors, in that they are coupled to G proteins and sodium and calcium channels permitting neural stimulation. Each receptor is capable of interacting with various classes of xenobiotics, of varying sizes. The pH of the xenobiotic determines sour (acid taste), whereas sodium or potassium concentrations determine salty taste. Many xenobiotics such as sugars, glycols, aldehydes, ketones, amides, amino acids, inorganic salts of lead, and bretylium activate the sweet receptors. Bitter taste results from long-chain organic substances containing nitrogen, or alkaloids, including quinine, strychnine, caffeine, and nicotine.[13,79] The threshold for bitter receptor stimulation is several orders of magnitudes lower than other taste receptors.[13] Umami taste is a more recently accepted primary taste, best defined as a pleasant savory taste. The primary xenobiotic that stimulates umami receptor is glutamate, such as monosodium-L-glutamate. Umami receptor stimulation is enhanced by 5'-ribonucleotide monophosphates such as inosine and guanosine.[205] Salivary proteins, such as zinc containing gustin and ebnerin, are important in the regulation of taste sensation.[86,90,110,172] These molecules serve as binding proteins and growth factors for the regeneration of taste receptors. Taste is also affected significantly by the appreciation of aromas or odors and, to a lesser extent, by visual perception.[162]

Classification of Gustatory Dysfunction
Types of gustatory dysfunction include *ageusia*, the inability to perceive taste; *hypogeusia*, the diminished sensitivity of taste; and *dysgeusia*, the distortion of normal taste. There are several variations of *dysgeusia*, such as *cacogeusia*, which is a perceived foul, perverted, or metallic taste.[77,119] Taste impairment is commonly related to direct damage to the taste receptors, adverse effects on their regeneration, or effects on receptor mechanisms.[87] These effects result from a xenobiotic, disease, aging, and nutritional disorders (Table 25–3).[72,79,152,183] Any abnormality that interferes with either the direct contact of a xenobiotic with the gustatory cells of the tongue or cranial nerves VII, IX, or X dramatically affects taste.[161] Most common forms of xenobiotic-induced dysgeusia are related to direct effects on the taste receptor site or effects related to receptor mechanisms such as G proteins, adenylate cyclase, and calcium channels.[106] Other forms of dysgeusia result from direct stimulation of chemical receptors by xenobiotics.[79,86]

TABLE 25–3 Xenobiotics Responsible for Alterations of Taste

Hypogeusia/Ageusia	Dysgeusia	Metallic Taste
Local	**Local**	**ACE inhibitors**
Chemical and thermal burns	Chemical burn	Acetaldehyde
Radiation therapy	Radiation therapy	Allopurinol
Systemic	**Systemic**	Arsenicals
ACE inhibitors	ACE inhibitors	Cadmium
Amiloride	Adriamycin	Ciguatoxin
Amrinone	Amphotericin B	Copper
Carbon monoxide	Botulism (in recovery)	*Coprinus* spp
Cocaine	Carbamazepine	Dipyridamole
Dimethylsulfoxide	Dimethylsulfoxide	Disulfiram
Gasoline	5-Fluorouracil	Ethambutol
Hydrochlorothiazide	Griseofulvin	Ferrous salts
Methylthiouracil	Isotretinoin	Flurazepam
Nitroglycerin	Levodopa	Iodine
NSAIDs	Nicotine	Lead
Penicillamine	Nifedipine	Levamisole
Propranolol	NSAIDs	Lithium
Pyrethrins	Phenylthiourea (hereditary)	Mercury
Smoking	Quinine	Methotrexate
Spironolactone	Zinc deficiency	Metformin
Triazolam		Metoclopramide
		Metronidazole
		Pentamidine
		Pine nuts
		Procaine penicillin
		Propafenone
		Snake venom
		Tetracycline

ACE = angiotensin-converting enzyme; NSAID = nonsteroidal antiinflammatory drug.

Angiotensin-converting enzyme (ACE) inhibitors commonly cause gustatory impairment, usually hypogeusia and dysgeusia.[19,74,121,203] Angiotensin-converting enzyme inhibitors work by inhibiting zinc-dependent ACE, and chelating zinc from taste receptors and salivary proteins results in gustatory dysfunction. Calcium channel blockers act by inhibiting calcium channels of the taste receptor mechanisms.[79] Many diuretics cause zinc depletion by enhancing zinc elimination in the urine,[79] whereas furosemide and spironolactone may also chelate zinc. Numerous xenobiotics also cause gustatory dysfunction through variable degrees of zinc chelation: amrinone, ethambutol, hydralazine, methyldopa, the nonsteroidal antiinflammatory drugs (NSAIDs), antithyroid medications, penicillamine, and phenytoin.[79,86,204] Arsenic, mercury, chromium, and lead either lead to chelation of zinc or replace zinc in salivary proteins because of a higher level of affinity. Chemotherapeutics and colchicine inhibit cellular division and taste receptor regeneration. The oral antiseptic chlorhexidine directly alters taste receptor function.[62] Acetazolamide causes cacogeusia when carbonated beverages are consumed. The exact mechanism is unclear, but is postulated to be a result of the inhibition of carbonic anhydrase causing carbon dioxide accumulation and an increased tissue bicarbonate.[86,99,124]

HEARING
Anatomy and Physiology
Normal hearing begins when sound waves are captured by the external auricle, traverse the external auditory canal, and are conducted to the tympanic membrane, the 3 auditory ossicles of the middle ear, and move (although dampened) through the oval window to the perilymph in the scala vestibuli

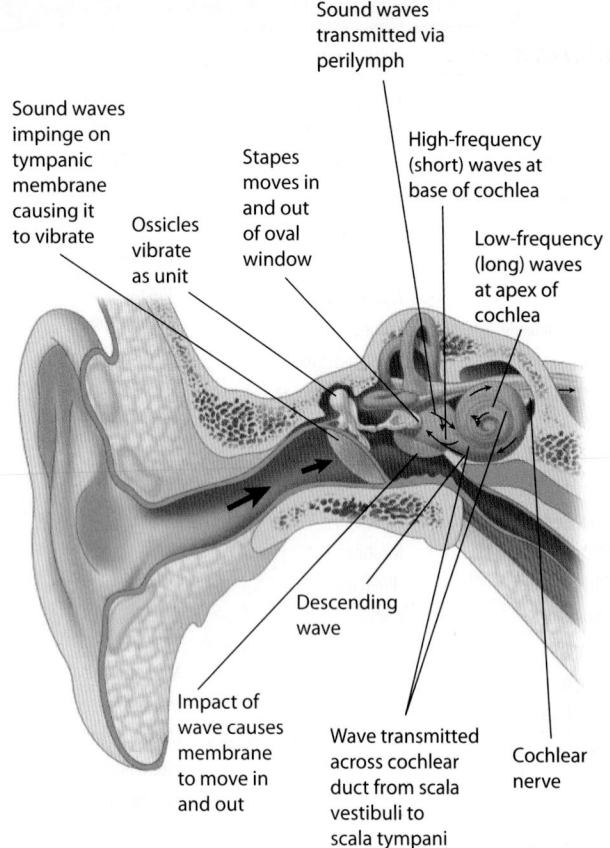

FIGURE 25–1. Pathways of sound conduction in the ear.

contain crosslinked stereocilia projections that detect transmitted shear forces, which lead to the influx of potassium from the endolymph through opened potassium channels.[46,112] Depolarization of the hair cells results in calcium influx and neurotransmitter release to the cochlear nerve. Repetitive movements of the stereocilia will amplify the specific sound signals. Neurologic signals from the cochlear nerve are conducted to the cochlear nucleus of the pons; bilateral projections are then sent to the superior olivary nucleus of the midbrain, nuclei of lateral lemnisci, inferior colliculus, medial geniculate body of the thalamus, and then to the auditory cortex of the temporal lobe.[178] Interruption or damage to any part of the hearing mechanism will lead to auditory impairment.

The anatomy and physiology of the cochlea and its importance in the biomechanics of hearing are reviewed in order to better understand the potential for xenobiotic injury. The word *cochlea* is derived from the Greek word *kochlias*, meaning snail, and describes its general structure—a 2.5-turn, spirally wound tube. The cochlea is further divided into 3 inner tubular structures: the upper tube or scala vestibuli, the middle tube or cochlear duct, and the lower tube or scala tympani. The scala vestibuli and the scala tympani contain the perilymph fluid. The cochlear duct contains endolymph fluid, the Reissner membrane at the roof, and the organ of Corti.[178] The cochlear fluids serve multiple functions: to conduct sound waves to the hair cells; to provide nutrients for and remove waste from the cells lining the cochlear duct; to control pressure distribution in the cochlea; and to maintain an electrochemical gradient for the function of the hair cells. The sodium concentration of the perilymph is similar to that of the extracellular fluid, and the potassium concentration of the endolymph is similar to that of the intracellular fluid.[60] Any significant alterations of the sodium or potassium concentrations will depress the cochlear potential and function. The stria vascularis controls the production of the cochlear fluids and the repolarization of the hair cells, and maintains the electrochemical gradient between the endolymph and the perilymph. The stria vascularis contains a high concentration of the oxidative enzymes, Na+,K+-ATPase, adenylate cyclase, and carbonic anhydrase, which are all highly susceptible to xenobiotics.[21,92,159]

Although human speech is composed of sounds in the frequency of 250 to 3,000 Hz, humans can normally detect sounds in the frequency range of 20 to 20,000 Hz.[136] The cochlea is a "tuned" structure with varying width and stiffness, such that different regions receive different sound waves. The stiffer

of the cochlea (Figs. 25–1 and 25–2). The sound wave is then transferred through the Reissner membrane at the roof of the cochlear duct, to the endolymph and the organ of Corti.[58,178] The specialized hair cells of the organ of Corti convert mechanical waves into neurologic signals. The hair cells

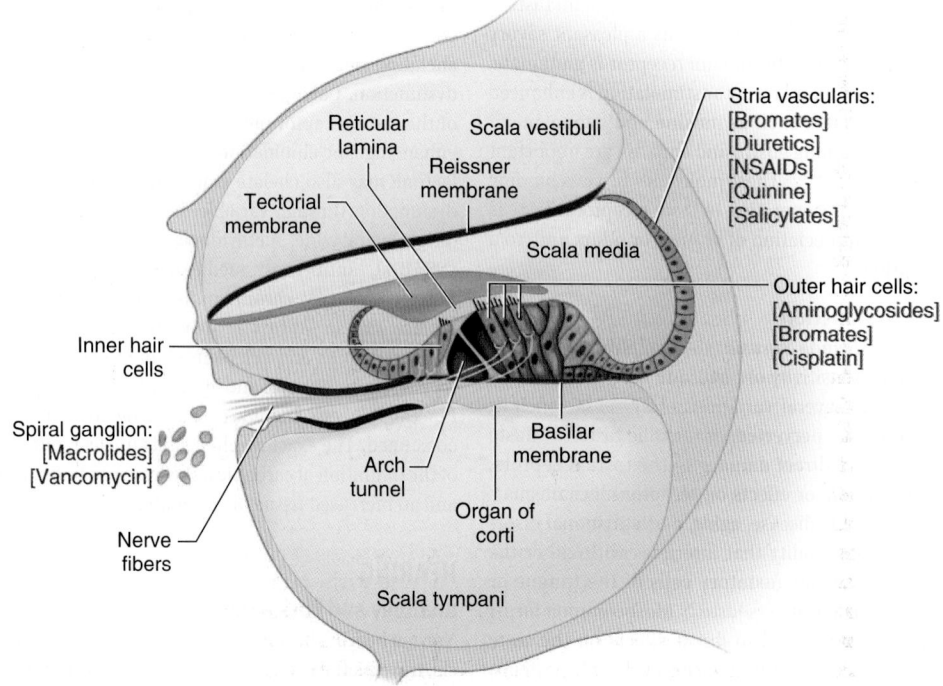

FIGURE 25–2. Cross-section of the organ of Corti showing sites of xenobiotic effect.

and wider base of the cochlea serves as a receptacle for higher-frequency sounds, whereas the apex is responsible for receiving the lower-frequency sounds.[58] Because various regions of the cochlea are susceptible to different forms of injury, audiologic testing is tailored specifically to each patient.[29]

Xenobiotic-Induced Ototoxicity

Ototoxicity includes effects on the cochlear and vestibular system. This section focuses on cochlear toxicity. Quinine and salicylates were widely recognized in the 1800s and streptomycin in the 1940s as causes of ototoxicity.[92,154] Drugs of abuse such as cocaine and heroin also cause hearing loss.[36,40,133,165,167,173,182] Several hundred xenobiotics are implicated as causes of either reversible or irreversible ototoxicity (Table 25–4).[23,96,104,130] Ototoxic xenobiotics primarily affect 2 different sites in the cochlea: the organ of Corti—specifically the outer hair cells—and the stria vascularis. Because of the limited regenerative capacity of the sensory hair cells and other supporting cells, when significant cellular damage occurs, the loss is often permanent.[50,58,92,176] Although cell death of the outer hair cells from inflammation and necrosis is expected when sufficient insults occur, apoptotic cell death is now postulated to be a major mechanism of ototoxicity from certain xenobiotics such as cisplatin and aminoglycosides.[21,23,47,92,96,151] Inhibition of caspases and calpain associated with apoptosis of the hair cells decreases ototoxicity from cisplatin and aminoglycosides in animals.[151,175] Heat shock proteins are endogenous molecules that respond to cellular stress and inhibit apoptosis. Xenobiotics, such as celestrol, that can up-regulate heat shock proteins prevent cisplatin and aminoglycoside toxicity in animal models.[43,64] Further studies are required to demonstrate clinical utility. Evidence supports the concept that otic injury is potentiated by loud noises. Although the actual cellular mechanisms for many forms of ototoxicity remain unclear,[200] some of the mechanisms are known.[69] Loop diuretics, such as furosemide, bumetanide, and ethacrynic acid, cause physiologic dysfunction and edema at the stria vascularis, resulting in reversible hearing loss.[92,117,194] The underlying mechanisms are the inhibition of potassium pumps and G proteins associated with adenylate cyclase.[9] Studies of loop diuretics demonstrate decreased potassium activity in the endolymph and a decreased endocochlear potential.[156] Permanent hearing loss associated with furosemide and ethacrynic acid is also reported, and appears to be related to direct interference with oxidative metabolism in the outer hair cells.[105,117,166]

Salicylates are a well-known cause of ototoxicity. Aspirin (acetylsalicylic acid)-induced hearing impairment was first reported in 1877.[100] Salicylate-induced hearing loss is generally a loss of 20 to 40 decibels (dB) and reversible.[18,90] Animal studies demonstrate immediate hearing impairment with the use of high doses of salicylates.[17,118,119,143] The mechanism of salicylate-induced ototoxicity is unclear, although multiple factors are postulated. Salicylates and other NSAIDs inhibit cyclooxygenase, which converts arachidonic acid to prostaglandin G_2 and prostaglandin H_2. These effects interfere with Na^+,K^+-ATPase pump function at the stria vascularis, and also decrease cochlear blood flow.[31,53,100] A reversible decrease in outer hair cell turgor secondary to membrane permeability changes impair otoacoustic emissions.[142,146] In support of these theories, pretreatment of

animals with leukotriene antagonists and α-adrenergic receptor antagonists attenuates or prevents salicylate-induced ototoxicity.[100]

Nonsteroidal antiinflammatory drugs and quinine also cause reversible hearing loss, particularly at the higher frequencies.[33,92] Occasionally, quinine-induced hearing loss is permanent.[92,160] The primary mechanism is related to prostaglandin inhibition.[100] Quinine inhibits the enzyme phospholipase A_2, which converts phospholipids to arachidonic acid. Quinine also inhibits calcium channels that interact with prostaglandins.[100]

Certain chemotherapeutics, such as cisplatin, vinblastine, and vincristine, cause permanent ototoxicity.[92] Cisplatin is the most ototoxic of the group, with clinically apparent hearing loss noted in 30% to 70% of the patients receiving doses of 50 to 100 mg/m². Other platinum derivatives such as carboplatin and oxaliplatin are less ototoxic than cisplatin. These chemotherapeutics typically damage the outer hair cells and also affect the stria vascularis.[92] The underlying mechanisms are related to the inhibition of adenylate cyclase in the stria vascularis, the inhibition of protein synthesis, and the formation of oxygen free radicals.[9,92,166] The generation of oxygen free radicals and the depletion of antioxidants result in the irreversible damage to the hair cells.[56] Furthermore, cranial radiation will cause synergistic toxicity if radiation precedes cisplatin therapy. Various antioxidants and free radical scavengers prevent cisplatin-induced ototoxicity in animals, perhaps preventing oxidative injury–induced apoptosis to hair cells.[110,125,148,151,155,180,198] Amifostine, a precursor to a thiol free radical scavenger, prevents cisplatin-induced nephrotoxicity, does not prevent cisplatin-induced ototoxicity.[158,193]

The aminoglycosides are best known for their association with irreversible ototoxicity,[141] but they are not concentrated in the cochlea. The endolymph concentration of gentamicin is approximately 10% of that in the serum. Neomycin and kanamycin are the most ototoxic, although all aminoglycosides are potentially toxic.[105] With the development of the newer aminoglycosides and therapeutic drug monitoring, the incidence of aminoglycoside-related ototoxicity is decreasing. The reported rates of ototoxicity for the more commonly used aminoglycosides gentamicin and tobramycin are between 5% and 8%.[116] In China, where aminoglycosides are readily available as nonprescription medications, as much as 66% of deafness is directly related to aminoglycoside toxicity.[67,112] Several uncommon genetic mutations that predispose to aminoglycoside-induced ototoxicity are identified, including A1555G and C1494T mutations.[61,81] The genetic transmission appears to be maternal via mitochondrial DNA, and the defects increase aminoglycoside binding to mitochondrial 12S ribosomal RNA.[61] These patients may experience rapid and severe hearing loss compared with normal people with a similar aminoglycoside exposure.[151]

Several mechanisms of aminoglycoside ototoxicity are postulated, including antagonism of calcium channels of the outer hair cells of the cochlea, blocking transduction of the hair cells and resulting in acute, reversible hearing deficits as well as binding to polyphosphoinositides of cell membranes to alter their functions. Polyphosphoinositides are essential for the generation of the second messengers diacylglycerol and inositol triphosphate and their ultimate cellular function, for the maintenance of lipid membrane structure and permeability, and as a source for arachidonic acid.[92,151] However, the most important mechanism is that aminoglycosides interact with transitional metal cations such as iron and copper via the Fenton or Fentonlike reaction to generate free radicals, damaging the hair cells. Aminoglycosides inhibit aconitase in the mitochondria and cause the accumulation of cations including iron that increases free radical generation. Aminoglycosides also inhibit ornithine decarboxylase, which is important for cellular recovery following an injury and makes the cell more susceptible to toxicity.[159] The outer hair cells of the cochlea are increasingly susceptible to aminoglycosides, and damage progresses from the inner row of the outer hair cells to the basal turn of the cochlea and, ultimately, to the apex.[4,7,105,151]

The risks of ototoxicity are increased with a duration of therapy of more than 10 days, concomitant use of other ototoxic xenobiotics, and the development of elevated serum concentrations.[7,59,157] There is no evidence that

TABLE 25–4	Etiologies of Xenobiotic-Induced Hearing Loss
Reversible	**Irreversible**
Antimicrobials: chloroquine, erythromycin, quinine	Aminoglycosides
	Bromates
Carbon monoxide	Chemotherapeutics: bleomycin, cisplatin, nitrogen mustard, vincristine, vinblastine
Cocaine	
Diuretics: acetazolamide, bumetanide, ethacrynic acid, furosemide, mannitol	Hydrocarbons: styrene, toluene, xylene
	Metals: arsenic, lead, mercury
Nonsteroidal antiinflammatory drugs	Opioids (infrequently)
Opioids (frequently)	
Salicylates	

single daily dosing of aminoglycosides alters the risk of ototoxicity.[138,191] Loop diuretics increase aminoglycoside toxicity by increasing aminoglycoside penetration into the endolymph. In animal models, certain free radical scavengers, such as glutathione, amifostine, and deferoxamine, decrease aminoglycoside-induced ototoxicity.[70,160,181,188,192] Fosfomycin, a phosphonic antibiotic, has limited efficacy in reducing aminoglycoside-induced ototoxicity.[135] Leupeptin and Z-DEVD-FMK, calpain and caspase inhibitors, respectively, that affect the apoptotic pathway, decrease ototoxicity in animal models.[34,69,170,175] Further studies are required to determine their applicability to humans. Salicylates, which act as free radical scavengers at therapeutic concentrations, prevent gentamicin ototoxicity in animals. Two randomized human trials using concomitant salicylate therapy at 1.5 and 3 g/d significantly attenuated gentamicin-induced ototoxicity.[12,171] Gastric adverse effects, including bleeding, were also more common in the salicylate group. Confirmation of these findings and determining safer alternatives are warranted.

Erythromycin, vancomycin, and their respective analogs are ototoxic. There are a number of reports of hearing loss following erythromycin therapy in humans and an animal study supporting the ototoxic potential. Most deficits in humans are transient, although several cases of permanent hearing loss are reported.[22,25] The mechanisms of toxicity remain unclear, although the proposed effects are on the central auditory pathways. Erythromycin-induced hearing loss occurs at both lower and higher frequencies for speech, allowing for recognition in the early stages of ototoxicity.[25] Similarly, both reversible and irreversible ototoxicities from the newer macrolide antibiotics clarithromycin and azithromycin are reported.[83,123] However, a large retrospective epidemiologic study failed to demonstrate hearing loss with macrolide antibiotics.[54]

The evidence for vancomycin-induced ototoxicity is less convincing. Although numerous cases of presumed vancomycin-related ototoxicity were reported, impurities with initial vancomycin production, and concomitant use of other ototoxic antibiotics and xenobiotics were common, and the lack of audiometric studies lead to complicated conclusions.[25] In limited animal studies, vancomycin alone does not induce ototoxicity, but it increases ototoxicity when administered concomitantly with an aminoglycoside.[24,113,190] A recent retrospective found an increase in hearing loss with vancomycin usage; the study did not find an association with trough vancomycin concentrations and some patients had concomitant ototoxicity xenobiotics.[63] Currently, there are inadequate information on the ototoxicity of other glycopeptide antibiotics similar to vancomycin such as teicoplanin, televancin, and daptomycin.

Bromates are among the most extensively studied ototoxic xenobiotics.[33,39,115,144] Bromates are used in hair "neutralizers," bread preservatives, and as fuses in explosive devices.[93,144,184] Following bromate administration the stria vascularis and hair cells of the organ of Corti are irreversibly damaged.[144] Substantial exposure to bromates also causes acute kidney injury, which decreases bromate elimination and, in turn, increases its ototoxic potential.[93,144]

It is intriguing that xenobiotics, such as the bromates, loop diuretics, cisplatin, and aminoglycosides, primarily affect both the cochlea and the kidneys. One possible explanation is that the stria vascularis and the renal tubules have similar functions in maintaining electrochemical gradients.[135,136] However, renal tubules regenerate, whereas damage to the hair cells and the stria vascularis of the cochlea is more likely to be permanent. Membrane transporters such as copper-transporter-1 (CTR1) and organic cation transporter 2 (OCT2) are important in the movement of xenobiotics such as cisplatin into cells. Although CTR1 is expressed in many types of cells, OCT2 expression is limited to renal, cochlear, and neural cells and may be critical to cellular toxicity.[37] Targeting the effects of OCT2 has the potential to limit both renal and cochlear toxicity.[199]

Sudden hearing loss is reported with recreational drug use, particularly with cocaine and opioids. For cocaine, the mechanism of injury is presumed to be related to cochlear hemorrhage and hypoxia subsequent to vasoconstriction.[40,133,182] Although other mechanisms such as a direct effect on the potassium channels in the hair cells and sodium channels of the auditory nerve are

postulated, they are not well elucidated in animal models. Concomitant opioid use and adulterants should be evaluated. Various opioids, including heroin, methadone, and hydrocodone, are associated with hearing loss.[36,165,167,173] Neither the route of use nor the presence of adulterants such as quinine can adequately explain the hearing loss. Most cases of opioid-associated hearing loss are reversible, but some are permanent. The mechanisms of opioid-associated hearing loss are unclear. Cases that involved the use of naloxone did not reverse hearing loss, which suggests a different mechanism from the well-known opioid effect that causes respiratory depression.[131,195] Several cases of opioid-acetaminophen–induced hearing loss responded well to cochlear implantation suggesting the site of injury involving the cochlea sparing the auditory nerve.[16,65,134,195] Hypoperfusion of the vestibulocochlear system secondary to opioid-induced vasospasm or vasculitis is postulated to be the cause of injury.[36,134,165,173,195] Another potential mechanism is the stimulation of opioid receptors in the cochlea, which inhibits adenylate cyclase activity, leading to hearing loss.[57] Various opioid receptors are identified in the cochlea, such as in the inner hair cells, outer hair cells, and the spiral ganglion. Others postulate that opioids have potential roles as neurotransmitters or neuromodulators that affect auditory function.[98]

Other xenobiotics implicated as ototoxins are carbon monoxide, lead, arsenic, mercury, toluene, xylene, and styrene.[89,177] However, both human and animal data are quite limited. Carbon disulfide, carbon tetrachloride, and trichloroethylene are also suspected of being ototoxic, but toxicity has not been demonstrated in humans.[89,167] Because exposures to xenobiotics are frequently occupational, they are of great concern as they may potentiate or be additive to other types of occupational hearing impairments.[102,149]

High-frequency hearing is most vulnerable, and early or limited impairment are often not noticeable unless audiometry, especially at 8,000 kHz and above, is performed.[189] These hearing tests are performed in infants using the measurement of auditory brain stem response.[14]

Noise-Induced Hearing Impairment

Noise-induced hearing impairment was recognized for hundreds of years, but became a great concern and increasingly prevalent with the industrial revolution and the discovery of gunpowder.[54] Some of the anatomic changes in the organ of Corti and the audiometric features of noise-induced hearing impairment were well described by 1900.[2,3,120] Unfortunately, few longitudinal studies on noise-induced hearing impairment are performed.

Although noises of sufficient magnitude cause hearing impairment with limited exposure, most noise-induced hearing losses result from preventable prolonged cumulative occupational exposure. The National Institute for Occupational Safety and Health has estimated that up to 1.7 million workers in the United States between 50 and 59 years of age have significant occupation-related hearing loss.[135] Noise is defined as any unwanted sound, which can be further characterized by duration, time pattern (continuous, intermittent, or impulsive), frequency, and intensity. Although loud sounds from concerts and personal listening devices are not typically classified as noise, they are included as noise for the purpose of this discussion. The intensity is measured in sound pressure levels (SPLs) and expressed in a logarithmic scale in decibels (dB). The intensity of a normal conversation is approximately 65 dB (Table 25–5).[135] The risk of noise-induced hearing loss is related to cumulative duration of exposure, intensity, and individual susceptibility.[132,139,197] Much of the risk assessment of noise-induced hearing loss is inexact. Most authorities agree that sounds with maximal intensity below 75 to 80 dB will not cause hearing impairment, regardless of the duration of exposure.[132] At higher intensity, the risk of hearing impairment increases with increased duration of exposure. Continued occupational exposure at 90 to 94 dB typically causes some high-frequency hearing loss in approximately 10 years.[2,139] Further exposure results in hearing loss in the lower frequency range. The Occupational Safety and Health Administration (OSHA) established guidelines for permissible occupational noise exposure based on an analysis of the average intensity and duration of exposure (Table 25–6).[2,197]

The pathophysiology of noise-induced hearing impairment is related to an excessive energy impact on the cochlea, but the exact biochemical

TABLE 25–5	Typical Sound Levels on the Decibel Scale
Sound	**Decibels**
Weakest sound that humans can detect	10
Quiet bedroom, soft whisper	20
Broadcast studio	25–30
Insulated lounge	50
Normal conversation	65
Television-audio	70
Vacuum cleaner	80
Machine press, subway car (35 mph)	95
Spray painting, snowmobile	105
Power saw	110
Maximum volume of MP3 players	100–115
Loud rock concert, car horn	115
Armored personnel carrier; ear pain begins	120
Jet plane engine, gunshot	145
Highest sound level that can occur	194

changes are unclear. Apoptotic death of the hair cells is demonstrated and inhibition of apoptotic pathways mitigates noise-induced toxicity in animal models. A limited exposure to excessive noise results in a temporary hearing impairment or temporary threshold shift with a duration of hours to weeks. However, prolonged exposure results in a permanent threshold shift or hearing impairment.[3,58,197] Initially, outer hair cells are lost, but more significant exposures result in damage to both inner and outer hair cells and all supporting structures in the organ of Corti. Cochlear nerve fibers degenerate after hair cell damage.[58,197] The section of the cochlea most at risk from loud noises is at the region of 9 to 13 mm (total length is 32 mm).[120] This region is responsible for hearing at the range of 3,000 to 6,000 kHz, corresponding to the typical noise-induced hearing loss pattern.

Much of the clinical assessment and monitoring of noise-induced hearing loss is based on pure tone hearing loss, demonstrating an audiometric deficit at 3,000 to 6,000 kHz.[136,139,197] Although human speech is composed

TABLE 25–6	OSHA Standard for Permissible Noise Exposure
Decibels A[a]	**Duration of Exposure per Day in Hours**
85	16
90	8
92	6
95	4
97	3
100	2
102	1.5
105	1
110	0.5
115	≤0.25

[a]Decibels using the A-scale filter.

mainly of low frequency sounds, the ability to perceive the higher frequency sounds is extremely important in speech recognition. For this reason, the major impairment in patients with noise-induced hearing loss is an inability to discriminate speech, particularly from background noise.[2,45] Currently, the science of the investigation of speech discrimination is limited with extensive areas for research.

Blast injury to the ear results from exposure to sound waves of extremely short duration but very high intensity, usually greater than 140 dB. Military personnel are particularly at risk.[32,140,186,189] Hearing loss from blast injury is related to rupture of the tympanic membrane, disruption of the ossicles, temporary cochlear dysfunction, and permanent cochlear dysfunction from labyrinthine fistulae and basilar membrane rupture.[30] When a large tympanic membrane rupture or disruption of the ossicles occurs, surgical intervention is often required to treat hearing impairment.[30]

Prevention of any type of noise-induced hearing loss remains the best solution. Various hearing protection devices are available if the noise exposure cannot be reduced. Better monitoring and more longitudinal studies are required on noise-induced hearing loss. Exposures to xenobiotics that impair hearing have synergistic effects with noise-induced hearing loss.[102,104] These factors should be addressed when noise exposure is evaluated. Furthermore, noise exposure is not limited to the workplace. Significant noise exposure occurs at home or from leisure activities, such as the use of power tools, loud music, and ambient exposure.[15,41,80,139] The impact of noise exposure outside of the workplace has only recently attracted the attention of investigators.

Tinnitus

Tinnitus is the sensation of sound not resulting from mechanoacoustic or electric signals. Virtually all humans experience tinnitus during their lives. The exact mechanism or mechanisms resulting in tinnitus are largely unknown.[163] Tinnitus is not necessarily associated with hearing loss. Several theories are proposed, but none is completely satisfactory. Tinnitus may result from spontaneous neurologic discharges when the hair cells or cochlear nerve is injured. Altered sound perception results from local or central effects when feedback mechanisms are interrupted.[48,55,95,119] Severing the cochlear nerve terminates tinnitus in less than half of affected patients, suggesting important central mechanisms.[10] Furthermore, certain etiologies of tinnitus, such as migraine headache and temporal lobe seizures, do not affect hearing directly. N-methyl-D-aspartate (NMDA) glutamate receptor activation (and enhanced cochlear signal transmission) is implicated as a mechanism for tinnitus in animal models; NMDA receptor activation results from cyclooxygenase inhibition or neurologic injuries.[82,142] Xenobiotics, including salicylates, cause hair cell dysfunction and modify neurotransmission centrally in both the cochlear nucleus and the inferior colliculus.[71,196] Although the probable sites involved in tinnitus are classified as peripheral (external ear, middle ear, or cochlear {CN VIII}), central, or extra-auditory (vascular, nasopharyngeal), some etiologies affect peripheral and central sites, and many etiologies remain unknown.[38,55,119]

Numerous xenobiotics are associated with tinnitus (Table 25–7), but the incidence is probably low and the implied relationships are usually supported only by case reports.[35,168,169] It is probable that the xenobiotics associated with hearing loss affect cochlear function, whereas those that produce tinnitus without hearing loss probably act on signal transmission at the cochlea and in the central nervous system. Xenobiotics that frequently produce tinnitus include streptomycin, neomycin, indomethacin, doxycycline, ethacrynic acid, furosemide, heavy metals, and high doses of caffeine.[75,168,169] Only a few xenobiotics, such as quinine and salicylates, consistently cause tinnitus at toxic doses.[17,55] These 2 xenobiotics also serve as examples of how the presence of tinnitus may be an indicator of xenobiotic toxicity and useful clinically.

Tinnitus associated with salicylates usually begins when serum concentrations are in the high therapeutic or low toxic range of approximately 20 to 40 mg/dL.[126] Membrane permeability changes cause a loss of outer hair cell turgor in the organ of Corti, which impairs acoustic emissions, explaining tinnitus to some extent.[142,143,146] N-Methyl-d-aspartate receptor

TABLE 25–7   Xenobiotics That Cause Tinnitus

β-Adrenergic antagonists

Antidepressants: amoxapine, cyclic antidepressants, lithium, tranylcypromine

Antiepileptics: carbamazepine

Antifungals: amphotericin B

Antihistamines

Antimicrobials: aminoglycosides, clindamycin, dapsone, metronidazole, sulfa derivatives, tetracyclines, thiabendazole, vancomycin

Antiparasitics: chloroquine, hydroxychloroquine

Antipsychotics: haloperidol, molindone

Bromates

Chemotherapeutics: 6-aminonicotinamide, cisplatin, methotrexate, nitrogen mustard, vinblastine

Cinchona alkaloids: quinine, quinidine

Diuretics: bumetanide, ethacrynic acid, furosemide

Hydrocarbons: benzene

Local anesthetics: bupivacaine, lidocaine, mepivacaine

Nonsteroidal antiinflammatory drugs

Oral contraceptives

Salicylates

Sympathomimetics: albuterol, caffeine, metaproterenol, methylphenidate, theophylline

---

activation from cyclooxygenase inhibition also causes tinnitus.[142] Before the wide availability of serum salicylate measurements, physicians treating gout or rheumatoid arthritis often titrated the salicylate dosage until tinnitus developed.[126] Tinnitus and other signs and symptoms of salicylism (Chap. 37) should be sufficient for physicians to diagnose salicylate toxicity before serum salicylate concentrations are available. However, tinnitus often is not evident in patients with hearing impairment despite significantly elevated salicylate concentrations.[126] The classic constellation of symptoms of quinine and salicylate toxicity, called cinchonism, includes nausea, vomiting, tinnitus, and visual disturbances.[4,28,129] Because serum quinine concentrations are not readily available, symptoms of quinine toxicity define the clinical diagnosis (Chap. 55).[179]

SUMMARY

- Numerous xenobiotics commonly affect the sense of smell, taste, and hearing, thus causing significant morbidity.
- Some of the events are predictable, whereas others will require monitoring and appropriate testing.
- Current knowledge about the pathophysiology of xenobiotics and these special organs at the molecular level is rapidly expanding.
- Although no definitive antidote is available for the prevention or treatment of xenobiotic-induced ototoxicity in humans, substantial progress has been achieved in both in vitro and in vivo animal models.

REFERENCES

1. Adelson L, Sunshine I. Fatal hydrogen sulfide poisoning. Report of three cases occurring in a sewer. *Arch Pathol.* 1966;81:375-380.
2. Alberti PW. Noise-induced hearing loss. *BMJ.* 1992;304:522.
3. Alberti PW. Occupational hearing loss. In: Ballenger JJ, ed. *Diseases of the Nose, Throat, Ear, Head, and Neck.* 14th ed. Philadelphia, PA: Lea & Febiger; 1991:1053-1068.
4. Alvan G, et al. Reversible hearing impairment related to quinine blood concentration in guinea pigs. *Life Sci.* 1989;45:751-755.
5. Amoore JE, Hautala E. Odor as an aid to chemical safety: odor thresholds compared with threshold limit values and volatilities for 214 industrial chemicals in air and water diluted. *J Appl Toxicol.* 1983;3:272-290.
6. Amoore JE. Olfactory genetics and anosmia. In: Beidler LM, ed. *Handbook of Sensory Physiology.* Vol 4. Chemical Senses, Part I. Berlin: Springer-Verlag; 1971:145-156.
7. Assael BM, et al. Ototoxicity of aminoglycoside antibiotics in infants and children. *Pediatr Infect Dis.* 1982;1:357-365.
8. Audeau FM, et al. Hydrogen sulfide poisoning: associated with pelt processing. *N Z Med J.* 1985;98:145-147.
9. Bagger-Sjoback D, et al. Characteristics and drug responses of cochlear and vestibular adenylate cyclase. *Arch Otorhinolaryngol.* 1980;228:217-222.
10. Barrs DM, Brackmann DE. Translabyrinthine nerve section: effect on tinnitus. *J Laryngol Otolaryngol.* 1984;98(suppl 9):287-293.
11. Beidler LM. Renewal of cells within taste buds. *J Cell Biol.* 1965;27:263-272.
12. Behnoud F, et al. Can aspirin protect or at least attenuate gentamicin ototoxicity in humans. *Saudi Med J.* 2009;30:1165-1169.
13. Behrens M, Meyerhof W. Gustatory and extragustatory functions of mammalian taste receptors. *Physiol Behav.* 2011;105:4-13.
14. Bergstorm L, Thompson PL. Ototoxicity. In: Brown RD, Daigneault EA, eds. *Pharmacology of Hearing: Experimental and Clinical Basis.* New York, NY: Wiley; 1981:119-134.
15. Bess FH, Poynor RE. Noise-induced hearing loss and snowmobiles. *Arch Otolaryngol.* 1974;99:45-51.
16. Blakley BW, Schilling H. Deafness associated with acetaminophen and codeine abuse. *J Otolaryngol Head Neck Surg.* 2008;37:507-509.
17. Boettcher FA, et al. Effects of sodium salicylate on evoked-response measures of hearing. *Hear Res.* 1989;42:129-142.
18. Boettcher FA, Salvi RJ. Salicylate ototoxicity: review and synthesis. *Am J Otolaryngol.* 1991;12:33-47.
19. Boyd O. Captopril-induced taste disturbance. *Lancet.* 1993;342:304.
20. Brown KS, Robinette RR. No simple pattern of inheritance in ability to smell solutions of cyanide. *Nature.* 1967;215:406-408.
21. Brown RD, et al. Ototoxicity drugs and noise. In: Evered D, Lawrenson G, eds. *Tinnitus.* Ciba Foundation Symposium 85. London: Pitman; 1981:151-171.
22. Brummett RE. Ototoxicity of erythromycin and analogues. *Otolaryngol Clin North Am.* 1993;26:811-819.
23. Brummett RE. Ototoxicity of vancomycin and analogues. *Otolaryngol Clin North Am.* 1993;26:821-827.
24. Brummett RE, et al. Augmented gentamicin ototoxicity induced by vancomycin in guinea pigs. *Arch Otolaryngol Head Neck Surg.* 1990;116:61-64.
25. Brummett RE, et al. Cochlear damage resulting from kanamycin and furosemide. *Acta Otolaryngol.* 1975;80:86-92.
26. Buckland ME, Cunningham AM. Alterations in the neurotrophic factors BDNE, GDNF and CNTF in the regenerating olfactory system. *Ann N Y Acad Sci.* 1998;855:260-265.
27. Burnett WW, et al. Hydrogen sulfide poisoning: review of 5 years' experience. *CMAJ.* 1977;117:1277-1280.
28. Burst JCM, Richter RW. Quinine amblyopia related to heroin addiction. *Ann Intern Med.* 1971;74:84-86.
29. Campbell KCM, Durrant J. Audiologic monitoring for ototoxicity. *Otolaryngol Clin North Am.* 1993;26:903-914.
30. Casler JD, et al. Treatment of blast injury to the ear. *Ann Otol Rhinol Laryngol.* 1989;98:13-22.
31. Cazals Y, et al. Acute effects of noradrenaline related vasoactive agents on the ototoxicity of aspirin: an experimental study in guinea pigs. *Hear Res.* 1988;36:89-96.
32. Chait R, et al. Blast injury of the ear: historical perspective. *Ann Otol Rhinol Laryngol.* 1989;98:9-12.
33. Chapman P. Naproxen and sudden hearing loss. *J Laryngol Otol.* 1982;96:163-166.
34. Chen Y, et al. Aspirin attenuates gentamicin ototoxicity: from the laboratory to the clinic. *Hear Res.* 2007;226:178-182.
35. Chiu JJ, et al. The detrimental effects of potassium bromate and thioglycolate on auditory brainstem response of guinea pig. *Chin J Physiol.* 2000;30:91-96.
36. Christenson BJ, Marjala ARP. Two cases of sudden sensorineural hearing loss after methadone overdose. *Ann Pharmacother.* 2010;44:207-210.
37. Ciarimboli G, et al. Organic cation transporter 2 mediates cisplatin-induced oto- and nephrotoxicity and is a target for protective interventions. *Am J Pathol.* 2010;176:1169-1180.
38. Ciba Foundation Symposium 85. A central or peripheral source of tinnitus. In: Evered D, Lawrenson G, eds. *Tinnitus.* London: Putnam; 1981:279-294.
39. Ciba Foundation Symposium 85. Appendix I: Definition and classification of tinnitus. In: Evered D, Lawrenson G, eds. *Tinnitus.* London: Pitman; 1981:300-302.
40. Ciorba A, et al. Considerations on the physiopathological mechanism of inner ear damage induced by intravenous cocaine abuse: cues from a case report. *Auris Nasus Larynx.* 2009;36:213-217.
41. Clark WW. Noise exposure from leisure activities. *J Acoust Soc Am.* 1991;90:175-181.
42. Cone TE Jr. Diagnosis and treatment: some diseases, syndromes, and conditions associated with an unusual odor. *Pediatrics.* 1968;41:993-995.
43. Cunningham LL, Brandon CS. Heat shock inhibits both aminoglycoside- and cisplatin-induced sensory hair cell death. *JARO.* 2006;7:299-307.
44. Davidson TM. The loss of smell. *Emerg Med.* 1988;20:104-116.
45. Davignon DD, Leshowitz BH. The speech-in-noise test: a new approach to the assessment of communication capability of elderly persons. *Int J Aging Hum Dev.* 1986;23:149-160.
46. Davis H. Advances in the neurophysiology and neuroanatomy of the cochlea. *J Acoust Soc Am.* 1962;34:1377-1385.
47. Devarajan P, et al. Cisplatin-induced apoptosis in auditory cells: role of death receptor and mitochondrial pathways. *Hear Res.* 2002;174:45-54.
48. Doty RL. A review of olfactory dysfunctions in man. *Am J Otolaryngol.* 1979;1:57-79.
49. Drewnowski A. Genetics of taste and smell. *World Rev Nutr Diet.* 1990;63:194-208.

50. Duckert LG, Rubel EW. Current concepts in hair regeneration. *Otolaryngol Clin North Am.* 1993;26:873-901.

51. Eggermont JJ. On the pathophysiology of tinnitus: a review and a peripheral model. *Hear Res.* 1990;48:111-123.

52. Emmett EA. Parosmia and hyposmia induced by solvent exposure. *Br J Ind Med.* 1976;3:196-198.

53. Escoubet B, et al. Prostaglandin synthesis by the cochlea or the guinea pig. Influence of aspirin, gentamicin, and acoustic stimulation. *Prostaglandins.* 1985;29:589-599.

54. Etminan M, et al. Risk of sensorineural hearing loss with macrolide antibiotics: a nested case-control study. *Laryngoscope.* 2016;127:229-232.

55. Evans EF. Chairman's closing remarks. In: Evered D, Lawrenson G, eds. *Tinnitus.* Ciba Foundation Symposium 85. London: Putman; 1981:295-302.

56. Evans P, Halliwel B. Free radicals and hearing. Cause, consequence, and criteria. *Ann N Y Acad Sci.* 1999;884:19-40.

57. Eybalin M, et al. Opioid receptors inhibit the adenylate cyclase in guinea pig cochlear. *Brain Res.* 1987;421:226-342.

58. Falk SA. Pathophysiological responses of the auditory organ to excessive noise. In: Lee DHK, Falk HL, Geiger SR, eds. *Handbook of Physiology: Reactions to Environmental Agents.* Bethesda, MD: American Physiological Society; 1977:17-30.

59. Fee WE Jr. Aminoglycoside ototoxicity in the human. *Laryngoscope.* 1980;90 (suppl 24):1-19.

60. Feldman AM. Cochlear fluids: physiology, biochemistry, and pharmacology. In: Brown RD, Daigneault EA, eds. *Pharmacology of Hearing. Experimental and Clinical Basis.* New York, NY: Wiley; 1981:81-97.

61. Fischel-Ghodsian N. Genetic factors in aminoglycoside toxicity. *Pharmacogenomics.* 2005;6:27-36.

62. Flotra L, et al. Side effects of chlorhexidine mouth washes. *J Dent Res.* 1971;79:119-125.

63. Forouzesh A, et al. Vancomycin otoxicity: a reevaluation in an era of increasing doses. *Antimicrob Agents Chemother.* 2009;53:483-486.

64. Francis SP, et al. Celastrol inhibits aminoglycoside-induced ototoxicity via heat shock protein 32. *Cell Death Dis.* 2011;2:e195-e206.

65. Freeman SR, et al. The association of codeine, macrocytosis and bilateral sudden or rapidly progressive profound sensorineural deafness. *Acta Otolaryngol.* 2009;129:1061-1066.

66. Froloff N, et al. Multiple human taste receptor sites: a molecular modeling approach. *Chem Senses.* 1996;21:425-445.

67. Fu DM. Survey of 1583 deaf mutes. *Qinghai Med J.* 1985;1:105-112.

68. Fukumoto Y, et al. Smell ability to solution of potassium-cyanide and its inheritance. *Jpn J Hum Genet.* 1957;2:7-16.

69. Gao W. Role of neurotrophins and lectins in prevention of ototoxicity. *Ann N Y Acad Sci.* 1999;884:312-327.

70. Garetz SL, et al. Attenuation of gentamicin ototoxicity by glutathione in the guinea pig in vivo. *Hear Res.* 1994;77:81-87.

71. Gerken GM. Central tinnitus and lateral inhibition: an auditory brainstem model. *Hear Res.* 1996;97:75-83.

72. Glover J, et al. Changes in taste associated with intravenous administration pentamidine. *J Assoc Nurses AIDS Care.* 1995;6:43-48.

73. Goldfrank LR, et al. Teaching the recognition of odors. *Ann Emerg Med.* 1982;11:684-686.

74. Gomez HJ, et al. Enalapril: a review of human pharmacology. *Drugs.* 1985;30 (suppl 1):13-24.

75. Goodey RJ. Drugs in the treatment of tinnitus. In: Evered D, Lawrenson G, eds. *Tinnitus.* Ciba Foundation Symposium 85. London: Putnam; 1981:263-278.

76. Gordon AS, et al. The effect of chronic cocaine abuse on human olfaction. *Arch Otolaryngol Head Neck Surg.* 1990;116:1415-1418.

77. Gordon CB. Practical approach to the loss of smell. *Am Fam Physician.* 1982;26:191-193.

78. Gorman W. The sense of smell. *Eye Ear Nose Throat.* 1964;43:54-58.

79. Griffin JP. Drug-induced disorder of taste. *Adv Drug React Rev.* 1992;11:229-239.

80. Grumet GW. Pandemonium in the modern hospital. *N Engl J Med.* 1993;322:433-437.

81. Guan MX, et al. A biochemical basis for the inherited susceptibility to aminoglycoside ototoxicity. *Hum Mol Genet.* 2000;9:1787-1793.

82. Guitton MJ, et al. Salicylate induces tinnitus through activation of cochlear NMDA receptors. *J Neurosci.* 2003;23:3944-3952.

83. Hajiioannou JK, et al. Clarithromycin induced reversible sensorineural hearing loss. *B-ENT.* 2011;7:127-130.

84. Hastings L. Sensory neurotoxicology: use of the olfactory system in the assessment of toxicity. *Neurotoxicol Teratol.* 1990;12:455-459.

85. Henkin RI, et al. Hypogeusia, dysgeusia, hyposmia, and dysosmia following influenza-like infection. *Ann Otol Rhinol Laryngol.* 1975;84:672-682.

86. Henkin RI, et al. A zinc protein isolated from human parotid saliva. *Proc Natl Acad Sci U S A.* 1975;72:488-492.

87. Henkin RI. Concepts of therapy in taste and smell dysfunction: repair of sensory receptor functions as primary treatment. In: Kurihara K, Suzuki N, Ogawa H, eds. *Olfaction and Taste.* Tokyo: Springer-Verlag; 1994:568-570.

88. Henkin RI. Drug-induced taste and smell disorders. Incidence, mechanisms and management related primarily to treatment of sensory receptor dysfunction. *Drug Saf.* 1994;11:318-377.

89. Hetu R, et al. Non-acoustic environmental factor influences on occupational hearing impairment: a preliminary discussion. Paper presented at the Second International Conference on the Combined Effects of Environmental Factors, Kanazama, Japan; 1986:17-31.

90. Heyneman CA. Zinc deficiency and taste disorders. *Ann Pharmacother.* 1996;30:186-187.

91. Hotz P, et al. Smell or taste disturbances, neurological symptoms, and hydrocarbon exposure. *Int Arch Occup Environ Health.* 1992;63:525-530.

92. Huang MY, Schacht J. Drug-induced ototoxicity: pathogenesis and prevention. *Med Toxicol.* 1989;4:452-467.

93. Hymes LC, et al. Bromate poisoning from hair permanent preparations. *Pediatrics.* 1985;76:975-978.

94. Jardini L, et al. Auditory changes associated with moderate blood salicylate levels. *Rheumatol Rehabil.* 1978;14:233-236.

95. Jastreboff PJ. Phantom auditory perception (tinnitus): mechanisms of generation and perception. *Neurosci Res.* 1990;8:221-254.

96. Jobe PC, Brown RD. Auditory pharmacology. *Trends Pharmacol Sci.* 1980;1:202-206.

97. Jojart G. Sense of smell after gentamicin nose-drops. *Lancet.* 1992;339:313.

98. Jongkamonwiwat N, et al. The existence of opioid receptors in the cochlea of guinea pigs. *Eur J Neurosci.* 2006;23:2701-2711.

99. Joyce PW. Taste disturbance with acetazolamide. *Lancet.* 1990;336:1446.

100. Jung TTK, et al. Ototoxicity of salicylate, nonsteroidal anti-inflammatory drugs, and quinine. *Otolaryngol Clin North Am.* 1993;26:791-810.

101. Kare MR, Mattes RD. A selective overview of the chemical senses. *Nutr Rev.* 1990;48:39-48.

102. Keeve JP. Ototoxic drugs and the workplace. *Am Fam Physician.* 1988;38:177-181.

103. Kirk RL, Stenhouse NS. Ability to smell solutions of potassium cyanide. *Nature.* 1953;171:698-699.

104. Kisiel DL, Bobbin RP. Miscellaneous ototoxic agents. In: Brown RD, Daigneault EA, eds. *Pharmacology of Hearing: Experimental and Clinical Basis.* New York, NY: Wiley; 1981:231-269.

105. Koegel L. Ototoxicity: a contemporary review of aminoglycosides, loop diuretics, acetylsalicylic acid, quinine, erythromycin, and cis-platinum. *Am J Otolaryngol.* 1985;6:190-199.

106. Kusakabe Y, et al. GUST27 and closely related G-protein-coupled receptors are localized in taste buds together with G_i-protein alpha-subunit. *Chem Senses.* 1996;21:335-340.

107. Laing DG, Francis GW. The capacity of humans to identify odors in mixtures. *Physiol Behav.* 1989;46:809-814.

108. Leopold DA, et al. Fish-odor syndrome presenting as dysosmia. *Arch Otolaryngol Head Neck Surg.* 1990;116:354-355.

109. Li G, et al. Salicylate protects hearing and kidney function from cisplatin toxicity without compromising its oncolytic action. *Lab Invest.* 2002;82:585-596.

110. Li XJ, Snyder SH. Molecular cloning of ebnerin, a von Ebner's gland protein associated with taste buds. *J Biol Chem.* 1995;270:17674-17679.

111. Lim DJ. Functional structure of the organ of Corti: a review. *Hear Res.* 1986;22:117-146.

112. Lu YF. Cause of 611 deaf mutes in schools for deaf children in Shanghai. *Shanghai Med J.* 1987;10:159.

113. Lutz H, et al. Ototoxicity of vancomycin: an experimental study in guinea pigs. *ORL J Otorhinolaryngol Relat Spec.* 1991;53:273-278.

114. Mann NM. Management of smell and taste problems. *Cleve Clin J Med.* 2002;69:329-336.

115. Matsumoto I, et al. Hearing loss following potassium bromate: two case reports. *Otolaryngol Head Neck Surg.* 1980;88:625-629.

116. Matz GJ. Aminoglycoside cochlear ototoxicity. *Otolaryngol Clin North Am.* 1993;26:705-736.

117. Matz GJ. The ototoxic effects of ethacrynic acid in man and animals. *Laryngoscope.* 1976;86:1065-1086.

118. McFadden D, Plattsmier HS. Aspirin abolishes spontaneous otoacoustic emissions. *J Acoust Soc Am.* 1984;76:443-448.

119. McFadden D. *Tinnitus: Facts, Theories, and Treatment.* Washington, DC: National Academy Press; 1982:10-24.

120. McGill TJ, Schuknecht HF. Human cochlear changes in noise induced hearing loss. *Laryngoscope.* 1976;86:1293-1302.

121. McNeil JJ, et al. Taste loss associated with oral captopril treatment. *Br Med J.* 1979;15:1555-1556.

122. Meyerhoff WL. Physiology of the nose and paranasal sinuses. In: Paparella MM, Schumrick DA, eds. *Otolaryngology: Basic Sciences and Related Disciplines.* Vol. 1. Philadelphia, PA: WB Saunders; 1980:308-311.

123. Mick P, Westerberg BD. Sensorineural hearing loss as a probable serious adverse drug reaction associated with low-dose oral azithromycin. *J Otolaryngol.* 2007;36:257-263.

124. Miller LG, Miller SM. Altered taste secondary to acetazolamide. *J Fam Pract.* 1990;31:199-200.

125. Minami SB, et al. Antioxidant protection in a new animal model of cisplatin-induced ototoxicity. *Hear Res.* 2004;198:137-143.

126. Mongan E, et al. Tinnitus as an indication of therapeutic serum salicylate levels. *JAMA.* 1973;226:142-145.

127. Mott AE, Leopold DA. Disorders of taste and smell. *Med Clin North Am.* 1991;75:1321-1353.

128. Muldoon LL, et al. Delayed administration of sodium thiosulfate in animal models reduces platinum ototoxicity without reduction of antitumor activity. *Clin Cancer Res.* 2000;6:309-315.

129. Myers EN, Bernstein JM. Salicylate ototoxicity. *Arch Otolaryngol.* 1965;82:483-493.

130. Nadol JB Jr. Hearing loss. *N Engl J Med*. 1993;329:1092-1102.

131. Nair EL, et al. The impact of sudden hearing loss secondary to heroin overdose on fitting outcomes. *Am J Audiol*. 2010;19:86-90.

132. National Institutes of Health. Noise and hearing loss. Consensus Development Conference statement. *JAMA*. 1990;263:3185-3190.

133. Nicoucar K, et al. Intralabyrinthine haemorrhage following cocaine consumption. *Acta Otolarngol*. 2005;125:899-901.

134. Oh AK, et al. Deafness associated with abuse of hydrocodone/acetaminophen. *Neurology*. 2000;54:2345.

135. Ohtani I, et al. Mechanism of protective effect of fosfomycin against aminoglycoside ototoxicity. *Auris Nasus Larynx*. 1984;11:119-124.

136. Olishifski JB. Occupational hearing loss, noise, and hearing conservation. In: Zenz C, ed. *Occupational Medicine: Principles and Practical Applications*. Chicago: Year Book; 1988:274-323.

137. Patterson PM, Lauder BA. The incidence and probable inheritance of "smell blindness." *J Hered*. 1948;39:295-297.

138. Peloquin CA, et al. Aminoglycoside toxicity: daily versus thrice-weekly dosing for treatment of mycobacterial diseases. *Clin Infect Dis*. 2004;38:1538-1544.

139. Phaneur R, Hetu R. An epidemiological perspective of the causes of hearing loss among industrial workers. *J Otolaryngol*. 1990;19:31-40.

140. Phillips YY, Zajtchuk JT. Blast injuries of the ear in military operations. *Ann Otol Rhinol Laryngol*. 1989;98:3-4.

141. Prazma J. Ototoxicity of aminoglycoside antibiotics. In: Brown RD, Daigneault EA, eds. *Pharmacology of Hearing: Experimental and Clinical Basis*. New York, NY: Wiley; 1981:155-193.

142. Puel JL. Cochlear NMDA receptor blockade prevents salicylate-induced tinnitus. *B-ENT*. 2007;3(suppl 7):19-22.

143. Puel JL, Guitton MJ. Salicylate-induced tinnitus: molecular mechanisms and modulation by anxiety. *Prog Brain Res*. 2007;166:141-146.

144. Quick CA, et al. Deafness and renal failure due to potassium bromate poisoning. *Arch Otolaryngol*. 1975;101:494-495.

145. Quick CA, et al. The relationship between cochlea and kidney. *Laryngoscope*. 1973;83:1469-1482.

146. Ramsden RT, et al. Electrocochleographic changes in acute salicylate overdosage. *J Laryngol Otol*. 1985;99:1269-1273.

147. Razani J, et al. Odor sensitivity is impaired in HIV-positive cognitively impaired patients. *Physiol Behav*. 1996;59:877-881.

148. Reser D, et al. L- and D-methionine provide equivalent long-term protection against CDDP-induced ototoxicity in vivo, with partial in vitro and in vivo retention of antineoplastic activity. *Neurotoxicology*. 1999;20:731-748.

149. Riggs LC, et al. Ototoxicity resulting from combined administration of cisplatin and gentamicin. *Laryngoscope*. 1996;106:401-406.

150. Roche RJ, et al. Quinine induces reversible high-tone hearing loss. *Br J Clin Pharmacol*. 1990;29:780-782.

151. Roland PS. New developments in our understanding of ototoxicity. *Ear Nose Throat J*. 2004;83.15-17.

152. Rollin H. Drug-related gustatory disorders. *Ann Otolaryngol*. 1978;87:37-42.

153. Rose CS, et al. Olfactory impairment after chronic occupational cadmium exposure. *J Occup Med*. 1992;34:600-605.

154. Rutka J, Alberti PW. Toxic and drug-induced disorders in otolaryngology. *Otolaryngol Clin North Am*. 1984;17:761-774.

155. Rybak LP, et al. Dose dependent protection by lipoic acid against cisplatin-induced ototoxicity in rats: antioxidant defense system. *Toxicol Sci*. 1999;47:195-202.

156. Rybak LP. Ototoxicity of loop diuretics. *Otolaryngol Clin North Am*. 1993;26:829-844.

157. Rybak MJ, et al. Prospective evaluation of the effect of an aminoglycoside dosing regimen on rates of observed nephrotoxicity and ototoxicity. *Antimicrob Agents Chemother*. 1999;43:1549-1555.

158. Santini V, Giles FJ. The potential of amifostine: from cytoprotective to therapeutic agent. *Hematologia*. 1999;84:1035-1042.

159. Schacht J. Biochemical basis of aminoglycoside ototoxicity. *Otolaryngol Clin North Am*. 1993;26:845-856.

160. Schacht J. Molecular mechanisms of drug-induced hearing loss. *Hear Res*. 1986;22:297-304.

161. Schiffman SS. Taste and smell in disease (part 1). *N Engl J Med*. 1983;308:1275-1279.

162. Schiffman SS. Taste and smell in disease (part 2). *N Engl J Med*. 1983;308:1337-1343.

163. Schleuning AJ. Management of the patient with tinnitus. *Med Clin North Am*. 1991;75:1225-1237.

164. Schneider BA. Anosmia: verification and etiologies. *Ann Otolaryngnol*. 1972;81:272-277.

165. Schrock A, et al. Sudden sensorineural hearing loss after heroin injection. *Eur Arch Otorhinolaryngol*. 2008;265:603-606.

166. Schweitzer VG. Ototoxicity of chemotherapeutic agents. *Otolaryngol Clin North Am*. 1993;26:759-789.

167. Schweitzer VG, et al. Sudden bilateral sensorineural hearing loss following polysubstance narcotic overdose. *J Am Acad Audiol*. 2011;22:208-214.

168. Seidman MD, Jacobson GP. Update on tinnitus. *Otolaryngol Clin North Am*. 1996;29:455-465.

169. Seligmann H, et al. Drug-induced tinnitus and other hearing disorders. *Drug Saf*. 1996;14:198-212.

170. Sha SH, et al. Aspirin to prevent gentamicin-induced hearing loss. *N Engl J Med*. 2006;354:1856-1857.

171. Sha SH, Schacht J. Salicylate attenuates gentamicin-induced ototoxicity. *Lab Invest*. 1999;79:807-813.

172. Shatzman AR, Henkin RI. Metal-binding characteristics of the parotid salivary protein gustin. *Biochim Biophys Acta*. 1980;623:107-118.

173. Shaw KA, et al. Methadone, another cause of opioid-associated hearing loss: a case report. *J Emerg Med*. 2011;41:635-639.

174. Shelley WB. A diagnosis you can smell. *Emerg Med*. 1992;24:232-235.

175. Shimizu A, et al. Cisplatin and caspase inhibitors protect vestibular sensory cells from gentamicin ototoxicity. *Acta Otolaryngol*. 2003;123:459-465.

176. Shulman A. The cochleovestibular system/ototoxicity/clinical issues. *Ann N Y Acad Sci*. 1999;884:433-436.

177. Shusterman DJ, Sheedy JE. Occupational and environmental disorders of the special senses. *Occup Med*. 1992;7:515-542.

178. Silverstein H, et al. Diagnosis and management of hearing loss. *Clin Symp*. 1994;44:1-32.

179. Smilkstein MJ, et al. Acute toxic blindness: unrecognized quinine poisoning. *Ann Emerg Med*. 1987;16:98-101.

180. Smoorenburg GF, et al. Protection and spontaneous recovery from cisplatin-induced hearing loss. *Ann N Y Acad Sci*. 1999;884:192-210.

181. Song BB, Schacht J. Variable efficacy of radical scavengers and iron chelators to attenuate gentamicin ototoxicity in guinea pig in vivo. *Hear Res*. 1996;94:87-93.

182. Stenner M, et al. Sudden bilateral sensorineural hearing loss after intravenous cocaine injection: a case report and review of the literature. *Laryngoscope*. 2009;119:2441-2443.

183. Stevens JC, et al. Taste sensitivity and aging: high incidence of decline revealed by repeated threshold. *Chem Senses*. 1995;20:451-459.

184. Stewart TH, et al. An outbreak of food-poisoning due to a flour improver, potassium bromate. *South Afr Med J*. 1969;43:200-202.

185. Stine R, et al. Hydrogen sulfide intoxication. *Ann Intern Med*. 1976;85:756-758.

186. Sullivan P. MD launches study to determine amount of job-related hearing loss in military. *CMAJ*. 1992;146:2061-2062.

187. Sumner D. Post-traumatic anosmia. *Brain*. 1964;87:107-120.

188. Takumida M, Anniko M. Brain-derived neurotrophic factor and nitric oxide synthase inhibitor protect the vestibular organ gentamicin ototoxicity. *Acta Otolaryngol*. 2002;122:10-15.

189. Tange RA, et al. The importance of high-tone audiometry in monitoring for ototoxicity. *Arch Otorhinolaryngol*. 1985;242:77-81.

190. Tange RA, et al. An experimental study of vancomycin induced cochlear damage. *Arch Otorhinolaryngol*. 1989;246:67-70.

191. Turnidge MB. Pharmacodynamics and dosing of aminoglycosides. *Infect Dis Clin North Am*. 2003;17:503-528.

192. Unal OF, et al. Prevention of gentamicin induced ototoxicity by trimetazidine in animal model. *Int J Pediatr Otorhinolaryngol*. 2005;69:193-199.

193. van As JW, et al. Medical interventions for the prevention of platinum-induced hearing loss in children with cancer. *Cochrane Database Syst Rev*. 2016;9:CD009219.

194. Verdel BM, et al. Drug-related nephrotoxic and ototoxic reactions—a link through a predictive mechanistic commonality. *Drug Saf*. 2008;31:877-884.

195. Vorasubin N, et al. Methadone-induced bilateral severe sensorineural hearing loss. *Am J Otolaryngol*. 2013;34:735-738.

196. Wallhauser-Frank E, et al. Salicylate alters 2-DG uptake in the auditory system: a model for tinnitus? *Neuroreport*. 1996;7:1585-1588.

197. Ward WD. Noise-induced hearing loss. In: Northern JL, ed. *Hearing Disorder*. 2nd ed. Boston: Little, Brown; 1984:143-152.

198. Watanabe KI, et al. Nitric oxide synthase inhibitor suppresses the ototoxic side effects of cisplatin in guinea pig. *Anticancer Drugs*. 2000;11:401-406.

199. Wensing KU, Ciarimboli G. Saving ears and kidneys from cisplatin. *Anticancer Res*. 2013;33:4183-4188.

200. Willems PJ. Genetic causes of hearing loss. *N Engl J Med*. 2000;342:1101-1109.

201. Wright HN. Characterization of olfactory dysfunction. *Arch Otolaryngol Head Neck Surg*. 1987;113:163-168.

202. Wysocki CJ, Gilbert AN. The National Geographic Smell Survey: the effects of age are heterogenous. *Ann N Y Acad Sci*. 1989;561:12-28.

203. Zazgornick J, et al. Captopril induced dysgeusia [letter]. *Lancet*. 1993;341:1542.

204. Zeller JA, et al. Ageusia as an adverse effect of phenytoin. *Lancet*. 1998;351:1101.

205. Zhang F, et al. Molecular mechanism for the umami taste synergism. *Proc Natl Acad Sci U S A*. 2008;105:20930-20934.

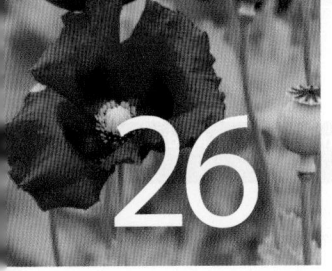

26 PSYCHIATRIC PRINCIPLES

Andrea M. Kondracke, Justin M. Lewin, Cathy A. Kondas, and Erin A. Zerbo

Psychiatric symptoms are often the cause of, or the effect of many toxicologic-presentations. Suicide attempts and aggressive behaviors are commonly associated with toxicity and can be uniquely difficult to assess and manage in the emergency department. Patient factors, clinician bias, and a lack of coordination of care exacerbate the difficulties and make evaluating and treating patients with psychiatric symptoms uniquely challenging in the medical setting. Patients are unable or unwilling to communicate adequately. They are frequently disorganized, psychotic, and engaged in self-injurious and/or dangerous behaviors. Mental illness, personality disorders, delirium, intoxication and withdrawal are frequently the underlying etiology of these behaviors and can interfere with treatment. The combative, threatening, and/or violent patient requires special consideration as the safety of the patient and staff is imminently jeopardized. The individual's medical condition and/or behavior can be life threatening, disruptive, and/or destructive. Patient behaviors are viewed dichotomously as deliberate, totally "out of control," and irrational. The truth is more complex, with some aspects occurring within the awareness and control of the patient and other aspects either unknown, out of the patient's control, and/or overwhelming to the patient. Coordination with and availability of psychiatric care is difficult and inaccessible.

Substances of abuse, overdose, and toxicity or adverse effects of psychiatric medications are the most obvious commonalities between the fields of psychiatry and toxicology. However, psychiatric symptoms overshadow other toxic or metabolic conditions and are confused for primary mental illnesses. In addition, the adverse effects or toxicity of xenobiotics mimics various symptoms of mental illness. Given the increased rates of suicide attempts and substance abuse among people with severe mental illness, distinguishing cause and effect is complex.

This chapter will review some of the special considerations that should be recognized when dealing with the overlap between psychiatry and toxicology. The chapter will start with an overview of the capacity assessment and its formal components. Then there is a discussion of the components of the medical evaluation of psychiatric patients for admission to a psychiatric facility. The third section is devoted to suicide and the suicidal or self-injurious patient. And finally substance use disorders are addressed. Principles of workplace violence and the violent patient will we addressed in Special Considerations: SC4.

CAPACITY ASSESSMENT

"Decision-making capacity is the ability to understand relevant information and to appreciate the reasonably foreseeable consequences of the decision."[3] Every consent form requires documentation of some aspects of a capacity assessment. Physicians are legally and ethically obligated to obtain informed consent for treatment and procedures. The initial presumption when evaluating capacity is that all people have decisional capacity.[2] Depriving a patient of his or her decision-making rights is a serious infringement on his or her liberties that has legal and ethical implications. Yet, only a patient with capacity can legally consent to medical treatment. Allowing a patient without capacity to consent to medical treatment is also problematic and has legal and ethical implications.

Physicians are constantly evaluating capacity, although they are not always cognizant of this fact. Capacity assessments are done quickly and implicitly in every patient encounter. Physicians ask themselves, "Can my patient make a decision?" "Does my patient understand the seriousness of the illness?" "Does the patient understand the treatment being offered and why?" "Does the individual understand the implications of the treatment and/or the implications of refusing the treatment?" "Does this patient have a problem that is interfering with his or her ability to understand or make a good decision?" If the patient appears to be making a poor decision, the physician may ask, "Why is the patient making this decision?" These are essential questions in patient care, a fundamental part of shared decision making and the basis of the capacity assessment.[27]

It is when there are impasses, ambiguity, or murky ethical situations that a patient's capacity comes into question, such as when a patient refuses a treatment that is clearly beneficial or life-sustaining. Another example occurs when a patient refuses treatment in the setting of a recent suicide attempt, such as refusing a treatment for a potentially lethal ingestion. In these scenarios, having a systematic approach to assessing capacity and good documentation is necessary.

It is important to note that capacity assessments occur at a specific moment in time regarding a specific medical decision. The assessment is not a "global" determination that persists throughout the hospitalization but rather it is a temporary determination that requires reassessment as factors change with time and/or situation. Capacity fluctuates with a change in the patient's mental status, medical or psychiatric condition, the time of day, amount of pain, level of anxiety, perceived support, recent medication administration, or in the context of withdrawal from a xenobiotic.

When assistance from a psychiatry consultant is requested, the primary physician should first perform his or her own capacity assessment. This should be done clearly and in the patient's native language. The physician should take into consideration the patient's health literacy, level of education, and cultural background. The information should be tailored to the patient's ability to understand. For example, it is not productive to refer to percentages to describe outcomes with a patient who has never learned basic math. The physician should be certain to address the medical condition, the procedure, the risks and benefits, and the option of "doing nothing."

The patient must engage in the evaluation. Refusal to engage indicates a lack of capacity by default.

The general legal standard for capacity requires assessment of 4 basic skills. They should be clearly documented.[2]

1. Communicate a Choice

The patient must clearly indicate a preference or choice. This choice should be consistent long enough for the choice to be implemented. The physician could ask the question, "Have you decided what you would like to do?" A patient with capacity can alter their decision over time for a variety of logical reasons such as changes in their medical condition or as additional information becomes available. However, when an individual changes his or her decision repeatedly or is unable to come to a decision despite sufficient time and information, it suggests the individual lacks capacity to make that specific decision. These cases often occur in patients who have a high degree of ambivalence, have poor short-term memory, a thought disorder, or who are delirious.

2. Understand Relevant Information

The patient must comprehend the fundamental information communicated by the care team.[3] The physician could ask, "Can you tell me about your medical problems?" "Can you tell me the procedure that is being offered to you?" "What are the risks and benefits?" This portion is preferably done by the primary physician who best understands the nuances of the procedure.

Often physicians assume that if the patient repeats these factors adequately, that is, the risks, benefits, and alternatives, then the patient has capacity and the assessment is complete; however, this is not always the case. The patient should be able to understand and manipulate the information independently, which can be demonstrated by asking the patient to paraphrase the physician's explanations rather than repeat verbatim. Difficulties in this domain can arise from deficits in attention, intelligence, or memory.

3. Appreciate the Situation and Its Consequences

The patient must be able to incorporate the relevant information. The medical condition in question must be acknowledged, and the individual must demonstrate awareness that the risks and benefits being discussed apply to him or her specifically, and will have implications in the individual's life. The physician can ask, "How will this procedure affect you?" If a patient is unable to answer this question, then he or she does not demonstrate capacity. A statement such as "The doctors say I could die from a heart attack if I do not get this stent placed right now, but I know that's not going to happen to me" would call the patient's capacity into question. Difficulties in this area often arise from denial, mistrust of the physician, cognitive or affective impairment, or delusional/paranoid thought processes.

4. Reason About Treatment Options

The patient must be able to demonstrate how, in a logical progression, he or she arrived at the decision. This is a synthesis of all the other requirements. The physician should ask, "How did you come to this decision?" "Why are you willing or unwilling to have the procedure?" The patient should be able to compare treatment options and consequences, and be able to explain how he or she arrived at the decision, including the reasoning involved. Patients can make "unreasonable," "wrong," or "bad" decisions and still have capacity; poor judgment is not equivalent to a lack of capacity. Furthermore, despite the physician's best intentions, every attempt should be made to honor a patient's decision if he or she meets the threshold for capacity. The patient's autonomy should prevail. Difficulties in this domain often occur in patients with delirium, dementia, extreme phobia, panic, anxiety, psychosis, depression, or anger.

If the patient is unable to perform one or more of these steps then he or she lacks capacity. Once a patient has been deemed to lack capacity he or she should be so informed. An assessment of why the patient lacks capacity should follow. Then, every effort to restore capacity and, as such, patient autonomy, should be attempted. For example, a patient with a substance use disorder who is experiencing withdrawal and therefore demands to leave the hospital and unwilling to participate in any discussion would lack capacity. Treatment of an individual's withdrawal will result in significant relief and rapid re-establishment of capacity. A patient experiencing opioid withdrawal feels the need to leave the hospital to use heroin; a dose of methadone to relieve withdrawal symptoms will allow this patient to participate in capacity evaluation and provide a rationally articulate reason for his or her choice, and it often leads to a more reasonable decision to continue the recommended treatment. On the other hand, in a patient who lacks capacity due to an irreversible process such as dementia, capacity cannot be restored.

When a patient is determined to lack capacity in life-threatening situations, physicians need to treat the patient over patient objection. The physician should continue to consider the patient's autonomy.[2] Efforts should always be made to impose the least restrictive measures while still providing appropriate care.

When patients lack capacity, every effort to find an alternative decision maker should be made. When there is no designated health care proxy and family members are not in agreement about what treatment choice the patient would want if he or she had the capacity to make that decision, most states have determined a specific hierarchy to identify which family member should make the decision.[3]

The hierarchy is state dependent. For example, in New York State, the alternative decision maker is determined by the Family Healthcare Decision Act of 2010 which states the hierarchy as: spouse or domestic partner, adult child, parent, adult sibling, friend, or extended family".[19]

TABLE 26–1	MacArthur Competence Assessment Tool—A Modified Overview[34]

Interview Process (15–20 minutes):
- Clinician discloses patient's disorder, recommended treatment, risks, benefits, and alternative treatments
- Patient expresses a treatment choice and explains how the choice was made

Questions embedded in the interview process assess patient's abilities in 3 areas:

1. Understanding
- Ask the patient to paraphrase what has been disclosed about the disorder, the recommended treatment, and the risks/benefits.
- If a patient demonstrates poor understanding, redisclose the information and reassess. (If a patient wasn't paying attention or found the concepts unfamiliar, his or her understanding should improve with redisclosure.)

2. Appreciation
- Does the patient acknowledge that the information applies to him or her? That treatment might have at least some benefit?
- A reasonable difference of opinion is permissible; however, if a patient's opinion is derived from delusional or distorted perceptions, these patients are lacking appreciation.

3. Reasoning
- Has the patient expressed a preference? What are his or her explanations for making that choice? Does he or she mention any consequences of treatment alternatives, how alternatives compare, or any thoughts about consequences besides those offered in the disclosure? Does the patient's final choice follow logically from the explanation?
- If the patient is not able to logically explain how he or she arrived at a choice, or is inconsistent in the choice, this indicates a failure of reasoning.

Although it is important to know what a capacity assessment is, it is equally important to understand its limitations. It does not determine what, if any, treatment should be initiated. It is not a psychiatric evaluation, nor is it a judgment of soundness.

A well-researched scale for determining decisional capacity is the MacArthur Competence Assessment Tool for Treatment (MacCAT-T), which is a semi-structured interview that requires 15 to 20 minutes to administer and is designed for use in a clinical setting (Table 26–1).[34]

Complexities of Capacity Determination in Clinical Settings

An important concept is the *sliding scale* of capacity, which has been supported by both expert consensus guidelines and the legal system. This "sliding scale" concept indicates that the threshold for deeming a patient to lack capacity changes depending upon the seriousness of the consequences. Refusing life- or limb-saving procedures requires the patient to demonstrate a very high level of understanding and reasoning. On the other hand, even if a patient shows limitations in one of the 4 basic skills during a capacity assessment and the risks of refusal are low, then the patient is thought to have capacity and the patient's autonomy prevails.

Decisional capacity is often part of a larger question about how to proceed with treatment for a particular patient. Once a patient is found to lack capacity, ethical questions arise about the appropriateness and practicality of imposing treatment. For example, should a patient who is refusing a necessary blood draw be sedated for the procedure? Sedating a patient has its own inherent risks, and psychological distress to the patient cannot be discounted. In these situations, it is often helpful to have a discussion involving the psychiatrist, and a general consensus can usually be reached weighing the risks and benefits of proceeding with treatment against a patient's will. In cases of life-threatening refusal of treatment, how to proceed is usually clear, but physicians often encounter situations in which the medical necessity of an intervention is urgent but not emergent. For example, for a patient who needs an amputation for an infected limb that is currently stable but will inevitably proceed to sepsis, the physician has a responsibility to petition the court for treatment over objection. These cases require a team approach involving psychiatry, risk management, legal services, and bioethics.

MEDICAL EVALUATION OF THE PSYCHIATRIC PATIENT PRIOR TO ADMISSION TO A PSYCHIATRIC FACILITY

Not all patients who present with psychiatric symptoms have mental illness. Intoxication, withdrawal syndromes, medical illness, metabolic abnormalities, organic brain, seizure, and dementia often present with symptoms that mimic mental illness. The psychiatric patient is often unwilling or unable to fully cooperate, creating substantial difficulty in obtaining a comprehensive medical history.

Behavioral disturbances also present unique challenges to diagnostic assessment. Patients are often unwilling or unable to fully cooperate, making it difficult to obtain a comprehensive medical history.

Emergency medicine physicians are often asked to "medically clear" patients for transfer to psychiatric units or psychiatric facilities. These evaluations are challenging because there are no universal standards. In fact, the very term is misleading and can lead to the omission of important details of the patient's medical history.

The purpose of "medical clearance" requested by evaluating psychiatrist is to:

1. determine if the patient has a serious medical condition that would make admission to a psychiatric hospital unsafe;
2. assess and treat any acute medical issue necessitating urgent or emergent intervention; and
3. help differentiate between an organic illness, a xenobiotic-induced disorder, and a primary mental illness as the cause of psychiatric symptoms.

The presence of either of the first 2 could well obviate the need for psychiatric admission and compromise or invalidate the accuracy of psychiatric assessment.[46] The evaluation should include a history and a thorough physical examination, including neurologic and mental status examination.

Some signs that suggest a medical cause of psychiatric symptoms include new onset of symptoms in a patient older than 40, abnormal vital signs, recent memory loss, or clouded sensorium.[25] Signs and symptoms that require further evaluation include abnormal vital signs, delirium, altered cognition, or an abnormal physical examination. Certain demographics are identified as high risk for medical instability: the elderly or very young, patients with substance abuse, abnormal movements, abrupt onset of symptoms, and patients with no prior psychiatric history. Patients with physical trauma and those with preexisting medical disorders or current medical complaints warrant special attention as well.[33]

Although the psychiatrist often requests routine laboratory testing for medical clearance, a number of studies demonstrate that selective testing based on history and physical examination is the correct and most cost-effective strategy. There is a strong consensus among physicians that routine laboratory testing is unnecessary, and without any clinical suspicion, the probability of false positive laboratory results begins to outweigh true positives.[10,24] The American College of Emergency Physicians provides a level B recommendation that diagnostic evaluation be directed by the history and physical examination, and that routine laboratory testing is low yield and not necessary as part of the emergency department assessment.[46]

The American Psychiatry Association and American Diabetes Association practice guidelines for starting patients on long-term second-generation antipsychotics include obtaining baseline fasting plasma glucose and fasting lipid as these medications are known to cause the metabolic syndrome and/or diabetes. Although these guidelines are not applicable to the emergency department setting, it is helpful to be aware of them.

The American College of Emergency Physicians also provides a level C recommendation against routine urine toxicology testing and blood alcohol concentrations in alert, awake and cooperative patients, and specifies that transfer to psychiatric care should not be delayed to await collection of samples for toxicologic analysis.[46] However, from the psychiatrist's perspective, this testing is time-sensitive and can change psychiatric management and disposition considerably. If the emergency physician knows the patient will

be transferred for psychiatric care and suspects substance abuse, it is helpful to obtain toxicologic results as early as possible.

Another important and common issue is acute intoxication with ethanol. At what point is it acceptable and appropriate to "medically clear" the patient for psychiatric evaluation? There are no evidence-based data to support that patients regain decision-making capacity at a particular blood alcohol concentration. Depending upon tolerance, cognition varies widely, and patients often develop ethanol withdrawal while significantly elevated blood alcohol concentrations persist.[22] Therefore, The American College of Emergency Physicians provides a level C recommendation that the patient's cognitive abilities be the basis on which the psychiatric assessment is initiated. A period of observation can be used to see if psychiatric symptoms resolve with resolution of intoxication, at which point the need for a psychiatric assessment can be revisited.[46]

Psychiatric facilities have varying degrees of capacity to care for medical conditions. Some facilities have onsite internal medicine providers and the ability to care for chronic or non-acute medical conditions. However, many do not. A shortcoming of psychiatric facilities is that few have the ability to care for either complicated acute or chronic medical illnesses. They often do not have adequate nursing capabilities or available equipment to care for patients with enhanced nursing need such as tracheostomies, tube feeding, intravenous fluids or medications, or supplemental oxygen. Therefore, emergency physicians are asked to identify a patient's disabilities. Knowing the limitations of these facilities can enhance the relationship between emergency physicians and psychiatrists, and ultimately help to facilitate transfers. In addition, EMTALA (Emergency Medical Treatment and Labor Act) requires that psychiatric patients with medical problems be transferred to a psychiatric facility that is equipped to handle the patient's medical problems.

SUICIDE AND SELF-INJURIOUS BEHAVIOR
Epidemiology
The term *suicide* refers to self-inflicted death with either explicit or implicit evidence that the person intended to die. Suicide has been the tenth leading cause of death each year in the United States since 2008, and accounted for 44,193 deaths in 2015.[17] It was the second leading cause of death among 10 to 34 year-olds in 2015, and accounts for 15.1% of deaths in this age group annually. Suicide accomplished in a variety of settings and by a variety of means, is associated with psychiatric-disorders and/or substance abuse, especially ethanol, and is frequently accomplished using psychoactive xenobiotics alone or in combination. Self-poisoning accounts for more than 70% of all serious suicide attempts.[50]

Suicidal Ideations
Suicidal thoughts and behaviors are common. The lifetime prevalence of adults having "seriously considered" suicide is 9.2%, whereas 3.1% report having formulated a plan, and 2.7% make a suicide attempt.[32,52] Given less than a third of individuals who have seriously considered suicide in their lifetime ultimately make a suicide attempt, studies have searched for unique risk factors that contribute to the transition from suicidal ideations to attempting suicide.[32,49,54] Given that the act of suicide is a statistically rare event in the overall population, it is difficult to definitively predict who will complete suicide. There are no proven formalized risk assessment tools. However, there are risk factors that are associated with an increase in the likelihood that an individual will attempt suicide, and there are some that are modifiable (Tables 26–2 and 26–3). The identification of modifiable risk factors provides opportunities for interventions. Additionally, there are protective factors that mitigate the risk for suicide, and it is important to assess for the presence or absence of these factors in determining the overall risk for suicide in a patient.

It is worth noting here that not all self-inflicted injuries are suicide attempts. Many of these are suicidal gestures or self-injurious behaviors. It is worth noting the explicit terminology here.

TABLE 26–2   Hierarchy of Factors Associated With an Increased Risk for Suicide

Psychiatric Risk Factors	Neurological and Medical Factors	Sociodemographic Factors	Genetic and Familial Factors
Major depressive disorder	Multiple sclerosis	Access to firearms	Family history of suicide (particularly in first-degree relatives)
Bipolar disorder	Huntington disease	Caucasian race	
Schizophrenia	Brain and spinal cord injury	Male sex (suicide completion)	Family history of mental illness, including substance use disorders
Alcohol use disorder	Seizure disorders	Female sex (suicide attempts)	
Other substance use disorders	Malignant neoplasms	Widowed, divorced, or single marital status, particularly among elderly men	
Alcohol intoxication	HIV/AIDS		
Personality disorders	Chronic pain syndromes	Elderly age group	
Bulimia or anorexia nervosa	Functional impairment	Adolescent and young adult age groups	
Post-traumatic stress disorder	Low concentration of serotonin metabolite 5-hydroxyindoleacetic acid (5-HIAA) in cerebrospinal fluid—(Research)	Gay, lesbian, or bisexual orientation	
Helplessness		Recent lack of social support (including living alone)	
Hopelessness		Unemployment	
Impulsivity		Decrease in socioeconomic status	
Aggression, including violence against others		Domestic partner violence	
Agitation		Recent stressful life event	
Factors related to current or past suicidal behavior:		Childhood sexual abuse	
Prior suicide attempts		Childhood physical abuse	
Suicidal ideation			
Suicidal plans			
Suicidal intent and lethality			

Self-Injury and Suicide Attempts

Self-injurious behavior refers to the self-infliction of painful, destructive, or injurious acts *without* the intent to die. An example is the superficial cutting that occurs in a patient with a borderline personality disorder, which is actually a coping mechanism that provides psychological relief; one hypothesis is that relief is mediated by the endogenous release of opioids.[62]

Suicide gesture refers to an attempt that is not felt to be medically serious, and often implies that the patient is making a "cry for help" rather than an attempt to die; such a *gesture* can still result in death, even if unintentional.

A **suicide attempt** refers to self-inflicted injury with a nonfatal outcome accompanied by either explicit or implicit evidence that the person intended to die. A medically serious suicide attempt is likely to be a more robust marker of successful suicide risk. As defined in the literature, **"serious" suicide attempts** meet one of the following criteria:

1. treatment in a specialized unit (such as an intensive care unit),
2. surgery under general anesthesia,
3. medical treatment beyond orogastric lavage, activated charcoal, or routine neurologic observation,
4. method with high risk of fatality (such as hanging or firearm), or
5. hospital admission longer than 24 hours.[6]

Those people who make serious attempts similarly tend to share with completers a higher rate of serious mental illness such as schizophrenia, bipolar disorder, or severe major depressive disorder.[6]

Suicidal or self-injurious patients are often encountered in emergency departments. Approximately 60% to 70% of all nonfatal self-inflicted injuries seen in an emergency department are the result of a suicide attempt, and an emergency department visit for self-harm is predictive of a completed suicide in the future.[13,61] In fact, based on a review of 90 studies on emergency department presentations for nonfatal self-injury, 16% of individuals will self-harm within the year, and up to 2% will die by suicide.[38,53,61] The average annual number of emergency department visits for attempted suicide and self-injury is increasing; from 2001 to 2014, the age-adjusted annual rates increased by ~35%. Sixty percent of all nonfatal self-injury presentations are by women. Self-poisoning is the most common method of self-injury (51%), followed by cutting or piercing (24%), and will be discussed further in the next section.[18]

Self-Poisonings

According to the most recent data from the National Electronic Injury Surveillance System (NEISS), there were 469,096 nonfatal self-injury cases treated in the United States emergency departments in 2014. Of these nonfatal self-injuries, self-poisoning was identified as the most common method of self-injury (51% of the cases). However, it should be noted that these data did not distinguish suicide attempts from self-injurious behaviors.

In the 16 states participating in the National Violent Death Reporting System in 2009, self-poisoning was the third leading method of suicide (following firearms and hanging/suffocation).[47] Detailed data from 2005 to 2007 indicates that 75% of individuals poisoned themselves with a substance (either illicit or licit, including alcohol) as opposed to other types of poison such as carbon monoxide. Seventy percent of individuals ingested just one "drug type," defined as prescription drugs versus nonprescription drugs versus alcohol/illicit drugs. Out of poisoning deaths due to a single "drug type," 80% were due to prescription drugs such as opioids, benzodiazepines, or antidepressants, and 10% were due to nonprescription drugs such as acetaminophen. When individuals consumed more than one "drug type," 45% involved alcohol or illicit drugs as part of the combination.[17,47,51]

There is a large body of literature about self-poisoning in the United Kingdom, and their data indicate proportionally higher death rates among poisonings with cyclic antidepressants versus selective serotonin reuptake inhibitors, which is not surprising given the cardiac toxicity of cyclic antidepressants. Venlafaxine, a serotonin-norepinephrine reuptake inhibitor, is more toxic in overdose than selective serotonin reuptake inhibitors. Poisoning deaths with atypical antipsychotics such as clozapine, olanzapine, and quetiapine were increasing, especially as of the early 2000s.[29]

TABLE 26–3   Factors Associated With Protective Effects for Suicide

Children in the home

Effective clinical care for mental, physical, and substance use disorders

Family and community support (connectedness)

Positive social support

Pregnancy

Religious beliefs and cultural practices

Skills in problem solving and conflict resolution

TABLE 26–4   Case Presentation: Suspected Self-Poisoning

	Case		Evolution		Disposition
Patient course	Patient found in the community; unresponsive	Patient monitored in the emergency department; vital signs stable; still unresponsive	Patient lethargic but cooperative; answers simple questions	Patient fully awake and alert	Evaluation complete
Treatment course	Prehospital	Triage medical assessment	Observation and monitoring	Formal psychiatric evaluation	Treatment planning

Physician course	Patient identification
	Search for prescription drugs, drug paraphernalia
	Assessment of cardiac and respiratory function
		Orogastric lavage (?)
		Activated charcoal (?)
		Diagnostic testing (blood studies, electrocardiography, urine toxicology)
		Contact collateral sources for history
		Prior records
			Focused psychiatric assessment:
			   elopement
			   aggressive behavior
			   decisional capacity
			   addressing confidentiality
			   immediate suicide risk
				Comprehensive psychiatric assessment:
				   diagnostic interviewing
				   risk factors
				   future risk
					Treatments:
					   medication
					   hospitalization
					   substance abuse
					   counseling
					   crisis intervention
					   family therapy

Table 26–4 depicts a case of suspected self-poisoning from the starting point of prehospital care through the completion of a comprehensive assessment and treatment planning.

Completed Suicide

While the annual rates of completed and attempted suicide continue to rise, there are distinguishing patterns between suicide attempts and completed suicides.[15,16] In 2015, men accounted for approximately 77% of completed suicides in the United States, with a majority by use of firearms (55.6% of male suicides), followed by suffocation (26.9%) then self-poisoning (10%). Men commit suicide at more than 3 times the rate than that of women, 21.76 deaths per 100,000 population versus 6.27 deaths per 100,000 population, respectively. In comparison, women's most common method of completed suicide was self-poisoning (33.4%), followed by firearms (30.5%), then suffocation (26.7%).[18] Given the lethal potential of a firearm and the broad-range of lethality from self-poisoning, one theory to explain the higher rate of suicide by males is their preferential use of firearms when compared to females who use self-poisoning methods more often. This theory is further supported by the fact that females attempt suicide at a higher rate than men.[17,43]

Ninety percent of suicide completers and attempters meet criteria for a diagnosable psychiatric illness, 70% have mood disorders, and 30% have alcohol abuse or dependence.[37] On average, one-third of suicide decedents test positive for alcohol, and 65% of them have a blood alcohol concentration higher than 80 mg/dL.[43]

Many individuals who complete suicide do so with the first attempt. Yet, a prior suicide attempt is still the strongest predictor of a future completed suicide.[36,55]

Initial Psychiatric Management

In every case of suspected self-poisoning, a thorough psychiatric assessment is warranted. It is helpful to call a psychiatric consult immediately after medical stabilization, even if the patient is unable to communicate, because important information such as pill bottles, ambulance call reports, and the ability to call the patient's family and outside providers are lost if the consult is delayed. It is helpful to the psychiatrist if serum drug concentrations are obtained for medications of which the patient has access. For example, valproic acid and/or lithium concentrations should be obtained if these were prescribed to the patient or a family member. Obtaining concentrations allows to investigate potential medications used in self-poisoning, as well as to determine compliance.

An early, focused assessment by the emergency physician is necessary to ascertain elopement risk and continued dangerous behavior. Subacute residual central nervous system effects of ingestions, such as confusion, disinhibition, fatigue, and fear, predispose patients to wander or elope. The patient should be searched for weapons, pills, and other potentially harmful materials to prevent additional self-harm or ingestion in the hospital. A high level of supervision should be maintained, and a patient should not be allowed to leave or be left unattended until an adequate assessment of the patient's mental status is completed. Depending on the architecture and organization of the emergency department and its personnel, it may be sufficient to place the patient in an open area in the direct line of sight of the medical staff. If such an arrangement is not possible, or if the patient is agitated and disruptive, it may be necessary to separate the patient from the general population. Under these circumstances, an individual aide should be assigned to observe the patient on a one-to-one basis and remain located within an arm's length of the patient at all times. In extreme cases when all else has failed, physical restraints are necessary to prevent further injury to both the patient and the staff. The need for such measures requires serial reassessment for their necessity.

A more detailed psychiatric assessment should be done as early as possible in the hospital stay as it is critical to address specific clinical concerns. Both history taking and collateral contacts help to establish the patient's baseline and mental status prior to the event. It is often difficult to differentiate a xenobiotic-induced delirium from mental illness. If the patient's cognitive functioning is impaired by xenobiotics, then critical historical details are often unreliable or unattainable.[8,20] Patient reports about intended overdose or self-harm should be documented in the record, because it is particularly important information to consider when patients become guarded and evasive after returning to baseline mental status. It should also be understood that predictable and transient disturbances in mood and perception result from many xenobiotics, and therefore a patient's initial reports while under the influence of the xenobiotic are often ephemeral.[8] The determination that the patient is stable is not solely established on the basis of blood concentrations of xenobiotic and/or ancillary medical tests, but rather when the emergency physician or medical toxicologist deems it appropriate.[39]

The physician cannot solely attribute altered mental status to poisoning or toxicity. Other toxic–metabolic and structural conditions coexist with, and/or masquerade as, toxicity; they must, therefore, be considered and systematically excluded.

Special Issues of Capacity in Suicide and Self-Poisonings

The emergency exception to the doctrine of informed consent also applies in circumstances where attempted suicide is suspected. The emergency exception permits detention, medication over objection, and necessary medical care until psychiatric assessment can be accomplished. This includes collecting information from collateral sources without the patient's consent. Even after management of the immediate medical emergency and resolution of toxicity, suspected self-injury is sufficient evidence of impaired decisional capacity for the emergency physician to detain a patient for further psychiatric assessment. The emergency physician should document the patient's objections in the medical record and indicate the basis for the determination of diminished capacity. After the patient is medically stabilized a full psychiatric assessment and formal capacity assessment by a psychiatrist can be initiated.

Comprehensive Psychiatric Assessment

The goal of comprehensive psychiatric assessment is to

1. characterize the nature of the attempt and any ongoing suicidal ideation that might be present,
2. explore risk factors for another suicide attempt, and
3. formulate a diagnostic impression.

These 3 elements help to determine the level of risk and guide immediate treatment and disposition planning.[68]

The best understanding of suicide at this time is that it results from intrinsic vulnerability factors interacting with external circumstances, which can be termed the "stress vulnerability." Intrinsic vulnerability is conferred by a variety of traits such as impulsivity or conditions such as depression, anxiety, low self-esteem, low self-efficacy, loneliness, and hopelessness. External factors include stressful life events, access to lethal means, and a host of other factors, positive and negative. Poor interpersonal problem-solving skills and a perceived lack of problem-solving ability also appear to increase risk.[23]

Assessing Suicide Attempts and Suicidal Ideation

The core of the suicide risk assessment is a detailed discussion of the patient's suicide attempt and any ongoing suicidal thoughts and urges. It is important to establish rapport and introduce these topics in an appropriate context in order to improve the patient's candor. This evaluation requires significant time and skillful interviewing, for which there is no substitute. This approach will enhance both the therapeutic quality of the interview and its reliability.

The clinician should explore the exact details of the attempt, including precipitating factors that may have begun days or weeks prior to the actual act. It is critical to determine the level of actual and intended lethality, along with the seriousness of the intent. Why did the patient make an attempt on that day or time? Understanding the patient's thought process can help to gauge the extent of impulsivity versus planning involved in the attempt. One approach to assess the level of impulsivity involved in a suicide attempt is to determine the time between the patient's first suicidal thought with a plan and intent, and the actual attempt. Signs of premeditation and planning are concerning, such as extensive researching on methods of suicide, organizing one's affairs (giving away possessions, ensuring a will is updated), or writing goodbye messages. It is crucial to determine if the patient expected to be found, and if any effort was made to notify someone about the impending attempt such as a phone call, Internet posting, or text message. How was the patient discovered, and by whom? A patient who overdoses alone in a hotel room is very different from someone who overdoses in the bedroom while the family is at home. Current feelings about surviving should also be assessed: Is the patient relieved, indifferent, or upset to be alive? Is there currently active or passive suicidal ideation? How forthcoming does the patient appear to be when discussing this? Other important information includes prior suicide attempts and their lethality and circumstances, the frequency and duration of suicidal ideation in the past, prior psychiatric treatment, prior and current medication trials, and a detailed substance abuse history. Psychological factors such as reactivity to positive and negative external events and subjective distress are also important to explore. The social history should focus on interpersonal conflict, stressors within romantic or family relationships, and employment or financial concerns. Current support systems or lack thereof are important to note, as are feelings of isolation and abandonment, which can all be contributing factors.[40]

The communication of suicidal ideas either directly or indirectly should not be misconstrued as a "cry for help" and hence evidence of lower risk. Communication is probably related to the degree of preoccupation with morbid thoughts and to personality characteristics that predispose individuals to revealing their thoughts to various degrees.[44] In psychological autopsy studies, approximately 50% to 70% of those who completed suicides gave some warning of their intention, and 30% to 40% disclosed a direct and specific intent to kill themselves.[5,59]

Although every aspect of suicide risk is not fully understood, it is known that an individual is at 50 to 100 times higher risk of suicide within the first 12 months after an episode of self-harm compared with the general population. About one-half of all people who commit suicide have a history of self-harm, and this increases to 60% in the juvenile population.[1] Although assessing the risk of suicide is difficult because there is no "typical" suicidal patient, there is at least one suicide scale that has demonstrated validity: the Columbia-Suicide Severity Rating Scale.[56] However, this scale requires training to administer and is too lengthy to be administered in an emergency department.

Psychiatric Illness and Suicide

One major consideration in suicide risk assessment is the occurrence of severe mental illness, most commonly affective illnesses (eg, major depressive disorder or bipolar disorder) and psychotic illnesses (eg, schizophrenia or schizoaffective disorder). Suicide risk for individuals with severe mental illness is 20 to 40 times higher than it is for the general population.[45] Psychological autopsy studies, which focus historically on the decedent's intentions and mental state prior to death, consistently reveal major psychiatric illness to be a factor in suicide and present in 93% of adult suicides.[41,45,57,60] This is also true of those who make medically serious suicide attempts.[7,41] In particular, prospective cohort studies and retrospective case–control investigations reveal clinical depression and bipolar disorder to dramatically increase suicide risk.[35,44,67] For mood disorders, factors correlated with current suicidality include current depression, severe anxiety, anhedonia, panic, insomnia, ambivalence, and active alcohol abuse.[44]

A number of avenues of inquiry suggest that violent suicide attempts are associated with a persistent deficiency in brain serotonin concentrations. Impulsive types of aggression and impulsive suicidal behavior are linked to serotonergic dysfunction in prefrontal cortical regions of the brain.[21] This deficiency is measured in the postmortem brain and cerebrospinal fluid analyses of suicide victims and survivors of violent attempts as compared to nonviolent attempts and to other patients. Hopelessness has also received a significant amount of study as a potential predictor of suicide; unfortunately, it appears to have a high sensitivity but a low specificity.[7] However, identifying hopelessness does provide for an intervention.

After mood disorders, chronic alcoholism is the most commonly reported disorder and is present in approximately 20% of cases. Moreover, alcoholic patients who also experience episodes of depression are at a higher risk for suicide than patients who present with either disorder separately. There are considerable data that other types of substance use such as heroin, cocaine, or polydrug use also increase the risk of suicidality when psychiatric illness is present, and this seems to be especially true in depressive or dysphoric mood disorders (unipolar, bipolar II, and mixed types of bipolar I disorders).[9,66] As a result, any assessment conducted on a patient with a substance use history must include an examination of symptoms of major depression or bipolar illness.[28,70]

Patients with schizophrenia are at risk for suicide at rates comparable to major depression and are 20 times more likely to attempt suicide than the general population.[65] Approximately 50% of patients with schizophrenia will attempt suicide and 13% of schizophrenic patients will successfully complete suicide.[11,65] Additionally, between 5% and 18% of patients with severe borderline personality disorder (especially those patients with comorbid depression) ultimately kill themselves.[30,41,64]

The ability to treat psychiatric disorders such as mood disorders, schizophrenia, borderline personality disorder, and alcoholism suggests that most suicides are preventable. Indeed, a suicide prevention program designed for general practitioners in Sweden demonstrated evidence for prevention based on the detection and treatment of depression.[58] The Centers for Disease Control and Prevention reported that psychiatric problems in US emergency departments represented approximately 3% of visits, which is significantly lower than the national psychiatric rate of 20% to 28%.[14] This suggests that psychiatric illness is underdiagnosed in the emergency department. Consequently, emergency physicians must enhance the comprehensive nature of their psychiatric screening to identify suicidality and concomitant mental disorders in patients presenting with self-injury.

Treatment

Following a comprehensive psychiatric assessment, the next step is deciding on treatment alternatives. Any patient who has made a suicide attempt must be considered to be at risk for another attempt, and some further intervention is warranted. The risk of a subsequent lethal attempt is approximately 1% per year over the first 10 years. The risk is highest during the first year. Suicide is most commonly a symptom of an underlying disease process, so the goal is to diagnose and treat the underlying disease in the setting that is the least restrictive while also ensuring safety for the patient. The treatment alternatives available will depend on the psychiatric sophistication of staff available to the emergency department at any given time. This section describes the commonly used interventions in the emergency department; they can be employed singly or in combination.

Psychotropic medications are used acutely in the treatment of severe anxiety or psychosis; however, in the case of antidepressants, several weeks are required for therapeutic effect, so their immediate use is not indicated in the emergency department. However, if the patient is to be discharged to the community with follow-up, it is reasonable for a psychiatrist to start an antidepressant in the emergency department setting. There are concerns about prescribing medications with relatively high potential for lethality in overdose, such as the cyclic antidepressants and nonselective monoamine oxidase inhibitors, to persons who have recently attempted suicide. However, the selective serotonin reuptake inhibitors are first-line treatment for depression and are relatively safe in overdose.

In 2007, the US Food and Drug Administration (FDA) ordered that all antidepressants should include a black box warning stating that there is an increased risk of suicidality in children, adolescents, and adults younger than 24 years of age. This risk was not increased in adults 25 to 64 years of age, and was actually decreased in adults older than 65 years of age. Further studies confirm this age-related difference.[12,63] Proposed explanations include an ascertainment bias, activation and/or akathisia as an adverse event in the first few weeks, or increased energy prior to improvement in mood resulting in increased ability to carry out suicidal plans. Nonetheless, the FDA and other authors emphasize that untreated depression also carries a risk of suicide, and treatment options should be carefully weighed with regard to their risks and benefits. Therefore, we recommend against the initiation of antidepressant therapy by the nonpsychiatric physician unless a tight linkage can be made between discharge and immediate (within days) aftercare by either a community outreach team or a crisis clinic.

Patients with depressive disorders can suffer from significant anxiety, overwhelming situational stressors such as job loss, new financial hardship, bereavement, or divorce. The prescription of a short course (days to weeks) of a benzodiazepine provides significant relief to the patient in crisis. Yet again, close psychiatric follow-up is essential.

After the patient's immediate symptoms have been treated, the next treatment decision is determining the setting in which further treatment may safely be provided. Not all patients with suicidal ideation or even significant attempts necessarily require hospitalization, and there is still a substantial stigma attached to psychiatric hospitalization. In general, hospitalization should be used if less restrictive measures cannot ensure the patient's safety. If significant doubt exists about the safety of outpatient treatment, then the patient should be placed in observation in the emergency department, admitted to a general hospital with close nursing supervision, or admitted to a psychiatric unit. "Holding beds," now available in some larger psychiatric emergency departments, are ideal for this purpose. There are localities with crisis outreach services that follow the patient after emergency department discharge and provide appropriate monitoring and continuity of care.

Patients most likely to respond to interventions in the emergency department are individuals who were stable, but as a result of some external event,

find their way of life threatened. This acute change results in a painful state of anxiety and causes mobilization of some combination of adaptive and maladaptive coping strategies. Finally, a second event, the precipitant, intensifies the anxiety to the point that the patient cannot tolerate the instability and is thrown into crisis. The patient then feels desperate, immobilized or vulnerable to various strong impulses including the impulse to run away, strike out at someone else, or kill him- or herself. Reality testing is preserved, and no major psychiatric syndrome is present. The patient accurately perceives his or her situation, understands that the current reaction is a psychological problem, and is highly motivated to obtain help. The crisis lasts for hours or weeks prior to the emergency department presentation and will ultimately resolve. Such patients respond well to crisis intervention and actually undergo some positive development in the course of treatment.

By contrast, patients whose condition has been deteriorating for some time in the absence of significant stressors, and who appear on examination to be suffering from severe depressive symptoms, are unlikely to benefit rapidly from supportive techniques. If such patients present with suicidal ideation or attempts, it will be difficult, though not impossible, to manage them outside the hospital.

Outpatient settings have the advantage of maintaining the patient's functional status as much as possible. Work and child care responsibilities, financial obligations, and social relationships are not disrupted. Unnecessary regression is halted. The patient assumes more responsibility for his or her outcome, and independence helps preserve self-esteem. These individuals remain closer to and more engaged with the people and situations with whom and with which they must learn to cope. Their morale can rapidly improve by the combination of support, planning, and modest early treatment successes.

However, in some cases, these same factors are disadvantageous. Routine tasks seem overwhelming. High levels of conflict render major relationships at least temporarily unworkable. Inpatient settings offer the advantage of respite, high levels of structure, more intensive professional and peer support, constant supervision, and, usually, more rapid pharmacologic and psychosocial intervention.

The choice of inpatient or outpatient setting will depend on the balance of strengths and weaknesses of the patient, the involvement and competence of family or friends, the availability of a therapist in the community, and the ongoing stresses in the patient's life. This decision is best made by a psychiatrist. Because a psychiatrist is not always present in many facilities, a trained mental health professional should optimally be on call to every emergency department. This may be a psychiatric social worker, nurse clinician, or psychologist. When such services are not available, it is appropriate to detain patients in the emergency department until a practitioner with specific competence is available or to transfer the patient to another facility for evaluation. Every state has laws that provide for the involuntary commitment of the mentally ill under circumstances that vary from state to state (Chap. 138). Any acute, deliberately self-injurious behavior would generally qualify. Chronic, repetitive dangerous behavior that is not deliberate, such as frequent unintentional opioid, alcohol, sedative–hypnotic, or illicit "recreational" psychoactive drug overdoses, warrants careful evaluation. In the absence of psychiatric illness, involuntary treatment is usually not necessary, but should be considered carefully if a patient appears unable to achieve self-care. The practitioner should be familiar with the criteria for commitment and the classes of health care professionals so empowered under state law.

There are other treatment interventions that can be provided in the emergency setting, including crisis intervention, substance abuse counseling, and family therapy. A single session in the emergency department is often sufficient to defuse a crisis or to spur the drug-abusing patient to seek help. Intervention initiated in the emergency department then continued as an outpatient setting.

Crisis intervention is a brief, highly focused therapy that seeks to deconstruct how a crisis occurred, with the intent of examining the patient's role. Often, patients have distorted perceptions of the crisis, and a gentle "correction" of catastrophic thinking is helpful. The crisis is presented to the patient as an unfortunate and perhaps tragic experience that the patient can overcome. Ideally, the patient should have a relief of symptoms and learn how crises may be avoided in the future. This insight intervention will likely fail for patients with severe depression because of the presence of profound hopelessness. It is most successful for patients who give a history of high functioning just prior to the crisis.

"Contracting for safety" was a popular technique in the past, and consists of patients being asked whether they can remain safe and agree not to engage in self-harm. However, there are no empirical data to show that it is effective, and in court cases it is not protective in terms of liability for the clinician. It is not recognized as part of the standard of care for the suicidal patient, and if anything, it seems to provide the clinician with a false sense of security. Its use is not recommended except as a technique to engage in a larger discussion of a safety plan that delineates scenarios the patient might face after leaving the hospital, and possible coping strategies.[31]

SUBSTANCE USE DISORDERS

Substance use disorders are characterized by compulsive drug seeking and drug taking in a setting of loss of control, continued use despite negative consequences, and functional impairment in several domains of a person's life. They are highly comorbid with suicidality, violence, and mental illness as described above in previous sections. Prevalence rates of substance use in the emergency department range from 9% to 47%, depending on the sample.[26] Emergency physicians and medical toxicologists are in a unique

position to identify substance use disorders and refer patients to additional treatment services. There is an extensive array of evidence-based treatment for substance use disorders, but less than 10% of persons with substance use disorders in the United States receive substance abuse treatment. There are increasing efforts to combat this. For example, the American College of Surgeons' Committee on Trauma (ACS-COT) now requires level I and II trauma centers to identify problem drinkers and level I centers must employ SBIRT (Screening Brief Intervention, and Referral to Treatment).[69]

DSM-5 Diagnoses

The psychiatrist's diagnostic handbook, the *Diagnostic and Statistical Manual of Mental Disorders* (DSM), codifies various diagnoses involving the use of substances. The latest version is the fifth edition, DSM-5, which was released in 2013.[4] Although previous versions of the DSM differentiated "substance abuse" and "substance dependence," the DSM-5 combines these categories into an overarching "substance use disorder" diagnosis with mild, moderate, and severe specifiers. Table 26–5 shows the criteria for an alcohol use disorder, and the reader can use this as a template to substitute other substances of abuse as well.

Neurobiology of Substance Use Disorders

It is helpful for the emergency physician to be able to recognize the signs and symptoms of a substance use disorder. Although the DSM-5 criteria are straightforward, many patients are not forthcoming and do not share the

---

TABLE 26–5　DSM-5: Criteria for Alcohol Use Disorder (2013)

Alcohol Use Disorder

Diagnostic Criteria

A. A problematic pattern of alcohol use leading to clinically significant impairment or distress, as manifested by at least two of the following, occurring within a 12-month period:
1. Alcohol is often taken in larger amounts or over a longer period than was intended.
2. There is a persistent desire or unsuccessful efforts to cut down or control alcohol use.
3. A great deal of time is spent in activities necessary to obtain alcohol, use alcohol, or recover from its effects.
4. Craving, or a strong desire or urge to use alcohol.
5. Recurrent alcohol use resulting in a failure to fulfill major role obligations at work, school, or home.
6. Continued alcohol use despite having persistent or recurrent social or interpersonal problems caused or exacerbated by the effects of alcohol.
7. Important social, occupational, or recreational activities are given up or reduced because of alcohol use.
8. Recurrent alcohol use in situations in which it is physically hazardous.
9. Alcohol use is continued despite knowledge of having a persistent or recurrent physical or psychological problem that is likely to have been caused or exacerbated by alcohol.
10. Tolerance, as defined by either of the following:
    a. A need for markedly increased amounts of alcohol to achieve intoxication or desired effect.
    b. A markedly diminished effect with continued use of the same amount of alcohol.
11. Withdrawal, as manifested by either of the following:
    a. The characteristic withdrawal syndrome for alcohol (refer to Criteria A and B of the criteria set for alcohol withdrawal).
    b. Alcohol (or a closely related substance, such as a benzodiazepine) is taken to relieve or avoid withdrawal symptoms.

Specify if:
- **In early remission:** After full criteria for alcohol use disorder were previously met, none of the criteria for alcohol use disorder have been met for at least 3 months but for less than 12 months (with the exception that Criterion A4, "Craving, or a strong desire or urge to use alcohol," may be met).
- **In sustained remission:** After full criteria for alcohol use disorder were previously met, none of the criteria for alcohol use disorder have been met at any time during a period of 12 months or longer (with the exception that Criterion A4, "Craving, or a strong desire or urge to use alcohol," may be met).

Specify if:
- **In a controlled environment:** This additional specifier is used if the individual is in an environment where access to alcohol is restricted.

Code based on current severity: Note for ICD-10-CM codes: If an alcohol intoxication, alcohol withdrawal, or another alcohol-induced mental disorder is also present, do not use the codes below for alcohol use disorder. Instead, the comorbid alcohol use disorder is indicated in the 4th character of the alcohol-induced disorder code (see the coding note for alcohol intoxication, alcohol withdrawal, or a specific alcohol-induced mental disorder). For example, if there is comorbid alcohol intoxication and alcohol use disorder, only the alcohol intoxication code is given, with the 4th character indicating whether the comorbid alcohol use disorder is mild, moderate, or severe: F10.129 for mild alcohol use disorder with alcohol intoxication or F10.229 for a moderate or severe alcohol use disorder with alcohol intoxication.

Specify current severity:
- **305.00 (F10.10) Mild:** Presence of 2–3 symptoms.
- **303.90 (F10.20) Moderate:** Presence of 4–5 symptoms.
- **303.90 (F10.20) Severe:** Presence of 6 or more symptoms.

extent of their drug use and its effect on their lives. In those cases, one can look for inconsistencies in either the history or the presentation. Denial is often prominent. For example, a patient might present intoxicated with an arm injury, but is unconcerned and dismissive about the incident when no longer intoxicated. One would expect a patient to demonstrate appropriate concern, rather than just "wanting to leave."

One of the more vexing aspects of substance-dependent patients is the frequency with which they minimize the dangerousness of their actions or the severity of their presentation. This can be interpreted as a sign of prefrontal cortex dysfunction due to the addiction. The patient is incorrectly processing risks and benefits, and is increasingly driven to compulsive drug use at the cost of natural rewards such as food, sex, love, or safety. Initial drug use results in relaxation, euphoria, stress relief, or a variety of other psychological effects, as mediated by the dopaminergic "reward pathway." It was traditionally taught that dopamine release in this pathway was synonymous with experiencing "pleasure," but it has become apparent that the function of dopamine is more accurately portrayed as indicating "salience" (or importance). A burst of dopamine in this pathway confers enhanced salience onto a particular stimulus or aspect of the environment, which means that this stimulus now appears more important and there is greater motivation to pay attention to it. One can see how this works well as a survival system, with natural rewards such as food and sex resulting in increased dopamine and subsequently greater salience. Drugs of abuse essentially "hijack" this pathway by directly producing supra-physiologic increases in dopamine that far exceeds the dopaminergic response to natural rewards.[42]

However, activity in the reward pathway only explains the acute effects of drugs and does not explain why someone's behavior changes so drastically as the individual becomes addicted. The cravings and compulsive behavior that occur in addiction result from glutamate-mediated circuits that develop in the prefrontal cortex and establish aberrant connections to the limbic system. Affected areas include the orbitofrontal cortex, which regulates salience attribution, and the anterior cingulate gyrus, which regulates inhibitory control. Late-stage addiction is characterized by derangements in these areas of the prefrontal cortex, which results in an increased salience for drugs of abuse combined with a reduced ability to inhibit impulsive behavior. It is a resulting "perfect storm": the person is extremely motivated to find and use drugs, and unable to stop or inhibit this behavior. Environmental "triggers" established by conditioning subsequently act to induce powerful states of craving and increased motivation to find and use a particular drug.[42]

Despite our sophistication in describing the neurobiology of addiction, it can be challenging for an individual clinician to act accordingly when dealing with an addicted patient; we are used to assuming that behavior is voluntary, especially if a person is coherent and oriented. It can be difficult to recall that a patient who is hostile and in denial actually has true neurobiological dysfunction, not unlike a patient with dementia or psychosis. Unfortunately, our current civil commitment laws have not "caught up" with this neurobiological understanding, and we do not hospitalize severely addicted patients against their will even if there are multiple presentations of intoxication or withdrawal and it is clear the patient is suffering substantially. However, some institutions have committed these types of patients and have shown some impressive outcomes.[48]

Treatment

Substance abuse treatment is ultimately an intermediate (weeks to months) to long-term (months to years) intervention. However, there are powerful initial steps that the emergency physician can take. Central among these is confronting the patient about the medical consequences of substance use. This can take the form of discussion only, or the physician can invite the patient to examine clinical laboratory results or view remarkable clinical diagnostic findings (hepatomegaly, repeated fractures from falls, liver enzyme abnormalities, or evidence of "silent" past myocardial infarction). There is little to be lost from a respectful but blunt confrontation of the patient's deterioration, and the patient may listen to a physician rather than family or friends. "Physician advice" in this manner is shown to be useful for patients who do

not yet meet criteria for a substance use disorder, and therefore still have sufficient control of their substance use to make a logical decision about the risks versus benefits of continued use.

Patients who are further along the addictive spectrum and who display behavioral or physiologic signs of moderate–severe substance use disorders are much less likely to curb their substance use in the face of adverse medical sequelae. For these patients, more intensive intervention is warranted, often in the form of a consultation. For most hospitals, this type of consultation would be fulfilled by a psychiatrist, but some institutions have a separate substance abuse consult service. Ideally, all patients suspected to have a substance use disorder should be referred to some type of aftercare when possible: inpatient or outpatient detoxification, inpatient or outpatient rehabilitation, or even follow-up with primary care.

In a busy emergency department, this can be quite cumbersome logistically, depending on the demographics of the patient population and the percentage of patients suspected to have a substance use disorder. Regulatory agencies at the state and federal levels are increasingly mandating substance abuse screening, brief interventions, and referrals (SBIRT), much like ACS-COT for trauma surgeons, and it is hoped this will result in increased resources for additional ancillary staff to assist with such tasks.

It is helpful to note that peer counseling is particularly useful in addictive disorders, and community 12-step programs like Narcotics Anonymous (NA) and Alcoholics Anonymous (AA) are ubiquitous worldwide. Alcoholics Anonymous has its own website and specific phone lines in some cities that are staffed by AA members with the express purpose of orienting potential new members and assisting them in attending their first meeting. Even if there is insufficient infrastructure in the emergency department to provide the more intensive intervention that might be needed for a substance-using patient, the physician can at least refer directly to AA. Patients with repeated presentations for substance intoxication/withdrawal should be considered for a higher level of care, since they may be demonstrating the inability to care for themselves. Such a decision would be made in conjunction with the psychiatrist and would have to comply with the local civil commitment laws. Finally, it is important to note that substance abuse treatment is quite effective, and that coerced treatment has been found to be just as effective as voluntary treatment. Given the remarkably high comorbidity of substance use disorders in the emergency department setting, it behooves us to attempt to connect these patients with the appropriate treatment.

SUMMARY

- Capacity assessment should be approached systematically, and such an approach is helpful in more complex situations. A "sliding scale" is a useful concept; when refusing an intervention would have serious consequences, a patient is held to a higher standard to demonstrate capacity.
- "Medical clearance" does not have a standard protocol, but in general the ED assessment should be guided by the history and physical examination.
- Both violent and suicidal behavior in the emergency department are the cause or the effect of many toxicologic presentations.
- It is incumbent on all emergency physicians to screen patients for psychiatric emergency presentations as part of a comprehensive screening for self-harm.
- Identifying risk factors for suicide and aggression can aid the clinician in employing preventive or early intervention strategies in the ED.
- Important risk factors for both suicidal and violent behavior include history of the behavior, comorbid mental illness, drug and alcohol intoxication, and young age.
- Mental status examination for suicidality should focus on extrinsic factors such as current ideation, intent, lethality of plan, current life stressors, as well as intrinsic vulnerability factors such as comorbid mental illness, feelings of hopelessness, and impulsivity.
- In terms of violence risk assessment, drug and alcohol intoxication, mental illness, and psychiatric medication noncompliance (alone or in

combination) are robust predictors of aggressive behavior in the ED and other inpatient settings.

■ Substance use disorders are highly prevalent in patients who present with psychiatric issues in the ED, and there are possibilities for identification and referral even in busy ED settings.

Acknowledgment

Kishor Malavade, MD, Mark R. Serper, PhD, Michael H. Allen, MD, Wendy Rives, MD (deceased), Brett R. Goldberg, PhD, and Cherie Elfenbein, MD, contributed to this chapter in previous editions.

REFERENCES

1. Anderson CA. Temperature and aggression: ubiquitous effects of heat on occurrence of human violence. *Psychol Bull.* 1989;106:74-96.
2. Appelbaum PS. Clinical practice. Assessment of patients' competence to consent to treatment. *N Engl J Med.* 2007;357:1834-1840.
3. Appelbaum PS, Grisso T. Assessing patients' capacities to consent to treatment. *N Engl J Med.* 1988;319:1635-1638.
4. American Psychiatric Association. *Diagnostic and Statistical Manual of Mental Disorders.* 5th ed. Arlington, VA: American Psychiatric Association; 2013.
5. Barraclough B, et al. A hundred cases of suicide: clinical aspects. *Br J Psychiatry.* 1974;125:355-373.
6. Beautrais AL, et al. Prevalence and comorbidity of mental disorders in persons making serious suicide attempts: a case-control study. *Am J Psychiatry.* 1996;153:1009-1014.
7. Beck AT, et al. Hopelessness and eventual suicide: a 10-year prospective study of patients hospitalized with suicidal ideation. *Am J Psychiatry.* 1985;142:559-563.
8. Bentur Y, et al. Toxicological features of deliberate self-poisonings. *Hum Exp Toxicol.* 2004;23:331-337.
9. Borges G, et al. Associations of substance use, abuse, and dependence with subsequent suicidal behavior. *Am J Epidemiol.* 2000;151:781-789.
10. Broderick KB, et al. Emergency physician practices and requirements regarding the medical screening examination of psychiatric patients. *Acad Emerg Med.* 2002;9:88-92.
11. Carmel H, Hunter M. Compliance with training in managing assaultive behavior and injuries from inpatient violence. *Hosp Community Psychiatry* 1990;41:558-560.
12. Carpenter DJ, et al. Meta-analysis of efficacy and treatment-emergent suicidality in adults by psychiatric indication and age subgroup following initiation of paroxetine therapy: a complete set of randomized placebo-controlled trials. *J Clin Psychiatry.* 2011;72:1503-1514.
13. Centers for Disease Control and Prevention. Nonfatal self-inflicted injuries treated in hospital emergency departments—United States, 2000. *MMWR Morb Mortal Wkly Rep.* 2002;51:436-438.
14. Centers for Disease Control and Prevention. Web-based Injury Statistics Query and Reporting System (WISQARS) [online]. 2005.
15. Centers for Disease Control and Prevention. Homicides and suicides—National Violent Death Reporting System, United States, 2003-2004. *MMWR Morb Mortal Wkly Rep.* 2006;55:721-724.
16. Centers for Disease Control and Prevention. Toxicology testing and results for suicide victims—13 states, 2004. *MMWR Morb Mprtal Wkly Rep.* 2006;55:1245-1248.
17. Centers for Disease Control and Prevention. Web-based Injury Statistics Query and Reporting System (WISQARS) [online]. 2010.
18. Centers for Disease Control and Prevention. Web-based Injury Statistics Query and Reporting System (WISQARS) [online]. 2014-2015.
19. Collier R. New York enacts surrogate decision-making legislation for incapacitated patients. *CMAJ.* 2010;182:E331-E332.
20. Crome P. The toxicity of drugs used for suicide. *Acta Psychiatr Scand Suppl.* 1993;371:33-37.
21. Davidson RJ, et al. Dysfunction in the neural circuitry of emotion regulation—a possible prelude to violence. *Science.* 2000;289:591-594.
22. Dhossche D, Rubinstein J. Drug detection in a suburban psychiatric emergency room. *Ann Clin Psychiatry.* 1996;8:59-69.
23. Dieserud G, et al. Toward an integrative model of suicide attempt: a cognitive psychological approach. *Suicide Life Threat Behav.* 2001;31:153-168.
24. Dolan JG, Mushlin AI. Routine laboratory testing for medical disorders in psychiatric inpatients. *Arch Intern Med.* 1985;145:2085-2088.
25. Dubin WR. Rapid tranquilization: antipsychotics or benzodiazepines? *J Clin Psychiatry.* 1988;49(suppl):5-12.
26. el-Guebaly N, et al. Substance abuse and the emergency room: programmatic implications. *J Addict Dis.* 1998;17:21-40.
27. Etchells E, et al. Assessment of patient capacity to consent to treatment. *J Gen Intern Med.* 1999;14:27-34.
28. Fawcett J, et al. Time-related predictors of suicide in major affective disorder. *Am J Psychiatry.* 1990;147:1189-1194.
29. Flanagan RJ. Fatal toxicity of drugs used in psychiatry. *Hum Psychopharmacol* 2008; 23 Suppl 1:43-51.
30. Frances A, Blumenthal SJ. Personality as a predictor of youthful suicide. In: Davidson L, Linnoila M, eds. *Report of the Secretary's Task Force on Youth Suicide. Volume 2: Risk Factors for Youth Suicide.* Rockville, MD: Alcohol, Drug Abuse, and Mental Health Administration; 1989:160-171.
31. Garvey KA, et al. Contracting for safety with patients: clinical practice and forensic implications. *J Am Acad Psychiatry Law* 2009;37:363-370.
32. Glenn CR, Nock MK. Improving the short-term prediction of suicidal behavior. *Am J Prev Med.* 2014;47:S176-S180.
33. Gregory RJ, et al. Medical screening in the emergency department for psychiatric admissions: a procedural analysis. *Gen Hosp Psychiatry.* 2004;26:405-410.
34. Grisso T, et al. The MacCAT-T: a clinical tool to assess patients' capacities to make treatment decisions. *Psychiatr Serv.* 1997;48:1415-1419.
35. Hagnell O, et al. Suicide rates in the Lundby study: mental illness as a risk factor for suicide. *Neuropsychobiology.* 1981;7:248-253.
36. Harris EC, Barraclough B. Suicide as an outcome for mental disorders. A meta-analysis. *Br J Psychiatry.* 1997;170:205-228.
37. Haw C, et al. Psychiatric and personality disorders in deliberate self-harm patients. *Br J Psychiatry.* 2001;178:48-54.
38. Hawton K, Fagg J. Suicide, and other causes of death, following attempted suicide. *Br J Psychiatry.* 1988;152:359-366.
39. Henry JA. A fatal toxicity index for antidepressant poisoning. *Acta Psychiatr Scand Suppl.* 1989;354:37-45.
40. Hirschfeld RM, Russell JM. Assessment and treatment of suicidal patients. *N Engl J Med.* 1997;337:910-915.
41. Inskip HM, et al. Lifetime risk of suicide for affective disorder, alcoholism and schizophrenia. *Br J Psychiatry.* 1998;172:35-37.
42. Kalivas PW, Volkow ND. The neural basis of addiction: a pathology of motivation and choice. *Am J Psychiatry.* 2005;162:1403-1413.
43. Karch DL, et al. Surveillance for violent deaths—National Violent Death Reporting System, 16 states, 2009. *MMWR Surveill Summ.* 2012;61:1-43.
44. Kessler RC, et al. Prevalence of and risk factors for lifetime suicide attempts in the National Comorbidity Survey. *Arch Gen Psychiatry.* 1999;56:617-626.
45. Kochanek KD, et al. Deaths: final data for 2002. *Natl Vital Stat Rep.* 2004;53:1-115.
46. Lukens TW, et al. Clinical policy: critical issues in the diagnosis and management of the adult psychiatric patient in the emergency department. *Ann Emerg Med.* 2006;47:79-99.
47. Lyons BH, et al. Surveillance for violent deaths—National Violent Death Reporting System, 17 States, 2013. *MMWR Surveill Summ.* 2016;65:1-42.
48. McCormack RP, et al. Commitment to assessment and treatment: comprehensive care for patients gravely disabled by alcohol use disorders. *Lancet.* 2013;382:995-997.
49. McFeeters D, et al. Patterns of stressful life events: distinguishing suicide ideators from suicide attempters. *J Affect Disord.* 2015;175:192-198.
50. Moscicki EK. Identification of suicide risk factors using epidemiologic studies. *Psychiatr Clin North Am.* 1997;20:499-517.
51. National Center for Injury Prevention and Control (US), Division of Violence Prevention. Suicides due to alcohol and/or drug overdose; a data brief from the National Violent Death Reporting System. Washington, DC: US Department of Health & Human Services; 2011.
52. Nock MK, et al. Cross-national prevalence and risk factors for suicidal ideation, plans and attempts. *Br J Psychiatry.* 2008;192:98-105.
53. Owens D, et al. Fatal and non-fatal repetition of self-harm. Systematic review. *Br J Psychiatry.* 2002;181:193-199.
54. Pan YJ, et al. Socioeconomic disadvantage, mental disorders and risk of 12-month suicide ideation and attempt in the National Comorbidity Survey Replication (NCS-R) in US. *Soc Psychiatry Psychiatr Epidemiol.* 2013;48:71-79.
55. Pokorny A.D.. Prediction of suicide in psychiatric patients. Report of a prospective study. *Arch Gen Psychiatry.* 1983;40:249-257.
56. Posner K, et al. The Columbia-Suicide Severity Rating Scale: initial validity and internal consistency findings from three multisite studies with adolescents and adults. *Am J Psychiatry.* 2011;168:1266-1277.
57. Rich CL, et al. San Diego suicide study. I. Young vs old subjects. *Arch Gen Psychiatry.* 1986;43:577-582.
58. Rihmer Z, et al. Depression and suicide on Gotland. An intensive study of all suicides before and after a depression-training programme for general practitioners. *J Affect Disord.* 1995;35:147-152.
59. Robins E, et al. The communication of suicidal intent: a study of 134 consecutive cases of successful (completed) suicide. *Am J Psychiatry.* 1959;115:724-733.
60. Robins E, et al. Some clinical considerations in the prevention of suicide based on a study of 134 successful suicides. *Am J Public Health Nations Health.* 1959;49:888-899.
61. Ryan J, et al. Suicide rate following attendance at an accident and emergency department with deliberate self harm. *J Accid Emerg Med.* 1996;13:101-104.
62. Stanley B, Siever LJ. The interpersonal dimension of borderline personality disorder: toward a neuropeptide model. *Am J Psychiatry.* 2010;167:24-39.
63. Stone M, et al. Risk of suicidality in clinical trials of antidepressants in adults: analysis of proprietary data submitted to US Food and Drug Administration. *BMJ.* 2009;339:b2880.
64. Stone MH. The course of borderline personality disorder. In: Tasman A, Hales R, Frances AJ, eds. *Review of Psychiatry.* Vol. 8. Washington, DC: American Psychiatric Press; 1987:103-122.

65. Tandon RJ, Michael D. Suicidal behavior in schizophrenia: diagnosis, neurobiology, and treatment implications. *Curr Opin Psychiatry*. 2003;16:193-197.

66. Tondo L, et al. Suicide attempts in major affective disorder patients with comorbid substance use disorders. *J Clin Psychiatry*. 1999;60(suppl 2):63-69; discussion 75-66, 113-116.

67. US Department of Commerce. Statistical Abstracts of the United States, 116th ed. 1996.

68. US Department of Health and Human Services. The Surgeon General's call to action to prevent suicide. 1999.

69. Vaca FE, Winn D. The basics of alcohol screening, brief intervention and referral to treatment in the emergency department. *West J Emerg Med*. 2007;8:88-92.

70. Vijayakumar L, Rajkumar S. Are risk factors for suicide universal? A case-control study in India. *Acta Psychiatr Scand*. 1999;99:407-411.

SC4

PATIENT VIOLENCE

Andrea M. Kondracke, Justin M. Lewin, Cathy A. Kondas, and Erin A. Zerbo

The aggressive and/or violent patient presents unique challenges. Like suicidal patients, aggressive individuals are difficult to treat and they tend to elicit strong negative reactions in hospital personnel ranging from anger to fear.[42] Workplace violence is unfortunately commonplace within the health care setting, and is particularly prominent in the inpatient psychiatry ward and emergency department settings.[20] Of the approximately 24,000 annual workplace assaults occurring between the years of 2011 and 2013 in the United States, approximately 75% were within the health care and social service settings.[37] The prevalence of verbal and physical assaults reported by emergency nurses within a 12-month period is as high as 100% and 82%, respectively.[34] Additionally, a survey of emergency physicians within the state of Michigan showed that 25% of emergency physicians reported being a target of physical assault within 12 months.[27] These statistics on workplace violence in health care settings are likely underestimates as events are often underreported to health care supervisors and administrators. Workplace violence occurs so frequently that there is a perception among health care workers that violence is "the norm" and an expected part of their job.[44]

Workplace violence is classified into 4 broad categories that are dependent on the relationship of the perpetrator to the workplace. In type I, which accounts for approximately 80% of workplace homicides, there is not an association between the two. These incidents are generally motivated by theft, with hospitals and pharmacies being susceptible because of their abundance of opioids, equipment, and money. However, this type of violence is no more likely to be experienced in health care settings. Preventive measures include environmental security measures such as metal detectors. In type II, the most common type in the hospital setting, the perpetrator is a patient or customer. In general, these acts of violence occur while workers are performing basic work functions. An example of this would be an intoxicated patient who punches a nurse while obtaining vital signs. In type III, the perpetrator is a current or former employee. In type IV, the perpetrator has a personal relationship with a specific employee but not with the institution.[41] The most common types of hospital violence are incidents of aggression against objects in the hospital (57%), violence directed against the hospital staff (28%), and violence directed against other patients (14%).[43]

In one study of violence in the emergency department, directors of emergency medicine residency programs were surveyed as to the frequency of verbal threats, physical attacks, and the presence of weaponry in the area. Of the 127 institutions surveyed, 74.7% of the residency directors responded; 41 (32%) reported receiving at least one verbal threat each day; 23 (18%) reported that weapons were displayed as a threat at least once each month. Fifty-five program directors (43%) noted that a physical attack on medical staff members occurred at least once a month.[29]

These studies underscore the need for timely identification of the potentially violent patient, as well as appropriate management for this diagnostically heterogeneous group.[13] The assessment and management of the violent patient should include provisions for patient and staff safety as well as a thorough search for the underlying cause of violent behavior.[23,42]

The section below addresses the differential diagnosis of violent behavior, predictions of violence, the pharmacotherapy for the treatment of aggressive and/or agitated behavior, and the use of seclusion and physical restraint. It also provides an overview of potential risk factors for violent behavior.

Differential Diagnosis

There are many causes of violent behavior; some are social, medical, or biological in nature. The most common characteristic of the violent patient is alteration in mental status. Factors such as metabolic derangements, exposure to xenobiotics (both licit and illicit), withdrawal syndromes, seizures, head trauma, stroke, psychosis, cognitive impairment, and personality disorder all predispose a patient to aggression and violence. Additionally, patients with severe pain, delirium, or extreme anxiety often respond to the efforts of emergency personnel with resistance, hostility, or overt aggression.

The stress-vulnerability model suggests that violence should be considered as the outcome of a dynamic interaction among numerous factors both intrinsic and extrinsic to the individual. Although education theoretically provides alternatives to violence, xenobiotic-induced delirium will render any education ineffective because delirium prevents patients from reasoning or exercising impulse control. Once confused, the patient often misinterprets health care efforts in a paranoid manner, and becomes violent under circumstances that would not normally be sufficient to provoke a violent outburst in that individual. Some patients, on the other hand, come from cultures in which aggressive behavior is more acceptable and/or expected, and these patients require little stress or provocation before responding in what is often perceived as aggression by Western cultural standards.

Prediction of Violence

Although there is a high expectation that violence is predictable, there are no proven predictors of violence. Prior history of violence is postulated as a risk factor for future violence. Patients in police custody are involved in 29% of shootings in emergency departments.[37] Predicting violent behavior based on medical diagnosis (eg, patients with HIV) is unfruitful and leads to bias or discrimination. Other factors such as personality disorders, mental illness, dementia, and substance abuse are areas that need further study.[42] Studies of emergency department violence show the following risk factors: the presence of guns, area of gang activity, low socioeconomic status, and interacting with patients who were recently given bad news.[37]

There are several structured approaches to violence risk assessment.[46] Examples are the Psychopathy Checklist–Revised (PCL-R); Historical Clinical Risk Management–20 (HCR-20); Classification of Violence Risk (COVR); Violence Risk Appraisal Guide (VRAG).[46] Structured approaches tend to have better efficacy for predicting violence than an unstructured approach. However, they also have many shortcomings: the sensitivities and specificities tend to hover around 0.7 and they are time consuming and require specific training to administer, rendering them impractical in the emergency department setting.[16]

Substance Use and Violence

The association between substance use and violence is well established. Alcohol is found in the offender, the victim, or both in one-half to two-thirds of homicides and serious assaults.[9,38] Substance use is seldom the sole cause, but it contributes to violence in a number of ways. Substance use interacts with other physiologic, cognitive, psychological, situational, and cultural factors including any underlying mental illness. A tripartite model for substance-related violence is described:[18,19]

1. systemic violence related to the sale and distribution of drugs,
2. economic compulsive violence associated with profit-oriented criminal activity to maintain the expenses of an individual's drug habit, and
3. psychopharmacologic violence resulting from the direct effects of the particular xenobiotic.

Toxicity causes disinhibition, impulsivity, perceptual disturbance, paranoia, irritability, misinterpretation, affective instability, and/or confusion. For example, synthetic cannabinoids, synthetic cathinones, and phencyclidine are well known to cause agitation, which is often accompanied by violent and uncontrollable behavior.

Withdrawal syndromes also promote aggressive behavior for a multitude of reasons, including physical discomfort, anticipatory anxiety, irritability as a direct result of withdrawal, and withdrawal-related delirium. Patients experiencing any of these symptoms have the potential to become aggressive, verbally abusive, or threatening. Prompt recognition of these syndromes and immediate treatment will prevent some aggressive outbursts or escalation to assaultive behaviors. Well-known xenobiotics that cause irritability and associated behaviors in withdrawal include ethanol, benzodiazepines, and opioids. Because drug use is often concealed, is difficult to ascertain on clinical grounds, and frequently contributes to violent behavior, urine and blood toxicologic studies are useful in enhancing the understanding and long-term treatment of some patients.[8]

Mental Illness and Violence

The relationship between mental illness and violence is also complex. The impact of present-day media and the counteracting efforts made to destigmatize mental illness often confound this issue. There are several studies showing an association between mental illness and increased risk for violence.[38] In one large epidemiologic study, the prevalence of violence for those without mental illness was 2%, whereas schizophrenia was associated with an 8% rate of violent behavior. But, of all respondents reporting violent behaviors, 42% had a substance use disorder. In patients with schizophrenia, having a co-occurring substance use disorder more than tripled the rate of violence.[45] However, based on a cohort study from the Netherlands, most of the common mental disorders were associated with violence until adjusting for violent victimization, negative life events, and social supports. Then the association of violence with most mental disorders was negligible, with the exception of substance use disorders, which retain a strong association with violent behavior.[45]

In addition to substance abuse and severe mental illnesses, researchers have consistently found a greater prevalence of personality disorders among individuals who become violent in an inpatient setting as compared to nonviolent inpatients.[7] Antisocial personality disorder is the condition most strongly associated with both substance use and aggression. Patients with either borderline or antisocial personality disorders are at risk for violent behavior as a result of chronic poor impulse control and impaired frustration tolerance in the context of poor coping skills.

Although persons with psychotic disorders are not generally aggressive, there are aspects of their psychosis that place them at risk for aggressive behavior. Hallucinations lead to aggression, such as when patients explicitly follow the instructions of a violent command auditory hallucination. Paranoid ideation that leads an individual to believe that she or he is at imminent risk of bodily harm ("They're trying to kill me"), sexual victimization ("Men and women are raping me"), or humiliation ("Everyone is laughing at me") or feeling physically trapped are examples of thoughts that lead psychotic patients to be aggressive.

Alternative Etiologies

Delirium from any underlying condition is a cause of aggression. Patients are often suddenly confused, frightened, or frankly psychotic as a result of impaired perception. Violence risk is also associated with cognitive dysfunction such as traumatic brain injury and dementia. These patients are unable to engage in a rational manner and verbal de-escalation is often futile.

Additional Factors in Aggressive Behavior

Many of the factors correlated with aggression are easy to observe and monitor in the hospital, yet some additional factors are not so easy to detect. One study found that most violent incidents in the hospital occur on Mondays and Fridays, and others have postulated that there is a seasonal variation of violence, with violence occurring more often in extreme temperatures.[10] There is an increase in the frequency of assaults by inpatients during the winter months, and it is hypothesized that increased population density, cold temperature, and less sunlight during the day could account for the increased violence. This finding is in contrast to the literature on outpatient violence, which has reported greater incidence of violence during the warmer months.[2] However, this same review conceded that any extreme temperature could evoke aggressive urges and frustration.

Although it is unclear whether cold temperatures provoke aggression to the same extent as hot temperatures, it does seem clear that overcrowding and social stressors, long wait times, and inadequate food supplies can lead to violent behavior.

Assessment of the Violent Patient

The comprehensive evaluation of the violent patient include a complete physical examination with the intent of revealing the underlying cause of the violent behavior as well as ensuring the discovery of secondary patient injuries. It is important to attempt to differentiate toxicity or withdrawal, cognitive impairment, delirium, and mental illness as treatment differs depending on etiology. Recommended laboratory analyses include blood chemistries (glucose, electrolytes), a complete blood count, liver function tests, renal function tests, thyroid function tests, and urinalysis. The need for lumbar puncture and/or neuroimaging is best guided by clinical history and physical examination.

Treatment

There are 3 main approaches to controlling aggressive behavior in order of escalation: First and foremost, there is verbal de-escalation. When this has failed, medical anxiolysis and sedation will be the next approach. Finally, under the most extreme circumstances where there is significant risk for harming self or others, the use of physical restraints are indicated.

Verbal De-escalation

Because of several high-profile deaths involving restraints, there is a continued focus on advancing techniques and training in de-escalation. These are now paramount to the treatment of agitation and violence in the medical setting. These techniques use both verbal and nonverbal communication, and include talking to a patient, building rapport, listening and understanding in a calm and compassionate manner, using a calm voice, making eye contact, and focusing on the person and not the behavior.

Many hospitals have behavioral response teams. At our institution, the creation of a crisis management team has proven to be a very successful way of intervening and avoiding the escalation of a violent situation. The purpose of these teams is to respond, assess, protect, and treat the patient with behavioral disturbances. The teams are generally multidisciplinary in nature and consist of mental health, medical, and security professionals. The members should have specialized training in evaluation, conflict resolution, and de-escalation techniques. Team members should possess good personal control, verbal and nonverbal engagement skills, and learn when and how to intervene while ensuring a safe environment. There is a balance between autonomy and limit-setting.

Psychopharmacologic Interventions

The goal of acute pharmacologic intervention for agitated or violent behavior is to target the suspected cause of the agitation while regaining behavioral control and ensuring safety. Targeting the underlying cause reduces the likelihood of recurrent agitation even after the sedating effects of the medications have diminished. Sedation alone may frighten and/or anger the patient and does not address the underlying etiology of the problematic behavior. For example, the patient in ethanol withdrawal presenting with agitation would benefit from a benzodiazepine, whereas, an antipsychotic could be detrimental and lead to unnecessary side effects (Chap. 77).

Given that the goals of treatment are specific to the suspected etiology of agitation, the formerly used term of "chemical restraints" has fallen out of favor. Chemical restraint is defined as "chemical measures for confining a patient's bodily movements, thereby preventing injury to self or others and reducing agitation."[12] Given that aggression results from multiple etiologies, there is much debate about the specific sedative and route of administration that should be used. Overall, studies show that both benzodiazepines and antipsychotics result in rapid control of agitation and aggression.[6,14,24,28]

Haloperidol is safely used in the treatment of agitation and aggression in patients with psychoses and delirium.[1,6,14,28] It can be administered orally, intravenously, or intramuscularly. Dosing intervals range from 30 minutes to 2 hours, with a usual regimen of haloperidol 5 mg given every 30 to 60 minutes; most patients respond after one to 3 doses. Older studies indicated that the dose of haloperidol needed to achieve sedation rarely exceeded a total of 50 mg in acute management, but it is unusual that more than 20 mg is needed.[31,32] It is important to take the individual patient into consideration. For example, in elderly and/or medically compromised patients, behavioral control is often achieved at doses as little as 1 to 2 mg. During a behavioral crisis, most psychiatrists would switch to a second-generation antipsychotic such as olanzapine or add a mood stabilizer such as valproic acid rather than continue to titrate haloperidol because of escalating risks of side effects as haloperidol dose is increased (such as extrapyramidal symptoms and QT interval prolongation).

Droperidol is an older antipsychotic used in United States since the 1960s. It is widely used in Europe for treatment of acute and chronic psychoses as it has sedating properties.[25] Droperidol is rarely used as an antipsychotic in the United States. Several studies compared the use of droperidol with alternatives to treat acute agitation, and evidence overall supports its use as a first-line treatment option for acute agitation. When compared to both haloperidol and olanzapine, droperidol had comparable efficacy in sedation on first administration of medication while having a lower risk of participants needing additional sedating medications after 60 minutes.[25] Although midazolam is proven to induce adequate sedation more rapidly than droperidol, 15 versus 30 minutes, respectively, midazolam also has a significantly higher rate of needing rescue medication for sedation, when compared to droperidol, 50% versus 10%, respectively.[33] Droperidol is taken orally at doses from 5 to 20 mg every 4 to 6 hours as needed; given intramuscularly at doses up to 10 mg every 4 to 6 hours as needed; or intravenously at doses of 5 to 15 mg every 4 to 6 hours as needed[25] (Chap. 67).

Various benzodiazepines are quite effective for sedation; their use has been examined in patients with psychoses, stimulant toxicity, sedative–hypnotic and alcohol withdrawal, and postoperative agitation.[17,35] Diazepam is given intravenously (IV) 5 to 10 mg, with rapid repeat dosing titrated to desired effect. Because diazepam is poorly absorbed from intramuscular (IM) sites, its preferred route of administration is either IV or oral. Lorazepam 1 to 2 mg or midazolam 5 to 10 mg is given orally or parenterally and repeated at 15- or 30-minute intervals, respectively, until the patient is calm. Midazolam is frequently used in the emergency department because of its rapid onset of action and short duration of effect of 1 to 4 hours, but it has a significant amnestic effect. Diazepam has a rapid onset of action intravenously and has a prolonged duration of action. The disadvantage of lorazepam is its delay to effect, which limits the rapidity of clinical response.

A 2016 systematic review and meta-analysis aimed to compare the use of benzodiazepines, antipsychotics, and a combination of these 2 classes in the treatment of agitated patients in the emergency department. The investigators' aim was to determine which of these pharmacologic approaches were more effective, measured by the proportion of individuals who remain sedated at 15 to 20 minutes and the need for repeat sedation,

as well as which approaches were safer, as determined by the proportion of reported adverse events. This systematic review concluded that a larger portion of patients remained sedated with therapeutic combination (use of both benzodiazepine and antipsychotic) compared to benzodiazepines alone. Additionally, antipsychotic monotherapy and combinations both required fewer repeated administrations for sedation than benzodiazepines alone. Benzodiazepine monotherapy was also associated with a higher incidence of adverse events than the antipsychotics alone or combinations.[26] We recommend the use of antipsychotic monotherapy in the presumed agitated psychosis in those primarily calm enough to be cared for by a psychiatrist with limited likelihood of a consequential toxicologic problem, whereas toxicologists treating undifferentiated episodes of toxicity and agitation prefer midazolam, diazepam or lorazepam. When appropriate regimens of monotherapy are initiated in these two scenarios and fail, a combination of benzodiazepines and antipsychotics is reasonable.

There are multiple indications for the use of ketamine within the field of medicine, including a potential treatment for major depressive disorders, as well as use in the emergency department as sedation for procedures and for intubation. Ketamine is an antagonist of the glutamate N-methyl-D-aspartate (NMDA) receptor that is a dissociative anesthetic, which provides both analgesia and amnesia.[47] There is some recent interest in the potential use of ketamine for acute agitation in the emergency department setting and in the prehospital setting.[30,40] In a retrospective cohort study, 32 cases of acute agitation in the emergency department were treated with ketamine and monitored for vital sign changes and the need for rescue sedating medications within 3 hours of ketamine administration. This study found that 62.5% of cases required additional sedating medications within 3 hours of initial ketamine administration. The authors hypothesized that the reason that the effects of ketamine on agitation were not sustained were unrelated to the underlying causes of the agitation. However, there were 8 cases where the subject received multiple doses of an antipsychotic or benzodiazepine without resolution of agitation, but on receiving a single dose of ketamine, no further medication for agitation was required for at least another 3 hours. This may indicate a unique role for ketamine as a potential alternative medication for agitation when the agitation is refractory to traditional pharmacologic interventions. In addition to examining the efficacy, this study also investigated the safety of using ketamine for agitation in the emergency department setting. Based on pre- and postadministration vital signs, there were mild increases in systolic blood pressure and heart rate but none of any clinical significance, and there were no cases of oxygen desaturation.[22] In 2017, a single-center, prospective, observational study compared the time to a defined reduction in agitation scores, rate of medication redosing, vital sign changes, and adverse events in agitated individuals in the emergency department receiving ketamine, benzodiazepines, and haloperidol, alone or in combination. This prospective study showed that the ketamine group had more patients who were no longer agitated at 5, 10, and 15 minutes after receiving medication. The ketamine group had similar rates of redosing, changes in vital signs, and adverse events compared to the benzodiazepine and haloperidol groups.[39] The findings in the 2 studies mentioned above are in stark contrast to a few studies on the prehospital administration of ketamine to treat agitation, which reported intubation rates between 39% and 63%.[11,36] In addition, a case series on prehospital use of ketamine for agitation showed that 3 of 13 patients (23%) developed hypoxia and another patient developed laryngospasm.[5] Given the conflicting and limited data on its safety in treating agitation, ketamine is not recommended as a first-line therapy to treat agitation in the emergency department setting, and physicians should use caution when using ketamine given concerns for significant adverse events which means evaluation for airway compromise and resuscitative preparedness (Chap. 83).

If a patient is agitated in the context of alcohol intoxication, we recommend antipsychotics and we suggest that benzodiazepines should be avoided because of the potential to cause additive respiratory depression. In contrast, benzodiazepines have a unique role in the treatment of agitation secondary to cocaine toxicity (Chap. 75 and Antidotes in Depth: A26). Antipsychotics, particularly low-potency antipsychotics (such as chlorpromazine), lower the seizure threshold in animals, so their use for patients with cocaine/amphetamine toxicity or alcohol/sedative–hypnotic withdrawal is not recommended.

There is special concern about sedation and respiratory depression with IM olanzapine, given that 8 fatalities were reported in the European literature when olanzapine was used in excessive dosages or combined with benzodiazepines and/or other antipsychotics. Although significant comorbidities were present in the patients who died, we now recommended against using IM olanzapine with other CNS depressants.[4] In general, concerns regarding respiratory depression mandate careful observation and monitoring of patients receiving sedation with any xenobiotic (Chap. 67).

Physical Restraint

Isolation and mechanical restraints are also used in the treatment of violent behavior. Isolation or seclusion can help to diminish environmental stimuli and thereby reduce hyperreactivity. However, a few aspects are worth mentioning: Because seclusion is defined by a condition of very limited interactive and environmental cues, it is not indicated for patients with unstable medical conditions, delirium, dementia, self-injurious behavior such as cutting or head banging, or those who are experiencing extrapyramidal reactions as a consequence of antipsychotics such as an acute dystonic reaction.[15] Mechanical restraint is used to prevent patient and staff injury, although it does occasionally lead to patient and staff injury itself.[3,21] All facilities should have clear, written policy guidelines for restraint that address monitoring, documentation, and provisions for patient comfort. Frequent reassessment of the patient and documentation of the need for continued restraint are essential and should be performed according to state law. However recommendations are that patients be constantly observed while being physically restrained or in seclusion. Attention is necessary to assess excessive restraint and excessive straining which may lead to sudden cardiac death.

See Tables SC4–1 and SC4–2 for violence warning signs and the S.A.F.E.S.T. Approach.

In conclusion, aggressive and violent behaviors are commonplace in the health care setting, with particularly high incidence of violence toward nursing assistants and nurses, and within the emergency department settings and inpatient psychiatric wards. Some aggressive behavior is attributable to the direct pharmacologic effects of xenobiotics, but probably represents only a modest fraction. Substance use is often implicated in violent behavior in the community, it can occur as a coincidental part of the lifestyle of violent individuals, and both substance use and violence are related to common underlying characteristics such as a personality disorder.

SUMMARY

Some ways of mitigating environmental risk factors in the hospital setting include:

- metal detectors and screening patients for weapons,
- ensuring adequate staff to patient ratios,
- early identification of potentially violent patients,
- ensure that staff and patient care are not compromised by overcrowding.
- workplace violence policy and prevention program,
- regular training in preventive measures, and
- violence prevention program and a designated "behavioral crisis response team."

TABLE SC4–1	Violence Warning Signs
Agitated movements	
Body posturing, rapid/shallow breathing	
Clenched fists	
Loud vocalizations	
Pacing	
Staring	
Striking at inanimate objects	
Threatening statements	

TABLE SC4–2	S.A.F.E.S.T. Approach
Spacing	Maintain a safe distance
	Allow both patient and you to have equal access to the door (but you should be closest)
	Do not touch the patient
Appearance	Maintain empathetic and professional detachment
	Use one primary person to build rapport
	Have security available as a show of strength
Focus	Watch the patient's hands
	Look for potential weapons
	Watch for escalating agitation
Exchange	Attempt to de-escalate by use of calm/continuous talking
	Avoid punitive or judgmental statements
	Use good listening skills
	Elicit patient cooperation by targeting the current problem
Stabilization	By the least restrictive and most appropriate approach(s) possible:
	Physical restraints
	Sedation (benzodiazepines)
	Antipsychotics
Treatment	Treat underlying cause
	May need to treat involuntarily

Data from FitzGerald D: S.A.F.E.S.T. Approach. *Tactical Intervention Guided Emergency Response (TIGER) Textbook*; 2003.

REFERENCES

1. Adams F. Neuropsychiatric evaluation and treatment of delirium in the critically ill cancer patient. *Cancer Bull.* 1984;36:156-160.
2. Anderson CA. Temperature and aggression: ubiquitous effects of heat on occurrence of human violence. *Psychol Bull.* 1989;106:74-96.
3. Bak J, et al. Mechanical restraint—which interventions prevent episodes of mechanical restraint?- a systematic review. *Perspect Psychiatr Care.* 2012;48:83-94.
4. Battaglia J. Pharmacological management of acute agitation. *Drugs.* 2005;65:1207-1222.
5. Burnett AM, et al. The emergency department experience with prehospital ketamine: a case series of 13 patients. *Prehosp Emerg Care.* 2012;16:553-559.
6. Carter G, et al. Repeated self-poisoning: increasing severity of self-harm as a predictor of subsequent suicide. *Br J Psychiatry.* 2005;186:253-257.
7. Centers for Disease Control and Prevention. Suicide in the United States. 2013.
8. Chermack ST, et al. Treatment needs of men and women with violence problems in substance use disorder treatment. *Subst Use Misuse.* 2009;44:1236-1262.
9. Clinton JE, et al. Haloperidol for sedation of disruptive emergency patients. *Ann Emerg Med.* 1987;16:319-322.
10. Coldwell JB, Naismith LJ. Violent incidents in special hospitals. *Br J Psychiatry.* 1989;154:270.
11. Cole JB, et al. A prospective study of ketamine versus haloperidol for severe prehospital agitation. *Clin Toxicol (Phila).* 2016;54:556-562.
12. De Fruyt J, Demyttenaere K. Rapid tranquilization: new approaches in the emergency treatment of behavioral disturbances. *Eur Psychiatry.* 2004;19:243-249.
13. DeLeo, et al. Self-directed violence. In: Krug EG, et al, eds. *World Report on Violence and Health.* Geneva: World Health Organization; 2002:183-212.
14. Dubin WR. Rapid tranquilization: antipsychotics or benzodiazepines? *J Clin Psychiatry.* 1988;49(suppl):5-12.
15. Dubin WR, Lion JR. Clinician Safety. Task Force Report No. 33. Washington, DC, 1992.
16. Fazel S, et al. Use of risk assessment instruments to predict violence and antisocial behaviour in 73 samples involving 24 827 people: systematic review and meta-analysis. *BMJ.* 2012;345:e4692.
17. Garza-Trevino ES, et al. Efficacy of combinations of intramuscular antipsychotics and sedative-hypnotics for control of psychotic agitation. *Am J Psychiatry.* 1989;146:1598-1601.
18. Goldfrank LR, Hoffman RS. The cardiovascular effects of cocaine. *Ann Emerg Med.* 1991;20:165-175.
19. Goldstein P. The drugs-violence nexus: a tripartite conceptual framework. *J Drug Iss.* 1986;15:493-506.
20. Gomaa AE, et al. Occupational traumatic injuries among workers in health care facilities—United States, 2012-2014. *MMWR Morb Mortal Wkly Rep.* 2015;64:405-410.

21. Hankin CS, et al. Agitation in the inpatient psychiatric setting: a review of clinical presentation, burden, and treatment. *J Psychiatr Pract.* 2011;17:170-185.

22. Hopper AB, et al. Ketamine use for acute agitation in the emergency department. *J Emerg Med.* 2015;48:712-719.

23. James A, et al. Violence and aggression in the emergency department. *Emerg Med J.* 2006;23:431-434.

24. Kessler RC, et al. Prevalence of and risk factors for lifetime suicide attempts in the National Comorbidity Survey. *Arch Gen Psychiatry.* 1999;56:617-626.

25. Khokhar MA, Rathbone J. Droperidol for psychosis-induced aggression or agitation. *Cochrane Database Syst Rev.* 2016;12:CD002830.

26. Korczak V, et al. Chemical agents for the sedation of agitated patients in the ED: a systematic review. *Am J Emerg Med.* 2016;34:2426-2431.

27. Kowalenko T, et al. Workplace violence: a survey of emergency physicians in the state of Michigan. *Ann Emerg Med.* 2005;46:142-147.

28. Lam JN, et al. The relationship between patients' gender and violence leading to staff injuries. *Psychiatr Serv.* 2000;51:1167-1170.

29. Lavoie FW, et al. Emergency department violence in United States teaching hospitals. *Ann Emerg Med.* 1988;17:1227-1233.

30. Le Cong M, et al. Ketamine sedation for patients with acute agitation and psychiatric illness requiring aeromedical retrieval. *Emerg Med J.* 2012;29:335-337.

31. Lenehan GP, et al. Use of haloperidol in the management of agitated or violent, alcohol-intoxicated patients in the emergency department: a pilot study. *J Emerg Nurs.* 1985;11:72-79.

32. Lerner Y, et al. Acute high-dose parenteral haloperidol treatment of psychosis. *Am J Psychiatry.* 1979;136:1061-1064.

33. Martel M, et al. Management of acute undifferentiated agitation in the emergency department: a randomized double-blind trial of droperidol, ziprasidone, and midazolam. *Acad Emerg Med.* 2005;12:1167-1172.

34. May DD, Grubbs LM. The extent, nature, and precipitating factors of nurse assault among three groups of registered nurses in a regional medical center. *J Emerg Nurs.* 2002;28:11-17.

35. Modell JG, et al. Inpatient clinical trial of lorazepam for the management of manic agitation. *J Clin Psychopharmacol.* 1985;5:109-113.

36. Olives TD, et al. Intubation of profoundly agitated patients treated with prehospital ketamine. *Prehosp Disaster Med.* 2016;31:593-602.

37. Phillips JP. Workplace violence against health care workers in the United States. *N Engl J Med.* 2016;374:1661-1669.

38. Rich CL, et al. San Diego suicide study. I. Young vs old subjects. *Arch Gen Psychiatry.* 1986;43:577-582.

39. Riddell J, et al. Ketamine as a first-line treatment for severely agitated emergency department patients. *Am J Emerg Med.* 2017;35:1000-1004.

40. Roberts JR, Geeting GK. Intramuscular ketamine for the rapid tranquilization of the uncontrollable, violent, and dangerous adult patient. *J Trauma.* 2001;51:1008-1010.

41. Rugala EA, Isaacs AR. Workplace violence: issues in response, Critical Incident Response Group, National Center for the Analysis of Violent Crime, FBI Academy, 2003.

42. Serper M, Bergman A. *Psychotic Violence: Methods, Motives, Madness.* New York, NY: International University Press Inc; 2003.

43. Soliman AE, Reza H. Risk factors and correlates of violence among acutely ill adult psychiatric inpatients. *Psychiatr Serv.* 2001;52:75-80.

44. Stene J, et al. Workplace violence in the emergency department: giving staff the tools and support to report. *Perm J.* 2015;19:e113-e117.

45. Ten Have M, et al. The association between common mental disorders and violence: to what extent is it influenced by prior victimization, negative life events and low levels of social support? *Psychol Med.* 2014;44:1485-1498.

46. Welsh EB, et al. Situational variables related to aggression in institutional settings. *Aggression Violent Behav.* 2013;18:792-796.

47. Wolff K, Winstock AR. Ketamine: from medicine to misuse. *CNS Drugs.* 2006;20:199-218.

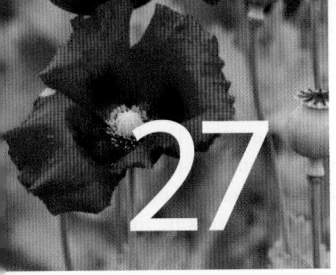

27 RENAL PRINCIPLES

Marc Ghannoum and David S. Goldfarb

ANATOMY AND BASIC PHYSIOLOGY

The kidneys lie in the paravertebral grooves at the level of the T12 to L3 vertebrae. The medial margin of each is concave, whereas the lateral margins are convex, giving the organ a bean-shaped appearance. In the adult, each kidney measures 10 to 12 cm in length, 5 to 7.5 cm in width, and 2.5 to 3.0 cm in thickness. In an adult man, each kidney weighs 125 to 170 g; in an adult woman, each kidney weighs 115 to 155 g.

On the medial surface of the kidney is the hilum, through which the renal artery, vein, renal pelvis, a nerve plexus, and lymphatics pass. On the convex surface, the kidney is surrounded by a fibrous capsule, which protects it, and a fatty capsule with a fibroareolar capsule called the *renal fascia*, which offers further protection and serves to anchor it in place.

The arterial supply begins with the renal arteries, which are direct branches of the aorta. On entering the hilum, the arteries subdivide into branches supplying the 5 major segments of each kidney: the apical pole, the anterosuperior segment, the anteroinferior segment, the posterior segment, and the inferior pole. These arteries subsequently divide within each segment to become lobar arteries. In turn, these vessels give rise to arcuate arteries that diverge into the sharply branching interlobular arteries, and then the afferent arterioles that directly supply the glomerular capillary tufts. The capillaries are then drained by the efferent arterioles, and peritubular capillaries, which also supply the vasa recta. Eventually, all are combined into the renal veins, which empty into the inferior vena cava.

The cut surface of the kidney reveals a pale outer rim and a dark inner region corresponding to the cortex and medulla, respectively. The cortex is 1 cm thick and surrounds the base of each medullary pyramid. The medulla consists of between 8 and 18 cone-shaped areas called *medullary pyramids*; the apex of each area forms a papilla containing the ends of the collecting ducts. Urine empties from each papilla into a calyx, and the calyces join together to form the renal pelvis. Urine is drained from the pelvis into the ureters and, subsequently, into the urinary bladder.

The kidneys serve 3 major functions: (1) homeostasis of fluids, acid–base balance, and electrolytes; (2) excretion of nitrogen, as urea, and other waste products; and (3) endocrine production such as 1,25-dihydroxy vitamin D, renin, and erythropoietin.

The kidneys maintain the constancy of the extracellular fluid by creating an ultrafiltrate of the plasma that is virtually free of cells and larger macromolecules, and then processing that filtrate, reclaiming what the body needs and letting the rest escape as urine. Every 24 hours, the adult's glomeruli filter nearly 180 L of water (total body water is ~25–60 L) and 25,000 mEq of sodium (total body Na^+ content is 1,200–2,800 mEq). Under normal circumstances, the kidneys regulate salt and water excretion, depending on intake and extrarenal losses. Only approximately 1% of the filtered water and 0.5% to 1% of the filtered Na^+ are excreted.

Renal function begins with filtration of plasma at the glomerulus, a highly permeable capillary network connecting 2 arterioles in series. The relative constriction or dilation of these vessels normally controls the glomerular filtration rate (GFR). The glomerular capillaries are lined with endothelial cells, and encased by specialized epithelial cells called podocytes. The filtration barrier consists of the filtration slits, the connections between adjoining podocytes, and the glomerular basement membrane, the layers between the podocytes and endothelial cells. Under healthy circumstances, the filtration fraction—the proportion of renal plasma that is filtered into the Bowman space, the potential space surrounding the glomerular capillary tuft—is approximately 20%. Plasma water crosses the filter, along with electrolytes, small solutes such as glucose, amino acids, lactate, and urea; blood cells and most of the larger proteins, including albumin and globulins, do not typically cross the filter, although recent observations suggest that more plasma proteins, including albumin, than previously thought are filtered and reclaimed by the proximal tubule. The filtrate then enters the tubules, the serial segments of which have varying roles to metabolize, reabsorb, and secrete various solutes.

The proximal tubule performs the bulk of reabsorption, isotonically reclaiming 65% to 70% of the filtrate. It has 3 segments, called S1, S2, and S3. Distal to the proximal tubule is the hairpin turn of the thin limb of the loop of Henle, a segment important in maintaining the corticomedullary concentration gradient, which is important for urinary concentration and dilution. The thick ascending limb of the loop of Henle follows, which also influences concentration and dilution of the urine and plays an important role in the balance of Na^+, Ca^{2+}, and Mg^{2+}. The distal convoluted tubules also reabsorb Na^+ and Ca^{2+} and are joined by the connecting tubules to form the collecting ducts. These segments are relatively "tight" epithelia, allowing the establishment of gradients of solute concentration from blood to urine or vice versa. These distal segments are where the fine-tuning of excretion and reclamation of water, urea, K^+, and H^+ occurs.

Given the importance of sodium balance to maintenance of cardiac preload and cardiac output, it is reasonable to consider sodium reabsorption, which occurs to an extent in every segment, as the kidney's most important role. Sodium reabsorption in the proximal tubule occurs both via both paracellular transport and transcellular transport. The former occurs in response to hydrostatic and oncotic pressures between the peritubular capillaries and the tubule, while the latter is mediated by a Na^+–H^+ exchanger stimulated by angiotensin II. In the distal tubule, hormones such as aldosterone, and a variety of kinases, control sodium transport.

Control of water balance includes urinary dilution or urinary concentration depending on the clinical circumstance. When dilution is appropriate, the ascending limb of the loop of Henle absorbs solute without water. This action produces a dilute tubular fluid and makes the medullary interstitium hypertonic. Suppression of the antidiuretic hormone (ADH; or vasopressin) leads to disappearance of water pores called aquaporins from the collecting duct; electrolyte-free water is then excreted. When urinary concentration is appropriate, ADH stimulates the appearance of aquaporins, allowing water to move from the tubule lumen into the interstitium, to minimize loss of electrolyte-free water.

The kidneys also regulate the balance of K^+ and H^+ (which are secreted by the distal nephron under the influence of aldosterone), and Ca^{2+} and phosphate via circulating parathyroid hormone, activated vitamin D, and fibroblast growth factor 23. The tubules also are capable of secretion of many solutes, including drugs such as diuretics, uric acid, and other organic anions.

XENOBIOTICS AND THE KIDNEYS

Xenobiotics affect kidney function in various ways and, conversely, renal disease influences their pharmacokinetics, which sometimes leads to dangerous overdosing and potential toxicity. In this case, kidney failure, whether acute or chronic, reduces the clearance of xenobiotics eliminated by the kidneys. The ideal dosing of drugs such as gabapentin, digoxin, baclofen, and vancomycin must be reduced several-fold in patients with advanced kidney failure compared to those with intact kidney function. Some xenobiotics are potentially toxic in patients with kidney impairment while being relatively benign in patients with normal GFR. This is the case for gadolinium-based contrast used for magnetic resonance imaging, which carries the risk of nephrogenic systemic fibrosis.[55]

Hemodialysis or peritoneal dialysis further complicates pharmacokinetics and drug dosing; in particular, the elimination of many antimicrobials are severely altered in critically ill patients with kidney failure, whether acute or chronic. In this setting, the risk of underdosing with subsequent therapeutic failure and breakthrough resistance acquired by microorganisms occasionally surpasses that of drug accumulation. A notable example is fluconazole: the required dosage in patients undergoing continuous renal replacement therapy even surpasses the drug requirement in patients with intact kidney function.[58] For those drugs of which a substantial fraction is removed by hemodialysis, drug re-dosing after dialysis is often recommended. The use of therapeutic guides is encouraged to ensure proper drug prescription in patients with a history of kidney disease.[16]

Many xenobiotics cause or aggravate renal dysfunction. The kidneys are particularly susceptible to toxic injury for 4 reasons: (1) they receive 20% to 25% of cardiac output, yet make up less than 1% of total body mass (~300 grams in a 70 kg man), implying a relatively large exposure to circulating xenobiotics; (2) they are metabolically active, and thus vulnerable to xenobiotics that disrupt metabolism or are activated by metabolism, such as acetaminophen (APAP); (3) they remove water from the glomerular filtrate, which increases the tubular concentration of xenobiotics; and (4) the glomeruli and interstitium are susceptible to attack by the immune system. Many factors, such as renal perfusion, affect an individual's reaction to a particular nephrotoxin.[3] Clinicians should be aware of these factors so as to minimize the adverse effect of a toxic exposure.

Xenobiotics can affect any part of the nephron (Fig. 27–1), although not every type of toxic renal exposure will result in loss of GFR. The following

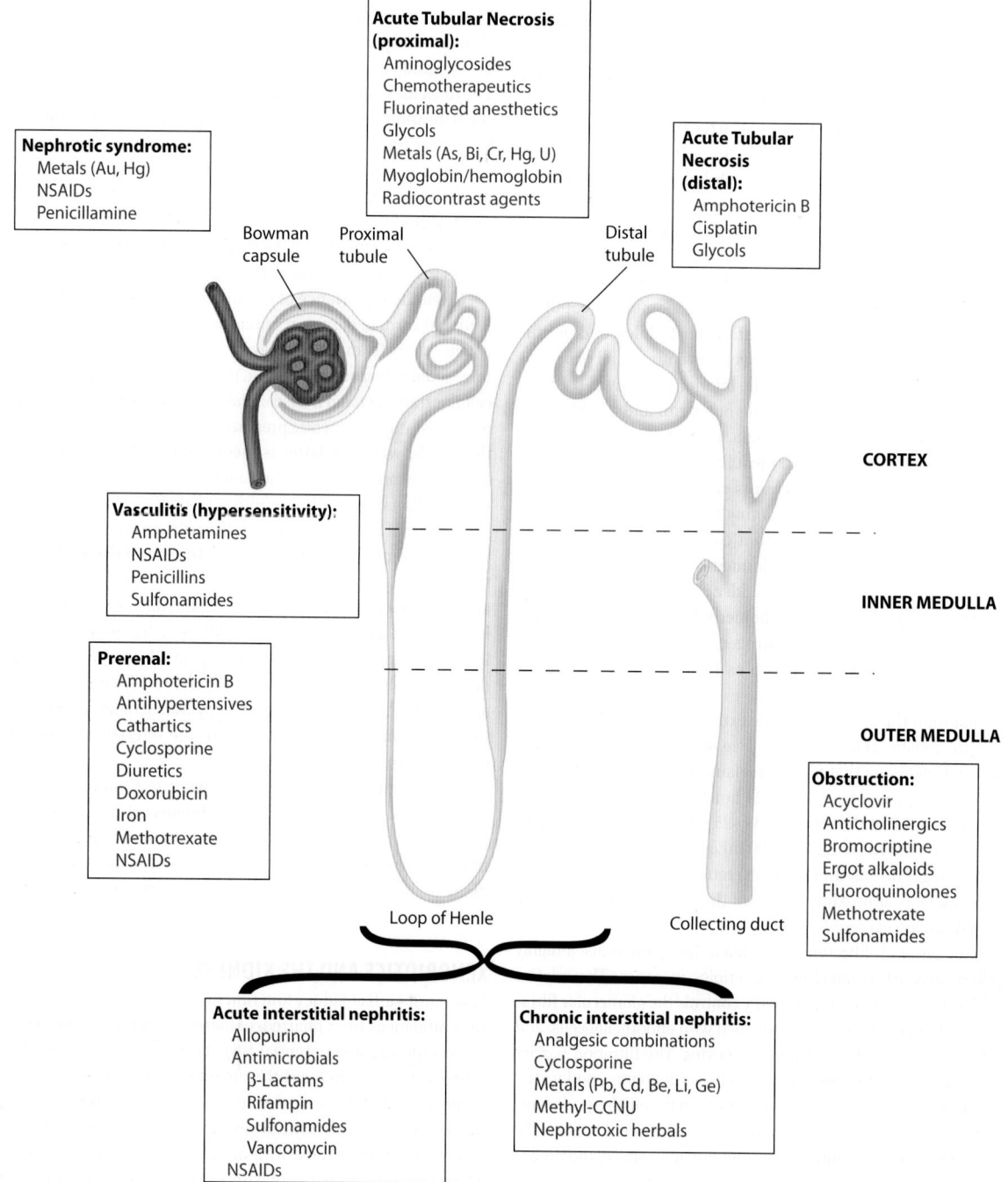

FIGURE 27–1. Schematic showing the major nephrotoxic processes and the sites on the nephron that xenobiotics chiefly affect. NSAIDs = nonsteroidal antiinflammatory drugs.

will be described: (1) acute kidney injury, (2) chronic kidney disease, and (3) functional kidney disorders.

Acute Kidney Injury

Acute kidney injury (AKI; formerly called "acute renal failure") relates to an abrupt decline in renal function that impairs the capacity of the kidney to maintain metabolic balance. Several definitions of AKI now exist, although they will likely be revised with the advent of newer and more specific biomarkers of kidney injury. The Kidney Disease: Improving Global Outcomes (KDIGO) clinical practice guidelines introduced staging criteria for AKI, based on prior work from the Acute Dialysis Quality Initiative (ADQI) and the Acute Kidney Injury Network (AKIN) (Table 27–1). The 3 traditional, main categories of AKI are prerenal, postrenal, and intrinsic AKI.

Prerenal AKI

Prerenal AKI implies impaired renal perfusion, which occurs with volume depletion, systemic vasodilation, heart failure, or preglomerular vasoconstriction. Renal hypoperfusion initiates a sequence of events leading to renal salt and water reabsorption.[3] Renin is released, causing production of angiotensin II, which enhances proximal tubular sodium reabsorption and stimulates adrenal aldosterone release, thus increasing distal sodium reabsorption. Therefore, prerenal AKI is usually accompanied by low urinary sodium excretion. Release of ADH increases water retention, manifested by a high urine osmolality. Histologically, the kidney appears normal.

Any toxic exposure that compromises renal perfusion potentially contributes to prerenal AKI, including bleeding (eg, from overdose of anticoagulants), volume depletion (diuretics, cathartics, or emetics), cardiac dysfunction (β-adrenergic antagonists), or hypotension from any cause.[53] Nonsteroidal antiinflammatory drugs (NSAIDs) lower the filtration rate by inhibiting production of vasodilatory prostaglandins in the afferent arteriole. Angiotensin-converting enzyme inhibitors (ACEIs) and angiotensin receptor blockers (ARBs) reduce the vasoconstrictive effect of angiotensin II on the efferent arteriole and can both cause prerenal AKI, especially in the setting of volume contraction. Finally, cardiotoxins, such as doxorubicin, cause severe heart failure (Fig. 27–1). Calcineurin inhibitors (cyclosporine, tacrolimus) also cause prerenal vasoconstriction by their effect on both afferent and efferent arterioles, possibly induced by endothelin. Calcineurin nephrotoxicity is

usually dose-dependent and especially occurs when trough concentrations remain supratherapeutic for an extended period of time. Nephrotoxicity is often reversible after temporary discontinuation or decrease in the calcineurin dose if identified relatively quickly.

Prerenal AKI is also caused by the hepatorenal syndrome, which is characterized by progressive renal hypoperfusion in the context of severe acute or chronic liver failure. In this setting, marked constriction of the renal arterial vasculature coexists with profound systemic and splanchnic hypotension, caused by several circulating mediators, including angiotensin, norepinephrine, vasopressin, endothelin, and isoprostane F_2.[50] That the cause of AKI is extrarenal is best illustrated by the fact that the histology of a kidney from a patient with hepatorenal syndrome is completely normal. The prognosis of the hepatorenal syndrome is entirely dependent on the recovery of liver function.

Finally, the entity known as the abdominal compartment syndrome is a potential cause of renal hypoperfusion.[9] Abdominal compartment syndrome is usually defined as new organ dysfunction induced by intraabdominal hypertension and occurs when the intraabdominal pressure exceeds 20 mm Hg, especially if sustained. The abdominal compartment syndrome is caused by several entities, but usually requires some abdominal event, especially with concomitant aggressive fluid resuscitation. Surgical decompression is life-saving in this context.

Renal AKI

Renal AKI implies intrinsic damage to the renal parenchyma, which is divided into vascular, glomerular, and tubulointerstitial etiologies.

Vascular etiologies of AKI include vasculitis, malignant hypertension, atheroemboli, scleroderma, and hemolytic-uremic syndrome or thrombotic thrombocytopenic purpura (HUS/TTP), the latter of which is sometimes associated with use of certain xenobiotics (Table 27–2).

Glomerular diseases infrequently cause acute AKI, but more commonly either a chronic or subacute decline in kidney function. Glomerular lesions either present with the nephrotic or nephritic syndrome. A nephritic pattern is associated with histological inflammation, an active urine sediment with proteinuria and hematuria, and impaired kidney function. Hypertension is common. The nephrotic syndrome is characterized by massive proteinuria (>3.5 g/day), hypoalbuminemia, hyperlipidemia, and pitting pedal edema that usually prompts the patient to seek medical attention. Although the relationships between these findings are not completely understood, the underlying event is injury to the glomerular barrier that normally prevents macromolecules from passing from the capillary lumen into the urinary space.

Xenobiotics induce nephrotic syndrome (Table 27–3) in 2 ways. First, they release antigens into the blood, which leads to antigen–antibody complex formation after the immune response is elicited. These complexes such as those of gold salts subsequently deposit in the glomerular basement membrane, thereby changing its properties[19] (Fig. 27–2). Second, they upset the immunoregulatory balance.

Kidney biopsy will permit identification of the characteristic pathologic pattern, which includes but is not limited to minimal glomerular change disease, membranous glomerulopathy, or focal segmental glomerulosclerosis. Hypoalbuminemia usually is worse than urinary excretion of albumin would suggest, as a result of tubular metabolism of filtered protein. The tubules also retain sodium, causing expansion of the extracellular space and edema.

TABLE 27–1	Kidney Disease Improving: Global Outcomes (KDIGO) Staging Criteria of Acute Kidney Injury (AKI)
Stage 1	Creatinine of 1.5–1.9 times baseline OR ≥0.3 mg/dL (≥26.5 μmol/L) increase in the serum creatinine OR Urine output <0.5 mL/kg/h for 6–12 hours
Stage 2	Creatinine of 2.0–2.9 times baseline increase in the serum creatinine OR Urine output <0.5 mL/kg/h for ≥12 hours
Stage 3	Creatinine of 3.0 times baseline increase in the serum creatinine OR Increase in serum creatinine to ≥4.0 mg/dL (≥353.6 μmol/L) OR Urine output of <0.3 mL/kg/h for ≥ 24 hours OR Anuria for ≥12 hours OR Initiation of renal replacement therapy OR In patients <18 years, decrease in estimated GFR to <35 mL/min per 1.73 m²

TABLE 27–2	Xenobiotics Most Commonly Causing Thrombotic Microangiopathy
Calcineurins inhibitors (cyclosporine, tacrolimus)	Prasugrel
Cisplatin	Quinine
Clopidogrel	Ticagrelor
Gemcitabine	Ticlopidine
Mitomycin C	

TABLE 27–3	Xenobiotics Most Commonly Causing Nephrotic Syndrome
Anabolic steroids	
Antimicrobials (cefixime, rifampicin)	
Captopril	
Chemotherapeutics (bevacizumab, sunitinib, sorafenib)	
Drugs of abuse (heroin, cocaine)	
Insect venom	
Interferon α	
Metals (Au, Hg, Li)	
Nonsteroidal antiinflammatory drugs	
Pamidronate	
Penicillamine	
Probenecid	
Sirolimus	

TABLE 27–4	Xenobiotics Most Commonly Causing Acute Tubular Necrosis
Acetaminophen	
Aluminum phosphide	
Antibacterials (aminoglycosides, ciprofloxacin, levofloxacin, colistin)	
Antifungals (amphotericin B, pentamidine)	
Antivirals (acyclovir, foscarnet, ritonavir, tenofovir, cidofovir, adefovir)	
Chemotherapeutics (cisplatin, ifosfamide, mithramycin, streptozotocin)	
Deferoxamine	
Etidronate	
Grass carp gallbladder	
Halothane	
Metals (As, Bi, Cr, Hg, U)	
Mushrooms (*Amanita* {especially *A. smithiana*}), *Cortinarius* spp)	
Non-protein colloids (mannitol, hydroxyethyl starches, dextran)	
Paraquat, diquat	
Radiocontrast agents (iodinated contrast, gadolinium)	

The glomerular lesion will progress to end-stage renal disease (ESRD) if the pathologic process continues.

The major causes of acute tubulointerstitial diseases include acute tubular necrosis (ATN), acute interstitial nephritis (AIN), and tumor lysis syndrome. Although there is controversy about how a tubular lesion leads to glomerular shutdown, it is generally felt that tubular obstruction, back-leak of filtrate across injured epithelium, renal hypoperfusion, and decreased glomerular filtering surface combine to impair glomerular filtration.[5,60] Additionally, filtration pressure is diminished by neutrophil infiltration into the interstitium and vasa recta. Evidence also suggests that prolonged medullary ischemia, perhaps caused by an imbalance in the production of vasoconstrictors such as endothelin and vasodilators such as nitric oxide, is important in prolonging the renal dysfunction after the tubular injury develops.[32]

Acute tubular necrosis is the most common cause of AKI in hospitalized patients (Table 27–4). Acute tubular necrosis is manifested pathologically by patchy necrosis of the tubular epithelium and occlusion of the lumen by casts and cellular debris (Fig. 27–3). Clinically, ATN presents as a rapid deterioration of kidney function. Muddy brown casts or renal tubular cells are typically seen in the urinary sediment, but hematuria and leukocyturia are unusual. Disorders of metabolic balance, such as hyperkalemia and metabolic acidosis, are also common. The abrupt fall in GFR usually leads to positive sodium and water balance.[39]

Acute tubular necrosis occurs following an ischemic or toxic injury.[5,46,60] Direct toxicity accounts for approximately 35% of all cases of ATN. Xenobiotics affect different segments of the renal tubules; for example, uranium and other heavy metals react with the proximal tubule and amphotericin the distal tubule (Fig. 27–1).[49] Certain xenobiotics cause a sudden or progressive decrease in GFR with concomitant prominent tubular wasting for electrolytes, though mechanisms of injury vary; this is the case of ifosfamide,[20] amphotericin B,[49] aminoglycosides,[48] pentamidine,[37] and cisplatin.[11] Poisoning also leads to ischemic tubular necrosis if hypotension or cardiac failure causes prolonged ischemia of nephron segments (proximal straight tubule and inner medullary collecting duct) that are particularly vulnerable to hypoxia. Patients who receive significant amounts of certain colloids (specifically mannitol, dextran, or hydroxyethyl starch)[13] occasionally develop AKI, characterized by tubular vacuolization or "osmotic nephrosis." Iodinated contrast causes AKI by mediating medullary vasoconstriction and inducing reactive oxygen species in tubules, despite recent studies questioning

FIGURE 27–2. Membranous glomerulonephropathy (secondary to gold), a cause of nephrotic syndrome. Globally thickened glomerular capillaries (✓) and interstitial foam cells (↗) are seen. Hematoxylin and eosin stain, ×450. *(Used with permission from Dr. Rabia Mir.)*

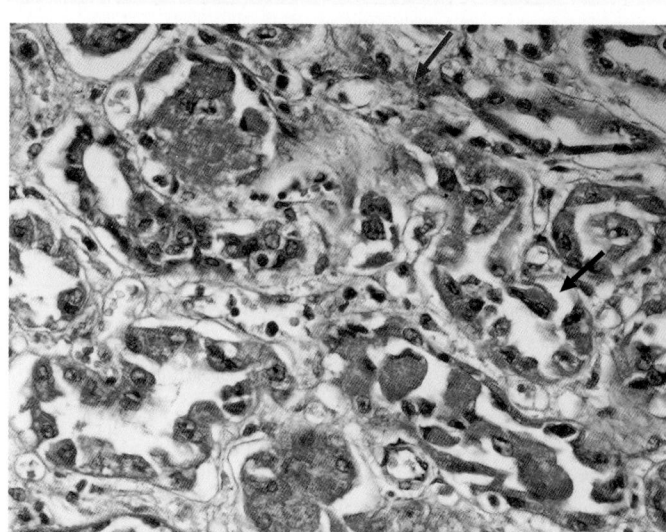

FIGURE 27–3. Acute tubular necrosis (secondary to mercury). Proximal tubular epithelial necrosis (✓) and sloughing are associated with interstitial edema (↗). Hematoxylin and eosin stain, ×450. *(Used with permission from Dr. Rabia Mir.)*

TABLE 27–5 Xenobiotics Most Commonly Causing Rhabdomyolysis

Alcohol
Antipsychotics
Carbon monoxide
Colchicine
Doxylamine
Drugs of abuse (heroin, cocaine, amphetamines, D-lysergic acid diethylamide, phencyclidine, synthetic cannabinoids)
HMG Co-A inhibitors (especially when prescribed with fibrates)
Monoclonal antibodies (rituximab, adalimumab)
Mushroom: *Tricholoma equestre*
Selective serotonin reuptake inhibitors
Snake and insect venoms
Xenobiotics causing hypokalemia or hypophosphatemia
Xenobiotics causing prolonged central nervous system depression (immobilization) or seizures
Zidovudine

TABLE 27–6 Differentiation Between Prerenal Acute Kidney Injury and Acute Tubular Necrosis

	Prerenal Acute Kidney Injury	Acute Tubular Necrosis
Fractional excretion of sodium (FE$_{Na}$)	<1%	>2%
Fractional excretion of urea (FE$_{Urea}$)	<35%	>50%
Serum urea/creatinine	>20	10–15
Urine osmolality	>400 mOsm/kg H$_2$O	Equivalent to plasma (*isosthenuric*)
Urine sodium	<20 mEq/L	>40 mEq/L
Urine sediment	Bland	Muddy "dirty" brown casts

the existence of this phenomenon. Whatever the clinical pattern of rapidly declining renal function, all forms of ATN usually present with oliguria, aside from toxicity to aminoglycosides that can present as non-oliguric ATN.[7]

Pigmenturia (myoglobinuria following rhabdomyolysis or hemoglobinuria from massive hemolysis) is another cause of tubular injury and necrosis by precipitating in the tubular lumen.[5,59] Myoglobin is normally excreted without causing toxicity. A study of patients with rhabdomyolysis suggests that the concentration of myoglobin in the urine affects the development of AKI.[59] If myoglobin inspissates in the tubular lumen because of renal hypoperfusion and high urinary concentration, it dissociates in the relatively acidic environment as H$^+$ is secreted, releasing tubulotoxic hematin. This toxicity stems from the iron-catalyzing production of oxygen free radicals.

Rhabdomyolysis is most often caused by direct muscle injury following trauma or prolonged immobilization (Table 27–5). Any poisoning causing extended unconsciousness (eg, opioids and sedative–hypnotics), hyperthermia (neuroleptic malignant syndrome), excessive muscle contraction (cocaine, amphetamines),[14,41] or tonic–clonic seizures (alcohol withdrawal, theophylline, isoniazid) may lead to muscle breakdown.[6] Other xenobiotics are directly myotoxic in some individuals, such as alcohol,[27] β-hydroxy-β-methylglutaryl coenzyme A (HMG-CoA) reductase inhibitors (statins),[23] carbon monoxide, copper sulfate, and zinc phosphate.[36,57] Rhabdomyolysis can also occur after extensive bee or wasp stings[26] or fire ant bites.[29] Hypokalemia and hypophosphatemia (eg, following diuretics and laxatives abuse) can also induce rhabdomyolysis. Synthetic cannabinoids are associated with an atypical form of acute kidney injury, sometimes accompanied by rhabdomyolysis.[8,41]

Hemoglobinuria follows hemolysis, which is caused by a number of xenobiotics, including snake and spider venoms, cresol, dapsone, phenol, aniline, arsine, stibine, naphthalene, dichromate, and methylene chloride. Sensitivity reactions to drugs (hydralazine, quinine) can also cause hemolysis.[28] The pathophysiology of hemoglobinuric ATN resembles that of myoglobinuria. The pigment deposits in the tubules and dissociates, causing necrosis to occur.[6] Volume depletion and acidosis precipitate the disorder; therefore, volume expansion and alkalinization help prevent kidney injury.

Differentiation of ATN from prerenal AKI is often clinically difficult, especially in critically ill patients; Table 27–6 illustrates empiric criteria to separate them, although there are numerous exceptions to these. These exceptions should always be correlated with clinical status. For example, fractional sodium excretion (the proportion of filtered sodium that appears in the urine, FE$_{Na}$) can be paradoxically high in prerenal AKI associated with metabolic alkalosis, diuretics, or adrenal insufficiency (Table 27–7), and in patients with chronic kidney disease. FE$_{Na}$ can also be low in renal AKI secondary to rhabdomyolysis or contrast-induced AKI.[39] Furthermore,

distinction between both entities is difficult when there is exposure to xenobiotics capable of affecting the kidneys in various ways. Nonsteroidal antiinflammatory drugs, for example, can cause prerenal AKI, ATN, acute interstitial nephritis, analgesic nephropathy, or membranous nephropathy.

The other major tubulointerstitial cause of AKI is AIN (Table 27–8), which is characteristically distinguished from ATN by a dense cellular infiltrate separating tubular structures on renal biopsy (Fig. 27–4). Nearly all cases of acute interstitial nephritis are caused by hypersensitivity.[38,47] Commonly implicated xenobiotics are antibiotics, proton-pump inhibitors, and NSAIDs. The diagnosis may be clear and kidney biopsy not necessary if kidney failure follows exposure to culpable xenobiotics and is accompanied by classic manifestations of systemic allergy such as fever, rash, or eosinophilia, although only 10% of patients typically present with this classic triad.[43] Flank pain or arthralgia may also be present. Unlike those with ATN, many patients with AIN have hematuria and

TABLE 27–7 Calculations

Fractional Na$^+$ excretion (FE$_{Na}$) = $\dfrac{([Na^+]_{urine}/[Na^+]_{plasma}) \times 100}{([Creat]_{urine}/[Creat]_{plasma})}$

Fractional Urea excretion (FE$_{Urea}$) = $\dfrac{([Urea]_{urine}/[Urea]_{plasma}) \times 100}{([Creat]_{urine}/[Creat]_{plasma})}$

Creatinine clearance (by urine collection) = $\dfrac{([Creat]_{urine} \times urine\ flow)}{([Creat]_{plasma})}$

Cockroft-Gault formula

Estimated creatinine clearance = $\dfrac{(140 - age) \times ideal\ body\ weight}{(72 \times [Creat]_{plasma})(\times 0.85\ if\ female)}$

MDRD formula

Estimated glomerular filtration rate = $\dfrac{186 \times [Creat]_{plasma}^{-1.154} \times Age^{-0.203}}{(\times 0.74\ if\ female) \times (1.21\ if\ African\ American)}$

CKD-EPI formula:
Estimated glomerular filtration rate = $141 \times min(Scr/\kappa, 1)^\alpha \times max(Scr/\kappa, 1)^{-1.209} \times 0.993^{Age} \times 1.018$ [if female], 1.159 [if black], where Scr is serum creatinine, κ is 0.7 for females and 0.9 for males, α is −0.329 for females and −0.411 for males, min indicates the minimum of Scr/κ or 1, and max indicates the maximum of Scr/κ or 1. In this table, the multiplication factors for race and sex are incorporated into the intercept, which results in different intercepts for age and sex combinations.[33]

Units: urine flow (mL/min), creatinine concentration (mg/dL), weight (kg), age (years). N.B. these formulae are only applicable in a steady state (ie, if renal function is stable). MDRD = Modification of Diet in Renal Disease.

TABLE 27–8	Xenobiotics Most Commonly Causing Acute Interstitial Nephritis

Allopurinol
Antiepileptics (carbamazepine, phenobarbital, phenytoin)
Antimicrobials (β-lactams, especially methicillin and cloxacillin, fluoroquinolones, sulfonamides, vancomycin, rifampin, nitrofurantoin, aminoglycosides, tetracyclines, colistin)
Azathioprine
Chinese herbs (*Stephania tetrandra, Magnolia officinalis*)
Diuretics (furosemide, thiazides)
H₁-antagonists (cimetidine, ranitidine)
Nonsteroidal antiinflammatory drugs (including selective cyclooxygenase-2 inhibitors)
Proton-pump inhibitors
Sulfinpyrazone
Zoledronate

TABLE 27–9	Xenobiotics Most Commonly Causing Postrenal Acute Kidney Injury

Bladder Dysfunction	Crystals	Retroperitoneal Fibrosis
Anticholinergics (antihistamines, atropine, cyclic antidepressants, scopolamine)	Acyclovir	β-Adrenergic antagonists
	Antiretroviral (indinavir, nelfinavir, -saquinavir, atazanavir)	Bromocriptine
Antipsychotics (butyrophenones, phenothiazines)	Ciprofloxacin	Herbals (*Stephania* spp, *Aristolochia* spp)
	Diethylene glycol	Hydralazine
Bromocriptine	Ethylene glycol	Methyldopa
Central nervous system depressants	Fluorinated anesthetics	Methysergide
	Fluoroquinolones	Pergolide
	Hemoglobin, myoglobin	
	Melamine	
	Methotrexate	
	Phenylbutazone	
	Sulfonamides	
	Vitamin C	

leukocyturia,[45] and sometimes eosinophiluria; however these tests have limited diagnostic utility.[43] The development of AIN is not dose-dependent and usually improves after cessation of the offending xenobiotic, although corticosteroids hasten recovery in severe cases.[15]

Tumor lysis syndrome also affects the tubulointerstitium and usually occurs following chemotherapy for large bulky lymphoproliferative, but not solid, tumors.[40] The incidence of tumor lysis has decreased with better pretherapeutic hydration and premedication with allopurinol or rasburicase.

Postrenal AKI

Postrenal AKI implies obstruction of urine flow anywhere from the renal pelvis to the urethra. An inclusive definition could classify obstruction of tubules due to crystals as postrenal AKI as well. Regardless of the cause of urinary tract obstruction, there are characteristic histologic and pathophysiologic alterations in the kidney: tubular dilation, predominantly in the distal tubule and collecting ducts, occurs initially and glomerular structure is preserved; subsequently dilation of the Bowman space occurs, and finally periglomerular fibrosis develops. Tubular function is impaired such that concentrating ability, potassium secretory function, and urinary acidification mechanisms are all altered.[56]

Urinary tract obstruction should always be considered when the kidneys fail rapidly. Acute kidney injury due to obstruction is divided into lower tract obstruction, which occurs at the bladder outlet, or upper tract obstruction,

occurring above the ureterovesical junctions. Lower tract obstruction occurs most frequently in men due to prostatic hypertrophy or prostate cancer, and in women due to cervical or endometrial cancer. Upper tract obstruction causing AKI is less frequent as it requires obstruction of both kidneys or ureters, unless the patient has a solitary kidney. Usually there is a history of abdominal or genitourinary cancer, or of kidney stones. Sudden anuria is a classical but rare feature of obstructive nephropathy; alternating phases of oliguria and polyuria are more common. Continued production of urine in the presence of obstruction leads to distension of the urinary tract above the blockage, manifesting as hydroureter or hydronephrosis. Calyceal dilation is common. Likewise, obstruction of the bladder outlet or urethra distends the bladder.

Xenobiotics are a common cause of obstruction (Table 27–9). Most such xenobiotics do so by impairing contraction of the bladder through anticholinergic action (atropine, antidepressants). Rarely, certain xenobiotics, particularly methysergide,[54] cause retroperitoneal fibrosis and ureteral constriction. Finally, a few xenobiotics lead to crystalluria and intratubular obstruction

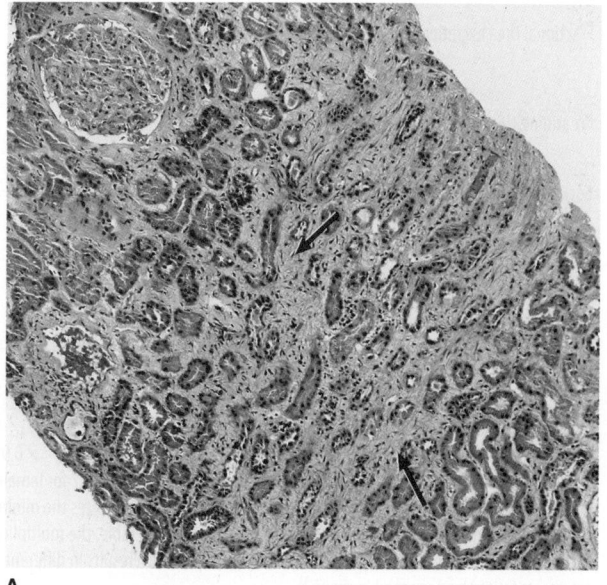
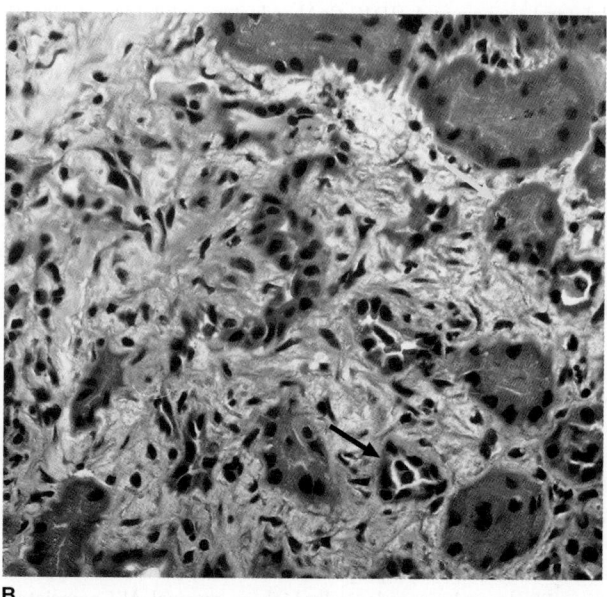

FIGURE 27–4. Acute interstitial nephritis (secondary to rifampin). Interstitial edema and patchy lymphocyte, plasma cell, and eosinophil infiltration occur without fibrosis ( ). Tubular epithelium shows degenerative and regenerative changes ( ) and mononuclear cell infiltration (tubulitis) ( ). (**A**) Hematoxylin and eosin stain × 112; (**B**) Hematoxylin and eosin stain, ×450. *(Used with permission from Dr. Rabia Mir.)*

(eg, oxalosis in ethylene glycol poisoning[35]). Sometimes the xenobiotic itself forms precipitates (sulfonamides, protease inhibitors such as atazanavir, or methotrexate).[22,44,51]

Patients who present with acutely deteriorating kidney function often represent a difficult diagnostic challenge. Not only are there 3 major etiologic categories, each category has several subdivisions; and more than one factor may be present. For example, a patient with an opioid overdose may have neurogenic hypotension (prerenal), together with muscle necrosis causing myoglobinuric AKI (intrinsic renal), and opioid-induced urinary retention (postrenal). Because renal, prerenal, and postrenal processes are not mutually exclusive and require different interventions, all 3 should always be considered, even when one appears to be the most obvious cause of the kidney failure.

Chronic Kidney Disease

Chronic kidney disease (CKD) refers to a disease process of a minimum duration of 3 months that causes a progressive decline of renal function. There is usually a gradual rise in blood urea nitrogen (BUN) and serum creatinine concentration as the GFR falls; unless advanced, there are often no clinical manifestations other than hypertension and nocturia (indicating loss of urinary concentrating ability). Classification of various stages of CKD, presently endorsed by KDIGO, is presented in Table 27–10.

Throughout the world, most cases of CKD are caused by diabetes, hypertension, or glomerulonephritis. Nevertheless, many xenobiotics are implicated as nephrotoxins in long-term exposures. The most common lesion of nephrotoxic CKD is chronic interstitial nephritis (Fig. 27–5), which involves destruction of tubules over a prolonged period,[12] with tubular atrophy, fibrosis, and a variable cellular infiltrate (Fig. 27–5), sometimes accompanied by papillary necrosis. This process then leads to ureteral colic via papillary sloughing. Acute interstitial nephritis progresses to chronic interstitial nephritis, if exposure is prolonged.[41] Analgesic nephropathy was a common etiology of CKD until certain analgesics (such as phenacetin) were discontinued.[36] Chronic interstitial nephritis presents with mild to moderate proteinuria that remains well under the nephrotic range. Unlike other chronic renal disorders, it is characterized by failure of the diseased tubules to adapt to the renal impairment, resulting in metabolic imbalances such as hyperchloremic metabolic acidosis, sodium wasting, and hyperkalemia early in the disease course.[10] Anemia is frequently observed.

Tenofovir, used in the treatment of HIV and hepatitis B, is associated with AKI with a risk of progressive CKD, attributed to mitochondrial DNA depletion and dysfunction of oxidative phosphorylation dysfunction.[42] The development of a tenofovir prodrug, tenofovir alafenamide, or TAF, achieves a higher intracellular concentration of the active metabolite tenofovir-diphosphate in the relevant immune cells. A much lower dose and lower plasma concentrations are required, and the prodrug fails to enter proximal

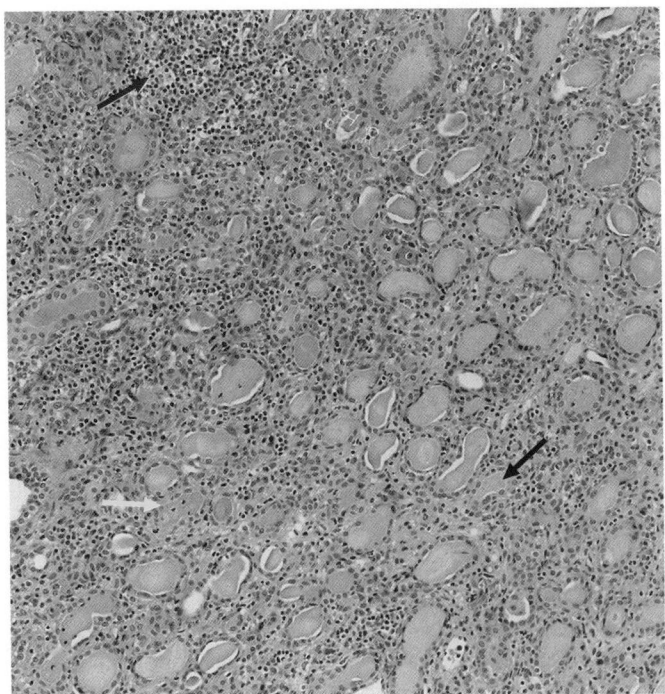

FIGURE 27–5. Chronic interstitial nephritis (secondary to NSAIDs). Interstitial fibrosis (—), lymphocytic infiltration (↗), and tubular atrophy (↙). Hematoxylin and eosin stain, ×225. *(Used with permission from Dr. Rabia Mir.)*

tubule cells. These properties of the prodrug offer the potential for important renal sparing benefit.[1]

Functional Toxic Renal Disorders

Although most toxic renal injury results in decreased renal function, certain functional disorders upset systemic balance despite normal GFR in anatomically normal kidneys. Three examples are presented here: renal tubular acidosis (RTA), syndrome of inappropriate secretion of ADH (SIADH), and diabetes insipidus (DI).

Renal tubular acidosis is a loss of ability to reclaim the filtered bicarbonate (proximal type 2 RTA) or a decreased ability to secrete protons and generate new bicarbonate to replace that lost in buffering the daily acid load (distal type I RTA). In either case, there is a non-anion gap hyperchloremic metabolic acidosis (Chap. 12).[31]

The primary defect in distal RTA (also called type 1 RTA) involves the decreased secretion of protons (H[+]) from the intercalated cells of the distal tubule. This results most frequently from a defect in the H[+]-translocating adenosine triphosphatase (ATPase) on the luminal surface of these cells. Less frequently occurring mechanisms include abnormalities of the chloride–bicarbonate exchanger, which is responsible for returning bicarbonate generated within the cell to the systemic circulation.[31] Amphotericin B and some analgesics cause a distal RTA by allowing secreted H[+] to leak back into the tubular cells.[49]

The primary defect in proximal type 2 RTA is variable and impairs reabsorption of sodium bicarbonate. Normally, the Na[+]-H[+] exchanger in the luminal membrane (NHE3), the Na[+],K[+]-ATPase in the basolateral membrane, and the enzyme carbonic anhydrase are the key systems necessary for proximal tubular bicarbonate reabsorption. Exit of sodium bicarbonate at the basolateral membrane requires the sodium-bicarbonate cotransporter NBC. If one or more of these mechanisms becomes disordered, then the resorptive capacity of the proximal tubule is diminished. Proximal RTA often occurs as part of the Fanconi syndrome, a generalized failure of proximal tubular transport (proximal RTA plus amino-aciduria, glycosuria, and hyperphosphaturia). Xenobiotics associated with type 2 RTA include aminoglycosides, lead, ifosfamide, mercury, and carbonic anhydrase inhibitors such as acetazolamide.[21]

Stage	GFR	Description
TABLE 27–10		**Classification of Chronic Kidney Disease as Defined by the Kidney Disease Outcomes Quality Initiative and Modified and Endorsed by the Kidney Disease: Improving Global Outcomes**
1	≥90	Any kidney damage with normal or ↑ in GFR
2	60–89	Kidney damage with mild ↓ in GFR
3a	45–59	Mild to moderate ↓ in GFR
3b	30–44	Moderate to severe ↓ in GFR
4	15–29	Severe ↓ in GFR
5	<15 or on dialysis	Kidney failure

GFR = glomerular filtration rate, determined by the 2009 CKD-EPI creatinine equation.

Reproduced with permission from Eckardt KU, Berns JS, Rocco MV, Kasiske BL. Definition and classification of CKD: the debate should be about patient prognosis--a position statement from KDOQI and KDIGO. *Am J Kidney Dis.* 2009;June;53(6):915-920.

What was once known as type 3 RTA is recognized to be a combination of features of both distal and proximal RTA and affects infants as part of an autosomal recessive syndrome. Carbonic anhydrase inhibitors affect the enzyme in both the proximal and distal tubules. Type 4 RTA is caused by a deficiency of aldosterone or by tubular resistance to its action. It most often occurs in adult patients with both diabetes and CKD who have hyporeninemic hypoaldosteronism. Hyperkalemia is the most prominent electrolyte disturbance while the metabolic acidosis, attributed to the ability of K^+ to inhibit glutaminase, the rate-limiting step of ammoniagenesis, is usually mild. The findings of Type 4 RTA most often occur as the result of treatment of hypertension and chronic kidney disease with angiotensin converting enzyme inhibitors, angiotensin receptor blockers, and mineralocorticoid receptor antagonists.[18] Nonsteroidal antiinflammatory drugs often cause hyperkalemia with or without metabolic acidosis through similar mechanisms.[25]

The syndrome of inappropriate secretion of ADH occurs when the posterior pituitary gland or abnormal, unregulated sources such as malignancies secrete ADH despite the absence of physiologic conditions that normally stimulate ADH secretion.[17] The usual stimulus for ADH release in normal, daily physiology is elevated plasma osmolality as the result of a temporary decreased availability of electrolyte-free water. The ADH release occurs as well despite normal serum osmolality when pathologic contraction of the effective arterial blood volume occurs (eg, volume depletion, congestive heart failure, cirrhosis). Antidiuretic hormone primarily affects the collecting tubule and causes increased water reabsorption by increasing the water permeability of the collecting duct by causing movement of aquaporins from intracellular lysosomes to the apical membranes. This effect of ADH leads to the main clinical manifestations of SIADH, namely, hyponatremia in the setting of euvolemia, accompanied by inappropriately concentrated urine (as reflected in a failure to decrease urine osmolality to 50–100 mOsm/kg). Although this manifestation most often occurs as a complication of intracranial lesions or from ectopic ADH production by a tumor or a diseased lung, many xenobiotics (eg, carbamazepine, chlorpropamide, antidepressants, vincristine, opioids, methylenedioxymethamphetamine {MDMA}) can also cause inappropriate ADH release (Chap. 12).

Diabetes insipidus (DI) is the inability of the kidneys to maximally concentrate the urine and retain water leading to inappropriate loss of urine. Its 2 causes are the absence of pituitary ADH secretion (central DI) or the absence of an appropriate renal response to ADH stimulation (nephrogenic DI).[4] Diabetes insipidus typically presents with polyuria or hypernatremia if water intake is limited in the presence of inappropriately dilute urine. Central DI can be due to autoimmune destruction of the pituitary or trauma but often is the result of a space-occupying lesion affecting the posterior pituitary. Nephrogenic diabetes insipidus (NDI) is caused by a variety of factors, including genetic disorders, kidney failure, disease states, or electrolyte perturbations, but xenobiotics are often implicated. Lithium, demeclocycline, foscarnet, and clozapine are drugs that can cause this syndrome (Chap. 12). Nephrogenic DI from lithium exposure is thought to result from impaired aquaporin-2 synthesis and transport despite normal ADH binding to vasopressin type 2 receptors at the basolateral membranes of the collecting ducts.[4]

PATIENT EVALUATION

Evaluation of a patient with suspected toxic renal injury should include consideration of extrarenal as well as renal factors. The response of the kidney to xenobiotics is affected by baseline renal function, renal blood flow, and the presence of urinary tract obstruction, all of which must be evaluated.

History

A history of kidney disease or conditions that affect the kidney (eg, diabetes, hypertension, cardiovascular disease, kidney stones, urinary tract infection, prior chemotherapy) should be noted. Pertinent family history of kidney disease, glomerulopathy, kidney stones, and polycystic kidney disease needs to be recorded. Flank pain, hematuria, urine discoloration, or an abnormal pattern of urine output are important findings. Acute loss of kidney function

is often suspected if urine output decreases, although this is a late sign and not universal. The patient's intravascular volume status affects renal perfusion. Thus, a recent history of heart disease, vomiting, or diarrhea is important. Symptoms of kidney failure are usually only present when severe but include anorexia, nausea and vomiting, tachypnea, chest pain (from uremic pericarditis), leg cramps, fatigue, edema, bleeding (from uremic platelet dysfunction), and mental status changes. Systemic symptoms such as arthralgias, weight loss, and fever suggest vasculitis.

All current xenobiotics should be evaluated for potential renal effects.[52] The patient's intake of ethanol and drugs of abuse, as well as intake of natural products and medicinal herbs, should be explored. A careful occupational history and assessment of hobbies and lifestyle are crucial, with emphasis on exposure to nephrotoxic xenobiotics.

Physical Examination

The patient's hemodynamic status should be carefully assessed. Postural changes in pulse and blood pressure, and either engorgement or decreased filling of the neck veins, may provide useful information about the intravascular volume, but seldom are they sensitive or specific. The skin should be examined for lesions. Funduscopy may reveal evidence of chronic hypertension or diabetes. All aspects of cardiac function should be noted, including presence or absence of a pericardial rub and edema. New-onset bluish lesions of toes suggest recent cholesterol emboli. Injuries or scars in the suprapubic area or evidence of past urologic or retroperitoneal surgery suggest obstruction, as does a palpable or percussible bladder. Asterixis and cognitive impairment is often present in late stages of uremic encephalopathy.

Laboratory Evaluation

Although history and physical examination are essential to identify nephrotoxic injury, laboratory testing is indispensable to confirm the degree of renal dysfunction. The initial approach to a patient with renal disease usually combines both assessment of GFR and urinalysis. Both are noninvasive, inexpensive, and have considerable predictive value for patients with renal disease.

Because creatinine is freely filtered by the glomerulus and not significantly reabsorbed or metabolized in the tubule, serum creatinine concentration is used as the preeminent marker of overall kidney function; because a small proportion of total excreted creatinine in urine appears as the result of tubular secretion, creatinine clearance always overestimates GFR. As the kidneys fail, creatinine concentration increases. However, the relationship between its concentration and GFR is hyperbolic, not linear; therefore, a small initial elevation in serum concentration denotes a large decrease in kidney function. By the time the serum creatinine concentration exceeds the upper limit of normal, GFR is reduced by up to 50%. Furthermore, creatinine secretion becomes a significantly greater proportion of creatinine excretion as GFR fails. Renal hypoperfusion and prerenal states are associated with a disproportionate rise in urea in comparison with the rise in creatinine, because urea is partially reabsorbed in the proximal tubule along with salt and water.[39] However, this often-cited increase in the BUN–creatinine ratio may fail to occur in patients with chronic kidney disease, including the elderly. There are other limitations of their use as markers of renal injury; decreased production of urea (starvation or liver failure) or creatinine (amputation, muscle wasting) may result in a normal BUN or creatinine in the presence of significant renal impairment. Certain xenobiotics alter measured concentrations of urea and creatinine in the absence of any change in renal function.[12] The most obvious is exogenous creatine taken to build muscle mass. Drugs that block renal creatinine secretion, such as cimetidine and trimethoprim, also increase serum creatinine. The BUN is raised independently of renal function by corticosteroids (increased protein catabolism), and tetracycline.

Recently, more sensitive serum or urine markers of early AKI have been proposed, such as serum cystatin C, urinary kidney injury molecule-1, neutrophil gelatinase–associated lipocalin (NGAL), and N-acetyl-β-glucosaminidase. Early studies suggest they help discriminate between ATN and prerenal AKI although they are costly and unavailable in most centers.[2,10]

Renal function is best evaluated by nuclear medicine (DTPA or MAG3 nuclear scan) and inulin clearance but these tests are impractical and expensive.

In patients with stable chronic kidney disease, a more precise estimation of the glomerular filtration rate is available. All laboratories today report an estimated GFR (eGFR), which has been validated in several populations of people with chronic kidney disease (Table 27–10). Most laboratories still report an estimate derived from the Modification of Diet in Renal Disease study (MDRD), while most research reports estimates derived from the CKD-EPI formula.[33,34] Twenty-four-hour urine collections to calculate creatinine clearance are occasionally done when low or high muscle mass are suspected to cause inaccuracies in estimates of GFR. Using any of these measurements in AKI is not helpful, as the accuracy of the measurement of clearance implies a steady state. Changing GFR during a clearance time period distorts the resulting estimation. There is also a lag period between changes in kidney function and changes in BUN or creatinine concentrations. An extreme example would be a patient undergoing bilateral nephrectomy: although GFR immediately postoperatively equals 0 mL/min, the increase in serum creatinine will only be evident after a few hours. Any clearance calculation would yield an estimated GFR very different from true GFR. In general, a patient with AKI and rapidly increasing creatinine concentration should be managed as if GFR were less than 10 mL/min until serum creatinine concentration stabilizes and GFR can more accurately be estimated. Estimation of GFR is most important in prescribing drugs. Because much of the relevant pharmacology literature pre-dates the current equations used to estimate GFR, many recommendations for drug dosing are still based on the Cockcroft–Gault formula, which estimates creatinine clearance.

Most patients presenting with AKI should have their urine examined. Standard automated dipsticks will detect albumin and glucose. The presence of a positive dipstick for blood when the urine contains no or few RBCs suggests either rhabdomyolysis or hemolysis. A simple urine spot test may help discriminate prerenal azotemia from ATN (Table 27–6); this is suggested by a fractional sodium excretion below 1% and urine osmolality above 400 mOsm/kg. Direct microscopic examination of the urine sediment also provides useful clues.[24] Dysmorphic red cells suggest glomerular hematuria but are neither sensitive nor specific. If acute interstitial nephritis is a consideration, a fresh urine sample should be stained for eosinophils, though frequently these cells are absent.[43] Calcium oxalate crystalluria is suggestive of exposure to xenobiotics such as ethylene glycol and vitamin C.[30]

Measurement of postvoiding residual urine volume, preferably by suprapubic ultrasonography or by passage of a urinary catheter with complete bladder emptying, can demonstrate lower urinary tract obstruction; if the volume is in excess of 75 to 100 mL, then bladder dysfunction or obstruction should be suspected. Among the many radiologic studies used in patients with kidney diseases, renal ultrasonography is the most useful and is indicated in all patients with AKI or CKD of unknown etiology; postrenal AKI is suggested by obstruction of the urinary tree, characteristically by swelling of one or 2 kidneys (hydronephrosis).[56] Asymmetry between kidney diameters is suggestive of renal artery stenosis. Cortex thinning and a poorly differentiated corticomedullary junction are consistent with long-standing kidney failure of any etiology. When the etiology of kidney disease remains elusive, a percutaneous renal biopsy will establish the final diagnosis. Table 27–11 summarizes the diverse nephrotoxic effects of various metals.

TABLE 27–11	Nephrotoxic Effects of Metals						
	Toxic ATN	Shock ATN	Hemolysis	Acute Interstitial Nephritis	Chronic Interstitial Nephritis	Tubular Dysfunction	Nephrotic Syndrome
Antimony	+						
Arsenic	+++	+++	++	+	+		
Barium	+						
Beryllium					++		
Bismuth	++					+	+
Cadmium					+++	+++	
Chromium	+++						
Copper		+	+				
Gadolinium	+						
Germanium					+		
Gold	+						+++
Iron		++			+		
Lead	+		+		+++	+++	
Lithium	+				+++	++	+
Mercury	+++	+				+	+
Platinum	++				++	++	
Silicon							+
Silver	+						
Thallium	+			+			
Uranium	+						

+++ = common; + = uncommon. ATN = acute tubular necrosis.

The absence of a +, ++ or +++ indicates no evidence of this effect.

SUMMARY

- The kidneys act as primary defenders against harmful xenobiotics entering the bloodstream.
- The environment, the workplace, and, especially, the administration of medications represent potential sources of nephrotoxicity. Consequently, it is important to determine, by history and observation, to which xenobiotics a patient was exposed and to be aware of their potential to harm the kidneys.
- It is equally crucial to work the other way when a patient presents with renal dysfunction: review all xenobiotics, both conventional and complementary, all xenobiotic exposures, and any conditions that can adversely affect the kidneys.

REFERENCES

1. Achhra AC, et al. Chronic kidney disease and antiretroviral therapy in HIV-positive individuals: recent developments. *Curr HIV/AIDS Rep.* 2016;13:149-157.
2. Alge JL, Arthur JM. Biomarkers of AKI: a review of mechanistic relevance and potential therapeutic implications. *Clin J Am Soc Nephrol.* 2015;10:147-155.
3. Badr KF, Ichikawa I. Prerenal failure: a deleterious shift from renal compensation to decompensation. *N Engl J Med.* 1988;319:623-629.
4. Bockenhauer D, Bichet DG. Pathophysiology, diagnosis and management of nephrogenic diabetes insipidus. *Nat Rev Nephrol.* 2015;11:576-588.
5. Bonventre JV, Yang L. Cellular pathophysiology of ischemic acute kidney injury. *J Clin Invest.* 2011;121:4210-4221.
6. Bosch X, et al. Rhabdomyolysis and acute kidney injury. *N Engl J Med.* 2009;361:62-72.
7. Boyer A, et al. Aminoglycosides in septic shock: an overview, with specific consideration given to their nephrotoxic risk. *Drug Saf.* 2013;36:217-230.
8. Centers for Disease Control and Prevention. Acute kidney injury associated with synthetic cannabinoid use—multiple states, 2012. *MMWR Morb Mortal Wkly Rep.* 2013;62:93-98.
9. De Waele JJ, et al. Understanding abdominal compartment syndrome. *Intensive Care Med.* 2016;42:1068-1070.
10. Doi K, et al. Mild elevation of urinary biomarkers in prerenal acute kidney injury. *Kidney Int.* 2012;82:1114-1120.
11. dos Santos NA, et al. Cisplatin-induced nephrotoxicity and targets of nephroprotection: an update. *Arch Toxicol.* 2012;86:1233-1250.
12. Ducharme MP, et al. Drug-induced alterations in serum creatinine concentrations. *Ann Pharmacother.* 1993;27:622-633.
13. Gadallah MF, et al. Case report: mannitol nephrotoxicity syndrome: role of hemodialysis and postulate of mechanisms. *Am J Med Sci.* 1995;309:219-222.
14. Goel N, et al. Cocaine and kidney injury: a kaleidoscope of pathology. *Clin Kidney J.* 2014;7:513-517.
15. Gonzalez E, et al. Early steroid treatment improves the recovery of renal function in patients with drug-induced acute interstitial nephritis. *Kidney Int.* 2008;73:940-946.
16. Aronoff GR, et al. *Drug Prescribing in Renal Failure: Dosing Guidelines for Adults and Children.* 5th ed. Philadelphia, PA: American College of Physicians; 2007.
17. Grant P, et al. The diagnosis and management of inpatient hyponatraemia and SIADH. *Eur J Clin Invest.* 2015;45:888-894.
18. Haas CS, et al. Renal tubular acidosis type IV in hyperkalaemic patients—a fairy tale or reality? *Clin Endocrinol (Oxf).* 2013;78:706-711.
19. Hall CL. Gold nephropathy. *Nephron.* 1988;50:265-272.
20. Hanly LN, et al. *N*-Acetylcysteine as a novel prophylactic treatment for ifosfamide-induced nephrotoxicity in children: translational pharmacokinetics. *J Clin Pharmacol.* 2012;52:55-64.
21. Haque SK, et al. Proximal renal tubular acidosis: a not so rare disorder of multiple etiologies. *Nephrol Dial Transplant.* 2012;27:4273-4287.
22. Hara M, et al. Atazanavir nephrotoxicity. *Clin Kidney J.* 2015;8:137-142.
23. Hill MD, Bilbao JM. Case of the month: February 1999—54 year old man with severe muscle weakness. *Brain Pathol.* 1999;9:607-608.
24. Kanbay M, et al. Acute tubular necrosis and pre-renal acute kidney injury: utility of urine microscopy in their evaluation—a systematic review. *Int Urol Nephrol.* 2010;42:425-433.
25. Kim S, Joo KW. Electrolyte and acid-base disturbances associated with non-steroidal anti-inflammatory drugs. *Electrolyte Blood Press.* 2007;5:116-125.
26. Kim YO, et al. Severe rhabdomyolysis and acute renal failure due to multiple wasp stings. *Nephrol Dial Transplant.* 2003;18:1235.
27. Klinkerfuss G, et al. A spectrum of myopathy associated with alcoholism. II. Light and electron microscopic observations. *Ann Intern Med.* 1967;67:493-510.
28. Kojouri K, et al. Quinine-associated thrombotic thrombocytopenic purpura-hemolytic uremic syndrome: frequency, clinical features, and long-term outcomes. *Ann Intern Med.* 2001;135:1047-1051.
29. Koya S, et al. Rhabdomyolysis and acute renal failure after fire ant bites. *J Gen Intern Med.* 2007;22:145-147.
30. Kraut JA, Kurtz I. Toxic alcohol ingestions: clinical features, diagnosis, and management. *Clin J Am Soc Nephrol.* 2008;3:208-225.
31. Laing CM, Unwin RJ. Renal tubular acidosis. *J Nephrol.* 2006;19(suppl 9):S46-S52.
32. Legrand M, et al. Renal hypoxia and dysoxia after reperfusion of the ischemic kidney. *Mol Med.* 2008;14:502-516.
33. Levey AS, et al. A new equation to estimate glomerular filtration rate. *Ann Intern Med.* 2009;150:604-612.
34. Levey AS, et al. GFR estimation: from physiology to public health. *Am J Kidney Dis.* 2014;63:820-834.
35. McMartin K. Are calcium oxalate crystals involved in the mechanism of acute renal failure in ethylene glycol poisoning? *Clin Toxicol (Phila).* 2009;47:859-869.
36. Melli G, et al. Rhabdomyolysis: an evaluation of 475 hospitalized patients. *Medicine (Baltimore).* 2005;84:377-385.
37. Miller RF, et al. Acute renal failure after nebulised pentamidine. *Lancet.* 1989;1:1271-1272.
38. Nast CC. Medication-induced interstitial nephritis in the 21st century. *Adv Chronic Kidney Dis.* 2017;24:72-79.
39. Pahwa AK, Sperati CJ. Urinary fractional excretion indices in the evaluation of acute kidney injury. *J Hosp Med.* 2016;11:77-80.
40. Pearson-Stuttard B, et al. Acute kidney injury from tumour lysis syndrome and urate crystalluria. *Br J Haematol.* 2015;170:444.
41. Pendergraft WF 3rd, et al. Nephrotoxic effects of common and emerging drugs of abuse. *Clin J Am Soc Nephrol.* 2014;9:1996-2005.
42. Perazella MA. Tenofovir-induced kidney disease: an acquired renal tubular mitochondriopathy. *Kidney Int.* 2010;78:1060-1063.
43. Perazella MA, Markowitz GS. Drug-induced acute interstitial nephritis. *Nat Rev Nephrol.* 2010;6:461-470.
44. Perazella MA, Moeckel GW. Nephrotoxicity from chemotherapeutic agents: clinical manifestations, pathobiology, and prevention/therapy. *Semin Nephrol.* 2010;30:570-581.
45. Perazella MA. Clinical approach to diagnosing acute and chronic tubulointerstitial disease. *Adv Chronic Kidney Dis.* 2017;24:57-63.
46. Rabb H, et al. Inflammation in AKI: current understanding, key questions, and knowledge gaps. *J Am Soc Nephrol.* 2016;27:371-379.
47. Raghavan R, Shawar S. Mechanisms of drug-induced interstitial nephritis. *Adv Chronic Kidney Dis.* 2017;24:64-71.
48. Rybak MJ, et al. Prospective evaluation of the effect of an aminoglycoside dosing regimen on rates of observed nephrotoxicity and ototoxicity. *Antimicrob Agents Chemother.* 1999;43:1549-1555.
49. Safdar A, et al. Drug-induced nephrotoxicity caused by amphotericin B lipid complex and liposomal amphotericin B: a review and meta-analysis. *Medicine (Baltimore).* 2010;89:236-244.
50. Salerno F, et al. Diagnosis, treatment and survival of patients with hepatorenal syndrome: a survey on daily medical practice. *J Hepatol.* 2011;55:1241-1248.
51. Shrishrimal K, Wesson J. Sulfamethoxazole crystalluria. *Am J Kidney Dis.* 2011;58:492-493.
52. Singh AP, et al. Animal models of acute renal failure. *Pharmacol Rep.* 2012;64:31-44.
53. Srisawat N, et al. Modern classification of acute kidney injury. *Blood Purif.* 2010;29:300-307.
54. Stecker JF Jr, et al. Retroperitoneal fibrosis and ergot derivatives. *J Urol.* 1974;112:30-32.
55. Swaminathan S, Shah SV. New insights into nephrogenic systemic fibrosis. *J Am Soc Nephrol.* 2007;18:2636-2643.
56. Truong LD, et al. Obstructive uropathy. *Contrib Nephrol.* 2011;169:311-326.
57. Wolff E. Carbon monoxide poisoning with severe myonecrosis and acute renal failure. *Am J Emerg Med.* 1994;12:347-349.
58. Yagasaki K, et al. Pharmacokinetics and the most suitable dosing regimen of fluconazole in critically ill patients receiving continuous hemodiafiltration. *Intensive Care Med.* 2003;29:1844-1848.
59. Zager RA. Rhabdomyolysis and myohemoglobinuric acute renal failure. *Kidney Int.* 1996;49:314-326.
60. Zuk A, Bonventre JV. Acute kidney injury. *Annu Rev Med.* 2016;67:293-307.

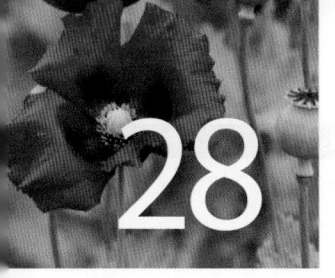

28 RESPIRATORY PRINCIPLES

Andrew Stolbach and Robert S. Hoffman

The primary function of the lungs is gas exchange. Specifically, this involves the transport of oxygen (O_2) into the blood, and the elimination of carbon dioxide (CO_2) from the blood. In addition, the lungs serve as minor organs of metabolism and elimination for a number of xenobiotics, a source of insensible water loss, and a means of temperature regulation. Air is conducted through proximal airways, made up of columnar epithelium and mucin-secreting goblet cells. Oxygen exchange occurs in distal airways, through type I pneumocytes, which make up most of alveolar surface area. Type II pneumocytes, which secrete surfactant, take up less pulmonary surface area.

Cellular oxygen use is dependent on many factors, including respiratory drive; percentage of oxygen in inspired air; airway patency; chest wall and pulmonary compliance; diffusing capacity; ventilation–perfusion mismatch; hemoglobin content; hemoglobin oxygen loading and unloading; cellular oxygen uptake; and cardiac output. Xenobiotics have the unique ability to impair each of these factors necessary for oxygen use and result in respiratory dysfunction (Table 28–1). This chapter illustrates how xenobiotics interact with the mechanisms of gas exchange and oxygen use. Discussion of chronic occupational lung injury is beyond the scope of this text; the reader is referred to a number of reviews for further information.[5]

PULMONARY MANIFESTATIONS OF XENOBIOTIC EXPOSURES

Respiratory Drive

Respiratory rate and depth are regulated by the need to maintain a normal partial pressure of carbon dioxide (PCO_2) and pH. Most of the control for ventilation occurs at the level of the medulla, although it is modulated both by involuntary input from the pons and voluntary input from the higher cortices. Changes in PCO_2 are measured primarily by a central chemoreceptor, which measures cerebralspinal fluid pH, and secondarily by peripheral chemoreceptors in the carotid and aortic bodies, which measure PCO_2. Input with regard to partial pressure of oxygen (PO_2) is obtained from carotid and aortic chemoreceptors. Stretch receptors in the chest relay information about pulmonary dynamics, such as the volume and pressure.

Xenobiotics affect respiratory drive in one of several ways: direct suppression of the respiratory center; alteration in the response of chemoreceptors to changes in PCO_2; direct stimulation of the respiratory center; increase in metabolic demands such as those resulting from agitation or fever, which, in turn, increases total body oxygen consumption; or indirectly, as a result of the creation of acid–base disorders. For example, opioids (Chap. 36) depress respiration by decreasing the responsiveness of chemoreceptors to CO_2 and by direct suppression of the pontine and medullary respiratory centers.[36,87,113] Any xenobiotic that causes a decreased respiratory drive or a decreased level of consciousness can produce bradypnea (a decreased respiratory rate), hypopnea (a decreased tidal volume), or both, resulting in absolute or relative hypoventilation (Chap. 3).

Methylxanthines and sympathomimetics increase both respiratory drive and oxygen consumption. Salicylates produce hyperventilation by both central and peripheral effects via respiratory alkalosis and metabolic acidosis. The net consequence of increased respiratory drive, increased oxygen consumption, or metabolic acidosis is the generation of tachypnea (an elevated respiratory rate), hyperpnea (an increased tidal volume), or both. Either alone or in combination, tachypnea and hyperpnea produce hyperventilation. Tables 28–2 and 28–3 both list xenobiotics that commonly produce hypoventilation and hyperventilation.

Decreased FiO$_2$

Barometric pressure at sea level ranges near 760 mm Hg. At this pressure, 21% of ambient air is composed of oxygen (the fraction of inspired oxygen {FiO_2} = 21%), and, after subtracting for the water vapor normally present in the lungs, the alveolar partial pressure of oxygen (PAO_2) is about 150 mm Hg. Any reduction in FiO_2 decreases the PAO_2, thereby producing signs and symptoms of hypoxemia (a low arterial partial pressure of oxygen {PaO_2}). At an FiO_2 of 12% to 16%, patients experience tachypnea, tachycardia, headache, mild confusion, and impaired coordination. A further decrease to an FiO_2 of 10% to 14% produces severe fatigue and cognitive impairment and when the FiO_2 decreases to between 6% and 10%, nausea, vomiting, and lethargy develop. An FiO_2 less than 6% is incompatible with life.[66]

TABLE 28–1	Respiration as a Target of Common Xenobiotics	
Location	**Mechanism of Effect**	**Common Xenobiotics**
Oxygen displacement	Simple asphyxiation	Carbon dioxide
Respiratory center	Direct stimulation	Methylxanthines
	Inhibition	Sedatives
	Indirect stimulation	Salicylates
Chest wall	Muscular weakness	Botulinum toxin
	Muscular rigidity	Fentanyl
Oropharynx	Angioedema	ACE inhibitor angioedema
	Obstruction	
Trachea	Barotrauma	Nitrous oxide (N_2O)
	Tissue destruction	Caustics
Larynx	Laryngospasm	Caustics
Bronchioles	Acute bronchospasm	Chemical irritant
	Delayed bronchospasm	Allergens
Alveoli/interstitial	Alveolar permeability (ARDS)	Smoke inhalation
	Alveolar hemorrhage	Bleomycin
	Diffuse airspace filling	Nitrogen dioxide (NO_2)
	Direct tissue destruction (primary or secondary)	Phosgene
	Fat embolism syndrome	Intravenous lipid emulsion
	Multifocal airspace filling	Intravenous drug use (septic emboli)
	Hypersensitivity pneumonitis	*Actinomycetes* spp
	Lymphocytic infiltrates or granulomas	Immune checkpoint inhibitors
	Metal pneumonitis	$ZnCl_2$ fume
	Pulmonary surfactant disruption	Hydrocarbons
	Pulmonary fibrosis	Paraquat (late)
Pulmonary vessels	Vasculitis	Levamisole
Pleura	Pleural plaque	Asbestos
Hilar lymph nodes	Calcification	Silica
	Lymphadenopathy	Phenytoin

TABLE 28–2	Xenobiotics Producing Hypoventilation
Baclofen	
Barbiturates	
Botulinum toxin	
Carbamates	
Clonidine	
Colchicine	
Conium maculatum (poison hemlock)	
Cyclic antidepressants	
Elapid venom	
Ethanol	
Ethylene glycol	
γ-Hydroxybutyrate and analogs	
Isopropanol	
Methanol	
Neuromuscular blockers	
Nicotine	
Opioids	
Organic phosphorus compounds	
Sedative–hypnotics	
Strychnine	
Tetanus toxin	
Tetrodotoxin	
Xenobiotic induced electrolyte abnormalities	

This effect on PAO_2 is typically observed as elevation increases above sea level, because while FiO_2 remains 21%, barometric pressure falls. At 18,000 feet, barometric pressure is only 380 mm Hg, and the PAO_2 falls to below 70 mm Hg. At 63,000 feet, the barometric pressure falls to 47 mm Hg, a level where the PAO_2 equals 0 mm Hg. Although it is important to remember this relationship, altitude-induced decreases in PAO_2 are rarely important in clinical medicine, even in commercial airline flights, in which the cabins are pressurized to a maximum of several thousand feet above sea level. However, in closed or low-lying spaces, oxygen is replaced or displaced by other gases that have no intrinsic toxicity. Common examples of these gases, referred to as simple asphyxiants (Table 28–4), are found alone or in combination with more toxic gases. Because they have little or no toxicity other than their ability to replace oxygen, removal of the victim from exposure and administration of supplemental oxygen are curative if permanent injury as a consequence of hypoxia has not already developed (Chap. 121).

TABLE 28–3	Xenobiotics Producing Hyperventilation	
Amphetamines	Isopropanol
Anticholinergics	Methanol
Camphor	Metformin
Carbon monoxide	Methemoglobin inducers
Cocaine	Methylxanthines
Cyanide	Nucleoside reverse transcriptase inhibitors
Dinitrophenol	Paraldehyde
Ethanol (ketoacidosis)	Pentachlorophenol
Ethylene glycol	Phenformin
Gyromitra spp (Mushroom)	Progesterone
Hydrogen sulfide	Salicylates
Iron	Sodium monofluoroacetate
Isoniazid	

TABLE 28–4	Examples of Simple Asphyxiants	
Argon	Hydrogen
Carbon dioxide	Methane
Ethane	Nitrogen
Helium	Propane

The potential magnitude of toxicity from simple asphyxiants is best exemplified by disasters in Cameroon near Lake Mounoun and Lake Nyos, in 1984 and 1986, respectively. Following an earthquake, Lake Nyos, a volcanic lake, released a cloud of CO_2 gas of approximately one-quarter million tons. Because CO_2 is 1.5 times heavier than air, the gas cloud flowed into the surrounding low-lying valleys, killing by asphyxia more than 1700 people, and affecting countless more people because of hypoxia. Most survivors recovered without complications.[11,40] Smaller-scale, but equally serious, toxicity from CO_2 results from improper handling of dry ice or release into a closed space.[42,47]

Chest Wall

Hypoventilation can result from a decrease in either respiratory rate or tidal volume. Thus, even when the stimulus to breathe is normal, adequate ventilation is dependent on the coordination and function of the muscles of the diaphragm and chest wall. Changes in this function can result in hypoventilation by 2 separate mechanisms; both muscle weakness and muscle rigidity impair the patient's ability to expand the chest wall. Some examples of toxicologic causes of muscle weakness include botulinum toxin,[97] electrolyte abnormalities, such as hypokalemia,[59,114] or hypermagnesemia,[2,33] organic phosphorus compounds,[77,98] and neuromuscular blockers.[15,52] Patients with hypoventilation caused by muscle weakness respond well to assisted ventilation and correction of the underlying problem (Chaps. 12, 38, 66, and 111). Chest-wall rigidity impairing ventilation can occur in strychnine poisoning,[17,57,64] tetanus,[24,57,103] and fentanyl use[23,25] (Chaps. 36 and 114). Often these patients are difficult to ventilate despite endotracheal intubation and therefore require muscle relaxants, neuromuscular blockers, or naloxone (for fentanyl).

Airway Patency

The airway can be compromised in several ways. As a patient's mental status becomes impaired, the airway is often obstructed by the tongue.[44] Alternatively, the presence of vomitus, or aspiration of activated charcoal or a foreign body, directly obstructs the trachea or major bronchi with resultant hypoxia.[54,72,90] Obstruction also results from increased secretions produced during organic phosphorus compound poisoning. Laryngospasm occurs either as a manifestation of systemic reactions, such as anaphylaxis, as a result of edema from thermal or caustic injury (Chaps. 103 and 120), or as a direct response to an irritant gas (Chap. 121). Similarly, if the tongue becomes swollen in response to thermal or caustic injury or toxic exposure to plants such as Dieffenbachia spp, or as a result of angioedema from drugs such as angiotensin-converting enzyme inhibitors, airway obstruction results (Chaps. 61, 103, 118, and 120).[36] Regardless of the mechanism, upper airway obstruction produces hypoventilation, hypoxemia, and hypercapnia (hypercarbia) with the persistence of a normal alveolar–arterial (A–a) gradient (see discussion of A–a gradients). Upper airway obstruction is often acute and severe and requires immediate therapy to prevent further clinical compromise. Bronchospasm, a common manifestation of anaphylaxis, also results from exposure to pyrolyzed cocaine,[96] smoke, irritant gases[46] (Table 28–5), dust (eg, cotton in byssinosis), or as a result of work-related asthma[63] and hypersensitivity pneumonitis[120] (Chaps. 120 and 121).

Pressure Phenomenon

Pneumothorax is an example of airway collapse caused by barotrauma, which more commonly results from the manner of administration of illicit

TABLE 28–5	Examples of Irritant Gases
Ammonia	Isocyanates
Chloramine	Nitrogen dioxide
Chlorine	Ozone
Chloroacetophenone	Phosgene
Chlorobenzylidene-malononitrile	Phosphine
Fluorine	Sulfur dioxide
Hydrogen chloride	

xenobiotics than from actual drug overdose. Barotrauma also results from nasal insufflation or inhalation of drugs. This form of barotrauma occurs most often in cocaine (particularly in the form of "crack") and marijuana users, who either smoke or insufflate these xenobiotics and then perform prolonged Valsalva or Mueller maneuvers in an attempt to enhance the effects of these xenobiotics (Chaps. 74 and 75).[13,100,116] The increased airway pressure leads to rupture of an alveolar bleb, and free air dissects along the peribronchial paths into the mediastinum and pleural cavities. Nitrous oxide abuse also causes barotrauma.[55] Siphoning of nitrous oxide from low-pressure tanks meant for inhalation is not typically associated with barotrauma. By contrast, inhalation of nitrous oxide, used as a propellant in whipped cream cans, generates tremendous pressure that sometimes results in severe barotrauma (Chaps. 65 and 81).

Ventilation–Perfusion Mismatch

Ventilation–perfusion (V/Q) mismatch is manifested at the extremes by aeration of the lung without arterial blood supply (as in pulmonary embolism from injected contaminants) and by a normal blood supply to the lung without any ventilation. Impaired blood supply to a normal lung and normal blood supply to an inadequately ventilated lung constitute an infinite number of gradations that exist between the extremes. The normal response to regional variations in ventilation is to shunt blood away from an area of lung poorly ventilated, thereby preferentially delivering blood to an area of the lung where gas exchange is more efficient. A hypoxia-induced reduction in local nitric oxide production appears to be responsible for the regional vasoconstriction that occurs.[1] This effect, commonly known as hypoxic pulmonary vasoconstriction, is best described in patients with chronic obstructive lung disease and facilitates compensation for the V/Q mismatch associated with that disorder. It is unclear whether xenobiotic-induced alterations in pulmonary nitric oxide production are significant determinants in the V/Q mismatch that occurs in poisoning.

In toxicology, V/Q mismatch most commonly results from perfusion of an abnormally ventilated lung that results from aspiration of gastric contents, a frequent complication of many types of poisoning.[54,78] Although alterations in consciousness and loss of protective airway reflexes are predisposing factors, certain xenobiotics, such as hydrocarbons, directly result in aspiration pneumonitis because of their specific characteristics of high volatility, low viscosity, and low surface tension (Chap. 105).

The diagnosis of aspiration pneumonitis often relies on chest radiography for confirmation. The location of the infiltrate depends on the patient's position when the aspiration occurred. Most commonly, aspiration occurs in the right mainstem bronchus, because the angle with the carina is not as acute as it is for entry into the left mainstem bronchus. When aspiration occurs in the supine position, the subsequent infiltrate is usually manifest in the posterior segments of the upper lobe and superior segments of the lower lobe. Aspiration typically involves vomitus; however, secretions, activated charcoal, teeth, dentures, food, and other foreign bodies are also frequently aspirated.

Diffusing Capacity Abnormalities

Severe impairment in diffusing capacity commonly results from local injury to the lungs in disorders such as interstitial pneumonia, aspiration, toxic inhalations, and near drowning, and from systemic effects of sepsis, trauma, and various other medical disorders.[10] When this process is acute and associated with clinical criteria, including crackles, hypoxemia, and bilateral infiltrates on a chest radiograph demonstrating a normal heart size, it has been historically referred to as *noncardiogenic pulmonary edema* or, *acute lung injury* (ALI).[10] The most severe manifestation of these processes was described as acute respiratory distress syndrome (ARDS). However, a task force of pulmonary specialists determined that all of these conditions are best classified as gradations of ARDS. According to the 2012 Berlin definition, ARDS consists of bilateral pulmonary infiltrates (by radiography or computed tomography), which occur within 7 days of an inciting event and are not explained by heart failure or fluid overload. Severity of ARDS is determined by the PaO_2/FiO_2 ratio. Acute respiratory distress syndrome is classified as mild (200 mm Hg $< PaO_2/FiO_2 \leq$ 300 mm Hg), moderate (100 mm Hg $< PaO_2/FiO_2 \leq$ 200 mm Hg), and severe ($PaO_2/FiO_2 \leq$ 100 mm Hg). Cases that once were described as ALI now fit under the mild ARDS classification.

Throughout this chapter and text, this newer nomenclature will be used. Using the older definition, it was estimated that 150,000 Americans developed ARDS annually, many as a result of xenobiotics; severe ARDS has a fatality rate approximating 50%.[4,35]

Commonly, patients are chronically exposed to xenobiotics associated with reduced diffusing capacity by smoking tobacco and other xenobiotics or working with asbestos, silica, and coal, which slowly causes pulmonary fibrosis or promotes emphysema. Chronically smoked cocaine is also recognized to alter pulmonary function.[104] Acutely, ARDS from opioids, salicylates, or phosgene and delayed severe fibrosis from paraquat causes profound alterations in diffusion (Chaps. 36, 37, 109, and 126).[82,91,121] Associated parenchymal damage is almost always present and causes both reduction in lung volumes and V/Q mismatch. Intravenous injection of talc, a common contaminant found in drugs of abuse,[85] and septic emboli from right-sided endocarditis[83,102] result in isolated vascular defects with reduction in diffusion capacity. Similarly, cocaine-induced pulmonary artery spasm obstructs vascular channels and alters pulmonary function, creating V/Q mismatch.[29]

Acute respiratory distress syndrome commonly occurs in cases of poisoning. The edema fluid (and the resulting hypoxia, pulmonary crackles, and radiographic abnormalities) develops in part because of increased permeability of the alveolar and capillary basement membrane.[22,26,91] Proteinaceous fluid leaks from the capillaries into the alveoli and interstitium of the lung. Several mechanisms are proposed as the cause of ARDS, although no single unifying mechanism exists for all of the xenobiotics implicated. Acute respiratory distress syndrome results from exposure to xenobiotics that produce hypoventilation by at least 3 different mechanisms: (1) hypoxia injures the vascular endothelial cells, (2) autoregulatory vascular redistribution causes localized capillary hypertension, or (3) alveolar microtrauma occurs as alveolar units collapse, only to be reopened suddenly during reventilation.[91] These and other events activate neutrophils and release inflammatory cytokines.[3,112] Other xenobiotics are directly toxic to the capillary epithelial cells or are at least partly responsible for the release of vasoactive substances.[3] The effects of salicylates and other nonsteroidal antiinflammatory drugs are most likely mediated via effects on prostaglandin synthesis. Finally, sympathomimetic stimulants occasionally cause "neurogenic" pulmonary edema, which is likely mediated by massive catecholamine discharge. Elevated catecholamine concentrations are also noted in experimental opioid overdose, possibly representing support for a link between hypoxia, hypercarbia, and the catecholamine hypothesis of ARDS.[76]

In the 1880s, William Osler described "oedema of left lung" in a morphine user. The opioids are still among the most common causes of ARDS (Chap. 36), but it is now recognized that there are many types of xenobiotics that can cause or are associated with ARDS, such as the sedative–hypnotics, salicylates, cocaine, carbon monoxide, diuretics, and calcium channel blockers (Table 28–6).[30,32,34,38,39,45,48,51,58,86,88,101,102,121] The route of xenobiotic administration is not usually the determining factor; ARDS results from oral, intravenous, and inhalational exposures. Because the source of the problem is increased pulmonary capillary permeability, patients with ARDS have a

TABLE 28–6	Common Xenobiotic Causes of Acute Respiratory Distress Syndrome
Amiodarone	Ethchlorvynol
Amphetamines	Irritant gases
Amphotericin	Lidocaine
Bleomycin	Opioids
Calcium channel blockers	Protamine
Carbon monoxide	Salicylates
Cocaine	Sedative–hypnotics
Colchicine	Smoke inhalation
Cyclic antidepressants	Streptokinase
Cytosine arabinoside	Vinca alkaloids

normal pulmonary-capillary wedge pressure, unlike patients with cardiogenic pulmonary edema.

True cardiogenic pulmonary edema also occurs as the result of poisoning. Etiologies for this phenomenon include the ingestion of xenobiotics with negative inotropy (eg, β-adrenergic antagonists, type IA antidysrhythmics), myocardial ischemia, dysrhythmia, or infarction (cocaine). Because many overdoses are mixed overdoses, the distinction between cardiogenic pulmonary edema and ARDS is often difficult to establish by physical examination and requires invasive monitoring techniques.

Although the treatments for cardiogenic pulmonary edema and ARDS have many similarities, critical aspects of the therapy differ; therefore, an accurate diagnosis must be established. Most diagnostic tests are not helpful in differentiating between the 2 diseases. Physical examination reveals the presence of crackles with both entities. An S3 gallop, if present, suggests a cardiac cause, but its absence does not establish the diagnosis of ARDS. In both entities, the arterial blood–gas analysis demonstrates hypoxia and chest radiography shows perihilar, basilar, or diffuse alveolar infiltrates. However, the presence of "vascular redistribution" on chest radiography is suggestive of a cardiogenic etiology; a normal-sized heart is more commonly associated with ARDS, whereas an enlarged heart is more typical of cardiogenic pulmonary edema. The diagnostic tests that are useful in establishing the correct diagnosis include echocardiography, transcutaneous bioimpedance, pulmonary artery catheter pressure measurements, and radionuclide ventriculography ("gated-pool" scan). Although the radionuclide scan accurately measures cardiac output, it is not routinely available in the emergency department or intensive care unit and usually requires the transport of a critically ill patient to the nuclear medicine suite. Although echocardiography is easily performed as a portable "bedside" technique, it is less sensitive and less specific for determinations of cardiac output. Therefore, the most definitive diagnostic procedure in the emergency setting is the insertion of a pulmonary artery catheter for hemodynamic monitoring. Cardiogenic pulmonary edema results from an elevated left-atrial filling pressure (elevated pulmonary-capillary wedge pressure) and a decreased cardiac output. In patients with ARDS, the pulmonary artery wedge pressure and the cardiac output are normal. Although not specifically well investigated in poisoning, experiences with transcutaneous bioimpedance measurements of cardiac output show promise for this portable noninvasive technique.[10,27,75,79]

The basic treatment for ARDS is supportive care while the xenobiotic is eliminated and healing occurs in the pulmonary capillaries.[3,61] The most important specific therapeutic intervention in patients with ARDS requiring mechanical ventilation involves the use of low tidal-volume ventilation (≤6 mL/kg predicted body weight).[1,43,112]

This results in reduced airway pressures, which seem to decrease the chance for alveolar distension and subsequent injury. The efficacy of jet ventilators or membrane oxygenators is inadequately studied. Some studies suggest a potential role for extracorporeal membrane oxygenation in the

treatment of ARDS.[56] Positive end-expiratory pressure (PEEP), which likely derives its benefit from keeping alveoli open, is considered an essential component in the management of ARDS.[31,43]

Positive end-expiratory pressure should be maintained in the range of 5 to 12 cm H_2O, to maintain a PO_2 of at least 55 mm Hg, or an oxygen saturation of 88%, with an inspired oxygen concentration of ≤40%. Although in cases of grave lung injury, higher PEEP settings are often required, they come with an increased incidence of pneumothorax or hypotension. Also, while an increase in PEEP typically results in a modest increase in PO_2, it causes a larger decrease in venous return and decreased cardiac output. Therefore, with each change in PEEP, the resulting increase (or perhaps decrease) in oxygen delivery to the body should be determined.[4]

A conservative fluid strategy improves oxygenation and decreases length of stay in the intensive care unit without increasing the incidence of shock or the need for hemodialysis. A conservative fluid management strategy is recommended for patients with ARDS who are not in shock, have not been in shock for at least 12 hours, and do not have other reasons to require liberal fluid administration.[115]

Hemoglobin and Chemical Asphyxiants

Disorders of hemoglobin oxygen content, and of hemoglobin loading and unloading, result in cellular hypoxia, which, in turn, results in hyperventilation. Anemia is a common complication of the infectious diseases associated with injection drug use. In addition, many xenobiotics result in hemolysis or direct bone marrow suppression. Among the latter group are the metals, lead, benzene, and ethanol. Hemolysis also occurs in individuals exposed to lead, copper, or arsine gas, and in patients with glucose-6-phosphate dehydrogenase deficiency exposed to oxidants (Chap. 20).

The oxygen-carrying capacity of blood declines in almost direct proportion to hemoglobin content,[106] as seen in Fig. 28–1. As shown in Fig. 28–1A, under most normal conditions the dissolved oxygen content of the blood contributes little; thus, the last portion of the equation can be eliminated. Anemia resulting in a decrease of the hemoglobin content to 7.5 g/dL (a hematocrit of ~22%) decreases the oxygen content of the blood to about 10.2 mL O_2/dL (Fig. 28–1B). Because central cyanosis is only visible with a concentration of reduced deoxyhemoglobin of at least 5 g/dL, unless an

Oxygen content (O_2 content) = hemoglobin bound oxygen + dissolved oxygen

A. Normal conditions: hemoglobin (Hb) = 15 g/dL; PO_2 = 100 mm Hg, oxygen saturation (O_2 sat) = 95%

O_2 (content = (Hb)(O_2 sat) (constant) + (another constant)(PO_2)
= (Hb)(O_2 sat)(1.39 mL O_2/g%) + (0.003 mL O_2/dL/mm Hg)(PO_2)
= (15 g/dL)(95%)(1.39 mL O_2/g%) + (0.003 mL O_2/dL/mm Hg)(100 mm Hg)
= (19.8 mL O_2/dL) + (0.3 mL O_2/dL)
= **20.1 mL O_2/dL = 20.1 vol%**

B. Anemia: Hb = 7.5 g/dL; PO_2 = 100 mm Hg, O_2 Sat = 95%

O_2 content = (Hb)(O_2 sat)(1.39 mL O_2/g%) + (0.003 mL O_2/dL/mm Hg)(PO_2)
= (7.5 g/dL)(95%)(1.39 mL O_2/g%) + (0.003 mL O_2/dL/mm Hg)(100 mm Hg)
= (9.9 mL O_2/dL) + (0.3 mL O_2/dL)
= **10.2 mL O_2/dL = 10.2 vol%**

C. Hyperbaric oxygen: Hb = 15 g/dL; PO_2 = 1500 mm Hg, O_2 Sat = 100%

O_2 content = (Hb)(O_2 sat)(1.39 mL O_2/g%) + (0.003 mL O_2/dL/mm Hg)(PO_2)
= (15 g/dL)(100%)(1.39 mL O_2/g%) + (0.003 mL O_2/dL/mm Hg)(1500 mm Hg)
= (20.9 mL O_2/dL) + (4.5 mL O_2/dL)
= **25.4 mL O_2/dL = 25.4 vol%**

FIGURE 28–1. Examples of calculations of the oxygen content of the blood under various conditions.

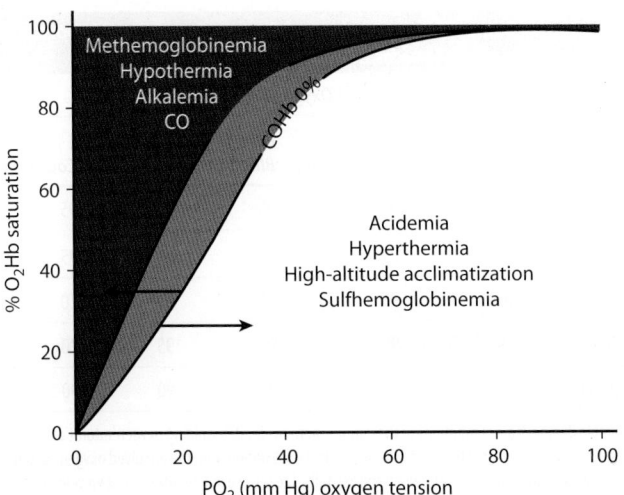

FIGURE 28–2. Oxyhemoglobin dissociation curve at 98.6°F (37°C) and pH 7.40. Hematocrit does not alter this relationship.

abnormal hemoglobin concentration is present, anemia significantly impairs oxygen-carrying capacity without the development of this common physical manifestation (Chap. 124).

By contrast, as the PO_2 reaches higher values (as in hyperbaric oxygen chambers), the dissolved oxygen content becomes significant and of therapeutic value, particularly when the oxygen-carrying content of hemoglobin is compromised. The PO_2 corresponding to an FiO_2 of 100% at 1 atm is approximately 575 mm Hg. By contrast, with hyperbaric oxygen at 3 atm and 100% oxygen, PO_2 values in excess of 1500 mm Hg can be achieved.[66] Under these conditions, the dissolved oxygen content of the blood rises dramatically (to as much as 4.5 mL O_2/dL) and becomes adequate to sustain life, even in the absence of any contribution from hemoglobin (Fig. 28–1C).

The chemical asphyxiants that produce methemoglobin, carboxyhemoglobin, and sulfhemoglobin interfere with oxygen loading and/or unloading to various degrees. Methemoglobin inhibits oxygen loading, producing cyanosis unresponsive to supplemental oxygen (Chap. 124). In addition, the oxyhemoglobin dissociation curve is shifted to the left, interfering with unloading (Fig. 28–2). Carboxyhemoglobin has similar effects on oxygen loading and unloading, but carboxyhemoglobin is not associated with cyanosis (Chap. 122). Although sulfhemoglobin also impairs oxygen loading, it shifts the oxyhemoglobin saturation curve to the right, favoring unloading of the remaining normal hemoglobin. Cyanide, hydrogen sulfide, and sodium azide primarily affect oxygen use by interfering with the cytochrome oxidase system (Chap. 123).

Cardiac Output

Any xenobiotic that causes a decreased cardiac output or hypotension has the potential to result in tissue hypoxia and tachypnea. This occurs most frequently with overdoses of β-adrenergic antagonists and calcium channel blockers, antidysrhythmics, cyclic antidepressants, and phenothiazines (Chap. 16).

Asthma and Occupational Exposures

Usually considered a cause of morbidity more than mortality, work-related asthma is frequently encountered by the practitioner. The pathophysiology of these illnesses is still being elucidated, and likely results from both immunoglobulin (Ig) E and non–IgE-related mechanisms.[16]

Work-related asthma is typically divided into 3 distinct clinical entities:

1. Work-aggravated asthma: Preexisting asthma worsened by allergens in the workplace.
2. Occupational asthma: Asthma caused by workplace exposure and not factors outside the workplace. There is a latency period between the symptoms and the first exposure, possibly as long as several years.
3. Reactive airway dysfunction syndrome (RADS): Asthma caused by nonimmunogenic stimuli in the workplace, occurring for the first time within 24 hours of exposure to an inhaled irritant xenobiotic.[6,21,111]

Occupational exposures are thought to be responsible for a substantial proportion of adult-onset asthma, estimated at 10% to 25% in one international prospective study.[20]

A large number of xenobiotics and occupations are associated with the development of work-aggravated and work-related asthma. Because researchers rely on surveys and interviews, the latency period between exposure and symptoms makes identification of these associations a challenge.

Many high-molecular-weight xenobiotics, usually plant or animal derived, are known etiologies, such as arthropod- and mite-related materials, latex, flour, molds, endotoxins, and biological enzymes. Lower-molecular-weight xenobiotics associated with work-related asthma include isocyanates (used in spray paints and foam manufacturing), cleaning agents, anhydrides, amines, dyes, and glues. For more information on specific xenobiotics, see Chap. 121.

In one study, the following occupations were found, in decreasing order, to be associated with the development of occupational asthma: printing, woodworking, nursing, agriculture and forestry, cleaning and caretaking, and electrical processors.[60]

By contrast to occupational asthma and work-aggravated asthma, the latency period between exposure and symptoms in RADS is short or absent, so it is typically easier for the health care professional to identify the precipitant from history. Xenobiotics frequently associated with RADS include cleaning agents (including chlorine, hypochlorite, ammonia, and chloramines), solvents, toluene diisocyanate, acids, alkali, nitrogen oxides, smoke, and diesel exhaust.[49,99]

APPROACH TO RESPIRATORY DYSFUNCTION IN THE POISONED PATIENT

The initial assessment of each patient must involve the evaluation of upper airway patency. Adequacy of ventilation should then be determined. If concomitant injury is suspected, then care must be taken to protect the cervical spine. When airway patency is in question, maneuvers to establish and protect the airway are of prime importance. Often this simply involves repositioning the chin, jaw, or head, or suctioning secretions or vomitus from the airway. However, insertion of an oral or nasopharyngeal airway, or nasopharyngeal or endotracheal intubation, or surgical cricothyroidotomy should be performed as clinically indicated. After the airway is secured, high-flow supplemental oxygen should be provided if needed and the depth, rate, and rhythm of respirations evaluated. An acceptable tidal breath is one that transports 10 to 15 mL of air/kg of body weight.[4]

Hypoventilation that results from an inadequate respiratory rate or tidal volume is arbitrarily defined as an arterial PCO_2 higher than 44 mm Hg and leads to hypoxia and ventilatory failure if uncorrected.[117] The symptoms of hypoxia and or hypercarbia are nonspecific and resemble toxicity from many xenobiotics. Initially, patients appear restless and confused. Signs of sympathetic discharge, such as tachycardia and diaphoresis, are commonly noted. Later, patients complain of headache, only to become sedated and subsequently comatose, as further deterioration occurs. These signs and symptoms are often nonspecific. We recommend early determination of oxygenation and ventilation when there is concern for respiratory failure in patients following xenobiotic overdose. Arterial blood gas and pulse oximetry are used to identify hypoxia, whereas capnography and blood gas (venous or arterial) are usually reasonable surrogates for determining ventilation.

A trial of naloxone, hypertonic dextrose, and thiamine is indicated for the patient with an altered mental status and or respiratory compromise when these etiologies are not otherwise easily clinically excluded (Chap. 4). Because opioid overdose and hypoglycemia are rapidly reversible, potential causes of respiratory failure, these diagnoses should be addressed before most other interventions are considered. Failure to identify and reverse these conditions will result in unnecessary diagnostic and therapeutic interventions in addition to irreversible neurologic sequelae.

Once an acceptable airway is established the remainder of the evaluation can proceed. A rapid assessment of the remainder of the vital signs (Chap. 3) should then occur. Obtaining a history and physical examination, measured oxygen saturation, measured ventilation, and chest radiography are sufficient to determine the diagnosis of pulmonary pathology in most cases. However, adjuncts, such as measurement of negative inspiratory force (NIF), invasive hemodynamic monitoring, evaluation of the arterial–venous oxygen difference, xenon ventilation and technetium scanning, and computed tomographic scanning are frequently required.

History

A directed history must include questions on the nature, onset, and duration of symptoms; substance use and abuse; home and occupational exposures; and underlying pulmonary pathology. If the patient has a significant degree of respiratory compromise, most or all of the history will have to be obtained from friends, relatives, paramedics, coworkers, or others.

Physical Examination

The physical evaluation must include a detailed assessment of depth, rate, and rhythm of respirations, use of accessory muscles, direct evaluation of the oropharynx, position of the trachea, and presence and quality of breathing sounds. Skin, nail bed, and conjunctival color must be observed for pallor or cyanosis. Funduscopic examination is a useful adjunct to the examination. Papilledema occurs in the presence of acute hypercapnia, but is neither sensitive nor specific for that diagnosis. Additionally, because cyanide poisoning interferes with oxygen delivery to tissue, the venous oxygen saturation remains high. During the funduscopic examination, this classically appears as arterialization of the retinal veins, in which the veins take on a color more characteristic of arteries (Chap. 123). A general assessment of muscle tone, with a specific emphasis on ocular and neck muscles, will give clues to weakness or rigidity syndromes that interfere with respiration. When in doubt, a determination of the negative inspiratory force will provide a rapid, objective, quantifiable bedside assessment of respiratory strength.

Pulse Oximetry

Pulse oximeters widely accepted as rapid, noninvasive indicators of hemoglobin oxygen saturation. As defined, hemoglobin–oxygen saturation is the ratio of oxyhemoglobin to total hemoglobin. By using 2 light-emitting diodes, the pulse oximeter is able to measure absorbance at the peak wavelengths for oxyhemoglobin and deoxyhemoglobin (typically at 940 and 660 nm). Thus, the ratio of oxyhemoglobin to oxyhemoglobin plus deoxyhemoglobin (total hemoglobin) is calculated. The clinician then estimates the PO_2 from the oxygen saturation.

Limitations of this approach require elaboration. Because the oxyhemoglobin dissociation curve becomes quite flat above 90% saturation (Fig. 28–2), small changes in saturation greater than 90% represent very large changes in PO_2. Thus, a decrease from 97% saturation to 95% saturation represents a substantial decrease in PO_2. Although a low saturation is an early indicator of hypoxic hypoxia, this is only one of many causes of tissue hypoxia. If total hemoglobin is low, then the oxygen-carrying capacity is inadequate even with excellent saturation (Fig. 28–1). Dyshemoglobinemias, such as carboxyhemoglobin, methemoglobin, and possibly sulfhemoglobin, interfere with the accuracy of pulse oximeter determinations and are of particular concern in the poisoned patient. Specifically, using a standard pulse oximeter, the presence of elevated levels of methemoglobin will tend to make the saturation determined by pulse oximetry approach 84% to 86% (Chap. 124).[8,83] Carboxyhemoglobin is falsely interpreted by the pulse oximeter as mostly oxyhemoglobin; thus, readings tend to appear normal even with significant carbon monoxide poisoning (Table 28–7).[107] Accurate response by the pulse oximeter also requires adequate blood pressure, lack of strong venous pulsations (as might occur in a patient with tricuspid regurgitation),

TABLE 28–7	Sample Interpretations of Oxygen Saturations Reported by Various Sources of Measurement			
	Percent Oxygen Saturation			
Condition	**PO$_2$ (mm Hg)**	**Arterial Blood Gas**	**Pulse Oximeter**	**Cooximeter**
Normal	95	95	95	95
Anemia	95	95	95	95*
Methemoglobinemia (30%)	95	95	85	70
Carboxyhemoglobinemia (30%)	95	95	95	70
Hypoxemia	60	90	90	90

The table demonstrates limitations of the various methods for determining oxygen saturation (O_2 saturation). The arterial blood gas calculates the O_2 saturation from the dissolved oxygen content (PO_2) and becomes abnormal only when the PO_2 falls. The pulse oximeter uses only 2 wavelengths of light and produces substantial errors in the presence of a dyshemoglobinemia. Because the cooximeter uses more wavelengths of light than the pulse oximeter, it can correctly identify the presence of carboxyhemoglobin and methemoglobin. The cooximeter has the additional advantage (*) of measuring the total hemoglobin and oxygen content, so that it is useful in the setting of anemia. All techniques are acceptable for the assessment of hypoxemia.

translucent nails (some shades of nail polish interfere), absence of circulating dyes (methylene blue), and a near-normal temperature. If the pulse oximeter does not produce an accurate reading, then an arterial blood gas should be obtained to assess oxygenation. Finally, we are often more interested in PCO_2 than PO_2, which is not a direct measure of ventilation. The pulse oximeter gives no information with regard to PCO_2. Although the pulse oximeter gives early clues to the presence of hypoxic hypoxia, extrapolation of oxygen saturation to standard arterial blood–gas values is problematic because of the many possible sources of error.

Pulse cooximeters (noninvasive spectral analysis cooximeter), designed to measure carboxyhemoglobin and methemoglobin, in addition to hemoglobin oxygen saturation, are now part of many clinical practices. Although these devices held promise to facilitate early, noninvasive diagnosis of carbon monoxide poisoning and methemoglobinemia, their utility is limited at best. A volunteer study, sponsored by the manufacturer of the device, demonstrated the ability to measure carboxyhemoglobin with an uncertainty of ±2% within the range of 0% to 15% and methemoglobin with an uncertainty of 0.5% within the range of 0% to 12%.[7] In a large study of screening for carboxyhemoglobin, the noninvasive cooximeter was 94% sensitive (95% confidence interval {CI}: 71%–100%) and 77% specific (95% CI: 75%–79%) for identification of a carboxyhemoglobin rate above 6.6%.[95] Other authors found high rates of false negatives when using the noninvasive cooximeter to screen for carbon monoxide poisoning.[105] A recent consensus group concluded that based on available data, these devices should not be used.[119]

Because of these limitations, the best role for this device is as a rapid screening tool perhaps best used in the prehospital setting. Positive results should be confirmed with a blood carboxyhemoglobin concentration, as should normal results whenever carbon monoxide poisoning is highly suspected, or when the result from the device is not consistent with the clinical appearance of the patient.

Capnography

Capnography is the noninvasive measurement of PCO_2 from the airway. Both the numerical value of CO_2 and the shape of the tracing, the capnogram, provide information to the clinician (Fig. 28–3). Measurements are obtained constantly during inhalation and exhalation. End-tidal CO_2 (EtCO$_2$) is the maximum partial pressure of CO_2 at the end of exhalation. End-tidal CO_2 underestimates $PaCO_2$ because exhaled air consists mostly of CO_2-poor air from dead space, in addition to air expired from alveoli. Anatomic dead space, always present, is from the nonventilated upper airways, whereas

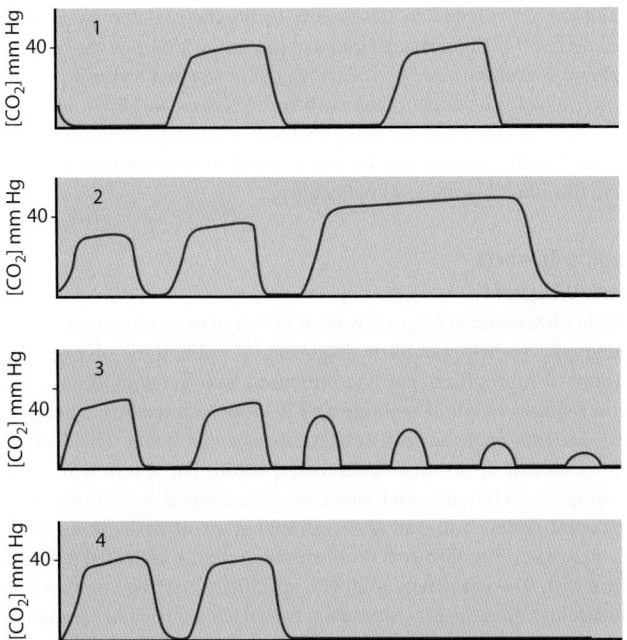

FIGURE 28–3. Capnograms. (1) Normal capnogram. (2) Bradypnea and hypoventilation. The tidal volumes are the same as (1) but the rate is slowing down. (3) Hypopnea and hypoventilation. The amplitude of the waveforms is decreasing. (4) Complete laryngospasm or apnea. After initial waveforms, there is no expired CO_2.

physiologic dead space results from underperfused areas of the lung. Therefore, a high $EtCO_2$ always correlates with an elevated $PaCO_2$, whereas a low value is potentially spurious. In patients without pulmonary disease, $EtCO_2$ is 2 to 5 mm Hg less than $PaCO_2$.[80] In nonintubated emergency department patients with metabolic acidosis, the mean difference was 6 mm Hg.[9] End-tidal CO_2 can be used to confirm endotracheal intubation, monitor endotracheal tube placement, monitor patients during procedural sedation, and assess patients with pulmonary illness. End-tidal CO_2 is also used as a tool to assess ventilation in patients obtunded from a xenobiotic (Fig. 28–3).[28] Although not considered as accurate a reflection of PCO_2 as endotracheal $EtCO_2$, noninvasive $EtCO_2$, would theoretically be the modality best used in nonintubated sedative-poisoned patients who are at risk for hypoventilation. Unfortunately, in a prospective cohort of patients poisoned with respiratory depressants, noninvasive $EtCO_2$ ≥50 mm Hg predicted complications of hypoventilation with only 46% sensitivity and 86% specificity.[108] Therefore, elevated noninvasive $EtCO_2$ predicts complications when elevated but cannot exclude complications when nonelevated.

Analytical Adjuncts

Blood Gas Analysis

Arterial blood gas analysis is an easy and rapid means of evaluating both acid–base status and gas exchange. Attention must be paid to the method for determining oxygen saturation, specifically whether it is measured or calculated from the PO_2. If the measured O_2 saturation is lower than would be predicted from the PO_2 (the calculated O_2 saturation), then the presence of an abnormal hemoglobin concentration (such as carboxyhemoglobin or methemoglobin) must be suspected. A normal calculated O_2 saturation does not exclude these disorders (see Use of the Cooximeter).

Because it is easier to obtain, venous blood gas analysis is often used as a substitute for arterial blood gas analysis.[18] In comparison with arterial values, venous pH and PO_2 are lower, whereas PCO_2 is higher. Errors can be introduced by increased muscle activity of the extremity being tested (seizures). In most cases, a venous blood gas can be used to evaluate PCO_2 and pH, but not PO_2. However, mixed venous blood (defined as right-heart blood) is required for accurate determination of the arterial–venous

oxygen extraction and is an excellent indicator of acid–base status, cardiovascular function, and oxygen use. Unfortunately, a central venous catheter is required for sampling. When performing a peripheral venous blood gas analysis, it is usually assumed that this is only an approximation of mixed venous blood.

The arterial PO_2 is generally considered adequate only if it lies within the flat portion at the upper right of the sigmoidal-shaped oxyhemoglobin dissociation curve (Fig. 28–2). That portion of the curve includes the PO_2 range from 60 to 100 mm Hg, which corresponds to oxygen saturations higher than 90%. As mentioned earlier, within this flat portion, there can be discernible changes in PO_2 with little change in oxygen saturation. For instance, an arterial PO_2 of 80 mm Hg corresponds roughly to an oxygen saturation of 95%. If the PO_2 falls to 60 mm Hg, then the oxygen saturation falls to 90%. This insignificant decrease in the oxygen-carrying capacity of the blood is of minimal clinical concern. However, if the PO_2 falls another 20 mm Hg, then there is a more significant reduction in oxygen saturation, to approximately 70%. Thus, changes in PO_2 higher than 60 mm Hg are usually not of acute therapeutic significance, because the O_2 saturation is higher than 90%. However, these changes are frequently of diagnostic significance.

An exception to this concept applies to the patient who is under metabolic stress, as might result from low cardiac output, impaired vascular flow, anemia, or dyshemoglobinemia. Under these circumstances, even the modest gain achieved by increasing both dissolved oxygen content and hemoglobin saturation higher than 90% is desirable, as discussed earlier (see Hemoglobin and Chemical Asphyxiants). Also, even if a PO_2 higher than 60 mm Hg or an O_2 saturation higher than 90% is considered acceptable in most acute settings, it is rarely desirable to achieve greater values over concerns for oxygen toxicity.

Significance of a Decreased PO_2

In a patient with a diminished PO_2, 5 clinically relevant mechanisms for the hypoxemia should be considered: (1) alveolar hypoventilation, (2) V/Q mismatch, (3) shunting, (4) diffusion abnormality, and, rarely, (5) a decrease in FiO_2. In most clinical circumstances, diffusion defects cannot be distinguished from V/Q mismatch. Usually the responsible mechanism can be identified by calculating the A–a oxygen gradient. In patients with alveolar hypoventilation, the A–a gradient is completely normal (≤15 mm Hg when breathing room air). Patients with V/Q mismatch have an A–a gradient that is increased but that normalizes when 100% oxygen is administered for at least 20 minutes. A normal A–a gradient is defined as less than 100 mm Hg on 100% oxygen. The arterial PO_2 on 100% oxygen reaches approximately 575 mm Hg. By contrast, a patient with a shunt will also have an increased A–a gradient while breathing room air, but when 100% oxygen is administered, the arterial PO_2 falls to substantially less than 575 mm Hg and the A–a gradient does not normalize. Finally, in the case of a patient with hypoxia resulting from breathing in an environment in which the FiO_2 is less than 21%, the PO_2 should correct rapidly when the patient is removed from the environment or supplemental oxygen is delivered.

In general, a low PO_2 can be improved by supplying supplemental oxygen. Although in this instance the patient's laboratory values are improved, the underlying process persists. It is important to remember that the laboratory correlate of hypoventilation is hypercapnia on the arterial blood–gas analysis. If hypercapnia is associated with acidemia, then assisted ventilation is recommended, regardless of whether the PO_2 corrects with supplemental oxygen.

Use of the Cooximeter

Routine analysis of an arterial blood gas yields a measured pH, a measured PO_2, and a measured PCO_2. Ordinarily, the serum bicarbonate, base excess, and percent oxygen saturation of hemoglobin are all calculated values. The oxygen saturation is of clinical significance because it usually correlates with the oxygen content of the blood; thus, the oxygen available to the tissues. However, implied in this relationship is a normal amount of functional hemoglobin. Because the oxygen saturation is calculated from the measured

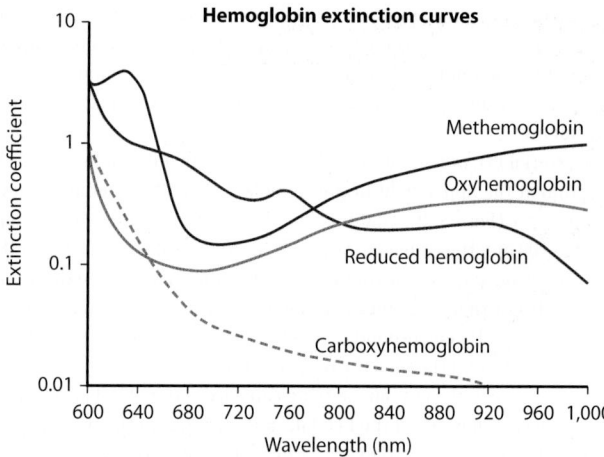

FIGURE 28–4. Cooximetry curves for normal and abnormal hemoglobin variants. Transmitted light absorbance spectra are shown for 4 hemoglobin species: oxyhemoglobin, reduced (deoxy) hemoglobin, carboxyhemoglobin, and methemoglobin.

PO$_2$ using the oxyhemoglobin dissociation curve, it represents only the saturation of normal hemoglobin. Thus, in the presence of even a small percentage of abnormal hemoglobin, the calculated oxygen saturation overestimates the total oxygen content of the blood. For example, a patient with a PO$_2$ of 95 mm Hg has a calculated oxygen saturation of 95%. If the patient also has a 30% methemoglobinemia, only 70% of the total hemoglobin is saturated to 95% and the actual saturation is only 67%. This gap is clinically important because hemoglobin saturations of less than 90% do not provide adequate oxygen delivery to the tissues.

As discussed above, despite the development of bedside noninvasive pulse-cooximetry, most clinicians still depend on laboratory cooximeters for measurement of carboxyhemoglobin and methemoglobin. Most cooximeters spectrophotometrically measure total hemoglobin, oxyhemoglobin, deoxyhemoglobin, carboxyhemoglobin, and methemoglobin. Newer models also measure fetal hemoglobin and sulfhemoglobin (Fig. 28–4). The resultant saturation is a measured oxygen saturation of the total hemoglobin by including all measured hemoglobin variants, and thus correlates with the total oxygen content of the blood.

The difference between measured and calculated oxygen saturation represents the percentage of abnormal hemoglobin present. This gap is helpful in the diagnosis of methemoglobin and carboxyhemoglobin, and is useful in assessing the adequacy of therapy for these disorders. Common indications for cooximetry include cyanosis that is unresponsive to oxygen (methemoglobin and sulfhemoglobin), known use of methemoglobin-forming xenobiotics (benzocaine, dapsone), smoke inhalation (carboxyhemoglobin and possibly methemoglobin), and evaluation of therapy for cyanide toxicity (methemoglobin).

Like so many other tools, the cooximeter is not perfect. Its biggest limitation occurs when dealing with uncommon hemoglobins. Older cooximeters use 4 wavelengths of light and have the ability to define only 4 hemoglobin variants. Consequently, rare dyshemoglobinemias, such as sulfhemoglobin, are misinterpreted as one or a combination of the 4 common hemoglobin variants, giving erroneous results. This phenomenon is commonly noted in neonates in whom fetal hemoglobin was interpreted as carboxyhemoglobin.[110,118] Although this error rarely adds greater than 10% to the true carboxyhemoglobin value, this amount is significant because of the difficulties in assessing the cognitive status of infants possibly exposed to carbon monoxide. Newer cooximeters use at least 6 wavelengths of light and are designed to measure fetal hemoglobin and sulfhemoglobin directly, avoiding these interference problems.[53] Another source of interference with cooximetry is the use of hydroxocobalamin, which has a deep red color. Hydroxocobalamin

administration resulted in falsely low carboxyhemoglobin by laboratory cooximetry.[73,84,120] Clinicians should use caution in interpreting carboxyhemoglobin concentrations in patients who have received hydroxocobalamin. When available, a sample obtained before hydroxocobalamin administration should be sent for cooximeter analysis. Additionally, cooximeters tend to inconsistently interpret low levels (<2.5%) of carboxyhemoglobin.[74] Fortunately, this rarely has clinical implications.

Imaging Adjuncts
Bedside Ultrasound
Bedside ultrasound is frequently used in lieu of or as an adjunct to chest radiography to help establish diagnoses of pulmonary edema, pleural effusion, compromised cardiac function, and pneumothorax. Ultrasound requires operator training and is more technically challenging in obese patients or those with subcutaneous emphysema. The diagnostic performance of ultrasound is discussed below. For a review of specific sonographic techniques and signs, we recommend a resource-focused ultrasound review.[41] In one observational study of patients in ICU, the presence of anterior diffuse B lines with lung sliding indicated pulmonary edema with 97% sensitivity and 95% specificity.[70] When combined with echocardiography, the presence of decreased left ventricular ejection fraction can help determine whether lung edema is cardiogenic or the result of ARDS. Ultrasound can reliably diagnose pneumothorax, as well. The combination of abolished lung sliding (extremely sensitive) with anterior A-lines strongly suggests pneumothorax. The presence of a "lung point" is pathognomonic for the condition. When these 3 signs were observed together, ultrasound had 88% sensitivity and 100% specificity in identifying pneumothorax in ICU patients.[71] In a prospective study of healthy volunteers and ARDS patients, ultrasound was 92% sensitive and 93% specific for identification of pleural effusion, compared to 42% sensitivity and 90% specificity for auscultation.[69]

Chest Radiography
Radiographic detection of a pneumothorax or pneumomediastinum, cardiogenic pulmonary edema, ARDS, aspiration pneumonitis, or the presence of a foreign body is crucial, but can usually be delayed until the initial evaluation is completed. Confirmation of endotracheal tube placement is necessary but initially can be ascertained by auscultating bilateral breath sounds following compression of a bag–valve–mask, or using a variety of marketed devices such as EtCO$_2$ detectors designed to help confirm tube placement. For patients with occupational disorders, chest radiography is essential to confirm and stage exposures to asbestos, silica, coal, and other causes of pneumoconiosis (Chap. 8).

Pulmonary Function Tests
Formal pulmonary function tests are seldom indicated in acute poisoning. However, bedside tests are helpful to predict respiratory failure in patients with suspected respiratory muscle weakness, such as that occurring from botulinum toxin, elapid venom, inhibitors of acetylcholinesterase, nicotine, and others. The determination of the maximum inspiratory pressure (MIP; sometimes referred to as "negative inspiratory force" {NIF}) identifies subclinical diaphragmatic weakness. In patients with primary neurologic conditions, a MIP of worse (closer to zero) than negative 30 cm H$_2$O is predictive of respiratory failure.[65] Although poor effort also results in an abnormal value, a normal value excludes respiratory muscle weakness. The test should be performed serially, at least every 2 to 4 hours following initial presentation, to identify changes in patient condition.

THERAPEUTIC OPTIONS
Supplemental Oxygen
Supplemental oxygen is indicated for all patients with suspected or confirmed respiratory insufficiency. Although it is generally advisable to begin

with high flow (12 L/min) via a nonrebreather mask, administering lower concentrations of oxygen is reasonable in more stable patients. Supplemental oxygen should be titrated to the minimum flow rate required to achieve adequate oxygen saturation. High-flow nasal oxygen (HFNO) systems deliver heated, humidified oxygen at flow rates up to 60 L/min.[68] These devices reduce dead space and increase oxygen delivery compared to conventional nasal cannulae. They are associated with improved user comfort and reduced minute ventilation requirement. High-flow nasal oxygen likely has its greatest benefit in patients who are hypoxic but not hypercapnic.

Pulse oximetry is a good modality for monitoring oxygenation, especially if used in conjunction with $EtCO_2$ recognizing the limitations of both modalities. An arterial blood gas should be obtained if there is concern that pulse oximetry saturation and the $EtCO_2$ are not reflective of the true saturation. Hyperbaric oxygen is indicated for carbon monoxide poisoning and rarely other exposures (Antidotes in Depth: A40).

Initially, there should be limited concern over worsening hypercapnia in patients with chronic obstructive pulmonary disease and respiratory failure. This concern should not deter clinicians from providing needed oxygen, because many of these patients will require intubation for their hypoventilation. It is important to appreciate that supplemental oxygen will improve hypoxia but not hypercarbia.

Additional respiratory support can be offered from bilevel positive airway pressure (BiPAP). Some experimental evidence supports the use of BiPAP for patients with acute respiratory dysfunction in the emergency department.[89] Although this technique is useful in overdosed patients, it should be considered only as a temporizing measure for patients who are expected to recover rapidly, or while preparing for intubation.

Intubation

Most sedative–hypnotic-poisoned patients are managed without intubation. However, in a large retrospective review of poisoned patients, sedative–hypnotics and opioids were still the first and second largest categories of exposures treated with endotracheal intubation.[12] After the decision for mechanical ventilation is made, the route needs to be selected. We recommend oral intubation because it permits the use of a larger endotracheal tube—usually 8 mm or even larger in adults—than does nasal intubation. If the patient later needs bronchoscopy, then it can be performed through the endotracheal tube. Some data suggest that bronchoscopy with bronchoalveolar lavage is of both diagnostic[109] and therapeutic[62] benefit for selected poisoned patients. Fiberoptic devices facilitate oral intubation in difficult cases, making nasotracheal intubation almost obsolete. However, an advantage of nasotracheal intubation over oral intubation is that orogastric lavage is performed more easily when the oral cavity is unimpeded. After the trachea is intubated, the tube should be checked to ensure that it is correctly positioned.

All patients who overdose and show signs or symptoms of respiratory insufficiency should have chest radiography performed. Unfortunately, intubated patients usually have portable radiography performed and the carina is frequently difficult to visualize because of the poor quality of the study. When seen, the carina is visualized between T5 and T7 in most patients. Thus, the tip of the endotracheal tube should be above T5 for proper (safe) placement. When portable chest radiography is obtained, the patient's neck is often either extended or flexed, altering the location of the endotracheal tube tip. For this reason, it is essential to note the position of the neck during radiography, because the tip of the endotracheal tube will move up (with flexion) or down (with extension) by almost 2 cm.[14]

Mechanical Ventilation

After a patient is intubated for ventilatory support, the respirator mode is selected. Patients with pure hypoventilation usually require a controlled fixed rate that is easily adjusted based on pulse oximetry, $EtCO_2$, and/or serial venous or arterial blood–gas analyses. Patients with pulmonary

parenchymal processes, such as ARDS or pneumonia, usually do best when placed on either assist control (AC) or intermittent mechanical ventilation (IMV) mode. Both of these modes are volume-controlled, meaning the clinicians set a volume and a minimal rate. In each of these modes, the patient is able to take additional breaths. In AC, the additional patient breaths trigger a ventilator-delivered breath at the preset tidal volume. With the IMV mode, the tidal volume of extra patient-initiated breaths is determined by the patient. This lowers mean airway pressure, which theoretically reduces the risk of barotrauma and hemodynamic compromise. Although the lower airway pressures associated with IMV are desirable, many authorities recommend the use of the assist mode because it eliminates the patient's work of breathing.[61]

The next step is to determine the appropriate FiO_2 to be delivered to the patient. A number of approaches are available to assist with this decision. One simple approach is to intubate a patient, control breathing, administer 100% oxygen, and decrease to an FiO_2 of less than 50% as quickly as possible in an attempt to prevent oxygen toxicity.[3] Although the toxic effects of oxygen are well known for paraquat (Chap. 109), evidence suggests that oxygen is an important mediator of other xenobiotic-induced pulmonary injuries such as with iron.[50] A PO_2 of at least 55 mm Hg or a measured oxygen saturation greater than 88% is generally acceptable, although many clinicians feel more comfortable establishing a "buffer" against deterioration by increasing the PO_2 to greater than 60 mm Hg.[1,112] In most patients, tidal volumes should be set on the order of 6 mL/kg/breath. These lower, "protective" tidal volumes cause less barotrauma, lung injury, and cytokine release. Lower tidal volumes decrease mortality and ventilator days for patients with ARDS and to improve clinical outcomes in patients without ARDS.[1,81] If oxygenation cannot be maintained with FiO_2 at or less than 50%, PEEP should be used, with careful reassessment of serial arterial blood–gas analyses, changes in effective compliance, and hemodynamic data with each increment in PEEP.

Pharmacologic Interventions: Antidotes

Only a few antidotes have a significant role in reversing xenobiotic-induced respiratory dysfunction. Naloxone has the greatest role. Respiratory stimulants were historically used to treat sedative poisoning, but this practice lost favor because of limited efficacy and the occurrence of adverse effects, such as seizures.[94] Recent authors reported the use of doxapram to stimulate ventilation in alcohol and GHB-poisoned patients.[92,93] However, because these poisonings can be managed almost universally safely by conservative non-pharmacologic means, the use of stimulants cannot be recommended at this time. Atropine and pralidoxime are useful for respiratory dysfunction from cholinesterase inhibitors (Antidotes in Depth: A35 and A36, and Chap. 111). Elapid antivenom (A39) and botulinum antitoxin (A6) are rarely used but may be lifesaving in the appropriate clinical scenario. Neostigmine and sugammadex reverse muscle weakness from nondepolarizing neuromuscular blockers (Chap. 66). More commonly, clinicians are required to treat bronchospasm from exposure to pulmonary irritants. The use of β_2-selective adrenergic-agonist bronchodilators are effective in these patients.[37] Although the role of corticosteroids remains controversial, they are reasonable adjuncts.[3]

When treating patients with bronchospasm from one of the work-related asthma syndromes, it is reasonable that management should be similar to that of any patient with pulmonary bronchospasm, such as emphasizing inhaled bronchodilators and corticosteroids (Fig. 28–5).

An inhaled solution of 2% sodium bicarbonate often provides symptomatic relief for patients with pulmonary exposure to hydrogen chloride or to chlorine (Antidotes in Depth: A5).

Exogenous nitric oxide was evaluated for a variety of pulmonary conditions. Specifically, indications investigated for nitric oxide include as a bronchodilator,[19] a means to reverse hypoxic pulmonary vasoconstriction,[3] and as treatment for ARDS.[2] Unfortunately, controlled studies fail to demonstrate a benefit for nitric oxide in patients with ARDS.[3,112] Similarly, the

Two 30-year-old patients who overdosed were brought to the ED. Each had ingested substantial amounts of barbiturates and diazepam. An arterial blood gas drawn from patient 1 while he was breathing room air revealed a pH of 7.18, PCO_2 of 70 mm Hg, PO_2 of 50 mm Hg, and a calculated bicarbonate of 24 mEq/L. An arterial blood gas drawn from patient 2, also breathing room air, revealed a pH of 7.31 PCO_2 of 50 mm Hg, PO_2 of 50 mm Hg, and a calculated bicarbonate of 25 mEq/L. Quick analysis showed that patient 1 was hypercapnic with a significant respiratory acidosis. Patient 2 did not appear as ill; his PCO_2 was not very elevated and his pH was not significantly reduced. The A–a gradients were calculated to be 12.5 mm Hg for patient 1 and 37.5 mm Hg for patient 2.

A. Arterial PCO_2 approximates alveolar PCO_2 and is substituted as:

$$PAO_2 = PiO_2 - \frac{PCO_2}{R}$$

$$PiO_2 = (FiO_2)(PB - PH_2O)$$

where PAO_2 is alveolar PO_2, PiO_2 is partial pressure of inspired O_2, $PaCO_2$ is arterial PCO_2, and R is the respiratory exchange ratio. Therefore:

$$PAO_2 = [(FiO_2)(PB - PH_2O)] - \frac{PCO_2}{R}$$

where FiO_2 is the inspired O_2 fraction PH_2O is water vapor pressure, and PB is barometric pressure. On room air at sea level, FiO_2 = 21%. At steady state, R = 0.8. At sea level, PB = 760 mm Hg, and PH_2O = 47 mm Hg. Therefore:

$$PAO_2 = [(FiO_2)(PB - PH_2O)] - \frac{PCO_2}{R}$$

$$= [(0.21)(760 - 47)] - \frac{PCO_2}{R}$$

$$= 150 - [(1.25)(PCO_2)]$$

Because the A–a gradient is equal to $PAO_2 - PaO_2$ it can be expressed as:

$$150 - [(1.25)(PCO_2)] - PaO_2 \text{ or } 150 - [(1.25)(PCO_2) + PaO_2]$$

A normal A–a gradient on room air is 10–15 mm Hg, but this increases with age. A rough estimate of the normal A–a gradient is one-third the patient's age.

B. Referring to the two overdosed patients above, the A–a gradient for patient 1 is:

$$150 - [(1.25)(70) + 50] = 12.5 \text{ mm Hg}$$

This calculation reveals a normal gradient, indicating that the etiology for hypoxemia and hypoventilation is extrinsic to the lung itself. In patient 2, the A–a gradient is:

$$150 - [(1.25)(50) + 50] = 37.5 \text{ mm Hg}$$

This abnormally high A–a gradient is consistent with the aspiration which was pneumonia seen on the patient's chest radiograph.

FIGURE 28–5. (A) Derivation of the definition of alveolar–arterial (A–a) oxygen gradients. **(B)** Applying the A–a gradients.

results are disappointing for corticosteroids, surfactants, and a variety of antiinflammatory drugs.[4,112]

SUMMARY

- Xenobiotics adversely affect tissue oxygenation at every step required for ventilation, oxygen delivery, and cellular respiration.
- Hypoxia and hypercarbia should be addressed as soon as they are suspected clinically. The use of supplemental oxygen or assisted ventilation should not be delayed.
- Although the clinical manifestations of hypoxia are constant regardless of etiology, the history, physical examination, and diagnostic testing often help to identify the specific mechanism of hypoxia.
- Invasive and noninvasive measures of oxygenation and ventilation should be used to assess response to therapy and need for further therapy. Clinicians should familiarize themselves with the strengths and limitations of pulse oximetry, end-tidal carbon dioxide capnography, venous and arterial blood–gas analyses, and cooximetry.
- In most cases of xenobiotic-induced respiratory depression, general supportive measures are favored over specific antidotal therapy.

REFERENCES

1. Acute Respiratory Distress Syndrome Network; Brower RG, et al. Ventilation with lower tidal volumes as compared with traditional tidal volumes for acute lung injury and the acute respiratory distress syndrome. *N Engl J Med.* 2000;342:1301-1308.
2. Adnot S, et al. NO in the lung. *Respir Physiol.* 1995;101:109-120.
3. Albertson TE, et al. The pharmacology and toxicology—of three new biologic agents used in pulmonary medicine. *J Toxicol Clin Toxicol.* 1995;33:427-438.
4. Artigas A, et al. The American-European Consensus-Conference on ARDS, part 2. Ventilatory, pharmacologic, supportive therapy, study design strategies and issues related to recovery and remodeling. *Intensive Care Med.* 1998;24:378-398.
5. Balmes JR. Occupational lung diseases. In: LaDou J, ed. *Current Occupational and Environmental Medicine.* 4th ed. New York, NY: McGraw-Hill; 2007:310-333.
6. Banks DE, Jalloul A. Occupational asthma, work-related asthma, and reactive airways dysfunction syndrome. *Curr Opin Pulm Med.* 2007;13:131-136.
7. Barker SJ, et al. Measurement of carboxyhemoglobin and methemoglobin by pulse oximetry: a human volunteer study. *Anesthesiology.* 2006;105:892-897.
8. Barker SJ, et al. Effects of methemoglobinemia on pulse oximetry and mixed venous oximetry. *Anesthesiology.* 1989;70:112-117.
9. Barton CW, Wang ES. Correlation of end-tidal CO_2 measurements to arterial $PaCO_2$ in nonintubated patients. *Ann Emerg Med.* 1994;23:560-563.
10. Baumann BM, et al. Cardiac and hemodynamic assessment of patients with cocaine-associated chest pain syndromes. *J Toxicol Clin Toxicol.* 2000;38:283-290.
11. Baxter PJ, et al. Lake Nyos disaster, Cameroon, 1986: the medical effects of large scale emission of carbon dioxide? *BMJ.* 1989;298:1437-1441.
12. Beauchamp GA, et al. Endotracheal intubation for toxicology exposures: a retrospective review of Toxicology Investigators Consortium (ToxIC) Cases. *J Emerg Med.* 2016;51:382-284.
13. Birrer RB, Calderon J. Pneumothorax, pneumomediastinum, and pneumopericardium following Valsalva's maneuver during marijuana smoking. *N Y State J Med.* 1984;84:619-620.
14. Blanc VF, Tremblay NA. The complications of tracheal intubation: a new classification with a review of the literature. *Anesth Analg.* 1974;53:202-213.
15. Book WJ, et al. Adverse effects of depolarizing neuromuscular blocking agents. Incidence, prevention and management. *Drug Saf.* 1994;10:331-349.
16. Boulet LP, et al. New insights into occupational asthma. *Curr Opin Allergy Clin Immunol.* 2007;7:96-101.
17. Boyd RE, et al. Strychnine poisoning. Recovery from profound lactic acidosis, hyperthermia, and rhabdomyolysis. *Am J Med.* 1983;74:507-512.
18. Brandenburg MA, Dire DJ. Comparison of arterial and venous blood gas values in the initial emergency department evaluation of patients with diabetic ketoacidosis. *Ann Emerg Med.* 1998;31:459-465.
19. Brett SJ, Evans TW. Nitric oxide: physiological roles and therapeutic implications in the lung. *Br J Hosp Med (Lond).* 1996;55:487-490.
20. Brooks SM. An approach to patients suspected of having an occupational pulmonary disease. *Clin Chest Med.* 1981;2:171-178.
21. Brooks SM, et al. Reactive airways dysfunction syndrome (RADS). Persistent asthma syndrome after high level irritant exposures. *Chest.* 1985;88:376-384.
22. Byrne K, Sugerman HJ. Experimental and clinical assessment of lung injury by measurement of extravascular lung water and transcapillary protein flux in ARDS: a review of current techniques. *J Surg Res.* 1988;44:185-203.
23. Caspi J, et al. Delayed respiratory depression following fentanyl anesthesia for cardiac surgery. *Crit Care Med.* 1988;16:238-240.
24. Cherubin CE. Epidemiology of tetanus in narcotic addicts. *N Y State J Med.* 1970;70:267-271.
25. Christian CM 2nd, et al. Postoperative rigidity following fentanyl anesthesia. *Anesthesiology.* 1983;58:275-277.
26. Cope DK, et al. Pulmonary capillary pressure: a review. *Crit Care Med.* 1992;20:1043-1056.
27. Cotter G, et al. Accurate, noninvasive continuous monitoring of cardiac output by whole-body electrical bioimpedance. *Chest.* 2004;125:1431-1440.
28. Davis DP, Patel RJ. Noninvasive capnometry for continuous monitoring of mental status: a tale of 2 patients. *Am J Emerg Med.* 2006;24:752-754.
29. Delaney K, Hoffman RS. Pulmonary infarction associated with crack cocaine use in a previously healthy 23-year-old woman. *Am J Med.* 1991;91:92-94.
30. Duberstein JL, Kaufman DM. A clinical study of an epidemic of heroin intoxication and heroin-induced pulmonary edema. *Am J Med.* 1971;51:704-714.
31. Esteban A, et al. Characteristics and outcomes in adult patients receiving mechanical ventilation: a 28-day international study. *JAMA.* 2002;287:345-355.
32. Ettinger NA, Albin RJ. A review of the respiratory effects of smoking cocaine. *Am J Med.* 1989;87:664-668.

33. Fassler CA, et al. Magnesium toxicity as a cause of hypotension and hypoventilation. Occurrence in patients with normal renal function. *Arch Intern Med.* 1985;145:1604-1606.

34. Fein A, et al. Carbon monoxide effect on alveolar epithelial permeability. *Chest.* 1980;78:726-731.

35. Ferguson ND, et al. Acute respiratory distress syndrome: the Berlin definition. *JAMA.* 2012;307:2526-2533.

36. Finley CJ, et al. Angiotensin-converting enzyme inhibitor-induced angioedema: still unrecognized. *Am J Emerg Med.* 1992;10:550-552.

37. Flury KE, et al. Airway obstruction due to inhalation of ammonia. *Mayo Clin Proc.* 1983;58:389-393.

38. Frand UI, et al. Heroin-induced pulmonary edema. Sequential studies of pulmonary function. *Ann Intern Med.* 1972;77:29-35.

39. Frand UI, et al. Methadone-induced pulmonary edema. *Ann Intern Med.* 1972;76:975-979.

40. Freeth SJ. Lake Nyos disaster. *BMJ.* 1989;299:513.

41. Gargani L, Volpicelli G. How I do it: lung ultrasound. *Cardiovasc Ultrasound.* 2014;12:25.

42. Gill JR, et al. Environmental gas displacement: three accidental deaths in the workplace. *Am J Forensic Med Pathol.* 2002;23:26-30.

43. Girard TD, Bernard GR. Mechanical ventilation in ARDS: a state of the art review. *Chest.* 2007;131:921-929.

44. Glassroth J, et al. The impact of substance abuse on the respiratory system. *Chest.* 1987;91:596-602.

45. Glauser FL, et al. Ethchlorvynol (Placidyl)-induced pulmonary edema. *Ann Intern Med.* 1976;84:46-48.

46. Griffith DE, Levin JL. Respiratory effects of outdoor air pollution. *Postgrad Med.* 1989;86:111-116.

47. Halpern P, et al. Exposure to extremely high concentrations of carbon dioxide: a clinical description of a mass casualty incident. *Ann Emerg Med.* 2004;43:196-199.

48. Heffner JE, Sahn SA. Salicylate-induced pulmonary edema. Clinical features and prognosis. *Ann Intern Med.* 1981;95:405-409.

49. Henneberger PK, et al. Work-related reactive airways dysfunction syndrome cases from surveillance in selected US states. *J Occup Environ Med.* 2003;45:360-368.

50. Howland MA. Risks of parenteral deferoxamine for acute iron poisoning. *J Toxicol Clin Toxicol.* 1996;34:491-497.

51. Humbert VH Jr, et al. Noncardiogenic pulmonary edema complicating massive diltiazem overdose. *Chest.* 1991;99:258-259.

52. Hunter JM. New neuromuscular blocking drugs. *N Engl J Med.* 1995;332:1691-1699.

53. IL 682 Co-oximeter system operators manual [brochure]. Rev 5, November 2003.

54. Isbister GK, et al. Aspiration pneumonitis in an overdose-population: frequency, predictors, and outcomes. *Crit Care Med.* 2004;32:88-93.

55. Joseph WL, et al. Pulmonary and cardiovascular implications of drug addiction. *Ann Thorac Surg.* 1973;15:263-274.

56. Katz NM, et al. Venovenous extracorporeal membrane-oxygenation for noncardiogenic pulmonary edema after coronary bypass surgery. *Ann Thorac Surg.* 1988;46:462-464.

57. King WW, Cave DR. Use of esmolol to control autonomic instability of tetanus. *Am J Med.* 1991;91:425-428.

58. Klein MD. Noncardiogenic pulmonary edema following hydrochlorothiazide-ingestion. *Ann Emerg Med.* 1987;16:901-903.

59. Knochel JP. Neuromuscular manifestations of electrolyte disorders. *Am J Med.* 1982;72:521-535.

60. Kogevinas M, et al. Exposure to substances in the workplace and new-onset asthma: an international prospective population-based study (ECRHS-II). *Lancet.* 2007;370:336-341.

61. Kollef MH, Schuster DP. The acute respiratory distress syndrome. *N Engl J Med.* 1995;332:27-37.

62. Kulling P. Hospital treatment of victims exposed to combustion products. *Toxicol Lett.* 1992;64-65:283-289.

63. Lam S, Chan-Yeung M. Occupational asthma: natural history, evaluation and management. *Occup Med.* 1987;2:373-381.

64. Lambert JR, et al. Management of acute strychnine poisoning. *CMAJ.* 1981;124:1268-1270.

65. Lawn ND, et al. Anticipating mechanical ventilation in Guillain-Barré Syndrome. *Arch Neurol.* 2001;58:893-898.

66. Leach RM. Hyperbaric oxygen therapy. *BMJ.* 1998;317:1140-1143.

67. Leeman M. The pulmonary circulation in acute lung injury: a review of some recent advances. *Intensive Care Med.* 1991;17:254-260.

68. Levy SD, et al. High-Flow oxygen therapy and other inhaled therapies in intensive care units. *Lancet.* 2016;387:1867-1878.

69. Lichtenstein D, et al. Comparative diagnostic performances of auscultation, chest radiography, and lung ultrasonography in acute respiratory distress syndrome. *Anesthesiology.* 2004;100:9-15.

70. Lichtenstein D, Mézière G. Relevance of lung ultrasound in the diagnosis of acute respiratory failure. The BLUE-protocol. *Chest.* 2008;134:117-125.

71. Lichtenstein DA. BLUE-protocol and FALLS-protocol: two applications of lung ultrasound in the critically ill. *Chest.* 2015;147:1659-1670.

72. Little JW, Smith LH. Pulmonary aspiration. *West J Med.* 1979;131:122-129.

73. Livshits Z, et al. Falsely low carboxyhemoglobin level after hydroxocobalamin therapy. *N Engl J Med.* 2012;367:1270-1271.

74. Mahoney JJ, et al. Measurement of carboxyhemoglobin and total hemoglobin by five specialized spectrophotometers (CO-oximeters) in comparison with reference methods. *Clin Chem.* 1993;39:1693-1700.

75. Middleton PM, Davies SR. Noninvasive hemodynamic monitoring in the emergency department. *Curr Opin Crit Care.* 2011;17:342-350.

76. Mills CA, et al. Cardiovascular effects of fentanyl reversal by naloxone at varying arterial carbon dioxide tensions in dogs. *Anesth Analg.* 1988;67:730-736.

77. Minton NA, Murray VS. A review of organophosphate poisoning. *Med Toxicol Adverse Drug Exp.* 1988;3:350-375.

78. Moll J, et al. Incidence of aspiration pneumonia in intubated patients receiving activated charcoal. *J Emerg Med.* 1999;17:279-283.

79. Moshkovitz Y, et al. Recent developments in cardiac output determination by bioimpedance: comparison with invasive cardiac output and potential cardiovascular applications. *Curr Opin Cardiol.* 2004;19:229-237.

80. Nagler J, Krauss B. Capnography: a valuable tool for airway management. *Emerg Med Clin North Am.* 2008;26:881-897.

81. Neto AS, et al. Association between use of lung-protective ventilation with lower tidal volumes and clinical outcomes among patients without acute respiratory distress syndrome: a meta-analysis. *JAMA.* 2012;308:1651-1659.

82. Onyeama HP, Oehme FW. A literature review of paraquat toxicity. *Vet Hum Toxicol.* 1984;26:494-502.

83. Osei C, et al. Septic pulmonary infarction: clinical and radiographic manifestations in 11 patients. *Mt Sinai J Med.* 1979;46:145-148.

84. Pace R, et al. Effects of hydroxocobalamin on carboxyhemoglobin measured under physiologic and pathologic conditions. *Clin Toxicol (Phila).* 2014;52:647-650.

85. Pare JA, et al. Pulmonary "mainline" granulomatosis: talcosis of intravenous methadone abuse. *Medicine (Baltimore).* 1979;58:229-239.

86. Parsons PE. Respiratory failure as a result of drugs, overdoses, and poisonings. *Clin Chest Med.* 1994;15:93-102.

87. Pentiah P, et al. Interactions of morphine sulfate and sodium salicylate on respiration in cats. *J Pharmacol Exp Ther.* 1966;154:110-118.

88. Persky VW, Goldfrank LR. Methadone overdoses in a New York City hospital. *JACEP.* 1976;5:111-113.

89. Pollack C Jr, et al. Feasibility study of the use of bilevel positive airway pressure for respiratory support in the emergency department. *Ann Emerg Med.* 1996;27:189-192.

90. Pollack MM, et al. Aspiration of activated charcoal and gastric contents. *Ann Emerg Med.* 1981;10:528-529.

91. Reed CR, Glauser FL. Drug-induced noncardiogenic pulmonary edema. *Chest.* 1991;100:1120-1124.

92. Richards JR, et al. Doxapram reversal of suspected gamma-hydroxybutyrate-induced Coma. *Am J Emerg Med.* 2017;35:517.

93. Richards JR, et al. Treatment of ethanol poisoning and associated hypoventilation with doxapram. *Am J Emerg Med.* 2016;34:2253.e1-2253.e2.

94. Richards RK. Analeptics: pharmacologic background and clinical use in barbiturate poisoning. *Neurology.* 1959;4:228-233.

95. Roth D, et al. Accuracy of noninvasive multiwave pulse oximetry compared with carboxyhemoglobin from blood gas analysis in unselected emergency department patients. *Ann Emerg Med.* 2011;58:74-79.

96. Rubin RB, Neugarten J. Cocaine-associated asthma. *Am J Med.* 1990;88:438-439.

97. Schmidt-Nowara WW, et al. Early and late pulmonary complications of botulism. *Arch Intern Med.* 1983;143:451-456.

98. Senanayake N, Karalliedde L. Neurotoxic effects of organophosphorus insecticides. An intermediate syndrome. *N Engl J Med.* 1987;316:761-763.

99. Shakeri MS, et al. Which agents cause reactive airways dysfunction syndrome (RADS)? A systematic review. *Occup Med (Lond).* 2008;58:205-211.

100. Shesser R, et al. Pneumomediastinum and pneumothorax after inhaling alkaloidal cocaine. *Ann Emerg Med.* 1981;10:213-215.

101. Sklar J, Timms RM. Codeine-induced pulmonary edema. *Chest.* 1977;72:230-231.

102. Stern WZ. Roentgenographic aspects of narcotic addiction. *JAMA.* 1976;236:963-965.

103. Sun KO, et al. Management of tetanus: a review of 18 cases. *J R Soc Med.* 1994;87:135-137.

104. Thadani PV. NIDA conference report on cardiopulmonary complications of "crack" cocaine use. Clinical manifestations and pathophysiology. *Chest.* 1996;110:1072-1076.

105. Touger M, et al. Performance of the RAD-57 pulse co-oximeter compared with standard laboratory carboxyhemoglobin measurement. *Ann Emerg Med.* 2012;56:382-388.

106. Treacher DF, Leach RM. Oxygen transport-1. Basic principles. *BMJ.* 1998;317:1302-1306.

107. Vegfors M, Lennmarken C. Carboxyhaemoglobinaemia and pulse oximetry. *Br J Anaesth.* 1991;66:625-626.

108. Viglino D, et al. Noninvasive end tidal CO_2 is unhelpful in the prediction of complications in deliberate drug poisoning. *Ann Emerg Med.* 2016;68:62-70.

109. Vijayan VK, et al. Bronchoalveolar lavage study in victims of toxic gas leak at Bhopal. *Indian J Med Res.* 1989;90:407-414.

110. Vreman HJ, et al. Interference of fetal hemoglobin with the spectrophotometric measurement of carboxyhemoglobin. *Clin Chem.* 1988;34:975-977.

111. Wagner GR, Wegman DH. Occupational asthma: prevention by definition. *Am J Ind Med.* 1998;33:427-429.

112. Ware LB, Matthay MA. The acute respiratory distress syndrome. *N Engl J Med.* 2000;342:1334-1349.

113. Weil JV, et al. Diminished ventilatory response to hypoxia and hypercapnia after morphine in normal man. *N Engl J Med.* 1975;292:1103-1106.

114. Wetherill SF, et al. Acute renal failure associated with barium-chloride poisoning. *Ann Intern Med.* 1981;95:187-188.

115. Wiedemann HP, et al. National Heart, Lung, and Blood Institute Acute Respiratory Distress Syndrome (ARDS) Clinical Trials Network: comparison of two fluid-management strategies in acute lung injury. *N Engl J Med.* 2006;354:2564-2575.

116. Wiener MD, Putman CE. Pain in the chest in a user of cocaine. *JAMA.* 1987;258:2087-2088.

117. Williams AJ. ABC of oxygen: assessing and interpreting arterial blood gases and acid-base balance. *BMJ.* 1998;317:1213-1216.

118. Wimberley PD, et al. Accurate measurements of hemoglobin oxygen saturation, and fractions of carboxyhemoglobin and methemoglobin in fetal blood using radiometer OSM3: corrections for fetal hemoglobin fraction and pH. *Scand J Clin Lab Invest Suppl.* 1990;203:235-239.

119. Wolf SJ, et al. Clinical policy: critical issues in the evaluation and management of adult patients presenting to the emergency department with acute carbon monoxide poisoning. *Ann Emerg Med.* 2017;69:98-107.

120. Woodard ED, et al. Outbreak of hypersensitivity pneumonitis in an industrial setting. *JAMA.* 1988;259:1965-1969.

121. Zimmerman GA, Clemmer TP. Acute respiratory failure during therapy for salicylate intoxication. *Ann Emerg Med.* 1981;10:104-106.

29 THERMOREGULATORY PRINCIPLES

Susi U. Vassallo and Kathleen A. Delaney

Despite exposure to wide fluctuations of environmental temperatures, human body temperature is maintained within a narrow range.[16,120] Elevation or depression of body temperature occurs when (1) thermoregulatory mechanisms are overwhelmed by exposure to extremes of environmental heat or cold; (2) endogenous heat production is either inadequate, resulting in hypothermia, or exceeds the physiologic capacity for dissipation, resulting in hyperthermia; or (3) disease processes or xenobiotic effects interfere with normal thermoregulatory responses to heat or cold exposure.

METHODS OF HEAT TRANSFER

Heat is transferred to or away from the body through radiation, conduction, convection, and evaporation. *Radiation* involves the transfer of heat from an object to the environment and from warm objects in the environment to another object, for example, from the sun to a body. *Conduction* involves the transfer of heat to solid or liquid media in direct contact with the body. Water immersion conducts significant amounts of heat away from the body. This effect facilitates cooling in a swimming pool on a hot summer day and hypothermia despite moderate ambient temperatures when an individual is wet on a rainy day. The amount of heat lost through conduction and radiation depends on the temperature gradient between the skin and its surroundings; cutaneous blood flow; and insulation such as subcutaneous fat, hair, clothing.[134] In the respiratory tract, heat is lost by conduction to water vapor or gas. In animals unable to sweat, this represents the primary method of heat loss. The amount of heat lost through the respiratory tract depends on the temperature gradient between inspired air and the environment and the rate and depth of breathing.[134] *Convection* is the transfer of heat to the air surrounding the body. Wind velocity and ambient air temperature are the major determinants of convective heat loss. *Evaporation* is the process of vaporization of water, such as that in sweat. Large amounts of heat are dissipated from the skin during this process, resulting in cooling. Ambient temperature, rate of sweating, air velocity, and relative humidity are important factors in determining how much heat is lost through evaporation. On a very hot and humid day, sweat pours off an exercising person, rather than evaporating and initiating heat loss. In very warm environments, thermal gradients are reversed, leading to transfer of heat to the body by radiation, conduction, or convection.[143]

PHYSIOLOGY OF THERMOREGULATION

In a human not affected by xenobiotics or disease, stimulation of peripheral and hypothalamic temperature-sensitive neurons results in autonomic, somatic, and behavioral responses that lead to the dissipation or conservation of heat. Thermoregulation is the complex physiologic process that serves to maintain hypothalamic temperature within a narrow range of $98.6 \pm 0.8°F$ $(37 \pm 0.4°C)$, known as the *set point*.[120] This hypothalamic set point is influenced by factors such as diurnal variation, the menstrual cycle, and others. Maintaining, raising, or lowering the set point results in many outwardly visible physiologic manifestations of thermoregulation such as sweating, shivering, flushing, or panting. In the central nervous system (CNS), thermosensitive neurons are located predominantly in the preoptic area of the anterior hypothalamus, but to a lesser extent in the posterior hypothalamus. These neurons are divided into those that are hot, cold sensitive, or temperature insensitive. Approximately 30% of preoptic neurons are warm sensitive. These increase their firing rate during warming and decrease their firing rate during cooling.[28] Warming of the hypothalamus in conscious animals results in vasodilation, hyperventilation, salivation, and increases in evaporative water loss, as well as a reduction of cold-induced shivering

and vasoconstriction.[120] Cooling of the hypothalamus in conscious animals causes shivering, vasoconstriction, and increased metabolic rate even if the environment is hot.[113] How these temperature-sensitive neurons of the hypothalamus detect temperature changes and affect neuronal transmission is unclear. Altered action potential initiation and propagation caused by temperature-dependent membrane potential changes are associated with the ratios of Na^+ to Ca^{2+} that alter neuronal excitability and neurotransmitter release, or effect on the Na^+,K^+-ATPase (adenosine triphosphatase) pump.[134] Xenobiotics that increase intracellular cyclic adenosine monophosphate (cAMP) concentrations increase the thermosensitivity of warm-sensitive neurons.[28] In the brain stem, warm- and cold-sensitive neurons are located in the medullary reticular formation, where information from cutaneous receptors, spinal cord, and preoptic area of the anterior hypothalamus is integrated.[125]

The spinal cord is thermosensitive. Heat- and cold-sensitive ascending spinal impulses are conducted in the spinothalamic tract. As in the hypothalamus, local heating or cooling of the spinal cord results in thermoregulatory responses.[120] In addition to the hypothalamus, brain stem, and spinal cord, there is evidence of thermosensitivity in the deep abdominal viscera.[110,120,209] Intraabdominal heating or cooling results in thermoregulatory responses. Cold- and warm-sensitive afferent impulses are recorded from the splanchnic nerves in animals.[110,211] Finally, the skin also contains heat and cold thermosensitive neurons. Whereas cold receptors are free nerve endings that protrude into the basal epidermis, warm-sensitive receptors protrude into the dermis.[119,121] Cutaneous thermoreceptor output is affected by the absolute temperature of the skin, rate of temperature change, and area of stimulation.[120] Cutaneous cold receptors are A-δ and C nociceptor afferent fibers. A-δ fibers are small-diameter, thinly myelinated fibers that conduct at 5 to 30 m/sec, and C fibers are small-diameter, unmyelinated fibers that conduct at 0.5 to 2 m/sec.[115] Afferents from heat receptors are primarily C fibers. Cutaneous thermoreceptive neurons respond to external temperature change as well as rate of temperature change, sending early warning to the CNS via afferent impulses, allowing rapid and transient thermoregulatory responses before brain temperature changes (Fig. 29–1). It is important to emphasize that thermoregulatory responses as described above are affected by xenobiotics and disease processes.

Vasomotor and Sweat Gland Function

Vasomotor responses to thermoregulatory input differ according to location. The normal thermoregulatory response to heat stress is mediated primarily by heat-sensitive neurons in the hypothalamus. In healthy individuals without impairment of vasodilatory mechanisms by xenobiotics, active vasodilation in the extremities occurs under noradrenergic control; increasing sympathetic stimulation results in vasoconstriction, and decreasing sympathetic stimulation results in vasodilation. Vasodilation in the head, trunk, and proximal limbs is not a result of decreased sympathetic tone; instead, it is a result of an active process involving the central nervous system and the peripheral cholinergic sudomotor nerves and the local effects of temperature on venomotor tone. Sweat glands release local transmitters, such as vasoactive intestinal polypeptide (VIP) or bradykinins, and vasodilation results. Areas of the body such as the forehead, where sweating is most prominent during heat stress, correspond to areas where active vasodilation is greatest. The neurotransmitters involved in the regulation of relationships between vasodilation and sweating as a response to heat stress are not fully elucidated in humans, but animal evidence suggests the presence of specific vasodilator nerves.[120]

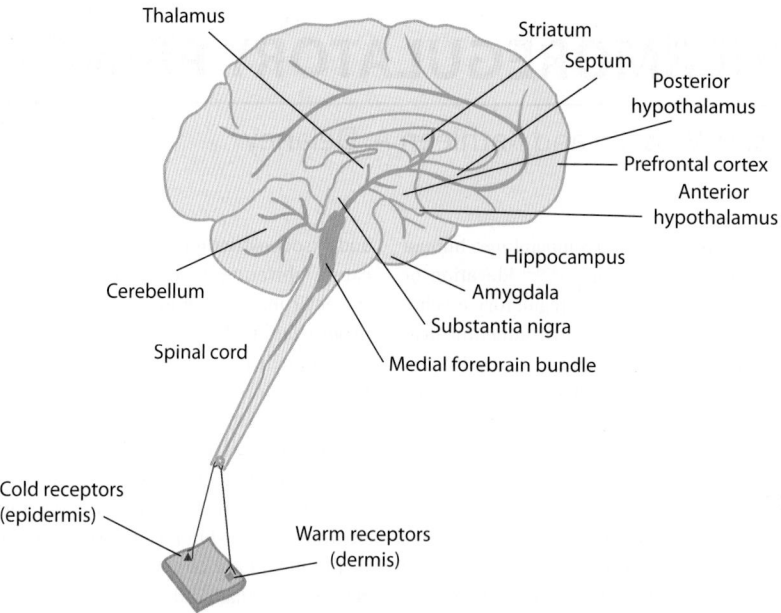

FIGURE 29–1. A representation of the response of cutaneous thermoreceptive neurons to external temperature change as an early warning to the central nervous system.

Sweat glands are controlled by postganglionic nerve fibers, which are cholinergic, and large amounts of acetylcholinesterase as well as other peptides modulate neural transmission.[125,126]

Neurotransmitters and Thermoregulation

The neurotransmitters involved in thermoregulation include serotonin, norepinephrine, acetylcholine, dopamine, prostaglandins, β-endorphins, and intrinsic hypothalamic peptides such as arginine vasopressin, adrenocorticotropic hormone (ACTH) thyrotropin-releasing hormone (TRH), and melanocyte-stimulating hormone (MSH).[50,199] Studies on the effects of individual neurotransmitters in thermoregulation yield contradictory results, depending on the animal species and the route of administration of the exogenous neurotransmitter. However, epidemiologic studies demonstrate that patients taking xenobiotics affecting these neurotransmitters are at greater risk for heat illness. In the laboratory, refinements in techniques of microinjection of neurotransmitters into the hypothalamus of animals, rather than intraventricular instillation, have elucidated microanatomic sites where neurotransmitters are active. More research is needed, however, because interspecies variations and theoretical differences in response to exogenous versus endogenous peptides make this area of study complex. There is ample clinical and epidemiologic evidence that xenobiotics that affect the neurotransmitters listed above influence the ability to thermoregulate.

Apomorphine is a mixed dopamine agonist that causes hypothermia in animals; studies using selective D_1- and D_2-receptor agonists and antagonists demonstrate the hypothermic effect of apomorphine as a result of its effects on D_2 receptors, with some modulation by D_1 receptors in the hypothalamus.[179] Stimulation of D_2 receptors mediate the hypothermia induced by the peptide sauvagine.[30] Stimulation of D_3 by specific agonists caused hypothermia in an animal model.[180,181] The link between dopamine D_2 receptors and norepinephrine receptors in the hypothalamus leads to vasodilation and hypothermia. The effect of clozapine in producing hypothermia in rats is caused by D_1 and D_3 stimulation.[180,220] Lesser-known peptides are also involved in thermoregulation. For example, neuropeptide Y is an amino acid neurotransmitter that occurs in high concentrations in the preoptic area of the anterior hypothalamus. Administration of neuropeptide Y caused a reduction in core temperature when administered with adrenergic receptor antagonists such as prazosin, an α_1-adrenergic antagonist; propranolol, a β-adrenergic antagonist; and clonidine, a central α_2-adrenergic agonist.[84,218] Temperature regulation is complicated as both central and peripheral mechanisms are involved. The results of studies of temperature changes induced in animal models by the administration of xenobiotics frequently vary depending on the ambient temperature at which the experiment is performed, and on the species of animal. The α_2-adrenergic agonist clonidine induced a dose-dependent significant increase in temperature of rats kept at high ambient temperature. This effect was mediated by the α_2-adrenergic postsynaptic receptors. The administration of an α_1-adrenergic antagonist and a central α_2-adrenergic agonist reduced the rise in temperature. The β_2-adrenergic agonist clenbuterol-induced hyperthermia is mediated by β-adrenergic receptors. However, the hyperthermic effect of clenbuterol may result from secondary α_2-adrenergic agonist stimulation centrally, perhaps from the norepinephrine release that results from β-adrenergic stimulation. In support of this is that the α_2-adrenergic antagonists block the increase in temperature caused by clenbuterol.[184]

Studies on muscarinic receptors demonstrate involvement of muscarinic M_2 and M_3 receptors in the production of hypothermia when agonists to these receptors are administered centrally.[221] Blockers of ATP-sensitive K^+ channels can reverse the effect of cholinomimetic drugs in producing hypothermia.[206]

XENOBIOTIC EFFECTS ON THERMOREGULATION

Many xenobiotics have pharmacologic effects that interfere with thermoregulatory responses (Tables 29–1 and 29–2).[168,170,252] α-Adrenergic agonists prevent vasodilation in response to heat stress. Increased endogenous heat production in the setting of increased motor activity occurs during exercise and also occurs in patients manifesting cocaine or amphetamine toxicity. Life-threatening hyperthermia is associated with the use of these xenobiotics. Whereas adrenergic antagonists and calcium channel blockers diminish the cardiac reserve available to compensate for heat-induced vasodilation, diuretics decrease cardiac reserve through their effects on intravascular volume.[63] β-Adrenergic antagonists also interfere with the capacity to maintain normothermia under conditions of cold stress, possibly related to their interference with the mobilization of substrates required for thermogenesis.[170] Opioids and diverse sedative–hypnotics depress hypothalamic function and predispose to hypothermia.[85] Carbon monoxide poisoning must also be considered in hypothermic patients. Organic phosphorus compounds and other xenobiotics that cause cholinergic stimulation cause hypothermia by stimulation of inappropriate sweating and possibly through depression of the endogenous use of calorigenic substrates.[170] Xenobiotics with anticholinergic effects decrease sweating and predispose to hyperthermia, which is of particular concern during environmental heat exposure or exercise.

TABLE 29–1	Effects of Xenobiotics That Predispose to Hyperthermia

I. Impaired cutaneous heat loss
- A. Vasoconstriction through α-adrenergic stimulation
  - Amphetamines
  - Cocaine
  - Ephedrine
  - Phenylpropanolamine
  - Pseudoephedrine
- B. Sweat gland dysfunction
  - Antihistamines
  - Antimuscarinics
  - Cyclic antidepressants
  - Topiramate
  - Zonisamide

II. Myocardial depression
- A. Decreased cardiac output
  - Antidysrhythmics
  - β-Adrenergic antagonists
  - Calcium channel blockers
- B. Reduced cardiac filling by salt and water depletion
  - Diuretics
  - Ethanol

III. Hypothalamic depression
- Antipsychotics

IV. Impaired behavioral response
- Cocaine
- Ethanol
- Opioids
- Phencyclidine
- Sedative–hypnotics

V. Uncoupling of oxidative phosphorylation
- Dinitrophenol
- Pentachlorophenol
- Salicylates

VI. Increased muscle activity through agitation, seizures, or rigidity
- Amphetamines
- Caffeine
- Cocaine
- Isoniazid
- Lithium
- Monoamine oxidase inhibitors
- Phencyclidine
- Serotonin toxicity
- Strychnine
- Thyroid hormone excess

VII. Dystonia
- Antipsychotics
- Neuroleptic Malignant Syndrome (NMS)

VIII. Withdrawal
- Dopamine agonists
- Ethanol
- Sedative–hypnotics

TABLE 29–2	Effects of Xenobiotics That Predispose to Hypothermia

Impaired nonshivering thermogenesis
- β-Adrenergic antagonists
- Cholinergics
- Hypoglycemics

Impaired perception of cold
- Carbon monoxide
- Ethanol
- Hypoglycemics
- Opioids
- Sedative–hypnotics

Impaired shivering by hypothalamic depression
- Antipsychotics
- Carbon monoxide
- Ethanol
- General anesthetics
- Opioids
- Sedative–hypnotics

Impaired vasoconstriction
- α-Adrenergic antagonists
- Antipsychotics
- Ethanol

to the antidopamine effect. Effects on cold tolerance are attributed to their α-adrenergic antagonist effects, which prevent vasoconstriction in response to cold stress.[169] In addition, hyperthermia associated with severe extrapyramidal rigidity occurs in patients taking antipsychotics.[161] This rigidity is attributed to the dopamine-blocking effects of this class of drugs.

The Effects of Ethanol

Ethanol is the xenobiotic most commonly related to the occurrence of hypothermia by virtue of its effects on CNS depression, vasodilation, and blunting of behavioral responses to cold. However, thermoregulatory dysfunction associated with ethanol intoxication is undoubtedly more complex.

In animal models, ethanol leads to hypothermia, the extent of which is partly dependent on ambient temperature.[194,212,213] In mice, as the dose of ethanol increased, body temperature decreased, and the rate of this decline in body temperature was faster at higher ethanol doses.[190] The decline in body temperature could be reversed by increasing ambient temperature; increasing ambient temperature to 96.8°F (36°C) caused an immediate rise in the body temperature.[190] The poikilothermic effect of ethanol was not a result of hypoglycemia. Poikilothermia is the variation in body temperature greater than ±3.6°F (±2°C) on exposure to environmental temperature changes. Rats treated with equipotent amounts of pentobarbital showed the same effects on body temperature as rats treated with ethanol, suggesting a similar central mechanism of CNS depression resulting in altered thermoregulation.[190]

Numerous mechanisms are involved in the ethanol-induced depression of CNS function.[215] Genetic factors influence the role of ethanol in the production of hypothermia. Mice are selectively bred for genetic sensitivity or insensitivity to acute ethanol-induced hypothermia, and the differences appear to be mediated by the serotonergic systems.[86,100,185,190] Cyclo His-Pro DKP, another neurotransmitter that is found in many animal species, acts at the preoptic-anterior hypothalamus to modulate body temperature. Exogenous administration of this neuropeptide produced a dose-dependent decrease in ethanol-induced hypothermia. Attenuation of hypothermia resulted from passive immunization with Cyclo His-Pro DKP antibody.[37,130] Ethanol effects appears to be mediated through modulation of endogenous opioid peptides because high-dose (10 mg/kg) naloxone reverses ethanol-induced hypothermia in animals.[202]

Pharmacokinetic characteristics of ethanol metabolism change in the presence of hypothermia. Hypothermic piglets infused with ethanol showed slower ethanol metabolism and a smaller volume of distribution (V_d) and, as

Phenothiazines appear to interfere with normal response to both heat and cold. Severe hyperthermia associated with the absence of sweating is frequently described in patients using phenothiazines and is a consequence of their anticholinergic effects.[222,264] In addition, phenothiazines have central effects interfering with the hypothalamus, commonly although incompletely attributed

a result, higher ethanol concentrations than normothermic control piglets. Ethanol elimination and metabolism decreased as temperature fell.[148]

Tolerance develops to the effect of ethanol-induced hypothermia in all species.[88,194] The degree of tolerance is proportional to the dose and duration of treatment with ethanol and is not explained by the increased rate of metabolism with chronic exposure.[134] Age is a factor in the development of tolerance; older animals do not display the same degree of tolerance to the hypothermic effects of chronic ethanol administration as do younger animals.[187,202,262] The development of tolerance to ethanol-induced hypothermia is affected by genetic factors. Experimentally, tolerance to ethanol-induced hypothermia increases the incorporation of certain amino acids into proteins in the rat brain. The formation of new proteins in ethanol-tolerant rats suggests stimulation of gene expression associated with ethanol tolerance.[134,255] Upregulation of the in N-methyl-D-aspartate (NMDA) receptors are also implicated in the development of ethanol tolerance. In addition, altered nicotinamide adenine dinucleotide (NADH) oxidation to NAD$^+$, diminishes blood flow to the liver, or slows metabolism through the microsomal enzyme system.[215]

Hypothermia alters the breath–ethanol partition in the alveolus, and the temperature of expired breath alters breath–ethanol analysis results. In patients with mild hypothermia, breath–ethanol analysis results in lower values by 7.3% per degree centigrade (or 1.8°F) decrease in body temperature.[91] Whether breath–ethanol analysis is also affected by hyperthermia remains to be studied.[91]

DISEASE PROCESSES AND THERMOREGULATION

Many disease processes interfere with normal thermoregulation, limiting an individual's capacity to prevent hypothermia or hyperthermia. Extensive dermatologic disease or cutaneous burns impair sweating and vasomotor responses to heat stress.[34] Patients with autonomic disturbances secondary to diabetes mellitus or peripheral vascular disease also have altered vasomotor responses that impair vasodilation and sweating.[236] Extensive surgical dressings preclude the evaporation of sweat in an otherwise normal patient. Heat-stressed persons with poor cardiac reserve and lower cardiac output are not able to sustain skin blood flow rates high enough to maintain normothermia.[77,240] Intense motor activity leads to excessive heat production in all patients, particularly those with Parkinson disease or hyperthyroidism. Patients with agitated delirium or seizures also have significantly elevated rates of endogenous heat production. Hypothalamic injury caused by cerebrovascular accidents, trauma, or infection disturb thermoregulation.[76,165] Hypothalamic dysfunction leads to high, unremitting fevers and insufficient stimulation of heat loss mechanisms such as sweating. Hypothalamic damage predisposes to hypothermia by interference with centrally mediated heat conservation.[76,165,223,224] Fever, the normal response to stimulation of the hypothalamus by pyrogens, results in an elevated physiologic temperature set point and is a disadvantage in the heat-stressed individual[120] (Table 29–3).

HYPOTHERMIA

Epidemiology

Hypothermia is defined as a lowering of the core body temperature to below 95°F (<35°C). Between 2003 and 2013, there were 13,419 hypothermia-related deaths for the United States overall. The Centers for Disease Control and Prevention defines these deaths as those with an underlying or contributing cause of death from exposure to excessive natural cold[45] (Table 29–3).

Alaska, Montana, Wyoming, and New Mexico had the greatest overall death rates from hypothermia. States with milder climates and rapid fluctuations in temperature, such as North and South Carolina, and western states, such as Arizona, with high elevations and cold nighttime temperatures also report hypothermia-related deaths.[44]

Response to Cold

The normal physiologic response to cold is initiated by stimulation of cold-sensitive neurons in the skin, so that the onset of the body response to cold occurs before cooling of central blood. Cold-sensitive neurons in the skin send afferent impulses to the hypothalamus, resulting in shivering and

TABLE 29–3	Factors Predisposing to Hypothermia
Advanced age	**Immobilization**
Decreased ability to shiver	Central nervous system dysfunction illness
Decreased metabolic rate	Spinal cord injury
Decreased temperature discrimination	Trauma
Reduced peripheral blood flow	**Medical Diseases**
Central nervous system depression	Hepatic failure
Cerebrovascular accident	Sepsis
Ethanol	Uremia
Hypothalamic dysfunction	**Nutritional**
Infection	Glycogen depletion
Xenobiotics, diverse	Hypoglycemia
Endocrine	Starvation
Adrenal insufficiency	Thiamine deficiency
Diabetic ketoacidosis	**Social**
Hyperosmolar coma	Failure to use indoor heating
Hypopituitarism	Homelessness
Hypothyroidism	Inadequate indoor heating
Environmental	Poverty
Homelessness	Social isolation
Unintentional exposure to	

piloerection. Shivering is the main thermoregulatory response to cold in humans, except in neonates, in whom nonshivering thermogenesis prevails. Shivering is initiated in the posterior hypothalamus when impulses from cold-sensitive thermoreceptors are integrated in the anterior hypothalamus and communicated to the posterior hypothalamus or when cold-sensitive neurons in the posterior hypothalamus are activated directly. Efferent stimuli from the posterior hypothalamus travel through the midbrain tegmentum, pons, and lateral medullary reticular formation to the motor pathways of the tectospinal and rubrospinal tracts, resulting in shivering.[19] A mechanism of stimulation of shivering that usually occurs later when core temperature drops is the local cooling of the spinal cord, which leads to shivering by increasing excitability of motor neurons.

Heat produced without muscle contraction is known as nonshivering thermogenesis.[32,120] Nonshivering thermogenesis is mediated by the sympathetic nervous system.[54] Catecholamines activate adenyl cyclase, increasing cAMP, resulting in mobilization of fat and glucose stores (β-adrenergic receptors).[171,217] Nonshivering thermogenesis is blocked by α-adrenergic receptor antagonism and increased by administration of norepinephrine. Brown adipose tissue is the most important site of nonshivering thermogenesis. In humans, brown fat is found primarily in neonates, although in cold-acclimatized people, small amounts are found on autopsy.[32] Brown adipose tissue functions as a thermoregulatory effector organ, producing heat by the oxidation of fatty acids when the tissue is stimulated by norepinephrine.[36]

In addition to shivering and nonshivering thermogenesis, efferent sympathetic fibers from the hypothalamus stimulate peripheral vasoconstriction (α-adrenergic receptors). Piloerection and vasoconstriction result in decreased heat loss from the body. Intense vasoconstriction shunts blood away from the periphery to the core and antidiuretic hormone antagonism results in increased urine output and hemoconcentration.

Several disease processes commonly result in an inability to maintain a normal body temperature in a cool environment (Table 29–3).[65,163]

Underlying Illness in Hypothermia

Evaluations to determine the presence of underlying diseases are often difficult in a patient with hypothermia.[67,89,163] The mental status is not usually significantly abnormal until the temperature falls below 90°F (32.2°C). If normal mental status is not regained when the temperature reaches 90°F (32.2°C) during rewarming, underlying CNS structural, toxic, or metabolic problems

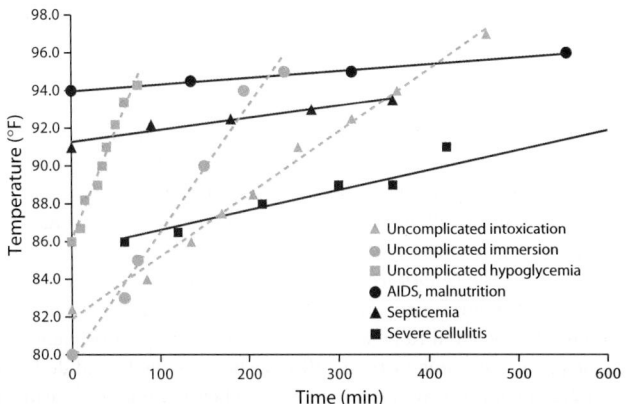

FIGURE 29-2. Relation of rewarming rate to underlying illness. *(Reproduced with permission from Delaney KA, Vassallo SU, Larkin GL, et al. Rewarming rates in urban patients with hypothermia: prediction of underlying infection. Acad Emerg Med, 2006 Sep;13(9):913-921.)*

are probable.[67,89,163,207] Failure of the patient to rewarm quickly suggests the presence of underlying disease[67] (Fig. 29-2). In one study, whereas hypothermic patients without underlying disease are reported to rewarm at a rate of 1.0°F/h to 3.7°F/h (0.6°C/h–2.1°C/h) (average, 2.1°F/h; 1.2°C/h), patients with significant underlying disease (sepsis, gastrointestinal hemorrhage, diabetic ketoacidosis, pulmonary embolus, myocardial infarction) warmed at a rate of 0.25°F/h to 1.8°F/h (0.1°C/h–1.0°C/h) (average, 1°F/h; 0.6°C/h).[67,258]

Alteration of Pharmacology in Hypothermia

The pharmacology of certain xenobiotics is altered in the setting of hypothermia. In hypothermic piglets, the V_d and the clearance of fentanyl are decreased.[149] Similarly, in piglets given gentamicin, the V_d and clearance rate decreased in direct proportion to the decrease in cardiac output and glomerular filtration rate (GFR).[147] Hypothermic puppies given intravenous (IV) lidocaine showed slower rates of disappearance of the drug than when normothermic.[186] Humans and animals given propranolol showed a reduced V_d and decreased total body clearance, resulting in higher than expected propranolol concentrations.[175,176,192] Decreased hepatic metabolism of propranolol during hypothermia is demonstrated in vitro.[176] Hypothermia prolongs neuromuscular blockade with *d*-tubocurarine[111] and increases neuromuscular blockade with suxamethonium.[262] Phenobarbital metabolism and V_d decreased with hypothermia in children.[133] The lethal dose of digoxin was doubled in hypothermic dogs.[17] Digoxinlike substances are present during hypothermia.[124]

Reasons for altered metabolism in hypothermia include delayed distribution of the drug and altered enzyme function with temperature and pH changes. Cardiac output decreases, leading to decreased liver perfusion and decreased delivery of drug to hepatic microsomal enzymes.[111,136-138,200] Plasma volume decreases as free water moves intracellularly, causing hemoconcentration and further decreasing organ perfusion.[112] Biliary excretion of atropine, procaine, and sulfanilamide decreases in vitro.[136-138] In vitro, the activity of metabolic pathways, including acetylation and hydrolysis, decrease with cooling.[136,137]

These same metabolic changes occur in therapeutic hypothermia. Hypothermia is induced for its neuroprotective effects but requires attention to alterations in pharmacokinetics and pharmacodynamics of xenobiotics administered during hypothermia. Physiological changes during induced hypothermia are similar to those of unintentional hypothermia and include slowed enzymatic reactions, vasoconstriction, decreased-cardiac output, and hemoconcentration. Studies support a decrease in the V_d of pancuronium, midazolam, morphine, and gentamicin.[64] Clearance of xenobiotics is affected by organ perfusion, enzyme activity, and xenobiotic characteristics such as the degree of protein binding and the pK_a. Hepatic and renal clearance is affected by regional blood flow, which is decreased during hypothermia. In general, the decrease in the V_d and the decrease in clearance

result in increased serum xenobiotic concentrations.[64] Experimental studies in animals demonstrate a 25% increase in fentanyl concentrations at a core temperature of 32°C.[92] Concurrent-supportive modalities during hypothermia such as cardiopulmonary bypass or extracorporeal membrane oxygenation (ECMO) further alter the kinetics of xenobiotics during hypothermia.[260] In neonates, asphyxia treated with induced hypothermia presents the additional complication of rapidly changing neonatal physiology and the effects of supportive measures such as ECMO.[64]

Clinical Findings

The clinical effects of hypothermia are related to the membrane depressant effects of cold, which result in ionic and electrical conduction disturbances in the brain, heart, peripheral nerves, and other major organs[123] (Table 29-4). Cold tissues are protected by decreases in tissue oxygen requirements. As body temperature decreases, metabolic activity declines at a rate of approximately 7% per 1.8°F (1°C).[263] This effect provides significant protection to vital organs despite the potentially deleterious effects of membrane suppression.

Effects on the CNS are temperature dependent. However, predicting the temperature of the patient based on the clinical presentation is unreliable.[31,33,71] The patient with mild hypothermia (90°F–95°F; 32.2°C–35°C) may have a relatively normal clinical appearance. Ataxia, clumsiness, slowed response to stimuli, and dysarthria are common.[89] As cooling continues, the mental status

TABLE 29-4	Physiologic and Clinical Manifestations of Hypothermia

Cardiovascular
Normal, decreased, or increased cardiac output
Normal heart rate or tachycardia 20 to shivering, then bradycardia as severity of hypothermia increases
Vasoconstriction and central shunting of blood

Electrocardiogram
Prolongation of intervals (PR, QRS and QT)
Atrial fibrillation
Increased ventricular irritability
J-point elevation ("Osborn waves")

Central nervous system
Mild: 90°F–95°F (32°C–35°C)
    Normal mental status or slightly slowed
Moderate: 80°F–90°F (27°C–32°C)
    Lethargic but verbally responsive
Severe: 68°F–80°F (20°C–27°C)
    Unlikely to respond verbally or purposefully to noxious stimuli
Profound: <68°F (<20°C)
    Unresponsive; appears dead

Gastrointestinal tract
Decreased motility
Depressed hepatic metabolism

Hematologic
Hemoconcentration
Left shift of oxyhemoglobin dissociation curve

Kidneys
Cold-induced diuresis (antidiuretic hormone antagonism)

Lungs
Hyperventilation to hypoventilation with increasing hypothermia
Bronchorrhea

Metabolic
Metabolic acidosis
Increased glycogenolysis
Increased serum free fatty acids
Normal thyroid and adrenal function

slowly deteriorates. In moderate hypothermia (80°F–90°F; 27°C–32.2°C), the patient is usually lethargic but still likely to respond verbally. In severe hypothermia (68°F–80°F; 20°C–26.6°C), the patient is unlikely to respond verbally but will react purposefully to noxious stimuli.[89,116] With profound hypothermia (<68°F; <20°C), the patient is unresponsive to stimuli. The patient "appears dead".[116] However, standard criteria for brain death do not apply to hypothermic patients. The hypothermia itself protects against cerebral hypoxic damage.[123] Temperature drop inhibits the release of the excitatory neurotransmitter glutamate and attenuates the release of dopamine in animal models of brain ischemia, suggesting a protective effect of hypothermia in brain injury.[39] Cerebrospinal fluid (CSF) glutamate concentrations were lower in patients showing benefit from mild induced hypothermia after brain injury compared with brain-injured patients kept normothermic.[173]

Patients have survived with body temperatures as low as 48.2°F (9°C).[93] Vigorous resuscitation is required for these patients. This approach leads to hours of cardiopulmonary resuscitation (CPR) of hypothermic patients with ventricular fibrillation, ventricular tachycardia, or asystole but is sometimes successful in resuscitating patients initially presumed to be dead.[238]

For field rescue work, the Swiss distinguish between 5 stages of hypothermia and provide guidelines for rescue in dangerous environmental conditions. These stages are based on the degree of consciousness, the presence or absence of shivering, cardiac activity, and core temperature.[33,75] The adage that a patient cannot be considered dead until the patient is warm and dead is further refined by the Swiss guidelines for field rescue attempts under avalanche conditions.

The cardiac and hemodynamic effects of cold correlate closely with body temperature. As cooling begins, there is a transient increase in cardiac output. Tachycardia develops secondary to shivering and sympathetic stimulation. At about 81°F (27.2°C), shivering ceases. Bradycardia develops with maintenance of a normal cardiac stroke volume.[35,67] This bradycardia is responsible for the decreased myocardial oxygen demand, which is protective in the setting of hypothermia.[35] In profound hypothermia, bradycardia may progress to asystole and death.

Unlike cerebral circulation, where autoregulation is preserved during cooling, coronary autoregulation is disturbed during hypothermia, and the myocardium is at risk of compromise.[142] Attempts to maximize myocardial oxygenation through administration of oxygen and volume replacement to increase diastolic filling pressures are recommended.

The initial response to cold is hyperventilation; however, as temperature continues to decrease, hypoventilation develops, which infrequently progresses to apnea and death. In animal models, this is attributed to cold-induced failure of phrenic nerve conduction.[142]

The Cardiac Rhythm Disturbances

The most common electrocardiographic (ECG) abnormality in hypothermia is generalized, progressive depression of myocardial conduction. The PR, QRS, and QT intervals all prolong, and increasingly profound hypothermia leads to gradual progression to asystole.[74,251] Ventricular fibrillation occurs in an irritable myocardium most commonly at temperatures less than 86°F (30°C), resulting in a high O_2 consumption dysrhythmia. Atrial fibrillation is the most common dysrhythmia occurring in the presence of hypothermia.[90,201,253] Shivering is not always clinically evident, but the characteristic fine muscular tremor frequently produces a mechanical artifact in the baseline of the ECG.[78] A deflection occurring at the junction of the QRS and ST segment is invariably present in patients with temperatures <86°F (<30°C) (Fig. 29–3). First described in a single patient in 1938, the J-point deflection is commonly known as the *Osborn wave*.[79,203,247] The J-point deflection, thought to be a "current of injury" associated with CO_2 retention under hypothermic conditions, was believed to be a poor prognostic sign.[203] Subsequent study does not support any prognostic significance because the J-point deflection is invariably found in hypothermic patients when multiple ECG leads are obtained.[78,79,201,249,253] The size of the J-point deflection increases as body temperature decreases.[219,282] Atrial dysrhythmias that occur in the absence of underlying heart disease invariably disappear solely with rewarming.

Management

After blood specimens are drawn, the hypothermic patient in whom hypoglycemia is present should be given 0.5 to 1.0 g of dextrose/kg of body weight as $D_{50}W$ (50% dextrose in water in adults or $D_{20}W$ or $D_{10}W$ as appropriate for children) and at least 100 mg of IV thiamine. If hypoglycemia is the cause of the hypothermia, the response to dextrose is usually dramatic, heralded by the onset of shivering and rapid return to normal body temperature. Wernicke encephalopathy is uncommon but is associated with mild hypothermia; thermoregulation and normal ocular motion typically returns after the initiation of thiamine therapy.[57]

Hypothermia shifts the oxygen dissociation curve to the left (Chap. 28), resulting in decreased oxygen unloading to tissues; therefore, oxygen administration is reasonable.[66] If clinically indicated, endotracheal intubation should be performed for airway protection or inadequate ventilation or oxygenation.[60] However, there are rare case reports of ventricular fibrillation occurring during endotracheal intubation.[14,99,116,204] Every effort should be made to limit patient activity and stimulation during the acute rewarming period because activity increases myocardial oxygen demand or alters myocardial temperature gradients, increasing the risk of iatrogenic ventricular fibrillation. Although pulmonary artery catheters and central venous lines are typically inserted in clinically unstable patients they should be avoided unless absolutely essential so as not to precipitate ventricular dysrhythmias.[114,157,248] If a central venous catheter is considered necessary, it should not be allowed to touch the endocardium.[250] Patients who develop ventricular fibrillation or asystole are difficult to manage because of the many supportive therapies required at once and the often lengthy resuscitation efforts. In these instances, CPR should be initiated and the patient intubated and ventilated to maintain a pH of 7.40, uncorrected for temperature.[66] Active internal rewarming (see later discussion) should be instituted in the

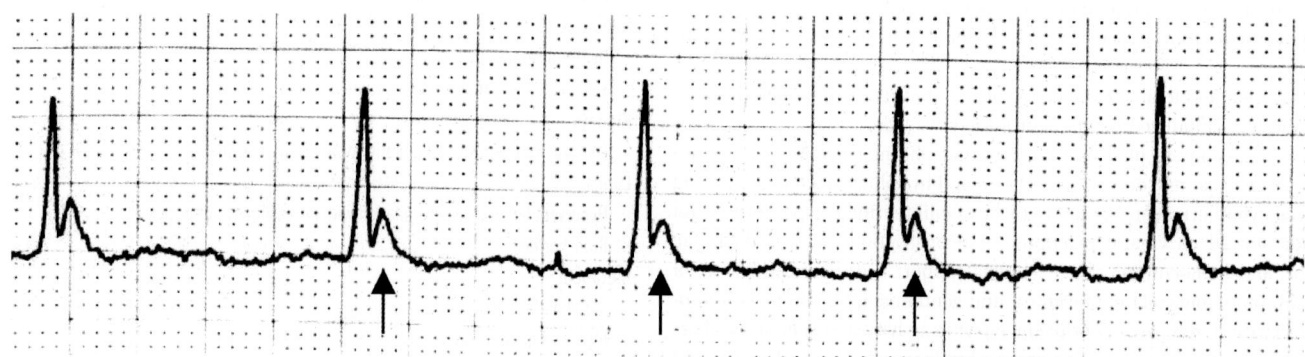

FIGURE 29–3. A characteristic electrocardiographic finding in a patient with profound hypothermia. The terminal phase of the QRS complex shows a typical elevation of the J-point Osborn wave (↑). *(Adapted from the research performed by Susi Vassallo, MD and Kathleen A. Delaney, MD.)*

patient in cardiac arrest because standard therapy for ventricular fibrillation or asystole are often unsuccessful until rewarming is achieved. There is a risk of toxicity if multiple doses of drugs are administered in the hypothermic patient in whom drug metabolism is altered and circulation is arrested. However, based on current research discussed later, it is reasonable to incorporate pharmacotherapy into the management of hypothermic cardiac arrest. A vasopressor, either epinephrine or vasopressin, is reasonable to increase the coronary perfusion pressure. Amiodarone or lidocaine should be administered if ventricular fibrillation is present. Defibrillation in humans is often not successful until the temperature exceeds 86°F (30°C); however, defibrillation can be successfully accomplished in animals and patients with temperatures of less than 86°F (30°C).[6,14,61,261] A reasonable approach is that if defibrillation is unsuccessful below 86°F (30°C), defibrillation should not be attempted again until the patient is warmed several degrees centigrade. Pneumatically powered devices capable of mechanical chest compression and cardiopulmonary bypass are appropriate and safe during prolonged hypothermic cardiopulmonary arrests.[14,53,239,248]

Arterial Blood Gas Physiochemistry in Hypothermia

Assessment of the adequacy of ventilation and oxygenation in the hypothermic patient often poses a dilemma to clinicians because the chemical effects of cold on arterial pH and blood gases lead to confusion in the interpretation of arterial blood gas values. Cold inhibits the dissociation of water molecules, causing pH to increase as cooling occurs. In vitro, the pH change of blood as it is cooled increases parallel to the pH change of neutral water. The partial pressures of CO_2 and O_2 decrease as cooling occurs even as the blood content of those gases remains unchanged. Blood in a syringe taken from a patient whose body temperature is 98.6°F (37°C) yields a pH of 7.40 and a PCO_2 of 40 mm Hg in the blood gas machine at 98.6°F (37°C) but yields a pH of 7.72 and a PCO_2 of 14 mm Hg if the blood is cooled to 61°F (16°C) and the values are measured at that temperature. Specially calibrated laboratory equipment, not routinely available, is required to measure blood gas values directly at other than normal body temperature. A patient whose body temperature is 61°F (16°C) and whose actual in vivo blood gas values are a pH of 7.72 and PCO_2 of 14 mm Hg will have a pH of 7.40 and PCO_2 of 40 mm Hg when the blood is warmed to 98.6°F (37°C) and measured in the standard laboratory blood gas machine. Because the machine measures pH and blood gas pressures only in blood warmed to 98.6°F (37°C) (the uncorrected values), the actual in vivo values in hypothermic patients can be approximated using mathematically derived corrected values. Because the pH of neutrality has also increased, it is unclear what clinical meanings these corrected values have. The uncorrected values indicate what the pH and PCO_2 would be if the patient were normothermic. At first glance, the clinician might be content to learn that a hypothermic patient at 61°F (16°C) has a corrected pH of 7.47 and PCO_2 of 40 mm Hg. However, the uncorrected values in the blood gas machine at 98.6°F (37°C) of pH of 7.18 and PCO_2 of 111 mm Hg indicate that the patient has a significant respiratory acidosis. Attempts to maintain a corrected pH of 7.40 will lead to hypoventilation and risk alveolar collapse and impairment of oxygenation. The preponderance of evidence in the anesthesia and cardiovascular surgery literature suggests that maintenance of ventilation is associated with a decreased incidence of myocardial injury and a decreased incidence of ventricular fibrillation.[66] Thus, the pH and PCO_2 blood gas values should be left uncorrected after the blood sample is warmed in the blood gas machine and interpreted in the same way as in a normothermic patient.[66]

Hypotension

When hypotension occurs in a patient with hypothermia, it is possibly a result of the presence of bradycardia and volume depletion. However, hypotension is a predictor of infection, particularly when associated with a slow rewarming rate.[67] In hypothermia, salt and water depletion occurs as a result of a variety of mechanisms, including central shunting of blood by vasoconstriction and cold-induced diuresis. Cold diuresis occurs when increases in central blood volume result in inhibition of the release of antidiuretic

hormone. Impairment of renal enzyme activity and decreased renal tubular reabsorption contribute to the large quantities of dilute urine known as cold diuresis.[112,116,157,263] An infusion of 0.9% NaCl should be given to expand intravascular volume. Urine output is an important indicator of organ perfusion and the adequacy of intravascular volume in hypothermic patients, although the initial cold diuresis leads to underestimation of fluid needs.[263]

The best means to effect resuscitation of a hypothermic victim in ventricular fibrillation is controversial. The most recent recommendations of the American Heart Association (AHA) for the treatment of cardiac arrest when the core body temperature is below 86°F (<30°C) states that the administration of a vasopressor or antidysrhythmic according to standard Advanced Cardiac Life Support algorithm concurrent with rewarming is reasonable.[7,156] A meta-analysis of animal studies of antidysrhythmic and vasopressor therapy for ventricular fibrillation in the setting of hypothermia found that there was significant improvement in the return of spontaneous circulation (ROSC) in animals that received epinephrine or vasopressin.[261] In this report, the authors could not identify a benefit to the use of amiodarone administered without a vasopressor. They postulated that this is most likely due to the improvement in coronary perfusion pressure caused by vasopressors during cardiac arrest.[261] The benefit of amiodarone in profound hypothermia is probably limited but is reasonable and as there are no other options indicated.

Epinephrine and Vasopressin

The administration of vasopressin to pigs in hypothermic cardiac arrest increased coronary perfusion pressure and improved defibrillation success.[228] In a pig model, when warmed thoracic lavage was used, vasopressin increased coronary perfusion pressure and increased the 1-hour survival.[229] In this study, the administration of 0.9% NaCl resulted in zero episodes of successful defibrillation, but all 8 vasopressin-treated pigs had restoration of spontaneous circulation after electrical defibrillation and had improved short-term survival. The whole-body temperature was not increased, but the authors postulated that myocardial warming occurred.[228] In another study in which epinephrine was given to one group of pigs and vasopressin to another, increased coronary perfusion pressure and ROSC resulted in both groups.[152,153] In contrast, body temperature significantly increased during CPR with thoracic lavage, and epinephrine increased coronary perfusion pressure, but no improvement in ROSC occurred.[150] The length of time of cardiac arrest, the doses of drug, and the efforts to rewarm differed in these studies. A 19-year-old patient who had a prolonged hypothermic cardiopulmonary arrest showed no improvement after 2 mg of epinephrine but had immediate restoration of spontaneous circulation after the administration of vasopressin.[244] Interactions with epinephrine, vasopressin, and ischemia during CPR are complex and incompletely understood.[153,261]

Amiodarone

Amiodarone is recommended in the current AHA algorithm for ventricular fibrillation in normothermia.[7] In one study comparing the use of amiodarone, bretylium, and placebo in a hypothermic dog model, amiodarone showed no statistical improvement in causing ROSC.[242] There was no significant difference among the groups; only one of 10 amiodarone-treated dogs demonstrated ROSC versus 3 of 10 in the placebo group and 4 of 10 in the bretylium-treated dogs.[267] However, in a study in which hypothermic dogs in ventricular fibrillation were treated with epinephrine before administration of 10 mg/kg of amiodarone, there was a significantly higher rate of ROSC.[261] It is therefore reasonable to administer amiodarone with epinephrine for ventricular fibrillation in patients with hypothermia.

Dopamine

Dopamine increases cardiac output, mean arterial pressure, heart rate, and stroke volume in dogs cooled to 77°F (25°C) and stabilizes pulmonary arterial wedge pressure.[191] In a canine hypothermia model, dopamine infusions provided some protection from ventricular fibrillation. Dopamine lowered the temperature at which ventricular fibrillation occurred and reduced the incidence of ventricular fibrillation, as did infusion of norepinephrine.[9] The added benefit of dopamine in hypothermia results from its renal and splanchnic vasodilating properties, increasing renal perfusion and supporting urine output.[102] Dopamine increases myocardial oxygen demand and decreases peripheral perfusion, potentially detrimental effects in hypothermic patients.[9] For this reason, dopamine is not indicated in profoundly compromised patients with hypothermia.

Rewarming

Three types of rewarming modalities are used in the management of hypothermic patients.[56,79]

Passive external rewarming involves covering the patient with blankets and protecting the patient from further heat loss. Passive external rewarming uses the patient's own endogenous heat production for rewarming and is most successful in healthy patients with mild to moderate hypothermia whose capacity for endogenous heat production is intact.[115] Passive external rewarming is reported to be successful in hypothermic patients with temperatures as low as 69°F (20.6°C).[246,253,259] Advocates of passive external rewarming argue that it allows vasoconstriction to persist and decreases the afterdrop and shock from vasodilation associated with active skin rewarming.[115,182,246]

Active external rewarming involves the external application of heat to the patient. There is disagreement about the possible detrimental effects of active external rewarming. For example, skin warming leads to a physiologically detrimental suppression of shivering.[115] Acute vasodilation of peripheral vessels could cause hypotension and an increased peripheral demand on the persistently cold myocardium. The return of cold blood from the extremities to the heart is suggested to exacerbate intramyocardial temperature gradients, which could cause ventricular irritability during hypothermia. However, in pigs, blood returning to the heart was found to be warm before warming of central organs occurred.[103]

Afterdrop is the continuing decrease in temperature after rewarming begins. There is no evidence that it actually occurs in humans.[243] In one study of 33 patients with core temperature below 82.4°F (<28°C), no patient experienced afterdrop during peripheral rewarming.[214]

There is no evidence of pooling of blood in the periphery nor of increased flow during surface rewarming.[167,225,257] Flow studies in the hand, arm, calf, and foot demonstrate that afterdrop has already occurred and is completed before any increase in blood flow occurs in the limbs.[179,286] Initial experiments demonstrating afterdrop reflected continued cooling of central structures before heat from external sources reached the core and are no longer considered relevant to the human resuscitation.[103,167,257]

Mortality rates for active external rewarming are frequently reported to be higher than for passive external rewarming,[210] but case selection is not controlled in these series. Sicker patients with stable cardiac rhythms who fail to rewarm passively and are then actively rewarmed have a higher mortality rate directly correlated with their underlying disease rather than by the method of therapy.[67] Selection of either passive or active external rewarming in treatment of mild to moderate hypothermic patients with perfusing cardiac rhythms does not appear to influence the prognosis as much as the presence or absence of underlying disease.[67,128,182,258] In our experience, active external rewarming has not resulted in death except in patients with severe underlying disease.[67]

Active internal rewarming involves attempts to increase central core temperature directly by warming the heart before the extremities or periphery. Minimally invasive modalities of active internal rewarming include the administration of heated, humidified oxygen delivered by face mask or endotracheal tube[117] and gastric lavage with warmed fluids. More invasive modalities, procedures that are fundamental to the rewarming controversy, include peritoneal lavage with warmed dialysate[132,195] and the rerouting of blood through external blood-rewarming equipment via cardiopulmonary or femoral–femoral bypass and hemodialysis.[38,122,188] Heparin-coated bypass systems are available that avoid systemic anticoagulation, thus decreasing the risk of bleeding complications. It is suggested that extracorporeal venovenous rewarming and continuous arteriovenous rewarming show improved rewarming rates compared with standard techniques such as saline lavage of the bladder, stomach, or peritoneal cavity.[96] Extracorporeal methods of active internal rewarming should be reserved for severely hypothermic patients (<80°F or <27°C) or those with unstable cardiac rhythms (ventricular fibrillation, ventricular tachycardia, or asystole) attributed to hypothermia.[6,65,113] In patients with stable rhythms, studies are essential to resolve the debate over the merits of passive or active external rewarming versus active internal rewarming. Transcutaneous pacing was successful in improving hemodynamic parameters and speeding rewarming in an animal model.[76]

Many patients with temperatures below 86°F (30°C) were successfully treated with passive external rewarming with, at most, the addition of warm, humidified oxygen.[67,235,259] Patient temperature correlates poorly with outcome.[6,61,155,251] Treatment recommendations should never be based solely on temperature as the stability of the vital signs, the cardiac rhythm, and the underlying cause of hypothermia are much more critical considerations in management.

Hyperkalemia is not described as a consequence of rewarming.[60] In all of the evidence collected with regard to hyperkalemia, this abnormality was present as a consequence of the hypothermia and not the rewarming.[116,171,226]

Prognosis in Hypothermia

Except in cases of profound hypothermia,[116] the prognosis is most closely correlated with the presence or absence of underlying disease.[128,182,198,258,259] In patients with hypothermia alone, in the absence of underlying disease, the mortality rate is 0% to 10%. In the presence of a severe underlying disease such as sepsis, the mortality rate is much greater.[67] Morbidity results from associated frostbite and trauma.

Prolonged cardiopulmonary arrest and absolute temperature are not predictive of poor outcome.[6,61,155,248,251] In severely hypothermic patients, profound hyperkalemia ([K⁺] >10 mEq/L) is associated with unsuccessful resuscitation.[116,171,226]

Frostbite

Hypothermia is sometimes accompanied by frostbite when patients are exposed to environmental temperatures that are lower than 20°F (6.7°C).[183] Frostbite should be managed by rapid rewarming of the frozen part of the affected person. The extremity involved is placed in warm water (100°F–108°F; 38°C–43°C) for 30 minutes. The water temperature must be maintained and corrected because the frozen extremity will cool the water in the basin.

The amputation rate is decreased with the use of iloprost, a prostacyclin. The dose is 2 ng/mL per minute for 6 hours each day for 5 days.[40] Parenteral analgesics are frequently necessary because the rewarming process is often painful. Frostbitten areas should never be rubbed because the tissue is particularly sensitive to trauma.

HYPERTHERMIA

Definition of Heatstroke

Heatstroke is defined by a rectal temperature greater than 105.5°F (40.8°C) in the setting of a neurologic disturbance manifested by mental status changes, including confusion, delirium, stupor, coma, or convulsions.[143] However, temperature measurements typically occur post cooling efforts and the site of the temperature measurement does not adequately reflect core temperature. Another definition of heatstroke is "a form of hyperthermia associated with systemic inflammatory response syndrome leading to multiorgan dysfunction in which encephalopathy predominates."[26,160]

Although the absence of sweating was once thought to be an essential component of the definition of heatstroke,[51,196] many patients with heatstroke maintain the ability to sweat.[59,172,232,254] The presence or absence of sweating at the time of collapse is not a part of the clinical diagnosis of heatstroke.[172] If maximal heat loss mechanisms are in play, the patient will be sweating but the heat loss mechanisms are simply inadequate to keep up with heat stress. Temperature criteria cannot be absolute because information regarding the patient's temperature is rarely available at the time of onset of heatstroke. In some instances, the temperature will not be measured for several hours, during which time cooling will commonly have been instituted or occurred spontaneously.[140,141] When appropriate environmental conditions prevail, the diagnosis of heatstroke should be made liberally. Autopsy findings demonstrate extensive diffuse tissue injury.[73] In the establishment of the cause of death, the forensic literature emphasizes the need to consider the circumstances of death, environmental temperatures and the victim's coexisting medical conditions and medications that predispose to heatstroke.[73]

Epidemiology of Heatstroke

Hundreds of people die annually of heatstroke in the United States, 80% of whom are older than age 50 years.[41] Heat waves or extended periods of high temperatures kill more people than any other weather-related event in the United States.[62] Midwestern and southern states experience the highest temperatures and the highest numbers of heat stress hospitalizations. When counting heat-related fatalities, the number is underestimated if only death certificates are included in which hyperthermia is listed as the underlying cause of death. Including hyperthermia as a contributing factor to death increased the total number of heat-related deaths by 54% from 1993 to 2003; several studies show mortality rates from heatstroke to be 5.6% to 80%.[13,42,43] Thousands of other victims survive with significant heat-related morbidity. The high morbidity and mortality of heatstroke markedly contrast with those of profound hypothermia, in which the prognosis is related not to the temperature itself but to the underlying etiology. The overall prognosis in heatstroke depends primarily on how long the body temperature is elevated before cooling, the maximum temperature reached, and the affected individual's premorbid health.[25]

Thermoregulation and Heat Stress

The normal thermoregulatory response to heat stress is mediated primarily by heat-sensitive neurons in the hypothalamus. Increased body core temperature results in active dilation of cutaneous vessels, and skin blood flow increases.[120,217] Because increased skin blood flow is attained primarily by an increase in heart rate and stroke volume, the capacity to increase cardiac output is critical to cooling. Compensatory shifting of blood flow from the splanchnic and renal vessels to the skin further increases skin blood flow.[127] The combination of vasodilation, increased skin blood flow, and increased sweating results in heat loss through convection and evaporation. Salt and water depletion that occurs after profuse sweating increases plasma osmolarity. Heat-sensitive neurons in the preoptic anterior hypothalamus are inhibited by locally increased osmolarity and by input from distal hepatoportal osmoreceptors. The inhibition of heat sensitive neurons results in decreased heat dissipation response.[50,199]

Types of Heatstroke

Heatstroke is commonly divided into 2 types, exertional and nonexertional. Nonexertional, or classic, heatstroke describes heatstroke occurring in the absence of extreme exercise. Nonexertional heatstroke is most commonly described during heat waves to excess wearing clothing that causes heat retention (lower evaporation), and the victims are predominantly those persons least able to tolerate heat: infants,[12] older adults,[55,232] individuals with psychiatric disorders, and chronically ill individuals.

Exertional heatstroke occurs as a result of increased motor activity. It occurs in young, healthy individuals who are exercising or in individuals whose increased motor activity results from other causes, such as seizures or agitation. Often a period of significant heat stress in exercising individuals precedes the development of heatstroke. Military recruits who develop heatstroke sometimes present to the camp infirmary with vague complaints before collapse.[232] Published studies of heatstroke in miners, athletes, and military recruits describe several precipitating factors in heatstroke, including fatigue associated with a recent deficit in sleep, poor physical conditioning, a recent febrile illness, recent heat-related symptoms such as thirst or weakness, relative volume depletion, failure to allow for acclimatization or inability to acclimatize, and obesity. Symptoms of nausea, weakness, headache, diarrhea, or irritability often precede the development of heatstroke. A rapid onset of symptoms and acute loss of consciousness are frequently reported as the heatstroke, the preceding period of heat stress, and insidious symptoms often go unrecognized. Although exertional heatstroke is more likely to occur during intense exertion in a hot, humid

environment, it also occurs with moderately intense exercise early in the morning, when environmental conditions are not recognized as a thermoregulatory stress.[10]

Differential Diagnosis of Hyperthermia

In addition to exposure and exertion, conditions that predispose to severe hyperthermia include primary hypothalamic lesions, intracranial hemorrhage, agitation, alcohol and sedative–hypnotic withdrawal, seizures, and the use of therapeutic and illicit xenobiotics (Table 29–5).[101,105,107,151,174,245] Heatstroke occurs with the medical use of amphetamines to treat attention-deficit hyperactivity disorder, and the use of amphetamines as a party drug at dance events called raves. Mortality from cocaine overdose

TABLE 29–5 Differential Diagnosis of Hyperthermia

I. Increased heat production

Increased muscle activity
- Agitation
- Catatonia
- Ethanol withdrawal
- Exercise
- Infectious diseases
- Malignant hyperthermia
- Monoamine oxidase inhibitor drug interactions
- Neuroleptic malignant syndrome
- Parkinson disease
- Sedative–hypnotic withdrawal
- Seizures
- Serotonin toxicity
- Xenobiotics

Increased metabolic rate
- Hyperthyroidism
- Pheochromocytoma
- Sympathomimetics

II. Impaired heat loss

Environmental
- Heat
- Humidity
- Lack of acclimatization

Social disadvantage
- Confinement to bed
- Top floor apartments
- Isolation
- Lack of air conditioning
- Closed windows
- Poverty

Medical illness
- Cardiac insufficiency
- Central nervous system dysfunction
- Diabetes
- Hypertension
- Pulmonary

Salt and water depletion

Fatigue

Limited behavioral response
- Extremes of age
- Intellectual disability
- Psychiatric impairment
- Xenobiotics

increases in high ambient temperature. The mean daily number of deaths from cocaine overdose was 33% higher when the ambient temperature exceeded 88°F (31°C).[186]

Serotonin Toxicity

Serotonin toxicity, results from excess stimulation of the serotonin receptors, primarily the 5-HT$_{1A}$ subtype.[103] Treatment focuses on control of hyperthermia by using aggressive cooling; muscle relaxation, primarily by using benzodiazepines; or, in severe cases, endotracheal intubation and paralysis (Chap. 69).

Malignant Hyperthermia

Malignant hyperthermia is a very rare disorder, that is associated with a congenital disturbance of calcium regulation in striated muscle. Malignant hyperthermia was first reported in 1960. Ten deaths occurred in a single family after general anesthesia.[72] Exposure to anesthetics, depolarizing muscle relaxants, or rarely, severe exertion precipitates uncontrolled calcium efflux from the sarcoplasmic reticulum, leading to severe muscle rigidity and hyperthermia[108] The clinical setting of severe muscle rigidity and hyperthermia after general anesthesia usually is adequate to define the syndrome (Chap. 66).

Neuroleptic Malignant Syndrome

Neuroleptic malignant syndrome, a severe extrapyramidal syndrome associated with muscle rigidity, autonomic dysfunction, and altered mental status, was first described in 1968.[68] This disorder develops during the administration of antipsychotics or the withdrawal of dopaminergic xenobiotics. Increased muscle tone because of dopaminergic blockade of the striatum as well as central altered hypothalamic thermoregulation leads to hyperthermia.[118] Neuroleptic malignant syndrome must be distinguished from the much more common cases of classical or exertional heatstroke (Chap. 67).

These medical conditions, serotonin toxicity, malignant hyperthermia, and neuroleptic malignant syndrome are distinguished by the patient's history of present illness, physical examination, clinical presentation including the time course of illness, and the environmental conditions.

Inflammatory Mediators in Heatstroke

The response to heat stress is a coordinated interplay between the mediators of inflammation, including endothelial cells, leukocytes, inflammatory cytokines, and endotoxins.[160] These are important mediators of the systemic immune response. However, in heatstroke, they are responsible for systemic inflammation and activation of the coagulation cascade, similar to the systemic inflammatory response syndrome (SIRS). Many proinflammatory cytokines are identified in heatstroke, including tumor necrosis factor (TNF); interleukins-2, -6, -8, -10, and -12; interferon-α and -β; and granulocyte colony–stimulating factors.[24] In one study of 18 heatstroke patients, circulating cytokine concentrations correlated with clinical indices of heatstroke severity.[129,160] Cooling delays the release of interleukin-1β, interleukin-6, and TNF in vitro. Studies in hyperthermic animals focus on the modulation of the mediators of inflammation as possible future adjuncts to cooling. In another study, recombinant human activated protein C provided cytoprotection by decreasing release of inflammatory cytokines but did not improve survival.[27] Whole-body cooling restored appropriate concentrations of cardiac tissue protein associated with loss of structural integrity of the cardiac myocytes and reversed cardiac dysfunction.[47]

Heat stress causes increased gene transcription of heat shock proteins, which render the organism more resistant to heat injury, protecting cells from injury and increasing cell survival. Heat shock protein 72 is protective against injury from heat stress,[97] and the extent of protection correlates with the concentration of heat shock protein.[126,168]

During exercise, splanchnic hypoperfusion increases the translocation of bacteria from the gut into the bloodstream, establishing the cascade of inflammation and injury that perpetuates tissue injury after normothermia is established.[83]

Pathophysiologic Characteristics of Heatstroke

In heatstroke, hypotension and tachycardia are caused by a number of factors. Patients with heatstroke often have a reduced plasma volume secondary to salt and water depletion. Peripheral pooling of blood is associated with an increase in cutaneous blood flow from 0.5 to 7 or 8 L/min.[127,217] In addition, patients often manifest primary myocardial insufficiency.[144] Clinically, patients exhibit either a hypo- or hyperdynamic circulatory response. The observed circulatory response to heat stress is a function of the patient's cardiac reserve, volume status, and degree of myocardial heat injury. The hyperdynamic condition is characterized by increased cardiac index and decreased systemic vascular resistance.[197] These hemodynamic characteristics occur in patients who are able to maintain a significantly increased cardiac output in response to the circulatory demand of heat stress.

Volume-depleted patients and those patients with primary myocardial insufficiency exhibit a hypodynamic response. These patients have a decreased cardiac index and increased systemic vascular resistance.[197,241] Whether pulmonary vascular resistance is affected is unclear. High central venous pressures (CVPs) were found in some patients, with evidence of right heart failure and right heart dilation on autopsy.[172] These findings led to the suggestion that pulmonary vascular resistance was elevated.[197] In 22 of 34 patients with heatstroke, CVPs were greater than 3 cm H$_2$O. Twelve patients had a CVP of 0 cm H$_2$O, and 10 had a CVP that exceeded 10 cm H$_2$O. The authors cautioned against injudicious infusion of large quantities of IV fluids that result in complications of congestive heart failure and fluid overload. In the study, only 3 patients required more than 2 L of 0.9% sodium chloride solution during cooling. Crystalloid infusion ranged from 500 to 2500 mL, and none of the patients developed problems associated with fluid overload.[230]

A study of compromised elderly patients with heatstroke using pulmonary artery catheters showed that pulmonary vascular resistance was low or normal. Pulmonary capillary wedge pressures were not elevated.[240] A study of 13 cases of heatstroke in pilgrims to Mecca, Saudi Arabia, monitored with pulmonary artery catheters demonstrated a good correlation of CVP with pulmonary capillary wedge pressures.[3] Serial ECGs in 51 of these pilgrims with heatstroke showed normal sinus rhythm in 25%, sinus tachycardia in 52%, atrial fibrillation in 16%, and sinus bradycardia in 6%. ST-segment depression and other ST segment and T wave changes were reported. The QT interval showed no abnormality.[3] Electrocardiographic changes suggestive of acute coronary syndrome occur, yet normal coronary arteries are noted on coronary catheterization.[1] In some patients, echocardiography showed pericardial effusions and regional wall motion abnormalities, asymmetric septal hypertrophy, right ventricular dilation, and left ventricular dilation with impaired function.[4]

Autopsy studies of the heart demonstrate right heart dilation, pericardial effusions, interstitial edema, degeneration and necrosis of myocardial fibers, and subendocardial hemorrhages. Postmortem examination of the lungs revealed vascular congestion, pleural effusions, and parenchymal hemorrhages.[172,197]

Gastrointestinal hemorrhage, vomiting, and diarrhea occur frequently.[232] At autopsy, edema and hemorrhage of the bowel wall occur.[46] These changes are partly a result of the regional ischemia of splanchnic blood vessels and resultant hypoperfusion and hypoxia. Increased bowel wall edema and bleeding predispose to the release of bacteria into the bloodstream from the gut, causing focal microvascular changes in the intestinal villi, leading to bowel wall anoxia and further injury.[26] Liver injury occurs commonly and is not clinically manifest until the second or third day after the temperature increase.[140,232] Centrilobular changes, such as widening of central veins and adjacent sinusoids and pooling of blood, and varying degrees of hepatocellular degeneration are demonstrated on liver biopsy. Repeat biopsies demonstrated that these changes resolve as the patient recovers.[140] In other cases, only congestion and fatty infiltration are reported (Chap. 21).[46]

Neuropsychiatric impairment is, by definition, present in all cases of heatstroke, and the duration of altered consciousness correlates significantly with mortality.[11,232] Autopsy studies demonstrate a variety of structural and microscopic CNS injuries. Edema and venous congestion are evident. The number of cortical neurons is reduced, with concomitant glial proliferation.

Cerebellar Purkinje cell deterioration is marked. The hypothalamus appears to be relatively spared, with limited edema of the neuronal nuclei. Hemorrhages occur throughout the brain.[46,172,232] Carotid artery vasoconstriction occurs in response to heating in an in vitro model using the carotid arteries of rabbits to elucidate the mechanism of ischemia and injury in heatstroke.[189] Heatstroke-induced cerebral ischemia is associated with increased glutamate release, activation of cerebral dopaminergic neurons causing dopamine overload, and gliosis. These changes are attenuated by induction of hypothermia in an animal model.[49]

Reports of magnetic resonance imaging (MRI) of brains of patients recovering from heatstroke describe radiographic findings, including hemorrhagic and ischemic abnormalities of the cerebrum and cerebellum, delayed cerebellar atrophy, central pontine myelinolysis, vascular infarcts, and medial thalamic lesions, which correspond anatomically to the paraventricular nucleus. The paraventricular nucleus is involved with core temperature regulation via the hypothalamic–pituitary–adrenal axis.[18] The clinical symptoms of dysphagia, quadriparesis, wasting, extrapyramidal syndrome, and pancerebellar syndrome have corresponding MRI findings.[5] Persistent cerebellar dysfunction occurs, as does lower motor neuron damage, manifested by areflexia and muscle wasting.[69,158] Abnormal nerve conduction studies are documented.[135] Higher cortical functions are spared in survivors or are reversible when they occur.[82,162,178] Permanent neurologic sequelae are correlated with the degree and duration of hyperthermia.

Acute kidney injury (AKI) was a major cause of death in heatstroke victims before the advent of hemodialysis.[227,254] In addition to the direct effects of heat, volume depletion, and hypotension, myoglobinuria secondary to rhabdomyolysis results in further renal tubular injury. This is especially common in an agitated or exercising patient.[52,101,205] The mechanism by which myoglobin contributes to AKI remains controversial. At autopsy, the kidneys are enlarged, with extensive petechial hemorrhage.[205] Acute tubular necrosis is demonstrated on biopsy. In exertional heatstroke with AKI, renal hemodynamics are compromised because of increased vasoconstrictive hormones, such as catecholamines, renin, aldosterone, and endothelin-1, and decreased vasodilatory hormones, such as prostaglandin E_2.[164]

Bleeding is associated with significant morbidity and mortality in many cases of heatstroke. The etiology of coagulation disturbances in patients with heatstroke appear to be multifactorial. Elevation of the prothrombin time occurs within 30 minutes of temperature elevation and is attributed to direct heat injury of clotting factors.[15] Liver damage significantly contributes to the coagulation disturbances, although this does not manifest as rapidly.[15,190,208] Two patients with severe liver failure secondary to heatstroke received liver transplantation; both died after chronic rejection.[219] A third patient with extensive liver cell necrosis as a consequence of heatstroke was referred for liver transplantation but recovered completely with supportive therapy.[98] Evidence of diffuse capillary basement membrane injury is demonstrable by electron microscopy and is thought to precipitate consumptive coagulopathy in severe cases of heatstroke.[46,237] Thrombocytopenia is very common and occurs within 30 minutes of onset of heatstroke, frequently in the absence of other evidence of disseminated intravascular coagulation. Direct thermal injury leading to decreased platelet survival and megakaryocyte damage plays a role (Table 29–6).[172,190]

Clinical Findings in Heatstroke

Clinical evaluation of a hyperthermic patient begins with careful assessment of the vital signs. Vital sign abnormalities commonly include tachycardia with heart rates greater than 130 beats/min, hypotension, and tachypnea with the respiratory rates often above 30 breaths/min. Most importantly, temperature is elevated. After cooling, there is often a secondary rise in temperature that suggests persistent disturbances central hypothalmic dysregulation.[172]

Neurologic examination reveals a confused, delirious, comatose, or seizing patient. Pupils are normal, fixed and dilated, or pinpoint. Decerebrate or decorticate posturing is sometimes present. Muscle tone is increased, normal, or flaccid. The skin is often hot and dry, or diaphoretic. Nasal and oropharyngeal bleeding presents as a consequence of the acute coagulopathy.

TABLE 29–6	Physiologic and Clinical Manifestations of Heatstroke

Cardiovascular
  Hypodynamic in elderly adults
  Hyperdynamic in young, healthy individuals
  Electrocardiogram
    Nonspecific
    Widening of QRS because of an underlying abnormality (cocaine toxicity, hyperkalemia associated with rhabdomyolysis)

Central nervous system
  Altered mental status
    Irritability, confusion, ataxia, seizures, coma
    Weakness, dizziness, headache
    Plantar extension, pupillary abnormalities, decorticate posturing
  Electroencephalogram
    Normal or diffuse slowing
  Cerebrospinal fluid
    Normal or increased protein
    Lymphocytosis

Gastrointestinal
  Vomiting, diarrhea, hematemesis

Hematologic
  Bleeding diathesis
    Prolonged PT and PTT
    Disseminated intravascular coagulation
    Thrombocytopenia
    Petechiae
    Purpura
  Leukocytosis

Hepatic
  Hepatic insufficiency at 12–36 hours
  Elevated AST, ALT, LDH

Metabolic
  Metabolic acidosis and respiratory alkalosis
  Electrolyte disturbance
    Hypernatremia
    Hypokalemia
    Hypocalcemia
    Hypophosphatemia

Muscle
  Rhabdomyolysis
  Elevated CPK

Renal
  Decreased renal perfusion
  Myoglobinuria
  Proteinuria
  Oliguria
  Acute tubular necrosis
  Interstitial necrosis

ALT = alanine aminotransferase; AST = aspartate aminotransferase; CPK = creatine phosphokinase; LDH = lactate dehydrogenase; PT = prothrombin time; PTT = partial thromboplastin time.

Examination of the lungs is often nonspecific, although heatstroke victims are at risk of acute respiratory distress syndrome (ARDS) as a primary event associated with capillary endothelial damage or after overly aggressive fluid resuscitation. Aspiration secondary to seizures occurs. Cardiac auscultation reveals a flow murmur secondary to high cardiac output or a right ventricular gallop. Neck vein distension indicates increased central venous pressure. Jaundice suggests hepatic injury and occurs on the second or third day after the onset of heatstroke.[48] Gross gastrointestinal bleeding is sometimes present. A petechial rash develops, probably secondary to capillary endothelial damage.

Laboratory findings of severe hyperthermia include lactate dehydrogenase (LDH) elevation as a consequence of diffuse tissue injury. Early rises in alanine aminotransferase (ALT) and aspartate aminotransferase (AST), which peak at 48 hours, are indicators of the liver damage that occurs during heatstroke.[140] Muscle enzymes were elevated in all patients in a study of exertional heatstroke[232] and in 86% of patients in one study of nonexertional heatstroke.[106] Nonspecific ST- and T-wave changes on ECG are common. Myocardial enzyme elevation occurs and correlates with ECG changes.[141] Results of lumbar puncture are nonspecific, are often normal, and often demonstrate elevated CSF protein and a lymphocytosis.[232]

Other laboratory parameters are affected by heatstroke. Salt and water depletion leads to hemoconcentration in patients exposed to elevated temperatures for a period of time. Hypokalemia is common, with potassium deficits as great as 500 mEq occurring during the early period of heat exposure. Arterial blood gas analysis typically shows a respiratory alkalosis secondary to direct stimulation of the respiratory center by heat or a metabolic acidosis with an elevated lactate concentration.[59,232] Metabolic acidosis is the most frequent acid–base disturbance, either alone or part of a mixed picture. The prevalence of metabolic acidosis correlates with the degree of hyperthermia; 95% of patients demonstrated metabolic acidosis when the body temperature exceeded 107.6°F (42°C).[24]

Hypophosphatemia is common and is attributed to respiratory alkalosis, which causes intracellular shifts of phosphate. However, 8 of 10 heatstroke patients developed hypophosphatemia, and none was alkalemic.[23] The hypophosphatemia in these patients was associated with increased phosphaturia and decreased tubular reabsorption of phosphorus, a finding that reversed after cooling.[145] Renal tubular damage leads to phosphate depletion.[109] In contrast, phosphate and potassium are elevated when significant muscle injury occurs. Calcium is normal or low, the latter secondary to binding to damaged muscle tissue. Later, hypercalcemia occurs, possibly as a result of release of this bound calcium.[94,166]

Significant alterations occur in lymphocyte subsets in heatstroke victims. One study reported an increased ratio of T-suppressor to T-cytotoxic cells, as well as increased natural killer cells. There was a significant decrease in the percentages of T and B cells and T-helper cells. These changes correlate with the degree of hyperthermia.[21,159] Catecholamines are increased in heatstroke[2] and affect the distribution of the lymphocyte subsets.[25] It is possible that the increased susceptibility to infection described in heatstroke and the alterations in lymphocyte populations are related.[21]

Effects of Xenobiotics in Heatstroke

Xenobiotics predispose the individual to heatstroke by 2 primary mechanisms: increased production of heat as a result of xenobiotic action and interference with the body's ability to dissipate heat because of pharmacologic or toxicologic effects on thermoregulation (Table 29–5). Xenobiotic interactions also cause life-threatening increases in temperature, such as the combination of monoamine oxidase inhibitors with meperidine or dextromethorphan resulting in serotonin toxicity.

During heat stress, vasodilation leads to increased cutaneous blood flow requiring an increased cardiac output to maintain blood pressure. Parasympathetic stimulation results in increased sudomotor activation. Xenobiotics that impair these physiologic mechanisms for heat dissipation predispose the individual to heatstroke. Xenobiotics with anticholinergic effects, such as antihistamines, cyclic antidepressants, and antipsychotics, interfere with sweating. Heatstroke as a result of oligohidrosis is reported for zonisamide and topiramate.[146-193] The mechanism is postulated to concern the inhibition of carbonic anhydrase, an enzyme associated with eccrine sweat gland function. Sympathomimetics stimulate α-adrenergic receptors, impairing vasodilation. Antihypertensives and antianginals (most notably calcium channel antagonists and β-adrenergic antagonists) with negative inotropic

and chronotropic effects impair the ability of the heart to meet the output requirements of increased skin blood flow. Diuretic-induced salt and water depletion also limits cardiac output. Antipsychotics cause hypothalamic depression and are anticholinergic, altering the normal CNS response to heat stress. Finally, xenobiotics such as ethanol, opioids, and sedative–hypnotics impair normal behavioral responses, and heat-related discomfort may go unnoticed.

Heatstroke and Subsequent Heat Intolerance

Whether heatstroke victims are subsequently unable to adapt to exercise in a hot environment remains unclear. Is the heatstroke victim genetically predisposed to heat intolerance, or does heatstroke occur as a result of environmental and host factors? Several studies suggest that heatstroke leads to persistent heat intolerance. These studies often use a single heat intolerance test.[81,231,233,234] A study of 10 previous heatstroke victims showed no difference in acclimatization responses, thermoregulation, whole-body sodium and potassium balance, sweat gland function, and blood values when compared with control participants.[10] The rate of recovery from exertional heatstroke probably differs among individuals. In this study, one of 10 patients was found to have recurrent heat intolerance 12 months after the study.[10] Resolution of heat intolerance was delayed for 5 months in an individual who had experienced heatstroke twice.[139]

The effects of xenobiotics on acclimatization requires a sound understanding of the physiology of heat loss mechanisms in humans. Xenobiotics and medical conditions affect the ability to acclimatize. The physiological effectiveness of heat loss is critical to maintenance of normal body temperature. There are reports of the effects of drugs on the ability to acclimatize to heat.[104] Hyoscine produced a 43% depression in sweat rate in this report, retarding the development of acclimatization. Salicylates do not affect the hyperthermia of exercise. Acclimatization studies in humans most often use young and healthy exercising subjects.

Treatment of Heatstroke

Management must focus on the early recognition of hyperthermia. Rapid cooling is the first priority and is associated with improved outcomes. Cooling that is delayed allowing body temperatures to remain above 102.2°F (38.9°C) for more than 30 minutes is associated with a high morbidity and mortality. In one report of the Chicago heat wave of 1995, only one patient of 58 victims was cooled within 30 minutes, resulting in an in-hospital mortality rate of 21% and an additional 28% mortality rate within 1 year.[70] Cooling by covering in ice water was twice as rapid in lowering the core temperature as was cooling by using an evaporative spray.[10] Ice water immersion results in faster cooling compared with all of the evaporative cooling methods in some studies.[39,58,87,95,154] A report of endovascular cooling using a heat exchange balloon catheter demonstrated dangerously lengthy cooling times and inadequate cooling measures.[177]

Successful treatment requires adequate preparation. Equipment needed for rapid cooling should always be readily available in the emergency department and includes fans, ice, and tubs for immersion. En route to the hospital, the patient should be soaked in water and ice to begin rapid and aggressive cooling. Respiration and cardiovascular status should be stabilized and monitored. The cause of the heatstroke should be determined and appropriate measures initiated immediately. Xenobiotics, such as antihistamines, butyrophenones, and phenothiazines, and physical restraints that interfere with heat dissipation, such as straitjackets, are contraindicated.[107] A patient who is hyperthermic in the setting of ethanol or sedative–hypnotic withdrawal should be treated with a benzodiazepine.[106] The patient should never be confined to a small, unventilated seclusion room. Adequate cooling, hydration, sedation, and electrolytes and substrate repletion should be ensured.[105]

In the emergency department, appropriate laboratory studies should be performed and an IV line inserted. A rectal probe should be placed for continuous temperature monitoring. The patient should be immersed in an ice bath with a fan blowing over the patient if possible.

Agitation, seizures, and cardiac dysrhythmias must be managed while cooling is accomplished. Benzodiazepines are the treatment of choice for agitation and seizures. Hypotension should be treated with fluids and cooling. Volume repletion should be monitored carefully by parameters such as blood pressure, pulse, and urine output. As the temperature returns to normal, the hypotension will resolve if significant volume deficits are not present.[51,143,144] In patients with myoglobinuria, an attempt should be made to increase renal blood flow and urine output. The use of sodium bicarbonate and mannitol in the prevention of acute tubular necrosis in these cases is not routinely recommended.[80,94,216]

Phenothiazines and butyrophenones should not be used because they depress an already altered mental status, produce hepatotoxicity in a compromised liver, lower the seizure threshold,[20] cause acute dystonic reactions, exacerbate hypotension, and interfere with thermoregulation and cooling by affecting the hypothalamus. When shivering occurs during cooling, we recommend the judicious use of a benzodiazepine. In addition, benzodiazepines treat ethanol and sedative–hypnotic withdrawal and cocaine toxicity, common causes of hyperthermia.

There is no role for antipyretics in the management of heatstroke. Aspirin and acetaminophen lower temperature by reducing the hypothalamic set point, which is only altered in a patient febrile from inflammation or endogenous pyrogens.[72,120] Heatstroke occurs when cooling mechanisms are overwhelmed. The hypothalamic thermoregulatory set point is not disturbed.[16]

Dantrolene is the preferred drug in the treatment of malignant hyperthermia (Antidotes in Depth: A24).[131,256] It acts directly on skeletal muscle and either inhibits the release of calcium or increases calcium uptake through the sarcoplasmic reticulum.[29] Its usefulness has not been demonstrated in other conditions associated with hyperthermia, and there is no evidence to support its administration for other conditions.[8] In a prospective, randomized, double-blind, placebo-controlled study of 52 patients with heatstroke, IV dantrolene at 2 mg/kg of body weight did not alter cooling time.[22] There was no significant difference in the mean number of hospital days necessitated by heatstroke victims who received dantrolene and cooling versus those who received cooling alone. The dopamine agonists bromocriptine and amantadine sometimes administered as part of the treatment of neuroleptic malignant syndrome are not indicated in the management of classical or exertional heatstroke (Table 29–7).

TABLE 29–7 Management of Heatstroke

Preparation
  Ice and cooling fans available in emergency department
  Monitor weather reports
  Alert media
On arrival
  Rapid cooling-monitor with rectal probe
    Clear airway and administer oxygen
    Cover with ice and water-soaked sheets
    Stabilize respiratory and cardiovascular status
    Cool as rapidly as possible
  Intravenous access
    Dextrose (0.5–1.0 g/kg) and 100 mg of thiamine as clinically indicated
    Benzodiazepines for agitation, shivering, seizures
  Continuous monitoring
    Remove from ice bath at 101-102°F (38.3-38.8°C)
    Watch for rebound hyperthermia
  Cautions
    Antipsychotics contraindicated because of serious adverse effects
    Antipyretics do not work
    Dantrolene is not indicated
    Cooling blankets alone are inadequate

SUMMARY

- Xenobiotics disturb normal thermoregulation, and it leads to the abnormal conditions of hyperthermia or hypothermia. These disturbances of homeostasis present significant clinical management challenges.
- Hypothermia and heatstroke are preventable conditions.
- Immediate and aggressive cooling is imperative in heatstroke. Near-normal body temperature should be achieved within 30 minutes from onset of heatstroke.
- Rewarming of the patient with hypothermia and a stable cardiac rhythm can often be successfully accomplished with patience and without extracorporeal methods.
- Many xenobiotics increase the risk to patients when the heat index is excessive and the very medications used to treat their chronic diseases increase their risks of heat-related morbidity and mortality.
- Climate change causing increasingly hot weather demands systemic national preventive health efforts municipal preparedness and public education efforts to prevent deaths during increasingly hot conditions.

REFERENCES

1. Akhtar MJ, et al. Electrocardiographic abnormalities in patients with heat stroke. *Chest.* 1993;104:411-414.
2. al-Hadramy MS, Ali F. Catecholamines in heat stroke. *Mil Med.* 1989;154:263-264.
3. al-Harthi SS, et al. Hemodynamic changes and intravascular hydration state in heat stroke. *Ann Saudi Med.* 1989;9:378-383.
4. al-Harthi SS, et al. Non-invasive evaluation of cardiac abnormalities in heat stroke pilgrims. *Int J Cardiol.* 1992;37:151-154.
5. Albukrek D, et al. Heat-stroke-induced cerebellar atrophy: clinical course, CT and MRI findings. *Neuroradiology.* 1997;39:195-197.
6. Althaus U, et al. Management of profound accidental hypothermia with cardiorespiratory arrest. *Ann Surg.* 1982;195:492-495.
7. American Heart Association. 2015. https://eccguidelines.heart.org/index.php/circulation/cpr-ecc-guidelines-2/part-10-special-circumstances-of-resuscitation/. Accessed September 5, 2017.
8. Amsterdam JT, et al. Dantrolene sodium for treatment of heatstroke victims: lack of efficacy in a canine model. *Am J Emerg Med.* 1986;4:399-405.
9. Angelakos ET, Daniels JB. Effect of catecholamine infusions on lethal hypothermic temperatures in dogs. *J Appl Physiol.* 1969;26:194-196.
10. Armstrong LE, et al. Time course of recovery and heat acclimation ability of prior exertional heatstroke patients. *Med Sci Sports Exerc.* 1990;22:36-48.
11. Austin MG, Berry JW. Observations on one hundred cases of heatstroke. *JAMA.* 1956;161:1525-1529.
12. Bacon C, et al. Heatstroke in well-wrapped infants. *Lancet.* 1979;1:422-425.
13. Basu R, Samet JM. Relation between elevated ambient temperature and mortality: a review of the epidemiologic evidence. *Epidemiol Rev.* 2002;24:190-202.
14. Baumgartner FJ, et al. Cardiopulmonary bypass for resuscitation of patients with accidental hypothermia and cardiac arrest. *Can J Surg.* 1992;35:184-187.
15. Beard ME, Hickton CM. Haemostasis in heat stroke. *Br J Haematol.* 1982;52:269-274.
16. Bernheim HA, et al. Fever: pathogenesis, pathophysiology, and purpose. *Ann Intern Med.* 1979;91:261-270.
17. Beyda EJ, et al. Effect of hypothermia on tolerance of dogs to digitalis. *Circ Res.* 1961;9:129-135.
18. Bhatnagar S, Dallman MF. The paraventricular nucleus of the thalamus alters rhythms in core temperature and energy balance in a state-dependent manner. *Brain Res.* 1999;851:66-75.
19. Birzis L, Hemingway A. Descending brain stem connections controlling shivering in cat. *J Neurophysiol.* 1956;19:37-43.
20. Blum K, et al. Enhancement of alcohol withdrawal convulsions in mice by haloperidol. *Clin Toxicol.* 1976;9:427-434.
21. Bouchama A, et al. Distribution of peripheral blood leukocytes in acute heatstroke. *J Appl Physiol.* 1992;73:405-409.
22. Bouchama A, et al. Ineffectiveness of dantrolene sodium in the treatment of heatstroke. *Crit Care Med.* 1991;19:176-180.
23. Bouchama A, et al. Mechanisms of hypophosphatemia in humans with heatstroke. *J Appl Physiol.* 1991;71:328-332.
24. Bouchama A, De Vol EB. Acid-base alterations in heatstroke. *Intensive Care Med.* 2001;27:680-685.
25. Bouchama A, et al. Prognostic factors in heat wave related deaths: a meta-analysis. *Arch Intern Med.* 2007;167:2170-2176.
26. Bouchama A, Knochel JP. Heat stroke. *N Engl J Med.* 2002;346:1978-1988.
27. Bouchama A, et al. Recombinant activated protein C attenuates endothelial injury and inhibits procoagulant microparticles release in baboon heatstroke. *Arterioscler Thromb Vasc Biol.* 2008;28:1318-1325.

28. Boulant JA. Hypothalamic neurons. Mechanisms of sensitivity to temperature. *Ann N Y Acad Sci.* 1998;856:108-115.

29. Britt BA. Dantrolene. *Can Anaesth Soc J.* 1984;31:61-75.

30. Broccardo M, Improta G. Sauvagine-induced hypothermia: evidence for an interaction with the dopaminergic system. *Eur J Pharmacol.* 1994;258:179-184.

31. Brown DJ, et al. Accidental hypothermia. *N Engl J Med.* 2012;367:1930-1938.

32. Bruck K. Non-shivering thermogenesis and brown adipose tissue in relation to age, and their integration in the thermoregulatory system. In: Lindberg O, ed. *Brown Adipose Tissue.* New York, NY: Elsevier; 1970:117-154.

33. Brugger H, et al. Resuscitation of avalanche victims: evidence-based guidelines of the international commission for mountain emergency medicine (ICAR MEDCOM): intended for physicians and other advanced life support personnel. *Resuscitation.* 2013;84:539-546.

34. Buchwald I, Davis PJ. Scleroderma with fatal heat stroke. *JAMA.* 1967;201:270-271.

35. Buckberg GD, et al. Studies of the effects of hypothermia on regional myocardial blood flow and metabolism during cardiopulmonary bypass. I. The adequately perfused beating, fibrillating, and arrested heart. *J Thorac Cardiovasc Surg.* 1977;73:87-94.

36. Cannon B, et al. Brown adipose tissue. More than an effector of thermogenesis? *Ann N Y Acad Sci.* 1998;856:171-187.

37. Carlton J, et al. Attenuation of alcohol-induced hypothermia by cyclo (His-Pro) and its analogs. *Neuropeptides.* 1995;28:351-355.

38. Carr ME Jr, Wolfert AI. Rewarming by hemodialysis for hypothermia: failure of heparin to prevent DIC. *J Emerg Med.* 1988;6:277-280.

39. Casa DJ, et al. Cold water immersion: the gold standard for exertional heatstroke treatment. *Exerc Sport Sci Rev.* 2007;35:141-149.

40. Cauchy E, et al. A controlled trial of a prostacyclin and rt-PA in the treatment of severe frostbite. *N Engl J Med.* 2011;364:189-190.

41. Centers for Disease Control Prevention. Heat-related illnesses and deaths— United States, 1994-1995. *MMWR Morb Mortal Wkly Rep.* 1995;44:465-468.

42. Centers for Disease Control and Prevention. Heat-related deaths—Chicago, Illinois, 1996-2001, and United States, 1979-1999. *MMWR Morb Mortal Wkly Rep.* 2003;52:610-613.

43. Centers for Disease Control and Prevention. Impact of heat waves on mortality— Rome, Italy, June–August 2003. *MMWR Morb Mortal Wkly Rep.* 2004;53:369-371.

44. Centers for Disease Control and Prevention. Hypothermia-related deaths—United States, 2003-2004. *MMWR Morb Mortal Wkly Rep.* 2005;54:173-175.

45. Centers for Disease Control and Prevention. Hypothermia related deaths. Wisconsin 2014 and United States, 2003-2013. *MMWR Morb Mortal Wkly Rep.* 2015;64:141-143.

46. Chao TC, et al. Acute heat stroke deaths. *Pathology.* 1981;13:145-156.

47. Cheng BC, et al. Body cooling causes normalization of cardiac protein expression and function in a rat heatstroke model. *J Proteome Res.* 2008;7:4935-4945.

48. Chobanian SJ. Jaundice occurring after resolution of heat stroke. *Ann Emerg Med.* 1983;12:102-103.

49. Chou YT, et al. Hypothermia attenuates cerebral dopamine overloading and gliosis in rats with heatstroke. *Neurosci Lett.* 2003;336:5-8.

50. Clark WG, Lipton JM. Brain and pituitary peptides in thermoregulation. *Pharmacol Ther.* 1983;22:249-297.

51. Clowes GH Jr, O'Donnell TF Jr. Heat stroke. *N Engl J Med.* 1974;291:564-567.

52. Cogen FC, et al. Phencyclidine-associated acute rhabdomyolysis. *Ann Intern Med.* 1978;88:210-212.

53. Cohen DJ, et al. Resuscitation of the hypothermic patient. *Am J Emerg Med.* 1988;6:475-478.

54. Collins KJ. The autonomic nervous system and the regulation of body temperature. In: Bannister R, ed. *Autonomic Failure: A Textbook of Clinical Disorders of the Autonomic Nervous System.* 3rd ed. New York, NY: Oxford University Press; 1992:212-230.

55. Collins KJ, Exton-Smith AN. 1983 Henderson Award Lecture. Thermal homeostasis in old age. *J Am Geriatr Soc.* 1983;31:519-524.

56. Collis ML, et al. Accidental hypothermia: an experimental study of practical rewarming methods. *Aviat Space Environ Med.* 1977;48:625-632.

57. Cooper KE, Ferguson AV. Thermoregulation and hypothermia in the elderly. In: Pozos RS, Wittmers LE, eds. *The Nature and Treatment of Hypothermia.* Minneapolis: University of Minnesota Press; 1983:165-181.

58. Costrini A. Emergency treatment of exertional heatstroke and comparison of whole body cooling techniques. *Med Sci Sports Exerc.* 1990;22:15-18.

59. Costrini AM, et al. Cardiovascular and metabolic manifestations of heat stroke and severe heat exhaustion. *Am J Med.* 1979;66:296-302.

60. Danzl DF, et al. Multicenter hypothermia survey. *Ann Emerg Med.* 1987;16:1042-1055.

61. DaVee TS, Reineberg EJ. Extreme hypothermia and ventricular fibrillation. *Ann Emerg Med.* 1980;9:100-102.

62. Davis RE, et al. Changing heat-related mortality in the United States. *Environ Health Perspect.* 2003;111:1712-1718.

63. de Garavilla L, et al. Adverse effects of dietary and furosemide-induced sodium depletion on thermoregulation. *Aviat Space Environ Med.* 1990;61:1012-1017.

64. de Haan TR, et al. Pharmacokinetics and pharmacodynamics of medication in asphyxiated newborns during controlled hypothermia. The PharmaCool multicenter study. *BMC Pediatr.* 2012;12:45.

65. Delaney KA. Hypothermic sudden death. In: Paradis NA, et al, eds. *Cardiac Arrest.* Baltimore, MD: Williams and Wilkins; 1996:745-760.

66. Delaney KA, et al. Assessment of acid-base disturbances in hypothermia and their physiologic consequences. *Ann Emerg Med.* 1989;18:72-82.

67. Delaney KA, et al. Rewarming rates in urban patients with hypothermia: prediction of underlying infection. *Acad Emerg Med.* 2006;13:913-921.

68. Delay J, Deniker P. Drug-induced extrapyramidal syndromes. In: Vinkin PJ, Bruyn GW, eds. *Handbook of Clinical Neurology: Diseases of the Basal Ganglia.* Amsterdam: North Holland; 1969:248-266.

69. Delgado G, et al. Spinal cord lesions in heat stroke. *J Neurol Neurosurg Psychiatry.* 1985;48:1065-1067.

70. Dematte JE, et al. Near-fatal heat stroke during the 1995 heat wave in Chicago. *Ann Intern Med.* 1998;129:173-181.

71. Deslarzes T, et al. An evaluation of the Swiss staging model for hypothermia using case reports from the literature. *Scand J Trauma Resusc Emerg Med.* 2016;24:16.

72. Dinarello CA, Wolff SM. Pathogenesis of fever in man. *N Engl J Med.* 1978;298:607-612.

73. Donoghue ER, et al. Criteria for the diagnosis of heat-related deaths: National Association of Medical Examiners. Position paper. National Association of Medical Examiners Ad Hoc Committee on the Definition of Heat-Related Fatalities. *Am J Forensic Med Pathol.* 1997;18:11-14.

74. Durakovic Z, et al. The corrected Q-T interval in the elderly with urban hypothermia. *Coll Antropol.* 1999;23:683-690.

75. Durrer B, et al. The medical on-site treatment of hypothermia: ICAR-MEDCOM recommendation. *High Alt Med Biol.* 2003;4:99-103.

76. el-Gamal N, Frank SM. Perioperative thermoregulatory dysfunction in a patient with a previous traumatic hypothalamic injury. *Anesth Analg.* 1995;80:1245-1247.

77. el-Sherif N, et al. The effect of acute thermal stress on general and pulmonary hemodynamics in the cardiac patient. *Am Heart J.* 1970;79:305-317.

78. Emslie-Smith D. Accidental hypothermia; a common condition with a pathognomic electrocardiogram. *Lancet.* 1958;2:492-495.

79. Emslie-Smith D, et al. The significance of changes in the electrocardiogram in hypothermia. *Br Heart J.* 1959;21:343-351.

80. Eneas JF, et al. The effect of infusion of mannitol-sodium bicarbonate on the clinical course of myoglobinuria. *Arch Intern Med.* 1979;139:801-805.

81. Epstein Y, et al. Role of surface area-to-mass ratio and work efficiency in heat intolerance. *J Appl Physiol.* 1983;54:831-836.

82. Eshel GM, Safar P. The role of the central nervous system in heatstroke: reversible profound depression of cerebral activity in a primate model. *Aviat Space Environ Med.* 2002;73:327-332; discussion 333-334.

83. Eshel GM, et al. The role of the gut in the pathogenesis of death due to hyperthermia. *Am J Forensic Med Pathol.* 2001;22:100-104.

84. Esteban J, et al. Central administration of neuropeptide Y induces hypothermia in mice. Possible interaction with central noradrenergic systems. *Life Sci.* 1989;45:2395-2400.

85. Fell RH, et al. Severe hypothermia as a result of barbiturate overdose complicated by cardiac arrest. *Lancet.* 1968;1:392-394.

86. Feller DJ, et al. Serotonin and genetic differences in sensitivity and tolerance to ethanol hypothermia. *Psychopharmacology (Berl).* 1993;112:331-338.

87. Ferris EB, et al. Heat stroke: clinical and chemical observations on 44 cases. *J Clin Invest.* 1937;17:249-262.

88. Finn DA, et al. Temperature dependence of ethanol depression in rats. *Psychopharmacology (Berl).* 1986;90:185-189.

89. Fischbeck KH, Simon RP. Neurological manifestations of accidental hypothermia. *Ann Neurol.* 1981;10:384-387.

90. Fleming PR, Muir FH. Electrocardiographic changes in induced hypothermia in man. *Br Heart J.* 1957;19:59-66.

91. Fox GR, Hayward JS. Effect of hypothermia on breath-alcohol analysis. *J Forensic Sci.* 1987;32:320-325.

92. Fritz HG, et al. The effect of mild hypothermia on plasma fentanyl concentration and biotransformation in juvenile pigs. *Anesth Analg.* 2005;100:996-1002.

93. Fruehan AE. Accidental hypothermia. Report of eight cases of subnormal body temperature due to exposure. *Arch Intern Med.* 1960;106:218-229.

94. Gabow PA, et al. The spectrum of rhabdomyolysis. *Medicine (Baltimore).* 1982;61:141-152.

95. Gaffin SL, et al. Cooling methods for heatstroke victims. *Ann Intern Med.* 2000;132:678.

96. Gentilello LM, et al. Continuous arteriovenous rewarming: rapid reversal of hypothermia in critically ill patients. *J Trauma.* 1992;32:316-325; discussion 325-327.

97. Gibson OR, et al. Isothermic and fixed-intensity heat acclimation methods elicit equal increases in Hsp72 mRNA. *Scand J Med Sci Sports.* 2015;25(suppl 1):259-268.

98. Giercksky T, et al. Severe liver failure in exertional heat stroke. *Scand J Gastroenterol.* 1999;34:824-827.

99. Gillen JP, et al. Ventricular fibrillation during orotracheal intubation of hypothermic dogs. *Ann Emerg Med.* 1986;15:412-416.

100. Gilliam DM, Collins AC. Concentration-dependent effects of ethanol in long-sleep and short-sleep mice. *Alcohol Clin Exp Res.* 1983;7:337-342.

101. Ginsberg MD, et al. Amphetamine intoxication with coagulopathy, hyperthermia, and reversible renal failure. A syndrome resembling heatstroke. *Ann Intern Med.* 1970;73:81-85.

102. Goldberg LI. Cardiovascular and renal actions of dopamine: potential clinical applications. *Pharmacol Rev.* 1972;24:1-29.

103. Golden FSC, Hervey GR. The "after-drop" and death after rescue from immersion in cold water. In: Adam JM, ed. *Hypothermia Ashore and Afloat.* Aberdeen, TX: Aberdeen University Press; 1981:37-56.

104. Goldsmith R, et al. Effects of drugs on heat acclimatization by controlled hyperthermia. *J Appl Physiol.* 1967;22:301-304.

105. Graham BS, et al. Nonexertional heatstroke. Physiologic management and cooling in 14 patients. *Arch Intern Med.* 1986;146:87-90.

106. Greenblatt DJ, et al. Fatal hyperthermia following haloperidol therapy of sedative-hypnotic withdrawal. *J Clin Psychiatry.* 1978;39:673-675.

107. Greenland P, Southwick WH. Hyperthermia associated with chlorpromazine and full-sheet restraint. *Am J Psychiatry.* 1978;135:1234-1235.

108. Gronert GA. Controversies in malignant hyperthermia. *Anesthesiology.* 1983;59:273-274.

109. Guntupalli KK, et al. Effects of induced total-body hyperthermia on phosphorus metabolism in humans. *Am J Med.* 1984;77:250-254.

110. Gupta BN, et al. Cold-sensitive afferents from the abdomen. *Pflugers Arch.* 1979;380:203-204.

111. Ham J, et al. Pharmacokinetics and pharmacodynamics of D-tubocurarine during hypothermia in the cat. *Anesthesiology.* 1978;49:324-329.

112. Hamlet MP. Fluid shifts in hypothermia. In: Pozos RS, Wittmers LE, eds. *The Nature and Treatment of Hypothermia.* Minneapolis: University of Minnesota Press; 1983:94-99.

113. Hammel HT. Regulation of internal body temperature. *Annu Rev Physiol.* 1968;30:641-710.

114. Harari A, et al. Haemodynamic study of prolonged deep accidental hypothermia. *Eur J Intensive Care Med.* 1975;1:65-70.

115. Harnett RM, et al. A review of the literature concerning resuscitation from hypothermia: part I—the problem and general approaches. *Aviat Space Environ Med.* 1983;54:425-434.

116. Hauty MG, et al. Prognostic factors in severe accidental hypothermia: experience from the Mt. Hood tragedy. *J Trauma.* 1987;27:1107-1112.

117. Hayward JS, Steinman AM. Accidental hypothermia: an experimental study of inhalation rewarming. *Aviat Space Environ Med.* 1975;46:1236-1240.

118. Heiman-Patterson TD. Neuroleptic malignant syndrome and malignant hyperthermia. Important issues for the medical consultant. *Med Clin North Am.* 1993;77:477-492.

119. Hensel H. Cutaneous thermoreceptors. In: Hensel H, ed. *Handbook of Sensory Physiology.* Berlin: Springer-Verlag; 1972:79-110.

120. Hensel H. Neural processes in thermoregulation. *Physiol Rev.* 1973;53:948-1017.

121. Hensel H, et al. Structure and function of cold receptors. *Pflugers Arch.* 1974;352:1-10.

122. Hernandez E, et al. Hemodialysis for treatment of accidental hypothermia. *Nephron.* 1993;63:214-216.

123. Hochachka PW. Defense strategies against hypoxia and hypothermia. *Science.* 1986;231:234-241.

124. Hoffman RS, et al. Endogenous Digitalis-like factors in hypothermic patients. *Gen Intern Med Clin Innov.* 2016;1:67-70.

125. Hori T, Harada Y. Responses of midbrain raphe neurons to local temperature. *Pflugers Arch.* 1976;364:205-207.

126. Hsu SF, et al. Heat shock protein 72 may improve hypotension by increasing cardiac mechanical efficiency and arterial elastance in heatstroke rats. *Int J Cardiol.* 2016;219:63-69.

127. Hubbard RW. The role of exercise in the etiology of exertional heatstroke. *Med Sci Sports Exerc.* 1990;22:2-5.

128. Hudson LD, Conn RD. Accidental hypothermia. Associated diagnoses and prognosis in a common problem. *JAMA.* 1974;227:37-40.

129. Huisse MG, et al. Leukocyte activation: the link between inflammation and coagulation during heatstroke. A study of patients during the 2003 heat wave in Paris. *Crit Care Med.* 2008;36:2288-2295.

130. Jacobs JJ, et al. Cyclo (His-Pro): mapping hypothalamic sites for its hypothermic action. *Brain Res.* 1982;250:205-209.

131. Jardon OM. Physiologic stress, heat stroke, malignant hyperthermia—a perspective. *Mil Med.* 1982;147:8-14.

132. Jessen K, Hagelsten JO. Peritoneal dialysis in the treatment of profound accidental hypothermia. *Aviat Space Environ Med.* 1978;49:426-429.

133. Kadar D, et al. The fate of phenobarbitone in children in hypothermia and at normal body temperature. *Can Anaesth Soc J.* 1982;29:16-23.

134. Kalant H, Le AD. Effects of ethanol on thermoregulation. *Pharmacol Ther.* 1983;23:313-364.

135. Kalita J, Misra UK. Neurophysiological studies in a patient with heat stroke. *J Neurol.* 2001;248:993-995.

136. Kalser SC, et al. Drug metabolism in hypothermia. Uptake, metabolism and excretion of C14-procaine by the isolated, perfused rat liver. *J Pharmacol Exp Ther.* 1968;164:396-404.

137. Kalser SC, et al. Drug metabolism in hypothermia. Uptake, metabolism and excretion of S35-sulfanilamide by the isolated, perfused rat liver. *J Pharmacol Exp Ther.* 1968;159:389-398.

138. Kalser SC, et al. Drug metabolism in hypothermia. II. C 14-atropine uptake, metabolism and excretion by the isolated, perfused rat liver. *J Pharmacol Exp Ther.* 1965;147:260-269.

139. Keren G, et al. Temporary heat intolerance in a heatstroke patient. *Aviat Space Environ Med.* 1981;52:116-117.

140. Kew M, et al. Liver damage in heatstroke. *Am J Med.* 1970;49:192-202.

141. Kew MC, et al. The heart in heatstroke. *Am Heart J.* 1969;77:324-335.

142. Kiley JP, et al. The effect of hypothermia on central neural control of respiration. *Respir Physiol.* 1984;58:295-312.

143. Knochel JP. Environmental heat illness. An eclectic review. *Arch Intern Med.* 1974;133:841-864.

144. Knochel JP, et al. The renal, cardiovascular, hematologic and serum electrolyte abnormalities of heat stroke. *Am J Med.* 1961;30:299-309.

145. Knochel JP, Caskey JH. The mechanism of hypophosphatemia in acute heat stroke. *JAMA.* 1977;238:425-426.

146. Knudsen JF, et al. Oligohidrosis and fever in pediatric patients treated with zonisamide. *Pediatr Neurol.* 2003;28:184-189.

147. Koren G, et al. Influence of hypothermia on the pharmacokinetics of gentamicin and theophylline in piglets. *Crit Care Med.* 1985;13:844-847.

148. Koren G, et al. Effect of hypothermia on the pharmacokinetics of ethanol in piglets. *Ann Emerg Med.* 1989;18:118-121.

149. Koren G, et al. The influence of hypothermia on the disposition of fentanyl—human and animal studies. *Eur J Clin Pharmacol.* 1987;32:373-376.

150. Kornberger E, et al. Effects of epinephrine in a pig model of hypothermic cardiac arrest and closed-chest cardiopulmonary resuscitation combined with active rewarming. *Resuscitation.* 2001;50:301-308.

151. Krisko I, et al. Severe hyperpyrexia due to tranylcypromine-amphetamine toxicity. *Ann Intern Med.* 1969;70:559-564.

152. Krismer AC, et al. Cardiopulmonary resuscitation during severe hypothermia in pigs: does epinephrine or vasopressin increase coronary perfusion pressure? *Anesth Analg.* 2000;90:69-73.

153. Krismer AC, et al. Vasopressin during cardiopulmonary resuscitation: a progress report. *Crit Care Med.* 2004;32:S432-S435.

154. Laskowski LK, et al. Ice water submersion for rapid cooling in severe drug-induced hyperthermia. *Clin Toxicol (Phila).* 2015;53:181-184.

155. Laufman H. Profound accidental hypothermia. *JAMA.* 1951;147:1201-1212.

156. Lavonas EJ, et al. Part 10: Special circumstances of resuscitation: 2015 American Heart Association guidelines update for cardiopulmonary resuscitation and emergency cardiovascular care. *Circulation.* 2015;132(Suppl 2):S501-S18.

157. Ledingham IM, Mone JG. Treatment of accidental hypothermia: a prospective clinical study. *Br Med J.* 1980;280:1102-1105.

158. Lefkowitz D, et al. Cerebellar syndrome following neuroleptic induced heat stroke. *J Neurol Neurosurg Psychiatry.* 1983;46:183-185.

159. Leon LR, Bouchama A. Heat stroke. *Compr Physiol.* 2015;5:611-647.

160. Leon LR, Helwig BG. Role of endotoxin and cytokines in the systemic inflammatory response to heat injury. *Front Biosci (Schol Ed).* 2010;2:916-938.

161. Levinson DF, Simpson GM. Neuroleptic-induced extrapyramidal symptoms with fever. Heterogeneity of the "neuroleptic malignant syndrome." *Arch Gen Psychiatry.* 1986;43:839-848.

162. Lew HL, et al. Rehabilitation of a patient with heat stroke: a case report. *Am J Phys Med Rehabil.* 2002;81:629-632.

163. Lewin S, et al. Infections in hypothermic patients. *Arch Intern Med.* 1981;141:920-925.

164. Lin YF, et al. Vasoactive mediators and renal haemodynamics in exertional heat stroke complicated by acute renal failure. *QJM.* 2003;96:193-201.

165. Lipton JM, et al. Thermoregulatory disorders after removal of a craniopharyngioma from the third cerebral ventricle. *Brain Res Bull.* 1981;7:369-373.

166. Llach F, et al. The pathophysiology of altered calcium metabolism in rhabdomyolysis-induced acute renal failure. Interactions of parathyroid hormone, 25-hydroxycholecalciferol, and 1,25-dihydroxycholecalciferol. *N Engl J Med.* 1981;305:117-123.

167. Lloyd EL. The cause of death after rescue. *Int J Sports Med.* 1992;13:196-199.

168. Lomax P. Neuropharmacological aspects of thermoregulation. In: Pozos RS, Wittmers LE, eds. *The Nature and Treatment of Hypothermia.* Minneapolis: University of Minnesota Press; 1983:81-94.

169. MacKenzie MA, et al. Poikilothermia in man: pathophysiology and clinical implications. *Medicine (Baltimore).* 1991;70:257-268.

170. Maickel RP. Interaction of drugs with autonomic nervous function and thermoregulation. *Fed Proc.* 1970;29:1973-1979.

171. Mair P, et al. Prognostic markers in patients with severe accidental hypothermia and cardiocirculatory arrest. *Resuscitation.* 1994;27:47-54.

172. Malamud N, et al. Heatstroke: a clinicopathologic study of 125 fatal cases. *Milit Surg.* 1946;99:397-444.

173. Marion DW, et al. Treatment of traumatic brain injury with moderate hypothermia. *N Engl J Med.* 1997;336:540-546.

174. McAllister RG Jr. Fever, tachycardia, and hypertension with acute catatonic schizophrenia. *Arch Intern Med.* 1978;138:1154-1156.

175. McAllister RG Jr, et al. Effects of hypothermia on propranolol kinetics. *Clin Pharmacol Ther.* 1979;25:1-7.

176. McAllister RG Jr, Tan TG. Effect of hypothermia on drug metabolism. In vitro studies with propranolol and verapamil. *Pharmacology.* 1980;20:95-100.

177. Megarbane B, et al. Endovascular hypothermia for heat stroke: a case report. *Intensive Care Med.* 2004;30:170.

178. Mehta AC, Baker RN. Persistent neurological deficits in heat stroke. *Neurology.* 1970;20:336-340.

179. Menon MK, et al. Influence of D-1 receptor system on the D-2 receptor-mediated hypothermic response in mice. *Life Sci.* 1988;43:871-881.

180. Millan MJ, et al. Evidence that dopamine D3 receptors participate in clozapine-induced hypothermia. *Eur J Pharmacol.* 1995;280:225-229.

181. Millan MJ, et al. S 14297, a novel selective ligand at cloned human dopamine D3 receptors, blocks 7-OH-DPAT-induced hypothermia in rats. *Eur J Pharmacol*. 1994;260:R3-R5.

182. Miller JW, et al. Urban accidental hypothermia: 135 cases. *Ann Emerg Med*. 1980;9:456-461.

183. Mills W. Accidental hypothermia. In: Pozos RS, Wittmers LE, eds. *The Nature and Treatment of Hypothermia*. Minneapolis: University of Minnesota Press; 1983:182-193.

184. Mogilnicka E, et al. Clonidine and a beta-agonists induce hyperthermia in rats at high ambient temperature. *J Neural Transm*. 1985;63:223-235.

185. Moore JA, Kakihana R. Ethanol-induced hypothermia in mice: influence of genotype on development of tolerance. *Life Sci*. 1978;23:2331-2337.

186. Morishima HO, et al. Body temperature and disappearance of lidocaine in newborn puppies. *Anesth Analg*. 1971;50:938-942.

187. Murphy MT, Lipton JM. Effects of alcohol on thermoregulation in aged monkeys. *Exp Gerontol*. 1983;18:19-27.

188. Murray PT, Fellner SK. Efficacy of hemodialysis in rewarming accidental hypothermia victims. *J Am Soc Nephrol*. 1994;5:422-423.

189. Mustafa S, et al. Hyperthermia-induced vasoconstriction of the carotid artery, a possible causative factor of heatstroke. *J Appl Physiol*. 2004;96:1875-1878.

190. Myers RD. Alcohol's effect on body temperature: hypothermia, hyperthermia or poikilothermia? *Brain Res Bull*. 1981;7:209-220.

191. Nicodemus HF, et al. Hemodynamic effects of inotropes during hypothermia and rapid rewarming. *Crit Care Med*. 1981;9:325-328.

192. Nicodemus HF, et al. Lidocaine/propranolol: hemodynamic effects during hypothermia and rewarming. *J Surg Res*. 1981;30:6-13.

193. Nieto-Barrera M, et al. [Anhidrosis and hyperthermia associated with treatment with topiramate]. *Rev Neurol (Paris)*. 2002;34:114-116.

194. Nikki P, et al. Effect of ethanol on body temperature, postanaesthetic shivering and tissue monoamines in halothane-anaesthetized rats. *Ann Med Exp Biol Fenn*. 1971;49:157-161.

195. O'Connor JP. Use of peritoneal dialysis in severely hypothermic patients. *Ann Emerg Med*. 1986;15:104-105.

196. O'Donnell TF Jr. Acute heat stroke. Epidemiologic, biochemical, renal, and coagulation studies. *JAMA*. 1975;234:824-828.

197. O'Donnell TF Jr, Clowes GH Jr. The circulatory abnormalities of heat stroke. *N Engl J Med*. 1972;287:734-737.

198. O'Keeffe KM. Accidental hypothermia: a review of 62 cases. *JACEP*. 1977;6:491-496.

199. Ogawa T, Low PA. Autonomic regulation of temperature and sweating. In: Low PA, ed. *Autonomic Disorders: Evaluation and Management*. Boston, MA: Little, Brown; 1993:79-91.

200. Ohmura A, et al. Effects of hypocarbia and normocarbia on cardiovascular dynamics and regional circulation in the hypothermic dog. *Anesthesiology*. 1979;50:293-298.

201. Okada M. The cardiac rhythm in accidental hypothermia. *J Electrocardiol*. 1984;17:123-128.

202. Okuliczkorayn I, et al. Tolerance to hypothermia and hypnotic action of ethanol in 3 and 14 months old rats. *Pharmacol Res*. 1992;25:63-64.

203. Osborn JJ. Experimental hypothermia; respiratory and blood pH changes in relation to cardiac function. *Am J Physiol*. 1953;175:389-398.

204. Osborne L, et al. Survival after prolonged cardiac arrest and accidental hypothermia. *Br Med J (Clin Res Ed)*. 1984;289:881-882.

205. Patel R, et al. Myoglobinuric acute renal failure in phencyclidine overdose: report of observations in eight cases. *Ann Emerg Med*. 1980;9:549-553.

206. Patel S, Hutson PH. Hypothermia induced by cholinomimetic drugs is blocked by galanin: possible involvement of ATP-sensitive K$^+$ channels. *Eur J Pharmacol*. 1994;255:25-32.

207. Paton BC. Accidental hypothermia. *Pharmacol Ther*. 1983;22:331-377.

208. Perchick JS, et al. Disseminated intravascular coagulation in heat stroke. Response to heparin therapy. *JAMA*. 1975;231:480-483.

209. Rawson RO, Quick KP. Evidence of deep-body thermoreceptor response to intra-abdominal heating of the ewe. *J Appl Physiol*. 1970;28:813-820.

210. Reuler JB. Hypothermia: pathophysiology, clinical settings, and management. *Ann Intern Med*. 1978;89:519-527.

211. Riedel W. Warm receptors in the dorsal abdominal wall of the rabbit. *Pflugers Arch*. 1976;361:205-206.

212. Ritzmann RF, Tabakoff B. Body temperature in mice: a quantitative measure of alcohol tolerance and physical dependence. *J Pharmacol Exp Ther*. 1976;199:158-170.

213. Ritzmann RF, Tabakoff B. Dissociation of alcohol tolerance and dependence. *Nature*. 1976;263:418-420.

214. Roggla M, et al. Severe accidental hypothermia with or without hemodynamic instability: rewarming without the use of extracorporeal circulation. *Wien Klin Wochenschr*. 2002;114:315-320.

215. Romm E, Collins AC. Body temperature influences on ethanol elimination rate. *Alcohol*. 1987;4:189-198.

216. Ron D, et al. Prevention of acute renal failure in traumatic rhabdomyolysis. *Arch Intern Med*. 1984;144:277-280.

217. Rowell LB. Cardiovascular aspects of human thermoregulation. *Circ Res*. 1983;52:367-379.

218. Ruiz de Elvira MC, Coen CW. Centrally administered neuropeptide Y enhances the hypothermia induced by peripheral administration of adrenoceptor antagonists. *Peptides*. 1990;11:963-967.

219. Saissy JM. Liver transplantation in a case of fulminant liver failure after exertion. *Intensive Care Med*. 1996;22:831.

220. Salmi P, et al. Antagonism by SCH 23390 of clozapine-induced hypothermia in the rat. *Eur J Pharmacol*. 1994;253:67-73.

221. Sanchez C, Lembol HL. The involvement of muscarinic receptor subtypes in the mediation of hypothermia, tremor, and salivation in male mice. *Pharmacol Toxicol*. 1994;74:35-39.

222. Sarnquist F, Larson CP Jr. Drug-induced heat stroke. *Anesthesiology*. 1973;39:348-350.

223. Satinoff E. Impaired recovery from hypothermia after anterior hypothalamic lesions in hibernators. *Science*. 1965;148:399-400.

224. Satinoff E. Disruption of hibernation caused by hypothalamic lesions. *Science*. 1967;155:1031-1033.

225. Savard GK, et al. Peripheral blood flow during rewarming from mild hypothermia in humans. *J Appl Physiol*. 1985;58:4-13.

226. Schaller MD, et al. Hyperkalemia. A prognostic factor during acute severe hypothermia. *JAMA*. 1990;264:1842-1845.

227. Schrier RW, et al. Nephropathy associated with heat stress and exercise. *Ann Intern Med*. 1967;67:356-376.

228. Schwarz B, et al. Vasopressin improves survival in a pig model of hypothermic cardiopulmonary resuscitation. *Crit Care Med*. 2002;30:1311-1314.

229. Schwarz B, et al. Neither vasopressin nor amiodarone improve CPR outcome in an animal model of hypothermic cardiac arrest. *Acta Anaesthesiol Scand*. 2003;47:1114-1118.

230. Seraj MA, et al. Are heat stroke patients fluid depleted? Importance of monitoring central venous pressure as a simple guideline for fluid therapy. *Resuscitation*. 1991;21:33-39.

231. Shapiro Y, et al. Heat intolerance in former heatstroke patients. *Ann Intern Med*. 1979;90:913-916.

232. Shibolet S, et al. Heatstroke: its clinical picture and mechanism in 36 cases. *Q J Med*. 1967;36:525-548.

233. Shvartz E, et al. Heat acclimation, physical fitness, and responses to exercise in temperate and hot environments. *J Appl Physiol*. 1977;43:678-683.

234. Shvartz E, et al. Prediction of heat tolerance from heart rate and rectal temperature in a temperate environment. *J Appl Physiol*. 1977;43:684-688.

235. Silfvast T, Pettila V. Outcome from severe accidental hypothermia in Southern Finland—a 10-year review. *Resuscitation*. 2003;59:285-290.

236. Smith CJ, Johnson JM. Responses to hyperthermia. Optimizing heat dissipation by convection and evaporation: neural control of skin blood flow and sweating in humans. *Auton Neurosci*. 2016;196:25-36.

237. Sohal RS, et al. Heat stroke. An electron microscopic study of endothelial cell damage and disseminated intravascular coagulation. *Arch Intern Med*. 1968;122:43-47.

238. Southwick FS, Dalglish PH Jr. Recovery after prolonged asystolic cardiac arrest in profound hypothermia. A case report and literature review. *JAMA*. 1980;243:1250-1253.

239. Splittgerber FH, et al. Partial cardiopulmonary bypass for core rewarming in profound accidental hypothermia. *Am Surg*. 1986;52:407-412.

240. Sprung CL. Hemodynamic alterations of heat stroke in the elderly. *Chest*. 1979;75:362-366.

241. Sprung CL, et al. The metabolic and respiratory alterations of heat stroke. *Arch Intern Med*. 1980;140:665-669.

242. Stoner J, et al. Amiodarone and bretylium in the treatment of hypothermic ventricular fibrillation in a canine model. *Acad Emerg Med*. 2003;10:187-191.

243. Strapazzon G, et al. Accidental hypothermia. *N Engl J Med*. 2013;368:681-682.

244. Sumann G, et al. Cardiopulmonary resuscitation after near drowning and hypothermia: restoration of spontaneous circulation after vasopressin. *Acta Anaesthesiol Scand*. 2003;47:363-365.

245. Tavel ME, et al. A critical analysis of mortality associated with delirium tremens. Review of 39 fatalities in a 9-year period. *Am J Med Sci*. 1961;242:18-29.

246. Tolman KG, Cohen A. Accidental hypothermia. *CMAJ*. 1970;103:1357-1361.

247. Tomaszewski W. Changements electrocardiographiques. Ovserves chez un homme mort de froid. *Arch Mal Coeur*. 1938;31:525-528.

248. Towne WD, et al. Intractable ventricular fibrillation associated with profound accidental hypothermia—successful treatment with partial cardiopulmonary bypass. *N Engl J Med*. 1972;287:1135-1136.

249. Trevino A, et al. The characteristic electrocardiogram of accidental hypothermia. *Arch Intern Med*. 1971;127:470-473.

250. Truscott DG, et al. Accidental profound hypothermia. Successful resuscitation by core rewarming and assisted circulation. *Arch Surg*. 1973;106:216-218.

251. Tysinger DS Jr, et al. The electrocardiogram of dogs surviving 1.5 degrees centigrade. *Am Heart J*. 1955;50:816-822.

252. Vassallo SU, Delaney KA. Pharmacologic effects on thermoregulation: mechanisms of drug-related heatstroke. *J Toxicol Clin Toxicol*. 1989;27:199-224.

253. Vassallo SU, et al. A prospective evaluation of the electrocardiographic manifestations of hypothermia. *Acad Emerg Med*. 1999;6:1121-1126.

254. Vertel RM, Knochel JP. Acute renal failure due to heat injury. An analysis of ten cases associated with a high incidence of myoglobinuria. *Am J Med*. 1967;43:435-451.

255. Walczak DD. Biochemical correlates of alcohol tolerance: role of cerebral protein synthesis. University of Toronto.

256. Ward A, et al. Dantrolene. A review of its pharmacodynamic and pharmacokinetic properties and therapeutic use in malignant hyperthermia, the neuroleptic malignant syndrome and an update of its use in muscle spasticity. *Drugs*. 1986;32:130-168.

257. Webb P. Afterdrop of body temperature during rewarming: an alternative explanation. *J Appl Physiol.* 1986;60:385-390.

258. Weyman AE, et al. Accidental hypothermia in an alcoholic population. *Am J Med.* 1974;56:13-21.

259. White JD. Hypothermia: the Bellevue Experience. *Ann Emerg Med.* 1982;11:417-424.

260. Wildschut ED, et al. Effect of hypothermia and extracorporeal life support on drug disposition in neonates. *Semin Fetal Neonatal Med.* 2013;18:23-27.

261. Wira CR, et al. Anti-arrhythmic and vasopressor medications for the treatment of ventricular fibrillation in severe hypothermia: a systematic review of the literature. *Resuscitation.* 2008;78:21-29.

262. Wislicki L. Effects of hypothermia and hyperthermia on the action of neuromuscular blocking agents. I. Suxamethonium. *Arch Int Pharmacodyn Ther.* 1960;126:68-78.

263. Wong KC. Physiology and pharmacology of hypothermia. *West J Med.* 1983;138:227-232.

264. Zelman S, Guillan R. Heat stroke in phenothiazine-treated patients: a report of three fatalities. *Am J Psychiatry.* 1970;126:1787-1790.

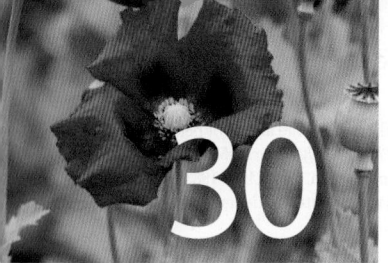

30

REPRODUCTIVE AND PERINATAL PRINCIPLES

Jeffrey S. Fine

Reproductive and perinatal principles in toxicology are often derived from basic science studies and are applied cautiously to clinical practice. This chapter reviews several principles of reproductive medicine that have implications for toxicology, including the physiology of pregnancy and placental xenobiotic transfer, the effects of xenobiotics on the developing fetus and the neonate, and the management of poisoning or overdose in pregnant women.

One of the most dramatic effects of exposure to a xenobiotic during pregnancy is the birth of a child with congenital malformations. Teratology, the study of birth defects, has principally been concerned with the study of physical malformations. A broader view of teratology includes "developmental" teratogens—xenobiotics that induce structural malformations, metabolic or physiologic dysfunction, or psychological or behavioral alterations or deficits in the offspring, either at or after birth.[291] Only 4% to 6% of birth defects are attributable to known pharmaceuticals or occupational and environmental exposures.[291,302]

Some reproductive effects of xenobiotics occur before conception. Female germ cells are formed in utero; adverse effects from xenobiotic exposure theoretically occur from the time of a woman's own intrauterine development to the end of her reproductive years. An example of a xenobiotic that had both teratogenic and reproductive effects is diethylstilbestrol (DES), which was most notable for causing vaginal or cervical adenocarcinoma (or both) in some women who were exposed to DES in utero and which also had adverse effects on fertility and pregnancy outcome in the same cohort of women exposed in utero.[239,263]

Men generally receive less attention with respect to reproductive risks. Male gametes are formed after puberty; only from that time on are they susceptible to xenobiotic injury. An example of a xenobiotic affecting male reproduction is dibromochloropropane, which reduces spermatogenesis and, consequently, fertility. In general, much less is known about the paternal contribution to teratogenesis.[63,130,152]

Occupational exposures to xenobiotics are potentially important but are often poorly defined. In 2015, there were approximately 43 million women of reproductive age in the workforce.[331] Although approximately 90,000 chemicals are used commercially in the United States, only a few thousand of them have been specifically evaluated for reproductive toxicity. Many xenobiotics have teratogenic effects when tested in animal models, but there are relatively few well-defined human teratogens (Table 30–1).[302] Thus, most tested xenobiotics do not appear to present a human teratogenic risk, but most xenobiotics have not been tested. Some of the presumed safe xenobiotics have other reproductive, nonteratogenic toxicities. Several excellent reviews and online resources are available.[39,106,266,302,325]

Another type of xenobiotic exposure for a pregnant woman is intentional overdose. Although a xenobiotic taken in overdose can have direct toxicity to the fetus, fetal toxicity frequently results from maternal pulmonary or hemodynamic compromise, further emphasizing the critical interdependency of the maternal–fetal dyad.

Xenobiotic exposures before and during pregnancy can have effects throughout gestation and also extend into and beyond the newborn period. In addition, the effects of xenobiotic administration in the perinatal period and the special case of delivering xenobiotics to an infant via breast milk deserve particular consideration.

PHYSIOLOGIC CHANGES DURING PREGNANCY THAT AFFECT DRUG PHARMACOKINETICS

Many physical and physiologic changes that occur during pregnancy affect both the absorption and distribution of xenobiotics in the pregnant woman and consequently potentially affect the amount of xenobiotics delivered to the fetus.[21]

Delayed gastric emptying, decreased gastrointestinal (GI) motility, and increased transit time through the GI tract occur during pregnancy. These changes result in delayed but more complete GI absorption of xenobiotics and, consequently, lower peak plasma concentrations which may be consequential in an adverse manner. Because blood flow to the skin and mucous membranes is increased, absorption from dermal exposure is increased. Similarly, absorption of inhaled xenobiotics is increased because of increased tidal volume and decreased residual lung volume.

An increased free xenobiotic concentration in the pregnant woman can be caused by several factors during the later stages of pregnancy a decreased plasma albumin, increased binding competition, and decreased hepatic biotransformation. Fat stores increase throughout pregnancy and are maximal at about 30 weeks; near term, free fatty acids are released, and along with them the lipophilic xenobiotics that have accumulated in the lipid compartment are released. The increased concentration of circulating free fatty acids leads to competition with circulating free xenobiotics for binding sites on albumin.

Other factors leading to decreased free xenobiotic concentrations, early in pregnancy, are increased fat stores, as well as the increased plasma and extracellular fluid volume, which lead to a greater volume of distribution. Increased renal blood flow and glomerular filtration may or can result in increased renal elimination.

Cardiac output increases throughout pregnancy, with the placenta receiving a gradually increasing proportion of total blood volume. Xenobiotic delivery to the placenta therefore increases over the course of pregnancy.

These processes interact dynamically, and it is difficult to predict their net effect. The concentrations of many xenobiotics, such as lithium, gentamicin, and carbamazepine, decrease during pregnancy even if the dose administered is unchanged.[110]

Although not specifically related to the physiologic changes occurring during pregnancy, the fetus can also be exposed to xenobiotics that had accumulated in adipose tissue before pregnancy. For example, typical retinoid malformations occurred in a baby born to a woman whose pregnancy began one year after she discontinued the use of etretinate (retinoic acid), a medication that is used to treat severe psoriasis, congenital ichthyosis acne, and several other disorders of keratinization which may have clinical implications.[179]

XENOBIOTIC EXPOSURE IN PREGNANT WOMEN

Exposure to xenobiotics during pregnancy is common. At some time during pregnancy, as many as 90% of pregnant women take prescription or nonprescription medications other than vitamins, mineral supplements, and iron. The most commonly used are analgesics, antipyretics, antimicrobials, antihistamines, vitamin B_6 and antiemetics.[73,74,198,250,310,328] In addition, use of caffeine, tobacco, and alcohol is common. Some pregnant women use xenobiotics to treat a preexisting chronic disease such as epilepsy or a newly diagnosed

TABLE 30–1	Known and Possible Human Teratogens	
Xenobiotic	**Reported Effects**	**Comments**
Alkylating agents (eg, busulfan, chlorambucil, cyclophosphamide, mechlorethamine, nitrogen mustard)	Growth retardation, cleft palate, microphthalmia, hypoplastic ovaries, cloudy corneas, renal agenesis, malformations of digits, cardiac defects, other anomalies	10%–50% malformation rate, depending on the agent. Cyclophosphamide-induced damage requires cytochrome P450 oxidation.
Aminopterin, methotrexate (amethopterin)	Hydro- or microcephaly; meningoencephalocele; anencephaly; abnormal cranial ossification; cerebral hypoplasia; growth retardation; eye, ear, and nose malformations; cleft palate; malformed extremities or fingers; reduction in derivatives of first branchial arch; developmental delay	Folate antagonists inhibit dihydrofolate reductase. High rate of malformations.
Amiodarone	Transient neonatal hypothyroidism, with or without goiter; hyperthyroidism	Amiodarone contains 39% iodine by weight. Small to moderate risk from 10 weeks to term for thyroid dysfunction.
Androgens	Virilization of the female external genitalia: clitoromegaly, labioscrotal fusion	Dose dependent. Stimulates growth of sex steroid receptor–containing tissue.
Angiotensin-converting enzyme inhibitors and angiotensin II type 1 receptors blockers	Fetal or neonatal death, prematurity, oligohydramnios, neonatal anuria, IUGR, secondary skull hypoplasia, limb contractures, pulmonary hypoplasia	Significant risk of effects related to chronic fetal hypotension during second or third trimester. If used during early pregnancy, can be switched during first trimester.
Carbamazepine	Upslanting palpebral fissures, epicanthal folds, short nose with long philtrum, fingernail hypoplasia, developmental delay, NTD	1% risk for NTD. Risk of other malformations is unquantified. Risk is increased in setting of therapy with multiple antiepileptics, particularly valproic acid. Mechanism involves an epoxide intermediate. High-dose folate is recommended to prevent NTDs.
Carbon monoxide	Cerebral atrophy, intellectual disability, microcephaly, convulsions, spastic disorders, intrauterine death	With severe maternal poisoning, high risk for neurologic sequelae.
Cocaine	IUGR, microcephaly, neurobehavioral abnormalities, vascular disruptive phenomenon (limb amputation, cerebral infarction, visceral or urinary tract abnormalities)	Vascular disruptive effects because of decreased uterine blood flow and fetal vascular effects from first trimester through the end of pregnancy.
Diazepam	Cleft palate	Controversial association, probably low risk.
Diethylstilbestrol (DES)	*Female offspring:* vaginal adenosis, clear cell adenocarcinoma of the vagina, irregular menses, reduced pregnancy rates, increased rate of preterm deliveries, increased perinatal mortality and spontaneous abortion *Male offspring:* epididymal cysts, cryptorchidism, hypogonadism, diminished spermatogenesis	A synthetic nonsteroidal estrogen that stimulates estrogen receptor–containing tissue. 40%–70% risk of morphologic changes in vaginal epithelium. Risk of carcinoma is approximately one in 1,000 for exposure before the 18th gestational week. Most patients exposed to DES in utero can conceive and deliver normal children.
Ethanol	FAS: pre- or postnatal growth retardation, intellectual disability, fine motor dysfunction, hyperactivity, microcephaly, maxillary hypoplasia, short palpebral fissures, hypoplastic philtrum, thinned upper lips, joint, digit anomalies	Neither a threshold for effects nor a safe dose has been identified. Partial expression or other congenital anomalies. Increased incidence of spontaneous abortion, premature delivery, and stillbirth; neonatal withdrawal.
Fluconazole	Craniosynostosis, orbital hypoplasia, humeral radial synostosis, femoral bowing	Risk related to high-dose (400–800 mg/d), chronic, parenteral use. Single 150-mg oral dose probably safe.
Iodine and iodine-containing products	Thyroid hypoplasia after the eighth week of development	High doses of radioiodine isotopes can additionally produce cell death and mitotic delay. Tissue- and organ-specific damage depends on the specific radioisotope, dose, distribution, metabolism, and localization.
Lead	Lower scores on developmental tests	Higher risk when maternal lead is >10 mcg/dL.
Lithium carbonate	Ebstein anomaly	Controversial association. Low risk.
Methimazole	Aplasia cutis, skull hypoplasia, dystrophic nails, nipple abnormalities, hypo- or hyperthyroidism	Small risk of anomalies or goiter with first trimester exposure. Hypothyroidism risk after 10 weeks of gestation.
Methyl mercury, mercuric sulfide	Normal appearance at birth; cerebral palsylike syndrome after several months; microcephaly, intellectual disability, cerebellar symptoms, eye or dental anomalies	Inhibits enzymes, particularly those with sulfhydryl groups. In acute poisoning, the fetus is 4–10 times more sensitive than an adult.
Methylene blue (intraamniotic injection)	Hemolytic anemia, neonatal jaundice, possible intestinal atresia,	Used to identify twin amniotic sacs during amniocentesis.
Misoprostol	Vascular disruptive phenomena (eg, limb reduction defects); Moebius syndrome (paralysis of sixth and seventh facial nerves)	Synthetic prostaglandin E_1 analog. Effects observed in women after unsuccessful attempts to terminate pregnancy.

(Continued)

TABLE 30–1	Known and Possible Human Teratogens (Continued)	
Xenobiotic	**Reported Effects**	**Comments**
Mycophenolate mofetil	Microtia, orofacial cleft, coloboma, hypertelorism, micrognathia, conotruncal CHD, agenesis of the corpus callosum, esophageal atresia, digital hypoplasia	Immunosuppressive xenobiotic used in transplant recipients, inhibits inosine monophosphate dehydrogenase and blocks de novo purine synthesis in T and B lymphocytes.
Oxazolidine-2,4-diones (trimethadione, paramethadione)	Fetal trimethadione syndrome: V-shaped eyebrows; low-set ears with anteriorly folded helix; high-arched palate; irregular teeth; CNS anomalies; severe developmental delay; cardiovascular, genitourinary, and other anomalies	An 83% risk of at least one major malformation with any exposure; 32% die. Characteristic facial features are associated with chronic exposure.
Paroxetine	Cardiovascular malformations, mostly VSD and ASD	Possible small (1%) increased risk. Possible risk with other SSRIs has not been quantified.
Penicillamine	Cutis laxa, hyperflexibility of joints	Copper chelator—copper deficiency inhibits collagen synthesis or maturation. Few case reports; low risk.
Phenytoin	Fetal hydantoin syndrome: microcephaly, intellectual disability, cleft lip or palate, hypoplastic nails or phalanges, characteristic facies—low nasal bridge, inner epicanthal folds, ptosis, strabismus, hypertelorism, low-set ears, wide mouth	Effects seen with chronic exposure. A 5%–10% risk of typical syndrome, 30% risk of partial syndrome. Risks confounded by those associated with epilepsy itself and use of other antiepileptics.
Polychlorinated biphenyls	Cola-colored children; pigmentation of gums, nails, and groin; hypoplastic, deformed nails; IUGR; abnormal skull calcifications	Cytotoxic xenobiotic. Body residue can affect subsequent offspring for up to 4 years after exposure. Most cases followed high consumption of PCB-contaminated rice oil; 4%–20% of offspring were affected.
Progestins (eg, ethisterone, norethindrone)	Masculinization of female external genitalia	Progestogens are converted into androgens or have weak androgenic activity. Stimulate or interfere with sex steroid receptors. Effects occur only after exposure to high doses of some testosterone-derived progestins in <1% of those exposed. Oral contraceptives containing these agents are not thought to present teratogenic risk.
Quinine	Hypoplasia of eighth nerve, deafness, abortion	Effects related to high doses used as abortifacients.
Radiation, ionizing	Microcephaly, intellectual disability, eye anomalies, growth retardation, visceral malformations	Significant doses of radiation from diagnostic or therapeutic sources produce cell death and mitotic delay. There is no measurable risk with x-ray exposures of 5 rads or less at any stage of pregnancy.
Retinoids (isotretinoin, etretinate, high-dose vitamin A)	Spontaneous abortions; micro- or hydrocephalus; deformities of cranium, ears, face, heart, limbs, liver	Retinoids can cause direct cytotoxicity, alter apoptosis, and inhibit migration of neural crest cells. For isotretinoin, 38% risk of malformations; 80% are CNS malformations. Effects are associated with vitamin A doses of 25,000–100,000 units/day. Exposures below 10,000 IU/day present no risk to fetuses. Topical retinoids are not considered a reproductive risk.
Smoking	Placental lesions, IUGR, increased perinatal mortality, increased risk of SIDS, neurobehavioral effects such as learning deficits and hyperactivity.	Possible mechanisms include vasoconstriction (nicotine effect); hypoxia secondary to hypoperfusion, CO, and CN; and altered development of neurons and neural pathways via stimulation of nicotinic acetylcholine receptors.
Streptomycin	Hearing loss	Rare reports.
Tetracycline	Yellow, gray-brown, or brown staining of deciduous teeth, hypoplastic tooth enamel	Effects seen after 4 months of gestation because tetracyclines must interact with calcified tissue.
Thalidomide	Limb phocomelia, amelia, hypoplasia, congenital heart defects, renal malformations, cryptorchidism, abducens paralysis, deafness, microtia, anotia	~20% risk for exposure during days 34–50 of gestation.
Trimethoprim	NTD, oral clefts, hypospadias, and cardiovascular defects	~1% risk of NTD for first trimester exposure. Mechanism is folic acid inhibition.
Valproic acid	Spina bifida, ASD, cleft palate, hypospadias, polydactyly, craniosynostosis, cognitive deficits	Risk for spina bifida is ~1%, but the risk for dysmorphic facies is greater. Risk is confounded by risks associated with epilepsy itself or use of other anticonvulsants.
Vitamin D	Possible association with supravalvular aortic stenosis, elfin facies, and intellectual disability	Large doses of vitamin D disrupt cellular calcium regulation. Genetic susceptibility plays a role.
Warfarin	Fetal warfarin syndrome: nasal hypoplasia, chondrodysplasia punctata, brachydactyly, skull defects, abnormal ears, malformed eyes, CNS malformations, microcephaly, hydrocephalus, skeletal deformities, intellectual disability, spasticity	10%–25% risk of malformation for first trimester exposure, 3% risk of hemorrhage, 8% risk of stillbirth. Bleeding is an unlikely explanation for effects produced in the first trimester. CNS defects occur during the second or third trimesters and are related to bleeding.

ASD = atrial septal defect; CHD = congestive heart disease; CN = cyanide; CNS = central nervous system; CO = carbon monoxide; FAS = fetal alcohol syndrome; IUGR = intrauterine growth restriction; NSAID = nonsteroidal antiinflammatory drug; NTD = neural tube defect; PCB = polychlorinated biphenyl; SIDS = sudden infant death syndrome; SSRI = selective serotonin reuptake inhibitor; VSD = ventricular septal defect.

Data from Brent RL. Environmental causes of human congenital malformations: The pediatrician's role in dealing with these complex clinical problems caused by a multiplicity of environmental and genetic factors. *Pediatrics.* 2004;113:957-968; Nulman I, et al. Teratogenic drugs and chemicals in humans. In: Koren G, ed. Medication Safety in Pregnancy and Breastfeeding. New York: McGraw-Hill; 2007:21-30; and Polifka JE, Friedman JM. Medical genetics: 1. Clinical teratology in the age of genomics. *CMAJ.* 2002;167:265-273.

disease such as deep vein thrombosis. Many women use various prescription and nonprescription xenobiotics before recognizing that they are pregnant.

Following the international experience with thalidomide in the 1960s that identified a high frequency of congenital malformations associated with its use, the US Food and Drug Administration (FDA) decided there was a need for guidance to prescribers regarding the use of medications during pregnancy. In 1979, the FDA began to require pharmaceutical manufacturers to label their products with respect to use in pregnancy and introduced the ABCDX classification scheme familiar to most practitioners in the United States.[332] Classification systems similar to the former FDA system were developed in Sweden and Australia.[272,289]

The intent of those classification systems was to inform practitioners about the nature of the available evidence regarding risk in pregnancy. However, the ABCDX system was criticized for a number of reasons—the manufacturer assigned the risk category, there was no requirement for additional research, and there was no requirement to update the label when new information became available.[6]

One of the most significant problems with the ABCDX system is the general impression among health care practitioners that the letter categories indicated teratogenic risk with a hierarchy of harmful effects and an equivalence of risk within each category.[82,296,297] For example, a category C medication was generally considered riskier than a category B medication in pregnancy even though category C was the default category for medications about which there was little or no specific human information available and for which the risk was unknown. Approximately 90% of medications were classified as category C.[193]

In addition, there was significant discordance between the use-in-pregnancy labeling and the teratogenic risk as determined by clinical teratologists.[5,193] Manufacturers labeled certain medications as category X (contraindicated in pregnancy) even when there was only limited information associating the medication with any adverse fetal or neonatal effects. For example, oral contraceptives carried a category X classification even though they are not considered teratogenic; the category X was assigned because there was no indication for use of oral contraceptives in pregnancy.[176] Certain medications that carried a category D (high-risk) classification might have caused problems only at certain times during pregnancy or in particular circumstances. In several reports, approximately 6% of pregnant women were prescribed medications that were categorized as D or X and 1% were prescribed medications that are considered teratogenic.[5,13,193] Even medications that have been classified as category D or X sometimes had only a very low risk of teratogenicity or other adverse effects, and exposure to these xenobiotics, even during the first trimester, would not necessarily have been an indication to terminate a pregnancy.[86]

The difficulty regarding appropriate drug labeling reflects many complex questions regarding the use of medications during pregnancy. How should animal data in general be evaluated? How should animal data be extrapolated to humans? How should the teratogenic risk be defined and quantified for any particular xenobiotic? How should the risk of not treating a particular disease be compared with the risk of using a particular medication to treat that disease? Finally, how should the answers to these questions be communicated to practitioners and the public?[297]

In an attempt to address many of these problems, the FDA organized a taskforce in 1998 to propose changes to the labeling of medications for use in pregnancy and lactation.[142,176] The changes, referred to as the "Pregnancy and Lactation Labeling Rule" (PLLR), were initially published in 2008, finalized in 2014, and took effect in 2015 with full implementation expected by 2020.[334] The new PLLR requires "the removal of pregnancy categories A, B, C, D, and X from all human and prescription drug and product labeling" and specifies the content and format for new labels. This content requires (1) a concise description and estimate of the risk of structural teratogenesis, fetal or infant mortality, and impaired growth or physiologic function; (2) details of animal and human data, in particular information from registries, cohort studies, and case–control studies; and (3) clinical considerations such as risk of the disease (treated or untreated) versus risk of the medication, need for dose adjustment in pregnancy, adverse drug reactions specific to pregnancy, monitoring of drug use and effect, effects on labor and delivery, and neonatal complications. The PLLR also requires detailed information with regard to medication use during lactation (previously referred to as the "nursing mothers" section) as well as a new section that describes medication effects on both female and male fertility. There is also a requirement to update the label as new information becomes available that could make the label "inaccurate, false, or misleading."

The new labels will be completely phased in by 2020. Drugs approved after 2015 must use the new labeling format. Drugs released after 2001 will have the newly formatted labels phased in over several years. Drugs approved and released prior to 2001 will not be required to use the new format but will be required to eliminate any reference to a previously assigned letter from the ABCDX system. Considering that the new FDA labels are being phased in over several years, the editors have decided to retain the ABCDX designation in other chapters for this edition.

Specific current information on individual xenobiotics can be obtained from local and regional teratogen information services and published books,[39,302] some of which also have online versions.[228,266,325] *Motherisk* is a Canadian program that uses accumulated evidence and experience to advise women about their actual risk of using a particular medication or being exposed to a particular xenobiotic in a current or planned pregnancy.[227,228]

Although most women are primarily concerned about the teratogenic effects of medications, in utero exposure to therapeutic medications has other pharmacologic effects on newborn infants, such as hyperbilirubinemia or withdrawal syndromes.[39,78]

Estimates of substance use in pregnancy vary tremendously, depending on the geographic location, practice environment, patient population, and screening method. In the National Survey on Drug Use and Health, approximately 16% of pregnant women smoked cigarettes, 11% drank ethanol, 5% used marijuana, 0.25% used cocaine, and 0.1% used heroin.[285] Women tend to decrease their exposure to xenobiotics after they know they are pregnant.[33,150,153]

PLACENTAL REGULATION OF XENOBIOTIC TRANSFER TO FETUSES

With respect to the transfer of xenobiotics from mother to fetus, the placenta functions in a manner similar to other lipoprotein membranes. Most xenobiotics enter the fetal circulation by passive diffusion down a concentration gradient across the placental membranes. The characteristics of a substance that favor this passive diffusion are low molecular weight (LMW), lipid solubility, neutral polarity, and low protein binding.[9] Polar molecules and ions are transported through interstitial pores.[9]

Xenobiotics with a MW greater than 1,000 Da do not diffuse passively across the placenta, and this characteristic is used to therapeutic advantage. For example, warfarin (MW, 1,000 Da) easily crosses the placenta and causes specific fetal malformations.[342] However, heparin (MW, 15,000 Da), which is too large to cross the placenta, is not teratogenic and, consequently, is the preferred anticoagulant during pregnancy. Most medications have MWs between 250 and 400 Da and easily cross the placenta. For example, thiopental is highly lipid soluble and crosses the placenta rapidly. Fetal plasma concentrations reach maternal concentrations within a few minutes. Neuromuscular blockers such as vecuronium are more polar and cross the placenta slowly.[9]

Although ionization is a limiting factor for diffusion, some highly charged molecules will diffuse across the placenta. Valproic acid (pK_a of 4.7) is nearly completely ionized at physiologic pH, yet there is rapid equilibration across the placental membrane. The small amount of xenobiotic that exists in the nonionized form rapidly crosses the placenta, and as the equilibrium is reestablished, an additional, small amount of nonionized xenobiotic becomes available for diffusion.[9]

Fetal blood pH changes during gestation. Embryonic intracellular pH is high relative to the intracellular pH of the pregnant woman. During this developmental stage, weak acids diffuse across the placenta to the embryo and remain there because of "ion trapping." Many teratogens, such as valproic acid, trimethadione, phenytoin, thalidomide, warfarin, and isotretinoin, are weak acids. Although ion trapping does not explain the mechanism of teratogenesis, it explains how xenobiotics accumulate in an embryo. Late in gestation, the fetal blood is 0.10 to 0.15 pH units more acidic than the maternal blood; this pH differential permits weakly basic xenobiotics to concentrate in the fetus during this period.[9]

The relative concentrations of protein-binding sites in the pregnant woman and fetus also have an impact on the extent of xenobiotic transfer to the fetus. As maternal free fatty acid concentrations increase near term, these fatty acids displace xenobiotics such as valproic acid or diazepam from maternal protein-binding sites and make more free xenobiotic available for transfer to the fetus.[9] Fetal albumin concentrations increase during gestation and exceed maternal albumin concentrations by term. Because the fetus does not have high concentrations of free fatty acids to compete for protein-binding sites, these sites are available for binding the xenobiotics. At birth, when neonatal free fatty acid concentrations increase 2- to 3-fold, they displace stored xenobiotic from the binding protein. In the cases of valproic acid and diazepam, the elevated concentrations of free xenobiotic have adverse effects on the newborn infant.[114,151,236,265]

The placenta also affects xenobiotic presentation to the fetus by ion trapping and xenobiotic metabolism. The placenta blocks the transfer of some positively charged ions such as cadmium and mercury[125] and actually accumulates them. This barrier does not necessarily protect the fetus, however, because these metal ions interfere with normal placental function and lead to placental necrosis and subsequent fetal death.

Beyond diffusion, specific transporters are found on both the fetal and maternal sides of the placenta. Transporters from the ATP-binding class (ABC) and the solute carrier class (SLC) have been identified.[46] These transporters help to deliver maternal solutes to the fetus and help the fetus to eliminate metabolic byproducts. They are also involved in the delivery of xenobiotics to the fetus.

The placenta contains xenobiotic-metabolizing enzymes capable of performing both phase I and phase II reactions (Chaps. 11 and 21). CYP1A1 is the primary CYP enzyme found in the placenta.[46] However, the concentration of biotransforming enzymes in the placenta is significantly lower than that in the liver, and it is unlikely that the level of enzymatic activity is protective

for the fetus.[230] Moreover, the fetus is exposed to reactive intermediates that form during these processes.

Placental transfer of xenobiotics has a positive effect as it permits delivery of desired therapies to the fetus. For example, if a fetus is found to have a supraventricular tachycardia or atrial flutter, digoxin given to the mother treats the tachydysrhythmia in the fetus.[145,231-234]

EFFECTS OF XENOBIOTICS ON THE DEVELOPING ORGANISM

A basic premise of teratogenicity is that the particular toxic effects of a xenobiotic are determined by the stage of development of the embryo or fetus.[38] Although the fertilized ovum is generally thought to be resistant to toxic insult before implantation,[37] xenobiotics in the fallopian or uterine secretions prevent implantation of the embryo. Xenobiotic exposure leading to cell loss or chromosomal abnormalities also leads to loss of the embryo, possibly even before pregnancy is detected. If the preimplantation embryo survives a xenobiotic exposure, the functional cells usually proceed to normal development.[298] Teratogens that act in such a manner elicit an "all-or-none response"; that is, the exposed embryo will either die or go on to normal development.

The dose–response curve of an environmental xenobiotic demonstrates *deterministic* (threshold) or *stochastic* (no threshold) effects.[38] Mutagenic and carcinogenic events are stochastic phenomena. Teratogenesis is a deterministic phenomenon with a threshold dose below which no effects occur. As the dose of the teratogen increases above the threshold, the magnitude of the effect increases. The effects might be the number of offspring that die or develop malformations or the extent or severity of malformations. Radiation has both deterministic effects (eg, microcephaly and growth retardation) and stochastic effects (induction of leukemia). Strictly speaking, teratogenic effects are those that occur at doses that do not cause maternal toxicity because maternal toxicity itself might be responsible for an observed adverse or teratogenic effect on the developing organism.[37]

Organogenesis occurs during the embryonic stage of development between days 18 and 60 of gestation. Most gross malformations are determined before day 36, although genitourinary and craniofacial anomalies occur later.[37] The period of susceptibility to teratogenic effects varies for each organ system (Fig. 30–1). For instance, the palate has a very short

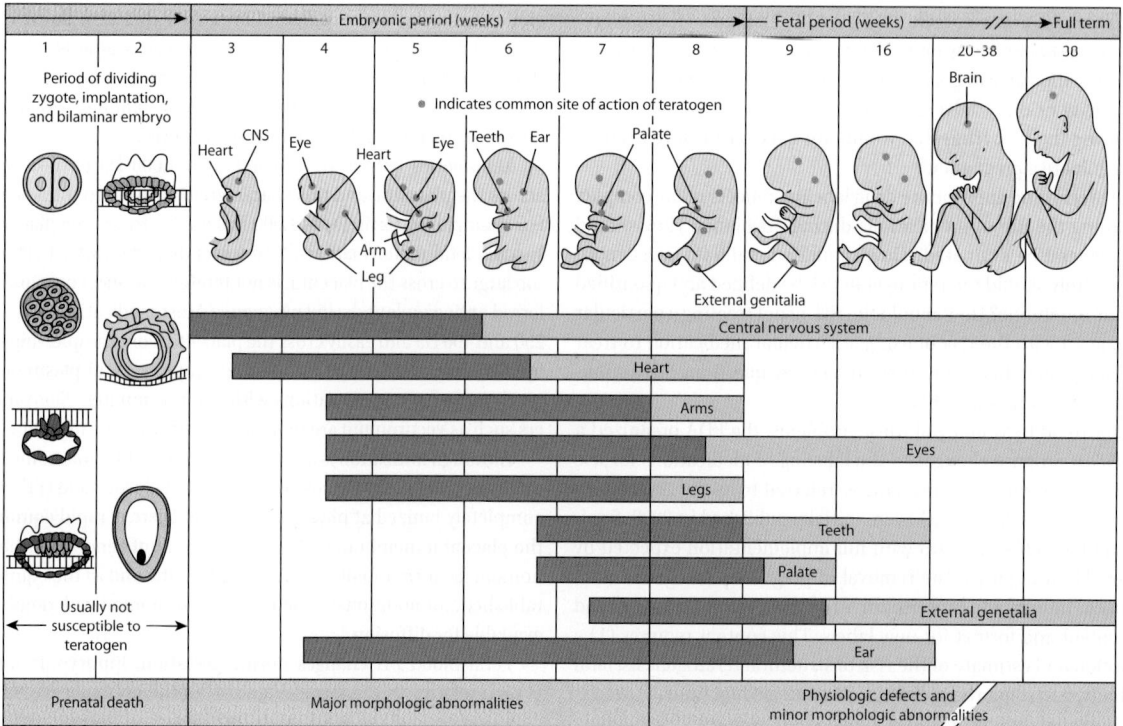

FIGURE 30–1. Critical periods of human prenatal development. *(Modified with permission from Moore KL, Persaud TVN, Torehia MG. Before We Are Born: Essentials of Embryology and Birth Defects, 8th ed. Philadelphia, PA: Saunders; 2013.)*

period of sensitivity, lasting approximately 3 weeks, whereas the complete development of the central nervous system (CNS), including neurogenesis and differentiation, arborization, synaptogenesis and synaptic organization, and myelinization and gliogenesis, remains susceptible throughout the fetal period and into the neonatal period and infancy.

Theoretically, knowing the exact time of teratogen exposure during gestation would allow prediction of a teratogenic effect; this is true in animal models, where the dose and time of exposure can be strictly controlled. It is also true for thalidomide in which different limb anomalies are specifically related to exposures on particular days of gestation.[337] In many clinical situations, for xenobiotics administered either for a short course or chronically, relating teratogenicity to a particular xenobiotic exposure is difficult because the exact time of conception and the exact time of exposure are unknown. This is particularly true when the primary exposure precedes the identification of pregnancy but there is secondary or ongoing exposure during pregnancy as xenobiotics are redistributed from tissue storage sites.[179]

During the fetal period, formed organs continue their cellular differentiation and grow to functional maturity. Exposure to xenobiotics such as cigarettes and their toxic constituents during this period generally leads to growth retardation. Teratogenic malformations or death occur as a result of disruption or destruction of growing organs, as has resulted from exposure to angiotensin-converting enzyme inhibitors and angiotensin II, type I receptor blockers during the second and third trimesters.[45]

Another concern during the fetal period is the initiation of carcinogenesis. Significant cellular replication and proliferation lead to a dramatic growth in size of the organism. At the same time, when the fetus is exposed to xenobiotics, development of biotransformation systems expose the organism to reactive metabolites that also initiate tumor formation. Some tumors, such as neuroblastoma, appear so early in postnatal life that their prenatal origin is likely. In pregnant rats given ethylnitrosourea during the embryonic period, lethal or teratogenic effects occur.[267] If ethylnitrosourea is administered during the fetal period, there is an increased incidence of tumors in the offspring. Clear cell vaginal and cervical adenocarcinomas occur in the female offspring of women exposed to diethylstilbestrol (DES) during pregnancy.[263]

MECHANISMS OF TERATOGENESIS

Cytotoxicity is one mechanism of teratogenesis and is the characteristic result of exposure to alkylating or chemotherapeutic agents. Aminopterin, for example, inhibits dihydrofolate reductase activity and leads to suppression of mitosis and cell death. If exposure to a cytotoxic xenobiotic occurs very early in development, the conceptus can die, but sublethal exposure during organogenesis can result in maldevelopment of particular structures. There is evidence that after cell death, the remaining cells in an affected region try to repair the damage caused by the missing cellular elements. This "restorative growth" can lead to uncoordinated growth and exacerbate the original malformation.

In the case of cytotoxic agents, the mechanism of action is understood, although it is not always clear why particular xenobiotics affect particular structures. With other xenobiotics, the structural effects have a clearer relationship to the site of action. For instance, when corticosteroids are administered in large doses to some experimental animals during the period of organogenesis, malformations of the palate occur. Glucocorticoid receptors are found in high concentrations in the palate of the developing mouse embryo.[259] Corticosteroid exposure had previously been thought to cause cleft palate in humans at a low frequency,[251,301] but recent work suggests there is no association between corticosteroid exposure and cleft palate.[25,307]

Caloric deficiency is not considered teratogenic during the period of organogenesis; however, specific nutritional or vitamin deficiencies are. In particular, there is an increased incidence of neural tube defects (anencephaly and spina bifida) associated with dietary folate deficiency, although the specific mechanism of teratogenesis is unknown. To ensure that all women of childbearing age have adequate folate stores by the time they become pregnant and during their pregnancy and to reduce the number of severe birth defects, it is important for women of childbearing age to have folate supplementation either as vitamin or dietary supplements even before they become pregnant. Because fortification of grain products is considered critical to help accomplish this goal, the FDA requires US manufacturers to add folic acid to enriched breads, cereals, flours, corn meals, pastas, rice, and other grain products.[244]

Ethanol affects fetuses both directly and indirectly. The craniofacial malformations that occur in fetal alcohol syndrome (FAS) probably result from the effects of ethanol during the period of organogenesis. Growth retardation results from direct effects of ethanol on fetal growth or from indirect effects resulting from ethanol-induced maternal nutritional deficiencies.

MANAGEMENT OF ACUTE POISONING IN PREGNANT WOMEN

For most women, pregnancy and the postpartum period are a period of emotional happiness. However, women have a lifetime prevalence of depression that is 2 to 3 times higher than men, and for some women, psychiatric illness during pregnancy, particularly depression and anxiety, represents a significant comorbidity. A new first episode or recurrence of major depression occurs in approximately 3% to 5% of pregnant women and 1% to 6% of women in the postpartum period; an additional 5% to 6% of women during pregnancy and the postpartum period will have minor symptoms of depression.[188] Overall, these rates of depression are about the same in pregnant and nonpregnant women; however, during the postpartum period, the onset of new episodes of depression are higher than for nonpregnant women. Pregnant teenagers are also at higher risk of depression during pregnancy.[191]

Postpartum "baby blues" are common, typically involve relatively mild symptoms including mood swings, irritability, anxiety, and crying spells, and generally resolve by 2 weeks after delivery.[199] Postpartum blues do not include suicidal ideation. True depression is manifested by feelings of hopelessness or helplessness and include suicidal ideation. Postpartum psychosis, typically associated with bipolar disorder, is uncommon, but it represents a true psychiatric emergency because there is a high risk of suicide, infanticide, or both.[28]

Risk factors for perinatal depression include an unplanned pregnancy, ambivalence about the pregnancy, poor social support, marital difficulties, adverse life events, and chronic stressors such as financial problems.[61,181,338] Of substantial importance is a personal or family history of depression, particularly previous perinatal depression. Discontinuation of antidepressant therapy represents a significant risk for relapse of disease, although relapse is possible even while a woman is receiving an antidepressant. Additional risk factors for depression include miscarriage, stillbirth, and preterm delivery.[293]

Depression in pregnancy has adverse effects on both the mother and the fetus.[32,316] For the pregnant woman, adverse effects include noncompliance with prenatal care; self-medication with tobacco, ethanol, and both licit and illicit xenobiotics drugs; poor sleep; poor appetite; and poor weight gain. In addition, there is an increased risk of spontaneous abortion, preeclampsia, preterm delivery, and fetal growth retardation. For many of these outcomes, it is difficult to differentiate the contributions from multiple confounding and interacting factors, including psychopathology, socioeconomic status, acute and chronic stressors, smoking, and the use of ethanol and other drugs of abuse.

One of the most extreme outcomes of depression is suicide. Suicidal ideation occurs in about 5% of pregnant women in community samples and up to 20% in women with underlying psychiatric illness.[111,191,240] Even so, suicide and suicide attempts during pregnancy are uncommon. Each year a small number of women die during pregnancy or the postpartum period; 1% to 5% of these pregnancy-related deaths are the result of suicide.[51,72,245] Between 2% and 12% of women who attempt or commit suicide are pregnant.[161,164,257] Overall, completed suicide occurs less frequently during pregnancy.[14,191,212] Psychiatric illness, including previous suicide attempts, predisposes to suicide attempts in pregnancy. Acute stressors leading to impulsive acts account for most of the uncompleted suicide attempts; these reasons include loss of a lover, economic crisis, prior loss of children, an unwanted pregnancy, and desire for an abortion.[68,187,350]

Women who complete suicide typically have more severe psychiatric illness. In particular, these women are likely to use more violent means of suicide such as hanging or self-inflicted gunshot wounds, although poisonings are a significant contributor to these deaths.[90,245] In addition, substance and ethanol use are significant contributing factors in many cases; additionally, some pregnancy-related deaths are secondary to complications of substance use, such as overdose.[245] Initiation of child protection proceedings, particularly in the setting of maternal substance use, is an additional risk factor for postpartum suicide.[245] Some suicides follow pregnancy-related or neonatal complications.[90]

Ingestion of xenobiotics is the most common method of attempted suicide during pregnancy and the postpartum period.[61,109,257,261] There are approximately 7,000 xenobiotic exposures in pregnant women reported to the AAPCC annually, which account for approximately 2% of the exposures in adolescent and adult females of childbearing age (Chap. 130). The patterns of xenobiotic exposure are similar to those of adolescent and adult exposures in general with analgesics being the most common exposure. A similar pattern has also been reported for a California sample.[218] Some of these xenobiotic exposures are attempts to terminate pregnancy (Chap. 19).[257] As with most poisonings overall, the severity of poisoning in pregnant women is typically minor.[240,245]

In one US national sample, 1,659 pregnant women had poisoning-related hospitalizations, representing 0.04% of all hospitalized pregnant women and approximately 10% of injury-related admissions of pregnant women. A total of 244 of these women (15%) delivered their babies during these poisoning-related hospitalizations.[173] In a Swedish cohort, there was a higher rate of miscarriage than expected.[102]

In national samples from both the United States and England, approximately 2% to 3% of deaths in pregnancy and the immediate postpartum period follow suicidal poisoning.[51,245] The AAPCC reports approximately 2 deaths per year in pregnant women, which represents approximately 2 per 1,000 AAPCC-reported adolescent and adult deaths overall, 4 per 1,000 deaths in adolescent and adult women, and approximately 3 deaths per 10,000 (0.03%) xenobiotic exposures in pregnancy (Chap. 130). In a combined Hungarian series of pregnant women who had suicidal poisonings, 19 of 1,044 (1.8%) died.[69]

Any woman who attempts suicide during pregnancy or the postpartum period should have a psychiatric evaluation after she is medically stabilized. In particular, a growing number of specialized units or teams focus on pregnant and postpartum women and attempt to keep women and infants together in the postpartum period.[199,245]

Managing any acute overdose during pregnancy provokes discussion of several questions. Is the general management different? Do altered metabolism and pharmacokinetics increase or decrease the woman's risk of morbidity or mortality from a xenobiotic overdose? Is the fetus at risk of poisoning from a maternal overdose? Is there a teratogenic risk to the fetus from an acute overdose or poisoning? Is the use of an antidote contraindicated or should use be modified? When should a potentially viable fetus be emergently delivered to prevent toxicity? When should termination of a pregnancy be recommended?

As described earlier, physiologic changes during pregnancy affect pharmacokinetics; xenobiotics taken in overdose also have unpredictable toxicokinetics. In any significant overdose during pregnancy, pregnancy-related alterations in pharmacokinetics are unlikely to protect the woman from significant morbidity or mortality.

Although a single high-dose exposure to a xenobiotic during the period of organogenesis might seem analogous to an experimental model to induce teratogenesis, most xenobiotics ingested as a single, acute overdose do not induce physical deformities.[70] Antiepileptics are teratogenic and sometime are ingested in suicide gestures or attempts, but their teratogenicity is probably more directly related to chronic exposure. Acute acetaminophen (APAP) toxicity in the first trimester leads to an increased risk of spontaneous abortion,[270] suggesting a teratogenic effect similar to the all-or-none response described earlier. In general, however, it is extremely difficult to

ascribe teratogenicity to a particular xenobiotic exposure based on a single case report. There is, for example, a report of multiple severe congenital malformations in the stillborn fetus of a woman who overdosed on isoniazid during the 12th week of pregnancy.[185] However, because the background incidence of congenital malformations is 3% to 6%, it is almost impossible to determine for a single individual whether a particular exposure is the etiology of observed malformations.[71] The Budapest Registry of Self-Poisoned Patients uses this construct to screen for possible teratogenic effects of xenobiotics in overdose.[69,70] Considering the successful outcome of most pregnancies that progress to term after an acute overdose, it is very unlikely that the small risk of teratogenesis would lead to a recommendation for termination of pregnancy after an acute overdose of most xenobiotics.[86]

In general, any condition that leads to a severe metabolic derangement in a pregnant woman is likely to have an adverse impact on her developing fetus. Therefore, the management of overdose in a pregnant woman usually follows the principles outlined in Chap. 4, with close attention paid to the airway, oxygenation, and hemodynamic stability. The use of naloxone or dextrose has not been specifically assessed in pregnancy, but clinicians should be guided by the same considerations raised in managing the nonpregnant patient with alterations in respiratory or neurologic function. Opioid-induced respiratory failure in a pregnant patient will lead to fetal hypoxia and adverse effects; opioid withdrawal in a pregnant woman, whether induced by abstinence or the use of naloxone, can adversely affect the fetus or the pregnancy. Consideration of the benefits and risks of the use of naloxone for an opioid-poisoned woman in respiratory distress or coma suggests that reduced morbidity, for both the mother and fetus, is achieved by the use of carefully titrated doses of naloxone to minimize the likelihood of maternal withdrawal (Chap. 36 and Antidotes in Depth: A4).

Gastrointestinal decontamination is frequently a part of the early management of acute poisoning in nonpregnant patients. Gastric lavage is not specifically contraindicated for pregnant patients, and the usual concerns about airway management apply.

There is no specific contraindication to the use of activated charcoal in a pregnant woman. There is limited evidence for a role for whole-bowel irrigation (WBI) in the management of pregnant patients with certain xenobiotic exposures, for example, in the treatment of iron overdose in pregnancy.[335] The use of oral polyethylene glycol-electrolyte solution (PEG) is safe in pregnant women.[237]

There have been no clinical trials on the use of antidotes in pregnant women in the context of acute poisoning. Deferoxamine is studied to treat chronic iron overload in pregnant women, and there is supportive data for this medication. Because there are no reports of adverse fetal effects from antidotal treatment of a poisoned pregnant woman, the benefit of antidotal therapy will almost invariably outweighs the risk of use in pregnancy. Conversely, in at least one case, withholding deferoxamine therapy contributed to the death of both a woman and her fetus.[207,320]

ACETAMINOPHEN

Acetaminophen is the most common analgesic and antipyretic used during pregnancy and is also one of the most common xenobiotic overdoses during pregnancy. There are 3 published series of acute APAP overdose during all trimesters of pregnancy[220,221,270] in addition to multiple case reports. Overall, most pregnant women who continue their pregnancies recover from an APAP ingestion without adverse effects to themselves or their babies.

Twenty-eight women with first trimester exposures who continued their pregnancies are reported.[221,270] Nineteen women, 5 of whom had toxic serum APAP concentrations, delivered full-term infants. One woman with severe hepatotoxicity died along with the fetus. Eight women had spontaneous abortions; 5 of these 8 had toxic serum concentrations and received NAC (one within 8 hours and 4 between 12 and 17 hours after ingestion).

Thirty-two women with second-trimester exposures who continued their pregnancies are reported.[105,197,221,270,275,317] Twenty-seven women, 7 of whom had toxic serum APAP concentrations, delivered full-term infants. One woman developed fulminant hepatic failure and underwent liver transplant at 20 weeks' gestation; the infant developed severe complications in utero, and the woman terminated the pregnancy at 23 weeks. Two women, one with a nontoxic serum concentration and one who developed hepatotoxicity, delivered premature infants. Two women with nontoxic serum APAP concentrations had spontaneous abortions probably unrelated to the overdose.

Fifty-five women with third trimester exposures who continued their pregnancies are reported.[20,47,66,107,126,141,172,184,221,256,270,274,279,281,287,322,340] Forty-two women, 15 of whom had toxic serum APAP concentrations, delivered full-term infants. Eleven women delivered premature infants. Five of them had toxic serum APAP concentrations and hepatotoxicity, 4 had toxic serum APAP concentrations without hepatotoxicity, and 2 had nontoxic serum APAP concentrations. Two women with severe hepatotoxicity delivered still-born infants who also showed signs of hepatotoxicity and one woman with severe hepatotoxicity delivered an infant who died at 34 hours of life.

There are also several case reports of adverse pregnancy outcome in the setting of chronic use of APAP or acute overdose associated with chronic substance use.[52,141,174,200,270,327] It is difficult to interpret these reports with respect to specific APAP effect because of the confounders of chronic disease, chronic APAP use, and the use of additional medications and substances.

Although APAP at recommended doses is considered safe in pregnancy,[189] in overdose, it puts the developing fetus at risk. As the cases demonstrate, APAP crosses the placenta to reach the fetus. The cases suggest an increased risk of spontaneous abortion after overdose during the first trimester, particularly in the setting of toxic serum APAP concentrations and delayed NAC therapy.[270] The cases also suggest that overdose during the first trimester can lead to late sequelae, for instance, premature labor.

Some experimental work might explain early pregnancy loss after overdose. Acetaminophen prevented the development of preimplantation (2-cell stage) mouse embryos in culture, an effect that was not associated with alterations in glutathione concentrations,[182] and led to abnormal neuropore development in cultured rat embryos.[315] These data suggest that APAP is directly toxic to the immature organism. However, other work reported that similar embryotoxic effects were associated with reductions in glutathione concentrations[346] and that *N*-acetyl-*p*-benzoquinoneimine (NAPQI) produced nonspecific toxicity when added to the rat embryo culture medium.[315]

The fetal liver has some ability to metabolize APAP to a reactive intermediate in vitro. Cytochrome P450 (CYP) activity was detected in intact hepatocytes, as well as in microsomal fractions isolated from the livers of fetuses aborted between 18 and 23 weeks of gestation. This fetal hepatic CYP activity increased between 18 and 23 weeks (the only period studied) but was maximally only 10% of the activity of hepatocytes isolated from adults after brain death.[277] In 2 clinical cases, cysteine and mercapturate conjugates were identified in newborns exposed to APAP in utero, suggesting that the fetus and neonate metabolize APAP through the CYP system.[184] These data suggest that the fetus in utero and the neonate generate a toxic metabolite. The clinical cases suggest that the fetal liver is susceptible to injury, although whether this fetal hepatotoxicity is related to fetal APAP toxicity, maternal toxicity, or postmortem changes is unclear.

This CYP activity has not been further characterized. However, CYP2E1, one of the cytochromes responsible for APAP metabolism, is present in human fetal tissues as early as 16 weeks of gestation.[225] CYP3A4 and CYP1A2 are also involved in APAP metabolism but are not present in fetal liver. CYP3A7 is a functional fetal form of the CYP3 family, but its metabolic activity with respect to APAP is unstudied.[127]

The clinical cases help address several questions regarding management of overdose during the third trimester (Table 30–2). Eight women whose pregnancies were all at less than 36 weeks of gestation developed hepatotoxicity. Two infants died in utero and one infant died on the second day of life with evidence of hepatotoxicity. The other 5 infants experienced problems associated with prematurity but did not develop obvious hepatotoxicity. One of these 5 infants had 4 exchange transfusions to treat a cord acetaminophen concentration of 76 mcg/mL and had an unexplained death at 3 months of age. Five women whose pregnancies were all at 36 or more weeks of gestation

did not develop hepatotoxicity. One infant had 2 exchange transfusions to treat a cord acetaminophen concentration of 217 mcg/mL and did not develop hepatotoxicity but died of sudden infant death syndrome (SIDS) at 5 months of age. One infant received intravenous (IV) NAC and had a transient elevation of aspartate aminotransferase (AST) and prothrombin time. Two infants were not treated, and both did well, although one had a transient elevation of AST. One infant was born 6 weeks after the overdose and was normal.

Taken together these cases suggest that when there is maternal hepatotoxicity there is a moderate risk of fetal hepatotoxicity and fetal morbidity. There is also a moderate risk of prematurity delivery.

Urgent delivery is often recommended in the setting of severe maternal hepatotoxicity that is associated with fetal distress. Although a fetus with prolonged exposure to APAP in utero is at risk of developing severe hepatotoxicity, not all at-risk infants have been affected. The contribution of gestational age, maternal disease state, or other maternal factors to fetal or neonatal toxicity is unknown. Although there are insufficient case data to suggest that APAP overdose per se is an indication for urgent delivery, some authorities recommend urgent delivery when the maternal serum APAP concentration is in the toxic range but hepatotoxicity has not yet developed.[324] The clinical cases also suggest that significant APAP overdose with or without associated hepatotoxicity can precipitate premature labor and that even women with nontoxic serum concentrations are at an increased risk.

In 2 cases, exchange transfusion was used to treat the exposed neonate. In both cases, the APAP half-life was prolonged, and in neither case was this affected by the transfusion. Disturbingly, these 2 infants had unexplained deaths at several months of age. There are currently no data to support the use of exchange transfusion as therapy for elevated serum APAP concentrations in a neonate.

A pregnant woman with acute toxic APAP ingestion should be treated with NAC (Chap. 33 and Antidotes in Depth: A3). This therapy is intended to treat the mother. Maternal hepatotoxicity and delayed NAC therapy are associated with fetal toxicity;[270] whether NAC therapy can prevent later sequelae such as premature delivery is unclear. Although NAC did not cross the sheep placenta in vivo[299] and the perfused human placenta in vitro, NAC was found in cord blood after it was administered to 4 mothers before delivery.[141] Even if NAC does cross the placenta, whether it can prevent fetal hepatotoxicity is unknown because not all exposed fetuses develop hepatotoxicity.

Use of APAP during pregnancy may be associated with other risks. One area of concern is the association of prenatal exposure to APAP with the development of childhood asthma. Several meta-analyses have reviewed many of the published studies.[57,91,93] Many of those studies were criticized for lack of control of potential confounders such as the stage of pregnancy, dose and frequency of use, variable definitions of asthma, and the different childhood age groups considered. One of the biggest concerns is the possible confounding by indication because why a pregnant woman took acetaminophen, whether for a respiratory tract infection or for back pain for example, may be important as a predictor. Notwithstanding these concerns, the meta-analyses report a positive association between prenatal exposure to APAP and childhood wheezing and/or asthma with an OR of approximately 1.28-1.5.

IRON

Intentional iron exposures during pregnancy are reported; maternal toxicity is generally greater than fetal toxicity. In 2 cases, normal babies were delivered, although the mothers died.[247,268] In another case, the mother had severe iron toxicity with metabolic acidosis, shock, kidney failure, and disseminated intravascular coagulation but was not treated with deferoxamine because of concerns about its teratogenic risks. Instead, the mother received an exchange transfusion followed 45 minutes later by a spontaneous abortion of the 16-week fetus.[207,320] Neonatal and cord blood iron concentrations were not elevated. In several cases, pregnant women who had signs and symptoms of iron poisoning and elevated serum iron concentrations were treated with deferoxamine and subsequently delivered normal babies.[30,162,177,262,292,330]

TABLE 30–2   Reported Cases of Third Trimester APAP Overdose

Gestational Age (wk)	Maternal APAP Concentration (mcg/mL)(time[a])	Maternal AST Peak (IU/L) (time[a])	Infant APAP Concentration (mcg/mL)(time[a])	Infant Hepatotoxicity (Yes/No)	Comment	Reference
27	0 (36 hours)	1,226 (36 hours)	ND	No	C/S for fetal distress. Infant: mild respiratory distress syndrome.	107
27–28	56 (16 hours)	6,226 (96 hours)	ND	Yes	Ingestion over 24 hours. No fetal movements at presentation. PO NAC started at 20 hours. Induced labor at 4 days. Infant: stillborn with diffuse hepatic necrosis. Hepatic APAP 250 mcg/g.	126
29	160 (10 hours)	4,300 (50 hours)	76 (16 hours, cord)	No	Ingestion of aspirin, caffeine, and quinine followed 17 hours later by APAP. Presented in labor. Treated with oral methionine. Spontaneous delivery at 16 hours. Infant: moderate hyaline membrane disease. Peak AST of 86 IU/L (cord). Four whole-blood exchange transfusions. Discharged home at 54 days of life. Died at 106 days; no apparent cause.	184, 322
30	55 (18 hours)	4,000 (48 hours)	ND	ND	Maternal chorioamnionitis with delivery at 31 weeks. Respiratory distress syndrome and hyperbilirubinemia.	256
31	40 (26 hours)	13,320 (60 hours)	41 (27)	Yes	APAP only, C/S for fetal distress one hour after initial maternal evaluation. Infant's birth weight was 1,620 g. Apgar scores 0, 0, 1.[b] Infant died at 34 hours of life. Mother died at 34 hours postingestion. No autopsy of mother or child.	340
32	448 (12 hours)	5,269 (48 hours)	0 (84 hours, cord)	No	IV NAC started at 12 hours. Induced delivery at 84 hours. Infant: transient hypoglycemia, mild respiratory distress, mild jaundice. Peak AST of 56 IU/L (day 1 of life).	221, 279
32	166 (4 hours)	"Normal"	ND	ND	Vaginal delivery at term without complications.	66
33	135 (28 hours)	6,237 (66 hours)	330 (3 days, cord)	Yes	Oral NAC at 12 hours. Fetal death at 2 days; spontaneous delivery at 3 days. Infant: stillborn with diffuse hepatic necrosis.	270
36	280 (3–4 hours)	"Normal"	217 (6–7 hours, cord)	No	Ingestion of APAP, ethanol, barbiturates. Elective C/S at 6–7 hours. Infant: double-volume exchange transfusion at 18 hours. Discharge at 40 days, "cot death" at 157 days.	274
36	200 (5 hours)	25 (24 hours)	ND	No	Oral NAC (? time). Infant: spontaneous delivery 6 weeks after ingestion. Normal neonatal course.	47
38	216 (4 hours)	"Normal"	13 (17 hours, cord)	No	NAC (? route). Infant: normal neonatal course.	172, 281
"Term"	147 (9 hours)	28 (9 hours)	133 (9 hours, 4 hours of life)	No	Infant PT of 44 at 4 hours of life. IV NAC. No problems. AST of 86 IU/L at 4 hours of life.	20
Term?	89 (11 hours)	326 (35 hours)	144 (11 hours, 4 hours of life)	No	Mother presented in labor at 6 hours. Infant received IV NAC at 4 hours of life. AST of 55 IU/L at 4 hours of life.	287

[a]Time after maternal ingestion. [b]Apgar scores are at 1, 5, and 10 minutes.

APAP = acetaminophen; AST = aspartate aminotransferase; C/S = cesarean section; IV = intravenous; NAC = N-acetylcysteine; ND = not done or not reported; PO = oral; PT = prothrombin time.

Although the placenta transports iron to the fetus efficiently,[19] it also blocks the transfer of large quantities of iron. In a sheep model of iron poisoning, only a small amount of iron was transferred across the placenta despite significantly elevated serum iron concentrations.[67]

Deferoxamine is an effective antidote for iron poisoning (Chap. 45 and Antidotes in Depth: A7), but it is reported to be a teratogen that causes skeletal deformities and abnormalities of ossification when given to pregnant rabbits at high doses. A rat model observed similar effects but only with doses of deferoxamine that caused maternal toxicity.[34] Experimentally, in sheep, deferoxamine was minimally transported across the placenta;[67] therefore, the reported fetal effects could be secondary to chelation of essential nutrients (eg, trace metals) on the maternal side of the placenta.[324]

In clinical case reports of iron overdose for which deferoxamine was used, there have been no adverse effects on the fetus, although most have been either second or third trimester poisonings.[30,162,177,247,262,292,330] In a case series of 49 patients with iron poisoning during pregnancy, few of the patients exhibited any clinical toxicity other than vomiting and diarrhea; 25 received deferoxamine, most by the oral route.[219] One woman with a first trimester overdose, 8 women with second trimester overdoses, and 12 women with third trimester overdoses were treated with deferoxamine and subsequently delivered full-term infants. One infant whose mother overdosed at 30 weeks of gestation had webbed fingers on one hand. One woman who overdosed at 20 weeks had minimal clinical toxicity, received deferoxamine, and delivered a 2.5-kg male infant at 34 weeks of gestation. One woman with a first trimester overdose and 2 women with second trimester overdoses elected to terminate their pregnancies.

Further support for the safe use of deferoxamine in pregnancy is the experience with its use for pregnant women with thalassemia major. For many years, deferoxamine has been administered as part of the therapy for posttransfusion iron overload without adverse effects.[305] Considering the potentially fatal nature of severe iron poisoning, deferoxamine should be administered when signs and symptoms indicate significant poisoning.

Iron overdose is one of the few specific indications for WBI, because iron is not adsorbed to activated charcoal (Antidotes in Depth: A1 and A2). A case report demonstrated elimination of pill fragments after treatment of a pregnant woman with WBI.[335]

CARBON MONOXIDE

Carbon monoxide is the leading cause of unintentional poisoning fatalities in the United States. In contrast to iron and most other xenobiotics, when pregnant women are exposed to carbon monoxide, the fetus is at greater risk of toxicity than the mother. There are reports of both the mother and fetus dying; the mother surviving but the fetus dying; and both the mother and fetus surviving but with an adverse neonatal outcome, primarily brain damage resembling that seen after severe cerebral ischemia.[48,65,169,194,208,242,335,353] Similar clinical effects are also observed in animal models.[83,115,195]

The case literature suggests an increased risk of poor fetal outcome with clinically severe maternal poisoning or significantly elevated carboxyhemoglobin concentrations.[169,242] Women with minimal symptoms or low concentrations of carboxyhemoglobin have a low risk of fetal toxicity, but a lower limit of exposure without effect has not been specifically defined.[169]

In animal models, under experimental conditions, the fetus has a carboxyhemoglobin concentration 10% to 15% higher than the mother.[135,195] After exposure to carbon monoxide, the fetus achieves peak carboxyhemoglobin concentrations 58% higher than those achieved by the mother at steady state, and the time to peak concentration is also delayed compared with that of the mother. Similarly, the elimination of carbon monoxide occurs more slowly in the fetus than in the mother.[135,194,195] One case report describes such a phenomenon: after one hour of supplemental oxygen, the maternal carboxyhemoglobin concentration was 7% and the fetal carboxyhemoglobin concentration was 61% at the time of death in utero.[88]

Carbon monoxide leads to fetal hypoxia by several mechanisms: (1) maternal carboxyhemoglobin leads to a decrease in the oxygen content of maternal blood, and therefore less oxygen is delivered across the placenta to the fetus, which normally has an arterial PO_2 of only 20 to 30 mm Hg; (2) fetal carboxyhemoglobin causes a decrease in fetal PO_2; (3) carbon monoxide shifts the oxyhemoglobin dissociation curve to the left and decreases the release of oxygen to the fetal tissues (an exacerbation of the physiologic left shift found with normal fetal hemoglobin); and (4) carbon monoxide inhibits cytochrome oxidase or other mitochondrial functions.

The treatment for severe carbon monoxide poisoning is hyperbaric oxygen therapy (HBO) (Chap. 122 and Antidotes in Depth: A40). There are questions about the use of HBO in pregnant women because animal models suggest HBO adversely affects the embryo or fetus.[98,226,290,323] The applicability of these animal models to humans is difficult to assess; many of the animal models used hyperbaric conditions of greater pressures and duration than those clinically used for humans.

Hyperbaric oxygen therapy has been used therapeutically for carbon monoxide poisoning in pregnancy with good results reported, although there are limited data on the long-term follow-up of the children.[41,97,108,120,136,169,336] One large series reported 44 women who were exposed to carbon monoxide during pregnancy and were treated with HBO, regardless of clinical severity or gestational age: 33 had term births, one had a premature delivery 22 weeks after HBO during an episode of maternal fever, 2 had spontaneous miscarriages (one 12 hours after severe poisoning and one 15 days after mild poisoning), one delivered a child with Down syndrome, one had an elective abortion, and 6 were lost to follow-up.[88] Details regarding trimester of exposure, maternal carboxyhemoglobin concentration, and severity of symptoms are not available, making it difficult to interpret the reported adverse outcomes. Although HBO appears to be safe for pregnant women and seems to present little risk to the fetus, it is not clear whether HBO can prevent carbon monoxide–related fetal toxicity.

Hyperbaric oxygen is appropriate therapy for any pregnant woman exposed to carbon monoxide with an elevated serum carboxyhemoglobin concentration or evidence of fetal distress. To allow the fetal carboxyhemoglobin to be eliminated, if HBO therapy is not available, 100% oxygen is recommended for all pregnant women for 5 times as long as the time needed for her carboxyhemoglobin concentration to return to the normal range.[194]

Thus, if a pregnant woman's carboxyhemoglobin concentration returns to normal in one hour, she should continue to receive 100% oxygen for at least 5 hours.

SUBSTANCE USE DURING PREGNANCY

Substance use during pregnancy leads to complex medical and psychosocial effects for the pregnant woman as well as the fetus and newborn infant. With the increased use of cocaine during the latter half of the 1980s and 1990s, there was great interest in determining the effects of cocaine use during pregnancy. As research in this area progressed, many of the critical methodologic issues related to substance use research were highlighted.[99,149,186,238,354]

Substance-using women often have multiple risk factors for adverse pregnancy outcomes, such as low socioeconomic status, polysubstance use, ethanol and cigarette use, sexually transmitted infections, AIDS, malnutrition, and lack of prenatal care. Lack of prenatal care is highly correlated with premature birth, and smoking is associated with spontaneous abortion, growth retardation, and SIDS.[158,348] Other factors not specifically related to substance use such as age, race, gravidity, and prior pregnancies also affect pregnancy outcome. Each of these factors represents a significant potential confounding variable when the effects of a particular xenobiotic such as ethanol or opioids are evaluated during pregnancy and must be controlled for in research design. Many of these factors are also significant confounders in evaluation of postnatal growth and development.

Bias can occur in the selection of study subjects. For example, if all the patients are selected from an inner-city public hospital obstetrics service, minorities may be over-represented. On the other hand, if all the patients are selected from substance-using populations of rural Vermont or West Virginia, minorities may be under-represented. There may be significant differences in socioeconomic status or genetics. If cohorts are followed over a long time, study subjects are frequently lost to follow-up. The ones who continue may be more motivated or may have more problems that need attention?

Categorizing patients into substance-use groups is difficult. Self-reporting of substance use is frequently unreliable or inaccurate and making determinations about the nature, frequency, quantity (dose), or timing (with respect to gestation) of xenobiotic exposure is difficult. Because substance users frequently use multiple xenobiotics, it is difficult to categorize subjects into particular xenobiotic-use groups, and patients using different xenobiotics can be inadvertently grouped together. In fact, there probably are no actual xenobiotic-free control groups.

When urine drug screens are used to identify substance users, there is a high probability of false negatives because drug screens reflect only recent use. This factor is particularly important because substance use tends to decrease later in pregnancy and a negative urine drug screen in the third trimester or at delivery will fail to identify a woman who was using xenobiotics early in pregnancy. Testing for xenobiotics in hair or meconium can improve the accuracy of the analysis with regard to the entire pregnancy.[35,167]

Another bias involves selection of infants who are exposed to xenobiotics. Evaluating newborns who are "at risk," show signs of substance withdrawal, or have positive urine drug screens will miss some exposed infants. When research concerns the neurobehavioral development of children exposed in utero to substances, it is important that the examiners performing the evaluation be blinded to the infants' xenobiotic exposure category. Finally, there is bias against publishing research that shows a negative or nonsignificant effect.[168]

Ethanol

Approximately 9% of pregnant women (200,000) 15 to 44 years of age report consuming ethanol during the previous month, 4.6% (100,000) report binge drinking, and 0.8% (20,000) report heavy drinking. Of nonpregnant women 15 to 44 years of age, about 55% report consuming ethanol during the previous month, 30% report binge drinking, and 6% report heavy drinking.[286] The highest prevalence of drinking is during the first trimester and decreases in the second and third trimesters. These numbers are consistent with the CDC estimate of a 7.3% risk of an ethanol-exposed pregnancy.[119]

Chronic ethanol use during pregnancy produces a constellation of fetal effects. *Fetal alcohol spectrum disorders* (FASD) is an umbrella term describing the range of effects that can occur in an individual whose mother drank ethanol during pregnancy.[29,311]

The most severe effects occur in the FAS which is characterized by (1) intrauterine or postnatal growth retardation; (2) intellectual disability or behavioral abnormalities; and (3) facial dysmorphogenesis, particularly microcephaly, short palpebral fissures, epicanthal folds, maxillary hypoplasia, cleft palate, a hypoplastic philtrum, and micrognathia.[29,206] A child can be diagnosed with FAS even when a history of regular gestational ethanol use cannot be confirmed.

In an attempt to formalize diagnostic criteria for FAS and other gestational ethanol-related effects, the Institute of Medicine proposed some additional descriptors that are in common use and which have been refined.[143,318] *Partial FAS* is applied to a child with some of the characteristic facial features and with growth retardation, neurodevelopmental abnormalities, or other behavioral problems. *Alcohol-related birth defects* (ARBD) are congenital anomalies other than the characteristic facial features described earlier, for example, cleft palate, which sometimes occurs with regular gestational ethanol use. *Alcohol-related neurodevelopmental disorder* (ARND) describes neurodevelopmental abnormalities or other behavioral problems, which sometimes occur with regular gestational alcohol use.

Differential expression of the syndrome reflects the effects of varying quantities of ethanol ingested at critical periods specific for particular effects. The craniofacial anomalies probably represent teratogenic effects during organogenesis but some CNS abnormalities and growth retardation result from adverse effects later in gestation.

There is considerable controversy about what amount of ethanol consumption causes FASD.[235,243] Some researchers believe that FASD is a result of alcoholism—chronic regular use or frequent binging—rather than to low concentrations of gestational ethanol exposure, no matter how little or how infrequent.[2,118] A high level of consumption would be in the range of 50 to 100 mL of 100% ethanol (4–6 "standard" drinks of hard liquor) regularly throughout pregnancy[318] or binge drinking (at least 5 standard drinks per occasion), with a significantly elevated peak blood ethanol concentration.[101,215] However there are reports of behavioral abnormalities associated with the consumption of as little as one drink per week.[312] In this regard, neither a no-effect amount nor a safe amount of ethanol use in pregnancy has been determined,[156] and therefore the US Surgeon General recommends no ethanol consumption during pregnancy.[246]

The incidence of FAS in the United States is reported as 0.3 to 0.8 per 1,000 children when measured by passive surveillance and record review.[103] In-person expert assessment of a community-based school-age sample reported an incidence of 6 to 9 per 1,000 children.[214] This means that several hundred children with FAS and several thousand with fetal ethanol effects will be born each year; thus, ethanol use is considered the leading preventable cause of intellectual disability in this country.[318] Although the primary determinant of FAS and its effects is the amount of maternal ethanol consumption, there is some evidence that paternal ethanol exposure plays a contributing role.[1]

Ethanol use during pregnancy leads to an increased incidence of spontaneous abortion, premature deliveries, stillbirths,[205] neonatal ethanol withdrawal,[26,241] and possibly carcinogenesis.[163] Infants can be irritable or hypertonic and can have problems with habituation and arousal. Long-term behavioral and intellectual effects include decreased IQ, learning disabilities, memory deficits, speech and language disorders, hyperactivity, and dysfunctional behavior in school.[213,312,319]

Autopsies of children with FAS demonstrate malformations of gray and white matter, a failure of certain regions such as the corpus callosum to develop, a failure of certain cells such as the cerebellar astrocytes to migrate, and a tendency for tissue in certain regions to die.[96] The mechanisms of ethanol-induced teratogenesis are not fully elucidated.[27,128] Much of the work in animals has focused on the developing nervous system, where ethanol adversely affects nerve cell growth, differentiation, and migration, particularly in areas of the neocortex, hippocampus, sensory nucleus, and cerebellum.[123,321]

Several mechanisms are potential contributors to the effects of ethanol.[117,222] Ethanol interferes with a number of different growth factors that affect neuronal migration and development.[349] In addition, ethanol interferes with the development and function of both serotonin and N-methyl-D-aspartate (NMDA) receptors. Ethanol, or possibly its metabolite acetaldehyde, also causes cell necrosis directly or through the generation of free radicals and excessive apoptosis.[60,96,132] In particular, craniofacial abnormalities could be related to apoptosis of neural crest cells through the formation of free radicals, a deficiency of retinoic acid, or the altered expression of homeobox genes that regulate growth and development.[321]

One integrative model of ethanol-induced teratogenesis proposes that sociobehavioral risk factors, such as drinking behavior, smoking behavior, low socioeconomic status, and cultural or ethnic influences, create provocative biologic conditions, such as high peak blood ethanol concentrations, circulating tobacco constituents, and undernutrition. These provocative factors exacerbate fetal vulnerability to potential teratogenic mechanisms, such as ethanol-related hypoxia or free radical–induced cell damage.[3]

Opioids

Opioid use in pregnancy remains a significant cause of both maternal and neonatal morbidity. Over the past 2 decades, use and misuse of opioids, particularly prescription opioids, has been spiraling upward in the United States. Of women 15 to 44 years of age, 25% to 40% are prescribed opioids, in particular hydrocodone, codeine, and oxycodone.[7] These prescription rates are higher for women insured by Medicaid compared to private insurance and for women living in the south compared to the northeast. Similarly, opioid prescription rates for pregnant women are also high, ranging from 10% in a Veterans Administration sample, to 14% in a commercial insurance sample, to 29% in a Medicaid sample.[23,76,89,171] Again there are significant regional (state to state) variations as well as urban versus rural differences in these prescribing patterns during pregnancy that reflect general trends in opioid prescribing.[76,339] Hydrocodone, codeine, and oxycodone are also the primary opioids prescribed during pregnancy.

Past month surveys provide a different perspective. Approximately 21,000 pregnant women 15 to 44 years of age report illicit and prescription opioid misuse and abuse (approximately 0.2% of pregnant women report heroin use, 0.8% report the illicit use of prescription analgesics, and approximately 0.1% report the use of oxycodone).[284,286,309]

Pregnant opioid users are at increased risk for many medical complications of pregnancy, such as hepatitis, sepsis, endocarditis, sexually transmitted infections, and AIDS, and at increased risk for obstetric complications, such as miscarriage, premature delivery, or stillbirth.[99,116] Some of the obstetric complications are related to associated risk factors in addition to the opioid use. Maternal opioid use most commonly affects fetal growth.[99,116,354] There is an increased incidence of low birth weight in babies born to opioid-using mothers compared with control participants, and the effect is greater for heroin than for methadone.

There is extensive clinical experience with Medication Assisted Therapy (MAT) with methadone maintenance during pregnancy. Compared with untreated heroin use, methadone maintenance during pregnancy is associated with better obstetric care, decreased risk of maternal withdrawal, increased fetal growth, decreased fetal mortality, decreased risk of HIV infection, and increased likelihood that a child will be discharged home with his or her parents.[154] Women who receive low-dose methadone and good prenatal care are at increased risk for pregnancy-related complications but have birth outcomes similar to nonusers.[99]

Just as alternative opioid replacement strategies with buprenorphine were introduced for opioid users in general, buprenorphine is more frequently being used during pregnancy especially for women maintained on buprenorphine before becoming pregnant. In one large trial, obstetric outcomes were similar after buprenorphine treatment compared with methadone although more women in the buprenorphine arm dropped out of the study because they did not feel well during the induction of therapy.[154,155] Similar results regarding obstetric outcomes were reported in one study primarily looking at neonatal abstinence syndrome (NAS).[42] In another large cohort of women on MAT, a small number of women switched from buprenorphine to methadone for a variety of reasons, but some birth outcomes such as gestational age and birth weight were a little better in the buprenorphine group.[224] One group in Australia reported the use of implantable naltrexone in pregnant patients after opioid detoxification.[146,147]

The most significant acute neonatal complication of opioid use during pregnancy is the NAS, which is characterized by hyperirritability; GI dysfunction; respiratory distress; and vague autonomic effects, including yawning, sneezing, mottling, and fever.[144] Myoclonic jerks or seizures also signify neurologic irritability. Withdrawing infants are recognizable by their extreme jitteriness despite efforts at consolation. Approximately 50% to 90% of chronic opioid-exposed newborns show some signs of NAS.[99,154]

Just as opioid use and misuse has increased among the general population overall and pregnant women in particular, so has the frequency of NAS increased in the United States and abroad. In the United States, between 2000 and 2012 the rate of NAS increased from 1.2 per 1,000 to 5.8 per 1,000 live births.[253,255] Again there is significant regional variation. The rate of NAS varied from a low of 0.7 per 1,000 births in Hawaii to 33.4 per 1,000 in West Virginia[165] and is more prevalent in rural compared to urban areas.[339] In 2012, the average cost of hospitalization was $66,700 for a baby with NAS and $93,400 for a baby with NAS treated pharmacologically as compared to $3500 for an uncomplicated term newborn. Considering that approximately 4% of neonatal ICU days overall and in some centers as much as 40% to 50% of neonatal ICU days are attributed to babies with NAS, much of this cost is related to an increased number of infants admitted to NICUs for therapy and to prolonged lengths of stay for treatment.[329] Approximately 80% of the 2012 aggregate cost of 1.5 billion dollars was covered by Medicaid.

The Neonatal alcohol abstinence syndrome typically occurs within one week of birth. Heroin withdrawal usually occurs within the first 24 hours whereas methadone and buprenorphine withdrawal usually occur within 2 to 3 days of delivery. The onset of methadone withdrawal is delayed compared to heroin because methadone has a larger volume of distribution and slower metabolism in the neonate and therefore an increased half-life. The onset and severity of methadone withdrawal may be related to the absolute neonatal serum concentration or possibly to the rate of decline in concentration.[80,175] In one study, methadone withdrawal occurred when the plasma concentration fell below 0.06 mg/mL.[278]

As mentioned previously, the onset and severity of withdrawal is related to which opioids were used; which other prescription medications or substances were used; how much of these prescription medications or other substances was used long-term; how much was used near the time of delivery; the character of the labor; whether analgesics or anesthetics were used; and the maturity, nutrition, and medical condition of the neonate.[77] Acute NAS generally last from days to weeks but as many as 80% of infants were reported to have recurrence of some symptoms such as restlessness, agitation, tremors, wakefulness, hyperphagia, colic, or vomiting for 3 to 6 months.[54] In general, the incidence and severity of withdrawal are greater from methadone than from either heroin or buprenorphine.[144]

In general, babies who are extremely irritable; have feeding difficulties, diarrhea, or significant tremors; or cry continuously should receive pharmacological therapy.[144] The severity of withdrawal as measured by a standardized scoring scale is typically used to determine the need for therapy; several scales are in use although none has been validated.[99,192] Although most hospitals have treatment protocols for NAS, there is significant variation in their use.[31,254] Reducing this variation by training staff to apply these scores in a consistent manner leads to reductions in length of treatment, length of hospital stay, and total dose of opioid administered.[18]

Severe NAS often require pharmacologic therapy, and the typical approach was to provide care in a NICU. However, considering that treatment of withdrawal is recommended to begin with swaddling or tightly wrapping the infant, minimal handling or stimulation, and demand feeding, all in a quiet and comforting environment, the NICU is increasingly being seen as a less-than-ideal environment to provide care. In fact, this phase of

treatment is generally neither standardized nor controlled in clinical trials of pharmacologic therapy.[122]

In one center where a standardized approach to treatment based on a rooming-in model with increased family involvement was implemented on an inpatient non-NICU ward, the proportion of infants treated with morphine decreased from 46% to 27% and the morphine dose decreased from 13.7 mg to 6.6 mg per infant.[137] In addition, the length of stay (LOS) decreased from 16.9 to 12.3 days and the average cost decreased from $19,737 to $8,755 per treated infant. This center also used a standardized treatment and weaning protocol. In another center using a similar approach, the proportion of infants treated decreased from 98% to 14%, the average LOS decreased from 22.4 days to 5.9 days, and the average cost decreased from $44,824 to $10,259 per infant.[121] In contrast to almost every other study that uses the original or modified version of the Finnegan neonatal abstinence scoring system to determine the need for pharmacologic therapy, this group developed a score focused only on what might be considered an infant's primary needs—the ability to eat, sleep, and be consoled. Pharmacologic therapy was instituted only if maximal nonpharmacologic intervention was unsuccessful and these primary needs could not be fulfilled.

Opioid agonists such as morphine, methadone, buprenorphine, tincture of opium, and paregoric; sedative–hypnotics such as diazepam and phenobarbital; and clonidine have all been used both individually and in various combinations to treat withdrawal. Most centers primarily use oral morphine to treat withdrawal because it is a short-acting pure opioid agonist and the formulation has no additives.[260] Buprenorphine is being increasingly explored as a primary treatment option. Clonidine and phenobarbital are typically used as adjunctive therapies. Few well-controlled trials have evaluated the relative efficacy of various approaches or examined long-term effects of therapy.[248,249]

At one center, sublingual buprenorphine was compared to oral morphine.[154,155] In these trials, buprenorphine was associated with a 5- to 15-day (18%–46%) decreased length of opioid treatment (LOT) and an 11- to 19-day (29%–36%) decreased length of stay (LOS). In one trial comparing buprenorphine to methadone, both the average LOT and the average LOS were both approximately 4.5 days less in the buprenorphine group. In this study, the LOT for buprenorphine was shorter than the LOT in 2 of the 3 buprenorphine versus morphine studies. It is hard to know exactly how to compare these findings, considering that the studies have different patient populations and different treatment algorithms, and that regardless of the opioid chosen the LOT and LOS can decrease in association with standardized opioid treatment and weaning protocols as well as with a standardized and intensified approach to nonpharmacologic intervention. Nonetheless, the evidence suggests that the LOT and LOS are both shorter after buprenorphine compared to either morphine or methadone.

Five percent to 7% of babies showing signs of withdrawal experience seizures, generally by 10 days after birth.[134] Seizures occur more frequently after methadone withdrawal than after heroin withdrawal. These seizures do not necessarily predispose to idiopathic epilepsy; in one small study, children who had withdrawal seizures were without seizures and had normal neurologic examination findings and psychometric testing at one-year follow-up.[81]

Opioid agonists are more effective at preventing withdrawal seizures from heroin or methadone than phenobarbital or diazepam are.[134,157] However, sedative–hypnotics are commonly abused by pregnant heroin users or pregnant women maintained on methadone. Therefore sedative–hypnotic withdrawal seizures can contribute to the overall neonatal abstinence symptomatology, and for this reason, many treatment protocols include the use phenobarbital as a treatment adjunct.

Infants of opioid-using mothers have a 2 to 3 times increased risk for SIDS compared with control participants.[158,159] Proposed mechanisms include a decreased medullary responsiveness to CO_2 or some condition related to the postnatal environment.[99]

Although young children born to opioid users do not seem to have significant differences in behavior compared to control participants, older children have increased learning problems and school dysfunction particularly related to behavior difficulties.[354]

Cocaine

Approximately 0.1% of pregnant women in the United States between the ages of 15 and 44 years report previous-month use of cocaine; for 2016, this represented only 1,000 women.[286] This is in contrast to approximately 431,000 female cocaine users between the ages of 15 and 44 years who reported previous-month use for the same period. Compared to the numbers reported during the cocaine epidemic of the 1990s, this is a significant reduction in exposure. Nonetheless, the number of children exposed to cocaine in utero over the past 30 years has been estimated at 7.5 million.[50] The consequences of cocaine use during pregnancy have been extensively reviewed.[139,178,210,258]

The incidence of abruptio placentae may be significant when related to acute cocaine use.[303] Some uncommon perinatal problems include seizures, cerebral infarctions, and intraventricular hemorrhage.[58,258]

Cocaine use is significantly related to decreases in gestational age, birth weight, length, and head circumference, although these growth parameters generally correct by several years of age.[178,210] In addition, these growth effects are exacerbated by concomitant ethanol, tobacco, and opioid use.[178,210] Good prenatal care can mitigate many of these adverse effects of cocaine.[201,269,354]

Significant congenital malformations were reported among some infants who were exposed to cocaine in utero, specifically genitourinary malformations, cardiovascular malformations, and limb-reduction defects.[44,106] However, in one large population-based study, there was no increase in the incidence of malformations.[209]

Teratogenic effects are observed in animal models of in utero cocaine exposure. Decreased maternal and fetal weight gain and an increased frequency of fetal resorption were demonstrated in rats[95]; sporadic physical anomalies are also observed.[59] Teratogenic effects similar to those observed in humans were reported in mice, including bony defects of the skull, cryptorchidism, hydronephrosis, ileal atresia, cardiac defects, limb deformities, and eye abnormalities.[100,202,203,223] Cocaine caused hemorrhage and edema of the extremities and, subsequently, limb-reduction defects in rats when administered during midgestation in the postorganogenic period.[343]

The perinatal effects of cocaine are probably mediated through a vascular mechanism. Cocaine administration in the pregnant ovine model causes increased uterine vascular resistance, decreased uterine blood flow, increased fetal heart rate and arterial blood pressure, and decreased fetal PO_2 and O_2 content.[17,351] Similar effects are reported in rats.[252] Fetal hypoxia causes rupture of fetal blood vessels and infarction in developing organ systems such as the genitourinary system[56,223,308] or the CNS.[53,79,344] Hyperthermia or direct effects of cocaine in the fetus could exacerbate these effects.[36] Limb-reduction defects similar to those attributed to cocaine are produced after mechanical clamping of the uterine vessels.[36,345] A developing concept is that after vasospasm and ischemia, reperfusion occurs with the generation of oxygen free radicals and subsequent injury.[351,352]

Despite the reported malformations and a possible mechanism neither the human epidemiology nor the effects observed in animal models suggest a specific teratogenic syndrome. The risk of a significant malformation from prenatal cocaine exposure is low, but the effect, if one occurs, could be severe.[37,84,106]

One of the greatest concerns about prenatal cocaine exposure is the potential adverse effect on the developing child, and this is an intensive area of epidemiologic research. The most common findings in early infancy are lability of behavior and autonomic regulation; decreased alertness and orientation; and abnormal reflexes, tone, and motor maturity. However, many studies show no effect, especially after controlling for confounding variables.[94,178,210] For some children, effects manifest in later infancy as difficulty with information processing and learning. For school-age children, observed cognitive deficits are often related to the home environment even for children who showed some of the typical neonatal behaviors.[104,178,210] Nonetheless, there is evidence of impairment in modulating attention and impulsivity, which makes handling unfamiliar, complex, and stressful tasks

more difficult,[178,210,216] and these effects are also observed in animal models of prenatal cocaine exposure.[84,129,190,313]

The mechanism of neurotoxicity is not specifically elucidated. As described earlier, for many of the maternal and fetal physical defects, cocaine has direct toxicity, or alternatively, effects could be mediated through hypoxia or oxygen free radicals. Because cocaine interferes with neurotransmitter reuptake, it is likely that cocaine also disrupts normal neural ontogeny by interfering with the trophic functions of neurotransmitters on the developing brain, in particular dysfunction of signal transduction via the dopamine D_1 receptor.[129,190,217] These mechanisms are important in the etiology of neurobehavioral effects.

BREASTFEEDING

In the United States, breastfeeding is the recommended method of infant nutrition because it offers nutritional, immunologic, and psychological benefits without additional costs. Many women use prescription and nonprescription xenobiotics while breastfeeding and are concerned about the possible ill effects on their infants of these xenobiotics in the breast milk. This concern extends to the possible exposure of infants to occupational and environmental xenobiotics via breast milk.[276,295] The response to many of these concerns can be determined by the answer to the following question: Does the risk to an infant from a xenobiotic exposure via breast milk exceed the benefit of being breastfed?[183]

Pharmacokinetic factors determine the amount of xenobiotic available for transfer from maternal plasma into breast milk; only free xenobiotic can traverse the mammary alveolar membrane. Most xenobiotics are transported by passive diffusion. A few xenobiotics, such as ethanol and lithium, are transported through aqueous-filled pores. The factors that determine how well a xenobiotic diffuses across the membrane are similar to those for other biologic membranes such as the placenta: MW, lipid solubility, and degree of ionization.

Large-molecular-weight xenobiotics, such as heparin and insulin, do not pass into breast milk. Lipid solubility is important not only for diffusion but also for xenobiotic accumulation in breast milk because breast milk is rich in fat, especially breast milk that is produced in the postcolostral period (~3–4 days postpartum). With a pH near 7.0, breast milk is slightly more acidic than plasma. Consequently, xenobiotics that are weak acids in plasma exist largely as ionized molecules and cannot be easily transported into milk. Conversely, xenobiotics that are weak bases exist in plasma largely as nonionized molecules and are available for transport into breast milk. In breast milk, ionization of the weak base xenobiotics occurs, and the xenobiotics are concentrated as a result of ion trapping. In other words, xenobiotics that are weak bases could concentrate in breast milk. Whereas sulfacetamide (pK_a of 5.4, a weak acid) has a concentration in plasma 10 times its concentration in breast milk, sulfanilamide (pK_a of 10.4, a weak base) is found in equal concentrations in both plasma and breast milk.[183]

The net effect of these physiologic processes is expressed in the milk-to-plasma (M/P) ratio. Xenobiotics with higher M/P ratios have relatively greater concentrations in breast milk. The M/P ratio does not, however, reflect the absolute concentration of a xenobiotic in the breast milk, and a xenobiotic with a high M/P *ratio* is not necessarily found at a high *concentration* in the breast milk. For example, morphine has an M/P ratio of 2.46 (is concentrated in breast milk), but only 0.4% of a maternal dose is excreted into the breast milk.[16] In general, for most xenobiotics, approximately 1% to 2% of the maternally administered dose is presented to the infant in breast milk.[183]

The M/P ratio has several limitations. It does not account for differences in xenobiotic concentration that result from (1) repeat or chronic dosing, (2) breastfeeding at different times relative to maternal xenobiotic dosing, (3) differences in milk production during the day or even during a particular breastfeeding session, (4) the time postpartum (days, weeks, or months) when the measurement is made, and (5) maternal disease.

While being cognizant of the limitations, a spot breast milk xenobiotic concentration or a concentration estimate based on the M/P ratio allows a simplistic estimation of the quantity of xenobiotic to which an infant is exposed, assuming a constant breast milk concentration:

Infant dose = Breast milk concentration × Amount consumed

The effect of this dose on the infant depends on the bioavailability of the xenobiotic in breast milk, the pharmacokinetic parameters that determine xenobiotic concentrations in the infant, and the infant's receptor sensitivity to the xenobiotic. These parameters are often different in neonates than in adults and could lead to xenobiotic accumulation; generally, absorption is greater, but metabolism and clearance are reduced.[15] These effects are exaggerated in premature infants.[264,273] The amount of most xenobiotics delivered to infants in breast milk is usually adequately metabolized and eliminated.[183]

Many of the above considerations are theoretical, and the number of specifically contraindicated xenobiotics is quite small.[283] Published guidelines on the advisability of breastfeeding during periods of maternal therapy are generally based on the expected effects of full doses in the infant or on case reports of adverse occurrences. Interestingly, when the reports of adverse effects were reviewed, 37% of cases were in infants younger than 2 weeks, 63% were in infants younger than 1 month, and 78% were in infants younger than 2 months; 18% were in infants 2 to 6 months old; and only 4% were in infants older than 6 months.[12] It seems, therefore, that adverse effects are most likely to be observed in the first few weeks of life, when an infant's metabolic capacity is significantly less than that of an older infant, child, or adult.[8,75]

For most xenobiotics, a risk-to-benefit analysis must be made. For example, lithium is transferred in breast milk and leads to measurable, although subtherapeutic, serum concentrations in a breastfed infant. Although the effects of such exposure to lithium are unknown, many practitioners believe that the benefit of treating a mother's bipolar illness outweighs the potential risk to the infant.[183,294] There is also a small increased risk of carcinogenicity associated with exposure to some environmental xenobiotics through breast milk.[276]

Similarly, the breastfed infant of a woman who smokes is exposed to nicotine and other tobacco constituents, both by inhalation and via breast milk. Although such a child is at increased risk for respiratory illness as a result of exposure to tobacco smoke, some of the risk may be mitigated by breastfeeding.[271,283]

In most cases, women do not need to stop breastfeeding while using pharmaceuticals, such as most common antibiotics. However, "compatibility" with breastfeeding is generally based on a lack of reported adverse effects, which reflects limited clinical experience with a particular xenobiotic in breastfeeding patients. Therefore, in the setting of limited information, exposure to a xenobiotic through breast milk should be regarded as a small potential risk, and the infant should receive appropriate medical follow-up. Not all "compatible" medications are safe in all situations. For instance, phenobarbital can produce CNS depression in an infant if the mother's serum concentration is in the high therapeutic or supratherapeutic range, which often occurs while dosage adjustments are being made. Such a concentration may or may not produce CNS depression in the mother. Nalidixic acid, nitrofurantoin, sulfapyridine, and sulfisoxazole, although generally safe, can cause hemolysis in a breastfed infant with glucose-6-phosphate dehydrogenase deficiency.

When women use substances postpartum, there is delivery of some xenobiotic to the infant via breast milk, and there are rare case reports of infants experiencing adverse effects.[55] Because of these possible direct effects on the baby, as well as the detrimental effects on the physical and emotional health of the mother and on the caregiving environment, the use of substances such as cocaine, methamphetamine, and heroin during the breastfeeding period is discouraged, and women actively using substances are discouraged from breastfeeding.[283] However, women who are or have been abstinent from substance use and are participating in a treatment program are generally encouraged to breastfeed their infants.[4,183]

Although ethanol is not specifically contraindicated for breastfeeding mothers, decreased milk production and adverse effects in infants are noted with maternal consumption of large amounts of ethanol.

Questions sometimes arise regarding possible lead exposure during breastfeeding. Lead crosses into breast milk from blood and is the most likely source of lead exposure for most breastfeeding infants.[196] Approximately 1% of US women between the ages of 15 and 49 years have blood lead concentrations greater than 5 mcg/dL.[92] Some estimates suggest that breast milk concentrations are less than 3% of the maternal blood lead; therefore, if the maternal lead concentration is 5 mcg/dL, then the amount of lead delivered to the infant could be 1.5 mcg/L of breast milk.[124,170] This represents a relatively small exposure. In a sample of breastfed babies from one US city, the mean infant lead concentration was less than 3 mcg/dL, the highest concentration was 8 mcg/dL, and only 7.8% of values were greater than 5 mcg/dL.[196] The current consensus is that the benefits of breastfeeding outweigh the relatively small exposure to lead in breast milk.[347] Blood lead screening for most women is not recommended.

There are, however, some subpopulations of pregnant women at increased risk of elevated environmental lead exposure for whom blood lead screening is recommended. Risk factors for significant lead exposure in pregnant women include recent immigration, pica practices, occupational exposure, poor nutritional status, culturally specific practices such as the use of traditional remedies or imported cosmetics, and the use of traditional lead-glazed pottery for cooking and storing as well as those involved with renovation or remodeling in older homes.[92]

All women should have an assessment of risk for environmental lead exposure. Women at increased risk should have blood lead screening. When possible, pregnant and postpartum women with blood lead concentrations of 5 mcg/dL or higher should be removed from occupational or environmental lead sources and discouraged from practices or activities that result in increased exposure.[92] In addition, some evidence suggests that dietary supplementation of calcium can reduce the mobilization of lead in postpartum women.[133] In cases of elevated maternal lead concentrations, decisions regarding breastfeeding should be made on an individual basis.

In 2007, after the death of a breastfeeding 13-day-old infant whose mother was using codeine, the US FDA issued a public health advisory regarding the use of codeine by breastfeeding women.[333] In the initial case, the mother was found to be compound heterozygous for a *CYP2D6*2A* allele and a *CYP2D6*2x2* gene duplication and therefore an "ultrametabolizer" of codeine.[166] In other words, codeine was metabolized to morphine at an exaggerated rate, and the infant ingested a high dose of morphine via the breast milk. The ultrametabolizer phenotype is present in up to 10% of whites and up to 30% of Ethiopians, North Africans, and Saudi Arabians.[333] In addition, both the mother and the infant were homozygous for the *UGT2B7*2* allele, which leads to elevated concentrations of morphine-6-glucuronide, an active metabolite.

Another decreased-function gene variant of *ABCB1* has a role in this codeine toxicity. *ABCB1* codes for a P-glycoprotein involved in transporting morphine out of the CNS. Decreased gene function would lead to increased accumulation of morphine in the CNS and potentially increased toxicity.[306]

Decisions on breastfeeding should be made with the informed involvement of the woman; her physicians; and when necessary, a consultant with special expertise in this field. Guidelines are available from several sources.[39,183]

TOXICOLOGIC PROBLEMS IN NEONATES

Physiologic differences between adults and newborn infants affect xenobiotic absorption, distribution, and metabolism.[15,160,341] Appropriate administration of xenobiotics to newborn infants therefore requires an understanding of the appropriate developmental state for medication dosing and pharmacokinetics. Even so, approximately 8% of all medication doses administered in NICUs are up to 10 times greater or lesser than the dose ordered,[64] and as many as 30% of newborns in NICUs sustain adverse drug effects, some of which are life threatening or fatal.[16] Pharmacokinetic differences between adults and newborns account for some cases of unanticipated xenobiotic toxicity that occur in newborn infants.

Gastrointestinal absorption of xenobiotics in neonates is generally slower than in adults.[15,160,341] This delay is related to decreased gastric acid secretion, decreased gastric emptying and transit time, and decreased pancreatic enzyme activity. The GI environment of newborns and young infants allows the growth of *Clostridium botulinum* and the subsequent development of infant botulism (Chap. 38). Infantile botulism is reported in infants several weeks of age.[148,326]

Although it is uncommon, cutaneous absorption of xenobiotics is sometimes a route of toxic exposure in a newborn.[87,282] Aniline dyes used for marking diapers are absorbed, causing methemoglobinemia,[282] and contaminated diapers were responsible for one epidemic of mercury poisoning.[22] The absorption of hexachlorophene antiseptic wash has led to neurotoxicity with marked vacuolization of myelin seen microscopically.[180,211,304] The dermal application of antiseptic ethanol has caused hemorrhagic necrosis of the skin of some premature infants. Iodine antiseptics have led to hypothyroidism in mature newborns.[49] An increased potential for absorption and toxicity has followed the application of corticosteroids[112,280] and boric acid[85] to the skin of children with cutaneous disorders.

Other routes of exposure have led to clinical poisoning. Several children inhaled talcum powder and died from acute respiratory distress syndrome.[40,229] Inhalation of mercury from incubator thermometers is a potential risk.[11] One child died after the ophthalmic instillation of cyclopentolate hydrochloride.[24]

Because of differences in total body water and fat compared with adults, the distribution of absorbed xenobiotics differs in neonates.[15,160,341] Water represents 80% of body weight in a full-term baby compared with 60% in an adult. Approximately 20% of a term baby's body weight is fat compared with only 3% in a premature baby. The increased volume of water means that the volume of distribution for some water-soluble xenobiotics, such as theophylline and phenobarbital, is increased.

Protein binding of xenobiotics is lower in newborns compared with adults: the serum concentration of proteins is lower, there are fewer receptor sites that become saturated at lower xenobiotic concentrations, and binding sites have decreased binding affinity.[15,160,341] Protein binding has potential relevance with respect to bilirubin, an endogenous metabolite that at very high concentrations causes kernicterus; bilirubin competes with exogenously administered xenobiotics for protein binding sites. In vitro, certain xenobiotics, such as sulfonamides and ceftriaxone, displace bilirubin from protein receptor sites, which might increase the risk of kernicterus, although this has not been clinically demonstrated. Conversely, bilirubin itself displaces other xenobiotics, such as phenobarbital or phenytoin, leading to increased plasma xenobiotic concentrations.

Newborn infants have decreased hepatic metabolic capacity compared with adults, which can lead to xenobiotic toxicity.[15,160] For example, caffeine, used in the treatment of neonatal apnea, has an extremely prolonged half-life in newborns because CYP1A2 has only 5% of the normal adult activity.[15] Except for CYP1A2, most of the CYP isoenzymes reach approximately 25% of adult activity in newborns by about 1 month of age.

Two disease clusters related to immature metabolic function are described. The "gasping baby syndrome," characterized by gasping respirations, metabolic acidosis, hypotension, CNS depression, convulsions, kidney failure, and occasionally death, is attributed to high concentrations of benzyl alcohol and benzoic acid in the plasma of affected infants.[10,43,113] Benzyl alcohol, a bacteriostatic, was added to IV flush solutions and accumulated in newborns after repetitive doses. The high concentrations of benzoic acid could not be further metabolized to hippuric acid by the immature liver. Immature glucuronidation in neonates is responsible for the "gray-baby syndrome" after high doses of chloramphenicol (Chaps. 31, 46 and 54).[138]

The umbilical vessels are a common site of vascular access in sick neonates. Because blood drains into the portal vein, it is possible that IV medications experience a "first-pass" effect, although whether this route of xenobiotic administration affects metabolism or clearance has not been well studied. Most functions of the kidney, including glomerular filtration rate (GFR) and tubular secretion, are relatively immature at birth;[15] the GFR

of a newborn is approximately 30% of that of an adult. Xenobiotics such as aminoglycosides and digoxin are excreted unchanged by the kidney and therefore depend on glomerular filtration for clearance. Dosing of these xenobiotics in a newborn must account for these differences.

An interesting association has been made periodically over the years between the use of erythromycin, particularly in the first 2 weeks of life, and idiopathic hypertrophic pyloric stenosis.[62,140,204,288,314] Although erythromycin is known to interact with motilin receptors in the antrum of the stomach, no specific etiology has been defined.[131]

Very little specific information is available to guide clinicians in the management of xenobiotic poisoning in newborn infants. In the case of cutaneous exposure to a xenobiotic, absorption is probably already complete by the time toxicity is noted. Nonetheless, the xenobiotic should be discontinued and the skin surface should be decontaminated. In the case of oral exposure, gastrointestinal decontamination is not generally performed in neonates, and neonates are at increased risk of fluid, electrolyte, and thermoregulatory problems after gastric lavage or the use of cathartics. Multiple-dose activated charcoal was used in a 1.4-kg, 2-week-old premature infant to treat iatrogenic theophylline toxicity.[300] Hemodialysis, hemoperfusion, and exchange transfusion can be used in neonates to treat xenobiotic toxicity but require care in specialized units that experience with these extra-corporeal modalities (Chaps. 6 and 31).

SUMMARY

- Human embryos and fetuses are exposed to xenobiotics through the placenta of the pregnant woman; the neonates are exposed to xenobiotics via breast milk.
- Xenobiotic effects on developing humans include both congenital malformations as well as neurobehavioral abnormalities that manifest later in life.
- The use of xenobiotics in a pregnant or breastfeeding woman is a complex area of medical practice and presents clinicians with potentially difficult management decisions regarding the benefit of therapy to the mother and the risk to the mother or fetus of xenobiotic exposure.
- The goal is to optimize benefit for both the mother and the child but at least to minimize the risk to the fetus. In almost all cases, the primary approach is to fully and appropriately treat the mother.
- Appropriate management of many of the potential problems is facilitated by the coordinated efforts of obstetricians, perinatologists, neonatologists, pediatricians, and toxicologists.

REFERENCES

1. Abel E. Paternal contribution to fetal alcohol syndrome. *Addict Biol.* 2004;9:127-133.
2. Abel EL. Fetal alcohol syndrome: a cautionary note. *Curr Pharm Des.* 2006;12:1521-1529.
3. Abel EL, Hannigan JH. Maternal risk factors in fetal alcohol syndrome: provocative and permissive influences. *Neurotoxicol Teratol.* 1995;17:445-462.
4. Jansson LM, Academy of Breastfeeding Medicine Protocol C. ABM clinical protocol #21: Guidelines for breastfeeding and the drug-dependent woman. *Breastfeed Med.* 2009;4:225-228.
5. Adam MP, et al. Evolving knowledge of the teratogenicity of medications in human pregnancy. *Am J Med Genet C Semin Med Genet.* 2011;157C:175-182.
6. Addis A, et al. Risk classification systems for drug use during pregnancy: are they a reliable source of information? *Drug Saf.* 2000;23:245-253.
7. Ailes EC, et al. Opioid prescription claims among women of reproductive age—United States, 2008-2012. *MMWR Morb Mortal Wkly Rep.* 2015;64:37-41.
8. Alcorn J, McNamara PJ. Pharmacokinetics in the newborn. *Adv Drug Deliv Rev.* 2003;55:667-686.
9. Allegaert K, et al. Physicochemical and structural properties regulating placental drug transfer. In: Polin RA, eds. *Fetal and Neonatal Physiology*, Vol 1. 5th ed. Philadelphia, PA: Elsevier; 2017:208-221.
10. American Academy of Pediatrics. Benzyl alcohol: toxic agent in neonatal units. *Pediatrics.* 1983;72:356-358.
11. American Academy of Pediatrics. Mercury vapor contamination of infant incubators: a potential hazard. *Pediatrics.* 1984;67:637.
12. Anderson PO, et al. Adverse drug reactions in breastfed infants: less than imagined. *Clin Pediatr (Phila).* 2003;42:325-340.
13. Andrade SE, et al. Use of prescription medications with a potential for fetal harm among pregnant women. *Pharmacoepidemiol Drug Saf.* 2006;15:546-554.

14. Appleby L. Suicide during pregnancy and in the first postnatal year. *BMJ.* 1991;302:137-140.

15. Aranda JV, et al. Developmental pharmacology. In: Fanaroff AA, Martin RJ, eds. *Neonatal-Perinatal Medicine*, Vol 1. St. Louis, MO: Mosby; 2002:144-166.

16. Aranda JV, et al. Epidemiology of adverse drug reactions in the newborn. *Dev Pharmacol Ther.* 1982;5:173-184.

17. Arbeille P, et al. Effect of long-term cocaine administration to pregnant ewes on fetal hemodynamics, oxygenation, and growth. *Obstet Gynecol.* 1997;90:795-802.

18. Asti L, et al. A quality improvement project to reduce length of stay for neonatal abstinence syndrome. *Pediatrics.* 2015;135:e1494-e1500.

19. Atkinson DE, et al. Placental transfer. In: Neill JD, ed. *Knobil and Neill's Physiology of Reproduction*, Vol 2. Amsterdam: Elsevier; 2006:2787-2827.

20. Aw MM, et al. Neonatal paracetamol poisoning. *Arch Dis Child Fetal Neonatal Ed.* 1999;81:F78.

21. Backburn ST. Pharmacology and pharmacokinetics during the perinatal period. In: Backburn ST, ed. *Maternal, Fetal, & Neonatal Physiology*. 4th ed. St. Louis, MO: Elsevier; 2012:183-215.

22. Banzaw TM. Mercury poisoning in Argentine babies linked to diapers. *Pediatrics.* 1981;67:637.

23. Bateman BT, et al. Patterns of opioid utilization in pregnancy in a large cohort of commercial insurance beneficiaries in the United States. *Anesthesiology.* 2014;120:1216-1224.

24. Bauser CR, et al. Systemic cyclopentolate (Cyclogyl) toxicity in the newborn infant. *J Pediatr.* 1973;82:501.

25. Bay Bjorn AM, et al. Use of corticosteroids in early pregnancy is not associated with risk of oral clefts and other congenital malformations in offspring. *Am J Ther.* 2014;21:73-80.

26. Beattie JO. Transplacental alcohol intoxication. *Alcohol Alcohol.* 1986;21:163-166.

27. Becker HC, et al. Teratogenic actions of ethanol in the mouse: a minireview. *Pharmacol Biochem Behav.* 1996;55:501-513.

28. Bergink V, Kushner SA. Postpartum psychosis. In: Galbally M, et al, eds. *Psychopharmacology and Pregnancy: Treatment Efficacy, Risks, and Guidelines*. Heidelverg: Springer; 2014:139-149.

29. Bertrand J, et al. *Fetal Alcohol Syndrome: Guidelines for Referral and Diagnosis*. Atlanta, GA, Centers for Disease Control and Prevention; 2004.

30. Blanc P, et al. Deferoxamine treatment of acute iron intoxication in pregnancy. *Obstet Gynecol.* 1984;64:12S-14S.

31. Bogen DL, et al. Wide variation found in care of opioid-exposed newborns. *Acad Pediatr.* 2017;17:374-380.

32. Bonari L, et al. Perinatal risks of untreated depression during pregnancy. *Can J Psychiatry.* 2004;49:726-735.

33. Bonati M, Fellin G. Changes in smoking and drinking behaviour before and during pregnancy in Italian mothers: implications for public health intervention. ICGDUP (Italian Collaborative Group on Drug Use in Pregnancy). *Int J Epidemiol.* 1991;20:927-932.

34. Bosque MA, et al. Assessment of the developmental toxicity of deferoxamine in mice. *Arch Toxicol.* 1995;69:467-471.

35. Boumba VA, et al. Hair as a biological indicator of drug use, drug abuse or chronic exposure to environmental toxicants. *Int J Toxicol.* 2006;25:143-163.

36. Brent RL. Relationship between uterine vascular clamping, vascular disruption syndrome, and cocaine teratogenicity. *Teratology.* 1990;41:757-760.

37. Brent RL. The application of the principles of toxicology and teratology in evaluating the risks of new drugs for treatment of drug addiction in women of reproductive age. *NIDA Res Monogr.* 1995;149:130-184.

38. Brent RL. Environmental causes of human congenital malformations: the pediatrician's role in dealing with these complex clinical problems caused by a multiplicity of environmental and genetic factors. *Pediatrics.* 2004;113:957-968.

39. Briggs GG, et al. *Drugs in Pregnancy and Lactation: A Reference Guide to Fetal and Neonatal Risk*. 11th ed. Philadelphia, PA: Lippincott, Williams & Williams; 2017.

40. Brouillette F, Weber ML. Massive aspiration of talcum powder by an infant. *Can Med Assoc J.* 1978;119:354-355.

41. Brown DB, et al. Hyperbaric oxygen treatment for carbon monoxide poisoning in pregnancy: a case report. *Aviat Space Environ Med.* 1992;63:1011-1014.

42. Brown MS, et al. Methadone versus morphine for treatment of neonatal abstinence syndrome: a prospective randomized clinical trial. *J Perinatol.* 2015;35:278-283.

43. Brown WJ, et al. Fatal benzyl alcohol poisoning in a neonatal intensive care unit. *Lancet.* 1982;1:1250.

44. Buehler BA, et al. Teratogenic potential of cocaine. *Semin Perinatol.* 1996;20:93-98.

45. Bullo M, et al. Pregnancy outcome following exposure to angiotensin-converting enzyme inhibitors or angiotensin receptor antagonists: a systematic review. *Hypertension.* 2012;60:444-450.

46. Burcham PC. Chemicals and the unborn. In: Burcham PC, ed. *An Introduction to Toxicology*. London: Springer; 2014:189-220.

47. Byer AJ, et al. Acetaminophen overdose in the third trimester of pregnancy. *JAMA.* 1982;247:3114-3115.

48. Caravati EM, et al. Fetal toxicity associated with maternal carbon monoxide poisoning. *Ann Emerg Med.* 1988;17:714-717.

49. Chabrolle JP, Rossier A. Goitre and hypothyroidism in the newborn after cutaneous absorption of iodine. *Arch Dis Child.* 1978;53:495-498.

50. Chae SM, Covington CY. Biobehavioral outcomes in adolescents and young adults prenatally exposed to cocaine: evidence from animal models. *Biol Res Nurs.* 2009;10:318-330.

51. Chang J, et al. Homicide: a leading cause of injury deaths among pregnant and postpartum women in the United States, 1991-1999. *Am J Public Health.* 2005;95:471-477.

52. Char VC, et al. Letter: Polyhydramnios and neonatal renal failure—a possible association with maternal acetaminophen ingestion. *J Pediatr.* 1975;86:638-639.

53. Chasnoff IJ, et al. Perinatal cerebral infarction and maternal cocaine use. *J Pediatr.* 1986;108:456-459.

54. Chasnoff IJ, et al. Early growth patterns of methadone-addicted infants. *Am J Dis Child.* 1980;134:1049-1051.

55. Chasnoff IJ, et al. Cocaine intoxication in a breast-fed infant. *Pediatrics.* 1987;80:836-838.

56. Chavez GF, et al. Maternal cocaine use during early pregnancy as a risk factor for congenital urogenital anomalies. *JAMA.* 1989;262:795-798.

57. Cheelo M, et al. Paracetamol exposure in pregnancy and early childhood and development of childhood asthma: a systematic review and meta-analysis. *Arch Dis Child.* 2015;100:81-89.

58. Chiriboga CA. Neurological correlates of fetal cocaine exposure. *Ann N Y Acad Sci.* 1998;846:109-125.

59. Church MW, et al. Dose-dependent consequences of cocaine on pregnancy outcome in the Long-Evans rat. *Neurotoxicol Teratol.* 1988;10:51-58.

60. Cohen-Kerem R, Koren G. Antioxidants and fetal protection against ethanol teratogenicity. I. Review of the experimental data and implications to humans. *Neurotoxicol Teratol.* 2003;25:1-9.

61. Comtois KA, et al. Psychiatric risk factors associated with postpartum suicide attempt in Washington State, 1992-2001. *Am J Obstet Gynecol.* 2008;199:120.e1-120.e5.

62. Cooper WO, et al. Very early exposure to erythromycin and infantile hypertrophic pyloric stenosis. *Arch Pediatr Adolesc Med.* 2002;156:647-650.

63. Cordier S. Evidence for a role of paternal exposures in developmental toxicity. *Basic Clin Pharmacol Toxicol.* 2008;102:176-181.

64. Cotten CM, et al. Pharmacology in neonatal care. In: Merenstein GB, Gardner SL, eds. *Handbook of Neonatal Intensive Care*. 6th ed. St. Louis, MO: Mosby Elsevier; 2006:184.

65. Cramer CR. Fetal death due to accidental maternal carbon monoxide poisoning. *J Toxicol Clin Toxicol.* 1982;19:297-301.

66. Crowell C, et al. Caring for the mother, concentrating on the fetus: intravenous N-acetylcysteine in pregnancy. *Am J Emerg Med.* 2008;26:735.e1-735.e2.

67. Curry SC, et al. An ovine model of maternal iron poisoning in pregnancy. *Ann Emerg Med.* 1990;19:632-638.

68. Czeizel A, Lendvay A. Attempted suicide and pregnancy. *Am J Obstet Gynecol.* 1989;161:497.

69. Czeizel AE. Attempted suicide and pregnancy. *J Inj Violence Res.* 2011;3:45-54.

70. Czeizel AE, et al. Self-poisoning during pregnancy as a model for teratogenic risk estimation of drugs. *Toxicol Ind Health.* 2008;24:11-28.

71. Czeizel AE, et al. Teratologic evaluation of 178 infants born to mothers who attempted suicide by drugs during pregnancy. *Obstet Gynecol.* 1997;90:195-201.

72. Dannenberg AL, et al. Homicide and other injuries as causes of maternal death in New York City, 1987 through 1991. *Am J Obstet Gynecol.* 1995;172:1557-1564.

73. Daw JR, et al. Prescription drug use during pregnancy in developed countries: a systematic review. *Pharmacoepidemiol Drug Saf.* 2011;20:895-902.

74. Daw JR, et al. Prescription drug use in pregnancy: a retrospective, population-based study in British Columbia, Canada (2001-2006). *Clin Ther.* 2012;34:239-249.e2.

75. de Wildt SN. Profound changes in drug metabolism enzymes and possible effects on drug therapy in neonates and children. *Expert Opin Drug Metab Toxicol.* 2011;7:935-948.

76. Desai RJ, et al. Increase in prescription opioid use during pregnancy among Medicaid-enrolled women. *Obstet Gynecol.* 2014;123:997-1002.

77. Desmond MM, Wilson GS. Neonatal abstinence syndrome: recognition and diagnosis. *Addict Dis.* 1975;2:113-121.

78. Diav-Citrin O, Koren G. Direct drug toxicity to the fetus. In: Koren G, ed. *Medication Safety in Pregnancy and Breastfeeding*. New York, NY: McGraw-Hill; 2007:85-119.

79. Dixon SD, Bejar R. Echoencephalographic findings in neonates associated with maternal cocaine and methamphetamine use: incidence and clinical correlates. *J Pediatr.* 1989;115:770-778.

80. Doberczak TM, et al. Relationship between maternal methadone dosage, maternal-neonatal methadone levels, and neonatal withdrawal. *Obstet Gynecol.* 1993;81:936-940.

81. Doberczak TM, et al. One-year follow-up of infants with abstinence-associated seizures. *Arch Neurol.* 1988;45:649-653.

82. Doering PL, et al. Review of pregnancy labeling of prescription drugs: is the current system adequate to inform of risks? *Am J Obstet Gynecol.* 2002;187:333-339.

83. Dominick MA, Carson TL. Effects of carbon monoxide exposure on pregnant sows and their fetuses. *Am J Vet Res.* 1983;44:35-40.

84. Dow-Edwards D. Comparability of human and animal studies of developmental cocaine exposure. *NIDA Res Monogr.* 1996;164:146-174.

85. Ducey J, Williams DB. Transcutaneous absorption of boric acid. *J Pediatr.* 1953;43:644-651.

86. Einarson A. The way women perceive teratogenic risk: how it can influence decision making during pregnancy regarding drug use or abortion of an unwanted pregnancy. In: Koren G, ed. *Medication Safety in Pregnancy and Breastfeeding*. New York, NY: McGraw-Hill; 2007:295-307.

87. Elhassani SB. Neonatal poisoning: causes, manifestations, prevention, and management. *South Med J.* 1986;79:1535-1543.

88. Elkharrat D, et al. Acute carbon monoxide intoxication and hyperbaric oxygen in pregnancy. *Intensive Care Med.* 1991;17:289-292.

89. Epstein RA, et al. Increasing pregnancy-related use of prescribed opioid analgesics. *Ann Epidemiol.* 2013;23:498-503.

90. Esscher A, et al. Suicides during pregnancy and 1 year postpartum in Sweden, 1980-2007. *Br J Psychiatry* 2016;208:462-469.

91. Etminan M, et al. Acetaminophen use and the risk of asthma in children and adults: a systematic review and metaanalysis. *Chest.* 2009;136:1316-1323.

92. Ettinger AS, Wengrovitz AG. Guidelines for the identification and management of lead exposure in pregnant and lactating women. http://www.cdc.gov/nceh/lead/publications/LeadandPregnancy2010.pdf. Published 2010. Accessed July 7, 2013.

93. Eyers S, et al. Paracetamol in pregnancy and the risk of wheezing in offspring: a systematic review and meta-analysis. *Clin Exp Allergy.* 2011;41:482-489.

94. Eyler FD, Behnke M. Early development of infants exposed to drugs prenatally. *Clin Perinatol.* 1999;26:107-150, vii.

95. Fantel AG, Macphail BJ. The teratogenicity of cocaine. *Teratology.* 1982;26:17-19.

96. Farber NB, Olney JW. Drugs of abuse that cause developing neurons to commit suicide. *Brain Res Dev Brain Res.* 2003;147:37-45.

97. Farrow JR, et al. Fetal death due to nonlethal maternal carbon monoxide poisoning. *J Forensic Sci.* 1990;35:1448-1452.

98. Ferm VH. Teratogenic effects of hyperbaric oxygen. *Proc Soc Exp Biol Med.* 1964;116:975-976.

99. Finnegan LP, Kandall SR. Maternal and neonatal effects of alcohol and drugs. In: Lowinson JH, et al, eds. *Substance Abuse: A Comprehensive Textbook.* 4th ed. Philadelphia, PA: Lippincott Williams & Wilkins; 2005:805-839.

100. Finnell RH, et al. Preliminary evidence for a cocaine-induced embryopathy in mice. *Toxicol Appl Pharmacol.* 1990;103:228-237.

101. Flak AL, et al. The association of mild, moderate, and binge prenatal alcohol exposure and child neuropsychological outcomes: a meta-analysis. *Alcohol Clin Exp Res.* 2014;38:214-226.

102. Flint C, et al. Pregnancy outcome after suicide attempt by drug use: a Danish population-based study. *Acta Obstet Gynecol Scand.* 2002;81:516-522.

103. Fox DJ, et al. Fetal alcohol syndrome among children aged 7-9 years—Arizona, Colorado, and New York, 2010. *MMWR Morb Mortal Wkly Rep.* 2015;64:54-57.

104. Frank DA, et al. Growth, development, and behavior in early childhood following prenatal cocaine exposure: a systematic review. *JAMA.* 2001;285:1613-1625.

105. Franko KR, et al. Accidental acetaminophen overdose results in liver transplant during second trimester of pregnancy: a case report. *Transplant Proc.* 2013;45:2063-2065.

106. Friedman JM, Polifka JE. *Teratogenic Effects of Drugs: A Resource for Clinicians (TERIS).* Baltimore, MD: Johns Hopkins University Press; 2000.

107. Friedman S, et al. Cesarean section after maternal acetaminophen overdose. *Anesth Analg.* 1993;77:632-634.

108. Gabrielli A, Layon AJ. Carbon monoxide intoxication during pregnancy: a case presentation and pathophysiologic discussion, with emphasis on molecular mechanisms. *J Clin Anesth* 1995;7:82-87.

109. Gandhi SG, et al. Maternal and neonatal outcomes after attempted suicide. *Obstet Gynecol.* 2006;107:984-990.

110. Gedeon C, Koren G. Gestational changes in drug disposition in the maternal-fetal unit. In: Koren G, ed. *Medication Safety in Pregnancy and Breastfeeding.* New York, NY: McGraw-Hill; 2007:5-11.

111. Gelaye B, et al. Suicidal ideation in pregnancy: an epidemiologic review. *Arch Womens Ment Health.* 2016;19:741-751.

112. Gemme G, et al. Picture of the month. Cushing's syndrome due to topical corticosteroids. *Am J Dis Child.* 1984;138:987-988.

113. Gershanik J, et al. The gasping syndrome and benzyl alcohol poisoning. *N Engl J Med.* 1982;307:1384-1388.

114. Gillberg C. "Floppy infant syndrome" and maternal diazepam. *Lancet.* 1977;2:244.

115. Ginsberg MD, Myers RE. Fetal brain injury after maternal carbon monoxide intoxication. Clinical and neuropathologic aspects. *Neurology.* 1976;26:15-23.

116. Glantz JC, Woods JR. Cocaine, heroin, and phencyclidine: obstetric perspectives. *Clin Obstet Gynecol.* 1993;36:279-301.

117. Goodlett CR, Horn KH. Mechanisms of alcohol-induced damage to the developing nervous system. *Alcohol Res Health.* 2001;25:175-184.

118. Gray R, Henderson J. Review of the Fetal Effects of Prenatal Alcohol Exposure, National Perinatal Epidemiology Unit, University of Oxford, 2006.

119. Green PP, et al. Vital signs: alcohol-exposed pregnancies—United States, 2011-2013. *MMWR Morb Mortal Wkly Rep.* 2016;65:91-97.

120. Greingor JL, et al. Acute carbon monoxide intoxication during pregnancy. One case report and review of the literature. *Emerg Med J.* 2001;18:399-401.

121. Grossman MR, et al. An initiative to improve the quality of care of infants with neonatal abstinence syndrome. *Pediatrics.* 2017;139.

122. Grossman MR, et al. Neonatal abstinence syndrome: time for a reappraisal. *Hosp Pediatr.* 2017;7:115-116.

123. Guerri C. Neuroanatomical and neurophysiological mechanisms involved in central nervous system dysfunctions induced by prenatal alcohol exposure. *Alcohol Clin Exp Res.* 1998;22:304-312.

124. Gulson BL, et al. Relationships of lead in breast milk to lead in blood, urine, and diet of the infant and mother. *Environ Health Perspect.* 1998;106:667-674.

125. Gundacker C, Hengstschlager M. The role of the placenta in fetal exposure to heavy metals. *Wien Med Wochenschr.* 2012;162:201-206.

126. Haibach H, et al. Acetaminophen overdose with fetal demise. *Am J Clin Pathol.* 1984;82:240-242.

127. Hakkola J, et al. Developmental expression of cytochrome P450 enzymes in human liver. *Pharmacol Toxicol.* 1998;82:209-217.

128. Hannigan JH. What research with animals is telling us about alcohol-related neurodevelopmental disorder. *Pharmacol Biochem Behav.* 1996;55:489-499.

129. Harvey JA. Cocaine effects on the developing brain: current status. *Neurosci Biobehav Rev.* 2004;27:751-764.

130. Haschek WM, et al. Male reproductive system. In: Haschek WM, et al, eds. *Toxicologic Pathology.* London: Academic Press; 2010:553-597.

131. Hauben M, Amsden GW. The association of erythromycin and infantile hypertrophic pyloric stenosis: causal or coincidental? *Drug Saf.* 2002;25:929-942.

132. Henderson GI, et al. Ethanol, oxidative stress, reactive aldehydes, and the fetus. *Front Biosci.* 1999;4:D541-D550.

133. Hernandez-Avila M, et al. Dietary calcium supplements to lower blood lead levels in lactating women: a randomized placebo-controlled trial. *Epidemiology.* 2003;14:206-212.

134. Herzlinger RA, et al. Neonatal seizures associated with narcotic withdrawal. *J Pediatr.* 1977;91:638-641.

135. Hill EP, et al. Carbon monoxide exchanges between the human fetus and mother: a mathematical model. *Am J Physiol.* 1977;232:H311-H323.

136. Hollander DI, et al. Hyperbaric oxygen therapy for the treatment of acute carbon monoxide poisoning in pregnancy. A case report. *J Reprod Med.* 1987;32:615-617.

137. Holmes AV, et al. Rooming-in to treat neonatal abstinence syndrome: improved family-centered care at lower cost. *Pediatrics.* 2016;137.

138. Holt D, et al. Chloramphenicol toxicity. *Adverse Drug React Toxicol Rev.* 1993;12:83-95.

139. Holzman C, Paneth N. Maternal cocaine use during pregnancy and perinatal outcomes. *Epidemiol Rev.* 1994;16:315-334.

140. Honein MA, et al. Infantile hypertrophic pyloric stenosis after pertussis prophylaxis with erythromycin: a case review and cohort study. *Lancet.* 1999;354:2101-2105.

141. Horowitz RS, et al. Placental transfer of *N*-acetylcysteine following human maternal acetaminophen toxicity. *J Toxicol Clin Toxicol.* 1997;35:447-451.

142. Howard TB, et al. Monitoring for teratogenic signals: pregnancy registries and surveillance methods. *Am J Med Genet C Semin Med Genet.* 2011;157:209-214.

143. Hoyme HE, et al. A practical clinical approach to diagnosis of fetal alcohol spectrum disorders: clarification of the 1996 institute of medicine criteria. *Pediatrics.* 2005;115:39-47.

144. Hudak ML, Tan RC. Neonatal drug withdrawal. *Pediatrics.* 2012;129:e540-e560.

145. Hui L, Bianchi DW. Prenatal pharmacotherapy for fetal anomalies: a 2011 update. *Prenat Diagn.* 2011;31:735-743.

146. Hulse GK, et al. Methadone maintenance vs. implantable naltrexone treatment in the pregnant heroin user. *Int J Gynaecol Obstet.* 2004;85:170-171.

147. Hulse GK, et al. Obstetric and neonatal outcomes associated with maternal naltrexone exposure. *Aust N Z J Obstet Gynaecol.* 2001;41:424-428.

148. Hurst DL, Marsh WW. Early severe infantile botulism. *J Pediatr.* 1993;122:909-911.

149. Hutchings DE. The puzzle of cocaine's effects following maternal use during pregnancy: are there reconcilable differences? *Neurotoxicol Teratol.* 1993;15:281-286.

150. Ihlen BM, et al. Changes in the use of intoxicants after onset of pregnancy. *Br J Addict.* 1990;85:1627-1631.

151. Jager-Roman E, et al. Fetal growth, major malformations, and minor anomalies in infants born to women receiving valproic acid. *J Pediatr.* 1986;108:997-1004.

152. Janssen S. Male reproductive toxicology. In: Ladou J, Harrison RJ, eds. *Current Diagnosis & Treatment: Occupational & Environmental Medicine.* 5th ed. New York, NY: McGraw-Hill; 2014:450-462.

153. Johnson SF, et al. Changes in alcohol, cigarette, and recreational drug use during pregnancy: implications for intervention. *Am J Epidemiol.* 1987;126:695-702.

154. Jones HE, et al. Methadone and buprenorphine for the management of opioid dependence in pregnancy. *Drugs.* 2012;72:747-757.

155. Jones HE, et al. Neonatal abstinence syndrome after methadone or buprenorphine exposure. *N Engl J Med.* 2010;363:2320-2331.

156. Jones KL, Chambers CD. What really causes FAS? A different perspective. *Teratology.* 1999;60:249-250.

157. Kandall SR, et al. Opiate v CNS depressant therapy in neonatal drug abstinence syndrome. *Am J Dis Child.* 1983;137:378-382.

158. Kandall SR, Gaines J. Maternal substance use and subsequent sudden infant death syndrome (SIDS) in offspring. *Neurotoxicol Teratol.* 1991;13:235-240.

159. Kandall SR, et al. Relationship of maternal substance abuse to subsequent sudden infant death syndrome in offspring. *J Pediatr.* 1993;123:120-126.

160. Kearns GL, et al. Developmental pharmacology—drug disposition, action, and therapy in infants and children. *N Engl J Med.* 2003;349:1157-1167.

161. Khalifeh H, et al. Suicide in perinatal and non-perinatal women in contact with psychiatric services: 15 year findings from a UK national inquiry. *Lancet Psychiatry.* 2016;3:233-242.

162. Khoury S, et al. Deferoxamine treatment for acute iron intoxication in pregnancy. *Acta Obstet Gynecol Scand.* 1995;74:756-757.

163. Kiess W, et al. Fetal alcohol syndrome and malignant disease. *Eur J Pediatr.* 1984;143:160-161.
164. Kleiner GJ, Greston WM. Suicide during pregnancy. In: Cherry SH, Merkatz IR, eds. *Complications of Pregnancy: Medical, Surgical, Gynecologic, Psychosocial, and Perinatal.* Baltimore, MD: William & Wilkins; 1991:269-89.
165. Ko JY, et al. Incidence of neonatal abstinence syndrome—28 states, 1999-2013. *MMWR Morb Mortal Wkly Rep.* 2016;65:799-802.
166. Koren G, et al. Pharmacogenetics of morphine poisoning in a breastfed neonate of a codeine-prescribed mother. *Lancet.* 2006;368:704.
167. Koren G, et al. Estimation of fetal exposure to drugs of abuse, environmental tobacco smoke, and ethanol. *Ther Drug Monit.* 2002;24:23-25.
168. Koren G, et al. Bias against the null hypothesis: the reproductive hazards of cocaine. *Lancet.* 1989;2:1440-1442.
169. Koren G, et al. A multicenter, prospective study of fetal outcome following accidental carbon monoxide poisoning in pregnancy. *Reprod Toxicol.* 1991;5:397-403.
170. Kosnett MJ, et al. Recommendations for medical management of adult lead exposure. *Environ Health Perspect.* 2007;115:463-471.
171. Kroll-Desrosiers AR, et al. Receipt of prescription opioids in a national sample of pregnant Veterans receiving Veterans Health Administration care. *Womens Health Issues.* 2016;26:240-246.
172. Kumar A, et al. Paracetamol overdose in children. *Scott Med J.* 1990;35:106-107.
173. Kuo C, et al. Injury hospitalizations of pregnant women in the United States, 2002. *Am J Obstet Gynecol.* 2007;196:161.e1-161.e6.
174. Kurzel RB. Can acetaminophen excess result in maternal and fetal toxicity? *South Med J.* 1990;83:953-955.
175. Kuschel CA, et al. Can methadone concentrations predict the severity of withdrawal in infants at risk of neonatal abstinence syndrome? *Arch Dis Child Fetal Neonatal Ed.* 2004;89:F390-F393.
176. Kweder SL. Drugs and biologics in pregnancy and breastfeeding: FDA in the 21st century. *Birth Defects Res A Clin Mol Teratol.* 2008;82:605-609.
177. Lacoste H, et al. Acute iron intoxication in pregnancy: case report and review of the literature. *Obstet Gynecol.* 1992;80:500-501.
178. Lambert BL, Bauer CR. Developmental and behavioral consequences of prenatal cocaine exposure: a review. *J Perinatol.* 2012;32:819-828.
179. Lammer EJ. A phenocopy of the retinoic acid embryopathy following maternal use of etretinate that ended one year before conception. *Teratology.* 1988;37:42.
180. Lampert P, et al. Hexachlorophene encephalopathy. *Acta Neuropathol.* 1973;23:326-333.
181. Lancaster CA, et al. Risk factors for depressive symptoms during pregnancy: a systematic review. *Am J Obstet Gynecol.* 2010;202:5-14.
182. Laub DN, et al. Effects of acetaminophen on preimplantation embryo glutathione concentration and development in vivo and in vitro. *Toxicol Sci.* 2000;56:150-155.
183. Lawrence RA, Lawrence RM. *Breastfeeding: A Guide for the Medical Profession.* 8th ed. Philadelphia, PA: Elsevier; 2016.
184. Lederman S, et al. Neonatal paracetamol poisoning: treatment by exchange transfusion. *Arch Dis Child.* 1983;58:631-633.
185. Lenke RR, et al. Severe fetal deformities associated with ingestion of excessive isoniazid in early pregnancy. *Acta Obstet Gynecol Scand.* 1985;64:281-282.
186. Lester BM, et al. Studies of cocaine-exposed human infants. *NIDA Res Monogr.* 1996;164:175-210.
187. Lester D, Beck AT. Attempted suicide and pregnancy. *Am J Obstet Gynecol.* 1988;158:1084-1085.
188. Lewis AJ. Depression in pregnancy and child development: understanding the mechanisms of transmission. In: Galbally M, et al, eds. *Psychopharmacology and Pregnancy: Treatment Efficacy, Risks, and Guidelines.* Heidelberg: Springer; 2014:47-65.
189. Li DK, et al. Exposure to non-steroidal anti-inflammatory drugs during pregnancy and risk of miscarriage: population based cohort study. *BMJ.* 2003;327:368.
190. Lidow MS. Consequences of prenatal cocaine exposure in nonhuman primates. *Brain Res Dev Brain Res.* 2003;147:23-36.
191. Lindahl V, et al. Prevalence of suicidality during pregnancy and the postpartum. *Arch Womens Ment Health.* 2005;8:77-87.
192. Lipsitz PJ. A proposed narcotic withdrawal score for use with newborn infants. A pragmatic evaluation of its efficacy. *Clin Pediatr (Phila).* 1975;14:592-594.
193. Lo WY, Friedman JM. Teratogenicity of recently introduced medications in human pregnancy. *Obstet Gynecol.* 2002;100:465-473.
194. Longo LD. The biological effects of carbon monoxide on the pregnant woman, fetus, and newborn infant. *Am J Obstet Gynecol.* 1977;129:69-103.
195. Longo LD, Hill EP. Carbon monoxide uptake and elimination in fetal and maternal sheep. *Am J Physiol.* 1977;232:H324-H330.
196. Lozoff B, et al. Higher infant blood lead levels with longer duration of breastfeeding. *J Pediatr.* 2009;155:663-667.
197. Ludmir J, et al. Maternal acetaminophen overdose at 15 weeks of gestation. *Obstet Gynecol.* 1986;67:750-751.
198. Lupattelli A, et al. Medication use in pregnancy: a cross-sectional, multinational web-based study. *BMJ Open.* 2014;4:e004365.
199. Lusskin SI, et al. Perinatal depression: hiding in plain sight. *Can J Psychiatry.* 2007;52:479-488.
200. Maalouf EF, et al. Arthrogryposis multiplex congenita and bilateral mid-brain infarction following maternal overdose of co-proxamol. *Eur J Paediatr Neurol.* 1997;1:183-186.
201. MacGregor SN, et al. Cocaine abuse during pregnancy: correlation between prenatal care and perinatal outcome. *Obstet Gynecol.* 1989;74:882-885.
202. Mahalik MP, et al. Teratogenic potential of cocaine hydrochloride in CF-1 mice. *J Pharm Sci.* 1980;69:703-706.
203. Mahalik MP, Hitner HW. Antagonism of cocaine-induced fetal anomalies by prazosin and diltiazem in mice. *Reprod Toxicol.* 1992;6:161-169.
204. Mahon BE, et al. Maternal and infant use of erythromycin and other macrolide antibiotics as risk factors for infantile hypertrophic pyloric stenosis. *J Pediatr.* 2001;139:380-384.
205. Makarechian N, et al. Association between moderate alcohol consumption during pregnancy and spontaneous abortion, stillbirth and premature birth: a meta-analysis. In: Koren G, ed. *Medication Safety in Pregnancy and Breastfeeding.* New York, NY: McGraw-Hill, 2007.
206. Manning MA, Eugene Hoyme H. Fetal alcohol spectrum disorders: a practical clinical approach to diagnosis. *Neurosci Biobehav Rev.* 2007;31:230-238.
207. Manoguerra AS. Iron poisoning: report of a fatal case in an adult. *Am J Hosp Pharm.* 1976;33:1088-1090.
208. Margulies JL. Acute carbon monoxide poisoning during pregnancy. *Am J Emerg Med.* 1986;4:516-519.
209. Martin ML, et al. Trends in rates of multiple vascular disruption defects, Atlanta, 1968-1989: is there evidence of a cocaine teratogenic epidemic? *Teratology.* 1992;45:647-653.
210. Martin MM, et al. Cocaine-induced neurodevelopmental deficits and underlying mechanisms. *Birth Defects Res C Embryo Today.* 2016;108:147-173.
211. Martin-Bouyer G, et al. Outbreak of accidental hexachlorophene poisoning in France. *Lancet.* 1982;1:91-95.
212. Marzuk PM, et al. Lower risk of suicide during pregnancy. *Am J Psychiatry* 1997;154:122-123.
213. Mattson SN, Riley EP. A review of the neurobehavioral deficits in children with fetal alcohol syndrome or prenatal exposure to alcohol. *Alcohol Clin Exp Res.* 1998;22:279-294.
214. May PA, et al. Prevalence and characteristics of fetal alcohol spectrum disorders. *Pediatrics.* 2014;134:855-866.
215. May PA, et al. Maternal alcohol consumption producing fetal alcohol spectrum disorders (FASD): quantity, frequency, and timing of drinking. *Drug Alcohol Depend.* 2013;133:502-512.
216. Mayes LC, et al. Regulation of arousal and attention in preschool children exposed to cocaine prenatally. *Ann N Y Acad Sci.* 1998;846:126-143.
217. McCarthy DM, et al. Effects of prenatal exposure to cocaine on brain structure and function. *Prog Brain Res.* 2014;211:277-289.
218. McClure CK, et al. The epidemiology of acute poisonings in women of reproductive age and during pregnancy, California, 2000-2004. *Matern Child Health J.* 2011;15:964-973.
219. McElhatton PR, et al. The consequences of iron overdose and its treatment with desferrioxamine in pregnancy. *Hum Exp Toxicol.* 1991;10:251-259.
220. McElhatton PR, et al. Paracetamol overdose in pregnancy: analysis of the outcomes of 300 cases referred to the Teratology Information Service. *Reprod Toxicol.* 1997;11:85-94.
221. McElhatton PR, et al. Paracetamol poisoning in pregnancy: an analysis of the outcomes of cases referred to the Teratology Information Service of the National Poisons Information Service. *Hum Exp Toxicol.* 1990;9:147-153.
222. Medina AE. Fetal alcohol spectrum disorders and abnormal neuronal plasticity. *Neuroscientist.* 2011;17:274-287.
223. Mehanny SZ, et al. Teratogenic effect of cocaine and diazepam in CF1 mice. *Teratology.* 1991;43:11-17.
224. Meyer MC, et al. Methadone and buprenorphine for opioid dependence during pregnancy: a retrospective cohort study. *J Addict Med.* 2015;9:81-86.
225. Miller MS, et al. Drug metabolic enzymes in developmental toxicology. *Fundam Appl Toxicol.* 1996;34:165-175.
226. Miller PD, et al. Effect of hyperbaric oxygen on cardiogenesis in the rat. *Biol Neonate.* 1971;17:44-52.
227. Moretti ME. Motherisk: the Toronto model for counseling in reproductive toxicology. In: Koren G, ed. *Medication Safety in Pregnancy and Breastfeeding.* New York, NY: McGraw-Hill; 2007:295-307.
228. Motherisk. http://www.motherisk.org. Accessed April 1, 2017.
229. Motomatsu K, et al. Two infant deaths after inhaling baby powder. *Chest.* 1979;75:448-450.
230. Myllynen P, et al. The fate and effects of xenobiotics in human placenta. *Expert Opin Drug Metab Toxicol.* 2007;3:331-346.
231. Namouz-Haddad S, Koren G. Fetal pharmacotherapy 1: prenatal glucocorticoids. *J Obstet Gynaecol Can.* 2013;35:920-922.
232. Namouz-Haddad S, Koren G. Fetal pharmacotherapy 2: fetal arrhythmia. *J Obstet Gynaecol Can.* 2013;35:1023-1027.
233. Namouz-Haddad S, Koren G. Fetal pharmacotherapy 3: magnesium sulfate. *J Obstet Gynaecol Can.* 2013;35:1101-1104.
234. Namouz-Haddad S, Koren G. Fetal pharmacotherapy 4: fetal thyroid disorders. *J Obstet Gynaecol Can.* 2014;36:60-63.
235. Nathanson V, et al. Is it all right for women to drink small amounts of alcohol in pregnancy? No. *BMJ.* 2007;335:857.
236. Nau H, et al. Valproic acid in the perinatal period: decreased maternal serum protein binding results in fetal accumulation and neonatal displacement of the drug and some metabolites. *J Pediatr.* 1984;104:627-634.

237. Neri I, et al. Polyethylene glycol electrolyte solution (Isocolan) for constipation during pregnancy: an observational open-label study. *J Midwifery Womens Health.* 2004;49:355-358.

238. Neuspiel DR. Behavior in cocaine-exposed infants and children: association versus causality. *Drug Alcohol Depend.* 1994;36:101-107.

239. Newbold RR, et al. Adverse effects of the model environmental estrogen diethylstilbestrol are transmitted to subsequent generations. *Endocrinology.* 2006;147:S11-S17.

240. Newport DJ, et al. Suicidal ideation in pregnancy: assessment and clinical implications. *Arch Womens Ment Health.* 2007;10:181-187.

241. Nichols MM. Acute alcohol withdrawal syndrome in a newborn. *Am J Dis Child.* 1967;113:714-715.

242. Norman CA, Halton DM. Is carbon monoxide a workplace teratogen? A review and evaluation of the literature. *Ann Occup Hyg.* 1990;34:335-347.

243. O'Brien P. Is it all right for women to drink small amounts of alcohol in pregnancy? Yes. *BMJ.* 2007;335:856.

244. Oakley GP Jr. Folic acid-preventable spina bifida: a good start but much to be done. *Am J Prev Med.* 2010;38:569-570.

245. Oates M, Cantwell R. Deaths from psychiatric causes. In: Centre for Maternal and Child Enquiries (CMACE): *Saving Mothers' Lives: Reviewing Maternal Deaths to Make Motherhood Safer–2006-2008. The Eighth Report of the Confidential Enquiries into Maternal Deaths in the United Kingdom. BJOG.* 2011;118(suppl 1):133-144.

246. Office of the Surgeon General. *U.S. Surgeon General Releases Advisory on Alcohol Use in Pregnancy.* Washington, DC: US Department of Health and Human Services; 2005.

247. Olenmark M, et al. Fatal iron intoxication in late pregnancy. *J Toxicol Clin Toxicol.* 1987;25:347-359.

248. Osborn DA, et al. Opiate treatment for opiate withdrawal in newborn infants. *Cochrane Database Syst Rev.* 2010:CD002059.

249. Osborn DA, et al. Sedatives for opiate withdrawal in newborn infants. *Cochrane Database Syst Rev.* 2010:CD002053.

250. Palmsten K, et al. The most commonly dispensed prescription medications among pregnant women enrolled in the U.S. Medicaid Program. *Obstet Gynecol.* 2015;126:465-473.

251. Park-Wyelie L, et al. Birth defects after maternal exposure to corticosteroids: prospective controlled cohort study and a meta-analysis of epidemiological studies. In: Koren G, ed. *Medication Safety in Pregnancy and Breastfeeding.* New York, NY: McGraw-Hill; 2007:541-548.

252. Patel TG, et al. Cocaine decreases uteroplacental blood flow in the rat. *Neurotoxicol Teratol.* 1999;21:559-565.

253. Patrick SW, et al. Prescription opioid epidemic and infant outcomes. *Pediatrics.* 2015;135:842-850.

254. Patrick SW, et al. Variation in treatment of neonatal abstinence syndrome in US children's hospitals, 2004-2011. *J Perinatol.* 2014;34:867-872.

255. Patrick SW, et al. Neonatal abstinence syndrome and associated health care expenditures: United States, 2000-2009. *JAMA.* 2012;307:1934-1940.

256. Payen C, et al. Intoxication par le paracétamol chez la femme enceinte: à propos d'un cas. *Arch Pediatr.* 2011;18:1100-1102.

257. Perrone J, Hoffman RS. Toxic ingestions in pregnancy: abortifacient use in a case series of pregnant overdose patients. *Acad Emerg Med.* 1997;4:206-209.

258. Plessinger MA, Woods JR. Cocaine in pregnancy. Recent data on maternal and fetal risks. *Obstet Gynecol Clin North Am.* 1998;25:99-118.

259. Pratt R, Salomon DS. Biochemical basis for the teratogenic effects of glucocorticoids. In: Juchau MR, ed. *The Biochemical Basis of Chemical Teratogenesis.* New York, NY: Elsevier/North Holland; 1981:179-199.

260. Provincial Council for Maternal and Child Health. Neonatal Abstinence Syndrome Clinical Guideline. http://www.pcmch.on.ca/health-care-providers/maternity-care/pcmch-strategies-and-initiatives/neonatal-abstinence-syndrome/. Last accessed July 23, 2018.

261. Rayburn W, et al. Drug overdose during pregnancy: an overview from a metropolitan poison control center. *Obstet Gynecol.* 1984;64:611-614.

262. Rayburn WF, et al. Iron overdose during pregnancy: successful therapy with deferoxamine. *Am J Obstet Gynecol.* 1983;147:717-718.

263. Reed CE, Fenton SE. Exposure to diethylstilbestrol during sensitive life stages: a legacy of heritable health effects. *Birth Defects Res C Embryo Today.* 2013;99:134-146.

264. Reed MD, Besunder JB. Developmental pharmacology: ontogenic basis of drug disposition. *Pediatr Clin North Am.* 1989;36:1053-1074.

265. Rementeria JL, Bhatt K. Withdrawal symptoms in neonates from intrauterine exposure to diazepam. *J Pediatr.* 1977;90:123-126.

266. Reprotox. http://www.reprotox.org. Accessed April 1, 2017.

267. Rice JM, Donovan PJ. Mutagenesis and carcinogenesis. In: Fabro S, Scialli AR, eds. *Drug and Chemical Action in Pregnancy.* New York, NY: Marcel Dekker; 1986:205-236.

268. Richards R, Brooks SE. Ferrous sulphate poisoning in pregnancy (with afibrinogenaemia as a complication). *West Indian Med J.* 1966;15:134-140.

269. Richardson GA, Day NL. Maternal and neonatal effects of moderate cocaine use during pregnancy. *Neurotoxicol Teratol.* 1991;13:455-460.

270. Riggs BS, et al. Acute acetaminophen overdose during pregnancy. *Obstet Gynecol.* 1989;74:247-253.

271. Riordan J. Drugs and breastfeeding. In: Riordan J, Auerbach KG, eds. *Breastfeeding and Human Lactation.* 2nd ed. Sudbury, Ontario, Canada: Jones & Bartlett; 1999:163-219.

272. Ritchie H, Bolton P. The Australian categorisation of risk of drug use in pregnancy. *Aust Fam Physician.* 2000;29:237-241.

273. Rivera-Calimlim L. The significance of drugs in breast milk. Pharmacokinetic considerations. *Clin Perinatol.* 1987;14:51-70.

274. Roberts I, et al. Paracetamol metabolites in the neonate following maternal overdose. *Br J Clin Pharmacol.* 1984;18:201-206.

275. Robertson RG, et al. Acetaminophen overdose in the second trimester of pregnancy. *J Fam Pract.* 1986;23:267-268.

276. Rogan WJ. Breastfeeding in the workplace. *Occup Med (Lond).* 1986;1:411-413.

277. Rollins DE, et al. Acetaminophen: potentially toxic metabolite formed by human fetal and adult liver microsomes and isolated fetal liver cells. *Science.* 1979;205:1414-1416.

278. Rosen TS, Pippenger CE. Pharmacologic observations on the neonatal withdrawal syndrome. *J Pediatr.* 1976;88:1044-1048.

279. Rosevear SK, Hope PL. Favourable neonatal outcome following maternal paracetamol overdose and severe fetal distress. Case report. *Br J Obstet Gynaecol.* 1989;96:491-493.

280. Ruiz-Maldonado R, et al. Cushing's syndrome after topical application of corticosteroids. *Am J Dis Child.* 1982;136:274-275.

281. Ruthnum P, Goel KM. ABC of poisoning: paracetamol. *Br Med J (Clin Res Ed).* 1984;289:1538-1539.

282. Rutter N. Percutaneous drug absorption in the newborn: hazards and uses. *Clin Perinatol.* 1987;14:911-930.

283. Sachs HC; Committee on Drugs. The transfer of drugs and therapeutics into human breast milk: an update on selected topics. *Pediatrics.* 2013;132:e796-e809.

284. SAMHSA Center for Behavioral Health Statistics and Quality. National Survey on Drug Use and Health, 2007-2010. http://www.samhsa.gov/data/NSDUH/2k10Results Tables/NSDUHTables2010R/HTM/Sect6peTabs55to107.htm-Tab6.74B. Published 2010. Accessed June 8, 2017.

285. SAMHSA Center for Behavioral Health Statistics and Quality. National Survey on Drug Use and Health, 2007-2010. http://www.samhsa.gov/data/NSDUH/2k10Results Tables/NSDUHTables2010R/HTM/Sect6peTabs55to107.htm-Tab6.74B. Published 2012. Accessed April 7, 2017.

286. SAMHSA Center for Behavioral Health Statistics and Quality. 2015 National Survey on Drug Use and Health: Detailed Tables. https://http://www.samhsa.gov/data/sites/default/files/NSDUH-DetTabs-2016/NSDUH-DetTabs-2016.htm-tab6-65A. Published 2017. Accessed September 28, 2017.

287. Sancewicz-Pach K, et al. Suicidal paracetamol poisoning of a pregnant woman just before a delivery. *Przegl Lek.* 1999;56:459-462.

288. SanFilippo JA. Infantile hypertrophic pyloric stenosis related to ingestion of erythromycine estolate: a report of five cases. *J Pediatr Surg.* 1976;11:177-180.

289. Sannerstedt R, et al. Drugs during pregnancy: an issue of risk classification and information to prescribers. *Drug Saf.* 1996;14:69-77.

290. Sapunar D, et al. Effects of hyperbaric oxygen on rat embryos. *Biol Neonate.* 1993;63:360-369.

291. Schardein JL. *Chemically Induced Birth Defects.* 3rd ed. New York, NY: Marcel Dekker; 2000.

292. Schauben JL, et al. Iron poisoning: report of three cases and a review of therapeutic intervention. *J Emerg Med.* 1990;8:309-319.

293. Schiff MA, Grossman DC. Adverse perinatal outcomes and risk for postpartum suicide attempt in Washington State, 1987-2001. *Pediatrics.* 2006;118:e669-e675.

294. Schou M. Lithium treatment during pregnancy, delivery, and lactation: an update. *J Clin Psychiatry* 1990;51:410-413.

295. Schreiber JS. Parents worried about breast milk contamination. What is best for baby? *Pediatr Clin North Am.* 2001;48:1113-1127, viii.

296. Scialli AR. Identifying teratogens: the tyranny of lists. *Reprod Toxicol.* 1997;11:555-559.

297. Scialli AR, et al. Communicating risks during pregnancy: a workshop on the use of data from animal developmental toxicity studies in pregnancy labels for drugs. *Birth Defects Res A Clin Mol Teratol.* 2004;70:7-12.

298. Scialli AR, Fabro S. The stage dependence of reproductive toxicology. In: Fabro S, Scialli AR, eds. *Drug and Chemical Action in Pregnancy.* New York, NY: Marcel Dekker; 1986:191-204.

299. Selden BS, et al. Transplacental transport of N-acetylcysteine in an ovine model. *Ann Emerg Med.* 1991;20:1069-1072.

300. Shannon M, et al. Multiple dose activated charcoal for theophylline poisoning in young infants. *Pediatrics.* 1987;80:368-370.

301. Shepard TH, et al. Update on new developments in the study of human teratogens. *Teratology.* 2002;65:153-161.

302. Shepard TH, Lemire RJ. *Catalog of Teratogenic Agents.* 13th ed. Baltimore, MD: Johns Hopkins University Press; 2010.

303. Shiono PH, et al. The impact of cocaine and marijuana use on low birth weight and preterm birth: a multicenter study. *Am J Obstet Gynecol.* 1995;172:19-27.

304. Shuman RM, et al. Neurotoxicity of hexachlorophene in humans. II. A clinicopathological study of 46 premature infants. *Arch Neurol.* 1975;32:320-325.

305. Singer ST, Vichinsky EP. Deferoxamine treatment during pregnancy: is it harmful? *Am J Hematol.* 1999;60:24-26.

306. Sistonen J, et al. Prediction of codeine toxicity in infants and their mothers using a novel combination of maternal genetic markers. *Clin Pharmacol Ther.* 2012;91:692-699.

307. Skuladottir H, et al. Corticosteroid use and risk of orofacial clefts. *Birth Defects Res A Clin Mol Teratol.* 2014;100:499-506.

308. Slutsker L. Risks associated with cocaine use during pregnancy. *Obstet Gynecol.* 1992;79:778-789.

309. Smith K, Lipari RN. Women of childbearing age and opioids. *The CBHSQ Report: January 17, 2017.* Center for Behavioral Health Statistics and Quality, Substance Abuse and Mental Health Services Administration, Rockville, MD.
310. Smolina K, et al. Trends and determinants of prescription drug use during pregnancy and postpartum in British Columbia, 2002-2011: a population-based cohort study. *PLoS One.* 2015;10:e0128312.
311. Sokol RJ, et al. Fetal alcohol spectrum disorder. *JAMA.* 2003;290:2996-2999.
312. Sood B, et al. Prenatal alcohol exposure and childhood behavior at age 6 to 7 years: I. dose-response effect. *Pediatrics.* 2001;108:E34.
313. Spear LP, et al. Animal behavior models. Increased sensitivity to stressors and other environmental experiences after prenatal cocaine exposure. *Ann N Y Acad Sci.* 1998;846:76-88.
314. Stang H. Pyloric stenosis associated with erythromycin ingested through breastmilk. *Minn Med.* 1986;69:669-670, 682.
315. Stark KL, et al. Dysmorphogenesis elicited by microinjected acetaminophen analogs and metabolites in rat embryos cultured in vitro. *J Pharmacol Exp Ther.* 1990;255:74-82.
316. Stein A, et al. Effects of perinatal mental disorders on the fetus and child. *Lancet.* 2014;384:1800-1819.
317. Stokes IM. Paracetamol overdose in the second trimester of pregnancy. Case report. *Br J Obstet Gynaecol.* 1984;91:286-288.
318. Stratton K, et al, eds. *Fetal Alcohol Syndrome: Diagnosis, Epidemiology, Prevention, and Treatment.* Washington, DC: Committee to Study Fetal Alcohol Syndrome, Institute of Medicine, National Academy Press; 1996.
319. Streissguth AP, O'Malley K. Neuropsychiatric implications and long-term consequences of fetal alcohol spectrum disorders. *Semin Clin Neuropsychiatry.* 2000;5:177-190.
320. Strom RL, et al. Fatal iron poisoning in a pregnant female. *Minn Med.* 1976;59:483-489.
321. Sulik KK. Genesis of alcohol-induced craniofacial dysmorphism. *Exp Biol Med (Maywood).* 2005;230:366-375.
322. Taney J, et al. Placental abruption with delayed fetal compromise in maternal acetaminophen toxicity. *Obstet Gynecol.* 2017;130:159-162.
323. Telford IR, et al. Hyperbaric oxygen causes fetal wastage in rats. *Lancet.* 1969;2:220-221.
324. Tenenbein M. Poisoning in pregnancy. In: Koren G, ed. *Maternal-Fetal Toxicology: A Clinician's Guide.* 3rd ed. New York, NY: Marcel Dekker; 2001.
325. TERIS (Teratogen Information System). http://depts.washington.edu/terisdb/ Accessed April 1, 2017.
326. Thilo EH, et al. Infant botulism at 1 week of age: report of two cases. *Pediatrics.* 1993;92:151-153.
327. Thornton SL, Minns AB. Unintentional chronic acetaminophen poisoning during pregnancy resulting in liver transplantation. *J Med Toxicol.* 2012;8:176-178.
328. Thorpe PG, et al. Medications in the first trimester of pregnancy: most common exposures and critical gaps in understanding fetal risk. *Pharmacoepidemiol Drug Saf.* 2013;22:1013-1018.
329. Tolia VN, et al. Increasing incidence of the neonatal abstinence syndrome in U.S. neonatal ICUs. *N Engl J Med.* 2015;372:2118-2126.
330. Turk J, et al. Successful therapy of iron intoxication in pregnancy with intravenous deferoxamine and whole bowel irrigation. *Vet Hum Toxicol.* 1993;35:441-444.
331. US Census Bureau American FactFinder. American Community Survey: Table B23001. Sex by age by employment status for the population 16 years and over. 2015.
332. US Food and Drug Administration. Labeling and prescription drug advertising: content and format for labeling for human prescription drugs. *Fed Regist.* 1979;44.
333. US Food and Drug Administration. Use of codeine products in nursing mothers—questions and answers. http://www.fda.gov/Drugs/DrugSafety/PostmarketDrugSafetyInformationforPatientsandProviders/ucm118113.htm. Published 2007. Accessed March 20, 2013.
334. US Food and Drug Administration. Pregnancy and lactation labeling (drugs) final rule. https://http://www.fda.gov/Drugs/DevelopmentApprovalProcess/DevelopmentResources/Labeling/ucm093307.htm. Published 2014. Accessed Jul 17, 2017.
335. Van Ameyde KJ, Tenenbein M. Whole bowel irrigation during pregnancy. *Am J Obstet Gynecol.* 1989;160:646-647.
336. Van Hoesen KB, et al. Should hyperbaric oxygen be used to treat the pregnant patient for acute carbon monoxide poisoning? A case report and literature review. *JAMA.* 1989;261:1039-1043.
337. Vargesson N. Thalidomide-induced teratogenesis: history and mechanisms. *Birth Defects Res C Embryo Today.* 2015;105:140-156.
338. Vesga-Lopez O, et al. Psychiatric disorders in pregnant and postpartum women in the United States. *Arch Gen Psychiatry.* 2008;65:805-815.
339. Villapiano NL, et al. Rural and urban differences in neonatal abstinence syndrome and maternal opioid use, 2004 to 2013. *JAMA Pediatr.* 2017;171:194-196.
340. Wang PH, et al. Acetaminophen poisoning in late pregnancy. A case report. *J Reprod Med.* 1997;42:367-371.
341. Ward RM, Lugo RA. Drug therapy in the newborn. In: MacDonald MG, et al, eds. *Avery's Neonatology: Pathophysiology & Management of the Newborn.* 6th ed. Philadelphia, PA: Lippincott Williams & Wilkins; 2005:1507-1556.
342. Warkany J. Warfarin embryopathy. *Teratology.* 1976;14:205-209.
343. Webster WS, Brown-Woodman PD. Cocaine as a cause of congenital malformations of vascular origin: experimental evidence in the rat. *Teratology.* 1990;41:689-697.
344. Webster WS, et al. Fetal brain damage in the rat following prenatal exposure to cocaine. *Neurotoxicol Teratol.* 1991;13:621-626.
345. Webster WS, et al. Uterine trauma and limb defects. *Teratology.* 1987;35:253-260.
346. Weeks BS, et al. Acetaminophen toxicity to cultured rat embryos. *Teratog Carcinog Mutagen.* 1990;10:361-371.
347. Weitzman M, Kursmark M. Breast-feeding and child lead exposure: a cause for concern. *J Pediatr.* 2009;155:610-611.
348. Werler MM. Teratogen update: smoking and reproductive outcomes. *Teratology.* 1997;55:382-388.
349. West JR, et al. Fetal alcohol syndrome: the vulnerability of the developing brain and possible mechanisms of damage. *Metab Brain Dis.* 1994;9:291-322.
350. Whitlock FA, Edwards JE. Pregnancy and attempted suicide. *Compr Psychiatry.* 1968;9:1-12.
351. Woods JR. Maternal and transplacental effects of cocaine. *Ann N Y Acad Sci.* 1998;846:1-11.
352. Woods JR, et al. An introduction to reactive oxygen species and their possible roles in substance abuse. *Obstet Gynecol Clin North Am.* 1998;25:219-236.
353. Woody RC, Brewster MA. Telencephalic dysgenesis associated with presumptive maternal carbon monoxide intoxication in the first trimester of pregnancy. *J Toxicol Clin Toxicol.* 1990;28:467-475.
354. Zuckerman B, et al. Overview of the effects of abuse and drugs on pregnancy and offspring. *NIDA Res Monogr.* 1995;149:16-38.

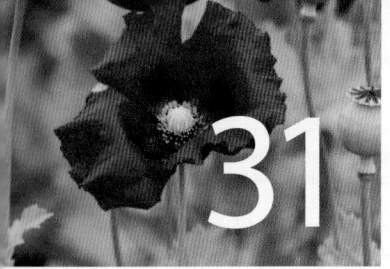

31 PEDIATRIC PRINCIPLES

Elizabeth Q. Hines and Jeffrey S. Fine

Poisoning remains a significant but preventable cause of pediatric injury. Phone calls to poison control centers regarding pediatric exposures are more frequent than those regarding any other age group. Pediatricians have been leaders for 60 years in helping to establish and promote the study of medical toxicology, supporting the use of regional poison control centers and promoting the principles of poison prevention. Although the basic approaches to the medical management of toxicologic problems outlined in Chaps. 3 and 4 are generally applicable to both children and adults, some issues such as child abuse by poisoning are of particular concern. This chapter provides a perspective on the application of generally accepted toxicologic principles to children.

EPIDEMIOLOGY

To understand the magnitude of pediatric poisoning and its impact, epidemiologists examine multiple parameters, such as exposure, morbidity, mortality, and cost; however, these parameters are often difficult to measure accurately. An important source of information on the extent and effects of poisoning exposures in the United States is the American Association of Poison Control Centers' (AAPCC's) National Poison Data System. Every year, the AAPCC compiles standardized data collected from poison control centers throughout the United States; the 2015 annual review includes information submitted by 55 regional poison control centers. In the following discussion, comments on AAPCC data refer to cumulative information from the previous 5 published reports covering the years 2011 to 2015 (Chap. 130).

Each year, the AAPCC reports approximately 1.1 million potentially toxic exposures in young children from birth to 6 years of age that account for almost half (48%) of all reported exposures in the AAPCC database. Pediatric exposures involving all children and adolescents younger than 19 years account for 61% of all reported exposures. Of the reported pediatric exposures in children and adolescents, young children (younger than 6 years) account for 78%, school-age children (between 6 and 12 years) account for 10%, and adolescents (between 13 and 19 years of age) account for 12%. Females represent 43% of the reported poisoning exposures in young children and 58% of the reported exposures among adolescents.

Among the AAPCC-reported xenobiotic exposures in young children, 99% are coded as unintentional. There is some controversy regarding the use of the term *unintentional* with respect to childhood poisoning. A toddler quite purposefully *intends* to ingest a substance but does *not intend* to injure or harm him- or herself. *Unsupervised* is a term preferred by some epidemiologists to better describe the etiology of these exposures.[110] In contrast, 39% of reported adolescent exposures are coded as unintentional, and 56% of adolescent exposures are coded as intentional. This shift in intentionality is due to an increased frequency of adolescent intentional substance use, abuse, and suicidal exposures. This high frequency of intentional poisoning in adolescents has been reported by others.[36,141,183]

Table 31–1 shows the leading causes of AAPCC-reported exposures in children under 6 years. Exposures in this age group include xenobiotics that are commonly found around the house, such as cleaning products, cosmetics, plants, hydrocarbons, and insecticides as well as pharmaceuticals. It is important to understand that Table 31–1 lists the most commonly reported *exposures*, but that not all of these *reported* exposures are *confirmed* exposures and not even all *confirmed exposures* lead to serious morbidity or mortality. For example, children are most frequently exposed to cosmetic products; however, the amount ingested is typically small and most cosmetics manufactured in the United States are nontoxic, making the outcome of exposure minor.

Clinically significant exposures are unusual in children younger than 6 months. When they do occur, they most commonly result from the inadvertent administration of an incorrect drug or drug dose by a parent,[23,62,110,126] intentional administration of a drug by a parent or sibling,[45,78] or passive exposure (eg, to the smoke of "crack" cocaine or phencyclidine).[17,77,128,158,191] Any poisoning in a child younger than one year of age should be carefully evaluated for possible child abuse or neglect (see later discussion).[78]

Several characteristics typically associated with ingestions by young children differentiate them from ingestions by adolescents or adults: (a) they are without suicidal intent; (b) there is usually only one xenobiotic involved; (c) the xenobiotics are usually nontoxic; (d) the amount is usually small; and (e) toddlers usually present for evaluation relatively soon after the ingestion is discovered, generally within 1 to 2 hours. The peak age for childhood poisoning is between 1 and 3 years.[23,31,110,155] Unintentional ingestion is unusual after age 5 years although when it occurs it is sometimes the result of mistakenly consuming a xenobiotic from a mislabeled container.[26] Some intentional ingestions between the ages of 5 and 9 years result from intrafamilial stress or suicidal intent. After age 9 years and through adolescence, overdose or poisoning frequently results from either suicidal gestures or suicidal attempts or from the adverse effects of alcohol or substance use. This previously discussed age-dependent shift in intentionality toward substance use and abuse and suicide is associated with a significant change in outcome. Only 1% of exposed children under 6 years have a recorded outcome as moderate, major, or death compared to 17% of adolescents (Table 31–2).

The peak age for hospitalizing young children exposed to xenobiotics is between 1 and 3 years, reflecting the peak age of exposure. Whereas hospitalization of children younger than age 2 years typically results from exposure to nonpharmaceutical xenobiotics, children older than 2 years as well as adolescents are more commonly exposed to pharmaceuticals.[55,63,183] Adolescents are also thought to be more frequently hospitalized than children after exposure to xenobiotics but this is a subject of debate.[63] This is a result of the need for medical management and, often, psychiatric hospitalization. As many as 30% of children who experience one ingestion will experience a repeat ingestion; adolescents are particularly prone to recidivism.[63,86] Children who ingest poisons are also at a greater risk for other types of injuries.[15,53]

Another source of data related to poisoning morbidity is the National Electronic Injury Surveillance System (NEISS) online database maintained by the US Centers for Disease Control and Prevention (CDC), which provides information on emergency department (ED) visits and hospitalizations.[32] For the period 2005 to 2014, the CDC estimates approximately 45,000 ED visits and 3,400 hospitalizations (8%) per year for young children 0 to 5 years who are exposed to a xenobiotic. Children 6 to 12 years old account for approximately 10,000 ED visits and 1,000 hospitalizations (10%) per year and adolescents 13 to 19 years old account for approximately 109,000 ED visits and 21,000 hospitalizations (19%) per year.

In a published review of NEISS data related to medication exposures in young children, approximately one-half of the ED visits were the result of unsupervised medication exposures and one-half were the result of adverse drug events after caregiver medication administration.[110] Approximately one-half of the medications were prescription pharmaceuticals and the other half were over-the-counter products. The most commonly involved prescription medication categories were opioids, benzodiazepines, antidepressants, beta adrenergic antagonists, and amphetamines. Ninety-two percent of all over-the-counter exposures involved acetaminophen (APAP), cough and cold products, ibuprofen, and diphenhydramine. The admission

TABLE 31–1	Average Annual Totals for the Most Common Pediatric Xenobiotic Exposures Reported to the American Association of Poison Control Centers (2011–2015)[a,b]

Age Younger Than 6 Years

Category	Number of Exposures
Cosmetics and personal care products	154,459
Cleaning substances	116,366
Analgesics	104,870
Topical preparations	67,231
Vitamins	49,005
Antihistamines	45,323
Insecticides, pesticides, and rodenticides	36,353
Plants	29,603
Gastrointestinal preparations	29,377
Antimicrobials	28,836

Ages 6–12 Years

Category	Number of Exposures
Cosmetics and personal care products	9,342
Analgesics	8,657
Antihistamines	7,160
Vitamins	6,504
Cleaning substances	5,867
Bites and envenomations	5,759
Plants	5,051
Stimulants and street drugs	4,968
Cough and cold preparations	4,743
Cardiovascular pharmaceuticals	4,045

Ages 13–19 Years

Category	Number of Exposures
Analgesics	23,064
Antidepressants	9,225
Sedative–hypnotics	7,286
Stimulants and street drugs	7,267
Cough and cold preparations	6,478
Cleaning substances	6,394
Antihistamines	6,130
Cosmetics and personal care products	6,051
Bites and envenomations	4,743
Anticonvulsants	2,554

[a]See Chap. 130 for references and discussion. [b]Does not include the American Association of Poison Control Centers' category "foreign bodies."

TABLE 31–2	Outcome of Reported Pediatric Xenobiotic Exposures (2011–2015)[a]

	Effects (% of Reported Exposures)[b,c]			
Age (years)	Minor or None	Moderate	Major	Death
0–5	99	0.97	0.08	0.003
6–12	97	3	0.18	0.007
13–19	83	15	1.5	0.04
All children and adolescents 0–19	97	2.8	0.26	0.008

[a]See Chap. 130 for references and discussion. [b]Approximate percentage. [c]*Minor* is minimal signs and symptoms, often not requiring therapy or had no follow-up; *moderate* is more pronounced, prolonged, or systemic signs and symptoms, often requiring therapy; and *major* is life-threatening signs and symptoms.

rate in this population was 18.5% for unsupervised ingestions and 6.0% for caregiver-administered medication events.

Although the AAPCC reports overall outcome related to age, it does not specifically stratify outcome of exposure to individual xenobiotics by age. In a multiyear review published in 1992, the AAPCC did report the xenobiotics that caused the greatest number of major and fatal effects in young children. The categories associated with the greatest number of major effects included cleaning substances, cardiovascular drugs, hydrocarbons, sedative/hypnotics, and antidepressants.[107] A more recent study reported a shift in the substances with highest morbidity requiring pediatric intensive care unit (PICU) admissions. PICU admissions following unintentional ingestions were more frequently due to buprenorphine/naloxone, cardiac medications, and alpha-2-agonists. However, PICU admissions following intentional ingestions were due to medications from 43 different drug classes; patients frequently took their own medications, over-the-counter medications, or substances they obtained from a friend often with suicidal intent.[54]

Other national and international reports of hospitalized patients include a similar distribution of xenobiotic exposures that cause significant morbidity and hospitalizations.[4,10,33,197] However, in rural areas of many developing countries, kerosene and pesticides are the leading causes of xenobiotic-related hospitalizations, and the spectrum of pharmaceutical exposures is often different (Chap. 136).[2,72,74,127,134,136]

Poisoning accounts for approximately 2% of young childhood and 7% of adolescent injury-related deaths in the United States.[32] Based on information from death certificates filed in state vital statistics offices as well as demographic information provided by funeral directors, the CDC reports 1023 poisoning deaths in children younger than 6 years of age from 2005 to 2014 for an average of about 102 per year. These deaths represent a 78% decrease from the 456 deaths reported by the CDC in 1959.[31] There are several factors responsible for this decrease, including improved poisoning prevention strategies such as child-resistant closures and improved medical care. In addition, some industrial or pharmaceutical products previously found around the home have been replaced with less toxic products or were reformulated to safer concentrations.[28] It is also possible that there has been a decrease in reporting (Chap. 130).

Although the AAPCC data provide a remarkable amount of epidemiologic information, there are questions about the accuracy of the data.[75,76,190] For example, as mentioned earlier, the CDC reported 1023 poisoning-related deaths in children younger than 6 years of age from 2005 to 2014. During the same period, the AAPCC reported 253 deaths in young children. A primary weakness of the AAPCC data is due to its voluntary reporting method of ascertainment and it must be recognized that many significant poisonings go unreported to poison control centers. In Rhode Island, only 45 of 369 poisoning deaths were reported to the regional poison control center[105] (Chap. 130).

According to the 2013 AAPCC National Poison Database System pediatric fatality review, 47% of the reported pediatric fatalities resulted from unintentional exposures. Of these 47% were environmental exposures, mostly carbon monoxide poisoning, 40% were xenobiotic ingestions, and 10% were therapeutic errors.[111] Fifty-three percent of AAPCC-reported pediatric fatalities were the result of intentional exposures primarily related to substance use, abuse, and suicidal intent.

There are some significant etiologic differences between children and adolescents, particularly with regard to the lethality of xenobiotics. According to the 2013 NPDS pediatric fatality review, the xenobiotics causing the greatest number of childhood deaths were carbon monoxide, household products (gasoline, batteries, cleaners, laundry detergent, lamp oils), and pharmaceuticals, with opiates (buprenorphine and methadone) accounting for 10% of the unintentional childhood deaths. In contrast, the xenobiotics causing the greatest number of adolescent deaths were "designer drugs" (psychogenic phenylethylamines and synthetic cannabinoids), prescription opioids (methadone, oxycodone, hydrocodone, buprenorphine), and antidepressants. Unfortunately, there is an increasing trend in exposures of adolescents to these substances, and although the overall number of actual deaths from use, abuse, and suicide remain too small to comment on statistically, they are of concern.

The most notable difference between the xenobiotics causing pediatric morbidity and mortality today and studies from the 1960s and 1970s is that salicylates are no longer a leading cause of reported poisoning morbidity and mortality.[40,44] This change is likely related to a combination of factors, including federal regulations requiring child-resistant closures, the 81-mg dose form replacing higher doses as the most common formulation of aspirin prescribed, as well as the overall decreased use of aspirin in children (Chap. 37).[18,38,84,129,147]

Poisoning also has an economic cost. An ED visit for a poisoned child costs $1,077, on average, while the mean charge for hospitalization is $11,792, which can vary significantly based on the length of stay and outcome. Based on the estimated number of poisoned children seen in the ED each year, the total US health care cost for emergency care would be estimated as $162.3 million dollars.[131] According to the CDC in 2010, for fatal poisonings of children and adolescents, the average medical cost was approximately $6,000, but the average work loss cost was $1.9 million for a total cost of $1.9 billion.[32]

BEHAVIORAL, ENVIRONMENTAL, AND PHYSICAL ISSUES

An oversimplification of the etiology of childhood poisonings would be the formulation that unsupervised toddlers exploring their environment inadvertently ingest xenobiotics. However, this approach ignores the complex interplay of factors that contribute to most ingestions in children.

One approach to understanding injury causation uses the Haddon Matrix.[73] Applying this model to poisoning, there are 3 interacting factors: the patient (host), the xenobiotic (agent), and the environment. These factors interact during 3 phases: preinjury, injury, and postinjury. The factors themselves contribute to the likelihood, nature, magnitude of, and host response to an injury. Modification of these factors helps reduce the frequency or severity of an injury.

For example, if a 2-year-old child finds a tablet there is a risk of ingestion. Storing the tablets in a child-resistant container (CRC) or storing the container out of reach can help to reduce the risk of ingestion. In this case, both the agent and the environment are modified in the preinjury phase. However, both of these strategies are considered active prevention strategies, as they require the caregiver to actively replace the top back on the container or actively place the container back on a high shelf. Another method of preinjury prevention involves passive prevention. For example, if the tablet is an iron-containing multivitamin, limiting the amount of iron in each tablet would make the formulation of the product safer overall. In this regard, the availability of a safer product is passive for the user but active for the manufacturer or for regulators.[29]

The injury phase covers both the ingestion and the initial pathophysiologic host response. Again, particular factors determine the nature and extent of injury. Continuing the example above, if the tablet is a 325-mg APAP tablet, the ingestion will not lead to injury. However, if the tablet is a 0.2-mg clonidine tablet, there is a higher likelihood of toxicity.

The postinjury phase is concerned with both the ongoing host response and the medical management of the patient who is poisoned. In this phase, it would be determined whether the 2-year-old child with a clonidine ingestion is manifesting signs of toxicity, such as coma or hypotension; whether the child requires treatment with activated charcoal (AC), intravenous (IV) fluid, or naloxone; and whether the child requires hospital admission.

This paradigm is only a model. In reality, it is often difficult to examine any individual factor independently, and the relative contributions of these factors are not well defined. Nonetheless, consideration of the individual factors of host, agent, and environment allows us to focus on several relevant aspects of poisoning in children.

Childhood and adolescence are times of tremendous growth and development.[205] Some of these physical and social changes place children and teenagers at increased risk for poisonings. By 7 months of age, an infant can sit up and can pivot to grab an object; by 9 to 10 months of age, most infants can creep and crawl; by 15 months of age, most toddlers are walking quite competently and eagerly exploring. Between 9 and 12 months of age, a skillful pincer grasp with the thumb and forefinger develops that allows the child to pick up small objects. Throughout this period, one of the child's primary sensory experiences is sucking on or gumming objects that are placed in the mouth. Thus, the combination of 3 developmental skills—the ability to move around the home and depart the immediate view of a guardian, the ability to pick up and manipulate small objects, and the tendency of children to put things in their mouths—places them at risk for poisoning.

As children develop socially, they desire to become more like their parents and they tend to imitate behaviors such as taking medicine or using mouthwash. Children are typically taught that medicine is good for them when they are sick. Many children's medicines are sweetened and flavored to make them more palatable, and many parents inappropriately encourage their children to take medicines by telling them "it tastes like candy." Children are observed "making tea" from plants or "making pizza" with mushrooms from the yard.[26]

As children become more mobile, agile, and curious, xenobiotics that were previously outside their reach become accessible even when stored in difficult-to-reach places. Evidence suggests that some parents underestimate the developmental skills of their children.[53] Although 87% of parents believe unintentional injuries and poisonings are preventable, only 68% actually take action such as using safety belts or car seats. These parents also consider "being careful" as an effective preventive action and only 10% take any action toward removing or securing poisons.[52] Unfortunately, a primary motivator to shift parental perception of risk and precipitate action occurs only after a child poisoning event or a near miss when it is too late. Additionally, there is often the risk of perceived safety if an event is not associated with any morbidity.[66,130]

As previously discussed, some of the reasons why a child ingests a pill are that it is there, it looks and maybe tastes like candy or food, or the child is mimicking the behavior of a parent who ingests medicines or vitamins to cure illness and improve health. However, these reasons may not be sufficient to explain why xenobiotic exposures occur. Another aspect of poisoning that must be considered is the interaction between the child's temperament and the social environment.

Many authors have tried to identify psychosocial predictors for childhood poisoning in general and for repeat poisoning in particular.[21,56,87,90,173] As many as 30% of children repeatedly ingest xenobiotics, frequently the same xenobiotic. Factors associated with single and repeat episodes of childhood poisoning include hyperactivity, impulsive risk-taking behavior, rebelliousness, and negativistic attitude. Other factors seem to be associated more with the quality of supervision by parents or guardians, who themselves are experiencing medical illnesses, depression, or social isolation.[90] Finally, a stressful environment or a major social problem also contributes.[167,174]

With regard to the xenobiotic, a number of issues affect the preinjury and injury phases, and modification of any one of the interacting factors of host, xenobiotic, or environment potentially prevents or reduces the severity of injury. By decreasing the inherent toxicity of household products available around the house, the likelihood of injury is reduced after exposure to one of these products. For example, less toxic rodenticides such as warfarin replaced more toxic ones such as thallium or sodium monofluoroacetate and relatively nontoxic paradichlorobenzene mothballs have largely replaced the relatively more toxic camphor-containing mothballs.

It is also possible to reduce the likelihood of ingestion by making a xenobiotic unpalatable. Denatonium benzoate is an aversive bitter xenobiotic that is added to some liquids such as windshield washer fluid and antifreeze to prevent unintentional poisoning.[85] However, some trials show that whereas older children respond negatively to these xenobiotics with the first taste, younger children have already ingested 1 to 2 teaspoonfuls before being deterred by the bitter flavor.[20,166] This is an important consideration because even a small amount of a xenobiotic such as methanol can be toxic (see later discussion). The actual efficacy of denatonium benzoate in poison prevention is largely unstudied.[148]

The problem of unintentional ingestions is compounded by poison "look-alikes," xenobiotics that resemble candy or food products.[57] Some common examples are ferrous sulfate tablets and vitamins that look like common candies and fuel oils that come in cans resembling soft drink containers. Many shampoos and dishwashing detergents are given lemon or strawberry scents and have pictures of fruits on the labels. More recently changes in marijuana legalization across the country have led to more edible marijuana products coming to the market. Children easily confuse marijuana cookies and candies with their traditional counterparts. In states where these products are legally sold, the number of poisoned children is climbing.[19,188] Children are not always able to distinguish poison "look-alikes" from real candies, fruits, and sodas, and they may be attracted to bright colors, pleasant smells, and appealing packages. Eliminating these "look-alikes" might prevent some unintentional ingestions.

Probably the most significant changes to xenobiotics themselves have occurred in the physical characteristics with regard to packaging and dispensing of pharmaceuticals and some other xenobiotics with child-resistant closures mandated by the Poison Prevention Packaging Act of 1970 (Chap. 1).[29,39] According to the act, "child-resistant" means that the packaging must be effective at preventing 85% of children from opening the package and yet allow 90% of adults to open the package. This legislation is credited with causing a significant reduction in morbidity and mortality caused by poisoning from aspirin and other regulated products, although this analysis was challenged.[38,146,186] Child-resistant closures are also credited with reducing the number of toxic exposures to kerosene.[101]

Although child-resistant containers are a significant deterrent to unintentional ingestions in toddlers, they are not completely effective; by definition, they allow 15% of children to gain access. Problems include the dispensing of pharmaceuticals in nonresistant containers, not properly closing child-resistant containers, leaving pharmaceuticals out of the child-resistant container, and transferring products to a different nonresistant container.[30,172] Up to 70% of potentially toxic pharmaceuticals are stored in non–child-resistant or in improperly functioning child-resistant containers. Several studies identified poor functioning of the closures when there is sticky liquid or pill residue around the top or in the screw threads of the child-resistant container.[86,94,195] A false sense of security associated with these closures leads some parents to be less compulsive regarding safe storage of the containers.[66,130] A double barrier, such as a unit-dose dispenser within a child-resistant container or a blister pack, is recommended for a few pharmaceuticals associated with significant poisonings such as iron and antidepressants.[94] Recently, flow restrictor valves were voluntarily added to some over-the-counter analgesic liquid products to help decrease the volume of liquid dispensed when the child-resistant closure is not fully secured or the child is able to breach the closure mechanism.[109]

In 1997, the Food and Drug Administration (FDA) issued a regulation to package products with 30 mg or more of elemental iron per tablet in unit-dose packages such as blister packs.[59] The intent of this regulation was to reduce the likelihood of iron poisoning in children. Even before this regulation was instituted, the number of fatal childhood iron ingestions declined significantly; therefore, it is not known how much if any of the decrease was related to the mandated packaging changes. In any case, the rule was overturned in 2003, when it was determined that the FDA did not have the statutory authority to regulate a drug for the purpose of poison prevention.[60] As yet there is no evidence of a resurgence of iron-related fatalities.

A discussion of containers and storage naturally leads to a consideration of the third factor in the injury-causation model discussed earlier, the environment, which is particularly important in the preinjury and the injury phases. Approximately 80% of childhood pharmaceutical ingestions occur at home; most of the remainder occurs at the homes of grandparents, other relatives, and friends. At home, the medicine usually belongs either to the child or to a parent, although a significant number of medications, both at home and away from home, belong to a grandparent.[86,106] Grandparents, other relatives, and family friends without children at home often do not obtain or retain medications in child-resistant containers and are not as attentive to safe storage practices. Poison prevention education directed to these groups is particularly helpful.[119]

Medications are frequently kept in the kitchen or bedroom while they are being used.[86,195] In the kitchen, medications are stored in the refrigerator, on the table, or on the counter; in the bedroom, medications are left on a dresser or bedside table. A parent's or grandparent's belongings are another location where medications are commonly found. Interestingly, there are no significant differences in the storage practices in the homes of children who ingest and those who do not ingest medicines, so storage practices alone cannot predict the likelihood of childhood poisoning.[173,195]

One important caveat relates to the storage of nonpharmaceutical xenobiotics, particularly those in liquid form. These types of xenobiotics should never be transferred for storage to familiar household containers, such as food jars or wine or soda bottles; stored in areas low to the ground such as beneath sinks; or kept in cabinets that do not have child-resistant locks. Both children and adults have been unintentionally exposed to xenobiotics, such as sodium hydroxide, pesticides, hydrocarbons, and potassium cyanide, that were stored in bottles in the refrigerator.[182] Many of the kerosene exposures reported from developing countries occur because the kerosene is stored in water bottles, jugs, or other containers in easily accessible locations. When the weather is hot, children mistake the clear liquid kerosene for water.[1,2,165]

HISTORY OF THE INGESTION

The appropriate management of any poisoned patient is influenced by the history of the exposure. Except in rare cases of child abuse, parents or guardians generally provide information to the fullest extent possible. As a rule, in the case of children, the xenobiotic and time of ingestion are known. However, the reported number of pills or volume of liquid ingested is rarely accurate.[80,150] Clues to the amount ingested are the number of pills or volume of liquid in a bottle before and after an ingestion, the number of pills set out on the night table, or the area of a spot of liquid after a spill. When symptoms are suggestive of poisoning but the history is inadequate, information about possible exposure outside of the home, such as with a babysitter, grandparent, friend, or other relative, should be obtained because approximately 15% of childhood poisonings occur outside the home.[86,138]

In contrast, many adolescents are not forthcoming when relating the history of an intentional ingestion, especially when they are depressed, suicidal, or concerned about the response of their guardian or parent. When caring for these patients, the clinician must use the history provided but should remain skeptical about the reported type and number of xenobiotics ingested, as well as the time of ingestion.

When a child is suspected of being the victim of abuse or intentionally poisoned by a parent or guardian, the health care provider must ensure that (a) the history of the poisoning remains consistent over time and among people providing the details of the event, (b) the child's clinical presentation is consistent with the history of the poisoning, and (c) the reported actions are consistent with the child's developmental level.

GASTROINTESTINAL DECONTAMINATION

Chapter 5 is devoted to a complete discussion of gastrointestinal (GI) decontamination. This section reiterates and emphasizes only a few important points.

As described earlier, children generally ingest small quantities of a single xenobiotic. For most of these ingestions, gastric emptying is unnecessary. Some examples of nontoxic ingestions are eating a crayon or the leaf of a jade plant, licking the cap of a household bleach container, or swallowing 2 adult-strength APAP tablets.

Orogastric lavage is a method of gastric emptying occasionally indicated for the most serious ingestions. Orogastric lavage typically requires a very large bore 40-French tube in order to guarantee that the interior diameter and side-port holes are large enough to allow pill fragments to effectively pass back out through the tube. Small children, however, cannot generally tolerate such a large orogastric lavage tube, and a smaller tube is unlikely to be effective for removing large pills or fragments from the stomach of a small child. Additionally, placement of an orogastric tube is an unpleasant and frightening procedure for an infant or child. There is a risk of local trauma from tube placement, and there is the potential for more serious injury such as esophageal perforation. Also, many children vomit during placement of an orogastric tube, increasing the risk for aspiration. Therefore, the use of orogastric lavage is practically limited to adolescents with large potentially fatal ingestions. Orogastric lavage should never be used as a form of punishment or as a form of education. The patient should be intubated to protect the airway before orogastric lavage if the patient has a diminished gag reflex or a depressed level of consciousness.

Historically, administration of syrup of ipecac to poisoned patients was considered a primary emergency intervention and the availability of syrup of ipecac in the home was a primary tenet of pediatric anticipatory guidance. Since 2004 the American Academy of Pediatrics, the American Academy of Clinical Toxicology, and the European Association of Poison Control Centers and Clinical Toxicologists have all recommended against the use because of its unproven benefit, its adverse effects, and its abuse potential.[6,8]

Activated charcoal (AC) is a current mainstay of poison treatment in EDs.[5,37] Children will generally drink AC when coaxed to do so if the AC is disguised in a baby bottle or soft drink container or sweetened with juice or sorbitol.[192] A nasogastric or orogastric tube should rarely ever be inserted to administer AC in an awake patient. Placement of the tube, the presence of AC in the stomach, the effects of the xenobiotic, all may make the child vomit, making aspiration of AC or stomach contents a risk. For AC to be used safely in a patient who is comatose and who does not have a gag reflex, the patient should be intubated and the airway protected first, prior to insertion of an orogastric tube. Because of these risks, AC alone is unnecessary for a nontoxic or minimally toxic ingestion.

METHODS OF ENHANCED ELIMINATION

For consequential poisoning with xenobiotics such as methanol, ethylene glycol, salicylates, lithium, and theophylline, hemodialysis is the optimal technique to enhance elimination. It is feasible to perform these extracorporeal techniques on newborns or small infants in appropriately equipped centers with dedicated personnel. The primary limiting factor is the ability to obtain vascular access.[124,177,178] However, even large centers that routinely do hemodialysis in children will periodically not be able to manage very small infants. Peritoneal dialysis was used for the treatment of ethanol intoxication in a child,[71] but this technique is not recommended.

Exchange transfusion is occasionally used to enhance xenobiotic elimination. This technique is potentially useful for a xenobiotic with a small volume of distribution when multiple-dose AC cannot be administered, the xenobiotic is poorly adsorbed to AC, and when access to specialized hemodialysis or hemoperfusion is not readily available. Exchange transfusion was used successfully for poisoning by salicylates[50,117] and theophylline.[16,135,161] Another xenobiotic for which exchange transfusion is a potential therapeutic alternative is chloral hydrate.[11]

TABLE 31–3	Xenobiotics That Cause Severe Toxicity to an Infant After a Small Adult Dose, a Single Pill, or a Small Volume

β-Adrenergic antagonists (sustained release)

Benzocaine

Bupropion

Caffeine (Powdered)

Calcium channel blockers (sustained release)

Camphor

Caustics (sodium hydroxide)

Chloroquine

Clonidine

Cyclic antidepressants

Cycloplegics (ophthalmic)

Diphenoxylate and atropine (Lomotil)

Ethylene glycol

Imidazolines (nasal spray)

Methanol

Methyl salicylate (oil of wintergreen)

Nicotine (liquid)

Opioids

Pesticides (organophosphates and carbamates, phosphides, and tetramine)

Phenothiazines

Quinine

Sulfonylureas

Theophylline

XENOBIOTICS THAT ARE TOXIC IN SMALL QUANTITIES

When children ingest even small quantities of toxic xenobiotics, they are potentially ingesting relatively large doses because of their small size. There are a number of xenobiotics that cause significant toxicity or rarely death with as little as one pill or one teaspoonful.[14,104] Table 31–3 lists these xenobiotics.

XENOBIOTICS THAT CAUSE DELAYED TOXICITY IN CHILDREN

Several xenobiotics warrant particular concern because their effects are frequently significantly delayed. Classic examples are atropine–diphenoxylate (Lomotil)[22,42,118] and sulfonylurea antidiabetics such as glipizide.[69,139,180] Both of these xenobiotics have the potential to cause serious morbidity with initial symptoms or recurrence of symptoms delayed by as many as 24 hours after ingestion.

Children with real or possible ingestions of Lomotil or a sulfonylurea should be admitted for observation and monitoring even if they are initially asymptomatic (Chaps. 36 and 47). With the advent of new modified-release formulations of calcium channel blockers and β-adrenergic antagonists, concern for delayed toxicity and possibly death has become even greater.[126]

XENOBIOTICS THAT CAUSE UNUSUAL OR IDIOSYNCRATIC REACTIONS IN NEONATES OR CHILDREN

Benzyl Alcohol: Gasping Syndrome

Benzyl alcohol is a preservative added to some liquid pharmaceutical preparations (Chap. 46). IV flush solutions containing benzyl alcohol were implicated as the cause of the "gasping syndrome" in sick newborns; the syndrome includes severe metabolic acidosis, encephalopathy, respiratory depression, and gasping.[7] The association was made when elevated concentrations of benzoic acid and hippuric acid—metabolites of benzyl alcohol—were found in infants with this syndrome.[27,65]

Chloramphenicol: Gray Baby Syndrome

Chloramphenicol is a broad-spectrum antibiotic that was used in children because of its activity against *Haemophilus influenzae*. It was largely replaced by other antibiotics in the United States because of its association with aplastic anemia. When administered at high doses, chloramphenicol is associated with the "gray baby syndrome," which includes abdominal distension, vomiting, metabolic acidosis, progressive pallid cyanosis, irregular respirations, hypothermia, hypotension, and vasomotor collapse. Although these effects occur primarily in premature newborn infants, they also occur in older children and adults (Chap. 54).

Gray baby syndrome is associated with serum chloramphenicol concentrations greater than 100 mg/L. Increased chloramphenicol concentrations result from (a) inadequate conjugation of chloramphenicol with glucuronic acid because of inadequate activity of glucuronyl transferase in the newborn liver and (b) decreased renal elimination of unconjugated chloramphenicol. The exact mechanism of toxicity is unknown; there is speculation that free radicals produced during the metabolism of chloramphenicol may interfere with mitochondrial function.[82]

Ethanol: Hypoglycemia

Ethanol is a major constituent of many liquid preparations, such as mouthwash, vanilla flavoring, perfume, and hand sanitizers. Besides its well-known sedative–hypnotic effects, ethanol poisoning in children is associated with hypoglycemia. Typical ethanol metabolism to acetic acid results in a shift to higher NADH:NAD$^+$ ratio. This redox state favors the conversion of pyruvate to lactate, diverting pyruvate away from the Krebs cycle and gluconeogenesis. This decreased source of energy and glucose is poorly tolerated in children, especially because of reduced hepatic glycogen stores. Ethanol-induced hypoglycemia increases the risk for seizure and exacerbation of other CNS effects induced by ethanol poisoning. There does not seem to be a definite blood alcohol concentration threshold for the development of hypoglycemia, which has been reported with blood alcohol concentrations as low as 20 mg/dL[41] (Chap. 76).

Imidazolines and Clonidine: Central Nervous System Effects

Imidazolines such as tetrahydrozoline, oxymetazoline, xylometazoline, and naphazoline are nonprescription sympathomimetics used as nasal decongestants and conjunctival vasoconstrictors (Chap. 49). Clonidine is an imidazoline derivative used as an antihypertensive (Chap. 61). In small children, these xenobiotics cause severe central nervous system (CNS) depression, respiratory depression, bradycardia, miosis, and hypotension.[13,116,193] The presumed mechanism of action is by stimulation of central α_2-adrenergic and imidazole receptors. Although naloxone has been reported to reverse some of the CNS effects of clonidine, there are no reports of its successful use with the other imidazolines (Chap. 61).

HISTORICAL POISONINGS

There have been numerous times throughout history that children have been disproportionately affected by a toxicologic mass casualty incident.

Aniline Dye

In 1886, Rayner first described a series of newborn children on his maternity ward appearing dusky in color and somewhat limp. Six months later when a second series of newborns presented, he linked the symptoms to a delivery of diapers that were freshly stamped with aniline dye.[89] The dye was absorbed through the newborn skin causing symptoms of what is now known as methemoglobinemia. Despite reports and warnings, aniline continued to be used as a diaper marking dye for decades.[83,89,137] Today, we continue to see pediatric aniline-dye-induced methemoglobinemia from contaminated Indian Holi festival dyes and shoe dyes as well.[132,170]

Sulfanilamide Elixir

In the late 1930s, the antibiotic medication sulfanilamide was used to treat infections such as streptococcal pharyngitis. Because of a demand for a liquid preparation, an elixir was rushed to market without adequate testing. Sulfanilamide itself is poorly soluble and many of the typical diluents were inadequate; however diethylene glycol functioned well as a solvent and was sweet tasting. Unfortunately diethylene glycol is severely toxic and causes acute kidney injury.[64] The use of diethylene glycol as a diluent for sulfanilamide caused more than 100 deaths including many children.[12,187] As a result and to avoid similar tragedies, the Food,

Drug, and Cosmetic Act was passed in 1938 that requires animal testing of new drugs and data submission to the FDA before marketing to the public.

Unfortunately diethylene glycol continues to be used sporadically around the world with the same tragic effects. In 1996, in Haiti, there were 85 deaths of 109 children treated for acute kidney injury associated with the use of diethylene glycol–contaminated APAP syrup.[133] Again in 1998, in India, 33 out of 36 children who presented with acute kidney injury died after ingesting diethylene glycol–containing cough expectorant.[169] Whether use of diethylene glycol in these cases despite available information regarding its toxicity was out of ignorance or related to unethical financial corruption has not been resolved.

Melamine

Melamine has widespread uses, most commonly in the plastic dinnerware industry. In the trace quantities that may leach from dinnerware into food to be eaten, melamine is generally considered not toxic. However, in 2008, in China, an outbreak of infantile urolithiasis was associated with melamine-containing powdered infant formula.

The protein content of food is measured based on its nitrogen content. Melamine is more than 60% nitrogen by weight, and by adding melamine to a dry powdered formula the apparent protein content is falsely elevated. Unfortunately, some Chinese formulas were measuring more than 6,000 ppm melamine compared to less than 1 ppm in a comparable US product.[171] More than 294,000 Chinese children were affected, leading to 51,900 hospitalizations and 6 deaths.

MEDICATION ERRORS

Ever since the publication of the Institute of Medicine's report titled *To Err Is Human* in 1999, increasing attention is being paid to the issue of medical errors in medicine.[95] Although most of the research regarding medication errors has focused on adults (Chap. 134), this problem also affects children. Remarks in this section are generally limited to the pediatric literature.

Approximately 276,600 exposures each year are classified by the AAPCC as therapeutic errors. For 2011 to 2015, there were a total of 7 deaths attributed to therapeutic errors. Of children younger than the age of 6 years, approximately 40% of the errors resulting in severe injury or death occurred in children younger than the age of 1 year.[184]

Medication errors occur at any phase of a process that includes ordering, order transcription, pharmacy dispensing, preparation and administration of the medication, and monitoring of medication effects. In fact, the same types of errors occur at multiple points in the process. Table 31–4 provides some examples of errors.

TABLE 31–4 Examples of Medication Errors

1. **Wrong drug.** In one nursery, an epidemic mimicking neonatal sepsis was caused when racemic epinephrine was inadvertently administered instead of vitamin E because both drugs were manufactured by the same company, distributed in nearly identical bottles, and stored near each other inside the nursery refrigerator.[176]

2. **Wrong drug formulation.** Acetaminophen suppositories (120 mg) were ordered for a toddler, but adult-strength suppositories (650 mg) were distributed and administered every 4 hours. The child developed hepatotoxicity requiring hospitalization and therapy (Chap. 33).

3. **Wrong dose.** A 1-kg premature infant required sedation for a diagnostic study. A high dose of chloral hydrate, 100 mg/kg, was miscalculated to be 1 g (1,000 mg) instead of 100 mg. The child had a cardiopulmonary arrest and died. When drugs require milligram per kilogram dosing, it is easy to make decimal mistakes in the calculation or in the transcription.

4. **Wrong route.** A 17-month-old girl with a central venous line (CVL) and a gastrostomy tube required an upper gastrointestinal series. Barium sulfate was inadvertently injected into the CVL instead of the gastrostomy tube. The patient had several episodes of vomiting and developed fever and rigors but ultimately recovered.[175]

5. **Wrong dose.** A patient had the dose of cyclosporine changed from 10 mg to 7 mg twice daily. The child received 70 mg (0.7 mL of solution) instead of 7 mg (0.07 mL). When the prescription was refilled, the parents received a 5-mL syringe to use instead of a 1-mL syringe they had used previously.[46]

Most of the analyses of medication errors have occurred in inpatient settings. The reported frequencies of medication errors vary widely—from 0.47% to 5.7% of written orders and from 0.51 to 157 per 1,000 patient-days.[58,81,88,91,153]

The variance largely depends on whether the definition of "error" does or does not include prescribing errors, regardless of whether or not they are corrected, and whether potential, or only actual, adverse drug events are included. The reported frequencies also vary depending on whether there is active case finding or whether there is only voluntary reporting.

In a 2001 study of pediatric inpatients in which orders were actively monitored for a 6-week period, 5.7% of 10,778 prescriptions had errors in the order for the medication, transcription of the order, dispensing or administration of the medication, or monitoring of medication effects (56 per 100 admissions, 157 per 1,000 patient-days).[91] Overall, 1.1% of these errors could have *potentially* caused an adverse effect (10 per 100 admissions, 29 per 1,000 patient-days). Eighty-four percent of the errors occurred during the ordering or transcription phase, so most of the errors were intercepted and corrected before drug administration. There were 26 true adverse drug events, but only 5 were considered preventable errors (0.05%, 0.52 per 100 admissions, 1.8 per 1,000 patient-days). Although the overall error rate was similar to that reported by the same group in a study of adults, the rate of errors that could *potentially* have caused harm was 3 times greater; 41% of the potentially harmful errors were not intercepted. However, one review suggests that the prescription error rate is higher in adults than in children.[103]

Generally, error rates are higher in intensive care units, where the sickest patients are cared for; such patients often receive multiple medications with complex administration regimens.[58,81,91,140,153,185,194] Results similar to those from inpatient settings are reported in pediatric EDs.[99,159]

Children are at increased risk of a medication error for several reasons: (a) someone other than the child administers the medication, so there is little opportunity to prevent or limit drug administration; (b) a young child cannot warn practitioners about possible problems such as allergies; (c) a young child cannot inform practitioners when he or she is experiencing an adverse event; (d) medication ordering and administration in children frequently requires dose calculations; (e) inexperienced practitioners are uncomfortable with pediatric dosing or related calculations; and (f) incorrect measurement or dilution of concentrated stock solutions may yield a small volume, which is not perceived as containing a relatively large dose of medication.[34,46,67]

One of the most common errors is prescription, preparation, or administration of an incorrect dose, particularly in children, for whom almost every prescription requires knowledge of the patient's weight and a calculation of a weight-based dose.[91,100,102] In addition, even the milligram per kilogram dose varies depending on the age of the patient or the diagnosis. Although pediatric doses are generally determined on a milligram per kilogram basis, if the weight is recorded in pounds and this weight is used in the calculation, there will be a built-in 2-fold error. Calculation errors also occur when drug preparation requires dilution of a concentrated stock solution or special compounding.[184] Further confusion arises when *mg* is written as or misinterpreted as mcg or μg in a calculation or vice versa.[43]

When an extra zero is added or a required zero is omitted from calculations, written or verbal prescriptions, or in dispensed and administered medications, a 10-fold error occurs. These large errors are common and result in significant under- or overdosing; 10-fold errors are reported in testing scenarios, case series, and case reports.[46,49,96,97,100,140,144,149,153] These errors are of particular concern because the risk of toxicity generally increases with significant overdose.

Because the causes of medication error are numerous and complex, the solutions must be multifaceted and interdisciplinary. The approach to the problem is contained within the field of human factors research and potentially requires changes in individual factors such as knowledge; environmental factors such as interruptions; and system problems such as how medications are ordered, stocked, and dispensed (Chap. 134).[95,179,189]

Pediatric critical care areas, including the ED, benefit from having precalculated weight-based dosing charts available for resuscitation medications

and for other commonly prescribed medications; this is a recommendation of the American Heart Association.[9] Many clinical units have developed their own dosing schemes. Commercial products, such as the Broselow–Luten system, are also available and reduce the number of medication errors in simulated[3,112,113,160] and actual resuscitations.[152] There is some controversy related to the ability of these length-based commercial products to accurately predict the weights of American children because of the growing obesity epidemic. However, most resuscitation medications should be dosed on ideal body weight as estimated by these length-based tools when a patient's clinical status precludes obtaining an accurate weight.[114] Additionally, international populations, depending on their development status, also vary from the length-based weight predictions set forth by the Broselow–Luten system.[125]

The previous discussion was almost exclusively related to hospital-based medication use, but significant errors also occur in outpatient settings. Antipyretics are among the most frequently recommended medications for children. Although significant toxicity after unintentional ingestions in toddlers is now rare, administration of multiple supratherapeutic doses of APAP is common and can cause significant hepatotoxicity.[98]

In fact, many parents have difficulty calculating the appropriate dose of APAP and measuring out the appropriate amount after it is calculated despite having received instructions and graduated cups or oral-dosing syringes.[70,115,121,168] In a simulated encounter, only 11% of medical students were able to identify a pediatric APAP dosing error even when provided with appropriate history, actual product used, and dosing instructions.[51] Relevant factors related to these errors include the characteristics of the instructions regarding medication measurement and administration, the health literacy and health numeracy of caregivers, and the accuracy of different measuring devices (Chap. 129).

Two of the most commonly used measuring devices are also the most inaccurate—the teaspoon and the graduated cup.[154,200] The household teaspoon is not standardized for volume and can easily be confused with a household tablespoon.[115] Acetaminophen and ibuprofen elixirs are typically packaged with a graduated cup for administration even though graduated syringes are considered the most accurate of the measuring instruments available and are recommended by the AAP for young children. In addition, over-the-counter products are sold with inconsistencies between the dosing instructions and the measuring device.[202] In other words, the instructions may describe mL measurement when the measuring device has teaspoon graduations or vice versa.

Health literacy and health numeracy are becoming increasingly understood factors with regard to the safe and effective delivery of health care in general and the reduction of the rate of medical errors in particular. Health literacy plays a key role in a caregiver's ability to read and understand instructions about and labels on prescriptions and nonprescription medications.[164] The labels on medication containers are not standardized with respect to the layout and placement of information or the use of abbreviations or units of measure, may be printed in small fonts that are physically difficult to read, and difficult to understand by people with lower health literacy or limited English proficiency.[108,201,202] Instructions for medication administration have the same problems. Visual cues using pictograms in the instructions or color-coded or premarked syringes are practical ways to improve the accuracy of parental medication dosing (Chap. 129).[61,198,199]

INTENTIONAL POISONING AND CHILD ABUSE

Intentional poisoning of children is a rare, but significant, form of child abuse. As previously discussed, the majority of unintentional childhood poisonings have no or only mild effects. However, the risk of morbidity or mortality from "malicious" intentional poisoning is as high as 20% to 30%.[47,78,181] In 1967, Kempe described the "battered child" as a syndrome of classic physical injuries, including long bone fractures, subdural hematomas, and nutritional wasting, that placed the young child at risk for death.[92] This early description also defined child abuse by poisoning as the intentional administration of a drug or the exposure of a child to a natural gas or toxic substance.

Today, there are 4 primary scenarios of child abuse by poisoning: (a) medical child abuse (previously *Munchausen syndrome by proxy*); (b) disciplinary/behavioral modification; (c) drug-assisted sexual assault; and (d) attempted homicide.[48]

In 1977, the term *Munchausen syndrome by proxy* was first used to describe a condition in which a parent or guardian falsifies medical evidence of nonexistent disease(s) or creates the signs and symptoms of disease in a child (factitious illness).[122,123,151] For example, the first 2 published cases involved (a) a case of adulterated urine used to simulate disease and (b) a case of repetitive salt poisoning used to produce symptoms of hypernatremic disease, which ultimately proved fatal. This intentional poisoning of a child, although typically a manifestation of the parent's complex psychiatric illness, is today considered medical child abuse regardless of underlying intent.[24,68,156]

These children suffer both from the symptoms related to the poisoning itself as well as from multiple medical evaluations, frequent hospitalizations, invasive medical procedures, diagnostic testing, and unneeded therapy. Rarely these children die. Since the parent is the caregiver and historian as well as the perpetrator, a prerequisite for this challenging diagnosis is a low index of suspicion.[78] Several warning signals help suggest a diagnosis of medical child abuse (Table 31–5).

Typically, patients present with 4 main categories of illness: (a) metabolic derangements (eg, salt or water ingestion), (b) gastrointestinal symptoms (eg, laxative or syrup of ipecac poisoning), (c) hemorrhagic disease (eg, warfarins), or (d) neurologic symptoms (central nervous system depression or excitation). Despite the historic prevalence of these types of poisonings, this is a partial list because any xenobiotic could be used to poison a child as was seen in 2 recent studies, where the National Poison Data System (NPDS) if not already used in this chapter was queried for childhood cases coded as "malicious" intent. There were approximately 160 cases per year of malicious administration involving pharmaceuticals and 450 cases per year involving the malicious administration of nonpharmaceuticals. The median age of exposure was 1.5 years (pharmaceuticals) and 3 years (nonpharmaceuticals). The most commonly reported pharmaceutical categories included analgesics, stimulants/street drugs, sedatives/hypnotics, cough and cold products, and ethanol. The most commonly reported nonpharmaceutical categories included cleaning products, cosmetic products, and pesticides.[203,204]

Intentional poisoning is associated with other forms of abuse; approximately 20% of poisoned children have evidence of physical abuse.[47,78] Of children presenting to EDs after presumed unintentional poisoning, 36% had previous ED visits for trauma, 7% for poisoning, 6% for both trauma and poisoning, and 1.4% for failure to thrive. At the time of the visit, only 7% were evaluated for possible abuse, and 2.7% were considered neglected.[78] These data do not prove an association between poisoning and physical trauma; however, in some children, repeat episodes of trauma or poisoning could signal a significant intrafamilial stress or neglect. As previously discussed, almost all of the reported young childhood poison exposures are recorded as unintentional ingestions typical of exploratory behavior; however, some of these exposures are likely due to neglect. Although medical neglect is difficult to define, it should be considered every time a caregiver has failed to provide adequate supervision to prevent a xenobiotic exposure,[78,196] with particular attention paid to cases involving repeated exposures, endangerment, or exposure to illicit substances and drugs of abuse.[48]

In households where legal and illegal substances are present and used, a chaotic environment leads to poor supervision and increased risk of exposure to these substances. Exposure occurs via side-stream/secondhand exposure,[17,77,128,157,191] unintentional ingestion,[93,145] and rectal administration,[142] as well as through breast milk.[35] Children have been given doses of alcohol, methadone, and other xenobiotics to quiet them or to prevent withdrawal.[44,79,143] There are reports of babysitters blowing marijuana smoke into babies' faces to "get them high" or to quiet them.[158]

Siblings of children evaluated and treated for poisoning also suffer from medical child abuse. In addition, significant psychiatric problems are manifest by the victim, parents, and siblings.[25,120,156,162]

Child abuse or neglect must be part of the differential diagnosis of any case of childhood poisoning. Intentional poisoning should be considered and evaluated for[78,79]

- An "ingestion" in a child younger than one year
- A case with a confusing history or presentation
- A child with signs and symptoms inconsistent with the history (lacks biologic/chronologic plausibility)
- A child with a previous poisoning or a child whose siblings were previously evaluated for poisoning
- A child with a previous presentation for a rare or unexplained medical condition
- A child with apnea, unexplained seizures, currently defined as brief resolved unexplained events (BRUE) previously called or an apparent life-threatening events (ALTE)
- A massive ingestion by a small child
- An ingestion of multiple xenobiotics by a small child
- An exposure to substances of abuse
- An intoxication with a xenobiotic to which a child could or would not typically have access
- "Accidental ingestions" in a school-age child
- A history of previous trauma, child abuse, or neglect
- Sudden infant death syndrome or an unexplained death

These considerations of child abuse notwithstanding, rare diseases do occur. One child's rare inherited metabolic disorder, methyl malonic acidemia, was misdiagnosed as ethylene glycol poisoning because the chromatographic appearance of the metabolite propionic acid was similar to that of ethylene glycol.[163]

SUMMARY

- Young children and adolescents are frequently exposed to potentially toxic xenobiotics; fortunately, most childhood exposures are ingestions of nonpoisonous xenobiotics or small nontoxic quantities of potentially toxic xenobiotics.
- When a child sustains a significant toxic exposure, management follows general toxicologic principles.
- Although most childhood exposures are unintentional, the clinician should be alert to the possibility of intentional poisoning of a child with pharmaceutical or household products.
- The normal development of children places them at risk for unintentional ingestions. A chaotic home environment or a disorganized social structure augments these risks.

TABLE 31–5	Medical Child Abuse: Suggestive Characteristics in Clinical Situations

1. The child has a persistent or recurrent illness that cannot be explained.
2. The history of disease or results of diagnostic tests are inconsistent with the general health and appearance of the child.
3. The signs and symptoms cause the mature clinician to remark, "I've never seen anything like this before!"
4. The signs and symptoms do not occur when the child is separated from the parent.
5. The parent is particularly attentive and refuses to leave the child's bedside even for a few minutes.
6. The parent develops particularly close relations with hospital staff.
7. The parent seems less worried than the physician about the child's condition.
8. Treatments are not tolerated (eg, intravenous lines fall out frequently, prescribed medications lead to vomiting).
9. The proposed diagnosis is a rare disease.
10. "Seizures" are unwitnessed by medical staff and reportedly do not respond to any treatment.
11. The parent has a complicated medical or psychiatric history.
12. The parent is or was associated with the health care field.

Data from Meadow R. Munchausen syndrome by proxy. *Arch Dis Child*. 1982 Feb;57(2):92-98.

- Small size puts children at increased risks for medication dosing and dispensing errors, and their immature metabolic processes leads to unexpected toxicity from pharmaceuticals.
- Toxicologists should encourage parents to provide as safe a home environment as possible to prevent unintentional ingestions and must encourage practitioners to exercise special vigilance when administering medications to children.

REFERENCES

1. Abu-Ekteish F. Kerosene poisoning in children: a report from northern Jordan. *Trop Doct.* 2002;32:27-29.
2. Adejuyigbe EA, et al. Childhood poisoning at the Obafemi Awolowo University Teaching Hospital, Ile-Ife, Nigeria. *Niger J Med.* 2002;11:183-186.
3. Agarwal S, et al. Comparing the utility of a standard pediatric resuscitation cart with a pediatric resuscitation cart based on the Broselow tape: a randomized, controlled, crossover trial involving simulated resuscitation scenarios. *Pediatrics.* 2005;116:e326-e333.
4. Ahmed A, et al. Poisoning emergency visits among children: a 3-year retrospective study in Qatar. *BMC Pediatr.* 2015;15:104.
5. American Academy of Clinical Toxicology; European Association of Poisons Centres and Clinical Toxicologists. Position statement and practice guidelines on the use of multi-dose activated charcoal in the treatment of acute poisoning. *J Toxicol Clin Toxicol.* 1999;37:731-751.
6. American Academy of Clinical Toxicology; European Association of Poisons Centres and Clinical Toxicologists. Position paper: Ipecac syrup. *J Toxicol Clin Toxicol.* 2004;42:133-143.
7. American Academy of Pediatrics. Benzyl alcohol: toxic agent in neonatal units. *Pediatrics.* 1983;72:356-358.
8. American Academy of Pediatrics. Poison treatment in the home. American Academy of Pediatrics Committee on Injury, Violence, and Poison Prevention. *Pediatrics.* 2003;112:1182-1185.
9. American Heart Association. PALS Provider Manual 2016.
10. Andiran N, Sarikayalar F. Pattern of acute poisonings in childhood in Ankara: what has changed in twenty years? *Turk J Pediatr.* 2004;46:147-152.
11. Anyebuno MA, Rosenfeld CR. Chloral hydrate toxicity in a term infant. *Dev Pharmacol Ther.* 1991;17:116-120.
12. Ballentine C. Taste of raspberries, taste of death: The 1937 elixir sulfanilimide incident. *FDA Consumer Magazine.* https://http://www.fda.gov/aboutfda/whatwedo/history/productregulation/sulfanilamidedisaster/. Published 1981. Accessed May 22, 2017.
13. Bamshad MJ, Wasserman GS. Pediatric clonidine intoxications. *Vet Hum Toxicol.* 1990;32:220-223.
14. Bar-Oz B, et al. Medications that can be fatal for a toddler with one tablet or teaspoonful: a 2004 update. *Paediatr Drugs.* 2004;6:123-126.
15. Baraff LJ, et al. The relationship of poison center contact and injury in children 2 to 6 years old. *Ann Emerg Med.* 1992;21:153-157.
16. Barazarte V, et al. Exchange transfusion in a case of severe theophylline poisoning. *Vet Hum Toxicol.* 1992;34:524.
17. Bateman DA, Heagarty MC. Passive freebase cocaine ("crack") inhalation by infants and toddlers. *Am J Dis Child.* 1989;143:25-27.
18. Belay ED, et al. Reye's syndrome in the United States from 1981 through 1997. *N Engl J Med.* 1999;340:1377-1382.
19. Berger E. Legal marijuana and pediatric exposure pot edibles implicated in spike in child emergency department visits. *Ann Emerg Med.* 2014;64:A19-A21.
20. Berning CK, et al. Research on the effectiveness of denatonium benzoate as a deterrent to liquid detergent ingestion by children. *Fundam Appl Toxicol.* 1982;2:44-48.
21. Bithoney WG, et al. Childhood ingestions as symptoms of family distress. *Am J Dis Child.* 1985;139:456-459.
22. Block SM, et al. Lomotil poisoning in children: two case reports. *S Afr Med J.* 1977;51:553-554.
23. Bond GR, et al. The growing impact of pediatric pharmaceutical poisoning. *J Pediatr.* 2012;160:265-270 e261.
24. Bools C, et al. Munchausen syndrome by proxy: a study of psychopathology. *Child Abuse Negl.* 1994;18:773-788.
25. Bools CN, et al. Co-morbidity associated with fabricated illness (Munchausen syndrome by proxy). *Arch Dis Child.* 1992;67:77-79.
26. Brayden RM, et al. Behavioral antecedents of pediatric poisonings. *Clin Pediatr (Phila).* 1993;32:30-35.
27. Brown WJ, et al. Fatal benzyl alcohol poisoning in a neonatal intensive care unit. *Lancet.* 1982;1:1250.
28. Budnitz DS, Lovegrove MC. The last mile: taking the final steps in preventing pediatric pharmaceutical poisonings. *J Pediatr.* 2012;160:190-192.
29. Budnitz DS, Salis S. Preventing medication overdoses in young children: an opportunity for harm elimination. *Pediatrics.* 2011;127:e1597-e1599.
30. Centers for Disease Control. Unintentional poisoning among young children—United States. *MMWR Morb Mortal Wkly Rep.* 1983;32:117-118.
31. Centers for Disease Control. Update: childhood poisonings—United States. *MMWR Morb Mortal Wkly Rep.* 1985;34:117-118.
32. Centers for Disease Control and Prevention—National Center for Injury Prevention and Control. Web-based Injury Statistics Query and Reporting System (WISQARS). http://www.cdc.gov/ncipc/wisqars. Published 2017. Accessed May 29, 2017.
33. Chan TY, et al. Epidemiology of poisoning in the New Territories south of Hong Kong. *Hum Exp Toxicol.* 1997;16:204-207.
34. Chappell K, Newman C. Potential tenfold drug overdoses on a neonatal unit. *Arch Dis Child Fetal Neonatal Ed.* 2004;89:F483-F484.
35. Chasnoff IJ, et al. Cocaine intoxication in a breast-fed infant. *Pediatrics.* 1987;80:836-838.
36. Cheng TL, et al. The spectrum of intoxication and poisonings among adolescents: surveillance in an urban population. *Inj Prev.* 2006;12:129-132.
37. Chyka PA, Seger D. Position statement: single-dose activated charcoal. American Academy of Clinical Toxicology; European Association of Poisons Centres and Clinical Toxicologists. *J Toxicol Clin Toxicol.* 1997;35:721-741.
38. Clarke A, Walton WW. Effect of safety packaging on aspirin ingestion by children. *Pediatrics.* 1979;63:687-693.
39. Consumer Product Safety Commission. Poison Prevention Packaging Act of 1970, 15 U.S.C. 1471-1476.
40. Craft AW. Circumstances surrounding deaths from accidental poisoning 1974-80. *Arch Dis Child.* 1983;58:544-546.
41. Cummins LH. Hypoglycemia and convulsions in children following alcohol ingestion. *J Pediatr.* 1961;58:23-26.
42. Cutler EA, et al. Delayed cardiopulmonary arrest after Lomotil ingestion. *Pediatrics.* 1980;65:157-158.
43. Dart RC, Rumack BH. Intravenous acetaminophen in the United States: iatrogenic dosing errors. *Pediatrics.* 2012;129:349-353.
44. Deeths TM, Breeden JT. Poisoning in children—a statistical study of 1,057 cases. *J Pediatr.* 1971;78:299-305.
45. Densen-Gerber J. The forensic pathology of drug-related child abuse. *Leg Med Annu.* 1978:135-147.
46. Diav-Citrin O, et al. Medication errors in paediatrics: a case report and systematic review of risk factors. *Paediatr Drugs.* 2000;2:239-242.
47. Dine MS, McGovern ME. Intentional poisoning of children—an overlooked category of child abuse: report of seven cases and review of the literature. *Pediatrics.* 1982;70:32-35.
48. Dinis-Oliveira RJ, Magalhaes T. Children intoxications: what is abuse and what is not abuse. *Trauma Violence Abuse.* 2013;14:113-132.
49. Doherty C, Mc Donnell C. Tenfold medication errors: 5 years' experience at a university-affiliated pediatric hospital. *Pediatrics.* 2012;129:916-924.
50. Done AK, Otterness LJ. Exchange transfusion in the treatment of oil of wintergreen (methyl salicylate) poisoning. *J Pediatr.* 1956;18:80-85.
51. Dudas RA, Barone MA. Can medical students identify a potentially serious acetaminophen dosing error in a simulated encounter? a case control study. *BMC Med Educ* 2015;15:13.
52. Eichelberger MR, et al. Parental attitudes and knowledge of child safety. A national survey. *Am J Dis Child.* 1990;144:714-720.
53. Eriksson M, et al. Accidental poisoning in pre-school children in the Stockholm area. Medical, psychosocial and preventive aspects. *Acta Paediatr Scand Suppl.* 1979;275:96-101.
54. Even KM, et al. Poisonings requiring admission to the pediatric intensive care unit: a 5-year review. *Clin Toxicol (Phila).* 2014;52:519-524.
55. Ferguson JA, et al. Some epidemiological observations on medicinal and non-medicinal poisoning in preschool children. *J Epidemiol Community Health.* 1992;46:207-210.
56. Flagler SL, Wright L. Recurrent poisoning in children: a review. *J Pediatr Psychol.* 1987;12:631-641.
57. Flomenbaum NE, Howland MA. Pretty poison. *Emerg Med.* 1986;4:69-84.
58. Folli HL, et al. Medication error prevention by clinical pharmacists in two children's hospitals. *Pediatrics.* 1987;79:718-722.
59. Food and Drug Administration. Iron-containing supplements and drugs: label warning statements and unit-dose packaging requirements, 21 CFR Parts 101, 111, and 310. *Fed Regist.* 1997;62:2218-2250.
60. Food and Drug Administration. Iron-containing supplements and drugs; label warning statements and unit-dose packaging requirements; removal of regulations for unit-dose packaging requirements for dietary supplements and drugs. Final rule; removal of regulatory provisions in response to court order. *Fed Regist.* 2003;68:59714-59715.
61. Frush KS, et al. Evaluation of a method to reduce over-the-counter medication dosing error. *Arch Pediatr Adolesc Med.* 2004;158:620-624.
62. Gaudreault P, et al. Poison exposures and use of ipecac in children less than 1 year old. *Ann Emerg Med.* 1986;15:808-810.
63. Gauvin F, et al. Hospitalizations for pediatric intoxication in Washington State, 1987-1997. *Arch Pediatr Adolesc Med.* 2001;155:1105-1110.
64. Geiling EMK, Cannon PR. Pathologic effects of elixir of sulfanilamide (diethylene glycol) poisoning a clinical and experimental correlation: final report. *JAMA.* 1938;111:919-926.
65. Gershanik J, et al. The gasping syndrome and benzyl alcohol poisoning. *N Engl J Med.* 1982;307:1384-1388.
66. Gibbs L, et al. Understanding parental motivators and barriers to uptake of child poison safety strategies: a qualitative study. *Inj Prev* 2005;11:373-377.
67. Goldmann D, Kaushal R. Time to tackle the tough issues in patient safety. *Pediatrics.* 2002;110:823-826.

68. Gray J, Bentovim A. Illness induction syndrome: paper I—a series of 41 children from 37 families identified at the Great Ormond Street Hospital for Children NHS Trust. *Child Abuse Negl.* 1996;20:655-673.

69. Greenberg B, et al. Chlorpropamide poisoning. *Pediatrics.* 1968;41:145-147.

70. Gribetz B, Cronley SA. Underdosing of acetaminophen by parents. *Pediatrics.* 1987;80:630-633.

71. Grubbauer HM, Schwarz R. Peritoneal dialysis in alcohol intoxication in a child. *Arch Toxicol.* 1980;43:317-320.

72. Gupta S, et al. Trends in poisoning in children: experience at a large referral teaching hospital. *Natl Med J India.* 1998;11:166-168.

73. Haddon W Jr. Advances in the epidemiology of injuries as a basis for public policy. *Public Health Rep.* 1980;95:411-421.

74. Hamid MH, et al. Acute poisoning in children. *J Coll Physicians Surg Pak.* 2005;15:805-808.

75. Hamilton RJ, Goldfrank LR. Poison center data and the Pollyanna phenomenon. *J Toxicol Clin Toxicol.* 1997;35:21-23.

76. Harchelroad F, et al. Treated vs reported toxic exposures: discrepancies between a poison control center and a member hospital. *Vet Hum Toxicol.* 1990;32:156-159.

77. Heidemann SM, Goetting MG. Passive inhalation of cocaine by infants. *Henry Ford Hosp Med J.* 1990;38:252-254.

78. Henretig FM, et al. Child abuse by poisoning. In: Reece RM, Christian CW, eds. *Child Abuse: Medical Diagnosis and Management.* 3rd ed. Elk Grove Village, IL: American Academy of Pediatrics; 2009:549-599.

79. Hickson GB, et al. Parental administration of chemical agents: a cause of apparent life-threatening events. *Pediatrics.* 1989;83:772-776.

80. Hitchings AW, et al. Determining the volume of toxic liquid ingestions in adults: accuracy of estimates by healthcare professionals and members of the public. *Clin Toxicol (Phila).* 2013;51:77-82.

81. Holdsworth MT, et al. Incidence and impact of adverse drug events in pediatric inpatients. *Arch Pediatr Adolesc Med.* 2003;157:60-65.

82. Holt D, et al. Chloramphenicol toxicity. *Adverse Drug React Toxicol Rev.* 1993;12:83-95.

83. Howarth BE. Epidemic of aniline methaemoglobinaemia in newborn babies. *Lancet.* 1951;1:934-935.

84. Hurwitz ES. Reye's syndrome. *Epidemiol Rev.* 1989;11:249-253.

85. Jackson MH, Payne HA. Bittering agents: their potential application in reducing ingestions of engine coolants and windshield wash. *Vet Hum Toxicol.* 1995;37:323-326.

86. Jacobson BJ, et al. Accidental ingestions of oral prescription drugs: a multicenter survey. *Am J Public Health.* 1989;79:853-856.

87. Jones JG. The child accident repeater: a review. *Clin Pediatr (Phila).* 1980;19:284-288.

88. Juntti-Patinen L, Neuvonen PJ. Drug-related deaths in a university central hospital. *Eur J Clin Pharmacol.* 2002;58:479-482.

89. Kagan BM, et al. Cyanosis in premature infants due to aniline dye intoxication. *J Pediatr.* 1949;34:574-578.

90. Katrivanou A, et al. Psychopathology and behavioural trends of children with accidental poisoning. *J Psychosom Res.* 2004;57:95-101.

91. Kaushal R, et al. Medication errors and adverse drug events in pediatric inpatients. *JAMA.* 2001;285:2114-2120.

92. Kempe CH, et al. The battered-child syndrome. *JAMA.* 1962;181:17-24.

93. Kharasch S, et al. Esophagitis, epiglottitis, and cocaine alkaloid ("crack"): "accidental" poisoning or child abuse? *Pediatrics.* 1990;86:117-119.

94. King WD, Palmisano PA. Ingestion of prescription drugs by children: an epidemiologic study. *South Med J.* 1989;82:1468-1471, 1478.

95. Kohn LT, eds. *To Err Is Human: Building a Safer Health System.* Washington, DC: Committee on Quality of Health Care in America, Institute of Medicine, National Academy Press; 1999.

96. Koren G, et al. Errors in computing drug doses. *Can Med Assoc J.* 1983;129:721-723.

97. Koren G, Haslam RH. Pediatric medication errors: predicting and preventing tenfold disasters. *J Clin Pharmacol.* 1994;34:1043-1045.

98. Kozer E, et al. A prospective study of multiple supratherapeutic acetaminophen doses in febrile children. *Vet Hum Toxicol.* 2002;44:106-109.

99. Kozer E, et al. Variables associated with medication errors in pediatric emergency medicine. *Pediatrics.* 2002;110:737-742.

100. Kozer E, et al. Prospective observational study on the incidence of medication errors during simulated resuscitation in a paediatric emergency department. *BMJ.* 2004;329:1321.

101. Krug A, et al. The impact of child-resistant containers on the incidence of paraffin (kerosene) ingestion in children. *S Afr Med J.* 1994;84:730-734.

102. Lesar TS. Errors in the use of medication dosage equations. *Arch Pediatr Adolesc Med.* 1998;152:340-344.

103. Lewis PJ, et al. Prevalence, incidence and nature of prescribing errors in hospital inpatients: a systematic review. *Drug Saf.* 2009;32:379-389.

104. Liebelt EL, Shannon MW. Small doses, big problems: a selected review of highly toxic common medications. *Pediatr Emerg Care.* 1993;9:292-297.

105. Linakis JG, Frederick KA. Poisoning deaths not reported to the regional poison control center. *Ann Emerg Med.* 1993;22:1822-1828.

106. Litovitz T, et al. Prescription drug ingestions in children: whose drug? *Vet Hum Toxicol.* 1986;28:14-15.

107. Litovitz T, Manoguerra A. Comparison of pediatric poisoning hazards: an analysis of 3.8 million exposure incidents. A report from the American Association of Poison Control Centers. *Pediatrics.* 1992;89:999-1006.

108. Lokker N, et al. Parental misinterpretations of over-the-counter pediatric cough and cold medication labels. *Pediatrics.* 2009;123:1464-1471.

109. Lovegrove MC, et al. Efficacy of flow restrictors in limiting access of liquid medications by young children. *J Pediatr.* 2013;163:1134-1139.e1.

110. Lovegrove MC, et al. Emergency hospitalizations for unsupervised prescription medication ingestions by young children. *Pediatrics.* 2014;134:e1009-e1016.

111. Lowry JA, et al. Pediatric fatality review of the 2013 National Poison Database System (NPDS): focus on intent. *Clin Toxicol (Phila).* 2015;53:79-81.

112. Lubitz DS, et al. A rapid method for estimating weight and resuscitation drug dosages from length in the pediatric age group. *Ann Emerg Med.* 1988;17:576-581.

113. Luten RC, et al. Length-based endotracheal tube and emergency equipment in pediatrics. *Ann Emerg Med.* 1992;21:900-904.

114. Luten RC, et al. The use of the Broselow tape in pediatric resuscitation. *Acad Emerg Med.* 2007;14:500-501; author reply 501-502.

115. Madlon-Kay DJ, Mosch FS. Liquid medication dosing errors. *J Fam Pract.* 2000;49:741-744.

116. Mahieu LM, et al. Imidazoline intoxication in children. *Eur J Pediatr.* 1993;152:944-946.

117. Manikian A, et al. Exchange transfusion in severe infant salicylism. *Vet Hum Toxicol.* 2002;44:224-227.

118. McCarron MM, et al. Diphenoxylate-atropine (Lomotil) overdose in children: an update (report of eight cases and review of the literature). *Pediatrics.* 1991;87:694-700.

119. McFee RB, Caraccio TR. "Hang Up Your Pocketbook"—an easy intervention for the granny syndrome: grandparents as a risk factor in unintentional pediatric exposures to pharmaceuticals. *J Am Osteopath Assoc.* 2006;106:405-411.

120. McGuire TL, Feldman KW. Psychologic morbidity of children subjected to Munchausen syndrome by proxy. *Pediatrics.* 1989;83:289-292.

121. McMahon SR, et al. Parents can dose liquid medication accurately. *Pediatrics.* 1997;100:330-333.

122. Meadow R. Munchausen syndrome by proxy. The hinterland of child abuse. *Lancet.* 1977;2:343-345.

123. Meadow R. Munchausen syndrome by proxy. *Arch Dis Child.* 1982;57:92-98.

124. Medley SR. Acute dialysis children. In: Lerma EV, Weir MR, eds. *Henrich's Principles and Practice of Dialysis.* 5th ed. Philadelphia, PA: Wolters Kluwer; 2017:634-646.

125. Meguerdichian MJ, Clapper TC. The Broselow tape as an effective medication dosing instrument: a review of the literature. *J Pediatr Nurs.* 2012;27:416-420.

126. Miller MA, et al. Delayed clinical decompensation and death after pediatric nifedipine overdose. *Am J Emerg Med.* 2007;25:197-198.

127. Mintegi S, et al. International epidemiological differences in acute poisonings in pediatric emergency departments [published online ahead of print January 24, 2017]. *Pediatr Emerg Care.* doi:10.1097/PEC.0000000000001031.

128. Mirchandani HG, et al. Passive inhalation of free-base cocaine ("crack") smoke by infants. *Arch Pathol Lab Med.* 1991;115:494-498.

129. Monto AS. The disappearance of Reye's syndrome—a public health triumph. *N Engl J Med.* 1999;340:1423-1424.

130. Morrongiello BA, Kiriakou S. Mothers' home-safety practices for preventing six types of childhood injuries: what do they do, and why? *J Pediatr Psychol.* 2004;29:285-297.

131. Nalliah RP, et al. Children in the United States make close to 200,000 emergency department visits due to poisoning each year. *Pediatr Emerg Care.* 2014;30:453-457.

132. Noronha N, et al. The painted shoes. *BMJ Case Rep.* 2015;2015.

133. O'Brien KL, et al. Epidemic of pediatric deaths from acute renal failure caused by diethylene glycol poisoning. Acute Renal Failure Investigation Team. *JAMA.* 1998;279:1175-1180.

134. Oguche S, et al. Pattern of hospital admissions of children with poisoning in the Sudano-Sahelian North eastern Nigeria. *Niger J Clin Pract* 2007;10:111-115.

135. Osborn HH, et al. Theophylline toxicity in a premature neonate—elimination kinetics of exchange transfusion. *J Toxicol Clin Toxicol.* 1993;31:639-644.

136. Paudyal BP. Poisoning: pattern and profile of admitted cases in a hospital in central Nepal. *JNMA J Nepal Med Assoc.* 2005;44:92-96.

137. Pickup JD, Eeles J. Cyanosis in newborn babies caused by aniline-dye poisoning. *Lancet.* 1953;265:118.

138. Polakoff JM, et al. The environment away from home as a source of potential poisoning. *Am J Dis Child.* 1984;138:1014-1017.

139. Quadrani DA, et al. Five year retrospective evaluation of sulfonylurea ingestion in children. *J Toxicol Clin Toxicol.* 1996;34:267-270.

140. Raju TN, et al. Medication errors in neonatal and paediatric intensive-care units. *Lancet.* 1989;2:374-376.

141. Ramisetty-Mikler S, et al. Poisoning hospitalizations among Texas adolescents: age and gender differences in intentional and unintentional injury. *Tex Med.* 2005;101:64-71.

142. Reinhart MA. Child abuse: cocaine absorption by rectal administration. *Clin Pediatr (Phila).* 1990:357.

143. Richards RG, Cravey RH. Infanticide due to ethanolism. *J Analyt Toxicol.* 1978;2:60-61.

144. Rieder MJ, et al. Tenfold errors in drug dosage. *CMAJ.* 1988;139:12-13.

145. Riggs D, Weibley RE. Acute hemorrhagic diarrhea and cardiovascular collapse in a young child owing to environmentally acquired cocaine. *Pediatr Emerg Care.* 1991;7:154-155.

146. Rodgers GB. The safety effects of child-resistant packaging for oral prescription drugs. Two decades of experience. *JAMA.* 1996;275:1661-1665.

147. Rodgers GB. The effectiveness of child-resistant packaging for aspirin. *Arch Pediatr Adolesc Med.* 2002;156:929-933.

148. Rodgers GC Jr, Tenenbein M. The role of aversive bittering agents in the prevention of pediatric poisonings. *Pediatrics.* 1994;93:68-69.

149. Romano MJ, Dinh A. A 1000-fold overdose of clonidine caused by a compounding error in a 5-year-old child with attention-deficit/hyperactivity disorder. *Pediatrics.* 2001;108:471-472.

150. Ros SP, McMannis SI. Are parents accurate in their assessment of fluid volumes? *Pediatr Emerg Care.* 1991;7:204-205.

151. Rosenberg DA. Munchausen syndrome by proxy. In: Reece RM, Christian CW, eds. *Child Abuse: Medical Diagnosis and Management.* 3rd ed. Elk Grove Village, IL: American Academy of Pediatrics; 2009:513-547.

152. Rosenbluth G, Wilson SD. Pediatric and neonatal patients are particularly vulnerable to epinephrine dosing errors. *Ann Emerg Med.* 2010;56:704-705; author reply 705.

153. Ross LM, et al. Medication errors in a paediatric teaching hospital in the UK: five years operational experience. *Arch Dis Child.* 2000;83:492-497.

154. Ryu GS, Lee YJ. Analysis of liquid medication dose errors made by patients and caregivers using alternative measuring devices. *J Manag Care Pharm.* 2012;18:439-445.

155. Schillie SF, et al. Medication overdoses leading to emergency department visits among children. *Am J Prev Med.* 2009;37:181-187.

156. Schreier H. Munchausen by proxy. *Curr Probl Pediatr Adolesc Health Care.* 2004;34:126-143.

157. Schwartz RH, Einhorn A. PCP intoxication in seven young children. *Pediatr Emerg Care.* 1986;2:238-241.

158. Schwartz RH, et al. Intoxication of young children with marijuana: a form of amusement for "pot"-smoking teenage girls. *Am J Dis Child.* 1986;140:326.

159. Selbst SM, et al. Preventing medical errors in pediatric emergency medicine. *Pediatr Emerg Care.* 2004;20:702-709.

160. Shah AN, et al. Effect of an intervention standardization system on pediatric dosing and equipment size determination: a crossover trial involving simulated resuscitation events. *Arch Pediatr Adolesc Med.* 2003;157:229-236.

161. Shannon M, et al. Exchange transfusion in the treatment of severe theophylline poisoning. *Pediatrics.* 1992;89:145-147.

162. Shaw RJ, et al. Factitious disorder by proxy: pediatric condition falsification. *Harv Rev Psychiatry.* 2008;16:215-224.

163. Shoemaker JD, et al. Misidentification of propionic acid as ethylene glycol in a patient with methylmalonic acidemia. *J Pediatr.* 1992;120:417-421.

164. Shone LP. Health literacy and health policy. *Acad Pediatr.* 2012;12:253-254.

165. Shotar AM. Kerosene poisoning in childhood: a 6-year prospective study at the Princess Rahmat Teaching Hospital. *Neuro Endocrinol Lett.* 2005;26:835-838.

166. Sibert JR, Frude N. Bittering agents in the prevention of accidental poisoning: children's reactions to denatonium benzoate (Bitrex). *Arch Emerg Med.* 1991;8:1-7.

167. Sibert R. Stress in families of children who have ingested poisons. *Br Med J.* 1975;3:87-89.

168. Simon HK, Weinkle DA. Over-the-counter medications. Do parents give what they intend to give? *Arch Pediatr Adolesc Med.* 1997;151:654-656.

169. Singh J, et al. Diethylene glycol poisoning in Gurgaon, India, 1998. *Bull World Health Organ.* 2001;79:88-95.

170. Singh J, et al. Acquired methemoglobinemia due to contaminated Holi colors—a rare but preventable complication. *Indian J Pediatr.* 2013;80:351-352.

171. Skinner CG, et al. Melamine toxicity. *J Med Toxicol.* 2010;6:50-55.

172. Slagle MA, et al. Pharmacists' use of safety caps on refilled prescriptions. *Am Pharm.* 1994;NS34:37-40.

173. Sobel R. Traditional safety measures and accidental poisoning in childhood. *Pediatrics.* 1969;44(suppl):811-816.

174. Sobel R. The psychiatric implications of accidental poisoning in childhood. *Pediatr Clin North Am.* 1970;17:653-685.

175. Soghoian S, et al. Unintentional i.v. injection of barium sulfate in a child. *Am J Health Syst Pharm.* 2010;67:734-736.

176. Solomon SL, et al. Medication errors with inhalant epinephrine mimicking an epidemic of neonatal sepsis. *N Engl J Med.* 1984;310:166-170.

177. Sousa CN, et al. Haemodialysis for children under the age of two years. *J Ren Care.* 2008;34:9-13.

178. Stein D. Infant Hemodialysis. In: Nissenson AR, Fine RN, eds. *Handbook of Dialysis Therapy.* 5th ed. Philadelphia, PA: Elsevier; 2017:877-881.

179. Stucky ER. Prevention of medication errors in the pediatric inpatient setting. *Pediatrics.* 2003;112:431-436.

180. Szlatenyi CS, et al. Delayed hypoglycemia in a child after ingestion of a single glipizide tablet. *Ann Emerg Med.* 1998;31:773-776.

181. Tenenbein M. Pediatric toxicology: current controversies and recent advances. *Curr Probl Pediatr.* 1986;16:185-233.

182. Thompson JN. Corrosive esophageal injuries. I. A study of nine cases of concurrent accidental caustic ingestion. *Laryngoscope.* 1987;97:1060-1068.

183. Trinkoff AM, Baker SP. Poisoning hospitalizations and deaths from solids and liquids among children and teenagers. *Am J Public Health.* 1986;76:657-660.

184. Tzimenatos L, Bond GR. Severe injury or death in young children from therapeutic errors: a summary of 238 cases from the American Association of Poison Control Centers. *Clin Toxicol (Phila).* 2009;47:348-354.

185. Vincer MJ, et al. Drug errors and incidents in a neonatal intensive care unit. A quality assurance activity. *Am J Dis Child.* 1989;143:737-740.

186. Viscusi WK. Consumer behavior and the safety effects of product safety regulation. *J Law Econ.* 1985;28:527-554.

187. Wallace H. Deaths due to elixir of sulfanilamide-massengill: report of secretary of agriculture submitted in response to house resolution 352 of Nov. 18, 1937, and senate resolution 194 of Nov. 16, 1937. *JAMA.* 1937;109:1985-1988.

188. Wang GS, et al. Association of unintentional pediatric exposures with decriminalization of marijuana in the United States. *Ann Emerg Med.* 2014;63:684-689.

189. Wears R, Leape LL. Human error in emergency medicine. *Ann Emerg Med.* 1999;34:370-372.

190. Weisman RS, Goldfrank L. Poison center numbers. *J Toxicol Clin Toxicol.* 1991;29:553-557.

191. Welch MJ, Correa GA. PCP intoxication in young children and infants. *Clin Pediatr (Phila).* 1980;19:510-514.

192. West L. Innovative approaches to the administration of activated charcoal in pediatric toxic ingestions. *Pediatr Nurs.* 1997;23:616-619.

193. Wiley JF 2nd, et al. Clonidine poisoning in young children. *J Pediatr.* 1990;116:654-658.

194. Wilson DG, et al. Medication errors in paediatric practice: insights from a continuous quality improvement approach. *Eur J Pediatr.* 1998;157:769-774.

195. Wiseman HM, et al. Accidental poisoning in childhood: a multicentre survey. 2. The role of packaging in accidents involving medications. *Hum Toxicol.* 1987;6:303-314.

196. Wood JN, et al. Evaluation and referral for child maltreatment in pediatric poisoning victims. *Child Abuse Negl.* 2012;36:362-369.

197. Woolf A, et al. Costs of poison-related hospitalizations at an urban teaching hospital for children. *Arch Pediatr Adolesc Med.* 1997;151:719-723.

198. Yin HS, et al. Randomized controlled trial of a pictogram-based intervention to reduce liquid medication dosing errors and improve adherence among caregivers of young children. *Arch Pediatr Adolesc Med.* 2008;162:814-822.

199. Yin HS, et al. Use of a pictographic diagram to decrease parent dosing errors with infant acetaminophen: a health literacy perspective. *Acad Pediatr.* 2011;11:50-57.

200. Yin HS, et al. Parents' medication administration errors: role of dosing instruments and health literacy. *Arch Pediatr Adolesc Med.* 2010;164:181-186.

201. Yin HS, et al. Health literacy assessment of labeling of pediatric nonprescription medications: examination of characteristics that may impair parent understanding. *Acad Pediatr.* 2012;12:288-296.

202. Yin HS, et al. Evaluation of consistency in dosing directions and measuring devices for pediatric nonprescription liquid medications. *JAMA.* 2010;304:2595-2602.

203. Yin S. Malicious use of pharmaceuticals in children. *J Pediatr.* 2010;157:832-836.e1.

204. Yin S. Malicious use of nonpharmaceuticals in children. *Child Abuse Negl.* 2011;35:924-929.

205. Zuckerman BS, Duby JC. Developmental approach to injury prevention. *Pediatr Clin North Am.* 1985;32:17-29.

CASE STUDY 6

History A 78-year-old man presents to the emergency department after his family found him to be acutely confused. The family states that he was in his usual state of health until one day prior to presentation. The patient had not complained of nausea, vomiting, diarrhea, or abdominal pain. The family is unaware of any new medications that the patient might have been prescribed or any new exposures.

Physical Examination On presentation to the emergency department, the patient appeared confused and disoriented. Blood pressure, 140/70 mmHg, pulse, 115 beats/min, respiratory rate, 26 breaths/min; oxygen saturation, 94% on room air, and tympanic temperature 38.2°C (100.8°F). The physical examination demonstrated dry mucous membranes and clear lung sounds with crackles at the bases; his neurologic examination was nonfocal. He was not following commands, but appeared to be moving all extremities with equal strength.

Initial Management Given the elevated temperature and the confusion, the medical team was concerned that the patient's delirium had an infectious etiology the point of care glucose was normal, and they ordered a noncontrast head CT, chest radiograph, venous blood gas with a lactate concentration, basic metabolic panel, hepatic function tests, a complete blood count, urinalysis, and blood and urine cultures. The patient was empirically started on broad-spectrum antibiotics; and 1 L of 0.9% sodium chloride solution was administered intravenously over 30 minutes. Pertinent laboratory results included a urinalysis with 1+ leukocyte esterase and trace ketones and basic metabolic panel with an anion gap of 18 mEq/L. The blood gas analysis revealed a pH 7.46, PCO_2 22 mm Hg, HCO_3^- 14 mEq/L, and lactate 3.5 mmol/L.

What Is the Differential Diagnosis? Confusion and delirium are common reasons for elderly patients to present to the emergency department. Often, an infection is the etiology for the acute onset of delirium. However, older patients often suffer from several chronic conditions, and are taking multiple medications, enhancing the risk of drug-induced adverse effects, including drug-induced delirium. Furthermore, some patients have underlying dementia and can inadvertently take too much of their own medication (Chap. 32).

In recent years, there has been an increase in the prevalence of illicit substance abuse and prescription drug misuse in the older population, which, along with alcohol misuse, may be clinically unrecognized. In patients who present with confusion, elevated temperature, tachycardia, and hypertension, it is important consider ethanol withdrawal in the differential diagnosis (Chap. 77). A full drug history should include prescription and nonprescription items, and non-oral drugs, including drug-releasing patches. Numerous drugs are available as transdermal patches, and incorrect use, such as application of multiple patches, can lead to toxicity. Therefore, the patient must fully undress and be placed in a gown for a thorough physical evaluation. Anticholinergic patches are common as a treatment for vertigo and motion sickness (Chap. 49). Patients who have signs of anticholinergic toxicity can present with an altered sensorium and an elevated temperature, which can initially be mistaken for sepsis.

What Clinical and Laboratory Analyses Help Explain the Causes of This Patient's Presentation? A geriatric patient who presents with confusion should be evaluated for medical causes of delirium. A thorough patient history and physical examination can frequently reveal the cause of the patient's altered mental status and, therefore, should direct the laboratory evaluation. In general, the physician should order serum electrolytes and glucose urinalysis, blood and urine cultures, and a chest radiograph in patients with fever, as well as an electrocardiogram. In patients who have an unexplained altered mental status, a lumbar puncture is indicated to evaluate for meningitis and encephalitis. If no obvious infection is found to explain delirium, and there is inadequate reason to diagnose anticholinergic toxicity, a salicylate concentration should be ordered (Chap. 37).

Chronic salicylate toxicity is much more frequently missed than acute toxicity. Often, elderly patients with chronic salicylism are misdiagnosed with a delirium that is undifferentiated or of unclear etiology and admitted with a diagnosis such as delirium of unclear etiology, resulting in a significant delay in initiating the appropriate therapy. The mortality associated with chronic salicylate toxicity is higher than acute salicylate toxicity. Therefore, in elderly patients who present with a new delirium of unclear etiology, the physician should closely review of the anion gap and blood gas; for example, this patient's mixed picture of metabolic acidosis and respiratory alkalosis might point to potential salicylate toxicity (Chap. 7).

Further Diagnosis and Treatment In this patient, a presumptive diagnosis of urosepsis was initially made. The patient was admitted to the hospital and was continued on antibiotics. After being in the hospital for 2 days, the patient was persistently agitated and delirious, at which point a neurology consult was obtained. At that time, the family revealed that the patient had been complaining of worsening arthritis pain and had been taking aspirin to treat the pain. A salicylate concentration was ordered, and it was found to be significantly elevated at 58 mg/dL. The patient received a sodium bicarbonate bolus and was started on a sodium bicarbonate infusion was begun (Antidotes in depth: A5). In view of the patient's altered mental status, a nephrology consult was also obtained and the patient underwent dialysis (Chap. 6). The patient improved, his mental status cleared, and he was discharged home. The family and the patient were counseled regarding safe practices for storage and administration of medication.

32 GERIATRIC PRINCIPLES

Michael E. Stern, Judith C. Ahronheim, and Mary Ann Howland

PREVALENCE, LETHALITY, AND UNDERRECOGNITION OF TOXIC EXPOSURE

The population is aging steadily across the world. In the United States, people older than 65 years of age comprise an increasing proportion of the population at large (14.5%), and those 85 years and older represent the fastest growing segment of the population.[3] The elderly also comprise an increasing proportion of patients cared for in multiple medical settings, not the least of which is the emergency department (ED) setting. As a result of continuing advances in health education, technology, and pharmacotherapy, many people are living longer. Long life is associated with an increased disease burden. The aging of the "baby boomer" generation (people born between 1946 and 1964) is rapidly changing the medical landscape. Compared with all other age groups, patients 65 years of age and older account for 16% of the total population of patients who visit an ED, one-third of ED ambulance arrivals, and the highest proportion of patients in EDs triaged as emergent.[32] Moreover, this population represents the highest number of hospital and intensive care unit admissions.[159]

Although the elderly account for only a small minority of toxicologic exposures, when exposed, they have a high overall mortality rate. Among exposures reported to the American Association of Poison Control Centers (AAPCC), the fatality ratio for adults (ie, number of cases divided by number of deaths) exhibits a bimodal pattern, declining after age 30 until age 60, when it again rises (Chap. 130).

The factors associated with the increased fatality ratio after age 60 are complex, but are likely due in part to physiologic vulnerability. The geriatric population is physiologically heterogeneous, encumbering research that seeks to differentiate "normal" senescence from changes that occur as a result of disease. This heterogeneity is pertinent to clinical response to xenobiotics, variability of pharmacokinetics, and recovery from exogenous insults, such as adverse drug effects and toxicologic emergencies.

Exposures reported to the AAPCC underestimate the serious consequences for elderly people exposed to xenobiotics that are toxic or potentially toxic. Data from the National Electronic Injury Surveillance System–Cooperative Adverse Drug Event Surveillance Project (NEISS-CADES) indicate that patients aged 65 years and older accounted for 25% of estimated visits related to adverse drug events (ADEs), with almost 50% of such visits requiring hospitalization or prolonged monitoring in the ED during 2004–2005.[20] Furthermore, the incidence of ADEs increases steeply from age 65 years through the tenth decade of life.[20] More recent NEISS-CADES data indicate that almost 50% of elders who required emergency hospitalization as a result of ADEs are 80 years of age or older.[19] Finally, the problem is likely even greater than the NEISS-CADES study suggests, because their data did not capture ADEs in patients treated or dying outside of EDs, ADEs that could only have been recognized after admission, or that were erroneously diagnosed as non–drug-related problems. A better understanding of the specific contributions of overall disease burden in elderly patients and, in particular, the role of high-risk medications to ED presentations of geriatric syndromes, will also produce data that more accurately reflect the scope of the problem.[86]

In one study, 7 specific pharmaceuticals were selected from the AAPCC database for analysis based on their prevalent use and potential toxicity from 1995 through 2002. These pharmaceuticals were theophylline, digoxin, benzodiazepines, cyclic antidepressants (CAs), calcium channel blockers, acetaminophen (APAP), and salicylates.[154] The death rate from intentional or unintentional exposure to these 7 pharmaceuticals increased by 35% for each decade of life after age 19 years. Although prescribing patterns change over time, most of these drugs, as well as many others, continue to pose problems for patients in the latest decades of life.[20,82] Problems such as these have been accompanied by continuous and longstanding input from geriatric organizations and professionals,[162] and a series of published guidelines with regard to prescribing, namely the "Beers Criteria" governing potentially inappropriate medications (PIMs)[8,15] and "STOPP/START."[64,139] Still, there remains a limited understanding of PIMs across all provider types, that continues to result in increased morbidity and mortality in geriatric patients. For example, despite cautionary guidelines, benzodiazepine prescribing for older adults in both ambulatory clinics and EDs did not change from 2001 to 2010, and in the oldest individuals, aged 85 and older, who are at highest risk of adverse events, there was an increase in benzodiazepine use.[126] Providers other than geriatricians, by whom and toward whom these guidelines were developed and directed, often lack knowledge of their existence. To that end, several organizations have made efforts to promulgate the published criteria for a broader number of practitioners.[4,56,156]

Toxic exposures in the elderly are underrecognized in the clinical setting for a number of reasons. First, because of pharmacokinetic and pharmacodynamic changes that occur with aging,[11,44] a standard adult dose, even when associated with a "therapeutic" serum concentration, can produce an unexpected, serious effect that goes unrecognized by the clinician. Second, the presentation of disease, including xenobiotic toxicity, is often deemed "atypical" in the elderly,[94] although in geriatric practice, many "atypical" presentations constitute classic geriatric syndromes. Geriatric syndromes include, among others, falls[123] and delirium,[91] which have a multiplicity of causes, but in the elderly are common presenting signs of xenobiotic toxicity. In the case of falls, sedative–hypnotics, opioids, antipsychotics, antidepressants, and certain cardiovascular medications are among the most often implicated.[60,145,155,179] Even the antidementia cholinesterase inhibitors are implicated (though less commonly) because of their potential to cause bradycardia in patients at risk.[144] If the patient is cognitively impaired and the fall is unwitnessed, when the immediate consequences of the fall are addressed (eg, fracture or rhabdomyolysis), the xenobiotic or other primary etiology causing it is often neglected.[109] Delirium, likewise, is a common presentation of xenobiotic toxicity.[78,91] A large variety of xenobiotics cause mental status changes that are mistakenly attributed to non–xenobiotic-related causes in the elderly.[173] Conversely, altered mental status as a manifestation of delirium frequently goes unrecognized[88,120] or misdiagnosed, for example, as Alzheimer disease or psychiatric illness.[151] A striking case of drug-induced mental status changes is represented by a previously normal 66-year-old man who developed psychosis and attempted suicide after taking increasing doses of dextromethorphan-containing cough syrup for a respiratory infection. The patient was treated with psychiatric medications, and several months elapsed before providers realized that his behavior was xenobiotic-induced rather than due to a primary psychiatric condition.[128]

Finally, in some circumstances, the presentation of drug toxicity is delayed in elderly individuals. Drugs with long half-lives often take days to reach a steady state and hence do not achieve peak effects until days after the drug therapy is initiated. In some older patients, the active metabolite of flurazepam, desalkylflurazepam, has a half-life of up to 100 hours or longer, which requires weeks to achieve a steady state.[72] When peak effects are delayed in this manner, xenobiotic toxicities are easily mistaken for non–xenobiotic-related illnesses.

Table 32–1 lists xenobiotics commonly responsible for toxicity in the elderly.

TABLE 32–1	Xenobiotics That Pose an Increased Risk of Toxicity in the Elderly[a]

Anticholinergics and antispasmodics
Anticoagulants and platelet inhibitors
Antidepressants
Antidiabetics
Antipsychotics
Antiparkinsons
Benzodiazepines and other sedative–hypnotics
Cardiovascular medications
    β-Adrenergic antagonists
    Calcium channel blockers
    Digoxin
    Peripheral α_1-adrenergic receptor antagonists
Ethanol
Magnesium- and phosphate-containing laxatives
Metoclopramide
Nonsteroidal antiinflammatory drugs
Opioids
Proton-pump inhibitors (chronic use)
Salicylates
Skeletal muscle relaxants

[a]List is consistent with "Beers" Criteria for which recommendations regarding caution are "strong," as supported by "moderate" quality of evidence or greater.[8]

PHARMACOKINETICS

Age-related pharmacokinetic changes have important clinical implications for elderly patients, with certain processes having greater or more consistent impact (eg, renal elimination) than others.

Absorption

In general, absorption of xenobiotics does not decline significantly with age, but specific examples serve to highlight some age-associated impact. For example, a decline in gastric alcohol dehydrogenase activity increases the bioavailability of ingested ethanol in the elderly.[147] The decline in this enzyme is attributed to an increased incidence of gastric atrophy that occurs with age, and which is associated with underlying *Helicobacter pylori* infection, an increase in antiparietal cell antibodies, and age-associated decline in gastric blood flow and overall mucosal function.[50,169,205] Whether age-related changes occur in metabolic enzymes that are present in the intestines, brain, kidneys, and other organ systems and what impact such changes have on drug disposition and drug interactions remain open questions. The precise

contributions of age-related changes in the gastric and intestinal tract (eg, alteration in gastric pH and a decrease in small bowel surface area) to xenobiotic absorption are not adequately determined. Delayed gastric emptying leads to delayed intestinal absorption of certain xenobiotics, but changes in direct absorption of pharmaceuticals are not substantial enough to have an important clinical impact on overall bioavailability. Xenobiotic-to-xenobiotic interactions likely play the main role in decreased bioavailability in the elderly.

P-glycoprotein (P-gp), a transmembrane transport protein involved in xenobiotic interactions and movement in the kidneys, intestines, and other organs, has been widely studied. Limited research on the impact of aging suggests a decline in P-gp activity, but this has not been a consistent finding.[18,191] Studies more consistently demonstrate an age-associated diminished P-gp expression at the blood–brain barrier,[13,33,186,192,193] a decrease that is inversely related to the degree of amyloid in the brain.[33,192,193] This suggests that diminished P-gp activity is associated with reduced efflux of beta-amyloid protein, leading to its accumulation in the brain, arguably playing a role in the pathogenesis of Alzheimer disease. Positron emission tomography (PET) studies of normal humans and those with Alzheimer disease, using radiolabeled verapamil, a P-gp substrate, demonstrate decreased P-gp activity as represented by increased volume of distribution of verapamil in the brain.[13,185,186] Noting that the altered pharmacokinetics in such studies resembles that of P-gp inhibition of xenobiotics explored in therapeutic drug research (eg, to enhance CNS penetration of antiepileptics in refractory seizures), researchers raise the possibility that an age-associated reduction in P-gp activity could also be responsible for enhanced CNS effects of various xenobiotics in the elderly.[185] More research is needed to explore the neurotoxic implications of chronic P-gp deficiency,[33,109] as well as its role in enhanced sensitivity that elderly patients exhibit to numerous xenobiotics, an enduring problem accounting for a very high proportion of ADEs in that population, with serious clinical ramifications.

Distribution

Age-related alterations in body composition affects xenobiotic disposition in later life (Table 32–2). For example, lean muscle mass and total body water decline, and the fat-to-lean ratio increases with advancing age.[108,137] Thus, highly lipid-soluble xenobiotics tend to have an increased volume of distribution (V_d). As a result, there is often a delay before steady state is reached, and peak effect and toxicity typically occur later than expected, as demonstrated with amiodarone and certain benzodiazepines. In contrast, xenobiotics that distribute in water, such as ethanol, have a smaller V_d, leading to higher peak concentrations and potential toxicity. This accounts, at least in part, for the more pronounced peak effect of ethanol in the elderly and for the increased blood alcohol concentration (BAC) attained in an older adult who drinks an equivalent amount of ethanol compared to a younger person.[180,189]

TABLE 32–2	Pharmacokinetic Considerations in the Elderly		
	Young	Elderly	Effect on Kinetics
Fat (% of body weight)	15	↑30	↑V_d for xenobiotics distributing to fat (amitriptyline, diazepam)
Intracellular water (% of body weight)	42	↓30	↓V_d for water soluble xenobiotics
Muscle (% of body weight)	17	↓12	↓V_d for xenobiotics distributing into lean tissue (APAP, caffeine, digoxin, ethanol)
Albumin (g/dL)	≥4	↓With acute or chronic illness	↑Free concentrations of xenobiotics if >90% bound to albumin, especially in overdose; interpretation of serum concentration altered
Liver	Normal	↓Size ↓Hepatic blood flow	Liver enzymes not predictive of compromise; concentrations of xenobiotics with high extraction (propranolol, triazolam) may increase; ↓hepatic oxidation (diazepam, chlordiazepoxide)
Kidney	Normal	↓Renal blood flow ↓GFR ↓Tubular secretion	↑Accumulation (lithium, aminoglycosides, N-acetyl procainamide, ACE inhibitors, cimetidine, digoxin, opioid metabolites)

ACE = angiotensin-converting enzyme; APAP = acetaminophen; GFR = glomerular filtration rate; V_d = volume of distribution.

Protein reserve diminishes with age as a consequence of decreased muscle mass and decreased protein synthesis.[150] Although serum albumin concentration remains in the normal range in healthy elderly individuals,[26] elderly people are more likely to experience a rapid decrease in albumin concentrations when experiencing acute or chronic illness or when their protein intake diminishes.[45,203] A decline in serum protein concentration increases the free or active fraction of xenobiotics that are otherwise highly protein bound. Free xenobiotic is able to travel more readily to the liver and kidney for metabolism or excretion, so a gradual change in the serum protein concentration is unlikely to lead to a change in the patient's overall response to the xenobiotic. However, these changes are clinically important for interpreting serum concentrations of highly protein-bound xenobiotics. Clinical laboratories typically measure total xenobiotic concentrations, which include both free and bound xenobiotic. Because most xenobiotic is bound, the reported value reflects mostly bound xenobiotic; therefore, the total xenobiotic concentration often is in the therapeutic range even though the active unbound fraction is actually elevated. Phenytoin, which is highly bound to albumin, serves as an illustrative example. If the serum concentration of phenytoin is reported as subtherapeutic, the physician might order a dose increase even though the free fraction of phenytoin actually is in the therapeutic range. With a dose increase, the free or active fraction increases to toxic concentrations. Basic xenobiotics are not bound to albumin but to α1-acid glycoprotein, an acute-phase reactant that tends to increase, rather than decrease, with age.[1] However, the increase attributed to age is most likely related to underlying disease. These unpredictable changes would be expected to have the reverse effect on the ratio of bound to unbound xenobiotic in any laboratory report. However, the correlation between clinical effect and free xenobiotic concentrations requires further study because of the complex factors involved—for example, alterations in V_d, tissue-specific xenobiotic concentrations, changes to the number of protein-binding sites, and the contribution of other serum proteins to xenobiotic binding.

Hepatic Metabolism

The nature of age-associated changes in hepatic metabolism and their impact on xenobiotic elimination is controversial. A decline in functional hepatocyte number occurs with age. This reduction in liver mass is accompanied by a decrease in hepatic blood flow,[200] which results in decreased efficiency of hepatic extraction. Drugs with a high extraction ratio are dependent on liver blood flow and are most affected (eg, lidocaine; propranolol). This diminished hepatic extraction results in delayed clearance of xenobiotics, particularly those that undergo extensive first-pass hepatic metabolism when orally administered, thus increasing their potential toxicity (eg, calcium channel blockers, certain beta adrenergic antagonists, morphine). Enzymatic processes themselves are less predictable.[104] Aging appears to affect the synthetic enzymatic phase 2 reactions (conjugation) less than the nonsynthetic hepatic biotransformation phase 1 reactions (eg, oxidative, others) (Chap. 11). There is substantial genetic variability among cytochrome P450 enzymes, making it difficult to interpret studies of age-related alterations in phase 1. Studies that account for confounding factors that could affect those enzymes, such as concurrent xenobiotics or cigarette smoking, or that account for isoenzyme genotype, fail to fully demonstrate an age-related change in hepatic oxidative enzyme function.[17]

Hepatic conjugation does not decline significantly with age, so xenobiotics such as lorazepam and temazepam that are metabolized by these processes do not have prolonged elimination half-lives. In contrast, xenobiotics such as diazepam and flurazepam, which are metabolized by hepatic oxidative enzymes, are eliminated more slowly with age.[72] Similar to many oxidized xenobiotics, metabolites of diazepam and flurazepam are active, undergo further metabolism, and remain in circulation after the parent xenobiotic has been metabolized. The active metabolites of some xenobiotics, such as opioids, are renally eliminated, and excretion is prolonged because of an age-related decline in kidney function (Table 32–3).

Regardless of duration of action, however, benzodiazepines, opioids, and various other xenobiotics must be used with caution in the elderly because

TABLE 32–3	Xenobiotics with Narrow Therapeutic-to-Toxic Ratios and Potential for Accumulation in the Presence of Diminished Kidney Function

Anticoagulants
    Apixaban
    Dabigatran
    Heparins (low-molecular-weight)
    Rivaroxaban
Antimicrobials
    Aminoglycosides
    Imipenem
    Pyrazinamide
    Vancomycin
Digoxin
DPP-4 inhibitors (Gliptins)
Gabapentin
Glyburide
Lithium
Metformin
Methotrexate
Nonsteroidal antiinflammatory drugs
Opioids with active metabolites that cause toxicity
    Morphine (morphine 6-glucuronide): respiratory depression, oversedation (morphine 3 glucuronide): neuroexcitation
    Codeine (morphine)
    Hydromorphone (hydromorphone 3-glucuronide): potential for neuroexcitation
    Meperidine (normeperidine: neuroexcitation, seizures)
Procainamide (N-acetyl procainamide metabolites)
Salicylates

of their enhanced effect even at low doses and even at onset of action (see Pharmacodynamics, below).

Renal Function and Occult Reduction in Glomerular Filtration Rate

The most consistent age-associated pharmacokinetic change is a decline in glomerular filtration rate (GFR). Glomerular filtration rate declines, on the average, by 50% between the ages of 30 and 80 years,[48,157] with an accelerated decline in the last decades of life.[124,157] However, serum creatinine does not rise in parallel with the reduction of GFR, because lean body muscle mass, the source of serum creatinine, declines with age.[108,137] Therefore, serum creatinine is an unreliable marker of renal function in older adults and cannot be expected to accurately predict the renal elimination of xenobiotics or their metabolites in the elderly.

Numerous authors have reviewed the large body of existing research regarding age-related renal changes, and the limitations of cross-sectional and longitudinal data of healthy and nonhealthy subjects.[11,49,69] Studies focus on measured or estimated glomerular filtration rate,[48,124,157] microanatomy of cadaver kidneys,[69] biopsy of kidneys from healthy older organ donors,[158] and anti-aging gene expression.[52] Still, because of the heterogeneity of the aging population, research has not yet identified a precise "senescent" change separate from changes due to disease. For example, despite a virtual universality of "nephrosclerosis"[69] among those older than 85 years, this complex of anatomic and histologic findings does not correlate with declines in GFR.[158]

Because it is impractical, often difficult, and arguably of questionable value to measure GFR before instituting therapy with a renally excreted xenobiotic, clinicians commonly (eGFR) using age-adjusted formulas based on serum creatinine, or on cystatin C, a nonmuscle-based protein.[36,118] However, age-related declines in GFR are not universal, and limited data from longitudinal studies suggest that as many as 33% of elderly individuals do not experience this age-related decline.[122,157] Modifications of predictive formulas to correct for body surface area[89,165] and obesity[198] are offered to better reflect kidney function, but anthropomorphic measurements are unreliable in the elderly,[105,170] and physiologic variability is great. Conversely, predictive formulas could significantly overestimate actual GFR in chronically ill, debilitated elderly people, including those with chronic kidney disease (CKD),[112] or inappropriately label robust older adults as having a potentially progressive form of CKD when they do not.[68] Current consensus guidelines for estimating GFR play a large role in research studies and in predicting outcomes in adults with chronic kidney disease,[90,118] but their accuracy in the oldest subjects has been criticized, given the paucity of studies involving or focusing on elderly subjects,[68,146] and remains controversial.[68,119] To overcome the limitations inherent in using an age-heterogeneous cohort, alternate methods of estimating GFR have been offered, based on a cohort of apparently healthy subjects 70 years of age and older (mean age 78).[146,160] An estimate using such a cohort would arguably incorporate age-appropriate normative values for serum creatinine and cystatin C, both of which exhibit non-GFR alterations that would be more prevalent in an elderly population.

The pertinent question here, however, is how to make decisions about "renal" dosing for elderly patients, whether they are apparently healthy or appear ill and debilitated. To this end, a practical approach is called for.

We suggest that the clinician:

1. Recognize that mild to moderate reduced kidney function in the elderly is typically occult, masked by a normal or even low serum creatinine. This problem is enhanced in older adults who are frail or chronically ill.

2. Exercise great caution when prescribing maintenance doses of renally eliminated medications that have a narrow therapeutic index (Table 32–3).

3. Follow therapeutic concentrations of renally excreted xenobiotics when appropriate and available, recognizing that "trough" concentrations are only accurate once steady state is reached, and a steady state will be unexpectedly delayed in an elderly patient whose reduced kidney function is occult.

Failure to exercise caution in these cases is an important iatrogenic cause of toxicity.[117]

PHARMACODYNAMICS

Pharmacodynamic factors also affect a patient's response to a particular xenobiotic. In general, age-related physiologic changes in target or nontarget organs lead to increased sensitivity to most xenobiotics, although sensitivity to some xenobiotics is also decreased. For example, experimental evidence demonstrates that the sensitivity of the β-adrenergic receptor declines with aging, leading to a diminished response to both β-adrenergic agonists and antagonists.[39,58,190] However, these experimental findings are not necessarily demonstrated clinically.[9,10] Observed enhanced sensitivity to xenobiotics is probably due to altered pharmacokinetics in many, if not most, cases.[75] Proving that enhanced sensitivity is related to altered pharmacodynamics would require demonstrating that the concentration of xenobiotic at the tissue site was not increased as the result of diminished elimination. Nonetheless, the clinical response to many xenobiotics is altered in diverse ways among the elderly, because of age-related changes and the presence of disease in the target or a nontarget organ.[35,75] Table 32–4 provides examples of pathologic or physiologic changes that frequently occur in the elderly and disorders that are worsened or unmasked by xenobiotics.

UNINTENTIONAL POISONING, ADVERSE DRUG EVENTS, AND THERAPEUTIC ERRORS

Although the elderly account for numerically far fewer reported poisonings overall, the exposure rate per 100,000 population remains substantial (Chap. 130). The contribution of adverse drug events (ADEs) and therapeutic errors pose a particular problem for older patients and are an important part of poisoning analysis.[154]

The incidence of ADEs among adults increases steadily with age; it is at least twice as high among those aged 65 years and older compared to younger patients,[20] and is highest of all in those aged 80 years and older.[20,84] An ADE refers to "an unwanted event that occurs with normal, prescribed, labeled or

TABLE 32–4	Pathophysiologic Disorders Exacerbated or Unmasked by Xenobiotics in the Elderly[a]	
Disorder or Alteration	**Drug**	**Possible Outcome**
ADH secretion (increased)	Antipsychotics, SSRIs	Hyponatremia
Androgenic hormones (decreased in men)	Digoxin, spironolactone	Gynecomastia
Baroreceptor dysfunction, venous insufficiency	Antipsychotics, diuretics, TCAs, α₁-adrenergic antagonists	Orthostatic hypotension
Bladder dysfunction	Diuretics, α₁-adrenergic antagonists	Incontinence
Cardiac disease	Thiazolidinediones	Congestive heart failure
Dementia	Sedatives, anticholinergics, many others	Confusion
Gastritis (atrophic)	NSAIDs, salicylates	Gastric hemorrhage
Immobility, cathartic bowel	Anticholinergics, cholinesterase inhibitors opioids, CCBs	Constipation; fecal impaction
Nodal disease (sinus or AV)	β-Adrenergic antagonists, CCBs, digoxin	Bradycardia
Parkinson disease; Lewy body dementia	Antipsychotics, metoclopramide	Parkinsonism
Prostatic hyperplasia	Anticholinergics, CAs, disopyramide	Urinary retention
Thermoregulation, disordered	Antipsychotics	Hypo- or hyperthermia
Venous insufficiency	CCBs, gabapentin	Edema

[a]Disorder often preclinical before drug started.

ADH = antidiuretic hormone; AV = atrioventricular; CCB = calcium channel blocker; DPP-4 = dipeptidyl peptidase-4; NSAID = nonsteroidal antiinflammatory drug; SSRI = selective serotonin reuptake inhibitor; CA = cyclic antidepressants.

recommended use of the drug" (Chap. 134). Adverse drug events are more likely to be serious in the elderly than in younger adults. Serious ADEs, that is, those resulting in death, hospitalization, life-threatening outcome, disability, or other serious outcomes, are most prevalent among people 85 years of age and older.[23] Adverse drug events in persons older than 60 years are often the result of therapeutic errors.[37,47,82] A therapeutic error is defined as "an unintentional deviation from a proper therapeutic regimen that results in the wrong dose, incorrect route of administration, administration to the wrong person, or administration of the wrong substance"; therapeutic errors also include "unintentional administration of drugs or foods that are known to interact" (Chap. 134). In the NEISS-CADES study, unintentional overdoses (defined as "excessive doses or supratherapeutic drug effects") accounted for 65.7% of ADE-related hospitalizations in older adults.[19]

Many serious ADEs reported in elderly patients are potentially preventable.[76,77,100] The NEISS-CADES data reveal that drugs requiring careful outpatient monitoring are disproportionately represented among ED visits attributed to unintentional drug overdose.[19,21] Data from 2007 to 2009 indicate that warfarin, insulins, antiplatelet drugs, and antidiabetics accounted for an estimated 67% of ADE-related hospitalizations in people 65 years of age and older, with digoxin and anticonvulsants contributing another 5.2%.[21] Furthermore, ADEs, many of which are preventable, are common shortly after hospital discharge.[100]

For certain medications, ADEs are often best prevented by not prescribing them to vulnerable patients (or if essential, prescribing with great caution and careful monitoring), and by cautioning against their use if they are available without prescription. Criteria that guide clinicians regarding PIMs in elderly patients are periodically updated, and serve to enable the prescribing clinician to appraise the regimen in the context of the patient's concurrent diagnoses and then alert the prescriber to more appropriate treatment choices. Although PIMs cause numerically fewer ADEs than more frequently prescribed xenobiotics,[19,21] consensus as well as evidence exist that they are still strongly associated with adverse outcomes in elderly patients, including hospitalization and mortality.[61,99,114] Potentially inappropriate medications are also linked to enhanced risk of specific ADEs. For example, the elderly are at enhanced risk of severe upper gastrointestinal (GI) bleeding[199] and adverse cardiovascular outcomes due to NSAIDs.[187] Although this could be explained partly by increased exposure to and regular use of these drugs for chronic conditions, older adults are particularly vulnerable because of underlying atrophic gastritis, and silent or overt cardiovascular disease, respectively, which can be unmasked by exposure to the NSAID. Similarly, elderly diabetics are at enhanced risk of developing heart failure from certain antidiabetics. For example, thiazolidinediones, which promote fluid retention by enhancing renal sodium absorption, are contraindicated in advanced heart failure but can unmask abnormal cardiac function in elderly patients with apparently silent disease.[136,167] The elderly are also at greater risk of prolonged hypoglycemia from certain sulfonylureas, particularly glyburide.[166] Age-related mechanisms to explain this vulnerability to glyburide include a decreased counterregulatory hormonal response to xenobiotic-induced hypoglycemia,[131] inappropriate stimulation of insulin if hypoglycemia is present,[174] or reduced excretion of a renally eliminated active metabolite of glyburide.[97] Last, but not least, anticholinergics are also problematic, causing confusion in patients with preclinical or overt dementia, and, particularly in men, causing urinary retention due to underlying BPH.[99] Other age-related factors involved in enhanced susceptibility to ADEs are given in Tables 32–2 and 32–4.

Precautionary admonitions notwithstanding, guidelines are meant to enhance physician prescribing choices and in no way replace rigorous clinical judgement in any individual patient.

In contrast to serious consequences of therapeutic errors or unintentional overdoses, serious reactions occur even with appropriate doses of certain medications. An important example is the neuroleptic malignant syndrome (NMS), which is potentially life threatening. Although the risk of developing NMS has not been linked to advanced age per se,[29] antipsychotics are often prescribed to frail elderly, such as those with dementia, and NMS can be overlooked in a patient with comorbidities that could obscure a precise diagnosis, such as cerebrovascular events, heat stroke, or antipsychotic sensitivity syndrome,[29] or be diagnosed as akinetic crisis, which it closely resembles.[141] However, the clinical distinction is less important than the need for the prescriber to exercise extreme caution before using antipsychotics in patients at high risk such as those with Parkinson disease or Lewy body dementia.[65,164]

ADVERSE DRUG EVENTS: RECOGNIZING RISK AND AVOIDING PITFALLS

In addition to physiologic changes that influence xenobiotic disposition or effect, multiple factors contribute to the high risk of ADEs in older adults. Importantly, many of these factors can be foreseen and prevented, and are reviewed in detail here.

Complicated Medication Regimens and Polypharmacy

A complicated medication regimen reduces adherence, increases errors, and increases the risk of potentially important xenobiotic interactions.[24,133] Older adults take more prescription and nonprescription xenobiotics than any other patient group,[73,101] and the likelihood of experiencing an ADE increases with the increasing number of xenobiotics taken.[86] The problem is amplified by the common practice of pharmacies to fill an ongoing prescription of a particular medication with different brands over time; this diversity is expected but often problematic, and it is not necessarily accompanied by an adequate discussion with the patient or caregiver, or in the case of a mail

order pharmacy, by highlighting the change. The new drug will differ in size, shape, or color from the medication previously dispensed, sometimes also appearing similar or identical to a different medication of the patient's regimen, and medication errors can occur. The same problem occurs when a generic version of the prescribed medication is replaced with the proprietary name. These complexities are compounded by involvement of multiple providers,[178] complex medication scheduling, long-term use, underlying cognitive dysfunction, poor vision, and lack of assistance or monitoring in medication administration.

Comorbidity—Overt and Subclinical

Concurrent disease in target or nontarget organs alters the patient's sensitivity to a xenobiotic, resulting in a serious ADE, which is possible even when the patient is given a standard or previously used dose. Coexistent disease is often subclinical, and the patient's enhanced sensitivity will not be anticipated. For example, a patient with subclinical Alzheimer disease whose cognitive function is overtly normal can often acutely develop delirium or symptoms of dementia when given standard doses of such drugs as sedative–hypnotics or cyclic antidepressants. Adverse drug events commonly manifest as delirium.[63] Delirium is a medical emergency and an important cause of ED visits by the elderly.[88] Unfortunately, ED physicians often fail to correctly diagnose delirium,[70,78] despite the fact that the one-year mortality rate is similar to that observed with acute myocardial infarction and sepsis. Furthermore, the delirium often remains undiagnosed by the hospital physician, perhaps because many if not most elderly with delirium have a "hypoactive" presentation, characterized by sedation and reduced psychomotor activity.[79]

A large variety of symptoms occur when unrecognized disease is worsened or unmasked by xenobiotics (Table 32-4).

Prescriber Lack of Knowledge

Another factor contributing to ADEs is the physician's lack of knowledge with regard to the principles of geriatric prescribing.[55,80,93,115,142] In addition to prescribing inappropriate doses or increasing the dose too rapidly, clinicians often prescribe drugs considered potentially inappropriate for the elderly at any dose, such as cyclic antidepressants, anticholinergics, and long-acting benzodiazepines.[8] Although such medications are useful in certain circumstances, appropriate caution and monitoring is essential. At a minimum, and particularly in the case of PIMs, it is reasonable to attend to specific risk factors outlined here and elsewhere in an effort to prevent ADEs.

Prescribing New Medications Too Soon: Learning From History

Very often, clinicians are unduly ready to prescribe medications newly on the market, despite available alternatives. Pharmaceuticals recently approved by the Food and Drug Administration (FDA) are sometimes promoted as being safer than older ones, but problems often become apparent only after marketing and use by large numbers of patients. Many examples are illustrative. Gatifloxacin, a renally eliminated fluoroquinolone, was removed from the market only after several years of use when it was finally linked to both hypoglycemia and hyperglycemia in large numbers of elderly subjects.[74,143] The hypnotic zolpidem was marketed as a safe alternative to benzodiazepines for the elderly, but was soon reported to cause comparable problems, including confusion, global amnesia, memory loss, and falls.[194,196] Benzodiazepines themselves represented an apparent improvement over earlier sedative hypnotics, such as barbiturates, chloral hydrate, and meprobamate, which have narrow therapeutic indices as well as important pharmacokinetic interactions. Fundamentally, however, the intrinsic properties of any new sedating medication should be anticipated to create significant problems in those at risk. Analogously, newly approved anticoagulants, despite apparent theoretical advantages, predictably confer an enhanced bleeding risk in elderly patients due to high-risk occult pathologies, risk of falling, problems inherent in the renal route of elimination, and pharmacodynamic, and in some cases, pharmacokinetic interactions. For example, low-molecular-weight heparins were expected to be safer than unfractionated heparin but therapeutic monitoring requires measurement of antifactor Xa activity, which is not as readily available as standard tests that guided dosing of older anticoagulants;

hence, therapeutic monitoring is usually not performed.[84] Low-molecular-weight heparins are eliminated by the kidneys, and repeated doses lead to progressive anticoagulation when GFR is below the level needed for adequate clearance,[34,121] a degree of CKD that is often overlooked in elderly patients.[87] Reported cases of serious, unexpected enoxaparin-induced bleeding occur in elderly patients who are receiving "standard," not age-appropriate, dosing.[183,188] Similarly, the release of dabigatran, a renally eliminated direct thrombin inhibitor approved in 2010, was soon followed by many reports of severe GI bleeding and hemorrhagic stroke in the United States,[171,181] and internationally.[83] The latter source specifically noted the preponderance of elderly patients in the reports. This finding is consistent with its use in atrial fibrillation, which is most prevalent among the elderly and for which dabigatran was approved. It is premature to conclude that the lack of monitoring or failure to adjust for occult CKD is a cause; however, the clinical trial supporting approval of dabigatran, which randomized subjects with mean age of 71 years, specifically excluded those with estimated GFR less than or equal to 30 mL/min.[40] Similar pharmacokinetics apply to the new class of anticoagulants, the direct factor Xa inhibitors (eg, apixaban, rivaroxaban), and bleeding that was identified in a largely elderly population[41] should surprise no one. Importantly, anticoagulants in general remain among the most important causes of ADEs, therapeutic errors, and hospitalizations.[19,82] In order to reduce untoward bleeding in the elderly, who are at highest risk, it is essential for clinicians to be mindful of the possible presence of occult CKD when elimination is via the renal route, the presence of lesions with the potential to bleed, and the possibility of pharmacodynamic and pharmacokinetic interactions, and should be prepared to perform therapeutic monitoring if appropriate and available.

Inadequate Research on Geriatric Subjects in Premarketing Studies

It is not surprising that ADEs are first noted following FDA approval in the postmarketing period when actual patients (as opposed to carefully selected research subjects) are exposed to the new medication, because their effects are often inadequately studied in the elderly, generally comprising low numbers in clinical trials.[14,22,116] The nature of research itself is also relevant. When subjects are young adults and disease free, pharmacokinetic profiles do not reflect patterns of medication disposition characteristic of geriatric patients. Pharmacokinetic testing is sometimes limited to a one-time dose, and frequently the evaluation takes place over a short period of time. On average, approximately 5 half-lives of a xenobiotic are necessary to achieve steady-state concentrations (Chap. 9). Thus, a xenobiotic with a half-life of 24 hours will not reach a steady state for 5 days, and in the presence of prolonged elimination associated with age-related factors, a steady state will not be reached for substantially longer. As a result, even if elderly subjects are included in a drug trial, the ultimate effect might not be appreciated during testing intervals designed for younger patients. Even when a substantial number of subjects older than 60 years are enrolled in a clinical trial, a much smaller proportion of patients older than 70 years is included.[14,116,161] Furthermore, the heterogeneity of elderly subjects themselves makes it even more difficult to draw conclusions and make clinical assumptions across the entire group of "elderly" reported in studies. At a minimum, research should endeavor to identify subgroup age cohorts when conceptualizing care approaches and applying research design and analysis to geriatric patients.

Adverse events from xenobiotics that are studied in the elderly or others with chronic illness are typically less obvious in the presence of a comorbidity in the population at risk. The cyclooxygenase-2 (COX-2) inhibitor rofecoxib (Vioxx) was withdrawn from the market in 2004 after it was shown to increase the risk of myocardial infarction and stroke, especially in older adults.[51] Based on the complex actions of COX-1 and COX-2 in many tissues, the possibility existed that COX-2 inhibition increased cardiovascular morbidity, for example, by leaving COX-1–mediated platelet aggregation unopposed while inhibiting prostacyclin-induced vasodilation or by leading to fluid retention and increased blood pressure via renal mechanisms.[81,148] Because the elderly typically have one or more chronic illnesses[35] as well as occult disease, extra vigilance is required when new xenobiotics are given,

and clinicians and clinical investigators must be very mindful of the theoretical possibilities of adverse outcomes.

In view of the vulnerability of older patients to many medications, the FDA requires that sponsors of new drug applications present effectiveness and safety data for important demographic subgroups, including the elderly, in their FDA submission data.[30] However, exceptions to the rule are allowed. For example, when studies include insufficient numbers of subjects older than 65 years to determine whether the elderly respond differently to the medication, the labeling must state this, but the statement is a poor substitute for providing actual efficacy and safety data.[38] Unfortunately, geriatric recommendations in the package insert are often insufficiently specific to provide guidance for medications commonly used in this population.[172] International guidelines, likewise, have had limited adherence and impact on the proportion of older adults in clinical trials, even for diseases most common in the elderly.[14]

Medication/Xenobiotic Interactions—Provider Factors

Drugs, such as anticoagulants, digoxin, diuretics, and many others commonly prescribed in the elderly, are frequently involved in serious drug interactions.[86] This situation is complicated by the frequency with which elderly patients, who often have multisystem disease, visit multiple physicians, who prescribe medications without specific knowledge of, or attention to, the remainder of the patient's medication regimen, thereby increasing the risk of inappropriate combinations.[71,177] In addition to lack of communication among providers, one physician often prescribes a medication to treat the side effect of a different one that was previously prescribed by another provider without ever making the connection as to the cause. This usually unnecessary and potentially dangerous practice is tantamount to a "prescribing cascade" that results in iatrogenic polypharmacy. Problems also arise when patients obtain prescriptions from more than one pharmacy.[125] Warfarin is a particular problem, owing to its narrow therapeutic index and numerous xenobiotic interactions, the potential for which is often ignored at the point of care.[66] Examples of such prescribing oversights, include, among others, antibiotics such as ciprofloxacin, clarithromycin, and trimethoprim/sulfamethoxazole.

Herbal preparations also interact with prescription pharmaceuticals.[92] The use of herbal preparations has increased substantially in recent years, but few patients voluntarily report use of these or other nonprescribed therapies to their physicians, and too often physicians fail to inquire specifically about such "alternative" or "complementary" therapies. These xenobiotics are commonly used by elderly patients,[149] in whom targeted symptoms or illness often occur. For example, gingko is promoted for memory, hawthorn leaf for cardiovascular disease, saw palmetto for benign prostatic hyperplasia (BPH), and St John's wort for depression; all of these can interact with prescription medications or cause adverse reactions on their own. Poisonings, herb–drug interactions, and other problems related to herbal preparations are discussed further in Chap. 43.

Nonprescription pharmaceuticals also cause serious adverse effects and participate in also drug food interactions.[134] Approximately 40% of older adults take one or more nonprescription in addition to prescription medications and dietary supplements,[149] and some lead to problems. For example, excessive use of magnesium-containing preparations frequently causes severe toxicity in older individuals.[62,140] Impaired GFR, decreased GI motility, and other medical comorbidities are just 3 risk factors that potentiate magnesium toxicity in the elderly. The source of magnesium in these cases include the cathartics that contain magnesium hydroxide (Milk of Magnesia) and magnesium citrate, antacid preparations, and magnesium sulfate (Epsom salts).[62] Likewise, sodium phosphate formulations harm kidney function in certain elderly patients despite normal baseline creatinine,[103] leading the FDA to issue warnings about dosage for patients at risk, including those 55 years of age and older.[183] Virtually all of the most popular nonprescription medications are more likely to produce problems in the elderly than in younger patients, including GI bleeding (aspirin and other NSAIDs), enhanced warfarin sensitivity (cimetidine), confusion and urinary retention (anticholinergic antihistamines/sleep aids), and cardiovascular symptoms (pseudoephedrine). Furthermore, increasing numbers of prescription medications have switched to nonprescription status, compounding the problem.[42,138]

Outdated and discontinued medications are an additional problem for the elderly, who often retain unused or partially used products in their homes for decades or continue to request prescription renewals when safer or more effective alternatives are available. Patients often are unwilling to change or physicians continue to renew the prescription without sufficiently reevaluating the patient or to consider safer new alternatives. Potential examples include digoxin and theophylline, which were responsible for large numbers of adverse events diagnosed in EDs,[19,20] as well as sedating antihistamines, other anticholinergics, and diazepam.

Other Patient Factors

Other age-related factors increase the risk of unintentional poisonings in geriatric patients; impaired vision, hearing, and memory lead to misunderstanding or an inability to follow directions concerning the use of prescription and nonprescription medications. Dementia is another important risk factor in unintentional poisonings. These patients are reported to have twice the incidence of unintentional poisonings compared to those without dementia.[132] In addition to cognitive impairment, patients with dementia sometimes exhibit abnormal feeding behaviors leading to toxic ingestions.[197]

SUICIDE AND INTENTIONAL POISONINGS

The risk of suicide in men increases with age in a bimodal distribution, rising steadily after age 70 years. By age 85 years, the age-adjusted rate among men was 48 suicides per 100,000 in 2015.[31] White men have a substantially higher risk of suicide than age-matched cohorts among the African American population. Native American and Alaskan Native men comprise another high-risk group; however, after age 55 years, the numbers in those groups are too small to make meaningful comparisons.[31] In women, the suicide rate peaks in midlife and then declines. Notably, however, among adults of all races and age groups combined, women have a much lower rate of suicide than men, a gender difference that exists in virtually all regions of the world.[201] In the United States, among those 65 and older, the suicide rate in women was 5.1 per 100,000 in 2015, as compared to 31.0 for men.[31]

Methods of suicides differ by gender, however.[25] In the United States, the proportion of suicides by poisoning is much lower among men than women at all ages.[31] Firearms account for far more suicide-related deaths than do poisonings or other methods, particularly among men, in whom the proportion of deaths due to firearms increases steadily after age 60 years. Among men 70 years and older in 2015, more than 80% of suicides were due to firearms, compared to 7% attributed to poisons.[31] Among the few women 70 years and older who commit suicide, 35% of suicides were attributed to firearms, and 35% to poisons.[31] Geographic and cultural factors also determine the method of suicide. In countries other than the United States, firearms are much less frequently used to commit suicide at any age, with suicide by oral overdose, toxic inhalation, or hanging comprising a much greater proportion.[5,175] Among the elderly, limited data suggest that the pattern of xenobiotics responsible for suicidal deaths is changing because selective serotonin reuptake inhibitors are increasingly prescribed for depression instead of older antidepressants.[27] In the United States, higher suicide rates are associated with greater use of cyclic antidepressants than SSRIs or other, newer antidepressants,[67] which could be related to the greater lethality of cyclic antidepressants in overdose, or poorer tolerability leading to nonadherence and enhanced suicide risk. In a Swedish study examining autopsy-confirmed suicides that included analysis of legal xenobiotics, the incidence of suicidal fatalities attributed to benzodiazepines was reported to be increasing despite a marked decrease in benzodiazepine prescriptions.[28] Overdose of benzodiazepines is rarely fatal unless it is accompanied by alcohol or another xenobiotic or a serious medical condition.[53] However, the likelihood of fatality from an overdose of benzodiazepine taken alone increases markedly with each decade of life,[154] perhaps because benzodiazepines in frail elderly people commonly lead to secondary morbidity and mortality from

aspiration pneumonia, falls including hip fracture and traumatic intracranial hemorrhage, and other medical complications that are the proximate cause of death in the case of overdose.

Notably, flunitrazepam and nitrazepam, the 2 most frequently implicated in single benzodiazepine suicides in Sweden,[28] are not available in the United States. However, single-drug suicides are reported with other benzodiazepines that are available, such as flurazepam, triazolam, diazepam, and oxazepam.[28,127,130]

SUBSTANCE ABUSE IN THE ELDERLY

Substance abuse declines with age[57] but is important to consider in older adults under relevant clinical circumstances. Abuse of alcohol or other xenobiotics frequently is the continuation of long-term habits, or in some individuals begins later in life.[102] Alcohol is the most common substance of abuse in people older than 65 years, but surveys demonstrate an increase in illicit xenobiotic use and prescription drug misuse among older adults in recent years.[12,129,202] As increasing numbers of people enter the later decades of life (including those with past history of abuse disorders), illicit and nonmedical use is expected to increase still further. Unfortunately, a strong case can be made that middle-aged substance abusers have an "accelerated rate of biologic aging" than their nonabusing peers[98] and are less likely to survive into old age, or will be frailer than their same-age peers.

One could argue that frailty could hamper a person's acquisition of illicit substances, but analgesics are among the most commonly prescribed group of medications among elderly people, second only to cardiovascular medications. In a 2003 survey of community residing elderly, 23%, 21%, and 52% of those aged 65 to 74, 75 to 84, and 85 and older, respectively, had some exposure to opioids.[135] More recently, the Office of Inspector General (OIG) reported that 32% of Medicare part D beneficiaries received at least one prescription schedule II or III medications in 2014.[129] The OIG report, which does not state how many beneficiaries were older than 65 years, also noted an increase in fraud complaints involving incidents of "questionable" billing and prescribing, raising a concern that patients were receiving unnecessary opioids or that diversion of these controlled substances was occurring.[129]

Although only a small proportion of people who take opioids are likely to abuse them, concern exists that long-term use could ensue once a prescription is written, even for procedures such as low-risk surgery.[6] In a recent study of Medicare Part D insurance claims, 14.9% of 92,882 hospitalized beneficiaries with no recent opioid use had a new opioid claim within 7 days after hospitalization; of these, 72.3% were aged 65 years or older, and one-third of the older beneficiaries had a claim 90 days postdischarge.[95] In a separate study of 1,808,355 Medicare Part D beneficiaries prescribed opioids, 34.6%, 14.2%, and 11.9% filled prescriptions from 2, 3, and 4 or more separate providers, respectively.[96]

Another recent misused medication among older adults is the antidiarrheal loperamide, a poorly absorbed, nonprescription synthetic opioid, and a popular alternative to prescription opioids. A study of trends in intentional loperamide abuse and misuse between 2010 and 2015 revealed that 14.8% (257) of 1,736 exposures were in patients older than 60 years, of which 62 were suspected suicide attempts, with 2 resulting in fatalities.[184]

Substance abuse in late life is probably underrecognized and underreported.[152,204] In a 5-year study of patients admitted to a level I trauma unit, among those 65 years of age or older (average age approximately 75 years) who underwent toxicologic screening, a positive BAC was present in 11% (mean concentration 163 mg/dL) and a positive urine drug screen in 48.3%.[54] Sixty-nine percent had a BAC greater than 80 mg/dL, which is consistent with other studies of elderly patients presenting to trauma facilities, in which a large majority have a BAC of 80 mg/dL or above.[163,204] Such results, although similarly found in nonelderly trauma patients,[54,204] have different implications in the older adult. As a result of physiologic and pharmacologic changes discussed earlier, the elderly have greater risks on cognitive and motor function, despite a smaller amount of ethanol ingested,[180,189] Also, while many are injured as drivers in motor vehicle crashes, the majority have serious trauma due to falling.[54]

Among elderly trauma patients who are screened for and have positive urine toxicology, opioids and sedatives are most commonly found,[54,163,204] all of which, like ethanol, are more likely to impair older than younger adults at a given dose. As both medical and recreational marijuana use is becoming legalized and decriminalized across the country, it is logical to ask whether older users might be more seriously affected, whether as drivers, or as those who fall. No research to date has focused on this question but clinicians, patients, and family members are well advised to exercise caution.

According to data from the National Survey of Drug Use and Health (NSDUH), from 2002 to 2014 the proportion of adults aged 50 to 64 years who reported cannabis use in the past month increased from 1.1% to 6.1%, and among those aged 65 years and older from 0.3 to 1.3%.[12] These increases were higher than for any age group; among all age groups combined, the increase was 35% compared to 333% for those aged 50 to 64 years and 455% for the oldest group. Although synthetic cannabinoids and marijuana, where available, are increasingly considered as alternative treatments for conditions such as chemotherapy-induced nausea and vomiting, and muscle spasticity associated with multiple sclerosis,[43,113,168] both medical and recreational marijuana could have more deleterious consequences for older as compared to younger adults. In addition to unwanted cognitive effects, of particular concern are physiologic responses to marijuana that can secondarily affect vulnerable organ systems, notably producing cardiovascular and cerebrovascular problems (Chap. 74).

Substance Withdrawal

Some caveats are in order when it comes to the older alcoholic patient at risk for withdrawal. Studies suggesting a longer duration or greater severity of the syndrome in the elderly are criticized for their small size, retrospective nature, and absence of middle-aged comparison groups.[106] However, vigilance is essential because delayed assessment and intervention will lead to greater morbidity.[59] Furthermore, because of an age-related decreased physiologic reserve, the adverse physiologic effects of ethanol withdrawal such as elevated blood pressure, sustained tachycardia, and delirium will have a more profoundly negative impact on the elderly. For treatment of withdrawal, some clinicians recommend shorter-acting benzodiazepines, such as lorazepam rather than chlordiazepoxide,[153] because the latter and its metabolites are particularly long acting in the elderly, leading to progressive and excessive sedation as the drug and metabolites accumulate. Long-acting benzodiazepines, moreover, are more often associated with injury, including fractures, than short-acting benzodiazepines.[176] Regardless of which benzodiazepine is used for alcohol withdrawal, careful monitoring with symptom-triggered dosing is preferable to a fixed-dose schedule in elderly patients, as in all other patients being treated for ethanol withdrawal.

Symptoms of withdrawal from other xenobiotics, for example, benzodiazepines, opioids, baclofen, carisoprodol, and cognitive enhancers such as cholinesterase inhibitors, are mistaken for nonxenobiotic manifestations. The medication itself, even judiciously prescribed and monitored, will result in withdrawal symptoms, if the patient makes an uninformed decision to discontinue the medication, forgets to take it, or is unable to refill the prescription in a timely fashion. The failure to consider use of these xenobiotics, whether illicit, nonprescription, or prescription, will have serious consequences. If a careful history is not elicited, withdrawal from these xenobiotics will be missed or misdiagnosed as due to another disease process and be inappropriately managed as a result. Given the ongoing "graying" of the population, greater vigilance and screening will be needed upon presentation to the hospital and reassessed upon admission as an inpatient.

MANAGEMENT

Management decisions must be made with the foregoing principles in mind. Gastrointestinal (GI) decontamination should proceed as in younger patients. However, because constipation is a more frequent problem in the elderly, when multiple-dose activated charcoal is used, particular attention must be paid to GI function and motility. The specific precautions and contraindications in the basic management and GI decontamination detailed in Chap. 5 are particularly pertinent for the geriatric population.

The presence of clinical or preclinical congestive heart failure or CKD will increase the risk of fluid overload when sodium bicarbonate is used. In the elderly, extracorporeal removal is often indicated earlier in cases of salicylate, lithium, or metformin poisoning, in which elimination will be hampered by a decreased GFR.

A situation that often goes unrecognized in geriatric patients is the problem of ethanol or other substance withdrawal syndromes. Because elderly patients are typically not perceived as substance abusers, or because a physician evaluating an unfamiliar patient is not aware of the patient's chronic use of prescribed benzodiazepines or opioids, the possibility of withdrawal is frequently neglected when unanticipated complications occur during hospitalization. Under updated Geriatric Trauma Management Guidelines,[7] every geriatric trauma patient should be assessed for ethanol use as a cause of delirium. By extrapolation, alcohol withdrawal detection should increase in this particularly vulnerable trauma population.

Strategies to limit unintentional toxic exposures in elderly patients with cognitive or sensory impairment should be similar to those used in young children, who are also at high risk of ingesting toxic xenobiotics or pharmaceuticals prescribed for others in the household (Chap. 129). The strategies should include the removal of potentially dangerous and unnecessary xenobiotics from the patient's environment. A recognition of and reliance on the important role that Emergency Medical Services (EMS) prehospital personnel play in the acquisition of all xenobiotics (whether illicit, prescription, or nonprescription) from the home of a community-dwelling older patient cannot be overstated. Emergency Medical Services often represents a unique opportunity for a medical provider to gain vital information that could impact the diagnosis and management of a toxicologic emergency in the elderly. The physician should request that the patient or caregiver bring all medications to the office in the original bottles. The physician should then make an effort to limit the number of medications prescribed or to seek alternative medications with a safer therapeutic index or appropriate geriatric safety profile. For patients who are unable to reliably take their own medications, administration and control of the medications ultimately becomes the responsibility of the caregiver rather than the patient. Usually the patient's capabilities are obvious, but early dementia can be very subtle, so a caregiver who accompanies the patient should always be involved in the prescribing and counseling encounter.

CRITERIA FOR ADMISSION AND TIMING OF DISCHARGE

When geriatric patients are evaluated in the ED for poisonings or serious ADEs, the need for hospital admission should be weighed carefully against the known hazards of hospitalization for the elderly.[46] The physician should be particularly alert to certain situations that might mandate admission, including unexplained mental status changes, overdose of a prescribed medication with a prolonged duration of action, or evidence of inadequate home care or elder abuse/neglect, such as poor hygiene or unexplained injury.

When there is concern that the established caregivers at home are abusing or neglecting the patient, the patient requires further observation, removal from the environment, and possibly hospitalization. Signs of actual physical abuse will be more obvious than signs of neglect[110]; however, neglect is more prevalent than physical abuse.[2] Vulnerable elderly who are physically disabled or cognitively impaired are often brought to the hospital because of presumed illness, but the source of the problem may actually be the caregiver. The caregiver, frequently but not necessarily a family member, could be depleting the patient's funds for personal use. Patients may become ill because funds were diverted from the purchase of food or because the patient's prescription drugs were sold on the street. More direct abuse infrequently takes the form of intentional poisoning or oversedation of the patient by overdose of the patient's own prescription drugs, or selling the patient's medications (diversion) or withholding them, resulting in clinical deterioration. Provision for follow-up care, such as an alternative place to live and guardian appointment, is essential because abuse and neglect are associated with serious outcomes.[111]

Unresolved mental status changes require close observation and hospitalization. Elderly patients who are confused or unable to walk are sometimes mistakenly assumed to be chronically impaired. However, incomplete explanation of an altered mental status or physical impairment should prompt careful inquiry into the patient's baseline functional status. Poor function should never be assumed to be "normal aging." Many very elderly patients are cognitively normal, physically robust, and independent in all activities of daily living.

A patient whose problems are attributed to overdose with or due to bioaccumulation of a long-acting medication requires prolonged monitoring. Because the duration of action frequently is markedly prolonged among geriatric patients, a higher degree of vigilance is required. An important example is chlordiazepoxide, which is commonly used for alcohol withdrawal and exhibits a very long half-life in older patients, especially after repeated dosing. The ultra–long-acting sulfonylurea chlorpropamide, rarely used today, but others such as glyburide cause relatively prolonged hypoglycemia compared with other insulin secretagogues, as noted above.

In conclusion, a better understanding of core geriatric emergency medicine principles—including physiologic changes of aging, effects of comorbid disease, cognitive dysfunction, atypical clinical presentations, geriatric syndromes, and the impact of polypharmacy—will advance the goal of providing improved and more humanistic care for older adults with toxicologic emergencies that will ultimately transcend age, leading to improvements in the care for all in need.

SUMMARY

- Older patients account for only a small fraction of total poisoning victims, but when poisoned, they have a high mortality rate.
- The elderly are much more likely to experience serious ADEs as a consequence of both appropriate and inappropriate use of medications.
- Always consider ADEs as the potential etiology of a medical or traumatic presentation to the hospital.
- Attention to risk factors for ADEs is essential in this vulnerable population.
- Important risk factors include pharmacokinetic and pharmacodynamic changes; the presence of overt or subclinical disease, including dementia; patient and provider error; suicide risk; complex medication; and a general lack of knowledge about the principles of prescribing for the geriatric population.

REFERENCES

1. Abernethy DR, Kerzner L. Age effects on alpha-1-acid glycoprotein concentration and imipramine plasma protein binding. *J Am Geriatr Soc.* 1984;32:705-708.
2. Acierno R, et al. Prevalence and correlates of emotional, physical, sexual, and financial abuse and potential neglect in the United States: the National Elder Mistreatment Study. *Am J Public Health.* 2010;100:292-297.
3. The Administration on Aging. A profile of older Americans: 2015. U.S. Department of Health and Human Services. https://aoa.acl.gov/aging_statistics/Profile/2015/docs/2015-Profile.pdf. Published 2015. Accessed February 25, 2017.
4. AGS Choosing Wisely Workgroup. American Geriatrics Society identifies another five things that healthcare providers and patients should question. *J Am Geriatr Soc.* 2014;62:950-960.
5. Ajdacic-Gross V, et al. Methods of suicide: international suicide patterns derived from the WHO mortality database. *Bull World Health Organ.* 2008;86:726-732.
6. Alam A, et al. Long-term analgesic use after low-risk surgery. A retrospective cohort study. *Arch Intern Med.* 2012;172:425-430.
7. American College of Surgeons. Committee on Trauma. Trauma Quality Improvement Program (TQIP) geriatric trauma management guidelines. https://www.facs.org/~/media/files/quality%20programs/trauma/tqip/geriatric%20guide%20tqip.ashx. Accessed February 22, 2017.
8. American Geriatrics Society 2015 Beers Criteria Update Expert Panel. American Geriatrics Society 2015 Beers Criteria for potentially inappropriate medications use in older adults. *J Am Geriatr Soc.* 2015;63:2227-2246.
9. Aronow W. Postinfarction use of beta blockers in elderly patients. *Drugs Aging.* 1997;11:424-432.
10. Aronow WS. Office management of hypertension in older persons. *Am J Med.* 2011;124:498-500.
11. Aymanns C, et al. Review on pharmacokinetics and pharmacodynamics and the aging kidney. *Clin J Am Soc Nephrol.* 2010;5:314-327.
12. Azofeifa A, et al. National Estimates of Marijuana Use and Related Indicators—National Survey on Drug Use and Health, United States, 2002-2014. *MMWR Surveill Summ.* 2016;65(No.SS-11):1-25. https://www.cdc.gov/mmwr/volumes/65/ss/ss6511a1.htm. Accessed March 7, 2017.
13. Bartels AL, et al. Blood-brain barrier *P*-glycoprotein function decreases in specific brain regions with aging: a possible role in progressive neurodegeneration. *Neurobiol Aging.* 2009;30:1818-1824.
14. Beers E, et al. Participation of older people in preauthorization trials of recently approved medicines. *J Am Geriatr Soc.* 2014;62:1883-1890.
15. Beers MH. Explicit criteria for determining potentially inappropriate medication use by the elderly: an update. *Arch Intern Med.* 1997;157:1531-1536.
16. Boyer EW, Shannon M. The serotonin syndrome. *N Engl J Med.* 2005;352:1112-1120.
17. Brenner SS, et al. Influence of age and cytochrome P450 2C9 genotype on the steady-state disposition of diclofenac and celecoxib. *Clin Pharmacokinet.* 2003;42:283-292.
18. Brenner SS, Klotz U. *P*-Glycoprotein function in the elderly. *Eur J Clin Pharmacol.* 2004;60:97-102.
19. Budnitz DS, et al. Emergency hospitalizations for adverse drug events in older Americans. *N Engl J Med.* 2011;365:2002-2012.
20. Budnitz DS, et al. National surveillance of emergency department visits for outpatient adverse drug events. *JAMA.* 2006;296:1858-1866.
21. Budnitz DS, et al. Medication use leading to emergency department visits for adverse drug events in older adults. *Ann Intern Med.* 2007;147:755-765.
22. Bugeja G, et al. Exclusion of elderly people from clinical research: a descriptive study of published reports. *Br Med J.* 1997;315:1059.
23. Burke LB, et al. Geriatric drug use and adverse drug event reporting in 1990: a descriptive analysis of the two national data bases. *Annu Rev Gerontol Geriatr.* 1992;12:1-28.
24. Butkiewicz M, et al. Drug-drug interaction profiles of medication regimens extracted from a de-identified electronic medical records system. *AMIA Summits on Translational Science Proceedings.* 2016;2016:33-40. https://www.ncbi.nlm.nih.gov/pmc/articles/PMC5001747/pdf/2382866.pdf. Accessed February 8, 2017.
25. Callanan VJ, Davis MS. Gender differences in suicide methods. *Soc Psychiatry Psychiatr Epidemiol.* 2012;47:857-869.
26. Campion EW, et al. The effect of age on serum albumin in healthy males: report from the Normative Aging Study. *J Gerontol.* 1988;43:M18-M20.
27. Carlsten A, et al. Suicides by drug poisoning among the elderly in Sweden 1969-1996. *Soc Psychiatry Psychiatr Epidemiol.* 1999;34:609-614.
28. Carlsten A, et al. The role of benzodiazepines in elderly suicides. *Scand J Public Health.* 2003;31:224-228.
29. Caroff SN, et al. Neuroleptic malignant syndrome in elderly patients. *Expert Rev Neurother.* 2007;7:423-431.
30. Center for Drug Evaluation and Research. *Guidance for Industry: Content and Format for Geriatric Labeling, October 2001.* http://www.fda.gov/downloads/Drugs/GuidanceComplianceRegulatoryInformation/Guidances/UCM075062.pdf. Accessed March 7, 2017.
31. Centers for Disease Control and Prevention. *Injury Prevention & Control: Data & Statistics (WISQARS) Fatal Injury Reports.* http://www.cdc.gov/injury/wisqars/fatal_injury_reports.html. Accessed March 27, 2017.
32. Centers for Disease Control and Prevention. National Center for Health Statistics. National Hospital Ambulatory Medical Care Survey: 2013 emergency department summary tables. https://www.cdc.gov/nchs/data/ahcd/nhamcs_emergency/2013_ed_web_tables.pdf. Accessed March 27, 2017.
33. Chiu C, et al. *P*-Glycoprotein expression and amyloid accumulation in human aging and Alzheimer's disease: preliminary observations. *Neurobiol Aging.* 2015;36:2475-2482.
34. Chow SL, et al. Correlation of antifactor Xa concentrations with renal function in patients on enoxaparin. *J Clin Pharmacol.* 2003;43:586-590.
35. Cigolle CT, et al. Geriatric conditions and disability: the Health and Retirement Study. *Ann Intern Med.* 2007;147:156-164.
36. CKD-EPI. Chronic Kidney Disease Epidemiology Collaboration. Cystatin C based equations. http://ckdepi.org/equations/cystatin-c-based-equations/. Last updated July 2014. Accessed February 25, 2017.
37. Cobaugh DJ, Krenzelok EP. Adverse drug reactions and therapeutic errors in older adults: a hazard factor analysis of poison center data. *Am J Health Syst Pharm.* 2006;63:2228-2234.
38. Code of Federal Regulations. 21 CFR 201.57(c)(9)(v)(B)(1).
39. Connolly MJ, et al. Impaired bronchodilator response to albuterol in healthy elderly men and women. *Chest.* 1995;108:401-406.
40. Connolly SJ, et al, for the Randomized Evaluation of Long-Term Anticoagulation Therapy Investigators. Dabigatran versus warfarin in patients with atrial fibrillation. *N Engl J Med.* 2009;361:1139-1151.
41. Connolly SJ, et al. for the ANNEXA-4 Investigators. Andexanet alfa for acute major bleeding associated with factor Xa inhibitors. *N Engl J Med.* 2016;375:1131-1141.
42. Consumer Healthcare Products Association. Ingredients & dosages transferred from Rx-to-OTC status (or new OTC approvals) by the Food and Drug Administration since 1975. http://www.chpa.org/SwitchFAQs.aspx. Published February 8, 2017. Accessed February 25, 2017.
43. Corey-Bloom J, et al. Smoked cannabis for spasticity in multiple sclerosis: a randomized, placebo-controlled trial. *CMAJ.* 2012;184:1143-1150.
44. Corsonello A, et al. Age-related pharmacokinetic and pharmacodynamic changes and related risk of adverse drug reactions. *Curr Med Chem.* 2010;17:571-584.

45. Covinsky KE, et al. Serum albumin concentration and clinical assessments of nutritional status in hospitalized older people: different sides of different coins? *J Am Geriatr Soc.* 2002;50:631-637.

46. Creditor MC. Hazards of hospitalization of the elderly. *Ann Intern Med.* 1993;118:219-223.

47. Crouch BI, Caravati EM. Poisoning in older adults: a 5-year experience of US poison control centers. *Ann Pharmacother.* 2004;38:2005-2011.

48. Davies DF, Shock NW. Age changes in glomerular filtration rate: effective renal plasma flow and tubular excretory capacity in adult males. *J Clin Invest.* 1950;29:496-507.

49. Delanaye P, Glassock RJ. Glomerular filtration rate and aging: another longitudinal study—a long time coming! *Nephron.* 2015;131:1-4.

50. Dooley CP, et al. Prevalence of *Helicobacter pylori* infection and histologic gastritis in asymptomatic persons. *N Engl J Med.* 1989;321:1562-1566.

51. Drazen JM. Cox-2 inhibitors—a lesson in unexpected problems. *N Engl J Med.* 2005;352:1131-1132.

52. Drew DA, et al. Association between soluble klotho and change in kidney function: the Health Aging and Body Composition Study. *J Am Soc Nephrol.* 2017;28:1859-1866.

53. Drummer OH, Ranson DL. Sudden death and benzodiazepines. *Am J Forensic Med Pathol.* 1996;17:336-342.

54. Ekeh AP, et al. The prevalence of positive drug and alcohol screens in elderly trauma patients. *Subst Abus.* 2014;35:51-55.

55. Ferry ME, et al. Physicians' lack of knowledge of prescribing for the elderly: a study in primary care physicians in Pennsylvania. *J Am Geriatr Soc.* 1985;33:616-625.

56. Fick DM, Resnick B. 2012 Beers Criteria update: how should practicing nurses use the criteria? *J Gerontol Nurs.* 2012;38:3-5.

57. Fink A, et al. Alcohol-related problems in older persons: determinants, consequences and screening. *Arch Intern Med.* 1996;156:1150-1156.

58. Fitzergald JD. Age-related effects of beta blockers and hypertension. *J Cardiovasc Pharmacol.* 1988;12(suppl):S83-S92.

59. Foy A, et al. The course of alcohol withdrawal in a general hospital. *Q J Med.* 1997;90:253-261.

60. French DD, et al. Outpatient medications and hip fractures in the US. *Drugs Aging.* 2005;22:877-885.

61. Fu AZ, et al. Inappropriate medication use and health outcomes in the elderly. *J Am Geriatr Soc.* 2004;52:1934-1939.

62. Fung MC, et al. Hypermagnesemia. Elderly over-the-counter drug users at risk. *Arch Fam Med.* 1995;4:718-723.

63. Gallagher P, Lavan AH. Predicting risk of adverse drug reactions in older adults. *Ther Adv Drug Saf.* 2016;7:11-22.

64. Gallagher P, et al. STOPP (Screening Tool of Older Person's Prescriptions) and START (Screening Tool to Alert Doctors to Right Treatment) consensus validation. *Int J Clin Pharmacol Ther.* 2008;46:72-83.

65. Gaugler JE, et al. Characteristics of patients misdiagnosed with Alzheimer's disease and their medication use: an analysis of the NACC-UDS database. *BMC Geriatr.* 2013;13:137. http://bmcgeriatr.biomedcentral.com/articles/10.1186/1471-2318-13-137. Accessed February 26, 2017.

66. Ghaswalla PK, et al. Warfarin-antibiotic interactions in older adults of an outpatient anticoagulant clinic. *Am J Geriatr Pharmacother.* 2012;10:352-360.

67. Gibbons RD, et al. The relationship between antidepressant medication use and rate of suicide. *Arch Gen Psychiatry.* 2005;62:165-172.

68. Glassock R, et al. An age-calibrated classification of chronic kidney disease. *JAMA.* 2015;314:559-560.

69. Glassock RJ, Rule AD. The implications of anatomical and functional changes of the aging kidney: with an emphasis on the glomeruli. *Kidney Int.* 2012;82:270-277.

70. Gower LEJ, Gatewood MO, Kang CS. Emergency department management of delirium in the elderly. *West J Emerg Med.* 2012;13:194-201.

71. Green JL, et al. Is the number of prescribing physicians an independent risk factor for adverse drug events in an elderly outpatient population? *Am J Geriatr Pharmacother.* 2007;5:31-39.

72. Greenblatt DJ, et al. Kinetics and clinical effects of flurazepam in young and elderly noninsomniacs. *Clin Pharmacol Ther.* 1981;30:475-486.

73. Gu Q, et al. Prescription drug use continues to increase: U.S. prescription drug data for 2007-2008. NCHS Data Brief No. 42 September 2010. Centers for Disease Control, National Center for Health Statistics. https://www.cdc.gov/nchs/data/databriefs/db42.pdf.

74. Gurwitz JH. Serious adverse drug effects—seeing the trees through the forest. *N Engl J Med.* 2006;354:1413-1415.

75. Gurwitz JH, Avorn J. The ambiguous relation between aging and adverse drug reactions. *Ann Intern Med.* 1991;114:956-966.

76. Gurwitz JH, et al. Incidence and preventability of adverse drug events among older persons in the ambulatory setting. *JAMA.* 2003;289:1107-1116.

77. Gurwitz JH, et al. The incidence of adverse drug events in two large academic long-term care facilities. *Am J Med.* 2005;118:251-258.

78. Han JH, Wilber ST. Altered mental status in older patients in the emergency department. *Clin Geriatr Med.* 2013;29:101-136.

79. Han JH, et al. Delirium in older emergency department patients: recognition, risk factors, and psychomotor subtypes. *Acad Emerg Med.* 2009;16:193-200.

80. Hastings S, et al. Quality of pharmacotherapy and outcomes for older veterans discharged from the emergency department. *J Am Geriatr Soc.* 2008;56:875-880.

81. Hawkey CJ. COX-2 inhibitors. *Lancet.* 1999;353:307-314.

82. Hayes BD, et al. Causes of therapeutic errors in older adults: evaluation of National Poison Center data. *J Am Geriatr Soc.* 2009;57:653-658.

83. Health Sciences Authority (Singapore). Bleeding events associated with dabigatran etexilate (Pradaxa®): recommendation to use with caution in the elderly and renally impaired patients. http://www.hsa.gov.sg/publish/hsaportal/en/health_products_regulation/safety_information/product_safety_alerts/safety_alerts_2011/bleeding_events_associated.html. Accessed March 11, 2013.

84. Hirsh J, et al. Parenteral anticoagulants. *Chest.* 2008;133(suppl):141S-159S.

85. Hogan DB. Long-term efficacy and toxicity of cholinesterase inhibitors in the treatment of Alzheimer disease. *Can J Psychiatry.* 2014;59:618-623.

86. Hohl CM, et al. Polypharmacy, adverse drug-related events, and potential adverse drug interactions in elderly patients presenting to an emergency department. *Ann Emerg Med.* 2001;38:666-671.

87. Hulot JS, et al. Dosing strategy in patients with renal failure receiving enoxaparin for the treatment of non-ST-segment elevation in acute coronary syndrome. *Clin Pharmacol Ther.* 2005;77:542-552.

88. Hustey FM, et al. The prevalence and documentation of impaired mental status in elderly emergency department patients. *Ann Emerg Med.* 2002;39:248-253.

89. Ibrahim H, et al. An alternative formula to the Cockcroft-Gault and the modification of diet in renal diseases formulas in predicting GFR in individuals with type 1 diabetes. *J Am Soc Nephrol.* 2005;16:1051-1060.

90. Inker LA, et al; CKD-EPI Investigators. Estimating glomerular filtration rate from serum creatinine and cystatin C. *N Engl J Med.* 2012;367:20-29.

91. Inouye SK, et al. Delirium. In: Halter JB, eds. *Hazzard's Geriatric Medicine and Gerontology.* 7th ed. New York, NY: McGraw-Hill; 2017. http://accessmedicine.mhmedical.com.lproxy.nymc.edu/content.aspx?bookid=1923&sectionid=143987225. Accessed March 28, 2017.

92. Izzo AA, Ernst E. Interactions between herbal medicines and prescribed drugs. An updated systemic review. *Drugs.* 2009;69:1777-1798.

93. Jackson SHD, et al. Optimization of drug prescribing. *Br J Clin Pharmacol.* 2004;57:231-236.

94. Jarrett PG, et al. Illness presentation in elderly patients. *Arch Intern Med.* 1995;155:1060-1064.

95. Jena AB, et al. Hospital prescribing of opioids to medicare beneficiaries. *JAMA Intern Med.* 2016;176:990-997.

96. Jena AB, et al. Opioid prescribing by multiple providers in Medicare: retrospective observational study of insurance claims. *BMJ.* 2014;348:g1393.

97. Jonsson A, et al. Effects and serum levels of glibenclamide and its active effects and serum levels of glibenclamide and its active metabolites in patients with type 2 diabetes. *Diabetes Obes Metab.* 2001;3:403-409.

98. Kalapatapu RK, Sullivan MA. Prescription use disorders in older adults. *Am J Addict.* 2010;19:515-522.

99. Kalisch Ellett LM, et al. Multiple anticholinergic medication use and risk of hospital admission for confusion or dementia. *J Am Geriatr Soc.* 2014;62:1916-1922.

100. Kanaan AO, et al. Adverse drug events after hospital discharge in older adults: types, severity, and involvement of Beers Criteria medications. *J Am Geriatr Soc.* 2013;61:1894-1899.

101. Kaufman DW, et al. Recent patterns of medication use in the ambulatory adult population in the United States. The Slone Survey. *JAMA.* 2002;287:337-344.

102. Kausch O. Cocaine abuse in the elderly: a series of three case reports. *J Nerv Ment Dis.* 2002;190:562-565.

103. Khurana A, et al. The effect of oral sodium phosphate drug products on renal function in adults undergoing bowel endoscopy. *Arch Intern Med.* 2008;168:593-597.

104. Kinirons MT, Crome P. Clinical pharmacokinetics considerations in the elderly. An update. *Clin Pharmacokinet.* 1997;33:302-312.

105. Kirk SFL, et al. Are the measures used to calculate BMI accurate and valid for the use in older people? *J Human Nutr Dietetics.* 2003;16:365-370.

106. Kramer KL, et al. Managing alcohol withdrawal in the elderly. *Drugs Aging.* 1999;14:409-425.

107. Kruse W. Problems and pitfalls in the use of benzodiazepines in the elderly. *Drug Saf.* 1990;5:328-344.

108. Kyle UG, et al. Total body mass, fat mass, fat-free mass, and skeletal muscle in older people: cross-sectional differences in 60 year-old persons. *J Am Geriatr Soc.* 2001;49:1633-1640.

109. Lacher SE, et al. P-Glycoprotein transport of neurotoxic pesticides. *J Pharmacol Exp Ther.* 2015;355:99-107.

110. Lachs M, Pillemer K. Abuse and neglect of elderly persons. *N Engl J Med.* 1995;332:437-443.

111. Lachs MS, et al. The mortality of elder mistreatment. *JAMA.* 1998;280:428-432.

112. Lamb EJ, et al. Estimation of glomerular filtration rate in older patients with chronic renal insufficiency: is the modification of diet in renal disease formula an improvement? *J Am Geriatr Soc.* 2003;51:1012-1017.

113. Langford RM, et al. A double-blind, randomized, placebo-controlled, parallel-group study of THC/CBD oromucosal spray in combination with the existing treatment regimen, in the relief of central neuropathic pain in patients with multiple sclerosis. *J Neurol.* 2013;260:984-997.

114. Lau DT, et al. Hospitalization and death associated with potentially inappropriate medication prescriptions among elderly nursing home residents. *Arch Intern Med.* 2005;165:68-74.

115. Lavan AH, et al. Methods to reduce prescribing errors in elderly patients with multimorbidity. *Clin Interv Aging.* 2016;11:857-866.

116. Lee PY, et al. Representation of elderly persons and women in published randomized trials of acute coronary syndromes. *JAMA.* 2001;286:708-713.

117. Lesar TS, et al. Factors related to errors in medication prescribing. *JAMA.* 1997;277:312-317.

118. Levey AS, et al. GFR estimation: from physiology to public health. *Am J Kidney Dis.* 2014;63:820-834.

119. Levey AS, et al. Chronic kidney disease in older people. *JAMA.* 2015;314:557-558.

120. Lewis LM, et al. Unrecognized delirium in ED geriatric patients. *Am J Emerg Med.* 1995;13:142-145.

121. Lim W, et al. Meta-analysis: low-molecular-weight heparin and bleeding in patients with severe renal insufficiency. *Ann Intern Med.* 2006;144:673-684.

122. Lindeman R, et al. Longitudinal studies on the rate of decline in renal function with age. *J Am Geriatr Soc.* 1985;33:278-285.

123. Lord SR. Falls. In: Halter JB, et al. eds. *Hazzard's Geriatric Medicine and Gerontology.* 7th ed. New York, NY: McGraw-Hill; 2017. http://accessmedicine.mhmedical.com.lproxy.nymc.edu/content.aspx?bookid=1923&sectionid=143987225. Accessed March 28, 2017.

124. Malmgren L, et al. Declining estimated glomerular fitration rate and its association with mortality and comorbidity over 10 years in elderly women. *Nephron.* 2015;130:245-255.

125. Marcum ZA, et al. Effect of multiple pharmacy use on medication adherence and drug-drug interactions in older adults with Medicare part D. *J Am Geriatr Soc.* 2014;62:244-252.

126. Marra EM, et al. Benzodiazepine prescribing in older adults in U.S. Ambulatory Clinics and emergency departments (2001-10). *J Am Geriatr Soc.* 2015;63:2074-2081.

127. Martello S, et al. Acute flurazepam intoxication: a case report. *Am J Forensic Med Pathol.* 2006;27:55-57.

128. Matin N, et al. Dextromethorphan-induced near-fatal suicide attempt in a slow metabolizer at cytochrome P450 2D6. *Am J Geriatr Pharmacother.* 2007;5:162-165.

129. Maxwell A. Office of Evaluation and Inspections, Office of Inspector General, Department of Health and Human Services. Opioid use among seniors—issues and emerging trends. 2015. OIG analysis of Medicare Part D data, 2015. https://oig.hhs.gov/testimony/docs/2016/maxwell0216.pdf. Accessed February 27, 2017.

130. McIntyre IM, et al. A fatality due to flurazepam. *J Forensic Sci.* 1994;39:1571-1574.

131. Meneilly GS, et al. Counterregulatory hormone responses to hypoglycemia in the elderly patient with diabetes. *Diabetes.* 1994;43:403-410.

132. Mitchell RJ, et al. Dementia and intentional and unintentional poisoning in older people: a 10 year review of hospitalization records in New South Wales, Australia. *Int Psychogeriatr.* 2015;27:1757-1768. Erratum 2015;27:2015.

133. Monane M, et al. The effects of initial drug choice and comorbidity on antihypertensive therapy compliance: results from a population-based study in the elderly. *Am J Hypertens.* 1997;10(7, pt 1):697-704.

134. Moore N, et al. Adverse drug reactions and drug-drug interactions with over-the-counter NSAIDs. *Ther Clin Risk Manag.* 2015;112:1061-1075.

135. Moxey ED, et al. Prescription drug use in the elderly: a descriptive analysis. *Health Care Financ Rev.* 2003;24:127-141.

136. Nesto RW, et al. Thiazolinedione use, fluid retention, and congestive heart failure—a consensus statement from the American Heart Association and American Diabetes Association. *Circulation.* 2003;108:2941-2948.

137. Novak LP. Aging, total body potassium, fat-free mass, and cell mass in males and females between ages 18 and 85 years. *J Gerontol.* 1972;27:428-443.

138. Oliver E. An overview of the US regulatory system for OTC products. GlaxoSmithKline Consumer Healthcare. *Regul Rapporteur.* 2013;10:4-9. https://embed.topra.org/sites/default/files/regrapart/1/4954/2013-3-regulatory-rapporteur-overview-us-otc.pdf. Accessed March 19, 2017.

139. O'Mahony D, et al. STOPP/START criteria for potentially inappropriate prescribing in older people: version 2. *Age Ageing.* 2015;44:213-218.

140. Onishi S, Yoshino S. Cathartic-induced fatal hypermagnesemia in the elderly. *Intern Med.* 2006;45:207-210.

141. Onofrj M, et al. Emergencies in parkinsonism: akinetic crisis, life-threatening dyskinesias, and polyneuropathy during L-Dopa gel treatment. *Parkinsonism Relat Disord.* 2009;15(suppl 3):S233-S236.

142. Papaioannou A, et al. Assessment of adherence to renal dosing guidelines in long-term care facilities. *J Am Geriatr Soc.* 2000;48:1470-1473.

143. Park-Wyllie LY, et al. Outpatient gatifloxacin therapy and dysglycemia in older adults. *N Engl J Med.* 2006;354:1352-1361.

144. Park-Wyllie LY, et al. Cholinesterase inhibitors and hospitalization for bradycardia: a population-based study. *PLoS Med.* 2009;6:e1000157.

145. Payne RA, et al. Association between prescribing cardiovascular and psychotropic medications and hospital admission for falls or fractures. *Drugs Aging.* 2013;30:247-254.

146. Pottel H, et al. Estimating glomerular filtration rate for the full age spectrum from serum creatinine and cystatin C. *Nephrol Dial Transplant.* 2016;31:1-11.

147. Pozzato G, et al. Ethanol metabolism and aging: the role of "first pass metabolism" and gastric alcohol dehydrogenase activity. *J Gerontol.* 1995;50:B135-B141.

148. Psaty BM, Furberg CD. COX-2 inhibitors—lessons in drug safety. *N Engl J Med.* 2005;352:1133-1135.

149. Qato DM, et al. Changes in prescription and over-the-counter medication and dietary supplement use among older adults in the United States, 2005 vs 2011. *JAMA Intern Med.* 2016;176:473-482.

150. Rattan SI, et al. Protein synthesis, posttranslational modifications, and aging. *Ann N Y Acad Sci.* 1992;663:48-62.

151. Reeves RR, et al. Inappropriate psychiatric admission of elderly patients with unrecognized delirium. *South Med J.* 2010;103:111-115.

152. Reid MC, et al. Physician awareness of alcohol use disorders among older patients. *J Gen Intern Med.* 1998;13:729-734.

153. Rigler SK. Alcoholism in the elderly. *Am Fam Physician.* 2000;61:1710-1716.

154. Rogers JJ, Heard K. Does age matter? Comparing case fatality rates for selected poisonings reported to U.S. poison centers. *Clin Toxicol.* 2007;45:705-708.

155. Rolita L, et al. Greater number of narcotic analgesic prescriptions for osteoarthritis is associated with falls and fractures in elderly adults. *J Am Geriatr Soc.* 2013;61:335-340.

156. Rosenberg MS, et al. Geriatric emergency department guidelines. American College of Emergency Physicians; American Geriatrics Society; Emergency Nurses Association; Society for Academic Emergency Medicine; Geriatric Emergency Department Guidelines Task Force. *Ann Emerg Med.* 2014;63:e7-e25.

157. Rowe J, et al. The effect of age on creatinine clearance in men: a cross-sectional and longitudinal study. *J Gerontol.* 1976;31:155-163.

158. Rule AD, et al. The association between age and nephrosclerosis on renal biopsy among health adults. *Ann Internal Med.* 2010;152:561-567.

159. Samaras N, et al. Older patients in the emergency department: a review. *Ann Emerg Med.* 2010;56:261-269.

160. Schaeffner ES, et al. Two novel equations to estimate kidney function in persons aged 70 years or older. *Ann Intern Med.* 2012;157:471-481.

161. Scher KS, Murria A. Under-representation of older adults in cancer registration trials: known problem, little progress. *J Clin Oncol.* 2012;30:2036-2038.

162. Scott IA, et al. Minimizing inappropriate medications in older populations: a 10-step conceptual framework. *Am J Med.* 2012;125:529-537.

163. Selway JS, et al. Alcohol use and testing among older trauma victims in Maryland. *J Trauma.* 2008;62:442-446.

164. Shea YF, Chu LW. Neuroleptic malignant syndrome caused by quetiapine in an elderly man with Lewy body dementia. *J Am Geriatr Soc.* 2016;64:e55-e56.

165. Shoker A, et al. Performance of creatinine clearance equations on the original Cockcroft-Gault population. *Clin Nephrol.* 2006;66:89-97.

166. Shorr RI, et al. Individual sulfonylureas and serious hypoglycemia in older people. *J Am Geriatr Soc.* 1996;44:751-755.

167. Singh S, et al. Thiazolinediones and heart failure. *Diabetes Care.* 2007;30:2148-2153.

168. Smith LA, et al. Cannabinoids for nausea and vomiting in adults with cancer receiving chemotherapy. *Cochrane Database Syst Rev.* 2015;issue11:CD009464.

169. Sonnenberg A, Genta RM. Changes in the gastric mucosa with aging. *Clin Gastroenterol Hepatol.* 2015;13:2276-2281.

170. Sorkin JD, et al. Longitudinal change in height of men and women: implications for interpretation of the body mass index. *Am J Epidemiol.* 1999;150:969-976.

171. Southworth MR, et al. Dabigatran and postmarketing reports of bleeding. *N Engl J Med.* 2013;368:1272-1274.

172. Steinmetz KL, et al. Assessment of geriatric information on the drug label for commonly prescribed drugs in older people. *J Am Geriatr Soc.* 2005;53:891-894.

173. Svenson J. Obtundation in the elderly patient. *Am J Emerg Med.* 1987;5:524-527.

174. Szoke E, et al. Effects of glimepiride and glyburide on glucose counterregulation and recovery from hypoglycemia. *Metabolism.* 2006;55:78-83.

175. Tadros G, Salib E. Age and methods of fatal self harm (FSH). Is there a link? *Int J Geriatr Psychiatry.* 2000;15:848-852.

176. Tamblyn RM, et al. A 5-year prospective assessment of the risk associated with individual benzodiazepines and doses in new elderly users. *J Am Geriatr Soc.* 2005;53:233-241.

177. Tamblyn RM, et al. Do too many cooks spoil the broth? Multiple physician involvement in medical management of elderly patients and potentially inappropriate drug combinations. *CMAJ.* 1996;154:1177-1184.

178. Thorpe JM, et al. Dual health care system use and high-risk prescribing in patients with dementia: a national cohort study. *Ann Intern Med.* 2017;166:157-163.

179. Tinetti ME. Preventing falls in older persons. *N Engl J Med.* 2003;348:42-49.

180. Tupler LA, et al. Alcohol pharmacodynamics in young-elderly adults contrasted with young and middle-aged subjects. *Psychopharmacology (Berlin).* 1995;118:460-470.

181. U.S. Food and Drug Administration. Drug Safety Communication: update on the risk for serious bleeding events with the anticoagulant Pradaxa (dabigatran). http://www.fda.gov/Drugs/DrugSafety/ucm282724.htm. Accessed March 27, 2017.

182. U.S. Food and Drug Administration. FDA Drug Safety Communication: FDA warns of possible harm from exceeding recommended dose of over-the-counter sodium phosphate products to treat constipation. https://www.fda.gov/Drugs/DrugSafety/ucm380757.htm. Published January 8, 2014. Accessed February 27, 2017.

183. Vadnerkar A, Brensilver JM. Enoxaparin-associated spontaneous retroperitoneal hematoma in elderly patients with impaired creatinine clearance: a report of two cases. *J Am Geriatr Soc.* 2004;52:477-479.

184. Vakkalanka JP, et al. Epidemiologic trends in loperamide abuse and misuse. *Ann Emerg Med.* 2017;69:73-78.

185. Van Assema DM, et al. Blood-brain barrier *P*-glycoprotein function in Alzheimer's disease. *Brain.* 2012;135(pt 1):181-189.

186. Van Assema, DME, et al. *P*-Glycoprotein function at the blood-brain barrier: effects of age and gender. *Mol Imaging Biol.* 2012;14:771-776.

187. Varas-Lorenzo C, et al. Myocardial infarction and individual nonsteroidal anti-inflammatory drugs meta-analysis of observational studies. *Pharmacoepidemiol Drug Saf.* 2013;22:559-570.

188. Vaya A, et al. Enoxaparin-related fatal spontaneous retroperitoneal hematoma in the elderly. *Thromb Res.* 2003;110:69-71.

189. Vestal RE, et al. Aging and ethanol metabolism. *Clin Pharmacol Ther.* 1977;21:343-354.

190. Vestal RE, et al. Reduced beta-adrenoceptor sensitivity in the elderly. *Clin Pharmacol Ther.* 1979;26:181-186.

191. Vilas-Boas V, et al. *P*-Glycoprotein activity in human Caucasian male lymphocytes does not follow its increased expression during aging. *Cytometry A.* 2011;79:912-919.

192. Vogelgesang S, et al. Deposition of Alzheimer's beta-amyloid is inversely correlated with *P*-glycoprotein expression in the brains of elderly non-demented humans. *Pharmacogenetics.* 2002;12:535-541.

193. Vogelgesang S, et al. The role of *P*-glycoprotein in cerebral amyloid angiopathy; implications for the early pathogenesis of Alzheimer's disease. *Curr Alzheimer Res.* 2004;1:121-125.

194. Wagner AK, et al. Benzodiazepine use and hip fractures in the elderly. Who is at greatest risk? *Arch Intern Med.* 2004;164:1567-1572.

195. Wallis WE, et al. Hypoglycemia masquerading as cerebrovascular disease (hypoglycemic hemiplegia). *Ann Neurol.* 1985;18:510-512.

196. Wang PS, et al. Zolpidem use and hip fractures in older people. *J Am Geriatr Soc.* 2001;49:1685-1690.

197. Welker JA, Zaloga GP. Pine oil ingestion. A common cause of poisoning. *Chest.* 1999;116:1822-1826.

198. Winter MA, et al. Impact of various body weights and serum creatinine concentrations on the bias and accuracy of the Cockcroft-Gault equation. *Pharmacotherapy.* 2012;32:604-612.

199. Wolfe MM, et al. Gastrointestinal toxicity of nonsteroidal anti-inflammatory agents. *N Engl J Med.* 1999;340:1888-1899.

200. Woodhouse KW, Wynne HA. Age-related changes in liver size and hepatic blood flow: the influence on drug metabolism in the elderly. *Clin Pharmacokinet.* 1988;15:287-294.

201. World Health Organization. World Health Statistics 2016. Monitoring Health for the Sustainable Development Goals. http://www.who.int/gho/publications/world_health_statistics/2016/EN_WHS2016_TOC.pdf. Published 2016. Accessed February 27, 2017.

202. Wu L, Blazer DG. Illicit and nonmedical drug use among older adults: a review. *J Aging Health.* 2011;23:481-504. http://www.ncbi.nlm.nih.gov/pmc/articles/PMC3097242/pdf/nihms288551.pdf. Accessed February 28, 2017.

203. Young VR. Amino acids and proteins in relation to the nutrition of elderly people. *Age Ageing.* 1990;19:S10-S24.

204. Zautcke JL, et al. Geriatric trauma in the state of Illinois: substance use and injury patterns. *Am J Emerg Med.* 2002;20:14-17.

205. Zhang Y, et al. Gastric parietal cell antibiodies, *Helicobacter pylori* infection and chronic atrophic gastritis: evidence from a large population based study in Germany. *Cancer Epidemiol Biomarkers Prev.* 2013;22:821-826.

33 ACETAMINOPHEN

Robert G. Hendrickson and Nathanael J. McKeown

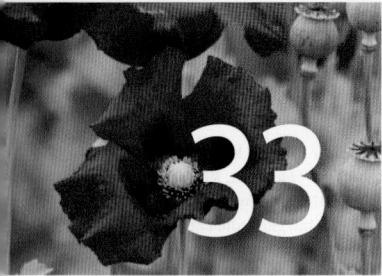

MW	= 151 Da
Therapeutic serum concentration	= 10–30 mcg/mL
	= 66–199 µmol/L

HISTORY AND EPIDEMIOLOGY

By the late 1800s, both phenacetin and acetanilide were used as analgesics and antipyretics, but their acceptance was limited by significant side effects, including methemoglobinemia. N-Acetyl-p-aminophenol is a major metabolite of phenacetin and acetanilide and is responsible for both analgesia and antipyresis. N-acetyl-p-aminophenol was synthesized in 1878 and has a low risk of causing methemoglobinemia. N-Acetyl-p-aminophenol is abbreviated as APAP (N-**a**cetyl-p-**a**mino**p**henol) and is referred to as acetaminophen (N-**acet**yl-para**aminophen**ol) in the United States, Canada, Japan, and several other countries and as paracetamol (**para**-**acet**yl**am**inophen**ol**) in most other areas of the globe. These terms are all acronyms of the chemical name. Acetaminophen was first used clinically in the United States and the United Kingdom in the mid 1950s, but its widespread acceptance was delayed until the 1970s because of concerns of the toxicities of its precursors. Acetaminophen has since proved to be a remarkably safe medication at appropriate dosage, which has led to its popularity. Acetaminophen is available in myriad single-medication dose formulations and delivery systems and in a variety of combinations with opioids, other analgesics, sedatives, decongestants, expectorants, and antihistamines.[205] The diversity and wide availability of APAP products dictate that the potential for APAP toxicity be evaluated not only after identified ingestions but also after exposure to unknown or multiple xenobiotics in settings of intentional overdose, abuse, and therapeutic misadventures.

Despite enormous experience with APAP toxicity, many controversies and challenges remain unresolved. New formulations and analogs are being introduced, including multiple extended-release and transmucosal formulations that will require reassessments of the available knowledge.[129,261] To best understand the continuing evolution in the approach to APAP toxicity, it is critical to start with certain fundamental principles and then to apply these principles to both typical and atypical presentations in which APAP toxicity must be evaluated.

PHARMACOLOGY

Acetaminophen is an analgesic and antipyretic with weak peripheral antiinflammatory and antiplatelet properties. Analgesic activity is reported at a serum [APAP] of 10 mcg/mL and antipyretic activity at 4 to 18 mcg/mL.[379]

Acetaminophen has a unique mechanism of action among the analgesic antipyretics. Most of the nonsteroidal antiinflammatory drugs (NSAIDs) occupy the cyclooxygenase (COX) binding site on the enzyme prostaglandin H_2 synthase (PGH_2) and prevent arachidonic acid from physically entering the site and being converted to prostaglandin H_2. Acetaminophen also inhibits prostaglandin H_2 production but does so indirectly by reducing a heme on the peroxidase (POX) portion of the PGH_2,[223] and indirectly inhibiting COX activation.[14,217] In this way, APAP function is highly dependent on cellular location and intracellular conditions.[254] Acetaminophen strongly inhibits prostaglandin synthesis where concentrations of POX and arachidonic acid ("peroxide tone") are low, such as in the brain.[114] In conditions of high peroxide tone, such as inflammatory cells (macrophages) and platelets, prostaglandin synthesis is less affected by APAP,[14,45,126,217,245,254] although this is not universal.[16] This dissociation explains the strong central antipyretic and analgesic effect of APAP but weak peripheral antiinflammatory and antiplatelet effects. Functionally, APAP predominantly acts as a central indirect inhibitor of COX-2 enzymes,[156,243] with some mild peripheral COX-2 inhibition[206] and minimal COX-1 inhibition (Chap. 35).[59]

Antipyresis and analgesia are predominantly mediated by this central indirect COX-2 inhibition and the resulting decrease in prostaglandin E_2 (PGE_2) synthesis.[110,126,189,245] Additional analgesic effects are mediated by serotoninergic, opioid, cannabinoid, and transient receptor potential vanilloid cation channel subfamily V member 1 (TPRV1) receptors.[219] Stimulation of descending serotonergic pathways is demonstrated in rats[42] and humans,[126,260] and the analgesic effect of APAP is inhibited by several serotonin antagonists or serotonin depletion.[8,260,262,300] In rats, the analgesic effect of APAP is attenuated by opioid receptor antagonists.[54,263,301] However, APAP binds poorly to opioid receptors,[276-278] and the exact opioid mechanism remains unexplained.[301] Activation of the central or peripheral endogenous cannabinoid system, potentially from an APAP metabolite,[158] is theorized but remains controversial.[32,81,138,253] Finally, activation of TPRV1 receptors by a lipoamino metabolite of APAP, and the resulting activation of T-type calcium channels was demonstrated in mice and contributes to analgesia.[179]

PHARMACOKINETICS

After ingestion of a therapeutic dose, immediate-release APAP is rapidly absorbed from the small intestine with a time to peak [APAP] of approximately 30 minutes for liquid formulations and 45 minutes for tablet formulations.[10,95,116] Extended-release APAP has a time to peak of 1 to 2 hours but is almost entirely absorbed by 4 hours.[98] The time to peak is delayed by food[95] and coingestion of opioids or antimuscarinics.[137] The oral bioavailability is 60% to 98%,[281] and the volume of distribution (V_d) is 1 L/kg.[10,11] Peak [APAP] after recommended doses typically ranges from 8 to 20 mcg/mL.[10,116] After administration of 20 to 25 mg/kg of rectal suppositories, the peak [APAP] ranges from 4.1 to 13.6 mcg/mL, the time to peak [APAP] is 2 to 4 hours (range, 0.4–8 hours), and the bioavailability is 30% to 40%.[22,39,136] Acetaminophen is available in the intravenous (IV) form in many countries as well as a prodrug (eg, propacetamol) in the United Kingdom. The time to peak of the IV formulations are immediate (< 15 minutes). In adults, peak [APAP] after a 1-g infusion is approximately 30 mcg/mL and after a 2-g infusion is approximately 75 mcg/mL with a large range of 31 to 161 mcg/mL.[7,113,133,259] Acetaminophen enters the cerebrospinal fluid within 15 minutes after IV dosing and within 45 minutes after oral or rectal doses.[326] Whereas the V_d is higher in both pregnant women and neonates, clearance rates are higher in pregnant women and lower in neonates.[6,7,193] Acetaminophen has total protein binding of 10%

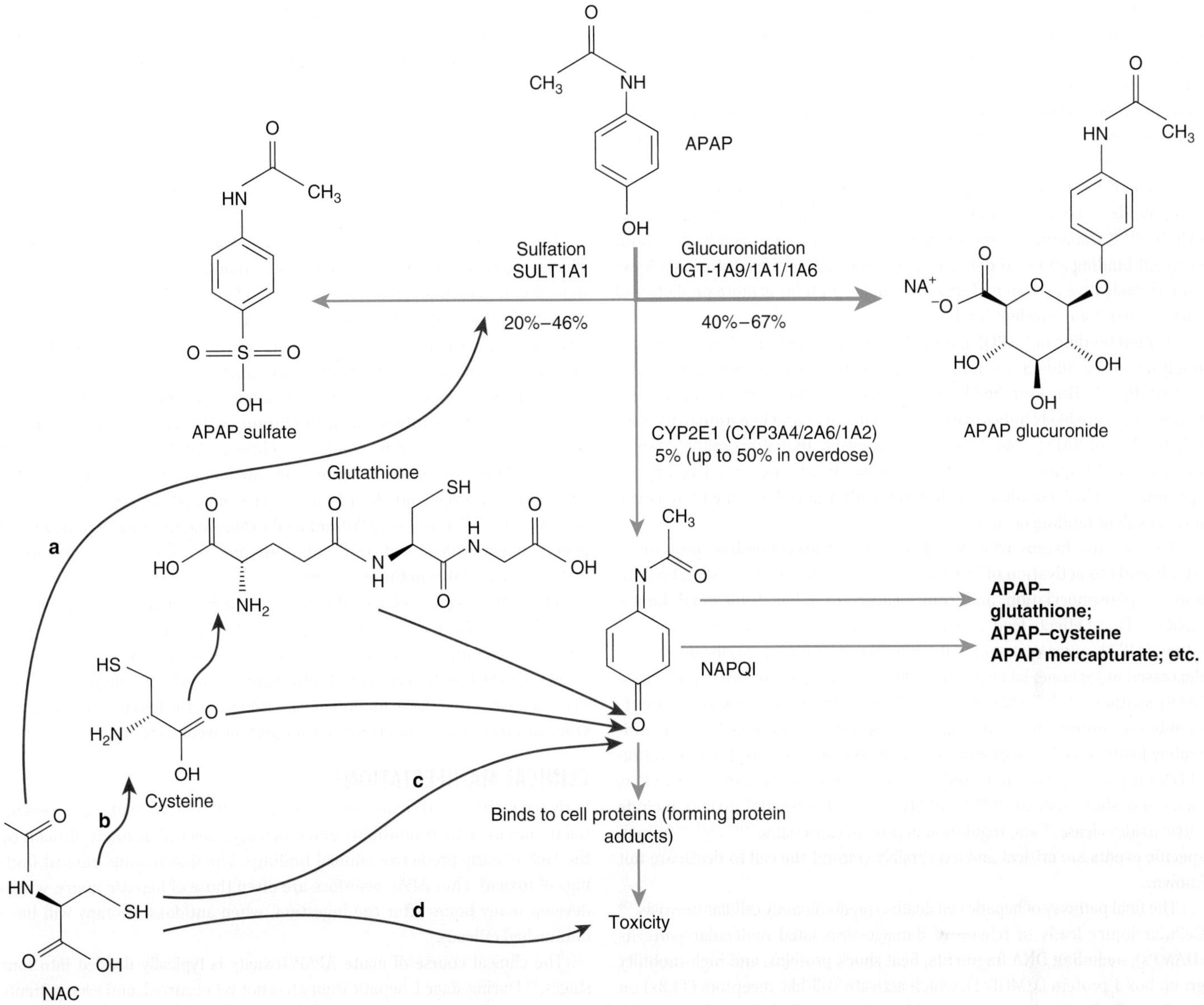

FIGURE 33–1. Important routes of acetaminophen (APAP) metabolism in humans and mechanisms of *N*-acetylcysteine (NAC) hepatoprotection. *N*-acetylcysteine augments sulfation (*a*), NAC is a glutathione (GSH) precursor (*b*), NAC is a GSH substitute (*c*), and NAC improves multiorgan function (*d*) during hepatic failure and possibly limits the extent of hepatocyte injury. APAP = *N*-acetyl-*p*-aminophenol; NAPQI = *N*-acetyl-*p*-benzoquinoneimine.

to 30% that does not change in overdose.[234] Acetaminophen crosses the placenta and enters breast milk in small amounts (< 2% of ingested dose).[208,250]

After absorption, approximately 90% of APAP normally undergoes hepatic conjugation with glucuronide (40%–67%), mostly via UGT1A9/1A1/1A6, and sulfate (20%–46%), mostly via SULT1A1, to form inactive metabolites, which are eliminated in the urine.[71] A small fraction of unchanged APAP (< 5%) and other minor metabolites reach the urine.[237] The remaining fraction, approximately 5% in therapeutic doses, is oxidized by CYP2E1 (and, to a lesser extent, CYP3A4, CYP2A6, and CYP1A2),[146,222] resulting in the formation of *N*-acetyl-*p*-benzoquinoneimine (NAPQI).[70] Glutathione (GSH) quickly combines with NAPQI,[236] and the resulting complexes are converted to nontoxic cysteine or mercaptate conjugates, which are eliminated in the urine (Fig. 33–1).[233,237] The elimination half-life of APAP is approximately 2 to 3 hours after a nontoxic dose[5,270] but is prolonged in patients who develop hepatotoxicity.[270]

TOXICOKINETICS

After most oral overdoses, the majority of APAP absorption occurs within 2 hours, and peak plasma concentrations generally occur within 4 hours. Later peaks or double peaks are occasionally documented in overdoses and have generally occurred after large ingestions (> 50 g) with or without coingested antimuscarinics.[38,154,340,368] After overdose, NAPQI production is largely

the result of activity of the CYP2E1 enzyme,[142,146] and the amount of NAPQI formed is increased out of proportion to the APAP dose and accounts for up to 20% to 50% of metabolism in patients with hepatotoxicity.[271] Contributions of CYP1A2, CYP3A4, and CYP2A6 to the production of NAPQI in humans are small and insignificant in most cases but depend on individual host factors and dosage.[146,256,280,359] After clinically significant overdose, nontoxic sulfation metabolism of APAP becomes saturated.[2,186,284] Rates of metabolism through glucuronidation are highly variable, increase proportionately in overdose, and are not saturatable in humans (Fig. 33–1).[24,90,186,267,284]

The toxicokinetics of IV APAP are largely unknown. Doses of 15 mg/kg, 75 mg/kg, and 146 mg/kg produce [APAP] of 10 mcg/mL, 35 mcg/mL, and 117 mcg/mL, respectively, at 4 hours, with half-lives ranging from 2 to 6 hours.[27,68,87]

PATHOPHYSIOLOGY

The safety of appropriate APAP dosing results from the availability of electron donors such as reduced GSH and other thiol (S-H)-containing compounds. After therapeutic APAP dosing, GSH supply and turnover far exceed that required to detoxify NAPQI. With ample GSH supply, NAPQI is largely bound by GSH, and no toxicity occurs, although NAPQI-cysteine protein adducts do form within the liver, and some are released into the serum within hours.[152,232,251] After overdose, the rate and quantity of NAPQI formation outstrip supply and turnover of GSH, resulting in the release of NAPQI within the cell. N-acetyl-p-benzoquinoneimine then rapidly binds to hepatocyte constituents, including the cysteine portion of intramitochondrial proteins, producing protein adducts within the liver. In animal experiments, hepatotoxicity becomes evident only when hepatic [GSH] decreases to 30% of baseline or below.[236]

When NAPQI formation overwhelms the supply of thiol-containing compounds, it covalently binds[142,266] and arylates proteins throughout the cell,[67,172,174,266] inducing a series of events that result in cell death.[54,67,174] Both covalent binding and GSH deficiency are necessary for hepatotoxicity; however, the selective arylation of specific cellular proteins is more predictive of toxicity than total covalent binding.[67,163,167]

Protein binding of NAPQI and the formation of protein adducts does not imply toxicity as adducts are formed and detected in the serum at a therapeutic [APAP].[151,251] However, highly elevated concentrations of protein adducts in the serum are likely indicative of cellular necrosis and hepatotoxicity. Protein binding of NAPQI leads to a cascade of events that alters mitochondrial function and impairs cell defenses against endogenous reactive oxygen species.[174,285] This cascade is ameliorated with N-acetylcysteine (NAC) even after covalent binding occurs.[50,120,167,285]

The cascade begins with NAPQI binding to mitochondrial proteins,[384] which leads to activation of MAP kinases (eg, MLK-3, RIP-1, ASK-1, GSK3B) and[82,393] phosphorylation and translocation of c-Jun N-terminal kinase (JNK).[384] These effects lead to opening of mitochondrial permeability transition (MPT) pores, causing mitochondrial membrane permeability,[283,285] decreased mitochondrial respiration, and decreased adenosine triphosphate (ATP) synthesis.[96,283] Furthermore, MPT opening leads to release of intermembrane proteins (endonuclease G, apoptosis inducing factor) and ultimately leads to DNA fragmentation[72] and cellular necrosis. Fragmentation of DNA is partially caused by inhibition of topoisomerase 2-α[25,321] as well as calcium dyshomeostasis.[240,360,361] Additional mechanisms of toxicity include nitric oxide release[298] and regulation of protein expression.[35,163,164,283,297] Which specific events are critical and irreversibly commit the cell to death are not known.

The final pathway of hepatic cell death is predominantly cellular necrosis.[135] Cellular injury leads to release of damage-associated molecular patterns (DAMPs), including DNA fragments, heat shock proteins, and high-mobility group box 1 protein (HMGB-1), which activate Toll-like receptors (TLRs) on Kupffer cells, leading to further cytokine release, and nitric oxide release.[298] Some of the intracellular components that are released from necrotic cells are biomarkers of hepatic injury and include aspartate aminotransferase (AST), alanine aminotransferase (ALT), microRNA 122 (miRNA-122), HMGB-1, keratin-18 protein (K-18), and protein adducts.[12,13,92,152,209] Apoptosis occurs early in APAP toxicity[221,265,282] or after activation of the immune system in response to cellular necrosis[1,12] but is not likely the major mechanism of cellular toxicity. Macrophages, neutrophils, and inflammatory cells infiltrate after necrosis[160,162,196,199] followed by a cascade of inflammatory cytokines such as interleukin (IL) 1, IL-6, IL-8, leukotrienes, Toll-like receptor-9 (TLR-9),[220] and monocyte chemotactic protein-1 (MCP-1).[166,167,196,213,220,274] Cellular infiltration contributes to further hepatocellular destruction[213] but is not necessary for hepatic injury.[72,199] Hepatocyte recovery, repair, and proliferation are modulated by inflammatory mediators, cellular infiltration, and bile acids. The balance of necrosis and regeneration is an important area of current research.[36,37,165]

Hepatotoxicity initially and most profoundly occurs in hepatic zone III (centrilobular) because this zone is the area with the largest concentration of oxidative metabolism (CYP2E1; Fig. 21–1). In more severe hepatotoxicity, necrosis extends into zones II and I, destroying the entire hepatic parenchyma.

Kidney injury after acute overdose is typically acute tubular necrosis that is most likely caused by local production of NAPQI by renal CYP2E1 enzymes.[47,144,159] However, several other nephrotoxic mechanisms are proposed.[143] Conversion of APAP and hepatically derived APAP–GSH[239] to nephrotoxic

p-aminophenol[58] and p-benzoquinone are demonstrated in animal models.[227] N-acetyl-p-benzoquinoneimine formation via renal COX-2 and prostaglandin-mediated renal medullary ischemia[273] are also suspected of contributing to chronic analgesic nephropathy from APAP alone or in combination with other analgesics.[115,299] In patients with hepatic failure, volume depletion and hepatorenal syndrome are the most important contributory cofactors.[378] Dose-related renal potassium wasting[255,369] after acute APAP overdose is caused by APAP-induced renal vasoconstriction due to COX inhibition, a NAC effect, or both.[255]

Direct injury to organs other than the liver and kidney is rarely reported. The mechanism of early central nervous system (CNS) depression after APAP ingestion is undefined, but theoretical mechanisms include serotonin and opioid effects as well as APAP-induced CNS GSH depletion.[56] Early after massive APAP ingestion, metabolic acidosis and elevated lactate result from alterations in mitochondrial respiratory function.[53,107,114,327,350] Rare cases of metabolic acidosis with 5-oxoprolinemia and 5-oxoprolinuria are reported and are more likely in women with chronic APAP use and chronic kidney disease.[49,111,157] In this rare condition, chronic APAP use combined with acute oxidative stress and inflammatory mediators lead to an alteration of the γ-glutamyl cycle and elevations of γ-glutamylcysteine and 5-oxoproline (Fig. 33–2).[49,157,212] Cases of APAP-induced oxoprolinemia may be indicative of genetic polymorphisms of GSH synthetase and 5-oxoprolinase, and genetic testing is reasonable in these patients.[212]

The remaining sequelae of severe toxicity are secondary effects of fulminant hepatic failure rather than direct APAP effects, and the pathophysiology of these complex multisystem problems is well described.[204] The ability of NAC to ameliorate secondary multiorgan failure via extrahepatic mechanisms suggests that the oxidation of vital thiols and the loss of normal microvascular function are important components of secondary organ failure.[141,177]

CLINICAL MANIFESTATIONS

Early recognition and treatment of patients with APAP poisoning are essential to minimize their morbidity and mortality. This task is made difficult by the lack of early predictive clinical findings. The first reliable clinical findings of toxicity after APAP overdose are often those of hepatic injury, which develop many hours after the ingestion, when antidotal therapy will have diminished efficacy.

The clinical course of acute APAP toxicity is typically divided into four stages.[291] During stage I, hepatic injury has not yet occurred, and even patients who ultimately develop severe hepatotoxicity are often asymptomatic. Clinical findings, when present, are nonspecific and include nausea, vomiting, malaise, pallor, and diaphoresis. Laboratory indices of hepatic function are normal. In cases of massive overdose, a decreased level of consciousness,[100,131,188,290,327,348] metabolic acidosis, and even death[43,325] may occur during this stage in the absence of clinical findings of hepatotoxicity.[43,112,188,290,318,392] The metabolic acidosis is associated with elevated lactate concentrations[131,188,231,290,318,327,377,391] and is caused by inhibition of electron transport by APAP, NAPQI, or both.[106,107,131,318] These clinical findings should never be attributed to APAP alone without thorough evaluation for other possible causes.

Stage II represents the onset of hepatic injury, which occurs in fewer than 5% of those who overdose.[334] The AST is the most sensitive widely available measure to detect the onset of hepatotoxicity, and [AST] abnormalities always precede evidence of actual hepatic dysfunction (prolonged prothrombin time {PT}, international normalized ratio {INR}, elevated bilirubin concentration, hypoglycemia, encephalopathy, and metabolic acidosis). When stage II occurs, [AST] elevation most commonly begins within 24 hours after ingestion and is nearly universal by 36 hours.[132,323] In the most severely poisoned patients, AST may increase as early as 12 hours after ingestion.[132,323] The ALT begin to elevate shortly after the AST, but they peak at similar concentrations, and AST decreases earlier than the [ALT]. Of note, both AST and [ALT] are markers of hepatotoxicity, but because [AST] rises and decreases earlier than [ALT], we recommend using AST for detecting early hepatotoxicity and for determining hepatic recovery. In all other cases, AST and ALT are interchangeable and are described generically as aminotransferases in this chapter.

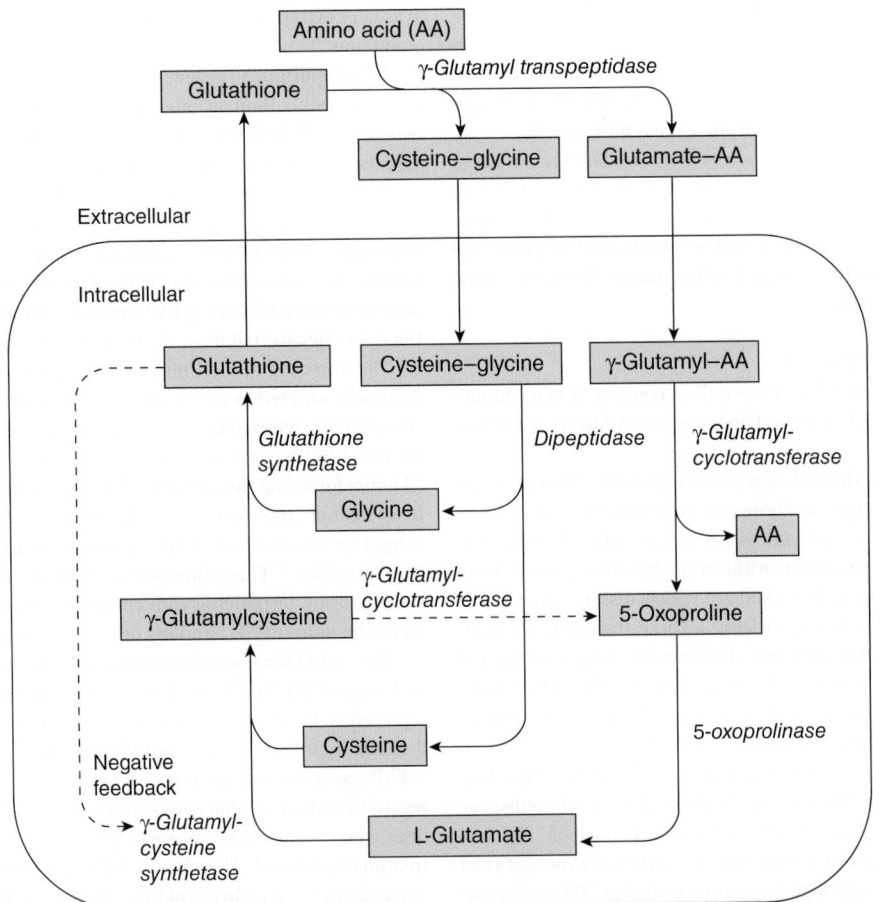

FIGURE 33–2. γ-Glutamyl cycle. The γ-glutamyl cycle is the primary pathway for glutathione synthesis and degradation. In rare cases, or massive acetaminophen (APAP) use combined with acute oxidative stress may lead to decreased glutathione concentrations, which via a feedback loop, increases γ-glutamylcysteine concentrations, which is then converted to 5-oxoproline, leading to acidosis and elevated 5-oxoproline concentrations. *(Reproduced with permission from Duewall JL, Fenves AZ, Richey DS, et al. 5-Oxoproline (pyroglutamic) acidosis associated with chronic acetaminophen use. Proc (Bayl Univ Med Cent) 2010 Jan;23(1):19-20.)*

Concentrations of APAP-protein adducts (APAP-CYS) become detectable within hours of ingestion,[170] peak with AST, and have an elimination half-life of about 27 hours.[77,170] Symptoms and signs during stage II vary with the severity of hepatic injury. Acetaminophen-induced *hepatotoxicity* is defined as a peak [AST] or [ALT] above 1,000 IU/L. Although lower peak concentrations of [AST] or [ALT] represent some injury to hepatic tissue, they rarely have any clinical relevance.

Stage III, defined as the time of maximal hepatotoxicity, most commonly occurs between 72 and 96 hours after ingestion. The clinical manifestations of stage III include fulminant hepatic failure with encephalopathy and coma, and, rarely, hemorrhage. Results of laboratory studies are variable; AST and ALT concentrations above 10,000 IU/L are common, even in patients without other evidence of hepatic failure. Much more important than the degree of [aminotransferase] elevation, abnormalities of PT and INR, glucose, lactate, creatinine, and pH are essential determinants of prognosis and treatment.

Renal function abnormalities are rare (< 1%) overall,[62,272,372] but they occur in as many as 25% of patients with significant hepatotoxicity[153,272] and in 50% to 80% of those with hepatic failure.[195,287,378] Renal abnormalities are more common after repeated excessive dosing[195] and in adolescents and older adults.[46,62,226,241] After acute ingestions, elevations of serum creatinine typically occur between 2 and 5 days after ingestion, peak on days 5 to 7 (range, 3–16 days),[372] and normalize over 1 month.[226] When severe acute kidney injury (AKI) necessitating hemodialysis occurs, it nearly always occurs in patients with marked hepatic injury. Patients with hepatorenal syndrome are commonly treated with continuous renal replacement therapy, and among those who survive, kidney failure generally resolves within 1 month.[211,287] Infrequently, mild AKI occurs without elevations in [aminotransferase].[4,46,66,104]

Fatalities from fulminant hepatic failure generally occur between 3 and 5 days after an acute overdose. Death results from either single or combined complications of multiorgan failure, including acute respiratory distress syndrome, sepsis, cerebral edema, or, rarely, hemorrhage. Patients who survive this period reach stage IV, defined as the recovery phase. Survivors have complete hepatic regeneration, and no cases of chronic hepatic dysfunction are reported. The rate of recovery varies; in most cases, [AST], pH, PT, and INR, and [lactate] are normal by 7 days in survivors of acute overdoses. [Alanine Aminotransferases] remains elevated longer than [AST], and creatinine may be elevated for more than 1 month. The recovery time is much longer in severely poisoned patients, and hepatic histologic abnormalities potentially persist for months.[207,225,264]

DIAGNOSTIC TESTING

Assessing the Risk of Toxicity

Principles Guiding the Diagnostic Approach

Most patients with APAP exposures do not develop toxicity, and the overall mortality rate after acute APAP ingestion is less than 0.5%.[334] However, APAP is now the leading cause of acute liver failure (ALF) in the United States and much of the developed world.[195] To maintain the seemingly divergent goals of avoiding the enormous cost of overtreatment while minimizing patient risk, clinicians must understand the basis for and sensitivity of current toxicity screening methods. A discussion of the diagnostic approach follows.

When evaluating risk, it is useful to separate different categories of APAP exposure. There is an extensive body of experience and literature on acute overdose in typical circumstances, permitting a systematic approach with demonstrated efficacy. For issues related to repeated supratherapeutic APAP dosing, uncertain circumstances, new APAP formulations, and many other permutations, there is an important conceptual framework for decision making but little in the way of validated strategies. For these challenges, the central concepts and one approach are presented here, with the understanding that the challenges continue to evolve and that more than one approach may have validity.

The ideal model for determining risk after APAP overdose would assess the individual's metabolic enzyme activity (CYP2E1, UDP-glucuronyl transferase, and sulfotransferase activity), the amount and rate of NAPQI formation, the availability of hepatic GSH, early markers of cellular disruption, and the balance of NAPQI formation and hepatic GSH turnover. At present, none of these measures is available to clinicians.

Risk Determination After Acute Overdose

Determining risk in a patient with acute overdose consists of determining the initial risk based on dosing history and then potentially further risk stratifying with serum [APAP].

Acute overdose usually is defined as a single ingestion, although many patients actually overdose incrementally over a brief period of time. For purposes of this discussion, an *acute overdose* is somewhat arbitrarily defined as one in which the entire ingestion occurs within a single 4-hour period. Doses of 7.5 g in an adult or 150 mg/kg in a child are widely disseminated as the lowest acute dose capable of causing toxicity.[271] These standards are likely quite conservative but have stood the test of time as sensitive markers and are corroborated with human data.[370,395] However, it is more likely that doses of at least 12 g (~150 mg/kg) in an adult or 200 to 350 mg/kg in a child are necessary to cause hepatotoxicity in most patients.[238,365,370]

The adult standard is less controversial than that for children because massive ingestions, unreliable histories, and factors that might predispose to toxicity occur primarily in adults, justifying continued use of 7.5 g as a screening amount to avoid missing serious toxicity. In patients younger than 6 years of age, with unintentional ingestions, use of a higher 200-mg/kg cutoff is reasonable[57,85,238,352] and is likely appropriate but is incompletely studied.

The dose history should be used in the assessment of risk only if there is reliable corroboration or direct validation. Although the amount ingested by history linearly correlates with risk of toxicity and an [APAP] over the treatment line,[26,370,395,102,200] historic information is not sufficiently reliable in every patient to exclude significant ingestion, particularly in patients with the intent of self-harm.[102,200,395] Reported ingested doses of 6 g, 13 g, 30 g, and 50 g infer a risk of about 5%, 10%, 50%, and 90%, respectively, that the [APAP] will be above the treatment line.[102] However, suicidal patients with ingestions who do not confirm an ingestion of APAP have a measurable concentration in 1.4% to 8.4% of cases[15,216] and a concentration over the treatment line in 0.2% to 2.2%.[15,216] Therefore, when the history suggests possible risk, the patient should be further assessed with measurement of a serum [APAP].

Interpretation of [APAP] after acute exposures is based on an adaptation of the Rumack-Matthew nomogram (Fig. 33–3).[293] The original nomogram was based on the observation that untreated patients who subsequently developed an [AST] above 1,000 IU/L could be separated from those who did not on the basis of their initial [APAP]. A nomogram was constructed that plotted the initial concentration versus time since ingestion, and a discriminatory line was drawn to separate patients who developed hepatotoxicity from those who did not. The initial discriminatory line stretched from an [APAP] of 300 mcg/mL at 4 hours to 50 mcg/mL at 12 hours but was lowered to between 200 mcg/mL at 4 hours and 50 mcg/mL at 12 hours after evaluation of additional patients.[293] The half-life of APAP was not a factor in the development of the nomogram, and the slope of the treatment line is based on empirical clinical data and does not reflect any discriminatory APAP half-life or APAP kinetics.[293] The nomogram is designed and validated using a single value obtained at or greater than 4 hours after ingestion to allow for complete APAP absorption. Although patients who develop hepatotoxicity typically have APAP half-lives greater than 4 hours,[270,329] plotting multiple points on the nomogram or using an APAP half-life to determine risk is not adequately studied and has significant limitations.[185,338] The nomogram

was later extrapolated to 24 hours using the same slope of the original nomogram line.[293]

It is important to realize that the line was based on [aminotransferase] elevation rather than on hepatic failure or death, and it was chosen to be very sensitive, with little regard to specificity. Without antidotal therapy, only 60% of those with an initial APAP above this original line will develop hepatotoxicity as defined by [aminotransferases] above 1,000 IU/L, but the risk of hepatotoxicity is not the same for all such patients. Elevated [aminotransferase] develops in virtually all untreated patients with [APAP] far above the line, and serious hepatic dysfunction occurs frequently; the incidence of hepatotoxicity among patients with an [APAP] immediately above the line is very low, and the risk of hepatic failure or death is far less.[272,328]

The line used in the United States runs parallel to the original but was arbitrarily lowered by 25% to add even greater sensitivity.[291,293] The lower line, subsequently referred to as the *treatment line* or *150 line*, starts at a concentration of 150 mcg/mL at 4 hours following ingestion and ends at 4.7 mcg/mL 24 hours following the overdose. The treatment line is one of the most sensitive screening tools used in medicine. The incidence of nomogram failures using this line in the United States is only 1% to 3% (depending on time to treatment).[293] These infrequent "failures" result from inaccurate ingestion histories, or patients with currently undefined risk factors for toxicity, including unique GSH handling or CYP enzyme activities.[230,293]

The United Kingdom uses a single nomogram line starting at 100 mcg/mL at 4 hours ("100 line") for all acute APAP ingestions.[122] This single 100 line replaced a two-tiered treatment protocol that treated low-risk patients if either their [APAP] exceeded the "200 line" or high risk patients if their [APAP] exceeded the "100 line."[373] The change was motivated by concern with regard to a small number of patients with an [APAP] between the 100 and 200 lines who developed hepatotoxicity[23,48,89,293,337,373] and a desire to simplify the treatment protocol. The change led to an increase in adult and pediatric admissions,[20,248] anaphylactoid reactions to NAC, and millions of additional dollars in treatment costs.[19]

Based on these observations and more than 25 years of use, the 150 line is adequate in nearly all cases and is reliable when rigorously followed. When using the APAP nomogram, it is essential to precisely define the time window during which APAP ingestion occurred and, if the time is unknown, to use the *earliest possible time* as the time of ingestion. Using this approach, patients with an [APAP] below the treatment line, even if only slightly so, do not require further evaluation or treatment for acute APAP overdose. Reports of patients developing hepatotoxicity with an [APAP] below the treatment line are exceedingly rare, and risks are estimated as less than 1% risk of hepatotoxicity and less than 0.05% of liver failure.[23,293] This also applies to most patients with factors that predispose them to APAP-induced hepatotoxicity. There is adequate experience with acute APAP overdose in the settings of potentially predisposing factors such as chronic heavy ethanol use, chronic medication with CYP-inducing xenobiotics, and inadequate nutrition to recommend that no special approach is required in such cases. Further study is needed to determine if rare events, such as acute APAP ingestion in the setting of chronic isoniazid (INH) use,[105,244,390] might uniquely predispose patients to toxicity and require alteration of this approach.

The goal should be to determine an [APAP] at the earliest point at which it will be meaningful in decision making. Therefore, measurement of an [APAP] 4 hours after ingestion or as soon as possible thereafter is used to confirm the patient's risk of toxicity and thus the need to initiate NAC. Although it is optimal to start NAC therapy as soon as possible after confirmation of risk, NAC is nearly 100% effective if started before 8 hours after ingestion.[328,333] This allows clinicians some leeway to wait for the laboratory results before starting therapy in patients in whom the history of ingestion suggests that the 4-hour [APAP] will fall below the treatment line. However, it should be noted that delaying NAC therapy longer than 8 hours after ingestion increases the patient's risk. If there is any concern about the availability of an [APAP] before this time, then treatment with NAC should be initiated. In such cases, the [APAP] still should be determined as soon as possible. When the results become available, they should be interpreted according to

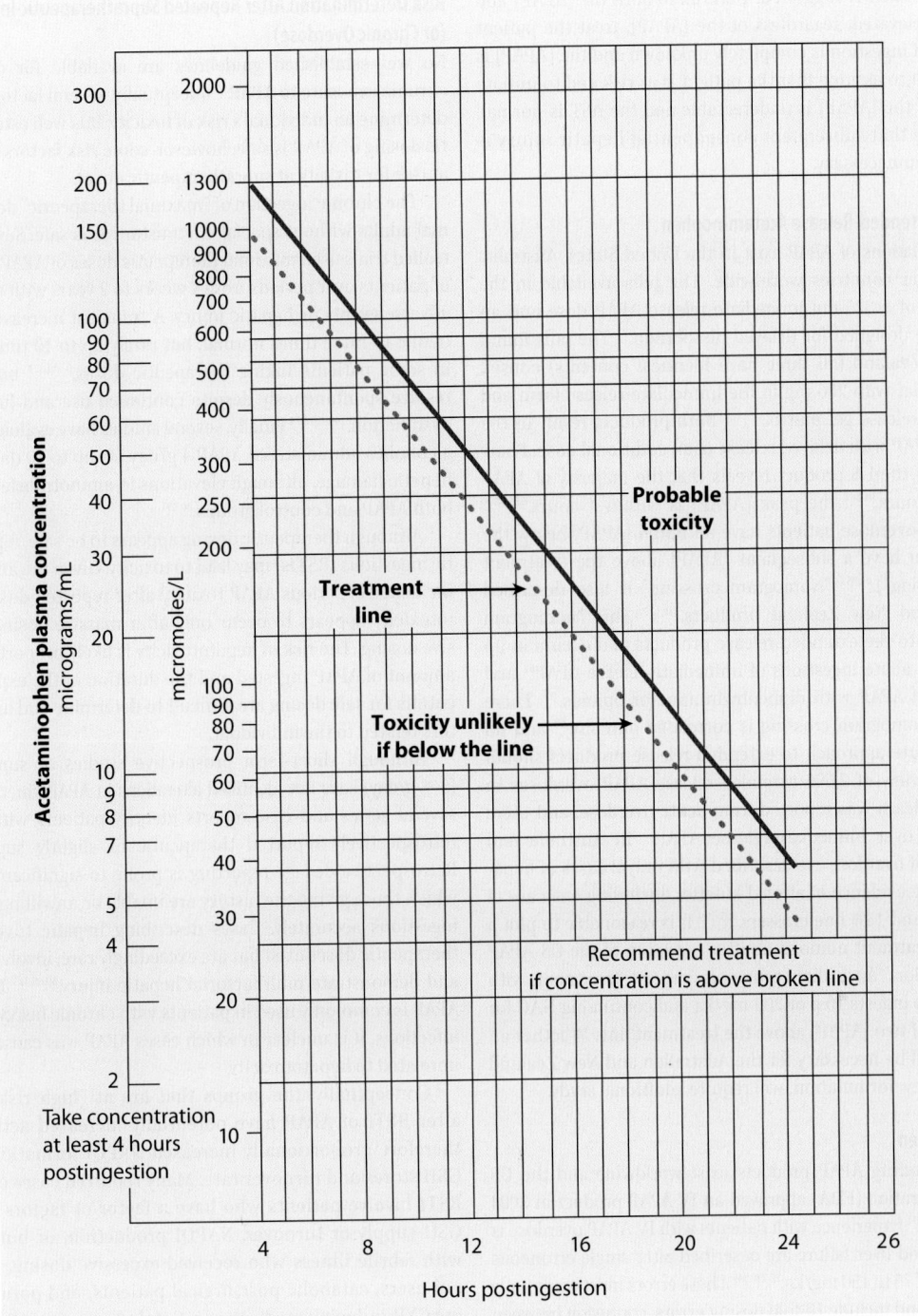

FIGURE 33–3. Rumack-Matthew nomogram (reconstructed) for determining the risk of acetaminophen (APAP)-induced hepatoxicity after a single acute ingestion. Serum [APAP] above the treatment line on the nomogram indicates the need for *N*-acetylcysteine therapy. *(Reproduced with permission from Tintinalli JE, Stapczynski S, Ma OJ, et al. Tintinalli's Emergency Medicine: A Comprehensive Study Guide, 8th ed. New York, NY: McGraw-Hill Education; 2016.)*

the treatment line on the APAP nomogram and NAC either continued or discontinued on the basis of this result. In the unusual circumstance in which no determination of an [APAP] can ever be obtained, evidence of possible risk by history alone is sufficient to initiate and complete a course of NAC therapy postingestion.

Early Measurement of [APAP]
Measurement of the [APAP] between 2 and 4 hours after ingestion is only helpful to exclude ingestion of APAP. If an [APAP] is undetectable in this time frame, significant APAP overdose is likely excluded.[387] However, an [APAP] that is detectable between 2 and 4 hours cannot be definitively interpreted and, unless undetectable, mandates repeat testing at 4 hours. An [APAP]

before 2 hours should not be interpreted because of several cases of low or undetectable [APAP] in this time period with a resulting 4-hour [APAP] over the treatment line.[118,347]

Determination of Risk When the Acetaminophen Nomogram Is Not Applicable
Risk Determination When Time of Ingestion Is Unknown
With careful questioning of the patient, family, and others, it is almost always possible to establish a time window during which the APAP ingestion must have occurred. The *earliest possible time* of ingestion ("worst-case scenario") is used for risk-determination purposes. If this time window cannot be established or is so broad that it encompasses a span of more than 24 hours,

then the following approach is suggested. Determine both the [APAP] and [AST]. If the [AST] is elevated, regardless of the [APAP], treat the patient with NAC. If the time of ingestion is completely unknown and the [APAP] is detectable, it is prudent to assume that the patient is at risk and to initiate treatment with NAC. If the [APAP] is undetectable and the AST is normal, there is little evidence that subsequent consequential hepatic injury is possible,[325] and NAC is unnecessary.

Risk Assessment After Extended-Release Acetaminophen

Extended-release formulations of APAP exist in the United States, Australia, New Zealand, and other countries worldwide. The pills available in the United States consists of a 325-mg immediate-release APAP dose and an additional 325-mg dose designed for delayed dissolution.[83] The pills found in Australia and New Zealand (all three have identical contents) consist of a 665-mg bilayer tablet with 206 mg in the immediate-release form and 459 mg in a sustained-release gel matrix.[127,128] Both products result in the immediate release of APAP with delayed release of an additional dose. Pharmacokinetic analysis of the US product reveals that the majority of APAP is absorbed within 4 hours,[98,363] the peak [APAP] is within 4 hours,[61,98,349] and a small number of overdose patients have an initial [APAP] below the treatment line but then have a subsequent [APAP] above the treatment line ("nomogram crossing").[61,363] "Nomogram crossing" is also described with the Australian and New Zealand products.[128,129] This "nomogram crossing" is not unique to the extended-release products and occurs in up to 10% of patients with acute ingestions of immediate-release APAP[52] and those with ingestions of APAP with diphenhydramine or opioids.[184] There is little evidence that nomogram crossing is correlated outcome[83] and no evidence that an alternate approach to extended-release products should be used. In a 9-year review of 2,596 extended-release APAP overdoses in the United States, one death was reported from acute overdose, and there was no increased risk over immediate-release APAP.[76] In Australia and New Zealand, 48 cases of overdose are described with only 2 cases of hepatotoxicity, but with some evidence of altered kinetics, including one case of a double-hump [APAP] and 15% line crossers.[127-129] It is reasonable to plot a single [APAP] on the treatment nomogram after ingestion of the US APAP extended-release ingestion. Australian protocols suggest treatment with NAC for any patient who ingests 10 g or 200 mg/kg and continuing NAC for patients who have one of two [APAP] above the treatment line. Whether an alternative approach will be necessary for the Australian and New Zealand products, or any other new formulation, will require additional study.

Intravenous Acetaminophen

Several IV APAP and prodrug APAP products exist worldwide and the US Food and Drug Administration (FDA) approved an IV APAP product in 2004 (IV APAP, 1 g in 100 mL).[130] Experience with patients with IV APAP overdose is limited. Hepatotoxicity and liver failure are described after single erroneous supratherapeutic doses of 75 to 150 mg/kg.[27,130,249] These errors most commonly occur in young children and include 10-fold dosing errors, confusion between mg and mL, and incorrect route (oral product given intravenously).[28,130] Cases of hepatotoxicity with liver failure are reported after repeated therapeutic dosing (59–77 mg/kg/d) in severely catabolic patients over 3 to 5 days.[202,315]

Although the nomogram is extensively studied in patients with oral APAP ingestion, there is no evidence for its use in those with IV overdose. Intravenous administration of APAP leads to a higher initial [APAP] and higher bioavailability than oral use and should theoretically expose the liver to less APAP.[87] Both routes lead to similar 4-hour [APAP],[7,10,87] and cases of hepatotoxicity and liver failure have occurred in patients whose [APAP] was well below the treatment line.[27,87] Given the limited data and that iatrogenic errors are usually quantifiable, it seems reasonable to treat a patient with NAC if he or she was exposed to more than 60 mg/kg of IV APAP in a single dose and to treat until the [APAP] is undetectable. Finally, it is also reasonable to treat patients receiving multiple therapeutic doses of IV APAP with NAC if there is evidence of hepatotoxicity or if there is evidence of APAP accumulation (eg, the [APAP] is above therapeutic concentrations that are expected for the last dose).[130,315,202]

Risk Determination After Repeated Supratherapeutic Ingestions (or Chronic Overdose)

No well-established guidelines are available for determining risk after chronic exposure to APAP. Conceptually, several factors must be evaluated to determine an individual's risk of toxicity. It is well established that therapeutic dosing of APAP is safe; however, some risk factors put individual patients at risk for toxicity at supratherapeutic doses.

The chronic ingestion of "maximal therapeutic" doses (3–4 g/day) in normal adults without special circumstances is safe. Several randomized, controlled trials used maximal therapeutic doses of APAP (4 g/day) in thousands of patients over periods from 4 weeks to 2 years with no reported increase in adverse events or hepatic injury. A transient increase in aminotransferases of one to three times normal, but rarely up to 10 times normal, is detected in some patients taking therapeutic doses,[3,149,374] but these abnormalities resolve spontaneously despite continued use and have not led to hepatic dysfunction.[149,191,374] Finally, several studies have evaluated abstaining chronic alcoholics administered APAP 4 g/day for up to 10 days with no evidence of hepatic damage, although elevations in aminotransferases were detected in both APAP and control groups.[80,191]

Although therapeutic dosing appears to be safe, repeated supratherapeutic ingestions (RSTIs) may lead to toxicity. Given the amount of APAP use, the incidence of serious APAP toxicity after repeated doses is small, and hepatotoxicity appears to occur only after massive dosing or prolonged excessive dosing. The risk of hepatotoxicity is likely proportional to both the total amount of APAP ingested and the duration of the exposure; however, exact cutoffs for safe dosing are difficult to determine and are likely subject to factors related to the individual.

Although short-term prospective studies of supratherapeutic dosing (6–8 g/day) have not identified alterations in APAP kinetics or hepatotoxicity,[119] several series and case reports identify patients with hepatotoxicity who retrospectively reported therapeutic or slightly supratherapeutic doses. Retrospective dosage reporting is prone to significant errors and issues in which those giving the history are unable or unwilling to report or estimate ingestions accurately. Cases describing hepatic toxicity after in-hospital therapeutic doses exist but are exceedingly rare, involve unusual risk factors, and demonstrate multifactorial hepatic injury.[60,65,315] Furthermore, because APAP is commonly used in patients with chronic heavy ethanol use and viral infections, it is unclear in which cases APAP was causative, contributory, or unrelated to hepatotoxicity.

Conceptually, the groups that are at "high risk" for hepatotoxicity after RSTI of APAP have potentially increased activity of CYP2E1 and therefore proportionally increased NAPQI formation or have decreased GSH stores and turnover rate. Many reported cases of APAP toxicity from RSTI involve patients who have a factor or factors that influence their GSH supply or turnover, NAPQI production, or both, including infants with febrile illness who received excessive dosing, chronic heavy ethanol users, catabolic postsurgical patients, and patients chronically taking CYP-inducing medications. Catabolic states enhance CYP2E1 activity and shunt hepatic metabolism to gluconeogenesis, leading to decreased glucose precursors for glucuronidation and subsequent increased production of NAPQI.

There is significant individual variability in genetic factors that are usually unknown to the clinician that increase or decrease the risk of toxicity.[24] A small subset of patients are able to ingest large amounts of APAP chronically without hepatotoxicity, possible because of increased ability to detoxify NAPQI (increased GSH-S-transferase P and NADPH quinone 1 activity) and decreased NAPQI production (reduced CYP2E1 activity and distribution).[24,103]

To determine the need for NAC, evaluate the patient's risk based on dosing history and other risk factors and then use limited laboratory testing that consists of an [APAP] and [AST], with additional testing as indicated by these results and other clinical features. The objective is to identify the two conditions that warrant NAC therapy—remaining APAP yet to be metabolized and potentially serious hepatic injury.

Role of History and Physical Examination in Repeated Supratherapeutic Ingestions

The first consideration when evaluating a patient with a history of repeated supratherapeutic APAP dosing is the presence or absence of signs or symptoms of hepatotoxicity. Regardless of risk factors or dosing history, such findings should prompt treatment with NAC and laboratory evaluation. This is particularly important because most reported cases of serious toxicity after repeated dosing are symptomatic for more than 24 hours before diagnosis, and earlier treatment improves outcome.

In asymptomatic patients, a reasonable approach is to perform laboratory evaluation for those who have ingested more than 200 mg/kg/day (or 10 g/day, whichever is less) in a 24-hour period or more than 150 mg/kg/day (or 6 g/day, whichever is less) in a 48-hour period.[80,84,218] In children younger than 6 years of age, laboratory evaluation is reasonable if the reported ingestion is more than 100 mg/kg/day during a 72-hour period or longer.

Several factors or characteristics place patients at higher risk for APAP toxicity from repeated supratherapeutic dosing. Theoretical high-risk factors include chronic heavy ethanol use; chronic ingestion of INH; febrile illnesses in infants and young children; and malnutrition, catabolic states (eg, post-surgical), AIDS, and anorexia. In some cases, animal or basic science studies show evidence of increased risk, and there have been multiple anecdotal reports of toxicity at slightly supratherapeutic doses.

Role of Laboratory Evaluation in Repeated Supratherapeutic Ingestions

After a patient is determined to be at risk, the [APAP] and [AST] should be determined. These should be interpreted using the concept that a patient is at risk of hepatotoxicity if there is evidence of hepatic injury (elevation of [AST]) or there remains enough APAP to produce further hepatic damage.

Using the strategy described here, patients with an elevated AST are considered at risk, regardless of their [APAP]. An [APAP] is useful in patients with a normal [AST] as a tool to determine only whether sufficient APAP remains to lead to subsequent NAPQI formation and delayed hepatotoxicity. In many cases, the [AST] is normal, and the [APAP] is undetectable, obviating the need for NAC. If the AST is normal, then the patient is considered at risk if the [APAP] is 10 mcg/mL or above.

Higher thresholds for nontreatment, such as an [APAP] below 30 mcg/mL or an [AST] twice as high as normal, have been suggested but have not been studied, and their sensitivity is unknown. The multiplicative sum of the [APAP] and the higher of the [AST] or the [ALT] (< 1,500 mg/L*IU/L) predicts a low likelihood of hepatotoxicity in patients treated with NAC.[329,381] This tool is less conservative than the method described and should not be used to determine the need for NAC, but it has some use in prognosticating risk after NAC is started.

Patients who develop a highly elevated [AST] after chronic APAP overdose should be treated and further evaluated with laboratory tests to assess hepatotoxicity and prognosis ([creatinine], PT, INR, pH, [phosphate], and [lactate]). Initial elevations of INR or creatinine are markers of poor prognosis in RSTI of APAP.[5]

The measurement of APAP protein adducts in urine is described and theoretically could quantify NAPQI production in the liver. It is also suggested that adduct concentration identifies APAP-induced hepatotoxicity in undifferentiated patients with an elevated AST; however, adducts are elevated after both therapeutic and RSTI APAP ingestions and a clear defining value has not been determined.[133] In addition, the test remains largely unavailable and is insufficiently studied.[88,167,242] Several other biomarkers, including miRNA-122, nK18, and acetylated HMGB-1, have been tested in acute overdoses, but their utility in RSTI is unclear.[92]

Patients who are identified as at risk, with either an elevated [AST] *or* an elevated [APAP], should be treated with NAC.

Risk Determination After Acetaminophen Exposure in Children

Serious hepatotoxicity or death after acute APAP overdose is extremely rare in children.[292,352] Predominant theories[6] for resistance to toxicity include a relative hepatoprotection in children because of increased sulfation capacity[233]

or differences in the characteristics of childhood poisonings, including smaller ingested doses, overestimation of liquid doses, and unique formulations (pediatric elixirs contain propylene glycol, which inhibits CYP2E1).[178,354] This has led some to suggest higher screening values and a higher nomogram line for children.[40] However, no significant change in NAPQI production is demonstrated in children, and a more liberal approach to children's acute APAP ingestions is inadequately studied and not recommended. After repeated supratherapeutic APAP dosing, there is no evidence that children are relatively protected. Hepatic injury after supratherapeutic APAP is likely exceedingly rare in children.[198] However, infants and children with acute febrile illnesses comprise one of the few groups in which toxicity after repeated excessive dosing is well described.[270] Common sources of dosing errors include substitution of adult for pediatric preparations, overzealous dosing by amount or frequency in attempts to maximize effect, and failure to read the label and dose carefully.[257,270] Age younger than 2 years is an independent risk factor for development of toxicity.[176] These rare cases of toxicity in febrile children with repeated supratherapeutic dosing likely reflect that these children constitute the most common setting for pediatric APAP use and that children are at greater relative risk for excessive dosing because of their size. Although logically one can argue that inflammatory oxidant stress and short-term fasting during febrile infectious illnesses affect oxidative drug metabolism and decrease GSH supply, these relationships are complex and not well defined. Of the reported cases of repeated supratherapeutic APAP dosing in children with hepatic injury, the cause was likely an isolated infectious illness in some, APAP in others, and a combination of the two in still others.

Risk Determination After Acetaminophen Exposure in Pregnancy

The initial risk of toxicity in a pregnant woman is similar to that of a nonpregnant patient with a few exceptions. No alteration of the treatment line is necessary. In fact, there are no reported cases of fetal or maternal toxicity in women with an [APAP] below the treatment line[228] or in those treated with NAC within 10 hours of an acute ingestion.[286] However, there is controversy in assessing the risk of fetal toxicity after the mother is determined to be at risk. To better understand the issues, a review of maternal–fetal physiology and pharmacokinetics related to APAP and NAC is necessary.

Acetaminophen crosses the human placenta,[208,247,288] and an [APAP] in fetuses is similar to maternal serum concentrations within hours after ingestion.[247,288] Fetal metabolism of APAP probably is inefficient but is not completely understood. Sulfation is the primary method of metabolism of APAP in fetuses, but sulfation capacity decreases in the second half of pregnancy.[2] Oxidative metabolism of APAP occurs in the second and third trimesters but is slower than in adults, and glucuronidation is undetectable until 23 weeks of gestation.[289] Cytochrome P450 enzymes (CYPs) that are capable of oxidizing APAP are present in fetuses as early as 18 weeks gestation.[289] However, the activity of these enzymes is less than 10% that of adult enzymes at 18 weeks of gestation and increases to only 20% activity at 23 weeks.[289] How the opposing forces of decreased overall metabolism of APAP and decreased NAPQI formation impact fetal risk is unclear.

The mechanism of fetal risk in women with APAP toxicity and the degree of fetal toxicity that is attributable to fetal metabolism of APAP or to maternal illness are unclear. In clinical case series, the majority of pregnant women who overdose on APAP have uneventful pregnancies.[228,286] Pregnant women who develop APAP toxicity in the first trimester have an increased risk of spontaneous abortion,[286] fetal demise is described in the second trimester,[117,355] and those who develop APAP toxicity after about 20 weeks of gestation have a potential risk of fetal hepatotoxicity because of fetal metabolism.[117] However, reports of third-trimester fetal hepatotoxicity are rare[228,286] and are only associated with severe maternal toxicity.[286,367] The factors associated with poor fetal outcome after a large APAP overdose are delayed treatment with NAC and young gestational age.

The decision to treat a pregnant woman with NAC requires evaluation of the known efficacy and beneficial effects as well as the adverse events of NAC for both the fetus and the mother. Every indication suggests that NAC is both safe and effective in treating the mother,[286] but there are inadequate data to evaluate efficacy in fetuses, although fetal outcome is generally excellent after maternal treatment with NAC.[286] Given that NAC is safely used in many pregnancies[228,286] and fetal mortality is linked to delays to treatment, NAC should be initiated in pregnant women who meet the same criteria as nonpregnant patients. The necessary length of NAC therapy is difficult to determine. The 21-hour IV protocol probably is the most commonly recommended NAC protocol used for pregnant women worldwide; however, there is a paucity of published experience supporting NAC treatment courses shorter than the oral 72-hour protocol (Chap. 31).[228,286]

Ethanol and Risk Determination

The effects of ethanol on APAP toxicity are complex and are best described by clearly separating experimental animal data from actual human overdose experience, acute ethanol use from chronic heavy ethanol use or alcoholism, and single from repeated supratherapeutic APAP dosing. Ethanol use itself is difficult to define, and many studies use different definitions. For the purpose of this section, the term *chronic heavy ethanol use* is defined as a person who ingests a mean of greater than two to three standard ethanol-containing drinks per day.[309] Moderate ethanol use is defined as a mean of one to two standard ethanol-containing beverages per day. The term *alcoholic* will be used to define people whom either self-define as alcoholics or are identified as an alcoholic by the CAGE questionnaire, the Michigan Alcohol Screening Test, or a similar screen.[86,190,192]

Although not entirely consistent, both animal and human data suggest that acute ethanol coingestion with APAP is hepatoprotective. Ethanol coingestion decreases NAPQI formation presumably by inhibiting CYP2E1 in both humans[357,358] and animals.[302,358] In large retrospective evaluations of overdoses, acute ethanol ingestion independently decreases the risk of severe hepatotoxicity in chronic heavy ethanol users[309] and in nonchronic heavy ethanol users[328] but did not significantly decrease the risk of hepatotoxicity ([ALT] > 1,000 IU/L) in a smaller prospective study.[371]

However, chronic ethanol administration increases the risk of hepatotoxicity from APAP dosing in animals.[362,394] This is due to induction of CYP2E1 metabolism after the ethanol is metabolized,[356] resulting in increased NAPQI formation, as well as decreased mitochondrial GSH supply impairing hepatocyte protection and regeneration.[394]

After *acute APAP overdose*, chronic heavy alcohol users who have not coingested ethanol are at a slightly increased risk; however, this elevated risk is of little clinical importance given the sensitivity of the treatment line.[335] There is no credible evidence that chronic heavy alcohol use should alter the approach after an acute APAP overdose using the treatment line. In fact, the treatment line was developed with clinical data that included chronic heavy ethanol users.[270,291] Given the paucity of data linking chronic heavy ethanol use to nomogram failures, the treatment line is adequately sensitive for screening after an acute APAP overdose, regardless of the patient's history of chronic heavy ethanol use.

The relationship between chronic heavy ethanol use and *chronic APAP use* is complex. Patients with chronic heavy ethanol use and repeated supratherapeutic APAP dosing have developed hepatotoxicity. Complicating these reports are the clinical challenges of obtaining accurate histories in chronic heavy ethanol users, failure to exclude non-APAP causes of hepatotoxicity, and other factors. Alcoholics are at higher risk of both using supratherapeutic doses of APAP and using combinations of multiple APAP-containing products.[314] In contrast, prospective evidence demonstrates minimal risk of hepatotoxicity in alcoholic patients who ingest therapeutic doses of APAP.[18,147,190,192] In prospective trials of ingestion of 4 g/day of APAP or placebo in chronic moderate to heavy ethanol users for up to 10 days, no clinically relevant increases in [AST] versus placebo were identified.[18,86,147,190,192] However, it should be noted that in studies involving persons who abuse alcohol, mild elevations of an [AST] (< 120 IU/L) were noted in 40% of both study and control participants, and more significant increases (> 120 IU/L, or three times normal) were noted in 4% to 6% of participants.[171,173] In addition, in all studies, a small group of patients developed significant increases in [AST], but most were unchanged. Patients who develop elevated [AST] after therapeutic dosing who are then rechallenged with additional APAP develop similar

increases in [AST],[147] implying that individual factors are likely more important than the chronic heavy ethanol use itself.

CYP Inducers and Risk Determination

Isoniazid is an inducer of CYP2E1 that has been theorized to proportionally increase the production of NAPQI from APAP. Similarly, several other medications, including phenytoin, carbamazepine, and phenobarbital, are theorized to increase APAP toxicity because of nonspecific CYP induction or induction of other CYPs. None of these antiepileptics induces CYP2E1, although there is some evidence that they increase NAPQI formation in cultured human hepatocyte and animal models, possibly through inhibition of glucuronidation.[99,236] However, clinical experience suggests that there is no need to change the approach to these patients.

Risk Assessment of Hepatotoxicity When the Diagnosis is Uncertain

In some cases, patients present with, or develop, hepatotoxicity with no clear ingestion history. Because APAP is the most common cause of ALF, the most reasonable approach to patients with evidence of liver failure or highly elevated aminotransferase concentrations is to consider them at risk of APAP-induced ALF even with an undetectable [APAP]. Other common causes of acute elevations of [aminotransferase] should be considered, including rhabdomyolysis and hepatotoxicity related to hypoperfusion or hypoxemia.

Up to 20% of adult and up to 50% of pediatric patients with ALF have an undetermined cause. Several biomarkers differentiate APAP ALF from other causes but are not yet clinically available. Protein adduct measurements have some utility in determining cases of adult APAP ALF, but they are not clinically available and have poor sensitivity and specificity in pediatric ALF.[9] The pattern of laboratory tests suggest that ALF is from APAP but are not absolutely diagnostic.[229] Cases of APAP ALF tend to have higher [AST] and [ALT] and lower [bilirubin] than other common causes of ALF.[9]

Assessing Actual Toxicity: Critical Components of the Diagnostic Approach

Initial Testing

[APAP] should be measured in patients with acute APAP overdose and no evident hepatotoxicity, but no other initial laboratory assessment is required. AST should be measured in patients who are considered to be at risk for APAP toxicity according to the nomogram or history (in the case of repeated supratherapeutic dosing) or in those suspected of already having mild hepatotoxicity by history and physical examination.

Unless evidence of serious hepatotoxicity is present, the [AST] is a sufficient indication of hepatic conditions, and no additional testing is initially needed. [ALT] increases after [AST] and is not necessary to determine early toxicity. Death of hepatocytes, resulting in release of measurable hepatic enzymes, precedes all cases of serious hepatic dysfunction. Mild AKI rarely occurs without hepatotoxicity;[46] however, at least minimal elevation of the [AST] generally precedes evidence of clinically significant nephrotoxicity.[4,56] Exceptions are rare,[46,182] and routine screening of kidney function in the absence of an elevated [AST] is probably unnecessary.

Acetaminophen overdose often leads to minor prolongation of PT even without causing hepatotoxicity.[376] This most commonly occurs between 4 and 24 hours after ingestion and is the result of NAPQI-related inhibition of vitamin K–dependent γ-carboxylation of factors II, VII, IX, and X.[353,376] These minor prolongations (resulting in a PT that usually is less than twice control) are rarely clinically relevant, are not evidence of hepatotoxicity, and should not be used as prognostic factors or indications for NAC treatment. In fact, treatment with NAC also prolongs PT[171,187] by interfering with the PT assay, by reversing an APAP/NAPQI effect,[353] or by direct NAC effects.[353]

Ongoing Monitoring and Testing

If no initial elevation of AST is noted, then repeated determination of AST alone—without other biochemical testing—is sufficient to exclude the development of hepatotoxicity. The [AST] should be determined before the end of the protocol or every 24 hours if using a longer protocol. If an elevated [AST] is noted, then PT, INR, and [creatinine] should be measured and repeated every 24 hours or more frequently if clinically indicated. Results of other hepatic tests, such as plasma γ-glutamyl transferase (GGT), alkaline phosphatase, lactate dehydrogenase, and bilirubin, which are useful when determining the cause of hepatic abnormalities, will be abnormal in cases of serious APAP-induced hepatotoxicity but provide little additional useful information if the cause is certain (Chap. 21).

If evidence of hepatic failure is noted, then careful monitoring of blood glucose, pH, PT, INR, creatinine, lactate, and phosphate concentrations are important in assessing extrahepatic organ toxicity and are vital in assessing hepatic function and the patient's potential need for hepatic transplant (see Assessing Prognosis). In addition, meticulous bedside evaluation is necessary to determine and document vital signs, neurologic status, and evidence of bleeding.

Role of Biomarkers and Risk Determination

Although the risk of hepatotoxicity is generally low when NAC is started in the appropriate timeframe, there are cases in which risk assessment is difficult or impossible. In cases with unknown time of ingestions, late presenters, or multiple (staggered) ingestions, it may not be possible to accurately determine risk, and the current practice is to proceed conservatively. However, the conservative practice of treatment with NAC for unclear risk scenarios carries with it a risk of adverse reactions to NAC (which are more common in these scenarios) as well as excessive health care resource management. In these cases, use of a biomarker allows for targeted therapy to select individuals at high risk of adverse outcomes or allow early and safe discharge of well and low-risk groups. Although these biomarkers will be discussed here, none is currently rapidly clinically available for use and data are insufficient to recommend their use.

Protein Adducts

Protein adducts indicate intracellular binding of NAPQI to hepatocyte proteins[88,168,275] and can be determined experimentally. While there is a bedside tool in development, protein adducts are inadequately studied to be currently useful in risk assessment. After over-exposure to APAP, NAPQI is not immediately bound to GSH and is released within the cell to bind with the cysteine components on proteins. One of these protein-APAP adducts is 3-(cysteinyl-S-yl)-APAP. However, hepatic toxicity from APAP requires not only protein binding, and therefore protein adducts, but an inflammatory cascade to produce cell necrosis.[44] Therefore, protein adducts are signs of NAPQI binding, but not necessarily of toxicity. Animals exposed to APAP overdose develop elevated concentrations of serum protein adducts.[41,152,167]

In humans with therapeutic dosing of APAP, protein adducts are usually detected in small quantities in the blood (< 0.5 nmol/mL), likely from intrahepatic protein binding followed by hepatic cellular turnover or protein adduct export from the cell. However, some patients with therapeutic dosing have concentrations of up to 1.0 nmol/mL.[152] In humans after overdose, protein adducts are released into the serum and largely parallel the [aminotransferase] in their time course. Peak concentrations are detected in 2 to 3 days and decrease with an elimination half-life of 27 hours (41 hours with kidney failure);[77] however, protein adducts remain detectable for up to 2 weeks.[169] A protein adduct concentration above 1.0 nmol/mL is suggested as being consistent with an acute APAP overdose, but this recommendation requires further validation.[152]

Plasma GSH can be measured or approximated using [GGT] but have an uncertain relationship to hepatic GSH availability.[314,339]

Micro RNA

Micro RNAs (miRNAs) are small, noncoding RNAs that regulate cell proteins by repressing mRNA.[209] miRNA-122 is the most abundant hepatic microRNA and is specific to the liver.[209] In human studies, miRNA-122 increases before other markers, such as ALT, and is actively released from hepatocytes before cell lysis.[92,210] The [miRNA-122] correlates with peak [ALT][13] and peak INR.[13]

In patients with acute APAP overdose whose initial [ALT] is normal and in patients who are treated within 8 hours, [miRNA-122] is higher in those who develop hepatic injury,[13] suggesting that it may be useful in differentiating low-risk patients from high-risk patients earlier than other markers.

High-Mobility Group Box-1

Another biomarker, HMGB-1, is passively released by hepatocytes during necrosis. HMGB-1 targets TLRs and initiates an inflammatory cascade that leads to cell necrosis or apoptosis. This biomarker is elevated in patients with APAP hepatotoxicity but not in those without hepatotoxicity, rises earlier than the [ALT],[92] and correlates with both peak [ALT] and INR. An acetylated form of HMGB-1 is secreted as an inflammatory mediator by macrophages and monocytes and increases only in patients with APAP toxicity who later either meet transplant criteria (King's College criteria {KCC}), die, or receive a hepatic transplant. This biomarker requires further study but has promise as an earlier marker for more intensive treatment or for transplant.[12]

Keratin-18

Keratin-18 (K18, or nK18 {necrosis K18}) is an epithelial and hepatic cell filament protein that is released passively during cell necrosis. Caspase-cleaved K18 (aK18, or apoptosis K18) fragments are released passively during apoptosis. The [K18] is elevated in patients who develop hepatotoxicity, even before [ALT] elevation.[13,91]

MANAGEMENT

Gastrointestinal Decontamination

In cases of very early presentation or coingestion of xenobiotics that delay gastrointestinal (GI) absorption, gastric emptying is appropriate for some patients. In general, however, gastric emptying is not appropriate for patients with isolated APAP overdose because of the very rapid GI absorption of APAP and the availability of an effective and safe antidote.

Administration of activated charcoal (AC) shortly after APAP ingestion decreases the number of patients who have an [APAP] above the treatment line.[51,102] Although AC is most effective when given within the first 1 to 2 hours after APAP ingestion, it is reasonable to give AC at later times provided there are no contraindications.[102,344,345] Interactions between AC and orally administered NAC are likely clinically unimportant. In the majority of cases, there should be no interaction because GI absorption of APAP, and therefore the necessity to give AC, is complete by 4 hours after ingestion, and NAC typically is administered between 4 and 8 hours after ingestion. As a result, there is generally no difficulty separating the doses. If delayed or repeated AC dosing is indicated because of suspected delayed absorption or coingestants, then a strategy using an IV NAC protocol is recommended. Alternatively, oral NAC and AC doses may be separated by 1 to 2 hours, with NAC given the priority for the first dose because time to administration of NAC correlates with risk of hepatotoxicity.[328,333] N-Acetylcysteine is absorbed high in the GI tract and is not likely to interact with AC if they are not administered simultaneously.

Supportive Care

General supportive care consists primarily of managing the hepatic injury, AKI, and other manifestations. Treatment of these problems is based on general principles and is not APAP dependent. Discussion of the management of hepatic failure is clearly beyond the scope of this chapter, but certain aspects deserve mention. Monitoring for and treatment of hypoglycemia are critical because hypoglycemia is one of the most readily treatable of the life-threatening effects of hepatic failure. If adequate viable hepatocytes are present, vitamin K produces some improvement in coagulopathy; thus, trial dosing is reasonable as hepatic injury develops and as it resolves. Administration of fresh-frozen plasma (FFP) and prothrombin complex concentrates (PCCs) should be based on specific indications rather than PT and INR alone. Hemorrhage is rare in APAP-induced hepatic failure, and correction of coagulopathy should only be necessary for procedures and life-threatening bleeding. Supportive therapies for cerebral edema, including cooling, hypertonic saline, elevation of the head, and support of the cerebral perfusion pressure, are all indicated.

Antidotal Therapy with *N*-Acetylcysteine

Mechanism of Action of *N*-Acetylcysteine. Conceptually, it is helpful to think of NAC as serving three distinct roles. During the metabolism of APAP to NAPQI, NAC *prevents toxicity* by limiting the formation of NAPQI. More important, it *increases the capacity to detoxify* NAPQI that is formed (Fig. 33–1). In fulminant hepatic failure, NAC *treats toxicity* through nonspecific mechanisms that preserve multiorgan function (Antidotes in Depth: A3).

N-Acetylcysteine prevents toxicity mostly by serving as a GSH precursor[197] and as a GSH substitute,[320] combining with NAPQI and being converted to cysteine and mercaptate conjugates.[53,48] *N*-Acetylcysteine also supplies cysteine as a substrate for sulfation, allowing less metabolism by oxidation to NAPQI.[330] Each of these preventive mechanisms must be in place early, and none is of benefit after NAPQI has initiated cell injury. Time is required to saturate nontoxic metabolism, form excessive NAPQI, deplete GSH, and overcome GSH production; thus, there is a window of opportunity after exposure to an APAP overdose during which NAC is initiated before the onset of hepatic injury without any loss of efficacy. Based on large clinical trials, NAC efficacy is nearly complete as long as it is initiated within 8 hours of an acute overdose.[180,328,332,333] However, the relationship between the time to administration of NAC and the risk of hepatotoxicity is a continuous variable. The risk of hepatotoxicity begins to increase at 6 hours for patients with an [APAP] greater than 600 mcg/mL and is closer to 8 hours for patients with an [APAP] just over the treatment line.[328,346] For this reason, NAC therapy should be initiated as soon as possible after 4 hours and not delayed past 8 hours.

Several observations illustrate the effectiveness of NAC by other mechanisms of action even after NAPQI formation and binding. *N*-Acetylcysteine actually reverses NAPQI oxidation in an in vitro human hepatocyte model,[221] and even after cell injury is initiated, NAC diminishes hepatocyte injury.[49] Most significantly, a prospective, randomized trial found that even after fulminant hepatic failure was evident, IV NAC diminished the need for vasopressors and the incidences of cerebral edema and death.[177] In this study, despite improved organ function and survival in the NAC-treated group, there was no apparent difference in the degree of hepatic injury, implying that much of the benefit of NAC in this setting is not derived from hepatic effects. Whether based on its nonspecific antioxidant effects, its increase in oxygen delivery and utilization, its ability to enhance GSH supply and mitochondrial ATP production, or its role in mediating microvascular tone,[93,140,173,296,343,366,367] *N*-Acetylcysteine improves function in several organs affected by multisystem failure.[93,364] In fact, NAC preserves cerebral blood flow and perfusion in the setting of cerebral edema[375] more effectively than traditional therapies such as mannitol and hyperventilation, which may produce detrimental adverse effects.

Although NAC has a defined role in preventing and treating APAP-induced hepatic injury, its role in treating APAP-induced AKI is less clear. When used early after ingestion in animals, NAC produces a small reduction in kidney injury.[239,331] In retrospective reviews of human data, NAC has little effect on kidney injury[90] but does not appear to be harmful.[241] However, few data are available to recommend NAC therapy in treating isolated AKI or after resolution of hepatic injury.

N-Acetylcysteine Administration. *N*-Acetylcysteine is administered via the oral or IV routes and in protocols that have historically varied in length. The most common regimens are a 12-hour IV infusion, a 21-hour IV infusion, and a 72-hour oral dosing protocol. However, the concept of a set-length protocol is obsolete. Conceptually, practitioners should start NAC when the patient is at risk of toxicity, continue NAC while the patient remains at risk or has hepatotoxicity, and stop NAC when that risk or toxicity is gone. Most institutions now use either oral or IV NAC in a variable length protocol, using indicators of patient toxicity rather than a set protocol length.[148]

With the exception of established hepatic failure, for which only the IV route has been investigated,[177] the IV and oral routes of NAC are equally efficacious in preventing or treating APAP toxicity.[51,269] In brief, whereas IV NAC

is associated with rare but severe anaphylactoid reactions and medication errors,[145] oral NAC is associated with a greater than 20% risk of vomiting. There are three scenarios in which IV NAC is preferentially recommended: (1) APAP toxicity in pregnant women, (2) APAP-induced hepatic failure, and (3) intractable vomiting preventing oral treatment.

Duration of *N*-Acetylcysteine Treatment. Known mechanisms of action and the observation that all studied durations of NAC are effective when started within 8 hours[51] suggest that all courses of treatment currently published are effective when NAC is used for its early preventive actions. There is some suggestion that there is a slightly decreased risk of hepatotoxicity if IV NAC, as opposed to oral NAC, is used before 10 hours after the ingestion, but this remains controversial.[386] Results from use of the traditional 21-hour IV NAC protocol, the 48-hour and 36-hour IV NAC protocols studied in the United States,[336] one 20-hour protocol,[389] a 12-hour protocol,[21] and other "short-course" dosing protocols[34,33,382] indicate that these therapies are likely safe and effective in these low-risk scenarios.[351,388]

It is important to realize that even in low-risk patients (those treated within 8 hours), regardless of the protocol length (12, 21, 36, 48, or 72 hours) or route of delivery, NAC therapy should be continued until APAP metabolism is complete (the [APAP] is below detection) and there are no signs of hepatotoxicity.

With this concept in mind, it is reasonable to *shorten* a set course of NAC if the patient is at low risk and the above criteria are met ([APAP] undetectable, [AST] normal, PT/INR less than twice normal, and no encephalopathy).[33,85,328] This approach is conceptually reasonable and is aimed at decreasing unnecessary therapy as there is no evidence that prolonged NAC is helpful and there is one animal study that suggested that prolonged NAC inhibits hepatic recovery;[385] however, adequate studies have not definitively confirmed its safety.[319,328]

N-Acetylcysteine therapy should be continued *beyond* the prescribed "protocol length" if there is evidence of hepatic injury ([AST] > 1,000 IU/L, PT/INR greater than twice normal, or encephalopathy is present) or APAP metabolism is incomplete the ([APAP] detectable). This likely will not be an issue in the vast majority of cases because the [ALT] of approximately half of all NAC-treated patients with an [APAP] above the treatment line will remain below 100 IU/L, and only 4% of patients treated with NAC develop hepatotoxicity ([ALT] > 1,000 IU/L).[21,332] The IV NAC dosing protocol that has proved beneficial in patients with hepatic failure is the same initial dosing as the traditional IV protocol but with the third IV infusion continued until there is resolution of hepatic failure. These observations suggest that rather than a single duration of therapy for all patients, it is appropriate to extend treatment protocols based on the clinical course of the patient.[85]

After NAC therapy is extended beyond a set-length protocol, the decision to discontinue therapy should be entirely based on the patient's condition. For patients who develop hepatic failure, we recommend continuing IV NAC until the PT or INR is below twice normal and encephalopathy, if present, is resolved.[218] For patients without hepatic failure but with an elevated [AST], we recommend continuing NAC until hepatic abnormalities improve (eg, [AST] is decreasing and < 1,000 IU/L or the [AST]/[ALT] ratio < 0.4).[229] The [AST] should be used to determine whether to stop NAC, as the [AST] decreases earlier upon recovery than [ALT] (half-life of 15 h for [AST] and 40 h for [ALT]).[78]

Assessing Risk of Hepatotoxicity

Most patients who are treated with NAC do not develop hepatotoxicity and have short hospital stays; a small percentage develop hepatotoxicity and an even smaller group develop hepatic failure. It is helpful to predict the risk of hepatotoxicity based on initial findings to direct the intensity of monitoring and therapy (see Dose Adjustment) and patient disposition.

In general, both the time from ingestion to the initiation of NAC and the [APAP] are directly proportional to the patient's risk of developing hepatotoxicity and hepatic failure.[305,328,333] Even in patients treated early after their ingestion, the risk of hepatotoxicity is significant if their [APAP] is highly elevated.[224,293] In patients who are treated with NAC, the risk of hepatotoxicity increases from below 5% to about 10% if the [APAP] is over the "300 line" and to 20% to 40% if over the "500 line."[55,224] Using these principles, a nomogram is used to determine the risk of hepatotoxicity on patient arrival. Unfortunately, this only predicts the risk of a peak [aminotransferase] above 1,000 IU/L and cannot determine the risk of death or need for transplantation. The multiplicative sum of the AST (or ALT) and the [APAP] also predicts hepatotoxicity (sensitivity of 91% and specificity of 63% if the sum is > 1,500 mg/L*IU/L).[329] Acetylated HMGB-1 is a promising biomarker for detecting patients who will go on to have severe hepatic failure and may become useful for early prognostication, but it requires further study.[12] In initial human studies, acet-HMGB-1 increased only in patients who later met the KCC for hepatic transplant, received a transplant, or died.[12]

Dose Adjustment

In rare cases, patients with massive ingestions with or without antimuscarinic coingestants have a highly elevated [APAP] for prolonged periods or secondary elevations of the [APAP].[97,100,154,313,368] Several of these patients developed hepatotoxicity despite early (< 6 hours) IV NAC therapy,[55,100,154,224,313,368] raising the question of whether the traditional IV NAC infusion (6.25 mg/kg/h) provides enough NAC for these rare patients with a late elevated [APAP] or massive ingestions. Patients who are treated with NAC within 8 hours have a risk of hepatotoxicity that increases linearly with increasing [APAP] with abrupt increases in risk at the 300 line and 500 line and an increase in risk of coagulopathy at the 900 line, suggesting increased NAC dosing at these intervals is appropriate.[55] In these rare patients, we recommend treating with greater amounts of NAC when prolonged, massive [APAP] is evident.[313,341] No data exist to determine which, if any, alternative NAC dosing strategy is superior. For a detailed description of increased dosing for massive ingestions, highly elevated [APAP], and prolonged elevations of [APAP], see Antidotes in Depth: A3. A brief synopsis is described below and is based on calculations that use logical inferences, but none of these concepts has been studied and should not be considered standard therapy.[224,294]

The following is reasonable give a patient who presents with an [APAP] above the "500" line the traditional IV NAC dosing in addition to traditional oral NAC dosing. In the event a patient cannot take the oral NAC (eg, somnolent, coingestion of a caustic), we recommend the IV loading dose followed by the 4-hour dose (12.5mg/kg/h) for the duration of the treatment regimen. In the event a patient presents later than 8 hours and the [APAP] is above the theoretical 500 line, then we also recommend the IV loading dose followed by 12.5 mg/kg/h for the duration of the treatment regimen.

Hepatic Transplantation

Hepatic transplantation increases survival for a select group of severely ill patients who have APAP-induced fulminant hepatic failure.[125,218] Tremendous improvements in transplantation and supportive hepatic care have increased immediate survival rates after hepatic transplantation to 69% to 83% with 3- to 5-year survival rates of 50% to 66%,[29,181,279,317,322] respectively, which is similar to transplant survival for other causes of acute hepatic failure. Patients who meet criteria for transplant but do not receive an organ have survival rates of 25% to 40%.[94,195,306]

Concerns that patients who receive transplants for APAP-induced fulminant hepatic failure will have lower survival rates and be unable to maintain posttransplant medication regimens have resulted in the majority of patients not being listed for transplant.[29,322] However, those who meet psychosocial criteria for transplantation have high rates of survival,[29,69,218,322] and only 12% later die from intentional rejection or suicide attempts.[26] Techniques that allow subtotal hepatectomy with transplantation and eventual weaning of immunosuppressants have demonstrated high 5-year survival rates (63%) and allow for higher rates of transplantation if further studies support these findings.[215,279]

Assessing Prognosis

Determining a patient's prognosis and predicting patients who require transplantation early in the course of the disease is an important area of current research.

TABLE 33–1 King's College Criteria

Either of the following historically predicted a survival rate <20% and the need for immediate transplantation, currently the survival rate for these patients is 25-40% without transplantation.

1. Arterial pH <7.3 or [lactate] >3.0 mmol/L after fluid resuscitation

OR

2. All of the following:
   a. [Creatinine] >3.3 mg/dL
   b. Prothrombin time >100 sec (or international normalized ratio >6.5)
   c. Grade III or IV encephalopathy (somnolence to stupor, responsive to verbal stimuli, confusion, gross disorientation)

The most commonly used prognosticator of mortality is the KCC (Table 33–1), which was developed and validated on patients with APAP-induced fulminant hepatic failure. The criteria include a serum pH below 7.30 after fluid resuscitation or the combination of creatinine above 3.3 mg/dL, PT above 100 sec (INR > 6.5 is commonly used), and grade III or IV encephalopathy. The survival rate of patients who meet the KCC but are not transplanted is 25% to 40%.[17,29,63,74,76,94,125,195,305] Survival rates have significantly increased since the original studies, likely because of the utilization of prolonged NAC therapy and improved supportive care for patients with acute hepatic failure.[124,306]

When determining the KCC, interpretation of PT and INR must include awareness of concurrent NAC therapy as well as therapy with vitamin K, PCCs, factor VII, and FFP. The use of vitamin K, if effective, implies that transplant is unnecessary because viable liver remains. If vitamin K is ineffective, then PT and INR can be used, as discussed in the previous paragraph. Transfusion of exogenous clotting factors, such as FFP or PCCs, alters interpretation because the resulting improvement in PT and INR does not indicate improvement in hepatic function. The prognostic importance of monitoring PT and INR in this setting suggests that FFP should be given only for evidence of bleeding, with risk of bleeding from known concomitant trauma, or before invasive procedures, and not based merely on the PT or INR.

A [lactate] above 3.5 mmol/L at a median of 55 hours after APAP ingestion or [lactate] above 3.0 mmol/L after fluid resuscitation is both a sensitive and specific predictor of patient death without transplant.[30,79] Additional studies confirmed [lactate] as an independent predictor of prognosis but suggest that it does not add significantly to the KCC.[63,311] Others have confirmed a lower specificity than initially reported.[124,311] Using a higher cutoff (> 4.7 mmol/L) has a high sensitivity (98%) and negative predictive value (NPV) (95%), but moderate specificity (58%) for determining death or transplant.[63,311]

Unfortunately, patients often meet the KCC and lactate criteria quite late in their course of disease, so these criteria are not useful as early predictors or as standards for transfer to a facility that performs hepatic transplant. General factors that are associated with increased mortality include unintentional overdose, repeated supratherapeutic dosing, and delays to receiving NAC therapy.[73,75] Additional predictors of severity of hepatic toxicity in patients treated with NAC include a rapid doubling of the [AST] or [ALT] (doubling < 8 hours)[132] and an [AST] or [ALT] reaching 1,000 IU/L within 20 hours of NAC treatment.[117] Several attempts at determining early predictors of death or the need for transplant have proven to be no more effective than the KCC, including serum [phosphate] on day 2,[31,308] Model for Endstage Liver Disease (MELD) score of 32 or above,[63,214,312] serum Gc-globulin,[203,304] factor V concentration,[161,258] factor VIII:V ratio,[258,269] worsening day 4 PT and INR,[139] and PT (in seconds) larger than the number of hours since ingestion.[246]

An Acute Physiology and Chronic Health Evaluation (APACHE) II score above 15 in patients with isolated APAP ingestions is as specific as the above KCC criteria and slightly more sensitive.[63,235] These criteria are beneficial in determining whether to transfer a patient to a transplant center because the score is easily calculated, is sensitive, and is available within the first day of admission; however, confounders such as coingestants decrease its utility. Furthermore, an APACHE II score above 60 identifies additional patients with multiorgan dysfunction who require transplantation.[29]

TABLE 33–2 Prediction of Death or Transplant in 125 Patients With Acetaminophen-Induced Liver Failure[63]

Score	Sensitivity (%)	Specificity (%)	PPV	NPV
King's College Criteria	47	83	0.70	0.65
Acute Physiology and Chronic Health Evaluation II (>12)	67	76	0.69	0.75
Sequential Organ Failure Assessment (>12)	67	80	0.74	0.74
Model for Endstage Liver Disease (>32)	89	25	0.49	0.77
[Lactate] (>3.3 mmol/L)	91	52	0.69	0.83

NPV = negative predictive value; PPV = positive predictive value.

Several measurements of organ failure are postulated as indications for transfer to a regional transplant center from a nontransplant facility. The Sequential Organ Failure Assessment (SOFA) score higher than 7 within the first 96 hours after *acute* overdose and evidence of the systemic inflammatory response syndrome both predict increased mortality (a 100% sensitivity and a 74% to 77% specificity).[74] Conversely, a patient with a SOFA score of 7 or less during the first 96 hours after *acute* overdose has a low mortality risk (< 2%), low risk of requiring renal replacement therapy (< 4%), and low risk of requiring intracranial pressure monitoring (< 2%).[74] Additionally, a SOFA score below 6 after RSTI of APAP predicts survival and a low risk of the need for renal replacement therapy or intracranial pressure monitoring (< 10%).[76]

The KCC, APACHE II, SOFA, and MELD scores, as well as serum [lactate] 12 hours after admission, are all helpful in making patient decisions.[63] The MELD score (> 32) and [lactate] (> 4.7 mmol/L) are the most sensitive to determine death or transplant in APAP-induced hepatic failure. These scores predict high mortality and the need for a higher level of care (Table 33–2), but the most specific scores are the KCC, APACHE II (> 11), and SOFA (> 12). These are most helpful in determining patients who need transplant (Table 33–2).

The multiplicative sum of the [APAP] and the higher of the AST or ALT (> 1,500 mg/dL*IU/L) is highly sensitive at predicting coagulopathy (INR > 2) in patients treated with NAC,[64] although specificity is only 57% (81% in patients treated longer than 8 hours after ingestion).[329,381] The Psi parameter, which uses the [APAP] and time to NAC, is useful for predicting hepatotoxicity (sensitivity, 97%; specificity, 92%; likelihood risk (LR), 11.4), but its usefulness in predicting coagulopathy is limited (sensitivity, 71%; specificity, 85%; LR, 4.8).[64]

Acetylated HMGB-1 is a biomarker that is released as a proinflammatory mediator from monocytes and macrophages and in one small study was highly correlated with patients who met transplantation criteria or died.[12]

All of these studies are promising, but will require validation before clinical use is postulated.

Additional Elimination Techniques

Several clinical scenarios benefit from increasing clearance of APAP from the body. Indications early after APAP overdose include patients with an exceedingly high [APAP] who are at high risk of hepatotoxicity despite NAC therapy as well as those with hyperlactatemia and metabolic acidosis. Later in the course of APAP toxicity, elimination techniques are used to remove the remaining [APAP] in patients who are imminently receiving a hepatic transplant or for removal of toxins related to hepatic failure (Table 33–3).

Hemodialysis

Both intermittent hemodialysis and continuous venovenous hemodialysis increase elimination of APAP. Intermittent hemodialysis has been used early after overdose to eliminate a highly elevated [APAP], typically above

TABLE 33–3 Management of Patients at Risk for APAP Toxicity

1. Start NAC on patients at risk of hepatotoxicity:
   a. In acute overdose, plot a single [APAP] on the nomogram using the earliest possible time of ingestion. If the plot is over the treatment line, initiate NAC
      i. If patient is at risk for massive and prolonged exposure to APAP (eg, ingestion > 30 g and/or coingested antimuscarinics), higher-dose NAC therapy is reasonable
   b. In RSTI, if [AST] is elevated, initiate NAC
   c. If AST is normal and [APAP] > 10 mcg/mL, initiate NAC
   d. If patient has evidence of liver failure (encephalopathy, INR/prothrombin time elevation), transfer to liver transplant center
2. Initiate IV NAC or rarely oral NAC.
3. Laboratory evaluation at 20 to 24 hours (20 hours if IV NAC is used, 20–24 hours if PO NAC is used). Continue NAC on patients who remain at risk of toxicity or have developed toxicity.
   a. If patient remains at risk of toxicity ([APAP] detectable) or if toxicity is evident ([AST] elevated), then continue NAC for 16–24 hours more
   b. If the [APAP] at 20 to 24 hours is very elevated, consider higher dose NAC therapy
4. Continue laboratory evaluation every 16–24 hours.
5. Stop NAC when the patient is no longer at risk of toxicity:
   a. If liver failure was evident, continue NAC until INR < 2, encephalopathy resolves, and the [APAP] is undetectable
   b. If liver failure was not evident, but the [AST] was elevated, then continue NAC until the [AST] has decreased to < 1,000 IU/L, no evidence of liver failure, and the [APAP] is undetectable

AST = aspartate aminotransferase; INR = international normalized ratio; IV = intravenous; NAC = N-acetylcysteine; PO = oral; RSTI = repeated supratherapeutic ingestion.

500 mcg/mL[108,134,327,377] and in patients with slow clearance of APAP late after overdose.[383] A systematic review suggests hemodialysis for patients with altered mental status, elevated [lactate], or metabolic acidosis with an [APAP] greater than 700 mcg/mL or for an [APAP] greater than 900 mcg/mL if the patient is treated with NAC. Furthermore, they recommend hemodialysis for an [APAP] greater than 1,000 mcg/mL regardless of therapy.[123] Clearance averages 150 to 300 mL/min.[108,134,327,383] In several cases, hemodialysis has removed gram quantities of APAP (4–20 g),[327] and the amount that hemodialysis removes varies directly with the [APAP].[108,327,383] Hemodialysis reduces the APAP elimination half-life by approximately 50% to 80%[134,252,327,383] and has an extraction ratio of 50% to 80%.[134,327,380,383]

Hemodialysis also removes NAC with a clearance (CL$_{HD}$) of 114mL/kg/h and an extraction ratio of 50% to 76%.[155,327] We recommend doubling NAC infusion rates during hemodialysis to compensate.[134,155,327] Hemodialysis does not remove APAP protein adducts.[77]

N-Acetylcysteine clearance during CVVH (CL$_{CVVH}$) is 42 mL/kg/h with an extraction ratio of 13%.[155,377] In one case, CVVH removed 24 g of APAP over 16 hours.[377] No dosing adjustment is likely necessary during CVVH.[77,155]

Plasmapheresis and Plasma Exchange

Plasmapheresis removes small amounts (5%) of APAP with therapeutic dosing, but few data exist with regard to overdose.[109] Plasmapheresis is useful in patients with ALF to correct coagulopathy, but it does not reliably correct encephalopathy.[324]

Exchange transfusion was used in one 1.22-kg neonate who had an [APAP] of 75 mcg/mL after maternal oral overdose and subsequent delivery.[201] Exchange transfusion eliminated a portion of total APAP as evidenced by a reduced [APAP] and a rebound [APAP] after transfusion. For example, in one exchange of 210 mL blood (1.22 kg patient), the serum [APAP] decreased from 32 mcg/mL to zero and then rebounded to 30 mcg/mL.[201]

Liver Dialysis

Liver dialysis devices include extracorporeal albumin dialysis (eg, molecular adsorbent recirculation system {MARS}), fractionated plasma separation and adsorption, and single-pass albumin dialysis (SPAD). The MARS system is used as a bridge to transplantation, for hemodynamic stabilization before hepatic transplant, or as a bridge to spontaneous recovery in patients with APAP-induced hepatic failure. Although MARS improves encephalopathy,[316] cerebral blood flow,[307] hemodynamics (increases in systemic vascular resistance, mean arterial pressure, and decreases in cardiac index and pulse),[194,310] and intracranial pressure,[342] a meta-analysis concluded that MARS has no effect on mortality in multiple causes of ALF.[183] One report notes complete removal of APAP from the blood. The ([APAP] decreased from 40 mcg/mL to 0 mcg/mL from inflow to outflow) during MARS with a rebound [APAP], suggesting that MARS improves APAP clearance.[121]

Fractionated plasma separation, albumin adsorption, and hemodialysis is also used as a bridge to transplantation but is relatively unstudied in APAP induced acute hepatic failure. Fractionated plasma separation, albumin adsorption, and hemodialysis (eg, Prometheus system) produces higher clearance of ammonia than MARS but does not improve hemodynamics.[194]

Single-pass albumin dialysis is venovenous hemodialysis with a dialysate containing 4.4% albumin. Single-pass albumin dialysis (SPAD) more effectively clears ammonia than MARS,[303] but there were no changes in hemodynamics or encephalopathy after therapy with SPAD in one study of patients with acute hepatic failure.[175]

We recommend treatment with MARS, if available, in patients with fulminant hepatic failure who meet clinical criteria for transplantation or high mortality (eg, KCC) regardless of whether or not they will be transplanted.

SUMMARY

■ The decision to treat a patient with an acute APAP overdose requires plotting a single [APAP] onto the modified Rumack-Matthew nomogram and treating patients with NAC if the [APAP] plots above the treatment "150" line.

■ We recommend treating patients with NAC after RSTIs of APAP if their [AST] is greater than normal or their [APAP] is detectable.

■ The KCC identify patients with high mortality and is an indication for evaluation for hepatic transplantation.

■ Following massive ingestions of APAP, after NAC therapy is started, an informed decision should be made when to stop NAC: which requires an assessment of the [AST] and [APAP], that the risk of developing toxicity is low ([APAP] is undetectable and [AST] is normal), and any toxicity that occurred has now resolved ([AST] has decreased and is near normal and there is no evidence of hepatic failure). This method may result in NAC therapy that is either shorter or longer than the traditional protocol length.

Acknowledgment

Martin J. Smilkstein, MD, and Kenneth Bizovi, MD, contributed to this chapter in previous editions.

REFERENCES

1. Adebayo D, et al. Mechanistic biomarkers in acute liver injury: are we there yet? *J Hepatol.* 2012;56:1003-1005.
2. Adjei AA, et al. Interindividual variability in acetaminophen sulfation by human fetal liver: implications for pharmacogenetic investigations of drug-induced birth defects. *Birth Defects Res A Clin Mol Teratol.* 2008;82:155-165.
3. Ahlers S, et al. Aminotransferase levels in relation to short-term use of acetaminophen four grams daily in postoperative cardiothoracic patients in the intensive care unit. *Anaesth Intensive Care.* 2011;39:1056-1063.
4. Akca S, et al. Isolated acute renal failure due to paracetamol intoxication in an alcoholic patient. *Nephron.* 1999;83:270-271.
5. Alhelail MA, et al. Clinical course of repeated supratherapeutic ingestion of acetaminophen. *Clin Toxicol (Phila).* 2011;4:713-718.
6. Allegaert K, van den Anker J. Pharmacokinetics and pharmacodynamics of intravenous acetaminophen in neonates. *Exp Rev Clin Pharmacol.* 2011;4:713-718.
7. Allegaert K, et al. Paracetamol pharmacokinetics and metabolism in young women. *BMC Anesthesiol.* 2015;15:163.
8. Alloui A, et al. Paracetamol exerts a spinal, tropisetron-reversible, antinociceptive effect in an inflammatory pain model in rats. *Eur J Pharmacol.* 2002;443:71-77.
9. Alonso EM, et al.; Pediatric Acute Liver failure Study Group. Acetaminophen adducts detected in serum of pediatric patients with acute liver failure. *J Pediatr Gastroenterol Nutr.* 2015;61:102-107.
10. Ameer B, et al. Absolute and relative bioavailability of oral acetaminophen preparations. *J Pharm Sci.* 1983;72:955-958.
11. Andreasen PB, Hutter L. Paracetamol (acetaminophen) clearance in patients with cirrhosis of the liver. *Acta Med Scand.* 1979;624:99-105.
12. Antoine DJ, et al. Molecular forms of HMGB1 and keratin-18 as mechanistic biomarkers for mode of cell death and prognosis during clinical acetaminophen hepatotoxicity. *J Hepatol.* 2012;56:1070-1079.
13. Antoine DJ, et al. Mechanistic biomarkers provide early and sensitive detection of acetaminophen-induced acute liver injury at first presentation to hospital. *Hepatology.* 2013;58:777-787.
14. Aronoff DM, et al. New insights into the mechanism of action of acetaminophen: its clinical pharmacologic characteristics reflect its inhibition of the two prostaglandin H2 synthases. *Clin Pharmacol Ther.* 2006;79:9-19.
15. Ashbourne JF, et al. Value of rapid screening for acetaminophen in all patients with intentional drug overdose. *Ann Emerg Med.* 1989;18:1035-1038.
16. Ayoub SS, et al. Inhibition of the diclofenac-induced cyclooxygenase-2 activity by paracetamol in cultured macrophages is not related to the intracellular lipid hydroperoxide tone. *Fund Clin Pharmacol.* 2011;25:186-190.
17. Bailey B, et al. Fulminant hepatic failure secondary to acetaminophen poisoning: a systematic review and meta-analysis of prognostic criteria determining the need for liver transplantation. *Crit Care Med.* 2003;31:299-305.
18. Bartels S, et al. Are recommended doses of acetaminophen hepatotoxic for recently abstinent alcoholics? A randomized trial. *Clin Toxicol (Phila).* 2008;46:243-249.
19. Bateman DN, et al. Effect of the UK's revised paracetamol poisoning management guidelines on admissions, adverse reactions and costs of treatment. *Br J Clin Pharmacol.* 2014;78:610-618.
20. Bateman DN, et al. Impact of reducing the threshold for acetylcysteine treatment in acute paracetamol poisoning: the recent United Kingdom experience. *Clin Toxicol (Phila).* 2014;52:868-872.
21. Bateman DN, et al. Reduction of adverse effects from intravenous acetylcysteine treatment for paracetamol poisoning: a randomised controlled trial. *Lancet.* 2014; 383:697-704.
22. Beck DH, et al. The pharmacokinetics and analgesic efficacy of larger dose rectal acetaminophen (40 mg/kg) in adults: a double-blinded, randomized study. *Anesth Analg.* 2000;90:431-436.
23. Beer C, et al. Liver unit admission following paracetamol overdose with concentrations below current UK treatment thresholds. *QJM.* 2007;100:93-96.
24. Ben-Shachar R, et al. The biochemistry of acetaminophen hepatotoxicity and rescue: a mathematical model. *Theor Biol Med Model.* 2012;9:55.
25. Bender RP, et al. Acetyl-benzoquinone imine, the toxic metabolite of acetaminophen, is a topoisomerase poison II. *Biochemistry.* 2004;43:3731-3739.
26. Bentur Y, et al. Reliability of history of acetaminophen ingestion in intentional drug overdose patients. *Hum Exp Toxicol.* 2011;30:44-50.
27. Beringer RM, et al. Intravenous paracetamol overdose: two case reports and a change to national treatment guidelines. *Arch Dis Child.* 2011;96:307-308.
28. Berling I, et al. Intravenous paracetamol toxicity in a malnourished child. *Clin Toxicol (Phila).* 2012;50:74-76.
29. Bernal W, et al. Use and outcome of liver transplantation in acetaminophen-induced acute liver failure. *Hepatology.* 1998;27:1050-1055.
30. Bernal W, et al. Blood lactate as an early predictor of outcome in paracetamol-induced acute liver failure: a cohort study. *Lancet.* 2002;359:558-563.
31. Bernal W, Wendon J. More on serum phosphate and prognosis of acute liver failure. *Hepatology.* 2003;38:533-534.
32. Bertolini A, et al. Paracetamol: new vistas of an old drug. *CNS Drug Rev.* 2006;12: 250-275.
33. Betten DP, et al. A prospective evaluation of shortened course oral *N*-acetylcysteine for the treatment of acute acetaminophen poisoning. *Ann Emerg Med.* 2007;50:272-279.
34. Betten DP, et al. A retrospective evaluation of shortened-duration oral *N*-acetylcysteine for the treatment of acetaminophen poisoning. *J Med Toxicol.* 2009;5:183-190.
35. Beyer RP, et al. Multicenter study of acetaminophen hepatotoxicity reveals the importance of biological endpoints in genomic analyses. *Toxicol Sci.* 2007;99:326-337.
36. Bhushan B, et al. Role of bile acids in liver injury and regeneration following acetaminophen overdose. *Am J Pathol.* 2013;183:1518-1526.
37. Bhushan B, et al. Pro-regenerative signaling after acetaminophen-induced acute liver injury in mice identified using a novel incremental dose model. *Am J Pathol.* 2014;184:3013-3025.
38. Bihari S, et al. Delayed and prolonged elevated serum paracetamol level after an overdose—possible causes and implications. *Crit Care Resus.* 2011;13:275-277.
39. Birmingham PK, et al. Twenty-four-hour pharmacokinetics of rectal acetaminophen in children: an old drug with new recommendations. *Anesthesiology.* 1997;87:244-252.
40. Bond GR, et al. Acetaminophen ingestion in childhood: cost and relative risk of alternative referral strategies. *J Toxicol Clin Toxicol.* 1994;32:513-525.
41. Bond GR. Acetaminophen protein adducts: a review. *Clin Toxicol (Phila).* 2009;47:2-7.
42. Bonnefont J, et al. Orally administered paracetamol does not act locally in the rat formalin test: evidence for a supraspinal, serotonin-dependent antinociceptive mechanism. *Anesthesiology.* 2003;99:976-981.
43. Bourdeaux C, et al. Death from paracetamol overdose despite appropriate treatment with *N*-acetylcysteine. *Emerg Med J.* 2007;24:e31.

44. Bourdi M, et al. Protection against acetaminophen-induced liver injury and lethality by interleukin role of inducible nitric oxide synthase. *Hepatology.* 2002;10:289-298.

45. Boutaud O, et al. Determinants of the cellular specificity of acetaminophen as an inhibitor of prostaglandin H(2) synthases. *Proc Natl Acad Sci U S A.* 2002;99:7130-7135.

46. Boutis K, Shannon M. Nephrotoxicity after acute severe acetaminophen poisoning in adolescents. *J Toxicol Clin Toxicol.* 2001;39:441-445.

47. Breen K, et al. In situ formation of the acetaminophen metabolite covalently bound in kidneys and lung: supportive evidence provided by total hepatectomy. *Biochem Pharmacol.* 1982;31:115-116.

48. Bridger S, et al. Lesson of the week: deaths from low dose paracetamol poisoning. *Br Med J.* 1998;316:1724-1725.

49. Brooker G, et al. High anion gap metabolic acidosis secondary to pyroglutamic aciduria (5-oxoprolinuria): association with prescription drugs and malnutrition. *Ann Clin Biochem.* 2007;44:406-409.

50. Bruno MK, et al. Antidotal effectiveness of N-acetylcysteine in reversing acetaminophen-induced hepatotoxicity: enhancement of the proteolysis of arylated proteins. *Biochem Pharmacol.* 1988;37:4319-4325.

51. Buckley NA, et al. Activated charcoal reduces the need for N-acetylcysteine treatment after acetaminophen (paracetamol) overdose. *J Toxicol Clin Toxicol.* 1999;37: 753-757.

52. Buckley NA, et al. Oral or intravenous N-acetylcysteine: which is the treatment of choice for acetaminophen (paracetamol) poisoning? *J Toxicol Clin Toxicol.* 1999;37: 759-767.

53. Buckpitt AR, et al. Varying effects of sulfhydryl nucleophiles on acetaminophen oxidation and sulfhydryl adduct formation. *Biochem Pharmacol.* 1979;28:2941-2946.

54. Bujalska M. Effect of nonselective and selective opioid receptors antagonists on antinociceptive action of acetaminophen. *Pol J Pharmacol.* 2004;56:539-545.

55. Cairney DG, et al. Plasma paracetamol concentration at hospital presentation has a dose-dependent relationship with liver injury despite prompt treatment with intravenous acetylcysteine. *Clin Toxicol (Phila).* 2016;54:405-410.

56. Campbell NR, et al. Renal impairment associated with an acute paracetamol overdose in the absence of hepatotoxicity. *Postgrad Med J.* 1992;68:116-118.

57. Caravati EM. Unintentional acetaminophen ingestion in children and the potential for hepatotoxicity. *J Toxicol Clin Toxicol.* 2000;38:291-296.

58. Carpenter HM, Mudge GH. Acetaminophen nephrotoxicity: studies on renal acetylation and deacetylation. *J Pharmacol Exp Ther.* 1981;218:161-167.

59. Catella-Lawson F, et al. Cyclooxygenase inhibitors and the antiplatelet effects of aspirin. *N Engl J Med.* 2001;345:1809-1817.

60. Ceelie I, et al. Acute liver failure after recommended doses of acetaminophen in patients with myopathies. *Crit Care Med.* 2011;39:678-682.

61. Cetaruk EW, et al. Tylenol extended relief overdose. *Ann Emerg Med.* 1997;30:104-108.

62. Chen YG, et al. Risk of acute kidney injury and long-term outcome in patients with acetaminophen intoxication: a nationwide population-based retrospective cohort study. *Medicine (Baltimore).* 2015;94:e2040.

63. Cholongitas E, et al. Comparison of the sequential organ failure assessment score with the King's College Hospital Criteria and the Model for End-Stage Liver Disease Score for the prognosis of acetaminophen-induced acute liver failure. *Liver Transpl.* 2012;18:405-412.

64. Chomchai S, Chomchai C. Predicting acute acetaminophen hepatotoxicity with acetaminophen-aminotransferase multiplication product and the Psi parameter. *Clin Toxicol (Phila).* 2014;52:506-511.

65. Claridge LC, et al. Acute liver failure after administration of paracetamol at the maximum recommended daily dose in adults. *BMJ* c6764. 2010;341.

66. Cobden I, et al. Paracetamol-induced acute renal failure in the absence of fulminant liver damage. *Br Med J.* 1982;284:21-22.

67. Cohen SD, Khairallah EA. Selective protein arylation and acetaminophen-induced hepatotoxicity. *Drug Metab Rev.* 1997;29:59-77.

68. Cook SF, et al. Population pharmacokinetics of intravenous paracetamol (acetaminophen) in preterm and term neonates: model development and external evaluation. *Clin Pharmacokinet.* 2016;55:107-119.

69. Cooper SC, et al. Outcomes of liver transplantation for paracetamol (acetaminophen)-induced hepatic failure. *Liver Transpl.* 2009;15:1351-1357.

70. Corcoran GB, et al. Evidence that acetaminophen and N-hydroxyacetaminophen form a common arylating intermediate, N-acetyl-p-benzoquinoneimine. *Mol Pharmacol.* 1980;18:536-542.

71. Court MH DS, et al. Interindividual variability in acetaminophen glucuronidation by human liver microsomes: identification of relevant acetaminophen UDP-glucuronosyltransferase isoforms. *J Pharm Exp Ther.* 2001;299:998-1006.

72. Cover C, et al. Pathophysiological role of the acute inflammatory response during acetaminophen hepatotoxicity. *Toxicol Appl Pharmacol.* 2006;216:98-107.

73. Craig DGN, et al. Overdose pattern and outcome in paracetamol-induced acute severe hepatotoxicity. *Br Pharm.* 2011;71:273-282.

74. Craig DGN, et al. The systemic inflammatory response syndrome and sequential organ failure assessment scores are effective triage markers following paracetamol (acetaminophen) overdose. *Aliment Pharmacol Ther.* 2011;34:219-228.

75. Craig DGN, et al. Staggered overdose pattern and delay to hospital presentation are associated with adverse outcomes following paracetamol-induced hepatotoxicity. *Br Pharm.* 2012;73:285-294.

76. Craig DGN, et al. The sequential organ failure assessment (SOFA) score is an effective triage marker following staggered paracetamol (acetaminophen) overdose. *Aliment Pharmacol Ther.* 2012;35:1408-1415.

77. Curry SC, et al. Prolonged acetaminophen-protein adduct elimination during renal failure, lack of adduct removal by hemodiafiltration, and urinary adduct concentrations after acetaminophen overdose. *J Med Toxicol.* 2015;11:169-178.

78. Curtis RM, Sivilotti ML. A descriptive analysis of aspartate and alanine aminotransferase rise and fall following acetaminophen overdose. *Clin Toxicol (Phila).* 2015;53:849-855.

79. Dabos KJ, et al. A biochemical prognostic model of outcome in paracetamol-induced acute liver injury. *Transplantation.* 2005;80:1712-1717.

80. Daly FF, et al. Prospective evaluation of repeated supratherapeutic acetaminophen (paracetamol) ingestion. *Ann Emerg Med.* 2004;44:393-398.

81. Dani M, et al. The local antinociceptive effects of paracetamol in neuropathic pain are mediated by cannabinoid receptors. *Eur J Pharm.* 2007;573:214-215.

82. Dara L, et al. Receptor interacting protein kinase 1 mediates murine acetaminophen toxicity independent of the necrosome and not through necroptosis. *Hepatology.* 2015;62:1847-1857.

83. Dart RC, et al. The safety profile of sustained release paracetamol during therapeutic use and following overdose. *Drug Saf.* 2005;28:1045-1056.

84. Dart RC, et al. Acetaminophen poisoning: an evidence-based consensus guideline for out-of-hospital management. *Clin Toxicol (Phila).* 2006;44:1-18.

85. Dart RC, Rumack BH. Patient-tailored acetylcysteine administration. *Ann Emerg Med.* 2007;50:280-281.

86. Dart RC, et al. The effects of paracetamol (acetaminophen) on hepatic tests in patients who chronically abuse alcohol—a randomized study. *Alim Pharmacol Ther.* 2010;32:478-486.

87. Dart RC, Rumack BH. Intravenous acetaminophen in the United States: iatrogenic dosing errors. *Pediatrics.* 2012;129:349-353.

88. Davern TJ, et al. Measurement of serum acetaminophen-protein adducts in patients with acute liver failure. *Gastroenterology.* 2006;130:687-694.

89. Davie A. Acetaminophen poisoning and liver function [letter]. *N Engl J Med.* 1994; 331:1310.

90. Davis M, et al. Paracetamol overdose in man: relationship between pattern of urinary metabolites and severity of liver damage. *Q J Med.* 1976;45:181-191.

91. Dear JW, Antoine DJ. Stratification of paracetamol overdose patients using new toxicity biomarkers: current candidates and future challenges. *Expert Rev Clin Pharmacol.* 2014;7:181-189.

92. Dear JW, et al. Early detection of paracetamol toxicity using circulating liver microRNA and markers of cell necrosis. *Br J Clin Pharmacol.* 2014;77:904-905.

93. Devlin J, et al. N-acetylcysteine improves indocyanine green extraction and oxygen transport during hepatic dysfunction. *Crit Care Med.* 1997;25:236-242.

94. Ding GK, Buckley NA. Evidence and consequences of spectrum bias in studies of criteria for liver transplant in paracetamol hepatotoxicity. *QJM.* 2008;101:723-729.

95. Divoll M, et al. Effect of food on acetaminophen absorption in young and elderly subjects. *J Clin Pharmacol.* 1982;22:571-576.

96. Donnelly PG, et al. Inhibition of mitochondrial respiration in vivo is an early event in acetaminophen-induced hepatotoxicity. *Arch Toxicol.* 1994;68:110-118.

97. Dougherty PP, Klein-Schwartz W. Unexpected late rise in plasma acetaminophen concentrations with change in risk stratification in acute acetaminophen overdoses. *J Emerg Med.* 2012;43:58-63.

98. Douglas DR, et al. A pharmacokinetic comparison of acetaminophen products (Tylenol Extended Relief vs regular Tylenol). *Acad Emerg Med.* 1996;3:740-744.

99. Douidar SM, Ahmed AE. A novel mechanism for the enhancement of acetaminophen hepatotoxicity by phenobarbital. *J Pharmacol Exp Ther.* 1987;240:578-583.

100. Doyon S, Klein-Schwartz W. Hepatotoxicity Despite early administration of intravenous N-acetylcysteine for acute acetaminophen overdose. *Acad Emerg Med.* 2009;16:34-39.

101. Duewall JL, et al. 5-Oxoproline (pyroglutamic) acidosis associated with chronic acetaminophen use. *Proc (Bayl Univ Med Cent).* 2010;23:19-20.

102. Duffull SB, Isbister GK. Predicting the requirement for N-acetylcysteine in paracetamol poisoning from reported dose. *Clin Toxicol (Phila).* 2013;51:772-776.

103. Eakins R, et al. Adaptation to acetaminophen exposure elicits major changes in expression and distribution of the hepatic proteome. *Sci Rep.* 2015;5:16423.

104. Eguia L, Materson BJ. Acetaminophen-related acute renal failure without fulminant liver failure. *Pharmacotherapy.* 1997;17:363-370.

105. Epstein MM, et al. Inhibition of the metabolism of paracetamol by isoniazid. *Br J Clin Pharmacol.* 1991;31:139-142.

106. Esterline RL, Ji S. Metabolic alterations resulting from the inhibition of mitochondrial respiration by acetaminophen in vivo. *Biochem Pharmacol.* 1989;38:2390-2392.

107. Esterline RL, et al. Reversible and irreversible inhibition of hepatic mitochondrial respiration by acetaminophen and its toxic metabolite, N-acetyl-p-benzoquinoneimine (NAPQI). *Biochem Pharmacol.* 1989;38:2387-2390.

108. Farid NR, et al. Haemodialysis in paracetamol self-poisoning. *Lancet.* 1972;2:396-398.

109. Fauvelle F, et al. Diclofenac, paracetamol, and vidarabine removal during plasma exchange in polyarteritis nodosa patients. *Biopharm Drug Dispo.* 1991;12:411-424.

110. Feldberg W, Gupta K. Pyrogen fever and prostaglandin-like activity in cerebrospinal fluid. *J Physiol.* 1973;228:41-53.

111. Fenves AZ, et al. Increased anion gap metabolic acidosis as a result of 5-oxoproline (pyrogluatamic acid): a role for acetaminophen. *Clin J Am Soc Nephrol.* 2006;1:441-447.

112. Flanagan RJ, Mant TGK. Coma and metabolic acidosis early in severe acute paracetamol poisoning. *Hum Toxicol.* 1986;5:256-259.

113. Flouvat B, et al. Bioequivalence study comparing a new paracetamol solution for injection and propacetamol after single intravenous infusion in healthy subjects. *Int J Clin Pharm Ther.* 2004;42:50-57.

114. Flower R, Vane J. Inhibition of prostaglandin synthetase in brain explains the anti-pyretic activity of paracetamol (4-acetamidophenol). *Nature.* 1972;240:410-411.

115. Fored CM, et al. Acetaminophen, aspirin, and chronic renal failure. *N Engl J Med.* 2001;345:1801-1808.

116. Forrest JAH, et al. Clinical pharmacokinetics of paracetamol. *Clin Pharm.* 1982;7:93-107.

117. Franko KR, et al. Accidental acetaminophen overdose results in liver transplant during second trimester of pregnancy: a case report. *Transplant Proc.* 2013;45:2063-2065.

118. Froberg BA, et al. Negative predictive value of acetaminophen concentrations within four hours of ingestion. *Acad Emerg Med.* 2013;20:1072-1075.

119. Gelotte CK, et al. Clinical features of a repeat dose multiple-day pharmacokinetics trial of acetaminophen at 4, 6, and 8 g/day. *J Toxicol Clin Toxicol.* 2003;41:726.

120. Gerber JG, et al. Effect of *N*-acetylcysteine on hepatic covalent binding of paracetamol (acetaminophen). *Lancet.* 1977;1:657-658.

121. Geus H, et al. Enhanced paracetamol clearance with molecular adsorbents recirculating system (MARS) in severe autointoxication. *Blood Purif.* 2010;30:118-119.

122. Gosselin S, et al. Treating acetaminophen overdose: thresholds, costs and uncertainties. *Clin Toxicol.* 2013;51:130-133.

123. Gosselin S, et al. Extracorporeal treatment for acetaminophen poisoning: recommendations from the EXTRIP workgroup. *Clin Toxicol (Phila).* 2014;52:856-867.

124. Gow PJ, et al. Time to review the selection criteria for transplantation in paracetamol-induced fulminant hepatic failure? *Liver Transplant.* 2007;13:1762-1763.

125. Grady JG, et al. Early indicators of prognosis in fulminant hepatic failure. *Gastroenterology.* 1989;97:439-445.

126. Graham GG, Kieran FS. Mechanism of action of paracetamol. *Am J Ther.* 2005;12:46-55.

127. Graudins A, et al. Early presentation following overdose of modified-release paracetamol (Panadol Osteo) with biphasic and prolonged paracetamol absorption. *N Z J Med.* 2009;122:64-71.

128. Graudins A, et al. Overdose with modified-release paracetamol results in delayed and prolonged absorption of paracetamol. *Intern Med J.* 2010;40:72-76.

129. Graudins A. Overdose with modified-release paracetamol (Panadol Osteo(R)) presenting to a metropolitan emergency medicine network: a case series. *Emerg Med Australas.* 2014;26:398-402.

130. Gray T, et al. Intravenous paracetamol—an international perspective of toxicity. *Clin Toxicol.* 2011;49:150-152.

131. Gray TA, et al. Hyperlactataemia and metabolic acidosis following paracetamol overdose. *Q J Med.* 1987;65:811-821.

132. Green TJ, et al. When do the aminotransferases rise after acute acetaminophen overdose? *Clin Toxicol.* 2010;48:787-792.

133. Gregoire N, et al. Safety and pharmacokinetics of paracetamol following intravenous administration of 5 g during the first 24 h with a 2-g starting dose. *Clin Pharm Ther.* 2007;81:401-405.

134. Grunbaum AM, et al. Acetaminophen and *N*-acetylcysteine dialysance during hemodialysis for massive ingestion [abstract]. *Clin Toxicol.* 2013;51:270-271.

135. Gujral JS, et al. Mode of cell death after acetaminophen overdose in mice: apoptosis or oncotic necrosis? *Toxicol Sci.* 2002;67:322-328.

136. Hahn TW, et al. Pharmacokinetics of rectal paracetamol after repeated dosing in children. *Br J Anaesth.* 2000;85:512-519.

137. Halcomb S, et al. Pharmacokinetic effects of diphenhydramine or oxycodone in simulated acetaminophen overdose. *Acad Emerg Med.* 2005;12:169-172.

138. Haller VL, et al. Non-cannabinoid CB1, non-cannabinoid CB2 antinociceptive effects of several novel compounds in the PPQ stretch test in mice. *Eur J Pharm.* 2006;546:60-68.

139. Harrison PM, et al. Serial prothrombin time as prognostic indicator in paracetamol induced fulminant hepatic failure. *Br Med J.* 1990;310:964-966.

140. Harrison PM, et al. Improved outcome of paracetamol-induced fulminant hepatic failure by late administration of acetylcysteine. *Lancet.* 1990;335:1572-1573.

141. Harrison PM, et al. Improvement by acetylcysteine of hemodynamics and oxygen transport in fulminant hepatic failure. *N Engl J Med.* 1991;324:1852-1857.

142. Hart SG, et al. Evidence against deacetylation and for cytochrome P450-mediated activation in acetaminophen-induced nephrotoxicity in the CD-1 mouse. *Toxicol Appl Pharmacol.* 1991;107:1-15.

143. Hart SG, et al. Acetaminophen nephrotoxicity in CD-1 mice. Evidence of a role for in situ activation in selective covalent binding and toxicity *Toxicol Appl Pharmacol.* 1994;126:216-275.

144. Hart SG, et al. Acetaminophen nephrotoxicity in CD-1 mice. I. Evidence of a role for in situ activation in selective covalent binding and toxicity. *Toxicol Appl Pharmacol.* 1994:267-275.

145. Hayes BD, et al. Frequency of medication errors with intravenous acetylcysteine for acetaminophen overdose. *Ann Pharmacother.* 2008;42:766-770.

146. Hazai E, et al. Reduction of toxic metabolite formation of acetaminophen. *Biochem Biophys Res Commun.* 2002;291:1089-1094.

147. Heard K, et al. A randomized trial to determine the change in alanine aminotransferase during 10 days of paracetamol (acetaminophen) administration in subjects who consume moderate amounts of alcohol. *Aliment Pharmacol Ther.* 2007;26:283-290.

148. Heard K. A multicenter comparison of the safety of oral versus intravenous acetylcysteine for treatment of acetaminophen overdose. *Clin Toxicol.* 2010;48:424-430.

149. Heard K, et al. A randomized, placebo-controlled trial to determine the course of aminotransferase elevation during prolonged acetaminophen administration. *BMC Pharmacol Toxicol.* 2014;15:39.

150. Heard K, et al. A single-arm clinical trial of a 48-hour intravenous *N*-acetylcysteine protocol for treatment of acetaminophen poisoning. *Clin Toxicol (Phila).* 2014;52:512-518.

151. Heard K, et al. Paracetamol (acetaminophen) protein adduct concentrations during therapeutic dosing. *Br J Clin Pharmacol.* 2016;81:562-568.

152. Heard KJ, et al. Acetaminophen-cysteine adducts during therapeutic dosing and following overdose. *BMC Gastroenterol.* 2011;11:1-9.

153. Hedeland RL, et al. Early predictors of severe acetaminophen-induced hepatotoxicity in a paediatric population referred to a tertiary paediatric department. *Acta Paediatr.* 2014;103:1179-1186.

154. Hendrickson RG, et al. Bactrian ("double hump") acetaminophen pharmacokinetics: a case series and review of the literature. *J Med Toxicol.* 2010;6:337-344.

155. Hernandez SH, et al. The pharmacokinetics and extracorporeal removal of *N*-acetylcysteine during renal replacement therapies. *Clin Toxicol.* 2015;53:941-949.

156. Hinz B, et al. Acetaminophen (paracetamol) is a selective cyclooxygenase-2 inhibitor in man. *FASEB J.* 2007;22:383-390.

157. Hodgman MJ, et al. Profound metabolic acidosis and oxoprolinuria in an adult. *J Med Toxicol.* 2007;3:119-124.

158. Hogestatt ED, et al. Conversion of acetaminophen to the bioactive N-acylphenolamine AM404 via fatty acid amide hydrolase-dependent arachidonic acid conjugation in the nervous system. *Biol Chem.* 2006;280:31405-31412.

159. Hoivik DJ, et al. Gender-related differences in susceptibility to acetaminophen-induced protein arylation and nephrotoxicity on the CD-1 mouse. *Toxicol Appl Pharmacol.* 1995;130:257-271.

160. Ishida Y, et al. Opposite roles of neutrophils and macrophages in the pathogenesis of acetaminophen-induced acute liver injury. *Eur J Immunol.* 2006;36:1028-1038.

161. Izumi S, et al. Coagulation factor V levels as a prognostic indicator in fulminant hepatic failure. *Hepatology.* 1996;23:1507-1511.

162. Jaeschke H. How relevant are neutrophils for acetaminophen hepatotoxicity? *Hepatology.* 2006;43:1191-1194.

163. Jaeschke H, Bajt ML. Intracellular signaling mechanisms of acetaminophen-induced liver cell death. *Toxicol Sci.* 2006;89:31-41.

164. Jaeschke H, Liu J. Neutrophil depletion protects against murine acetaminophen hepatotoxicity: another perspective. *Hepatology.* 2007;45:1588-1589.

165. Jaeschke H, et al. Acetaminophen hepatotoxicity and repair: the role of sterile inflammation and innate immunity. *Liver Int.* 2012;32:8-20.

166. James L, et al. Cytokines and toxicity in acetaminophen overdose. *J Clin Pharm.* 2005;45:1165-1171.

167. James LP, et al. Effect of *N*-acetylcysteine on acetaminophen toxicity in mice: relationship to reactive nitrogen and cytokine formation. *Toxicol Sci.* 2003;75:458-467.

168. James LP, et al. Detection of acetaminophen protein adducts in children with acute liver failure of indetermined cause. *Pediatrics.* 2006;118:e676-e681.

169. James LP, et al. Pharmacokinetics of acetaminophen-protein adducts in adults with acetaminophen overdose and acute liver failure. *Drug Metab Dispos.* 2009;37:1779-1784.

170. James LP, et al. Acetaminophen protein adduct formation following low-dose acetaminophen exposure: comparison of immediate-release vs extended-release formulations. *Eur J Clin Pharmacol.* 2013;69:851-857.

171. Jepsen S, Hansen AB. The influence of *N*-acetylcysteine on the measurement of prothrombin time and activated partial thromboplastin time in healthy subjects. *Scand J Clin Lab Invest.* 1994;54:543-547.

172. Jollow DJ, et al. Acetaminophen-induced hepatic necrosis. II Role of covalent binding in vivo. *J Pharmacol Exp Ther.* 1973;187:195-212.

173. Jones AL. Mechanism of action and value of *N*-acetylcysteine in the treatment of early and late acetaminophen poisoning: a critical review. *J Toxicol Clin Toxicol.* 1998;36:277-285.

174. Josephy PD. The molecular toxicology of acetaminophen. *Drug Metab Rev.* 2005;37:581-594.

175. Karvellas CJ, et al. A case-control study of single-pass albumin dialysis for acetaminophen-induced acute liver failure. *Blood Purif.* 2009;28:151-158.

176. Kearns GL, et al. Acetaminophen intoxication during treatment: what you don't know can hurt you. *Clin Pediatr.* 2000;39:133-144.

177. Keays R, et al. Intravenous acetylcysteine in paracetamol induced fulminant hepatic failure: a prospective controlled trial. *BMJ.* 1991;303:1026-1029.

178. Kelava T, et al. Influence of small doses of various drug vehicles on acetaminophen-induced liver injury. *Can J Physiol Pharmacol.* 2010;88:960-967.

179. Kerckhove N, et al. Ca(v)3.2 calcium channels: the key protagonist in the supraspinal effect of paracetamol. *Pain.* 2014;155:764-772.

180. Kerr F, et al. The Australasian Clinical Toxicology Investigators Collaboration randomized trial of different loading infusion rates of *N*-acetylcysteine. *Ann Emerg Med.* 2005;45:402-408.

181. Khan LR, et al. Long-term outcome following liver transplantation for paracetamol overdose. *Transplant Int.* 2010;23:524-529.

182. Kher K, Makker S. Acute renal failure due to acetaminophen ingestion without concurrent hepatotoxicity. *Am J Med.* 1987;82:1280-1281.

183. Khuroo MS, et al. Molecular adsorbent recirculating system for acute and acute-on-chronic liver failure: a meta-analysis. *Liver Tranpl.* 2004;10:1099-1106.

184. Kirschner RI, et al. Nomogram line crossing after acetaminophen combination product overdose. *Clin Toxicol (Phila).* 2016;54:40-46.

185. Kobrinsky NO, et al. Treatment of advanced malignancies with high-dose acetaminophen. *Cancer Invest.* 1996;14:202-210.

186. Kostrubsky SE, et al. Phenobarbital and phenytoin increased acetaminophen hepatotoxicity due to inhibition of UDP-glucuronosyltransferases in cultured human hepatocytes. *Toxicol Sci.* 2005;87:146-155.

187. Koterba AP, et al. Coagulation protein function. II Influence of thiols upon acetaldehyde effects. *Alcohol.* 1995;12:49-57.

188. Koulouris Z, et al. Metabolic acidosis and coma following a severe acetaminophen overdose. *Ann Pharmacother.* 1999;33:1191-1194.

189. Kozer E, et al. The association between acetaminophen concentration in the cerebrospinal fluids and temperature decline in febrile infants. *Ther Drug Monit.* 2007;29:819-823.

190. Kuffner EK, et al. Effect of maximal daily doses of acetaminophen on the liver of alcoholic patients: a randomized, double-blind, placebo-controlled trial. *Arch Intern Med.* 2001;161:2247-2252.

191. Kuffner EK, et al. Retrospective analysis of transient elevations in alanine aminotransferase during long-term treatment with acetaminophen in osteoarthritis clinical trials. *Curr Med Res Opin.* 2006;22:2137-2148.

192. Kuffner EK, et al. The effect of acetaminophen (four grams a day for three consecutive days) on hepatic test in alcoholic patients—a multicenter randomized study. *BMC Med.* 2007;5:13-22.

193. Kulo A, et al. Pharmacokinetics of a loading dose of intravenous paracetamol post caesarean delivery. *Int J Obstet Anesth.* 2012;21:125-128.

194. Laleman W, et al. Effect of the molecular adsorbent recirculating system and Prmetheus devices on systemic haemodynamics and vasoactive agents in patients with acute-on-chronic alcoholic liver failure. *Crit Care.* 2006;10:R108.

195. Larson AM, et al. Acetaminophen-induced acute liver failure: results of a United States multicenter, prospective study. *Hepatology.* 2005;42:1364-1372.

196. Laskin DL, et al. Modulation of macrophage functioning abrogates the acute hepatotoxicity of acetaminophen. *Hepatology.* 1995;21:1045-1050.

197. Lauterburg BH, et al. Mechanism of action of *N*-acetylcysteine in the protection against the hepatotoxicity of acetaminophen in rats in vivo. *J Clin Invest.* 1983;71:980-991.

198. Lavonas EJ, et al. Therapeutic acetaminophen is not associated with liver injury in children: a systematic review. *Pediatrics.* 2010;126:e1430-e1394.

199. Lawson JA, et al. The hepatic inflammatory response after acetaminophen overdose: role of neutrophils. *Toxicol Sci.* 2000;54:509-516.

200. Leang Y, et al. Reported ingested dose of paracetamol as a predictor of risk following paracetamol overdose. *Eur J Clin Pharmacol.* 2014;70:1513-1518.

201. Lederman S, et al. Neonatal paracetamol poisoning: treatment by exchange transfusion. *Arch Dis Child.* 1983;58:631-633.

202. Lee PJ, et al. Possible hepatotoxicity associated with intravenous acetaminophen in a 36-year-old female patient. *P T.* 2015;40:123-132.

203. Lee WH, et al. Predicting survival in fulminant hepatic failure using serum Gc protein concentrations. *Hepatology.* 1995;21:101-105.

204. Lee WM. Acute liver failure. *N Engl J Med.* 1993;329:135-138.

205. Lee WM. Acetaminophen toxicity: changing perceptions on a social/medical issue. *Hepatology.* 2007;46:966-970.

206. Lee YS, et al. Acetaminophen selectively suppresses peripheral prostaglandin E2 release and increases COX-2 gene expression in a clinical model of acute inflammation. *Pain.* 2007;129:279-286.

207. Lesna M, et al. Evaluation of paracetamol-induced damage in liver biopsies. *Virchows Arch Pathol.* 1976;370:333-344.

208. Levy G, et al. Evidence of placental transfer of acetaminophen [letter]. *Pediatrics.* 1974;55:895.

209. Lewis PJ, et al. Circulating microRNAs as potential markers of human drug-induced liver injury. *Hepatology.* 2011;54:1767-1776.

210. Lewis PJ, et al. Serum microRNA biomarkers for drug-induced liver injury. *Clin Pharmacol Ther.* 2012;92:291-293.

211. Lines SW, et al. The outcomes of critically ill patients with combined severe acute liver and kidney injury secondary to paracetamol toxicity requiring renal replacement therapy. *Ren Fail.* 2011;33:785-788.

212. Liss DB, et al. What is the clinical significance of 5-oxoproline (pyroglutamic acid) in high anion gap metabolic acidosis following paracetamol (acetaminophen) exposure? *Clin Toxicol (Phila).* 2013;51:817-827.

213. Liu ZX, et al. Neutrophil depletion protects against murine acetaminophen hepatotoxicity. *Hepatology.* 2006;43:1220-1230.

214. Llado L, et al. Is MELD really the definitive score for liver allocation? *Liver Transpl.* 2002;8:795-798.

215. Lodge JPA, et al. Emergency subtotal hepatectomy: a new concept for acetaminophen-induced acute liver failure: temporary hepatic support by auxiliary orthotopic liver transplantation enables long-term success. *Ann Surg.* 2008;247:238-249.

216. Lucanie R, et al. Utility of acetaminophen screening in unsuspected suicidal ingestions. *Vet Hum Toxicol.* 2002;44:171-173.

217. Lucas R, et al. Cellular mechanisms of acetaminophen: role of cyclooxygenase. *FASEB J.* 2005;19:635-637.

218. Makin AJ, et al. A 7-year experience of severe acetaminophen-induced hepatotoxicity. *Gastroenterology.* 1995;109:1907-1916.

219. Mallet C, et al. TRPV1 in brain is involved in acetaminophen-induced antinociception. *PLoS One.* 2010;5.

220. Manakkat Vijay GK, et al. Neutrophil Toll-Like receptor 9 expression and the systemic inflammatory response in acetaminophen-induced acute liver failure. *Crit Care Med.* 2016;44:43-53.

221. Manov I, et al. *N*-acetylcysteine does not protect HepG2 cells against acetaminophen-induced apoptosis. *Basic Clin Pharmacol Toxicol.* 2004;94:213-225.

222. Manyike PT, et al. Contribution of CYP2E1 and CYP3A to acetaminophen reactive metabolite formation. *Clin Pharmacol Ther.* 2000;67:275-282.

223. Markey CM, et al. Quantitative studies of hydroperoxide reduction by prostaglandin H synthase. *J Biol Chem.* 1987;13:6266-6279.

224. Marks DJB, et al. Outcomes from massive paracetamol overdose: a retrospective observational study. *Br J Clin Pharmacol.* 2017;83:1263-1272.

225. Mathew J, et al. Non-parenchymal cell responses in paracetamol (acetaminophen)-induced liver injury. *J Hepatol.* 1994;20:537-541.

226. Mazer M, Perrone J. Acetaminophen-induced nephrotoxicity: pathophysiology, clinical manifestations, and management. *J Med Toxicol.* 2008;4:2-6.

227. McCrae TA, et al. Evaluation of 3-(cysteine-S-yl) acetaminophen in the nephrotoxicity of acetaminophen in rats. *Toxicologist.* 1989;9:47.

228. McElhatton PR, et al. Paracetamol overdose in pregnancy analysis of the outcomes of 300 cases referred to the Teratology Information Service. *Reprod Toxicol.* 1997;11:85-94.

229. McGovern AJ, et al. Can AST/ALT ratio indicate recovery after acute paracetamol poisoning? *Clin Toxicol.* 2015;53:164-167.

230. McQuade DJ, et al. Paracetamol toxicity: what would be the implications of a change in UK treatment guidelines? *Eur J Clin Pharmacol.* 2012;68:1541-1547.

231. Mendoza CD, et al. Coma, metabolic acidosis and normal liver function in a child with a large serum acetaminophen level. *Ann Emerg Med.* 2006;48:637.

232. Milesi-Halle A, et al. Indocyanine green clearance varies as a function of *N*-acetylcysteine treatment in a murine model of acetaminophen toxicity. *Chem Biol Interact.* 2011;189:222-229.

233. Miller RP, et al. Acetaminophen elimination kinetics in neonates, children, and adults. *Clin Pharmacol Ther.* 1976;19:676-684.

234. Milligan TP, et al. Studies on paracetamol binding to serum proteins. *Ann Clin Biochem.* 1994;31:492-496.

235. Mitchell I, et al. Earlier identification of patients at risk from acetaminophen-induced acute liver failure. *Crit Care Med.* 1998;26:279-284.

236. Mitchell JR, et al. Acetaminophen-induced hepatic necrosis. IV Protective role of glutathione. *J Pharmacol Exp Ther.* 1973;187:185-194.

237. Mitchell JR, et al. Acetaminophen-induced hepatic injury: protective role of glutathione in man and rationale for therapy. *Clin Pharmacol Ther.* 1974;16:676-684.

238. Mohler CR, et al. Prospective evaluation of mild to moderate pediatric acetaminophen exposures. *Ann Emerg Med.* 2000;35:239-244.

239. Moller-Hartmann W, Siegers CP. Nephrotoxicity of paracetamol in the rate-mechanistic and therapeutic aspects. *J Appl Toxicol.* 1991;11:141-146.

240. Moore M, et al. The toxicity of acetaminophen and *N*-acetyl-*p*-benzoquinoneimine in isolated hepatocytes is associated with thiol depletion and increased cytosolic Ca2+. *J Biol Chem.* 1985;260:13035-13040.

241. Mour G, et al. Acute renal dysfunction in acetaminophen poisoning. *Ren Fail.* 2005;27:381-383.

242. Muldrew KL, et al. Determination of acetaminophen-protein adducts in mouse liver and serum and human serum after hepatotoxic doses of acetaminophen using high-performance liquid chromatography with electrochemical detection. *Drug Metab Disp.* 2002;30:446-451.

243. Murakami M, et al. Regulation of prostaglandin E2 biosynthesis by membrane-associated prostaglandin E2 synthase that acts in concert with cyclooxygenase-2. *J Biol Chem.* 2000;276:32783-32792.

244. Murphy R, et al. Severe acetaminophen toxicity in a patient receiving isoniazid. *Ann Intern Med.* 1990;113:799-800.

245. Muth-Selbach U, et al. Acetaminophen inhibits spinal prostaglandin E2 release after peripheral noxious stimulation. *Anesthesiology.* 1999;91:231-239.

246. Mutimer DJ, et al. Serious paracetamol poisoning and the results of liver transplantation. *Gut.* 1994;35:809-814.

247. Naga Rani MA, et al. Placental transfer of paracetamol. *J Indian Med Assoc.* 1989;87:182-183.

248. Narayan H, et al. Disproportionate effect on child admissions of the change in Medicines and Healthcare Products Regulatory Agency guidance for management of paracetamol poisoning: an analysis of hospital admissions for paracetamol overdose in England and Scotland. *Br J Clin Pharmacol.* 2015;80:1458-1463.

249. Nevin DG, Shung J. Intravenous paracetamol overdose in a preterm infant during anesthesia. *Pediatr Anesthes.* 2010:105-114.

250. Notarianni L, et al. Passage of paracetamol into breast milk and its subsequent metabolism by the neonate. *Br J Clin Pharmacol.* 1987;24:63-67.

251. O'Malley GF, et al. Protein-derived acetaminophen-cysteine can be detected after repeated supratherapeutic ingestion of acetaminophen in the absence of hepatotoxicity. *J Med Toxicol.* 2015;11:317-320.

252. Oie S, et al. Effect of hemodialysis on kinetics of acetaminophen elimination by anephric patients. *Clin Pharamcol Ther.* 1975;18:68-686.

253. Ottani A, et al. The analgesic activity of paracetamol is prevented by the blockade of cannabinoid CB1 receptors. *Eur J Pharm.* 2006;531:280-281.

254. Ouellet M, Percival MD. Mechanism of acetaminophen inhibition of cyclooxygenase isoforms. *Arch Biochem Biophys.* 2001;387:273-280.

255. Pakravan N, et al. Effect of acute paracetamol overdose on changes in serum and urine electrolytes. *Br J Clin Pharm.* 2007;64:824-832.

256. Patten PE, et al. Cytochrome P450 enzymes involved in acetaminophen activation by rat and human liver microsomes and their kinetics. *Chem Res Toxicol.* 1993;6:511-518.

257. American Academy of Pediatrics. Acetaminophen toxicity in children. *Pediatrics.* 2001;108:1020-1024.

258. Pereira L, et al. Coagulation factor V and VII/V ratio as predictors of outcome in paracetamol induced fulminant hepatic failure: relation to other prognostic indicators. *Gut.* 1992;33:98-102.

259. Pettersson PH, et al. Early bioavailability of paracetamol after oral or intravenous administration. *Acta Anaesthesiol Scand.* 2004;48:867-870.

260. Pickering G, et al. Analgesic effect of acetaminophen in humans: first evidence of a central serotonergic mechanism. *Clin Pharmacol Ther.* 2006;79:371-378.

261. Pickering G, et al. A new transmucous-buccal formulation of acetaminophen for acute traumatic pain: a non-inferiority, randomized, double-blind, clinical trial. *Pain Physician.* 2015;18:249-257.

262. Pini L, et al. The antinociceptive action of paracetamol is associated with changes in the serotonergic system in the rat brain. *Eur J Pharm.* 1996;308:31-40.

263. Pini L, et al. Naloxone-reversible antinociception by paracetamol in the rat. *J Pharmacol Exp Ther.* 1997;280:934-940.

264. Portmann B, et al. Histopathological changes in the liver following a paracetamol overdose: correlation with clinical and biochemical parameters. *J Pathol.* 1975;117:169-181.

265. Possamai LA, et al. Character and temporal evolution of apoptosis in acetaminophen-induced acute liver failure. *Crit Care Med.* 2013;41:2543-2550.

266. Potter WZ, et al. Acetaminophen induced hepatic necrosis III: Cytochrome P450 mediated covalent binding in vitro. *J Pharmacol Exp Ther.* 1973;187:203-210.

267. Prescott L. Drug conjugation in clinical toxicology. *Biochem Soc Trans.* 1984;12:96-99.

269. Prescott L. Oral or intravenous N-acetylcysteine for acetaminophen poisoning? *Ann Emerg Med.* 2005;45:409-413.

270. Prescott LF, et al. Plasma-paracetamol half-life and hepatic necrosis in patients with paracetamol overdosage. *Lancet.* 1971;1:519-522.

271. Prescott LF. Kinetics and metabolism of paracetamol and phenacetin. *Br J Clin Pharmacol.* 198010(suppl 2):291S-298S.

272. Prescott LF. Paracetamol overdosage: pharmacological considerations and clinical management. *Drugs.* 1983;25:290-314.

273. Prescott LF, et al. The comparative effects of paracetamol and indomethacin on renal function in health female volunteers. *Br J Clin Pharmacol.* 1990;29:403-412.

274. Pu S, et al. Loss of 5-lipoxygenase activity protects mice against paracetamol-induced liver toxicity. *Br J Pharmacol.* 2016;173:66-76.

275. Pumford NR, et al. Immunochemical quantitation of 3-(Cystein-S-yl) acetaminophen adducts in serum and liver proteins of acetaminophen-treated mice. *J Pharmacol Exp Ther.* 1989;248:190-196.

276. Raffa R, et al. Discovery of "self-synergistic" spinal/supraspinal antinociception produced by acetaminophen (paracetamol). *J Pharmacol Exp Ther.* 2000;295:291-294.

277. Raffa R, et al. Opioid receptors and acetaminophen (paracetamol). *Eur J Pharmacol.* 2004;503:209-210.

278. Raffa RB, Codd EE. Lack of binding of acetaminophen to 5-HT receptor or uptake sites (or eleven other binding/uptake assays). *Life Sci.* 1996;59:PL37-40.

279. Rajput I, et al. Subtotal hepatectomy and whole graft auxiliary transplantation for acetaminophen-associated acute liver failure. *HPB (Oxford).* 2014;16:220-228.

280. Raucy JL, et al. Acetaminophen activation by human liver cytochromes P-450 IIE1 and P-450 IA2. *Arch Biochem Biophys.* 1989;271:270-283.

281. Rawlins MD, et al. Pharmacokinetics of paracetamol after intravenous and oral administration. *Eur J Clin Pharmacol.* 1977;11:283-286.

282. Ray SD, et al. Protection of acetaminophen-induced hepatocellular apoptosis and necrosis by cholesteryl hemisuccinate pretreatment. *J Pharmacol Exp Ther.* 1996;279:1470-1483.

283. Raza H, John A. Differential cytotoxicity of acetaminophen in mouse macrophage J774.2 and human hepatoma HepG2 Cells: protection by diallyl sulfide. *PLoS One.* 2015;10:e0145965.

284. Reddyhoff D, et al. Timescale analysis of a mathematical model of acetaminophen metabolism and toxicity. *J Theor Biol.* 2015;386:132-146.

285. Reid AB, et al. Mechanisms of acetaminophen-induced hepatotoxicity: role of oxidative stress and mitochondrial permeability transition in freshly isolated mouse hepatocytes. *J Pharmacol Exp Ther.* 2004;311:855-863.

286. Riggs BS, et al. Acute acetaminophen overdose during pregnancy. *Obstet Gynecol.* 1989;74:247-253.

287. Riordan A, et al. Acute kidney injury in patients admitted to a liver intensive therapy unit with paracetamol-induced hepatotoxicity. *Nephrol Dial Transplant.* 2011;26:3501-3508.

288. Roberts I, et al. Paracetamol metabolites in the neonate following maternal overdose. *Br J Clin Pharmacol.* 1984;18:201-206.

289. Rollins DE, et al. Acetaminophen: potentially toxic metabolite formed by human fetal and adult liver microsomes and isolated fetal liver cells. *Science.* 1979;205:1414-1416.

290. Roth B, et al. Early metabolic acidosis and coma after acetaminophen ingestion. *Ann Emerg Med.* 1999;33:452-456.

291. Rumack BH, et al. Acetaminophen over-dose. 662 cases with evaluation of oral acetylcysteine treatment. *Arch Intern Med.* 1981;141:380-385.

292. Rumack BH. Acetaminophen overdose in young children: treatment and effects of alcohol and other additional ingestants in 417 cases. *Am J Dis Child.* 1984;138:428-433.

293. Rumack BH. Acetaminophen hepatotoxicity: the first 35 years. *J Toxicol Clin Toxicol.* 2002;40:3-20.

294. Rumack BH, Bateman DN. Acetaminophen and acetylcysteine dose and duration: past, present, and future. *Clin Toxicol (Phila).* 2012;50:91-98.

296. Saito C, et al. Novel mechanisms of protection against acetaminophen hepatotoxicity in mice by glutathione and N-acetylcysteine. *Hepatology.* 2010;51:246-254.

297. Salhanick SD, et al. Hyperbaric oxygen reduces acetaminophen toxicity and increases HIF-1alpha expression. *Acad Emerg Med.* 2006;13:707-714.

298. Salhanick SD, et al. Endothelially derived nitric oxide affects the severity of early acetaminophen-induced hepatic injury in mice. *Acad Emerg Med.* 2006;13:479-485.

299. Sandler DP. Analgesic use and chronic renal disease. *N Engl J Med.* 1989;320:399-404.

300. Sandrini M, et al. Differential involvement of central B and 5-HT receptor subtypes in the antinociceptive effect of paracetamol. *Inflamm Res.* 2003;52:347-352.

301. Sandrini M, et al. Effect of acute and repeated administration of paracetamol on opioidergic and serotonergic systems in rats. *Inflamm Res.* 2007;56:139-142.

302. Sato C, Lieber CS. Mechanism of the preventive effect of ethanol on acetaminophen-induced hepatotoxicity. *J Pharmacol Exp Ther.* 1981;218:811-815.

303. Sauer IM, et al. In vitro comparison of the molecular adsorbent recirculation system (MARS) and single-pass albumin dialysis (SPAD). *Hepatology.* 2004;39:1408-1414.

304. Schiodt FV, et al. Admission levels of serum Gc-globulin: predictive value in fulminant hepatic failure. *Hepatology.* 1996;23:713-718.

305. Schiodt FV, et al. Prediction of hepatic encephalopathy in paracetamol overdose: a prospective and validated study. *Scand J Gastroenterol.* 1999;7:723-728.

306. Schiodt FV, et al. Gc-globulin and prognosis in acute liver failure. *Liver Transpl.* 2005;11:1223-1227.

307. Schmidt LE, et al. Cerebral blood flow velocity increases during a single treatment with the molecular adsorbents recirculating system in patients with acute on chronic liver failure. *Liver Transpl.* 2001;7:709-712.

308. Schmidt LE, Dalhoff K. Serum phosphate is an early predictor of outcome in severe acetaminophen-induced hepatotoxicity. *Hepatology.* 2002;36:659-665.

309. Schmidt LE, et al. Acute versus chronic alcohol consumption in acetaminophen-induced hepatotoxicity. *Hepatology.* 2002;35:876-882.

310. Schmidt LE, et al. Systemic hemodynamic effects of treatment with the molecular adsorbents recirculating system in patients with hyperacute liver failure: a prospective controlled trial. *Liver Transpl.* 2003;9:290-297.

311. Schmidt LE, Larson FS. Prognostic implications of hyperlactatemia, multiple organ failure and systemic inflammatory response syndrome in patients with acetaminophen-induced acute liver failure. *Crit Care Med.* 2006;34:337-343.

312. Schmidt LE, Larsen FS. MELD score as a predictor of liver failure and death in patients with acetaminophen-induced liver failure. *Hepatology.* 2007;45:789-796.

313. Schwartz EA, et al. Development of hepatic failure despite use of intravenous acetylcysteine after a massive ingestion of acetaminophen and diphenhydramine. *Ann Emerg Med.* 2009;54:421-423.

314. Seifert CF, Anderson DC. Acetaminophen usage patterns and concentrations of glutathione and gamma-glutamyl transferase in alcoholic subjects. *Pharmacotherapy.* 2007;27:1473-1482.

315. Seifert SA, et al. Acute hepatotoxicity associated with therapeutic doses of intravenous acetaminophen. *Clin Toxicol (Phila).* 2016;54:282-285.

316. Sen S, et al. Pathophysiological effects of albumin dialysis in acute-on-chronic liver failure: a randomized controlled study. *Liver Transpl.* 2004;10:1109-1119.

317. Serper M, et al. Risk factors, clinical presentation, and outcomes in overdose with acetaminophen alone or with combination products: results From the Acute Liver Failure Study Group. *J Clin Gastroenterol.* 2016;50:85-91.

318. Shah AD, et al. Understanding lactic acidosis in paracetamol (acetaminophen) poisoning. *Br J Clin Pharmacol.* 2010;71:20-28.

319. Shah NL, Gordon FD. N-acetylcysteine for acetaminophen overdose: when enough is enough. *Hepatology.* 2007;46:939-941.

320. Shayani-Jam H, Nematollahi D. Electrochemical evidences in oxidation of acetaminophen in the presence of glutathione and *N*-acetylcysteine. *Chem Commun.* 2010;46:409-411.

321. Shen W, et al. Acetaminophen-induced cytotoxicity in cultured mouse hepatocytes: effects of Ca2+-endonuclease, repair DNA, and glutathione depletion inhibitors on DNA fragmentation and cell death. *Toxicol Appl Pharmacol.* 1992;112:34-40.

322. Simpson KJ, et al. The utilization of liver transplantation in the management of acute liver failure: comparison between acetaminophen and non-acetaminophen etiologies. *Liver Transplant.* 2009;15:600-609.

323. Singer AJ, et al. The temporal profile of increased transaminase levels in patients with acetaminophen-induced liver dysfunction. *Ann Emerg Med.* 1995;26:49-53.

324. Singer AL, et al. Role of plasmapheresis in the management of acute hepatic failure in children. *Ann Surg.* 2001;234:418-424.

325. Singer PP, et al. Acute fatal acetaminophen overdose without liver necrosis. *J Forens Sci.* 2007;52:992-994.

326. Singla NK, et al. Plasma and cerebrospinal fluid pharmacokinetic parameters after single-dose administration of intravenous, oral, or rectal acetaminophen. *Pain Pract.* 2012;12:523-532.

327. Sivilotti ML, et al. Antidote removal during haemodialysis for massive acetaminophen overdose. *Clin Toxicol (Phila).* 2013;51:855-863.

328. Sivilotti MLA, et al. A risk quantification instrument for acute acetaminophen overdose patients treated with *N*-acetylcysteine. *Ann Emerg Med.* 2005;46:263-271.

329. Sivilotti MLA, et al. Multiplying the serum aminotransferase by the acetaminophen concentration to predict toxicity following overdose. *Clin Toxicol (Phila).* 2010; 793-799.

330. Slattery JT, et al. Dose-dependent pharmacokinetics of acetaminophen: evidence of glutathione depletion in humans. *Clin Pharmacol Ther.* 1987;41:413-418.

331. Slitt AL, et al. Standard of care may not protect against acetaminophen-induced nephrotoxicity. *Basic Clin Pharm Toxicol.* 2004;95:247-248.

332. Smilkstein MJ, et al. Acetaminophen overdose: how critical is the delay to *N*-acetylcysteine [abstract]? *Vet Hum Toxicol.* 1987;29:486.

333. Smilkstein MJ, et al. Efficacy of oral *N*-acetylcysteine in the treatment of acetaminophen overdose. *N Engl J Med.* 1988;319:1557-1562.

334. Smilkstein MJ, et al. Efficacy of oral *N*-acetylcysteine in the treatment of acetaminophen overdose: analysis of the national multicenter study. *N Engl J Med.* 1988;3190: 1976-1985.

335. Smilkstein MJ, et al. *N*-Acetylcysteine in the treatment of acetaminophen overdose. *N Engl J Med.* 1989;320:1418.

336. Smilkstein MJ, et al. Acetaminophen overdose: a 48-hour intravenous *N*-acetylcysteine treatment protocol. *Ann Emerg Med.* 1991;20:1058-1063.

337. Smilkstein MJ, et al. Acetaminophen poisoning and liver function. *N Engl J Med.* 1994;330:1310-1311.

338. Smilkstein MJ, Rumack BH. Elimination half-life as a predictor of acetaminophen-induced hepatotoxicity [abstract]. *Vet Hum Toxicol.* 1994;36:377.

339. Smith CV, et al. Compartmentation of glutathione: implications for the study of toxicity and disease. *Toxicol Appl Pharmacol.* 1996;140:1-12.

340. Smith SW, et al. Acetaminophen overdose with altered acetaminophen pharmacokinetics and hepatotoxicity associated with premature cessation of intravenous *N*-acetylcysteine therapy. *Ann Pharmacother.* 2008;42:1333-1339.

341. Smith SW, et al. Acetaminophen overdose with altered acetaminophen pharmacokinetics and hepatotoxicity associated with premature cessation of intravenous *N*-acetylcysteine therapy. *Ann Pharmacother.* 2008;42:1333-1339.

342. Sorkine P, et al. Role of the molecular adsorbent recycling system (MARS) in the treatment of patients with acute exacerbation of chronic liver failure. *Crit Care Med.* 2001;29:1332-1336.

343. Spies CD, et al. Influence of *N*-acetylcysteine on indirect indicators of tissue oxygenation in septic shock patients: results from a prospective, randomized, double-blind study. *Crit Care Med.* 1994;22:1738-1746.

344. Spiller HA, et al. A prospective evaluation of the effect of activated charcoal before oral *N*-acetylcysteine in acetaminophen overdose. *Ann Emerg Med.* 1994;23:519-523.

345. Spiller HA, et al. Efficacy of activated charcoal administered more than four hours after acetaminophen overdose. *J Emerg Med.* 2006;30:1-5.

346. Spyker D, et al. Response surface analysis of acetaminophen (APAP) overdose hepatotoxicity—unmasking the data. *Clin Pharmacol Ther* 2003;73:27.

347. Spyres MB, et al. Limitations of the evidence supporting use of undetectable acetaminophen levels obtained <4 hours post-ingestion to rule out toxicity. *Clin Toxicol (Phila).* 2017;55:366.

348. Steelman R, et al. Metabolic acidosis and coma in a child with acetaminophen toxicity. *Clin Pediatr.* 2004;43:201-203.

349. Stork CM, et al. Pharmacokinetics of extended relief vs regular release Tylenol in simulated human overdose. *J Toxicol Clin Toxicol.* 1996;34:157-162.

350. Strubelt O, Younes M. The toxicological relevance of paracetamol-induced inhibition of hepatic respiration and ATP depletion. *Biochem Pharmacol.* 1992;44:163-170.

351. Taylor SE. Acetaminophen intoxication and length of treatment: how long is long enough? A comment. *Pharmacotherapy.* 2004;24:694-696.

352. Tenenbein M. Acetaminophen: the 150 mg/kg myth. *J Toxicol Clin Toxicol.* 2004;42:145-148.

353. Thijssen HH, et al. Paracetamol (acetaminophen) warfarin interaction: NAPQI, the toxic metabolite of paracetamol, is an inhibitor of enzymes in the vitamin K cycle. *Thromb Haemost.* 2004;92:797-802.

354. Thomsen MS, et al. Cytochrome P4502E1 inhibition by propylene glycol prevents acetaminophen (paracetamol) hepatotoxicity in mice without cytochrome P4501A2 inhibition. *Pharmacol Toxicol.* 1995;76:395-399.

355. Thornton SL, Minns AB. Unintentional chronic acetaminophen poisoning during pregnancy resulting in liver transplantation. *J Med Toxicol.* 2012;8:176-178.

356. Thummel K, et al. Ethanol and production of the hepatotoxic metabolite of acetaminophen in healthy adults. *Clin Pharmacol Ther.* 2000;67:591-599.

357. Thummel KE, et al. Mechanism by which ethanol diminishes the hepatotoxicity of acetaminophen. *J Pharmacol Exp Ther.* 1988;245:129-136.

358. Thummel KE, et al. Effect of ethanol on hepatotoxicity of acetaminophen in mice and on reactive metabolite formation by mouse and human liver microsomes. *Toxicol Appl Pharmacol.* 1989;100:391-397.

359. Thummel KE, et al. Oxidation of acetaminophen to N-acetyl-p-benzoquinone imine by human CYP3A4. *Biochem Pharmacol.* 1993;45:1563-1569.

360. Tirmenstein MA, Nelson SD. Subcellular binding and effects on calcium homeostasis produced by acetaminophen and a non-hepatotoxic regioisomer 3-hydroxyacetoanilide in mouse liver. *J Biol Chem.* 1989;264:9814-9819.

361. Tirmenstein MA, Nelson SD. Acetaminophen-induced oxidation of protein thiols: contributions of impaired thiol-metabolizing enzymes and the breakdown of adenosine nucleotides. *J Biol Chem.* 1990;265:3059-3065.

362. Tredger JM, et al. Effects of ethanol ingestion on the metabolism of a hepatotoxic dose or paracetamol in mice. *Xenobiotica.* 1986;16:661-670.

363. Vassallo S, et al. Use of the Rumack-Matthew nomogram in cases of extended-release acetaminophen toxicity. *Ann Intern Med* 940. 1996;125.

364. Vaughan D, et al. Deciphering the oxyradical inflammation Rosetta stone: O2-NO, OONO-, polymorphonuclear neutrophils, poly(ADP-ribose) synthetase, systemic inflammatory response syndrome, and multiple organ dysfunction syndrome. *Crit Care Med.* 1999;27:1666-1669.

365. Villeneuve E, et al. Four-hour acetaminophen concentration estimation after ingested dose based on pharmacokinetic models. *Clin Toxicol (Phila).* 2014;52:556-560.

366. Walsh TS, et al. The effect of *N*-acetylcysteine on oxygen transport and uptake in patients with fulminant hepatic failure. *Hepatology.* 1998;27:1332-1340.

367. Walsh TS, Lee A. *N*-acetylcysteine administration in the critically ill. *Intensive Care Med.* 1999;25:432-434.

368. Wang GS, et al. Hepatic failure despite early acetylcysteine following large acetaminophen-diphenhydramine overdose. *Pediatrics.* 2011;127:e1077-e1080.

369. Waring WS, et al. Acute acetaminophen overdose is associated with dose-dependent hypokalemia: a prospective study of 331 patients. *Basic Clin Pharm Toxicol.* 2007;102: 325-328.

370. Waring WS, et al. Does the patient history predict hepatotoxicity after acute paracetamol overdose? *Q J Med.* 2008;101:121-125.

371. Waring WS, et al. Acute ethanol coingestion confers a lower risk of hepatotoxicity after deliberate acetaminophen overdose. *Acad Emerg Med.* 2008;15:54-58.

372. Waring WS, et al. Delayed onset of acute renal failure after significant paracetamol overdose. *Hum Exp Toxicol.* 2010;29:63-68.

373. Waring WS. Criteria for acetylcysteine treatment and clinical outcomes after paracetamol poisoning. *Exp Rev Clin Pharmacol.* 2012;5:311-318.

374. Watkins PB, et al. Aminotransferase elevations in healthy adults receiving 4 grams of acetaminophen daily. *JAMA.* 2006;296:87-93.

375. Wendon JA, et al. Cerebral blood flow and metabolism in fulminant liver failure. *Hepatology.* 1994;19:1407-1413.

376. Whyte IM, et al. Acetaminophen causes an increased international normalized ratio by reducing functional factor VII. *Ther Drug Monit.* 2000;22:742-748.

377. Wiegand TJ, et al. Massive acetaminophen ingestion with early metabolic acidosis and coma: treatment with IV NAC and continuous venovenous hemodiafiltration. *Clin Toxicol.* 2010;48:156-159.

378. Wilkinson SP, et al. Frequency of renal impairment in paracetamol overdose compared with other causes of acute liver damage. *J Clin Pharmacol.* 1977;30:220-224.

379. Wilson JT, et al. Efficacy, disposition, and pharmacodynamics of aspirin, acetaminophen and choline salicylate in young febrile children. *Ther Drug Monit.* 1982;4: 147-180.

380. Winchester JF, et al. Extracorporeal treatment of salicylate or acetaminophen poisoning—is there a role? *Arch Intern Med.* 1981;141:370-374.

381. Wong A, et al. External validation of the paracetamol-aminotransferase multiplication product to predict hepatotoxicity from paracetamol overdose. *Clin Toxicol (Phila).* 2015;53:807-814.

382. Woo OF, et al. Shorter duration of oral *N*-Acetylcysteine therapy for acute acetaminophen overdose. *Ann Emerg Med.* 2000;35:363-368.

383. Wu ML, et al. Hemodialysis as adjunctive therapy for severe acetaminophen poisoning: a case report. *Chin Taipei.* 1999;62:907-913.

384. Xie Y, et al. Mechanisms of acetaminophen-induced cell death in primary human hepatocytes. *Toxicol Appl Pharmacol.* 2014;279:266-274.

385. Yang R, et al. Prolonged treatment with *N*-acetylcysteine delays liver recovery from acetaminophen hepatotoxicity. *Crit Care R55.* 2009;13.

386. Yarema MC, et al. Comparison of the 20-hour intravenous and 72-hour oral acetylcysteine protocols for the treatment of acute acetaminophen poisoning. *Ann Emerg Med.* 2009;54:606-614.

387. Yarema MC, et al. Can a serum acetaminophen concentration obtained less than 4 hours post-ingestion determine which patients do not require treatment with acetylcysteine? *Clin Toxicol (Phila).* 2017;55:102-108.

388. Yip L, et al. Intravenous administration of oral *N*-acetylcysteine. *Crit Care Med.* 1998;26:40-43.

389. Yip L, Dart RC. A 20-hour treatment for acute acetaminophen overdose. *N Engl J Med.* 2003;348:2471-2472.

390. Zand R, et al. Inhibition and induction of cytochrome P4502E1-catalyzed oxidation by isoniazid in humans. *Clin Pharmacol Ther.* 1993;54:142-149.

391. Zein JG, et al. Early anion gap metabolic acidosis in acetaminophen overdose. *Am J Emerg Med.* 2010;28:798-802.

392. Zezulka A, Wright N. Severe metabolic acidosis early in paracetamol poisoning. *Br Med J.* 1982;285:851-852.

393. Zhang YF, et al. Role of receptor interacting protein (RIP)1 on apoptosis-inducing factor-mediated necroptosis during acetaminophen-evoked acute liver failure in mice. *Toxicol Lett.* 2014;225:445-453.

394. Zhao P, et al. Selective mitochondrial glutathione depletion by ethanol enhances acetaminophen toxicity in rat liver. *Hepatology.* 2002;36:326-335.

395. Zyoud SH, et al. Reliability of the reported ingested dose of acetaminophen for predicting the risk of toxicity in acetaminophen overdose patients. *Pharmacoepidemiol Drug Saf.* 2012;21:207-213.

N-ACETYLCYSTEINE

Robert G. Hendrickson and Mary Ann Howland

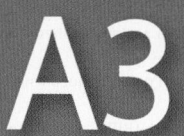

N-Acetylcysteine

Glutathione

Methionine   Cysteamine

INTRODUCTION

N-Acetylcysteine (NAC) is the cornerstone of therapy for patients with potentially lethal acetaminophen (APAP) overdoses. If administered early, NAC can prevent APAP-induced hepatotoxicity. If administered after the onset of hepatotoxicity, NAC improves outcomes and decreases mortality. *N*-Acetylcysteine appears to also limit hepatotoxicity from other xenobiotics that result in glutathione (GSH) depletion and free radical formation, such as cyclopeptide-containing mushrooms, carbon tetrachloride, chloroform, pennyroyal oil, clove oil, and possibly liver failure from chronic valproic acid use. Finally, NAC is routinely useful in the management of adults with fulminant hepatic failure caused by nontoxicologic etiologies.[20,36,64,76,82,84,96,145,149,165]

HISTORY

Shortly after the first case of APAP hepatotoxicity was reported, Mitchell et al described the protective effect of GSH.[94] Prescott[106] first suggested NAC for APAP poisoning in 1974. Early experiments demonstrated that NAC could prevent APAP-induced hepatotoxicity in mice and that the oral (PO) and intravenous (IV) routes were equally efficacious when treatment was initiated early after ingestion.[102] Several groups[106,110,118] performed human research with PO and IV NAC in the 1970s. The US Food and Drug Administration (FDA) approved NAC for PO use in 1985, for IV use in 2004; an effervescent tablet was approved for PO use in 2016.

PHARMACOLOGY

Chemistry

N-Acetylcysteine is a thiol-containing (R-SH) compound that increases intracellular cysteine concentrations by deacetylating into cysteine as well as causing release of intracellular protein- and membrane-bound cysteine.[175] The amino acids cysteine, glycine, and glutamate are used to synthesize GSH, the primary intracellular antioxidant.

Related Xenobiotics

Cysteamine, methionine, and NAC, which are all GSH precursors or substitutes, have been used successfully to prevent hepatotoxicity, but cysteamine and methionine both produce more adverse effects than NAC, and methionine is less effective than NAC. Therefore, NAC has emerged as the preferred treatment.[109,136,156,157]

Both liposomal NAC and NAC amide have been studied in animals and are being developed with the intent of increasing intracellular delivery of NAC and decreasing adverse effects.[8,73,153] *N*-Acetylcysteine amide is an NAC molecule with the carboxyl group replaced by an amide.

Mechanism of Action

N-Acetylcysteine has several distinct roles in the treatment of APAP poisoning. Early after ingestion when APAP is being metabolized to *N*-acetyl benzoquinoneimine (NAPQI), NAC prevents toxicity by rapidly detoxifying NAPQI. After hepatotoxicity is evident, NAC decreases toxicity through several nonspecific mechanisms, including free radical scavenging, increasing oxygen delivery, increased mitochondrial adenosine triphosphate (ATP) production, antioxidant effects, and alteration of microvascular tone.

N-Acetylcysteine effectively prevents APAP-induced hepatotoxicity if it is administered before GSH stores are depleted to 30% of normal. This level of depletion occurs approximately 6 to 8 hours after toxic APAP ingestion.[110,116] In this preventive role, NAC acts primarily as a precursor for the synthesis of GSH.[78] The availability of cysteine is the rate-limiting step in the synthesis of GSH, and NAC is effective in replenishing diminished supplies of both cysteine and GSH. In this way, NAC concentration ([NAC]) has a direct relationship with the amount of NAPQI detoxified and therefore higher [NAPQI] (and presumably [APAP] require higher [NAC]). Additional minor mechanisms of NAC in preventing hepatotoxicity include acting as a substrate for sulfation,[135] as an intracellular GSH substitute by directly binding to NAPQI,[27] and by enhancing the reduction of NAPQI to APAP.[79,132]

After NAPQI covalently binds to hepatocytes and other tissues,[116] NAC modulates the subsequent cascade of inflammatory events in a variety of ways.[53,146] *N*-Acetylcysteine may act directly as an antioxidant or as a precursor to GSH.[122] Glutathione protects cells against electrophilic compounds by acting as both a reducing agent and an antioxidant. *N*-Acetylcysteine improves oxygen delivery[40,53,142,160,161] and utilization in extrahepatic organs such as the brain, heart, and kidney, probably by improving blood flow in the microvasculature, although the exact mechanism is unclear. In addition, NAC increases hepatic mitochondrial ATP production in mice[124] and demonstrates a suppressive action on macrophages, neutrophils, leukocyte endothelial cell adhesion, and cytokines.[76]

Pharmacokinetics and Pharmacodynamics

When NAC is present in plasma it exists reduced or oxidized state, either free or bound to plasma proteins or with other thiols and -SH groups resulting in the formation of mixed disulfides such as NAC–cysteine.[111] *N*-Acetylcysteine has a relatively small volume of distribution (0.5 L/kg), and protein binding is 83%. *N*-Acetylcysteine is metabolized to many sulfur-containing compounds such as cysteine, GSH, methionine, cystine, and disulfides, as well as conjugates of electrophilic compounds, that are not routinely measured.[101,111] Thus, the pharmacodynamic study of NAC is complex. In addition, the pharmacokinetics of NAC are complicated based on whether total or free NAC is being measured.[111]

Pharmacokinetics of Oral *N*-Acetylcysteine

Oral NAC is rapidly absorbed, but its bioavailability is low (10%–30%) because of significant first-pass metabolism.[101,111] The mean time to peak serum concentration is 1.4 ± 0.7 hours. The mean elimination half-life is 2.5 ± 0.6 hours and is linear with increasing dose up to 3,200 mg/m²/day given as a single daily dose. Intersubject serum NAC concentrations vary tenfold.[101] Chronic administration leads to a decrease in peak plasma concentration (C_{max}) from 8.9 mg/L (55 µmol/L) at the end of 1 month to 5.1 mg/L (31 µmol/L) at the end of 6 months.[101]

Conflicting in vitro[30,74,123] and in vivo[26,44,99,114] data regarding the concomitant use of PO NAC and activated charcoal suggest that the resultant bioavailability of NAC is either decreased or unchanged. This interaction is likely of limited clinical importance, and PO or IV NAC can be initiated without concern for activated charcoal interaction (Chap. 33).

The effervescent NAC formulation (when dissolved in water) has a mean time to peak serum concentration of 1.8 hours with similar peak concentration and area under the plasma drug concentration versus time curve (AUC) as an equivalent dose of the PO NAC solution.[3,49]

Pharmacokinetics of Intravenous *N*-Acetylcysteine

When only free NAC was analyzed, healthy volunteers given 600 mg of IV NAC achieved peak serum NAC C_{max} 49 mg/L (300 µmol/L) with a half-life of 2.27 hours compared with a C_{max} of 2.6 mg/L (16 µmol/L) after 600 mg PO.[23] Serum concentrations after IV administration of an initial loading dose of 150 mg/kg over 15 minutes reach approximately 500 mg/L (3,075 µmol/L).[111] A steady-state serum concentration of 35 mg/L (10–90 mg/L) is reached in approximately 12 hours with the standard IV protocol.[111] Several alternative protocols exist with variable kinetics. In general, slower loading doses lead to lower peak [NAC],[65,167] and shorter protocols (eg, 12 hour protocol)[19] lead to lower 20-hour [NAC] than longer protocols.[29] Approximately 30% of NAC is eliminated renally.

When in the blood, IV and PO NAC have a similar half-life (2–2.5 hours). This half-life is increased in the setting of severe liver failure or end-stage kidney disease because of a reduction in clearance.[68,98]

Intravenous versus Oral Administration

As in the case of many issues related to APAP toxicity, the choice of PO versus IV NAC is complex. The available information suggests that each has advantages and disadvantages, and that one is more appropriate than the other in certain settings. Because no controlled studies have compared IV with PO NAC, conclusions about the relative benefit of each are difficult.

With the exception of fulminant hepatic failure, for which only the IV route has been investigated, IV and PO NAC administration are equally efficacious in treating patients with APAP toxicity.[108] Some data suggest that IV NAC is slightly more efficacious when given less than 12 hours after an overdose and that PO NAC is more efficacious when given after 16 hours after overdose; however, this study compared patient groups that differed by decade of treatment and by country. It remains unclear if these differences are true or clinically relevant.[107,170] In addition, any difference in outcome for patients who are treated after 16 hours almost certainly is related to the duration and total dose of NAC therapy rather than the route itself. The route of NAC should not be a factor when considering efficacy.

Although the route of NAC does not affect efficacy, rarely, in massive APAP overdoses with highly elevated [APAP] and altered kinetics, the dose of NAC in the traditional three-bag system appears to be inadequate to bind to the NAPQI that is produced. This rare scenario is an issue of the dose of NAC, not the route of NAC. *N*-Acetylcysteine must be supplied in a quantity that is consistent with the amount of NAPQI that is being produced, and the traditional IV NAC three-bag system's 6.25 mg/kg/h will need to be increased or PO NAC dosing used in these cases.

The decision of which route to use should not be affected by questions of efficacy but should depend on the rate of adverse events, safety, availability, and ease of use. Safety is the best understood of these issues. Nausea and vomiting occurs in up to 20% of patients treated with PO NAC compared with

7% with the traditional three-bag IV NAC protocol.[55] Diarrhea and headache are prevalent, but there is no credible evidence of more serious complications resulting from PO NAC. Reports of skin rash and unusual complications are rare. In contrast, IV NAC is associated with a 14% to 18%[19,72] rate of anaphylactoid reactions, although rates of 2% to 6% are reported in retrospective trials.[62,69,164,173] Several alternative IV NAC protocols report lower rates of anaphylactic reactions that required treatment when compared with the traditional three-bag protocol.[19,65,167] Most anaphylactic reactions are mild and include rash, flushing, nausea, and vomiting.[19,72,126,174] Anaphylactoid reactions are severe in approximately 1% of cases,[19,72,172] and in rare instances lead to hypotension and death.[9,13,18,56,95] Anaphylactoid reactions are attributed to both the dose and concentration of NAC and are caused by a non–IgE-mediated release of histamine from mast cells and mononucleocytes.[32] Acetaminophen inhibits mast cell histamine release; therefore, a higher APAP concentration at the time of NAC delivery decreases the risk of anaphylactoid reactions.[32,128,162] The anaphylactoid reaction rate is decreased by using a more dilute NAC solution[62,69,72,173] and by slowing NAC infusions in some studies.[26] In one prospective study, prolongation of the 150-mg/kg loading infusion from 15 to 60 minutes did not decrease the anaphylactoid rate significantly (from 18% to 14%),[72] but another prospective study that used a lower dose (100 mg/kg) and slower infusion (2 hours) decreased anaphylactoid reactions significantly (31% to 5%) compared with 150 mg/kg infused over 15 minutes.[19]

Minor reactions, such as rash, generally do not require treatment, rarely recur, and do not preclude administration of subsequent NAC doses.[12,137,176] Even when urticaria, angioedema, and respiratory symptoms develop, they usually are easily treated, and NAC can be subsequently restarted with a very low incidence of recurrence.[12,103,126,176] Although proper dosing of IV NAC is very safe, it nevertheless is less safe than PO NAC because of the possibility of severe anaphylactoid reactions, the risk of dosing errors,[54,56,95] and the possibility of incomplete or delayed treatment because of anaphylactoid reactions.[19]

Intravenous NAC is dosed using a complex three-bag preparation system (see Dosing and Administration section later) that has led to an up to 33% error rate, including 19% of patients having a greater than 1-hour interruption of NAC.[54] Attempts at simplifying this system are described, but are not adequately studied for general use[19,65,133,167] (Table A3–1).

Additional safety concerns involve dosing for both small children and obese adults. The IV NAC dosing regimen includes a milligrams per kilogram dose in a fixed water volume, leading to variability of IV NAC concentration.[25,62] This leads to a large solute-free water administration in children, with the potential for hyponatremic seizures.[147] The high [NAC] in obese adults potentially risks an increased rate of anaphylactoid reactions. Thus, alternative dosing strategies were developed for children (constant 3% concentration)[25] and obese adults (ceiling weight of 100 kg; see Dosing) are utilized.[43]

The main disadvantages of the PO NAC formulation are the high rate of vomiting and the concern that vomiting delays therapy.[107] Delays in administration of NAC are correlated with an increased risk of hepatotoxicity.[136] The IV route has a lower rate of vomiting than PO NAC and may decrease the use of antiemetics, which are associated with altered mental status, and a higher rate of [ALT] elevation.[19] A potential disadvantage of PO NAC is that its absorption is delayed up to 1 hour compared with IV NAC.[60] Finally, PO NAC doses are difficult to administer to patients with altered mental status because of aspiration risks; IV NAC offers a distinct advantage in these instances.

One theoretical, albeit unproven, advantage of PO NAC early in the course of toxicity is that direct delivery via the portal circulation yields a higher concentration of NAC in the target compartment of toxicity, the liver. Because of this first-pass clearance, PO NAC results in circulating NAC 20- to 30-fold lower than after IV dosing, suggesting that most PO NAC is taken up by the liver.[23,60] However, an elevated serum NAC concentration may be an advantage of IV NAC administration when the liver is not the only target organ of NAC, such as liver failure accompanied by cerebral edema or in pregnancy.

TABLE A3–1 Three-Bag Method Dosage Guide for *N*-Acetylcysteine by Weight for Patients Weighing ≥ 40 kg[a]

Body Weight		Loading Dose (150 mg/kg in 200 mL D₅W over 60 minutes)	Second Dose (50 mg/kg in 500 mL D₅W over 4 hours)	Third Dose (100 mg/kg in 1000 mL D₅W over 16 hours)
(kg)	(lb)	*N*-Acetylcysteine 20% (mL)[b]	*N*-Acetylcysteine 20% (mL)[b]	*N*-Acetylcysteine 20% (mL)[b]
100	220	75	25	50
90	198	67.5	22.5	45
80	176	60	20	40
70	154	52.5	17.5	35
60	132	45	15	30
50	110	37.5	12.5	25
40	88	30	10	20

[a]The total volume administered should be adjusted for patients weighing < 40 kg and for those requiring fluid restriction. [b]Acetadote (acetylcysteine) is available in 30-mL (200-mg/mL) single-dose glass vials. D₅W = 5% dextrose in water.

Several economic analyses conclud that IV NAC is less expensive than PO NAC,[90,92] but others conclud the opposite.[80] However, the majority of cost is associated with length of hospital stay, and because none of these studies have taken into account that many patients treated with PO NAC now receive shorter courses than 72 hours,[22,35] the studies do not represent current use.

Before the availability of the current IV formulation in the United States, the PO formulation was used intravenously with an excellent safety profile[42,69,173] and without published evidence of infectious or febrile consequences.[42,69] We recommend against the IV use for this purpose, but note that it was historically effective and necessary in cases in which only the PO formulation was available and the patient had intractable vomiting or APAP-induced fulminant hepatic failure.[5]

Specific Indications for Intravenous *N*-Acetylcysteine

In addition to decisions based on cost, duration, safety, and ease of use, three situations exist for which the available information suggests IV NAC is preferable to PO NAC: (1) fulminant hepatic failure, (2) inability to tolerate PO NAC, and (3) APAP poisoning in pregnancy. Each of these requires further study for validation, but all three seem well supported by current information.

Fulminant hepatic failure is an important indication for IV NAC. Intravenous is the only route that has been studied in liver failure.[71] Although PO NAC may be effective, it has not been formally studied. Second, evidence that (some or all of) the benefit of NAC in liver failure is extrahepatic suggests that IV NAC is preferable.[52] Intravenous NAC results in higher serum [NAC], which presumably leads to more NAC delivery to critical organs. Finally, concomitant gastrointestinal bleeding, use of lactulose, and other factors make IV NAC more practical.

Common indications for IV NAC include patients with very high [APAP] who are approaching or are more than 6 to 8 hours from the time of ingestion as well as those who are unable to tolerate PO NAC after a brief aggressive trial of antiemetic therapy. Use of IV NAC is recommended to prevent further delays and resultant loss of NAC efficacy, even without proof that continued vomiting significantly limits NAC absorption.

The most controversial indication for IV NAC use is during pregnancy. Administration of IV NAC to the mother has the theoretical advantage of increased delivery to the fetus over PO NAC use. Intravenous administration circumvents first-pass metabolism, presumably exposing the fetal circulation to higher maternal serum concentrations. Some studies suggest that placental transfer of NAC to the fetus is limited.[67,130] However, one case series found that the NAC concentration in cord or neonatal blood after PO maternal NAC administration equaled the NAC concentration that is achieved in patients treated with PO NAC.[63] Of course, an equivalent serum [NAC] does not prove adequacy of therapy. Unlike the neonates studied, patients treated with PO NAC have extensive first-pass hepatic uptake before NAC entry into the serum, in which [NAC] was measured.[23,60] Whether serum [NAC] in the neonates studied reflects any significant hepatic NAC delivery is uncertain.

ROLE IN ACETAMINOPHEN TOXICITY

In acute overdose, treatment with NAC should be initiated if the serum [APAP] is plotted on or above the treatment line on the Rumack-Matthew nomogram or the patient's history suggests an acute APAP ingestion of 150 mg/kg or greater and the results of blood tests will not be available within 8 hours of ingestion. In patients with chronic APAP ingestions, treatment with NAC should be initiated if either aspartate aminotransferase (AST) is above normal, or the [APAP] is higher than expected given the dose and time (Chap. 33).

Intravenous NAC is approved by the FDA for treatment of potentially hepatotoxic quantity of APAP within 8 to 10 hours after ingestion. Both the PO liquid formulation and the newer PO effervescent formulation are approved for use in a 72-hour protocol for APAP toxicity.[3]

ROLE IN NONACETAMINOPHEN POISONING

Diverse investigations of NAC as a treatment for a number of xenobiotics associated with free radical or reactive metabolite toxicity are reported. Some of these xenobiotics include acrylonitrile, amatoxins, cadmium, chloroform, carbon tetrachloride, cyclophosphamide, 1,2-dichloropropane, doxorubicin, eugenol, pulegone, ricin, and zidovudine. *N*-Acetylcysteine has not been studied well enough for any of these xenobiotics in humans to definitively recommend it as a therapeutic intervention. However, the best evidence supports the use of NAC in cases of acute exposures to cyclopeptide-containing mushrooms and carbon tetrachloride.[31,45,47,158] *N*-Acetylcysteine also decreased cisplatin-induced nephrotoxicity in both rats and human cell cultures, although in vivo human data are sparse.[10,125] *N*-Acetylcysteine is reasonable in cases of acute pennyroyal oil (ie, pulegone) or clove oil (eg, eugenol) ingestions based on their similarities to APAP-induced hepatotoxicity. Both pulegone and eugenol are converted to reactive metabolites that deplete GSH, leading to centrilobular hepatic necrosis.[151,152] *N*-Acetylcysteine may be effective in treating patients with hepatotoxicity from chronic valproate use, given the evidence that the 2,4-diene valproic acid metabolite acts as an electrophile and reduces hepatic GSH. However, there is no evidence that NAC is effective in treating patients with acute valproate toxicity and no evidence or theoretical efficacy in treating valproate-induced hyperammonemia. In animal studies, NAC increases the excretion of several metals and other elements, including boron, cadmium, chromium, cobalt, gold, and methylmercury.[14,16,31,57] The clinical usefulness of this effect remains unclear. *N*-Acetylcysteine reduced hepatic graft failure when used during organ procurement for hepatic transplant.[34]

N-Acetylcysteine was studied as an oncologic chemopreventive and antineoplastic[6,39,97,125] as well as for lung injury,[38,39] cardiac injury,[139,140] myocardial infarction,[46] multiorgan failure from trauma and sepsis,[50,113,127,141] traumatic brain or spine injury,[15,150,172] chronic obstructive pulmonary disease,[144] ifosfamide-induced nephrotoxicity,[51] postcardiac surgery,[87] hepatorenal syndrome,[61] *Helicobacter pylori* infections,[88] necrotizing enterocolitis,[148] sickle cell disease,[100] and bipolar disorder.[21] Rescue NAC therapy was also studied with high-dose APAP (> 20 g/m^2) used as chemotherapy in patients with select advanced malignancies.[75,97,166]

N-Acetylcysteine was extensively studied to determine its effects on IV contrast-induced nephropathy. Pretreatment with either PO or IV formulations was also been studied before angiography with mixed results. Absolute creatinine change in the positive studies remains quite small and is typically below 0.2 mg/dL.[48,77,83] Large randomized trials found no reduction in the risk of nephrotoxicity after intravascular angiographic procedures[2] or in emergency department computed tomography,[155] and current knowledge suggests that NAC is ineffective for these indications.[2,48,77,155]

N-Acetylcysteine was studied in the treatment of patients with non–APAP-related acute liver failure with mixed results. In a randomized trial in adults, NAC improved transplant-free survival in early non–APAP-related acute liver failure (eg, mild encephalopathy) but had no effect in those with severe encephalopathy.[82] A more recent study of patients with acute liver failure noted a significantly higher transplant-free survival rate in patients who received NAC compared with historical control participants.[36] Although another study using historic control participants suggests that NAC improves survival in children with non–APAP-related acute liver failure,[76] a prospective randomized study showed no difference in 1-year survival rates and a lower 1-year transplant-free survival rate, particularly in children younger than 2 years of age.[143]

N-Acetylcysteine is used in cases of cyclopeptide-containing mushroom poisoning, particularly poisoning with *Amanita phalloides*. *N*-Acetylcysteine therapy for amatoxin poisoning is largely based on the similarity of toxicity of amatoxin to APAP, specifically delayed onset of centrilobular hepatic necrosis. Decreases in intracellular GSH stores were identified in isolated rat hepatocytes that were exposed by amanita extracts,[70] leading to the reasonable conclusion that supplying the tissue with thiols decreases toxicity. In retrospective studies, patients treated with NAC had lower mortality rates than those treated with supportive care;[45] however, in animal studies, NAC has little effect on hepatotoxicity.[154]

We recommend the use of NAC in the treatment of xenobiotic hepatotoxicity associated with free radical or reactive metabolite toxicity. The evidence is limited, but the toxicity of xenobiotic associated hepatoxicity is consequential and the minimal risk of NAC merits utilization.

ADVERSE EVENTS AND SAFETY ISSUES

Liquid or effervescent NAC cause nausea, vomiting, flatus, diarrhea, gastroesophageal reflux, and dysgeusia; generalized urticaria occurs rarely. Generalized anaphylactoid reactions described after IV NAC dosing[19,18,37,89] are not noted after PO therapy and are likely related to rate, concentration, or high serum [NAC].[17]

Although the IV route ensures delivery, rate-related anaphylactoid reactions occur in 14% to 18% of patients,[19,72,167] and up to one-third of patients have the infusion stopped because of reactions.[19,54,86] Most reactions are mild (6%) or moderate (10%) such as cutaneous reactions, nausea, and vomiting; severe reactions such as bronchospasm, hypotension, and angioedema are rare (1%).[19,65] Anaphylactoid reactions are more common in patients with lower [APAP] (25% if APAP is < 150 mcg/mL) than in those with high [APAP] (3% if APAP is > 300 mcg/mL)[128,162] because APAP decreases histamine release from mononucleocytes and mast cells in a dose-dependent manner.[32]

If hypotension, dyspnea, wheezing, flushing, or erythema occurs, then NAC should be stopped. Adverse reactions, confined to flushing and erythema, are usually transient, and we recommend continuing NAC with meticulous monitoring for systemic symptoms that indicate the need to stop the NAC. Urticaria can be managed with diphenhydramine with the same precautions.[12] Iatrogenic overdoses with IV NAC resulted in severe reactions, including hypotension, hemolysis, cerebral edema, seizures, and death.[9,13,56,89,95]

After the reaction resolves, we recommend carefully restarting NAC at a slower rate after 1 hour, assuming NAC is still indicated. If the reaction persists or worsens, IV NAC should be discontinued and a switch to PO NAC is recommended. We recommend against stopping NAC because of mild anaphylactoid reactions because there is evidence of poor outcomes in patients who are undertreated with NAC in these scenarios.[86] Intravenous NAC decreases clotting factors and increases the prothrombin time in healthy volunteers and overdose patients without evidence of hepatic damage.[66,85,104,163] This effect occurs within the first hour, stabilizes after 16 hours of continuous IV NAC, and rapidly returns to normal when the infusion is stopped.[66] International normalized ratio (INR) elevations are mild and are typically below 1.5 to 2.0. Because the INR is used as a marker of the severity of toxicity and is one of the criteria for transplantation, this adverse effect of NAC should always be considered when evaluating the patient's condition. An elevated INR that remains below 2 without other indicators of hepatic damage is probably related to the NAC.

There is little experience with the use of the effervescent NAC tablets in APAP toxicity. There is one case of throat edema in a patient who directly ingested an effervescent tablet.[171] Although no cases of fluid overload or hypernatremia have been reported, the Cetylev PO effervescent tablet contains 438 mg of sodium per 2.5-g tablet, which equates to 7 g of sodium during the first day of treatment for a 60-kg patient. Caution should be exercised and the PO effervescent tablet avoided when treating small children and patients with sodium restriction.

SAFETY IN PREGNANCY AND NEONATES

Untreated APAP toxicity is a far greater threat to fetuses than is NAC treatment.[33,115] *N*-Acetylcysteine traverses the human placenta and produces cord blood concentrations comparable to maternal blood concentrations.[63] For treatment of pregnant patients with APAP toxicity, IV NAC (not PO NAC) has the advantage of assuring fetal delivery of NAC because of reduction of the first pass metabolism. *N*-Acetylcysteine is FDA Pregnancy Category B.

Limited data exist with regard to the management of neonatal APAP toxicity,[11,81,117,131] although IV and PO NAC have been used safely.[1,11] No adverse events were observed when preterm newborns were treated with IV NAC (Chaps. 30 and 33).[1,7,105] The elimination half-life of NAC in preterm neonates was 11 hours compared with 5.6 hours in adults.[7] When treating neonates, IV administration has the advantage of assuring adequate antidotal delivery and has been administered without adverse effects.[7,105,165]

DOSING AND ADMINISTRATION

The standard IV NAC protocol is a loading dose of 150 mg/kg up to a maximum of 15 g in 200 mL of 5% dextrose in water (D$_5$W) (for adults) infused over 60 minutes followed by a first maintenance dose of 50 mg/kg up to a maximum of 5 g in 500 mL D$_5$W (for adults) infused over 4 hours followed by a second maintenance dose of 100 mg/kg up to a maximum of 10 g in 1,000 mL D$_5$W (for adults) infused over 16 hours (6.25 mg/kg/h) (Tables A3–1 and A3–4).

When NAC is administered either as the liquid formulation or the dissolved effervescent tablet, the patient should receive a 140-mg/kg loading dose either orally or by enteral tube. Starting 4 hours after the loading dose, 70 mg/kg should be given every 4 hours, for an additional 17 doses, for a total dose of 1,330 mg/kg. The liquid formulation should be diluted to 5% and can be mixed with a soft drink to enhance palatability (Tables A3–2 and A3–3). The effervescent tablets are dissolved in either 150 mL or 300 mL of water depending on the dose.[3] If any dose is vomited within 1 hour of administration, then we recommend repeating the dose or using the IV route. Antiemetics (eg, metoclopramide or ondansetron) are reasonable to ensure absorption; however, one study noted an increased rate in aminotransferase elevation in patients who were randomized to ondansetron.[19] Whether this is an ondansetron-specific association, an effect of decreased gastric emptying, or another association is unknown.

Several other regimens, including 48-hour IV, 36-hour IV, 12-hour IV, 36-hour PO, and 20-hour PO protocols, are described; however, none of these has been adequately studied for general use (Chap. 33).[19,35,133,137,167,168]

Three protocols have been developed with the intent of decreasing peak [NAC] and decreasing adverse effects, particularly anaphylactoid

TABLE A3–2   Calculating the Loading Dose of Oral *N*-Acetylcysteine Solution[a]

Body Weight					
(kg)	(lb)	*N*-Acetylcysteine (g)	mL of 20% N-Acetylcysteine Oral Solution	Diluent (mL)	5% Solution (Total mL)
100–109	220–240	15	75	225	300
90–99	198–218	14	70	210	280
80–89	176–196	13	65	195	260
70–79	154–174	11	55	165	220
60–69	132–152	10	50	150	200
50–59	110–130	8	40	120	160
40–49	88–108	7	35	105	140
30–39	66–86	6	30	90	120
20–29	44–64	4	20	60	80

[a]If the patient weighs < 20 kg (usually patients younger than 6 years), calculate the dose of *N*-Acetylcysteine. Each milliliter of 20% *N*-Acetylcysteine solution contains 200 mg of *N*-Acetylcysteine. The loading dose is 140 mg per kilogram of body weight. Three mL of diluent is added to each milliliter of 20% *N*-Acetylcysteine solution. Do not decrease the proportion of diluent.

reactions. The SNAP protocol infuses an initial 100 mg/kg over 2 hours and then 200 mg/kg over 10 hours.[19] In a randomized controlled trial, this protocol decreased severe anaphylactoid rates from 31% with the traditional IV NAC "three-bag" protocol to 5%. Although the study was not large enough to prove equivalent efficacy, hepatotoxicity rates were similar (2% SNAP protocol versus 3% IV NAC "three-bag" protocol).[19] Another protocol infused 200 mg/kg over 4 hours and then 100 mg/kg over 16 hours, and found a lower rate of anaphylactic reactions (4.3% versus 10%) and no difference in hepatotoxicity.[167] A third group suggested infusing 200 mg/kg at the time of presentation and over a variable time (4–9 h) and then 100 mg/kg over 16 hours but had a high rate of overtreatment.[65] Although these protocols seem to decrease adverse events and severe anaphylactic reactions, their efficacy has not been studied against the standard protocol. It is not known precisely how much NAC is needed early after overdose when [APAP] are high, and there remains concern that protocols that reduce the initial dose or rate of NAC loading will not be matching early [NAC] with early [NAPQI].

Conceptually, NAC therapy should be started if the patient is at risk of toxicity, continued as long as is necessary, and it should be stopped when the patient is no longer at risk of toxicity.[169] For a detailed description of the indications for treating APAP toxicity with NAC, see Chap. 33. Briefly, in acute overdoses (from 4–24 h after ingestion), NAC therapy should be initiated if the initial APAP concentration falls above the treatment line of the Rumack-Matthew nomogram. In acute overdoses when the patient arrives more than 24 hours after ingestion, we recommend starting NAC if the APAP concentration is detectable or if the [AST] is elevated. In repeated supratherapeutic ingestions, NAC therapy should be initiated if *either* the APAP concentration is detectable *or* the AST is elevated (Chap. 33).

After the protocol is initiated, an [APAP] and [AST] are evaluated before the end of the NAC infusion (<20 hours for IV NAC) or at 24 hours (for PO NAC). If a shortened protocol is being used (eg, SNAP), then an [APAP] and [AST] should be evaluated at the end of the infusion. If the [APAP] is undetectable and the [AST] is normal, then we recommend discontinuing NAC. NAC beyond the "protocol length" if the [APAP] remains detectable or the [AST] is significantly elevated. There are no data to support what degree of AST elevation should be used as a cutoff for treatment. We recommend continuing the NAC protocol until the [APAP] is undetectable; there is no evidence of hepatic failure; and the [AST], if it was elevated, has significantly decreased. There is no validated criteria to define a significant decrease in [AST], but two consecutive decreasing values, an [AST] less than 1,000 IU/L,

TABLE A3–3   Calculating the Maintenance Dose of Oral *N*-Acetylcysteine Solution[a]

Body Weight					
(kg)	(lb)	*N*-Acetylcysteine (g)	20% N-Acetylcysteine Oral Solution (mL)	Diluent (mL)	5% Solution (Total mL)
100–109	220–240	7.5	37	113	150
90–99	198–218	7	35	105	140
80–89	176–196	6.5	33	97	130
70–79	154–174	5.5	28	82	110
60–69	132–152	5	25	75	100
50–59	110–130	4	20	60	80
40–49	88–108	3.5	18	52	70
30–39	66–86	3	15	45	60
20–29	44–64	2	10	30	40

[a]If the patient weighs < 20 kg (usually patients younger than 6 years), calculate the dose of *N*-Acetylcysteine. Each milliliter of 20% *N*-Acetylcysteine solution contains 200 mg of *N*-Acetylcysteine. The maintenance dose is 70 mg/kg. Three mL of diluent is added to each milliliter of 20% *N*-Acetylcysteine solution. Do not decrease the proportion of diluent.

TABLE A3–4	Three-Bag Method Dosage Guide for *N*-Acetylcysteine by Weight for Patients Weighing < 40 kg[a]						
Body Weight		Loading Dose (150 mg/kg over 60 minutes)		Second Dose (50 mg/kg over 4 hours)		Third Dose (100 mg/kg over 16 hours)	
(kg)	(lb)	N-Acetylcysteine 20% (mL)	D₅W (mL)[b]	N-Acetylcysteine 20% (mL)[b]	D₅W (mL)	N-Acetylcysteine 20% (mL)[b]	D₅W (mL)
30	66	22.5	100	7.5	250	15	500
25	55	18.75	100	6.25	250	12.5	500
20	44	15	60	5	140	10	280
15	33	11.25	45	3.75	105	7.5	210
10	22	7.5	30	2.5	70	5	140

[a]Acetadote (*N*-Acetylcysteine) is hyperosmolar (2,600 mOsm/L) and is compatible with D₅W, one-half normal saline (0.45% sodium chloride injection), and water for injection. [b]Acetadote is available in 30-mL (200-mg/mL) single-dose glass vials.

D₅W = 5% dextrose in water.

or an [AST]/[ALT] ratio of 0.4 or are reasonable and are commonly used.[93] If hepatic failure intervenes, then IV NAC is recommended at 6.25 mg/kg/h and continued until the patient has a normal mental status (or recovery from hepatic encephalopathy)[53] and the patient's INR decreases below 2.0 or until the patient receives a liver transplant.[24,34,52,71]

For the rare patient who ingests exceptionally large doses of APAP or who has prolonged and significantly elevated [APAP] consideration should be given to treating with greater amounts of NAC when prolonged, massive APAP concentrations are evident.[41,58,91,129,138] The rationale for increasing NAC dosing include that the IV infusion rate (6.25 mg/kg/h) was derived to treat a 16-g ingestion of APAP.[119] Although it is effective for most patients who ingest APAP, an ingestion that is several times larger than 16 g may require additional NAC. In addition, published cases of patients who have developed hepatotoxicity despite early NAC therapy have ingested more than 16 g of APAP and were treated with the IV (6.25 mg/kg/h) infusion.[41,91,129,138] There are no reported early NAC failures with the PO protocol, which may be attributed to its higher dose (17.5 mg/kg/h) and duration. Finally, the risk of hepatotoxicity increases incrementally if the [APAP] is above the "300 line," the "450 line," and the "600 line" when treated with the traditional three-bag method (6.25 mg/kg/h IV NAC infusion),[28,91] suggesting that these are reasonable indications for increased dosing or additional therapy.

No data exist to determine which, if any, alternative NAC dosing strategy is effective; however, it seems reasonable to increase NAC dosing if the hepatic exposure to APAP (and therefore NAPQI) is prolonged and massive. Several strategies are theorized, but none were studied. The following is reasonable:

We recommend that any patient who presents with an [APAP] above the "500" line receive the traditional IV NAC dosing in addition to traditional PO NAC dosing. In the event a patient cannot take the PO NAC (eg, somnolent, caustic coingestion), we recommend that the patient should receive the IV loading dose followed by the 4-hour dose (12.5 mg/kg/h) for the duration of the treatment regimen. In the event a patient presents later than 8 hours and the [APAP] is above the theoretical 500 line, then we recommend that the IV loading dose is followed by 12.5 mg/kg/h for the duration of the treatment regimen.

N-Acetylcysteine is efficiently removed by hemodialysis (clearance = 114 mL/kg/min; extraction ratio = 50%–76%),[59,134] and we suggest doubling NAC infusion rates during hemodialysis to compensate.[59,134] *N*-Acetylcysteine clearance during continuous venovenous hemodialysis (CVVHD) is 42 mL/kg/h with an extraction ratio of only 13%, so recommend against dosing adjustment during CVVHD.[59] Although there are few studies on NAC dosing in obese patients, it is reasonable to limit PO and IV NAC dosing using a maximum weight of 100 kg, given that patients who are larger than 100 kg have an equivalent hepatic volume and similar ingestion amounts as patients who weigh less than 100 kg. Although dosing with a maximum weight is logical and the IV NAC package insert now reflects dosing with a maximum weight of 100 kg, it has not yet been adequately studied in obese humans.[112,159]

Previously, dosing information for IV NAC was unavailable for patients weighing less than 40 kg, and problems with osmolarity, sodium concentrations, and fluid requirements became apparent when improper dilutions were used. The package insert now gives specific information for dosing in these patients (Table A3–4).

The IV dosing of NAC is complicated because three different preparations must be prepared with each based on weight. A retrospective study estimated that there was a 33% medication error rate in the preparation and delivery of IV NAC.[54] To limit these errors, Tables A3–1 and A3–4 from the package insert, which give the appropriate doses and dilutions for adults and patients weigh less than 40 kg, should be used.[1] In addition, the following website has a dosage calculator: http://acetadote.com/dosecalc.php.

The effervescent PO formulation comes in 2.5-g and 500-mg tablets, which are lemon-mint flavored to increase palatability, and requires mixing the tablets into variable amounts of water, depending on the dose. Tables are provided in the package insert. Dosing is limited to 100 kg. Dosing for 1- to 19-kg patients requires dissolving 5 g (two 2.5-g tablets) in 100 mL of water and then calculating the volume given based on the 50-mg/mL solution (eg, 140 mg/kg × 10 kg = 1,400 mg; 1,400 mg × 1 mL/50 mg = 28 mL).[3]

FORMULATION

N-Acetylcysteine is available as a 20% concentration in 30-mL single-dose vials designed for dilution before IV administration. *N*-Acetylcysteine liquid for PO administration is available in 10-mL vials of 10% and 20% for PO administration and should also be diluted before administration. *N*-Acetylcysteine is also available as 500-mg and 2.5-g PO effervescent tablets (Cetylev), which are dissolved in water before PO ingestion.

SUMMARY

- *N*-Acetylcysteine is the primary antidote for APAP toxicity.
- We recommend NAC use in cyclopeptide containing mushroom toxicity (eg, *A. phalloides*), carbon tetrachloride, and pulegone toxicity (pennyroyal oil).
- *N*-Acetylcysteine should be started if there is significant risk of toxicity and stopped when the risk of toxicity is gone and any toxicity that had occurred is resolving.
- Oral and IV NAC have essentially equivalent efficacy.
- Intravenous NAC has approximately an 18% risk of anaphylactoid reactions, most of which are mild, and PO NAC has a 20% risk of vomiting.
- Higher doses of NAC are reasonable for cases of massive ingestion or cases in which a prolonged high [APAP] is present.

Acknowledgment

Martin Jay Smilkstein, MD, contributed to this Antidote in Depth in a previous edition.

REFERENCES

1. Acetadote package insert. http://acetadotecom/homephp. Accessed June 15, 2017.
2. Acetylcysteine for Prevention of Renal Outcomes in Patients Undergoing Coronary and Peripheral Vascular Angiography: Main Results From the Randomized Acetylcysteine for Contrast-Induced Nephropathy Trial (ACT). *Circulation*. 2011;124:1250-1259.
3. US Food and Drug Administration. Cetylev™ prescribing information. https://wwwaccessdatafdagov/drugsatfda_docs/label/2016/207916s000lblpdf. Accessed June 15, 2017.
4. Aab A, et al. Testing hadronic interactions at ultrahigh energies with air showers measured by the Pierre Auger Observatory. *Phys Rev Lett*. 2016;117:192001.
5. Aaboud M, et al. Measurement of the inelastic proton-proton cross section at sqrt[s]= 13 TeV with the ATLAS detector at the LHC. *Phys Rev Lett*. 2016;117:182002.
6. Agarwal A, et al. *N*-acetyl-cysteine promotes angiostatin production and vascular collapse in an orthotopic model of breast cancer. *Am J Pathol*. 2004;164:1683-1696.
7. Ahola T, et al. Pharmacokinetics of intravenous *N*-acetylcysteine in pre-term new-born infants. *Eur J Clin Pharmacol*. 1999;55:645-650.
8. Alipour M, et al. Therapeutic effect of liposomal-*N*-acetylcysteine against acetaminophen-induced hepatotoxicity. *J Drug Target*. 2013;21:466-473.
9. Appelboam AV. Fatal anaphylactoid reaction to *N*-acetylcysteine: caution in patients with asthma. *Emerg Med J*. 2002;19:594-595.
10. Appenroth D, et al. Beneficial effect of acetylcysteine on cisplatin nephrotoxicity in rats. *J Appl Toxicol*. 1993;13:189-192.
11. Aw MM, et al. Neonatal paracetamol poisoning. *Arch Dis Child Fetal Neonatal Ed*. 1999;81:F77-F77.
12. Bailey B, McGuigan MA. Management of anaphylactoid reactions to intravenous *N*-acetylcysteine. *Ann Emerg Med*. 1998;31:710-715.
13. Bailey B, et al. Status epilepticus after a massive intravenous *N*-acetylcysteine overdose leading to intracranial hypertension and death. *Ann Emerg Med*. 2004;44:401-406.
14. Ballatori N, et al. *N*-acetylcysteine as an antidote in methylmercury poisoning. *Environ Health Perspect*. 1998;106:267-271.
15. Baltzer WI, et al. Randomized, blinded, placebo-controlled clinical trial of *N*-acetylcysteine in dogs with spinal cord trauma from acute intervertebral disc disease. *Spine*. 2008;33:1397-1402.
16. Banner W, et al. Experimental chelation therapy in chromium, lead, and boron intoxication with *N*-acetylcysteine and other compounds. *Toxicol Appl Pharmacol*. 1986;83:142-147.
17. Barrett KE, et al. Histamine secretion induced by *N*-acetyl cysteine. *Agents Actions*. 1985;16:144-146.
18. Bateman DN, et al. Adverse reactions to *N*-acetylcysteine. *Hum Toxicol*. 1984;3:393-398.
19. Bateman DN, et al. Reduction of adverse effects from intravenous acetylcysteine treatment for paracetamol poisoning: a randomised controlled trial. *Lancet*. 2014;383:697-704.
20. Ben-Ari Z, et al. *N*-acetylcysteine in acute hepatic failure (non-paracetamol-induced). *Hepatogastroenterology*. 2000;47:786-789.
21. Berk M, et al. The promise of *N*-acetylcysteine in neuropsychiatry. *Trends Pharmacol Sci*. 2013;34:167-177.
22. Betten DP, et al. A retrospective evaluation of shortened-duration oral *N*-acetylcysteine for the treatment of acetaminophen poisoning. *J Med Toxicol*. 2009;5:183-190.
23. Borgström L, et al. Pharmacokinetics of *N*-acetylcysteine in man. *Eur J Clin Pharmacol*. 1986;31:217-222.
24. Bromley PN, et al. Effects of intraoperative *N*-acetylcysteine in orthotopic liver transplantation. *Br J Anaesth*. 1995;75:352-354.
25. Brush DE, Boyer EW. Intravenous *N*-acetylcysteine for children. *Pediatr Emerg Care*. 2004;20:649-650.
26. Buckley NA, et al. Activated charcoal reduces the need for *N*-acetylcysteine treatment after acetaminophen (paracetamol) overdose. *J Toxicol Clin Toxicol*. 1999;37:753-757.
27. Buckpitt AR, et al. Varying effects of sulfhydryl nucleophiles on acetaminophen oxidation and sulfhydryl adduct formation. *Biochem Pharmacol*. 1979;28:2941-2946.
28. Cairney DG, et al. Plasma paracetamol concentration at hospital presentation has a dose-dependent relationship with liver injury despite prompt treatment with intravenous acetylcysteine. *Clin Toxicol (Phila)*. 2016;54:405-410.
29. Chiew AL, et al. Evidence for the changing regimens of acetylcysteine. *Br J Clin Pharmacol*. 2016;81:471-481.
30. Chinouth RW, et al. *N*-acetylcysteine adsorption by activated charcoal. *Vet Hum Toxicol*. 1980;22:392-394.
31. Chyka PA, et al. Utility of acetylcysteine in treating poisonings and adverse drug reactions. *Drug Saf*. 2000;22:123-148.
32. Coulson J, Thompson JP. Paracetamol (acetaminophen) attenuates in vitro mast cell and peripheral blood mononucleocyte cell histamine release induced by *N*-acetylcysteine. *Clini Toxicol (Phila)*. 2010;48:111-114.
33. Crowell C, et al. Caring for the mother, concentrating on the fetus: intravenous *N*-acetylcysteine in pregnancy. *Am J Emerg Med*. 2008;26:735.e731-735.e732.
34. D'Amico F, et al. Use of *N*-acetylcysteine during liver procurement: a prospective randomized controlled study. *Liver Transpl*. 2012;19:135-144.
35. Dart RC, Rumack BH. Patient-tailored acetylcysteine administration. *Ann Emerg Med*. 2007;50:280-281.
36. Darweesh SK, et al. Effect of *N*-acetylcysteine on mortality and liver transplantation rate in non-acetaminophen-induced acute liver failure: a multicenter study. *Cling Drug Invest*. 2017;37:473-482.
37. Dawson AH, et al. Adverse reactions to *N*-acetylcysteine during treatment for paracetamol poisoning. *Med J Aust*. 1989;150:329-331.
38. De Backer WA, et al. *N*-acetylcysteine pretreatment of cardiac surgery patients influences plasma neutrophil elastase and neutrophil influx in bronchoalveolar lavage fluid. *Intensive Care Med*. 1996;22:900-908.
39. De Flora S, et al. Chemopreventive properties and mechanisms of *N*-acetylcysteine. The experimental background. *J Cell Biochem*. 1995;59:33-41.
40. Devlin J, et al. *N*-acetylcysteine improves indocyanine green extraction and oxygen transport during hepatic dysfunction. *Crit Care Med*. 1997;25:236-242.
41. Doyon S, Klein-Schwartz W. Hepatotoxicity despite early administration of intravenous *N*-acetylcysteine for acute acetaminophen overdose. *Acad Emerg Med*. 2009;16:34-39.
42. Dribben WH, et al. Stability and microbiology of inhalant *N*-acetylcysteine used as an intravenous solution for the treatment of acetaminophen poisoning. *Ann Emerg Med*. 2003;42:9-13.
43. Duncan R. New recommendation for *N*-acetylcysteine dosing may reduce incidence of adverse effects. *Emerg Med J*. 2006;23:584-584.
44. Ekins BR, et al. The effect of activated charcoal on *N*-acetylcysteine absorption in normal subjects. *Am J Emerg Med*. 1987;5:483-487.
45. Enjalbert F, et al. Treatment of amatoxin poisoning: 20-year retrospective analysis. *J Toxicol Clin Toxicol*. 2002;40:715-757.
46. Eshraghi A, et al. Evaluating the effect of intracoronary *N*-acetylcysteine on platelet activation markers after primary percutaneous coronary intervention in patients with ST-elevation myocardial infarction. *Am J Ther*. 2016;23:e44-e51.
47. Flanagan RJ, Meredith TJ. Use of *N*-acetylcysteine in clinical toxicology. *Am J Med*. 1991;91:S131-S139.
48. Gonzales DA, et al. A meta-analysis of *N*-acetylcysteine in contrast-induced nephrotoxicity: unsupervised clustering to resolve heterogeneity. *BMC Med*. 2007;5.
49. Greene SC, et al. Effervescent *N*-acetylcysteine tablets versus oral solution *N*-acetylcysteine in fasting healthy adults: an open-label, randomized, single-dose, crossover, relative bioavailability study. *Curr Ther Res*. 2016;83:1-7.
50. Gundersen Y, et al. *N*-acetylcysteine administered as part of the immediate post-traumatic resuscitation regimen does not significantly influence initiation of inflammatory responses or subsequent endotoxin hyporesponsiveness. *Resuscitation*. 2005;64:377-382.
51. Hanly LN, et al. *N*-acetylcysteine as a novel prophylactic treatment for ifosfamide-induced nephrotoxicity in children: translational pharmacokinetics. *J Clin Pharmacol*. 2012;52:55-64.
52. Harrison PM, et al. Improved outcome of paracetamol-induced fulminant hepatic failure by late administration of acetylcysteine. *Lancet*. 1990;335:1572-1573.
53. Harrison PM, et al. Improvement by acetylcysteine of hemodynamics and oxygen transport in fulminant hepatic failure. *N Engl J Med*. 1991;324:1852-1857.
54. Hayes BD, et al. Frequency of medication errors with intravenous acetylcysteine for acetaminophen overdose. *Ann Pharmacother*. 2008;42:766-770.
55. Heard K. A multicenter comparison of the safety of oral versus intravenous acetylcysteine for treatment of acetaminophen overdose. *Clin Toxicol (Phila)*. 2010;48:424-430.
56. Heard K, Schaeffer TH. Massive acetylcysteine overdose associated with cerebral edema and seizures. *Clin Toxicol (Phila)*. 2011;49:423-425.
57. Henderson PHT, Shum S. *N*-acetylcysteine therapy of acute heavy metal poisoning in mice. *Vet Hum Toxicol*. 1985;53:941-949.
58. Hendrickson RG, et al. Bactrian ("double hump") acetaminophen pharmacokinetics: a case series and review of the literature. *J Med Toxicol*. 2010;6:337-344.
59. Hernandez SH, et al. The pharmacokinetics and extracorporeal removal of *N*-acetylcysteine during renal replacement therapies. *Clin Toxicol (Phila)*. 2015;53:941-949.
60. Holdiness MR. Clinical pharmacokinetics of *N*-acetylcysteine. *Clin Pharmacokinet*. 1991;20:123-134.
61. Holt S, et al. Improvement in renal function in hepatorenal syndrome with *N*-acetylcysteine. *Lancet*. 1999;353:294-295.
62. Horowitz BZ, et al. Not so fast! *Ann Emerg Med*. 2006;47:122-123.
63. Horowitz RS, et al. Placental transfer of *N*-acetylcysteine following human maternal acetaminophen toxicity. *J Toxicol Clin Toxicol*. 1997;35:447-451.
64. Hu J, et al. Efficacy and safety of acetylcysteine in "non-acetaminophen" acute liver failure: a meta-analysis of prospective clinical trials. *Clin Res Hepatol Gastroenterol*. 2015;39:594-599.
65. Isbister GK, et al. A prospective observational study of a novel 2-phase infusion protocol for the administration of acetylcysteine in paracetamol poisoning. *Clin Toxicol (Phila)*. 2016;54:120-126.
66. Jepsen S, Hansen AB. The influence of *N*-acetylcysteine on the measurement of prothrombin time and activated partial thromboplastin time in healthy subjects. *Scand J Clin Lab Invest*. 1994;54:543-547.
67. Johnson D, et al. Transfer of *N*-acetylcysteine by the human placenta. *Vet Hum Toxicol*. 1993;35:365.
68. Jones AL, et al. Pharmacokinetics of *N*-acetylcysteine are altered in patients with chronic liver disease. *Aliment Pharmacol Ther*. 1997;11:787-791.
69. Kao LW, et al. What is the rate of adverse events after oral *N*-acetylcysteine administered by the intravenous route to patients with suspected acetaminophen poisoning? *Ann Emerg Med*. 2003;42:741-750.

70. Kawaji A, et al. In vitro toxicity test of poisonous mushroom extracts with isolated rat hepatocytes. *J Toxicol Sc.* 1990;15:145-156.

71. Keays R, et al. Intravenous acetylcysteine in paracetamol induced fulminant hepatic failure: a prospective controlled trial. *BMJ.* 1991;303:1026-1029.

72. Kerr F, et al. The Australasian Clinical Toxicology Investigators Collaboration randomized trial of different loading infusion rates of *N*-acetylcysteine. *Ann Emerg Med.* 2005;45:402-408.

73. Khayyat A, et al. *N*-acetylcysteine amide, a promising antidote for acetaminophen toxicity. *Toxicol Lett.* 2016;241:133-142.

74. Klein-Schwartz W, Oderda GM. Adsorption of oral antidotes for acetaminophen poisoning (methionine and *N*-acetylcysteine) by activated charcoal. *Clin Toxicol* 1981;18:283-290.

75. Kobrinsky NL, et al. Treatment of advanced malignancies with high-dose acetaminophen and *N*-acetylcysteine rescue. *Cancer Invest.* 1996;14:202-210.

76. Kortsalioudaki C, et al. Safety and efficacy of *N*-acetylcysteine in children with non-acetaminophen-induced acute liver failure. *Liver Transpl.* 2007;14:25-30.

77. Kshirsagar AV. *N*-acetylcysteine for the prevention of radiocontrast induced nephropathy: a meta-analysis of prospective controlled trials. *J Am Soc Nephrol.* 2004;15:761-769.

78. Lauterburg BH, et al. Mechanism of action of *N*-acetylcysteine in the protection against the hepatotoxicity of acetaminophen in rats in vivo. *J Clin Invest.* 1983;71:980-991.

79. Lauterburg BH, Velez ME. Glutathione deficiency in alcoholics: risk factor for paracetamol hepatotoxicity. *Gut.* 1988;29:1153-1157.

80. Lavonas EJ, et al. Intravenous administration of *N*-acetylcysteine: oral and parenteral formulations are both acceptable. *Ann Emerg Med.* 2005;45:223-224.

81. Lederman S, et al. Neonatal paracetamol poisoning: treatment by exchange transfusion. *Arch Dis Child* 1983;58:631-633.

82. Lee WM, et al. Intravenous *N*-acetylcysteine improves transplant-free survival in early stage non-acetaminophen acute liver failure. *Gastroenterology.* 2009;137:856-864.e851.

83. Loomba RS, et al. Role of *N*-acetylcysteine to prevent contrast-induced nephropathy. *Am J Ther.* 2016;23:e172-e183.

84. Lovat R, Preiser J-C. Antioxidant therapy in intensive care. *Curr Opin Crit Care.* 2003;9:266-270.

85. Lucena MI, et al. The administration of *N*-acetylcysteine causes a decrease in prothrombin time in patients with paracetamol overdose but without evidence of liver impairment. *Eur J Gastroenterol Hepatol.* 2005;17:59-63.

86. Lucyk SN, et al. Outcomes of patients with premature discontinuation of the 21-h intravenous *N*-acetylcysteine protocol after acute acetaminophen overdose. *J Emerg Med.* 2016;50:629-637.

87. Mahmoud KM, Ammar AS. Effect of *N*-acetylcysteine on cardiac injury and oxidative stress after abdominal aortic aneurysm repair: a randomized controlled trial. *Acta Anaesthesiol Scand.* 2011;55:1015-1021.

88. Makipour K, Friedenberg FK. The potential role of *N*-acetylcysteine for the treatment of *Helicobacter pylori*. *J Clin Gastroenterol.* 2011;45:841-843.

89. Mant TG, et al. Adverse reactions to acetylcysteine and effects of overdose. *BMJ.* 1984;289:217-219.

90. Marchetti A, Rossiter R. Managing acute acetaminophen poisoning with oral versus intravenous *N*-acetylcysteine: a provider-perspective cost analysis. *J Med Econ.* 2009;12:384-391.

91. Marks DJB, et al. Outcomes from massive paracetamol overdose: a retrospective observational study. *Br J Clin Pharmacol.* 2017;83:1263-1272.

92. Martello JL, et al. Cost minimization analysis comparing enteral *N*-acetylcysteine to intravenous acetylcysteine in the management of acute acetaminophen toxicity. *Clin Toxicol (Phila).* 2010;48:79-83.

93. McGovern AJ, et al. Can AST/ALT ratio indicate recovery after acute paracetamol poisoning? *Clin Toxicol (Phila).* 2015;53:164-167.

94. Mitchell JR, et al. Acetaminophen-induced hepatic injury: Protective role of glutathione in man and rationale for therapy. *Clin Pharmacol Ther.* 1974;16:676-684.

95. Mullins ME, Vitkovitsky IV. Hemolysis and hemolytic uremic syndrome following five-fold *N*-acetylcysteine overdose. *Clin Toxicol (Phila).* 2011;49:755-759.

96. Nabi T, et al. Role of *N*-acetylcysteine treatment in non-acetaminophen-induced acute liver failure: a prospective study. *Saudi J Gastroenterol.* 2017;23:169-175.

97. Neuwelt AJ, et al. Preclinical high-dose acetaminophen with *N*-acetylcysteine rescue enhances the efficacy of cisplatin chemotherapy in atypical teratoid rhabdoid tumors. *Pediatr Blood Cancer.* 2013;61:120-127.

98. Nolin TD, et al. Multiple-dose pharmacokinetics and pharmacodynamics of *n*-acetylcysteine in patients with end-stage renal disease. *Clin J Am Soc Nephrol.* 2010;5:1588-1594.

99. North DS, et al. Effect of activated charcoal administration on acetylcysteine serum levels in humans. *Am J Hosp Pharm.* 1981;38:1022-1024.

100. Nur E, et al. *N*-acetylcysteine reduces oxidative stress in sickle cell patients. *Ann Hematol.* 2012;91:1097-1105.

101. Pendyala L, Creaven PJ. Pharmacokinetic and pharmacodynamic studies of *N*-acetylcysteine, a potential chemopreventive agent during a phase I trial. *Cancer Epidemiol Biomarkers Prev.* 1995;4:245-251.

102. Piperno E. Reversal of experimental paracetamol toxicosis with *N*-acetylcysteine. *Lancet.* 1976;308:738-739.

103. Pizon AF, LoVecchio F. Adverse reaction from use of intravenous *N*-acetylcysteine. *J Emerg Med.* 2006;31:434-435.

104. Pizon AF, et al. The in vitro effect of *n*-acetylcysteine on prothrombin Time in plasma samples from healthy subjects. *Acad Emerg Med.* 2011;18:351-354.

105. Porta R, et al. Lack of toxicity after paracetamol overdose in an extremely preterm neonate. *Eur J Clin Pharmacol.* 2012;68:901-902.

106. Prescott L. Successful treatment of severe paracetamol overdosage with cysteamine. *Lancet.* 1974;303:588-592.

107. Prescott L. Oral or intravenous *N*-acetylcysteine for acetaminophen poisoning? *Ann Emerg Med.* 2005;45:409-413.

108. Prescott L. Oral or intravenous *N*-acetylcysteine for acetaminophen poisoning? *Ann Emerg Med.* 2005;45:409-413.

109. Prescott LF, et al. Cysteamine, methionine, and penicillamine in the treatment of paracetamol poisoning. *Lancet.* 1976;308:109-113.

110. Prescott LF, et al. Intravenous *N*-acetylcysteine: the treatment of choice for paracetamol poisoning. *BMJ.* 1979;2:1097-1100.

111. Prescott LF, et al. The disposition and kinetics of intravenous *N*-acetylcysteine in patients with paracetamol overdosage. *Eur J Clin Pharmacol.* 1989;37:501-506.

112. Radosevich JJ, et al. Hepatotoxicity in obese versus nonobese patients with acetaminophen poisoning who are treated with intravenous *N*-acetylcysteine. *Am J Ther.* 2016;23:e714-e719.

113. Rank N, et al. *N*-acetylcysteine increases liver blood flow and improves liver function in septic shock patients: results of a prospective, randomized, double-blind study. *Crit Care Med.* 2000;28:3799-3807.

114. Renzi FP, et al. Concomitant use of activated charcoal and *N*-acetylcysteine. *Ann Emerg Med.* 1985;14:568-572.

115. Riggs BS, et al: Acute acetaminophen overdose during pregnancy. *Obstet Gynecol.* 1989;74:247-253.

116. Roberts DW, et al. Immunohistochemical localization and quantification of the 3-(cystein-S-yl)-acetaminophen protein adduct in acetaminophen hepatotoxicity. *Am J Pathol.* 1991;138:359-371.

117. Roberts I, et al. Paracetamol metabolites in the neonate following maternal overdose. *Br J Clin Pharmacol.* 1984;18:201-206.

118. Rumack BH, Peterson RG. Acetaminophen overdose: incidence, diagnosis, and management in 416 patients. *Pediatrics.* 1978;62(5 pt 2 suppl):898-903.

119. Rumack BH, Bateman DN. Acetaminophen and acetylcysteine dose and duration: past, present and future. *Clin Toxicol (Phila).* 2012;50:91-98.

122. Rushworth GF, Megson IL. Existing and potential therapeutic uses for *N*-acetylcysteine: the need for conversion to intracellular glutathione for antioxidant benefits. *Pharmacol Ther.* 2014;141:150-159.

123. Rybolt TR, et al. In vitro coadsorption of acetaminophen and *N*-acetylcysteine onto activated carbon powder. *J Pharm Sci.* 1986;75:904-906.

124. Saito C, et al. Novel mechanisms of protection against acetaminophen hepatotoxicity in mice by glutathione and *N*-acetylcysteine. *Hepatology.* 2010;51:246-254.

125. Sajadi MM, et al. Correlation between circulating HIV-1 RNA and broad HIV-1 neutralizing antibody activity. *J Acquir Immune Defic Syndr.* 2011;57:9-15.

126. Sandilands EA, Bateman DN. Adverse reactions associated with acetylcysteine. *Clin Toxicol (Phila).* 2009;47:81-88.

127. Schaller G, et al. Effects of *N*-acetylcysteine against systemic and renal hemodynamic effects of endotoxin in healthy humans. *Crit Care Med.* 2007;35:1869-1875.

128. Schmidt LE. Identification of patients at risk of anaphylactoid reactions to *N*-acetylcysteine in the treatment of paracetamol overdose. *Clin Toxicol (Phila).* 2013;51:467-472.

129. Schwartz EA, et al. Development of hepatic failure despite use of intravenous acetylcysteine after a massive ingestion of acetaminophen and diphenhydramine. *Ann Emerg Med.* 2009;54:421-423.

130. Selden BS, et al. Transplacental transport of *N*-acetylcysteine in an ovine model. *Ann Emerg Med.* 1991;20:1069-1072.

131. Sharma A HM, et al. The dilemma of NAC therapy in a premature infant. *J Toxicol Clin Toxicol.* 2000;38:57.

132. Shayani-Jam H, Nematollahi D. Electrochemical evidences in oxidation of acetaminophen in the presence of glutathione and *N*-acetylcysteine. *Chem Commun.* 2010;46:409-411.

133. Shen F, et al. A dosing regimen for immediate *N*-acetylcysteine treatment for acute paracetamol overdose. *Clin Toxicol (Phila).* 2011;49:643-647.

134. Sivilotti ML, et al. Antidote removal during haemodialysis for massive acetaminophen overdose. *Clin Toxicol (Phila).* 2013;51:855-863.

135. Slattery JT, et al. Dose-dependent pharmacokinetics of acetaminophen: Evidence of glutathione depletion in humans. *Clin Pharmacol Ther.* 1987;41:413-418.

136. Smilkstein MJ, et al. Efficacy of oral *N*-acetylcysteine in the treatment of acetaminophen overdose: analysis of the national multicenter study. *N Engl J Med.* 1988;3190:1976-1985.

137. Smilkstein MJ, et al. Acetaminophen overdose: a 48-hour intravenous *N*-acetylcysteine treatment protocol. *Ann Emerg Med.* 1991;20:1058-1063.

138. Smith SW, et al. Acetaminophen overdose with altered acetaminophen pharmacokinetics and hepatotoxicity associated with premature cessation of intravenous *N*-acetylcysteine therapy. *Ann Pharmacother.* 2008;42:1333-1339.

139. Sochman J. *N*-acetylcysteine in acute cardiology: 10 years later: what do we know and what would we like to know?! *J Am Coll Cardiol.* 2002;39:1422-1428.

140. Šochman J, et al. Infarct size limitation: acute *N*-acetylcysteine defense (ISLAND) trial. Start of the study. *Int J Cardiol.* 1995;49:181-182.

141. Spapen HD, et al. Effects of *N*-acetylcysteine on microalbuminuria and organ failure in acute severe sepsis. *Chest.* 2005;127:1413-1419.

142. Spies CD, et al. Influence of *N*-acetylcysteine on indirect indicators of tissue oxygenation in septic shock patients: results from a prospective, randomized, double-blind study. *Crit Care Med.* 1994;22:1738-1746.

143. Squires RH, et al. Intravenous *N*-acetylcysteine in pediatric patients with nonacetaminophen acute liver failure: a placebo-controlled clinical trial. *Hepatology.* 2013;57:1542-1549.

144. Stav D, Raz M. Effect of *N*-acetylcysteine on air trapping in COPD. *Chest.* 2009;136: 381-386.

145. Stravitz RT, et al. Intensive care of patients with acute liver failure: recommendations of the U.S. Acute Liver Failure Study Group. *Crit Care Med.* 2007;35:2498-2508.

146. Stravitz RT, et al. Effects of *N*-acetylcysteine on cytokines in non-acetaminophen acute liver failure: potential mechanism of improvement in transplant-free survival. *Liver Int.* 2013;33:1324-1331.

147. Sung L, et al. Dilution of Intravenous *N*-acetylcysteine as a cause of hyponatremia. *Pediatrics.* 1997;100:389-389.

148. Tayman C, et al. *N*-acetylcysteine may prevent severe intestinal damage in necrotizing enterocolitis. *J Pediatr Surg.* 2012;47:540-550.

149. Teriaky A. The role of *N*-acetylcysteine in the treatment of non-acetaminophen acute liver failure. *Saudi J Gastroenterol.* 2017;23:131-132.

150. Thomale U-W, et al. The effect of *N*-acetylcysteine on posttraumatic changes after controlled cortical impact in rats. *Intensive Care Med.* 2005;32:149-155.

151. Thomassen D, et al. Reactive intermediates in the oxidation of menthofuran by cytochromes P-450. *Chem Res Toxicol.* 1992;5:123-130.

152. Thompson D, et al. Formation of glutathione conjugates during oxidation of eugenol by microsomal fractions of rat liver and lung. *Biochem Pharmacol.* 1990;39:1587-1595.

153. Tobwala S, et al. Comparative evaluation of *N*-acetylcysteine and N-acetylcysteineamide in acetaminophen-induced hepatotoxicity in human hepatoma HepaRG cells. *Exp Biol Med (Maywood).* 2015;240:261-272.

154. Tong TC, et al. Comparative treatment of α-amanitin poisoning with *N*-acetylcysteine, benzylpenicillin, cimetidine, thioctic acid, and silybin in a murine model. *Ann Emerg Med.* 2007;50:282-288.

155. Traub SJ, et al. *N*-acetylcysteine plus intravenous fluids versus intravenous fluids alone to prevent contrast-induced nephropathy in emergency computed tomography. *Ann Emerg Med.* 2013;62:511-520.e525.

156. Vale JA. Treatment of acetaminophen poisoning. *Arch Intern Med.* 1981;141:394.

157. Vale JA, Wheeler DC. Anaphylactoid reactions to acetylcysteine. *Lancet.* 1982;320:988.

158. Valles EG, et al. N-acetyl cysteine is an early but also a late preventive agent against carbon tetrachloride-induced liver necrosis. *Toxicol Lett.* 1994;71:87-95.

159. Varney SM, et al Acetylcysteine for acetaminophen overdose in patients who weigh >100 kg. *Am J Ther.* 2014;21:159-163.

160. Walsh TS, et al. The effect of *N*-acetylcysteine on oxygen transport and uptake in patients with fulminant hepatic failure. *Hepatology.* 1998;27:1332-1340.

161. Walsh TS, Lee A. *N*-acetylcysteine administration in the critically ill. *Intensive Care Med.* 1999;25:432-434.

162. Waring WS, et al. Lower incidence of anaphylactoid reactions to *N*-acetylcysteine in patients with high acetaminophen concentrations after overdose. *Clin Toxicol (Phila).* 2008;46:496-500.

163. Wasserman GS, Garg U. Intravenous administration of *N*-acetylcysteine: interference with coagulopathy testing. *Ann Emerg Med.* 2004;44:546-547.

164. Whyte IM, et al. Safety and efficacy of intravenous *N*-acetylcysteine for acetaminophen overdose: analysis of the Hunter Area Toxicology Service (HATS) database. *Curr Med Res Opin.* 2007;23:2359-2368.

165. Wiest DB, et al. Antenatal pharmacokinetics and placental transfer of *N*-acetylcysteine in chorioamnionitis for fetal neuroprotection. *J Pediatr.* 2014;165:672-677 e672.

166. Wolchok JD, et al. Phase I trial of high dose paracetamol and carmustine in patients with metastatic melanoma. *Melanoma Res.* 2003;13:189-196.

167. Wong A, Graudins A. Simplification of the standard three-bag intravenous acetylcysteine regimen for paracetamol poisoning results in a lower incidence of adverse drug reactions. *Clin Toxicol (Phila).* 2016;54:115-119.

168. Woo OF, et al. Shorter duration of oral *N*-acetylcysteine therapy for acute acetaminophen overdose. *Ann Emerg Med.* 2000;35:363-368.

169. Yang R, et al. Prolonged treatment with *N*-acetylcysteine delays liver recovery from acetaminophen hepatotoxicity. *Crit Care.* 2009;13:R55.

170. Yarema MC, et al. Comparison of the 20-hour intravenous and 72-hour oral acetylcysteine protocols for the treatment of acute acetaminophen poisoning. *Ann Emerg Med.* 2009;54:606-614.

171. Yeniocak S, et al. Acute severe respiratory distress secondary to misuse of an *N*-acetylcysteine effervescent tablet. *Am J Emerg Med.* 2010;28:842.e845-842.e846.

172. Yi J-H, et al. Early, transient increase in complexin I and complexin II in the cerebral cortex following traumatic brain injury is attenuated by *N*-acetylcysteine. *J Neurotrauma.* 2006;23:86-96.

173. Yip L, et al. Intravenous administration of oral *N*-acetylcysteine. *Crit Care Med.* 1998;26:40-43.

174. Yip L, Dart RC. A 20-hour treatment for acute acetaminophen overdose. *N Engl J Med.* 2003;348:2471-2472.

175. Zhou J, et al. Intravenous administration of stable-labeled *N*-acetylcysteine demonstrates an indirect mechanism for boosting glutathione and improving redox status. *J Pharm Sci.* 2015;104:2619-2626.

176. Zyoud SH, et al. Incidence of adverse drug reactions induced by *N*-acetylcysteine in patients with acetaminophen overdose. *Hum Exp Toxicol.* 2010;29:153-160.

COLCHICINE, PODOPHYLLIN, AND THE VINCA ALKALOIDS

Cynthia D. Santos and Capt. Joshua G. Schier

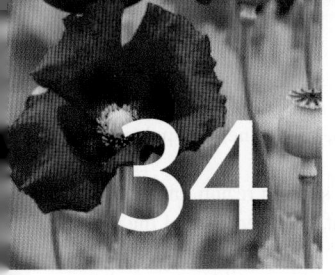

Colchicine

Podophyllotoxin

Vinblastine: R₁ = CH₃
Vincristine: R₁ = CHO

Colchicine, podophyllotoxin, and the vinca alkaloids exert their primary toxicity by binding to tubulin and interfering with microtubule structure and function. The ubiquitous nature of microtubules within human cells and the heavy reliance on them for maintenance of normal cell functions present numerous opportunities for these xenobiotics to cause dysfunction at a cellular, organ, and organ system level in a dose-dependent fashion. This chapter discusses the history, pharmacology, pharmacokinetics, toxicokinetics, pathophysiology, toxic dose, clinical manifestations, diagnostic testing and management of toxicity resulting from these xenobiotics both during therapeutic use and in the overdose setting. Because some information is limited, not all of the aforementioned topics will be discussed for each xenobiotic.

COLCHICINE

History

The origins of colchicine and its history in poisoning can be traced back to Greek mythology. Medea was the evil daughter (and a known poisoner) of the king of Colchis, a country that lay east of the Black Sea in Asia Minor. After being betrayed by her husband Jason (of Jason and the Argonauts), she killed their children and her husband's lover. Medea used plants of the Liliaceae family, of which *Colchicum autumnale* is a member, to poison her victims.[20,132,172] The use of colchicum for medicinal purposes is reported in *Pedanius Dioscorides De Materia Medica*, an ancient medical text, written in the first century A.D.,[132] and subsequently in the 6th century A.D. by Alexander of Tralles, who recommended it for treating arthritic conditions.[110] However, colchicum fell out of favor, perhaps because of its pronounced gastrointestinal (GI) effects, until it was introduced for "dropsy" and various other nonrheumatic conditions in 1763.[20,172] In the late 18th century, a colchicum-containing product known as *Eau Medicinale* appeared, which reportedly had strong antigout effects.[172] Colchicine, the active alkaloidal component in colchicum, was isolated in 1820 and rapidly became popular as an antigout medication.[132,172] Benjamin Franklin reportedly had gout and is credited with introducing colchicine in the United States.[132] Colchicine

is still used in the acute treatment and prevention of gout and is used in other disorders, including amyloidosis, Behçet's syndrome, familial Mediterranean fever, pericarditis, arthritis, pulmonary fibrosis, vasculitis, biliary cirrhosis, pseudogout, certain spondyloarthropathies, calcinosis, and scleroderma.[11,20,121,125] Systematic data supporting the efficacy of colchicine therapy in many of these other diseases are lacking.

Colchicine is derived from two plants of the Liliaceae family, *C. autumnale* (autumn crocus, meadow saffron, wild saffron, naked lady, son-before-the-father) and *Gloriosa superba* (glory lily).[172] The autumn crocus contains different amounts of colchicine by weight, depending on the plant part (bulb, 0.8%; flowers, 0.1%; seeds, 0.8%; and the corm or underground stem, 0.6%).[110,132,151] Colchicine concentrations within the plant peak during the summer months.[132] The leaves of *C. autumnale* closely resemble those of the *Allium ursinum* or wild garlic and are mistaken for them.[39,40,98] The tubers of *G. superba* were confused with *Ipomoea batatas* (sweet potatoes) in one report[172] (Chap. 118).

There is a dearth of good epidemiologic data on colchicine poisoning. The American Association of Poison Control Centers records several hundred overall exposures annually (Chap. 130). The majority of these exposures are in adults and are categorized as unintentional. Of the cases with a recorded outcome, approximately 10% have evidence of moderate or major toxicity or resulted in death.[36] A limited number of cases are caused by intentional suicidal ingestions with colchicine and therapeutic colchicine administration has contributed to adverse health effects, and in some cases death, among hospitalized patients (probably related to failure to adjust dosing for renal impairment).[147] At least 50 adverse events (23 of which were fatalities) were linked to the use of intravenous (IV) colchicine.[4] The United States Food and Drug Administration ordered companies to stop the marketing of unapproved injectable drug compounds containing colchicine in 2009.[4] Serious questions remain about the utility of colchicine in light of its extremely narrow therapeutic index.

Pharmacology

Colchicine is a potent inhibitor of microtubule formation and function that interferes with cellular mitosis, intracellular transport mechanisms, and maintenance of cell structure and shape.[125,172] The ubiquitous presence of microtubules in cells throughout the body presents a wide variety of targets for colchicine in poisoning.[125,172] Colchicine accumulates in leukocytes and has inhibitory effects on leukocyte adhesiveness, ameboid motility, mobilization, lysosome degranulation, and chemotaxis.[20,44,53,167] At doses used clinically, colchicine inhibits neutrophil and synovial cell release of chemotactic glycoproteins.[174,194] Colchicine also inhibits microtubule polymerization, which disrupts inflammatory cell-mediated chemotaxis and phagocytosis.[178] It reduces expression of adhesion molecules on endothelial and white blood cells (WBCs) and affects polymorphonuclear cell cytokine production.[9,21,144] Colchicine also acts as a competitive antagonist at GABA_A receptors.[216]

Pharmacokinetics and Toxicokinetics

Colchicine is rapidly absorbed in the jejunum and ileum and has a bioavailability generally between 25% and 50%.[172,182] It is highly lipid soluble[172] with a volume of distribution that ranges from 2.2 to 12 L/kg, and is reported to increase to 21 L/kg in overdose.[172,175,176,205] Colchicine binding to plasma proteins approaches 50%.[143,172] Protein binding is principally to albumin, although some binding to α₁-acid-glycoprotein and other lipoproteins is reported.[182] During the first several hours after acute overdose, colchicine is sequestered in white and red blood cells (RBCs) in concentrations 5 to 10 times higher than serum.[182] Peak serum concentrations after ingestion occur between 1 to 3 hours.[125] Toxic effects usually do not occur with concentrations less than 3 ng/mL.[79,143,212]

Colchicine is primarily metabolized through the liver with up to 20% of the ingested dose excreted unchanged in the urine.[108,172,205] Colchicine undergoes demethylation by CYP3A4.[108,125,157,203] Detoxification mainly occurs through deacetylation, demethylation, biliary secretion, and excretion in the stool.[108,125,141,180,182,203] Enterohepatic recirculation of colchicine occurs.[3,157,172]

Studies reporting on the serum colchicine elimination half-lives range from 9 to 108 minutes.[14,95,172,182,213] On closer examination, however, these times probably more accurately reflect a rapid initial distribution phase. The drug undergoes a more delayed terminal elimination phase, which ranges from 1.7 to 30 hours, depending on the individual compartment model used to estimate elimination and the amount of colchicine absorbed.[3,82,176,180,182,205] These values are on the same order as, and probably reflect the tubulin–colchicine complex disassociation time.[157] Individuals with end-stage kidney disease and liver cirrhosis have elimination half-lives that are prolonged up to 10-fold.[125] Colchicine remains in measurable quantities in certain tissues for a long time, as evidenced by its detection in WBCs after 10 days and in urine 7 to 10 days after exposure.[77,172] Colchicine crosses the placenta and is secreted in breast milk, but it is not dialyzable.[125] Postmortem examination of colchicine-poisoned patients reveals high concentrations within the bone marrow, testicles, spleen, kidney, lung, brain, and heart.[175]

Drug Interactions

Colchicine metabolism is susceptible to drug interactions. Because colchicine is detoxified by CYP3A4, blood concentrations are susceptible to xenobiotics that alter the function of this enzyme, such as erythromycin, clarithromycin, and grapefruit juice.[45,70,87,125] In particular, coadministration of clarithromycin and colchicine, especially in patients with chronic kidney disease, increases the risk of fatal interaction.[6,107] P-glycoprotein (P-gp) expels and clears colchicine, and drugs that inhibit P-gp directly affect the amount of colchicine eliminated and hence toxicity.[157] For example, cyclosporine increases colchicine toxicity.[75] Coadministration of colchicine with statin or fibrate drugs, cyclosporine, ketoconazole, ritonavir, verapamil ER, diltiazem ER, fluindione (vitamin K antagonist) and nephrotoxic xenobiotics such as nonsteroidal antiinflammatory drugs and angiotensin-converting enzyme inhibitors has resulted in colchicine poisoning.[204,208] Concomitant administration of P-gp or CYP3A4 inhibitors and colchicine should be avoided in patients with abnormal renal or hepatic function. If treatment with a P-gp or a strong CYP3A4 inhibitor is required in patients taking colchicine with normal renal or hepatic function, a dose reduction or temporary cessation of colchicine treatment should be considered.[5,204,208]

Pathophysiology

Microtubules play a vital role in cellular mitosis and possess a high amount of dynamic instability.[17,76,116,188] Microtubules are made up of tubulin protein subunits, of which three are known to exist: α, β, and γ.[116,139,188] These structures are highly dynamic with α-β tubulin heterodimers, constantly being added at one end and removed at the other.[116,117] Microtubules undergo two forms of dynamic behavior: dynamic instability, in which microtubule ends switch between growth and shortening phases, and treadmilling, in which there is a net growth (addition of heterodimers) at one end and a shortening (loss) at the other.[25] Assembly and polymerization dynamics are regulated by additional proteins known as stabilizing microtubule-associated proteins (MAPs) and destabilizing MAPs.[25] These dynamic behaviors and a resultant equilibrium are needed for multiple cell functions, including cell support, transport, and mitotic spindle formation for cell replication.[116] Xenobiotics that bind to specific regions on tubulin can interfere with microtubule structure and function, thereby possibly causing mitotic dysfunction and arrest.[139,188] This leads to cellular dysfunction and death.[188] Xenobiotics that target microtubules can be generally divided into two categories:

polymerization inhibitors (ie, vinca alkaloids, colchicine) and polymerization promoters (ie, taxanes, laulimalides).[25]

Colchicine binds to a tubulin dimer at a specific region known as the *colchicine-binding domain*, which is located at the interphase of the α and β subunits of the tubulin heterodimer.[25,99] This binding is relatively slow, temperature dependent, and generally irreversible, resulting in an alteration of the protein's secondary structure.[99,116,131] Colchicine binds at a second reversible but lower affinity site on tubulin.[116,131] Current evidence suggests that the colchicine–tubulin complex binds to the microtubule ends and prevents further growth by sterically blocking further addition of dimers.[25] Conformational changes in the tubulin and colchicine complex also result as colchicine concentrations increase, which weakens the lateral bonds at the microtubule end.[25,175] Lateral and longitudinal interactions between dimers within a microtubule help stabilize the structure. The number of colchicine–tubulin dimers incorporated into the microtubule determines the stability of the microtubule ends.[25] All of these processes prevent adequate binding of the next tubulin subunit and result in cessation of microtubule growth.[139,188] Whereas at low concentrations, colchicine arrests microtubule growth, at high concentrations, colchicine actually causes microtubule depolymerization through disassociation of tubulin dimers.[25]

These conformational changes ultimately result in disassembly of the microtubule spindle in metaphase of cellular mitosis, cellular dysfunction, and death.[81,99,116,163,183] The effects of colchicine are dose dependent, with high concentrations inhibiting further microtubule polymerization, as well as inducing depolymerization of already formed microtubules.[128] Low concentrations can simply affect new microtubule formation and have no effect on preestablished polymer mass.[128] Colchicine also inhibits microtubule-mediated intracellular granule transport.[20,125]

Toxic Dose

The toxic dose for colchicine is not well established. An early case series suggested that patients with ingestions of greater than 0.8 mg/kg uniformly died and those with ingestions above 0.5 mg/kg but less than 0.8 mg/kg would survive if given supportive care.[28] This information was based on a limited series of patients and is not necessarily generalizable.[148] More recent literature suggests that severe toxicity and even death occurs with doses smaller than 0.5 mg/kg, and conversely, some patients survive ingestions reported to be in excess of 0.8 mg/kg.[71,145,148] This inability to accurately quantify the toxic dose in humans is likely due in great part to difficulty in dose estimation from the patient's history and significant advances in supportive care. Furthermore, many comorbid conditions (eg, kidney disease) and other pharmaceuticals, which when coadministered can enhance colchicine's adverse health effects; this complicates the determination of a minimal toxic dose.

Clinical Presentation

The clinical findings among colchicine poisoned patients are commonly described as triphasic (Table 34–1).[103] GI irritant effects, such as nausea, vomiting, abdominal distress, and diarrhea, occur within several hours after an overdose[38,69] and lead to severe volume depletion.[106,148,150] This first stage usually persists for 12 to 24 hours after ingestion.[106,136] The second stage is characterized by widespread organ system dysfunction, particularly the bone marrow, and lasts for several days.[71,148,150] The final phase is characterized by recovery or death, and the progression is usually defined within 1 week.[103,106]

After overdose, the hematopoietic effects of colchicine are characterized by an initial peripheral leukocytosis, which is often as high as 30,000/mm³. This is followed by a profound leukopenia, which is classically lower than 1,000/mm³. It is commonly accompanied by pancytopenia, usually beginning 48 to 72 hours after overdose.[82,153] The hematopoietic manifestations occur as a result of colchicine's effects on bone marrow cell division.[138,215] A rebound leukocytosis and recovery of all cell lines occur if the patient survives.

Colchicine toxicity is associated with the development of dysrhythmias and cardiac arrest.[84,103] Complete AV block occurred in a child who ingested 0.4 to 0.5 mg/kg.[78] In a rabbit model, colchicine results in a dose–dependent reduction in effective refractory period while maintaining a stable

Phase	Timeᵃ	Signs and Symptoms	Therapy or Follow-Up
TABLE 34–1		**Colchicine Poisoning: Common Clinical Findings, Timing of Onset, and Treatment**	
I	0–24 h	Nausea, vomiting, diarrhea	Antiemetics
			GI decontamination for early presentation
		Salt and water depletion	IV fluids
		Leukocytosis	Close observation for leukopenia for 24 h
II	1–7 days	Risk of sudden cardiac death (24–48 h)	ICU admission and appropriate resuscitation
		Pancytopenia	G-CSF
		Acute kidney injury	Hemodialysis
		Sepsis	Antibiotics
		ARDS	Oxygen, mechanical ventilation
		Electrolyte imbalances	Repletion as needed
		Rhabdomyolysis	IV fluids, hemodialysis
III	>7 days	Alopecia (sometimes delayed 2–3 wk)	Follow-up within 1–2 mo
		Myopathy, neuropathy, or myoneuropathy	EMG testing, biopsy, and neurologic follow-up as needed

ᵃThe interval time course is not absolute, and overlap of symptom presentations occurs.

ARDS = acute respiratory distress syndrome; EMG = electromyography; G-CSF = granulocyte-colony stimulating factor; GI = gastrointestinal; ICU = intensive care unit; IV = intravenous.

repolarization period and increased inducibility of ventricular fibrillation.[84] Sudden cardiovascular collapse from colchicine typically occurs between 24 to 36 hours after ingestion.[138,148] Profound hypovolemia and shock contribute to this collapse,[148] but colchicine has direct toxic effects on skeletal and cardiac muscle, causing rhabdomyolysis.[31,149,210]

Myopathy,[220] neuropathy,[12,128] and a combined myoneuropathy[10,55,124,193] result from both long-term therapy and acute poisoning.[128] A combined myoneuropathy is reported more often, with myopathy dominating the clinical picture.[124] The myoneuropathy is often initially misdiagnosed as polymyositis or uremic neuropathy (caused by coexistent acute or chronic kidney disease).[124] Myoneuropathy usually develops in the context of chronic, therapeutic dosing in patients with some baseline renal impairment,[124] although it is reported to occur in the presence of normal renal function as well.[170] Patients present with proximal limb weakness, distal sensory abnormalities, distal areflexia, and nerve conduction problems consistent with an axonal neuropathy.[124,165] A small amount of myelin degeneration is reported on autopsy, which suggests a myelinopathic component.[37] The myopathy is characterized by vacuolar changes on biopsy and accompanied by lysosome accumulation.[10,74,124,226] Elevated serum creatine kinase activity is present concurrently with symptoms.[124,150] Weakness usually resolves within several weeks of drug discontinuation.[124] Myopathy has also occurred with concomitant use of hydroxymethylglutaryl–coenzyme A reductase inhibitors (statins) in patients with chronic kidney disease.[7] Myopathy symptoms typically resolve within 4 to 6 weeks, or in some patients, up to 6 to 8 months.[220]

Acute respiratory distress syndrome (ARDS) occurs with colchicine toxicity.[102,141] The cause is not well understood but probably results from several factors, including respiratory muscle weakness, multisystem organ failure, and possibly direct pulmonary toxicity.[61,136,141,187,202] Other indirect effects of colchicine include acute kidney injury and various electrolyte abnormalities.[128]

Alopecia, which is usually reversible, is a well-described complication that occurs 2 to 3 weeks after poisoning in survivors.[82,131] Dermatologic complications range in severity from epithelial cell atypia to toxic epidermal necrolysis.[81,179]

Neurologic effects, including delirium, stupor, coma, delayed encephalopathy, and seizures, are reported in colchicine poisoning.[88,153,216]

Other reported complications of colchicine poisoning include bilateral adrenal hemorrhage,[199] disseminated intravascular coagulation,[189] pancreatitis,[207] and liver dysfunction.[150]

Although uncommon, poisoning from IV colchicine administration has occurred. Clinical and laboratory manifestations are similar to those that occur after oral overdose, including multisystem organ dysfunction and cytopenias.[47]

Colchicine does not appear to be a significant human teratogen, but the limited work on this subject is not definitive.[65]

Testing

Colchicine concentrations in body fluids are not available in a clinically relevant fashion and have no well-established correlation with severity of illness. However, effective steady-state serum concentrations for treatment of patients with various illnesses are reported as 0.5 to 3.0 ng/mL.[143] Concentrations greater than 3.0 ng/mL are associated with toxicity depending on the clinical situation, and concentrations greater than 24 ng/mL are definitely associated with poisoning.[79,143,212,222] Serum concentrations do not correlate well with the amount of xenobiotic ingested in massive oral overdose settings.[64] Initial laboratory monitoring should include a complete blood count (CBC), serum electrolytes, renal and liver function tests, creatine kinase, phosphate, calcium, magnesium, prothrombin time, activated partial thromboplastin time, and urinalysis. Other laboratory studies, such as a troponin, arterial blood gases, lactate, fibrinogen, and fibrin split products, are helpful in guiding care if cardiotoxicity, ARDS, or coagulopathies, respectively, are present. If cardiotoxicity is present or suspected, serial troponin concentrations (every 6–12 hours) are recommended. There is an association between increasing concentrations and cardiovascular collapse.[85,210] An electrocardiogram and chest radiograph should also be obtained. Serial CBCs are reasonable (at least every 12 hours) to evaluate for the development of depression in cell lines. Bile appears to be the biological matrix of choice for postmortem testing, probably because of normal postmortem biological processes that can increase blood colchicine concentration.[23,152] One colchicine-associated fatality who had a premortem blood colchicine concentration of 50 ng/mL also had a postmortem femoral blood concentration of 137 ng/mL and a bile concentration greater than 600 ng/mL.[222] Another reported a postmortem blood concentration of 60 ng/mL.[2] Two IV colchicine-associated fatalities had postmortem blood colchicine concentrations of 32 and 44 ng/mL.[47]

Management

Treatment for patients with colchicine toxicity is mainly supportive, which includes IV fluid replacement, vasopressor use, hemodialysis (for acute kidney injury, not for toxin removal), antibiotics for suspected secondary infection, colony-stimulating factors, and adjunctive respiratory therapy (endotracheal intubation, positive end-expiratory pressure) as indicated. Consultation with nephrology and hematology specialists should be obtained in the case of impaired renal function or evidence of hematologic toxicity. In severe, refractory poisoning, it is reasonable to attempt options such as intraaortic balloon pump therapy and extracorporeal membrane oxygenation therapy.[160]

Because most patients with an acute oral colchicine overdose present several hours after their ingestion, vomiting has already begun, and the utility of GI decontamination is inadequately defined. However, given the extensive morbidity and mortality associated with colchicine overdose, orogastric lavage is most helpful and is reasonable in patients presenting within 1 to 2 hours of potentially life-threatening ingestions, who have no contraindications, are not already vomiting, and for which the physician is proficient in the procedure.[1,30,209] A dose of activated charcoal (AC) is recommended after lavage or in its place if lavage is not appropriate or possible. Because limited evidence supports that colchicine undergoes some enterohepatic recirculation, administration of a single dose of AC to a patient presenting to a health care facility beyond 2 hours after ingestion is recommended if no contraindications exist. Multiple-dose activated charcoal (MDAC) is also recommended in these patients as well for the same reason in that the absorption of colchicine is one of the most beneficial interventions for this exceptionally grave poisoning.[3,172] The delay in presentation to a health care facility coupled with the fact that patients often have GI symptoms such as vomiting significantly complicates using MDAC. Antiemetic medications will control emesis and facilitate AC administration.

Experimental colchicine-specific antibodies can restore colchicine-affected tubulin activity in animal models of colchicine poisoning[166] and was successfully used in a single human case of severe colchicine poisoning.[16] In colchicine-poisoned rats, anticolchicine Fab fragments caused a rapid 7.1-fold increase in serum colchicine concentration followed by increased urinary excretion of both colchicine and Fab anticolchicine. The increased urinary excretion of these fragments was associated with reversal of colchicine-induced diarrhea.[16,166] In the single human case report, administration of anticolchicine Fab fragments 40 hours after a 0.96-mg/kg colchicine ingestion was temporally associated with a dramatic improvement in clinical and hemodynamic status. This improvement was also associated with a significant increase in serum colchicine concentrations, which suggests a redistribution of drug into the intravascular space.[16] Unfortunately, this therapy is not commercially available.

Granulocyte-colony stimulating factor (G-CSF) is useful in the treatment of patients with colchicine-induced leukopenia and thrombocytopenia.[59,97,119,225] The dose of G-CSF, the dosing frequency, and the route of administration were variable in the reported cases.[59,97,119,225] Administration of G-CSF is recommended if the patient begins to manifest evidence of leukopenia. Dosing should be in accordance with the manufacturer's instructions.

Hemodialysis and hemoperfusion are not viable options for patients with colchicine poisoning based on its large volume of distribution, but hemodialysis is required if renal failure is present.[19,26,27,175,176,205,215] The use of whole-blood and plasma exchange for patients presenting with lethal-dose colchicine exposures was tried, but evidence of efficacy is lacking, and it is not recommended for routine care.[160]

Because of the significant morbidity and mortality associated with colchicine toxicity, all symptomatic patients with suspected or known overdoses should be admitted to the hospital for observation. Because these patients have a risk of sudden cardiovascular collapse within the first 24 to 48 hours,[148] intensive care unit monitoring is recommended for at least this initial time period. A troponin concentration is recommended every 6 to 12 hours during this period because increasing results suggest an increased risk of cardiotoxicity and cardiovascular collapse.[85,210] Blood cell counts should be followed at least daily to watch for cytopenias. Poisoned patients manifest GI signs and symptoms within several hours of ingestion and should be observed for at least 8 to 12 hours. Patients who do not manifest GI signs and symptoms within that time period after ingestion are unlikely to be significantly poisoned.

PODOPHYLLUM RESIN OR PODOPHYLLIN

History

Podophyllin is the name often used to refer to a resin extract from the rhizomes and roots of certain plants of the genus *Podophyllum*.[63,91] Examples include the North American perennial *Podophyllum peltatum* (mayapple or mandrake), the related Indian species *Podophyllum emodi*, and the Taiwanese *Podophyllum pleianthum*[63] (Chap. 118). It is more descriptive to refer to it as podophyllum resin.[63,91] Podophyllum resin, or podophyllin, contains at least 16 active compounds.[49,63,91] These include a variety of lignins and flavonols, including podophyllotoxin, picropodophyllin, α- and β-pellatins, desoxypodophyllotoxin, and quercetin.[46,49,63,91] Podophyllotoxin, a component of podophyllin, is a potent microtubular poison, similar to colchicine, and causes similar effects in overdose.[63]

The first reported modern era medicinal use of podophyllin preparations was as a laxative in the 19th century.[46,49,168] Its cathartic properties, as well as its potential toxicity, were noted as early as 1890, when the first fatality from podophyllin was recorded.[190,219] Podophyllin was used to treat individuals with a variety of other health issues, including liver disease, scrofula, syphilis, warts, and cancer.[63] Etoposide and teniposide are semisynthetic derivatives of podophyllotoxin used as chemotherapeutics.[63]

Poisoning usually is caused by systemic absorption after topical application, after ingestion of the resin or plant, and after consumption of a commercial preparation of the extract. Systemic toxicity is described after unintentional dispensing of the incorrect herb, as well as after ingestion of herbal preparations containing podophyllin.[50,51,68]

Pharmacology

Podophyllin is primarily used in modern pharmacopeia as a topical treatment for patients with verruca vulgaris and condyloma acuminatum.[46,127] The active ingredient is believed to be podophyllotoxin.[63,201] Podophyllotoxin exists in the plant as a β-D-glucoside.[190] Numerous synthetic and semisynthetic derivatives of podophyllotoxin exist; however, the most important are probably the chemotherapeutics etoposide and teniopside.[63] The antitumor effect of etoposide and teniposide results from their interaction with topoisomerase II and free radical production, leading to DNA strand breakage, an effect not shared by podophyllin and colchicine.[43,63] Use of etoposide and teniposide leads to a cessation of cell growth in the late S or early G2 phase of the cell cycle.[43,63,86] Further discussion of these xenobiotics can be found in the Chap. 50.

Pharmacokinetics and Toxicokinetics

Very limited information exists regarding the pharmacokinetics (absorption, distribution, metabolism, and elimination) of podophyllin as a preparation or for its major active ingredient, podophyllotoxin. Podophyllotoxin is highly lipid soluble and easily crosses cell membranes.[89,156,190]

Absorption of podophyllotoxin was measured in seven men after application of various amounts of a 0.5% ethanol podophyllotoxin preparation for condylomata acuminata.[211] Peak serum concentrations of 1 to 17 ng/mL were achieved within 1 to 2 hours after topical administration of doses ranging from 0.1 to 1.5 mL (0.5–7.5 mg).[211] Patients treated with less than or equal to 0.05 mL had no detectable podophyllotoxin in their serum. Topical administration of 0.1 mL yielded peak serum concentrations up to 5 ng/mL within 1 to 2 hours and up to 3 ng/mL at 4 hours. Topical administration of 1.5 mL yielded peak serum concentrations ranging from 5 to 9 ng/mL within 1 to 2 hours, concentrations of 5 to 7 ng/mL at 4 hours, 3 to 4.5 ng/mL at 8 hours, and 3.5 ng/mL at 12 hours.[211]

Pathophysiology

The components of podophyllin have numerous actions within the cell, including inhibition of purine synthesis, inhibition of purine incorporation into RNA, reduction of cytochrome oxidase and succinoxidase activity, and inhibition of microtubule structure and function.[46,86,214] Podophyllotoxin causes its toxicity similar to colchicine[63,221] because it is able to bind to tubulin subunits and interfere with subsequent microtubule structure and function.[63,221] Interestingly, radiolabeled podophyllotoxin inhibits colchicine binding to tubulin, suggesting that their binding sites overlap.[63] Podophyllotoxin binds more rapidly than colchicine, and binding is reversible in contrast to colchicine.[63] Podophyllotoxin also inhibits fast axoplasmic transport similar to colchicine by interference with microtubule structure and function.[165,208] Many other compounds, such as the vinca alkaloids, cryptophycins, and halichondrins, also inhibit microtubule polymerization in a similar manner.[117]

Toxic Dose

The minimum toxic dose associated with podophyllin ingestion is unknown. Limited information on the situations surrounding the few case reports of podophyllin poisoning that do exist does not provide sufficient detail from which to estimate it.

Clinical Presentation

Poisoning is described after ingestion,[42] as well as after absorption from topical application of podophyllin.[137,142] Toxicity also is reported after IV administration of podophyllotoxin[94] and ingestion of mandrake root or herbal remedies containing podophyllin.[68,83,219] Nausea, vomiting, abdominal pain, and diarrhea usually begin within several hours after ingestion.[137,142,196] Symptoms of poisoning is often delayed for 12 hours or more after topical exposure to podophyllin and are typically caused by improper usage (excessive topical exposure, interruption in skin integrity, or failure to remove the preparation after a short time period).[137,140,190] Initial clinical findings are not necessarily dictated by the route of exposure.[137]

Alterations in central and peripheral nervous system function tend to predominate in podophyllin toxicity. Patients present with confusion, obtundation, or coma.[56,68,142,196,201] Permanent encephalopathy and cerebral atrophy occurred in some cases.[123]

Delirium and both auditory and visual hallucinations have occurred during the initial presentation.[57,80,198] Patients developed paresthesias, lost deep tendon reflexes, and developed a Babinski sign.[52,68,158,190] Cranial nerve involvement, including diploplia,[49] nystagmus,[56] dysmetria,[52] dysconjugate gaze,[198] and facial nerve paralysis,[57] are all reported. Patients who recover from the initial event are at risk of developing a peripheral sensorimotor axonopathy.[52,56,190] The reported duration for recovery from podophyllin-induced axonopathy is variable but is likely to take several months.[56,68,142,156] Dorsal radiculopathy[89] and autonomic neuropathy are reported.[127] A myelopathic component in the neuropathy is reported.[51]

Hematologic toxicity from podophyllin most likely results from its antimitotic effects. A review of the limited literature suggests that it is similar to colchicine but is not nearly as consistent in its pattern, severity, and frequency. An initial leukocytosis[173,190] commonly occurs after poisoning, which is followed by leukopenia, thrombocytopenia, or generalized pancytopenia.[127,190] In patients who recover, cell lines tend to reach their nadir within 4 to 7 days after exposure.[173,196]

Other complications of poisoning include fever,[140] ileus,[80,140,198] elevated liver function test results,[196] hyperbilirubinemia,[104] coagulopathy,[104] seizures,[57,181] and acute kidney injury.[140,218] Teratogenic effects resulting from exposure during pregnancy are reported.[49,118]

Testing

Podophyllin or podophyllotoxin concentrations are not readily available. Routine testing for suspected or known podophyllin poisoning should include routine laboratory tests and other targeted testing as needed. Serial cell blood counts should be obtained in cases of poisoning to evaluate for pancytopenia.

Management

Management primarily consists of supportive and symptomatic care. If the patient presents within the first several hours of ingestion, a dose of AC is reasonable. Any topically applied podophyllin should be removed and the area thoroughly cleansed. Patients either progress to multisystem organ dysfunction and death or recover with supportive care. Blood cell counts should be monitored similarly to colchicine poisoning (at least daily).

A few case reports of treatment with extracorporeal elimination techniques exist. These reports include resin hemoperfusion[101] and charcoal hemperfusion.[142,190] The role these procedures played in the patients' clinical courses is unclear. As a result, given the lack of evidence and potential risk, they cannot be routinely recommended at this time.

Patients with significant ingestions of podophyllin develop GI symptoms within a few hours,[52,83,104,158,218,219] but patients have also presented with primarily neurologic symptoms, such as confusion or obtundation.[42,46,80,137] The onset of toxicity is reported to be delayed as long as 12 hours after ingestion.[42,46,56,68] Dermal exposure results in even further delayed onset of toxicity because systemic absorption is delayed and symptom onset is more insidious.[173,190,198] Patients should therefore be observed for the onset of toxicity for at least 12 hours after ingestion and at least 24 hours after dermal exposures. We recommended that asymptomatic patients with unintentional exposures and good follow-up who are discharged after 12 to 24 hours have scheduled follow-up with a primary care physician and a repeat cell blood count within 24 hours.

VINCRISTINE AND VINBLASTINE
History

More than 150 different alkaloidal compounds have been isolated from the periwinkle plant (*Catharanthus roseus*), most of which were used throughout history to manage illness from a variety of medical disorders, including cancer, scurvy, diabetes, toothache, and hypertension.[223] Among these 150 are about 20 different compounds that have antineoplastic activity. Vincristine and vinblastine are pharmaceuticals derived from compounds in the periwinkle plant and are among the most commonly used vinca alkaloid derivatives in medicine.[171] They are typically used as part of a chemotherapy regimen for various cancers. The two chemotherapeutics are administered intravenously and should never be administered intrathecally. Intrathecal administration of vinblastine or vincristine is always the result of an error, is a neurosurgical emergency, and is associated with life-threatening complications (Special Considerations: SC7 and SC8).[8] There are a few case reports of intramuscular administration of these antineoplastics, but they will not be discussed because there are so few, and readers are referred to the actual publications for further information.[15,164] Although other vinca derivatives exist, some have oral formulations and share similar modes of action (causing microtubule dysfunction); however, this section focuses primarily on vincristine and vinblastine. Regardless, the pathophysiology of disease, clinical manifestations of illness, and management of poisoning from similar compounds and the plant itself[223] are similar to those of vincristine and vinblastine.

Pathophysiology

Vincristine and vinblastine are used specifically for the treatment of patients with leukemias, lymphomas, and certain solid tumors. Their mechanism of activity is similar to the mechanisms of activity of colchicine, podophyllotoxin, and the taxoids (eg, paclitaxel, docetaxel).[62,161] These chemotherapeutics disrupt microtubule assembly from tubulin subunits by either preventing their formation or depolymerization, both of which are necessary for routine cell maintenance. Vinblastine binds to the β-subunit of the tubulin heterodimer at a specific region known as the *vinblastine binding site*.[163] Microtubules are responsible for several basic cellular functions, including cell division, axonal transport of nutrients and organelles, and cellular movement. Mitotic metaphase arrest is commonly observed because of the inability to form spindle fibers from the microtubules. Cell death quickly ensues as a result of the interruption of these homeostatic functions, accounting for the clinical manifestations.

The mechanism of neurotoxicity is not well understood but is related to inhibition of microtubular synthesis, which leads to axonal degeneration in the peripheral nervous system.[90,159] A brain biopsy of a patient with a vincristine-related death showed neurotubular dissociation, which is characteristic of vincristine damage in experimental animals.[32,34,54,66]

A single study demonstrated in mice poisoned with a vinca derivative that administration of murine monoclonal antibodies active against vinca alkaloids is protective and significantly improved survival.[93]

Genetic polymorphisms are associated with the development of vincristine-associated neuropathy. A mutation in the *CEP72* gene,[66] which encodes for a protein involved in microtubule formation, and reduced expression of the genes that encode for CYP3A5 are associated with vincristine-induced peripheral neuropathy.[32]

Pharmacokinetics

After IV administration, vincristine is rapidly distributed to tissue stores and highly bound to proteins and RBCs.[41] The capacity of vincristine to be bound by plasma proteins ranges from 50% to 80%.[169] In more than 50% of children given IV vincristine, serum concentrations were not detected 4 hours after administration.[146] The vinca alkaloids are primarily eliminated through the liver. Patients with hepatic dysfunction are susceptible to toxicity. Elimination of vincristine occurs via the hepatobiliary system,[41] and it has a terminal plasma half-life of about 24 hours.[155] Vincristine overdose is the most frequently reported antineoplastic overdose in the literature. This is because there are at least four different potential inappropriate ways to dose and administer vincristine, including confusing it with vinblastine, misinterpreting the dose, administering it by the wrong route, and confusing two different-strength vials. The normal dose of vincristine is 0.06 mg/kg, and a single dose should not exceed 2 mg for either an adult or child.

Drug Interactions

Administration of itraconazole with therapeutic doses of intravenously administered vincristine cause toxicity because of at least two primary reasons: (1) itraconazole-induced inhibition of certain cytochrome P450 enzymes (most likely the CYP3A subfamily) delays vincristine metabolism in vivo, and (2) inhibition of P-gp–mediated efflux of vincristine from inside cells, where it then accumulates.[13] Coadministration of other azole antifungals, cyclosporine, isoniazid, erythromycin, mitomycin C, phenytoin, and nifedipine are also implicated in vincristine toxicity for the same aforementioned reasons.[67,185,186] Azole antifungals exacerbate vinblastine-related hyponatremia in children.[228]

Toxic Dose

The minimum toxic doses associated with adverse health effects from a single dose of vincristine and vinblastine are not well established. However, chemotherapeutic regimens tend to keep single doses at or below 2 mg to decrease the likelihood of peripheral neuropathy. Unfortunately, toxicity occurs with cumulative dosing over time, as that typically occurs with chemotherapeutic regimens. Peripheral neuropathy tends to begin after a cumulative dose (administered over multiple sessions, not all at once) of 30 to 40 mg.[24]

Clinical Presentation

Despite their similarity in structure, vincristine and vinblastine differ in their clinical toxicity. Vincristine produces less bone marrow suppression and more neurotoxicity than does vinblastine. During the therapeutic use of vincristine, myelosuppression occurs in only 5% to 10% of patients.[105] However, this effect is common in the overdose setting, and when it occurs, the need for replacement blood products and concern for overwhelming infection is apparent.[130] The decrease in cell counts begins within the first week and lasts for up to 3 weeks. Other manifestations of acute vincristine toxicity are mucositis, central nervous system disorders, and syndrome of inappropriate antidiuretic hormone (SIADH).

Central nervous system disorders are varied and unusual during therapeutic vincristine therapy because of its poor penetrance of the blood–brain barrier. They are, however, more common when there is delayed elimination, damage to the blood brain–barrier, overdose, or inadvertent intrathecal administration. Generalized seizures from toxicity or secondary effects generally occur from 1 to 7 days after exposure.[109,115,120,197] Other manifestations are depression, agitation, insomnia, and hallucinations. Vincristine stimulation of the hypothalamus appears to be responsible for the fevers and SIADH noted in overdosed patients.[177] The fevers begin 24 hours after exposure and last 6 to 96 hours. Serum electrolytes need to be monitored, typically for 10 days.

Autonomic dysfunction is observed, and it commonly includes ileus, constipation, and abdominal pain. Paraparesis, paraplegia, atony of the bladder, cranial nerve palsies (specifically ptosis) hypertension, and hypotension also occur.[67,73,120,227]

Ascending peripheral neuropathies occur after inadvertent large ingestions and during routine chemotherapy. The risk is limited somewhat by keeping the total for a single dose below 2 mg.[191] Neuropathy appears after an overdose, starting at about 2 weeks and lasting for 6 to 7 weeks. Paresthesias, neuritic pain, ataxia, bone pain, wrist drop, foot drop, involvement of cranial nerves III to VII and X, and diminished reflexes are observed.[217] Cranial nerve III involvement, manifesting as bilateral ptosis, was reported in several cases of vincristine toxicity in children.[100,162] The incidence of paresthesia increases with dose and is reported to be 56% in patients treated at doses between 12.5 and 25 mcg/kg.[105] At a dose of 75 mcg/kg, the incidence of patients with a sensory disorder increased by sixfold. The loss of reflexes, the earliest and most consistent sign of vincristine neuropathy, is maximal at 17 days after a single massive dose. Muscular weakness is a limiting point in therapy and typically involves the distal dorsiflexors of the extremities, although laryngeal involvement is also reported.[126,184] These severe neurologic symptoms may be reversed by either withholding therapy or reducing the dosage upon manifestation of these findings.[126] Unlike the vinca alkaloids, Taxol-induced

peripheral neuropathy is predominantly sensory and resolves faster with discontinuation.[129] This is because of the different effects on microtubule assembly by these xenobiotics.

Vincristine-induced myocardial infarctions are reported, but their cause is not understood.[134,192,200,224] Although rare, vincristine administration is associated with an allergic-type cutaneous reaction.[154]

Testing

Vincristine and vinblastine testing is not readily available at most hospitals. Organ-specific toxicity is evaluated through the use of routinely available laboratory tests (eg, cell blood count, electrolytes, renal and liver function tests).

Management

Generalized seizures are a life-threatening complication of vincristine or vinblastine overdose. Treatment with benzodiazepines is usually successful and is the recommended front-line antiepileptic intervention, although phenytoin was used successfully in a patient with barbiturate hypersensitivity.[120] Prophylactic phenobarbital and benzodiazepines were used to prevent seizures in two patients.[48,122] Supportive and symptomatic care is recommended for organ specific toxicity as needed.[48] Monitoring daily blood counts is recommended daily, and G-CSF is used to treat neutropenia.[48,130,197] Of note is that the RBC response from the use of erythropoietin is limited because of the induction of metaphase arrest in the erythroblasts.[135]

The symptoms of acute toxicity usually last for 3 to 7 days, and the neurologic sequelae lasts for months. Nerve conduction studies are helpful in assessing the extent of any clinical signs and symptoms of peripheral neuropathy.

Clinical findings of a peripheral neuropathy appears after an excessive dose or after multiple small doses in which the cumulative dose exceeds 30 to 40 mg.[24] Treatment for this condition is variable and includes pain and paresthesia management, including opioids, nonsteroidal antiinflammatory drugs, tricyclic antidepressants, vitamin E, gabapentin, and lamotrigine.[24] In a controlled clinical trial for vincristine-induced peripheral neuropathy, glutamic acid therapy had limited efficacy. Patients receiving vincristine therapy were given glutamic acid as 500 mg orally 3 times a day.[113] There was a decreased incidence in loss of the Achilles tendon reflex and a delayed onset of paresthesias in the glutamic acid–treated group. No reported adverse effects with glutamic acid were observed in this investigation. Animal studies involving the administration of glutamic and aspartic acid to mice poisoned with either vinblastine or vincristine demonstrate increased survival and decreased sensorimotor peripheral neuropathy.[33,60,112] The mechanisms of these observed effects with glutamic acid remain unclear, but several authors have suggested the ability of glutamic acid to competitively inhibit a common cellular transport mechanism for vincristine,[29,58] its ability to assist in the stabilization of tubulin and promote its polymerization into microtubules,[35,96] and the ability of glutamic acid to improve cellular metabolism by overcoming the inhibition in the tricarboxylic acid cycle.[72,114] Although the role of glutamic acid in acute toxicity needs further study, it is not harmful and is reasonable to try in this setting. Glutamic acid is given as 500 mg orally three times a day and continued until the serum vincristine concentration is below toxicity.[113] L-Glutamic acid is the preferred stereoisomer because it is biologically active, and this product is available as a powder from various distributors in the United States. Case reports document success in treating bilateral ptosis with combinations of pyridoxine and pyridostigmine[162] or pyridoxine and thiamine.[100] These therapies are also reasonable to institute.

Leucovorin shortens the course of vincristine-induced peripheral neuropathy[92] and myelosuppression.[122] The mechanism is attributed to the ability of leucovorin to overcome a vincristine-mediated block of dihydrofolate reductase and thymidine synthetase (Antidotes in Depth: A12).[92] However, neither leucovorin[18,111,206] nor pyridoxine[111] was definitely shown to be effective. Therefore, there is insufficient evidence from which to make a recommendation regarding its use as a therapy at this time. An initial experimental investigation evaluating the efficacy of antibody therapy to limit vinca alkaloid toxicity shows promise.[93] Unfortunately, vinca alkaloid specific antibodies for human poisoning are not commercially available.

The rapid distribution and high protein binding characteristics of vincristine favor early intervention and methods other than hemodialysis. Double-volume exchange transfusion was performed at 6 hours postexposure in three children who were overdosed with 7.5 mg/m² of IV vincristine.[122] This procedure replaced approximately 90% of the circulating blood volume by exchanging twice the patient's blood volume. Of the two survivors, their respective postexchange serum vincristine concentrations were 57% and 71% lower than their preexchange concentrations. The amount of vincristine removed was not determined. Although these patients developed peripheral neuropathies, myelosuppression, and autonomic instability, the author noted that the duration of illness was shorter than previously reported. Thus, based on the pharmacokinetic profile of vincristine and these two reports, exchange transfusion in children is the preferred method of enhanced elimination when the patient presents soon after the administration of the drug, and plasmapheresis is the preferred method in adults.

Plasmapheresis was attempted with vinca alkaloid overdoses.[130,169] In an 18-year-old patient who received two 8-mg IV doses of vincristine at 12-hour intervals, the procedure was performed 6 hours after the second dose, and 1.5 times the plasma volume was plasmapheresed.[169] Postplasmapheresis serum vincristine concentration was 23% lower than the starting concentration. The patient survived with myelosuppression, neurotoxicity, and SIADH.

One case of IV vinblastine overdose was reported to be successfully managed with plasma exchange procedures performed at 4 hours and 18 hours after vinblastine administration, resulting in markedly less toxicity than what was expected.[195]

Patients receiving an overdose of vincristine intravenously should be admitted to a cardiac-monitored bed and observed for 24 to 72 hours.[133] If patients remain asymptomatic during the observation period, they can be discharged with follow-up for bone marrow suppression and SIADH; otherwise, depending on the patient's clinical condition, continual observation for progression of neurologic symptoms is warranted.[22]

SUMMARY

- Colchicine toxicity is evident several hours after ingestion and consists of severe nausea, vomiting, diarrhea, and abdominal pain followed by pancytopenia several days later. Colchicine-poisoned patients have a higher risk of sudden cardiac death, especially during the period between 24 and 36 hours after ingestion; increasing serial troponin concentrations in these patients suggest a higher risk of cardiovascular complications. Podophyllum toxicity is less pronounced compared with colchicine and occurs after dermal application (Table 34–2).
- Early GI decontamination and supportive treatment are the hallmarks of therapy for all colchicine and podophyllin exposure because there are no commercially available and proven antidotes.
- Excessive doses of intravenously administered vincristine or vinblastine cause severe toxicity and are managed with supportive and symptomatic care as well.
- Although definitive data confirming clinical benefit is lacking, exchange transfusion, plasmapheresis, and plasma exchange are reasonable in severely poisoned patients as soon as possible; any potential efficacy likely decreases as the interval from exposure to treatment initiation increases.

TABLE 34–2	Comparison of Antimitotic Overdose			
	Colchicine	**Podophyllum Resin**	**Vincristine**	**Vinblastine**
Route of exposure	PO	PO and cutaneous	IV	IV
Initial symptoms	GI effects,[a] neurologic effects (obtundation, confusion, delirium, seizures, myoneuropathy, areflexia)	GI effects,[a] fever, neurologic effects (obtundation, confusion, delirium, paresthesias, lost reflexes, cranial nerve involvement)	GI effects,[a] fever, neurologic effects (depression, agitation, delirium, paresthesias, muscle weakness, lost reflexes, cranial nerve involvement)	GI effects,[a] fever, myalgias, neurologic effects (but *less* than vincristine)
Initial symptom onset	Several hours after ingestion; delayed onset beyond 12 h very unlikely	Several hours after ingestion; delayed presentation (past 12 h) is possible, especially after cutaneous exposure	Usually within 24–48 h	Usually within 24–48 h
Hematologic effects	Leukocytosis (24–48 h after ingestion); pancytopenia (beginning 48–72 h after ingestion)	Similar to colchicine; however, not well characterized and reported less frequently	Occurs but *decreased* severity compared with vinblastine	Myelosuppression; *increased* severity compared with vincristine
CNS effects	Late (48–72 h after ingestion); obtundation, confusion, and lethargy secondary to progression of MSD	Can be early (<12 h after ingestion); typically occur later or secondary to progression of MSD	Variable; cranial neuropathies; seizures; obtundation, confusion, and lethargy; also occur because of progression of MSD	Occurs but *decreased* severity compared with vincristine
Delayed PNS effects	Myoneuropathy most common (can also occur early); reported most often in chronic colchicine users with kidney dysfunction	Peripheral sensorimotor axonopathy	Autonomic and ascending peripheral neuropathy; *increased* severity compared with vinblastine	Autonomic and peripheral neuropathy; *decreased* severity compared with vincristine
Clinical course	Recovery or MSD and death	Recovery or MSD and death	Recovery or MSD and death; SIADH	Recovery or MSD and death; SIADH
Management	Supportive; GI decontamination (activated charcoal, orogastric lavage for life-threatening ingestions if within 1–2 h, no contraindications present, and provider is proficient in the procedure); G-CSF for neutropenia	Supportive; GI decontamination (activated charcoal) for oral exposures and skin decontamination for cutaneous exposures	Primarily supportive; G-CSF for neutropenia. For treatment of intrathecal overdoses, see Special Considerations: SC7	Primarily supportive; G-CSF for neutropenia; exchange transfusion, plasmapheresis or plasma exchange are reasonable for severe toxicity. For treatment of intrathecal overdoses, see Special Considerations: SC7

[a]Nausea, vomiting, diarrhea, and abdominal discomfort.

CNS = central nervous system; G-CSF = granulocyte-colony stimulating factor; GI = gastrointestinal; IV = intravenous; MSD = multisystem organ dysfunction; PNS = peripheral nervous system; PO = oral; SIADH = syndrome of inappropriate antidiuretic hormone secretion.

Disclaimer

The findings and conclusions in this article are those of the authors and do not necessarily represent the views of the Centers for Disease Control and Prevention or the Agency for Toxic Substances and Disease Registry.

Acknowledgement

Richard Wang, DO, contributed to this chapter in a previous edition.

REFERENCES

1. Activated charcoal adsorbs colchicine but does not replace gastric lavage. *Prescrire Int.* 2011;20:54.
2. Abe E, et al. A novel LC-ESI-MS-MS method for sensitive quantification of colchicine in human plasma: application to two case reports. *J Anal Toxicol.* 2006;30:210-215.
3. Achtert G, et al. Pharmacokinetics/bioavailability of colchicine in healthy male volunteers. *Eur J Drug Metab Pharmacokinet.* 1989;14:317-322.
4. US Food and Drug Administration. FDA takes action to stop the marketing of unapproved injectable drugs containing colchicine. 2008. https://www.fda.gov/Drugs/GuidanceComplianceRegulatoryInformation/EnforcementActivitiesbyFDA/SelectedEnforcementActionsonUnapprovedDrugs/ucm119642.htm. Accessed May 28, 2008.
5. US Food and Drug Administration. Information for Healthcare Professionals: New Safety Information for Colchicine (marketed as Colcrys). 2013. http://www.fda.gov/Drugs/DrugSafety/PostmarketDrugSafetyInformationforPatientsandProviders/DrugSafetyInformationforHeathcareProfessionals/ucm174315.htm. Accessed January 18, 2017.
6. Akdag I, et al. Acute colchicine intoxication during clarithromycin administration in patients with chronic renal failure. *J Nephrol.* 2006;19:515-517.
7. Alayli G, et al. Acute myopathy in a patient with concomitant use of pravastatin and colchicine. *Ann Pharmacother.* 2005;39:1358-1361.
8. Alcaraz A, et al. Intrathecal vincristine: fatal myeloencephalopathy despite cerebrospinal fluid perfusion. *J Toxicol Clin Toxicol.* 2002;40:557-561.
9. Allen JN, et al. Colchicine has opposite effects on interleukin-1 beta and tumor necrosis factor-alpha production. *Am J Physiol.* 1991;261(4 Pt 1):L315-321.
10. Altiparmak MR, et al. Colchicine neuromyopathy: a report of six cases. *Clin Exp Rheumatol.* 2002;20(4 suppl 26):S13-16.
11. Angulo P, Lindor KD. Management of primary biliary cirrhosis and autoimmune cholangitis. *Clin Liver Dis.* 1998;2:333-351, ix.
12. Angunawela RM, Fernando HA. Acute ascending polyneuropathy and dermatitis following poisoning by tubers of *Gloriosa superba. Ceylon Med J.* 1971;16:233-235.
13. Ariffin H, et al. Severe vincristine neurotoxicity with concomitant use of itraconazole. *J Paediatr Child Health.* 2003;39:638-639.
14. Back A, et al. Distribution of radioactive colchicine in some organs of normal and tumor-bearing mice. *Proc Soc Exp Biol Med.* 1951;77:667-669.
15. Barzdo M, et al. Erroneous administration of vinblastine. *Pharm World Sci.* 2009;31:362-364.
16. Baud FJ, et al. Brief report: treatment of severe colchicine overdose with colchicine-specific Fab fragments. *N Engl J Med.* 1995;332:642-645.
17. Bayley PM, Martin SR. Microtubule dynamic instability: some possible physical mechanisms and their implications. *Biochem Soc Trans.* 1991;19:1023-1028.
18. Beer M, et al. Vincristine overdose: treatment with and without leucovorin rescue. *Cancer Treat Rep.* 1983;67:746-747.
19. Ben-Chetrit E, et al. Colchicine clearance by high-flux polysulfone dialyzers. *Arthritis Rheum.* 1998;41:749-750.
20. Ben-Chetrit E, Levy M. Colchicine: 1998 update. *Semin Arthritis Rheum.* 1998;28: 48-59.
21. Ben-Chetrit E, Navon P. Colchicine-induced leukopenia in a patient with familial Mediterranean fever: the cause and a possible approach. *Clin Exp Rheumatol.* 2003;21 (4 suppl 30):S38-40.
22. Berenson MP. Recovery after inadvertent massive overdosage of vincristine (NSC-67574). *Cancer Chemother Rep.* 1971;55:525-526.
23. Beyer J DO, Maurer HH. Analysis of toxic alkaloids in body samples. *Forensic Sci Int.* 2009;185:1-9.
24. Bhagra A, Rao RD. Chemotherapy-induced neuropathy. *Curr Oncol Rep.* 2007;9: 290-299.
25. Bhattacharyya B, et al. Anti-mitotic activity of colchicine and the structural basis for its interaction with tubulin. *Med Res Rev.* 2008;28:155-183.
26. Bismuth C. Biological valuation of extra-corporeal techniques in acute poisoning. *Acta Clin Belg Suppl.* 1990;13:20-28.
27. Bismuth C, et al. Biological evaluation of hemoperfusion in acute poisoning. *Clin Toxicol.* 1981;18:1213-1223.
28. Bismuth C, et al. [Medullary aplasia after acute colchicine poisoning. 20 cases]. *Nouv Presse Med.* 1977;6:1625-1629.
29. Bleyer WA, et al. Uptake and binding of vincristine by murine leukemia cells. *Biochem Pharmacol.* 1975;24:633-639.
30. Bond GR. The role of activated charcoal and gastric emptying in gastrointestinal decontamination: a state-of-the-art review. *Ann Emerg Med.* 2002;39:273-286.
31. Boomershine KH. Colchicine-induced rhabdomyolysis. *Ann Pharmacother.* 2002; 36:824-826.
32. Bosilkovska M, et al. Severe Vincristine-induced neuropathic pain in a CYP3A nonexpressor with reduced CYP3A4/5 activity: case study. *Clin Ther.* 2016;38:216-220.
33. Boyle FM, et al. Glutamate ameliorates experimental vincristine neuropathy. *J Pharmacol Exp Ther.* 1996;279:410-415.
34. Bradley WG, et al. The neuromyopathy of vincristine in man. Clinical, electrophysiological and pathological studies. *J Neurol Sci.* 1970;10:107-131.
35. Brady ST. Basic properties of fast axonal transport and the role of fast axonal transport in axonal growth. In: Elam JS, et al. ed. *Axonal Transport in Neuronal Growth and Regeneration.* New York, NY: Plenum; 1984:13-27.
36. Bronstein AC, et al. 2010 Annual Report of the American Association of Poison Control Centers' National Poison Data System (NPDS): 28th annual report. *Clin Toxicol (Phila).* 2011;49:910-941.
37. Brown WO SL. Effects of colchicine on human tissues. *Am J Clin Pathol.* 1945;15:189-195.
38. Bruns BJ. Colchicine toxicity. *Australas Ann Med.* 1968;17:341-344.
39. Brvar M, et al. Acute poisoning with autumn crocus (*Colchicum autumnale* L.). *Wien Klin Wochenschr.* 2004;116:205-208.
40. Brvar M, et al. Case report: fatal poisoning with Colchicum autumnale. *Crit Care.* 2004;8:R56-59.
41. Calabresi P CB. Antineoplastic agents. In: Goodman LS LL, et al. eds. *The pharmacological basis of therapeutics.* 9th ed. New York, NY: McGraw-Hill; 1996:1224-1287.
42. Campbell AN. Accidental poisoning with podophyllin. *Lancet.* 1980;1:206-207.
43. Canel C, et al. Podophyllotoxin. *Phytochemistry.* 2000;54:115-120.
44. Caner JE. Colchicine inhibition of chemotaxis. *Arthritis Rheum.* 1965;8:757-764.
45. Caraco Y, et al. Acute colchicine intoxication—possible role of erythromycin administration. *J Rheumatol.* 1992;19:494-496.
46. Cassidy DE, et al. Podophyllum toxicity: a report of a fatal case and a review of the literature. *J Toxicol Clin Toxicol.* 1982;19:35-44.
47. Centers for Disease Control and Prevention. Deaths from intravenous colchicine resulting from a compounding pharmacy error—Oregon and Washington, 2007. *MMWR Morb Mortal Wkly Rep.* 2007;56:1050-1052.
48. Chae L, et al. Overdose of vincristine: experience with a patient. *J Korean Med Sci.* 1998;13:334-338.
49. Chamberlain MJ, et al. Medical memoranda. Toxic effect of podophyllum application in pregnancy. *Br Med J.* 1972;3:391-392.
50. Chan TY, Critchley JA. The spectrum of poisonings in Hong Kong: an overview. *Vet Hum Toxicol.* 1994;36:135-137.
51. Chang MH, et al. Reversible myeloneuropathy resulting from podophyllin intoxication: an electrophysiological follow up. *J Neurol Neurosurg Psychiatry.* 1992;55:235-236.
52. Chang MH, et al. Acute ataxic sensory neuronopathy resulting from podophyllin intoxication. *Muscle Nerve.* 1992;15:513-514.
53. Chappey ON, et al. Colchicine disposition in human leukocytes after single and multiple oral administration. *Clin Pharmacol Ther.* 1993;54:360-367.
54. Cho ES, et al. Neurotoxicology of vincristine in the cat. Morphological study. *Arch Toxicol.* 1983;52:83-90.
55. Choi SS, et al. Colchicine-induced myopathy and neuropathy. *Hong Kong Med J.* 1999;5:204-207.
56. Clark AN, Parsonage MJ. A case of podophyllum poisoning with involvement of the nervous system. *Br Med J.* 1957;2:1155-1157.
57. Coruh M, Argun G. Podophyllin poisoning. A case report. *Turk J Pediatr.* 1965;7:100-103.
58. Creasey WA, et al. Colchicine, vinblastine and griseofulvin. Pharmacological studies with human leukocytes. *Biochem Pharmacol.* 1971;20:1579-1588.
59. Critchley JA, et al. Granulocyte-colony stimulating factor in the treatment of colchicine poisoning. *Hum Exp Toxicol.* 1997;16:229-232.
60. Cutts JH. Effects of other agents on the biologic responses to vincaleukoblastine. *Biochem Pharmacol.* 1964;13:421-431.
61. Davies HO, et al. Massive overdose of colchicine. *CMAJ.* 1988;138:335-336.
62. Deconti RC CW. Clinical aspects of the dimeric Catharan-thus alakaloids. In: Taylor WI FN, ed. *The Catharanthus Alkaloids: Botany, Chemistry, Pharmacology and Clinical Use.* New York, NY: Marcel Dekker; 1975:237-278.
63. Desbene S, Giorgi-Renault S. Drugs that inhibit tubulin polymerization: the particular case of podophyllotoxin and analogues. *Curr Med Chem Anticancer Agents.* 2002;2:71-90.
64. Deveaux M, et al. Colchicine poisoning: case report of two suicides. *Forensic Sci Int.* 2004;143:219-222.
65. Diav-Citrin O, et al. Pregnancy outcome after in utero exposure to colchicine. *Am J Obstet Gynecol.* 2010;203:144 e141-146.
66. Diouf B, et al. Association of an inherited genetic variant with vincristine-related peripheral neuropathy in children with acute lymphoblastic leukemia. *JAMA.* 2015;313:815-823.
67. Dixi G, et al. Vincristine induced cranial neuropathy. *J Assoc Physicians India.* 2012;60:56-58.
68. Dobb GJ, Edis RH. Coma and neuropathy after ingestion of herbal laxative containing podophyllin. *Med J Aust.* 1984;140:495-496.
69. Dodds AJ, et al. Colchicine overdose. *Med J Aust.* 1978;2:91-92.
70. Dogukan A, et al. Acute fatal colchicine intoxication in a patient on continuous ambulatory peritoneal dialysis (CAPD). Possible role of clarithromycin administration. *Clin Nephrol.* 2001;55:181-182.
71. Dominguez de Villota E, et al. Colchicine overdose: an unusual origin of multiorgan failure. *Crit Care Med.* 1979;7:278-279.
72. Dorr RT FW. *Cancer Chemotherapy Handbook.* New York, NY: Elsevier; 1980.

73. Duman O, et al. Treatment of vincristine-induced cranial polyneuropathy. *J Pediatr Hematol Oncol.* 2005;27:241-242.

74. Dupont P, et al. Colchicine myoneuropathy in a renal transplant patient. *Transpl Int.* 2002;15:374-376.

75. Eleftheriou G, et al. Colchicine-induced toxicity in a heart transplant patient with chronic renal failure. *Clin Toxicol (Phila).* 2008;46:827-830.

76. Erickson HP, O'Brien ET. Microtubule dynamic instability and GTP hydrolysis. *Annu Rev Biophys Biomol Struct.* 1992;21:145-166.

77. Ertel NH. Measurement of colchicine in urine and peripheral leukocytes [abstract]. *Clin Res.* 1971;19:348.

78. Ertuğrul İ, et al. Acute colchicine intoxication complicated with complete AV block. *Turk J Pediatr.* 2015;57:398-400.

79. Ferron GM, et al. Oral absorption characteristics and pharmacokinetics of colchicine in healthy volunteers after single and multiple doses. *J Clin Pharmacol.* 1996;36:874-883.

80. Filley CM, et al. Neurologic manifestations of podophyllin toxicity. *Neurology.* 1982;32:308-311.

81. Finger JE, Headington JT. Colchicine-induced epithelial atypia. *Am J Clin Pathol.* 1963;40:605-609.

82. Folpini A, Furfori P. Colchicine toxicity—clinical features and treatment. Massive overdose case report. *J Toxicol Clin Toxicol.* 1995;33:71-77.

83. Frasca T, et al. Mandrake toxicity. A case of mistaken identity. *Arch Intern Med.* 1997;157:2007-2009.

84. Frommeyer G, et al. Colchicine Increases ventricular vulnerability in an experimental whole-heart model. *Basic Clin Pharmacol Toxicol.* 2017;120:505-508.

85. Gaze DC, Collinson PO. Cardiac troponins as biomarkers of drug- and toxin-induced cardiac toxicity and cardioprotection. *Expert Opin Drug Metab Toxicol.* 2005;1:715-725.

86. Georgatsos JG, Karemfyllis T. Action of podophyllic acid on malignant tumors. II. Effects of podophyllic acid ethyl hydrazide on the incorporation of precursors into the nucleic acids of mouse mammary tumors and livers in vivo. *Biochem Pharmacol.* 1968;17:1489-1492.

87. Goldbart A, et al. Near fatal acute colchicine intoxication in a child. A case report. *Eur J Pediatr.* 2000;159:895-897.

88. Gooneratne IK, et al. Toxic encephalopathy due to colchicine—*Gloriosa superba* poisoning. *Pract Neurol.* 2014;14:357-359.

89. Gorin F, et al. Dorsal radiculopathy resulting from podophyllin toxicity. *Neurology.* 1989;39:607-608.

90. Green LS, et al. Axonal transport disturbances in vincristine-induced peripheral neuropathy. *Ann Neurol.* 1977;1:255-262.

91. Gruber M. Podophyllum versus podophyllin. *J Am Acad Dermatol.* 1984;10(2 Pt 1):302-303.

92. Grush OC, Morgan SK. Folinic acid rescue for vincristine toxicity. *Clin Toxicol.* 1979;14:71-78.

93. Gutowski MC, et al. Reduction of toxicity of a vinca alkaloid by an anti-vinca alkaloid antibody. *Cancer Invest.* 1995;13:370-374.

94. Savel H. Clinical experience with intravenous podophyllotoxin. *Proc Am Assoc Cancer Res.* 1964;5:56.

95. Halkin H, et al. Colchicine kinetics in patients with familial Mediterranean fever. *Clin Pharmacol Ther.* 1980;28:82-87.

96. Hamel E, Lin CM. Glutamate-induced polymerization of tubulin: characteristics of the reaction and application to the large-scale purification of tubulin. *Arch Biochem Biophys.* 1981;209:29-40.

97. Harris R, et al. Colchicine-induced bone marrow suppression: treatment with granulocyte colony-stimulating factor. *J Emerg Med.* 2000;18:435-440.

98. Hartung EF. History of the use of colchicum and related medicaments in gout; with suggestions for further research. *Ann Rheum Dis.* 1954;13:190-200.

99. Hastie SB. Interactions of colchicine with tubulin. *Pharmacol Ther.* 1991;51:377-401.

100. Hatzipantelis E, et al. Bilateral eyelid ptosis, attributed to vincristine, treated successfully with pyridoxine and thiamine in a child with acute lymphoblastic leukemia. *Toxicol Int.* 2015;22:162-164.

101. Heath A, et al. Treatment of podophyllin poisoning with resin hemoperfusion. *Hum Toxicol.* 1982;1:373-378.

102. Hill RN, et al. Letter: Adult respiratory distress syndrome associated with colchicine intoxication. *Ann Intern Med.* 1975;83:523-524.

103. Hobson CH, Rankin AP. A fatal colchicine overdose. *Anaesth Intensive Care.* 1986;14:453-455.

104. Holdright DR, Jahangiri M. Accidental poisoning with podophyllin. *Hum Exp Toxicol.* 1990;9:55-56.

105. Holland JF, et al. Vincristine treatment of advanced cancer: a cooperative study of 392 cases. *Cancer Res.* 1973;33:1258-1264.

106. Hood RL. Colchicine poisoning. *J Emerg Med.* 1994;12:171-177.

107. Hung IF, et al. Fatal interaction between clarithromycin and colchicine in patients with renal insufficiency: a retrospective study. *Clin Infect Dis.* 2005;41:291-300.

108. Hunter AL, Klaassen CD. Biliary excretion of colchicine. *J Pharmacol Exp Ther.* 1975;192:605-617.

109. Hurwitz RL, et al. Reversible encephalopathy and seizures as a result of conventional vincristine administration. *Med Pediatr Oncol.* 1988;16:216-219.

110. Insel PA. Analgesic-antipyretics and antiinflammatory agents: drug employed in the treatment of rheumatoid arthritis and gout. In: Gilman AG, et al, ed. *Goodman and Gilman's The Pharmacological Basis of Therapeutics.* New York, NY: MacMillan; 1990:674-676.

111. Jackson DV Jr, et al. Clinical trial of folinic acid to reduce vincristine neurotoxicity. *Cancer Chemother Pharmacol.* 1986;17:281-284.

112. Jackson DV Jr, et al. Improved tolerance of vincristine by glutamic acid. A preliminary report. *J Neurooncol.* 1984;2:219-222.

113. Jackson DV, et al. Amelioration of vincristine neurotoxicity by glutamic acid. *Am J Med.* 1988;84:1016-1022.

114. Jef R. Vinblastine. In: Jef R, ed. *Martindale: The Extra Pharmacopoeia.* London: Pharmaceutical Press; 1989:655-657.

115. Johnson FL, et al. Seizures associated with vincristine sulfate therapy. *J Pediatr.* 1973;82:699-702.

116. Jordan A, et al. Tubulin as a target for anticancer drugs: agents which interact with the mitotic spindle. *Med Res Rev.* 1998;18:259-296.

117. Jordan MA. Mechanism of action of antitumor drugs that interact with microtubules and tubulin. *Curr Med Chem Anticancer Agents.* 2002;2:1-17.

118. Karol MD, et al. Podophyllum: suspected teratogenicity from topical application. *Clin Toxicol.* 1980;16:283-286.

119. Katz R, et al. Use of granulocyte colony-stimulating factor in the treatment of pancytopenia secondary to colchicine overdose. *Ann Pharmacother.* 1992;26:1087-1088.

120. Kaufman IA, et al. Overdosage with vincristine. *J Pediatr.* 1976;89:671-674.

121. Kim KY, et al. A literature review of the epidemiology and treatment of acute gout. *Clin Ther.* 2003;25:1593-1617.

122. Kosmidis HV, et al. Vincristine overdose: experience with 3 patients. *Pediatr Hematol Oncol.* 1991;8:171-178.

123. Kumar M, et al. Permanent neurological sequelae following accidental podophyllin ingestion. *J Child Neurol.* 2012;27:209-210.

124. Kuncl RW, et al. Colchicine myopathy and neuropathy. *N Engl J Med.* 1987;316:1562-1568.

125. Lange U, et al. Current aspects of colchicine therapy—classical indications and new therapeutic uses. *Eur J Med Res.* 2001;6:150-160.

126. Legha SS. Vincristine neurotoxicity. Pathophysiology and management. *Med Toxicol.* 1986;1:421-427.

127. Leslie KO, Shitamoto B. The bone marrow in systemic podophyllin toxicity. *Am J Clin Pathol.* 1982;77:478-480.

128. Levy M, et al. Colchicine: a state-of-the-art review. *Pharmacotherapy.* 1991;11:196-211.

129. Lipton RB, et al. Taxol produces a predominantly sensory neuropathy. *Neurology.* 1989;39:368-373.

130. Lotz JP, et al. Overdosage of vinorelbine in a woman with metastatic non-small-cell lung carcinoma. *Ann Oncol.* 1997;8:714-715.

131. Luduena RF, Roach MC. Tubulin sulfhydryl groups as probes and targets for antimitotic and antimicrotubule agents. *Pharmacol Ther.* 1991;49:133-152.

132. Mack RB. Achilles and his evil squeeze. Colchicine poisoning. *N C Med J.* 1991; 52:581-583.

133. Maeda K, et al. A massive dose of vincristine. *Jpn J Clin Oncol.* 1987;17:247-253.

134. Mandel EM, et al. Vincristine-induced myocardial infarction. *Cancer.* 1975;36:1979-1982.

135. Marmont AM. Selective metaphasic arrest of erythroblasts by vincristine in patients receiving high doses of recombinant human erythropoietin for myelosuppressive anemia. *Leukemia.* 1992;(6 suppl 4):167-170.

136. Maxwell MJ, et al. Accidental colchicine overdose. A case report and literature review. *Emerg Med J.* 2002;19:265-267.

137. McGuigan M. Toxicology of topical therapy. *Clin Dermatol.* 1989;7:32-37.

138. McIntyre IM, et al. Death following colchicine poisoning. *J Forensic Sci.* 1994;39:280-286.

139. Melki R, et al. Cold depolymerization of microtubules to double rings: geometric stabilization of assemblies. *Biochemistry.* 1989;28:9143-9152.

140. Miller RA. Podophyllin. *Int J Dermatol.* 1985;24:491-498.

141. Milne ST, Meek PD. Fatal colchicine overdose: report of a case and review of the literature. *Am J Emerg Med.* 1998;16:603-608.

142. Moher LM, Maurer SA. Podophyllum toxicity: case report and literature review. *J Fam Pract.* 1979;9:237-240.

143. Molad Y. Update on colchicine and its mechanism of action. *Curr Rheumatol Rep.* 2002;4:252-256.

144. Molad Y RJ, et al. A new mode of action for an old drug: colchicine decreases surface expression of adhesion molecules on both neutrophils (PMNs) and endothelium (abstract). *Arthritis Rheum.* 1992;35(suppl):S35.

145. Montiel V, et al. Multiple organ failure after an overdose of less than 0.4 mg/kg of colchicine: role of coingestants and drugs during intensive care management. *Clin Toxicol (Phila).* 2010;48:845-848.

146. Morasca L, et al. Duration of cytotoxic activity of vincristine in the blood of leukemic children. *Eur J Cancer.* 1969;5:79-80.

147. Mullins M, et al. Unrecognized fatalities related to colchicine in hospitalized patients. *Clin Toxicol (Phila).* 2011;49:648-652.

148. Mullins ME, et al. Fatal cardiovascular collapse following acute colchicine ingestion. *J Toxicol Clin Toxicol.* 2000;38:51-54.

149. Mullins ME, et al. Troponin I as a marker of cardiac toxicity in acute colchicine overdose. *Am J Emerg Med.* 2000;18:743-744.

150. Murray SS, et al. Acute toxicity after excessive ingestion of colchicine. *Mayo Clin Proc.* 1983;58:528-532.

151. Muzaffar A, Brossi A. Chemistry of colchicine. *Pharmacol Ther.* 1991;49:105-109.

152. Nagesh KR MM, et al. Suicidal plant poisoning with *Colchicum autumnale*. *J Forensic and Legal Med.* 2011;2011:285-287.

153. Naidus RM, et al. Colchicine toxicity: a multisystem disease. *Arch Intern Med.* 1977;137:394-396.

154. Nakashima H, et al. Cutaneous reaction induced by vincristine. *Br J Dermatol.* 2005;153:225-226.

155. Nelson RL. The comparative clinical pharmacology and pharmacokinetics of vindesine, vincristine, and vinblastine in human patients with cancer. *Med Pediatr Oncol.* 1982;10:115-127.

156. Ng TH, et al. Encephalopathy and neuropathy following ingestion of a Chinese herbal broth containing podophyllin. *J Neurol Sci.* 1991;101:107-113.

157. Niel E, Scherrmann JM. Colchicine today. *Joint Bone Spine.* 2006;73:672-678.

158. O'Mahony S, et al. Neuropathy due to podophyllin intoxication. *J Neurol.* 1990; 237:110-112.

159. Ochs S WR. Comparison of the block of fast axoplasmic transport in mammalian nerve by vincristine, vinblastine, and desacetyl vinblastine amide sulfate (DVA). *Proc Am Assoc Cancer Res.* 1975;16:70-75.

160. Ozdemir R, et al. Fatal poisoning in children: acute colchicine intoxication and new treatment approaches. *Clin Toxicol (Phila).* 2011;49:739-743.

161. Dustin P. Microtubule poisons. *Microtubules.* Berlin: Springer-Verlag; 1984:447-449.

162. Palkar AH, et al. Vincristine-induced neuropathy presenting as ptosis and ophthalmoplegia in a 2-year-old boy. *J Pediatr Ophthalmol Strabismus.* 2015;52 Online:34-37.

163. Panda D, et al. Kinetic stabilization of microtubule dynamics at steady state in vitro by substoichiometric concentrations of tubulin-colchicine complex. *Biochemistry.* 1995;34:9921-9929.

164. Patiroglu T, et al. Accidental intramuscular overdose administration of vincristine. *Drug Chem Toxicol.* 2012;35:232-234.

165. Paulson JC, McClure WO. Inhibition of axoplasmic transport by colchicine, podophyllotoxin, and vinblastine: an effect on microtubules. *Ann N Y Acad Sci.* 1975;253:517-527.

166. Peake PW, et al. Fab fragments of ovine antibody to colchicine enhance its clearance in the rat. *Clin Toxicol (Phila).* 2015;53:427-432.

167. Phelps P. Appearance of chemotactic activity following intra-articular injection of monosodium urate crystals: effect of colchicine. *J Lab Clin Med.* 1970;76:622-631.

168. Phillips RA, et al. Cathartics and the sodium pump. *Nature.* 1965;206:1367-1368.

169. Pierga JY, et al. Favourable outcome after plasmapheresis for vincristine overdose. *Lancet.* 1992;340:185.

170. Pirzada NA, et al. Colchicine induced neuromyopathy in a patient with normal renal function. *J Clin Rheumatol.* 2001;7:374-376.

171. Prakash V, Timasheff SN. Mechanism of interaction of vinca alkaloids with tubulin: catharanthine and vindoline. *Biochemistry.* 1991;30:873-880.

172. Putterman C, et al. Colchicine intoxication: clinical pharmacology, risk factors, features, and management. *Semin Arthritis Rheum.* 1991;21:143-155.

173. Rate RG, et al. Podophyllin toxicity. *Ann Intern Med.* 1979;90:723.

174. Roberts WN, et al. Colchicine in acute gout. Reassessment of risks and benefits. *JAMA.* 1987;257:1920-1922.

175. Rochdi M, et al. Toxicokinetics of colchicine in humans: analysis of tissue, plasma and urine data in ten cases. *Hum Exp Toxicol.* 1992;11:510-516.

176. Rochdi M, et al. Pharmacokinetics and absolute bioavailability of colchicine after i.v. and oral administration in healthy human volunteers and elderly subjects. *Eur J Clin Pharmacol.* 1994;46:351-354.

177. Rosenthal S, Kaufman S. Vincristine neurotoxicity. *Ann Intern Med.* 1974;80:733-737.

178. Rott KT, Agudelo CA. Gout. *JAMA.* 2003;289:2857-2860.

179. Roujeau JC, et al. Toxic epidermal necrolysis (Lyell syndrome). *J Am Acad Dermatol.* 1990;23(6 Pt 1):1039-1058.

180. Rudi J, et al. Plasma kinetics and biliary excretion of colchicine in patients with chronic liver disease after oral administration of a single dose and after long-term treatment. *Scand J Gastroenterol.* 1994;29:346-351.

181. Rudrappa S, Vijaydeva L. Podophyllin poisoning. *Indian Pediatr.* 2002;39:598-599.

182. Sabouraud A, et al. Pharmacokinetics of colchicine: a review of experimental and clinical data. *Z Gastroenterol.* 1992;(30 suppl 1):35-39.

183. Sackett DL, Varma JK. Molecular mechanism of colchicine action: induced local unfolding of beta-tubulin. *Biochemistry.* 1993;32:13560-13565.

184. Sandler SG, et al. Vincristine-induced neuropathy. A clinical study of fifty leukemic patients. *Neurology.* 1969;19:367-374.

185. Sathiapalan RK, et al. Vincristine-itraconazole interaction: cause for increasing concern. *J Pediatr Hematol Oncol.* 2002;24:591.

186. Sathiapalan RK, El-Solh H. Enhanced vincristine neurotoxicity from drug interactions: case report and review of literature. *Pediatr Hematol Oncol.* 2001;18:543-546.

187. Sauder P, et al. Haemodynamic studies in eight cases of acute colchicine poisoning. *Hum Toxicol.* 1983;2:169-173.

188. Shi Q, et al. Recent progress in the development of tubulin inhibitors as antimitotic antitumor agents. *Curr Pharm Des.* 1998;4:219-248.

189. Simons RJ, Kingma DW. Fatal colchicine toxicity. *Am J Med.* 1989;86:356-357.

190. Slater GE, et al. Podophyllin poisoning. Systemic toxicity following cutaneous application. *Obstet Gynecol.* 1978;52:94-96.

191. Slimowitz R. Thoughts on a medical disaster. *Am J Health Syst Pharm.* 1995;52:1464-1465.

192. Somers G, et al. Letter: Myocardial infarction: a complication of vincristine treatment? *Lancet.* 1976;2:690.

193. Soto O, Hedley-Whyte ET. Case records of the Massachusetts General Hospital. Weekly clinicopathological exercises. Case 33-2003. A 37-year-old man with a history of alcohol and drug abuse and sudden onset of leg weakness. *N Engl J Med.* 2003;349:1656-1663.

194. Spilbert I, et al. Urate crystal-induced chemotactic factor: isolation and partial characterization. *J Clin Invest.* 1976;58:815-819.

195. Spiller M, et al. A case of vinblastine overdose managed with plasma exchange. *Pediatr Blood Cancer.* 2005;45:344-346.

196. Stoehr GP, et al. Systemic complications of local podophyllin therapy. *Ann Intern Med.* 1978;89:362-363.

197. Stones DK. Vincristine overdosage in paediatric patients. *Med Pediatr Oncol.* 1998;30:193.

198. Stoudemire A, et al. Delirium induced by topical application of podophyllin: a case report. *Am J Psychiatry.* 1981;138:1505-1506.

199. Stringfellow HF, et al. Waterhouse-Friderichsen syndrome resulting from colchicine overdose. *J R Soc Med.* 1993;86:680.

200. Subar M, Muggia FM. Apparent myocardial ischemia associated with vinblastine administration. *Cancer Treat Rep.* 1986;70:690-691.

201. Sullivan M, et al. Toxicology of podophyllin. *Proc Soc Exp Biol Med.* 1951;77:269-272.

202. Tanios MA, et al. Severe respiratory muscle weakness related to long-term colchicine therapy. *Respir Care.* 2004;49:189-191.

203. Tateishi T, et al. Colchicine biotransformation by human liver microsomes. Identification of CYP3A4 as the major isoform responsible for colchicine demethylation. *Biochem Pharmacol.* 1997;53:111-116.

204. Terkeltaub RA, et al. Novel evidence-based colchicine dose-reduction algorithm to predict and prevent colchicine toxicity in the presence of cytochrome P450 3A4/P-glycoprotein inhibitors. *Arthritis Rheum.* 2011;63:2226-2237.

205. Thomas G, et al. Zero-order absorption and linear disposition of oral colchicine in healthy volunteers. *Eur J Clin Pharmacol.* 1989;37:79-84.

206. Thomas LL, et al. Massive vincristine overdose: failure of leucovorin to reduce toxicity. *Cancer Treat Rep.* 1982;66:1967-1969.

207. Ting JY. Acute pancreatitis related to therapeutic dosing with colchicine: a case report. *J Med Case Rep.* 2007;1:64.

208. Unknown. Colchicine: serious interactions. *Rev Prescrire.* 2008;28:2008.

209. Vale JA. Position statement: gastric lavage. American Academy of Clinical Toxicology; European Association of Poisons Centres and Clinical Toxicologists. *J Toxicol Clin Toxicol.* 1997;35:711-719.

210. van Heyningen C, Watson ID. Troponin for prediction of cardiovascular collapse in acute colchicine overdose. *Emerg Med J.* 2005;22:599-600.

211. von Krogh G. Podophyllotoxin in serum: absorption subsequent to three-day repeated applications of a 0.5% ethanolic preparation on condylomata acuminata. *Sex Transm Dis.* 1982;9:26-33.

212. Wallace SL, Ertel NH. Plasma levels of colchicine after oral administration of a single dose. *Metabolism.* 1973;22:749-753.

213. Wallace SL, et al. Colchicine plasma levels. Implications as to pharmacology and mechanism of action. *Am J Med.* 1970;48:443-448.

214. Waravdekar VS, et al. Enzyme changes induced in normal and malignant tissues with chemical agents. V. Effect of acetylpodophyllotoxin-omega-pyridinium chloride on uricase, adenosine deaminase, nucleoside phosphorylase, and glutamic dehydrogenase activities. *J Natl Cancer Inst.* 1955;16:99-105.

215. Weakley-Jones B, et al. Colchicine poisoning: case report of two homicides. *Am J Forensic Med Pathol.* 2001;22:203-206.

216. Weiner JL, et al. Colchicine is a competitive antagonist at human recombinant gamma-aminobutyric acid A receptors. *J Pharmacol Exp Ther.* 1998;284:95-102.

217. Weiss HD, et al. Neurotoxicity of commonly used antineoplastic agents (first of two parts). *N Engl J Med.* 1974;291:75-81.

218. West WM, et al. Fatal podophyllin ingestion. *South Med J.* 1982;75:1269-1270.

219. WH D. Fatal podophyllum poisoning. *Med Rec.* 1890;37:409.

220. Wilbur K, Makowsky M. Colchicine myotoxicity: case reports and literature review. *Pharmacotherapy.* 2004;24:1784-1792.

221. Wisniewski H, et al. Effects of mitotic spindle inhibitors on neurotubules and neurofilaments in anterior horn cells. *J Cell Biol.* 1968;38:224-229.

222. Wollersen H, et al. Accidental fatal ingestion of colchicine-containing leaves—toxicological and histological findings. *Leg Med (Tokyo).* 2009;(11 suppl 1):S498-499.

223. Wu ML, et al. Severe bone marrow depression induced by an anticancer herb Cantharanthus roseus. *J Toxicol Clin Toxicol.* 2004;42:667-671.

224. Yancey RS, Talpaz M. Vindesine-associated angina and ECG changes. *Cancer Treat Rep.* 1982;66:587-589.

225. Yoon KH. Colchicine induced toxicity and pancytopenia at usual doses and treatment with granulocyte colony-stimulating factor. *J Rheumatol.* 2001;28:1199-1200.

226. Younger DS, et al. Colchicine-induced myopathy and neuropathy. *Neurology.* 1991;41:943.

227. Zeng G, et al. Paraplegia and paraparesis from intrathecal methotrexate and cytarabine contaminated with trace amounts of vincristine in China during 2007. *J Clin Oncol.* 2011;29:1765-1770.

228. Zhong LP, et al. Antifungal azoles exacerbate vinblastine-related hyponatremia in ALL children. *Zhongguo Shi Yan Xue Ye Xue Za Zhi.* 2014;22:1386-1390.

35 NONSTEROIDAL ANTIINFLAMMATORY DRUGS

William J. Holubek

HISTORY AND EPIDEMIOLOGY

In the 1950s, the only treatment for rheumatoid arthritis included high-dose aspirin and gold therapy (chrysotherapy). While searching for new compounds that were chemically nonsteroidal and had antiinflammatory properties, Dr. Stewart Adams filed a patent for "Antiinflammatory Agents" in 1961. One of the compounds in this list was 2-(4-isobutylphenyl) propionic acid, which today we call ibuprofen. This discovery created a new class of drugs designated as non-steroidal antiinflammatory drugs (NSAIDs).[36] Ibuprofen was initially marketed in the United Kingdom in 1969 and was introduced to the US market in 1974. Ibuprofen became available without a prescription in the United States in 1984.

In addition to the numerous benefits of NSAIDs, some deleterious and life-threatening effects are associated with both their therapeutic use and overdose. In an attempt to circumvent some of these adverse effects, selective cyclooxygenase-2 (COX-2) inhibitors were developed, and in 1999, the first selective COX-2 inhibitor, rofecoxib, was approved by the US Food and Drug Administration (FDA), but it was withdrawn from the market in 2004 after postmarketing surveillance concluded that an increase in myocardial infarctions and cerebrovascular accidents were associated with its use.

Nonsteroidal antiinflammatory drugs are considered among the most commonly used and prescribed nonprescription medications in the world.[12,72] An estimated one in seven patients with rheumatologic diseases is given a prescription for NSAIDs, and another one in five people in the United States uses NSAIDs for acute common complaints.[94]

Ibuprofen, naproxen, and ketoprofen are currently the only nonprescription NSAIDs in the United States. Nonsteroidal antiinflammatory drugs are also contained in cough and cold preparations and in prescription combination drugs (eg, ibuprofen with hydrocodone) and are occasionally found as adulterants in herbal preparations.[61]

The American Association of Poison Control Centers (AAPCC) compiles data regarding potentially toxic exposures called into participating poison centers throughout the United States using the National Poison Data System (NPDS) (Chap. 130). The AAPCC Annual Report lists NSAIDs among the top 25 substances associated with the largest number of fatalities.

The term *NSAID* used in this chapter does not refer to salicylates, which are unique members of the NSAID class and are covered in Chap. 37.

PHARMACOLOGY

These chemically heterogeneous compounds are divided into carboxylic acid and enolic acid derivatives and COX-2 selective inhibitors (Table 35–1). They all share the ability to inhibit prostaglandin (PG) synthesis. Prostaglandin synthesis begins with the activation of phospholipases (commonly, phospholipase A_2) that cleave phospholipids in the cell membrane to form arachidonic acid (AA). Arachidonic acid is metabolized by PG endoperoxide G/H synthase, otherwise known as COX, to form many eicosanoids, including PGs and the prostanoids, prostacyclin (PGI_2) and thromboxane A_2 (TXA_2). Arachidonic acid is also metabolized by lipoxygenase (LOX) to form hydroperoxy eicosatetraenoic acid (HPETE), which is converted to many different leukotrienes (LTs) that are involved in creating a proinflammatory environment (Fig. 35–1).

The COX enzyme responsible for PG production exists in two isoforms termed *COX-1* and *COX-2*. The isoform COX-1 is constitutively expressed by virtually all cells throughout the body but is the only isoform found within platelets. This enzyme produces eicosanoids that govern "housekeeping" functions, including vascular homeostasis and hemostasis, gastric cytoprotection, and renal blood flow (RBF) and function.[11,75] Conversely, COX-2 is rapidly induced (within 1–3 hours) in inflamed tissue and infiltrating cells (largely endothelial cells) by laminar shear or mechanical stress and cytokines and produces PGs that are responsible for creating the classic inflammatory response with clinical symptoms of warmth, pain, redness, and swelling. Cyclooxygenase-2 is also upregulated by several cytokines, growth factors, and tumor promoters involved with cellular differentiation and mitogenesis, suggesting a role in cancer development.[11,31,81]

Glucocorticoids inhibit phospholipase A (PLA) and downregulate the induced expression of COX-2, which decreases the production of eicosanoids and PGs, respectively, but oral steroids are clinically not the first choice for an antiinflammatory drug regimen given their extensive adverse side effect profile, which includes osteoporosis, hyperglycemia, hypertension, glaucoma, muscle weakness, fluid retention, and mood swings. Most NSAIDs nonselectively inhibit the COX enzymes in a competitive or time-dependent, reversible manner, unlike salicylates, which irreversibly acetylate COX (Chap. 37). Inhibiting COX-1 can interrupt tissue homeostasis, leading to deleterious clinical effects. In what may seem advantageous, some NSAIDs (eg, etodolac, meloxicam, and nimesulide) preferentially inhibit COX-2 over COX-1, while others were specifically designed to selectively inhibit COX-2 (eg, celebrex).[92] As will be discussed later in this chapter, many of the selective COX-2 inhibitors (sometimes referred to as *coxibs*) were removed from the market in the United States because of their increased risk of adverse cardiovascular events.

Nonsteroidal antiinflammatory drugs do not inhibit the LOX enzyme or the production of LTs; however, some data suggest that blocking the COX enzymes allows AA to be shunted toward the LOX pathway, increasing the production of proinflammatory and chemotactic-vasoactive LTs.[34,52,81,94]

PHARMACOKINETICS AND TOXICOKINETICS

Most NSAIDs are organic acids with extensive protein binding (95%–99%) and small volumes of distribution of approximately 0.1 to 0.2 L/kg. Oral absorption of most NSAIDs occurs rapidly and near completely, resulting in bioavailabilities above 80%. Time to achieve peak plasma concentrations vary widely (Table 35–1).[34]

Taken at therapeutic doses, most NSAIDs widely distribute throughout the body, penetrate inflamed joints, and obtain synovial fluid concentrations about half of plasma concentration, such as ibuprofen, naproxen, and piroxicam. However, some NSAIDs achieve synovial fluid concentrations equal to or greater than their plasma concentrations, such as indomethacin and tolmetin. Dermal preparations of NSAIDs (commonly diclofenac) achieve therapeutic concentrations in localized tissue while maintaining low plasma concentrations.[56] Ketorolac and diclofenac have topical activity and are used in ophthalmologic solutions.[34] Antiinflammatory drugs have the ability to cross the blood–brain barrier, but the specific pharmacologic and physicochemical properties facilitating this ability are not well defined.[3,53]

The plasma elimination half-life in therapeutic dosing varies from as short as 1 to 2 hours for diclofenac and ibuprofen to 50 to 60 hours for oxaprozin and piroxicam (Table 35–1). Most NSAIDs undergo hepatic metabolism with renal excretion of metabolites; however, diclofenac undergoes extensive first-pass metabolism with an oral bioavailability of about 50%, but indomethacin and ketorolac are excreted 10% to 20% unchanged in the urine. Variable amounts of NSAIDs are recovered in the feces.[34]

The kinetics of NSAIDs change in the setting of an overdose. Therapeutic and supratherapeutic doses of naproxen (250 mg–4 g) result in the same half-life and time to peak plasma concentration, but the clearance and volume of distribution increase proportionately.[64,74] When plasma protein binding of naproxen becomes saturated, the free drug concentration increases more rapidly than the total drug concentration, resulting in increased urinary

TABLE 35–1	Classes and Pharmacology of Selected Nonsteroidal Antiinflammatory Drugs[9,17,29,34,53,62]			
	Time to Peak Plasma Concentration (hours)	Half-Life (hours)	Pharmacokinetics	Unique Features
CARBOXYLIC ACIDS				
Acetic Acids				
Diclofenac[a,b]	2–3	1–2	First-pass effect; hepatic metabolism (CYP2C 9)	Decreases leukocyte arachidonic acid concentration; topical activity; hepatotoxic
Etodolac	1	7	Hepatic metabolism	Inhibits leukocyte motility; coronary vasoconstrictor effect
Indomethacin	1–2	2.5	Demethylation (50%)	Poor antiinflammatory effect; topical activity
Ketorolac	<1	4–6	Urinary excretion	For parenteral use also
Sulindac	1–2	7	Active metabolite with a half-life of 18 h	Prodrug; hepatotoxic
Tolmetin	<1	5	Hepatic metabolism	Accumulates in synovia
Fenamic Acids				
Meclofenamate	0.5–2.0	2–3	Urinary excretion (~70%); active metabolite	Seizures; GI inflammation
Mefenamic acid	2–4	3–4	Urinary excretion (50%)	Seizures; prostaglandin antagonist
Propionic Acids				
Fenoprofen	2	2–3	Decreased oral absorption (~85%)	Increased CSF concentration
Flurbiprofen	1–2	6	Urinary excretion unchanged (~20%)	Increased CSF concentration
Ibuprofen[c,d]	<0.5	2–4	Hepatic metabolism; urinary excretion	Also formulated for parenteral use
Indobufen[e]	2	6–7	Urinary excretion (70%–80%)	In Europe, used as prophylaxis for thrombus formation
Ketoprofen[c]	1–2	2	Hepatic metabolism; urinary excretion	Bradykinin antagonist; stabilizes lysosomal membranes
Naproxen[c]	1	14	Increased half-life with kidney dysfunction	Inhibitory effect on leukocytes; prolonged platelet inhibition
Oxaprozin	3–6	40–60	Hepatic metabolism	Once-daily administration
Salicylates (Chap. 37)				
ENOLIC ACIDS				
Oxicams				
Meloxicam[a]	5–10	15–20	Hepatic metabolism (CYP2C9)	High COX-2 selectivity
Nabumetone	3–6	24	Hepatic metabolism; active metabolites	Prodrug
Piroxicam	3–5	45–50	Hepatic metabolism (CYP2C9)	Inhibits neutrophil activation
Pyrazolone				
Phenylbutazone[e]	2	54–99	Hepatic metabolism; active metabolites	Irreversible agranulocytosis; aplastic anemia
CYCLOOXGENASE-2 SELECTIVE INHIBITORS[f]				
Celecoxib	2–4	6–12	Hepatic metabolism (CYP2C9)	Inhibits CYP2D6
Nimesulide[e]	1–3	2–5	Urinary excretion (60%); active metabolites	Inhibits neutrophil activation

[a]COX-2 preferential. [b]Available in combination with misoprostol. [c]Nonprescription. [d]Available in combination with oxycodone and hydrocodone. [e]Not available in the United States for humans. [f]Rofecoxib (Vioxx) and valdecoxib (Bextra) are no longer available.

COX = cyclooxygenase; CSF = cerebrospinal fluid; GI = gastrointestinal.

excretion.[74] Overdoses of oral ibuprofen do not appear to prolong its elimination half-life.[37,54,95]

PATHOPHYSIOLOGY

Gastrointestinal (GI) toxicity is the most common adverse effect from NSAID use (Table 35–2). Normally, the COX-1 enzyme expressed in the gastric epithelial cells leads to the production of PGs (PGE_2 and PGI_2), which are responsible for maintaining GI mucosal integrity by increasing cytoprotective mucous production, decreasing stomach acid production, and enhancing mucosal blood flow. Antiinflammatory drugs inhibit the production of these cytoprotective PGs, as well as the platelet aggregatory TXA_2, and they also have a direct cytotoxic or local irritation effect, increasing the risk of gastric and duodenal ulcers, perforations, and hemorrhage.[24,68,72] Although various enteric coated formulations were created to reduce NSAID contact with the gastric mucosa,

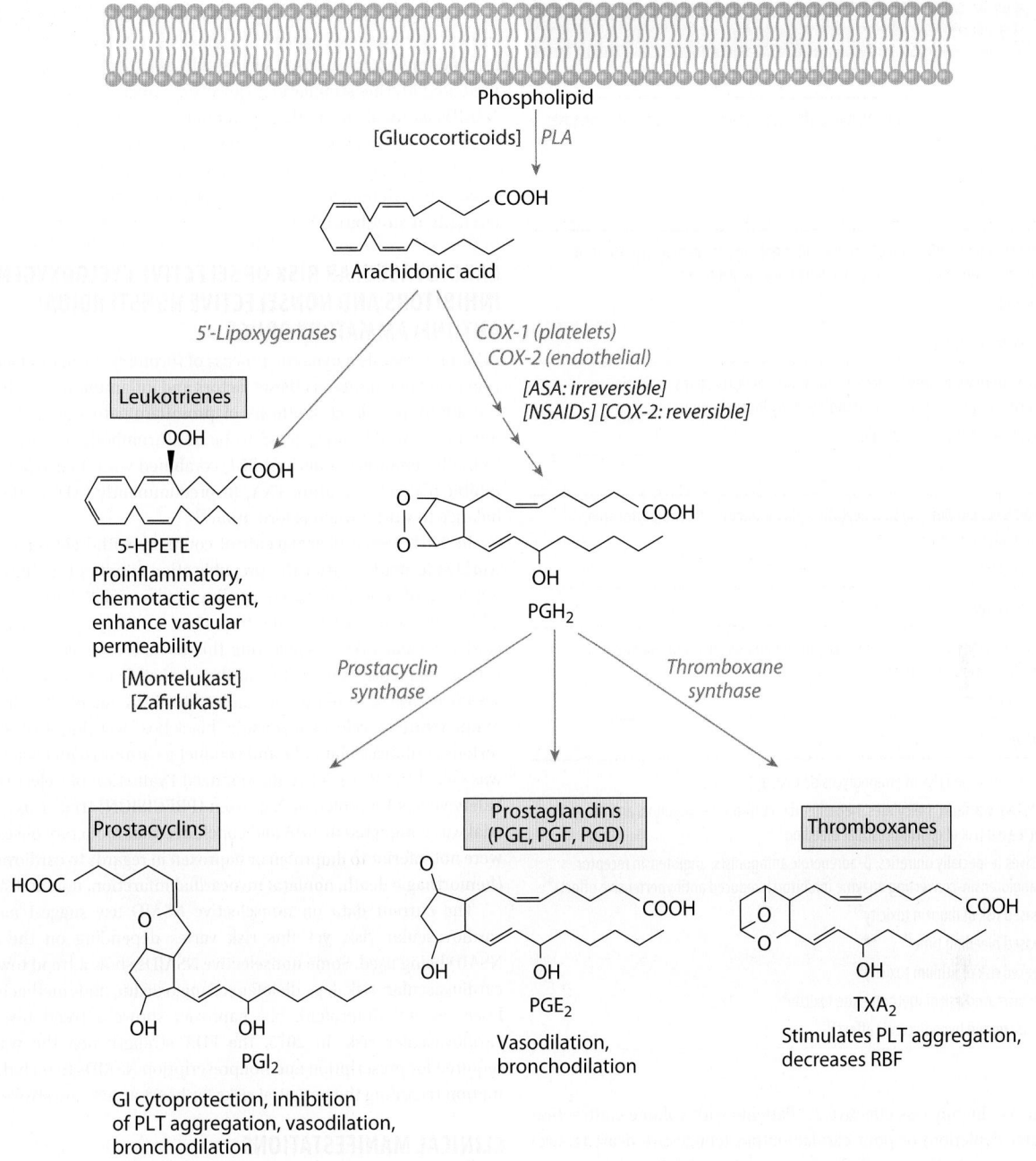

FIGURE 35-1. Arachidonic acid (AA) metabolism. This figure also illustrates some of the major differences between cyclooxygenase-1 (COX-1) and cyclooxygenase-2 (COX-2). Phospholipase A (PLA) is stimulated by physical, chemical, inflammatory, and mitogenic stimuli and releases AA from cell membranes. The COX-1 enzyme synthesizes prostaglandins (PGs) that maintain cellular and vascular homeostasis. The COX-2 enzyme produces PGs within activated macrophages and endothelial cells that accompany inflammation. Whereas nonsteroidal antiinflammatory drugs (NSAIDs) reversibly inhibit both COX isoforms, selective COX-2 inhibitors inhibit the COX-2 isoform. Some authors suggest that inhibiting the COX enzymes shunts AA metabolism toward the production of chemotactic-vasoactive leukotrienes. Glucocorticoids inhibit PLA and down regulate induced expression of COX-2. ASA = acetylsalicylic acid; 5-HPETE, hydroperoxy eicosatetraenoic acid; GI = gastrointestinal; PGI_2 = prostacyclin; PGD = prostaglandin D; PGE_2 = prostaglandin E; PGF = prostaglandin F; PGH_2 = prostaglandin H_2; PLT = platelet; RBF = renal blood flow; TXA_2 = thromboxane.

no significant reduction in GI adverse events resulted.[34] Esophageal and small intestinal ulcers and strictures are also associated with NSAID use. Small intestinal diaphragms (or webs) are concentric weblike septa arising from submucosal fibrosis that eventually cause a small bowel obstruction. These diaphragms rarely occur but are considered pathognomonic for NSAID use.[24]

Selective COX-2 inhibitors decrease the incidence of significant GI toxicity compared with some nonselective NSAIDs, a benefit that is lost in patients concomitantly taking warfarin or low-dose aspirin.[4,13,31,93] Although *Helicobacter pylori* and NSAID use both individually increase the risk of gastroduodenal ulcers, there are conflicting data regarding the relationship between the two, given the wide array of study designs, individual responses to infection and

treatments, and different gastric acid suppressants. However, current evidence suggests that the risk of GI toxicity and peptic ulcer disease is decreased by eradicating *H. pylori* in NSAID users and NSAID-naïve users.[12,19,24,72,86]

The kidney produces locally homeostatic PGs largely via COX-1, including PGI_2, PGE_2, and PGD_2, that maintain adequate glomerular filtration rate (GFR) and RBF and function by augmenting renal vasodilation, inhibiting sodium chloride absorption, and antagonizing the action of antidiuretic hormone (vasopressin). Antiinflammatory drugs oppose this homeostatic renal vasodilation and augment sodium reabsorption, blunting the antihypertensive effect of thiazide and loop diuretics. Antiinflammatory drugs also decrease renin synthesis, a mechanism shared by β-adrenergic antagonists, rendering this

TABLE 35–2 Selected Adverse Effects of Nonsteroidal Antiinflammatory Drugs

Gastrointestinal

Acute: dyspepsia, ulceration, perforation, hemorrhage, elevated hepatic aminotransferases, hepatocellular injury (rare)
Chronic: same as above

Renal

Acute: acute kidney failure, fluid and electrolyte retention, hyperkalemia, hypertension interstitial nephritis, nephrotic syndrome, papillary necrosis, azotemia
Chronic: same as above

Hypersensitivity or Pulmonary

Acute: asthma exacerbation, anaphylactoid and anaphylactic reactions, urticaria, angioedema, acute respiratory distress syndrome, drug-induced lupus
Chronic: angioedema, drug-induced lupus

Hematologic

Acute: increased bleeding time, agranulocytosis, aplastic anemia, thrombocytopenia, neutropenia, hemolytic anemia
Chronic: same as above

Central Nervous System

Acute: headache, dizziness, lethargy, coma, aseptic meningitis, delirium, cognitive dysfunction, hallucinations, psychosis
Chronic: same as above

Drug Interactions

Aminoglycosides: increased risk of aminoglycoside toxicity[77]
Anticoagulants (eg, warfarin, salicylates, heparins, direct thrombin inhibitors and Xa inhibitors): increased risk of gastrointestinal bleeding[11,75]
Antihypertensives (especially diuretics, β-adrenergic antagonists, angiotensin receptor blockers and angiotensin-converting enzyme inhibitors): reduced antihypertensive effects[94]
Digoxin: increased risk of digoxin toxicity[85]
Ethanol: increased bleeding time[75]
Lithium: increased risk of lithium toxicity[67]
Methotrexate: increased risk of methotrexate toxicity[67]
Sulfonylureas: increased hypoglycemic effect[83]

antihypertensive therapy less effective.[31,94] Patients with volume contraction (salt and water depletion) or poor cardiac output (congestive heart failure) have elevated concentrations of renal vasoconstrictor substances from stimulation of both the renin–angiotensin–aldosterone axis and the sympathetic nervous system, so NSAID use in these patients inhibits the synthesis of compensatory vasodilatory PGs, resulting in unopposed renal vasoconstriction and causing decreased RBF and GFR. This effect leads to medullary ischemia and possibly acute kidney injury (AKI), particularly in older adults.[70] This vasoconstrictive effect is also associated with COX-2 selective inhibitors and appears to be reversible upon discontinuation of therapy.[60,70,94]

Normal platelet function depends partly on endothelial-derived PGI_2 (largely via constitutively expressed COX-1), which blocks platelet activation and causes vasodilation, allowing blood to flow freely within vessels. At the site of vascular injury, platelets are activated by binding to collagen-bound von Willebrand factor and synthesize and release TXA_2, a potent platelet stimulator and vasoconstrictor. The antiplatelet activity of NSAIDs stems from their ability to inhibit COX-1, thereby inhibiting platelet-stimulating TXA_2 synthesis. Selective COX-2 inhibitors also decrease PGI_2 and TXA_2 synthesis but affect TXA_2 synthesis to a lesser degree, creating a more prothrombotic environment, which is the predominant theory of how selective COX-2 inhibitors increase the risk of adverse cardiovascular events (see later for further discussion).[75]

Prostaglandins play a major role during the initiation of parturition. Administration of exogenous $PGF_{2\alpha}$ and PGE_2 is used to induce uterine activity, and indomethacin was used successfully as a tocolytic agent by blunting PG-mediated uterine stimulation. However, a major clinical drawback in using NSAIDs as tocolytics is their potential to cause premature constriction or closure of the ductus arteriosus in utero. Vasodilatory PGs are required to keep the fetal ductus arteriosus patent, and inhibiting these PGs causes fetal ductal constriction, leading to pulmonary hypertension and persistent fetal circulation after birth.[58]

CARDIOVASCULAR RISK OF SELECTIVE CYCLOOXYGENASE-2 INHIBITORS AND NONSELECTIVE NONSTEROIDAL ANTIINFLAMMATORY DRUGS

Atherosclerosis is a dynamic process of thrombus formation and inflammation involving numerous tissue factors and inflammatory mediators.[32] Given the ability to inhibit synthesis of proinflammatory PGs, selective COX-2 inhibitors would be expected to be antithrombotic; however, their ability to inhibit endothelial-derived PGI_2 combined with their relative inability to inhibit platelet-activating TXA_2 (a predominantly COX-1 effect) shifts the balance toward thrombus formation.[59]

In 2004, Merck pharmaceutical company withdrew rofecoxib from the worldwide market given the prepublication results of a study demonstrating an undisputed elevated cardiovascular risk.[15] Several other studies addressing selective COX-2 inhibitors had similarly increased risk of adverse cardiovascular events, suggesting this to be a class effect.[27,66,82] Valdecoxib was subsequently removed from the market, leaving celecoxib as the only selective COX-2 inhibitor available. The FDA mandated that Pfizer, the manufacturer of celecoxib, include "black box" warnings to customers of the serious cardiovascular risks and conduct a cardiovascular safety trial, which was called the Prospective Randomized Evaluation of Celecoxib Integrated Safety versus Ibuprofen or Naproxen (PRECISION) trial. This noninferiority trial was completed in 2016 and concluded that moderate doses of celecoxib were not inferior to ibuprofen or naproxen in regards to cardiovascular death (hemorrhagic death, nonfatal myocardial infarction, nonfatal stroke).[65,82]

The current data on nonselective NSAID use suggest an increase in cardiovascular risk, yet this risk varies depending on the nonselective NSAID being used. Some nonselective NSAIDs show a trend toward elevated cardiovascular risk (eg, diclofenac, meloxicam, indomethacin, and, to a lesser extent, ibuprofen), but naproxen shows a trend toward minimal cardiovascular risk. In 2015, the FDA strengthened the warning labels required for prescription and nonprescription NSAIDs to include more information regarding the potential risks for heart attack and stroke.[21,33,55,78,91]

CLINICAL MANIFESTATIONS

Nonsteroidal antiinflammatory drugs are a heterogeneous class of drugs, some carrying a unique toxicity profile. Fortunately, most nonselective NSAIDs behave similarly in overdose, although much of the medical literature specifically describes ibuprofen. Regardless of the particular NSAID ingested, symptoms typically manifest within 4 hours after ingestion.[37-39,51,54,90]

Initial clinical manifestations are usually mild and predominantly include GI symptoms, such as nausea, vomiting, or abdominal pain, or neurologic symptoms, such as drowsiness, headache, tinnitus, blurred vision, diplopia, and dizziness. More moderate and severe findings are rare and include coma, seizures, central nervous system (CNS) depression, metabolic acidosis, hypotension, hypothermia, rhabdomyolysis, electrolyte imbalances, cardiac dysrhythmias, and AKI.[20,37,38,51,54,90] Massive NSAID ingestions lead to multisystem organ failure and death.[22,43,80,89,95]

Neurologic Effects

The neurologic effects of NSAID use vary from the mild drowsiness, headache, and dizziness with therapeutic dosing to the more life-threatening CNS depression, coma, and seizures in overdose. The mechanism associated with the decreased level of consciousness is unknown; however, several animal studies suggest a relationship with opioid receptors, and a human case report documents a dramatic return of consciousness in a child after intravenous (IV) administration of high-dose naloxone.[28] Other reported neurologic manifestations of toxicity include optic neuritis, amblyopia, color blindness, transient diplopia, other visual disturbances, transient loss of hearing, acute psychosis, and cognitive dysfunction.[40,67]

Drug-induced aseptic meningitis is reported with several NSAIDs, including tolmetin, rofecoxib, naproxen, sulindac, piroxicam, and diclofenac, but ibuprofen is more commonly implicated, perhaps because of its widespread use. The incidence of developing aseptic meningitis is unknown but thought to be very low. Clinical findings appear shortly after exposure and are similar to infectious meningitis, including fever and chills, headache, meningeal signs, nausea, vomiting, and altered mental status. Additionally, patients also display symptoms consistent with an allergic reaction, such as erythema, face edema, and conjunctivitis. Cerebrospinal fluid findings include pleocytosis (mainly neutrophils), elevated protein, normal or low glucose, and negative cultures. Studies suggest an allergic mechanism behind NSAID-induced aseptic meningitis because it appears to occur with select NSAIDs and not the whole class, it is not dose-dependent, and symptoms present much quicker with reexposure. An immunologic mechanism is also suggested because it appears to be more common in patients with systemic lupus erythematosus (SLE) or mixed connective tissue disease.[1,40,63,67]

Some studies describe a condition termed "medication overuse headache" in patients who regularly take NSAIDs for migraine or tension-type headaches and whose headaches resolve after discontinuation of NSAIDs.[1] Muscle twitching and generalized tonic-clonic seizures are described with mefenamic acid overdose and usually occur within 7 hours after ingestion.[2] Seizures are also associated with ibuprofen overdose,[69] although the specific mechanism is unknown.

Renal and Electrolyte Effects

Both acute overdose and chronic therapeutic dosing of NSAIDs have deleterious effects on kidney function, most of which are reversible. These include sodium retention and edema, hyperkalemia, AKI, membranous nephropathy, nephrotic syndrome, interstitial nephritis, and both acute and chronic renal papillary necrosis.[40,71,94] The incidence of developing these serious side effects is about 1% to 5% of those exposed but approaches 20% in patients with comorbidities, such as congestive heart failure, volume depletion, diabetes mellitus, underlying kidney disease, SLE, cirrhosis, diuretic therapy, and advanced age.[41,52] There is also growing concern over the potential development of AKI with NSAID use in patients who are concurrently taking multiple antihypertensive medications, such as diuretics, angiotensin-converting enzyme inhibitors, and angiotensin receptor blockers.[49]

Acute tubulointerstitial nephritis (ATIN) is one of the more common forms of NSAID-induced renal impairment, occurring with short-term therapeutic dosing.[25,52] Many cases of ATIN probably go undiagnosed because clinical symptoms usually do not appear until significant renal impairment occurs.[25,73] Significant elevations in blood urea nitrogen (azotemia) occur in older patients within 5 to 7 days of initiating NSAID therapy and usually return to baseline within 2 weeks of discontinuation.[35]

Analgesic abuse nephropathy is a condition whose pathogenesis is not well defined, but it develops from excessive, chronic therapeutic consumption of NSAIDs. This results in AKI manifested by renal papillary necrosis, often requiring hemodialysis.[79,94] Analgesic abuse nephropathy was originally described with the use of analgesic combinations including phenacetin and aspirin in addition to caffeine and has decreased in prevalence after the removal of phenacetin from many world markets.

Anion gap metabolic acidosis, with and without AKI, complicates many acute, massive ibuprofen ingestions and is often profound.[26,43,95,96] The cause of the acidosis in this setting is most likely multifactorial, involving profound hypotension and tissue hypoperfusion with elevated lactate concentrations and the accumulation of ibuprofen and its two major metabolites, all weak acids.[51] An elevated anion gap metabolic acidosis with elevated lactate concentrations is also described after naproxen overdose, suggesting this to be a class effect given that all NSAIDs are acid derivatives.[14]

Use of NSAIDs by pregnant women is associated with reversible oligohydramnios and is used therapeutically as a treatment modality for polyhydramnios. Decreased fetal urine output and neonatal acute and chronic kidney failure, including transient oligoanuria, are associated with gestational NSAID use, commonly indomethacin.[6,30,45]

Gastrointestinal Effects

Adverse GI effects from acute and chronic NSAID use range from mild dyspepsia to ulcer formation, which can lead to life-threatening GI hemorrhage and perforation. Factors that influence the risk of developing symptoms include number, duration, and dose of NSAID; concomitant usage of an anticoagulant, antiplatelet, steroid, or selective serotonin reuptake inhibitor; age; prior history of ulcer; *H. pylori* status; and comorbidities.[76]

Dyspepsia is the most common adverse GI effect, occurring in up to 60% of patients, but most patients with dyspepsia do not have ulcers. Studies suggest 20% to 30% of chronic NSAID users have ulcers, although many are asymptomatic and clinically insignificant. To help prevent the development of ulcers associated with NSAID therapy, concomitant use of misoprostol (a PGE_1 analog), an H_2-receptor antagonist, or a proton pump inhibitor (PPI) is often used; however, PPIs are superior for both preventing and healing gastroduodenal ulcers resulting from chronic NSAID therapy.[72,76] The annual incidence of developing a symptomatic or clinical significant upper GI ulcer is 2.5% to 4.5%, but that of developing a perforation, hemorrhage, or obstruction is 1% to 1.5%.[76] The relative risk of developing gastroduodenal perforation, ulcer, or hemorrhage during chronic, therapeutic NSAID therapy ranges from 2.7 to 5.4, with ketorolac posing the greatest risk.[68,88] Acute NSAID overdoses cause bloody emesis; fecal occult blood loss; and severe, life-threatening GI hemorrhage.

Nonsteroidal antiinflammatory drug–induced hepatotoxicity is a well-known adverse effect that prompted the removal of several NSAIDs from the market. Hepatotoxicity occurs with an incidence of less than 0.1% and can be quite difficult to diagnose because many patients on chronic NSAID therapy have underlying conditions, such as SLE or rheumatoid arthritis, that cause hepatotoxicity. NSAID-induced hepatotoxicity is an idiosyncratic reaction primarily causing hepatocellular injury and does not depend on the chemical class. Diclofenac and sulindac are most commonly implicated.[87]

Immunologic and Dermatologic Effects

The nonimmunologic anaphylactoid and the IgE-mediated anaphylactic reactions that are reported with the use of NSAIDs are clinically indistinguishable from one another, producing flushing, urticaria, bronchospasm, edema, and hypotension. Evidence for anaphylactic reactions includes the presence of NSAID-specific IgE antibodies, positive wheal-and-flare skin reactions, and lack of cross-reactivity with oral challenges of aspirin and other NSAIDs.[8] The proposed mechanism of NSAID-induced anaphylactoid reactions involves the inhibition of COX-1, which not only inhibits the production of PGE_2 (which causes bronchodilation and inhibits the release of histamine from mast cells and basophils) but also shunts the AA metabolism to increased production of bronchoconstricting LTs.

The term *aspirin-sensitive asthmatic* is a bit of a misnomer because it refers to anaphylactoid reactions that occur with any COX-1–inhibiting NSAID, not only aspirin. Selective COX-2 inhibitors cause similar clinical reactions but with an unclear mechanism. There is little cross-reactivity between NSAIDs and selective COX-2 inhibitors, and reports of reactions to one COX-2 inhibitor and not another suggest a predominant IgE-mediated mechanism.[8,47,84]

The most common skin reactions include angioedema and facial swelling, urticaria and pruritus, bullous eruptions, and photosensitivity. Although rare, toxic epidermal necrolysis and Stevens-Johnson syndrome are reported.[40]

Hematologic Effects

As a class, NSAIDs are frequently implicated in the development of drug-induced thrombocytopenia and cause adverse effects on most other cell lines and function, including agranulocytosis, aplastic anemia, hemolytic anemia, methemoglobinemia, and pancytopenia.[5,23,40,46,62] Specifically, phenylbutazone in chronic, therapeutic doses was associated with agranulocytosis and aplastic anemia,[80] prompting its removal from the US market in the 1970s. The inhibitory effect of NSAIDs on granulocyte adherence, activation, and phagocytosis, in addition to the potential for masking signs and symptoms, is suggested as the mechanism responsible for the association between NSAID use and necrotizing fasciitis.[42]

The ability of a particular type of NSAID to inhibit platelet aggregation and affect bleeding time depends on the dose and half-life because NSAIDs reversibly inhibit COX. One dose of ibuprofen prolongs the bleeding time within 2 hours and persists for up to 12 hours; however, this increase in bleeding time usually remains within the upper limit of normal range. This is in contrast to aspirin, which irreversibly inhibits COX, and typically doubles the bleeding time within 12 hours, returning to normal within 24 to 48 hours.[75] Compared with placebo, flurbiprofen and indobufen clinically inhibit platelet function, thereby decreasing vascular reocclusion after angioplasty and preventing thromboembolic complications.[10,16] The concern over whether ketorolac has clinically significant effects on postoperative bleeding remains controversial depending on the surgical procedure and patient population.[18]

Nonsteroidal antiinflammatory drug use potentiates bleeding in patients already at higher risk. These patients include those with thrombocytopenia, coagulation factor deficiencies, or von Willebrand disease and those ingesting alcohol or on warfarin therapy.[75]

Cardiovascular Effects

Although no evidence supports a direct cardiotoxic effect of NSAIDs or their metabolites, acute and massive NSAID overdoses are complicated by persistent and severe hypotension; myocardial ischemia; and cardiac conduction abnormalities and dysrhythmias, including bradycardia, ventricular tachycardia or fibrillation, and prolonged QT interval.[26,43,95] The cause of these findings is yet to be elucidated, although these effects are reported only in severely ill patients with acid–base abnormalities and multisystem organ involvement (see Cardiovascular Risk earlier).

Pulmonary Effects

Although there is no evidence of direct pulmonary toxicity, some case reports describe the development of acute respiratory distress syndrome similar to the clinical manifestations of salicylate toxicity, suggesting an NSAID class mechanism–based process.[26,43,50,57] Although chest radiographic findings such as bilateral pulmonary infiltrates appear to resolve rapidly, one study reported persistent clinical abnormalities associated with exertional dyspnea 1 month later (see Immunologic Effects earlier).[57]

DIAGNOSTIC TESTING

Serum concentrations of most NSAIDs can be determined but usually only by a specialty laboratory requiring several days to report results. Although ibuprofen nomograms were constructed in an attempt to correlate serum concentrations with clinical toxicity,[37,44] the utility of these nomograms proved limited.[39,54]

We recommend obtaining laboratory measurements, including complete blood count, serum electrolytes, blood urea nitrogen, and creatinine, for all symptomatic patients, patients with intentional ingestions, ibuprofen ingestion of greater than 400 mg/kg in a child, or ibuprofen ingestion of greater than 6 g in an adult.[39] For patients presenting with significant neurologic effects, such as CNS depression, further evaluation of acid–base and ventilatory status by blood gas, hepatic aminotransferases, and prothrombin time are recommended. A computed tomography scan of the head and a lumbar puncture is clinically indicated in cases of suspected aseptic meningitis or when structural or infectious etiologies are suspected. An acetaminophen (APAP) concentration should always be determined in patients with intentional ingestions and in patients presenting with an unclear history because many people mistake APAP for NSAIDs and many variably compounded analgesics because of confusing labeling

and packaging or unawareness that they are completely different types of analgesics. For similar reasons, obtaining a salicylate concentration is reasonable.

MANAGEMENT

Management of a patient with an NSAID overdose is largely supportive and guided by the clinical signs and symptoms. Most asymptomatic patients with intentional overdose and those with normal vital signs require observation for 4 to 6 hours and a serum APAP concentration before being medically cleared. Children with ibuprofen ingestions of less than 100 mg/kg can be observed at home, but those who ingest greater than 400 mg/kg are at high risk for toxicity and require medical evaluation.[39] We recommend GI decontamination with activated charcoal (AC) for asymptomatic patients with the potential for a large ingestion, symptomatic patients, and children with a history of ibuprofen ingestion greater than 400 mg/kg.[39,48] Given that serum concentration of ibuprofen continues to increase after the time of emergency department arrival in patients with massive overdose, AC can be administered immediately. For patients with massive overdoses of sustained-release preparations, gastric lavage followed by AC and subsequent multiple-dose AC is reasonable.[95]

Patients who develop severe, life-threatening manifestations usually present with lethargy or unresponsiveness.[26,43,57,69,95] Aggressive, supportive care is indicated in these patients, including stabilization of the airway and IV fluid therapy. An early electrocardiogram is essential to detect any significant electrolyte abnormalities or conduction disturbances. Electrolyte imbalances should be corrected and sodium bicarbonate therapy administered for life-threatening metabolic acidosis. Hypotension should be treated initially with IV fluid therapy followed by direct-acting vasopressors if necessary. Electrocardiograms should be monitored for the development of any life-threatening electrolyte imbalances or cardiac conduction abnormalities.

Given their high protein binding and low volumes of distribution, NSAIDs are not amenable to extracorporeal removal techniques and thus, we recommend not to perform hemodialysis to remove an NSAID; however, in cases of refractory metabolic acidosis or AKI, hemodialysis or continuous renal replacement therapies are useful to correct the acid–base status.[7,50] Patients with seizures, which are characteristic of mefenamic acid overdose,[2] should be treated with IV benzodiazepines.

SUMMARY

- Antiinflammatory drugs are among the most commonly used drugs in the world.
- Most patients with NSAID overdoses develop nonspecific symptoms, including nausea and abdominal discomfort, requiring little clinical management other than psychiatric assessment.
- Gastrointestinal decontamination is recommended in patients with large intentional ingestions.
- In all cases of intentional NSAID ingestion, APAP coingestion should be excluded.

REFERENCES

1. Auriel E, et al. Nonsteroidal anti-inflammatory drugs exposure and the central nervous system. *Handb Clin Neurol.* 2014;119:577-584.
2. Balali-Mood M, et al. Mefenamic acid overdosage. *Lancet Lond Engl.* 1981;1:1354-1356.
3. Bannwarth B, et al. Clinical pharmacokinetics of nonsteroidal anti-inflammatory drugs in the cerebrospinal fluid. *Biomed Pharmacother.* 1989;43:121-126.
4. Battistella M, et al. Risk of upper gastrointestinal hemorrhage in warfarin users treated with nonselective NSAIDs or COX-2 inhibitors. *Arch Intern Med.* 2005;165:189-192.
5. van den Bemt PMLA, et al. Drug-induced immune thrombocytopenia. *Drug Saf.* 2004;27:1243-1252.
6. Benini D, et al. In utero exposure to nonsteroidal anti-inflammatory drugs: neonatal renal failure. *Pediatr Nephrol Berl Ger.* 2004;19:232-234.
7. Bennett RR, et al. Acute oliguric renal failure due to ibuprofen overdose. *South Med J.* 1985;78:490-491.
8. Berkes EA. Anaphylactic and anaphylactoid reactions to aspirin and other NSAIDs. *Clin Rev Allergy Immunol.* 2003;24:137-147.

9. Bernareggi A. Clinical pharmacokinetics of nimesulide. *Clin Pharmacokinet.* 1998;35: 247-274.

10. Bhana N, McClellan KJ. Indobufen: an updated review of its use in the management of atherothrombosis. *Drugs Aging.* 2001;18:369-388.

11. Bjorkman DJ. The effect of aspirin and nonsteroidal anti-inflammatory drugs on prostaglandins. *Am J Med.* 1998;105(suppl 1):8S-12S.

12. Bjorkman DJ. Current status of nonsteroidal anti-inflammatory drug (NSAID) use in the United States: risk factors and frequency of complications. *Am J Med.* 1999;107:3-8.

13. Bombardier C, et al. Comparison of upper gastrointestinal toxicity of rofecoxib and naproxen in patients with rheumatoid arthritis. *N Engl J Med.* 2000;343:1520-1528.

14. Bortone E, et al. Triphasic waves associated with acute naproxen overdose: a case report. *Clin EEG Electroencephalogr.* 1998;29:142-145.

15. Bresalier RS, et al. Cardiovascular events associated with rofecoxib in a colorectal adenoma chemoprevention trial. *N Engl J Med.* 2005;352:1092-1102.

16. Brochier ML. Evaluation of flurbiprofen for prevention of reinfarction and reocclusion after successful thrombolysis or angioplasty in acute myocardial infarction. The Flurbiprofen French Trial. *Eur Heart J.* 1993;14:951-957.

17. Capone ML, et al. Clinical pharmacology of platelet, monocyte, and vascular cyclooxygenase inhibition by naproxen and low-dose aspirin in healthy subjects. *Circulation.* 2004;109:1468-1471.

18. Chan DK, Parikh SR. Perioperative ketorolac increases post-tonsillectomy hemorrhage in adults but not children. *Laryngoscope.* 2014;124:1789-1793.

19. Chan FKL. NSAID-induced peptic ulcers and *Helicobacter pylori* infection: implications for patient management. *Drug Saf.* 2005;28:287-300.

20. Chelluri L, Jastremski MS. Coma caused by ibuprofen overdose. *Crit Care Med.* 1986;14:1078-1079.

21. US Food and Drug Administration. Consumer Updates. FDA Strengthens Warning of Heart Attack and Stroke Risk for Non-Steroidal Anti-Inflammatory Drugs. https://www.fda.gov/forconsumers/consumerupdates/ucm453610.htm. Accessed April 30, 2017.

22. Court H, Volans GN. Poisoning after overdose with non-steroidal anti-inflammatory drugs. *Adverse Drug React Acute Poisoning Rev.* 1984;3:1-21.

23. Cramer RL, et al. Agranulocytosis associated with etodolac. *Ann Pharmacother.* 1994;28:458-460.

24. Cryer B, Kimmey MB. Gastrointestinal side effects of nonsteroidal anti-inflammatory drugs. *Am J Med.* 1998;105:20S-30S.

25. Dixit MP, et al. Non-steroidal anti-inflammatory drugs-associated acute interstitial nephritis with granular tubular basement membrane deposits. *Pediatr Nephrol Berl Ger.* 2008;23:145-148.

26. Downie A, et al. Severe metabolic acidosis complicating massive ibuprofen overdose. *Postrad Med J.* 1993;69:575-577.

27. Drazen JM. COX-2 inhibitors—a lesson in unexpected problems. *N Engl J Med.* 2005; 352:1131-1132.

28. Easley RB, Altemeier WA. Central nervous system manifestations of an ibuprofen overdose reversed by naloxone. *Pediatr Emerg Care.* 2000;16:39-41.

29. Edlund A, et al. Coronary flow regulation in patients with ischemic heart disease: release of purines and prostacyclin and the effect of inhibitors of prostaglandin formation. *Circulation.* 1985;71:1113-1120.

30. Fieni S, et al. Oligohydramnios and fetal renal sonographic appearances related to prostaglandin synthetase inhibitors. A case report. *Fetal Diagn Ther.* 2004;19:224-227.

31. FitzGerald GA, Patrono C. The coxibs, selective inhibitors of cyclooxygenase-2. *N Engl J Med.* 2001;345:433-442.

32. Furie B, Furie BC. Mechanisms of thrombus formation. *N Engl J Med.* 2008;359:938-949.

33. Graham DY, et al. Gastric adaptation. Studies in humans during continuous aspirin administration. *Gastroenterology.* 1988;95:327-333.

34. Grosser T, et al. Anti-inflammatory, antipyretic, and analgesic agents; pharmacotherapy of gout. In: Brunton LL, et al, eds. *Goodman & Gilman's: The Pharmacological Basis of Therapeutics.* 12th ed. New York, NY: McGraw-Hill Education; 2011.

35. Gurwitz JH, et al. Nonsteroidal anti-inflammatory drug-associated azotemia in the very old. *JAMA.* 1990;264:471-475.

36. Halford GM, et al. 50th anniversary of the discovery of ibuprofen: an interview with Dr Stewart Adams. *Platelets.* 2012;23:415-422.

37. Hall AH, et al. Ibuprofen overdose: 126 cases. *Ann Emerg Med.* 1986;15:1308-1313.

38. Hall AH, et al. Ibuprofen overdose—a prospective study. *West J Med.* 1988;148: 653-656.

39. Hall AH, et al. Ibuprofen overdose in adults. *J Toxicol Clin Toxicol.* 1992;30:23-37.

40. Halpern SM, et al. Ibuprofen toxicity. A review of adverse reactions and overdose. *Adverse Drug React Toxicol Rev.* 1993;12:107-128.

41. Harirforoosh S, Jamali F. Renal adverse effects of nonsteroidal anti-inflammatory drugs. *Expert Opin Drug Saf.* 2009;8:669-681.

42. Holder EP, et al. Nonsteroidal anti-inflammatory drugs and necrotising fasciitis. An update. *Drug Saf.* 1997;17:369-373.

43. Holubek W, et al. A report of two deaths from massive ibuprofen ingestion. *J. Med. Toxicol.* 2007;3:52-55.

44. Jenkinson ML, et al. The relationship between plasma ibuprofen concentrations and toxicity in acute ibuprofen overdose. *Hum Toxicol.* 1988;7:319-324.

45. Kaplan BS, et al. Renal failure in the neonate associated with in utero exposure to nonsteroidal anti-inflammatory agents. *Pediatr Nephrol Berl Ger.* 1994;8:700-704.

46. Kaushik P, et al. Celecoxib-induced methemoglobinemia. *Ann Pharmacother.* 2004; 38:1635-1638.

47. Kelkar PS, et al. Urticaria and angioedema from cyclooxygenase-2 inhibitors. *J Rheumatol.* 2001;28:2553-2554.

48. Lapatto-Reiniluoto O, et al. Effect of activated charcoal alone or given after gastric lavage in reducing the absorption of diazepam, ibuprofen and citalopram. *Br J Clin Pharmacol.* 1999;48:148-153.

49. Lapi F, et al. Concurrent use of diuretics, angiotensin converting enzyme inhibitors, and angiotensin receptor blockers with non-steroidal anti-inflammatory drugs and risk of acute kidney injury: nested case-control study. *BMJ.* 2013;346:e8525.

50. Le HT, et al. Ibuprofen overdose complicated by renal failure, adult respiratory distress syndrome, and metabolic acidosis. *J Toxicol Clin Toxicol.* 1994;32:315-320.

51. Linden CH, Townsend PL. Metabolic acidosis after acute ibuprofen overdosage. *J Pediatr.* 1987;111(6 Pt 1):922-925.

52. Marasco WA, et al. Ibuprofen-associated renal dysfunction. Pathophysiologic mechanisms of acute renal failure, hyperkalemia, tubular necrosis, and proteinuria. *Arch Intern Med.* 1987;147:2107-2116.

53. Matoga M, et al. Influence of molecular lipophilicity on the diffusion of arylpropionate non-steroidal anti-inflammatory drugs into the cerebrospinal fluid. *Arzneimittelforschung.* 1999;49:477-482.

54. McElwee NE, et al. A prospective, population-based study of acute ibuprofen overdose: complications are rare and routine serum levels not warranted. *Ann Emerg Med.* 1990;19:657-662.

55. McGettigan P, Henry D. Cardiovascular risk and inhibition of cyclooxygenase: a systematic review of the observational studies of selective and nonselective inhibitors of cyclooxygenase 2. *JAMA.* 2006;296:1633-1644.

56. McPherson ML, Cimino NM. Topical NSAID formulations. *Pain Med Malden Mass.* 2013;14(suppl 1):S35-S39.

57. Menzies DG, et al. Fulminant hyperkalaemia and multiple complications following ibuprofen overdose. *Med Toxicol Adverse Drug Exp.* 1989;4:468-471.

58. Moise KJ, et al. Indomethacin in the treatment of premature labor. Effects on the fetal ductus arteriosus. *N Engl J Med.* 1988;319:327-331.

59. Mukherjee D, et al. Risk of cardiovascular events associated with selective COX-2 inhibitors. *JAMA.* 2001;286:954-959.

60. Murray MD, Brater DC. Adverse effects of nonsteroidal anti-inflammatory drugs on renal function. *Ann Intern Med.* 1990;112:559-560.

61. Nelson L, et al. Aplastic anemia induced by an adulterated herbal medication. *J Toxicol Clin Toxicol.* 1995;33:467-470.

62. Newton TA, Rose SR. Poisoning with equine phenylbutazone in a racetrack worker. *Ann Emerg Med.* 1991;20:204-207.

63. Nguyen HT, Juurlink DN. Recurrent ibuprofen-induced aseptic meningitis. *Ann Pharmacother.* 2004;38:408-410.

64. Niazi SK, et al. Dose dependent pharmacokinetics of naproxen in man. *Biopharm Drug Dispos.* 1996;17:355-361.

65. Nissen SE, et al. Cardiovascular safety of celecoxib, naproxen, or ibuprofen for arthritis. *N Engl J Med.* 2016;375:2519-2529.

66. Nussmeier NA, et al. Complications of the COX-2 inhibitors parecoxib and valdecoxib after cardiac surgery. *N Engl J Med.* 2005;352:1081-1091.

67. O'Brien WM, Bagby GF. Rare adverse reactions to nonsteroidal antiinflammatory drugs. 4. *J Rheumatol.* 1985;12:785-790.

68. Ofman JJ, et al. A metaanalysis of severe upper gastrointestinal complications of nonsteroidal antiinflammatory drugs. *J Rheumatol.* 2002;29:804-812.

69. Oker EE, et al. Serious toxicity in a young child due to ibuprofen. *Acad Emerg Med.* 2000;7:821-823.

70. Perazella MA, Eras J. Are selective COX-2 inhibitors nephrotoxic? *Am J Kidney Dis.* 2000;35:937-940.

71. Radford MG, et al. Reversible membranous nephropathy associated with the use of nonsteroidal anti-inflammatory drugs. *JAMA.* 1996;276:466-469.

72. Raskin JB. Gastrointestinal effects of nonsteroidal anti-inflammatory therapy. *Am J Med.* 1999;106(suppl 5):3S-12S.

73. Rossert J. Drug-induced acute interstitial nephritis. *Kidney Int.* 2001;60:804-817.

74. Runkel R, et al. Pharmacokinetics of naproxen overdoses. *Clin Pharmacol Ther.* 1976; 20:269-277.

75. Schafer AI. Effects of nonsteroidal anti-inflammatory therapy on platelets. *Am J Med.* 1999;106(suppl 5):25S-36S.

76. Scheiman JM. NSAID-induced gastrointestinal injury: a focused update for clinicians. *J Clin Gastroenterol.* 2016;50:5-10.

77. Scott CS, et al. Renal failure and vestibular toxicity in an adolescent with cystic fibrosis receiving gentamicin and standard-dose ibuprofen. *Pediatr Pulmonol.* 2001;31:314-316.

78. Scott PA, et al. Non-steroidal anti-inflammatory drugs and myocardial infarctions: comparative systematic review of evidence from observational studies and randomised controlled trials. *Ann Rheum Dis.* 2007;66:1296-1304.

79. Segasothy M, et al. Chronic renal disease and papillary necrosis associated with the long-term use of nonsteroidal anti-inflammatory drugs as the sole or predominant analgesic. *Am J Kidney.* 1994;24:17-24.

80. Smolinske SC, et al. Toxic effects of nonsteroidal anti-inflammatory drugs in overdose. An overview of recent evidence on clinical effects and dose-response relationships. *Drug Saf.* 1990;5:252-274.

81. Smyth EM, et al. Lipid-Derived autacoids: eicosanoids and platelet-activating Factor. In: Brunton LL, et al, eds. *Goodman & Gilman's: The Pharmacological Basis of Therapeutics.* 12th ed. New York, NY: McGraw-Hill Education; 2011.

82. Solomon SD, et al. Cardiovascular risk associated with celecoxib in a clinical trial for colorectal adenoma prevention. *N Engl J Med.* 2005;352:1071-1080.

83. Sone H, et al. Ibuprofen-related hypoglycemia in a patient receiving sulfonylurea. *Ann Intern Med.* 2001;134:344.

84. Stevenson DD. Anaphylactic and anaphylactoid reactions to aspirin and other nonsteroidal anti-inflammatory drugs. *Immunology Allergy Clin North Am.* 2001; 21:745-768.

85. Stöllberger C, Finsterer J. Nonsteroidal anti-inflammatory drugs in patients with cardio- or cerebrovascular disorders. *Z Kardiol.* 2003;92:721-729.

86. Tang C-L, et al. Eradication of *Helicobacter pylori* infection reduces the incidence of peptic ulcer disease in patients using nonsteroidal anti-inflammatory drugs: a meta-analysis. *Helicobacter.* 2012;17:286-296.

87. Tolman KG. Hepatotoxicity of non-narcotic analgesics. *Am J Med.* 1998;105(suppl 1B): 13S-19S.

88. Traversa G, et al. Gastroduodenal toxicity of different nonsteroidal antiinflammatory drugs. *Epidemiol Camb Mass.* 1995;6:49-54.

89. Vale JA, Meredith TJ. Acute poisoning due to non-steroidal anti-inflammatory drugs. Clinical features and management. *Med Toxicol.* 1986;1:12-31.

90. Volans G, et al. Ibuprofen overdose. *Int J Clin Pract Suppl.* 2003:54-60.

91. Waksman JC, et al. Nonselective nonsteroidal antiinflammatory drugs and cardiovascular risk: are they safe? *Ann Pharmacother.* 2007;41:1163-1173.

92. Warner TD, et al. Nonsteroid drug selectivities for cyclo-oxygenase-1 rather than cyclo-oxygenase-2 are associated with human gastrointestinal toxicity: a full in vitro analysis. *Proc Natl Acad Sci U S A.* 1999;96:7563-7568.

93. Weideman RA, et al. Risks of clinically significant upper gastrointestinal events with etodolac and naproxen: a historical cohort analysis. *Gastroenterology.* 2004;127:1322-1328.

94. Whelton A. Nephrotoxicity of nonsteroidal anti-inflammatory drugs: physiologic foundations and clinical implications. *Am J Med.* 1999;106(5B):13S-24S.

95. Wood DM, et al. Fatality after deliberate ingestion of sustained-release ibuprofen: a case report. *Crit Care Lond Engl.* 2006;10:R44.

96. Zuckerman GB, Uy CC. Shock, metabolic acidosis, and coma following ibuprofen overdose in a child. *Ann Pharmacother.* 1995;29:869-871.

36 OPIOIDS

Lewis S. Nelson and Dean Olsen

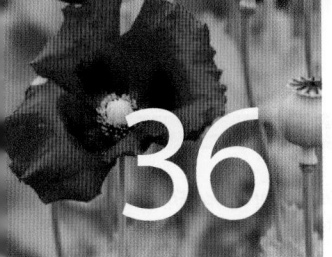

Morphine

Opioids are among the oldest therapies in our pharmacopeia, and clinicians recognize their universal utility to limit human distress from pain. Although opioids are widely used as potent analgesics, they have the potential for abuse because of their psychoactive properties. Although the therapeutic and toxic doses are difficult to predict because of the development of tolerance with chronic use, the primary adverse events from excessive dosing are respiratory depression and sedation.

HISTORY AND EPIDEMIOLOGY

The medicinal value of opium, the dried extract of the poppy plant *Papaver somniferum*, was first recorded circa 1500 B.C. in the Ebers papyrus. Raw opium is composed of at least 10% morphine, but extensive variability exists depending on the environment in which the poppy is grown.[109] Although reformulated as laudanum (deodorized tincture of opium; 10 mg morphine/mL) by Paracelsus, paregoric (camphorated tincture of opium; 0.4 mg morphine/mL), Dover's powder (pulvis Doveri), and Godfrey's cordial in later centuries, the contents remained largely the same: phenanthrene poppy derivatives, such as morphine and codeine. Over the centuries since the Ebers papyrus, opium and its components have been used in two distinct manners: medically to produce profound analgesia and nonmedically to produce psychoactive effects.

Currently, the widest clinical application of opioids is for acute or chronic pain relief. Opioids are available in various formulations that allow administration by virtually any route: epidural, inhalational, intranasal, intrathecal, oral, parenteral (ie, subcutaneous {SC}, intravenous {IV}, intramuscular {IM}), rectal, transdermal, and transmucosal. Patients also benefit from several of the presumed nonanalgesic effects produced by certain opioids. For example, codeine and hydrocodone are widely used as antitussives and loperamide as an antidiarrheal.

Morphine was isolated from opium by Armand Séquin in 1804. Charles Alder Wright synthesized heroin from morphine in 1874. Ironically, the development and marketing of heroin as an antitussive agent by Bayer, the German pharmaceutical company, in 1898 legitimized the medicinal role of heroin.[193] Subsequently, various xenobiotics with opioidlike effects were marketed, each promoted for its presumed advantages over morphine. However, in general, the purported advantages of such medications have fallen short of expectations, particularly with regard to their potential for abuse and addiction.

Unfortunately, the history of opium and its derivatives is marred by humankind's endless quest for xenobiotics that produce pleasurable effects. Opium smoking was so problematic in China by the 1830s that the Chinese government attempted to prohibit the importation of opium by the British East India Company. This act led to two Opium Wars between China and Britain. China eventually accepted the importation and sale of the drug and was forced to turn over Hong Kong to British rule. The euphoric and addictive potential of the opioids is immortalized in the works of several famous writers, such as Thomas de Quincey (*Confessions of an English Opium Eater*, 1821),

Samuel Coleridge (*The Rime of the Ancient Mariner*, 1798), and Elizabeth Barrett Browning (*Aurora Leigh*, 1856).

Because of mounting concerns of addiction and overdose in the United States, the Harrison Narcotics Tax Act, enacted in 1914, made nonanalgesic use of opioids illegal. Since that time and despite extensive legislative and other efforts, recreational and habitual use of heroin and other opioids have remained epidemic in the United States and worldwide and currently are one of the leading causes of death in the United States.

Prescription opioids have until recently accounted for approximately 75% of all opioid-related deaths in the US. In 2009, deaths from prescription drugs, mainly opioids, first exceeded those from motor vehicle crashes.[27] From 2000 to 2015, the rate of deaths from drug overdoses increased 137%, including a 200% increase in the rate of overdose deaths involving opioids (opioid analgesics and heroin).[173]

Current data demonstrate that the United States' opioid epidemic includes two distinct but interrelated trends: a 20-year increase in overdose deaths involving prescription opioid analgesics and a recent surge in illicit opioid overdose deaths, driven largely by heroin and other illicit opioids.[173] Beginning around 2013, the rate of drug overdose deaths involving synthetic opioids increased sharply, driven principally by nonpharmaceutical fentanyl, fentanyl analogs, and novel opioid agonists (U47700 and others). All of these opioids are manufactured in illegal laboratories, primarily in China and Mexico, and imported into the United States more readily than heroin. These illicit opioids are either used to adulterate heroin or are, used to create counterfeit prescription opioid pills, which complicates the attribution of the cause of death in heroin decedents.[77,173,174]

Over the past decade, the realization that opioid analgesics are subject to extensive abuse has led to the development of newer formulations of existing opioids that theoretically reduced abuse potential.[32] The use of "tamper-resistant formulations" was emphasized as an approach to reduce the abuser's ability to crush or dissolve the tablet for insufflation or injection, respectively.[177] Although renamed "abuse deterrent formulations" (ADFs), the true clinical benefit of such formulations in reducing abuse is not known. Descriptions of the means to subvert the deterrence mechanism are widely described on the internet. Because the majority of patients who develop addiction or hyperalgesia ingest intact tablets, ADFs are highly unlikely to beneficially impact these adverse outcome. Although primarily a concern with extended-release or long-acting opioid formulations because of their greater content of opioid, abuse-deterrent immediate-release formulations were recently introduced to address this concern.[102]

The terminology used in this chapter recognizes the broad range of xenobiotics commonly considered to be opiumlike. The term *opiate* specifically refers to the alkaloids naturally derived directly from the opium poppy: morphine; codeine; and, to some extent, thebaine and noscapine. *Opioids* are a much broader class of xenobiotics that are capable of either producing opiumlike effects or binding to opioid receptors. A *semisynthetic opioid*, such as heroin or oxycodone, is created by chemical modification of an opiate. A *synthetic opioid* is a chemical, not derived from an opiate, that is capable of binding to an opioid receptor and producing opioid effects clinically. Synthetic opioids, such as methadone and fentanyl, bear little apparent structural similarity to the opiates. Opioids also include the naturally occurring animal-derived opioid peptides such as endorphin and nociceptin/orphanin FQ. The term *narcotic* refers to sleep-inducing xenobiotics and initially was used to connote the opioids. However, law enforcement and the public currently use the term to indicate any illicit psychoactive substance, including, paradoxically, cocaine. The term *opioid* as used hereafter encompasses the opioids and the opiates.

PHARMACOLOGY

Opioid-Receptor Subtypes

Despite nearly a century of opioid studies, the existence of specific opioid receptors was not proposed until the mid-20th century. Beckett and Casy noted a pronounced stereospecificity of existing opioids (only the L-isomer is active) and postulated that the drug needed to "fit" into a receptor.[11] In 1963, after studies on the clinical interactions of nalorphine and morphine, the theory of receptor dualism[196] postulated the existence of two classes of opioid receptors. Such opioid binding sites were not demonstrated experimentally until 1973.[159] Intensive experimental scrutiny using selective agonists and antagonists continues to permit refinement of receptor classification. The current, widely accepted schema postulates the coexistence of three major classes of opioid receptors, each with multiple subtypes, and several poorly defined minor classes.

Initially, the reason such an elaborate system of receptors existed was unclear because no endogenous ligand could be identified. However, evidence for the existence of such endogenous ligands was uncovered in 1975 with the discovery of metenkephalin and leuenkephalin[129] and the subsequent identification of β-endorphin and dynorphin. As a group, these endogenous ligands for the opioid receptors are called *endorphins* (*endo*genous m*orphine*). Each is a five–amino acid peptide cleaved from a larger precursor peptide: proenkephalin, proopiomelanocortin, and prodynorphin, respectively. Additionally, a minor related endogenous opioid (nociceptin/orphanin FQ) and its receptor ORL are described.

All three major opioid receptors have been cloned and sequenced. Each consists of seven transmembrane segments, an amino terminus, and a carboxy terminus. Significant sequence homology exists between the transmembrane regions of opioid receptors and those of other members of the guanosine triphosphate (GTP)–binding protein (G-protein)–binding receptor superfamily. However, the extracellular and intracellular segments differ from one another. These nonhomologous segments probably represent the ligand-binding and signal transduction regions, respectively, which would be expected to differ among the three classes of receptors. The individual receptors have distinct distribution patterns within the central nervous system (CNS) and peripherally on nerve endings within various tissues, mediating unique but not entirely understood clinical effects. Until recently, researchers used varying combinations of agonists and antagonists to pharmacologically distinguish between the different receptor subtypes. However, knockout mice (ie, mutant mice lacking the genes for an individual opioid receptor) promise new insights into this complex subject.[72]

Because multiple opioid receptors exist and each elicits a different effect, determining the receptor to which an opioid preferentially binds should allow prediction of the clinical effect of the opioid. However, binding typically is not limited to one receptor type, and the relative affinity of an opioid for differing receptors accounts for the clinical effects (Table 36–1). Even the endogenous opioid peptides exhibit substantial crossover among the receptors.

Although the familiar pharmacologic nomenclature derived from the Greek alphabet is used throughout this textbook, the International Union of Pharmacology (IUPHAR) Committee on Receptor Nomenclature has twice recommended a nomenclature change from the original Greek symbol system to make opioid receptor names more consistent with those of other neurotransmitter systems.[220] In the first new schema, the receptors were denoted by their endogenous ligand (*opioid peptide* [OP]), with a subscript identifying their chronologic order of discovery.[52] The δ receptor was renamed OP_1, the κ receptor was renamed OP_2, and the μ receptor was renamed OP_3. However, adoption of this nomenclature met with significant resistance, presumably because of problems that would arise when merging previously published work that had used the Greek symbol nomenclature. The currently proposed nomenclature suggests the addition of a single letter in front of the OP designation and the elimination of the number. In this schema, the μ receptor is identified as MOP. In addition, the latest iteration formally recognizes the nociceptin/orphanin FQ or NOP receptor as a fourth receptor family.

TABLE 36–1	**Clinical Effects Related to Opioid Receptors**		
1996 Conventional Name	Proposed IUPHAR Name	IUPHAR Name	Important Clinical Effects of Receptor Agonists
$μ_1$	OP_{3a}	MOP	Supraspinal analgesia / Peripheral analgesia / Sedation / Euphoria / Prolactin release
$μ_2$	OP_{3b}	MOP	Spinal analgesia / Respiratory depression / Physical dependence / Gastrointestinal dysmotility / Pruritus / Bradycardia / Growth hormone release
$κ_1$	OP_{2a}	KOP	Spinal analgesia / Miosis / Diuresis
$κ_2$	OP_{2b}	KOP	Psychotomimesis / Dysphoria
$κ_3$	OP_{2b}	KOP	Supraspinal analgesia
δ	OP_1	DOP	Spinal and supraspinal analgesia / Modulation of μ-receptor function / Inhibit release of dopamine
Nociceptin/ orphanin FQ	OP_4	NOP	Anxiolysis / Analgesia

IUPHAR = International Union of Pharmacology Committee on Receptor Nomenclature.

Mu Receptor (μ, MOP, OP_3)

The early identification of the μ receptor as the morphine binding site gave this receptor its designation.[135] Although many exogenous xenobiotics produce supraspinal analgesia via μ receptors, the endogenous ligand is elusive. Nearly all of the recognized endogenous opioids have some affinity for the μ receptor, although none is selective for the receptor. Endomorphin-1 and -2 are nonpeptide ligands present in brain that may represent the endogenous ligand.

Experimentally, two subtypes ($μ_1$ and $μ_2$) are well defined, although currently no xenobiotics have sufficient selectivity to make this dichotomy clinically relevant. Experiments with knockout mice suggest that both subtypes derive from the same gene and that either posttranslational changes or local cellular effects subsequently differentiate them. The $μ_1$ subtype is responsible for supraspinal (brain) analgesia and for the euphoria sometimes engendered by these xenobiotics. Although stimulation of the $μ_2$ subtype produces spinal-level analgesia, it also produces respiratory depression. Predictably, μ receptors are found in the medullary cough center, peripherally in the gastrointestinal (GI) tract, and on various sensory nerve endings, including the articular surfaces (see analgesia under Clinical Manifestations later). All of the currently available μ agonists have some activity at the $μ_2$ receptor and therefore produce some degree of respiratory compromise. This localization of μ receptors to regions of the brain involved in analgesia (periaqueductal gray, nucleus raphe magnus, medial thalamus), euphoria and reward (mesolimbic system), and respiratory function (medulla) is expected.[89]

Kappa Receptor (κ, KOP, OP_2)

Although dynorphins now are known to be the endogenous ligands for these receptors, originally, they were identified by their ability to bind ketocyclazocine and thus were labeled κ.[135] These receptors exist predominantly in the spinal cords of higher animals, but they also are found in the antinociceptive regions of the brain and the substantia nigra. Stimulation is responsible for spinal analgesia, miosis, and diuresis (via inhibition of antidiuretic hormone release). κ-receptor stimulation is not associated with significant respiratory depression or constipation. The receptor currently is subclassified into three subtypes. The $κ_1$ receptor subtype is responsible for spinal analgesia. This analgesia is not reversed by μ-selective antagonists,[143] supporting the role of κ receptors as independent mediators of analgesia. Although the function of the $κ_2$ receptor subtype is largely unknown, stimulation of cerebral $κ_2$ receptors by xenobiotics such as pentazocine and salvinorin A produces psychotomimesis in distinction to the euphoria evoked by μ agonists.[186] The $κ_3$ receptor subtype is found throughout the brain and participates in supraspinal analgesia. This receptor is primarily responsible for the action of nalorphine, an agonist–antagonist opioid. Nalbuphine, another agonist–antagonist, exerts its analgesic effect via both $κ_1$ and $κ_3$ agonism, although both nalorphine and nalbuphine are antagonists to morphine at the μ receptor.[161]

Delta Receptor (δ, DOP, OP_1)

Little is known about δ receptors, although the enkephalins are their endogenous ligands. Opioid peptides identified in the skin and brain of *Phyllomedusa* frogs, termed *dermorphin* and *deltorphin*, respectively, are potent agonists at the δ receptor. δ receptors have important in spinal and supraspinal analgesia (probably via a noncompetitive interaction with the μ receptor) and in cough suppression. δ receptors mediate dopamine release from the nigrostriatal pathway, where they modulate the motor activity associated with amphetamine.[90] Conversely these receptors do not modulate dopamine in the mesolimbic tracts and have only a slight behavioral reinforcing role. Subpopulations, specifically $δ_1$ and $δ_2$, are postulated based on in vitro studies but presently are not confirmed in vivo.[220]

Nociceptin/Orphanin FQ Receptor (ORL_1, NOP, OP_4)

The ORL_1 receptor was identified in 1994 based on sequence homology during screening for opioid-receptor genes with DNA libraries. It has a similar distribution pattern in the brain and uses similar transduction mechanisms as the other opioid-receptor subtypes. It binds many different opioid agonists and antagonists. Its insensitivity to antagonism by naloxone, often considered the sine qua non of opioid character, delayed its acceptance as an opioid-receptor subtype. Simultaneous identification of an endogenous ligand, called *nociceptin* by the French investigators and *orphanin* FQ by the Swiss investigators, allowed the designation OP_4. A clinical role has not yet been defined, but anxiolytic and analgesic properties are described.[38]

Opioid-Receptor Signal Transduction Mechanisms

Figure 36–1 illustrates opioid-receptor signal transduction mechanisms. Research on the mechanisms by which an opioid receptor induces an effect continues to produce confusing and often contradictory results. Despite the initial theory that each receptor subtype is linked to a specific transduction mechanism, individual receptor subtypes use one or more mechanisms, depending on several factors, including receptor localization (eg, presynaptic versus postsynaptic). As noted, all opioid-receptor subtypes are members of a superfamily of membrane-bound receptors that are coupled to G proteins.[220] The G proteins are responsible for signaling the cell that the receptor is activated and for initiating the desired cellular effects. The G proteins are generally of the pertussis toxin-sensitive, inhibitory subtype known as G_i or G_o, although coupling to a cholera toxin-sensitive, excitatory G_s subtype is described. Regardless of subsequent effect, the G proteins consist of three conjoined subunits, α, β, and γ. The βγ subunit is liberated upon GTP binding to the subunit. When the α subunit dissociates from the βγ subunit, it modifies specific effector systems, such as phospholipase C or adenylate cyclase, or directly affect a channel or transport protein. Guanidine triphosphate subsequently is hydrolyzed by a GTPase intrinsic to the α subunit, which prompts its reassociation with the βγ subunit and termination of the receptor-mediated effect.

CLINICAL MANIFESTATIONS

Table 36–2 outlines the clinical effects of opioids.

Therapeutic Effects of Opioids
Analgesia and Euphoria

Although classical teaching attributes opioid analgesia solely to the brain, opioids actually modulate cerebral cortical pain perception at supraspinal, spinal, and peripheral levels. The regional distribution of the opioid receptors confirms that μ receptors are responsible for most of the analgesic effects of morphine within the brain. They are found in highest concentration within areas of the brain classically associated with analgesia—the periaqueductal gray, nucleus raphe magnus, locus ceruleus, and medial thalamus. Microelectrode-induced electrical stimulation of these areas[167] or iontophoretic application of agonists into these regions results in profound analgesia.[13] Specifically, enhancement of inhibitory outflow from these supraspinal areas to the sensory nuclei of the spinal cord (dorsal roots) dampens nociceptive neurotransmission. Additionally, inactivation of the μ-opioid–receptor gene in embryonic mouse cells results in offspring that are insensitive to morphine analgesia.[136]

Blockade of the *N*-methyl-D-aspartate (NMDA) receptor, a mediator of excitatory neurotransmission, enhances the analgesic effects of μ-opioid agonists and reduces the development of tolerance (see Dextromethorphan later).[1] Even more intriguing is the finding that low-dose naloxone (0.25 mcg/kg/h) actually improves the efficacy of morphine analgesia.[69] Administration of higher dose, but still low-dose, naloxone (1 mcg/kg/h) obliterated its opioid-sparing effect. Although undefined, the mechanism may be related to selective inhibition of G_s-coupled excitatory opioid receptors by extremely low concentrations of opioid-receptor antagonist.[39,40]

Xenobiotics with strong binding affinity for δ receptors in humans, when given intrathecally, produce significantly more analgesia than morphine administered similarly. Indeed, the use of spinal and epidural opioid analgesia is predicated on the direct administration of opioid near the κ and δ receptors in the spinal cord. Agonist–antagonist opioids, with agonist affinity for the κ receptor and antagonist effects at the μ receptor, maintain analgesic efficacy.

Communication between the immune system and the peripheral sensory nerves occurs in areas of tissue inflammation. In response to inflammatory mediators, such as interleukin-1, immune cells locally release opioid peptides, which bind and activate peripheral opioid receptors on sensory nerve terminals.[221] Agonism at these receptors reduces afferent pain neurotransmission and inhibits the release of other proinflammatory compounds, such as substance P.[199] Intraarticular morphine (1 mg) administered to patients after arthroscopic knee surgery produces significant, long-lasting analgesia that is prevented with intraarticular naloxone.[198] The clinical analgesic effect of 5 mg of intraarticular morphine is equivalent to 5 mg of morphine given IM.[31] Intraarticular analgesia is mediated by local μ receptors.[63]

Antitussive

Codeine and dextromethorphan are two opioids with a suggestion of cough-suppressant activity. Cough suppression is not likely mediated via the $μ_1$ opioid receptor because the ability of other opioids to suppress the medullary cough centers is not correlated with their analgesic effect. Various models suggest that cough suppression occurs via agonism of the $μ_2$ or κ opioid receptors or antagonism of the δ opioid receptor and that the σ or NMDA receptors also are involved.[205]

Nontherapeutic and Adverse Effects of Opioids
Abuse and Addiction

Addiction is defined as a maladaptive pattern of substance use leading to clinically significant impairment or distress. Opioid use disorder (OUD, which replaced the term opioid dependence in the *Diagnostic and Statistical Manual of Mental Disorders,* 5th edition) is defined as a problematic pattern of opioid use leading to clinically significant impairment or distress.[3] Both definitions are determined by a number of diagnostic criteria, including

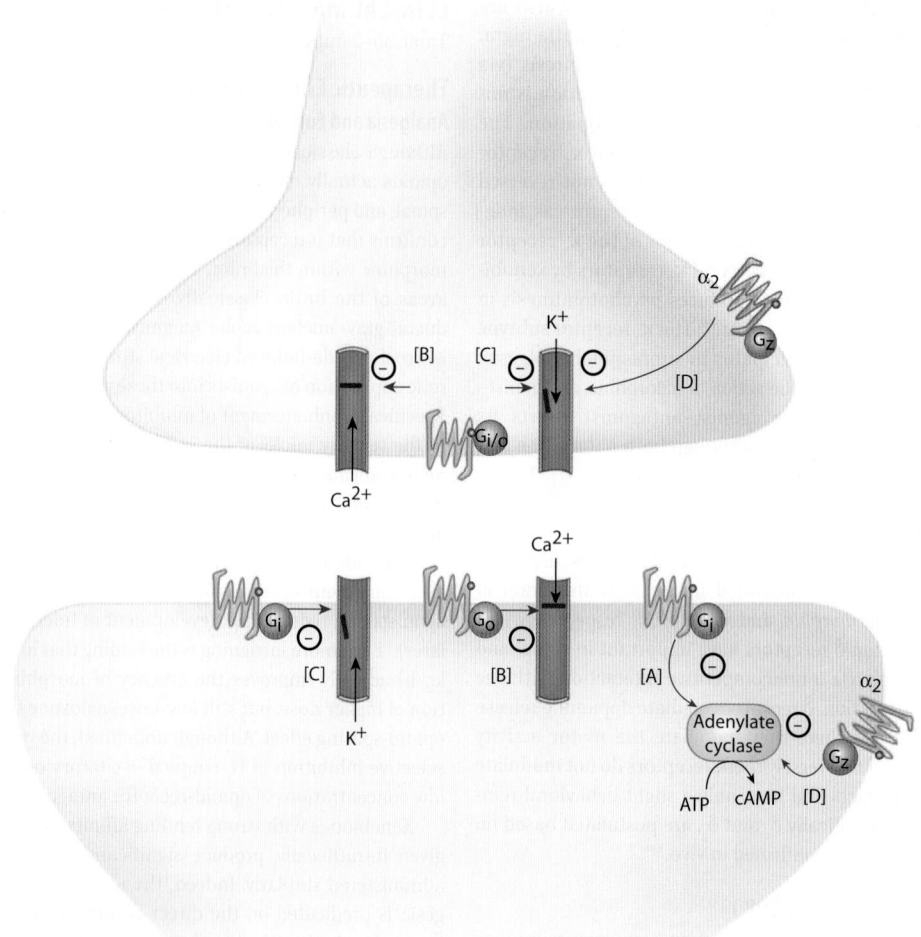

FIGURE 36–1. Opioid-receptor signal transduction mechanisms. Upon binding of an opioid agonist to an opioid receptor, the respective G protein is activated. G proteins (**A**) reduce the capacity of adenylate cyclase to produce cyclic adenosine monophosphate (cAMP); (**B**) close calcium channels that reduce the signal to release neurotransmitters; or (**C**) open potassium channels and hyperpolarize the cell, which indirectly reduces cell activity. Each mechanism is found coupled to each receptor subtype, depending on the location of the receptor (pre- or postsynaptic), and the neuron within the brain (see text). Note that α_2 receptors (**D**) mediate similar effects using a different G protein (G_z).

Adenylate cyclase/cAMP (A). Inhibition of adenylate cyclase activity by G_i or G_o is the classic mechanism for postsynaptic signal transduction invoked by the inhibitory μ receptors. However, this same mechanism is are identified in cells bearing either δ or κ receptors. Activation of cAMP production by adenylate cyclase, with subsequent activation of protein kinase A, occurs after exposure to very-low-dose opioid agonists and produces excitatory, antianalgesic effects.[44]

Calcium (Ca²⁺) channels (B). Presynaptic μ receptors inhibit norepinephrine release from the nerve terminals of cells of the rat cerebral cortex. Adenylate cyclase is not the modulator for these receptors because inhibition of norepinephrine release is not enhanced by increasing intracellular cAMP levels by various methods. Opioid-induced blockade is, however, prevented by increased intracellular calcium concentrations that are induced either by calcium ionophores, which increase membrane permeability to calcium, or by increasing the extracellular calcium concentration. This implies a role for opioid-induced closure of N-type calcium channels, presumably via a G_o protein. Reduced intraterminal concentrations of calcium prevent the neurotransmitter-laden vesicles from binding to the terminal membrane and releasing their contents. Nerve terminals containing dopamine have an analogous relationship with inhibitory κ receptors, as do acetylcholine-bearing neurons with opioid receptors.

Potassium(K⁺) channels (C). Increased conductance through a potassium channel, generally mediated by G_i or G_o, results in membrane hyperpolarization with reduced neuronal excitability. Alternatively, protein kinase A–mediated reduction in membrane potassium conductance enhances neuronal excitability.

tolerance, withdrawal, and deleterious social consequences of opioid use (Table 36–3). Both addiction and OUD share a complicated relationship with, and often overlap, depression and occur in at least 5% of patient using classical definitions and may occur in as many as 40%.[146] This wide range is related to the difficulty of diagnosing misuse, abuse, and OUD in this patient population and inconsistent definitions of misuse and abuse between studies.[30]

Opioid abuse or therapeutic misuse dramatically increases addiction and overdose. Although media reports highlight the abuse of prescription opioids by sports figures and other personalities, such use had simultaneously reached epidemic levels in rural regions of the country where heroin is difficult to obtain. Many of these patients develop an opioid use disorder, particularly addiction, through initial use for therapeutic purposes and then are unable to discontinue their use.

The abuse and addiction liabilities of semisynthetic opioids, based on their subjective profile, are generally similar.[222] Although many users initially receive oxycodone or hydrocodone as analgesics, the majority of abusers obtain the drugs illicitly or from friends.[17,83] Significant efforts by regulatory agencies enhance the understanding and reduce the adverse consequences of opioid use. This includes efforts such as those at the U.S. Food and Drug Administration (FDA) through Risk Evaluation and Mitigation Strategies (REMS), individual states through prescription drug monitoring programs,[158] law enforcement at local and national levels, insurers and pharmacy benefit managers, and the drug manufacturers.[80,216] Physicians and pharmacists have been charged criminally for inappropriate prescribing and dispensing, respectively, for patients with the intent to sell or abuse these drugs.[80]

TABLE 36–2	Clinical Effects of Opioids
Cardiovascular	Bradycardia
	Orthostatic hypotension
	Peripheral vasodilation
Dermatologic	Flushing (histamine)
	Pruritus
Endocrinologic	Reduced antidiuretic hormone release
	Increased prolactin release
	Reduced gonadotrophin release
Gastrointestinal	Increased anal sphincter tone
	Increased biliary tract pressure
	Reduced gastric acid secretion
	Reduced motility (constipation)
Neurologic	Analgesia
	Antitussive
	Euphoria
	Sedation, coma
	Seizures (meperidine, propoxyphene)
Ophthalmic	Miosis
Pulmonary	Acute respiratory distress syndrome
	Bronchospasm (histamine)
	Respiratory depression

It is increasingly clear that the prescribing behavior of physicians has been a driver of the widespread misuse of opioids occurring over the past 2 decades. The reasons for such changes are complex but include a mixture of regulatory, sociological, and financial pressures. Data to support the safety and efficacy of opioids for the management of chronic pain are very limited.

TABLE 36–3	Criteria for Opioid Use Disorder[3]

A problematic pattern of opioid use leading to clinically significant impairment or distress, as manifested by at least two of the following, occurring within a 12-month period:

1. Opioids are often taken in larger amounts or over a longer period than was intended.
2. There is a persistent desire or unsuccessful efforts to cut down or control opioid use.
3. A great deal of time is spent in activities necessary to obtain the opioid, use the opioid, or recover from its effects.
4. Craving, or a strong desire or urge to use opioids.
5. Recurrent opioid use resulting in a failure to fulfill major role obligations at work, school, or home.
6. Continued opioid use despite having persistent or recurrent social or interpersonal problems caused or exacerbated by the effects of opioids.
7. Important social, occupational, or recreational activities are given up or reduced because of opioid use.
8. Recurrent opioid use in situations in which it is physically hazardous.
9. Continued opioid use despite knowledge of having a persistent or recurrent physical or psychological problem that is likely to have been caused or exacerbated by the substance.
10. Tolerance, as defined by either of the following:
    - A need for markedly increased amounts of opioids to achieve intoxication or desired effect
    - A markedly diminished effect with continued use of the same amount of an opioid

Note: This criterion is not considered to be met for those taking opioids solely under appropriate medical supervision.

11. Withdrawal, as manifested by either of the following:
    - The characteristic opioid withdrawal syndrome (refer to Criteria A and B of the criteria set for opioid withdrawal).
    - Opioids (or a closely related substance) are taken to relieve or avoid withdrawal symptoms.

Almost all studies of the long-term use of opioids study periods of use measured in weeks, although in clinical practice patients receive opioid therapy for years. Despite a lack of data, many physicians prescribe opioids for the treatment of chronic nonterminal pain, which results in high rates of OUD. In response to this, the Centers for Disease Control and Prevention has issued guidelines for treatment of chronic pain that encourage alternative medications and therapies initially, discussion of risks of addiction with the patient, use of short-acting opioids, periodic pain and function reassessment, screening for use disorder and diversion, and dispensing of naloxone to patients at risk for overdose.[55]

There is an association between opioids prescribed for acute pain and the development of long-term opioid use.[10,24,33,97,184] Although long-term use reflects ongoing pain, hyperalgesia, dependence, or addiction, the lack of data to support continued beneficial effect compared with harm raises concern. One study suggests the intensity of a physician's opioid prescribing in the emergency department (ED) setting is positively associated with the probability that a patient will become a long-term opioid user over the subsequent 12 months.[10] Another concluded that the likelihood of chronic opioid use after receipt of an opioid prescription increases most sharply in the first days of therapy, particularly after 5 days or 1 month of opioids prescribed.[173] This association was also noted in patients prescribed opioids for postoperative pain with 6% of opioid-naïve patients undergoing both minor and major surgical procedures continuing to use opioids after 90 days after surgery.[21] These studies support the theory that OUD often begins through an initial exposure to a physician-prescribed opioid and that some individuals are "programmed" to have greater reward from and more difficulty discontinuing the use of opioids. The risk of long-term opioid use should be factored into the risk–benefit analysis when considering even short-term opioid therapy.

The pleasurable effects of many xenobiotics used by humans are mediated by the release of dopamine in the mesolimbic system. This final common pathway is shared by all opioids that activate the μ–δ receptor complex in the ventral tegmental area, which, in turn, indirectly promotes dopamine release in the mesolimbic region. Opioids also have a direct reinforcing effect on their self-administration through μ receptors within the mesolimbic system.[88]

The sense of well-being and euphoria associated with strenuous exercise appears to be mediated by endogenous opioid peptides and μ receptors. This so-called "runner's high" is reversible with naloxone.[183] Naloxone reverses euphoria or even produces dysphoria in nonexercising, highly trained athletes.[45,104] Even in normal individuals, high-dose naloxone (4 mg/kg) produces dysphoria.[34]

Exogenous opioids do not induce uniform psychological effects. Some of the exogenous opioids, particularly those that are highly lipophilic such as heroin, are euphorigenic, but morphine is largely devoid of such pleasurable effects.[191] However, morphine administration results in analgesia, anxiolysis, and sedation. Although heroin has little affinity for opioid receptors and must be deacetylated to morphine for effect, these seemingly incompatible properties likely are related to pharmacokinetic differences in blood–brain barrier penetration.[155] Chronic users note that fentanyl produces effects that are subjectively similar to those of heroin.[125] This effect offers an explanation of the higher prevalence of fentanyl, as opposed to other accessible opioids, as an abused drug by anesthesiologists,[15,224] as well as the burgeoning appearance of fentanyl and its analogs as a heroin substitute in the community.[174] In distinction, certain opioids, such as pentazocine, produce dysphoria, an effect that is related to their affinity for κ or σ receptors.

Hyperalgesia

Chronic use of opioid analgesics is associated with hyperalgesia, or a heightened sensitivity to pain.[35] This effect was described decades ago in methadone-maintained patients[92] and is again recognized because of the increased use of chronic opioid therapy for pain.[22] Clinically, hyperalgesia manifests as the need for increasing doses of analgesics to mitigate pain, and it occurs as part of or is confused with the development of tolerance. Conceptually, as opposed to tolerance, which is the progressive failure of a drug to adequately treat the pain, hyperalgesia is the intrinsic increase in the degree of pain in response to an analgesic. The exact mechanisms for the development of opioid-induced hyperalgesia are still not clearly understood. The treatment for hyperalgesia should include weaning from opioids and providing alternative modalities of pain relief.

Miosis

Stimulation of parasympathetic pupilloconstrictor neurons in the Edinger-Westphal nucleus of the oculomotor nerve by morphine produces miosis. Additionally, morphine increases firing of pupilloconstrictor neurons to light,[127] which increases the sensitivity of the light reflex through central reinforcement.[228] Although sectioning of the optic nerve blunts morphine-induced miosis, the consensual reflex in the denervated eye is enhanced by morphine. Because opioids classically mediate inhibitory neurotransmission, hyperpolarization of sympathetic nerves or of inhibitory neurons to the parasympathetic neurons (removal of inhibition) ultimately mediate the classic "pinpoint pupil" associated with opioid use.

Not all patients using opioids present with miosis. Meperidine has a lesser miotic effect than other conventional opioids, and propoxyphene use does not result in miosis.[74] Use of opioids with predominantly κ-agonist effects, such as pentazocine, may not result in miosis. Mydriasis occurs in some severely poisoned patients secondary to hypoxic brain injury. Additionally, concomitant drug use or the presence of adulterants will potentially alter pupillary findings. For example, the combination of heroin and cocaine ("speedball") produces virtually any size pupil, depending on the relative contribution by each xenobiotic. Similarly, patients ingesting diphenoxylate and atropine (Lomotil) or those using scopolamine-adulterated heroin typically develop mydriasis.[84]

Gastrointestinal

Historically, the morphine analog apomorphine was used as a rapidly acting emetic whose clinical use was limited by its tendency to depress the patient's level of consciousness. Emesis induced by apomorphine is mediated through agonism at D_2 receptor subtypes within the chemoreceptor trigger zone of the medulla. Many opioids, particularly morphine, produce significant nausea and vomiting when used therapeutically.[29] Whether these effects are inhibited by naloxone is not clearly established, but they likely are not.

Although loperamide is widely used therapeutically to manage diarrhea, opioid-induced constipation is frequently a bothersome side effect of both medical and nonmedical use of opioids. Constipation, mediated by μ_2 receptors within the smooth muscle of the intestinal wall,[96] is ameliorated by oral naloxone. Provided the first-pass hepatic glucuronidative capacity is not exceeded (at doses of ~6 mg), enteral naloxone is poorly bioavailable and thus induces few, if any, opioid withdrawal symptoms.[142] Methylnaltrexone and naloxegol are bioavailable, "peripherally restricted" opioids that do not cross the blood–brain barrier except in overdose. Although they antagonize the effects of opioids on the GI tract opioid receptor,[17,200] the opioid withdrawal syndrome only occurs rarely (Antidotes in Depth: A4).[141] Lubiprostone is a bicyclic fatty acid derived from prostaglandin E_1 (PGE_1) metabolite that increases fluid secretion in the GI tract. Lubiprostone, methylnaltrexone and naloxegol, are approved by the FDA for treatment of opioid-induced constipation in patients with noncancer pain.[151]

Movement Disorders

Patients infrequently experience acute muscular rigidity with rapid IV injection of certain high-potency opioids, especially fentanyl and its derivatives.[203] This condition is particularly prominent during induction of anesthesia and in neonates.[65] The rigidity primarily involves the trunk and impairs chest wall movement sufficiently to exacerbate hypoventilation. Chest wall rigidity contributes to the lethality associated with epidemics of fentanyl-adulterated or fentanyl-substituted heroin. Although the mechanism of muscle rigidity is unclear, it is likely related to blockade of dopamine receptors in the basal ganglia. Other postulated mechanisms include γ-aminobutyric acid (GABA) antagonism and NMDA agonism. Opioid antagonists generally are therapeutic but do produce adverse hemodynamic effects, withdrawal phenomena,

or uncontrollable pain, depending on the situation.[65] Also, rapid escalation of methadone doses can result in the development of choreoathetoid movements.[14]

Endocrine

Chronic use of opioids is associated with hypofunction of the hypothalamic–pituitary–gonadal axis by binding to hypothalamic opioid receptors and decreasing the secretion of gonadotropin-releasing hormone.[18] Clinical findings include reduced libido, erectile dysfunction, hot flashes, and depression, as well as anemia, hair loss, and osteopenia.[181] Additionally, both men and women may have infertility. Furthermore, opioids reduce the release of corticotropin releasing hormone from the hypothalamus, leading to a reduction of adrenocorticotropic hormone (ACTH) release from the pituitary. This reduces adrenal function, and clinically relevant adrenal insufficiency occurs.[18] In addition, prolactin concentrations commonly rise and lead to gynecomastia.[166]

Hearing Loss

Although relatively rare, rapidly progressive sensorineural hearing loss occurs in heavy users of opioid analgesics.[93] This effect is associated with most opioids, including hydrocodone, oxycodone, and methadone. The mechanism remains unknown, and suggested causes include ischemia, genetic predisposition, direct cochlear toxicity, and hypersensitization that manifests upon reexposure after a period of opioid abstinence.[185] Most patients recover after abstinence, although some are only successfully treated with cochlear implants.[93]

Toxic and Life-Threatening Effects of Opioids

When used appropriately for medical purposes, opioids are generally safe and effective. However, excessive use in terms of dose or duration results in adverse consequences. Most adverse or toxic effects are predictable based on opioid pharmacodynamics (eg, respiratory depression), although several opioids produce unexpected "nonopioid" responses. Determining that a patient has opioid toxicity is generally more important than identifying the specific opioid involved. Notwithstanding some minor variations, patients poisoned by all available opioids predictably develop a constellation of signs, known as the *opioid toxic syndrome* (Chap. 3). Mental status depression, hypoventilation, miosis, and hypoperistalsis are the classic elements.

Respiratory Depression

Experimental use of various opioid agonists and antagonists consistently implicates μ_2 receptors in the respiratory depressant effects of morphine.[186] Through these receptors, opioid agonists reduce ventilation by diminishing the sensitivity of the medullary chemoreceptors to hypercapnea.[227] In addition to loss of hypercarbic stimulation, opioids depress the ventilatory response to hypoxia.[126] The combined loss of hypercarbic and hypoxic drive leaves virtually no stimulus to breathe, and apnea ensues. Equianalgesic doses of the available opioid agonists produce approximately the same degree of respiratory depression.[59,187] This is supported by experiments in MOR-deficient knockout mice.[171] Patients chronically exposed to opioid agonists, such as those on methadone maintenance, experience chronic hypoventilation, although tolerance to loss of hypercarbic drive develops over several months.[133] However, such patients never develop complete tolerance to loss of hypoxic stimulation.[175] Although some opioids, notably the agonist–antagonists and partial agonists, typically demonstrate a ceiling effect on respiratory depression, such sparing generally occurs at the expense of analgesic potency and is incomplete. The different activity profiles likely are a result of differential activities at the opioid-receptor subtypes. That is, agonist–antagonists are predominantly κ-receptor agonists and either partial agonists or antagonists at μ sites, and partial agonists produce only limited agonism at the μ opioid receptor.

It is important to recognize that ventilatory depression results from a reduction in either respiratory rate or tidal volume. Thus, although respiratory rate is more accessible for clinical measurement, it is not an ideal index of ventilatory depression. In fact, morphine-induced respiratory depression in humans initially is related more closely to changes in tidal volume.[187] Large doses of opioids also result in a reduction of respiratory rate.

Respiratory depression is the primary cause of death after therapeutic use or overdose. Common reasons for iatrogenic overdose include a failure to appreciate the importance of genetic polymorphisms (see Codeine), sleep apnea, drug interactions, active metabolites (see Morphine), or the complicated pharmacokinetics of the long-acting and extended-release opioids.[153] In a population-based cohort study, higher doses of opioid analgesics were associated with increased overdose risk, and much of the risk at higher doses appears to be associated with co-prescribed benzodiazepines.[51]

Pulmonary and Acute Respiratory Distress Syndrome

Reports linking opioids with the development of acute pulmonary abnormalities became common in the 1960s, although the first report was made by William Osler in 1880.[156] Almost all opioids are implicated, and opioid-related acute respiratory distress syndrome (ARDS) is reported in diverse clinical situations. Typically, the patient regains normal ventilation after a period of profound respiratory depression, either spontaneously or after the administration of an opioid antagonist, and over the subsequent several minutes to hours develops hypoxemia and crackles on auscultation. Occasionally, classic frothy, pink sputum is present in the patient's airway or in the endotracheal tube of an intubated patient. Decedents often have what is described as a "foam cone" of frothy material extruding from their nose and mouth.[53] Acute lung injury (currently known as ARDS) was described in 71 (48%) of 149 hospitalized heroin overdose patients in New York City,[57] although the current incidence in this patient group appears to be lower. The outcome generally depends on comorbid conditions and the delay to adequate care. Acute respiratory distress syndrome occurs as an isolated finding or in the setting of multisystem organ damage.

No single mechanism can be consistently invoked in the genesis of opioid-associated ARDS. However, several prominent theories are each well supported by experimental data. Rather than causing ARDS, naloxone sometimes unmasks the clinical findings of ARDS that were not apparent because an adequate physical examination could not be performed until breathing was restored. Other evidentiary cases involve surgical patients given naloxone postoperatively who subsequently awoke with clinical signs of ARDS. In addition to presumably receiving the naloxone for ventilatory compromise or hypoxia, these patients received multiple intraoperative medications, further obscuring the etiology.[163] Although naloxone ordinarily is safe when appropriately administered to nonopioid-tolerant individuals, the production of acute opioid withdrawal is often linked with "naloxone-induced" ARDS. In this situation, as in patients with "neurogenic" pulmonary edema, massive sympathetic discharge from the CNS occurs and produces "cardiogenic" pulmonary edema from the acute effects of catecholamines on the myocardium. In a series of experiments, precipitated opioid withdrawal in nontolerant dogs was associated with dramatic cardiovascular changes and abrupt elevation of serum catecholamine concentrations.[144,145] The effects were more dramatic in dogs with an elevated PCO_2 than in those with a normal or low PCO_2, suggesting the potential benefit of adequately ventilating patients before opioid reversal with naloxone. Similar effects occur in humans undergoing ultrarapid opioid detoxification (UROD; see later).[62]

Even though abrupt precipitation of withdrawal by naloxone contributes to the development of ARDS, it cannot be the sole etiology. Alveolar filling was noted in 50% to 90% of the postmortem examinations performed on heroin overdose patients, many of whom were declared dead before arrival to medical care and thus never received naloxone.[87,91] In addition, neither naloxone nor any other opioid antagonist was available when Osler and others described their initial cases of pulmonary edema, now termed ARDS. Alternatively, the negative intrathoracic pressure generated by attempted inspiration against a closed glottis creates a large pressure gradient across the alveolar membrane and draws fluid into the alveolar space. This mechanical effect, also known as the *Müller maneuver*, was invoked as the cause of ventilator-associated ARDS before the advent of demand ventilators and neuromuscular blockers. In the setting of opioid overdose, glottic laxity prevents

adequate air entry during inspiration. This effect is especially prominent at the time of naloxone administration, in which case breathing will reinstitute before the return of adequate upper airway function.

Cardiovascular

Arteriolar and venous dilation secondary to opioid use results in a mild reduction in blood pressure.[225] This effect is clinically useful for treatment of patients with acute cardiogenic pulmonary edema. However, although patients typically do not develop significant supine hypotension, orthostatic changes in blood pressure and pulse routinely occur. Bradycardia is unusual, although a reduction in heart rate is common as a result of the associated reduction in CNS stimulation. Opioid-induced hypotension is mediated by histamine release, although induction of histamine release does not appear to occur through interaction with an opioid receptor. It is related to the nonspecific ability of certain xenobiotics to activate mast cell G proteins[9] and induce degranulation of histamine-containing vesicles. Many opioids share this ability, which is conferred by the presence of a positive charge on a hydrophobic molecule. Accordingly, not all opioids are equivalent in their ability to release histamine.[9] After administration of one of four different opioids to 60 healthy patients, meperidine produced the most hypotension and elevation of serum histamine concentrations; fentanyl produced the least.[67] The combination of H_1 and H_2 antagonists is effective in ameliorating the hemodynamic effects of opioids in humans.[160]

Adulterants and coingestants often produce significant cardiovascular toxicity. For example, quinine-adulterated heroin is associated with dysrhythmias. Cocaine, surreptitiously added to heroin, often causes significant myocardial ischemia or infarction. Similarly, concern that naloxone administration may "unmask" cocaine toxicity in patients simultaneously using cocaine and heroin ("speedball") probably is warranted but rarely is demonstrated unequivocally.

Certain opioids at therapeutic concentrations, particularly methadone, interfere with normal cardiac repolarization and produce QT interval prolongation, an effect that predisposes to the development of torsade de pointes.[122,152] Many patients who receive methadone experience minor increases in QT interval, although a small percentage of patients experience a substantial increase to more than 500 ms.[122] Methadone prolongs the QT interval via interactions with cardiac K^+ channels.[113]

Seizures

Seizures are a rare complication of therapeutic use of most opioids. In patients with acute opioid overdose, seizures most likely are caused by hypoxia. However, experimental models demonstrate a proconvulsant effect of morphine that potentiates the convulsant effect of other xenobiotics.[234] These effects are variably inhibited by naloxone, suggesting the involvement of a mechanism other than opioid receptor binding. In humans, morphine-induced seizures are reported in neonates and are reversed by naloxone,[42] although opioid withdrawal seizures in neonates are more common.

Seizures should be anticipated in patients with meperidine, tapentadol, or tramadol toxicity. The ability of fentanyl and its analogs to induce seizures is controversial. They are used to activate epileptiform activity for localization in patients with temporal lobe epilepsy who are undergoing surgical exploration.[140] However, electroencephalography performed on patients undergoing fentanyl anesthesia did not identify seizure activity even though the clinical assessment suggested that approximately one-third of them had seizures.[192] The rigidity and myoclonus associated with fentanyl use are frequently misinterpreted as a seizure.

SPECIFIC OPIOIDS

The vast majority of opioid-poisoned patients follow predictable clinical courses that can be anticipated based on an understanding of opioid receptor pharmacology. However, certain opioids taken in overdose produce atypical manifestations. Therefore, careful clinical assessment and institution of empiric therapy usually are necessary to ensure proper management (Table 36–4).

TABLE 36–4   Classification, Potency, and Characteristics of Opioids and Opioid Antagonists

Opioid	Type[a]	Derivation	Analgesic Dose (mg) (via route, equivalent to 10 mg of morphine SC[b])	Comments[a,c]
Buprenorphine	PA	Semisynthetic	0.3 IM	Medication assisted therapy requires 6–16 mg/day (contains naloxone)
Butorphanol	AA	Semisynthetic	2 IM	
Codeine	Ag	Natural	60 PO	Often combined with acetaminophen; requires demethylation to morphine by CYP2D6
Dextromethorphan	NEC	Semisynthetic	Nonanalgesic (10–30 PO)	Antitussive; psychotomimetic via NMDA receptor
Diphenoxylate	Ag	Synthetic	Nonanalgesic (2.5 PO)	Antidiarrheal, combined with atropine; difenoxin is potent metabolite
Fentanyl	Ag	Synthetic	0.75 IM	Very short acting (<1 h)
Fentanyl analogs	Ag	Synthetic	Variable, but high potency	Examples include furanyl fentanyl and carfentanil
Heroin	Ag	Semisynthetic	5 SC	Used therapeutically in some countries; Schedule I medication in the United States
Hydrocodone	Ag	Semisynthetic	1IM, 2PO	
Hydromorphone	Ag	Semisynthetic	1.3 SC	
Levorphanol	Ag	Semisynthetic	2 SC or IM	
Loperamide	Ag	Synthetic	Nonanalgesic (2 PO)	Antidiarrheal; abuse; P-glycoprotein substrate
Meperidine	Ag	Synthetic	75 SC or IM	Seizures caused by metabolite accumulation
Methadone	Ag	Synthetic	10 IM	Very long acting (24 h)
Methylnaltrexone	Ant	Synthetic	Nonanalgesic (8–12 SC); 15PO	Peripherally acting antagonist; reverses opioid-induced constipation
Morphine	Ag	Natural	10 SC or IM	
Naglexol	Ant	Synthetic	Nonanalgesic (25 PO)	Peripherally acting antagonist; reverses opioid constipation; P-glycoprotein substrate
Nalbuphine	AA	Semisynthetic	10 IM	
Naloxone	Ant	Semisynthetic	Nonanalgesic (0.04 IV or IM)	Short-acting antagonist (0.5 h)
Naltrexone	Ant	Semisynthetic	Nonanalgesic (50 PO)	Very long-acting antagonist (24 h)
Oxycodone	Ag	Semisynthetic	5 PO	Often combined with acetaminophen; OxyContin is extended release
Oxymorphone	Ag	Semisynthetic	1 SC	
Paregoric	Ag	Natural	25 mL PO	Tincture of opium (0.4 mg/mL)
Pentazocine	AA	Semisynthetic	50 SC	Psychotomimetic via receptor
Tapentadol	Ag	Synthetic	50 PO	Seizures
Tramadol	Ag	Synthetic	50–100 PO	Seizures possible with therapeutic dosing

[a]Agonist–antagonists, partial agonists, and antagonists may cause withdrawal in tolerant individuals. [b]Typical dose (mg) for xenobiotics without analgesic effects is given in parentheses. [c]Duration of therapeutic clinical effect 3–6 h unless noted; likely to be exaggerated in overdose.

AA = agonist antagonist (κ agonist, μ antagonist); Ag = full agonist (μ₁, μ₂, κ); Ant = full antagonist (μ₁, μ₂, κ antagonist); IM = intramuscular; IV = intravenous; NEC = not easily classified; NMDA = N-methyl-D-aspartate; PA = partial agonist (μ₁, μ₂ agonist, κ antagonist); PO = oral; SC = subcutaneous.

Morphine and Codeine

Morphine is poorly bioavailable by the oral route because of extensive first-pass elimination. Morphine is hepatically metabolized primarily to morphine-3-glucuronide (M3G) and, to a lesser extent, to morphine-6-glucuronide (M6G), both of which are cleared renally. Unlike M3G, which is essentially devoid of activity, M6G has μ-agonist effects in the CNS.[25] However, M6G administered peripherally is significantly less potent as an analgesic than is morphine.[188] The polar glucuronide has a limited ability to cross the blood–brain barrier, and P-glycoprotein is capable of expelling M6G from the cerebrospinal fluid. The relative potency of morphine and M6G in the brain is incompletely defined, but the metabolite is generally considered to be several-fold more potent.[5]

This explains why caution is required when administering morphine to patients with kidney failure.

Codeine itself is an inactive opioid agonist, and it requires metabolic activation by O-demethylation to morphine by CYP2D6 (Fig. 36–2). This typically represents a minor metabolic pathway for codeine metabolism. N-demethylation into norcodeine by CYP3A4 and glucuronidation is more prevalent but produces inactive metabolites. The need for conversion to morphine explains why approximately 5% to 7% of white patients, who are devoid of CYP2D6 function, cannot derive an analgesic response from codeine.[101,124] An increasingly recognized phenomenon is that ultrarapid CYP2D6 metabolizers produce unexpectedly large amounts of morphine from codeine, with resulting life-threatening opioid toxicity.[70,164]

Heroin

Heroin is 3,6-diacetylmorphine, and its exogenous synthesis is performed relatively easily from morphine and acetic anhydride. Heroin has a lower affinity for the μ opioid receptor than does morphine, but it is rapidly metabolized by plasma cholinesterase and liver human carboxylesterase (hCE)-2 to 6-monoacetylmorphine, a more potent μ agonist than morphine (Fig. 36–2).[182] Users claim that heroin has an enhanced euphorigenic effect, often described as a "rush." This effect likely is related to the enhanced blood–brain barrier penetration that results from the additional organic functional groups of heroin and its subsequent metabolic activation within the CNS. Interestingly, cocaine and heroin compete for metabolism by plasma cholinesterase and the two human liver carboxylesterases hCE-1 and hCE-2. This interaction has pharmacokinetic and clinical consequences in patients who "speedball."[12,110]

Heroin is available in two distinct chemical forms: base or salt. The hydrochloride salt form typically is a white or beige powder and was the common form of heroin available before the 1980s.[108] Its high water solubility allows simple IV administration. Heroin base, on the other hand, now is the more prevalent form of heroin in most regions of the world. It often is brown or black. "Black tar heroin" is one appellation referring to an impure South American import available in the United States. Because heroin base is virtually insoluble in water, IV administration requires either heating the heroin until it liquefies or mixing it with acid. Alternatively, because the alkaloidal form is heat stable, smoking or "chasing the dragon" is sometimes used as an alternative route. Street-level heroin base frequently contains caffeine or barbiturates,[108] which improves the sublimation of heroin and enhances the yield.[99]

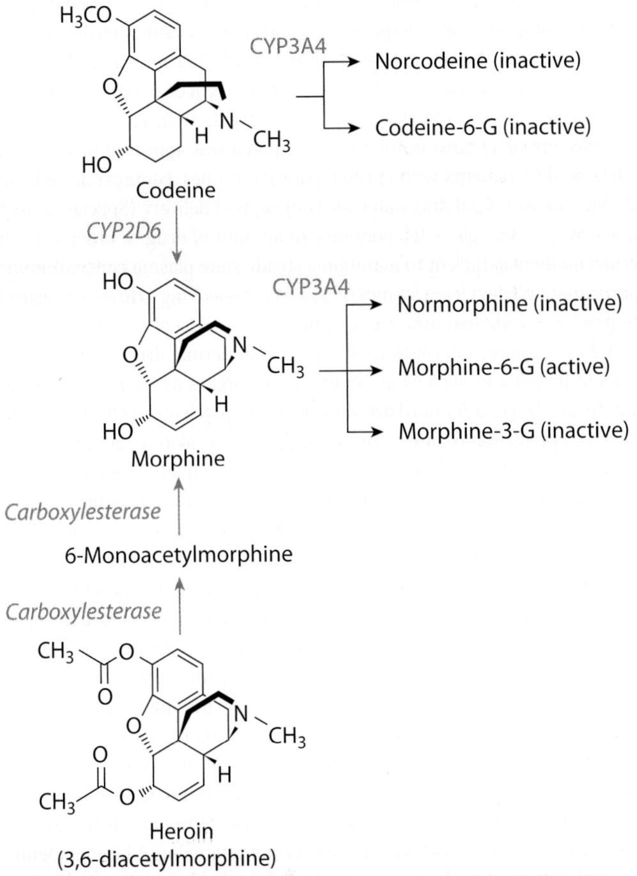

FIGURE 36–2. Opiate and opioid metabolism. Codeine is *O*-methylated to morphine, *N*-demethylated to norcodeine, or glucuronidated to codeine-6-glucuronide (codeine-6-G). Morphine is *N*-demethylated to normorphine or glucuronidated to either morphine-3-glucuronide (morphine-3-G) or morphine-6-glucuronide (morphine-6-G). Heroin is converted to morphine by a two-step process involving plasma cholinesterase and two human liver carboxylesterases known as human carboxylesterase-1 and human carboxylesterase-2.

Widespread IV use has led to many significant direct and indirect medical complications, particularly hepatitis, endocarditis and AIDS, in addition to fatal and nonfatal overdose. Nearly two-thirds of all long-term (longer than 10 years) heroin users in Australia have overdosed on heroin.[47] Among recent-onset heroin users, 23% have overdosed on heroin, and 48% were present when someone else overdosed.[79] Risk factors for fatality after heroin use include the concomitant use of other drugs of abuse, particularly ethanol; recent abstinence, as occurs during incarceration, during which time opioid tolerance has waned;[180] and perhaps unanticipated fluctuations in the concentration or purity of the available heroin.[46,169]

Because most overdoses occur in experienced heroin users and about half occur in the company of other users,[47] the prescribing of naloxone to heroin users for bystander administration is an increasingly available form of harm reduction. Naloxone access for opioid overdose rescue is one of the US Department of Health and Human Services' three priority areas for responding to the opioid crisis,[208] and access to community program-based naloxone distribution for potential overdose bystanders exists in at least 30 states since initial efforts in the late 1990s.[230] Bystanders include people who also use opioids or a friend or family member of a person at risk for overdose. Most community-based naloxone distribution programs provide education on overdose prevention by instructing potential rescuers to recognize known signs of overdose. Naloxone can also be administered by a first responder, such as police or firefighter.

Much of the data proffered to support this practice look at the proportion of those trained that use naloxone within a given time period[137] (maximum potential lives saved) rather than outcomes of overdosed patients with and without bystander intervention. It is possible that many of the patients who receive naloxone did not need the antidote for survival, but that does not mitigate the potential benefit of bystander administration. However, although community-based naloxone distribution programs have gained much momentum in recent years, the cost– and risk–benefit of this practice still remain inadequately understood.[26] For example, despite the acknowledged injection skills of the other users in the "shooting gallery," their judgment likely is impaired. In one survey, summoning an ambulance was the initial response to overdose of a companion in only 14% of cases.[48] A survey of heroin users suggested they lacked an understanding of the pharmacology of naloxone, which might lead to inappropriate behaviors regarding both heroin and naloxone administration.[179] The Peltzman effect describes the beneficial effect of a public health intervention is offset by other risk-taking behavior, in this case perhaps using larger doses of opioid (Antidotes in Depth: A4 and Special Considerations: SC6).[162]

Recognition of the efficacy of intranasal heroin administration, or snorting, has fostered a resurgence of heroin use, particularly in suburban communities. The reason for this trend is likely related to falling supplies of the prescription opioids. People already misusing or addicted to prescription opioids are acquiring heroin, which is more available and less expensive, as a substitute, but heroin carries distinct risks.[32] It is also widely suggested that the increasing purity of the available heroin renders it more suitable for intranasal use. However, because intranasal administration of a mixture of 3% heroin in lactose produces clinical and pharmacokinetic effects similar to an equivalent dose administered IM, the relationship between heroin purity and price and intranasal use is uncertain.[36,172] Needle avoidance certainly is important, reducing the risk of transmission of various infectious diseases, including HIV. Heroin smoking has also increased in popularity in the United States, albeit not to the extent in other countries (see "Chasing the Dragon" later). In addition, users of prescription drugs such as oxycodone or hydrocodone often change to heroin as the supplies of prescription opioids tighten and prices rise.[106] As such, a component of the recent increase in heroin overdose deaths is likely due to the lack of availability and increased cost of prescription opioids.[173] Celebrities and blogs have popularized intranasal heroin use as a "safe" alternative to IV use. Although intranasal use is less dangerous than IV use from an infectious disease perspective, it is clear that both fatal overdose and drug dependency remain common.[209]

Adulterants, Contaminants, and "Heroin" Substitutes

Retail (street-level) heroin almost always contains adulterants or contaminants, which are differentiated by the intent of their admixture. Adulterants typically are benign because inflicting harm on the consumer with their addition would be economically and socially unwise, although adulterants occasionally are responsible for epidemic death. Most heroin overdose decedents do not have serum morphine concentrations that substantially differ from those of living users, raising the possibility that the individual death is related to an adulterant or contaminant.[49]

Historically, alkaloids, such as quinine and strychnine, were used to adulterate heroin to mimic the bitter taste of heroin and to mislead clients. Quinine was initially added in a poorly reasoned attempt to quell an epidemic of malaria among IV heroin users in New York City in the 1930s.[87] That quinine adulteration was common is demonstrated by the common practice of urine screening for quinine as a surrogate marker for heroin use. However, quinine was implicated as a causative factor in an epidemic of heroin-related deaths in the District of Columbia between 1979 and 1982. Toxicity attributed to quinine in heroin users includes cardiac dysrhythmias (Chap. 55), amblyopia, and thrombocytopenia. Quinine adulteration currently is much less common than it was in the past. Trend analysis of illicit wholesale and street-level heroin adulteration over a 12-year period in Denmark revealed that although caffeine, acetaminophen, methaqualone, and phenobarbital all were prevalent adulterants, quinine was not found.[108] Analysis of US heroin samples revealed the presence of procaine, quinine, caffeine, acetaminophen, mannitol lactose, and diphenhydramine in significant quantities.[20] Many other adulterants or contaminants, including thallium, lead, sugars, chalk, brick dust, powdered milk, starch, cocaine, and amphetamines, have been reported.[2]

Poisoning by scopolamine-tainted heroin reached epidemic levels in the northeastern United States in 1995.[84] Exposed patients presented with acute psychosis and anticholinergic signs. Several patients were treated with physostigmine, with excellent therapeutic results.

Clenbuterol, a β_2-adrenergic agonist with a rapid onset and long duration of action, was found to be a contaminant in street heroin in the Eastern United States in early 2005. Users rapidly developed nausea, chest pain, palpitations, dyspnea, and tremor. Physical findings included significant tachycardia and hypotension, as well as hyperglycemia, hypokalemia, and increased lactate concentrations on laboratory evaluation, and a few fatalities occurred.[95,233] The initial patients were thought to be cyanide poisoned. Several patients were treated with β-adrenergic antagonists or calcium channel blockers and potassium supplementation with good results.

"Chasing the Dragon"

Intravenous injection and insufflation are the preferred means of heroin self-administration in the United States. In other countries, including the Netherlands, the United Kingdom, and Spain, a prevalent method is "chasing the dragon" whereby users inhale the white pyrolysate that is generated by heating heroin base on aluminum foil using a handheld flame. This means of administration produces heroin pharmacokinetics similar to those observed after IV administration.[89] Chasing the dragon is not a new phenomenon, but it has gained acceptance among both IV heroin users and drug-naïve individuals. The reasons for this shift are diverse but probably are related to the avoidance of injection drug use with its concomitant infectious risks.

In the early 1980s, a group of individuals who smoked heroin in the Netherlands developed spongiform leukoencephalopathy. Since the initial report, similar cases were reported in other parts of Europe and in the United States.[123,131] Initial findings typically occur within 2 weeks of use and include bradykinesia, ataxia, abulia (inability to make decisions), and speech abnormalities. Of those whose symptoms did not progress, about half recovered. However, in others, progression to spastic paraparesis, pseudobulbar palsy, or hypotonia occurred over several weeks. Approximately half of individuals in this group do not develop further deficits or improve, but death occurs in approximately 25% of reported cases. The prominent symmetric cerebellar and cerebral white matter destruction noted on brain computed tomography and magnetic resonance imaging corresponds to that noted at necropsy.[116,154]

The syndrome has the characteristics of a point-source toxic exposure, but no culpable contaminants were identified, although aluminum concentrations were frequently elevated.[64] A component or pyrolysis product unique to certain batches of "heroin" is possible.[19] Treatment is largely supportive. Based on the finding of regional mitochondrial dysfunction on functional brain imaging and an elevated brain lactate concentration, supplementation with coenzyme Q 300 mg four times a day has purported benefit and is a reasonable treatment, but it has not undergone controlled study.[123]

Oxycodone, Hydrocodone, Hydromorphone, and Oxymorphone

These semisynthetic opioids are widely used to treat acute and chronic pain. For acute pain, several are sold in fixed combination with acetaminophen (eg, Percocet {oxycodone}, Vicodin {hydrocodone}), raising concerns about the complications of acetaminophen hepatotoxicity as the dose of opioid is escalated. Most are available in extended-release formulations that contain a large quantity of opioid intended to be released over many hours. Up until recently, those intent on abuse were able to crush the tablet, which destroys the controlled-release matrix and liberates large amounts of insufflatable or injectable opioid. New abuse deterrent formulation (ADF) standards required now of all extended release opioids make physical or chemical tampering difficult, limiting but not preventing this practice.[177] Abuse can still occur by ingesting intact pills, which can provide a cumulative amount of opioid.

Fentanyl and Its Analogs

Fentanyl is a short-acting opioid agonist that has approximately 50 to 100 times the potency of morphine. It is well absorbed by the transmucosal route, accounting for its use in the form of a "lozenge" or spray. Fentanyl is widely abused as a heroin substitute (intentionally or unintentionally because of adulteration).[15] Experienced heroin users cannot easily differentiate fentanyl from heroin, although in one study, heroin was noted to provide a more intense "rush."[125] There are thousands of deaths attributed to the illicit use of pharmaceutical fentanyl across North America.

Transdermal fentanyl in the form of a patch was approved in 1991 and is widely used by patients with chronic pain syndromes. Fentanyl has adequate solubility in both lipid and water for transdermal delivery (Special Considerations: SC3)[120] A single patch contains an amount of drug to provide a transdermal gradient sufficient to maintain a steady-state plasma concentration for approximately 3 days (eg, a 50-mcg/h patch contains 5 mg). However, even after the patch is considered exhausted, approximately 50% of the total initial fentanyl dose remains. Interindividual variation in dermal drug penetration and errors in proper use, such as use of excessive patches or warming of the skin, leads to an iatrogenic fentanyl overdose. Fentanyl patch misuse and abuse occur either by application of one or more patches to the skin or by withdrawal or extraction of the fentanyl from the reservoir for subsequent administration.[207]

Historically, the largest spontaneous and self-limited fentanyl epidemics, which included more than 1,000 deaths, occurred between 2005 and 2007 primarily in the Philadelphia, Chicago, and Detroit regions because of surreptitiously adulterated or substituted heroin. Fentanyl was identified by postmortem urine and blood testing or through analysis of unused drug found on either the decedent or persons with whom the decedent shared drugs.[28]

Regional epidemics of heroin substitutes with "superpotent" activity occasionally produce a dramatic increase in "heroin-related" fatalities. Epidemic deaths among heroin users first appeared in Orange County, California, in 1979 and were traced to α-methylfentanyl sold under the brand name China White.[121] Similar epidemics of China White poisoning occurred in Pittsburgh in 1988 and in Philadelphia in 1992, although the adulterant in these cases was 3-methylfentanyl, another potent analog. A later epidemic in New York City marked the reappearance of 3-methylfentanyl under the brand name Tango and Cash. Typically, patients present comatose and apneic, with no opioids detected on routine blood and urine analysis. In such cases, unsuspecting users had administered their usual "dose of heroin," measured in 25-mg "bags" that contained variable amounts of the fentanyl analog. Because of the exceptional potency of this fentanyl analog (as much as 10,000 times greater than that of morphine), users rapidly developed apnea.

Deaths caused by fentanyl sharply increased in late 2013. During this time period, the fentanyl prescription rate remained relatively stable, suggesting diversion of pharmaceutical fentanyl was not the etiology. Through law enforcement intelligence, it became clear that this increase resulted from the growing availability of nonpharmaceutical (illicitly produced) fentanyl.[77,173,174] In 2015, there was a further sharp increase in opioid fatalities attributable to novel fentanyl analogs, such as acetyl fentanyl, butyryl fentanyl, furanyl fentanyl, and carfentanil (Fig. 36–3). Each of these analogs contains functional groups substituted onto fentanyl that not only changes the pharmacologic effects but also allows the illicit drug to both temporarily skirt controlled substances laws and remain undetectable on traditional opioid immunoassay tests.[148] These highly potent opioids are imported, often through the mail, from synthetic laboratories, primarily in China, in small batches that readily evade detection by law enforcement. Other novel "research" opioids, including compounds such as MT-45, and AH-7921, U-47700, U-50488, which are not fentanyl derivatives, are also associated with significant public health and medical consequences.[148,157,173] Although unconfirmed, the xenobiotic used by Russian authorities to overcome terrorists and subdue a hostage situation in Moscow in October 2002 was carfentanil,[226] a potent μ-receptor agonist that is also used as a positron emission tomography scan radioligand.

Although fentanyl is a more potent opioid agonist than heroin, the dose of naloxone required to reverse respiratory depression is similar to that of clinically equivalent doses of other common opioids.[206] This is because the binding affinity (K_d) of fentanyl at the μ opioid receptor is similar to that of both morphine and naloxone.[128,218] The responsiveness of the fentanyl analogs to reversal by naloxone appears to be pharmacologically similar,[149] but in the clinical setting, it is very difficult to predict. Given the unpredictability of dosing and the extreme potency of the illicit opioids, administration of a large dose, either in absolute or relative terms, should reasonably be expected to require higher than normal doses of naloxone for reversal (Antidotes in Depth: A4).[128]

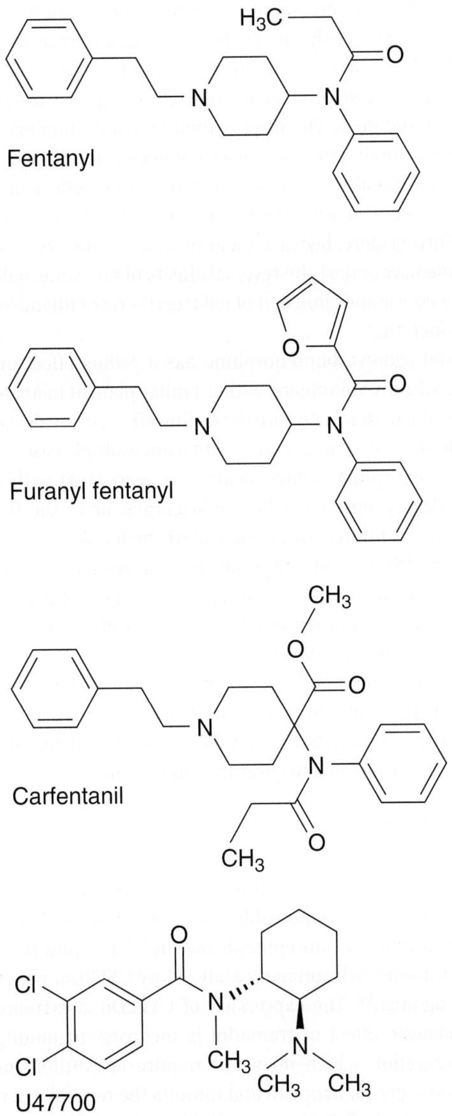

Xenobiotics Used in Medication Assisted Therapy: Methadone and Buprenorphine

Two contrasting approaches to the management of patients with chronic opioid use exist: (1) detoxification and abstinence and (2) maintenance therapy. Detoxification probably is most appropriate for patients motivated or compelled to discontinue opioid use and remain abstinent. It is usually performed by tapered withdrawal of an opioid agonist. Maintenance therapy includes use of a long-acting opioid antagonist, such as naltrexone, to pharmacologically block the effects of additional opioid use. Greater success in reducing recurrent opioid use is achieved through medication-assisted therapy (MAT), which is essentially maintenance therapy using opioid substitution.[25]

Methadone

Methadone is a synthetic μ-opioid–receptor agonist used both for treatment of chronic pain and as MAT for opioid dependence. Although therapeutic use of methadone, whether for pain or MAT, is generally safe, rapid dose escalation during induction of therapy rarely unintentionally result in toxicity and fatal respiratory depression.[25] This adverse effect is generally the result of the combination of variable pharmacokinetics (unpredictable but generally long half-life) and the time lag for the development of tolerance.

Methadone has been routinely available in many cities for MAT since the 1960s through methadone maintenance treatment programs (MMTPs).[54] In MMTPs, the abused opioid (historically heroin) is replaced by methadone, which is legal, pure, oral, and long acting. Methadone allows patients to abstain from activities associated with procurement and administration of the abused opioid and eliminates much of the morbidity and mortality associated with illicit drug use. Although often successful in achieving opioid abstinence, some methadone users continue to use heroin, other opioids, and other xenobiotics.[112]

Primarily because of its low cost compared with other extended-release opioids, until about 2007, methadone was increasingly used in the treatment of chronic pain.[66] Because such policies led to disproportionate adverse effects in patients receiving Medicaid and a safety warning about methadone issued by the FDA in 2006,[66] many such practices were abandoned. Despite accounting for only 1% of opioid prescriptions in 2014, methadone was implicated in approximately 23% of prescription opioid deaths that year.[66] The majority of methadone-related decedents used methadone for pain indications not as part of MAT.[107]

Methadone is administered as a chiral mixture of (R,S)-methadone. In humans, methadone metabolism is mediated by several cytochrome P450 (CYP) isozymes, mainly CYP3A4 and CYP2B6 and to a lesser extent CYP2D6. CYP2B6 demonstrates stereoselectivity toward (S)-methadone.[73] In vivo data show that CYP2B6 slow metabolizer status is associated with high (S)-, but not serum (R)-methadone concentrations.[41] (R)-methadone is used in Germany and is both more effective and safer than the chiral mixture or the (S) enantiomer because the former is largely devoid of QT effects and is the enantiomer that binds to opioid receptors, but it is not available in the United States at the present time.

Methadone predictably and in a concentration-dependent fashion produces QT interval prolongation because of blockade of the hERG (human ether-a-gogo related gene) channel.[134] In the human heart, the hERG voltage-gated potassium channel mediates the rapidly activating delayed rectifier current (Chap. 15). Blocking potassium efflux from the cardiac myocyte prolongs cellular repolarization, prolonging the QT interval. Syncope and

FIGURE 36–3. Structural design of novel fentanyl analogs (furanyl fentanyl and carfentanil) and the novel "research" opioid U-47700.

sudden death caused by ventricular dysrhythmias (eg, torsade de pointes) are the result. Genetic factors in the metabolism of methadone[58] and baseline QT status at the initiation of methadone therapy underlie and potentially predict adverse effects. In clinical trials, QT interval prolongation was greater in individuals who were CYP2B6 slow metabolizers, and this population had higher (S)-methadone concentrations.[58] (S)-methadone binding to hERG is twofold greater than that of (R)-methadone.[103]

A major difficulty is identification of individuals who are at risk for life-threatening dysrhythmias from methadone-induced QT interval prolongation. Expert-derived guidelines recommend questioning patients about intrinsic heart disease or dysrhythmias, counseling patients initiating methadone therapy, and obtaining a pretreatment electrocardiogram (ECG) and a follow-up ECG at 30 days and yearly.[122] Patients who receive methadone doses of greater than 100 mg/day necessitate more frequent ECGs, particularly after dose escalation or change in comorbid disease staus.[122] Although these guidelines are disputed by some and limited data exist on the utility of the ECG as a screening test for persons at risk for torsade de pointes from methadone, given its low cost, easy availability, and minimal invasiveness, we agree with the guideline recommendations.[111]

Methadone abuse and unintentional overdose is often related to the manner in which MMTPs dispense the drug.[107] Most patients attending MMTPs are given doses of methadone greater than needed to simply prevent withdrawal and to prevent surreptitious heroin or other opioid use.[201] Additionally, most MMTPs provide their established patients with sufficient methadone to last through a weekend or holiday without the need to revisit the program. This combination of dose and quantity permits diversion of portions of the dose without the attendant risk of opioid withdrawal. Furthermore, home storage of this surplus drug in inappropriate containers, such as juice containers or baby bottles,[85] is a cause of unintentional methadone ingestion by children. Such events should be anticipated because methadone is frequently formulated as a palatable liquid, and it is not always stored in child-resistant containers. The primary reason for distribution as a liquid, as opposed to the pill form given to patients with chronic pain syndromes, is to ensure dosing compliance while being dispensed at the MMTP. Unfortunately, death is frequent in children who overdose.[129] Since 2007, the overdose death rate has declined and is associated with actions aimed at reducing methadone use for pain. In 2006, the FDA issued warnings about the risks of prescribing methadone for pain.[107]

Buprenorphine

Because prescription of methadone for medication assisted therapy is restricted to federally licensed MMTPs, it is inaccessible and inconvenient for many patients. Buprenorphine was approved in 2000 for MAT for office-based prescribing in patients with opioid addiction. It is administered daily at home, providing a more attractive alternative for patients than daily MMTP visits, and it substantially broadened the potential for obtaining outpatient MAT. However, because of the initial limitations on patient volume (which was subsequently expanded), the requirement for physician certification, and possibly the hesitation on the part of community physicians to welcome patients with substance use disorder into their practices, many of the benefits of office-based buprenorphine therapy over methadone are not yet realized.

Buprenorphine, a partial μ-opioid agonist, in doses of 8 to 16 mg sublingually, is effective at suppressing both opioid withdrawal symptoms and the covert use of illicit drugs. Buprenorphine, although abused, has a substantially better safety profile than methadone. That is, buprenorphine overdose is associated with markedly less respiratory depression than full agonists such as methadone. Because there is no reported effect on the QT interval, patients on methadone with concerning QT interval prolongation are offered the opportunity to switch to buprenorphine. Reasons for refusal are multifactorial and include the potential to precipitate withdrawal symptoms at induction, loss of the pleasant effects of methadone, and the reluctance of prescribers to escalate dosing regimens.[98]

Buprenorphine competes with the extant opioid for the μ receptor; thus, administration of initial doses of buprenorphine in patients taking methadone for medication assisted therapy or who are dependent on any other opioid can be complicated by opioid withdrawal. For this reason, the initial dose of buprenorphine is often administered in the presence of a physician and only when the patient is in mild to moderate withdrawal. Buprenorphine cessation results in a mild withdrawal syndrome and for this reason should be an advantage in opioid detoxification programs.[6] Buprenorphine is available as a sublingual (SL) tablets or sublingual or buccal films containing both buprenorphine and naloxone (Suboxone), which is added to prevent IV use.

At therapeutic doses, buprenorphine produces nearly complete occupancy of the μ opioid receptors, and its receptor affinity is sufficiently strong that it prevents other opioids from binding.[82] Although naloxone prevents the clinical effects of buprenorphine, the reversal of respiratory effects by naloxone appears to be related in a nonlinear fashion. Relatively low bolus doses of IV naloxone have no effect on the respiratory depression induced by buprenorphine, but high doses (5–10 mg) caused only partial reversal of the respiratory effects of buprenorphine. More recently, data in healthy volunteers suggest a bell-shaped dose response to naloxone.[176,215] Although doses that would reverse other opioids were ineffective (0.2–0.4 mg), increasing the dose of naloxone to 2 to 4 mg caused full reversal of buprenorphine respiratory depression. However, the onset of reversal is usually slower than occurs when antagonizing other opioids.[215] Further increasing the naloxone dose to 5 to 7 mg caused a decline in reversal activity and increased the degree of respiratory depression. The reasons for this are unclear. Therefore, it is recommended that the reversal of respiratory depression be treated with a starting dose that is slightly higher than that used to reverse other opioids and increased slowly and titrated to reversal of respiratory depression. For example, a starting dose of naloxone of 0.02 mg/kg, or 1 mg in an adult, is a reasonable initial dose. The dose is then increased incrementally, not to exceed a dose of about 5 mg for concern of decreasing efficacy of naloxone. Because of the difficulty in prediction of naloxone's effect in treatment of buprenorphine-induced respiratory depression, all patients should be closely monitored. Furthermore, because sedation and respiratory depression from buprenorphine may outlast the reversal effects of naloxone, boluses or short infusions or a continuous infusion of naloxone is recommended to maintain respiratory function.[78]

As a partial agonist, buprenorphine has a ceiling effect on respiratory depression in healthy volunteers, with a similar plateau in analgesic effect.[43] However, in some patients, despite the ceiling effect, clinically consequential respiratory depression does occur.[210] Data from multiple case series indicate that most buprenorphine-related deaths are associated with concomitant use of other drugs, most often benzodiazepines, or to the IV injection of crushed tablets.[210] Children are at particularly high risk.[23]

The higher affinity (lower K_d) and partial agonism of buprenorphine should allow it to function as an antagonist to the respiratory depressant effects of heroin and improve spontaneous respiration. Although administration of sublingual buprenorphine for opioid overdose is reportedly successful in some case reports,[229] there is not enough evidence to recommend this practice at this time. In fact, some reported deaths involved patients given buprenorphine tablets intravenously by fellow drug abusers for the treatment of heroin-induced respiratory depression.[16]

Other Unique Opioids
Tramadol and Tapentadol

Tramadol and tapentadol are synthetic analgesics with both opioid and nonopioid mechanisms responsible for their clinical effects. Tramadol is a reuptake inhibitor of norepinephrine and 5-HT, and it has an active metabolite, O-desmethyltramadol catalyzed by CYP2D6, which is a μ opioid receptor agonist.[165] The expression of CYP2D6 is extremely variable. Thus, the analgesic effect of tramadol is inconsistent among individual patients. Tapentadol, which does not require activation, has relatively strong μ-opioid receptor agonism and inhibits the reuptake of norepinephrine but not serotonin.[86] Both are available in immediate- and extended-release formulations.

A large number of spontaneous reports to the FDA describe therapeutic use of tramadol resulting in seizures, particularly on the first day of therapy. However, epidemiologic studies have not confirmed this association.[71] Tramadol-related seizures are not responsive to naloxone but are suppressed with benzodiazepines. In fact, the prescribing information cautions against using naloxone in patients with tramadol overdose because the risk of seizure is increased in animal models. Correspondingly, one patient in a prospective series had a seizure that was temporally related to naloxone administration.[196] Acute overdose of tramadol is generally considered non–life threatening, and most fatalities were associated with polysubstance overdose. Ultrarapid metabolizers at CYP2D6 will develop complications at conventional doses.[61] Patients using monoamine oxidase inhibitors (MAOIs) are at risk for development of serotonin toxicity after use of tramadol.

Tramadol abuse is reported. Data indicate an increase in tramadol inquires in recent years, and tramadol was the second most common drug inquired about on a user-based website next to oxycodone.[232] In August 2014, tramadol was moved to Schedule IV of the US Controlled Substances Act, reflecting its potential for abuse and diversion. In a review of physician drug abuse in several states, tramadol was the second most frequent opioid reported.[190,212] Opioid abusers recognized tramadol as an opioid only when given in an amount that was six times the therapeutic dose, but at this dose, they did not develop opioidlike clinical effects such as miosis. Patients develop typical opioid manifestations after a large overdose. Significant respiratory depression is uncommon and should respond to naloxone.[196] Hypoglycemia is associated with therapeutic use of tramadol, and it is reasonable to admit all patients with tramadol-induced hypoglycemia because of the uncertainty of continuing risk.[68] Generally, urine drug screening for drugs of abuse is negative for opioids in tramadol-using patients. Tapentadol is relatively new to the market, and although its abuse potential remains concerning and case reports exist,[115] there are insufficient epidemiologic data to identify diversion or abuse.[50]

Diphenoxylate

Although diphenoxylate is structurally similar to meperidine, its extreme insolubility limits absorption from the GI tract. This factor enhances its use as an antidiarrheal, which presumably occurs via a local opioid effect at the GI μ receptor. However, there is significant systemic absorption of the standard adult formulation with resulting toxicity in children, and all such exposures in children should be deemed consequential. Diphenoxylate is formulated with a small dose (0.025 mg) of atropine (as Lomotil), both to enhance its antidiarrheal effect and to discourage illicit use.

Because both components of Lomotil are absorbed and their pharmacokinetic profiles differ somewhat, a biphasic clinical syndrome is occasionally noted.[138] Patients typically manifest atropine poisoning (anticholinergic syndrome), either independently or concomitantly with the opioid effects of diphenoxylate. Delayed, prolonged, or recurrent toxicity is common and is classically related to the delayed gastric emptying effects inherent to both opioids and anticholinergics. However, these effects are more likely explained by the accumulation of the hepatic metabolite difenoxin, which is a significantly more potent opioid than diphenoxylate and possesses a longer serum half-life. Still, the relevance of gastroparesis is highlighted by the retrieval of Lomotil pills by gastric lavage as late as 27 hours postingestion.

A review of 36 pediatric reports of diphenoxylate overdoses found that although naloxone was effective in reversing the opioid toxicity, recurrence of CNS and respiratory depression was common.[138] This series included a patient with an asymptomatic presentation 8 hours postingestion who was observed for several hours and then discharged. This patient returned to the ED 18 hours postingestion with marked signs of atropinism. In this same series, children with delayed onset of respiratory depression and other opioid effects were reported, and others describe cardiopulmonary arrest 12 hours postingestion. Naloxone infusion is indicated for patients with recurrent signs of opioid toxicity. Because of the delayed and possibly severe consequences, all individuals with potentially significant ingestions should be admitted for monitored observation in the hospital.

Loperamide

Loperamide is another insoluble meperidine analog that is used to treat diarrhea and is available over the counter as a nonprescription medication. At therapeutic doses, it inhibits peristaltic activity through agonism of μ opioid receptors, calcium channel blockade, calmodulin inhibition, and decreasing paracellular permeability in the large intestine.[8,197] At therapeutic dosing (< 16 mg/day), loperamide is essentially devoid of central opioid effects because transporter protein P-glycoprotein actively facilitates removal of the drug from the gut and the CNS.[213,217] However, larger than recommended doses overcome these mechanisms, enabling CNS penetration and affording relief of opioid withdrawal symptoms or even opioidlike euphoria and psychotropic effects. These effects are facilitated by coingestion of a P-glycoprotein inhibitor. Central nervous system and respiratory depression are reported after therapeutic oral dosing in infants.[130] Since 2010, loperamide exposures misuse and abuse continue to increase in the United States because prescription opioids are costly and becoming less accessible.[214] Loperamide was initially placed in Schedule II, down scheduled to Schedule V in 1977, and descheduled in 1982.[212] Because it is not tracked as a controlled substance, the true extent of use, diversion, and abuse are largely unavailable. As people with OUD search for alternatives to self-treat opioid dependence and withdrawal symptoms, loperamide is becoming more popular as an easily available inexpensive option.

Deaths are reported at the high doses required for CNS effects (70–400 mg) and are associated with respiratory depression cardiotoxicity.[60,197] Loperamide inhibits human cardiac sodium channels and inhibits delayed-rectifier potassium currents in vitro. Correspondingly, both QRS prolongation and polymorphic ventricular tachycardia are reported after overdose.[60,197] Inhibition of calcium channel function likely contributes to its cardiac toxicity in overdose. Naloxone should be administered to reverse consequential respiratory depression associated with loperamide overdose.[60] In patients who present with wide complex dysrhythmias and polymorphic ventricular tachycardia, it is reasonable to use sodium bicarbonate and magnesium sulfate, as potentially preventive measures but primary treatment is electrical cardioversion. However, data on the optimal treatment of cardiotoxicity associated with loperamide overdose are very limited.

Dextromethorphan

Dextromethorphan is devoid of analgesic properties altogether, even though it is the optical isomer of levorphanol, a potent opioid analgesic. Based on this structural relationship, dextromethorphan is commonly considered an opioid, although its receptor pharmacology is much more complex. At high doses, dextromethorphan binds to opioid receptors to produce miosis, respiratory depression, and CNS depression, which are at least partially reversed by naloxone. Binding to the phencyclidine (PCP) site on the NMDA receptor, with subsequent inhibition of calcium influx through this receptor-linked ion channel, causes sedation. This same activity accounts for its antiepileptic properties and for its neuroprotective effects in ischemic brain injury. Because NMDA receptor blockade both reduces hyperalgesia and enhances the analgesic effects of μ-opioid agonists, combination therapy with morphine and dextromethorphan is increasingly studied and used.[114,119]

Blockade of presynaptic serotonin reuptake by dextromethorphan causes the serotonin toxicity in patients receiving MAOIs or other serotonergics.[194] Movement disorders, described as choreoathetoid or dystonialike, occasionally occur and presumably result from alteration of dopaminergic neurotransmission. Dextrorphan, the active O-demethylation metabolite of dextromethorphan, is produced by CYP2D6, an enzyme with a well-described genetic polymorphism.[7] Whereas patients with the "extensive metabolizer" polymorphism appear to experience more drug-related psychoactive effects, poor metabolizers experience more adverse effects related to the parent compound.[237]

Dextromethorphan is available without prescription in cold preparations, primarily because of its presumed lack of significant addictive potential. Despite this, the prevalence of use among high school students was high but decreased recently.[195] Common street names include "DXM," "dex," and "roboshots." Users often have expectations of euphoria and hallucinations, but a dysphoria comparable to that of PCP commonly ensues. Reports of substantial cold medicine consumption raise concerns, including acetaminophen poisoning, opioid dependency, and bromide toxicity.[100] This last concern relates to the common formulation of dextromethorphan as the hydrobromide salt. At times, the first clue is an elevated serum chloride concentration when measured on certain autoanalyzers (Chaps. 7 and 12).

Meperidine

Meperidine was previously widely used for treatment of chronic and acute pain syndromes. Its use was dramatically reduced and is either closely monitored in many institutions or eliminated because of its adverse risk–benefit profile. Meperidine produces clinical manifestations typical of the other opioids and may lead to greater euphoria caused by its blockade of presynaptic serotonin reuptake.[236] This most consequential nonopioid-receptor effect causes serotonin toxicity, characterized by muscle rigidity, hyperthermia, and altered mental status, particularly in patients using MAOIs (Chap. 71). Normeperidine, a toxic, renally eliminated hepatic metabolite, accumulates in patients receiving chronic high-dose meperidine therapy, such as those with sickle cell disease or cancer or in those with chronic kidney disease.[204] Normeperidine causes excitatory neurotoxicity, which manifests as delirium, tremor, myoclonus, or seizures. Based on animal studies and human evidence, the seizures do not respond to naloxone.[75]

DIAGNOSTIC TESTING

Laboratory Considerations

Opioid-poisoned patients are particularly appropriate for a rapid clinical diagnosis because of the unique characteristics of the opioid toxic syndrome. Additionally, even in situations in which the assay results are available rapidly, the fact that several distinct classes of opioids and nonopioids produce similar opioid effects limits the use of laboratory tests, such as immunoassays, that rely on structural features to identify xenobiotics. Furthermore, because opioids are chemically detectable long after their clinical effects have dissipated, assay results cannot be considered in isolation but rather viewed in the clinical context. Several well-described problems with laboratory testing of opioids are described later and in Chap. 7.

Cross-Reactivity

Many opioids share significant structural similarities, such as morphine and oxycodone or methadone and propoxyphene (Fig. 36–4). Because most clinical assays depend on structural features for identification, structurally similar xenobiotics are frequently detected in lieu of the desired one. Whether a similar xenobiotic is noted by the assay depends on the sensitivity and specificity of the assay and the serum concentration of the xenobiotic. Some cross-reactivities are predictable, such as that of hydrocodone with morphine, on a variety of screening tests. Other cross-reactivities are less predictable, as in the case of the cross-reaction of dextromethorphan and the PCP component of the fluorescence polarization immunoassay (Abbott TDx),[178] a widely used drug abuse screening test (Chap. 7).[200]

Congeners and Adulterants

Commercial opiate assays, which are usually specific for morphine (a metabolite of heroin), do not readily detect most of the semisynthetic and synthetic opioids. Epidemic fatalities involving fentanyl derivatives remained unexplained despite obvious opioid toxicity until the ultrapotent fentanyl analog α-methylfentanyl (although initially misidentified as 3-methylfentanyl) was identified by more sophisticated testing.[121,135] Oxycodone, hydrocodone, and other common morphine derivatives have variable detectability by different opioid screens and generally only when in high concentrations.[132] Currently, because of the public health threat of fentanyl analogs and other potent opioids, reference and forensic laboratories have markedly expanded their detection capabilities by using advanced technologies such as tandem mass spectroscopy.[148]

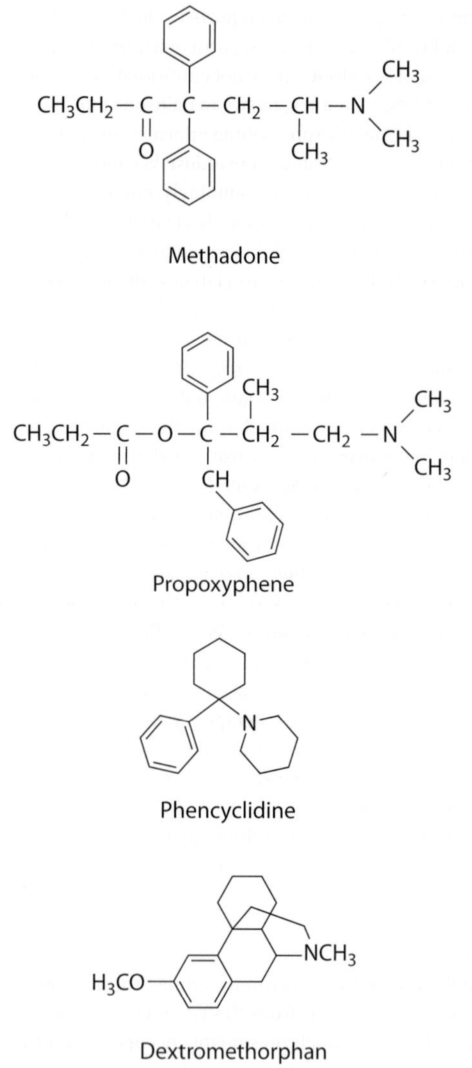

FIGURE 36–4. Structural similarity between methadone and propoxyphene and between phencyclidine and dextromethorphan.

Drug Metabolism

A fascinating dilemma often arises in patients who ingest moderate to large amounts of poppy seeds.[118] These seeds, which are widely used for culinary purposes, are derived from poppy plants and contain both morphine and codeine. After ingestion of a single poppy seed bagel, patients infrequently develop elevated serum morphine and codeine concentrations and test positive for morphine.[147,170] Because the presence of morphine on a drug abuse screen supports illicit heroin use, the implications are substantial. Federal workplace testing regulations thus require corroboration of a positive morphine assay with assessment of another heroin metabolite, 6-monoacetylmorphine, before reporting a positive result.[150,219] Humans readily deacetylate heroin, which is diacetylmorphine but cannot acetylate morphine and therefore cannot synthesize 6-monoacetylmorphine.

Similar problems occur in patients taking therapeutic doses of codeine. Because codeine is demethylated to morphine by CYP2D6, a morphine screen will be positive as a result of metabolism and not structural cross-reactivity.[71] Thus, determination of the serum codeine or 6-monoacetylmorphine concentration is necessary in these patients. Determination of the serum codeine concentration is not foolproof, however, because codeine is present in opium, which is used to synthesize heroin.

Forensic Testing

Decision making regarding the cause of death in the presence of systemic opioids often is complex.[44] Variables that often are incompletely defined contribute substantially to the difficulty in attributing or not attributing the cause of death to the opioid. These variables include the specifics regarding the timing of exposure, the preexisting degree of sensitivity or tolerance, the role of cointoxicants (including parent opioid metabolites), and postmortem redistribution and metabolism.[56,112] Techniques to help further elucidate the likely cause of death include the application of postmortem pharmacogenetic principles[105] and the use of alternative specimens (Chap. 140).

MANAGEMENT

The consequential effects of acute opioid poisoning are CNS and respiratory depression. Although early support of ventilation and oxygenation is generally sufficient to prevent death, prolonged use of bag-valve-mask ventilation and endotracheal intubation can often be avoided by cautious administration of an opioid antagonist. Opioid antagonists, such as naloxone, competitively inhibit binding of opioid agonists to opioid receptors, allowing the patient to resume spontaneous respiration. Naloxone competes at all receptor subtypes, although not equally, and is effective at reversing almost all adverse effects mediated through opioid receptors (Antidotes in Depth: A4).

Because many clinical findings associated with opioid poisoning are nonspecific, the diagnosis requires clinical acumen. Differentiating acute opioid poisoning from other etiologies with similar clinical presentations is challenging. Patients manifesting findings of opioid poisoning, found in an appropriate environment, or with characteristic physical clues such as fresh needle marks require little corroborating evidence. However, subtle presentations of opioid poisoning are encountered, and other xenobiotics can simulate opioid poisoning. Hypoglycemia, hypoxia, and hypothermia result in clinical manifestations that share features with opioid poisoning and often exist concomitantly. Many other xenobiotics are rapidly identifiable with routinely available, point-of-care testing, but their existence does not exclude opioid poisoning. Other xenobiotics responsible for similar clinical presentations include clonidine, PCP, phenothiazines, and sedative–hypnotics (primarily benzodiazepines). In such patients, clinical evidence usually is available to assist in diagnosis. For example, nystagmus nearly always is noted in PCP-toxic patients, hypotension or ECG) abnormalities in phenothiazine-poisoned patients, and coma with virtually normal vital signs in patients poisoned by benzodiazepines. Most difficult to differentiate on clinical grounds is toxicity produced by the centrally acting antihypertensives such as clonidine (see later and Chap. 61). Additionally, myriad traumatic, metabolic, and infectious etiologies may occur simultaneously and must always be evaluated appropriately.

Antidote Administration

The goal of naloxone therapy is not necessarily complete restoration of normal consciousness; rather, the goal is reinstitution of adequate spontaneous ventilation. Because precipitation of withdrawal is potentially detrimental and often unpredictable, we recommend administering the lowest practical naloxone dose initially, with rapid escalation as warranted by the clinical situation. Most patients respond to 0.04 of naloxone administered IV,[117] although the requirement for ventilatory assistance is often slightly prolonged because the onset will be slower than with larger doses. We recommend repeating this dose for several doses at 3-minute intervals, as needed for persistent findings, with escalation up to 0.4-mg and 2-mg doses.[37] Infrequently if the presumption of opioid overdose persists repetitive bolus doses of naloxone of 2 mg up to a total of 10 mg is indicated. In patients who do not respond to high doses, opioid-induced hypoventilation is excluded (Antidotes in Depth: A4). Administration in this fashion usually avoids endotracheal intubation and allows for timely identification of patients with nonopioid causes of their clinical condition yet diminishes the risk of precipitation of acute opioid withdrawal. Subcutaneous administration allows for smoother arousal than the high-dose IV route, but is unpredictable in onset and prolonged in offset.[223] Prolonged effectiveness of naloxone by the SC route can be a considerable disadvantage if a withdrawal syndrome develops or if discharge from the ED is dependent on the duration of effect of the antagonist, so we recommend IV dosing and titration to effect whenever feasible (Antidotes in Depth: A4).

In the absence of a confirmatory history or diagnostic clinical findings, the cautious empiric and titrated administration of naloxone will be both diagnostic and therapeutic. Naloxone, even at extremely high doses, has an excellent safety profile in opioid-naïve patients receiving the medication for nonopioid-related indications, such as spinal cord injury or acute ischemic stroke. However, administration of naloxone to opioid-dependent patients often results in adverse effects; specifically, precipitation of an acute withdrawal syndrome should be anticipated. The resultant agitation, hypertension, and tachycardia produce significant distress for the patient and complicate management for the clinical staff and occasionally is life threatening. Additionally, emesis, a common feature of acute opioid withdrawal, is particularly hazardous in patients who do not rapidly regain consciousness after naloxone administration. For example, patients with concomitant ethanol or sedative–hypnotic exposure and those with head trauma are at substantial risk for pulmonary aspiration of vomitus if their airways are unprotected.

Identification of patients likely to respond to naloxone conceivably would reduce the unnecessary and potentially dangerous precipitation of withdrawal in opioid-dependent patients. Routine prehospital administration of naloxone to all patients with subjectively assessed altered mental status or respiratory depression was not beneficial in 92% of patients.[235] Alternatively, although not perfectly sensitive, a respiratory rate of 12 breaths/min or less in an unconscious patient presenting via emergency medical services best predicted a response to naloxone.[94] In contrast, neither respiratory rate below 8 breaths/min nor coma was able to predict a response to naloxone in hospitalized patients.[231] It is unclear whether the discrepancy between the latter two studies is a result of the demographics of the patient groups or whether patients with prehospital opioid overdose present differently than patients with iatrogenic poisoning. Regardless, relying on the respiratory rate to assess the need for ventilatory support or naloxone administration is not ideal because hypoventilation secondary to hypopnea may precede that caused by bradypnea.[168,189]

The decision to discharge a patient who awakens appropriately after naloxone administration is based on practical considerations. Patients presenting with profound hypoventilation or hypoxia are at risk for development of ARDS or posthypoxic encephalopathy. We recommend observing these patients for at least 24 hours in a medical setting. Based on the pharmacokinetics of naloxone, patients manifesting only moderate signs of opioid poisoning who remain normal for at least 2 hours after a standard parenteral dose of naloxone are likely safe to discharge (Antidotes in Depth: A4). Patients requiring larger doses of naloxone should be observed longer, although 6 hours should generally be sufficient. Patients with uncontrolled drug use or after a suicide attempt often need psychosocial interventions before discharge from the ED. Patients who have used methadone or an extended-release opioid formulation often require continuous infusion of naloxone or administration of a long-acting opioid antagonist is indicated to maintain adequate ventilation. Patients receiving a naloxone infusion should be maintained for 12 to 24 hours and then observed an additional 4 to 6 hours after discontinuation of the naloxone infusion (Antidotes in Depth: A4).

Patients with recurrent or profound poisoning by long-acting opioids, such as methadone, or patients with large GI burdens (eg, "body packers" or those taking extended-release preparations) often require continuous infusion of naloxone to ensure continued adequate ventilation (Table 36–5). An hourly infusion rate of two-thirds of the initial reversal dose of naloxone is usually sufficient to prevent recurrence.[78] Titration of the dose is often necessary as indicated by the clinical situation. Although repetitive bolus dosing of naloxone is effective, it is labor intensive and subject to error.

Despite the availability of long-acting opioid antagonists (eg, naltrexone) that theoretically permit single-dose reversal of methadone poisoning, the attendant risk of precipitating an unrelenting withdrawal syndrome hinders their use as antidotes for initial opioid reversal. We recommend against their use for opioid overdose in almost all circumstances. However, these opioid antagonists have a clinical role in the maintenance of consciousness and ventilation in opioid-poisoned patients already awakened by naloxone who are not experiencing opioid withdrawal. Prolonged observation and perhaps antidote readministration will be required to match the pharmacokinetic

TABLE 36–5	Recommended Use of a Naloxone Infusion

1. If a naloxone bolus (start with 0.04 mg IV and titrate) is successful, for those determined to need an infusion administer two-thirds of the effective bolus dose per hour by IV infusion; frequently reassess the patient's respiratory status.
2. If respiratory depression is not reversed after the initial bolus dose:
   Increase dose slowly and titrate to reversal of respiratory depression. Administer up to 10 mg of naloxone as an IV bolus.
   If the patient does not respond, do not initiate an infusion.
   AND prepare for
   Intubation of the patient, as clinically indicated.
3. If the patient develops withdrawal after the bolus dose:
   Allow the effects of the bolus to abate.
   If respiratory depression recurs, administer half of the initial bolus dose and begin an IV infusion at two-thirds of the new bolus dose per hour. Frequently reassess the patient's respiratory status.
4. If the patient develops withdrawal signs or symptoms during the infusion:
   Stop the infusion until the withdrawal symptoms abate.
   Restart the infusion at half the initial rate; frequently reassess the patient's respiratory status.
   Exclude withdrawal from other xenobiotics.
5. If the patient develops respiratory depression during the infusion:
   Readminister half of the initial bolus and repeat until reversal occurs.
   Increase the infusion by half of the initial rate; frequently reassess the patient's respiratory status.
   Exclude continued absorption, readministration of opioid, and other etiologies as the cause of the respiratory depression.

IV = intravenous.

parameters of the agonist and antagonist. For example, it is reasonable to give well children who ingest short-acting opioids a long-acting opioid antagonist such as naltrexone because they are not expected to develop delayed opioid toxicity beyond the duration of the antagonist. However, the same caveats remain regarding the need for extended hospital observation periods if ingestion of methadone or other long-acting opioids is suspected.

Body Packers

In an attempt to transport illicit drugs from one country to another, body packers ingest large numbers of multiple-wrapped packages of concentrated cocaine or heroin. When the authorities discover such individuals or when individuals in custody become ill, they may be brought to a hospital for evaluation and management. Although these patients generally are asymptomatic on arrival, they are at risk for delayed, prolonged, or lethal poisoning as a consequence of packet rupture.[211] In the past, determining the country of origin of the current journey was nearly diagnostic of packet content. However, because most of the heroin imported into the United States now originates from South America, which is also the major source of imported cocaine, the discernment from cocaine on this basis is impossible. Given the current greater revenue potential of heroin, the majority of body packers carry heroin (Special Considerations: SC5).[76]

Rapid and Ultrarapid Opioid Detoxification

The concept of antagonist-precipitated opioid withdrawal is promoted extensively as a "cure" for opioid dependency, particularly heroin and oxycodone, but has fallen out of favor in recent years. Rather than slow, deliberate withdrawal or detoxification from opioids over several weeks, antagonist-precipitated withdrawal occurs over several hours or days.[81] The purported advantage of this technique is a reduced risk of relapse to opioid use because the duration of discomfort is reduced and a more rapid transition to naltrexone maintenance can be achieved. Although most studies find some beneficial short-term results, relapse to drug use is very common.[139] Rapid opioid detoxification techniques are usually offered by outpatient clinics and typically consist of naloxone- or naltrexone-precipitated opioid withdrawal tempered with varying amounts of clonidine, benzodiazepines, antiemetics, or other drugs. Ultrarapid opioid detoxification uses a similar concept but involves the use of deep

sedation or general anesthesia for greater patient control and comfort. The risks of these techniques are not fully defined, but are of substantial concern. Massive catecholamine release, ARDS, acute kidney injury, and thyroid hormone suppression does occur after UROD, and many patients still manifest opioid withdrawal 48 hours after the procedure. As with other forms of opioid detoxification, the loss of tolerance after successful completion of the program paradoxically increases the likelihood of death from heroin overdose if these individuals relapse. That is, recrudescence of opioid use in predetoxification quantities is likely to result in overdose.[202] Both techniques are costly; UROD under anesthesia commonly costs thousands of dollars. We agree with the professional medical organizations involved in addiction management that have publicly expressed concern for this form of detoxification.[4]

SUMMARY

- Opioid poisonings, both intentional and unintentional, remain major causes of drug-related morbidity and mortality.
- Although the therapeutic and toxic doses are difficult to predict because of the development of tolerance with chronic use, the primary adverse event from excessive dosing is respiratory depression.
- Mechanical ventilation, or administration of a short-acting opioid antagonist such as naloxone, are adequate initial therapies. Naloxone dosing requires cautious escalation.
- An appreciation of the pharmacologic differences among the various opioids allows for the identification and appropriate management of patients poisoned or otherwise adversely affected by these xenobiotics.

REFERENCES

1. Aicher SA, et al. Co-localization of mu opioid receptor and N-methyl-D-aspartate receptor in the trigeminal dorsal horn. *J Pain.* 2002;3:203-210.
2. Akhgari M, et al. Street level heroin, an overview on its components and adulterants. In: Preedy V, ed. *Neuropathology of Drug Addictions and Substance misuse.* Vol 3. 1st ed. New York, NY: Elsevier; 2016:863-877.
3. American Psychiatric Association. *Diagnostic and Statistical Manual of Mental Disorders.* 5th ed. Arlington, VA: American Psychiatric Publishing; 2013.
4. American Society of Addiction Medicine. Public Policy Statement on Rapid and Ultra Rapid Opioid Detoxification. http://www.asam.org/advocacy/find-a-policy-statement/view-policy-statement/public-policy-statements/2011/12/15/rapid-and-ultra-rapid-opioid-detoxification.
5. Andersen G, et al. Relationships among morphine metabolism, pain and side effects during long-term treatment: An update. *J Pain Symptom Manage.* 2003;25:74-91.
6. Assadi SM, et al. Opioid detoxification using high doses of buprenorphine in 24 hours: a randomized, double blind, controlled clinical trial. *J Subst Abuse Treat.* 2004;27:75-82.
7. Bailey B, et al. Discrepancy between CYP2D6 phenotype and genotype derived from post-mortem dextromethorphan blood level. *Forensic Sci Int.* 2000;110:61-70.
8. Baker DE. Loperamide: A pharmacological review. *Rev Gastroenterol Disord.* 2007;7(suppl 3):S11-S18.
9. Barke KE, Hough LB. Opiates, mast cells and histamine release. *Life Sci.* 1993;53:1391-1399.
10. Barnett ML, et al. Opioid-prescribing patterns of emergency physicians and risk of long-term use. *N Engl J Med.* 2017;376:663-673.
11. Beckett AH, Casy AF. Synthetic analgesics: stereochemical considerations. *J Pharm Pharmacol.* 1954;6:986-1001.
12. Bencharit S, et al. Structural basis of heroin and cocaine metabolism by a promiscuous human drug-processing enzyme. *Nat Struct Biol.* 2003;10:349-356.
13. Bodnar RJ, et al. Role of mu 1-opiate receptors in supraspinal opiate analgesia: a microinjection study. *Brain Res.* 1988;447:25-34.
14. Bonnet U, et al. Choreoathetoid movements associated with rapid adjustment to methadone. *Pharmacopsychiatry.* 1998;31:143-145.
15. Booth JV, et al. Substance abuse among physicians: a survey of academic anesthesiology programs. *Anesth Analg.* 2002;95:1024-1030.
16. Boyd J, et al. Serious overdoses involving buprenorphine in Helsinki. *Acta Anaesthesiol Scand.* 2003;47:1031-1033.
17. Brands B, et al. Prescription opioid abuse in patients presenting for methadone maintenance treatment. *Drug Alcohol Depend.* 2004;73:199-207.
18. Brennan MJ. The effect of opioid therapy on endocrine function. *Am J Med.* 2013;126(3 suppl 1):S12-S18.
19. Brenneisen R, Hasler F. GC/MS determination of pyrolysis products from diacetylmorphine and adulterants of street heroin samples. *J Forensic Sci.* 2002;47:885-888.
20. Broseus J, et al. The cutting of cocaine and heroin: a critical review. *Forensic Sci Int.* 2016;262:73-83.
21. Brummett CM, et al. New persistent opioid use after minor and major surgical procedures in US adults. *JAMA Surg.* 2017:e170504.

22. Brush DE. Complications of long-term opioid therapy for management of chronic pain: the paradox of opioid-induced hyperalgesia. *J Med Toxicol.* 2012;8:387-392.

23. Budnitz DS, et al. Notes from the field: pediatric emergency department visits for buprenorphine/naloxone ingestion—United States, 2008-2015. *MMWR Morb Mortal Wkly Rep.* 2016;65:1148-1149.

24. Butler MM, et al. Emergency department prescription opioids as an initial exposure preceding addiction. *Ann Emerg Med.* 2016;68:202-208.

25. Center for Substance Abuse Prevention. *Methadone-Associated Mortality: Report of a National Assessment.* Rockville, MD: US Department of Health and Human Services, Substance Abuse and Mental Health Services Administration, Center for Substance Abuse Treatment; 2004.

26. Centers for Disease Control and Prevention (CDC). Community-based opioid overdose prevention programs providing naloxone—United States, 2010. *MMWR Morb Mortal Wkly Rep.* 2012;61:101-105.

27. Centers for Disease Control and Prevention (CDC). Drug overdose deaths—Florida, 2003-2009. *MMWR Morb Mortal Wkly Rep.* 2011;60:869-872.

28. Centers for Disease Control and Prevention (CDC). Nonpharmaceutical fentanyl-related deaths—multiple states, April 2005-March 2007. *MMWR Morb Mortal Wkly Rep.* 2008;57:793-796.

29. Cepeda MS, et al. Incidence of nausea and vomiting in outpatients undergoing general anesthesia in relation to selection of intraoperative opioid. *J Clin Anesth.* 1996;8:324-328.

30. Cheatle MD. Prescription opioid misuse, abuse, morbidity, and mortality: balancing effective pain management and safety. *Pain Med.* 2015;16(suppl 1):S3-S8.

31. Christensen O, et al. Analgesic effect of intraarticular morphine. A controlled, randomised and double-blind study. *Acta Anaesthesiol Scand.* 1996;40:842-846.

32. Cicero TJ, et al. Effect of abuse-deterrent formulation of OxyContin. *N Engl J Med.* 2012;367:187-189.

33. Clarke H, et al. Rates and risk factors for prolonged opioid use after major surgery: population based cohort study. *BMJ.* 2014;348:g1251.

34. Cohen MR, et al. Behavioural effects after high dose naloxone administration to normal volunteers. *Lancet.* 1981;2:1110-1110.

35. Compton P, et al. Hyperalgesia in heroin dependent patients and the effects of opioid substitution therapy. *J Pain.* 2012;13:401-409.

36. Cone EJ, et al. Pharmacokinetics and pharmacodynamics of intranasal snorted heroin. *J Anal Toxicol.* 1993;17:327-337.

37. Connors NJ, Nelson LS. The evolution of recommended naloxone dosing for opioid overdose by medical specialty. *J Med Toxicol.* 2016;12:276-281.

38. Courteix C, et al. Evidence for an exclusive antinociceptive effect of nociceptin/orphanin FQ, an endogenous ligand for the ORL1 receptor, in two animal models of neuropathic pain. *Pain.* 2004;110:236-245.

39. Crain SM, Shen KF. Antagonists of excitatory opioid receptor functions enhance morphine's analgesic potency and attenuate opioid tolerance/dependence liability. *Pain.* 2000;84:121-131.

40. Crain SM, Shen KF. Modulation of opioid analgesia, tolerance and dependence by gs-coupled, GM1 ganglioside-regulated opioid receptor functions. *Trends Pharmacol Sci.* 1998;19:358-365.

41. Crettol S, et al. Methadone enantiomer plasma levels, CYP2B6, CYP2C19, and CYP2C9 genotypes, and response to treatment. *Clin Pharmacol Ther.* 2005;78:593-604.

42. da Silva O, et al. Seizure and electroencephalographic changes in the newborn period induced by opiates and corrected by naloxone infusion. *J Perinatol.* 1999;19:120-123.

43. Dahan A, et al. Buprenorphine induces ceiling in respiratory depression but not in analgesia. *Br J Anaesth.* 2006;96:627-632.

44. Daldrup T. A forensic toxicological dilemma: the interpretation of post-mortem concentrations of central acting analgesics. *Forensic Sci Int.* 2004;142:157-160.

45. Daniel M, et al. Opiate receptor blockade by naltrexone and mood state after acute physical activity. *Br J Sports Med.* 1992;26:111-115.

46. Darke S, et al. Fluctuations in heroin purity and the incidence of fatal heroin overdose. *Drug Alcohol Depend.* 1999;54:155-161.

47. Darke S, et al. Overdose among heroin users in Sydney, Australia: I. prevalence and correlates of non-fatal overdose. *Addiction.* 1996;91:405-411.

48. Darke S, et al. Overdose among heroin users in Sydney, Australia: II. Responses to overdose. *Addiction.* 1996;91:413-417.

49. Darke S, et al. A comparison of blood toxicology of heroin-related deaths and current heroin users in Sydney, Australia. *Drug Alcohol Depend.* 1997;47:45-53.

50. Dart RC, et al. Assessment of the abuse of tapentadol immediate release: the first 24 months. *J Opioid Manag.* 2012;8:395-402.

51. Dasgupta N, et al. Cohort study of the impact of high-dose opioid analgesics on overdose mortality. *Pain Med.* 2016;17:85-98.

52. Dhawan BN, et al. International union of pharmacology. XII. Classification of opioid receptors. *Pharmacol Rev.* 1996;48:567-592.

53. Dinis-Oliveira RJ, et al. "Foam cone" exuding from the mouth and nostrils following heroin overdose. *Toxicol Mech Methods.* 2012;22:159-160.

54. Dole VP, Nyswander M. A medical treatment for diacetylmorphine (heroin) addiction. A clinical trial with methadone hydrochloride. *JAMA.* 1965;193:646-650.

55. Dowell D, et al. CDC guideline for prescribing opioids for chronic pain—United States, 2016. *MMWR Recomm Rep.* 2016;65:1-49.

56. Drummer OH. Postmortem toxicology of drugs of abuse. *Forensic Sci Int.* 2004;142:101-113.

57. Duberstein JL, Kaufman DM. A clinical study of an epidemic of heroin intoxication and heroin-induced pulmonary edema. *Am J Med.* 1971;51:704-714.

58. Eap CB, et al. Stereoselective block of hERG channel by (S)-methadone and QT interval prolongation in CYP2B6 slow metabolizers. *Clin Pharmacol Ther.* 2007;81:719-728.

59. Eckenhoff JE, Oech SR. The effects of narcotics and antagonists upon respiration and circulation in man. A review. *Clin Pharmacol Ther.* 1960;1:483-524.

60. Eggleston W, et al. Loperamide abuse associated with cardiac dysrhythmia and death. *Ann Emerg Med.* 2017;69:83-86.

61. Elkalioubie A, et al. Near-fatal tramadol cardiotoxicity in a CYP2D6 ultrarapid metabolizer. *Eur J Clin Pharmacol.* 2011;67:855-858.

62. Elman I, et al. Ultrarapid opioid detoxification: effects on cardiopulmonary physiology, stress hormones and clinical outcomes. *Drug Alcohol Depend.* 2001;61:163-172.

63. Elvenes J, et al. Expression of functional mu-opioid receptors in human osteoarthritic cartilage and chondrocytes. *Biochem Biophys Res Commun.* 2003;311:202-207.

64. Exley C, et al. Elevated urinary aluminium in current and past users of illicit heroin. *Addict Biol.* 2007;12:197-199.

65. Fahnenstich H, et al. Fentanyl-induced chest wall rigidity and laryngospasm in preterm and term infants. *Crit Care Med.* 2000;28:836-839.

66. Faul M, et al. Methadone prescribing and overdose and the association with medicaid preferred drug list policies—United States, 2007-2014. *MMWR Morb Mortal Wkly Rep.* 2017;66:320-323.

67. Flacke JW, et al. Histamine release by four narcotics: a double-blind study in humans. *Anesth Analg.* 1987;66:723-730.

68. Fournier JP, et al. Tramadol use and the risk of hospitalization for hypoglycemia in patients with noncancer pain. *JAMA Intern Med.* 2015;175:186-193.

69. Gan TJ, et al. Opioid-sparing effects of a low-dose infusion of naloxone in patient-administered morphine sulfate. *Anesthesiology.* 1997;87:1075-1081.

70. Gasche Y, et al. Codeine intoxication associated with ultrarapid CYP2D6 metabolism. *N Engl J Med.* 2004;351:2827-2831.

71. Gasse C, et al. Incidence of first-time idiopathic seizures in users of tramadol. *Pharmacotherapy.* 2000;20:629-634.

72. Gavériaux-Ruff C, Kieffer BL. Opioid receptor genes inactivated in mice: the highlights. *Neuropeptides.* 2002;36:62-71.

73. Gerber JG, et al. Stereoselective metabolism of methadone N-demethylation by cytochrome P4502B6 and 2C19. *Chirality.* 2004;16:36-44.

74. Ghoneim MM, et al. Comparison of four opioid analgesics as supplements to nitrous oxide anesthesia. *Anesth Analg.* 1984;63:405-412.

75. Gilbert PE, Martin WR. Antagonism of the convulsant effects of heroin, d-propoxyphene, meperidine, normeperidine and thebaine by naloxone in mice. *J Pharmacol Exp Ther.* 1975;192:538-541.

76. Gill JR, Graham SM. Ten years of "body packers" in New York City: 50 deaths. *J Forensic Sci.* 2002;47:843-846.

77. Gladden RM, et al. Fentanyl law enforcement submissions and increases in synthetic opioid-involved overdose deaths - 27 states, 2013-2014. *MMWR Morb Mortal Wkly Rep.* 2016;65:837-843.

78. Goldfrank L, et al. A dosing nomogram for continuous infusion intravenous naloxone. *Ann Emerg Med.* 1986;15:566-570.

79. Gossop M, et al. Frequency of non-fatal heroin overdose: survey of heroin users recruited in non-clinical settings. *BMJ.* 1996;313:402.

80. Government Accounting Office. OxyContin abuse and diversion and efforts to address the problem: highlights of a government report. *J Pain Palliat Care Pharmacother.* 2004;18:109-113.

81. Gowing L, et al. Opioid antagonists under heavy sedation or anaesthesia for opioid withdrawal. *Cochrane Database Syst Rev.* 2006;(2):CD002022.

82. Greenwald MK, et al. Effects of buprenorphine maintenance dose on mu-opioid receptor availability, plasma concentrations, and antagonist blockade in heroin-dependent volunteers. *Neuropsychopharmacology.* 2003;28:2000-2009.

83. Gugelmann HM, Nelson LS. The prescription opioid epidemic: repercussions on pediatric emergency medicine. *Pediatr Emerg Med.* 2012;13:260-268.

84. Hamilton RJ, et al. A descriptive study of an epidemic of poisoning caused by heroin adulterated with scopolamine. *J Toxicol Clin Toxicol.* 2000;38:597-608.

85. Harkin K, et al. Storing methadone in babies' bottles puts young children at risk. *BMJ.* 1999;318:329-330.

86. Hartrick CT, Rozek RJ. Tapentadol in pain management: a mu-opioid receptor agonist and noradrenaline reuptake inhibitor. *CNS Drugs.* 2011;25:359-370.

87. Helpern M, Rho YM. Deaths from narcotism in New York City. Incidence, circumstances, and postmortem findings. *N Y State J Med.* 1966;66:2391-2408.

88. Hemby SE, et al. The effects of intravenous heroin administration on extracellular nucleus accumbens dopamine concentrations as determined by in vivo microdialysis. *J Pharmacol Exp Ther.* 1995;273:591-598.

89. Hendriks VM, et al. Heroin self-administration by means of "chasing the dragon": pharmacodynamics and bioavailability of inhaled heroin. *Eur Neuropsychopharmacol.* 2001;11:241-252.

90. Henriksen G, Willoch F. Imaging of opioid receptors in the central nervous system. *Brain.* 2008;131(Pt 5):1171-1196.

91. Hine CH, et al. Analysis of fatalities from acute narcotism in a major urban area. *J Forensic Sci.* 1982;27:372-384.

92. Ho A, Dole VP. Pain perception in drug-free and in methadone-maintained human ex-addicts. *Proc Soc Exp Biol Med.* 1979;162:392-395.

93. Ho T, et al. Hydrocodone use and sensorineural hearing loss. *Pain Physician.* 2007;10:467-472.

94. Hoffman JR, et al. The empiric use of naloxone in patients with altered mental status: a reappraisal. *Ann Emerg Med.* 1991;20:246-252.

95. Hoffman RS, et al; Clenbuterol Study Investigators. A descriptive study of an outbreak of clenbuterol-containing heroin. *Ann Emerg Med.* 2008;52:548-553.

96. Holzer P. Opioids and opioid receptors in the enteric nervous system: from a problem in opioid analgesia to a possible new prokinetic therapy in humans. *Neurosci Lett.* 2004;361:192-195.

97. Hoppe JA, et al. Association of emergency department opioid initiation with recurrent opioid use. *Ann Emerg Med.* 2015;65:493-499.e4.

98. Hser YI, et al. Treatment retention among patients randomized to buprenorphine/ naloxone compared to methadone in a multi-site trial. *Addiction.* 2014;109:79-87.

99. Huizer H. Analytical studies on illicit heroin. V. efficacy of volatilization during heroin smoking. *Pharm Weekbl Sci.* 1987;9:203-211.

100. Hung YM. Bromide intoxication by the combination of bromide-containing over-the-counter drug and dextromethorphan hydrobromide. *Hum Exp Toxicol.* 2003;22:459-461.

101. Ingelman-Sundberg M. Genetic polymorphisms of cytochrome P450 2D6 (CYP2D6): clinical consequences, evolutionary aspects and functional diversity. *Pharmacogenomics J.* 2005;5:6-13.

102. Inspirion Delivery Sciences L, ed. Roxybound package insert. Valley Cottage, NY; 2017.

103. Inturrisi CE. Pharmacology of methadone and its isomers. *Minerva Anestesiol.* 2005;71:435-437.

104. Janal MN, et al. Pain sensitivity, mood and plasma endocrine levels in man following long-distance running: effects of naloxone. *Pain.* 1984;19:13-25.

105. Jannetto PJ, et al. Pharmacogenomics as molecular autopsy for postmortem forensic toxicology: genotyping cytochrome P450 2D6 for oxycodone cases. *J Anal Toxicol.* 2002;26:438-447.

106. Jones CM. Heroin use and heroin use risk behaviors among nonmedical users of prescription opioid pain relievers—United States, 2002-2004 and 2008-2010. *Drug Alcohol Depend.* 2013;132:95-100.

107. Jones CM, et al. Trends in methadone distribution for pain treatment, methadone diversion, and overdose deaths—United States, 2002-2014. *MMWR Morb Mortal Wkly Rep.* 2016;65:667-671.

108. Kaa E. Impurities, adulterants and diluents of illicit heroin. changes during a 12-year period. *Forensic Sci Int.* 1994;64:171-179.

109. Kalant H. Opium revisited: a brief review of its nature, composition, non-medical use and relative risks. *Addiction.* 1997;92:267-277.

110. Kamendulis LM, et al. Metabolism of cocaine and heroin is catalyzed by the same human liver carboxylesterases. *J Pharmacol Exp Ther.* 1996;279:713-717.

111. Kao D, et al. Trends in reporting methadone-associated cardiac arrhythmia, 1997-2011: an analysis of registry data. *Ann Intern Med.* 2013;158:735-740.

112. Karch SB, Stephens BG. Toxicology and pathology of deaths related to methadone: retrospective review. *West J Med.* 2000;172:11-14.

113. Katchman AN, et al. Influence of opioid agonists on cardiac human ether-a-go-go-related gene K(+) currents. *J Pharmacol Exp Ther.* 2002;303:688-694.

114. Katz NP. MorphiDex (MS:DM) double-blind, multiple-dose studies in chronic pain patients. *J Pain Symptom Manage.* 2000;19(1 suppl):S37-41.

115. Kemp W, et al. Death due to apparent intravenous injection of tapentadol. *J Forensic Sci.* 2013;58:288-291.

116. Keogh CF, et al. Neuroimaging features of heroin inhalation toxicity: "chasing the dragon." *AJR Am J Roentgenol.* 2003;180:847-850.

117. Kim HK, Nelson LS. Reversal of opioid-induced ventilatory depression using low-dose naloxone (0.04 mg): a case series. *J Med Toxicol.* 2016;12:107-110.

118. King MA, et al. Poppy tea and the baker's first seizure. *Lancet.* 1997;350:716-716.

119. King MR, et al. Perioperative dextromethorphan as an adjunct for postoperative pain: a meta-analysis of randomized controlled trials. *Anesthesiology.* 2016;124:696-705.

120. Kornick CA, et al. Benefit-risk assessment of transdermal fentanyl for the treatment of chronic pain. *Drug Saf.* 2003;26:951-973.

121. Kram TC, et al. Behind the identification of china white. *Anal Chem.* 1981;53:1386.

122. Krantz MJ, et al. QTc interval screening in methadone treatment. *Ann Intern Med.* 2009;150:387-395.

123. Kriegstein AR, et al. Leukoencephalopathy and raised brain lactate from heroin vapor inhalation (chasing the dragon). *Neurology.* 1999;53:1765-1773.

124. Lötsch J, et al. Genetic predictors of the clinical response to opioid analgesics: clinical utility and future perspectives. *Clin Pharmacokinet.* 2004;43:983-1013.

125. LaBarbera M, Wolfe T. Characteristics, attitudes and implications of fentanyl use based on reports from self-identified fentanyl users. *J Psychoactive Drugs.* 1983;15:293-301.

126. Lalley PM. Opioidergic and dopaminergic modulation of respiration. *Respir Physiol Neurobiol.* 2008;164:160-167.

127. Lee HK, Wang SC. Mechanism of morphine-induced miosis in the dog. *J Pharmacol Exp Ther.* 1975;192:415-431.

128. Leysen JE, et al. [3H]sufentanil, a superior ligand for mu-opiate receptors: binding properties and regional distribution in rat brain and spinal cord. *Eur J Pharmacol.* 1983;87:209-225.

129. Li L, et al. Fatal methadone poisoning in children: Maryland 1992-1996. *Subst Use Misuse.* 2000;35:1141-1148.

130. Litovitz T, et al. Surveillance of loperamide ingestions: an analysis of 216 poison center reports. *J Toxicol Clin Toxicol.* 1997;35:11-19.

131. Long H, et al. A fatal case of spongiform leukoencephalopathy linked to chasing the dragon. *J Toxicol Clin Toxicol.* 2003;41:887-891.

132. Magnani B, Kwong T. Urine drug testing for pain management. *Clin Lab Med.* 2012;32:379-390.

133. Marks CE, Goldring RM. Chronic hypercapnia during methadone maintenance. *Am Rev Respir Dis.* 1973;108:1088-1093.

134. Martell BA, et al. Impact of methadone treatment on cardiac repolarization and conduction in opioid users. *Am J Cardiol.* 2005;95:915-918.

135. Martin WR, et al. The effects of morphine- and nalorphine- like drugs in the nondependent and morphine-dependent chronic spinal dog. *J Pharmacol Exp Ther.* 1976;197:517-532.

136. Matthes HW, et al. Loss of morphine-induced analgesia, reward effect and withdrawal symptoms in mice lacking the mu-opioid-receptor gene. *Nature.* 1996;383:819-823.

137. McAuley A, et al. Exploring the life-saving potential of naloxone: a systematic review and descriptive meta-analysis of take home naloxone (THN) programmes for opioid users. *Int J Drug Policy.* 2015;26:1183-1188.

138. McCarron MM, et al. Diphenoxylate-atropine (Lomotil) overdose in children: an update (report of eight cases and review of the literature). *Pediatrics.* 1991;87:694-700.

139. McGregor C, et al. A comparison of antagonist-precipitated withdrawal under anesthesia to standard inpatient withdrawal as a precursor to maintenance naltrexone treatment in heroin users: outcomes at 6 and 12 months. *Drug Alcohol Depend.* 2002;68:5-14.

140. McGuire G, et al. Activation of electrocorticographic activity with remifentanil and alfentanil during neurosurgical excision of epileptogenic focus. *Br J Anaesth.* 2003;91:651-655.

141. McNicol E, et al. Efficacy and safety of mu-opioid antagonists in the treatment of opioid-induced bowel dysfunction: systematic review and meta-analysis of randomized controlled trials. *Pain Med.* 2008;9:634-659.

142. Meissner W, et al. Oral naloxone reverses opioid-associated constipation. *Pain.* 2000;84:105-109.

143. Millan MJ, et al. Kappa-opioid receptor-mediated antinociception in the rat. II. supraspinal in addition to spinal sites of action. *J Pharmacol Exp Ther.* 1989;251:342-350.

144. Mills CA, et al. Narcotic reversal in hypercapnic dogs: comparison of naloxone and nalbuphine. *Can J Anaesth.* 1990;37:238-244.

145. Mills CA, et al. Cardiovascular effects of fentanyl reversal by naloxone at varying arterial carbon dioxide tensions in dogs. *Anesth Analg.* 1988;67:730-736.

146. Minozzi S, et al. Development of dependence following treatment with opioid analgesics for pain relief: a systematic review. *Addiction.* 2013;108:688-698.

147. Moeller MR, et al. Poppy seed consumption and toxicological analysis of blood and urine samples. *Forensic Sci Int.* 2004;143:183-186.

148. Mohr AL, et al. Analysis of novel synthetic opioids U-47700, U-50488 and furanyl fentanyl by LC-MS/MS in postmortem casework. *J Anal Toxicol.* 2016;40:709-717.

149. Moresco A, et al. Use of naloxone to reverse carfentanil citrate-induced hypoxemia and cardiopulmonary depression in rocky mountain wapiti (cervus elaphus nelsoni). *J Zoo Wildl Med.* 2001;32:81-89.

150. Mulé S J, Casella GA. Rendering the poppy-seed defense defenseless: identification of 6-monoacetylmorphine in urine by gas chromatography/mass spectroscopy. *Clin Chem.* 1988;34:1427-1430.

151. Nelson AD, Camilleri M. Opioid-induced constipation: advances and clinical guidance. *Ther Adv Chronic Dis.* 2016;7:121-134.

152. Nelson LS. Toxicologic myocardial sensitization. *J Toxicol Clin Toxicol.* 2002;40:867-879.

153. Niesters M, et al. Opioid-induced respiratory depression in paediatrics: a review of case reports. *Br J Anaesth.* 2013;110:175-182.

154. Offiah C, Hall E. Heroin-induced leukoencephalopathy: characterization using MRI, diffusion-weighted imaging, and MR spectroscopy. *Clin Radiol.* 2008;63:146-152.

155. Oldendorf WH, et al. Blood-brain barrier: penetration of morphine, codeine, heroin, and methadone after carotid injection. *Science.* 1972;178:984-986.

156. Osler W. Oedema of the left lung-morphia poisoning. *Montreal Gen Hosp Rep.* 1880;1:291-293.

157. Papsun D, et al. Analysis of MT-45, a novel synthetic opioid, in human whole blood by LC-MS-MS and its identification in a drug-related death. *J Anal Toxicol.* 2016;40:313-317.

158. Perrone J, et al. Prescribing practices, knowledge, and use of prescription drug monitoring programs (PDMP) by a national sample of medical toxicologists, 2012. *J Med Toxicol.* 2012;8:341-352.

159. Pert CB, Snyder SH. Opiate receptor: demonstration in nervous tissue. *Science.* 1973;179:1011-1014.

160. Philbin DM, et al. The use of H1 and H2 histamine antagonists with morphine anesthesia: a double-blind study. *Anesthesiology.* 1981;55:292-296.

161. Pick CG, et al. Nalbuphine, a mixed kappa 1 and kappa 3 analgesic in mice. *J Pharmacol Exp Ther.* 1992;262:1044-1050.

162. Prasad V, Jena AB. The Peltzman effect and compensatory markers in medicine. *Healthc (Amst).* 2014;2:170-172.

163. Prough DS, et al. Acute pulmonary edema in healthy teenagers following conservative doses of intravenous naloxone. *Anesthesiology.* 1984;60:485-486.

164. Racoosin JA, et al. New evidence about an old drug—risk with codeine after adenotonsillectomy. *N Engl J Med.* 2013;368:2155-2157.

165. Raffa RB, et al. Mechanistic and functional differentiation of tapentadol and tramadol. *Expert Opin Pharmacother.* 2012;13:1437-1449.

166. Rhodin A, et al. Opioid endocrinopathy: a clinical problem in patients with chronic pain and long-term oral opioid treatment. *Clin J Pain.* 2010;26:374-380.

167. Richardson DE, Akil H. Pain reduction by electrical brain stimulation in man. Part 1: Acute administration in periaqueductal and periventricular sites. *J Neurosurg.* 1977;47:178-183.

168. Rigg JR, Rondi P. Changes in rib cage and diaphragm contribution to ventilation after morphine. *Anesthesiology.* 1981;55:507-514.

169. Risser D, et al. Quality of heroin and heroin-related deaths from 1987 to 1995 in Vienna, Austria. *Addiction.* 2000;95:375-382.

170. Rohrig TP, Moore C. The determination of morphine in urine and oral fluid following ingestion of poppy seeds. *J Anal Toxicol.* 2003;27:449-452.

171. Romberg R, et al. Comparison of morphine-6-glucuronide and morphine on respiratory depressant and antinociceptive responses in wild type and mu-opioid receptor deficient mice. *Br J Anaesth.* 2003;91:862-870.

172. Rook EJ, et al. Pharmacokinetics and pharmacokinetic variability of heroin and its metabolites: review of the literature. *Curr Clin Pharmacol.* 2006;1:109-118.

173. Rudd RA, et al. Increases in drug and opioid overdose deaths—United States, 2000-2014. *MMWR Morb Mortal Wkly Rep.* 2016;64:1378-1382.

174. Rudd RA, et al. Increases in drug and opioid-involved overdose deaths—United States, 2010-2015. *MMWR Morb Mortal Wkly Rep.* 2016;65:1445-1452.

175. Santiago TV, et al. Control of breathing during methadone addiction. *Am J Med.* 1977;62:347-354.

176. Sarton E, et al. Naloxone reversal of opioid-induced respiratory depression with special emphasis on the partial agonist/antagonist buprenorphine. *Adv Exp Med Biol.* 2008;605:486-491.

177. Schaeffer T. Abuse-deterrent formulations, an evolving technology against the abuse and misuse of opioid analgesics. *J Med Toxicol.* 2012;8:400-407.

178. Schier J. Avoid unfavorable consequences: dextromethorphan can bring about a false-positive phencyclidine urine drug screen. *J Emerg Med.* 2000;18:379-381.

179. Seal KH, et al. Attitudes about prescribing take-home naloxone to injection drug users for the management of heroin overdose: a survey of street-recruited injectors in the San Francisco Bay Area. *J Urban Health.* 2003;80:291-301.

180. Seaman SR, et al. Mortality from overdose among injecting drug users recently released from prison: database linkage study. *BMJ.* 1998;316:426-428.

181. Seftel AD. Re: opioid-induced androgen deficiency (OPIAD). *J Urol.* 2013;189:251.

182. Selley DE, et al. Mu opioid receptor-mediated G-protein activation by heroin metabolites: evidence for greater efficacy of 6-monoacetylmorphine compared with morphine. *Biochem Pharmacol.* 2001;62:447-455.

183. Sgherza AL, et al. Effect of naloxone on perceived exertion and exercise capacity during maximal cycle ergometry. *J Appl Physiol.* 2002;93:2023-2028.

184. Shah A, et al. Characteristics of initial prescription episodes and likelihood of long-term opioid use—United States, 2006-2015. *MMWR Morb Mortal Wkly Rep.* 2017;66:265-269.

185. Shaw KA, et al. Methadone, another cause of opioid-associated hearing loss: a case report. *J Emerg Med.* 2011;41:635-639.

186. Sheffler DJ, et al. The magic mint hallucinogen finds a molecular target in the kappa opioid receptor. *Trends Pharmacol Sci.* 2003;24:107-109.

187. Shook JE, et al. Differential roles of opioid receptors in respiration, respiratory disease, and opiate-induced respiratory depression. *Am Rev Respir Dis.* 1990;142:895-909.

188. Skarke C, et al. Analgesic effects of morphine and morphine-6-glucuronide in a transcutaneous electrical pain model in healthy volunteers. *Clin Pharmacol Ther.* 2003;73:107-121.

189. Skarke C, et al. Respiratory and miotic effects of morphine in healthy volunteers when P-glycoprotein is blocked by quinidine. *Clin Pharmacol Ther.* 2003;74:303-311.

190. Skipper GE, et al. Tramadol abuse and dependence among physicians. *JAMA.* 2004;292:1818-1819.

191. Smith GM, Beecher HK. Subjective effects of heroin and morphine in normal subjects. *J Pharmacol Exp Ther.* 1962;136:47-52.

192. Smith NT, et al. Seizures during opioid anesthetic induction—are they opioid-induced rigidity? *Anesthesiology.* 1989;71:852-862.

193. Sneader W. The discovery of heroin. *Lancet.* 1998;352:1697-1699.

194. Sovner R, Wolfe J. Interaction between dextromethorphan and monoamine oxidase inhibitor therapy with isocarboxazid. *N Engl J Med.* 1988;319:1671.

195. Spangler DC, et al. Dextromethorphan: a case study on addressing abuse of a safe and effective drug. *Subst Abuse Treat Prev Policy.* 2016;11:22.

196. Spiller HA, et al. Prospective multicenter evaluation of tramadol exposure. *J Toxicol Clin Toxicol.* 1997;35:361-364.

197. Stanciu CN, et al. Loperamide, the "poor man's methadone": brief review. *J Psychoactive Drugs.* 2017;49:18-21.

198. Stein C, et al. Analgesic effect of intraarticular morphine after arthroscopic knee surgery. *N Engl J Med.* 1991;325:1123-1126.

199. Stein C, et al. Attacking pain at its source: new perspectives on opioids. *Nat Med.* 2003;9:1003-1008.

200. Storrow AB, et al. The dextromethorphan defense: dextromethorphan and the opioid screen. *Acad Emerg Med.* 1995;2:791-794.

201. Strain EC, et al. Moderate- vs high-dose methadone in the treatment of opioid dependence: a randomized trial. *JAMA.* 1999;281:1000-1005.

202. Strang J, et al. Loss of tolerance and overdose mortality after inpatient opiate detoxification: follow up study. *BMJ.* 2003;326:959-960.

203. Streisand JB, et al. Fentanyl-induced rigidity and unconsciousness in human volunteers. incidence, duration, and plasma concentrations. *Anesthesiology.* 1993;78:629-634.

204. Szeto HH, et al. Accumulation of normeperidine, an active metabolite of meperidine, in patients with renal failure of cancer. *Ann Intern Med.* 1977;86:738-741.

205. Takahama K, Shirasaki T. Central and peripheral mechanisms of narcotic antitussives: codeine-sensitive and -resistant coughs. *Cough.* 2007;3:8.

206. Takahashi M, et al. Naloxone reversal of opioid anesthesia revisited: clinical evaluation and plasma concentration analysis of continuous naloxone infusion after anesthesia with high-dose fentanyl. *J Anesth.* 2004;18:1-8.

207. Tharp AM, et al. Fatal intravenous fentanyl abuse: four cases involving extraction of fentanyl from transdermal patches. *Am J Forensic Med Pathol.* 2004;25:178-181.

208. The US Department of Health and Human Services. HHS takes strong steps to address opioid-drug related overdose, death and dependence. http://www.hhs.gov/about/news/2015/03/26/hhs-takes-strong-steps-to-address-opioid-drug-related-overdose-death-and-dependence.html. Accessed May 11, 2017.

209. Thiblin I, et al. Fatal intoxication as a consequence of intranasal administration (snorting) or pulmonary inhalation (smoking) of heroin. *Forensic Sci Int.* 2004;139:241-247.

210. Tracqui A, et al. Buprenorphine-related deaths among drug addicts in France: a report on 20 fatalities. *J Anal Toxicol.* 1998;22:430-434.

211. Traub SJ, et al. Body packing—the internal concealment of illicit drugs. *N Engl J Med.* 2003;349:2519-2526.

212. United States Department of Justice, Diversion Control Division. *Scheduling Actions Controlled Substances Regulated Chemicals.* May 2017:80.

213. Upton RN. Cerebral uptake of drugs in humans. *Clin Exp Pharmacol Physiol.* 2007;34:695-701.

214. Vakkalanka JP, et al. Epidemiologic trends in loperamide abuse and misuse. *Ann Emerg Med.* 2017;69:73-78.

215. van Dorp E, et al. Naloxone reversal of buprenorphine-induced respiratory depression. *Anesthesiology.* 2006;105:51-57.

216. Van Zee A. The promotion and marketing of oxycontin: commercial triumph, public health tragedy. *Am J Public Health.* 2009;99:221-227.

217. Vandenbossche J, et al. Loperamide and P-glycoprotein inhibition: assessment of the clinical relevance. *J Pharm Pharmacol.* 2010;62:401-412.

218. Villiger JW, Ray et al. Characteristics of [3H]fentanyl binding to the opiate receptor. *Neuropharmacology.* 1983;22:447-452.

219. von Euler M, et al. Interpretation of the presence of 6-monoacetylmorphine in the absence of morphine-3-glucuronide in urine samples: evidence of heroin abuse. *Ther Drug Monit.* 2003;25:645-648.

220. Waldhoer M, et al. Opioid receptors. *Annu Rev Biochem.* 2004;73:953-990.

221. Walker JS. Anti-inflammatory effects of opioids. *Adv Exp Med Biol.* 2003;521:148-160.

222. Walsh SL, et al. The relative abuse liability of oral oxycodone, hydrocodone and hydromorphone assessed in prescription opioid abusers. *Drug Alcohol Depend.* 2008;98:191-202.

223. Wanger K, et al. Intravenous vs subcutaneous naloxone for out-of-hospital management of presumed opioid overdose. *Acad Emerg Med.* 1998;5:293-299.

224. Ward CF, et al. Drug abuse in anesthesia training programs. A survey: 1970 through 1980. *JAMA.* 1983;250:922-925.

225. Ward JM, et al. Effects of morphine on the peripheral vascular response to sympathetic stimulation. *Am J Cardiol.* 1972;29:659-666.

226. Wax PM, et al. Unexpected gas casualties in Moscow: a medical toxicology perspective. *Ann Emerg Med.* 2003;41:700-705.

227. Weil JV, et al. Diminished ventilatory response to hypoxia and hypercapnia after morphine in normal man. *N Engl J Med.* 1975;292:1103-1106.

228. Weinhold LL, Bigelow GE. Opioid miosis: effects of lighting intensity and monocular and binocular exposure. *Drug Alcohol Depend.* 1993;31:177-181.

229. Welsh C, et al. A case of heroin overdose reversed by sublingually administered buprenorphine/naloxone (suboxone). *Addiction.* 2008;103:1226-1228.

230. Wheeler E, et al; Centers for Disease Control and Prevention (CDC). Opioid overdose prevention programs providing naloxone to laypersons—United States, 2014. *MMWR Morb Mortal Wkly Rep.* 2015;64:631-635.

231. Whipple JK, et al. Difficulties in diagnosing narcotic overdoses in hospitalized patients. *Ann Pharmacother.* 1994;28:446-450.

232. Wightman RS, et al. Comparative analysis of opioid queries on erowid.org: an opportunity to advance harm reduction. *Subst Use Misuse.* 2017:1-5.

233. Wingert WE, et al. Detection of clenbuterol in heroin users in twelve postmortem cases at the Philadelphia medical examiner's office. *J Anal Toxicol.* 2008;32:522-528.

234. Yajima Y, et al. Effects of differential modulation of mu-, delta- and kappa-opioid systems on bicuculline-induced convulsions in the mouse. *Brain Res.* 2000;862:120-126.

235. Yealy DM, et al. The safety of prehospital naloxone administration by paramedics. *Ann Emerg Med.* 1990;19:902-905.

236. Zacny JP, Gutierrez S. Characterizing the subjective, psychomotor, and physiological effects of oral oxycodone in non-drug-abusing volunteers. *Psychopharmacology (Berl).* 2003;170:242-254.

237. Zawertailo LA, et al. Psychotropic effects of dextromethorphan are altered by the CYP2D6 polymorphism: a pilot study. *J Clin Psychopharmacol.* 1998;18:332-337.

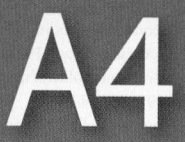

A4 OPIOID ANTAGONISTS

Lewis S. Nelson and Mary Ann Howland

Morphine

Naloxone

Naltrexone

Nalmefene

INTRODUCTION

Naloxone, naltrexone, and methylnaltrexone are pure competitive opioid antagonists at the mu (μ), kappa (κ), and delta (δ) receptors. Opioid antagonists prevent the actions of opioid agonists, reverse the effects of both endogenous and exogenous opioids, and cause opioid withdrawal in opioid-dependent patients. Naloxone is the primary opioid antagonist used to reverse respiratory depression in patients manifesting opioid toxicity. The parenteral dose should be titrated to maintain adequate airway reflexes and ventilation. By titrating the dose, in small increments based on clinical response, abrupt opioid withdrawal should be prevented. This

titrated low dose method of administration limits withdrawal-induced adverse effects, such as vomiting and the potential for aspiration pneumonitis, and a surge in catecholamines with the potential for cardiac dysrhythmias and the acute respiratory distress syndrome (ARDS). Because of its poor oral bioavailability, oral naloxone was previously suggested as treatment for patients with opioid-induced constipation. Methylnaltrexone, a parenteral medication, and naloxegol, an oral formulation, are effective in reversing opioid-induced constipation without inducing opioid withdrawal. This is because their central nervous system (CNS) entry is restricted. Naltrexone is used both orally and intramuscularly in patients after opioid detoxification to maintain opioid abstinence and as an adjunct to achieve ethanol abstinence.

HISTORY

The understanding of structure–activity relationships led to the synthesis of many new molecules in the hope of producing potent opioid agonists free of abuse potential. Although this goal is not yet realized, opioid antagonists and partial agonists resulted from these investigations. N-Allylnorcodeine was the first opioid antagonist synthesized (in 1915), and N-allylnormorphine (nalorphine) was synthesized in the 1940s.[40,82] Nalorphine was recognized as having both agonist and antagonist effects in 1954. Naloxone was synthesized in 1960, and naltrexone in 1963. The synthesis of opioid antagonists that are unable to cross the blood–brain barrier (sometimes called peripherally restricted) allowed patients receiving long-term opioid analgesics to avoid opioid-induced constipation, one of the most uncomfortable side effects associated with opioid therapy. Since the mid-1990s and the reappearance of the opioid epidemic of the 21st century, there has been a steady increase in the use of naloxone that is prescribed or directly dispensed to users of any opioid who are at risk of overdose as well as for administration by bystanders.[14]

PHARMACOLOGY

Chemistry

Minor structural alterations are used to convert an agonist into an antagonist. The substitution of the N-methyl group on morphine by a larger functional group led to nalorphine and converted the agonist levorphanol to the antagonist levallorphan.[38] Naloxone and naltrexone are derivatives of oxymorphone with antagonist properties resulting from addition of organic or other functional groups.[38,42]

Mechanism of Action

The mu receptors are responsible for analgesia, sedation, miosis, euphoria, respiratory depression, and decreased gastrointestinal (GI) motility. Kappa receptors are responsible for spinal analgesia, miosis, dysphoria, anxiety, nightmares, and hallucinations. Delta receptors are responsible for analgesia and hunger. The currently available opioid receptor antagonists are most potent at the mu receptor, with higher doses required to affect the kappa and delta receptors. They all bind to the opioid receptor in a competitive fashion, preventing the binding of agonists, partial agonists, or mixed agonist–antagonists without producing any independent action.

Pharmacokinetics

Naloxone and naltrexone differ primarily in their pharmacokinetics. Naltrexone has a longer duration of action and sufficient oral bioavailability to produce systemic effects. At therapeutic doses, methylnaltrexone is relatively effectively excluded from the CNS and only produces peripheral effects in overdose. Selective antagonists for mu, kappa, and delta are available experimentally and are undergoing investigation.

The oral bioavailability of naloxone is less than 2%,[30,76] rectal bioavailability is 15%,[76] and the sublingual bioavailability is only 10%.[8] The bioavailability of a concentrated intranasal naloxone formulation is approximately 44% that of naloxone administered by the intramuscular (IM) route.[1] In the same study, the apparent half-life of 4 mg of the 40 mg/mL formulation sprayed into one or both nostrils was approximately 2.1 hour compared with 1.24 hour for 0.4 mg administered IM into the thigh. In contrast, naloxone is well absorbed by all parenteral routes of administration. The approximate onset of action with the various routes of administration are as follows: intralingual, 30 seconds; intravenous (IV), 1 to 2 minutes; endotracheal, 60 seconds; intranasal, 3.4 minutes; inhalational (nebulized), 5 minutes; subcutaneous (SC), 5.5 minutes; and IM, 6 minutes.[26,44,62,91] The distribution half-life is rapid (~5 minutes) because of its high lipid solubility. Protein binding is low,[1] and the volume of distribution (V_d) is 0.8 to 2.64 L/kg.[34]

An IV naloxone dose of 13 mcg/kg (~1 mg in an 80-kg opioid-naïve adult) occupies approximately 50% of the available opioid receptors.[57] The duration of action of naloxone is approximately 20 to 90 minutes and depends on the dose and route of administration of naloxone and the rates of elimination of the agonist and naloxone.[8,28,85] Naloxone is hepatically metabolized to several compounds, including a glucuronide conjugate. The elimination half-life after IV administration is 60 to 90 minutes in adults and approximately two to three times longer in neonates.

Naltrexone is rapidly absorbed with an oral bioavailability of 5% to 60% because of extensive first pass effects, and peak serum concentrations occur at 1 hour.[37] Distribution is rapid, with a V_d of approximately 15 L/kg and low protein binding.[48] Naltrexone is metabolized in the liver to β-naltrexol (major metabolite with 2%–8% activity) and 2-hydroxy,3-methoxy-β-naltrexol and undergoes an enterohepatic cycle.[54,89] The plasma elimination half-lives are 4 hours for naltrexone and 13 hours for β-naltrexol, with a terminal phase of elimination of 96 hours and 18 hours, respectively.[87] The terminal elimination half-life corresponds most closely with the clinical effects of naltrexone.[51] Naltrexone for extended-release injectable suspension (Vivitrol, Alkermes) displays an initial peak concentration at approximately 2 hours after injection; a second peak 2 to 3 days later; and approximately 14 days after dosing, the concentration slowly declines over the subsequent month.[4]

Methylnaltrexone is a quaternary amine methylated derivative of naltrexone that is peripherally restricted because of its poor lipid solubility and limited ability to cross the blood–brain barrier.[99] After SC administration, peak serum concentrations occur in about 30 minutes. The drug has a V_d of 1.1 L/kg and is minimally protein bound (11%–15%). Although there are several metabolites, 85% of the drug is eliminated unchanged in the urine.[99]

Naloxegol is an orally bioavailable, pegylated derivative of naloxone. Pegylation reduces its ability to cross the blood–brain barrier and allows its removal by the P-glycoprotein efflux pump. Peak serum concentration occurs at about 2 hours. Elimination is primarily through CYP3A4 metabolism, and the half-life is 6 to 11 hours.

Pharmacodynamics

In the proper doses, pure opioid antagonists reverse all of the effects at the mu, kappa, and delta receptors of endogenous and exogenous opioid agonists. Buprenorphine, a partial agonist that behaves clinically like an antagonist in opioid dependent people, has a very high affinity for and slow rate of dissociation from the mu receptor.[65] Actions of opioid agonists that are not mediated by interaction with opioid receptors, such as direct mast cell liberation of histamine and the potassium channel blocking effects of methadone, are not reversed by these antagonists.[5] Chest wall rigidity from rapid fentanyl infusion is usually reversed with naloxone.[19] Opioid-induced seizures in animals, such as from propoxyphene, are antagonized by opioid antagonists, although seizures caused by meperidine (normeperidine) and tramadol are not.[33] The benefit of naloxone for opioid-induced seizures in humans is less clear. A report of two newborns

who developed seizures associated with fentanyl and morphine infusion demonstrated abrupt clinical and electroencephalographic resolution after administration of naloxone.[22]

Opioids operate bimodally on opioid receptors.[20] At very low concentrations, mu opioid receptor agonism is excitatory and increases pain. This antianalgesic effect of opioids is modulated through a G_s protein and usually is less important clinically than the well-known inhibitory actions that result from coupling to a G_o protein at usual analgesic doses. For this reason, extremely low doses of opioid antagonists (ie, 0.25 mcg/kg/h of naloxone) enhance the analgesic potency of opioids, including morphine, methadone, and buprenorphine.[21,32] Naloxone also attenuates or prevents the development of tolerance and dependence.[32] Coadministration of these very low doses of antagonists with the opioid also limits opioid-induced adverse effects such as nausea, vomiting, constipation, and pruritus.[99]

Opioid antagonists reverse the effects of endogenous opioid peptides, including endorphins, dynorphins, and enkephalins with variable effectiveness. Endogenous opioids are found in tissues throughout the body and work in concert with other neurotransmitter systems to modulate many physiologic effects.[29,84] For instance, during shock, the release of circulating endorphins produces an inhibition of central sympathetic tone by stimulating kappa receptors within the locus coeruleus, resulting in vasodilation. Vagal tone is also enhanced through stimulation of opioid receptors in the nucleus ambiguus. Naloxone continues to be explored in resuscitation from cardiac arrest,[71] which appears to be related to its effects at the delta-opioid receptor. The data do not support its routine administration at this time.[55,64]

ROLE IN OPIOID TOXICITY

Naloxone use by medical personnel for the management of patients with opioid toxicity has evolved over the past 50 years. Initial studies found the use of naloxone to be relatively safe and highly effective in awakening opioid-toxic patients.[43,97] Although once recommended to be administered empirically to nearly every patient with a depressed level of consciousness and respiratory depression,[41] as complications of precipitated opioid withdrawal in opioid-dependent patients became more apparent, such aggressive use diminished dramatically.[9] Currently, the empiric parenteral dose that we recommend for all opioid-dependent patients is 0.04 mg,[18] although in nondependent patients, higher doses are administered without concern for precipitating withdrawal. The goal of reversal of opioid toxicity is to improve the patient's ventilation while avoiding withdrawal (see later discussion).

Take-home naloxone distribution and naloxone prescribing for bystander administration in addition to programs for nonmedical first responders continue to significantly expand around the world.[90] The majority of the naloxone available for community-based use is intended for administration by the intranasal route.[3,7] Increasing the availability of naloxone leads to an increased rate of reversal from opioid-induced unresponsiveness, although the absolute numbers and rates of preventing death are unknown.[94] However, debates exist on best approaches to this public health attempt at harm reduction (see Adverse Effects and Safety Issues). See further discussion in Special Considerations: SC6 on harm reduction.

ROLE IN MAINTENANCE OF OPIOID ABSTINENCE

Opioid dependence is managed either by substitution of the primary opioid, typically heroin or a prescription opioid, with methadone or buprenorphine or by detoxification and subsequent abstinence. Maintenance of abstinence is facilitated by the administration of daily or depot formulations of naltrexone.[74] This is of particular importance in patients whose opioid tolerance has waned because of abstinence, whether voluntary or forced, such as in the immediate period after incarceration.[50]

Before naltrexone is administered for abstinence maintenance, the patient must be weaned from opioid dependence and be a willing participant. Naloxone should be administered intravenously to confirm that the patient is no longer opioid dependent and is therefore safe for naltrexone administration. With naloxone, opioid withdrawal, if it occurs, will be short lived instead of prolonged as it is after the administration of naltrexone. Prolonged treatment with naltrexone (and naloxone) results in upregulation and supersensitivity of opioid receptors.[75] Although the clinical implications are undefined, concern should be heightened for enhanced clinical response to an opioid after resumption of opioid use in patients who discontinue naltrexone therapy.

ROLE IN ETHANOL ABSTINENCE

Naltrexone, particularly the IM depot form, is used as adjunctive therapy in ethanol dependence based on the theory that the endogenous opioid system modulates ethanol intake.[13,81] Naltrexone reduces ethanol craving, the number of drinking days, and relapse rates.[52,68] Naltrexone induces moderate to severe nausea in 15% of patients, possibly as a result of alterations in endogenous opioid tone induced by prolonged ethanol ingestion.

OTHER USES

Poorly orally bioavailable opioid antagonists (eg, naloxone) and peripherally restricted opioid antagonists (eg, methylnaltrexone) are used to prevent or treat the constipation occurring as a side effect of opioid use, whether for pain management or addiction therapy.[11] Evacuation resulted from methylnaltrexone, within 4 hours, and naloxegol, within 6 hours, but the beneficial effect was small by absolute standards, and the drugs are expensive.[15,80]

Opioid antagonists are sometimes used in the management of overdoses with nonopioids such as ethanol,[25] clonidine,[73] captopril,[86] and valproic acid.[79] In none of these instances is the reported improvement as dramatic or consistent as in the reversal of an opioid. The mechanisms for each of these, although undefined, is suggested to relate to reversal of endogenous opioid peptides at opioid receptors.

Naloxone was used to reverse the effects of endogenous opioid peptides in patients with septic shock, although the results were variable.[24] Treatment is often ineffective and will result in adverse effects in patients who are opioid tolerant.

Opioid antagonists at low doses are used for treatment of morphine-induced pruritus resulting from systemic or epidural exposure and for treat of pruritus associated with cholestasis.[61,66]

ADVERSE EFFECTS AND SAFETY ISSUES

Pure opioid antagonists produce no clinical effects in opioid-naïve or nondependent patients even when administered in massive doses (grams) in a spinal cord injury study.[10] Although in another study when naloxone was administered to opioid-naïve patients in large doses (2 mg/kg), a variety of symptoms, including anxiety, difficulty concentrating, sadness, irritability, sweating, and GI manifestations were reported.[2] Some of these findings lasted for a few days.

When patients dependent on opioid agonists are exposed to opioid antagonists, agonist–antagonists, or partial agonists, they exhibit opioid withdrawal, including yawning, lacrimation, diaphoresis, rhinorrhea, piloerection, mydriasis, vomiting, diarrhea, myalgias, mild elevations in heart rate and blood pressure, and insomnia. Antagonist-precipitated withdrawal also sometimes results in an "overshoot" phenomenon, from a transient increase in circulating catecholamines, resulting in hyperventilation, tachycardia, and hypertension.[47]

Under these circumstances, there is a potential for related withdrawal-related complications. In the cardiovascular system, myocardial ischemia and infarction, myocardial stunning (takotsubo, stress cardiomyopathy), heart failure, hypertension, and dysrhythmia are rarely reported.[46] In the CNS, agitation should be expected and is occasionally profound, and seizures, although rare, may occur. Delirium, although rarely reported in patients withdrawing because of opioid abstinence, occur during precipitated opioid withdrawal.[35]

In the lungs, case reports describe acute respiratory distress syndrome (ARDS) in association with naloxone administration, almost uniformly in opioid-dependent patients.[67,72] The clinical complexities of the setting make it difficult to analyze and attribute these adverse effects solely to naloxone.[12] Adult respiratory distress syndrome occurs after heroin overdose in the absence of naloxone,[27] making the exact contribution of naloxone unclear. Rather, in certain patients, naloxone likely unmasks ARDS previously induced by the opioid but unrecognized because of the patient's concomitant opioid-induced respiratory depression.

If the patient's airway is unprotected during withdrawal and vomiting occurs, aspiration pneumonitis may complicate the recovery.[17] Given the frequency of polysubstance abuse and overdose associated with altered consciousness, the risk of precipitating withdrawal-associated vomiting should always be a concern.

These severe manifestations of precipitated opioid withdrawal also occur with ultra-rapid opioid detoxification and are associated with fatalities occurring in the postdetoxification period.[39] This rapid form of deliberate detoxification differs significantly from the opioid withdrawal associated with volitional opioid abstinence (Chap. 14).

Many of the adverse effects observed in patients with precipitated opioid withdrawal are the result of excessive circulating catecholamines. The catecholamine response to naloxone is significantly greater in dogs with hypercapnia compared with those that are normocapnic or hypocapnic.[59] Although not studied in humans, this highlights the potential ability of manual ventilation before the administration of naloxone to ameliorate the aforementioned complications.

Resedation is a function of the relatively short duration of action of the opioid antagonist compared with the opioid agonist. Most opioid agonists have durations of action longer than that of naloxone and shorter than that of naltrexone (with the exception of methadone). A long duration of action is advantageous when the antagonist is used to promote abstinence (naltrexone) but is undesired when inappropriately administered to an opioid-dependent patient (see Observation Period After Antagonist Administration).

Unmasking underlying cocaine or other stimulant toxicity may explain some of the cardiac dysrhythmias that develop after naloxone-induced opioid reversal in a patient simultaneously using both opioids and stimulants (Chaps. 73 and 75).[58]

Antagonists stimulate the release of hormones from the pituitary, resulting in increased concentrations of luteinizing hormone, follicle-stimulating hormone, and adrenocorticotropic hormone and stimulate the release of prolactin in women.[69]

Observation Period After Antagonist Administration

What constitutes an appropriate observation period after antagonist administration depends on many factors. After IV bolus naloxone at doses less than 2 mg, observation for 2 hours is typically adequate to determine whether sedation and respiratory depression will return as the naloxone effect diminishes and the initial opioid effects return. Therefore, although the matched pharmacokinetics of heroin and naloxone suggest potential utility for this practice, the high frequency of methadone, extended-release prescription opioids, transdermal fentanyl, and novel opioids such as the fentanyl derivatives in many communities raises concern for this practice.[49] That is, the pharmacokinetic mismatch between naloxone and these other opioids would expectedly result in recurrent opioid toxicity from long acting and extended release opioids.[88]

Although no fatalities were identified in death certificate searches after the rapid prehospital release of patients who were administered naloxone after presumably overdosing with heroin, these studies are limited by the use of heroin primarily, and not methadone, the potential for incomplete follow-up, the low death rate following heroin overdose and the minimization of the nonfatal consequences of resedation.[16,88,95] In clinical practice, it is common for patients with opioid overdose to receive repetitive doses of naloxone, raising questions about the safety of releasing patients before transport.[16,95] Additionally, the benefit of the observation period in the emergency department permits harm reduction education, recognition of suicidal ideation, evaluation and referral for long-term addiction treatment, and initiation of preventive intervention (Chap. 36 and Special Considerations: SC6).

Similarly, patients discontinued from a continuous naloxone infusion or those who received large total initial doses of naloxone by any route, including intranasal, typically necessitate subsequent observation for at least 4 hours, and perhaps 6 hours, to ensure that respiratory depression or sedation does not recur. Observation should be meticulous and include periodic direct assessment of arousability and ventilatory rate and effort, as well as continuous pulse oximetry off supplemental oxygen. Optimally, continuous capnometry should be used.

Management of Iatrogenic Withdrawal

Excessive administration of an opioid antagonist to an opioid-dependent patient will predictably result in opioid withdrawal. When induced by naloxone, all that is generally required is protecting the patient from harm and reassuring the patient that the effects will be short lived. Supportive care is valuable during the transient withdrawal. After inadvertent administration of naltrexone, the expected duration of the withdrawal syndrome generally mandates the use of pharmacologic intervention.[31,53] Overcoming the opioid receptor antagonism is difficult, but if used in titrated doses, fentanyl or morphine is often successful. Fentanyl has the advantage over morphine of causing less histamine release. Although the use of buprenorphine was only indirectly studied in this role,[83] it has several potential advantages, including high receptor affinity, long duration of action, low risk of oversedation and the possibility of converting to long term buprenophine treatment. If only moderate withdrawal is present, the administration of metoclopramide, clonidine, or a benzodiazepine is usually adequate.[46]

PREGNANCY AND LACTATION

Naloxone and naltrexone are pregnancy Category C medications. A risk-to-benefit analysis must be performed for pregnant women, particularly those who are opioid tolerant, and their newborns. Inducing opioid withdrawal in the mother probably will induce withdrawal in the fetus and should be avoided. Similarly, administering naloxone (or naltrexone) to newborns of opioid-tolerant mothers may induce neonatal withdrawal and should be used cautiously (Chaps. 30, 31, and 36).[60]

DOSING AND ADMINISTRATION

Before administration of naloxone, the patient should receive adequate ventilation to ensure that the patient is not hypercapnic (see Adverse Effects and Safety Issues). The initial dose of antagonist is dependent on the dose of agonist, the amount that reaches the brain, and the relative binding affinity of the agonist and antagonist at the opioid receptors. The presently available antagonists have a greater affinity for the mu receptor than for the kappa or delta receptors. Some opioids, such as buprenorphine, require greater than expected doses of antagonist to reverse the effects at the mu receptor and exhibit a bell-shaped response to naloxone (see later).[85,96] The duration of action of the antagonist depends on many drug and patient variables, such as the dose and the clearance of both antagonist and agonist.[63]

A dose of naloxone 0.4 mg IV will reverse the respiratory depressant effects of most opioids and is an appropriate starting dose in non–opioid-dependent patients. However, this dose in an opioid-dependent patient usually produces withdrawal, which should be avoided if possible. The goal is to produce a spontaneously and adequately ventilating patient without precipitating significant or abrupt opioid withdrawal. Therefore, 0.04 mg IV is a reasonable starting dose in most patients, with incremental increases by 0.04 mg, while supporting the patient's ventilation and oxygenation, up to a dose of 0.12 mg. The readily available 0.4 mg/mL formulation of parenteral naloxone can be diluted with 9 mL of 0.9% sodium chloride for a total volume of 10 mL, yielding a concentration of 0.04 mg/mL. In those without response, increasing by 0.2 or 0.4 mg up to a dose of 2 mg is a reasonable approach.[9] Dosing beyond 2 mg for those who have an opioid toxidrome is often suggested by 2 mg additional doses, even up to 10 mg,[9] but this is not prospectively validated and rarely required. In situations in which an ultra-potent opioid, often a fentanyl derivative, has been administered, there are reports of response after very large naloxone doses of 10 mg. Whether this

is due to the relatively large dose or unique receptor kinetics of these opioids is unknown, but this practice seems reasonable. Failure of the patient to respond to 8 to 10 mg of naloxone suggests that a conventional opioid is not responsible for the respiratory depression and sedation, an additional respiratory depressant is present, or the patient has hypoxic encephalopathy. In this latter situation, pupillary dilation may help in the assessment.

The dose in children without opioid dependence is essentially the same as for adults (ie, 0.1 mg/kg to the adult dose of 2 mg). However, for those with opioid dependence and the possibility of precipitated withdrawal or recrudescence of severe underlying pain, a more gentle reversal with 0.04 mg, with concomitant supportive care, is warranted. Although both the adult and pediatric doses recommended here are lower than those conventionally suggested in other references, the availability of safe and effective interim ventilatory therapy permits these lower doses and lowers the acceptable risk of precipitating withdrawal (Chaps. 4 and 36).

When 1 mg of naloxone is administered IV, it prevents the action of 25 mg of IV heroin for 1 hour; 50 mg of oral naltrexone antagonizes this dose of heroin for 24 hours, 100 mg of oral naltrexone has a blocking effect for 48 hours, and 150 mg of oral naltrexone is effective for 72 hours.[54]

The use of low doses of IV naloxone to reverse opioid overdose prolongs the time to improvement of ventilation, and during this period, assisted ventilation is appropriate. The same limitation exists with SC naloxone administration, and the absorbed dose is more difficult to titrate than when administered IV.[91] Naloxone is also administered intranasally, although this route results in the delivery of unpredictable doses. In the prehospital setting, the time to onset of clinical effect of intranasal naloxone is comparable to that of IV or IM naloxone, largely because of the delay in obtaining IV access and slow absorption, respectively.[6,44] Intranasal naloxone is not recommended as first-line treatment by health care providers in hospitals but is reasonable for prehospital providers when other routes of administration are unavailable or undesirable.[45] Nebulized naloxone (2 mg is mixed with 3 mL of 0.9% sodium chloride solution) has similar limitations in dose accuracy and is further limited in patients with severe ventilatory depression, the group most in need of naloxone. Although reports suggest successful use of nebulized naloxone, patients with opioid overdose are not optimal candidates for inhalation therapy because of both the poor respiratory effort and to the likelihood of over- or underdosing of naloxone.[92] Although needleless delivery is a clear prehospital advantage,[56] the lack of the ability to titrate substantially reduces the usefulness of intranasal or nebulized naloxone in the hospital.

Evaluation for the redevelopment of respiratory depression after naloxone administration requires nearly continuous monitoring. This is significantly more likely to occur after an extended-release or long-acting opioid and is increasingly a concern with the unique fentanyl derivatives that currently appear as adulterants in the illicit opioid supply.[78] Resedation should be treated with either repeated dosing of the antagonist or, in some cases, such as after a long-acting opioid agonist, with another bolus followed by a continuous infusion of naloxone.[78] Two-thirds of the total bolus dose of naloxone that resulted in reversal, when given hourly, usually maintains the desired effect.[36] Titration upward or downward is easily accomplished as necessary to both maintain adequate ventilation and avoid withdrawal. A continuous infusion of naloxone is not a substitute for continued vigilance. A period of 12 to 24 hours often is chosen for observation based on the presumed opioid, the route of administration, and the dosage form (sustained release). Body packers are a unique subset of patients who, because of the reservoir of drug in the GI tract, require individualized antagonist management strategies (Special Considerations: SC5).

Use of longer acting opioid antagonists, such as naltrexone, places the patient at substantial risk for protracted withdrawal syndromes. The use of a long-acting opioid antagonist in acute care situations should be reserved for carefully considered special indications, such as unintentional exposures to short acting opioids in nondependent patients, together with extended periods of observation or careful follow-up. An oral dose of 150 mg of naltrexone generally lasts 48 to 72 hours and should be adequate as an antidote for the majority of patients with opioid toxicity.[51] As noted, this drug should not be administered to a patient with opioid dependence. Discharge of patients with opioid toxicity after successful administration of a long-acting opioid antagonist, although theoretically attractive, is not well studied. There are concerns about attempts by patients to overcome the opioid antagonism by administering high doses of opioid agonist,[39] with subsequent respiratory depression as the effect of the antagonist wanes.

Naltrexone is administered orally in a variety of dosage schedules for treatment of opioid dependence. A common dosing regimen is 50 mg/day Monday through Friday and 100 mg on Saturdays. Alternatively, 100 mg every other day or 150 mg every third day can be administered. The IM extended-release suspension is injected monthly at a recommended dose of 380 mg.

Methylnaltrexone SC dosing for opioid-induced constipation is weight based.[98] The dose is 0.15 mg/kg for patients who weigh less than 38 kg and more than 114 kg. For patients who weigh between 38 and less than 62 kg, 8 mg is administered, and for those between 62 and 114 kg, 12 mg is provided. Dosing for patients with stage 4 or 5 chronic kidney disease is established at half the standard recommended dose.

Naloxegol tablets should be swallowed whole and not be crushed or chewed. The daily dose is 25 mg once in the morning at least 1 hour before or 2 hours after a meal, and the dose halved in patients who develop signs and symptoms of opioid withdrawal with the higher dose. The starting dosage for patients with a stage 4 or 5 kidney disease is 12.5 mg once daily.

Alvimopan is approved by the US Food and Drug Administration for the management of postoperative ileus in the hospital setting and is not indicated for outpatient or long-term use. It is contraindicated in patients who have taken opioids for more than 7 days. The dose is 12 mg orally 0.5 to 5 hours preoperatively. The day after surgery, the maintenance dose is 12 mg twice a day. The total maximum number of doses is 15 during hospitalization.

Buprenorphine

Naloxone reverses the respiratory depressant effects of buprenorphine in a unique dose–response curve.[23,70,85,96] Bolus doses of naloxone of 2 to 3 mg followed by a continuous infusion of 4 mg/h in adults were able to fully reverse the respiratory depression associated with IV buprenorphine administered in a total dose of 0.2 and 0.4 mg over 1 hour.[85] Reversal was not apparent until about 45 to 60 minutes after the infusion. A reappearance of respiratory depression occurred when the naloxone infusion was stopped because the distribution of naloxone out of the brain and its subsequent elimination from the body are much faster than those of buprenorphine. Consistent with the unique response curve, doses of naloxone greater than 4 mg/h actually led to the redevelopment of respiratory depression. It is postulated that buprenorphine has differential effects on the mu opioid receptor subtypes (Chap. 36), with agonist activity at low doses and antagonist action at high doses. Therefore, excess naloxone antagonizes the opioid antagonistic effects of high dose buprenorphine and worsens the respiratory depression.

Interestingly, there is support for the use of buprenorphine to manage patients with opioid overdose.[93,100] Perhaps not surprisingly, the antagonistic effects of buprenorphine are not dose related, and the maximal effects occurring at 1 mg IM (which equates to about 0.4 mg sublingually).[77] Given the partial agonist effects of buprenorphine, the resulting withdrawal syndrome is less severe than that after a pure opioid antagonist.[77] This practice requires additional study before recommending its use.

FORMULATION AND ACQUISITION

Naloxone (Narcan) for IV, IM, or SC administration is available in concentrations of 0.4 and 1 mg/mL, with and without parabens in 1- and 2-mL ampoules, vials, and syringes and in 10-mL multidose vials with parabens. Naloxone is frequently diluted in 0.9% sodium chloride solution or 5% dextrose to facilitate continuous IV infusion. Naloxone is stable in 0.9% sodium chloride solution at a variety of concentrations for up to 24 hours. An auto-injector containing 2 mg of naloxone is available. Intranasal formulations vary and include the use of the 1-mg/mL solution with a mucosal atomizer device (MAD) and a 2-mg/0.1 mL (20 mg/mL concentration) and 4-mg/0.1 mL (40 mg/mL concentration) naloxone administration device.

Naltrexone is available as a 50-mg capsule-shaped tablet. It is also available as a 380-mg vial for reconstitution with a carboxymethylcellulose and polysorbate diluent to form an injectable suspension intended for monthly IM administration.[4]

Methylnaltrexone is available as a 12-mg/0.6-mL solution for SC injection.[67]

Naloxegol is available as an oral tablet, in 12.5 mg and 25 mg strengths.

SUMMARY

- Naloxone and naltrexone are pure competitive opioid antagonists at the mu (μ), kappa (κ), and delta (δ) receptors.
- Methylnaltrexone (parenteral) and naloxegol (oral) are peripherally acting opioid antagonists used to counteract opioid induced constipation and do not have CNS effects except in overdose.
- Naloxone is the primary opioid antagonist used to reverse respiratory depression in patients manifesting opioid toxicity.
- A titrated low-dose method of IV administration, starting at 0.04 mg in an adult, limits withdrawal-induced adverse effects, such as vomiting and the potential for aspiration pneumonitis, and a surge in catecholamines with the potential for cardiac dysrhythmias and ARDS.
- Naltrexone is used orally for patients after opioid detoxification to maintain opioid abstinence and as an adjunct to achieve ethanol abstinence. It is used in specific circumstances to prevent recurrent opioid toxicity in nondependent patients with otherwise uncomplicated opioid overdoses.
- Intranasal naloxone is increasingly used by bystanders for the emergency reversal of patients with opioid-induced CNS and respiratory depression.

REFERENCES

1. Adapt Pharma, Inc. Narcan (Naloxone Hydrochloride) Nasal Spray Prescribing Information. 2017:1-17. http://www.narcannasalspray.com/pdf/NARCAN-Prescribing-Information.pdf.
2. Akorn, Inc. Naloxone Hydrochloride Injection, USP. 2017:1-11. https://dailymed.nlm.nih.gov/dailymed/getFile.cfm?setid=747e602c-93f9-4723-a899-4c1c55c35ef8&type=pdf.
3. Albert S, et al. Project Lazarus: community-based overdose prevention in rural North Carolina. *Pain Med*. 2011;12(suppl 2):S77-S85.
4. Alkermes, Inc. Vivitrol (Naltrexone for Extended Release Injectable Suspension). 2015:1-11.
5. Barke KE, Hough LB. Opiates, mast cells and histamine release. *Life Sci*. 1993;53:1391-1399.
6. Barton ED, et al. Efficacy of intranasal naloxone as a needleless alternative for treatment of opioid overdose in the prehospital setting. *J Emerg Med*. 2005;29:265-271.
7. Beletsky L, et al. Prevention of fatal opioid overdose. *JAMA*. 2012;308:1863-1864.
8. Berkowitz BA. The relationship of pharmacokinetics to pharmacological activity: morphine, methadone and naloxone. *Clin Pharmacokinet*. 1976;1:219-230.
9. Boyer EW. Management of opioid analgesic overdose. *N Engl J Med*. 2012;367:146-155.
10. Bracken MB, et al. A randomized, controlled trial of methylprednisolone or naloxone in the treatment of acute spinal-cord injury. Results of the Second National Acute Spinal Cord Injury Study. *N Engl J Med*. 1990;322:1405-1411.
11. Brock C, et al. Opioid-induced bowel dysfunction: pathophysiology and management. *Drugs*. 2012;72:1847-1865.
12. Buajordet I, et al. Adverse events after naloxone treatment of episodes of suspected acute opioid overdose. *Eur J Emerg Med*. 2004;11:19-23.
13. Candidate SS, et al. A systematic review of naltrexone for attenuating alcohol consumption in women with alcohol use disorders. *Alcohol Clin Exp Res*. 2017;41:466-472.
14. Centers for Disease Control and Prevention (CDC). Community-based opioid overdose prevention programs providing naloxone—United States, 2010. *MMWR Morbidity and Mortality Weekly Report*. 2012;61:101-105.
15. Chey WD, et al. Naloxegol for opioid-induced constipation in patients with noncancer pain. *N Engl J Med*. 2014;370:2387-2396.
16. Christenson J, et al. Early discharge of patients with presumed opioid overdose: development of a clinical prediction rule. *Acad Emerg Med*. 2000;7:1110-1118.
17. Clarke SFJ, et al. Naloxone in opioid poisoning: walking the tightrope. *Emerg Med J*. 2005;22:612-616.
18. Connors NJ, Nelson LS. The evolution of recommended naloxone dosing for opioid overdose by medical specialty. *J Med Toxicol*. 2016;12:414-415.
19. Coruh B, et al. Fentanyl-induced chest wall rigidity. *Chest*. 2013;143:1145-1146.

20. Crain SM, Shen KF. Antagonists of excitatory opioid receptor functions enhance morphine's analgesic potency and attenuate opioid tolerance/dependence liability. *Pain.* 2000;84:121-131.

21. Cruciani RA, et al. Ultra-low dose oral naltrexone decreases side effects and potentiates the effect of methadone. *J Pain Symptom Manage.* 2003;25:491-494.

22. da Silva O, et al. Seizure and electroencephalographic changes in the newborn period induced by opiates and corrected by naloxone infusion. *J Perinatol.* 1999;19:120-123.

23. Dahan A. Opioid-induced respiratory effects: new data on buprenorphine. *Palliat Med.* 2006;20(8 suppl):3-8.

24. DeMaria A, et al. Naloxone versus placebo in treatment of septic shock. *Lancet.* 1985;1:1363-1365.

25. Dole VP, et al. Arousal of ethanol-intoxicated comatose patients with naloxone. *Alcohol Clin Exp Res.* 1982;6:275-279.

26. Dowling J, et al. Population pharmacokinetics of intravenous, intramuscular, and intranasal naloxone in human volunteers. *Ther Drug Monit.* 2008;30:490-496.

27. Duberstein JL, Kaufman DM. A clinical study of an epidemic of heroin intoxication and heroin-induced pulmonary edema. *Am J Med.* 1971;51:704-714.

28. Evans JM, et al. Degree and duration of reversal by naloxone of effects of morphine in conscious subjects. *Br Med J.* 1974;2:589-591.

29. Faden AI, et al. Endorphins in experimental spinal injury: therapeutic effect of naloxone. *Ann Neurol.* 1981;10:326-332.

30. Fishman J, et al. Disposition of naloxone-7,8,3H in normal and narcotic-dependent men. *J Pharmacol Exp Ther.* 1973;187:575-580.

31. Fishman M. Precipitated withdrawal during maintenance opioid blockade with extended release naltrexone. *Addiction.* 2008;103:1399-1401.

32. Gan TJ, et al. Opioid-sparing effects of a low-dose infusion of naloxone in patient-administered morphine sulfate. *Anesthesiology.* 1997;87:1075-1081.

33. Gilbert PE, Martin WR. Antagonism of the convulsant effects of heroin, d-propoxyphene, meperidine, normeperidine and thebaine by naloxone in mice. *J Pharmacol Exp Ther.* 1975;192:538-541.

34. Glass PS, et al. Comparison of potency and duration of action of nalmefene and naloxone. *Anesth Analg.* 1994;78:536-541.

35. Golden SA, Sakhrani DL. Unexpected delirium during rapid opioid detoxification (ROD). *J Addict Dis.* 2004;23:65-75.

36. Goldfrank L, et al. A dosing nomogram for continuous infusion intravenous naloxone. *Ann Emerg Med.* 1986;15:566-570.

37. Gonzalez JP, Brogden RN. Naltrexone. A review of its pharmacodynamic and pharmacokinetic properties and therapeutic efficacy in the management of opioid dependence. *Drugs.* 1988;35:192-213.

38. Goodman AJ, et al. Mu opioid receptor antagonists: recent developments. *ChemMedChem.* 2007;2:1552-1570.

39. Hamilton RJ, et al. Complications of ultrarapid opioid detoxification with subcutaneous naltrexone pellets. *Acad Emerg Med.* 2002;9:63-68.

40. Hart ER, McCawley EL. The pharmacology of *N*-allylnormorphine as compared with morphine. *J Pharmacol Exp Ther.* 1944;82:339-348.

41. Hoffman JR, et al. The empiric use of naloxone in patients with altered mental status: a reappraisal. *Ann Emerg Med.* 1991;20:246-252.

42. Kane BE, et al. Molecular recognition of opioid receptor ligands. *Drug Addiction.* 2008:585-608.

43. Kaplan JL, et al. Double-blind, randomized study of nalmefene and naloxone in emergency department patients with suspected narcotic overdose. *Ann Emerg Med.* 1999;34:42-50.

44. Kelly A-M, et al. Randomised trial of intranasal versus intramuscular naloxone in prehospital treatment for suspected opioid overdose. *Med J Aust.* 2005;182:24-27.

45. Kerr D, et al. Intranasal naloxone for the treatment of suspected heroin overdose. *Addiction.* 2008;103:379-386.

46. Kienbaum P, et al. Sympathetic neural activation evoked by mu-receptor blockade in patients addicted to opioids is abolished by intravenous clonidine. *Anesthesiology.* 2002;96:346-351.

47. Kienbaum P, et al. Profound increase in epinephrine concentration in plasma and cardiovascular stimulation after mu-opioid receptor blockade in opioid-addicted patients during barbiturate-induced anesthesia for acute detoxification. *Anesthesiology.* 1998;88:1154-1161.

48. Kogan MJ, et al. Estimation of the systemic availability and other pharmacokinetic parameters of naltrexone in man after acute and chronic oral administration. *Res Commun Chem Pathol Pharmacol.* 1977;18:29-34.

49. Kolinsky D, et al. Is a prehospital treat and release protocol for opioid overdose safe? *J Emerg Med.* 2017;52:52-58.

50. Lee JD, et al. Extended-release naltrexone to prevent opioid relapse in criminal justice offenders. *N Engl J Med.* 2016;374:1232-1242.

51. Lee MC, et al. Duration of occupancy of opiate receptors by naltrexone. *J Nucl Med.* 1988;29:1207-1211.

52. Lin S-K. Pharmacological means of reducing human drug dependence: a selective and narrative review of the clinical literature. *Br J Clin Pharmacol.* 2014;77:242-252.

53. Lubman D, et al. Emergency management of inadvertent accelerated opiate withdrawal in dependent opiate users. *Drug Alcohol Rev.* 2003;22:433-436.

54. Mallinckrodt, Inc. Naltrexone Hydrochloride Prescribing Information. 2015:1-17. http://www2.mallinckrodt.com/WorkArea/DownloadAsset.aspx?id=1943.

55. Martins HS, et al. Effects of terlipressin and naloxone compared with epinephrine in a rat model of asphyxia-induced cardiac arrest. *Clinics (Sao Paulo).* 2013;68:1146-1151.

56. McDermott C, Collins NC. Prehospital medication administration: a randomised study comparing intranasal and intravenous routes. *Emerg Med Int.* 2012;2012:1-6.

57. Melichar JK, et al. Naloxone displacement at opioid receptor sites measured in vivo in the human brain. *Eur J Pharmacol.* 2003;459:217-219.

58. Merigian KS. Cocaine-induced ventricular arrhythmias and rapid atrial fibrillation temporally related to naloxone administration. *Am J Emerg Med.* 1993;11:96-97.

59. Mills CA, et al. Cardiovascular effects of fentanyl reversal by naloxone at varying arterial carbon dioxide tensions in dogs. *Anesth Analg.* 1988;67:730-736.

60. Moe-Byrne T, et al. Naloxone for opiate-exposed newborn infants. *Cochrane Database Syst Rev.* 2012;2:CD003483.

61. Murphy JD, et al. Analgesic efficacy of intravenous naloxone for the treatment of postoperative pruritus: a meta-analysis. *J Opioid Manag.* 2011;7:321-327.

62. Mycyk M. Nebulized naloxone gently and effectively reverses methadone intoxication. *J Emerg Med.* 2003;24:185-187.

63. Olofsen E, et al. Naloxone reversal of morphine- and morphine-6-glucuronide-induced respiratory depression in healthy volunteers: a mechanism-based pharmacokinetic-pharmacodynamic modeling study. *Anesthesiology.* 2010;112:1417-1427.

64. Partownavid P, et al. Involvement of opioid receptors in the lipid rescue of bupivacaine-induced cardiotoxicity. *Anesth Analg.* 2015;121:340-347.

65. Pasternak GW. Multiple opiate receptors: déjà vu all over again. *Neuropharmacology.* 2004;47(suppl 1):312-323.

66. Phan NQ, et al. Antipruritic treatment with systemic μ-opioid receptor antagonists: a review. *J Am Acad Dermatol.* 2010;63:680-688.

67. Prough DS, et al. Acute pulmonary edema in healthy teenagers following conservative doses of intravenous naloxone. *Anesthesiology.* 1984;60:485-486.

68. Rösner S, et al. Opioid antagonists for alcohol dependence. *Cochrane Database Syst Rev.* 2010:CD001867.

69. Russell JA, et al. Reduced hypothalamo-pituitary-adrenal axis stress responses in late pregnancy: central opioid inhibition and noradrenergic mechanisms. *Ann NY Acad Sci.* 2008;1148:428-438.

70. Sarton E, et al. Naloxone reversal of opioid-induced respiratory depression with special emphasis on the partial agonist/antagonist buprenorphine. *Adv Exp Med Bio.* 2008;605:486-491.

71. Saybolt MD, et al. Naloxone in cardiac arrest with suspected opioid overdoses. *Resuscitation.* 2010;81:42-46.

72. Schwartz JA, Koenigsberg MD. Naloxone-induced pulmonary edema. *Ann Emerg Med.* 1987;16:1294-1296.

73. Seger DL. Clonidine toxicity revisited. *J Toxicol Clin Toxicol.* 2002;40:145-155.

74. Sigmon SC, et al. Opioid detoxification and naltrexone induction strategies: recommendations for clinical practice. *Am J Drug Alcohol Abuse.* 2012;38:187-199.

75. Sirohi S, et al. Mu-opioid receptor up-regulation and functional supersensitivity are independent of antagonist efficacy. *J Pharmacol Exp Ther.* 2007;323:701-707.

76. Smith K, et al. Low absolute bioavailability of oral naloxone in healthy subjects. *Int J Clin Pharmacol Ther.* 2012;50:360-367.

77. Strain EC, et al. Buprenorphine effects in methadone-maintained volunteers: effects at two hours after methadone. *J Pharmacol Exp Ther.* 1995;272:628-638.

78. Sutter ME, et al. Fatal fentanyl: one pill can kill. *Acad Emerg Med.* 2017;24:106-113.

79. Thanacoody HKR. Chronic valproic acid intoxication: reversal by naloxone. *Emerg Med J.* 2007;24:677-678.

80. Thomas J, et al. Methylnaltrexone for opioid-induced constipation in advanced illness. *N Engl J Med.* 2008;358:2332-2343.

81. Thorsell A. The μ-opioid receptor and treatment response to naltrexone. *Alcohol Alcohol.* 2013;48:402-408.

82. Unna K. Antagonistic effect of *N*-allyl-normorphine upon morphine. *J Pharmacol Exp Ther.* 1943;79:28-31.

83. Urban V, Sullivan R. Buprenorphine rescue from naltrexone-induced opioid withdrawal during relatively rapid detoxification from high-dose methadone: a novel approach. *Psychiatry (Edgmont).* 2008;5:56-58.

84. van den Berg MH, et al. Endogenous opioid peptides and blood pressure regulation during controlled, stepwise hemorrhagic hypotension. *Circ Shock.* 1991;35:102-108.

85. van Dorp E, et al. Naloxone reversal of buprenorphine-induced respiratory depression. *Anesthesiology.* 2006;105:51-57.

86. Varon J, Duncan SR. Naloxone reversal of hypotension due to captopril overdose. *Ann Emerg Med.* 1991;20:1125-1127.

87. Verebey K, et al. Naltrexone: disposition, metabolism, and effects after acute and chronic dosing. *Clin Pharmacol Ther.* 1976;20:315-328.

88. Vilke GM, et al. Assessment for deaths in out-of-hospital heroin overdose patients treated with naloxone who refuse transport. *Acad Emerg Med.* 2003;10:893-896.

89. Wall ME, et al. Metabolism and disposition of naltrexone in man after oral and intravenous administration. *Drug Metabolism and Disposition.* 1981;9:369-375.

90. Walley AY. Opioid overdose prevention and naloxone rescue kits: what we know and what we don't know. *Addict Sci Clin Pract.* 2017;12:4.

91. Wanger K, et al. Intravenous vs subcutaneous naloxone for out-of-hospital management of presumed opioid overdose. *Acad Emerg Med*. 1998;5:293-299.

92. Weber JM, et al. Can nebulized naloxone be used safely and effectively by emergency medical services for suspected opioid overdose? *Prehosp Emerg Care*. 2012;16:289-292.

93. Welsh C, et al. A case of heroin overdose reversed by sublingually administered buprenorphine/naloxone (Suboxone). *Addiction*. 2008;103:1226-1228.

94. Wheeler E, et al. Opioid overdose prevention programs providing naloxone to laypersons—United States, 2014. *MMWR Morbidity and Mortality Weekly Report*. 2015;64:631-635.

95. Willman MW, et al. Do heroin overdose patients require observation after receiving naloxone? *Clin Toxicol (Phila)*. 2016;55:308.

96. Yassen A, et al. Mechanism-based pharmacokinetic-pharmacodynamic modelling of the reversal of buprenorphine-induced respiratory depression by naloxone: a study in healthy volunteers. *Clin Pharmacokinet*. 2007;46:965-980.

97. Yealy DM, et al. The safety of prehospital naloxone administration by paramedics. *Ann Emerg Med*. 1990;19:902-905.

98. Yuan CS, et al. Methylnaltrexone for reversal of constipation due to chronic methadone use: a randomized controlled trial. *JAMA*. 2000;283:367-372.

99. Yuan CS. Tolerability, Gut effects, and pharmacokinetics of methylnaltrexone following repeated intravenous administration in humans. *J Clin Pharmacol*. 2005;45:538-546.

100. Zamani N, Hassanian-Moghaddam H. Intravenous buprenorphine: a substitute for naloxone in methadone-overdosed patients? *Ann Emerg Med*. 2017;69:737-739.

Special Considerations

INTERNAL CONCEALMENT OF XENOBIOTICS

Jane M. Prosser

Internal concealment of illicit xenobiotics is a significant concern for local and international police efforts as well as medical and public health practitioners. There are two distinct categories of concealment colloquially known as "body stuffers" and "body packers." The term *body stuffer* refers to individuals who hide xenobiotics in a body cavity or ingest them in an attempt to avoid discovery. The xenobiotics are concealed in an unplanned manner and are often poorly wrapped. The term *body packer* refers to individuals who conceal xenobiotics, typically in large quantities, in a premeditated fashion almost exclusively for the purposes of international smuggling.

BODY PACKERS

Internal concealment of xenobiotics for the purpose of smuggling was first reported in Canada in 1973. A 21-year-old man presented with a small bowel obstruction as a result of swallowing a condom filled with hashish. He had swallowed the condom to transport it into Canada after a trip to Lebanon.[21] Internal xenobiotic smuggling subsequently became a worldwide problem as increased surveillance at international borders made conventional transportation of illegal xenobiotics more difficult. Improved detection of smugglers also increased the number of patients brought to the attention of health care providers. Unfortunately, in attempts to evade enhanced detection, pregnant women and children as young as 6 years of age have been used as body packers.[7,13,16]

Airline and airport personnel are trained to identify people who may be body packers. Suspicious behavior includes not eating or drinking on the airplane, abnormal behavior while going through customs, and overt signs of xenobiotic toxicity.[82,94]

Composition of Packages

Body packers typically swallow large numbers of well-prepared packages, each filled with substantial amounts of xenobiotic. Although ingestion is common, packets are also sometimes concealed by insertion into the vagina and rectum.[22,99] The most frequently smuggled cargo is either heroin or cocaine, but other xenobiotics are also reported (Table SC5–1). Body packers often swallow 50 to 100 packages, and ingestion of as many as 500 is reported.[100] Each package typically contains from 0.5 to 10 g of xenobiotic. Therefore, one person may carry as much as 1.5 kg of xenobiotic.[89] Lethal doses of cocaine and heroin are not well characterized. For reference, death from cocaine toxicity is reported after ingestion of as little as 2 to 3 g,[77] and the lethal dose of oral heroin in an opioid-naïve person is above 300 mg.[30] As such, each packet should be considered to contain a potentially lethal dose.

TABLE SC5–1	Xenobiotics Associated With Internal Concealment

Cannabis[58,89]

Cocaine powder and liquid[20,78]

Crack cocaine[78]

Hashish and hashish oil[72]

Heroin[31,49]

Methamphetamine[40,58]

Methylenedioxymethamphetamine (ecstasy)[92]

Prescription drugs[79]

Oxycodone[7]

A number of materials have been used for xenobiotic packaging. Some, such as latex, are used as wrappers. Others such as carbon paper and aluminum foil are used to change the radiodensity and decrease the likelihood of detection with diagnostic and forensic imaging studies. Packages have been made using plastic bags, plastic wrap, condoms, finger cots, balloons, cellophane, wax, tape, rubber gloves, surgical ligatures, paraffin, and fiberglass.[11,32,39,62,73]

Initial reports suggested a high rate of complications caused by packaging failure.[62] However, advances in the technology of packet construction have decreased rates of rupture.[73] A typical packet in current use is composed of a core of compacted xenobiotic covered by several layers of latex and encased in an outer wax coating.[94] More recently, the transport of xenobiotic in liquid form was reported.[10,68]

Important historical details include the number and contents of packets, the type of wrapping, the time of ingestion, and any associated symptoms. Body packers, as well as those financing and receiving the packages, generally know exactly how many packets are being carried. However, the individual are often reluctant to give an accurate clinical history to the health care provider or legal authorities.

Bioavailability

The oral bioavailability of cocaine hydrochloride is approximately 30% to 40%, which is similar to intranasal administration.[26,104] Rectal and vaginal bioavailability of cocaine hydrochloride and the oral, rectal, and vaginal bioavailability of crack cocaine have not been studied.

Oral exposure to heroin results in rapid first-pass metabolism to morphine[34] and can be considered a morphine prodrug.[26,46] The peak concentrations after 10 mg of oral heroin are similar to those expected from 10 mg of oral morphine.[7] The rectal bioavailability of morphine has a 1:1 ratio with oral administration. Although heroin is rectally bioavailable,[81] one study examining the bioavailability after rectal suppository administration in two opioid-dependent patients found it to be approximately 50% less than the oral bioavailability.[36]

Clinical Manifestations

Body packers undergoing medical examination may be asymptomatic, may have classic cocaine or opioid toxidromes, may have a mixed presentation, or may present with life-threatening manifestations of xenobiotic toxicity or mechanical bowel obstruction or perforation. Physical examination should be thorough, with a focus on findings related to these clinical manifestations (Chaps. 36 and 75).

When packets are too large to pass or malaligned, obstruction occurs at any point in the gastrointestinal (GI) tract. Individuals carrying packets containing opioids appear to be at higher risk of GI obstruction, even with intact packets.[33] The reason for this is unclear, but it may be related to microperforation of the package or contamination of the outside of the package during manufacture, resulting in opioid-induced GI stasis. Patients with a history of abdominal surgery also appear be at increased risk of obstruction.[19,44] GI perforation and peritonitis can result if the obstruction is untreated.[19] Dysphagia,[14] esophageal perforation and mediastinitis,[44,47] gastric ulcers,[66] gastric hemorrhage,[23,44] esophageal obstruction,[52] hematochezia,[96] incarcerated hernias,[90] uterine ischemia,[14] and septic shock[33] have resulted after packet rupture.

Laboratory Evaluation

Drug screening results are difficult to interpret. Although generally, a positive result should raise concern for a ruptured packet, positive results may also be due to external contamination of the packet during preparation from a microperforation or from prior xenobiotic utilization. Thus, some patients with packets that appear externally intact will have a positive urine drug screen.[33,63] The rate of positive screens in asymptomatic patients is reported to be as great as 52% to 72%.[20,23] Screening typically correlates closely with the drug carried,[32] but it is potentially misleading in that some patients transporting any xenobiotic will ingest opioids for the purpose of slowing GI transit time.[69] Additionally, some patients carry a combination of xenobiotics, known as "double breasting."[33]

A subsequent urine drug screen is particularly useful in the setting of a patient with an initially negative screening result. An initially negative result that later becomes positive suggests a ruptured packet and is an indication for very close monitoring or surgical removal. This is of particular concern in the setting of a cocaine body packer when a change from a negative to a positive screening result might indicate the potential for a precipitous decline.

Radiographic Evaluation

All suspected body packers should undergo radiographic evaluation. Abdominal radiographs have a detection sensitivity of 75% to 95%, but this success in recognition varies based on the number of packets and their methodology of construction.[11,61,98] Packets can be visualized as multiple radiodense foreign bodies (Fig. 8–8). The "double-condom sign" is a lucent ring surrounding the packet and results from air trapped between layered wrappings.[74] The "rosettelike" sign results from the air trapped in the knot when the condom or balloon is tied.[87] Caution must be used when interpreting plain radiographic studies. In one series, 19% of patients had false-negative radiographs, with one patient subsequently passing 135 packets.[62] False-positive results are also reported because of constipation,[51] intraabdominal calcifications,[95] and bladder stones.[105] Oral contrast administration is suggested by some to increase the sensitivity of plain radiography.[31,43,60]

Computed tomography (CT) scanning has a higher sensitivity than plain radiography,[38,54,85] with sensitivities reported to range from 96% to 100% (Figs. SC5–1 and SC5–2).[1,29,107] Although abdominal radiography is frequently used in airports as an initial screening test, CT is preferred in the hospital given this higher sensitivity. Noncontrast CT is the preferred modality because contrast may obscure packets.[75] Although likely to identify patients with multiple packets, a false-negative contrast CT scan after whole-bowel irrigation (WBI) was reported in a body packer who subsequently passed a single packet per rectum.[37] Retrospective review of the CT could not identify the packet. Recent studies suggest that even low-dose CT scans are quite accurate.[83] One study found a difference in Hounsfield units (HU) between packets containing cocaine (–219 HU) and heroin (–520 HU), suggesting that CT scanning can also potentially distinguish among package contents. However, other authors report a lack of utility of this measurement because of variations in drug formulation, compression, and packing materials.[56,102] Smaller slice size may aid in detection of smaller packets and use of lung windows in addition to traditional abdominal windows may also improve detection rates.[5,6] Ingestion of liquid cocaine can result in "jigsaw" pattern describing the interface of gas between packets visualized on CT scan.[68]

Ultrasonography may be another useful screening tool to reduce radiation exposure, particularly for evaluation of women of childbearing age. However, its utility has only been evaluated in a few small case series.[12,42,64] In one series of patients arrested on suspicion of body packing at an international airport, ultrasound examination correctly identified 40 of 42 body packers with positive plain radiographs. The two false-negative results occurred when packets were located low in the rectum.[67] Although potentially useful as a screening tool, particularly for patients in whom CT has increased risk, such as pregnant patients, it cannot definitively exclude packets.

Magnetic resonance imaging (MRI) is used less commonly than CT. However, MRI is able to detect the presence of packets, although it is less reliable in determining the number of packets.[41] Magnetic resonance imaging

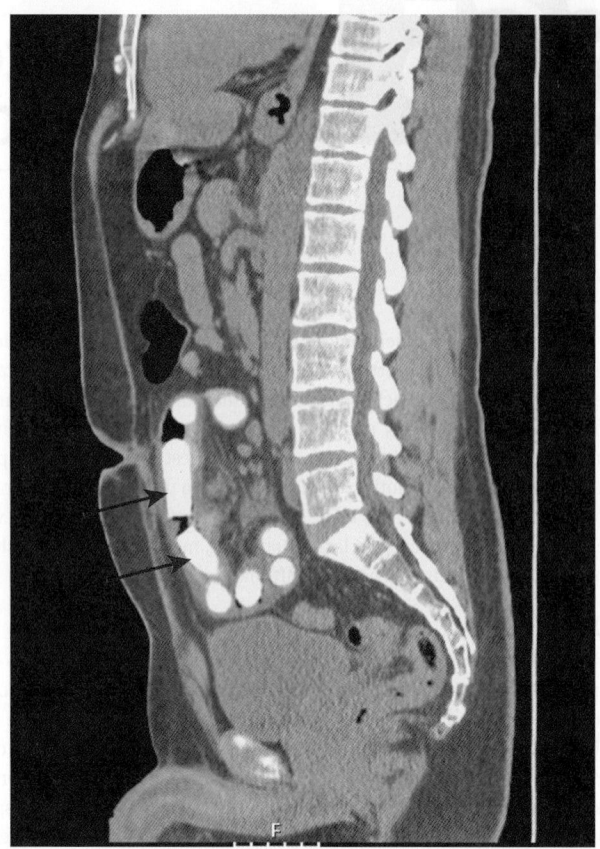

FIGURE SC5–1. Computed tomography (sagittal view) of the abdomen showing packets in the intestine. *(Used with permission from The Fellowship in Medical Toxicology, New York University School of Medicine, New York City Poison Center.)*

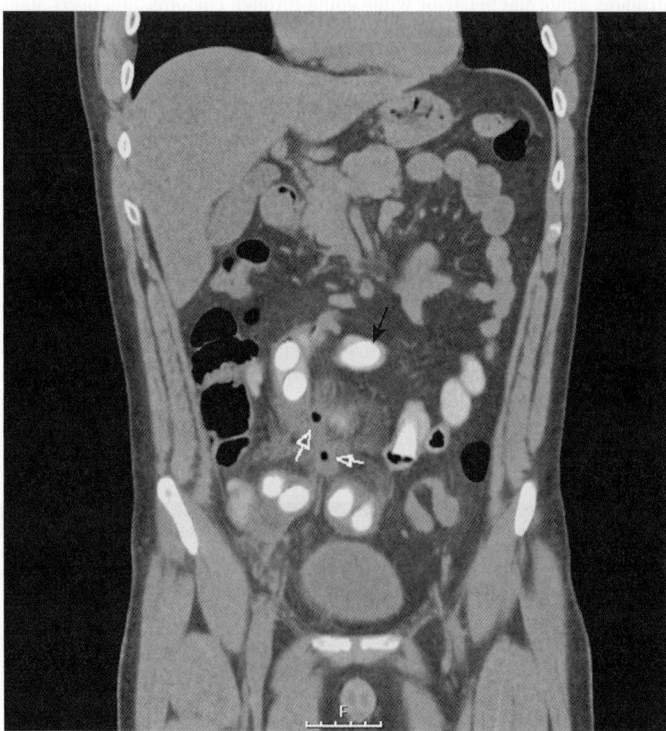

FIGURE SC5–2. Computed tomography (coronal view) of the abdomen showing packets associated with free air (lower two arrows) caused by bowel perforation. *(Used with permission from The Fellowship in Medical Toxicology, New York University School of Medicine, New York City Poison Center.)*

may be useful for diagnosis in cases when there is concern about radiation exposure.[8] Pregnant women have been used as body packers because of hesitation from customs officials and health care providers to obtain radiographs. However, the average radiation dose of 100 milliards from an abdominal radiograph is much less than the threshold thought to induce fetal malformations. Abdominal radiography, ultrasonography, and MRI may be useful screening tools in pregnant women who are suspected body packers because none presents significant risk to fetuses. When considering CT, as in any situation, practitioners must ensure that patient's health and safety are the foremost concerns, and in each case, the risk of exposure to radiation must be weighed against the risks of undiagnosed internal concealment of xenobiotics.

Management

All patients suspected of internal concealment of drugs should be closely monitored during evaluation. This should include blood pressure, heart rate, pulse oximetry, and continuous carbon dioxide monitoring, as well as direct visualization of the patient.

Gastrointestinal decontamination is a vital element in the management of body packers. Initially, surgical intervention was thought to be necessary in all body packers secondary to perceived high rates of toxicity and death.[28,89] The incidence of life-threatening complications has decreased due in part to both better packaging[62,73] and to increased rates of detection of asymptomatic carriers. Currently, a more conservative nonsurgical approach is suggested for asymptomatic patients[94] and is supported by a several large series (Fig. SC5–3).[3,4,9,11,20,62,82,98,100]

Treatment with activated charcoal (AC) is frequently suggested based on the fact that cocaine and heroin are both well adsorbed to AC.[59] However, there are no data showing actual benefit. Furthermore, AC may be detrimental if contamination of the peritoneal cavity occurs after GI rupture or during surgery or if it obscures visualization should endoscopy become indicated. Therefore, the risks and benefits must be weighed in each patient. Activated charcoal is of questionable value for cocaine packers given the higher risk of the need for surgical intervention. Also, it is not likely to improve the

outcome of symptomatic heroin body packers because these patients can be successfully managed with opioid antagonists and mechanical ventilation. Despite these risks and given the potential benefit of AC, we feel the use of AC is reasonable.

The utility of WBI to enhance elimination is generally accepted but has not been rigorously evaluated. There is a theoretical concern that polyethylene glycol could increase the water solubility of heroin should rupture occur[98] and that it may decrease the adsorption of cocaine to AC should AC be given.[59] Given the lack of in vitro data to support these risks[25] and its generally accepted benefit, WBI is recommended to decrease intestinal transit time (Antidotes in Depth: A2). We recommend not to perform orogastric lavage because packets are too large to fit through holes in the lavage tube.

Cathartics are sometimes recommended for GI decontamination. Although oil-based cathartics were frequently used in the past,[11,61] a non–oil-based medication such as magnesium citrate is preferred. Paraffin oil may dissolve some packet wrappers, potentially resulting in drug toxicity.[101] Use of promotility xenobiotics, such as metoclopramide and erythromycin, is reported,[97] but these are unlikely to add significantly to the use of WBI. Enemas and manual disimpaction should be avoided or used with great caution because packet rupture may occur.[48,55]

Treatment of symptomatic patients depends on the nature of the xenobiotic ingested. Patients manifesting opioid toxicity should be treated with the opioid antagonist naloxone by intravenous bolus and infusion and mechanical ventilation if necessary. Opioid antagonists also improve GI motility (Antidotes in Depth: A4). Surgical decontamination is generally not indicated for opioid poisoning because optimal medical therapy should be adequate.

Rupture of a cocaine packet, however, is a life-threatening emergency that requires aggressive medical and surgical therapy (Chap. 75). Benzodiazepines or other sedative-hypnotics such as propofol are recommended as temporizing measures, but surgical intervention for packet removal should be performed emergently in body packers with *any* sign of cocaine or amphetamine toxicity. Indications for surgery include, but are not limited to only hypertension, tachycardia, agitation or other alteration in mental status, myocardial ischemia, bowel ischemia, seizures, respiratory distress but also to the transition of a urine drug screen result from negative to positive.

Surgical removal of the packets is also the therapy of choice in the case of mechanical obstruction from any xenobiotic-containing packet.[39,71,86] Surgical removal may not be definitive; in one series, 6 of 70 patients were found to have retained packets postoperatively.[19] Also, emergent surgical removal is associated with a high rate of postoperative infection and fascial dehiscence for reasons that are not well understood.[18,19,86] Endoscopy[80,83,98] and proctoscopy[35] have been used successfully for removal of packets. However, caution must be used because attempted endoscopic removal can cause packet rupture and resultant toxicity.[89] Endoscopic removal should be reserved for cases in which a few packets are retained after failure of conservative management.

It is essential to ensure the passage of all packets before discharging a patient from medical care. Packets are reported to remain even in patients with clear rectal effluent after WBI.[43] After negative abdominal radiographs are obtained, a confirmatory study should be done using CT. However, these modalities do not have 100% sensitivity, and retained packets may be present.[37] It is therefore recommended that patients be observed for 24 hours after the passage of three packet-free stools[11] and negative confirmatory CT. Complete GI decontamination must be ensured before releasing the patient from close medical observation.

BODY STUFFERS

Body stuffers usually present for health care when they are taken into custody by law enforcement officers. Typically, the person has hastily ingested the xenobiotic or inserted it into the rectum or vagina to hide the evidence from the police. Because the person was not planning to conceal the xenobiotic, the xenobiotic is likely unwrapped, as in the case

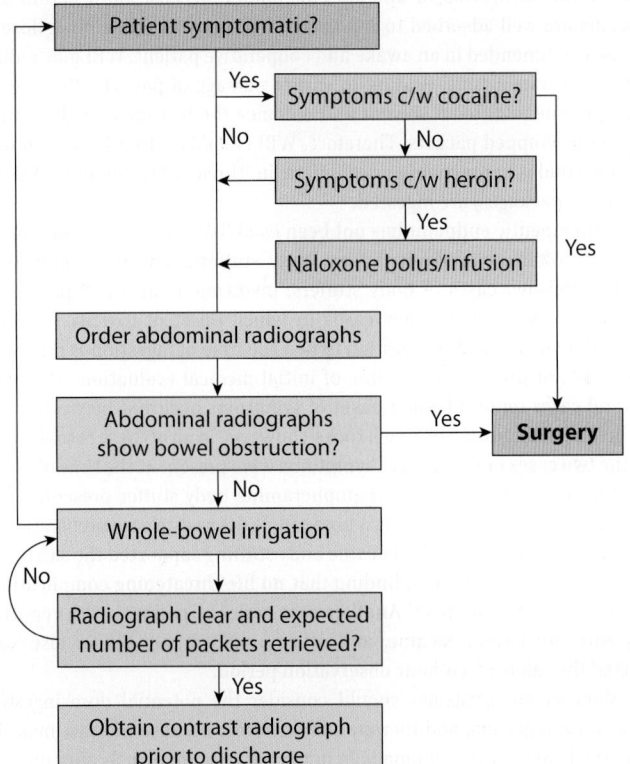

FIGURE SC5–3. Algorithm for managing cocaine or heroin body packers.

of crack cocaine "rocks,"[65] or poorly wrapped in materials intended for distribution.

Pertinent historical information includes time of ingestion, xenobiotic, amount ingested, packaging, and symptoms consistent with xenobiotic ingestion. Unfortunately, an accurate history is often difficult to obtain. Patients who are recent arrestees are prone to anticipate a secondary gain of delay to incarceration by reporting the ingestion of drugs; alternatively, some individuals deny ingestion to avoid prosecution. Complicating the clinical picture is the possibility that law enforcement officers may assume internal concealment of illicit substances when they are unable to find a substance after the arrest.

Composition of Packages

Because xenobiotics are typically transported locally in plastic bags, condoms,[88] balloons,[15] glassine envelopes, aluminum foil,[79] or crack vials,[43] these are the most frequently reported wrappers. Reported amounts vary from one dose to up to 30 packages of unspecified dose.[49] Cocaine, either in crack rocks or the hydrochloride salt form, are most commonly ingested,[78] but other xenobiotics are also reported (Table SC5–1). Typically, the xenobiotics are ingested although other routes of exposure include the external auditory canal, rectum, and vagina.[53,57,93]

The importance of obtaining a precise history related to packaging material is highlighted by an in vitro study examining the effects of packet construction, medium used for dissolution, and pH on release of cocaine from drug packets. Cocaine was released almost immediately from paper packaging and least readily from condoms. Cellophane packing led to intermediate concentrations compared with paper and condom wrappers. When packets were double or triple wrapped in cellophane, decreased concentrations were noted. All packets released more xenobiotic in an acidic medium.[2]

Clinical Manifestations

After oral ingestion of drug packets or crack rocks, toxicity is most frequently absent or mild.[49,50] However, although most case series report low rates of complications, both significant toxicity and death occur.[27,45,50,69] The time of onset of clinical effects in body stuffers is typically within several hours.[1,49,50] After the ingestion of cocaine in crack vials, the onset of toxicity was delayed by 3 to 4 hours.[43]

Most body stuffers reported in the literature had symptom onset within 6 hours of ingestion. Initial effects can occur 6 hours after ingestion; however, in nearly all reported cases, these patients displayed some manifestations at the time of initial medical contact. Two exceptions are noted in the literature. A 50-year-old woman reported ingesting xenobiotics at the time of incarceration. Seven hours later, a prison physician noted normal pulse and mental status, and she was placed in her cell to be observed by staff members every half hour. Prison staff documentation noted that she was "correct" and sat up 30 minutes before being found dead in the cell 11 hours after the time of ingestion. Postmortem examination revealed an open cocaine packet in the intestine.[70] A patient who placed methamphetamine in a plastic bag with a small hole in an attempt to create a sustained-release mechanism presented for abdominal pain 10 hours later. This patient remained without findings of methamphetamine intoxication until 42 hours after ingestion.[40]

Laboratory Evaluation

Laboratory xenobiotic testing is difficult to interpret in body stuffers because these patients are often habitual substance users. Thus, a positive drug screen result could be equally indicative of either prior use or current toxicity or both. Likewise, a negative result does not exclude recent ingestion or leaking packages. One study of 50 suspected body stuffers found that urine drug screening correctly classified the presence or absence of packets only 57% of the time.[61] Several authors report toxicity or death occurring in the presence of a negative urine screen result despite symptoms consistent with packet contents.[33,40] One explanation is that patients may die of drug toxicity before substantial urinary excretion occurs.

Radiographic Evaluation

Although detection of stuffed xenobiotics is possible by diagnostic imaging studies, the sensitivity is very poor.[24,49,61] Plastic bags, crack vials, and staples (enclosing plastic bags) are rarely visualized.[49] In one series of patients with crack vial ingestions, only 2 of 23 of abdominal radiographs were positive[43] in patients who subsequently passed vials. In two other series of cocaine body stuffers, all plain radiographs were negative.[50,88] Computed tomography scanning may identify some packets missed on radiographs, but the sensitivity has not been investigated and missed packets are reported with CT scanners as well.[24] Therefore, imaging is not likely to be clinically useful in these patients.

Management

Body stuffers who exhibit xenobiotic toxicity should be managed according to standard principles for managing that xenobiotic or suspected xenobiotic (Chaps. 36 and 75).

Patients with GI complaints should be evaluated for ileus or obstruction. Removal of packets has been performed by endoscopy[17,49,76] but is useful only for a small number of packets because each package requires an additional passage of the endoscope. Endoscopy should be used with extreme caution because it may cause packet rupture with subsequent toxicity or aspiration of the packet with airway obstruction.[89] Bronchoscopic removal of pieces of a balloon wrapping in the airway was successful in one patient after attempted orogastric lavage led to balloon aspiration.[15] Use of colonoscopy[82] is also reported but carries a risk of rupture similar to that associated with upper endoscopy. The need for surgical intervention was reported in only one case. This patient presented with a complaint of epigastric pain 3 days after ingesting a large plastic bag filled with 15 to 20 smaller bags of cocaine. He showed no signs of cocaine toxicity but required surgical removal because the bag was still retained in the stomach 4 days postingestion.[24]

Management of asymptomatic body stuffers has not been rigorously evaluated. Treatment with AC and WBI is often advocated for high-risk patients. Although these methods have not been proven to reduce morbidity or mortality, they offer theoretical benefits.[43,49,50,88] Activated charcoal may reduce the absorption of liberated xenobiotic because both heroin and cocaine are well adsorbed to AC. Given this theoretical benefit, a dose of AC is recommended in an awake and cooperative patient. WBI may reduce intestinal transit time, leading to earlier passage of packets. However, it may provide additional solvent and enhance the leakage and absorption of poorly wrapped packets. Therefore, WBI is unlikely to offer any clinical benefits and is not recommended unless life-threatening amounts of xenobiotic (in packages) are ingested.

A therapeutic endpoint has not been established in part because packages are often not recovered from body stuffers. Review of more than 1,000 published cases of body stuffers, involving a variety of packaging methods, reveals only a few cases in which onset of toxicity occurred more than 6 hours after ingestion (when the time of ingestion is reported) and was not present at the time of initial medical evaluation. There are several cases reported when onset of symptoms occurred between 8 and 10 hours postingestion of "crack rocks"; however, in all of these cases (except in the two cases noted earlier), symptoms were present at the time of initial health care contact.[17,76] A methamphetamine body stuffer presented in a delayed manner after ingesting a homemade delayed-release preparation.[103] A retrospective review after cocaine body stuffing supported the safety of a 6-hour observation period, finding that no life-threatening complications occurred in 106 patients.[67] Another case series of patients with reported exposure to heroin, cocaine, and other unknown substances also supported the safety of a 6-hour observation period.[106]

Management strategies should consider the potential dose ingested, time since ingestion, and therapy administered. Because the vast majority of patients remain asymptomatic or develop symptoms shortly after medical contact, it is reasonable to observe asymptomatic patients for 6 hours.

Because rare patients may have more delayed presentations, patients who have ingested large, potentially lethal doses or those who refuse AC should be observed for longer periods of time in a closely monitored setting. Multiple stools devoid of packages or a lack of symptoms after 24 hours are reasonable end points for monitoring these patients.

LEGAL PRINCIPLES

Because clinical errors have the potential for life-threatening consequences, it is essential to evaluate patients within the context of their unique medical, social, ethical, and legal settings. It is important to remember there may be significant motivation to deny ingestion altogether or conceivably secondary gain from overreporting the dose to delay incarceration. Often, patients refuse medical care either as an assertion of innocence or over concerns that evidence produced might be incriminatory.

In the United States, patients have a legal right to refuse care if they are competent to do so. This includes body stuffers and body packers who are under arrest. Patients with decisional capacity cannot be forced to take AC, WBI, any other form of therapy or diagnostic procedure. In this scenario, lower risk procedures may be acceptable to patients over more definitive tests; for example, a pregnant woman suspected of body packing may be agreeable to ultrasonography over CT scan given its lower risk. If in police custody, however, the individual may be kept in the hospital for an extended observation period. This strategy maintains the patient's medical autonomy and ensures clinical stability. If signs of life-threatening toxicity subsequently develop, the patient will most likely have lost decisional capacity, and therapy and management can proceed as medically necessary.

If a body packer who is not in legal custody presents for medical care, physicians face an ethical dilemma. Calling the authorities is a violation of the patient's right to confidentiality. However, possession of large amounts of drugs may theoretically endanger the hospital staff because criminal elements expect drug delivery. Consultation with hospital legal counsel, risk management, and the ethics committee are recommended in this situation (Chap. 138).

SUMMARY

- Patients with intestinal concealment of xenobiotic present diagnostic, therapeutic, ethical, and medicolegal challenges.
- History, laboratory, and radiologic studies must be interpreted with caution.
- Conservative management is preferred for asymptomatic body packers with vigilant observation.
- Management strategies should focus on the needs of each individual patient and the xenobiotic ingested.
- A complex patient physician relationship is common and must be effectively transformed into a trusting relationship to ensure reliable and high-quality care.

REFERENCES

1. Ab Hamid S, et al. Characteristic imaging features of body packers: a pictorial essay. *Jpn J Radiol*. 2012;30:386-392.
2. Aks SE, et al. Cocaine liberation from body packets in an in vitro model. *Ann Emerg Med*. 1992;21:1321-1325.
3. Alfa-Wali M, et al. Assessment of the management outcomes of body packers. *ANZ J Surg*. 2016;86:821-825.
4. Alipour-faz A, et al. Assessing the epidemiological data and management methods of body pacers admitted to a referral center in Iran. *Medicine*. 2016;95:1-5.
5. Asha SE, Cooke A. Sensitivity and specificity of emergency physicians and trainees for identifying internally concealed drug packages on abdominal computed tomography scan: do lung windows improve accuracy? *J Emerg Med*. 2015;49:268-273.
6. Bahrami-Motlagh H, et al. Added value of lung window in detecting drug mules on non-contrast abdominal computed tomography. *Radiol Med*. 2016;121:472-477.
7. Beno S, et al. Pediatric body packing: drug smuggling reaches a new low. *Pediatr Emerg Care*. 2005;21:744-746.
8. Bulakci M, et al. Detection of body packing by magnetic resonance imaging: a new diagnostic tool? *Abdom Imaging*. 2013;38:436-441.
9. Bulstrode N, et al. The outcome of drug smuggling by "body packers"—the British experience. *Ann R Coll Surg Engl*. 2002;84:35-38.
10. Burillo-Putze G, et al. Liquid cocaine body packers. *Clin Toxicol*. 2012;50:522-524.
11. Caruana DS, et al. Cocaine-packet ingestion. Diagnosis, management, and natural history. *Ann Intern Med*. 1984;100:73-74.
12. Cengel F, et al. The role of ultrasonography in the imaging of body packers comparison with CT: a prospective study. *Abdom Imaging*. 2015;40:2143-2151.
13. Chakrabarty A, et al. Smuggling contraband drugs using paediatric "body packers." *Arch Dis Child*. 2006;91:51.
14. Choudhary AM, et al. Endoscopic removal of a cocaine packet from the stomach. *J Clin Gastroenterol*. 1998;27:155-156.
15. Cobaugh DJ, et al. Cocaine balloon aspiration: successful removal with bronchoscopy. *Am J Emerg Med*. 1997;15:544-546.
16. Cordero DR, et al. Cocaine body packing in pregnancy. *Ann Emerg Med*. 2006;48:323-325.
17. Cranston PE, et al. CT of crack cocaine ingestion. *J Comput Assist Tomogr*. 1992;16:560-563.
18. de Bakker JK, et al. Body packers: a plea for conservative treatment. *Langenbecks Arch Surg*. 2012;397:125-130.
19. de Beer SA, et al. Surgery for body packing in the Caribbean: a retrospective study of 70 patients. *World J Surg*. 2008;32:281-285.
20. de Prost N, et al. Prognosis of cocaine body-packers. *Intensive Care Med*. 2005;31:955-958.
21. Deitel M, Syed AK. Intestinal obstruction by an unusual foreign body. *Can Med Assoc J*. 1973;109:211-212.
22. Diamant-Berger O, et al. Intracorporeal concealment of narcotics. Experience of medicolegal emergencies at the Hotel-Dieu Hospital in Paris: 100 cases. *Presse Med*. 1988;17:107-110.
23. Duenas-Laita A, et al. Body packing. *N Engl J Med*. 2004;350:1260-1261; author reply 1260-1261.
24. Eng JG, et al. False-negative abdominal CT scan in a cocaine body stuffer. *Am J Emerg Med*. 1999;17:702-704.
25. Farmer JW, Chan SB. Whole body irrigation for contraband bodypackers. *J Clin Gastroenterol*. 2003;37:147-150.
26. Fattinger K, et al. Nasal mucosal versus gastrointestinal absorption of nasally administered cocaine. *Eur J Clin Pharmacol*. 2000;56:305-310.
27. Fineschi V, et al. The cocaine "body stuffer" syndrome: a fatal case. *Forensic Sci Int*. 2002;126:7-10.
28. Fishbain DA, Wetli CV. Cocaine intoxication, delirium, and death in a body packer. *Ann Emerg Med*. 1981;10:531-532.
29. Flach PM, et al. "Drug mules" as a radiological challenge: sensitivity and specificity in identifying internal cocaine in body packers, body pushers and body stuffers by computed tomography, plain radiography and Lodox. *Eur J Radiol*. 2012;81:2518-2526.
30. Gable RS. Comparison of acute lethal toxicity of commonly abused psychoactive substances. *Addiction*. 2004;99:686-696.
31. Gherardi R, et al. A cocaine body packer with normal abdominal plain radiograms. Value of drug detection in urine and contrast study of the bowel. *Am J Forensic Med Pathol*. 1990;11:154-157.
32. Gherardi RK, et al. Detection of drugs in the urine of body-packers. *Lancet*. 1988;1:1076-1078.
33. Gill JR, Graham SM. Ten years of "body packers" in New York City: 50 deaths. *J Forensic Sci*. 2002;47:843-846.
34. Girardin F, et al. Pharmacokinetics of high doses of intramuscular and oral heroin in narcotic addicts. *Clin Pharmacol Ther*. 2003;74:341-352.
35. Glass JM, Scott HJ. "Surgical mules": the smuggling of drugs in the gastrointestinal tract. *J R Soc Med*. 1995;88:450-453.
36. Gyr E, et al. Pharmacodynamics and pharmacokinetics of intravenously, orally and rectally administered diacetylmorphine in opioid dependents, a two-patient pilot study within a heroin-assisted treatment program. *Int J Clin Pharmacol Ther*. 2000;38:486-491.
37. Hahn I-H, et al. Contrast CT scan fails to detect the last heroin packet. *J Emerg Med*. 2004;27:279-283.
38. Hartoko TJ, et al. The body packer syndrome: cocaine smuggling in the gastrointestinal tract. *Klin Wochenschr*. 1988;66:1116-1120.
39. Hassanian-Moghaddam H, Abolmasoumi Z. Consequence of body packing of illicit drugs. *Arch Iran Med*. 2007;10:20-23.
40. Hendrickson RG, et al. "Parachuting" meth: a novel delivery method for methamphetamine and delayed-onset toxicity from "body stuffing." *Clin Toxicol*. 2006;44:379-382.
41. Hergan K, et al. Drug smuggling by body packing: what radiologists should know about it. *Eur Radiol*. 2004;14:736-742.
42. Hierholzer J, et al. Drug smuggling by ingested cocaine-filled packages: conventional x-ray and ultrasound. *Abdom Imaging*. 1995;20:333-338.
43. Hoffman RS, et al. Prospective evaluation of "crack-vial" ingestions. *Vet Hum Toxicol*. 1990;32:164-167.
44. Hutchins KD, et al. Heroin body packing: three fatal cases of intestinal perforation. *J Forensic Sci*. 2000;45:42-47.
45. Introna F Jr, Smialek JE. The "mini-packer" syndrome. Fatal ingestion of drug containers in Baltimore, Maryland. *Am J Forensic Med Pathol*. 1989;10:21-24.
46. Inturrisi CE, et al. The pharmacokinetics of heroin in patients with chronic pain. *N Engl J Med*. 1984;310:1213-1217.
47. Johnson JA, Landreneau RJ. Esophageal obstruction and mediastinitis: a hard pill to swallow for drug smugglers. *Am Surg*. 1991;57:723-726.

48. Jonsson S, et al. Acute cocaine poisoning. Importance of treating seizures and acidosis. *Am J Med.* 1983;75:1061-1064.

49. Jordan MT, et al. A five-year review of the medical outcome of heroin body stuffers. *J Emerg Med.* 2009;36:250-256.

50. June R, et al. Medical outcome of cocaine bodystuffers. *J Emerg Med.* 2000;18:221-224.

51. Karhunen PJ, et al. Pitfalls in the diagnosis of drug smuggler's abdomen. *J Forensic Sci.* 1991;36:397-402.

52. Karkos PD, et al. An unusual foreign body in the oesophagus. The body packer syndrome. *Eur Arch Otorhinolaryngol.* 2005;262:154-156.

53. Kashani J, Ruha A-M. Methamphetamine toxicity secondary to intravaginal body stuffing. *J Toxicol Clin Toxicol.* 2004;42:987-989.

54. Kersschot EA, et al. Roentgenographical detection of cocaine smuggling in the alimentary tract. *Rofo.* 1985;142:295-298.

55. Koehler SA, et al. The risk of body packing: a case of a fatal cocaine overdose. *Forensic Sci Int.* 2005;151:81-84.

56. Laberke PJ, et al. Systematic evaluation of radiation dose reduction in CT studies of body packers: accuracy down to submillisievert levels. *Am J Roentgenol.* 2016;206:740-746.

57. Lopez HH, et al. Cannabis: accidental peroral intoxication. The hashish smuggler roentogenographically unmasked. *JAMA.* 1974;227:1041-1042.

58. Low VHS, Dillon EK. Agony of the ecstasy: report of five cases of MDMA smuggling. *Australas Radiol.* 2005;49:400-403.

59. Makosiej FJ, et al. An in vitro evaluation of cocaine hydrochloride adsorption by activated charcoal and desorption upon addition of polyethylene glycol electrolyte lavage solution. *J Toxicol Clin Toxicol.* 1993;31:381-395.

60. Marc B, et al. The cocaine body-packer syndrome: evaluation of a method of contrast study of the bowel. *J Forensic Sci.* 1990;35:345-355.

61. Marc B, et al. Managing drug dealers who swallow the evidence. *BMJ.* 1989;299:1082.

62. McCarron MM, Wood JD. The cocaine "body packer" syndrome. Diagnosis and treatment. *JAMA.* 1983;250:1417-1420.

63. Meatherall RC, Warren RJ. High urinary cannabinoids from a hashish body packer. *J Anal Toxicol.* 1993;17:439-440.

64. Meijer R, Bots ML. Detection of intestinal drug containers by ultrasound scanning: an airport screening tool? *Eur Radiol.* 2003;13:1312-1315.

65. Merigian KS, et al. Adrenergic crisis from crack cocaine ingestion: report of five cases. *J Emerg Med.* 1994;12:485-490.

66. Miller JS, et al. Giant gastric ulcer in a body packer. *J Trauma.* 1998;45:617-619.

67. Moreira M, et al. Validation of a 6-hour observation period for cocaine body stuffers. *Am J Emerg Med.* 2001;29:299-303

68. Mozes O, et al. Radiographic features of intracorporeally smuggled liquid cocaine. *A Forensic Sci Med Pathol.* 2014;10:535-542.

69. Nihira M, et al. Urinalysis of body packers in Japan. *J Anal Toxicol.* 1998;22:61-65.

70. Norfolk GA. The fatal case of a cocaine body-stuffer and a literature review—towards evidence based management. *J Forensic Leg Med.* 2007;14:49-52.

71. Olmedo R, et al. Is surgical decontamination definitive treatment of "body-packers"? *Am J Emerg Med.* 2001;19:593-596.

72. Pamilo M, et al. Narcotic smuggling and radiography of the gastrointestinal tract. *Acta Radiol Diagn.* 1986;27:213-216.

73. Pidoto RR, et al. A new method of packaging cocaine for international traffic and implications for the management of cocaine body packers. *J Emerg Med.* 2002;23:149-153.

74. Pinsky MF, et al. Narcotic smuggling: the double condom sign. *J Can Assoc Radiol.* 1978;29:79-81.

75. Pinto A, et al. Radiological and practical aspects of body packing. *Br J Radiol.* 2014;87:1-8.

76. Pollack CV, et al. Two crack cocaine body stuffers. *Ann Emerg Med.* 1992;21:1370-1380.

77. Price KR. Fatal cocaine poisoning. *J Forensic Sci Soc.* 1974;14:329-333.

78. Puschel K, et al. Analysis of 683 drug packages seized from "body stuffers." *Forensic Sci Int.* 2004;140:109-111.

79. Roberts JR, et al. The bodystuffer syndrome: a clandestine form of drug overdose. *Am J Emerg Med.* 1986;4:24-27.

80. Robinson T, et al. Body smuggling of illicit drugs: two cases requiring surgical intervention. *Surgery.* 1993;113:709-711.

81. Rook EJ, et al. Pharmacokinetics and pharmacokinetic variability of heroin and its metabolites: review of the literature. *Curr Clin Pharmacol.* 2006;1:109-118.

82. Schaper A, et al. Surgical treatment in cocaine body packers and body pushers. *Int J Colorectal Dis.* 2007;22:1531-1535.

83. Schultz B, et al. Body packers on your examination table: how helpful are plan x-ray images? A definitive low-dose CT protocol as a diagnosis tool for body packers. *Clin Radiol.* 2014;69:e525-530.

84. Sherman A, Zingler BM. Successful endoscopic retrieval of a cocaine packet from the stomach. *Gastrointest Endosc.* 1990;36:152-154.

85. Shahnazi M, et al. Comparison of abdominal computed tomography with and without oral contrast in diagnosis of body packers and body stuffers. *Clin Toxicol.* 2015;53:596-603.

86. Silverberg D, et al. Surgery for "body packers"—a 15-year experience. *World J Surg.* 2006;30:541-546.

87. Sinner WN. The gastrointestinal tract as a vehicle for drug smuggling. *Gastrointest Radiol.* 1981;6:319-323.

88. Sporer KA, Firestone J. Clinical course of crack cocaine body stuffers. *Ann Emerg Med.* 1997;29:596-601.

89. Suarez CA, et al. Cocaine-condom ingestion. Surgical treatment. *JAMA.* 1977;238:1391-1392.

90. Swan MC, et al. Cocaine by internal mail: two surgical cases. *J R Soc Med.* 2003;96:188-189.

91. Taheri MS, et al. Swallowed opium packets: CT diagnosis. *Abdom Imaging.* 2008;33:262-266.

92. Takekawa K, et al. Methamphetamine body packer: acute poisoning death due to massive leaking of methamphetamine. *J Forensic Sci.* 2007;52:1219-1222.

93. Thompson AC, Terry RM. Cannabis-resin foreign body in the ear. *N Engl J Med.* 1989;320:1758.

94. Traub SJ, et al. Packing—the internal concealment of illicit drugs. *N Engl J Med.* 2003;349:2519-2526.

95. Traub SJ, et al. False-positive abdominal radiography in a body packer resulting from intraabdominal calcifications. *Am J Emerg Med.* 2003;21:607-608.

96. Traub SJ, et al. Pediatric "body packing." *Arch Pediatr Adolesc Med.* 2003;157:174-177.

97. Traub SJ, et al. Use of pharmaceutical promotility agents in the treatment of body packers. *Am J Emerg Med.* 2003;21:511-512.

98. Utecht MJ, et al. Heroin body packers. *J Emerg Med.* 1993;11:33-40.

99. van der Vlies CH, Busch OR. Images in clinical medicine. An intraabdominal cyst. *N Engl J Med.* 2007;357:e6.

100. van Geloven AA, et al. Bodypacking—an increasing problem in The Netherlands: conservative or surgical treatment? *Eur J Surg.* 2002;168:404-409.

101. Visser L, et al. Do not give paraffin to packers. *Lancet.* 1998;352:1352.

102. Wackerle B, et al. Detection of narcotic-containing packages in "body-packers" using imaging procedures. Studies in vitro and in vivo. *Rofo.* 1986;145:274-277.

103. West PL, et al. Methamphetamine body stuffers: an observational case series. *Ann Emerg Med.* 2010;55:190-197.

104. Wilkinson P, et al. Intranasal and oral cocaine kinetics. *Clin Pharmacol Ther.* 1980;27:386-394.

105. Wilogren J. Misdiagnosis lead to man's handcuffing, suit claims. *The New York Times.* December 6, 1998:62.

106. Yamamoto T, et al. Management of body stuffers presenting to the emergency department. *Eur J Emerg Med.* 2016;23:425-429.

107. Yang RM, et al. Heroin body packing: clearly discerning drug packets using CT. *South Med J.* 2009;102:470-475.

SC6

PREVENTION, TREATMENT, AND HARM REDUCTION APPROACHES TO OPIOID OVERDOSES

Daniel Schatz and Joshua D. Lee

INTRODUCTION

Opioid-related deaths rates in the United States continue to rise. A decades-long US prescription drug epidemic persists, driven by high rates of per capita opioid analgesic dispensing, and is now paired with a growing availability of illicit heroin, fentanyl, and fentanyl derivatives. Rates of opioid use disorders, opioid treatment admissions, opioid-related emergency department (ED) and hospital admissions, and overdose mortality have all steadily increased since 1990.[8] In 2012, the Centers for Disease Control and Prevention (CDC) reported that for every unintentional overdose death related to an opioid analgesic, 9 people were admitted for substance abuse treatment, 35 visited EDs, 161 reported drug abuse or dependence, and 461 reported nonmedical uses of opioid analgesics.[10] Recent federal and state reform efforts seek to bolster a public health response to opioid use disorders and overdose deaths.[14,50] The availability and dissemination of core evidence-based interventions that treat and prevent overdose events and fatalities, however, has not kept pace with the number of persons using, suffering harm, and dying from opioids.

Evidence for, and policies supporting core community-based overdose interventions, which are harm reduction education and counseling, and naloxone distribution and administration, are reviewed here. Overdose outcomes associated with opioid use disorder treatment, including opioid use disorder treatments with agonist (methadone, buprenorphine) and antagonist (naltrexone) pharmacotherapies and counseling-only modalities, are addressed. Larger policy efforts and national practice guidelines with important implications for overdose prevention, including state prescription monitoring requirements and recently published CDC guidelines for the use of opioid analgesia for nonmalignant chronic pain are emphasized.

EPIDEMIOLOGY

Overdose Rates

Opioid use in the US has grown steadily since the 1990s, largely because of widespread and routine opioid analgesic prescribing. As of 2014, of 47,055 total US unintentional poisoning deaths, 18,893 were attributed to opioid analgesics and 10,574 to heroin.[9] Heroin availability and related problems appear to be accelerating, and heroin "markets" have expanded to all large US metropolitan areas as well as a substantial proportion of rural counties. More recently, novel opioids, such as U-47700 and W-18, and illicit fentanyl analogs, such as carfentanil, have entered street heroin formulations. This appears to drive local micro-epidemics and significant increases in overdose death rates.[13,35]

Risk Factors

"Opioid overdose" generally refers to oversedation, hypoventilation, and anoxia stemming from an excessive dose of an opioid agonist alone or in combination with other central nervous system depressants. Established risk factors for opioid overdose include:[48,49]

- Persons with opioid dependence, particularly after periods of reduced use, resulting in loss of tolerance (after detoxification, release from incarceration, cessation of recovery treatment)
- People who inject opioids
- People who use prescription opioids, particularly those taking higher doses

- People who use opioids in combination with other sedating xenobiotics
- People who use opioids and have medical conditions such as HIV, liver or lung disease or depression
- Household members, including children, of people in possession of opioids (including prescription opioids)
- People with obstructive sleep apnea

Primary and secondary prevention efforts may target any or all of these risk factors, such as increased access to evidence-based treatments and harm reduction interventions at release from correctional facilities; public and medical practice regulatory reforms designed to lower rates and doses of opioid prescribing for painful conditions; or reducing the coadministration of other substances, particularly benzodiazepines, alcohol, and cocaine.

NALOXONE AND HARM REDUCTION APPROACHES TO OVERDOSE PREVENTION AND OVERDOSE REVERSAL

Naloxone administration is the principal overdose intervention taught to at-risk opioid users, persons in treatment, and family members, as well as first responders. Naloxone pharmacokinetics and naloxone efficacy for overdose are discussed in Chapter 36, Antidotes in Depth: A4, and Special Considerations: SC5.

Community-Based Effectiveness

Most opioid overdoses occur in the setting of a bystander and often in a private location.[23,39] Because of the time-dependent nature of the development of hypoxic brain injury as well as the rapidity and effectiveness of naloxone, many educational initiatives aim to reach those most likely to be in first contact with the patient. Education generally consists of overdose prevention; rapid recognition; and appropriate response, including timely administration of naloxone, rescue breathing or cardiopulmonary resuscitation, recovery positioning, and emergency medical services (EMS) activation. Despite variability in education duration (10 minutes to 1 hour) and educator qualifications,[11] the feasibility of naloxone programs was demonstrated in a variety of populations, including laypersons.[24] Although no randomized controlled trial exists, several cohort studies demonstrate effectiveness of community-based opioid overdose programs in the rates of opioid-related deaths. A prospective cohort study in Massachusetts found adjusted opioid overdose death rate ratios of 0.54 and 0.73 for communities with high degrees of opioid overdose program implementation (more than 100 participants per 100,000 population) and low degrees of implementation (1–100 participants per 100,000 population), respectively, compared with communities without any overdose program.[47] A Chicago-based study observed a 10% to 20% reduction in heroin overdose-related deaths after implementation of a naloxone education program.[29] In a meta-analysis, 11 of 18 programs reported 100% survival rates after naloxone administration; the remaining programs showed survival rates varying from 83% to 96%. The reduced survival rates were thought to be due to unknown outcomes, which may have included death, and time to administration of naloxone.[11]

Controversies Regarding Naloxone

Although naloxone has proven efficacy, both under ideal conditions and in the community, controversy still exists. One common objection to increasing the supply of naloxone is that it will allow users to feel more comfortable with drug use, ultimately leading to paradoxical increased use and risk-taking behavior. Such effects have been seen following previous public health safety projects, such as seatbelt use and football helmets.[1,37] However, this has not occurred in communities where naloxone programs were initiated. In fact, several communities where naloxone programs exist observed decreased drug use.[29,46] Another common concern is that when naloxone is given, there is no perceived need to activate 911, a critical component of overdose response. Activation of EMS has had mixed results despite pre- and postnaloxone education.[11] In one study, 71% cited "fear of police involvement" as the primary reason for not activating 911, and 20% thought medical intervention was unnecessary.[6] In New York City, EMS was activated 74% of the time by naloxone-trained laypersons,[38] which is similar to a 68% activation rate in a prior New York City study involving those without naloxone education.[45] Another concern is the inappropriate administration of naloxone by laypersons, especially if under the influence of an opioid or other xenobiotic, but studies have shown that trained laypersons are able to recognize opioid overdose and safely and appropriately administer naloxone.[5]

Policies Regarding Naloxone

Many reforms and efforts are being undertaken to increase the availability, prescribing, and administration of naloxone. One target for reform is decreasing the liability concern at the prescriber and dispensing levels. In an effort to lower these barriers, many states have given prescribers immunity or are allowing third-party or standing prescriptions (ie, prescribing to someone other than the patient). Many states have expanded administration regulations to include nonmedical providers or laypersons. Although the laws regarding prescribing naloxone vary from state to state, many are moving toward pharmacist dispensing without a prescription ("behind the counter") or non-prescription availability without personal identification, although this latter ability falls under federal jurisdiction. Good Samaritan laws, which exist in almost all states, are an effort to increase administration of naloxone and activation of EMS by laypersons without fear of legal repercussions.[31] More recently, the Comprehensive Addiction and Recovery Act of 2016 (CARA 2016) put forth measures to increase the availability and training of naloxone use to first responders.[50]

Safe Injection Sites and Medical Heroin Interventions

Although controversial and to date prohibited in the United States, safe injection sites are becoming more prevalent internationally.[34] Heroin-assisted treatment (HAT) appears to be an effective intervention in terms of higher treatment retention both in European[16,25] and Canadian studies.[41] The Vancouver-based North American Opioid Medication Initiative (NAOMI) trial[41] randomized 226 adult current and chronic heroin injectors with a history of prior methadone maintenance to (1) injectable diacetylmorphine (DAM, heroin) or hydromorphone or (2) methadone maintenance treatment. Retention in the treatment arm (HAT) was 87.8% compared with 54.1% for methadone. Eleven overdoses occurred in the 115 patients randomized to HAT across more than 70,000 injection events versus no overdoses on methadone; 10 of these received naloxone, and all events resolved without any further negative sequela.[33] Increased patient satisfaction[26] and higher self-reported health-related quality of life[18] likely contributed to the increased HAT retention rates. Importantly, HAT was also associated with lower self-reported rates of criminal activity and superior cost-effectiveness.[32]

Opioid Treatment as Overdose Prevention

Opioid use disorder treatment is itself intended to reduce illicit opioid use and prevent harm and death. Treatment effects associated with methadone, buprenorphine, and to some extent naltrexone include prevention of overdoses; reduced rates of communicable disease transmission and injection drug use; improved function and quality of life; and lower health and societal costs, including reduced criminal behavior and incarceration. The direct impact of opioid treatments on overdose event rates, however, can be difficult when examining individual or aggregate clinical trial results or when looking at overall ecologic trends, as opposed to estimating effects on overall

crude mortality rates. There are also crucial differences in medication-based treatments and counseling-only approaches; the later likely contribute to higher rates of overdose after relapse.

Methadone and Buprenorphine

Mu opioid receptor agonist maintenance treatments with methadone (a full agonist) or buprenorphine (a partial agonist) are both the basic evidence-based, first-line treatments for an active opioid use disorders.[30] An active opioid user, who is tolerant to opioids, can be inducted onto either medication and thereafter titrated to and maintained on a maintenance dose that blocks or partly blocks the activity of further administered opioids. Maintenance opioid therapy allows the patient to retain acceptable levels of energy, cognition, and daily function, with reduced cravings and urges for illicit opioids. Buprenorphine maintenance can be delivered in an office-based setting, and both opioids can be used as directly observed therapy in a licensed opioid treatment program (or methadone maintenance program). Buprenorphine and methadone treatment can be blended with specialty addiction treatment in detoxification units; residential rehabilitation centers; or as part of intensive outpatient therapy, in which either medication can be combined with more intensive counseling. Systematic reviews, meta-analyses, and epidemiologic studies consistently find associations between exposure and retention in methadone maintenance with lower mortality rates compared with opioid-dependent individuals who discontinue such treatment.[7,12,43,51] Overdose rates fell in France and Baltimore, MD, during recent periods of methadone and buprenorphine treatment expansion.[3,22,42] Despite these clear trends favoring a treatment effect, individual randomized treatment trials have typically not been designed or powered to specifically estimate effects on overdose rates, making precise estimates of agonist treatment effects on opioid overdoses unavailable.[27,28]

Extended-Release Naltrexone

Extended-release naltrexone (XR-NTX) is a more recently Food and Drug Administration–approved (2010) therapy for opioid use disorder, specifically for the prevention of opioid relapse after detoxification.[2] The extended-release, monthly, intramuscular depot formulation is designed to improve adherence to naltrexone therapy. Previously, naltrexone was approved and available as a daily oral tablet, which had limited or no effectiveness because of nonadherence. Extended-release naltrexone is an opioid relapse-prevention approach to treatment; a patient must be detoxified and opioid free at the time of induction. The naltrexone blockade then renders usual doses of opioid analgesics or heroin ineffective and noneuphoric. The pivotal efficacy of the NTX trial had no overdose events (fatal or nonfatal) in either the XR-NTX or placebo arms.[20] A subsequent XR-NTX effectiveness trial focused on a forensic adult outpatient population and found a lower rate of a combined fatal and nonfatal overdose outcome among XR-NTX participants compared with the treatment-as-usual control arm.[21]

Counseling-Only Treatments

Contrary to opioid pharmacotherapy treatments, detoxifying from opioids and graduation to further residential or outpatient counseling-only modalities elevates the acute risk of overdose.[44] There are some practical advantages to counseling-only opioid addiction treatments. There are minimal requirements for a licensed medical provider or prescriber to be a member of the program staff, which is often composed primarily of addiction counselors. Patient preference for a "drug-free" recovery is respected. There is some evidence of effectiveness for various psychosocial counseling approaches for long-term recovery versus no treatment or drop-outs.[40] However, many studies show opioid relapse, overdose, and death occur at higher rates in counseling-only treatments over both the short and long terms compared with medication maintenance approaches.[51] Furthermore, acutely weaning and lowering the tolerance of an opioid-dependent user in a controlled environment (eg, jail, hospital, detoxification facility, inpatient rehabilitation), followed by return to the community, is an important overdose risk factor and arguably worse for patients than no treatment and continued illicit opioid use.[44] Counseling-only approaches to opioid treatment continue to be widespread and in many parts of the United States and rapid access is essential to prevent recurrent overdoses. Increasing rates of medication treatment is a leading public health concern.[14] Recent federal initiatives to expand the availability of opioid treatment medications recognize that counseling-only approaches to the opioid overdose epidemic are inadequate and potentially counterproductive.

Opioid Policies and Practice Reforms in the United States

Currently, extensive attention is being paid to the opioid epidemic and overdose rates by lawmakers and administrators at local, state, and federal levels. Overall efforts to reduce the volume and supply of opioid analgesics have important implications for overdose prevention. Prescriber practice reforms and regulatory efforts aimed at reducing individual opioid analgesic prescribing, state prescription monitoring programs, and the recent Drug Enforcement Agency upscheduling of hydrocodone to a Class II controlled substance may all contribute to lower opioid prescribing and overdose rates.[17,19,36] More peripherally, states with regulated medical marijuana and cannabis legalization laws report lower rates of opioid overdose.[4] These findings could represent unmeasured confounders, such as provider or payor policies, or an intriguing hypothesis that among chronic pain patients or the general population, increased cannabis use reduces exposure to opioids. An overriding public health aim regarding opioid use is to reduce harm and limit overdose risk, and these types of policies will require continuous evaluation and revision. The routine prescription of potent opioid analgesics for non-malignant chronic pain by US providers should end as described in the 2016 CDC practice guidelines.[15]

SUMMARY

- The US opioid and opioid overdose epidemic has recently generated unprecedented media, policy, and patient advocacy attention. Drug poisonings in the US, the majority of which are now opioid related, are a leading cause of preventable death in young adults, and in comparison, now exceed the number of US annual automobile-related fatalities or breast cancer deaths.
- Preventing death in the setting of an overdose event involves immediate and sustained reversal of opioid agonist mediated hypoxia, hypoventilation, and oversedation, which is accomplished with basic life support, naloxone administration, and the activation of EMS.
- There is evidence that regional public health and harm reduction efforts to increase naloxone availability and training in overdose recognition and reversal are effective. Widespread expansion of these programs remains warranted.
- Secondary prevention of overdose events among opioid-dependent persons also hinges on improved and expanded access to evidence-based treatments for opioid use disorders, principally methadone and buprenorphine maintenance.
- Primary prevention of overall opioid use is of critical importance, given that a majority of opioid overdose deaths remain linked to prescription analgesics, and most current heroin users have initiated opioid use with opioid medications.
- Practice guidelines regarding both the management of acute and chronic pain are increasingly adamant that opioid analgesia should be used selectively in as few patients as possible, limited in dose and duration, and not as a primary treatment of chronic pain.

REFERENCES

1. Abdukadirov S. The Unintended Consequences of Safety Regulation. June 4, 2013. https://ssrn.com/abstract=2343923 or http://dx.doi.org/10.2139/ssrn.2343923.
2. Alkermes, PLC. VIVITROL® (naltrexone for extended-release injectable suspension) Intramuscular. https://www.accessdata.fda.gov/drugsatfda_docs/label/2010/021897s015lbl.pdf.
3. Auriacombe M, et al. French field experience with buprenorphine. *Am J Addict.* 2004;13(suppl 1):S17-S28.
4. Bachhuber MA, et al. Medical cannabis laws and opioid analgesic overdose mortality in the United States, 1999-2010. *JAMA Intern Med.* 2014;174:1668-1673.
5. Bazazi AR, et al. Preventing opiate overdose deaths: examining objections to take-home naloxone. *J Health Care Poor Underserved.* 2010;21:1108-1113.
6. Bennett AS, et al. Characteristics of an overdose prevention, response, and naloxone distribution program in Pittsburgh and Allegheny County, Pennsylvania. *J Urban Health.* 2011;88:1020-1030.
7. Caplehorn JR, et al. Methadone maintenance and addicts' risk of fatal heroin overdose. *Subst Use Misuse.* 1996;31:177-196.
8. Centers for Disease Control and Prevention. Wide-ranging Online Data for Epidemiologic Research (WONDER), Multiple-Cause-of-Death file, 2000–2014. http://www.cdc.gov/nchs/data/health_policy/AADR_drug_poisoning_involving_OA_Heroin_US_2000-2014.pdf. Accessed May 1, 2017.
9. Centers for Disease Control and Prevention, National Center for Health Statistics, National Vital Statistics System, Mortality File. (2015). Number and Age-Adjusted Rates of Drug-poisoning Deaths Involving Opioid Analgesics and Heroin: United States, 2000–2014. Atlanta, GA: Centers for Disease Control and Prevention. http://www.cdc.gov/nchs/data/health_policy/AADR_drug_poisoning_involving_OA_Heroin_US_2000-2014.pdf.
10. Centers for Disease Control and Prevention. CDC grand rounds: prescription drug overdoses—a U.S. epidemic. *MMWR Morb Mortal Wkly Rep.* 2012;61:10-13.
11. Clark AK, et al. A systematic review of community opioid overdose prevention and naloxone distribution programs. *J Addict Med.* 2014;8:153-163.
12. Clausen T, et al. Mortality among opiate users: opioid maintenance therapy, age and causes of death. *Addiction.* 2009;104:1356-1362.
13. DeMio T. OD crisis: flying blind in search of killer heroin's source. *Cincinnati Inquirer,* August 26, 2016. http://www.cincinnati.com/story/news/2016/08/25/od-crisis-flying-blind-search-killer-heroins-source/89339560.
14. US Department of Health and Human Services. HHS announces new actions to combat opioid epidemic [press release]. http://www.hhs.gov/about/news/2016/07/06/hhs-announces-new-actions-combat-opioid-epidemic.html.
15. Dowell D, et al. CDC guideline for prescribing opioids for chronic pain—United States, 2016. *JAMA.* 2016;315:1624-1645.
16. Haasen C, et al. Heroin-assisted treatment for opioid dependence: randomised controlled trial. *Br J Psychiatry.* 2007;191:55-62.
17. Haynes A, et al. Trends in analgesic exposures reported to Texas Poison Centers following increased regulation of hydrocodone. *Clin Toxicol.* 2016;54:434-440.
18. Karow A, et al. Quality of life under maintenance treatment with heroin versus methadone in patients with opioid dependence. *Drug Alcohol Depend.* 2010;112: 209-215.
19. Kennedy-Hendricks A, et al. Opioid overdose deaths and Florida's crackdown on pill mills. *Am J Public Health.* 2016;106:291-297.
20. Krupitsky E, et al. Injectable extended-release naltrexone for opioid dependence: a double-blind, placebo-controlled, multicentre randomised trial. *Lancet.* 2011;377:1506-1513.
21. Lee JD, et al. Extended-release naltrexone to prevent opioid relapse in criminal justice offenders. *N Engl J Med.* 2016;374:1232-1242.
22. Lepère B, et al. [Reduction in the number of lethal heroin overdoses in France since 1994. Focus on substitution treatments]. *Ann Med Interne (Paris).* 2001;152(suppl 3): IS5-IS12.
23. Levy B, et al. Recognition and response to opioid overdose deaths-New Mexico, 2012. *Drug Alcohol Depend.* 2016;167:29-35.
24. Lim JK, et al. Prescribe to prevent: overdose prevention and naloxone rescue kits for prescribers and pharmacists. *J Addict Med.* 2016;10:300-308.
25. March JC, et al; PEPSA team. Controlled trial of prescribed heroin in the treatment of opioid addiction. *J Subst Abuse Treat.* 2006;31:203-211.
26. Marchand KI, et al. Client satisfaction among participants in a randomized trial comparing oral methadone and injectable diacetylmorphine for long-term opioid-dependency. *BMC Health Serv Res.* 2011;11:174.
27. Mattick RP, et al. Methadone maintenance therapy versus no opioid replacement therapy for opioid dependence. *Cochrane Database Syst Rev.* 2009:CD002209.
28. Mattick RP, et al. Buprenorphine maintenance versus placebo or methadone maintenance for opioid dependence. *Cochrane Database Syst Rev.* 2014:CD002207.
29. Maxwell S, et al. Prescribing naloxone to actively injecting heroin users: a program to reduce heroin overdose deaths. *J Addict Dis.* 2006;25:89-96.
30. National Institute of Drug Abuse. Principles of Drug Addiction Treatment: A Research-Based Guide; Third Edition. https://www.drugabuse.gov/publications/principles-drug-addiction-treatment-research-based-guide-third-edition/evidence-based-approaches-to-drug-addiction-treatment/pharmacotherapies.
31. Network for Public Health Law. Legal Interventions to Reduce Overdose Mortality: Naloxone Access and Overdose Good Samaritan Laws. https://www.networkforphl.org/_asset/qz5pvn/network-naloxone-10-4.pdf. Accessed September 22, 2016.
32. Nosyk B, et al. Cost-effectiveness of diacetylmorphine versus methadone for chronic opioid dependence refractory to treatment. *CMAJ.* 2012;184:E317-E328.
33. Oviedo-Joekes E, et al. Diacetylmorphine versus methadone for the treatment of opioid addiction. *N Engl J Med.* 2009;361:777-786.
34. Oviedo-Joekes E, et al. Scientific and political challenges in North America's first randomized controlled trial of heroin-assisted treatment for severe heroin addiction: rationale and design of the NAOMI study. *Clin Trials.* 2009;6:261-271.
35. Paone D, et al. Unintentional drug poisoning (overdose) deaths involving heroin and/or fentanyl in New York City, 2000–2015. New York City Department of Health and

Mental Hygiene, Epi Data Brief, August 2016, No. 74. https://www1.nyc.gov/assets/doh/downloads/pdf/epi/databrief74.pdf.

36. Patrick SW, et al. Implementation of prescription drug monitoring programs associated with reductions in opioid-related death rates. *Health Aff (Millwood).* 2016;35:1324-1332.

37. Peltzman S. The effects of automobile safety regulation. *J Political Econ.* 1975;4:677-726.

38. Piper TM, et al. Evaluation of a naloxone distribution and administration program in New York City. *Subst Use Misuse.* 2008;43:858-870.

39. Powis B, et al. Self-reported overdose among injecting drug users in London: extent and nature of the problem. *Addiction.* 1999;94:471-478.

40. Ravndal E, Amundsen EJ. Mortality among drug users after discharge from inpatient treatment: an 8-year prospective study. *Drug Alcohol Depend.* 2010;108:65-69.

41. Schechter M, et al. North American Opiate Medication Initiative (NAOMI): multi-centre, randomized controlled trial of heroin-assisted therapy for treatment-refractory injection opiate users. Canada, Ottawa: Canadian Institutes of Health Research; 2006.

42. Schwartz RP, et al. Opioid agonist treatments and heroin overdose deaths in Baltimore, Maryland, 1995-2009. *Am J Public Health.* 2013;103:917-922.

43. Sordo L, et al. Mortality risk during and after opioid substitution treatment: systematic review and meta-analysis of cohort studies. *BMJ.* 2017;357:j1550.

44. Strang J, et al. Loss of tolerance and overdose mortality after inpatient opiate detoxification: follow up study. *BMJ.* 2003;326:959-960.

45. Tracy M, et al. Circumstances of witnessed drug overdose in New York City: implications for intervention. *Drug Alcohol Depend.* 2005;79:181-190.

46. Wagner KD, et al. Evaluation of an overdose prevention and response training programme for injection drug users in the Skid Row area of Los Angeles, CA. *Int J Drug Policy.* 2010;21:186-193.

47. Walley AY, et al. Opioid overdose rates and implementation of overdose education and nasal naloxone distribution in Massachusetts: interrupted time series analysis. *BMJ.* 2013;346:f174.

48. Wilder CM, et al. Risk factors for opioid overdose and awareness of overdose risk among veterans prescribed chronic opioids for addiction or pain. *J Addictive Dis.* 2016;35:42-51.

49. World Health Organization. Information Sheet on Opioid Overdose. November 2014. http://www.who.int/substance_abuse/information-sheet/en/.

50. United States Congress. Comprehensive Addiction Recovery Act 2016.

51. Zanis DA, Woody GE. One-year mortality rates following methadone treatment discharge. *Drug Alcohol Depend.* 1998;52:257-260.

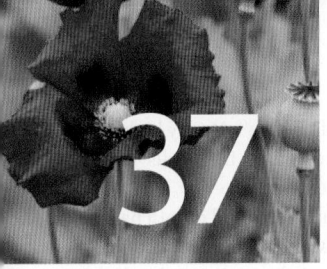

37 SALICYLATES

Daniel M. Lugassy

Acetylsalicylic acid

Methyl salicylic acid

Salicylic Acid

MW = 138 Da

Therapeutic serum concentration = 15–30 mg/dL

= 1.1–2.2 mmol/L

HISTORY AND EPIDEMIOLOGY

The Ancient Egyptians recognized the pain-relieving effects of concoctions made from myrtle and willow leaves. Hippocrates was among the first reported to use willow bark and leaves from the *Salix* species to relieve fever, but it was not until 1829 that the glycoside salicin was extracted from the willow bark and used as an antipyretic. Seven years later, salicylic acid was isolated, and by the late 1800s, it was being used to treat gout, rheumatic fever, and elevated body temperature. The less irritating acetylated salicylate compound was first synthesized in 1833, and in 1899, acetylsalicylic acid was commercially introduced as aspirin by Bayer. With that, the modern era of aspirin therapy and salicylate toxicity began.

The American Association of Poison Control Centers (AAPCC) National Poison Data System (NPDS) collects and reports annual exposure data in the United States. Analgesics, which include both aspirin and acetaminophen (APAP), continue to rank first among pharmaceuticals most frequently reported in human exposures (Chap. 130). Salicylate toxicity and fatalities have long been a major toxicological concern. From the 1950s to 1970s, salicylates were the leading cause of fatal childhood poisoning. The association with Reye syndrome, safer packaging, and the increased use of nonsteroidal antiinflammatory drugs (NSAIDs), APAP, and other alternatives to aspirin decreased the incidence of unintentional salicylate poisoning. In the annual 2015 NPDS review of fatalities, 18 cases of death were documented from single substance acetylsalicylic acid exposures and another 31 fatalities included acetylsalicylic acid as part of the exposure (Chap. 130).[93] A query of the same NPDS database for single-agent aspirin poisoning deaths occurring from 2008 to 2012 yielded 83 cases in which death was coded as a direct consequence of aspirin poisoning.[45] Despite decline in general use, it is still imperative that clinicians are adept at early recognition and swift management of patients with salicylate overdose.

Aspirin and other salicylate-containing products continue to be some of the most common prescription and nonprescription xenobiotics used by the general public. Since landmark trials demonstrated the inhibition of platelet function by aspirin in the 1970s, its use became the standard of care for cardiovascular disease prevention and treatment. Subsequent investigations demonstrated potential benefits of aspirin in primary and secondary prevention of myocardial infarction, colon cancer, and transient ischemic attack. Its antiinflammatory properties continue to make it an active investigational xenobiotic for cancer.[1] Thus salicylates continue to be readily available and will continue to lead to significant morbidity and mortality in overdose.

PHARMACOLOGY

Aspirin and other salicylates have analgesic, antiinflammatory, and antipyretic properties, a combination of traits shared by all of the NSAIDs (Chap. 35). Most of the beneficial effects of NSAIDs result from their inhibition of cyclooxygenase (COX). This enzyme enables the synthesis of prostaglandins, which in turn mediate inflammation and fever.[110,136] Contributing to the antiinflammatory effects and independent of the effects on prostaglandins, salicylates and other NSAIDs also directly inhibit neutrophils.[10] There are two types of salicylic acid esters, phenolic esters such as aspirin and carboxylic acid esters, including methyl salicylate, phenyl salicylate, and glycosalicylate.[27] Most of the studies of salicylate metabolism involve aspirin.[27] There is an implicit assumption that all members of the salicylate class have similar properties after being converted to salicylic acid.

Salicylates and NSAIDs are purportedly most effective in treating the pain accompanying inflammation and tissue injury. Such pain is elicited by prostaglandins liberated by bradykinin and other cytokines. Fever is also mediated by cytokines such as interleukins (IL-1β, IL-6), α and β interferons, and tumor necrosis factor-α, all of which increase synthesis of prostaglandin E_2. In turn, this inflammatory mediator increases cyclic adenosine monophosphate (cAMP), which triggers the hypothalamus to elevate the body temperature set point, resulting in increased heat generation and decreased heat loss.[116]

Because platelets cannot regenerate COX-1, a daily dose of as little as 30 mg of aspirin inhibits COX-1 for the 8- to 12-day lifespan of the platelet.[116] Adverse effects of aspirin and some NSAIDs related to alteration of COX include gastrointestinal (GI) ulcerations and bleeding, interference with platelet adherence,[117] and a variety of metabolic and organ-specific effects described later in this chapter.

To achieve an antiinflammatory effect for patients with chronic conditions such as rheumatoid arthritis, in the past, salicylates were prescribed in doses sufficient to achieve a serum salicylate concentration between 15 and 30 mg/dL, which is considered the therapeutic range. Concentrations higher than 30 mg/dL are typically associated with signs and symptoms of toxicity.

PHARMACOKINETICS

Aspirin is rapidly absorbed from the stomach. The pK_a of aspirin is 3.5, and the majority is nonionized (ie, acetylsalicylic acid) in the strongly acidic stomach (pH 1–2).[27,59] Although absorption of acetylsalicylate is less efficient in the small bowel because of its higher pH, it is substantial and rapid due to the large surface area of the small intestine increases the solubility of acetylsalicylate.[90,91] After ingestion of therapeutic doses of immediate-release acetylsalicylate, therapeutic serum concentrations are achieved in 30 minutes, and maximum concentrations are often attained in less than 1 hour.[27]

The plasma half-life of acetylsalicylate is about 15 minutes because it is rapidly hydrolyzed to salicylate. The apparent half-life for salicylate is about 2 to 3 hours at antiplatelet doses and increases to 12 hours at antiinflammatory doses demonstrating dose dependent elimination.[95] Aspirin undergoes biotransformation in the liver and is then eliminated by the kidneys. The apparent volume of distribution (V_d) increases from 0.2 L/kg at low concentrations to 0.3 to 0.5 L/kg at higher concentrations.[78,79,127]

TOXICOKINETICS

In overdose, several factors contribute to variable pharmacokinetics and present very challenging obstacles to effectively managing patients poisoned with salicylates. The dose contributes to the magnitude and duration of toxicity, but other important factors include the formulation, rate of gastric emptying, alterations in gastric pH (eg, proton pump inhibitors, H_2 antagonists) bezoar formation, hepatic and renal function, and both the serum and urine pH.

There is a decrease in protein (albumin) binding from 90% at therapeutic concentrations to less than 75% at toxic concentrations caused by saturation of protein binding sites.[2,12,34] Salicylates have substantially longer apparent half-lives at toxic concentrations than at therapeutic concentrations, varying from 2 to 4 hours at therapeutic concentrations to as long as 20 hours at toxic concentrations.[29,79] The dosage form of salicylates (eg, effervescent, enteric coated) influences the absorption rate.[115,118,145] Therapeutic doses of enteric-coated tablets produce peak serum concentrations at 4 to 6 hours after ingestion, and in overdose, the reported peak is delayed up to 24 hours after ingestion.[35,145] Delayed absorption of immediate-release aspirin results from salicylate-induced pylorospasm or pharmacobezoar formation.[12,115,122]

Salicylates are conjugated with glycine and glucuronides in the liver and are eliminated by the kidneys. Approximately 10% of salicylates are excreted in the urine as free salicylic acid, 75% as salicyluric acid, 10% as salicylic phenolic glucuronides, 5% as acylglucuronides, and 1% as gentisic acid (Fig. 37–1).[116] As the concentration of salicylates increases, two of the five pathways of elimination—those for salicyluric acid and the salicylic phenolic glucuronide—become saturated and exhibit zero-order kinetics. As a result of this saturation, overall salicylate elimination changes from first-order kinetics to zero-order kinetics (Chap. 9).[78,79] In a healthy adult, these altered saturation kinetics typically occur after as little as 1 to 2 g of acute aspirin ingestion.[79]

When administered chronically, a small increase in dosage or a small decrease in metabolism or elimination results in substantial increases in serum salicylate concentrations and the risk of toxicity.[69] At very high serum concentrations, salicylate elimination again resembles first-order elimination as an increasing fraction undergoes renal clearance.

Free salicylic acid is filtered through the glomerulus and is both passively reabsorbed and actively secreted from the proximal tubules. More than 30% of an ingested salicylate dose is eliminated in alkaline urine and as little as 2% in acidic urine.[140] Salicylate conjugates (glycine and glucuronides) are filtered and secreted by the proximal tubules; salicylate conjugates are not reabsorbed across renal tubular cells because of limited lipid solubility, and the amount eliminated depends on the glomerular filtration rate and proximal tubule secretion but not urine pH. Protein-binding abnormalities, urine and plasma pH variations, and delayed absorption all influence both the maximum salicylate concentration and the rate of decline.[91,115]

Other Forms of Salicylate

Topical Salicylate, Methyl Salicylate (Oil of Wintergreen), and Salicylic Acid

Topical salicylates, which are used as keratolytics (salicylic acid) or as rubefacients (≤30% methyl salicylate), are rarely responsible for salicylate poisoning when used in their intended manner because absorption through normal skin is very slow. However, particularly in children, extensive application of topical preparations containing methyl salicylate result in poisoning.[15,143] After 30 minutes of contact time, only 1.5% to 2.0% of a dose is absorbed, and even after 10 hours of contact with the methyl salicylate, only 12% to 20% of the salicylate is systemically absorbed.[15] Heat, occlusive dressings, young age, inflammation, certain body areas with enhanced absorption, and psoriasis may increase topical salicylate absorption.[18,133,137] In one case report, scrotal exposure to methyl salicylate caused significant salicylate toxicity with a delayed diagnosis.[133] In a study of healthy volunteers, a profound effect of

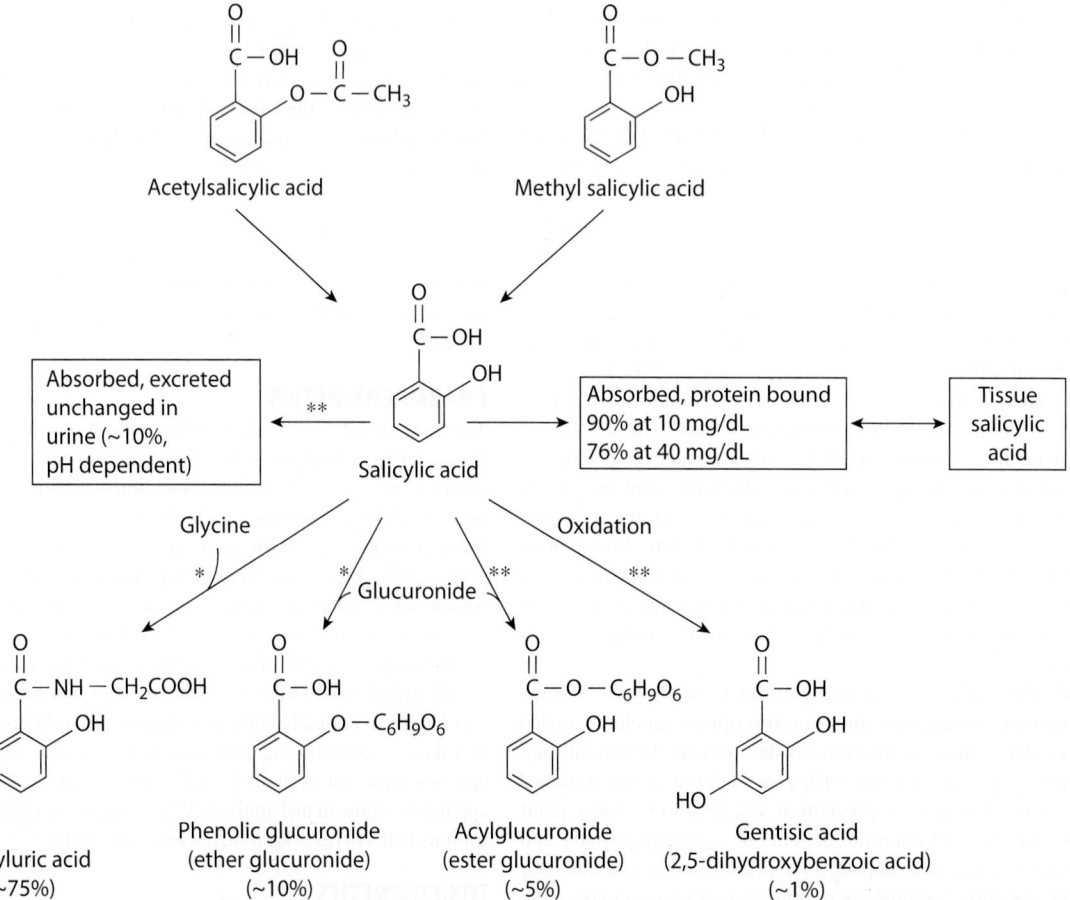

FIGURE 37–1. Salicylic acid metabolism. At excessive doses, the four mechanisms of salicylic acid metabolism are overloaded, leading to increased tissue binding, decreased protein binding, and increased excretion of unconjugated salicylic acid. *Asterisk* (C*) indicates Michaelis-Menten kinetics; *double asterisk* (**) indicates first-order kinetics.

transdermal absorption of methyl salicylate was demonstrated from exercise and heat exposure, with a threefold increase in the systemic availability of salicylate.[26]

Ingestion of methyl salicylate is potentially disastrous because 1 mL of 98% oil of wintergreen contains an equivalent quantity of salicylate as 1.4 g of aspirin. The minimum toxic salicylate dose of approximately 150 mg/kg body weight can almost be achieved with 1 mL of oil of wintergreen, which represents 140 mg/kg of salicylates for a 10-kg child. In Hong Kong, medicated oils containing methyl salicylate accounted for 48% of acute salicylate poisoning cases treated in one hospital.[17] Methyl salicylate is rapidly absorbed from the GI tract, and much, but not all, of the ester is rapidly hydrolyzed to free salicylate. Despite rapid and complete absorption, serum concentrations of salicylates are much less than predicted after ingestion of methyl salicylate containing cream compared with oil of wintergreen.[143] Vomiting is common, along with abdominal discomfort. The onset of symptoms usually occurs within 2 hours of ingestion.[18] Patients with methyl salicylate toxicity have died in less than 6 hours, emphasizing the need for early determinations of salicylate concentrations in addition to frequent testing after such exposures.

Clinicians should be aware of the danger associated with powder formulations of salicylate that are simply mixed with water or juice before ingestion. In a small retrospective study, these powder formulations appeared less likely to have delayed peak serum salicylate concentrations compared with tablet formulations.[120]

Bismuth Subsalicylate

Bismuth subsalicylate, which is available in several nonprescription formulations, releases salicylate in the GI tract, where it is subsequently absorbed. Each milliliter of common liquid preparations of bismuth subsalicylate contains 8.7 mg of salicylic acid.[40] After a large therapeutic dose (60 mL), peak salicylate concentrations reach 4 mg/dL at 1.8 hours after ingestion.[40] Patients with diarrhea and infants with colic using large quantities of bismuth subsalicylate are at increased risk for developing salicylate toxicity.[138] Chronic use should also raise concerns for bismuth toxicity (Chap. 87).

PATHOPHYSIOLOGY

Aspirin has a pKa of 3.5, but as mentioned earlier, it is rapidly hydrolyzed to salicylic acid, which has a pKa of 2.97. Salicylic acid at physiologic pH exists predominantly in a charged (ionized) state (Chap. 9). But in overdose, as the serum pH falls, more salicylate shifts toward a nonionized (uncharged) salicylic acid form that readily permeates across lipid bilayers and cell membranes. This is an important effect in that it allows salicylic acid to enter cells exerting its toxic effects across a wide variety of organs and is discussed later as a target for management.

Acid–Base and Metabolic Effects

Salicylate interferes with the citric acid cycle, which limits production of adenosine triphosphate (ATP).[67] It also uncouples oxidative phosphorylation, causing accumulation of pyruvic and lactic acids and releasing energy as heat (Chap. 11).[73] Salicylate induced increases in fatty acid metabolism generates ketone bodies, including β-hydroxybutyric acid, acetoacetic acid, and acetone. Toxic concentrations of salicylate impair renal hemodynamics, leading to the accumulation of inorganic acids. The net result of all of these metabolic processes is an anion gap metabolic acidosis in which the unmeasured anions include salicylate and its metabolites, lactate, ketoacids, and inorganic acids (Chap. 12).

The salicylate effect on glucose metabolism is variable and depends on the severity and phase of toxicity. Salicylate administration in mice increases glycogenolysis and results in hyperglycemia.[125] Early adrenergic effects of acute salicylate toxicity stimulate epinephrine and glucagon release, enhancing glycogenolysis as well as gluconeogenesis. But salicylate inhibits alanine and aspartate aminotransferase, and both enzymes provide key amino acid substrates for gluconeogenesis. Hypoglycemia also results from the combined effect of increased energy demands, depletion of glycogen stores, and decreased gluconeogenesis.[112]

Salicylate-poisoned mice had dramatic increases in serum lactate concentration compared with control mice, likely because of increased glycogenolysis and anaerobic glycolysis to compensate partly for the energy loss caused by uncoupling of oxidative phosphorylation, (Chap. 11).[56,89] There was also a marked increase in oxygen consumption in mice even with low salicylate concentrations, highlighting the importance of salicylate-induced uncoupling of oxidative phosphorylation which is the cause of increased body temperature.[57] Several investigations examined the etiology of uncoupling of oxidative phosphorylation in salicylate poisoning. By using intact or fragmented mitochondria, it was demonstrated that increasing concentrations of salicylate result in decreased phosphate uptake and a concomitant decrease in the phosphate/oxygen (P/O) ratio.[89,101] The impaired P/O ratio demonstrates the inefficiency of ATP production by illustrating that the rate of phosphate incorporation into ATP per molecule falls despite oxygen consumed during oxidative phosphorylation. Salicylates reduce lipogenesis by blocking the incorporation of acetate into free fatty acids and increase peripheral fatty acid metabolism as an energy source. This salicylate-induced increased fatty acid metabolism generates ketones, including β-hydroxybutyric acid, acetoacetic acid, and acetone.

Neurologic Effects

The central nervous system (CNS) effects are the most visible and most consequential clinical effects in salicylate-poisoned patients. With increasing CNS salicylate concentrations, neuronal energy depletion likely develops as salicylate uncouples neuronal and glial oxidative phosphorylation.[89] Several other mechanisms also likely contribute to the neurotoxic effects of salicylates. Salicylate also causes release of apoptosis-inducing factor (AIF) or cytochrome C, triggers p38 mitogen-activated protein kinase, and activates glial caspase-3, which are responsible for programmed neuronal cell apoptosis.[113] It is likely that in addition to severe cellular acidosis, these effects lead to neuronal dysfunction and ultimately cerebral edema.

Salicylate poisoning reportedly produces clinical discordance between serum and cerebrospinal fluid (CSF) glucose concentrations.[112] Despite normal serum glucose concentrations, CSF glucose concentration decreased 33% in salicylate-poisoned mice compared with control mice.[134] In other words, the rate of CSF glucose use exceeded the rate of supply even in the presence of a normal serum glucose concentration. This hypoglycorrhachia demonstrates that altered glucose metabolism and transport plays a role in the deleterious neurologic effects of the neuroglycopenia resulting from salicylate poisoning. Salicylate-poisoned mice have lower CSF glucose concentrations than control mice but can maintain similar concentrations of ATP by enhanced glycolysis. Administration of dextrose in these salicylate-poisoned mice suppressed clinical signs of toxicity underlying the importance of providing supplemental glucose despite normal serum concentrations as discussed later in the management of toxicity.[134]

Hepatic Effects

Hepatic injury from either acute or chronic overdose of salicylate is rare. Although the hepatocyte is the location of its toxic effects on several metabolic pathways such as glycogenolysis and the Krebs cycle, other concurrent coingestants and causes should be evaluated if there is a clinically significant elevation of aminotransferases or bilirubin concentration or signs of acute liver failure.[148]

An unavoidable historical link exists between the hepatic encephalopathy in Reye syndrome and aspirin. A buildup of fatty acids in the hepatocyte resulting in microvesicular steatosis is characteristic of Reye syndrome. This occurs through salicylate depletion of intrahepatocyte coenzyme A (Co-A), in which fatty acids entering the hepatocyte cytoplasm cannot be transported into the mitochondria for β-oxidation. Although this mechanism is only suggestive in the relationship between aspirin and Reye syndrome, it is clear from epidemiologic evidence that aspirin is an essential cofactor among others in the development of this syndrome.[48]

Otolaryngologic Effects

The molecular mechanism of salicylate ototoxicity is not completely understood but appears to be multifactorial. Inhibition of cochlear COX by salicylate increases arachidonate, enabling calcium flux and neural excitatory effects of N-methyl-D-aspartic acid (NMDA) on cochlear spinal ganglion neurons.[107,108,121] Also, the prevention of prostaglandin synthesis interferes with the Na+, K+-adenosine triphosphatase (ATPase) pump in the stria vascularis, and the vasoconstriction decreases cochlear blood flow.[13,16,38,64] Membrane permeability changes cause a loss of outer hair cell turgor in the organ of Corti, which impairs otoacoustic emissions.[107,109] A more complete description of the pathophysiology of salicylate-induced ototoxicity and sensorineural alterations as well as comparisons with the patterns of other ototoxic xenobiotics is found in Chap. 25.

Pulmonary Effects

Salicylates have very potent stimulatory effects on respiratory drive via several mechanisms. Direct stimulation of the medullary respiratory neurons produces hyperpnea and tachypnea even at therapeutic concentrations. In fact, in a human trial, salicylates decreased the number and duration of apneic events in patients with sleep apnea.[103] Increased sensitivity to PCO_2 and pH further increases ventilation. Carotid body and peripheral arterial chemoreceptor stimulation also contribute to salicylate-induced hyperventilation.[87]

Some patients with either acute or chronic salicylism develop acute respiratory distress syndrome (ARDS). It is often a sign of severe and advanced toxicity and can be lethal. One study[114] that summarized data from nearly 400 consecutive cases of salicylate toxicity reported in the literature[4,54,132,141] concluded that ARDS occurred in approximately 7% of cases. The development of ARDS in salicylate poisoning is associated with a history of cigarette smoking, chronic overdose, metabolic acidosis, and neurologic symptoms at the time of arrival.[97]

Although the exact etiology of salicylate-induced ARDS is unclear, as with other causes, ARDS results from increased pulmonary capillary permeability and subsequent exudation of high-protein edema fluid into the interstitial or alveolar spaces.[60] Adrenergic excess in salicylate poisoning may injure the hypothalamus, leading to a shift in blood from the systemic to the pulmonary circulation because of a loss of left ventricular compliance with left atrial and pulmonary capillary hypertension (Chap. 16). Additionally, the resulting hypoxia produces pulmonary arterial hypertension and a local release of vasoactive substances, worsening ARDS.[61] Unventilated salicylate-poisoned sheep were more likely to develop ARDS compared with a mechanically ventilated control group, suggesting that the mechanical stress of prolonged and severe hyperventilation is a significant contributing factor to this complication.[83]

Gastrointestinal Effects

Salicylate disrupts the mucosal barrier that normally protects the gastric lining from the extremely acidic contents of the stomach. Gastrointestinal injuries leading to ulcers or bleeding are among the most common adverse effects from therapeutic use of aspirin, but in acute overdose, the most common manifestations result from local gastric irritation presenting with nausea and vomiting. Emesis is triggered both by local mucosal irritation and central stimulation of the chemoreceptor trigger zone.[11] Hemorrhagic gastritis, decreased gastric motility, and pylorospasm result from the direct gastric irritant effects of salicylates.[118]

Renal Effects

The kidneys play a major role in the excretion of salicylate and its metabolites. Although some believe that salicylates are nephrotoxic, the majority of experimental evidence does not strongly support this notion.[25,36,102] Most of the adverse renal effects historically associated with salicylates occurred with use of combination products such as aspirin–phenacetin–caffeine tablets and were likely caused by the phenacetin.[36] Renal papillary necrosis and chronic interstitial nephritis, initially characterized by reduced tubular function and reduced concentrating ability, rarely occur in adults using salicylates unless they have chronic illnesses that already compromise renal function.

Volume losses in patients with salicylate toxicity that develop from hyperventilation and hyperthermia also cause prerenal acute kidney injury (AKI). The kidneys also respond to salicylate poisoning by excreting an increased solute load, including large quantities of bicarbonate, sodium, potassium, and organic acids.[5] Rarely, salicylates also induce a Fanconilike syndrome with generalized proximal tubular dysfunction characterized by glucosuria (despite normal serum glucose), proteinuria, aminoaciduria, and uric acid wasting.[135]

Hematologic Effects

The hematologic effects of salicylate poisoning include hypoprothrombinemia and platelet dysfunction.[100] The platelet dysfunction, caused by irreversible acetylation of COX-1 and COX-2, prevents the formation of thromboxane A_2, which is normally responsible for platelet aggregation. Although the platelets are numerically and morphologically intact, they are unresponsive to thrombogenic stimulation. At supratherapeutic doses, salicylate decreases the plasma concentration of the γ-carboxyglutamate containing coagulation factors and an accumulation of microsomal substrates for vitamin K–dependent carboxylase in the liver and lung.[119] The result of this interruption of vitamin K cycling is similar to that of warfarin,[99] leading to hypoprothrombinemia (factor II) as well as decreases in factors VII, IX, and X (Chap. 58).

CLINICAL MANIFESTATIONS OF SALICYLATE POISONING

The following sections describe the typical clinical manifestations that follow toxic exposures to salicylates. The natural course of acute ingestions begins with nonspecific GI symptoms, early tachypnea caused by direct central respiratory stimulation, development of an anion gap metabolic acidosis, and several minor neurologic sequelae. As the acidosis worsens, clinical effects progress and invariably evolve to severe CNS toxicity. Hyperthermia, cerebral edema, coagulopathy, ARDS, and severe acidemia are the gravest clinical consequences and are often preterminal events. Cerebral edema is often seen at autopsy in those who succumb to salicylate toxicity.

The earliest signs and symptoms of salicylate toxicity, which include nausea, vomiting, diaphoresis, and tinnitus, typically develop within 1 to 2 hours of acute ingestion.[13,46] But the type of salicylate-containing preparation, comorbidities, coingestants, and compromise in renal or hepatic function potentially delay the onset of symptoms up to 24 hours after exposure.[118] Case reports of enteric-coated aspirin tablet ingestions demonstrate delays in symptom onset and time to initial detectable salicylate concentration, with peak salicylate concentrations reported to occur 2 to 3 days after initial exposure.[32,145]

Acute Salicylate Poisoning

Salicylates are extremely irritating to the GI mucosa; early vomiting after ingestion are a warning sign of a potentially clinically significant ingestion. Emesis occurs both by direct GI irritation and from salicylate-induced stimulation of the chemoreceptor trigger zone.[11] Pylorospasm, delayed gastric emptying, and decreased GI motility complicate toxicity by altering absorption kinetics. Hemorrhagic gastritis also occurs, likely as a consequence of severe emesis and alteration of protective mucosal GI barriers.

The initial evaluation of a patient suspected of salicylate poisoning must start with a thorough assessment of the respiratory rate and depth. Subtle tachypnea or hyperpnea should not be overlooked because if missed, they will delay the initiation of appropriate laboratory analysis and management. Direct central stimulation of the respiratory center increases minute volume ventilation, determined by the product of respiratory rate and tidal volume. A primary respiratory alkalosis predominates initially, although an anion gap metabolic acidosis begins to develop early in the course of salicylate toxicity. By the time a symptomatic adult patient presents to the hospital after a salicylate overdose, a mixed acid–base disturbance is often prominent.[46] This latter finding includes two primary processes, respiratory alkalosis and metabolic acidosis, and is discernible by arterial blood gas (ABG) or venous blood gas (VBG) and serum electrolyte analyses. In one study of 66 salicylate-poisoned adults, 22% had respiratory alkalosis, and 56% had mixed respiratory alkalosis and metabolic acidosis.[46]

TABLE 37–1	Progressive Acid-Base Stages of Salicylate Poisoning

Early: Respiratory alkalosis, alkalemia, and alkaluria

Intermediate: Respiratory alkalosis, metabolic acidosis, alkalemia, and aciduria

Late: Metabolic acidosis with either a respiratory alkalosis or respiratory acidosis, acidemia, and aciduria

On presentation, salicylate-poisoned adults who demonstrate respiratory acidosis should alert the clinician to the fact that systemic toxicity is severe. This patient will likely be late in the clinical course of poisoning and have salicylate induced ARDS, fatigue from hyperventilating for a prolonged period of time, or CNS depression (from either salicylate itself or coingestants). These broad variations of clinical toxicity can be divided into three general time frames based on rapidly available laboratory testing. The progressive stages salicylate poisoning are demonstrated in Table 37–1.

Mixed overdoses are common; in one study, one-third of patients with a presumed primary salicylate overdose took other xenobiotics.[46] Benzodiazepines, barbiturates, alcohol, and cyclic antidepressants all blunt the centrally induced hyperventilatory response to salicylates, resulting in either actual respiratory acidosis (PCO_2 >40 mm Hg) or metabolic acidosis without some respiratory compensation (PCO_2 <40 mm Hg but inappropriately high for the concomitant degree of metabolic acidosis). In both adults and children, the development of respiratory acidosis occurs as salicylate poisoning progresses. The combination of metabolic and respiratory acidosis in a salicylate poisoning results in severe and worsening acidemia that is an exceedingly grave situation and almost invariably is a preterminal event.[105]

When clinical and radiographic manifestations of ARDS are observed in the setting of salicylate toxicity, the following conditions should be considered: aspiration pneumonitis, viral and bacterial infections, neurogenic ARDS, and salicylate-induced ARDS (Chap. 28).[61,68] In 111 consecutive patients with peak salicylate concentrations above 30 mg/dL, ARDS occurred in 35% of patients older than 30 years of age and none of the 55 patients younger than 16 years of age. The average arterial blood pH was 7.37 in the six adult patients with ARDS and 7.46 in the 30 adults without ARDS. There was no significant difference in salicylate concentrations, which were approximately 57 mg/dL in both groups.[141] In a 2-year review of all salicylate deaths in Ontario, Canada, 59% of 39 autopsies revealed pulmonary pathology, mostly "pulmonary edema" (ARDS).[86]

Although hyperventilation is centrally mediated, patients may develop a spectrum of CNS abnormalities that includes confusion, agitation, and lethargy and then ultimately seizures and coma. Human and animal evidence suggests that hypoglycorrhachia despite euglycemia contributes to the neurotoxic effects. Stupor, coma, and delirium may be reversed by the administration of dextrose in children and adults with salicylate toxicity and normal serum glucose concentrations. In one report, a child underwent lumbar puncture, and CSF analysis demonstrated no detectable glucose despite a normal peripheral glucose.[24] The most severe neurologic clinical findings are likely associated with the development of cerebral edema and portend a poor prognosis. Excluding effects on ventilation, signs of neurologic toxicity, even if mild, should be of great concern.

Tinnitus, a subjective sensation of ringing or hissing with or without hearing loss, loss of absolute acoustic sensitivity, and alterations of perceived sounds are the three effects resulting from exposure to large doses of salicylates.[16] The pattern of salicylate-induced auditory sensorineural alterations is different than that of other ototoxic xenobiotics.[16] Tinnitus is a demonstrable manifestation of CNS toxicity even without alterations in mental status. As CNS salicylate concentrations increase, tinnitus is rapidly followed by diminished auditory acuity that sometimes leads to deafness.[13] As acute toxicity progresses, other CNS effects include vertigo, hyperactivity, agitation, delirium, hallucinations, lethargy, seizures, and stupor. Coma is rare and is generally a late finding occurring in severe acute poisoning or mixed overdoses.[4,147]

Paratonia, extreme muscle rigidity, is reported in severe salicylate poisoning pre- and postmortem, and the rigidity, it was unresponsive to

TABLE 37–2	Differential Characteristics of Acute and Chronic Salicylate Poisoning	
	Acute	**Chronic**
Age	Younger	Older
Etiology	Overdose usually intentional	Therapeutic misadventures; iatrogenic
Diagnosis	Easily recognized (absent coingestion)	Frequently unrecognized
Other diseases	None	Underlying disorders (especially chronic pain conditions)
Suicidal ideation	Typical	Atypical
Serum concentrations	Marked elevation	Intermediate elevation
Mortality	Uncommon when recognized and properly treated	More common due to delayed recognition

succinylcholine in a single case report.[86,111] Decreased ATP production, impaired glycolysis, increased lactate, and uncoupling of muscular oxidative phosphorylation likely contribute to this phenomenon. This excess neuromuscular activity leads to rhabdomyolysis acute tubular necrosis and, most concerning, hyperthermia, which is typically a preterminal condition.[77,89,90]

Chronic Salicylate Poisoning

Chronic salicylate poisoning most typically occurs in older adults as a result of unintentional overdosing on salicylates used for primary and secondary prevention of cardiovascular disorders and osteoarthritis in addition to analgesia and as an antipyretic[5,30,69] (Table 37–2). Presenting signs and symptoms of chronic salicylate poisoning can be similar to those of acute toxicity and include nausea and vomiting, hearing loss and tinnitus, dyspnea and hyperventilation, tachycardia, hyperthermia, and neurologic manifestations (eg, confusion, delirium, agitation, hyperactivity, slurred speech, hallucinations, seizures, coma).[4,33,76] Although there is considerable overlap with acute salicylate poisoning, the slow, insidious onset of chronic poisoning in older adults frequently causes delayed recognition of the true cause of the patient's presentation.[4,46,75]

On occasion, ill patients who have chronic salicylate poisoning are misdiagnosed as having delirium, dementia, or encephalopathy of undetermined origin; or diseases such as sepsis (fever of unknown origin), alcoholic ketoacidosis, respiratory failure, or cardiopulmonary disease.[4,6,21,37] Unfortunately, many of the signs and symptoms of chronic salicylate toxicity were mistakenly attributed to the illness for which the salicylates were administered.[21,129] In one report, despite an extensive evaluation during a first hospitalization for ARDS, chronic salicylism was not diagnosed until a second hospitalization for the same respiratory symptoms.[23] This case highlights the need to include chronic salicylism in the differential for ARDS with or without neurologic symptoms.

In a study of 73 consecutive adults hospitalized with salicylate poisoning, 27% were not correctly diagnosed for as long as 72 hours after admission.[4] In this group, 60% of the patients had a neurologic consultation before the diagnosis of salicylism was established. When diagnosis is delayed in older adults, the morbidity and mortality associated with salicylate poisoning are high. The mortality rate was reported to be as high as 25% in the 1970s,[4] and there are no data to suggest that survival after delayed diagnosis is substantially better today.

EVALUATION AND DIAGNOSTIC TESTING

The most commonly reported route of exposure is from the acute ingestion of aspirin, which, as mentioned earlier, has a very short serum half-life of about 15 minutes during which time it is rapidly converted to salicylate. The symptoms of toxicity are due to the systemic effects of salicylate and not the parent compound. Systemic toxicity is concerning after the following exposures: ingestions of 150 mg/kg or 6.5 g of aspirin, whichever is less; ingestion of greater than a lick or taste of oil of wintergreen (98% methyl salicylate) by children younger than 6 years of age; and more than 4 mL of oil of wintergreen by patients 6 years of age and older.[22] These patients as well as those with significant topical exposures and signs of toxicity should be promptly evaluated for salicylate toxicity.

The initial approach to a patient suspected of salicylate toxicity should include a serum salicylate concentration. It is very important to recognize that other laboratory assays such as an ABG or VBG, electrolytes to determine anion gap, the presence of serum or urine ketones, and a lactate concentration are often sufficient to uncover an unrecognized salicylate poisoning. It also is important to evaluate renal and hepatic function because dysfunction in either will exacerbate toxicokinetic effects in patients with acute or chronic exposures.

Elevated anion gaps are caused by increases in unmeasured anions that are primarily salicylate but also related to increases in lactic acid, ketoacids, and daily endogenous dietary acids. Contributing factors to the rise in the anion gap discussed earlier include volume loss from vomiting, AKI, and increased metabolic energic production.

Several studies demonstrate that empiric serum salicylate concentrations are not required as part of a general toxicologic evaluation in patients with acute self-poisoning. Routine salicylate testing is likely unnecessary without a history of salicylate ingestion, an inability to obtain a valid history (altered mental status), or clinical features of salicylate poisoning.[19,51,144] One retrospective study also demonstrated that screening for salicylism is not needed in the absence of an elevated anion gap.[124] Although an anion gap metabolic acidosis is likely found in most cases of salicylate toxicity, severe salicylism is rarely reported to falsely elevate serum chloride, bringing the anion gap closer to a normal range.[62]

One explanation for the falsely elevated chloride concentrations comes from laboratory misinterpretation of salicylate ions for chloride ions that leads to a falsely lowered anion gap.[70] Additionally, a renal tubular acidosis can occur in salicylate poisoning, resulting in metabolic acidosis with a normal anion gap.[142] Several case reports demonstrate low or normal anion gaps in patients with significant salicylate toxicity; therefore, a normal anion gap should not rule out salicylate poisoning.[8,70]

Although it is wise to curtail empiric testing, clinicians should likely err on the side of ordering a salicylate concentration if there is any clinical concern because the morbidity and mortality are significantly increased with delays in recognition and management. Many of the signs and symptoms of salicylate toxicity are vague and often mistakenly attributed to another illness with disastrous consequences. In the review of all salicylate deaths in Ontario, Canada, in 1983 and 1984, the author noted that in six of the 23 (26%) patients who arrived alert, no salicylate determination was identified in the medical record, and that probably neither the diagnosis nor the severity of the salicylate poisoning was recognized.[86]

Salicylate Analysis

Serum salicylate concentrations are relatively easy to obtain in most hospital laboratories today. Several methods are available for determining serum salicylate concentrations. The Trinder assay was once the most popular method for the measurement of salicylate in serum by using spectrophotometric analysis. Trinder's reagent contains mercuric chloride and hydrochloric acid used to precipitate serum proteins. The measured absorbance at 540 nm of a ferric ion–salicylate complex allows for accurate determination of the serum salicylate concentration. Historically, there have been several bedside urine qualitative test (ie, mercuric chloride, ferric chloride) used to assess for the presence of salicylate. Both the Trinder reaction and the bedside tests have limited utility today in modern centers because of poor specificity and chemical hazards and are no longer permissible in the United States under the federal Clinical Laboratory Improvement Amendments (CLIA).

Serum salicylate concentrations are commonly reported in mg/dL in the United States, but confusion can arise because values can also be reported in mg/L and mcg/mL. Reporting salicylate concentrations as mg/L when the clinician is accustomed to receiving results as mg/dL or inadvertently reporting actual mg/L (before internal laboratory conversion) produces

erroneous results. Such misinterpretations[52] suggest a toxic salicylate concentration in a patient whose serum salicylate concentration is actually within the therapeutic range (eg, "165 mg/L" instead of "16.5 mg/dL"). Most errors can be identified before initiation of aggressive therapy, such as hemodialysis (HD), by determining whether the reported salicylate concentration is consistent with the clinical presentation and ABG or VBG results and, when time permits, repeating the salicylate determination with appropriate consideration for methodology and conversion calculations.[52] Using the earlier example, a patient with a serum salicylate concentration of 165 mg/dL would undoubtedly show clinical signs of salicylate toxicity and have a profound acid–base abnormality, but a patient with a concentration of 165 mg/L would likely be asymptomatic.

It should also be noted that several clinical scenarios and xenobiotic exposures are recognized to cause false-positive or falsely elevated true salicylate concentrations. Depending on the assay, medications that reportedly interfered with accurate salicylate measurement include thioridazine, promethazine, prochlorperazine, chlorpromazine, N-acetylcysteine, and cysteamine.[9] Significantly falsely elevated serum salicylate concentrations are well recognized after diflunisal overdose.[31,128] Hyperbilirubinemia can create clinically significant false-positive results in neonates and adults.[9,14] Interestingly, hyperlipidemia can also cause significant interference and false elevation of serum salicylate concentrations.[20] If there is concern for false salicylate concentrations, clinicians should contact laboratory personnel, who often have information regarding instrument-specific recognized interferences for each assay as published by the manufacturer. Several techniques are used to determine a true salicylate concentration in the setting of a known interference. One of the most sensitive and specific assays now available is an automated immunoassay based on specific antisalicylate antiserum with fluorescence polarization immunoassay (FPIA) detection technology.[9]

Interpretation of Serum Salicylate Concentrations and Correlation with Toxicity

The recommended therapeutic concentration of salicylate is 10 to 30 mg/dL, but this varies by indication. Antiinflammatory dosing usually is advised to be on the higher end of this spectrum, but analgesic effects occur as low as 5 to 10 mg/dL. Serum concentrations above 30 mg/dL are usually not found unless there is a supratherapeutic, acute, or chronic toxic exposure. Initial salicylate concentrations do not correlate with severe outcomes in salicylate poisoning.[123]

The correlation of serum salicylate concentrations and clinical toxicity is often poor and dependent on several factors. A concurrent arterial or venous blood pH should be determined when a serum salicylate concentration is obtained because in the presence of acidemia, more salicylic acid leaves the blood and enters the CSF and other tissues (Fig. 37–2), increasing

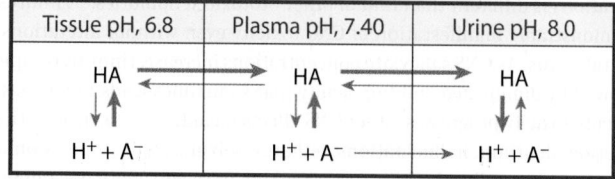

FIGURE 37–2. Rationale for alkalinization. Alkalinization of the plasma with respect to the tissues and alkalinization of the urine with respect to plasma shifts the equilibrium to the plasma and urine and away from the tissues, including the brain. This equilibrium shift results in "ion trapping."[129]

the toxicity. A decreasing serum salicylate concentration is difficult to interpret in isolation because it may reflect either an increased tissue distribution with increasing toxicity or an increased clearance with decreasing toxicity. Clinical correlation is required. For example, a decreasing serum salicylate concentration accompanied by a decreasing or low blood pH should be presumed to reflect a serious or worsening situation, not a benign or improving one. Patients with chronic toxicity demonstrate more significant clinical effects at lower concentrations compared with acute toxicity given the increased distribution over time into tissue compartments and specifically the CNS.

Although impractical clinically, salicylate concentrations in the CSF are likely the most accurate measure of toxicity, directly correlating with death in a rat model.[57] Animals that were lethally poisoned with salicylate were comatose and died from seizures. The time to death after salicylate administration varied greatly as did the blood, muscle, and liver salicylate concentrations. However, regardless of the time of death and the concentrations in blood, muscle, or liver, all animals died with a consistently narrow range of CSF salicylate concentrations.[57] Inhalation of CO_2 (lowering serum pH) in a rat resulted in a precipitous decrease in serum salicylate concentrations, which returned to baseline rapidly after the discontinuation of CO_2.[56] This suggests that the salicylate redistributed into tissue during the period of induced respiratory acidosis and reequilibrated after its correction. After administration of radiolabeled salicylate to cats, autoradiographs of the brain visually and objectively documented the profound effect that acidemia has on the distribution of salicylate into the brain.[49]

Before serum assays were readily available, physicians who prescribed aspirin would advise patients to take repeated doses until tinnitus occurred and then "back off" a little to maintain this "steady state." Tinnitus and the subsequent reversible hearing loss typically occur at serum salicylate concentrations of 20 to 45 mg/dL.[13,16,94] This prompted investigations into whether salicylate-induced tinnitus could be used as an indicator of serum salicylate concentration and toxicity. Unfortunately, some patients with therapeutic concentrations of salicylates had tinnitus, and many with higher or toxic concentrations had no tinnitus. In a study of 94 patients with salicylate concentrations above 30 mg/dL on one or more occasions, tinnitus only correlated with serum salicylate concentrations in 30%; 55% had no tinnitus, although audiologic testing results were usually abnormal regardless of the patient's perception of presence or absence of tinnitus.[53] Thus, although symptomatic ototoxicity is a helpful warning sign of salicylate toxicity when present, it is too nonspecific and too insensitive to serve as an indicator of serum salicylate concentrations. Severe outcomes in salicylate poisoning were associated with increased respiratory rate, older age, and lactate concentrations above 2.25 mmol/L.[123]

MANAGEMENT

The management of patients with salicylate poisoning is aimed at supporting vital signs and organ function, preventing or limiting ongoing exposure from the gut or skin, and enhancing elimination of salicylate that has already entered the systemic circulation. It is imperative to understand that there is no true antidote for salicylate toxicity; no xenobiotic can combat the clinical toxicity demonstrated in consequential exposures. Hemodialysis, as discussed later, aims to remove salicylate from the tissues but may not correct severe organ toxicity such as ARDS or cerebral edema and can therefore not guarantee survival after severe toxicity occurs.[41,88] Rather, all therapies are better at preventing tissue injury than treating it.

It is imperative to understand that the primary toxicity of salicylate is on the CNS, and the amount of salicylate in the brain is a function of pH with acidemia enhancing CNS penetration of the drug. Management strategies strive to create concentration gradients and pH conditions that favor exit of salicylate from the CNS and other tissues and enhanced renal elimination.

Gastrointestinal Decontamination and Use of Activated Charcoal

The use of orogastric lavage and activated charcoal (AC) is discussed in Chap. 5 and Antidotes in Depth: A1. Their effects on the absorption and

elimination of salicylates have been extensively studied. In vitro studies demonstrate that each gram of AC maximally adsorbs approximately 550 mg of salicylic acid.[80,96] In humans, AC reduces the absorption of therapeutic doses of aspirin by 50% to 80%, effectively adsorbing aspirin released from enteric-coated and sustained-release preparations in addition to immediate-release tablets.[80] Presumably, the sooner AC is given after salicylate ingestion, the more effective it will be in reducing absorption. A 10:1 ratio of AC to ingested salicylate appears to result in maximal efficacy but is often impractical given the fact that ingestions of salicylate often reach 20- to 30-g amounts or more. Although peak serum concentrations are markedly decreased from predicted concentrations, aspirin desorption from the aspirin–AC complex in the alkaline milieu of the small bowel potentially diminishes the impact of AC on total absorption.[43,84,96] The addition of a cathartic to the initial dose of AC was abandoned for most xenobiotics, but a benefit of adding sorbitol to AC in preventing salicylate absorption was demonstrated in one study.[71]

Repetitive or multiple-dose AC (MDAC) is recommended to achieve desired ratios of AC to salicylate (and probably limits desorption), which reportedly reduces the concentration of initially absorbed salicylate to only 15% to 20%.[43] Multiple dose activated charcoal prevents absorption of unabsorbed salicylates over that achieved by single-dose AC.[7,55,58] Thus, the use of MDAC to decrease GI absorption of salicylates is recommended, particularly if a pharmacobezoar or extended-release preparation is suspected, barring contraindications (Antidotes in Depth: A1).

The value of MDAC in enhancing salicylate elimination through GI dialysis is considered controversial by some.[3,63] In one volunteer study of a 2,800-mg dose of aspirin followed by 25 g of AC at 4, 6, 8, and 10 hours after ingestion, the total amount of salicylate excreted from the body increased by 9% to 18% but was not considered statistically significant.[72] Efficacy is likely greater in an overdose situation, when more unbound salicylate is available because of decreased protein binding. However, in another study of the effects of MDAC on the clearance of high-dose intravenous (IV) aspirin in a porcine model, MDAC did not enhance the clearance of salicylates under conditions when the venous bicarbonate was kept at 15 mEq/L or less and urine pH kept at 7.5 or less.[63] In contrast to the findings of both of these studies, two children with salicylate overdoses were successfully treated with MDAC given every 4 hours for 36 hours, but it is unclear whether the predominant role of MDAC was to prevent absorption or enhance elimination.[139] Overall, the administration of two to four properly timed doses of AC is recommended. The administration of AC or MDAC must be balanced against risks of vomiting and aspiration, especially in patients with altered mental status and unprotected airways (Chap. 5).

In theory, whole-bowel irrigation (WBI) with polyethylene glycol electrolyte lavage solution (PEG-ELS) in addition to AC reduces absorption, particularly for enteric-coated aspirin preparations.[131] However, in an experimental model, WBI and MDAC did not increase the clearance of absorbed salicylate.[84]

Fluid Replacement

There is a need to differentiate between restoration of fluid and electrolyte balance in salicylate-poisoned patients and increasing the fluid load presented to the kidneys in an attempt to achieve "forced diuresis." Fluid losses in patients with salicylate poisoning are prominent, especially in children, and can be attributed to hyperventilation, vomiting, fever, a hypermetabolic state, polyuria, cathartic administration, and perspiration.[5,130] For all of these reasons, the patient's volume status must be adequately assessed and corrected if necessary along with any glucose and electrolyte abnormalities. As in other cases, accurate management of volume status in poisoned patients may require invasive or noninvasive monitoring of central venous pressures, especially in patients with cardiac disease, ARDS, or AKI.

Increasing fluids beyond restoration of fluid balance to achieve forced diuresis is a practice that was inappropriately promoted in the past. Although forced diuresis theoretically increases renal tubular flow and reduces the urine tubular cell diffusion gradient for reabsorption, renal excretion of salicylate depends much more on urine pH than on flow rate, and use of forced diuresis under any circumstances is not effective regardless of whether diuretics, osmotic agents, or large fluid volumes are used to achieve the diuresis.[104] Although renal salicylate clearance varies in direct proportion to flow rate, its relation to pH is logarithmic.[66,75] In summary, although fluid imbalance must be corrected, forced diuresis does little more than oral fluids to enhance elimination over a 24-hour period[104] and subjects the patient to the hazards of fluid overload and is therefore not recommended.

Serum and Urine Alkalinization

The cornerstone of the management of patients with salicylate toxicity is to shift salicylate out of the brain and tissues into the serum, where elimination through the kidneys can then occur. Alkalinization of the serum with respect to the tissues and alkalinization of the urine with respect to the serum accomplishes this goal by facilitating the movement and "ion trapping" of salicylate into the serum and the urine (Fig. 37–2). Alkalinization of the serum by a substance that does not easily cross the blood–brain barrier such as intravenously administered sodium bicarbonate reduces the fraction of salicylate in the nonionized form and increases the pH gradient with the CSF. This both prevents entry and helps remove salicylate from the CNS.[49,55-57,129]

Serum alkalinization with IV sodium bicarbonate is recommended for all symptomatic patients whose serum salicylate concentrations exceed the therapeutic range and for clinically suspected cases of salicylism until a salicylate concentration and simultaneously obtained blood pH are available to guide treatment. Patients on therapeutic regimens of salicylates who feel well with salicylate concentrations of 30 to 40 mg/dL and who do not manifest toxicity do not require intervention.

Alkalinization is typically achieved with a bolus of 1 to 2 mEq/kg of sodium bicarbonate IV followed by an infusion of 3 ampules of sodium bicarbonate (132 mEq) in 1 L of 5% dextrose in water administered at 1.5 to 2.0 times the maintenance fluid range. Urine pH should be maintained at 7.5 to 8.0, and hypokalemia must be corrected (see later discussion) to achieve maximum urinary alkalinization. The volume load should remain modest while previous losses are repleted (Antidotes in Depth: A5).

Oral bicarbonate administration should never be substituted for IV bicarbonate to achieve alkalinization because the oral route potentially increases salicylate absorption from the GI tract by enhancing dissolution. Hyperventilation alone should not be relied on, and IV sodium bicarbonate should be used for alkalinization.

Urine Alkalinization

Because salicylic acid is a weak acid (pK$_a$ of 2.97), it is ionized in an alkaline milieu and theoretically can be "trapped" there. This occurs because there is no specific uptake mechanism in the kidney for salicylate ion, and passive reabsorption of a charged molecule is very limited. Thus, alkalinization of the urine (defined as a pH of 7.5 or greater) with sodium bicarbonate results in enhanced excretion of the ionized salicylate ion (Fig. 37–2).

Alkalinization of the urine is recommended as a first-line treatment for patients with moderately severe salicylate poisoning who do not meet the criteria for HD.[106,134] It is also recommended for salicylate-poisoned patients who require HD while preparations are being made to perform HD. Although salicylic acid is almost completely ionized within physiologic pH limits, small changes in pH obtained by alkalinization have substantial changes in the relative amount of salicylate in the charged form.

Regardless of the reason for the change in serum pH, renal excretion of salicylate is very dependent on urinary pH.[66,104,140] Alkalinization increases free salicylate secretion from the proximal tubule but does not affect renal elimination of salicylate conjugates. Alkalinizing the urine from a pH of 5 to 8 logarithmically increased renal salicylate clearance from 1.3 to 100 mL/min (Fig. 37–3).[66,92] Assuming an overdose V$_d$ of 0.5 L/kg, this increased clearance would decrease the salicylate half-life from 310 to 4 hours. However, in reality, alkalinizing the urine from a pH of 5 to 8 has a more modest effect on serum salicylate clearance.[104]

Although the administration of acetazolamide, a noncompetitive carbonic anhydrase inhibitor, results in the formation of bicarbonate rich

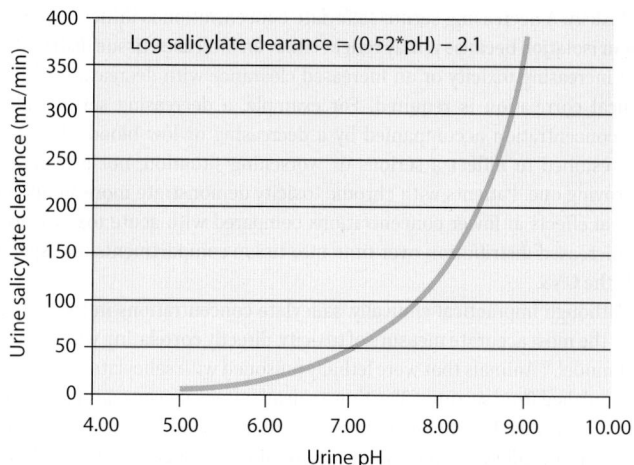

FIGURE 37–3. The relationship between urine pH and urine salicylate clearance. This curve was adapted from a logarithmic relationship determined by Kallen in patients with salicylate poisoning. It illustrates the need to substantially increase urine pH above 7 to impact elimination.[66]

alkaline urine, it also causes a metabolic acidosis and acidemia.[42,55,56] This latter effect of acetazolamide is usually self-limited and mild but nevertheless increases the concentration of freely diffusible nonionized molecules of salicylic acid, thereby increasing the V$_d$ and most probably enhancing the penetrance of salicylate into the CNS.[56,79]

Hypokalemia is a common complication of salicylate poisoning and sodium bicarbonate therapy and can prevent urinary alkalinization unless corrected. In the presence of hypokalemia, the renal tubules reabsorb potassium ions in exchange for hydrogen ions, preventing urinary alkalinization. If urinary alkalinization cannot be achieved easily, hypokalemia, excretion of organic acids, and salt and water depletion are the likely reasons for failure. Calcium concentrations should be monitored because decreases in both ionized[30] and total serum calcium[44] are also complications of bicarbonate therapy.

Glucose Supplementation

As discussed earlier, salicylate poisoning significantly alters glucose metabolism, transport, and relative requirements. Clinically, this is relevant in that the presence of a normal serum glucose concentration may not be reflective of a normal CSF glucose concentration. The neurotoxicity of salicylism could be partly caused by this hypoglycorrhachia. Dextrose administration alone has reversed acute delirium associated with salicylate toxicity.[23,24,69,74] It is therefore recommended to liberally administer dextrose to all patients with altered mental status in salicylate toxicity regardless of their serum glucose concentration. A bolus of 0.5 to 1 g/kg of dextrose with additional doses or even continuous infusion is recommended for patients being treated for severe salicylate toxicity.

Extracorporeal Removal

Indications for HD include severe salicylate poisoning, altered mental status, ARDS requiring supplemental oxygen, standard therapy is deemed to be failing regardless of the salicylate concentration, salicylate concentrations above 100 mg/dL, and salicylate concentrations above 90 mg/dL with impaired renal function[65] (Table 37–3). It is reasonable when a patient cannot tolerate the increased solute load that results from alkalinization or large-volume infusions necessary. Failure to tolerate such therapy can be anticipated if the patient has initial symptoms that are consistent with severe salicylate toxicity or has a history of congestive heart failure or chronic kidney disease.

In most instances, intermittent HD is the preferred method but hemoperfusion (HP) and continuous renal replacement therapies are appropriate when no HD is available.[65] Hemodialysis will not only clear the salicylate but also rapidly correct fluid, electrolyte, and acid–base disorders that will not be corrected by HP alone. The combination of HD and HP in series is feasible and theoretically may be useful for treating patients with severe or

TABLE 37–3	Indications for Hemodialysis in Patients with Salicylate Poisoning

General Recommendation
- Intermittent hemodialysis is the preferred modality.

Indications
ECTR is recommended if *any* of the following are met:
- Salicylate concentration ≥100 mg/dL (≥7.2 mmol/L)
- Salicylate concentration ≥90 mg/dL (≥6.5 mmol/L) in the presence of impaired kidney function
- Altered mental status
- New hypoxemia requiring supplemental oxygen
- If standard therapy (eg, supportive measures, bicarbonate) fails and:
  - Salicylate concentration ≥90 mg/dL (≥6.5 mmol/L)
  - Salicylate concentration ≥80 mg/dL (≥5.8 mmol/L) in the presence of impaired kidney function
  - If the systemic pH is ≤7.20

Hemodialysis should be continued until
- There is clear clinical improvement is apparent *and*
- Salicylate concentration <19 mg/dL (1.4 mmol/L) *or*
- Hemodialysis was performed for a period of at least 4–6 h when salicylate concentrations are not readily available

Modified with permission from Juurlink DN, Gosselin S, Kielstein JT, et al. Extracorporeal Treatment for Salicylate Poisoning: Systematic Review and Recommendations From the EXTRIP Workgroup. *Ann Emerg Med.* 2015 Aug;66(2):165-181.

mixed overdoses,[28] but it is rarely used. A rapid reduction of serum salicylate concentrations in severely poisoned patients was described with the use of continuous renal replacement therapy, a technique that may be valuable for patients who are too unstable to undergo HD or when HD is unavailable (Chap. 6).[146] There is only one published clinical experience with sustained low-efficiency dialysis for salicylate toxicity, which demonstrated similar clearance rates to other continuous extracorporeal therapies.[81] Exchange transfusion is recommended in neonates when HD is unavailable.[65]

While the patient is awaiting HD, alkalinization of serum and urine is recommended using sodium bicarbonate therapy. During HD, it is unnecessary to continue bicarbonate therapy because it will be provided by HD. It is prudent to reinstitute bicarbonate therapy after HD is completed, especially if patients are still symptomatic or serum salicylate concentrations are pending.

Nephrology consultation should be sought early and liberally to anticipate and prevent avoidable morbidity and mortality. Despite the well-recognized benefit of extracorporeal removal of salicylates in severe toxicity, delays in initiating HD remain a potentially preventable cause of death despite repeated calls over many years for prompt HD for patients with salicylate poisoning.[41,88]

In Table 37–3, impaired kidney function can be defined as advanced chronic kidney disease, AKI, when baseline not available, elevated creatinine of greater than 2 mg/dL in adults or 1.5 mg/dL in older adults, children with no baseline creatinine concentration, a serum creatinine greater than twice the upper limit of normal for age and sex or the presence of oligo- or anuria for more than 6 hours, regardless of serum creatinine concentration.[65]

The initiation of HD should not be considered definitive treatment because patients often still have a significant GI burden of salicylate, resulting in continued absorption. Even with early and multiple runs of HD, patients may still succumb to this poisoning, particularly if salicylate is still being absorbed from the GI tract into the blood.[88]

Sedation, Intubation, and Mechanical Ventilation Risks

Salicylate-poisoned patients have a significantly increased minute ventilation rate brought about by both tachypnea and hyperpnea, often exceeding 20 to 30 L/min. Any decrease in minute ventilation increases the PCO_2 and decreases the pH. This shifts salicylate into the CNS, exacerbating toxicity. Thus, extreme caution must be used with chemical sedation, intubation, and initiation of mechanical ventilation.

Although induced hyperventilation may effectively increase the blood pH in certain patients, endotracheal intubation followed by assisted ventilation

of a salicylate-poisoned patient poses particular risks if it is not meticulously performed. Although early endotracheal intubation to maintain hyperventilation will aid in the management of patients whose respiratory efforts are faltering, health care providers must maintain appropriate hypocarbia through hyperventilation. Ventilator settings that result in an increase in the patient's PCO_2 relative to premechanical ventilation will produce relative respiratory acidosis even if serum pH remains in the alkalemic range.

In a search of a poison control center database of patients with salicylate poisoning between 2001 and 2007, seven patients were identified with salicylate concentrations above 50 mg/dL who had both premechanical ventilation and postmechanical ventilation data. All seven had postmechanical ventilation pH values below 7.4, and five of the six for whom recorded PCO_2 values were available had postmechanical ventilation PCO_2 values above 50 mm Hg, suggesting substantial hypoventilation. Two of the seven patients died after intubation, and one sustained neurologic injury. Inadequate mechanical ventilation of patients with salicylate poisoning was associated with respiratory acidosis, a decrease in the serum pH, and an abrupt clinical deterioration.[126] Even when achieved, however, respiratory alkalosis sustained by hyperventilation (assisted or unassisted) alone should never be considered a substitute for use of either sodium bicarbonate (to achieve both alkalemia and alkalinuria) or HD (when indicated).

If sedation is required, although there is no clear choice of preferred sedative, the goals are to minimize respiratory depression and use the minimum amount required for desired sedation. If intubation is deemed necessary, which it often is in severe toxicity or multidrug ingestions, the following steps should be taken to optimize before, during, and after intubation conditions. The goal should be to maintain or exceed minute ventilation rates that were present before intubation. Before intubation, an attempt should be made to optimize serum alkalinization by administering a 2-mEq/kg bolus of sodium bicarbonate. Preparations should be made to minimize the time the patient will spend with apnea or decreased ventilation by considering an awake intubation. The provider most experienced in intubation should be present as well as any adjunct materials to increase first-pass success. An intensivist, respiratory technician, or other mechanical ventilator expert should be consulted to help match preintubation minute ventilation. After mechanical ventilation has begun, frequent blood gas monitoring should be obtained and ventilator settings adjusted as needed.[126] One report suggested the use of ketamine for awake intubation, thereby minimizing the hypoventilation associated with rapid-sequence intubation.[39]

If mechanical ventilation has already occurred or is planned in patients with salicylate toxicity, emergent nephrology consult is indicated for HD if not previously obtained.[126] In a retrospective single poison control center investigation of patients[85] in which symptoms, severity, and indications for HD cannot be reliably obtained,[50] patients who had salicylate concentrations above 50 mg/dL and were intubated demonstrated high rates of mortality when no HD was performed; in 56 cases, the overall survival rate was 73.2%, but without HD and a peak salicylate concentration above 50 mg/dL, only 56% survived, and no patients survived without HD when above 80 mg/dL.

Serum Salicylate Concentration and pH Monitoring

Careful observation of the patient, correlation of the serum salicylate concentrations with blood pH, and repeat determinations of serum salicylate concentrations every 2 to 4 hours are essential until the patient is clinically improving and has a low serum salicylate concentration in the presence of a normal or high blood pH. In all cases, after a presumed peak serum salicylate concentration is reached, at least one additional serum concentration should be obtained several hours later. Analyses should be obtained more frequently in managing seriously ill patients to assess the efficacy of treatment and the possible need for HD.

Pediatric Considerations

The predominant primary respiratory alkalosis that initially characterizes salicylate poisoning in adults either does not occur or is often transient in young children.[47,129] This likely results from the limited ventilatory reserve of small children that prevents the same degree of sustained hyperpnea as occurs in adults. The typical acidemia noted in seriously poisoned children led some investigators in the past to incorrectly suggest that pediatric salicylate poisoning produces only metabolic acidosis. Although after a significant salicylate exposure, some children present with a mixed acid–base disturbance and a normal or high pH, most present with acidemia,[47] suggesting the need for more urgent intervention because the protective effect of alkalemia on CNS penetration of salicylate is already lost. Although not routinely recommended, exchange transfusion effectively removes large quantities of salicylate in infants too small to undergo emergent HD without extensive delays.[82]

Pregnancy

Considered a rare event, salicylate poisoning during pregnancy poses a particular hazard to fetuses because of the acid–base and hematologic characteristics of fetuses and placental circulation. Salicylates cross the placenta and are present in higher concentrations in a fetus than in the mother. The respiratory stimulation that occurs in the mother after toxic exposures does not occur in the fetus, which has a decreased capacity to buffer acid. The ability of a fetus to metabolize and excrete salicylates is also less than in the mother. In addition to its toxic effects on the mother, including coagulation abnormalities, acid–base disturbances, tachypnea, and hypoglycemia, repeated exposure to salicylates late in gestation displaces bilirubin from protein binding sites in the fetus, causing kernicterus.

A case report described fetal demise in a woman who claimed to ingest 50 aspirin tablets per day for several weeks during the third trimester of pregnancy. This raises concerns that a fetus is at greater risk from salicylate exposures than is the mother. The need for emergent delivery of near-term fetuses of salicylate-poisoned mothers should be evaluated on a case-by-case basis (Chap. 30).[98]

SUMMARY

- The clinical presentation of a patient with a salicylate overdose is best characterized by an early onset of nausea, vomiting, abdominal pain, tinnitus, and lethargy.
- The combination of a primary respiratory alkalosis and a primary metabolic acidosis with net alkalemia constitutes the classic early acid–base abnormality of salicylate poisoning in the adult.
- Initial efforts in managing patients with salicylate poisoning include restoration of intravascular volume, the provision of dextrose, the use of AC to limit absorption, and urinary alkalinization to enhance renal elimination of salicylate.
- Hemodialysis is indicated in patients with significant salicylate toxicity (eg, altered mental status, ARDS, AKI, or the inability to administer sodium bicarbonate) and significantly elevated salicylate concentrations.
- It is essential to maintain alkalemia to prevent CNS penetration of salicylate. As such, sedation and mechanical ventilation can be rapidly lethal if they impair minute ventilation, causing a rise in PCO_2 and a fall in pH.

Acknowledgment

Neal E. Flomenbaum, MD; Eddy A. Bresnitz, MD; Donald Feinfeld, MD (deceased); and Lorraine Hartnett, MD, contributed to this chapter in previous editions.

REFERENCES

1. Algra AM, Rothwell PM. Effects of regular aspirin on long-term cancer incidence and metastasis: a systematic comparison of evidence from observational studies versus randomized trials. *Lancet Oncol.* 2012;13:518-527.
2. Alvan G, et al. High unbound fraction of salicylate in plasma during intoxication. *Br J Clin Pharmacol.* 1981;11:625-626.
3. American Academy of Clinical Toxicology. Position statement and practice guidelines on the use of multi-dose activated charcoal in the treatment of acute poisoning. American Academy of Clinical Toxicology; European Association of Poisons Centres and Clinical Toxicologists. *J Toxicol Clin Toxicol.* 1999;37:731-751.
4. Anderson RJ, et al. Unrecognized adult salicylate intoxication. *Ann Intern Med.* 1976;85:745-748.
5. Arena FP, et al. Salicylate-induced hypoglycemia and ketoacidosis in a nondiabetic adult. *Arch Intern Med.* 1978;138:1153-1154.
6. Bailey RB, Jones SR. Chronic salicylate intoxication. A common cause of morbidity in the elderly. *J Am Geriatr Soc.* 1989;37:556-561.
7. Barone JA. Evaluation of the effects of multiple-dose activated charcoal on the absorption of orally administered salicylate in a simulated toxic ingestion model. *Ann Emerg Med.* 1988;17:34-37.
8. Bauer S, Darracq MA. Salicylate toxicity in the absence of anion gap metabolic acidosis. *Am J Emerg Med.* 2016;34:1328 e1321-1323.
9. Berkovitch M, et al. False-high blood salicylate levels in neonates with hyperbilirubinemia. *Ther Drug Monit.* 2000;22:757-761.
10. Bertolini A, et al. Dual acting anti-inflammatory drugs: a reappraisal. *Pharmacol Res.* 2001;44:437-450.
11. Bhargava KP, et al. The mechanism of the emetic action of sodium salicylate. *Br J Pharmacol Chemother.* 1963;21:45-50.
12. Borga O, et al. Protein binding of salicylate in uremic and normal plasma. *Clin Pharmacol Ther.* 1976;20:464-475.
13. Brien JA. Ototoxicity associated with salicylates. A brief review. *Drug Saf.* 1993;9:143-148.
14. Broughton A, et al. Bilirubin interference with a salicylate assay performed on an Olympus analyser. *Ann Clin Biochem.* 2000;37(Pt 3):408-410.
15. Brubacher JR, Hoffman RS. Salicylism from topical salicylates: review of the literature. *J Toxicol Clin Toxicol.* 1996;34:431-436.
16. Cazals Y. Auditory sensori-neural alterations induced by salicylate. *Prog Neurobiol.* 2000;62:583-631.
17. Chan TY. Medicated oils and severe salicylate poisoning: quantifying the risk based on methyl salicylate content and bottle size. *Vet Hum Toxicol.* 1996;38:133-134.
18. Chan TY. Potential dangers from topical preparations containing methyl salicylate. *Hum Exp Toxicol.* 1996;15:747-750.
19. Chan TY, et al. The clinical value of screening for salicylates in acute poisoning. *Vet Hum Toxicol.* 1995;37:37-38.
20. Charlton NP, et al. Falsely elevated salicylate levels. *J Med Toxicol.* 2008;4:310-311.
21. Chui PT. Anesthesia in a patient with undiagnosed salicylate poisoning presenting as intraabdominal sepsis. *J Clin Anesth.* 1999;11:251-253.
22. Chyka PA, et al. Salicylate poisoning: an evidence-based consensus guideline for out-of-hospital management. *Clin Toxicol (Phila).* 2007;45:95-131.
23. Cohen DL, et al. Chronic salicylism resulting in noncardiogenic pulmonary edema requiring hemodialysis. *Am J Kidney Dis.* 2000;36:E20.
24. Cotton EK, Fahlberg VI. Hypoglycemia with salicylate poisoning. A report of two cases. *Am J Dis Child.* 1964;108:171-173.
25. D'Agati V. Does aspirin cause acute or chronic renal failure in experimental animals and in humans? *Am J Kidney Dis.* 1996;28:S24-S29.
26. Danon A, et al. Effect of exercise and heat exposure on percutaneous absorption of methyl salicylate. *Eur J Clin Pharmacol.* 1986;31:49-52.
27. Davison C. Salicylate metabolism in man. *Ann N Y Acad Sci.* 1971;179:249-268.
28. De Broe ME, et al. Clinical experience with prolonged combined hemoperfusion-hemodialysis treatment of severe poisoning. *Artif Organs.* 1981;5:59-66.
29. Done AK. Salicylate intoxication. Significance of measurements of salicylate in blood in cases of acute ingestion. *Pediatrics.* 1960;26:800-807.
30. Done AK, Temple AR. Treatment of salicylate poisoning. *Mod Treat.* 1971;8: 528-551.
31. Duffens KR, et al. Falsely elevated salicylate levels due to diflunisal overdose. *J Emerg Med.* 1987;5:499-503.
32. Dulaney A, Kerns W. Delayed peak salicylate level following intentional overdose. *Clin Toxicol.* 2010;48:610.
33. Durnas C, Cusack BJ. Salicylate intoxication in the elderly. Recognition and recommendations on how to prevent it. *Drugs Aging.* 1992;2:20-34.
34. Ekstrand R, et al. Concentration dependent plasma protein binding of salicylate in rheumatoid patients. *Clin Pharmacokinet.* 1979;4:137-143.
35. Elko C, Von Derau K. Salicylate undetected for 8 hours after enteric-coated aspirin overdose. *Clin Toxicol.* 2001;39:482-483.
36. Emkey RD. Aspirin and renal disease. *Am J Med.* 1983;74:97-9101.
37. English M, et al. Chronic salicylate poisoning and severe malaria. *Lancet.* 1996;347:1736-1737.
38. Escoubet B, et al. Prostaglandin synthesis by the cochlea of the guinea pig. Influence of aspirin, gentamicin, and acoustic stimulation. *Prostaglandins.* 1985;29:589-599.
39. Farmer BF, et al. Ketamine and midazolam for procedural sedation prevents respiratory depression in life-threatening aspirin toxicity. *Clin Toxicol.* 2013;51:367-368.
40. Feldman S, et al. Salicylate absorption from a bismuth subsalicylate preparation. *Clin Pharmacol Ther.* 1981;29:788-792.
41. Fertel BS, et al. The underutilization of hemodialysis in patients with salicylate poisoning. *Kidney Int.* 2009;75:1349-1353.
42. Feuerstein RC, et al. The use of acetazolamide in the therapy of salicylate poisoning. *Pediatrics.* 1960;25:215-227.
43. Filippone GA, et al. Reversible adsorption (desorption) of aspirin from activated charcoal. *Arch Intern Med.* 1987;147:1390-1392.
44. Fox GN. Hypocalcemia complicating bicarbonate therapy for salicylate poisoning. *West J Med.* 1984;141:108-109.
45. Frischtak HL, et al. Clinical characteristics of fatal salicylate poisonings. *Clin Toxicol.* 2015;53:236.

46. Gabow PA, et al. Acid-base disturbances in the salicylate-intoxicated adult. *Arch Intern Med.* 1978;138:1481-1484.

47. Gaudreault P, et al. The relative severity of acute versus chronic salicylate poisoning in children: a clinical comparison. *Pediatrics.* 1982;70:566-569.

48. Glasgow JF. Reye's syndrome: the case for a causal link with aspirin. *Drug Saf.* 2006;29:1111-1121.

49. Goldberg MA, et al. The effects of carbon dioxide on the entry and accumulation of drugs in the central nervous system. *J Pharmacol Exp Ther.* 1961;131:308-318.

50. Gosselin S, et al. Intubation and salicylate overdose. *Am J Emerg Med.* 2017;35:1193.

51. Graham CA, et al. Paracetamol and salicylate testing: routinely required for all over-dose patients? *Eur J Emerg Med.* 2006;13:26-28.

52. Hahn IH, et al. Errors in reporting salicylate levels. *Acad Emerg Med.* 2000;7:1336-1337.

53. Halla JT, et al. Symptomatic salicylate ototoxicity: a useful indicator of serum salicylate concentration? *Ann Rheum Dis.* 1991;50:682-684.

54. Heffner JE, Sahn SA. Salicylate-induced pulmonary edema. Clinical features and prognosis. *Ann Intern Med.* 1981;95:405-409.

55. Heller I, et al. Significant metabolic acidosis induced by acetazolamide. Not a rare complication. *Arch Intern Med.* 1985;145:1815-1817.

56. Hill JB. Experimental salicylate poisoning: observations on the effects of altering blood pH on tissue and plasma salicylate concentrations. *Pediatrics.* 1971;47:658-665.

57. Hill JB. Salicylate intoxication. *N Engl J Med.* 1973;288:1110-1113.

58. Hillman RJ, Prescott LF. Treatment of salicylate poisoning with repeated oral charcoal. *Br Med J (Clin Res Ed).* 1985;291:1472.

59. Hogben CA, et al. Absorption of drugs from the stomach. II. The human. *J Pharmacol Exp Ther.* 1957;120:540-545.

60. Hormaechea E, et al. Hypovolemia, pulmonary edema and protein changes in severe salicylate poisoning. *Am J Med.* 1979;66:1046-1050.

61. Hrnicek G, et al. Pulmonary edema and salicylate intoxication. *JAMA.* 1974;230:866-867.

62. Jacob J, Lavonas EJ. Falsely normal anion gap in severe salicylate poisoning caused by laboratory interference. *Ann Emerg Med.* 2011;58:280-281.

63. Johnson D, et al. Effect of multiple-dose activated charcoal on the clearance of high-dose intravenous aspirin in a porcine model. *Ann Emerg Med.* 1995;26:569-574.

64. Jung TT, et al. Ototoxicity of salicylate, nonsteroidal antiinflammatory drugs, and quinine. *Otolaryngol Clin North Am.* 1993;26:791-810.

65. Juurlink DN, et al. Extracorporeal treatment for salicylate poisoning: systematic review and recommendations from the EXTRIP Workgroup. *Ann Emerg Med.* 2015;66:165-181.

66. Kallen RJ, et al. Hemodialysis in children: technique, kinetic aspects related to varying body size, and application to salicylate intoxication, acute renal failure and some other disorders. *Medicine (Baltimore).* 1966;45:1-50.

67. Kaplan EH, et al. Effects of salicylate and other benzoates on oxidative enzymes of the tricarboxylic acid cycle in rat tissue homogenates. *Arch Biochem Biophys.* 1954;51:47-61.

68. Karliner JS. Noncardiogenic forms of pulmonary edema. *Circulation.* 1972;46:212-215.

69. Karsh J. Adverse reactions and interactions with aspirin. Considerations in the treatment of the elderly patient. *Drug Saf.* 1990;5:317-327.

70. Kaul V, et al. Negative anion gap metabolic acidosis in salicylate overdose—a zebra! *Am J Emerg Med.* 2013;31:1536 e1533-1534.

71. Keller RE, et al. Contribution of sorbitol combined with activated charcoal in prevention of salicylate absorption. *Ann Emerg Med.* 1990;19:654-656.

72. Kirshenbaum LA, et al. Does multiple-dose charcoal therapy enhance salicylate excretion? *Arch Intern Med.* 1990;150:1281-1283.

73. Krebs HG, et al. Hyperlactatemia and lactic acidosis. *Essays Med Biochem.* 1975;1:81-103.

74. Kuzak N, et al. Reversal of salicylate-induced euglycemic delirium with dextrose. *Clin Toxicol (Phila).* 2007;45:526-529.

75. Lawson AA, et al. Forced diuresis in the treatment of acute salicylate poisoning in adults. *Q J Med.* 1969;38:31-48.

76. Lemesh RA. Accidental chronic salicylate intoxication in an elderly patient: major morbidity despite early recognition. *Vet Hum Toxicol.* 1993;35:34-36.

77. Leventhal LJ, et al. Salicylate-induced rhabdomyolysis. *Am J Emerg Med.* 1989;7:409-410.

78. Levy G. Clinical pharmacokinetics of aspirin. *Pediatrics.* 1978;62(5 Pt 2 suppl):867-872.

79. Levy G. Pharmacokinetics of salicylate elimination in man. *J Pharm Sci.* 1965;54:959-967.

80. Levy G, Tsuchiya T. Effect of activated charcoal on aspirin absorption in man. Part I. *Clin Pharmacol Ther.* 1972;13:317-322.

81. Lund B, et al. Efficacy of sustained low-efficiency dialysis in the treatment of salicylate toxicity. *Nephrol Dial Transplant.* 2005;20(7):1483-1484.

82. Manikian A, et al. Exchange transfusion in severe infant salicylism. *Vet Hum Toxicol.* 2002;44:224-227.

83. Mascheroni D, et al. Acute respiratory failure following pharmacologically induced hyperventilation: an experimental animal study. *Intensive Care Med.* 1988;15:8-14.

84. Mayer AL, et al. Multiple-dose charcoal and whole-bowel irrigation do not increase clearance of absorbed salicylate. *Arch Intern Med.* 1992;152:393-396.

85. McCabe DJ, Lu JJ. The association of hemodialysis and survival in intubated salicylate-poisoned patients. *Am J Emerg Med.* 2017;35:899-903.

86. McGuigan MA. A two-year review of salicylate deaths in Ontario. *Arch Intern Med.* 1987;147:510-512.

87. McQueen DS, et al. Arterial chemoreceptor involvement in salicylate-induced hyperventilation in rats. *Br J Pharmacol.* 1989;98:413-424.

88. Minns AB, et al. Death due to acute salicylate intoxication despite dialysis. *J Emerg Med.* 2011;40:515-517.

89. Miyahara JT, Karler R. Effect of salicylate on oxidative phosphorylation and respiration of mitochondrial fragments. *Biochem J.* 1965;97:194-198.

90. Montgomery H, et al. Salicylate intoxication causing a severe systemic inflammatory response and rhabdomyolysis. *Am J Emerg Med.* 1994;12:531-532.

91. Montgomery PR, et al. Salicylate metabolism: effects of age and sex in adults. *Clin Pharmacol Ther.* 1986;39:571-576.

92. Morgan AG, Polak A. The excretion of salicylate in salicylate poisoning. *Clin Sci.* 1971;41:475-484.

93. Mowry JB, et al. 2015 Annual Report of the American Association of Poison Control Centers' National Poison Data System (NPDS): 33rd Annual Report. *Clin Toxicol (Phila).* 2016;54:924-1109.

94. Myers EN, et al. Salicylate ototoxicity: a clinical study. *N Engl J Med.* 1965;273:587-590.

95. Needs CJ, Brooks PM. Clinical pharmacokinetics of the salicylates. *Clin Pharmacokinet.* 1985;10:164-177.

96. Neuvonen PJ, et al. Reduction of absorption of digoxin, phenytoin and aspirin by activated charcoal in man. *Eur J Clin Pharmacol.* 1978;13:213-218.

97. Niehoff JM, Baltatzis PA. Adult respiratory distress syndrome induced by salicylate toxicity. *Postgrad Med.* 1985;78:117-119, 123.

98. Palatnick W, Tenenbein M. Aspirin poisoning during pregnancy: increased fetal sensitivity. *Am J Perinatol.* 1998;15:39-41.

99. Park BK, Leck JB. On the mechanism of salicylate-induced hypothrombinaemia. *J Pharm Pharmacol.* 1981;33:25-28.

100. Patrono C, et al. Antiplatelet drugs: American College of Chest Physicians Evidence-Based Clinical Practice Guidelines (8th Edition). *Chest.* 2008;133:233.

101. Penniall R. The effects of salicylic acid on the respiratory activity of mitochondria. *Biochim Biophys Acta.* 1958;30:247-251.

102. Phillips BM, et al. Does aspirin play a role in analgesic nephropathy? *Aust N Z J Med.* 1976;6(suppl 1):48-53.

103. Pillar G, et al. Amelioration of sleep apnea by salicylate-induced hyperventilation. *Am Rev Respir Dis.* 1992;146:711-715.

104. Prescott LF, et al. Diuresis or urinary alkalinisation for salicylate poisoning? *Br Med J (Clin Res Ed).* 1982;285:1383-1386.

105. Proudfoot AT, Brown SS. Acidaemia and salicylate poisoning in adults. *Br Med J.* 1969;2:547-550.

106. Proudfoot AT, et al. Position paper on urine alkalinization. *J Toxicol Clin Toxicol.* 2004;42:1-26.

107. Puel J-L, Guitton MJ. Salicylate-induced tinnitus: molecular mechanisms and modulation by anxiety. *Prog Brain Res.* 2007;166:141-146.

108. Puel JL. Cochlear NMDA receptor blockade prevents salicylate-induced tinnitus. *B-ENT.* 2007;3(suppl 7):19-22.

109. Ramsden RT, et al. Electrocochleographic changes in acute salicylate overdosage. *J Laryngol Otol.* 1985;99:1269-1273.

110. Rao P, Knaus EE. Evolution of nonsteroidal anti-inflammatory drugs (NSAIDs): cyclooxygenase (COX) inhibition and beyond. *J Pharm Pharm Sci.* 2008;11:81s-110s.

111. Rao RB. Paratonia (rapid rigor mortis) in salicylate (ASA) poisoning. *Clin Toxicol.* 1999;37:605-606.

112. Raschke R, et al. Refractory hypoglycemia secondary to topical salicylate intoxication. *Arch Intern Med.* 1991;151:591-593.

113. Rauschka H, et al. Acute cerebral white matter damage in lethal salicylate intoxication. *Neurotoxicology.* 2007;28:33-37.

114. Reed CR, Glauser FL. Drug-induced noncardiogenic pulmonary edema. *Chest.* 1991;100:1120-1124.

115. Rivera W, et al. Delayed salicylate toxicity at 35 hours without early manifestations following a single salicylate ingestion. *Ann Pharmacother.* 2004;38:1186-1188.

116. Roberts LJ, Morrow JD. Analgesic-antipyretic and antiinflammatory agents and drugs emplyoed in the treatment of gout. In: Goodman LS, et al, eds: *Goodman & Gilman's the Pharmacological Basis of Therapeutics.* 10th ed. New York, NY: McGraw-Hill; 2001:687-731.

117. Roberts MS, et al. Implications of hepatic and extrahepatic metabolism of aspirin in selective inhibition of platelet cyclooxygenase. *N Engl J Med.* 1985;312:1388-1389.

118. Romankiewicz JA, Reidenberg MM. Factors that modify drug absorption. *Ration Drug Ther.* 1978;12:1-5.

119. Roncaglioni MC, et al. The vitamin K-antagonism of salicylate and warfarin. *Thromb Res.* 1986;42:727-736.

120. Rose SR, et al. Absorption of salicylate powders versus tablets following overdose: a poison center observational study. *Clin Toxicol (Phila).* 2016;54:857-861.

121. Ruel J, et al. Salicylate enables cochlear arachidonic-acid-sensitive NMDA receptor responses. *J Neurosci.* 2008;28:7313-7323.

122. Salhanick S, et al. Aspirin bezoar proven by upper endoscopy. *Clin Toxicol.* 2002;40:688.

123. Shively RM, et al. Acute salicylate poisoning: risk factors for severe outcome. *Clin Toxicol (Phila).* 2017;55:175-180.

124. Sporer KA, Khayam-Bashi H. Acetaminophen and salicylate serum levels in patients with suicidal ingestion or altered mental status. *Am J Emerg Med.* 1996;14(5):443-446.

125. Sproull DH. The glycogenolytic action of sodium salicylate. *Br J Pharmacol Chemother.* 1954;9:121-124.

126. Stolbach AI, et al. Mechanical ventilation was associated with acidemia in a case series of salicylate-poisoned patients. *Acad Emerg Med*. 2008;15:866-869.

127. Swintosky JV. Illustrations and pharmaceutical interpretations of first order drug elimination rate from the bloodstream. *J Am Pharm Assoc Am Pharm Assoc*. 1956;45:395-400.

128. Szucs PA, et al. Pseudosalicylate poisoning: falsely elevated salicylate levels in an overdose of diflunisal. *Am J Emerg Med*. 2000;18:641-642.

129. Temple AR. Acute and chronic effects of aspirin toxicity and their treatment. *Arch Intern Med*. 1981;141:364-369.

130. Temple AR, et al. Salicylate poisoning complicated by fluid retention. *Clin Toxicol*. 1976;9:61-68.

131. Tenenbein M. Whole bowel irrigation as gastrointestinal decontamination procedure after acute poisoning. *Med Toxicol Adverse Drug Exp*. 1988;3:77-84.

132. Thisted B, et al. Acute salicylate self-poisoning in 177 consecutive patients treated in ICU. *Acta Anaesthesiol Scand*. 1987;31:312-316.

133. Thompson TM, et al. Salicylate toxicity from genital exposure to a methylsalicylate-containing rubefacient. *West J Emerg Med*. 2016;17:181-183.

134. Thurston JH, et al. Reduced brain glucose with normal plasma glucose in salicylate poisoning. *J Clin Invest*. 1970;49:2139-2145.

135. Tsimihodimos V, et al. Salicylate-induced proximal tubular dysfunction. *Am J Kidney Dis*. 2007;50:463-467.

136. Vane JR, Botting RM. The mechanism of action of aspirin. *Thromb Res*. 2003;110:255-258.

137. Vazquez Martinez JL, et al. Unrecognized Transcutaneous Severe Salicylate Intoxication in an Infant. *Pediatr Emerg Care*. 2015;31:e8.

138. Vernace MA, et al. Chronic salicylate toxicity due to consumption of over-the-counter bismuth subsalicylate. *Am J Med*. 1994;97:308-309.

139. Vertrees JE, et al. Repeated oral administration of activated charcoal for treating aspirin overdose in young children. *Pediatrics*. 1990;85:594-598.

140. Vree TB, et al. Effect of urinary pH on the pharmacokinetics of salicylic acid, with its glycine and glucuronide conjugates in human. *Int J Clin Pharmacol Ther*. 1994;32:550-558.

141. Walters JS, et al. Salicylate-induced pulmonary edema. *Radiology*. 1983;146:289-293.

142. Watanabe T. Normal anion gap metabolic acidosis in salicylate overdose. *Am J Emerg Med*. 2016;34:2457-2458.

143. Wolowich WR, et al. Plasma salicylate from methyl salicylate cream compared to oil of wintergreen. *J Toxicol Clin Toxicol*. 2003;41:355-358.

144. Wood DM, et al. Measuring plasma salicylate concentrations in all patients with drug overdose or altered consciousness: is it necessary? *Emerg Med J*. 2005;22:401-403.

145. Wortzman DJ, Grunfeld A. Delayed absorption following enteric-coated aspirin overdose. *Ann Emerg Med*. 1987;16:434-436.

146. Wrathall G, et al. Three case reports of the use of haemodiafiltration in the treatment of salicylate overdose. *Hum Exp Toxicol*. 2001;20:491-495.

147. Yip L, Dart et al. Concepts and controversies in salicylate toxicity. *Emerg Med Clin North Am*. 1994;12:351-364.

148. Zimmerman HJ. Effects of aspirin and acetaminophen on the liver. *Arch Intern Med*. 1981;141(3 Spec No):333-342.

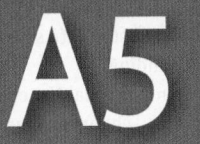

Antidotes in Depth

A5

SODIUM BICARBONATE

Paul M. Wax and Ashley Haynes

INTRODUCTION

Sodium bicarbonate is a nonspecific antidote that is effective in the treatment of a variety of poisonings by means of a number of distinct mechanisms (Table A5–1). However, the support for its use in these settings is predominantly based on animal evidence, case reports, and consensus.[13] It is most commonly used in toxicology as a treatment for patients with cyclic antidepressant (CA) and salicylate poisonings. Sodium bicarbonate also has a role in the treatment of phenobarbital, chlorpropamide, and chlorophenoxy herbicide poisonings and wide-complex tachydysrhythmias induced by Na^+ channel blocking type IA and IC antidysrhythmics and cocaine. Correcting the life-threatening acidemia induced by cyanide, methanol, and ethylene glycol metabolism and enhancing formate elimination are other important indications for sodium bicarbonate.

PHARMACOLOGY

Sodium bicarbonate has a molecular weight of 84 Da. It is supplied in solution at approximately pH 8.0 (pH limits range from 7.0 to 8.5). The onset of action of intravenous (IV) sodium bicarbonate is rapid with a duration of action of 8 to 10 minutes.[3] Sodium bicarbonate increases plasma bicarbonate and buffers excess hydrogen ion.[35] In normal individuals, the distribution volume for bicarbonate salts is approximately twice the extracellular fluid (ECF) volume.[46,103] The apparent bicarbonate space (ABS) proportionally increases in severe acidemia, leading to higher bicarbonate requirements.[41] Canine studies demonstrated that this effect is not due to the acidemia per se but due to the tight correlation of extracellular bicarbonate concentrations with the ABS.[1] Low bicarbonate concentrations increase the apparent volume of distribution in a highly dynamic manner.[1] Human studies, in which the ABS is described by the equation $ABS = (0.36 + 2.44/[HCO_3^-]) \times$ weight (kg) appear to support this concept.[90]

ALTERED INTERACTION BETWEEN XENOBIOTIC AND SODIUM CHANNEL

The most important role of sodium bicarbonate in toxicology is the ability to reverse potentially fatal cardiotoxic effects of myocardial Na^+ channel blockers such as CAs and other type IA and IC antidysrhythmics.[19] Its mechanism of action in these cases results from both an increase in $[Na^+]$ and a change in the proportion of the Na^+ channel blocker that is ionized, resulting in an altered distribution away from its channel.[95] Use of sodium bicarbonate for myocardial Na^+ channel blocker overdose developed as an extension of sodium lactate use in the treatment of patients with toxicity from type IA antidysrhythmics. Noting similarities in electrocardiographic (ECG) findings between hyperkalemia and quinidine toxicity (ie, QRS widening), investigators in the 1950s began to use sodium lactate (which is rapidly metabolized in the liver to sodium bicarbonate) to treat quinidine and procainamide toxicity.[6,12,111] In a canine model, quinidine-induced ECG changes and hypotension were consistently reversed by infusion of sodium lactate.[11] Clinical experience confirmed this benefit.[12] Similar efficacy in the treatment of patients with procainamide cardiotoxicity was also reported.[111]

The introduction of CAs during the 1960s yielded reports of conduction disturbances, dysrhythmias, and hypotension occurring in overdose. Extending the use of sodium lactate for the type I antidysrhythmics to CA poisoning, uncontrolled observations in the 1970s showed a decrease in mortality rate from 15% to less than 3%.[42] In 1976, sodium bicarbonate was successful in a pediatric series of CA-induced dysrhythmias.[20] In this series, 9 of 12 children who developed multifocal premature ventricular contractions, ventricular tachycardia, or heart block reverted to normal sinus rhythm with sodium bicarbonate therapy alone. An early canine experiment of amitriptyline-poisoning demonstrated resolution of dysrhythmias upon blood alkalinization to a blood pH above 7.40.[20]

An improved understanding of the mechanism and utility of sodium bicarbonate came from a series of animal experiments during the 1980s. In amitriptyline-poisoned dogs, sodium bicarbonate reversed conduction disturbances and ventricular dysrhythmias and suppressed ventricular ectopy.[74] When comparing sodium bicarbonate, respiratory alkalemia (hyperventilation), hypertonic (3%) sodium chloride, and lidocaine, both sodium bicarbonate and hyperventilation proved most efficacious in reversing ventricular dysrhythmias and narrowing QRS prolongation.

In desipramine-poisoned rats, the isolated use of either hypertonic sodium chloride or sodium bicarbonate was effective in decreasing QRS duration.[80] Both sodium bicarbonate and hypertonic sodium chloride also increased mean arterial pressure, but hyperventilation or direct intravascular volume repletion with mannitol did not. In further studies both in vivo and on isolated cardiac tissue, alkalinization and increased sodium concentration improved CA effects on cardiac conduction.[95,96] Although respiratory alkalemia and hypertonic sodium chloride each independently improved conduction velocity, this effect was greatest when sodium bicarbonate was administered.

Another study on amitriptyline-poisoned rats demonstrated that treatment with hypertonic sodium bicarbonate was associated with shorter QRS interval, longer duration of sinus rhythm, and increased survival rates.[57] Sodium bicarbonate works independently of initial blood pH. Animal studies show that cardiac conduction improves after treatment with sodium bicarbonate or hypertonic sodium chloride in both normal and acidemic animals.[80] Clinically, CA-poisoned patients who were already alkalemic responded to repeat doses of sodium bicarbonate.[71]

Although several authors suggested that the efficacy of sodium bicarbonate is modulated via a pH-dependent change in plasma protein binding that decreases the proportion of free drug,[21,62] further study failed to support this hypothesis.[83] The administration of large doses of a binding protein α_1-acid glycoprotein (AAG) (to which CAs show significant affinity) to desipramine-poisoned rats only minimally decreased cardiotoxicity. Although the addition of AAG increased the concentrations of total desipramine and protein-bound desipramine in the serum, the concentration of active free desipramine did not decline significantly. A redistribution of CA from peripheral sites prevented lowering of free desipramine concentration.[83] The persistence of other CA-associated toxicities, antimuscarinic effects and seizures, also argues against changes in protein-binding modulating toxicity. In vitro

TABLE A5–1	Sodium Bicarbonate: Mechanisms, Site of Action, and Uses in Toxicology	
Mechanism	**Site of Action**	**Uses**
Alters interaction between the xenobiotic and Na⁺ channel	Heart	β-Adrenergic antagonists with MSA
		Amantadine
		Bupropion
		Carbamazepine
		Chloroquine
		Citalopram
		Cocaine
		Cyclic antidepressants
		Dimenhydrinate
		Diphenhydramine
		Disopyramide
		Encainide
		Flecainide
		Fluoxetine
		Hydroxychloroquine
		Lamotrigine
		Mesoridazine
		Orphenadrine
		Procainamide
		Propafenone
		Propoxyphene
		Quinidine
		Quinine
		Thioridazine
		Venlafaxine
Alters xenobiotic ionization leading to altered tissue distribution	Retina	Formic acid
	Brain	Phenobarbital
		Salicylates
Alters xenobiotic ionization leading to enhanced xenobiotic elimination	Kidneys	Chlorophenoxy herbicides
		Chlorpropamide
		Diflunisal
		Fluoride
		Formic acid
		Methotrexate
		Phenobarbital
		Salicylates
		Uranium
Corrects life-threatening acidemia	Metabolic	Cyanide
		Ethylene glycol
		Metformin
		Methanol
Increases xenobiotic solubility	Kidneys	DAMPA
		Methotrexate
Neutralization	Lungs	Chlorine gas, HCl
Maintenance of chelator effect	Kidneys	Dimercaprol (BAL)–metal
Prevents ferrihemate release from myoglobin	Kidneys	Drug-induced rhabdomyolysis
Shifts potassium into cells		Drug-induced hyperkalemia

BAL = British anti-Lewisite; DAMPA = methotrexate metabolite 4-amino-4-deoxy-10-methylpteroic acid; MSA = membrane-stabilizing activity acebutolol, betaxolol, carvedilol, metoprolol, oxprenolol, propranolol.

studies performed in plasma protein-free bath further substantiate sodium bicarbonate's efficacy independent of plasma protein binding.[95]

Sodium bicarbonate has a crucial antidotal role in myocardial Na⁺ channel blocker poisoning by increasing the number of open Na⁺ channels, thereby partially reversing fast Na⁺ channel blockade. This decreases QRS prolongation and reduces life-threatening cardiovascular toxicity such as ventricular dysrhythmias and hypotension.[74,80,95] The animal evidence supports two distinct and additive mechanisms for this effect: a pH-dependent effect and a sodium-dependent effect. The pH-dependent effect increases the fraction of the more freely diffusible nonionized xenobiotic. Both the ionized xenobiotic and the nonionized forms are able to bind to the Na⁺ channel, but assuming myocardial Na⁺ channel blockers act like local anesthetics, it is estimated that 90% of the block results from the ionized form. Increase the nonionized fraction limits the quantity of xenobiotic available to bind to the Na⁺ channel. The sodium-dependent effect increases the availability of Na⁺ ions to pass through the open channels. Decreased ionization should not significantly decrease the rate of CA elimination because of the small contribution of renal pathways to overall CA elimination (<5%). Sodium displaces flecainide and likely other Na⁺ channel blocking drugs from the channel itself.[88]

Although anecdotal accounts support the efficacy of sodium bicarbonate in treating CA cardiotoxicity in humans,[50] these reports are uncontrolled observations; controlled studies are unavailable. In one of the largest retrospective observational studies involving 91 patients who received sodium bicarbonate after CA overdose, QRS complex widening corrected in 39 of 49 patients who had QRS durations above 120 ms, and hypotension corrected within 1 hour in 20 of 21 patients who had systolic blood pressures below 90 mm Hg.[51] Use of sodium bicarbonate was not associated with any complications in this study.

Prospective validation of treatment criteria for use of sodium bicarbonate after CA overdose have not been performed. Recommended indications are conduction delays (QRS complex duration above 100 ms or a right bundle branch block), wide-complex tachydysrhythmias, and hypotension.[63] Because studies demonstrate a critical threshold QRS complex duration (160 ms or greater) at which ventricular dysrhythmias significantly increase in propensity,[16] it seems reasonable that narrowing the QRS complex duration through use of sodium bicarbonate or hyperventilation prevents the development of dysrhythmias. Practice patterns vary considerably with regard to the use of sodium bicarbonate when the QRS complex duration is below 160 ms.[100] Although sodium bicarbonate has no proven efficacy in either the treatment or prophylaxis of CA-induced seizures, seizures often produce acidemia, which rapidly increases the risks of conduction disturbances and ventricular dysrhythmias.[107] Administering sodium bicarbonate when the QRS complex duration is 100 ms or greater establishes a theoretical margin of safety in the event the patient suddenly deteriorates without adding significant demonstrable risk. When the QRS complex duration is below 100 ms, given the minimal risk of seizures or dysrhythmias, we recommend not to administer prophylactic sodium bicarbonate.[101] In patients exhibiting a type I Brugada ECG pattern (right bundle branch block with downsloping ST segment elevation in V1–V3) and QRS complex widening after CA ingestion, sodium bicarbonate administration narrows the QRS complex. Depending on the nature of the patient's intrinsic channel and degree of acquired channelopathy, the unmasked Brugada pattern may or may not reverse (Chap. 15).[9,56,65]

Because cardiotoxicity often worsens during the first few hours after ingestion, we recommend sodium bicarbonate therapy be initiated immediately if the QRS interval is greater than 100 ms. Because CA-induced hypotension responds to sodium bicarbonate, we recommend hypotension be treated with prompt sodium bicarbonate therapy. In CA-poisoned patients who present with altered mental status or seizures without QRS complex widening or hypotension, we recommend not to give sodium bicarbonate.

Because the potential benefits of alkalinization in CA overdose usually outweigh the risks, we recommend sodium bicarbonate be administered regardless of whether the patient has an acidemic or normal pH.

The time to resolution of conduction abnormalities during continuous bicarbonate infusion varies significantly, ranging from several hours to several days.[64,101] Potential ongoing or delayed absorption because of antimuscarinic CA properties, CA pharmacologic preparations, coingestants, and other factors may play into this. In a case of poisoning from modified-release amitriptyline, sodium bicarbonate was required on multiple occasions over 110 hours after the initial ingestion to reverse ongoing Na^+ channel conduction disturbances.[75] It is reasonable to discontinue sodium bicarbonate infusion upon hemodynamic improvement and resolution of cardiac conduction abnormalities and altered mental status, although controlled data supporting such an approach are lacking.

Sodium bicarbonate is useful in treating patients with cardiotoxicity from other myocardial Na^+ channel blockers that present with widened QRS complexes, dysrhythmias, and hypotension. Isolated case reports provide the bulk of the evidence in these situations. The utility of sodium bicarbonate in treating patients with type IA and IC antidysrhythmics, diphenhydramine, quinine, cocaine, and others is demonstrated.[15,30,33,91,93,102,111]

Use of sodium bicarbonate in the treatment of patients with overdoses of amantadine, a xenobiotic with multiple myocardial channel effects, was suggested, but concurrent hypokalemia limits its use.[98] Although the usefulness of sodium bicarbonate in reversing QRS complex widening is occasionally observed during fluoxetine and citalopram overdose,[22,34,43] Na^+ channel disturbances are uncommon in most cases of selective serotonin reuptake inhibitor (SSRI) overdose. Routine use of alkalinization therapy in SSRI toxicity is not recommended, as it might risk worsening QT interval prolongation by promoting hypokalemia. It is reasonable to administer sodium bicarbonate in the management of patients with other ingestions associated with type IA–like cardiac conduction abnormalities and dysrhythmias, such as carbamazepine, lamotrigine, and the phenothiazines thioridazine and mesoridazine.[47] Case reports regarding bupropion toxicity have been mixed, with some demonstrating no response to sodium bicarbonate,[2,32,112] but others support its use.[38] The reported lack of efficacy of sodium bicarbonate in reversing QRS complex prolongation caused by bupropion poisoning is due to prolongation of QRS complex by an alternate mechanism.[112] Bupropion contributes to QRS prolongation because of reduction of cardiac intercellular coupling (ie, inhibition of gap junction communication), as opposed to Na^+ channel blockade.[25] Given that the potential benefit may outweigh the risks, it is reasonable to use sodium bicarbonate in the setting of bupropion toxicity.

Cocaine, a local anesthetic with membrane-stabilizing properties resembling other type I antidysrhythmics, causes similar conduction disturbances. In several canine models of cocaine toxicity, sodium bicarbonate successfully reversed cocaine-induced QRS complex prolongation[10,78] and improved myocardial function.[113] Of interest, sodium loading by itself failed to produce a benefit. Similar findings were demonstrated in cocaine-treated guinea pig hearts.[114] Patients with cocaine-induced cardiotoxicity responded to treatment with sodium bicarbonate.[55,77,110] In many of these cases, simultaneous treatment with sedation, active cooling, and hyperventilation confounds the interpretation of the benefit of sodium bicarbonate; however, given its mechanism of action, we recommend its use.

ALTERED XENOBIOTIC IONIZATION TO ALTER DISTRIBUTION AND ENHANCE ELIMINATION

Salicylates

Although there is no known specific antidote, judicious sodium bicarbonate use is recommended in the treatment of salicylate toxicity. Through its ability to alter the concentration gradient of the ionized and nonionized fractions of salicylates, sodium bicarbonate decreases tissue (eg, CNS) concentrations of salicylates and enhances urinary elimination of salicylates.[86]

Salicylate is a weak acid with a pK_a of 3.0. As pH increases, the ionized proportion increases. Because of the presence of polar groups, ionized molecules penetrate lipid-soluble membranes less efficiently than do nonionized molecules. Consequently, when the ionized forms predominate, weak

acids such as salicylates accumulate in an alkaline milieu, such as an alkaline urine (Fig. 37-2).[68,105]

Although alkalinizing the urine to increase salicylate elimination is an important intervention in the treatment of patients with salicylate poisoning, increasing the serum pH in patients with severe salicylism proves even more consequential by protecting the brain from a lethal central nervous system (CNS) salicylate burden. In these patients, using sodium bicarbonate to "trap" salicylate in the blood by keeping it out of the brain decreases the likelihood of clinical deterioration. Salicylate lethality is directly related to primary CNS dysfunction, which in turn corresponds to a "critical brain salicylate concentration."[49] At physiologic pH, at which a very small proportion of the salicylate is in the nonionized form, a small change in pH is associated with a significant change in amount of nonionized molecules. For example, whereas at a pH of 7.40, 0.004% of the salicylate molecules are in the nonionized form, at a pH of 7.20, 0.008%, of the salicylate is in the nonionized form. In experimental models, lowering the blood pH produced a shift of salicylate into the tissues.[23] Hence, acidemia in patients with significant salicylate poisonings is devastating. In salicylate-poisoned rats, increasing the blood pH with sodium bicarbonate produced a shift in salicylate out of the tissues and into the blood.[48] This change in salicylate distribution did not result from enhanced urinary excretion because occlusion of the renal pedicles failed to alter these results.

Enhancing the elimination of salicylate by trapping ionized salicylate in the urine is also beneficial. Salicylate elimination at therapeutic concentrations is predominantly through first-order hepatic metabolism. At these low concentrations, without alkalinization, only approximately 10% to 20% of salicylate is eliminated unchanged in the urine. With increasing concentrations, enzyme saturation occurs (Michaelis-Menten kinetics); thus, a larger percentage of elimination occurs as unchanged free salicylate. Under these conditions, in an alkaline urine, urinary excretion of free salicylate becomes even more significant, accounting for 60% to 85% of total elimination.[44,89] The relationship between salicylate clearance and urine pH—log(Salicylate clearance) = [(0.52 × pH) – 2.1][54]—would suggest that increasing urine pH from 5.0 to 8.0 could increase the amount of salicylate cleared by almost 40-fold.

The exact mechanism of pH-dependent salicylate elimination has generated controversy. The pH-dependent increase in urinary elimination initially was ascribed to "ion trapping," which is the filtering of both ionized and nonionized salicylate while reabsorbing only the nonionized salicylate.[99] However, limiting reabsorption of the ionizable fraction of filtered salicylate cannot be the primary mechanism responsible for enhanced elimination produced by sodium bicarbonate.[66] Because the quantitative difference between the percentage of molecules trapped in the ionized form at a pH of 5.0 (99% ionized) and a pH of 8.0 (99.999% ionized) is small, decreases in tubular reabsorption cannot fully explain the rapid increase in urinary elimination seen at a pH above 7.0.

"Diffusion theory" offers a reasonable alternative explanation. Fick's law of diffusion states that the rate of flow of a diffusing substance is proportional to its concentration gradient. At a higher urinary pH, a greater proportion of secreted nonionized molecules quickly becomes ionized upon entering the alkaline environment, and more salicylate (ie, nonionized salicylate) must pass from the peritubular fluid into the urine in an attempt to reach equilibrium with the nonionized fraction. In fact, as long as nonionized molecules are rapidly converted to ionized molecules in the urine, equilibrium in the alkaline milieu will never be achieved. The concentration gradient of peritubular nonionized salicylates to urinary nonionized salicylates continues to increase with increasing urinary pH. Hence, increased tubular diffusion, not decreased reabsorption, probably accounts for most of the increase in salicylate elimination observed in the alkaline urine.[66]

We recommend sodium bicarbonate in the treatment of salicylate poisoning for most patients with evidence of significant systemic toxicity. Relative contraindications to sodium bicarbonate use include severe acute kidney injury (AKI) or chronic kidney disease (CKD) and acute respiratory distress syndrome.[54] Dosing recommendations depend on the acid–base considerations. We recommend alkalinization be started with a continuous sodium bicarbonate infusion of 150 mEq in 1 L of dextrose in water (D_5W) at 150 to 200 mL/h (or about twice the maintenance requirements in a child). Continued titration with sodium bicarbonate over 4 to 8 hours is recommended until the urinary pH reaches 7.5 to 8.0.[106,108] For patients with low serum bicarbonate, IV administration of 1 to 2 mEq of sodium bicarbonate per kilogram of body weight is recommended.[108] The addition of the dextrose is important because salicylate toxicity causes hypoglycemia.[108] Achieving a urinary pH of 8.0 is difficult but is the goal. Fastidious attention to the patient's changing acid–base status is required. Blood pH should not rise above 7.55 to prevent complications of alkalemia, although some clinicians would accept a ceiling of 7.60, depending on the risk–benefit circumstances.[51,61,97,100] In hypokalemic patients, the kidneys preferentially reabsorb potassium in exchange for hydrogen ions. Urinary alkalinization will be unsuccessful as long as hydrogen ions are excreted into the urine. Thus, concurrent potassium supplementation to achieve and maintain normokalemia is required to alkalinize the urine.[115]

Phenobarbital

Although cardiopulmonary support is the most critical intervention in the treatment of patients with severe phenobarbital overdose, sodium bicarbonate is a useful adjunct to general supportive care. The utility of sodium bicarbonate is particularly important considering the long plasma half-life (~100 hours) of phenobarbital. Phenobarbital is a weak acid (pK_a of 7.24) that undergoes significant renal elimination. As in the case of salicylates, alkalinization of the blood and urine reduces the severity and duration of toxicity. In a study of mice, the median anesthetic dose for mice receiving phenobarbital increased by 20% with the addition of sufficient sodium bicarbonate to increase the blood pH from 7.23 to 7.41, demonstrating decreased tissue concentrations associated with increased pH.[109] Animal evidence extrapolated to humans suggests that phenobarbital-poisoned patients in deep coma might develop a respiratory acidosis secondary to hypoventilation, with the acidemia enhancing the phenobarbital transfer into the brain, thus worsening CNS and respiratory depression. Alternatively, increasing the pH with bicarbonate, ventilatory support, or both would enhance the phenobarbital efflux from brain, thus lessening toxicity. Given phenobarbital's relatively high pK_a, significant urinary phenobarbital accumulation is evident only when urinary pH is increased above 7.5.[14] As the pH approaches 8.0, a threefold increase in urinary elimination occurs. The urine-to-serum ratio of phenobarbital, although much higher in alkaline urine than in acidic urine, remains less than unity, thereby suggesting less of a role for tubular secretion than in salicylate poisoning.

Clinical studies examining the role of alkalinization in phenobarbital poisoning are inadequately designed. Many are poorly controlled and fail to examine the effects of alkalinization, independent of coadministered diuretic therapy. In one uncontrolled study with phenobarbital overdoses, a 59% to 67% decrease in the duration of unconsciousness in patients occurred in patients administered alkali compared with nonrandomized control participants.[70] In other older studies, treatment with sodium lactate and urea reduced mortality and frequency of tracheotomy to 50% of control participants, enhanced elimination, and shortened coma.[60,73] In a later human volunteer study, urinary alkalinization with sodium bicarbonate in addition to hydration was associated with a decrease in phenobarbital elimination half-life from 148 to 47 hours.[39] However, this beneficial effect was less than the effect achieved by multiple-dose activated charcoal (MDAC), which reduced the half-life to 19 hours. In a nonrandomized study of phenobarbital-poisoned patients comparing urinary alkalinization alone, MDAC alone, and both methods together, both the phenobarbital half-life decreased most rapidly and the clinical course improved most rapidly in the group of patients who received MDAC alone.[69] Interesting, the combination approach proved inferior to MDAC alone but was better than alkalinization alone. The authors speculated that when both treatments were used together, the increased ionization of phenobarbital resulting from sodium bicarbonate infusion might have decreased the efficacy of MDAC. Although these studies suggest that

MDAC is more efficacious than urinary alkalinization in the treatment of phenobarbital-poisoned patients, in patients with contraindications to MDAC, it is reasonable to alkalinize the urine.

We do not currently recommend sodium bicarbonate therapy in the treatment of patients with ingestions of other barbiturates, such as pentobarbital and secobarbital, which either have a pK_a above 8.0 or are predominantly eliminated hepatically.

Methotrexate

Urinary alkalinization with sodium bicarbonate in addition to hydration is routinely used during high-dose methotrexate cancer chemotherapy therapy to achieve a urine pH of 7.0 or greater prior to methotrexate administration.[105] Methotrexate is predominantly eliminated unchanged in the urine. Unfortunately, methotrexate, as well as its metabolites DAMPA (4-amino-4-deoxy-10-methylpteroic acid) and 7-hydroxymethotrexate, are poorly water soluble in acidic urine. Under these conditions, tubular precipitation of the methotrexate occurs, leading to AKI and decreased elimination, increasing the likelihood of methotrexate toxicity. Administration of sodium bicarbonate (as well as intensive hydration) during high-dose methotrexate infusions increases methotrexate solubility and the elimination of methotrexate and its metabolites.[29,94] Formal studies in which chemotherapy was dosed per body surface have included bicarbonate infusions up to 200 mL/m^2/h for 8 hours with 5.4 gm/m^2 commencing 1 hour before methotrexate infusion.[87] In practice, alkalization is typically maintained with intravenous sodium bicarbonate 50-150 mEq/L to achieve adequate urine flow and alkalinization until leucovorin administration ceases. In the setting of methotrexate toxicity, it is reasonable to provide sodium bicarbonate 150 mEq in 1 L of dextrose in water (D_5W) at 150 to 250 mL/h, in a manner similar to salicylate toxicity until methotrexate has cleared.

Chlorophenoxy Herbicides

Alkalinization is recommended in the treatment of patients with poisonings from weed killers that contain chlorophenoxy compounds, such as 2,4-dichlorophenoxyacetic acid (2,4-D) or 2-(4-chloro-2-methylphenoxy) propionic acid (MCPP).[85] Poisoning results in muscle weakness, peripheral neuropathy, coma, hyperthermia, and acidemia. These compounds are weak acids (pK_a of 2.6 and 3.8 for 2,4-D and MCPP, respectively) that are excreted largely unchanged in the urine. In an uncontrolled case series of 41 patients poisoned with a variety of chlorophenoxy herbicides, 19 of whom received sodium bicarbonate, alkaline diuresis significantly reduced the half-life of each by enhancing renal elimination.[36] In one patient, resolution of hyperthermia and metabolic acidosis and improvement in mental status were associated with a transient elevation of serum concentration, perhaps reflecting chlorophenoxy compound redistribution from the tissues into the more alkalemic blood. The limited data suggest that the increased ionized fractions of the weak-acid chlorophenoxy compounds produced by alkalinization is trapped in both the blood and the urine as demonstrated both with salicylates and phenobarbital. Although data are limited to case reports, it is reasonable to administer sodium bicarbonate because of evidence that its use shortens the duration of effect.

CORRECTION OF LIFE-THREATENING METABOLIC ACIDOSIS

Some toxins cause an accumulation of acid byproducts leading to metabolic acidosis. Unchecked, metabolic acidosis leading to acidemia has important physiologic consequences. These are complex and depend on multiple other factors as well, including compensatory mechanisms, with the most severe effects involving the cardiovascular system.[31] When blood pH decreases from 7.40 to 7.20, cardiac output increases because of increased catecholamine concentrations, but when below 7.10 to 7.20, a decrease in cardiac output ensues.[58] Other cardiovascular effects include increased propensity for dysrhythmias, decreased systemic vascular tone, and pulmonary vasoconstriction.[58] The respiratory system suffers from increased respiratory stimulus and increased work of breathing. Additionally, 2,3-DPG (2,3-diphosphoglycerate) decreases, leading to a rightward shift of the oxygen dissociation curve and decreased release of oxygen to the tissues. Further consequences include cerebral vasodilation, hyperkalemia, hypercalcemia, increased renal oxygen demand and diuresis, decreased splanchnic perfusion with delayed gastric emptying, impaired platelet aggregation, and coagulopathy.[31,58]

Treatment of metabolic acidosis is largely aimed at treating the underlying cause. However, because the effects of persistent acidemia are severe, sodium bicarbonate is reasonable to administer to correct the acidemia in toxic alcohols and metformin toxicity.

Toxic Alcohols
Sodium bicarbonate has two important roles in treating patients with toxic alcohol ingestions. As an immediate temporizing measure, it is reasonable to consider administration of sodium bicarbonate to treat the life-threatening acidemia associated with methanol and ethylene glycol ingestions. In rats poisoned with ethylene glycol, the administration of sodium bicarbonate alone resulted in a fourfold increase in the median lethal dose.[17] Clinically, titrating the endogenous acid with bicarbonate greatly assists in reversing the consequences of severe acidemia, such as hemodynamic instability and multiorgan dysfunction.

The second role of bicarbonate in the treatment of toxic alcohol poisoning involves its ability to favorably alter the distribution and elimination of certain toxic metabolites.[92] In cases of methanol poisoning, the proportion of ionized formic acid is increased by administering bicarbonate, thereby trapping formic acid in the blood compartment.[53,67] Consequently, decreased visual toxicity results from removal of the toxic metabolite from the eyes. In cases of formic acid (pK_a of 3.7) ingestion, sodium bicarbonate decreases tissue penetration of the formic acid and enhances urinary elimination.[72]

Early treatment of acidemia with sodium bicarbonate is recommended in cases of methanol and ethylene glycol poisoning.[46,59] Sodium bicarbonate therapy should be administered to toxic alcohol-poisoned patients with an arterial pH below 7.30.[7,8] More than 400 to 600 mEq of sodium bicarbonate may be required in the first few hours.[52] In cases of ethylene glycol toxicity, sodium bicarbonate administration worsens hypocalcemia, so the serum calcium concentration should be monitored. Combating the acidemia, however, is not the mainstay of therapy, and concurrent administration of IV fomepizole or ethanol and evaluation for hemodialysis are almost always indicated.

Metformin
Metformin toxicity, either from overdose or therapeutic use in the setting of AKI or CKD, causes severe, life-threatening metabolic acidemia with an elevated lactate concentration. The use of high-dose sodium bicarbonate to correct the metabolic acidosis, as well as extracorporeal removal of the metformin, is recommended in these cases.[26,45] Although an exact threshold for initiating sodium bicarbonate is not well-defined, it would be reasonable to initiate this in severe acidosis, similar to that of other causes of acidosis (pH <7.10, serum bicarbonate <10 mmol/L).[58]

NEUTRALIZATION
Chlorine Gas
Nebulized sodium bicarbonate serves as a useful adjunct in the treatment of patients with pulmonary injuries resulting from chlorine gas inhalation.[5,27] Inhaled sodium bicarbonate neutralizes the hydrochloric acid that is formed when the chlorine gas reacts with the water in the respiratory tree. Although oral sodium bicarbonate is not recommended for neutralizing acid ingestions because of the problems associated with the exothermic reaction and production of carbon dioxide in the relatively closed gastrointestinal tract, the rapid exchange of air in the lungs with the environment facilitates heat dissipation. In a sheep model of chlorine inhalation, animals treated with 4% nebulized sodium bicarbonate solution demonstrated a higher PO_2 and lower PCO_2 than did the 0.9% sodium chloride treated animals.[28] There was no difference, however, in 24-hour mortality rate or pulmonary histopathology. In a retrospective review, 86 patients with chlorine gas inhalation were treated with nebulized sodium bicarbonate.[18] Sixty-nine patients were sent

home from the emergency department, 53 of whom had clearly improved. In a more recent study, 44 patients who were diagnosed with reactive airway dysfunction syndrome after an acute exposure to chlorine gas were randomized to receive either nebulized sodium bicarbonate (4 mL of 4.2% sodium bicarbonate solution) or nebulized placebo.[5] Both groups also received IV corticosteroids and inhaled β_2-adrenergic agonists. Compared with the placebo group, the nebulized sodium bicarbonate group had significantly higher forced expiratory volume in 1 second (FEV_1) values at 120 and 240 minutes and scored significantly higher on a posttreatment quality of life questionnaire. In patients experiencing reactive airway symptoms, it is reasonable to treat with a nebulized solution of 4 mL of 3.75% to 4.2% sodium bicarbonate solution in addition to humidified oxygen and inhaled β_2-adrenergic agonists. Nebulized sodium bicarbonate failed to demonstrate a benefit in the treatment of chloramine gas exposure.[79]

OTHER INDICATIONS
Adverse effects and safety concerns are associated with the dissociation of the dimercaprol (British anti-Lewisite {BAL}) metal binding that occurs in acid urine. Because dissociation of the BAL–metal chelate occurs in acidic urine, it is recommended to alkalinize the urine of patients receiving BAL with hypertonic sodium bicarbonate to a pH of 7.5 to 8.0 to prevent renal liberation of the metal.[24]

Sodium bicarbonate provides a renal protection benefit after exposure to depleted uranium. Animal studies suggest that sodium bicarbonate in conjunction with a chelator such as deferiprone accelerates uranium excretion and reduces uranium nephrotoxicity and thus it is reasonable to administer.[40]

ADVERSE EFFECTS AND SAFETY ISSUES
The use of sodium bicarbonate has associated risks. Excessive alkalemia (with adverse effects upon respiratory physiology), hypernatremia, fluid overload, hypokalemia, and hypocalcemia occur.[37,61,80,89,99] The package insert urges caution in patients with congestive heart failure, severe renal insufficiency, and preexisting edema with sodium retention.[4] Regarding its use to treat salicylism, early on, patients with pure respiratory alkalosis often have alkaluria and alkalemia and do not require urinary alkalinization. Young children who rapidly develop metabolic acidosis often require alkalinization but should be at less risk for complications of this therapy.[76] However, because hypertonic sodium bicarbonate causes hypernatremia, decreased cerebrospinal fluid pressure, and possible intracranial hemorrhage in children younger than 2 years of age, the 4.2% solution is preferred in these patients.[4] Extravasation causes local tissue damage.[4] Dobutamine and norepinephrine are incompatible with sodium bicarbonate solutions, and calcium solutions cause precipitation.

PREGNANCY AND LACTATION
According to the Food and Drug Administration (FDA), sodium bicarbonate is a Category C drug. The World Health Organization rates sodium bicarbonate as compatible with breastfeeding.

DOSING AND ADMINISTRATION
For the treatment of QRS complex prolongation in the setting of myocardial sodium channel poisoning, we recommend administration of 1 to 2 mEq/kg of sodium bicarbonate IV as a bolus over a period of 1 to 2 minutes.[81] Greater amounts, totaling as much as 35 mEq/kg over hours of resuscitation, are sometimes required to treat patients with recurrent unstable ventricular dysrhythmias.[84] Similar boluses should be repeated as needed to achieve a blood pH of 7.50 to 7.55.[82,104] Because sodium bicarbonate has a brief duration of effect, a continuous infusion usually is required after the initial IV boluses. The treatment endpoint is the narrowing of the QRS interval. Excessive alkalemia (pH >7.55) and hypernatremia should be avoided. To prepare a sodium bicarbonate infusion, three 50-mL ampules of 8.4% or 7.5% solution should be placed in 1 L of 5% D_5W and run at twice maintenance with frequent evaluation of the QRS duration, potassium concentration, and pH, depending on the fluid requirements and blood pressure of the patient. Frequent evaluation of

the fluid status should be performed to avoid precipitating pulmonary edema. An optimal duration of therapy has not been established.

For the treatment of patients with salicylate poisoning, sodium bicarbonate should be administered by bolus or infusion using the dosing strategies described earlier to achieve a serum pH of 7.45–7.55, until the with a goal of a urinary pH of 8.0. Careful and frequent monitoring of the urinary pH and serum potassium concentration is critical to ensure optimal treatment. In salicylate-poisoned patients with altered mental status, aggressive administration of sodium bicarbonate is required to ensure that the serum pH is greater than at least 7.40 to 7.45 although not exceed pH 7.55.

FORMULATIONS

The most commonly used sodium bicarbonate preparations are an 8.4% solution (1 M) containing 1 mEq each of sodium and bicarbonate ions per milliliter (calculated osmolarity of 2,000 mOsm/L) and a 7.5% solution containing 0.892 mEq each of sodium and bicarbonate ions per milliliter (calculated osmolarity of 1,786 mOsm/L). Fifty-milliliter ampules of the 8.4% and 7.5% solutions therefore contain 50 and 44.6 mEq of sodium bicarbonate, respectively. The common infant formulation is a 4.2% solution packaged as a 10-mL injectable ampule. This yields 5 mEq per container (0.5 mEq each of sodium and bicarbonate ions per milliliters). According to the package insert, the FDA-approved indications for sodium bicarbonate include the "treatment of certain drug intoxications, including barbiturates (where dissociation of the barbiturate-protein complex is desired), in poisoning by salicylates or methyl alcohol, and in hemolytic reactions requiring alkalinization of the urine to diminish nephrotoxicity of blood pigments. Urinary alkalinization is also used in methotrexate therapy to prevent nephrotoxicity."

SUMMARY

- Sodium bicarbonate remains an important treatment of a wide variety of xenobiotic exposures.
- Sodium bicarbonate is effective in patients poisoned by myocardial sodium channel blockers by providing sodium through its effects on drug ionization and subsequent diffusion from the sodium channel binding site.
- Sodium bicarbonate is effective for salicylates, phenobarbital, methotrexate, and other weak acids because of its ability to "ion trap" in blood or urine compartments and mitigate target organ accumulation.
- Nebulized sodium bicarbonate administration is reasonable in neutralizing inhaled acids such as chlorine gas.

REFERENCES

1. Adrogue HJ, et al. Influence of steady-state alterations in acid-base equilibrium on the fate of administered bicarbonate in the dog. *J Clin Invest.* 1983;71:867-883.
2. Al-Abri SA, et al. Delayed bupropion cardiotoxicity associated with elevated serum concentrations of bupropion but not hydroxybupropion. *Clin Toxicol (Phila).* 2013;51:1230-1234.
3. Sodium Bicarbonate monograph. Lexicomp Inc. Accessed May 12, 2017.
4. Anonymous.Sodiumbicarbonatepackageinsert.https://dailymed.nlm.nih.gov/dailymed/drugInfo.cfm?setid=86137340-55c3-4ed2-8166-2fb2779ca759. Accessed April 1, 2017.
5. Aslan S, et al. The effect of nebulized NaHCO3 treatment on "RADS" due to chlorine gas inhalation. *Inhal Toxicol.* 2006;18:895-900.
6. Bailey DJ Jr. Cardiotoxic effects of quinidine and their treatment. *Arch Intern Med.* 1960;105:13-22.
7. Barceloux DG, et al; American Academy of Clinical Toxicology Ad Hoc Committee on the Treatment Guidelines for Methanol P. American Academy of Clinical Toxicology practice guidelines on the treatment of methanol poisoning. *J Toxicol Clin Toxicol.* 2002;40:415-446.
8. Barceloux DG, et al. American Academy of Clinical Toxicology Practice Guidelines on the Treatment of Ethylene Glycol Poisoning. Ad Hoc Committee. *J Toxicol Clin Toxicol.* 1999;37:537-560.
9. Bebarta VS, Waksman JC. Amitriptyline-induced Brugada pattern fails to respond to sodium bicarbonate. *Clin Toxicol (Phila).* 2007;45:186-188.
10. Beckman KJ, et al. Hemodynamic and electrophysiological actions of cocaine. Effects of sodium bicarbonate as an antidote in dogs. *Circulation.* 1991;83:1799-1807.
11. Bellet S, et al. The reversal of cardiotoxic effects of quinidine by molar sodium lactate: an experimental study. *Am J Med Sci.* 1959;237:165-176 passim.
12. Bellet S, Wasserman F. The effects of molar sodium lactate in reversing the cardiotoxic effect of hyperpotassemia. *AMA Arch Intern Med.* 1957;100:565-581.
13. Blackman K, et al. Plasma alkalinization for tricyclic antidepressant toxicity: a systematic review. *Emerg Med (Fremantle).* 2001;13:204-210.
14. Bloomer HA. A critical evaluation of diuresis in the treatment of barbiturate intoxication. *J Lab Clin Med.* 1966;67:898-905.
15. Bodenhamer JE, Smilkstein MJ. Delayed cardiotoxicity following quinine overdose: a case report. *J Emerg Med.* 1993;11:279-285.
16. Boehnert MT, Lovejoy FH Jr. Value of the QRS duration versus the serum drug level in predicting seizures and ventricular arrhythmias after an acute overdose of tricyclic antidepressants. *N Engl J Med.* 1985;313:474-479.
17. Borden TA, Bidwell CD. Treatment of acute ethylene glycol poisoning in rats. *Invest Urol.* 1968;6:205-210.
18. Bosse GM. Nebulized sodium bicarbonate in the treatment of chlorine gas inhalation. *J Toxicol Clin Toxicol.* 1994;32:233-241.
19. Bradberry SM, et al. Management of the cardiovascular complications of tricyclic antidepressant poisoning: role of sodium bicarbonate. *Toxicol Rev.* 2005;24:195-204.
20. Brown TC. Sodium bicarbonate treatment for tricyclic antidepressant arrhythmias in children. *Med J Aust.* 1976;2:380-382.
21. Brown TC, et al. The use of sodium bicarbonate in the treatment of tricyclic antidepressant-induced arrhythmias. *Anaesth Intensive Care.* 1973;1:203-210.
22. Brucculeri M, et al. Reversal of citalopram-induced junctional bradycardia with intravenous sodium bicarbonate. *Pharmacotherapy.* 2005;25:119-122.
23. Buchanan N, et al. Experimental salicylate intoxication in young baboons. A preliminary report. *J Pediatr.* 1975;86:225-232.
24. Byrns MC, Penning TM. *Environmental Toxicology: Carcinogens and Heavy Metals.* In: Brunton LL, Hilal-Dandan R, Knollmann BC. eds. Goodman & Gilman's: The Pharmacological Basis of Therapeutics, 12ed. New York, NY:Macmillan, 2011.
25. Caillier B, et al. QRS widening and QT prolongation under bupropion: a unique cardiac electrophysiological profile. *Fundam Clin Pharmacol.* 2012;26:599-608.
26. Calello DP, et al. Extracorporeal treatment for metformin poisoning: systematic review and recommendations from the Extracorporeal Treatments in Poisoning Workgroup. *Crit Care Med.* 2015;43:1716-1730.
27. Cevik Y, et al. Mass casualties from acute inhalation of chlorine gas. *South Med J.* 2009;102:1209-1213.
28. Chisholm C, et al. Effect of hydration on sodium bicarbonate therapy for chlorine inhalation injuries [abstract]. *Ann Emerg Med.* 1988;18:466.
29. Christensen ML, et al. Effect of hydration on methotrexate plasma concentrations in children with acute lymphocytic leukemia. *J Clin Oncol.* 1988;6:797-801.
30. Cole JB, et al. Wide complex tachycardia in a pediatric diphenhydramine overdose treated with sodium bicarbonate. *Pediatr Emerg Care.* 2011;27:1175-1177.
31. Curley GF, Laffey JG. Acidosis in the critically ill—balancing risks and benefits to optimize outcome. *Crit Care.* 2014;18:129.
32. Curry SC, et al. Intraventricular conduction delay after bupropion overdose. *J Emerg Med.* 2005;29:299-305.
33. D'Alessandro LC, et al. Life-threatening flecainide intoxication in a young child secondary to medication error. *Ann Pharmacother.* 2009;43:1522-1527.
34. Engebretsen KM, et al. Cardiotoxicity and late onset seizures with citalopram overdose. *J Emerg Med.* 2003;25:163-166.
35. Fernandez PC, et al. The concept of bicarbonate distribution space: the crucial role of body buffers. *Kidney Int.* 1989;36:747-752.
36. Flanagan RJ, et al. Alkaline diuresis for acute poisoning with chlorophenoxy herbicides and ioxynil. *Lancet.* 1990;335:454-458.
37. Fox GN. Hypocalcemia complicating bicarbonate therapy for salicylate poisoning. *West J Med.* 1984;141:108-109.
38. Franco V. Wide complex tachycardia after bupropion overdose. *Am J Emerg Med.* 2015;33:1540 e1543-1545.
39. Frenia ML, et al. Multiple-dose activated charcoal compared to urinary alkalinization for the enhancement of phenobarbital elimination. *J Toxicol Clin Toxicol.* 1996;34:169-175.
40. Fukuda S, et al. The effects of bicarbonate and its combination with chelating agents used for the removal of depleted uranium in rats. *Hemoglobin.* 2008;32:191-198.
41. Garella S, et al. Severity of metabolic acidosis as a determinant of bicarbonate requirements. *N Engl J Med.* 1973;289:121-126.
42. Gaultier M. Sodium bicarbonate and tricyclic-antidepressant poisoning. *Lancet.* 1976;2:1258.
43. Graudins A, et al. Fluoxetine-induced cardiotoxicity with response to bicarbonate therapy. *Am J Emerg Med.* 1997;15:501-503.
44. Gutman A, et al. A study, by simultaneous clearance techniques, of salicylate excretion in man: effect of alkalinization of the urine by bicarbonate administration; effect of probenecid. *J Clin Invest.* 1955;34:711-721.
45. Harvey B, et al. Severe lactic acidosis complicating metformin overdose successfully treated with high-volume venovenous hemofiltration and aggressive alkalinization. *Pediatr Crit Care Med.* 2005;6:598-601.
46. Herken W, Rietbrock N. The influence of blood-pH on ionization, distribution, and toxicity of formic acid. *Naunyn Schmiedebergs Arch Exp Pathol Pharmakol.* 1968;260:142-143.
47. Herold TJ. Lamotrigine as a possible cause of QRS prolongation in a patient with known seizure disorder. *CJEM.* 2006;8:361-364.

48. Hill JB. Experimental salicylate poisoning: observations on the effects of altering blood pH on tissue and plasma salicylate concentrations. *Pediatrics.* 1971;47:658-665.

49. Hill JB. Salicylate intoxication. *N Engl J Med.* 1973;288:1110-1113.

50. Hoffman JR, McElroy CR. Bicarbonate therapy for dysrhythmia and hypotension in tricyclic antidepressant overdose. *West J Med.* 1981;134:60-64.

51. Hoffman JR, et al. Effect of hypertonic sodium bicarbonate in the treatment of moderate-to-severe cyclic antidepressant overdose. *Am J Emerg Med.* 1993;11:336-341.

52. Jacobsen D, McMartin KE. Methanol and ethylene glycol poisonings. Mechanism of toxicity, clinical course, diagnosis and treatment. *Med Toxicol.* 1986;1:309-334.

53. Jacobsen D, et al. Methanol and formate kinetics in late diagnosed methanol intoxication. *Med Toxicol Adverse Drug Exp.* 1988;3:418-423.

54. Kallen RJ, et al. Hemodialysis in children: technique, kinetic aspects related to varying body size, and application to salicylate intoxication, acute renal failure and some other disorders. *Medicine (Baltimore).* 1966;45:1-50.

55. Kerns W 2nd, et al. Cocaine-induced wide complex dysrhythmia. *J Emerg Med.* 1997;15:321-329.

56. Kim HS, et al. Unresponsive Male. *Ann Emerg Med.* 2017;69:552-561.

57. Knudsen K, Abrahamsson J. Epinephrine and sodium bicarbonate independently and additively increase survival in experimental amitriptyline poisoning. *Crit Care Med.* 1997;25:669-674.

58. Kraut JA, Madias NE. Metabolic acidosis: pathophysiology, diagnosis and management. *Nat Rev Nephrol.* 2010;6:274-285.

59. Kulig K DJ, et al. Toxic effects of methanol, ethylene glycol, and isopropyl alcohol. *Topics Emerg Med.* 1984;6:14-29.

60. Lassen N. Treatment of severe acute barbiturate poisoning by forced diuresis and alkalinization of the urine. *Lancet.* 1960;2:338-342.

61. Lawson AA. Forced diuresis in the treatment of acute salicylate poisoning in adults. *Q J Med.* 1969;38:31-48.

62. Levitt MA, et al. Amitriptyline plasma protein binding: effect of plasma pH and relevance to clinical overdose. *Am J Emerg Med.* 1986;4:121-125.

63. Liebelt EL. Targeted management strategies for cardiovascular toxicity from tricyclic antidepressant overdose: the pivotal role for alkalinization and sodium loading. *Pediatr Emerg Care.* 1998;14:293-298.

64. Liebelt EL, et al. Serial electrocardiogram changes in acute tricyclic antidepressant overdoses. *Crit Care Med.* 1997;25:1721-1726.

65. Littmann L, et al. Brugada-type electrocardiographic pattern induced by cocaine. *Mayo Clin Proc.* 2000;75:845-849.

66. Macpherson CR, et al. The excretion of salicylate. *Br J Pharmacol Chemother.* 1955;10:484-489.

67. Martin-Amat G, et al. Methanol poisoning: ocular toxicity produced by formate. *Toxicol Appl Pharmacol.* 1978;45:201-208.

68. Milne MD, et al. Non-ionic diffusion and the excretion of weak acids and bases. *Am J Med.* 1958;24:709-729.

69. Mohammed Ebid AH A-RH. Pharmacokinetics of phenobarbital during certain enhanced elimination modalities to evaluate their clinical efficacy in management of drug overdose. *Ther Drug Monit.* 2001;23:209-216.

70. Mollaret P, et al. Treatment of acute barbiturate intoxication through plasmatic and urinary alkalinization. *Presse Med.* 1959;67:1435-1437.

71. Molloy DW, et al. Use of sodium bicarbonate to treat tricyclic antidepressant-induced arrhythmias in a patient with alkalosis. *Can Med Assoc J.* 1984;130:1457-1459.

72. Moore DF, et al. Folinic acid and enhanced renal elimination in formic acid intoxication. *J Toxicol Clin Toxicol.* 1994;32:199-204.

73. Myschetzky A, Lassen NA. Osmotic diuresis and alkalinization of the urine in the treatment of severe acute barbiturate intoxication. *Dan Med Bull.* 1963;10:104-108.

74. Nattel S, Mittleman M. Treatment of ventricular tachyarrhythmias resulting from amitriptyline toxicity in dogs. *J Pharmacol Exp Ther.* 1984;231:430-435.

75. O'Connor N, et al. Prolonged clinical effects in modified-release amitriptyline poisoning. *Clin Toxicol (Phila).* 2006;44:77-80.

76. Oliver TK Jr, Dyer ME. The prompt treatment of salicylism with sodium bicarbonate. *AMA J Dis Child.* 1960;99:553-565.

77. Ortega-Carnicer J, et al. Aborted sudden death, transient Brugada pattern, and wide QRS dysrhythmias after massive cocaine ingestion. *J Electrocardiol.* 2001;34:345-349.

78. Parker RB, et al. Comparative effects of sodium bicarbonate and sodium chloride on reversing cocaine-induced changes in the electrocardiogram. *J Cardiovasc Pharmacol.* 1999;34:864-869.

79. Pascuzzi TA, Storrow AB. Mass casualties from acute inhalation of chloramine gas. *Mil Med.* 1998;163:102-104.

80. Pentel P, Benowitz N. Efficacy and mechanism of action of sodium bicarbonate in the treatment of desipramine toxicity in rats. *J Pharmacol Exp Ther.* 1984;230:12-19.

81. Pentel PR, Benowitz NL. Tricyclic antidepressant poisoning. Management of arrhythmias. *Med Toxicol.* 1986;1:101-121.

82. Pentel PR, et al. Effect of hypertonic sodium bicarbonate on encainide overdose. *Am J Cardiol.* 1986;57:878-880.

83. Pentel PR, Keyler DE. Effects of high dose alpha-1-acid glycoprotein on desipramine toxicity in rats. *J Pharmacol Exp Ther.* 1988;246:1061-1066.

84. Pierog JE, et al. Tricyclic antidepressant toxicity treated with massive sodium bicarbonate. *Am J Emerg Med.* 2009;27:1168 e1163-1167.

85. Prescott LF, et al. Treatment of severe 2,4-D and mecoprop intoxication with alkaline diuresis. *Br J Clin Pharmacol.* 1979;7:111-116.

86. Proudfoot AT, et al. Does urine alkalinization increase salicylate elimination? If so, why? *Toxicol Rev.* 2003;22:129-136.

87. Proudfoot AT, et al. Position paper on urine alkalinization. *J Toxicol Clin Toxicol.* 2004;42:1-26.

88. Ranger S, et al. Modulation of flecainide's cardiac sodium channel blocking actions by extracellular sodium: a possible cellular mechanism for the action of sodium salts in flecainide cardiotoxicity. *J Pharmacol Exp Ther.* 1993;264:1160-1167.

89. Reimold EW, et al. Salicylate poisoning. Comparison of acetazolamide administration and alkaline diuresis in the treatment of experimental salicylate intoxication in puppies. *Am J Dis Child.* 1973;125:668-674.

90. Repetto HA, Penna R. Apparent bicarbonate space in children. *ScientificWorldJournal.* 2006;6:148-153.

91. Richards JR, et al. Treatment of cocaine cardiovascular toxicity: a systematic review. *Clin Toxicol (Phila).* 2016;54:345-364.

92. Roe O IC. Methanol poisoning. Its clinical course, pathogenesis and treatment. *Acta Med Scand.* 1946;126(suppl 182):S1-S253.

93. Salerno DM, et al. Reversal of flecainide-induced ventricular arrhythmia by hypertonic sodium bicarbonate in dogs. *Am J Emerg Med.* 1995;13:285-293.

94. Sand TE, Jacobsen S. Effect of urine pH and flow on renal clearance of methotrexate. *Eur J Clin Pharmacol.* 1981;19:453-456.

95. Sasyniuk BI, Jhamandas V. Mechanism of reversal of toxic effects of amitriptyline on cardiac Purkinje fibers by sodium bicarbonate. *J Pharmacol Exp Ther.* 1984;231:387-394.

96. Sasyniuk BI, et al. Experimental amitriptyline intoxication: treatment of cardiac toxicity with sodium bicarbonate. *Ann Emerg Med.* 1986;15:1052-1059.

97. Savege TM, et al. Treatment of severe salicylate poisoning by forced alkaline diuresis. *Br Med J.* 1969;1:35-36.

98. Schwartz M, et al. Cardiotoxicity after massive amantadine overdose. *J Med Toxicol.* 2008;4:173-179.

99. Segar WE. The critically ill child: salicylate intoxication. *Pediatrics.* 1969;44:440-444.

100. Seger DL, et al. Variability of recommendations for serum alkalinization in tricyclic antidepressant overdose: a survey of U.S. Poison Center medical directors. *J Toxicol Clin Toxicol.* 2003;41:331-338.

101. Shannon MW. Duration of QRS disturbances after severe tricyclic antidepressant intoxication. *J Toxicol Clin Toxicol.* 1992;30:377-386.

102. Sharma AN, et al. Diphenhydramine-induced wide complex dysrhythmia responds to treatment with sodium bicarbonate. *Am J Emerg Med.* 2003;21:212-215.

103. Singer RB, et al. The acute effects in man of rapid intravenous infusion of hypertonic sodium bicarbonate solution. I. Changes in acid-base balance and distribution of the excess buffer base. *Medicine (Baltimore).* 1955;34:51-95.

104. Smilkstein MJ. Reviewing cyclic antidepressant cardiotoxicity: wheat and chaff. *J Emerg Med.* 1990;8:645-648.

105. Smith SW, Nelson LS. Case files of the New York City Poison Control Center: antidotal strategies for the management of methotrexate toxicity. *J Med Toxicol.* 2008;4:132-140.

106. Snodgrass W, et al. Salicylate toxicity following therapeutic doses in young children. *Clin Toxicol.* 1981;18:247-259.

107. Taboulet P, et al. Cardiovascular repercussions of seizures during cyclic antidepressant poisoning. *J Toxicol Clin Toxicol.* 1995;33:205-211.

108. Temple AR. Acute and chronic effects of aspirin toxicity and their treatment. *Arch Intern Med.* 1981;141(3 Spec No):364-369.

109. Waddell WJ, Butler TC. The distribution and excretion of phenobarbital. *J Clin Invest.* 1957;36:1217-1226.

110. Wang RY. pH-dependent cocaine-induced cardiotoxicity. *Am J Emerg Med.* 1999;17:364-369.

111. Wasserman F, et al. Successful treatment of quinidine and procaine amide intoxication; report of three cases. *N Engl J Med.* 1958;259:797-802.

112. Wills BK, Zell et al. Bupropion-associated QRS prolongation unresponsive to sodium bicarbonate therapy. *Am J Ther.* 2009;16:193-196.

113. Wilson LD, Shelat C. Electrophysiologic and hemodynamic effects of sodium bicarbonate in a canine model of severe cocaine intoxication. *J Toxicol Clin Toxicol.* 2003;41:777-788.

114. Winecoff AP, et al. Reversal of the electrocardiographic effects of cocaine by lidocaine. Part 1. Comparison with sodium bicarbonate and quinidine. *Pharmacotherapy.* 1994;14:698-703.

115. Yip L, et al. Concepts and controversies in salicylate toxicity. *Emerg Med Clin North Am.* 1994;12:351-364.

38

BOTULISM

Howard L. Geyer

HISTORY AND EPIDEMIOLOGY

Botulism, a potentially fatal neuroparalytic illness, results from exposure to botulinum neurotoxin (BoNT), which is produced by the bacterium *Clostridium botulinum* and other *Clostridium* species. The earliest cases of botulism were described in Europe in 1735 and were attributed to improperly preserved German sausage; the name of the disease alludes to this association because *botulus* is the Latin word for *sausage*. Emile van Ermengem identified the causative organism in 1897 and named it *Bacillus botulinum*; it was later renamed *Clostridium botulinum*.[25] These gram-positive, spore-forming bacteria produce eight serotypes of BoNT, denoted A through H.[88,134]

In adults, most cases result from ingestion of toxin in contaminated food, but in infants, most cases result from consumption of bacterial spores that proliferate and produce toxin in the gastrointestinal (GI) tract. Less common forms of botulism include wound botulism, in which spores are inoculated into a wound and locally produce toxin, and inhalational botulism caused by aerosolized BoNT, which potentially can be used as a weapon of bioterrorism.

Botulism outbreaks occur throughout the world[149] and have been reported from such diverse areas as Uganda,[179] Iran,[137] Japan,[128] Thailand,[96] Pakistan,[93] Australia,[113] France,[1] Portugal,[103] Poland,[58] Greenland,[82] Chile,[12] and Canada.[123] In 2016, a total of 150 laboratory-confirmed cases and 10 probable cases of botulism were reported to the US Centers for Disease Control and Prevention (CDC).[39] Foodborne botulism constituted 14% of cases, infant botulism 73% of cases, and wound botulism 12%. In this analysis, toxin type A accounted for 83% of cases of foodborne botulism, with the remainder split between type A and type B (27% each). Toxin type A was responsible in at least 88% of cases of wound botulism, and infant botulism was caused by toxin type A in 36% and to toxin type B in 59% of cases. Two deaths from foodborne botulism were reported in 2016.[39] The case fatality rate has improved for all botulism toxin types, probably caused by increasing awareness of the condition and consequent earlier diagnosis, appropriate and early use of antitoxin, and better and more accessible life support techniques.

In the past 50 years, home-processed food has accounted for 65% of outbreaks, with commercial food processing constituting only 7% of reported cases; in the remaining outbreaks, the origin is unknown.[45] Common home-canning errors responsible for botulism include failure to use a pressure cooker and allowing food to putrefy at room temperature. Minimally processed foods such as soft cheeses lack sufficient quantities of intrinsic barriers to BoNT production, such as salt and acidifying agents.[143] These foods become high-risk sources of botulism when refrigeration standards are violated. The US Food and Drug Administration (FDA) continuously reviews recommendations for appropriate measures to process such foods.[168,169]

Awareness of evolving trends and unusual presentations or locations of botulism permits the establishment of preventive education programs. Outbreaks of botulism have been associated with specialty foods consumed by different ethnic groups, such as chopped garlic in soy oil by Chinese in Vancouver, British Columbia;[123,163] uneviscerated salted fish—called *kapchunka*—eaten by Russian immigrants in New York City;[36,167] and the same fish—called *faseikh*—eaten in Egypt.[182] The incidence of botulism is high in Alaska where traditional foods include fermented fish and fish eggs, seal, beaver, and whale; between 2001 and 2014, one-third of cases of foodborne botulism in the United States occurred in Alaska. Approximately 90% of toxin type E outbreaks have occurred in Alaska because of home-processed fish or meat

from marine animals,[52,107,181] and one incident occurred in New Jersey.[37] In the 1990s, three cases of botulism involved members of a Native American church after they ingested a ceremonial tea made from the buttons of dried, alkaline-ground peyote cactus that were stored for 2 months in a water-filled refrigerated jar. The resultant alkaline and anaerobic milieu presumably fostered the growth of toxin from naturally occurring spores.[83] In 1996, eight cases of foodborne botulism in Italy were linked to mascarpone cream cheese eaten either alone or in tiramisu contaminated with BoNT type A.[14] Other outbreaks have been linked to mushrooms bottled in a restaurant,[38] home-canned bamboo shoots,[44,47] home-pickled eggs,[48] commercial carrot juice,[40] commercially processed chili sauce,[41] home-prepared tofu,[42,49] improperly stored potato soup,[51] and improperly jarred pesto.[31]

Larger outbreaks are especially concerning. In April 2015, 29 patients in Ohio developed botulism (25 laboratory-confirmed cases and 4 probable cases) after consuming home-canned potatoes at a church potluck meal; one died of respiratory failure.[114] In June 2016, 31 male inmates in a medium-security federal correctional institution in Mississippi developed botulism after drinking "pruno," an illicit alcohol made by the prisoners;[115] similar preparations were responsible for four prior outbreaks in prisons in California, Utah, and Arizona.[43,180,186] Twenty-four patients were hospitalized and nine required mechanical ventilation, but none died. This botulism outbreak was the largest in the United States since 1978, when 32 people were affected after eating at a New Mexico country club.[35]

Among cases attributed to commercial food processing, vegetables (peppers, beans, mushrooms, tomatoes, and beets, with or without meat) were thought to be the causative agents in approximately 70%, meat in 17%, and fish in 13% of cases.[45] Although only 4% of foodborne botulism is associated with food purchased in restaurants, restaurant-related outbreaks usually affect large numbers of individuals.[107]

Of 29 laboratory-confirmed cases of foodborne botulism in 2016, there were three multi-case outbreaks, each involving two or three patients.[39] Among hundreds of reports of botulism from 1975 to 1988 involving more than 400 persons, approximately 70% involved only one person, 20% involved two persons, and only 10% involved more than two persons, yielding a mean of 2.7 cases per outbreak.[185] Single affected patients were more severely ill, with 85% requiring intubation compared with only 42% requiring intubation in multi-person outbreaks, presumably because diagnosis in the index case leads to more rapid therapeutic intervention for associated cases.

Infant botulism is more common in certain geographic areas than in others presumably because of higher concentrations of botulinum spores in soil. Raw honey is a potential source of spores.[124] Most affected infants are younger than 6 months of age. Of 128 confirmed cases reported in 2014, most were from California (38%), New Jersey (8%), Maryland (7%), Pennsylvania (6%), or Texas (5%). The median age was 17 weeks (range, 2–54 weeks), and 46% were female. No US deaths from infant botulism were reported in 2014.[39] With appropriate support and treatment, a favorable outcome is achieved in the majority of cases.

In 2016, 24 cases of wound botulism were confirmed in the United States; 15 of these cases occurred in California. Age ranged from 25 to 68 years, with a median of 45 years, and 29% were women. Patients continue to be almost exclusively injection drug users.[39]

In ways unimaginable when the first edition of this book was published, medical and public health realities associated with terrorism in the 21st century unfortunately have resulted in increased relevance of botulism to medical practitioners (Chaps. 126 and 127). The advent of therapeutic BoNT injections has raised other concerns regarding potential adverse consequences.[10]

BACTERIOLOGY

The genus *Clostridium* comprises a group of four spore-forming anaerobic gram-positive bacillary species that produce eight different neurotoxic proteins. *C. botulinum* produces all BoNT serotypes A through H, *C. baratii* produces toxin type F, *C. butyricum* produces toxin type E, and *C. argentinense* (sometimes considered a subgroup of *C. botulinum*) produces toxin type G.[88] Some strains produce two different toxin types. Most cases of botulism result from BoNT types A, B, E, or F.[39,65,170] Reports of cases caused by BoNT type F have increased in recent years in parallel with improved ability of laboratories to detect *C. baratii* and other clostridial species producing toxin type F. The seven types A to G were recognized for over 40 years until in 2014 when a new toxin was identified in an infant with botulism and was designated type H.[21]

Clostridial species are ubiquitous, and the bacteria and spores are present in soil, seawater, and air.[160] Genomic sequence analysis shows that multiple toxin subtypes exist within each of the eight main types A through H; for example, there are eight subtypes of type A, designated A1 through A8.[88] In the United States, toxin type A is found in soil west of the Mississippi;[106] type B is found east of the Mississippi, particularly in the Allegheny range; and type E is found in the Pacific northwest and the Great Lakes states.[46,160] Toxin types A and B typically are found in poorly processed meats and vegetables. Toxin type E is commonly found in raw or fermented marine fish and mammals. Toxin types C and D cause disease in birds and mammals. Toxin type G has not been associated with naturally occurring disease. Although the different botulinum toxins differ in the cellular molecules they target, their ultimate pathophysiology and clinical syndromes are identical.

All botulinum spores are dormant and highly resistant to damage. They withstand boiling at 212°F (100°C) for hours, although they usually are destroyed by 30 minutes of moist heat at 248°F (120°C). Factors that promote germination of spores in food are pH greater than 4.5, sodium chloride content less than 3.5%, and low nitrite concentration. Most viable organisms produce toxin in an anaerobic milieu with temperatures greater than 80.6°F (27°C), although some strains produce toxins even when conditions are not optimal. Clostridia produce toxin type E at temperatures as low as 41°F (5°C). To prevent spore germination, acidifying agents such as phosphoric or citric acid are added to canned or bottled foods that have a low acid content, such as green beans, corn, beets, asparagus, chili peppers, mushrooms, spinach, figs, olives, and certain nonacidic tomatoes. Unlike the spores, the toxin itself is heat labile and is destroyed by heating to 176°F (80°C) for 30 minutes or to 212°F (100°C) for 10 minutes. At high altitudes, where the boiling point of water may be as low as 202.5°F (94.7°C), boiling for a full 30 minutes is prudent to ensure that the toxin is destroyed. Under high-altitude conditions, pressure cooking at 13 to 14 lb of pressure often is necessary to achieve appropriate temperatures to destroy the toxin in a timely fashion.

Foods contaminated with *C. botulinum* toxin types A and B often look or smell putrefied because of the action of proteolytic enzymes.[81] In contrast, because toxin type E organisms are saccharolytic and not proteolytic, foods contaminated with toxin type E typically look and taste normal.[17]

PHARMACOKINETICS AND TOXICOKINETICS

BoNT is the most potent toxin known. The LD_{50} for mice is 3 million molecules injected intraperitoneally. The human oral lethal dose is 1 mcg.[147]

Foodborne botulism results from ingestion of preformed BoNT from food contaminated with *Clostridium* spores. The toxin is complexed to associated proteins (hemagglutinins and a nontoxic nonhemagglutin)[88] that protect it from the acidic and proteolytic environment in the stomach. In the intestine, the alkaline pH dissociates the toxin from the associated proteins, allowing for subsequent absorption into the bloodstream.[121] Because the toxin is often demonstrated only in the stool, determining the percentage of the toxin actually absorbed is difficult.[64,67] The median incubation period for all patients is 1 day, but it ranges from 0 to 7 days for toxin type A, 0 to 5 days for toxin type B, and 0 to 2 days for toxin type E.[185]

Infant botulism does not result from ingestion of preformed BoNT but rather from ingestion of *C. botulinum* spores, which germinate in the GI tract and produce toxin. The immaturity of the bacterial flora in the infant GI tract facilitates colonization by the organisms. Adults with altered GI tracts (eg, those who have undergone gastric bypass or are taking proton pump inhibitors or H_2 antagonists) also rarely develop botulism in the same way, with the onset of symptoms typically following ingestion by 1 or 2 months. Cases of foodborne infant botulism associated with home-canned food have been reportedly extremely rarely.[6,105]

In wound botulism, spores proliferate in a wound or abscess and locally elaborate toxin. The incubation period is typically less than 2 weeks, but delays as long as 51 days are reported.[86]

The duration of action of the BoNT types varies depending on the components of the neurotransmitter release apparatus that are disrupted (see Pathophysiology). It is unclear whether the persistence of clinical effect results from the individual cleavage target, the intraneuronal biological half-life of the toxin, or both. Current evidence indicating intraneuronal toxin metabolism or elimination is inadequate.

PATHOPHYSIOLOGY

Botulinum neurotoxin is produced as a protein consisting of a single polypeptide chain with a molecular weight of 900 kDa, which includes a 750-kDa nontoxic protein and a 150-kDa neurotoxic component. To become fully active, the single-chain polypeptide 150-kDa neurotoxin must undergo proteolytic cleavage to generate a dichain structure consisting of a 100-kDa heavy chain linked by a disulfide bond to a 50-kDa light chain. The dichain form of the molecule is responsible for all clinical manifestations.[29,84] Both the single polypeptide chain toxin and the dichain form are resistant to GI degradation.[108]

The ingested toxin binds to serotype-specific receptors on the mucosal surfaces of gastric and small intestinal epithelial cells, where endocytosis is followed by transcytosis, permitting release of the toxin on the serosal (basolateral) cell surface.[100,142] The dichain form travels intravascularly to peripheral cholinergic nerve terminals, where it binds rapidly and irreversibly to the cell membrane and is taken up by endocytosis. The heavy chain is responsible for cell-specific membrane binding to acetylcholine-containing neurons (Fig. 38–1). Botulinum neurotoxin use dual host receptors to achieve their high affinity; whereas BoNT A binds a ganglioside and synaptic vesicle glycoprotein 2, BoNT B uses synaptotagmin. This mechanism allows rapid toxin entry via synaptic vesicles. The subsequent acidification of the synaptic vesicle lumen triggers the heavy chain N-terminal domain to form a channel to facilitate translocation of the light chain into the cytosol.[97]

When inside the cell, the light chain acts as a zinc-dependent endopeptidase to cleave presynaptic membrane polypeptides that are essential components of the soluble *N*-ethylmaleimide-sensitive factor attachment receptor (SNARE) apparatus that subserves acetylcholine exocytosis, thereby inhibiting release.[147] Botulinum neurotoxin types specifically cleave different proteins belonging to the SNARE family, and these differences are one possible reason for their variable toxicity.[155] SNARE proteins targeted by proteolysis include vesicle-associated membrane protein (VAMP) called synaptobrevin which is localized on synaptic vesicles, syntaxin found on the presynaptic membrane, and synaptosomal-associated protein (SNAP)-25, which is attached to syntaxin and to the presynaptic membrane. Toxin types A and E cleave SNAP-25; types B, D, F, and G act on VAMP/synaptobrevin; and type C cleaves both syntaxin and SNAP-25 (Fig. 38–1).[100] All BoNT types impair transmission at acetylcholine-dependent synapses in the peripheral nervous system, but cholinergic synapses in the central nervous system are not thought to be affected. Very high concentrations of BoNT also impair release of other neurotransmitters, including norepinephrine and serotonin.[80] Botulinum neurotoxin also exerts effects via mechanisms other than cleavage of SNARE proteins, possibly including apoptosis or gene expression.[112]

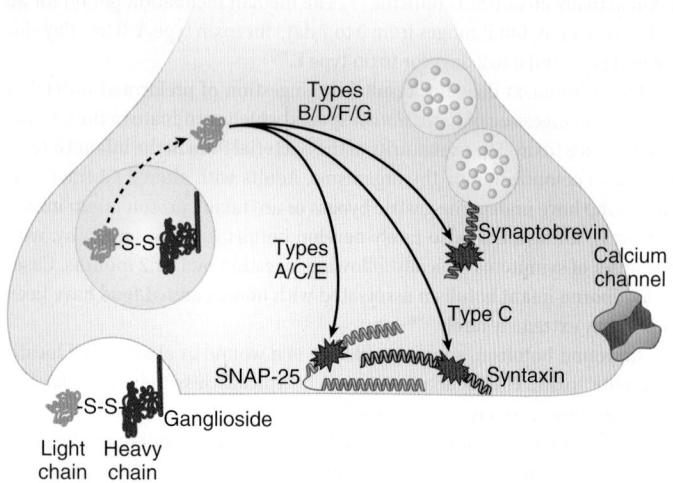

FIGURE 38–1. Botulinum toxins consist of two peptides linked by disulfide bonds. The heavy chain is responsible for specific binding to acetylcholine (ACh)-containing neurons. After binding to the cell surface, the entire complex undergoes endocytosis and subsequent translocation of the light chain into the nerve cell cytoplasm. The light chain contains a zinc-requiring endopeptidase that cleaves soluble *N*-ethylmaleimide sensitive factor (NSF) attachment protein receptor (SNARE) proteins belonging to the docking–fusion complex required for neuroexocytosis of ACh. These proteins may be associated with the synaptic vesicles (v-SNARE) or with their targets on the presynaptic membrane (t-SNARE). Botulinum neurotoxin types A and E proteolyze the t-SNARE protein known as synaptosomal-associated protein (SNAP)-25, and BoNT type C cleaves both SNAP-25 and syntaxin, which is attached to SNAP-25 and to the presynaptic membrane. Botulinum neurotoxin types B, D, F, and G target the v-SNARE protein VAMP/synapto synaptobrevin. As a result of cleavage of these components of the docking complex by the endopeptidase, ACh is not released and neuromuscular transmission is impaired.

CLINICAL MANIFESTATIONS

Foodborne Botulism

Although botulism is the most dreaded of all food poisonings, the initial phase of the disease often is so subtle that it goes unnoticed. Botulism frequently is misdiagnosed on the first visit to a health care provider.[32] When GI effects are striking and food poisoning is suspected, the differential diagnosis should include other acute poisonings, such as metals; plants; mushrooms; and the common bacterial, viral, and parasitic agents discussed in Chap. 39.

The onset of symptoms typically occurs the day after ingestion. Early GI signs and symptoms of botulism include nausea, vomiting, abdominal distension, and pain. A time lag (from 12 hours to several days but usually not more than 24 hours) typically occurs before neurologic signs and symptoms appear. Common findings include diplopia (often horizontal); blurred vision with impaired accommodation; and bilaterally symmetric flaccid paralysis, which typically begins in cranial muscles and descends to the limbs. Constipation caused by smooth muscle involvement is frequent, and urinary retention and ileus also occur. Anticholinergiclike effects such as dry mouth, dysphagia, and dysarthria or dysphonia (manifested by a nasal quality to the voice) occur, and many patients exhibit fixed mydriatic pupils with ptosis. Deep tendon reflexes are usually reduced or absent. Hypotension and bradycardia sometimes develop, but temperature regulation is normal.

Severe weakness of respiratory muscles necessitates intubation and mechanical ventilation. Approximately 67% of botulism patients with toxin type A require intubation compared with 52% of patients with toxin type B and 39% with toxin type E.[185]

Importantly, mental status and sensation remain normal. These findings, along with the absence of tachycardia, distinguish botulism from the anticholinergic syndrome, which shares many initial features with botulism.

The differential diagnosis of botulism includes a variety of toxicologic and nontoxicologic conditions (Table 38–1). All of these disorders have weakness as a prominent feature, but many are readily differentiated from botulism based on their time course or a history of exposure. The most difficult and frequently encountered diagnostic challenge is differentiating

TABLE 38–1A	Toxicologic Differential Diagnosis of Botulism
Xenobiotic Exposure	**Typical Associated Findings**
Aminoglycosides	Paralysis (usually in a patient with myasthenia gravis or other neuromuscular disorders)
Anticholinergics	Mydriasis, vasodilation, fever, tachycardia, ileus, dry mucosa, urinary retention, altered mental status
Batrachotoxin (eg, poison dart frog)	Paralysis almost instantaneous, cardiac arrest
Buckthorn (*Karwinskia humboldtiana*)	Rapidly progressive ascending paralytic neuropathy with quadriplegia
Carbon monoxide	Headache, nausea, altered mental status, tachypnea, elevated carboxyhemoglobin level
Conotoxin (cone snails)	Burning, itching, and edema at site of sting; circumoral paresthesias; nausea; facial muscle paralysis, ptosis, sialorrhea; respiratory and cardiac arrest
Depolarizing and nondepolarizing neuromuscular blockers (eg, curare, succinylcholine, rocuronium, vecuronium)	Paralysis without sedation or sensory involvement
Diphtheria	Exudative pharyngitis, cardiac manifestations, hypotension, demyelinating neuropathy with cranial nerve involvement (late)
Bungarotoxin (Elapids: kraits, coral snakes, sea snakes)	Cramps, fasciculations, tremor, salivation, nausea, vomiting followed by bulbar palsy and paralysis including slurred speech, diplopia, ptosis, dysphagia, dyspnea, respiratory compromise
Organic phosphorus compounds, carbamates	Salivation, lacrimation, urination, defecation, miosis, fasciculations, bronchorrhea, delayed neuropathy
Paralytic shellfish poisoning (saxitoxin, neosaxitoxin)	Incubation <1 h, dysesthesias, paresthesias, dysphagia, respiratory paralysis
Tetrodotoxin (pufferfish, blue-ringed octopus, *Taricha* newts)	Nausea, diarrhea; circumoral paresthesias, dizziness, hypotension, bradycardia. When severe: hypersalivation, cyanosis, diaphoresis, dysphagia, anarthria.
Thallium	Alopecia, painful ascending sensory neuropathy, constipation, cranial neuropathy, Mees lines

TABLE 38–1B Nontoxicologic Differential Diagnosis of Botulism

Condition	Typical Associated Findings
Electrolyte abnormalities	
• Hyperkalemia	Fatigue, dyspnea, palpitations, nausea, vomiting, paresthesias
• Hypokalemia	Fatigue, exercise intolerance, myalgia, dyspnea, palpitations or dysrhythmia
• Hypermagnesemia	Hyporeflexia, facial paresthesias, respiratory depression, hypotension, bradycardia, ileus, diffuse flushing, nausea, vomiting
Encephalitis	Fever, altered mental status, seizures; CSF showing elevated protein and pleocytosis
Food "poisoning" (other bacterial)	Rapid onset of disease; absence of cranial nerve findings
Guillain-Barré syndrome or acute inflammatory demyelinating polyneuropathy (and Miller Fisher variant)	Areflexia, paresthesias, ataxia, CSF showing elevated protein without pleocytosis, slowed nerve conduction velocity; ophthalmoparesis in Miller Fisher syndrome
Hypokalemic periodic paralysis	Proximal muscle weakness; no cranial nerve involvement or sensory findings
Inflammatory or infectious myelopathy and polyradiculopathy	Complete (transverse) or incomplete spinal syndrome with paraparesis or sensory level or sensory signs; possible sphincter dysfunction or back pain; may be preceded by viral illness; CSF pleocytosis and elevated protein
Lambert-Eaton myasthenic syndrome	Neoplasm (especially small cell lung cancer), limb weakness exceeding ocular or bulbar weakness, increased strength after sustained contractions; postexercise facilitation on repetitive nerve stimulation; antibodies to voltage-gated calcium channels
Myasthenia gravis	Aggravation of fatigue with exercise, fluctuating weakness, acetylcholine receptor or muscle-specific (MuSK) antibodies, positive edrophonium test, decremental response on high-frequency repetitive nerve stimulation
Poliomyelitis	Fever, GI symptoms, asymmetric weakness; CSF showing elevated protein and pleocytosis
Polymyositis	Insidious onset; proximal limb weakness; dysphagia; muscle tenderness sometimes present; elevated creatine kinase, aldolase, C-reactive protein, and ESR; fibrillations and sharp waves on electromyography
Stroke	Asymmetric weakness, abnormal brain imaging
Tetanus	Rigidity; cranial nerves usually normal
Tick paralysis (Dermacentor spp)	Rapidly evolving paralysis, ptosis, absence of paresthesias; normal CSF analysis, presence of an embedded tick with resolution upon removal

CSF = cerebrospinal fluid; ESR = erythrocyte sedimentation rate; GI = gastrointestinal.

between botulism and the Miller Fisher variant of Guillain-Barré syndrome (Table 38–2). Because physicians so rarely encounter botulism (especially compared with other much more common disorders in the differential diagnosis), initiation of appropriate management often is significantly delayed. The index case of an epidemic or an isolated case often is misdiagnosed at a stage when the risk of morbidity and mortality still could be substantially diminished. This is particularly true of toxin type E botulism, which typically initially causes much more prominent GI signs than neurologic signs.[17]

Infant Botulism
First described in California in 1976, several thousand cases of infant botulism have now been confirmed across the world,[9,85,90] from all inhabited continents except Africa.[70] Interestingly, 95% of reported cases occur in the United States.[56,130] In 2016, 47 of 150 laboratory-confirmed cases occurred in California.[39] Aggressive surveillance and educational efforts have been practiced in that state since 1976, which may help to explain the disproportionate distribution of reported cases.[8]

TABLE 38–2 Differentiating Botulism from Guillain-Barré Syndrome

	Botulism	Guillain-Barré Syndrome	Miller Fisher Variant of Guillain-Barré Syndrome
Fever	Absent (except in wound botulism)	Occasionally present	Occasionally present
Pupils	Dilated or unreactive (50%)	Normal	Normal
Ophthalmoparesis	Present (early)	May be present (late)	Present (early)
Paralysis	Descending	Ascending (classically, but not necessarily)	Descending
Deep tendon reflexes	Diminished	Absent	Absent
Ataxia	Absent	Often present	Present
Paresthesias	Absent	Present	Present
CSF protein	Normal	Elevated (late)	Elevated (late)

CSF = cerebrospinal fluid.

Infant botulism is the most common form of botulism in the United States, and virtually all cases are caused by BoNT type A or B. Affected children are younger than 1 year (median, 15 weeks) and characteristically have normal gestation and birth. The first signs of infant botulism are constipation; difficulty with feeding, sucking, and swallowing; a feeble cry; and diffusely decreased muscle tone ("floppy baby").[50] The hypotonia is particularly apparent in the limbs and neck. Ophthalmoplegia, loss of facial grimacing, dysphagia, diminished gag reflex, poor anal sphincter tone, and respiratory failure are often present, but fever does not occur. Mydriasis typically is present. The differential diagnosis of infant botulism initially includes salt and water depletion, failure to thrive, sepsis, and a viral syndrome. Because the toxin in infant botulism is absorbed gradually as it is produced, the onset of clinical manifestations commonly is less abrupt than in severe cases of foodborne botulism, which are caused by large amounts of preformed toxin absorbed over a brief period of time.

Infant botulism results from ingestion of *C. botulinum* organisms in food or following the inhalation or ingestion of organism-laden aerosolized dust. Many cases occur near construction sites or soil disruption for other reasons, or in children of parents who work in construction, farming, plant nursery, or plumbing.[63] A number of factors determine a child's susceptibility to development of botulism. Although bile acids and gastric acid in the GI tract inhibit clostridial growth in older children and adults, gastric acidity is reduced in the infant during the first few months of life.[109] Also, some infants are deficient in immunologic mechanisms for spore control, resulting in a permissive environment for spore germination and toxin development within their GI tracts with subsequent absorption. Approximately 70% of infant botulism cases occur in breastfed infants, even though only 45% to 50% of all infants are breastfed. Formula-fed infants are rapidly colonized by *Coliforme* spp, *Enterococcus* spp, and *Bacteroides* spp, which inhibit *C. botulinum* proliferation; conversely, the absence of these typical organisms in breastfed infants facilitates *C. botulinum* multiplication.[85]

Epidemiologic studies in Europe found that ingestion of honey was associated with 59% of cases of infant botulism.[15] When *C. botulinum* spores were isolated from honey implicated in cases of infant botulism, the same toxin type was isolated from the infant and, as expected, no preformed toxin was isolated from the honey.[9] It is possible that pollen and nectar carried by worker bees results in contamination of honey with spores of *Clostridia* found in soil.[124] In addition, the oxidative metabolism of *Bacillus alvei*, another common contaminant of honey, may promote spore germination by creating a anaerobic microenvironment.[121] Honey is the only food generally considered likely to be a risk factor for infant botulism,[9] although a 2001 report from the United Kingdom implicated an infant formula.[28]

Previous studies suggested a correlation between the presence of both *C. botulinum* organisms and toxin and sudden infant death syndrome (SIDS).[8,161] However, in a prospective study of 248 infants with SIDS, *C. botulinum* was not found in the stool cultures of any of the children.[33]

Patients with infant botulism must be managed in the hospital, preferably in a pediatric intensive care unit, at least for the first week, when the risk of respiratory arrest is greatest. In one study, approximately 80% of children with botulism required intubation for reduced vital capacity on pulmonary function testing, and 25% of these children had frank respiratory compromise.[148] In a group of 57 affected infants aged 18 days to 7 months managed during the decade ending in the mid-1980s, 77% were intubated, and 68% required mechanical ventilation. In the subsequent decade, investigators from the same institution found that 37 of 60 (62%) infants required endotracheal intubation (for a mean duration of 21 days).[4] The apparent decrease in intubations and complications was ascribed to better understanding of disease progression and closer observation of patients. However, a similar study at another institution revealed that 13 of 24 (54%) infants admitted between 1985 and 1994 required ventilatory support, compared to 15 of 20 (75%) infants admitted in the subsequent decade.[171] All but one patient in this study required nasogastric feeding. In one series, younger patients were more likely to require mechanical ventilation.[127] Airway complications of intubation such as stridor, granuloma formation, and subglottic stenosis are common, yet tracheotomy is infrequently required.[4] The survival rate in infant botulism is approximately 98% and most patients are discharged home from the hospital.[127,148]

Wound Botulism

The first recorded case of wound botulism occurred in 1943 and was reported in 1951.[59] The classic presentation of wound botulism involves a motor vehicle crash resulting in a deep muscle laceration, crush injury, or compound fracture treated with open reduction. The wound typically is dirty and associated with inadequate débridement, subsequent purulent drainage, and local tenderness, although in some cases, the wound appears clean and uninfected. Four to 18 days later, cranial nerve palsies and other neurologic findings typical of botulism appear.[119] Other manifestations characteristic of food-related botulism, such as GI symptoms, usually are absent.

In wound botulism, an abscess, sinusitis, or other tissue infection harbors the Clostridial organisms. Recognition of botulism as a potential complication of wound infections is essential for appropriate early and aggressive therapy. In one analysis, fever was present in only 7% of patients with wound botulism.[77]

The CDC identified 24 cases of wound botulism in the United States in 2014.[39] Botulinum neurotoxin type A accounted for 88% of the cases.[39] Use of heroin, particularly subcutaneous injection ("skin popping") of black tar heroin, is associated with an increased risk of wound botulism.[53,132,183] This association appears to be related, at least in part, to the physical characteristics of black tar heroin such as its viscosity, its potential to facilitate anaerobic growth and spore germination, and its ability to devitalize tissue or inhibit wound resolution.[20] Wound botulism also is reported in association with subcutaneous,[138] intraveneous,[164] and intranasal[98,139] cocaine use. The first case of wound botulism with BoNT type E was reported in 2007, affecting a drug user in Sweden.[13]

Adult Intestinal Colonization Botulism

Although GI colonization is the typical pathogenic mechanism responsible for infant botulism, it is rare in adults. Prior to 1997, only 15 cases were reported.[79,117] Patients invariably have anatomic or functional GI abnormalities. Risk factors favoring organism persistence and *C. botulinum* colonization include achlorhydria (surgically or pharmacologically induced), previous intestinal surgery, and probably recent antibiotic therapy. These factors compromise the gastric and bile acid barrier, gut flora, and motility, thus allowing spore germination, altered bacterial growth, and toxin development.

Cases of adult infectious botulism are reported in patients with Crohn disease after ileal bypass surgery,[79] jejunoileal bypass for obesity,[73,116] gastroduodenostomy,[116] vagotomy and pyloroplasty,[116] and necrotic volvulus.[107] In such hosts, botulism results from the ingestion of food contaminated with *C. botulinum* organisms and no preformed toxin, with intraluminal elaboration of toxin occurring in vivo.[56]

In one case of adult intestinal colonization botulism, a high concentration of endogenously produced antibody to toxin type A was identified.[79] This finding highlights a distinct characteristic of this form of botulism, because endogenous antitoxin immunity does not develop in patients with foodborne botulism.[147]

Iatrogenic Botulism

Botulinum toxins are used therapeutically in the treatment of a variety of disorders. Three preparations of BoNT type A are available in the United States: onabotulinumtoxinA (Botox), abobotulinumtoxinA (Dysport), and incobotulinumtoxinA (Xeomin). Botulinum neurotoxin type B is available as rimabotulinumtoxinB (Myobloc). All are approved by the FDA for treatment of cervical dystonia and upper limb spasticity; onabotulinumtoxinA is also approved for lower limb spasticity. OnabotulinumtoxinA and incobotulinumtoxinA are also indicated for treatment of blepharospasm. Additionally, onabotulinumtoxinA is approved for strabismus, chronic migraine, severe axillary hyperhidrosis inadequately managed by topical therapies, and detrusor overactivity associated with a neurologic condition. All three formulations of BoNT type A are approved for cosmetic purposes. Botulinum neurotoxin is also used off-label for a variety of neurologic and non-neuro-logic conditions. In Japan and the United Kingdom, a preparation of BoNT type F is available.[154] Some studies suggest that animals receiving BoNT type F have more transient and reversible weakness than that associated with types A and B.[26]

A 2016 practice guideline update by the American Academy of Neurology assessed the level of evidence of the four BoNT products for various neurologic indications. Based on the evidence, the authors issued Level A recommendations (denoting an intervention that should be offered) for treatment of cervical dystonia with abobotulinumtoxinA or rimabotulinumtoxinB; treatment of upper limb spasticity with abobotulinumtoxinA, incobotulinumtoxinA, or onabotulinumtoxinA; treatment of lower limb spasticity with abobotulinumtoxinA or onabotulinumtoxinA; and treatment of chronic migraine with onabotulinumtoxinA.[159]

Botulinum neurotoxin is thought to exert its therapeutic effect in most cases by temporarily weakening muscles whose overactivity results in the clinical condition. Doses range widely depending on the size of the muscles to be treated, the severity of the muscular contraction, and the commercial preparation of the toxin. The injected toxin blocks the local neuromuscular junction by inhibiting release of acetylcholine. The "chemodenervated" muscles recover within 2 to 4 months as nerve transmission is restored through sprouting of new nerve endings and formation of functional connections at motor endplates,[2,147] necessitating repeated injections of BoNT for sustained clinical efficacy.

Doses of BoNT are measured in functional units corresponding to the median intraperitoneal lethal dose (LD_{50}) in female Swiss-Webster mice weighing 18 to 20 g.[131] The units of each marketed pharmaceutical are distinctly different, which has led to inadvertent overdosing.[175] The potential for confusion is substantial when switching between products because their relative potencies are quite different.[125,144,151] Attempts to establish precise lethal doses of BoNT are complicated by the lack of human data, use of varying formulations of toxin by different investigators, changes in manufacturing processes, and factual errors in the published literature.[29] One group of investigators estimated that "lethal amounts of crystalline type A toxin for a 70-kg human would be approximately 0.09 to 0.15 mcg intravenously or intramuscularly, 0.70 to 0.90 mcg inhalationally, and 70 mcg orally,"[10] but it is unclear whether these values can be applied reliably to any currently available commercial product.

In a series of 139 patients with cervical dystonia randomized to treatment with BoNT type A or BoNT type B, no difference in efficacy was found between serotypes; the groups were also equivalent in frequency of adverse effects such as neck pain and neck weakness, but dry mouth and dysphagia were more common in the group treated with BoNT type B.[57]

After repeated injections of therapeutic doses of BoNT, patients develop neutralizing antibodies that would limit the subsequent efficacy of the toxins; this prompts switching to a different toxin type. In 1998, the formulation of Botox was changed to reduce the amount of potentially antigenic protein from 25 ng of neurotoxin complex protein per 100 units to 5 ng of complex protein per 100 units, and studies in patients with cervical dystonia demonstrate a sixfold lower rate of development of anti-BoNT antibodies with the newer formulation.[89] For Xeomin, the protein content is 0.6 ng per 100 units; Dysport contains 4.35 ng of protein per 500-unit vial (ie, 0.87 ng per 100 units).

Although one early marketing assumption was that the neurotoxin does not diffuse from the injection site, BoNT can diffuse into adjacent tissues and produce local adverse effects.[141] Systemic manifestations are of concern when an inadvertent, excessive, or misdirected dose of toxin is administered or in the setting of a neuromuscular disorder that may be previously undiagnosed, as in one case in which injection of BoNT type A unmasked Lambert-Eaton myasthenic syndrome (LEMS).[66] In addition, a number of studies demonstrate that even appropriately injected doses result in neuromuscular junction abnormalities throughout the body, occasionally producing autonomic dysfunction without muscle weakness.[75,101,126] Several cases of iatrogenic botulismlike symptoms, including diplopia and severe generalized muscle weakness with widespread electromyographic (EMG) abnormalities,

resulted from therapeutic or cosmetic use of intramuscular BoNT injections.[18,24,69,172,187] A 2008 report raised the possibility that BoNT type A undergoes retrograde axonal transport and transcytosis to afferent neurons,[5] suggesting a potential mechanism for such generalized effects. However, the reproducibility and clinical significance of these findings have yet to be established.

In a much publicized case from late 2004, four patients in Florida developed paralysis after being injected with BoNT type A. An FDA investigation revealed that these patients were injected by an unlicensed physician who obtained raw toxin (not approved for medical purposes) and administered it at a dose 2,000 to 100,000 times greater than that used in clinical practice.[3] These events were not believed to be relevant to the use of approved pharmaceutical BoNT. In February 2008, the FDA issued an Early Communication stating that it was reviewing safety data on BoNT after receiving reports of hospitalization or death in patients injected with these therapies, mostly in children treated for spasticity associated with cerebral palsy.[173] In 2009, the FDA mandated changes to the prescribing information for the BoNT products, requiring a Boxed Warning highlighting the possibility of potentially life-threatening effects distant from the injection site; a Risk Evaluation and Mitigation Strategy, including a medication guide to help patients understand the risks and benefits of the botulinum neurotoxin; and changes of the drug names to underscore differences between the potencies of the individual products and the lack of interchangeability among them.[175]

Inhalational Botulism

Inhaled BoNT is estimated to be 100 times more potent than ingested BoNT; a single gram of toxin, if disseminated evenly, could kill more than 1 million people.[10] A 1962 report from West Germany described three veterinary workers who inhaled BoNT type A from the fur of animals they were handling; on the third day after exposure, they developed mucus in the throat, dysphagia, and dizziness, and on the next day, they developed ophthalmoparesis, mydriasis, dysarthria, gait dysfunction, and weakness.[10] Use of aerosolized BoNT as a bioweapon has been attempted by terrorists in Japan, and both the Soviet Union and Iraq developed BoNT as part of biological warfare programs (Chap. 127).[10,61,188]

DIAGNOSTIC TESTING

The CDC case definition for foodborne botulism is established in a patient with a neurologic disorder manifested by diplopia, blurred vision, bulbar weakness, or symmetric paralysis in whom:

- Botulinum neurotoxin is detected in serum, stool, or implicated food samples or
- *C. botulinum* is isolated from stool *or*
- A clinically compatible case is epidemiologically linked to a laboratory-confirmed case of botulism[46]

Routine laboratory studies, including cerebrospinal fluid analysis, are normal in patients with botulism but are usually performed to exclude other etiologies. Specific tests can be helpful in diagnosing botulism.

Edrophonium Testing

Edrophonium is a rapidly acting cholinesterase inhibitor of short duration that is useful in the diagnosis of myasthenia gravis. It is occasionally used to differentiate myasthenia gravis from botulism. This drug inhibits the metabolism of acetylcholine located in synapses, permitting continued binding with the reduced number of postsynaptic acetylcholine receptors in myasthenia gravis.

A syringe containing 10 mg of edrophonium is prepared, and then a test dose of 1 to 2 mg is administered intravenously. A positive result (ie, supportive of myasthenia gravis) consists of dramatic improvement in the strength of weak muscles within 30 to 60 seconds and lasting 3 to 5 minutes. If there is no effect, the remainder of the edrophonium is given and the same effect sought. Ideally, a second syringe is filled with saline and the test performed

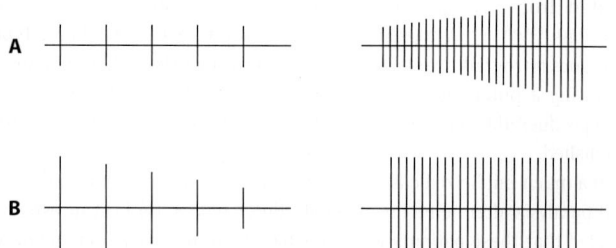

FIGURE 38–2. Schematic representations of repetitive nerve stimulation at low (5/sec) and high (50/sec) frequencies. In botulism (**A**), stimulation produces a small muscle action potential that is facilitated (increases in amplitude) by repetitive stimulation at higher frequencies. This effect (which, although classic, is not found in all cases of botulism) results from increased acetylcholine release with high-frequency stimulation because of intracellular calcium accumulation. In contrast, myasthenia gravis (**B**) is associated with a normal muscle action potential amplitude and a decremental response at low-frequency stimulation with a normal response at high-frequency stimulation. Myasthenia gravis, a disorder of the muscle endplate, produces this decremental response at low frequencies because the natural reduction in acetylcholine response with subsequent stimulation falls below threshold.

under double-blind conditions to ensure accurate assessment and remove the potential of a placebo effect.

Because release of acetylcholine is impaired in botulism, preventing its catabolism with an anticholinesterase medication typically has little clinical benefit, but a weaker effect is occasionally observed if some neurons maintain the ability to release acetylcholine. Thus, in rare cases, early in the course of botulism, injection of edrophonium results in limited improvement in strength, but this is far less dramatic than the improvement that occurs in patients with myasthenia gravis.[136]

Electrophysiologic Testing

In all forms of botulism, sensory nerve action potentials are normal. Motor potentials in severely affected muscles typically are reduced in amplitude, but conduction velocity is not affected. Repetitive nerve stimulation at high frequencies would be expected to result in an increment of the amplitude of the motor potential, given the presynaptic localization of the defect, but this finding is neither sensitive nor specific; it also is more common in disease caused by BoNT type B than with type A.[55,110] A marked incremental response with high-frequency repetitive stimulation is more likely to suggest LEMS than botulism. Likewise, a decremental response to low-frequency repetitive nerve stimulation is characteristic of LEMS but is not consistently present in botulism.[110]

The needle EMG examination in botulism is characterized by low-amplitude, short-duration motor unit action potentials (MUAPs) caused by blockade of neuromuscular transmission in many muscle fibers (Fig. 38–2).

Polyphasic MUAPs are also common. Recruitment is usually normal but is reduced in severely affected muscles if all muscle fibers of a motor unit are blocked. Spontaneous activity, including positive sharp waves and fibrillation potentials, is often seen. Single-fiber EMG is useful in demonstrating abnormal neuromuscular transmission; for patients who cannot control voluntary muscle activation (eg, as infants), stimulated jitter analysis is proposed but is not universally available.[129,177]

Although these electrodiagnostic abnormalities support the diagnosis of botulism, there are no pathognomonic electrophysiologic findings. Nerve conduction studies and EMG are most useful for excluding alternative diagnoses, including Guillain-Barré syndrome and other neuropathies (both demyelinating and axonal), poliomyelitis, myasthenia gravis, and myopathies. Occasionally, muscle biopsy is necessary to exclude a myopathic process.[110]

Laboratory Testing

If foodborne botulism is suspected, samples of serum, stool, vomitus, gastric contents, and suspected foods should be subjected to anaerobic culture (for *C. botulinum*) and mouse bioassay (for BoNT) (Table 38–3). A list of the patient's medications should accompany each sample to exclude other xenobiotics that might interfere with the assay (eg, pyridostigmine) or be toxic to the mice. The serum samples must be collected before initiation of antitoxin therapy. When wound botulism is considered, serum, stool, exudate, débrided tissue, and swab samples should be collected. For infant botulism, feces and serum samples also should be obtained. In infants who are constipated, an enema with nonbacteriostatic sterile water will facilitate collection. All enema fluid and stool should be sent for analysis. The specimens should be refrigerated (not frozen) and examined as soon as possible after collection. Detailed information on specimen collection and examination is available online from the CDC (https://www.cdc.gov/botulism/pdf/bot-manual.pdf).[45]

In the mouse lethality assay, which remains the gold standard for diagnosis, the sample (serum, stool, or food) is injected intraperitoneally into mice, which are then observed for development of signs of botulism. Control mice are injected with the sample as well as antitoxin. This test is very sensitive, with a detection limit of 0.01 ng/mL of sample eluate. However, it is laborious and expensive, and a positive result is often delayed for several days, reducing its usefulness in early diagnosis of botulism.[104] Alternative methods for detecting BoNT, including immunologic methods (eg, enzyme-linked immunosorbent assay, endopeptidase assays, and analysis of synaptic activity in neuronal cell cultures) have been used successfully.[23,135,140,158]

Clostridium botulinum can be cultured under strict anaerobic conditions. Stool specimens are incubated anaerobically and then subcultured on egg yolk agar to assess for lipase production, although this test is not specific as other clostridia also produce lipase. Various protocols using polymerase chain reaction and probe hybridization to detect and identify *C. botulinum* are described but are not widely applied in clinical practice.[94,104]

TABLE 38–3	Epidemiologic and Laboratory Assessment of Botulism[a]			
Classification	**Foodborne**	**Infant**	**Wound**	**Adult Intestinal Colonization**
BoNT type	A, B, E, F, G in humans; C, D in animals	A, B, C, F, H	A, B	A
Route	Ingestion of toxin	Ingestion of bacteria and spores	Wound, abscess (sinusitis)	Ingestion of bacteria and spores
Specimens	Stool: positive for bacteria/spores and toxin	Stool: positive for bacteria/spores and toxin for up to 8 wk after recovery	Wound site: Gram stain, aerobic and anaerobic cultures; positive for bacteria/spores	Stool: positive for bacteria/spores and toxin
BoNT in serum	Yes	Yes (but low sensitivity)	Yes	Yes
Bacteria/spores[a] in food	Yes	Yes	Not applicable	Yes
BoNT in food	Yes	No	Not applicable	No

[a]"Bacteria/spores" refers to *C. botulinum*.

BoNT = botulinum toxin.

MANAGEMENT
Supportive Care
Respiratory compromise is the usual cause of death from botulism. To prevent or treat this complication, hospital admission of the patient and of all individuals with suspected exposure is mandatory. Careful continuous monitoring of respiratory status using parameters such as vital capacity, peak expiratory flow rate, negative inspiratory force (NIF), pulse oximetry, end-tidal CO_2, and the presence or absence of a gag reflex is essential to determine the need for intubation if a patient begins to manifest signs of bulbar paralysis.[148] The NIF is the most reliable, readily obtainable test for determining the need for intubation. When suspicion of botulism is high and the vital capacity is less than 20 mL/kg or the NIF is poorer than –30 cm H_2O, intubation is generally indicated.[102,118]

Reverse Trendelenburg positioning at 20 to 25 degrees with cervical support has been suggested to be beneficial by enhancing diaphragmatic function. In theory, this approach would reduce the risk of aspiration while decreasing the pressure of abdominal viscera on the diaphragm, with resultant improvement in ventilatory effort. However, its clinical application to seriously ill patients has not been validated.[10]

In addition to attention to respiratory issues, patients require nutrition (enteral or parenteral), prompt recognition and treatment of secondary infections, and prophylaxis against deep vein thromboses.

Gastrointestinal Decontamination
Removal of the spores and toxin from the gut should be attempted. Although most patients present after a substantial time delay, the bacteria or BoNT (or both) can still be present hours or even days later. Activated charcoal is recommended as a routine part of supportive care because in vitro it adsorbs BoNT type A and probably also the other BoNT types.[76] Gastric lavage or emesis should be initiated only for an asymptomatic person who has very recently ingested a known contaminated food. If a cathartic is chosen, sorbitol is preferable because other cathartics such as magnesium salts potentially exacerbate neuromuscular blockade. Theoretically, whole-bowel irrigation has a role in decontamination, particularly if there is concern about initiating emesis, but interventions other than activated charcoal have not been evaluated under these circumstances.

Wound Care
Thorough wound débridement is the most critical aspect in the management of wound botulism and should be performed promptly.[86,107] Antibiotic therapy alone is inadequate, as evidenced by several case reports of disease despite antibiotic therapy. Penicillin G is one of many drugs with excellent in vitro antimicrobial efficacy against C. botulinum and is useful for wound management.[165] However, penicillin has no role in the management of botulism caused by preformed toxin nor does it prevent gut spores from germinating. For these reasons, penicillin is not considered useful in infant and adult infectious botulism, and it is not by itself adequate for wound botulism. We recommend against using medications that interfere with neuromuscular transmission, such as aminoglycoside[146] and fluoroquinolone antibiotics[91] and clindamycin.[150]

Guanidine, Dalfampridine, and 3,4-Diaminopyridine
Guanidine is no longer recommended for treatment of botulism because its merits were not substantiated.[68,92] (See previous editions of this text for a more extensive discussion.) Several studies[145] and case reports[62] have proposed that dalfampridine (4-aminopyridine) and 3,4-diaminopyridine are effective in improving neuromuscular transmission by enhancing acetylcholine release from the motor nerve terminal. In a rat BoNT type A model of botulism, 3,4-diaminopyridine restored neuromuscular function and enhanced animal survival.[156] Results in humans have been mostly disheartening,[60,157] but given the promising animal data and the apparent response in some patients,[74] along with the effectiveness in patients with LEMS, further investigative efforts may prove fruitful. Dalfampridine (Ampyra) is FDA approved to improve walking in patients with multiple sclerosis, but its potential to induce seizures at therapeutic doses limits its clinical usefulness. The fact that 3,4-diaminopyridine does not substantially cross the blood–brain barrier, resulting in limited central nervous system manifestations, makes this xenobiotic appropriate for further investigation, but cannot be recommended for routine use at the current time.

Botulinum Antitoxin
Since the 1960s, passive immunization with antitoxin has been used to neutralize unbound BoNT. In the United States, botulinum antitoxin (BAT) is available for adults and children older than 1 year through the CDC, the Alaska Division of Public Health, and the California Department of Public Health. State public health officials can obtain the antitoxin through the CDC by calling 770-488-7100. In 2013, the FDA approved a heptavalent BAT containing equine-derived antibody to botulinum toxin types A through G. It currently is the only BAT available in the United States for the treatment of botulism in adults and for cases of infant botulism caused by nerve toxins other than types A and B.[174]

Because of the rarity and severity of botulism, randomized controlled studies of antitoxin in humans are neither feasible nor ethical. The current heptavalent BAT was shown to increase survival in guinea pig and rhesus macaque animal models.[22] In a CDC analysis of an open-label observational study involving 109 patients with suspected or confirmed botulism, treatment with BAT within 2 days of symptom onset was associated with a shorter length of hospitalization (13.7 days less), shorter duration in intensive care unit (6.6 days less), and shorter duration of mechanical ventilation (11.8 days less) compared with patients treated later.[22] Because of the benefit of earlier treatment, physicians should contact their state health department at the time the diagnosis of botulism is first suspected to expedite obtaining antitoxin from the CDC.

In a review of 132 cases of type A foodborne botulism from 1984 (when only trivalent antitoxin was available), a lower fatality rate and a shorter course of illness were demonstrated for patients who received the antitoxin, even after controlling for age and incubation period.[166] The earlier a patient received antitoxin, the shorter was the clinical course. In addition, no respiratory arrests occurred more than 5 hours after antitoxin was administered. Two studies on the use of antitoxin in the presence of wound botulism demonstrated that the longer the delay to antitoxin administration, the more prolonged the requirement for ventilatory support and the poorer the outcome.[54]

Serum, stool, and gastric aspirate samples should be collected before administration of antitoxin. In adults (17 years and older), the entire vial of botulinal antitoxin should be given intravenously as a 1:10 vol/vol dilution in 0.9% sodium chloride at rate of 0.5 mL/min for 30 minutes, optionally increasing to 1 mL/min for 30 minutes and then 2 mL/min if tolerated. In children 1 to 17 years of age, the dose and infusion rate are modified based on body weight; in infants (younger than 1 year), the dose is 10% of the adult dose and infusion rate is based on body weight.[22] Premedication with corticosteroids and antihistamines is reasonable in children and in patients with a suspected history of reaction to equine-derived products. Epinephrine and diphenhydramine should be readily available to treat anaphylaxis or hypersensitivity reactions.[22] The overall rate of adverse reactions, including hypersensitivity and serum sickness,[27] to equine-derived BATs is reported as 9% to 17%, with an incidence of anaphylaxis as high as 1.9%.[17,120] However, because BAT is despeciated, the risk of such reactions likely is lower.

The antitoxin neutralizes only unbound toxin; consequently, it can prevent paralysis but does not affect already paralyzed muscles.[72] Because of the potential lethality of foodborne botulism, the antitoxin should be given to patients in whom the diagnosis is suspected; treatment should not be delayed while awaiting laboratory confirmation of the diagnosis. In the event of a potential outbreak of foodborne botulism, asymptomatic individuals should be closely monitored for early signs of illness so that antitoxin can be administered promptly[153] (Antidotes in Depth: A6).

Treatment of Infant Botulism

Similar to adults, infants with botulism require intensive care, with meticulous monitoring for respiratory compromise and autonomic dysfunction.[133] Constipation can be severe.

In October 2003, the FDA licensed human-derived botulism antitoxin antibodies as botulism immune globulin (BabyBIG) for treatment of infant botulism types A and B.[7] A randomized trial of 122 cases of infant botulism showed that treatment with intravenous botulism immune globulin significantly reduced the length of hospital stay and intensive care, duration of mechanical ventilation and tube or intravenous feeding, and cost of hospitalization relative to placebo without causing serious adverse effects.[11,71] Similar results were seen in a 2007 retrospective chart review.[176] BabyBIG is available from the California Department of Health Services Infant Botulism Treatment and Prevention Program (510-231-7600; http://www.infantbotulism.org).[34]

Prevention

Measures used to prevent infant botulism include limiting exposure to spores by thoroughly washing foods and objects that might be placed in a child's mouth. In addition, honey should not be given to infants younger than 6 months of age.

Vaccination strategies are under investigation, including several recombinant vaccines that have shown promise in protecting against botulism in animal and human trials.[19,160] Future approaches may include treatments that inhibit BoNT trafficking or promote toxin clearance or acetylcholine potentiation, among other mechanisms.[16,95]

PROGNOSIS

The prolonged and variable period of recovery that occurs after exposure to BoNT is directly related to the extent of neuromuscular blockade and neurogenic atrophy as well as the regeneration rates of nerve endings and presynaptic membranes.[111] If the patient has excellent respiratory support during the acute phase and receives adequate parenteral nutrition, residual neurologic disability may not occur. Although the initial course sometimes is protracted, near-total functional recovery can follow within several months to 1 year. Common long-term sequelae include dysgeusia, dry mouth, constipation, dyspepsia, arthralgia, exertional dyspnea, tachycardia, and easy fatigability.

The status of 13 patients who survived a toxin type B botulinum outbreak was characterized 2 years later by persistent dyspnea and fatigue, although surprisingly, pulmonary function test results had returned to normal in all patients.[184] Inspiratory muscle weakness persisted in 4 of 13 patients. Maximal oxygen consumption and maximal workload during exercise were diminished in all patients, and all had more rapid shallow breathing and a higher dyspnea score than controls. The reasons for premature exercise termination may be multifactorial. Although persistent respiratory muscle weakness may be an explanation, most dyspnea and fatigue appeared to be related to reduced cardiovascular fitness, leg fatigue, and diminished nutrition.[184]

A 2007 case-control series reported long-term outcomes in 217 adults with foodborne botulism in the Republic of Georgia. Six patients died; the remaining 211 were interviewed a median of 4.3 years after onset of disease. They were significantly more likely than control participants to report ongoing fatigue, dizziness, weakness, dry mouth, difficulty lifting things, and difficulty breathing with moderate exertion.[78]

PREGNANCY

At least eight cases of botulism occurring during pregnancy are reported.[30] None of the neonates had neurologic evidence of botulism, though two (one with a heroin-abusing mother) had complications apparently unrelated to the botulism.[122,162] The large molecular weight of the neurotoxin (150 kDa) makes passive diffusion through the placenta unlikely, and experimental results in rabbits attest that this does not take place.[87] Appropriate care of the affected mother and preparation for maternal complications of delivery appear to ensure the best potential outcome for the infant.

All commercially available BoNT products are FDA Pregnancy Category C. Published case reports regarding therapeutic use of BoNT during pregnancy mostly describe uncomplicated births, although two miscarriages have been reported. In a review of 137 prospective pregnancies in the Allergan safety database of women treated with onabotulinumtoxinA during pregnancy or within 3 months before pregnancy, 79% resulted in live births, of which 2.7% were associated with fetal defects. These prevalence rates are said to be similar to those in the general population.[30]

It is unknown whether BoNT is excreted in breast milk.

EPIDEMIOLOGIC AND THERAPEUTIC ASSISTANCE

Whenever botulism is suspected or proven, the local health department should be contacted. The health department should report to the CDC Emergency Operations Center at 770-488-7100. The CDC can provide or facilitate diagnostic, consultative, and laboratory testing services, access to BAT, and assistance in epidemiologic investigations. All foods that are potentially responsible for the illness should be refrigerated and preserved for epidemiologic investigation. The merits of this surveillance and antitoxin release system were demonstrated in Argentina,[178] where the CDC assisted in establishing nation-specific principles, including local stocking of antitoxin and establishing mechanisms for distribution, emergency identification, response, and laboratory confirmation of suspected cases. Expansion of this system to other nations will enhance worldwide botulism surveillance for foodborne botulism and for potential terrorist dissemination of BoNT.[152]

SUMMARY

- Most cases of botulism in the United States affect infants younger than 6 months of age. Because of an epidemiologic association, honey should not be given to babies younger than 1 year of age.
- Most cases of foodborne botulism relate to food processed at home under improper conditions.
- Treatment of botulism should not be delayed while awaiting laboratory confirmation in patients presenting with diplopia, blurred vision, bulbar weakness, or symmetric paralysis.
- BabyBIG, a botulism immune globulin, is available for treatment of infant botulism types A and B, and there is a heptavalent BAT against serotypes A through G for infants with botulism caused by other BoNT types and for noninfants. Treatment should not be delayed while laboratory diagnosis is pending.

Acknowledgment

Neal E. Flomenbaum, MD, contributed to this chapter in previous editions.

REFERENCES

1. Abgueguen P, et al. Nine cases of foodborne botulism type B in France and literature review. *Eur J Clin Microbiol Infect Dis.* 2003;22:749-752.
2. Alderson K, et al. Botulinum-induced alteration of nerve-muscle interactions in the human orbicularis oculi following treatment for blepharospasm. *Neurology.* 1991;41:1800-1800.
3. Allergan I. Allergan's BOTOX—botulinum toxin type A—not the cause of botulism in Florida patients. 2004. http://www.cosmeticsurgery-news.com/article2334.html. Accessed January 16, 2017.
4. Anderson TD, et al. Airway complications of infant botulism: ten-year experience with 60 cases. *Otolaryngol Head Neck Surg.* 2002;126:234-239.
5. Antonucci F, et al. Long-distance retrograde effects of botulinum neurotoxin A. *J Neurosci.* 2008;28:3689-3696.
6. Armada M, et al. Foodborne botulism in a six-month-old infant caused by home-canned baby food. *Ann Emerg Med.* 2003;42:226-229.
7. Arnon SS. Creation and development of the public service orphan drug human botulism immune globulin. *Pediatrics.* 2007;119:785-789.
8. Arnon SS. Infant botulism. In: Feigin RD, Cherry JD, eds. *Textbook of Pediatric Infectious Diseases.* 4th ed. Philadelphia, PA: WB Saunders; 1998:1570-1577.
9. Arnon SS, et al. Honey and other environmental risk factors for infant botulism. *J Pediatr.* 1979;94:331-336.
10. Arnon SS, et al. Botulinum toxin as a biological weapon. *JAMA.* 2001;285:1059.

11. Arnon SS, et al. Human botulism immune globulin for the treatment of infant botulism. *N Engl J Med.* 2006;354:462-471.

12. Arriagada SD, et al. [Infant botulism: case report and review]. *Rev Chilena Infectol.* 2009;26:162-167.

13. Artin I, et al. First case of type E wound botulism diagnosed using real-time PCR. *J Clin Microbiol.* 2007;45:3589-3594.

14. Aureli P, et al. An outbreak in Italy of botulism associated with a dessert made with mascarpone cream cheese. *Eur J Epidemiol.* 2000;16:913-918.

15. Aureli P, et al. Infant botulism and honey in Europe: a commentary. *Pediatr Infect Dis J.* 2002;21:866-868.

16. Azarnia Tehran D, et al. A novel inhibitor prevents the peripheral neuroparalysis of botulinum neurotoxins. *Sci Rep.* 2015;5:17513.

17. Badhey H, et al. Two fatal cases of type E adult food-borne botulism with early symptoms and terminal neurologic signs. *J Clin Microbiol.* 1986;23:616-618.

18. Bakheit AM, et al. Generalised botulism-like syndrome after intramuscular injections of botulinum toxin type A: a report of two cases. *J Neurol Neurosurg Psychiatry.* 1997;62:198-198.

19. Baldwin MR, et al. Subunit vaccine against the seven serotypes of botulism. *Infect Immun.* 2007;76:1314-1318.

20. Bamberger J. Wound botulism associated with black tar heroin. *JAMA.* 1998;280:1479.

21. Barash JR, Arnon SS. A novel strain of *Clostridium botulinum* that produces type B and type H botulinum toxins. *J Infect Dis.* 2014;209:183-191.

22. BAT® [Botulism Antitoxin Heptavalent (A, B, C, D, E, F, G)—(Equine)] [prescribing information]. Winnipeg, Canada: Cangene Corporation; 2015.

23. Beske PH, et al. Botulinum and tetanus neurotoxin-induced blockade of synaptic transmission in networked cultures of human and rodent neurons. *Toxicol Sci.* 2016;149:503-515.

24. Bhatia KP, et al. Generalised muscular weakness after botulinum toxin injections for dystonia: a report of three cases. *J Neurol Neurosurg Psychiatry.* 1999;67:90-93.

25. Bieri PL. Botulinum neurotoxin. In: Spencer PS, et al, eds. *Experimental and Clinical Neurotoxicology.* 2nd ed. New York, NY: Oxford University Press; 2000:xl.

26. Billante CR, et al. Comparison of neuromuscular blockade and recovery with botulinum toxins A and F. *Muscle Nerve.* 2002;26:395-403.

27. Black RE, Gunn RA. Hypersensitivity reactions associated with botulinal antitoxin. *Am J Med.* 1980;69:567-570.

28. Brett MM, et al. A case of infant botulism with a possible link to infant formula milk powder: evidence for the presence of more than one strain of *Clostridium botulinum* in clinical specimens and food. *J Med Microbiol.* 2005;54(Pt 8):769-776.

29. Brin MF, Blitzer A. Botulinum toxin: dangerous terminology errors. *J Royal Soc Med.* 1993;86:493-494.

30. Brin MF, et al. Pregnancy outcomes following exposure to onabotulinumtoxinA. *Pharmacoepidemiol Drug Saf.* 2016;25:179-187.

31. Burke P, et al. Outbreak of foodborne botulism associated with improperly jarred pesto—Ohio and California, 2014. *MMWR Morb Mortal Wkly Rep.* 2016;65:175-177.

32. Burningham MD, et al. Wound botulism. *Ann Emerg Med.* 1994;24:1184-1187.

33. Byard RW, et al. *Clostridium botulinum* and sudden infant death syndrome: a 10 year prospective study. *J Paediatr Child Health.* 1992;28:156-157.

34. California Department of Health Services. Infant Botulism Treatment and Prevention Program. http://www.infantbotulism.org. Accessed January 17, 2017.

35. Centers for Disease Control. Botulism—New Mexico. *MMWR Morb Mortal Wkly Rep.* 1978;27:138.

36. Centers for Disease Control. International outbreak of type E botulism associated with ungutted, salted whitefish. *MMWR Morb Mortal Wkly Rep.* 1987;36:812-813.

37. Centers for Disease Control. Outbreak of type E botulism associated with an uneviscerated, salt-cured fish product—New Jersey, 1992. *MMWR Morb Mortal Wkly Rep.* 1992;41:521-522.

38. Centers for Disease Control. Restaurant-associated botulism from mushrooms bottled in-house—Vancouver, British Columbia, Canada. *MMWR Morb Mortal Wkly Rep.* 1987;36:103.

39. Centers for Disease Control and Prevention. Botulism Annual Summary, 2016. https://www.cdc.gov/botulism/pdf/Botulism-2016-SUMMARY-508.pdf. Accessed May 16, 2018.

40. Centers for Disease Control and Prevention. Botulism associated with commercial carrot juice—Georgia and Florida, September 2006. *MMWR Morb Mortal Wkly Rep.* 2006;55:1098-1099.

41. Centers for Disease Control and Prevention. Botulism associated with commercially canned chili sauce—Texas and Indiana, July 2007. *MMWR Morb Mortal Wkly Rep.* 2007;56:767-769.

42. Centers for Disease Control and Prevention. Botulism associated with home-fermented tofu in two Chinese immigrants—New York City, March-April 2012. *MMWR Morb Mortal Wkly Rep.* 2013;62:529-532.

43. Centers for Disease Control and Prevention. Botulism from drinking prison-made illicit alcohol—Utah 2011. *MMWR Morb Mortal Wkly Rep.* 2012;61:782-784.

44. Centers for Disease Control and Prevention. Botulism from home-canned bamboo shoots—Nan Province, Thailand, March 2006. *MMWR Morb Mortal Wkly Rep.* 2006;55:389-392.

45. Centers for Disease Control and Prevention. Botulism in the United States, 1899–1996. Handbook for Epidemiologists, Clinicians and Laboratory Workers. 1998. https://www.cdc.gov/botulism/pdf/bot-manual.pdf. Accessed January 16, 2017.

46. Centers for Disease Control and Prevention. Case definitions for infectious conditions under public health surveillance. *MMWR Recomm Rep.* 1997;46(Rr-10):1-55.

47. Centers for Disease Control and Prevention. Foodborne botulism associated with home-canned bamboo shoots—Thailand, 1998. *MMWR Morb Mortal Wkly Rep.* 1999;48:437-439.

48. Centers for Disease Control and Prevention. Foodborne botulism from eating home-pickled eggs—Illinois, 1997. *MMWR Morb Mortal Wkly Rep.* 2000;49:778-780.

49. Centers for Disease Control and Prevention. Foodborne botulism from home-prepared fermented tofu—California, 2006. *MMWR Morb Mortal Wkly Rep.* 2007;56:96-97.

50. Centers for Disease Control and Prevention. Infant botulism—New York City, 2001-2002. *MMWR Morb Mortal Wkly Rep.* 2003;52:21-24.

51. Centers for Disease Control and Prevention. Notes from the field: botulism caused by consumption of commercially produced potato soups stored improperly—Ohio and Georgia, 2011. *MMWR Morb Mortal Wkly Rep.* 2011;60:890.

52. Centers for Disease Control and Prevention. Outbreak of botulism type E associated with eating a beached whale—Western Alaska, July 2002. *MMWR Morb Mortal Wkly Rep.* 2003;52:24-26.

53. Centers for Disease Control and Prevention. Wound botulism among black tar heroin users—Washington, 2003. *MMWR Morb Mortal Wkly Rep.* 2003;52:885-886.

54. Chang GY, Ganguly G. Early antitoxin treatment in wound botulism results in better outcome. *Eur Neurol.* 2003;49:151-153.

55. Cherington M. Electrophysiologic methods as an aid in diagnosis of botulism: a review. *Muscle Nerve.* 1982;5:S28-29.

56. Cochran DP, Appleton RE. Infant botulism—is it that rare? *Dev Med Child Neurol.* 2008;37:274-278.

57. Comella CL, et al. Comparison of botulinum toxin serotypes A and B for the treatment of cervical dystonia. *Neurology.* 2005;65:1423-1429.

58. Czerwinski M, et al. Foodborne botulism in Poland in 2014. *Przegl Epidemiol.* 2016;70:217-223.

59. Davis JB, et al. *Clostridium botulinum* in a fatal wound infection. *JAMA.* 1951;146:646-648.

60. Davis LE, et al. Human type A botulism and treatment with 3,4-diaminopyridine. *Electromyogr Clin Neurophysiol.* 1992;32:379-383.

61. Dembek ZF, et al. Botulinum toxin. In: Lenhart MK, et al, eds. *Medical Aspects of Biological Warfare.* Washington, DC: US Department of the Army, Office of the Surgeon General and the Borden Institute; 2007:337-353.

62. Dock M, et al. [Treatment of severe botulism with 3,4-diaminopyridine]. *Presse Med.* 2002;31:601-602.

63. Domingo RM, et al. Infant botulism: two recent cases and literature review. *J Child Neurol.* 2008;23:1336-1346.

64. Dowell VR. Coproexamination for botulinal toxin and *Clostridium botulinum. JAMA.* 1977;238:1829.

65. Dykes JK, et al. Investigation of the first case of botulism caused by *Clostridium butyricum* type E toxin in the United States. *J Clin Microbiol.* 2015;53:3363-3365.

66. Erbguth F, et al. Systemic effect of local botulinum toxin injections unmasks subclinical Lambert-Eaton myasthenic syndrome. *J Neurol Neurosurg Psychiatry.* 1993;56:1235-1236.

67. Fach P, et al. PCR and gene probe identification of botulinum neurotoxin A-, B-, E-, F-, and G-producing *Clostridium* spp. and evaluation in food samples. *Appl Environ Microbiol.* 1995;61:389-392.

68. Faich GA, et al. Failure of guanidine therapy in botulism A. *N Engl J Med.* 1971;285:773-776.

69. Fan KL, et al. Delayed antitoxin treatment of two adult patients with botulism after cosmetic injection of botulinum type A toxin. *J Emerg Med.* 2016;51:677-679.

70. Fenicia L, Anniballi F. Infant botulism. *Ann Ist Super Sanita.* 2009;45:134-146.

71. Frankovich TL, Arnon SS. Clinical trial of botulism immune globulin for infant botulism. *West J Med.* 1991;154:103.

72. Franz DR, et al. Efficacy of prophylactic and therapeutic administration of antitoxin for inhalation botulism. In: DasGupta BR, ed. *Botulinum and Tetanus Neurotoxins.* New York, NY: Plenum Press; 1993:473-476.

73. Freedman M, et al. Botulism in a patient with jejunoileal bypass. *Ann Neurol.* 1986;20:641-643.

74. Friggeri A, et al. 3,4-Diaminopyridine may improve neuromuscular block during botulism. *Crit Care.* 2013;17:449.

75. Girlanda P, et al. Botulinum toxin therapy: distant effects on neuromuscular transmission and autonomic nervous system. *J Neurol Neurosurg Psychiatry.* 1992;55:844-845.

76. Gomez HF, et al. Adsorption of botulinum toxin to activated charcoal with a mouse bioassay. *Ann Emerg Med.* 1995;25:818-822.

77. Gonzales y Tucker RD, Frazee B. View from the front lines: an emergency medicine perspective on clostridial infections in injection drug users. *Anaerobe.* 2014;30:108-115.

78. Gottlieb SL, et al. Long-term outcomes of 217 botulism cases in the Republic of Georgia. *Clin Infect Dis.* 2007;45:174-180.

79. Griffin PM, et al. Endogenous antibody production to botulinum toxin in an adult with intestinal colonization botulism and underlying Crohn's disease. *J Infect Dis.* 1997;175:633-637.

80. Habermann E, Dreyer F. Clostridial neurotoxins: handling and action at the cellular and molecular level. *Curr Top Microbiol Immunol.* 1986;129:93-179.

81. Hallett M. One man's poison—clinical applications of botulinum toxin. *N Engl J Med.* 1999;341:118-120.

82. Hammer TH, et al. Fatal outbreak of botulism in Greenland. *Infect Dis (Lond).* 2015;47:190-194.

83. Hashimoto H, et al. Botulism from peyote. *N Engl J Med.* 1998;339:203-204.

84. Hatheway CL. Toxigenic clostridia. *Clin Microbiol Rev.* 1990;3:66-98.

85. Hentges DJ. The intestinal flora and infant botulism. *Clin Infect Dis.* 1979;1:668-673.

86. Hikes DC, Manoli A. Wound botulism. *J Trauma.* 1981;21:68-71.

87. Hildebrand, et al. Distribution and particle size of type A botulinum toxin in body fluids of intravenously injected rabbits. *Proc Soc Exp Biol Med.* 1961;107:284-289.

88. Hill KK, et al. Genetic diversity within the botulinum neurotoxin-producing bacteria and their neurotoxins. *Toxicon.* 2015;107(Pt A):2-8.

89. Jankovic J, et al. Comparison of efficacy and immunogenicity of original versus current botulinum toxin in cervical dystonia. *Neurology.* 2003;60:1186-1188.

90. Johnson RO, et al. Diagnosis and management of infant botulism. *Am J Dis Child.* 1979;133:586-593.

91. Jones SC, et al. Fluoroquinolone-associated myasthenia gravis exacerbation: evaluation of postmarketing reports from the US FDA adverse event reporting system and a literature review. *Drug Saf.* 2011;34:839-847.

92. Kaplan JE, et al. Botulism, type A, and treatment with guanidine. *Ann Neurol.* 1979;6:69-71.

93. Khan MR, et al. Botulism in children: a diagnostic dilemma in developing countries. *J Coll Physicians Surg Pak.* 2013;23:443-444.

94. Kirchner S, et al. Pentaplexed quantitative real-time PCR assay for the simultaneous detection and quantification of botulinum neurotoxin-producing clostridia in food and clinical samples. *Appl Environ Microbiol.* 2010;76:4387-4395.

95. Kiris E, et al. Recent advances in botulinum neurotoxin inhibitor development. *Curr Top Med Chem.* 2014;14:2044-2061.

96. Kongsaengdao S, et al. An outbreak of botulism in Thailand: clinical manifestations and management of severe respiratory failure. *Clin Infect Dis.* 2006;43:1247-1256.

97. Kroken AR, et al. Entry of botulinum neurotoxin subtypes A1 and A2 into neurons. *Infect Immun.* 2017;85:1-15.

98. Kudrow DB, et al. Botulism associated with *Clostridium botulinum* sinusitis after intranasal cocaine abuse. *Ann Intern Med.* 1988;109:984-985.

99. Lalli G, et al. The journey of tetanus and botulinum neurotoxins in neurons. *Trends in Microbiology.* 2003;11:431-437.

100. Lange DJ, et al. Distant effects of local injection of botulinum toxin. *Muscle Nerve.* 1987;10:552-555.

101. Lawn ND, et al. Anticipating mechanical ventilation in Guillain-Barré syndrome. *Arch Neurol.* 2001;58:893-898.

102. Lecour H. Food-borne botulism. A review of 13 outbreaks. *Arch Intern Med.* 1988;148:578-580.

103. Lindstrom M, Korkeala H. Laboratory diagnostics of botulism. *Clin Microbiol Rev.* 2006;19:298-314.

104. Lonati D, et al. Fatal course of foodborne botulism in an eight-month old infant. *Pediatr Rep.* 2011;3:e31.

105. MacDonald KL. Type A botulism from sauteed onions. Clinical and epidemiologic observations. *JAMA.* 1985;253:1275-1278.

106. MacDonald KL, et al. The changing epidemiology of adult botulism in the United States. *Am J Epidemiol.* 1986;124:794-799.

107. Maksymowych AB, Simpson LL. Binding and transcytosis of botulinum neurotoxin by polarized human colon carcinoma cells. *J Biol Chem.* 1998;273:21950-21957.

108. Maples HD, et al. Special pharmacokinetic and pharmacodynamic considerations in children. In: Burton ME SL, et al, ed. *Applied Pharmacokinetics and Pharmacodynamics: Principles of Therapeutic Drug Monitoring.* 4th ed. Philadelphia, PA: Lippincott Williams & Wilkins; 2005:213-230.

109. Maselli RA, Bakshi N. Botulism. *Muscle Nerve.* 2000;23:1137-1144.

110. Maselli RA, et al. Cluster of wound botulism in California: clinical, electrophysiologic, and pathologic study. *Muscle Nerve.* 1997;20:1284-1295.

111. Matak I, Lackovic Z. Botulinum neurotoxin type A: actions beyond SNAP-25? *Toxicology.* 2015;335:79-84.

112. May ML, et al. Infant botulism in Australia: availability of human botulinum antitoxin for treatment. *Med J Aust.* 2010;193:614-615.

113. McCarty CL, et al. Large outbreak of botulism associated with a church potluck meal—Ohio, 2015. *MMWR Morb Mortal Wkly Rep.* 2015;64:802-803.

114. McCrickard L, et al. Notes from the field: botulism outbreak from drinking prison-made illicit alcohol in a federal correctional facility—Mississippi, June 2016. *MMWR Morb Mortal Wkly Rep.* 2017;65:1491-1492.

115. McCroskey LM, Hatheway CL. Laboratory findings in four cases of adult botulism suggest colonization of the intestinal tract. *J Clin Microbiol.* 1988;26:1052-1054.

116. McCroskey LM, et al. Type F botulism due to neurotoxigenic *Clostridium baratii* from an unknown source in an adult. *J Clin Microbiol.* 1991;29:2618-2620.

117. Mehta S. Neuromuscular disease causing acute respiratory failure. *Respir Care.* 2006;51:1016-1021; discussion 1021-1013.

118. Merson MH, Dowell VR. Epidemiologic, clinical and laboratory aspects of wound botulism. *N Engl J Med.* 1973;289:1005-1010.

119. Metzger JF, Lewis GE. Human-derived immune globulins for the treatment of botulism. *Clin Infect Dis.* 1979;1:689-692.

120. Montecucco C, et al. Botulinum neurotoxins: mechanism of action and therapeutic applications. *Mol Med Today.* 1996;2:418-424.

121. Morrison GA, et al. Botulism in a pregnant intravenous drug abuser. *Anaesthesia.* 2006;61:57-60.

123. Morse DL, et al. Garlic-in-oil associated botulism: episode leads to product modification. *Am J Public Health.* 1990;80:1372-1373.

124. Nakano H, et al. Multiplication of *Clostridium botulinum* in dead honey-bees and bee pupae, a likely source of heavy contamination of honey. *International J Food Microbiol.* 1994;21:247-252.

125. Odergren T, et al. A double blind, randomised, parallel group study to investigate the dose equivalence of Dysport and Botox in the treatment of cervical dystonia. *J Neurol Neurosurg Psychiatry.* 1998;64:6-12.

126. Oiney RK, et al. Neuromuscular effects distant from the site of botulinum neurotoxin injection. *Neurology.* 1988;38:1780-1780.

127. Opila T, et al. Trends in outcomes and hospitalization charges of infant botulism in the United States: a comparative analysis between Kids' Inpatient Database and National Inpatient Sample. *Pediatr Neurol.* 2017;67:53-58.

128. Otofuji T, et al. A food-poisoning incident caused by *Clostridium botulinum* toxin A in Japan. *Epidemiol Infect.* 1987;99:167-172.

129. Padua L, et al. Neurophysiological assessment in the diagnosis of botulism: usefulness of single-fiber EMG. *Muscle Nerve.* 1999;22:1388-1392.

130. Paisley JW, et al. A second case of infant botulism type F caused by Clostridium baratii. *Pediatr Infect Dis J.* 1995;14:912-914.

131. Parish JL. Commercial preparations and handling of botulinum toxin type A and type B. *Clin Dermatol.* 2003;21:481-484.

132. Passaro DJ. Wound botulism associated with black tar heroin among injecting drug users. *JAMA.* 1998;279:859.

133. Patural H, et al. Infant botulism intoxication and autonomic nervous system dysfunction. *Anaerobe.* 2009;15:197-200.

134. Peck MW, et al. Historical perspectives and guidelines for botulinum neurotoxin subtype nomenclature. *Toxins.* 2017;9.

135. Pellett S. Progress in cell based assays for botulinum neurotoxin detection. *Current Topics in Microbiol Immunol.* 2013;364:257-285.

136. Pickett JB. AAEE case report #16: Botulism. *Muscle Nerve.* 1988;11:1201-1205.

137. Pourshafie MR, et al. An outbreak of food-borne botulism associated with contaminated locally made cheese in Iran. *Scand J Infect Dis.* 1998;30:92-94.

138. Rapoport S, Watkins PB. Descending paralysis resulting from occult wound botulism. *Ann Neurol.* 1984;16:359-361.

139. Roblot F, et al. Botulism in patients who inhale cocaine: the first cases in France. *Clin Infect Dis.* 2006;43:e51-e52.

140. Rosen O, et al. Early, real-time medical diagnosis of botulism by endopeptidase-mass spectrometry. *Clin Infect Dis.* 2015;61:e58-61.

141. Ross MH, et al. Treatment of occupational cramp with botulinum toxin: diffusion of toxin to adjacent noninjected muscles. *Muscle Nerve.* 1997;20:593-598.

142. Rummel A. The long journey of botulinum neurotoxins into the synapse. *Toxicon.* 2015;107(Pt A):9-24.

143. Sacks HS. The botulism hazard. *Ann Intern Med.* 1997;126:918.

144. Sampaio C, et al. DYSBOT: a single-blind, randomized parallel study to determine whether any differences can be detected in the efficacy and tolerability of two formulations of botulinum toxin type A—Dysport and Botox—assuming a ratio of 4:1. *Mov Disord.* 1997;12:1013-1018.

145. Sanders DB, et al. A randomized trial of 3,4-diaminopyridine in Lambert-Eaton myasthenic syndrome. *Neurology.* 2000;54:603-603.

146. Santos JI, et al. Potentiation of *Clostridium botulinum* toxin aminoglycoside antibiotics: clinical and laboratory observations. *Pediatrics.* 1981;68:50-54.

147. Schantz EJ, Johnson EA. Properties and use of botulinum toxin and other microbial neurotoxins in medicine. *Microbiol Rev.* 1992;56:80-99.

148. Schmidt-Nowara WW, et al. Early and late pulmonary complications of botulism. *Arch Intern Med.* 1983;143:451-456.

149. Schmidt RD, Schmidt TW. Infant botulism: a case series and review of the literature. *J Emerg Med.* 1992;10:713-718.

150. Schulze J, et al. Clindamycin and nicotinic neuromuscular transmission. *Lancet.* 1999;354:1792-1793.

151. Scott AB, Suzuki D. Systemic toxicity of botulinum toxin by intramuscular injection in the monkey. *Mov Disord.* 1988;3:333-335.

152. Shapiro RL, et al. Botulism surveillance and emergency response. A public health strategy for a global challenge. *JAMA.* 1997;278:433-435.

153. Shapiro RL, et al. Botulism in the United States: a clinical and epidemiologic review. *Ann Intern Med.* 1998;129:221-228.

154. Sheean GL, Lees AJ. Botulinum toxin F in the treatment of torticollis clinically resistant to botulinum toxin A. *J Neurol Neurosurg Psychiatry.* 1995;59:601-607.

155. Sheridan RE. Gating and permeability of ion channels produced by botulinum toxin types A and E in PC12 cell membranes. *Toxicon.* 1998;36:703-717.

156. Siegel LS, et al. Effect of 3,4-diaminopyridine on the survival of mice injected with botulinum neurotoxin type A, B, E, or F. *Toxicol Appl Pharmacol.* 1986;84:255-263.

157. Siegel LS, Price JI. Ineffectiveness of 3,4-diaminopyridine as a therapy for type C botulism. *Toxicon.* 1987;25:1015-1018.

158. Simon S, et al. Recommended immunological strategies to screen for botulinum neurotoxin-containing samples. *Toxins.* 2015;7:5011-5034.

159. Simpson DM, et al. Practice guideline update summary: botulinum neurotoxin for the treatment of blepharospasm, cervical dystonia, adult spasticity, and headache: report of the Guideline Development Subcommittee of the American Academy of Neurology. *Neurology.* 2016;86:1818-1826.

160. Smith LA, Rusnak JM. Botulinum neurotoxin vaccines: past, present, and future. *Crit Rev Immunol.* 2007;27:303-318.

161. Sonnabend OR, et al. Continuous microbiological and pathological study of 70 sudden and unexpected infant deaths: toxigenic intestinal *Clostridium botulinum* infection in 9 cases of sudden infant death syndrome. *Lancet.* 1985;325:237-241.

162. St Clair EH, et al. Letter: observations of an infant born to a mother with botulism. *J Pediatr.* 1975;87:658.

163. St Louis ME, et al. Botulism from chopped garlic: delayed recognition of a major outbreak. *Ann Intern Med.* 1988;108:363-368.

164. Swedberg J, et al. Wound botulism. *West J Med.* 1987;147:335-338.

165. Swenson JM, et al. Susceptibility of *Clostridium botulinum* to thirteen antimicrobial agents. *Antimicrob Agents Chemother.* 1980;18:13-19.

166. Tacket CO, et al. Equine antitoxin use and other factors that predict outcome in type A foodborne botulism. *Am J Med.* 1984;76:794-798.

167. Telzak EE, et al. An international outbreak of type E botulism due to uneviscerated fish. *J Infect Dis.* 1990;161:340-342.

168. Townes JM. The botulism hazard. *Ann Intern Med.* 1997;126:919.

169. Townes JM. An outbreak of type A botulism associated with a commercial cheese sauce. *Ann Intern Med.* 1996;125:558.

170. Trehard H, et al. A cluster of three cases of botulism due to *Clostridium baratii* type F, France, August 2015. *Euro Surveill.* 2016;21.

171. Tseng-Ong L, Mitchell WG. Infant botulism: 20 years' experience at a single institution. *J Child Neurol.* 2007;22:1333-1337.

172. Tugnoli V, et al. Botulism-like syndrome after botulinum toxin type A injections for focal hyperhidrosis. *Br J Dermatol.* 2002;147:808-809.

173. US Food and Drug Administration. Early communication about an ongoing safety review of Botox and Botox Cosmetic (botulinum toxin type A) and Myobloc (botulinum toxin type B). 2008. http://www.fda.gov/Drugs/DrugSafety/PostmarketDrugSafetyInformationforPatientsandProviders/DrugSafetyInformationforHeathcareProfessionals/ucm070366.htm. Accessed January 16, 2017.

174. US Food and Drug Administration. FDA approves first Botulism Antitoxin for use in neutralizing all seven known botulinum nerve toxin serotypes. 2013. http://www.fda.gov/NewsEvents/Newsroom/PressAnnouncements/ucm345128.htm. Accessed January 16, 2017.

175. US Food and Drug Administration. Information for Healthcare Professionals: OnabotulinumtoxinA (marketed as Botox/Botox Cosmetic), AbobotulinumtoxinA (marketed as Dysport) and RimabotulinumtoxinB (marketed as Myobloc). 2009. http://www.fda.gov/Drugs/DrugSafety/PostmarketDrugSafetyInformationforPatientsandProviders/DrugSafetyInformationforHeathcareProfessionals/ucm174949.htm. Accessed January 16, 2017.

176. Underwood K, et al. Infant botulism: a 30-year experience spanning the introduction of botulism immune globulin intravenous in the intensive care unit at Childrens Hospital Los Angeles. *Pediatrics.* 2007;120:e1380-e1385.

177. Verma S, Lin J. Stimulated jitter analysis for the evaluation of neuromuscular junction disorders in children. *Muscle Nerve.* 2016;53:471-472.

178. Villar RG, et al. Outbreak of type A botulism and development of a botulism surveillance and antitoxin release system in Argentina. *JAMA.* 1999;281:1334-1338, 1340.

179. Viray MA, et al. Outbreak of type A foodborne botulism at a boarding school, Uganda, 2008. *Epidemiol Infect.* 2014;142:2297-2301.

180. Vugia DJ, et al. Botulism from drinking pruno. *Emerg Infect Dis.* 2009;15:69-71.

181. Wainwright RB, et al. Food-borne botulism in Alaska, 1947-1985: epidemiology and clinical findings. *J Infect Dis.* 1988;157:1158-1162.

182. Weber JT, et al. A massive outbreak of type E botulism associated with traditional salted fish in Cairo. *J Infect Dis.* 1993;167:451-454.

183. Werner SB, et al. Wound botulism in California, 1951–1998: recent epidemic in heroin injectors. *Clin Infect Dis.* 2000;31:1018-1024.

184. Wilcox P, et al. Long-term follow-up of symptoms, pulmonary function, respiratory muscle strength, and exercise performance after botulism. *Am Rev Respir Dis.* 1989;139:157-163.

185. Woodruff BA, et al. Clinical and laboratory comparison of botulism from toxin types A, B, and E in the United States, 1975-1988. *J Infect Dis.* 1992;166:1281-1286.

186. Yasmin S, et al. Outbreak of botulism after consumption of illicit prison-brewed alcohol in a maximum security prison—Arizona, 2012. *J Correct Health Care.* 2015;21:327-334.

187. You G, et al. Rapidly progressive muscle paralysis and acute respiratory failure following endoscopic botulinum toxin injection. *ACG Case Rep J.* 2016;3:e166.

188. Zilinskas RA. Iraq's biological weapons. *JAMA.* 1997;278:418.

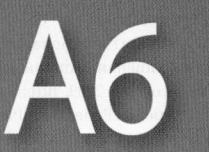

Antidotes in Depth

A6

BOTULINUM ANTITOXIN

Silas W. Smith and Howard L. Geyer

INTRODUCTION

Antidotal therapies for adult and infant *Clostridium botulinum* infection are available as equine- and human-derived immunoglobulin antitoxins. Antitoxins are beneficial for most clinical forms of botulism, although their utility is restricted to limiting disease progression rather than to reversing clinical manifestations.

HISTORY

Beginning in the 1930s, a formalin-inactivated toxoid against botulinum neurotoxin was first tested in humans, and in 1946, a bivalent (against types A and B) formaldehyde-inactivated toxoid was deployed by the Department of Defense as prophylaxis for at-risk individuals during the US Offensive Biological Warfare Program.[56,65] Before 1999, an equine trivalent antitoxin (BAT-ABE) was used to treat botulism.[13] From 1999 to 2010, equine-derived, licensed bivalent botulinum antitoxin AB (BAT-AB) and investigational monovalent serotype E botulinum antitoxin (BAT-E) were available in the United States as immunoglobulin preparations. Patients with presumed wound botulism received BAT-AB. BAT-AB and BAT-E antitoxins were coadministered to patients with foodborne botulism. On March 13, 2010, equine heptavalent botulinum antitoxin (H-BAT, NP-018), an investigational new drug sponsored by the Centers for Disease Control and Prevention (CDC), replaced licensed bivalent BAT-AB and investigational BAT-E.[16] Effective November 30, 2011, the CDC also stopped providing the investigational pentavalent (ABCDE) botulinum toxoid (PBT) for vaccination of workers at risk for occupational exposure.[17] Botulism Immune Globulin Intravenous (Human) (BIG-IV), or BabyBIG was created by the California Department of Health Services (CDHS) in 1991 to treat infants affected by type A or type B botulism; it received Food and Drug Administration (FDA) approval in 2003.[2,27] On March 22, 2013, the FDA approved H-BAT, equine Botulism Antitoxin Heptavalent (A, B, C, D, E, F, G), which is currently available.

PHARMACOLOGY

Chemistry and Preparation

A toxoid is an inactivated form of a bacterial toxin. An antitoxin is an antibody or antibody fragment capable of neutralizing a toxin. Multiple injections of formalin-inactivated toxoid are required over months to effectively immunize horses against botulinum toxin and to produce equine-derived antitoxins.[37] The resultant antibotulinum immunoglobulin requires several purification and preparation steps.[30] Heptavalent botulism antitoxin is produced by pooling plasma from horses immunized with seven specific botulinum toxoid types (A–G) followed by pepsin digestion and blending of the seven unique serotype antitoxins into a heptavalent product.[11] The antitoxin potencies for botulism serotypes A to G in H-BAT are provided in Table A6–1. By convention, 1 IU of BAT neutralizes 10,000 mouse intraperitoneal median lethal doses ($MIPLD_{50}$) of toxin types A, B, C, D, and F and 1,000 $MIPLD_{50}$ of toxin type E (the IU for type G remains undefined).[15] As the equine H-BAT is "despeciated" by pepsin enzymatic cleavage to remove the Fc fragment portion, the resultant product is composed of 90% or greater Fab and $F(ab')_2$ immunoglobulin fragments and less than 2% intact immunoglobulin G (IgG).[16] This decreases the risk of immediate hypersensitivity reactions and serum sickness.

Human whole IgG BIG-IV was formerly produced from pooled adult plasma collected from human donors immunized multiple times with

PBT (A-E).[45,61] The current purified immunoglobulin is derived from cold ethanol precipitation of pooled adult plasma from persons who were immunized with a recombinant botulinum vaccine for serotypes A and B (rBV A/B) followed by a number of purification steps to inactivate and/or remove infectious agents.[34] The reconstituted product (2 mL containing 50 ± 10 mg immunoglobulin in each milliliter) is primarily IgG, with trace amounts of IgA and IgM, and contains greater than or equal to 15 IU/mL anti-type A toxin activity and greater than or equal to 4 IU/mL anti-type B toxin activity; antibody titers against botulinum neurotoxins C, D, and E are undetermined.[27,34]

Mechanism of Action

Current antitoxins (whether equine or human derived) bind to and neutralize free botulinum toxin.[13] Thus, antitoxins are ineffective against toxin bound to presynaptic acetylcholine release sites, toxin endocytosed by peripheral neuronal cells, and intracellular botulinum toxin light chain endopeptidase activity.[9] Affected presynaptic endplates must regenerate to regain function.

Pharmacokinetics and Pharmacodynamics

Antidotal antibody fragments {eg, $(F(ab')_2$, $F(ab')$, and single-chain variable fragments (scFvs)} demonstrate shortened half-lives in vivo compared with whole immunoglobulins.[39] Improved renal clearance and uptake by vascular endothelium and surrounding tissues contributes to this effect.[50] Although linking fragments to polyethylene glycol (PEG) can extend the half-life,[19] this methodology remains investigational. Half-lives for antitoxin types A, B, and E were 6.5, 7.6, and 5.3 days, respectively, in a patient provided whole intact IgG trivalent antitoxin.[29] Because H-BAT contains primarily Fab and $F(ab')_2$ immunoglobulin fragments and minimal intact whole IgG, administration of H-BAT antitoxin yields shorter half-lives which are on the order of hours (Table A6–1). These half-lives generally increase in a nonlinear fashion when two vials were administered (Table A6–1). The total volume of distribution ranges from 1,465 mL (anti-D) to 14,172 mL (anti-E) and tends to increase with multiple vials.[12] The more rapid clearance of Fab and $F(ab')_2$ fragments compared with whole IgG, infrequently necessitates repeat H-BAT dosing in patients with wound or intestinal colonization or other cases in which in situ botulinum toxin production continues after antitoxin clearance.[16] Indeed, recurrence of paralysis was reported after H-BAT therapy in a patient with persistent type F intestinal colonization.[24] Given the neutralization parameters provided by each IU of BAT as indicated previously, the antitoxin in H-BAT would offset a total amount of toxin ranging from 5.1×10^6 $MIPLD_{50}$ of botulinum E toxin to 4.5×10^7 $MIPLD_{50}$ of botulinum A toxin (Table A6–1).[54] These values would be anticipated to provide significant neutralization, because patient serum botulinum toxin concentrations in foodborne botulism are usually less than 10 $MIPLD_{50}$/mL and rarely exceed 32 $MIPLD_{50}$/mL using a plasma volume of 3,000 mL reported previously.[3,29,53] However, in isolated outbreaks, botulinum toxin concentrations in adult serum samples collected less than 18 hours after exposure are reported to be as high as 160 $MIPLD_{50}$/mL.[5] Other extremely rare cases have yielded human serum botulinum toxin concentrations of type A of 1,800 $MIPLD_{50}$/mL.[54] Nevertheless, even with these elevated exposures, the reported H-BAT maximum concentration values[12] after single-vial administration are anticipated to sufficiently neutralize 26,900 $MIPLD_{50}$/mL of botulinum A toxin, 19,000 $MIPLD_{50}$/mL of botulinum B toxin, 22,600 $MIPLD_{50}$/mL of botulinum C toxin, 8,100 $MIPLD_{50}$/mL of botulinum D toxin, 940 $MIPLD_{50}$/mL of botulinum E toxin, and 23,700 $MIPLD_{50}$/mL of botulinum F toxin (Table A6–1).

TABLE A6–1	Botulinum Antitoxin Parameters						
				Antitoxin Serotype			
	A	B	C	D	E	F	G
Heptavalent Botulinum Antitoxin (H-BAT)							
Antitoxin potency (IU per vial)	4,500	3,300	3,000	600	5,100	3,000	600
Anticipated neutralization (MIPLD$_{50}$)	4.5×10^7	3.3×10^7	3.0×10^7	6.0×10^6	5.1×10^6	3.0×10^7	Undefined
Maximum concentration values (IU/mL), one-vial administration	2.69	1.90	2.26	0.81	0.94	2.37	0.59
Maximum concentration values (MIPLD$_{50}$/mL)	2.69×10^4	1.90×10^4	2.26×10^4	8.1×10^3	9.4×10^2	2.37×10^4	Undefined
Maximum concentration values (IU/mL), 1-vial administration	6.23	4.28	4.89	1.60	1.75	4.29	1.19
Maximum concentration values (MIPLD$_{50}$/mL)	6.23×10^4	4.28×10^4	4.89×10^4	1.60×10^4	1.75×10^3	4.29×10^4	Undefined
Half-life (h), one-vial administration	8.64	34.2	29.6	7.51	7.75	14.1	11.7
Half-life (h), two-vial administration	10.2	57.1	45.6	7.77	7.32	18.2	14.7
Volume of distribution, one-vial administration	3,637	9,607	6,066	1,465	14,172	3,413	2,372
Volume of distribution, two-vial administration	3,993	14,865	8,486	1,653	11,596	4,334	3,063
Botulism Immune Globulin Intravenous (Human) (BabyBIG-IV)							
Potency (IU/mL)[a]	15	4					
Anticipated neutralization (MIPLD$_{50}$)	1.5×10^5	4×10^4					
Half-life (days)	28	28					
Bivalent botulinum antitoxin AB (BAT-AB) (for historical comparison)							
Antitoxin potency (IU)	7,500	5,500					
Monovalent serotype E botulinum antitoxin (BAT-E) (for historical comparison)							
Antitoxin potency (IU)					5,000		
Equine trivalent antitoxin (BAT-ABE) (for historical comparison)							
Antitoxin potency (IU)	7,500	5,500			8,500		

[a]The reconstituted vial contains a total of 2 mL.

MIPLD$_{50}$ = mouse intraperitoneal median lethal dose.

Data from references 12, 24, 27, 32, 34, 49, and 54.

A second vial would provide even greater protection (Table A6–1). This might be warranted in particularly severe exposures because circulating neutralizing antibody concentrations and botulinum toxin interactions are nonlinear and lead to a more efficacious, disproportional increase in botulinum toxin neutralization when antibody concentrations are increased.[38,53] Although anticipating or interpreting absolute neutralization efficacy is inexact because of numerous factors, one study that measured four patients' serum antitoxin concentrations after trivalent antitoxin (BAT-ABE) administration determined that the patients' measured antitoxin titers would retain the capability to neutralize 1,500, 1,000, and 12 times the anticipated toxin concentrations of types A, B, and E, respectively.[29]

A new botulinum neurotoxin "type H" recovered from a naturally occurring infant botulism case raised concern because it was unable to be neutralized by available monovalent botulinum neurotoxin types (A–G) or a heptavalent antitoxin product.[6,21] Botulinum neurotoxin "type H" shares sequence homology with the botulinum neurotoxin type A1 heavy chain binding domain and the botulinum neurotoxin F5 light chain enzymatic domain. Subsequent mouse bioassay and neuronal cell-based assays demonstrated that commercial H-BAT provides complete neutralization of botulinum neurotoxin "type H" at exposures of 100 MIPLD$_{50}$/mL and complete neutralization with a single exception at 2,000 MIPLD$_{50}$/mL.[38] Given that serum botulinum toxin concentrations in foodborne botulism rarely exceed 32 MIPLD$_{50}$/mL, one H-BAT vial is anticipated to be sufficient to treat most botulism type H cases and bivalent strain cases (a strain that produces dual, distinct botulinum neurotoxins).[29,38]

The half-life of BIG-IV is approximately 28 days.[34] BabyBIG Lot 2 anti-A titers were 0.5371 ± 0.2134 IU/mL on day 1 after administration, declining to 0.0193 ± 0.0141 IU/mL by week 20.[34] Because 1 IU neutralizes 10,000 mouse intraperitoneal median lethal doses (MIPLD$_{50}$) of botulinum toxin A, this yields approximate neutralization titers of 5,370 MIPLD$_{50}$/mL on day 1 and 193 MIPLD$_{50}$/mL by week 20.[15,34] Thus, a single infusion is anticipated to neutralize all botulinum toxin that might be absorbed from an infant's colon for several months.[4]

Related Agents

To properly interpret earlier botulism studies, it is important to recall that the previously available, equine BAT-AB antitoxin contained 7,500 IU of anti-A antitoxin and 5,500 IU of anti-B antitoxin.[49] Monovalent serotype E botulinum antitoxin contained 5,000 IU of antitoxin. Trivalent antitoxin (BAT-ABE), contained 7,500 IU anti-A, 5,500 IU anti-B, and 8,500 IU anti-E antitoxins.[32] Investigational, whole and fragment-derived monoclonal antibodies that are raised in murine and equine species against type A and B are also being explored.[37,39] Investigational PBT vaccine, combining individual monovalent toxoids, was initially manufactured by Parke Davis more than 50 years ago and was subsequently produced by the Michigan Department of Public Health under contract from the US Army.[26,55]

The US Department of Defense Medical Countermeasure Systems-Joint Vaccine Acquisition Program (MCS-JVAP) manages the development pipeline for the lead replacement vaccine—recombinant botulinum vaccine (rBV A/B)—which is intended to protect adults 18 to 55 years old against botulism type A (subtype A1) and type B (subtype B1).[28,52] Other monoclonal antibodies, small peptides and peptide mimetics, receptor mimics and antagonists, endosome modulators, and endopeptidase inhibitors are being explored for botulism treatment.[1]

ANTITOXIN ROLE IN ADULT BOTULISM

Rigorous adult morbidity and mortality studies are difficult to perform because the rarity of botulism, varied exposure and presentation, delayed recognition when bound toxin is no longer scavengable by antitoxin, and inconsistent clinical care. Given the delay involved in confirmatory testing by the CDC or public health laboratories, which could decrease the window of opportunity for antitoxin reversal potential, the decision to administer H-BAT is often made on the basis of empirical clinical and epidemiologic grounds. Earlier disease recognition and an organized public health approach consisting of surveillance, emergency notification, stocking, a release and distribution system, and laboratory confirmation appear to be responsible for decreasing morbidity and increasing survival after typical foodborne botulism.[51,64] Simian experiments demonstrate reduced mortality with antitoxin administration.[43] Early antitoxin administration appears to be a critical factor affecting clinical course and outcome. In a 1963 type E outbreak, all three patients who died failed to receive antitoxin, but three of five who received BAT survived.[35] Trivalent equine antitoxin decreased the fatality rate of botulinum A poisoning in a case series of 132 patients from 1973 to 1980.[59] The mortality rate was 10% in patients receiving antitoxin within 24 hours after onset, 15% in those who received antitoxin more than 24 hours after onset, and 46% in those without antitoxin administration. Age over 60 years and being an index patient conferred a greater mortality risk; a shorter incubation period of less than 36 hours (a likely measure of toxin dose) increased duration of hospitalization, mechanical ventilation, and time to sustained improvement.[59] The case-fatality rate was 3.5% in patients with type E botulism who were provided antitoxin and 28.9% for untreated control participants from previous years, although the utilization of supportive measures was uncontrolled.[33] In a retrospective review of 29 patients admitted between 1991 and 2005 with type A and a single case of type B wound botulism, a delay in antitoxin administration correlated with increased length of intensive care unit (ICU) stay.[44] In 20 patients with type A wound botulism treated from 1991 to 1998, those who received antitoxin within 12 hours of presentation required mechanical ventilation 57% of the time for a median duration of 11 days compared with those who failed to received antitoxin within 12 hours in whom 85% required mechanical ventilation for a median duration of 54 days.[48] Again, a shorter time to presentation heralded more severe disease (respiratory failure). A third wound botulism series (types A and B) with seven patients confirmed the importance of early therapy. Those receiving antitoxin more than 8 days from symptom onset or not at all (1 case) had worse outcomes compared with those receiving it within 4 days of symptom onset, including need for persistent mechanical ventilation (40%), bedridden (100%), inability to discharge to home setting (100%), and prolonged hospital course.[18] In an uncontrolled, retrospective review of 205 cases of foodborne botulinum (predominantly type E) in Canada from 1985 to 2005, patients receiving antitoxin experienced a median hospital length of stay of 5 days, which was significantly shorter than the group that did not receive antitoxin (median length of stay, 11 days).[36]

An earlier despeciated heptavalent botulism immune globulin (dBIG), which was prepared by the University of Minnesota under US Army contract, was deployed in the 1991 Egyptian type E botulism outbreak.[30] In a 2006 Thailand type A outbreak, a heptavalent antitoxin was administered to 20 patients 5 days after toxin ingestion when respiratory failure was already present. Mechanical ventilation and hospital duration were shorter compared with a historical study, and there were no deaths in those receiving antitoxin.[68] In a 2011 Utah prison botulism outbreak caused by potato-based pruno (prison-brewed alcohol), H-BAT was administered to eight patients a median of 12 hours after emergency department (ED) arrival and 73.3 hours after exposure.[67] Three patients required intubation; all survived.[67] Heptavalent botulism antitoxin was used in a separate prison botulism outbreak in Arizona in 2012 in eight inmates who also had consumed potato-based pruno.[70] Incubation periods ranged from 10 to 67 hours. All patients received antitoxin within 24 hours of hospital admission, seven required intubation and percutaneous endoscopic gastrostomies, and none died.[70] In the largest US botulism outbreak in nearly 40 years, which resulted from home-canned potato salad at a church potluck meal, 25 of 29 confirmed or probable cases received heptavalent botulinum antitoxin (H-BAT); 11 required intubation and mechanical intubation; and 1 patient died of respiratory failure shortly after arriving at the ED.[40]

The absolute time frame for efficacy remains undetermined. In 109 patients treated under the CDC open-label protocol, H-BAT administration within 2 days after symptom onset (compared with longer than 2 days) was associated with clinically significant, shorter mean durations of hospitalization (12.4 versus 26.1 days), ICU utilization (9.2 versus 15.8 days), and mechanical ventilation (11.6 versus 23.4 days).[12] However, circulating toxin can persist for long periods in patients with foodborne botulism. One study reported toxin detection in almost 20% of serum specimens taken greater than or equal to 10 days after toxin ingestion.[69] Furthermore, persistent, viable organisms or spores were present in stools 40% of the time at 10 days or more after toxin ingestion. A review of laboratory-confirmed botulism cases in Alaska from 1959 to 2007 demonstrated that toxin could be recovered in patients' sera up to 11 days after ingestion, but no serum specimens collected after antitoxin administration tested positive.[23] In one case, toxin was detected in serum 12 days after the onset of descending paralysis.[22] Another patient in a multinational foodborne outbreak had toxin detected at 25 days after symptom onset.[54] Other isolated cases detail detectible circulating toxin as late as 3.5 weeks after contaminated food consumption.[20] Botulinum toxin–associated ileus can result in conditions conducive for continued absorption and prolonged toxin exposure. In other scenarios, contaminated wounds and orthopedic hardware can harbor *Clostridia* species despite antibiotic therapy.[60] Collectively, these factors suggest that H-BAT could still provide clinical benefit in patients with delayed presentations or disease recognition, in whom gastrointestinal or circulating toxin presents a persistent risk. Indeed, one report documented improvement when H-BAT was administered 48 hours after admission and many days after consumption of type-unspecified, botulism-contaminated canned corn.[31] Clinically significant improvement (weaning from mechanical ventilation and resumption of feeding) was documented in a case of BIG-IV administered 13 days after onset of infant botulism.[10] Botulinal antitoxins are also provided in cases of iatrogenic botulism.[57] In two patients with cosmetic iatrogenic botulism type A, administration of monovalent type A antitoxin as late as 7 and 9 days after the onset of weakness and bulbar symptoms improved symptoms.[25] Based on these limited data, it would be reasonable to provide BAT in delayed scenarios.

Botulism poisoning does not appear to induce protective immunity or decrease morbidity or mortality associated with subsequent exposure in food or wound botulism.[7,13,71] Thus, retreatment with antitoxin is required upon reexposure or in recurrent cases.

ANTITOXIN ROLE IN INFANT BOTULISM

BabyBIG is approved for treatment of patients younger than 1 year of age with infant botulism caused by toxin type A or B. BabyBIG is no longer derived from human donors vaccinated with PBT (A–E), only those immunized with recombinant botulinum vaccine for serotypes A and B. Thus, H-BAT is required to treat infants with non–type A or B botulism. In a double-blind and subsequent open-label trial, treatment with BabyBIG-IV significantly reduced the overall length of hospital and intensive care stay, the duration of mechanical ventilation, tube and intravenous (IV) feeding, and the cost of hospitalization.[2,4] A retrospective review of 67 ICU patients with type A or B botulinum toxin from 1976 to 2005 found clinically significant decreases in length of hospital stay, ICU stay, and mechanical ventilation in patients who received BabyBIG-IV and those who did not.[62] Another retrospective review of patients with type A or B botulinum toxin from 1985 to 2005 reported a significant decrease in length of stay a reduced need for nasogastric feeding and duration of tracheal intubation in infants treated with botulism immune globulin.[71]

Bivalent BAT-AB and other equine derived products were rarely used in infants because of concern for anaphylaxis, lifelong hypersensitivity, and unclear efficacy.[15] However, in situations when BabyBIG-IV was unavailable because of lack of access or cost, BAT-AB treatment within 5 days of symptom onset significantly reduced overall hospital and ICU stays, duration of mechanical ventilation, tube feedings, and incidence of sepsis.[63]

ADVERSE EFFECTS AND SAFETY ISSUES

Despite purification, inactivation, and filtration measures, potential transmission of bloodborne infectious agents from animal or human donors (pooled equine or human plasma) may still occur. Treatment with whole equine-derived antitoxins risks hypersensitivity reactions and serum sickness.[49] Early rates of adverse reactions during the first decade during which BAT was available (1967–1977) ranged from 9% to 21%.[8,42] The reported rates of anaphylaxis and serum sickness were 1.9% and 3.7%, respectively.[8] However, the doses of antitoxin were larger than those subsequently used. Heptavalent botulism antitoxin despeciation further decreases, but does not eliminate this risk. Heptavalent botulism immune globulin (dBIG) produced adverse reactions in 10 of 45 patients when used in one botulism type E outbreak.[30] These included nine "mild" reactions (local skin reactions, 6; pruritus, 1; urticaria, 1; shivering, 1) and one episode of "suggested serum sickness" without additional detail. The incidence of adverse effects of dBIG was similar to other internationally available antitoxins.[30] Healthy participants administered H-BAT in clinical trials (56 total, of whom 20 received two vials) reported headache, pruritus, nausea, and urticaria at rates of 9%, 5%, 5%, and 5%, respectively.[12] Two moderate allergic reactions required treatment. Eleven subjects produced anti-BAT antibodies. The open-label CDC observation study revealed adverse reactions in 10% of 228 assessable patients: pyrexia (4%), rash (2%), chills (1%), nausea (1%), and edema (1%).[12] There were no immediate hypersensitivity reactions, one cardiac arrest, and one episode of serum sickness. Heptavalent botulism antitoxin contains maltose, which can interfere with certain non–glucose-specific blood glucose monitoring systems and falsely elevated glucose readings.[12]

Hypersensitivity reactions might also occur to human BIG-IV, although this was not reported in clinical trials.[34] Human BIG is contraindicated in patients with a prior history of severe reactions to other human immunoglobulin preparations.[34] Patients with selective immunoglobulin A deficiency have the potential to develop antibodies to immunoglobulin A and could have anaphylactic reactions to subsequent administration of blood products that contain immunoglobulin A. The most commonly reported adverse reaction was a mild, transient erythematous rash on the face or trunk. Kidney function should be assessed and monitored; if compromised, BabyBIG-IV is administered at minimum concentration and rate of infusion. The prescribing information warns of adverse events from immune globulin therapy, including aseptic meningitis, hemolytic anemia, thrombosis, transfusion-related acute lung injury, and hyperviscosity, although these are unreported with the Human BIG-IV immune globulin product.[34] Administration of live-virus vaccines (ie, measles, mumps, rubella, and varicella) utilization should be delayed for 3 or more months after BabyBIG-IV treatment because of concerns of loss of immunization efficacy.

PREGNANCY AND LACTATION

Although there is limited information regarding H-BAT use in pregnancy, whole equine bivalent and trivalent antitoxins have been previously administered without apparent harm to the mother or the fetus.[14,41,46,47,58] Pregnancy is not a contraindication to H-BAT. Given the morbidity and mortality of botulism, maternal treatment benefits would presumably exceed risks of harm, although all decisions are ultimately made on a case-by-case basis. The breast milk distribution of heptavalent botulism antitoxin is unknown.

DOSING AND ADMINISTRATION

Close monitoring; medications, including epinephrine, diphenhydramine, and corticosteroids; therapeutic modalities; and practitioners who are capable of diagnosing and treating anaphylactic or anaphylactoid reactions (including intubation competence) should be immediately available before and during antitoxin administration.

Botulism Antitoxin Heptavalent (A, B, C, D, E, F, and G)

Unlike prior equine-derived products, H-BAT does not require routine sensitivity testing before administration. In patients at risk for hypersensitivity reactions—those with previous therapy with an equine-derived antivenom or antitoxin or a history of hypersensitivity to horses, asthma, or hay fever—H-BAT administration is begun at the lowest rate achievable (<0.01 mL/min) and monitored.[12] Three separate dosing strategies are recommended for adults, pediatric patients (1–17 years of age), and infants younger than 1 year of age. The adult dose is one vial. The vial is diluted 1:10 in 0.9% sodium chloride and administered intravenously via an optional 15-micron in-line filter. Barring any infusion-related safety concerns, the initial rate is 0.5 mL/min for the first 30 minutes, which is increased to 1 mL/min for the next 30 minutes and then to 2 mL/min until completion of the infusion. For pediatric patients, the dose is a percentage of the adult (one vial) dose calculated according to the dosing rule summarized in the package insert. For pediatric patients with a body weight of 30 kg or less, the percentage of the adult dose to administer is equal to twice the body weight (in kilograms); for patients with a body weight greater than 30 kg, the percentage of the adult dose to administer equals the weight (in kilograms) + 30.[12] This rule yields the recommended percentages of the adult dose to administer for pediatric weight intervals from 10 to greater than 55 kg reproduced in the package insert.[12] Without ever exceeding the adult rates, the infusion is initiated at a rate of 0.01 mL/kg/min for the first 30 minutes, which is increased 0.01 mL/kg/min every 30 minutes, to a maximum infusion rate of 0.03 mL/kg/min until completion. Infants (younger than 1 year of age) receive 10% of the adult dose regardless of body weight. The infusion is initiated at a rate of 0.01 mL/kg/min for the first 30 minutes, which is increased 0.01 mL/kg/min every 30 minutes, to a maximum infusion rate of 0.03 mL/kg/min until completion.

Botulism Immune Globulin Intravenous (Human)

The lyophilized product is reconstituted with 2 mL of Sterile Water for Injection USP, to obtain a 50 mg/mL human BIG-IV solution. The vial should not be shaken because this causes foaming. Infusion should begin within 2 hours of reconstitution. A dedicated IV line using low volume tubing and a constant infusion pump are used to provide 75 mg/kg (1.5 mL/kg of reconstituted 50-mg/mL BIG-IV solution). The BIG-IV solution can be "piggybacked" into a preexisting line if it contains Sodium Chloride Injection USP, 2.5% dextrose in water, 5% dextrose in water, 10% dextrose in water, or 20% dextrose in water (with or without added sodium chloride). If a preexisting line must be used, BIG-IV should not be diluted more than 1:2 with any of these solutions.[34] Human BIG-IV is administered at an initial rate of 25 mg/kg/h (0.5 mL/kg/h of reconstituted 50-mg/mL BIG-IV solution) for the first 15 minutes, which is then increased to 50 mg/kg/hr (1 mL/kg/hr of reconstituted 50 mg/mL BIG-IV solution), for a total infusion time of 97.5 minutes at the recommended dose.

Other Immunoglobulins

In regions where whole, equine-derived antitoxins are still available, it is important to note that these products required sensitivity testing and potential desensitization, and the package inserts should be consulted for specific procedural details for dosing and administration, particularly because titers and volumes may differ by brand.[49] For prophylaxis, the recommended dose of BAT-AB for an individual ate food suspected of being infected with *C. botulinum* depends on the amount of food eaten and is 1,500 to 7,500 IU of anti-type A and 1,100 to 5,500 IU of anti-type B intramuscularly (20%–100%

of one vial). This initial therapy was followed in 12 to 24 hours by the injection of a second vial if any signs or symptoms of botulism developed.[49] In addition, 1,000 IU to 5,000 IU (20% to 100% of one vial) of investigational anti-type E, based on the estimated ingested quantity of botulinum toxin, was used for type E outbreaks.[66] The BAT-AB and BAT-E treatment doses were one vial of antitoxin diluted 1:10 (vol/vol) in 0.9% sodium chloride solution and administered slowly intravenously over 30 to 60 minutes.[32,49] Subsequent doses could be provided intravenously every 2 to 4 hours if progression of clinical findings occurs. The BAT-AB and BAT-E are administered separately.

FORMULATION AND ACQUISITION

Heptavalent botulism antitoxin is supplied in either 20-mL or 50-mL single-dose vials. Despite variable vial filling of 10 to 22 mL/vial, the amount of A to G antitoxin contained per vial is fixed: more than 4,500 IU of anti-A, more than 3,300 IU of anti-B, more than 3,000 IU of anti-C, more than 600 IU of anti-D, more than 5,100 IU of anti-E, more than 3,000 IU of anti-F, and more than 600 IU of anti-G.[12] The bulk material contains approximately 30 to 70 mg/mL of protein. Heptavalent botulism antitoxin contains 10% maltose and 0.03% polysorbate 80. Heptavalent botulism antitoxin is stored frozen at or below 5°F (−15°C) until used. Thawed H-BAT must be maintained at 36° to 46°F (2°–8°C) and used within 36 months or until 48 months from the manufacture date, whichever occurs earliest. Heptavalent botulism antitoxin should not be refrozen. Frozen H-BAT can be thawed in a refrigerator at 36° to 46°F (2°–8°C) over approximately 14 hours. Rapid thawing can be achieved by placing at room temperature for 1 hour followed by a water bath at 98.6°F (37°C) until thawed. Reconstituted H-BAT may be stored refrigerated for use within 8 to 10 hours.

BabyBIG is formulated as a single-use, solvent-detergent-treated, sterile vial containing 100 ± 20 mg of lyophilized immunoglobin (primarily IgG with trace amounts of IgA and IgM), stabilized with 5% sucrose and 1% albumin (human), without preservative and supplied with 2 mL of Sterile Water for Injection USP for reconstitution.[27,34]

Bivalent BAT-AB, which may be available outside of the United States, must be maintained at 2° to 8°C (35°–46°F) and not frozen. It contains phenol 0.4% as a preservative.

Clinicians who suspect botulism should immediately call their local or state health department's emergency 24-hour telephone service to request release of BAT and comply with legal reporting requirements; a single case is considered a public health emergency. When local and state public health authorities are unavailable, the CDC Emergency Operations Center telephone contact is 770-488-7100. The CDC controls H-BAT distribution from stocks located throughout a national network of decentralized Quarantine Stations. The California Infant Botulism Treatment and Prevention Program (510-231-7600) maintains the supply of BabyBIG for infant botulism treatment. The Biomedical Advanced Research and Development Authority (BARDA) within the US Department of Health and Human Services has obtained approximately 120,000 H-BAT doses for the Strategic National Stockpile (SNS), with anticipated completion of delivery of 80,000 additional doses by 2018.[65] The CDC released 50 doses of H-BAT from the SNS to Ohio during a large outbreak from home-canned potato salad.[40]

SUMMARY

- In conjunction with frequent clinical assessments and aggressive supportive care of respiratory, gastric, and urinary function, BAT decreases morbidity and mortality after typical foodborne or wound botulism.
- Preliminary data suggest that early administration of licensed H-BAT decreases duration of hospitalization, ICU utilization, and mechanical ventilation.
- Licensed BabyBIG-IV provides effective treatment for infant botulism.
- Early consultation with local and state health departments, the CDC Emergency Operations Center (770-488-7100), or a regional poison control center (or other comparable agencies in other parts of the world) should occur to rapidly access effective therapeutic modalities and diagnostic tests for botulism.

REFERENCES

1. Anniballi F, et al. New targets in the search for preventive and therapeutic agents for botulism. *Expert Rev Anti Infect Ther*. 2014;12:1075-1086.
2. Arnon SS. Creation and development of the public service orphan drug human botulism immune globulin. *Pediatrics*. 2007;119:785-789.
3. Arnon SS, et al. Botulinum toxin as a biological weapon: medical and public health management. *JAMA*. 2001;285:1059-1070.
4. Arnon SS, et al. Human botulism immune globulin for the treatment of infant botulism. *N Engl J Med*. 2006;354:462-471.
5. Ball AP, et al. Human botulism caused by *Clostridium botulinum* type E: the Birmingham outbreak. *Q J Med*. 1979;48:473-491.
6. Barash JR, Arnon SS. A novel strain of *Clostridium botulinum* that produces type B and type H botulinum toxins. *J Infect Dis*. 2014;209:183-191.
7. Bilusic M, et al. Recurrent bulbar paralysis caused by botulinum toxin type B. *Clin Infect Dis*. 2008;46:e72-e74.
8. Black RE, Gunn RA. Hypersensitivity reactions associated with botulinal antitoxin. *Am J Med*. 1980;69:567-570.
9. Cai S, Singh BR. Strategies to design inhibitors of *Clostridium botulinum* neurotoxins. *Infect Disord Drug Targets*. 2007;7:47-57.
10. Campbell AJ, et al. Effective treatment of infant botulism on day 13 after symptom onset with human botulism antitoxin. *J Paediatr Child Health*. 2017;53:416-418.
11. Safety Study of 7 Botulinum Antitoxin Serotypes Derived from Horses (NCT00360737). http://clinicaltrials.gov/ct2/show/NCT00360737. Accessed August 27, 2012.
12. Cangene Corporation/ Prescribing Information. BAT, Botulism Antitoxin Heptavalent (A, B, C, D, E, F, G)—(Equine) Sterile Solution for Injection. Winnipeg, Canada: Cangene Corporation; 2017.
13. Castrodale L. Botulism in Alaska. A guide for physicians and health care providers. 2011 Update. Anchorage, Alaska: Alaska Department of Health and Social Services; 2011, http://www.epi.hss.state.ak.us/id/botulism/Botulism.pdf. Accessed August 27, 2012.
14. Centers for Disease Control and Prevention (CDC). Wound botulism—California, 1995. *MMWR Morb Mortal Wkly Rep*. 1995;44:889-892.
15. Centers for Disease Control and Prevention (CDC). *Botulism in the United States, 1899-1996. Handbook for Epidemiologists, Clinicians, and Laboratory Workers*. Atlanta, GA: Centers for Disease Control and Prevention; 1998.
16. Centers for Disease Control and Prevention (CDC). Investigational heptavalent botulinum antitoxin (HBAT) to replace licensed botulinum antitoxin AB and investigational botulinum antitoxin E. *MMWR Morb Mortal Wkly Rep*. 2010;59:299.
17. Centers for Disease Control and Prevention (CDC). Notice of CDC's discontinuation of investigational pentavalent (ABCDE) botulinum toxoid vaccine for workers at risk for occupational exposure to botulinum toxins. *MMWR Morb Mortal Wkly Rep*. 2011;60:1454-1455.
18. Chang GY, Ganguly G. Early antitoxin treatment in wound botulism results in better outcome. *Eur Neurol*. 2003;49:151-153.
19. Chapman AP. PEGylated antibodies and antibody fragments for improved therapy: a review. *Adv Drug Deliv Rev*. 2002;54:531-545.
20. Donadio JA, et al. Diagnosis and treatment of botulism. *J Infect Dis*. 1971;124:108-112.
21. Dover N, et al. Molecular characterization of a novel botulinum neurotoxin type H gene. *J Infect Dis*. 2014;209:192-202.
22. Elder A, et al. Translocation of inhaled ultrafine manganese oxide particles to the central nervous system. *Environ Health Perspect*. 2006;114:1172-1178.
23. Fagan RP, et al. Persistence of botulinum toxin in patients' serum: Alaska, 1959-2007. *J Infect Dis*. 2009;199:1029-1031.
24. Fagan RP, et al. Initial recovery and rebound of type f intestinal colonization botulism after administration of investigational heptavalent botulinum antitoxin. *Clin Infect Dis*. 2011;53:e125-128.
25. Fan KL, et al. Delayed antitoxin treatment of two adult patients with botulism after cosmetic injection of botulinum type A toxin. *J Emerg Med*. 2016;51:677-679.
26. Fiock MA, et al. Studies on immunity to toxins of *Clostridium botulinum*. IX. Immunologic response of man to purified ABCDE botulinum toxoid. *J Immunol*. 1963;90:697-702.
27. Food and Drug Administration: Summary Basis of Approval. Botulism Immune Globulin Intravenous (Human) (BIG-IV). California Department of Health Services Botulism Immune Globulin Intravenous (Human) (BIG-IV) Biologics License Application; 2003. http://www.fda.gov/downloads/biologicsbloodvaccines/bloodbloodproducts/approvedproducts/licensedproductsblas/fractionatedplasmaproducts/ucm117169.pdf. Accessed August 24, 2012.
28. Hart MK, et al. Advanced development of the rF1V and rBV A/B vaccines: progress and challenges. *Adv Prev Med*. 2012;2012:731604.
29. Hatheway CH, et al. Antitoxin levels in botulism patients treated with trivalent equine botulism antitoxin to toxin types A, B, and E. *J Infect Dis*. 1984;150:407-412.
30. Hibbs RG, et al. Experience with the use of an investigational F(ab')2 heptavalent botulism immune globulin of equine origin during an outbreak of type E botulism in Egypt. *Clin Infect Dis*. 1996;23:337-340.
31. Hill SE, et al. Foodborne botulism treated with heptavalent botulism antitoxin. *Ann Pharmacother*. 2013;47:e12.
32. Horowitz BZ. Type E botulism. *Clin Toxicol*. 2010;48:880-895.
33. Iida H. Specific antitoxin therapy in type E botulism. *Jpn J Med Sci Biol*. 1963;16:311-313.

34. Infant Botulism Treatment and Prevention Program, California Department of Public Health: BabyBIG [Botulism Immune Globulin Intravenous (Human) (BIG-IV)] Lyophilized Powder for Reconstitution and Injection [prescribing information]. Richmond, CA: California Department of Public Health; 2016.

35. Koenig MG, et al. Clinical and laboratory observations on type E botulism in man. *Medicine.* 1964;43:517-545.

36. Leclair D, et al. Foodborne botulism in Canada, 1985-2005. *Emerg Infect Dis.* 2013;19:961-968.

37. Li D, et al. New equine antitoxins to botulinum neurotoxins serotypes A and B. *Biologicals.* 2012;40:240-246.

38. Maslanka SE, et al. A Novel Botulinum neurotoxin, previously reported as serotype H, has a hybrid-like structure with regions of similarity to the structures of serotypes A and F and is neutralized with serotype A antitoxin. *J Infect Dis.* 2016;213:379-385.

39. Mazuet C, et al. Characterization of botulinum neurotoxin type A neutralizing monoclonal antibodies and influence of their half-lives on therapeutic activity. *PloS One.* 2010;5:e12416.

40. McCarty CL, et al. Large Outbreak of Botulism Associated with a Church Potluck Meal—Ohio, 2015. *MMWR Morb Mortal Wkly Rep.* 2015;64:802-803.

41. McLaughlin J, Funk B. New Recommendations for Use of Heptavalent Botulinum Antitoxin (H-BAT). State of Alaska Epidemiology Bulletin. Bulletin No. 5: March 3, 2010.

42. Merson MH, et al. Current trends in botulism in the United States. *JAMA.* 1974; 229:1305-1308.

43. Oberst FW, et al. Evaluation of botulinum antitoxin, supportive therapy, and artificial respiration in monkeys with experimental botulism. *Clin Pharmacol Ther.* 1968;9:209-214.

44. Offerman SR, et al. Wound botulism in injection drug users: time to antitoxin correlates with intensive care unit length of stay. *West J Emerg Med.* 2009;10:251-256.

45. Pickett J, et al. Syndrome of botulism in infancy: clinical and electrophysiologic study. *N Engl J Med.* 1976;295:770-772.

46. Polo JM, et al. Botulism and pregnancy. *Lancet.* 1996;348:195.

47. Robin L, et al. Botulism in a pregnant women. *N Engl J Med.* 1996;335:823-824.

48. Sandrock CE, Murin S. Clinical predictors of respiratory failure and long-term outcome in black tar heroin-associated wound botulism. *Chest.* 2001;120:562-566.

49. Sanofi Pasteur Limited. Botulism Antitoxin Bivalent (Equine) Types A and B. Package Insert R2-0705 USA. Toronto, Canada: Sanofi Pasteur Limited; 2005.

50. Sevcik C, et al. Initial volume of a drug before it reaches the volume of distribution: pharmacokinetics of F(ab')2 antivenoms and other drugs. *Toxicon.* 2007;50:653-665.

51. Shapiro RL, et al. Botulism surveillance and emergency response. A public health strategy for a global challenge. *JAMA.* 1997;278:433-435.

52. Shearer JD, et al. Preclinical safety assessment of recombinant botulinum vaccine A/B (rBV A/B). *Vaccine.* 2012;30:1917-1926.

53. Shearer JD, et al. Botulinum neurotoxin neutralizing activity of immune globulin (IG) purified from clinical volunteers vaccinated with recombinant botulinum vaccine (rBV A/B). *Vaccine.* 2010;28:7313-7318.

54. Sheth AN, et al. International outbreak of severe botulism with prolonged toxemia caused by commercial carrot juice. *Clin Infect Dis.* 2008;47:1245-1251.

55. Smith LA. Botulism and vaccines for its prevention. *Vaccine.* 2009;27(suppl 4):D33-D39.

56. Smith LA, Rusnak JM. Botulinum neurotoxin vaccines: past, present, and future. *Crit Rev Immunol.* 2007;27:303-318.

57. Souayah N, et al. Severe botulism after focal injection of botulinum toxin. *Neurology.* 2006;67:1855-1856.

58. St. Clair EH, et al. Observations of an infant born to a mother with botulism. *J Pediatr.* 1975;87:658.

59. Tacket CO, et al. Equine antitoxin use and other factors that predict outcome in type A foodborne botulism. *Am J Med.* 1984;76:794-798.

60. Taylor SM, et al. Wound botulism complicating internal fixation of a complex radial fracture. *J Clin Microbiol.* 2010;48:650-653.

61. Thilo EH, et al. Infant botulism at 1 week of age: report of two cases. *Pediatrics.* 1993;92:151-153.

62. Underwood K, et al. Infant botulism: a 30-year experience spanning the introduction of botulism immune globulin intravenous in the intensive care unit at Childrens Hospital Los Angeles. *Pediatrics.* 2007;120:e1380-e1385.

63. Vanella de Cuetos EE, et al. Equine botulinum antitoxin for the treatment of infant botulism. *Clin Vaccine Immunol.* 2011;18:1845-1849.

64. Villar RG, et al. Outbreak of type A botulism and development of a botulism surveillance and antitoxin release system in Argentina. *JAMA.* 1999;281:1334-1338, 1340.

65. Webb RP, et al. Botulinum neurotoxin. In: Morse SA, ed. *Bioterrorism.* Rijeka, Croatia: Intech; 2012.

66. Weber JT, et al. A massive outbreak of type E botulism associated with traditional salted fish in Cairo. *J Infect Dis.* 1993;167:451-454.

67. Williams BT, et al. Emergency department identification and critical care management of a Utah prison botulism outbreak. *Ann Emerg Med.* 2014;64:26-31.

68. Witoonpanich R, et al. Survival analysis for respiratory failure in patients with foodborne botulism. *Clin Toxicol (Phila).* 2010;48:177-183.

69. Woodruff BA, et al. Clinical and laboratory comparison of botulism from toxin types A, B, and E in the United States, 1975-1988. *J Infect Dis.* 1992;166:1281-1286.

70. Yasmin S, et al. Outbreak of botulism after consumption of illicit prison-brewed alcohol in a maximum security prison—Arizona, 2012. *J Correct Health Care.* 2015;21:327-334.

71. Yuan J, et al. Recurrent wound botulism among injection drug users in California. *Clin Infect Dis.* 2011;52:862-866.

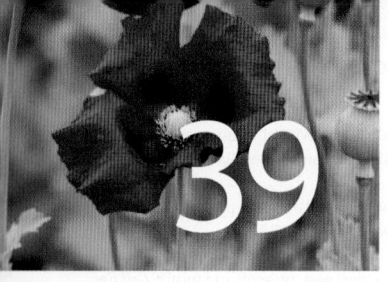

39 FOOD POISONING

Laura J. Fil and Michael G. Tunik

Each year in the United States known foodborne pathogens are responsible for approximately 30.7 million illnesses, 228,144 hospitalizations, and 2,612 deaths.[47] It is estimated that foodborne illness costs an annual burden to the American society of 36 billion dollars, which is estimated to be an average cost burden per illness of $3,630.[143] Worldwide food distribution, large-scale national food preparation and distribution networks, limited food regulatory practices, and corporate greed place everyone at risk. Food poisoning causes morbidity and mortality by one or more of the following mechanisms: (bacteria, viruses and parasites) that can be transmitted in food; toxins that are produced by organisms, can be consumed in food; and xenobiotics can be inadvertently or purposefully used to contaminate food and ultimately be ingested.

This chapter is organized into four major types of food poisoning: foodborne poisoning with neurologic effects, food poisoning with gastrointestinal (GI) symptoms, foodborne poisoning with anaphylaxislike effects, and food poisoning used for bioterrorism.

HISTORY AND EPIDEMIOLOGY

In the United States, viruses are the most responsible cause of foodborne outbreaks (82%) followed by bacteria (12%), and parasites (6%). Norovirus was the most common cause of single, confirmed etiology outbreaks (54%). The bacteria that caused the largest number of food poisonings were *Salmonella* spp, *Clostridium perfringens, Staphylococcus aureus* enterotoxin, and *Shigella* spp. The estimated annual number of episodes of foodborne pathogen related illness, hospitalization and death in the United States is shown in Table 39–1.[48]

Globally, researchers estimated foodborne pathogens were found to cause 582 million cases of illnesses annually. The leading cause of foodborne illness was norovirus (125 million cases) followed by campylobacter (96 million). Most important, around 43% of the disease burden from contaminated food occurred in children younger than 5 years of age, who make up 9% of the population.[110]

In the past decade, large numbers of people have also had food poisoning because of purposeful placement of chemicals in food.[51]

Many foodborne illnesses result in long-term sequelae to the GI, immune, nervous, respiratory, renal, cardiovascular, endocrine, and hepatic systems.[14]

FOODBORNE POISONING WITH NEUROLOGIC SYMPTOMS

The differential diagnosis of patients with foodborne poisoning presenting with neurologic symptoms is vast (Tables 39–2 and 39–3). The sources of many of these cases are ichthyosarcotoxic, involving toxins from the muscles, viscera, skin, gonads, and mucous surfaces of the fish; rarely, toxicity follows consumption of the fish blood or skeleton. Most episodes of poisoning are not species specific, although particular forms of toxicity from Tetraodontiformes (puffer fish), Gymnothoraces (moray eel), and newts (*Taricha* and other species) are recognized.

In cases of ciguatera poisoning, the major symptoms usually are neurotoxic, and the GI symptoms are minor. Knowing where the fish was caught often helps establish a diagnosis, but refrigerated transport of foods and rapid worldwide travel can complicate the assessment. Travelers to Caribbean, Pacific, and Canary islands, as well as those traveling within the United States, have experienced ciguatera poisoning.[119,155] In geographically disparate regions of Canada,[161] individuals have experienced domoic acid poisoning caused by ingestion of cultivated mussels from Prince Edward Island.

In the differential diagnosis of foodborne poisons presenting with neurologic findings, activities other than eating must always be considered. In particular, sport divers often perform their activities in high-risk areas such as Florida, California, and Hawaii and often during the high-risk periods from May through August. In the process, they may sustain a sting from a stingray tail, or laceration (from a deltoid or pectoral fin spine of a lionfish or stonefish) that can cause consequential marine toxicity (Chap. 116). Scientists have found that the chance of encountering numerous bacterial pathogens harmful to both human and marine life was cut in half near seagrass meadows. Swimmers and divers can limit disease by choosing waters rich in seagrass meadows.[165]

Ciguatera Poisoning

Ciguatera poisoning is one of the most commonly reported forms of vertebrate fishborne poisonings in the United States, accounting for almost half of the reported cases.[85] Ciguatoxins are lipid soluble, polyether compounds consisting of 13 to 14 rings fused by ether linkages into a rigid ladder-like structure (Fig. 39–1). Ciguatera poisoning is endemic to warm water, bottom-dwelling reef fish living around the globe between 35° North and 35° South latitude, which includes tropical areas such as the Indian Ocean, the South Pacific, and the Caribbean. Hawaii and Florida report 90% of all cases occurring in the United States, most commonly from May through August.[125] The incidence and geographical distribution of ciguatera are increasing because of increased fish trade and consumption, international tourism, and climate changes.

TABLE 39–1	Estimated Annual Number of Episodes of Illness, Hospitalizations and Death Caused by Pathogens Transmitted Commonly by Food in the United States (2014)[48]		
Pathogen	Total Mean Episodes	Total Mean Hospitalizations	Total Mean Deaths
BACTERIA			
Bacillus cereus	62,623	20	0
Campylobacter spp.	1,322,137	13,240	119
Clostridium botulinum	56	42	9
Clostridium perfringens	969,342	439	26
*STEC O157**	96,534	3,268	31
Listeria monocytogenes	1,662	1,520	266
Salmonella spp.	1,229,007	23,128	452
S. enterica	5,752	623	0
Shigella spp.	494,908	5,491	38
Staphylococcus spp.	241,994	1,067	6
Streptococcus Group A	11,257	1	0
Vibrio vulnificus	207	202	77
Vibrio parahaemolyticus	44,950	129	5
Yersinia enterocolitica	116,706	637	34
PARASITES			
Cryptosporidium spp.	748,123	210	46
Giardia intestinalis	1,221,564	225	34
Trichinella	162	6	0
VIRUSES			
Astrovirus	3,090,384	17,430	5
Hepatitis A	35,769	2,255	171
Norovirus	20,865,958	56,013	571
Rotavirus	3,090,384	69,721	32

*STEC = shiga toxin producing Escherichia coli.

TABLE 39–2	Differential Diagnosis of Possible Foodborne Poisoning Presenting with Neurologic Findings[a]

Anticholinergic poisoning
Bacterial food poisoning
Botulism
Dinoflagellates (brevetoxin, saxitoxin)
Marine food poisoning (ciguatoxin, tetrodotoxin)
Metals (arsenic, lead, mercury)
Monosodium glutamate
Mushrooms (*Amanita* spp, *Gyromitra* spp)
Organic phosphorus compounds

[a]Altered mental status, motor weakness, and sensory changes.

More than 500 fish species have caused human cases of ciguatera poisoning, with the barracuda, sea bass, parrot fish, red snapper, grouper, amber jack, kingfish, and sturgeon the most common sources. The common factor is the comparably large size of the fish involved.

Large fish (1.5–3.0 kg or more) become vectors of ciguatera poisoning in accordance with complex feeding patterns inherent in aquatic life. This traditional teaching is challenged by a recent study. The lack of relationship between toxicity and size observed for most of the species and families from the six islands in French Polynesia suggests that fish size cannot be used as an efficient predictor of fish toxicity.[75] Ciguatoxin is found in blue-green algae, protozoa, and the free algae dinoflagellates. These plankton members of the phylum Protozoa are single-celled, motile, flagellated, pigmented organisms thriving through photosynthesis. Photosynthetic dinoflagellates such as *Gambierdiscus toxicus* and bacteria within the dinoflagellates are the origins of ciguatoxin.[66,97,130] Dinoflagellates are the main nutritional source for small herbivorous fish, which, in turn, are the major food source for larger carnivorous fish, thereby increasing the ciguatoxin concentrations in the flesh, adipose tissue, and viscera of larger and larger fish.[12]

Ciguatoxin is heat stable, lipid soluble, acid stable, odorless, and tasteless. When purified, the toxin is a large (molecular weight, 1,100 Da) complex ester that does not harm the fish but is stored in its tissues.[125,131] The molecule binds to voltage-sensitive sodium channels in diverse tissues and increases the sodium permeability of the channel.[191] The ciguatoxins cause hyperpolarization and a shift in the voltage dependence of channel activation, which opens the sodium channels. Ciguatoxins bind selectively to a particular binding site on the neuron's voltage-sensitive sodium channel protein.[129]

Multiple ciguatoxins are identified in the same fish, perhaps explaining the variability of symptoms and differing severity.[130] People can be affected after eating fresh or frozen fish that was prepared by all common methods: boiling, baking, frying, stewing, or broiling. The appearance, taste, and smell of the ciguatoxic fish are usually unremarkable. The majority of symptomatic episodes begin 2 to 6 hours after ingestion, 75% within 12 hours, and 96% within 24 hours.[12] Symptoms include acute onset of diaphoresis; headaches, abdominal pain with cramps, nausea, or vomiting; profuse watery diarrhea; and a constellation of dramatic neurologic symptoms.[209] A sensation of loose or painful teeth is reported. Typically, peripheral dysesthesias and paresthesias predominate. Watery eyes, tingling, and numbness of the tongue, lips, throat, and perioral area occur. A strange metallic taste is frequently reported as is a reversal of temperature discrimination, the pathophysiology of which remains to be elucidated.[34] Myalgias, most often in the lower extremities; arthralgias; ataxia; and weakness are commonly experienced.[12]

Dysuria[81] and symptoms of dyspareunia and vaginal and pelvic discomfort are reported to occur in some women after sexual intercourse with men who are ciguatoxic and whose semen contains the toxin.[118] Vertigo, seizures, and visual disturbances (eg, blurred vision, scotomata, and transient blindness) are reported.

Bradycardia and orthostatic hypotension are described.[77] The GI symptoms usually subside within 24 to 48 hours; however, cardiovascular and neurologic symptoms typically persist for several days to weeks, depending

TABLE 39–3	Foodborne Neurologic Toxicity (Primary Presenting Symptoms)						
Disease	**Toxin**	**Toxin Source and Mechanism**[**]	**Onset**	**Duration**	**Findings**	**Therapy**	**Diagnosis**
Ciguatera	Ciguatoxin	Large reef fish: amber jack, barracuda, snapper, parrot, sea bass, moray **Increased sodium channel permeability	2–24 h	Days-weeks	Paresthesias, nausea; vomiting, diarrhea, temperature reversal	Mannitol, amitriptyline	Clinical, mouse bioassay, immunoassay
Tetrodotoxin	Tetrodotoxin	Puffer fish, *fugu*, blue-ringed octopus, newts, horseshoe crab Dinoflagellate **Blocks sodium channel	Minutes to hours	Days	Paresthesias, respiratory depression, hypotension	Respiratory support	Clinical
Neurotoxic shell-fish poisoning	Brevetoxin	Mussels, clams, scallops, oysters, *Ptychodiscus brevis*: "red tide" **Increased sodium channel permeability	15 min to 18 h	Days	Bronchospasm, temperature reversal, nausea; vomiting, diarrhea, paresthesias	Bronchodilators	Clinical, mouse bioassay of food, HPLC
Paralytic shellfish poisoning	Saxitoxin	Mussels, clams, scallops, oysters, *Protogonyaulax catenella*, *Protogonyaulax tamarensis* **Decreases sodium channel permeability	30 min	Days	Respiratory depression, paresthesias, nausea, vomiting, diarrhea	Respiratory support	Clinical, mouse bioassay of food, HPLC
Amnestic shellfish poisoning	Domoic acid	Mussels, possibly other shellfish; *Nitzschia pungens* **Excitatory neurotoxicity	15 min to 38 h	Years	Amnesia, nausea; vomiting, diarrhea, paresthesias, respiratory depression	Respiratory support	Clinical, mouse bioassay of food, HPLC
Botulism	Botulinum toxin	Home-canned foods, honey, corn syrups, *Clostridium botulinum* **Binds presynaptically, blocks acetylcholine release	12–72 h	Weeks	Vomiting, diarrhea, respiratory depression, initial cranial nerve paralysis followed by a symmetric descending paralysis of the motor and autonomic nerves	Antitoxin, respiratory support	Clinical, immunoassay, serologic, bacteriologic

HPLC = high-pressure liquid chromatography.

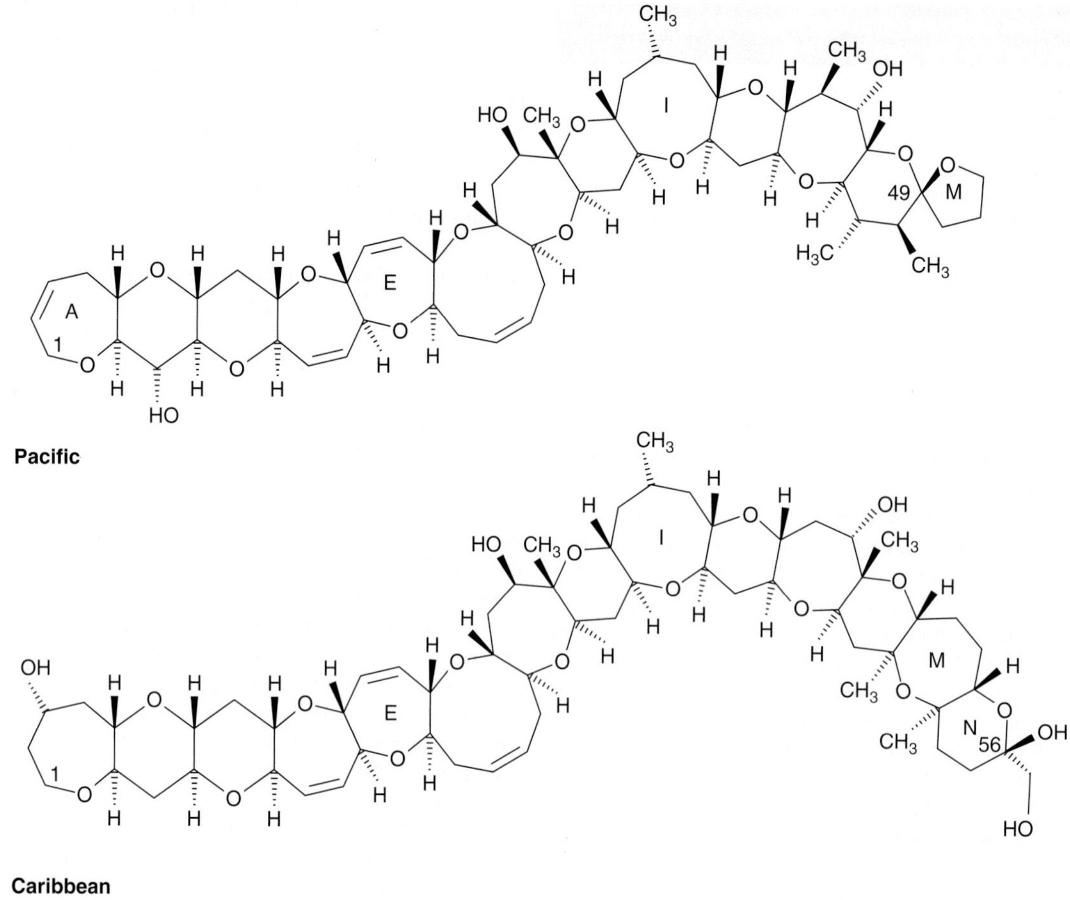

FIGURE 39-1. The structure of Pacific and Caribbean ciguatoxins. *Source: Food and Agriculture Organization of the United Nations. 2004, Marine Biotoxins; FAO Food and Nutrition Paper 80. http://www.fao.org/docrep/007/y5486e/y5486e00.htm. Reproduced with permission.*

on the amount of toxin ingested. Delayed effects include protracted itching and hiccoughs. Ciguatoxin is transmitted in breast milk[23] and can cross the placenta.[159]

Although deaths are reported, internationally, none have been documented in the United States.[85] When it occurs, death is a result of respiratory paralysis and seizures not managed with adequate life support. One study showed that the main contributory factors associated with death were the consumption of ciguatoxin-rich fish parts (viscera and head) in larger amounts, ingestion of the ciguatoxic fish species (eg, barracuda, sea bass, red snapper, grouper), ingestion of reef fish collected after storms, and ultimately individual susceptibility.[52]

The Food and Drug Administration' (FDA's) and Ciguatoxin (CTX) fish testing procedure is performed in an analytical laboratory setting and uses a two-tiered protocol involving: (1) in vitro mouse neuroblastoma (N2a) cell assay as a semiquantitative screen for toxicity consistent with CTX mode of action and (2) liquid chromatography tandem–mass spectrometry (LC-MS/MS) for molecular confirmation of CTX. To date, there is no commercially available, rapid, cost-effective, fish-testing product that has been demonstrated by independent investigations to provide CTX detection in seafood with adequate reliability or accuracy.

Laboratory testing is not readily available, and it often takes days to weeks to receive the result. A useful approach to diagnosis and management includes laboratory testing to exclude other possible etiologies and determine the need for, or extent of, specific therapeutic interventions.

Initial treatment for victims of ciguatoxin poisoning includes standard supportive care for a toxic ingestion.[209] In most patients, elimination of the toxin is accelerated if vomiting (40%) and diarrhea (70%) have occurred. Administration of activated charcoal has benefit for patients who are not vomiting. In patients with significant GI fluid loss through vomiting,

diarrhea, or both, intravenous (IV) fluid and electrolyte repletion are essential. The orthostatic hypotension responds to IV fluids and α-adrenergic agonists. Symptomatic bradycardia is treated with atropine.[73]

Intravenous mannitol is reported to alleviate neurologic and muscular dysfunctional symptoms associated with ciguatera; however, GI symptoms are not ameliorated.[158,160] An in vivo study showed that there was no change in neuronal swelling when ciguatera-poisoned cells were treated with mannitol but did show some prevention of the membrane depolarization and repetitive firing of action potentials induced by ciguatera.[19] Despite these findings, one prospective randomized control trial, mannitol failed to produce any greater improvement in symptoms than did IV normal saline solution. This study is a randomized double-blinded control trial to answer this question. Most of the previous data on the use of mannitol in ciguatera poisoning was either obtained in an uncontrolled or randomized but nonblinded fashion or is the result of case reports.[179] Mannitol should be used with caution because it causes hypotension. Vascular reexpansion and cardiovascular stability should be initial treatment priorities. Mannitol works by inhibiting the ciguatoxin-induced opening of sodium channels on the neuron membranes or reducing the neural edema via an osmotic gradient and is recommended in the hemodynamically stable patient. The search for a treatment for ciguatera poisoning that has minimal side effects and is easily accessible is ongoing. Two cases were reported of symptomatic patients exposed to ciguatera who were successfully treated with pregabalin.[30] There is limited evidence for the efficacy of pregabalin.[30]

Admission to the hospital for cautious supportive care is essential when the diagnosis is uncertain or when volume depletion or any consequential manifestations are present (Tables 39–2 and 39–3). The etiology of the symptoms must be rapidly identified to provide specific therapy, if available. Diaphoresis is a common clinical finding and an important factor in the differential diagnosis. Late in the course of ciguatera poisoning, amitriptyline 25 mg orally twice daily helps alleviate symptoms,[27] which have been reported to persist up to 1 year. Patients recovering from ciguatera should avoid alcohol and nuts for 3 to 6 months if their consumption exacerbates symptoms.

Ciguateralike Poisoning

Moray, conger, and anguillid eels carry a ciguatoxinlike neurotoxin in their viscera, muscles, and gonads that does not affect the eel itself. The toxin is a complex ester that is structurally very similar to ciguatoxin and is heat stable.[154] Individuals who eat these eels can infrequently manifest neurotoxic symptoms similar to ciguatoxin or show signs of cholinergic toxicity, such as hypersalivation, nausea, vomiting, and diarrhea. Shortness of breath, mucosal erythema, and cutaneous eruptions also occur. These findings are present in addition to the neurotoxic symptoms.[90] Management is supportive. Death is related to the complications of neurotoxicity, such as seizures and respiratory paralysis.

Shellfish Poisoning

Healthy mollusks living between 30° North and 30° South latitude ingest and filter large quantities of dinoflagellates. These dinoflagellates are the major source of available ocean food during the "non-R" months (May through August) in the northern hemisphere. During this time, these dinoflagellates are responsible for the "red tides" that occur from California to Alaska, from New England to the St. Lawrence, and across the west coast of Europe.[137] The number of toxic dinoflagellates in these "red tides" is often so overwhelming that birds and fish die, and humans who walk along the beach experience respiratory symptoms caused by aerosolized toxin.[140]

Ingestion of shellfish, including oysters, clams, mussels, and scallops, contaminated by dinoflagellates or algae causes neurotoxic, paralytic, and amnestic syndromes. The dinoflagellates most frequently implicated are *Karenia brevis* (originally named *Gymnodinium breve* in 1948, renamed *Ptychodiscus brevis* in 1979, and reclassified again to the current nomenclature in 2000). The diatoms causing neurotoxic shellfish poisoning (NSP) include *Protogonyaulax catanella* and *Protogonyaulax tamarensis*, which cause paralytic shellfish poisoning, and *Nitzschia pungens*, the diatom implicated in amnestic shellfish poisoning. Proliferation of these diatoms cause a red tide, but shellfish poisoning occurs even in the absence of this extreme proliferation.

Paralytic shellfish poisoning is caused by saxitoxin. Saxitoxin blocks the voltage-sensitive sodium channel in a manner identical to tetrodotoxin (TTX; see later). The shellfish implicated usually are clams, oysters, mussels, and scallops, but poisoning has occurred through consumption of crustaceans, gastropods, and fish. In the summer of 2013, a saxitoxin outbreak was identified among 31 individuals in the who consumed green mussels in the Philippines. The symptoms in these individuals ranged from circumoral and extremity numbness to dizziness and lightheadedness. One adult and one child died secondary to cardiorespiratory arrest.[56]

The higher the number of affected shellfish consumed, the more severe the symptoms. Symptoms usually occur within 30 minutes of ingestion. Neurologic effects predominate and include paresthesias and numbness of the mouth and extremities, a sensation of floating, headache, ataxia, vertigo, muscle weakness, paralysis, and cranial nerve dysfunction manifested by dysphagia, dysarthria, dysphonia, and transient blindness. Gastrointestinal symptoms are less common and include nausea, vomiting, abdominal pain, and diarrhea. Fatalities occur as a result of respiratory failure, usually within the first 12 hours after symptom onset. Muscle weakness often persists for weeks.

Treatment is supportive. Early intervention for respiratory failure is indicated. Orogastric lavage and cathartics were used to remove unabsorbed toxin from the GI tract and were not efficacious and thus are not recommended.[31,127,145,183] Activated charcoal is reasonable if vomiting has not occurred. Antibodies against saxitoxin have reversed cardiorespiratory failure in animals,[16] but this therapy is not yet available for humans. Assays for saxitoxin include a mouse bioassay, enzyme-linked immunosorbent assay (ELISA), and high-performance liquid chromatography (HPLC). High-performance liquid chromatography is demonstrated to result in good interlaboratory accuracy,[203] but the differences in saxitoxin derivatives make standardization of an analytic test difficult.[11,121]

Neurotoxic shellfish poisoning is caused by brevetoxin. Brevetoxin, which is produced by *K. brevis* (previously *Gymnodium brevis*, and subsequently *P. brevis*), is a lipid-soluble, heat-stable polyether toxin similar to ciguatoxin. It acts by stimulating sodium flux through the sodium channels of both nerve and muscle.[8,35] Similar to paralytic shellfish poisoning, the shellfish implicated usually are clams, oysters, mussels, and other filter feeders. Neurotoxic shellfish poisoning is characterized by gastroenteric manifestations with associated neurologic symptoms. Gastrointestinal symptoms include abdominal pain, nausea, vomiting, diarrhea, and rectal burning. Neurologic features include paresthesias, reversal of hot and cold temperature sensation, myalgias, vertigo, and ataxia. Other effects include headache, malaise, tremor, dysphagia, bradycardia, decreased reflexes, and mydriasis. Paralysis does not occur. Bradycardia and mydriasis are not commonly present in an individual patent. The incubation period is 3 hours (range, 15 minutes–18 hours). Gastrointestinal and neurologic symptoms appear simultaneously. Other manifestations of brevetoxin poisoning include mucosal irritation, cough, and bronchospasm, which occur when *P. brevis* is aerosolized by wave action during red tides. The duration of effects averages 17 hours (range, 1–72 hours).[145]

Brevetoxins are identified by mouse bioassay; ELISA; and, more recently, antibody radioimmunoassay and reconstituted sodium channels. (Reconstitution is when a purified membrane protein is incorporated into a membrane bilayer and the reconstituted channel is then used as a tool for the measurement of specific toxin binding.[163,200]) Treatment is supportive, and severe respiratory depression is very uncommon. Therapy includes removal of the patient from the environment and the administration of bronchodilators. An antagonist to brevetoxin named brevenal has been discovered and is in the early research phase as a potential therapy.[82] Neurotoxic shellfish poisoning is not fatal.

Amnestic shellfish poisoning is caused by domoic acid, which is produced by the diatom a *N. pungens*. Domoic acid is structurally similar to glutamic acid, kainic acid, and aspartic acid (Fig. 39–2). Because of this structural similarity, domoic acid interacts with the glutamate receptors on nerve cell terminals. Glutamate is the principal neuroexcitatory transmitter in the brain and is necessary for synaptic transmission (Chap. 13). However, excessive glutamate is associated with neurodegeneration, seizures, and apoptosis.[124]

The most extensively documented human outbreak occurred in Canada in 1987, when 107 individuals who had consumed mussels harvested from cultivated river estuaries on Prince Edward Island were affected.[161] Other human outbreaks have occurred due to a similar diatom—*Pseudonitzschia australis*—which has been isolated in shellfish from other areas.[74] Pelican deaths caused by domoic acid–laden anchovies were reported in 1991 and Canada instituted monitoring for domoic acid after this outbreak.[197] The death of 400 sea lions in California in 1998 was linked to domoic acid from the same diatom.[180]

Amnestic shellfish poisoning is characterized by GI symptoms of nausea, vomiting, abdominal cramps, diarrhea, and neurologic symptoms of memory loss and, less frequently, coma, seizures, hemiparesis, ophthalmoplegia,

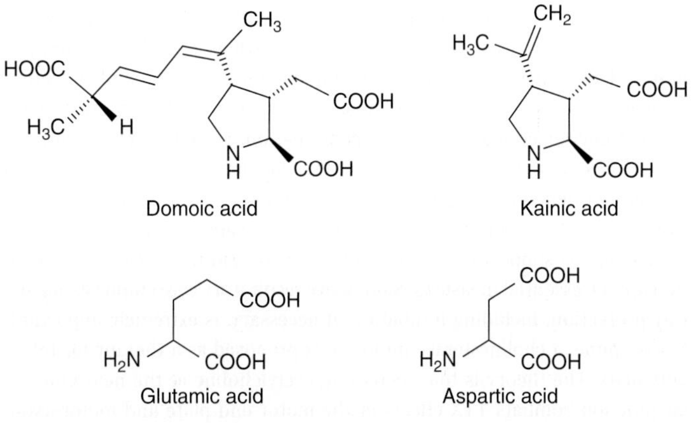

FIGURE 39–2. Comparison of the chemical structures of domoic acid, kainic acid, glutamic acid, and aspartic acid.[121]

purposeless chewing, and grimacing. Other signs and symptoms include hemodynamic instability and cardiac dysrhythmias. Symptoms typically begin 5 hours (range, 15 minutes–38 hours) after ingestion of mussels. The mortality rate is 2%, with death most frequently occurring in older patients, who experience more severe neurologic symptoms. Ten percent of victims have long-term antegrade memory deficits, as well as motor and sensory neuropathy. Postmortem examinations revealed neuronal damage in the hippocampus and amygdala.[195] Animal studies show that domoic acid can cross the placenta.[138]

Tetrodotoxin Poisoning

This type of fish poisoning involves only the order Tetraodontiformes. Although this order of fish is not restricted geographically, it is eaten most frequently in Japan, California, Africa, South America, and Australia.[90] Cases also occurred in Florida and New Jersey, as well as Europe, the Mediterranean, and Bangladesh. Approximately 100 freshwater and saltwater species exist in this order, including a number of pufferlike fish such as the globe fish, balloon fish, blowfish, and toad fish.[147] Tetrodotoxin (TTX) found in these fish is also isolated from the blue-ringed octopus[71] and the gastropod mollusk[211] and are responsible for fatalities from ingestion of horseshoe crab eggs.[102] Certain TTX-containing newts (*Taricha*, notophthalmus, triturus, and cynops), particularly *Taricha granulosa*, found in Oregon, California, and southern Alaska, are reportedly fatal when ingested. Most newts and salamanders with bright colors and rough skins contain toxins.[28] In Japan, *fugu* (a local variety of puffer fish) is considered a delicacy, but special licensing is required to prepare this exceedingly toxic fish. In 1989, the US FDA legalized the importation of puffer fish. However, before exportation from Japan, the fish must be laboratory tested and certified by two Japanese organizations to be free of TTX.[49]

Tetrodotoxin is a heat-stable, water-soluble nonprotein found mainly in the fish skin, liver, ovary, intestine, and possibly muscle.[90,175] The ovary has a high concentration of the toxin and is most poisonous if eaten during the spawning season. Tetrodotoxin is detected by mouse bioassay. It is unstable when heated to 212°F (100°C) in acid, distinguishing it from saxitoxin. Tetrodotoxin from fish is detected using fluorescent spectrometry[11] or from the urine of poisoned patients using a combination of immunoaffinity chromatography and fluorometric HPLC.[105]

Similar to saxitoxin, TTX is produced by marine bacteria and likely accumulate in animals higher on the food chain that consume these bacteria.[151] Accumulation of toxins, primarily in the skin, of two species of Asian puffer fish is documented. Whether this accumulation of toxin is simply an evolutionary adaptation, to remove a toxic substance, or one that has evolutionary advantages of protection is unclear.[150]

Neurotoxicity is produced by inhibition of sodium channels and blockade of neuromuscular transmission. The sodium channel is blocked from the external surface of the neuron by the TTX molecule, which contains a guanidinium group that fits into the external orifice of the sodium channel. This causes external "plugging" of the sodium channel, although the gating mechanism remains functional.[148,149]

Effects of TTX poisoning typically occur within minutes of ingestion. Headache, diaphoresis, dysesthesias, and paresthesias of the lips, tongue, mouth, face, fingers, and toes evolve rapidly. Buccal bullae and salivation develop. Dysphagia, dysarthria, nausea, vomiting, and abdominal pain ensue. Generalized malaise, loss of coordination, weakness, fasciculations, and an ascending paralysis (with risk of respiratory paralysis) occur in 4 to 24 hours. Other cranial nerves are involved. In more severe toxicity, hypotension is present. In some studies, the mortality rate approaches 50%.[186]

Therapy is supportive. Removal of the toxin and prevention of absorption are the essential measures. Supportive respiratory care emphasizing airway protection, including intubation, if necessary, is extremely important. Neostigmine, a cholinesterase inhibitor, is proposed as a therapy for tetrodotoxicity. The theory is that increasing acetylcholine at the neuromuscular junction combats TTX effects at the motor end plate and motor axon. Although this sounds promising, a recent literature review found the data insufficient to make an evidence-based recommendation.[132]

Clostridium botulinum

In 2015, the CDC reported 39 cases of laboratory-confirmed foodborne botulism and 141 cases of infant botulism.[50] Home-canned fruits and vegetables, as well as commercial fish products, are among the common foods causing botulism. The incubation period usually is 12 to 36 hours; typical signs and symptoms include some initial GI symptoms followed by malaise, fatigue, diplopia, dysphagia, and rapid development of small muscle incoordination.[122] In botulism, the toxin is irreversibly bound to the structures within the nerve terminal, where it impairs the presynaptic release of acetylcholine.[115] A patient's survival depends on rapidly diagnosing botulism and immediate initiation of aggressive respiratory therapy. Establishing the diagnosis early makes it possible to treat the "sentinel" or index patient and also others who consumed the contaminated food with antitoxin before their developing signs and symptoms (Chap. 38 and Antidotes in Depth: A6). The differential diagnosis of botulism includes myasthenia gravis, atypical Guillain-Barré syndrome, tick-induced paralysis, and certain chemical ingestions (Tables 39–1 and 39–2).

PREVENTION OF MARINE FOODBORNE DISEASE

Careful evaluation of the symptoms and meticulous reporting to local and state health departments, as well as to the US Centers for Disease Control and Prevention (CDC), will allow for more precise analysis of epidemics of poisoning from contaminated or poisonous food or fish. Many states and countries have developed rigorous health codes with regard to harvesting certain species of fish in certain areas at certain times.

Some examples of actions taken by state, federal, and foreign health agencies in controlling epidemics of seafood-borne food poisoning are the following: The health code of Miami, Florida, prohibits the sale of barracuda and warns against eating fillets from large and potentially toxic fish containing ciguatoxin. A 3,230-km stretch of the Massachusetts coastline was noted to be unsafe for shellfish harvesting because of a red tide bloom. The National Oceanic and Atmospheric Administration's Fisheries Service along with the FDA declared a health emergency and confiscated shellfish harvested in this area and prohibited the marketing, export, and serving of shellfish.[33] The Japanese closely regulate preparation and selling of the puffer fish (fugu), requiring that preparers receive special training and licensing. The sale of fugu is now also permitted under strict control in the United States as well. The Canadian government identifies and registers the location and time of harvesting of mussels, and mussels are tested for the presence of domoic acid.[74,161]

Less Common Poisonings
Echinoderms

The sea urchin usually causes toxicity by contact with its spinous processes, but this Caribbean delicacy is also toxic upon ingestion. When the sea urchin is prepared as food, the venom-containing gonads should be removed because they contain an acetylcholine-like substance that causes the cholinergic syndrome of profuse salivation, abdominal pain, nausea, vomiting, and diarrhea.

Haff Disease

The consumption of cooked seafood can potentially lead to a syndrome of myalgias and rhabdomyolysis. This syndrome is termed Haff disease, after an outbreak occurred in the 1920s in approximately 1,000 persons living along the Koenigsberg Haff, an inlet of the Baltic Sea. The actual etiology of Haff disease is unknown, but it is suspected that the causative agent is similar to a palytoxin (potent vasoconstrictor). Treatment is hydration with intravenous fluids.[63]

FOOD POISONING ASSOCIATED WITH DIARRHEA

The initial differential diagnosis for acute diarrhea involves several etiologies: infectious (bacterial, viral, parasitic, and fungal), structural (including surgical), metabolic, functional, inflammatory, toxin induced, and food induced. The differential diagnosis is described in greater detail in Chap. 18.

An elevated temperature is caused by invasive organisms, including *Salmonella* spp, *Shigella* spp, *Campylobacter* spp, invasive *E. coli*, *Vibrio parahaemolyticus*, and *Yersinia* spp, as well as some viruses. Episodes of acute gastroenteritis not typically associated with fever are caused by organisms producing toxins, including *S. aureus*, *Bacillus cereus*, *Clostridium perfringens*, enterotoxigenic *E. coli*, and viruses.[4]

Fecal leukocytes typically are found in patients with invasive shigellosis, salmonellosis, *Campylobacter* enteritis, typhoid fever, invasive *E. coli* colitis, *V. parahaemolyticus*, *Yersinia enterocolitica*, and inflammatory bowel disease. In all of these conditions, except typhoid fever, the leukocytes are primarily polymorphonuclear; in typhoid fever, they are mononuclear. No stool leukocytes are noted in cholera, viral diarrheas, noninvasive *E. coli* diarrhea, or nonspecific diarrhea.[95]

The timing of diarrheal onset after exposure or the incubation period is useful in differentiating the cause. Extremely short incubation periods of less than 6 hours are typical for *Staphylococcus* spp, *B. cereus* (type I), enterotoxigenic *E. coli*,[4,134,194] and preformed enterotoxins, as well as roundworm larval ingestions. Intermediate incubation periods of 8 to 24 hours are found with *C. perfringens*, *B. cereus* (type II enterotoxin), enteroinvasive *E. coli*,[64,142] and *Salmonella*. Longer incubation periods occur in other bacterial causes of acute gastroenteritis (Table 39–4).

The three most likely etiologies of diarrhea are infectious, xenobiotics (chemicals found in an organism, not normally present, frequently a pollutant or contaminant), and foodborne. These three etiologies are not mutually exclusive. The differential diagnosis must be established among these groups. When the time from exposure to onset of symptoms is brief, all of the nonbacterial infectious etiologies (viral, parasitic, fungal, and algal), except

for upper GI invasion by roundworm larvae, can be eliminated and the possibility of a bacterial etiology with enterotoxin production becomes more likely (Table 39–4).[4,24]

Epidemiology

Epidemiologic analysis is of immediate importance, particularly when GI diseases strike more than one person in a group. The questions raised in Table 39–5 should be answered.[174] If available, an infectious disease consultant or infection control officer should be called for assistance. Alternatively, assistance from state and local health departments should be sought. Often, only the CDC or state health department has the resources to investigate and confirm a presumptive diagnosis in an outbreak. Sophisticated techniques such as toxin detection, matching the organism in the food by phage type with a food handler, matching an organism by phage type with other persons, isolating 10 or more organisms per gram of implicated food,[64,68] or polymerase chain reaction (PCR) identification of bacterial or plasmid DNA are potentially useful, although generally not possible using the laboratory and personnel available in most hospitals.[32,39,83] Structural, metabolic, and functional causes often can be eliminated. As in these diseases, neither a significant grouping of cases nor a limited clinical history is characteristic. Foodborne parasites such as *Trichinella spiralis* (trichinosis), *Toxoplasma gondii* (toxoplasmosis), and *G. lamblia* (giardiasis) must be considered, although acute GI symptoms are not usually prominent.

Salmonella Species

Salmonella enterica infections are of great concern in the United States. Two particular outbreaks define very special problems. In the 1980s, recurrent

		Symptoms							
Etiology	**Onset**	**A**	**V**	**Di**	**Dy**	**F**	**Source**	**Pathogenesis**	**Therapy**
Staphylococcus spp	2–6 h	+	+	+	−	−	Prepared foods: meats, pastries, salads	Heat-stable enterotoxin	Fluid and electrolyte resuscitation
Bacillus cereus									
Type I	1–6 h	+	+	+	−	−	Fried rice	Heat-labile toxin	Fluid and electrolyte resuscitation
Type II	12 h	+	−	+	−	−	Meats, vegetables	Heat-labile toxin	
Anisakiasis	1–12 h	+	+	−	−	−	Raw fish, sushi, (Eustrongyloides), minnows, salmon, cod, herring, squid, tuna	Intestinal larvae	Endoscopy, laparotomy removal
Clostridium perfringens	8–24 h	+	±	+	±	−	Poultry, heat-processed meats	Heat-labile enterotoxin	Fluid and electrolyte resuscitation
Salmonella spp	8–24 h	±	±	+	±	+	Poultry, egg	Bacteria, endotoxin (bacteremia)	Antibiotics
Escherichia coli									
Enterotoxigenic	<6 h	+	±	+	−	+	Enteric contact		Fluid and electrolyte resuscitation
Invasive	24–72 h	+	−	+	+	+	Raw produce	Bacteria (invasive)	Antibiotics
Hemorrhagic	24–72 h	+	+	+	+	±	Under cooked beef, unpasteurized milk	Shiga toxin heat stable	Fluid and electrolyte resuscitation and hematologic (blood transfusion) support
Vibrio cholerae	24–72 h	±	±	+	−	±	Water, food enteric contact	Heat labile enterotoxin	Fluid and electrolyte resuscitation, antibiotics
Shigella spp	24–72 h	+	±	+	+	±	Institutional food handler, household, preschool, enteric contact	Endotoxin Shiga toxin	Antibiotics
Campylobacter jejuni	1–7 d	+	+	+	±	+	Milk, poultry, unchlorinated water	Bacteria, heat labile enterotoxin	Antibiotics
Yersinia spp	1–7 d	+	+	+	±	+	Pork, milk, pets	Bacteria, enterotoxin	Antibiotics

TABLE 39–4 Foodborne Infections: Gastrointestinal (Time of Onset and Primary Presenting Symptom)

A = abdominal pain; Di = diarrhea; Dy = dysentery; F = fever; V = vomiting.

TABLE 39–5 Epidemiologic Analysis of Gastrointestinal Disease

1. Is the occurrence of the disease in a large group significant enough to be consistent with foodborne disease (two or more cases)?
2. Is the symptomatology in affected individuals well defined and similar?
3. Are the onset, time, and duration of illness similar among affected group members (incubation)?
4. What are the possible modes of transmission (eg, contact, food, water)?
5. Is there a relationship between the time of exposure of the group and the mode of transmission?
6. Do attack rates differ for age, gender, or occupation?
7. Can it be determined which foods were served and to whom? Can the items that were not eaten by those who did not become ill be identified?
8. What is the food-specific attack rate?
9. How was the food procured? How was it stored?
10. Was cooking technique adequate?
11. Was personal hygiene acceptable?
12. Was there animal contamination?

outbreaks associated with grade A eggs or food containing such eggs occurred. In the past, such outbreaks of *Salmonella* enteritis were attributed to infection of the egg with *Salmonella* (from the GI tract of the chicken) through cracks in the shell. More recently, outbreaks involved noncracked, nonsoiled eggs.[144] In these cases, presumably, the *Salmonella* has infected the eggs before the shell was formed. In either case, people who consume raw or undercooked eggs are at most risk for *Salmonella* enteritis. Raw eggs are standard ingredients of chocolate mousse, hollandaise sauce, eggnog, Caesar salads, and homemade ice cream. Whole, partially cooked eggs are problematic when eaten sunny side up or poached.[45] The second group of outbreaks was associated with raw milk,[164] which has become very popular in certain communities. Inadequate microwave cooking also causes small outbreaks.[68] These outbreaks are of great concern because they frequently involve multiple drug-resistant *Salmonella* infections.[58] Drinking pasteurized milk is not absolutely protective. An outbreak of salmonellosis resulting in more than 16,000 culture-proven cases was traced to one Illinois dairy. The probable cause of the outbreak was a transfer line connecting raw and pasteurized milk containment tanks.[171]

The contamination of food that is widely distributed places thousands at risk. An outbreak of *Salmonella* food poisoning from peanut butter caused 529 confirmed illnesses in 48 states and Canada, 116 hospitalizations, and possibly 8 deaths.[44] The CDC estimates that the proportion of *Salmonella* infections that are confirmed by laboratory testing is 3% of the total, so that the estimated magnitude of infected people affected by this type of contamination incident is more than 15,000 individuals annually. News reports state that the peanut butter contamination with *Salmonella* was suspected; however, the peanut butter was then nationally distributed before confirmatory testing resulted.[93,94] The ethical and public health implications of maintaining meticulous standards are highlighted by this epidemic.

Additional concern developed over the widespread use of antibiotics in animal feed, responsible for meats, poultry, and manure-fertilized vegetables now frequently containing resistant bacterial strains to which virtually the entire population is exposed.[58,171]

The diagnosis of *Salmonella* infection is made through culture of the stool. The treatment of *Salmonella* is fluid and, electrolyte resuscitation, and antibiotics (ciprofloxacin or alternatively azithromycin).[112]

FOODBORNE POISONING ASSOCIATED WITH MULTIORGAN SYSTEM DYSFUNCTION

The hemolytic uremic syndrome (HUS) is frequently caused by a bacterial gastroenteritis. The most commonly responsible organism is *E. coli* O157:H7.[87] Other bacteria and xenobiotics cause the same findings. Typical laboratory findings in HUS include microangiopathic hemolytic anemia, thrombocytopenia, and acute kidney injury (AKI).

Hemolytic uremic syndrome begins with a prodrome of diarrhea 90% of the time. The diarrhea lasts for 3 to 4 days and frequently becomes bloody.

Abdominal pain caused by colitis is common, and vomiting, altered mental status (irritability or lethargy), pallor, and low-grade fever frequently occur. At presentation, many patients have oliguria or anuria, and 10% of children have a generalized seizure at HUS onset.[182]

Hemolytic uremic syndrome is frequently associated with enterohemorrhagic *E. coli* (EHEC) or *E. coli* O157:H7 with postdiarrheal HUS.[29,136,156,157,169,206] Food products from cattle (ground beef, milk, yogurt, cheese) and water contaminated with fecal material are EHEC sources.[62,139] Contaminated water used in gardens and unpasteurized apple cider have caused bloody diarrhea and HUS as a result of EHEC.[18,57]

Enterohemorrhagic *E. coli*, including *E. coli* O157:H7, produces a toxin similar to that produced by *Shigella dysenteriae* type I, referred to as Shigalike toxin (SLT) or verotoxin.[24] The proposed mechanism for SLT damage is intestinal absorption, bloodstream access to renal glomerular endothelium, intracellular adsorption via glycolipid receptors, ribosomal inactivation, and cell death.[193] In animal models, organ damage is more severe if endothelial cells have high concentrations of globotriaosylceramide receptors, which have a high binding affinity for Shiga toxin. Other organs with these receptors include the kidney, GI, and central nervous systems, which explain the pattern of organ damage in children with HUS. Endothelial cell damage and other pathologic processes, including platelet and leukocyte activation, triggering of the coagulation cascade, and the production of cytokines, occur.[104,202] Types of SLT exist as SLT-1, SLT-2, and additional variants of SLT-2 structure are identified.[20]

Detection of *E. coli* O157:H7 through stool culture early in the course of disease is useful. The recovery of organisms decreases after the first week of illness.[193] *Escherichia coli* O157:H7 almost always produces SLT; therefore, if stool cultures are negative, enzyme immunoassay (EIA) and PCR tests can be used to detect SLT in the stool when *E. coli* can no longer be identified by culture.[32]

Treatment of HUS should focus on meticulous supportive care, with fluid and electrolyte balance the priority. Dialysis should be instituted early for azotemia, hyperkalemia, acidemia, and fluid overload. Red blood cells and platelet transfusions are required. It is reasonable to treat hypertension with short-acting calcium channel blockers (nifedipine 0.25–0.5 mg/kg/dose orally) and seizures with benzodiazepines. Plasmapheresis was in nondiarrheal HUS and in recurrent HUS after renal transplantation. Anti–SLT-2 antibodies protected mice from SLT-2 toxicity, but IV immunoglobulin with SLT-2 activity did not improve outcome in children with HUS. A double-blind, placebo-controlled study on the use of synthetic SLT receptors attached to an oral carrier found that mortality or serious morbidity of HUS syndrome did not change as a result.[199]

The mortality rate from HUS with good supportive care is approximately 5%; another 5% of victims have end-stage kidney disease or cerebral ischemic events and chronic neurologic impairment. Prolonged anuria (longer than 1 week), oliguria (longer than 2 weeks), or severe extrarenal disease serve as markers for higher mortality and morbidity.[162]

There is some evidence that early treatment with antibiotics increases the risk of development HUS in children with *E. coli* O157:H7 infections.[187] An earlier meta-analysis and randomized trial did not find this association.[166,172] Because of this concern, it is not typically recommended to treat patients with clinical or epidemiologic presentations consistent with *E. coli* O157:H7 infections (crampy abdominal pain, bloody diarrhea, regional outbreak) until a definitive pathogen can be identified.[196]

Approximately 10% of the cases of HUS are not caused by SLT-producing bacteria or streptococci and are classified as atypical. Atypical HUS has a poor prognosis, with death rates as high as 25% and progression to end-stage kidney disease in half of the patients.[153]

Strategies to prevent the spread of *E. coli* O157:H7 and subsequent HUS include public education on the importance of thorough cooking of beef to a "well-done" temperature of 170°F (77°C), pasteurization of milk and apple cider, and thorough cleaning of vegetables. Public health measures include education of clinicians to consider *E. coli* O157:H7 in patients with bloody diarrhea and ensuring the routine capability of microbiology laboratories to culture *E. coli* O157:H7 and provide for EIA or PCR determination of SLT.

Public health departments should provide active surveillance systems to identify early outbreaks of *E. coli* O157:H7 infection.

Staphylococcus Species

In cases of suspected food poisoning with a short incubation period, the physician should first assess the risk for staphylococcal causes. The usual foods associated with staphylococcal toxin production include milk products and other proteinaceous foods, cream-filled baked goods, potato and chicken salads, sausages, ham, tongue, and gravy. Pie crust can act as an insulator, maintaining the temperature of the cream filling and occasionally permitting toxin production even during refrigeration.[6] A routine assessment must be made for the presence of lesions on the hands or nose of any food handlers involved. Unfortunately, carriers of enterotoxigenic staphylococci are difficult to recognize because they usually lack lesions and appear healthy.[96] A fixed association between a particular food and an illness would be most helpful epidemiologically but rarely occurs clinically. Factors such as environment, host resistance, nature of the agent, and dose make the results surprisingly variable.

Although patients with staphylococcal food poisoning rarely have significant temperature elevations, 16% of 2,992 documented cases in a published review had a subjective sense of fever.[96] Abdominal pain, nausea followed by vomiting, and diarrhea dominate the clinical findings. Diarrhea does not occur in the absence of nausea and vomiting. The mean incubation period is 4.4 hours with a mean duration of illness of 20 hours. Two staphylococcal enterotoxin food poisoning incidents involving large numbers of people are reported. At a public event in Brazil in 1998, half of the 8,000 people who attended had nausea, emesis, diarrhea, abdominal pain, and dizziness within hours of consuming food. Of the ill patients, 2,000 overwhelmed the capacity of local emergency departments; 396 (20%) were admitted, including 81 to intensive care units; and 16 young children and older adults died.[185] In another report, 328 individuals became ill with symptoms of diarrhea, vomiting, dizziness, chills, and headache after eating cheese or milk.[182] In both reports, staphylococcus enterotoxin was found in the food consumed.

Most enterotoxins are produced by *S. aureus* coagulase–positive species. The enterotoxins initiate an inflammatory response in GI mucosal cells and lead to cell destruction. The enterotoxins also result in sudden effects on the emesis center in the brain and diverse other organ systems. Discrimination of unique *S. aureus* isolates from those found in foodborne outbreaks is established using restriction fragment length polymorphism analysis by pulsed-field gel electrophoresis and PCR techniques.[207] The illness usually lasts for 24 to 48 hours. The treatment is supportive care with hydration and electrolyte repletion.[188]

Bacillus cereus

Another foodborne toxin that produces GI effects is associated with eating reheated fried rice. *Bacillus cereus* type I is the causative organism, and bacterial overgrowth and toxin production causes consequential early onset nausea and vomiting.[2] Infrequently, this toxin causes liver failure.[135] *Bacillus cereus* type II has a delayed onset of similar GI effects including diarrhea.[76] The diagnosis of *B. cereus* infection is made through culture of the stool. The treatment of *B. cereus* is fluid and electrolyte resuscitation, and antibiotics (including ciprofloxacin or vancomycin).[25]

Campylobacter jejuni

Campylobacter jejuni is a major cause of bacterial enteritis. The organism is most commonly isolated in children younger than 5 years and in adults 20 to 40 years of age. *Campylobacter* enteritis outbreaks are more common in the summer months in temperate climates. Although most cases of *Campylobacter* enteritis are sporadic, outbreaks are associated with contaminated food and water. The most frequent sources of *Campylobacter* spp in food are raw or undercooked poultry products[70] and unpasteurized milk.[189] Birds are a common reservoir, and small outbreaks are associated with contamination of milk by birds pecking on milk-container tops.[189] Contaminated water supplies are also frequent sources of *Campylobacter enteritis* involving large numbers

of individuals.[22] *Campylobacter jejuni* is heat labile; cooking of food, pasteurization of milk, and chlorination of water prevent human transmission.

The incubation period for *Campylobacter* enteritis varies from 1 to 7 days (mean, 3 days). Typical symptoms include diarrhea, abdominal cramps, and fever. Other symptoms include headache, vomiting, excessive gas, and malaise. The diarrhea contains gross blood, and leukocytes are frequently present on microscopic examination.[95] Illness usually lasts 5 to 6 days (range, 1–8 days). Rarely, symptoms last for several weeks. Severely affected individuals present with lower GI hemorrhage, abdominal pain mimicking appendicitis, a typhoidlike syndrome, reactive polyarthritis (Reiter syndrome), or meningitis. Guillain-Barré is associated with the disease with an incidence of less than 1 in 1,000 cases.[3] The organism is detected using PCR identification techniques.[79] Treatment is supportive and consists of volume resuscitation and antibiotics for the more severe cases.[4]

Group A *Streptococcus*

Bacterial infections not usually associated with food or food handling are nevertheless occasionally transmitted by food or food handling. Transmission of streptococci in food prepared by an individual with streptococcal pharyngitis is demonstrated.[60] A Swedish food handler caused 153 people to become ill with streptococcal pharyngitis when his infected finger wound contaminated a layer cake served at a birthday party.[9]

Yersinia enterocolitica

Yersinia enterocolitica causes enteritis most frequently in children and young adults. Typical clinical features include fever, abdominal pain, and diarrhea, which usually contains mucus and blood.[10,192,204] Other associated findings include nausea, vomiting, anorexia, and weight loss. The incubation period is 1 to 7 days or more. Less common features include prolonged enteritis, reactive polyarthritis, pharyngeal and hepatic involvement, and rash. *Yersinia* is a common pathogen in many animals, including dogs and pigs. Sources of human infection include milk products, raw pork products, infected household pets, and person-to-person transmission.[26,89,123] The diagnosis is based on cultures of food, stool, blood, and, less frequently, skin abscesses, pharyngeal cultures, or cultures from other organ tissues (mesenteric lymph nodes, liver). *Yersinia* is identified by PCR.[103] Patients receiving the chelator deferoxamine (Antidotes in Depth: A7) frequently acquire *Yersinia* infections because the deferoxamine–iron complex acts as a siderophore for organism growth. Therapy is usually supportive, but patients with invasive disease (eg, bacteremia, bacterial arthritis) should be treated with IV antibiotics. Fluoroquinolones and third-generation cephalosporins are highly bacteriocidal against *Yersinia* spp.

Listeria monocytogenes

Listeriosis transmitted by food usually occurs in pregnant women and their fetuses, older adults, and immunocompromised individuals using corticosteroids or with malignancies, diabetes mellitus, kidney disease, or HIV infection.[17,41,43,178] Typical food sources include undercooked chicken and unpasteurized milk as well as soft cheeses such as feta, queso fresco, queso blanco, queso panela, blue cheese, and brie. Individuals at risk should avoid the usual sources and should be evaluated for listeriosis if typical symptoms of fever, severe headache, muscle aches, and pharyngitis develop. Treatment with IV ampicillin and aminoglycoside, or trimethoprim–sulfamethoxazole is indicated for systemic *Listeria* infections.

Xenobiotic-Induced Diseases

In addition to the aforementioned saxitoxin, tetrodotoxin, domoic acid, and ciguatoxin, many other xenobiotics contaminate our food sources. Careful assessment for possible foodborne pesticide poisoning is essential. For example, aldicarb contamination has occurred in hydroponically grown vegetables and watermelons contaminated with pesticides.[86] Eating malathion-contaminated chapatti and wheat flour resulted in 60 poisonings, including a death in one outbreak[54] (Chap. 110). Insecticides, rodenticides, arsenic, lead, or fluoride preparations can be mistaken for a food ingredient. These poisonings usually have a rapid onset of signs and symptoms after exposure.

The possibility of unintentional acute metal salt ingestion must also be evaluated. This type of poisoning most typically occurs when very acidic fruit punch is served in metal-lined containers. Antimony, zinc, copper, tin, or cadmium in a container are dissolved in an acidic food or juice medium.

Mushroom-Induced Disease

Some species produce major GI effects. *Amanita phalloides*, the most poisonous mushroom, usually causes GI symptoms as well as hepatotoxic effects with a delay to clinical manifestations. The rapid onset of symptoms suggests some of the gastroenterotoxic mushrooms, but this is not always true as in the case of *Amanita smithiana*, which has an early GI phase followed later by acute kidney injury (Chap. 117).

Intestinal Parasitic Infections

The popularity of eating raw fish, or sushi, led to an increase in reported intestinal parasitic infections. Etiologic agents are roundworms (*Eustrongyloides anisakis*) and fish tapeworms (*Diphyllobothrium* spp). Symptoms of anisakiasis are either upper intestinal (occur 1–12 hours after eating) or lower intestinal (delayed for days or weeks). Typical symptoms include nausea, vomiting, and severe crampy abdominal pain; with intestinal perforation, severe pain, rebound, and guarding occur. A dietary history of eating raw fish is needed to establish diagnosis and therapy. Visual inspection of the larvae (on endoscopy, laparotomy, or pathologic examination) is useful. Treatment of intestinal infection involves surgical or laparoscopic removal. *Anisakis simplex* and *Pseudoterranova decipiens* are Anisakidae that are found in several types of consumed raw fish, including mackerel, cod, herring, rockfish, salmon, yellow fin tuna, and squid. Reliable methods of preventing ingestion of live anisakid larvae are freezing at −4°F (−20°C) for 60 hours or cooking at 140°F (60°C) for 5 minutes.[38,111,133,170,176,210]

Diphyllobothriasis (fish tapeworm disease) is caused by eating uncooked fish such as herring, salmon, pike, and whitefish that harbor the parasite. The symptoms are less acute than with intestinal roundworm ingestions and usually begin 1 to 2 weeks after ingestion.[37] Signs and symptoms include nausea, vomiting, abdominal cramping, flatulence, abdominal distension, diarrhea, and megaloblastic anemia due to vitamin B_{12} deficiency. The diagnosis is based on a history of ingesting raw fish and on identification of the tapeworm proglottids in stool. Treatment with niclosamide, praziquantel, or paromomycin usually is effective.[42]

Monosodium Glutamate

This clinical presentation is misnamed "Chinese restaurant syndrome" because it results from the ingestion of monosodium glutamate (MSG), which has multicultural use in the preparation of many foods. Monosodium glutamate (regarded as "safe" by the FDA) can cause other acute and bizarre neurologic symptoms. Affected individuals present with a burning sensation of the upper torso, facial pressure, headache, flushing, chest pain, nausea and vomiting, and, infrequently, life-threatening bronchospasm[4] and angioedema.[190] The intensity and duration of symptoms are generally dose related but with significant variation in individual responses to the amount ingested.[177,212] Monosodium glutamate causes "shudder attacks" or a seizure-like syndrome in young children. Absorption is more rapid after fasting, and the typical burning symptoms rapidly spread over the back, neck, shoulders, abdomen, and occasionally the thighs. Gastrointestinal symptoms are rarely prominent and symptoms can usually be prevented by prior ingestion of food. When symptoms do occur, they tend to last approximately 1 hour. Monosodium glutamate is also marketed as an effective flavor enhancer.[15] Many sausages and canned soups contain large doses of MSG.

There is evidence that humans have a unique taste receptor for glutamate.[114] This explains its ability to act as a flavor enhancer for foods. Glutamate is also an excitatory neurotransmitter that can stimulate central nervous system neurons through activation of glutamate receptors and be the explanation for some of the neurologic symptoms described with ingestion.[213]

Animal studies in which MSG was administered perorally in doses similar to average human intake or intake of extreme users showed that MSG led to disturbances in metabolism affecting insulin, fatty acids, and triglycerides in serum. Monosodium glutamate also affected several genes implicated in adipocytes differentiation. It elevated aminotransferase concentrations and bile synthesis and led to oxidative stress in the liver and to pathological changes in ovaries and fallopian tubes. These more recent findings will lead to further understanding of MSG and its safety in long-term use.[100]

Anaphylaxis and Anaphylactoid Presentations

Some foods and foodborne toxins cause allergic or anaphylacticlike manifestations,[106] also sometimes referred to as "restaurant syndromes"[181] (Table 39–6). The similarity of these syndromes complicates a patient's future approach to safe eating. Isolating the precipitant is essential so that the risk can be effectively assessed. Manufacturers of processed foods should provide an unambiguous listing of ingredients on package labels. Sensitive

TABLE 39–6	Symptoms of Foodborne Toxicity			
	Onset	Symptoms or Signs	Cause	Therapy
Anaphylaxis (anaphylactoid)	Minutes to hours	Urticaria, angioedema, bronchospasm, hypotension, cardiorespiratory arrest	Allergens—nuts, eggs, milk, fish, shellfish, peanuts, soy	Oxygen, epinephrine, β_2-adrenergic agonist, corticosteroids, fluid and electrolyte resuscitation, H_1, H_2 histamine antagonists, avoidance
Monosodium glutamate (MSG)	Minutes	Flushing, hypotension, palpitations, facial pressure, headaches, rhinitis, bronchospasm, shivering	Flavor enhancer of foods	Oxygen, β_2-adrenergic agonists, fluid and electrolyte resuscitation, avoidance
Metabisulfites	Minutes	Flushing, hypotension, bronchospasm	Preservative in wines, salad (bars), fruit juice, shrimp	See Anaphylaxis; avoidance
Scombroid	Minutes to hours	Flushing, hypotension, urticaria, headache, pruritus, gastrointestinal symptoms	Large fish—poorly refrigerated; tuna, bonito, albacore, mackerel, mahi mahi (histamine)	Histamine (H_1, H_2) antagonists
Tyramine	Minutes to hours	Headache, hypertension	Wines, aged cheeses that contain tyramine (INH or MAOI) increases risk	Avoidance
Tartrazine	Hours	Urticaria, angioedema, bronchospasm	Yellow coloring food additive	See Anaphylaxis; avoidance

INH = isoniazid; MAOI = monoamine oxide inhibitor.

individuals (or in the cases of children, their parents) must be rigorously attentive.[173,215] Those who experience severe reactions should make sure that epinephrine and antihistamines are always available immediately. Attempts to prevent allergic reactions to dairy products by avoiding dairy-containing foods may fail. Nondairy foods are still periodically processed in equipment used for dairy products or contain flavor enhancers of a dairy origin (eg, partially hydrolyzed sodium caseinate), both of which cause morbidity and mortality in allergic individuals.[78] Individuals with known food allergies do not always carry prescribed autoinjectable epinephrine syringes, in some cases from a belief that the allergen is easily identifiable and avoidable.[106] Food additives that cause anaphylactic or anaphylactoid reactions include antibiotics, aspartame, butylated hydroxyanisole, butylated hydroxytoluene, nitrates or nitrites, sulfites, and paraben esters.[128] Regulation of these preservatives is limited, and xenobiotics such as sulfites are so ubiquitous that predicting which guacamole, cider, vinegar, fresh or dried fruits, wines, or beers contain these sensitizing xenobiotics may be impossible.

Scombroid Poisoning

Scombroid poisoning originally was described with the Scombridae fish (including the large dark-meat marine tuna, albacore, bonito, mackerel, and skipjack). However, the most commonly ingested vectors identified by the CDC are nonscombroid fish, such as mahi mahi and amber jack. All of the implicated fish species live in temperate or tropical waters. Ingestion of bluefish and tilapia is associated with scombroid poisoning.[67,152] The incidence of this disease is probably far greater than was originally perceived. This type of poisoning differs from other fishborne causes of illness in that it is entirely preventable if the fish is properly stored after removal from the water.

Scombroid poisoning can result from eating cooked, smoked, canned, or raw fish. The implicated fish all have a high concentration of histidine in their dark meat. *Morganella morganii, E. coli,* and *Klebsiella pneumoniae,* commonly found on the surface of the fish, contain a histidine decarboxylase enzyme that acts on a warm (not refrigerated), freshly killed fish, converting histidine to histamine, saurine, and other heat-stable substances. Although saurine was suggested as the causative toxin, chromatographic analysis demonstrates that histamine is found as histamine phosphate and saurine is merely histamine hydrochloride.[72,146] The term *saurine* originated from saury, a Japanese dried fish delicacy often associated with scombroid poisoning. The extent of spoilage usually correlates with histamine concentrations. Histamine concentrations in healthy fish are less than 0.1 mg/100 g fish meat. In fish left at room temperature, the concentration rapidly increases, reaching toxic concentrations of 100 mg/100 g fish within 12 hours.

The appearance, taste, and smell of the fish are usually unremarkable.[7] Rarely, the skin has an abnormal "honeycombing" character or a pungent, peppery taste that is a clue to its toxicity. Within minutes to hours after eating the fish, the individual experiences numbness, tingling, or a burning sensation of the mouth; dysphagia; headache; and, of particular significance for scombroid poisoning, a unique flush characterized by an intense diffuse erythema of the face, neck, and upper torso.[107] Rarely, pruritus, urticaria, angioedema, or bronchospasm ensues. Nausea, vomiting, dizziness, palpitations, abdominal pain, diarrhea, and prostration may develop.[55,61,80,107,141]

The prognosis is good with appropriate supportive care and parenteral antihistamines such as diphenhydramine. Histamine (H_2)-receptor antagonists such as cimetidine or ranitidine are also reasonable to administer because they can also be useful in alleviating GI symptoms.[21] Toxic substance removal using orogastric suctioning or adsorption from the gut by activated charcoal are reportedly used, but no randomized trials demonstrate benefit over treatment with antihistamines. Inhaled β_2-adrenergic agonists and epinephrine are necessary if bronchospasm is prominent. Although rare, another concern with scombroid toxicity is coronary vasospasm.[5,59] Patients usually show significant improvement within a few hours.

Elevated serum or urine histamine concentrations can confirm the diagnosis but are clinically unnecessary. If any uncooked fish remains, isolation of causative bacteria from the flesh is suggestive but not diagnostic. A capillary electrophoretic assay makes rapid histamine detection possible.[96]

Histamine concentrations greater than 50 mg/100 g fish meat are considered hazardous by the FDA; in Europe, the concentrations are 100 to 200 mg/100 g.[99] Research demonstrates that human subjects can tolerate up to 180 mg of pure histamine orally without noticeable effects.[5] Isoniazid increases the severity of the reaction to scombroid fish by inhibiting enzymes that metabolize histamine.[99,201]

Patients should be reassured that they are not allergic to fish if other individuals experience a similar reaction while eating the same fish at the same time or if any remaining fish can be preserved and tested for elevated histamine concentrations. If this information is not available, then an anaphylactic reaction to the fish cannot be excluded. Table 39–6 represents the differential diagnosis of flushing, bronchospasm, and headache. Because many people often consume alcohol with fish, alcohol is an independent variable.

The differential diagnosis of the scombrotoxic flush apart from a disulfiramlike reaction includes ingestion of niacin or nicotinic acid, pheochromocytoma and carcinoid syndrome. The history and clinical evolution usually establish the diagnosis quickly.

Global Food Distribution: Illegal Food Additives

The United States imports food from all over the world, year round. Approximately 19% of the food consumed in the United States is imported. An analysis of outbreak data from 1996 to 2014 shows 195 outbreak investigations implicated an imported food, resulting in about 11,000 illnesses, about 1,000 hospitalizations, and 19 deaths. The number of outbreaks associated with an imported food has increased from an average of 3 per year (1996–2000) to an average of 18 per year (2009–2014).[84] Xenobiotics are given to animals to increase their health and growth. Clenbuterol, a β_2 agonist, was administered to cattle raised for human consumption. Clenbuterol causes toxicity in humans who eat contaminated animal meat. Tachycardia, tremors, nausea, epigastric pain, headache, muscle pain, and diarrhea were present in 50 poisoned patients. Other findings included hypertension, hypokalemia, and leukocytosis.[168] No deaths are reported. The use of antibiotics, β_2 agonists, and other growth enhancers continues, despite safety concerns and laws against their use, because these practices increase yield and profit.

The globalization of food supplies and international agricultural trade has created a new global threat—the apparent purposeful contamination of food for profit. In 2008, almost 300,000 children in China were affected by melamine contamination of milk. Of these, 50,000 were hospitalized, and 6 reported deaths occurred.

The melamine-contaminated milk was sold in China as powdered infant formula, with more than 22 brands containing melamine. The contamination was not limited to China because melamine has been found in candy, chocolate, cookies, and biscuits sold in the United States, likely because of the adulteration of milk used in preparation of these products.

Melamine is a non-nutritious, nitrogen-containing compound, usually used in glues, plastics, and fertilizers. To increase profits, milk sold in China was previously diluted, causing protein malnutrition in children. Because the nitrogen content of milk (a surrogate measure for protein content) is now carefully monitored to detect dilution and to prevent another episode of malnutrition, melamine was added to increase the measured nitrogen content and hide the dilution. This purposeful addition of melamine is suspected to be the cause of the melamine contamination of powdered milk in China.

Melamine and its metabolite cyanuric acid are excreted in the kidneys. Kidney stones containing melamine and uric acid were found in 13 children with acute kidney injury who had consumed melamine containing milk formula.[88,205] Both melamine and cyanuric acid appear necessary to cause kidney stones in animals. The combination alone caused renal crystals in cats.[164] Melamine found in wheat gluten was added to pet food in 2007 resulted in thousands of complaints and dozens of suspected animal deaths in the United States.

The melamine milk contamination is one of the largest reported deliberate food adulteration incidents. It affected about 300,000 Chinese infants and young children and caused 6 deaths.[51,101]

In India, 22 children were killed after becoming poisoned when eating their school lunch. It was discovered that the cooking oil was being kept in a container previously used for monocrotophos, a water-soluble organophosphate.[92,126]

Food products from all over the world find their way into our foods. Increased vigilance by the agencies responsible for food safety, both in countries where the food originates and in countries that import the food, is needed to prevent other events such as the melamine contaminations. Chapter 2 discusses numerous other foodborne toxicologic outbreaks.

Vegetables and Plants

Plants and vegetables produce clinical signs and symptoms that are associated with diverse presentations often are involved in food poisoning.[91,108,109,115,117] Edible plants and plant products that are poorly cooked or prepared or contaminated result in poisoning. Extensive discussion of this is found in Chap. 118. The development of genetically modified plants has led many to be concerned about both the long- and short-term health effects. Currently, animal data are being collected, and no definitive conclusions about health effects have been made.

FOOD POISONING AND BIOTERRORISM

The threat of terrorist assaults is discussed in Chaps. 126 and 127. The use of food as a vehicle for intentional contamination with the intent of causing mass suffering or death has already occurred in the United States.[46,113,198] In the first report, 12 laboratory workers had GI signs and symptoms, primarily severe diarrhea, after consuming food purposefully contaminated with *Shigella dysenteriae* type II served in a staff break room.[113] Four workers were hospitalized; none had reported long-term sequelae. This *Shigella* strain rarely causes endemic disease. Nevertheless an identical strain, identified by pulsed-field gel electrophoresis, was found in eight of the 12 symptomatic workers, as well as in the pastries served in the break room and in the laboratory stock culture of *S. dysenteriae*. This finding suggests purposeful poisoning of food eaten by laboratory personnel. The person responsible and the motive remain unknown.

The second case series describes a large community outbreak of food poisoning caused by *Salmonella typhimurium*.[198] The outbreak occurred in the Dalles, Oregon, area during the fall of 1984; a total of 751 people developed *Salmonella* gastroenteritis. The outbreak was traced to the intentional contamination of restaurant salad bars and coffee creamer by members of a religious commune using a culture of *S. typhimurium* purchased before the outbreak of food poisoning. A criminal investigation found a *Salmonella* culture on the religious commune grounds that contained *S. typhimurium* identical to the *Salmonella* strain found in the food poisoning victims. It was identified by using antibiotic sensitivity, biochemical testing, and DNA restriction endonuclease digestion of plasmid DNA. Only after more than 1 year of investigation was this *Salmonella* outbreak linked to terrorist activity. Reasons for the delay in identifying the outbreak as a purposeful food poisoning included (1) no apparent motive; (2) no claim of responsibility; (3) no pattern of unusual behavior in the restaurants; (4) no disgruntled restaurant employees identified; (5) multiple time points for contamination indicated by epidemic exposure curves, suggesting a sustained source of contamination and not a single act; (6) no previous event of similar nature as a reference; (7) the likeliness of other possibilities (eg, repeated unintentional contamination by restaurant workers); and (8) fear that the publicity necessary to aid the investigation might generate copycat criminal activity.

Publication of the event was delayed by almost 10 years out of fear of unintentionally encouraging copycat activity. On the other hand, use of biological weapons by the Japanese cult Aum Shinrikyo appears to have motivated authorities to release this publication in the hopes of quickly identifying similar deliberate food poisoning patterns in the future.

A third report describes a disgruntled employee who contaminated 200 lb of meat at a supermarket with a nicotine-containing insecticide.[46] Ninety-two people became ill, and four sought medical care. Signs and symptoms included vomiting, abdominal pain, rectal bleeding, and one case of atrial tachycardia.

There are multiple reports of deliberate food poisoning with tetramine.[53,214] In one particular case of human greed, a Chinese restaurant owner poisoned the food in his neighbor's restaurant with tetramine. Tetramine or tetramethylenedisulfotetramine is a highly lethal neurotoxic rodenticide, once used worldwide, now illegal in the United States. The snack shop owner caused hundreds to become ill and 38 deaths by spiking his competitor's breakfast offerings (fried dough sticks, sesame cakes, and sticky rice balls). Tetramethylenedisulfotetramine is an odorless and tasteless white crystal that is water soluble. The mechanism of action is noncompetitive irreversible binding to the chloride channel on the γ-aminobutyric acid receptor complex, which blocks the influx of chloride and alters the neurons potential. It is referred to as a "cage convulsant" because of its globular structure. Severe toxicity presents with tachycardia, dysrhythmias, agitation, status epilepticus, and coma. Immediate or early treatment with sodium-(RS)-2,3-dimercaptopropane-1-sulfonate (DMPS) and pyridoxine (vitamin B_6) (A15) appears to be effective in a mouse model.[13,65,208]

The capacity of foodborne xenobiotics that are easy to obtain and disburse to infect large numbers of people is clearly exemplified by two specific outbreaks: (1) the purposeful *Salmonella* outbreak in Oregon and (2) the apparently unintentional *Salmonella* outbreak that resulted in more than 16,000 culture-proven cases traced to contamination in an Illinois dairy. The probable cause of the outbreak was a contaminated transfer pipe connecting the raw and pasteurized milk containment tanks.[171] These events emphasize the vulnerability of our food supply and the importance of ensuring its safety and security.

PREVENTION OF FOODBORNE ILLNESS

The incidence of foodborne disease has increased over the years and has resulted in a major public health problem on the global level. The current methods for detecting foodborne pathogens are inefficient. This has led to the research and development of rapid detection methods.

The three major types of rapid detection methods are biosensor-based, nucleic acid–based, and immunological-based methods. Biosensor detection methods use an analytical device that contains a bioreceptor and transducer. The transducer converts the biological interactions into a measurable electrical signal. Examples of biosensor based methods are optical, electrochemical, and mass-based biosensors. Nucleic acid–based detection methods work by detecting specific DNA or RNA in the pathogen. An example of this test is the PCR, immunological-based methods detect foodborne pathogens based on antibody–antigen interactions, whereby a particular antibody binds to the specific antigen. An example of an immunological based detection method is ELISA.

In general, the rapid detection methods are more efficient and sensitive than the conventional detection methods. Rapid detection methods may be a very useful way of preventing foodborne disease in the future. Currently, implementing special equipment and training personnel along with high costs have thwarted comprehensive application of rapid detection methods at this time.[120]

SUMMARY

- The diverse etiologies of food poisoning involve almost all aspects of toxicology.
- Our concerns center around the natural toxicity of plants or animals, the contamination of which can occur in the field, during factory processing, subsequent transport and distribution, or during home preparation or storage.
- Whether these events are intentional or unintentional, they alter our approaches to general nutrition and society.
- Issues in food safety include the governmental role in food preparation and protection, bacteria such as *Salmonella* and *E. coli* 0157:H7, prions in Creutzfeldt-Jacob disease (bovine encephalopathy), and genetically altered materials such as corn.
- Future discussions of food poisonings and interpretations of the importance of these problems may dramatically alter our food sources and their preparation and monitoring.

REFERENCES

1. Ackman DM, et al. Reptile-associated salmonellosis in New York State. *Pediatr Infect Dis J.* 1995;14:955.
2. Agata N, et al. Production of *Bacillus cereus* emetic toxin (cereulide) in various foods. *Int J Food Microbiol.* 2002;73:23.
3. Allos BM. *Campylobacter jejuni* infections: update on emerging issues and trends. *Clin Infect Dis.* 2001;32:1201.
4. American Medical Association, American Nurses Association-American Nurses Foundation, Centers for Disease Control and Prevention, et al. Diagnosis and management of foodborne illnesses: a primer for physicians and other health care professionals. *MMWR Morbid Mortal Wkly Rep.* 2004;53:1.
5. Anastasius M, Yiannikas J. Scombroid fish poisoning illness and coronary artery vasospasm. *Australas Med J.* 2015;8:96.6.
6. Anunciacao LL, et al. Production of staphylococcal enterotoxin A in cream-filled cake. *Int J Food Microbiol.* 1995;26:259.
7. Arnold SH, Brown WD. Histamine (?) toxicity from fish products. *Adv Food Res.* 1978;24:113.
8. Asai S, et al. The site of action of *Ptychodiscus brevis* toxin within the parasympathetic axonal sodium channel h gate in airway smooth muscle. *J Allergy Clin Immunol.* 1984;73:824.
9. Asteberg I, et al. A food-borne streptococcal sore throat outbreak in a small community. *Scand J Infect Dis.* 2006;38:988–994.
10. Attwood SE, et al. Yersinia infection and acute abdominal pain. *Lancet.* 1987;1:529.
11. Baden DG, et al. Marine toxins. In: deWolff FA, Vinken PJ, eds. *Handbook of Clinical Neurology: Intoxication of the Nervous System.* Amsterdam: Elsevier; 1994:141-175.
12. Bagnis R, et al. Clinical observations on 3,009 cases of ciguatera (fish poisoning) in the South Pacific. *Am J Trop Med Hyg.* 1979;28:1067.
13. Barrueto F Jr, et al. Status epilepticus from an illegally imported Chinese rodenticide: "tetramine." *J Toxicol Clin Toxicol.* 2003;41:991-994.
14. Batz MB, et al. Long-term consequences of foodborne infections. *Infect Dis Clin North Am.* 2013;27:599.
15. Bellisle F. Effects of monosodium glutamate on human food palatability. *Ann N Y Acad Sci.* 1998;855:438.
16. Benton BJ, et al. Reversal of saxitoxin-induced cardiorespiratory failure by a burro-raised alpha-STX antibody and oxygen therapy. *Toxicol Appl Pharmacol.* 1994;124:39.
17. Berenguer J, et al. Listeriosis in patients infected with human immunodeficiency virus. *Rev Infect Dis.* 1991;13:115.
18. Besser RE, et al. An outbreak of diarrhea and hemolytic uremic syndrome from *Escherichia coli* O157:H7 in fresh-pressed apple cider. *JAMA.* 1993;269:2217.
19. Birinyi-Strachan L, et al. Neuroprotectant effects of iso-osmolar D-mannitol to prevent Pacific ciguatoxin-1 induced alterations in neuronal excitability: a comparison with other osmotic agents and free radical scavengers. *Neuropharmacology.* 2005 Oct; 49:669-86.
20. Bitzan M, et al. The role of *Escherichia coli* O 157 infections in the classical (enteropathic) haemolytic uraemic syndrome: results of a Central European, multicentre study. *Epidemiol Infect.* 1993;110:183.
21. Blakesley ML. Scombroid poisoning: prompt resolution of symptoms with cimetidine. *Ann Emerg Med.* 1983;12:104.
22. Blaser MJ, Reller LB. *Campylobacter* enteritis. *N Engl J Med.* 1981;305:1444-1452.
23. Blythe DG, de Sylva DP. Mother's milk turns toxic following fish feast. *JAMA.* 1990;264:2074.
24. Bokete TN, et al. Shiga-like toxin-producing *Escherichia coli* in Seattle children: a prospective study. *Gastroenterology.* 1993;105:1724.
25. Bottone EJ. *Bacillus cereus*, a volatile human pathogen. *Clin Microbiol Rev.* 2010;23:382.
26. Bottone EJ. *Yersinia enterocolitica*: the charisma continues. *Clin Microbiol Rev.* 1997;10:257.
27. Bowman PB. Amitriptyline and ciguatera. *Med J Aust.* 1984;140:802.
28. Bradley SG, Klika LJ. A fatal poisoning from the Oregon rough-skinned newt (*Taricha granulosa*). *JAMA.* 1981;246:247.
29. Brandt JR, et al. *Escherichia coli* O 157:H7-associated hemolytic-uremic syndrome after ingestion of contaminated hamburgers. *J Pediatr.* 1994;125:519.
30. Brett J, Murnion B. Pregabalin to treat ciguatera fish poisoning. *Clin Toxicol.* 2015;53:588.
31. Brett MM. Food poisoning associated with biotoxins in fish and shellfish. *Curr Opin Infect Dis.* 2003;16:461.
32. Brian MJ, et al. Polymerase chain reaction for diagnosis of enterohemorrhagic *Escherichia coli* infection and hemolytic-uremic syndrome. *J Clin Microbiol.* 1992;30:1801.
33. Buchanan S. Red tide triggers New England shellfish fishery failure determination. National Oceanic and Atmospheric Administration. http://www.publicaffairs.noaa.gov/releases2005/jun05/noaa05-r121.html.
34. Cameron J, Capra MF. The basis of the paradoxical disturbance of temperature perception in ciguatera poisoning. *J Toxicol Clin Toxicol.* 1993;31:571.
35. Catterall WA, et al. Molecular properties of the sodium channel: a receptor for multiple neurotoxins: *Bull Soc Pathol Exot.* 1992;85:481.
36. Centers for Disease Control and Prevention (CDC). Vital Signs: Multistate Foodborne Outbreaks—United States, 2010–2014. *MMWR Morb Mortal Wkly Rep.* 2015;64: 1221-1225.
37. Centers for Disease Control and Prevention. Diphyllobothriasis associated with salmon. *MMWR Morb Mortal Wkly Rep.* 1981;30:331-338.
38. Centers for Disease Control and Prevention. Intestinal perforation caused by larval Eustrongylides—Maryland. *MMWR Morb Mortal Wkly Rep.* 1982;31:383.
39. Centers for Disease Control and Prevention. Surveillance for epidemics—United States. *MMWR Morb Mortal Wkly Rep.* 1989;38:694.
40. Centers for Disease Control and Prevention. Scombroid fish poisoning—Illinois, South Carolina. *MMWR Morb Mortal Wkly Rep.* 1989;38:140.
41. Centers for Disease Control and Prevention. Update: foodborne listeriosis—United States, 1988–1990. *MMWR Morb Mortal Wkly Rep.* 1992;41:251, 257.
42. Centers for Disease Control and Prevention. Drugs for parasitic infections. *Med Lett Drugs Ther.* 1998;40:1.
43. Centers for Disease Control and Prevention. Multistate outbreak of listeriosis—United States, 1998. *MMWR Morb Mortal Wkly Rep.* 1998;47:1085.
44. The Centers for Disease Control and Prevention. Multistate outbreak of Salmonella infections associated with peanut butter and peanut butter–containing products—United States, 2008–2009. https://www.cdc.gov/mmwr/preview/mmwrhtml/mm58e0129a1.htm.
45. Centers for Disease Control and Prevention. Outbreaks of Salmonella serotype enteritidis infection associated with eating raw or undercooked shell eggs—United States, 1996–1998. *MMWR Morb Mortal Wkly Rep.* 2000;49:73.
46. Centers for Disease Control and Prevention. Nicotine poisoning after ingestion of contaminated ground beef—Michigan, 2003. *MMWR Morb Mortal Wkly Rep.* 2003;52:413.
47. Centers for Disease Control and Prevention (CDC). Multistate outbreak of Salmonella infections associated with peanut butter and peanut butter–containing products—United States, 2008-2009. *MMWR Morb Mortal Wkly Rep.* 2009 Feb 6;58:85-90.
48. Centers for Disease Control and Prevention (CDC). Surveillance for Foodborne Disease Outbreaks, United States, 2014, Annual Report. Atlanta, Georgia: US Department of Health and Human Services, CDC, 2016. https://www.cdc.gov/foodsafety/pdfs/foodborne-outbreaks-annual-report-2014-508.pdf. Last accessed May 21, 2018.
49. Centers for Disease Control and Prevention. Tetrodotoxin poisoning outbreak from imported dried puffer fish—Minneapolis, Minnesota, 2014. *MMWR Morb Mortal Wkly Rep.* 2015;63:1222.
50. Centers for Disease Control and Prevention (CDC). Botulism Annual Summary, 2015. Atlanta, Georgia: US Department of Health and Human Services, CDC, 2017.
51. Chan EY, et al. Public-health risks of melamine in milk products. *Lancet.* 2008;372: 1444-1445.
52. Chan TY. Characteristic features and contributory factors in fatal ciguatera fish poisoning—implications for prevention and public education. *Am J Tio Med Hyg.* 2016;94:704.
53. Chau CM, et al. Tetramine poisoning. *Hong Kong Med J.* 2005;11:511-4.
54. Chaudhry R, et al. A foodborne outbreak of organophosphate poisoning. *Br Med J. (Clin Res Ed).* 1998;317:268.
55. Chen KT, Malison MD. Outbreak of scombroid fish poisoning, Taiwan. *Am J Public Health.* 1987;77:1335.
56. Ching PK, et al. Lethal paralytic shellfish poisoning from consumption of green mussel broth, Western Samar, Philippines, August 2013. *Western Pac Surveill Response J.* 2015;6:22-26.
57. Cieslak PR, et al. *Escherichia coli* O157:H7 infection from a manured garden. *Lancet.* 1993;342:367.
58. Cody SH, et al. Two outbreaks of multidrug-resistant *Salmonella* serotype typhimurium DT104 infections linked to raw-milk cheese in Northern California. *JAMA.* 1999;281:1805.
59. Cucunato M, et al. Acute coronary syndrome and scombroid syndrome. *Int J Cardiol.* 2015;187:317.
60. Decker MD, et al. Food-borne streptococcal pharyngitis in a hospital pediatrics clinic. *JAMA.* 1985;253:679.
61. Demoncheaux J-P, et al. A large outbreak of scombroid fish poisoning associated with eating yellowfin tuna (*Thunnus albacares*) at a military mass catering in Dakar, Senegal. *Epidemiol Infect.* 2012;140:1008-1012.
62. Deschenes G, et al. Cluster of cases of haemolytic uraemic syndrome due to unpasteurised cheese. *Pediatr Nephrol.* 1996;10:203.
63. Diaz JH. Global incidence of rhabdomyolysis after cooked seafood consumption (Haff disease). *Clin Toxicol.* 2015;53:421.
64. DuPont HL, et al. Pathogenesis of *Escherichia coli* diarrhea. *N Engl J Med.* 1971;285:1.
65. Eckholm E. Man admits poisoning food in rival's shop, killing 38 in China. *The New York Times.* 2002; A.5. http://query.nytimes.com/gst/abstract.html?res=F40E11FE3E540C7B8DDDA00894DA404482.
66. Endean R, et al. Apparent relationships between toxins elaborated by the cyanobacterium *Trichodesmium erythraeum* and those present in the flesh of the narrow-barred Spanish mackerel *Scomberomorus commersoni*. *Toxicon.* 1993;31:1155.
67. Etkind P, et al. Bluefish-associated scombroid poisoning. An example of the expanding spectrum of food poisoning from seafood. *JAMA.* 1987;258:3409.
68. Evans MR, et al. Salmonella outbreak from microwave cooked food. *Epidemiol Infect.* 1995;115:227.
69. FAO. Ciguatera Fish Poisoning. In Marine Biotoxins; *FAO Food and Nutrition Paper 80*; Food and Agriculture Organization of the United Nations: Rome, Italy; 2004:185-218.
70. Finch MJ, Blake PA. Foodborne outbreaks of campylobacteriosis: the United States experience, 1980–1982. *Am J Epidemiol.* 1985;122:262.

71. Flachsenberger WA. Respiratory failure and lethal hypotension due to blue-ringed octopus and tetrodotoxin envenomation observed and counteracted in animal models. *J Toxicol Clin Toxicol.* 1986;24:485.

72. Foo LY. Scombroid poisoning. Isolation and identification of "saurine." *J Sci Food Agric.* 1976;27:807.

73. Friedman MA, et al. An updated review of ciguatera fish poisoning: clinical, epidemiological, environmental and public health management. *Mar Drugs.* 2017;14;15:pii: E72.

74. Fritz L, et al. An outbreak of domoic acid poisoning attributed to the pinnate diatom pseudonitzchia australis. *J Phycol.* 1992;28:439-442.

75. Gaboriau M, et al. Ciguatera fish toxicity in French Polynesia: size does not always matter. *Toxicon.* 2014;84C:41-50.

76. Gaulin C, et al. An outbreak of *Bacillus cereus* implicating a part-time banquet caterer. *Can J Public Health.* 2002;93:353.

77. Geller RJ, Benowitz NL. Orthostatic hypotension in ciguatera fish poisoning. *Arch Intern Med.* 1992;152:2131.

78. Gern JE, Yang et al. Allergic reactions to milk-contaminated "nondairy" products. *N Engl J Med.* 1991;324:976.

79. Giesendorf BA, Quint WG. Detection and identification of *Campylobacter* spp. using the polymerase chain reaction. *Cell Mol Biol* (Noisy-le-grand). 1995;41:625.

80. Gilbert RJ, et al. Scombrotoxic fish poisoning: features of the first 50 incidents to be reported in Britain (1976–9). *Br Med J.* 1980;281:71.

81. Gillespie NC, et al. Ciguatera in Australia. Occurrence, clinical features, pathophysiology and management. *Med J Aust.* 1986;145:584.

82. Gold EP, et al. Brevenal, a brevetoxin antagonist from *Karenia brevis*, binds to a previously unreported site on mammalian sodium channels. *Harmful Algae.* 22013;26:12.

83. Goossens H, et al. Investigation of an outbreak of *Campylobacter upsaliensis* in day care centers in Brussels: analysis of relationships among isolates by phenotypic and genotypic typing methods. *J Infect Dis.* 1995;172:1298.

84. Gould LH, et al. Outbreaks of disease associated with food imported into the United States, 1996–2014. *Emerg Infect Dis.* 2017;23:525-528.

85. Gould H, et al. Surveillance for foodborne disease outbreaks—United States, 2009–2010. *MMWR.* 2013;62:41-47.

86. Green MA, et al. An outbreak of watermelon-borne pesticide toxicity. *Am J Public Health.* 1987;77:1431.

87. Griffin PM, Tauxe RV. The epidemiology of infections caused by *Escherichia coli* O157:H7, other enterohemorrhagic E. coli, and the associated hemolytic uremic syndrome. *Epidemiol Rev.* 1991;13:60.

88. Guan N, et al. Melamine-contaminated powdered formula and urolithiasis in young children. *N Engl J Med.* 2009;360:1067-1074.

89. Gutman LT, et al. An inter-familial outbreak of *Yersinia enterocolitica* enteritis. *N Engl J Med.* 1973;288:1372.

90. Halstead BW, Halstead LG. *Poisonous and Venomous Marine Animals of the World.* Rev. ed. Princeton, NJ: Darwin Press; 1978.

91. Hardin JW, Arena JM. *Human Poisoning from Native and Cultivated Plants.* Chapel Hill, NC: Duke University Press; 1969:69-73.

92. Harris G, Kumar H. Contaminated lunches kill 22 Children in India. *The New York Times.* http://www.nytimes.com/2013/07/18/world/asia/children-die-from-tainted-lunches-at-indian-school.html.

93. Harris G. Peanut products sent out before tests. *The New York Times.* http://www.nytimes.com/2009/02/12/health/policy/12peanut.html?_r=0.

94. Harris G. Salmonella was found at peanut plant before. *The New York Times.* 2009. http://www.nytimes.com/2009/01/28/us/29Peanut.html?_r=1&scp=1&sq=salmonella%20peanut%20butter&st=cse.

95. Harris JC, et al. Fecal leukocytes in diarrheal illness. *Ann Intern Med.* 1972;76:697.

96. Holmberg SD, Blake PA. Staphylococcal food poisoning in the United States. New facts and old misconceptions. *JAMA.* 1984;251:487.

97. Holmes MJ, et al. Strain dependent production of ciguatoxin precursors (gambiertoxins) by *Gambierdiscus toxicus* (Dinophyceae) in culture. *Toxicon.* 1991;29:761.

98. Hui JY, Taylor SL. Inhibition of in vivo histamine metabolism in rats by foodborne and pharmacologic inhibitors of diamine oxidase, histamine *N*-methyltransferase, and monoamine oxidase. *Toxicol Appl Pharmacol.* 1985;81:241.

99. Hungerford J. Scombroid poisoning a review. *Toxicon.* 2010;56:231-243.

100. Husarova V, Ostatnikova D. Monosodium glutamate toxic effects and their implications for human intake: a review. *JMED Res.* 2013.

101. Ingelfinger JR. Melamine and the global implications of food contamination. *N Engl J Med.* 2008;359:2745-2748.

102. Kanchanapongkul J, Krittayapoositpot P. An epidemic of tetrodotoxin poisoning following ingestion of the horseshoe crab *Carcinoscorpius rotundicauda*. *Southeast Asian J Trop Med Public Health.* 1995;26:364.

103. Kapperud G, et al. Detection of pathogenic *Yersinia enterocolitica* in foods and water by immunomagnetic separation, nested polymerase chain reactions, and colorimetric detection of amplified DNA. *Appl Environ Microbiol.* 1993;59:2938.

104. Karpman D, et al. Cytokines in childhood hemolytic uremic syndrome and thrombotic thrombocytopenic purpura. *Pediatr Nephrol.* 1995;9:694.

105. Kawatsu K, et al. Application of immunoaffinity chromatography for detection of tetrodotoxin from urine samples of poisoned patients. *Toxicon.* 1999;37:325.

106. Kemp SF, et al. Anaphylaxis. A review of 266 cases. *Arch Intern Med.* 1995;155:1749.

107. Kim R. Flushing syndrome due to mahimahi (scombroid fish) poisoning. *Arch Dermatol.* 1979;115:963.

108. Kingsbury JM. *Poisonous Plants of the United States and Canada.* Englewood Cliffs, NJ: Prentice Hall; 1964.

109. Kingsbury JM. Phytotoxicology. I. Major problems associated with poisonous plants. *Clin Pharmacol Ther.* 1969;10:163.

110. Kirk MD, et al. World Health Organization estimates of the global and regional disease burden of 22 foodborne bacterial, protozoal, and viral diseases, 2010: A Data Synthesis. *PLoS Med.* 2015;12.

111. Kliks MM. Human anisakiasis: an update. *JAMA.* 1986;255:2605.

112. Kman NE, Werman HA. Disorders presenting primarily with diarrhea. In: Tintanelli J, et al. eds. *Tintanelli's Emergency Medicine: A Comprehensive Study Guide.* 7th ed. New York, NY: McGraw-Hill; 2016. http://accessemergencymedicine.mhmedical.com/content.aspx?bookid=1658&sectionid=109429982.

113. Kolavic SA, et al. An outbreak of *Shigella* dysenteriae type 2 among laboratory workers due to intentional food contamination. *JAMA.* 1997;278:396.

114. Kurihara K, Kashiwayanagi M. Physiological studies on umami taste. *J Nutr.* 2000;130:931S-934S.

115. Lamanna C, Carr CJ. The botulinal, tetanal, and enterostaphylococcal toxins: a review. *Clin Pharmacol Ther.* 1967;8:286.

116. Lampe KF, McCann MA. *AMA Handbook of Poisonous and Injurious Plants.* Chicago, IL: American Medical Association; 1985.

117. Lampe KF. Rhododendrons, mountain laurel, and mad honey. *JAMA.* 1988;259:2009.

118. Lange WR, et al. Can ciguatera be a sexually transmitted disease? *J Toxicol Clin Toxicol.* 1989;27:193.

119. Lange WR, et al. Travel and ciguatera fish poisoning. *Arch Intern Med.* 1992;152:2049.

120. Law JW, et al. Rapid Methods for the detection of foodborne bacterial pathogens: principles, applications, advantages and limitations. *Frontiers Microbiol.* 2015;5.

121. Laycock MV, et al. Isolation and purification procedures for the preparation of paralytic shellfish poisoning toxin standards. *Nat Toxins.* 1994;2:175.

122. Lecour H, et al. Food-borne botulism. A review of 13 outbreaks. *Arch Intern Med.* 1988;148:578-580.

123. Lee LA, et al. *Yersinia enterocolitica* O:3 infections in infants and children, associated with the household preparation of chitterlings. *N Engl J Med.* 1990;322:984.

124. Lefebvre KA, Robertso A. Domoic acid and human exposure risks: *a review, Toxicon.* 2009;56:218.

125. Lehane L, Lewis RJ. Ciguatera: recent advances but the risk remains. *Int J Food Microbiol.* 2000;61:91.

126. Leiken JB. Intentional food poisoning. *Chicago Medicine.* 2014. https://www.clintox.org/documents/WMDSIG/Intentional_Food_Poisoning_published.pdf.

127. Levin RE. Paralytic shellfish toxins: their origin, characteristics and methods of detection: a review. *J Food Biochem.* 1991;15:405-417.

128. Levine AS, et al. Food technology. A primer for physicians. *N Engl J Med.* 1985;312:628.

129. Lewis RJ, et al. Purification and characterization of ciguatoxins from moray eel (*Lycodontis javanicus*, Muraenidae). *Toxicon.* 1991;29:1115-1127.

130. Lewis RJ, Sellin M. Multiple ciguatoxins in the flesh of fish. *Toxicon.* 1992;30:915.

131. Lewis RJ, Holmes MJ. Origin and transfer of toxins involved in ciguatera. *Comp Biochem Physiol C.* 1993;106:615.

132. Liu SH, et al. Is neostigmine effective in severe pufferfish-associated tetrodotoxin poisoning? *Clin Toxicol.* 2015;53:13.

133. Lopez-Serrano MC, et al. Gastroallergic anisakiasis: findings in 22 patients. *J Gastroenterol Hepatol.* 2000;15:503.

134. Lumish RM, et al. Heat-labile enterotoxigenic *Escherichia coli* induced diarrhea aboard a Miami-based cruise ship. *Am J Epidemiol.* 1980;111:432-436.

135. Mahler H, et al. Fulminant liver failure in association with the emetic toxin of *Bacillus cereus.* *N Engl J Med.* 1997;336:1142-1148.

136. Martin DL, et al. The epidemiology and clinical aspects of the hemolytic uremic syndrome in Minnesota. *N Engl J Med.* 1990;323:1161-1167.

137. Massachusetts Department of Health. The red tide—a public health emergency. *N Engl J Med.* 1973;288:1126-1127.

138. Maucher J, Ramsdell J. Maternal-fetal transfer of domoic acid in rats at two gestational time points. *Environ. Health Perspec.* 2007;115:1743.

139. McCarthy TA, et al. Hemolytic-uremic syndrome and *Escherichia coli* O121 at a lake in Connecticut, 1999. *Pediatrics.* 2001;108:E59.

140. McCollum JP, et al. An epidemic of mussel poisoning in North-East England. *Lancet.* 1968;2:767-770.

141. Merson MH, et al. Scombroid fish poisoning. Outbreak traced to commercially canned tuna fish. *JAMA.* 1974;228:1268-1269.

142. Merson MH, et al. Travelers' diarrhea in Mexico. A prospective study of physicians and family members attending a congress. *N Engl J Med.* 1976;294:1299-1305.

143. Minor T, et al. The per case and total annual costs of foodborne illness in the United States. *Risk Anal.* 2015;35: 1125.

144. Mishu B, et al. *Salmonella enteritidis* gastroenteritis transmitted by intact chicken eggs. *Ann Intern Med.* 1991;115:190-194.

145. Morris PD, et al. Clinical and epidemiological features of neurotoxic shellfish poisoning in North Carolina. *Am J Public Health.* 1991;81:471-474.

146. Morrow JD, et al. Evidence that histamine is the causative toxin of scombroid-fish poisoning. *N Engl J Med.* 1991;324:716-720.

147. Mosher HS, et al. Tarichatoxin–tetrodotoxin: a potent neurotoxin. *Science*. 1964;144: 1100-1110.

148. Narahashi T. Mechanism of action of tetrodotoxin and saxitoxin on excitable membranes. *Fed Proc*. 1972;31:1124-1132.

149. Narahashi T. Tetrodotoxin—a brief history. *Proc Jpn Acad Ser B*. 2008;84:147-154.

150. Ngy L, et al. Occurrence of paralytic shellfish toxins in Cambodian Mekong pufferfish *Tetraodon turgidus*: selective toxin accumulation in the skin. *Toxicon*. 2008;51:280-288.

151. Noguchi T, et al. TTX accumulation in pufferfish. *Comp Biochem Physiol D*. 2006;1:145-152.

152. Nordt SP, Pomeranz D. Scombroid poisoning from tilapia. *Am J Emerg Med*. 2016; 34:339.

153. Noris M, Remuzzi G. Atypical hemolytic-uremic syndrome. *N Engl J Med*. 2009;361:1676.

154. Nukina M, et al. Two interchangeable forms of ciguatoxin. *Toxicon*. 1984;22:169-176.

155. Nunez D, et al. Outbreak of ciguatera food poisoning by consumption of amberjack (*Seriola* spp.) in the Canary Islands, May 2012. *Euro Surveill*. 2012;17:7.

156. Orr P, et al. An outbreak of diarrhea due to verotoxin-producing *Escherichia coli* in the Canadian Northwest Territories. *Scand J Infect Dis*. 1994;26:675-684.

157. Ostroff SM, et al. Infections with *Escherichia coli* O157:H7 in Washington State. The first year of statewide disease surveillance. *JAMA*. 1989;262:355-359.

158. Palafox NA, et al. Successful treatment of ciguatera fish poisoning with intravenous mannitol. *JAMA*. 1988;259:2740-2742.

159. Pearn J, et al. Ciguatera and pregnancy. *Med J Aust*. 1982;1:57-58.

160. Pearn JH, et al. Ciguatera and mannitol: experience with a new treatment regimen. *Med J Aust*. 1989;151:77-80.

161. Perl TM, et al. An outbreak of toxic encephalopathy caused by eating mussels contaminated with domoic acid. *N Engl J Med*. 1990;322:1775-1780.

162. Pickering LK, et al. Hemolytic-uremic syndrome and enterohemorrhagic *Escherichia coli*. *Pediatr Infect Dis J*. 1994;13:459-476.

163. Poli MA, et al. Radioimmunoassay for PbTx-2-type brevetoxins: epitope specificity of two anti-PbTx sera. *J AOAC Int*. 1995;78:538-542.

164. Potter ME, et al. Unpasteurized milk. The hazards of a health fetish. *JAMA*. 1984;252:2048-2052.

165. Price M. Underwater grasslands can cut concentrations of harmful bacteria in half. *Science Magazine. 2017*. http://www.sciencemag.org/news/2017/02/underwater-grasslands-can-cut-concentrations-harmful-bacteria-half.

166. Proulx F, et al. Randomized, controlled trial of antibiotic therapy for *Escherichia coli* O157:H7 enteritis. *J Pediatr*. 1992;121:299-303.

167. Puschner B, et al. Assessment of melamine and cyanuric acid toxicity in cats. *J Vet Diagn Invest*. 2007;19:616-624.

168. Ramos F, et al. Proposed guidelines for clenbuterol food poisoning. *Am J Med*. 2004;117:362.

169. Rowe PC, et al. Epidemiology of hemolytic-uremic syndrome in Canadian children from 1986 to 1988. The Canadian Pediatric Kidney Disease Reference Centre. *J Pediatr*. 1991;119:218-224.

170. Ruttenberg M. Safe sushi. *N Engl J Med*. 1989;321:900-901.

171. Ryan CA, et al. Massive outbreak of antimicrobial-resistant salmonellosis traced to pasteurized milk. *JAMA*. 1987;258:3269-3274.

172. Safdar N, et al. Risk of hemolytic uremic syndrome after antibiotic treatment of Escherichia coli O157:H7 enteritis: a meta-analysis. *JAMA*. 2002;288:996-1001.

173. Sampson HA, et al. Fatal and near-fatal anaphylactic reactions to food in children and adolescents. *N Engl J Med*. 1992;327:380-384.

174. Sartwell PE. *Maxcy-Rosenau Preventive Medicine and Public Health*. 10th ed. Norwalk, CT: Appleton & Lange; 1992.

175. Schantz EJ, Johnson EA. Properties and use of botulinum toxin and other microbial neurotoxins in medicine. *Microbiol Rev*. 1992;56:80-99.

176. Schantz PM. The dangers of eating raw fish. *N Engl J Med*. 1989;320:1143-1145.

177. Schaumburg HH, et al. Monosodium L-glutamate: its pharmacology and role in the Chinese restaurant syndrome. *Science*. 1969;163:826-828.

178. Schlech WF III. Foodborne listeriosis. *Clin Infect Dis*. 2000;31:770-775.

179. Schnorf H, et al. Ciguatera fish poisoning: a double-blind randomized trial of mannitol therapy. *Neurology*. 2002;58:873-880.

180. Scholin CA, et al. Mortality of sea lions along the central California coast linked to a toxic diatom bloom. *Nature*. 2000;403:80-84.

181. Settipane GA. The restaurant syndromes. *Arch Intern Med*. 1986;146:2129-2130.

182. Siegler RL, et al. A 20-year population-based study of postdiarrheal hemolytic uremic syndrome in Utah. *Pediatrics*. 1994;94:35-40.

183. Sierra-Beltran AP, et al. An overview of the marine food poisoning in Mexico. *Toxicon*. 1998;36:1493-1502.

184. Simeao Do Carmo L, et al. Food poisoning due to enterotoxigenic strains of Staphylococcus present in Minas cheese and raw milk in Brazil. *Food Microbial*. 2002;19:9-14.

185. Simeao Do Carmo LS, et al. A case study of a massive staphylococcal food poisoning incident. *Foodborne Pathog Dis*. 2004;1:241-246.

186. Sims JK, Ostman DC. Pufferfish poisoning: emergency diagnosis and management of mild human tetrodotoxication. *Ann Emerg Med*. 1986;15:1094-1098.

187. Smith KE, et al. Antibiotic treatment of *Escherichia coli* O157 infection and the risk of hemolytic uremic syndrome, Minnesota. *Pediatr Infect Dis J*. 2012;31:37-41.

188. Smith LM, Simon AM. Food and waterborne illnesses. In: Tintanelli J, et al, eds. *Tintanelli's Emergency Medicine: A Comprehensive Study Guide*. 7th ed. New York, NY: McGraw-Hill; 2016. http://accessemergencymedicine.mhmedical.com/content.aspx?bookid=1658&sectionid=109435875.

189. Southern JP, et al. Bird attack on milk bottles: possible mode of transmission of *Campylobacter jejuni* to man. *Lancet*. 1990;336:1425-1427.

190. Squire EN Jr. Angio-oedema and monosodium glutamate. *Lancet*. 1987;1:988.

191. Swift AE, Swift TR. Ciguatera. *J Toxicol Clin Toxicol*. 1993;31:1-29.

192. Tacket CO, et al. An outbreak of *Yersinia enterocolitica* infections caused by contaminated tofu (soybean curd). *Am J Epidemiol*. 1985;121:705-711.

193. Tarr PI, et al. *Escherichia coli* O157:H7 and the hemolytic uremic syndrome: importance of early cultures in establishing the etiology. *J Infect Dis*. 1990;162:553-556.

194. Taylor WR, et al. A foodborne outbreak of enterotoxigenic *Escherichia coli* diarrhea. *N Engl J Med*. 1982;306:1093-1095.

195. Teitelbaum JS, et al. Neurologic sequelae of domoic acid intoxication due to the ingestion of contaminated mussels. *N Engl J Med*. 1990;322:1781-1787.

196. Thomas DE, Elliot EJ. Interventions for preventing diarrhea-associated hemolytic uremic syndrome: systematic review. *BMC Public Health*. 2013;13:799.

197. Todd E. Domoic acid and amnesic shellfish poisoning: a review. *J Food Prot*. 1993;56:68-83.

198. Torok TJ, et al. A large community outbreak of salmonellosis caused by intentional contamination of restaurant salad bars. *JAMA*. 1997;278:389-395.

199. Trachtman H, et al. Effect of an oral *Shiga* toxin-binding agent on diarrhea-associated hemolytic uremic syndrome in children: a randomized controlled trial. *JAMA*. 2003;290:1337-1344.

200. Trainer VL, et al. Detection of marine toxins using reconstituted sodium channels. *J AOAC Int*. 1995;78:570-573.

201. Uragoda CG, Kottegoda SR. Adverse reactions to isoniazid on ingestion of fish with a high histamine content. *Tubercle*. 1977;58:83-89.

202. van de Kar NC, et al. The fibrinolytic system in the hemolytic uremic syndrome: in vivo and in vitro studies. *Pediatr Res*. 1994;36:257-264.

203. van Egmond HP, et al. Paralytic shellfish poison reference materials: an intercomparison of methods for the determination of saxitoxin. *Food Addit Contam*. 1994;11:39-56.

204. Vantrappen G, et al. *Yersinia* enteritis. *Med Clin North Am*. 1982;66:639-653.

205. Gao J, Wang F, Kuang X. Assessment of chronic renal injury from melamine-associated pediatric urolithiasis: an eighteen-month prospective cohort study. *Ann Saudi Med*. 2016;36:252-257.

206. Waters JR, et al. Infection caused by *Escherichia coli* O157:H7 in Alberta, Canada, and in Scotland: a five-year review, 1987-1991. *Clin Infect Dis*. 1994;19:834-843.

207. Wei HL, Chiou CS. Molecular subtyping of *Staphylococcus aureus* from an outbreak associated with a food handler. *Epidemiol Infect*. 2002;128:15-20.

208. Whitlow KS, et al. Tetramethylenedisulfotetramine: old agent and new terror. *Ann Emerg Med*. 2005;45:609-613.

209. Withers NW. Ciguatera fish poisoning. *Annu Rev Med*. 1982;33:97-111.

210. Wittner M, et al. Eustrongylidiasis—a parasitic infection acquired by eating sushi. *N Engl J Med*. 1989;320:1124-1126.

211. Yang CC, et al. An outbreak of tetrodotoxin poisoning following gastropod mollusc consumption. *Hum Exp Toxicol*. 1995;14:446-450.

212. Yang WH, et al. The monosodium glutamate symptom complex: assessment in a double-blind, placebo-controlled, randomized study. *J Allergy Clin Immunol*. 1997;99:757-762.

213. Yu L, et al. Potent protection of ferulic acid against excitotoxic effects of maternal intragastric administration of monosodium glutamate at a late stage of pregnancy on developing mouse fetal brain. *Eur Neuropsychopharmacol*. 2006;16:170-177.

214. Zhang Y, et al. Tetramine poisoning: a case report and review of the literature. *Forensic Sci Int*. 2011;204.

215. Yunginger JW, et al. Fatal food-induced anaphylaxis. *JAMA*. 1988;260:1450-1452.

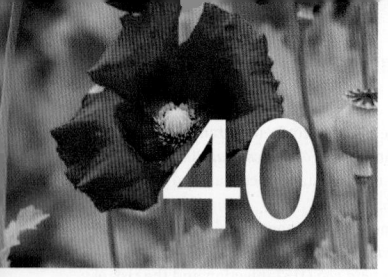

40 DIETING XENOBIOTICS AND REGIMENS

Jeanna M. Marraffa

OH
NH—CH₃
CH₃

Ephedrine

INTRODUCTION AND HISTORY

Obesity is a worldwide epidemic, and the United States has the largest proportion of a national population of overweight and obese individuals. According to the World Health Organization, 67.3% of the US population older than 18 years of age has a body mass index (BMI) of 25 or greater. The only country that has a larger proportion is the United Arab Emirates.[135] The majority of countries in the world have demonstrated a doubling to quadrupling of those with obesity in the past 30 years.[61] Some estimates predict that nearly 38% of the world's adult population will be overweight and 20% will be obese by 2030.[61,66] Even more alarming, the incidence of obesity in children between the ages of 6 and 19 years has tripled in the past 30 years. In one systematic review, there was a strong association between childhood obesity and adult obesity. Eighty percent of obese adolescents were obese into adulthood.[117] Although there are conflicting data, it is clear that obesity results in excess mortality.[39,40] In 2009, the Centers for Disease Control and Prevention reported more than 110,000 deaths caused by obesity in the United States. Mortality is a proven increase for every 5 kg/m² higher than a BMI of greater than 25 kg/m² with a reduction of median survival of 8 to 10 years in those with a BMI between 40 and 45 kg/m².[103] Obesity is linked to numerous health risks, including type 2 diabetes, hypertension, coronary heart disease,[10,18] metabolic syndrome,[133] fatty liver, and low back pain.[114] Obesity is considered a leading preventable health risk, second only to cigarette smoking with a large economic impact costing upward of $147 billion annually.[21]

Americans spend upward of $60 billion per year on weight loss therapies. Pharmacologic interventions typically result in a 5% to 10% weight loss, although a return to baseline upon drug cessation is common.[32,109] Surgical interventions consistently achieve substantial weight loss, causing up to a 30% reduction in weight, but they are associated with numerous and varied complications.[26]

One of the earliest accounts of weight loss therapy dates back to 10th century Spain. King Sancho I, who was obese, underwent successful treatment with a "theriaca" thought to contain plants and possibly opioids, administered with wine and oil. In addition, he was closely supervised and treated by a physician.[60]

Weight loss xenobiotics (Table 40–1) are available as prescription medications (lorcaserin, phentermine, phentermine/topiramate, bupropion/naltrexone, phendimetrazine, orlistat, and liraglutide), nonprescription dietary supplements (*Citrus aurantium*, chitosan, *Garcinia cambogia*, caffeine), and nonprescription diet aids (orlistat). Numerous other prescription medications, including thyroid medications and metformin, have been used on an off-label basis for weight loss. Numerous xenobiotics are promoted as weight loss aids, many with no proven efficacy and some with serious toxicity.

The history of dieting xenobiotics is checkered. A number of weight loss therapies were withdrawn or banned by the Food and Drug Administration (FDA) because of serious adverse health effects (Table 40–2). Phenylpropanolamine (PPA),[27] fenfluramine/phentermine,[27] and sibutramine[63] were withdrawn from the US market. The endocannabinoid receptor inverse agonist (rimonabant) never reached the US market but was withdrawn in Europe

after its use was associated with serious dysphoria.[106] γ-Hydroxybutyric acid (GHB) and its congeners were initially sold as dietary supplements (Chap. 80) and promoted to body builders as a means to "convert fat into muscle" as a result of increasing growth hormone. Because of toxicity and its association with drug-facilitated sexual assault, GHB is strictly controlled as a Schedule I drug, with limited availability as a schedule III drug for narcolepsy (sodium oxybate: Xyrem). Clenbuterol is a long-acting β₂-adrenergic agonist. Because of the stimulant properties and lipolytic effects, clenbuterol is abused by body builders and others as a stimulant and anoretic.[57,138] Despite at least one meta-analysis demonstrating that that β-human chorionic gonadotropin (β-HCG) was without efficacy in the treatment of obesity,[75] injectable beta-HCG continues to be sold for weight loss, with the potential for significant harm.[74]

Since 2012, the prescription pharmaceutical market has developed, and the FDA approved numerous new medications. Phentermine/topiramate, lorcaserin, bupropion/naltrexone, liraglutide, and orlistat are all available in the United States. Pharmacologically different, they show modest promise, at best in the weight loss drug armamentarium. There is ongoing research both for existing and novel pharmaceutical approaches for weight loss and will likely be presented to the FDA for new drug approval or labeling changes to include weight loss. Despite numerous innovative pharmacologic approaches and advancements, there will likely be no perfect, ideal weight loss drug.

PHARMACOLOGY

The hypothalamus is the key site in the brain that regulates food intake, energy expenditure, satiety, and metabolism. It also integrates endocrine signaling to meet the energy demand.[83] The hormonal endocrine regulation of appetite continues to be extensively investigated. Dieting xenobiotics can be divided into classes based on one or more of the following mechanisms or action: (1) appetite suppression (*anorectics*), (2) alteration of food absorption or elimination, or (3) increased energy expenditure. Sympathomimetics, serotonergics, dinitrophenol, and bupropion/naltrexone all work pharmacologically on the hypothalamus to induce weight loss. Dinitrophenol is a mitochondrial uncoupler, thereby resulting in an increasing energy expenditure.[71] Glucagon-like peptide-1 (GLP-1) agonists, such as liraglutide, act on the hypothalamus and suppress appetite.[17]

Endocannabinoid receptor antagonists bind to CB1 endocannabinoid receptors in the brain and in the intestines, liver, pancreas, adipose tissue, and skeletal muscle. Antagonizing central CB1 receptors has a negative effect on the reward pathway in the mesolimbic system as well as decreasing appetite via the hypothalamus.[30] Leptin is secreted from fat proportionate to the amount of lipids contained in the adipocyte, with women secreting more leptin than men. Leptin acts on the hypothalamus to decrease food intake, enhancing the metabolic rate and energy expenditure. Ghrelin is secreted by the stomach, and concentrations increase after fasting and just before meals. Ghrelin stimulates the hypothalamus and stimulates food intake. Glucagon-like peptide-1 enhances glucose-induced insulin secretion while suppressing glucagon release (Fig. 40–1).[17,33] Most humans have metabolically active brown adipose tissue containing both brown and beige adipocytes. Under conditions of obesity, there appears to be inhibition of brown and beige adipocytes. Although very early in research, beige adipocytes may be a potential therapeutic target for obesity.[115]

SYMPATHOMIMETICS

Although controversial, certain sympathomimetic amines still carry official indications for short-term weight reduction (Table 40–3). Sympathomimetic amines share a β-phenylethylamine parent structure and include phentermine,

TABLE 40–1	Weight Loss Xenobiotics			

Drug or Supplement[a]	Mechanism of Action	Regulation Status, DEA Schedule	Adverse Effects or Contraindications[b]
Sympathomimetics			
Bitter orange extract (*Citrus aurantium*)	Contains synephrine and octopamine; increases thermogenesis and lipolysis	Dietary supplement	Hypertension, cerebral ischemia, myocardial ischemia, prolonged QT interval
Bupropion/naltrexone	Increased release of norepinephrine; synergistic effect of midbrain dopamine	Nonscheduled prescription drug	Tachycardia; hypertension; seizures. Opioid withdrawal in tolerant patients
Diethylpropion	Increased release of norepinephrine and dopamine	Schedule IV	Dry mouth, tremor, insomnia, headache, agitation, palpitations, hypertension, stroke, dysrhythmias; contraindications: monoamine oxidase inhibitor use within 14 days, glaucoma, hyperthyroidism
Guarana (*Paullinia cupana*)	Contains caffeine, which may increase thermogenesis	Dietary supplement	Nausea, vomiting, insomnia, diuresis, anxiety, palpitations
Mazindol	Increased release of norepinephrine and dopamine	Schedule IV	Dry mouth, tremor, insomnia, headache, agitation, palpitations, hypertension, stroke, dysrhythmias; contraindications: monoamine oxidase inhibitor use within 14 days, glaucoma, hyperthyroidism
Phentermine	Increased release of norepinephrine and dopamine	Schedule IV	Similar to diethylpropion
Phentermine/topiramate	Increased release of norepinephrine and dopamine (phentermine); exact mechanism of action for topiramate remains speculative	Schedule IV	Phentermine: similar to diethylpropion. Topiramate: central nervous system depression; ataxia; non–anion gap metabolic acidosis; kidney stones. Contraindication: first trimester pregnancy
Raspberry ketone	Structurally similar to synephrine; increases thermogenesis and lipolysis	Dietary supplement	Nausea, vomiting, insomnia, hypertension, tachycardia, anxiety, palpitations
Serotonergics			
Lorcaserin (Belviq)	Selective agonist at 5-HT$_{2C}$	Schedule IV	Dizziness, headache, nausea; serotonin toxicity possible after overdose
GLP-1 Agonists			
Albiglutide, Dulaglutide, Exenatide, Liraglutide	GLP-1 analog	Nonscheduled prescription medication	Nausea, diarrhea. Potential: hypoglycemia
GI Agents			
Chitosan	Insoluble marine fiber that binds dietary fat	Dietary supplement	Decreased absorption of fat-soluble vitamins. Contraindications: shellfish allergy
Orlistat	Inhibits gastric and pancreatic lipases	Prescription and nonprescription medication	Abdominal pain, oily stool, fecal urgency or incontinence; fat-soluble vitamin loss. Contraindications: cholestasis, chronic malabsorption
Fibers and Other Supplements			
Chromium picolinate	Improves blood glucose and lipids; produces fat loss (unproven)	Dietary supplement	Dermatitis, hepatitis, possibly mutagenic in high doses
Garcinia cambogia	Increases fat oxidation (unproven)	Dietary supplement	None reported
Glucomannan	Expands in stomach to increase satiety	Dietary supplement	GI obstruction with tablet form. Contraindications: abnormal GI anatomy

[a]Trade names and botanical names are given in parentheses. [b]All xenobiotics are contraindicated during pregnancy and lactation.

GI = gastrointestinal; GLP-1 = glucagon-like peptide-1; MAOI = monamine oxidase inhibitor; 5-HT$_{2c}$ = serotonin receptor.

diethylpropion, and mazindol, which are Schedule IV drugs and carry warnings that advise prescribers to limit use to only a few weeks. Phentermine/topiramate extended release (Qsymia) is indicated for long-term use.[5,9] Regardless of their source and legal status, sympathomimetics generally share a spectrum of toxicity and produce adverse effects similar to amphetamines (Chap. 73). Both PPA and ephedra were popular sympathomimetics used in weight loss products, and were both fraught with significant toxicity and are no longer available. Reported toxicity associated with PPA generally results from hypertension.[95] A comprehensive review of more than 100 case reports of adverse drug effects involving PPA revealed 24 intracranial hemorrhages, 8 seizures, and 8 fatalities between 1965 and 1990.[71] Ephedra (*Ephedra sinica*), or Ma-huang, is a

TABLE 40–2	High-Risk Xenobiotics Unapproved or Withdrawn by the US Food and Drug Administration		
Drug or Supplement[a]	Mechanism of Action	Regulation Status, DEA Schedule, or Withdrawal Date	Adverse Effects or Contraindications
Amphetamine	Increased release of norepinephrine and dopamine	Schedule II	Sympathomimetic effects, psychosis, dependence
Benzphetamine	Increased release of norepinephrine and dopamine	Schedule III	Sympathomimetic effects, psychosis, dependence
Caffeine	β_2-Adrenergic agonist activity; increased energy expenditure	Never approved	Nausea, vomiting, tachycardia, wide pulse pressure, hypokalemia, hyperglycemia, anion gap metabolic acidosis
Clenbuterol	β_2-Adrenergic agonist activity	Never approved	Tachycardia, headache, nausea, vomiting; may be prolonged
Dexfenfluramine	Promotes central serotonin release and inhibits its reuptake	Withdrawn September 1997	Valvular heart disease, primary pulmonary hypertension
Dieter's teas (senna, cascara, aloe, buckthorn)	Stimulant laxative herbs that promote colonic evacuation	FDA required label warning, June 1995	Diarrhea, vomiting, nausea, abdominal cramps, electrolyte disorders, dependence
Dinitrophenol	Alters metabolism by uncoupling oxidative phosphorylation	Never approved; available on the Internet	Hyperthermia, cataracts, hepatotoxicity, skin rash, peripheral neuropathy
Ephedra sinica (Ma-huang)	Increased release of NE and dopamine	Banned by FDA, April 2004	Sympathomimetic effects, psychosis
Fenfluramine	Increased release and decreased reuptake of serotonin	Withdrawn September 1997	Valvular heart disease, primary pulmonary hypertension
Guar gum	Hygroscopic polysaccharide swells in stomach, producing early satiety	Banned by FDA, July 1990	Esophageal and small bowel obstruction, fatalities
β-Human chorionic gonadotrophin	Unknown	Never approved	Coronary artery dissection
LipoKinetix (sodium usniate, norephedrine, 3,5-diiodothyronine, yohimbine, caffeine)	Unknown	FDA warning, November 2001	Acute hepatitis
Phendimetrazine	Increased release of NE and dopamine	Schedule III	Sympathomimetic effects, psychosis
Phenylpropanolamine	α_1-Adrenergic agonist	Withdrawn November 2000	Sympathomimetic effects, headache, hypertension, myocardial infarction, intracranial hemorrhage
Rimonabant	Endocannabinoid receptor inverse partial agonist	Never approved in the United States; withdrawn from European market in 2011	Anxiety, nausea, diarrhea, dizziness; increased suicidality and depression
Salicylate (willow bark)	Uncoupler of oxidative phosphorylation	Never approved	Nausea, vomiting, tinnitus, tachycardia, altered mental status, anion gap metabolic acidosis (see chapter)
Sibutramine	Inhibits reuptake of serotonin and norepinephrine	Withdrawn October 2010	Increase in cardiovascular toxicity; increase in nonfatal myocardial infarction; increase in nonfatal stroke

[a]Trade names or botanical names as appropriate are given in parentheses.

DEA = Drug Enforcement Administration; FDA = Food and Drug Administration; NE = norepinephrine.

plant that contains six sympathomimetic amines, known collectively as *ephedra alkaloids*. The FDA banned ephedra-containing products in 2004 because of cases of serious cardiovascular toxicity[54] and acute hepatitis.[86]

Pharmacology

Sympathomimetic amines that act at α- and β-adrenergic receptors are clinically effective in promoting weight loss but have numerous side effects that limit their clinical use. Soon after its introduction as a pharmaceutical for nasal congestion in the 1930s, the prototype sympathomimetic drug amphetamine (Fig. 40–2) was noted to cause weight loss (Chap. 73). The weight loss effect of amphetamine was also readily apparent in early animal studies, although tolerance to the anorectic effects was also noted.[125] The primary mechanism of action of the weight loss effects of

sympathomimetics is central nervous system (CNS) stimulation, resulting from increased release of norepinephrine and dopamine.[121] The effects include direct suppression of the appetite center in the hypothalamus and reduced taste and olfactory acuity, leading to decreased interest in food. Increased energy and euphoriant effects of the stimulants also contribute to weight loss. However, tachyphylaxis occurs, and the rate of weight loss diminishes within a few weeks of initiating therapy.[35] Significant side effects and abuse potential severely limit the therapeutic use of this class.

Adverse Effects

The absence of polar hydroxyl groups from a sympathomimetic amine increases its lipophilicity; therefore, unsubstituted or predominantly alkyl group substituted compounds such as amphetamine, ephedrine, and PPA

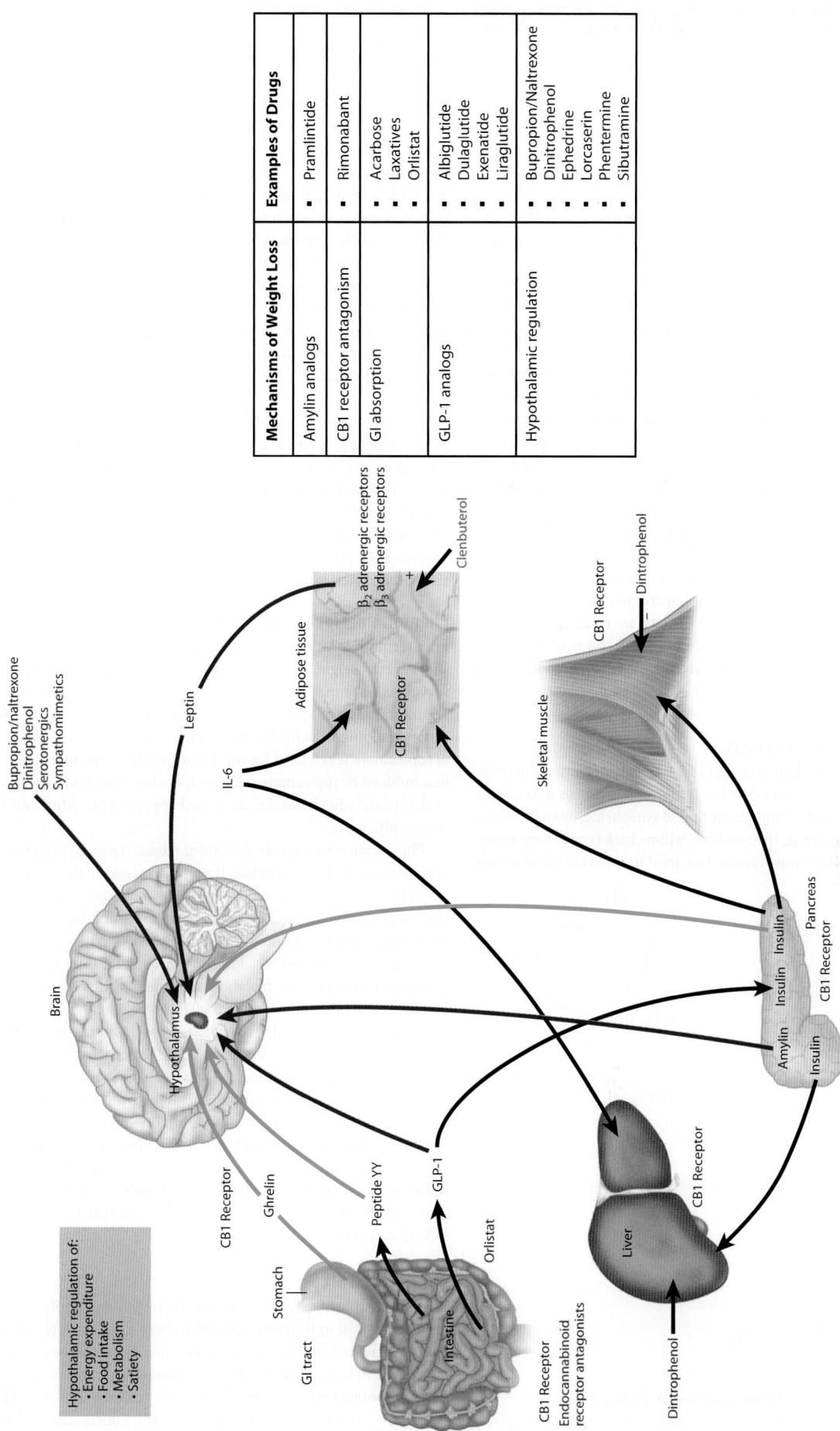

Mechanisms of Weight Loss	Examples of Drugs
Amylin analogs	• Pramlintide
CB1 receptor antagonism	• Rimonabant
GI absorption	• Acarbose • Laxatives • Orlistat
GLP-1 analogs	• Albiglutide • Dulaglutide • Exenatide • Liraglutide
Hypothalamic regulation	• Bupropion/Naltrexone • Dinitrophenol • Ephedrine • Lorcaserin • Phentermine • Sibutramine

FIGURE 40–1. Endocrine and neuroendocrine pathways of obesity and weight loss regimens. Systems regulating food ingestion and energy balance are interconnected and regulated. The hypothalamus regulates food intake, satiety, energy expenditure, and metabolism. Adipose tissue functions for glucose uptake and conversion; lipogenesis and lipolysis; β oxidation of fatty acids; and release of leptin, adiponectin, and interleukin-6 (Il-6), all of which regulate energy balance. CB1 = endocannabinoid receptor; GI = gastrointestinal; GLP-1 = glucagon-like peptide 1; Red text: *Suggests a negative effect or antagonist effect;* Green text: *Suggests a positive effect or agonist effect;* Black arrow: *normal cause/effect;* Green arrow: *increases hunger;* Red arrow: *promotes satiety;* Green text: *promotes satiety;* Black arrow: *normal cause/effect and + if promotes positive effects and - if promotes negative effects.*

TABLE 40–3	Defining Overweight and Obesity in the United States	
Age	Overweight	Obese
2–19 y of age	BMI between 85th and 95th percentiles[a]	BMI ≥95th percentile[a]
≥20 y of age	BMI ≥25 but <30	BMI ≥30

[a]From the Centers for Disease Control and Prevention's sex-specific body mass index (BMI) for age growth charts

Data from Ogden CL, Flegal KM. Changes in terminology for childhood overweight and obesity. *Natl Health Stat Report.* 2010 Jun 25;(25):1-5.

have greater CNS activity. Mild cardiovascular and CNS stimulant effects include headache, tremor, sweating, palpitations, and insomnia. More severe effects that may occur after overdose of sympathomimetic amines include anxiety, agitation, psychosis, seizures, palpitations, and chest pain.[127,129]

Hypertension is common after overdose and occasionally after therapeutic use. Patients present with confusion and altered mental status as a result of hypertensive encephalopathy. Reflex bradycardia after exposure to xenobiotics with predominantly α-adrenergic agonist effects often accompanies the hypertension and provides a clue to the diagnosis. Children are at especially high risk for hypertensive episodes because of the relatively significant dose per kilogram of body weight from even a single tablet. Other manifestations include chest pain, palpitations, tachycardia, hypertension, syncope, coronary vasospasm, mania, psychosis, and convulsions.[94]

Clinically significant hypertension should be treated with a rapid acting, easily titratable vasodilator such as nicardipine or phentolamine. Analogous to the management of cocaine toxicity, we recommend against the use of β-adrenergic antagonists avoided because the resultant unopposed α-adrenergic agonist effects may lead to greater vasoconstriction and hypertension.[4] Agitation, tachycardia, and seizures should be treated initially with benzodiazepines.

Herbal Sympathomimetic Products

Since ephedra was banned, herbal weight loss supplements have been reformulated. Many now contain an extract of bitter orange (*Citrus aurantium*), a natural source of the sympathomimetic amine synephrine, often in combination with caffeine, guarana, theophylline, willow bark (containing salicylates), diuretics, and other constituents. The dried fruit peel of bitter orange

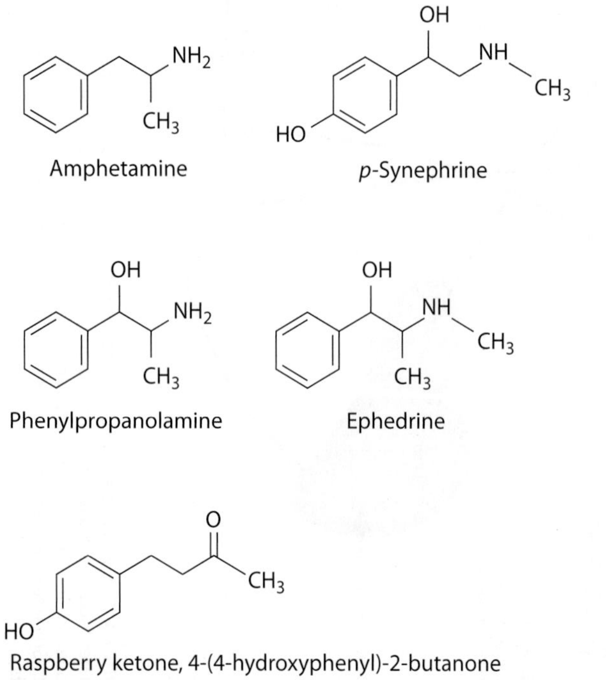

FIGURE 40–2. Sympathomimetic amines formerly and currently used for weight loss.

is a traditional remedy for gastrointestinal (GI) ailments. The predominant constituents, *p*-synephrine (Fig. 40–2) and octopamine, are structurally similar to epinephrine and norepinephrine. The isomer *m*-synephrine (phenylephrine) is used extensively as a vasopressor and nasal decongestant. Although the physiologic actions of synephrine are not fully characterized, it appears to interact with amine receptors in the brain and acts at peripheral α₁-adrenergic receptors, resulting in vasoconstriction and increased blood pressure.[44,124] Some evidence indicates that synephrine also has both β_2 and β_3-adrenergic agonist activity,[19,82,105] which could increase lipolysis. β_3-Adrenergic agonists have remarkable antiobesity effects in rodents;[137] however, effects in humans are not as profound.

Nearly 2% of 4,140 Californians surveyed had used a *C. aurantium*–containing product several times a week. Despite the study of more than 350 participants that concluded that *C. aurantium* did not produce changes in blood pressure or heart rate and was without significant adverse effects,[123] there are numerous case reports describing toxicity. Tachydsrhythmias,[38] cerebral ischemia,[13] QT prolongation,[88] and myocardial infarction[82,91] are all reported.

Raspberry ketone, 4-(4-hydroxyphenyl)-2-butanone, is promoted to induce weight loss and is available as a supplement. Structurally similar to synephrine, its purported effects on weight loss are similar. The amount of raspberry ketone in a typical dose of a dietary supplement is equal to the amount derived from 40 kg of raspberries. The effect on weight loss and adipose tissue remains unclear.[85,94] There has been only one report of toxicity described in the literature, and clinical effects are consistent with other sympathomimetics.[126]

Phentermine/Topiramate

Phentermine is a sympathomimetic that retains an FDA indication for short-term weight loss. It increases release of norepinephrine, which serves as an appetite suppressant via the effects on the hypothalamus. Topiramate is available for a variety of conditions, including seizure disorders and migraine headaches. Weight loss is a demonstrated side effect of topiramate when used for these indications.[67] The mechanism of weight loss induced by topiramate remains speculative and is likely a combination of decreased caloric intake, increased energy expenditure, and decreased energy efficiency.[5,45]

Phentermine/topiramate controlled release (Qsymia) is approved for long-term management of weight loss. If, within 24 weeks of therapy initiation, there is less than a 5% decrease in body weight, therapy should be terminated.[25] The clinical trials evaluating the efficacy of phentermine/topiramate were short-term studies performed in approximately 4,000 patients.[5,9,45] In all of these trials, there was a substantial decline in body fat (upward of 10%) as well as improvement in other metabolic parameters, including lipid control and glucose regulation. Cardiovascular effects reveal mild increases in heart rate at therapeutic dosing.[129] There appears to be an increased risk of congenital malformations, particularly orofacial clefts, when this drug was taken during the first trimester of pregnancy.[43] Topiramate is a carbonic anhydrase inhibitor, and electrolyte abnormalities, including hyperchloremia, hypokalemia, and decreased bicarbonate resulting in non–anion gap metabolic acidosis are commonly associated with use.[113] Overdose of topiramate causes CNS depression, ataxia, seizures and laboratory abnormalities noted above.[14] Although there have been no documented cases of overdose of this combination product, its toxicity can be extrapolated from the known toxicities of the individual components.

SEROTONERGICS

Xenobiotics that affect central release and reuptake of serotonin are approved for a number of indications, including depression, anxiety, nicotine dependency, migraine headache, and premenstrual dysphoric syndrome. Serotonin is believed to have a role in appetite suppression, which is due to the effect on the hypothalamic serotonin 5-HT₂C receptor, as well as the 5-HT₁A, 5-HT₁B, and 5-HT₆ receptors.[52,53] Serotonin receptor effects also enhance energy expenditure. Use of serotonin agonists for weight loss is associated with cardiac valvulopathy (5-HT$_{2B}$ receptor), hallucinations (5-HT$_{2A}$ receptor), and pulmonary hypertension (5-HT$_{1B}$), and serotonin toxicity. The serotonergics dexfenfluramine (Redux), fenfluramine (Pondimin), and sibutramine were all removed from the US market because of significant cardiac toxicity.[1,15,63]

Lorcaserin (Belviq) is a selective agonist at the 5-HT$_{2C}$ receptor.[36,79] This novel selectivity for the 5-HT$_{2C}$ receptor results in weight loss with a decreased incidence of toxicity compared with other serotonergics.[53] Lorcaserin neither stimulates the release of norepinephrine, dopamine, or serotonin, nor does it inhibit the reuptake of these neurotransmitters.[53]

Lorcaserin 10 mg twice daily resulted in a significant reduction in body fat after 52 weeks of therapy in 3,182 participants that was maintained for 1 year.[120] No increase in the incidence of cardiac valvulopathy was demonstrated in the 2-year follow-up in the participants receiving lorcarserin.[120] A recent study[80] described 44 patients with exposures to lorcaserin, 30 of whom had unintentional exposures.[14] There were no major adverse outcomes or death reported, and the majority of adverse events included agitation or irritability, diaphoresis, drowsiness, tachycardia, and muscle rigidity consistent with serotonergic toxicity. Management of the toxic effects mediated by serotonin receptors should address the specific clinical effects. Benzodiazepines are recommended for tachycardia and hypertension that occurs in the setting of psychomotor agitation. Rapid identification and management of serotonin toxicity are essential to prevent associated morbidity and mortality (Chap. 69).

XENOBIOTICS THAT ALTER FOOD ABSORPTION, METABOLISM, AND ELIMINATION

Fat Absorption Blockers

Orlistat was approved by the FDA in 1999 for treatment of obesity. It is also available as nonprescription medication. Orlistat abuse should be assessed in patients presenting with related adverse events. Orlistat is the only FDA-approved drug that alters the absorption, distribution, and metabolism of food. Orlistat is a potent inhibitor of gastric and pancreatic lipase, thus reducing lipolysis and increasing fecal fat excretion.[20] The drug is not systemically absorbed but exerts its effects locally in the GI tract. It inhibits hydrolysis of dietary triglycerides and reduces absorption of the products of lipolysis, monoglycerides, and free fatty acids. Several clinical trials demonstrate that orlistat reduces GI fat absorption by as much as 30%.[140] When taken in association with a calorie-restricted diet, weight loss of approximately 10% body weight can be achieved in 1 year.[118]

Orlistat should be taken only in conjunction with meals that have a high fat content; it should not be consumed in the absence of food intake. Adverse effects correlate with the amount of dietary fat consumption and include abdominal pain, oily stool, fecal incontinence, fecal urgency, flatus, and increased defecation. Systemic effects are rare because of the lack of systemic absorption.[37,94] Liver toxicity manifesting as cholestatic, jaundice, and centrilobular necrosis are reported,[84,107] although the mechanism is unknown. In a cohort of nearly 16,000 patients in England, there were reports of aminotransferase elevations but no cases of serious hepatotoxicity. Two of the cases were deemed as causally related to orlistat, and one had evidence of initial aminotransferase elevation and elevation on rechallenge.[97] Concomitant use of natural fibers (6 g of psyllium mucilloid dissolved in water) is proposed reduce the GI side effects of orlistat. Because orlistat reduces absorption of fat-soluble food constituents, daily ingestion of a multivitamin supplement containing vitamins A, D, and K, and β-carotene is advised to prevent resultant deficiency. Pancreatitis[3] and oxalate nephropathy[117] are rarely reported after orlistat use. There are no reported intentional overdoses of orlistat. There are limited data regarding unintentional pediatric exposure to orlistat, and the toxicity appears to be limited to mild GI effects.[92] In overdose and/or misuse, treatment should be responsive to clinical manifestations.

Dietary Fibers

Glucomannan, a dietary fiber consisting of glucose and mannose, is derived from konjac root, a traditional Japanese food. Edible forms of glucomannan include konjac jelly and konjac flour, which are mixed with liquid before ingestion. Purified glucomannan is available in capsule form and is found in various proprietary products marketed for weight loss. On contact with water, glucomannan swells to approximately 200 times its original dry volume, turning into a viscous liquid. It lowers blood cholesterol and glucose concentrations and decreases systolic blood pressure,[7,129] but significant weight loss benefits are not demonstrated.[68] Following several reports of esophageal obstruction, glucomannan tablets were withdrawn from the market in Australia in 1985.[55] Serious adverse effects are not described with encapsulated glucomannan, presumably because slower dissolution allows for GI transit before expansion. Glucomannan capsules are available as a nutritional supplement in the United States, although adequate safety and efficacy studies have not been published.

Dinitrophenol

Dinitrophenol

One of the earliest attempts at a pharmaceutical treatment for obesity was 2,4-dinitrophenol (DNP), which was popularized as a weight loss adjuvant in the 1930s.[49,98] This chemical, which is used in dyes, wood preservatives, herbicides, and explosives, was never approved as a pharmaceutical. Dinitrophenol was legally available as a dietary supplement before enactment of the US Federal Food, Drug, and Cosmetic Act of 1938 and thus remained legal. Dinitrophenol is readily available in capsules or tablets and can be purchased online.[59,98] By increasing metabolic energy expenditure, it reportedly produces weight loss of 1 to 2 lb per week in doses of 200 to 300 mg per day.[25,46,49] Dinitrophenol increases metabolic work by uncoupling oxidative phosphorylation in the mitochondria. Through this mechanism, the hydrogen ion gradient that facilitates adenosine triphosphate (ATP) synthesis is disrupted, and ATP production is arrested, although oxidative metabolism in the citric acid cycle continues (Chap. 11). This mechanism results in inefficient substrate utilization, and the resulting energy loss is dissipated as heat. This wastes calories but also increases temperature and, occasionally, life-threatening hyperthermia occurs.[79] In fact, DNP was reportedly administered to Russian soldiers during World War II to keep them warm during winter battles.[49] Symptoms related to DNP toxicity include malaise, rashes, headache, diaphoresis, thirst, peripheral neuropathy,[100] and dyspnea. Acute toxic effects include hyperthermia, hepatotoxicity, agranulocytosis, respiratory failure, coma, and death.[59,70,138] Delayed-onset cataracts were a frequent and serious complication of DNP use.[11]

Epidemic use of DNP occurred in Texas in the 1980s when industrial DNP was used at a physician's weight loss center. The physician distributed DNP under the trade name Mitcal. The fatality of a wrestler after an intentional overdose in 1984 led a Texas court to prohibit the practice.[70] Dinitrophenol continues to reappear as a weight loss treatment,[98] and cases of serious toxicity are reported.[46,49] Management should emphasize rapid cooling (Chap. 29). Benzodiazepines should also be used as an adjunct therapy for management of agitation and seizures.

Endocannabinoid Receptor Antagonists and Inverse Agonists

In the past 15 years, the endocannabinoid system (ECS) and its involvement in weight loss sparked excitement and potential for novel xenobiotics. Endocannabinoids, which are the natural ligand for the cannabinoid receptor, have diverse effects on metabolic functions.[58] The ECS contributes to the regulation of food intake, body weight, and energy balance, and it may have a role in inflammation and neuropathic pain.[64,108,132,136] It has long been known that tetrahydrocannabinol, the active principle in marijuana (*Cannabis sativa*), stimulates appetite and is an effective antiemetic[22,96] (Chap. 74).

Several CB1 receptor antagonists and inverse agonists showed promise in both animal and human studies of weight loss. Rimonabant was approved for therapeutic use in Europe, and clinical trials in the United States were performed. Clinical studies note that these xenobiotics showed a significant and sustained reduction in body weight.[104] There was also improvement in insulin resistance with a decline in plasma leptin, insulin, and free fatty acid concentrations, presumably caused by the upregulation of the peripheral ECS system in diabetes.[56,106] In the clinical trials, there was a significant increase in adverse events, including anxiety and depression in the rimonabant groups. This led to a delay in the FDA approval of this product for therapeutic use. Shortly after approval in Europe, it became evident that the effects of anxiety and depression were far greater than initially expected. Rimonabant was never approved by the FDA, and other phase III studies, including those involving other endocannabinoid receptor inverse agonists (eg, taranabant), were terminated early because of a range of dose-related GI, nervous, psychiatric, cutaneous, and vascular side effects.[6,102] Rimonabant was removed from the European market after only 2 years.[81] Centrally acting CB1 antagonists proved to have an unfavorable risk–benefit relationship. However, peripherally acting CB1 antagonists have promise for weight loss, and further research is ongoing.[34,51] Current animal research uses AM4113, a central CB1 neutral antagonist for weight loss as well as nicotine dependence apparently without the psychiatric effects.[50] It remains unclear what role that CB1 receptor antagonists will play in the weight loss drug therapeutics.

Naltrexone/Bupropion

Bupropion/naltrexone (Contrave) was FDA approved in late 2014.[131] The mechanisms by which naltrexone/bupropion cause weight loss is incompletely understood.[131] Proopiomelanocortin (POMC)-producing neurons in the hypothalamus are stimulated with bupropion, and naltrexone inhibits the opioid-mediated POMC autoinhibition. This combination of stimulation and inhibition of the negative feedback loop on POMC neurons is believed to facilitate ongoing weight loss. Additionally, it is believed that there is synergism with naltrexone and bupropion in midbrain dopamine areas resulting in decreased food intake, presumably through modulation of mesolimbic reward systems.[48,65,132] The synergistic effect has shown good results in sustainable weight loss.[48,131]

The FDA mandated a clinical trial evaluating cardiovascular risk of naltrexone SR 32 mg/bupropion SR 360 mg in participants with underlying cardiovascular risk factors. The study reported less than a twofold increase in cardiovascular risk. However, it was terminated before completion, and it is impossible to confirm the lack of increased cardiovascular toxicity in susceptible patients.[90,111]

Adverse events from this product result from the known toxicity of each individual xenobiotic. Naltrexone is generally expected to be safe and well tolerated in opioid-naïve patients; however, it will cause prolonged opioid withdrawal symptoms in opioid-tolerant patients and will significantly reduce the efficacy of opioids if they are required[141] (Antidotes in Depth: A4). Bupropion toxicity is well described in the literature. Seizures occur with bupropion doses greater than 450 mg/day.[28,112] The amount of bupropion available in this formulation is of particular concern as is the potential for misuse or overdose. Bupropion toxicity is discussed in detail in Chap. 69.

Liraglutide

Glucagon-like peptide-1 is produced in the brain and distal intestine. During a meal, GLP-1 concentrations increase and remain elevated for several hours. Glucagon-like peptide-1 inhibits food intake, inhibits glucagon secretion, decreases gastric acid secretion, and delays gastric emptying.[17] Glucagon-like peptide-1 analogs have been FDA-approved pharmaceuticals for type 2 diabetes for several years with only one agent receiving weight loss as an approved indication for use. There are currently four GLP-1 analogs available in the United States (liraglutide, exenatide, dulaglutide, and albiglutide).

Liraglutide (Saxenda), a GLP-1 analog, previously on the US market for the treatment of type 2 diabetes, received FDA approval in late 2014 for weight loss. Liraglutide (3 mg) resulted in at least a 5% reduction of body weight in 63.2% of study participants compared with 27.1% in the control group. A total of 33.1% of participants demonstrated a greater than 10% reduction in body weight compared with 10.6% of control participants over the 56-week study period.[100] The drug was well tolerated with nausea and diarrhea being the most common adverse events.[29,100] In the participants who had adverse events during the clinical trials, nausea was reported in 40% of the participants, diarrhea in 20%, and vomiting in 16%.[100]

Although there are no documented overdoses of the 3-mg liraglutide formulation, there have been many reports of overdose with the other, lower doses formulations used in type 2 diabetes. In one case of intentional overdose of 72-mg liraglutide, mild GI toxicity predominated, and significant hypoglycemia was absent.[87] An inadvertent dosing error of 18 mg/day for 7 months in a 67-year-old male patient with type 2 diabetes only resulted in nausea, vomiting, and diarrhea.[12]

Alternative Pharmaceutical Approaches

In an attempt to find the "perfect" therapeutic alternative for weight loss, there is a desire to use currently approved xenobiotics for weight loss. Similar to topiramate, xenobiotics that are known to cause weight loss at therapeutic doses such as metformin, bupropion, and zonisamide continue to be investigated for both labeled and off-label use. Combination therapy aimed at multiple systems may prove efficacious. Although these xenobiotics provide a beneficial weight loss, each of them has its own inherent toxicities. Metformin can cause a metabolic acidosis with elevated lactate concentration, particularly in patients with underlying kidney dysfunction and after large intentional overdoses (Chap. 47). Zonisamide, an adjunct antiepileptic that is not used commonly, is associated with adverse events, including CNS depression and hypersensitivity (Chap. 48).[89,139]

HYPOCALORIC DIETS AND CATHARTIC OR EMETIC ABUSE

Starvation, as well as abuse of laxatives, syrup of ipecac, diuretics, and anorectics, has led to morbidity and mortality, often in young patients.[28,112] The potential for fad diets and laxative abuse should be evaluated in young people with unexplained salt and water depletion, syncope, hypokalemia, and metabolic alkalosis. A variety of extreme calorie-restricted diets resulting in profound weight loss were very popular in the late 1970s, but reports of a possible association between these diets and sudden death followed.[100] Myocardial atrophy was a consistent finding on autopsy. Torsade de pointes and other ventricular dysrhythmias may have occurred as a result of hypokalemia,[141] and protein-calorie malnutrition is proposed as a cause of death.[29,87,100]

After the negative reports and FDA warnings, the enthusiasm for liquid protein diets waned. Several current diets (Atkin's plan, South Beach diet) advocate intake of high protein, high fat, and low carbohydrates while allowing unlimited amounts of meat, fish, eggs, and cheese. Lack of carbohydrates induces ketosis, which results in salt and water depletion, giving the user the appearance of rapid weight loss. With rehydration and resumption of a normal diet, weight gain generally occurs. In addition, salt and water depletion causes orthostatic hypotension and ureterolithiasis. Atherosclerosis and hypercholesterolemia occur as a result of substitution of high-calorie, high fat foods for carbohydrates. Despite the rapid initial weight loss with these diets, when carbohydrates are reintroduced, weight gain occurs rapidly and significantly.[32] Regardless of the type of diet, there is no clinically relevant weight loss or maintenance of weight loss over the long term.[41,47,72]

Dieter's teas that contain combinations of herbal laxatives, including senna and *Cascara sagrada*, can produce profound diarrhea, salt and water depletion, and particular hypokalemia. They are associated with sudden death, presumably as a result of cardiac dysrhythmias. Despite FDA warnings of the dangers of these weight loss regimens, dieter's teas remain available in retail stores that sell nutritional supplements and are easily accessible to adolescents.

Chronic laxative use can result in an atonic colon ("cathartic bowel") and development of tolerance, with the subsequent need to increase dosing to achieve catharsis.[87] Various test methods can be used to detect laxative abuse. Phenolphthalein can be detected as a pink or red coloration to stool or urine after alkalinization. Colonoscopy reveals the benign, pathogno-monic "melanosis coli," the dark staining of the colonic mucosa secondary to anthraquinone laxative abuse. The combination of misuse or abuse of laxatives in conjunction with orlistat has the potential to cause severe diarrhea and subsequent fluid and electrolyte imbalances. Now that orlistat is readily available, there is a greater likelihood of being added to prescription weight loss regimens with or without the providers knowledge.[83] Syrup of ipecac was chronically used to induce emesis by patients with eating disorders, such as bulimia nervosa, leading to the development of cardiomyopathy, subsequent dysrhythmias, and death.[42,93] Emetine, a component of syrup of ipecac, was the alkaloid responsible for the severe cardiomyopathy. In 2003, an FDA advisory committee recommended that the nonprescription drug status of syrup of ipecac be rescinded because of its use by patients with bulimic disorders. Syrup of ipecac is no longer produced in the United States.

OTHER HERBAL REMEDIES

Several herbal approaches for weight loss have resulted in serious toxicity. In France, germander (*Teucrium chamaedrys*) supplements taken for weight loss resulted in seven cases of hepatotoxicity.[72] A "slimming regimen" first prescribed in a weight loss clinic in Belgium produced an epidemic of progressive kidney disease, known as Chinese herb nephropathy, when botanical misidentification led to the substitution of *Stephania tetrandra* with the nephrotoxic plant *Aristolochia fangji*.[128] The toxic constituent, identified as aristolochic acid, is implicated in numerous cases of kidney failure and urothelial carcinoma.[77] A case of profound digitalis toxicity occurred with a laxative regimen contaminated with *Digitalis lanata*.[119] Contamination of herbal products remains a concern today because of the lack of standardization of manufacturing processes. Until regulation of herbal products is improved and manufacturing practices worldwide are standardized, sporadic reports of herb-related toxicity likely will continue (Chap. 43).

FUTURE TARGETS FOR XENOBIOTIC DEVELOPMENT

Despite all of the advances in pharmacotherapy and surgical interventions, success remains limited. The ideal therapeutic intervention has yet to be identified, and combination therapy needs be addressed rigorously with caution. Ongoing investigation into the mechanisms and pathways that mediate appetite and energy balance continues. The hormonal endocrine regulation has provided promise and remains an area for future investigation and drug development.[84] Based on history, it is impossible to predict if any of these investigations will result in the creation and approval of new pharmaceutical agents available in the weight loss drug armamentarium.

NONPHARMACOLOGIC INTERVENTIONS

Although not a specific toxicologic concern, surgical and other nonpharmacologic interventions are included in the management of obesity. Vagus nerve stimulators have been studied and do show a reduction in body fat.[8,73]

Surgical interventions to manage obesity have increased in frequency over the past years and may provide a long-term solution for obesity. In 2013, there were approximately 460,000 surgical procedures performed.[78] Roux-en-Y gastric bypass, laparoscopic adjustable banding, and biliary-pancreatico diversion with duodenal switch are the most commonly described techniques.[2,8,78]

Sleeve gastrectomy is easier than Roux-en-Y and has been associated with fewer adverse events and similar efficacy.[78] The long-term body weight reduction is significantly better in bariatric surgery compared with standard medical treatment;[16,31,62,78] however, there are significant postoperative complications that do occur. The health of these patients is of particular concern because absorption of vitamins, minerals, and drugs is altered.[26,68,101,110] The pharmacokinetic properties of existing and newly initiated medications of orally administered medications are altered.[101,110] Evaluation of drug properties should be examined closely before initiation in this patient population. Despite the risks of the surgical procedures, the Centers for Medicare and Medicaid Services (CMS) agree that surgical intervention is necessary for patients with a BMI of 35 or greater who have at least one comorbidity and have been unsuccessful with medical treatment for obesity.

SUMMARY

- Obesity is a major health concern and a significant cause of preventable diseases and sequelae. Unproven weight loss modalities are associated with treatment failure and the potential for significant adverse events.
- Typical pharmaceutical weight loss strategies include:
  - Sympathomimetics
    - Tachyphylaxis occurs within weeks
    - Hypertension; tachycardia; anxiety
    - Cerebral ischemia; myocardial ischemia
  - Serotonergics
    - Dizziness, headache, nausea
    - Serotonin toxicity possible after overdose
  - GLP-1 analogs
    - Nausea, vomiting, diarrhea
    - Hypoglycemia possible after overdose
  - GI agents (orlistat)
    - Abdominal pain, nausea, vomiting, fecal incontinence, fat-soluble vitamin loss
  - Risks from caloric restriction, laxatives, unapproved therapies include:
    - Dinitrophenol: hyperthermia; high anion gap metabolic acidosis, and death
    - Beta-HCG: coronary artery dissection
    - Clenbuterol: tachycardia, wide pulse pressure hypotension, hypokalemia, anion gap metabolic acidosis
    - Laxatives or calorie restrictions: electrolyte disturbances; atonic colon
- Some common themes exist. Combination drug therapy likely provides the best weight loss, and toxicity from proven and unproven treatments remains a significant concern.
- Clinicians should be aware of the lack of regulation of most available diet remedies and should report adverse events involving these products to poison control centers and to the FDA MedWatch system so that appropriate regulatory actions can be taken to prevent further instances of toxicity.

Acknowledgment

Christine Haller, MD, and Jeanmarie Perrone, MD, contributed to this chapter in previous editions.

REFERENCES

1. Abenhaim L, et al. Appetite-suppressant drugs and the risk of primary pulmonary hypertension. International Primary Pulmonary Hypertension Study Group. *N Engl J Med.* 1996;335:609-616.
2. Adams TD, et al. Long-term mortality after gastric bypass surgery. *N Engl J Med.* 2007;357:753-761.
3. Ahmad FA, Mahmud S. Acute pancreatitis following orlistat therapy: report of two cases. *JOP J Pancreas.* 2010;11:61-63.
4. Albertson TE, et al. TOX-ACLS: toxicologic-oriented advanced cardiac life support. *Ann Emerg Med.* 2001;37(4 Suppl):S78-90.
5. Allison DB, et al. Controlled-release phentermine/topiramate in severely obese adults: a randomized controlled trial (EQUIP). *Obes Silver Spring Md.* 2012;20:330-342.
6. Aronne LJ, et al. A clinical trial assessing the safety and efficacy of taranabant, a CB1R inverse agonist, in obese and overweight patients: a high-dose study. *Int J Obes.* 2010;34:919-935.
7. Arvill A, Bodin L. Effect of short-term ingestion of konjac glucomannan on serum cholesterol in healthy men. *Am J Clin Nutr.* 1995;61:585-589.
8. Attenello F, et al. Theoretical Basis of Vagus Nerve Stimulation. *Prog Neurol Surg.* 2015;29:20-28.
9. Bays HE, Gadde KM. Phentermine/topiramate for weight reduction and treatment of adverse metabolic consequences in obesity. *Drugs Today Barc Spain. 1998.* 2011;47:903-914.
10. Bibbins-Domingo K, et al. Adolescent overweight and future adult coronary heart disease. *N Engl J Med.* 2007;357:2371-2379.
11. Boardman WW. Rapidly developing cataracts after dinitrophenol. *Calif West Med.* 1935;43:118-119.

12. Bode SFN, et al. 10-Fold liraglutide overdose over 7 months resulted only in minor side-effects. *J Clin Pharmacol.* 2013;53:785-786.

13. Bouchard NC, et al. Ischemic stroke associated with use of an ephedra-free dietary supplement containing synephrine. *Mayo Clin Proc.* 2005;80:541-545.

14. Brandt C, et al. Topiramate overdose: a case report of a patient with extremely high topiramate serum concentrations and nonconvulsive status epilepticus. *Epilepsia.* 2010;51:1090-1093.

15. Brenot F, et al. Primary pulmonary hypertension and fenfluramine use. *Br Heart J.* 1993;70:537-541.

16. Bult MJF, et al. Surgical treatment of obesity. *Eur J Endocrinol Eur Fed Endocr Soc.* 2008;158:135-145.

17. Burcelin R, Gourdy P. Harnessing glucagon-like peptide-1 receptor agonists for the pharmacological treatment of overweight and obesity. *Obes Rev Off J Int Assoc Study Obes.* September 2016.

18. Capewell S, Critchley JA. Adolescent overweight and coronary heart disease. *N Engl J Med.* 2008;358:1521; author reply 1522.

19. Carpéné C, et al. Selective activation of beta3-adrenoceptors by octopamine: comparative studies in mammalian fat cells. *Naunyn Schmiedebergs Arch Pharmacol.* 1999;359:310-321.

20. Carrière F, et al. Inhibition of gastrointestinal lipolysis by Orlistat during digestion of test meals in healthy volunteers. *Am J Physiol Gastrointest Liver Physiol.* 2001;281:G16-28.

21. Centers for Disease Control and Prevention, Public Health Service, U.S. Department Health. Adult Obesity Causes and Consequences. www.cdc.gov/obesity/adult/causes.html. Accessed November 7, 2016.

22. Chaput J-P, Tremblay A. Current and novel approaches to the drug therapy of obesity. *Eur J Clin Pharmacol.* 2006;62:793-803.

23. Clifton PM, et al. Long term weight maintenance after advice to consume low carbohydrate, higher protein diets--a systematic review and meta analysis. *Nutr Metab Cardiovasc Dis.* 2014;24:224-235.

24. Colman E. Dinitrophenol and obesity: an early twentieth-century regulatory dilemma. *Regul Toxicol Pharmacol RTP.* 2007;48:115-117.

25. Colman E, et al. The FDA's assessment of two drugs for chronic weight management. *N Engl J Med.* 2012;367:1577-1579.

26. Colquitt JL, et al. Surgery for weight loss in adults. In: *Cochrane Database of Systematic Reviews.* John Wiley & Sons, Ltd; 2014. http://onlinelibrary.wiley.com/doi/10.1002/14651858.CD003641.pub4/abstract. Accessed September 27, 2016.

27. Connolly HM, et al. Valvular heart disease associated with fenfluramine-phentermine. *N Engl J Med.* 1997;337:581-588.

28. Davidson J. Seizures and bupropion: a review. *J Clin Psychiatry.* 1989;50:256-261.

29. Davies MJ, et al. Efficacy of Liraglutide for Weight Loss Among Patients With Type 2 Diabetes: The SCALE Diabetes Randomized Clinical Trial. *JAMA.* 2015;314:687-699.

30. Di Marzo V, Matias I. Endocannabinoid control of food intake and energy balance. *Nat Neurosci.* 2005;8:585-589.

31. Dixon JB, et al. Adjustable gastric banding and conventional therapy for type 2 diabetes: a randomized controlled trial. *JAMA.* 2008;299:316-323.

32. Eckel RH. Clinical practice. Nonsurgical management of obesity in adults. *N Engl J Med.* 2008;358:1941-1950.

33. Elmquist JK, Scherer PE. The cover. Neuroendocrine and endocrine pathways of obesity. *JAMA.* 2012;308:1070-1071.

34. Engeli S. Central and peripheral cannabinoid receptors as therapeutic targets in the control of food intake and body weight. *Handb Exp Pharmacol.* 2012;357-381.

35. Fernstrom JD, Choi S. The development of tolerance to drugs that suppress food intake. *Pharmacol Ther.* 2008;117:105-122.

36. Fidler MC, et al. A one-year randomized trial of lorcaserin for weight loss in obese and overweight adults: the BLOSSOM trial. *J Clin Endocrinol Metab.* 2011;96:3067-3077.

37. Filippatos TD, et al. Orlistat-associated adverse effects and drug interactions: a critical review. *Drug Saf.* 2008;31:53-65.

38. Firenzuoli F, et al. Adverse reaction to an adrenergic herbal extract (Citrus aurantium). *Phytomedicine Int J Phytother Phytopharm.* 2005;12:247-248.

39. Flegal KM, et al. Prevalence of obesity and trends in the distribution of body mass index among US adults, 1999-2010. *JAMA.* 2012;307:491-497.

40. Flegal KM, et al. Sources of differences in estimates of obesity-associated deaths from first National Health and Nutrition Examination Survey (NHANES I) hazard ratios. *Am J Clin Nutr.* 2010;91:519-527.

41. Freedhoff Y, Hall KD. Weight loss diet studies: we need help not hype. *Lancet.* 2016;388:849-851.

42. Friedman EJ. Death from ipecac intoxication in a patient with anorexia nervosa. *Am J Psychiatry.* 1984;141:702-703.

43. Friedrich MJ. Studies probe mechanisms that have a role in obesity-associated morbidities. *JAMA.* 2012;308:1077-1079.

44. Fugh-Berman A, Myers A. Citrus aurantium, an ingredient of dietary supplements marketed for weight loss: current status of clinical and basic research. *Exp Biol Med Maywood NJ.* 2004;229:698-704.

45. Gadde KM, et al. Effects of low-dose, controlled-release, phentermine plus topiramate combination on weight and associated comorbidities in overweight and obese adults (CONQUER): a randomised, placebo-controlled, phase 3 trial. *Lancet Lond Engl.* 2011;377:1341-1352.

46. Goldgof M, et al. The chemical uncoupler 2,4-dinitrophenol (DNP) protects against diet-induced obesity and improves energy homeostasis in mice at thermoneutrality. *J Biol Chem.* 2014;289:19341-19350.

47. Greenberg I, et al; DIRECT Group. Adherence and success in long-term weight loss diets: the dietary intervention randomized controlled trial (DIRECT). *J Am Coll Nutr.* 2009;28:159-168.

48. Greenway FL, et al. Effect of naltrexone plus bupropion on weight loss in overweight and obese adults (COR-I): a multicentre, randomised, double-blind, placebo-controlled, phase 3 trial. *Lancet Lond Engl.* 2010;376:595-605.

49. Grundlingh J, et al. 2,4-dinitrophenol (DNP): a weight loss agent with significant acute toxicity and risk of death. *J Med Toxicol Off J Am Coll Med Toxicol.* 2011;7:205-212.

50. Gueye AB, et al. The CB1 Neutral Antagonist AM4113 Retains the Therapeutic Efficacy of the Inverse Agonist Rimonabant for Nicotine Dependence and Weight Loss with Better Psychiatric Tolerability. *Int J Neuropsychopharmacol.* 2016;19.

51. Guijarro A, et al. Sustained weight loss after Roux-en-Y gastric bypass is characterized by down regulation of endocannabinoids and mitochondrial function. *Ann Surg.* 2008;247:779-790.

52. Halford JCG, et al. Serotonergic anti-obesity agents: past experience and future prospects. *Drugs.* 2011;71:2247-2255.

53. Halford JCG, Harrold JA. 5-HT(2C) receptor agonists and the control of appetite. *Handb Exp Pharmacol.* 2012;:349-356.

54. Haller CA, Benowitz NL. Adverse cardiovascular and central nervous system events associated with dietary supplements containing ephedra alkaloids. *N Engl J Med.* 2000;343:1833-1838.

55. Henry DA, et al. Glucomannan and risk of oesophageal obstruction. *Br Med J Clin Res Ed.* 1986;292:591-592.

56. Heppenstall C, et al. Relationships between glucose, energy intake and dietary composition in obese adults with type 2 diabetes receiving the cannabinoid 1 (CB1) receptor antagonist, rimonabant. *Nutr J.* 2012;11:50.

57. Hoffman RJ, et al. Clenbuterol ingestion causing prolonged tachycardia, hypokalemia, and hypophosphatemia with confirmation by quantitative levels. *J Toxicol Clin Toxicol.* 2001;39:339-344.

58. Hoffstedt J, et al. Adipose tissue adiponectin production and adiponectin serum concentration in human obesity and insulin resistance. *J Clin Endocrinol Metab.* 2004;89:1391-1396.

59. Holborow A, et al. Beware the yellow slimming pill: fatal 2,4-dinitrophenol overdose. *BMJ Case Rep.* 2016;2016.

60. Hopkins KD, Lehmann ED. Successful medical treatment of obesity in 10th century Spain. *Lancet Lond Engl.* 1995;346:452.

61. Hruby A, Hu FB. The epidemiology of obesity: a big picture. *PharmacoEconomics.* 2015;33:673-689.

62. Inge TH, et al. Weight loss and health status 3 years after bariatric surgery in adolescents. *N Engl J Med.* 2016;374:113-123.

63. James WPT, et al. Effect of sibutramine on cardiovascular outcomes in overweight and obese subjects. *N Engl J Med.* 2010;363:905-917.

64. Jhaveri MD, et al. Endocannabinoid metabolism and uptake: novel targets for neuropathic and inflammatory pain. *Br J Pharmacol.* 2007;152:624-632.

65. Katsiki N, et al. Naltrexone sustained-release (SR) + bupropion SR combination therapy for the treatment of obesity: "a new kid on the block"? *Ann Med.* 2011;43:249-258.

66. Kelly T, et al. Global burden of obesity in 2005 and projections to 2030. *Int J Obes.* 2008;32:1431-1437.

67. Khandalavala B, Spangler M. Weight loss of 172 lb with topiramate in a patient with migraine headaches. *Am J Health-Syst Pharm AJHP Off J Am Soc Health-Syst Pharm.* 2012;69:367-368.

68. Klockhoff H, et al. Faster absorption of ethanol and higher peak concentration in women after gastric bypass surgery. *Br J Clin Pharmacol.* 2002;54:587-591.

69. Kraemer WJ, et al. Effect of adding exercise to a diet containing glucomannan. *Metabolism.* 2007;56:1149-1158.

70. Kurt TL, et al. Dinitrophenol in weight loss: the poison center and public health safety. *Vet Hum Toxicol.* 1986;28:574-575.

71. Lake CR, et al. Adverse drug effects attributed to phenylpropanolamine: a review of 142 case reports. *Am J Med.* 1990;89:195-208.

72. Larrey D, et al. Hepatitis after germander (Teucrium chamaedrys) administration: another instance of herbal medicine hepatotoxicity. *Ann Intern Med.* 1992;117:129-132.

73. Lebovitz HE. Interventional treatment of obesity and diabetes: an interim report on gastric electrical stimulation. *Rev Endocr Metab Disord.* 2016;17:73-80.

74. Lempereur M, et al. Spontaneous coronary artery dissection associated with β-HCG injections and fibromuscular dysplasia. *Can J Cardiol.* 2014;30:464.e1-3.

75. Lijesen GK, et al. The effect of human chorionic gonadotropin (HCG) in the treatment of obesity by means of the Simeons therapy: a criteria-based meta-analysis. *Br J Clin Pharmacol.* 1995;40:237-243.

76. Liu D, et al. The mitochondrial uncoupler DNP triggers brain cell mTOR signaling network reprogramming and CREB pathway up-regulation. *J Neurochem.* 2015;134:677-692.

77. Lord GM, et al. Urothelial malignant disease and Chinese herbal nephropathy. *Lancet Lond Engl.* 2001;358:1515-1516.

78. Makaronidis JM, Batterham RL. Potential Mechanisms Mediating Sustained Weight Loss Following Roux-en-Y Gastric Bypass and Sleeve Gastrectomy. *Endocrinol Metab Clin North Am.* 2016;45:539-552.

79. Martin CK, et al. Lorcaserin, a 5-HT(2C) receptor agonist, reduces body weight by decreasing energy intake without influencing energy expenditure. *J Clin Endocrinol Metab.* 2011;96:837-845.

80. Mcelhatton T. Clinical Effects and Outcomes Following Lorcaserin Ingestion. *Clin Toxicol Phila Pa.* 2015;53:756.

81. McNaughton R, et al. An investigation into drug products withdrawn from the EU market between 2002 and 2011 for safety reasons and the evidence used to support the decision-making. *BMJ Open.* 2014;4:e004221.

82. Mercader J, et al. Isopropylnorsynephrine is a stronger lipolytic agent in human adipocytes than synephrine and other amines present in Citrus aurantium. *J Physiol Biochem.* 2011;67:443-452.

83. Merlino DJ, et al. Gut-Brain Endocrine Axes in Weight Regulation and Obesity Pharmacotherapy. *J Clin Med.* 2014;3:763-794.

84. Montero JL, et al. Orlistat associated subacute hepatic failure. *J Hepatol.* 2001;34:173.

85. Morimoto C, et al. Anti-obese action of raspberry ketone. *Life Sci.* 2005;77:194-204.

86. Nadir A, et al. Acute hepatitis associated with the use of a Chinese herbal product, ma-huang. *Am J Gastroenterol.* 1996;91:1436-1438.

87. Nakanishi R, et al. Attempted suicide with liraglutide overdose did not induce hypoglycemia. *Diabetes Res Clin Pract.* 2013;99:e3-e4.

88. Nasir JM, et al. Exercise-induced syncope associated with QT prolongation and ephedra-free Xenadrine. *Mayo Clin Proc.* 2004;79:1059-1062.

89. Neuman MG, et al. Predicting possible zonisamide hypersensitivity syndrome. *Exp Dermatol.* 2008;17:1045-1051.

90. Nissen SE, et al. Effect of naltrexone-bupropion on major adverse cardiovascular events in overweight and obese patients with cardiovascular risk factors: a randomized clinical trial. *JAMA.* 2016;315:990-1004.

91. Nykamp DL, et al. Possible association of acute lateral-wall myocardial infarction and bitter orange supplement. *Ann Pharmacother.* 2004;38:812-816.

92. O'Connor MB. An orlistat "overdose" in a child. *Ir J Med Sci.* 2010;179:315.

93. Palmer EP, Guay AT. Reversible myopathy secondary to abuse of ipecac in patients with major eating disorders. *N Engl J Med.* 1985;313:1457-1459.

94. Park KS. Raspberry ketone increases both lipolysis and fatty acid oxidation in 3T3-L1 adipocytes. *Planta Med.* 2010;76:1654-1658.

95. Pentel P. Toxicity of over-the-counter stimulants. *JAMA.* 1984;252:1898-1903.

96. Perkins JM, Davis SN. Endocannabinoid system overactivity and the metabolic syndrome: prospects for treatment. *Curr Diab Rep.* 2008;8:12-19.

97. Perrio MJ, et al. The safety profiles of orlistat and sibutramine: results of prescription-event monitoring studies in England. *Obes Silver Spring Md.* 2007;15:2712-2722.

98. Petróczi A, et al. Russian roulette with unlicensed fat-burner drug 2,4-dinitrophenol (DNP): evidence from a multidisciplinary study of the internet, bodybuilding supplements and DNP users. *Subst Abuse Treat Prev Policy.* 2015;10.

99. Phillips L, Singer MA. Peripheral neuropathy due to dinitrophenol used for weight loss: something old, something new. *Neurology.* 2013;80:773-774.

100. Pi-Sunyer X, et al. A randomized, controlled trial of 3.0 mg of liraglutide in weight management. *N Engl J Med.* 2015;373:11-22.

101. Ponsky TA, et al. Alterations in gastrointestinal physiology after Roux-en-Y gastric bypass. *J Am Coll Surg.* 2005;201:125-131.

102. Proietto J, et al. A clinical trial assessing the safety and efficacy of the CB1R inverse agonist taranabant in obese and overweight patients: low-dose study. *Int J Obes.* 2010;34:1243-1254.

103. Prospective Studies Collaboration. Body-mass index and cause-specific mortality in 900 000 adults: collaborative analyses of 57 prospective studies. *Lancet.* 2009;373:1083-1096.

104. Ravinet Trillou C, et al. CB1 cannabinoid receptor knockout in mice leads to leanness, resistance to diet-induced obesity and enhanced leptin sensitivity. *Int J Obes Relat Metab Disord J Int Assoc Study Obes.* 2004;28:640-648.

105. Rosenbaum M. Obesity. *N Engl J Med.* 338:555.

106. Ruilope LM, et al. Effect of rimonabant on blood pressure in overweight/obese patients with/without co-morbidities: analysis of pooled RIO study results. *J Hypertens.* 2008;26:357-367.

107. Sall D, et al. Orlistat-induced fulminant hepatic failure. *Clin Obes.* 2014;4:342-347.

108. Sanger GJ. Endocannabinoids and the gastrointestinal tract: what are the key questions? *Br J Pharmacol.* 2007;152:663-670.

109. Saunders KH, et al. Pharmacotherapy for Obesity. *Endocrinol Metab Clin North Am.* 2016;45:521-538.

110. Seaman JS, et al. Dissolution of common psychiatric medications in a Roux-en-Y gastric bypass model. *Psychosomatics.* 2005;46:250-253.

111. Sharfstein JM, Psaty BM. Evaluation of the cardiovascular risk of naltrexone-bupropion: a study interrupted. *JAMA.* 2016;315:984-986.

112. Shepherd G, et al. Intentional bupropion overdoses. *J Emerg Med.* 2004;27:147-151.

113. Shiber JR. Severe non-anion gap metabolic acidosis induced by topiramate: a case report. *J Emerg Med.* 2010;38:494-496.

114. Shiri R, et al. The association between obesity and the prevalence of low back pain in young adults: the Cardiovascular Risk in Young Finns Study. *Am J Epidemiol.* 2008;167:1110-1119.

115. Sidossis L, Kajimura S. Brown and beige fat in humans: thermogenic adipocytes that control energy and glucose homeostasis. *J Clin Invest.* 2015;125:478-486.

116. Simmonds M, et al. Predicting adult obesity from childhood obesity: a systematic review and meta-analysis. *Obes Rev Off J Int Assoc Study Obes.* 2016;17:95-107.

117. Singh A, et al. Acute oxalate nephropathy associated with orlistat, a gastrointestinal lipase inhibitor. *Am J Kidney Dis Off J Natl Kidney Found.* 2007;49:153-157.

118. Sjöström L, et al. Randomised placebo-controlled trial of orlistat for weight loss and prevention of weight regain in obese patients. European Multicentre Orlistat Study Group. *Lancet Lond Engl.* 1998;352:167-172.

119. Slifman NR, et al. Contamination of botanical dietary supplements by Digitalis lanata. *N Engl J Med.* 1998;339:806-811.

120. Smith SR, et al. Multicenter, placebo-controlled trial of lorcaserin for weight management. *N Engl J Med.* 2010;363:245-256.

121. Spedding M, et al. Neural control of dieting. *Nature.* 1996;380:488.

122. Stephanie A. Diamond. Determination of the Effect of Raspberry Ketone on Markers of Obesity in High-fat Fed C57BL/6 Male Mice. 2015.

123. Stohs SJ, et al. A review of the human clinical studies involving Citrus aurantium (bitter orange) extract and its primary protoalkaloid p-synephrine. *Int J Med Sci.* 2012;9:527-538.

124. Stohs SJ, et al. A review of the receptor-binding properties of p-synephrine as related to its pharmacological effects. *Oxid Med Cell Longev.* 2011;2011:482973.

125. Tainter ML. Actions of benzedrine and propadrine in control of obesity. *J Nutr.* 1944;27:89-105. Abstract.

126. Takematsu, M, et al. Berries that weren't that sweet after all...A case of raspberry ketone intoxication. *Clin Toxicol Phila Pa.* 2013;51:284.

127. Traub SJ, et al. Dietary supplements containing ephedra alkaloids. *N Engl J Med.* 2001;344:1096; author reply 1096-1097.

128. Vanherweghem JL, et al. Rapidly progressive interstitial renal fibrosis in young women: association with slimming regimen including Chinese herbs. *Lancet Lond Engl.* 1993;341:387-391.

129. Vorsanger MH, et al. Cardiovascular effects of the new weight loss agents. *J Am Coll Cardiol.* 2016;68:849-859.

130. Vuksan V, et al. Konjac-mannan (glucomannan) improves glycemia and other associated risk factors for coronary heart disease in type 2 diabetes. A randomized controlled metabolic trial. *Diabetes Care.* 1999;22:913-919.

131. Wadden TA, et al. Weight loss with naltrexone SR/bupropion SR combination therapy as an adjunct to behavior modification: the COR-BMOD trial. *Obes Silver Spring Md.* 2011;19:110-120.

132. Wang J, Ueda N. Role of the endocannabinoid system in metabolic control. *Curr Opin Nephrol Hypertens.* 2008;17:1-10.

133. Weiss R, et al. Obesity dynamics and cardiovascular risk factor stability in obese adolescents. *Pediatr Diabetes.* 2009;10:360-367.

134. de Wolff FA, et al. Experience with a screening method for laxative abuse. *Hum Toxicol.* 1983;2:385-389.

135. World Health Organization Global Health Observatory Data Repository. http://apps.who.int/gho/data/node.main.A897A?lang=en.

136. Wright KL, et al. Cannabinoid CB2 receptors in the gastrointestinal tract: a regulatory system in states of inflammation. *Br J Pharmacol.* 2008;153:263-270.

137. Xiao C, et al. Anti-obesity and metabolic efficacy of the β3-adrenergic agonist, CL316243, in mice at thermoneutrality compared to 22°C. *Obes Silver Spring Md.* 2015;23:1450-1459.

138. Yen M, Ewald MB. Toxicity of Weight Loss Agents. *J Med Toxicol.* 2012;8:145-152.

139. Zaccara G, et al. Drug safety evaluation of zonisamide for the treatment of epilepsy. *Expert Opin Drug Saf.* 2011;10:623-631.

140. Zhi J, et al. Review of limited systemic absorption of orlistat, a lipase inhibitor, in healthy human volunteers. *J Clin Pharmacol.* 1995;35:1103-1108.

141. Zylstra M, et al. Iatrogenic Opioid-withdrawal Induced by Contrave. *J Clin Toxicol.* 2016;06.

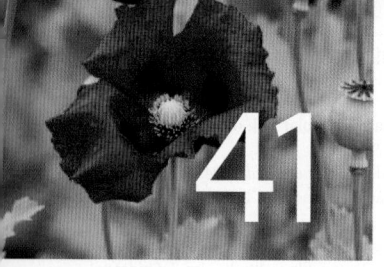

41 ATHLETIC PERFORMANCE ENHANCERS

Susi U. Vassallo

HISTORY AND EPIDEMIOLOGY

Interest in extraordinary athletic achievement fuels the modern-day science of performance enhancement in sports. The desire to improve athletic performance in a scientific manner is a relatively recent development. At one time, the focus on maximizing human physical and mental potential centered on the importance of manual work and military service. The role of sport was inconsequential, except for its potential in improving military preparedness.[95] Today, "sports doping" refers to the use of a prohibited xenobiotic to enhance athletic performance. The word *doping* comes from the Dutch word *doop*, a viscous opium juice used by the ancient Greeks.[32,128]

Controversy surrounding the systematic use of performance enhancing xenobiotics by the participating athletes has marred many sporting events. Since the International Olympic Committee (IOC) began testing during the 1968 Olympic games, prominent athletes have been sanctioned and stripped of their Olympic medals because they tested positive for banned xenobiotics. However, from a public health perspective, the use of performance-enhancing xenobiotics among athletes of all ages and abilities is a far more serious concern than the highly publicized cases involving world-class athletes. The majority of studies on the epidemiology of performance enhancing xenobiotics have investigated androgenic anabolic steroid use. *Androgenic* means masculinizing, and *anabolic* means tissue building. An *anabolic process* stimulates protein synthesis, promotes nitrogen deposition in lean body mass, and decreases protein breakdown. Studies of high school students document that 6.6% of male seniors have used anabolic steroids, and 35% of these individuals were not involved in organized athletics.[35] Others find rates of androgenic steroid use begins at age 10 years old and ranges from 3% to 19% of all adolescents.[102,114,156,174,229]

PRINCIPLES

Performance enhancers are classified in several ways. Some categorize performance enhancers according to the expected effects. For example, some xenobiotics increase muscle mass; others decrease recovery time, increase energy, or mask the presence of other xenobiotics. However, many xenobiotics frequently have several expected and unexpected effects. For example, diuretics are used to mask the presence of other xenobiotics by producing dilute urine, or they are used to reduce weight. Clenbuterol is an anabolic xenobiotic, but it also is a stimulant because of its β_2-adrenergic agonist effects. Depending on the xenobiotic, it is used either during training to improve future performance or during competition to improve immediate results or for weight loss.[32]

According to the 2017 World Anti-Doping Agency (WADA) World Anti-Doping Code, a xenobiotic or method constitutes doping and can be added to the Prohibited List if it is a masking xenobiotic or if it meets two of the following three criteria: it enhances performance, its use presents a risk to the athlete's health, and it is contrary to the spirit of sport[1] (Table 41–1).

Some of the prohibited xenobiotics are used to treat legitimate medical conditions of athletes.[1] Athletes with documented medical conditions requiring the use of a prohibited substance or method may request a therapeutic use exemption (TUE). For example, the use of an inhaled β-adrenergic agonist in low doses other than albuterol, salbutamol, or formoterol in an athlete with documented asthma requires a TUE.[1]

ANABOLIC XENOBIOTICS

Anabolic Androgenic Steroids

Anabolic-androgenic steroids (AASs) increase muscle mass and lean body weight and cause nitrogen retention.[148] The androgenic effects of steroids are responsible for male appearance and secondary sexual characteristics such

TABLE 41–1	Abbreviated Summary of World Anti-Doping Agency 2017 Prohibited List[1]

Substances (S) and Methods (M) Prohibited at All Times (In and Out of Competition)

S0. Any pharmacological substance with no current approval for therapeutic use

S1. Anabolic Agents
  Anabolic androgenic steroids
  Other anabolic agents
    Clenbuterol
    Selective androgen receptor modulators

S2. Peptide Hormone, Growth Factors, Related Agents, and Mimetics
  Erythropoiesis stimulation agents
  Chorionic gonadotropin and luteinizing hormone
  Corticotropins
  Growth hormone
Additional prohibited growth factors: affecting muscle, tendon or ligament protein synthesis/degradation, energy utilization, regenerative capacity, or fiber type switching

S3. β_2-Adrenergic Agonists
  Except inhaled salbutamol, formoterol, and salmeterol with urinary concentration limits

S4. Hormone Antagonists and Metabolic Modulators
  Aromatase inhibitors
  Selective estrogen receptor modulators
  Antiestrogens
  Myostatin modulators
  Metabolic modulators
    Insulins
    Peroxisome proliferator activated receptor delta agonist and AMP activate protein kinase axis agonists
    Meldonium

S5. Diuretics and Other Masking Agents
  Desmopressin, probenecid, plasma expanders, glycerol intravenous administration of albumin, dextran, hydroxyethyl starch, and mannitol
  Exception: ophthalmic use of carbonic anhydrase inhibitors

Prohibited Methods

M1. Manipulation of Blood and Blood Components

M2. Chemical and Physical Manipulation
  Tampering with samples
  Intravenous infusions

M3. Gene Doping: The transfer of polymers of nucleic acids or analogues, the use of normal or genetically modified cells

Substances (S) and Methods (M) Prohibited in Competition
In addition to the above, the following categories are prohibited only in competition:

S6. Stimulants

S7. Narcotics

S8. Cannabinoids: natural (marijuana) or cannabimimetics eg, "spice," JWH-018, JWH-073, HU-210

S9. Glucocorticosteroids; all are prohibited when administered by oral, intravenous, intramuscular, or rectal routes

Substances Prohibited in Particular (P) Sports

P1. Alcohol in competition. Detection by analysis of breath and or blood. Threshold is 0.10 g/L (air sports, archery, automobile, powerboating).

P2. β-Adrenergic Antagonists

TABLE 41–2	Synthetic Testosterone Derivatives/Anabolic Androgenic Steroids: Generic Nomenclature[1]	
17α-Alkyl Derivatives (Oral)	*17β-Ester Derivatives (Parenteral)*	*Testosterone Preparations (Topical)*
Ethylestrenol	Boldenone	Buccal gel, sublingual
Fluoxymesterone	Nandrolone decanoate	Dermal gel, ointment
Methandrostenolone	Nandrolone	Transdermal reservoir patch
Methyltestosterone	phenpropionate	
Oxandrolone	Testosterone esters	
Oxymetholone	Testosterone cypionate	
Stanozolol	Testosterone enanthate	
	Testosterone ester combination	
	Testosterone propionate	
	Trenbolone	

as increased growth of body hair and deepening of the voice. Testosterone is the prototypical androgen, and most AASs are synthetic testosterone derivatives. The WADA categorizes AASs into two groups: exogenous, referring to substances that are not ordinarily capable of being produced by the body naturally, and endogenous, referring to those capable of being produced by the body naturally. As such, there is sometimes discordance in categorization schemes with other governing entities. In this chapter, the term *anabolic steroid* means any xenobiotic, chemically and pharmacologically related to testosterone, other than estrogens, progestins, corticosteroids, and dehydroepiandrosterone (DHEA).

In the 1970s and 1980s, federal regulation of anabolic steroids was under the direction of the Food and Drug Administration (FDA). Because of increasing media reports on the use of AASs in sports, particularly by high school students and amateur athletes, Congress enacted the Anabolic Steroid Control Act of 1990, which amended the Controlled Substances Act and placed anabolic steroids in Schedule III. Schedule III implies that a drug has a currently accepted medical use in the United States and has less potential for abuse than the drugs categorized as Schedule I or II. The Anabolic Steroid Control Act of 2004 added certain steroid precursors, such as androstenedione and dihydrotestosterone, to the list of controlled substances that are considered illegal without a prescription. However, DHEA is exempted. Possession of androstenedione or other metabolic precursors called *prohormone drugs* is considered a federal crime. Nevertheless, AASs are still available illicitly via the Internet from international marketers, veterinary pharmaceutical companies, and some legitimate US manufacturers (Table 41–2).

Antiestrogens and Antiandrogens

In male athletes using androgens, avoiding the unwanted side effects of feminization, such as gynecomastia, or in female athletes, avoiding masculinization and features such as facial hair and deepening voice, requires manipulation of the metabolic pathways of androgen metabolism. Creating a xenobiotic that completely dissociates the desired from the unwanted effects has not been possible. However, xenobiotics with properties capable of manipulating metabolic pathways associated with undesirable side effects are divided into four main groups, all on the Prohibited List.

1. Aromatase inhibitors such as anastrozole and aminoglutethimide prevent the conversion of androstenedione and testosterone into estrogen.
2. The antiestrogen clomiphene blocks estrogen receptors in the hypothalamus, opposing the negative feedback of estrogen, causing an increase in gonadotropin-releasing hormone, thereby increasing testosterone release.
3. Selective estrogen receptor modulators (SERMs) such as tamoxifen and raloxifene bind to estrogen receptors and exhibit agonist or antagonist effects at the estrogen receptors. By indirectly increasing gonadotropin

release, SERMs restore endogenous testosterone production upon discontinuation of AASs.[181]
4. Selective androgen receptor modulators (SARMs) are nonsteroidal tissue selective *anabolic* xenobiotics. Selective androgen receptor modulators are neither aromatized nor substrates for 5α-reductase, nor do they undergo the same metabolic pathways as testosterone. Therefore, they have fewer unwanted androgenic side effects compared with testosterone.[77,212]

Administration

In the 1990s, approximately 50% of AASs were taken orally; the remainder were administered by intramuscular (IM) injection, with one-fourth of IM users sharing needles.[57] In the same era, one-third of the and syringes exchanged in a needle-exchange program in Wales were used for AAS injections.[164] Unlike therapeutically indicated regimens, which consist of fixed doses at regular intervals, athletes typically use AASs in cycles of 6 to 8 weeks.[15] For example, the athlete may use steroids for 2 months and then abstain for 2 months. This *cycling* of steroid use is based on the athlete's individual preferences and not on any validated protocol. *Stacking* implies combining the use of several AASs at one time, often with both oral and IM administration. To prevent *plateauing,* or developing tolerance, to any one AAS, some athletes use an average of five different AASs simultaneously on a cycle. The doses used are frequently hundreds of times in excess of scientifically-based therapeutic recommendations.[6,228] *Pyramiding* implies starting the AASs at a low dose, increasing the dose many times, and then tapering once again. Whereas fat-soluble steroids typically require several months to be totally eliminated, water-soluble steroids require only days to weeks to be cleared by the kidney. Water-soluble testosterone esters are used for "bridging therapy." *Bridging* refers to the practice of halting the administration of long-lasting alkylated testosterone formulations so that urine analyses at a specific time offer no evidence of use, but injections of shorter acting testosterone esters are used to replace the orally administered alkylated formulations. This strategy, which was used extensively in the German Democratic Republic, is documented in a review of the subject based on extensive research of previously classified records.[69] Clearance profiles for testosterone congeners were determined for each athlete. In general, the daily injection of testosterone esters was used when termination of the more readily detectable synthetic alkylated testosterone derivatives was necessary to avoid a positive doping test. These daily injections of testosterone propionate were halted 4 to 5 days before competition. Corrupt officials involved in doping were sure that the values would decrease to acceptable concentrations in time for the event based on the science of athletes' clearance of testosterone esters.[69]

Clinical Manifestations of Anabolic-Androgenic Steroid Use
Cancer

An association between AAS use and the development of cancer is observed in experimental animals.[183] Testicular and prostatic carcinomas are reported in more frequent users of anabolic-androgenic steroids.[64,75,182] Hepatocellular carcinoma,[101,157] cholangiocarcinoma,[15] Wilms tumor, and renal cell carcinoma are also reported in young AAS users.[34,173] The relationship between the dose of AASs and cancer is unknown.

Cardiovascular

Cardiac complications include acute myocardial infarction, venous thromboembolism, and sudden cardiac arrest due to lethal dysrhythmias.[11,67,90,97,143] Autopsy examination of the heart often reveals biventricular hypertrophy, extensive myocardial fibrosis, and contraction-band necrosis.[219] Myofibrillar disorganization as well as hypertrophy of the interventricular septum and left ventricle are present.[129] Compared with nonusers, anabolic androgenic steroid users demonstrated reduced left ventricular systolic and diastolic function and more coronary artery plaque volume. There is a dose dependent association with the coronary atherosclerotic burden. Intense training and use of AASs impair diastolic function by increasing left ventricular wall thickness.[16] Animal models and in vitro myocardial cell studies show similar pathologic changes.[50,113,144,211,218,219] Doppler echocardiography shows that several years after strength athletes discontinue using AASs, excessive concentric left ventricular hypertrophy remains. Growth hormone (GH) appears to potentiate the effects of AASs and further increase concentric remodeling of the left ventricle.[106] In addition to direct myocardial injury, vasospasm or thrombosis occurs.[144] Alkylated androgens lower the concentration of high-density lipoprotein (HDL) cholesterol and increases platelet aggregation.[6,67] Thromboembolic complications include pulmonary embolus,[54,76] stroke,[109,110] carotid arterial occlusion,[121] cerebral sinus thrombosis,[118] poststeroid balance disorder,[29] and popliteal artery entrapment.[125]

Dermatologic and Gingival

Cutaneous side effects are common and include keloid formation, sebaceous cysts, comedones, seborrheic furunculosis, folliculitis, and striae.[195] Acne is associated with steroid use and sometimes is referred to as "gymnasium acne."[43,166] A common triad of acne, striae, and gynecomastia occurs. The production of sebum is an androgen-dependent process, and dihydrotestosterone is active in sebaceous glands.[15] Gingival hyperplasia is reported.[158]

Endocrine

Conversion of AASs to estradiol in peripheral tissues results in feminization of male athletes. Gynecomastia is sometimes irreversible. Anabolic androgenic steroids use causes negative feedback inhibition of gonadotropin-releasing hormone, luteinizing hormone, and follicle-stimulating hormone from the hypothalamus. This process results in testicular atrophy and decreased spermatogenesis, which is often reversible. In women, menstrual irregularities and breast atrophy are reported.[15]

Hepatic

Hepatic subcapsular hematoma with hemorrhage is reported.[194] Peliosis hepatis, a condition of blood-filled sinuses in the liver that results in fatal hepatic rupture, occurs most commonly with the use of alkylated androgens and often does not improve when androgen use is stopped.[17,94,201,226] This condition is not associated with the dose or duration of treatment.[15,64,204] Cyproterone acetate is a chlorinated progesterone derivative that inhibits 5α-reductase and reportedly causes hepatotoxicity.[15,74,79]

Infectious

Local complications from injection include septic joints,[63] cutaneous abscess,[139,177] and *Candida albicans* endophthalmitis.[227] Injection of AASs using contaminated needles has led to transmission of infectious diseases such as human immunodeficiency virus and hepatitis B and C.[155,159,176,196,200] Severe varicella is reported in a long-term AAS user.[100]

Musculoskeletal

Supraphysiologic doses of testosterone, when combined with strength training, increase muscle strength and size.[26] The most common musculoskeletal complications of steroid use are tendon and ligament rupture.[70,92,122,127]

Neuropsychiatric

Distractibility, depression or mania, delirium, irritability, insomnia, hostility, anxiety, mood lability, and aggressiveness ("roid rage") may occur.[21,71,170,171,210] These neuropsychiatric effects do not appear to correlate with serum AAS concentrations.[198,210] Withdrawal symptoms from AAS include decreased libido, fatigue, and myalgias.[108,230]

Specific Anabolic Xenobiotics

Dehydroepiandrosterone

Dehydroepiandrosterone (DHEA) is a precursor to testosterone (Fig. 41–1). Because it is produced endogenously, DHEA most commonly is not categorized as an AAS. However, DHEA is weakly anabolic and weakly androgenic. Although banned by the FDA in 1996, this xenobiotic subsequently

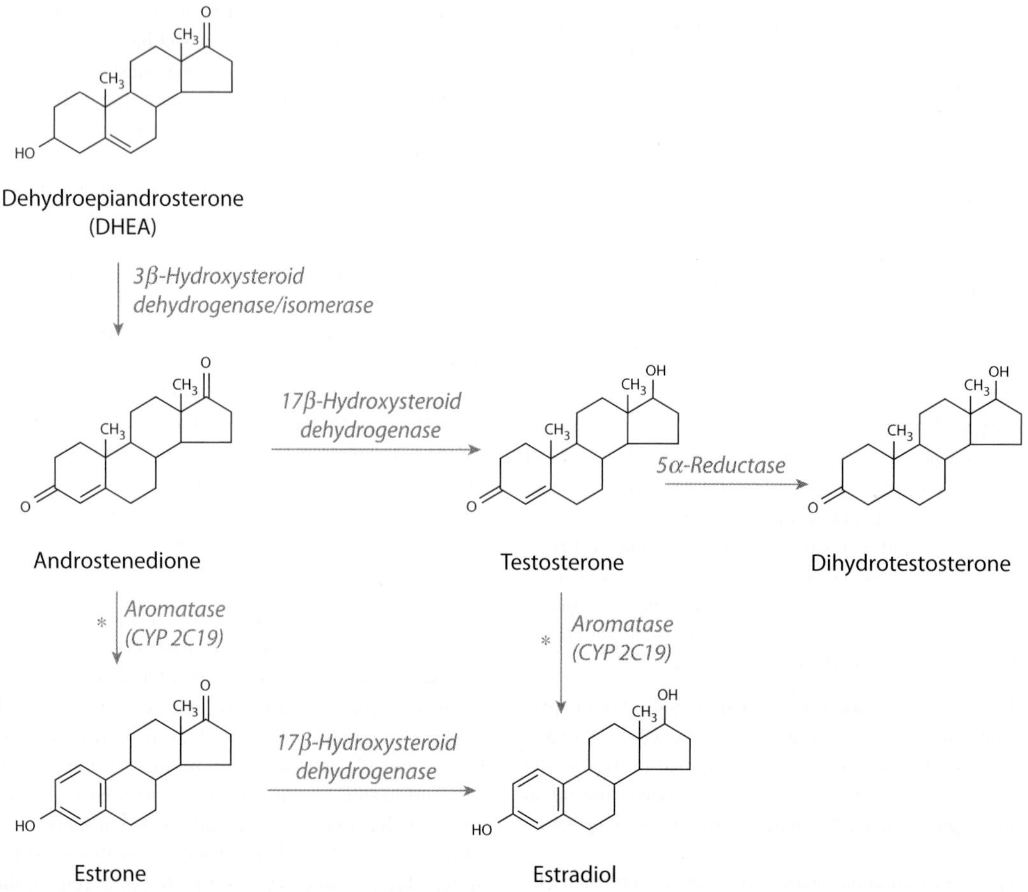

FIGURE 41–1. Metabolic pathway of the transformation of Dehydroepiandrosterone (DHEA) to androgens and estrogens. Anastrozole and aminogluthemide inhibit aromatase *(asterisk)*, thus blocking feminization after the utilization of androgens.

was marketed as a nutritional supplement and is available for purchase without a prescription.[80] Dehydroepiandrosterone is converted to androstenedione and then to testosterone by the enzyme 17β-hydroxysteroid dehydrogenase.[96,128,131] Administration of androstenedione in dosages of 300 mg/d increases testosterone and estradiol concentrations in some men and women.[124] Women with adrenal insufficiency given DHEA replacement at a dose of 50 mg/d orally for 4 months demonstrated increased serum concentrations of DHEA, androstenedione, testosterone, and dihydrotestosterone. Serum total and HDL cholesterol concentrations simultaneously decreased. Some women experienced androgenic side effects, including greasy skin, acne, and hirsutism.[14] Sense of well-being and sexuality increased in men and women after 4 months of treatment.[14,149] The neuropsychiatric effects of DHEA have been demonstrated in animals. Increased hypothalamic serotonin, anxiolytic effects, antagonism at the γ-aminobutyric acid type A (GABA$_A$) receptor, and agonism at the N-methyl-D-aspartate receptor (NMDA) are demonstrated.[14,132,145]

Clenbuterol

Clenbuterol is a β$_2$-adrenergic agonist that decreases fat deposition and prevents protein breakdown in animal models.[10,41,93] Clenbuterol is also a potent *nutrient partitioning agent*, a term implying it increases the amount of muscle and decreases the amount of fat produced per pound of feed given to cattle and other animals.[71,180] Clenbuterol increases the glycolytic capacity of muscle and causes hypertrophy, enhancing the growth of fast-twitch fibers (Chap. 63).[133,232] Use of clenbuterol in cattle farming is illegal in many countries. Nevertheless, the consumption of veal liver contaminated with clenbuterol has resulted in sympathomimetic symptoms and positive urine test results in affected individuals.[186] Clenbuterol is composed of a racemic mixture of (+) and (−) stereoisomers, eliminated in urine in approximately equal amounts. As clenbuterol accumulates in animal meat, stereoisomer ratios change over time, and (−) clenbuterol is depleted. By analyzing urinary ratios of clenbuterol stereoisomers, it is possible to differentiate administration of therapeutic clenbuterol preparations from inadvertent ingestion of clenbuterol in meat products.[215] The enantiomeric composition of clenbuterol from meat is different than the composition of clenbuterol from drugs. Analytic techniques relying on stereoselectivity can identify the source of the clenbuterol, whether it is ingested in meat or as a drug preparation. Tourists returning from Mexico and China are found to have traces of clenbuterol in their urine.[161]

PEPTIDES AND GLYCOPROTEIN HORMONES

Creatine

Creatine is an amino acid formed by combining the amino acids methionine, arginine, and glycine. It is synthesized naturally by the liver, kidneys, and pancreas. Creatine is found in protein-containing foods such as meat and fish. In its phosphorylated form, it is involved in the rapid resynthesis of adenosine triphosphate (ATP) from adenosine diphosphate (ADP) by acting as a substrate to donate phosphorus.[208] Because ATP is the immediate source of energy for muscle contraction, creatine is used by athletes to increase energy during short, high-intensity exercise.[222] Exceptional athletes have admitted to using creatine as part of their training nutritional regimen, leading to interest by athletes at all levels. Numerous studies demonstrate improved performance with creatine supplementation, particularly in sports requiring short, high-intensity effort.[28,35,116,142,222] Creatine is found in skeletal muscle and in the heart, brain, and kidneys. Two-thirds of creatine is stored primarily as phosphorylated creatine and the remainder as free creatine.[18] Consuming carbohydrates with creatine supplements increases total creatine and phosphorylated creatine stores in skeletal muscle.[18] This process explains why creatine is marketed in combination with carbohydrate. Human endogenous creatine production is 1 g/d, and normal diets containing meat and fish offer another 1 to 2 g/d as dietary intake. One to two grams of creatine is eliminated daily by irreversible conversion to creatinine.[225] Creatine is not currently on the WADA prohibited list 2017.[1]

Creatine supplementation is most commonly accomplished with creatine monohydrate. A dose of 20 to 25 g/d can increase the skeletal muscle total creatine concentration by 20%.[87,98] Creatine stores do not increase in some individuals despite creatine supplementation. Creatine uptake in skeletal muscle occurs via the creatine transporter proteins at the sarcolemma. Creatine transporter expression and activity, as well as exercise and training, influence the uptake of creatine and the effect of creatine loading on athletic performance.[202,203,205]

One adverse effect of creatine supplementation is weight gain, which is thought to result primarily from water retention.[87,142] However, evidence indicates that net protein increase is partially responsible for the weight gain associated with long-term creatine use.[104] Diarrhea was the most commonly reported side effect of creatine use in one study of 52 male college athletes. Other complaints were muscle cramping and dehydration, although many participants had no complaints.[104]

Creatine supplementation increases urinary creatine and creatinine excretion and may increase serum creatinine concentrations by 20%.[87,105] Long- and short-term creatine supplementation does not appear to have an adverse effect on kidney function.[168,169] One patient who had been taking creatine 5 g/d for 4 weeks developed interstitial nephritis that improved with cessation of creatine use. Whether ingestion of creatine caused the nephritis is unknown.[115] A young man with focal segmental glomerular sclerosis developed an elevated creatinine concentration and decreased glomerular filtration rate when creatine supplementation was started. The values returned to baseline upon cessation of creatine supplementation.[175] The possibility of developing decreased kidney function is a theoretical concern. Ingestion of large amounts of creatine results in formation of the carcinogenic substance N-nitrososarcosine, which induces esophageal cancer in rats.[12,13]

Human Growth Hormone

Human growth hormone (hGH) is an anabolic peptide hormone secreted by the anterior pituitary gland. It stimulates protein synthesis and increases growth and muscle mass in children. Recombinant hGH (rhGH) became available in 1984. It is commonly used therapeutically for children with GH deficiency in daily doses of 5 to 26 mcg/kg body weight.[223]

Growth hormone secretion is stimulated by GH-releasing hormone and is inhibited by somatostatin. Growth hormone receptors are found in many tissues, including the liver. Binding of hGH to hepatic receptors causes secretion of insulinlike growth factor-1 (IGF-1), which has potent anabolic effects and is the mediator for many of the actions of hGH.

Release of hGH, which occurs mainly during sleep, occurs in a pulsatile manner. Exercise stimulates hGH release, and more intense exercise causes proportionately more hGH release.[31,47,209] Amino acids such as ornithine, L-arginine, tryptophan, and L-lysine increase hGH release through an unknown mechanism and often are ingested for this purpose.[47,89]

By causing nitrogen retention and increased movement of amino acids into tissue, hGH stimulates protein synthesis and tissue growth. The effects on increasing muscle mass and size are demonstrated in GH-deficient individuals. Some studies do not support an increase in strength secondary to the increase in muscle size in athletes,[45,130] but others demonstrate lean body mass, strength, and power increases. Growth hormone improves muscle and cardiac function, increases red blood cell (RBC) mass and oxygen-carrying capacity, stimulates lipolysis, normalizes serum lipid concentrations, and decreases subcutaneous fat. It also improves mood and sense of well-being.[45,46,91,188,209,223]

Growth hormone is used by athletes for its anabolic potential. As a xenobiotic of abuse, it is particularly attractive because laboratory detection is difficult. In one survey, 12% of people in gyms used hGH for body building.[62] In another survey of adolescents, 5% of 10th-grade boys had used hGH.[179] It may be sold illicitly as recombinant hGH.

Administration of hGH often cause myalgias, arthralgias, carpal tunnel syndrome, and edema. The effects of hGH on skeletal growth depend on the user's age. In preadolescents, excessive hGH cause increased bony growth and gigantism. In adults, excessive hGH cause acromegaly.[217,219] Growth hormone causes glucose intolerance and hyperglycemia. Skin changes, such as increased melanocytic nevi and altered skin texture, occur.[167] Lipid profiles are adversely affected. High-density lipoprotein concentrations are decreased, a change associated with increased risk of coronary artery disease.[233] Because hGH must be given parenterally, there is risk of transmission of infection.[130] The illicit sale of cadaveric human pituitary-derived GH is associated with a risk of Creutzfeldt-Jakob disease.[53] Long-term users of hGH are at increased risk for prostate cancer because of the complications associated with IGF-1[80] (see later).

Testing for hGH is plagued by the difficulties inherent in testing for exogenous peptide doping in general—the identical amino acid sequences of both rhGH and hGH; the fluctuating, pulsatile secretion; short half-life; and variation in normal concentration depending on sleep as well as stress and exercise status. Unlike the ability to use the differing pattern of *N*-linked glycosylation in human erythropoietin (hEPO) produced in human kidneys to distinguish it from recombinant human erythropoietin (rhEPO) produced in hamsters, hGH has no *N*-linked glycosylation sites to facilitate differentiation.

The detection of GH relies primarily on the detection of hGH-dependent factors through which hGH exerts its effect, such as IGF-1 and IGF binding proteins, as well as other markers of bone growth and turnover, such as the *N*-terminal extension peptide of procollagen type III.[8,172] The isoform approach refers to the measurement of the various forms of GH. Whereas rhGH is primarily a 22-kDa monomeric form, pituitary hGH contains multiple isoforms. In athletes using rhGH, endogenous hGH with its multiple isoforms is suppressed through negative feedback on the pituitary. Therefore, the 22-kDa form characteristic of rhGH becomes predominant. The ratio of isoforms, as measured by immunoassay, changes.

Insulinlike Growth Factor-1

Insulinlike growth factor-1 is a peptide chain structurally related to insulin. A recombinant form is available.[84-86] Parenteral administration of IGF-1 is approved for clinical treatment of dwarfism and insulin resistance. Children who develop antibodies to rhGH often respond to IGF-1.

The primary stimulus for release of IGF-1 is hGH, although insulin, DHEA, and nutrition play a role. The actions of IGF-1 can be classified as either anabolic or insulinlike.[185] The effects of GH are primarily mediated by IGF-1. Insulinlike growth factor-1 is produced in the liver and many other cell types. Insulinlike growth factor-1 binds principally to the type I IGF receptor, which has 40% homology with the insulin receptor and a similar tyrosine kinase subunit. Although IGF-1 also binds to insulin receptors, it has only 1% of insulin affinity for the insulin receptor and actually increases glucose utilization by causing the movement of glucose into cells, increasing amino acid uptake and stimulating protein synthesis.

Side effects are similar to those associated with use of GH and include acromegaly. Other effects include headache, jaw pain, edema, and alterations in lipid profiles. A potentially serious side effect of IGF-1 is hypoglycemia. High endogenous plasma IGF-1 concentrations are associated with an increased risk for prostate cancer.[39]

Few studies on the efficacy of IGF-1 in improving the conditioning of athletes are available. Insulinlike growth factor-1 is preferred by female athletes because it does not cause virilization.[209]

Insulin

Insulin is used by body builders for its anabolic properties. Of 20 self-identified AAS users in a single gym, 25% who had no medical reason to take insulin reported using it to increase muscle mass.[178] These individuals stated that they had injected insulin from 20 to 60 times over the 6 months before the study.[174] Their practice was to inject 10 units of regular insulin and then eat sugar-containing foods after injection. As expected, hypoglycemia is reported in body builders using insulin.[60,99,175]

Insulin inhibits proteolysis and promotes growth by stimulating movement of glucose and amino acids into muscle and fat cells. It increases the synthesis of glycogen, fatty acids, and proteins (Chap. 47).[49]

Meldonium

Meldonium inhibits the carnitine transporter type 2, thereby reducing L-carnitine biosynthesis and transport. Long-term meldonium treatment may be beneficial by improving energy metabolism during hypoxia. This is the benefit that athletes seek. Meldonium improves glucose utilization. In one high-profile case, the athlete said that she was using meldonium to treat her prediabetes state; however, it is a banned substance, and the athlete was sanctioned.[48,126]

Human Chorionic Gonadotropin

In men, the glycoprotein hCG stimulates testicular steroidogenesis. In women, hCG is secreted by the placenta during pregnancy. It sometimes used by male athletes to prevent testicular atrophy during and after androgen administration.[111] Analysis of hCG in 740 urinary specimens of male athletes revealed abnormal concentrations in 21 individuals. This finding prompted the IOC ban on hCG use in 1987.[111] Presently, distinguishing exogenous hCG administration from hCG production in early pregnancy is under study.[117]

Very small amounts of hCG are normally present in men and nonpregnant women. Currently, measurement is made by immunoassay. The decision limit, the concentration at which the test result is considered positive, is set at 5 IU/mL urine. Trophoblastic tumors and nontrophoblastic tumors can increase hCG concentrations, and this possibility must be considered in the evaluation of elevated urinary hCG concentration.[117] Administration of hCG causes an increase in the total testosterone and epitestosterone produced.

OXYGEN TRANSPORT

Erythropoietin

Human erythropoietin is a hormone that, through a receptor-mediated mechanism, induces erythropoiesis by stimulating stem cells. Erythropoietin has been available since 1988 as rhEPO, and its use in international competition has been prohibited since 1990. Although hEPO is produced primarily by the kidneys, rhEPO is produced in hamsters;[56] this results in differing glycosylation patterns, an important piece in the laboratory detection of EPO in sports doping.

Because EPO increases exercise capacity and hemoglobin production, it is used by athletes, often with additional iron supplementation. The clinical effects of increased hemoglobin occur several days after administration.[73,160] Erythropoietin increases maximal oxygen uptake by 6% to 7%, an effect that lasts approximately 2 weeks after rhEPO administration is completed.[59]

Erythropoietin analogs such as darbepoetin are *erythropoiesis-stimulating proteins*, differing from EPO by five amino acids. Darbepoetin has a much longer half-life and can be injected weekly. Another protein, known as *synthetic erythropoiesis protein*, has a similar protein structure to EPO. The protein polymers created in this molecule have less immunogenicity, fewer biologic contaminants, and more predictable pharmacokinetics.[162]

Human EPO is secreted primarily by the kidney, although some is produced by the liver. The mean apparent half-lives of rhEPO are 4.5 hours after intravenous (IV) administration and 25 hours after subcutaneous administration.[187]

Erythropoietin enhances endothelial activation and platelet reactivity and increases systolic blood pressure during submaximal exercise.[25,207] These effects, in addition to the increase in hemoglobin, increase the risk of thromboembolic events, hypertension, and hyperviscosity syndromes.[25,141,160] Nineteen Belgian and Dutch cyclists died of uncertain causes between 1987 and 1990.[58] Increases in hematocrit subsequent to EPO use are believed to have contributed to these deaths.

An EPO overdose occurred in a patient who self-administered 10,000 units/d for an unknown period of time as a result of a dosing error. The patient presented to the hospital with confusion, a plethoric appearance, blackened toes, decreased pulses, and a hematocrit of 72%. Emergent erythropheresis was performed and resulted in rapid reduction of hematocrit and improvement in the patient's condition.[231] Another report of deliberate daily self-administration of an unknown dose of rhEPO resulted in a hematocrit of 70%. The patient was treated emergently with phlebotomy and IV hydration and improved.[33]

Testing for Erythropoietin

Erythropoietin is directly measured by a monoclonal anti-EPO antibody test, which does not distinguish between endogenously produced and exogenously administered recombinant EPO. Therefore, tracking indirect methods of EPO detection are used, such as measurement of hemoglobin or hematocrit. The isoelectric focusing double immunoblotting detection strategy is the WADA-accredited strategy.[42]

Previously, some sports-governing bodies, such as the International Cycling Federation and the International Skiing Federation, selected a hematocrit of 50% in men and 47% in women as the action level above which an athlete may be disqualified for presumed EPO use. However, normal hematocrit values vary greatly among athletes. Several studies have shown that hematocrits above the action values of 50% in men and 47% in women are common in athletes. From 3% to 6% of athletes who did not use EPO had hematocrits greater than 50%.[224] Of athletes living and training at altitudes between 2,000 and 3,000 m above sea level, 20.5% had hematocrit values higher than 50%.[224] Other studies confirm the increased hematocrits of athletes training at altitudes of 1,000 to 6,000 m.[23,190-192]

Although many endurance athletes have increased blood volume, the hematocrit may be lowered because of the increased plasma volume, which exceeds the RBC volume. This dilutional pseudoanemia is sometimes called *sports anemia*.[197] Additionally, hematocrit measurements are affected by hydration status, posture (upright versus supine), and nutrition, and they demonstrate an approximately 3% diurnal variation.[190] Because of natural variations among individuals, postural effects, and the ease of manipulation through saline infusion, indirect detection of EPO use by hematocrit measurement is fraught with potential for error.[160]

Several methods have been studied to detect the use of rhEPO by athletes. The ratio between serum soluble transferrin receptors (sTfr) and ferritin was used as an indirect method for detection of EPO use. The sTfr is released from RBC progenitors. Erythropoietin stimulates erythropoiesis and causes an increase in sTfr and a decrease in ferritin.[78] Individuals with other causes of polycythemia or accelerated erythropoiesis also can exhibit increased ratios and be falsely accused of EPO use. An increased hematocrit with sTfr greater than 10 mcg/mL and sTfr-to-serum protein ratio greater than 153 has been proposed as an indirect measurement of EPO use.[12]

State-of-the-art detection of EPO doping is accomplished by two techniques: isoelectric focusing and immunoblotting performed on urine samples. The two isoforms of EPO, recombinant and endogenous, have different glycosylation patterns and glycan sizes, resulting in differing molecular charges.[42,162] An immunoblotting procedure takes advantage of these different net charges, and the proteins can be separated by their charges when they are placed in an electric field.[123] Subsequently, by isoelectric focusing, this method obtains an image of EPO patterns in the urine.[123] World Anti-Doping Agency considers a positive urine test result by this method definitive, even without the blood testing of indirect markers.[42]

Because of the structural similarity of darbepoetin to EPO, these detection techniques also are effective for darbopoietin.[162]

STIMULANTS
Caffeine

Caffeine is a central nervous system stimulant that causes a feeling of decreased fatigue and increases endurance performance (Chap. 63).[61,163] These changes may occur through several different mechanisms, including increased calcium permeability in the sarcoplasmic reticulum and enhanced contractility of muscle, phosphodiesterase inhibition and subsequent increased cyclic nucleotides, adenosine blockade leading to blood vessel dilation, and inhibited lipolysis.

Amphetamines

The beneficial effects of amphetamines in sports result from their ability to mask fatigue and pain.[51] Initial studies done in soldiers showed that they could march longer and ignore pain when taking amphetamines

(Chap. 73).[217] In one study in college students, resting and maximal heart rate, strength, acceleration, and anaerobic capacity increased. However, although the perception of fatigue decreased, lactic acid continued to accumulate, and maximal oxygen consumption was unchanged.[40] Other studies show no significant effects on exercise performance.[107]

Sodium Bicarbonate

Sodium bicarbonate loading, known as "soda loading," has a long history of use in horse racing.[19] Sodium bicarbonate buffers the metabolic acidosis associated with an elevated lactate caused by exercise, thereby delaying fatigue and enhancing performance.[81,199]

During high-intensity exercise, metabolism becomes anaerobic, and lactic acid is produced. Intracellular acidosis is suggested to contribute to muscle fatigue by reducing the sensitivity of the muscle contractile apparatus to calcium.[165] Several studies demonstrated improved performance in running when sodium bicarbonate was ingested 2 to 3 hours before competition.[44,184] The study dose was 0.2 to 0.3 g/kg body weight of sodium bicarbonate, approximately 160 mEq of sodium bicarbonate per day. The effects of sodium bicarbonate are greatest when periods of exercise last longer than 4 minutes because anaerobic metabolism contributes more to total energy production and energy from aerobic metabolism diminishes.[72,80,81] Adverse effects of bicarbonate loading include diarrhea, abdominal pain, and the possibility of hypernatremia.

Contrary to this theory, an animal model demonstrated that intracellular acidosis associated with lactate production reversed muscle fatigue.[7,165] Previously, intracellular acidosis was thought to contribute to muscle fatigue by reducing the sensitivity of the muscle contractile apparatus to calcium, decreasing the force of muscle contraction. However, the mechanism of excitation-contraction is complex. Because it permeates membranes easily, chloride is an important ion in maintaining and stabilizing the muscle fiber resting membrane potential at normal pH. Because of this, a large sodium current is needed to overcome membrane stabilization and produce an action potential. In the case of intracellular acidosis, the permeability of the membrane to the chloride ion is reduced, the resting membrane potential is no longer stabilized, and less inward sodium influx is needed to produce an action potential. The excitability of the muscle T-tubule system is therefore increased by acidosis, protecting against muscle fatigue.[165]

DIURETICS

The WADA bans nonmedical diuretic use.[1] Diuretics are used in sports in which the athlete must achieve a certain weight to compete in discrete weight classes. In addition to weight loss, body builders find that diuretic use gives greater definition to the physique as the skin draws tightly around the muscles.[3] In one report, a professional body builder attempted to lose weight using diuretics, including bumetanide and spironolactone as well as potassium supplements. He presented with hyperkalemia and hypotension (Chap. 12).[3] Diuretics also result in increased urine production, thereby diluting the urine and making the detection of other banned xenobiotics more difficult.[36,52]

LABORATORY DETECTION

Enormous amounts of energy and money are expended to determine the presence or absence of performance-enhancing xenobiotics.[213] Analysis of samples on the international level is performed by a limited number of accredited laboratories. The majority of tests are performed on urine, with careful procedural requirements regarding handling of samples. Attention must be paid to proper storage of specimens because bacterial metabolism may increase urinary steroid concentrations.[27,55] Upon arrival of a sample at the testing laboratory, the integrity of the sample is checked, including the code, seal, visual appearance, density, and pH. Registration of the sample is completed, and the sample is divided into two aliquots. All testing is done on the first aliquot, and any positive results are confirmed on the second aliquot. The aliquots are commonly referred to as sample A and sample B. Sample preparation is difficult and time consuming.

The complexity of the laboratory testing and continuous attempts to evade detection is illustrated in the discovery of an AAS previously undetectable by standard sport doping tests of urine. In the following situation, there was no preexisting reference data for the unknown xenobiotic. In the summer of 2003, a used syringe was provided anonymously to the US antidoping authority. Through a painstaking process of analyses, a previously unrecognized chemical in the syringe was identified as a derivative of the AAS norbolethone, a known reference compound, leading to the discovery, synthesis, and detection of tetrahydrogestrinone (THG), a new chemical unknown as a pharmaceutical or veterinary compound.[38] Doping control analysis is forever challenged by new xenobiotics.[213]

Capillary Gas Chromatography–Mass Spectrometry

Capillary gas chromatography allows the determination of approximately 95% of all doping positive results. Gas chromatography typically is combined with mass spectrometry for detection of the majority of substances.[153,213] Analysis of the urine by gas chromatography–mass spectrophotometry (GC-MS) is the current standard for detection of AASs.[36] Such analysis relies on a large amount of previously derived reference data (Chap. 7).[38]

Testosterone-to-Epitestosterone Ratio

Gas chromatography–mass spectrophotometry cannot distinguish endogenous testosterone from pharmaceutically derived exogenous testosterone. Therefore, other methods of detection are needed. One way of detecting the use of exogenous testosterone is to measure the testosterone-to-epitestosterone (T/E) ratio.[221] Epitestosterone is not a metabolite of testosterone, but it is a 17-α epimer, differing from testosterone only in the configuration of the hydroxyl group on C-17. Men produce 30 times more testosterone than epitestosterone; however, 1% of testosterone and 30% of epitestosterone are excreted unchanged in the urine. Therefore, the normal T/E ratio in the urine is about 1:1.[206]

A T/E ratio less than 4:1 is considered acceptable; a T/E ratio greater than 4:1 is considered evidence of doping using testosterone. To maintain a normal T/E ratio, athletes self-administer both testosterone and epitestosterone.[37]

The overall pattern of the T/E ratio over time is important. Athletes subjected to testing will have previous measurements of their T/E ratios on record with antidoping authorities, or additional tests may be obtained to establish a pattern of T/E ratios. These results are plotted against time. The mean, standard deviation, and confidence values are calculated.[37] The confidence values of three or more samples taken over months will be less than 60% unless the athlete is using testosterone.[34] Sudden variations in an athlete's pattern of T/E ratios over time is a cause for further testing.

A steroid profile is measured on all urine samples. It consists of the urinary concentrations of testosterone, epitestosterone, androsterone, etiocholanolone, 5a-androstane-3a,17β-diol, and 5β-androstane-3a,17β-diol, together with the specific gravity of the urine sample. Further ratios are calculated to detect multiple forms of steroid doping.[1]

In one high-profile doping case in which the T/E ratio was elevated, the athlete suggested that ethanol consumption the previous night caused the elevated T/E ratio. In this regard, there is evidence that at very high doses; for example, 2 g/kg, ethanol increases the T/E ratio, although the T/E ratio did not exceed 6:1.[4,5] This effect of ethanol is more pronounced in women and is limited to 8 hours postingestion of ethanol. The mechanism of this effect of ethanol is that it increases the NADH-to-NAD+ ratio, and many steroid oxidation–reduction reactions are dependent on the relative abundance of NADH to NAD+.[65] Ketoconazole inhibits testosterone synthesis and causes a decrease in the T/E ratio within 6 hours of administration.[112]

Isotope Ratio Mass Spectrometry

Carbon is made up of six protons and six neutrons, giving it an atomic weight of 12 (^{12}C). Sometimes carbon has an extra neutron, giving it an atomic weight of 13 (^{13}C). Carbon is derived from carbon dioxide in the atmosphere. Warm climate plants, such as soy, process carbon dioxide differently than other plants, using different photosynthetic pathways for carbon dioxide fixation, causing the depletion of ^{13}C.[189] Pharmaceutical testosterone is made from plant sterols, primarily soy plants, and therefore has less ^{13}C isotope

than endogenous testosterone, made in the body from a typical human diet based in corn and not soy. This difference in isotope ratios is measured by isotope ratio mass spectrometry. An athlete's natural carbon makeup is determined by analysis of an endogenous reference compound such as the testosterone precursor cholesterol. Cholesterol may be called an "autostandard" because it represents the athlete's ^{13}C/^{12}C ratio.[24] Finally, it is the difference between the ratio of the athlete's ^{13}C/^{12}C ratio and an international standard ratio that is measured and reported.[2] Values are negative because both endogenous and pharmaceutical testosterone contain less ^{13}C than the international standard.[88]

Insulin

Laboratory detection methods for insulin are not yet standardized and accredited by WADA. Therefore, athletes are not currently tested for insulin use. The technology for testing for insulin uses immunoaffinity purification followed by liquid chromatography–tandem mass spectrometry to identify analytes including urinary metabolites of insulin.[216] When insulin is modified to improve its receptor selectivity or give it other favorable properties, the change in molecular weight or amino acid profile from human insulin makes it detectable by GC-MS.[216]

Masking Xenobiotics

Any chemical or physical manipulation done with the purpose of altering the integrity of a urine or blood sample is prohibited by WADA.[1] For example, use of IV fluids for dilution of the sample, or urine substitution, is prohibited. Some xenobiotics are added to the urine for the sole purpose of interfering with urine testing and are easily detected. Examples include "Klear," which is 90% methanol, and Golden Seal tea, which produces colored urine.[32] Other commercially available products include "Xxtra Clean," which contains pyridinium chlorochromate, and "Urine Luck," which contains glutaraldehyde.

Niacin is used to alter urine test results, although there is no evidence it is effective for this purpose. There are reports of niacin toxicity, including skin reactions such as itching, flushing, and burning, when niacin is used for this purpose.[146,147] More serious effects, including nausea, elevated liver enzymes, hypoglycemia, and anion gap metabolic acidosis, are reported as a result of ingesting niacin in large amounts, in the 2.5 to 5.5 g range over 1 to 2 days.[146,147]

A significant issue in the analysis of urine for the presence of prohibited peptides such as rhEPO is the masking potential of proteases surreptitiously added to urine specimens slated for doping analysis. The proteases are packaged in "grains" known as protease granules or "rice grains" and placed in the urethra.[212] Upon urination for the purpose of providing a specimen for doping analysis, the grain flows with urine into the specimen cup. The proteases, including trypsin, chymotrypsin, and papain, quickly degrade renally excreted peptides, most notably EPO, making them undetectable. By the process of autolysis, proteases themselves become undetectable over time. In one report, urine with elevated protease concentrations greater than 15 mcg/mL underwent further analysis to identify urinary proteins such as albumin.[212] Normally, the presence of urinary proteins creates the image of a visible band by gel electrophoresis. However, the urine with elevated protease activity will demonstrate something called *trace of burning*, a term indicating an absence of proteins.[214]

In this report, suspicious specimens were subjected to further testing using liquid chromatography–mass spectrometry. After further molecular sequencing of derived proteins, human proteases can be distinguished from nonhuman proteases, such as bovine chymotrypsin or papain. The addition of a protease inhibitor to urine samples immediately after collection is suggested as a future strategy to limit the effectiveness of protease addition as a masking method.[214]

In approximately 15% of urine samples performed in antidoping laboratories, there is no endogenous or rhEPO detectable by immunoelectrophoresis.[120] Undetectable EPO occurs more commonly in competition, the "competition effect." This is due in part to circumstances unrelated to doping, such as physiological variation in EPO production, gender, and very low or very high urine specific gravity. However, doping with exogenous EPO and inhibition of endogenous hEPO production or addition of proteases are other possible causes. Strenuous effort causes a shift in the isoforms of EPO, yielding a more basic isoelectric point, a result known as "effort" urine.[119] Urine samples deemed suspicious do not necessarily result in a positive doping test result.[120,212]

The list of prohibited masking xenobiotics includes diuretics; epitestosterone; probenecid; plasma expanders such as albumin, dextran, and hydroxymethyl starch; and α-reductase inhibitors such as finasteride and dutasteride.[1] Probenecid blocks urinary excretion of the glucuronide conjugates of AAS.

Gene Doping

The discovery of the genetic codes for some diseases has made gene therapy of medical conditions, such as muscular dystrophy, a reality. It is now conceivable that this technology can be used to enhance athletic performance. Gene doping is included on the WADA 2017 Prohibited List.[1] Gene doping is defined as "the non-therapeutic use of cells, genes, genetic elements, or of the modulation of gene expression, having the capacity to enhance athlete performance."[1] For example, insertion of a gene sequence could produce a desired effect, such as large muscles or increased body production of potentially advantageous substances such as testosterone or GH. In animal models, genes for EPO lead to erythropoiesis, and genes for IGF-1 produce increased muscle size and strength.[22] Myostatin, which belongs to a family of proteins that control growth and differentiation of tissues in the body, inhibits skeletal muscle growth.[103,193] Mutations of the myostatin gene may result in muscle hypertrophy. In dogs, the athletic performance of racing whippets is enhanced in animals with a myostatin gene mutation.[152] In humans, a report of an extremely muscular baby born with a mutation in the myostatin gene illustrates the potential effect of gene alterations on athletic performance. The mother of this infant was a professional athlete, and other members of the family were known for their strength.[193] This was a natural genetic mutation. Transcription regulators such as AMP-activated protein kinase (AMPK) are exercise mimetics and increase muscle endurance when administered orally in animal models.[83,154] Influencing the expression of the transcription factor peroxisome proliferator-activated receptor-δ (PPAR-δ), a nuclear hormone receptor hormone protein, leads to increased formation of slow twitch skeletal muscle. Angiotensin II receptor blockers such as telmisartan influence both the AMPK pathway and upregulate PPAR-δ, expression improving muscle performance.[66]

Athlete's Biological Passport

A significant development in the detection of blood transfusion, known as blood doping, is the development of a longitudinal record of an athlete's RBC parameters called the *athlete's biological passport*. This is individualized longitudinal monitoring that tests blood for markers of doping. Because of this record of athletes' biomarkers, athletes are more sophisticated and use very small amounts of blood-boosting xenobiotics. Such blood manipulation causes changes in gene expression that may be detected. The detection of plasticizer metabolites from blood storage and alteration of gene expression resulting from infusion of autologous blood are proposed adjuncts to detection of autologous blood transfusion.[150,151] The observation of physiological parameters over time has made it easier to detect use of performance-enhancing agents.[20]

Neurocognitive Enhancement

Improvement in brain function and mental agility is an element of performance enhancement receiving increasing study. Students report improving academic productivity as the motivation for use of stimulants. Those using methylphenidate and amphetamine have reported positive effects on working memory, delayed memory, and processing speed in learning. Whereas also limit cognitive flexibility. There is a wide dosing range for individual stimulants to increase cognitive performance. At this time, the effect of these xenobiotics on learning requires extensive study.[140]

Nutritional studies are reported to demonstrate the positive effects of fruit flavonoid supplementation. Blueberries and other berries in the diet enhance are suggested to enhance memory both with acute and chronic diet inclusion in both animals and human subjects.[9,30]

Enhancement of neurocognitive performance using vitamins and minerals is a new area of study.

PERFORMANCE ENHANCEMENT AND SUDDEN DEATH IN ATHLETES

Many unexpected deaths in certain groups of young competitors have occurred in the absence of obvious medical or traumatic causes. In some of these cases, the use of performance-enhancing drugs was linked to the deaths. The use of EPO, introduced in Europe in 1987, is suggested to have contributed to the large number of deaths in young European endurance athletes over the next several years.[82] In young healthy athletes experiencing cerebrovascular events or myocardial infarction, the temporal link between the use of cocaine, ephedrine, or performance enhancers such as AASs suggests a role for these xenobiotics as precipitants of these adverse events. Nevertheless, the leading cause of nontraumatic sudden death in young athletes is most often associated with cardiac anomalies. In autopsy studies of athletes in the United States with congenital sudden death, hypertrophic cardiomyopathy is the most common structural abnormality, accounting for more than one-third of the cardiac arrests followed by coronary artery anomalies.[134-138] In Italy, dysrhythmogenic right ventricular cardiomyopathy is implicated in one-fourth of these deaths.[68,220] Medical causes of sudden death other than cardiac causes include heat stroke (Chap. 29), sickle cell trait, and asthma.

SUMMARY

- Although the press spotlights a few world-class athletes, the majority of individuals using performance-enhancing substances are not in the public view. Some individuals experience adverse consequences.
- Knowledgeable clinicians identify these health effects when they occur and educate susceptible individuals on the health risks of using performance-enhancing substances.
- Continuous development and refinement of antidoping laboratory methods broadly benefit our understanding of the physiology of exercise.
- WADA is the international body responsible for coordinating antidoping efforts nationally and internationally, and as such, the WADA Prohibited List sets the standard for methods and substances barred in sports.

REFERENCES

1. Agency of World Anti-Doping. WADA. The 2017 prohibited list. https://www.wada-ama.org/sites/default/files/resources/files/2016-09-29_-_wada_prohibited_list_2017_eng_final.pdf. Accessed September 27, 2017.
2. Aguilera R, et al. Detection of testosterone misuse: comparison of two chromatographic sample preparation methods for gas chromatographic-combustion/isotope ratio mass spectrometric analysis. *J Chromatogr B Biomed Appl.* 1996;687:43-53.
3. al-Zaki T, Taibot-Stern J. A bodybuilder with diuretic abuse presenting with symptomatic hypotension and hyperkalemia. *Am J Emerg Med.* 1996;14:96-98.
4. Albeiroti S, et al. Influence of low and moderate alcohol consumption on urinary testosterone/epitestosterone ratio. *Am J Clin Pathol.* 2017;147:S179.
5. Albeiroti S, et al. The influence of small doses of ethanol on the urinary testosterone to epitestosterone ratio in men and women. *Drug Test Anal.* 2017 Jul 3. [Epub ahead of print]
6. Alen M, et al. Response of serum hormones to androgen administration in power athletes. *Med Sci Sports Exerc.* 1985;17:354-359.
7. Allen D, Westerblad H. Physiology. Lactic acid—the latest performance-enhancing drug. *Science.* 2004;305:1112-1113.
8. Anderson LJ, et al. Use of growth hormone, IGF-I, and insulin for anabolic purpose: pharmacological basis, methods of detection, and adverse effects. *Mol Cell Endocrinol.* 2017;7207:30337-30334.
9. Andres-Lacueva C, et al. Anthocyanins in aged blueberry-fed rats are found centrally and may enhance memory. *Nutr Neurosci.* 2005;8:111-120.
10. Anonymous. Muscling in on clenbuterol. *Lancet.* 1992;340:403.
11. Appleby M, et al. Myocardial infarction, hyperkalaemia and ventricular tachycardia in a young male body-builder. *Int J Cardiol.* 1994;44:171-174.

12. Archer MC. Use of oral creatine to enhance athletic performance and its potential side effects. *Clin J Sport Med.* 1999;9:119.
13. Archer MC, et al. Environmental nitroso compounds: reaction of nitrite with creatine and creatinine. *Science.* 1971;174:1341-1343.
14. Arlt W, et al. Dehydroepiandrosterone replacement in women with adrenal insufficiency. *N Engl J Med.* 1999;341:1013-1020.
15. Bagatell CJ, Bremner WJ. Androgens in men—uses and abuses. *N Engl J Med.* 1996;334:707-714.
16. Baggish AL, et al. Cardiovascular toxicity of illicit anabolic-androgenic steroid use. *Circulation.* 2017;135:1991-2002.
17. Bagheri SA, Boyer JL. Peliosis hepatis associated with androgenic-anabolic steroid therapy. A severe form of hepatic injury. *Ann Intern Med.* 1974;81:610-618.
18. Balsom PD, et al. Creatine in humans with special reference to creatine supplementation. *Sports Med.* 1994;18:268-280.
19. Ban BD. Sodium bicarbonate: speed catalyst or just plain baking soda. *J Am Vet Med Assoc.* 1994;204:1300-1302.
20. Banfi G. Limits and pitfalls of Athlete's Biological Passport. *Clin Chem Lab Med.* 2011;49:1417-1421.
21. Barker S. Oxymethalone and aggression. *Br J Psychiatry.* 1987;151:564.
22. Barton-Davis ER, et al. Viral mediated expression of insulin-like growth factor I blocks the aging-related loss of skeletal muscle function. *Proc Natl Acad Sci U S A.* 1998;95:15603-15607.
23. Beard JL, et al. Iron deficiency anemia and steady-state work performance at high altitude. *J Appl Physiol.* 1988;64:1878-1884.
24. Becchi M, et al. Gas chromatography/combustion/isotope-ratio mass spectrometry analysis of urinary steroids to detect misuse of testosterone in sport. *Rapid Commun Mass Spectrom.* 1994;8:304-308.
25. Berglund B, Ekblom B. Effect of recombinant human erythropoietin treatment on blood pressure and some haematological parameters in healthy men. *J Intern Med.* 1991;229:125-130.
26. Bhasin S, et al. The effects of supraphysiologic doses of testosterone on muscle size and strength in normal men. *N Engl J Med.* 1996;335:1-7.
27. Bilton RF. Microbial production of testosterone. *Lancet.* 1995;345:1186-1187.
28. Birch R, et al. The influence of dietary creatine supplementation on performance during repeated bouts of maximal isokinetic cycling in man. *Eur J Appl Physiol Occup Physiol.* 1994;69:268-276.
29. Bochnia M, et al. Poststeroid balance disorder—a case report in a body builder. *Int J Sports Med.* 1999;20:407-409.
30. Boespflug EL, et al. Enhanced neural activation with blueberry supplementation in mild cognitive impairment. *Nutr Neurosci.* 2017;1-9.
31. Borer KT. The effects of exercise on growth. *Sports Med.* 1995;20:375-397.
32. Bowers LD. Athletic drug testing. *Clin Sports Med.* 1998;17:299-318.
33. Brown KR, et al. Recombinant erythropoietin overdose. *Am J Emerg Med.* 1993;11:619-621.
34. Bryden AA, et al. Anabolic steroid abuse and renal-cell carcinoma. *Lancet.* 1995;346:1306-1307.
35. Casey A, et al. Creatine ingestion favorably affects performance and muscle metabolism during maximal exercise in humans. *Am J Physiol.* 1996;271:E31-37.
36. Catlin DH, et al. Testing urine for drugs. *Ann Biol Clin (Paris).* 1992;50:359-366.
37. Catlin DH, et al. Issues in detecting abuse of xenobiotic anabolic steroids and testosterone by analysis of athletes' urine. *Clin Chem.* 1997;43:1280-1288.
38. Catlin DH, et al. Tetrahydrogestrinone: discovery, synthesis, and detection in urine. *Rapid Commun Mass Spectrom.* 2004;18:1245-1049.
39. Chan JM, et al. Plasma insulin-like growth factor-I and prostate cancer risk: a prospective study. *Science.* 1998;279:563-566.
40. Chandler JV, Blair SN. The effect of amphetamines on selected physiological components related to athletic success. *Med Sci Sports Exerc.* 1980;12:65-69.
41. Choo JJ, et al. Anabolic effects of clenbuterol on skeletal muscle are mediated by beta 2-adrenoceptor activation. *Am J Physiol.* 1992;263:E50-56.
42. Citartan M, et al. Monitoring recombinant human erythropoietin abuse among athletes. *Biosens Bioelectron.* 2015;63:86-98.
43. Collins P, Cotterill JA. Gymnasium acne. *Clin Exp Dermatol.* 1995;20:509.
44. Costill DL, et al. Acid-base balance during repeated bouts of exercise: influence of HCO3. *Int J Sports Med.* 1984;5:228-231.
45. Crist DM, et al. Body composition response to exogenous GH during training in highly conditioned adults. *J Appl Physiol.* 1988;65:579-584.
46. Cuneo RC, et al. Growth hormone treatment in growth hormone-deficient adults. I. Effects on muscle mass and strength. *J Appl Physiol.* 1991;70:688-694.
47. Cuttler L. The regulation of growth hormone secretion. *Endocrinol Metab Clin North Am.* 1996;25:541-571.
48. Dambrova M, et al. Pharmacological effects of meldonium: biochemical mechanisms and biomarkers of cardiometabolic activity. *Pharmacol Res.* 2016;113:771-780.
49. Dawson RT, Harrison MW. Use of insulin as an anabolic agent. *Br J Sports Med.* 1997;31:259.
50. De Piccoli B, et al. Anabolic steroid use in body builders: an echocardiographic study of left ventricle morphology and function. *Int J Sports Med.* 1991;12:408-412.
51. Dekhuijzen PN, et al. Athletes and doping: effects of drugs on the respiratory system. *Thorax.* 1999;54:1041-1046.
52. Delbeke FT, Debackere M. The influence of diuretics on the excretion and metabolism of doping agents—V. Dimefline. *J Pharm Biomed Anal.* 1991;9:23-28.
53. Deyssig R, Frisch H. Self-administration of cadaveric growth hormone in power athletes. *Lancet.* 1993;341:768-769.
54. Dickerman RD, et al. Cardiovascular complications and anabolic steroids. *Eur Heart J.* 1996;17:1912.
55. Donike M, et al. *Recent advances in doping analysis.* Köln: Sport and Buch Strauss; 1996.
56. Dou P, et al. Rapid and high-resolution glycoform profiling of recombinant human erythropoietin by capillary isoelectric focusing with whole column imaging detection. *J Chromatogr A.* 2008;1190:372-376.
57. DuRant RH, et al. Use of multiple drugs among adolescents who use anabolic steroids. *N Engl J Med.* 1993;328:922-926.
58. Eicher ER. Better dead than second. *J Lab Clin Med.* 1992;120:359-360.
59. Ekblom B, Berglund B. Effect of erythropoietin administration on maximal aerobic power. *Scand J Med Sci Sports.* 1991;1:88-93.
60. Elkin SL, et al. Bodybuilders find it easy to obtain insulin to help them in training. *BMJ.* 1997;314:1280.
61. Essig D, et al. Effects of caffeine ingestion on utilization of muscle glycogen and lipid during leg ergometer cycling. *Int J Sports Med.* 1980;1:86-90.
62. Evans NA. Gym and tonic: a profile of 100 male steroid users. *Br J Sports Med.* 1997;31:54-58.
63. Evans NA. Local complications of self administered anabolic steroid injections. *Br J Sports Med.* 1997;31:349-350.
64. Falk H, et al. Hepatic angiosarcoma associated with androgenic-anabolic steroids. *Lancet.* 1979;2:1120-1123.
65. Falk O, et al. Effect of ethanol on the ratio between testosterone and epitestosterone in urine. *Clin Chem.* 1988;34:1462-1464.
66. Feng X, et al. Angiotensin II receptor blocker telmisartan enhances running endurance of skeletal muscle through activation of the PPAR-delta/AMPK pathway. *J Cell Mol Med.* 2011;15:1572-1581.
67. Ferenchick G, et al. Androgenic-anabolic steroid abuse and platelet aggregation: a pilot study in weight lifters. *Am J Med Sci.* 1992;303:78-82.
68. Finocchiaro G, et al. Etiology of sudden death in sports: insights from a United Kingdom regional registry. *J Am Coll Cardiol.* 2016;67:2108-2115.
69. Franke WW, Berendonk B. Hormonal doping and androgenization of athletes: a secret program of the German Democratic Republic government. *Clin Chem.* 1997;43:1262-1279.
70. Freeman BJ, Rooker GD. Spontaneous rupture of the anterior cruciate ligament after anabolic steroids. *Br J Sports Med.* 1995;29:274-275.
71. Freidl KE, Moore RJ. Clenbuterol, ma huang, caffeine, L-carnitine, and growth hormone releasers. *Natl Strength Condition Assoc.* 1992:35.
72. Freis T, et al. Effect of sodium bicarbonate on prolonged running performance: a randomized, double-blind, cross-over study. *PLoS One.* 2017;12:e0182158.
73. Fried W, et al. Observations on regulation of erythropoiesis during prolonged periods of hypoxia. *Blood.* 1970;36:607-616.
74. Friedman G, et al. Fatal fulminant hepatic failure due to cyproterone acetate. *Dig Dis Sci.* 1999;44:1362-1363.
75. Froehner M, et al. Intratesticular leiomyosarcoma in a young man after high dose doping with Oral-Turinabol: a case report. *Cancer.* 1999;86:1571-1575.
76. Gaede JT, Montine TJ. Massive pulmonary embolus and anabolic steroid abuse. *JAMA.* 1992;267:2328-2329.
77. Gao W, Dalton JT. Ockham's razor and selective androgen receptor modulators (SARMs): are we overlooking the role of 5alpha-reductase? *Mol Interv.* 2007;7:10-13.
78. Gareau R, et al. Transferrin soluble receptor: a possible probe for detection of erythropoietin abuse by athletes. *Horm Metab Res.* 1994;26:311-312.
79. Garty BZ, et al. Cirrhosis in a child with hypothalamic syndrome and central precocious puberty treated with cyproterone acetate. *Eur J Pediatr.* 1999;158:367-370.
80. Ghaphery NA. Performance-enhancing drugs. *Orthop Clin North Am.* 1995;26:433-442.
81. Gledhill N. Bicarbonate ingestion and anaerobic performance. *Sports Med.* 1984;1:177-180.
82. Gnarpe H, Gnarpe J. Increasing prevalence of specific antibodies to *Chlamydia pneumoniae* in Sweden. *Lancet.* 1993;341:381.
83. Goodyear LJ. The exercise pill—too good to be true? *N Engl J Med.* 2008;359:1842-1844.
84. Guha N. Assays for GH, IGF-I, and IGF binding protein-3. *Methods Mol Biol.* 2013;1065:117-128.
85. Guha N, et al. Insulin-like growth factor-I (IGF-I) misuse in athletes and potential methods for detection. *Anal Bioanal Chem.* 2013;405:9669-9683.
86. Guha N, et al. Biochemical markers of recombinant human insulin-like growth factor-I (rhIGF-I)/rhIGF binding protein-3 (rhIGFBP-3) misuse in athletes. *Drug Test Anal.* 2013;5:843-849.
87. Harris RC, et al. Elevation of creatine in resting and exercised muscle of normal subjects by creatine supplementation. *Clin Sci (Lond).* 1992;83:367-374.
88. Hatton CK. Beyond sports-doping headlines: the science of laboratory tests for performance-enhancing drugs. *Pediatr Clin North Am.* 2007;54:713-733, xi.
89. Haupt HA. Anabolic steroids and growth hormone. *Am J Sports Med.* 1993;21:468-474.
90. Hausmann R, et al. Performance enhancing drugs (doping agents) and sudden death—a case report and review of the literature. *Int J Legal Med.* 1998;111:261-264.

91. Healy ML, Russell-Jones D. Growth hormone and sport: abuse, potential benefits, and difficulties in detection. *Br J Sports Med.* 1997;31:267-268.

92. Hill JA, et al. The athletic polydrug abuse phenomenon. A case report. *Am J Sports Med.* 1983;11:269-271.

93. Hinkle RT, et al. Skeletal muscle hypertrophy and anti-atrophy effects of clenbuterol are mediated by the beta2-adrenergic receptor. *Muscle Nerve.* 2002;25:729-734.

94. Hirose H, et al. Fatal splenic rupture in anabolic steroid-induced peliosis in a patient with myelodysplastic syndrome. *Br J Haematol.* 1991;78:128-129.

95. Hoberman JM. *Mortal Engines: The Science of Performance and the Dehumanization of Sport.* The Free Press; 1992.

96. Horton R, Tait JF. Androstenedione production and interconversion rates measured in peripheral blood and studies on the possible site of its conversion to testosterone. *J Clin Invest.* 1966;45:301-313.

97. Huie MJ. An acute myocardial infarction occurring in an anabolic steroid user. *Med Sci Sports Exerc.* 1994;26:408-413.

98. Hultman E, et al. Muscle creatine loading in men. *J Appl Physiol.* 1996;81:232-237.

99. Ip EJ, et al. Weightlifting's risky new trend: a case series of 41 insulin users. *Curr Sports Med Rep.* 2012;11:176-179.

100. Johnson AS, et al. Severe chickenpox in anabolic steroid user. *Lancet.* 1995;345: 1447-1448.

101. Johnson FL, et al. Association of androgenic-anabolic steroid therapy with development of hepatocellular carcinoma. *Lancet.* 1972;2:1273-1276.

102. Johnson MD. Anabolic steroid use in adolescent athletes. *Pediatr Clin North Am.* 1990;37:1111-1123.

103. Joulia-Ekaza D, Cabello G. The myostatin gene: physiology and pharmacological relevance. *Curr Opin Pharmacol.* 2007;7:310-315.

104. Juhn MS, et al. Oral creatine supplementation in male collegiate athletes: a survey of dosing habits and side effects. *J Am Diet Assoc.* 1999;99:593-595.

105. Juhn MS, Tarnopolsky M. Oral creatine supplementation and athletic performance: a critical review. *Clin J Sport Med.* 1998;8:286-297.

106. Karila TA, et al. Anabolic androgenic steroids produce dose-dependent increase in left ventricular mass in power athletes, and this effect is potentiated by concomitant use of growth hormone. *Int J Sports Med.* 2003;24:337-343.

107. Karpovich PV. Effect of amphetamine sulfate on athletic performance. *JAMA.* 1959; 170:558-561.

108. Kashkin KB, Kleber HD. Hooked on hormones? An anabolic steroid addiction hypothesis. *JAMA.* 1989;262:3166-3170.

109. Kennedy MC. Anabolic steroid abuse and toxicology. *Aust N Z J Med.* 1992;22:374-381.

110. Kennedy MC, et al. Myocardial infarction and cerebral haemorrhage in a young body builder taking anabolic steroids. *Aust N Z J Med.* 1993;23:713.

111. Kicman AT, et al. Human chorionic gonadotrophin and sport. *Br J Sports Med.* 1991; 25:73-80.

112. Kicman AT, et al. Potential use of ketoconazole in a dynamic endocrine test to differentiate between biological outliers and testosterone use by athletes. *Clin Chem.* 1993;39:1798-1803.

113. Kinson GA, et al. Influences of anabolic androgens on cardiac growth and metabolism in the rat. *Can J Physiol Pharmacol.* 1991;69:1698-1704.

114. Korkia P. Use of anabolic steroids has been reported by 9% of men attending gymnasiums. *BMJ.* 1996;313:1009.

115. Koshy KM, et al. Interstitial nephritis in a patient taking creatine. *N Engl J Med.* 1999; 340:814-815.

116. Kreider RB. Effects of creatine supplementation on performance and training adaptations. *Mol Cell Biochem.* 2003;244:89-94.

117. Kuuranne T, et al. Analysis of human chorionic gonadotropin (hCG): application of routine immunological methods for initial testing and confirmation analysis in doping control. *Drug Test Anal.* 2013;5:614-618.

118. Lage JM, et al. Cyclist's doping associated with cerebral sinus thrombosis. *Neurology.* 2002;58:665.

119. Lamon S, et al. Effects of exercise on the isoelectric patterns of erythropoietin. *Clin J Sport Med.* 2009;19:311-315.

120. Lamon S, et al. Possible origins of undetectable EPO in urine samples. *Clin Chim Acta.* 2007;385:61-66.

121. Laroche GP. Steroid anabolic drugs and arterial complications in an athlete—a case history. *Angiology.* 1990;41:964-969.

122. Laseter JT, Russell JA. Anabolic steroid-induced tendon pathology: a review of the literature. *Med Sci Sports Exerc.* 1991;23:1-3.

123. Lasne F, et al. Detection of isoelectric profiles of erythropoietin in urine: differentiation of natural and administered recombinant hormones. *Anal Biochem.* 2002;311: 119-126.

124. Leder BZ, et al. Oral androstenedione administration and serum testosterone concentrations in young men. *JAMA.* 2000;283:779-782.

125. Lepori M, et al. The popliteal-artery entrapment syndrome in a patient using anabolic steroids. *N Engl J Med.* 2002;346:1254-1255.

126. Liepinsh E, Dambrova M. The unusual pharmacokinetics of meldonium: implications for doping. *Pharmacol Res.* 2016;111:100.

127. Liow RY, Tavares S. Bilateral rupture of the quadriceps tendon associated with anabolic steroids. *Br J Sports Med.* 1995;29:77-79.

128. Longcope C, et al. Conversion of blood androgens to estrogens in normal adult men and women. *J Clin Invest.* 1969;48:2191-2201.

129. Luke JL, et al. Sudden cardiac death during exercise in a weight lifter using anabolic androgenic steroids: pathological and toxicological findings. *J Forensic Sci.* 1990; 35: 1441-1447.

130. Macintyre JG. Growth hormone and athletes. *Sports Med.* 1987;4:129-142.

131. Mahesh VB, Greenblatt RB. In vivo conversion of dehydroepiandrosterone and androstenedione to testosterone in human. *Acta Endocrinol.* 1962;41:400-406.

132. Majewska MD, et al. The neurosteroid dehydroepiandrosterone sulfate is an allosteric antagonist of the GABAA receptor. *Brain Res.* 1990;526:143-146.

133. Maltin CA, et al. The effect of a growth promoting drug, clenbuterol, on fibre frequency and area in hind limb muscles from young male rats. *Biosci Rep.* 1986;6:293-299.

134. Maron BJ. Sudden death in young athletes. *N Engl J Med.* 2003;349:1064-1075.

135. Maron BJ. Risk stratification and role of implantable defibrillators for prevention of sudden death in patients with hypertrophic cardiomyopathy. *Circ J.* 2010;74:2271-2282.

136. Maron BJ, et al. Global epidemiology and demographics of commotio cordis. *Heart Rhythm.* 2011;8:1969-1971.

137. Maron BJ, et al. Causes of sudden death in competitive athletes. *J Am Coll Cardiol.* 1986;7:204-214.

138. Maron BJ, et al. Incidence of cardiovascular sudden deaths in Minnesota high school athletes. *Heart Rhythm.* 2013;10:374-347.

139. Maropis C, Yesalis CE. Intramuscular abscess. Another anabolic steroid danger. *Physician Sports Med.* 1994;22:105-107.

140. Marraccini ME, et al. Neurocognitive enhancement or impairment? A systematic meta-analysis of prescription stimulant effects on processing speed, decision-making, planning, and cognitive perseveration. *Exp Clin Psychopharmacol.* 2016;24:269-284.

141. Maschio G. Erythropoietin and systemic hypertension. *Nephrol Dial Transplant.* 1995;10(suppl 2):74-79.

142. McNaughton LR, et al. The effects of creatine supplementation on high-intensity exercise performance in elite performers. *Eur J Appl Physiol Occup Physiol.* 1998;78:236-240.

143. McNutt RA, et al. Acute myocardial infarction in a 22-year-old world class weight lifter using anabolic steroids. *Am J Cardiol.* 1988;62:164.

144. Melchert RB, et al. The effect of anabolic-androgenic steroids on primary myocardial cell cultures. *Med Sci Sports Exerc.* 1992;24:206-212.

145. Melchior CL, Ritzmann RF. Dehydroepiandrosterone is an anxiolytic in mice on the plus maze. *Pharmacol Biochem Behav.* 1994;47:437-441.

146. Mendoza C. Use of niacin in attempts to defeat urine drug testing-five states, January-September 2006. *MMWR Morb Mortal Wkly Rep.* 2007;56:365-366.

147. Mittal MK, et al. Toxicity from the use of niacin to beat urine drug screening. *Ann Emerg Med.* 2007;50:587-590.

148. Mooradian AD, et al. Biological actions of androgens. *Endocr Rev.* 1987;8:1-28.

149. Morales AJ, et al. Effects of replacement dose of dehydroepiandrosterone in men and women of advancing age. *J Clin Endocrinol Metab.* 1994;78:1360-1367.

150. Morkeberg J. Detection of autologous blood transfusions in athletes: a historical perspective. *Transfus Med Rev.* 2012;26:199-208.

151. Morkeberg J, et al. Detecting autologous blood transfusions: a comparison of three passport approaches and four blood markers. *Scand J Med Sci Sports.* 2011;21:235-243.

152. Mosher DS, et al. A mutation in the myostatin gene increases muscle mass and enhances racing performance in heterozygote dogs. *PLoS Genet.* 2007;3:e79.

153. Muller RK, et al. Introduction to the application of capillary gas chromatography of performance-enhancing drugs in doping control. *J Chromatogr A.* 1999;843:275-285.

154. Narkar VA, et al. AMPK and PPARdelta agonists are exercise mimetics. *Cell.* 2008; 134:405-415.

155. Nemechek PM. Anabolic steroid users—another potential risk group for HIV infection. *N Engl J Med.* 1991;325:357.

156. Nicholls AR, et al. Children's first experience of taking anabolic-androgenic steroids CAN occur before their 10th birthday: a systematic review identifying 9 factors that Predicted doping among young people. *Front Psychol.* 2017;8:1015.

157. Overly WL, et al. Androgens and hepatocellular carcinoma in an athlete. *Ann Intern Med.* 1984;100:158-159.

158. Ozcelik O, et al. The effects of anabolic androgenic steroid abuse on gingival tissues. *J Periodontol.* 2006;77:1104-1109.

159. Parana R, et al. Intravenous vitamin complexes used in sporting activities and transmission of HCV in Brazil. *Am J Gastroenterol.* 1999;94:857-858.

160. Parisotto R, et al. A novel method utilising markers of altered erythropoiesis for the detection of recombinant human erythropoietin abuse in athletes. *Haematologica.* 2000;85:564-572.

161. Parr MK, et al. Distinction of clenbuterol intake from drug or contaminated food of animal origin in a controlled administration trial—the potential of enantiomeric separation for doping control analysis. *Food Addit Contam Part A Chem Anal Control Expo Risk Assess.* 2017;34:525-535.

162. Pascual JA, et al. Recombinant erythropoietin and analogues: a challenge for doping control. *Ther Drug Monit.* 2004;26:175-179.

163. Pasman WJ, et al. The effect of different dosages of caffeine on endurance performance time. *Int J Sports Med.* 1995;16:225-230.

164. Pates R, Temple D. *The Use of Anabolic Steroids in Wales.* Cardiff, Wales: Welsh Committee on Drug Misuse; 1992.

165. Pedersen TH, et al. Intracellular acidosis enhances the excitability of working muscle. *Science*. 2004;305:1144-1147.

166. Pierard GE. [Image of the month. Gymnasium acne: a fulminant doping acne]. *Rev Med Liege*. 1998;53:441-443.

167. Pierard-Franchimont C, et al. Mechanical properties of skin in recombinant human growth factor abusers among adult bodybuilders. *Dermatology*. 1996;192:389-392.

168. Poortmans JR, et al. Effect of short-term creatine supplementation on renal responses in men. *Eur J Appl Physiol Occup Physiol*. 1997;76:566-567.

169. Poortmans JR, Francaux M. Long-term oral creatine supplementation does not impair renal function in healthy athletes. *Med Sci Sports Exerc*. 1999;31:1108-1110.

170. Pope HG, Katz DL. Affective and psychotic symptoms associated with anabolic steroid use. *Am J Psychiatry*. 1988;145:487-490.

171. Pope HG, Katz DL. Psychiatric and medical effects of anabolic-androgenic steroid use: a controlled study of 160 athletes. *Arch Gen Psychiatry*. 1994;51:375-382.

172. Powrie JK, et al. Detection of growth hormone abuse in sport. *Growth Horm IGF Res*. 2007;17:220-226.

173. Prat J, et al. Wilms tumor in an adult associated with androgen abuse. *JAMA*. 1977;237:2322-2323.

174. Radakovich J, et al. Rate of anabolic-androgenic steroid use among students in junior high school. *J Am Board Fam Pract*. 1993;6:341-345.

175. Reverter JL, et al. Self-induced insulin hypoglycemia in a bodybuilder. *Arch Intern Med*. 1994;154:225-226.

176. Rich JD, et al. The infectious complications of anabolic-androgenic steroid injection. *Int J Sports Med*. 1999;20:563-566.

177. Rich JD, et al. Abscess related to anabolic-androgenic steroid injection. *Med Sci Sports Exerc*. 1999;31:207-209.

178. Rich JD, et al. Insulin use by bodybuilders *JAMA*. 1998;279:1613-1614.

179. Rickert VI, et al. Human growth hormone: a new substance of abuse among adolescents? *Clin Pediatr (Phila)*. 1992;31:723-726.

180. Ricks CA, et al. Use of a beta-agonist to alter fat and muscle deposition in steers. *J Anim Sci*. 1984;59:1247-1255.

181. Riggs BL, Hartmann LC. Selective estrogen-receptor modulators—mechanisms of action and application to clinical practice. *N Engl J Med*. 2003;348:618-629.

182. Roberts JT, Essenhigh DM. Adenocarcinoma of prostate in 40-year-old body-builder. *Lancet*. 1986;2:742.

183. Rosner F, Khan MT. Renal cell carcinoma following prolonged testosterone therapy. *Arch Intern Med*. 1992;152:426, 429.

184. Rupp JC, et al. Effect of sodium-bicarbonate ingestion on blood and muscle pH and exercise performance. *Med Sci Sports Exerc*. 1983;15:115-115.

185. Russell-Jones DL, Umpleby M. Protein anabolic action of insulin, growth hormone and insulin-like growth factor I. *Eur J Endocrinol*. 1996;135:631-642.

186. Salleras L, et al. Epidemiologic study of an outbreak of clenbuterol poisoning in Catalonia, Spain. *Public Health Rep*. 1995;110:338-342.

187. Salmonson T, et al. The pharmacokinetics of recombinant human erythropoietin after intravenous and subcutaneous administration to healthy subjects. *Br J Clin Pharmacol*. 1990;29:709-713.

188. Salomon F, et al. The effects of treatment with recombinant human growth hormone on body composition and metabolism in adults with growth hormone deficiency. *N Engl J Med*. 1989;321:1797-1803.

189. Saudan C, et al. Testosterone and doping control. *Br J Sports Med*. 2006;40(suppl 1): i21-24.

190. Schmidt W, et al. How valid is the determination of hematocrit values to detect blood manipulations? *Int J Sports Med*. 2000;21:133-138.

191. Schmidt W, et al. Blood gas transport properties in endurance-trained athletes living at different altitudes. *Int J Sports Med*. 1990;11:15-21.

192. Schmidt W, et al. Effects of chronic hypoxia and exercise on plasma erythropoietin in high-altitude residents. *J Appl Physiol*. 1993;74:1874-1878.

193. Schuelke M, et al. Myostatin mutation associated with gross muscle hypertrophy in a child. *N Engl J Med*. 2004;350:2682-2688.

194. Schumacher J, et al. Large hepatic hematoma and intraabdominal hemorrhage associated with abuse of anabolic steroids. *N Engl J Med*. 1999;340:1123-1124.

195. Scott MJ Jr, et al. Linear keloids resulting from abuse of anabolic androgenic steroid drugs. *Cutis*. 1994;53:41-43.

196. Scott MJ, Scott MJ Jr. HIV infection associated with injections of anabolic steroids. *JAMA*. 1989;262:207-208.

197. Shaskey DJ, Green GA. Sports haematology. *Sports Med*. 2000;29:27-38.

198. Shiozawa Z, et al. Cerebral hemorrhagic infarction associated with anabolic steroid therapy for hypoplastic anemia. *Angiology*. 1986;37:725-730.

199. Siegler JC, et al. Mechanistic insights into the efficacy of sodium bicarbonate supplementation to improve athletic performance. *Sports Med Open*. 2016;2:41.

200. Sklarek HM, et al. AIDS in a bodybuilder using anabolic steroids. *N Engl J Med*. 1984;311:1701.

201. Smathers RL, et al. Computed tomography of fatal hepatic rupture due to peliosis hepatis. *J Comput Assist Tomogr*. 1984;8:768-769.

202. Snow RJ, Murphy RM. Creatine and the creatine transporter: a review. *Mol Cell Biochem*. 2001;224:169-181.

203. Snow RJ, Murphy RM. Factors influencing creatine loading into human skeletal muscle. *Exerc Sport Sci Rev*. 2003;31:154-158.

204. Soe KL, et al. Liver pathology associated with the use of anabolic-androgenic steroids. *Liver*. 1992;12:73-79.

205. Speer O, et al. Creatine transporters: a reappraisal. *Mol Cell Biochem*. 2004;256-257: 407-424.

206. Starka L. Epitestosterone. *J Steroid Biochem Mol Biol*. 2003;87:27-34.

207. Stohlawetz PJ, et al. Effects of erythropoietin on platelet reactivity and thrombopoiesis in humans. *Blood*. 2000;95:2983-2989.

208. Stricker PR. Other ergogenic agents. *Clin Sports Med*. 1998;17:283-297.

209. Sturmi JE, Diorio DJ. Anabolic agents. *Clin Sports Med*. 1998;17:261-282.

210. Su TP, et al. Neuropsychiatric effects of anabolic steroids in male normal volunteers. *JAMA*. 1993;269:2760-2764.

211. Takala TE, et al. Effects of training and anabolic steroids on collagen synthesis in dog heart. *Eur J Appl Physiol Occup Physiol*. 1991;62:1-6.

212. Thevis M, et al. New drugs and methods of doping and manipulation. *Drug Discov Today*. 2008;13:59-66.

213. Thevis M, et al. Annual banned-substance review: analytical approaches in human sports drug testing. *Drug Test Anal*. 2015;7:1-20.

214. Thevis M, et al. Proteases in doping control analysis. *Int J Sports Med*. 2007;28:545-549.

215. Thevis M, et al. Does the analysis of the enantiomeric composition of clenbuterol in human urine enable the differentiation of illicit clenbuterol administration from food contamination in sports drug testing? *Rapid Commun Mass Spectrom*. 2013;27:507-512.

216. Thevis M, et al. Mass spectrometric determination of insulins and their degradation products in sports drug testing. *Mass Spectrom Rev*. 2008;27:35-50.

217. Tyler DB. The effect of amphetamine sulfate and some barbiturates on the fatigue produced by prolonged wakefulness. *Am J Physiol*. 1947;150:253-262.

218. Urhausen A, et al. Are the cardiac effects of anabolic steroid abuse in strength athletes reversible? *Heart*. 2004;90:496-501.

219. Urhausen A, et al. One- and two-dimensional echocardiography in bodybuilders using anabolic steroids. *Eur J Appl Physiol Occup Physiol*. 1989;58:633-640.

220. Van Camp SP, et al. Nontraumatic sports death in high school and college athletes. *Med Sci Sports Exerc*. 1995;27:641-647.

221. van de Kerkhof DH, et al. Evaluation of testosterone/epitestosterone ratio influential factors as determined in doping analysis. *J Anal Toxicol*. 2000;24:102-115.

222. van Loon LJ, et al. Effects of creatine loading and prolonged creatine supplementation on body composition, fuel selection, sprint and endurance performance in humans. *Clin Sci (Lond)*. 2003;104:153-162.

223. Vance ML, Mauras N. Growth hormone therapy in adults and children. *N Engl J Med*. 1999;341:1206-1216.

224. Vergouwen PC, et al. Haematocrit in elite athletes. *Int J Sports Med*. 1999;20:538-541.

225. Walker JB. Creatine: biosynthesis, regulation, and function. *Adv Enzymol Rel Areas Mol Biol*. 1979;50:177-242.

226. Walter E, Mockel J. Images in clinical medicine. Peliosis hepatis. *N Engl J Med*. 1997;337:1603.

227. Widder RA, et al. Candida albicans endophthalmitis after anabolic steroid abuse. *Lancet*. 1995;345:330-331.

228. Wilson JD. Androgen abuse by athletes. *Endocr Rev*. 1988;9:181-199.

229. Yesalis CE, et al. Trends in anabolic-androgenic steroid use among adolescents. *Arch Pediatr Adolesc Med*. 1997;151:1197-1206.

230. Yesalis CE, et al. Anabolic steroid use: indications of habituation among adolescents. *J Drug Educ*. 1989;19:103-116.

231. Zelman G, et al. Erythropoietin overdose treated with emergency erythropheresis. *J Toxicol Clin Toxicol*. 1999;37:602-603.

232. Zeman RJ, et al. Slow to fast alterations in skeletal muscle fibers caused by clenbuterol, a beta 2-receptor agonist. *Am J Physiol*. 1988;254:E726-E732.

233. Zuliani U, et al. Effects of anabolic steroids, testosterone, and HGH on blood lipids and echocardiographic parameters in body builders. *Int J Sports Med*. 1989;10:62-66.

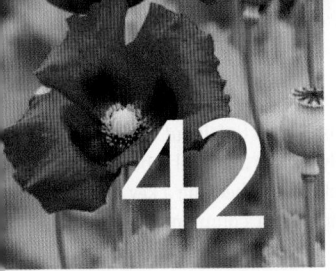

42 ESSENTIAL OILS

Lauren Kornreich Shawn

INTRODUCTION

Essential oils are a class of volatile oils that are extracted through steam distillation or are cold pressed from the leaves, flowers, bark, wood, fruit, or peel of a single parent plant. The term *essential* refers to the essence of a plant rather than an indispensable component of the oil or a vital biologic function. These compounds are a mixture of complex hydrocarbons that give the oil its aroma and potential therapeutic properties and that occasionally cause toxicity. More than 500 essential oils exist and are typically categorized into five chemical groups: terpenes, quinines, substituted benzenes, aromatic/aliphatic esters, and phenols and aromatic/aliphatic alcohols.

HISTORY AND EPIDEMIOLOGY

The potential for toxicity arises from several aspects of oil production, use, and regulation. These oils are not under regulation by the US Food and Drug Administration (FDA); therefore, there is no standard for manufacturing, leading to variability in active ingredients and adulterants with each producer. Furthermore, there is no standardized nomenclature for many of these herbs or for the exact chemical composition of a specific oil. Even with the strictest production guidelines, oils vary by the environment the plant was grown in and by part of the plant primarily used in production. Sometimes these differences are used to confer a particular property to the oil in terms of aroma or perceived therapeutic benefit.

Therapeutic use of essential oils can be traced back thousands of years in history to the ancient Greeks and ancient Egyptians, and it is also described in biblical writings. The first documents detailing an actual distillation process date back to the ninth century, when such oils were imported into Europe from the Middle East.[185] By the 16th century, concepts of separating fatty oils and essential oils from aromatic water became more defined, and oils were used frequently for fragrance, flavoring, and medicinal purposes. By the 19th century, these processes became industrialized, and specific chemicals could be identified and mass produced. Essential oils fell out of favor in the early 20th century as new medications and a desire for modernization developed. However, in the latter part of the 20th century, resurgence in interest and use of essential oils developed as many people deemed natural products to be safer and more environmentally benign. This chapter highlights some of the most commonly used oils for medicinal purposes that also have the greatest potential for toxicity.

Absinthe

Thujone

History

Artemisia absinthium is more commonly known as wormwood because of its use as an anthelmintic in ancient times. It is a member of the Compositae family, which also includes ragweed, chrysanthemums, marigolds, and daisies.[164] Absinthe is a liqueur composed of ethanol, oil of wormwood, and various other herbs, and it is known for its green color and bitter taste. It became a favorite among the artists and poets of Paris during the city's Belle Époque in the 19th century. Bohemian society enjoyed the drink by pouring water on top of a sugar cube that was suspended over a glass of absinthe. The addition of sugar water not only made the drink more palatable but also enhanced the herbal aroma and green coloration, which was referred to as the "louche effect."[120] This ritual was commonly performed in the early evening, and thus the "green hour" was akin to a Parisian "happy hour."[12]

The earliest recorded use of wormwood is found in the Ebers papyrus, which covers writings from 3550 to 1550 B.C. in Egypt.[12] During the first century A.D., Pliny described the anthelmintic properties of wormwood in *Historia Naturalis*. Dioscorides' *De Materia Medica*, which was considered an authoritative medical text through the Middle Ages, described the ability of wormwood not only to treat intestinal worms but also to repel fleas and other pests with topical application.[12] For millennia, available wine was commonly fortified with wormwood, and the formulation is still known today, albeit in much more dilute concentrations, as vermouth (derived from the German word for wormwood, *Wermut*).[139]

Absinthe was first distilled in Switzerland but came to prominence during the early 19th century, with Pernod's distillery in France.[120] During the French-Algerian wars of the 19th century, absinthe was used medicinally by the French troops to ward off infection and prevent dysentery.[119] Subsequently, the returning troops introduced the drink to French society. As early as 1850, descriptions of toxicity were documented. By the 1910s, many countries had made it illegal. In the 20th century, thujone was discovered to be the toxic component of absinthe. Absinthe is still available as Pernod, a formulation that is free of thujone. However, thujone-containing absinthe, as well as recipes for making it at home, can be obtained on the Internet.

Pharmacology

The bitter taste and anthelmintic properties come from the lactones absinthin and anabsinthin.[164] However, the toxicity of wormwood is due to its thujone content. Thujone is a monoterpene ketone that exists in α- and β-diastereoisomeric forms. Oil of wormwood may contain up to 70% thujone (α- and β-thujone).[164] The amount of the β isomer often exceeds that of α-thujone but is less toxic.[96] After oral absorption, both isomers undergo species specific hydroxylation reactions by the cytochrome (CYP) P450 enzymes and are subsequently glucuronidated and renally eliminated.[96] α-Thujone is metabolized primarily to 7-hydroxy α-thujone by CYP3A4 in humans, but there are at least six other metabolites, some of which are more prominent in other animal models.[95] The 7-hydroxy metabolite achieves a higher concentration in the brain, but it is less potent in binding the γ-aminobutyric acid (GABA)$_A$ receptor and is less toxic compared with its parent compound.[96]

Pathophysiology

α-Thujone is the more toxic of the two isomers and is a noncompetitive GABA$_A$ receptor antagonist, similar to picrotoxin.[96] This antagonism causes neuroexcitation, which results in hallucinations or seizures in a dose-dependent fashion. Ethanol enhances GABA activity and has a protective effect by reducing seizures in mice.[96] In the 1970s, it was speculated that thujone mediated the psychotropic effects of absinthe via cannabinoid receptors. However, further research demonstrated that despite low affinity for the CB1 and CB2 receptors, thujone failed to evoke any chemical signaling from binding.[132] Currently, research suggests that the psychotropic effects are mediated by the ability of α-thujone to desensitize the 5-HT$_3$ receptor.[53]

Thujones induce the synthesis of 5-aminolevulinic acid synthetase, leading to increased porphyrin production.[23] Individuals with defects in heme synthesis develop a porphyrialike syndrome upon ingestion of thujones. Some have speculated that Vincent Van Gogh had porphyria secondary to ingestion of absinthe and other volatile oils.

Clinical Features

Clinical features of acute toxicity are similar to those of ethanol intoxication, including euphoria and confusion, which can progress to restlessness, visual hallucinations, and delirium. Seizures have also occurred. Studies in 19th-century France revealed that the oil of wormwood component in absinthe, rather than the ethanol or other aromatic herbs, was responsible for auditory and visual hallucinations and seizures in humans and dogs.[6] Absinthism was recognized as a disease distinct from alcoholism as early as 1850s. It was characterized by delirium, hallucinations, tremors, and seizures. Although thujone is the purported xenobiotic in the development of these symptoms, the patients also drank excessive amounts of ethanol, so differentiating this syndrome from chronic sequelae of alcoholism is difficult.[6]

Rhabdomyolysis and acute kidney injury (AKI) are also reported after ingestion of oil of wormwood intended for preparation as absinthe.[186] The etiology of the rhabdomyolysis is unknown.

Camphor

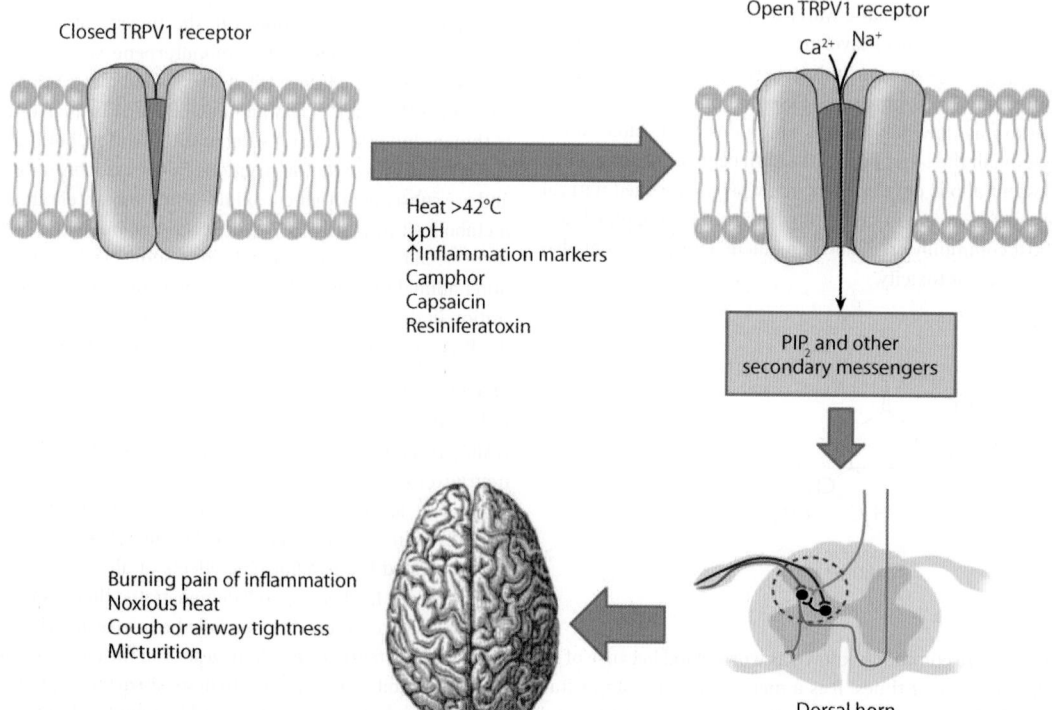

History

Originally derived from the bark of the camphor tree (*Cinnamomum camphora*), camphor has been widely used for centuries. It was described in writings from Marco Polo's visits to China, and in the 16th century it was referred to as the "balsam of disease."[13] Camphor has been used as an abortifacient, a contraceptive, a cold remedy, an aphrodisiac, an *anti*aphrodisiac, a lactation suppressor, and an antiseptic.[10,83] In the late 19th and early 20th centuries, it was also regarded as a cardiac stimulant and used extensively to treat congestive heart failure and cardiovascular compromise during influenza outbreaks.[60,78,81,127,129] By the 1920s, studies demonstrated that camphor was not

an effective cardiovascular stimulant, and its use began to fall out of favor.[129] In the 20th century, camphor was predominantly used as a topical rubefacient to provide local analgesia and antipruritic effects. It also became a key ingredient in paregoric (camphorated tincture of opium), a common household remedy for diarrhea and cough used until 1970. Throughout the 20th century, camphor was also available as a nonprescription remedy in the forms of camphorated oil, which was 20% camphor in cottonseed oil, and spirits of camphor, which was 10% camphor in alcohol. Toxicity occurred in cases in which camphorated oil was mistaken for castor oil and ingested in large amounts.[13,40,179] In 1982, the FDA limited any product from containing more than 11% camphor and banned camphorated oil after numerous reports of significant morbidity and mortality. It was also used extensively as a moth repellant. Today, camphor is found in topical products such as Vick's Vapo-Rub and Tiger Balm. Despite restrictions on its sale by the FDA, concentrated camphor products are still found in the United States. They are illegally sold in various communities for use as pesticides and medicinal remedies.[111]

Pharmacology

Camphor is a bicyclic monoterpene ketone that is rapidly absorbed from the gastrointestinal (GI) tract. Serum concentrations are detected within 15 minutes of ingestion.[144,149] It is also readily absorbed from the skin and mucous membranes.[111] It also crosses the placenta and blood–brain barrier.[149] A detectable concentration was found in amniotic fluid 20 hours after maternal ingestion.[149] Camphor is very lipophilic with a large volume of distribution. It is metabolized in the liver by CYP2A6 to 5-exo-hydroxycamphor, but other studies using animal models have cited 5-endo-hydroxycamphor and 3-hydroxycamphor as significant metabolites.[85,152,179] These metabolites then undergo glucuronidation and are excreted in the urine.[152]

Pathophysiology

The mechanism for seizures is still unknown. Camphor desensitizes the transient receptor potential vanilloid subtype 1 (TRPV1) channel, a nonspecific cation channel that mediates thermosensation and nociception in the peripheral nervous system (Fig. 42–1).[191] Currently, there are seven known

FIGURE 42–1. The transient receptor potential vanilloid subtype 1 (TRPV1) receptor is a nonspecific cation channel that is located on the skin and bladder, in the peripheral nociceptors and the dorsal horn of the spinal cord, and in the airway. Stimulation by heat, acidemia, and inflammation increases its activity; camphor, capsaicin, and resiniferatoxin are direct agonists. When open, TRPV1 stimulates intracellular signaling via PIP_2 to relay sensation of burning pain, noxious heat, airway tightness, and micturition.

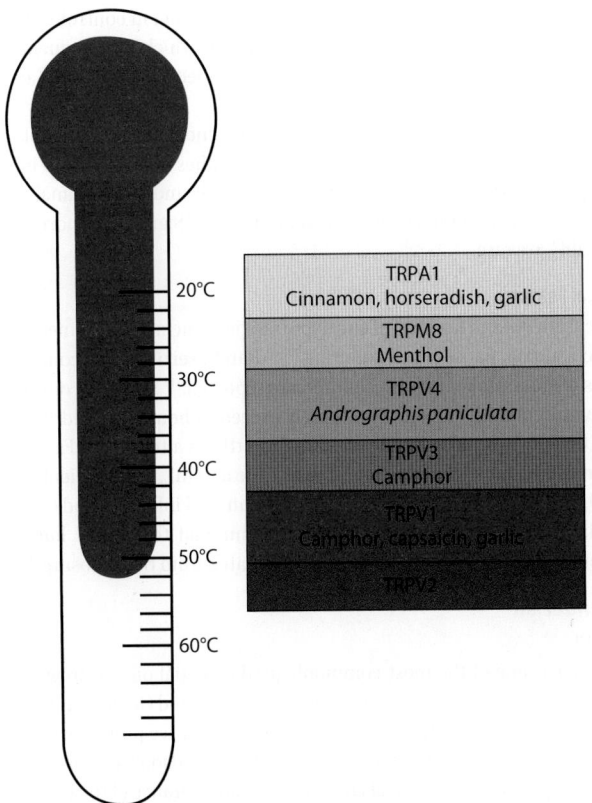

FIGURE 42–2. Schematic of the seven known mammalian thermo–transient receptor potential (TRP) channels based on their temperature threshold for activation. Certain natural xenobiotics can activate these receptors, which may lead to burning or heat sensation. Transient receptor potential A1 cation channel subfamily M member 8 (TRPM8) mediates cold sensation in sensory neurons. Menthol and eucalyptus' cooling and analgesic effects are thought to be caused by TRPM8 activation. Camphor desensitizes TRP vanilloid subtype 1 (TRPV1), which could explain the initial hot and then cool sensation when applied to skin. Camphor antagonizes TRPA1, which may mediate its antitussive effects.

transient receptors (of 27 known receptors within the family) that perceive temperatures ranging from noxious heat to noxious cold, depending on the type or combination of receptors activated (Fig. 42–2).[138,141,184] These receptors are primarily expressed by small-diameter sensory neurons of the dorsal root ganglion and trigeminal nerves.[18] Similar to other topical analgesics with effects on these channels, it is postulated that desensitization mediates the analgesic and cooling effect of topical camphor products. Transient receptor potential A1, with TRPA1, is also implicated as an important part in the production of cough. Camphor's antitussive effects are presumed to be through the desensitization of TRPV1 and antagonism of TRPA1 (Fig. 42–2).[76,131] There are TRPV1 receptors found in the central nervous system (CNS), but it is unknown whether they are implicated in the CNS effect of camphor toxicity. Autopsies of human case reports and animal studies demonstrate neuronal necrosis and degeneration on pathology, but the mechanism of action remains elusive.[166]

Hepatotoxicity is also reported and can range from a mild elevation in aminotransferase concentrations to fulminant hepatic failure. Children are more susceptible to hepatotoxicity because they have relatively immature liver enzymes and glucuronidation systems. The hepatotoxicity presents similarly to Reye syndrome with vomiting, rapid neurologic deterioration to coma, and hepatomegaly, but it does not have the same characteristic findings on biopsy.[103]

Clinical Features

Camphor toxicity is reported after nasal, topical, inhalational, and oral administration.[40,60,144,162,173,182] Gastrointestinal signs and symptoms developed within 5 to 90 minutes after ingestion.[14] Case reports of delayed onset

of symptoms are complicated by unknown time of ingestion or concomitant illness.[128] In a retrospective review of 182 cases, no patient developed symptoms more than 6 hours after ingestion.[83] Two grams of camphor can cause significant toxicity in adults when ingested, and children have died from as little as 0.7 to 1 g of 20% camphorated oil (1 tsp).[39,166] Other reports describe children having seizures but surviving after ingesting 0.5 to 6 g of camphor.[158]

Generally, the first effects are related to GI irritation and include nausea and vomiting, although patients who were exposed via topical or inhalational administration rarely have GI symptoms. Patients complain of feeling warm, faint, and vertiginous and have headaches.[104] Severe effects and findings include confusion, agitation, delirium, and hallucinations.[47,60,173] Seizures are common and usually develop within minutes to a few hours of exposure.[134] Status epilepticus is reported.[47,111]

Clove Oil

OH
OCH₃

CH₂

Eugenol

History

Clove oil is extracted from the plant *Syzygium aromaticum*, also known as *Eugenia aromatica*. This evergreen plant is native to the Maluku islands of Indonesia (traditionally known as the Spice Islands). Its dried, unopened buds are known as cloves, a descriptive name derived from the Latin word *clavus*, meaning nail. During the Chinese Han dynasty, subjects were required to chew cloves to mask bad breath when appearing before the emperor. In medieval and Renaissance Europe, cloves were considered to be a valuable commodity. They were used for flavoring and fragrance, as well as for medicinal purposes, and that tradition remains intact today. The first recorded medicinal use of cloves in Western society is found in *The Practice of Physic*, which was written in French in the 1640s and translated into English in 1687.[45] Clove oil is commonly mixed with zinc oxide as a sealant in dentistry, a practice that dates as early as 1873.[98] Clove oil is still used to alleviate toothaches, and one study found it just as effective as topical benzocaine for analgesia.[3]

Pharmacology

Typically, clove oil contains 60% to 90% eugenol, which is the primary active component. Eugenol undergoes sulfonation and glucuronidation in the liver, with a minor pathway involving the CYP enzymes to form a reactive intermediate that requires glutathione for proper elimination.[177]

Pathophysiology

The anesthetic properties of eugenol are mediated by blockade of various ion currents in nerves. This was initially demonstrated by the ability to block conduction of action potentials in frog sciatic nerves.[115] Given the structural similarity to capsaicin, studies sought to determine if the effects were mediated by a common mechanism. Studies of rat dorsal root ganglion cells suggest that eugenol acts in both a capsaicin receptor mediated pathway and by an independent pathway.[136] Capsaicin requires the TRPV1 receptor to inhibit voltage-gated calcium channels to desensitize peripheral nociceptors, but eugenol does not (Fig. 42–1).[122,135] Eugenol also inhibits voltage-gated sodium channels independently of TRPV1, and this likely mediates its anesthetic effects.[140] Eugenol similarly blocks voltage-gated potassium channels in neurons, which suggests a possible mechanism for the irritating effects of eugenol because potassium efflux is required to terminate action potentials and neurotransmitter release.[125]

Studies with rat hepatocytes demonstrated that eugenol causes glutathione depletion and subsequent hepatotoxicity in a dose- and time-dependent manner. The loss of glutathione occurred before the onset of cell death in these studies.[177] Furthermore, N-acetylcysteine (NAC) was able to prevent glutathione depletion and cell death. Eugenol inhibits prostaglandin synthetase, which would support the claims for its use as an antiinflammatory xenobiotic in dentistry.[98]

Clinical Features

There are several reports of allergic reactions and local irritation when eugenol zinc oxide was used for dental procedures.[17,116,156] There are fewer case reports of systemic toxicity from other forms of exposure. However, infants and children ingesting clove oil are reported to develop depressed mental status, anion gap metabolic acidosis, and hepatotoxicity complicated by coagulopathy and hypoglycemia.[27,68,89,102,121]

A single case report described a 24-year-old woman who developed permanent infraorbital anesthesia and anhidrosis after spilling a small amount of clove oil on her face in an attempt to relieve a toothache.[99]

Acute respiratory distress syndrome (ARDS) is reported with intravenous (IV) administration of clove oil. Similar findings of perivascular, interstitial, and alveolar edema are found in animal studies. The proposed mechanism is oxidant mediated, but this has not been verified.[112,189]

Eucalyptus Oil

Eucalyptol

History

Oil of eucalyptus is derived primarily from *Eucalyptus globulus*, a tree native to Australia. Eighteenth-century British explorers noted that the aboriginal people traditionally used eucalyptus as a fever remedy, so they brought it to England for further examination. The introduction of eucalyptus oil to the West led to an increased demand because it was increasingly used to treat the symptoms of the common cold and influenza. The oil was believed to be so effective that there were public campaigns to grow the trees in areas of Europe stricken with malaria and other infectious diseases. Great effort was made to determine how best to cultivate these plants in the colder, damper European environment.[8,150] In the 19th and early 20th centuries, eucalyptus oil was a common household remedy for coughs and fevers, and it was also used as an antiseptic.[44] It was even reported as effective in treating hemorrhage, burns, and diabetes.[9,165,178]

Pharmacology

Eucalyptus oil contains almost 70% eucalyptol, a monoterpene cyclic ether also known as 1,8-cineole. It is rapidly absorbed from the GI tract and metabolized by CYP3A4 and CYP3A5, to the 2-hydroxy and 3-hydroxy metabolites.[61]

Pathophysiology

Eucalyptus inhibits potassium-induced contractions of airway smooth muscles causing a myorelaxant effect, thus alleviating some patient's upper respiratory irritation.[126] However, eucalyptus also potentiates acetylcholine-induced contractions of the trachea in vitro, possibly by inhibiting acetylcholinesterase.[126] This finding would explain the upper respiratory irritation that commonly plagues workers who process eucalyptus trees for papers and other materials. Eucalyptol inhibits monocytes from producing several cytokines, particularly tumor necrosis factor (TNF)-α and interleukin (IL)-1β, from being produced.[106] It also suppresses arachidonic acid metabolism. These findings underlie the ability of eucalyptol to control

mucous hypersecretion; making it a potential adjunct in controlling asthma and chronic obstructive pulmonary disease, for which it is frequently used as an alternative medicine.[105,106,188] The cooling effects of eucalyptus are likely mediated by TRPM8 (Fig. 42–2).[30,174]

The mechanism of toxicity has yet to be elucidated. Eucalyptol affects the autonomic nervous system, but animal studies are difficult to interpret because mice seem relatively insensitive to the oil, and other animals require extremely high amounts to achieve toxic effect.[51,70] Significant morbidity and mortality are rare.

Clinical Features

Typical effects and findings of eucalyptus toxicity include drowsiness, slurred speech, ataxia, nausea, and vomiting.[72,169] Rarely, seizures and coma occur.[84] Cases of status epilepticus in children are reported.[117] Symptom onset is usually within minutes to hours and rarely exceeds 4 hours. In children, significant toxicity is reported after ingesting as little as a teaspoon. Fatalities are reported in adults who have ingested as little as 4 mL, but a patient survived a 120- to 200-mL ingestion after receiving mannitol infusions and dialysis.[72,84] Inhalational and dermal exposures have minimal toxicity as long as the patient is promptly removed or decontaminated from the exposure.[169]

Lavender Oil
History

Lavender is one of the most commonly used essential oils for fragrance and aromatherapy.[34] It was used by the ancient Romans and Greeks for its believed antimicrobial, carminative, sedative, and antidepressive properties. The oil is produced by steam distillation of the flower heads and foliage of the *Lavandula* species. However, the chemical composition and fragrance of the oil are determined by the proportion of flowers distilled within a particular batch.

There are four commonly used lavenders: *Lavandula latifolia*, a Mediterranean variety; *Lavandula angustifolia*, commonly known as English lavender (or *L. officinalis*); *Lavandula stoechas*, commonly known as French lavender; and *Lavandula x intermedia*, which is a sterile cross fertilization between *L. latifolia* and *L. angustifolia*.[34] The lavenders generally have the same major chemical constituents in their oils and ethnobotanical history, but some species have specific therapeutic benefits ascribed to them. For example, *L. stoechas* was traditionally used as a headache remedy, *L. latifolia* as an abortifacient, and *L. angustifolia* as a diuretic.[34] However, many of these effects, regardless of species used, have never been substantiated in the medical and scientific literature. Lavender oil is most commonly used in aromatherapy to enhance mood, decrease anxiety, or control pain. Most studies demonstrating improved pain control, decreased anxiety, or improved mood were small studies or poorly controlled. Silexin is an oral preparation of *L. agustifolia* that is sold as an anxiolytic in Germany. It is made under a standardized manufacturing process to decrease contaminants and increase the linalyl acetate concentration. Studies show it be noninferior to lorazepam or paroxetine in treatment of various anxiety disorders.[107,108]

Pharmacology

The main components of lavender oil are linalool, linalyl acetate, 1,8-cineole, β-ocimene, terpinen-4-ol, and camphor.[34] The proportion of each within a given batch of oil depends on the plant used and type of distillation. Plants with smaller camphor components, such as *L. angustifolia*, are used more for fragrance and cosmetic purposes because their aroma is considered to be more pleasant. Plants with higher camphor content are traditionally used for insect repellant and antimicrobial uses.

Linalool and linalyl acetate are the components believed to be responsible for the neuropsychiatric effects of lavender oil, specifically sedative and narcotic effects. These compounds are rapidly absorbed through the skin and can reach peak serum concentrations as soon as 19 minutes postexposure.[34,101] Studies in mice show that lavender oil acts on serotonin receptors, rather than GABA receptors, and this underlies its anxiolytic effects.[37,159] A single study involving positron emission tomography scans of people taking Silexin show the 5HT1$_A$ receptor as a likely binding site.[16] Linalool inhibits both nicotinic receptor–mediated acetylcholine release and glutamate release.[145,160]

Lavandula angustifolia has activity against methicillin-resistant *Staphylococcus aureus* and vancomycin-resistant *Enterococcus faecalis* as well as other bacteria.[190] Its potential as an antimicrobial and preservative in cosmetics is demonstrated.[118] Further research suggests that the linalool in lavender oil is responsible for its antimicrobial properties. Linalool was found to have a synergistic effect when added to other essential oils with known antimicrobial properties such as tea tree oil and bergamot.[93]

Pathophysiology

Lavender oil is very allergenic. Linalool is not electrophilic or chemically reactive, suggesting it would not be a contact allergen.[86] Linalyl acetate has an electrophilic center and is a weak allergen in studies.[163] However, both of these compounds immediately oxidize when exposed to air, generating hydroperoxides, which are strong allergens. This oxidation occurs regardless of whether pure linalool, linalyl acetate, or lavender oil is used.[86,163]

Several case series report the development of gynecomastia in prepubertal boys using lavender oil.[22,56,92,109] All the children in these reports had extensive endocrine evaluations, with no abnormalities detected, and in each case, the gynecomastia resolved when lavender oil was discontinued. Body washes and colognes containing lavender oil were frequently implicated as the source of exposure.[56,92] In vitro data showed that lavender oil elicits a dose-dependent increase in estrogen responsivity and antiandrogenic activity in breast cancer cell cultures, similar to the effects of estradiol.[92,109]

Clinical Features

The predominant clinical feature of exposure is contact dermatitis. Unexplained or "idiopathic" gynecomastia in prepubertal boys with negative endocrine evaluations should prompt questions regarding the use of these essential oils.

Nutmeg Oil

Myristicin

History

Nutmeg and mace originate from the evergreen tree *Myristica fragans*, which is native to the Maluku islands of Indonesia (Spice Islands) and was imported to Europe as early as the mid-12th century.[73,161] However, today, nutmeg is more commonly imported to the United States from Malaysia, Grenada, Trinidad, and other parts of the Caribbean.[161] The name *nutmeg* refers to the seed of the tree, which looks like a glossy brown nut. Mace is derived from the scarlet-colored aril that encloses the seed.

Although nutmeg is a common household spice and flavoring agent, it has been used for centuries for various ailments, including digestive disorders, cholera, rheumatic disease, psychiatric disorders, and pain.[73] Mace was used as an aphrodisiac, and nutmeg was commonly used in Europe and North America, albeit ineffectually, as an emmenagogue and abortifacient.[146] Indeed, most of the cases of nutmeg poisoning in the early 20th century were due to women attempting to terminate pregnancies or induce menses.[82] However, most cases of toxicity today are caused by people using nutmeg as a natural high.[1,33,143,155] The first reported case of nutmeg poisoning is attributed to Lobel, who described delirium in a pregnant woman who ingested 10 or 12 nutmeg seeds in 1576.[33] In 1832, the famous scientist Purkinje demonstrated the toxicity of nutmeg by ingesting seeds, causing delirium and then stupor.[82]

Pharmacology

The nutmeg seed yields 7% to 16% volatile oil, 4% to 8% of which is myristicin.[87] Myristicin is believed to be the psychoactive component of the oil, but some studies have brought that into question. It was initially hypothesized that myristicin was metabolized to the amphetamine derivative 3-methoxy-4,5-methylenedioxyamphetamine (MMDA) by the addition of ammonia to the allyl side chain. Elemicin, another main ingredient of the volatile oil, is metabolized to 3,4,5-trimethoxyamphetamine (TMA).[157] This was further supported by detection of MMDA by thin-layer chromatography of rat liver incubated with myristicin.[25] However, in vivo studies could neither replicate these results nor find evidence of the amphetamine derivatives. Gas chromatography of urine from rats and humans exposed to nutmeg, pure myristicin, or elemicin did not detect MMDA, TMA, or evidence of the original compounds.[21] However, other metabolites were found, suggesting extensive liver metabolism. It was later determined that CYP3A4 and CYP1A2 were primarily involved in the formation of the main metabolite of myristicin, 5-allyl-1-methoxy-2,3-dihydroxybenzene.[193]

Pathophysiology

Studies in mice suggest that nutmeg and fresh myristicin are monoamine oxidase inhibitors (MAOIs) but that excessive doses could reverse that effect.[181] However, nutmeg was less potent than known MAOIs on the market at the time. In the 1960s, nutmeg was studied as a possible antidepressant in five patients with mixed results, but a formal trial of nutmeg as a psychiatric medication was never conducted.[181] Data from an in vitro study show that nutmeg stimulates the cannabinoid system by inhibiting enzymes that degrade the body's own endocannabinoids. This study also demonstrated that nutmeg did not bind directly to cannabinoid receptors, serotonergic receptors, dopamine receptors, GABA receptors, or adrenergic receptors. The authors proposed that enzyme inhibition mediates the cannabinoidlike effects that occur in exposed patientss.[69]

Animal data show that nutmeg can induce tachycardia and increase the speed of conduction through the atrioventricular node in the acute setting, but chronic exposure caused bradycardia[154] The exact mechanism for this is unknown.

Cats appear to be exquisitely sensitive to nutmeg and develop not only acute mental status changes with nutmeg exposure but also liver damage, leading to hepatic encephalopathy.[180] This has not been reported in humans.

Clinical Features

Tachycardia, nausea, and dry mouth are common in acute exposures. Some patients develop GI distress and vomiting. Central nervous system effects and findings range from giddiness to a sense of detachment or impending doom to hallucinations and delusions.[1,11,46,82,142] Nutmeg ingestion rarely causes significant morbidity or mortality. Only two deaths have been reported. In 1887, an 8-year-old boy became comatose after ingesting two nutmegs and died the next day; however, he also received a wide variety of analeptics that likely were more harmful than the initial exposure.[33] The other case involved a detectable serum myristicin concentration on autopsy of a 55-year-old woman who had a toxic serum concentration of flunitrazepam and whose stomach contents smelled strongly of nutmeg.[170] It is unclear if the nutmeg contributed to her death. Several retrospective studies from poison control center data did not show any deaths or life-threatening toxicity. Of those hospitalized, the majority of patients had taken other drugs in addition to the nutmeg, complicating the clinical picture.[33,67] A single report describes seizures and altered mental status requiring intubation in a patient who intentionally ingested 39 g of ground nutmeg as a suicide attempt.[71]

Pennyroyal Oil

Pulegone

History

Oil of pennyroyal is derived from the plant *Mentha pulegium* from the Labiatae family. It has a mintlike odor and is still used as a flavoring and fragrance agent in foods and cosmetics. Its initial use was as a flea repellant. Pulegium is derived from the word *pulex*, which is Latin for flea.[80] Pennyroyal has been used for centuries as an emmemagogue and abortifacient, and most reported toxicities were from women ingesting large quantities to induce these effects. Dioscorides listed pennyroyal as an abortifacient in his *Da Materia Medica*, and the Greek playwright Aristophanes made frequent reference to it in his plays.[148] Women still occasionally use pennyroyal for these purposes today.

Pharmacology

The primary active ingredient in pennyroyal is pulegone, a monoterpene. In particular, $R(+)$-pulegone is the active isomer.[79] Pulegone is metabolized by the CYP450 enzymes into several metabolites, including menthofuran, which is thought to be the metabolite primarily responsible for hepatotoxicity, although other reactive intermediates are also implicated.[80,175]

Pathophysiology

In animal studies, pennyroyal causes centrilobular hepatic necrosis.[79] In a rat model, pulegone depletes glutathione in hepatocytes and in the plasma. Furthermore, hepatotoxicity is significantly increased in glutathione-depleted animals. However, another unknown reactive metabolite is also implicated because blocking the CYP450 system prevents glutathione depletion. Menthofuran had a minimal effect on glutathione concentrations in the plasma and liver, and its ability to cause hepatotoxicity was not affected by glutathione depletion, suggesting a role on another reactive metabolite.[176]

$R(+)$-Pulegone also causes necrosis in lung epithelium, but the mechanism remains unknown.[79] In addition, $R(+)$-pulegone decreases inward current from L-type calcium channels and blocks the inward rectifying potassium channels on the rat myocardium.[50]

Clinical Features

Common initial signs and symptoms are nausea, abdominal pain, and vomiting, often occurring within a few hours of exposure.[7] Central nervous system toxicity, including seizures and coma, develop in severe cases.[24,62] Ingestion of as little as 5 mL is implicated in severe CNS toxicity. However, in most cases, ingestion of 10 mL is primarily associated with GI symptoms and mild CNS symptoms such as dizziness and lethargy. Fatal cases involving liver failure, kidney failure, and disseminated intravascular coagulation occurred with ingestion of 15 mL, but these often involve large amounts or multiple doses over a short period of time.[2,172,183] In reported cases, patients either ingested a tea brewed from the leaves of *M. pulegium*, a tablet containing the herb, oil of pennyroyal, or essence of pennyroyal, which is an alcoholic preparation.[24,38,62,77] Most cases of severe toxicity involved women ingesting large amounts of the herb to induce an abortion; however, two cases involved confusing the leaves of *M. pulegium* for nontoxic mint leaves to make tea.[15]

Peppermint Oil

Menthol

History

Menthol or peppermint oil is one of the most commonly used flavoring agents in the world. It is derived from the distillation of leaves of the *Mentha piperita* herb, which is native to Europe and parts of Asia but easily grows in North America as well.[130] Before World War II, menthol was primarily exported from China and Japan, but as those trade routes became disrupted during and after the war; Brazil became the predominant exporter.[63] Peppermint flavor is common in oral care products, candies, cosmetics, pharmaceuticals, and beverages. Pure crystalline menthol was extracted from plants and introduced as a medicine in the 19th century. In the late 19th century, its use in upper respiratory illness was described, but the author cautioned that more information was needed to "become familiar with its actions and know its limitations."[64] However, menthol is still used today for many remedies with little supporting data. It is sold as an herbal remedy for pruritus, GI disorders such as irritable bowel syndrome, and cough and cold symptoms, as well as a topical analgesic.[192] Pure distilled peppermint oil is more expensive and primarily produced by the United States for toothpaste and other dental care products. Corn mint oil, also known for its minty scent and flavor, is derived from *Mentha arvensis* and contains 70% to 80% menthol. However, menthol derived from this plant has a more herbaceous flavor and is less commonly used commercially.[63]

Pharmacology

There are eight pairs of stereoisomers that exist for menthol, given its three asymmetric carbons on the central ring of the structure. However, only the (−) menthol form is found in nature and is the most potent.[63] Peppermint oil typically contains 30% to 55% menthol.[90]

Menthol is very lipid soluble and easily absorbed through the skin. Menthol is rapidly metabolized by the CYP450 system to primarily to *p*-menthane-3,8 diol and then glucuronidated and eliminated in the urine.[63] Menthol is a moderate inhibitor of CYP3A4, but its effects on the metabolism of other drugs such as the dihydropyridine calcium channel blockers are not clear.[59] In human pharmacokinetic studies, only glucuronidated menthol is detected in urine in ranges of 45% to 46% of the menthol ingested.[75] The plasma half-life of menthol glucuronide was determined to be 56.2 minutes and 42.6 minutes, respectively, when mint teas and candies were used.[75]

Pathophysiology

In the late 19th century, It was hypothesized that the cooling effects of menthol involved stimulation of a thermoreceptor. Many years later, two independent studies demonstrated the TRP cation channel subfamily M member 8 (TRPM8) is activated by both menthol and thermal stimuli in the cool to cold range of 46° to 82°F (8°–28°C) (Fig. 42–2).[141] This receptor TRPM8 is a member of the TRP family of excitatory ion channels (the same receptor family as TRPV1).[18] Menthol and cold stimuli increase intracellular calcium, which leads to depolarization and generation of an action potential. Some data suggest that the analgesic properties of menthol are mediated by its effects on sodium channels.[74]

Menthol was investigated as an adjunct to irritable bowel syndrome therapy. In vitro data with isolated animal ileum and jejunum tissue show that menthol reduces contractions by reducing calcium influx, even when such tissue was exposed to acetylcholine, histamine, and serotonin.[94] The proposed mechanism of action is L-type calcium channel blockade.[4] However, another study shows that menthol is a nicotinic receptor antagonist in the gastric mucosa, also causing smooth muscle relaxation.[5] In some countries, menthol is sold in an acid-resistant preparation as a carminative for irritable bowel symptoms. Menthol and peppermint oil both inhibit 5-HT$_3$ receptors in vitro as well as reduce serotonin-induced contractions of rat ileum, which could mediate some of the antiemetic effects.[90]

Menthol is commonly used to relieve the symptoms of upper respiratory infections, in particular rhinitis. However, despite the sensation of improved airflow and decreased congestion, menthol actually causes increased nasal congestion.[64,65] Inhalation of menthol, camphor, or eucalyptus did not decrease nasal resistance to airflow even though all of the participants reported an increased sensation of airflow.[29] Similar results were found for nasal menthol lozenges.[66]

Clinical Features

Application of menthol to skin or mucosa causes the sensation of coolness or warmth. Case reports regarding menthol toxicity are rare. One report pertains to Olbas oil, which contains 35% menthol. In addition to 35% eucalyptus oil, and other oils in smaller amounts. In this report, the child developed ataxia, nystagmus, and altered mental status.[137] A case report describes ARDS developing in a patient after an intentional IV injection of 5 mL of peppermint oil in a suicide attempt. Symptoms began within 2 hours of the exposure. Bronchoscopy and bronchoalveolar lavage did not show signs of aspiration or fat embolism as the etiology of the ARDS, suggesting direct cytotoxic injury from the peppermint oil.[19]

Pine Oil

α-Pinene

History

Pine oil is commonly used as a household cleaner, varnish, and polish. In the past, it had medicinal uses as an expectorant and topical liniment. Turpentine is an oleoresin solvent—a mixture of pine oils and resins distilled from the tree genus *Pinus*. Pine oil is also distilled from the same trees but does not include any resins. Turpentine is used as a degreaser and paint thinner. Pine oil is commonly found in Pine-Sol and similar household cleaners. These cleaners typically include 20% pine oil, 6% to 10% isopropyl alcohol, and other hydrocarbons.

Pharmacology

The lethal dose is in the range of 60 to 120 g in adults.[114] The major terpene is α-terpine. The major metabolite is bornyl acetate, which is produced by the enzymatic processes of hydration, hydroxylation, rearrangement, acetylation, and reduction in the liver.[114] The metabolites are excreted through the kidneys and lungs. Pine oil is readily absorbed, and clinical effects usually occur within 2 to 3 hours postingestion.[110]

Pathophysiology

Pine oil and turpentine are volatile hydrocarbon compounds with low viscosity. Aspiration and inhalational injury are common when low-viscosity hydrocarbons are ingested or inhaled (Chap. 105). Animals injected with pine oil develop ARDS, but the mechanism is unknown.[167,168]

Clinical Features

The most common reported symptoms are impaired mentation, psychomotor agitation, delirium, headache, nausea, ataxia, and GI distress. Gastrointestinal irritation and gastritis are reported, but actual perforation or high-grade lesions have not been found.[41] Acute kidney injury is also reported.[114] An isolated case report of hemorrhagic cystitis occurring after a patient ingested turpentine for several days to treat a cold has been described.[113] Fatalities are rare but are more likely to occur when the patient is an older adult.[187] The most severe outcomes involve an aspiration pneumonitis that can progress to ARDS or a secondary pneumonia.[26,110]

Tea Tree Oil
History

Tea tree oil is derived from the distillation of leaves of *Melaleuca alternifolia*, a plant that is native to Australia. The *Melaleuca* genus belongs to the Myrtaceae family and contains more than 230 species. The international standard for tea tree oil does not specify which *Melaleuca* species must be used but rather dictates a certain chemical content.[31] Traditionally,

M. alternifolia has been the primary source for the oil. Nevertheless, synonyms and ambiguous naming of various oils and plants make it difficult to identify the primary plant product. Tea tree oil is also known as melaleuca oil or ti tree oil in many cases. Furthermore, ti tree is the Maori and Samoan common name for plants of the *Cordyline* genus, a completely different plant.[31] There are oils from other *Melaleuca* species on the market that possess different chemical properties from that of tea tree oil, further complicating matters. Tea trees can also be known as paperbark trees, but paperbark oil may refer to oil from another type *Melaleuca* tree or even a nonrelated tree such as *Leptospermum* species.

The first reported use of *M. alternifolia* was in Australian Aborigines. Crushed leaves were inhaled to treat coughs and cold symptoms, and poultices of the leaves were applied to wounds. Oral histories describe swimming or bathing in healing lakes composed of decaying fallen tea tree leaves as a treatment for a variety of ailments.[31] The oil itself was not distilled until the 20th century, at which time it was touted as an antibacterial agent. Commercial production began after medicinal properties of the oil were first reported in the 1920s. Production slowed after World War II, presumably because of the increased use of antibiotics and decreased desire to use natural products. Renewed interest in the oil began in the 1970s, and production increased as well as became more standardized.

Pharmacology

Data on safety and toxicity are scant. Pharmacokinetic and pharmacodynamic data are limited. Animal studies and case reports of human poisoning demonstrate toxicity with oral exposure. The median lethal dose for rats is 1.9 to 2.6 mL/kg, and rats dosed 1.5 mL/kg appeared lethargic and ataxic.[31]

Tea tree oil is composed of terpene hydrocarbons and contains more than 100 components.[31] There can be variability in the composition of oils sold on the market, but there is an international standard stipulating that tea tree oil should contain at least 30% terpinen-4-ol, which is believed to be the primary antimicrobial agent and less than 15% 1,8-cineole, which is believed to be primarily responsible for the irritating properties.[31] There are other hydrocarbons found in tea tree oil that help make up its specific chemotype for the standard but are less involved in the presumed medicinal properties.

Pathophysiology

Tea tree oil is predominately used as a topical antiseptic, and its antimicrobial effects are the most studied use of the oil. It is bactericidal, but its mechanism of action is only partly elucidated. Tea tree oil, as a lipophilic hydrocarbon, disrupts the membranes of liposome model systems, supporting the hypothesis that it kills bacteria by disrupting their cell membranes.[43] Tea tree oil does not cause bacteria to lyse per se but makes them more susceptible to lysis when exposed to a hypertonic medium, or at least it causes an inability to recover from leakage of intracellular contents over time. This is demonstrated by leakage of potassium ions and 260-nm light-absorbing material (a marker of leakage of cytoplasm contents) in *S. aureus* and *Escherichia coli*.[32,42] Tea tree oil also inhibits respiration in *S. aureus*.[32,43] The hydrocarbons 1,8-cineole and terpinen-4-ol were primarily responsible for this phenomena.[32] Although 1,8-cineole was initially thought not to play a role in the antimicrobial activity of the oil, it seems to penetrate and disrupt the cellular membranes of bacteria. Terpinen-4-ol and α-terpineol have the greatest antimicrobial activity.

Tea tree oil also has antiinflammatory effects. Specifically, it inhibits lipopolysaccharide-induced production of the inflammatory mediators TNF-α, IL-1α, IL-10, and prostaglandin E$_2$ by monocytes in vitro.[88]

Clinical Manifestations

Skin irritation and allergic reactions are common effects with topical exposure. The allergic reactions are hypothesized to occur after the oil has undergone significant oxidation.[153] The hydrocarbon 1,8-cineole is implicated as the main irritating component, but there are few data to support this theory. In some of the cases of prepubertal gynecomastia reported in boys exposed to lavender oil, the patients were also exposed to tea tree oil.[92] However, it has not been demonstrated that tea tree oil affects the endocrine system. When ingested, tea tree oil commonly causes drowsiness, ataxia, and slurred speech. Case reports of children unintentionally ingesting a 100% concentration of tea tree oil show symptoms developing within 30 minutes of exposure. One child had resolution of symptoms within 5 hours, and another had to be intubated but had improvement in neurologic symptoms within 10 hours.[54,100,134] A case report describes using surfactant to treat an 18-month-old boy who developed ARDS after an unintentional ingestion of 100% tea tree oil. The child did well and was able to extubated by hospital day 3.[147] Surfactant has been used in cases of aspiration pneumonitis in children (Chap. 105). In all reported cases of pediatric and adult oral poisoning, patients responded well to supportive care alone; no deaths are reported.[54,100,134]

Oil of Wintergreen

Methyl salicylate

History

Oil of wintergreen was originally derived from *Gaultheria procumbens*, or the Eastern teaberry, which is a fragrant ground cover plant found in North America. The leaves were steamed and distilled to produce the oil that was used topically to relieve the symptoms of rheumatism. Oil of wintergreen is also obtained from the twigs of sweet birch, or *Betula lenta*. The active ingredient in oil of wintergreen is methyl salicylate, which has a pleasant, minty smell and taste, posing a significant hazard to children. Pure oil of wintergreen contains at least 98% methyl salicylate, but most commercial preparations of methyl salicylate contain far less.[57] The FDA regulations require that any drug containing more than 5% methyl salicylate have a warning against using it other than as a topical agent and keeping it out of the reach of children.[48] Oil of wintergreen has been used as a fragrance and flavoring agent in foods and household products.[97] It is also found in topical preparations worldwide, such as Tiger Balm and Ben-Gay, which are used to treat inflammation and myalgias. In many Asian countries, topical oils with benign, poetic names such as red flower oil and white flower oil contain high concentrations of methyl salicylate and are quite toxic when ingested.[35,36] Further confusing consumers and practitioners, there are many other names for this essential oil, including checkerberry oil, sweet birch oil, mountain tea, teaberry, groundberry oil, gaultheria oil, and spicewood oil.[57]

The first reported case of toxicity occurred in 1832, when six soldiers used the oil to flavor their tea.[55] The seminal case series was reported in the 1930s in which 43 exposures were tabulated, 20 involved children younger than the age of 4 years and had a 75% fatality rate.[171] The smallest lethal dose in this series was 4 mL of oil of wintergreen, and 6 mL was reported to be a lethal dose in a 21-year-old man.

Pharmacology

Methyl salicylate is absorbed both from the GI tract and transdermally. Normally, only 12% to 20% of topical salicylate is absorbed from the skin after 10 hours of application.[151] Heat, inflamed or broken skin, and prolonged use of occlusive dressings increase absorption.[28,91,133] Children have died after topical application.[28] Children are presumed to be at greater risk for toxicity because of their higher surface area–to–weight ratio and more permeable skin. After it has been absorbed, methyl salicylate enters the circulation and is transported to the liver, where it undergoes hydrolysis to form salicylic acid.[49] Methyl salicylate is a carboxylic acid ester. Most of the studies of salicylate metabolism involve aspirin, which is a phenolic ester. It is assumed that all forms of salicylate have similar properties after they are converted to

salicylic acid. The salicylic acid undergoes conjugation with glycine and glucuronic acid, forming salicyluric acid, salicyl acyl, and phenolic glucuronide. Salicylates then undergo renal elimination in the forms of salicyluric acid (75%), free salicylic acid (10%), salicylic phenol (10%) acyl (5%) glucuronides, and gentisic acid (<1%).[20,49,123,124]

Pathophysiology

Five milliliters (1 tsp) of oil of wintergreen is equivalent in salicylate content to 7 g of aspirin, which has been a fatal amount in some reported cases.[57] An extensive discussion of salicylate pathophysiology is given in Chap. 37.

Clinical Features

An overdose of methyl salicylate presents similarly to that of other salicylates such as aspirin. Salicylate poisoning is characterized by diaphoresis, nausea, vomiting, tinnitus, hyperpnea, and tachypnea. Mental status changes represent severe toxicity. Symptom onset is typically within a few hours given rapid absorption of the oil. Severe toxicity is associated with seizures, cerebral edema, ARDS, coma, and death. Further details on evaluation and management can be found in Chap. 37.

DIAGNOSTIC TESTING

Laboratory testing is of little utility in most essential oil toxicity, and the patient's clinical status will determine which tests are indicated. Some essential oil exposures do require specific studies, and they are listed below. Generally, blood or urine concentrations of the active ingredients are not available in a meaningful time frame and cannot and should not guide management. Patients who present with altered mental status or seizures warrant a complete evaluation that includes a rapid assessment of glucose, basic metabolic studies, a head computed tomography scan, and lumbar puncture for serious potential structural, infectious, or metabolic etiologies as guided by the history and examination. In patients who present with respiratory distress, chest radiographs, and continuous pulse oximetry are warranted.

- **Absinthe:** Laboratory studies should include a complete blood count (CBC), chemistry panel, creatine phosphokinase concentration, and glucose monitoring in patients who present with seizures. Urinalysis should be performed to evaluate for myoglobinuria.
- **Pennyroyal Oil:** A CBC and liver function studies, including the aminotransferases, bilirubin, prothrombin time, and partial thromboplastin time, and a β-human chorionic gonadotropin in women are indicated because many women ingest pennyroyal oil to terminate unwanted pregnancies.
- **Oil of wintergreen:** Serum salicylate concentrations, blood gas, serum potassium concentration, and urine pH initially should be sent every 1 to 2 hours to determine extent of toxicity and need for treatment (Chap. 37).

TREATMENT

The mainstay of treatment of symptomatic essential oil toxicity is supportive care, including monitoring of vital signs, IV fluids, and supplemental oxygen as needed. A dose of activated charcoal is reasonable in alert patients with an intact airway, but if there is a concern for seizures, activated charcoal should be withheld or deferred until the airway is protected. Dermal exposures should be properly decontaminated to prevent further absorption. Benzodiazepines are the mainstay of treatment in patients who present with agitation and seizures. A case report of unintentional eucalyptus poisoning in an elderly woman demonstrated naloxone as a potential antidote for lethargy and respiratory depression. There is not enough evidence to recommend routine use of naloxone in essential oil intoxications.[58]

A few of the essential oils require specific treatment:

- **Absinthe:** Rhabdomyolysis should be treated with IV fluids.
- **Camphor:** Most patients need supportive care with a focus on airway and circulatory management as well as aggressive treatment of seizures. Barbiturates are frequently cited as a first-line treatment of seizures based on one animal study that demonstrated decreased

neuronal damage with administration of pentobarbital.[166] However, it is likely that appropriate use of benzodiazepines would be just as effective. Given the risk of seizures and altered mental status, inducing emesis is not recommended. There is no proof of any benefit with orogastric lavage, and the rapid absorption of camphor from the GI tract decreases its likelihood of utility. The molecular weight and lipophilic nature of camphor indicates that it would likely be absorbed by activated charcoal. One animal study that underdosed the amount of activated charcoal as well gave subtoxic doses of camphor indicated that activated charcoal was not effective.[52] There have been no further studies examining this issue; however, given the risk of aspiration from emesis and seizure, activated charcoal should only be administered in patients with massive life-threatening ingestions and protected airways (Chap. 102).

■ **Clove oil:** In patients who exhibit signs of hepatotoxicity, it is reasonable to administer NAC. Although no definitive studies on NAC use in this patient population are available, the evidence that NAC is protective in the rat model, combined with the safety profile of NAC, warrant its use in the setting of eugenol-induced hepatotoxicity.[177]

■ **Pennyroyal oil:** One case of ingestion of a potentially fatal amount of pennyroyal was successfully treated with NAC.[7] Given in vitro studies showing glutathione depletion, it is recommended to administer NAC in cases of pennyroyal-induced hepatotoxicity. Because there is no established dosing regimen, using the same regimen used for acetaminophen toxicity would be reasonable.[176]

■ **Oil of wintergreen:** Alkalization with sodium bicarbonate and hemodialysis are indicated in cases of severe toxicity. Exchange transfusion was used successfully in children with life-threatening toxicity after methyl salicylate overdose (Chap. 37).[57]

SUMMARY

■ Essential oils are used as an alternative form of medical therapy.
■ These oils contain mixtures of complex hydrocarbons that are potentially toxic.
■ Cutaneous use of these products in moderation is associated with minimal toxicity. However, ingestion, prolonged inhalation, or excessive topical use causes significant morbidity and mortality.
■ Patients and health care providers should have open dialogues about the therapeutic use of these products and any concerning exposures should be referred to the regional poison control centers for guidance in management.

Acknowledgment

Sara Eliza Halcomb, MD, contributed to this chapter in previous editions.

REFERENCES

1. Akesson HO, Walinder J. Nutmeg intoxication. *Lancet.* 1965;1:1271-1272.
2. Allen WT. Note on a case of supposed poisoning by pennyroyal. *The Lancet.* 1897;149:1022-1023.
3. Alqareer A, et al. The effect of clove and benzocaine versus placebo as topical anesthetics. *J Dent.* 2006;34:747-750.
4. Amato A, et al. Effects of menthol on circular smooth muscle of human colon: analysis of the mechanism of action. *Eur J Pharmacol.* 2014;740:295-301.
5. Amato A, et al. Involvement of cholinergic nicotinic receptors in the menthol-induced gastric relaxation. *Eur J Pharmacol.* 2014;745:129-134.
6. Amory R. Experiments and observations on absinth and absinthism. *Boston Med Surg J.* 1868;78:68-71.
7. Anderson IB, et al. Pennyroyal toxicity: measurement of toxic metabolite levels in two cases and review of the literature. *Ann Intern Med.* 1996;124:726.
8. Anonymous. The eucalyptus and the Roman campagna. *Br Med J.* 1880;1:866-867.
9. Anonymous. Eucalyptus in the treatment of diabetes. *Br Med J.* 1902;1:1295-1296.
10. Anonymous. Oil of camphor in purulent peritonitis. *Br Med J.* 1911;2:764.
11. Anonymous. Nutmeg poisoning. *Br Med J.* 1959;2:1466-1467.
12. Arnold WN. Absinthe. *Scientific American.* 1989;260:112-117.
13. Aronow R. Camphor poisoning. *JAMA.* 1976;235:1260-1260.
14. Aronow R, Spigiel RW. Implications of camphor poisoning—therapeutic and administrative. *Drug Intell Clin Pharm.* 1976;10:631-634.
15. Bakerink JA, et al. Multiple organ failure after ingestion of pennyroyal oil from herbal tea in two infants. *Pediatrics.* 1996;98:944-947.
16. Baldinger P, et al. Effects of Silexan on the serotonin-1A receptor and microstructure of the human brain: a randomized, placebo-controlled, double-blind, cross-over study with molecular and structural neuroimaging. *Int J Neuropsychopharmacol.* 2014;18.
17. Barkin ME, Boyd JP, Cohen S. Acute allergic reaction to eugenol. *Oral Surg Oral Med Oral Pathol.* 1984;57:441-442.
18. Baylie RL, et al. Inhibition of the cardiac L-type calcium channel current by the TRPM8 agonist, (−)-menthol. *J Physiol Pharmacol.* 2010;61:543-550.
19. Behrends M, et al. Acute lung injury after peppermint oil injection. *Anesth Analg.* 2005;101:1160-1162.
20. Belsito D, et al. A toxicologic and dermatologic assessment of salicylates when used as fragrance ingredients. *Food Chem Toxicol.* 2007;45:S318-S361.
21. Beyer J, et al. Abuse of nutmeg (Myristica fragrans Houtt.): studies on the metabolism and the toxicologic detection of its ingredients elemicin, myristicin, and safrole in rat and human urine using gas chromatography/mass spectrometry. *Ther Drug Monit.* 2006;28:568-575.
22. Block SL. The possible link between gynecomastia, topical lavender, and tea tree oil. *Pediatr Ann.* 2012;41:56-58.
23. Bonkovsky HL, et al. Porphyrogenic properties of the terpenes camphor, pinene, and thujone—(with a note on historic implications for absinthe and the illness of Van Gogh, Vincent). *Biochem Pharmacol.* 1992;43:2359-2368.
24. Braithwaite PF. A case of poisoning by pennyroyal: recovery. *Br Med J.* 1906;2:865.
25. Braun U, Kalbhen DA. Evidence for the biogenic formation of amphetamine derivatives from components of nutmeg. *Pharmacology.* 1973;9:312-316.
26. Brook MP, et al. Pine oil cleaner ingestion. *Ann Emerg Med.* 1989;18:391-395.
27. Brown SA, et al. Disseminated intravascular coagulation and hepatocellular necrosis due to clove oil. *Blood Coagul Fibrinolysis.* 1992;3:665-668.
28. Brubacher JR, Hoffman RS. Salicylism from topical salicylates: review of the literature. *J Toxicol Clin Toxicol.* 1996;34:431-436.
29. Burrow A, et al. The effects of camphor, eucalyptus and menthol vapor on nasal resistance to air-flow and nasal sensation. *Acta Oto-Laryngolog.* 1983;96:157-161.
30. Caceres AI, et al. TRPM8 mediates the anti-inflammatory effects of eucalyptol. *Br J Pharmacol.* 2017.
31. Carson CF, et al. Melaleuca alternifolia (tea tree) oil: a review of antimicrobial and other medicinal properties. *Clin Microbiol Rev.* 2006;19:50.
32. Carson CF, et al. Mechanism of action of Melaleuca alternifolia (tea tree) oil on Staphylococcus aureus determined by time-kill, lysis, leakage, and salt tolerance assays and electron microscopy. *Antimicrob Agents Chemother.* 2002;46:1914-1920.
33. Carstairs SD, Cantrell FL. The spice of life: an analysis of nutmeg exposures in California. *Clin Toxicol.* 2011;49:177-180.
34. Cavanagh HMA, Wilkinson JN. Biological activities of lavender essential oil. *Phytother Res.* 2002;16:301-308.
35. Chan TYK. Medicated oils and severe salicylate poisoning: quantifying the risk based on methyl salicylate content and bottle size. *Vet Hum Toxicol.* 1996;38:133-134.
36. Chan TYK. Ingestion of medicated oils by adults: the risk of severe salicylate poisoning is related to the packaging of these products. *Hum Exp Toxicol.* 2002;21:171-174.
37. Chioca LR, et al. Anxiolytic-like effect of lavender essential oil inhalation in mice: participation of serotonergic but not GABAA/benzodiazepine neurotransmission. *J Ethnopharmacol.* 2013;147:412-418.
38. Ciganda C, Laborde A. Herbal infusions used for induced abortion. *J Toxicol Clin Toxicol.* 2003;41:235-239.
39. Clark TL. Fatal case of camphor poisoning. *Br Med J.* 1924;1:467.
40. Clark TL. Fatal case of camphor poisoning. *Br Med J.* 1924;1924:467-467.
41. Cording CJ, et al. A fatality due to accidental PineSol (TM) ingestion. *J Anal Toxicol.* 2000;24:664-667.
42. Cox SD, et al. Tea tree oil causes K+ leakage and inhibits respiration in Escherichia coli. *Lett Appl Microbiol.* 1998;26:355-358.
43. Cox SD, et al. The mode of antimicrobial action of the essential oil of Melaleuca alternifolia (tea tree oil). *J Appl Microbiol.* 2000;88:170-175.
44. Curgenven JB. Eucalyptus in scarlet fever. *Br Med J.* 1889;2:921.
45. Curtis EK. In pursuit of palliation: oil of cloves in the art of dentistry. *Bull Hist Dent.* 1990;38:9-14.
46. Cushny AR. Nutmeg poisoning. *Proc R Soc Med.* 1908;1(Ther Pharmacol Sect):39-44.
47. Davies R. A fatal case of camphor-poisoning. *Br Med J.* 1887;1:726.
48. Davis JE. Are one or two dangerous? Methyl salicylate exposure in toddlers. *J Emerg Med.* 2007;32:63-69.
49. Davison C, et al. Metabolism and toxicity of methyl salicylate. *J Pharmacol Exp Ther.* 1961;132:207.
50. de Cerqueira SVS, et al. R(+)-pulegone impairs Ca2+ homeostasis and causes negative inotropism in mammalian myocardium. *Eur J Pharmacol.* 2011;672:135-142.
51. De Vincenzi M, et al. Constituents of aromatic plants: eucalyptol. *Fitoterapia.* 2002;73:269-275.
52. Dean BS, et al. In vivo evaluation of the adsorptive capacity of activated-charcoal for camphor. *Vet Hum Toxicol.* 1992;34:297-299.
53. Deiml T, et al. alpha-thujone reduces 5-HT3 receptor activity by an effect on the agonist-induced desensitization. *Neuropharmacology.* 2004;46:192-201.
54. Del Beccaro MA. Melaleuca oil poisoning in a 17-month-old. *Vet Hum Toxicol.* 1995;37:557-558.

55. Diamond EF, Deyoung VR. Acute poisoning with oil of wintergreen treated by exchange transfusion. *Ama J Dis Child*. 1958;95:309-310.

56. Diaz A, et al. Prepubertal gynecomastia and chronic lavender exposure: report of three cases. *J Pediatr Endocrinol Metab*. 2016;29:103-107.

57. Done AK, Otterness LJ. Exchange transfusion in the treatment of oil of wintergreen (methyl salicylate) poisoning. *Pediatrics*. 1956;18:80-85.

58. Doshi D, et al. A novel use of naloxone as a treatment for eucalyptus oil induced central nervous system depression. *Clin Toxicol (Phila)*. 2011;49:768.

59. Dresser GK, et al. Evaluation of peppermint oil and ascorbyl palmitate as inhibitors of cytochrome P4503A4 activity in vitro and in vivo. *Clin Pharmacol Ther*. 2002;72: 247-255.

60. American Academy of Pediatrics. Committee on Drugs. Camphor—who needs it. *Pediatrics*. 1978;62:404-406.

61. Duisken M, et al. Metabolism of 1.8-cineole by human cytochrome P450 enzymes: identification of a new hydroxylated metabolite. *Biochimica Biophys Acta*. 2005;1722: 304-311.

62. Early DF. Pennyroyal—a rare cause of epilepsy. *Lancet*. 1961;2:580.

63. Eccles R. Menthol and related cooling compounds. *J Pharm Pharmacol*. 1994; 46:618-630.

64. Eccles R. Menthol: effects on nasal sensation of airflow and the drive to breathe. *Curr Allergy Asthma Rep*. 2003;3:210-214.

65. Eccles R, et al. The effects of menthol isomers on nasal sensation of air-flow. *Clin Otolaryngol*. 1988;13:25-29.

66. Eccles R, et al. The effects of oral-administration of (–)-menthol on nasal resistance to air-flow and nasal sensation of air-flow in subjects suffering from nasal congestion associated with the common cold. *J Pharm Pharmacol*. 1990;42:652-654.

67. Ehrenpreis JE, et al. Nutmeg poisonings: a retrospective review of 10 years experience from the Illinois Poison Center, 2001-2011. *J Med Toxicol*. 2014;10:148-151.

68. Eisen JS, et al. N-acetylcysteine for the treatment of clove oil-induced fulminant hepatic failure. *J Toxicol Clin Toxicol*. 2004;42:89-92.

69. El-Alfy AT, et al. Indirect modulation of the endocannabinoid system by specific fractions of nutmeg total extract. *Pharm Biol*. 2016;54:2933-2938.

70. Ferreira-da-Silva FW, et al. Effects of 1,8-cineole on electrophysiological parameters of neurons of the rat superior cervical ganglion. *Clin Exp Pharmacol Physiol*. 2009; 36:1068-1073.

71. Flam B, et al. Seizures associated with intentional severe nutmeg intoxication. *Clin Toxicol (Phila)*. 2015;53:917.

72. Foggie WE. Eucalyptus oil poisoning. *Br Med J*. 1911;1:359-360.

73. Forrest JE, Heacock RA. Nutmeg and mace—psychotropic spices from Myristica fragrans. *Lloydia*. 1972;35:440-449.

74. Gaudioso C, et al. Menthol pain relief through cumulative inactivation of voltage-gated sodium channels. *Pain*. 2012;153:473-484.

75. Gelal A, et al. Disposition kinetics and effects of menthol. *Clin Pharmacol Ther*. 1999; 66:128-135.

76. Geppetti P, et al. Camphor, an old cough remedy with a new mechanism. *Am J Respir Crit Care Med*. 2012;185:342; author reply 343.

77. Girling J. Poisoning by pennyroyal. *Br Med J*. 1887;1:1214.

78. Giuseppi PL. Camphor in acute influenzal bronchitis and bronchopneumonia. *Br Med J*. 1918;2:716.

79. Gordon WP, et al. Hepatotoxicity and pulmonary toxicity of pennyroyal oil and its constituent terpenes in the mouse. *Toxicol Appl Pharmacol*. 1982;65:413-424.

80. Gordon WP, et al. The metabolism of the abortifacient terpene, (r)-(+)-pulegone, to a proximate toxin, menthofuran. *Drug Metab Dispos*. 1987;15:589-594.

81. Gorman AD. Subcutaneous injections of camphor. *Br Med J*. 1920;1:828.

82. Green RC, Jr. Nutmeg poisoning. *Va Med Mon (1918)*. 1959;86:586-590.

83. Greene Rr IAC. The effect of camphor in oil on lactation. *JAMA*. 1938;110:641-642.

84. Gurr FW, Scroggie JG. Eucalyptus oil poisoning treated by dialysis and mannitol infusion. *Australas Ann Med*. 1965;14:238.

85. Gyoubu K, Miyazawa M. In vitro metabolism of (–)-camphor using human liver microsomes and CYP2A6. *Biol Pharm Bull*. 2007;30:230-233.

86. Hagvall L, et al. Lavender oil lacks natural protection against autoxidation, forming strong contact allergens on air exposure. *Contact Dermatitis*. 2008;59:143-150.

87. Hallstrom H, Thuvander A. Toxicological evaluation of myristicin. *Natural Toxins*. 1997;5:186-192.

88. Hart PH, et al. Terpinen-4-ol, the main component of the essential oil of Melaleuca alternifolia (tea tree oil), suppresses inflammatory mediator production by activated human monocytes. *Inflamm Res*. 2000;49:619-626.

89. Hartnoll G, et al. Near-fatal ingestion of oil of cloves. *Arch Dis Child*. 1993;69:392-393.

90. Heimes K, et al. Mode of action of peppermint oil and (–)-menthol with respect to 5-HT3 receptor subtypes: binding studies, cation uptake by receptor channels and contraction of isolated rat ileum. *Phytother Res*. 2011;25:702-708.

91. Heng MCY. Local necrosis and interstitial nephritis due to topical methyl salicylate and menthol. *Cutis*. 1987;39:442-444.

92. Henley DV, et al. Brief report—prepubertal gynecomastia linked to lavender and tea tree oils. *N Engl J Med*. 2007;356:479-485.

93. Herman A, et al. Linalool affects the antimicrobial efficacy of essential oils. *Curr Microbiol*. 2016;72:165-172.

94. Hills JM, Aaronson PI. The mechanism of action of peppermint oil on gastrointestinal smooth muscle. An analysis using patch clamp electrophysiology and isolated tissue pharmacology in rabbit and guinea pig. *Gastroenterology*. 1991;101:55-65.

95. Hold KM, et al. Detoxification of alpha- and beta-thujones (the active ingredients of absinthe): site specificity and species differences in cytochrome P450 oxidation in vitro and in vivo. *Chem Res Toxicol*. 2001;14:589-595.

96. Hold KM, et al. Alpha-thujone (the active component of absinthe): gamma-aminobutyric acid type A receptor modulation and metabolic detoxification. *Proc Natl Acad Sci U S A*. 2000;97:3826-3831.

97. Howrie DL, et al. Candy flavoring as a source of salicylate poisoning. *Pediatrics*. 1985; 75:869-871.

98. Hume WR. The pharmacological and toxicological properties of zinc oxide-eugenol. *J Am Dent Assoc*. 1986;113:789-791.

99. Isaacs G. Permanent local anaesthesia and anhidrosis after clove oil spillage. *Lancet*. 1983;1:882.

100. Jacobs MR, Hornfeldt CS. Melaleuca oil poisoning. *J Toxicol Clin Toxicol*. 1994;32: 461-464.

101. Jager W, et al. Percutaneous-absorption of lavender oil from a massage oil. *J Soc Cosmet Chem*. 1992;43:49-54.

102. Janes SEJ, et al. Essential oil poisoning: N-acetylcysteine for eugenol-induced hepatic failure and analysis of a national database. *Eur J Pediatr*. 2005;164:520-522.

103. Jimenez JF, et al. Chronic camphor ingestion mimicking Reyes syndrome. *Gastroenterology*. 1983;84:394-398.

104. Johnson G. Another case of poisoning by homeopathic solution of camphor. *Br Med J*. 1875;1:171.

105. Juergens UR, et al. Anti-inflammatory activity of 1.8-cineol (eucalyptol) in bronchial asthma: a double-blind placebo-controlled trial. *Respir Med*. 2003;97:250-256.

106. Juergens UR, et al. Inhibition of cytokine production and arachidonic acid metabolism by eucalyptol (1.8-cineole) in human blood monocytes in vitro. *Eur J Med Res*. 1998;3:508-510.

107. Kasper S. An orally administered lavandula oil preparation (Silexan) for anxiety disorder and related conditions: an evidence based review. *Int J Psychiatry Clin Pract*. 2013;17(suppl 1):15-22.

108. Kasper S, et al. Lavender oil preparation Silexan is effective in generalized anxiety disorder—a randomized, double-blind comparison to placebo and paroxetine. *Int J Neuropsychopharmacol*. 2014;17:859-869.

109. Kemper KJ, et al. Prepubertal gynecomastia linked to lavender and tea tree oils. *N Engl J Med*. 2007;356:2541-2542.

110. Khan AJ, et al. Turpentine oil inhalation leading to lung necrosis and empyema in a toddler. *Pediatr Emerg Care*. 2006;22:355-357.

111. Khine H, et al. A cluster of children with seizures caused by camphor poisoning. *Pediatrics*. 2009;123:1269-1272.

112. Kirsch CM, et al. Noncardiogenic pulmonary edema due to the intravenous administration of clove oil. *Thorax*. 1990;45:235-236.

113. Klein FA, Hackler RH. Hemorrhagic cystitis associated with turpentine ingestion. *Urology*. 1980;16:187-187.

114. Koppel C, et al. Acute poisoning with pine oil—metabolism of monoterpenes. *Archives of Toxicology*. 1981;49:73-78.

115. Kozam G. Effect of eugenol on nerve transmission. *Oral Surg Oral Med Oral Pathol*. 1977;44:799-805.

116. Kozam G, Mantell GM. Effect of eugenol on oral mucous membranes. *J Dent Res*. 1978;57:954-957.

117. Kumar KJ, et al. Eucalyptus oil poisoning. *Toxicol Int*. 2015;22:170-171.

118. Kunicka-Styczynska A, et al. Antimicrobial activity of lavender, tea tree and lemon oils in cosmetic preservative systems. *J Appl Microbiol*. 2009;107:1903-1911.

119. Lachenmeier DW. Wormwood (Artemisia absinthium L.)-A curious plant with both neurotoxic and neuroprotective properties? *J Ethnopharmacol*. 2010;131:224-227.

120. Lachenmeier DW, et al. Absinthe, a spirit drink—its history and future from a toxicological-analytical and food regulatory point of view. *Deutsche Lebensmittel-Rundschau*. 2004;100:117-129.

121. Lane BW, et al. Clove oil ingestion in an infant. *Hum Exp Toxicol*. 1991;10:291-294.

122. Lee MH, et al. Eugenol inhibits calcium currents in dental afferent neurons. *J Dent Res*. 2005;84:848-851.

123. Levy G. Clinical pharmacokinetics of aspirin. *Pediatrics*. 1978;62(5 Pt 2 suppl): 867-872.

124. Levy G, Tsuchiya T. Salicylate accumulation kinetics in man. *N Engl J Med*. 1972;287:425-432.

125. Li HY, et al. Eugenol inhibits K+ currents in trigeminal ganglion neurons. *J Dent Res*. 2007;86:898-902.

126. Lima FJB, et al. The essential oil of Eucalyptus tereticornis, and its constituents alpha- and beta-pinene, potentiate acetylcholine-induced contractions in isolated rat trachea. *Fitoterapia*. 2010;81:649-655.

127. Long FWD. Treatment of influenza with camphor. *Br Med J*. 1891;2:477.

128. Manoguerra AS, et al. Camphor poisoning: an evidence-based practice guideline for out-of-hospital management. *Clin Toxicol*. 2006;44:357-370.

129. Martin D, et al. Dermal absorption of camphor, menthol, and methyl salicylate in humans. *J Clin Pharmacol*. 2004;44:1151-1157.

130. McKay DL, Blumberg JB. A review of the bioactivity and potential health benefits of peppermint tea (Mentha piperita L.). *Phytother Res.* 2006;20:619-633.

131. McLeod RL, et al. TRPV1 antagonists as potential antitussive agents. *Lung.* 2008;186 (suppl 1):S59-S65.

132. Meschler JP, Howlett AC. Thujone exhibits low affinity for cannabinoid receptors but fails to evoke cannabimimetic responses. *Pharmacol Biochem Behav.* 1999; 62:473-480.

133. Morra P, et al. Serum concentrations of salicylic acid following topically applied salicylate derivatives. *Ann Pharmacother.* 1996;30:935-940.

134. Morris MC, et al. Ingestion of tea tree oil (Melaleuca oil) by a 4-year-old boy. *Pediatr Emerg Care.* 2003;19:169-171.

135. O'Neill J, et al. Unravelling the mystery of capsaicin: a tool to understand and treat pain. *Pharmacol Rev.* 2012;64:939-971.

136. Ohkubo T, Kitamura K. Eugenol activates Ca2+ permeable currents in rat dorsal root ganglion cells. *J Dent Res.* 1997;76:1737-1744.

137. Omullane NM, et al. Adverse CNS effects of menthol-containing Olbas oil. *Lancet.* 1982; 1:1121-1121.

138. Palkar R, et al. The molecular and cellular basis of thermosensation in mammals. *Curr Opin Neurobiol.* 2015;34:14-19.

139. Panesar PS, et al. Vermouth: technology of production and quality characteristics. *Adv Food Nutr Res.* 2011;63:251-283.

140. Park CK, et al. Eugenol inhibits sodium currents in dental afferent neurons. *J Dent Res.* 2006;85:900-904.

141. Patel T, et al. Menthol: a refreshing look at this ancient compound. *J Am Acad Dermatol.* 2007;57:873-878.

142. Payne RB. Nutmeg intoxication. *N Engl J Med.* 1963;269:36-39.

143. Payne RB. Nutmeg intoxication. *N Engl J Med.* 1963;269:36.

144. Phelan WJ. Camphor poisoning—over-counter dangers. *Pediatrics.* 1976;57:428-431.

145. Re L, et al. Linalool modifies the nicotinic receptor-ion channel kinetics at the mouse neuromuscular junction. *Pharmacol Res.* 2000;42:177-182.

146. Rees JH. Nutmeg poisoning. *Practitioner.* 1964;193:80-83.

147. Richards DB, et al. Pediatric tea tree oil aspiration treated with surfactant in the emergency department. *Pediatr Emerg Care.* 2015;31:279-280.

148. Riddle JM, Estes JW. Oral contraceptives in ancient and medieval times. *Am Scientist.* 1992;80:226-233.

149. Riggs J, et al. Camphorated oil intoxication in pregnancy—report of a case. *Obstet Gynecol.* 1965;25:255-258.

150. Roberts C. The eucalyptus in the campagna. *Br Med J.* 1880;1:949-950.

151. Roberts MS, et al. Topical bioavailability of methyl salicylate. *Aust N Z J Med.* 1982; 12:303-305.

152. Robertson JS, Hussain M. Metabolism of camphors and related compounds. *Biochem J.* 1969;113:57-65.

153. Rudback J, et al. Alpha-terpinene, an antioxidant in tea tree oil, autoxidizes rapidly to skin allergens on air exposure. *Chem Res Toxicol.* 2012;25:713-721.

154. Saleh M, et al. Acute and chronic effects of a nutmeg extract on the toad heart. *Pharmacol Biochem Behav.* 1989;32:83-86.

155. Sangalli BC, Chiang W. Toxicology of nutmeg abuse. *J Toxicol Clin Toxicol.* 2000;38: 671-678.

156. Sarrami N, et al. Adverse reactions associated with the use of eugenol in dentistry. *Br Dent J.* 2002;193:257-259.

157. Shulgin AT. Composition of myristicin fraction from oil of nutmeg. *Nature.* 1963; 197:379.

158. Siegel E, Wason S. Camphor toxicity. *Pediatr Clin North Am.* 1986;33:375-379.

159. Silenieks LB, et al. Silexan, an essential oil from flowers of Lavandula angustifolia, is not recognized as benzodiazepine-like in rats trained to discriminate a diazepam cue. *Phytomedicine.* 2013;20:172-177.

160. Silva Brum LF, et al. Effects of linalool on glutamate release and uptake in mouse cortical synaptosomes. *Neurochem Res.* 2001;26:191-194.

161. Sjoholm A, et al. Acute nutmeg intoxication. *J Intern Med.* 1998;243:329-331.

162. Skoglund RR, et al. Prolonged seizures due to contact and inhalation exposure to camphor—case report. *Clin Pediatr.* 1977;16:901-902.

163. Skold M, et al. Autoxidation of linalyl acetate, the main component of lavender oil, creates potent contact allergens. *Contact Dermatitis.* 2008;58:9-14.

164. Skyles AJ, Sweet BV. Wormwood. *Am J Health-Syst Pharm.* 2004;61:239.

165. Slack AB, MacMahon JJP. Eucalyptus ointment for burns. *Br Med J.* 1940;2:805.

166. Smith AG, Margolis G. Camphor poisoning; anatomical and pharmacologic study; report of a fatal case; experimental investigation of protective action of barbiturate. *Am J Pathol.* 1954;30:857-869.

167. Sperling F, et al. Acute effects of turpentine vapor on rats and mice. *Toxicol Appl Pharmacol.* 1967;10:8-20.

168. Sperling F, Marcus WL. Turpentine-induced histological changes in isolated rat and guinea pig lungs. *Arch Int Pharmacodyn Ther.* 1968;175:330.

169. Spoerke DG, et al. Eucalyptus oil—14 cases of exposure. *Vet Hum Toxicol.* 1989;31:166-168.

170. Stein U, et al. Nutmeg (myristicin) poisoning—report on a fatal case and a series of cases recorded by a poison information centre. *Forensic Sci Int.* 2001;118:87-90.

171. Stevenson CS. Oil of wintergreen (methyl salicylate) poisoning report of three cases, one with autopsy, and a review of the literature. *Am J Med Sci.* 1937;193:772-788.

172. Sullivan JB, et al. Pennyroyal oil poisoning and hepatotoxicity. *JAMA.* 1979;242: 2873-2874.

173. Summers GD. Case of camphor poisoning. *Br Med J.* 1947;2:1009.

174. Takaishi M, et al. 1,8-cineole, a TRPM8 agonist, is a novel natural antagonist of human TRPA1. *Mol Pain.* 2012;8:86.

175. Thomassen D, et al. Partial characterization of biliary metabolites of pulegone by tandem mass-spectrometry—detection of glucuronide, glutathione, and glutathionyl glucuronide conjugates. *Drug Metabolism and Disposition.* 1991; 19: 997-1003.

176. Thomassen D, et al. Menthofuran-dependent and independent aspects of pulegone hepatotoxicity— roles of glutathione. *J Pharmacol Exp Ther.* 1990;253:567-572.

177. Thompson DC, et al. Metabolism and cytotoxicity of eugenol in isolated rat hepatocytes. *Chem Biol Interact.* 1991;77:137-147.

178. Todd-White A. Tincture of eucalyptus in haemorrhage. *Br Med J.* 1908;2:81.

179. Trestrail JH, Spartz ME. Camphorated and castor-oil confusion and its toxic results. *Clin Toxicol.* 1977;11:151-158.

180. Truitt EB Jr. The pharmacology of myristicin and nutmeg. *Psychopharmacol Bull.* 1967;4:14.

181. Truitt EB Jr, et al. Evidence of monoamine oxidase inhibition by myristicin and nutmeg. *Proc Soc Exp Biol Med.* 1963;112:647-650.

182. Uc A, et al. Camphor hepatotoxicity. *South Med J.* 2000;93:596-598.

183. Vallance WB. Pennyroyal poisoning—a fatal case. *Lancet.* 1955;2:850-851.

184. Vay L, et al. The thermo-TRP ion channel family: properties and therapeutic implications. *Br J Pharmacol.* 2012;165:787-801.

185. Vigan M. Essential oils: renewal of interest and toxicity. *Eur J Dermatol.* 2010;20: 685-692.

186. Weisbord SD, et al. Poison on line—acute renal failure caused by oil of wormwood purchased through the Internet. *N Engl J Med.* 1997;337:825-827.

187. Welker JA, Zaloga GP. Pine oil ingestion—a common cause of poisoning. *Chest.* 1999;116:1822-1826.

188. Worth H, et al. Concomitant therapy with Cineole (Eucalyptole) reduces exacerbations in COPD: a placebo-controlled double-blind trial. *Respir Res.* 2009;10.

189. Wright SE, et al. Intravenous eugenol causes hemorrhagic lung edema in rats—proposed oxidant mechanisms. *J Lab Clin Med.* 1995;125:257-264.

190. Wu PA, James WD. Lavender. *Dermatitis.* 2011;22:344-347.

191. Xu H, et al. Camphor activates and strongly desensitizes the transient receptor potential vanilloid subtype 1 channel in a vanilloid-independent mechanism. *J Neurosci.* 2005;25:8924-8937.

192. Yosipovitch G, et al. Effect of topically applied menthol on thermal, pain and itch sensations and biophysical properties of the skin. *Arc Dermatol Res.* 1996;288: 245-248.

193. Yun CH, et al. Roles of human liver cytochrome P450 3A4 and 1A2 enzymes in the oxidation of myristicin. *Toxicol Lett.* 2003;137:143-150.

43 PLANT- AND ANIMAL-DERIVED DIETARY SUPPLEMENTS

Lindsay M. Fox

INTRODUCTION

Dietary supplements include vitamins, minerals, plant- and animal-derived preparations, amino acids, and a variety of other "natural" and "traditional" remedies with established history of use. Within the United States regulatory context, dietary supplements are distinct from *medications* because this term is reserved for drugs approved by the US Food and Drug Administration (FDA), which are regulated more rigorously in terms of safety and effectiveness. Although these products are distinct from medications, they contain xenobiotics that have many physiologic effects on the human body.

Many dietary supplements sold in the United States are based on diverse traditional healing practices from around the world, and they are often derived from plant and animal sources.

The study of plant- and animal-derived dietary supplements is complicated by the lack of standardized nomenclature. A variety of common, proprietary, and botanical names can cause confusion. A single plant preparation often has many common names, in addition to its botanical name. For example, *Datura stramonium* is also known as Jamestown weed, jimson weed, angel's trumpet, devil's apple, thornapple, apple of Peru, and tolguacha. Likewise, one common name for a plant refers to several plants. "Mandrake" refers not only to the belladonna-alkaloid–containing *Mandragora officinarum* but also the podophyllum-containing *Podophyllum peltatum*. Thus, accurate classification of plant- and animal-derived dietary supplements is difficult and often confusing. Using both common and botanical names, when possible, allows for more precise communication.

This chapter discusses the history, epidemiology, and regulation of plant- and animal-derived dietary supplements. Pharmacologic principles related to products derived from plants and animal sources are considered, as well as issues related to adulteration and contamination of supposedly natural products. The toxicities of select examples of plant- and animal-derived dietary supplements will be discussed. It is beyond the scope of this chapter to evaluate the effectiveness of dietary supplements for their purported uses. Reported traditional indications are mentioned in some cases to provide context without implying that the evidence for or against purported indications for these products was evaluated.

HISTORY AND EPIDEMIOLOGY

Since ancient times, people of nearly all cultures have used plant- and animal-derived dietary supplements to treat disease and promote health. A 60,000-year-old Iraqi burial site contained eight different medicinal plants.[104] The Egyptian Ebers papyrus, written circa 1500 B.C., lists 160 medicinal plants and their intended uses, including the use of salicin-containing willow bark to treat pain.[33] The Hippocratic Corpus, compiled around 400 B.C., contains many descriptions of herbs, including a number of recipes for plant-based gynecologic remedies; it prescribes the use of a likely extinct silphium plant to "create a wind in the womb" to induce abortion or expel a dead fetus.[108] In the first century A.D., the Greek physician Dioscorides wrote *De Materia Medica*, which described the indications for use of more than 600 plant- and animal-derived preparations, many of which are still used by herbalists today.[106] China's *Shennong Bencaojing*, or *Divine Farmer's Materia Medica*, first inked around 200 A.D., discusses hundreds of herbs, such as cannabis, ma huang (ephedra), and ginger.

During the Scientific Revolution, scientists began to isolate purified extracts of plant products for use as medicinals, and many modern pharmaceuticals are still derived from plant products. In 1806, a French pharmacist isolated a substance from the *Papaver somniferum* plant that he named morphine, after Morpheus, the Greek god of dreams.[117] In 1828, the active ingredient of the willow bark, salicin, was identified,[33] after which it began to be used to treat rheumatic fever. In 1897, acetylsalicylic acid was synthesized by scientists at Bayer, and it quickly became one of the most commonly used medications around the world.[33] The original name, aspirin (*a* cetyl-*spiric* acid), was derived from *Spiraea*, the plant genus from which salicylic acid once was prepared. *Artemisia annua* (sweet Annie, qing hao) was first described as a treatment for malaria (periodic fever) in China in 168 B.C.[62] In 1971, the active parent compound artemisinin was isolated by Chinese investigators. Artesunate, an artemisinin, is now recommended by the World Health Organization as the first-line treatment for severe *Plasmodium falciparum* malaria.[3] Between 1981 and 2014, 25% of new drugs approved in the United States were derived from plant or animal products found in nature, and an additional 10% were synthetic mimics designed in the image of molecules found in nature.[83]

In the current era, naturopaths, traditional healers, shamans, and a multitude of sometimes dubious websites offer plant- and animal-derived dietary supplements for medicinal purposes, and the products they sell are unfortunately often highly unreliable and potentially injurious. An estimated 5% of children and 18% of adults in the United States use nonvitamin, nonmineral dietary supplements, many of which are plant- and animal-derived dietary supplements.[58] Dietary supplements are estimated to contribute to 23,000 emergency department visits in the United States per year.[47] Consumers buy dietary supplements from offices of complementary and alternative medicine practitioners, health food stores, grocery stores, pharmacies, drug stores, gasoline stations, mail order companies, and the Internet. United States dietary supplement sales were estimated at $6.4 billion in 2014, representing direct sales of $3.1 billion, natural and health food sales of $2.2 billion, and $1.1 billion from mass-market retailers.[103] For more than a decade, dietary supplement sales have increased every year, with a 6.8% increase in 2014.[103] Similarly, worldwide plant- and animal-derived dietary supplement usage continues to grow. The current global supplements and remedies market was valued at $62 billion in 2012, and it is predicted to reach $115 billion by 2020.[49]

REGULATION OF DIETARY SUPPLEMENTS

In the United State, all dietary supplements are loosely regulated by the FDA. They are classified as a type of dietary supplement, meaning that they are considered nutrients with nondrug status.[58] Therefore, dietary supplements are not subject to the same rigorous standards as pharmaceutical products. There is little to no premarketing testing to assure quality and safety. Existing regulations are relatively weak, and those that exist are inadequately enforced. Enforcement relies heavily on a postmarketing surveillance approach to identify dangerous or contaminated products after consumers have suffered adverse consequences. As a result, American consumers are exposed to untested, unproven products that sometimes contain harmful ingredients, dangerous contaminants, or unlisted adulterants.

Current regulation of dietary supplements in the United States was defined in large part by the Dietary Supplement Health and Education Act of 1994 (DSHEA), which limited the authority of the FDA to regulate products categorized as dietary supplements.[13,58] Dietary supplements according to the DSHEA include vitamins, minerals, plant- and animal-derived products, amino acids, and any product that was sold as a "supplement" before October 15, 1994. After October 15, 1994, any new ingredient intended for use in dietary supplements requires notification and approval by the FDA at least 75 days in advance of marketing. The FDA must review and determine whether the proposed ingredient is expected to be safe under the intended conditions for use. However, because most ingredients contained in dietary supplements were in use before 1994, the vast majority of dietary supplements are not subject to even this weakened premarket safety evaluation. Note that there is no requirement to show effectiveness, a typical expectation associated with approval of pharmaceuticals. The DSHEA allows dietary supplement vendors to make structure or function claims, suggesting that a particular compound or ingredient may promote health or well-being. However, the DHSEA does not allow claims that a supplement treats or cures disease, except in the specific case of a vitamin or nutrient treating the disease state associated with a particular nutritional deficiency. Substantiation of these claims is required only if challenged by regulators. In 1999, the FDA implemented new dietary supplement labeling rules. According to these rules, all dietary supplement labels must provide a statement of identity (eg, ginseng), net quantity of contents (eg, 60 capsules), structure–function claims with disclaimers that the product has not been evaluated by the FDA, directions for use, supplements fact panel (list of serving size, amount, and active ingredients), other ingredients list, and name and place of business of manufacturer, packer, or distributor. The Dietary Supplement & Nonprescription Drug Consumer Protection Act was passed in 2006 and requires companies producing dietary supplements to track serious adverse events and report them to the FDA within 15 days of knowledge that the serious adverse events occurred.[13] In 2007, the FDA updated the Current Good Manufacturing Practice regulations for dietary supplements, and these regulations require that dietary supplements are produced in a consistent manner and that producers ensure quality standards for identity, purity, strength, and composition.[13] The FDA Food Safety Modernization Act was passed in 2010 and enhances the ability of the FDA to recall both foods and dietary supplements.[13]

After marketing, if the FDA determines that a manufactured dietary supplement is unsafe or in violation of regulations, the agency can warn the public, suggest changes to make the supplement safer, recall the product, or ban the product. The FDA can exercise these powers if adverse effects occur during postmarketing surveillance, if there is evidence of adulteration or contamination, if products are mislabeled or make false claims, or if the company is not following good manufacturing practices.[13] The FDA banned or recalled dietary supplement products because of safety concerns identified in postmarketing surveillance on numerous occasions. In July 2001, the FDA warned dietary supplement manufacturers to stop marketing products containing aristolochic acid (AA) because of the potential for nephrotoxicity[87] and to remove comfrey-containing products from the market because of the potential for hepatotoxicity caused by pyrrolizidine alkaloids (PAs).[71] In November 2001, the FDA warned the manufacturer of LipoKinetix (containing phenylpropanolamine, caffeine, yohimbine, diiodothyronine, sodium usniate) to remove the supplement from the marketplace because of reports of associated hepatotoxicity.[42] In 2002, the FDA warned consumers and health care professionals of the risk of hepatotoxicity associated with the use of kava-containing products.[40] However, the FDA did not ban kava-containing products in the United States. In 2004, the FDA banned all sales of dietary supplements containing ephedra because of the risk of serious cardiovascular toxicity.[38] Other examples of dietary supplement products or ingredients that were recalled or banned by the FDA include 14 different Hydroxycut products in 2009, 1,3-dimethlyamylamine in 2011, and OxyElite Pro and Aegeline in 2013.[13]

Although dietary supplements are not to be advertised for the treatment of disease without the approval of the FDA, research suggests that they often are. A study determined that 81% of websites marketing dietary supplements made one or more health claims without approval from the FDA, and of these sites, 55% made specific claim to treat, prevent, or cure a specific disease.[81]

In addition, two studies suggest that many dietary supplements do not even contain appreciable quantities of the listed herb. In one study of 54 ginseng products, 60% of those analyzed contained pharmacologically insignificant amounts of ginseng, and 25% contained no ginsenosides.[73] A study of echinacea preparations determined that 10% of preparations contained no measurable echinacea, the assayed species was consistent with labeled content in 52% of the sample, and only 43% met the quality standard described by

the label.[48] Perhaps more concerning than the insufficient quantities of herbs are the unlisted ingredients that contaminate and adulterate some dietary supplements. Metals and pharmaceutical compounds often taint these preparations, as is discussed in more detail later in the sections on contamination and adulteration of plant- and animal-derived dietary supplements.

The FDA has released data suggesting that its regulations alone are insufficient in ensuring the safety of dietary supplements sold in the United States. Between 2008 and 2012, the FDA found violations of manufacturing rules in nearly half of the 450 dietary supplement firms it inspected.[109] One in four inspected companies had violations serious enough to warrant release of an FDA warning letter that could result in a significant enforcement action such as halting production and distribution. The FDA also believes that adverse events associated with dietary supplements are significantly underreported by manufacturers even though it is required by law.[76] Even after a product is identified as unsafe, it can be a challenge for the FDA to take action to remove the product. It took more than a decade for the FDA to remove ephedra-containing products from the market even though they had caused hundreds of deaths and thousands of adverse reactions.[76]

Several studies have attempted to determine how US hospitals regulate dietary supplements use in their facilities.[4,9,27,46] Many hospitals do not have formal policies governing the use of dietary supplements in their facilities. Some hospitals ban dietary supplements, but most allow them as long as they were ordered by an authorized prescriber. Some concerns include difficulties in identifying products (particularly "home supply" products) and uncertainty about appropriate dosing, efficacy, safety, and consistency, as well as the potential for herb–xenobiotic interactions. Facilities struggle to balance patient-centered care with the legal, medical, and ethical concerns about the efficacy, safety, and cost of dietary supplements.[12,46]

In essence, regulation of dietary supplements has shifted from a poorly regulated food product into a unique category between a conventional food product and a drug. This has served to fuel the debate on both sides: those who view dietary supplements as more similar to food groups (eg, chamomile tea) and want less government regulation and others who argue that dietary supplements contain pharmacologically active drugs (eg, ephedra) that require greater regulation.[77,82]

PHARMACOLOGIC PRINCIPLES

The pharmacologic activity of dietary supplements is classified by five active constituent classes: volatile oils, resins, alkaloids, glycosides, and fixed oils.[105]

Volatile oils are aromatic plant ingredients (Table 43–1). They are also called ethereal or essential oils because they evaporate at room temperatures and have an odor, which is generally pleasant. Many are mucous membrane irritants and have central nervous system (CNS) activity. Examples of herbs containing volatile oils include pennyroyal oil (*Mentha pulegium*), catnip (*Nepeta cataria*), chamomile (*Matricaria chamomilla*), and garlic (*Allium sativum*) (Chap. 42).

Resins are complex chemical mixtures of acrid resins, resin alcohols, resinol, tannols, esters, and resenes. These substances are often strong gastrointestinal (GI) irritants. Examples of resin-containing herbs include dandelion (*Taraxacum officinale*), elder (*Sambucus* spp), and black cohosh root (*Cimicifuga racemosa*).

Alkaloids are a heterogeneous group of alkaline and nitrogenous compounds. The alkaloid compound usually is found throughout the plant. This class consists of many pharmacologically active and toxic compounds. Examples of alkaloid-containing herbs include aconitum (*Aconitum napellus*), goldenseal (*Hydrastis canadensis*), and Jimson weed (*Datura stramonium*).

Glycosides are esters that contain a sugar component (glycol) and a nonsugar (aglycone), which yields one or more sugars during hydrolysis. They include the anthraquinones, saponins, cyanogenic glycosides, and lactone glycosides. The anthraquinones (senna {*Cassia acutifolia*} and aloe {*Aloe vera*}) are irritant cathartics. Saponins (licorice {*Glycyrrhiza lepidota*} and ginseng {*Panax ginseng* and *P. quinquefolius*}) are mucous membrane irritants, cause hemolysis, and have steroid activity. Cyanogenic glycosides found in apricot, cherry, and peach pits release cyanide. Lactone glycosides

TABLE 43–1	Selected Dietary Supplements, Popular Use, and Potential Toxicities				
Herbal	**Scientific Name**	**Other Common Names**	**Traditional and Popular Usage**	**Active or Toxic Ingredient(s)**	**Adverse Effects**
Aconite	*Aconitum napellus, Aconitum kusnezoffii, Aconitum carmichaelii*	Monkshood, wolfsbane caowu, chuanwu, bushi	Topical analgesic, neuralgia, asthma, heart disease, arthritis	Aconite alkaloids (C19 diterpenoid esters), aconitine	GI upset, dysrhythmias
Alfalfa	*Medicago sativa*		Arthritis, diabetes	L-Canavanine	Lupus, pancytopenia
Aloe	*Aloe vera* and other species	Cape, Zanzibar, Socotrine, Curacao, Carrisyn	Heals wounds, emollient, laxative, abortifacient	Anthraquinones, barbaloin, isobarbaloin	GI upset, dermatitis, hepatitis
Apricot pits	*Prunus armeniaca*	—	(Laetrile) cancer remedy	Amygdalin	Cyanide poisoning
Aristolochia	*Aristolochia clematis, Aristolochia reticulata, Aristolochia fangchi*	Birthwort, heartwort, fangchi	Uterine stimulant, cancer treatment, antibacterial	Aristolochic acid	Nephrotoxicity, renal cancer, bladder cancer, retroperitoneal fibrosis
Astragalus	*Astragalus membranaceus*	Huang qi, milk vetch root	Immune booster, HIV, cancer, antioxidant, increase endurance	Astrogalasides, trigonoside, and flavonoid constituent	Alters effectiveness of immunosuppressives (eg, steroids, cyclosporine)
Atractylis	*Atractylis gummifera*	Piney thistle	Chewing gum, antipyretic, diuretic, gastrointestinal remedy	Potassium atractylate and gummiferin	Hepatotoxicity, altered mental status, seizures, vomiting, hypoglycemia
Autumn crocus	*Colchicum autumnale*	Crocus, fall crocus, meadow saffron, mysteria, vellorita	Gout, rheumatism, prostate, hepatic disease, cancer, gonorrhea	Colchicine	GI upset, kidney disease, agranulocytosis
Bee pollen, royal jelly	Derived from *Apis mellifera*	—	Increase stamina, athletic ability, longevity	Pollen mixture containing hyperallergenic plant pollen or fungi contamination	Allergic reactions
Bee venom	Derived from *Apis mellifera*	—	Immunomodulator	Phospholipase A2 and mellitin, hyaluronidases	Allergic reactions
Betel nut	*Areca catechu*	Areca nut, pinlang, pinang	Stimulant	Arecoline	Bronchospasm; chronic use associated with leukoplakia and oropharyngeal squamous cell carcinoma
Bitter orange	*Citrus aurantium*	Changcao, *Fructus aurantii*, green orange, kijitsu, Seville orange, sour orange, Zhi shi	Dyspepsia, increase appetite weight loss	Synephrine	Myocardial infarction, stroke, ephedrine-like effects
Black cohosh	*Cimicifuga racemosa*	Black snakeroot, squawroot, bugbane, baneberry	Abortifacient, menstrual irregularity, astringent, dyspepsia	Triterpene glycosides	Dizziness, nausea, vomiting, headache
Blue cohosh	*Caulophyllum thalictroides*	Squaw root, papoose root, blue ginseng	Abortifacient, dysmenorrhea, antispasmodic	*N*-methylcytisine (2.5% the potency of nicotine)	Nicotinic toxicity
Boneset	*Eupatorium perfoliatum*	Thoroughwort, vegetable antimony, feverwort	Antipyretic	Pyrrolizidine alkaloids	Hepatotoxicity, dermatitis, milk sickness
Borage	*Borago officinalis*	Bee plant, bee bread	Diuretic, antidepressant, antiinflammatory	Pyrrolizidine alkaloids, amabiline	Hepatotoxicity
Boron		Boron	Topical astringent, wound remedy	Boron	Dermatitis, GI upset, kidney toxicity and hepatotoxicity, seizures, coma
Broom	*Cytisus scoparius*	Scotch broom, Bannal, broom top	Cathartic, diuretic, induce labor, drug of abuse	L-Sparteine	Nicotinic toxicity
Buchu	*Agathosma betulina*	Bookoo, buku, diosma, bucku, bucco	Diuretic, stimulant, carminative, urine infections, insect repellent	Diosmin, hesperidin, pulegone	Hepatotoxicity
Buckthorn	*Rhamnus frangula*		Laxative	Anthraquinones	Diarrhea, weakness
Burdock root	*Arctium lappa, Arctium minus*	Great burdock, gobo, lappa, beggar's button, hareburr, niu bang zi	Diuretic, choleretic, induce sweating, skin disorders, burn remedy, diabetes treatment	Atropine (contamination with belladonna alkaloids during harvesting)	Anticholinergic toxicity
Caapi	*Banisteriopsis caapi*	Ayahuasca, yage	Used to increase bioavailability of DMT in other plants as part of ayahuasca ritual	Harmine, harmaline, tetrahydroharmine	Serotonin toxicity, hallucinations
Cantharidin	*Cantharis vesicatoria* beetle	Spanish fly, blister beetles	Aphrodisiac, abortifacient, blood purifier	Terpenoid: cantharidin	GI upset, urinary tract and skin irritant, kidney toxicity
Carp bile (raw)	*Ctenopharyngodon idellus, Cyprinus carpio*	Grass carp, common carp	Improve visual acuity and health	Cyprinol, C27 bile alcohol	Hepatitis, kidney failure

(Continued)

TABLE 43–1	Selected Dietary Supplements, Popular Use, and Potential Toxicities *(Continued)*				
Herbal	**Scientific Name**	**Other Common Names**	**Traditional and Popular Usage**	**Active or Toxic Ingredient(s)**	**Adverse Effects**
Cascara	*Rhamnus purshiana*	Cascara sagrada	Laxative	Anthraquinones	Diarrhea, weakness
Catnip	*Nepeta cataria*	Cataria, catnep, catmint	Indigestion, colic, sedative, euphoriant, headaches, emmenagogue	Nepetalactone	Sedation
Chacruna	*Psychotria viridis*	Chacruna	Ingested as part of ayahuasca ritual	DMT	Serotonin toxicity
Ch'an Su	*Bufo bufo gargarizans, Bufo bufo melanosticus*	Stone, lovestone, black stone, rock hard, chuan wu, kyushin	Topical anesthetic, aphrodisiac, cardiac disease	Bufodienolides, bufotenin	Dysrhythmias, hallucinations
Chamomile	*Matricaria chamomilla, Chamaemelum nobile*	Manzanilla	Digestive disorders, skin disorders, cramps	Allergens	Contact dermatitis, allergic reactions
Chaparral	*Larrea tridentata*	Creosote bush, greasewood, hediondilla	Bronchitis, analgesic, anti-aging, cancer	Nondihydroguaiaretic acid	Hepatotoxicity (chronic)
Chuen-Lin	*Coptis chinensis, Coptis japonicum*	Golden thread, Huang-Lien, Ma-Huang	Infant tonic	Berberine: displaces bilirubin from protein	Neonatal hyperbilirubinemia
Cinchona Bark	*Cinchona succirubra, Cinchona calisaya, Cinchona ledgeriana*	Red bark, Peruvian bark, Jesuit bark, China bark, Cinchona bark, quinaquina, fever tree	Malaria, fever, indigestion, cancer hemorrhoids, varicose veins, abortifacient	Quinine	Cinchonism: GI complaints, tinnitus, visual symptoms, cardiovascular toxicity, CNS toxicity
Clove	*Syzygium aromaticum*	Caryophyllum	Expectorant, antiemetic, counterirritant, antiseptic, carminative euphoriant	Eugenol (4-allyl-2-methoxyphenol)	Pulmonary toxicity (cigarettes)
Coltsfoot	*Tussilago farfara*	Coughwort, horsehoof, kuandong hua	Throat irritation, asthma, bronchitis, cough	Pyrrolizidine alkaloids: tussilagin, senkirkine	Allergy, hepatotoxicity
Comfrey	*Symphytum officinale, Symphytum spp, S. x uplandicum*	Knitbone, bruisewort, blackwort, slippery root, Russian comfrey	Ulcers, hemorrhoids, bronchitis, burns, sprains, swelling, bruises	Pyrrolizidine alkaloids: symphytine, echimidine, lasiocarpine	Hepatotoxicity
Compound Q	*Trichosanthes kirilowii*	Gualougen, GLQ-223, Chinese cucumber root	Fevers, swelling, expectorant, abortifacient, diabetes, AIDS	Trichosanthin	Pulmonary injury (ARDS), cerebral edema, cerebral hemorrhage, seizures, fevers
Dong Quai	*Angelica polymorpha*	Tang kuei, dang gui	Blood purifier, dysmenorrhea, improve circulation	Coumarin, psoralens, safrole in essential oil	Anticoagulant effects, photodermatitis, possible carcinogen in oil
Echinacea	*Echinacea angustifolia, Echinacea purpurea*	American cone flower, purple cone flower, snakeroot	Infections, immunostimulant	Echinacoside	CYP1A2 inhibitor
Elder	*Sambucus* spp	Elderberry, sweet elder, sambucus	Diuretic, laxative, astringent, cancer	Isoquercitrin cyanogenic glycoside: sambunigrin in leaves	GI upset, weakness if uncooked leaves ingested
Ephedra	*Ephedra* spp	Ma-huang, Mormon tea, yellow horse, desert tea, squaw tea, sea grape	Stimulant, bronchospasm	Ephedrine, pseudoephedrine	Headache, insomnia, dizziness, palpitations, seizures, stroke, myocardial infarction
Evening primrose	*Oenothera biennis*	Oil of evening primrose	Coronary disease, multiple sclerosis, cancer, diabetes rheumatoid arthritis, premenstrual syndrome	Cis-γ-linoleic acid	Seizures
Fennel	*Foeniculum vulgare*	Common, sweet, or bitter fennel	Gastroenteritis, expectorant, emmenagogue, stimulate lactation	Volatile oils: transanethole, fenchone; estrogens: dianethole, photoanethole	Ingestion of volatile oils: vomiting, seizures, pulmonary injury (ARDS), dermatitis, estrogen effects
Fenugreek	*Trigonella foenumgraecum*	Bird's foot, Greek hay seed	Expectorant, demulcent, anti-inflammatory, emmenagogue, galactogogue, diabetes	4-Hydroxyisoleucine	Hypoglycemia, hypokalemia
Feverfew	*Tanacetum parthenium*	Featherfew, altamisa, bachelor's button, featherfoil, febrifuge plant, midsummer daisy, nosebleed, wild quinine	Migraine headache, menstrual pain, asthma, dermatitis, arthritis, antipyretic, abortifacient	Parthenolide	Oral ulcerations, "post-feverfew syndrome," rebound of migraine symptoms, anxiety, insomnia following cessation of chronic use
Fo-Ti	*Polygonum multiflorum*	Climbing knotwood, he shou-wu	Scrofula, cancer, constipation therapy, promote longevity	Anthraquinones: chrysophanol, emodin, rhein	Cathartic

(Continued)

TABLE 43–1　Selected Dietary Supplements, Popular Use, and Potential Toxicities (Continued)

Herbal	Scientific Name	Other Common Names	Traditional and Popular Usage	Active or Toxic Ingredient(s)	Adverse Effects
Foxglove	Digitalis purpurea, Digitalis lanata, Digitalis lutea, Digitalis spp	Purple foxglove, throatwort, fairy finger, fairy cap, lady's thimble, scotch mercury, witch's bells, dead man's bells	Asthma, sedative, diuretic or cardiotonic, wounds and burns (India)	Cardioactive steroids (eg, digitoxin, gitoxin, digoxin, digitalin, gitaloxin)	Blurred vision, GI upset, dizziness, muscle weakness, tremors, dysrhythmias
Garcinia	Garcinia cambogia	Brindleberry, hydroxycitric acid	Weight loss	Hydroxycitric acid	Hypoglycemia in diabetics
Garlic	Allium sativum	Allium, stinking rose, rustic treacle, nectar of the gods, da suan	Infections, coronary artery disease, hypertension	Alliin, Ajoene	Contact dermatitis, gastroenteritis, antiplatelet effects
Germander	Teucrium chamaedrys	Wall germander	Antipyretic, abdominal disorders, wounds, diuretic, choleretic	Furano neoclerodane diterpenes	Hepatotoxicity
Ginger	Zingiber officinale		Carminative, diuretic, antiemetic, stimulant, motion sickness	Volatile oil, phenol, zingerone	Anticoagulant and antiplatelet effects
Ginkgo	Ginkgo biloba	Maidenhair tree, kew tree, tebonin, tanakan, rokan, kaveri	Asthma, chilblain, digestive aid, cerebral dysfunction	Ginkgo flavone glycosides and terpene lactones (ginkgolides and bilobalide)	Extracts: GI upset, headache, skin reaction; leaf: antiplatelet: allergic reactions
Ginseng	Panax ginseng, Panax quinquefolius, Panax pseudoginseng	Ren shen	Respiratory illnesses, gastrointestinal disorders, impotence, fatigue, stress, adaptogenic, external demulcent	Ginsenosides: panaxin, ginsenin	Ginseng abuse syndrome: elevated blood pressure, insomnia, anxiety and diarrhea
Glucomannan	Amorphophallus konjac	Konjac, konjac mannan	Weight-reducing agent: "grapefruit diet," increase viscosity, decrease gastric emptying	Polysaccharides	Esophageal and lower GI obstruction
Glucosamine	2-Amino-2-deoxyglucose	Chitosamine	Wound-healing polymer, antiarthritic	Glucosamine	Hepatotoxicity
Goat's rue	Galega officinalis	French lilac, French honeysuckle	Antidiabetic	Galegine, paragalegine	Hypoglycemia
Goji	Lycium barbarum, chinense	Wolfberry, gou qi zi	Protect liver, improve eyesight, enhance immune system	Carotenoids, lutein, atropine	Interaction with warfarin likely due to CYP2C9 inhibition
Goldenseal	Hydrastis canadensis	Orange root, yellow root, turmeric root	Astringent, GI disorders, dysmenorrhea	Berberine, hydrastine	GI upset, paralysis and respiratory failure
Gordolobo yerba	Senecio longiloba, Senecio aureu, Senecio vulgaris, Senecio spartoides	Groundsel, liferoot	Gargle, cough, emmenagogue	Pyrrolizidine alkaloids	Hepatotoxicity
Gotu Kola	Centella asiatica	Hydrocotyle, Indian pennywort, talepetrako	Wound healing, tonic, antibacterial	Asiaticoside, asiatic acid, madecassic acid	Contact dermatitis
Green tea	Camillia sinensis	Green tea	Antioxidant, weight loss, reduce cholesterol	Polyphenols (catechins and epigallocatechin gallate)	Hepatotoxicity from green tea extracts
Hawthorn	Crataegus oxyacantha, Crataegus laevigata, Crataegus monogyna	English hawthorn, haw, maybush, whitethorn	Hypertension, CHF, dysrhythmias, antispasmodic, sedative	Hyperoside, vitexin, procyanidin	Hypotension, sedation
Heliotrope	Crotalaria spectabilis, Heliotropium europaeum	Rattlebox, groundsel, viper's bugloss, bush tea	Cancer	Pyrrolizidine alkaloids	Hepatotoxicity
Henbane	Hyoscyamus niger	Fetid nightshade, poison tobacco, insane root, stinky nightshade	Sedative, analgesic, antispasmodic, asthma	Hyoscyamine, hyoscine	Anticholinergic toxicity
Holly	Ilex aquifolium, Ilex opaca, Ilex vomitoria	English holly, American holly, and yaupon	Tea, emetic, CNS stimulant, coronary artery disease	Saponins	GI upset
Horse Chestnut	Aesculus Hippocastanum	Horse chestnut, California buckeye, Ohio buckeye, buckeye	Arthritis, rheumatism, varicose veins, hemorrhoids	Esculin, nicotine, quercetin, quercitrin, rutin, saponin, shikimic acid	Fasciculations, weakness, incoordination, GI upset, paralysis, stupor
Hydrangea	Hydrangea arborescens, Hydrangea paniculata	Seven bark, wild hydrangea	Diuretic, stimulant, carminative, cystitis, renal calculi, asthma	Hydrangin, saponin	Dizziness, chest pain, GI upset
Iboga	Tabernanthe iboga	Ibogaine	Aphrodisiac, stimulant, hallucinogen, addiction treatment	Ibogaine	Hallucinations, prolonged QT, torsade de pointes

(Continued)

TABLE 43–1   Selected Dietary Supplements, Popular Use, and Potential Toxicities (*Continued*)

Herbal	Scientific Name	Other Common Names	Traditional and Popular Usage	Active or Toxic Ingredient(s)	Adverse Effects
Impila	*Callilepsis laureola*		Zulu traditional remedy	Potassium atractylatelike compound	Vomiting, hypoglycemia, centrilobular hepatic necrosis
Jalap	*Ipomoea purga*		Cathartic	Convolvulin	Profuse watery diarrhea
Jimsonweed	*Datura stramonium*	Datura, stramonium, apple of Peru, Jamestown weed, thornapple, tolguacha	Asthma	Atropine, scopolamine, hyoscyamine, stramonium	Anticholinergic toxicity
Kava kava	*Piper methysticum*	Awa, kava-kava, kew, tonga	Relaxation beverage, uterine relaxation headaches, colds, wounds, aphrodisiac	Kava lactones, flavokwain A and B	Mild euphoria, muscle weakness, skin discoloration, liver failure
Khat	*Catha edulis*	Qut, kat, chaat, Kus es Salahin, Tchaad, Gat	CNS stimulant, depression, fatigue, obesity, ulcers	Cathine, cathinone	Euphoria, dysphoria, stimulation, sedation, psychological dependence, leukoplakia
Kola nut	*Cola acuminata*	Botu cola, cola nut	Digestive aid, tonic, aphrodisiac, headache, diuretic	Caffeine, theobromine, kolanin	CNS stimulant
Kombucha	Mixture of bacteria and yeast	Manchurian tea	Memory loss, premenstrual syndrome, cancer	Unknown bacteria	Hepatotoxicity, metabolic acidosis
Kratom	*Mitragyna speciosa*	Ketum	Pain, opioid replacement, psychoactive effects	Mitragynine	Intrahepatic cholestasis, seizure, arrhythmia, impaired memory, coma
Licorice	*Glycyrrhiza glabra*	Spanish licorice, Russian licorice, gancao	Gastric irritation	Glycyrrhizin	Flaccidity weakness, dysrhythmias, hypokalemia, lethargy
Lipoic acid		α-Lipoic acid, thioctic acid	Antioxidant, diabetes, neuropathy, AIDS	Lipoic acid	Hypoglycemia
Lobelia	*Lobelia inflata*	Indian tobacco	Antispasmodic, respiratory stimulant, relaxant	Lobeline	Nicotine toxicity
Mace	*Myristica fragrans*	Mace, muscade, seed cover of nutmeg	Diarrhea, mouth sores, insomnia, rheumatism	Myristicin (methoxysafrole)	Hallucinations, GI upset
Mandrake	*Mandragora officinarum*		Hallucinogen	Atropine, scopolamine, hyoscyamine	Anticholinergic toxicity
Mate	*Ilex paraguayensis*	Paraguay tea	Stimulant	Caffeine	Methylxanthine toxicity
Mayapple	*Podophyllum peltatum* *P. hexandrum*	Mayapple, podophyllum	Emetic, cathartic, warts	Podophyllotoxin	GI upset, delirium, hallucinations, coma, cranial nerve abnormalities, peripheral sensorimotor axonopathy, hematologic toxicity, microtubule toxin
Mistletoe	*Viscum album, Phoradendron leucarpum*	Iscador	Antispasmodic, calmative, cancer, HIV	Viscotoxins, lectins	GI upset, bradycardia, delirium
Morning glory	*Ipomoea purpurea, Ipomoea violacea*	Heavenly blue, blue star, flying saucers	Hallucinogen	D-lysergic acid amide (ergine)	Hallucinations
Mugwort	*Artemisia vulgaris, Artemisia dracunculus, Artemisia lactiflora*	Felon herb, moxa, guizhou	Depression, dyspepsia, menstrual disorder, abortifacient	Lactones (sesquiterpenes)	Hallucinations allergic reaction (skin, pulmonary), vivid dreams
Nutmeg	*Myristica fragrans*	Mace, rou dou kou	Hallucinogen, abortifacient, aphrodisiac, GI disorders	Myristicin	Hallucinogen, GI upset
Oleander	*Nerium oleander*	Adelfa, laurier rose, rosa laurel, rose bay, rose francesca	Cardiac disorders, asthma, corns, cancer, epilepsy	Oleandrin, neriin, gentiobiosyl-oleandrin, odoroside A	GI upset, diarrhea, dysrhythmias
Ostrich fern	*Matteuccia struthipteris*	Fiddlehead fern	Laxative	Flavonoids	GI upset if eaten undercooked
Parsley	*Petroselinum crispum*	Rock parsley, garden parsley	Diuretic, uterine stimulant, abortifacient	Myristicin, apiol, furocoumarin, psoralen	Uterine stimulant, photosensitization
Passion flower	*Passiflora incarnata*	Passiflora, maypop	Insomnia, analgesic stimulant	Harmala alkaloids	Sedation
Pau d'Arco	*Tabebuia spp*	Ipe roxo, lapacho, taheebo tea	Tonic, "blood builder," cancer, HIV	Napthoquinone derivative: lapachol	GI upset anemia, bleeding
Pennyroyal oil	*Hedeoma pulegioides* *Mentha pulegium*	American pennyroyal, Squawmint, mosquito plant	Abortifacient, regulate menstruation, digestive tonic	Cyclohexanone: pulegone	Hepatotoxicity

(*Continued*)

TABLE 43–1 Selected Dietary Supplements, Popular Use, and Potential Toxicities *(Continued)*

Herbal	Scientific Name	Other Common Names	Traditional and Popular Usage	Active or Toxic Ingredient(s)	Adverse Effects
Periwinkle	*Catharanthus roseus*	Red periwinkle, Madagascar or Cape periwinkle, old maid, church-flower, ram-goat rose, "myrtle," magdalena	Hallucinogen, ocular inflammation, diabetes, hemorrhage, insect stings, cancers	Vincristine, vinblastine, indole alkaloid	GI upset, altered mental status, peripheral neuropathy, microtubule toxin
Pokeweed	*Phytolacca americana, Phytolacca decandra*	American nightshade, Cancer jalap, inkberry, poke, scoke	Arthritis, emetic, purgative	Saponins: phytolaccigenin, jaligonic acid, phytolaccagenic acid, pokeweed mitogen	Gastroenteritis, blurry vision, weakness, respiratory distress, seizures, leukocytosis
Rue	*Ruta graveolens*	Herb of grace, herb grass	Emmenagogue, antispasmodic, abortifacient	Furocoumarins, bergapten, xanthoxanthin	Photosensitization
Sage	*Salvia officinalis*	Garden sage, true sage, scarlet sage, meadow sage	Antiseptic, astringent, hormonal stimulant, carminative, abortifacient	Camphor, thujone	Seizures
St. John's wort	*Hypericum perforatum*	Klamath weed, John's wort, goatweed, sho-rengyo	Anxiety, depression, gastritis, insomnia, promote healing, HIV	Hyperforin, hypericin	Occasional photosensitization; interacts with many different drugs via induction of CYP3A4, CYP2B6, P-glycoprotein activity, as well as inhibition of monoamine oxidase
Salvia	*Salvia divinorum, Salvia miltiorrhizae*	Sierra mazateca, diviner's sage, magic mint, Maria pastora	Hallucinogen, renal disease	Salvinorum A, lithospermate B	Hallucinations
Sassafras	*Sassafras albidum*	Lauraceae	Stimulant, antispasmodic, purifier	Sassafras oil (80% Safrole)	Hepatotoxicity, carcinogen
Saw palmetto	*Serenoa repens*	Sabal, American dwarf palm tree, cabbage palm	Genitourinary disorders, increase sperm production, sexual vigor	5α-Reductase inhibitor	Diarrhea
Senna	*Cassia acutifolia, Cassia angustifolia*	Alexandrian senna	Stimulant, laxative, diet tea	Anthraquinone, glycosides (sennosides)	Diarrhea, CNS effects
Slippery elm	*Ulmus rubra, Ulmus fulva*	Elm, elm bark, red elm	Acne, boils, indigestion, abortifacient	Polysaccharide mucilage Oleoresin	Contact dermatitis
Soapwort	*Saponaria officinalis*	Bruisewort, bouncing bet, dog cloves, fuller's herb, latherwort	Acne, psoriasis, eczema, boils, natural soaps	Saponins	Intravenous: highly toxic Oral: none
Soy isoflavone	*Glycine max*		Menopausal symptoms, heart disease	Phytoestrogens: genistein, daidzein, glycitein	Carcinogen
Squill	*Urginea maritima, Urginea indica*	Sea onion Red Squill	Diuretic, emetic, cardiotonic, expectorant	Cardioactive steroid, scillaren A	Emesis, dysrhythmias
Syrian rue	*Peganum harmala*	Harmal, Espand, African rue, Mexican rue, Turkish rue	Antibiotic, anxiolytic, analgesic, emmenagogue, abortifacient, ayahuasca substitute, and as a protector against evil eye	Harmala alkaloids, quinazoline alkaloids	Serotonin toxicity, tremor, abortion
T'u-san-chi	*Gynura segetum*		Tea	Pyrrolizidine alkaloids	Hepatotoxicity
Tonka bean	*Dipteryx odorata, Dipteryx oppositifolia*	Tonquin bean, cumaru	Food, cosmetics	Coumarin	Anticoagulant effect
Tung seed	*Aleurites moluccana, Aleurites fordii*	Tung, candlenut, candleberry, barnish tree, balucanat, otaheite	Wood preservative (oil), purgative (oil), asthma treatment (seed)	Saponins, phytotoxins	GI upset, hyporeflexia, latex: dermatitis
Valerian	*Valeriana officinalis*	Radix valerianae, Indian Valerian, red valerian	Anxiety, insomnia, antispasmodic	Valepotriates, valerenic acid	Sedation
White cohosh	*Actaea alba, Actaea rubra*	Baneberry, snakeberry, doll's eyes, coralberry	Emmenagogue	Protoanemonin	Headache, GI upset, delirium, circulatory failure
White willow bark	*Salix alba*	Common willow, European willow	Fever, pain astringent	Salicin	Salicylate toxicity: GI upset, tachypnea, anion gap metabolic acidosis, tinnitus, CNS toxicity, hyperthermia, cerebral edema, ARDS, coagulopathy

(Continued)

TABLE 43–1	Selected Dietary Supplements, Popular Use, and Potential Toxicities *(Continued)*				
Herbal	*Scientific Name*	*Other Common Names*	*Traditional and Popular Usage*	*Active or Toxic Ingredient(s)*	*Adverse Effects*
Wild lettuce	*Lactuca virosa Lactuca sativa*	Lettuce opium, prickly lettuce	Sedative, cough suppressant, analgesic	Unknown	Sedative, potentiates other sedatives
Woodruff	*Galium odoratum*	Sweet woodruff	Wound healing, tonic, varicose veins, antispasmodic	Coumarin	Hepatotoxicity, bleeding
Wormwood	*Artemisia absinthium*	Absinthes	Sedative, analgesic, antihelminthic	Thujone	Psychosis, hallucinations, seizures
Yarrow	*Achillea millefolium*	Bloodwort, carpenter's grass, dog daisy, nosebleed	Heal wounds, viral symptoms, digestive disorder, diuretic	Unknown	Contact dermatitis
Yew	*Taxus baccata*	Yew	Antispasmodic, cancer remedy	Taxine	Dizziness, dry mouth, bradycardia, cardiac arrest
Yohimbe	*Pausinystalia yohimbe*	Yohimbi, yohimbehe	Body building, aphrodisiac, stimulant	Yohimbine	Hypertension, abdominal pain, weakness

ADHD = attention-deficit/hyperactivity disorder; ARDS = acute respiratory distress syndrome; CHF = congestive heart failure; CNS = central nervous system; DMT = dimethyltryptamine; GI = gastrointestinal; HIV = human immunodeficiency virus; LSD= lysergic acid diethylamide.

(tonka beans {*Dipteryx odorata*}) have anticoagulant activities. Cardiac glycosides defined as cardioactive steroids (Chap. 62) are found in foxglove (*Digitalis* spp) and oleander (*Nerium oleander*).

Fixed oils are esters of long-chain fatty acids and alcohols. Herbs containing fixed oils are generally used as emollients, demulcents, and bases for other products. Generally, they are the least active and least dangerous of all plant- and animal-derived dietary supplements. Examples include olive (*Olea europaea*) and peanut (*Arachis hypogaea*) oils.

PHARMACOKINETICS AND TOXICOKINETICS

For many dietary supplements, the details of absorption, distribution, metabolism, and excretion are poorly characterized. Many dietary supplements simply have not been studied rigorously. In addition, inadequately regulated manufacturing practices lead to a lack of consistency in dietary supplements. This lack of consistency poses challenges in attempts to research kinetics of plant- and animal-derived dietary supplements and limits the generalizability of results from the study of one product to other supposedly similar products. Contamination and adulteration further muddy efforts to document the therapeutic or toxic effects of a particular product. In addition, the inherent complexity and variation of the living organisms from which these preparations are derived creates unique considerations related to the pharmacokinetics and toxicokinetics of these products. This section describes considerations related to the pharmacokinetics and toxicokinetics of xenobiotics derived from complex, living organisms.

Dietary supplements are prepared using a variety of techniques, which introduces variation in the resulting product. The American Botanical Council describes a variety of methods for processing plants into dietary supplements, including decoction, infusion, tincture, liniment, poultice, essential oils, herbal infused oils, and percolation.[2] Herbalists extract xenobiotics from raw materials using water, oils, alcohols, or other solvents at different temperatures for varying lengths of time, leading to variation in content and concentration of xenobiotics that are available to be absorbed in the final product.

Some of the unique considerations relevant to understanding toxicokinetics and toxicodynamics of living organisms are illustrated through the example of the hepatotoxic PAs. The concentration of PA within a single species differs greatly depending on the environment in which a plant is grown.[60] The concentration of PA varies widely in different parts of the plant and is often higher in the roots and young shoots. The PA concentration of pepsin–comfrey capsules was found to vary from 270 mg/kg to 2,900 mg/kg, depending on whether leaves or roots were used as a source.[56] More than 600 different PA are recognized,[94] and an individual plant typically produces several different PAs, which vary greatly in toxicity. For example, in most *Senecio* species, the PA senecionine is

the backbone structure from which the seneciphylline, jacobine, and senkirkine PA are derived.[75] While a plant is alive, it bioconverts from one PA to another PA in response to environmental conditions, for example, in response to predation by herbivores.[75] Because certain PAs are much more toxic than others, the toxicity of an individual plant can change dynamically throughout the day. The production of PA also changes throughout the life cycle of a plant, often reaching peak shortly before flowering.[60] Even the death of a nearby PA-containing plant affects the PA content of the adjacent plants; for example, the PAs leached from rotting *Senecio jacobaea* plants are taken up by roots and translocated to leaves of nearby unrelated plant species.[86] There are many factors that create wide variation in the content and concentration of medicinally and toxicologically relevant xenobiotics contained in plants, reflecting the diversity of the natural world. This variation makes it difficult to predict the exact xenobiotics content without extensive testing of every individual dietary supplement product. After they have been absorbed, PAs are metabolized by cytochrome P450 monooxygenases in the liver to form highly reactive electrophilic metabolites that quickly adduct with nucleophilic groups in DNA and protein, explaining the predominance of hepatotoxicity.[34] However, a smaller amount of PAs are metabolized to less immediately reactive metabolites or bind to less nucleophilic groups and then are slowly released to act in other parts of the body. Therefore, some PAs are more likely to cause immediate liver damage and others more likely to persist over time and cause indolent damage to a variety of tissues.[34] Hydrolysis of ester bonds in PA leads to a nontoxic metabolite that is excreted by the kidney. Pyrrolizidine alkaloid toxicity is discussed in more detail later.

Because dietary supplements contain a multitude of biologically active compounds, one expects that these herb-derived compounds will have pharmacokinetic and pharmacodynamic interactions with one another, as well as with pharmaceutical products. These interactions are discussed in the next sections on pharmacologic interactions and pharmacologic synergy.

PHARMACOLOGIC INTERACTIONS

A major concern related to the use of dietary supplements is the potential for interactions with pharmaceutical products (Table 43–2). Survey research suggests that 15% of patients taking pharmaceutical products use herbal preparations concurrently, and many of these products pose a risk for pharmacologic interactions.[57] The risk is highest in pharmaceutical products with a narrow therapeutic index, such as warfarin and digoxin. Additionally, pharmacologic interactions are particularly problematic in patients taking daily medications when decreased xenobiotic concentrations lead to severe health consequences, such as antiviral medications for patients infected with HIV or immunosuppressant medications to prevent organ rejection in transplant patients.

TABLE 43–2   Selected Dietary Supplement–Drug Interactions

Herbal Preparation	Scientific Name	Reported Drug Interactions	Proposed Mechanisms
Danshen	*Salvia miltiorrhiza*	Increased risk of bleeding in patients on warfarin	Pharmacokinetic and pharmacodynamic mechanisms
Garlic	*Allium sativum*	Increased clotting time and INR in patients taking warfarin Decreased concentration of saquinavir	Pharmacokinetic effects via inhibition of CYP2E1 and induction of P-glycoprotein
Gingko	*Ginkgo biloba*	Enhanced sedative effects of trazadone and benzodiazepines; increased risk of bleeding in patients taking aspirin, warfarin, and NSAIDS Increased concentration of digoxin Increases or decreases effects of antihypertensives, depending on dose, duration, and xenobiotic Lowers seizure threshold, decreasing effectiveness of antiepileptics or increasing risk of seizure in drugs with proconvulsant effects Enhances the efficiency and reduce the extrapyramidal side effects of the classic antipsychotic haloperidol in patients with schizophrenia	Pharmacokinetic effects via induction of CYP2C19 activity and inhibition of intestinal and hepatic CYP3A4 activity Pharmacodynamic effects
Ginseng	*Panax ginseng*	Decreased INR in patients on warfarin Case reports of headache, tremulousness, and manic episodes in patients taking phenelzine	Both pharmacokinetic and pharmacodynamic effects
Kava	*Piper methysticum*	Enhances sedative effects of alcohol and benzodiazepines Increased "off" periods in patient on levodopa for Parkinson's disease	Pharmacodynamic effects via GABA agonism and dopamine antagonism Pharmacokinetic effects via inhibition of CYP2E1, CYP1A2, CYP2C9, CYP2C19, CYP2D6, CYP3A4, CYP4A9, and CYP4A11
Licorice	*Glycyrrhiza glabra*	Modulates metabolism of corticosteroids, leading to mineralocorticoid excess	Pharmacokinetic effects via both inhibition and/or induction of CYP3A activity depending on dose or duration; also inhibits 5α-, 5β-reductase, and 11β dehydrogenase
Piperine	*Piper nigrum Linn*, *Piper longum Linn*	Increased concentrations of propranolol, rifampin, spartein, theophylline, phenytoin	Pharmacokinetic effects via inhibition of P-glycoprotein and CYP3A4 in enterocytes and hepatocytes
St. John's wort	*Hypericum perforatum*	Decreases concentration of amitriptyline, nortriptyline, alprazolam, midazolam, ciclosporin, digoxin, imatinib, irinotecan, methadone, indinavir, nevirapine, quazepam, simvastatin, tacrolimus, irinotecan, finasteride Decreases effectiveness of oral contraceptives Decreases INR in patients taking warfarin Increases or decreases fexofenadine concentration depending on duration of treatment Increased risk of serotonin syndrome in patients taking SSRIs or other serotonergic agents Increased effect of clopidogrel on platelet aggregation in clopidogrel-resistant patients	Pharmacokinetic effects via induction of CYP3A4, CYP2E1, CYP2C19, and P-glycoprotein Pharmacodynamic effect via inhibition of monoamine reuptake, leading to interactions with antidepressants Also pharmacodynamics effects via inhibition of COX-1, leading to decreased platelet aggregation

COX = cyclooxygenase; GABA = γ-aminobutyric acid; INR = international normalized ratio; NSAID = nonsteroidal antiinflammatory drug.
Data from references 25, 26, 55, 57, 70.

Pharmacologic interactions with dietary supplements occur via a variety of pharmacokinetic and pharmacodynamics mechanisms. Concurrent use of dietary supplements and pharmaceutical products causes pharmacokinetic interactions that affect absorption, distribution, metabolism, and excretion of various pharmaceuticals by competing for binding at drug transport sites and drug metabolism enzymes. Herbal preparations also cause pharmacodynamic interactions through action at end-organ receptors. Therefore, some dietary supplements acutely amplify or attenuate the effects of pharmaceutical products. Additionally, prolonged use of some dietary supplements affects the cellular expression of enzyme or transport systems within a body, leading to the development of subacute or chronic interactions that sometimes differ in character from the initial acute pharmacologic interactions.

St. John's wort (*Hypericum perforatum*) is a common herbal preparation that exemplifies numerous pharmacokinetic and pharmacodynamics interactions (Fig. 43–1). St. John's wort interacts with more than 20 different pharmaceutical products in humans and causes clinically significant consequences.[25,55,57] Chronic use of St. John's wort induces P-glycoprotein (P-gp). P-glycoprotein is an efflux transporter located in the plasma membranes of a variety of tissues. Increased P-gp activity in the intestines leads to decreased absorption and increased excretion of a variety of pharmaceutical products. Chronic use of St. John's wort leads to decreased tissue concentrations of P-glycoprotein substrates.[55,57] St. John's wort also induces CYP3A4, CYP2E1, and CYP2C19, leading to increased metabolism of pharmaceutical products that are substrates for these enzymes.[57] Through induction of P-gp and CYP enzymes, St. John's wort use causes clinically significant pharmacokinetic interactions with a variety of pharmaceutical products. Concurrent use of St. John's wort and the immunosuppressant medication cyclosporin leads to subtherapeutic concentrations of cyclosporin and rejection of transplanted organs in multiple cases.[55] St. John's wort inhibits monoamine reuptake, increasing the levels of serotonin, norepinephrine, and dopamine in the synapse.[119] St. John's wort has precipitated serotonin toxicity when combined with medications affecting serotonin utilization in numerous cases.[55] St. John's wort increases the antiplatelet effects of clopidogrel via both pharmacokinetic and pharmacodynamics mechanisms. St. John's wort induces CYP3A4, which increases the activation of clopidogrel, a prodrug, to its active metabolite.[26,70] Coadministration St. John's wort was shown to increase

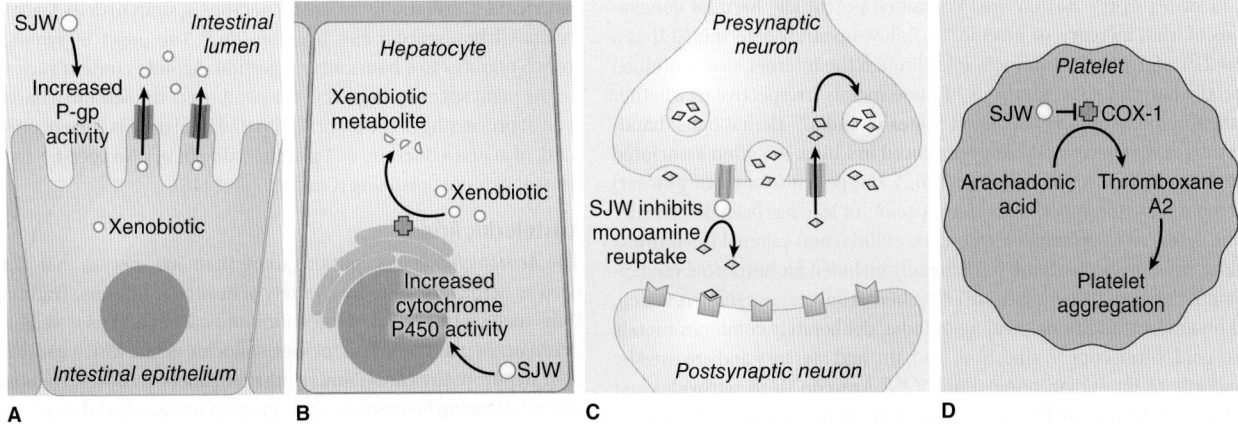

FIGURE 43–1. Mechanisms of pharmacokinetic and pharmacodynamic interactions involving St. Johns wort (SJW). (**A**) Induction of P-glycoprotein (P-gp) in the intestinal mucosa. St. John's wort induces activity of the efflux transporter P-gp, leading to decreased absorption and increased excretion of a variety of xenobiotics along the intestinal mucosa. (**B**) Induction of CYP enzymes in hepatocytes. St. John's wort induces activity of CYP2E1 and CYP2C19. Increased activity of CYP enzymes leads to increased metabolism of many different xenobiotics. (**C**) Inhibition of monoamine reuptake in synapse. St. John's wort inhibits reuptake of monoamines serotonin, norepinephrine, and dopamine, increasing the amount of these neurotransmitters in the synapse and increasing risk of serotonin toxicity when combined with other xenobiotics that act on the serotonin system. (**D**) Inhibition of cyclooxygenase-1 (COX-1) in platelets. St. John's wort inhibits COX-1, decreasing conversion of arachidonic acid to thromboxane A2 and inhibiting platelet aggregation, especially in combination with other antiplatelet agents.

platelet inhibition in clopidogrel nonresponders after coronary stent placement.[70] Hyperforin, a constituent of St. John's wort, inhibits cyclooxygenase-1 (COX-1) in platelets,[1] suggesting that the enhanced platelet inhibition in clopidogrel nonresponders may have been due to a synergy of pharmacokinetics (CYP3A4 induction) and pharmacodynamics (COX-1 inhibition).

PHARMACOLOGIC SYNERGY

Herbalists and traditional healers often suggest that the healing properties of plant- and animal-derived dietary supplements operate according to synergistic effects of multiple constituents that cannot be understood through a reductionist paradigm that focuses on the effects of a single active compound. Therefore, a whole plant is considered by some healers to be greater than the sum of its parts because the parts (ie, various xenobiotics) interact with one another to alter one another's pharmacologic effect. For example, the *Artemisia annua* plant contains artemisinin, from which the highly effective antimalarial drug artesunate was derived. Infusions of *A. annua* have been used for more than 1,000 years in China to treat symptoms related to malaria (periodic fever).[65] Traditionally prepared infusions of *A. annua* do not contain high enough concentrations of artemisinin to be effective against *P. falciparum*.[65] However, numerous in vitro and in vivo studies demonstrate that the dose of artemisinin necessary for effective activity against *P. falciparum* is much lower when administered in whole plant form than when artemisinin is used in isolation, possibly because of synergistic effects with flavonoids also contained in the plant.[65]

Herbalists often coadminister herbs, reasoning that different herbs work together in concert to have a greater effect or less toxicity than when administered alone. A well-described example of herbal synergy is the ayahuasca brew, which contains *Banisteriopsis caapi* and *Psychotria viridis*. The Quechua people administer ayahuasca in a traditional healing ceremony. According to the Quechua tradition, *B. caapi* is considered the spirit guide, and *P. viridis* is mixed to add light and color.[100] In fact, *B. caapi* contains harmala alkaloids that are monoamine oxidase inhibitors, increasing the oral bioavailability of the dimethyltryptamine (DMT) contained in *P. viridis* and collectively producing vivid hallucinations used in ceremonial rituals that neither plant could produce alone. Traditional Chinese medicine developed a detailed system based on synergy and describes four characteristics of medicinal preparations—the "principal" gives the primary therapeutic action, the "minister" amplifies the therapeutic action, the "assistant" decreases the toxicity of the preparation, and the "guide" helps bring the active xenobiotic to the proper location within the body.[116] The herbal preparation Xiao Chai Hu Tang, also

known as Sho-saiko-to, is a formula containing seven different herbs slows the progression of liver cirrhosis in clinical trials.[32,88,116] *Radix bupleuri* is considered the principal herb in the formula, with the other six herbs purported to serve various functions such as amplifying the therapeutic action of the principal herb or to reducing the toxicity of other herbs contained within the formula.[59] Preclinical research suggests that the effectiveness of the formula is greater when the herbs are used in combination than in isolation, suggesting the possibility of synergy.[88,116] More research is needed to elucidate whether traditional theories of synergy in plant- and animal-derived dietary supplements represent true pharmacokinetic or pharmacodynamics effects.

ADULTERATION WITH PHARMACEUTICAL PRODUCTS

The FDA released reports of more than 80 sexual enhancement dietary supplements that were adulterated with unlisted ingredients such as pharmaceutical products.[41] The FDA has also found that many plant- and animal-derived dietary supplements contain unlisted and potentially harmful ingredients. Weight loss, sexual enhancement, and body building products are most commonly implicated in cases of unlisted pharmaceutical adulterants.[39,41]

Patent medications are ready-made preparations used by traditional Chinese herbalists. Patent medications sometimes contain combinations of herbs and pharmaceutical medications, such as acetaminophen, aspirin, antihistamines, or corticosteroids.[22] Many of these adulterant pharmaceuticals are not listed on the packaging and sometimes are not even be approved for use in the United States.

For example, four cases of agranulocytosis followed consumption of *Chui Fong Tou Ku Wan*, a preparation that contains both aminopyrine (which is not approved for nonprescription sales in the United States) and phenylbutazone (which was withdrawn from the US market in the 1980s), neither of which is listed on the packaging.[93] Both aminopyrine and phenylbutazone are associated with agranulocytosis.

CONTAMINATION WITH METALS AND MINERALS

Metal and mineral poisonings from lead, cadmium, mercury, copper, selenium, zinc, and arsenic are associated with plant- and animal-derived dietary supplement usage.[19,21,30,92,98] High concentrations of these salts in the product sometimes result from contamination during the growing or manufacturing process of some plant- and animal-derived dietary supplements. Pay-loo-ah, a red and orange powder used by the Hmong people as a fever and rash remedy, was contaminated with lead.[17] In one study, 20% of surveyed Ayurvedic products produced in South Asia and sold on a nonprescription basis in stores in the Boston area contained potentially harmful concentrations of lead, mercury, or arsenic.[96] A follow-up study determined that a similar 21% of Ayurvedic products sold through the Internet also contained potentially harmful concentrations of these metals irrespective of whether manufacture occurred in the United States or India.[97] Herbal balls, hand-rolled mixtures of herbs and honey produced in China, are often associated with arsenic and mercury contamination.[37] Hai-ge-ten (clamshell powder) contamination with copper, chromium, arsenic, or lead has been described.[54] In some cases, as with cinnabar (mercuric sulfide) and calomel (mercurous chloride), these ingredients are intentionally included for purported medicinal benefit.[61] Ayurvedic remedies are either herbal only or *rasa shastra*, which, based on ancient traditional healing of India, deliberately combines metals such as gold, silver, copper, zinc, iron, lead, tin, and mercury and are used by the majority of the Indian population.[19,91,96,97] Azarcon (lead tetroxide) and greta (lead oxide) are used by an estimated Mexican families for treatment of *empacho*.[6,11] In Spanish, *empacho* means "blocked intestine," but it refers to any type of chronic digestive problem, including such diverse symptoms as constipation, diarrhea, nausea, vomiting, anorexia, apathy, and lethargy. Azarcon and greta are fine powders with total lead contents varying from 70% to more than 90%.[6,11] Treatment of metal toxicity in this context consists of ceasing consumption of the offending product and use of an appropriate chelator when indicated. For more information on toxicity of various metals, please see Chaps. 86, 93, and 95.

PATHOPHYSIOLOGY AND CLINICAL MANIFESTATIONS
Amygdalin
Amygdalin is a cyanogenic glycoside that is contained in many different plants, and it is most abundant in the seeds of several fruits from the *Rosaceae* family. The highest concentrations of amygdalin have been found in the seeds of familiar fruits such as green plums (10 mg/g), apricots (14 mg/g), black plums (mg/g), peaches (7 mg/g), and red cherries (4 mg/g).[10] Amygdalin is also known as laetrile and "vitamin B_{17}," although it is not a vitamin. Amygdalin in the form of laetrile has been advertised as a cancer treatment despite lack of evidence of effectiveness.[89] Amygdalin is enzymatically metabolized to form glucose, benzaldehyde, and hydrogen cyanide. The degree to which cyanide production occurs is unpredictable and varies based on temperature, acidity, and contribution of β-glucosidase enzymes from ingested plant matter, intestinal bacteria flora, and the tissue of exposed individual. Cyanide toxicity is more likely to occur after oral ingestion than after intravenous (IV) administration.[89] Cyanide inhibits multiple enzymes, including cytochrome oxidase. Inhibition of cytochrome oxidase disrupts oxidative phosphorylation within the electron transport chain and prevents cells from being able to use oxygen to produce adenosine triphosphate even when oxygen is available. Cyanide poisoning leads to acidosis, elevated lactate, and cardiovascular collapse. A 4-year-old child presented with cyanide toxicity after he received IV and oral "vitamin B_{17}."[99] For more information about cyanide poisoning, see Chap. 123 and Antidotes in Depth: A41 and A42.

Aconites
Aconites are derived from the roots of plants from the genus *Aconitum*. In China, aconite usually is derived from *Aconitum carmichaelii* (chuan wu) or *A. kuznezoffii* (caowu). In Europe and the United States, aconite is derived from *A. napellus*, commonly known as *monkshood* or *wolfsbane*. Aconites are traditionally used to treat fever and pain and to induce diuresis and diaphoresis. Aconite toxicity is caused by C19 diterpenoid-ester alkaloids, including aconitine, mesaconitine, and hypaconitine.[23] Aconitine binds to the open state of voltage-sensitive sodium channels in heart, nervous system, and muscles, leading to increased and prolonged sodium influx through these channels.[23] Paresthesias of the oral mucosa and entire body may be followed by nausea, vomiting, diarrhea, and hypersalivation and then by progressive skeletal muscle weakness. In the heart, the sodium channel effects of aconite poisoning lead to increased inotropy, delayed afterdepolarization, and early afterdepolarization, all of which cause a variety of dysrhythmias, including torsade de pointes, ventricular ectopics, ventricular tachycardia, and

ventricular fibrillation.[23,28] Central nervous system toxicity leads to centrally mediated bradycardia and hypotension.[23] The onset of symptoms occurs from 5 minutes to 4 hours after ingestion. Aconite content varies depending on the plant species, the part of the plant used, the season of harvest, and the type of processing of the plant. Estimated fatal dose is 2 mg of pure aconitine, 5 mL of aconite tincture, or 1 g of the wild plant.[23] No specific antidote exists to treat aconite poisoning (Chaps. 57 and 118).

Aristolochic Acids
The *Aristolochia* genus contains more than 500 species, many of which are used as herbal remedies by a variety of healing traditions. Traditional indications include treatment of infections and cancer and as a weight loss agent. *Aristolochia* plants contain toxic aristolochic acids, which cause aristolochic acid nephropathy (AAN) and urothelial cancer in dose-dependent fashion. The relationship between AA and kidney injury was first described in the early 1990s when an epidemic of kidney failure in more than 100 individuals in Belgium was linked to the use of *Aristolochia fangchi*, also known as birthwort, heart-wort, or fangchi, in a weight-loss regimen.[110,111] Since then, hundreds of cases of AAN were identified in more than 10 countries.[50,118] Aristolochic acids form covalent adducts with DNA, leading to dysfunction in DNA transcription and replication, ultimately causing cell cycle arrest.[74] Patients with AAN typically present with elevated serum creatinine, hypertension, anemia, glucosuria, proteinuria, white blood cell casts in the urine, and small kidneys with irregular cortical outlines on imaging.[74] A study of 300 patients with AAN in China described three different clinical presentations based on dose and duration of use.[118] Short-term, low-dose usage is associated with acute tubular dysfunction, which typically does not develop into end-stage renal disease (ESRD). Short-term, high-dose usage causes acute kidney injury, which generally progresses to ESRD over 1 to 7 years and sometimes leads to urothelial malignancy. Chronic use even at low levels frequently leads to ESRD within 2 years and poses an extremely high risk for urothelial cancer. A cumulative dose of more than 200 g of AA-containing compounds is suggested to pose a higher risk of urothelial carcinoma[84] (Chap. 27).

Artemisia, Absinthe, and Artesunate
Wormwood (*Artemisia absinthium*) extract has a long history of use for a variety of traditional medical indications, most prominently as an antihelminthic, and it is also the main ingredient in absinthe liquor. This volatile oil is a mixture of α- and β-thujone, which are monoterpene ketones.[67,68] Chronic absinthe use was formerly believed to cause "absinthism," characterized by psychosis, hallucinations, intellectual deterioration, and seizures, although now it is believed that these symptoms more likely resulted from alcoholism than wormwood itself.[67,68] Thujone causes seizures in research animals in a dose-dependent fashion, possibly through effects on γ-aminobutyric acid (GABA) receptors.[67,68] Consumption of absinthe liquor does not expose individuals to enough thujone to be likely to have a significant pharmacologic effect.[67,68] A case of wormwood-induced seizures, rhabdomyolysis, and acute kidney failure was described involving a patient who purchased from the Internet and consumed approximately 10 mL essential oil of wormwood, believing it was absinthe liquor.[114] Treatment remains supportive.

Sweet wormwood (*Artemisia annua*) has a very long history of use as an antimalarial and is the source for the pharmaceutical artesunate, an important antimalarial drug. Artemisia is also thought to have antiviral and anticancer activity. *A. annua* has a long history of use, with essentially no reports of major toxicity, and is therefore likely safe[65] (Chap. 55).

Betel Nut and Other Nicotinics
Betel (*Areca catechu*) is chewed by an estimated 200 million people worldwide for its euphoric effect. As an herb, it used as a digestive aid and as a treatment for cough and sore throat. Its active ingredient is arecoline, a direct-acting nicotinic agonist. The betel leaf also contains a phenolic volatile oil and an alkaloid capable of producing sympathomimetic reactions. Arecoline is a bronchoconstrictor, although weaker than methacholine, and sometimes exacerbate bronchospasm in patients with asthma chewing betel nut.[107] Treatment for betel nut toxicity is supportive. Long-term use of betel

nut is associated with leukoplakia and squamous cell carcinoma of the oral mucosa.[85] Many other herbal preparations have nicotinic effects. Examples of plants with nicotinic constituents include blue cohosh, broom, horse chestnut, lobelia, and tobacco.

Bufadienolides and Other Cardioactive Steroids

Ch'an Su, Kyushin, and "Love Stone" contain the secretions of the parotid and sebaceous glands of the toad *Bufo bufo gargarizans* or *Bufo melanosticus*.[15,63] Ch'an Su and Kyushin are traditional Chinese medicines used for the treatment of tonsillitis, sore throat, furuncle, palpitations, and cardiovascular diseases.[31] "Love Stone," also known as "Black Stone" and "Rock Hard," is an "aphrodisiac" intended for topical use.[18] Bufo toad extracts contains two groups of toxic compounds: digoxinlike cardioactive steroids consisting of bufadienolides, and the tryptamine alkaloid bufotenin. Clinical findings after ingestion are similar to those after cardioactive steroid poisoning, including GI effects and dysrhythmias. Several fatalities have been related to oral ingestion of Bufo toad extracts intended for use as topical aphrodisiacs,[18] as well as a fatality related to ch'an su that was mislabeled as a different preparation and unintentionally administered as a tea.[63] Severe toxic reactions and death are reported after mouthing toads, "licking," or eating an entire toad, or ingesting toad soup or toad eggs.[16] Assays for serum digoxin unreliably cross-react with bufadienolides but sometimes qualitatively assist in making a presumptive diagnosis.[18,63] For more information on cardioactive steroid poising, see Chap. 62 and Antidotes in Depth: A22.

Ephedra, Ephedrine, and Pseudoephedrine

Members of the genus *Ephedra* generally consist of erect evergreen plants resembling small shrubs. Common names include ma huang, sea grape, yellow horse, desert tea, squaw tea, and Mormon tea. *Ephedra* species have a long history of use as stimulants and for the management of bronchospasm. They contain the alkaloids ephedrine and pseudoephedrine among others.[52] In large doses, ephedrine causes nervousness, headache, insomnia, dizziness, hypertension, palpitations, skin flushing, tingling, vomiting, anxiety, restlessness, mania, and psychosis. Between 1995 and 1999, more than 1,000 cases of possible ephedra toxicity were reported to the FDA,[53,95] including many cases of serious cardiovascular events, such as stroke, myocardial infarction, and sudden death. In many cases when serious cardiovascular events occurred, the reported dose ingested appeared to be within the range recommended by the manufacturer's guidelines.[95] Analysis of commercially available ephedra products has demonstrated substantial variation in ephedrine, pseudoephedrine, and other ephedra alkaloid content both between brands and between lots of the same brand, with some products containing only 1 mg of ephedrine per unit dose, and other containing nearly 20 mg per unit dose.[52,95] Additionally, analysis of the ratios of alkaloids within these purportedly herbal products suggested that some were likely adulterated with pharmaceutical ephedrine.[52] In 2004, the FDA banned the sale of ephedra-containing dietary supplements, and the number of reported poisonings dropped precipitously after the ban was enforced.[120] However, other herbal preparations, such as bitter orange (*Citrus aurantia*), contain ephedralike alkaloids (synephrine), are still widely available, and may pose risk for cardiovascular events.[8] The treatment is similar to that for other CNS stimulants (Chap. 49).

Glycyrrhizin and Other Endocrine Disruptors

Licorice root from the *Glycyrrhiza glabra* plant is widely used as an ingredient in candies, lozenges, teas, and herbal preparations. The root contains a saponin glycoside, glycyrrhizin, that inhibits 11-β-hydroxysteroid dehydrogenase, decreasing conversion of cortisol to cortisone.[112] Chronic licorice consumption increases cortisol concentrations, which then act on renal mineralocorticoid receptors. Repeated consumption of licorice root causes a syndrome of mineralocorticoid excess with hypokalemia, sodium and water retention, peripheral edema, hypertension, and weakness.[112] Administration of 100 g of licorice by mouth over as little as 7 days resulted in decreased serum potassium concentrations below the normal range in previously healthy participants.[35] There are multiple reports of individuals experiencing cardiac dysrhythmias

or cardiac arrest in the context of chronic licorice consumption and profound hypokalemia.[29,36] *Serenoa repens*, commonly known as saw palmetto, interferes with estrogen and testosterone metabolism. It is sometimes used as a treatment for benign prostatic hypertrophy and alopecia. It has been associated with hot flashes followed by premature menarche in young girls.[78,80]

Harmala Alkaloids

Peganum harmala and *Banisteriopsis caapi* contain various pharmacologically active alkaloids; the most toxicologically relevant are the β-carboline alkaloids (also known as harmala alkaloids), such as harmine and harmaline.[79,90] *Peganum harmala* is used in the Middle East and northern Africa for numerous traditional indications such as an antibiotic, anxiolytic, analgesic, emmenagogue, and abortifacient and as a protector against evil eye.[72] *Banisteriopsis caapi* is used in combination with plants containing DMT (eg, *Psychotria viridis*) to produce a hallucinogenic state as part of a ethnobotanical hallucinogenic rituals, or ayahuasca ceremonies. High doses of β-carboline alkaloids produce confusion, hallucinations, psychomotor agitation, diffuse tremors, ataxia, vomiting, diarrhea, slight elevation of body temperature, and mild changes in heart rate and blood pressure.[44,79] Harmaline is approximately twice as toxic as harmine based on animal research.[72] Although content varies dramatically, a typical dose of ayahuasca contain approximately 100 to 200 mg of harmine and 20 to 40 mg of harmaline.[44,69] A typical dose of *P. harmala* is 3 to 8 g of seeds, containing approximately 120 to 350 mg of harmine and 170 to 450 mg of harmaline.[72,79] When consumed alone or as traditionally recommended, the alkaloids from *P. harmala* and *B. caapi* have a high therapeutic index, and even individuals who consume much larger than recommended quantities and require medical attention generally recover within several hours without long-term sequelae.[44,72,79] But the globalization of ayahuasca has produced a proliferation of inexperienced "shamans," some of whom are not trained in the traditional preparation of the ayahuasca brew, and sometimes add novel ingredients, leading to poor outcomes. Several fatalities related to ayahuasca are described in the medical literature. However, the cases in which details regarding the origin and content of the ayahuasca brew are available seem to suggest that severe intoxication and death have primarily resulted when inexperienced individuals prepare brews containing novel ingredients such as atropine, scopolamine, or nicotine or when nontraditional ingredients are substituted for traditional ingredients, for example when methoxy-*N*, *N*-dimethyltryptamine is used in place of DMT or when *P. harmala* is used in place of *B. caapi*.[44,69] In addition, the monoamine oxidase inhibition of β-carboline alkaloids poses risks for more severe serotonin toxicity when combined with other medications or drugs with serotonergic effects.[44] Management of β-carboline alkaloid toxicity is primarily supportive (Chaps. 69 and 71). For more information on psychoactive dietary supplement usage, see Table 43–3.

Kratom

Kratom (*Mitragyna speciosa*) is used as an analgesic, antidepressant, antidiarrheal, euphoriant, stimulant, and opioid replacement. Kratom contains the alkaloids mitragynine and 7-hydroxymitragynine, which are a mu-opioid receptor agonists, and additionally have activity on adrenergic, serotonergic, and dopaminergic receptors.[43] Mitragynine also appears to interfere with rectifier potassium currents, presenting a risk for sudden cardiac death.[106A] A study of mitragynine kinetics in 10 chronic kratom users found that 30 mg of mitragynine was enough to produce desired kratom effects without undesired side effects.[113] However, mitragynine concentration varies greatly in kratom products, and kratom users have been documented to use as much as 275 mg of mitragynine to produce desired effects.[113] The toxic and lethal doses of mitragynine are not well-defined. Kratom has potential for abuse given it's mu-opioid activity and sometimes produces a withdrawal syndrome when discontinued after chronic use.[43,66] However, despite kratom's opioid agonism, it has not been reported to cause respiratory depression.[66,113] Kratom use has been associated with hepatotoxicity, psychosis, seizure, coma, and death.[5,43] The United States Drug Enforcement Agency has considered classifying kratom as a controlled substance; however, at this time, it remains unscheduled and is regulated as a standard dietary supplement.

TABLE 43–3 Constituent Psychoactive Xenobiotics in Herbal Preparations

Labeled Ingredient	Scientific Name	Usage	Active Ingredients	Classification of Effect
Broom	Cytisus scoparius	Smoke for relaxation	L-Sparteine	Sedative
Caapi	Banisteriopsis caapi	Ingested in combination with other plants as part of ayahuasca ritual	Harmala alkaloids	Inhibits monoamine oxidase to increase bioavailability of DMT
California poppy	Eschscholzia californica	Smoke	Protopine, escholtzine, allocryptopine, californidine, chelirubine, sanguinarine, and macarpine	Euphoriant, sedative
Catnip	Nepeta cataria	Smoke or tea	Nepetalactone	Euphoriant
Ch'an Su	Bufo bufo gargarizans, Bufo bufo melanosticus	Smoke or lick	Bufotenin	Hallucinogen
Cinnamon	Cinnamomum camphora	Smoke, essential oil	Cinnamaldehyde	Stimulant
Chacruna	Psychotria viridis	Ingested as part of ayahuasca ritual	DMT	Hallucinogen
Clove	Syzgium aromaticum	Smoke in cigarette or "kreteks"	Eugenol	Euphoriant
Damiana	Turnera diffusa	Smoke	Unknown	Stimulant, hallucinogen
Hops	Humulus lupulus	Smoke or tea	Humulone, lupulone → methylbutenol	Sedative
Hydrangea	Hydrangea paniculata	Smoke	Hydrangin, saponin	Stimulant
Ibogaine	Tabernanthe iboga	Ingested	Ibogaine	Hallucinogen
Juniper	Juniperus macropoda	Smoke as hallucinogen	Unknown	Hallucinogen
Jurema	Mimosa hostilis	Smoke, tea or used as source for extraction DMT	DMT	Hallucinogen
Kava kava	Piper methysticum	Smoke or tea	Kava lactones	Hallucinogen
Kola nut	Cola acuminata	Smoke, tea, or capsules	Caffeine, theobromine, kolanin	Stimulant
Kratom	Mitragyna speciosa	Smoke, tea, or capsules	Mitragynine	Euphoriant, stimulant, opioid
Lobelia	Lobelia inflata	Smoke or tea	Lobeline	Euphoriant
Mandrake	Mandragora officinarum	Tea	Atropine, scopolamine	Hallucinogen
Mate	Ilex paraguayensis	Tea	Caffeine	Stimulant
Mormon tea	Ephedra nevadensis	Tea	Ephedrine	Stimulant
Morning glory	Ipomoea violacea	Ingest seeds	D-lysergic acid amide (ergine)	Hallucinogen
Nutmeg	Myristica fragrans	Tea	Myristicin	Hallucinogen
Passion flower	Passiflora incarnata	Smoke, tea, or capsules	Harmala alkaloids	Sedative
Periwinkle	Catharanthus roseus	Smoke or tea	Indole alkaloids	Hallucinogen
Prickly poppy	Argemone mexicana	Smoke	Protopine, bergerine, isoquinolones	Analgesic
Salvia	Salvia divinorum	Smoke, chew	Salvinorum A	Hallucinogen
Snakeroot	Rauwolfia serpentina	Smoke or tea	Reserpine	Tranquilizer
Syrian rue	Peganum harmala	Smoke, ingested	Harmala alkaloids, quinazoline alkaloids	Serotonin toxicity, abortifacient
Thorn apple	Datura stramonium	Smoke or tea	Atropine, scopolamine	Hallucinogen
Tobacco	Nicotiana spp	Smoke	Nicotine	Stimulant
Valerian	Valeriana officinalis	Tea or capsules	Chatinine, velerine alkaloids	Sedative
Wild lettuce	Lactuca sativa	Smoke	Unknown	Analgesic, sedative
Wormwood	Artemisia absinthium	Smoke, tea, spirits	Thujone	Analgesic
Yohimbe	Pausinystalia yohimbe	Smoke or tea	Yohimbine	Hallucinogen

DMT = dimethyltryptamine.

Pyrrolizidine Alkaloids and Other Hepatotoxins

The PAs are potent hepatotoxins that are estimated to be present in 3% of the world's flowering plants, among various diverse plant families.[102] Within the family Asteraceae, plants in the *Senecio* genus are responsible for numerous human poisonings when brewed in herbal teas or contaminating food products in diverse locations.[115] Within the family Fabaceae, plants in the *Crotalaria* genus have caused many cases of liver injury and death when brewed in bush tea in Jamaica and South Africa.[115] Within the family Boraginaceae, *Heliotropium* species caused thousands of poisonings when it contaminated wheat fields in Tajikistan and Afghanistan.[112] Also within the family Boraginaceae, plants within the *Symphytum* genus, commonly known as comfrey, cause poisonings when ingested as medicinal preparations or teas.[115] Numerous healing traditions throughout the world use plants that contain PAs. Many different PAs exist, which are classified into three categories based on structure: retronecine type, otonecine type, and platynecine type.[94] The retronecine types are the most toxic of the PAs.[94] Pyrrolizidine alkaloids contained in plants are protoxins that are activated by numerous hepatic cytochrome P450 isoenzymes to form highly reactive pyrrole esters, which then quickly form adducts with protein and DNA. Acute exposure to PAs causes a highly characteristic syndrome of hepatic sinusoidal hypertrophy and venous occlusion, resulting in hepatic sinusoidal obstruction syndrome, hepatomegaly, and cirrhosis[34] (Chap. 21). Chronic low-level exposure causes cirrhosis with a pathological profile that is difficult to distinguish from cirrhosis resulting from other causes, as well as pulmonary artery hypertension.[34] In addition, animal models and human cell cultures have demonstrated that PA metabolites bind to the gene encoding the tumor suppressor protein p53 and produce a wide variety of cancers in animal models, although definitive linkage to human cancers is not yet established.[34] It is recommended that daily intake of PA not exceed 7 ng/kg of dehydro-PAs per kilogram of body weight.[34]

Other herbs and extracts that have been associated with hepatotoxicity include black cohosh,[14] chaparral,[51,101] *Garcinia cambogia*,[45] germander,[14] green tea extract,[14,45] kava extract,[14] linoleic acid,[45] ma huang,[45] pennyroyal,[3,7] usnic acid,[45] and 1,3-dimethylamylamine.[45] In addition, products with the following names have been associated with liver toxicity: Herbalife,[45] Hydroxycut,[45] LipoKinetix,[45] and OxyELITE.[45]

Strychnine

The Chinese herbal preparation maqianzi is derived from the dried seeds of *Strychnos nux vomica* plant and is traditionally used in China to treat rheumatism and other musculoskeletal complaints. Maqianzi contains the alkaloids strychnine and brucine that compete with glycine for binding to glycinergic chloride channels, resulting in a loss of inhibition from the ventral horn of the spinal cord. Strychnine poisoning is characterized by involuntary generalized muscle contractions, respiratory and metabolic acidosis, rhabdomyolysis, and hyperthermia. The traditional recommended dose for maqianzi ranges from 0.3 to 1.2 g by mouth, and the processed seeds generally contain 1% to 2% strychnine.[24,64,121] A randomized placebo-controlled trial[64] of maqianzi with verified strychnine and brucine content found that eight participants of 60 who were administered standard treatment doses of maqianzi developed a "nux vomica response" characterized by "slight sweating, tongue rigidity, girdle sensation, and slight muscular twitch." An additional patient in this study had a more severe strychnine-like reaction that was not described in detail. This demonstrates there is overlap between the therapeutic dose and the toxic dose for this product. A woman who was reportedly administered 15 g of maqianzi developed muscle spasms and difficulty breathing, and her symptoms resolved within several hours,[24] For management of strychnine poisoning, see Chap. 114.

Tropane Alkaloids, Anticholinergics

Many plants contain the tropane alkaloids atropine (D,L-hyoscyamine), hyoscyamine, and scopolamine (L-hyoscine). They are sometimes used therapeutically for treatment of asthma and occasionally are mistakenly included in herbal teas.[20] Signs and symptoms of anticholinergic poisoning include mydriasis, diminished bowel sounds, urinary retention, dry mouth, flushed skin, tachycardia, and agitation. Mildly poisoned patients usually require only supportive care and sedation with IV benzodiazepines. More severe cases are treated with IV physostigmine (Antidotes in Depth: A11).

SUMMARY

- Plant- and animal-derived supplements are diverse products, many of which have a long history of traditional and cultural use.
- Plant- and animal-derived dietary supplement are poorly regulated and sometimes contain dangerous contaminants and adulterants.
- Plant- and animal-derived dietary supplements contain xenobiotics that are pharmacologically active and have the potential to cause toxicity and pharmacologic interactions.
- The physiologic and toxicologic effects of plant- and animal-derived supplements are diverse and often difficult to predict because of immense variation in the content and composition of these products.

Acknowledgment

Oliver Hung, MD; Mary Ann Howland, PhD; and Neal A. Lewin, MD, contributed to this chapter in previous editions.

REFERENCES

1. Albert D, et al. Hyperforin is a dual inhibitor of cyclooxygenase-1 and 5-lipoxygenase. *Biochem Pharmacol.* 2002;64:1767-1775.
2. American Botanical Council. Terminology—American Botanical Council. http://abc.herbalgram.org/site/PageServer?pagename=Terminology. Accessed April 18, 2017.
3. Anderson IB, et al. Pennyroyal toxicity: measurement of toxic metabolite levels in two cases and review of the literature. *Ann Intern Med.* 1996;124:726-734.
4. Ansani NT, et al. Hospital policies regarding herbal medicines. *Am J Health-Syst Pharm AJHP Off J Am Soc Health-Syst Pharm.* 2003;60:367-370.
5. Anwar M, et al. Notes from the field: Kratom (Mitragyna speciosa) exposures reported to poison centers—United States, 2010–2015. *MMWR Morb Mortal Wkly Rep.* 2016; 65:748-749.
6. Baer RD, Ackerman A. Toxic Mexican folk remedies for the treatment of empacho: the case of azarcon, greta, and albayalde. *J Ethnopharmacol.* 1988;24:31-39.
7. Bakerink JA, et al. Multiple organ failure after ingestion of pennyroyal oil from herbal tea in two infants. *Pediatrics.* 1996;98:944-947.
8. Bakhiya N, et al. Phytochemical compounds in sport nutrition: synephrine and hydroxycitric acid (HCA) as examples for evaluation of possible health risks. *Mol Nutr Food Res.* 2017;61.
9. Bazzie KL, et al. National survey of dietary supplement policies in acute care facilities. *Am J Health-Syst Pharm AJHP Off J Am Soc Health-Syst Pharm.* 2006;63:65-70.
10. Bolarinwa IF, et al. Amygdalin content of seeds, kernels and food products commercially-available in the UK. *Food Chem.* 2014;152:133-139.
11. Bose A, et al. Azarcón por empacho—another cause of lead toxicity. *Pediatrics.* 1983; 72:106-108.
12. Boyer E. Issues in the management of dietary supplement use among hospitalized patients. *J Med Toxicol Off J Am Coll Med Toxicol.* 2005;1:30-34.
13. Brown AC. An overview of herb and dietary supplement efficacy, safety and government regulations in the United States with suggested improvements. Part 1 of 5 series. *Food Chem Toxicol.* 2017;107(Pt A):449-471.
14. Brown AC. Liver toxicity related to herbs and dietary supplements: online table of case reports. Part 3 of 6. *Food Chem Toxicol.* 2016.
15. Brubacher JR, et al. Efficacy of digoxin specific Fab fragments (Digibind®) in the treatment of toad venom poisoning. *Toxicon.* 1999;37:931-942.
16. Brubacher JR, et al. Treatment of toad venom poisoning with digoxin-specific Fab fragments. *Chest.* 1996;110:1282-1288.
17. Centers for Disease Control and Prevention. Leads from the MMWR. Folk remedy-associated lead poisoning in Hmong children. *JAMA.* 1983;250:3149-3150.
18. Centers for Disease Control and Prevention (CDC). Deaths associated with a purported aphrodisiac—New York City, February 1993-May 1995. *MMWR Morb Mortal Wkly Rep.* 1995;44:853-855, 861.
19. Centers for Disease Control and Prevention (CDC). Lead poisoning associated with ayurvedic medications—five states, 2000-2003. *MMWR Morb Mortal Wkly Rep.* 2004; 53:582-584.
20. Chan JC, et al. Anticholinergic poisoning from Chinese herbal medicines. *Aust N Z J Med.* 1994;24:317-318.
21. Chan TY, et al. Chinese herbal medicines revisited: a Hong Kong perspective. *Lancet Lond Engl.* 1993;342:1532-1534.
22. Chan TY, Critchley JA. Usage and adverse effects of Chinese herbal medicines. *Hum Exp Toxicol.* 1996;15:5-12.

652   PART C • THE CLINICAL BASIS OF MEDICAL TOXICOLOGY

23. Chan TYK. Aconite poisoning. *Clin Toxicol*. 2009;47:279-285.
24. Chan TYK. Herbal medicine causing likely strychnine poisoning. *Hum Exp Toxicol*. 2002;21:467-468.
25. Chen X-W, et al. Herb-drug interactions and mechanistic and clinical considerations. *Curr Drug Metab*. 2012;13:640-651.
26. Choi JG, et al. A comprehensive review of recent studies on herb-drug interaction: a focus on pharmacodynamic interaction. *J Altern Complement Med*. 2016;22:262-279.
27. Cohen MH, et al. Emerging credentialing practices, malpractice liability policies, and guidelines governing complementary and alternative medical practices and dietary supplement recommendations: a descriptive study of 19 integrative health care centers in the United States. *Arch Intern Med*. 2005;165:289-295.
28. Coulson JM, et al. The management of ventricular dysrhythmia in aconite poisoning. *Clin Toxicol*. 2017;55:313-321.
29. Crean AM, et al. A sweet tooth as the root cause of cardiac arrest. *Can J Cardiol*. 2009;25:e357-358.
30. D'Arcy PF. Adverse reactions and interactions with herbal medicines. Part 1. Adverse reactions. *Adverse Drug React Toxicol Rev*. 1991;10:189-208.
31. Dasgupta A, et al. The Fab fragment of anti-digoxin antibody (digibind) binds digitoxin-like immunoreactive components of Chinese medicine Chan Su: monitoring the effect by measuring free digitoxin. *Clin Chim Acta*. 2001;309:91-95.
32. Deng G, et al. A single arm phase II study of a Far-Eastern traditional herbal formulation (sho-sai-ko-to or xiao-chai-hu-tang) in chronic hepatitis C patients. *J Ethnopharmacol*. 2011;136:83-87.
33. Desborough MJR, Keeling DM. The aspirin story—from willow to wonder drug. *Br J Haematol*. 2017;177:674-683.
34. Edgar JA, et al. Pyrrolizidine alkaloids: potential role in the etiology of cancers, pulmonary hypertension, congenital anomalies, and liver disease. *Chem Res Toxicol*. 2015;28:4-20.
35. Epstein MT, et al. Effect of eating liquorice on the renin-angiotensin aldosterone axis in normal subjects. *Br Med J*. 1977;1:488-490.
36. Eriksson JW, et al. Life-threatening ventricular tachycardia due to liquorice-induced hypokalaemia. *J Intern Med*. 1999;245:307-310.
37. Espinoza EO, et al. Arsenic and mercury in traditional Chinese herbal balls. *N Engl J Med*. 1995;333:803-804.
38. Food and Drug Administration. 2004—FDA acts to remove ephedra-containing dietary supplements from market. https://wayback.archive-it.org/7993/20170111185913/http://www.fda.gov/NewsEvents/Newsroom/PressAnnouncements/2004/ucm108379.htm. Accessed April 8, 2017.
39. Food and Drug Administration. Consumer updates—tainted products marketed as dietary supplements. https://www.fda.gov/ForConsumers/ConsumerUpdates/ucm236774.htm. Accessed July 21, 2017.
40. Food and Drug Administration. Consumers—consumer advisory: kava-containing dietary supplements may be associated with severe liver injury. https://www.fda.gov/food/resourcesforyou/consumers/ucm085482.htm. Accessed April 8, 2017.
41. Food and Drug Administration. Medication health fraud—more tainted sexual enhancement products. https://www.fda.gov/Drugs/ResourcesForYou/Consumers/BuyingUsingMedicineSafely/MedicationHealthFraud/ucm443502.htm. Accessed July 21, 2017.
42. Food and Drug Administration. Safety alerts for human medical products—Lipokinetix. https://wayback.archive-it.org/7993/20170112171530/http://www.fda.gov/Safety/MedWatch/SafetyInformation/SafetyAlertsforHumanMedicalProducts/ucm172824.htm. Accessed April 8, 2017.
43. Fluyau D, Revadigar N. Biochemical benefits, diagnosis, and clinical risks evaluation of kratom. *Front Psychiatry*. 2017;8.
44. Gable RS. Risk assessment of ritual use of oral dimethyltryptamine (DMT) and harmala alkaloids. *Addiction*. 2007;102:24-34.
45. García-Cortés M, et al. Hepatotoxicity by dietary supplements: a tabular listing and clinical characteristics. *Int J Mol Sci*. 2016;17:537.
46. Gardiner P, et al. Dietary supplements: inpatient policies in US children's hospitals. *Pediatrics*. 2008;121:e775-781.
47. Geller AI, et al. Emergency department visits for adverse events related to dietary supplements. *N Engl J Med*. 2015;373:1531-1540.
48. Gilroy CM, et al. Echinacea and truth in labeling. *Arch Intern Med*. 2003;163:699-704.
49. Global Industry Analysts, Inc. Herbal supplements and remedies—a global business report. http://www.strategyr.com/pressMCP-1081.asp.
50. Gökmen MR, et al. The epidemiology, diagnosis, and management of aristolochic acid nephropathy: a narrative review. *Ann Intern Med*. 2013;158:469-477.
51. Gordon DW. Chaparral ingestion: the broadening spectrum of liver injury caused by herbal medications. *JAMA*. 1995;273:489.
52. Gurley BJ, et al. Ephedrine-type alkaloid content of nutritional supplements containing ephedra sinica (ma-huang) as determined by high performance liquid chromatography. *J Pharm Sci*. 1998;87:1547-1553.
53. Haller CA, Benowitz NL. Adverse cardiovascular and central nervous system events associated with dietary supplements containing ephedra alkaloids. *N Engl J Med*. 2000;343:1833-1838.
54. Hill GJ, Hill S. Lead poisoning due to hai ge fen. *JAMA*. 1995;273:24-25.
55. Hu Z, et al. Herb-drug interactions: a literature review. *Drugs*. 2005;65:1239-1282.
56. Huxtable, RJ. The harmful potential of herbal and other plant products. *Drug Saf*. 1990;5:126-136.
57. Izzo AA, Ernst E. Interactions between herbal medicines and prescribed drugs: an updated systematic review. *Drugs*. 2009;69:1777-1798.
58. Job KM, et al. Herbal medicines: challenges in the modern world. Part 4. Canada and United States. *Expert Rev Clin Pharmacol*. 2016;9:1597-1609.
59. John Chen. Herbal monograph for xiao chai hu tang. http://www.acupuncturetoday.com/mpacms/at/article.php?id=31544. Accessed July 21, 2017.
60. Johnson AE, et al. Chemistry of toxic range plants. Variation in pyrrolizidine alkaloid content of Senecio, Amsinckia, and Crotalaria species. *J Agric Food Chem*. 1985;33:50-55.
61. Kang-Yum E, Oransky SH. Chinese patent medicine as a potential source of mercury poisoning. *Vet Hum Toxicol*. 1992;34:235-238.
62. Klayman DL. Qinghaosu (artemisinin): an antimalarial drug from China. *Science*. 1985;228:1049-1055.
63. Ko RJ, et al. Lethal ingestion of Chinese herbal tea containing ch'an su. *West J Med*. 1996;164:71-75.
64. Kong H-Y, et al. Safety of individual medication of Ma Qian Zi (semen strychni) based upon assessment of therapeutic effects of Guo's therapy against moderate fluorosis of bone. *J Tradit Chin Med Chung Tsa Chih Ying Wen Pan*. 2011;31:297-302.
65. van der Kooy F, Sullivan SE. The complexity of medicinal plants: the traditional Artemisia annua formulation, current status and future perspectives. *J Ethnopharmacol*. 2013;150:1-13.
66. Kruegel AC, Grundmann O. The medicinal chemistry and neuropharmacology of kratom: a preliminary discussion of a promising medicinal plant and analysis of its potential for abuse. *Neuropharmacology*. 2017;S0028-3908:30393-3.
67. Lachenmeier DW. Wormwood (Artemisia absinthium L.)—A curious plant with both neurotoxic and neuroprotective properties? *J Ethnopharmacol*. 2010;131:224-227.
68. Lachenmeier DW, et al. Absinthe—a review. *Crit Rev Food Sci Nutr*. 2006;46:365-377.
69. Lanaro R, et al. Ritualistic use of ayahuasca versus street use of similar substances seized by the police: a key factor involved in the potential for intoxications and overdose? *J Psychoactive Drugs*. 2015;47:132-139.
70. Lau WC, et al. The effect of St John's wort on the pharmacodynamic response of clopidogrel in hyporesponsive volunteers and patients: increased platelet inhibition by enhancement of CYP3A4 metabolic activity. *J Cardiovasc Pharmacol*. 2011;57:86-93.
71. Lewis C. Safety alerts & advisories—FDA advises dietary supplement manufacturers to remove comfrey products from the market. https://www.fda.gov/Food/RecallsOutbreaksEmergencies/SafetyAlertsAdvisories/ucm111219.htm. Accessed April 8, 2017.
72. Li S, et al. A review on traditional uses, phytochemistry, pharmacology, pharmacokinetics and toxicology of the genus Peganum. *J Ethnopharmacol*. 2017;203:127-162.
73. Liberti LE, Der Marderosian A. Evaluation of commercial ginseng products. *J Pharm Sci*. 1978;67:1487-1489.
74. Luciano RL, Perazella MA. Aristolochic acid nephropathy: epidemiology, clinical presentation, and treatment. *Drug Saf*. 2015;38:55-64.
75. Macel M. Attract and deter: a dual role for pyrrolizidine alkaloids in plant–insect interactions. *Phytochem Rev*. 2011;10:75-82.
76. Marcus DM, Grollman AP. The consequences of ineffective regulation of dietary supplements. *Arch Intern Med*. 2012;172:1035-1036.
77. McGuffin M. Should herbal medicines be regulated as drugs? *Clin Pharmacol Ther*. 2008;83:393-395.
78. Miroddi M, et al. Hot flashes in a young girl: a wake-up call concerning Serenoa repens use in children. *Pediatrics*. 2012;130:e1374-1376.
79. Moloudizargari M, et al. Pharmacological and therapeutic effects of Peganum harmala and its main alkaloids. *Pharmacogn Rev*. 2013;7:199.
80. Morabito P, et al. Serenoa repens as an endocrine disruptor in a 10-year-old young girl: a new case report. *Pharmacology*. 2015;96:41-43.
81. Morris CA. Internet marketing of herbal products. *JAMA*. 2003;290:1505.
82. Morrow JD. Why the United States still needs improved dietary supplement regulation and oversight. *Clin Pharmacol Ther*. 2008;83:391-393.
83. Newman DJ, Cragg GM. Natural products as sources of new drugs from 1981 to 2014. *J Nat Prod*. 2016;79:629-661.
84. Nortier JL, et al. Urothelial carcinoma associated with the use of a Chinese herb (Aristolochia fangchi). *N Engl J Med*. 2000;342:1686-1692.
85. Norton SA. Betel: consumption and consequences. *J Am Acad Dermatol*. 1998;38:81-88.
86. Nowak M, et al. Interspecific transfer of pyrrolizidine alkaloids: an unconsidered source of contaminations of phytopharmaceuticals and plant derived commodities. *Food Chem*. 2016;213:163-168.
87. Nutrition. Safety alerts & advisories—aristolochic acid: safety alert. https://www.fda.gov/food/recallsoutbreaksemergencies/safetyalertsadvisories/ucm095272.htm. Accessed April 8, 2017.
88. Oka H, et al. Prospective study of chemoprevention of hepatocellular carcinoma with Sho-saiko-to (TJ-9). *Cancer*. 1995;76:743-749.
89. PDQ Integrative, Alternative, and Complementary Therapies Editorial Board. Laetrile/Amygdalin (PDQ®): Health Professional Version. In: *PDQ Cancer Information Summaries*. Bethesda (MD): National Cancer Institute (US); 2002. http://www.ncbi.nlm.nih.gov/books/NBK65988/. Accessed April 27, 2017.
90. Pires APS, et al. Gas chromatographic analysis of dimethyltryptamine and β-carboline alkaloids in ayahuasca, an amazonian psychoactive plant beverage. *Phytochem Anal*. 2009;20:149-153.

91. Pontifex AH, Garg AK. Lead poisoning from an Asian Indian folk remedy. *Can Med Assoc J.* 1985;133:1227-1228.

92. Posadzki P, et al. Contamination and adulteration of herbal medicinal products (HMPs): an overview of systematic reviews. *Eur J Clin Pharmacol.* 2013;69:295-307.

93. Ridker PM. Toxic effects of herbal teas. *Arch Environ Health.* 1987;42:133-136.

94. Ruan J, et al. Metabolic activation of pyrrolizidine alkaloids: insights into the structural and enzymatic basis. *Chem Res Toxicol.* 2014;27:1030-1039.

95. Samenuk D, et al. Adverse cardiovascular events temporally associated with ma huang, an herbal source of ephedrine. *Mayo Clin Proc.* 2002;77:12-16.

96. Saper RB, et al. Heavy metal content of ayurvedic herbal medicine products. *JAMA.* 2004;292:2868-2873.

97. Saper RB, et al. Lead, mercury, and arsenic in US- and Indian-manufactured Ayurvedic medicines sold via the Internet. *JAMA.* 2008;300:915-923.

98. Sarma H, et al. Accumulation of heavy metals in selected medicinal plants. *Rev Environ Contam Toxicol.* 2011;214:63-86.

99. Sauer H, et al. Severe cyanide poisoning from an alternative medicine treatment with amygdalin and apricot kernels in a 4-year-old child. *Wien Med Wochenschr 1946.* 2015;165:185-188.

100. Schultes RE, Raffauf RF. *Vine of the Soul: Medicine Men, Their Plants and Rituals in the Colombian Amazonia.* Santa Fe, NM: Synergetic Press; 2004.

101. Sheikh NM. Chaparral-associated hepatotoxicity. *Arch Intern Med.* 1997;157:913.

102. Smith LW, Culvenor CCJ. Plant sources of hepatotoxic pyrrolizidine alkaloids. *J Nat Prod.* 1981;44:129-152.

103. Smith T, et al. Herbal dietary supplement sales in US increase 6.8% in 2014. *HerbalGram.* 2015;107:52-59.

104. Solecki RS. Shanidar IV, a Neanderthal flower burial in northern Iraq. *Science.* 1975;190:880-881.

105. Spoerke DG. Herbal medication: use and misuse. *Hosp Formul.* 1980:941-951.

106. Staub PO, et al. Back to the roots: a quantitative survey of herbal drugs in Dioscorides' De Materia Medica (ex Matthioli, 1568). *Phytomedicine.* 2016;23:1043-1052.

106a. Tay YL. Mitragynine and its potential blocking effects on specific cardiac potassium channels. *Toxicol Appl Pharmacol.* 2016;305:22-39.

107. Taylor RF, et al. Betel-nut chewing and asthma. *Lancet Lond Engl.* 1992;339:1134-1136.

108. Totelin L. When foods become remedies in ancient Greece: the curious case of garlic and other substances. *J Ethnopharmacol.* 2015;167:30-37.

109. Tsouderos T. Dietary supplements: manufacturing troubles widespread, FDA inspections show. chicagotribune.com. http://www.chicagotribune.com/lifestyles/health/ct-met-supplement-inspections-20120630-story.html. Accessed April 7, 2017.

110. Vanhaelen M, et al. Identification of aristolochic acid in Chinese herbs. *Lancet Lond Engl.* 1994;343:174.

111. Vanherweghem JL, et al. Rapidly progressive interstitial renal fibrosis in young women: association with slimming regimen including Chinese herbs. *Lancet Lond Engl.* 1993;341:387-391.

112. Walker BR, Edwards CR. Licorice-induced hypertension and syndromes of apparent mineralocorticoid excess. *Endocrinol Metab Clin North Am.* 1994;23:359-377.

113. Wananukul W, et al. Pharmacokinetics of mitragynine in man. *Drug Des Devel Ther.* 2015;9:2421-2429.

114. Weisbord SD, et al. Poison on line—acute renal failure caused by oil of wormwood purchased through the Internet. *N Engl J Med.* 1997;337:825-827.

115. Wiedenfeld H. Plants containing pyrrolizidine alkaloids: toxicity and problems. *Food Addit Contam Part Chem Anal Control Expo Risk Assess.* 2011;28:282-292.

116. Xue T. Synergy in traditional Chinese medicine. *Lancet Oncol.* 2016;17:e39.

117. Yaksh TL, Wallace MS. Opioids, analgesia, and pain management. In: Brunton LL, et al, eds. *Goodman & Gilman's: The Pharmacological Basis of Therapeutics.* 12th ed. New York, NY: McGraw-Hill Education; 2011.

118. Yang L, et al. Aristolochic acid nephropathy: variation in presentation and prognosis. *Nephrol Dial Transplant.* 2012;27:292-298.

119. Zanoli P. Role of hyperforin in the pharmacological activities of St. John's Wort. *CNS Drug Rev.* 2004;10:203-218.

120. Zell-Kanter M, et al. Reduction in ephedra poisonings after FDA ban. *N Engl J Med.* 2015;372:2172-2174.

121. Zeng Y, et al. Analysis of 32 toxic natural substances in herbal products by liquid chromatography quadrupole linear ion trap mass spectrometry. *J Pharm Biomed Anal.* 2015;115:169-173.

44 VITAMINS

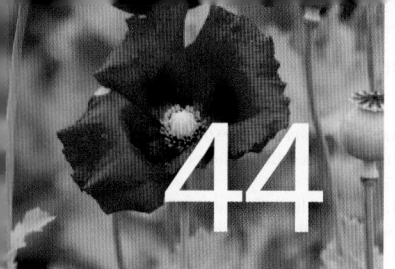

Beth Y. Ginsburg

Vitamins are essential for normal human growth and development.[5] By definition, a vitamin is a substance present in small amounts in natural foods, is necessary for normal metabolism, and the lack of which in the diet causes a deficiency disease.[46]

A standard North American diet is sufficient to prevent overt vitamin deficiency diseases.[71,82] However, suboptimal vitamin status is common in Western populations and is a risk factor for chronic diseases such as cardiovascular disease, cancer, and osteoporosis.[71,82] Groups at risk include older adults, hospitalized patients, alcohol-dependent individuals, pregnant women those with gastrointestinal disorders, those following gastric bypass interventions and other patients with poor nutritional status. The American Dietetic Association posits that the best strategy for promoting optimal health and reducing chronic disease is to choose a wide variety of nutrient-rich foods, and the use of supplements can help some people meet their nutritional needs.[167] Health care professionals should identify patients with poor nutrition or other reasons for increased vitamin needs and offer guidance on vitamin supplementation. It is suggested without evidence that because most people do not consume an optimal amount of vitamins by diet alone, adults should take vitamin and mineral supplements because the potential benefits likely outweigh any risk in the general population and may be particularly beneficial in older adults. The choice of supplement should reflect the patient's age, gender, stage of life, health status, risk factors, and family history and should involve physician guidance.[253]

National Health and Nutrition Examination Survey (NHANES) data collected from 2003 to 2006 demonstrate that dietary supplement use was reported by 49% of the population age 1 year and older, an increase of approximately 10% from NHANES data from 1988 to 1994, with 79% of users taking them daily for the previous 30 days.[22] Among adults and children, multivitamins and multiminerals (MVMMs) were the most commonly reported dietary supplement, with 33% of the population reporting use. The Council for Responsible Nutrition (CRN), a trade organization for the dietary supplement industry, has conducted yearly surveys since 2000 on the prevalence of dietary supplement use in the United States. Analysis of their data from 2007 to 2011 demonstrate an increased prevalence of dietary supplement use, 64% to 69% in adults, compared with previous NHANES surveys.[1] More recently, the CRN revealed in a 2015 report that the percentage of American adults taking dietary supplements has remained consistent at 68% from the years 2012 to 2015.[188] Ninety-eight percent of these dietary supplement users take vitamins and minerals, the most popular category of supplements, with the top five including a multivitamin (78%), vitamin D (32%), vitamin C (27%), calcium (24%), and vitamin B/B complex (18%). The CRN reported that the primary reasons given for supplement use are for overall health and wellness and to fill dietary nutrient gaps.[1] Current data suggest minimal, if any, risk associated with MVMM use at recommended daily intake levels in healthy people.[253] Unfortunately, many individuals share the mistaken beliefs that vitamin preparations provide extra energy or promote muscle growth and regularly ingest quantities of vitamins in great excess of the recommended dietary allowances (RDAs) (Table 44–1). The most commonly used MVMM preparations generally do not exceed 100% of the RDA, but excessive vitamin intake is more likely to occur in MVMM users who also take single vitamin supplements.[214] Excess vitamin intake also occurs in individuals taking an MVMM who eat a healthy diet that includes fortified foods and beverages.[182] Some vitamins are associated with consequential adverse effects when ingested in very large doses. Adverse effects also are associated with the use of some vitamins at the RDA or at amounts less than or approaching the established tolerable upper intake level (UL) in certain populations.

Individuals taking medications to reduce blood clotting, such as warfarin, should not take supplemental vitamin K because it is involved in blood clotting and reduces the effectiveness of warfarin and similar medications.

Vitamins was consistently among the 15 most common substance categories involved in human exposures reported to poison control centers in the United States and the sixth most common substance category in children 5 years old and younger, from 2011 to 2015 (Chap. 130). Vitamins were also among the top 25 substance categories with the greatest increase in serious exposures during this time period. However, vitamins were not among the substance categories associated with the largest number of fatalities.

Vitamins can be divided into two general classes. Most of the vitamins in the *water-soluble* class have minimal toxicity because they are stored to only a limited extent in the body. Thiamine, riboflavin, pantothenic acid, folic acid, and biotin are not reported to cause any toxicity after ingestion.[5] Vitamin B_{12} also is in the water-soluble class of vitamins. It exists in several forms and contains the mineral cobalt. Compounds with vitamin B_{12} activity are therefore given the group name of *cobalamins*. There is no toxicity associated with excess vitamin B_{12} intake via ingestion of food and supplements in healthy individuals.[124] Ascorbic acid (vitamin C), nicotinic acid (vitamin B_3), and pyridoxine (vitamin B_6) are water-soluble vitamins with associated toxicity syndromes. The *fat-soluble* vitamins bioaccumulate and therefore have toxic potentials that greatly exceed those of the water-soluble group. Vitamins A, D, and E (but not K) are associated with toxic syndromes after very large overdose or chronic overuse. The adverse effect secondary to vitamin K is limited to severe and sometimes fatal anaphylactoid reactions with rapid administration of the intravenous (IV) preparation.[80]

VITAMIN A

MW	= 272.43 Da
Therapeutic serum concentration	= 65–275 IU/dL
	16.6–83.3 mcg/dL

History and Epidemiology

Two independent groups discovered vitamin A in 1913.[171,193] They reported that animals fed an artificial diet with lard as the sole source of fat developed a nutritional deficiency characterized by xerophthalmia. They found that this deficiency could be corrected by adding to the diet a factor contained in butter, egg yolks, and cod liver oil. They named the substance "fat-soluble vitamin A." The chemical structure of vitamin A was determined in 1930.[135] Vitamin A is also found naturally in liver, fish, cheese, and whole milk. In the United States and other parts of the world, including some developing countries, many cereal, grain, dairy, and other products, as well as infant formulas, are fortified with vitamin A.[8,257]

Vitamin A toxicity occurs in people who ingest large doses of preformed vitamin A in their daily diets. Inuits in the 16th century recognized that ingestion of large amounts of polar bear liver caused a severe illness characterized by headaches and prostration.[81] Arctic explorers in the 1800s knew of the poisonous qualities of polar bear liver and described an acute illness after its ingestion.[90] Explorers also described a condition among the Inuit population known as *pibloktoq*, or "Arctic hysteria," characterized by depression,

TABLE 44–1	Recommended Dietary Daily Allowances or Adequate Daily Intakes					
Age (years)	Vitamin A (mcg RAE/IU)	Vitamin D (mcg/IU)[b,c]	Vitamin E (mg α-TA/IU)	Vitamin C (mg)	Vitamin B$_6$ (mg)	Niacin (mg NE)[a]
Infants						
0.0–0.5	400/1,300[a]	5/200[a]	4/4[a]	40[a]	0.1[a]	2[a]
0.5–1.0	500/1,700[a]	5/200[a]	5/5[a]	50[a]	0.3[a]	4[a]
Children						
1–3	300/990	5/200[a]	6/6	15	0.5	6
4–8	400/1,300	5/200[a]	7/7	25	0.6	8
Males						
9–13	600/2,000	5/200[a]	11/11	45	1	12
14–18	900/3,000	5/200[a]	15/15	75	1.3	16
19–50	900/3,000	5/200[a]	15/15	90	1.3	16
51–70	900/3,000	10/400[a]	15/15	90	1.7	16
>70	900/3,000	15/600[a]	15/15	90	1.7	16
Females						
9–13	600/2,000	5/200[a]	11/11	45	1.0	12
14–18	700/2,300	5/200[a]	15/15	65	1.2	14
19–50	700/2,300	5/200[a]	15/15	75	1.3	14
51–70	700/2,300	10/400[a]	15/15	75	1.5	14
>70	700/2,300	15/600[a]	15/15	75	1.5	14
Pregnant Women						
≤18	750/2,500	5/200[a]	15/15	80	1.9	18
19–50	770/2,500	5/200[a]	15/15	85	1.9	18
Lactating Women						
≤18	1,200/4,000	5/200[a]	19/19	115	2	17
19–50	1,300/4,300	5/200[a]	19/19	120	2	17

[a]These values represent the adequate daily intakes. Values without an [a] represent the recommended dietary daily allowances. [b], [c]

NE = niacin equivalent; RAE = retinol activity equivalents; α-TA = α-tocopherol acetate.

Data from Dietary Reference Intakes for Calcium, Phosphorous, Magnesium, Vitamin D, and Fluoride (1997); Dietary Reference Intakes for Thiamin, Riboflavin, Niacin, Vitamin B6, Folate, Vitamin B12, Pantothenic Acid, Biotin, and Choline (1998); Dietary Reference Intakes for Vitamin C, Vitamin E, Selenium, and Carotenoids (2000); Dietary Reference Intakes for Vitamin A, Vitamin K, Arsenic, Boron, Chromium, Copper, Iodine, Iron, Manganese, Molybdenum, Nickel, Silicon, Vanadium, and Zinc (2001); Dietary Reference Intakes for Water, Potassium, Sodium, Chloride, and Sulfate (2005); and Dietary Reference Intakes for Calcium and Vitamin D (2011). These reports may be accessed via www.nap.edu.

echolalia, insensitivity to extreme cold, and seizures, and believed it to be related to ingestion of polar bear liver and other organ meats.[197] Vitamin A toxicity was implicated in the etiology of pibloktoq because somatic and behavioral effects of vitamin A toxicity closely paralleled many of the symptoms reported in Inuit patients diagnosed with pibloktoq.[145] However, the toxic substance in polar bear liver was not identified as vitamin A until 1942.[215] The vitamin A content of polar bear liver is as high as 34,600 IU/g (10,400 RAE/g), supporting the view that vitamin A is the toxic factor in the liver.[217]

Vitamin A toxicity was reported in an adult who chronically ingested large amounts of beef liver,[123] as well as after ingestion of the liver of the grouper fish *Cephalopholis boenak*, which has a high content of vitamin A.[47] Ingestion of whale and seal liver, as well as the livers of large fish, such as shark, tuna, and sea bass, also is associated with development of vitamin A toxicity.

Vitamin A toxicity usually is not expected to occur after ingestion of large doses of provitamin A carotenoids. Vitamin A–induced hepatotoxicity and neurotoxicity were believed to have developed in an 18-year-old woman who maintained a diet nearly limited to foods rich in the carotenoid beta-carotene, including pumpkin, carrots, and laver (nori), for several years.[184] However, she also included an unspecified, although reportedly small, amount of fish, red meat, and liver in her diet.

Most reported cases of vitamin A toxicity result from inappropriate use of vitamin supplements.[24,27] In the United States, 28% of the population reported taking a dietary supplement containing vitamin A in 2003 to 2006.[22] Overall, vitamin A toxicity is not common with only 396 to 447 single exposures per year reported to United States poison control centers from 2011 to 2015. Of

these, most cases did not result in any outcome, and there were only nine or less moderate outcomes per year and one or no major outcomes per year.

Vitamin A is present in two forms. Preformed vitamin A as retinol is derived from retinyl esters, its storage form, in animal sources of food. Provitamin A carotenoids are vitamin A precursors and are found in plants. Among the carotenoids, beta-carotene is most efficiently made into retinol. The term *vitamin A* was classically only used to refer to the compound retinol. Currently, it is used to describe all retinoids, compounds chemically related to retinol that exhibit the biological activity of retinol. Retinol is converted in the body to the retinoids retinal and retinoic acid. Synthetic retinoids are developed via chemical modification of naturally occurring retinoids, often for a specific therapeutic purpose. Vitamin A activity is expressed in retinol activity equivalents (RAEs). One RAE corresponds to 1 mcg of retinol or 3.33 IU of vitamin A activity as retinol. One RAE also corresponds to 12 mcg of beta-carotene.

Vitamin A content varies widely among different food types. A 3-oz serving of cooked beef liver contains 30,325 IU (9,100 RAE) of vitamin A, and 1 cup of whole milk contains 305 IU (92 RAE) of vitamin A. Fish-liver oils, such as swordfish and black sea bass, have extremely large amounts of vitamin A, and some contain more than 180,000 IU (54,050 RAE) of vitamin A per gram of oil. Carotenoids are present in yellow and green fruits and vegetables. A raw carrot has a high beta-carotene content of approximately 20,250 IU (6,080 RAE). One half-cup serving of spinach contains approximately 7,400 IU (2,220 RAE) of beta-carotene, and an apricot or peach contains 500 to 600 IU (150-180 RAE). The average American diet provides about half of its daily vitamin A intake as carotenoids and about half as preformed vitamin A.[9]

The RDA of vitamin A is 900 mcg RAE/day (3,000 IU/day) for adult men and 700 mcg of RAE/day (2,300 IU/day) for women (Table 44–1).[85] The UL for adults is 3,000 mcg of RAE/day (9,900 IU/day).

As a group, retinoids have specific sites of action and varying degrees of biologic potency. Retinoic acid is primarily responsible for maintaining normal growth and differentiation of epithelial cells in mucus-secreting or keratinizing tissue.[165] Vitamin A deficiency results in the disappearance of goblet mucous cells and replacement of the normal epithelium with a stratified, keratinized epithelium. Dermal manifestations are the earliest to develop and include dry skin and hair and broken fingernails. In the cornea, hyperkeratization is called *xerophthalmia* and leads to permanent blindness. Alterations in the epithelial lining of other organ systems leads to increased susceptibility to respiratory infections, diarrhea, and urinary calculi. Vitamin A, in the form of 11-*cis*-retinal, plays a critical role in retinal function.[250] Deficiency results in *nyctalopia*, which is decreased vision in dim lighting, more commonly known as *night blindness*.

Vitamin A is prescribed for patients with specific dermatologic and ophthalmic conditions. Vitamin A toxicity often occurs in adults who continue to use the vitamin without medical supervision.[91]

Isotretinoin (Accutane), 13-*cis*-retinoic acid, is prescribed for treatment of severe cystic acne. Of concern is the teratogenicity associated with its use by pregnant women; therefore, it is contraindicated. There is no association between use of isotretinoin in men during the time of conception and birth defects. The iPLEDGE program is a mandatory United States Food and Drug Administration (FDA) Risk Evaluation and Mitigation Strategy for the distribution of isotretinoin that was initiated in 2006. Its goals are to inform prescribers, pharmacists, and patients about the serious risks of isotretinoin and safe-use conditions and to prevent fetal exposure to isotretinoin.[126] Components of the program include mandatory enrollment of male and female patients; documentation of a negative pregnancy test and birth control use; and prescriber, pharmacist, and patient education. The iPLEDGE program replaced the FDA's System to Manage Accutane-Related Teratogenicity (SMART) program that was initiated in 2002. Although both programs share many features, the SMART program was voluntary and did not include mandatory record keeping or reporting. A review after the implementation of the SMART program revealed an increase in the number of pregnant women prescribed isotretinoin compared with the previous year. It also revealed that prescribers were not providing adequate patient education regarding the risk of teratogenicity and that there was not compliance with essential portions of the pregnancy prevention program.[213]

All-trans-retinoic acid (ATRA), or tretinoin, is used as a differentiating chemotherapeutic in the treatment of acute promyelocytic leukemia (APL), a disease characterized by the accumulation of promyelocytic blasts in bone marrow caused by obstruction of differentiation of granulocytic cells.[148] All-trans-retinoic acid, in combination with anthracycline chemotherapy, improves the complete remission rate, often reported to be greater than 90%, and reduces the incidence of relapse to only 10% to 15% when used as maintenance therapy.[75] Acute promyelocytic leukemia differentiation syndrome (DS), previously known as ATRA syndrome or retinoic acid syndrome, is the main adverse effect and occurs in up 14% to 16% of patients who receive ATRA with an associated mortality rate of about 2%.[199] All-trans-retinoic acid also is used for the treatment of myelodysplastic syndrome and acute myelogenous leukemia.

Pharmacology, Pharmacokinetics, and Toxicokinetics

Absorption of vitamin A in the small intestine is nearly complete. However, some vitamin A is eliminated in the feces when large doses are taken. The majority of vitamin A is ingested as retinyl esters, the storage form of retinol.[165] Retinyl esters undergo enzymatic hydrolysis to retinol by digestive enzymes in the intestinal lumen and brush border of the intestinal epithelial wall. A small portion of retinol is absorbed directly into the circulation, where it is bound to retinol-binding protein (RBP) and transported to the liver. Most of the retinol is taken into intestinal epithelial cells by RBP.[190] Subsequently, retinol is reesterified and incorporated into chylomicrons, which are released into the blood and taken up by the Ito cells of the liver. After large oral doses,

significant amounts of retinyl esters coupled to chylomicrons circulate in association with low-density lipoprotein (LDL) and are delivered to the liver. Approximately 50% to 80% of the total vitamin A content of the body is stored in the liver as retinyl esters.[35] The liver releases vitamin A into the bloodstream to maintain a constant plasma retinol concentration and is thus delivered to tissues as needed.

Carotenoid absorption requires bile and absorbable fat in the stomach or intestine. These components combine with carotenoids to form mixed lipid micelles that move into the duodenal mucosal cells via passive diffusion. Most beta-carotene that is metabolized undergoes central cleavage via oxidation to form retinal, which is then reduced to retinol. Retinol is then esterified with fatty acids and incorporated into chylomicrons, which are transported to the bloodstream via the lymphatics for delivery to the liver. Massive doses of beta-carotene are rarely associated with vitamin A toxicity because of decreased efficiency in absorption secondary to saturation of dissolution in bulk lipid, micellar incorporation, and diffusion caused by a reduction in the concentration gradient.[196] Unabsorbed beta-carotene is excreted in the feces. In addition, there is a decrease in the rate of conversion of carotenoids to vitamin A.[63] Excess absorbed beta-carotene is incorporated with lipoproteins and released into the bloodstream via the lymphatics for delivery to the adipose tissue and adrenals for storage.

The normal serum retinol concentration is approximately 30 to 70 mcg/dL.[230] These concentrations are maintained at the expense of hepatic reserves when insufficient amounts of vitamin A are ingested. A normal adult liver contains enough vitamin A to fulfill the body's requirements for approximately 2 years.[177] Excessive intake of vitamin A is not initially reflected by elevated serum concentrations because vitamin A is soluble in fat but not in water. Instead, hepatic accumulation is increased. This storage system allows for cumulative toxic effects. Although no quantitative relationship exists between the magnitude of liver stores and serum concentrations of vitamin A, in chronic vitamin A toxicity, serum concentrations are generally higher than 3.49 μmol/L (95 mcg/dL).[27] Vitamin A has a half-life of 286 days.[233,255] Retinoids undergo a variety of metabolic and conjugation pathways and are subsequently eliminated in the feces, urine, or bile.

Pathophysiology

The mechanism of action for many of the toxic effects of vitamin A is at the nuclear level. Retinoic acid influences gene expression by combining with nuclear receptors.[165] Retinoids also influence expression of receptors for certain hormones and growth factors. Thus, they can influence the growth, differentiation, and function of target cells.[158]

In epithelial cells and fibroblasts, retinoids affect changes in nuclear transcription, resulting in enhanced production of proteins such as fibronectin and decreased production of other proteins such as collagenase.[163] Excessive concentrations of retinoids where goblet cells are present lead to the production of a thick mucin layer and inhibition of keratinization. In addition, lipoprotein membranes have increased permeability and decreased stability, resulting in extreme thinning of the epithelial tissue.

In vitro studies in bone demonstrate that high doses of vitamin A are capable of directly stimulating bone resorption and inhibiting bone formation leading to osteoporosis. This effect is secondary to increased osteoclast formation and activity and inhibition of osteoblast growth.[186]

Hepatotoxicity develops secondary to a single large acute overdose or ingestion of smaller doses if taken over a prolonged time.[91,142] A total of 90% of hepatic vitamin A stores are in the Ito, or fat-storing, cells of the liver, which are in the perisinusoidal space of Disse, and are responsible for maintaining normal hepatic architecture.[109,110] Ito cells undergo hypertrophy and hyperplasia as vitamin A storage increases.[142] This results in transdifferentiation of the Ito cell into a myofibroblast-like cell that secretes a variety of extracellular matrix components, leading to narrowing of the perisinusoidal space of Disse, obstruction to sinusoidal blood flow, and noncirrhotic portal hypertension (Fig. 44–1).[58,97,119,136,142,222] Continued ingestion of vitamin A and hepatic storage leads to obliteration of the space of Disse, sinusoidal barrier damage, perisinusoidal hepatocyte death, fibrosis, and cirrhosis (Chap. 21).[119,129,142,218]

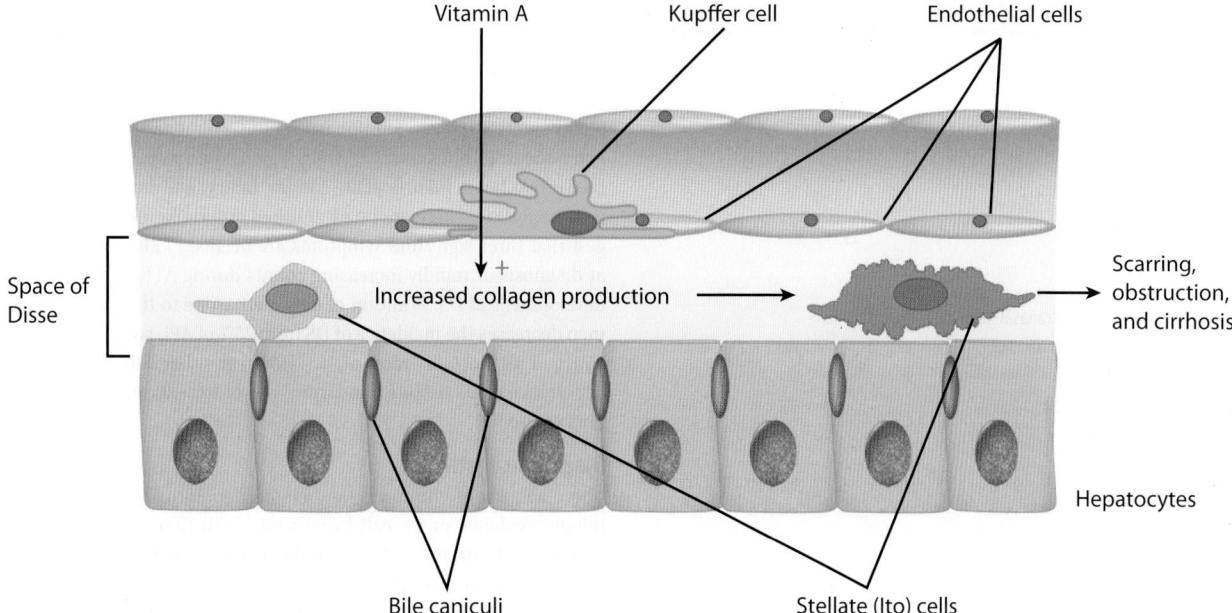

Vitamin A   Kupffer cell   Endothelial cells

Space of Disse

Increased collagen production

Scarring, obstruction, and cirrhosis

Hepatocytes

Bile caniculi   Stellate (Ito) cells

FIGURE 44–1. Schematic demonstration of hepatotoxicity resulting from excessive deposition of vitamin A in the Ito cells of the liver.

Vitamin A toxicity has long been thought to be the cause of the severe headaches and papilledema associated with idiopathic intracranial hypertension (IIH).[209] Increased concentrations of unbound retinol in the cerebral spinal fluid (CSF) of patients with IIH suggest that vitamin A is involved in the pathogenesis of IIH.[240,254] However, the mechanisms by which vitamin A leads to increased intracranial pressure (ICP) in IIH are not definitively known.[209] Unbound, circulating retinol and retinyl esters are proposed to interact with cell membranes and produce damage by membranolytic surface-active properties.[127] In the central nervous system (CNS), disruption of cell membrane integrity might lead to disruption of CSF outflow, thereby producing signs and symptoms consistent with IIH.[93,127,139,162] Vitamin A also can lead to intracranial hypertension via enhanced transcription of genes involved in CSF secretion or absorption.[102] Another explanation for the association of vitamin A with IIH involves the role of RBP as a signaling molecule altering CSF secretion or absorption.[155]

Clinical Manifestations

Clinical toxicity correlates well with total body vitamin A content, which is a function of both dose and duration of administration. A randomized double-blind trial, in which 390 women received 400,000 IU (120,000 RAE) of vitamin A as a single dose were compared with 380 women who received placebo, suggested that dosing at this level is well tolerated.[122] Doses of 100,000 IU (30,000 RAE) of vitamin A in infants aged 6 to 11 months and 200,000 IU (60,000 RAE) of vitamin A every 3 to 6 months for infants and children aged 12 to 60 months result in few adverse events.[26] The minimal dose required to produce toxicity in humans is not established. However, an animal study demonstrated a median lethal acute dose in monkeys of 560,000 IU (168,000 RAE) per kilogram of body weight.[161] In this study, all monkeys receiving more than 300,000 RAE/kg (999,000 IU/kg) died, but none died at a dose of 100,000 RAE/kg (333,000 IU/kg).

Vitamin A toxicity occurs more frequently secondary to chronic ingestions of vitamin A. Hepatotoxicity typically requires vitamin A ingestions of at least 50,000 to 100,000 IU/day (15,000 to 30,000 RAE/day) for months or years.[8,142] One study found that in patients with vitamin A-induced hepatotoxicity, the average daily vitamin A intake was higher in patients who developed cirrhosis (135,000 IU/day, 40,500 RAE/day) compared with patients who developed noncirrhotic liver disease (66,000 IU/day, 20,000 RAE/day).[89] However, case reports have documented hepatotoxicity resulting from vitamin A dosages as low as 25,000 IU/day (7,500 RAE/day),[91,142] a dosage widely available in nonprescription vitamin A preparations.

Symptoms of an acute massive overdose of vitamin A often develop within hours to 2 days after ingestion.[177] Initial signs and symptoms include headache, papilledema, scotoma, photophobia, seizures, anorexia, drowsiness, irritability, nausea, vomiting, abdominal pain, liver damage, and desquamation.[177] Nonspecific symptoms and manifestations include fatigue, fever, weight loss, edema, polydipsia, dysuria, hyperlipidemia, anemia, and menstrual abnormalities.

Chronic toxicity of vitamin A affects the skin, hair, bones, liver, and brain. The most common skin manifestations include xerosis, which is associated with pruritus and erythema, skin hyperfragility, and desquamation.[64,65,260] Retinoid toxicity causes hair thinning and even diffuse hair loss in 10% to 75% of patients.[84,95,138] In addition, the characteristics of the hair change after regrowth. Hair sometimes becomes permanently curly or kinky.[15] Nail changes include a shiny appearance, brittleness, softening, and loosening.[76] Dryness of mucous membranes develops with chapped lips and xerosis of nasal mucosa, which sometimes is associated with nasal bleeding.[55]

Hypercarotenemia develops when massive doses of beta-carotenes are ingested over several weeks. It manifests as a yellow-orange skin discoloration that can be differentiated from jaundice by the absence of scleral icterus and usually is not associated with morbidity.

Findings from epidemiologic studies are consistent with bone loss and a resulting increase in fracture risk. In northern Europe, the region with the highest incidence of osteoporotic fractures, dietary intake of vitamin A is high. A study of this population demonstrated that reduced bone density and increased risk of hip fracture correlate with vitamin A intake.[173] This finding is supported by other studies demonstrating an increased risk of hip fracture among women with elevated serum vitamin A concentrations and in women ingesting large daily amounts of vitamin A as supplements or in their diets.[78,191]

Other musculoskeletal findings include skeletal hyperostoses, most commonly affecting the vertebral bodies of thoracic vertebrae, extraspinal tendon and ligament calcifications, soft tissue ossification, cortical thickening of bone shafts, periosteal thickening, and bone demineralization.[55,177,179] Many of these findings are apparent on radiographs. Patients often complain of bone and joint pain and muscle stiffness or tenderness. Hypercalcemia, with low or normal parathyroid hormone (PTH) concentrations, likely results from increased osteoclast activity and bone resorption.[37] Patients with chronic kidney disease are at increased risk for developing hypercalcemia at vitamin A doses lower than usual toxic doses secondary to decreased renal metabolism of retinol. This complication occurred in an 8-year-old boy with chronic kidney disease after a dosage of 12,000 IU/day

TABLE 44–2	Xenobiotics Associated with Intracranial Hypertension

Antibiotics
- Ampicillin
- Minocycline
- Metronidazole
- Nalidixic acid
- Nitrofurantoin
- Sulfamethoxazole
- Tetracycline

Corticosteroid therapy (oral and intranasal) and cessation

Enflurane

Griseofulvin

Halothane

Ketamine

Lead

Lithium

Oral contraceptives and progestins

Phenothiazines

Phenytoin

Tubocurarine

Vitamin A

(3,600 RAE/day) for at least 2 years.[62] Premature epiphyseal closure in children is reported.[205] Teratogenic effects include interference with skeletal differentiation and growth.[37]

The degree of hepatotoxicity appears to correlate with the dose of vitamin A and chronicity of use. Hepatotoxicity occurs in humans after an acute ingestion of a massive dose of vitamin A (>600,000 IU or 180,000 RAE).[142] With large doses, cirrhosis develops and leads to portal hypertension, esophageal varices, jaundice, and ascites.[59,91,142] Hepatotoxicity is associated with elevations in bilirubin, aminotransferases, and alkaline phosphatase concentrations.

Idiopathic intracranial hypertension is characterized by elevated ICP in the absence of a structural anomaly. It occurs in patients with altered endocrine function, systemic diseases, or impaired cerebral venous drainage or ingestion of various xenobiotics, including excessive vitamin A (Table 44–2).[7] The syndrome is most common in young obese women, but the etiology remains unknown in most cases. The first case of IIH associated with vitamin A toxicity was described in 1954.[90] However, the symptoms were first described in 1856 by an Arctic explorer who noted vertigo and headache after eating polar bear liver.[229] Patients typically present with headache and visual disturbances, including sixth nerve palsies, visual field deficits, and blurred vision, and have a normal mental status. Despite severe papilledema, visual loss often is minimal. However, permanent blindness sometimes results from optic atrophy.[160] Other manifestations of neurotoxicity include ataxia, fatigue, depression, irritability, and psychosis.[33]

Isotretinoin is effective in the management of acne. However, its use is associated with teratogenicity. It is thought to interfere with cranial neural crest cells, which contribute to the development of both the ear and the conotruncal area of the heart, and may cause malformed or absent external ears or auditory canals and conotruncal heart defects.[144] Although studies do not show a teratogenic risk with topical preparations, case reports describe fetal malformations associated with topical preparation use during pregnancy.[19,42,131,156,228] In addition, mucocutaneous abnormalities, IIH, corneal opacities, hypercalcemia, hyperuricemia, musculoskeletal symptoms, liver function abnormalities, elevated triglyceride concentrations, and spontaneous abortion are reported.[12,83,89,106,107]

Acute promyelocytic leukemia differentiation syndrome (DS), previously known as ATRA syndrome, is the main adverse effect of treatment with ATRA. The pathophysiology of DS is not well understood but involves an inflammatory response. Proposed mechanisms include tissue infiltration of APL cells, particularly in the lungs but also in the liver, spleen, and heart, and leukocyte extravasation.[146] The onset of symptoms and manifestations is typically 2 to 21 days after initiation of ATRA.[199] The hallmarks of DS are fever and respiratory distress.[199,216] Other common signs and symptoms include an elevated white blood count, dyspnea, pulmonary edema, pulmonary infiltrates, and pleural and pericardial effusions.[199,216] Weight gain, bone pain, headache, hypotension, congestive heart failure, acute kidney injury, and hepatotoxicity occur less commonly.[199,216] There are no established criteria for diagnosis, but some suggest that three signs and symptoms are needed.[216] Elevated leukocyte counts at diagnosis or rapidly increasing counts during ATRA treatment predict the development of DS. Addition of dexamethasone to the ATRA treatment regimen decreases the incidence of DS from 25% of APL patients to approximately 15% and its mortality rate to 1%.[74] However, other data demonstrated a 17% occurrence of DS despite concurrent use of steroids, and not all authors support its use.[199,259]

Diagnostic Testing

The diagnosis of vitamin A–associated hepatotoxicity is supported by histologic evidence of Ito cell hyperplasia with fluorescent vacuoles on liver biopsy.[91] Laboratory testing should include serum electrolytes, including calcium, hepatic enzymes, a complete blood cell count, and a vitamin A concentration. Because the liver has a large storage capacity for excess vitamin A, hepatotoxicity occurs before an elevation in the serum concentration of vitamin A, which may be normal or even low, in the setting of an acute overdose. As the hepatic storage capacity is overwhelmed, the serum concentration rapidly rises in a nonlinear fashion. Further evaluation should be guided by the clinical presentation and the need to evaluate for other causes. It may include bone radiographs, computed tomography, magnetic resonance angiography and venography, and lumbar puncture.

Treatment

Management of a patient with a recent acute, large overdose of vitamin A should begin with gastrointestinal (GI) decontamination. This can be accomplished with a 50-g dose of activated charcoal. In extremely large overdoses that are expected to produce significant toxicity, it would be reasonable to perform gastric lavage if airway compromise is not a concern. Discontinuation of vitamin A and supportive care are the mainstays of treatment. Hypercalcemia should be treated in the usual manner with IV fluids, loop diuretics, calcitonin, bisphosphonates, and steroids, as needed depending on the severity.[32] Although most signs and symptoms of vitamin A toxicity resolve within 1 week after vitamin A discontinuation and treatment, papilledema, desquamation, and skeletal abnormalities sometimes persist for several months.

Idiopathic intracranial hypertension requires more aggressive therapy. Indications for treatment include visual field loss and symptoms of elevated ICP.[209] Acetazolamide, a carbonic anhydrase inhibitor, is the most commonly used treatment for IIH.[209] It is usually started at a dosage of 0.5 to 1 g/day and gradually increased until clinical improvement is seen to 3 to 4 g/day.[209] Acetazolamide has teratogenic effects in animals and is designated FDA Pregnancy Category C. Topiramate, a partial carbonic anhydrase inhibitor that is used in the treatment of migraine headaches and epilepsy, has demonstrated efficacy comparable to acetazolamide in the treatment of patients with IIH.[43] Furosemide is considered second-line treatment but is recommended in patients who cannot tolerate or receive acetazolamide.[36,209] The role of corticosteroids in the treatment of IIH is controversial, and they should not be used chronically for the treatment of papilledema.[36] However, a short course of high-dose corticosteroids is recommended in patients with acute visual loss from fulminant papilledema.[157] Lumbar puncture with CSF drainage is reasonable in patients with extremely high ICP but should be done in conjunction with a neurology consultation.

Treatment of APL DS involves prompt administration of corticosteroids, commonly dexamethasone 10 mg IV twice daily until symptoms resolve followed by a 2-week taper.[216] In patients with severe DS, an oncology consultation should be obtained to determine if ATRA should be discontinued or another chemotherapeutic, typically cytarabine, should be added to ATRA in patients with high white blood cell counts.[199] All-trans-retinoic acid can be reintroduced upon resolution of DS.

VITAMIN D

MW	= 384.62 Da
Therapeutic serum concentration	= 10–50 ng/mL

History and Epidemiology

Rickets, a disease of urban children living in temperate zones, was thought to result from the lack of a dietary factor or adequate sunshine. In 1919, two independent groups demonstrated that rickets could be prevented or cured by either the addition of cod liver oil to the diet or exposure to sunlight.[121,174] Vitamin D is found in cod liver oil and other foods, including butter, cheese, and cream, which contain 12 to 40 IU/100 g (0.3-1 mcg/100 g), eggs, which contain 25 IU/100 g (0.6 mcg/100 g), and fatty fish, such as salmon and mackerel, which contain 150 to 550 IU/100 g (4–14 mcg/100 g) and 1,100 IU/100 g (28 mcg/100 g), respectively. Some foods typically are fortified with vitamin D, including cereals, bread, and milk.[116] Many dietary supplements, such as multivitamins, contain vitamin D.

Rickets has been eliminated as a major public health concern in children in Europe and North America since the fortification of milk with vitamin D. Outbreaks of vitamin D poisoning subsequently occurred in Europe in the 1950s because of excessive fortification of milk and cereals to compensate for wartime nutritional deprivation of children.[60] This vitamin D poisoning led to a period of prohibition of vitamin D fortification of foods.[116] Subsequently, vitamin D supplementation resumed, and a study showed that milk and infant formulas rarely contain the amount of vitamin D stated on the label and may be either significantly underfortified or overfortified, leading to vitamin D deficiency or toxicity.[116] Vitamin D toxicity secondary to excessively fortified food and supplements continues to be a problem. In 2016, the Danish health authority recalled a vitamin D supplement that contained 75 times the recommended concentration of vitamin D.[18] At least 20 children had toxic serum concentrations of vitamin D, and more than half of these children had hypercalcemia.[219] Many cases of vitamin D toxicity result from continued supplementation of vitamin D and calcium initially prescribed for treatment of hypoparathyroidism, osteoporosis, or osteomalacia but inappropriately continued due among other reasons to inadequate patient physician communication.[57,150,200] Vitamin D toxicity is reported in dogs secondary to vitamin D_3 exposure in the form of rodenticides.[86]

Vitamin D deficiency should not occur in individuals who eat a well-balanced diet and are exposed to adequate sunlight. Casual exposure of cutaneous tissues to ultraviolet light during the summer months should produce adequate vitamin D storage for winter months.[103] Total body sun exposure provides the vitamin D equivalent of 10,000 IU/day (250 mcg/day); the body requires only a total vitamin D supply of 4,000 IU/day (100 mcg/day).[248] Breast-fed infants require supplemental vitamin D if they have limited exposure to sunlight because the vitamin D content of human milk is extremely low.[5] Other groups susceptible to vitamin D deficiency include older adults, vegans, persons with darkly pigmented skin, persons without adequate sunlight exposure such as those living in institutions and those who fastidiously employ sunblock.

The National Academy of Sciences issues dietary recommendations at the request of the governments of the United States and Canada. The IOM found that although average total vitamin D intake was below the median requirement in North Americans, average serum concentrations of vitamin D as 25-hydroxyvitamin D (25(OH)D) were above the 20 ng/mL (50 nmol/L) concentration that the IOM determined to be needed for good bone health. It suggested that sun exposure contributes meaningful amounts of vitamin D and that most of the population is meeting its needs for vitamin D.[50] Despite this finding, in 2010, the IOM revised its dietary reference intakes with an increase in the RDA for vitamin D across all age groups (Table 44–1). The new RDA assumes minimal sunlight exposure and is 600 IU/day (15 mcg/day) for nonelderly adults. The new RDA may lead to an increased number of persons taking vitamin D either by prescription or in the form of a dietary supplement. In addition, the IOM found that testing for vitamin D deficiency has become widespread.[50] However, the measurements or cutpoints of sufficiency or deficiency used by laboratories are not based on scientific studies, and there is no central regulatory authority determining which cutpoint should be used. The IOM found that many laboratories use an inappropriately high cutpoint for deficiency, thereby leading to an increased number of diagnoses of vitamin D deficiency and possibly persons taking unnecessary vitamin D supplements.

In 2014, a Canadian report questioned the accuracy of the IOM's calculations in determining the RDA for vitamin D.[246] Their statistical analysis of the same data used by the IOM estimated an RDA approximately 10-fold higher than that of the IOM, which they acknowledge is well above the established UL. The authors cited two studies conducted in northern Canada in areas with limited sun exposure, in which 10% to 15% of participants who were taking vitamin D supplements to ensure compliance with the RDA had 25(OH)D serum concentrations less than 50 nmol/L.[98,130] They suggest that if the IOM's calculations were accurate, this percentage should not exceed 2.5%. At this time, the IOM has not made any changes to its 2010 recommendations.

The use of vitamin D supplements to prevent and treat a variety of illnesses has increased substantially over the past decade.[105] Vitamin D deficiency is linked to autoimmune disease, cancer, cardiovascular disease, depression, dementia, infectious disease, musculoskeletal decline, and more.[105] However, the IOM concluded that vitamin D supplementation for indications other than musculoskeletal health is not supported by adequate scientific evidence.[50] Vitamin D is used for the prophylaxis and treatment of rickets, osteomalacia, and osteoporosis. It is also used for the treatment of hypoparathyroidism and skin conditions, including psoriasis.

Vitamin D is the name given to both ergocalciferol (vitamin D_2) and cholecalciferol (vitamin D_3). In humans, both forms of vitamin D have the same biologic potency although vitamin D_3 is typically recommended. One microgram of vitamin D is equivalent to 40 IU of vitamin D.

Pharmacology, Pharmacokinetics, and Toxicokinetics

Vitamin D itself is not biologically active and must go through extensive metabolism to an active form, whether it is ingested from a food source in the form of vitamin D_2 and D_3 or synthesized in the body. Vitamin D_3 is synthesized in the skin from 7-dehydrocholesterol (provitamin D_3) in a reaction catalyzed by ultraviolet B irradiation (Fig. 44–2).[150] Vitamin D_3 then is bound to vitamin D-binding protein, a protein that also binds vitamin D from the diet, and afterward enters the circulation. In the endoplasmic reticulum of the liver, vitamin D is metabolized to 25(OH)D by vitamin D-25-hydroxylase.[87] After forming, 25(OH)D is again bound to vitamin D-binding protein and transported to the proximal convoluted tubule in the kidney for hydroxylation to 1,25-dihydroxyvitamin D {1,25(OH)$_2$D}, or calcitriol, by 25(OH)D-1-α-hydroxylase.[87] This enzyme is subject to inhibition by increases in serum calcium. After forming formed, 1,25(OH)$_2$D is secreted back into circulation, bound to vitamin D–binding protein, and delivered to target cells where it binds to receptors.

Vitamin D might be more appropriately called a hormone rather than a vitamin because it is synthesized in the body, circulates in the blood, and then binds to receptors to evoke its biologic action. The primary role of vitamin D is regulation of calcium homeostasis via interactions with the intestines and bones. Protein-bound calcitriol is taken up by cells and then

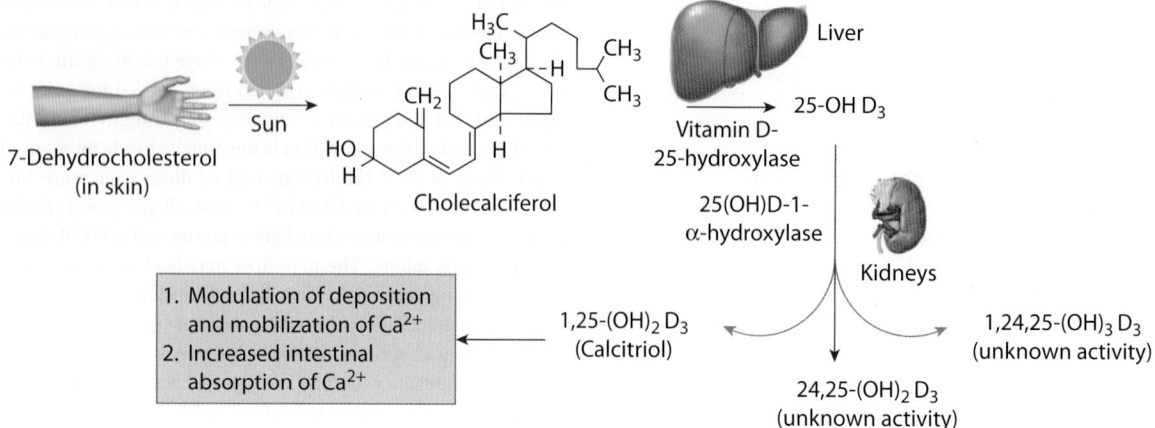

FIGURE 44–2. Schematic representation of the synthesis and physiologic response to vitamin D.

binds to a specific nuclear vitamin D receptor protein that, in turn, binds to regulatory sequences on chromosomal DNA.[150] The result is induction of gene transcription and translation of proteins that carry out the cellular functions of vitamin D. In the intestines, calcitriol increases the production of calcium binding proteins and plasma membrane calcium pump proteins, thereby increasing calcium absorption through the duodenum.[132] In the bone, calcitriol stimulates osteoclastic precursors to differentiate into mature osteoclasts.[115] Mature osteoclasts, together with PTH, lead to mobilization of calcium stores from bone, thereby raising serum concentrations of calcium. Given sufficient serum concentrations of calcium, calcitriol promotes bone mineralization by osteoblasts, resulting in increased deposition of calcium hydroxyapatite into the bone matrix.[115] Calcitriol also binds to a vitamin D receptor in the parathyroid glands, which leads to decreased synthesis and secretion of PTH.[185] The vitamin D receptor is present in most cells of the body, including lymphocytes, epidermal skin cells, and tumor cells.[221] The binding of calcitriol can inhibit proliferation and induce terminal differentiation.[203] Although the role of vitamin D is not elucidated in all cells, abnormalities present during vitamin D deficiency may help identify the function of vitamin D in various tissues.

Vitamin D deficiency results in hypocalcemia, leading to increased secretion of PTH, which acts to restore plasma calcium concentrations at the expense of bone. In children, this situation leads to rickets in which newly formed bone is not adequately mineralized and results in bone deformities and growth defects. Adults develop osteomalacia, a disease characterized by undermineralized bone matrix. Patients typically present with bone pain and tenderness and proximal muscle weakness. Bone deformities are limited to the advanced stages of disease.

The literature varies regarding the toxic dose of vitamin D, with little scientific data available for corroboration. The current upper level intake is set at 4,000 IU/day (100 mcg/day) for persons aged 9 years and older, with lower levels set for children younger than 9 years of age.[50] This is an increase compared to the previous UL of 2,000 IU/day (50 mcg/day).[248] There also are studies showing that dosages as high as 4,400 IU/day (110 mcg/day) and 100,000 IU (2,500 mcg) for 4 days did not result in adverse effects.[236,243,248] Case reports describe toxicity in the setting of vitamin D intake of 50,000 to 600,000 IU or, simply, doses in the milligram range, daily for prolonged periods.[57,96,159,200]

Pathophysiology

The hallmark of vitamin D toxicity is hypercalcemia. Vitamin D in the form of 1,25(OH)$_2$D promotes calcium absorption from the gut and mobilization of calcium from bone. Vitamin D toxicity is associated with a serum concentration of 25(OH)D 20 times higher than normal, whereas the concentration of 1,25(OH)$_2$D remains exceedingly variable.[87,201] 25-Hydroxyvitamin D mimics the action of 1,25(OH)$_2$D when it is present in excess and binds to receptors usually specific for 1,25(OH)$_2$D.[87,150] Alternatively, 25(OH)D, which has a higher affinity for vitamin D-binding protein compared with 1,25(OH)$_2$D,

preferentially binds to vitamin D-binding protein when it is present in elevated concentrations, displacing 1,25(OH)$_2$D and allowing it to circulate in an unbound form or loosely bound to albumin.[247] A study of patients with vitamin D toxicity who had normal or near normal total 1,25(OH)$_2$D concentrations had elevated free 1,25(OH)$_2$D concentrations.[201] The availability of 1,25(OH)$_2$D to its receptors likely is increased, resulting in vitamin D toxicity. These mechanisms explain how hypercalcemia occurs in cases of vitamin D toxicity despite inhibition of the conversion of 25(OH)D to 1,25(OH)$_2$D in the presence of increasing serum calcium concentrations.

Although hypercalcemia occurs with vitamin D supplementation, hypercalciuria and resultant nephrolithiasis do not necessarily occur. The degree of hypercalciuria that develops with vitamin D supplement use may not be sufficient to cause stone formation. Also, as serum calcium concentrations increase, inhibition of 25(OH)D-1-α-hydroxylase prevents the conversion of 25(OH)D to 1,25(OH)$_2$D, thereby limiting hypercalciuria and stone development.[94] However, this is not necessarily true when 25(OH)D concentrations are very high as occur in overdose. Nephrolithiasis is noted to occur with vitamin D supplementation in association with genetic mutations. When the gene for 1,25 dihydroxyvitamin D-24-hydroxylase cytochrome P450, *CYP24A1*, is mutated, the enzyme it codes for is inactivated, thereby preventing the conversion of 1,25(OH)$_2$D to the inactive calcitroic acid.[241] Individuals with one or two mutations of the gene develop hypercalcemia and hypercalciuria with stone formation, sometimes not presenting until adulthood. Compared with those with idiopathic stone formation, they have suppressed PTH concentrations, and high 1,25(OH)$_2$D concentrations. This mutation could account for the tendency of vitamin D to cause hypercalciuria and calcium stones in certain individuals.[94]

Clinical Manifestations

Patients with vitamin D toxicity present with signs and symptoms characteristic of hypercalcemia.[150] Early manifestations include weakness, fatigue, somnolence, irritability, headache, dizziness, muscle and bone pain, nausea, vomiting, abdominal cramps, and diarrhea or constipation (Chap. 12). As the calcium concentration increases, hypercalcemia induces polyuria and polydipsia. Diuresis results in salt and water depletion, further impairing calcium excretion. Although in some individuals, vitamin D supplementation can cause hypercalciuria, a known risk factor for nephrolithiasis,[53] a prospective analysis of three large cohort studies with multivariate adjustment for use of calcium supplements did not show any statistically significant association between vitamin D intake and risk of stone formation.[77] This finding is limited to chronic use and by a maximum mean total vitamin D intake of 1,317 IU/day, with a maximum mean dietary vitamin D intake of 410 IU/day and a maximum mean supplemental vitamin D dosage of 839 IU/day, across the three cohorts. A higher risk of nephrolithiasis with higher doses of vitamin D cannot be excluded. Severe hypercalcemia presents with ataxia, confusion, psychosis, seizures, coma, and acute kidney injury. In addition, cardiac dysrhythmias result from a shortened refractory period and slowed conduction. Findings on electrocardiography include increased PR intervals, widening of QRS complexes, QT interval shortening, and flattened T waves (Chap. 15).[187] Patients can develop metastatic calcification of the kidneys, blood vessels, myocardium, lung, and skin. Several patients with vitamin D toxicity have presented with anemia.[207,223] Proposed mechanisms for anemia include a direct effect of vitamin D on hematopoietic cells and inhibition of erythropoietin production.[207]

Diagnostic Testing

Vitamin D toxicity should be considered in patients presenting with signs and symptoms of hypercalcemia. In addition to an elevated serum calcium concentration, laboratory results reveal hyperphosphatemia given that vitamin D facilitates phosphate absorption in the small intestine, enhances its mobilization from bone, and decreases its excretion by the kidney.[164] The diagnosis should be suspected in children with nephrocalcinosis and hypercalciuria even if serum calcium and phosphorus concentrations are normal.[180] Serum 25(OH)D is measurable, but it is unlikely that results will be available quickly. According to the IOM, the desired 25(OH)D concentration range is 20 to 50 ng/mL.[50] The IOM also found that concentrations higher than 30 ng/mL were not consistently associated with increased benefit, and concentrations higher than 50 ng/mL may be cause for concern.

Management

Treatment of hypercalcemia in patients with vitamin D toxicity should include discontinuation of both vitamin D and calcium supplementation, maintenance of a low calcium diet, and administration of adequate volumes of oral or IV fluid to overcome dehydration and increase renal calcium clearance.[150] Many cases of hypercalcemia will respond to such supportive care. When patients are euvolemic, it is reasonable to add a loop diuretic in moderate cases of hypercalcemia requiring ongoing IV fluid administration. This helps prevent fluid overload and increases renal calcium clearance. However, electrolyte monitoring and replacement are necessary. Moderate to severe cases of hypercalcemia require additional treatment and should be managed like cases of moderate to severe hypercalcemia from other causes. Calcitonin is a hypocalcemic hormone secreted by the thyroid gland that decreases bone resorption by directly inhibiting osteoclast activity. It also reduces the serum calcium concentration by increasing renal calcium excretion. Salmon calcitonin is recommended at a dosage of 4 units/kg intramuscularly every 12 hours for up to 48 hours.[175,261] Calcitonin is more efficacious when administered with bisphosphonates, which also inhibit bone resorption via an effect on osteoclasts.[73] Pamidronate 90 mg IV over 2 hours or zoledronic acid 4 mg IV over 15 minutes is recommended.[149] Glucocorticoids decrease calcitriol production, thereby reducing serum calcium concentrations via a decrease in intestinal calcium absorption or inhibition of bone resorption.[137,238] It is reasonable to administer hydrocortisone 100 mg/day or prednisone 40 mg/day over 5 days to treat severe cases of hypercalcemia. Hemodialysis is reasonable in refractory cases of hypercalcemia.

ANTIOXIDANTS (VITAMINS E AND C)

The antioxidants include vitamins E and C and beta-carotene. During the 1990s, the concept that antioxidants had a protective effect against atherosclerosis and carcinogenesis was widely promoted. This notion was based on the "oxidative-modification hypothesis" of atherosclerosis, which proposes that atherogenesis is initiated by lipid peroxidation of LDL.[61] Unregulated or prolonged production of cellular oxidants leading to oxidant-induced DNA damage is thought to be responsible for carcinogenesis.[140] Epidemiologic evidence seems to support the use of antioxidants for these indications.[143,210,235] However, several prospective, randomized, placebo-controlled clinical trials, designed to test for the effect of antioxidant vitamins on cardiovascular disease and cancer, demonstrated that commonly used antioxidant regimens do not significantly reduce or prevent overall cardiovascular events or cancer.[40,100,101,112,189,263]

VITAMIN E

MW	= 430.69 Da
Therapeutic serum concentration	= 0.5–2.0 mg/dL

History and Epidemiology

The existence of vitamin E was first demonstrated in 1922 by researchers noting that female rats deficient in a dietary principle were unable to sustain a pregnancy.[69] Testicular lesions in male rats were described in deficiency states, and vitamin E was referred to as the "anti-sterility vitamin."[165] Vitamin E was first isolated from wheat-germ oil in 1936.[68] The richest sources of vitamin E include nuts, wheat germ, whole grains, and vegetable and seed oils, including soybean, corn, cottonseed, and safflower, and the products made from these oils. In general, animal products are poor sources of vitamin E. Human milk, in contrast to cow's milk, has sufficient vitamin E in the form of alpha-tocopherol to meet the needs of breastfed infants.[165]

Vitamin E is an essential nutrient. It is believed to be necessary for normal functioning of the nervous, reproductive, muscular, cardiovascular, and hematopoietic systems. Vitamin E includes eight naturally occurring compounds in two classes—tocopherols and tocotrienols—that have differing biologic activities. The most biologically active form is RRR-alpha-tocopherol, previously known as D-alpha-tocopherol, which is the most widely available form of vitamin E in food. A synthetic form of alpha-tocopherol, often used in vitamin supplements, contains a mixture of d and l isomers and is designated all-rac-alpha-tocopherol (previously d,l-alpha-tocopherol). One IU is equivalent to 1 mg of alpha-tocopherol acetate (alpha-TA).

Vitamin E supplementation should not be necessary in persons who consume a well-balanced diet. Vitamin E deficiency is found in patients with malabsorption syndromes, which occur in the presence of pancreatic insufficiency or hepatobiliary disease, such as biliary atresia.[34] Patients with abetalipoproteinemia are at risk for vitamin E deficiency.[20] In this rare disease, absorption and transport of vitamin E are impaired secondary to a lack of chylomicron and beta-lipoprotein formation. Manifestations of deficiency are variable but seem to have the most effect in organ systems that rely on vitamin E for normal functioning.[165] The clinical syndrome is primarily manifested by a peripheral neuropathy and spinocerebellar syndrome that improves with supplemental vitamin E.[176] Clinical findings include ophthalmoplegia, hyporeflexia, gait disturbances, and decreased sensitivity to vibration and proprioception.[34]

Use of vitamin E is proposed for a wide range of conditions. In most cases, scientific rationale for its use is lacking or is based on in vitro or animal data that are not validated in humans or are associated with equivocal results.[34] As examples, vitamin E is used for treatment of recurrent abortion, hemolytic anemias, claudication, wound healing, tardive dyskinesia, epilepsy, and acute respiratory distress syndrome. In addition, much research over the past decade has focused on the use of vitamin E for the prevention and treatment of cardiovascular disease and cancer, with disappointing results.[125]

Pharmacology, Pharmacokinetics, and Toxicokinetics

Vitamin E absorption is dependent on the ingestion and absorption of fat. The presence of bile also is essential. Vitamin E is passively absorbed in the intestinal tract into the lymphatic circulation by a nonsaturable process. Approximately 45% of a dose is absorbed in this manner and subsequently enters the bloodstream in chylomicrons, which are taken up by the liver. Vitamin E then is secreted back into the circulation, where it is primarily associated with LDL. Vitamin E is distributed to all tissues, with the greatest accumulation in adipose tissue, liver, and muscle.

The primary biologic function of vitamin E is as an antioxidant. It prevents damage to biologic membranes by protecting polyunsaturated fats within membrane phospholipids from oxidation.[41] It accomplishes this task by preferentially binding to peroxyl radicals and forming the corresponding organic hydroperoxide and tocopheroxyl radical, which, in turn interacts with other antioxidant compounds, such as ascorbic acid, thereby regenerating tocopherol. Vitamin E is responsible for cell growth and proliferation by combating the inhibitory effects of lipid peroxidation.[176] Vitamin E has a negative role in the regulation of cellular proliferation through its nonoxidant properties, such as inhibition of protein kinase C activity.[176]

Large amounts of vitamin E, ranging from 400 to 800 IU/day (400–800 mg/day) for months to years, were previously thought to be without apparent harm.[5] Vitamin E supplementation results in few obvious adverse effects, even at dosages as high as 3,200 mg/day (3,200 IU/day).[27] In several species, the oral median lethal dose was 2,000 mg/kg (2,000 IU/kg) or more, and significant adverse effects were observed only when daily doses were greater than 1,000 mg/kg (1,000 IU/kg), equivalent to 200 to 500 mg/kg (200–500 IU/kg) in humans.[177] However, a meta-analysis reveals that all-cause mortality increases at doses equal to or greater than 400 IU/day (400 mg/day).[178]

Pathophysiology

In vitro studies demonstrate that in high doses vitamin E may have a paradoxical prooxidant effect.[3,39,178] The prooxidant effect of vitamin E on LDLs is related to the production of alpha-tocopheroxyl radicals, which normally are inhibited by other antioxidants such as vitamin C. High doses of vitamin E displace other antioxidants, thereby disrupting the natural balance of the antioxidant system and increasing vulnerability to oxidative damage.[120] High doses of vitamin E inhibit human cytosolic glutathione S-transferases, enzymes that are active in the detoxification of xenobiotics and endogenous toxins.[245]

Clinical Manifestations

Gastrointestinal symptoms, including nausea and gastric distress, were reported in patients who had received vitamin E 2,000 to 2,500 IU/day (2,000–2,500 mg/day).[113,256] Diarrhea and abdominal cramps were reported in patients who received a dosage of 3,200 IU/day (3,200 mg/day).[11] Reports of other adverse effects, including fatigue, weakness, emotional changes, thrombophlebitis, increased serum creatinine concentration, and decreased thyroid hormone concentrations, are not reproduced in other case series or clinical trials.[177]

The most significant toxic effect of vitamin E, at dosages exceeding 1,000 IU/day (1,000 mg/day), is its ability to antagonize the effects of vitamin K.[5] Vitamin E increases the epoxidation of vitamin K to its inactive form, thereby increasing the vitamin K requirement several-fold.[13,28] Although high oral doses of vitamin E typically do not produce a coagulopathy in normal humans with adequate vitamin K stores, coagulopathy develops in vitamin K–deficient patients and patients taking warfarin.[13,28,51,72] Animal studies demonstrate that absorption of both vitamins A and K is impaired by large doses of vitamin E.[34,212]

VITAMIN C

MW	= 176.12 Da
Therapeutic serum concentration	= 0.4–2.0 mg/dL

History and Epidemiology

Vitamin C, also known as ascorbic acid, is employed as a preventive for the common cold. Interestingly, an extensive review of 14 studies of the role of vitamin C in the treatment of the common cold suggested that only eight were valid investigations, and none of the studies demonstrated any therapeutic benefit.[45] Its function as an antioxidant led to its use for the prevention and treatment of cardiovascular disease and cancer. Human data from clinical trials do not demonstrate that vitamin C significantly reduces or prevents overall cardiovascular events or cancer. Vitamin C may have a role as a reducing agent in the treatment of idiopathic methemoglobinemia (Chap. 124). However, it is less effective than standard treatment with methylene blue; therefore, it is not routinely indicated.[166] Vitamin C is popularly used to promote wound healing, treat cataracts, combat chronic degenerative diseases, counteract the effects of aging, increase mental attentiveness, and decrease stress.[51,177] However, little, if any, objective data demonstrate a benefit of treatment for any of these indications.[5] Vitamin C dietary supplements are commonly taken in dosages of 500 mg/day.

Vitamin C is used to prevent scurvy.[166] In 1747, James Lind, a physician in the British Royal Navy, analyzed the relationship between diet and scurvy and confirmed the protective and curative effects of citrus fruits. Vitamin C was isolated from cabbage in 1928 and subsequently shown in 1932 to be the active antiscorbutic factor in lemon juice. It was given the name *ascorbic acid* to indicate its role in preventing scurvy. Other dietary sources of vitamin C include tomatoes, strawberries, and potatoes. Today, those at risk for developing scurvy include older adults, alcoholics, chronic drug users, and others with inadequate diets, including infants fed formula diets with insufficient concentrations of vitamin C.[166] Symptoms include gingivitis, poor wound healing, bleeding, and petechiae and ecchymoses. Musculoskeletal signs and symptoms consisting of arthralgias, myalgias, hemarthroses, and muscular hematomas develop in 80% of cases.[70] Children experience severe pain in their lower limbs secondary to subperiosteal bleeding.[70]

Pharmacology, Pharmacokinetics, and Toxicokinetics

After ingestion, intestinal absorption of vitamin C occurs via an active transport system that is saturable.[211] Saturation occurs with ingestion of approximately 3 g/day. When given as a single oral dose, absorption decreases from 75% at 1 g to 20% at 5 g. Vitamin C is distributed from the plasma to all cells in the body. Tissue uptake is also a saturable process.[177] Metabolic degradation of vitamin C to oxalate accounts for 30% to 40% of oxalate excreted daily.[104] Because absorption and metabolic conversion are saturable, large ingestions of vitamin C should not significantly increase oxalate production.[227] Only a small amount of vitamin C is filtered through the glomeruli, and tubular resorption, a saturable process that competes with uric acid, usually is almost complete.[31] Plasma concentrations of vitamin C typically are maintained at approximately 1 mg/dL. The kidney efficiently eliminates excess vitamin C as unchanged ascorbic acid.

Vitamin C is a cofactor in several hydroxylation and amidation reactions by functioning as a reducing agent.[152,153] As a result, vitamin C plays an important role in the synthesis of collagen, carnitine, folinic acid, and norepinephrine. It also influences the processing of hormones such as oxytocin, antidiuretic hormone, and cholecystokinin. Vitamin C reduces iron from the ferric to the ferrous state in the stomach, thereby increasing intestinal absorption of iron. Vitamin C is involved in steroidogenesis in the adrenals. Vitamin C also has a prooxidant effect in vivo.[202] This effect is not believed to occur at dosages less than 500 mg/day but may occur in the setting of overdose.

Clinical Manifestations

The possibility of oxalate nephrolithiasis should not be a significant clinical concern.[89] Nevertheless, conflicting studies and reports exist regarding the association between vitamin C overdose and the development of oxalosis. A prospective study on the risk of kidney stones in men did not support an association between high daily vitamin C intake and stone formation.[54] This was also demonstrated in a study involving daily ingestion of 4 g of ascorbic acid for 5 days in healthy men in whom there was no increase in urinary oxalate excretion.[17] Another study demonstrated increased rates of oxalate absorption and endogenous synthesis contributing to hyperoxaluria, but this effect was found in individuals with a prior history of renal calcium oxalate stones and not in individuals without a prior history of calcium oxalate stones.[44] Some reports of high urine oxalate concentrations likely were erroneous because of conversion of ascorbate to oxalate in alkaline urine samples left standing after collection.[17,252] By contrast, other reports show an increase in urinary oxalate and calcium oxalate crystallization after ingestion of high doses of vitamin C in both stone formers and non-stone formers.[25,168] A recent report of a large prospective study over 11 years of men aged 45 to 79 years at baseline without prior history of renal stones demonstrated that high-dose vitamin C supplementation was associated with a dose-dependent twofold increase risk in development of first incident cases of kidney stones.[242] Individual case reports documenting the presence of oxalate stones in the setting of vitamin C overdose often have involved IV administration.[52,88,147,170,239,262] Oxalosis also is more likely to develop in patients with chronic kidney disease.[23,177] Gastrointestinal effects of high doses of vitamin C include localized esophagitis, given prolonged mucosal contact with ascorbic acid, and an osmotic diarrhea.[118,251]

VITAMIN B$_6$

MW	= 169 Da
Therapeutic serum concentration	= 3.6–18 ng/mL

History

Pyridoxine, pyridoxal, and pyridoxamine are related compounds that have the same physiologic properties. Although all three compounds are included in the term *vitamin B$_6$*, the vitamin is assigned the name *pyridoxine*. This vitamin was discovered in 1936 as the water-soluble factor whose deficiency was responsible for the development of dermatitis in rats.[166] In humans, deficiency is characterized by cheilosis, stomatitis, glossitis, blepharitis, and a seborrheic dermatitis around the eyes, nose, and mouth.[231] More important, pyridoxine deficiency is associated with seizures.

Pyridoxine is found in several foods, including meat, liver, whole-grain breads and cereals, soybeans, and vegetables.[166] Deficiency should not occur in humans who eat a well-balanced diet.[231]

In 2015, the American College of Obstetrics and Gynecology (ACOG) updated its recommendations on the treatment of nausea and vomiting of pregnancy (NVP) to include pyridoxine. According to ACOG, there is good and consistent scientific evidence (Level A) for the treatment of NVP with pyridoxine or pyridoxine plus doxylamine, and it is safe and effective and should be considered first-line pharmacotherapy.[4] Randomized controlled trials of pyridoxine compared with placebo show that pyridoxine is effective, compared with placebo, at reducing nausea and vomiting and that pyridoxine is effective at reducing severe vomiting but not mild vomiting.[220,249] However, a recent Cochrane review of randomized controlled trials found that pyridoxine improved nausea but did not decrease emesis.[169] In 2013, the FDA approved a delayed-release formulation of doxylamine and pyridoxine for the use in pregnant women with nausea and vomiting who do not respond to dietary and lifestyle changes.[232] A randomized controlled trial found that a delayed-release formulation of doxylamine and pyridoxine significantly improved NVP compared with placebo.[141] A retrospective analysis comparing pyridoxine to pyridoxine and doxylamine revealed that pyridoxine and doxylamine were more effective than pyridoxine alone in reducing NVP.[204]

This study did not compare pyridoxine and doxylamine to doxylamine alone. Doxylamine and pyridoxine are often recommended to be taken together individually in their nonprescription formulations because the combination formulation is expensive. The cause of NVP and the mechanism for how pyridoxine affects nausea are unknown.

Other historical uses of pyridoxine have included treatment of premenstrual syndrome and carpal tunnel syndrome.[2,66] High doses were suggested for treatment of schizophrenia and autism with variable results.[79,151]

Pharmacology

All forms of vitamin B$_6$ are well absorbed from the intestinal tract. Pyridoxine is rapidly metabolized to pyridoxal, pyridoxal phosphate (PLP), and 4-pyridoxic acid.[264] Pyridoxal phosphate accounts for approximately 60% of circulating vitamin B$_6$ and is the primary form that crosses cell membranes.[166] Most vitamin B$_6$ is renally excreted as 4-pyridoxic acid, with only 7% excreted unchanged in the urine.[166,264] Experiments in anephric rats demonstrate an up to 10-fold increase in susceptibility to pyridoxine-induced neurotoxicity, suggesting a need for caution when prescribing pyridoxine to patients with chronic kidney disease.[154]

Pyridoxal phosphate is the active form of vitamin B$_6$. It is a coenzyme required for the synthesis of γ-aminobutyric acid (GABA), an inhibitory neurotransmitter. Decreased GABA formation in the setting of pyridoxine deficiency contributes to seizures.[166] Isoniazid and other hydrazines inhibit the enzyme responsible for conversion of pyridoxine to PLP (Chap. 56 and Figs. 56–2 and 56–3).[117] In addition, isoniazid enhances the elimination of pyridoxine leading to neuropathy. Therefore, pyridoxine should be administered concomitantly with isoniazid to limit the development of peripheral neuropathy. Seizures resulting from isoniazid overdose often are successfully treated with pyridoxine (Antidotes in Depth: A15).

Pathophysiology

Ironically, both pyridoxine deficiency and pyridoxine toxicity are characterized by neurologic effects. Studies indicate that the mammalian peripheral sensory nervous system is vulnerable to large doses of pyridoxine.[224] Peripheral sensory nerves are vulnerable to circulating xenobiotics because of the permeability of their associated blood vessels.[224] Compared with the CNS, these nerves lack the blood–brain barrier. In addition, the nerves of the CNS are relatively shielded from pyridoxine toxicity because pyridoxine is transported into the CNS by a saturable mechanism.[224] In 1942, pyridoxine was recognized to cause severe weakness and pathological changes in peripheral nerves and dorsal root ganglia in dogs and rats.[14,234] Administration of IV pyridoxine 2 g/kg in two patients for the treatment of mushroom poisoning resulted in permanent dorsal root and sensory ganglia deficits.[6]

Clinical Manifestations

Chronic overdoses are associated with progressive sensory ataxia and severe distal impairment of proprioception and vibratory sensation. Reflexes are diminished or absent. Touch, pain, and temperature sensation are minimally impaired. These findings were first described in 1983 in a case series of seven patients who were taking pyridoxine 2 to 6 g/day for 2 to 40 months for premenstrual syndrome.[224] Nerve conduction and somatosensory studies in these patients showed dysfunction in the distal sensory peripheral nerves. Nerve biopsy showed widespread, nonspecific axonal degeneration. This syndrome was reported with pyridoxine doses as low as 200 mg/day.[198] Among 26 patients with elevated serum pyridoxine concentrations, the most common findings reported were numbness (96%), burning pain (49.9%), tingling (57.7%), balance difficulties (30.7%), and weakness (7.8%).[226] In most cases, symptoms gradually improved over several months with abstinence from pyridoxine. However, clinical manifestations sometimes progress for 2 to 3 weeks after pyridoxine discontinuation.[30]

Acute neurotoxicity occurs when a massive amount of pyridoxine is administered as a single dose or given over a few days.[6] Large overdoses of pyridoxine are associated with incoordination, ataxia, seizures, and death.[244]

NICOTINIC ACID

MW	= 123 Da
Therapeutic concentration	= Not determined

History

Nicotinic acid, or niacin, was discovered as an essential dietary component in the early 1900s.[92] A deficiency of this vitamin, also known as vitamin B$_3$, causes pellagra, which is characterized by dermatitis, diarrhea, and dementia. This disease was prevalent for centuries in countries that heavily relied on maize as a dietary staple until it was determined that pellagra could be prevented by increasing dietary intake of fresh eggs; milk; and fresh meat, including liver.[166] Other food sources of nicotinic acid include fish, poultry, nuts, legumes, and whole-grain and enriched breads and cereals. Supplementation of flour with nicotinic acid in 1939 probably is responsible for the near eradication of this disease in the United States. Chronic alcohol users still develop pellagra, likely secondary to malnutrition.[21,108]

Niacin was introduced as a treatment for hyperlipidemia in 1955.[10] Nicotinic acid reduces triglyceride synthesis, with a resultant drop in very-low-density lipoprotein cholesterol and LDL cholesterol and a rise in high-density-lipoprotein cholesterol.[92] Therapy usually is started with a single dose of 250 mg of the immediate-release formulation. The frequency of dose and total daily dose are gradually increased until a dose of 1.5 to 2.0 g/day, divided every 6 to 8 hours, is reached. If the LDL cholesterol concentration is not sufficiently decreased with this dosing regimen, then the dose is further increased up to a maximum dose of 6.0 g/day. Alternatively, an extended-release formulation is used with a starting dose of 500 mg. The dose is increased every 4 weeks based on effect and tolerance up to 1 to 2 g once daily. These doses of niacin are 100-fold higher than the amount necessary to meet adult nutritional needs.[208]

More recently, the nonmedicinal ingestion of niacin for altering or masking the results of urine testing for illicit drugs was noted.[16,181,206] However, there is no evidence that ingestion of niacin is capable of this effect.

Pharmacology, Pharmacokinetics, and Toxicokinetics

Nicotinic acid is well absorbed from the intestinal tract and is distributed to all tissues. With therapeutic dosing, little unchanged vitamin is excreted in the urine. When extremely high doses are ingested, the unchanged vitamin is the major urinary component. Nicotinic acid ultimately is converted to nicotinamide adenine dinucleotide (NAD$^+$) and nicotinamide adenine dinucleotide phosphate (NADP$^+$), which are the physiologically active forms of this vitamin. The reduced forms of NAD$^+$ and NADP$^+$, NADH and NADPH, respectively, act as coenzymes for proteins that catalyze oxidation-reduction reactions that are essential for tissue respiration.[166]

Clinical Manifestations

The most common adverse effect associated with niacin use is a vasodilatory cutaneous flushing described as a sense of warmth in the face, ears, neck, trunk, and less frequently in the extremities, lasting less than 1 to 2.5 hours.[128] Other symptoms include erythema, itching, and tingling. These effects occur at dosages of 0.5 to 1 g/day.[172] Symptoms commence within 15 to 30 minutes after ingestion of immediate-release niacin, 30 to 120 minutes after ingestion of extended-release niacin and at more variable times after ingestion of sustained-release niacin.[128] Symptoms are caused by the production of prostaglandin (PG) D$_2$ and E$_2$ via the G protein-coupled receptor, GPR109A.[29] Flushing occurs because of the predilection of the skin as a site of PG production after niacin ingestion.[237] PGD$_2$ and PGE$_2$ act on receptors DP$_1$ and EP$_{2/4}$ in dermal capillaries, causing vasodilation.[134] Vasodilatory adverse events occur in almost all of patients, particularly when given an immediate-release

form of niacin.[172] Many patients discontinue niacin use because of flushing. Long-term tolerance to flushing does develop with continued dosing of niacin, secondary to decreased PGD$_2$ output.[128]

Because rapid absorption of niacin is related to development of flushing, modified-release preparations of niacin were developed. A meta-analysis of 4,000 patients who used various time-release preparations of niacin showed that among the 70% of patients who experienced flushing, 85% used immediate-release niacin, 66% used extended-release niacin, and 26% used sustained-release niacin.[38] The modified-release preparations are more likely to produce GI adverse effects, such as epigastric distress, nausea, and diarrhea.[172] In addition, niacin-induced hepatotoxicity occurs more frequently and is more severe in patients treated with modified-release niacin rather than immediate-release niacin.[48,208] Elevated hepatic aminotransferases occur with dosages as low as 1 g/day, but signs of hepatic dysfunction occur at dosages of 2 to 3 g/day.[172] These patients have elevated serum bilirubin and ammonia concentrations and a prolonged prothrombin time. They develop fatigue, anorexia, nausea, vomiting, and jaundice. In most cases, liver function improves after niacin withdrawal.[67,172] Severe cases progress to fulminant hepatic failure and hepatic encephalopathy.[49,114,183] Niacin also causes amblyopia, hyperglycemia, hyperuricemia, coagulopathy, myopathy, and hyperpigmentation.[111] A 16-year-old boy who ingested 13 g of niacin over 48 hours developed metabolic acidosis, hypoglycemia, and coagulopathy and had elevated hepatic aminotransferases.[16] The patient also complained of severe myalgias and chest and abdominal pain. His signs and symptoms resolved after 5 days with IV fluid resuscitation and bicarbonate infusion.

Management

A dose of 325 mg of aspirin taken 30 minutes before ingestion of niacin diminishes flushing.[258] This is because aspirin inhibits cyclooxygenase, thereby decreasing production of PGs.

Other strategies for reducing flushing include dosing with meals and avoidance of alcohol, hot beverages, spicy foods, and hot baths or showers close to or after dosing.[56] Flushing is also decreased by starting at a low dose and gradually increasing to the full dose. Tolerance to flushing develops after several weeks, but flushing will recur if doses are missed.

Laropiprant, a PGD$_2$ antagonist at receptor DP$_1$, has demonstrated efficacy in numerous studies (phase 1, 2, and 3 trials) for reducing niacin-associated flushing.[128] In Europe, laropiprant was approved for use in 2008 in the form of a combined tablet, 1,000 mg of extended-release niacin with 20 mg laropiprant, and sold under the trade name Tredaptive. In 2008, the FDA did not give approval for a similar product with the trade name Cordaptive made by the same pharmaceutical company. In 2013, the HPS2-THRIVE (Heart Protection Study 2-Treatment of HDL to Reduce the Incidence of Vascular Events) collaborative group reported an increased incidence of myopathy among patients taking simvastatin plus extended-release niacin/laropiprant (ERN/LRPT) compared with those taking simvastatin plus placebo.[99] Also, ERN/LRPT in addition to statin therapy did not significantly reduce the risk of major vascular events in patients with well-controlled LDL-cholesterol concentrations. As a result, the study was halted, and production of Tredaptive ceased. Other findings included that 25.4% of participants taking ERN/LRPT stopped their randomized treatment compared with 16.6% taking placebo, mostly because of adverse dermatologic and GI effects.

In vitro studies demonstrate that methylnicotinate induces serotonin release from human platelets in addition to PGD$_2$ release from human mast cells.[194] Animal studies demonstrate the ability of various serotonin antagonists including cyproheptadine to inhibit the niacin-induced temperature increase, associated with flush, by 90%.[194] Flavonoids also were studied as a potential treatment for niacin flush because of their ability to inhibit both niacin-induced plasma PGD$_2$ and serotonin increase in a rat model.[195] In a small human study, a dietary supplement containing 150 mg of the flavanoid quercetin decreased the severity and longevity of erythema and burning sensation scores on a visual scale.[133]

SUMMARY

- Healthy adults consuming a well-balanced diet do not require vitamin supplementation.
- Vitamins are popularly believed to be a panacea and are commonly taken in supraphysiologic doses which produce serious adverse effects.
- Because the therapeutic index is large, toxicity generally does not develop unless very large doses are taken for sustained periods.
- Health care professionals should consider hypervitaminosis in the differential diagnosis when patients present with symptoms consistent with a vitamin toxicity syndrome.
- A thorough history, with emphasis on diet and underlying disease is essential before prescribing supplemental vitamins.

Acknowledgment

Richard J. Hamilton, MD, contributed to this chapter in previous editions.

REFERENCES

1. Dickson A, et al. Consumer usage and reasons for using dietary supplements: report of a series of surveys. *J Am Coll Nutr.* 2014;33:176-182.
2. Abraham G, Hargrove J. Effect of vitamin B 6 on premenstrual symptomatology in women with premenstrual tension syndrome: a double-blind crossover study. *Infertility.* 1980;3:155-165.
3. Abudu N, et al. Vitamins in human arteriosclerosis with emphasis on vitamin C and vitamin E. *Clin Chim Acta.* 2004;339:11-25.
4. Anonymous. Practice bulletin: nausea and vomiting of pregnancy. *Obstet Gynecol.* 2015;126:e12-e24.
5. Anonymous. Vitamin preparations as dietary supplements and as therapeutic agents. *JAMA.* 1987;257:1929-1936.
6. Albin R, et al. Acute sensory neuropathy from pyridoxine overdose. *Neurology.* 1987;37:1729-1732.
7. Allain H, Weintraub M. Drug-induced headache. *Ration Drug Ther.* 1980;14:1-6.
8. Allen L, Haskell M. Estimating the potential for vitamin A toxicity in women and young children. *J Nutr.* 2002;132:2907S-2919S.
9. Allowances CoRD. *Report of Food and Nutritional Board.* Washington, DC: National Academy of Sciences, National Research Council; 1989.
10. Altschul R, et al. Influence of nicotinic acid on serum cholesterol in man. *Arch Biochem Biophys.* 1955;54:558-559.
11. Anderson T, Reid D. A double-blind trial of vitamin E in angina pectoris. *Am J Clin Nutr.* 1974;27:1174-1178.
12. Anonymous. Adverse effects with isotretinoin. *FDA Drug Bull.* 1983;13:1-3.
13. Anonymous. Vitamin K, vitamin E and the coumarin drugs. *Nutr Rev.* 1982;40:180-181.
14. Antopol W, Tarlov I. Experimental study of the effects produced by large doses of vitamin B6. *J Neuropath Exp Neurol.* 1942;1:330-336.
15. Archer C, et al. Etretinate and acquired kinking of the hair. *Br J Dermatol.* 1987;12:239.
16. Arcinegas-Rodriguez S, et al. Metabolic acidosis, hypoglycemia, and severe myalgias: an attempt to mask urine drug screen results. *Pediatr Emerg Care.* 2011;27:315-317.
17. Auer B, et al. The effect of ascorbic acid ingestion on the biochemical and physicochemical risk factors associated with calcium oxalate kidney stone formation. *Clin Chem Lab Med.* 1998;36:143-147.
18. Authority Danish Health. Risk of severe intoxication with vitamin D drops. 2016. https://www.sst.dk/en/news/2016/risk-of-severe-intoxication-with-vitamin-d-drops. Accessed June 25, 2017.
19. Autret E, et al. Anophthalmia and agenesis of optic chiasma associated with adapalene gel in early pregnancy. *Lancet.* 1997;350:339.
20. Azizi E, et al. Abetalipoproteinemia treated with parenteral and oral vitamins A and E, and with medium chain triglycerides. *Acta Paediatr Scand.* 1978;67:797-801.
21. Badawy A. Pellagra and alcoholism: a biochemical perspective. *Alcohol Alcohol.* 2014;49: 238-250.
22. Bailey R, et al. Dietary supplement use in the United States, 2003-2006. *J Nutr.* 2011;141:261-266.
23. Balcke P, et al. Ascorbic acid aggravates secondary hyperoxalemia in patients on chronic hemodialysis. *Ann Intern Med.* 1984;101:344-345.
24. Bauernfeind J. *The Safe Use of Vitamin A: A Report of the International Vitamin A Consultative Group.* Washington, D.C.: Nutrition Foundation; 1980.
25. Baxmann A, et al. Effect of vitamin C supplements on urinary oxalate and pH in calcium stone-forming patients. *Kidney Int.* 2003;63:1066-1071.
26. Beaton G, et al. *Effectiveness of Vitamin A Supplementation in the Control of Young Child Morbidity and Mortality in Developing Countries. Nutrition Policy Discussion Paper No. 13.* Toronto, Canada: UN ACC/SCN;1993.
27. Bendich A, Langseth L. Safety of vitamin A. *Am J Clin Nutr.* 1989;49:358-371.
28. Bendich A, Machlin L. Safety of oral intake of vitamin E. *Am J Clin Nutr.* 1998;48:612-619.
29. Benyo Z, et al. GPR109A (PUMA-G/HM74A) mediates nicotinic acid-induced flushing. *J Clin Invest.* 2005;115:3634-3640.
30. Berger A, et al. Dose response, coasting, and differential fiber vulnerability in human toxic neuropathy: a prospective study of pyridoxine neurotoxicity. *Neurology.* 1992;42:1367-1370.
31. Berger L, et al. The effect of ascorbic acid on uric acid excretion with a commentary on the renal handling of ascorbic acid. *Am J Med.* 1977:71-76.
32. Bergman S, et al. Vitamin A-induced hypercalcemia: response to corticosteroids. *Nephron.* 1988;50:362-364.
33. Bernstein A, Leventhal-Rochon J. Neurotoxicity related to the use of topical tretinoin (Retin-A). *Ann Intern Med.* 1996;124:227-228.
34. Bieri J, et al. Medical uses of vitamin E. *N Engl J Med.* 1983;306:1063-1070.
35. Biesalski H, Nohr D. New aspects in vitamin A metabolism: the role of retinyl esters as systemic and local sources for retinol in mucous epithelia. *J Nutr.* 2004;134:3453S-3457S.
36. Binder D, et al. Idiopathic intracranial hypertension. *Neurosurgery.* 2004;54:538-552.
37. Binkley N, Krueger D. Hypervitaminosis A and bone. *Nutr Rev.* 2000;58:138-144.
38. Birjmohun R, et al. Efficacy and safety of high-density lipoprotein cholesterol-increasing compounds: a meta-analysis of randomized controlled trials. *J Am Coll Cardiol.* 2005;45: 185-197.
39. Bowry V, Stocker R. Tocopherol-mediated peroxidation. The prooxidant effect of vitamin E on the radical initiated oxidation of human low-density lipoprotein. *J Am Chem Soc.* 1993;115:6029-6044.
40. Brown B, Crowley J. Is there any hope for vitamin E? *JAMA.* 2005;293:1387-1390.
41. Burton G, et al. Is vitamin E the only lipid-soluble, chain-breaking antioxidant in human blood plasma and erythrocyte membranes? *Arch Biochem Biophys.* 1983;221:281-290.
42. Camera G, Pregliasco P. Ear malformation in baby born to mother using tretinoin cream. *Lancet.* 1992;339:687.
43. Celebisoy N, et al. Treatment of idiopathic intracranial hypertension: topiramate vs acetazolamide, an open-label study. *Acta Neurol Scand.* 2007;116:322-327.
44. Chai W, et al. Oxalate absorption and endogenous oxalate synthesis from ascorbate in calcium oxalate stone formers and non-stone formers. *Am J Kidney Dis.* 2004;44:1060-1069.
45. Chalmers T. Effect of ascorbic in the common cold: an evaluation of the evidence. *Am J Med.* 1975;58:532-536.
46. Chesney R. Modified vitamin D compounds in the treatment of certain bone diseases. In: Spiller G, ed: *Nutritional Pharmacology.* New York, NY: Alan R Liss; 1981:147-201.
47. Chiu Y, et al. Acute fish liver intoxication: report of three cases. *Changgeng Yi Xue Za Zhi.* 1999;22:468-473.
48. Christensen N, et al. Nicotinic acid treatment of hypercholesteremia: comparison of plain and sustained-action preparations and report of two cases of jaundice. *JAMA.* 1961;177:546-550.
49. Clementz G, Holmes A. Nicotinic acid-induced fulminant hepatic failure. *J Clin Gastroenterol.* 1989;9:582-584.
50. Committee IoMUS. *Dietary Reference Intakes for Calcium and Vitamin D.* Washington, DC; 2011.
51. Corrigan J. The effect of vitamin E on warfarin-induced vitamin K deficiency. *Ann NY Acad Sci.* 1982;393:361-368.
52. Cossey L, et al. Oxalate nephropathy and intravenous vitamin C. *Am J Kidney Dis.* 2013;61:1032-1035.
53. Curhan G, Taylor E. 24-h uric acid excretion and the risk of kidney stones. *Kidney Int.* 2008;73:489-496.
54. Curhan G, et al. A prospective study of the intake of vitamins C and B6 and the risk of kidney stones in men. *J Urol.* 1996;155:1847-1851.
55. David M, et al. Adverse effects of retinoids. *Med Toxicol.* 1988;3:273-288.
56. Davidson M. Niacin use and cutaneous flushing: mechanisms and strategies for prevention. *Am J Cardiol.* 2008;101:14B-19B.
57. Davies M, Adams P. The continuing risk of vitamin D intoxication. *Lancet.* 1978;2:621-623.
58. Davis B, et al. Retinol and extracellular collagen matrices modulate hepatic Ito cell collagen phenotype and cellular retinal binding protein levels. *J Biol Chem.* 1987;262:280-286.
59. Davis B, Vucic A. The effect of retinol on Ito cell proliferation in vitro. *Hepatology.* 1988;8:788-793.
60. DeLuca H. The vitamin D system in the regulation of calcium and phosphorus metabolism. *Nutr Rev.* 1979;37:161-193.
61. Diaz M, et al. Antioxidants and atherosclerotic heart disease. *N Engl J Med.* 1997;337:408-416.
62. Doireau V, et al. Vitamin A poisoning revealed by hypercalcemia in a child with kidney failure. *Arch Pediatr.* 1996;3:888-890.
63. Tee ES Jr. The medical importance of vitamin A and carotenoids (with particular reference to developing countries) and their determination. *Mal J Nutr.* 1995:179-230.
64. Elias P, Williams M. Retinoids, cancer and the skin. *Arch Dermatol.* 1981;117:160-280.
65. Ellis C, Voorhees J. Etretinate therapy. *J Am Acad Dermatol.* 1987;16:267-291.
66. Ellis J, et al. Therapy with vitamin B6 with and without surgery for treatment of patients having the idiopathic carpal tunnel syndrome. *Res Commun Chem Pathol Pharmacol.* 1981;33:331-344.
67. Etchason J, et al. Niacin-induced hepatitis: a potential side effect with low-dose time-release niacin. *Mayo Clin Proc.* 1991;66:23-28.
68. Evans H, et al. The isolation from wheat germ oil of an alcohol, α-tocopherol, having properties of vitamin E. *J Biol Chem.* 1936;113:329-332.

69. Evans H, Vishop K. On the relationship between fertility and nutrition. II. The ovulation rhythm in the rat on inadequate nutritional regimes. *J Metab Res*. 1922;1:319-356.

70. Fain O. Musculoskeletal manifestations of scurvy. *Joint Bone Spine*. 2005;72:124-128.

71. Fairfield K, Fletcher R.: Vitamins for chronic disease prevention in adults: scientific review. *JAMA*. 2002;287:3116-3126.

72. Farrell P, Bieri J. Megavitamin E supplementation in man. *Am J Clin Nutr*. 1975;18:1381-1386.

73. Fatemi S, et al. Effect of salmon calcitonin and etidronate on hypercalcemia of malignancy. *Calcif Tissue Int*. 1992;50:107-109.

74. Fenaux P, De Botton S. Retinoic acid syndrome: recognition, prevention, and management. *Drug Saf*. 1998;18:273-279.

75. Fenaux P, et al. Treatment of acute promyelocytic leukemia by retinoids. *Curr Top Microbiol Immunol*. 2007;313:101-128.

76. Ferguson M, et al. Severe nail dystrophy associated with retinoid therapy. *Lancet*. 1983;2.

77. Ferraro P, et al. Vitamin D intake and the risk of incident kidney stones. *J Urol*. 2017;197:405-409.

78. Feskanich D, et al. Vitamin A intake and hip fractures among postmenopausal women. *JAMA*. 2002;287:47-54.

79. Findling R, et al. High-dose pyridoxine and magnesium administration in children with autistic disorder: an absence of salutary effects in a double-blind, placebo-controlled study. *J Autism Dev Disord*. 1997;27:467-478.

80. Fiore L, et al. Anaphylactoid reactions to vitamin K. *J Thrombosis Thrombolysis*. 2001;11:175-183.

81. Fishman R. Polar bear liver, vitamin A, aquaporins, and pseudotumor cerebri. *Ann Neurol*. 2002;52:531-533.

82. Fletcher R, Fairfield K. Vitamins for chronic disease prevention in adults: clinical applications. *JAMA*. 2002;287:3127-3129.

83. Flynn W, et al. Pancreatitis associated with isotretinoin-induced hypertriglyceridemia. *Ann Intern Med*. 1987;106:63.

84. Foged E, Jocobson F. Side effects due to Ro-9359 (Tigason): a retrospective study. *Dermatologica*. 1982;164:395-403.

85. Food and Nutrition Board IoM, National Academies. Dietary Reference Intakes (DRIs): Recommended Dietary Allowances and Adequate Intakes, Vitamins. http://www.nationalacademies.org/hmd/Activities/Nutrition/SummaryDRIs/DRI-Tables.aspx. Accessed February 2. 2017.

86. Fooshee S, Forrester S. Hypercalcemia secondary to cholecalciferol rodenticide toxicosis in two dogs. *J Am Vet Med Assoc*. 1990;196:1265-1268.

87. Fraser D. Vitamin D. *Lancet*. 1995;345:4.

88. Friedman A, et al. Secondary oxalosis as a complication of parenteral alimentation in acute renal failure. *Am J Nephrol*. 1983;3:248-252.

89. Garewal H, Diplock A. How "safe" are antioxidant vitamins? *Drug Saf*. 1995;13:8-14.

90. Gerber A, et al. Vitamin A poisoning in adults with description of a case. *Am J Med*. 1954; 16:729-745.

91. Geubel A, et al. Liver damage caused by therapeutic vitamin A administration. Estimate of dose-related toxicity in 41 cases. *Gastroenterology*. 1991;100:1701-1709.

92. Gibbons L, et al. The prevalence of side effects with regular and sustained-release nicotinic acid. *Am J Med*. 1995;99:378-385.

93. Gjerris F, et al. Intracranial pressure, conductance to cerebrospinal fluid outflow, and cerebral blood flow in patients with benign intracranial hypertension (pseudotumor cerebri). *Ann Neurol*. 1985;17:158-162.

94. Goldfarb D. Does vitamin D supplementation cause kidney stones? *J Urol*. 2017;197:280-281.

95. Goldstein J, et al. Comparative effect of isotretinoin and etretinate on acne and sebaceous gland secretion. *J Am Acad Dermatol*. 1982;6:760-765.

96. Granado-Lorencio F, et al. Hypercalcemia, hypervitaminosis A and 3-epi-25-OH-D 3 levels after consumption of an "over the counter" vitamin D remedy. A case report. *Food Chem Toxicol*. 2012;50:2106-2108.

97. Grassnor A, Bachem M. Cellular sources of noncollagenous matrix proteins: role of fat-storing cells in fibrogenesis. *Semin Liver Dis*. 1990;10:30-45.

98. Greene-Finestone L, et al. 25-Hydroxyvitamin D in Canadian adults: biological, environmental, and behavioral correlates. *Osteoporos Int*. 2011;22:1389-1399.

99. HPS2-THRIVE Collaborative Group. HPS2-THRIVE randomized placebo-controlled trial in 25673 high-risk patients of ER niacin/laropiprant: trial design, pre-specified muscle and liver outcomes, and reasons for stopping study treatment. *Eur Heart J*. 2013;34: 1279-1291.

100. Heart Protection Study Collaborative Group. MRC/BHF Heart Protection Study of antioxidant vitamin supplementation in 20,536 "high-risk" individuals: a randomized placebo-controlled trial. *Lancet*. 2002;360:23-33.

101. Alpha-Tocopherol, Beta Carotene Cancer Prevention Study Group. The effect of vitamin E and beta carotene on the incidence of lung cancer and other cancers in male smokers. *N Engl J Med*. 1994;330:1029-1035.

102. Grzybowski D, et al. The role of vitamin A and its CSF metabolites in supporting a novel mechanism of idiopathic intracranial hypertension. *Cerebrospinal Fluid Res*. 2007;4(suppl 1):S44.

103. Haddad J. Vitamin D. Solar rays, the Milky Way or both? *N Engl J Med*. 1992;326:1213-1215.

104. Hagler L, Herman R. Oxalate metabolism. II. *Am J Clin Nutr*. 1973;26:882-889.

105. Haines S, Park S. Vitamin D supplementation: what's known, what to do, and what's needed. *Pharmacotherapy*. 2012;32:354-382.

106. Hall J. Vitamin A teratogenicity. *N Engl J Med*. 1984;311:797-798.

107. Hall J. Vitamin A. a newly recognized human teratogen—harbinger of things to come? *J Pediatr*. 1984;105:583-584.

108. Hariharasubramony A, et al. A case of alcohol-dependent syndrome and pellagra. *Int J Nutr Pharmacol Neurol Dis*. 2013;3:61-63.

109. Hendriks H, et al. Fat-storing cells: hyper- and hypovitaminosis A and the relationships with liver fibrosis. *Semin Liver Dis*. 1993;13:72-79.

110. Hendriks H, et al. Perisinusoidal fat-storing cells are the main vitamin A storage sites in rat liver. *Exp Cell Res*. 1985;160:138-149.

111. Henkin Y, et al. Niacin revisited: clinical observations on an important but underutilized drug. *Am J Med*. 1991;91:239-246.

112. Hennekens C, et al. Lack of effect of long-term supplementation with beta carotene on the incidence of malignant neoplasms and cardiovascular disease. *N Engl J Med*. 1996;334:1145-1149.

113. Hillman R. Tocopherol excess in man: creatinuria associated with prolonged ingestion. *Am J Clin Nutr*. 1957;5:597-600.

114. Hodis H. Acute hepatic failure associated with the use of low-dose sustained-release niacin. *JAMA*. 1990;264:181.

115. Holick M. Vitamin D: photobiology, metabolism, and clinical applications. In: DeGroot L, et al, eds: *Endocrinology*. 3rd ed. Philadelphia, PA: WB Saunders; 1995:990-1013.

116. Holick M, et al. The vitamin D content of fortified milk and infant formula. *N Engl J Med*. 1992;327:1637-1642.

117. Holtz P, Palm D. Pharmacological aspects of vitamin B 6. *Pharmacol Rev*. 1964;16:113-178.

118. Hoyt C. Diarrhea from vitamin C. *JAMA*. 1980;244:1674.

119. Hruban Z, et al. Ultrastructural changes in livers of two patients with hypervitaminosis A. *Am J Pathol*. 1974;76:451-468.

120. Huang H, Appel L. Supplementation of diets with alpha-tocopherol reduces serum concentrations of gamma- and delta-tocopherol in humans. *J Nutr*. 2003;133:3137-3140.

121. Huldschinsky K. Heilung von Rachitis durch Kunstliche Hohensonne. *Dtsch Med Wochenschr*. 1919;14:712-713.

122. Iliff P, et al. Tolerance of large doses of vitamin A given to mothers and their babies shortly after delivery. *Nutr Res*. 1999;129:1437-1446.

123. Inkeles S, et al. Hepatic and dermatologic manifestations of chronic hypervitaminosis A in adults. Report of two cases. *Am J Med*. 1986;80:491-496.

124. Institute of Medicine FaNB. *Dietary Reference Intakes: Thiamin, Riboflavin, Niacin, Vitamin B6, Folate, Vitamin B12, Pantothenic Acid, Biotin, and Choline*. Washington, DC; 1998.

125. Lonn E, et al; HOPE and HOPE-TOO Trial Investigators. Effects of long-term vitamin E supplementation on cardiovascular events and cancer: a randomized controlled trial. *JAMA*. 2005;293:1338-1347.

126. iPLEDGE. https://www.ipledgeprogram.com. Accessed March 30, 2017.

127. Jacobson M, et al. Serum vitamin A concentration is elevated in idiopathic intracranial hypertension. *Neurology*. 1999;53:1114-1118.

128. Jacobson T. A "hot" topic in dyslipidemia management—"hot to beat a flush": optimizing niacin tolerability to promote long-term treatment adherence and coronary disease prevention. *Mayo Clin Proc*. 2010;85:365-379.

129. Jacques E, et al. The histopathologic progression of vitamin A-induced hepatic injury. *Gastroenterology*. 1979;76:599-602.

130. Janz T, Pearson C. *Health at a Glance: Vitamin D Blood Levels of Canadians*. http://www.statcan.gc.ca/pub/82-624-x/2013001/article/11727-eng.htm.

131. Jick S, et al. First trimester topical tretinoid and congenital disorders. *Lancet*. 1993;341:1181-1182.

132. Johnson J, Kumar R. Renal and intestinal calcium transport. Role of vitamin D and vitamin D-dependent calcium binding proteins. *Semin Nephrol*. 1994;14:119-128.

133. Kalogeromitros D, et al. A quercetin containing supplement reduces niacin-induced flush in humans. *Int J Immunopathol Pharmacol*. 2008;21:509-514.

134. Kamanna V, et al. Nicotinic acid: recent developments. *Curr Opin Cardiol*. 2008;23:393-398.

135. Karner P, et al. Pflanzenfabstoffe, XXV: uber die Konstitution des Lycopins und Carotins. *Helv Chim Acta*. 1930;13:1084-1099.

136. Kent G, et al. Vitamin A containing lipocytes and formation of type III collagen in liver injury. *Proc Natl Acad Sci U S A*. 1976;73:3719-3722.

137. Kimberg D, et al. Effect of cortisone treatment on the active transport of calcium by the small intestine. *J Clin Invest*. 1971;50:1309-1321.

138. Kingston T, et al. Etretin therapy for severe psoriasis. *Arch Dermatol*. 1987;123:55-58.

139. Klar F, et al. Cerebrospinal fluid dynamics in patients with pseudotumor cerebri. *Neurosurgery*. 1979;5:208-216.

140. Klaunig J, Kamendulis L. The role of oxidative stress in carcinogenesis. *Annu Rev Pharmacol Toxicol*. 2004;44:239-267.

141. Koren G, et al. Effectiveness of delayed-release doxylamine and pyridoxine for nausea and vomiting of pregnancy: a randomized placebo controlled trial. *Am J Obstet Gynecol*. 2010;203:571.e571-571.e577.

142. Kowalski T, et al. Vitamin A hepatotoxicity. A cautionary note regarding 25,000 IU supplements. *Am J Med*. 1994;97:523-528.

143. Kushi L, et al. Intakes of vitamins A, C, E and postmenopausal breast cancer. The Iowa Women's Health Study. *Am J Epidemiol*. 1996;144:165-174.

144. Lammer E, et al. Retinoic acid embryopathy. *N Engl J Med*. 1985;313:837-841.

145. Landy D. Pibloktoq (hysteria) and Inuit nutrition: possible implication of hypervitaminosis A. *Soc Sci Med*. 1985;21:173-185.

146. Larson R, Tallman M. Retinoic acid syndrome: manifestations, pathogenesis, and treatment. *Best Pract Res Clin Haematol*. 2003;16:453-461.

147. Lawton J, et al. Acute oxalate nephropathy after massive ascorbic acid administration. *Arch Intern Med*. 1985;145:950-951.

148. Le-Coco F, et al. Acute promyelocytic leucemia: recent advances in diagnosis and management. *Semin Oncol*. 2008;35:401-409.

149. Lee D, Lee G. The use of pamidronate for hypercalcemia secondary to acute vitamin D intoxication. *Clin Toxicol*. 1998;36:719-721.

150. Lee K, et al. Iatrogenic vitamin D intoxication. Report of a case and review of vitamin D physiology. *Connecticut Med*. 1999;63:399-403.

151. Lerner V, et al. Vitamin B6 as add-on treatment in chronic schizophrenic and schizoaffective patients: a double-blind, placebo-controlled study. *J Clin Psychiatry*. 2002;63:54-58.

152. Levine M. New concepts in the biology and biochemistry of ascorbic acid. *N Engl J Med*. 1986;314:892-902.

153. Levine M, et al. In situ kinetics and ascorbic acid requirements. *World Rev Nutr Diet*. 1993;72:114-127.

154. Levine S, Saltzman A. Pyridoxine (vitamin B6) toxicity: enhancement by uremia in rats. *Food Chem Toxicol*. 2002;40:1449-1451.

155. Libien J, Blaner W. Retinol and retinol-binding protein in cerebrospinal fluid: can vitamin A take the "idiopathic" out of idiopathic intracranial hypertension? *J Neuroophthalmol*. 2007;27:253-257.

156. Lipson A, et al. Multiple congenital defects associated with maternal use of topical tretinoin. *Lancet*. 1993;341:1352-1353.

157. Liu G, et al. High-dose methylprednisolone and acetazolamide for visual loss in pseudotumor cerebri. *Am J Ophthalmol*. 1994;118:88-96.

158. Love J, Gudas L. Vitamin A, differentiation and cancer. *Curr Opin Cell Biol*. 1994;6:825-831.

159. Lowe H, et al. Vitamin D toxicity due to a commonly available "over the counter" remedy from the Dominican Republic. *J Clin Endocrinol Metab*. 2011;96:291-295.

160. Lysak W, Svien H. Long term follow-up on patients with diagnosis of pseudotumor cerebri. *J Neurol Surg*. 1966;25:284-287.

161. Macapinlac M, Olson J. A lethal hypervitaminosis A syndrome in young monkeys following a single intramuscular dose of a water-miscible preparation containing vitamins A, D 2 and E. *Int J Vitam Nutr Res*. 1981;51:331-341.

162. Malm J, et al. CSF hydrodynamics in idiopathic intracranial hypertension: a long-term study. *Neurology*. 1992;42:851-858.

163. Mangelsdorf D, et al. The retinoid receptors. In: Sporn M, et al, eds: *The Retinoids: Biology, Chemistry, Medicine*. 2nd ed. New York, NY: Raven Press; 1994:573-595.

164. Marcus R. Agents affecting calcification and bone turnover: calcium, phosphate, parathyroid hormone, vitamin D, calcitonin, and other compounds. In: Hardman J, et al, eds: *The Pharmacological Basis of Therapeutics*. 10th ed. New York, NY: McGraw-Hill; 2001: 1715-1752.

165. Marcus R, Coulston A. Fat-soluble vitamins: vitamins A, K, and E. In: Hardman J, et al, eds: *The Pharmacological Basis of Therapeutics*. 10th ed. New York, NY: McGraw-Hill; 2001: 1773-1791.

166. Marcus R, Coulston A. Water-soluble vitamins: the vitamin B complex and ascorbic acid. In: Hardman J, et al, eds: *The Pharmacological Basis of Therapeutics*. 10th ed. New York, NY: McGraw-Hill; 2001:1753-1771.

167. Marra M, Boyar A. Position of the American Dietetic Association: nutrient supplementation. *J Am Diet Assoc*. 2009;109:2073-2085.

168. Massey L, et al. Ascorbate increases human oxaluria and kidney stone risk. *J Nutr*. 2005;135:1673-1677.

169. Matthews A, et al. Interventions for nausea and vomiting in early pregnancy. *Cochrane Database of Syst Rev*. 2014.

170. McAllister C. Renal failure secondary to massive infusion of vitamin C. *JAMA*. 1984;252:1684.

171. McCollum E, Davis M. The necessity of certain lipids in the diet during growth. *J Biol Chem*. 1913;15:167-175.

172. McKenney J, et al. A comparison of the efficacy and toxic effects of sustained- vs immediate-release niacin in hypercholesterolemic patients. *JAMA*. 1994;271:672-677.

173. Melhus H, et al. Excessive dietary in-take of vitamin A is associated with reduced bone mineral density and increased risk for hip fracture. *Ann Intern Med*. 1998;129:770-778.

174. Mellanby E. An experimental investigation of rickets. *Lancet*. 1919;1:407-412.

175. Mete E, et al. Calcitonin therapy in vitamin D intoxication. *J Trop Pediatr*. 1997;43:241-242.

176. Meydani M. Vitamin E. *Lancet*. 1995;345:170-175.

177. Meyers D, et al. Safety of antioxidant vitamins. *Arch Intern Med*. 1996;156:925-935.

178. Miller EI, et al. Meta-analysis: high-dosage vitamin E supplementation may increase all-cause mortality. *Ann Intern Med*. 2005;142:37-46.

179. Mills C, Marks R. Adverse reactions to oral retinoids: an update. *Drug Saf*. 1993;9:280-290.

180. Misselwitz J, et al. Nephrocalcinosis, hypercalciuria and elevated serum levels of 1,25-dihydrovitamin D in children. *Acta Paediatr Scand*. 1990;79:637-643.

181. Mittal M, et al. Toxicity from the use of niacin to beat urine drug screening. *Ann Emerg Med*. 2007;50:587-590.

182. Mulholland C, Benford D. What is known about the safety of multivitamin-multimineral supplements for the generally healthy population? Theoretical basis for harm. *Am J Clin Nutr*. 2007;85:318S-322S.

183. Mullin G, et al. Fulminant hepatic failure after ingestion of sustained-release nicotinic acid. *Ann Intern Med*. 1989;111:253-255.

184. Nagai K, et al. Vitamin A toxicity secondary to excessive intake of yellow-green vegetables, liver and laver. *J Hepatol*. 1999;31:142-148.

185. Naveh-Many T, Silver J. Regulation of parathyroid hormone gene expression by hypocalcemia, hypercalcemia, and vitamin D in the rat. *J Clin Invest*. 1990;86:1313-1319.

186. Ng K, et al. Effect of retinoids on the growth, ultrastructure, and cytoskeletal structures of malignant rat osteoblasts. *Cancer Res*. 1985;45:5106-5113.

187. Nordt S, et al. Pharmacologic misadventure resulting in hypercalcemia from vitamin D intoxication. *J Emerg Med*. 2002;22:302-303.

188. Council for Responsible Nutrition. http://www.crnusa.org/CRNconsumersurvey/2015. Accessed January 30, 2017.

189. Omenn G, et al. Effects of a combination of beta-carotene and vitamin A on lung cancer and cardiovascular disease. *N Engl J Med*. 1996;334:1150-1155.

190. Ong D, et al. Cellular retinoid binding proteins. In: Sporn M, et al, eds: *The Retinoids: Biology, Chemistry, Medicine*. 2nd ed. New York, NY: Raven Press; 1994:283-317.

191. Opotowsky A, Bilezikian J. Serum vitamin A concentration and the risk of hip fracture among women 50 to 74 years old in the United States: a prospective analysis of the NHANESI follow-up study. *Am J Med*. 2004;117:169-174.

192. Oreffo R, et al. Effect of vitamin A on bone resorption: evidence for direct stimulation of isolated chicken osteoclasts by retinol and retinoic acid. *J Bone Miner Res*. 1988;3:203-209.

193. Osborne T, Mendel L. The relation of growth to the chemical constituents of the diet. *J Biol Chem*. 1913;15:311-326.

194. Papaliodis D, et al. Niacin-induced "flush" involves release of prostaglandin D2 from mast cells and serotonin from platelets: evidence from human cells in vitro and an animal model. *J Pharmacol Exp Ther*. 2008;327:665-672.

195. Papaliodis D, et al. The flavanoid luteolin inhibits niacin-induced flush. *Br J Pharmacol*. 2008;153:1382-1387.

196. Parker R. Absorption, metabolism, and transport of carotenoids. *FASEB J*. 1996;10:542-551.

197. Parker S. Eskimo psychopathology in the context of Eskimo personality and culture. *Am Anthropol*. 1962;64:76-96.

198. Parry G, Bredesen D. Sensory neuropathy with low dose pyridoxine. *Neurology*. 1985;35:1466-1468.

199. Patatanian E, Thompson D. Retinoic acid syndrome: a review. *J Clin Pharm Ther*. 2008;33: 331-338.

200. Paterson C. Vitamin-D poisoning. Survey of causes in 21 patients with hypercalcaemia. *Lancet*. 1980;1:1164-1165.

201. Pettifor J, et al. Serum levels of free 1,25-dihydroxyvitamin D in vitamin D toxicity. *Ann Intern Med*. 1995;122:511-513.

202. Podmore I, et al. Vitamin C exhibits pro-oxidant properties. *Nature*. 1998;392:559.

203. Pols H, et al. Vitamin D: a modulator of cell proliferation and differentiation. *J Steroid Biochem Mol Biol*. 1990;37:873-876.

204. Pope E, et al. Comparing pyridoxine and doxylamine succinate-pyridoxine HCl for nausea and vomiting of pregnancy: a matched, controlled cohort study. *J Clin Pharmacol*. 2015;55:809-814.

205. Prendiville J, et al. Premature epiphyseal closure—a complication of etretinate therapy in children. *J Am Acad Dermatol*. 1986;15:1259-1262.

206. Centers for Disease Control and Prevention (CDC). Use of niacin in attempts to defeat urine drug testing—five states, January-September 2006. *Morb Mortal Wkly Rep*. 2007; 56: 365-366.

207. Puig J, et al. Anemia secondary to vitamin D intoxication. *Ann Intern Med*. 1998;128:602-603.

208. Rader J, et al. Hepatic toxicity of unmodified and time-release preparations of niacin. *Am J Med*. 1992;92:77-81.

209. Randhawa S, Van Stavern G. Idiopathic intracranial hypertension (pseudotumor cerebri). *Curr Opin Ophthalmol*. 2008;19:445-453.

210. Rimm E, et al. Vitamin E consumption and the risk of coronary heart disease in men. *N Engl J Med*. 1993;328:1450-1456.

211. Rivers J. Safety of high-level vitamin C ingestion. *Ann NY Acad Sci*. 1987;498:445-454.

212. Roberts H. Perspective of vitamin E as therapy. *JAMA*. 1981;246:129-131.

213. Robertson J, et al. A survey of pregnant women using isotretinoin. *Birth Defects Res A Clin Mol Teratol*. 2005;73:881-887.

214. Rock C. Multivitamin-multimineral supplements: who uses them? *Am J Clin Nutr*. 2007; 85:277S-279S.

215. Rodahl K, Moore T. The vitamin A content and toxicity of polar bear and seal liver. *Biochem J*. 1943;37:166-169.

216. Rogers J, Yang D. Differentiation syndrome in patients with acute promyelocytic leukemia. *J Oncol Pharm Practice*. 2011;18:109-114.

217. Russel F. Vitamin A content of polar bear liver. *Toxicon*. 1966;5:61-62.

218. Russel R, et al. Hepatic injury from chronic hypervitaminosis A resulting in portal hypertension and as cites. *N Engl J Med*. 1974;291:435-440.

219. Rychla L. Danish health authority warns of toxic vitamin D product. 2016. http://cphpost.dk/news/danish-health-authority-warns-of-toxic-vitamin-d-product.html. Accessed June 25, 2017.

220. Sahakian V, et al. Vitamin B6 is effective therapy for nausea and vomiting of pregnancy: a randomized, double-blind placebo-controlled study. *Obstet Gynecol*. 1991;78:33-36.

221. Sandgren M, et al. Tissue distribution of the 1,25-dihydroxyvitamin D 3 receptor in the male rat. *Biochem Biophys Res Commun.* 1991;181:611-616.

222. Schafer S, et al. The synthesis of proteoglycans in fat storing cells of rat liver. *Hepatology.* 1987;7:680-687.

223. Scharfman W, Propp S. Anemia associated with vitamin D intoxication. *N Engl J Med.* 1956;255:1208-1212.

224. Schaumburg H, et al. Sensory neuropathy from pyridoxine abuse: a new megavitamin syndrome. *N Engl J Med.* 1983;309:445-448.

225. Scheven B, Hamilton N. Retinoic acid and 1,25-dihydroxyvitamin D 3 stimulate osteoclast formation by different mechanisms. *Bone.* 1990;11:53-59.

226. Scott K, et al. Elevated B6 levels and peripheral neuropathies. *Electromyogr Clin Neurophysiol.* 2008;48:219-223.

227. Sestili M. Possible adverse health effects of vitamin C and ascorbic acid. *Semin Oncol.* 1983;10:299-304.

228. Shapiro L, et al. Safety of first-trimester exposure to topical tretinoin: prospective cohort study. *Lancet.* 1997;350:1143-1144.

229. Sharieff G, Hanten K. Pseudotumor cerebri and hypercalcemia resulting from vitamin A toxicity. *Ann Emerg Med.* 1996;27:518-521.

230. Silverman A, et al. Hypervitaminosis A syndrome. A paradigm of retinoid side effects. *J Am Acad Dermatol.* 1987;16:1027-1039.

231. Skelton WI, Skelton N. Deficiency of vitamins A, B, C: something to watch for. *Postgrad Med.* 1990;87:293-310.

232. Slaughter S, et al. FDA approval of doxylamine-pyridoxine therapy for use in pregnancy. *N Engl J Med.* 2014;370:1081-1083.

233. Smith F, Goodman D. Vitamin A transport in human vitamin A toxicity. *N Engl J Med.* 1976;294:805-808.

234. Snodgrass R. Vitamin neurotoxicity. *Mol Neurobiol.* 1992;6:41-73.

235. Stampfer M, et al. Vitamin E consumption and the risk of coronary disease in women. *N Engl J Med.* 1993;328:1444-1449.

236. Stern P, et al. Demonstration that circulation 1,25-dihydroxyvitamin D is loosely regulated in normal children. *J Clin Invest.* 1981;68:1374-1377.

237. Stern R, et al. Tolerance to nicotinic acid flushing. *Clin Pharmacol Ther.* 1991;50:66-70.

238. Streck W, et al. Glucocorticoid effects in vitamin D intoxication. *Arch Intern Med.* 1979;139:974-977.

239. Swartz R, et al. Hyperoxaluria and renal insufficiency due to ascorbic acid administration during total parenteral nutrition. *Ann Intern Med.* 1984;100:530-531.

240. Tabassi A, et al. Serum and CSF vitamin A concentrations in idiopathic intracranial hypertension. *Neurology.* 2005;64:1893-1896.

241. Tebben P, et al. Vitamin D-mediated hypercalcemia: mechanisms, diagnosis, and treatment. *Endocr Rev.* 2016;37:521-547.

242. Thomas L, et al. Ascorbic acid supplements and kidney stone incidence among men: a prospective study. *JAMA Intern Med.* 2013;173:386-388.

243. Tjellesen L, et al. Serum concentration of vitamin D metabolites during treatment with vitamin D 2 and D 3 in normal premenopausal women. *Bone Miner.* 1986;1: 407-413.

244. Unna I. Studies of the toxicity and pharmacology of vitamin B 6 (2-methyl,3-hydroxy-4, 5- bis-pyridine). *Pharmacol Exp Ther.* 1940;70:400-407.

245. van Haaften R, et al. Inhibition of various glutathione S-transferase isoenzymes by RRR-alpha-tocopherol. *Toxicol In Vitro.* 2003;17:245-251.

246. Veugelers P, Ekwaru J. A statistical error in the estimation of the recommended dietary allowance for vitamin D. *Nutrients.* 2014;6:4472-4475.

247. Vieth R. The mechanisms of vitamin D toxicity. *Bone Miner.* 1990;11:267-272.

248. Vieth R. Vitamin D supplementation, 25-hydroxyvitamin D concentrations, and safety. *Am J Clin Nutr.* 1999;69:842-856.

249. Vutyavanich T, et al. Pyridoxine for nausea and vomiting of pregnancy: a randomized, double-blind, placebo-controlled trial. *Am J Obstet Gynecol.* 1995;173:881-884.

250. Wald G. The molecular basis of visual excitation. *Nature.* 1968;219:800-807.

251. Walta D, et al. Localized proximal esophagitis secondary to ascorbic acid ingestion and esophageal motility disorder. *Gastroenterology.* 1976;70:766-769.

252. Wandzilak T, et al. Effect of high dose vitamin C on urinary oxalate levels. *J Urol.* 1994;151:834-837.

253. Ward E. Addressing nutritional gaps with multivitamin and mineral supplements. *Nutr J.* 2014;13:72-82.

254. Warner J, et al. Retinol-binding protein and retinol analysis in cerebrospinal fluid and serum of patients with and without idiopathic intracranial hypertension. *J Neuroophthalmol.* 2007;27:258-262.

255. Weber F, et al. Reversible hepatotoxicity associated with hepatic vitamin A accumulation in a protein deficient patient. *Gastroenterology.* 1982;82:118-122.

256. Welch A. Lupus erythematosus: treatment by combined use of massive amounts of pantothenic acid and vitamin E. *Arch Dermatol Syphilol.* 1954;70:181-198.

257. West C, et al. Consequences of revised estimates of carotenoid bioefficacy for dietary control of vitamin A deficiency in developing countries. *J Nutr.* 2002;132: 2920S-2926S.

258. Whelan A, et al. The effect of aspirin on niacin-induced cutaneous reactions. *J Fam Pract.* 1992;34:165-168.

259. Wiley J, Firkin F. Reduction of pulmonary toxicity by prednisolone prophylaxis during all-transretinoic acid treatment of acute promyelocytic leukemia. *Leukemia.* 1995;9: 774-778.

260. Windhorst D, Nigra T. General clinical toxicology of oral retinoids. *J Am Acad Dermatol.* 1982;6:675-682.

261. Wisneski L. Salmon calcitonin in the acute management of hypercalcemia. *Calcif Tissue Int.* 1990;46:S26-S30.

262. Wong K, et al. Acute oxalate nephropathy after a massive intravenous dose of vitamin C. *Aust N Z J Med.* 1994;24:410-411.

263. Yusuf S, et al. Vitamin E supplementation and cardiovascular events in high-risk patients: the Heart Outcomes Prevention Evaluation Study Investigators. *N Engl J Med.* 2000;342:154-160.

264. Zempleni J, Kubler W. The utilization of intravenously infused pyridoxine in humans. *Clin Chim Acta.* 1994;229:27-36.

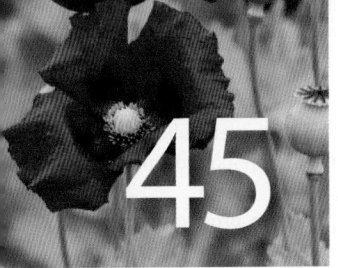

45 IRON

Jeanmarie Perrone

Iron

Molecular weight	= 55.85 Da
Serum normal concentration	= 80–180 mcg/dL
	= 14–32 μmol/L

INTRODUCTION

Iron poisoning has become uncommon. This success may underscore the importance of interventions gleaned from poison control center data and poison prevention advocacy. Blister packaging and smaller iron dosages, as well as education of parents and health care professionals have led to a great decline in iron-related morbidity. However, when significant iron poisonings do occur, clinicians must be aware of the nuances of presentation and diagnosis and be prepared to intervene if gastrointestinal (GI) toxic effects, acid–base disturbances, altered mental status, or hemodynamic compromise arise.

HISTORY AND EPIDEMIOLOGY

Iron salts such as ferrous sulfate have been used therapeutically for thousands of years and continue to be available, both with and without a prescription, for the prevention and treatment of iron deficiency anemia in patients of all ages. Despite this long history of use, the first reports of iron toxicity only occurred in the mid-20th century. Since then, numerous cases of iron poisoning and fatalities have been reported, mostly in children. In 1950, the manufacturer of "fersolate," an iron supplement, included a package warning: "Excessive doses of iron can be dangerous. Do not leave these tablets within reach of young children, who may eat them as sweets with harmful results."[78]

The incidence of iron exposures continued to increase in the 1980s, becoming the leading cause of poisoning deaths reported to poison control centers among young children in the 1990s (Chap. 130). This problem was highlighted in a case series of five toddlers with unintentional fatal exposure to prenatal vitamins containing iron.[11] The association between iron poisoning and prenatal vitamins highlights the availability of these potentially lethal medications in the homes of families with young children as an unintended consequence of more rigorous use of prenatal iron in pregnant women. A case-control study in Canada identified a fourfold increase in the risk of iron poisoning to the older sibling of a newborn during the first postpartum month.[38] The authors concluded that almost half of all hospital admissions of young children for iron poisoning could be prevented by safer storage of iron supplements in the year before and the year after the birth of a sibling.

In 1997, the Food and Drug Administration (FDA) mandated that all iron salt–containing preparations display warning labels regarding the dangers of pediatric iron poisoning. In addition to the warning labels, the FDA launched an educational campaign to alert caregivers and prescribers of the potential toxicity of iron supplements. The FDA also required unit dosing (blister packs) of prescriptions for preparations containing more than 30 mg of elemental iron and limitations on the number of pills dispensed. These efforts to prevent unintentional exposures dramatically decreased the incidence of poisoning and were pivotal in decreasing morbidity and mortality associated with iron poisoning.[73] However, in 2003, the FDA rescinded the blister packaging requirement in response to a lawsuit by the Nutritional Health Alliance charging that the FDA did not have jurisdiction over the packaging of dietary supplements.[20] Although isolated fatalities continue to occur, analysis of the Annual Reports from the National Poison Data System suggests the initial reduction in serious exposures from iron poisonings have been sustained (Chap. 130). Iron poisoning also occurs after ingestion of other iron salts used in industry, such as ferric chloride.[89]

PHARMACOLOGY, PHARMACOKINETICS, AND TOXICOKINETICS

Iron is an element critical to organ function. As a transition metal, iron readily accepts and donates electrons, shifting between the ferric (Fe^{3+}) and ferrous (Fe^{2+}) oxidation states (Chap. 10). This redox capacity illuminates the role of iron in multiple protein and enzyme complexes, including cytochromes and myoglobin, although it is principally incorporated into hemoglobin in erythrocytes. Whereas insufficient iron availability results in anemia, excess total-body iron results in hemochromatosis.

The body cannot directly excrete iron, so iron stores are regulated by controlling iron absorption from the GI tract. The absorption of iron salts (iron ions as Fe^{2+} or Fe^{3+}) occurs predominantly in the duodenum and is determined by the iron requirements of the body. In iron deficiency, iron absorption and uptake into intestinal mucosal cells increase from a normal 10% to 35% to as much as 80% to 95%. After uptake into the intestinal mucosal cells, iron is either stored as ferritin and lost when the cell is sloughed or released to transferrin, a serum iron binding protein. In therapeutic doses, some of these processes become saturated, and absorption into the intestinal cell is limited. However, in overdose, the oxidative effects of iron on GI mucosal cells lead to dysfunction of this regulatory balance, and passive absorption of iron increases down its concentration gradient (see Pathophysiology).[72] Iron ions are rapidly bound to circulating binding proteins, particularly transferrin. After transferrin is saturated with iron, "free" iron or non–transferrin-bound iron is widely distributed to the various organ systems, where it promotes damaging oxidative processes.

Iron supplements are available as the iron salts ferrous gluconate, ferrous sulfate, and ferrous fumarate and as the nonionic preparations carbonyl iron and polysaccharide iron. Additional sources of significant quantities of iron are vitamin preparations, especially prenatal vitamins (Table 45–1). Toxic effects of iron poisoning occur at doses of 10 to 20 mg/kg of elemental iron, which is defined as the amount of iron ion present in an iron salt (Table 45–1). Significant GI toxic effects occurred in human adult volunteers who ingested 10 to 20 mg/kg elemental iron.[9,47] In one volunteer study, six participants who ingested 20 mg/kg of elemental iron developed nausea and voluminous diarrhea within 2 hours, and five of the six participants had serum iron concentrations above 300 mcg/dL.[9]

In another study of human volunteers who ingested 5 to 10 mg/kg of elemental iron in the form of chewable iron-containing vitamins, peak serum iron concentrations occurred between 4.2 and 4.5 hours in all participants.[47] In overdose, peak concentrations of iron occur 2 to 6 hours after ingestion, depending on the iron preparation.[9,47] Chewable vitamins continue to entice children with their sweet taste and characteristic shapes, increasing the risk of significant exposure. Children's chewable multivitamins contain less iron per tablet (10–18 mg of elemental iron) than typical prenatal vitamins (65 mg of elemental iron). Iron toxicity still results when large quantities of chewable children's vitamins are ingested, but the therapeutic-to-toxic ratio is improved.[2] One animal study paradoxically demonstrates higher iron concentrations after ingestion of equivalent elemental iron doses of chewable versus solid iron tablets.[57] This finding was attributed, in part, to the limited gastric irritation associated with the chewable iron preparations, resulting in less vomiting.

The nonionic forms, carbonyl iron and iron polysaccharide appear to be less toxic after overdose than iron salts[69] despite their high elemental iron content.[42] Carbonyl iron is a form of elemental iron that is highly bioavailable

TABLE 45–1	Common Iron Formulations and Their Elemental Iron Content
Iron Formulation: Oral	**Elemental Iron (%)**
Ionic	
Ferrous chloride	28
Ferrous fumarate	33
Ferrous gluconate	12
Ferrous lactate	19
Ferrous sulfate	20
Nonionic[a]	
Carbonyl iron	98
Polysaccharide iron	46
Iron Formulation: Parenteral	
Ferric carboxymaltose	5
Ferric gluconate	1.25
Ferumoxytol	3
Iron dextran (low molecular weight)	5
Iron sucrose	2

[a]Although the nonionic iron formulations contain higher elemental iron content than ionic formulations, carbonyl iron and iron polysaccharide have better therapeutic-to-toxic ratios because of their limited gastrointestinal absorption rates.

in therapeutic doses compared with other forms of iron because of its very fine, spherical particle size (5 μm).[28] In a rat model of iron toxicity, carbonyl iron had a median lethal dose (LD_{50}) of 50 g/kg compared with an LD_{50} of 1.1 g/kg for ferrous sulfate.[84] No significant toxicity in humans exposed to carbonyl iron has been reported.[69] Iron polysaccharide contains approximately 46% elemental iron by weight. It is synthesized by neutralization of a ferric chloride carbohydrate solution. This form of iron also appears to have much lower toxicity than iron salts. The estimated LD_{50} in rats is more than 5 g/kg body weight. Retrospective poison control center data have failed to demonstrate significant toxicity from either of these products.[42]

Oral iron replacement is the primary treatment strategy for iron deficiency anemia; however, this may not be well tolerated or may be limited by absorption or ongoing bleeding. In contrast to oral iron, parenteral iron does significantly increase concentrations of hemoglobin, serum ferritin, and transferrin saturation. However, infusion of these iron formulations was historically associated with high rates of adverse events attributed to anaphylactoid reactions. It is postulated that early iron infusion events were related to the rapid release of large amounts of unbound iron causing severe toxicity. Subsequently, parenteral iron was complexed to high-molecular-weight dextran to stabilize and slow the release of iron and was widely administered to patients with kidney failure and chronic anemia, but measurable rates of adverse events persisted. More recently, iron combined with low-molecular-weight dextran was formulated and is a safer alternative. Newer parenteral formulations, including iron sucrose and sodium ferric gluconate, produce fewer adverse events.[19] A comparative analysis of nondialysis patients receiving intravenous (IV) iron for iron deficiency anemia further documented the highest risk of reactions in first exposures to iron dextran (including high- and low-molecular-weight formulations) and lowest with iron sucrose.[82] One case of self-poisoning by a nurse with IV iron infusion resulted in delayed hepatoxicity but no acute toxicity.[90]

PATHOPHYSIOLOGY

Iron participates in many oxidation reduction (redox) reactions. Iron catalyzes the generation of hydroxyl radicals intracellularly through the Fenton reaction and Haber-Weiss cycle and mediates its toxicologic effects as an inducer of oxidative stress and inhibitor of several key metabolic enzymes (Chap. 10). Reactive oxygen species oxidize membrane-bound lipids and cause loss of cellular integrity and tissue injury.[63,65]

The initial oxidative damage to the GI epithelium produced by iron-induced reactive oxygen species permits iron ions to enter the systemic circulation. A postmortem series of 11 patients who died from iron ingestion substantiated these findings with measurements of elevated iron concentrations in most major organs examined, including the stomach, liver, brain, heart, lung, small bowel, and kidney.[60] Congestion, edema, necrosis, and iron deposition in the gastric and intestinal mucosa, as well as hemorrhage and congestion in the lungs, are noted on postmortem examination.[32,49]

Iron ions disrupt critical cellular processes such as mitochondrial oxidative phosphorylation. Subsequent buildup of unused hydrogen ions usually incorporated into the synthesis of adenosine triphosphate leads to liberation of H⁺ and development of a metabolic acidosis (Chap. 11). In addition, absorption of iron from the GI tract leads to conversion of ferrous iron (Fe^{2+}) to ferric iron (Fe^{3+}). Ferric iron ions exceed the binding capacity of plasma, leading to formation of ferric hydroxide and release of three protons ($Fe^{3+} + 3H_2O \rightarrow Fe(OH)_3 + 3H^+$) further contributing to the acidosis.[63,72]

Decreased cardiac output contributes to shock in animals.[80,86] Although this finding is often attributed to decreased preload and relative bradycardia,[80] a direct negative inotropic effect of iron on the myocardium is also demonstrated in animal models.[3] Reports of early coagulopathy unrelated to hepatotoxicity[75] led to the identification of non–transferrin-bound iron as an inhibitor of thrombin formation and the reduction of the effect of thrombin on fibrinogen.[66]

CLINICAL MANIFESTATIONS

Classic teaching postulates five clinical stages of iron toxicity based on the pathophysiology of iron poisoning.[5,37,62] Although conceptually important, they are of limited benefit to clinicians managing poisoned patients. Although these stages are typically described in approximate postingestion time frames, a clinical stage should never be assigned based solely on the number of hours postingestion because patients do not necessarily follow the same temporal course through these stages.

The first stage of iron toxicity is characterized by nausea, vomiting, abdominal pain, and diarrhea. These "local" toxic effects of iron predominate, and subsequent salt and water depletion contribute to the ill appearance of the iron-poisoned patient. Intestinal ulceration, edema, transmural inflammation, and, in some extreme cases, small-bowel infarction and necrosis occur.[21,64] Hematemesis, melena, or hematochezia contribute to hemodynamic instability. Gastrointestinal symptoms and findings are prominent after significant overdose. Conversely, the absence of signs and symptoms, specifically vomiting, in the first 6 hours after ingestion, almost always excludes serious iron toxicity.

The second, or "latent," stage of iron poisoning commonly refers to the period 6 to 24 hours after ingestion when resolution of GI symptoms and findings occurs but overt systemic toxicity has not yet developed. Delineation of this stage likely evolved from early case reports of patients whose GI symptoms and findings had resolved before subsequent deterioration.[78] This second stage is not truly quiescent because cellular toxicity continues.[5] Although clinicians should be wary of patients who no longer have active GI complaints after iron overdose, most such patients have, in fact, recovered and are not in the latent phase. Patients in the latent phase generally have lethargy, tachycardia, or metabolic acidosis. They should be readily identifiable as clinically ill despite resolution of their GI symptoms. Patients who have remained well since ingestion and who have stable vital signs, a normal mental status, and a normal acid–base balance will have a benign clinical course.

Patients who progress to the third, or "shock," stage of iron poisoning have profound toxicity. This stage typically occurs in the first few hours after a massive (>60 mg/kg elemental iron) ingestion or as long as 12 to 24 hours after a more moderate (>40 mg/kg) ingestion. The cause of shock is likely multifactorial, resulting from one or more of these pathologic processes: hypovolemia, vasodilation, and poor cardiac output,[80,86] resulting in decreased tissue perfusion and a metabolic acidosis. Iron-induced coagulopathy worsens bleeding and hypovolemia.[75] Systemic toxicity produces central nervous system effects such as lethargy, hyperventilation, seizures, or coma. The fourth stage of iron poisoning is characterized by hepatic failure, which typically occurs 2 to 3 days after ingestion.[26] The hepatotoxicity is directly attributed to iron uptake by the reticuloendothelial system in the liver, where it causes oxidative damage.[24,88] The fifth stage of iron toxicity is rarely manifest. Gastric outlet obstruction, secondary to strictures and scarring from the initial GI injury, develops 2 to 8 weeks after ingestion.[23,31]

Patients treated for chronic iron overload are at increased risk for *Yersinia enterocolitica* infection. Iron is a required growth factor for *Y. enterocolitica*; however, the bacterium lacks the siderophore to solubilize and transport iron intracellularly. Because deferoxamine (DFO) is a siderophore, it fosters the growth of *Y. enterocolitica*. Deferoxamine may similarly facilitate growth and infection by ferrophilic organisms such as *Klebsiella* spp, *Vibrio* spp, *Aeromonas hydrophilia*, *Mucorales* spp, and other pathogens.[22,46,55,71] Thus, patients with chronic iron overload[12] or acute poisoning develop *Yersinia* infection or sepsis as a complication of iron poisoning or ironically DFO therapy.[52] *Yersinia* infection should be suspected in patients who experience abdominal pain, fever, and bloody diarrhea after resolution of iron toxicity. In this setting, cultures should be obtained, fluid and electrolyte repletion accomplished, and an appropriate antibiotic regimen initiated.

DIAGNOSTIC TESTING
Radiography
Iron is available in many forms, and the different preparations vary with respect to radiopacity on abdominal radiography.[70] Factors such as the time since ingestion and elemental iron content of the tablets are also important.[56,70] Liquid iron formulations and chewable iron tablets typically are not radiopaque.[16] A retrospective review of presumed iron ingestions in children revealed that abdominal radiographs were positive in only one of 30 patients who ingested chewable iron containing vitamin tablets.[16] Because adult tablet preparations have a higher elemental iron content and do not readily disperse, they tend to be more consistently radiopaque.[56] Finding radiopaque pills on an abdominal radiograph is helpful in guiding and evaluating the success of GI decontamination.[33] However, the absence of radiographic evidence of tablets is not a reliable indicator to exclude potential toxicity (Fig. 8–3).[56,59] Most patients with minimal symptoms should be managed without abdominal radiographs, given their lack of sensitivity. We recommend abdominal radiographs in patients with signs of severe poisoning to assess the quantity of retained tablets.

Laboratory Studies
Various laboratory studies are used as surrogate markers to assess the severity of iron poisoning. An anion gap metabolic acidosis and an elevated lactate concentration will develop in patients with serious iron ingestions. Serial blood counts and electrolyte measurements should be used to assess progression and response to volume replacement. Anemia will result from GI blood loss but may not be evident initially because of hemoconcentration secondary to plasma volume loss.

Although one small retrospective study of iron-poisoned children found that a white blood cell (WBC) count above 15,000/mm³ or a blood glucose concentration above 150 mg/dL was 100% predictive of iron concentration above 300 mcg/dL (a marker for clinical risk),[45] three subsequent similar studies were unable to validate this association.[13,44,59] In practice, an elevated WBC count or glucose concentration in the setting of a known or suspected iron ingestion should raise concern about an elevated serum iron concentration; however, assessment of the signs and symptoms of the patient is more reliable. Most important, a normal WBC count and glucose concentrations do not reliably exclude toxicity.

Although iron poisoning remains a clinical diagnosis, serum iron concentrations can be used effectively to gauge toxicity and the success of treatment.[5] In the previously mentioned human volunteer study of six adults who ingested 20 mg/kg of elemental iron, all six adults demonstrated

significant GI toxicity, and the four who required IV fluid resuscitation had peak serum iron concentrations in the range of 300 mcg/dL between 2 and 4 hours after ingestion.[9] Serum iron concentrations between 300 and 500 mcg/dL usually correlate with significant GI toxicity and modest systemic toxicity. Concentrations between 500 and 1,000 mcg/dL are associated with pronounced systemic toxicity and shock.[83] Concentrations above 1,000 mcg/dL are associated with significant morbidity and mortality.[83] Although elevated serum iron concentrations suggest the potential for significant toxicity, lower concentrations cannot be used to exclude the possibility of toxicity. A single serum iron concentration may not represent a peak concentration or may be falsely lowered by the presence of DFO interference in the colorimetric tests used routinely to measure iron. This inaccuracy in measurement can be avoided if the rarely available atomic absorption spectrometry technique is used.[25,30]

Total iron-binding capacity (TIBC) is a measurement of the total amount of iron that can be bound by transferrin in a given volume of serum.[18] Previously, clinical iron toxicity was thought not to occur if the serum iron concentration was less than the TIBC because insufficient circulating non–transferrin-bound iron was present to cause tissue damage. Although this is true, the error in interpretation results from the limitations of measuring TIBC values. Most important, the in vitro value of TIBC factitiously increases as a result of iron poisoning and thus has a tendency to apparently increase above a concurrently measured serum iron concentration.[9,77] Because of many confounding issues, the TIBC as currently determined has limited value in the assessment of iron-poisoned patients.

MANAGEMENT
Initial Approach
Following a significant ingestion, initial stabilization must include airway assessment and establishment of IV access. In the absence of coingestants, evidence of hematemesis or lethargy after an iron exposure is a manifestation of significant toxicity. Intravenous volume repletion should begin in any patient with a history of massive exposure (>60 mg/kg) or tachycardia, lethargy, or metabolic acidosis. In any lethargic patient at risk for further deterioration, early endotracheal intubation facilitates controlled GI decontamination. Abdominal radiography is recommended to estimate the iron burden in the GI tract given the caveats discussed earlier. Laboratory values, including chemistries, hemoglobin, iron concentration, coagulation, and hepatic profiles, should be obtained. An arterial or venous blood gas and a lactate concentration rapidly identify a metabolic acidosis. Patients who appear well and have had only one or two brief episodes of vomiting can be observed for 6 hours and then safely dispositioned. A serum iron concentration and most other laboratory testing are not indicated in patients who have minimal symptoms and normal vital signs.

Limiting Absorption
Gastrointestinal decontamination procedures should be initiated after stabilization. Adequate gastric emptying is critical after ingestion of xenobiotics, such as iron, that are not well adsorbed to activated charcoal. Because vomiting is a prominent early finding in patients with significant toxicity, induced emesis is not recommended. Orogastric lavage is more effective but often is of limited value because of the large size and poor solubility of most iron tablets; their ability to form adherent masses, bezoars, or concretions;[21,79] and their movement into the bowel several hours after ingestion.[39] The presence and location of radiopaque tablets on abdominal radiography can help guide early orogastric lavage in patients with suspected significant poisoning. Orogastric lavage (Antidotes in Depth: A2) will not be successful after iron tablets move past the pylorus, when WBI will be more appropriate and effective (Fig. 45–1).

Many strategies were used in the past in attempts to improve the efficacy of orogastric lavage. At the present time, no data support the use of oral DFO,[29,93,95] bicarbonate, phosphosoda, or magnesium.[72,88] Although some of these techniques demonstrate efficacy, avoidance of the associated risks mandates using only 0.9% sodium chloride solution or tap water for orogastric lavage.

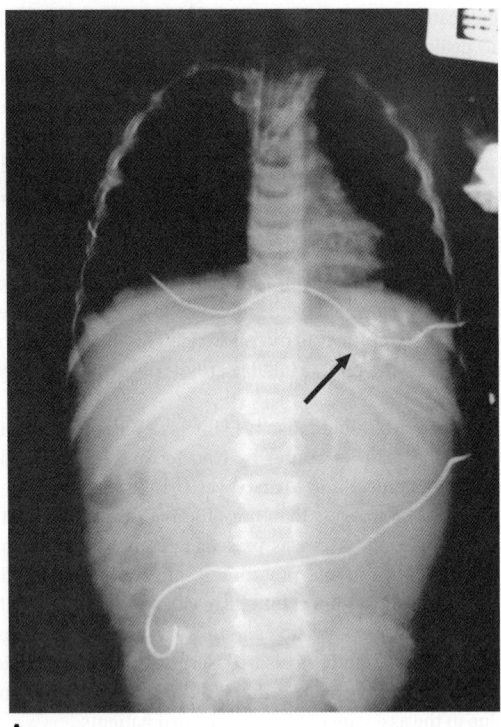 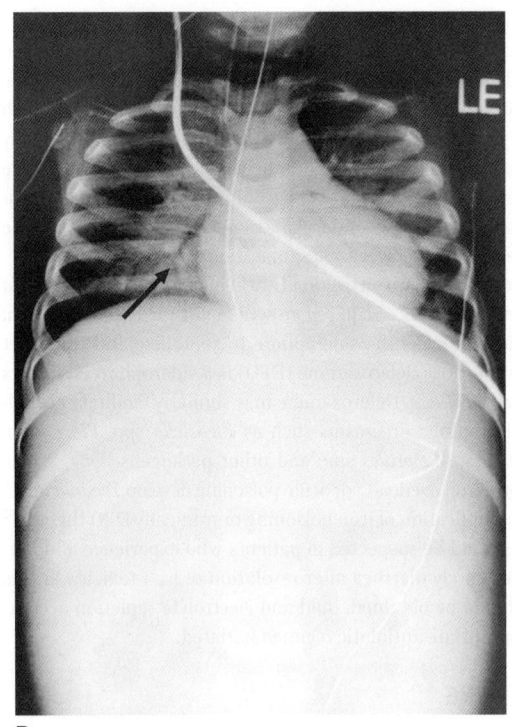

A   **B**

FIGURE 45–1. (**A**) A 17-month-old boy presented to the hospital with lethargy and hematemesis after a large ingestion of iron supplement tablets. Despite orogastric lavage and whole-bowel irrigation, iron tablets and fragments can be visualized in the stomach (➡) 4 hours after ingestion. (**B**) The same 17-month-old child 10 hours after ingestion. Persistent iron pills were removed from the stomach by gastrotomy. No further radiopaque fragments can be visualized; however, acute respiratory distress syndrome (➡) is now visible.

The value of WBI in patients with iron poisoning is supported primarily by case reports and one uncontrolled case series.[39,74] However, the rationale for WBI use is logical, especially considering the limitations of other gastric decontamination modalities. The usual dose of WBI with polyethylene glycol electrolyte lavage solution (PEG-ELS) is 500 mL/h in children and 2 L/h in adults. This rate is best achieved by starting slowly and increasing as tolerated, often using a nasogastric tube and an enteral feeding pump to administer large volumes. Antiemetics are recommended to treat nausea and vomiting. A large volume (44 L) of WBI was administered safely over a 5-day period to a child who had persistent iron tablets on serial abdominal radiographs[39] (Antidotes in Depth: A2 and Chap. 6).

For patients with life-threatening toxicity who demonstrate persistent iron in the GI tract despite orogastric lavage and WBI, it is reasonable to pursue upper endoscopy or gastrotomy and surgical removal of iron tablets adherent to the gastric mucosa.[21]

Deferoxamine

Deferoxamine has been available since the 1960s as a specific chelator for patients with acute iron overdose or chronic iron overload (eg, transfusion-dependent anemias). Deferoxamine, which is derived from culture of *Streptomyces pilosus*, has high affinity and specificity for iron. In the presence of ferric iron (Fe^{3+}), DFO forms the complex ferrioxamine, which is excreted by the kidneys,[40] usually imparting a reddish-brown color to the urine (Fig. 45–2). Deferoxamine chelates non–transferrin-bound iron and the iron transported between transferrin and ferritin[48,61] but not the iron present in transferrin, hemoglobin, or cytochromes.[4,40] Deferoxamine works by other mechanisms in addition to binding excess systemic iron. Because 100 mg of DFO chelates approximately 8.5 mg of ferric iron, recommended or typical therapeutic dosing of DFO does not produce significant excretion of chelated iron in the urine, yet it does often result in dramatic clinical benefits (Antidotes in Depth: A7). Sufficient evidence suggests that DFO can reach intracytoplasmic and mitochondrial non–transferrin-bound iron, thereby limiting intracellular iron toxicity.[48]

Deferoxamine is recommended for iron-poisoned patients with any of the following findings: repetitive vomiting, toxic appearance, lethargy,

hypotension accompanied by metabolic acidosis or signs of shock, and any patients with serum iron concentrations above 500 mcg/dL. Deferoxamine is initiated as an IV infusion, starting at 5 mg/kg/h and gradually increasing to a rate of 15 mg/kg/h. Hypotension is the rate-limiting factor as more rapid infusions are used.[34] After several hours of infusion at 15 mg/kg/h, the patient should be reassessed and the dose decreased to keep the maximum dose less than 6 to 8 g/24 hours. Patients who have concentrations below 500 mcg/dL

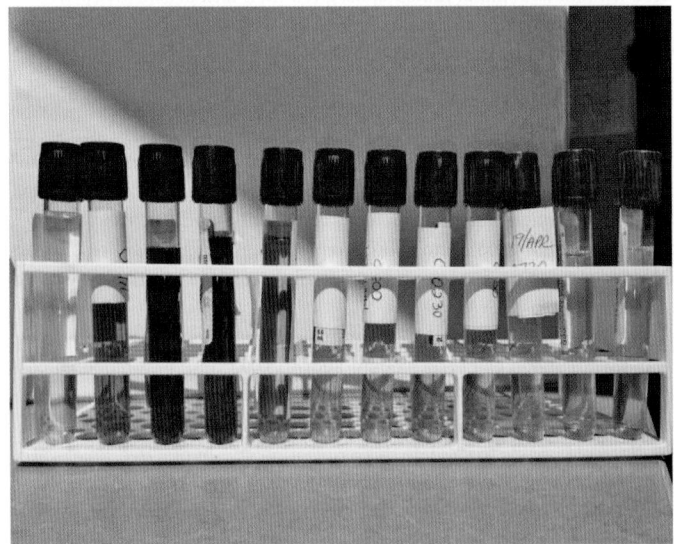

FIGURE 45–2. Sequential urine samples in a 22-year-old woman who may have ingested 180 tablets of ferrous sulfate (300 mg). She received 8 hours of deferoxamine at 15 mg/kg/h, 30 mg/kg/h for 2 hours, and then 15 mg/kg/h for 4 hours. The first serum iron concentration was 4,573 mcg/dL at 3 hours postingestion. The patient's first urine sample is on the left and then follow in sequence over a number of hours. *(Used with permission from Poison and Drug Information Service (PADIS). Alberta Health Services.)*

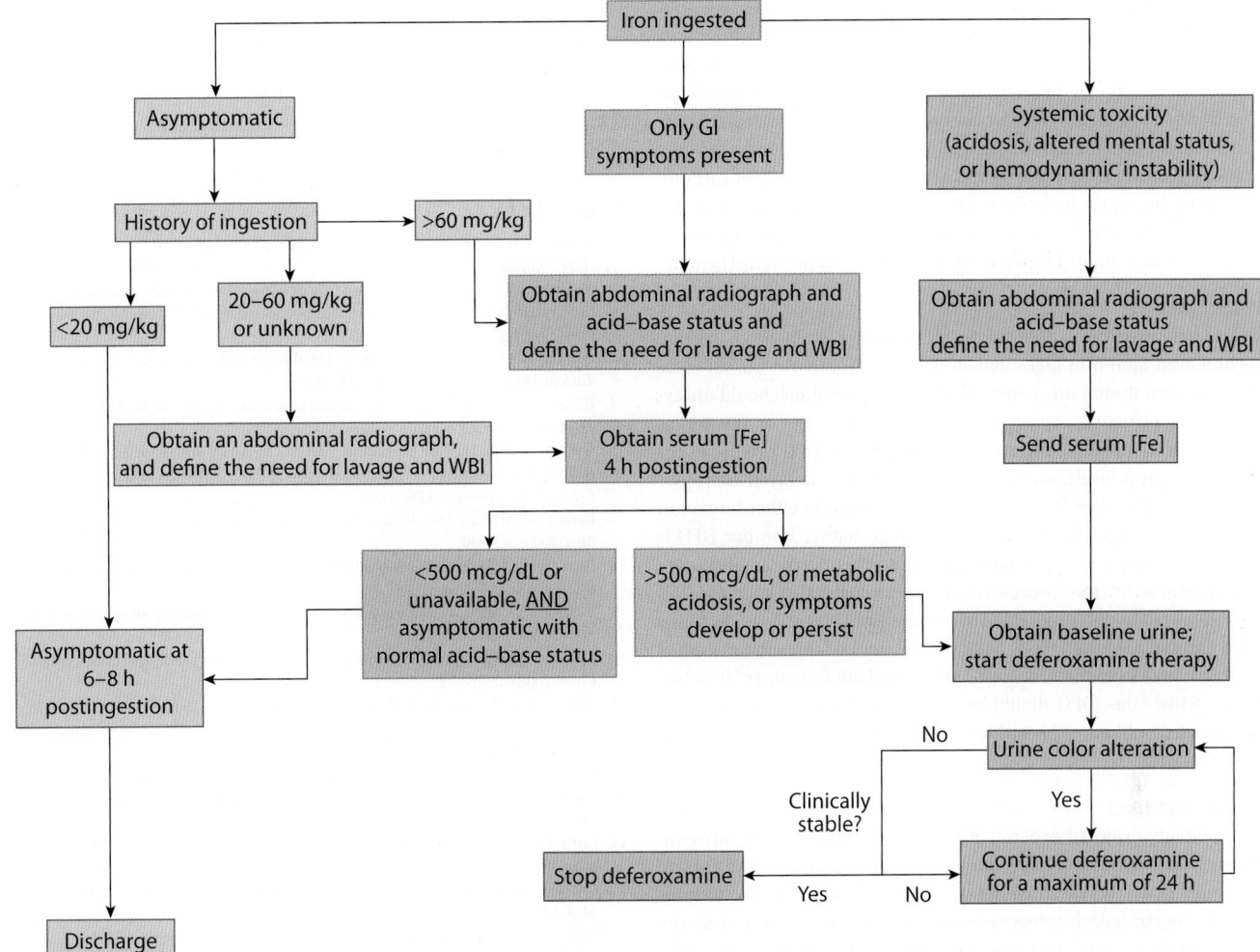

FIGURE 45–3. Algorithm for decision analysis after iron salt ingestion. GI = gastrointestinal; WBI = whole-bowel irrigation.

and who do not appear toxic should be treated supportively without administration of parenteral DFO (Fig. 45–3).

Clinicians have attempted to define the earliest clear endpoints for DFO therapy because of possible DFO toxicity. In one report, a urine iron-to-creatinine ratio (U_I/Cr) was used to determine if non–transferrin-bound iron excretion into the urine continued during DFO. This ratio is a more objective measure of the presence of ferrioxamine in the urine than the less reliable and more subjective use of urinary color change.[43,51] This method must be further studied clinically before its use can be advocated. Most authors agree that DFO therapy should be discontinued when the patient appears clinically well, the anion-gap acidosis has resolved, and urine color undergoes no further change.[53] The duration of DFO therapy should be limited to 24 hours to minimize risk of pulmonary toxicity. In patients with persistent signs and symptoms of serious toxicity after 24 hours of IV DFO, there is little evidence to define the risk or benefit for continuing DFO (Antidotes in Depth: A7).

Adverse Effects of Deferoxamine
Most adverse effects of DFO are reported in the setting of chronic administration for the treatment of hemochromatosis.[35,67] The same effects, such as acute respiratory distress syndrome (ARDS), are also described after treatment for acute iron overdose.[76] Four patients with serum iron concentrations ranging from 430 to 620 mcg/dL developed ARDS after IV administration of DFO for 32 to 72 hours.[76] An animal study revealed significantly increased pulmonary toxicity when high-dose DFO therapy was administered in the presence of high concentrations of oxygen (75%–80% FiO₂).[1] The authors suggested that this effect was mediated via an oxygen free radical mechanism (Antidotes in Depth: A7).

Experimental Therapies
Deferasirox is an oral iron chelator approved for the treatment of chronic iron overload and has been studied as a potential iron antidote in human volunteers. In a randomized, double-blind, placebo-controlled study, 5 mg/kg of iron was followed by deferasirox or placebo.[29] Deferasirox resulted in lower iron concentrations in the treated group. However, concerns included the possibility that deferasirox may increase the absorption of iron complex and that the deferasirox dosing may need to be too high in patients with large exposures to affect these results. Further study is warranted before this therapy can be recommended. Deferiprone is another oral iron chelator now approved for the treatment of refractory chronic iron overload secondary to thalassemia. Deferiprone combines with iron in a 3:1 ratio to form a stable complex that is excreted in the urine. Although deferiprone decreased the mortality rate in animal models of acute iron toxicity,[7,17] it has not yet been studied in acute iron poisoning.

Patient Disposition
Many patients who ingest iron do not develop significant toxic effects. Recommendations for hospital referral of toddlers who ingest iron range from those with potential exposures of 20 mg/kg up to 60 mg/kg.[5,43] These wide ranges probably result from the interpretation of retrospective studies in possibly "exposed" toddlers for whom the actual doses were estimated and serum values were not determined. Many authors suggest that doses were overestimated in patients who subsequently did not develop toxicity (Chap. 130). If a toddler remains asymptomatic or develops minimal or no GI manifestations after a 6-hour observation period in the emergency department, then discharge to an appropriate home situation is reasonable. Patients

who develop GI symptoms and signs of mild poisoning including vomiting and diarrhea can be observed with supportive care in an observation unit. Patients who manifest signs and symptoms of significant iron poisoning, such as metabolic acidosis, hemodynamic instability, or lethargy, should be monitored and treated in an intensive care unit. Hospital evaluation is recommended for any child with an estimated unintentional (unsupervised) ingestion of more than 20 mg/kg of elemental iron, except in the case of carbonyl iron. Children who appear well with unintentional ingestions between 10 and 20 mg/kg of elemental iron and only an isolated episode of vomiting should be closely followed at home in consultation with the poison control center.

Pregnant Patients

The use of iron to treat iron deficiency anemia during pregnancy has led to serious and even fatal iron ingestions in pregnant women.[8,41,58] In all cases of toxic exposures during pregnancy, maternal resuscitation should always be the primary objective, even if an antidote poses a real or theoretical risk to the fetus. Unproven concerns regarding possible DFO toxicity to the fetus have inappropriately, and at times, disastrously delayed therapy.[58] These fears about fetal DFO toxicity are not supported in either human or animal studies,[15,50] which have demonstrated that neither iron nor DFO is transferred to the fetus in appreciable quantities. An animal study demonstrated that fetal serum iron concentrations were not elevated and fetal DFO concentrations could not be detected in pregnant near-term ewes poisoned with iron and treated with DFO.[15] Fetal demise under these circumstances presumably results from maternal iron toxicity and not from direct iron toxicity to the fetus. Thus, DFO should be used to treat serious maternal iron poisoning and should never be withheld because of unfounded concern for fetal exposure to DFO.

Adjunctive Therapies

Another modality explored experimentally for treatment of iron intoxication is continuous arteriovenous hemofiltration (Chap. 6). In a study of five iron-poisoned dogs, increased elimination of ferrioxamine in the ultrafiltrate was demonstrated when increasing doses of DFO were infused into the arterial side of the system.[6] A variant of this approach was used successfully in an iron-poisoned toddler, who was treated with DFO and venovenous hemofiltration.[54] The authors demonstrated a decreasing serum iron concentration, and although a minimal concentration of iron was measured in the ultrafiltrate, the large volumes of dialysate used would remove significant amounts of iron. Theoretically, ferrioxamine in the blood could be dialyzable with current hemodialysis techniques (Chap. 6).

In toddlers with severe poisoning, exchange transfusion should be considered early to help physically remove all iron from the blood while replacing it with normal blood. Exchange transfusion in children is effective for poisonings such as aspirin or theophylline when the volume of xenobiotic distribution is small and removal from the blood compartment can be expected. Treatment with exchange transfusion has been suggested in iron poisoning based on early reports and in the successful treatment of an 18-month-old toddler with iron poisoning.[10] However, removal of blood volume must be performed cautiously because it can worsen hypotension in iron-poisoned patients with hemodynamic instability.

SUMMARY

- Iron is available in multiple formulations; prenatal vitamins, ferrous gluconate, ferrous fumarate, and ferrous sulfate are most toxic.
- Iron toxicity is determined by the amount of elemental iron ingested; signs and symptoms occur after ingestions of 20 mg/kg of elemental iron.
- Gastrointestinal decontamination, including orogastric lavage and WBI using PEG-ELS, are recommended when indicated because activated charcoal is ineffective in adsorbing iron.
- Abdominal radiography is recommended in determining the iron burden in the GI tract in those with large ingestions and those with symptoms. However, not all preparations are radiopaque.

- Gastrointestinal signs and symptoms of nausea, vomiting, diarrhea, hematemesis, and abdominal pain are prominent in iron poisoning.
- Systemic iron toxicity leads to metabolic acidosis, hypotension, coagulopathy, and multiorgan system failure.
- Diagnosis and treatment of shock and metabolic acidosis, as well as chelation with DFO, are critical.

REFERENCES

1. Adamson IY, et al. Pulmonary toxicity of deferoxamine in iron-poisoned mice. *Toxicol Appl Pharmacol*. 1993;120:13-19.
2. Anderson BD, et al. Retrospective analysis of ingestions of iron containing products in the United States: are there differences between chewable vitamins and adult preparations? *J Emerg Med*. 2000;19:255-258.
3. Artman M, et al. Depression of myocardial contractility in acute iron toxicity in rabbits. *Toxicol Appl Pharmacol*. 1982;66:329-337.
4. Balcerzak SP, et al. Mechanism of action of deferoxaminum on iron absorption. *Scand J Haematol*. 1966;3:205-212.
5. Banner W, Tong TG. Iron poisoning. *Pediatr Clin North Am*. 1986;33:393-409.
6. Banner W, et al. Continuous arteriovenous hemofiltration in experimental iron intoxication. *Crit Care Med*. 1989;17:1187-1190.
7. Berkovitch M, et al. The efficacy of oral deferiprone in acute iron poisoning. *Am J Emerg Med*. 2000;18:36-40.
8. Blanc P, et al. Deferoxamine treatment of acute iron intoxication in pregnancy. *Obstet Gynecol*. 1984;64(3 suppl):12S-14S.
9. Burkhart KK, et al. The rise in the total iron-binding capacity after iron overdose. *Ann Emerg Med*. 1991;20:532-535.
10. Carlsson M, et al. Severe iron intoxication treated with exchange transfusion. *Arch Dis Child*. 2008;93:321-322.
11. Centers for Disease Control and Prevention (CDC). Toddler deaths resulting from ingestion of iron supplements—Los Angeles, 1992-1993. *MMWR Morb Mortal Wkly Rep*. 1993;42:111-113.
12. Chiesa C, et al. Yersinia hepatic abscesses and iron overload. *JAMA*. 1987;257: 3230-3231.
13. Chyka PA, Butler AY. Assessment of acute iron poisoning by laboratory and clinical observations. *Am J Emerg Med*. 1993;11:99-103.
14. Corby DG, et al. Effect of orally administered magnesium hydroxide in experimental iron intoxication. *J Toxicol Clin Toxicol*. 23:489-499.
15. Curry SC, et al. An ovine model of maternal iron poisoning in pregnancy. *Ann Emerg Med*. 1990;19:632-638.
16. Everson GW, et al. Effectiveness of abdominal radiographs in visualizing chewable iron supplements following overdose. *Am J Emerg Med*. 1989;7:459-463.
17. Fassos FF, et al. Efficacy of deferiprone in the treatment of acute iron intoxication in rats. *J Toxicol Clin Toxicol*. 1996;34:279-287.
18. Finch CA, Huebers H. Perspectives in iron metabolism. *N Engl J Med*. 1982;306:1520-1528.
19. Fishbane S. Safety in iron management. *Am J Kidney Dis*. 2003;41(5 suppl):18-26.
20. Food and Drug Administration. Iron-containing supplements and drugs; label warning statements and unit-dose packaging requirements; removal of regulations for unit-dose packaging requirements for dietary supplements and drugs. Final rule; removal of regulatory provisions in response to court order. *Fed Regist*. 2003;68:59714-59715.
21. Foxford R, Goldfrank L. Gastrotomy—a surgical approach to iron overdose. *Ann Emerg Med*. 1985;14:1223-1226.
22. Fukushima T, et al. Direct evidence of iron uptake by the Gram-positive siderophore-shuttle mechanism without iron reduction. *ACS Chem Biol*. 2014;9:2092-2100.
23. Gandi RK, Robarts FH. Hour-glass stricture of the stomach and pyloric stenosis due to ferrous sulphate poisoning. *Br J Surg*. 1962;49:613-617.
24. Ganote CE, Nahara G. Acute ferrous sulfate hepatotoxicity in rats. An electron microscopic and biochemical study. *Lab Invest*. 1973;28:426-436.
25. Gevirtz NR, Wasserman LR. The measurement of iron and iron-binding capacity in plasma containing deferoxamine. *J Pediatr*. 1966;68:802-804.
26. Gleason WA, et al. Acute hepatic failure in severe iron poisoning. *J Pediatr*. 1979;95: 138-140.
27. Gomez HF, et al. Prevention of gastrointestinal iron absorption by chelation from an orally administered premixed deferoxamine/charcoal slurry. *Ann Emerg Med*. 1997;30: 587-592.
28. Gordeuk VR, et al. Carbonyl iron therapy for iron deficiency anemia. *Blood*. 1986;67: 745-752.
29. Griffith EA, et al. Effect of deferasirox on iron absorption in a randomized, placebo-controlled, crossover study in a human model of acute supratherapeutic iron ingestion. *Ann Emerg Med*. 58:69-73.
30. Helfer RE, Rodgerson DO. The effect of deferoxamine on the determination of serum iron and iron-binding capacity. *J Pediatr*. 1966;68:804-806.
31. Henretig FM, et al. Severe iron poisoning treated with enteral and intravenous deferoxamine. *Ann Emerg Med*. 1983;12:306-309.
32. Hoppe JO, et al. A review of the toxicity of iron compounds. *Am J Med Sci*. 1955;230: 558-571.
33. Hosking CS. Radiology in the management of acute iron poisoning. *Med J Aust*. 1969; 1:576-579.

34. Howland MA. Risks of parenteral deferoxamine for acute iron poisoning. *J Toxicol Clin Toxicol*. 1996;34:491-497.

35. Ioannides AS, Panisello JM. Acute respiratory distress syndrome in children with acute iron poisoning: the role of intravenous desferrioxamine. *Eur J Pediatr*. 2000;159:158-159.

36. Jackson TW, et al. The effect of oral deferoxamine on iron absorption in humans. *J Toxicol Clin Toxicol*. 1995;33:325-329.

37. Jagobs J, et al. Acute Iron Intoxication. *N Engl J Med*. 1965;273:1124-1127.

38. Juurlink DN, et al. Iron poisoning in young children: association with the birth of a sibling. *CMAJ*. 2003;168:1539-1542.

39. Kaczorowski JM, Wax PM. Five days of whole-bowel irrigation in a case of pediatric iron ingestion. *Ann Emerg Med*. 1996;27:258-263.

40. Keberle H. The biochemistry of desferrioxamine and its relation to iron metabolism. *Ann N Y Acad Sci*. 1964;119:758-768.

41. Khoury S, et al. Deferoxamine treatment for acute iron intoxication in pregnancy. *Acta Obstet Gynecol Scand*. 1995;74:756-757.

42. Klein-Schwartz W. Toxicity of polysaccharide—iron complex exposures reported to poison control centers. *Ann Pharmacother*. 2000;34:165-169.

43. Klein-Schwartz W, et al. Assessment of management guidelines. Acute iron ingestion. *Clin Pediatr (Phila)*. 1990;29:316-321.

44. Knasel AL, Collins-Barrow MD. Applicability of early indicators of iron toxicity. *J Natl Med Assoc*. 1986;78:1037-1040.

45. Lacouture PG, et al. Emergency assessment of severity in iron overdose by clinical and laboratory methods. *J Pediatr*. 1981;99:89-91.

46. Lin SH, et al. Fatal *Aeromonas hydrophila* bacteremia in a hemodialysis patient treated with deferoxamine. *Am J Kidney Dis*. 1996;27:733-735.

47. Ling LJ, et al. Absorption of iron after experimental overdose of chewable vitamins. *Am J Emerg Med*. 1991;9:24-26.

48. Lipschitz DA, et al. The site of action of desferrioxamine. *Br J Haematol*. 1971;20:395-404.

49. Luongo MA, Bjornson SS. The liver in ferrous sulfate poisoning; a report of three fatal cases in children and an experimental study. *N Engl J Med*. 1954;251:995-999.

50. McElhatton PR, et al. The consequences of iron overdose and its treatment with desferrioxamine in pregnancy. *Hum Exp Toxicol*. 1991;10:251-259.

51. McGuigan MA, et al. Qualitative deferoxamine color test for iron ingestion. *J Pediatr*. 1979;94:940-942.

52. Melby K, et al. Septicaemia due to *Yersinia* enterocolitica after oral overdoses of iron. *Br Med J (Clin Res Ed)*. 1982;285:467-468.

53. Mills KC, Curry SC. Acute iron poisoning. *Emerg Med Clin North Am*. 1994;12:397-413.

54. Milne C, Petros A. The use of haemofiltration for severe iron overdose. *Arch Dis Child*. 2010;95:482-483.

55. Neupane GP, Kim D-M. Comparison of the effects of deferasirox, deferiprone, and deferoxamine on the growth and virulence of *Vibrio vulnificus*. *Transfusion*. 2009;49:1762-1769.

56. Ng RC, et al. Iron poisoning: assessment of radiography in diagnosis and management. *Clin Pediatr (Phila)*. 1979;18:614-616.

57. Nordt SP, et al. Comparison of the toxicities of two iron formulations in a swine model. *Acad Emerg Med*. 1999;6:1104-1108.

58. Olenmark M, et al. Fatal iron intoxication in late pregnancy. *J Toxicol Clin Toxicol*. 1987;25:347-359.

59. Palatnick W, Tenenbein M. Leukocytosis, hyperglycemia, vomiting, and positive X-rays are not indicators of severity of iron overdose in adults. *Am J Emerg Med*. 1996;14:454-455.

60. Pestaner JP, et al. Ferrous sulfate toxicity a review of autopsy findings. *Biol Trace Elem Res*. 1999;69:191-198.

61. Propper R, Nathan D. Clinical removal of iron. *Annu Rev Med*. 1982;33:509-519.

62. Proudfoot AT, et al. Management of acute iron poisoning. *Med Toxicol*. 1986;1:83-100.

63. Reissmann KR, Coleman TJ. Acute intestinal iron intoxication II. Metabolic, respiratory and circulatory effects of absorbed iron salts. *Blood*. 1955;10:46-51.

64. Roberts RJ, et al. Acute iron intoxication with intestinal infarction managed in part by small bowel resection. *Clin Toxicol*. 1975;8:3-12.

65. Robotham JL, et al. Letter: iron poisoning: another energy crisis. *Lancet (London, England)*. 1974;2:664-665.

66. Rosenmund A, et al. Blood coagulation and acute iron toxicity. Reversible iron-induced inactivation of serine proteases in vitro. *J Lab Clin Med*. 1984;103:524-533.

67. Scanderbeg A, et al. Pulmonary syndrome and intravenous high-dose desferrioxamine. *Lancet*. 1990;336:1511.

68. Snyder BK, Clark RF. Effect of magnesium hydroxide administration on iron absorption after a supratherapeutic dose of ferrous sulfate in human volunteers: a randomized controlled trial. *Ann Emerg Med*. 1999;33:400-405.

69. Spiller HA, et al. Multi-center retrospective evaluation of carbonyl iron ingestions. *Vet Hum Toxicol*. 2002;44:28-29.

70. Staple TW, McAlister WH. Roentgenographic visualization of iron preparations in the gastrointestinal trace. *Radiology*. 1964;83:1051-1056.

71. Stintzi A, et al. Microbial iron transport via a siderophore shuttle: a membrane ion transport paradigm. *Proc Natl Acad Sci U S A*. 2000;97:10691-10696.

72. Tenenbein M. Toxicokinetics and toxicodynamics of iron poisoning. *Toxicol Lett*. 1998;102-103:653-656.

73. Tenenbein M. Unit-dose packaging of iron supplements and reduction of iron poisoning in young children. *Arch Pediatr Adolesc Med*. 2005;159:557-560.

74. Tenenbein M. Whole bowel irrigation in iron poisoning. *J Pediatr*. 1987;111:142-145.

75. Tenenbein M, Israels SJ. Early coagulopathy in severe iron poisoning. *J Pediatr*. 1988;113:695-697.

76. Tenenbein M, et al. Pulmonary toxic effects of continuous desferrioxamine administration in acute iron poisoning. *Lancet*. 1992;339:699-701.

77. Tenenbein M, Yatscoff RW. The total iron-binding capacity in iron poisoning. Is it useful? *Am J Dis Child*. 1991;145:437-439.

78. Thomson J. Ferrous sulphate poisoning. *Br Med J*. 1950;1:645-646.

79. Venturelli J, et al. Gastrotomy in the management of acute iron poisoning. *J Pediatr*. 1982;100:768-769.

80. Vernon DD, et al. Hemodynamic effects of experimental iron poisoning. *Ann Emerg Med*. 1989;18:863-866.

81. Wallace KL, et al. Effect of magnesium hydroxide on iron absorption following simulated mild iron overdose in human subjects. *Acad Emerg Med*. 1998;5:961-965.

82. Wang C, et al. Comparative risk of anaphylactic reactions associated with intravenous iron products. *J Am Med Assoc*. 2015;314:2062-2067.

83. Westlin WF. Deferoxamine as a chelating agent. *Clin Toxicol*. 1971;4:597-602.

84. Whittaker P, et al. Acute toxicity of carbonyl iron and sodium iron EDTA compared with ferrous sulfate in young rats. *Regul Toxicol Pharmacol*. 2002;36:280-286.

85. Whitten CF, et al. Studies in acute iron poisoning. II. Further observations on desferrioxamine in the treatment of acute experimental iron poisoning. *Pediatrics*. 1966;38:102-110.

86. Whitten CF, et al. Studies in acute iron poisoning III. The hemodynamic alterations in acute experimental iron poisoning. *Pediatr Res*. 1968;2:479-485.

87. Whitten CF, et al. Studies in acute iron poisoning. I. Desferrioxamine in the treatment of acute iron poisoning: clinical observations, experimental studies, and theoretical considerations. *Pediatrics*. 1965;36:322-335.

88. Witzleben CL, Chaffey NJ. Acute ferrous sulfate poisoning. A histochemical study of its effect on the liver. *Arch Pathol*. 1966;82:454-461.

89. Wu ML, et al. A fatal case of acute ferric chloride poisoning. *Vet Hum Toxicol*. 1998;40:31-34.

90. Yassin M, et al. A young adult with unintended acute intravenous iron intoxication treated with oral chelation: the use of liver FerriScan for diagnosing and monitoring tissue iron load. *Mediterr J Hematol Infect Dis*. 2017;9:e2017008.

DEFEROXAMINE

Mary Ann Howland

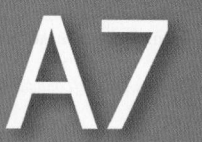

INTRODUCTION

Deferoxamine (DFO) is the parenteral chelator of choice for treatment of acute iron poisoning. Even though DFO has been used to treat patients with acute iron overdose for more than 60 years,[35] there is still much that is unknown. No controlled studies have evaluated the efficacy or dosing of DFO. Animal studies and case series from the 1960s and 1970s form the basis for current use of DFO. This information has been supplemented by case reports and clinical experience. Deferoxamine is also used for chelation of aluminum in patients with chronic kidney failure. The merits of DFO as a treatment strategy for acute iron overdose are discussed in Chap. 45 and for aluminum toxicity in Chap. 84.

HISTORY

The development of DFO (or desferrioxamine B) resulted from an analysis of the iron-containing metabolites of a species of *Actinomycetes*. Ferrioxamine is a brownish-red compound containing trivalent iron (ferric, Fe^{3+}) and three molecules of trihydroxamic acid isolated from the organism *Streptomyces pilosus*.[40] Deferoxamine is the colorless compound that results when the trivalent iron is chemically removed from ferrioxamine B (Fig. A7–1).[40]

PHARMACOLOGY

Chemistry

Deferoxamine is a water-soluble hexadentate chelator with a molecular weight of 561 Da. The commercial formulation is the mesylate salt with a

FIGURE A7–1. Ferrioxamine.

molecular weight of 657 Da. One mole of DFO binds 1 mole of Fe^{3+}; therefore, 100 mg DFO as the mesylate salt theoretically can bind 8.5 mg Fe^{3+}.

Deferoxamine has a much greater affinity constant for iron (10^{31}) and aluminum (10^{22}) than for zinc, copper, nickel, magnesium, or calcium (10^2–10^{14}).[40] Thus, at physiologic pH, DFO complexes almost exclusively with ferric iron.[30,91]

Related Chelators

Deferiprone, a bidentate oral iron chelator with a molecular weight of 139 Da, was approved by the US Food and Drug Administration (FDA) in 2011 for the treatment of iron overload in patients with thalassemia major in whom current treatment is inadequate.[26] Three moles of deferiprone are required to bind 1 mole of ferric ion to form a stable complex, which is excreted in the urine.[34] Inappropriate ratios of drug to iron are ineffective or even harmful because of the formation of potentially toxic intermediates.[34] Preliminary animal studies of the use of deferiprone in acute iron toxicity are contradictory.[10,25,38,41] A dose of 75 mg/kg deferiprone produces 60% of the total iron excretion that can be achieved with 50 mg/kg of DFO. All of the iron eliminated with deferiprone occurs in the urine, but DFO eliminates iron in the urine and feces.[45] In contrast to DFO, deferiprone is able to remove iron from transferrin and is often able to maintain normal iron stores in patients with chronic iron overload syndromes. Toxicity appears minimal, although some patients were required to stop deferiprone therapy to avoid iron deficiency. Adverse events include elevation of hepatic enzymes, gastrointestinal (GI) effects, arthralgia, and chromaturia. Because of embryofetal toxicity in animal studies, deferiprone is given an FDA pregnancy category D; DFO carries a boxed warning for neutropenia and agranulocytosis.[26] Deferiprone is now being combined with DFO because studies demonstrate additive or synergistic effects in chronic iron overload syndromes. It is hypothesized that deferiprone, because of its smaller size, can enter and chelate cardiac iron and then transfer it to DFO for elimination.[23,44,45,87]

Deferasirox, an oral iron chelator that was FDA approved in 2005, is indicated to treat chronic iron overload caused by blood transfusions or in patients with thalassemia major and elevated liver iron concentrations. Deferasirox, a tridentate ligand with a molecular weight of 373 Da, binds ferric iron in a 2:1 ratio. Deferasirox is lipid soluble with high protein binding (~99%). When bound to iron, the complex is predominantly eliminated in the feces. The serum half-life (19 ± 6.5 hours) is considerably longer than those of DFO and deferiprone (47–137 minutes). Preliminary studies demonstrate a comparable efficacy to DFO in patients with chronic iron overload.[86] One study using deferasirox in a human model of a modest supraphysiologic iron ingestion (only 5 mg/kg) demonstrated a reduction in serum iron concentrations when compared with placebo.[31] Concerns about achieving the effective dose ratio of deferasirox to iron of 2:1 and the effects of acidemia on the binding of deferasirox to iron in a large overdose limit its use.[60] In addition, similar to other oral chelators, concerns exist about increasing oral absorption of the deferasirox iron complex and the toxicity of this complex in an acute iron overdose.[24,69,78] Adverse events include boxed warnings for GI hemorrhage, kidney failure, and hepatic failure. Advanced age increases these risks.[24]

Mechanism of Action

Deferoxamine binds Fe^{3+} at the 3 N–OH sites, forming an octahedral iron complex (Fig. A7–1). When bound, the resultant ferrioxamine is very stable.

Deferoxamine benefits iron-poisoned patients by chelating non–transferrin-bound iron (previously referred to as "free iron"), iron in transit between transferrin and ferritin (labile chelatable iron pool),[4,34,49,71] and hemosiderin and ferritin while not directly affecting the iron of transferrin, hemoglobin, and cytochromes.[21,40] Although the binding affinity of DFO for iron is greater than the binding affinity of transferrin for iron, the slow pharmacokinetics of DFO prevent appreciable iron removal from transferrin. Deferoxamine binds non–transferrin-bound iron found in the plasma after transferrin saturation, which occurs acutely after an overdose or chronically in iron overload syndromes.[34] In vitro studies demonstrate that DFO chelates and inactivates cytoplasmic, lysosomal, and probably mitochondrial iron, preventing disruption of mitochondrial function and injury.[29,49] An in vitro study suggests that DFO gains access to cytosol and endosomes through endocytosis rather than passive diffusion.[29] In chronic iron overload, DFO slows the amount of iron that accumulates in the liver that would result in hepatic fibrosis.[21]

Pharmacokinetics and Pharmacodynamics

The volume of distribution of DFO ranges from 0.6 to 1.33 L/kg.[40,46,63] Because DFO is water soluble, entry into most cells is limited except for hepatocytes, in which facilitated uptake occurs.[67–69] The initial distribution half-life of DFO is 5 to 10 minutes.[43,77] The terminal elimination half-life of DFO is approximately 6 hours in healthy patients[2] but is approximately 3 hours in patients with thalassemia major. Deferoxamine is metabolized in the plasma to several metabolites (A-F), of which metabolite B is believed to be toxic.[40,46,63,65] Unchanged DFO undergoes glomerular filtration and tubular secretion.[53]

By comparison, ferrioxamine has a smaller volume of distribution than DFO. In nephrectomized dogs, the volume of distribution of ferrioxamine was calculated to be 19% of body weight compared with 50% of body weight for DFO.[40] This finding implies that DFO has a more extensive tissue distribution. The different pharmacokinetic characteristics are related to the potential for facilitated penetrance of the straight-chain molecule DFO compared with that of the octahedral ferrioxamine.[65] Experiments in dogs with normal kidney function demonstrate that intravenous (IV) ferrioxamine is entirely eliminated by the kidney within 5 hours via glomerular filtration and partial reabsorption.[38,53]

The pharmacokinetics of DFO and ferrioxamine differ in healthy compared with iron-overloaded patients. Whereas serum DFO concentrations in healthy patients are approximately twice the concentrations noted in patients with thalassemia major, ferrioxamine concentrations are five times greater in patients with thalassemia major compared with healthy patients.[40,79] The elimination of DFO occurs mostly by poorly identified plasma enzymes and to a lesser extent by biliary excretion into the feces.[21]

Deferoxamine is hemodialyzable. Deferoxamine can be administered during hemodialysis to remove ferrioxamine.[92] Hemodialysis,[15,77] particularly high-flux hemodialysis[84] and hemoperfusion,[15] are effective in ferrioxamine removal and are indicated in the treatment of patients with kidney failure. In one reported case, a child with a serum iron concentration of 3,906 mcg/dL received IV DFO at 15 mg/kg/h and underwent continuous venovenous hemofiltration; an iron concentration of 19 mcg/dL was eliminated in the dialysate fluid and 3,246 mcg/dL in the urine.[54]

ROLE IN IRON TOXICITY

Because of the limited amount of iron that can be chelated by DFO, aggressive GI decontamination and supportive measures should accompany its use in iron overdose, as discussed in Chap. 45.

Animal Studies

Guinea pigs given oral lethal doses of ferrous sulfate and oral DFO in a dose calculated to bind most of the iron showed dramatically improved survival rates.[55] Mortality rates in this study and in a swine study[20] were directly correlated with the delay to DFO administration.[55]

In two canine studies, dogs that received the iron–DFO complex orally had a 40% to 100% mortality rate.[91,92] When both oral and IV DFO were administered, the mortality rate was 67%.[90] A similar follow-up study demonstrated a 50% mortality rate in dogs given a lethal dose (225 mg/kg) of iron followed

by oral DFO (2.6 g) and IV DFO (0.75-1.5 mg/kg/min for 8-12 hours).[92] These studies discouraged further investigation in the use of oral DFO despite the more favorable results in other animal models.[5,36,55,83]

Early Human Use and History of Dosing Recommendations

In one of the earliest case series, 172 hemodynamically stable children who were not severely poisoned were treated with 5 to 10 g oral DFO and either 1 or 2 g intramuscular (IM) DFO every 3 to 12 hours.[90] Patients who were in shock or severely ill received 1 g of DFO IV at a maximum of 15 mg/kg/h every 4 to 12 hours for 2 to 3 days as necessary. Of the 28 patients who developed coma, shock, or both, three died. One of the three patients who died received late treatment with DFO.

This case series was expanded to 472 patients, and guidelines for DFO dosing were formulated as a result of this clinical experience.[89] The recommended initial dose of DFO was suggested as 1 g IM followed by 0.5 g at 4 and 8 hours later and then every 4 to 12 hours as necessary, not to exceed 6 g in 24 hours. For patients in shock, DFO was recommended at an initial dose not to exceed 1 g IV and a rate not to exceed 15 mg/kg/h followed 4 and 8 hours later by two 0.5-g doses for a total dosage not to exceed 6 g in 24 hours. These recommendations for total dosages were not scientifically developed and appear to be based on arbitrary assumptions. However, the manufacturer continues to recommend these doses.[21]

Intramuscular versus Intravenous Administration

Before 1976, IM DFO was the preferred route of administration, and IV DFO was reserved for patients in shock. However, when transfusion-induced iron overload was studied and IM and IV DFO administration were compared, IV DFO significantly enhanced urinary iron elimination.[72] This study provided compelling arguments against IM dosing, as did data showing higher peak and more stable DFO concentrations with IV infusions. A single patient was given 425 mg/kg IV over 24 hours without incident, although the increase in urinary iron excretion that occurred when the DFO dosage increased from 4 to 16 g/day appeared to be of limited benefit.

Duration of Dosing

The optimum duration of DFO administration is unknown. In canine models, serum iron concentrations peak within 3 to 5 hours and then decrease quickly as iron is transported out of the blood into the tissues.[85,93] In one human study, initial iron concentrations of approximately 500 mcg/dL decreased to approximately 100 mcg/dL within 12 hours.[47] Other case reports also suggest that most of the easily accessible iron is distributed out of the blood compartment within 24 hours.[22] Although severely poisoned patients have received DFO for more than 24 hours, pulmonary toxicity is associated with prolonged DFO infusions.[33,61,81] Intuitively, in patients with acute iron overdose, DFO should be administered early and for a shorter duration while the iron is easily accessible in the blood. In patients with chronic iron overload, prolonged infusions of smaller DFO doses will act as a sink and slowly remove iron from the limited labile pool and tissue stores.[37]

ROLE IN ALUMINUM TOXICITY

Patients with severe chronic kidney disease are at high risk for aluminum toxicity.[95] Acute aluminum toxicity resulting from bladder irrigations with alum for hemorrhagic cystitis is also reported.[64] Chronic aluminum toxicity is reported from the administration of aluminum salts as phosphate binders or from hemodialysis with a water source containing aluminum. Deferoxamine binds aluminum to form aluminoxamine, analogous to iron and ferrioxamine. The chelate is a 1:1 octahedral complex with aluminum.[95] Aluminoxamine is renally excreted. In patients with kidney insufficiency, hemodialysis (especially with a high-flux membrane) is effective in removing the aluminoxamine and should be used to prevent aluminum redistribution to the central nervous system (CNS) and other tissues.[57] The dosing of DFO is unclear but should be tailored to the patient's serum aluminum concentrations, symptoms, hemodialysis schedule, and response.[57] Periodic electroencephalographic monitoring is recommended. Deferoxamine dosages of 5 to 15 mg/kg/day, infused over several hours and 6 to 8 hours before a 3- to 4-hour run of high-flux hemodialysis, have been successful and maximize aluminoxamine removal without exacerbating adverse events.[57,74] The appropriate duration of this DFO dosing with hemodialysis is unknown and should be based on CNS symptoms, serum aluminum concentrations, and kidney function. The correlation of serum aluminum concentrations with toxicity is poorly defined and depends on the chronicity of aluminum exposure. Patients are treated with variable degrees of toxicity for several sessions infrequently (Chap. 84). The package insert states that dialysis patients with aluminum-associated encephalopathy who are treated with DFO may develop worsening neurologic function, dialysis dementia, or hypocalcemia with worsening hyperparathyroidism, but the standard treatment remains DFO with hemodialysis.[21,57]

ADVERSE EFFECTS

Deferoxamine administration to patients with acute iron overdose causes rate-related hypotension and systemic hypersensitivity reactions, pulmonary toxicity, and infection, as well as injection site reactions. Deferoxamine administration to patients with chronic iron overload causes auditory, ophthalmic, kidney and pulmonary toxicity, and infections.[9,13,37]

Significant hypotension was first noted in 1965 in two children who were administered approximately 80 to 150 mg/kg DFO IV over 15 minutes.[91] The mechanism for rate-related hypotension is not fully understood, although histamine release is at least partially implicated. Although elevated histamine concentrations were documented in a canine experiment, pretreatment with diphenhydramine was not protective.[92] Intravascular volume depletion caused by iron toxicity also contributes to hypotension. No experiment has determined the maximum safe rate of DFO administration. Adverse events of DFO, including tachycardia, hypotension, and shock, were reported with rapid infusion.[90] These complications resulted in the current recommendations for less rapid IV infusions of DFO not to exceed 15 mg/kg/h.[90-92] Currently suggested IV infusion rates are somewhat empirical because of the lack of robust evidence. Higher rates were administered successfully in critically ill patients when time was of the essence.[11,16,22]

Acute respiratory distress syndrome (ARDS) occurs in patients with acute iron overdoses who have received IV administration of DFO (15 mg/kg/h) therapy for more than 24 hours.[3,39,81] Usually, iron concentrations are normal in these patients within 24 hours, and the rationale for continued administration of DFO in these cases was not reported. Examination of the nontoxicologic literature reveals other instances of ARDS occurring in patients receiving continuous IV DFO for hemosiderosis and malignancies.[14,27,88] Administration of continuous IV doses of DFO for prolonged periods (>24 hours) was common to all of these patients. The mechanism for development of pulmonary toxicity after DFO is unknown. Pulmonary toxicity is theorized to result from excessive DFO chelation of intracellular iron and depletion of catalase, resulting in oxidant damage,[32] or generation of free radicals.[1]

Deferoxamine therapy rarely leads to infection with a number of organisms, including *Yersinia enterocolitica*, *Zygomycetes* spp, and *Aeromonas hydrophilia*. The virulence of these organisms is facilitated when the DFO–iron complex acts as a siderophore for their growth.[48,52,56] Most cases of septicemia occurred when DFO was used for treatment of aluminum toxicity in patients receiving chronic hemodialysis.[53] Several cases of *Yersinia* sepsis were reported after acute iron overdose and treatment with DFO.[52,56]

Ophthalmic toxicity characterized by decreased visual acuity and peripheral visual field deficits, night blindness, color blindness, and retinal pigmentary abnormalities has occurred in patients who received continuous IV DFO for thalassemia major and other nonacute iron and aluminum excess conditions.[8,12,19,59,62] Ototoxicity documented by audiograms indicated partial or total deafness.[65,66] However, neither ophthalmic toxicity nor ototoxicity is reported in the treatment of acute iron overdose treatment. When DFO is used in the absence of iron overload, zinc deficiency and decreases in serum ferritin, mean corpuscular volume, and hemoglobin develop.[42]

Infusion pump malfunctions have occasionally led to acute kidney injury (AKI) caused by IV DFO overdose. This overdose was successfully treated

with hemodialysis after failure of medical management.[17] One inadvertent overdose of IV DFO in a patient with severe iron overload associated with sickle cell β-thalassemia resulted in AKI within 12 to 18 hours. The patient received a planned 45 g (700 mg/kg) 96-hour infusion over 8 hours because of incorrect programming of the infusion pump. High-efficiency hemodialysis instituted after an 8-hour trial of IV hydration and mannitol was unsuccessful in restoring kidney function.[70]

PREGNANCY AND LACTATION

One literature review identified 61 cases of intentional iron overdose in pregnant women.[82] Serious iron toxicity with organ involvement was associated with spontaneous abortion, preterm delivery, and maternal death. There is no evidence to indicate that DFO is teratogenic.[82] Neither iron nor DFO appears to cross the ovine placenta.[18] A case report of a pregnant woman with thalassemia major and a review of 40 other pregnant patients with thalassemia treated extensively with DFO found no evidence of teratogenicity.[75] Thus, DFO should be administered to pregnant women with acute iron toxicity for the same indications as for nonpregnant women and is listed as FDA pregnancy category C. Excretion in breast milk is unknown.

DOSING AND ADMINISTRATION

The indications and dosage schedules for DFO administration are largely empirical.[6,73] Systemic toxicity associated with acute iron poisoning manifested by coma, shock, or metabolic acidosis warrants IV infusion of DFO. The duration of therapy should be limited to 24 hours to maximize effectiveness while minimizing the risk of pulmonary toxicity. Some investigators have suggested that more than the recommended dose of 15 mg/kg/h be infused during the first 24 hours for life-threatening iron toxicity, but this recommendation remains to be validated.[37] We recommend starting with 5 mg/kg/h and increasing after 15 minutes, if tolerated, to 15 mg/kg/h to minimize the risk of hypotension. In adults, after the first 1,000 mg is infused, the subsequent doses can be adjusted to infuse the remainder of the 6 to 8 g during the next 23 hours. How exactly this should be done is uncertain. Theoretically, an adult patient with significantly elevated serum iron concentrations (>1,000 mcg/dL) who is severely symptomatic might do better with continuing at a rate of 15 mg/kg/h if tolerated for the first several hours and then reducing the dose to limit the total 24-hour dose to 6 to 8 g. If after the first 1,000 mg the patient improves clinically, then it is reasonable to administer the remainder of the 5 g over the next 23 hours. In a 70-kg patient, this would be about 3 to 4 mg/kg/h for the next 23 hours. Dosing in obese patients is unknown; however, because DFO is water soluble, limiting the hourly dose in obese adults to 1,000 mg is reasonable. Although patients with mild toxicity can be treated with IM injections of 90 mg/kg of DFO (maximum of 1 g in children or 2 g in adults), this volume of antidote cannot be given IM with ease or painlessly in children.[21] Therefore, few clinicians administer IM DFO, with most preferring the IV route (Chap. 45). The total daily parenteral dose is limited by the infusion rate in children (if the manufacturer's recommendations are followed). Conservative recommendations in adults limit the dosage to 6 to 8 g/day. Although dosages as high as 16 g/day with diverse dosing regimens have been administered without incident, there are no data at this time to support this recommendation.[16,22,50,61,72,80]

URINARY COLOR CHANGE

To further define the role of DFO and the quantitative excretion of urinary iron, investigators studied urinary samples.[55] Several reviews of patients with acute iron poisoning who had received DFO[51,94] investigated the correlation between urinary iron concentrations and systemic toxicity. Most data suggest that the absence of a urine color change, often referred to as a *vin rose* color, after DFO administration indicates very little renal excretion of ferrioxamine.[28] However, unless a baseline urine color is obtained before DFO administration, post–DFO administration comparisons of urine color are unreliable. After DFO administration the *vin rose* color might not be appreciated despite severe iron toxicity or high serum iron concentrations

(Fig. 45–2).[76] No relationship between urinary iron excretion, clinical iron toxicity, and the effectiveness of DFO is established.

FORMULATION AND ACQUISITION

Deferoxamine mesylate is available in vials containing 500 mg or 2 g of sterile, lyophilized powder.[21] Adding 5 or 20 mL of sterile water for injection to either the 500-mg or the 2-g vial, respectively, results in an approximately 100-mg/mL solution. The drug must be completely dissolved before using. The resulting solution is isotonic, clear, and colorless to slightly yellow[21] and can be diluted further with 0.9% NaCl solution, dextrose in water, or Ringer lactate solution for IV administration. For IM administration, a smaller volume of solution is preferred. Adding 2 or 8 mL of sterile water for injection to the 500-mg or 2-g vial, respectively, results in a stronger yellow-colored solution containing approximately 200 mg/mL.

SUMMARY

- Deferoxamine is the parenteral chelator of choice for treatment of acute iron poisoning.
- No controlled studies have evaluated its efficacy or dosing.
- Deferoxamine should be administered intravenously.
- Early administration captures non–transferrin-bound iron still in the blood compartment.
- Administration for more than 24 hours after ingestion predisposes to ARDS.
- Deferoxamine is also used for chelation of aluminum in patients with chronic kidney failure.

REFERENCES

1. Adamson I, et al. Pulmonary toxicity of deferoxamine in iron-poisoned mice. *Toxicol Appl Pharmacol*. 1993;120:13-19.
2. Allain P, et al. Pharmacokinetics and renal elimination of desferrioxamine and ferrioxamine in healthy subjects and patients with hemochromatosis. *Br J Clin Pharmacol*. 1987;24:207-212.
3. Anderson KJ, Rivers PRA. Desferrioxamine in acute iron poisoning. *Lancet*. 1992;339:1602.
4. Balcerzak SP, et al. Mechanism of action of desferrioxamine on iron absorption. *Scand J Haematol*. 1966;3:205-212.
5. Banner W. Of iron and ancient mariners. *Ann Emerg Med*. 1997;30:687-688.
6. Banner W, Tong T. Iron poisoning. *Pediatr Clin North Am*. 1986;33:393-409.
7. Barman et al. Deferiprone. A review of its clinical potential in iron overload in beta-thalassaemia major and other trans-fusion-dependent diseases. *Drugs*. 1999;58:553-578.
8. Bene C, et al. Irreversible ocular toxicity from a single "challenge" dose of deferoxamine. *Clin Nephron*. 1989;31:45-48.
9. Bentur Y, et al. Deferoxamine (desferrioxamine), new toxicities for an old drug. *Drug Saf*. 1991;6:37-46.
10. Berkovitch M, et al. The efficacy of oral deferiprone in acute iron poisoning. *Am J Emerg Med*. 2000;18:36-40.
11. Berland Y, et al. Predictive value of desferrioxamine infusion test for bone aluminum deposit in hemodialyzed patients. *Nephron*. 1985;40:433-435.
12. Blake D, et al. Cerebral and ocular toxicity induced by desferrioxamine. *Q J Med*. 1985;219:345-355.
13. Botzenhardt S, et al. Safety profiles of iron chelators in young patients with haemoglobinopathies. *Eur J Haematol*. 2017;98:198-217.
14. Castriota Scanderberg A, et al. Pulmonary syndrome and intravenous high-dose desferrioxamine. *Lancet*. 1990;336:1511.
15. Chang TMS, Barne P. Effect of desferrioxamine on removal of aluminum and iron by coated charcoal hemoperfusion and hemodialysis. *Lancet*. 1983;2:1051-1053.
16. Cheney K, et al. Survival after a severe iron poisoning treated with intermittent infusions of deferoxamine. *J Toxicol Clin Toxicol*. 1995;33:61-66.
17. Cianciulli P, et al. Acute renal failure occurring during intravenous desferrioxamine therapy: recovery after haemodialysis. *Haematologica*. 1992;77:514-515.
18. Curry SC, et al. An ovine model of maternal iron poisoning in pregnancy. *Ann Emerg Med*. 1990;19:632-638.
19. Davies S, et al. Ocular toxicity of high-dose intravenous desferrioxamine. *Lancet*. 1983;2:181-184.
20. Dean B, et al. A study of iron complexation in a swine model. *Vet Hum Toxicol*. 1988;30:313-315.
21. Deferoxamine [package insert]. Lake Forest. IL: Hospira, Inc; 2018.
22. Douglas D, Smilkstein M. Deferoxamine-iron induced pulmonary injury and N-acetylcysteine. *J Toxicol Clin Toxicol*. 1995;33:495.
23. Evans P, et al. Mechanisms for the shuttling of plasma non-transferrin-bound iron (NTBI) onto deferoxamine by deferiprone. *Transl Res*. 2010;156:55-67.
24. Exjade [package insert]. East Hanover, NJ: Novartis Pharmaceuticals Corporation; 2016.
25. Fassos FF, Berkovitch M, Daneman N, et al. Efficacy of deferiprone in the treatment of acute iron intoxication in rats. *J Toxicol Clin Toxicol*. 1996;34:279-287.
26. Ferriprox (deferiprone) [package insert]. Rockville, MD: ApoPharma USA, Inc.; 2015.
27. Freedman M, et al. Pulmonary syndrome in patients with thalassemia major receiving intravenous deferoxamine infusions. *Am J Dis Child*. 1990;144:565-569.
28. Freeman DA, Manoguerra AS. Absence of urinary color change in severely iron poisoned child treated with deferoxamine [abstract]. *Vet Hum Toxicol*. 1981;23(suppl 1):49.
29. Glickstein H, et al. Intracellular labile iron pools as direct targets of iron chelators: a fluorescence study of chelator action in living cells. *Blood*. 2005;106:3242-3250.
30. Goodwin JF, Whitten CF. Chelation of ferrous sulfate solution by deferoxamine B. *Nature*. 1965;205:281-283.
31. Griffith E, et al. Effect of deferasirox on iron absorption in a randomized placebo controlled crossover study in a human model of acute supratherapeutic iron ingestion. *Ann Emerg Med*. 2011;58:69-73.
32. Helson L, et al. Desferrioxamine in acute iron poisoning. *Lancet*. 1992;339:1602-1603.
33. Henretig F, et al. Severe iron poisoning treated with enteral and intravenous deferoxamine. *Ann Emerg Med*. 1983;12:306-309.
34. Hershko C, et al. Pathophysiology of iron overload. *Ann N Y Acad Sci*. 1998;850:191-201.
35. Hoppe JO, et al. A review of the toxicity of iron compounds. *Am J Med Sci*. 1955;230:558-571.
36. Hoskin CS. A pharmacologic investigation of acute iron poisoning and its treatment. *Aust Paediatr J*. 1970;6:92-96.
37. Howland MA. Risks of parenteral deferoxamine. *J Toxicol Clin Toxicol*. 1996;34:491-497.
38. Hung O, et al. Deferiprone for acute iron poisoning [abstract]. *J Toxicol Clin Toxicol*. 1997;35:565.
39. Ioannides AS, Panisello JM. Acute respiratory distress syndrome in children with acute iron poisoning. The role of intravenous desferrioxamine. *Eur J Pediatr*. 2000;159:158-159.
40. Keberle M. The biochemistry of desferrioxamine and its relation to iron metabolism. *Ann N Y Acad Sci*. 1964;119:758-768.
41. Kontoghiorghes GJ. New concepts of iron and aluminum chelation therapy with oral L1 (deferiprone) and other chelators. *Analyst*. 1995;120:845-851.
42. Kontoghiorghes GJ, et al. Safety issues of iron chelation therapy in patients with normal range iron stores including thalassaemia, neurodegenerative, renal and infectious diseases. *Expert Opin Drug Saf*. 2010;9:201-206.
43. Kowdley K, Kaplan M. Iron chelation therapy with oral deferiprone—toxicity or lack of efficacy. *N Engl J Med*. 1998;339:468-469.
44. Kuo KH, Mrkobrada M. A systematic review and meta-analysis of deferiprone monotherapy and in combination with deferoxamine for reduction of iron overload in chronically transfused patients with β-thalassemia. *Hemoglobin*. 2014;38:409-421.
45. Kwiatkowski J. Oral iron chelators. *Hematol Oncol Clin North Am*. 2010;24:229-248.
46. Lee P, et al. Intravenous infusion pharmacokinetics of desferrioxamine in thalassemic patients. *Drug Metab Dispos*. 1993;21:640-644.
47. Leikin S, et al. Chelation therapy in acute iron poisoning. *J Pediatr*. 1969;71:425-430.
48. Lin S, et al. Fatal Aeromonas hydrophilia bacteremia in a hemodialysis patient treated with deferoxamine. *Am J Kidney Dis*. 1996;27:733-735.
49. Lipschitz D, et al. The site of action of desferrioxamine. *Br J Haematol*. 1971;20:395-404.
50. Lovejoy F. Chelation therapy in iron poisoning. *J Toxicol Clin Toxicol*. 1982;19:871-874.
51. McEnery J. Hospital management of acute iron ingestion. *Clin Toxicol*. 1971;4:603-613.
52. Melby K, et al. Septicemia due to *Yersinia enterocolitica* after oral doses of iron. *Br Med J*. 1982;285:487-488.
53. Mersko C, et al. Iron chelating therapy. *Crit Rev Clin Lab Sci*. 1988;26:303-340.
54. Milne C, Petros A. The use of haemofiltration for severe iron overdose. *Arch Dis Child*. 2010;95:482-483.
55. Moeschlin S, Schnider U. Treatment of primary and secondary hemochromatosis and acute iron poisoning with a new potent iron eliminating agent (desferrioxamine-B). *N Engl J Med*. 1963;269:57-66.
56. Mofenson HC, et al. Iron sepsis. *Yersinia enterocolitica* septicemia possibly caused by an overdose of iron. *N Engl J Med*. 1987;316:1092-1093.
57. Nakamura H, et al. Acute encephalopathy due to aluminum toxicity successfully treated by combined intravenous deferoxamine and hemodialysis. *J Clin Pharmacol*. 2000;40:296-300.
58. Olivieri NF, et al. Long-term safety and effectiveness of iron-chelation therapy with deferiprone for thalassemia major. *N Engl J Med*. 1998;339:417-423.
59. Olivieri N, et al. Visual and auditory neuro-toxicity in patients receiving subcutaneous deferoxamine infusions. *N Engl J Med*. 1986;314:869-873.
60. Parikh A, et al. Response to effect of deferasirox on iron absorption in a randomized placebo controlled crossover study in a human model of acute supratherapeutic iron ingestion. Letter to editor. *Ann Emerg Med*. 2011;58:219.
61. Peck M, et al. Use of high doses of deferoxamine (Desferal) in an adult patient with acute iron overdosage. *J Toxicol Clin Toxicol*. 1982;19:865-869.
62. Pengloan J, et al. Ocular toxicity after a single dose of desferrioxamine in two hemodialysis patients. *Nephron*. 1987;46:211-212.
63. Peter G, et al. Distribution and renal excretion of desferrioxamine and ferrioxamine in the dog and in the rat. *Biochem Pharmacol*. 1966;15:93-109.
64. Phelps K, et al. Encephalopathy after bladder irrigation with alum: case report and literature review. *Am J Med Soc*. 1999;318:185.
65. Porter JB, et al. A trial to investigate the relationship between DFO pharmacokinetics and metabolism and DFO-related toxicity. *Ann N Y Acad Sci*. 1998;30:483-487.

66. Porter JB, et al. Desferrioxamine ototoxicity. Evaluation of risk factors in thalassemic patients and guidelines for safe dosage. *Br J Haematol.* 1989;73:403-409.

67. Porter JB, et al. Recent insights into interactions of deferoxamine with cellular and plasma iron pools: Implications for clinical use. *Ann N Y Acad Sci.* 2005;1054:155-168.

68. Porter JB, Shah FT. Iron overload in thalassemia and related conditions: therapeutic goals and assessment of response to chelation therapies. *Hematol Oncol Clin North Am.* 2010;24:1109-1130.

69. Porter J, et al. Ethical issues and risk/benefit assessment of iron chelation therapy. Advances with deferiprone/deferoxamine combinations and concerns about the safety, efficacy and costs of deferasirox [letter to editor]. *Hemoglobin.* 2008;32:601-607.

70. Prasannan L, et al. Acute renal failure following deferoxamine overdose. *Pediatr Nephrol.* 2003;18:283-285.

71. Propper R, Nathan D. Clinical removal of iron. *Annu Rev Med.* 1982;33:509-519.

72. Propper R, et al. Reassessment of the use of desferrioxamine B in iron overload. *N Engl J Med.* 1976;294:1421-1423.

73. Robotham J, Lietman P. Acute iron poisoning. *Am J Dis Child.* 1980;134:875-879.

74. Sherrard D, et al. Precipitation of dialysis dementia by deferoxamine treatment of aluminum related bone disease. *Am J Kid Dis.* 1988;12:126-130.

75. Singer ST, Vichinsky EP. Deferoxamine treatment during pregnancy. Is it harmful? *Am J Hematol.* 1999;60:24-26.

76. Singhi SC, et al. Acute iron poisoning: clinical picture, intensive care needs and outcome. *Indian Pediatr.* 2003;40:1177-1182.

77. Stivelman J, et al. Kinetics and efficacy of deferoxamine in iron overloaded hemodialysis patients. *Kidney Int.* 1989;36:1125-1132.

78. Stumpf J. Deferasirox. *Am J Health Sys Pharm.* 2007;64:606-616.

79. Summers MR, et al. Studies in desferrioxamine and ferrioxamine metabolism in normal and iron loaded subjects. *Br J Haematol.* 1979;42:547-555.

80. Tenenbein M. Benefits of parenteral deferoxamine for acute iron poisoning. *J Toxicol Clin Toxicol.* 1996;34:485-489.

81. Tenenbein M, et al. Pulmonary toxic effects of continuous administration in acute iron poisoning. *Lancet.* 1992;339:699-701.

82. Tran T, et al. Intentional iron overdose in pregnancy—management and outcome. *J Emerg Med.* 2000;18:225-228.

83. Tripod JA. Pharmacologic comparison of the binding of iron and other metals. In: Gross F, ed. *Iron Metabolism. International Symposium on Iron Metabolism.* Berlin, Germany: Springer-Verlag; 1964:503-524.

84. Vasilakakis D, et al. Removal of aluminoxamine and ferrioxamine by charcoal hemoperfusion and hemodialysis. *Kidney Int.* 1992;41:1400-1407.

85. Vernon DD, et al. Hemodynamic effects of experimental iron poisoning. *Ann Emerg Med.* 1989;18:863-866.

86. Vichinsky E, et al. A randomised comparison of deferasirox versus deferoxamine for the treatment of transfusional iron overload in sickle cell disease. *Br J Haematol.* 2007;136:501-508.

87. Waalen J. More pieces to the iron chelation puzzle. *Transl Res.* 2010;156:53-54.

88. Weitman S, et al. Pulmonary toxicity of deferoxamine in children with advanced cancer. *J Natl Cancer Inst.* 1991;83:1834-1835.

89. Westlin W. Deferoxamine as a chelating agent. *Clin Toxicol.* 1971;4:597-602.

90. Westlin W. Deferoxamine in the treatment of acute iron poisoning. Clinical experiences with 172 children. *Clin Pediatr.* 1966;5:531-535.

91. Whitten C, et al. Studies in acute iron poisoning. Desferrioxamine in the treatment of acute iron poisoning—clinical observations, experimental studies and theoretical considerations. *Pediatrics.* 1965;36:322-335.

92. Whitten C, et al. Studies in acute iron poisoning. II. Further observations on deferoxamine in the treatment of acute experimental iron poisoning. *Pediatrics.* 1966;38:102-110.

93. Whitten CF, et al. Studies in acute iron poisoning III. The hemodynamic alterations in acute experimental iron poisoning. *Pediatr Res.* 1968;2:479-485.

94. Yatscoff RW, et al. An objective criterion for the cessation of deferoxamine therapy in the acutely poisoned patient. *J Toxicol Clin Toxicol.* 1991;29:1-10.

95. Yokel R. Aluminum chelation principles and recent advances. *Coord Chem Rev.* 2002;228:97-113.

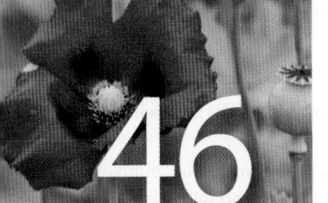

C. Pharmaceuticals

46

PHARMACEUTICAL ADDITIVES

Sean P. Nordt and Lisa E. Vivero

HISTORY AND EPIDEMIOLOGY

During the last century there were several outbreaks of toxicity in the United States associated with pharmaceutical additives (Chap. 2). The 1937 Massengill sulfanilamide disaster is the most notorious of these epidemics. Diethylene glycol, an excellent solvent and potent nephrotoxin, was substituted for the additives propylene glycol and glycerin in the liquid formulation of a new sulfanilamide antibiotic because of lower cost.[27,64,73] As a result, more than 100 people died from acute kidney failure.[27] Outbreaks of acute kidney failure occurred when diethylene glycol was used to solubilize acetaminophen in South Africa, Bangladesh, Nigeria, and Haiti, cough syrup in Panama, and teething powder in Nigera.[22,30,75,87,133,143]

In December 1983, a new parenteral vitamin E formulation (E-Ferol) was introduced. It contained 25 units/mL of α-tocopherol acetate, 9% polysorbate 80, 1% polysorbate 20, and water for injection. At the time, no premarketing testing was required for new formulations of an already approved drug. Several months after its release, a fatal syndrome in low-birth-weight infants, characterized by thrombocytopenia, acute kidney injury, cholestasis, hepatomegaly, and ascites, was described.[1,119] Thirty-eight deaths and 43 cases of severe symptoms were attributed to E-Ferol. Vitamin E was thought to be the cause and E-Ferol was recalled from the market 4 months after its release. It is now believed that the polysorbate emulsifiers were responsible.[1]

Although these additive-related occurrences are rare, relative to the frequency of pharmaceutical additive use, they illustrate the potential of pharmaceutical additive toxicity.

Pharmaceuticals are labeled specifically to focus attention on the active ingredient(s) of a product, thus giving the misimpression that additive ingredients are inert and unimportant. Additives, or excipients as they are more properly termed, are necessary to act as vehicles, add color, improve taste, provide consistency, enhance stability and solubility, and impart antimicrobial properties to medicinal formulations. Although it is true that most cases of excipient toxicity involve exposure to large quantities, or to prolonged or improper use, these adverse events are nonetheless related to the toxicologic properties of the excipient.

Prior to selecting the specific additives and quantity necessary for a drug formulation, the drug manufacturer must consider several factors, including the active ingredient's physical form, its solubility and stability, the desired final dosage form and route of administration, and compatibility with the dispensing container materials. Often, the same active ingredient requires different excipients to impart appropriate pharmacokinetic characteristics to different dosage forms, such as in long-acting and immediate-release formulations. Similarly, multiple-dose injection vials containing the same active ingredients as single-dose vials specifically require the addition of a bacteriostatic xenobiotic not necessary for single-dose vials.

Unlike requirements for active ingredients, there is no specific US Food and Drug Administration (FDA) approval system for pharmaceutical excipients. As such, the FDA determines the amount and type of data necessary to support the use of a specific excipient on a case-by-case basis. Under current practice, only excipients that were previously permitted for use in foods or pharmaceuticals are defined as *generally recognized as safe* (GRAS), or "GRAS listed." All components of a pharmaceutical product, including excipients, must be produced in accordance with current good manufacturing practice standards to ensure purity. The Safety Committee of the International Pharmaceutical Excipients Council developed guidelines for the toxicologic testing of new excipients.[172] Because of patent protection laws, it was

not until 1985 that manufacturers were required to provide a list of inactive ingredients contained in all pharmaceutical products. Although it is becoming easier to identify pharmaceutical additives in products, information on their effects and the mechanisms by which they cause adverse responses are often unknown or difficult to obtain.

This chapter summarizes the available literature on commonly used additives associated with direct toxicities (Table 46–1). Data on pharmacokinetics and mechanism of toxicity are presented when data are available. Although many additives are associated with hypersensitivity reactions, including anaphylaxis, these are not discussed because of their nonpharmacologic basis. However, excipients should always be considered as possibly causative in patients who develop hypersensitivity reactions.

BENZALKONIUM CHLORIDE

Benzalkonium chloride (BAC, BAK), or alkyldimethyl (phenylmethyl) ammonium chloride, is a quaternary ammonium cationic surfactant composed of a mixture of alkyl benzyl dimethyl ammonium chlorides. Although it is the most widely used ophthalmic preservative in the United States, it is also considered the most cytotoxic (Table 46–2).[96,104] Benzalkonium chloride is also used in otic and nasal formulations, and in some small-volume parenteral preparations. The antimicrobial activity of BAC includes gram-positive and gram-negative bacteria, and some viruses, fungi, and protozoa. Because of its rapid onset of action, good tissue penetration, and long duration of action, BAC is preferred over other preservatives. The concentration of BAC in ophthalmic medications usually ranges from 0.004% to 0.01%.[104] Strong BAC solutions (>0.1%) can be caustic (Chap. 103).

TABLE 46–1	Potential Systemic Toxicity of Various Pharmaceutical Excipients	
Cardiovascular		**Ophthalmic**
Chlorobutanol		Benzalkonium chloride
Propylene glycol		Chlorobutanol
Fluid and electrolyte		**Renal**
Polyethylene glycol		Polyethylene glycol
Propylene glycol		Propylene glycol
Sorbitol		
Gastrointestinal		
Sorbitol		
Neurologic		
Benzyl alcohol		
Chlorobutanol		
Polyethylene glycol		
Propylene glycol		

681

TABLE 46–2	Benzalkonium Chloride Concentrations of Common Ophthalmic Medications
Medication	**Percent**
Apraclonidine	0.01
Artificial tears	0.005–0.01
Betaxolol	0.01
Brimonidine/timolol	0.005
Carteolol	0.005
Ciprofloxacin	0.006
Cyclopentolate	0.01
Dexamethasone	0.01
Dorzolamide/timolol	0.0075
Gentamicin	0.01
Ketorolac	0.01
Levobunolol	0.004
Naphazoline	0.01
Ofloxacin	0.005
Phenylephrine	0.01
Pilocarpine	0.01
Polymyxin B sulfate/trimethoprim	0.004
Tetrahydrozoline	0.01
Timolol	0.01
Tobramycin	0.01
Tropicamide	0.01

Ophthalmic Toxicity

Corneal epithelial cells harvested from human cadavers within 12 hours of death were exposed to a medium containing 0.01% BAC.[168] The surfactant properties of BAC resulted in intracellular matrix dissolution and loss of epithelial superficial layers. Following exposure to the medium, mitotic activity ceased and degenerative changes to corneal epithelium were noted. During a 24-hour observation period, epithelial cell cytokinetic or mitotic activity did not occur. Patients with compromised corneal epithelia are at increased risk for the adverse effects of BAC.[168]

Two case reports demonstrate the potential toxicity of BAC and highlight the difficulty of diagnosing BAC toxicity. A 36-year-old woman complained of decreased vision when she inadvertently switched from Lensrins, a contact lens cleaning solution, to Dacriose, an isotonic boric acid solution preserved with BAC. After 3 days, she had inflammation, pain, and decreased visual acuity. Examination of the cornea revealed many superficial punctate erosions of the epithelium. An in vitro experiment identified significant binding of BAC to soft contact lenses.[59] In the second case, a 56-year-old man diagnosed with keratoconjunctivitis sicca was treated with topical antibiotics and artificial tears containing BAC. Following one year of continual use, the patient developed intractable pain, photophobia, and extensive breakdown of the corneal epithelium. Not suspecting the BAC-containing products, the patient continued to use the artificial tears solution for another 9 years despite continued pain and decreasing visual acuity. Replacement with a preservative-free saline solution resulted in resolution of pain, photophobia, and corneal changes.[104] Furthermore, there are newer ophthalmic medication preservatives available (eg, polyquaternium-1,

stabilized oxychloride complex, sodium perborate, Sof Zia), which in studies are less toxic than BAC.[4]

A case series of corneal endothelial injury following the inadvertent intraocular use of balanced salt solution (BSS) preserved with BAC instead of preservative-free BSS in 12 patients undergoing phacoemulsification, a surgical technique to remove cataract lenses. The BSS was instilled in the anterior chamber. The operating room had run out of preservative-free BSS and, unbeknownst to the surgeon, it was replaced with the BAC-containing BSS, which contained 0.013% BAC. This is in excess of recommended concentration for intraocular use and is associated with corneal endothelial injury and edema. Within 48 hours of instillation of the BSS, the visual acuity in all 12 patients was limited to only being able to count fingers at 2 feet. This persisted in 11 of the patients at a 6-month follow-up evaluation after the instillation of the BSS. One patient had improvement at 6 months of visual acuity to 20/120 and 20/30 without and with pinholes, respectively.[106]

Nasopharyngeal and Oropharyngeal Toxicity

Human adenoidal tissue was exposed to oxymetazoline nasal spray preserved with BAC at concentrations ranging from 0.005 to 0.15 mg/mL for 1 to 30 minutes.[16] Irregular and fractured epithelial cells occurred at all concentrations; however, these findings developed earlier and more frequently with the higher concentrations. The number of beating ciliary bodies also decreased as the duration and the concentrations increased. Benzalkonium chloride decreases the viscosity of the normal protective mucous lining of the naso- and oropharynx, resulting in cytotoxicity.

Administration of one of 3 nasal corticosteroid sprays (beclomethasone dipropionate, flunisolide, budesonide) preserved with either 0.031% or 0.022% BAC in the right nostril of rats twice daily for 21 days caused squamous cell metaplasia and a decrease in the number of goblet cells, cilia, and mucus.[17] No histologic changes occurred in rats receiving any of the preservative-free steroids or in tissue exposed to 0.9% sodium chloride solution administered into the left nostril as the control. Similarly, in another study, epithelial desquamation, inflammation, and edema occurred when 0.05% and 0.10% BAC was applied hourly to the nostrils of rats for 8 hours.[99] No lesions developed in the nostrils of rats receiving 0.01% BAC.

In an in vitro study, cultured human nasal epithelial cells were exposed to varying concentrations of BAC compared with another preservative, potassium sorbate (PS), with phosphate-buffered saline (PBS) as a control. Cell viability was greatly reduced at the higher concentrations of BAC compared with no decrease in cell viability in the PS or PBS groups. Additionally, at concentrations used clinically, loss of microvilli, destruction of cell membranes, and poor cytoskeletal alignment demonstrated by electron microscopy occurred.[84]

An in vitro study of human nasal mucosa exposed mucosa to either fluticasone or mometasone preserved with either BAC or PS at various concentrations with subsequent measure of ciliary beat frequency. Although PS did not affect ciliary beat frequency at any concentration, BAC adversely affected ciliary beat frequency. At lower concentrations, BAC slowed ciliary beat frequency and brought it to standstill at higher concentrations.[85] Another in vitro study in human nasal epithelial comparing budesonide, fluticasone propionate, azelastine hydrochloride, or levocabastine hydrochloride preserved with either BAC or PS at various concentrations showed similar results.[92]

Polyquaternium-1 (PQ), an alternative detergent preservative to BAC, is reported to be less toxic to various cell types. In an in vitro study of cultured human corneal and conjunctival cells exposed to various topical glaucoma medications preserved with either BAC with concentrations ranging from 0.001% to 0.005% or PQ 0.04% with other arms using BSS as "live" control and 70% methanol and 0.2% saponin as "dead" controls, PQ had less cytotoxicity to both cell types compared to BAC.[5] In an in vivo murine model comparing BAC concentrations 0.1% and 0.5% and PQ 0.1% and 0.5% to control BSS showed decreased tear production, increased corneal punctate lesions, increased in conjunctival injection, corneal neovascularization, and stromal inflammation in BAC compared to PQ and BSS.[100] It is important to note that both of these studies[5,100] involving PQ were funded by the manufacturer.

TABLE 46-3	Benzyl Alcohol Concentration of Common Medications		
Medication (concentration)		Percent	Benzyl Alcohol Dose (mg/dose volume)
Amiodarone (50 mg/mL)		2.0	60.6 mg/3 mL
Atracurium (10 mg/mL)		0.9	45 mg/5 mL
Bacteriostatic saline for injection		0.9	9 mg/mL
Bacteriostatic water for injection		0.9	9 mg/mL
Bumetanide (0.25 mg/mL)		1.0	40 mg/4 mL
Diazepam (5 mg/mL)		1.5	30 mg/2 mL
Enalaprilat (1.25 mg/mL)		0.9	9 mg/mL
Etoposide (20 mg/mL)		3.0	150 mg/5 mL
Glycopyrrolate (0.2 mg/mL)		0.9	9 mg/mL
Lorazepam (2 mg/mL, 4 mg/mL)		2.0	20 mg/mL
Methotrexate (25 mg/mL)		0.9	9 mg/mL
Midazolam (1 mg/mL, 5 mg/mL)		1.0	10 mg/mL
Prochlorperazine (5 mg/mL)		0.75	7.5 mg/mL

BENZYL ALCOHOL

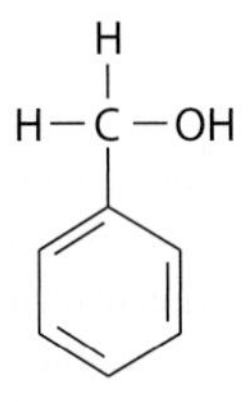

Benzyl alcohol (benzene methanol) is a colorless, oily liquid with a faint aromatic odor that is most commonly added to pharmaceuticals as a bacteriostatic (Table 46–3). In 1982, a "gasping" syndrome, which included hypotension, bradycardia, gasping respirations, hypotonia, progressive metabolic acidosis, seizures, cardiovascular collapse, and death, was first described in low-birth-weight neonates in intensive care units.[23,66] All the infants had received either bacteriostatic water or sodium chloride solution containing 0.9% benzyl alcohol to flush intravenous catheters or in parenteral medications reconstituted with bacteriostatic water or saline.[23,66] The syndrome occurred in infants who had received more than 99 mg/kg of benzyl alcohol (range, 99–234 mg/kg).[66] The World Health Organization (WHO) currently estimates the acceptable daily intake of benzyl alcohol to be not more than 5 mg/kg body weight.[25]

Pharmacokinetics

In adults, benzyl alcohol is oxidized to benzoic acid, conjugated in the liver with glycine, and excreted in the urine as hippuric acid. Preterm babies have a greater ability to metabolize benzyl alcohol to benzoic acid than do term babies, but are unable to convert benzoic acid to hippuric acid, probably because of glycine deficiency. This results in the accumulation of benzoic acid (Fig. 46–1).[66] A fatal case of metabolic acidosis was reported in a

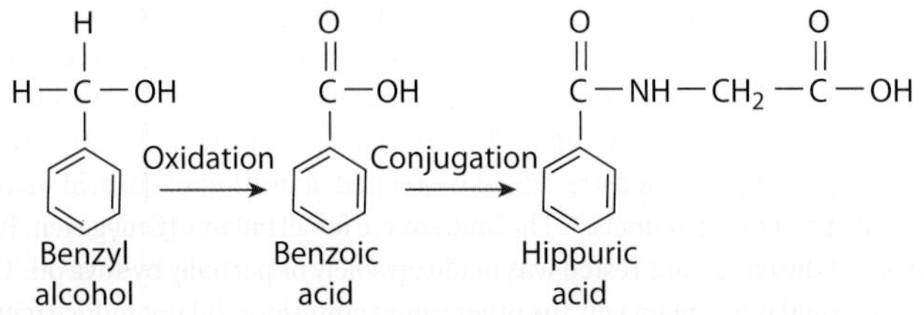

FIGURE 46-1. Oxidative metabolism of benzyl alcohol.

5-year-old girl who received 2.4 mg/kg/h diazepam preserved with benzyl alcohol for 36 hours to control status epilepticus. Elevated benzoic acid concentrations were identified in serum and urine samples. The estimated daily dosage of benzyl alcohol was 180 mg/kg.[66,107]

Neurologic Toxicity

Benzyl alcohol is believed to have a role in the increased frequency of cerebral intraventricular hemorrhages and mortality reported in very-low-birth-weight (VLBW) infants (weight <1,000 g) who received flush solutions preserved with benzyl alcohol.[83] An increased incidence of developmental delay and cerebral palsy was also noted in the same VLBW patients, suggesting a secondary damaging effect of benzyl alcohol.[14]

There are several case reports of transient paraplegia following the intrathecal or epidural administration of chemotherapeutics or analgesics containing benzyl alcohol as a preservative.[10,41,74,149] The local anesthetic effects are most likely responsible for the immediate paraparesis and limited duration of effects, rather than actual demyelination of nerve roots. In a rat study, lumbosacral dorsal root action potential amplitudes were measured after exposure to 0.9% or 1.5% benzyl alcohol solutions in either 0.9% sodium chloride solution or distilled water.[74] Rats exposed to all benzyl alcohol solutions for less than one minute had inhibited dorsal root action potentials. This was attributed to the local anesthetic effects of benzyl alcohol as function was 50% to 90% restored after rinsing the nerves with 0.9% sodium chloride solution. Chronic intrathecal exposure to benzyl alcohol 0.9% over 7 days resulted in scattered areas of demyelination and early remyelination. The 1.5% benzyl alcohol solution–exposed dorsal nerve roots showed greater changes, with widespread areas of demyelination and fatty degeneration of nerve fibers.

CHLOROBUTANOL

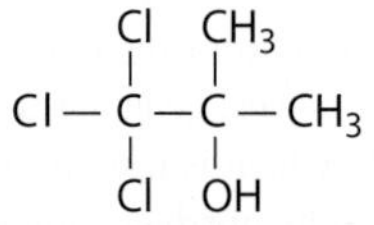

Chlorobutanol, or chlorbutol (1,1,1-trichloro-2-methyl-2-propanol), is available as volatile, white crystals with an odor of camphor. Chlorobutanol has antibacterial and antifungal properties and is widely used as a preservative in injectable, ophthalmic, otic, and cosmetic preparations at concentrations up to 0.5% (Table 46–4). Chlorobutanol also has mild sedative and local anesthetic properties and was formerly used therapeutically as a sedative–hypnotic.[20] The lethal human chlorobutanol dose is estimated to be 50 to 500 mg/kg.[128]

Central Nervous System Toxicity

Chlorobutanol has a chemical structure similar to trichloroethanol (Fig. 72–1), the active metabolite of chloral hydrate, and is believed to exhibit similar

TABLE 46-4	Chlorobutanol Concentrations of Common Medications		
Medication (concentration)		Percent	Chlorobutanol Dose (mg/dose volume)
Epinephrine injection (1 mg/mL)		0.5	1.5 mg/0.3 mL
Isoniazid injection (100 mg/mL)		0.25	7.5 mg/3 mL
Methadone injection (10 mg/mL)		0.5	5 mg/mL
Thiamine injection (100 mg/mL)		0.5	5 mg/mL
Pyridoxine (100 mg/mL)		0.5	5 mg/mL
Tobramycin ophthalmic ointment		0.5	—
Vasopressin (20 U/mL) injectable		0.5	2.5 mg/0.5 mL
Vitamin A injection (50,000 IU/mL)		0.5	5 mg/mL

pharmacologic properties. Central nervous system depression was reported in a 40-year-old alcoholic man who chronically abused Seducaps (formerly available in Australia and several other countries), a nonprescription hypnotic containing chlorobutanol as the active ingredient.[20] On admission to the emergency department, he had drowsiness, dysarthria, slurred speech, and occasional episodes of myoclonic movements. His peak serum chlorobutanol concentration was 100 mcg/mL, decreasing to 48 mcg/mL over 2 weeks, with a half-life of 3 days based on serial declining concentrations. This is similar to human volunteer pharmacokinetic data following oral administration of chlorobutanol demonstrating an elimination half-life of 10.3 ± 1.3 days.[170] His speech abnormality resolved after 4 weeks. Only chlorobutanol was detected in the patient's urine or serum. In a second case, a possible central nervous system depressant effect from chlorobutanol was suggested in a 19-year-old woman treated with high doses of intravenous morphine preserved with chlorobutanol.[47] She received approximately 90 mg/h of chlorobutanol for several days. Her peak serum chlorobutanol concentration was 83 mcg/mL, a concentration similar to that in the previous case report;[20] however, the coadministration of morphine precludes the effects being attributed to chlorobutanol alone.

Ketamine is neurotoxic when administered intrathecally to animals.[116,117] The potential neurotoxic effects of chlorobutanol as a preservative in ketamine compared with preservative-free ketamine was studied in rabbits.[117] Forty rabbits were given 0.3 mL intrathecally of either 1% preservative-free ketamine, 1% ketamine, 0.05% chlorobutanol, or 1% lidocaine as control. The rabbits were observed and hemodynamically monitored for 8 days and then euthanized. Histologic evaluation of the spinal cord as well as for blood–brain barrier lesions was performed. Seven of the 10 rabbits given intrathecal chlorobutanol showed both white and gray matter histologic changes as well as diffuse blood–brain barrier injury. No histologic changes were seen in either ketamine groups or the lidocaine group, and only one rabbit in each ketamine group had blood–brain barrier injury. These results suggest that chlorobutanol should not be administered intrathecally.[117]

A case series of 5 patients were given intra-arterial papaverine preserved with 0.5% chlorobutanol,[155] which is used to prevent cerebral vasospasm in patients with subarachnoid hemorrhage. Immediately after administration of papaverine in either the left, right, or bilateral anterior cerebral arteries, patients had an acute deterioration in neurologic status. Subsequent brain magnetic resonance imaging identified selective gray matter toxicity in the territories treated with papaverine. Postmortem brain histology in one patient also identified gray matter changes. The authors state the absence of white matter changes is not consistent with ischemic infarction but suggest direct toxic effect of either the papaverine or chlorobutanol. The manufacturer of the papaverine stated that no other reports had been made and the papaverine used came from 2 different lots; therefore, it is unclear if an unidentified independent variable caused these effects, but the authors caution using intra-arterial papaverine in patients with subarachnoid hemorrhage.[155]

Ophthalmic Toxicity

Chlorobutanol is a commonly used preservative in ophthalmic preparations and is less toxic to the eye than benzalkonium chloride.[132] Chlorobutanol increases the permeability of cells by impairing cell membrane structure.[168] An in vitro experiment using corneal epithelial cells harvested from human cadavers demonstrated arrested mitotic activity following chlorobutanol exposure.[168] At the commonly formulated concentration of 0.5%, chlorobutanol can cause eye irritation, most likely due to cellular contraction of epithelial microfilaments, cessation of normal cytokinesis, cell movement, and mitotic activity.[50] Degeneration of human corneal epithelial cells specifically manifested as membranous blebs, cytoplasmic swelling, and occasional breaks in the external cell membrane has also occurred at this concentration.[50]

LIPIDS

In general, there are 3 types of commercial intravenous lipid drug-delivery systems available: lipid emulsion, liposomal, and lipid complex (Table 46–5). Lipid emulsions are immiscible lipid droplets dispersed in an aqueous

TABLE 46–5 Lipid Carrier Formulations of Common Medications

Medication	Lipid Carrier
Amphotericin B	Lipid complex
Amphotericin B	Liposome
Bupivacaine	Liposome
Cytarabine	Liposome
Doxorubicin	Liposome (stealth)
Morphine sulfate	Liposome
Propofol	Emulsion

phase stabilized by an emulsifier (eg, egg, soy lecithin). Liposomes differ from emulsion lipid droplets in that they are vesicles composed of one or more concentric phospholipid bilayers surrounding an aqueous core. Lipophilic drugs are formulated for intravenous administration by partitioning them into the lipid phase of either an emulsion or liposome. Liposomes are capable of encapsulating hydrophilic xenobiotics within their aqueous core to exploit lipid pharmacokinetic properties.[162] Attaching a therapeutic drug to a lipid to form a lipid complex is another way to take advantage of lipid pharmacokinetics.

Lipid drug-delivery systems are biocompatible because of their similarity to endogenous cell membranes. They are created with stable lipid membranes resistant to hydrolysis or oxidation, to decrease toxicity, and to enhance therapeutic efficacy by altering drug pharmacokinetic and pharmacodynamic parameters. The biodistribution, and the rate of release and metabolism of a drug incorporated in a lipid drug-delivery system, is regulated by the type and concentration of oil and emulsifier used, pH, drug concentration dispersed in the medium, the size of the lipid particle, and the manufacturing process.[134,162] Intravenous formulations are usually isotonic and have a pH of 7 to 8.[162]

The rate of clearance of a lipid drug-delivery system from the blood depends on its physicochemical properties and the molecular weight of the emulsifier. Electrically charged lipid carriers are removed more rapidly than neutral particles.[26,134] Smaller lipid particle size and high-molecular-weight emulsifiers decrease clearance. "Stealth" liposome formulations incorporate a polyethylene glycol coating that prevents rapid detection and clearance of liposomes by the reticuloendothelial system, prolonging circulation time.[134] Active drug targeting is achieved by conjugating antibodies or vectors to side chains on the emulsifier.[26,134] For a therapeutic drug available in more than one lipid drug-delivery systems (eg, amphotericin B), it is important to note that any change in the lipid formulation can alter the pharmacokinetic, pharmacodynamic, and safety parameters of the drug; consequently, they are not equivalent dosage formulations (Chap. 54).

The physicochemical properties of lipid emulsions not only affect the therapeutic drugs carried by them, but the lipids themselves also have direct pharmacologic effects on the central nervous[182] and immune systems.[103] Lipid fatty acid mediators affect the membrane receptor channels of N-methyl-D-aspartate (NMDA) receptors, potentiating synaptic transmission.[120,122,136,165] Dogs given a medium-chain triglyceride emulsion intravenous infusion developed dose-related central nervous system metabolic and neurologic effects, accompanied by electroencephalographic changes consistent with encephalopathy observed when serum octanoate concentration reached 0.5 to 0.9 mM.[120] In an in vitro model, 3 of 9 lipid emulsions tested (Abbolipid, 20% soya and safflower oil; Intra-lipid, 20% soya oil; and Structolipid, 20% structured triglycerides) demonstrated a dose-related activation of cortical neuronal NMDA receptor channels.[182] The lipid source for all but one (Omegaven, 10% fish oil) of the emulsions tested was made up solely or partially by soya oil. The authors could not explain why the other 6 lipid emulsions did not induce membrane currents. Adequate control for the nonlipid constituent contribution of these emulsions is lacking. In another in vitro study, the same authors found that NMDA-induced neuronal currents are reduced by an unknown factor in the aqueous portion of Abbolipid.[183] This suggests that lipid emulsions pharmacologically enhance the anesthetic effect of hypnotics such as propofol. The clinical relevance of these studies remains to be determined.

Triglycerides in parenteral nutrition emulsions are implicated in altering the immune system, leading to an increased susceptibility to infection,[58,180] and altering lung function and hemodynamics in patients with acute respiratory distress syndrome.[103] Phospholipid activation of phospholipase A_2 may be an initiating cause.[58,103,180] However, it is not clear if these immunologic effects are a consequence of factors other than the lipid in the emulsion.

PARABENS

Methylparaben

The parabens, or parahydroxybenzoic acids, are a group of compounds widely employed as preservatives in cosmetics, food, and pharmaceuticals because of their bacteriostatic, fungistatic, and antioxidant properties (Table 46–6).[150] A survey conducted by the FDA identified the parabens as the second most common ingredients in cosmetic formulations, with water being the most common.[108] Parabens are often used in combination, because the presence of 2 or more parabens is synergistic.[107] Methylparabens and propylparabens are most commonly used.[150] Pharmaceutical paraben concentrations usually range from 0.1% to 0.3%.[144]

Widespread usage of parabens since the 1920s demonstrates a relatively low order of toxicity.[108] However, because of their allergenic potential they are currently considered less suitable for injectable and ophthalmic preparations.[144] Based on long-term animal studies, the WHO has set the total acceptable daily intake of ethylparabens, methylparabens, and propylparabens to be 10 mg/kg body weight.[144] In addition to allergic reactions, parabens have the potential to cause other adverse effects. Bilirubin displacement from albumin-binding sites occurred with administration of methylparaben- and propylparaben-preserved gentamicin when serum parabens concentrations were 3 to 15 mcg/mL.[43] Gentamicin alone has no

effect on bilirubin displacement.[109] Spermicidal activity was demonstrated in an in vitro study of human semen specimens exposed to local paraben concentrations of 1 to 8 mg/mL.[160] Possible interference with conception and potential adverse effects on fertility were not investigated in this paper. However, other investigators show a direct toxic effect of parabens on sperm mitochondrial function.[166] Sperm require an enormous amount of ATP to adequately fertilize ova.

Concerns have arisen regarding the potential estrogenic and anti-androgenic effects of the parabens and their common metabolite, p-hydroxybenzoic acid. Xenobiotics with these effects are commonly referred to as *endocrine disrupting substances*. It has been suggested that methylparaben is less toxic than butyl and benzyl-parabens with regard to oxidative stress and resultant cytotoxicity.[44,153] The clinical significance of these effects is not elucidated.[34,45,141,142,175] There is a focus on the role of parabens and the development of breast cancer due to the estrogenic effects of parabens. In a study of breast tissue following mastectomies of women with primary breast cancer, concentrations of parabens were highest in the axillary region compared to other more medial regions. These authors suggest there may be a role of using cosmetics and deodorants under the arm increasing local estrogenic effects on breast tissue.[12,77]

PHENOL

Phenol (carbolic acid, hydroxybenzene, phenylic acid, phenylic alcohol) is a commonly used preservative in injectable medications (Table 46–7). Phenol is a colorless to light pink, caustic liquid with a characteristic odor. When exposed to air and light, phenol turns a red or brown color.[40] Phenol exerts antimicrobial activity against a wide variety of microorganisms, bacteria, mycobacteria, and some fungi and viruses.[40] Phenol is well absorbed from the gastrointestinal tract, skin, and mucous membranes and is excreted in the urine as phenyl glucuronide and phenyl sulfate metabolites.[40] Although there are numerous reports of phenol toxicity following intentional ingestions or unintentional dermal exposures (Chap. 103), adverse reactions to its use as a pharmaceutical excipient are uncommon, most likely because of the small quantities used.[40]

Cutaneous Absorption

Systemic toxicity from cutaneous absorption of phenol is reported. Ventricular tachycardia was observed in an 11-year-old boy following application of a chemical peel solution containing 88% phenol in water and liquid soap. The solution was applied to 15% of his body surface area for the treatment of xeroderma pigmentosum. Immediately following the onset of the ventricular

TABLE 46–6	Paraben Concentrations of Common Medications and Doses		
Medication (concentration)		Percent	Paraben Dose (mg/dose volume)
Bupivacaine HCl injection[a]		0.1	1 mg/mL
Flumazenil injection (0.1 mg/mL)		0.2	4 mg/2 mL
Labetalol injection (5 mg/mL)		0.09	3.6 mg/4 mL
Lidocaine injection[a]		0.1	1 mg/mL
Methyldopa injection (50 mg/mL)		0.17	8.5 mg/5 mL
Naloxone injection (0.4 mg/mL)		0.2	2 mg/mL
Ondansetron injection (2 mg/mL)		0.14	2.7 mg/2mL
Pentazocine injection (30 mg/mL)		0.1	1 mg/mL
Sulfacetamide ophthalmic solution (100 mg/mL)		0.06	0.03 mg/drop

[a]Multidose vials of all strengths contain 0.1% paraben.

TABLE 46–7	Phenol Concentration of Common Medications	
Medication	Percent	Phenol Dose (mg/dose volume)
Antivenom (Crotaline)	0.25	25 (per vial)
Antivenom (*Micrurus fulvius*)	0.25	25 (per vial)
Pneumococcal 23 vaccine	0.25	1.25 mg/0.5 mL
Neostigmine methylsulfate injection[a]	0.45	4.5 mg/mL
Quinidine gluconate injection 80 mg/mL	0.25	25 mg/10 mL
Typhoid Vi vaccine	0.25	1.25 mg/0.5 mL

[a]Multidose vials of all strengths contain 0.45% phenol.

tachycardia, the phenol-treated areas were irrigated, an infusion of 0.9% sodium chloride solution was begun, and 2 intravenous lidocaine boluses were given followed by a lidocaine infusion. The dysrhythmia persisted for 3 hours. The urinary phenol concentration the following day was 58.9 mg/dL.[173] In a similar case, multifocal premature ventricular contractions were observed in a 10-year-old boy after application of a chemical peeling solution of 40% phenol, 0.8% croton oil in hexachlorophene soap, and water for the treatment of a giant hairy nevus.[181] The premature ventricular contractions were refractory to intravenous lidocaine but resolved with intravenous bretylium. No phenol concentrations were obtained to confirm systemic absorption. In a case series of 181 patients undergoing chemical face peeling with phenol-based solutions, 12 demonstrated cardiac dysrhythmias. This occurred more commonly in patients with comorbid diabetes mellitus, hypertension, or treatment with antidepressants.[101] Both lidocaine and propranolol treatment and pretreatment are reported to abate these dysrhythmias.[101] However, these are anecdotal reports and have not been formally studied sufficiently to support recommending their use.[21,70,169] Despite the risk of toxicity, phenol chemical peels are still used in some cases because phenol penetrates deep into tissues, providing both long-lasting and good cosmetic results. Most commonly, phenol chemical peels are used for deep acne scars and other severe skin disorders.

A 9-year-old girl sustained partial-thickness burns over 17% of her body following the topical administration of Creolin, which contains phenolic compounds. The Creolin was applied by her mother to delouse the patient. Creolin is not intended for human use and is generally used as deodorant cleanser for bathrooms, kennels, and barns. The child had 8 ounces poured onto her hair, which then flowed onto her neck, chest, back, left shoulder, and upper arm. Within minutes she became obtunded, requiring endotracheal intubation by paramedics. In the emergency department, she had sinus tachycardia with brief runs of ventricular tachycardia. She was decontaminated with soap and water, low-molecular-weight polyethylene glycol and ethanol. The patient experienced a mild elevation of hepatic aminotransferases and had dark-green–black urine while in the intensive care unit. This resolved and the patient was extubated and discharged to home on hospital day 4.[177]

Drowsiness, respiratory depression, and blue-colored urine were noted in a 6-month-old infant 12 hours after topical application of magenta paint over most of the body for seborrheic eczema.[146] Magenta paint (also known as Castellani paint) was widely used for seborrheic eczema and contained 4% phenol, magenta, boric acid, resorcinol, acetone, and ethanol. Further investigation found that phenol was detected in urine samples of 4 of 16 other infants with seborrheic eczema who had approximately 11% to 15% of their body surface area painted with magenta paint for 2 days.

POLYETHYLENE GLYCOL

Polyethylene glycols (PEGs; Carbowax, Macrogol) include several compounds with varying molecular weights (200–40,000 Da).[140] They are typically available as mixtures designated by a number denoting their average molecular weight. Polyethylene glycols are stable, hydrophilic substances, making them useful excipients for cosmetics and pharmaceuticals of all routes of administration (Table 46–8). Pegylation, a process that modifies the pharmacokinetics of therapeutic liposomes and proteins (eg, peginterferon-α), is the most recent application of PEG. At room temperature, PEGs with molecular weights less than 600 Da are clear, viscous liquids with a slight characteristic odor and bitter taste. Polyethylene glycols with molecular weights higher than 1,000 Da are soluble solids and range in consistency from pastes and waxy flakes to powders.[140] Commercially available products used for bowel-cleansing preparations and whole-bowel irrigation are solutions of PEG 3350 sometimes combined with electrolytes and known as PEG electrolyte lavage solution (Antidotes in Depth: A2).

The solid, high-molecular-weight PEGs are essentially nontoxic. Conversely, low-molecular-weight PEG exposures cause adverse effects similar to the chemically related toxic alcohols ethylene and diethylene glycol (Special Considerations: SC9).[30]

TABLE 46–8	Common Medications Containing PEG
Medication	*PEG Molecular Weight (Da)*
Etoposide injection	300
Lorazepam injection	400
Medroxyprogesterone depot	3,350
Mupirocin ointment	400, 3,350
PEG electrolyte lavage solution	3,350
Peginterferon α-2a	40,000

PEG = polyethylene glycol.

Pharmacokinetics

High-molecular-weight PEGs (>1,000 Da) are not significantly absorbed from the gastrointestinal tract, but low-molecular-weight PEGs are absorbed when taken orally.[49,156,157] Topical absorption also occurs when PEGs are applied to damaged skin.[24,163] Once in the systemic circulation, PEGs are mainly excreted unchanged in the urine;[49] however, low-molecular-weight PEGs (eg, PEG 300, PEG 400) are partially metabolized by alcohol dehydrogenase to hydroxyacid and diacid metabolites. The pharmacokinetics of intravenously administered PEG 3350 Da has not been studied; however, it did not appear to have any systemic effects when unintentionally given by this route.[145]

Nephrotoxicity

In rats fed various PEGs (200, 300, and 400) in their drinking water for 90 days, a solution of 8% PEG 200 produced renal tubular necrosis in all of the animals, followed by death within 15 days; however, a 4% PEG 200 solution resulted in only 2 of 9 rats dying within 80 days. A 16% PEG 400 solution killed all animals within 13 days; however, both 8% and 4% PEG 400 solutions had no observable effect except for a decrease in kidney weight when compared to control animals.[158] A canine study administering daily high-dose PEG 400 intravenously, up to 8.45 g/kg/day, failed to show serious renal toxicity. However, edema of kidney cells and increased glomerular volume occurred at these dosages, but were reversible.[105] Acute tubular necrosis was reported with oliguria, azotemia, and an anion gap metabolic acidosis following oral and topical exposures to low-molecular-weight PEGs (200 and 300). Acute kidney failure occurred in a 65-year-old man with a history of alcohol abuse and a seizure disorder after ingestion of the contents of a lava lamp containing 13% PEG 200.[51] About 48 hours after admission (approximately 50–72 hours post ingestion), the patient became oliguric with an anion gap metabolic acidosis and acute kidney failure. Blood sampling confirmed traces of the lava lamp fluid; none was detected in the urine. After clinical complications from ethanol withdrawal and aspiration pneumonitis, the patient was discharged 3 months later with residual kidney dysfunction attributed to the PEG component of the lamp contents. Acute tubular necrosis was noted at autopsy of 6 burn patients treated with a topical antibiotic cream in a PEG 300 base.[24,163] Mass spectrometry detected hydroxyacid and diacid metabolites in serum and urine samples. Oxalate crystals were seen in the urine of 2 cases. These effects were reproduced with the topical application of PEG for 7 days to rabbits with full-thickness skin defects.[163]

Neurotoxicity

There are reports of neurologic complications, such as paraplegia and transient bladder paralysis, following intrathecal corticosteroid injections containing 3% PEG as a vehicle.[15,19] In an in vitro experiment, rabbit vagus nerves were exposed to concentrations of PEG 3350 ranging from 3% to 40% for one hour.[15] A total of 3% and 10% PEG had no effect on nerve action potential amplitude or conduction velocity. Doses of 20% and 30% PEG significantly slowed nerve conduction and had varying effects on the amplitudes of action potentials. Forty percent PEG completely abolished action potentials. These changes were reversible and thought to be related to PEG-induced osmotic effects. The administration of PEG 1800 is a potential therapy for spinal cord injury by repairing damaged axons through cellular fusion of damaged cells following the short-term (2 minutes) application, in a guinea pig model. This increases compound action potential conduction.[154] Interestingly, administering a similar dose of PEG continuously for 25 minutes decreased compound action potentials approximately 64% in both damaged and nondamaged isolated mammalian spinal cords, suggesting dose-response toxicity.[38]

Another study in an ex vivo experiment of isolated injured spinal cords of Wistar rats showed combining hyperthermia (40°C) with various PEGs (400, 1000, and 2000) greatly improved compound action potential recovery compared to these PEGs at 25°C and 37°C. The lower-molecular-weight PEG 400 was the most effective. This occurs through PEG rapidly sealing damaged neuronal membranes.[95]

Fluid, Electrolyte, and Acid–Base Disturbances

Hyperosmolality was reported in 3 patients with burn surface areas ranging from 20% to 56% following repeated applications of Furacin, a topical antibiotic dressing containing 63% PEG 300, 32% PEG 4000, and 5% PEG 1000.[24] Polyethylene glycol produces an osmotic effect that is greater than expected for its molecular weight.[151] It is theorized that PEG increases osmolality by sequestering water through hydrogen binding, which reduces the availability of water to interact with solutes, thus increasing the chemical and osmotic activity of the solute. Hyperosmolality following the administration of a PEG-containing substance supports systemic PEG absorption.

Two cases of metabolic acidosis were reported following administration of therapeutic dosages of an intravenous nitrofurantoin solution containing PEG 300.[164] Similarly, an otherwise unexplained increased anion gap was reported in 3 patients being treated with a topical PEG-based burn cream.[24] Metabolism of the lower-molecular-weight PEGs by alcohol dehydrogenase to hydroxyacid and diacid metabolites explained the metabolic acidosis.[80]

PROPYLENE GLYCOL

$$\begin{array}{cc} OH & OH \\ | & | \\ CH_2 - CH & - CH_3 \end{array}$$

Propylene glycol (PG), or 1,2-propanediol, is a clear, colorless, odorless, sweet, viscous liquid employed in numerous pharmaceuticals (Table 46–9), foods, and cosmetics. Propylene glycol is used as a solvent and preservative with antiseptic properties similar to ethanol. The WHO has set the daily allowable intake of PG at a maximum of 25 mg/kg,[184] or 1.75 g/day for a 70-kg person.

Pharmacokinetics

Propylene glycol is rapidly absorbed from the gastrointestinal tract following oral administration and has a volume of distribution of approximately 0.6 L/kg.[118,160] When applied to intact epidermis, the absorption of PG is minimal. Percutaneous absorption occurs following application to damaged skin (eg, extensive burn surface areas). Approximately 12% to 45% of PG is excreted unchanged in the urine,[48] the remainder is hepatically metabolized sequentially by alcohol dehydrogenase to lactaldehyde, which is metabolized further by aldehyde dehydrogenase to lactic acid. Lactic acid is also formed by another metabolite, methylglyoxal.[131] Lactic acid is reduced to pyruvate catalyzed by lactate dehydrogenase.[131] The terminal half-life of propylene glycol is reported to be between 1.4 and 5.6 hours in adults and as long as 16.9 hours in neonates.[48,162]

Cardiovascular Toxicity

Intravenous preparations of phenytoin contain 40% PG to facilitate the dissolution of phenytoin. Nine years after intravenous phenytoin became available, several deaths were attributed to the rapid administration of phenytoin used for the treatment of cardiac dysrhythmias.[65,171,195]

Cardiovascular effects reported in these cases included hypotension, bradycardia, widening of the QRS complex, increased amplitude of T waves with occasional inversions, and transient ST segment elevations. Studies in cats[110] and calves[71] confirmed PG as the cardiotoxin. Bradycardia and depression of atrial conduction were not observed in cats pretreated with atropine, or in those with vagotomy following rapid intravenous infusion of PG, suggesting that these effects are vagally mediated.[110] Amplification of the QRS complex was noted in these same pretreated cats, also suggesting a direct cardiotoxic effect of PG. Similar results were reported in calves pretreated with atropine that received oxytetracycline in a PG vehicle.[71]

Neurotoxicity

Infants appear to have a decreased ability to clear PG when compared with older children and adults.[111] An increased frequency of seizures was reported in low-birth-weight infants who received 3 grams of PG daily in a parenteral multivitamin preparation.[111] Seizures developed in an 11-year-old boy receiving long-term oral therapy with vitamin D dissolved in PG.[8] Serum, electrolytes, and blood glucose were normal. Seizures abated after the product was discontinued. Propylene glycol possesses inebriating properties similar to ethanol. Central nervous system depression was reported following an intentional oral ingestion of a PG-containing product.[118]

A formerly available oral solution protease inhibitor amprenavir (Agenerase) had a black-box warning added to the product information for its high PG (550 mg/mL) vehicle content.[148] The recommended daily dosage of amprenavir supplied 1,650 mg/kg/day of PG. A 61-year-old man experienced visual hallucinations, disorientation, tinnitus, and vertigo after receiving a 750-mg dose (474 mg/kg PG) of amprenavir solution.[91]

Ototoxicity

Otic preparations contain up to 94% PG in solutions and 10% in suspensions as part of their vehicles.[54] In animal studies, application of high concentrations of PG (>10%) to the middle ear produced hearing impairment[124,125,178] and morphologic changes, including tympanic membrane perforation, middle ear adhesions, and cholesteatoma.[124,125,190] Although the effects of PG in the human middle ear have not been studied, all medications applied to the external ear canal are contraindicated in patients with perforated tympanic membranes.

Fluid, Electrolyte, and Acid–Base Disturbances

Patients receiving continuous or large intermittent quantities of medications containing PG develop high PG concentrations, particularly those with renal or hepatic insufficiency.[29,48] Propylene glycol–induced electrolyte and metabolic disturbances are evidenced by hyperosmolarity, and an elevated

TABLE 46–9	Propylene Glycol Concentration of Common Medications	
Medication (concentration)	Percent	Propylene Glycol Dose (g/dose volume)
Diazepam injection (5 mg/mL)	40	0.8 g/2 mL
Digoxin injection (250 mcg/mL)	40	0.8 g/2 mL
Etomidate (2mg/mL)	35	7 g/20 mL
Lorazepam injection (2 mg/mL, 4 mg/mL)	80	0.8 g/mL
Multivitamin injection	30	3 g/10 mL
Nitroglycerin injection (5 mg/mL)	30	3 g/10 mL
Pentobarbital sodium injection (50 mg/mL)	40	0.8 g/2 mL
Phenobarbital sodium injection (65 mg/mL, 130 mg/mL)	67.8	0.7 g/mL
Phenytoin injection (50 mg/mL)	40	0.8 g/2 mL
Trimethoprim-sulfamethoxazole injection (16–80 mg/mL)	40	2 g/5 mL

osmolar gap attributed to the osmotically active properties of PG. In most cases, both an elevated anion gap and elevated lactate concentration are present. Metabolic acidosis and hyperlactatemia result from PG metabolism.[28] These adverse effects are typically reported with intravenous preparations such as lorazepam,[7,76,86,192] diazepam,[186] etomidate,[174] nitroglycerin,[48] pentobarbital,[121] pediatric multivitamins,[67] and topical silver sulfadiazine.[13,55,98,185]

Systemic absorption of PG from topical application of silver sulfadiazine cream[55] resulted in hyperosmolality in patients with burn surface areas greater than 35% of their body.[13,55,98,185] In one study, 9 of 15 burn patients had osmolar gaps (>12) after application of the cream.[98] Similarly, a 3-year-old boy with extensive second- and third-degree burns over 60% body surface area developed a persistent elevated osmolar gap and metabolic acidosis with elevated lactate for approximately 20 days following application of silver sulfadiazine cream. Other potential etiologies were excluded. The osmolar gap and metabolic acidosis both resolved within 24 hours of discontinuing silver sulfadiazine.[185]

Hyperosmolarity occurred in 5 infants receiving a parenteral multivitamin that provided a daily PG dose of 3 g.[67] After 12 days, one premature infant had a PG concentration of 930 mg/dL and an osmolar gap of 136. Anion gap and lactic acid concentrations were normal. Eleven intubated children aged 1 to 15 months who were receiving continuous lorazepam infusions over 3 to 14 days accumulated serum PG concentrations of 17 to 226 mg/dL; however, increases in osmolar gap or serum lactate concentrations were not significantly different from baseline.[35] This was attributed to normal renal function and the low cumulative PG doses received (mean, 60 g).

A 72-year-old man died following the ingestion of the contents of a cold/hot therapy gel pack, which contained more than 99% of propylene glycol. Six hours after ingestion, he had an elevated osmolar gap accompanied by acute kidney injury. At 12 hours, he became comatose and an anion gap acidosis with a normal L-lactate concentration. He was found to have a very elevated D-lactate concentration, which was attributed to the PG ingestion. This patient had an extensive medical history and the course was complicated by multiorgan failure and death.[94]

Several small studies have found a strong correlation between elevated PG concentrations and increased osmolar gap measurements in critically ill patients receiving intravenous lorazepam and/or diazepam.[7,187,191,192] An osmolar gap greater than 10 is suggested as a marker for potential PG toxicity.[191] An osmolar gap of 20 corresponds to a serum PG concentration of approximately 48 mg/dL.[7] These authors provide a formula to estimate PG concentrations based on the osmolar gap: $[PG] = (-82.1 + [osmol\ gap \times 6.5])$. This equation should be used cautiously, as larger, more comprehensive studies are needed to validate it. In addition, elevated anion gap measurements and lactate concentrations occur. As PG toxicity mimics sepsis in these critically ill patients, sepsis should be excluded as the etiology of increased lactate, hypotension, and worsening renal function when considering PG toxicity. Hemodialysis is effective in removing PG and correcting acidemia. The administration of fomepizole should be considered with elevated PG concentrations to prevent further metabolism to lactic acid.[135,194]

Nephrotoxicity

Human proximal tubular cells exposed in vitro to PG concentrations of 500 to 2,000 mg/dL exhibited significant cellular injury and membrane damage within 15 minutes of exposure.[127] Repeated exposure for up to 6 days produced dose-dependent toxic effects at lower concentrations (76, 190, and 380 mg/dL).[126]

The chronic administration of PG contributes to proximal tubular cell damage and subsequent decreased kidney function. In a retrospective study of 8 patients who developed elevations in serum creatinine concentration while receiving continuous lorazepam infusions, serum creatinine rose within 3 to 60 days (median, 9 days).[192] The magnitude of serum creatinine rise was found to correlate with the serum PG concentration and duration of infusion. Serum creatinine decreased within 3 days of discontinuing the infusion. Patients with chronic kidney disease are at greater risk for accumulating PG because 45% of PG is eliminated unchanged by the kidneys;[48] the

remainder is metabolized by the liver. Caution should be used when prolonged administration of a PG-containing medication is necessary in the presence of renal or hepatic dysfunction.[127]

There are reports of propylene glycol–induced renal tubular necrosis. Daily PG vehicle dosages of 11 to 90 g/day over 14 days was associated with rising serum creatinine concentrations (0.7–2.1 mg/dL), elevated serum lactate concentrations, osmolar and anion gaps, and a serum PG concentration of 21 mg/dL.[193] Urine sediment analysis revealed numerous granular, muddy-brown-colored casts and no eosinophils, suggesting an acute renal tubular necrosis. Kidney biopsy and electron microscopy showed extensive dilation of the proximal renal tubules, with swollen epithelial cells and mitochondria. Numerous vacuoles containing debris were also noted. A kidney biopsy of another case with a serum PG concentration of 30 mg/dL showed disrupted brush borders of the proximal renal tubules after a sudden rise in serum creatinine concentration (3.1 mg/dL), nonoliguric kidney failure, and metabolic acidosis. This was attributed to an average daily PG dose of 70 g for 17 days.[76]

SORBITOL

Sorbitol (D-glucitol) is widely used in the pharmaceutical industry as a sweetener, moistening agent, and as a diluent (Table 46–10). Sorbitol occurs naturally in the ripe berries of many fruits, trees, and plants, and was first isolated in 1872 from the berries of the European mountain ash (Sorbus aucuparia).[129] It is particularly useful in chewable tablets because of its pleasant taste. In addition, it is widely used by the food industry in chewing gums, dietetic candies, foods, and enteral nutrition formulations. Sorbitol is approximately 50% to 60% as sweet as sucrose.[129]

Pharmacokinetics

Unlike sucrose, sorbitol is not readily fermented by oral microorganisms and is poorly absorbed from the gastrointestinal tract. Any absorbed sorbitol is metabolized in the liver to fructose and glucose.[129] Sorbitol has a caloric value of 4 kcal/g and is better tolerated by diabetics than sucrose; however, because some of it is metabolized to glucose, it is not unconditionally safe for people with diabetes and is obviously not "dietetic."[129]

TABLE 46–10	Common Medications Containing Sorbitol	
Medication (concentration)	**Percent**	**Sorbitol Dose (g/dose volume)**
Amantadine syrup (10 mg/mL)	64	6.4 g/10 mL
Calcium carbonate suspension (250 mg/mL)	28	1.4 g/5 mL
Carbamazepine syrup (20 mg/mL)	17	0.85 g/5 mL
Cimetidine syrup (60 mg/mL)	46	2.3 g/5 mL
Digoxin elixir (50 mcg/mL)	21	1 g/5 mL
Ferrous sulfate infant drops (15 mg/mL)	31	0.3 g/mL
Furosemide solution (8 mg/mL)	35	1.75 g/5 mL
Methadone HCl solution (1 mg/mL, 2 mg/mL)	14	0.7 g/5 mL
Potassium chloride solution (1.33 mEq/mL)	17.5	2.6 g/15 mL
Pseudoephedrine liquid (3 mg/mL, 6mg/mL)	35	1.75 g/5 mL

There is a concern of potentially fatal toxicity for individuals with hereditary fructose intolerance (HFI) receiving sorbitol-containing xenobiotics.[56] Hereditary fructose intolerance is an autosomal recessive disorder caused by a deficiency of fructose-1,6-bisphosphonate aldolase in the liver, kidney, cortex, and small intestine.[93] This results in the accumulation of fructose-1-phosphate, which prevents glycogen breakdown and glucose synthesis causing hypoglycemia. The prevalence of HFI is most commonly reported to be one in 20,000 persons, but can range between one in 11,000 and one in 100,000.[2,90,93]

There are reports of death following the prolonged administration of sorbitol, fructose, or sucrose in individuals with HFI.[39,152] Dietary exclusion of fructose, sucrose, and sorbitol prevents the adverse effects. This condition should not be confused with the more common disorder of dietary fructose intolerance, which is caused by a defect in the glucose-transport protein 5 system. This defect leads to the breakdown of fructose to carbon dioxide, hydrogen, and short-chain fatty acids by colonic bacteria, resulting in abdominal pain and bloating.[102] This latter syndrome is a potential cause of chronic abdominal pain in childhood.[69] Dietary fructose intolerance symptoms are minimized by limiting sorbitol, fructose, and sucrose in the diet.

Gastrointestinal Toxicity

In large dosages, sorbitol causes abdominal cramping, bloating, flatulence, vomiting, and diarrhea. Sorbitol exerts its cathartic effects by its osmotic properties, resulting in fluid shifts within the gastrointestinal tract. Iatrogenic osmotic diarrhea is reported following administration of many different liquid medication formulations containing sorbitol.[82,112] In a human volunteer study, 42 healthy adults ingested 10 g of a sorbitol solution. Sorbitol intolerance was detected in up to 55% of participants.[89] One theoretical explanation for why all participants did not experience the gastrointestinal adverse effects is unrecognized dietary fructose intolerance. Diarrhea resulting from sorbitol-containing medications is common and often overlooked as a possible etiology.[56,82] Ingestion of large quantities of sorbitol (>20 g/day in adults) is not recommended (Antidotes in Depth: A2).[129]

THIMEROSAL

Thimerosal (Merthiolate, Mercurothiolate), or sodium ethylmercurithiosalicylate, is an organic mercury compound that is approximately 49% elemental mercury (Hg°) by weight.[147,179] It is metabolized to ethylmercury and thiosalicylate. Thimerosal has a wide spectrum of antibacterial activity at concentrations ranging from 0.01% to 0.1%; however, higher concentrations are sometimes also used topically as an antiseptic.[123,147] Thimerosal has been widely used as a preservative since the 1930s in contact lens solutions, biologics, and vaccines, particularly those in multidose containers (Table 46–11). The use of thimerosal, which is necessary for the production process of some vaccines (eg, pertussis, influenza), leaves trace amounts in the final product.[11] High-dose thimerosal exposure resulted in neurotoxicity and nephrotoxicity. Although concerns exist regarding infant exposure to low-dose thimerosal through vaccinations and its effects on neurodevelopment, including possible links to causes of autism,[18] these concerns are unfounded (Chap. 95).[46]

Because specific guidelines for ethylmercury exposure have not been developed, regulatory guidelines for dietary methylmercury exposure were applied to monitor ethylmercury exposure from injected thimerosal-containing vaccines. Methylmercury is a similar, but more toxic, organic mercury compound (Chap. 95). Maximum daily recommended methylmercury exposures range from 0.1 mcg Hg/kg (US Environmental Protection Agency {EPA}) to 0.47 mcg Hg/kg (WHO).[3,32,37]

An FDA review of thimerosal-containing vaccines revealed that some infants, depending on the immunization schedule, vaccine formulations,

TABLE 46–11 Thimerosal Concentration of Common Medications

Medication	Percent	Dose (mg)
Injectable		
Antivenom (crotaline polyvalent immune) Fab	0.005	0.03 (per vial)
Antivenom (*Latrodectus mactans*)	0.01	0.25 (per vial)
Antivenom (*Micrurus fulvius*)	0.005	0.5 (per vial)
Diphtheria and tetanus toxoids[a]	Trace	<0.3 mcg
Influenza virus vaccine[b] (various)	0.01	0.025
Meningococcal vaccine-A/C/Y/W-135[b]	0.01	0.025
Topical		
Flurbiprofen ophthalmic solution	0.005	—
Neosporin (triple antibiotic) ophthalmic solution	0.001	—
Thimerosal tincture	0.1	—

[a]Trace defined by the US Food and Drug Administration as <1 mcg mercury each dose. [b]Multidose vials only.

and infant's weight, might be exceeding the EPA exposure limit of 0.1 mcg Hg/kg/day for methylmercury. Over the first 6 months of life, a total cumulative dose of up to 187.5 mcg Hg total from thimerosal-containing vaccines was possible. The US Public Health Service and the American Academy of Pediatrics jointly responded by recommending the preemptive reduction or removal of thimerosal from vaccines wherever possible.[3,31] The WHO and European regulatory bodies have similar recommendations.[57] To date, thimerosal has been removed from most US-licensed immunoglobulin products. All vaccines routinely recommended for children younger than 7 years are either thimerosal-free or contain only trace amounts (<0.5 mcg Hg/dose), with the exception of some inactivated influenza vaccines. Multidose vials requiring thimerosal preservative remain important for immunization programs in developing countries because of a lack of ability to consistently refrigerate vaccines. Although efforts continue to eliminate all sources of mercury exposure, complete elimination of thimerosal from all vaccines is unlikely in the near future.[11] When a thimerosal-containing vaccine is the only alternative, the benefits of vaccination far exceed any theoretical risk of mercury toxicity.[130]

Prior to thimerosal use in pharmaceuticals, evidence for its safety and effectiveness was provided in several animal species and in 22 humans.[139] Only limited data exist on infant mercury exposure from thimerosal-containing vaccines. Clinical studies that assess the effects of thimerosal exposure on neurodevelopment and renal and immunologic function are lacking. Based on a comprehensive review of epidemiologic data from the United States,[36,60,63,167,179] Denmark,[114,115] Sweden,[161] and the United Kingdom,[6,81] the Institute of Medicine's Immunization Safety Review Committee,[130] the Global Advisory Committee on Vaccine Safety,[189] and the European Agency for the Evaluation of Medicinal Products[52] have all concluded that no causal relationship exists between thimerosal-containing vaccines and autism. Continued surveillance of autistic spectrum disorders as thimerosal use declines will be conducted to evaluate any associated trends.

Pharmacokinetics

Limited pharmacokinetic data exist for thimerosal and ethylmercury. Once absorbed, thimerosal breaks down to form ethylmercury and thiosalicylate. Some ethylmercury further decomposes into inorganic mercury in the blood, and the remainder distributes into kidney and, to a lesser extent, brain tissue.[114,115] Because of its longer organic chain, ethylmercury is less stable and decomposes more rapidly than methylmercury, leaving less ethylmercury available to enter kidney and brain tissue.[114] Ethylmercury crosses the blood–brain barrier by passive diffusion.[115] Intracellular ethylmercury decomposes to inorganic mercury, which accumulates in kidney and brain tissues.[115] The half-life of thimerosal is estimated to be about 18 days.[115] Thimerosal is eliminated in the feces as inorganic mercury (Chap. 95).[138]

Mercury or Thimerosal Toxicity

Oral Administration

A case report described a 44-year-old man who ingested 5 g (83 mg/kg) of thimerosal in a suicide attempt; within 15 minutes, he began vomiting spontaneously. Gastric lavage was performed and chelation therapy begun with dimercaptopropane sulfonate. Gastroscopy revealed a hemorrhagic gastritis. Acute kidney injury was noted on the day of admission and persisted for 40 days. Four days after admission, the patient developed fever and a maculopapular exanthem attributed to thimerosal. The patient also developed an autonomic and ascending peripheral polyneuropathy that persisted for 13 days. Chelation therapy was continued for a total of 50 days with dimercaptopropane sulfonate followed by succimer. Elevated blood and urine mercury concentrations persisted for more than 140 days. The patient was discharged 148 days following the ingestion with only sensory defects in his toes. No other neurologic sequelae were noted.[137]

Oral absorption of thimerosal resulted in the fatal poisoning of an 18-month-old girl from the intra-otic instillation of a solution containing 0.1% thimerosal and 0.14% sodium borate. Tympanostomy tubes placed one year earlier allowed the irrigation solution to flow through the auditory tube into the nasopharynx, and subsequently to be swallowed and absorbed through the oral mucosa and gastrointestinal tract. A total of 1.2 L of solution (500 mg Hg) was instilled over a 4-week period, resulting in severe mercury poisoning. Four days after admission, the serum mercury concentration was 163 mcg/dL. The patient also received 1.7 g of boric acid. It is unclear what contribution, if any, the boric acid made to the serum mercury concentration. Chelation therapy with *N*-acetyl-D-penicillamine was initiated on day 51. Despite increased urinary mercury concentrations following administration of the *N*-acetyl-D-penicillamine, her neurologic function and blood mercury concentrations remained unchanged. The child died 3 months after admission. An autopsy was not performed.[147]

Intramuscular Administration

Urine mercury concentrations of 26 patients with hypogammaglobinemia, who received weekly intramuscular immunoglobulin G (IgG) replacement therapy preserved with 0.01% thimerosal, were studied. The dosages of IgG ranged from 25 to 50 mg/kg, containing 0.6 to 1.2 mg of mercury per dose.[72] The total estimated dose of mercury administered ranged from 4 to 734 mg over a period of 6 months to 17 years. Urine mercury concentrations were elevated in 19 patients, ranging from 31 to 75 mcg/L; however, no patients had clinical evidence of chronic mercury toxicity.[72]

Six cases of severe mercury poisoning resulting in 4 deaths were reported following the intramuscular administration of chloramphenicol preserved with thimerosal. A manufacturing error produced vials containing 510 mg of thimerosal (250 mg Hg) instead of 0.51 mg per vial. Two adults received 4 and 5.5 g of mercury each and 4 children received 0.2 to 1.8 g each. All 6 patients had extensive tissue necrosis at the site of injection. Fever, altered mental status, slurred speech, and ataxia were noted. Autopsy identified widespread degeneration and necrosis of the renal tubules; however, creatine kinase concentrations were not reported, so pigment-induced nephrotoxicity cannot be excluded. Elevated mercury concentrations were found in the injection site tissues, and in the kidneys, livers, and brains.[9]

Topical Administration

Thirteen infants were exposed to 9 to 48 topical applications of a 0.1% thimerosal tincture for the treatment of exomphalos. Analysis for elevated mercury concentrations was performed in 10 of 13 infants who unexpectedly died. Mercury concentrations were determined in various tissues from 6 of the infants. Mean tissue concentrations in fresh samples of liver, kidney, spleen, and heart ranged from 5,152 to 11,330 ppb, suggesting percutaneous absorption from these repeated topical applications.[53]

Ophthalmic Administration

Nine patients undergoing keratoplasty were exposed to a contact lens stored in a solution containing 0.002% thimerosal.[188] After 4 hours, the lens was removed and mercury concentrations of the aqueous humor and excised corneal tissues were determined. Mercury concentrations were elevated in both aqueous humor (range, 20–46 ng/mL higher) and corneal tissues (range, 0.6–14 ng/mL higher) as compared with eyes that had not been fitted with contact lenses. Only residual amounts of mercury remained on the contact lenses after 4 hours of wear. The authors noted that although the aqueous humor concentrations were in the same range as those measured in 10 patients with vision loss from systemic mercury poisoning (11–104 ng/mL), adverse effects did not occur.

A possible drug interaction between orally administered tetracyclines and thimerosal was reported to result in acute, varying degrees of eye irritation in contact lens wearers using thimerosal-containing contact lens solutions who started treatment with tetracycline.[42]

SUMMARY

- The benefits of pharmaceutical excipients include improved xenobiotic solubility, stability, and palatability, antimicrobial activity, the availability of various dosage forms, the provision of products with long-term storage, and the availability of multiple-dose packaging. Although excipients are essential and effective, they are suggested to possess no pharmacologic or toxicologic properties but are actually responsible for severe—and sometimes fatal—adverse effects.

- The toxicity of pharmaceutical excipients should be evaluated in patients requiring high doses or prolonged administration of any medication containing excipients, particularly those additives known to have toxicities.

- Under circumstances in which there is no option but to continue treating a patient with a particular xenobiotic, switching to a preservative-free product, or to another brand without the offending excipient, should obviate the need for discontinuation of an effective xenobiotic. In addition to inherent toxicities, many excipients are also responsible for allergic reactions.

- In the majority of cases, pharmaceutical excipients are safe and effective, and their benefits far exceed their potential for adverse effects when properly administered.

REFERENCES

1. Alade SL, et al. Polysorbate 80 and E-Ferol toxicity. *Pediatrics*. 1986;77:593-597.
2. Ali M, et al. Hereditary fructose intolerance. *J Med Genet*. 1998;35:353-365.
3. American Academy of Pediatrics, Committee on Infectious Diseases and Committee on Environmental Health. Thimerosal in vaccines—an interim report to clinicians (RE9935). *Pediatrics*. 1999;104:570-574.
4. Ammar DA, et al. Effects of benzalkonium chloride-preserved, Polyquad-preserved, and SofZia-preserved topical glaucoma medications on human ocular epithelial cells. *Adv Ther*. 2010;27:837-845.
5. Ammar DA, et al. Effects of benzalkonium chloride and Polyquad-preserved combination glaucoma medications on cultured human ocular surface cells. *Adv Ther*. 2011;28:501-510.
6. Andrews N, et al. Thimerosal exposure in infants and developmental disorders. A retrospective cohort study in the United Kingdom does not support a causal association. *Pediatrics*. 2004;114:584-591.
7. Arroliga AC, et al. Relationship of continuous infusion lorazepam to serum propylene glycol concentration in critically ill adults. *Crit Care Med*. 2004;32:1709-1714.
8. Arulanantham K, Genel M. Central nervous system toxicity associated with ingestion of propylene glycol. *J Pediatr*. 1978;93:515-516.
9. Axton JH. Six cases of poisoning after parenteral organic mercurial compound (Merthiolate). *Postgrad Med J*. 1972;48:417-421.
10. Bagshawe KD, et al. Intrathecal methotrexate. *Lancet*. 1969;2:1258.
11. Ball LK, et al. An assessment of thimerosal use in childhood vaccines. *Pediatrics*. 2001;107:1147-1154.
12. Barr L, et al. Measurement of paraben concentrations in human breast tissue at serial locations across the breast from axilla to sternum. *J Appl Toxicol*. 2012;32:219-232.
13. Bekeris L, et al. Propylene glycol as a cause of an elevated serum osmolality. *Am J Clin Pathol*. 1979;72:633-636.
14. Benda GI, et al. Benzyl alcohol toxicity. Impact on neurologic handicaps among surviving very-low-birth-weight infants. *Pediatrics*. 1986;77:507-512.
15. Benzon HT, et al. The effect of polyethylene glycol on mammalian nerve impulses. *Anesth Analg*. 1987;66:553-559.
16. Berg ØH, et al. The effect of a benzalkonium chloride-containing nasal spray on human respiratory mucosa in vitro as a function of concentration and time of action. *Pharmacol Toxicol*. 1995;76:245-249.

17. Berg ØH, et al. The effects of topical nasal steroids on rat respiratory mucosa in vivo, with special reference to benzalkonium chloride. *Allergy.* 1997;52:627-632.
18. Bernard S, et al. Autism. A novel form of mercury poisoning. *Med Hypotheses.* 2001;56:462-471.
19. Bernat JL. Intraspinal steroid therapy. *Neurology.* 1981;31:168-171.
20. Borody T, et al. Chlorobutanol toxicity and dependence. *Med J Aust.* 1979;1:288.
21. Botta SA, et al. Cardiac arrhythmias in phenol face peeling: a suggested protocol for prevention. *Aesth Plast Surg.* 1988;12:115-117.
22. Bowie MD, McKenzie D. Diethylene glycol poisoning in children. *S Afr Med J.* 1972;46:931-934.
23. Brown WJ, et al. Fatal benzyl alcohol poisoning in a neonatal intensive care unit. *Lancet.* 1982;1:1250.
24. Bruns DE, et al. Polyethylene glycol intoxication in burn patients. *Burns.* 1982;9:49-52.
25. Brunson EL. Benzyl alcohol. In: Rowe RC, et al, eds. *Handbook of Pharmaceutical Excipients.* 4th ed. Washington, DC: American Pharmaceutical Association; 2003:53-55.
26. Buszello K, Muller BW. Emulsions as drug delivery systems. In: Nielloud F, Marti-Mestres G, eds. *Drugs and the Pharmaceutical Sciences. Pharmaceutical Emulsions and Suspensions.* New York, NY: Marcel Dekker; 2000:191-224.
27. Calvery HO, Klumpp TG. The toxicity for human beings of diethylene glycol with sulfanilamide. *South Med J.* 1939;32:1105-1109.
28. Cate JC, Hedrick R. Propylene glycol intoxication and lactic acidosis. *N Engl J Med.* 1980;303:1237.
29. Cawley MJ. Short-term lorazepam infusion and concern for propylene glycol toxicity. Case report and review. *Pharmacotherapy.* 2001;21:1140-1144.
30. Centers for Disease Control and Prevention. Fatalities associated with ingestion of diethylene glycol-contaminated glycerin used to manufacture acetaminophen syrup—Haiti, November 1995–June 1996. *MMWR Morb Mortal Wkly Rep.* 1996;45:649-650.
31. Centers for Disease Control and Prevention. Recommendations regarding the use of vaccines that contain thimerosal as preservative. *MMWR Morb Mortal Wkly Rep.* 1999;48:996-998.
32. Centers for Disease Control and Prevention. Thimerosal in vaccines. A joint statement of the American Academy of Pediatrics and the Public Health Service. *MMWR Morb Mortal Wkly Rep.* 1999;48:563-565.
33. Chassany O, et al. Drug-induced diarrhoea. *Drug Saf.* 2000;22:53-72.
34. Chen J, et al. Antiandrogenic properties of parabens and other phenolic containing small molecules in personal care products. *Toxicol Appl Pharmacol.* 2007;221:278-284.
35. Chicella M, et al. Propylene glycol accumulation associated with continuous infusion of lorazepam in pediatric intensive care patients. *Crit Care Med.* 2002;30:2752-2756.
36. Clements CJ. The evidence for the safety of thiomersal in newborn and infant vaccines. *Vaccine.* 2004;22:1854-1861.
37. Clements CJ, et al. Thiomersal in vaccines. *Lancet.* 2000;355:1279-1280.
38. Cole A, Shi R. Prolonged focal application of polyethylene glycol induces conduction block in guinea pig spinal cord white matter. *Toxicol in Vitro.* 2005;19:215-220.
39. Collins J. Time for fructose solutions to go. *Lancet.* 1993;341:600.
40. Conway V, Mulski M. Phenol. In: Rowe RC, et al, eds. *Handbook of Pharmaceutical Excipients.* 4th ed. Washington, DC: American Pharmaceutical Association; 2003:426-428.
41. Craig DB, Habib GG. Flaccid paraparesis following obstetrical epidural anesthesia. Possible role of benzyl alcohol. *Anesth Analg.* 1977;56:219-221.
42. Crook TG, Freeman JJ. Reactions induced by the concurrent use of thimerosal and tetracycline. *Am J Optom Physiol Optics.* 1983;60:759-761.
43. Cukier JO, et al. The displacement of albumin bound bilirubin by gentamicin. *Pediatr Res.* 1974;8:399.
44. Dagher Z, et al. *p*-Hydroxybenzoate esters metabolism in MCF7 breast cancer cells. *Food Chem Toxicol.* 2012;50:4109-4114.
45. Darbre PD, Harvey PW. Paraben esters: review of recent studies of endocrine toxicity, absorption, esterase and human exposure, and discussion of potential human health risks. *J Appl Toxicol.* 2008;28:561-578.
46. Davidson PW, et al. Mercury exposure and child development outcomes. *Pediatrics.* 2004;113:1023-1029.
47. DeChristoforro R, et al. High-dose morphine complicated by chlorobutanol-somnolence. *Ann Intern Med.* 1983;98:335-336.
48. Demey HE, et al. Propylene glycol induced side effects during intravenous nitroglycerin therapy. *Intensive Care Med.* 1988;14:221-226.
49. DiPiro JT, et al. Absorption of polyethylene glycol after administration of a PEG-electrolyte lavage solution. *Clin Pharm.* 1986;5:153-155.
50. Epstein SP, et al. Comparative toxicity of preservatives on immortalized corneal and conjunctival epithelial cells. *J Ocul Pharmacol Ther.* 2009;25:113-119.
51. Erickson TB, et al. Acute renal toxicity after ingestion of lava light liquid. *Ann Emerg Med.* 1996;27:781-784.
52. European Agency for the Evaluation of Medicinal Products. EMEA public statement on thiomersal in vaccines for human use-recent evidence supports safety of thimerosal-containing vaccines. http://www.ema.europa.eu/docs/en_GB/document_library/Scientific_guideline/2009/09/WC500003904.pdf. Accessed May 15, 2014.
53. Fagan DG, et al. Organ mercury levels in infant with omphaloceles treated with organic mercurial antiseptic. *Arch Dis Child.* 1977;52:962-964.
54. FDA Center for Drug Evaluation and Research. Inactive ingredient guide (redacted) January 1996. http://www.fda.gov/cder/drug/iig/default.htm. Accessed February 24, 2005.
55. Fligner CL, et al. Hyperosmolality induced by propylene glycol, a complication of silver sulfadiazine therapy. *JAMA.* 1985;253:1606-1609.
56. Florence AT, Salole EG, eds. *Formulation Factors in Adverse Reactions.* London: Wright; 1990:11.
57. Freed GL, et al. Vaccine safety policy analysis in three European countries. The case of thimerosal. *Health Policy.* 2002;62:291-307.
58. Garnacho-Montero J, et al. Effects of three intravenous lipid emulsions on the survival and mononuclear phagocytes function of septic rats. *Nutrition.* 2002;18:751-754.
59. Gassett AR. Benzalkonium chloride toxicity to the human cornea. *Am J Ophthalmol.* 1977;84:169-171.
60. Geier DA, Geier MR. A comparative evaluation of the effects of MMR immunization and mercury doses from thimerosal-containing childhood vaccines on the population prevalence of autism. *Med Sci Monit.* 2004;10:PI33-PI39.
61. Geier DA, Geier MR. An assessment of the impact of thimerosal on childhood neurodevelopmental disorders. *Pediatr Rehabil.* 2003;6:97-102.
62. Geier DA, Geier MR. Thimerosal in childhood vaccines, neurodevelopmental disorders, and heart disease in the United States. *J Am Phys Surg.* 2003;8:6-11.
63. Geier MR, Geier DA. Neurodevelopmental disorders after thimerosal containing vaccines. A brief communication. *Exp Biol Med (Maywood).* 2003;228:660-664.
64. Geiling EM, Cannon PR. Pathologic effects of elixir of sulfanilamide (diethylene glycol) poisoning. *JAMA.* 1938;111:919-926.
65. Gellerman GL, Martinez C. Fatal ventricular fibrillation following intravenous sodium diphenylhydantoin therapy. *JAMA.* 1967;200:337-338.
66. Gershanik J, et al. The gasping syndrome and benzyl alcohol poisoning. *N Engl J Med.* 1982;307:1384-1388.
67. Glasgow AM, et al. Hyperosmolality in small infants due to propylene glycol. *Pediatrics.* 1983;72:353-355.
68. Glover ML, Reed MD. Propylene glycol. The safe diluent that continues to cause harm. *Pharmacotherapy.* 1996;16:690-693.
69. Gomara RE, et al. Fructose intolerance in children in children presenting with abdominal pain. *J Pediatr Gastroenterol Nutr.* 2008;47:303-308.
70. Gross BG. Cardiac arrhythmias during phenol face peeling. *Plast Reconstr Surg.* 1984;73:590-594.
71. Gross DR, et al. Cardiovascular effects of intravenous administration of propylene glycol and oxytetracycline in propylene glycol in calves. *Am J Vet Res.* 1979;40:783-791.
72. Haeney MR, et al. Long-term parenteral exposure to mercury in patients with hypogammaglobulinaemia. *Br Med J.* 1979;2:12-14.
73. Hagebusch OE. Necropsies of four patients following administration of elixir sulfanilamide—Massengill. *JAMA.* 1937;109:1537-1539.
74. Hahn AF, et al. Paraparesis following intrathecal chemotherapy. *Neurology.* 1983;33:1032-1038.
75. Hanif M, et al. Fatal renal failure by diethylene glycol in paracetamol elixir. The Bangladesh epidemic. *BMJ.* 1995;311:88-91.
76. Hansen L, et al. Development and evaluation of a guideline for monitoring propylene glycol toxicity in pediatric intensive care unit patients receiving continuous infusion lorazepam. *J Pediatr Pharmacol Ther.* 2015;20:367-372.
77. Harvey PW, Everett DJ. Parabens detection in different zones of the human breast: consideration of source and implications of findings. *J Appl Toxicol.* 2012;32:305-309.
78. Hayman M, et al. Acute tubular necrosis associated with propylene glycol from concomitant administration of intravenous lorazepam and trimethoprim-sulfamethoxazole. *Pharmacotherapy.* 2003;23:1190-1194.
79. Henley E. Sorbitol-based elixirs, diarrhea and enteral tube feeding. *Am Fam Physician.* 1997;55:2084-2086.
80. Herold DA, et al. Oxidation of polyethylene glycols by alcohol dehydrogenase. *Biochem Pharmacol.* 1989;38:73-76.
81. Heron J, Golding J; ALSPAC Study Team. Thimerosal exposure in infants and developmental disorders. A prospective cohort study in the United Kingdom does not support a causal association. *Pediatrics.* 2004;114:577-583.
82. Hill DB, et al. Osmotic diarrhea by sugar-free theophylline solution in critically ill patients. *J Parenter Enteral Nutr.* 1991;15:332-334.
83. Hiller JL, et al. Benzyl alcohol toxicity. Impact on mortality and intraventricular hemorrhage among very-low birth-weight infants. *Pediatrics.* 1986;77:500-506.
84. Ho CY, et al. In vitro effects of preservatives in nasal sprays on human nasal epithelial cells. *Am J Rhinol.* 2008;22:125-129.
85. Hofmann T, et al. Influence of preservatives and topical steroids on ciliary beat frequency in vitro. *Arch Otolaryngol Head Neck Surg.* 2004;130:440-445.
86. Horinek EL, et al. Propylene glycol accumulation in critically ill patients receiving continuous intravenous lorazepam infusions. *Ann Pharmacother.* 2009;43:1964-1971.
87. http://www.washingtonpost.com/wp-dyn/content/article/2009/02/06/AR2009020601160_2.html. Accessed May 15, 2014. Nigeria: 84 children dead from teething formula.
88. Hviid A, et al. Association between thimerosal containing vaccine and autism. *JAMA.* 2003;290:1763-1766.
89. Jain NK, et al. Sorbitol intolerance in adults. *Am J Gastroenterol.* 1985;80:678-681.
90. James CL, et al. Neonatal screening for HFI. Frequency of the most common mutant aldolase B allele (A149P) in the British population. *J Med Genet.* 1996;33:837-841.
91. James CW, et al. Central nervous system toxicity and amprenavir oral solution. *Ann Pharmacother.* 2001;35:174.

92. Jiao J, et al. The effect of topical corticosteroids, topical antihistamines, and preservatives on human ciliary beat frequency. *ORL J Otorhinolaryngol Relat Spec.* 2014;76:127-136.

93. Jorde LB, et al. Biochemical genetics. Disorders of metabolism. In: Jorde LB, et al, eds. *Medical Genetics.* 2nd ed. St. Louis, MO: Mosby; 2000:136-155.

94. Jorens PG, et al. Unusual D-lactic acid acidosis from propylene glycol metabolism in overdose. *J Toxicol Clin Toxicol.* 2004;42:163-169.

95. Kouhzaei S, et al. The neuroprotective ability of polyethylene glycol is affected by temperature in ex vivo spinal cord injury model. *J Membr Biol.* 2013;246:613-619.

96. Kibbe AH. Benzalkonium chloride. In: Rowe RC, et al, eds. *Handbook of Pharmaceutical Excipients.* 4th ed. Washington, DC: American Pharmaceutical Association; 2003:45-47.

97. Kibbe AH, Weller PJ. Thimerosal. In: Rowe RC, et al, eds. *Handbook of Pharmaceutical Excipients.* 4th ed. Washington, DC: American Pharmaceutical Association; 2003:648-650.

98. Kulick MI, et al. Hyperosmolality in the burn patient. Analysis of an osmolal discrepancy. *J Trauma.* 1980;20:223-228.

99. Kuoyama Y, et al. Nasal lesion induced by intranasal administration of benzalkonium chloride in rats. *J Toxicol Sci.* 1997;22:153-160.

100. Labbe A, et al. Comparison of toxicological profiles of benzalkonium chloride and polyquaternium-1: an experimental study. *J Ocul Pharmacol Ther.* 2006;22:267-278.

101. Landau M. Cardiac complications in deep chemical peels. *Dermatol Surg.* 2007;33:190-193.

102. Ledochowski M, et al. Fructose and sorbitol-reduced diet improves mood and gastrointestinal disturbances in fructose malabsorbers. *Scand J Gastroenterol.* 2000;35:1048-1052.

103. Lekka ME, et al. The impact of intravenous fat emulsion administration in acute lung injury. *Am J Respir Crit Care Med.* 2004;169:638-644.

104. Lemp MA, Zimmerman LE. Toxic endothelial degeneration in ocular surface disease treated with topical medications containing benzalkonium chloride. *Am J Ophthalmol.* 1988;105:670-673.

105. Li BQ, et al. Systemic toxicity and toxicokinetics of a high dose of polyethylene glycol 400 in dogs following intravenous injection. *Drug Chem Toxicol.* 2011;34:208.

106. Liu H, et al. Toxic endothelial cell destruction from intraocular benzalkonium chloride. *J Cataract Refract Surg.* 2001;27:1746-1750.

107. Lopez-Herce J, et al. Benzyl alcohol poisoning following diazepam intravenous infusion. *Ann Pharmacother.* 1995;29:632.

108. Lorenzetti OJ, Wernet TC. Topical parabens. Benefits and risks. *Dermatologica.* 1977;154:244-250.

109. Loria CJ, et al. Effect of antibiotic formulations in serum protein. Bilirubin interaction of newborn infants. *J Pediatr.* 1976;89:479-482.

110. Louis S, et al. The cardiovascular changes caused by intravenous Dilantin and its solvent. *Am Heart J.* 1967;74:523-529.

111. MacDonald MG, et al. Propylene glycol. Increased incidence of seizures in low-birth-weight infants. *Pediatrics.* 1987;79:622-625.

112. Madigan SM, et al. The solution was the problem. *Clin Nutr.* 2002;21:531-532.

113. Madsen KM, et al. Thimerosal and the occurrence of autism. Negative ecological evidence from Danish population-based data. *Pediatrics.* 2003;112:604-606.

114. Magos L. Neurotoxic character of thimerosal and the allometric extrapolation of adult clearance half-time to infants. *J Appl Toxicol.* 2003;23:263-269.

115. Magos L, et al. The comparative toxicology of ethyl and methylmercury. *Arch Toxicol.* 1985;57:260-297.

116. Malinovsky JM, et al. Ketamine and midazolam neurotoxicity in the rabbit. *Anesthesiology.* 1991;75:91-97.

117. Malinovsky JM, et al. Is ketamine or its preservative responsible for neurotoxicity in the rabbit? *Anesthesiology.* 1993;78:109-115.

118. Martin G, Finberg L. Propylene glycol. A potentially toxic vehicle in liquid dosage form. *J Pediatr.* 1970;77:877-878.

119. Martone WJ, et al. Illness with fatalities in premature infants. Association with intravenous vitamin E preparation, E-Ferol. *Pediatrics.* 1986;78:591-600.

120. Miles JM, et al. Metabolic and neurologic effects of an intravenous medium-chain triglyceride emulsion. *JPEN J Parenter Enteral Nutr.* 1991;15:37-41.

121. Miller MA, et al. Propylene glycol-induced lactic acidosis in a patient receiving continuous infusion pentobarbital. *Ann Pharmacother.* 2008;42:1502-1506.

122. Miller B, et al. Potentiation of NMDA receptor currents by arachidonic acid. *Nature.* 1992;355:722-725.

123. Möller H. Merthiolate allergy. A nationwide iatrogenic sensitization. *Acta Derm Venereol.* 1977;57:509-517.

124. Morizono T. Toxicity of ototopical drugs. Animal modeling. *Ann Otol Rhinol Laryngol Suppl.* 1990;148:42-45.

125. Morizono T, et al. Ototoxicity of propylene glycol in experimental animals. *Am J Otolaryngol.* 1980;1:393-399.

126. Morshed KM, et al. Propylene glycol-mediated injury in a primary cell culture of human proximal tubule cells. *Toxicol Sci.* 1998;46:410-417.

127. Morshed KM, et al. Acute toxicity of propylene glycol. An assessment using cultured proximal tubule cells of human origin. *Fundam Appl Toxicol.* 1994;23:38-43.

128. Nash RA. Chlorbutanol. In: Rowe RC, et al, eds. *Handbook of Pharmaceutical Excipients.* 4th ed. Washington, DC: American Pharmaceutical Association; 2003:141-143.

129. Nash RA. Sorbitol. In: Rowe RC, et al, eds. *Handbook of Pharmaceutical Excipients.* 4th ed. Washington, DC: American Pharmaceutical Association; 2003:596-599.

130. National Academy of Sciences, Immunization Safety Review Committee. Immunization safety review. Vaccines and autism. http://www.nap.edu/catalog.php?record_id=10997. Accessed May 15, 2014.

131. Neale BW, et al. Propylene glycol-induced lactic acidosis in a patient with normal renal function: a proposed mechanism and monitoring recommendations. *Ann Pharmacother.* 2005;39:1732-1736.

132. Neville R, et al. Preservative cytotoxicity to cultured corneal epithelial cells. *Curr Eye Res.* 1986;5:367-372.

133. Okuonghae HO, et al. Diethylene glycol poisoning in Nigerian children. *Ann Trop Paediatr.* 1992;12:235-238.

134. Papahadjopoulos D. Steric stabilization an overview. In: Janoff SA, ed. *Liposomes Rational Design.* New York, NY: Marcel Dekker; 1999:1-12.

135. Parker MG, et al. Removal of propylene glycol and correction of increased osmolar gap by hemodialysis in a patient on high dose lorazepam infusion therapy. *Intensive Care Med.* 2002;28:81-84.

136. Petrou S, et al. Structural requirements for charged lipid molecules to directly increase or suppresses K^+ channel activity in smooth muscle cells. *J Gen Physiol.* 1994;103:471-486.

137. Pfab R, et al. Clinical course of severe poisoning with thimerosal. *J Toxicol Clin Toxicol.* 1996;34:453-460.

138. Pichichero ME, et al. Mercury concentrations and metabolism in infants receiving vaccines containing thimerosal. A descriptive study. *Lancet.* 2002;360:1737-1741.

139. Powell HM, Jamieson WA. Merthiolate as a germicide. *Am J Hyg.* 1931;13:296-310.

140. Price JC. Polyethylene glycol. In: Rowe RC, et al, eds. *Handbook of Pharmaceutical Excipients.* 4th ed. Washington, DC: American Pharmaceutical Association; 2003:454-459.

141. Prusakiewicz JJ, et al. Parabens inhibit human skin estrogen sulfotransferase activity: possible link to paraben estrogenic effects. *Toxicology.* 2007;232:248-256.

142. Pugazhendhi D, et al. Oestrogenic activity of *p*-hydroxybenzoic acid (common metabolite of paraben esters) and methylparaben in human breast cancer cell lines. *J Appl Toxicol.* 2005;25:301-309.

143. Rentz ED, et al. Outbreak of acute renal failure in Panama in 2006: a case-control study. *Bull World Health Organ.* 2008;86:749-756.

144. Rieger MM. Methylparaben. In: Rowe RC, et al, eds. *Handbook of Pharmaceutical Excipients.* 4th ed. Washington, DC: American Pharmaceutical Association; 2003:390-394.

145. Rivera W, et al. Unintentional intravenous infusion of GoLYTELY in a 4-year-old girl. *Ann Pharmacother.* 2004;38:1183-1185.

146. Rogers SC, et al. Percutaneous absorption of phenol and methyl alcohol in magenta paint BPC. *Br J Dermatol.* 1978;98:559-560.

147. Rohyans J, et al. Mercury toxicity following Merthiolate ear irrigations. *J Pediatr.* 1984;104:311-313.

148. Rubin M. Dear health care professional. Agenerase [letter]. Research Triangle Park, NC: Glaxo Wellcome; 2000.

149. Saiki JH, et al. Paraplegia following intrathecal chemotherapy. *Cancer.* 1972;29:370-374.

150. Schamberg IL. Allergic contact dermatitis to methyl and propyl paraben. *Arch Dermatol.* 1967;95:626-328.

151. Schiller LR, et al. Osmotic effects of polyethylene glycol. *Gastroenterology.* 1988;94:933-941.

152. Schulte MJ, Lenz W. Fatal sorbitol infusion in patient with fructose sorbitol intolerance. *Lancet.* 1977;2:188.

153. Shah KH, Verma RJ. Butyl *p*-hydroxybenzoic acid induces oxidative stress in mice liver—an in vivo study. *Acta Pol Pharm.* 2011;68:875-879.

154. Shi R, Borgens RB. Acute repair of crushed guinea pig spinal cord by polyethylene glycol. *J Neurophysiol.* 1999;81:2406-2414.

155. Smith WS, et al. Neurotoxicity of intra-arterial papaverine preserved with chlorobutanol used for the treatment of cerebral vasospasm after aneurysmal subarachnoid hemorrhage. *Stroke.* 2004;35:2518-2522.

156. Smyth HF, et al. The toxicity of high-molecular-weight polyethylene glycols: chronic oral and parenteral administration. *J Am Pharm Assoc.* 1947;36:157-160.

157. Smyth HF, et al. The chronic oral toxicity of the polyethylene glycols. *J Am Pharm Assoc.* 1955;44;27-30.

158. Smyth HF, et al. The toxicology of the polyethylene glycols. *J Am Pharm Assoc (Wash).* 1950;39:349-354.

159. Song BL, et al. In vitro spermicidal activity of parabens against human spermatozoa. *Contraception.* 1989;39:331-335.

160. Speth PA, et al. Propylene glycol pharmacokinetics and effect after intravenous infusion in humans. *Ther Drug Monit.* 1987;9:255-258.

161. Stehr-Green P, et al. Autism and the thimerosal containing vaccines. Lack of consistent evidence for an association. *Am J Prev Med.* 2003;25:101-106.

162. Strickley RG. Solubilizing excipients in oral and injectable formulations. *Pharm Res.* 2004;21:201-230.

163. Sturgill BC, et al. Renal tubular necrosis in burn patients treated with topical polyethylene glycol. *Lab Invest.* 1982;46:81A.

164. Sweet AY. Fatality from intravenous nitrofurantoin. *Pediatrics.* 1958;22:1204.

165. Tabuchi S, et al. Lipid mediators modulate NMDA receptor currents in a *Xenopus* oocyte expression system. *Neurosci Lett.* 1997;237:13-16.

166. Tavares RS, et al. Parabens in male infertility—is there a mitochondrial connection. *Reprod Toxicol.* 2009;27:1-7.

167. Thompson WW, et al. Early thimerosal exposure and neuropsychological outcomes at 7 to 10 years. *N Engl J Med.* 2007;27;357:1281-1292.

168. Tripathi BJ, Tripathi RC. Cytotoxic effects of benzalkonium chloride and chlorobutanol on human corneal epithelial cells in vitro. *Lens Eye Toxic Res.* 1989;6:395-403.

169. Truppman ES, Ellenby JD. Major electrocardiographic changes during chemical peeling. *Plast Reconstr Surg.* 1979;63:44-48.

170. Tung C, et al. The pharmacokinetics of chlorobutanol in man. *Biopharm Drug Dispos.* 1982;3:321-378.

171. Unger AH, Sklaroff HJ. Fatalities following intravenous use of sodium diphenylhydantoin for cardiac arrhythmias. *JAMA.* 1967;200:35-36.

172. United States Pharmacopeial Convention. *United States Pharmacopeia 24/National Formulary 19.* Rockville, MD: United States Pharmacopeial Convention; 2000.

173. Unlu RE, et al. Phenol intoxication in a child. *J Craniofac Surg.* 2004;15:1010-1013.

174. Van de Wiele B, et al. Propylene glycol toxicity caused by prolonged infusion of etomidate. *J Neurosurg Anesthesiol.* 1995;7:259-262.

175. van Meeuwen JA, et al. Aromatase inhibiting and combined estrogenic effects of parabens and estrogenic effects of other additives in cosmetics. *Toxicol Appl Pharmacol.* 2008;230:372-382.

176. Vassalli L, et al. Propylene glycol-induced cholesteatoma in chinchilla middle ears. *Am J Otolaryngol.* 1988;9:180-188.

177. Vearrier D, et al. Phenol toxicology following cutaneous to creolin: a case report. *J Med Toxicol.* 2015;11:227-231.

178. Vernon J, et al. The ototoxic potential of propylene glycol in guinea pigs. *Arch Otolaryngol.* 1978;104:726-729.

179. Verstraeten T, et al. Safety of thimerosal-containing vaccines. A two-phased study of computerized health maintenance organization databases. *Pediatrics.* 2003;112:1039-1048.

180. Wanten GJ, et al. Parenteral administration of medium- but not long-chain lipid emulsions may increase the risk for infections by candida albicans. *Infect Immun.* 2002;70:6471-6474.

181. Warner MA, Harper JV. Cardiac dysrhythmias associated with chemical peeling with phenol. *Anesthesiology.* 1985;62:366-367.

182. Weigt HU, et al. Activation of neuronal N-methyl-D-aspartate receptor channels by lipid emulsions. *Anesth Analg.* 2002;94:331-337.

183. Weigt HU, et al. Lipid emulsions reduce NMDA-evoked currents. *Neuropharmacology.* 2004;47:373-380.

184. Weller PJ. Propylene glycol. In: Rowe RC, et al, eds. *Handbook of Pharmaceutical Excipients.* 4th ed. Washington, DC: American Pharmaceutical Association; 2003:521-523.

185. Willis MS, et al. Persistent lactic acidosis after chronic topical application of silver sulfadiazine in a pediatric burn patient: a review of the literature. *Int J Burn Trauma.* 2013;3:1-8.

186. Wilson KC, et al. Propylene glycol toxicity in a patient receiving intravenous diazepam. *N Engl J Med.* 2000;343:815.

187. Wilson KC, et al. Propylene glycol toxicity: a severe iatrogenic illness in ICU patients receiving IV benzodiazepines. A case series and prospective, observational pilot study. *Chest.* 2005;128:1674-1681.

188. Winder AF, et al. Penetration of mercury from ophthalmologic preservatives into the human eye. *Lancet.* 1980;2:237-239.

189. World Health Organization Global Advisory Committee on Vaccine Safety: Statement on thiomersal. http://www.who.int/vaccine_safety/committee/topics/thiomersal/en/. Accessed May 15, 2014.

190. Wright CG, et al. Tympanic membrane microstructure in experimental cholesteatoma. *Acta Otolaryngol.* 1991;111:101-111.

191. Yahwak JA, et al. Determination of a lorazepam dose threshold for using the osmol gap to monitor for propylene glycol toxicity. *Pharmacotherapy.* 2008;28:984-991.

192. Yaucher NE, et al. Propylene glycol-associated renal toxicity from lorazepam infusion. *Pharmacotherapy.* 2003;23:1094-1099.

193. Yorgin PD, et al. Propylene glycol-induced proximal tubule cell injury. *Am J Kidney Dis.* 1997;30:134-139.

194. Zar T, et al. Acute kidney injury, hyperosmolality and metabolic acidosis associated with lorazepam. *Nat Clin Pract Nephrol.* 2007;3:515-520.

195. Zoneraich S, et al. Sudden death following intravenous sodium diphenylhydantoin. *Am Heart J.* 1976;91:375-377.

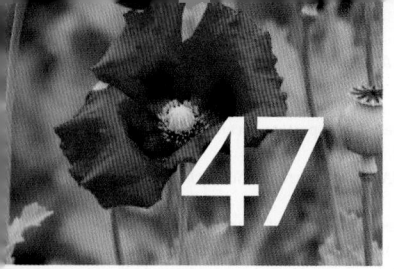

47 ANTIDIABETICS AND HYPOGLYCEMICS/ ANTIGLYCEMICS

George M. Bosse

Glucose	
MW	= 180 Da
Normal fasting range (plasma)	= 60–99 mg/dL
	= 3.3–5.6 mmol/L

HISTORY AND EPIDEMIOLOGY

Insulin first became available for use in 1922 after Banting and Best successfully treated diabetic patients using pancreatic extracts.[13] In an attempt to more closely simulate physiologic conditions, additional "designer" insulins with unique kinetic properties have been developed, including a rapid-acting insulin that mimics baseline (before meals) insulin secretion, known as lispro.[81,157] The hypoglycemic activity of a sulfonamide derivative used for typhoid fever was noted during World War II, and verified later in animals.[90] The sulfonylureas in use today are chemical modifications of that original sulfonamide compound. In the mid-1960s, the first-generation sulfonylureas were widely used. Newer second-generation drugs differ primarily in their potency.

Although insulin is widely used for treating diabetes mellitus, oral hypoglycemic exposures are more commonly reported to poison control centers than are insulin exposures, based on 15 years of data from 2001 to 2015 (Chap. 130). In an older review of 1,418 medication-related cases of hypoglycemia, sulfonylureas (especially the long-acting chlorpropamide and glyburide) alone or with a second hypoglycemic accounted for the largest percentage of cases (63%).[147] Only 18 of the sulfonylurea cases in this series involved intentional overdose. However, hypoglycemia is reported in as many as 20% of patients using sulfonylureas.[73] In a study of 99,628 emergency hospitalizations for adverse drug events in adults older than 65 years, 14% were due to insulin and 11% were due to oral hypoglycemics. The majority (95%) of the hospitalizations related to insulin and oral hypoglycemics were due to hypoglycemia.[24] Other causes of hypoglycemia are listed in Table 47–1.

The biguanides metformin and phenformin were developed as derivatives of *Galega officinalis*, the French lilac, recognized in medieval Europe as a treatment for diabetes mellitus.[11] Phenformin was removed from the US market in 1977 because of its association with life-threatening metabolic acidosis with an elevated lactate concentration.

Development of the α-glucosidase inhibitors began in the 1960s when an α-amylase inhibitor was isolated from wheat flour.[143] Acarbose was discovered more than 10 years later and approved for use in the United States in 1995. Troglitazone and repaglinide were approved for use in the United States in 1997. The US Food and Drug Administration subsequently directed the manufacturer of troglitazone to withdraw the product from the US market in 2000 because of associated liver toxicity. Exenatide, a synthetic form of a compound found in the saliva of the Gila monster, is an incretin mimetic. Incretin is a hormone that stimulates insulin secretion in response to meals. Liraglutide, dulaglutide, and albiglutide are synthetic analogs of human incretin. Other newer xenobiotics include the gliptins, the amylin analog pramlintide, and the sodium glucose co-transporter 2 (SGLT2) inhibitors.

PHARMACOLOGY

Insulin is synthesized as a precursor polypeptide in the β islet cells of the pancreas. Proteolytic processing results in the formation of proinsulin, which is cleaved, giving rise to C-peptide and insulin itself, a double-chain molecule containing 51 amino acid residues. Glucose concentration plays a major role in the regulation of insulin release.[132] Glucose is phosphorylated after transport into the β islet cell of the pancreas. Further metabolism of glucose-6-phosphate results in the formation of ATP. Adenosine triphosphate inhibition of the K^+ channel results in cell depolarization, inward calcium flux, and insulin release. After release, insulin binds to specific receptors on cell surfaces in insulin-sensitive tissues, particularly the hepatic, muscle, and adipose cells. The action of insulin on these cells involves various phosphorylation and dephosphorylation reactions.

Figure 47–1 depicts the chemical structures of noninsulin antidiabetics. The sulfonylureas stimulate the β cells of the pancreas to release insulin and are often referred to as insulin secretagogues. They are ineffective in type 1 diabetes mellitus that results from islet cell destruction (Fig. 47–2). This

TABLE 47–1	Xenobiotic and Non Toxicologic Causes of Hypoglycemia		
Artifactual	**Medical Conditions**	**Neoplasms**	Hypoglycin (Ackee)
Chronic myelogenous leukemia	Acquired immunodeficiency syndrome (AIDS)	Carcinomas (diverse extrapancreatic)	Indomethacin
Polycythemia vera	Alcoholism	Hematologic	Methylenecyclopropylglycine (Litchi)
Endocrine Disorders	Anorexia nervosa	Insulinoma	
Addison's disease	Autoimmune disorders	Mesenchymal	Pentamidine
Glucagon deficiency	Burns	Multiple endocrine adenopathy type 1	Propoxyphene
Graves disease	Diarrhea (childhood)	Sarcomas (retroperitoneal)	Quinidine
Panhypopituitarism (Sheehan syndrome)	Leucine sensitivity	**Reactive Hypoglycemia**	Quinine
Hepatic Disease	Muscular activity (excessive)	**Xenobiotics**	Ritodrine
Acute hepatic atrophy	Postgastric surgery (including gastric bypass)	β-Adrenergic antagonists	Salicylates
Carcinoma	Pregnancy	Alloxan	Streptozocin
Cirrhosis	Protein calorie malnutrition	Antidiabetics	Sulfonamides
Galactose or fructose intolerance	Rheumatoid arthritis	Cibenzoline	Vacor
Glycogen storage disease	Septicemia	Disopyramide	Valproic acid
Neoplasia	Shock	Ethanol	Venlafaxine
Kidney Disease	Systemic lupus erythematosus	Gatifloxacin	
Chronic hemodialysis			
Chronic kidney disease			

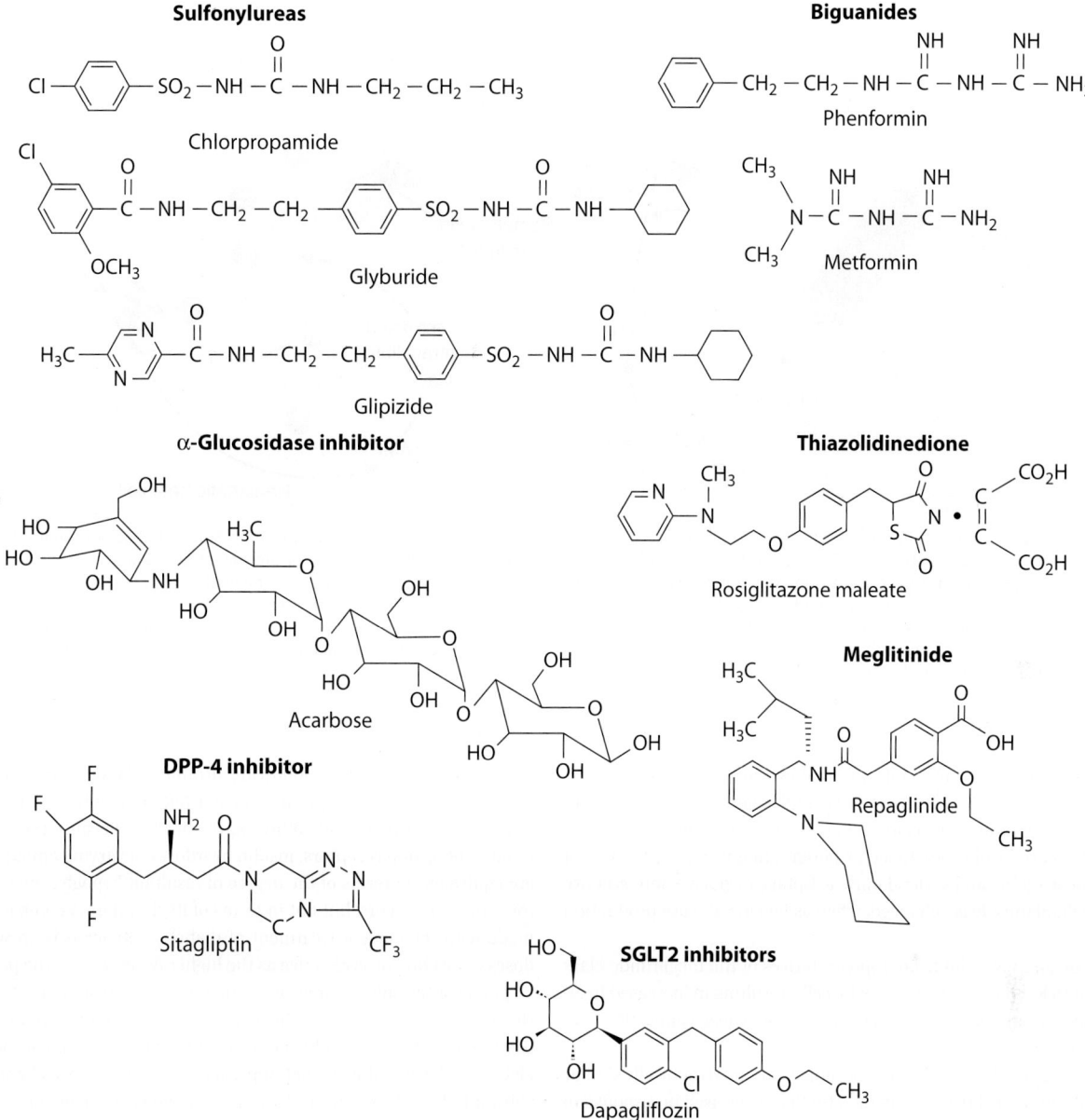

FIGURE 47–1. Chemical structures of representative oral antidiabetics. The glucagonlike peptide (GLP-1) analogs and amylin analogs are large polypeptides. Their structures are not shown here. SGLT2=sodium-glucose cotransporter; DPP-4 inhibitor=dipeptidylpeptidase-4 inhibitor.

stimulatory effect diminishes with chronic therapy. All the sulfonylureas bind to high-affinity receptor sensors on the pancreatic β cell membrane, resulting in closure of K⁺ channels.[49,60,61] Inhibition of potassium efflux mimics the effect of naturally elevated intracellular ATP and results in insulin release. High-affinity sulfonylurea receptors are also present within pancreatic β cells and are postulated to be either located on granular membranes or part of a regulatory exocytosis kinase. Binding to these receptors promotes exocytosis by direct interaction with secretory machinery not involving closure of the plasma membrane K⁺ channels.[49,60,61]

The linkage of 2 guanidine molecules forms the biguanides. Metformin is an oral biguanide approved for treatment of type 2 diabetes mellitus. It acts by several mechanisms, the most important of which involves the inhibition of mitochondrial complex I, which subsequently leads to activation of adenosine monophosphate activated protein kinase (AMPK). Adenosine monophosphate activated protein kinase activation is postulated to mediate antihyperglycemic effects, although alternative signaling pathways may be involved.[22]

Metformin has other actions that are independent of AMPK activation and result in beneficial as well as undesirable side effects.[71] These include induction of mitochondrial stress, suppression of glucagon signaling, and activation of autophagy. Metformin inhibits glycerophosphate dehydrogenase, which is important in the glycerophosphate shuttle and results in inhibition of gluconeogenesis. Alteration of intestinal microbiota by metformin occurs and plays a role in the uptake and utilization of glucose by the intestines. Metformin also increases levels of glucagonlike peptide-1 (GLP-1) and induces GLP-1 receptors. Glucagonlike peptide-1 is an incretin that is released in response to an oral glucose load; it enhances the release of insulin, delays gastric emptying, and reduces food intake. Glucose lowering by metformin can be summarized to occur by a combination of effects, which include inhibition of gluconeogenesis, decreased hepatic glucose output, enhanced peripheral glucose uptake, decreased fatty acid oxidation, and increased intestinal use of glucose.

Acarbose and miglitol are oligosaccharides that inhibit α-glucosidase enzymes such as glucoamylase, sucrase, and maltase in the brush border of the small intestine. As a result, postprandial elevations in blood glucose concentrations are blunted.[171] Delayed gastric emptying is another proposed mechanism for the antihyperglycemic effect of these oligosaccharides.[136]

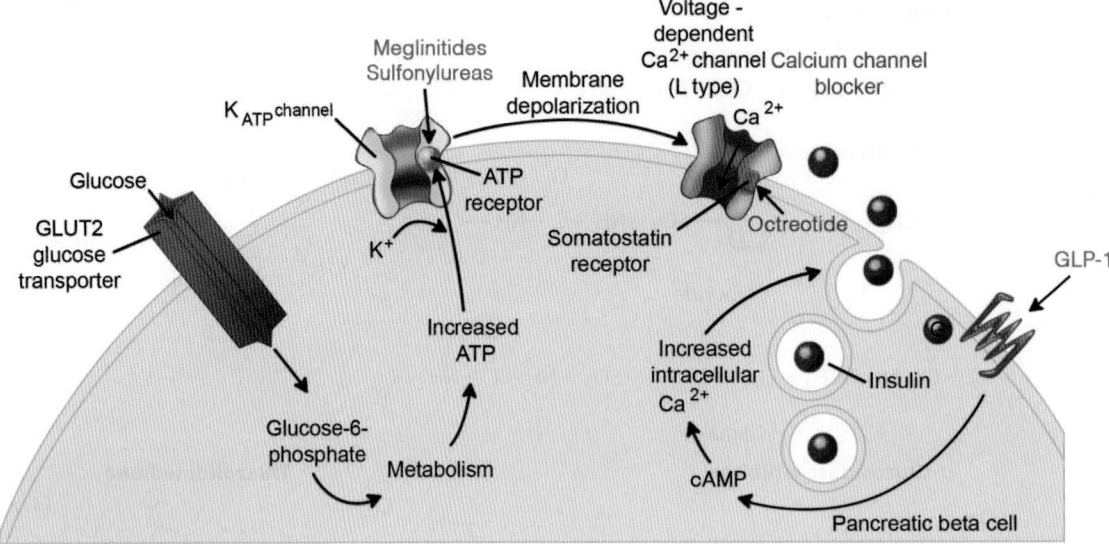

FIGURE 47–2. Under normal conditions, cells release insulin in response to elevation of intracellular ATP concentrations. Sulfonylureas potentiate the effects of ATP at its "sensor" on the ligand gated K⁺ channels and prevent efflux of K⁺. The subsequent rise in intracellular potential opens voltage-gated Ca²⁺ channels, which increases intracellular calcium concentration through a series of phosphorylation reactions. The increase in intracellular calcium results in the release of insulin. Release of insulin is also caused by binding of sulfonylureas to postulated receptor sites on regulatory exocytosis kinase and insulin granular membranes. Octreotide inhibits calcium entry through the Ca²⁺ channel, thereby inhibiting insulin release. GLP-1 acts on a G-protein coupled receptor, which results in accumulation of cAMP, and subsequent increased intracellular calcium stimulated insulin release. GLUT = membrane bound glucose transporter. GLP-1 = glucagonlike peptide-1; cAMP = cyclic adenosine monophosphatase.

Insulin resistance in patients with type 2 diabetes mellitus occurs because of secretion of biologically defective insulin molecules, circulating insulin antibodies, or target tissue defects in insulin action.[120] The thiazolidinedione derivatives decrease insulin resistance by potentiating insulin sensitivity in the liver, adipose tissue, and skeletal muscle. Uptake of glucose into adipose tissue and skeletal muscle is enhanced, whereas hepatic glucose production is reduced.[21,72]

Repaglinide and nateglinide are representatives of the meglitinide class that also bind to K⁺ channels on pancreatic cells, resulting in increased insulin secretion.[139] Compared to the sulfonylureas, the hypoglycemic effects of the meglitinides are shorter in duration.

Exenatide, liraglutide, dulaglutide, and albiglutide are structurally similar to glucagonlike peptide-1 (GLP-1), an incretin that is released in response to an oral glucose load. Glucagonlike peptide-1 enhances the release of insulin, delays gastric emptying, and reduces food intake. Glucagonlike peptide-1 is metabolized very rapidly, rendering it therapeutically ineffective. The GLP-1 analogs have much longer half-lives, rendering them useful in the treatment of type 2 diabetes mellitus.[165] Sitagliptin, saxagliptin, linagliptin, and alogliptin inhibit dipeptidyl peptidase-4 (DPP-4), the enzyme responsible for the inactivation of GLP-1.[3] Pramlintide is an amylin analog. Amylin is produced in the pancreatic β cell and acts in conjunction with insulin to inhibit gastric emptying, decrease postprandial glucagon secretion, and promote satiety.[91]

The kidneys contribute significantly to glucose homeostasis. The SGLT2 inhibitors are located mainly in the proximal tubule, and account for up to 90% of glucose absorption. The SGLT2 inhibitors, such as canagliflozin, block the reabsorption of glucose, with subsequent excretion into the urine.[50]

PHARMACOKINETICS AND TOXICOKINETICS

Pharmacokinetic parameters of the hypoglycemics are given in Tables 47–2 and 47–3. The onset and duration of action in therapeutic doses vary considerably among preparations. Insulin overdose usually occurs after administration by the subcutaneous or intramuscular route. As might be predicted based on slow onset and prolonged duration of action of some of the preparations, insulin overdose may result in delayed and prolonged hypoglycemia. However, hypoglycemia occurs with short-acting forms as well because of some unusual toxicokinetic features. Some of these unpredicted responses

are caused by a depot effect following intramuscular or subcutaneous administration, and poor absorption is further potentiated by the poor perfusion that occurs during periods of hypoglycemia.[112,156] Because there are a finite number of insulin receptors, insulin overdoses of varying amounts probably are equivalent in terms of the degree of resultant hypoglycemia once receptor saturation occurs, but not in terms of its duration. A comparison can be made with the current treatment of diabetic ketoacidosis, in which lower doses of insulin are as effective as the higher doses used in the past.[80]

Many of the sulfonylureas have long durations of action, which explains the unusually long period of hypoglycemia that occurs in both therapeutic use and overdose. Second-generation sulfonylureas (glimepiride, glipizide, glyburide) have half-lives that approach 24 hours and are characterized by substantial fecal excretion of the parent molecule. The sulfonylureas frequently cause hypoglycemia (Table 47–2). As with insulin, the sulfonylureas cause delayed onset of hypoglycemia following overdose.[121,134] The reason for the potential delayed onset of effects with sulfonylureas cannot be simply explained by known kinetic principles but could be related to counterregulatory mechanisms that fail over time.

Metformin metabolism is negligible, and the majority of an absorbed dose is actively secreted in the urine unchanged. With renal dysfunction, the clearance of metformin declines in proportion to the decline of creatinine clearance.[64] Plasma protein binding is negligible.[12] Repaglinide and nateglinide are prandial glucose regulators characterized by rapid onset and short duration of action. Overdose experience and toxicokinetic data for repaglinide are lacking. It is not clear whether hypoglycemia would be prolonged or delayed in onset following overdose. In one case of nateglinide overdose, hypoglycemia occurred early and was short lived.[114] Exenatide is available in an extended-release form, and dulaglutide and albiglutide are formulated such that these drugs are administered once weekly. The gliptins have long half-lives and cause pronounced inhibition of DPP-4, resulting in a long duration of action (approximately 24 hours) after therapeutic doses.[88] Pramlintide has a half-life of approximately 40 minutes when used in therapeutic doses.[32] The SGLT2 inhibitors have durations of action that allow for once-daily dosing.[43] The GLP-1 analogs and amylin analogs are large polypeptides; they represent the 2 classes of noninsulin antidiabetics that are only administered parenterally (subcutaneously).

TABLE 47–2   Characteristics of Noninsulin Antidiabetics

Xenobiotic	Duration of Action	Active Hepatic Metabolite	Active Urinary Excretory Product	Likelihood of Hypoglycemia in Overdose
I. Sulfonylureas				
First-generation				
Acetohexamide	12–18 h	(++)	(++)	H
Chlorpropamide	24–72 h	(+)	(++)	H
Tolazamide	10–24 h	(++)	(++)	H
Tolbutamide	6–12 h	(+)	(++)	H
Second-generation				
Glimepiride	24 h	(++)	(++)	H
Glipizide	16–24 h	(−)	(+)	H
Glyburide	18–24 h	(++)	(++)	H
II. Biguanides				
Metformin	12–24 h	(−)	(++)	L
Phenformin	6–8 h	(−)	(++)	L
III. α-Glucosidase Inhibitors				
Acarbose	2 h	(−)	(+)	L
Miglitol	2 h	(−)	(++)	L
IV. Thiazolidinedione Derivatives				
Pioglitazone	16–24 h	(++)	(++)	H
Rosiglitazone	12–24 h	(++)	(−)	H
V. Meglitinides				
Nateglinide	4–6 h	(++)	(+)	H
Repaglinide	1–3 h	(−)	(−)	H
VI. GLP-1 Analogs				
Exenatide	6–8 h	(−)	(−)	L
Liraglutide	24 h	(−)	(−)	L
Dulaglutide	1 wk	(−)	(−)	L
Albiglutide	1 wk	(−)	(−)	L
VII. DPP-4 inhibitors				
Sitagliptin	24 h	(−)	(++)	L
Saxagliptin	24 h	(++)	(++)	L
Linagliptin	24 h	(−)	(+)	L
Alogliptin	24 h	(++)	(++)	L
VIII. Amylin Analog				
Pramlintide	3 h	(−)	(−)	L
IX. SGLT-2 Inhibitors				
Canagliflozin	24 h	(−)	(−)	L
Dapagliflozin	24 h	(−)	(−)	L
Empagliflozin	24 h	(−)	(++)	L

(++) = Substantial; (+) = Limited; (−) = None/Negligible; H = High Likelihood; L = Low Likelihood.

GLP-1 analogs = glucagonlike peptide analogs; SLGLT2 = sodium-glucose cotransporter; DPP-4 inhibitor = dipeptidyl peptidase-4 inhibitor.

PATHOPHYSIOLOGY OF HYPOGLYCEMIA

To varying degrees, the antidiabetics all produce a nearly identical clinical condition of hypoglycemia. The etiologies of hypoglycemia are divided into 3 general categories:[54] physiologic or pathophysiologic conditions (Table 47–1), direct effects of various hypoglycemics (Tables 47–2 and 47–3), and potentiation of hypoglycemics by interactions with other xenobiotics (Table 47–4).

Hypoglycemia usually results in decreased insulin secretion, with production of alternate fuels, particularly ketones. Ketone production occurs as a result of fatty acid metabolism.[85] Nonketotic hypoglycemia can occur with hyperinsulinemia such as from an insulinoma.[123]

Central nervous system (CNS) symptoms predominate in hypoglycemia because the brain relies almost entirely on glucose as an energy source. However, during prolonged starvation, the brain can utilize ketones derived from free fatty acids. In contrast to the brain, other major organs such as the heart, liver, and skeletal muscle often function during hypoglycemia because they can use various fuel sources, particularly free fatty acids.[149]

Emphasis on tighter glucose control as a means of preventing microvascular effects carries with it an increased risk for hypoglycemia.[39,40] Regulation of glucose control to near-normal glucose concentrations, the characteristics of each individual's awareness of hypoglycemia, and the individual counterregulatory mechanisms define the frequency and intensity of

TABLE 47–3	Characteristics of Various Forms of Insulin		
Insulin	Onset of Action (hours)	Duration of Action (hours)	Peak Glycemic Response (hours)
Rapid Acting			
Aspart	0.25	3–5	0.75–1.5
Glulisine	0.5	<5	1.5–2
Lispro	0.25–0.5	<5	0.5–2.5
Short Acting			
Regular	0.5–1	5–8	2.5–5
Intermediate Acting			
Lente	1–3	18–24	6–14
NPH	1–2	18–24	6–14
Long Acting			
Detemir	1.5	24	No true peak
Glargine	1.1	24	No true peak
Ultralente	4–6	20–36	8–20

hypoglycemia.[148] The Diabetic Control and Complications Trial research group reported 62 episodes of blood glucose concentration less than 50 mg/dL with CNS manifestations requiring assistance for every 100 patient-years in patients undergoing an intensive insulin therapy regimen. This was in comparison to a conventional therapy group, which had 19 such episodes per 100 patient-years.[39,40] The intensive therapy group received 3 or more insulin injections per day or used a pump in an effort to achieve a glucose concentration as close to normal as possible, whereas the conventional therapy group received one or 2 daily insulin injections.

There has also been an emphasis in tighter control of glucose in critically ill patients, even in the absence of known diabetes mellitus. Hyperglycemia occurs in critically ill patients due to several mechanisms and is associated with increased mortality in patients with a variety of medical and surgical diagnoses.[82] In a study of critically ill surgical patients, tight control of glucose was associated with decreased morbidity and mortality.[169] However,

TABLE 47–4	Xenobiotics Known to React with Hypoglycemics Resulting in Hypoglycemia

β-Adrenergic antagonists
Angiotensin-converting enzyme (ACE) inhibitors
Allopurinol
Anabolic steroids
Chloramphenicol
Clofibrate
Disopyramide
Ethanol
Fluoroquinolones
Haloperidol
Methotrexate
Monoamine oxidase inhibitors
Pentamidine
Phenylbutazone
Probenecid
Quinine
Salicylates
Sulfonamide
Trimethoprim-sulfamethoxazole
Warfarin

such benefits in other studies are not always clearly replicated, and significant hypoglycemia is reported.[52,168]

The issue of tight glycemic control has to be analyzed with respect to various factors, such as old versus young age, outpatient versus critically ill (including surgical vs nonsurgical patients), microvascular versus macrovascular complications, and diabetic versus nondiabetic patients. Although benefits of tight glycemic control are demonstrable, these are often outweighed by the deleterious effects of hypoglycemia.[1,56,95,96,103]

The autonomic nervous system regulates glucagon and insulin secretion, glycogenolysis, lipolysis, and gluconeogenesis. β-Adrenergic antagonists affect all of these mechanisms and can result in hypoglycemia. β-Adrenergic antagonist–induced hypoglycemia is a particular risk[65] secondary to increased insulin half-life and reduced renal gluconeogenesis in the presence of renal dysfunction.[124] In addition, the clinical presentation of hypoglycemia may be muted when β-adrenergic antagonists are present because the expected autonomic responses of tachycardia, diaphoresis, and anxiety may not occur. Although this is assumed to be true, an adverse effect on hypoglycemic awareness could not be demonstrated in healthy volunteers given metoprolol, atenolol, and propranolol.[78]

The concept of hypoglycemia-associated autonomic failure in diabetes mellitus is well described.[37] Recurrent episodes of hypoglycemia result in autonomic failure by causing defective compensatory glucose counterregulation and subsequent hypoglycemic unawareness. As glucose concentrations fall, normal sensing mechanisms result in decreased insulin secretion and increased glucagon and epinephrine secretion. These counterregulatory defenses against hypoglycemia are defective in most people with type 1 diabetes mellitus and in many with type 2 diabetes mellitus. A comparison study was conducted in diabetes patients with hypoglycemia awareness and hypoglycemia unawareness, using positron emission tomography with radiolabeled fluorodeoxyglucose to measure changes in brain glucose kinetics.[47] Alterations in cortical responses to hypoglycemia were found in those with unawareness of hypoglycemia. This group also had significantly less epinephrine output in response to hypoglycemia.

Although various nonantidiabetic xenobiotics can cause hypoglycemia (Table 47–1), salicylates and ethanol are particularly notable for their unintended hypoglycemic effects. The mechanism of ethanol-induced hypoglycemia is discussed in Chap. 76. Salicylate inhibition of prostaglandin synthesis in the β cell of the pancreas is postulated to result in enhanced insulin secretion.[14] Salicylates may also cause hypoglycemia by mechanisms that do not involve enhanced insulin secretion. Hypoglycorrhachia in the presence of peripheral euglycemia was demonstrated in a mouse study,[164] and it correlates with reports in humans of reversal of euglycemic delirium after administration of dextrose.[84]

CLINICAL MANIFESTATIONS

Hypoglycemia and its secondary effects on the CNS (neuroglycopenia) are the most common adverse effects related to insulin and the sulfonylureas. It is essential to remember that hypoglycemia is primarily a clinical, not a numerical, disorder. Clinical hypoglycemia is the failure to maintain a CSF glucose concentration that prevents signs or symptoms of glucose deficiency. The clinical presentations of patients with hypoglycemia are extremely variable and it must be excluded as an etiology of any neuropsychiatric abnormality, whether persistent or transient, focal or generalized. The cerebral cortex usually is most severely affected. These findings are categorized below:[131]

- Delirium with subdued, confused, or agitated behavior.
- Coma with multifocal brain stem abnormalities, including decerebrate spasms and respiratory abnormalities, with preservation of the oculocephalic (doll's eyes), oculovestibular (cold-caloric), and pupillary responses.
- Focal neurologic deficits simulating a cerebrovascular accident (CVA) with or without the presence of coma. There are numerous reports[7,153] and series[145,170] of patients with focal neurologic deficits.
- Seizure activity (single, multiple, or status epilepticus).

These neuropsychiatric symptoms are usually reversible if the hypoglycemia is corrected promptly. The morbidity resulting from undiagnosed hypoglycemia is related partly to the etiology and partly to the duration and severity of the hypoglycemia. The etiologies of hypoglycemia encompass both severe diseases such as fulminant hepatic failure and benign problems such as a missed meal by an insulin-requiring diabetes patient or a patient on an oral antidiabetic. The literature with regard to outcome is difficult to interpret. Although a study of 125 emergency department (ED) cases of symptomatic hypoglycemia reported an 11% mortality rate,[99] only one death (0.8%) was attributed directly to hypoglycemia. In that same study, 9 patients (7.2%) presented with seizures (focal in one case), 3 patients (2.4%) presented with hemiparesis, and 4 survivors (3.2%) suffered residual neurologic deficits. In one tertiary care medical center, 1.2% of all admitted patients had numerical hypoglycemia (defined as a glucose concentration <50 mg/dL). The overall mortality was 27% for this group of 94 patients.[54] The longer and more profound the hypoglycemic episode, the more likely permanent CNS damage will occur.[10]

No absolute criteria available from the physical examination or history distinguish one form of metabolic coma from another. Moreover, all of the findings classically associated with hypoglycemia, such as tremor, sweating, tachycardia, confusion, coma, and seizures, are frequently absent.[69] The glycemic threshold is the glucose concentration below which clinical manifestations develop, a threshold that is host variable. In one study, the mean glycemic threshold for hypoglycemic symptoms was 78 mg/dL in patients with poorly controlled type 1 diabetes compared to 53 mg/dL in those without the disease.[17]

Many patients with well-controlled type 1 diabetes are unaware of hypoglycemia. It appears that even in the presence of numerical hypoglycemia, diabetes patients with near-normal glycosylated hemoglobin concentrations maintain near-normal glucose uptake by the brain, thereby preserving cerebral metabolism and limiting the response of counterregulatory hormones. The result of this limited response is unawareness of hypoglycemia.[17,19] A threshold is likely achieved below which the glucose concentration is inadequate, but this may be a concentration so close to that causing serious neuroglycopenia that patients have limited opportunity for corrective action.[19] Hypoglycemia unawareness is most likely in diabetes patients with chronic use of hypoglycemics because of hypoglycemia-associated autonomic failure.[37] Acute ingestion of hypoglycemics in nondiabetic patients typically would cause more classic signs and symptoms.

Sinus tachycardia, atrial fibrillation, and ventricular premature contractions are the most common dysrhythmias associated with hypoglycemia.[89,119] An outpouring of catecholamines in a response to hypoglycemia, transient electrolyte abnormalities, and underlying heart disease appear to be the most likely etiologies. Based on their mechanisms of action, both insulin and the sulfonylureas are expected to promote the shift of potassium into cells, and hypokalemia after insulin overdose is well documented.[9,156] Other cardiovascular manifestations including acute coronary syndromes rarely are the sole manifestations of hypoglycemia.[16,46,128] Increased release of catecholamines during hypoglycemia increases myocardial oxygen demand and decreases supply by causing coronary vasoconstriction, especially in patients with diabetes who are at increased risk of atherosclerosis. Hypoglycemia leads to catecholamine release which also causes cardiac repolarization abnormalities that contribute to atrial and ventricular dysrhythmias.[167]

Hypothermia often occurs in hypoglycemic patients.[55,77,158] If present, hypothermia usually is mild (90°F–95°F {32°C –35°C}), unless coexisting conditions such as environmental exposure, infection, head injury, or hypothyroidism are present. In a study comparing 2 groups of patients with depressed mental status, hypothermia was almost exclusively limited to the hypoglycemic patients; of these patients, 53% with demonstrated hypoglycemia showed hypothermia.[158] The central hypothalamic response to hypoglycemia stimulated by the sympathetic nervous system infrequently "overshoots" normal temperatures, resulting in hyperthermia following recovery.[33]

Besides decreasing glucose concentrations, the hypoglycemics can produce a number of adverse effects, both in overdose and in therapeutic doses.

Older sulfonylureas, predominantly chlorpropamide, cause a syndrome of inappropriate antidiuretic hormone secretion[75] and disulfiram-ethanol reactions.[129] These adverse effects are exceedingly uncommon with the newer second-generation sulfonylureas.

Hypoglycemia is at times delayed until 18 hours after lente insulin overdose,[112] persist for up to 53 hours after subcutaneous insulin glargine overdose,[23] and is reported to persist up to 6 days after ultralente insulin overdose.[100] Death after insulin overdose cannot be correlated directly with either the dose or preparation. Some patients have died with doses estimated in the hundreds of units, whereas others have survived doses in the thousands of units.[144] Mortality and morbidity likely correlate better with delay in recognition of the problem, duration of symptoms, onset of therapy, and type of complications, as opposed to the absolute degree of hypoglycemia or persistence of elevated insulin concentrations. In a retrospective study of insulin overdose, 7 of 17 cases (41%) developed recurrent hypoglycemia between 5 and 39 hours after overdose despite oral feeding and intravenous dextrose infusion ranging from 5 to 17 g of dextrose per hour.[156] A significant correlation was noted between the amount of insulin injected and the total amount of dextrose used for treatment. This is surprising because one would expect that the amount of dextrose infused would be independent of the dose of insulin following saturation of insulin receptors. Another study of intentional insulin overdose in 25 patients found no correlation between the insulin dose and the amount of administered dextrose.[109]

Insulin is a large polypeptide structure. Although one would expect significant degradation by gut enzymes if ingested, there is a report of hypoglycemia to as low as 25 mg/dL after ingestion of 3,000 units of a combination of aspart, lispro, and glargine.[159]

In a retrospective review of 40 patients with sulfonylurea overdoses, the time from ingestion to the onset of hypoglycemia, when known, was variable.[121] The longest delay was 21 hours after ingestion of glyburide and 48 hours after ingestion of chlorpropamide. In a retrospective poison control center review of 93 cases of sulfonylurea exposures in children, 25 patients (27%) developed hypoglycemia, with a time of onset ranging from 0.5 to 16 hours and a mean of 4.3 hours.[134] In a prospective poison control center study of sulfonylurea exposures in children, 56 of 185 (30%) patients developed hypoglycemia, with a time of onset ranging from 1 to 21 hours and a mean of 5.3 hours.[152] Single-tablet ingestions of chlorpropamide 250 mg, glipizide 5 mg, and glyburide 2.5 mg result in hypoglycemia in young children,[134] and the hypoglycemia is often delayed.[160] Hypoglycemia did not occur until 45 hours after ingestion of a 10-mg extended-release glipizide tablet in a 6-year-old child.[125]

Hypoglycemia is reported in a few cases of metformin overdose. In a 2-case series, metabolic acidosis with an elevated lactate concentration was evident on initial presentation.[162] Hypoglycemia was present initially in one of the cases but did not develop until 7 hours later in the second case. There is no mention of co-ingestants in these cases. Hypoglycemia is reported in a 15-year-old who presented 2 hours after ingestion of metformin and quetiapine.[4] Extensive laboratory investigation excluded insulin and sulfonylureas as causal. Hypoglycemia and metabolic acidosis with an elevated lactate concentration are reported in a case of overdose with metformin, atenolol, and diclofenac.[66] In a series of 36 metformin overdose cases, 2 patients developed hypoglycemia, and co-ingestants were not felt to be contributory.[107] Insufficient evidence supports the concept that metformin-associated hypoglycemia can develop in a patient who does not have metabolic acidosis. Because many patients receiving metformin also take sulfonylureas, hypoglycemia should be anticipated after overdose.

Despite limited overdose data, acarbose and miglitol are not likely to cause hypoglycemia based on their mechanism of action of inhibiting α-glucosidase. The most common adverse effects associated with therapeutic use of these xenobiotics are gastrointestinal, including nausea, bloating, abdominal pain, flatulence, and diarrhea. Elevated aminotransferase concentrations were noted after use of acarbose in clinical trials.[70] Most patients were asymptomatic, and the aminotransferase concentrations returned to normal after the drug was discontinued. The therapeutic use of acarbose in some cases reportedly led to hepatotoxicity that resolved after the drug was discontinued.[8,30]

Hypoglycemia would not be expected after thiazolidinedione overdose, despite limited overdose data. The most serious adverse effect of troglitazone is the development of liver toxicity with therapeutic doses, which in some cases was severe enough to require liver transplantation.[62,117] Liver toxicity related to therapeutic use of rosiglitazone[6,57] and pioglitazone is also reported.[98,101] Therapeutic use of pioglitazone and rosiglitazone may precipitate fluid retention in patients with congestive heart failure.[116] A meta-analysis concluded that rosiglitazone therapy is associated with an increased risk of myocardial infarction and death from cardiovascular causes.[118]

Hypoglycemia should be anticipated after repaglinide and nateglinide ingestion. Hypoglycemia is reported after nateglinide overdose,[114] and a case of intentionally self-induced hypoglycemia secondary to repaglinide is reported.[68] Hypoglycemia developed 14 hours postingestion in a case of repaglinide overdose.[51]

The GLP-1 analogs and gliptins are reported to have pharmacologic effects that are glucose-dependent.[58] This does not necessarily apply to the overdose situation, and hypoglycemia is uncommonly reported in such settings. "Severe hypoglycemia" was reported in a phase III clinical trial after inadvertent administration of 10 times the normal dose of exenatide. The specific glucose concentration is not noted in the report.[27] Injection of 90 mcg of exenatide in a 40-year-old and 1,800 mcg in a 46-year-old resulted in gastrointestinal symptoms but no hypoglycemia.[35,83] As a result of a transcription error, a 67-year-old received 18 mg liraglutide daily over a 7-month period. He had several hospitalizations for evaluation of nausea, vomiting, and diarrhea but never developed hypoglycemia.[15] A 33-year-old injected 72 mg of liraglutide and developed nausea and vomiting, but no hypoglycemia.[113]

An 86-year-old ingested 1,700 mg of sitagliptin in a suicide attempt and did not develop hypoglycemia during an overnight hospitalization.[59] A multicenter poison control center study reviewed 650 cases of gliptin exposure, with exclusion of co-ingestant cases.[141] Three of these reportedly developed hypoglycemia, although the description of these cases is not clear with respect to associated neuroglycopenia. The glucose concentrations were based on bedside testing, not on specimens sent to the laboratory.

There are limited overdose data with regard to amylin analogs. Pramlintide is used therapeutically in conjunction with insulin, and hypoglycemia in this setting is more likely than with insulin use alone.[91]

Therapeutic use of SGLT2 inhibitors results in euglycemic ketoacidosis.[161] This is one of the newest classes of drugs used for diabetes, with limited overdose data. Based on their pharmacology, inhibition of renal glucose reabsorption would not be expected to occur to a degree that would result in hypoglycemia.[38]

DIAGNOSTIC TESTING

Suspicion of hypoglycemia, particularly neuroglycopenia, is important in any patient with an abnormal neurologic examination. The most frequent reasons for failure to diagnose hypoglycemia and mismanaging patients are the erroneous conclusions that the patient is not hypoglycemic but rather is psychotic, epileptic, experiencing a CVA, or intoxicated because of an "odor of alcohol" on the breath (Chap. 76). Compounding the problem of misdiagnosis is the erroneous assumption that a single bolus of 0.5 to 1 g/kg of hypertonic dextrose will always be sufficient.

Plasma glucose concentrations, although generally accurate, are time consuming, so treatment should not be delayed pending the results of laboratory testing. Glucose reagent strip testing can be performed at the bedside. The sensitivity of these tests for detecting hypoglycemia is excellent, but these tests are not perfect. Several interfering substances may cause false elevations of bedside glucose reagent strip concentrations, including maltodextrin, acetaminophen, bilirubin, triglyceride, and uric acid.[48,79] Bedside glucose testing is discussed in more detail in Antidotes in Depth: A8.

Diagnostic studies other than determinations of glucose concentrations are often indicated, depending on the clinical situation. In some instances, determination of serum ethanol concentration is helpful in confirming alcohol as a contributing or sole etiologic factor. Analysis of BUN, creatinine, and eGFR (estimated glomerular filtration rate) indicates the presence of renal dysfunction as a causative factor of hypoglycemia. This commonly occurs in patients with diabetes taking insulin, who often develop renal dysfunction after they have had the disease for several years, with insulin half-life increasing as eGFR decreases. Measures of hepatic function will be a clue to liver disease as a cause of hypoglycemia, although liver disease will also be evident on physical examination. Seizures are commonly associated with hypoglycemia, but other studies, such as electrolytes, and imaging of the brain, are indicated if doubt about the etiology exists.

In the majority of overdose cases, laboratory testing for specific antidiabetics is not helpful. Exceptions might include malicious, surreptitious, or unintentional overdoses (discussed in the next section). Metformin concentrations vary and do not necessarily correlate with the clinical condition.[5,86,87]

For known diabetic patients in whom intentional, unintentional or malicious overdose is not suspected, the clinician must search diligently for the cause of hypoglycemia. Sometimes it is as simple as a missed meal in an insulin or oral antidiabetic user or an unusually strenuous exercise routine, but in many cases the cause cannot be clearly defined. Numerous medical conditions, as well as a variety of xenobiotics, are commonly involved (Table 47–1), and diagnostic testing must be individualized for each episode depending on the clinical suspicion. Diagnosing the etiology as "idiopathic" is never acceptable.

EVALUATION OF MALICIOUS, SURREPTITIOUS, OR UNINTENTIONAL INSULIN OVERDOSE

The physical examination will often provide helpful clues to the evaluation of a suspected malicious, surreptitious, or unintentional insulin overdose. A meticulous search will reveal a site that is erythematous, hemorrhagic, atypically boggy in nature, or even painful if the subcutaneous or intramuscular injection of insulin was particularly large. A simple unexplained needle puncture mark in the appropriate clinical setting suggests insulin injection.

An understanding of how the β cells of the pancreas secrete insulin in response to glucose concentrations in the blood is essential to understanding the investigation of fasting hypoglycemia.[36] When the plasma glucose concentration is less than 45 mg/dL, insulin secretion should be almost completely suppressed, so plasma insulin concentrations should be minimal or absent.[130] Moreover, insulin is secreted as proinsulin, which is cleaved in vivo to form insulin (a double-stranded peptide), and C-peptide, which are released into the blood in equimolar quantities. Insulin is biologically active, whereas proinsulin has limited activity, and C-peptide has no activity. Although insulin is normally cleared during hepatic transit, C-peptide is not. For this reason, C-peptide can be utilized as a quantitative marker of endogenous insulin secretion. In contrast, commercially available exogenous human insulin does not contain C-peptide fragments (Table 47–5). When plasma glucose concentration falls to hypoglycemic concentrations (usually <60 mg/dL), insulin concentration should fall to less than 6 μU/mL. If hypoglycemia is caused by exogenous insulin administration, plasma C-peptide concentrations should be less than 0.2 nmol/L in the presence of insulin concentrations that are substantially higher than insulin concentrations resulting from an insulinoma. With insulinoma, insulin concentrations generally are greater than 6 μU/mL in the presence of hypoglycemia. Insulinoma results in elevations of both C-peptide and insulin concentrations. Sulfonylurea overdose is expected to have similar effects, but concentrations in reported cases of sulfonylurea-induced hypoglycemia vary considerably.[44] In the face of uncertainty, sulfonylurea concentrations are available from reference laboratories. Animal insulin can be distinguished from human insulin by high-performance liquid chromatography.[63] However, this technique has limited use because of the virtually exclusive use of recombinant insulin at present.

TABLE 47–5	Laboratory Assessment of Fasting Hypoglycemia			
Clinical State	Insulin[a] (Serum) (µU/mL)	C-Peptide (Serum) (nmol/L)	Proinsulin Serum (pmol/L)	Antiinsulin Antibodies[b]
Normal	<6	<0.2	<5	–
Exogenous insulin	Very high	Low (suppressed)	Absent	Present[c]
Insulinoma	High	High	Present	Absent
Sulfonylurea ingestion[d]	High	High	Present	Absent
Autoimmune	Very high (artifact)	Low (or) high (artifact)	Present	Present
Decreased glucose production	Low	Low	Present	Absent
Neoplasia (non–β-cell)	Low	Low	Present	Absent

[a]Insulin concentrations are determined during fasting induced hypoglycemia at low concentrations, preferably <60 mg/dL of plasma glucose. [b]The antiinsulin antibodies produced spontaneously differ from those of treated (exposed to exogenous insulin) and those of untreated insulin-dependent diabetic patients. [c]The presence of antiinsulin antibodies occurs less frequently in those exposed only to human insulin. [d]Sulfonylurea ingestion is diagnosed by detection of the parent compound metabolites in serum or urine.

In summary, patients with exogenous insulin-induced hypoglycemia will have high insulin concentrations, the presence of insulin-binding antibodies (if chronic insulin users),[53] and low C-peptide concentrations. Those who have taken sulfonylureas will have high insulin concentrations, absent insulin-binding antibodies, high C-peptide concentrations, and the presence of urinary sulfonylurea metabolites (Table 47–5). The issues of evidence collection that are appropriate to document malicious or surreptitious use of insulin successfully are described (Chap. 138).[94]

MANAGEMENT

Treatment centers on the correction of hypoglycemia and the anticipation that hypoglycemia may recur. Symptomatic patients with hypoglycemia require immediate treatment with 0.5 to 1 g/kg hypertonic intravenous dextrose in the form of $D_{50}W$ in adults, $D_{25}W$ in children, and $D_{10}W$ in neonates. Occasionally, patients require a larger dose to achieve an initial response. If hypoglycemia is suspected but not confirmed, as in the absence of rapid reagent strip availability or when such readings are "borderline," dextrose should be administered. Theoretical risks are associated with use of hypertonic dextrose in the setting of acute cerebral ischemia, but failure to rapidly correct hypoglycemia will lead to deleterious neurologic effects. Appropriate emergency and toxicologic uses of hypertonic dextrose are covered in detail in Antidotes in Depth: A8.

We recommend not to use glucagon as an antihypoglycemic except in the uncommon situation where intravenous access cannot be obtained. Glucagon has a delay to onset of action and is ineffective in patients with depleted glycogen stores, as in the malnourished elderly, cancer patients, or alcoholics. Glucagon also stimulates insulin release from the pancreas, which is reported to lead to prolonged hypoglycemia in settings such as sulfonylurea ingestion and insulinoma.[163]

Numerous studies have evaluated approaches for treating insulin reactions with carbohydrates in tablet, solution, or gel forms in a well-defined diabetic population.[150] None of these forms is appropriate for the undifferentiated, possibly hypoglycemic patient if intravenous access is available, but should be carried by all diabetic patients.

A common occurrence involves symptomatic hypoglycemic patients who receive intravenous dextrose in the prehospital setting and subsequently refuse transport to the hospital. The authors of a retrospective review of 571 paramedic runs involving hypoglycemic patients concluded that out-of-hospital treatment of hypoglycemic diabetic patients is safe and effective even when transport is refused.[151] However, of the 159 patients who agreed to hospital transport, 40% were admitted. The admitted group was older than those released from the ED. The admission rate for transported patients on oral hypoglycemics was higher than those on insulin. The reasons for admission are not otherwise detailed. The authors of a prospective study involving 132 hypoglycemic diabetic patients who refused transport after therapy concluded that most such patients have good short-term outcome, but they still encouraged transport because of the risk of recurrent hypoglycemia.[108] One patient died in each of these 2 studies. A prospective study in 35 patients with 38 hypoglycemic events related to insulin use concluded that most patients were successfully treated in the prehospital setting without transport.[92] However, 2 patients developed recurrent hypoglycemia that they treated themselves, and one of these patients required placement in a long-term care facility for posthypoglycemic encephalopathy. We therefore recommend that all hypoglycemic patients should be transported to the ED.

Emesis, lavage, and catharsis are of limited benefit in the management of patients who overdose on hypoglycemics. The extensive affinity between chlorpropamide, tolazamide, tolbutamide, glyburide, glipizide, and activated charcoal is demonstrated in vitro.[76] The affinities ranged from 0.45 to 0.52 g/g activated charcoal at pH 7.5 and were higher at pH 4.9. Single-dose activated charcoal should be beneficial in the management of these overdoses. Although affinity studies are lacking for the other oral hypoglycemics, their chemical characteristics are such that single-dose activated charcoal is expected to be beneficial for these overdoses as well.

In patients who overdose on insulin, case reports describe the use of surgical excision of the injection site.[29,93,104] However, this technique has not been studied in a systematic fashion and we recommend against excision. Needle aspiration of a depot site is less invasive and can be performed, but intravenous dextrose should be sufficient in most cases.

MAINTAINING EUGLYCEMIA AFTER INITIAL CONTROL

After the patient is awake and alert, further therapy depends on the pharmacokinetics of the xenobiotic involved and pancreatic islet cell function. Some patients, particularly those with prolonged hypoglycemia, have persistent altered mental status despite euglycemia. Whether the event was unintentional or intentional with suicidal or homicidal intent must be determined. One problem associated with dextrose administration occurs in individuals who can produce insulin via glucose-stimulated insulin release (nondiabetic patients and those with type 2 diabetes mellitus), placing them at substantial risk for recurrent hypoglycemia. This complication occurs with insulin overdose but is particularly problematic with overdoses of sulfonylurea or meglitinide because these hypoglycemics stimulate insulin release. Treatment with hypertonic dextrose solutions can be expected to result in dramatic yet only transient increases in glucose concentrations, with a subsequent fall in plasma glucose concentration, possibly back to hypoglycemic concentrations.

For patients with diabetes who unintentionally inject an excessive amount of insulin and are not neuroglycopenic, feeding (carbohydrates and proteins) should be initiated and intravenous access maintained while avoiding routine dextrose infusion. In the event of recurrent symptomatic hypoglycemia, a hypertonic intravenous dextrose bolus followed by an infusion of D_5W is recommended. Overdose in the setting of suicidal or homicidal intent likely involves significant quantities of insulin. Nondiabetic patients are particularly prone to significant hypoglycemia because they lack insulin resistance. Feeding is recommended with a target of maintaining glucose concentrations in the 100- to 150-mg/dL range using a hypertonic dextrose infusion ($D_{10}W$ or greater) as needed based on serial measurements of plasma glucose concentrations.

Central venous lines should be used when a $D_{20}W$ or greater infusion is instituted, because hypertonic dextrose solutions are venous irritants and sclerosing to the vasculature. The presence of glycosuria is not an adequate indicator of euglycemia; frequent serial blood or reagent strip glucose concentrations should be obtained. The appropriate timing of glucose monitoring varies depending on the clinical situation. Mental status must be observed. As a rough guide, glucose monitoring every 1 to 2 hours after initial control is reasonable, with subsequent spacing of the intervals to once every 4 to 6 hours. Phosphate concentrations should be monitored because dextrose loading may lead to hypophosphatemia.[110] Potassium concentrations should be monitored because dextrose administration leads to hypokalemia in nondiabetic patients and rarely hyperkalemia in patients with impaired insulin secretion.[34] The duration of serial sampling depends on the stability of the patient, the underlying metabolic disorders, the extent of overdose, and the rate of improvement. When the patient begins to eat an adequate diet and the initial hypoglycemia is controlled, the plasma glucose concentration will rise, and the concentration and rate of dextrose infusion can be tapered. Many patients may actually develop significant hyperglycemia.

The therapeutic approach differs for patients who overdose on sulfonylureas or meglitinides. After initial control of hypoglycemia with hypertonic dextrose, feeding is again recommended. Intravenous access is necessary, but routine continuous dextrose infusion should be avoided. As with insulin overdose, frequent monitoring of glucose concentrations and mental status is critical. We recommend use of octreotide for recurrent hypoglycemia in this setting because of the significant risk of glucose-stimulated insulin release.

Octreotide, a semisynthetic long-acting analog of somatostatin with an intravenous half-life of 72 minutes, inhibits glucose-stimulated β cell insulin release via receptors coupled to G proteins on β islet cells.[18] Somatostatin is present in diverse tissues such as the hypothalamus, pancreas, and gastrointestinal tract. It alters the secretion of growth hormone and thyroid-stimulating hormone, gastrointestinal secretions, and the endocrine pancreas (glucagon and insulin).[137,138] Octreotide was compared to intravenous hypertonic dextrose and to diazoxide and concomitant dextrose in normal subjects brought to hypoglycemia using glipizide.[18] Fewer episodes of recurrent hypoglycemia occurred after octreotide therapy, and overall dextrose requirements were lower than in the dextrose-alone and dextrose-plus-diazoxide groups. Several successful clinical experiences with octreotide are reported with quinine-induced hypoglycemia resulting from malaria therapy,[127] insulinoma,[67] nesidioblastosis of infancy,[41] hypoglycemia related to therapeutic use of gliclazide,[20] and tolbutamide overdose.[18] In a retrospective study of 9 patients with hypoglycemia resulting from either glyburide or glipizide, octreotide effectively reduced the risk of recurrent hypoglycemia.[105] Despite limited evidence, octreotide would be expected to be effective in the treatment of recurrent hypoglycemia following overdose of all classes of non-insulin antidiabetics.

Octreotide appears to be relatively free of serious side effects. The most likely adverse effects are injection-site discomfort if it is administered subcutaneously and gastrointestinal symptoms such as nausea, bloating, diarrhea, and constipation.[97] Our suggested adult octreotide dose is 50 mcg subcutaneously every 6 hours (Antidotes in Depth: A9). The patient should be monitored for 12 to 24 hours after the last dose of octreotide. This observation will ensure that recurrence of hypoglycemia does not occur. Like octreotide, diazoxide is reportedly effective in patients with refractory sulfonylurea-induced hypoglycemia.[74,121] However, octreotide is the preferred therapy because diazoxide has the potential to cause hypotension, cerebrovascular compromise and myocardial infarction.[105]

ADMITTING PATIENTS TO THE HOSPITAL

The decision to admit a patient is complex, but several guidelines can be followed. Admission is usually required for hypoglycemia related to sulfonylureas, ethanol, starvation, hepatic failure, and renal dysfunction, and for hypoglycemia of unknown etiology. The decision to admit a patient often depends on finding an etiology for hypoglycemia, particularly in the setting of insulin use. In most cases, if a diabetic patient on therapeutic doses of insulin develops hypoglycemia after a missed meal, the patient can be discharged after a 4- to 6-hour observation period during which the individual eats a meal and remains asymptomatic with no evidence of hypoglycemia. Patients receiving therapeutic doses of insulin usually require inpatient evaluation of recurrent and unexplained hypoglycemic episodes. Patients with hypoglycemia after unintentional overdose with long-acting insulin should generally be admitted. Hospitalization is usually recommended after unintentional overdose with ultrashort-acting, short-acting, or intermediate-acting insulin if hypoglycemia is persistent or recurrent during a 4- to 6-hour observation period in the ED. Many factors are responsible for unintentional insulin overdose, such as patient error because of impaired vision, syringe structure, and prescription error when undiagnosed hospital admission is recommended. Admission is usually indicated for any patient, regardless of serum glucose concentration or presence or absence of symptoms, who intentionally overdoses on a sulfonylurea or any form of injected insulin, because delayed, profound, and protracted hypoglycemia is expected. Although intravenous insulin overdose is expected to result in more immediate symptoms, experience with this scenario is limited. Admission in this setting is generally advised unless short-acting insulin is involved. Glargine is expected to act like regular insulin when administered intravenously. It is long-acting when administered subcutaneously because of the formation of microprecipitates that are absorbed slowly. Hypoglycemia related to sulfonylurea use in any setting including a missed meal or a viral illness typically necessitates hospitalization.[25]

Patients with possible intentionally self-induced hypoglycemia should generally be admitted. Intentionally self-induced hypoglycemia is most commonly recognized by members of the medical profession. Administration of insulin to a nondiabetic child is a form of child abuse or an attempt at homicide[45] (Chap. 31). Children who have been given an inappropriate dose of insulin, as well as any patient who may be a victim of attempted homicide, should generally be admitted.

A 4- to 6-hour observation period is recommended after metformin overdose. Further observation or hospital admission is usually not required for patients who remain asymptomatic during this period with no evidence of metabolic acidosis, elevated lactate concentration, renal dysfunction, emesis, or hypoglycemia. Patients who overdose on α-glucosidase inhibitors are not expected to have delayed or serious systemic toxicity, and routine medical admission is unnecessary. There are limited data regarding the risk of hypoglycemia and other adverse events after thiazolidinedione ingestion. Based on the mechanism of action and existing clinical experience, hypoglycemia is possible but uncommon after unintentional thiazolidinedione overdose. Delayed onset of hypoglycemia or other serious clinical manifestations is unlikely. A 4- to 6-hour observation period after thiazolidinedione overdose is recommended. Meglitinides are expected to behave pharmacologically like sulfonylureas. For this reason alone, hospital admission after meglitinide overdose is generally advisable, even when the patient is asymptomatic. A 4- to 6-hour observation period is recommended after overdose of GLP-1 analogs, gliptins, amylin analogs, and SGLT2 inhibitors. Delayed onset of clinical manifestations is unlikely.

Children who unintentionally ingest one or more sulfonylurea tablets should generally be hospitalized for 24 hours. Although this recommendation may be controversial and some authors suggest shorter observation periods[26] or even home monitoring in some cases,[140] we believe that delayed hypoglycemic effects of sulfonylurea ingestion in children are well documented[134,152,160] and convincing enough to support admission in most cases. Asymptomatic children with single-tablet exposures to sulfonylureas are best managed without prophylactic intravenous dextrose, which could contribute to delayed onset of hypoglycemia.[26] Elevations in glucose concentrations stimulate insulin release by the pancreas. Such patients instead are best managed by early feeding, frequent checks of glucose concentrations, and observation of mental status.

METABOLIC ACIDOSIS WITH AN ELEVATED LACTATE CONCENTRATION

Throughout this chapter, the term *metabolic acidosis with an elevated lactate concentration* (MALA) is used rather than *metformin-associated lactic acidosis* or *metformin-induced metabolic acidosis*. The biochemical and pathophysiologic processes involving lactate are complex, but a few points are worth summarizing. An elevated lactate concentration occurs in various diseases and can be present in the absence of acidosis. The production of lactic acid does not result in a net increase in hydrogen ion concentration unless there is associated impairment of oxidative metabolism. Impaired oxidative metabolism leads to an increase in hydrogen ion production through the hydrolysis of ATP.[111] In a pig overdose model, metformin caused metabolic acidosis with an elevated lactate concentration, mitochondrial dysfunction, and inhibition of oxygen consumption. Infusion of lactic acid alone did not cause inhibition of oxygen consumption (Fig. 47-3).[133]

The biguanides are uniquely associated with the occurrence of MALA. Phenformin causes lactic acid production by several mechanisms, including interference with cellular aerobic metabolism and subsequent enhanced anaerobic metabolism. Phenformin suppresses hepatic gluconeogenesis

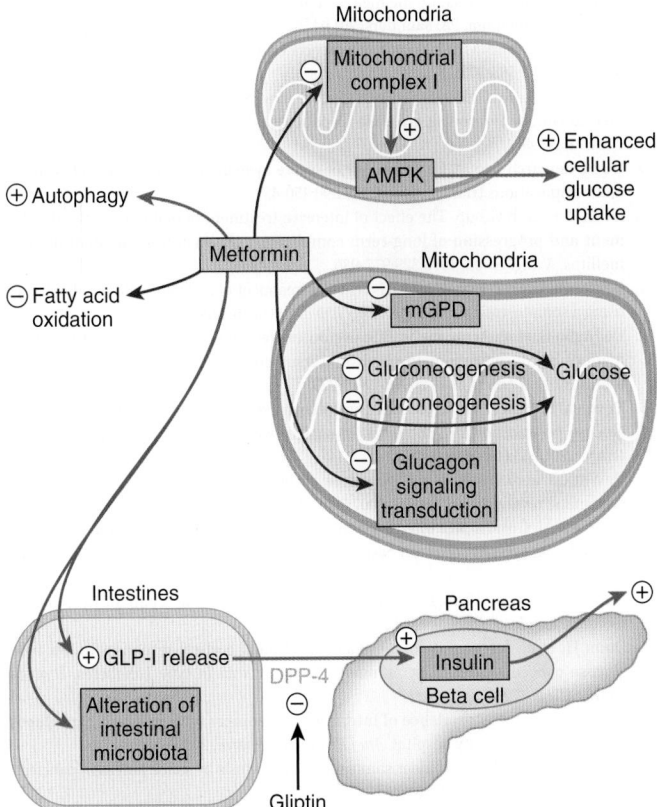

FIGURE 47–3. Metformin inhibits mitochondrial complex I, which activates adenosine monophosphate activated protein kinase (AMPK), resulting in enhanced cellular glucose uptake. Metformin also causes inhibition of mitochondrial glycerophosphate dehydrogenase (mGPD), leading to inhibition of gluconeogenesis. Inhibition of glucagon signaling transduction also leads to inhibition of gluconeogenesis. Metformin enhances glucagonlike peptide-1 (GLP-1) release from the intestines, and stimulates GLP-1 receptors on pancreatic beta islet cells, leading to enhanced insulin release. Gliptins enhance the effect of GLP-1 by inhibition of its inactivation by dipeptidyl peptidase-4. Other mechanisms of metformin include induction of autophagy, inhibition of fatty acid oxidation, and favorable alteration of intestinal microbiota.

from pyruvate and causes a decrease in hepatocellular pH, resulting in decreased lactate consumption and decreased hepatic lactate uptake. Metformin-associated metabolic acidosis with an elevated lactate concentration occurs 20 times less commonly than that occurring with phenformin. In isolated perfused rat liver, metformin inhibits both hepatic lactate uptake and conversion of lactate to glucose.[135] Metabolic acidosis with an elevated lactate concentration related to metformin usually occurs in the presence of an underlying condition, particularly renal dysfunction.[31] In this setting, increased tissue burden of metformin, which is renally eliminated, probably occurs. Other risk factors include cardiorespiratory insufficiency, septicemia, liver disease, a history of MALA, advanced age, alcohol abuse, and use of radiologic contrast media.[12,31] Iodinated contrast material induces acute renal dysfunction, leading to accumulation of metformin and subsequent risk of development of MALA. However, the risk of developing MALA after contrast administration is low in patients taking metformin who have normal renal function and no other risk factors.[102,115] The American College of Radiology recommends and we concur on the temporary discontinuation of metformin for 48 hours after administration of intravenous contrast media if the eGFR is less than 30 mL/min/1.73 m².[2]

Metabolic acidosis with an elevated lactate concentration occurs after acute metformin overdose[87,106,122,162] but is uncommon. In one case,[106] metabolic acidosis was not diagnosed until 14 hours after metformin overdose. The patient had early symptoms of repeated vomiting at 1 hour postingestion. The presence of early gastrointestinal symptoms prompted prolonged observation, allowing for the diagnosis of delayed-onset metabolic acidosis. Metabolic acidosis with an elevated lactate concentration occurred in 2 of 65 adult metformin exposures reported to a poison control center[154] and was not reported in a poison control center series of 55 pediatric metformin exposures.[155] In a retrospective review of 398 cases of acute metformin exposures from 2 poison control centers, MALA in 9.1% of single product overdose and in 0.7% of polypharmacy overdoses.[172] In a retrospective review, MALA was reported in 11 of 36 metformin overdose cases.[107] Acid–base data are detailed in only a few of these cases described as having severe toxicity; the lowest blood pH was 7.16.

A systematic review from the Cochrane Library concluded that therapeutic use of metformin is not associated with an increased risk of MALA compared with other antidiabetic treatments if no contraindications are present.[142] This erroneous conclusion was based on a review of prospective comparative trials and observational cohort studies. However, the risk of MALA in the setting of overdose or renal dysfunction was not assessed. Although MALA after overdose is not common, it does occur with sufficient frequency to require vigilance on the part of the treating physician. In this setting, metformin is clearly responsible for causing metabolic.[28] Case reports were not used in the Cochrane review, and a few cases of MALA in the setting of therapeutic use with no underlying risk factors are reported.[31,126,166]

It is difficult to predict outcome after metformin overdose. A retrospective literature review found no deaths in cases with a nadir serum pH greater than 6.9, a peak serum lactate concentration less than 25 mmol/L, or a peak serum metformin concentration less than 50 mcg/mL.[42] However, a retrospective review of intensive care unit patients with MALA found no association between metformin concentrations in survivors and nonsurvivors.[146] There was an association between mortality and lactate concentrations and pH.

Metformin-associated MALA is a potentially lethal condition. Recognition and awareness of this disorder are important. Symptoms are nonspecific and include abdominal pain, nausea, vomiting, malaise, myalgia, and dizziness. However, gastrointestinal symptoms are common adverse effects associated with therapeutic use of metformin and do not necessarily require discontinuation of the drug. More severe clinical manifestations of metformin-associated MALA include confusion, blindness, mental status depression, hypothermia, respiratory insufficiency, and hypotension. Serum metformin concentrations can be obtained as a diagnostic aid, but these not necessity correlate with the clinical condition in both the acute overdose setting and in the setting of therapeutic metformin use.[86,87]

Aggressive airway management and vasopressor therapy should be given as clinically indicated. Indications for use of intravenous sodium bicarbonate in critically ill patients with metabolic acidosis with an elevated lactate concentration of various etiologies are poorly defined and controversial. Rather than using an arterial pH cutoff, we recommend using sodium bicarbonate given evidence of impaired buffering capacity based on a serum bicarbonate threshold concentration of less than 5 mEq/L.

Metformin would be expected to be dialyzable based on its small size and limited protein binding. However, it has a large volume of distribution. A literature review concluded that metformin is moderately dialyzable, and extracorporeal treatment is recommended if either the blood lactate concentration is greater than 20 mmol/L, or the pH is less than or equal to 7.00, or standard therapies, including sodium bicarbonate, are not effective.[28] Even if metformin removal is inadequate, clinical improvement may occur due to correction of acid–base status.

SUMMARY

- Numerous xenobiotics and medical conditions may cause hypoglycemia.
- Hypoglycemia is the predominant adverse effect related to therapeutic use and overdose of many of the drugs used for treatment of diabetes mellitus.
- Various clinical manifestations, particularly neuropsychiatric, may occur and can be confused with conditions such as ethanol intoxication, psychosis, epilepsy, and cerebrovascular accidents.
- The potential for delayed and prolonged hypoglycemia must be recognized in overdose situations.
- Although several treatment options exist, rapid intravenous administration of dextrose is the most important measure.
- Octreotide is useful for patients with recurrent hypoglycemia following sulfonylurea or meglitinide overdose, and would be expected to be useful for the treatment of recurrent hypoglycemia following overdose with all other noninsulin antidiabetics.

REFERENCES

1. Abdelmalak BB, Lansang MC. Revisiting tight glycemic control in perioperative and critically ill patients: when one size may not fit all. *J Clin Anesth*. 2013;25:499-507.
2. ACR Manual on Contrast Media, V10.2, 2016. ACR Committee on Drugs and Contrast Media; American College of Radiology. Metformin; 45-47.
3. Ahren B. Dipeptidyl peptidase-4 inhibitors: clinical data and clinical implications. *Diabetes Care*. 2007;30:1344-1350.
4. Al-Abri SA, et al. Metformin overdose-induced hypoglycemia in the absence of other antidiabetic drugs. *Clin Toxicol (Phila)*. 2013;51:444-447.
5. Al-Jebawi AF, et al. Lactic acidosis with therapeutic metformin blood levels in a low-risk diabetic patient. *Diabetes Care*. 1998;21:1364-1365.
6. Al-Salman J, et al. Hepatocellular injury in a patient receiving rosiglitazone: a case report. *Ann Intern Med*. 2000;132:121-124.
7. Andrade R, et al. Hypoglycemic hemiplegic syndrome. *Ann Emerg Med*. 1984;13:529-531.
8. Andrade RJ, et al. Acarbose-associated hepatotoxicity. *Diabetes Care*. 1998;21:2029-2030.
9. Arem R, Zoghbi W. Insulin overdose in eight patients: insulin pharmacokinetics and review of the literature. *Medicine (Baltimore)*. 1985;64:323-332.
10. Arky RA, et al. Irreversible hypoglycemia. A complication of alcohol and insulin. *JAMA*. 1968;206:575-578.
11. Bailey CJ, Day C. Traditional plant medicines as treatments for diabetes. *Diabetes Care*. 1989;12:553-564.
12. Bailey CJ, Turner RC. Metformin. *N Engl J Med*. 1996;334:574-579.
13. Banting FG, et al. Pancreatic extracts in the treatment of diabetes mellitus: preliminary report. *CMAJ*. 1922;12:141-146.
14. Baron SH. Salicylates as hypoglycemic agents. *Diabetes Care*. 1982;5:64-71.
15. Bode SF, et al. *J Clin Pharm;[Letter to Editor]*. 2013;52:785-786.
16. Bowman CE, et al. Hypoglycaemia and angina. *Lancet*. 1985;1:639-640.
17. Boyle PJ, et al. Plasma glucose concentrations at the onset of hypoglycemic symptoms in patients with poorly controlled diabetes and in nondiabetics. *N Engl J Med*. 1988;318:1487-1492.
18. Boyle PJ, et al. Octreotide reverses hyperinsulinemia and prevents hypoglycemia induced by sulfonylurea overdoses. *J Clin Endocrinol Metab*. 1993;76:752-756.
19. Boyle PJ, et al. Brain glucose uptake and unawareness of hypoglycemia in patients with insulin-dependent diabetes mellitus. *N Engl J Med*. 1995;333:1726-1731.
20. Braatvedt GD. Octreotide for the treatment of sulphonylurea induced hypoglycaemia in type 2 diabetes. *N Z Med J*. 1997;110:189-190.
21. Bressler R, Johnson D. New pharmacological approaches to therapy of NIDDM. *Diabetes Care*. 1992;15:792-805.
22. Bridges HR, et al. Molecular features of biguanides required for targeting of mitochondrial respiratory complex I and activation of AMP-kinase. *BMC Biol*. 2016;14:65.
23. Brvar M, et al. Poisoning with insulin glargine [letter]. *Clin Toxicol*. 2005;43:219-220.
24. Budnitz DS, et al. Emergency hospitalizations for adverse drug events in older Americans. *N Engl J Med*. 2011;365:2002-2012.
25. Burge MR, et al. A prospective trial of risk factors for sulfonylurea-induced hypoglycemia in type 2 diabetes mellitus. *JAMA*. 1998;279:137-143.
26. Burkhart KK. When does hypoglycemia develop after sulfonylurea ingestion? *Ann Emerg Med*. 1998;31:771-772.
27. Calara F, et al. A randomized, open-label, crossover study examining the effect of injection site on bioavailability of exenatide (synthetic exendin-4). *Clin Ther*. 2005;27:210-215.
28. Calello DP, et al. Extracorporeal treatment for metformin poisoning: systemic review and recommendations from the extracorporeal treatments in poisoning workgroup. *Crit Care Med*. 2015;43:1716-1730.
29. Campbell IW, Ratcliffe JG. Suicidal insulin overdose managed by excision of insulin injection site. *Br Med J (Clin Res Ed)*. 1982;285:408-409.
30. Carrascosa M, et al. Acarbose-induced severe hepatotoxicity. *Lancet*. 1997;349:698-699.
31. Chan NN, et al. Metformin-associated lactic acidosis: a rare or very rare clinical entity. *Diabet Med*. 1999;16:273-281.
32. Chase HP, et al. Pramlintide lowered glucose excursions and was well tolerated in adolescents with type 1 diabetes: results from a randomized single-blind, placebo-controlled, crossover study. *J Pediatr*. 2009;155:369-373.
33. Chochinov R, Daughaday WH. Marked hyperthermia as a manifestation of hypoglycemia in long-standing diabetes mellitus. *Diabetes*. 1975;24:859-860.
34. Clark BA, Brown RS. Potassium homeostasis and hyperkalemic syndromes. *Endocrinol Metab Clin North Am*. 1997;26:553-573.
35. Cohen V, Teperikidis E. Acute exenatide (Byetta) poisoning was not associated with significant hypoglycemia. *Clin Toxicol*. 2008;46:346-347.
36. Cryer PE. Hypoglycemia. In: Melmed S, et al, eds. *Williams Textbook of Endocrinology*. 12th ed. Philadelphia, PA: Saunders; 2011:1552-1577.
37. Cryer PE. Mechanisms of hypoglycemia-associated autonomic failure in diabetes. *N Engl J Med*. 2013;369:363-372.
38. Davidson JA, Kuritzky L. Sodium glucose co-transporter 2 inhibitors and their mechanism for improving glycemia in patients with type 2 diabetes. *Postgrad Med*. 2014;126:33-48.
39. DCCT Research Group. Epidemiology of severe hypoglycemia in the diabetes control and complications trial. *Am J Med*. 1991;90:450-459.
40. DCCT Research Group. The effect of intensive treatment of diabetes on the development and progression of long-term complications in insulin-dependent diabetes mellitus. *N Engl J Med*. 1993;329:977-986.
41. Delemarre-van de Waal HA, et al. Long-term treatment of an infant with nesidioblastosis using a somatostatin analogue. *N Engl J Med*. 1987;316:222-223.
42. Dell'Aglio D, et al. Acute metformin overdose: examining serum pH, lactate level, and metformin concentrations in survivors versus nonsurvivors: a systematic review of literature. *Ann Emerg Med*. 2009;54:818-823.
43. Deviveni D, et al. Pharmacokinetics and pharmacodynamics of canagliflozin, a sodium glucose co-transporter 2 inhibitor, in subject with type 2 diabetes mellitus. *J Clin Pharm*. 2013;53:601-610.
44. DeWitt CR, et al. Insulin and C-peptide levels in sulfonylurea-induced hypoglycemia: a systematic review. *J Med Toxicol*. 2007;3:107-118.
45. Dine MS, McGovern ME. Intentional poisoning of children—an overlooked category of child abuse: report of seven cases and review of the literature. *Pediatrics*. 1982;70:32-35.
46. Duh E, Feinglos M. Hypoglycemia-induced angina pectoris in a patient with diabetes mellitus. *Ann Intern Med*. 1994;121:945-946.
47. Dunn JT, et al. Attenuation of amygdala and frontal cortical responses to low blood glucose concentration in asymptomatic hypoglycemia in type I diabetes. *Diabetes*. 2007;56:2766-2773.
48. Eastham JH, et al. Prevalence of interfering substances with point-of-care glucose testing in a community hospital. *Am J Health Syst Pharm*. 2009;66:167-170.
49. Eliasson L, et al. PKC-dependent stimulation of exocytosis by sulfonylureas in pancreatic beta cells. *Science*. 1996;271:813-815.
50. Elkinson S, Scott LJ. Canagliflozin: first global approval. *Drugs*. 2013;73:979-988.
51. Elling R, et al. Prolonged hypoglycemia after a suicidal ingestion of repaglinide with unexpected slow plasma elimination. *Clin Toxicol*. 2016;54:158-160.
52. Fahy BG, Coursin DB. Critical glucose control: the devil is in the details. *Mayo Clin Proc*. 2008;83:394-397.
53. Fineberg SE, et al. Immunogenicity of recombinant DNA human insulin. *Diabetologia*. 1983;25:465-469.
54. Fischer KF, et al. Hypoglycemia in hospitalized patients. Causes and outcomes. *N Engl J Med*. 1986;315:1245-1250.
55. Fitzgerald FT. Hypoglycemia and accidental hypothermia in an alcoholic population. *West J Med*. 1980;133:105-107.

56. Fullerton B, et al. Intensive glucose control versus conventional glucose control for type I diabetes mellitus (review). *The Cochrane Collaboration.* New York, NY: John Wiley & Sons, Ltd; 2016:1-3.

57. Forman LM, et al. Hepatic failure in a patient taking rosiglitazone. *Ann Intern Med.* 2000;132:118-121.

58. Furman BL. The development of Byetta (exenatide) from the venom of the Gila monster as an anti-diabetic agent. *Toxicon.* 2012;59:464-474.

59. Furukawa S, et al. Suicide attempt by an overdose of sitagliptin, an oral hypoglycemic agent: A case report and a review of the literature. *Endocrin J.* 2012;59:329-333.

60. Gaines KL, et al. Characterization of the sulfonylurea receptor on beta cell membranes. *J Biol Chem.* 1988;263:2589-2592.

61. Gerich JE. Oral hypoglycemic agents. *N Engl J Med.* 1989;321:1231-1245.

62. Gitlin N, et al. Two cases of severe clinical and histologic hepatotoxicity associated with troglitazone. *Ann Intern Med.* 1998;129:36-38.

63. Given BD, et al. Hypoglycemia due to surreptitious injection of insulin. Identification of insulin species by high-performance liquid chromatography. *Diabetes Care.* 1991;14:544-547.

64. Graham GG, et al. Clinical pharmacokinetics of metformin. *Clin Pharmacokinet.* 2011;50:81-98.

65. Grajower MM, et al. Hypoglycemia in chronic hemodialysis patients: association with propranolol use. *Nephron.* 1980;26:126-129.

66. Harvey B, et al. Severe lactic acidosis complicating metformin overdose successfully treated with high-volume venovenous hemofiltration and aggressive alkalinization. *Pediatr Crit Care Med.* 2005;6:598-601.

67. Hearn PR, et al. The use of SMS 201-995 (somatostatin analogue) in insulinomas. Additional case report and literature review. *Horm Res.* 1988;29:211-213.

68. Hirshberg B, et al. Repaglinide-induced factitious hypoglycemia. *J Clin Endocrinol Metab.* 2001;86:475-477.

69. Hoffman JR, et al. The empiric use of hyper-tonic dextrose in patients with altered mental status: a reappraisal. *Ann Emerg Med.* 1992;21:20-24.

70. Hollander P. Safety profile of acarbose an alpha-glucosidase inhibitor. *Drugs.* 1992;44(suppl 2):47-53.

71. Hur KY, Lee M. New mechanisms of metformin action: Focusing on mitochondria and the gut. *J Diabetes Investig.* 2015;6:600-609.

72. Iwamoto Y, et al. Effects of troglitazone: a new hypoglycemic agent in patients with NIDDM poorly controlled by diet therapy. *Diabetes Care.* 1996;19:151-156.

73. Jennings AM, et al. Symptomatic hypoglycemia in NIDDM patients treated with oral hypoglycemic agents. *Diabetes Care.* 1989;12:203-208.

74. Johnson SF, et al. Chlorpropamide-induced hypoglycemia: successful treatment with diazoxide. *Am J Med.* 1977;63:799-804.

75. Kadowaki T, et al. Chlorpropamide-induced hyponatremia: incidence and risk factors. *Diabetes Care.* 1983;6:468-471.

76. Kannisto H, Neuvonen PJ. Adsorption of sulfonylureas onto activated charcoal in vitro. *J Pharm Sci.* 1984;73:253-256.

77. Kedes LH, Field JB. Hypothermia: a clue to hypoglycemia. *N Engl J Med.* 1964;271:785-787.

78. Kerr D, et al. Beta-adrenoceptor blockade and hypoglycaemia. A randomised double-blind placebo controlled comparison of metoprolol CR atenolol and propranolol LA in normal subjects. *Br J Clin Pharmacol.* 1990;29:685-693.

79. Kirrane BM, et al. Unrecognized hypoglycemia due to maltodextrin interference with bedside glucometry. *J Med Toxicol.* 2009;5:20-23.

80. Kitabchi AE. Low-dose insulin therapy in diabetic ketoacidosis: fact or fiction? *Diabetes Metab Rev.* 1989;5:337-363.

81. Koivisto VA. The human insulin analogue insulin lispro. *Ann Intern Med.* 1998;30:260-266.

82. Krinsley JS. Association between hyperglycemia and increased hospital mortality in a heterogeneous population of critically ill patients. *Mayo Clin Proc.* 2003;78:1471-1478.

83. Krishnan L. No clinical harm from a massive exenatide overdose—a short report [letter to the editor]. *Clin Toxicol (Phila).* 2013;51:61.

84. Kuzak N, et al. Reversal of salicylate-induced euglycemic delirium with dextrose. *Clin Toxicology.* 2007;45:526-529.

85. Laffel L. Ketone bodies: a review of physiology, pathophysiology and application of monitoring to diabetes. *Diabetes Metab Res Rev.* 1999;15:412-426.

86. Lalau JD, et al. Role of metformin accumulation in metformin-associated lactic acidosis. *Diabetes Care.* 1995;18:779-784.

87. Lalau JD, et al. Consequences of metformin intoxication. *Diabetes Care.* 1998;21:2036-2037.

88. Langley AK, et al. Dipeptidyl peptidase IV inhibitors and the incretin system in type 2 diabetes mellitus. *Pharmacotherapy.* 2007;27:1163-1180.

89. Leak D, Starr P. The mechanism of arrhythmias during insulin-induced hypoglycemia. *Am J Heart.* 1962;63:688-691.

90. Lebovitz HE. The oral hypoglycemic agents. In: Porte D Jr, Sherwin RS, eds. *Ellenberg & Rifkin's Diabetes Mellitus.* 5th ed. Stamford, CT: Appleton & Lange; 1997:761-788.

91. Lee NJ, et al. Efficacy and harms of the hypoglycemic agent pramlintide in diabetes mellitus. *Ann Fam Med.* 2010;8:542-549.

92. Lerner EB, et al. Can paramedics safely treat and discharge hypoglycemic patients in the field? *Am J Emerg Med.* 2003;21:115-120.

93. Levine DF, Bulstrode C. Managing suicidal insulin overdose. *BMJ.* 1982;285:974-975.

94. Levy WJ, et al. Unusual problems for the physician in managing a hospital patient who received a malicious insulin overdose. *Neurosurgery.* 1985;17:992-996.

95. Lipska KJ, et al. Polypharmacy in the aging patient: a review of glycemic control in older adults with type 2 diabetes. *JAMA.* 2016;315:1034-1045.

96. Lipska KJ, et al. Potential overtreatment of diabetes mellitus in older adults with tight glycemic control. *JAMA.* 2015;175:356-362.

97. Longnecker SM. Somatostatin and octreotide: literature review and description of therapeutic activity in pancreatic neoplasia. *Drug Intell Clin Pharm.* 1988;22:99-106.

98. Maeda K. Hepatocellular injury in a patient receiving pioglitazone. *Ann Intern Med.* 2001;135:306.

99. Malouf R, Brust JC. Hypoglycemia: causes, neurological manifestations, and outcome. *Ann Neurol.* 1985;17:421-430.

100. Martin FI, et al. Attempted suicide by insulin overdose in insulin-requiring diabetics. *Med J Aust.* 1977;1:58-60.

101. May LD, et al. Mixed hepatocellular cholestatic liver injury after pioglitazone therapy. *Ann Intern Med.* 2002;136:449-452.

102. McCartney MM, et al. Metformin and contrast media—a dangerous combination? *Clin Radiol.* 1999;54:29-33.

103. McCoy RG, et al, et al. Intensive treatment and severe hypoglycemia among adults with type 2 diabetes. *JAMA Intern Med.* 2016;176:969-978.

104. McIntyre AS, et al. Local excision of subcutaneous fat in the management of insulin overdose. *Br J Surg.* 1986;73:538.

105. McLaughlin SA, et al. Octreotide: an antidote for sulfonylurea-induced hypoglycemia. *Ann Emerg Med.* 2000;36:133-138.

106. McLelland J. Recovery from metformin overdose. *Diabet Med.* 1985;2:410-411.

107. McNamara K, Isbister GK. Hyperlactataemia and clinical severity of acute metformin overdose. *Int Med J.* 2015;45:402-408.

108. Mechem CC, et al. The short-term outcome of hypoglycemic diabetic patients who refuse ambulance transport after out-of-hospital therapy. *Acad Emerg Med.* 1998;5:768-772.

109. Megarbane B, et al. Intentional overdose with insulin: prognostic factors and toxicokinetic/toxicodynamic profiles. *Crit Care.* 2007;11(R115);1-10.

110. Miller DW, Slovis CM. Hypophosphatemia in the emergency department therapeutics. *Am J Emerg Med.* 2000;18:457-461.

111. Mizock BA. Controversies in lactic acidosis—implications in critically ill patients. *JAMA.* 1987;258:497-501.

112. Munck O, Quaade F. Suicide attempted with insulin. *Dan Med Bull.* 1963;10:139-141.

113. Nakanishi R, et al. Attempted suicide with liraglutide overdose did not induce hypoglycemia. *Diabetes Rsch Clin Pract.* 2012;99:e3-e4.

114. Nakayama S, et al. Hypoglycemia following a nateglinide overdose in a suicide attempt [letter]. *Diabetes Care.* 2005;28:227.

115. Nawaz S, et al. Clinical risk associated with contrast angiography in metformin treated patients: a clinical review. *Clin Radiol.* 1998;53:342-344.

116. Nesto RW, et al. Thiazolidinedione use, fluid retention, and congestive heart failure: a consensus statement from the American Heart Association and American Diabetes Association: October 7, 2003. *Circulation.* 2003;108:2941-2948.

117. Neuschwander-Tetri BA, et al. Troglitazone-induced hepatic failure leading to liver transplantation. A case report. *Ann Intern Med.* 1998;129:38-41.

118. Nissen SE, Wolski K. Effect of rosiglitazone on the risk of myocardial infarction and death from cardiovascular causes. *N Engl J Med.* 2007;356:2457-2471.

119. Odeh M, et al. Transient atrial fibrillation precipitated by hypoglycemia. *Ann Emerg Med.* 1990;19:565-567.

120. Olefsky JM, Kruszynska YT. Insulin resistance. In: Porte JD, et al., eds. *Ellenberg & Rifkin's Diabetes Mellitus.* 6th ed. New York, NY: McGraw-Hill; 2003:367-400.

121. Palatnick W, et al. Clinical spectrum of sulfonylurea overdose and experience with diazoxide therapy. *Arch Intern Med.* 1991;151:1859-1862.

122. Palatnick W, et al. Severe lactic acidosis from acute metformin overdose [abstract]. *J Toxicol Clin Toxicol.* 1999;37:638-639.

123. Pallais JC, et al. Case 33-2012: a 34 year old woman with episodic paresthesias and altered mental status after childbirth. *N Engl J Med.* 2012;367:1637-1646.

124. Peitzman SJ, Agarwal BN. Spontaneous hypoglycemia in end-stage renal failure. *Nephron.* 1977;19:131-139.

125. Pelavin PI, et al. Extended-release glipizide overdose presenting with delayed hypoglycemia and treated with subcutaneous octreotide. *J Pediatr Endocrinol Metab.* 2009;22:171-175.

126. Pepper GM, Schwartz M. Lactic acidosis associated with glucophage use in man with normal renal and hepatic function. *Diabetes Care.* 1997;20:232-233.

127. Phillips RE, et al. Effectiveness of SMS 201–995, a synthetic long-acting somatostatin analogue in treatment of quinine-induced hyperinsulinaemia. *Lancet.* 1986;1:713-716.

128. Pladziewicz DS, Nesto RW. Hypoglycemia-induced silent myocardial ischemia. *Am J Cardiol.* 1989;63:1531-1532.

129. Podgainy H, Bressler R. Biochemical basis of the sulfonylurea-induced Antabuse syndrome. *Diabetes.* 1968;17:679-683.

130. Polonsky KS. A practical approach to fasting hypoglycemia. *N Engl J Med.* 1992;326:1020-1021.

131. Posner JB, et al. *Plum and Posner's Diagnosis of Stupor and Coma.* 4th ed. New York: Oxford University Press; 2007.

132. Powers AC. Diabetes mellitus. In: Fauci AS, et al, eds. *Harrison's Principles of Internal Medicine.* 17th ed. New York, NY: McGraw-Hill; 2008:2275-2304.

133. Protti A, et al. Metformin overdose, but not lactic acidosis *per se*, inhibits oxygen consumption in pigs. *Crit Care.* 2012;16:R75.

134. Quadrani DA, et al. Five-year retrospective evaluation of sulfonylurea ingestion in children. *J Toxicol Clin Toxicol.* 1996;34:267-270.

135. Radziuk J, et al. Effects of metformin on lactate uptake and gluconeogenesis in the perfused rat liver. *Diabetes.* 1997;46:1406-1413.

136. Ranganath L, et al. Delayed gastric emptying occurs following acarbose administration and is a further mechanism for its anti-hyperglycaemic effect. *Diabet Med.* 1998;15:120-124.

137. Reichlin S. Somatostatin (part I). *N Engl J Med.* 1983;309:1495-1501.

138. Reichlin S. Somatostatin (second of two parts). *N Engl J Med.* 1983;309:1556-1563.

139. Rendell MS, Kirchain WR. Pharmacotherapy of type 2 diabetes mellitus. *Ann Pharmacother.* 2000;34:878-895.

140. Robertson WO. Sulfonylurea ingestions: hospitalization not mandatory. *J Toxicol Clin Toxicol.* 1997;35:115-118.

141. Russel JL, et al. Clinical effects of exposure to DPP-4 inhibitors as reported to the national poison data system. *J Med Toxicol.* 2014;10:152-155.

142. Saltpeter S, et al. Risk of fatal and nonfatal lactic acidosis with metformin use in type 2 diabetes mellitus [systematic review]. Cochrane Metabolic and Endocrine Disorders Group. *Cochrane Database Syst Rev.* 2010;4:CD002967.

143. Salvatore T, Giugliano D. Pharmacokinetic-pharmacodynamic relationships of acarbose. *Clin Pharmacokinet.* 1996;30:94-106.

144. Samuels MH, Eckel RH. Massive insulin overdose: detailed studies of free insulin levels and glucose requirements. *J Toxicol Clin Toxicol.* 1989;27:157-168.

145. Seibert DG. Reversible decerebrate posturing secondary to hypoglycemia. *Am J Med.* 1985;78:1036-1037.

146. Seidowsky A, et al. Metformin-associated lactic acidosis: a prognostic and therapeutic study. *Crit Care Med.* 2009;37:2191-2196.

147. Seltzer HS. Drug-induced hypoglycemia. *Endocrin Metabol Clin N Amer.* 1989;18:163-183.

148. Service FJ. Hypoglycemic disorders. *N Engl J Med.* 1995;332:1144-1152.

149. Shulman GI, et al. Integrated fuel metabolism. In: Porte JD, et al, eds. *Ellenberg & Rifkin's Diabetes Mellitus.* 6th ed. New York, NY: McGraw-Hill; 2003:1-13.

150. Slama G, et al. The search for an optimized treatment of hypoglycemia. Carbohydrates in tablets, solution or gel for the correction of insulin reactions. *Arch Intern Med.* 1990;150:589-593.

151. Socransky SJ, et al. Out-of-hospital treatment of hypoglycemia: refusal of transport and patient outcome. *Acad Emerg Med.* 1998;5:1080-1085.

152. Spiller HA, et al. Prospective multicenter study of sulfonylurea ingestion in children. *J Pediatr.* 1997;131:141-146.

153. Spiller HA, et al. Hemiparesis and altered mental status in a child after glyburide ingestion. *J Emerg Med.* 1998;16:433-435.

154. Spiller HA, et al. Multicenter case series of adult metformin ingestion [abstract]. *J Toxicol Clin Toxicol.* 1999;37:639.

155. Spiller HA, et al. Multicenter case series of pediatric metformin ingestion. *Ann Pharmacother.* 2000;34:1385-1388.

156. Stapczynski JS, Haskell RJ. Duration of hypoglycemia and need for intravenous glucose following intentional overdoses of insulin. *Ann Emerg Med.* 1984;13:505-511.

157. Stocks AE. Insulin lispro: experience in a private practice setting. *Med J Aust.* 1999;170:364-367.

158. Strauch BS, et al. Hypothermia in hypoglycemia. *JAMA.* 1969;210:345-346.

159. Svingos RS, et al. Life-threatening hypoglycemia associated with intentional insulin ingestion. *Pharmacotherapy.* 2013;33:e28-e33.

160. Szlatenyi CS, et al. Delayed hypoglycemia in a child after ingestion of a single glipizide tablet. *Ann Emerg Med.* 1998;31:773-776.

161. Taylor SI, et al. SGLT2 inhibitors may predispose to ketoacidosis. *J Clin Endocrinol Metab.* 2015;100:2849-2852.

162. Teale KF, et al. The management of metformin overdose. *Anaesthesia.* 1998;53:698-701.

163. Thoma ME, et al. Persistent hypoglycemia and hyperinsulinemia: caution in using glucagon. *Am J Emerg Med.* 1996;14:99-101.

164. Thurston JH, et al. Reduced brain glucose with normal plasma glucose in salicylate poisoning. *J Clin Invest.* 1970;49:2139-2145.

165. Todd JF, Bloom SR. Incretins and other peptides in the treatment of diabetes. *Diabet Med.* 2007;24:223-232.

166. Tymms DJ, Leatherdale BA. Lactic acidosis due to metformin therapy in a low risk patient. *Postgrad Med J.* 1988;64:230-231.

167. Umpierrez G, Korytkowski M. Diabetic emergencies—ketoacidosis, hyperglycaemic hyperosmolar state and hypoglycaemia. *Nature Review Endocrin.* 2016;12:222-232.

168. Van den Berghe G, et al. Intensive insulin therapy in the medical ICU. *N Engl J Med.* 2006;354:449-461.

169. Van den Berghe G, et al. Intensive insulin therapy in critically ill patients. *N Engl J Med.* 2001;345:1359-1367.

170. Wallis WE, et al. Hypoglycemia masquerading as cerebrovascular disease (hypoglycemic hemiplegia). *Ann Neurol.* 1985;18:510-512.

171. Welborn TA. Acarbose, an alpha-glucosidase inhibitor for non-insulin-dependent diabetes. *Med J Aust.* 1998;168:76-78.

172. Wills BK, et al. Can acute overdose of metformin lead to lactic acidosis? *Am J Emerg Med.* 2010;28:857-861.

A8

DEXTROSE (D-GLUCOSE)

Vincent Nguyen and Larissa I. Velez

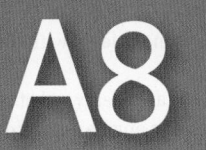

CH$_2$OH

OH

OH   OH

OH

Dextrose (D-glucose)

INTRODUCTION

Hypoglycemia is a common cause of altered mental status. Although classically associated with tachycardia, tremor, and diaphoresis, the predictive value of these manifestations is too low to be relied on.[25] As a result, all patients with altered consciousness require either rapid point-of-care testing of their glucose concentrations or empiric treatment for presumed hypoglycemia. When rapidly diagnosed and treated, hypoglycemic patients typically recover without sequelae. Delayed or incomplete therapy may lead to permanent neurologic dysfunction.

HISTORY

In 1891, Fisher performed the unbelievable feat of identifying the 16 possible different spatial configurations of aldohexose (C$_6$H$_{12}$O$_6$), the most prominent member being dextrose or D-glucose.[44] This discovery won him the 1902 Nobel Prize in chemistry. This chapter will use *dextrose* as the term for the antidote and *glucose* as the general term for aldohexose.[10] The diverse manifestations of hypoglycemia, and the treatment of severe cases with intravenous dextrose, have been appreciated for decades.[80]

Chemistry and Physiology

Sugar is the general term used for sweet carbohydrates that are used as food. Simple sugars are called monosaccharides and include glucose (also known as dextrose, as the L-isomer is hardly found in nature), fructose (also known as fruit sugar, the sweetest of them all) and galactose. The disaccharides include maltose, lactose, and sucrose (also known as table or granulated sugar).

Sugars (sucrose) are found in the tissues of most plants but are only present in sufficient concentrations for efficient extraction in sugarcane and sugar beet. Commercially, glucose is produced from the hydrolysis of starch. Several crops are the source of starch, with corn being the most common in the United States.

In humans, carbohydrates are absorbed and transported via 2 main systems. Sodium-dependent glucose transporters (SGLT1 through SGLT6) are responsible for the intestinal and renal glucose absorption.[20] Their discovery was the first description of the mechanism of "flux coupling" or co-transporting, in which transporting one substrate down its concentration gradient (sodium in this case) creates energy that is used to transport a second substrate against a concentration gradient (glucose). The SGLT2 inhibitors (commonly termed "gliflozins") are a family of drugs used to manage type 2 diabetes mellitus that inhibit SGLT2 in the proximal tubule of the nephron, resulting in glycosuria.[41,99,105,147] Glucose uptake transporters include GLUT1-GLUT14 and HMIT (H+/myoinositol transporter). Facilitative transporters move molecules down their concentration gradient. This facilitative diffusion process does not require energy. Binding of glucose to one of the GLUT receptors causes a conformational change that results in its translocation across the membrane.[64] GLUT4 is expressed in insulin-sensitive tissues and regulates whole-body glucose homeostasis.[96] Even in low substrate conditions such as in neurons and the placenta, the high affinity for glucose by GLUT3 facilitates transport.[12] The absorption of fructose in the small intestine is dependent on GLUT5.[16] The GLUT5 transporter has wide variability and is dependent on the amount of glucose ingested relative to the fructose. Decreased fructose absorption leads to abdominal bloating and osmotic diarrhea in susceptible individuals.[65]

Glucose delivered hematogenously to the liver, adipose tissue, and muscle cells is absorbed and stored as glycogen—under the influence of insulin—or used by all cells to produce adenosine triphosphate (ATP) and pyruvate via glycolysis. Hepatic glycogen can later be converted to glucose and returned to the blood when insulin is low or absent. In contrast, glycogen found in muscle and adipose cells is used internally and not released into the systemic circulation. Some glucose is converted to lactate by astrocytes, and then utilized as an energy source.[115,128,138] Finally, glucose is also directly used by intestinal cells and red blood cells.

Pharmacokinetics

Accurate prediction of the amount of dextrose required to effectively treat patients with hypoglycemia is complex. At equilibrium, 25 g of dextrose distributed in total body water in a 70-kg adult is calculated to increase the serum glucose concentration by about 60 mg/dL.[63] In the few clinical studies performed, the magnitude of glucose elevation after oral or IV dextrose loading was unpredictable. In one study, 25 g (50 mL) of D$_{50}$W administered to both diabetic and nondiabetic adults resulted in a mean blood glucose elevation of 166 mg/dL when measured in the opposite extremity 3 to 5 minutes after the bolus; however, the range of this elevation was between 37 and 370 mg/dL above baseline.[2] In a human model of insulin-induced hypoglycemia, oral administration of 10 or 20 g of dextrose increased the serum glucose concentration from 60 to 120 mg/dL over one hour.[148] Another study used 25 nondiabetic volunteers and administered 25 g of IV dextrose as D$_{50}$W. Glucose concentrations were then measured at 5, 15, 30, and 60 minutes. Volume of distribution formulas could not accurately predict postinfusion glucose concentrations. The serum glucose elevation was statistically significant from baseline at 5 and 15 minutes, with glucose concentrations returning to baseline at 30 minutes postinfusion.[9]

Two prehospital studies also evaluated the magnitude of glucose elevation in hypoglycemic patients after a 10-g dextrose bolus (100 mL of D$_{10}$W). Pretreatment mean serum glucose concentrations were 37 and 38 mg/dL, respectively. After the bolus, the median glucose concentrations were 91 and 98 mg/dL, respectively. Therefore, the median rise in serum glucose concentration was between 54 and 60 mg/dL.[60,71] In these studies, the time to measurement of serum glucose concentration after the bolus was not uniform, but the median time to testing was 8 minutes.

Pharmacodynamics

Adenosine triphosphate provides the metabolic energy that fuels all critical cellular processes in all organs. In the adult brain, the anaerobic and aerobic metabolism of glucose occurring through glycolysis and the citric acid cycle, respectively, are the primary sources of ATP (Chap. 11). Although the adult brain can use fatty acids, amino acids, lactate, and ketones as alternate substrates for ATP synthesis, these are not adequate to sustain normal cerebral function in the setting of glucose deprivation. In contrast, in fetal and neonatal brains, glucose is the only substrate for ATP production.[109,139]

Although a blood or serum glucose less than 60 mg/dL defines hypoglycemia, clinical hypoglycemia cannot be entirely predicted by strict numerical values. Rather, it is best defined by organ dysfunction in the setting of inadequate glucose concentrations. The onset of numerical hypoglycemia in both adults and children is often followed rapidly by global cerebral dysfunction, owing to neuroglycopenia. In individuals with diabetes, the density and sensitivity of neuronal insulin receptors vary as a function of glycemic control, such that diabetic patients with poor glycemic control have fewer and less sensitive neuronal insulin receptors and experience hypoglycemic symptoms at much higher blood concentrations of glucose than those who are normally euglycemic. An important study of diabetic patients demonstrated that the mean blood glucose concentration for symptomatic hypoglycemia in poorly controlled diabetic patients was 78 ± 5 mg/dL compared with 53 ± mg/dL in well-controlled patients.[13] This differential response to hypoglycemia is also described at higher glucose concentrations in poorly controlled versus intensely controlled diabetic patients.[67] Thus, in a subset of diabetics neuroglycopenia occurs despite "normal" peripheral blood glucose concentrations.[143] Additionally, a report described 2 patients with salicylate toxicity who presented with altered mentation that resolved after treatment with $D_{50}W$, despite normal serum glucose concentrations. The etiology was attributed to salicylate-induced neuroglycopenia.[76] The occurrence of low brain glucose concentrations despite normal serum glucose concentration is described in a rat model of salicylate toxicity.[132] In rare cases, glucose-consuming cancer cells can produce large amounts of lactate (Warburg effect), which is available as an alternate source of energy for the brain. Even in the presence of profound hypoglycemia, these patients remain asymptomatic.[38]

On the other hand, while *chronic hyperglycemia* causes the glycemic threshold at which counterregulatory response occurs to be reset to a higher glucose concentration, *repeated hypoglycemia* causes the glycemic threshold at which counterregulatory response occurs to be reset to a lower glucose concentration. Diabetic patients with repeated episodes of hypoglycemia—usually those subjected to tight control—will have neuroglycopenia *before* the appearance of autonomic warning signs such as sweating, palpitations, and anxiety. This condition, known as hypoglycemia-associated autonomic failure, often termed "hypoglycemia unawareness," results in prolonged exposure to low serum glucose concentrations.[24,69,102,111,129] The etiology of hypoglycemia unawareness is not completely understood. There is strong evidence from animal studies that the activity of neurons in the ventromedial hypothalamus (VMH) plays a critical role in initiating compensatory responses to hypoglycemia. The VMH is a key component of a complex glucose-sensing network.[89] Recurrent hypoglycemia lowers the glucose concentration at which these neurons are activated, giving the patients less time to react to hypoglycemia.[90] Risk factors include chronic exposure to low glucose concentrations, antecedent hypoglycemia, recurrent severe hypoglycemia, duration of diabetes, and the failure of counterregulatory hormones.[22,23,29]

Hypoglycemia causes a myriad of neuropsychiatric sequelae that are clinically indistinguishable from those of other toxic-metabolic, infectious, and structural brain injuries.[33,87,94,118,142,150] In a case series, presenting signs and symptoms of hypoglycemia included dizziness and tremulousness (8%); focal stroke syndromes (2%); movement disorders or seizures (7%); irritability, confusion, or bizarre behavior (30%); delirium, stupor, or coma (52%); and irreversible encephalopathy.[87] These incidences are similar to those in a case series of patients with insulinomas.[28] In cases of undifferentiated coma, both the absence of pupillary light reflex (sensitivity 83% and specificity 77%, positive predictive value {PPV} 70% and negative predictive value {NPV} 87%, likelihood ratio {LR} 3.56) and the presence of anisocoria (sensitivity 39% and specificity 96%, PPV 86 and NPV 70, LR 9) are helpful in diagnosing structural (intracerebral hemorrhage, subarachnoid hemorrhage, subdural hematoma, cerebral infarction, epidural hematoma) instead of metabolic causes (drug overdose, hypoglycemia, sepsis).[133] Hypoglycemic hemiplegia is a well-recognized, although rare, entity, and therein

lies the relevance of a serum glucose concentrations in patients with focal neurologic symptoms.[87]

The heart is partially dependent on glucose as an energy substrate. Hypoglycemia causes myocardial stress that manifests as angina and/or dysrhythmias. There are 2 mechanisms postulated for hypoglycemia-induced dysrhythmias. First, it causes potassium current inhibition, which results in QT interval prolongation.[98] This is aggravated by the systemic catecholamine response to hypoglycemia, which results in increased intracellular calcium, another dysrhythmogenic stimulus.[35,79,93,97,98,101] Nocturnal hypoglycemia is associated with the "dead in bed" syndrome. The postulated mechanisms are hypotonia of the respiratory muscles with an impaired awakening, mediated by orexin-A neurons, and QT interval prolongation and other dysrhythmogenic effects of hypoglycemia.[48,103] Orexins (hypocretins) are novel neuropeptides that play a role in the regulation of energy balances. They are highly excitatory neuropeptides that affect an organism's wakefulness. Repeated episodes of hypoglycemia result in adaptations in orexin-A, causing defective awakening and hypotonia of the upper airway muscles during sleep.[103] Finally, counterregulatory hormone responses to hypoglycemia are also impaired by sleep.[31,68]

ROLE IN HYPOGLYCEMIA
Empiric Treatment Considerations

The history and physical examination, although always important to ascertain, do not reliably detect hypoglycemic patients.[62] Tachycardia, diaphoresis, pallor, hypertension, tremors, hunger, and restlessness tend to predominate when the decline in blood glucose concentration is rapid. However, neuroglycopenia, even when severe, will not always trigger autonomic responses.[28] Signs and symptoms are further blunted or absent in the setting of concurrent use of β-adrenergic antagonists. Similarly, GABA agonists blunt autonomic nervous system, neuroendocrine, and metabolic counterregulatory responses to hypoglycemia, an effect that reportedly persists for days.[59] Central nervous system signs of neuroglycopenia are also nonspecific. They include visual disturbances, psychiatric disturbances, confusion, stupor, coma, seizures, and focal neurologic findings.[87,119] In children, sometimes the only sign of neuroglycopenia is lethargy or irritability.[153]

The bedside diagnosis of hypoglycemia is limited by the sensitivity and specificity of reagent strips, which do not have the reliability and accuracy of laboratory analysis.[104] Sensitivities of commonly available reagent strips for detection of hypoglycemia range between 92% and 97%.[18,19,66,78,86,117] The accuracy of these point-of-care testing methods is affected by the source of blood, whether arterial, venous, or capillary, and by the poor perfusion associated with shock and cardiac arrest.[8,21,34,47,70,75,77,85,130] A critical care unit study that evaluated patients in shock showed that 32% were incorrectly diagnosed as hypoglycemic when capillary blood was used. All these patients were either normoglycemic or hyperglycemic. Results of reagent strip tests of venous blood correlated well with laboratory results, correctly classifying all patients. No cases of hypoglycemia were missed.[8] Therefore, capillary determinations of glucose should be used with caution in the critically ill population, recognizing that false-positive detection of hypoglycemia might occur.[85] When feasible, laboratory measurements are preferred in these patient populations. A second best alternative is reagent strip testing using venous blood rather than capillary blood samples.

Several studies compared the accuracy of reagent strips for the detection of hypoglycemia from capillary and venous blood compared with the gold standard of the laboratory. Two studies, one with 97 subjects[47] and one with 270 subjects,[75] evaluated the agreement between reagent strip determinations of capillary and venous blood glucose concentrations in healthy euglycemic volunteers. In the larger study, 18% of subjects had a >15 mg/dL difference between capillary and venous reagent strip tests. In this study, capillary measurements were better correlated with the laboratory values. Whether these results have any clinical significance is not clear because none of the subjects were outside the euglycemic range. However, the results suggest that the capillary blood glucose test has greater accuracy in the euglycemic range and in healthy individuals.

The "safe" number at which no cases of symptomatic hypoglycemia are missed by reagent strip testing is a subject of debate because of the inherent risk of error from lack of sensitivity. In one study in which hypoglycemia was defined as a blood glucose concentration below 60 mg/dL, 2 of 33 hypoglycemic patients were not detected at the bedside. A cutoff of 90 mg/dL would have detected 100% of numerically hypoglycemic patients.[78] Based on these studies, it can be argued that a bedside reagent measurement of 90 mg/dL is a conservative cutoff for assurance of euglycemia in all patients.

With reagent strip testing, variations in hematocrit and the presence of isopropyl alcohol in the sample also alter the accuracy of the test.[11,52] In some specific tests, such as one using glucose dehydrogenase pyrroloquinolinequinone (GDH-PQQ), accuracy is affected by a number of interfering substances and xenobiotics, such as serum acetaminophen concentrations above 8 mg/dL, a serum bilirubin concentration above 20 mg/dL, a serum galactose concentration above 10 mg/dL, a maltose concentration above 16 mg/dL, a serum uric acid above 10 to 16 mg/dL, serum triglycerides above 5,000 mg/dL, and the presence of D-xylose in the sample. All of these result in falsely elevated glucose measurements.[37] There are also in vitro reports of interference with the use of intravenous lipid emulsion therapy as an antidote.[53] Notably, icodextrin, an ingredient in peritoneal dialysis, results in overestimation of glucose measurements because it is metabolized to maltose. In several case reports and at least 18 cases reported in a review, this resulted in excess insulin administration and subsequent hypoglycemia.[37,45,74,112] Glucose-monitoring systems that use the GDH-PQQ method should not be used in patients using icodextrin in the PD fluid.[134] Maltose is also contained in some immunoglobulin solutions, and the same interference is expected.[39,126] Glucose measurements by the GDH-PQQ and the amperometric methods are also affected by the hematocrit.[125,144] Whereas hematocrits lower than 20% result in a falsely elevated glucose measurements, hematocrits above 55% result in falsely low measured glucose concentrations.[37] In a retrospective review of patients admitted to a hospital over a 12-month period, 1.2% were identified as having interfering substances. Of these, 36% patients had active orders for insulin products. The most common interferences identified were a low hematocrit (44% of patients) and a high serum uric acid (29% of patients).[37]

One final consideration is in patients with salicylate toxicity (Chap. 37), in which serum glucose is not an accurate reflection of brain glucose concentrations.[131,132] Salicylate poisoning is a relatively uncommon cause for drug-induced hypoglycemia.[107,123] Salicylates uncouple oxidative phosphorylation, which results in increased intracellular glucose demands. Rarely, patients demonstrate symptoms of neuroglycopenia despite normal serum glucose concentrations. Dextrose administration reverses the signs and symptoms and likely improves survival.[76,131]

Recent advances in monitoring technology include continuous glucose monitoring, which uses a sensor placed under the skin that measures interstitial fluid glucose.[110] These sensors are generally accurate at normal glucose concentrations. However, in situations where the glucose is fluctuating, the interstitial glucose concentration lags for up to 15 minutes. Patients are encouraged to measure a capillary blood glucose before making treatment decisions.[149] Currently, there are no FDA-approved noninvasive glucose-measuring devices in the United States.[124] Table 47–1 summarizes xenobiotics and nontoxicologic conditions that are associated with hypoglycemia.

ROLE IN ETHANOL DISORDERS

Alcoholic ketoacidosis (AKA) is a metabolic emergency (Chap. 76). It occurs when malnourished chronic alcoholic patients cease or significantly decrease their food intake. This is often accompanied by vomiting. The result is salt and water depletion with an anion gap metabolic acidosis that is typically accompanied by a normal to low serum glucose (unlike diabetic ketoacidosis).[5] In children, hypoglycemia occasionally ensues after exposure to ethanol and other ethanol-containing products.[40,108] Newborns and young infants, present with irritability, feeding problems, lethargy, cyanosis, tachypnea, and/or hypothermia.[58]

The management of AKA consists of rehydration using isotonic, dextrose-containing solutions; parenteral thiamine administration; potassium replacement; and addressing the underlying medical problem that led to AKA (Chap. 76).[46]

ROLE IN SALICYLATE POISONING

Patients with salicylate toxicity demonstrate symptoms of neuroglycopenia despite normal serum glucose concentrations. Dextrose administration reverses these signs and symptoms of neuroglycopenia.[76] Chapter 37 provides an in-depth discussion of salicylate toxicity and its management.

ROLE IN CARDIOVASCULAR TOXICITY

High-dose insulin (HDI) is one of the cornerstones of management of patients with drug-induced cardiovascular toxicity. Insulin improves carbohydrate utilization by the cells and restores calcium fluxes. This improves cardiac contractility and allows for improved vascular tone.[92] The available data are strongest for calcium channel blocker toxicity, and there are also reports that describe benefits in cases of β-adrenergic antagonist toxicity.[81,154] The initial bolus of 1 unit/kg and subsequent infusion of 1 unit/kg/h of regular insulin must be supplemented with sufficient dextrose to maintain euglycemia. The use of continuous dextrose infusions with HDI is reviewed in Antidotes in Depth: A21.

Aluminum phosphide is a fumigant for grains that releases phosphine gas, which causes injury due to free radical formation. Deaths occur from both pulmonary (acute respiratory distress syndrome) and cardiac toxicity.[56] The management remains supportive, but in one report the use of HDI improved mortality (72.7% in conventional treatment vs 50% in the HIE group, $P = .03$).[57]

ROLE IN HYPERKALEMIA

Hyperkalemia occurs most commonly as a result of end-stage kidney disease. It also represents an adverse medication reaction. Intravenous insulin is used to redistribute potassium inside the cell. A dose of 0.1 Units/kg of regular insulin is usually followed by 25 g of IV 50% dextrose.[82,146] The onset of action for this intervention is less than 15 minutes and peaks at 30 to 60 minutes. This regimen results in an average serum potassium decrease of about 0.6 mEq/L.[146]

ADVERSE EFFECTS AND SAFETY ISSUES

The most serious complication associated with hypoglycemia is directly attributable to the failure to diagnose and treat it. Most complications due to the administration of concentrated IV dextrose are either clinically insignificant or exceedingly rare. Phlebitis and sclerosis of veins occurs. Tissue necrosis is reported after soft tissue extravasation of $D_{50}W$ and after inadvertent intraarterial injection.[7,30] Inappropriately large boluses of $D_{50}W$ in children are associated with seizures, brain hemorrhage, and hyperosmolar coma.[120] Anaphylactoid reactions are rarely reported after the administration of $D_{50}W$.[27] Iatrogenic exacerbation of Wernicke's encephalopathy with acute glucose or carbohydrate loading in the absence of adequate thiamine replacement was a once popular myth stemming from a single article reporting a handful of patients have had unrecognized Wernicke's encephalopathy before prolonged periods of glucose administration.[140,145] A single acute administration of dextrose does not appear to cause this effect.[54] Therefore, correction of hypoglycemia should never be delayed in order to administer thiamine (Antidotes in Depth: A27).[114]

Dilute dextrose solution should not be simultaneously infused through the same intravenous line as blood as it causes pseudoagglutination of erythrocytes. These solutions can also result in electrolyte dilution and excess intravascular volume.

An important consideration is the development of rebound hypoglycemia when dextrose is used typically to treat sulfonylurea-induced hypoglycemia, although this also occurs in other patients who received concentrated dextrose solutions as a bolus (Chap. 47). As mentioned above, serial measurements of glucose and close patient monitoring should follow any dextrose boluses.[91] Patients should also receive oral carbohydrates as soon as clinically safe and feasible.

Patients with prolonged or severe hypoglycemia frequently remain in a persistent state of altered consciousness despite normalization of blood glucose concentrations—a condition loosely defined as posthypoglycemic encephalopathy or hypoglycemic encephalopathy. The pathophysiology of hypoglycemic encephalopathy is poorly understood.[127] In large part because there is no generally accepted clinical definition, the clinical course, magnetic resonance imaging (MRI) findings, and overall outcomes are highly variable. Magnetic resonance imaging studies reported a broad spectrum of possible lesion patterns involving both gray and white brain matter.[6,72,83,88,95] Mortality rates of patients with posthypoglycemic encephalopathy reportedly range from 23.7% to 46%; however, survivors frequently recover with little or no disability.[151]

Concerns Regarding Elevated Blood Glucose Concentrations in Patients With Critical Illness

Hyperglycemia (and insulin resistance) is a common phenomenon after acute critical illness.[135] The evidence suggesting an association between high glucose concentrations on admission, persistent hyperglycemia, and high glucose variability and worse clinical outcomes is substantial.[4,32,61,73,84,100,106,121,152]

Although it is evident that hyperglycemia in critically ill patients is undesirable, the optimal blood glucose range is controversial. Initial trials suggested that intensive glucose control could reduce morbidity and mortality.[136,137] Subsequent trials did not confirm these findings, showing instead that targeting a blood glucose of 80 to 110 mg/dL increases the incidence of hypoglycemia,[42,43] which is independently associated with increased mortality.[113] The current literature supports moderate, early glucose control in most critical illnesses (goal glucose of 180 mg/dL) while avoiding hypoglycemia.[1,3,14,122,141]

PREGNANCY AND LACTATION

Dextrose is a pregnancy category C (IV) and A (oral), as studies do not exist regarding its safety to the fetus. Hypoglycemia is a serious concern for fetal and neonatal well-being, and the best evidence suggests that hypoglycemia in a pregnant woman should be approached in the same manner as in a nonpregnant patient.[55] Although there are no data regarding the use of hypertonic dextrose in lactation, it is unlikely to be a concern, because even if the concentration of glucose in subsequent breast milk is significantly increased, the effect will be transient.

Dosing and Administration

Patients with asymptomatic or minimally symptomatic hypoglycemia should be treated with oral carbohydrates (juice, milk, candy, or glucose tablets). For adults, we recommend a dose of 20 g which should result in symptomatic improvement in 15 to 20 minutes.[26] Because this improvement is transient and can result in reactive hypoglycemia, we also recommend that the initial glucose intake be followed by a more substantial meal whenever feasible. For the patient unable (coma, seizures) or unwilling (from neuroglycopenia) to receive oral glucose, the IV route must be used. In an adult, a bolus dose of 0.5 to 1.0 g/kg of IV dextrose is recommended. Similarly, the improvement in serum glucose concentration is transient, and the patient should be monitored closely for recurrence of hypoglycemia.[26] In common practice, a dextrose infusion follows the initial dextrose bolus, with the recognition that this supplies very little caloric content and is insufficient in most cases where glucose is being rapidly redistributed and utilized.[26]

Rapid increases in serum glucose are sufficient to stimulate insulin release from the pancreas and result in reactive (or rebound) hypoglycemia. Therefore, glucose concentrations must be closely followed after a bolus of concentrated dextrose solutions. This effect is exaggerated in patients, particularly those with normally functioning pancreatic islet cells, who have ingested sulfonylureas, which increase the glucose-responsive release of insulin by the islet cells.[49,50]

TABLE A8–1	Dosing of Dextrose for Symptomatic Hypoglycemia		
Age	Concentration	Bolus	Dose in mL/kg
Adult	$D_{50}W$ (50% = 0.5 g/mL)	0.5–1.0 g/kg	1–2
Child	$D_{25}W$ (25% = 0.25 g/mL)	0.5–1.0 g/kg	2–4
Infant	$D_{10}W$ (10% = 0.1 g/mL)	0.5–1.0 g/kg	5–10

In most cases, the rapid correction of hypoglycemia by the administration of 0.5 to 1.0 g/kg of concentrated IV dextrose (Table A8–1) immediately reverses the neurologic and cardiac effects caused by hypoglycemia. However, prolonged or severe hypoglycemia can result in permanent brain injury, myocardial infarction, and death.[17,36,95] Because of the myriad presentations of hypoglycemia, the difficulties inherent in making the clinical diagnosis, and the serious consequences of failure to treat the condition, the empirical administration of hypertonic dextrose to all patients with altered mental status was once a standard prehospital and emergency department practice.[15,62,63]

Formulation and Acquisition

Dextrose is available in multiple formulations between 2.5% and 70% for intravenous use. Concentrations greater than 10% should be infused via a central venous catheter, except in emergencies. Table A8–1 summarizes the most commonly available preparations.

SUMMARY

- Dextrose is an effective antidote for patients with hypoglycemia, an essential substrate for those with alcoholic ketoacidosis and an adjunct to maintain euglycemia during high-dose insulin therapy for cardiovascular drug toxicity.
- Hypoglycemia mimics many syndromes, producing diverse alterations in consciousness, including focal neurologic syndromes.
- The currently available reagent strips reliably demonstrate the absence of significant hypoglycemia at reading concentrations greater than 90 mg/dL. Profound neurologic impairment likely is not the result of hypoglycemia with such concentrations, even in diabetic patients.
- In patients with shock or cardiac arrest, testing venous blood is preferred over capillary blood.
- Dextrose should be administered to all patients with altered levels of consciousness and a serum glucose concentration <90 mg/dL by rapid testing methodology.
- Dextrose should be empirically administered to patients with altered levels of consciousness in the rare cases where bedside reagent strips are not readily available.

Acknowledgment
Kathleen A. Delaney contributed to this chapter in previous editions.

REFERENCES

1. Adams HP Jr, et al. Guidelines for the early management of adults with ischemic stroke: a guideline from the American Heart Association/American Stroke Association Stroke Council, Clinical Cardiology Council, Cardiovascular Radiology and Intervention Council, and the Atherosclerotic Peripheral Vascular Disease and Quality of Care Outcomes in Research Interdisciplinary Working Groups: the American Academy of Neurology affirms the value of this guideline as an educational tool for neurologists. *Stroke*. 2007;38:1655-1711.
2. Adler PM. Serum glucose changes after administration of 50% dextrose solution: pre- and in-hospital calculations. *Am J Emerg Med*. 1986;4:504-506.
3. Agus MS, et al. Tight glycemic control in critically ill children. *N Engl J Med*. 2017;376:729-741.
4. Ali NA, et al. Glucose variability and mortality in patients with sepsis. *Crit Care Med*. 2008;36:2316-2321.
5. Allison MG, McCurdy MT. Alcoholic metabolic emergencies. *Emerg Med Clin North Am*. 2014;32:293-301.
6. Aoki T, et al. Reversible hyperintensity lesion on diffusion-weighted MRI in hypoglycemic coma. *Neurology*. 2004;63:392-393.

7. Arad I, Benady S. Letter: Gangrene following intraumbilical injection of hypertonic glucose. *J Pediatr.* 1976;89:327-328.

8. Atkin SH, et al. Fingerstick glucose determination in shock. *Ann Intern Med.* 1991;114:1020-1024.

9. Balentine JR, et al. Effect of 50 milliliters of 50% dextrose in water administration on the blood sugar of euglycemic volunteers. *Acad Emerg Med.* 1998;5:691-694.

10. Baron DN, McIntyre N. Letter: glucose is dextrose is glucose. *Br Med J.* 1976;2:41-42.

11. Barreau PB, Buttery JE. The effect of the haematocrit value on the determination of glucose levels by reagent-strip methods. *Med J Aust.* 1987;147:286-288.

12. Bell GI, et al. Molecular biology of mammalian glucose transporters. *Diabetes Care.* 1990;13:198-208.

13. Boyle PJ, et al. Plasma glucose concentrations at the onset of hypoglycemic symptoms in patients with poorly controlled diabetes and in nondiabetics. *N Engl J Med.* 1988;318:1487-1492.

14. Broderick J, et al. Guidelines for the management of spontaneous intracerebral hemorrhage in adults: 2007 update: a guideline from the American Heart Association/American Stroke Association Stroke Council, High Blood Pressure Research Council, and the Quality of Care and Outcomes in Research Interdisciplinary Working Group. *Stroke.* 2007;38:2001-2023.

15. Browning RG, et al. 50% dextrose: antidote or toxin? *J Emerg Nurs.* 1990;16:342-349.

16. Buchs AE, et al. Characterization of GLUT5 domains responsible for fructose transport. *Endocrinology.* 1998;139:827-831.

17. Burns CM, et al. Patterns of cerebral injury and neurodevelopmental outcomes after symptomatic neonatal hypoglycemia. *Pediatrics.* 2008;122:65-74.

18. Cheeley RD, Joyce SM. A clinical comparison of the performance of four blood glucose reagent strips. *Am J Emerg Med.* 1990;8:11-15.

19. Choubtum L, et al. Accuracy of glucose meters in measuring low blood glucose levels. *J Med Assoc Thai.* 2002;85(suppl 4):S1104-S1110.

20. Crane RK. Intestinal absorption of sugars. *Physiol Rev.* 1960;40:789-825.

21. Critchell CD, et al. Accuracy of bedside capillary blood glucose measurements in critically ill patients. *Intensive Care Med.* 2007;33:2079-2084.

22. Cryer PE. Hypoglycemia-associated autonomic failure in diabetes. *Am J Physiol Endocrinol Metab.* 2001;281:E1115-E1121.

23. Cryer PE. Diverse causes of hypoglycemia-associated autonomic failure in diabetes. *N Engl J Med.* 2004;350:2272-2279.

24. Cryer PE. Hypoglycemia-associated autonomic failure in diabetes. *Handb Clin Neurol.* 2013;117:295-307.

25. Cryer PE. Mechanisms of hypoglycemia-associated autonomic failure in diabetes. *N Engl J Med.* 2013;369:362-372.

26. Cryer PE, et al. Evaluation and management of adult hypoglycemic disorders: an Endocrine Society Clinical Practice Guideline. *J Clin Endocrinol Metab.* 2009;94:709-728.

27. Czarny D, et al. Anaphylactoid reaction to 50% solution of dextrose. *Med J Aust.* 1980;2:255-258.

28. Daggett P, Nabarro J. Neurological aspects of insulinomas. *Postgrad Med J.* 1984;60:577-581.

29. Davis SN, et al. Effects of intensive therapy and antecedent hypoglycemia on counterregulatory responses to hypoglycemia in type 2 diabetes. *Diabetes.* 2009;58:701-709.

30. DeLorenzo RA, Vista JP. Another hazard of hypertonic dextrose. *Am J Emerg Med.* 1994;12:262-263.

31. Diabetes Research in Children Network Study G. Impaired overnight counterregulatory hormone responses to spontaneous hypoglycemia in children with type 1 diabetes. *Pediatr Diabetes.* 2007;8:199-205.

32. Dossett LA, et al. Blood glucose variability is associated with mortality in the surgical intensive care unit. *Am Surg.* 2008;74:679-685; discussion 685.

33. Duarte J, et al. Hypoglycemia presenting as acute tetraplegia. *Stroke.* 1993;24:143.

34. DuBose JJ, et al. Discrepancies between capillary glucose measurements and traditional laboratory assessments in both shock and non-shock states after trauma. *J Surg Res.* 2012;178:820-826.

35. Duh E, Feinglos M. Hypoglycemia-induced angina pectoris in a patient with diabetes mellitus. *Ann Intern Med.* 1994;121:945-946.

36. Duvanel CB, et al. Long-term effects of neonatal hypoglycemia on brain growth and psychomotor development in small-for-gestational-age preterm infants. *J Pediatr.* 1999;134:492-498.

37. Eastham JH, et al. Prevalence of interfering substances with point-of-care glucose testing in a community hospital. *Am J Health Syst Pharm.* 2009;66:167-170.

38. Elhomsy GC, et al. "Hyper-warburgism," a cause of asymptomatic hypoglycemia with lactic acidosis in a patient with non-Hodgkin's lymphoma. *J Clin Endocrinol Metab.* 2012;97:4311-4316.

39. Epstein JS, et al. Important drug information: immune globulin intravenous (human). *Int J Trauma Nurs.* 1999;5:139-140.

40. Ernst AA, et al. Ethanol ingestion and related hypoglycemia in a pediatric and adolescent emergency department population. *Acad Emerg Med.* 1996;3:46-49.

41. Faillie JL. Pharmacological aspects of the safety of gliflozins. *Pharmacol Res.* 2017;118:71-81.

42. Finfer S, et al. Intensive versus conventional glucose control in critically ill patients. *N Engl J Med.* 2009;360:1283-1297.

43. Finfer S, et al. Hypoglycemia and risk of death in critically ill patients. *N Engl J Med.* 2012;367:1108-1118.

44. Fischer E. Uber Die Configuration des Traubenzucker s. und seiner Isomeren [On the configuration of grape sugar and its isomers]. *Berichted. Deusch. Chem. Gesellsch.* 1891;24:1836-1845.

45. Flore K, Delanghe J. Icodextrin: a major problem for glucose dehydrogenase-based glucose point of care testing systems. *Acta Clin Belg.* 2006;61:351-354.

46. Fulop M. Alcoholic ketoacidosis. *Endocrinol Metab Clin North Am.* 1993;22:209-219.

47. Funk DL, et al. Comparison of capillary and venous glucose measurements in healthy volunteers. *Prehosp Emerg Care.* 2001;5:275-277.

48. Gill GV, et al. Cardiac arrhythmia and nocturnal hypoglycaemia in type 1 diabetes—the "dead in bed" syndrome revisited. *Diabetologia.* 2009;52:42-45.

49. Glatstein M, et al. Sulfonylurea intoxication at a tertiary care paediatric hospital. *Can J Clin Pharmacol.* 2010;17:e51-e56.

50. Glatstein M, et al. Octreotide for the treatment of sulfonylurea poisoning. *Clin Toxicol (Phila).* 2012;50:795-804.

51. Gray CS, et al. Glucose-potassium-insulin infusions in the management of post-stroke hyperglycaemia: the UK Glucose Insulin in Stroke Trial (GIST-UK). *Lancet Neurol.* 2007;6:397-406.

52. Grazaitis DM, Sexson WR. Erroneously high Dextrostix values caused by isopropyl alcohol. *Pediatrics.* 1980;66:221-223.

53. Grunbaum AM, et al. Analytical interferences resulting from intravenous lipid emulsion. *Clin Toxicol (Phila).* 2012;50:812-817.

54. Hack JB, Hoffman RS. Thiamine before glucose to prevent Wernicke encephalopathy: examining the conventional wisdom. *JAMA.* 1998;279:583-584.

55. Harris DL, et al. Dextrose gel for neonatal hypoglycaemia (the Sugar Babies Study): a randomised, double-blind, placebo-controlled trial. *Lancet.* 2013;382:2077-2083.

56. Hashemi-Domeneh B, et al. A review of aluminium phosphide poisoning and a flowchart to treat it. *Arh Hig Rada Toksikol.* 2016;67:183-193.

57. Hassanian-Moghaddam H, Zamani N. Therapeutic role of hyperinsulinemia/euglycemia in aluminum phosphide poisoning. *Medicine (Baltimore).* 2016;95:e4349.

58. Haymond MW. Hypoglycemia in infants and children. *Endocrinol Metab Clin North Am.* 1989;18:211-252.

59. Hedrington MS, et al. Effects of antecedent GABAA activation with alprazolam on counterregulatory responses to hypoglycemia in healthy humans. *Diabetes.* 2010;59:1074-1081.

60. Hern HG, et al. D10 in the treatment of prehospital hypoglycemia: a 24 month observational cohort study. *Prehosp Emerg Care.* 2017;21:63-67.

61. Hirshberg E, et al. Alterations in glucose homeostasis in the pediatric intensive care unit: hyperglycemia and glucose variability are associated with increased mortality and morbidity. *Pediatr Crit Care Med.* 2008;9:361-366.

62. Hoffman JR, et al. The empiric use of hypertonic dextrose in patients with altered mental status: a reappraisal. *Ann Emerg Med.* 1992;21:20-24.

63. Hoffman RS, Goldfrank LR. The poisoned patient with altered consciousness. Controversies in the use of a "coma cocktail." *JAMA.* 1995;274:562-569.

64. Hruz PW, Mueckler MM. Structural analysis of the GLUT1 facilitative glucose transporter (review). *Mol Membr Biol.* 2001;18:183-193.

65. Jones HF, et al. Intestinal fructose transport and malabsorption in humans. *Am J Physiol Gastrointest Liver Physiol.* 2011;300:G202-G206.

66. Jones JL, et al. Determination of prehospital blood glucose: a prospective, controlled study. *J Emerg Med.* 1992;10:679-682.

67. Jones TW, et al. Resistance to neuroglycopenia: an adaptive response during intensive insulin treatment of diabetes. *J Clin Endocrinol Metab.* 1997;82:1713-1718.

68. Jones TW, et al. Decreased epinephrine responses to hypoglycemia during sleep. *N Engl J Med.* 1998;338:1657-1662.

69. White JR. The Contribution of Medications to Hypoglycemia Unawareness. *Diabetes Spectrum* 2007;20:77-80. Last accessed May 31, 2018. http://spectrum.diabetesjournals.org/content/20/2/77.

70. Kanji S, et al. Reliability of point-of-care testing for glucose measurement in critically ill adults. *Crit Care Med.* 2005;33:2778-2785.

71. Kiefer MV, et al. Dextrose 10% in the treatment of out-of-hospital hypoglycemia. *Prehosp Disaster Med.* 2014;29:190-194.

72. Kim JH, Koh SB. Extensive white matter injury in hypoglycemic coma. *Neurology.* 2007;68:1074.

73. Krinsley JS. The severity of sepsis: yet another factor influencing glycemic control. *Crit Care.* 2008;12:194.

74. Kroll HR, Maher TR. Significant hypoglycemia secondary to icodextrin peritoneal dialysate in a diabetic patient. *Anesth Analg.* 2007;104:1473-1474, table of contents.

75. Kumar G, et al. Correlation of capillary and venous blood glucometry with laboratory determination. *Prehosp Emerg Care.* 2004;8:378-383.

76. Kuzak N, et al. Reversal of salicylate-induced euglycemic delirium with dextrose. *Clin Toxicol (Phila).* 2007;45:526-529.

77. Lacara T, et al. Comparison of point-of-care and laboratory glucose analysis in critically ill patients. *Am J Crit Care.* 2007;16:336-346; quiz 347.

78. Lavery RF, et al. A prospective evaluation of glucose reagent teststrips in the prehospital setting. *Am J Emerg Med.* 1991;9:304-308.

79. Leak D, Starr P. The mechanism of arrhythmias during insulin-induced hypoglycemia. *Am Heart J.* 1962;63:688-691.

80. Leyton O. Hypoglycaemia. *Proc R Soc Med.* 1926;19:47-50.

81. Lheureux PE, et al. Bench-to-bedside review: hyperinsulinaemia/euglycaemia therapy in the management of overdose of calcium-channel blockers. *Crit Care.* 2006;10:212.

82. Li T, Vijayan A. Insulin for the treatment of hyperkalemia: a double-edged sword? *Clin Kidney J.* 2014;7:239-241.

83. Lo L, et al. Diffusion-weighted MR imaging in early diagnosis and prognosis of hypoglycemia. *AJNR Am J Neuroradiol.* 2006;27:1222-1224.

84. Longstreth WT Jr, Inui TS. High blood glucose level on hospital admission and poor neurological recovery after cardiac arrest. *Ann Neurol.* 1984;15:59-63.

85. Lonjaret L, et al. Relative accuracy of arterial and capillary glucose meter measurements in critically ill patients. *Diabetes Metab.* 2012;38:230-235.

86. Maisels MJ, Lee CA. Chemstrip glucose test strips: correlation with true glucose values less than 80 mg/dl. *Crit Care Med.* 1983;11:293-295.

87. Malouf R, Brust JC. Hypoglycemia: causes, neurological manifestations, and outcome. *Ann Neurol.* 1985;17:421-430.

88. Maruya J, et al. Rapid improvement of diffusion-weighted imaging abnormalities after glucose infusion in hypoglycaemic coma. *J Neurol Neurosurg Psychiatry.* 2007;78:102-103.

89. McCrimmon R. The mechanisms that underlie glucose sensing during hypoglycaemia in diabetes. *Diabet Med.* 2008;25:513-522.

90. McCrimmon R. Glucose sensing during hypoglycemia: lessons from the lab. *Diabetes Care.* 2009;32:1357-1363.

91. McLaughlin SA, et al. Octreotide: an antidote for sulfonylurea-induced hypoglycemia. *Ann Emerg Med.* 2000;36:133-138.

92. Megarbane B, et al. The role of insulin and glucose (hyperinsulinaemia/euglycaemia) therapy in acute calcium channel antagonist and beta-blocker poisoning. *Toxicol Rev.* 2004;23:215-222.

93. Meinhold J, et al. Electrocardiographic changes during insulin-induced hypoglycemia in healthy subjects. *Horm Metab Res.* 1998;30:694-697.

94. Montgomery BM, Pinner CA. Transient hypoglycemic hemiplegia. *Arch Intern Med.* 1964;114:680-684.

95. Mori F, et al. Hypoglycemic encephalopathy with extensive lesions in the cerebral white matter. *Neuropathology.* 2006;26:147-152.

96. Mueckler M. Facilitative glucose transporters. *Eur J Biochem.* 1994;219:713-725.

97. Navarro-Gutierrez S, et al. Bradycardia related to hypoglycaemia. *Eur J Emerg Med.* 2003;10:331-333.

98. Nordin C. The case for hypoglycaemia as a proarrhythmic event: basic and clinical evidence. *Diabetologia.* 2010;53:1552-1561.

99. Novikov A, Vallon V. Sodium glucose cotransporter 2 inhibition in the diabetic kidney: an update. *Curr Opin Nephrol Hypertens.* 2016;25:50-58.

100. Nurmi J, et al. Early increase in blood glucose in patients resuscitated from out-of-hospital ventricular fibrillation predicts poor outcome. *Diabetes Care.* 2012;35:510-512.

101. Odeh M, et al. Transient atrial fibrillation precipitated by hypoglycemia. *Ann Emerg Med.* 1990;19:565-567.

102. Oyer DS. The science of hypoglycemia in patients with diabetes. *Curr Diabetes Rev.* 2013;9:195-208.

103. Parekh B. The mechanism of dead-in-bed syndrome and other sudden unexplained nocturnal deaths. *Curr Diabetes Rev.* 2009;5:210-215.

104. Petersen JR, et al. Comparison of POCT and central laboratory blood glucose results using arterial, capillary, and venous samples from MICU patients on a tight glycemic protocol. *Clin Chim Acta.* 2008;396:10-13.

105. Poulsen SB, et al. Sodium-glucose cotransport. *Curr Opin Nephrol Hypertens.* 2015;24:463-469.

106. Prisco L, et al. Early predictive factors on mortality in head injured patients: a retrospective analysis of 112 traumatic brain injured patients. *J Neurosurg Sci.* 2012;56:131-136.

107. Raschke R, et al. Refractory hypoglycemia secondary to topical salicylate intoxication. *Arch Intern Med.* 1991;151:591-593.

108. Rayar P, Ratnapalan S. Pediatric ingestions of household products containing ethanol: a review. *Clin Pediatr (Phila).* 2013;52:203-209.

109. Rehncrona S, et al. Brain lactic acidosis and ischemic cell damage: 1. Biochemistry and neurophysiology. *J Cereb Blood Flow Metab.* 1981;1:297-311.

110. Renard. Implantable glucose sensors for diabetes monitoring. *Minim Invasive Ther Allied Technol.* 2004;13:78-86.

111. Reno CM, et al. Defective counterregulation and hypoglycemia unawareness in diabetes: mechanisms and emerging treatments. *Endocrinol Metab Clin North Am.* 2013;42:15-38.

112. Riley SG, et al. Spurious hyperglycaemia and icodextrin in peritoneal dialysis fluid. *BMJ.* 2003;327:608-609.

113. Rosso C, et al. Intensive versus subcutaneous insulin in patients with hyperacute stroke: results from the randomized INSULINFARCT trial. *Stroke.* 2012;43:2343-2349.

114. Schabelman E, Kuo D. Glucose before thiamine for Wernicke encephalopathy: a literature review. *J Emerg Med.* 2012;42:488-494.

115. Schurr A. Lactate, glucose and energy metabolism in the ischemic brain (review). *Int J Mol Med.* 2002;10:131-136.

116. Scott JF, et al. Glucose potassium insulin infusions in the treatment of acute stroke patients with mild to moderate hyperglycemia: the Glucose Insulin in Stroke Trial (GIST). *Stroke.* 1999;30:793-799.

117. Scott PA, et al. Accuracy of reagent strips in detecting hypoglycemia in the emergency department. *Ann Emerg Med.* 1998;32:305-309.

118. Seibert DG. Reversible decerebrate posturing secondary to hypoglycemia. *Am J Med.* 1985;78:1036-1037.

119. Seltzer HS. Drug-induced hypoglycemia. A review of 1418 cases. *Endocrinol Metab Clin North Am.* 1989;18:163-183.

120. Shah A, et al. Hazards of pharmacological tests of growth hormone secretion in childhood. *BMJ.* 1992;304:173-174.

121. Siegelaar SE, et al. Mean glucose during ICU admission is related to mortality by a U-shaped curve in surgical and medical patients: a retrospective cohort study. *Crit Care.* 2010;14:R224.

122. Siraj ES, et al. Insulin dose and cardiovascular mortality in the ACCORD Trial. *Diabetes Care.* 2015;38:2000-2008.

123. Snodgrass WR. Salicylate toxicity. *Pediatr Clin North Am.* 1986;33:381-391.

124. So CF, et al. Recent advances in noninvasive glucose monitoring. *Med Devices (Auckl).* 2012;5:45-52.

125. Solnica B, et al. The effect of hematocrit on the results of measurements using glucose meters based on different techniques. *Clin Chem Lab Med.* 2012;50:361-365.

126. Souza SP, et al. False hyperglycemia induced by polivalent immunoglobulins. *Transplantation.* 2005;80:542-543.

127. Suh SW, et al. Hypoglycemia, brain energetics, and hypoglycemic neuronal death. *Glia.* 2007;55:1280-1286.

128. Tanaka M, et al. Role of lactate in the brain energy metabolism: revealed by bioradiography. *Neurosci Res.* 2004;48:13-20.

129. Tesfaye N, Seaquist ER. Neuroendocrine responses to hypoglycemia. *Ann N Y Acad Sci.* 2010;1212:12-28.

130. Thomas SH, et al. Accuracy of fingerstick glucose determination in patients receiving CPR. *South Med J.* 1994;87:1072-1075.

131. Thurston IH. Blood glucose: how reliable an indicator of brain glucose? *Hosp Pract.* 1976;11:123-130.

132. Thurston JH, et al. Reduced brain glucose with normal plasma glucose in salicylate poisoning. *J Clin Invest.* 1970;49:2139-2145.

133. Tokuda Y, et al. Pupillary evaluation for differential diagnosis of coma. *Postgrad Med J.* 2003;79:49-51.

134. Tsai CY, et al. False elevation of blood glucose levels measured by GDH-PQQ-based glucometers occurs during all daily dwells in peritoneal dialysis patients using icodextrin. *Perit Dial Int.* 2010;30:329-335.

135. Van den Berghe G, et al. Clinical review: intensive insulin therapy in critically ill patients: NICE-SUGAR or Leuven blood glucose target? *J Clin Endocrinol Metab.* 2009;94:3163-3170.

136. Van den Berghe G, et al. Intensive insulin therapy in the medical ICU. *N Engl J Med.* 2006;354:449-461.

137. van den Berghe G, et al. Intensive insulin therapy in critically ill patients. *N Engl J Med.* 2001;345:1359-1367.

138. van Hall G, et al. Blood lactate is an important energy source for the human brain. *J Cereb Blood Flow Metab.* 2009;29:1121-1129.

139. Vannucci RC, Yager JY. Glucose, lactic acid, and perinatal hypoxic-ischemic brain damage. *Pediatr Neurol.* 1992;8:3-12.

140. Villeneuve E, et al. There is no contraindication to emergent glucose administration. *Ann Emerg Med.* 2017;69:376-377.

141. Wagstaff AE, Cheung NW. Diabetes and hyperglycemia in the critical care setting: has the evidence for glycemic control vanished? (Or ... is going away?). *Curr Diab Rep.* 2014;14:444.

142. Wallis WE, et al. Hypoglycemia masquerading as cerebrovascular disease (hypoglycemic hemiplegia). *Ann Neurol.* 1985;18:510-512.

143. Wang HF, et al. Neuroglycopenia in an euglycaemic patient under intensive insulin therapy. *Anaesth Intensive Care.* 2010;38:1137-1138.

144. Watkinson PJ, et al. The effects of precision, haematocrit, pH and oxygen tension on point-of-care glucose measurement in critically ill patients: a prospective study. *Ann Clin Biochem.* 2012;49:144-151.

145. Watson AJ, et al. Acute Wernickes encephalopathy precipitated by glucose loading. *Ir J Med Sci.* 1981;150:301-303.

146. Weisberg LS. Management of severe hyperkalemia. *Crit Care Med.* 2008;36:3246-3251.

147. White JR Jr. Sodium glucose cotransporter 2 inhibitors. *Med Clin North Am.* 2015;99:131-143.

148. Wiethop BV, Cryer PE. Alanine and terbutaline in treatment of hypoglycemia in IDDM. *Diabetes Care.* 1993;16:1131-1136.

149. Wilhelm B, et al. Evaluation of CGMS during rapid blood glucose changes in patients with type 1 diabetes. *Diabetes Technol Ther.* 2006;8:146-155.

150. Winer JB, et al. A movement disorder as a presenting feature of recurrent hypoglycaemia. *Mov Disord.* 1990;5:176-177.

151. Witsch J, et al. Hypoglycemic encephalopathy: a case series and literature review on outcome determination. *J Neurol.* 2012;259:2172-2181.

152. Yaghi S, et al. The effect of admission hyperglycemia in stroke patients treated with thrombolysis. *Int J Neurosci.* 2012;122:637-640.

153. Yealy DM, Wolfson AB. Hypoglycemia. *Emerg Med Clin North Am.* 1989;7:837-848.

154. Yuan TH, et al. Insulin-glucose as adjunctive therapy for severe calcium channel antagonist poisoning. *J Toxicol Clin Toxicol.* 1999;37:463-474.

OCTREOTIDE

Silas W. Smith and Mary Ann Howland

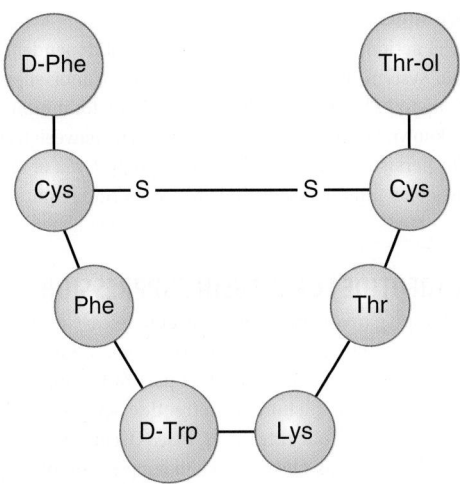

INTRODUCTION

Octreotide is a long-acting, synthetic octapeptide analog of somatostatin, a hormone that inhibits the release of numerous anterior pituitary and gastrointestinal hormones, including pancreatic insulin. It is the essential complement to dextrose (Antidotes in Depth: A8) for the treatment of refractory hypoglycemia induced by overdoses of inhibitors of insulin secretagogues such as sulfonylureas (and rarely the meglitinides) and quinine (and rarely other quinolones).

HISTORY

Somatostatin is a collective term for shorter fragments (SRIF-28, SRIF-25, and SRIF-14) cleaved from preprosomatostatin (116 amino acids) and prosomatostatin (92 amino acids).[17] In 1973 during the search for growth hormone–releasing factor, somatostatin was identified as a growth hormone inhibitor.[15] Somatostatin has far-reaching effects as a central nervous system (CNS) neurotransmitter and as a modulator of hormonal release.[64,75] The importance of somatostatin on insulin secretion led to the need to create an analog as a therapeutic tool, as somatostatin use is limited by its short duration of action. Octreotide was synthesized in 1982 in an effort to develop a longer-acting somatostatin analog.[7] Octreotide is currently approved by the FDA for the treatment of acromegaly, carcinoid tumors, and vasoactive intestinal peptide tumors. It is also used therapeutically for the treatment of pituitary adenomas, pancreatic islet cell tumors, portal hypertension, esophageal varices, and secretory diarrhea.[64]

PHARMACOLOGY
Mechanism of Action on Insulin Secretion

The effects of somatostatin are mediated by high-affinity binding to membrane receptors on target tissues. The six different known somatostatin receptor subtypes belong to a superfamily of G-protein coupled receptors and are identified and assigned numbers (SSTR1–SSTR5) according to their order of discovery, with SSTR2 having 2 splice variants (SSTR2A and SSTR2B).[17,23,76,88] By sequence homology, SSTR2, SSTR3, and SSTR5 belong to one group, which bind the classic somatostatin receptor ligands (SRLs), whereas SSTR1 and SSTR4 do not.[76] Somatostatin receptor type 2 (SSTR2) is

found in the brain, pituitary, stomach, liver, kidney, lung, intestine, spleen, thymus, uterus, prostate, and adrenal gland; SSTR5 is found in brain, pituitary, stomach, intestine, thyroid, and adrenal gland.[64,72,84,108] These varied SSTR targets underlie the use of SRLs in acromegaly; carcinoid, vasoactive intestinal peptide, and neuroendocrine tumors; portal hypertension; esophageal varices; and secretory diarrhea.[64] The pancreas contains all 5 subtypes, but SSTR5 is more prevalent in the β-cells and SSTR2 is more prevalent in the α-cells in mice.[108] In humans, SSTR2 is the functionally dominant somatostatin receptor in pancreatic β- and α-cells.[55,72]

Experiments in both healthy human volunteers and an isolated perfused canine pancreas model demonstrate the ability of somatostatin to inhibit glucose-stimulated insulin release.[2,36] In pancreatic β-cells that hypersecrete insulin through targeted mutagenesis of the sulfonylurea receptor, octreotide suppresses C-peptide, and insulin release.[46] Somatostatin inhibits insulin secretion by a G-protein–mediated decrease in calcium entry through voltage-dependent Ca^{2+} channels.[51] This is distinct from the site of action of sulfonylureas and diazoxide, which respectively open and close the ATP-sensitive K^+ (K_{ATP}) channel (Fig. 47–2).[31,66,79,97] Somatostatin, like epinephrine, stimulates a pertussis toxin–sensitive, G_i-coupled receptor that inhibits adenyl cyclase and production of cyclic adenosine monophosphate (cAMP) to decrease intracellular calcium and thereby reduce insulin secretion.[47] Simultaneous distal reduction in phosphorylation of specific proteins also reduces insulin secretion.[31,47,62] This latter mechanism is independent of Ca^{2+}.[31,47] In human pancreatic β- and α-cells, somatostatin agonism via SSTR2 hyperpolarizes human β-cells and decreases depolarization-evoked exocytosis in both α- and β-cells via several mechanisms.[55] There is an increased activation of K^+ channels such as the G-protein gated inward rectifying potassium (GIRK, Kir3.x) channel and others.[14,55] This effect is independent of the K_{ATP} channel, and thus it remains effective when the K_{ATP} channel is antagonized by a sulfonylurea. Somatostatin also appears to inhibit a depolarization leak current (mediated by an as yet unidentified channel). Furthermore, somatostatin reduces voltage-gated P/Q-type Ca^{2+} currents[55] and directly inhibits Ca^{2+} dependent insulin (and glucagon) exocytosis.[44,55] Thus, in α-cells, somatostatin SSTR2 stimulation leads to inhibition of glucagon secretion.[77] One additional mechanism involves β-cell activation of SSTR to decrease insulin gene promoter and/or transcription factor activity and thus reduce insulin biosynthesis.[31,113] The relative importance of all somatostatin mechanisms under various physiological conditions, somatostatin concentrations, and xenobiotics remains to be fully elucidated.

Octreotide, lanreotide, and vapreotide are somatostatin receptor ligands (SRLs) with high binding affinity for subtype SSTR2, a lower affinity for SSTR5 and SSTR3, and almost no affinity for SSTR1 and SSTR4.[64] Pasireotide is second-generation SRL characterized by significantly higher binding to SSTR5 (40 times), SSTR1 (30 times), and SSTR3 (5 times) and lower binding to SSTR2 (2.5 times less) compared to octreotide.[24] Octreotide and SRLs thus inhibit growth hormone, glucagon, and insulin release. Octreotide also suppresses the response of luteinizing hormone to gonadotropin-releasing hormone; decreases splanchnic blood flow; and inhibits the release of thyroid-stimulating hormone and the gastrointestinal signal transmitters serotonin, gastrin, vasoactive intestinal peptide, secretin, motilin, and pancreatic polypeptide.[66,75] The antiproliferative effects of octreotide in neuroendocrine tumors are mediated by SSTR regulation of the PI3K/Akt (MAP kinase) pathway and indirectly by inhibition of mitogenic growth factors and tumor angiogenesis.[101,104] Studies comparing octreotide to somatostatin in rats and monkeys demonstrate that octreotide is 1.3 times as potent as somatostatin in inhibiting insulin secretion. Likewise, compared with somatostatin, octreotide was 45 times more potent in inhibiting growth hormone secretion and 11 times more potent in inhibiting glucagon release.[7] Pasireotide was more efficacious than octreotide in preventing hypoglycemia in glyburide-treated rats.[93] Octreotide had no effect on the responses of adrenocorticotropin, cortisol, prolactin, luteinizing hormone, and follicle-stimulating hormone to insulin-induced hypoglycemia.[66] In contrast, growth hormone and thyroid hormone are significantly inhibited.[27,66,105]

Clinically, the ability of somatostatin to inhibit glucose- and glucagon-mediated insulin response was confirmed in a study of human volunteers.[36] Intravenous (IV) infusion of 1 g of tolbutamide over 2 minutes caused insulin concentrations to rise and serum glucose concentration to drop sharply. In the presence of somatostatin and tolbutamide, administration of IV glucagon caused a rise in glucose concentration without the expected subsequent glucose-stimulated rise in insulin. The effects of somatostatin were short-lived. Within 5 minutes of stopping the somatostatin, the insulin-releasing effects of tolbutamide continued, and within 15 minutes the serum glucose concentration fell. Peak insulin concentrations were achieved within 25 minutes. In another human volunteer study, somatostatin provided as a continuous infusion suppressed insulin secretion induced by glucagonlike peptide-1 (GLP-1) infusion.[94] Indeed, the efficacy of somatostatin (and later octreotide) in suppressing insulin secretion led to its utilization in the clinical insulin suppression test (IST) and in multiple pancreatic glycemic clamping technique experiments (with various glucose, insulin, and glucagon concentrations) in order to probe human physiology.[29,53,60,109] When measured in patients with sulfonylurea intentional overdose, octreotide also suppressed insulin concentrations.[41]

Related Xenobiotics

Lanreotide, vapreotide, and pasireotide are long-acting, FDA-approved SRLs.[24] Use of these pharmaceuticals in insulin secretagogue-induced hypoglycemia is unstudied in humans at this time and therefore cannot be recommended.

Pharmacokinetics

The pharmacokinetics of IV and subcutaneous (SC) octreotide were studied in 8 healthy adult volunteers.[61] Subjects received 25, 50, 100, and 200 mcg IV octreotide over 3 minutes and 50, 100, 200, and 400 mcg SC octreotide in random order. Following IV administration, the distribution half-life averaged 12 minutes, and the elimination half-life ranged from 72 ± 22 minutes to 98 ± 37 minutes. The apparent volume of distribution (V_d) of the central compartment was dose dependent and increased from approximately 5.7 L at 25, 50, and 100 mcg IV to 10 L at 200 mcg IV doses.[61] The V_d determined by area under the curve (AUC) ranged from 18 ± 6 L to 30 ± 30 L and showed no dose dependency.[61] Approximately 30% of elimination was renal, and this was reduced in the elderly and in those with chronic kidney disease.[75] After SC administration, bioavailability was 100%, and peak concentrations were achieved within 30 minutes with an absorption half-life of 5 to 12 minutes. The elimination half-life was 88 to 102 minutes. Peak serum concentrations after SC administration ranged from 2.4 ng/mL at doses of 50 mcg to 23.5 ng/mL at doses of 400 mcg. After IV administration, peak serum concentrations ranged from 9.6 ng/mL at doses of 50 mcg to 27.8 ng/mL at doses of 200 mcg.[61] To place these values in perspective, octreotide acetate binds SSTR2 with an affinity of approximately 1 ng/mL, but requires concentrations of 10 ng/mL to completely saturate the receptor.[112]

The pharmacokinetics in patients with pathologic conditions differ from the pharmacokinetics in healthy volunteers; patients with acromegaly achieve lower peak concentrations and a higher steady-state V_d.[75] In volunteer studies, octreotide pharmacokinetics differ in patients with kidney and liver disease, with increases in the area under the curve and decreased clearance.[54,78] The half-life prolongs to 2.5 hours (creatinine clearance, 40–60 mL/min), 3.0 hours (creatinine clearance, 10–39 mL/min), 3.1 hours (creatinine

clearance <10 mL/min), 3.4 hours (steatosis and nonalcoholic liver disease), and 3.7 hours (cirrhosis). The half-life in the elderly is prolonged by 46%.[75] In one case of maternal to fetal transfer of octreotide, the neonatal octreotide half-life was 350 minutes.[20] Out of concern that the site of injection could lead to variable efficacy due to absorptive differences, octreotide pharmacokinetics were studied in 16 volunteers. Each received 500-mcg SC octreotide in the extremity (arm) and abdomen; there were no statistically significant differences in octreotide plasma peak, AUC, or half-life.[83] It is important to note that octreotide kinetics are markedly different in the long-acting release (LAR) depot formulation, which is provided at 4-week intervals.

Pharmacodynamics

The duration of action of octreotide is variable and dependent on the outcome or organ system of interest. When used for tumor suppression, the duration lasts up to 12 hours.[75] The duration of action for inhibition of insulin secretion is unknown but presumed to be somewhere between 6 and 12 hours. When used for persistent hyperinsulinemic hypoglycemia of infancy (PHHI; also known as congenital hyperinsulinism), octreotide required continuous infusion.[81]

ROLE OF OCTREOTIDE FOR INSULIN SUPPRESSION

Octreotide inhibits glucose-stimulated insulin release.[2,36] Octreotide was studied in humans in several clinical conditions, including insulinomas and hypoglycemia of infancy, and is utilized as part of the insulin suppression test.[3,28,37,50,53,56,81,100] In most instances, octreotide suppressed insulin concentrations and glucose concentrations rose. Occasionally, worsening or refractory hypoglycemia was observed when suppression of α cell glucagon release outlasts suppression of β cell insulin release, despite appropriate catecholamine and cortisol counterregulatory response.[8,16,35,71,74,100] Another reason for variable effects in these conditions includes the absence of octreotide-susceptible SSTR receptor subtypes.[26]

Octreotide currently is used in toxicology for treatment of patients with hypoglycemia from insulin secretagogues. Controlled studies in rabbits given oral gliclazide demonstrate that a single dose of octreotide 50 or 100 mcg SC resulted in fewer hypoglycemic events and dextrose boluses, although single dosing did not eliminate hypoglycemia entirely.[45]

Octreotide efficacy for sulfonylurea-induced hypoglycemia was demonstrated in an early experimental study. Eight healthy volunteers were given 1.43 mg/kg glipizide orally and randomized to receive either a variable dextrose infusion to remain euglycemic, diazoxide 300 mg IV over 30 minutes and repeated every 4 hours with dextrose, or octreotide 30 ng/kg/min IV continuously.[11] Following glipizide administration, hypoglycemia of 50 mg/dL was achieved within 30 to 165 minutes.[11] Insulin concentrations in the diazoxide group were comparable with those in the glipizide group and were 4 to 5 times higher than in the octreotide group. Four of the 8 patients in the octreotide group did not require supplemental dextrose. At the fifth hour of the protocol, an IV bolus of 50 mL of 50% dextrose was given to the octreotide group to study the response to hyperglycemia. Approximately 6.5 hours was necessary for the serum glucose concentration to drop to 85 mg/dL, whereas only 3 hours was necessary in the dextrose and diazoxide groups.[11] This demonstrates that octreotide suppresses ability of hyperglycemia to result in the endogenous release of insulin. Diazoxide infusion was associated with higher norepinephrine concentrations, whereas epinephrine concentrations were similar in all groups.[11] All xenobiotics were stopped at 13 hours, and serum glucose concentrations fell to less than 65 mg/dL within 1.5 hours in subjects who received the dextrose and diazoxide, whereas the serum glucose concentrations remained greater than 65 mg/dL in 6 of the 8 octreotide subjects for the 4-hour observation period. Without additional octreotide, hypoglycemia recurred for as long as 30 hours after the initial glipizide administration. In 3 patients with sulfonylurea-induced hypoglycemia, insulin and C-peptide concentrations were appropriately suppressed following octreotide administration.[34] One prospective, randomized controlled trial of 40 hypoglycemic, poisoned patients who received a single octreotide 75-mcg dose SC demonstrated consistently higher glucose values for the duration for which octreotide would be expected to be effective (6–8 hours).[32] The failure to control for carbohydrate intake and combined exposure to insulin complicates interpretation of these results.

Multiple case studies, case series, and evidence-based reviews support the efficacy of octreotide following overdoses of chlorpropamide, glibenclamide, gliclazide, glimepiride, glipizide, glyburide, nateglinide, and tolbutamide.[1,12,13,19,21,25,30,34,38,39,41,42,59,67,69,73,85,92,107] These cases encompass both intentional and unintentional overdoses in children and adults with and without diabetes and with and without kidney dysfunction. In these case reports, therapeutic doses have ranged considerably, and the most frequent doses were 50 to 100 mcg SC repeated every 6 to 12 hours in the adult patients and 1 to 2 mcg/kg SC or IV as a starting dose in children and repeated every 6 hours as needed.[13,19,38]

The meglitinides (repaglinide, nateglinide, and mitiglinide) typically have a short duration of action and carry a low risk for hypoglycemia.[31,98] Nevertheless, hypoglycemia is reported in both overdose and with therapeutic meglitinide doses.[49,68,82] Octreotide, at doses of 75 to 100 mcg subcutaneously successfully treated meglitinide-induced hypoglycemia.[33,96]

Quinine is a quinoline antimalarial similar to chloroquine, halofantrine, hydroxychloroquine, and mefloquine.[31] Life-threatening hypoglycemia is a well-recognized complication of quinine treatment of *Plasmodium falciparum* malaria, and occasionally complicates therapy with other quinolines.[4,106] Intravenous chloroquine (800 mg infused over 3 hours) decreased blood glucose by 25% in healthy volunteers.[40] In a randomized, double-blinded study, hydroxychloroquine significantly increased insulin concentrations and lowered serum glucose in response to an oral glucose challenge.[95] Quinine (and its analogues) block the K_{ATP} channel in a dose-dependent fashion in an analogous manner to sulfonylureas.[9,43,79] In this setting, hypertonic dextrose and diazoxide therapy are frequently inadequate, with ensuing refractory hypoglycemia. In controlled studies of healthy volunteers, octreotide suppressed the release of insulin associated with quinine.[87] In an investigation of the potential hypoglycemia-sparing effect of octreotide given for treatment of quinine-induced hypoglycemia, healthy adults were given 50 mcg/h octreotide or placebo as a continuous IV infusion for 4 hours, followed at the first hour by infusion of a 490-mg quinine base.[86] In the control subjects, serum insulin concentrations rose and serum glucose concentrations fell significantly, whereas in the octreotide group, insulin concentrations fell and glucose concentrations remained constant. This effect of octreotide began within 30 minutes and persisted for 2 hours after octreotide was stopped. Octreotide was used successfully to treat refractory hypoglycemia in a woman receiving 600 mg quinine IV for malaria.[86] A subsequent treatment study[87] confirmed these findings and noted that a single octreotide (100 mcg) dose suppressed quinine-induced hypoglycemia within 15 minutes. Because quinolone antibiotics such as ciprofloxacin, levofloxacin, gatifloxacin, and nalidixic acid share a 4-quinolone nucleus with quinine, they are also infrequently associated with hypoglycemia due to K_{ATP} channel inhibition.[65] There are case reports of octreotide reversal of quinolone-associated hypoglycemia.[57]

The imidazolines such as clonidine, phentolamine, and yohimbine also inhibit the K_{ATP} channel.[31,89,90] This provides a mechanistic explanation for the rare hypoglycemia that occurs clinically with the imidazole antagonists.[52] Although not reported clinically, octreotide is a reasonable therapeutic approach for repeated episodes of imidazoline-associated hypoglycemia.

ADVERSE EFFECTS AND SAFETY ISSUES

Octreotide is generally well tolerated, but toxicologic experience is limited. Adverse reactions occurring with short-term administration usually are local or gastrointestinal such as nausea, abdominal cramps, diarrhea, fat malabsorption, and flatulence.[64] Stinging at the injection site occurs in approximately 7% of patients but rarely lasts more than 15 minutes.[110] Healthy adult volunteers receiving octreotide noted no side effects when given IV doses of 25 or 50 mcg or SC doses of 50 or 100 mcg. At higher doses, early transient nausea and later-appearing but longer-lasting diarrhea and

abdominal pain frequently occur.[60,61] Healthy adult volunteers were given IV bolus doses of octreotide as high as 1,000 mcg and infusion doses of 30,000 mcg over 20 minutes and 120,000 mcg over 8 hours without serious adverse effects. Single doses in healthy adult volunteers resulted in decreased biliary contractility and bile secretion.[75] Diarrhea (76%), abdominal pain/distention (29%), and dizziness (12%) were common features when healthy adult volunteers were given octreotide 0.5 mcg/min with a 25-mcg bolus.[53] Long-term octreotide therapy lasting weeks to months results in biliary tract abnormalities.[75,111] Octreotide use to reverse sulfonylurea-induced and episodic hypoglycemia rarely results in bradycardia, hypokalemia, hyperkalemia, anaphylactoid reactions, hypertension, and apnea.[1,6,18,25,102] Product information and clinical trials suggests the potential for acute cholecystitis, biliary abnormalities including sludge, stones, infections, and obstruction, cholestatic hepatitis, and pancreatitis.[10,50,75]

No side effects were noted in 7 small-for-gestational-age neonates given octreotide 8 to 18 mcg/kg/day for 9 to 45 days to treat PHHI.[81] In a combined single-arm, open-label clinical trial (5 patients) and observational registry study (19 patients) of octreotide administered for diazoxide-resistant PHHI, no severe adverse events related to octreotide were observed during an observation period of 695 patient-months.[50] Gallstones/sludge, vomiting, hyperglycemia, diarrhea/whitish stool, and elevation of alkaline phosphatase were the most common nonsevere side effects.[50] In a review of 428 infants prescribed 490 courses of octreotide primarily for chylothorax, pleural effusion, hypoglycemia, and gastrointestinal hemorrhage that did not control for indication, octreotide administration was associated with hypoglycemia (<40 mg/dL) in 2% of octreotide courses, hyperglycemia (>250 mg/dL) in 1% of octreotide courses, and necrotizing enterocolitis (NEC) in 2% of octreotide courses.[103]

Octreotide alters the balance among insulin, glucagon, and growth hormone. Serum glucose concentrations must be serially monitored. Hyperglycemia often occurs, but as noted above cases of hypoglycemia are also reported.[10] The package labeling states that symptomatic hypoglycemia occurs in patients with type I diabetes and their insulin requirements will likely be reduced.[75] The most likely explanation is suppression of counterregulatory hormones, in particular when glucagon suppression is more persistent than insulin suppression.[35,71,75] Long-term administration of octreotide or octreotide use in circumstances other than sulfonylurea-induced hypoglycemia is also associated with hypothyroidism, bradycardia and cardiac conduction abnormalities, worsening congestive heart failure and QT interval prolongation, pancreatitis, hypoxemia and pulmonary hypertension in premature neonates, NEC, altered fat absorption, hyperkalemia, and decreased vitamin B_{12} concentrations.[1,6,35,48,50,63,75,103]

Drug interactions are expected with xenobiotics that affect glucose regulation. Octreotide significantly decreases oral absorption of cyclosporine and increases the bioavailability of bromocriptine.[10] Because octreotide suppresses the activity of the cytochrome P450 enzymes, in particular CYP3A4, drugs with narrow therapeutic indices metabolized by these enzymes should be monitored more closely.[75] Total parenteral nutrition solutions are incompatible with octreotide because of the formation of a glycosyl octreotide conjugate.[10]

PREGNANCY AND LACTATION

Octreotide is considered a category B drug.[75] Maternal to fetal transfer of exogenous octreotide is documented.[20] Studies of octreotide excretion in breast milk are not reported. However, intravenous ^{111}In-labeled octreotide is taken up by breast tissue, and ^{111}In decreases in breast milk followed a biexponential pattern with a half-life of 0.45 to 4.9 days.[22]

DOSING AND ADMINISTRATION

No controlled trials have evaluated the optimal dose of octreotide for the management of sulfonylurea overdose. In adults, a dose of 50 mcg octreotide SC given every 6 hours is recommended for a total duration of 24 hours. In children, a dose of 4 to 5 mcg/kg/d SC divided every 6 hours, up to the adult dose, is recommended for initial therapy. This pediatric dose is derived from the literature on treatment of PHHI.[37] In situations where compromised peripheral blood flow is expected, octreotide is recommended to be administered IV in the same dose but every 4 hours instead of every 6 hours. An increase in the dose is occasionally required, and continuous octreotide infusions are utilized in refractory cases.[39,67]

While the optimal duration of octreotide therapy awaits definitive study, several principles and patient factors help guide management. The duration of action of every sulfonylurea except tolbutamide exceeds 12 hours, and this will be altered with extended-release formulations, sulfonylureas with enterohepatic recirculation, in overdose, and with coingestions or coadministrations.[32,85,91] The onset of hypoglycemia can be significantly delayed following ingestion (as late as 21 to 48 hours, depending upon the sulfonylurea), and hypoglycemic recurrence as late as 30 to 70 hours is reported in the literature.[58,80,85,99] In one cohort of type 2 diabetic patients with sulfonylurea-induced hypoglycemia, in-hospital recurrent hypoglycemia occurred in 36%.[13] Acute or chronic kidney dysfunction (whether intrinsic or secondary to insufficient perfusion as in cases of congestive heart failure), which can predispose to sulfonylurea-induced hypoglycemia in the first place, alters the elimination of both oral sulfonylureas and antidotal octreotide. A controlled animal study demonstrated the failure of single-dose octreotide to completely eliminate recurrent late (9–24 hour) hypoglycemic episodes.[45] Human experimental and pragmatic data demonstrate the inadequacy of a single or a few octreotide doses. In humans administered glipizide in a controlled fashion, after 13 hours, of continuously provided octreotide therapy, 2 of 8 subjects (25%) had glucose concentrations decrease more than 3 hours after stopping octreotide. Without ongoing octreotide, hypoglycemia persisted for as long as 30 hours and hyperinsulinemia persisted for greater than 16 hours after the initial glipizide administration.[11] Treatment failures (episodes of glucose <60 mg/dL) occurred in 10 of 22 patients (45%) in a prospective, randomized controlled trial employing only a single-dose octreotide strategy; 2 events occurred at 12 and 13 hours after octreotide administration.[32] In one case series, treatment failure (hypoglycemia) occurred 14 hours after the last dose of octreotide (more than 30 hours after glyburide ingestion), and an additional failure occurred 36 hours after a single dose of octreotide (40 hours after ingestion of extended-release glipizide).[69] In another case series of pediatric patients ingesting glipizide or glyburide, 4 of 5 experienced recurrence of hypoglycemia after octreotide dosing, at 6, 7, 10, and 17 hours.[18] Repeat octreotide was required in one of 5 adult type 2 diabetic patients treated for sulfonylurea-induced hypoglycemia.[13] In a separate case series, recurrent hypoglycemia was seen in 3 of 6 adult patients with sulfonylurea-induced hypoglycemia, despite octreotide administration.[34]

The available pharmacokinetic, animal, and human data suggest that one or 2 octreotide doses is likely to be insufficient, and that 24 hours to several days of therapy and/or observation will be required, depending on the particular xenobiotic, quantity of ingestion, coingestants, caloric intake, and individual patient factors. Regardless of the dosing strategy utilized, it is recommended that during octreotide therapy and for 12 to 24 hours following termination of octreotide therapy before discharge, all patients be carefully monitored for recurrent hypoglycemia with careful attention to mental status and frequent checks of glucose concentrations, particularly during sleep.[11] The potential for unrecognizable recurrent hypoglycemia during sleep necessitates that patients must not be discharged during a high-risk circadian phase (eg, evening or night), unless the patients are monitored for an adequate amount of time after completing octreotide therapy and after a dextrose challenge (which can increase the release of insulin). The ability to consume sufficient calories should be ensured. Other patients at risk for hypoglycemia unawareness (ie, defective glucose counterregulation and hypoglycemia without warning symptoms)[5] should also be carefully monitored for 12 to 24 hours following octreotide termination.

Both SC and IV administration are acceptable, although the usual route is SC, which is preferred because of the pharmacokinetic limitations of the IV route delineated above. The SC administration sites should be rotated. For IV infusion, octreotide can be diluted in sterile 0.9% sodium chloride solution or D_5W and infused over 15 to 30 minutes or by IV bolus over 3 minutes.[75]

Refrigeration of octreotide is recommended for prolonged storage, although octreotide is stable at room temperature for 14 days when protected from light. Active warming of refrigerated octreotide is not recommended, although passive warming to room temperature prior to administration is suggested to reduce the pain of SC administration.[70] Using the smallest volume possible also reduces the pain with SC administration. A depot formula designed to last for 4 weeks is available (Sandostatin LAR Depot). Although the depot formula is useful for patients with insulinomas, its duration of action far exceeds that of any insulin secretogogue, making it an unnecessary choice and therefore not recommended for the management of xenobiotic-induced hypoglycemia. Vapreotide, lanreotide, and pasireotide are somatostatin analogs that are available in the United States but are inappropriate for use in the setting of xenobiotic-induced insulin secretion.

FORMULATION AND ACQUISITION

Octreotide acetate injection is available in ampules and multidose vials ranging in concentration from 50 to 1,000 mcg/mL. The multidose vials contain phenol. It should not be confused with the long-acting LAR formulations.

SUMMARY

- The available evidence indicates that octreotide is useful for preventing the reoccurrence of hypoglycemia induced by the insulin secretagogues such as sulfonylureas (and rarely the meglitinides) and quinine (and rarely other quinolones).
- Octreotide is more effective and is better tolerated than diazoxide in suppressing insulin release.
- Octreotide is not a substitute for IV dextrose for the immediate treatment of hypoglycemia and does not decrease the need for frequent glucose assessments and assurance of sufficient caloric intake.
- Before discharge, the following should be ensured: the effects of octreotide have dissipated, the patient remains euglycemic following an adequate oral dextrose challenge, and there is a sufficiently prolonged observation time since ingestion to ensure that hypoglycemia will not occur in a fasting or sleeping patient.

REFERENCES

1. Adabala M, et al. Severe hyperkalaemia resulting from octreotide use in a haemodialysis patient. *Nephrol Dial Transplant.* 2010;25:3439-3442.
2. Alberti KG, et al. Inhibition of insulin secretion by somatostatin. *Lancet.* 1973;2:1299-1301.
3. Alberts AS, Falkson G. Rapid reversal of life-threatening hypoglycaemia with a somatostatin analogue (octreotide). A case report. *S Afr Med J.* 1988;74:75-76.
4. Assan R, et al. Mefloquine-associated hypoglycaemia in a cachectic AIDS patient. *Diabetes Metab.* 1995;21:54-58.
5. Bakatselos SO. Hypoglycemia unawareness. *Diabetes Res Clin Pract.* 2011;93(suppl 1):S92-S96.
6. Batra YK, et al. Octreotide-induced severe paradoxical hyperglycemia and bradycardia during subtotal pancreatectomy for congenital hyperinsulinism in an infant. *Paediatr Anaesth.* 2007;17:1117-1119.
7. Bauer W, et al. SMS 201-995: a very potent and selective octapeptide analogue of somatostatin with prolonged action. *Life Sci.* 1982;31:1133-1140.
8. Boden G, et al. Ineffectiveness of SMS 201-995 in severe hyperinsulinemia. *Diabetes Care.* 1988;11:664-668.
9. Bokvist K, et al. Block of ATP-regulated and Ca2(+)-activated K+ channels in mouse pancreatic beta-cells by external tetraethylammonium and quinine. *J Physiol.* 1990;423:327-342.
10. Borna RM, et al. Pharmacology of octreotide: clinical implications for anesthesiologists and associated risks. *Anesthesiol Clin.* 2017;35:327-339.
11. Boyle PJ, et al. Octreotide reverses hyperinsulinemia and prevents hypoglycemia induced by sulfonylurea overdoses. *J Clin Endocrinol Metab.* 1993;76:752-756.
12. Braatvedt GD. Octreotide for the treatment of sulphonylurea induced hypoglycaemia in type 2 diabetes. *N Z Med J.* 1997;110:189-190.
13. Braatvedt GD, et al. The clinical course of patients with type 2 diabetes presenting to the hospital with sulfonylurea-induced hypoglycemia. *Diabetes Technol Ther.* 2014;16:661-666.
14. Braun M. The somatostatin receptor in human pancreatic beta-cells. *Vitam Horm.* 2014;95:165-193.
15. Brazeau P, et al. Hypothalamic polypeptide that inhibits the secretion of immunoreactive pituitary growth hormone. *Science.* 1973;179:77-79.
16. Brunner JE, et al. Hypoglycemia after administration of somatostatin analog (SMS 201-995) in metastatic carcinoid. *Henry Ford Hosp Med J.* 1989;37:60-62.

17. Bruns C, et al. Molecular pharmacology of somatostatin-receptor subtypes. *Ann N Y Acad Sci.* 1994;733:138-146.
18. Calello D, et al. Octreotide for pediatric sulfonylurea overdose: review of 5 cases [abstract]. *Clin Toxicol.* 2005;43:671.
19. Calello DP, et al. Case files of the Medical Toxicology Fellowship Training Program at the Children's Hospital of Philadelphia: a pediatric exploratory sulfonylurea ingestion. *J Med Toxicol.* 2006;2:19-24.
20. Caron P, et al. Maternal-fetal transfer of octreotide. *N Engl J Med.* 1995;333:601-602.
21. Carr R, Zed PJ. Octreotide for sulfonylurea-induced hypoglycemia following overdose. *Ann Pharmacother.* 2002;36:1727-1732.
22. Castronovo FP Jr, et al. Radioactivity in breast milk following ^{111}In-octreotide. *Nucl Med Commun.* 2000;21:695-699.
23. Csaba Z, et al. Molecular mechanisms of somatostatin receptor trafficking. *J Mol Endocrinol.* 2012;48:R1-R12.
24. Cuevas-Ramos D, Fleseriu M. Pasireotide: a novel treatment for patients with acromegaly. *Drug Des Dev Ther.* 2016;10:227-239.
25. Curtis JA, Greenberg MI. Bradycardia and hyperkalemia associated with octreotide administration [abstract]. *Clin Toxicol.* 2006;44:498.
26. de Sa SV, et al. Somatostatin receptor subtype 5 (SSTR5) mRNA expression is related to histopathological features of cell proliferation in insulinomas. *Endocr Relat Cancer.* 2006;13:69-78.
27. del Pozo E, et al. Endocrine profile of a long-acting somatostatin derivative SMS 201-995. Study in normal volunteers following subcutaneous administration. *Acta Endocrinol (Copenh).* 1986;111:433-439.
28. Demirbilek H, et al. Clinical characteristics and phenotype-genotype analysis in Turkish patients with congenital hyperinsulinism; predominance of recessive KATP channel mutations. *Eur J Endocrinol.* 2014;170:885-892.
29. Djurhuus CB, et al. Effects of cortisol on lipolysis and regional interstitial glycerol levels in humans. *Am J Physiol Endocrinol Metab.* 2002;283:E172-E177.
30. Dougherty PP, Klein-Schwartz W. Octreotide's role in the management of sulfonylurea-induced hypoglycemia. *J Med Toxicol.* 2010;6:199-206.
31. Doyle ME, Egan JM. Pharmacological agents that directly modulate insulin secretion. *Pharmacol Rev.* 2003;55:105-131.
32. Fasano CJ, et al. Comparison of octreotide and standard therapy versus standard therapy alone for the treatment of sulfonylurea-induced hypoglycemia. *Ann Emerg Med.* 2008;51:400-406.
33. Fasano CJ, Rowden AK. Successful treatment of repaglinide-induced hypoglycemia with octreotide. *Am J Emerg Med.* 2009;27:756.e3-756.e4.
34. Fleseriu M, et al. Successful treatment of sulfonylurea-induced prolonged hypoglycemia with use of octreotide. *Endocr Pract.* 2006;12:635-640.
35. Gama R, et al. Octreotide exacerbated fasting hypoglycaemia in a patient with a pro-insulinoma; the glucostatic importance of pancreatic glucagon. *Clin Endocrinol (Oxf).* 1995;43:117-120; discussion 20-22.
36. Gerich JE, et al. Effect of somatostatin on plasma glucose and insulin responses to glucagon and tolbutamide in man. *J Clin Endocrinol Metab.* 1974;39:1057-1060.
37. Glaser B, et al. Persistent hyperinsulinemic hypoglycemia of infancy: long-term octreotide treatment without pancreatectomy. *J Pediatr.* 1993;123:644-650.
38. Glatstein M, et al. Sulfonylurea intoxication at a tertiary care paediatric hospital. *Can J Clin Pharmacol.* 2010;17:e51-e56.
39. Glatstein M, et al. Octreotide for the treatment of sulfonylurea poisoning. *Clin Toxicol (Phila).* 2012;50:795-804.
40. Goyal V, Bordia A. The hypoglycemic effect of chloroquine. *J Assoc Physicians India.* 1995;43:17-18.
41. Graudins A, et al. Diagnosis and treatment of sulfonylurea-induced hyperinsulinemic hypoglycemia. *Am J Emerg Med.* 1997;15:95-96.
42. Green RS, Palatnick W. Effectiveness of octreotide in a case of refractory sulfonylurea-induced hypoglycemia. *J Emerg Med.* 2003;25:283-287.
43. Gribble FM, et al. The antimalarial agent mefloquine inhibits ATP-sensitive K-channels. *Br J Pharmacol.* 2000;131:756-760.
44. Gromada J, et al. Somatostatin inhibits exocytosis in rat pancreatic alpha-cells by G(i2)-dependent activation of calcineurin and depriming of secretory granules. *J Physiol.* 2001;535:519-532.
45. Gul M, et al. The effectiveness of various doses of octreotide for sulfonylurea-induced hypoglycemia after overdose. *Adv Ther.* 2006;23:878-884.
46. Guo D, et al. Modeling congenital hyperinsulinism with ABCC8-deficient human embryonic stem cells generated by CRISPR/Cas9. *Sci Rep.* 2017;7:3156.
47. Hansen JB, et al. Inhibition of insulin secretion as a new drug target in the treatment of metabolic disorders. *Curr Med Chem.* 2004;11:1595-1615.
48. Healy ML, et al. Severe hypoglycaemia after long-acting octreotide in a patient with an unrecognized malignant insulinoma. *Intern Med J.* 2007;37:406-409.
49. Hirshberg B, et al. Repaglinide-induced factitious hypoglycemia. *J Clin Endocrinol Metab.* 2001;86:475-477.
50. Hosokawa Y, et al. Efficacy and safety of octreotide for the treatment of congenital hyperinsulinism: a prospective, open-label clinical trial and an observational study in Japan using a nationwide registry. *Endocr J.* 2017;64:867-880.
51. Hsu WH, et al. Somatostatin inhibits insulin secretion by a G-protein-mediated decrease in Ca2+ entry through voltage-dependent Ca2+ channels in the beta cell. *J Biol Chem.* 1991;266:837-843.
52. Huang C, et al. Hypoglycemia associated with clonidine testing for growth hormone deficiency. *J Pediatr.* 2001;139:323-324.
53. Hwu CM, et al. A comparison of insulin suppression tests performed with somatostatin and octreotide with particular reference to tolerability. *Diabetes Res Clin Pract.* 2001;51:187-193.
54. Jenkins SA, et al. Pharmacokinetics of octreotide in patients with cirrhosis and portal hypertension; relationship between the plasma levels of the analogue and the magnitude and duration of the reduction in corrected wedged hepatic venous pressure. *HPB Surg.* 1998;11:13-21.
55. Kailey B, et al. SSTR2 is the functionally dominant somatostatin receptor in human pancreatic beta- and alpha-cells. *Am J Physiol Endocrinol Metab.* 2012;303:E1107-E1116.
56. Kane C, et al. Therapy for persistent hyperinsulinemic hypoglycemia of infancy. Understanding the responsiveness of beta cells to diazoxide and somatostatin. *J Clin Invest.* 1997;100:1888-1893.
57. Kelesidis T, Canseco E. Quinolone-induced hypoglycemia: a life-threatening but potentially reversible side effect. *Am J Med.* 2010;123:e5-e6.
58. Klein-Schwartz W, et al. Treatment of sulfonylurea and insulin overdose. *Br J Clin Pharmacol.* 2016;81:496-504.
59. Krentz AJ, et al. Successful treatment of severe refractory sulfonylurea-induced hypoglycemia with octreotide. *Diabetes Care.* 1993;16:184-186.
60. Krentz AJ, et al. Octreotide: a long-acting inhibitor of endogenous hormone secretion for human metabolic investigations. *Metabolism.* 1994;43:24-31.
61. Kutz K, et al. Pharmacokinetics of SMS 201-995 in healthy subjects. *Scand J Gastroenterol Suppl.* 1986;119:65-72.
62. Lahlou H, et al. Molecular signaling of somatostatin receptors. *Ann N Y Acad Sci.* 2004;1014:121-131.
63. Laje P, et al. Necrotizing enterocolitis in neonates receiving octreotide for the management of congenital hyperinsulinism. *Pediatr Diabetes.* 2010;11:142-147.
64. Lamberts SW, et al. Octreotide. *N Engl J Med.* 1996;334:246-254.
65. Lewis RJ, Mohr JF 3rd. Dysglycaemias and fluoroquinolones. *Drug Saf.* 2008;31:283-292.
66. Lightman SL, et al. The effect of SMS 201-995, a long-acting somatostatin analogue, on anterior pituitary function in healthy male volunteers. *Scand J Gastroenterol Suppl.* 1986;119:84-95.
67. Llamado R, et al. Continuous octreotide infusion for sulfonylurea-induced hypoglycemia in a toddler. *J Emerg Med.* 2013;45:e209-e213.
68. Mafauzy M. Repaglinide versus glibenclamide treatment of Type 2 diabetes during Ramadan fasting. *Diabetes Res Clin Pract.* 2002;58:45-53.
69. McLaughlin SA, et al. Octreotide: an antidote for sulfonylurea-induced hypoglycemia. *Ann Emerg Med.* 2000;36:133-138.
70. Mercadante S. The role of octreotide in palliative care. *J Pain Symptom Manage.* 1994;9:406-411.
71. Mohnike K, et al. Long-term non-surgical therapy of severe persistent congenital hyperinsulinism with glucagon. *Horm Res.* 2008;70:59-64.
72. Moldovan S, et al. Somatostatin inhibits B-cell secretion via a subtype-2 somatostatin receptor in the isolated perfused human pancreas. *J Surg Res.* 1995;59:85-90.
73. Nakayama S, et al. Hypoglycemia following a nateglinide overdose in a suicide attempt. *Diabetes Care.* 2005;28:227-228.
74. Navascues I, et al. Severe hypoglycemia as a short-term side-effect of the somatostatin analog SMS 201-995 in insulin-dependent diabetes mellitus. *Horm Metab Res.* 1988;20:749-750.
75. Novartis Pharmaceuticals Corporation. Sandostatin® (octreotide acetate) injection [prescribing information]. East Hanover, NJ: Novartis Pharmaceuticals Corporation; 2012.
76. Olias G, et al. Regulation and function of somatostatin receptors. *J Neurochem.* 2004;89:1057-1091.
77. Orgaard A, Holst JJ. The role of somatostatin in GLP-1-induced inhibition of glucagon secretion in mice. *Diabetologia.* 2017;60:1731-1739.
78. Ottesen LH, et al. The pharmacokinetics of octreotide in cirrhosis and in healthy man. *J Hepatol.* 1997;26:1018-1025.
79. Pace CS, Tarvin JT. Somatostatin: mechanism of action in pancreatic islet beta-cells. *Diabetes.* 1981;30:836-842.
80. Palatnick W, et al. Clinical spectrum of sulfonylurea overdose and experience with diazoxide therapy. *Arch Intern Med.* 1991;151:1859-1862.
81. Pan S, et al. Experience of octreotide therapy for hyperinsulinemic hypoglycemia in neonates born small for gestational age: a case series. *Horm Res Paediatr.* 2015;84:383-387.
82. Papa G, et al. Safety of type 2 diabetes treatment with repaglinide compared with glibenclamide in elderly people: a randomized, open-label, two-period, cross-over trial. *Diabetes Care.* 2006;29:1918-1920.
83. Patel SR, et al. Comparison of the pharmacokinetics of octreotide injected at two subcutaneous sites. *J Natl Cancer Inst.* 1989;81:1926-1929.
84. Patel YC. Somatostatin and its receptor family. *Front Neuroendocrinol.* 1999;20:157-198.
85. Pelavin PI, et al. Extended-release glipizide overdose presenting with delayed hypoglycemia and treated with subcutaneous octreotide. *J Pediatr Endocrinol Metab.* 2009;22:171-175.
86. Phillips RE, et al. Hypoglycaemia and counterregulatory hormone responses in severe falciparum malaria: treatment with Sandostatin. *Q J Med.* 1993;86:233-240.
87. Phillips RE, et al. Effectiveness of SMS 201-995, a synthetic, long-acting somatostatin analogue, in treatment of quinine-induced hyperinsulinaemia. *Lancet.* 1986;1:713-716.

88. Pisarek H, et al. Expression of somatostatin receptor subtypes in human pituitary adenomas—immunohistochemical studies. *Endokrynol Pol.* 2009;60:240-251.

89. Plant TD, Henquin JC. Phentolamine and yohimbine inhibit ATP-sensitive K+ channels in mouse pancreatic beta-cells. *Br J Pharmacol.* 1990;101:115-120.

90. Plant TD, et al. Clonidine inhibits ATP-sensitive K+ channels in mouse pancreatic beta-cells. *Br J Pharmacol.* 1991;104:385-390.

91. Powers AC, D'Alessio D. Endocrine pancreas and pharmacotherapy of diabetes mellitus and hypoglycemia. In: Brunton LL, et al. eds. *Goodman & Gilman's The Pharmacological Basis of Therapeutics.* 12th ed. New York, NY: McGraw-Hill; 2011.

92. Rath S, et al. Octreotide in children with hypoglycaemia due to sulfonylurea ingestion. *J Paediatr Child Health.* 2008;44:383-384.

93. Schmid HA. Pasireotide (SOM230) prevents sulfonylurea-induced hypoglycemia in rats. *Exp Clin Endocrinol Diabetes.* 2015;123:193-197.

94. Shalev A, et al. Effects of glucagon-like peptide 1 (7-36 amide) on glucose kinetics during somatostatin-induced suppression of insulin secretion in healthy men. *Horm Res.* 1998;49:221-225.

95. Sheikhbahaie F, et al. The effect of hydroxychloroquine on glucose control and insulin resistance in the prediabetes condition. *Adv Biomed Res.* 2016;5:145.

96. Sherk DK, Bryant SM. Octreotide therapy for nateglinide-induced hypoglycemia. *Ann Emerg Med.* 2007;50:745-746.

97. Shyng S, et al. Regulation of KATP channel activity by diazoxide and MgADP. Distinct functions of the two nucleotide binding folds of the sulfonylurea receptor. *J Gen Physiol.* 1997;110:643-654.

98. Spiller HA, Sawyer TS. Toxicology of oral antidiabetic medications. *Am J Health Syst Pharm.* 2006;63:929-938.

99. Spiller HA, et al. Prospective multicenter study of sulfonylurea ingestion in children. *J Pediatr.* 1997;131:141-146.

100. Stehouwer CD, et al. Aggravation of hypoglycemia in insulinoma patients by the long-acting somatostatin analogue octreotide (Sandostatin). *Acta Endocrinol (Copenh).* 1989;121:34-40.

101. Strosberg J, Kvols L. Antiproliferative effect of somatostatin analogs in gastroentero-pancreatic neuroendocrine tumors. *World J Gastroenterol.* 2010;16:2963-2970.

102. Tenenbein MS, Tenenbein M. Anaphylactoid reaction to octreotide [abstract]. *Clin Toxicol.* 2006;44:707.

103. Testoni D, et al. Safety of octreotide in hospitalized infants. *Early Hum Dev.* 2015;91:387-392.

104. Theodoropoulou M, et al. Octreotide, a somatostatin analogue, mediates its antiproliferative action in pituitary tumor cells by altering phosphatidylinositol 3-kinase signaling and inducing Zac1 expression. *Cancer Res.* 2006;66:1576-1582.

105. Thornton PS, et al. Short- and long-term use of octreotide in the treatment of congenital hyperinsulinism. *J Pediatr.* 1993;123:637-643.

106. Unubol M, et al. Hypoglycemia induced by hydroxychloroquine in a patient treated for rheumatoid arthritis. *J Clin Rheumatol.* 2011;17:46-47.

107. Vallurupalli S. Safety of subcutaneous octreotide in patients with sulfonylurea-induced hypoglycemia and congestive heart failure. *Ann Pharmacother.* 2010;44:387-390.

108. van der Hoek J, et al. Novel subtype specific and universal somatostatin analogues: clinical potential and pitfalls. *Curr Pharm Des.* 2005;11:1573-1592.

109. Varghese RT, et al. Mechanisms underlying the pathogenesis of isolated impaired glucose tolerance in humans. *J Clin Endocrinol Metab.* 2016;101:4816-4824.

110. Verschoor L, et al. On the use of a new somatostatin analogue in the treatment of hypoglycaemia in patients with insulinoma. *Clin Endocrinol (Oxf).* 1986;25:555-560.

111. Wass JA, et al. Proceedings of the discussion, "Tolerability and safety of Sandostatin." *Metabolism.* 1992;41:80-82.

112. Woltering EA, et al. Effect of octreotide LAR dose and weight on octreotide blood levels in patients with neuroendocrine tumors. *Pancreas.* 2005;31:392-400.

113. Zhou G, et al. Negative regulation of pancreatic and duodenal homeobox-1 by somatostatin receptor subtype 5. *Mol Endocrinol.* 2012;26:1225-1234.

48 ANTIEPILEPTICS

Suzanne Doyon

HISTORY AND EPIDEMIOLOGY

Epilepsy affects 6 per 1,000 population in the United States.[54] More than 50 distinct epileptic syndromes are identified; they are categorized into partial (60%) and generalized (40%) epilepsies.[31] Partial epileptic seizures arise from localized cortical sites, and generalized epileptic seizures involve both cerebral hemispheres.[31]

Historically, seizures were treated by a variety of methods, including ketogenic diets, fluid restriction, and surgical excision of scars or irritable cortical foci.[118] The first truly effective antiepileptic therapy was introduced in 1857, when the administration of bromides was noted to sedate patients and significantly reduce their seizures.[118] Phenobarbital, a sedative–hypnotic, was first used to treat seizures in 1912. Most of the subsequently introduced antiepileptics, such as primidone (2-desoxyphenobarbital), had chemical structures similar to that of phenobarbital, and sedation was erroneously believed to be an essential component of antiepileptic therapy.

The search for nonsedating antiepileptics led to the introduction of phenytoin in 1938 and benzodiazepines, carbamazepine, and valproic acid (VPA) in the 1960s. These antiepileptics were the only medications available until the 1990s, when second-generation antiepileptics were introduced: gabapentin, lamotrigine, levetiracetam, oxcarbazepine, tiagabine, topiramate, felbamate, vigabatrin, lacosamide, and zonisamide.

Broad-spectrum antiepileptics are effective in the management of all seizure types. Narrow-spectrum antiepileptics are restricted to patients who have partial (localized) epilepsy with partial or secondarily generalized seizures.[54] Antiepileptics are also currently used for a host of disorders, including psychiatric illnesses, refractory pain, drug withdrawal syndromes, migraines, cluster headaches, spasms, and chronic cough. Based on reports, in 2009, the Food and Drug Administration issued a warning about increased risk of suicidal thoughts or actions following treatment with carbamazepine, lamotrigine, levetiracetam, oxcarbazepine, phenytoin, tiagabine, topiramate, valproic acid, and zonisamide.[25,50,88]

Carbamazepine, lamotrigine, oxcarbazepine, and valproic acid are associated with pregnancy complications such as preeclampsia, premature births, spontaneous abortions, and stillbirths.[8,12]

This chapter reviews the toxicity and management of overdoses with antiepileptics other than the benzodiazepines and barbiturates, which are discussed in Chap. 72.

PHARMACOLOGY

The mechanisms of action of antiepileptics include (1) sodium channel blockade; (2) calcium channel blockade; (3) blockade of excitatory amines; (4) GABA (gamma-aminobutyric acid) potentiation; and (5) binding to synaptic vesicle glycoprotein 2A (SV2A). Some antiepileptics have multiple mechanisms of action. Table 48–1 and Figs. 48–1 and 48–2 summarize these effects.

Voltage-gated Na$^+$ channels are fundamental units that evoke action potentials in neurons. These fast channels are large integral membrane proteins with an important alpha subunit and 2 smaller auxiliary beta subunits which act as modulators. Nine different Na$^+$ channels exist (Na$^+$ 1.1–1.9), each with a slightly different alpha subunit. Alpha subunits have multiple (up to 7) distinct binding sites. Carbamazepine, eslicarbazepine, lamotrigine, oxcarbazepine, phenytoin, rufinamide, topiramate, VPA, and zonisamide all bind to the batrachotoxin-binding site (or adjacent area) on alpha subunits of Na$^+$ channels. They close the internal gates, thereby preventing action potential propagation and decreasing repetitive firing.[58,125,198] At therapeutic concentrations, binding of antiepileptics to a Na$^+$ channel is largely selective. At toxic

concentrations, selectivity is lost, and both high-frequency and spontaneous sodium channels are blocked, including those found in cardiac tissue.[22,98,141,176] Lacosamide enhances slow inactivation of Na$^+$ channel (Fig. 48–1).[43]

Voltage-gated Ca^{2+} channels are multisubunit complexes that are broadly classified into high- and low-voltage groups. High-voltage Ca^{2+} channels include the L, N, P/Q, and R-type channels located primarily on presynaptic neurons; low-voltage Ca^{2+} include the T-type channels located on dendrites of thalamic neurons.[9] Gabapentin and pregabalin bind to the $\alpha_2\delta_1$ subunit of the high-voltage N-type Ca^{2+} channels, reducing the frequency of calcium fusion of synaptic vesicles to membranes and thereby reducing glutamate exocytosis.[60] Levetiracetam also inhibits N-type Ca^{2+} channels, but this is not its major mechanism of action.[114] Lamotrigine inhibits N- and P/Q-type Ca^{2+} channels.[190] Topiramate inhibits L-type Ca^{2+} channels; these channels are found on smooth and striated muscle cells, endocrine cells, and, importantly, cardiomyocytes. Finally, zonisamide inhibits T-type Ca^{2+} channels, thus reducing the neuronal pacemaker current (Fig. 48–1).[179]

Several excitatory amine receptors have been identified. They are located on the postsynaptic membrane and are glutamate-activated ligand-gated ion channels. N-methyl-D-aspartate (NMDA), kainate, and alpha-amino-3-hydroxy-5-methyl-4-isoxazolepropionic acid (AMPA) are the predominant excitatory amine receptors. When activated, these receptors allow for the influx of Na$^+$, K$^+$, and Ca^{2+} into cells. VPA competitively inhibits the NMDA receptor.[59] Topiramate inhibits the kainate receptor.[65] Perampanel, a third-generation antiepileptic, inhibits the AMPA receptor (Fig. 48–1).[23]

Synaptic vesicle glycoprotein 2A (SV2A) is a member of the superfamily of proteins called membrane transporters that are an integral part of secretory vesicles in neuronal tissue. Synaptic vesicular glycoprotein 2A plays an important role in seizure pathophysiology.[85] Levetiracetam binds to SV2A, inducing a conformational change in the protein that leads to inhibition of vesicular exocytosis of glutamate from the presynaptic neuron (Fig. 48–1).[110,116]

γ-Aminobutyric acid is an inhibitory neurotransmitter that is the target of antiepileptics, which often aim to increase concentrations of GABA in the synapse. Vigabatrin irreversibly inhibits GABA transaminase, the enzyme primarily responsible for GABA metabolism.[34] Valproic acid is reported to have similar effects.[139] Tiagabine inhibits the GABA transporter GAT-1 (also known as SLC6A1) and thereby prevents reuptake of GABA into presynaptic neurons.[11] Neither gabapentin nor pregabalin, despite their structural similarity to GABA, mimics GABA when iontophoretically applied to GABA neurons (Fig. 48–2).[129]

Lastly, ezogabine (retigabine in Europe) is a unique antiepileptic that opens voltage-gated K$^+$ channels and increases the M current, thereby hyperpolarizing the membrane.[117]

CARBAMAZEPINE

Carbamazepine is structurally related to the cyclic antidepressants. It is approved for the management of seizures and trigeminal neuralgia and is a pregnancy category D medication associated with kinked ribs and cleft palate.[14]

Pharmacokinetics and Toxicokinetics

Carbamazepine is lipophilic, with slow and unpredictable absorption after oral administration and rapid distribution to all tissues. Peak concentrations can be delayed postingestion up to 100 hours.[19,145] It is metabolized primarily by CYP3A4 to carbamazepine 10,11-epoxide, which is pharmacologically active. This quantifiable metabolite is further degraded by epoxide hydrolase to carbamazepine-diol, a largely inactive compound.[92] Carbamazepine is unique because it induces its own metabolism after 2 to 4 weeks. The

TABLE 48–1 Comparison of Mechanisms of Action of Antiepileptics

	Na⁺ Channel	Ca²⁺ Channel	GABA	GABA Transaminase	GABA Reuptake	NMDA AMPA kainate	Synaptic Vesicle Glycoprotein 2A	K⁺ Channel	Carbonic Anhydrase
Carbamazepine	Blocks							Potentiates?	
Eslicarbazepine acetate	Blocks	Blocks (T-type)							
Ezogabine								Potentiates	
Gabapentin		Blocks (N-type)							
Lacosamide	Blocks								
Lamotrigine	Blocks	Blocks (N-, P/Q-type)							
Levetiracetam		Blocks (N-type)					Binding		
Oxcarbazepine	Blocks								
Perampanel						Blocks (AMPA)			
Phenytoin/Fosphenytoin	Blocks								
Pregabalin		Blocks (N-type)							
Rufinamide	Blocks								
Stiripentol			Potentiates						
Tiagabine					Blocks				
Topiramate	Blocks	Blocks (L-type)	Potentiates			Blocks (kainate)			Blocks
Valproic acid	Blocks			Blocks		Blocks (NMDA)			
Vigabatrin				Blocks					
Zonisamide	Blocks	Blocks (T-type)							Blocks

GABA = γ-aminobutyric acid; NMDA = N-methyl-D-aspartate; AMPA = alpha-amino-3-hydroxyl-5-methyl-4-isoxazolepropionate.

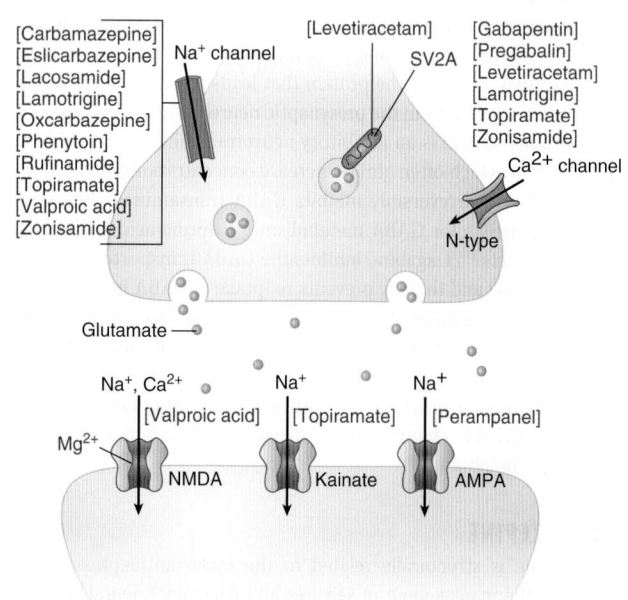

FIGURE 48–1. Excitatory neurons. In presynaptic neurons, carbamazepine, eslicarbazepine, lamotrigine, oxcarbazepine, phenytoin, rufinamide, topiramate, valproic acid and zonisamide all inhibit the Na⁺ channel, preventing the release of the excitatory neurotransmitter glutamate. Lacosamide binds differently and enhances slow inactivation, i.e. inhibitory effect. Gabapentin, lamotrigine, levetiracetam, pregabalin, topiramate, and zonisamide all inhibit the Ca²⁺ channel, preventing the release of glutamate. In post synaptic neurons, perampanel, topiramate, and valproic acid each inhibit a different excitatory receptor. AMPA=alpha-amino-3-hydroxy-5-methyl-4-isoxazolepropionic acid; NMDA = N-methyl-D-aspartate. SV2ₐ = Synaptic vesicle protein 2ₐ.

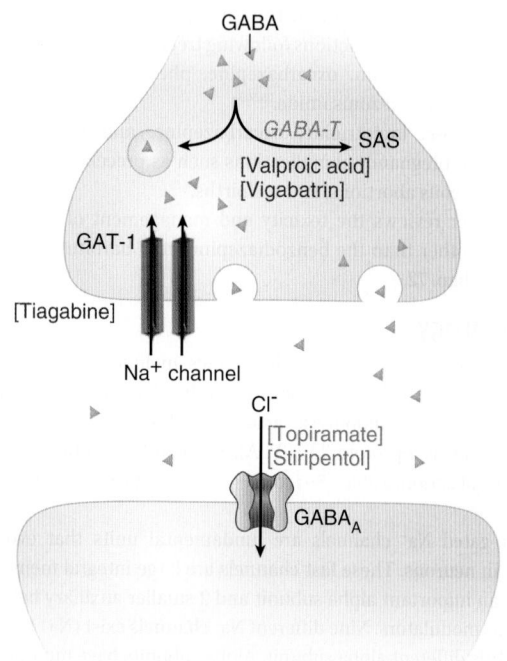

FIGURE 48–2. Inhibitory neurons. In presynaptic neurons, valproic acid and vigabatrin inhibit GABA metabolism; tiagabine inhibits its transporter; the end result is increased GABA in the synaptic cleft. In post synaptic neurons, stiripentol and topiramate modulate GABA_A receptors. GABA = γ-aminobutyric acid; GABA-T = GABA transaminase; GAT1 = GABA transporter; SAS = succinic acid semialdehyde.

TABLE 48–2	Pharmacokinetics of Antiepileptics After Oral Administration							
	Time to Max Serum Concentration (hours)	Therapeutic Serum Concentration		Volume of Distribution (L/kg)	Protein Binding (%)	Urinary Elimination Unchanged (%)	Active Metabolite	Elimination Half-Life (hours)
		(mg/L)	(μmol/L)					
Carbamazepine	6–8 IR 4–26 ER	4–12	17–51	0.8–1.8	75	1–2	CBZ10–11 epoxide	Acute 6–20; chronic 5–12
Eslicarbazepine	1–4	10–35		2.7	35	1	S-licarbazepine	20–40
Ezogabine	0.5–2	a	a	2–6	80	20	None	8
Gabapentin	2–3	2–20	12–117	0.6–08	0	100	None	5–9
Lacosamide	0.5–4	5–10	20–40?	0.6	15	40	None	12–13
Lamotrigine	1–3	3–15	12–58	0.1–1.4	55	10	None	15–35
Levetiracetam	1–2	10–46	60–240	0.6	0	95	None	6–8
Oxcarbazepine	1–5	1–3	4–12	0.7	67	1	10-hydroxy carbazepine	1–2
Perampanel	0.5–1.5	a	a	77	96	2	None	70–110
Phenobarbital	1–6	15–40	65–172	0.7	35–50	20–50	None	53–140
Phenytoin	5–24	10–20	40–79	0.6	>90	<5	None	6–60
Pregabalin	1–2	2–5	18–52	0.5	0	>90	None	5–7
Rufinamide	5–6	5–35	20–140	0.7–1.1	30	2	None	8–12
Tiagabine	0.5–2	0.02–0.2	0.027–0.27	1–1.3	95	<5	None	5–9
Topiramate	2–4	5–20	15–74	0.6–0.8	15	60	None	20–30
Valproic acid	1–24 in overdose	50–120	347–832	0.1–0.4	>90b	<5	None	5–18
Vigabatrin	1–2	0.8–36	155–619	0.8	0	100	None	6–8
Zonisamide	2–5	10–40	47–189	1.45	50	30	None	50–70

IR = immediate release; ER = extended release; CBZ = carbamazepine; aNot yet established; b = saturable.

elimination half-life is 25 to 65 hours at initiation of therapy and decreases to 12 to 17 hours with continued dosing.[42] Zero-order elimination kinetics are observed following large overdoses (Tables 48–2 and 48–3).[194]

Clinical Manifestations
Acute carbamazepine toxicity is characterized by neurologic and cardiovascular effects. The neurologic disturbances include nystagmus, ataxia, seizures, and coma.[19,75,115] Status epilepticus is reported.[168] Cardiovascular effects include sinus tachycardia, hypotension, myocardial depression, and, rarely, cardiac conduction abnormalities such as QRS complex and QT interval prolongation.[28,48,64] The toxicity of carbamazepine in children differs slightly from that in adults. Children experience a higher incidence of dystonic reactions, choreoathetosis, and seizures and have a lower incidence of ECG abnormalities.[166,175] Chronic carbamazepine overdose can result in headaches, diplopia, ataxia, and leukopenia.[155]

The incidence of carbamazepine-induced hyponatremia ranges from 1.8% to 40%. Increased antidiuretic hormone secretion (SIADH) or increased sensitivity of peripheral osmoreceptors to antidiuretic hormone are suggested mechanisms (Chap. 12).[99,186]

Diagnostic Testing
Therapeutic serum concentrations of carbamazepine are 4 to 12 mg/L. Carbamazepine-10,11-epoxide concentrations are 1 to 10 mg/L and can exceed 10 mg/L with therapeutic use of lamotrigine or VPA, secondary to epoxide hydrolase inhibition (Table 48–4). Electrolytes should be checked in patients with altered mental status because of the risk of hyponatremia.[99,186] Carbamazepine cross-reacts with some toxicology screening for tricyclic antidepressants (Chap. 68).[52]

Management
Rigorous supportive care underlies management. Multiple-dose activated charcoal is associated with improved outcomes in several studies and is recommended for to patients presenting with large overdoses, if there are no contraindications.[13,70,115] Seizures should be treated with benzodiazepines. Vasopressors should be used for hypotension that is refractory to fluids. Sodium bicarbonate is recommended if the QRS complex duration exceeds 100 milliseconds (ms).[48] Serial serum concentrations should be obtained owing to delays in peak concentrations. Extracorporeal drug removal is reasonable in cases of severe poisonings associated with intractable seizures or life-threatening dysrhythmias.[62] Intermittent hemodialysis (HD) is preferred.[62]

ESLICARBAZEPINE ACETATE
Eslicarbazepine acetate is a third-generation antiepileptic that belongs to the dibenzazepine family, which includes carbamazepine (first-generation) and oxcarbazepine (second-generation). It is a prodrug that is presystemically metabolized in the liver to S(+)-licarbazepine (95%) and R(–)-licarbazepine (5%).[162] S(+)-Licarbazepine is also the pharmacologically active metabolite of oxcarbazepine (Tables 48–2 and 48–3).[162] Eslicarbazepine is expected to be more effective than oxcarbazepine and is further discussed in the oxcarbazepine section.[162]

EZOGABINE
Ezogabine (Retigabine in Europe) is a recently approved antiepileptic. Hepatic hydrolysis/N-acetylation followed by glucuronidation are responsible for 50% to 65% of its metabolism. Uridine-diphosphate-glucuronosyltransferase

TABLE 48–3	Metabolism of Antiepileptics and Effects on CYP Enzymes		
	Metabolized by	**Induction**	**Inhibition**
Carbamazepine	3A4; 1A2; 2C8; 2C9;	2C9; 3A family	None
Eslicarbazepine acetate	Hydrolysis; UGT	Weak 3A4	2C9, 2C19
Ezogabine	N-acetylation	None	None
Gabapentin	None	None	None
Lacosamide	3A4, 2C9, 2C19	None	None
Lamotrigine	UGT	None	None
Levetiracetam	None	None	None
Oxcarbazepine	UGT	None	2C19, 3A4
Perampanel	3A4; UGT	Weak 3A4; 2B6	Weak 2C8; UGT
Phenobarbital	2C9; 2C19, 2E1	3A family	None
Phenytoin	2C9; 2C19; 3A4	2C family; 3A family	None
Pregabalin	None	None	None
Rufinamide	Hydrolysis; UGT	None	None
Tiagabine	3A4	None	None
Topiramate	None	None	2C19
Valproic acid	2C9; 2C19; UGT	None	2C19
Vigabatrin	None	None	None
Zonisamide	3A4; acetylation	None	None

UGT = uridine-diphosphate-glucuronosyltransferase.

(UGT1A4) is the principal isoenzyme involved.[200] It is associated with bluish skin discoloration (6%), maculopathy, urinary disorders, and QT prolongation (Tables 48–2 and 48–3).[127]

GABAPENTIN

Gabapentin is a narrow-spectrum antiepileptic approved for the management of seizures, postherpetic neuralgia, chronic neuropathic pain, migraine headaches, and restless leg syndrome.[54] Gabapentin can be misused and abused.[45] It is a category C medication with limited human data in pregnancy.[14]

Pharmacokinetics and Toxicokinetics

The bioavailability of gabapentin is approximately 60% in the therapeutic dose range. Absorption kinetics are dose-dependent, with decreasing bioavailability at increased dosage because of saturation of the L-amino acid transport system.[15,185] It has high water solubility but poor lipid solubility.[15] Dosage adjustments are necessary in patients with creatinine clearance or estimated glomerular filtration rate (eGFR) of 60 mL/min or less.[140] It is not metabolized by and does not affect the CYP450 system and has no significant interactions with other antiepileptics (Tables 48–2 and 48–3).[200]

Clinical Manifestations

Sedation, ataxia, movement disorders, slurred speech, and gastrointestinal (GI) symptoms are reported after acute gabapentin overdose.[78,95,193] Gabapentin withdrawal is characterized by agitation, confusion, tachycardia, and possibly seizures.[128]

Diagnostic Testing

Therapeutic serum concentrations of gabapentin are 2 to 20 mg/L. Because of its large therapeutic index, monitoring of serum gabapentin concentrations is not routinely necessary.[97]

Management

Treatment is largely supportive. Saturation of the transporter system limits GI absorption and movement across the blood–brain barrier.[15,185] Hemodialysis and hemoperfusion are not generally necessary, but up to 35% is removed by HD in anuric patients.[39,78] Gabapentin withdrawal does not respond well to administration of benzodiazepines and should be treated with tapering doses of gabapentin.[128]

LACOSAMIDE

Lacosamide is a functionalized amino acid with high water solubility.[97] It is a category C medication with limited data in human pregnancy.[14]

Pharmacokinetics and Toxicokinetics

Lacosamide is almost 100% bioavailable orally. It is predominantly excreted unchanged in the urine and 30% metabolized in liver (2C19).[82] Enzyme inducers such as carbamazepine and phenytoin can significantly reduce serum lacosamide concentrations (Tables 48–2 and 48–3).[82]

Diagnostic Testing

Lacosamide's therapeutic serum concentration is 5 to 10 mg/L.[82] Monitoring of concentration is not routinely recommended in overdose.

Clinical Manifestations

Gastrointestinal effects, QRS complex prolongation, dysrhythmias, intractable hypotension, and death are reported following acute overdose.[26,119] Prolongation of the QRS complex is reported following overdose of a mix of lacosamide and other Na+ channel blockers.[37,142]

Management

Electrocardiographic monitoring and supportive care are recommended. QRS complex prolongation responds to administration of sodium bicarbonate, and hypotension responds to administration of vasopressors making these reasonable therapeutics.[26,119]

LAMOTRIGINE

Lamotrigine is a phenyltriazine antiepileptic also approved for maintenance treatment of bipolar mood disorder.[82] It is a category C medication with limited human data in pregnancy.[14]

Pharmacokinetics and Toxicokinetics

The bioavailability of lamotrigine approaches 100%.[82] It is predominantly glucuronidated to lamotrigine-2-N-glucuronide.[82] The elimination half-life is approximately 25 hours but can be significantly reduced (12 hours) in the presence of phenytoin and carbamazepine.[199] The half-life is doubled by VPA, an enzyme inhibitor. Significantly reduced clearance of lamotrigine occurs in patients with Gilbert syndrome (syndrome of defective glucuronidation) (Tables 48–2 and 48–3).[198]

Clinical Manifestations

Neurologic and cardiovascular manifestations predominate following lamotrigine overdose. In large case series, seizures, central nervous system depression, agitation, myoclonus, and hyperreflexia were present.[134] Status epilepticus is reported.[109,141] Tachycardia, hypertension, and tachypnea are also frequently present along with QRS complex prolongation, Brugada-like ECG abnormalities, and third-degree heart block.[22,134,141,176] Chronic supratherapeutic dosing resulted in oculogyric crises in 4 patients.[188]

Diagnostic Testing

Therapeutic serum concentrations of lamotrigine are 2 to 15 mg/L.[82] Monitoring of concentration is not routinely recommended in overdose.

Management

Supportive care and cardiac monitoring should be provided. Lamotrigine-induced seizures respond to benzodiazepines.[134,191] Data on HD and hemoperfusion are not available. Intravenous lipid emulsion is not recommended owing to toxicity based on limited data (Antidotes in Depth: A23).[22,134]

TABLE 48–4   Antiepileptic Drug Interactions

	Toxicity Increased by	Anticonvulsant Effect Decreased by	Increases Concentrations of	Decreases Concentrations of
Carbamazepine	Allopurinol, amiodarone, cimetidine, danazol, diltiazem, fluoxetine, fluvoxamine, gemfibrozil, INH, ketoconazole, lamotrigine, macrolides, nefazodone, nicotine, propoxyphene, protease inhibitors, stiripentol, verapamil	Benzodiazepines, felbamate, isotretinoin, phenobarbital, phenytoin, primidone, succinimides, VPA	None	Doxycycline, felbamate, haloperidol, lamotrigine, OCPs, phenytoin, primidone, tiagabine, VPA, warfarin
Eslicarbazepine	None	CBZ, phenobarbital, phenytoin, topiramate	Phenytoin	CBZ, lamotrigine, topiramate, VPA
Ezogabine	None	CBZ, lamotrigine, phenobarbital, phenytoin	Phenobarbital	Lamotrigine
Gabapentin	Cimetidine	Antacids	Felbamate	None
Lamotrigine	Sertraline, VPA	CBZ, phenobarbital, phenytoin	CBZ epoxide	None
Levetiracetam	None	None	Phenytoin	None
Oxcarbazepine	None	CBZ, phenobarbital, phenytoin	Phenytoin	Lamotrigine, OCPs
Perampanel	None	CBZ, phenobarbital, phenytoin, oxcarbazepine, topiramate	Oxcarbazepine	CBZ, lamotrigine, VPA
Phenytoin	Allopurinol, amiodarone, chloramphenicol, chlorpheniramine, clarithromycin, cloxacillin, cimetidine, disulfiram, ethosuximide, felbamate, fluconazole, fluorouracil, fluoxetine, fluvoxamine, imipramine, INH, methylphenidate, metronidazole, miconazole, omeprazole, phenylbutazone, sulfonamides, ticlopidine, trimethoprim, tolbutamide, tolazamide, topiramate, VPA, warfarin	Antacids, antineoplastics CBZ, calcium, diazepam, diazoxide, ethanol (chronic), folic acid, influenza vaccine, loxapine, nitrofurantoin, phenobarbital, phenylbutazone, pyridoxine, rifampin, salicylates, sulfisoxazole, sucralfate, theophylline, tolbutamide, VPA, vigabatrin	Phenobarbital, primidone, warfarin	Amiodarone, CBZ, cardioactive steroids, corticosteroids, cyclosporine, disopyramide, dopamine, doxycycline, furosemide, haloperidol, influenza vaccine, levodopa, methadone, mexiletine, OCP, phenothiazines, quinidine, tacrolimus, theophylline, tiagabine, tolbutamide, VPA
Pregabalin	None	Gabapentin, oxcarbazepine	None	Tiagabine
Rufinamide	VPA	CBZ, phenobarbital, phenytoin	Phenytoin	CBZ, lamotrigine,
Tiagabine	None	CBZ, phenobarbital, phenytoin	None	VPA
Topiramate	None	CBZ, phenobarbital, phenytoin	Phenytoin	OCPs, cardioactive steroids
Valproic acid	Cimetidine, felbamate, ranitidine	Antacids, CBZ, chitosan, chlorpromazine, felbamate, INH, methotrexate, phenobarbital, phenytoin, primidone, salicylates	Felbamate, lamotrigine, phenobarbital, primidone	CBZ, tiagabine
Vigabatrin	None	None	None	Phenytoin
Zonisamide	None	CBZ, phenobarbital, phenytoin	?CBZ	-CBZ

CBZ = carbamazepine; INH = isoniazid; OCP = oral contraceptive pill; VPA = valproic acid.

LEVETIRACETAM

Levetiracetam is an enantioselective isomer (S) piracetam analogue antiepileptic that may also be effective in the treatment of traumatic brain injury.[71,82] It is a category C medication with limited human data in pregnancy.[14]

Pharmacokinetics and Toxicokinetics

The bioavailability of levetiracetam approaches 100%. The major metabolic pathway involves enzymatic hydrolysis of the acetamide group. This reaction occurs in the blood and is not dependent on hepatic CYP450 activity.[82] There are no active metabolites.[82] Dosage adjustments are necessary in patients with creatinine clearances or eGFR of 80 mL/min or less (Tables 48–2 and 48–3).[91,173]

Clinical Manifestations

Mild central nervous system (CNS) depression and ataxia were reported in one large case series.[104] Respiratory depression requiring intubation was occurred in one case report.[7] Chronic therapy is not associated with behavioral problems in adults but is associated with aggression and agitation in up to 20% of children.[73,123]

Diagnostic Testing

Therapeutic serum concentrations of levetiracetam are 12 to 46 mg/L. Because of its large therapeutic index, routine monitoring of serum levetiracetam concentrations is not necessary.[82]

Management

Supportive care should be provided. Extracorporeal removal treatment is not recommended.

OXCARBAZEPINE

Oxcarbazepine is an analog of carbamazepine that functions as a prodrug of licarbazepine, also known as monohydroxycarbazepine.[162] It is a category C medication with limited data in human pregnancy.[14]

Pharmacokinetics, Toxicokinetics

Oxcarbazepine has 100% bioavailability. Rate-limited presystemic ketoreduction rapidly metabolizes oxcarbazepine to licarbazepine, also known as monohydroxycarbazepine. Metabolism is skewed toward formation of S(+)-licarbazepine (80%), which is pharmacologically active.[162] Plasma elimination half-life of oxcarbazepine is 2 hours, and licarbazepine, 8 to 15 hours.[146] Oxcarbazepine minimally inhibits CYP3A4 but increases glucuronidation.[146,199] Licarbazepine concentrations are reduced by 25% in the presence of enzyme inducers such as carbamazepine and phenytoin (Tables 48–2 and 48–3).[146,200]

Clinical Manifestations
Central nervous system effects (lethargy, nystagmus, dizziness) and cardiovascular effects (tachycardia, hyper/hypotension) are reported after overdose.[148,170] In severe cases, coma, respiratory depression and seizures are noted.[170] The rate-limited enzymatic conversion to the active metabolite may limit toxicity; in some cases, serum concentrations of oxcarbazepine were very high (10-fold), while concentrations of S(+)- and R(−)-licarbazepine were low (2-fold).[56,148,187] In one large case series of acute overdoses, electrolyte abnormalities were rarely reported.[170] Oxcarbazepine is associated with drug-induced liver injury.[77]

Diagnostic Testing
Therapeutic serum concentrations of oxcarbazepine are 10 to 35 mg/L. Licarbazepine (monohydroxycarbazepine) serum concentrations are 3 to 35 mg/L.[112] Monitoring of concentrations is not routinely recommended in overdose. Electrolytes should be checked in patients with altered mental status because of the risk of hyponatremia (<135 mmol/L).[112]

Management
Rigorous supportive care underlies management. Hemodialysis (HD) does not increase the clearance of oxcarbazepine/10-hydroxycarbazepine, so HD is not recommended.[56]

PERAMPANEL
Perampanel is a recently approved antiepileptic with a unique mechanism of action. It is a noncompetitive (allosteric) AMPA receptor antagonist.[10] It has a favorable pharmacokinetic profile and an extremely long elimination half-life of 70 hours.[10] Perampanel's metabolism is induced by carbamazepine and phenytoin.[10] Therapeutic serum concentrations have not yet been established.[82] Lethargy and slurred speech were observed for 48 hours following one case report of a large overdose.[76] Supportive care and monitoring of mental status are recommended in overdose (Tables 48–2 and 48–3).

PHENYTOIN AND FOSPHENYTOIN
Phenytoin was first synthesized in 1908 but its antiepileptic properties were not discovered until 1938. It is a pregnancy category D medication, associated with the fetal hydantoin syndrome and cerebral hemorrhage in neonates.[14]

Fosphenytoin is a water-soluble phosphate ester prodrug of phenytoin. Advantages include more rapid administration, availability for intramuscular (IM) administration, and low potential for tissue injury at injection sites.[57]

Pharmacokinetics and Toxicokinetics
Phenytoin is rapidly distributed to all tissues following a 2-compartment model. Oral loading doses of 20 mg/kg yield therapeutic (>10 mg/L) serum concentrations at 5.6 ± 0.2 hours.[180] In cases of very large oral overdoses, GI absorption is altered and peak serum concentrations can be delayed for days.[24,29,61] Additionally, phenytoin occasionally forms concretions in the GI tract.[24,29]

Phenytoin is extensively bound to serum proteins, mainly albumin. Only the unbound free fraction is pharmacologically active. A significant fraction of phenytoin remains unbound in neonates, uremic patients, and other patients with hypoalbuminemia, such as patients in ICUs.[36]

Phenytoin is predominantly metabolized by CYP enzymes (2C9 and 2C19) to inactive metabolites, less than 1% is excreted unchanged in the urine. Its rate of elimination varies as a function of its concentration (ie, rate is nonlinear; Michaelis–Menten kinetics).[152] At phenytoin concentrations below 10 mg/L, elimination usually is first-order, and half-life is 6 and 24 hours. At higher concentrations, zero-order elimination occurs because of saturation of the hydroxylation reaction, and the apparent half-life increases to 20 to 105 hours (Chap. 9) (Tables 48–2 and 48–3).[46]

Fosphenytoin is metabolized by tissue and blood phosphatases to phenytoin, phosphate, and formaldehyde. The half-life of conversion of fosphenytoin to phenytoin is 7 to 15 minutes.[51] Although molar conversion is equivalent, differences in molecular mass necessitate a 1.5:1 conversion factor from fosphenytoin–phenytoin; for example, 1.5 g fosphenytoin sodium = 1 g phenytoin sodium.[113]

Clinical Manifestations
Acute phenytoin toxicity produces predominantly neurologic dysfunction, affecting the cerebellar and vestibular systems. Phenytoin concentrations greater than 15 mg/L are associated with nystagmus; concentrations greater than 30 mg/L are associated with ataxia and poor coordination; and concentrations exceeding 50 mg/L are associated with lethargy, slurred speech, and pyramidal and extrapyramidal manifestations.[29,131] Ophthalmoplegia, opsoclonus, and other focal neurologic deficits are also reported.[174] Cardiovascular instability, de novo seizures, and death following oral overdoses are rare.[174,197]

Intravenous overdose produces the same symptoms as oral overdose, with the addition of cardiotoxicity, hypotension, and dysrhythmias. These manifestations are usually attributed to the diluents propylene glycol (40%) and ethanol (10%).[41,46,67,132]

Metabolism of fosphenytoin releases phosphate and formaldehyde. Iatrogenic overdoses of fosphenytoin are associated with hyperphosphatemia, hypocalcemia, bradycardia, hypotension, and asystole.[90,102,124,154]

The purple glove syndrome is a serious complication of IV phenytoin or fosphenytoin administration whose incidence ranges from 1% to 6%.[57] Pathophysiology is unclear but appears to be related either to microextravasation or an unidentified procoagulant mechanism. Symptoms begin 2 to 12 hours after administration and include discoloration and edema distal to the site of administration.[18] Mild symptoms typically resolve over days, but when severe, lead to necrosis, possibly necessitating amputation.[57] The risk of purple glove syndrome associated with fosphenytoin is lower because of its water solubility.[57]

Chronic therapy results in gingival overgrowth in up to 20% of patients.[133] It is also associated with decreased ADH, osteomalacia, hepatotoxicity, and megaloblastic anemia.[161]

Diagnostic Testing
Serum phenytoin concentrations are 10 to 20 mg/L. Because of zero-order elimination, very high serum phenytoin concentrations often take days to return to the therapeutic range.[29,47,111]

Measurement of free phenytoin concentration is helpful in neonates, elderly, hypoalbuminemic, and uremic patients because it compares more reliably with the cerebrospinal fluid concentration.[36,69] Therapeutic free phenytoin concentrations are 1.0 to 2.1 mg/L.

Management
The treatment of patients with oral phenytoin overdoses is largely supportive. Oral multidose activated charcoal (MDAC) is recommended in severe overdoses presenting with profound coma.[5,165] Hemodialysis, charcoal hemoperfusion, plasmapheresis, and other extracorporeal techniques such as molecular adsorbents recirculating systems (MARS) is reasonable in severe cases with life-threatening cardiovascular instability or profound neurologic impairment.[5] All patients admitted to the hospital for oral phenytoin overdose require frequent neurologic assessments; routine cardiac monitoring is not necessary because of the low risk of cardiac toxicity following oral overdose.[44,197] Phenytoin-induced agranulocytosis can be treated successfully with administration of granulocyte colony–stimulating factor.[178]

Intravenous phenytoin is associated with hypotension, cardiac dysrhythmias, and dyskinesias. These are usually transient and resolve in 60 minutes. Stopping the phenytoin infusion for a few minutes and administering a bolus of 250 to 500 mL of 0.9% sodium chloride solution generally is sufficient to treat the hypotension. Restarting the infusion at half the initial rate is recommended.

Fosphenytoin IV overdose is associated with QT interval prolongation due to hyperphosphatemia and hypocalcemia. Electrolytes should be corrected immediately; HD may be required.[124] Dysrhythmias are reported and require prolonged periods of cardiopulmonary resuscitation.[102,154]

The management of extravasation is discussed in Special Considerations: SC8.

PREGABALIN

Pregabalin is an antiepileptic developed as a more potent analog of gabapentin. It is indicated in the management of seizures and neuropathic pain.[157] Pregabalin is abused and misused.[45,72,177] It is a category C medication with limited human data in pregnancy.[14]

Pharmacokinetics and Toxicokinetics

Pregabalin, unlike gabapentin, does not have a saturable GI transporter protein and is highly bioavailable, with rapid absorption. It is not protein-bound, and more than 90% is excreted unchanged in the urine.[151,199] Dose adjustments are necessary in patients with GFR less than 60 mL/min.[195] Pregabalin has no significant interactions with other antiepileptics except perhaps increasing the steady-state concentrations of tiagabine (Tables 48–2 and 48–3).[15]

Clinical Manifestations

Cerebellar dysfunction (including dizziness, ataxia, and nystagmus), tremors, twitching, and seizures are described after overdose.[83,130,143,164,195] Third-degree atrioventricular block, QT interval prolongation, encephalopathy, and respiratory failure are observed.[2,101,195] Peripheral edema, weight gain, and decompensated congestive heart failure occur with chronic therapy.[135]

Diagnostic Testing

Therapeutic concentrations of pregabalin are 2.8 to 8.3 mg/L.[82] Monitoring of concentration is not routinely recommended in overdose.

Management

Rigorous supportive care underlies management.[2,101,195] Cardiac monitoring is recommended. It is reasonable to utilize HD in patients with severe CKD.

RUFINAMIDE

Rufinamide is a recently approved antiepileptic. Therapeutic serum concentrations are 10 to 35 mg/L and metabolism is induced by carbamazepine and phenytoin (Tables 48–2 and 48–3). In clinical trials, the most frequently reported adverse events at high doses included lethargy, aggravated seizures, vomiting, and rashes.[192] There are no data on overdose.

TIAGABINE

Tiagabine inhibits GABA reuptake and is a category C medication with limited data in human pregnancy.[14]

Pharmacokinetics and Toxicokinetics

Tiagabine is quickly absorbed and has 90% bioavailability.[146] It is predominantly (98%) metabolized in the liver, via CYP3A4.[146] The elimination half-life is 8 hours and can be shortened to 2 to 3 hours in the presence of carbamazepine, phenytoin, or phenobarbital (Tables 48–2 and 48–3).[82]

Clinical Manifestations

In a large case series, lethargy, confusion, and tachycardia were observed following acute overdose.[171] Facial myoclonus (grimacing) and seizures are also reported.[21,169,171]

Diagnostic Testing

Therapeutic tiagabine concentrations are 0.02 to 0.2 mg/L.[82] Monitoring of concentration is not routinely recommended in overdose.

Management

Supportive care should be provided. Seizures respond to administration of benzodiazepines.[55,84,89,144] Status epilepticus resistant to benzodiazepines should be treated with barbiturates or propofol. Posturing and grimacing

are treated with benzodiazepines.[21] Hemodialysis will likely not be effective because of very high protein binding.

TOPIRAMATE

Topiramate is an antiepileptic approved for mood stabilizing and migraine prophylaxis.[54] Its sulfamate moiety weakly inhibits carbonic anhydrase, specifically the II and IV isoforms, present in the kidneys and CNS.[38] Topiramate is a pregnancy category D medication because of the risk of oral clefts.[14]

Pharmacokinetics and Toxicokinetics

Topiramate is 80% bioavailable.[146] Approximately 50% is excreted unchanged by the kidneys and the rest is metabolized in the liver, using yet-to-be identified CYP enzymes.[146] Elimination half-life is 20 to 30 hours (Tables 48–2 and 48–3).[120,146]

Clinical Manifestations

Lethargy, ataxia, nystagmus, myoclonus, hallucinations, coma, seizures, and status epilepticus are all reported following topiramate overdose.[100,193] Abnormal speech patterns and disturbances in verbal fluency appear at high concentrations.[121] In some overdoses, effects last for days.[107] Hyperchloremic non–anion gap metabolic acidosis results from inhibition of renal cortical carbonic anhydrase (lowest reported bicarbonate concentration, 12 mEq/L) along with hypocitraturia and high urine pH leading to formation of calcium phosphate stones.[66,86] The hyperchloremic metabolic acidosis typically appears within hours of ingestion and can persist for days.[27,49,149,184]

Chronic topiramate therapy is associated with acute bilateral secondary acute angle-closure glaucoma, acute bilateral myopia, and other visual problems in the first 2 weeks of therapy.[53] Additionally, chronic topiramate is associated with a risk of kidney stone in up to 1.5% of patients.[86]

Diagnostic Testing

Therapeutic concentrations of topiramate are 5 to 20 mg/L. Electrolytes should be evaluated for the presence of a hyperchloremia and metabolic acidosis.[86] Monitoring of concentration is not routinely recommended in overdose.

Management

Meticulous supportive care should be provided. Severe hyperchloremic metabolic acidosis (pH <7.2) should be treated with sodium bicarbonate 1 to 2 mEq/kg bolus intravenously and an infusion. Sodium bicarbonate impairs the antiepileptic effect of topiramate.[27,49] Intermittent HD can increase topiramate clearance 12-fold.[16,120] It is reasonable to consider intermittent HD in patients with life-threatening topiramate toxicity presenting with significant neurologic impairment, intractable electrolyte abnormalities, or anuria. Calcium phosphate stones should be treated with fluids, restriction of sodium intake, and possible supplementation with potassium citrate.[86]

VALPROIC ACID

Valproic acid (di-*n*-propylacetic acid {VPA}) is a simple branched-chain carboxylic acid antiepileptic that is also approved for treatment of mania associated with bipolar disorder and in migraine prophylaxis.[54] It is a category D drug in pregnancy and is associated with neural tube and facial defects.[14]

Pharmacokinetics, Toxicokinetics, and Pathophysiology

Valproic acid is well absorbed from the GI tract with a bioavailability of 90%. Peak concentrations usually are reached in 6 hours, except for enteric-coated and extended-release preparations, where peak concentrations can be delayed up to 24 hours.[46,93] Valproic acid is 90% protein bound at therapeutic concentrations. Protein binding can decrease to 15% when VPA concentrations increase as a result of saturation of binding sites (Tables 48–2 and 48–3).[63]

Valproic acid is predominantly metabolized in the liver, with less than 3% excreted unchanged in the urine.[183] Glucuronidation (50%), β-oxidation (40%), and ω-oxidation (10%) account for most of the hepatic metabolism of VPA.[160] β-Oxidation occurs in the mitochondrial matrix and starts with passive diffusion of VPA across the mitochondrial membrane and ends with

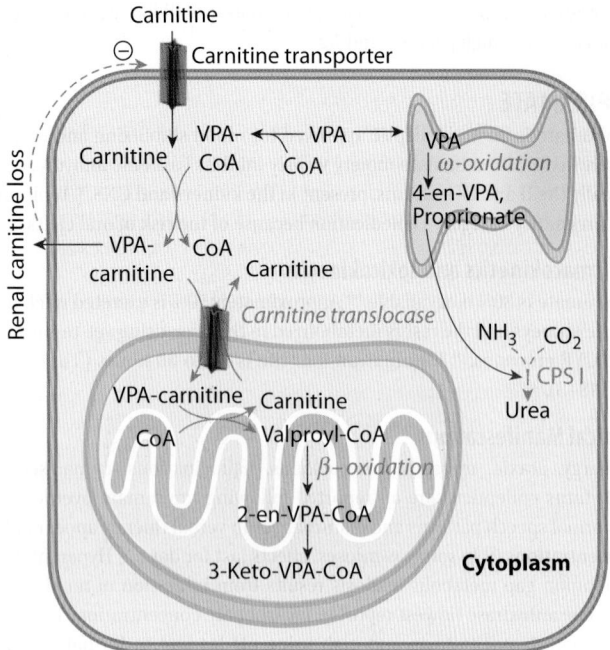

FIGURE 48–3. Valproic acid (VPA) metabolism by the hepatocyte. Valproic acid is linked to coenzyme A (CoA) by acyltransferase I and subsequently transferred to carnitine. Valproylcarnitine (VPA-carnitine) is shuttled into the mitochondrion, where, after transfer back to CoA by acyltransferase II, it undergoes β-oxidation, yielding several metabolites. These metabolites sequester CoA, preventing its use in the β-oxidation of other fatty acids. This process may lead to a Reyelike syndrome of hepatic steatosis. Alternatively, valproylcarnitine may diffuse from the cell and be renally eliminated, or it may inhibit cellular uptake of carnitine. In either case, the cellular depletion of carnitine shifts valproate metabolism toward microsomal ω-oxidation, which occurs in the endoplasmic reticulum. This pathway forms 4-en-valproate, a putative hepatotoxin. ω-Oxidation products and reduced N-acetylglutamate also interfere with carbamoylphosphate synthase I (CPS I), the initial step in the urea cycle, resulting in hyperammonemia.

the transport of metabolites in the opposite direction using acetyl-CoA and carnitine as transporters (Fig. 48–3 and Table 48–5).[106,181]

Mitochondrial β-oxidation of VPA depletes carnitine stores through various mechanisms. First, VPA increases carnitine excretion via formation of valproylcarnitine, which is renally excreted. Second, valproylcarnitine inhibits the adenosine triphosphate (ATP)–dependent carnitine transporter located on the plasma membrane. Third, VPA metabolites trap mitochondrial CoA. Mitochondrial CoA trapping decreases ATP production, which in turn negatively affects the carnitine transporter.[106,160,181] Reduced mitochondrial CoA activity decreases the formation of N-acetylglutamate, an obligatory cofactor for carbamoylphosphate synthetase I (CPSI). CPSI is the primary enzyme responsible for incorporation of ammonia into the urea cycle. The result is failure to metabolize ammonia and hyperammonemia. Hyperammonemia can injure muscle and brain tissue.[6,188]

Mitochondrial dysfunction, inhibition of β-oxidation, depletion of carnitine, depletion of acetyl-CoA, and possibly depletion of glutathione stores impair lipid metabolism and lead to fatty acid accumulation, steatosis, lysosomal leakage, formation of reactive oxygen species, and cytotoxicity histologically similar to Reye syndrome.[150,160]

Clinical Manifestations

Valproic acid toxicity is associated with neurologic symptoms and metabolic disturbances. Ataxia and lethargy are common.[63] In one large case series, patients with serum VPA concentrations greater than 850 mg/L manifested coma, respiratory depression, and hypotension.[167] Hypernatremia, hypocalcemia, and hyperammonemia are reported.[46,163,167] Anion gap metabolic acidosis is a poor prognostic sign. It results from accumulation of ketoacids, carboxylic, and propionic acid.[3,32,70] Bone marrow suppression occurs 3 to 5 days

after acute massive overdoses and is characterized by pancytopenia.[3,167] Pancreatitis, hepatotoxicity, and acute kidney injury are rare manifestations of acute toxicity.[3,32,94]

Chronic VPA therapy may lead to hepatotoxicity and microvesicular steatosis secondary to the aforementioned metabolic aberration in fatty acid metabolism.[17,40] Clinical findings vary from asymptomatic elevation of aminotransferase concentrations to fatal hepatitis.

Valproate-induced hyperammonemic encephalopathy is characterized by impaired consciousness with lethargy, focal or bilateral neurologic signs, and aggravated seizures. It is not always accompanied by elevated VPA concentrations or hepatotoxicity. The etiology is uncertain, but elevated ammonia concentrations coupled with elevated concentrations of some of the more neurotoxic VPA metabolites are likely responsible.[20,47,189]

Diagnostic Testing

Therapeutic serum concentrations of VPA are 50 to 100 mg/L.[82] Electrolytes should be monitored because of the risk of hypernatremia, hypocalcemia, elevated serum lactate, and hyperammonemia.[160]

Management

Rigorous supportive care should be provided. Activated charcoal is recommended in the initial management. Repetitive doses are reasonable in massive overdoses.

L-Carnitine is recommended to treat hyperammonemia or hepatotoxicity.[87,105,181] L-Carnitine depletion results in an accumulation of toxic metabolites and hyperammonemia. L-Carnitine loading dose is 100 mg/kg IV over 30 minutes (maximum, 6 g) followed by 15 mg/kg IV over 10 to 30 minutes every 4 hours until clinical improvement occurs. Whereas IV L-carnitine is preferred in symptomatic patients, oral carnitine is sufficient in asymptomatic patients (Antidotes in Depth: A10). Extracorporeal drug removal is recommended in cases of severe intoxication associated with VPA serum concentrations greater than 900 mg/L, coma, respiratory depression requiring intubation, or pH <7.1.[63] Intermittent HD is preferred.[63,163]

VIGABATRIN

Vigabatrin, or vinyl GABA, is a stereospecific irreversible inhibitor of GABA-transaminase.[54] It is a category C medication in pregnancy.[14]

Pharmacokinetics, Toxicokinetics

Vigabatrin is rapidly absorbed and has a 60% to 80% bioavailability.[14] Duration of action is 24 hours.[146] It is completely excreted unchanged in the urine.[146] Dosage adjustments are necessary in patients with creatinine clearance or eGFR less than 80 mL/min.[156] Drug interactions are not common (Tables 48–2 and 48–3).[146]

Clinical Manifestations

Agitation, coma, and psychosis are reported following acute ingestion.[33,103] Chronic toxicity may result in dizziness, tremor, depression, and psychosis.[103] The use of vigabatrin is associated with a risk of retinopathy and irreversible peripheral field defects, and permanent visual loss in up to 44% of patients.[82,158]

Diagnostic Testing

Therapeutic serum concentrations of vigabatrin are 0.8 to 36 mg/L.[82] Monitoring of concentration is not routinely recommended in overdose.

Management

Supportive care should be provided. Benzodiazepines are recommended for severe agitation. Visual defects may be irreversible.[82] Cases of mild vigabatrin-induced psychosis resolve on withdrawal of the medication.[103]

ZONISAMIDE

Zonisamide is a sulfonamide derivative. Similarly to topiramate, zonisamide inhibits carbonic anhydrase enzymes.[82] It is a category C medication in pregnancy.[14]

TABLE 48-5	Adverse Events Associated With Therapy		
	Common	*Serious*	*DRESS Syndrome*
Carbamazepine	Dizziness, sedation, blurred vision, ataxia, weight gain, nausea, leukopenia	Agranulocytosis (1/200,000), aplastic anemia (1/500,000), rash (10%), SJS (rare), hyponatremia (1.8%–40%)	Yes
Eslicarbazepine	Dizziness, sedation, nausea, ataxia, diplopia	Rash	Yes
Ezogabine	Skin and nail discoloration, dizziness, sedation, ataxia	Maculopathy, urinary disorders, QT interval prolongation	No
Gabapentin	Sedation, dizziness, mild weight gain, ataxia, behavioral effect (children)	None	No
Lamotrigine	Dizziness, blurred vision, insomnia, headache	Rash, SJS (1–3/1,000), hypersensitivity (rare), hepatotoxicity (rare)	Yes
Lacosamide	Dizziness, sedation, ataxia, nausea	Rash	No
Levetiracetam	Fatigue, irritability, anxiety, asthenia	Psychosis (rare)	Yes
Oxcarbazepine	Fatigue, dizziness, ataxia, diplopia, nausea, headache	Rash, SJS or TEN (0.5–6/million), hyponatremia (2.5%), anaphylaxis (rare)	Yes
Perampanel	Dizziness, sedation, ataxia	Psychiatric and behavioral problems	No
Phenytoin	Fatigue, dizziness, ataxia, nausea, headache, gingival hypertrophy, hirsutism, osteopenia	Rash, SJS or TEN (2–4/10,000), megaloblastic anemia (rare), hepatotoxicity (rare), lupuslike syndrome	Yes
Pregabalin	Sedation, weight gain, peripheral edema	Peripheral edema	No
Rufinamide	Sedation, dizziness, nausea, headache, diplopia	Rash	Possible
Tiagabine	Fatigue, dizziness, ataxia, somnolence, anxiety	Seizures	No
Topiramate	Sedation, ataxia, word-finding difficulty, slowed speech, difficulty concentrating, anorexia, weight loss, paresthesias, oligohidrosis (children)	Metabolic acidosis (3%), nephrolithiasis (1.5%), acute glaucoma (rare), heat stroke	No
Valproic acid	Sedation, ataxia, weight gain, nausea, tremor, hair loss	Hepatotoxicity (1/20,000), pancreatitis (1/3,000), thrombocytopenia, hyperammonemia, aplastic anemia (rare)	No
Vigabatrin	Fatigue, headache, dizziness, weight gain	Peripheral vision loss, psychosis	No
Zonisamide	Sedation, ataxia, difficulty concentrating, irritability, nausea, headache	Aplastic anemia, nephrolithiasis (0.2%–4%), rash (1%–2%), SJS or TEN (rare), heat stroke (rare)	No

DRESS = Drug Reaction with Eosinophilia and Systemic Symptoms; SJS = Stevens–Johnson syndrome; TEN = toxic epidermal necrolysis.

Pharmacokinetics, Toxicokinetics

Zonisamide is 65% bioavailable.[82] It is primarily metabolized by the liver via CYP3A4.[82] The elimination half-life is 60 hours.[82] Metabolism is increased by enzyme inducers such as carbamazepine and phenytoin (Tables 48-2 and 48-3).[200]

Clinical Manifestations

Symptoms include lethargy, coma, seizures, and hyperchloremic metabolic acidosis.[126] QT prolongation, hypotension, and cardiac arrest are reported.[74,126,182]

Diagnostic Testing

Therapeutic serum concentrations of zonisamide are 10 to 40 mg/L.[82] Low serum bicarbonate is occasionally present.[30,126] Monitoring of concentration is not routinely recommended in overdose.

Management

Supportive care is the mainstay of management.[126] Zonisamide is cleared via HD in chronically hemodialyzed patients.[81] There are no data in overdose and HD is not recommended.

DRUG-INDUCED HYPERSENSITIVITY SYNDROME (DIHS)

Drug-induced hypersensitivity syndrome (DIHS) is a severe adverse drug event first described in 1950.[79] Previously known as the anticonvulsant hypersensitivity syndrome or Drug Reaction with Eosinophilia and Systemic Symptoms (DRESS), there exists no current consensus on nomenclature. Drug-induced hypersensitivity syndrome is characterized by fever, morbilliform cutaneous eruption, and multiorgan manifestations.[79] The syndrome occurs in approximately one of every 1,000 to 10,000 uses of antiepileptics. The most commonly implicated antiepileptics are carbamazepine, phenytoin, phenobarbital, and lamotrigine but oxcarbazepine, levetiracetam, and rufinamide are also involved (Fig. 17-9).[68,136,153] The etiology of DIHS remains unknown but data suggest a genetic defect in drug metabolism (*HLA-A*3101* in Northern Europeans and Japanese individuals) or epigenetic disruption leading to reactivation of T cells that harbor latent herpesviruses (particularly HHV-6).[35,147]

Drug-induced hypersensitivity syndrome occurs most frequently within the first 2 months of therapy and is not related to dose or serum concentration. The pathophysiology is related to the accumulation of reactive arene oxide metabolites resulting from decreased epoxide hydrolase enzyme activity. These metabolites bind to macromolecules and cause cellular apoptosis and necrosis. They also form neoantigens that trigger T cell–mediated delayed (type IV) hypersensitivity reactions. Interestingly, the same metabolite is believed to cause other serious dermatologic reactions, such as Stevens–Johnson syndrome and toxic epidermal necrolysis (Chap. 17 and Fig. 17-6).[172]

Initial symptoms include fever (38°C–40°C) for 1 to 2 weeks followed by a diffuse, pruritic macular exanthem that spreads from face to trunk to extremities. Facial edema is common.[1] Mucositis is present in 30%, and tender lymphadenopathy in 75% of cases.[4,80] Multiorgan involvement usually occurs 1 to 2 weeks into the syndrome. The liver is the most frequently affected organ (>80% of cases), although involvement of the CNS (encephalitis), heart (myocarditis), lungs (pneumonitis), kidney (nephritis), and thyroid are possible. Liver disturbances range from mildly elevated aminotransferase concentrations to fulminant hepatic failure.[80] Eosinophilia (>2.0×10^9 eosinophils per L) and mononucleosis-type atypical lymphocytosis are common.[79,147] This syndrome is commonly mistaken for sepsis.[79] Fatality rates are reportedly as high as 5% to 10%.[80,136]

Skin biopsies reveal dense perivascular lymphocytic infiltration, with extravasated erythrocytes, eosinophils, and dermal edema.[79] Lymph node histology reveals benign hyperplasia or pseudolymphoma.[79] Other laboratory abnormalities include positive rheumatoid factor, antinuclear antibodies, anti–double-stranded DNA smooth muscle antibodies, cold agglutinins, and hypo- or hypergammaglobulinemia.[80] There is no reliable standard for the diagnosis of this syndrome, and separate diagnostic criteria have been developed by the European Registry for Severe Cutaneous Adverse Reaction and the Japanese Research Committee on Severe Cutaneous Adverse Reaction.[79] Prompt discontinuation of the offending antiepileptic is essential and benzodiazepines should be used temporarily to control seizures. Patients should be admitted to the intensive care or burn unit for fluid replacement, correction of electrolytes, warming environment, high caloric intake diet, prevention of bacterial or viral suprainfection, and appropriate skin care. Topical steroids should be applied for symptomatic relief.[137] Methylprednisolone 30 mg/kg is recommended. Intravenous immunoglobulin 2 g/kg over 5 days is recommended if patient fails to respond quickly to methylprednisolone.[80,122] Corticosteroids should be gradually tapered over 3 to 6 months.[35] Extracorporeal membrane oxygenation (ECMO), intraaortic balloon pump, and left ventricular–assist devices can be used to treat myocarditis, and organ transplantation is recommended in cases of intractable liver or heart failure.[35,108] The major cause of death is hepatic necrosis.[80]

In one case series, 90% of patients with this syndrome showed in vitro cross-reactivity to other aromatic antiepileptics.[96] Based on this evidence, avoidance of phenytoin, carbamazepine, phenobarbital, primidone, lamotrigine, levetiracetam, oxcarbazepine, and rufinamide is recommended; benzodiazepines, VPA, gabapentin, topiramate, and tiagabine are safe alternatives. Clinicians should report all cases of DIHS to the US Food and Drug Administration Adverse Event Reporting System (FAERS) (http://www.fda.gov/Drugs/GuidanceComplianceRegulatoryInformation/Surveillance/AdverseDrugEffects/ucm115894.htm).

SUMMARY

- All antiepileptics produce CNS symptoms in overdose; therefore, differentiation based on clinical findings is difficult. Lethargy, sedation, ataxia, and nystagmus occur after overdoses of almost all the antiepileptics.

- Coma occurs after substantial overdose of all antiepileptics with perhaps the exception of gabapentin. Seizures are possible following carbamazepine, lamotrigine, pregabalin, and zonisamide overdoses.

- Hemodynamic instability and abnormal ECGs are rare findings. Carbamazepine, lamotrigine, and possibly topiramate can cause QRS complex prolongation.

- Except for VPA overdoses, there are no specific antidotes or overdoses of antiepileptics. Supportive care alone usually yields beneficial outcomes.

- Patients with severe VPA overdoses or VPA-induced hyperammonemia should be treated with L-carnitine. Extracorporeal drug removal is rarely necessary.

REFERENCES

1. Aday AW, et al. Prevention as precipitant. *N Engl J Med.* 2016;375:471-475.
2. Aksakal E, et al. Complete atrioventricular block due to overdose of pregabalin. *Am J Emerg Med.* 2012;30:2101.e1-2101.e4.
3. Andersen GO, Ritland S. Life-threatening intoxication with sodium valproate. *J Toxicol Clin Toxicol.* 1995;33:279-284.
4. Ang CC, et al. Retrospective analysis of drug-induced hypersensitivity syndrome: a study of 27 patients. *J Am Acad Dermatol.* 2010;63:219-227.
5. Anseeuw K, et al., on behalf of the EXTRIP workgroup. Extracorporeal treatment in phenytoin poisoning; systematic review and recommendations from the EXTRIP (Extracorporeal Treatments in Poisoning) workgroup. *Am J Kidney Dis.* 2016;67:187-197.
6. Bachman C, et al. Ammonia toxicity to the brain and creatinine. *Mol Genet Metab.* 2004;81(suppl 1):S52-S57.
7. Barrueto F, et al. A case of levetiracetam (Keppra) poisoning with clinical and toxicokinetic data. *J Toxicol Clin Toxicol.* 2002;40:881-884.
8. Bech BH, et al. Use of antiepileptic drugs during pregnancy and risk of spontaneous abortion and stillbirths: population-based cohort study. *BMJ.* 2014;349:1-11.
9. Benarroch EE. Neuronal voltage-gated calcium channels: Brief overview of their function and clinical implications in neurology. *Neurology.* 2010;74:1310-1315.
10. Bialer M, White HS. Key factors in the discovery and development of new antiepileptic drugs. *Nat Rev.* 2010;9:68-82.
11. Borden LA, et al. Tiagabine, SK & F 89976-A, CI-966, and NNC-711 are selective for the cloned GABA transporter GAT-1. *European J Pharmacol.* 1994;269:219-224.
12. Borthen I, et al. Complications during pregnancy in women with epilepsy: population-based cohort study. *BJOG.* 2009;116:1736-1742.
13. Brahmi K, et al. Influence of activated charcoal on pharmacokinetics and clinical features of carbamazepine poisoning. *Am J Emerg Med.* 2006;24:440-443.
14. Briggs GG, et al., eds. *Drugs in Pregnancy and Lactation.* 7th ed. Philadelphia, PA: Lippincott, Williams & Wilkins; 2005.
15. Brockbrader HN, et al. A comparison of the pharmacokinetics and pharmacodynamics of pregabalin and gabapentin. *Clin Pharmacokinet.* 2010;49:661-669.
16. Browning L, et al. Possible removal of topiramate by continuous renal replacement therapy. *J Neurol Sci.* 2010;288:186-189.
17. Bryant AE, Dreifuss FE. Valproic acid hepatic fatalities: US experience since 1986. *Neurology.* 1996;46:465-469.
18. Burneo JG, et al. A prospective study of the incidence of the purple glove syndrome. *Epilepsia.* 2001;42:1156-1159.
19. Cameron RJ, et al. Efficacy of charcoal hemoperfusion in massive carbamazepine poisoning. *J Toxicol Clin Toxicol.* 2002;40:507-512.
20. Camilleri C, et al. Fatal cerebral edema after moderate valproic acid overdose. *Ann Emerg Med.* 2005;45:337-338.
21. Cantrell FL, et al. Intentional overdose with tiagabine: an unusual clinical presentation. *J Emerg Med.* 2004;27:271-272.
22. Castanares-Zapatero D, et al. Lipid emulsion as rescue therapy in lamotrigine overdose. *J Emerg Med.* 2012;42:48-51.
23. Ceolin L, et al. A novel anti-epileptic agent, perampanel, selectively inhibits AMPA receptor-mediated synaptic transmission in the hippocampus. *Neurochem Int.* 2012; 61:517-522.
24. Chaikin P, Adir J. Unusual absorption profile of phenytoin in a massive overdose case. *J Clin Pharmacol.* 1987;27:70-73.
25. Christensen J, et al. Epilepsy and risk of suicide: a population-based case-control study. *Lancet Neurol.* 2007;6:693-698.
26. Chu-Tan JL, et al. Cardiac sodium channel blockade after an intentional ingestion of lacosamide, cyclobenzaprine, and levetiracetam: case report. *Clin Toxicol.* 2015;53: 565-568.
27. Chung AM, Reed MD. Intentional topiramate ingestion in an adolescent female. *Ann Pharmacother.* 2004;38:1439-1442.
28. Ciszowski K, et al. The influence of carbamazepine plasma levels on blood pressure and some ECG parameters in patients with acute intoxication. *Przegl Lek.* 2007; 64:248-251.
29. Craig S. Phenytoin poisoning. *Neurocrit Care.* 2005;3:161-170.
30. Cross JH, et al. Safety and tolerability of zonisamide in paediatric patients with epilepsy. *Eur J Pediatr Neurol.* 2014;18:747-758.
31. Proposal for revised classification of epilepsies and epileptic syndromes. Commission on classification and terminology of the international league against epilepsy. *Epilepsia.* 1989;30:389-399.
32. Connacher AA, et al. Fatality due to massive overdose of sodium valproate. *Scott Med J.* 1987;32:85-86.
33. Davie MB, et al. Vigabatrin overdose. *Med J Aust.* 1996;165:403.
34. Davies JA. Mechanism of action of antiepileptic drugs. *Seizures.* 1995;4:267-271.
35. Descamps V, Ranger-Rogez S. DRESS syndrome. *Joint Bone Spine.* 2014;81:15-21.
36. DeSchoenmakere G, et al. Phenytoin intoxication in critically ill patients. *Am J Kidney Dis.* 2005;45:189-192.
37. DiGiorgio AC, et al. Ventricular tachycardia associated with lacosamide co-medication in drug-resistant epilepsy. *Epilepsy Behav Case Rep.* 2013;1:26-28
38. Dodgson SJ, et al. Topiramate as an inhibitor of carbonic anhydrase isoenzymes. *Epilepsia.* 2000;41(suppl):S35-S39.
39. Dogukan A, et al. Gabapentin-induced coma in a patient with renal failure. *Hemodial Int.* 2006;10:168-169.
40. Dreifuss FE, et al. Valproic acid hepatic fatalities. *Neurology.* 1989;39:201-207.
41. Earnest MP, et al. Complications of intravenous phenytoin for acute treatment of seizures. *JAMA.* 1983;249:762-765.
42. Eichelbaum M, et al. Plasma kinetics of carbamazepine and its epoxide metabolite in man after single and multiple doses. *Euro J Clin Pharmacol.* 1975;8:337-341.
43. Errington A, et al. The investigational anticonvulsant lacosamide selectively enhances slow inactivation of voltage-gated sodium channels. *Mol Pharmacol.* 2008;73:157-169.
44. Evers ML, et al. Cardiac monitoring after phenytoin overdose. *Heart Lung.* 1997; 26:325-328.
45. Evoy KE, et al. Abuse and misuse of pregabalin and gabapentin. *Drugs.* 2017;77:403-426.

46. Eyer F, et al. Acute valproate poisoning: pharmacokinetics, alterations of fatty acid metabolism and changes during therapy. *J Clin Psychopharmacol.* 2005;25:376-380.

47. Eyer F, et al. Treatment of severe intravenous phenytoin overdose with hemodialysis and hemoperfusion. *Med Sci Monit.* 2008;14:145-148.

48. Faisy C, et al. Carabamazepine-associated left ventricular dysfunction. *J Toxicol Clin Toxicol.* 2000;38:339-342.

49. Fakhoury T, et al. Topiramate overdose: clinical and laboratory features. *Epilepsy Behav.* 2002;3:185-189.

50. Food and Drug Administration. Suicidal behavior and ideation and antiepileptic drugs. https://www.fda.gov/drugs/drugsafety/postmarketdrugsafetyinformationfor patientsandproviders/ucm100190. Accessed September 28, 2017.

51. Fischer JH, et al. Fosphenytoin clinical pharmacokinetics and comparative advantages in acute treatment of seizures. *Clin Pharmacol.* 2003;42:33-58.

52. Fleishman A, Chiang VW. Carbamazepine overdose recognized by a tricyclic antidepressant assay. *Pediatrics.* 2001;107:176-177.

53. Fraunfelder FW, et al. Topiramate-associated acute bilateral secondary angle-closure glaucoma. *Ophthalmology.* 2004;111:109-111.

54. French JA, Pedley TA. Initial management of epilepsy. *N Engl J Med.* 2008;359:166-176.

55. Fulton JA, et al. Tiagabine overdose: a case of status epilepticus in a non-epileptic individual. *Clin Toxicol.* 2005;43:869-871.

56. Furlanat M, et al. Acute oxcarbazepine, benazepril and hydrochlorothiazide overdose with alcohol. *Ther Drug Monit.* 2006;28:267-268.

57. Garbovski LA, et al. Purple glove syndrome after phenytoin or fosphenytoin administration: review of reported cases and recommendations for prevention. *J Med Toxicol.* 2015;11:445-459.

58. Garnett WR. Clinical pharmacology of topiramate: a review. *Epilepsia.* 2000;41:61-65.

59. Gean PW, et al. Valproic acid suppresses the synaptic response mediated by the NMDA receptors in rat amygdala slices. *Brain Res Bull.* 1994;33:333-336.

60. Gee NS, et al. The novel anticonvulsant drug, gabapentin (Neurontin) binds to the 2 subunits of a calcium channel. *J Biol Chem.* 1996;271:5768-5776.

61. Ghannoum M, et al. Successful hemodialysis in a phenytoin overdose: case report and review of the literature. *Clin Nephrol.* 2010;74:59-64.

62. Ghannoum M, et al., on behalf of EXTRIP workgroup. Extracorporeal treatment for carbamazepine poisoning: systematic review and recommendations from the EXTRIP workgroup. *Clin Toxicol.* 2014;52:993-1004.

63. Ghannoum M, et al., on behalf of the EXTRIP workgroup. The extracorporeal treatment of valproic acid poisoning: systematic review and recommendations from the EXTRIP workgroup. *Clin Toxicol.* 2015;53:454-465.

64. Gheshlaghi F, et al. Relationship of cardiovascular complications with level of consciousness in patients with acute carbamazepine intoxication. *Med Arh.* 2012;66:9-11.

65. Gibbs JW, et al. Cellular actions of topiramate: blockade of kainate-evoked inward currents in cultured hippocampal neurons. *Epilepsia.* 2000;41(suppl 1):S10-S16.

66. Goldfarb DS. A woman with recurrent calcium phosphate kidney stones. *Clin J Am Nephrol.* 2012;7:1172-1178.

67. Goldschlager AW, Karliner JS. Ventricular standstill after intravenous diphenylhydantoin. *Am Heart J.* 1967;74:410-412.

68. Gomez-Zorilla S, et al. Levetiracetam-induced drug reaction with eosinophilia and systemic symptoms syndrome. *Ann Pharmacother.* 2012;46:e20.

69. Gordon MF, Gerstenblitt D. The use of free phenytoin levels in averting phenytoin toxicity. *N Y State J Med.* 1990;90:469-470.

70. Graudins A, et al. Massive overdose with controlled-release carbamazepine resulting in delayed peak serum concentrations and life-threatening toxicity. *Emerg Med.* 2002;14:89-94.

71. Grunewald R. Levetiracetam in treatment of idiopathic epilepsies. *Epilepsia.* 2005;46(suppl 9):154-160.

72. Guerrieri D, et al. Postmortem and toxicological findings in a series of furanylfentanyl-related deaths. *J Anal Toxicol.* 2016;41:242-249.

73. Halma E, et al. Behavioral side-effects of levetiracetam in children with epilepsy: a systematic review. *Seizure.* 2014;23:685-691.

74. Hofer KA, et al. Moderate toxic effects following acute zonisamide overdose. *Epilepsy Behav.* 2011;21:91-93.

75. Hojer J, et al. Clinical features in 28 consecutive cases of laboratory confirmed massive poisoning with carbamazepine alone. *J Toxicol Clin Toxicol.* 1993;31:449-458.

76. Hoppner A, et al. Clinical course of intoxication with new anticonvulsant drug perampanel. *Epileptic Disord.* 2013;15:362-362.

77. Hsu HF, Huang SY. Severe hepatitis associated with administration of oxcarbazepine. *Pediatr Int.* 2010;52:677-678.

78. Hung TY, et al. Gabapentin toxicity: an important cause of altered consciousness in patients with uraemia. *Emerg Med J.* 2008;25:178-179.

79. Husain Z, et al. DRESS syndrome Part I. Clinical perspectives. *J Am Acad Dermatol.* 2013;68:693.e1-693.e14.

80. Husain Z, et al. DRESS syndrome Part II. Management and therapeutics. *J Am Acad Dermatol.* 2013;68:709.

81. Ijiri Y, et al. Dialyzability of antiepileptic drug zonisamide in patients undergoing hemodialysis. *Epilepsia.* 2004;45:924-927.

82. Jacob S, Nair AB. An updated overview on therapeutic drug monitoring of recent antiepileptic drugs. *Drugs Res Dev.* 2016;16:303-316.

83. Jeong SH, et al. Transient positive horizontal head impulse test in pregabalin intoxication. *J Epilepsy Res.* 2015;5:101-103.

84. Jette N, et al. Tiagabine-induced nonconvulsive status epilepticus in an adolescent without epilepsy. *Neurology.* 2006;67:1514-1515.

85. Kaminski RM, et al. SV2A protein is a broad-spectrum anticonvulsant target: functional correlation between protein binding and seizure protection in models of both partial and generalized epilepsy. *Neuropharmacology.* 2008;54:715-720.

86. Kaplon DM, et al. Patients with and without prior urolithiasis have hypocitraturia and incident kidney stones while on topiramate. *Urology.* 2011;77:295-298.

87. Katiyar A, Aaron C. Case files of the Children's Hospital of Michigan regional poison control center: the use of carnitine for the management of acute valproic acid toxicity. *J Med Toxicol.* 2007;3:129-138.

88. Katz R. Briefing document of the July 10, 2008, advisory committee meeting to discuss antiepileptic drugs (AEDs) and suicidality. Memorandum. https://www.fda.gov/ohrms/dockets/ac/08/briefing/2008-4372b1-01-FDA-Katz.pdf. Accessed September 28, 2017.

89. Kazzi Z, et al. Seizures in a pediatric patient with tiagabine overdose. *J Med Toxicol.* 2006;2:160-162.

90. Keegan MT, et al. Hypocalcemia-like changes after administration of intravenous fosphenytoin. *Mayo Clinic Proc.* 2002;77:584-586.

91. Keppra [package insert]. Smyrna, GA: UCB Inc; 2009.

92. Kerr BM, et al. Human liver carbamazepine metabolism. Role of CYP3A4 and CYP2C8 in 10,11 epoxide formation. *Biochem Pharmacol.* 1994;47:1969-1979.

93. Khan E, et al. Sustained low-efficiency dialysis with filtration (SLEDD-f) in the management of acute sodium valproate intoxication. *Hemodial Int.* 2008;12:211-214.

94. Khoo SH, Layland MJ. Cerebral edema following acute sodium valproate overdose. *J Toxicol Clin Toxicol.* 1992;30:209-214.

95. Klein-Schwartz W, et al. Characterization of gabapentin overdose using a poison center case series. *J Toxicol Clin Toxicol.* 2003;41:11-15.

96. Knowles S, et al. Anticonvulsant hypersensitivity syndrome: an update. *Expert Opin Drug Saf.* 2012;11:767-778.

97. Krasowski MD. Therapeutic drug monitoring of the newer anti-epilepsy medications. *Pharmaceuticals.* 2010;3:1909-1935.

98. Krause LU, et al. Atrioventricular block following lacosamide intoxication. *Epilepsy.* 2011;20:725-727.

99. Kuz GM, Manssourian A. Carbamazepine-induced hyponatremia: assessment of risk factors. *Ann Pharmacother.* 2005;39:1943-1945.

100. Langman LJ, et al. Fatal acute topiramate toxicity. *J Anal Toxicol.* 2003;27:323-324.

101. Lee S. Pregabalin intoxication-induced encephalopathy with triphasic waves. *Epilepsy Behav.* 2012;25:170-173.

102. Leiber BL, Snodgrass WR. Cardiac arrest following large intravenous fosphenytoin overdose in an infant [abstract]. *J Toxicol Clin Toxicol.* 1998;36:473.

103. Levinson DF, Devinsky O. Psychiatric adverse events during vigabatrin therapy. *Neurology.* 1999;53:1503-1511.

104. Lewis JC, et al. An 11-year review of levetiracetam ingestions in children less than 6 years of age. *Clin Toxicol.* 2014;52:964-968.

105. L'Heureux PE, Hantson P. Carnitine in the treatment of valproic acid-induced toxicity. *J Pediatr.* 2011;158:802-807.

106. Li J, et al. Mitochondrial metabolism of valproic acid. *Biochemistry.* 1991;30:388-394.

107. Lin G, Lawrence R. Pediatric case report of topiramate toxicity. *Clin Toxicol.* 2006;44:67-69.

108. Lo MH, et al. Drug reaction with eosinophilia and systemic symptoms syndrome associated myocarditis: a survival experience after extracorporeal membrane oxygenation support. *J Clin Pharm Ther.* 2013;38:172-174.

109. Lofton AL, Klein-Schwartz W. Evaluation of lamotrigine toxicity reported to poison centers. *Ann Pharmacother.* 2004;38:1-5.

110. Loscher W, et al. Synaptic vesical glycoprotein 2A ligands in the treatment of epilepsy and beyond. *CNS Drugs.* 2016;30:1055-1077.

111. Lowry JA, et al. Unusual presentation of iatrogenic phenytoin toxicity in a newborn. *J Med Toxicol.* 2005;1:26-29.

112. Lu X, Wang X. Hyponatremia induced by antiepileptic drug in patients with epilepsy. *Expert Opinion Drug Safety.* 2017;16:77-87.

113. Luer M. Fosphenytoin. *Neurol Res.* 1998;20:178-182.

114. Lukyanetz EA, et al. Selective blockade of N type calcium channels by levetiracetam. *Epilepsia.* 2002;43:9-18.

115. Lurie Y, et al. Limited efficacy of gastrointestinal decontamination in severe slow-release carbamazepine overdose. *Ann Pharmacother.* 2007;41:1539-1543.

116. Lyseng-Williamson KA. Spotlight on levetiracetam in epilepsy. *CNS Drugs.* 2011;25:901-905.

117. Main MJ, et al. Modulation of KCNQ2/3 potassium channel by the novel anticonvulsant retigabine. *Mol Pharmacol.* 2000;58:253-262.

118. Magiorkinis E, et al. Highlights of the history of epilepsy: the last 200 years. *Epilepsy Res Treat.* 2014;2014:1-13.

119. Malissin I, et al. Fatal lacosamide poisoning in relation to cardiac conduction impairment and cardiovascular failure. *Clin Toxicol.* 2013;51:381-382.

120. Manitpisitkul P, et al. Pharmacokinetics of topiramate in patients with renal impairment, end-stage renal disease undergoing hemodialysis, or hepatic impairment. *Epilepsy Res.* 2014;108:891-901.

121. Marino SE, et al. The effect of topiramate plasma concentration on linguistic behavior, verbal recall and working memory. *Epilepsy Behav.* 2012;24:1-19.

122. Mayorga C, et al. Improvement of toxic epidermal necrolysis after the early administration of a single high dose of intravenous immunoglobulin. *Ann Allergy Asthma Immunol.* 2003;91:86-91.

123. Mbizvo JK, et al. Levetiracetam add-on for drug-resistant focal epilepsy: an updated Cochrane review (review). *Cochrane Database Syst Rev.* 2012;9:1-53.

124. McBride KD, et al. Hyperphosphatemia due to fosphenytoin in a pediatric ESRD patient. *Pediatr Nephrol.* 2005;20:1182-1185.

125. McLean MJ, Macdonald RL. Carbamazepine and 10,11-epoxycarbamazepine produce use- and voltage-dependent limitation of rapidly firing action potentials of mouse central neurons in cell culture. *J Pharmacol Exp Ther.* 1986;238:727-738.

126. McStay C, et al. Complete recovery after acute zonisamide overdose in adolescent female. *Pediatr Emerg Care.* 2018;34:e30-e31.

127. Medical Letter™. Ezogabine (Potiga) toxicity. *Med Lett Drugs Ther.* 2013;1430:1-2.

128. Mersfelder TL, Nichols WH. Gabapentin: abuse, dependence, and withdrawal. *Ann Pharmacother.* 2016;50:229-233.

129. Mico JA, Prieto R. Elucidating the mechanism of action of pregabalin: alpha(2) delta as a therapeutic target in anxiety. *CNS Drugs.* 2012;26:637-648.

130. Miljevic C, et al. A case of pregabalin intoxication. *Psychiatriki.* 2012;2392:162-165.

131. Miller MA, et al. Hemodialysis and hemoperfusion in a patient with an isolated phenytoin overdose. *Am J Emerg Med.* 2006;24:748-749.

132. Mixter CG, et al. Cardiac and peripheral vascular effects of diphenylhydantoin sodium. *Am J Cardiol.* 1966;17:332-338.

133. Mohan RPS, et al. Phenytoin-induced gingival enlargement: a dental awakening for patients with epilepsy. *BMJ Case Rep.* 2013;20131-2.

134. Moore PW, et al. A case series of patients with lamotrigine toxicity at one center from 2003 to 2012. *Clin Toxicol.* 2013;51:545-549.

135. Murphy N, et al. Decompensation of chronic congestive heart failure associated with pregabalin in patients with neuropathic pain. *J Card Fail.* 2007;13:227-229.

136. Nam YH, et al. Drug reaction with eosinophilia and systemic syndrome is not uncommon and show better clinical outcomes than generally recognised. *Allergol Immunopathol (Madr).* 2015;43:19-24.

137. Natkunaajah J, et al. Ten cases of drug reaction with eosinophilia and systemic symptoms (DRESS) treated with pulsed intravenous methylprednisolone. *Eur J Dermatol.* 2011;21:385-391.

138. National Kidney Disease Education program. Chronic kidney disease and drug dosing: information for providers. http://www.nkdep.nih.gov/professionals/drug-dosing-information.htm. Posted September 2009. Revised January 2010. Accessed March 2017.

139. Nau H, Loscher W. Valproic acid: brain and plasma levels of the drug and its metabolites, anticonvulsant effects, and GABA metabolism in mouse. *J Pharmacol Exp Ther.* 1982;220:654-659.

140. Neurontin [package insert]. New York, NY: Pfizer Inc; 2009.

141. Nogar JN, et al. Severe sodium channel blockade and cardiovascular collapse due to massive lamotrigine overdose. *J Toxicol Clin Toxicol.* 2011;49:854-857.

142. Novy J, et al. Lacosamide neurotoxicity associated with concomitant use of sodium channel-blocking antiepileptic drugs: a pharmacodynamic interaction? *Epilepsy.* 2011;20:20-23.

143. Olaizola I, et al. Pregabalin-associated acute psychosis and epileptiform EEG-changes. *Seizure.* 2006;15:208-210.

144. Ostovskiy D, et al. Tiagabine overdose can induce convulsive status epilepticus. *Epilepsia.* 2002;43:773-774.

145. Patel VH, et al. Delayed elevation in carbamazepine concentrations after overdose: a retrospective poison center study. *Am J Ther.* 2013;20:602-606.

146. Patsalos PN. Drug interactions with the newer antiepileptic drugs (AEDs)-part 1: pharmacokinetic and pharmacodynamic interactions between AEDs. *Clin Pharmacokinet.* 2013;52:927-966.

147. Pavlos R, et al. HLA and pharmacogenetics of drug sensitivity. *Pharmacogenomics.* 2012;13:1285-1306.

148. Pedrini M, et al. Acute oxcarbazepine overdose in an autistic boy. *Br Jour Clin Pharmacol.* 2009;67:579-581.

149. Philippi H, et al. Topiramate and metabolic acidosis in infants and toddlers. *Epilepsia.* 2002;43:744-747.

150. Pourahmad J, et al. A new approach on valproic acid induced hepatotoxicity: involvement of lysosomal membrane leakiness and cellular proteolysis. *Toxicol in Vitro.* 2012;26:545-551.

151. Randinitis EJ, et al. Pharmacokinetics of pregabalin in subjects with various degrees of renal function. *J Clin Pharmacol.* 2003;43:277-283.

152. Richens A, Dunlop A. Serum phenytoin levels in management of epilepsy. *Lancet.* 1975;2:247-248.

153. Roquin G, et al. First report of lamotrigine-induced drug rash with eosinophilia and systemic symptoms syndrome with pancreatitis. *Ann Pharmacother.* 2010;44: 1998-2000.

154. Rose R, et al. Fosphenytoin-induced bradyasystole arrest in an infant treated with charcoal hemofiltration [abstract]. *J Toxicol Clin Toxicol.* 1998;36:473.

155. Rush JA, Beran RG. Leucopenia as an adverse reaction to carbamazepine therapy. *Med J Aust.* 1984;140:426-428.

156. Sabril [package insert]. Cincinnati, OH: Lundbeck; 2016.

157. Schulze-Bonhage A. Pharmacokinetic and pharmacodynamic profile of pregabalin and its role in the treatment of epilepsy. *Expert Opinion Drug Metab Toxicol.* 2013;9:105-115.

158. Segott RC. Recommendations for visual evaluations of patients treated with vigabatrin. *Clin Opin Ophthalmol.* 2010;21:442-446.

159. Sikma MA, et al. Increased unbound drug fraction in acute carbamazepine intoxication: suitability and effectiveness of high-flux haemodialysis. *Intensive Care Med.* 2012;38:916-917.

160. Silva MFB, et al. Valproic acid metabolism and its effects on mitochondrial fatty acid oxidation: a review. *J Inherit Metab Dis.* 2008;31:205-216.

161. Singh CW, et al. Incidence and risk estimate of drug-induced agranulocytosis in Hong Kong Chinese. A population-based case-control study. *Pharmacoepidemiol Drug Saf.* 2017;26:248-255.

162. Singh RP, Asconape JJ. A review of eslicarbazepine acetate for the adjunctive treatment of partial-onset epilepsy. *J Central Nervous System Dis.* 2011;3:179-187.

163. Singh SM, et al. Extracorporeal management of valproic acid overdose: a large regional experience. *J Nephrol.* 2004;17:43-49.

164. Sjoberg G, Feychting K. Pregabalin overdose in adults and adolescents-experience in Sweden. *J Toxicol Clin Toxicol.* 2010;48:282.

165. Skinner CG, et al. Randomized controlled study on the use of multiple-dose activated charcoal in patients with supratherapeutic phenytoin levels. *J Toxicol Clin Toxicol.* 2012;50:764-769.

166. Soman P, et al. Dystonia—a rare manifestation of carbamazepine toxicity. *Postgrad Med J.* 1994;70:54-56.

167. Spiller HA, et al. Multicenter case series of valproic acid ingestion: serum concentrations and toxicity. *J Toxicol Clin Toxicol.* 2000;38:755-760.

168. Spiller HA, Carlisle RD. Status epilepticus after massive carbamazepine overdose. *J Toxicol Clin Toxicol.* 2002;40:81-90.

169. Spiller HA, et al. Retrospective evaluation of tiagabine overdoses. *J Toxicol Clin Toxicol.* 2005;43:855-859.

170. Spiller HA, et al. Thirteen years of oxcarbazepine exposures reported to US poison centers: 2000 to 2012. *Hum Experimental Toxicol.* 2016;35:1055-1059.

171. Spiller HA, et al. Review of toxicity and trends in the use of tiagabine as reported to US poison centers 2000 to 2012. *Hum Exp Toxicol.* 2016;35:109-113.

172. Stern RS. Exanthematous drug eruptions. *N Engl J Med.* 2012;366:2492-2501.

173. Stevens LA, et al on behalf of the Chronic Kidney Disease Epidemiology Collaboration (CKD-EPI). Comparison of drug dosing recommendations based on measured GFR and kidney function estimating equations. *Am J Kidney Dis.* 2010;55:660-670.

174. Stilman N, Masdeu JC. Incidence of seizures with phenytoin toxicity. *Neurology.* 1985;35:1769-1772.

175. Stremski ES, et al. Pediatric carbamazepine intoxication. *Ann Emerg Med.* 1995;25: 624-630.

176. Strimel WJ, et al. Brugada-like electrocardiographic pattern induced by lamotrigine toxicity. *Clin Neuropharmacol.* 2010;33:265-267.

177. Sundstrom M, et al. Patterns of drug abuse among drug users with regular and irregular attendance for treatment as detected by comprehensive UHPLC-HR-TOF-MS. *Drug Test Anal.* 2016;8:39-45.

178. Sung SF, et al. Charcoal hemoperfusion in an elderly man with life-threatening adverse reactions due to poor metabolism of phenytoin. *J Formos Med Assoc.* 2004;103:648-652.

179. Suzuki S, et al. Zonisamide blocks T-type calcium channel in cultured neurons of rat cerebral cortex. *Epilepsy Res.* 1992;12:21-27.

180. Swadron SP, et al. A comparison of phenytoin-loading techniques in the emergency department. *Acad Emerg Med.* 2004;11:244-252.

181. Sztajinkrycer MD. Valproic acid toxicity: overview and management. *J Toxicol Clin Toxicol.* 2002;40:789-801.

182. Sztajinkrycer et al. Acute zonisamide overdose: a death revisited. *Vet Hum Toxicol.* 2003;45:154-156.

183. Thanacoody RH. Extracorporeal elimination in acute valproic acid poisoning. *Clin Toxicol.* 2009;47:609-666.

184. Traub SJ, et al. Acute topiramate toxicity. *J Toxicol Clin Toxicol.* 2003;41:987-990.

185. Uchino H, et al. Transport of amino acid-related compounds mediated by L-type amino acid transporter 1 (LAT1): insight into the mechanisms of substrate recognition. *Mol Pharmacol.* 2002;61:729-737.

186. VanAmselvoort T, et al. Hyponatremia associated with carbamazepine and oxcarbazepine therapy: a review. *Epilepsia.* 1994;35:181-188.

187. VanOpstal M, et al. Severe overdosage with the antiepileptic drug oxcarbazepine. *Br J Pharmacol.* 2004;58:329-331.

188. Veerapandiyan A, et al. Oculogyric crises secondary to lamotrigine overdosage. *Epilepsia.* 2011;52:4-6.

189. Verrotti A, et al. Anticonvulsant hypersensitivity syndrome in children. *CNS Drugs.* 2002;16:197-205.

190. Wang SJ, et al. Inhibition of N type calcium current by lamotrigine in rat amygdala neurons. *Neuroreport.* 1996;7:3037-3040.

191. Waring WS. Lamotrigine overdose associated with generalised seizures [published online ahead of print February 16, 2009]. *BMJ Case Rep.*

192. Wheless JW, et al. Safety and tolerability of rufinamide in children with epilepsy: a pooled analysis of 7 clinical studies. *J Child Neurol.* 2009;24:1520-1525.

193. Wills B, et al. Clinical outcomes with newer anticonvulsant overdose: a poison center observational study. *J Med Toxicol.* 2014;10:254-260.
194. Winnicka RI, et al. Carbamazepine poisoning: elimination kinetics and quantitative relationship with carbamazepine 10,11 epoxide. *J Toxicol Clin Toxicol.* 2002;40:759-765.
195. Wood DM, et al. Significant pregabalin toxicity managed with supportive care alone. *J Med Toxicol.* 2010;6:435-437.
196. Wong PT, Teo WL. The effect of phenytoin on glutamate and GABA transport. *Neurochem Res.* 1986;11:1379-1382.
197. Wyte CD, Berk WA. Severe oral phenytoin overdose does not cause cardiovascular morbidity. *Ann Emerg Med.* 1991;20:508-512.
198. Xie X, et al. Interaction of the antiepileptic drug lamotrigine with recombinant rat brain type IIA Na⁺ channels in rat hippocampal neurons. *Pflugers Arch.* 1995;430:437-446.
199. Yoo L, et al. Treatment of pregabalin toxicity by hemodialysis in a patient with kidney failure. *Am J Kidney Dis.* 2009;54:1127-1130.
200. Zaccara G, Perucca E. Interactions between antiepileptic drugs and other drugs. *Epileptic Disord.* 2014;16:409-432.

L-CARNITINE

Mary Ann Howland

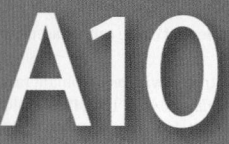

L-Carnitine

INTRODUCTION

L-Carnitine (levocarnitine) is an amino acid vital to the mitochondrial utilization of fatty acids. It is approved by the US Food and Drug Administration (FDA) for treatment of L-carnitine deficiency that either results from inborn errors of metabolism[31] or is associated with hemodialysis. L-Carnitine is also used to treat carnitine deficiency secondary to valproic acid or that associated with zidovudine (AZT)-induced mitochondrial myopathy.[11,12,21]

Based on the proposed mechanism of action of valproic acid–induced hyperammonemia and valproic acid–induced hepatic toxicity, L-carnitine should theoretically help with both of these conditions, but the data to support this are limited. Based on the available evidence, L-carnitine is recommended for patients with valproic acid–induced hyperammonemia and valproic acid–induced hepatic toxicity. Because of limited bioavailability, symptomatic patients should receive L-carnitine intravenously, with oral administration reserved for patients who are not acutely ill.

HISTORY

L-Carnitine is found in mammals, in many bacteria, and in very small amounts in most plants except for avocado and soy products.[44] Carnitine was first discovered in 1905 in extracts of muscle, and its name is derived from *carnis*, the Latin word for flesh.[22] Subsequently, its chemical formula and structure were identified, and in 1997, its enantiomeric properties were confirmed.[44] Carnitine was formerly known as vitamin BT.

PHARMACOLOGY

Chemistry

Carnitine is a water-soluble amino acid that exists in either the D- or L-form; however, the endogenous L isomer is the active form and which is used therapeutically. L-Carnitine has a molecular weight of 161 Da. At physiologic pH, L-carnitine contains both a positively charged quaternary nitrogen ion and a negatively charged carboxylic acid group.[16]

Mechanism of Action

Fatty acids provide 9 kcal/g and are important sources of human energy, particularly for the liver, heart, and skeletal muscle. The utilization of fatty acids as an energy source requires L-carnitine–mediated passage through both the outer and inner mitochondrial membranes to reach the mitochondrial matrix, where β-oxidation occurs (Figs. 11–10 and 48–3). Enzymes in the outer and inner mitochondrial membranes (carnitine palmitoyltransferase and carnitine acylcarnitine translocase) catalyze the synthesis, translocation, and regeneration of L-carnitine.[39] Binding of L-carnitine to fatty acids occurs through esterification at the hydroxyl group on the chiral carbon.[16] The L-carnitine regenerated in the mitochondrial matrix can also translocate in the opposite direction, from the matrix and through the inner membrane back to the intermembrane space. Acyl-coenzyme A (CoA) is transported by carnitine from the cytosol to the mitochondria and undergoes β-oxidation

in the mitochondrial matrix, generating acetyl-CoA, which then enters the tricarboxylic acid cycle for the generation of adenosine triphosphate (ATP).

L-Carnitine Homeostasis

Approximately 54% to 87% of the body stores of L-carnitine are derived from meat and dairy products in the diet; the remainder is endogenously synthesized from trimethyllysine.[44] This amino acid, found largely in skeletal muscle, is converted to trimethylammoniobutanoate (γ-butyrobetaine) and then carried to the liver and kidney for hydroxylation to L-carnitine.[22] Synthesis of L-carnitine in the liver and kidney occurs at a rate of approximately 2 μmol/kg/day and is regulated by the amount of diet-derived trimethyllysine.[22,44] L-Carnitine is filtered by the kidneys, and tubular reabsorption maintains serum L-carnitine concentrations in the normal range, which is approximately 40 to 50 μmol/L.[45]

Pharmacokinetics of Exogenous L-Carnitine

Carnitine pharmacokinetics are very complex and must take into consideration extensive interconversion between L-carnitine and acylcarnitine as well as multicompartmental nonlinear pharmacokinetic modeling.[45] The current understanding of L-carnitine pharmacokinetics is largely derived from 3 major studies.[10,20,54] L-Carnitine is not bound to plasma proteins. Its volume of distribution (V_d) of the central compartment (V_c) is 0.15 L/kg, approximating extracellular fluid volume. Its V_d is 0.7 L/kg. The data vary depending on whether a 2-compartment or 3-compartment model was used for the analysis. The α half-life was 0.6 to 0.7 hours, with a (terminal elimination) half-life of 10 to 23 hours, when a 3-compartment model was used,[54] but was 4 to 6.5 hours when a 2-compartment model was used.[20] The kidneys rapidly eliminate L-carnitine, and as the dose increases, renal clearance increases, reflecting saturation of renal reuptake by organic cation/carnitine transporter.[45] Baseline serum concentrations for L-carnitine are 40 μmol/L but increase to a peak concentration of 1,000 μmol/L after 2 g of L-carnitine are administered intravenously. Oral (PO) administration of 2 g produces peaks of only 15 to 70 μmol/L, demonstrating poor oral bioavailability. The time to peak concentrations after PO administration occurs at 2.5 to 7.0 hours, indicating slow uptake and release by intestinal mucosal cells. After a 2-g carnitine dose, PO absorption is rapidly saturated, and no further absorption occurs after administration of 6 g PO. After a radiolabeled dose, most L-carnitine is metabolized to trimethylamine N-oxide and butyrobetaine, with only approximately 4% to 8% remaining unchanged. The metabolites trimethylamine and trimethylamine N-oxide are theorized to accumulate after chronic high-dose PO therapy in patients with severely compromised kidney function because these metabolites are water soluble and are normally excreted in the urine.[10] Fecal excretion of L-carnitine is less than 1% of the total dose. Carnitor (L-carnitine) tablets are bioequivalent to the Carnitor PO solution, with a bioavailability of approximately 15%. After 4 days of dosing at 1,980 mg (6 × 330-mg tablets) twice daily or 2 g twice daily of the PO solution, the maximum serum concentration was 80 μmol/L.

ROLE IN VALPROIC ACID AND HYPERAMMONEMIA

Valproic acid causes hyperammonemia (>80 mcg/dL or >35 μmol/L) without predictability for causing symptoms or hepatic dysfunction.[2,4] Hyperammonemia and hepatic toxicity are both associated either with therapeutic dosing or an acute overdose. Depending on the study, as many as 35% of children receiving valproic acid develop hyperammonemia, often with corresponding reduced serum L-carnitine concentrations.[8,19,32,34] In the absence of hepatic dysfunction, the postulated mechanisms for hyperammonemia are unclear but are likely to result from interference with hepatic synthesis of urea or a small increase in ammonia production by the kidney.[33,55] Valproic acid, essentially a short-chain fatty acid, induces both carnitine and acetyl-CoA deficiencies by combining with L-carnitine as valproylcarnitine and with acetyl-CoA as valproyl-CoA. Ultimately, β-oxidation of all fatty acids is reduced, resulting in decreased energy production and accumulation of hepatic fatty acid stores. Valproylcarnitine inhibits the renal reabsorption of L-carnitine in experimental models.[38]

Valproic acid stimulates glutaminase, favoring glutamate uptake and ammonia release from the kidney. Glutamate dehydrogenase, acting on this glutamate, produces further ammonia in the conversion of this glutamate to α-ketoglutaric acid. In addition, the formation of valproyl-CoA in the mitochondria inhibits the synthesis of N-acetylglutamate synthase leading to reduced concentrations of hepatic N-acetylglutamate (NAGA). Without sufficient NAGA, a cofactor for carbamoyl phosphate synthetase I (CPS I), the synthesis of urea from ammonia in the liver is impaired and ammonia concentrations rise (Figs. 11–10 and 48–3).[1]

In humans taking valproic acid, L-carnitine supplementation reduces ammonia concentrations.[2,4,6,8,28,42,46,48,56] An early report suggests that supplementation of L-carnitine improved ammonia elimination (3–15 hours) compared with published controls (11–90 hours), although the difference was not statistically significant.[52,53] Subsequently, in one case report administration of L-carnitine along with discontinuation of the valproic acid resulted in rapid neurologic improvement and normalization of the EEG within 24 hours whereas the ammonia concentration decreased from 204 to 47 μmol/L within 6 hours.[46] And in another reported case, the ammonia concentration dropped from 256 to 124 μmol/L in 4 hours following L-carnitine administration.[40]

ROLE IN VALPROIC ACID–ASSOCIATED HEPATOTOXICITY

Valproic acid therapy is commonly associated with a transient dose-related asymptomatic increase in liver enzyme concentrations and a rare symptomatic, life-threatening, idiosyncratic hepatotoxicity similar to Reye syndrome.[50,51] Liver histology demonstrates microvesicular steatosis, similar to that described in both hypoglycin-induced Jamaican vomiting sickness (Chap. 118) and Reye syndrome. This occurrence presumably results from either L-carnitine or acetyl-CoA deficiency, which inhibit mitochondrial β-oxidation of valproic acid and other fatty acids, causing hepatocellular accumulation. One study compared valproic acid administration in mice bred to have decreased carnitine stores with normal mice and found that those with decreased carnitine stores developed microvesicular steatosis of the liver and demonstrated decreased mitochondrial oxidative capacity.[26]

Rat studies demonstrate that toxic doses of valproic acid over 7 days cause microvesicular steatosis, mitochondrial swelling, hyperammonemia, and hypocarnitinemia.[50] When coadministered with L-carnitine, the mitochondrial swelling, hyperammonemia, and carnitine concentrations were similar to control rats, and the microvesicular steatosis was reduced.[50] In one study in which rats were rendered carnitine deficient, the administration of carnitine decreased the concentration in plasma and urine of valproic acid metabolites associated with β-oxidation and increased the urinary concentration of the valproic acid glucuronide metabolite.[24]

The strongest evidence for the benefit of L-carnitine treatment in improving survival from valproic acid–induced hepatotoxicity comes from the retrospective analysis of patients identified by the International Registry for Adverse Reactions to valproic acid.[7] When 50 patients with acute, symptomatic hepatic dysfunction who were not treated with L-carnitine were compared with 42 similar patients treated with L-carnitine, only 10% of the untreated patients survived, but 48% of the L-carnitine–treated patients survived.[7] Early diagnosis, prompt discontinuance of valproic acid, and administration of intravenous (IV) rather than PO L-carnitine was associated with the greatest survival rate.[7] Most patients received 50 to 100 mg/kg/day of L-carnitine regardless of the route of administration.[7]

Acute valproic acid overdose rarely causes hepatotoxicity.[52] However, if a patient were to develop hepatotoxicity after a valproic acid overdose, we recommend the administration of L-carnitine.[25,27,28,37,41,47] The development of hepatotoxicity after a valproic acid overdose cannot be predicted, leading many authors to recommend administering prophylactic doses of L-carnitine to patients with severe overdoses, often defined by encephalopathy or a valproic acid concentration greater than 450 mg/L, with or without evidence of hepatotoxicity.[28,41,47,52] It is reasonable to administer L-carnitine to patients with encephalopathy, with or without hepatotoxicity, and in the setting of an acute overdose if the patient develops a metabolic acidosis. There is not enough evidence to recommend carnitine based solely on a valproic acid concentration.

L-CARNITINE CONCENTRATIONS

In the serum, 80% of L-carnitine is free, and approximately 20% is acylated.[15] In adults who eat all food groups and children older than 1 year of age, the normal serum concentration of free L-carnitine is 22 to 66 μmol/L and the total L-carnitine concentration is 28 to 84 μmol/L. Vegetarians have L-carnitine concentrations 12% to 30% lower than omnivores.[43]

Studies in patients taking valproic acid demonstrate decreases in both free and total serum L-carnitine concentrations[42] and decreases in both total and free muscle L-carnitine concentrations.[3]

Case studies demonstrate reduced serum free L-carnitine concentrations and abnormal valproic acid metabolite profiles that normalize with L-carnitine supplementation.[23,35,36] All of these data support the therapeutic use of L-carnitine and provide a potential mechanism for its beneficial effects in valproic acid–induced hepatotoxicity.

ADVERSE EFFECTS AND SAFETY ISSUES

L-Carnitine administration is well tolerated.[30,34] Transient nausea and vomiting are the most common side effects reported, with diarrhea and a fishy body odor noted at higher doses.[10] Following long-term high doses of L-carnitine in patients with severely compromised kidney function, the potentially toxic L-carnitine metabolites trimethylamine and methylamine N-oxide accumulate. The importance of trimethylamine and its metabolite dimethylamine accumulation may contribute to cognitive abnormalities and the fishy odor.[14] In a pharmacokinetic study after IV administration of 6 g of L-carnitine over 10 minutes, 2 of 6 subjects complained of transient visual blurring; one subject also complained of headache and lightheadedness. The manufacturer of L-carnitine has received case reports of convulsive episodes after L-carnitine use by patients with and without preexisting seizure disorders. No reports of seizures related to L-carnitine use can be found in the human literature.[57] The only data suggesting carnitine-related seizures are found in a rat model.[17]

There are no known contraindications to the use of L-carnitine. However, only the L isomer and not the racemic mixture should be used. The D-isomer is considered harmful and leads to depletion of L-carnitine in serum and in cardiac and skeletal muscles.[49] The D, L mixture interferes with mitochondrial utilization of L-carnitine and is associated with myastheniaalike symptoms and cardiac dysrhythmias.[49]

OVERDOSE OF L-CARNITINE

No cases of toxicity from overdose are reported, although large oral doses infrequently cause diarrhea.[10] The LD_{50} in rats is 5.4 g/kg IV and 19.2 g/kg PO.[10]

PREGNANCY AND LACTATION

L-Carnitine is considered FDA pregnancy category B. There is no information on excretion into breast milk.

DOSING AND ADMINISTRATION

The optimal dosing of L-carnitine for valproic acid–induced hyperammonemia or hepatotoxicity has not been established. Recommendations for IV L-carnitine administration to patients with acute metabolic disorders resulting from L-carnitine deficiency range from 50 to 500 mg/kg/day.[10,13]

In the setting of severe metabolic crisis, a loading dose equal to the daily dose is recommended to be given initially followed by the daily dose divided and administered every 4 hours, and never more than every 6 hours.[10] The 500 mg/kg/day dose was intended for children[9] and offers no maximum dose. After the IV loading dose, a maximal daily dose of 6 g is reasonable. The oral dosing of L-carnitine is 50 to 100 mg/kg/day up to 3 g/day and should be reserved for patients who are not acutely ill. In adults, this is achieved by providing 990 mg (3 × 330-mg tabs) 3 times a day.

For patients with an acute overdose of valproic acid and without hepatic enzyme abnormalities or symptomatic hyperammonemia, L-carnitine administration is reasonable to prevent hepatotoxicity, and enteral doses of 100 mg/kg/day divided every 8 hours up to 3 g/day are appropriate. For patients with valproic acid–induced symptomatic hepatotoxicity, symptomatic hyperammonemia, metabolic acidosis, or encephalopathy, IV L-carnitine is recommended at a dose of 100 mg/kg IV up to 6 g administered over 30 minutes as a loading dose followed by 15 mg/kg every 6 hours administered over 10 to 30 minutes.

FORMULATION AND ACQUISITION

L-Carnitine is available as a sterile injection for IV use in 1 g/5 mL single-dose vials.[10] L-Carnitine is supplied without a preservative. After the vial is opened, the unused portion should be discarded. L-Carnitine injection is compatible with and stable when mixed with 0.9% sodium chloride solution or lactated ringer solution in concentrations as high as 8 mg/mL for as long as 24 hours.[10] L-Carnitine is also available as 250- and 330-mg tablets; as an oral solution with artificial cherry flavoring, malic acid, sucrose syrup, and methylparaben and propylparaben as preservatives; and as sugar-free oral solutions at a concentration of 100 mg/mL that contain parabens and some also contain propylene glycol.[9] The PO solution does not require dilution but dilution in other drinks improves palatability by masking the taste. Slow consumption reduces gastrointestinal side effects.[10]

SUMMARY

- ■ L-Carnitine is recommended for patients with valproic acid–induced hyperammonemia, hepatotoxicity, metabolic acidosis, and encephalopathy.
  - • Symptomatic patients should receive intravenous L-carnitine, not the oral preparation.
  - • Asymptomatic patients should receive oral L-carnitine.

REFERENCES

1. Aires CC, et al. New insights on the mechanisms of valproate-induced hyperammonemia: inhibition of hepatic N-acetylglutamate synthase activity by valproyl-CoA. *J Hepatol.* 2011;55:426-434.
2. Altunbasak S, et al. Asymptomatic hyperammonemia in children treated with valproic acid. *J Child Neurol.* 1997;12:461-463.
3. Anil M, et al. Serum and muscle carnitine levels in epileptic children receiving sodium valproate. *J Child Neurol.* 2009;24:80-86.
4. Barrueto F Jr, Hack JB. Hyperammonemia and coma without hepatic dysfunction induced by valproate therapy. *Acad Emerg Med.* 2001;8:999-1001.
5. Berthelot-Moritz F, et al. Fatal sodium valproate poisoning. *Intensive Care Med.* 1997;23:599.
6. Beversdorf D, et al. Valproate induced encephalopathy treated with carnitine in an adult. *J Neurol Neurosurg Psychiatry.* 1996;61:211.
7. Bohan TP, et al. Effect of L-carnitine treatment for valproate-induced hepatotoxicity. *Neurology.* 2001;56:1405-1409.
8. Böhles H, et al. The effect of carnitine supplementation in valproate-induced hyperammonaemia. *Acta Paediatr.* 1996;85:446-449.
9. Carnitor (levocarnitine) tablets, Carnitor Oral Solution, and Carnitor SF Sugar Free Oral solution [package insert]. Gaithersburg, MD: Sigma-Tau; April 2015.
10. Carnitor (levocarnitine) Injection [product information]. Gaithersburg, MD: Sigma-Tau; April 2015.
11. Carter R, et al. Severe lactic acidosis in association with reverse transcriptase inhibitors with potential response to L-carnitine in a pediatric HIV positive patient. *AIDS Patient Care.* 2004;18:131-134.
12. Claessens Y, et al. Bench to bedside review: severe lactic acidosis in HIV patients treated with nucleoside analogue reverse transcriptase inhibitors. *Crit Care.* 2003;7:226-232.
13. De Vivo DC, et al. L-Carnitine supplementation in childhood epilepsy: current perspectives. *Epilepsia.* 1998;39:1216-1225.
14. Eknoyan G, et al. Practice recommendations for the use of L-carnitine in dialysis-related carnitine disorder. National Kidney Foundation Carnitine Consensus Conference. *Am J Kidney Dis.* 2003;41:868-876.
15. Evangeliou A, Vlassopoulos D. Carnitine metabolism and deficit—when supplementation is necessary? *Curr Pharm Biotechnol.* 2003;4:211-219.
16. Evans A. Dialysis-related carnitine disorder and levocarnitine pharmacology. *Am J Kidney Dis.* 2003;41(suppl):S13-S26.
17. Fariello RG, et al. Transient seizure activity induced by acetylcarnitine. *Neuropharmacology.* 1984;23:585-587.
18. Ferrari R, et al. Therapeutic effects of L-carnitine and propionyl-L-carnitine on cardiovascular disease: a review. *Ann N Y Acad Sci.* 2004;1033:79-91.
19. Hamed SA, Abdella MM. The risk of asymptomatic hyperammonemia in children with idiopathic epilepsy treated with valproate: relationship to blood carnitine status. *Epilepsy Res.* 2009;86:32-41.
20. Harper P, et al. Pharmacokinetics of intravenous and oral bolus doses of L-carnitine in healthy subjects. *Eur J Clin Pharmacol.* 1988;35:555-562.
21. Hoffman R, Currier J. Management of antiretroviral treatment related complications. *Infect Dis Clinics North Am.* 2007;21:103-132.
22. Hoppel C. The role of carnitine in normal and altered fatty acid metabolism. *Am J Kidney Dis.* 2003;41(suppl 4):S4-S12.
23. Ishikura H, et al. Valproic acid overdose and L-carnitine therapy. *J Anal Toxicol.* 1996;20:55-58.
24. Katayama H, et al. Effects of carnitine on valproic acid pharmacokinetics in rats. *J Pharm Sci.* 2016;105:3199-3204.
25. Katiyar A, Aaron C. Case files of the children's hospital of Michigan regional poison control center: the use of carnitine for the management of acute valproic acid toxicity. *J Med Toxicol.* 2007;3:129-138.
26. Knapp A, et al. Toxicity of valproic acid in mice with decreased plasma and tissue carnitine stores. *J Pharm Exp Ther.* 2008;324:568-575.
27. Laub MC, et al. Serum carnitine during valproic acid therapy. *Epilepsia.* 1986;27:559-562.
28. Lheureux P, Hantson P. Carnitine in the treatment of valproic acid induced toxicity. *Clin Toxicol.* 2009;47:101-111.
29. Longo N, et al. Disorders of carnitine transport and the carnitine cycle. *Am J Med Genet C Semin Med Genet.* 2006;142C:77-85.
30. LoVecchio F, et al. L-Carnitine was safely administered in the setting of valproic acid toxicity. *Am J Emerg Med.* 2005;23:321-322.
31. Magoulas PL, El-Hattab AW. Systemic primary carnitine deficiency: an overview of clinical manifestations, diagnosis, and management. *Orphanet J Rare Dis.* 2012;7:68.
32. Maldonado C, et al. Carnitine and/or acetylcarnitine deficiency as a cause of higher levels of ammonia. *Biomed Res Int.* 2016;2016:2920108.
33. Marini AM, et al. Hepatic and renal contributions to valproic acid-induced hyperammonemia. *Neurology.* 1988;38:365-371.
34. Mock CM, Schwetschenau KH. Levocarnitine for valproic-acid-induced hyperammonemic encephalopathy. *Am J Health Syst Pharm.* 2012;69:35-39.
35. Murakami K, et al. Alterations of urinary acetylcarnitine in valproate-treated rats: the effect of L-carnitine supplementation. *J Child Neurol.* 1992;7:404-407.
36. Murakami K, et al. Effect of L-carnitine supplementation on acute valproate intoxication. *Epilepsia.* 1996;37:687-689.
37. Murphy JV, et al. Hepatotoxic effects in a child receiving valproate and carnitine. *J Pediatr.* 1993;123:318-320.
38. Okamura N, et al. Involvement of recognition and interaction of carnitine transporter in the decrease of L-carnitine concentration induced by pivalic acid and valproic acid. *Pharm Res.* 2006;23:1729-1735.
39. Pande SV. Carnitine-acylcarnitine translocase deficiency. *Am J Med Sci.* 1999;318:22-27.
40. Papaseit E, et al. A case of acute valproic acid poisoning treated successfully with L-carnitine. *Eur J Emerg Med.* 2012;19:57-58.
41. Perrott J, et al. L-Carnitine for acute valproic acid overdose: a systematic review of published cases. *Ann Pharmacother.* 2010;44:1287-1293.
42. Raskind JY, El-Chaar M. The role of carnitine supplementation during valproic acid therapy. *Ann Pharmacother.* 2000;34:630-638.
43. Rebouche CJ. Carnitine function and requirements during the life cycle. *FASEB J.* 1992;6:3379-3386.
44. Rebouche CJ, Seim H. Carnitine metabolism and its regulation in microorganisms and mammals. *Annu Rev Nutr.* 1998;18:39-61.
45. Reuter S, Evans A. Carnitine and acylcarnitines. *Clin Pharmacokinet.* 2012;51:553-572.
46. Rigamonti A, et al. Valproate induced hyperammonemic encephalopathy successfully treated with levocarnitine. *J Clin Neurosci.* 2014;21:690-691.
47. Russell S. Carnitine as an antidote for acute valproate toxicity in children. *Curr Opin Pediatr.* 2007;19:206-210.
48. Segura-Bruna N, et al. Valproate induced hyperammonemic encephalopathy. *Acta Neurol Scand.* 2006;114:1-7.
49. Smith SW. Chiral toxicology: it's the same thing...only different. *Toxicol Sci.* 2009;110:4-30.
50. Sugimoto T, et al. Hepatotoxicity in rat following administration of valproic acid: effect of L-carnitine supplementation. *Epilepsia.* 1987;28:373-377.

51. Sugimoto T, et al. Reye-like syndrome associated with valproic acid. *Brain Dev.* 1983;5:334-337.

52. Sztajnkrycer M. Valproic acid toxicity: overview and management. *J Toxicol Clin Toxicol.* 2002;40:789-801.

53. Sztajnkrycer MD, et al. Valproate-induced hyperammonemia: preliminary evaluation of ammonia elimination with carnitine administration. *J Toxicol Clin Toxicol.* 2001;39:497.

54. Uematsu T, et al. Pharmacokinetics and safety of L-carnitine infused I.V. in healthy subjects. *Eur J Clin Pharmacol.* 1988;34:213-216.

55. Verrotti A, et al. Valproate-induced hyper-ammonemic encephalopathy. *Metab Brain Dis.* 2002;17:367-373.

56. Wadzinski J, et al. Valproate associated hyperammonemic encephalopathy. *J Am Board Fam Med.* 2007;20:499-502.

57. Zeiler FA, et al. Levocarnitine induced seizures in patients on valproic acid: A negative systematic review. *Seizure.* 2016;36:36-39.

History A 27-year-old man was found acting abnormally in a train station. When approached by police, he seemed to be hallucinating and answering questions inappropriately, for which emergency medical services was activated. When the paramedics arrived, they recorded: a blood pressure of 148/92 mm Hg, a pulse of 142 beats/min, and a respiratory rate of 16 breaths/min. They noted dilated pupils and disorientation, but did not comment on other abnormalities. An intravenous line was inserted, and the patient was given oxygen via nasal cannula at 4 L/min during transport to the hospital. No further history could be obtained.

Physical Examination On arrival to the hospital, the patient appeared to be a well-nourished, appropriately dressed man in significant distress. Vital signs were blood pressure, 152/92 mm Hg; pulse, 155 beats/min; respiratory rate, 22 breaths/min; rectal temperature, 99.4°F; oxygen saturation, 100% on nasal cannula at 4 L/min; and glucose, 117 mg/dL. Physical examination revealed a normal head without signs of trauma, the pupils were 7 to 8 mm and not reactive (Fig. CS7–1), and the extraocular muscles appeared normal. His neck was supple. His chest was clear to auscultation, and other than tachycardia, his heart sounds were normal. His abdomen was slightly distended and tender in the suprapubic area with absent bowel sounds. His skin was warm and dry. The neurologic examination was notable for good strength in all four extremities with intermittent myoclonic jerking, slight symmetrical hyperreflexia, and plantar flexion. He was mumbling incoherently, looking about the

room as if he were responding to external stimuli and could not answer questions.

Because the patient could not provide any history, his belongings were searched for possible information. Despite being well dressed, he had no wallet, cell phone, pills, or other useful information in his pockets, suggesting that perhaps the patient was surreptitiously drugged and then robbed.

Initial Management The patient was immediately attached to a cardiac monitor, and an electrocardiogram (ECG) was obtained. An intravenous line (IV) was inserted and the patient was rapidly given 1 L of 0.9% sodium chloride solution.

What Is the Differential Diagnosis? The patient's presentation is notable for hypertension, tachycardia, and tachypnea with dilated, nonreactive pupils, and hallucinations. The toxicologic differential diagnosis includes anticholinergics and antihistamines (Chap. 49), certain antipsychotics and antidepressants (Chaps. 67 and 68), ethanol and sedative–hypnotic withdrawal (Chap. 77), sympathomimetics such as amphetamines and cocaine (Chaps. 73 and 75), and hallucinogens (Chap. 79). However, a more detailed evaluation of the physical examination was suggestive of an anticholinergic toxic syndrome (Chap. 3 and Table 3–2) in that the skin was dry, the pupils were widely dilated and poorly responsive, the bowel sounds were diminished, and the bladder was distended. All of these findings were inconsistent with sympathomimetics, hallucinogens, and ethanol or sedative–hypnotic withdrawal. Although cyclic antidepressants and some antipsychotics

are potent anticholinergics, their toxicity is usually associated with hypotension and somnolence.

What Clinical and Laboratory Analyses Help Exclude Life-Threatening Causes of this Patient's Presentation? In patients with suspected anticholinergic toxicity, the single most consequential test is to obtain an ECG. The ECG is used primarily to identify signs of sodium channel blockade that are characteristic of cyclic antidepressant overdose (Chaps. 15 and 68) but also occur with some phenothiazine antipsychotics (Chap. 67), diphenhydramine (Chap. 49), type IA and IC antidysrhythmics (Chap. 57), cocaine (Chap. 75), and some other xenobiotics. A prolonged QRS complex duration would not only help provide a diagnosis in patients with TCA poisoning but would also indicate the need to intervene with hypertonic sodium bicarbonate (Antidotes in Depth: A5). The patient's ECG is shown in Fig. CS7–2.

Additional life-threatening conditions that might be anticipated in patients with anticholinergic toxicity include hyperthermia, seizures, and rhabdomyolysis. Blood samples were sent to the laboratory for a complete blood count, electrolytes, creatine phosphokinase, and concentrations of acetaminophen and ethanol.

Further Diagnosis and Treatment The combination of a clinical anticholinergic syndrome with subtle markers of sodium channel blockade and a normal blood pressure was most suggestive of diphenhydramine toxicity. Given that the patient was uncomfortable and unable to provide a history, a decision was made to administer physostigmine (Antidotes in Depth: A11). Atropine was brought to the bedside. One milligram of physostigmine was infused over 5 minutes. Over the next few minutes, the patient's pupils became smaller, and his heart rate dropped to 110 beats/min. He became calm, but his speech was still garbled and incoherent and his bowel sounds were quiet. A second dose of 1 mg of physostigmine was given over 5 minutes. Shortly thereafter, the patient's speech became clear, and he asked to drink water and use a urinal. He spontaneously voided 800 mL of clear urine. His blood pressure was 132/84 mm Hg, and his pulse was 98 beats/min.

He related that he had no medical history, no surgical history, and no allergies to medications and was not taking any prescription, nonprescription, or illicit drugs. The last thing he remembered was that he was early for his

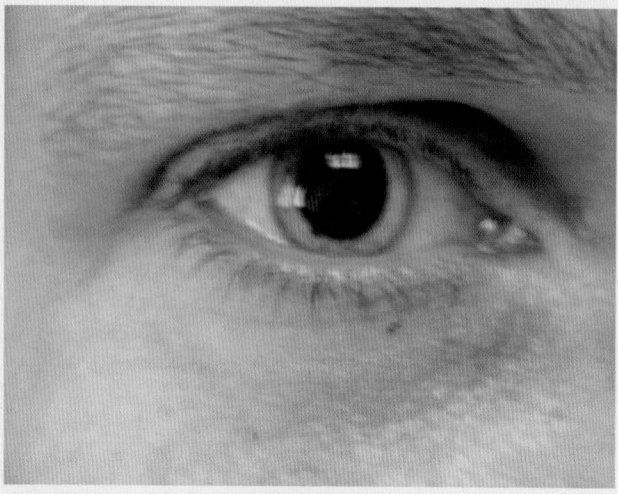

FIGURE CS7–1. The patient's right eye demonstrating a large and fixed pupil.

CASE STUDY 7 (CONTINUED)

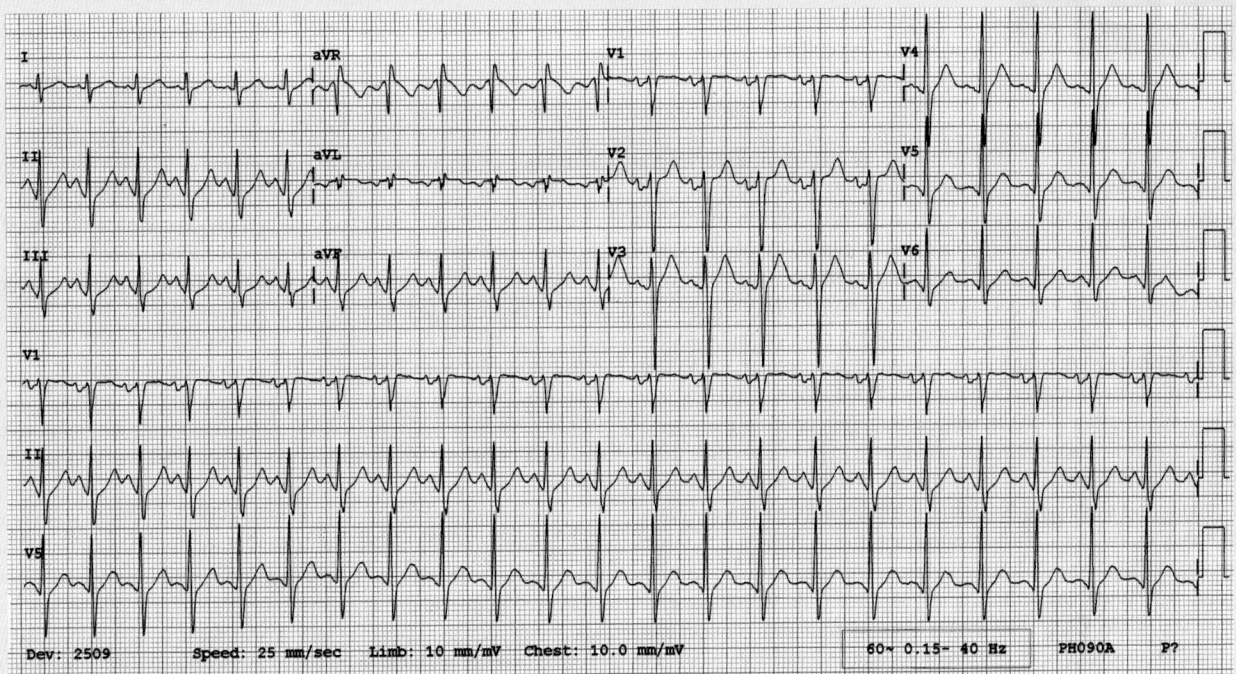

FIGURE CS7–2. Electrocardiogram showing sinus tachycardia with a QRS complex duration of 90 milliseconds (ms), a QT interval of 320 ms (QTc 506 ms), and findings consistent with early sodium channel blockade (an S wave in I and an R wave in aVR despite a relatively normal QRS complex duration).

train and went to the station bar for a drink with someone he met while waiting.

All of the patient's laboratory tests were within normal limits except for his blood ethanol concentration, which was 32 mg/dL.

The health care team was concerned about drug-facilitated robbery and had the department social worker meet with the patient. He was offered the opportunity for comprehensive testing as well as filing a report with the police, which he declined. He was observed for 8 hours and remained well, so he was discharged at his own request.

49 ANTIHISTAMINES AND DECONGESTANTS

Sophie Gosselin

Antihistamines and decongestants rank among the highest prescription and nonprescription xenobiotics used in the United States. In 2015, antihistamines and cough and cold preparations ranked respectively 6th and 12th in substance categories most frequently involved in human exposure–related calls to US Poison Control Centers. Antihistamines ranked 14th in categories associated with the largest number of fatalities in 2015 (Chap. 130).[113]

Popular beliefs suggests that expectorants or decongestants depress cough and relieve congestion, and antihistamines also promote sleep. In an effort to retain selected drugs on the nonprescription market, the US Food and Drug Administration (FDA) developed a nonprescription monograph rule allowing some medications in use before 1972 to remain on the market without new clinical trials. As such, many nonprescription decongestants, antihistamines, and expectorants remained available for children without adequate safety or efficacy data in younger age groups. Between the years 1998 and 2007, 8.7% of US parents surveyed reported to have used an antihistamine- or decongestant-containing remedy for their children younger than 12 years in the past week. The majority of these children were younger than 5 years. Pseudoephedrine, brompheniramine, and chlorpheniramine were the 3 most common ingredients used.[180]

Unwanted effects associated with their use posed significant public health problems, particularly in children. Fatality studies associated with nonprescription cough and cold medicines reported that although uncommon, most deaths involved nontherapeutic dosages, administration for sedation purposes, and use in children primarily younger than 2 years of age.[34] However, the causality of death by cough and cold medicine is often debated. The data needed to prove this relationship are often incomplete because of such factors as the lack of postmortem drug quantification.[134] In 2007, a group of pediatricians and pharmacists petitioned the FDA requesting a change in labeling for children younger than 6 years on the basis that safety was never demonstrated in this age group. This petition alerted the general public of the underestimated adverse effects of these xenobiotics.[144,168] In early 2008, the FDA Public Health Advisory announced that cough and cold products were not recommended for children younger than 2 years, and later that same year the Consumer Healthcare Products Association (CHPA), a trade group of generic drug manufacturers, announced that its members were voluntarily modifying product labels for cough and cold medicines to exclude children younger than 4 years.[173]

Despite their widespread use, many reviews of nonprescription medications for cough in adults and children found no evidence for the effectiveness.[155] Conclusions are similar regarding the use of antihistamines or decongestants in otitis media.[28] Moreover, many well-conducted studies of antihistamines in monotherapy or in combination with a decongestant for patients with upper respiratory illness reported a significant absence of overall symptom improvement.[155,178] It is also suggested that the majority of any perceived benefit of cough suppressants are due to the sensory impact of sweetness and the placebo effect as well as the concerning intent of using the known adverse effect of sedation as a therapeutic goal.[45]

A systematic review on the toxicity of common cough and cold remedies in children younger than 12 years concluded there is sufficient evidence of an unfavorable risk-to-benefit ratio to support measures aimed at restricting use of cough and cold medications in younger age groups.[74] As individuals seek to ameliorate the symptoms of an unpleasant illness, official restrictions in younger age groups have yielded concerns of increased off-label use of medicines intended for older age groups or substitution with other xenobiotics. Two analyses of both poison control center data and emergency department (ED) visits reported significant decreases in annual rates of both therapeutic medication errors and overall ED visits related to cough and cold medicines. However, the rate of unintentional ingestions did not change after the marketing revisions in 2007, implying that further efforts to increase packaging safety and parental education are needed.[88,101,148]

Despite many consumer-directed newsletter and media campaigns, the overall use in the general population seems constant. This is indicated by the rising sales in the category "cough- and cold-related" nonprescription medications between 2008 and 2011, reaching $4.2 billion in 2011, higher than analgesics ($2.7 billion).[29] A survey done in 2010 for CHPA found that 93% of US adults prefer to treat their minor ailments with nonprescription products before seeking professional care, and 85% would do the same for their children.[161]

Recreational use of antihistamines and decongestants was reported as early as the 1970s.[125] The popular "T's and blues," referring to the combination of pentazocine (Talwin) and the blue-colored antihistamine tripelennamine were used intravenously as a substitute for heroin. In 1983, when naloxone was included in pentazocine (Talwin NX), abuse patterns decreased.[10] Nonprescription sympathomimetics, such as pseudoephedrine, are also used as precursors in the illicit synthesis of methamphetamine. Although the rates of potential adverse events are perceived as low, the issue takes on added significance when the magnitude of the exposure rates for these xenobiotics is considered. In a survey of 2528 participants distributed across the United States, 4.5% of adult participants in 2006 reported taking pseudoephedrine within the past week compared with 8.1% in 2002, and 3.8% reported the use of diphenhydramine compared with 4.4% in 2002.[82,154] Both poison control center and clinical experience suggests that recreational use of antihistamines are increasing. Dextromethorphan-containing products are widely used for recreational purposes (Chap. 36).

Regardless of intent, exposures to these xenobiotics are relatively frequent, as illustrated by the number of calls received to the American Association of Poison Control Centers (AAPCC). Compilation of the National Poison Data System (NPDS) reports for the years 2000 to 2015 shows that the total number of exposure calls related to antihistamines has increased in the last 10 years, reaching 3.8% of calls and ranked eighth in the substance category with the greatest rate of exposure increase.[113] In contrast, both pediatric and adult cough and cold preparation–related calls have decreased since 2007 (Chap. 130).

In combination with each other, analgesics or antipyretics, antihistamines, and decongestants are easily accessible to the public. This availability perpetuates the widespread public impression that nonprescription xenobiotics are "safe" and contributes to their frequent use, misuse, and abuse.

ANTIHISTAMINES
History and Epidemiology
History

After the discovery of histamine, Bovet and other researchers at the Pasteur Institute attempted to synthesize antagonists to better understand its physiological role. In 1939, pyrilamine was found to be extremely effective in guinea pigs but not safe enough for humans. In 1941, phenbenzamine was the first antihistamine deemed suitable for clinical use.[157] Diphenhydramine was synthesized in 1943, and shortly after, in 1947, orphenadrine was derived. The more pronounced anticholinergic effects of the hydrochloride salt of orphenadrine explain its use in the treatment of Parkinson disease, and the citrate salt is used as a muscle relaxant. In the same years, Searle and Company, in Chicago, modified diphenhydramine to reduce drowsiness. Dimenhydrinate, the resulting 8-chlorotheophylline salt, serendipitously cured a patient of her long-standing motion sickness. This benefit was proven in a clinical trial in 1949, in which 25% of the troops crossing the Atlantic from New York who received a placebo experienced seasickness compared with only 4% of those receiving dimenhydrinate.[157]

Reports of adverse effects and toxicity were soon published. The first report of a death associated with diphenhydramine occurred in 1948.[14] However, in this patient, several other factors could have contributed to her demise. Deaths were also reported with methapyrilene, but given its frequent coingestion with propoxyphene or scopolamine and the variable postmortem serum concentrations reported, attribution of causality was difficult.[135] In the 1950s, more pediatric overdose cases were reported, and the resemblance to atropine poisoning was noted. At the time, treatment consisted of phenobarbital, "pressure respirations," and cooling with tepid water sponges.[132]

In the following decade, more than 5,000 compounds were synthesized by more than 500 chemists and tried for human use. Bovet was awarded the Nobel Prize in Physiology or Medicine in 1957 for his work related to the synthesis of compounds blocking the effects of bodily substances such as histamine.[16]

Cyclizine, a piperazine rather than a dimethylamine, was developed in the 1960s. It proved to be long acting and was used during the first manned flight to the moon by the National Aeronautic and Space Administration to control space sickness. It is no longer approved for use in the United States, although its derivative, hydroxyzine, remains in use.[157] In the 1970s, terfenadine was synthesized as a tranquilizer, but it lacked central nervous system (CNS) penetration. However, its peripheral antihistaminic effects proved useful. In 1989, more than 773 reactions to terfenadine were reported ranging from prolonged QT intervals to convulsions in supratherapeutic ingestions.[35] In 1992, the FDA issued a warning for the risk of torsade de pointes with terfenadine when administered with CYP3A4 inhibitors. Fexofenadine, its active metabolite, was marketed instead.[157]

None of the initial xenobiotics could antagonize histamine-induced gastric acid secretion, leading to the determination of the existence of more than one type of histamine receptors. The histamine receptor subtypes were identified as H_1 and H_2. The H_2 receptors were noted to be located in the stomach. Attempts to identify H_2 receptor antagonists identified guanylhistamine, a partial agonist, and initiated the understanding of the physiology of histamine receptors.[156]

Cimetidine was synthesized in 1972, but its binding to the heme moiety of the cytochrome P450 with resultant inhibition caused medication interactions as well as altered mental status.[175] Ranitidine, a less polar molecule, did not enter the CNS and did not interfere with the P450 cytochromes. It rapidly became one of the best-selling drugs and has remained so for many years.

Seeking to better understand the action of histamine in the CNS, animal studies in the early 1980s postulated the existence of another histamine receptor located presynaptically. The existence of a distinct H_3 receptor inhibiting the neuronal synthesis of histamine (autoreceptor) when stimulated was validated with the development of the selective agonist R-α-methylhistamine and antagonist thioperamide.[6] A fourth histamine receptor is now recognized. Its primary function seems to modulate inflammatory and immune responses as well as nociception.[71] The numerous functions of histamine and its receptors in the nervous system, immune system, and other organs are continually being appreciated. Trials are under way for the use of H_3 and H_4 histamine receptor antagonists in CNS cognitive disorder, Parkinson disease, rheumatoid arthritis, obesity, and allergic rhinitis treatments.[167,194]

Epidemiology

Antihistamines are available worldwide, and many do not require a prescription. These medications find widespread application in the treatment of conditions such as anaphylaxis, benign positional vertigo, dystonic reactions, hyperemesis gravidarum, gastroesophageal reflux disease, stress gastritis, and other histamine-mediated disorders. They are also used for their ability

to act on other receptors in the treatment of serotonin toxicity. Additionally, they are used for symptomatic relief of allergy symptoms as in allergic rhinitis, conjunctivitis, or urticaria and are included in many combination cough and cold preparations as discussed previously. First-generation antihistamines are widely available without prescription and are also marketed as sleep aids. These 2 factors contribute to their common ingestion in suicide attempts.[127] Second- and third-generation H_1 antihistamines are less frequently implicated in suicide attempts. Although reporting is not comprehensive, about one in 5 antihistamine-related exposures called to poison control centers are intentional. More than 42% of antihistamine exposures are related to confirmed diphenhydramine and 62% of those are from nonprescription sources (Chap. 130).

The H_2 antihistamines have a better safety profile in therapeutic and overdose situations.[111] Even though many references cite the possibility of bradydysrhythmias, hypotension, and cardiac arrest with massive ingestions or intravenous (IV) administration of H_2 antihistamines, these reports are rare. The incidence of adverse cardiovascular events with H_2 antihistamines is largely unknown. In the largest published review assessing 881 cases of solely cimetidine exposures, most were in children from 12 to 36 months of age, and 76% were unintentional in nature. No fatalities were observed.[91] A review of NPDS reports from 2001 to 2015 did not identify any fatalities from single-product ingestion of cimetidine or other H_2 antihistamines.[113] Only a few case reports of fatalities associated with acute exposures to H_2 antihistamines in adults can be found, mainly in forensic literature with little clinical information.[78]

Children seem to be at increased risk for antihistamine toxicity and most of the reported deaths in this age group involve diphenhydramine. Perhaps this is due to the ease of obtaining a toxic dose in milligrams per kilogram of body weight with very few tablets or liquid concentration in the commercial products available.[104,115]

Fatalities are also reported with other antihistamines, albeit often in combination with dextromethorphan and pseudoephedrine, making it difficult to attribute the cause of death to the antihistamine alone.[15] Liquid formulations and topical preparations are available and attractive to children, resulting in unintentional ingestions when accessible. First-generation antihistamines are also administered for their sedative properties by parents and prescribed by pediatricians for various purposes, including promoting recovery of sick children or as a relief for working parents.[2,120] However, the result of a randomized trial of diphenhydramine for this indication showed it was no more effective than placebo for nighttime awakenings or parental happiness.[109]

Pharmacology

Histamine Receptor Physiology

The H_1 receptors are located in the CNS, heart, vasculature, airways, sensory neurons, gastrointestinal (GI) smooth muscle, immune system, and adrenal medulla. Through H_1 receptors, histamine interacts with G proteins in the plasma membranes. Stimulation of H_1 receptors results in increased synthesis by phospholipases A_2 and C, inositol-1,4,5-triphosphate, and several diacylglycerols (DAGs) from phospholipids located in cell membranes. Inositol-1,4,5-triphosphate causes release of calcium, which then activates calcium-calmodulin–dependent myosin light-chain kinase, resulting in enhanced cross-bridging and smooth muscle contraction. The active and inactive forms of this receptor subtype are in equilibrium at baseline, and histamine shifts the equilibrium to the active conformation.[150]

The **H_1 receptors** are most commonly associated with mediation of inflammation. The other functions of histamine and the H_1 receptor include control of the sleep–wake cycle, cognition, memory, and endocrine homeostasis. The H_1 receptor stimulation also causes vasodilation, increases vascular permeability, and increases bronchoconstriction. Cardiac histamine H_1 receptor stimulation increases atrioventricular nodal conduction time.[36]

The **H_2 receptors** are located in cells of the gastric mucosa, heart, lung, CNS, uterus, and immune cells. The H_2 receptor stimulation is mediated by adenylate cyclase activation of cyclic adenosine monophosphate (cAMP)–dependent protein kinase in smooth muscle and in parietal cells of the stomach and results in increased gastric acidity through stimulation of the H^+,K^+-ATPase pump, causing release of H^+ into the gastric lumen. The action of histamine on the H_2 receptor increases sinus node automaticity, ventricular contraction force, and coronary flow as well as vascular permeability and mucus production in the airways.[71,150]

The **H_3 receptors** are found in neurons of the central and peripheral nervous systems, airways, and GI tract. The action of histamine on H_3 receptors of the CNS decreases further release of histamine, acetylcholine, dopamine, and serotonin. These receptors partly act to prevent excessive bronchoconstriction and are implicated in control of neurogenic inflammation and proinflammatory activity.[98]

The **H_4 receptors** are located in leukocytes, bone marrow, spleen, lung, liver, colon, and hippocampus. The H_4 receptor plays a role in the differentiation of myeloblasts and promyelocytes and in eosinophil chemotaxis.[98]

All 4 types of histamine receptors are heptahelical transmembrane molecules that transduce extracellular signals via G proteins to intracellular second-messenger systems.[150] Xenobiotics acting at each of the 4 histamine-modulated receptor sites are identified. To date, no H_3 or H_4 antihistamines are available for commercial clinical use (Fig. 49–1).

HISTAMINE RECEPTORS: INVERSE AGONISTS VERSUS ANTAGONISTS

All known H_1 histamine antagonists function as inverse agonists and are not simply reversible competitive antagonists. Rather than preventing the binding of histamine to its receptor as in a classical competitive antagonist model, these xenobiotics stabilize the inactive form of the histamine receptor and shift the equilibrium to this inactive conformation (Fig. 49–2).[150]

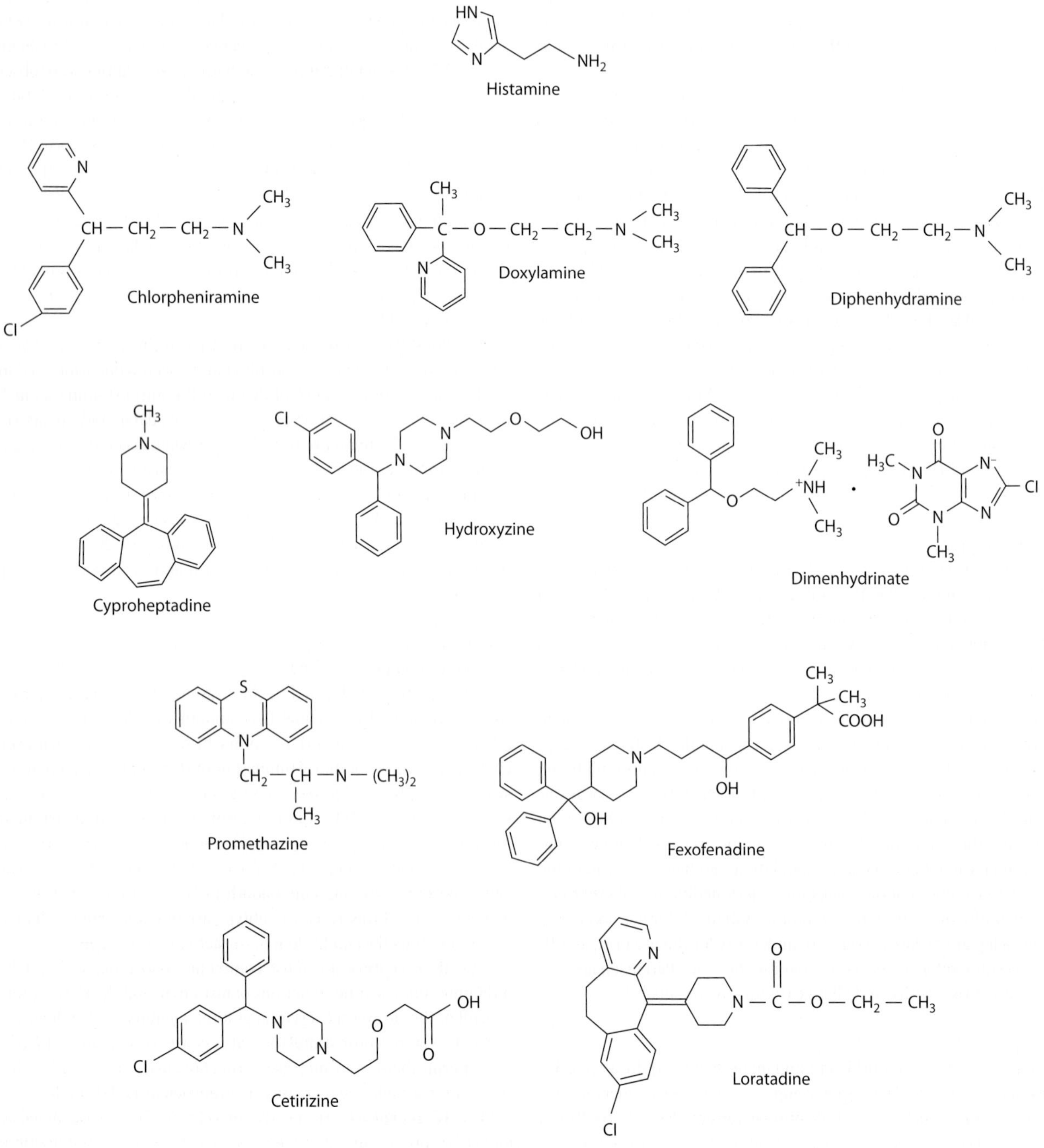

FIGURE 49–1. Structure of histamine and selected H_1 receptor antihistamines.

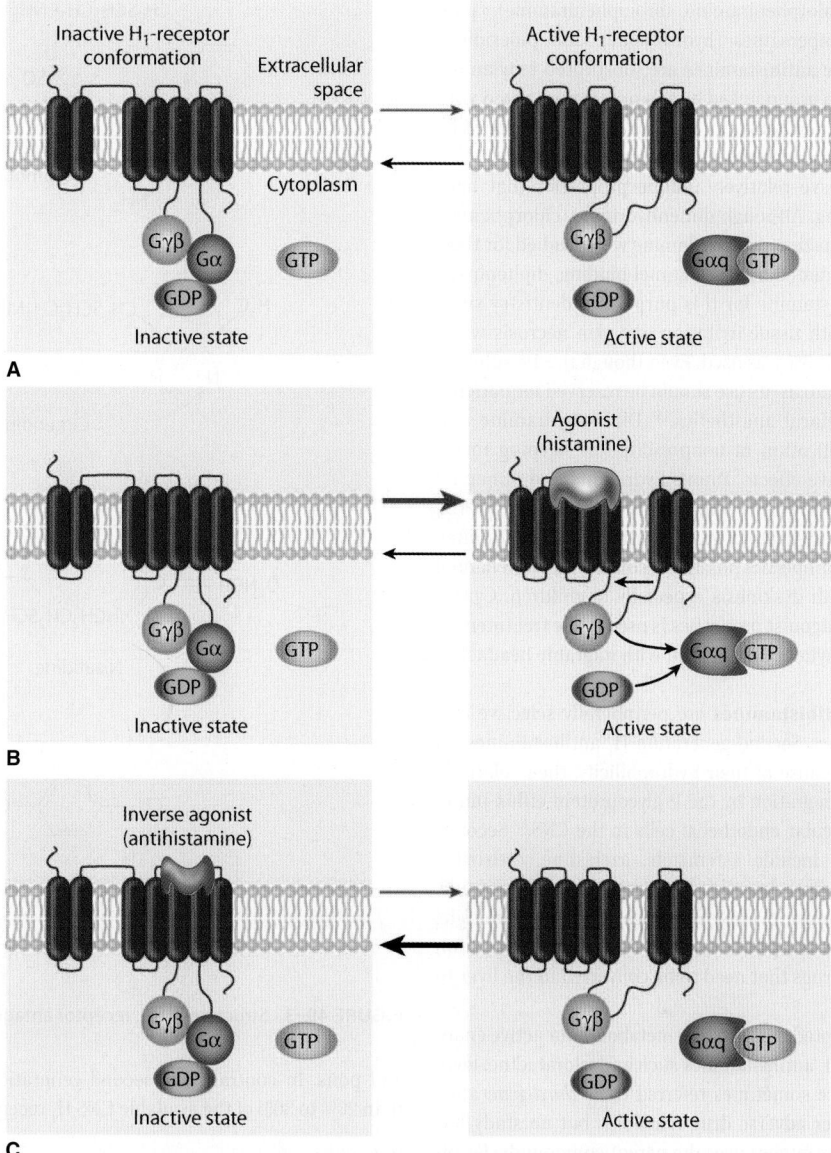

FIGURE 49-2. Action of histamine and antihistamines on the H_1 receptor. *Molecular basis of action of histamine and antihistamines.* (**A**) The inactive state of the histamine H_1 receptor is in equilibrium with the active state. (**B**) The agonist, histamine, has preferential affinity for the active state, stabilizes the receptor in this conformation, and shifts the equilibrium toward the active state. (**C**) An H_1 antihistamine (inverse agonist) has preferential affinity for the inactive state, stabilizes the receptor in this conformation, and shifts the equilibrium toward the inactive state. GDP = guanosine diphosphate; GTP = guanosine triphosphate. *(Reproduced with permission from Simons FE, Simons KJ. Histamine and H_1-antihistamines: celebrating a century of progress. J Allergy Clin Immunol. 2011 Dec;128(6):1139-1150.)*

However, for consistency with the medical literature and the current terminology for these xenobiotics, the terms *antihistamine* or *histamine antagonist* rather than *inverse agonist* are used.

H_1 Antihistamines

Antiallergic and antiinflammatory activities of the H_1 antihistamines involve multiple mechanisms. Inhibition of the release of mediators from mast cells or basophils involves a direct inhibitory effect on calcium ion channels, thereby reducing the inward calcium current activated when intracellular stores of calcium are depleted. Inhibition of the expression of cell adhesion molecules and eosinophil chemotaxis involves downregulation of the H_1 receptor–activated nuclear factor (κB), which binds to promoter or enhancer regions of genes that regulate the synthesis of proinflammatory cytokines and adhesion proteins.[150]

Another classification system of H_1 antihistamines stratifies them by sedating properties and ability to cross the blood–brain barrier and refers to them in terms of generations as they appeared into clinical use. Positron

emission tomography (PET) is now the standard method used to assess H_1 receptor occupancy of antihistamines in the CNS.[192]

First-generation H_1 antihistamines readily penetrate the blood–brain barrier and produce CNS effects, including sedation and performance impairment. Central effects of the first-generation H_1 antihistamines likely result from their high lipophilicity or lack of recognition by the P-glycoprotein efflux pump on the luminal surfaces of vascular endothelial cells in the CNS. First-generation H_1 antihistamines also bind to muscarinic, serotonin and to α-adrenergic receptors as well as cardiac ion channels. Their binding to the voltage-gated Na^+ channels produces use-dependent block because of their much higher affinity to the inactivated Na^+ channels, and their binding to the K^+ channels alters repolarization (Chap. 15).[25,150]

Six major classes of H_1 antihistamines are traditionally recognized based on molecular structure. The classes were initially populated by first-generation derivatives of ethylenediamine (mepyramine, tripelennamine), ethanolamine (diphenhydramine, doxylamine, orphenadrine, dimenhydrate), alkylamines (pheniramine, chlorpheniramine, brompheniramine), phenothiazines (promethazine), piperazines (hydroxyzine), and piperidines (azatadine). Many of the classic antihistamines are substituted ethylamine structures with a tertiary amino group linked by a 2- or 3-carbon chain with 2 aromatic groups. This structure differs from histamine by the absence of a primary amino group and the presence of a single aromatic moiety.

Some H_1 antihistamines have relatively unique properties that have led to special uses or marketing. Although dimenhydrinate, chlorpheniramine, cyproheptadine, promethazine, and pyrilamine were studied for their local anesthetic properties mediated by Na^+ channel binding, diphenhydramine is the most used antihistamine for this purpose in dentistry since the 1960s.[92] Concerns arose with tissue irritation and skin necrosis when diphenhydramine hydrochloride 5% was used. Even though the 1% solution produces erythema without necrosis, its use should be reserved for patients truly allergic to conventional local anesthetics.[153] Diphenhydramine and doxylamine find frequent application in nonprescription sleeping medications because of their sedative effects. Diphenhydramine and dimenhydrinate have relatively strong antimuscarinic activity and are used for the management of motion sickness. Oxatomide, a sedating H_1 antihistamine, possesses mast cell–stabilizing properties possibly mediated via Ca^{2+}-channel blockade and is associated with dyskinesia especially in children. Cyproheptadine which has 5-HT_2 antagonist properties is used in the treatment of serotonin toxicity and as prophylaxis for children with migraine headaches (Chap. 69).

Second-generation H_1 antihistamines are peripherally selective and have a higher therapeutic index. Second-generation H_1 antihistamines do not penetrate the CNS well because of their hydrophilicity, their relatively high molecular weight, and recognition by the P-glycoprotein efflux pump on the luminal surfaces of vascular endothelial cells in the CNS.[25] Second-generation H_1 antihistamines include astemizole, azelastine, cetirizine, ebastine, ketotifen, levocabastine, loratadine, mizolastine, olopatadine, and terfenadine. They have lower binding affinities for the cholinergic, α-adrenergic, and β-adrenergic receptor sites than do the first-generation antihistamines. Many are prodrugs that need to be converted in the liver to water-soluble metabolites.

Although not officially accepted terminology, metabolites or active enantiomers of second-generation H_1 antihistamines such as desloratadine, levocetirizine, and fexofenadine are sometimes referred to as *third-generation antihistamines*. They have fewer adverse drug reactions, but no study has confirmed their therapeutic advantages over the parent compounds. Fexofenadine, however, does not have the cardiac toxicity of its parent drug terfenadine. In a test of wheal suppression, which correlates better to receptor occupancy than plasma concentrations, fexofenadine had the earliest onset of action, and levocetirizine showed maximal inhibition at 3 and 6 hours.[57]

Cautious prescribing practices lead to a preference for second-generation H_1 antihistamines in patients whose activities are "safety critical" and would be affected by any psychomotor impairment (eg, those who operate motor vehicles).[64,103] In a randomized placebo-controlled driving simulator trial, 60 mg of fexofenadine did not interfere with driving performance. However, 50 mg of diphenhydramine produced poorer driving performance than ethanol (100 mg/dL). Of note, subjective feelings of drowsiness were not predictors of impairment.[185] Despite these findings, care must be exercised in the selection and use of second-generation H_1 antihistamines because some subjective or objective sedation still results from their use, especially if higher-than-recommended dosages are taken, and particularly with cetirizine.[38,138] Furthermore, a meta-analysis suggested that the differentiation between sedating and nonsedating H_1 antihistamines is subtle, with some studies lacking the methodology to correctly distinguish between medication adverse effects and the signs and symptoms of the condition being treated.[12,164] Overall, the relative incidence of anticholinergic and CNS adverse effects caused by second-generation H_1 antihistamines are similar to that produced by placebo.[38] Using recommended doses of antihistamines, PET scanning shows that first-generation antihistamines occupy more than 70% of the H_1 receptors in the frontal cortex, temporal cortex, hippocampus,

Famotidine

Cimetidine

Nizatidine

Ranitidine

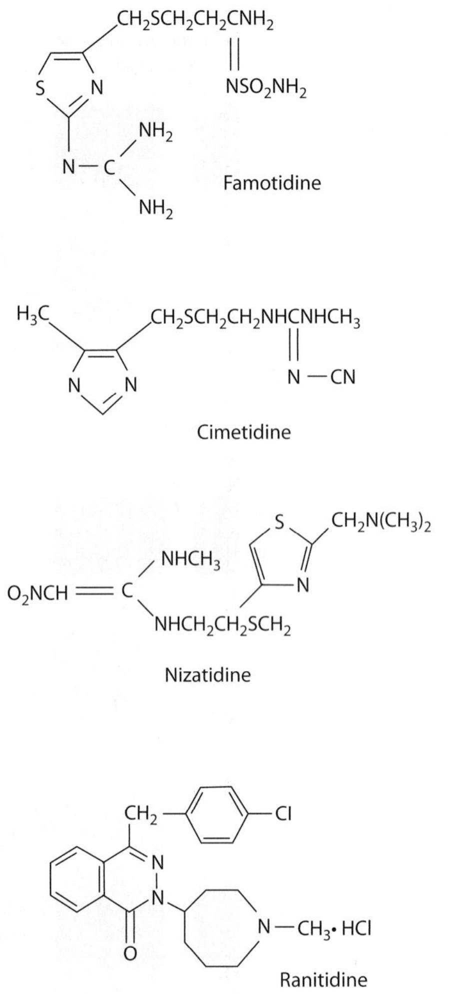

FIGURE 49–3. Structures of H_2 receptor antagonists.

and pons. In contrast, the second-generation antihistamines occupy less than 20% to 30% of the available CNS H_1 receptors.[163,164]

H_2 Antihistamines

These structural analogs of histamine are highly selective inhibitors of the H_2 receptor site. Cimetidine is the original antihistamine in this class; it includes the imidazole ring of histamine (Fig. 49–3). Although ranitidine and famotidine have a furan (ranitidine) or thiazole (famotidine) group instead, they retain significant structural similarity to histamine.

The effectiveness of H_2 antihistamines in the treatment of diseases caused by excessive gastric acid secretion is improved further by their concomitant alteration in the response of parietal cells to acetylcholine and gastrin, 2 other stimulants for gastric acid secretion (Fig. 49–4). Of note, H_2 antihistamines have little pharmacologic effect elsewhere in the body, and they have weak CNS penetration secondary to their hydrophilic properties.

H_3 Antihistamines

These xenobiotics are the focus of much research; however, none is currently commercially available.[194] Some prototypical drugs include ciproxifan, clobenpropit, pitolisant, and thioperamide. This category is further divided into the imidazole-based and non–imidazole-based series.[174] Because of nootropic (cognitive enhancement) and stimulant effects, it is suggested that H_3 antihistamines might play a future role in the treatment of attention deficit and hyperactivity disorder, narcolepsy, depression, or dementia. Pitolisant was granted orphan drug status in the European Union and United States. Its benefit in the treatment of narcolepsy is contested, and it is currently in clinical trials for Parkinson disease and schizophrenia.[143] Conessine, a herbal used in Ayurvedic medicine for dysentery, is also a selective H_3 antihistamine.[55,139]

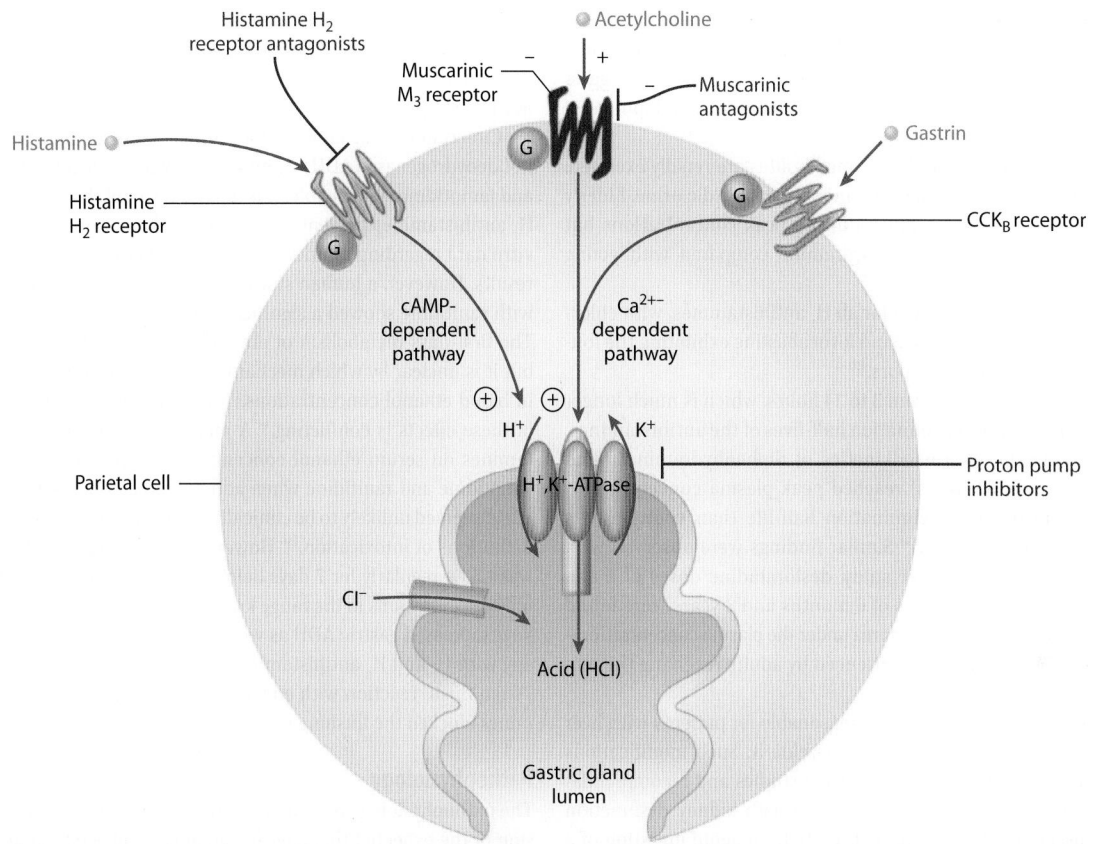

FIGURE 49–4. Schematic representation of a gastric parietal cell demonstrating the mechanism of hydrogen ion secretion into the lumen. Gastric acid is modulated by both the calcium-dependent and cyclic adenosine monophosphate (cAMP)–dependent pathway. Histamine binding to the H_2 receptor increases gastric acidity by increasing cAMP. Both acetylcholine and gastrin increase gastric acidity by increasing the influx of calcium. Whereas acetylcholine binds at the muscarinic 3 (M_3) receptor, gastrin binds the cholecystokinin B (CCK_B) receptor.

H_4 Antihistamines

No xenobiotics of this class are currently commercially available. Because of their association with mast cells and eosinophils, clinical trials of H_4 antagonists are studying their potential therapeutic benefit in the treatment of allergic rhinitis, asthma, and autoimmune disorders. The compounds with the most published information are JNJ 397588979 and JNJ 38518168, with efficacy in preclinical models of pruritus, dermatitis, asthma, and arthritis. Toreforant (JNJ 38518168) a histamine H_4 receptor antagonists showed promised in phase II studies in patients with rheumatoid arthritis treated with methotrexate.[167]

Atypical Antihistamines

Other xenobiotics are named atypical antihistamines because of their inhibitory effect on the enzyme histidine decarboxylase, which catalyzes the transformation of histidine to histamine as opposed to action on the H_1 receptor. Tritoqualine has been commercially available in Europe since the 1960s and is used for persistent allergic rhinitis.[126] To date, no case report of overdose with atypical antihistamines are published.

Pharmacokinetics and Toxicokinetics

H_1 Antihistamines

Absorption. The H_1 antihistamines are generally well absorbed after oral administration, and most achieve peak plasma concentrations within 2 to 3 hours. Although less well studied, dermal absorption appears to be consequential, especially with extensive or prolonged application to abnormal skin.[169] The maximum antihistaminic effect occurs several hours after peak serum concentrations. In supratherapeutic or overdose circumstances, absorption is often prolonged by the antimuscarinic effect on the GI tract.

Although ingestion is the usual route of exposure, rare cases of topical preparations containing diphenhydramine and promethazine cause agitation attributed to anticholinergic toxicity in children. Blood concentrations in these patients are often above the peak therapeutic concentration of 0.06 mg/L.[50,73,142,147,190] Many cases were associated with concomitant varicella infection, blurring the causality of the clinical findings attributed to topical diphenhydramine alone. Lumbar punctures were not done to exclude encephalitis, but symptoms improved with cessation of diphenhydramine. Several cases occurred after a bath, calling into question the role of peripheral vasodilation in increasing dermal absorption. Some patients had concomitant oral diphenhydramine therapy but none exceeding the recommended dose of 5 mg/kg/day. One death solely after exposure to topical diphenhydramine is reported in a child with eczema.[169] All cases of topical antihistamine-induced toxicity involved administration covering a significant body surface area of abnormal skin.

Distribution. Antihistamines are typically lipid soluble with variable octanol/water partition coefficients. They are also highly bound to plasma protein in therapeutic concentrations. The saturability of protein binding in toxic concentrations is largely unknown. The average volume of distribution is between 0.5 and 12 L/kg but extends to 30 L/kg with desloratadine.

Metabolism. Hepatic metabolism is the primary route of metabolism for antihistamines.[122] Cetirizine, fexofenadine, and levocetirizine are exceptions. A poor metabolizer phenotype of desloratadine is identified in both children and adults. In these individuals, the apparent half-life of desloratadine is 50 hours or more compared with the average population whose half-life is around 26 hours.[129] This variability does not appear to impact the safety profile of desloratadine. Many Asian patients acetylate therapeutic concentrations of diphenhydramine to a nontoxic metabolite twice as rapidly as Caucasian patients, making Asians much less sensitive to both the psychomotor and sedative effects.[159] Results of a study of 100 patients in a sample of 2074 antihistamine users reporting excessive daytime sleepiness after use of H_1 antihistamines (predominantly chlorpheniramine) suggest that the presence of the CYP2D6*10 allele is a risk factor for development of H_1 antihistamine–induced adverse drug reactions.[140]

Excretion. All antihistamines and their metabolites are renally excreted. Moreover, chlorpheniramine elimination is increased in acidic urine. Elderly adults (mean age, 69 years) had similar time to peak concentrations but longer elimination half-lives of diphenhydramine compared with young adults.[152]

Elimination half-life is quite varied for all H_1 antihistamines, with chlorpheniramine, hydroxyzine, azelastine, and levocabastine exhibiting the longest termination half-lives up to 24 hours.[150]

The duration of action ranges from 3 to 24 hours, which is much longer than predicted from the serum elimination half-lives of the antihistamines. One study addressing the pharmacokinetics of diphenhydramine found that children (mean age, 8.9 years) reached peak plasma concentrations faster and had a shorter mean elimination half-life than young adults for the same dosage per kilogram.[150] Similar findings were observed with hydroxyzine.[151] In another volunteer study, desloratadine doses of 1 and 1.25 mg in children between the ages of 6 months and 2 years were found to provide a single-dose target exposure (area under the plasma concentration–time curve) comparable with that experienced by adults receiving the recommended 5-mg dose.[58]

Modifications in therapeutic doses are reasonable for patients with liver or kidney dysfunction, young people, and the elderly. Such modifications often must be made empirically because formal studies and recommendations for many xenobiotics are lacking. Patients with kidney dysfunction are likely more susceptible to developing toxicity from acute ingestion of a second-generation antihistamine, and dose adjustment is recommended for cetirizine, desloratadine, fexofenadine, levocetirizine, and loratadine.[33]

Drug interactions. Recognized pharmacokinetic drug interactions involving the H_1 antihistamines are generally caused by modulation of CYP450 metabolism (most often CYP2D6 or CYP3A4) or via interference with active transport mechanisms such as P-glycoprotein or organic anion transporter polypeptide (OATP). The currently available second-generation H_1 antihistamines undergo fewer clinically relevant pharmacokinetic interactions than the first-generation H_1 antihistamines.[9,40]

H_2 Antihistamines

Absorption. Cimetidine is rapidly and completely absorbed after oral administration, but only 40% to 50% of ranitidine and famotidine are bioavailable with a peak concentration within 3 hours. All have reduced absorption when administered concomitantly with food.

Distribution. Cimetidine has a volume of distribution of approximately 2 L/kg. Famotidine and ranitidine have a variable volume of distribution in different age groups ranging from 1 to 4 L/kg. All have protein binding in the range of 15% to 25%.

Metabolism. Cimetidine has some hepatic metabolism (15%), but ranitidine and famotidine do not (<5%).

Excretion. Up to 70% of ranitidine is eliminated unchanged in the urine, and 10% is eliminated unchanged in the stool. Famotidine and cimetidine are also primarily renally excreted. Kidney excretion is lower for oral than for IV administration.

Elimination half-life. The elimination half-life in patients with normal kidney function is approximately 2 hours, but the half-life is substantially prolonged with impaired renal function (up to 10 hours) and in elderly adults (4 hours).

Interactions. Cimetidine is responsible for numerous drug–drug interactions because it inhibits cytochrome P450 activity, thereby impairing hepatic drug metabolism. It also reduces hepatic blood flow, resulting in decreased clearance of drugs that are highly extracted by the liver. None of the other currently available H_2 antihistamines inhibit the cytochrome P450 oxidase system.[105] Additionally, by altering gastric pH, cimetidine and all of the other

H_2 antagonists potentially alter the absorption of acid-labile xenobiotics. Finally, cimetidine and ranitidine are associated with myelosuppression, particularly when administered with xenobiotics capable of causing bone marrow suppression.[7]

Cimetidine is an inhibitor of ethanol-oxidizing activity of gastric alcohol dehydrogenase (ADH) in human enzymes, but inhibition by nizatidine and famotidine is negligible. It is likely a result of the thiazole group of these H_2 antihistamines preventing binding to the enzymatic substrate site.[160] In vitro data regarding ranitidine inhibition of gastric ADH yielded conflicting results. However, a human study comparing oral versus IV ethanol kinetics with ranitidine showed a significant reduction in first-pass metabolism.[19,65] The first-pass metabolism of ethanol is influenced by the gastric mucosa, but it is unclear by which mechanisms ranitidine might influence increases in blood ethanol concentrations.[118] The literature on the clinical relevance of these effects is conflicting.[18] A meta-analysis of the effect of H_2 antihistamines on serum ethanol concentrations reported small elevations with cimetidine and ranitidine when administered concurrently, but the overall effect seemed unlikely to be clinically significant related to the accepted legal definitions of intoxication.[186] However, a subsequent study when ranitidine was taken regularly for 7 days before drinking demonstrated elevated ethanol concentrations in the range known to impair driving skills.[5] Many Asians have increased gastric ADH as well as decreased ALDH-2.[119] Combined therapy with H_1 and H_2 antihistamines were investigated as a treatment for the "Asian flush" reaction with encouraging results. However, only H_2 antihistamines blocked the flushing reaction[110] (Table 49–1).

Pathophysiology

The pathophysiology of acute H_1 antihistamine overdose is largely an extension of the expected therapeutic and adverse effects. These effects are best classified in broad categories according to the type of receptors involved. Acute H_2 antihistamine toxicity is explained by a loss of selectivity for the gastric H_2 receptor and inhibition of the cardiac H_2 receptors responsible for positive chronotropy and inotropy.[84,189]

The pathophysiology of H_1 antihistamine abuse is thought to be multifactorial. Humans are reported to abuse dimenhydrinate and diphenhydramine for their euphoric and hallucinogenic effects as well as for their reported anxiolytic and anticholinergic properties.[61] Recreational ingestion up to 5 g is reported, although most common recreational doses used to experience euphoria and hallucinations average 1 g.[60] Promethazine often combined with codeine is widely abused in certain demographic groups.

However, animal studies of self-administration and conditioned place preferences suggest that antihistamines also have a rewarding potential independent of its euphoric effects, which increases with use. Dimenhydrinate abuse is linked to the stimulant effect of the 8-chlorotheophylline component but alone does not produce rewarding effects. However, diphenhydramine antagonizes muscarinic receptors, modulates serotonin function, enhances dopamine concentrations, and potentiates opioid receptors. It is now thought that the combination of diphenhydramine and the methylxanthine (8-chlorotheophylline) as in dimenhydrinate has a synergistic effect on the rewarding potential.[60] The dose–response for this to occur in humans remains to be studied. Older antihistamines such as chlorpheniramine are also selective serotonin receptor inhibitors, which might explain their nonmedical use (Table 49–2).[63]

Clinical Manifestations

H_1 Antihistamines

The toxic doses for each antihistamine are not well defined. The commonly cited threshold of toxicity of 3 to 5 times the therapeutic dose for first-generation antihistamines as well as cetirizine, loratadine, and fexofenadine originating from algorithms in various articles is not validated.[165] Extrapolating plasma concentrations to an ingested dose is not accurate in predicting clinical effects for diphenhydramine and doxylamine.[89,90] A dose-dependent relationship for diphenhydramine toxicity was published, indicating a high risk of seizures with ingestions above 1.5 g in adults.[130]

TABLE 49–1	Pharmacokinetics Properties of Commonly Used Antihistamines in the United States						
Antihistamine		Half-Life (h)[b]	Duration of Action (h)[a]	Hepatic Metabolism	Log D[c]	V_d (L/kg)[b]	Urinary Elimination (%)
H₁ antihistamines First-generation	Chlorpheniramine	12–43 (urine pH dependent)	24	Yes	1.13	5–7	30
	Cyproheptadine	N/A	4–6	Yes	4.93	N/A	72
	Diphenhydramine	3–14	12	Yes	1.92	3–4	4
	Doxylamine	10–11	N/A	Yes	1.15	2.7	N/A
	Hydroxyzine	13–27	24	Yes	2.21	13–31	15
	Promethazine	9–16	4–6	Yes	2.73	9–19	<1
Second-generation	Cetirizine	6.5–10	12–24	<40%	−0.02	0.58	70
	Desloratadine	21–27	>24	Yes	2.95	10–30	41
	Fexofenadine	9–20	12–24	<8%	2.68	12	11
	Levocetirizine	N/A	>24	<15%	−0.83	0.41	85
	Loratadine	3–20	24	Yes	6.23	26–32	
H₂ antihistamines	Cimetidine	2	6–10			1.4	35–60
	Ranitidine	2.1	12			1.6–2.4	69
	Nizatidine	1.3	24	Yes	N/A	1.2–1.8	61
	Famotidine	2.6	12			0.9–1.4	67

[a]Brunton LB, et al., eds: *Goodman & Gilman's The Pharmacological Basis of Therapeutics*. 11th ed. New York: McGraw-Hill; 2005. [b]Baselt RC. *Disposition of Toxic Drugs and Chemicals in Man*. 7th ed. Foster City, CA: Biomedical Publications; 2004. [c]Log D is the octanol/water partition coefficient at a pH of 7.

V_d = volume of distribution.

Data from Wilson CO, Beale JM, Block JH. *Wilson and Gisvold's Textbook of Organic Medicinal and Pharmaceutical Chemistry*, 12th ed. Baltimore, MD: Lippincott Williams & Wilkins; 2011.

Neurologic. Acute overdose of first-generation H₁ antihistamine usually results in the onset of toxicity within 2 hours. Dose–response effects account for the wide spectrum of altered mental status observed. Drowsiness that occurs in milder poisoning rapidly progresses to obtundation and seizures with larger ingestions. Compared with adults, children more commonly present with excitation, irritability, or ataxia as well as being more prone to having hallucinations or seizures.[8] Patients typically exhibit an anticholinergic syndrome, including mydriasis, tachycardia, hyperthermia, dry mucous membranes, urinary retention, diminished bowel sounds, and altered mental status such as disorientation and hallucinations. The skin appears flushed,

TABLE 49–2	Effects of H₁ Antihistamines		
Effects	Clinical Result	First Generation	Second Generation
Mast cell histamine inhibition	Decreased itching Decreased vascular permeability Vasodilation	Therapeutic	Therapeutic
Calcium channel blockade	Decreased mediator release	Therapeutic	Therapeutic
CNS antihistamine receptor occupancy	Sedation Impaired psychomotor performance	Marked effect in therapeutic and overdose	Minimal or no effect reported with cetirizine in overdose
CNS serotonin receptor antagonism	Increased appetite Weight gain	Occurs in therapeutic doses; no significance in overdose	No effect
Peripheral muscarinic receptor antagonism	Dry mucosa Decreased peristalsis Urinary retention Sinus tachycardia Mydriasis	Marked effect in overdose; minimal effect can occur at therapeutic doses	Minimal or no effect
Central muscarinic receptor antagonism	Agitation Delirium Hallucinations	Marked effect in overdose	No effect
α-Adrenergic receptors	Dizziness Hypotension	Marked effect in overdose; minimal effect can occur at therapeutic doses	No effect
Cardiac sodium and potassium channel blockers	Prolonged QRS complex Prolonged QT interval	Marked effect in overdose on Na⁺ channel	Minimal or no effect at therapeutic doses except terfenadine, astemizole on K⁺ channel

CNS = central nervous system.

warm, and dry. Hyperthermia occurs in severe cases and correlates with the extent of agitation, ambient temperature and humidity, and length of time during which the patient cannot dissipate heat because of anticholinergic-mediated reduction in sweating (Chap. 29).

Some patients with high therapeutic dosing or after overdose develop a central anticholinergic syndrome in which CNS anticholinergic effects, such as hallucinations, outlast peripheral anticholinergic effects. At a later stage of ingestion the lack of tachycardia, skin changes, or other peripheral anticholinergic manifestations complicates establishment of the correct diagnosis for antihistamine poisoned patients unless there is a clear exposure history.[56,184] Ingestion of second-generation H$_1$ or H$_2$ antihistamines usually does not result in significant CNS depression or anticholinergic effects except perhaps in pediatric patients or in adults with altered pharmacokinetic parameters. Although dry mouth and mydriasis are common adverse therapeutic effects, sedation is of the greatest concern.

Seizures occur at any point in time in the course of the poisoning but typically begin in the first few hours and represent severe toxicity. Chlorpheniramine is both a serotonin reuptake inhibitor and a postsynaptic 5-HT$_{1A}$ and 5-HT$_{2A}$ receptor agonist.[79] Agonism of 5-HT receptors is associated with seizures. All first-generation H$_1$ antihistamines produce seizures, although pheniramine seems to be more proconvulsant than others.[21] Up to 22% of drug-induced seizures in children are related to an antihistamine exposure, and diphenhydramine is a common cause of recreational drug–induced seizures.[1,52,166]

Mydriasis develops at both therapeutic and toxic doses, with most patients describing blurred vision or diplopia. Both vertical and horizontal nystagmus occur in patients with diphenhydramine overdose.[48]

In a review of 136 patients with diphenhydramine overdose, somnolence, lethargy, or coma occurred in approximately 55% of patients, and 15% experienced a catatonic stupor.[89] Several reports suggest that young children experience more respiratory complications, CNS stimulation, anticholinergic effects, and seizures than do adults.[115] In a placebo-controlled study comparing the CNS effects of the first- and second-generation H$_1$ antihistamines, the second-generation antihistamines caused less cognitive dysfunction and somnolence.[38,70] This finding was corroborated in the simulated driving model in which loratadine produced significantly less impairment than diphenhydramine.[64] Use of diphenhydramine compared with loratadine in a work setting results in significantly higher injury rates.[51] Observational postmarketing cohort studies conducted in England on large numbers of patients reported rates of sedation or drowsiness of fewer than 1% for desloratadine and levocetirizine.[95,96]

Cardiovascular. Sinus tachycardia is a consistent finding after overdose with an H$_1$ antihistamine with anticholinergic effects and can persist after other toxic manifestations and delirium have resolved. Both hypotension and hypertension occur.[100] These findings probably relate more to the patient's age, volume status, and vascular tone than to a specific class of antihistamines. Binding to cardiac ion channels results in prolongation of both the QRS complexes and QT intervals and are reported with most first-generation H$_1$ antihistamines at doses that are supratherapeutic.[27,92] Brugada-pattern electrocardiographic (ECG) changes are also reported.[99,193]

Cardiotoxicity observed with terfenadine and astemizole resulted from accumulation of the parent drug in cardiac tissue after inhibition of drug elimination (eg, terfenadine–ketoconazole interaction) and was potentially exacerbated by electrolyte (eg, Ca^{2+}) imbalances or concomitant use of another ion channel blocker.[13,69] Terfenadine and astemizole are no longer approved for use in the United States and many other countries. Second-generation H$_1$ antihistamines currently available are less dysrhythmogenic.[66,128] Rare cases of QT interval prolongation are reported in therapeutic situations but the incidence of dysrhythmias with second-generation H$_1$ antihistamines in overdose is unknown.[3] One study reported 6 cases of patients taking amiodarone with loratadine who presented with episodes of torsade de pointes and syncope. Amiodarone accumulation is reported with co-treatment with loratadine, and all patients made a full recovery after loratadine was stopped. Loratadine accumulation via CYP3A4 inhibition by amiodarone is

the mechanism suspected to explain this occurrence.[4] Prolongation of the QT interval is reported with cetirizine (mainly with kidney failure or large ingestions), but no cases are published with desloratadine or levocetirizine.[3]

Other. Rhabdomyolysis occurs in patients with extreme agitation or seizures after an H$_1$ antihistamine overdose.[53] Rhabdomyolysis is commonly noted in patients who overdose with doxylamine even in the absence of trauma or other common etiologies such as seizures, shock, or crush injuries. The mechanism remains undefined. A prospective study found that 87% of patients who ingested more than 20 mg/kg of doxylamine developed rhabdomyolysis, and this dose was the best predictor of this complication.[76] Another retrospective review found a dose of more than 13 mg/kg to be the only predictive factor of doxylamine-induced rhabdomyolysis.[86] Rhabdomyolysis is reported as a rare adverse event after diphenhydramine overdose.[47] One case of compartment syndrome following ingestion of diphenhydramine alone is published.[179] This complication more commonly occurs in association with other factors such as ethanol intoxication or immobilization. Creatine phosphokinase concentrations are reported as high as 262,000 IU/L without seizure activity.[42,47,85]

Unless complications such as aspiration or kidney failure develop, most patients are symptomatic for 24 to 48 hours with resolution of cardiac symptoms occurring before neurologic recovery. Anticholinergic delirium and residual sinus tachycardia can last a few days, but generally neither requires cardiac monitoring in intensive care settings. Other adverse effects that mostly occur in therapeutic use include pancytopenia and cholestatic jaundice (cetirizine), fixed-drug rash, urticaria, photosensitivity, hyperthermia, elevated aminotransferases, or agranulocytosis. Hypersensitivity reactions to antihistamines are exceptionally rare but are reported.[39] Postmortem findings are generally limited to pulmonary and visceral congestion, suggesting cardiogenic causes of death.[80]

Special populations. Elderly patients are more susceptible to adverse events because kidney and liver dysfunction delay antihistamine metabolism.[70] All H$_1$ antihistamines cross the placenta, and some are teratogenic in animals. First- and second-generation antihistamines fall into FDA categories B and C and should be individually addressed, avoiding or minimizing exposure when possible (Chap. 30). Because of their antimuscarinic effects, the first-generation antihistamines are generally contraindicated in patients with glaucoma or benign prostatic hypertrophy.

H$_2$ Antihistamines

These xenobiotics are well tolerated in overdose even after large ingestions. Patients uncommonly develop tachycardia, dilated and sluggishly reactive pupils, slurred speech, and confusion.[158,175] In a retrospective study of acute cimetidine overdoses, 8.9% of patients had symptoms related to the ingestion, and those with reported moderate medical outcomes had ingested cimetidine with suicidal intent. Severe dysrhythmias, including ventricular fibrillation and bradycardia leading to fatal cardiac arrest are reported following rapid IV infusion of cimetidine.[146] Deaths are reported in rare instances of large ingestion of cimetidine.[87]

Famotidine and ranitidine produce even fewer dose-related toxicities in overdose. In addition, they are less likely than cimetidine to induce or inhibit the CYP enzyme system, thereby producing fewer drug–drug interactions.[72]

Diagnostic Testing

The bedside diagnosis of antihistamine toxicity is a clinical one. Antihistamines cause false-positive results on several rapid urine drug screens by immunoassay for amphetamines (ranitidine), methadone (diphenhydramine, doxylamine), and phencyclidine (diphenhydramine, doxylamine). Cyproheptadine, diphenhydramine, and hydroxyzine also produce false-positive results to tricyclic antidepressants (TCAs) in serum immunoassays only.[162] Such results are of concern, particularly in children, and should always be confirmed if malicious intent is suspected.[136]

Comprehensive blood or urine analysis screening with liquid chromatography/mass spectroscopy (LC/MS) or gas chromatography/mass spectroscopy (GC/MS) provides antihistamine concentrations, but these are more useful in medicolegal or forensic situations. The turn-around time usually needed is unlikely to provide results at the time of initial assessment. Moreover, treatment is based on alleviation or correction of toxic signs or symptoms and should not depend on a concentration result that does not correlate with toxicity.[85,89,90] Measurement of antihistamine concentrations in body fluids is not readily available and is generally unnecessary for clinical assessment and management.

Several publications estimate the toxic diphenhydramine concentration in children to be approximately 5 mg/L. Fatal antihistamine concentrations are reported with great variability. However, as occurs in adults, toxic effects and fatalities are reported with lower concentrations. Considering diphenhydramine is subject to postmortem redistribution, it would be prudent to obtain blood samples as soon as possible to aid in determining the cause of death in fatalities involving these xenobiotics.[8]

Management
General Management
The initial management of a given exposure should begin with a consultation with a poison control center. Guidelines are published and validated with regard to the evidence-based out-of-hospital management of diphenhydramine and dimenhydrinate exposure and allow for home observation for any ingestion under 7.5 mg/kg in children younger than 6 years or under 300 mg or 7.5 mg/kg for adults and older children.[11,141] Other criteria for medical evaluation for other antihistamines vary according to local practices, but in general, ingestions of less than 5 times the maximal therapeutic dose is rarely toxic.

Patients presenting to hospitals after exposure of any antihistamine must be triaged and medically assessed quickly, generally within 30 minutes of arrival, because those who will develop severe complications are initially indistinguishable from those who will have a benign course, and the window for GI decontamination may soon elapse.

The individual should be attached to a cardiac monitor and observed for signs of Na^+ channel blockade (increased QRS complex duration), potassium channel blockade (prolonged QT interval), and related dysrhythmias, as well as for seizures. Intravenous access should be established and airway protection ensured.

Gastrointestinal decontamination is recommended with care to avoid aspiration in patients with large ingestions of first-generation H_1 antihistamines or early presentations but is generally not needed for H_2 antihistamines. The use of oral activated charcoal (AC), although more effective if administered early with regard to time of ingestion, is reasonable even after a delay for ingestion of large amounts that might reduce absorption time. Multiple-dose AC or whole-bowel irrigation (WBI) is usually not indicated. Neostigmine administration was used with success in drug-induced ileus, thus facilitating gut decontamination, but there is not enough evidence to routinely recommend this at the current time.[24]

Enhanced elimination techniques do not benefit the toxicity of these xenobiotics because of their large volumes of distribution, extensive protein binding, and absence of enterobiliary circulation. However, exceptional case reports are published using hemoperfusion and hemodialysis with resolution of the dysrhythmias previously unresponsive to treatment. These patients had ingested 20 mg/kg (adult) and 50 mg/kg (child) of diphenhydramine. All cases reported diphenhydramine concentrations in the fatal range. The mechanism proposed to explain these recoveries is that removal of diphenhydramine from the toxic compartment during extracorporeal treatment might have been enough to improve the distributive shock suspected to be from α-adrenergic blockade.[106,114,181] Unfortunately, no clearance data, only blood concentrations before and after dialysis, are reported, thus making conclusions on the efficacy of enhanced removal debatable and not recommended.

Assessment of the serum acetaminophen concentration is important because of its inclusion in many cough and cold products. Other laboratory studies should be obtained as indicated by history or physical signs and symptoms. Kidney function and creatine kinase should be obtained on

all patients, particularly in patients with seizures or doxylamine overdose. Serum pregnancy tests should be obtained in women of childbearing age. An ECG should be obtained on all patients during the initial assessment and repeated at regular intervals, particularly if physostigmine use is considered. Continuous ECG monitoring is preferable for high-risk patients such as those with altered mental status or large ingestions.

The patient's vital signs and mental status must be monitored. Serial assessments of the patient's vital signs, particularly temperature, and mental status should be made. The potential for clinical deterioration necessitates management of symptomatic patients in a monitored environment.

Specific Treatments
Sedation can increase the risk for aspiration. Intubation to secure the airway is recommended when excessive sedation compromises ventilation.

Seizures should be treated with an IV benzodiazepine such as 2 to 4 mg (0.05–0.1 mg/kg in children) of lorazepam, 2 to 5 mg (0.02 mg/kg in children) of midazolam, or 10 mg (0.2–0.5 mg/kg in children) of diazepam with repeated dosing as necessary.[49,75] Hypertonic saline (3%) was shown to be effective in diphenhydramine-induced seizures in an animal model, but there is not enough evidence to routinely recommend this at the current time.[68] Recurrent seizures refractory to benzodiazepines or hypertonic sodium bicarbonate (see below) should be treated with propofol or general anesthesia. Phenytoin use is discouraged as in most toxicologic-induced seizures.

Hypotension generally responds to isotonic fluids (0.9% sodium chloride solution or lactated Ringer solution). If the desired increase in blood pressure is not attained, hypertonic sodium bicarbonate therapy or vasopressors should be titrated to achieve an acceptable blood pressure. In one instance, cardiogenic shock and myocardial depression resulting from a 10-g ingestion of pyrilamine could only be reversed with an intraaortic balloon counterpulsation device.[54] This approach should rarely be needed.

The Na^+ channel blockade (type IA antidysrhythmic) properties of diphenhydramine and other antihistamines leads to wide-complex dysrhythmias that resemble those that occur after cyclic antidepressant overdose (Chap. 68). Hypertonic sodium bicarbonate reverses diphenhydramine or other antihistamine-associated conduction abnormalities (Antidotes in Depth: A5).[27,49,75,145]

Type IA (quinidine, procainamide, disopyramide), IC (flecainide), and III (amiodarone, sotalol) antidysrhythmics are contraindicated because of their capacity to prolong the QRS complex and the QT interval. The successful use of IV lipid emulsion is reported in several case reports, but its efficacy is debated because of other reports with no change in the patient's clinical condition. Because of the current equipoise in its possible efficacy and known adverse effects, its use is reasonable in cases of cardiovascular compromise refractory to standard treatments. The use of lipid emulsion is explained in more detail in another chapter (Antidotes in Depth: A23).

Rhabdomyolysis-associated nephrotoxicity should be prevented by early use of IV fluid, NaCl 0.9%, to produce a urine output of 1 to 3 mL/kg/h. Once established, antihistamine-induced rhabdomyolysis is treated with IV fluids.[121] Although urinary alkalinization is reportedly helpful to prevent myoglobin-induced nephrotoxicity, its usefulness is controversial and might be best reserved when urinary pH is lower than 6.5 (Antidotes in Depth: A5).[26] Serum potassium concentration and ECGs should be obtained to exclude significant hyperkalemia from muscle injury or acute kidney injury. Initial hypocalcemia caused by precipitation of phosphate from muscle breakdown should not be replaced unless dangerously low because calcium redistributes into the circulation in later phases.[121]

Hyperthermic patients should be monitored for the development of disseminated intravascular coagulation and other complications. Cooling via evaporative methods (tepid mist or cooling blanket or fan) is generally sufficient, but patients with severe hyperthermia should receive more rapid cooling using an ice bath (Chap. 29). The goal is to return the patient to a normothermic state as rapidly as possible. There is insufficient evidence to recommend therapeutic hypothermia in poisoned patients with antihistamines.

Agitation or psychosis generally responds readily to titration of a benzodiazepine. Although most commonly a direct central effect, other frequent causes of agitation such as urinary retention or bright lights shone into dilated eyes unable to react should not be forgotten. Physostigmine effectively reverses the peripheral or central anticholinergic syndrome and is recommended as a benzodiazepine-sparing strategy, but should only be administered after the initial cardiovascular toxicity, if present, has resolved or is no longer a possibility. It should be used with caution in an attempt to reverse coma or sedation caused by anticholinergic toxicity (Antidotes in Depth: A11).

In a retrospective comparison of physostigmine and benzodiazepines, physostigmine was safer and more effective for treating anticholinergic agitation and delirium.[22] Contraindications to physostigmine use include wide QRS complex or bradycardia noted by ECG, asthma, and pulmonary disease. The primary benefits of physostigmine use in patients with antihistamine overdose include restoration of GI motility, elimination of agitation, and possible obviation of the need for computed tomography (CT) scan or lumbar puncture if the patient regains a normal mental status and can provide a clear history. The anticipated benefits of physostigmine must outweigh the potential risks before its use.

Before physostigmine is administered, the patient should be attached to a cardiac monitor, and secure IV access should be established. Physostigmine (1–2 mg in adults; 0.5 mg in children) should be administered by IV bolus over 5 to 10 minutes with continuous monitoring of vital signs, ECG, breath sounds, and oxygen saturation by pulse oximetry. The initial dose of physostigmine can be repeated at 5- to 10-minute intervals if anticholinergic symptoms are not reversed and cholinergic symptoms such as salivation, diaphoresis, bradycardia, lacrimation, urination, or defecation do not develop. When improvement occurs as a result of physostigmine, repeated doses of physostigmine at 30- to 60-minute intervals are often necessary, taking into account the fact metabolism of the offending xenobiotic is occurring and that subsequent doses might need to be lowered to avoid cholinergic symptoms. Another alternative for confirmed central anticholinergic symptoms expected to last many hours could be the administration of oral anticholinesterases such as donepezil, tacrine, or rivastigmine.[37,117] They are noncompetitive reversible anticholinesterases, crossing the blood–brain barrier, with a longer duration of action than physostigmine. Continuous infusion of physostigmine is a reasonable option to reverse symptoms of anticholinergic toxicity but requires constant ICU level monitoring.[124] A dose of IV atropine should be available at the patient's bedside to treat cholinergic toxicity if it occurs. Although benzodiazepines can be used, excessive sedation with repetitive dosing presents undesirable effects.

DECONGESTANTS
History and Epidemiology
History

Decongestants are xenobiotics acting on α-adrenergic receptors, producing vasoconstriction, decreasing edema of mucous membranes, and improving bronchiolar air movement. Ma Huang, the horsetail plant of the Red Emperor, was used in China for at least 2,000 years before it was introduced into Western medicine in the late 19th century by Japanese researchers, who isolated the active ingredient from Ephedra plants. Ephedrine, the first xenobiotic of the sympathomimetic amine class to be used pharmaceutically, was first approved in 1926 by the Council of Pharmacy and Chemistry of the American Medical Association and was very popular in the treatment of asthma. Amphetamines were later synthesized to palliate to a shortage of Ephedra plant availability. Pseudoephedrine is a natural stereoisomer of ephedrine, and phenylephrine was introduced into clinical medicine in the 1930s and in 1949 replaced amphetamines in several compounds. Amphetamine was marketed as nasal decongestant (Benzedrine Inhaler), which was eventually withdrawn in the 1960s because of widespread abuse.

Imidazoline decongestants, on the other hand, were derived from piperazine compounds while investigating their use as uric acid remedies to combat gout. As more imidazolines were synthesized for gout treatment,

one of the compound, tolazoline, was found to have weak adrenergic blocking activity but its naphthyl analogue produced the reverse effect. Naphazoline was introduced in the 1940s as a decongestant. In the decades that followed, many imidazoline decongestants have been developed and tried for clinical use.[156]

Epidemiology

Despite many years of widespread decongestant use in the United States and sporadic case reports of adverse effects, the magnitude and public health significance of adverse effects of this class of medications was only relatively recently appreciated. From 1991 to 2000, the FDA received 22 spontaneous reports of hemorrhagic stroke associated with phenylpropanolamine (PPA) use, and more than 30 other cases were reported in the literature since 1979. Statistical analysis published in 2000 confirmed that PPA is an independent risk factor for hemorrhagic stroke in women.[23,83] The FDA recommended removal of PPA from the market in 2000 because of its association with intracranial hemorrhages. Many manufacturers took steps to remove or reformulate PPA-containing products well before the FDA rule-making process could be completed.

Fatality rates with decongestants suffer from the selection bias of case reporting as well as which xenobiotics are examined. One study addressing the cause of death in children did not include imidazoline derivatives in their search strategy but these xenobiotics might have been included in part of the cases assessed.[34] Despite these biases, studies report a positive association between fatalities in children younger than 2 years and pseudoephedrine-containing cough and cold medications resulting in high pseudoephedrine concentrations. Additional nonfatal adverse events also occurred in the children during that study period.[30]

The majority of reported exposures are unintentional. Data from the 2015 NDPS report shows that only one in 5 cough and cold preparation exposures are intentional.[113] In another study, postmortem analysis of unexpected infant fatalities yielded 10 deaths (ages 17 days–10 months) associated with the use of cough and cold medicines.[134] In response to new information and concerns, the FDA required labeling changes on medications aimed toward young children. In January 2012, the US Consumer Product Safety Commission proposed a new rule requiring child-resistant packaging for any nonprescription drug product containing the equivalent of 0.08 mg or more of an imidazoline in a single package.[172]

Recreational use of ephedrine-containing stimulants is common, and combinations of these xenobiotics with caffeine or other herbs may be marketed as "herbal ecstasy" (Chap. 43). The sale of dietary supplements containing Ephedra, Ma Huang, *Sida cordifolia*, and Pinellia (ephedrine alkaloids) was banned by the FDA in 2004 because of concerns over their cardiovascular effects, including hypertension, seizures, stroke, and dysrhythmias.[59] Companies challenged this rule in court, but it was finally upheld in 2006. Xenobiotics that contain chemically synthesized ephedrine, traditional Chinese herbal remedies, and herbal teas are not covered by the rule. Specific guidelines as to what constitutes a traditional remedy are still unclear and are currently under the FDA dietary supplement category.[171] Since then, many manufacturers have substituted ephedra by *Citrus aurantium*, whose principal ingredient is *p*-synephrine, and are marketing products as being "ephedra free."[133] The FDA ban on sales of ephedra had a significant reduction on the number of calls to poison control centers and in the number of death.[195]

Imidazoline abuse is also associated with strokes, although population incidences are not reported.[97] Of all the decongestants, only ephedrine and pseudoephedrine are on the list of xenobiotics monitored in competitive sports.[191] Phenylephrine and synephrine concentrations in urine are no longer monitored.

The Combat Methamphetamine Epidemic Act signed into law in March 2006 limited methamphetamine precursor availability and additional precautions in pharmacies such as dispensing limits for nonprescription quantities, requesting personal identification, and storage of the medications behind pharmacy counters. This aimed to reduce potential harm associated with these xenobiotics by closing loopholes contained in the

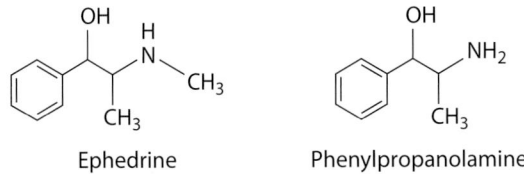

FIGURE 49-5. Structure of ephedrine and phenylpropanolamine decongestants.

TABLE 49-3	Effects of Decongestants		
	Therapeutic	Duration Action (h)	*Toxic*
Imidazolines			
Naphazoline	Nasal decongestant	8	Acute: hypertension followed by hypotension, bradycardia, hypoventilation, hypotonia, CNS depression, hallucinations
Oxymetazoline	Otorrhea reduction	6–7	
Tetrahydrozoline	Nasal decongestant	4–8	
Xylometazoline	Nasal decongestant	5–6	
			Chronic: mydriasis from ocular administration
Sympathomimetic			
Ephedrine	Nasal decongestant	3–5	Hypertension, tachycardia, insomnia, psychosis
Phenylephrine	Nasal decongestant, vasopressor	1	Hypertension, reflex bradycardia
Pseudoephedrine	Nasal decongestant	3–4	Hypertension, tachycardia, insomnia, psychosis

previous regulations.[170] The success of such stricter measures has yet to be quantified.[107,116,136] Travel and Internet purchases being more common, it can also be expected that individuals might present with toxicity from xenobiotics not otherwise available in their countries of residence.

Pharmacology

Decongestants are divided into 2 categories, sympathomimetic amines and imidazolines.

Sympathomimetics

The decongestants phenylephrine, pseudoephedrine, ephedrine, and PPA (Fig. 49–5) reduce nasal congestion by stimulating the α-adrenergic receptor sites on vascular smooth muscle.[77] Both α_1- and α_2-adrenergic receptor subtypes are linked to a Gq protein activating smooth muscle contraction via the IP_3 signal transduction pathway (Fig. 49–6). This process constricts dilated arterioles and reduces blood flow to engorged nasal vascular beds. The α-adrenergic mediated decrease in volume ultimately lowers resistance to airflow. Prolonged topical administration produces rebound congestion upon discontinuation; possible mechanisms include desensitization of receptors and mucosal damage. This damage is caused by α_2-adrenergic–mediated arteriolar constriction, resulting in decreased blood supply to the mucosa.

Phenylephrine is a direct α_1-adrenergic receptor agonist with very little β-adrenergic agonist activity at therapeutic doses. Pseudoephedrine and ephedrine are mixed-acting direct and indirect nonspecific $\alpha_{1,2}$-adrenergic and $\beta_{1,2}$-adrenergic receptor agonists. Pseudoephedrine is the D-isomer of ephedrine and has only up to 25% of the adrenergic receptor activity of ephedrine.[43] Phenylpropanolamine is an $\alpha_{1,2}$-adrenergic receptor agonist devoid of β-adrenergic receptor activity. Phenylpropanolamine both directly stimulates $\alpha_{1,2}$-adrenergic receptors and indirectly stimulates these receptors by causing norepinephrine release.

Imidazolines

The decongestant effects of the imidazoline class of xenobiotics results from their vasoconstrictive action as α-adrenergic agonists, with binding to α_2-adrenergic receptors on blood vessels. In addition, these medications

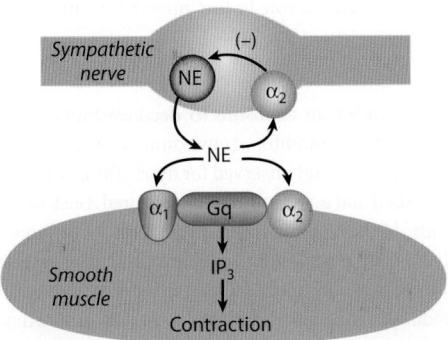

FIGURE 49-6. Mechanism of action of the α-adrenergic decongestants. The α-adrenergic decongestants stimulate postsynaptic α_1- and α_2-adrenergic receptors to increase the concentration of inositol triphosphate (IP_3), which mediates vasoconstriction of blood vessels and reduces swollen mucosa. The imidazoline decongestants also bind to postsynaptic α_2-adrenergic receptors on these blood vessels.

have high affinity for imidazoline receptors, which are located in the ventrolateral medulla and some peripheral tissues. Three classes of imidazoline receptors are recognized. Imidazoline$_1$ (I_1) receptors mediate the inhibitory actions of imidazoline xenobiotics to lower blood pressure. The imidazoline$_2$ (I_2) receptor is an important binding site for monoamine oxidase, and the imidazoline$_3$ (I_3) receptor regulates insulin secretion from pancreatic cells.[62] The imidazoline receptor field is in expansion as more physiological roles are found for these receptors, namely cell proliferation, regulation of body fat, inflammation, pain and opioid addiction, appetite, epilepsy, and neuroprotection. Table 49–3 summarizes the pharmacologic and toxic effect of available decongestants.

The imidazoline (I) category of direct sympathomimetic receptor agonists is generally reserved for topical application. The agonists in this class are used for their local effects in the nasal passages and the eyes. The more common medications include oxymetazoline, tetrahydrozoline, and naphazoline (Fig. 49–7). The α_1-adrenergic–mediated vasoconstriction is complemented by an additive effect of preferential binding to α_2-adrenergic receptors located on resistance vessels regulating blood flow. The imidazoline decongestants such as oxymetazoline and naphazoline are pure central and peripheral α_2-adrenergic receptor agonists; tetrahydrozoline stimulates α_2-adrenergic receptors and H_2 receptors. These medications are primarily used as nasal decongestants. Tetrahydrozoline is available without a prescription as an ophthalmic preparation to decrease conjunctival injection.

Selective α_2-adrenergic receptor agonists acting on nasal veins for decongestant effect are being developed to minimize toxicity and adverse effects associated with current nonselective decongestants affecting nasal veins and arteries.[31]

Pharmacokinetics and Toxicokinetics

Sympathomimetics

Phenylephrine and other decongestants of this class are pharmacologically active after topical or oral administration. Absorption from the GI tract is rapid, with peak blood concentrations occurring within 2 to 4 hours of ingestion. They have variable hepatic metabolism via monoamine oxidase and mainly renal elimination. Children have shorter elimination half-lives of pseudoephedrine than adults at doses under 60 mg. Urinary elimination of pseudoephedrine is pH dependent.[149] Pseudoephedrine is excreted in breast milk, but use during lactation is considered acceptable.

Toxic effects occur at therapeutic dosage in patients with altered pharmacokinetics such as those with end-stage kidney disease. A meta-analysis found a dose–response relationship between blood pressure and

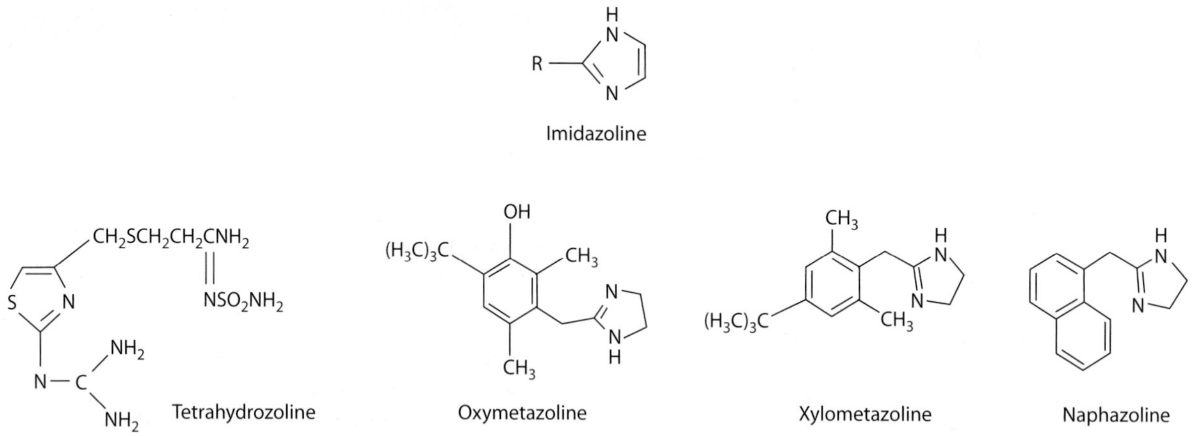

FIGURE 49–7. Structure of imidazoline and the imidazoline decongestants.

pseudoephedrine in therapeutic situations.[137] Toxic symptoms are an extension of the adverse effects and follow a similar dose–response curve.

Imidazolines

The imidazolines are rapidly absorbed from the GI tract and mucous membranes. Despite their use for many decades, their metabolism is poorly studied.[102] Their elimination half-lives are from 2 to 4 hours. All imidazoline preparations have a relatively rapid onset of action, with 60% of maximum effectiveness occurring after only 20 minutes. Oxymetazoline is the only medication with a duration of action more than 8 hours. The other preparations have an average duration of action of approximately 4 hours.

The toxicity of these medications follows a dose–response curve and accentuates the action on receptors. There is no information regarding modification of pharmacokinetics parameters in supratherapeutic conditions.

Pathophysiology

Sympathomimetic

Sympathomimetic decongestants cause their toxic effects via excessive stimulation of the adrenergic system and in effect produce signs and symptoms associated with the sympathomimetic toxidrome. Excessive vasoconstriction can result in end-organ damage to the brain, retina, heart, and kidneys.

Imidazolines

Imidazolines stimulate imidazoline receptors and produce a sympatholytic effect that in supratherapeutic conditions results in marked bradycardia and hypotension.

Clinical Manifestations

Sympathomimetics

Ingestions of less than 1 mg/kg of pseudoephedrine in children are reported to produce almost no toxicity and are generally managed conservatively without the need for hospital evaluation. A study of acute ingestions in children age 6 months to 5 years reported an absence of symptoms at doses lower than 120 mg and lethargy with doses above 360 mg.[188] Following a decongestant overdose of this class, most patients present with a sympathomimetic syndrome with CNS stimulation, hypertension, tachycardia, or reflex bradycardia in response to pure α_1-adrenergic agonist induced hypertension (Chap. 73). Approximately 4 to 5 times the recommended dose of pseudoephedrine is required to cause hypertension.[43,46] An increase in sinus dysrhythmias is reported in adults with ingestion of 120 mg of pseudoephedrine and moderate exercise.[17] Headache was the most common initial symptom (39%) reported by patients who later developed severe toxicity from PPA. In 45 patients who developed hypertensive encephalopathy from PPA ingestion, 24 patients developed intracranial hemorrhages, 15 developed seizures, and 6 died.[93] Seizures, myocardial infarction, bradycardia, atrial and ventricular dysrhythmias, ischemic bowel infarction, and cerebral hemorrhages are reported, even with therapeutic dosing.[23,182] In a review of 500 reports of

adverse reactions from patients who had ingested ephedrine and associated stimulants as dietary supplements, 8 fatalities from myocardial infarction and cerebral hemorrhage were reported.[123] Psychosis, agitation, and manic behavior are reported with acute ingestion.

Imidazolines

When ingested, the imidazoline decongestants naphazoline, oxymetazoline, tetrahydrozoline, and xylometazoline are potent central and peripheral α_2-adrenergic and imidazoline receptor agonists. In overdose, they cause CNS depression, and initial brief hypertension followed by hypotension, bradycardia, and respiratory depression similar to clonidine (Chap. 61).[67] Children are particularly sensitive to the effects of the imidazoline decongestants. Cases of acute stroke are reported in adults with naphazoline abuse.[32]

Rare cases of cardiomyopathy with apical ballooning (Takotsubo) are reported after large ingestion or chronic use of pseudoephedrine or oxymetazoline.[183,196] Acute respiratory distress syndrome from vasoconstriction of pulmonary vessels can also occur with both classes of decongestants. Reversible encephalopathy with bilateral posterior hemispheric edema on neuroimaging was reported after nonprescription use of pseudoephedrine albeit in a patient with an autoimmune disorder that might have been a predisposing factor.[44] Toxic effects usually resolve within 8 to 16 hours. However, they may persist for more than 24 hours if a sustained-release product is ingested.

Diagnostic Testing

The bedside diagnostic of decongestant toxicity is a clinical one. Sympathomimetic decongestants cause false-positive results for amphetamines on several rapid urine drug screens by immunoassay.[112] Comprehensive blood or urine analysis screening test by LC/MS or GC/MS can be obtained for research purposes, in child abuse, or in forensic studies to determine the cause of death. They have no role in the immediate clinical management of poisoned patients.

Management

Patients presenting after an exposure to decongestants should be triaged promptly and brought to a monitored environment. A cardiac monitor should be attached to the patient and observed for dysrhythmias. Intravenous access should be established and airway protection ensured. Gastrointestinal decontamination with AC is recommended in patients with large ingestions of pseudoephedrine if no contraindications are present. A retrospective study of xylometazoline ingestion in children reported toxicity above nasal or oral exposure exceeding 0.4 mg/kg body weight. Ingestions of more than 0.1 mg/kg of naphazoline or tetrahydrozoline produced severe toxicity in children. The decision to give AC in these instances should be made individually because liquid formulations are rapidly absorbed and might not be amenable to AC adsorption by the time of presentation.[176] Activated charcoal administration is reasonable even several hours after ingestion of sustained-release decongestant preparations. More than one dose of AC is reasonable to complete GI decontamination in massive ingestion of oral preparations, but multidose AC for enhanced elimination purposes has no role. Whole-bowel irrigation and renal-enhanced elimination techniques are not indicated.

Specific Treatment

Neurologic toxicity. Patients with extreme agitation, seizures, and psychosis should initially be treated with administration of oxygen and IV benzodiazepines, titrated upward to effect. A patient with a persisting headache, focal neurologic deficits, or abnormal neuropsychiatric findings after decongestant ingestion should be evaluated for cerebral hemorrhage by noncontrast head CT. If the timing of the imaging is delayed, reducing the sensitivity of this modality, subsequent lumbar puncture to exclude subarachnoid hemorrhage is reasonable based on clinical suspicion.

Respiratory toxicity. Children presenting with respiratory depression from imidazoline decongestants have responded to naloxone. These case reports are too few to establish the efficacy of this therapy. Nevertheless, the use of naloxone in imidazoline toxicity is reasonable and low risk in non–opioid-dependent patients.[20,81]

Cardiovascular toxicity. Tachycardia, palpitations, and hypertension that occur in mild sympathomimetic poisonings usually respond to benzodiazepines. For a patient who remains hypertensive or is believed to have chest pain of ischemic origin treatment with phentolamine, an α-adrenergic antagonist, or nicardipine is recommended. Labetalol has been proposed and used in some reported cases; however, because of its different affinity for α- and β-adrenergic receptors depending on the route of administration, its use is not recommended when coronary vasospasm is suspected.[177] Labetalol is a more potent β- than α-adrenergic receptor antagonist when given intravenously.[94,108] Beta-adrenergic antagonists should be avoided because of concern for unopposed α-adrenergic effects. An ECG is required, and any elevation of the ST segment warrants immediate consultation with a cardiologist.

Patients with ventricular dysrhythmias from sympathomimetic decongestants should be treated with standard doses of lidocaine or sodium bicarbonate (if the QRS complex is prolonged). The evidence for efficacy of amiodarone in this setting is still lacking.[41,131] Phenylpropanolamine causes hypertension with a reflex bradycardia and atrioventricular block that is responsive to standard doses of atropine. Atropine must be used with caution because it can cause a dangerous increase in blood pressure as the reflex bradycardia reverses. Therefore, a vasodilator such as phentolamine is recommended because the stimulus for the bradycardia is corrected with reversal of the hypertension.

Imidazoline-induced hypertension rarely requires therapy, but in the setting of symptomatic hypertension, a short-acting α-adrenergic antagonist such as phentolamine is reasonable.[187] However, the hypertension is generally transient and followed by hypotension. Initial antihypertensive therapy could exacerbate toxicity and should only be reserved for cases in which severe hypertension represents a true urgency for end-organ damage.

SUMMARY

- Within a few hours of ingestion of H$_1$ antihistamines, anticholinergic toxicity is expected.
- Cardiotoxicity via sodium channel blockade can be fatal and is treated with sodium bicarbonate.
- Physostigmine or other anticholinesterases are recommended to reverse anticholinergic effects of H$_1$ antihistamines.
- H$_2$ antihistamines rarely result in symptoms or signs of toxicity.
- Decongestants used for recreational purposes can be ingested in doses that produce toxic sympathomimetic effects.
- Patients with abnormal mental status or seizures should be investigated to exclude intracranial hemorrhages.
- Topical imidazoline decongestants can produce toxicity, typically in the form of hypotension and bradycardia.
- The treatment of patients with toxicity from sympathomimetic decongestants follows the same treatment guidelines as amphetamines and other sympathomimetics.

Acknowledgment

Anthony J. Tomassoni, MD, and Richard S. Weisman, PharmD, contributed to this chapter in previous editions.

REFERENCES

1. Alldredge BK, et al. Seizures associated with recreational drug abuse. *Neurology.* 1989;39:1037-1039.
2. Allotey P, et al. "Social medication" and the control of children: a qualitative study of over-the-counter medication among Australian children. *Pediatrics.* 2004;114:e378-e383.
3. Anonymous. Cetirizine and loratadine: minimal risk of QT prolongation. *Prescrire Int.* 2010;19:26-28.
4. Antonelli D, et al. Torsade de pointes in patients on chronic amiodarone treatment: contributing factors and drug interactions. *Isr Med Assoc J.* 2005;7:163-165.
5. Arora S, et al. Alcohol levels are increased in social drinkers receiving ranitidine. *Am J Gastroenterol.* 2000;95:208-213.
6. Arrang JM, et al. Highly potent and selective ligands for histamine H3-receptors. *Nature.* 1987;327:117-123.
7. Aymard JP, et al. Haematological adverse effects of histamine H2-receptor antagonists. *Med Toxicol Adverse Drug Exp* 1988;3:430-448.
8. Baker AM, et al. Fatal diphenhydramine intoxication in infants. *J Forensic Sci.* 2003;48:425-428.
9. Bartra J, et al. Interactions of the H1 antihistamines. *J Investig Allergol Clin Immunol.* 2006;16(suppl 1):29-36.
10. Baum C, et al. The impact of the addition of naloxone on the use and abuse of pentazocine. *Public Health Rep.* 1987;102:426-429.
11. Bebarta VS, et al. Validation of the American Association of Poison Control Centers out of hospital guideline for pediatric diphenhydramine ingestions. *Clin Toxicol (Phila).* 2010;48:559-562.
12. Bender BG, et al. Sedation and performance impairment of diphenhydramine and second-generation antihistamines: a meta-analysis. *J Allergy Clin Immunol.* 2003;111:770-776.
13. Berul CI, Morad M. Regulation of potassium channels by nonsedating antihistamines. *Circulation.* 1995;91:2220-2225.
14. Blackman NS, Hayes JC. Fatality associated with Benadryl therapy; report of a case. *J Allergy.* 1948;19:390-392.
15. Boland DM, et al. Fatal cold medication intoxication in an infant. *J Anal Toxicol.* 2003;27:523-526.
16. Bovet D. The relationships between isosterism and competitive phenomena in the field of drug therapy of the autonomic nervous system and that of the neuromuscular transmission. *Nobel Lectures, Physiology or Medicine 1942-1962,* vol 3. Amsterdam: Elsevier; 1964:553-577.
17. Bright TP, et al. Selected cardiac and metabolic responses to pseudoephedrine with exercise. *J Clin Pharmacol.* 1981;21(11-12, pt 1):488-492.
18. Brown J. Omeprazole, ranitidine and cimetidine have no effect on peak blood ethanol concentrations, first pass metabolism or area under the time-ethanol curve under "real-life" drinking conditions. *Aliment Pharmacol Ther.* 1998;12:141-145.
19. Brown AS, et al. Ranitidine increases the bioavailability of postprandial ethanol by the reduction of first pass metabolism. *Gut.* 1995;37:413-417.
20. Bucaretchi F, et al. [Acute exposure to imidazoline derivatives in children]. *J Pediatr (Rio J).* 2003;79:519-524.
21. Buckley NA, et al. Pheniramine—a much abused drug. *Med J Aust.* 1994;160:188-192.
22. Burns MJ, et al. A comparison of physostigmine and benzodiazepines for the treatment of anticholinergic poisoning. *Ann Emerg Med.* 2000;35:374-381.
23. Cantu C, et al. Stroke associated with sympathomimetics contained in over-the-counter cough and cold drugs. *Stroke.* 2003;34:1667-1672.
24. Chan B, et al. Use of neostigmine for the management of drug induced ileus in severe poisonings. *J Med Toxicol.* 2005;1:18-22.
25. Chen C, et al. P-Glycoprotein limits the brain penetration of nonsedating but not sedating H1-antagonists. *Drug Metab Dispos* 2003;31:312-318.
26. Cho YS, et al. Comparison of lactated Ringer's solution and 0.9% saline in the treatment of rhabdomyolysis induced by doxylamine intoxication. *Emerg Med J.* 2007;24:276-280.
27. Cole JB, et al. Wide complex tachycardia in a pediatric diphenhydramine overdose treated with sodium bicarbonate. *Pediatr Emerg Care.* 2011;27:1175-1177.
28. Coleman C, Moore M. Decongestants and antihistamines for acute otitis media in children. *Cochrane Database Syst Rev.* 2008:CD001727.
29. Consumer Healthcare Products Association. CHPA Press Room. OTC Sales by Category—2008-2011. 2012. http://www.chpa-info.org/pressroom/Sales_Category .aspx. Accessed August 12, 2012.
30. Centers for Disease Control and Prevention. Infant deaths associated with cough and cold medications—two states, 2005. *MMWR Morb Mortal Wkly Rep.* 2007;56:1-4.
31. Corboz MR, et al. Mechanism of decongestant activity of alpha 2-adrenoceptor agonists. *Pulm Pharmacol Ther.* 2008;21:449-454.
32. Costantino G, et al. Ischemic stroke in a man with naphazoline abuse history. *Am J Emerg Med.* 2007;25:983.e981-983.e982.
33. Criado PR, et al. Histamine, histamine receptors and antihistamines: new concepts. *An Bras Dermatol.* 2010;85:195-210.

34. Dart RC, et al. Pediatric fatalities associated with over the counter (nonprescription) cough and cold medications. *Ann Emerg Med.* 2009;53:411-417.

35. Davies AJ, et al. Cardiotoxic effect with convulsions in terfenadine overdose. *BMJ.* 1989;298:325.

36. Davila I, et al. Effect of H1 antihistamines upon the cardiovascular system. *J Investig Allergol Clin Immunol.* 2006;16(suppl 1):13-23.

37. Dawson A, et al. Tacrine in the treatment of anticholinergic poisoning. Abstracts of the European Association of Poisons Centres and Clinical Toxicologists XXIII International Congress #28. *Clin Toxicol (Phila).* 2003;41:383-564.

38. Day J. Pros and cons of the use of antihistamines in managing allergic rhinitis. *J Allergy Clin Immunol.* 1999;103(3, pt 2):S395-S399.

39. Demoly P, et al. Hypersensitivity to H1-antihistamines. *Allergy.* 2000;55:679-680.

40. Devillier P, et al. Clinical pharmacokinetics and pharmacodynamics of desloratadine, fexofenadine and levocetirizine: a comparative review. *Clin Pharmacokinet.* 2008;47:217-230.

41. DeWitt CR, et al. The effect of amiodarone pretreatment on survival of mice with cocaine toxicity. *J Med Toxicol.* 2005;1:11-18.

42. Do KD, et al. Exertional rhabdomyolysis in a bodybuilder following overexertion: a possible link to creatine overconsumption. *Clin J Sport Med.* 2007;17:78-79.

43. Drew CD, et al. Comparison of the effects of D-(−)-ephedrine and L-(+)-pseudoephedrine on the cardiovascular and respiratory systems in man. *Br J Clin Pharmacol.* 1978;6:221-225.

44. Ebbo M, et al. Posterior reversible encephalopathy syndrome induced by a cough and cold drug containing pseudoephedrine [in French]. *Rev Med Interne.* 2010;31:440-444.

45. Eccles R. Mechanisms of the placebo effect of sweet cough syrups. *Respir Physiol Neurobiol.* 2006;152:340-348.

46. Ekins BR, Spoerke DG Jr. An estimation of the toxicity of non-prescription diet aids from seventy exposure cases. *Vet Hum Toxicol.* 1983;25:81-85.

47. Emadian SM, et al. Rhabdomyolysis: a rare adverse effect of diphenhydramine overdose. *Am J Emerg Med.* 1996;14:574-576.

48. Etzel JV. Diphenhydramine-induced acute dystonia. *Pharmacotherapy.* 1994;14:492-496.

49. Farrell M, et al. Response of life threatening dimenhydrinate intoxication to sodium bicarbonate administration. *J Toxicol Clin Toxicol.* 1991;29:527-535.

50. Filloux F. Toxic encephalopathy caused by topically applied diphenhydramine. *J Pediatr.* 1986;108:1018-1020.

51. Finkle WD, et al. Increased risk of serious injury following an initial prescription for diphenhydramine. *Ann Allergy Asthma Immunol.* 2002;89:244-250.

52. Finklestein Y, et al. Drug-induced seizures in children presenting to the emergency department. Abstracts 2012 Annual Meeting of the North American Congress of Clinical Toxicology (NACCT) October 1-6, 2012 Las Vegas, NV, USA. Abstract # 227. *Clin Toxicol (Phila).* 2012;50:574-729.

53. Frankel D, et al. Non-traumatic rhabdomyolysis complicating antihistamine overdose. *J Toxicol Clin Toxicol.* 1993;31:493-496.

54. Freedberg RS, et al. Cardiogenic shock due to antihistamine overdose. Reversal with intra-aortic balloon counterpulsation. *JAMA.* 1987;257:660-661.

55. Garg S, Bhutani KK. Chromatographic analysis of Kutajarista—an ayurvedic polyherbal formulation. *Phytochem Anal.* 2008;19:323-328.

56. Garza MB, et al. Central anticholinergic syndrome from orphenadrine in a 3 year old. *Pediatr Emerg Care.* 2000;16:97-98.

57. Grant JA, et al. A double-blind, randomized, single-dose, crossover comparison of levocetirizine with ebastine, fexofenadine, loratadine, mizolastine, and placebo: suppression of histamine-induced wheal-and-flare response during 24 hours in healthy male subjects. *Ann Allergy Asthma Immunol.* 2002;88:190-197.

58. Gupta SK, et al. Desloratadine dose selection in children aged 6 months to 2 years: comparison of population pharmacokinetics between children and adults. *Br J Clin Pharmacol.* 2007;64:174-184.

59. Haller CA, Benowitz NL. Adverse cardiovascular and central nervous system events associated with dietary supplements containing ephedra alkaloids. *N Engl J Med.* 2000;343:1833-1838.

60. Halpert AG, et al. Dimenhydrinate produces a conditioned place preference in rats. *Pharmacol Biochem Behav.* 2003;75:173-179.

61. Halpert AG, et al. Mechanisms and abuse liability of the anti-histamine dimenhydrinate. *Neurosci Biobehav Rev.* 2002;26:61-67.

62. Head GA, Mayorov DN. Imidazoline receptors, novel agents and therapeutic potential. *Cardiovasc Hematol Agents Med Chem.* 2006;4:17-32.

63. Hellbom E. Chlorpheniramine, selective serotonin-reuptake inhibitors (SSRIs) and over-the-counter (OTC) treatment. *Med Hypotheses.* 2006;66:689-690.

64. Hennessy S, Strom BL. Nonsedating antihistamines should be preferred over sedating antihistamines in patients who drive. *Ann Intern Med.* 2000;132:405-407.

65. Hernandez-Munoz R, et al. Human gastric alcohol dehydrogenase: its inhibition by H2-receptor antagonists, and its effect on the bioavailability of ethanol. *Alcohol Clin Exp Res.* 1990;14:946-950.

66. Hey JA, et al. Cardiovascular profile of loratadine. *Clin Exp Allergy.* 1999;29(suppl 3):197-199.

67. Higgins G, et al. Pediatric poisoning from over-the-counter imidazoline-containing products. *Ann Emerg Med.* 1991;20:655-658.

68. Holger JS, et al. Physostigmine, sodium bicarbonate, or hypertonic saline to treat diphenhydramine toxicity. *Vet Hum Toxicol.* 2002;44:1-4.

69. Honig PK, et al. Terfenadine-ketoconazole interaction. Pharmacokinetic and electrocardiographic consequences. *JAMA.* 1993;269:1513-1518.

70. Horak F, Stübner UP. Comparative tolerability of second generation antihistamines. *Drug Saf.* 1999;20:385-401.

71. Huang J-F, Thurmond RL. The new biology of histamine receptors. *Curr Allergy Asthma Rep.* 2008;8:21-27.

72. Humphries TJ, Merritt GJ. Review article: drug interactions with agents used to treat acid-related diseases. *Aliment Pharmacol Ther.* 1999;13:18-26.

73. Huston RL, et al. Toxicity from topical administration of diphenhydramine in children. *Clin Pediatr (Phila).* 1990;29:542-545.

74. Isbister GK, et al. Restricting cough and cold medicines in children. *J Paediatr Child Health.* 2012;48:91-98.

75. Jang DH, et al. Status epilepticus and wide-complex tachycardia secondary to diphenhydramine overdose. *Clin Toxicol (Phila).* 2010;48:945-948.

76. Jo Y-I, et al. Risk factors for rhabdomyolysis following doxylamine overdose. *Hum Exp Toxicol.* 2007;26:617-621.

77. Johnson DA, Hricik JG. The pharmacology of α-adrenergic decongestants. *Pharmacotherapy.* 1993;13(6, pt II):110S-115S.

78. Jones GR, Singer PP. Rare fatality attributed to an overdose of cimetidine. *Can Soc Forensic Sci.* 2003;36:73-76.

79. Karamanakos PN. Can chlorpheniramine cause serotonin syndrome? *Singapore Med J.* 2007;48:482; author reply 483.

80. Karch SB. Diphenhydramine toxicity: comparisons of postmortem findings in diphenhydramine-, cocaine-, and heroin-related deaths. *Am J Forensic Med Pathol.* 1998;19:143-147.

81. Katar S, et al. Naloxone use in a newborn with apnea due to tetrahydrozoline intoxication. *Pediatr Int.* 2010;52:488-489.

82. Kaufman DW, et al. Recent patterns of medication use in the ambulatory adult population of the United States: the Slone survey. *JAMA.* 2002;287:337-344.

83. Kernan WN, et al. Phenylpropanolamine and the risk of hemorrhagic stroke. *N Engl J Med.* 2000;343:1826-1832.

84. Khankoeva AI, et al. Mechanisms of histamine-induced increase of calcium level in cardiomyocytes. A relative efficacy of histamine receptor blockers. *Bull Exp Biol Med.* 1997;123:357-359.

85. Khosla U, et al. Antihistamine-induced rhabdomyolysis. *South Med J.* 2003;96:1023-1026.

86. Kim HJ, et al. The associative factors of delayed-onset rhabdomyolysis in patients with doxylamine overdose. *Am J Emerg Med.* 2011;29:903-907.

87. King AR. Cardiac arrest and cimetidine. *Med J Aust.* 1981;1:139-140.

88. Klein-Schwartz W, et al. Impact of the voluntary withdrawal of over-the-counter cough and cold medications on pediatric ingestions reported to poison centers. *Pharmacoepidemiol Drug Saf.* 2010;19:819-824.

89. Koppel C, et al. Clinical symptomatology of diphenhydramine overdose: an evaluation of 136 cases in 1982 to 1985. *J Toxicol Clin Toxicol.* 1987;25:53-70.

90. Koppel C, et al. Poisoning with over-the-counter doxylamine preparations: an evaluation of 109 cases over the counter preparation. *Hum Toxicol.* 1987;6:355-359.

91. Krenzelok EP, et al. Cimetidine toxicity: an assessment of 881 cases. *Ann Emerg Med.* 1987;16:1217-1221.

92. Kuo CC, et al. Inhibition of Na(+) current by diphenhydramine and other diphenyl compounds: molecular determinants of selective binding to the inactivated channels. *Mol Pharmacol.* 2000;57:135-143.

93. Lake CR, et al. Adverse drug effects attributed to phenylpropanolamine: a review of 142 case reports. *Am J Med.* 1990;89:195-208.

94. Lalonde RL, et al. Labetalol pharmacokinetics and pharmacodynamics: evidence of stereoselective disposition. *Clin Pharmacol Ther.* 1990;48:509-519.

95. Layton D, et al. Examining the utilization and tolerability of the non-sedating antihistamine levocetirizine in England using prescription-event monitoring data. *Drug Saf.* 2011;34:1177-1189.

96. Layton D, et al. Examining the tolerability of the non-sedating antihistamine desloratadine: a prescription-event monitoring study in England. *Drug Saf.* 2009;32:169-179.

97. Leupold D, Wartenberg KE. Xylometazoline abuse induced ischemic stroke in a young adult. *Neurologist.* 2011;17:41-43.

98. Leurs R, et al. En route to new blockbuster anti-histamines: surveying the offspring of the expanding histamine receptor family. *Trends Pharmacol Sci.* 2011;32:250-257.

99. Levine M, Lovecchio F. Diphenhydramine-induced Brugada pattern. *Resuscitation.* 2010;81:503-504.

100. Llenas J, et al. Cardiotoxicity of histamine and the possible role of histamine in the arrhythmogenesis produced by certain antihistamines. *Drug Saf.* 1999;21(suppl 1):33-38.

101. Lokker N, et al. Parental misinterpretations of over-the-counter pediatric cough and cold medication labels. *Pediatrics.* 2009;123:1464-1471.

102. Mahajan MK, et al. In vitro metabolism of oxymetazoline: evidence for bioactivation to a reactive metabolite. *Drug Metab Dispos* 2011;39:693-702.

103. Mann RD, et al. Sedation with "non-sedating" antihistamines: four prescription-event monitoring studies in general practice. *Br Med J.* 2000;320:1184-1187.

104. Marinetti L, et al. Over-the-counter cold medications—postmortem findings in infants and the relationship to cause of death. *J Anal Toxicol.* 2005;29:738-743.

105. Martinez C, et al. Comparative in vitro and in vivo inhibition of cytochrome P450 CYP1A2, CYP2D6, and CYP3A by H2-receptor antagonists. *Clin Pharmacol Ther.* 1999;65:369-376.

106. McKeown NJ, et al. Survival after diphenhydramine ingestion with hemodialysis in a toddler. *J Med Toxicol.* 2011;7:147-150.

107. McKetin R, et al. A systematic review of methamphetamine precursor regulations. *Addiction.* 2011;106:1911-1924.

108. Mehvar R, Brocks DR. Stereospecific pharmacokinetics and pharmacodynamics of beta-adrenergic blockers in humans. *J Pharm Pharm Sci.* 2001;4:185-200.

109. Merenstein D, et al. The trial of infant response to diphenhydramine: the TIRED study—a randomized, controlled, patient-oriented trial. *Arch Pediatr Adolesc Med.* 2006;160:707-712.

110. Miller NS, et al. Histamine receptor antagonism of intolerance to alcohol in the Oriental population. *J Nerv Ment Dis.* 1987;175:661-667.

111. Mills JG, et al. The safety of ranitidine in over a decade of use. *Aliment Pharmacol Ther.* 1997;11:129-137.

112. Moeller KE, et al. Urine drug screening: practical guide for clinicians. *Mayo Clin Proc.* 2008;83:66-76.

113. Mowry JB, et al. 2015 Annual Report of the American Association of Poison Control Centers' National Poison Data System (NPDS): 33rd Annual Report. *Clin Toxicol (Phila).* 2016;54:924-1109.

114. Mullins ME, et al. Life-threatening diphenhydramine overdose treated with charcoal hemoperfusion and hemodialysis. *Ann Emerg Med.* 1999;33:104-107.

115. Nine JS, Rund CR. Fatality from diphenhydramine monointoxication: a case report and review of the infant, pediatric, and adult literature. *Am J Forensic Med Pathol.* 2006;27:36-41.

116. Nonnemaker J, et al. Are methamphetamine precursor control laws effective tools to fight the methamphetamine epidemic? *Health Econ.* 2011;20:519-531.

117. Noyan MA, et al. Donepezil for anticholinergic drug intoxication: a case report. *Prog Neuropsychopharmacol Biol Psychiatry.* 2003;27:885-887.

118. Oneta CM, et al. First pass metabolism of ethanol is strikingly influenced by the speed of gastric emptying. *Gut.* 1998;43:612-619.

119. Oroszi G, Goldman D. Alcoholism: genes and mechanisms. *Pharmacogenomics.* 2004;5:1037-1048.

120. Owens JA, et al. Medication use in the treatment of pediatric insomnia: results of a survey of community-based pediatricians. *Pediatrics.* 2003;111(5, pt 1):e628-e635.

121. Parekh R, et al. Rhabdomyolysis: advances in diagnosis and treatment. *Emerg Med Pract.* 2012;14:1-15; quiz 15.

122. Paton DM, Webster DR. Clinical pharmacokinetics of H1-receptor antagonists (the antihistamines). *Clin Pharmacokinet.* 1985;10:477-497.

123. Perrotta D, et al. Adverse events associated with ephedrine-containing products—Texas, December 1993-September 1995. *JAMA.* 1996;276:1711-1712.

124. Phillips M, et al. Physostigmine continuous infusion for the treatment of anticholinergic toxicity in combined diphenhydramine and bupropion overdose. Abstracts 2012 Annual Meeting of the North American Congress of Clinical Toxicology (NACCT) October 1-6, 2012 Las Vegas, NV, USA. *Clin Toxicol (Phila).* 2012;50:574-720.

125. Poklis A. T's and blues. *JAMA.* 1978;240:108.

126. Pradalier A, et al. Étude randomisée en double aveugle contre placebo de la tritoqualine hypostamine* dans la rhinite allergique perannuelle. *Revue Française d'Allergologie et d'Immunologie Clinique.* 2003;43:175-179.

127. Pragst F, et al. Poisonings with diphenhydramine—a survey of 68 clinical and 55 death cases. *Forensic Sci Int.* 2006;161:189-197.

128. Pratt C, et al. Cardiovascular safety of fexofenadine HCl. *Clin Exp Allergy.* 1999;29(suppl 3):212-216.

129. Prenner B, et al. Adult and paediatric poor metabolisers of desloratadine: an assessment of pharmacokinetics and safety. *Expert Opin Drug Saf.* 2006;5:211-223.

130. Radovanovic D, et al. Dose-dependent toxicity of diphenhydramine overdose. *Hum Exp Toxicol.* 2000;19:489-495.

131. Rakovec P, et al. Ventricular tachycardia induced by abuse of ephedrine in a young healthy woman. *Wien Klin Wochenschr.* 2006;118:558-561.

132. Reichelderfer TE, et al. Treatment of acute Benadryl (diphenhydramine hydrochloride) intoxication with severe central nervous system changes and recovery. *J Pediatr.* 1955;46:303-307.

133. Retamero C, et al. "Ephedra-free" diet pill-induced psychosis. *Psychosomatics.* 2011;52:579-582.

134. Rimsza ME, Newberry S. Unexpected infant deaths associated with use of cough and cold medications. *Pediatrics.* 2008;122:e318-e322.

135. Rives HF, et al. A fatal reaction to methapyrilene. *JAMA.* 1949;140:1022-1024.

136. Rogers SC, et al. Rapid urine drug screens: diphenhydramine and methadone cross-reactivity. *Pediatr Emerg Care.* 2010;26:665-666.

137. Salerno SM, et al. Effect of oral pseudoephedrine on blood pressure and heart rate: a meta-analysis. *Arch Intern Med.* 2005;165:1686-1694.

138. Salmun LM, et al. Loratadine versus cetirizine: assessment of somnolence and motivation during the workday. *Clin Ther.* 2000;22:573-582.

139. Santora VJ, et al. A new family of H3 receptor antagonists based on the natural product Conessine. *Bioorg Med Chem Lett.* 2008;18:1490-1494.

140. Saruwatari J, et al. Impact of CYP2D6*10 on H1-antihistamine-induced hypersomnia. *Eur J Clin Pharmacol.* 2006;62:995-1001.

141. Scharman EJ, et al. Diphenhydramine and dimenhydrinate poisoning: an evidence-based consensus guideline for out-of-hospital management. *Clin Toxicol (Phila).* 2006;44:205-223.

142. Schunk JE, Svendsen D. Diphenhydramine toxicity from combined oral and topical use. *Am J Dis Child.* 1988;142:1020-1021.

143. Schwartz JC. The histamine H3 receptor: from discovery to clinical trials with pitolisant. *Br J Pharmacol.* 2011;163:713-721.

144. Sharfstein JM, et al. Over the counter but no longer under the radar—pediatric cough and cold medications. *N Engl J Med.* 2007;357:2321-2324.

145. Sharma AN, et al. Diphenhydramine-induced wide complex dysrhythmia responds to treatment with sodium bicarbonate. *Am J Emerg Med.* 2003;21:212-215.

146. Shaw RG, et al. Cardiac arrest after intravenous injection of cimetidine. *Med J Aust.* 1980;2:629-630.

147. Shawn DH, McGuigan MA. Poisoning from dermal absorption of promethazine. *Can Med Assoc J.* 1984;130:1460-1461.

148. Shehab N, et al. Adverse events from cough and cold medications after a market withdrawal of products labeled for infants. *Pediatrics.* 2010;126:1100-1107.

149. Simons FE, et al. Pharmacokinetics of the orally administered decongestants pseudoephedrine and phenylpropanolamine in children. *J Pediatr.* 1996;129:729-734.

150. Simons FE, Simons KJ. Histamine and H1-antihistamines: celebrating a century of progress. *J Allergy Clin Immunol.* 2011;128:1139-1150.e1134.

151. Simons FE, et al. Pharmacokinetics and antipruritic effects of hydroxyzine in children with atopic dermatitis. *J Pediatr.* 1984;104:123-127.

152. Simons KJ, et al. Diphenhydramine: pharmacokinetics and pharmacodynamics in elderly adults, young adults, and children. *J Clin Pharmacol.* 1990;30:665-671.

153. Singer AJ, Hollander JE. Infiltration pain and local anesthetic effects of buffered vs plain 1% diphenhydramine. *Acad Emerg Med.* 1995;2:884-888.

154. Slone Epidemiology Center. *Patterns of Medication Use in the United States 2006.* Boston, MA: Slone Epidemiology Center at Boston University; 2006.

155. Smith SM, et al. Over-the-counter (OTC) medications for acute cough in children and adults in ambulatory settings. *Cochrane Database Syst Rev.* 2012;8:CD001831.

156. Sneader W. Hormones analogues. In: *Drug Discovery: A History.* Chap. 18. Chichester, UK: John Wiley & Sons; 2005:468.

157. Sneader W. Drugs originating from the screening of organic chemicals. In: *Drug Discovery: A History.* Chap. 28. Chichester, UK: John Wiley & Sons; 2005:468.

158. Sonnenblick M, et al. Neurological and psychiatric side effects of cimetidine—report of 3 cases with review of the literature. *Postgrad Med J.* 1982;58:415-418.

159. Spector R, et al. Diphenhydramine in Orientals and Caucasians. *Clin Pharmacol Ther.* 1980;28:229-234.

160. Stone CL, et al. Cimetidine inhibition of human gastric and liver alcohol dehydrogenase isoenzymes: identification of inhibitor complexes by kinetics and molecular modeling. *Biochemistry.* 1995;34:4008-4014.

161. Strategy One. *CHPA. Your Health at Hand: Perception of over-the-counter medicine in the U.S.* November 24, 2010.

162. Syed H, et al. Doxylamine toxicity: seizure, rhabdomyolysis and false positive urine drug screen for methadone. *BMJ Case Rep.* 2009;2009.

163. Tagawa M, et al. Neuroimaging of histamine H1-receptor occupancy in human brain by positron emission tomography (PET): a comparative study of ebastine, a second-generation antihistamine, and (+)-chlorpheniramine, a classical antihistamine. *Br J Clin Pharmacol.* 2008;52:501-509.

164. Tashiro M, et al. Roles of histamine in regulation of arousal and cognition: functional neuroimaging of histamine H1 receptors in human brain. *Life Sci.* 2002;72:409-414.

165. Ten Eick AP, et al. Safety of antihistamines in children. *Drug Saf.* 2001;24:119-147.

166. Thundiyil JG, et al. Evolving epidemiology of drug-induced seizures reported to a Poison Control Center System. *J Med Toxicol.* 2007;3:15-19.

167. Thurmond RL, et al. Toreforant, a histamine H4 receptor antagonist, in patients with active rheumatoid arthritis despite methotrexate therapy: results of 2 phase II studies. *J Rheumatol.* 2016;43:1637-1642.

168. Traynor K. FDA investigating nonprescription cough and cold products. *Am J Health Syst Pharm.* 2007;64:802-803.

169. Turner JW. Death of a child from topical diphenhydramine. *Am J Forensic Med Pathol.* 2009;30:380-381.

170. United States Department of Justice Drug Enforcement Administration. Combat Methamphetamine Epidemic Act of 2005. Public Law 109-177, 2006;257-277. http://www.deadiversion.usdoj.gov/meth/pl109_177.pdf. Accessed August 10, 2012.

171. United States Food and Drug Administration. Dietary supplements. Guidance documents. http://www.fda.gov/Food/GuidanceComplianceRegulatoryInformation/GuidanceDocuments/DietarySupplements/default.htm. Published 2011. Accessed January 30, 2013.

172. United States Food and Drug Administration. Products containing imidazolines equivalent of 0.08 milligrams or more. Consumer Product Safety Commission. Notice of proposed rulemaking. *Fed Regist.* 2012;77:3646.

173. United States Food and Drug Administration. Statement following CHPA's announcement on nonprescription over-the-counter cough and cold medicines in children. http://www.fda.gov/NewsEvents/Newsroom/PressAnnouncements/2008/ucm116964.htm. Published 2008. Accessed August 12, 2012.

174. Vaccaro WD, Sher R, Berlin M, et al. Novel histamine H3 receptor antagonists based on the 4-[(1*H*-imidazol-4-yl)methyl]piperidine scaffold. *Bioorg Med Chem Lett.* 2006; 16:395-399.

175. Van Sweden B, Kamphuisen HAC. Cimetidine neurotoxicity. EEG and behaviour aspects. *Eur Neurol.* 1984;23:300-305.

176. van Velzen AG, et al. A case series of xylometazoline overdose in children. *Clin Toxicol (Phila).* 2007;45:290-294.

177. Vanden Hoek TL, et al. Part 12: cardiac arrest in special situations: 2010 American Heart Association Guidelines for Cardiopulmonary Resuscitation and Emergency Cardiovascular Care. *Circulation.* 2010;122(suppl 3):S829-S861.

178. Vassilev ZP, et al. Safety and efficacy of over-the-counter cough and cold medicines for use in children. *Expert Opin Drug Saf.* 2010;9:233-242.

179. Vearrier D, Curtis JA. Case files of the medical toxicology fellowship at Drexel University. Rhabdomyolysis and compartment syndrome following acute diphenhydramine overdose. *J Med Toxicol.* 2011;7:213-219.

180. Vernacchio L, et al. Medication use among children <12 years of age in the United States: results from the Slone Survey. *Pediatrics.* 2009;124:446-454.

181. Viertel A, et al. Treatment of diphenhydramine intoxication with haemoperfusion. *Nephrol Dial Transplant.* 1994;9:1336-1338.

182. Wang NE, et al. Hypertensive crisis and NSTEMI after accidental overdose of sustained release pseudoephedrine: a case report. *Clin Toxicol (Phila).* 2008;46:922-923.

183. Wang R, et al. Apical ballooning syndrome secondary to nasal decongestant abuse. *Arq Bras Cardiol.* 2009;93:e75-e78.

184. Watemberg NM, et al. Central anticholinergic syndrome on therapeutic doses of cyproheptadine. *Pediatrics.* 1999;103:158-160.

185. Weiler JM, et al. Effects of fexofenadine, diphenhydramine, and alcohol on driving performance. A randomized, placebo-controlled trial in the Iowa driving simulator. *Ann Intern Med.* 2000;132:354-363.

186. Weinberg DS, et al. Effect of histamine-2 receptor antagonists on blood alcohol levels: a meta-analysis. *J Gen Intern Med.* 1998;13:594-599.

187. Wenzel S, et al. Course and therapy of intoxication with imidazoline derivate naphazoline. *Int J Pediatr Otorhinolaryngol.* 2004;68:979-983.

188. Wezorek C, et al. Pediatric pseudoephedrine ingestions: a retrospective study. *Vet Hum Toxicol.* 1991;33:362.

189. Wolff AA, Levi R. Histamine and cardiac arrhythmias. *Circ Res.* 1986;58:1-16.

190. Woodward GA, Baldassano RN. Topical diphenhydramine toxicity in a five year old with varicella. *Pediatr Emerg Care.* 1988;4:18-20.

191. World Anti Doping Agency. The 2012 Prohibited List International Standard. http://www.wada-ama.org/Documents/World_Anti-Doping_Program/WADP-Prohibited-list/2012/WADA_Prohibited_List_2012_EN.pdf. Published 2012. Accessed August 29, 2012.

192. Yanai K, et al. Positron emission tomography evaluation of sedative properties of antihistamines. *Expert Opin Drug Saf.* 2011;10:613-622.

193. Yap YG, et al. Drug-induced Brugada syndrome. *Europace.* 2009;11:989-994.

194. Yu F, et al. The future antihistamines: histamine H3 and H4 receptor ligands. *Adv Exp Med Biol.* 2010;709:125-140.

195. Zell-Kanter M, Leikin J. FDA's ban on ephedra results in plummeting calls to poison centers. 2012 Annual Meeting of the North American Congress of Clinical Toxicology (NACCT) October 1–6, 2012 Las Vegas, NV, USA. *Clin Toxicol (Phila).* 2012;50:637.

196. Zlotnick DM, Helisch A. Recurrent stress cardiomyopathy induced by Sudafed PE. *Ann Intern Med.* 2012;156:171-172.

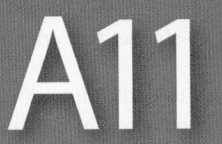

Antidotes in Depth

A11 PHYSOSTIGMINE SALICYLATE

Mary Ann Howland

INTRODUCTION

Physostigmine is a carbamate that reversibly inhibits cholinesterases in both the peripheral and central nervous system (CNS).[60] The tertiary amine structure of physostigmine permits CNS penetration and differentiates it from neostigmine and pyridostigmine, which are quaternary amines that have limited ability to enter the CNS. The inhibition of cholinesterases prevents the metabolism of acetylcholine, allowing acetylcholine to accumulate and antagonize the antimuscarinic effects of xenobiotics such as atropine, scopolamine, and diphenhydramine.[23,43,72] Although physostigmine previously was used as an antagonist to the antimuscarinic effects of cyclic antidepressants and phenothiazines, we currently recommend against this use because of a poor risk-to-benefit ratio, and the potential for exacerbation of life-threatening cardiotoxicity. Similarly, physostigmine has a poor risk-to-benefit ratio in the management of presumed γ-hydroxybutyric acid (GHB) and baclofen toxicity.[5,49,63,73] Atypical antipsychotics have complex pharmacologic effects. Although some atypical antipsychotics, such as quetiapine and olanzapine, have significant antimuscarinic side effects, the benefit of treating these anticholinergic effects with physostigmine must be weighed against the potential risks of exacerbating cardiotoxicity.[10,25,61,70]

HISTORY

The history of physostigmine dates back to antiquity and the Efik people of Old Calabar in Nigeria.[21,27,30,60] The chiefs in this area used a poisonous concoction made from the beans of an aquatic leguminous perennial plant found in the area to create a judicial test, the *esere ordeal*. *Esere* was the word used to represent both the bean and the ritual used to test the innocence or guilt of an accused person. The chiefs also believed that the *esere* had the power to detect and kill persons practicing witchcraft. Supposedly, innocent persons quickly swallowed the poison, which resulted in immediate emesis.[30] Vomiting allowed the innocent to survive without therapy or to be given an antidote of excrement in water. The guilty, however, hesitated swallowing, leading to speculation that sublingual absorption led to severe systemic symptoms without the benefit of vomiting. These persons were noted to develop mouth fasciculations and died foaming at the mouth. Daniell, a British medical officer stationed in Calabar, brought samples of the bean and the plant back to England in 1840.[30] John Balfour, a professor of medicine and botany at the Edinburgh Medical School, characterized the plant, which became known as *Physostigma venenosum Balfour* (family Leguminoseae), in 1857. The active alkaloid was isolated by Jobst and Hesse in 1864 and was named physostigmine. Independently, one year later Vee and Leven also isolated and named the active alkaloid eserine. This year also saw physostigmine's first antidotal use.[41]

Christison performed the first toxicologic studies, including self-experimentation with increasing doses of the seed. Fraser, Christison's student and successor, originated the concept of antagonism from his experiments with physostigmine and atropine. Fraser plotted the dose relationships between the effects of atropine versus physostigmine on various organs such as the eye and the heart, demonstrating the antidotal effects of atropine for the lethal effects of physostigmine.[21] Subsequent experiments with physostigmine led to the development of the theory of neurohumoral transmission.[27] By the 1930s, physostigmine was used as a miotic for patients with glaucoma, a treatment for myasthenia gravis, for reversal of the paralytic effects of curare, and an antidote for atropine and nicotinic insecticides.

PHARMACOLOGY
Chemistry

Physostigmine salicylate is the salicylate salt of physostigmine, a carbamate with a molecular weight of 275 Da. Figure A11–1 shows the general formula for carbamate cholinesterase inhibitors and the chemical structures of physostigmine ($C_{15}H_{21}O_2N_3$), a tertiary amine, and neostigmine, a quaternary amine. Naturally occurring physostigmine consists of a racemic mixture with the (–) isomer greater than 100 times more potent in inhibiting acetylcholinesterase.[56]

Mechanism of Action

Physostigmine is a reversible inhibitor of acetylcholinesterase. Similar to acetylcholine, physostigmine is a substrate for the cholinesterases (choline ester hydrolases), erythrocyte acetylcholinesterase, and plasma cholinesterase. Both acetylcholine and physostigmine bind to cholinesterases to form a complex, from which part of the complex known as the *leaving group* (ie, choline for acetylcholine) is removed, and the remaining acetylated (for acetylcholine) or carbamylated (for physostigmine) enzyme is hydrolyzed, regenerating the enzyme and freeing the acetate or carbamate groups, respectively (Figs. 110–2 and 110–3). For acetylcholine, the

A. General structure of carbamate inhibitors

B. Physostigmine

C. Neostigmine

FIGURE A11–1. (**A**) General formula for carbamate cholinesterase inhibitors. (**B**) Structure of physostigmine. (**C**) Structure of neostigmine.

755

process is extremely rapid, with a turnover time of 150 milliseconds. In contrast, the half-life for hydrolysis of the carbamylated enzyme is 15 to 30 minutes.[60] The I_{50} (molar concentration that inhibits 50% of the enzyme) of physostigmine is 2.3×10^{-7} mol/L (M) for acetylcholinesterase, which is much weaker than for other carbamates at 1×10^{-10} M and many organic phosphorus compounds at 1×10^{-11} M.[28] Only the S-isomer of physostigmine inhibits cholinesterases, with plasma cholinesterase slightly more sensitive than acetylcholinesterase.[4] Newer xenobiotics used in the treatment of Alzheimer disease[13] show selectivity for the CNS and for acetylcholinesterase. This group includes tacrine, donepezil, and galantamine, which are reversible cholinesterase inhibitors, and rivastigmine, considered a pseudo-irreversible or slowly reversible inhibitor. These pharmaceuticals and neostigmine[29] have undergone limited study for reversal of anticholinergic poisoning.[13,29,33,53]

Pharmacokinetics and Pharmacodynamics

Physostigmine is poorly absorbed orally, with a bioavailability of less than 5% to 12%.[1,46] Cholinesterases rapidly cleave the ester linkage, resulting in very little unaltered physostigmine elimination in the urine. Pharmacokinetic parameters after intravenous (IV) administration of 1.5 mg over 60 minutes in 9 patients with Alzheimer disease demonstrated the following: volume of distribution, 2.4 ± 0.6 L/kg; half-life, 16.4 ± 3.2 minutes; peak serum concentration, 3 ± 0.5 ng/mL; and clearance, 0.1 L/min/kg (7.7 L/min). There was a threefold interindividual variability in plasma physostigmine concentrations. Plasma cholinesterase concentrations demonstrated inhibition within 2 minutes of initiating the physostigmine infusion. The half-life of plasma cholinesterase inhibition was 83.7 ± 5.2 minutes, with full recovery within 3 hours of termination of physostigmine infusion. The effects on plasma cholinesterase inhibition lasted approximately 5 times longer than the half-life of physostigmine.[32] All patients experienced varying degrees of diaphoresis, nausea, vomiting, headache, and generalized fatigue despite pretreatment with 2.5 mg of methscopolamine.[3,32]

ROLE IN ANTIMUSCARINIC TOXICITY

Physostigmine was first used as an antidote in 1864 to counteract severe atropine poisoning.[41] Today its role is primarily in the treatment of antimuscarinic poisoning. More than 600 xenobiotics respond to physostigmine.[14] Anticholinergics fall into the categories of antimuscarinic (atropine, scopolamine, hyoscyamine, propantheline, benztropine, trihexyphenidyl), neuromuscular blockers (curare), and ganglionic blockers (trimethaphan). Other xenobiotics (antihistamines, antipsychotics, and antidepressants) have antimuscarinic properties that are not their primary therapeutic actions and are often considered adverse drug effects.

The clinical use of physostigmine has varied over time.[2,15,51,55,67] Owing to its ability to cause CNS arousal, physostigmine was used in the 1970s to reverse the CNS effects of a large number of antimuscarinics and used inappropriately to treat toxicity from nonantimuscarinics.[22,37,39,42,47] The success with regard to antimuscarinics is directly related to the inhibition of cholinesterase. The effects of physostigmine on nonantimuscarinic xenobiotics such as the benzodiazepines, opioids,[34,48,68] GHB,[5,63] and baclofen[50] result from either the direct action of acetylcholine on the reticular activating system or interdependence of central neurotransmitters.[42] Few serious adverse effects are reported.[66] However, asystole followed administration of physostigmine in 2 patients with tricyclic antidepressant (TCA) overdose, and others have also reported these findings.[44,52,62] In addition, animal experiments do not support the use of physostigmine for this overdose.[19,64,71] This occurrence led to the realization that toxicity from TCA is complex and consists of more than just antimuscarinic effects.[44] Cyclic antidepressant–induced sodium channel blockade causes myocardial depression, QRS complex prolongation, and ventricular dysrhythmias. Physostigmine augments vagal effects, thus contributing to decreased cardiac output and cardiac conduction defects. An extensive review of the literature concluded that the safety of physostigmine use for seizures or cardiotoxicity in the setting of cyclic antidepressant toxicity was difficult to predict and thus not recommended, and we agree.[59]

In most instances, risks of physostigmine use for xenobiotics that are not primarily antimuscarinic outweigh any benefit.

This analysis is certainly also true with regard to GHB (Chap. 80).[63] γ-Hydroxybutyric acid is often used concomitantly with other xenobiotics, and the clinical manifestations are highly variable.[73] Recovery from GHB typically occurs spontaneously within several hours (16 minutes to 6 hours).[8,9,17,35,63,65] Three patients in whom a presumptive diagnosis of GHB toxicity was made were treated with physostigmine.[8] The 3 patients had an improved mental status within 5 to 15 minutes. One of these patients relapsed and then fully awakened 40 minutes later. This patient was incontinent of feces, an adverse effect likely caused by the physostigmine.[8] All 3 of the patients were arousable before physostigmine use. Although anesthetic study of GHB in the 1970s is the rationale cited for the current use of physostigmine, it is illogical in the care of those who illicitly use GHB because of limited demonstrated benefit and significant undetermined risks.[26]

However, in cases of antimuscarinic overdose, physostigmine use clearly is beneficial.[7,51] A study of 52 patients showed that whereas benzodiazepines controlled agitation in 24% of patients and were ineffective in reversing delirium, physostigmine controlled agitation and reversed delirium in 96% and 87% of patients, respectively.[7] A shorter time to recovery after agitation was observed in those treated with physostigmine. No significant differences between these groups with regard to side effects or length of stay were noted.[7]

We recommend the use of physostigmine in the presence of peripheral or central antimuscarinic manifestations without evidence of significant QRS complex prolongation. Peripheral manifestations of an antimuscarinic include dry mucosa, dry skin, flushed face, mydriasis, hyperthermia, decreased bowel sounds, urinary retention, and tachycardia. Central manifestations include agitation, delirium, hallucinations, seizures, and coma.[20,24,36] The peripheral and central findings are usually present on clinical presentation.[1,6,11,16,18,28,54,58] Rarely, the central findings may persist longer than the peripheral findings, or be more prominent.

ADVERSE EFFECTS AND SAFETY ISSUES

An excess of physostigmine results in accumulation of acetylcholine at peripheral muscarinic receptors, nicotinic receptors (skeletal muscle, autonomic ganglia, adrenal glands), and CNS sites.[31] Muscarinic effects produce stimulation of smooth muscle and glandular secretions in the respiratory, gastrointestinal, and genitourinary tracts, and inhibition of contraction of most vascular smooth musculature.[2,40] Nicotinic effects are stimulatory at low doses and depressant at high doses. For example, acetylcholine excess at the neuromuscular junction produces fasciculations followed by weakness and paralysis. Its effect on the CNS results in anxiety, dizziness, tremors, confusion, ataxia, coma, and seizures.[31] Electroencephalograms demonstrate asynchronous discharges followed by higher voltage discharges and a pattern similar to tonic–clonic seizures.[31] The cardiovascular effects are dose dependent and directly related to the presence of the diverse muscarinic and nicotinic effects.[31] In addition to its inhibition of cholinesterase, physostigmine has a direct action on the nicotinic acetylcholine receptor ionic channel.[38,57]

Physostigmine toxicity results when physostigmine is used in the absence of antimuscarinic toxicity or when excess doses are administered relative to the antimuscarinic xenobiotic exposure. Patients overdosed with physostigmine should be managed with intensive supportive care, including mechanical ventilation if needed; IV atropine[69] titrated to reverse bronchial secretions; and, rarely, pralidoxime to reverse skeletal muscle effects.[12]

We do not recommend administering physostigmine to patients with reactive airway disease, peripheral vascular disease, intestinal or bladder obstruction, intraventricular conduction defects, and atrioventricular block or in patients receiving therapeutic doses of choline esters and succinycholine.[45,46] It is unclear why the package insert also lists diabetes as a contraindication and there is no reason to limit use for these patients if indicated clinically.[45] Drug interactions with cholinergic agonists (eg, ophthalmic pilocarpine); depolarizing neuromuscular blockers; or other anticholinesterases such as carbamates, organic phosphorus compounds, and pyridostigmine are expected to be additive clinical effects when taken concomitantly with physostigmine. The actions of xenobiotics metabolized by plasma cholinesterases such as cocaine, succinylcholine, or mivacurium are expected to be prolonged.

Physostigmine salicylate injection contains sodium metabisulfite as a preservative.[45] Sulfites may cause life-threatening anaphylactoid reactions in susceptible individuals.

PREGNANCY AND LACTATION

Physostigmine is US Food and Drug Administration pregnancy category C. Little information is available regarding the effects of physostigmine in pregnancy. Transient muscular weakness occurred in 10% to 20% of neonates whose mothers received anticholinesterase treatment for myasthenia gravis.[46] Physostigmine should only be given when the benefit clearly outweighs the risk. Safety in lactation is not established.

DOSING AND ADMINISTRATION

Prior to administration of physostigmine, the patient should be attached to a cardiac monitor and atropine placed at the bedside. The recommended dose of physostigmine is 1 to 2 mg in adults and 0.02 mg/kg (maximum, 0.5 mg/dose) in children intravenously infused over at least 5 minutes. The onset of action usually is within minutes.[28] It is reasonable to repeat this dose after 10 to 15 minutes if an adequate response is not achieved and muscarinic effects are not noted. Rapid administration is likely to cause bradycardia, hypersalivation leading to respiratory difficulty, and seizures. Although the half-life of physostigmine is approximately 16 minutes, its duration of action usually is much longer (often >1 hour) and is directly related to the duration of cholinesterase inhibition.[3] After reversal of anticholinergic symptoms, additional doses are recommended if clinical relapse occurs. The effective dose depends on the ingested dose and duration of action of the antimuscarinic xenobiotic. Although a total of 4 mg in divided doses usually is sufficient in most clinical situations,[20] significant interindividual variability exists. Atropine should be available at the bedside and titrated to effect should excessive cholinergic toxicity develop. A dose of atropine administered at half the physostigmine dose is recommended.

FORMULATION AND ACQUISITION

Physostigmine is available in 2-mL ampules containing 1 mg/mL of physostigmine salicylate. The vehicle contains sodium metabisulfite and benzyl alcohol.[45]

SUMMARY

- Physostigmine is used for the management of patients with an antimuscarinic syndrome, particularly those who have an agitated delirium and a normal QRS complex duration.
- In these patients, physostigmine has an excellent risk-to-benefit profile.

REFERENCES

1. Aquilonius S, Hartvig P. Clinical pharmacokinetics of cholinesterase inhibitors. *Clin Pharmacokinet.* 1986;11:236-249.
2. Arens AM, et al. Safety and effectiveness of physostigmine: a 10-year retrospective review. *Clin Toxicol (Phila).* 2018;56:101-107.
3. Asthana S, et al. Clinical pharmacokinetics of physostigmine in patients with Alzheimer's disease. *Clin Pharmacol Ther.* 1995;58:299-309.
4. Atack JR, et al. Comparative inhibitory effects of various physostigmine analogs against acetyl and butyrocholinesterases. *J Pharmacol Exp Ther.* 1989;249:194-202.
5. Bania TC, Chu J. Physostigmine does not effect arousal but produces toxicity in an animal model of severe-hydroxybutyrate intoxication. *Acad Emerg Med.* 2005;12:185-189.
6. Beaver KM, Gavin TJ. Treatment of acute anticholinergic poisoning with physostigmine. *Am J Emerg Med.* 1998;16:505-507.
7. Burns MJ, et al. A comparison of physostigmine and benzodiazepines for the treatment of anticholinergic poisoning. *Ann Emerg Med.* 2000;35:374-381.
8. Caldicott DGE, Kuhn M. Gamma-hydroxybutyrate overdose and physostigmine: teaching new tricks to an old drug? *Ann Emerg Med.* 2001;37:99-102.
9. Chin RL, et al. Clinical course of γ-hydroxy-butyrate overdose. *Ann Emerg Med.* 1998;31:716-722.
10. Cole JB, et al. Reversal of quetiapine-induced altered mental status with physostigmine: a case series. *Am J Emerg Med.* 2012;30:950-953.
11. Crowell EB, Ketchum JS. The treatment of scopolamine-induced delirium with physostigmine. *Clin Pharmacol Ther.* 1967;8:409-414.
12. Cumming G, et al. Treatment and recovery after massive overdose of physostigmine. *Lancet.* 1968;20:147-149.
13. Darreh-Shori T, et al. Long-lasting acetylcholinesterase splice variations in anticholinesterase-treated Alzheimer's disease patients. *J Neurochem.* 2004;88:1102-1113.
14. Daunderer M. Physostigmine salicylate as an antidote. *Int J Clin Pharmacol Ther Toxicol.* 1980;18:523-535.
15. Dawson AH, Buckley NA. Pharmacological management of anticholinergic delirium—theory, evidence and practice. *Br J Clin Pharmacol.* 2016;81:516-524.
16. Duvoisin R, Katz R. Reversal of central anticholinergic syndrome in man by physostigmine. *JAMA.* 1968;206:1963-1965.
17. Eckstein M, et al. Gamma-hydroxy-butyrate (GHB): report of a mass intoxication and review of the literature. *Prehosp Emerg Care.* 1999;3:357-361.
18. El-Yousef MK, et al. Reversal of antiparkinsonian drug toxicity by physostigmine: a controlled study. *Am J Psychiatry.* 1973;130:141-145.
19. Fleck C, Bräunlich H. Failure of physostigmine in intoxications with tricyclic antidepressants in rats. *Toxicology.* 1982;24:335-344.
20. Forrer GR, Miller JJ. Atropine coma—a somatic therapy in psychiatry. *Am J Psychiatry.* 1958;115:455-458.
21. Fraser TR. On the characters, action and therapeutic uses of the bean of Calabar. *Edinb Med J.* 1863;9:36-56;235-245.
22. Giannini AJ, Castellani S. A case of phenylcyclohexylpyrrolidine (PHP) intoxication treated with physostigmine. *J Toxicol Clin Toxicol.* 1982;19:505-508.
23. Glatstein MM, et al. Use of physostigmine for hallucinogenic plant poisoning in a teenager: case report and review of the literature. *Am J Ther.* 2012;19:384-388.
24. Goldfrank L, et al. Anticholinergic poisoning. *J Toxicol Clin Toxicol.* 1982;19:17-25.
25. Hail SL, et al. Successful management of olanzapine-induced anticholinergic agitation and delirium with a continuous intravenous infusion of physostigmine in a pediatric patient. *Clin Toxicol.* 2013;51:162-166.
26. Henderson RS, Holmes CM. Reversal of the anaesthetic action of sodium gamma-hydroxybutyrate. *Anaesth Intensive Care.* 1976;4:351-354.
27. Holmstedt BO. The ordeal bean of old Calabar: the pageant of *Physostigmine venenosum* in medicine. In: Swain T, ed. *Plants in the Development of Modern Medicine.* Cambridge, MA: Harvard University Press; 1975:303-360.
28. Holzgrate RE, et al. Reversal of postoperative reactions to scopolamine with physostigmine. *Anesth Analg.* 1973;52:921-925.
29. Isbister GK, et al. Treatment of anticholinergic-induced ileus with neostigmine. *Ann Emerg Med.* 2001;38:689-693.
30. Karczmar AG. History of the research with anticholinesterase agents. In: Karczmar AG, ed. *International Encyclopedia of Pharmacology and Therapeutics.* Vol I. Oxford: Pergamon Press; 1970:1-44.
31. Karczmar AG. Pharmacology of anticholinesterase agents. In: Karczmar AG, ed. *International Encyclopedia of Pharmacology and Therapeutics.* Vol I. Oxford: Pergamon Press; 1970:45, 363.
32. Knapp S, et al. Correlation between plasma physostigmine concentrations and percentage of acetylcholinesterase inhibition over time after controlled release of physostigmine in volunteer subjects. *Drug Metab Dispos.* 1991;19:400-404.
33. Krall WJ, et al. Cholinesterase inhibitors: a therapeutic strategy for Alzheimer disease. *Ann Pharmacother.* 1999;33:441-450.
34. Larson GF, et al. Physostigmine reversal of diazepam-induced depression. *Anesth Analg.* 1977;56:348-351.
35. Li J, et al. A tale of novel intoxication: seven cases of γ-hydroxybutyric acid overdose. *Ann Emerg Med.* 1998;31:723-728.
36. Longo VG. Behavioral and electroencephalographic effects of atropine and related compounds. *Pharmacol Rev.* 1966;18:965-996.
37. Manoguerra AS. Poisoning with tricyclic antidepressant drugs. *Clin Toxicol.* 1977;10:149-158.
38. Militante J, et al. Activation and block of the adult muscle-type nicotinic receptor by physostigmine: single-channel studies. *Mol Pharmacol.* 2008;74:764-776.
39. Nattel S, et al. Physostigmine in coma due to drug overdose. *Clin Pharmacol Ther.* 1979;25:96-102.
40. Nguyen TT, et al. Adverse events from physostigmine: an observational study. *Am J Emerg Med.* 2018;36:141-142.
41. Nickalls RWD, Nickalls EA. The first use of physostigmine in the treatment of atropine poisoning. *Anesthesiology.* 1988;43:776-779.
42. Nilsson E. Physostigmine treatment in various drug-induced intoxications. *Ann Clin Res.* 1982;14:165-172.
43. Padilla RB, Pollack ML. The use of physostigmine in diphenhydramine overdose. *Am J Emerg Med.* 2002;20:569-570.
44. Pentel P, Peterson CD. Asystole complicating physostigmine treatment of tricyclic antidepressant overdose. *Ann Emerg Med.* 1980;9:588-590.
45. Physostigmine Salicylate Injection [package insert]. Lake Forest, IL: Akorn; 2008.
46. Physostigmine Sulfate. *American Hospital Formulary Service (AHFS).* Bethesda, MD: American Society of Health-System Pharmacists; 2013.
47. Rumack BH. 707 cases of anticholinergic poisoning treated with physostigmine [abstract]. Presented at Annual Meeting of American Academy of Clinical Toxicology; Montreal, Quebec, Canada, 1975.

48. Rupreht J, et al. Physostigmine versus naloxone in heroin overdose. *J Toxicol Clin Toxicol.* 1983;21:387-397.

49. Saltuari L, et al. Failure of physostigmine in treatment of acute severe intrathecal baclofen intoxication. *N Engl J Med.* 1990;322:1533-1534.

50. Saulino M, et al. Best practices for intrathecal baclofen therapy: troubleshooting. *Neuromodulation.* 2016;19:632-641.

51. Schneir AB, et al. Complications of diagnostic physostigmine administration to emergency department patients. *Ann Emerg Med.* 2003;42:14-19.

52. Shannon M. Toxicology reviews: physostigmine. *Pediatr Emerg Care.* 1998;14:224-226.

53. Shepherd G, et al. Donepezil overdose: a tenfold dosing error. *Ann Pharmacother.* 1999;33:812-815.

54. Smiler BG, et al. Physostigmine reversal of scopolamine delirium in obstetric patients. *Am J Obstet.* 1973;116:326-329.

55. Smilkstein MJ. Physostigmine [editorial]. *J Emerg Med.* 1991;9:275-277.

56. Smith SW. Chiral toxicology: it's the same thing...only different. *Toxicol Sci.* 2009;110:4-30.

57. Somani SM, Dube SN. Physostigmine—an overview as pretreatment drug for organophosphate intoxication. *Int J Clin Pharmacol Ther Toxicol.* 1989;27:367-387.

58. Sopchak CA, et al. Central anticholinergic syndrome due to Jimson Weed physostigmine: therapy revisited? *J Toxicol Clin Toxicol.* 1998;36:42-45.

59. Suchard JR. Assessing physostigmine's contraindication in cyclic antidepressant ingestions. *J Emerg Med.* 2003;25:185-191.

60. Taylor P. Anticholinesterase agents. In: Brunton LL, ed. *Goodman & Gilman's The Pharmacological Basis of Therapeutics.* Chap 10. 12th ed. New York, NY: McGraw-Hill; 2011. http://accessmedicine.mhmedical.com.ezproxy.med.nyu.edu/content.aspx?bookid=374&Sectionid= 41266216. Accessed April 27, 2014.

61. Titier K, et al. Atypical antipsychotics: from potassium channels to torsade de pointes and sudden death. *Drug Saf.* 2005;28:35-51.

62. Tong T, et al. Tricyclic antidepressant overdose. *Drug Intel Clin Pharm.* 1976;10:711. http://journals.sagepub.com.ezproxy.med.nyu.edu/doi/pdf/10.1177/106002807601001209. Last accessed September 25, 2017.

63. Traub SJ, et al. Physostigmine as a treatment for gamma-hydroxybutyrate toxicity: a review. *J Toxicol Clin Toxicol.* 2002;40:781-787.

64. Vance MA, et al. Potentiation of tricyclic antidepressant toxicity by physostigmine in mice. *Clin Toxicol.* 1977;11:413-421.

65. Viera AJ, Yates SW. Toxic ingestion of gamma-hydroxybutyric acid. *South Med J.* 1999;92:404-405.

66. Walker WE, et al. Physostigmine—its use and abuse. *JACEP.* 1976;5:436-439.

67. Watkins JW, et al; Toxicology Investigators Consortium investigators. The use of physostigmine by toxicologists in anticholinergic toxicity. *J Med Toxicol.* 2015;11:179-184.

68. Weinstock M, et al. Effect of physostigmine on morphine-induced postoperative pain and somnolence. *Br J Anaesth.* 1982;54:429-443.

69. Weiss S. Persistence of action of physostigmine and the atropine physostigmine antagonism in animals and in man. *J Pharmacol Exp Ther.* 1925;27:181-188.

70. Weizberg M, et al. Altered mental status from olanzapine overdose treated with physostigmine. *Clin Toxicol.* 2006;44:319-325.

71. Wiezorek WD, Kästner I. Effects of physostigmine on acute toxicity of tricyclic antidepressants and benzodiazepines in mice and rats. *Arch Toxicol Suppl.* 1982;5:133-135.

72. Young SE, et al. Reversal of systemic toxic effects of scopolamine with physostigmine salicylate. *Am J Ophthalmol.* 1971;72:1136-1138.

73. Zvosec D, et al. Physostigmine for gamma-hydroxybutyrate coma: inefficacy, adverse events, and review. *Clin Toxicol.* 2007;45:261-265.

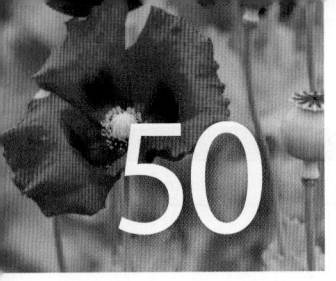

50 CHEMOTHERAPEUTICS

Richard Y. Wang

Chemotherapeutics or antineoplastics are a unique class of pharmaceuticals commonly used to kill cancer cells. The conventional chemotherapeutics are also toxic to noncancerous cells in the host, which makes an overdose of these pharmaceuticals a major concern to clinicians. Most overdoses from conventional chemotherapeutics are iatrogenic, and they involve misreading of the product label, and errors in dosing and transcription of orders (Chap. 134). A key element in these incidents is the lack of familiarity of the clinician with the use of these select pharmaceuticals. In the last several years, the use of chemotherapeutics has changed. For example, therapeutic indications now include other diseases, such as autoimmune diseases; the new chemotherapeutics target cancer cells and many of them are administered orally, and new delivery techniques are available. These new developments will increase the number and frequency of unintentional exposures and unintended dosing regimens, although the adoption of safety standards for the administration limits these errors (Chap. 134).[24,31]

Although overdoses of chemotherapeutics are infrequent, these events are of greater consequence than overdoses of many other xenobiotics because these drugs have a narrow therapeutic index. This is evident from surveillance data from poison control centers in the United States. From 1988 to 2015, the median annual number of people exposed to chemotherapeutics reported to US poison control centers was about 1200. In the last 10 years of data, the number of annual exposures to these chemotherapeutics went from 1649 in 2006 to 2039 in 2015 (Chap. 130). These exposures represent about 0.1–0.2% of pharmaceutical exposures, or 0.06–0.1% of all exposures annually reported to US poison control centers. Approximately two-thirds of the people exposed to chemotherapeutics in these reports were adults, one-fourth of the group were young children, and the remainder were adolescents. The annual trend for the proportion of exposures among adults and children remained at approximately 70% and 25%, respectively, from 2001 to 2015. Children and adolescents between the ages of 6 and 19 years accounted for approximately 6% of the population annually exposed, and this frequency did not change during these years. Although these differences among age groups might represent the incidence of cancer in these populations, further analysis is warranted to better define the reasons for these observations.

Among single exposures to chemotherapeutics reported to US poison control centers from 2007 to 2015, the annual percentage of unintentional exposures approached 90% and the annual percentage of exposures resulting in moderate or major severity in toxicity remained at approximately 6%. The mortality was about 0.2–0.3% of single exposures in this same period. These observations are attributed to the substantial toxicity of these chemotherapeutics. A prospective study on medication safety in the ambulatory chemotherapy setting demonstrated that potential adverse drug events from medical errors for chemotherapy orders were more likely to be serious than nonchemotherapy orders.[21] The prevalence of the exposure to chemotherapeutics is expected to continue increasing because of the increased availability of oral formulations[71] and their expanding therapeutic indications, but their severity is likely to fall as the immunotherapies become more widely utilized.

PATIENT-SPECIFIC FACTORS CONTRIBUTING TO TOXICITY

Aside from unintentional exposures, additional factors leading to increased toxicity associated with chemotherapeutics include age, sex, comorbidities, compromised host state, and diminished kidney and liver functions. Diminished hepatic clearance caused by altered enzyme expression is accounted for by age, sex, smoking status, and the concurrent use of other xenobiotics. Differences in sex contributes to varying pharmacokinetic parameters, including bioavailability, distribution, metabolism, and elimination. Women

treated with 5-fluorouracil (5-FU) for colon cancer had a twofold higher frequency of drug-related toxicity than men.[68] The manifestations included leukopenia, diarrhea, and stomatitis. Although the basis for this difference in toxicity between sexes is not known, it can result from a decreased 5-FU clearance in women.[74]

At an individual level, genetic polymorphisms can contribute to differences in xenobiotic response with resultant toxicity by altering targets, transporters, and enzyme complexes. Such variations are characterized for several enzymes that are involved in the metabolism of chemotherapeutics. Two examples of this type of toxicity include irinotecan used for the treatment of metastatic colon cancer and 5-fluorouracil used for the treatment of certain types of gastrointestinal (GI) and breast cancers. Irinotecan is a topoisomerase I inhibitor that works through its active metabolite, SN-38, which causes diarrhea and neutropenia at elevated concentrations.[70] A genetic variant of uridine diphosphate glucuronosyltransferase (UGT1A1) containing the T7 allele glucuronidates SN-38 at a slower rate than other variants, which results in increased SN-38 concentrations and increased toxicity.[3,29] Another example is 5-fluorouracil (5-FU), which is an antagonist to uracil, and it is inactivated by dihydropyrimidine dehydrogenase (DPD) in the liver (Chap. 51). The enzyme DPD metabolizes more than 80% of 5-FU to 5,6-dihydro-5-fluorouracil and alpha-fluoro-beta-alanine, and low or absent activity of this enzyme results in hematologic and GI toxicities from treatment with 5-FU or its prodrug capecitabine. The genetic variant DPYD*2A (rs3918290) of DPD is an inactive enzyme, and patients homozygous for this allele are at risk for severe toxicity and advised to seek an alternative therapeutic.[8] There are additional polymorphisms in metabolism associated with chemotherapeutics[19]; however, further work is necessary to define their clinical significance. Because of the narrow therapeutic index of the chemotherapeutics, the significance of such findings demonstrates the benefit of individual drug monitoring and genetic screening for use to maximize the therapeutic efficacy while limiting host toxicity.

CLASSES OF CHEMOTHERAPEUTICS

Most chemotherapeutics are grouped into one of 5 categories: alkylating agents, antibiotics, antimetabolites, antimitotics, and platinum-based complexes (Table 50–1). Some new chemotherapeutics target specific proteins located on the cell membrane, such as growth factor receptors, to inhibit the proliferation of tumor cells (Fig. 50–1).[36,50] These chemotherapeutics are categorized as monoclonal antibodies and protein kinase inhibitors based on their mechanisms of action. The antimetabolites are grouped by the substrates with which they interfere. Methotrexate is a folate antagonist; other nonchemotherapeutics with a similar mechanism, but lesser toxicity include trimethoprim and pyrimethamine. The antimitotics are plant alkaloids and they exert toxic effects by interrupting microtubule assembly. Others are naturally derived and include the antibiotics and the enzyme L-asparaginase, which is isolated from bacteria. The alkylating agents are more commonly used than other chemotherapeutics and cause covalent binding to nucleic acids, which inhibits DNA activity (Fig. 50–2). The more notable chemotherapeutics in this class, including those with similar activity, are the nitrogen mustards, nitrosoureas, and platinum-based complexes. The alkylating agents affect the cell at all phases in the cell cycle. Some xenobiotics are cell cycle phase–specific; that is, they affect the cell at only a specific phase in the cell cycle. For example, vincristine is M phase–specific and cytarabine is S phase–specific, in their sites of action. Other chemotherapeutics inhibit topoisomerase, which is necessary for DNA replication because it allows for reversible DNA strand breaks.

TABLE 50–1	Classification of Chemotherapeutics, Their Adverse Effects, and Antidotal Therapy			
Class	**Antineoplastic**	**Adverse Effects**	**Overdose**	**Antidotes**
Alkylating agents	Busulphan	Hyperpigmentation, pulmonary fibrosis, hyperuricemia	Myelosuppression	
	Dacarbazine	Hypotension, hepatocellular toxicity, influenzalike illness		
	Nitrogen mustards			
	Chlorambucil, cyclophosphamide, ifosfamide, mechlorethamine, melphalan	Hemorrhagic cystitis, encephalopathy, pulmonary fibrosis	Seizures, encephalopathy, myocardial necrosis, acute kidney injury, hyponatremia	MESNA; methylene blue
	Nitrosoureas			
	Carmustine, lomustine, semustine, streptozocin	Pulmonary fibrosis, hepatocellular toxicity, acute kidney injury	Myelosuppression (delayed onset and prolonged duration)	
	Procarbazine	Inhibition of monoamine oxidase (MAOI)		
	Temozolomide		Myelosuppression	
Antibiotics	Anthracycline			
	Daunorubicin, doxorubicin, epirubicin, idarubicin	Dilated congestive cardiomyopathy	Dysrhythmias, cardiomyopathy, CHF, myelosuppression	Dexrazoxane
	Bleomycin	Pulmonary fibrosis		
	Dactinomycin	Hepatocellular toxicity		
	Mitomycin C	Hemolytic uremic syndrome		
	Mitoxantrone	Dilated cardiomyopathy	Cardiomyopathy, CHF	None
Antimetabolites	Methotrexate	Mucositis, nausea, diarrhea, hepatocellular toxicity	Mucositis, myelosuppression, acute kidney injury	Folinic acid; Glucarpidase (carboxypeptidase-G_2)
	Purine analogs			
	Fludarabine	Encephalopathy, muscle weakness		
	Mercaptopurine	Hyperuricemia, pancreatitis, cholestasis	Myelosuppression, hepatocellular toxicity	
	Pentostatin	Hepatocellular toxicity		
	Thioguanine	Hyperuricemia		
	Pyrimidine analogs			
	Cytarabine	Acute respiratory distress syndrome, neuropathy, cerebellar ataxia		
	Fluorouracil, capecitabine	Cardiogenic shock, cardiomyopathy, cerebellar ataxia, diarrhea, mucositis, myelosuppression, neuropathy	Mucositis, myelosuppression, myocardial ischemia, cardiac conduction disorders	Uridine triacetate
Antimitotics	Taxanes			None
	Docetaxel, paclitaxel	GI perforation, peripheral neuropathy, dysrhythmias		
	Vinca alkaloids			
	Vinblastine, vincristine, vindesine	Peripheral neuropathy, hyponatremia (SIADH)	Encephalopathy, seizures, autonomic instability, paralytic ileus, myelosuppression	
Enzyme	L-Asparaginase	Hypersensitivity, pancreatitis, and coagulopathy	No reports	None
Monoclonal antibodies	Many: Gemtuzumab, trastuzumab	Hypersensitivity, specific to the site of action, and infection	No reports	None
Platinum-based complexes	Cisplatin, carboplatin, oxaliplatin	Acute kidney injury, peripheral neuropathy, hypomagnesemia, hypocalcemia, hyponatremia, ototoxicity, myelosuppression	Seizures, encephalopathy, ototoxicity, retinal toxicity, myelosuppression, peripheral neuropathy	Amifostine; thiosulfate
Protein kinase inhibitors	Many: Gefitinib, sorafenib, erlotinib	GI (nausea, diarrhea), acneiform rash (folliculitis), nail fragility, and xerosis (EGFR inhibitor), interstitial lung disease (erlotinib, gefitinib), hypertension (inhibitors of VEGF and PDGFR), hypothyroidism (sunitinib), and infection	Nausea, vomiting, facial rash, and edema	None
Topoisomerase inhibitor	Camptothecins	Neutropenia, mucositis, diarrhea, early onset cholinergic syndrome (irinotecan)	Myelosuppression	None
	Irinotecan			
	Topotecan			
	Epipodophyllotoxins			
	Etoposide, teniposide	CHF, hypotension		

CHF = congestive heart failure, EGFR = epidermal growth factor receptor; GI = gastrointestinal; MESNA= mercaptoethane sulfonate; MAOI = monoamine oxidase inhibitor; PDGFR = platelet-derived growth factor receptor; SIADH = syndrome of inappropriate antidiuretic hormone; VEGF = vascular endothelial growth factor.

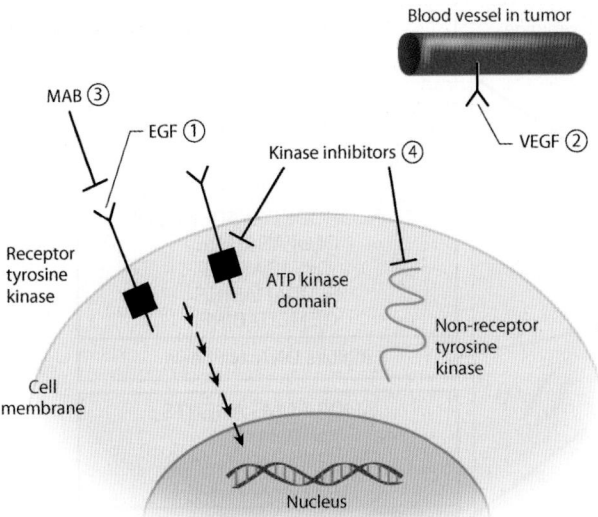

FIGURE 50–1. Sites of action of selected targeted agents. Tyrosine kinases initiate signal transduction pathways and production of transcription factors that are responsible for cellular processes, including proliferation, survival, angiogenesis, and progression. Growth factors, such as endothelial growth factor (EGF) and vascular endothelial growth factor (VEGF), bind and activate transmembrane tyrosine kinases by causing receptor dimerization and phosphorylation ①. VEGF promotes endothelial cell mitogenesis and migration, which leads to vascular proliferation ②. Tyrosine kinases are inhibited by monoclonal antibody (MAB) binding at the cell surface receptor site ③ or by kinase inhibitors at the adenine triphosphate (ATP) binding site or substrate-binding site, or causing a change in the conformation of the enzyme (NIB) ④.

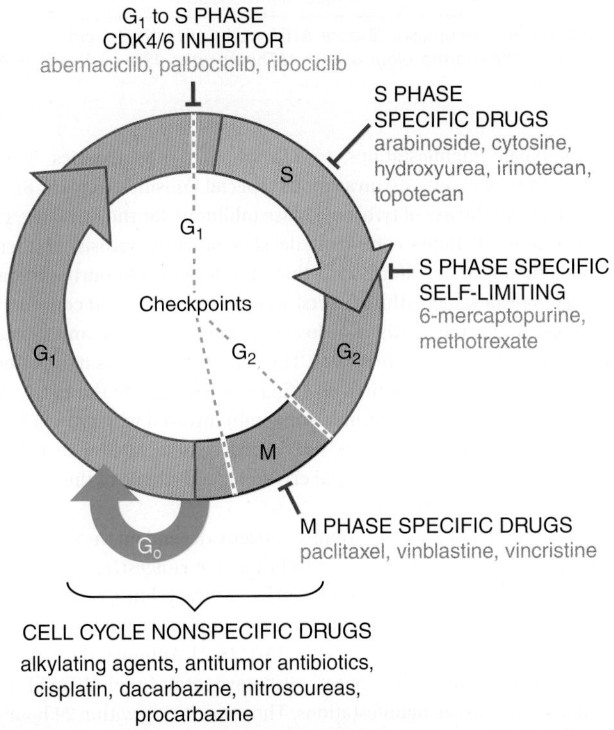

G₁ to S PHASE CDK4/6 INHIBITOR
abemaciclib, palbociclib, ribociclib

S PHASE SPECIFIC DRUGS
arabinoside, cytosine, hydroxyurea, irinotecan, topotecan

S PHASE SPECIFIC SELF-LIMITING
6-mercaptopurine, methotrexate

Checkpoints

G₁, G₂, S, M, G₀

M PHASE SPECIFIC DRUGS
paclitaxel, vinblastine, vincristine

CELL CYCLE NONSPECIFIC DRUGS
alkylating agents, antitumor antibiotics, cisplatin, dacarbazine, nitrosoureas, procarbazine

FIGURE 50–2. Cell cycle specificity of chemotherapeutics: selected class of cell style phase-specific chemotherapeutics and their sites of action in the cell cycle. Arrows represent the progression of the cell cycle by phases, G₀ (resting), G₁ (gap1), G₂ (gap2), M (mitosis), and S (DNA synthesis). *(Reproduced with permission from Brunton LL, Hilal-Dandan R, Knollmann BC. Goodman & Gilman's: The Pharmacological Basis of Therapeutics, 13th ed. New York, NY: McGraw Hill Education; 2018.)*

MECHANISMS OF ACTION

The mechanisms responsible for the cytotoxic effects of the chemotherapeutics are the disruption of cellular growth and proliferation (Chap. 23), which impairs DNA function by causing strand breaks, inhibiting strand relaxation, and serving as inhibitory analogs of essential cofactors and nitrogenous bases of nucleic acids (Fig. 50–3). For example, alkylating agents form reactive intermediates that covalently bind to nitrogenous bases on the DNA structure, which leads to the formation of strand breaks and mispairings. Cross-linkages between strands occurs with the nitrogen mustards because they contain 2 reactive chloroethyl side chains (Fig. 23–2). The planar anthracycline antibiotics intercalate with DNA, impair topoisomerase II activity, and cause DNA strand breaks through oxidative damage induced by a reactive semiquinone intermediate. The relaxation of DNA strands is impaired by topoisomerase I inhibitors, such as topotecan. Topotecan is derived from camptothecin, which is isolated from the tree *Camptotheca acuminata*. Single methyl transfer reactions and base pairings are essential activities during DNA synthesis that are affected by the antimetabolites, which include structural analogs to folate, pyrimidines, and purines.

Recent cancer therapy includes chemotherapeutics that limit cellular proliferation by inhibiting growth factor receptor activation and enhancing cell lysis by antibody-dependent cell-mediated cytotoxicity and complement-dependent cytotoxicity. Monoclonal antibodies to tumor cell surface antigens, such as CD20, CD22, and CD30, and the C1q complement are used to direct host defense mechanisms or deliver chemotherapeutics to these sites. For example, brentuximab vedotin is an antibody conjugated to the antimitotic agent, monomethyl auristatin E, and it is directed at CD30-positive tumor cells, which is common to lymphomas. Other antibody conjugates include radioactive isotopes (eg, Yttrium-90) and pseudomonas exotoxin A.[61] In addition to the above antigens, monoclonal antibodies against tumor growth factor receptors are available.

Tumor growth factors promote cell growth and proliferation (by angiogenesis). Their receptors located at the cell membrane are characterized for certain tumors, such as epidermal growth factor receptor (EGFR) found in lung, kidney, and gastrointestinal tumors, and human epidermal growth factor receptor 2 (HER2) in the breast. Vascular endothelial growth factor receptor (VEGFR) and platelet-derived growth factor receptor (PDGFR) are active in angiogenesis. Inactivation of these receptors is accomplished with therapeutic monoclonal antibodies (MAB) and protein kinase inhibitors. Monoclonal antibodies prevent the activation of these receptors by inhibiting substrate binding to the receptor located at the extracellular surface. Kinase inhibitors are considered to be small molecule therapeutics that impair the ATP activation of growth factor receptors, serine/tyrosine kinase inhibitors, mTOR kinase inhibitors, and certain signal transduction proteins responsible for tumor cell division and angiogenesis.

The disruption of the proliferation of keratinocytes, and intestinal epithelial cells at these tissue sites accounts for the anticipated toxic effects from the use of MABs and kinase inhibitors directed at EGFR. The therapeutic use of the protein kinase inhibitors of VEGFR and PDGFR, such as sunitinib and sorafenib, is associated with hypertension, which is attributed to endothelial dysfunction and diminished microvascular regrowth.

These monoclonal antibodies are derived from both human and chimeric (human and murine) sources, which contributes to the toxicity. The nomenclature scheme for this class of therapeutics is available elsewhere.[75] Immunologic responses to the presence of foreign proteins include rigors, nausea, vomiting, and rashes. Some organ-specific effects of varying antibodies include bone marrow, skin (via EGFR), kidney (hypomagnesemia via EGFR), gastrointestinal (via EFGR), and cardiac (via HER2, trastuzumab).

MANIFESTATIONS OF TOXICITY

The chemotherapeutics are primarily toxic to cells, with a high level of mitotic activity, such as hematopoietic and intestinal epithelial cells (Chap. 23). This characteristic feature accounts for their common clinical manifestations of toxicity, including mucositis, alopecia, and bone marrow suppression.

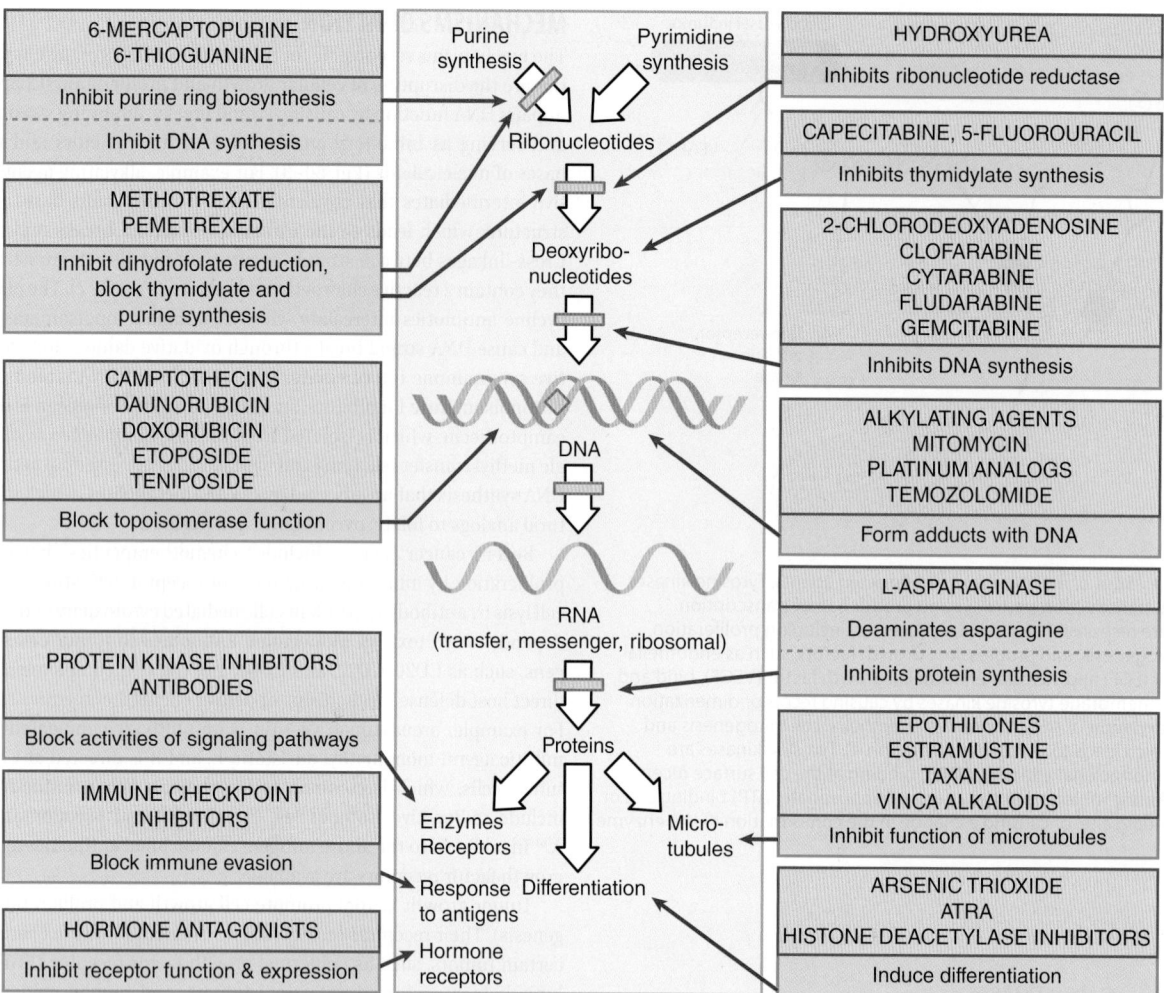

FIGURE 50–3. Summary of the mechanisms and sites of action of some chemotherapeutics useful in neoplastic disease. ATRA = all-*trans* retinoic acid. *(Reproduced with permission from Brunton LL, Hilal-Dandan R, Knollmann BC. Goodman & Gilman's: The Pharmacological Basis of Therapeutics, 13th ed. New York, NY: McGraw Hill Education; 2018.)*

They also cause protracted vomiting because they stimulate the chemoreceptor trigger zone in the medulla by vagal and sympathetic pathways either directly or indirectly through the GI tract. The likelihood for vomiting depends on the dose, the route of administration, and the type of chemotherapeutic. Although the onset of emesis typically occurs within 6 hours and lasts for 24 hours, delayed or persistent (>24 hours since administration) emesis occurs with cisplatin, cyclophosphamide, carboplatin, and doxorubicin. The factors attributed to acute or early onset of vomiting during therapy are serotonin ($5HT_3$ receptor) (primary) and dopamine (DA_2 receptor) mediated pathways. In contrast, persistent vomiting is attributed to various factors, including a tachykinin substance P (neurokinin {NK_1} receptor), local GI effects, and inflammation from cellular breakdown.

The time of onset for the other manifestations is typically in the first week following treatment, with mucositis preceding leukopenia, which varies depending on the chemotherapeutic and the dose. For example, the nadir and full recovery for neutropenia is about 10 to 14 days and 21 days, respectively, but more prolonged delays occur for busulfan and carmustine, and when higher doses are used. Anthracyclines and platinum-based complexes are likely to cause severe neutropenia, and methotrexate, 5-fluorouracil, bleomycin, and doxorubicin are likely to cause mucositis and severe dehydration because of the amount of GI fluid loss from diarrhea and vomiting. Death usually results from overwhelming sepsis as enteric organisms traverse compromised intestinal epithelium, enter the bloodstream, and attack a host with neutropenia from bone marrow suppression. Some of the unique manifestations of certain chemotherapeutics involve the skin, heart, central and peripheral nervous systems, and kidneys.

Dermatologic manifestations caused by chemotherapeutics include hypersensitivity reactions, extravasations (Special Considerations: SC8), and cytotoxicity from the use of tyrosine kinase inhibitors for the EGFR (eg, gefitinib, erlotinib).[77] Patients commonly develop pruritus, xerosis, erythema, and folliculitis or an acneiform rash that can desquamate during therapy. These reactions develop within the first week of treatment and continue for several weeks. The folliculitis is a dose-dependent response and typically resolves within weeks after treatment. The dermal response is more intense with monoclonal antibodies than the kinase inhibitors for the EFGR. The other kinase inhibitors (ie, sunitinib, sorafenib) involved with growth factor receptors for angiogenesis (ie, VEGFR, PDGFR) are associated with a "hand-foot" skin reaction, which is a painful erythema and edema of the palm and sole that leads to desquamation.

The cardiovascular manifestations of toxicity depend on the chemotherapeutic, and the common adverse effects include congestive heart failure (CHF), dysrhythmias, and hypertension. The anthracyclines, cyclophosphamide, 5-fluorouracil, and arsenic trioxide are examples of chemotherapeutics that cause cardiac toxicity (Tables 50–2, 15-1, 16-4). Although the anthracyclines classically produce late-onset cardiomyopathy (nonischemic), they also cause acute cardiac manifestations. Those occurring within 24 hours of therapy include dysrhythmias, ST segment and T wave changes on the electrocardiogram (ECG), diminished left ventricular ejection fraction (LVEF) leading to congestive heart failure, pericarditis, myocarditis, and sudden death.[7,57,58,65,76] Arsenic trioxide (As_2O_3) used for the treatment of acute promyelocytic leukemia causes dose-dependent prolongation of the QT interval and ventricular tachydysrhythmias, including torsade de pointes, during

TABLE 50–2	Cardiovascular Manifestations of Toxicity of Selected Chemotherapeutics	
Chemotherapeutic	Time of Onset Since Treatment	Manifestation
Anthracycline	<24 hours	Dysrhythmias, ST segment and T wave changes on ECG; diminished LVEF leading to CHF, pericarditis, myocarditis, and sudden death
	Months to years, typically at 1–4 months	Dilated congestive cardiomyopathy
Arsenic trioxide	Days	Prolongation of QT interval on ECG leading to ventricular tachydysrhythmias (torsade de pointes)
Cyclophosphamide	Days	CHF, hemorrhagic pericarditis, tamponade, and death
5-Fluorouracil	Hours to days	Myocardial ischemia, cardiac conduction disorders, and cardiogenic shock

CHF = congestive heart failure, ECG = electrocardiogram; LVEF = left ventricular ejection fraction.

the course of treatment.[5] Inorganic arsenic inhibits the slow (I_{Ks}) and rapid (I_{Kr}) delayed rectifier K^+ channels of ventricular myocytes, which impairs the efflux of potassium ions during ventricular repolarization (Chap. 86). These ECG changes tend to develop after several days of drug therapy, reverse upon discontinuation of the drug, and occur more frequently during intravenous than oral therapy because of the increased blood concentration of arsenic from the intravenous route of administration.[60] Patients at increased risk for cardiac conduction disorders during arsenic trioxide therapy include those with hypokalemia and hypomagnesemia, on medications that prolong the QT interval, and with underlying cardiac conduction disorders. Myocardial ischemia leading to cardiogenic shock occurs from the high-dose infusion of 5-fluorouracil.[69] The metabolite fluoroacetate is purported to cause endothelial damage and result in vasospasm.[4,25] Normalization of ECG findings, including diminished QRS complex voltage and abnormal ventricular wall motion, is expected by 48 hours after the discontinuation of infusion therapy.[13] Within a few days of exposure at high doses from therapy during bone marrow transplant or the overdose setting, cyclophosphamide causes CHF, hemorrhagic pericarditis, tamponade, and death at high doses. The cardiomyopathy from anthracyclines involves biventricular failure and its onset is variable, from months to years. Although this period is usually 1 to 4 months, it tends be longer for the less toxic anthracycline analogs.[22,32,62] Trastuzumab is associated with a slight increase in the incidence of CHF from diminished LVEF among patients previously treated with anthracyclines or with underlying heart disease.[23] A potential mechanism for the enhanced cardiac toxicity from the drug interaction is that trastuzumab disrupts the HER2-neuregulin compensatory response by the heart to the exposure to anthracyclines.[14] Lapatinib is another chemotherapeutic targeting HER2, but by inhibiting phosphorylation at the tyrosine kinase domain, and it slightly decreases LVEF.[47]

The neurologic toxicities of chemotherapeutics include central and peripheral manifestations. The acute manifestations of toxicity include alterations in mental status and seizures, which occur from the systemic administration of high doses of nitrogen mustards (cyclophosphamide, ifosfamide, and chlorambucil), nitrosoureas (lomustine), methotrexate, and vincristine. The inappropriate intrathecal administration of vincristine and methotrexate causes central nervous system toxicity (Special Considerations: SC7). Patients with prior seizure disorders, delayed drug clearance, and altered drug pharmacokinetics (eg, nephrotic syndrome)[55] are at increased risk for seizures. L-Asparaginase, 5-fluorouracil, and procarbazine are associated with alterations in mental status.[72] Cerebellar dysfunction is described in 5% of patients treated with 5-FU,[48] and high-frequency ototoxicity occurs

with cisplatin toxicity. The delayed-onset manifestations of neurotoxicity from chemotherapeutics include leukoencephalopathy and peripheral neuropathies. Leukoencephalopathy from methotrexate typically presents as a delayed onset of behavioral and progressive dementia and is irreversible. Peripheral neuropathy involving both sensory and motor findings is seen with the vinca alkaloids (vincristine) and bortezomib, whereas only sensory involvement is noted with cisplatin and paclitaxel.[39]

Kidney failure from tubulointerstitial pathology occurs from methotrexate, cisplatin, ifosfamide, or nitrosoureas in a dose-dependent manner. The nitrosoureas such as semustine can cause glomerular injury leading to sclerosis. Kidney damage is attributed to the formation of insoluble intratubular precipitates of drug metabolites (7-OH MTX metabolite for MTX) or reactive intermediates (cisplatin, nitrosoureas) that lead to cell death. The nitrosoureas also form isocyanates, which impair enzymes and contribute to irreversible kidney damage.[38] The onset, severity, and reversibility of kidney toxicity depend on the administered dose and the chemotherapeutic. For example, streptozocin is more nephrotoxic than the other nitrosoureas: semustine, lomustine, and carmustine. Patients at increased risk for worsening kidney function from these chemotherapeutics include those with prior kidney disease, increased age, salt and water depletion, hypotension, and concomitant use of nephrotoxic xenobiotics, such as aminoglycosides. Young children (<5 years old) are more vulnerable to ifosfamide-induced proximal tubular toxicity leading to urinary loss of phosphate and bicarbonate than older patients.[41,66] Also, patients with third space fluid, such as ascites and pleural effusions, and aciduria are at increased risk for MTX-induced kidney toxicity because of the prolonged half-life of the drug and the increased likelihood for the formation of insoluble precipitates in the renal tubules at a low urinary pH. The kidney failure from methotrexate, cispla and streptozocin typically presents within 1 to 2 weeks. Patients treated with semustine present with kidney compromise months to years following exposure.[73] Patients develop fluid and electrolyte abnormalities from the above chemotherapeutics, causing renal tubular disorders, and from vincristine, causing centrally mediated syndrome of inappropriate antidiuretic hormone secretion (SIADH) (Chaps. 12 and 34).

DIAGNOSTIC TESTING

The determination of a chemotherapeutic concentration in a clinical specimen is not routinely available, except for methotrexate. At certain research centers, the testing for specific xenobiotics such as busulfan,[64] cisplatin (platinum),[17] cyclophosphamide,[49] fluorouracil (α-fluoro-β-alanine),[49] ifosfamide,[49] and vincristine[15] are available. These concentrations are used to assist in confirming exposure and monitoring drug clearance, but should not be relied on to determine initial management because of the difficulty in obtaining these tests and ability to correlate the concentrations with clinical toxicity.

For certain chemotherapeutics, the presence of typical clinical manifestations strongly suggest their toxicity, for example, cisplatin (acute kidney injury and ototoxicity), vinca alkaloids (peripheral neuropathy, central autonomic instability) and SIADH, anthracyclines (CHF and dilated cardiomyopathy), ifosfamide (encephalopathy and seizures), and methotrexate (acute kidney injury, mucositis, and pancytopenia). The diagnosis of a patient with toxicity from these xenobiotics is based on a historical evidence for exposure, clinical manifestations, and laboratory findings that support toxicity or exposure. For patients presenting with delayed symptoms, the association between toxicity and exposure requires an increased level of awareness to establish the causation.[22] Additional studies should be performed to evaluate for specific disorders noted on the clinical examination, such as electromyography and nerve conduction studies for peripheral neuropathies, electroretinogram for retinopathies, and echocardiography for cardiac dysfunction.

GENERAL MANAGEMENT

The initial management of these patients includes stabilization of the hemodynamic status, decontamination, institution of antidotal therapy, and enhanced elimination. Maximal benefits from antidotes and enhanced elimination can be obtained through their timely institution. Hypotension typically results from salt and water depletion, cardiac dysfunction, or sepsis. It is reasonable to treat patients with myocardial ischemia from 5-FU with coronary vasodilators, such as nitrates and calcium channel blockers. Seizures are treated with benzodiazepines, and propofol. Encephalopathy from high-dose ifosfamide has been treated with methylene blue (adult: 50 mg intravenously {IV}) (Antidotes in Depth: A43).[46] Patients with blood dyscrasias, including neutropenia and thrombocytopenia, should be evaluated for gastrointestinal bleeding and infections. Those at risk for overwhelming sepsis should be started on broad-spectrum antibiotics and granulocyte colony stimulating factor as indicated. Oral activated charcoal is recommended for patients who present soon after an oral exposure to limit the gastrointestinal bioavailability of the agent. Repeat oral doses of activated charcoal are reasonable to enhance the clearance of methotrexate in patients with acute kidney injury.[20]

Patients with chemotherapeutic-related vomiting are typically difficult to manage. Combination therapy involving multiple antiemetics are needed to treat patients exposed to chemotherapeutics with high emetogenic potential (eg, cisplatin, doxorubicin, cyclophosphamide, lomustine) or excessive doses of chemotherapeutics with low emetogenic potential (eg, $5HT_3$ Vinca alkaloids, fluorouracil). Recommended therapies include serotonin receptor antagonists, corticosteroids, dopamine receptor antagonist, NK_1 receptor antagonist, or a benzodiazepine.[27] Serotonin receptor antagonists are effective for vomiting starting within 6 hours of exposure and are used with dexamethasone and a NK_1 receptor antagonist in patients with protracted vomiting. Once the serotonin receptors are saturated, additional doses are no longer effective. Neurokinin receptor antagonists used in combination with a corticosteroid, such as dexamethasone, are effective for managing delayed-onset vomiting, which can last for 5 days. Atypical antipsychotics (ie, olanzapine) and phenothiazines are reasonable to treat breakthrough vomiting. Benzodiazepines are reasonable in this setting, but they are most effective for the prevention of vomiting. A basic chemistry panel, complete blood count, urinalysis, and ECG should be obtained for patients with a significant overdose to evaluate toxicity and to establish baseline values. Pregnant women exposed to chemotherapeutics require individualized care that include consultations with an obstetrician-gynecologist, neonatologist, or a medical oncologist.[43,54] Information regarding the gestational age at the time of the exposure, and the name and class of the chemotherapeutic are important for this discussion.

The patient's peripheral blood count should be followed for up to 2 weeks after a chemotherapeutic is administered because of the delayed onset of myelosuppression.

Gastrointestinal fluid losses from vomiting, diarrhea, and mucosal ulcerations can lead to salt and water depletion, which should be treated with intravenous fluids. Intravenous fluids are important for patients with cisplatin and methotrexate toxicity to promote the renal elimination of toxic metabolites. Patients with cisplatin toxicity should be treated with 0.9% sodium chloride and an osmotic diuretic to maintain an adequate chloride gradient to promote the renal elimination of cisplatin. Urinary alkalinization is recommended for patients with MTX toxicity to limit the precipitation of drug metabolites in the renal tubules.

Antidotal therapy is available for only a few xenobiotics, including anthracyclines (dexrazoxane), methotrexate (leucovorin, glucarpidase), cisplatin (amifostine, thiosulfate), 5-FU or capecitabine (uridine triacetate), and ifosfamide (methylene blue, mercaptoethane sulfonate). These antidotes permit the use of higher doses of chemotherapeutics in cancer patients. However, patients with overdoses from chemotherapeutics also benefit from the use of these antidotes, which should be initiated soon after the decision to treat has been made. Additional information regarding them is found in Chap. 51 and Antidotes in Depth: A12, A13, A14, and A43.

Information on the use of enhanced elimination to remove these chemotherapeutics and their metabolites is limited to case reports in the literature. The effectiveness of these procedures is based on principles similar to other xenobiotics, including molecular size, extent of protein binding, and volume of distribution. Patients with diminished endogenous clearance from kidney failure or third spacing of fluid can benefit from these procedures as well. For example, cisplatin is highly protein bound and favored for removal by plasmapheresis, but patients with kidney failure also benefit from hemodialysis. Hemoperfusion was used for doxorubicin and it is recommended for use when it is available.[11,30,40,78] For the nitrogen mustards and the alkyl sulfonates, hemodialysis has been used. The early institution of these procedures can maximize the potential benefits to the patient.

The decision to use myeloid growth factors in patients with agranulocytosis depends on the severity and nature of the neutropenia, the anticipated speed of recovery, and the tumor type. Granulocyte-macrophage colony–stimulating factor (GM-CSF) was used for several patients with overdoses such as cisplatin, melphalan, bleomycin, fluorouracil, and methotrexate.[12,26,33-35,37,42,45,63] Typically, if promyelocytes and myelocytes are present in the bone marrow, neutrophil recovery will occur spontaneously in 4 to 7 days, following the withdrawal of the offending chemotherapeutic.[18] However, when granulopoiesis is completely absent, neutrophil recovery cannot be expected for at least 14 days. The use of granulocyte colony–stimulating factor (G-CSF) or GM-CSF accelerates neutrophil recovery during cytotoxic chemotherapy. When myeloid precursors are present in the bone marrow, G-CSF accelerates neutrophil recovery in 1 to 4 days. If myeloid precursors are absent, neutrophil recovery with G-CSF takes longer, but is still enhanced. Granulocyte macrophage colony-stimulating factor is specifically indicated for use in older adult patients with neutropenia following induction chemotherapy for acute myelogenous leukemia, in mobilization of progenitor cells into the peripheral compartment for leukapheresis, and in myeloid recovery following transplantation of peripheral blood progenitor cells or bone marrow transplantation.

The serum concentration of the chemotherapeutic should be below detection before institution of G-CSF to gain maximal response; typically, G-CSF is initiated within one to 3 days of the completion of the treatment cycle. The treatment with G-CSF is continued beyond the expected white blood cell (WBC) nadir for an approximately 2-week course, although it can be prolonged for CCNU (lomustine) overdoses because of direct toxicity to progenitor cells in the bone marrow (Chap. 23).[1,67] The absolute neutrophil count (ANC) is monitored twice a week to assess the response to G-CSF. Bone pain should be anticipated from the use of colony-stimulating factors, presumably because of the increase in cellularity in the marrow space. Additional expected side effects from GM-CSF therapy include myalgia, fevers, and pericarditis.

Granulocyte macrophage colony-stimulating factor produces a transient beneficial response in the WBCs in patients with aplastic anemia.[10] However, when the anemia is severe, the GM-CSF therapy is not effective. Another hematopoietic growth factor, erythropoietin, is approved for use in patients with anemia associated with cancer chemotherapy.[6,52] Although the purpose of this therapy is to decrease the need for red blood cell transfusions, it does not replace the need for red blood cell transfusion when indicated.

CHEMOTHERAPEUTICS IN THE WORKPLACE

Pharmacists, nurses, physicians, and others involved in the preparation and dispensing of chemotherapeutics, and those who may be exposed to the body fluids of patients treated with chemotherapeutics, are at increased risk for toxicity. Several studies demonstrate that chemotherapeutics are detected at the work environment and measured in workers,[28,53,56] and there is concern about the possible genotoxic effects from these exposures.[16,59] The worker adsorption of these xenobiotics occurs by either the dermal, inhalational, or gastrointestinal route. The factors determining the amount of worker exposure include the nature of the work, the amount of drug used, the frequency and duration of exposure, the physical and chemical nature of the drug, and the use of ventilated cabinets and personal protection equipment during the handling of these chemotherapeutics. The workplace guidelines for chemotherapeutics fall under the broader category of hazardous agents. National Institute for Occupational Safety and Health (NIOSH) defines a "drug" as a "hazardous agent" if it is carcinogenic, teratogenic, genotoxic, associated with developmental or reproductive toxicity, or toxic to organs at low dose. A sample list of drugs considered to be hazardous by NIOSH is available.[9]

Regulatory and workplace recommendations for exposure levels and the waste management of these xenobiotics are available from various agencies and organizations. These recommendations are limited in scope because only a small number of xenobiotics or adverse health effects have been adequately studied, and many xenobiotics do not meet the current definition for inclusion. US Environmental Protection Agency (Resource Conservation and Recovery Act, 40 CFR §§260–279)[51] regulates 9 chemotherapeutics (arsenic trioxide, chlorambucil, cyclophosphamide, daunorubicin, melphalan, mitomycin C, naphthylamine mustard, streptozocin, and uracil mustard) and the equipment and devices associated with their preparation or delivery, as well as their disposal, as hazardous waste.[51] The current recommendations for worker safety with these xenobiotics at the workplace include the proper management of the work environment (eg, storage, handling, preparation, administration, use of personal protection equipment, decontamination, and waste disposal) and the institution of a medical surveillance program with approved laboratory testing.[2,44,59]

SUMMARY

- The chemotherapeutics are a unique therapeutic class because their cytotoxicity is a direct effect.
- Most conventional chemotherapeutic overdoses are iatrogenic, involving misreading of the product label, and errors in dosing and transcription of orders (Chap. 134). A key element is the lack of familiarity of the health care provider with the use of these select xenobiotics.
- Clinical manifestations of chemotherapeutic toxicity depend on the mechanism of action, route of administration, and duration of exposure. The gut epithelium and hematopoietic cells are extremely susceptible to toxicity because of their high mitotic activity. They are important because their failure will lead to overwhelming sepsis and death.
- Treatment remains primarily supportive in nature. The early institution of cytoprotectants, such as leucovorin, glucarpidase for methotrexate, amifostine for cisplatin, uridine triacetate for 5-FU and capecitabine, and dexrazoxane for anthracyclines, as antidotal therapy in overdosed patients can limit further toxicity. However, further work is needed to better define their use in these situations.
- The best treatment for chemotherapeutic overdoses is prevention, which can be accomplished by maintaining a heightened awareness when working with these xenobiotics, educating the patient and health care provider regarding their use, and providing increased skilled and standardized care.

Disclaimer

The findings and conclusions in this chapter are those of the author and do not necessarily represent the official position of the Centers for Disease Control and Prevention.

REFERENCES

1. Abele M, et al. CCNU overdose during PCV chemotherapy for anaplastic astrocytoma. *J Neurol.* 1998;245:236-238.
2. American Society of Hospital Pharmacists. ASHP guidelines on handling hazardous drugs. *Am J Hosp Pharm.* 2006;63:1172-1193.
3. Ando Y, et al. Polymorphisms of UDP-glucuronosyltransferase gene and irinotecan toxicity: a pharmacogenetic analysis. *Cancer Res.* 2000;60:6921-6926.
4. Arellano M, et al. The anti-cancer drug 5-fluorouracil is metabolized by the isolated perfused rat liver and in rats into highly toxic fluoroacetate. *Br J Cancer.* 1998;77:79-86.
5. Au WY, Kwong YL. Arsenic trioxide: safety issues and their management. *Acta Pharmacol Sin.* 2008;29:296-304.
6. Bokemeyer C, et al. EORTC guidelines for the use of erythropoietic proteins in anaemic patients with cancer: 2006 update. *Eur J Cancer.* 2007;43:258-270.
7. Bristow MR. Toxic cardiomyopathy due to doxorubicin. *Hosp Pract (Off Ed).* 1982;17:101-108, 110-111.
8. Caudle KE, et al. Clinical Pharmacogenetics Implementation Consortium guidelines for dihydropyrimidine dehydrogenase genotype and fluoropyrimidine dosing. *Clin Pharmacol Ther.* 2013;94:640-645.
9. Centers for Disease Control and Prevention. NIOSH list of antineoplastic and other hazrdous drugs in healthcare settings. https://www.cdc.gov/niosh/topics/antineoplastic/pdf/hazardous-drugs-list_2016-161.pdf. Published 2016.
10. Champlin RE, et al. Treatment of refractory aplastic anemia with recombinant human granulocyte-macrophage-colony-stimulating factor. *Blood.* 1989;73:694-699.
11. Chodorowski Z, Sein Anand J. Air embolus as a complication of a haemoperfusion catheter removal after iatrogenic intoxication with doxorubicin—a case report [in Polish]. *Przegl Lek.* 2004;61:408-409.
12. Chu G, et al. Massive cisplatin overdose by accidental substitution for carboplatin. Toxicity and management. *Cancer.* 1993;72:3707-3714.
13. de Forni M, et al. Cardiotoxicity of high-dose continuous infusion fluorouracil: a prospective clinical study. *J Clin Oncol.* 1992;10:1795-1801.
14. de Korte MA, et al. [111]Indium-trastuzumab visualises myocardial human epidermal growth factor receptor 2 expression shortly after anthracycline treatment but not during heart failure: a clue to uncover the mechanisms of trastuzumab-related cardiotoxicity. *Eur J Cancer.* 2007;43:2046-2051.
15. Desai ZR, et al. Can severe vincristine neurotoxicity be prevented? *Cancer Chemother Pharmacol.* 1982;8:211-214.
16. El-Ebiary AA, et al. Evaluation of genotoxicity induced by exposure to antineoplastic drugs in lymphocytes of oncology nurses and pharmacists. *J Appl Toxicol.* 2013;33:196-201.
17. Erdlenbruch B, et al. Topical topic: accidental cisplatin overdose in a child: reversal of acute renal failure with sodium thiosulfate. *Med Pediatr Oncol.* 2002;38:349-352.
18. Fleischman RA. Southwestern Internal Medicine Conference: clinical use of hematopoietic growth factors. *Am J Med Sci.* 1993;305:248-273.
19. Flockhart DA, et al. Clinically available pharmacogenomics tests. *Clin Pharmacol Ther.* 2009;86:109-113.
20. Gadgil SD, et al. Effect of activated charcoal on the pharmacokinetics of high-dose methotrexate. *Cancer Treat Rep.* 1982;66:1169-1171.
21. Gandhi TK, et al. Medication safety in the ambulatory chemotherapy setting. *Cancer.* 2005;104:2477-2483.
22. Gbadamosi J, et al. Severe heart failure in a young multiple sclerosis patient. *J Neurol.* 2003;250:241-242.
23. Gianni L, et al. Treatment with trastuzumab for 1 year after adjuvant chemotherapy in patients with HER2-positive early breast cancer: a 4-year follow-up of a randomised controlled trial. *Lancet Oncol.* 2011;12:236-244.
24. Goldspiel B, et al. ASHP guidelines on preventing medication errors with chemotherapy and biotherapy. *Am J Health Syst Pharm.* 2015;72:e6-e35.
25. Gorgulu S, et al. A case of coronary spasm induced by 5-fluorouracil. *Acta Cardiol.* 2002;57:381-383.
26. Gratwohl A, et al. Emergency therapy with granulocyte-macrophage colony-stimulating factor (GM-CSF) [in German]. *Schweiz Med Wochenschr.* 1991;121:413-417.
27. Hesketh PJ, et al. Antiemetics: American Society of Clinical Oncology Focused Guideline Update. *J Clin Oncol.* 2016;34:381-386.
28. Hon CY, et al. Antineoplastic drug contamination in the urine of Canadian healthcare workers. *Int Arch Occup Environ Health.* 2015;88:933-941.
29. Innocenti F, et al. Epirubicin glucuronidation is catalyzed by human UDP-glucuronosyltransferase 2B7. *Drug Metab Dispos.* 2001;29:686-692.
30. Iwasaki T, et al. Regional pharmacokinetics of doxorubicin following hepatic arterial and portal venous administration: evaluation with hepatic venous isolation and charcoal hemoperfusion. *Cancer Res.* 1998;58:3339-3343.
31. Jacobson JO, et al. Revisions to the 2009 american society of clinical oncology/oncology nursing society chemotherapy administration safety standards: expanding the scope to include inpatient settings. *J Oncol Pract.* 2012;8:2-6.
32. Jensen BV, et al. Functional monitoring of anthracycline cardiotoxicity: a prospective, blinded, long-term observational study of outcome in 120 patients. *Ann Oncol.* 2002;13:699-709.
33. Jirillo A, et al. Accidental overdose of melphalan per os in a 69-year-old woman treated for advanced endometrial carcinoma. *Tumori.* 1998;84:611.
34. Jost LM. Overdose with melphalan (Alkeran): symptoms and treatment. A review [in German]. *Onkologie.* 1990;13:96-101.
35. Jung HK, et al. A case of massive cisplatin overdose managed by plasmapheresis. *Korean J Intern Med.* 1995;10:150-154.
36. Karamouzis MV, et al. Therapies directed against epidermal growth factor receptor in aerodigestive carcinomas. *JAMA.* 2007;298:70-82.
37. Kim IS, et al. Accidental overdose of multiple chemotherapeutic agents. *Korean J Intern Med.* 1989;4:171-173.
38. Kramer RA, et al. Effects of buthionine sulfoximine on the nephrotoxicity of 1-(2-chloroethyl)-3-(trans-4-methylcyclohexyl)-1-nitrosourea (MeCCNU). *J Pharmacol Exp Ther.* 1985;234:498-506.
39. Krarup-Hansen A, et al. Neuronal involvement in cisplatin neuropathy: prospective clinical and neurophysiological studies. *Brain.* 2007;130(pt 4):1076-1088.
40. Ku Y, et al. Clinical pilot study on high-dose intraarterial chemotherapy with direct hemoperfusion under hepatic venous isolation in patients with advanced hepatocellular carcinoma. *Surgery.* 1995;117:510-519.
41. Loebstein R, Koren G. Ifosfamide-induced nephrotoxicity in children: critical review of predictive risk factors. *Pediatrics.* 1998;101:E8.
42. McEvilly M, et al. Use of uridine triacetate for the management of fluorouracil overdose. *Am J Health Syst Pharm.* 2011;68:1806-1809.
43. Mir O, Berveiller P. Increased evidence for use of chemotherapy in pregnancy. *Lancet Oncol.* 2012;13:852-854.

44. OccupationalSafetyandHealthAdministration. Sec VI, Chapt II: Categorization of drugs as hazardous. TED 1-0.15A. OSHA Technical manual. http://www.osha.gov/dts/osta/otm/otm_vi/otm_vi_2.html#2. Published 1999.

45. Pecherstorfer M, et al. High-dose intravenous melphalan in a patient with multiple myeloma and oliguric renal failure. *Clin Investig.* 1994;72:522-525.

46. Pelgrims J, et al. Methylene blue in the treatment and prevention of ifosfamide-induced encephalopathy: report of 12 cases and a review of the literature. *Br J Cancer.* 2000;82:291-294.

47. Perez EA, et al. Cardiac safety of lapatinib: pooled analysis of 3689 patients enrolled in clinical trials. *Mayo Clin Proc.* 2008;83:679-686.

48. Pirzada NA, et al. Fluorouracil-induced neurotoxicity. *Ann Pharmacother.* 2000;34:35-38.

49. Poupeau C, et al. Pilot study of biological monitoring of four antineoplastic drugs among Canadian healthcare workers. *J Oncol Pharm Pract.* 2017;23:323-332.

50. Reichert JM, et al. Monoclonal antibody successes in the clinic. *Nat Biotechnol.* 2005;23:1073-1078.

51. Resource Conservation and Recovery Act. Resource Conservation and Recovery Act. 1996:260-279.

52. Rizzo JD, et al. Use of epoetin and darbepoetin in patients with cancer: 2007 American Society of Clinical Oncology/American Society of Hematology clinical practice guideline update. *J Clin Oncol.* 2008;26:132-149.

53. Sabatini L, et al. Biological monitoring of occupational exposure to antineoplastic drugs in hospital settings. *Med Lav.* 2012;103:394-401.

54. Salani R, et al. Cancer and pregnancy: an overview for obstetricians and gynecologists. *Am J Obstet Gynecol.* 2014;211:7-14.

55. Salloum E, et al. Chlorambucil-induced seizures. *Cancer.* 1997;79:1009-1013.

56. Schreiber C, et al. Uptake of antineoplastic agents in pharmacy personnel. Part II: study of work-related risk factors. *Int Arch Occup Environ Health.* 2003;76:11-16.

57. Schwartz CL, et al. Corrected QT interval prolongation in anthracycline-treated survivors of childhood cancer. *J Clin Oncol.* 1993;11:1906-1910.

58. Schwartz RG, et al. Congestive heart failure and left ventricular dysfunction complicating doxorubicin therapy. Seven-year experience using serial radionuclide angiocardiography. *Am J Med.* 1987;82:1109-1118.

59. Sessink PJ, Bos RP. Drugs hazardous to healthcare workers. Evaluation of methods for monitoring occupational exposure to cytostatic drugs. *Drug Saf.* 1999;20:347-359.

60. Siu CW, et al. Effects of oral arsenic trioxide therapy on QT intervals in patients with acute promyelocytic leukemia: implications for long-term cardiac safety. *Blood.* 2006;108:103-106.

61. Smaglo BG, et al. The development of immunoconjugates for targeted cancer therapy. *Nat Rev Clin Oncol.* 2014;11:637-648.

62. Stahl M, et al. Application of adjuvant chemotherapy in colorectal cancer—a survey in the region of Essen, Germany. *Onkologie.* 2005;28:7-10.

63. Steger GG, et al. GM-CSF in the treatment of a patient with severe methotrexate intoxication. *J Intern Med.* 1993;233:499-502.

64. Stein J, et al. Accidental busulfan overdose: enhanced drug clearance with hemodialysis in a child with Wiskott-Aldrich syndrome. *Bone Marrow Transplant.* 2001;27:551-553.

65. Steinberg JS, et al. Acute arrhythmogenicity of doxorubicin administration. *Cancer.* 1987;60:1213-1218.

66. Stohr W, et al. Ifosfamide-induced nephrotoxicity in 593 sarcoma patients: a report from the Late Effects Surveillance System. *Pediatr Blood Cancer.* 2007;48:447-452.

67. Trent KC, et al. Multiorgan failure associated with lomustine overdose. *Ann Pharmacother.* 1995;29:384-386.

68. Tsalic M, et al. Severe toxicity related to the 5-fluorouracil/leucovorin combination (the Mayo Clinic regimen): a prospective study in colorectal cancer patients. *Am J Clin Oncol.* 2003;26:103-106.

69. Tsavaris N, et al. Cardiotoxicity following different doses and schedules of 5-fluorouracil administration for malignancy—a survey of 427 patients. *Med Sci Monit.* 2002;8:PI51-PI57.

70. Wasserman E, et al. Severe CPT-11 toxicity in patients with Gilbert's syndrome: two case reports. *Ann Oncol.* 1997;8:1049-1051.

71. Weingart SN, et al. Medication errors involving oral chemotherapy. *Cancer.* 2010;116:2455-2464.

72. Weiss HD, et al. Neurotoxicity of commonly used antineoplastic agents (second of two parts). *N Engl J Med.* 1974;291:127-133.

73. Weiss RB, et al. Nephrotoxicity of semustine. *Cancer Treat Rep.* 1983;67:1105-1112.

74. Wettergren Y, et al. Pretherapeutic uracil and dihydrouracil levels of colorectal cancer patients are associated with sex and toxic side effects during adjuvant 5-fluorouracil-based chemotherapy. *Cancer.* 2012;118:2935-2943.

75. World Health Organization. International Nonproprietary Names (INN) for biological and biotechnological substances. http://www.who.int/medicines/services/inn/Bio-Rev2011.pdf. Published 2011. Accessed August 25, 2017.

76. Wortman JE, et al. Sudden death during doxorubicin administration. *Cancer.* 1979;44:1588-1591.

77. Wyatt AJ, et al. Cutaneous reactions to chemotherapy and their management. *Am J Clin Dermatol.* 2006;7:45-63.

78. Yoshida H, et al. Pharmacokinetics of doxorubicin and its active metabolite in patients with normal renal function and in patients on hemodialysis. *Cancer Chemother Pharmacol.* 1994;33:450-454.

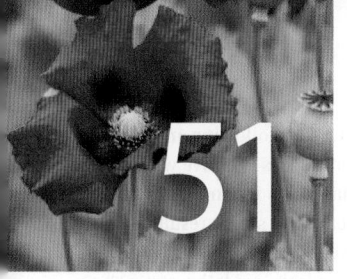

51 METHOTREXATE, 5-FLUOROURACIL, AND CAPECITABINE

Richard Y. Wang

Methotrexate and the fluoropyrimidines (5-fluorouracil and capecitabine) belong to the chemotherapeutic class of antimetabolites. Patients affected by these chemotherapeutics present with significant clinical toxicities that are potentially fatal. Clinicians must recognize these patients early and be prepared to provide immediate interventions that include specific antidotal therapies. The oral formulations of methotrexate and capecitabine present a risk for intentional or unintentional chemotherapeutics ingestion in the home.

METHOTREXATE

Methotrexate (MTX) is commonly used for a many malignant conditions. Its immunosuppressive activity also allows it to be used for rheumatoid arthritis, organ transplantation, psoriasis, trophoblastic diseases, and termination of pregnancy.[20,47]

Risk factors for MTX toxicity include impaired kidney function (primary route of drug elimination); third compartment spacing: ascites and pleural effusions; concurrent use of nephrotoxins, such as nonsteroidal antiinflammatory drugs (NSAIDs) and aminoglycosides[55] and certain intravenous radiologic contrast agents;[30,40] age; folate deficiency; and concurrent infection.[95] Methotrexate toxicity depends on the dose, but even more on the duration of exposure.

Pharmacology

The therapeutic and toxic effects of methotrexate are based on its ability to limit DNA and RNA syntheses by inhibiting dihydrofolate reductase (DHFR) and thymidylate synthetase (Fig. 51–1). Dihydrofolate reductase reduces folic acid first to dihydrofolate and then to tetrahydrofolate (FH_4), which serves

as an essential cofactor in the synthesis of purine nucleotides that are used in the synthesis of DNA and RNA. Methotrexate, a structural analog of folate, competitively inhibits DHFR by binding to the enzymatic site of action. Methotrexate polyglutamates are formed intracellularly by folylpolyglutamate synthetase and they also inhibit DHFR. The inhibition of DHFR diminishes reduced folate production, which is necessary for the formation of purine nucleotides. Reduced folates are also required by thymidyl synthetase to serve as methyl donors in the formation of thymidyl. Thymidyl is then used for DNA synthesis. In addition, thymidyl production is impaired by the direct inhibition of thymidylate synthetase by polyglutamated derivatives of methotrexate.

The antiinflammatory effect of MTX likely involves the following mechanisms: (1) inhibition of trans-methylation (by depletion of intracellular folate stores) which causes the death of T cells and inhibits the formation of polyamines (spermine and spermidine) that are involved in the inflammatory cascade, (2) reduction in intracellular concentration of glutathione, and (3) inhibition of intracellular 5-aminoimidazole-4-carboxamide ribonucleotide (AICAR) transformylase, which leads to increased extracellular concentration of adenosine through a series of steps (see below). Adenosine binds to the A_{2a} receptor located on the surface of leukocytes, and it affects selected functions, where it inhibits the syntheses of cytokines (TNF α) and complements produced by macrophages, and inhibits lymphocyte proliferation and migration to targeted sites.[23,69]

The de novo synthesis of purine nucleotides involves the formylation of the intermediate AICAR to formyl-AICAR by AICAR transformylase in the latter steps of the pathway. Formyl-AICAR proceeds to form inosine and then adenosine. The latter step is facilitated by adenosine deaminase. Adenosine is phosphorylated to AMP, ADP, and ATP. These phosphorylated species of adenosine can translocate to the extracellular compartment, where they are converted to adenosine. Polyglutamates of MTX inhibit AICAR transformylase, which causes an increase in the concentration of AICAR and then the inhibition of AMP and adenosine (via AICA ribonucleoside) deaminases.[74] The inhibition of these deaminases increases the intracellular concentrations of adenosine and its phosphorylated derivatives, and contributes to the movement of these products to the extracellular compartment.

The bioavailability of methotrexate is limited by a saturable intestinal absorption mechanism. At oral doses less than 30 mg/m², the absorption is 90% and the peak plasma MTX concentration is achieved at one to 2 hours. In children administered oral MTX, peak blood concentrations mean (SD) of MTX were 0.71 (0.17) µmol/L and 1.48 (0.46) µmol/L for doses at less than or equal to 10 and 30 mg/m², respectively.[92,98] In adults, MTX administered as an oral dose of 7.5 mg, 15 mg, or 50 mg achieved peak blood concentrations (mean, SD) of 0.48 (0.09) µmol/L , 0.84 (0.3) µmol/L, and 1.84 (0.70) µmol/L, respectively.[4,99] At oral doses greater than 30 mg/m², gut bioavailability significantly decreases. For example, at doses greater than 80 mg/m², the absorption is less than 10% to 20%.[14]

Methotrexate dosing regimens for chemotherapy are variable, but high-dose therapy is equal to or is greater than 1,000 mg/m². Conventional intravenous doses of up to 100 mg/m² are often administered without leucovorin rescue. Doses of 1,000 mg/m² are considered potentially lethal. Much higher doses (2,000–3,000 mg g/m²) can be given when MTX is followed by leucovorin "rescue" in order to prevent life-threatening toxicity. Mortality from high-dose MTX is approximately 6%, and occurs primarily when MTX concentrations are not monitored.[95,101]

Methotrexate has a triphasic plasma clearance. The initial plasma distribution half-life is short at 0.75 hours. The second half-life is 2 to 3.4 hours and represents renal clearance of the drug. The third phase has a half-life of

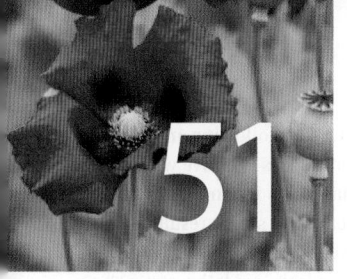

FIGURE 51–1. Mechanism of MTX toxicity. Methotrexate inhibits dihydrofolate reductase activity, which is necessary for DNA and RNA synthesis. Leucovorin bypasses blockade to allow for continued synthesis. MTX = methotrexate.

about 8 to 10.4 hours and represents tissue redistribution into the plasma. This third phase is prolonged in the setting of kidney failure and is associated with bone marrow and gastrointestinal (GI) toxicity. The volume of distribution is 0.6 to 0.9 L/kg and protein binding is 50%. Healthy kidneys eliminate 50% to 80% of MTX unchanged within 48 hours of administration. When the creatinine clearance is less than 60 mL/min, MTX clearance is delayed.[83,105] Ten percent to 30% of MTX is eliminated unchanged in the bile, which contributes to enterohepatic circulation of the chemotherapeutic. In the setting of kidney failure, the half-life of MTX is prolonged by the recirculation of MTX in the gut.

Hepatic aldehyde oxidase metabolizes a minor portion (<10%) of MTX to 7-hydroxy methotrexate (7-OH-MTX), which inhibits DHFR but to a lesser extent than MTX. Aldehyde oxidase is also found in renal tubules, but not in the glomerulus, and its contribution to the local production of 7-OH-MTX and kidney injury remains to be determined.[70] Another metabolite is 2,4-diamino-N(10)-methylpteroic acid (DAMPA), and it accounts for less than 5% of MTX. In the gut, bacterial carboxypeptidase acts on MTX to form DAMPA, which is reabsorbed into the blood compartment. Approximately 50% of -N(10) DAMPA is eliminated unchanged by the kidneys, and this metabolite is inactive at DHFR based on poor cellular uptake and inhibition of the enzyme when compared to MTX.[112]

Pathophysiology

At high doses, methotrexate and the insoluble drug metabolites 7-OH-MTX and DAMPA accumulate and precipitate in the renal tubules, causing reversible acute tubular necrosis. Methotrexate is one-tenth as soluble at a pH of 5.5 as it is at a pH of 7.5.[14,85] Expressed another way, the plasma concentration threshold for nephrotoxicity is 2.2 mmol/L when the urine pH is 5.5, and 22 mmol/L when the urine pH is 6.9. Thus, patients who are either inadequately hydrated or not alkalinized are at risk for acute kidney failure from high-dose MTX treatment.[3,48] Methotrexate is excreted unchanged in the urine by both glomerular filtration and active tubular secretion. A small amount of MTX is metabolized intracellularly to polyglutamate derivatives, which inhibit DHFR and thymidyl synthetase and are believed to be responsible for the persistent cytotoxic effect of MTX because they do not easily diffuse outside of the cell. The threshold concentration for MTX in plasma that inhibits DNA synthesis is lower for intestinal epithelial cells (0.005 μM/L) than for hematopoietic cells (0.01 μmol/L) by one order of magnitude.[20] Thus, patients with a significant exposure to MTX will develop GI toxicity before bone marrow toxicity.

The decreased production of reduced folates and diminished folate content in the hepatocyte likely contribute to injury, which leads to hepatic fibrosis from the stimulation of hepatic stellate cells by adenosine.[74,75] Patients on long-term therapy with MTX and elevated aminotransferases can develop hepatic fibrosis from persistent injury to the liver.

Clinical Manifestations

In the course of MTX therapy, a variety of disorders can occur, resulting from either increased patient susceptibility to toxicity or excessive administration. The clinical manifestations of MTX toxicity include stomatitis, esophagitis, kidney failure, myelosuppression, hepatitis, and central neurologic system dysfunction. In a group of 23 patients who received 45 courses of high-dose MTX therapy with leucovorin rescue, the most commonly observed signs included increased aspartate aminotransferase (AST) or alanine aminotransferase (ALT) (81%), nausea and vomiting (66%), mucositis (33%), dermatitis (18%), leukopenia (11%), thrombocytopenia (9%), and creatinine elevation (7%).[77]

Nausea and vomiting, considered rare from cancer therapy with MTX at 40 mg/m², typically begin 2 to 4 hours after high-dose therapy (1,000 mg/m²) and last for about 6 to 12 hours. Mucositis, characterized by mouth soreness, stomatitis, or diarrhea, usually occurs in the first week of therapy, and can last for 4 to 7 days. Other gastrointestinal effects resulting from MTX therapy include pharyngitis, anorexia, gastrointestinal hemorrhage, and toxic megacolon.[9] Hepatocellular toxicity, as defined by increased hepatic enzymes (AST, ALT), and hyperbilirubinemia occur with both acute and chronic therapies.[62,71,77] It is usually associated with high dose regimens, and

elevations in AST/ALT will begin within one to 3 days following an exposure to a significant dose of MTX. Laboratory abnormalities improve within 1 to 2 weeks of discontinuation of MTX. The mechanism is incompletely understood, but toxicity is attributed to reduced liver folate stores resulting from intracellular competition with polyglutamates of MTX for glutamyl conjugation in chronic exposures,[11] and cellular damage from oxidative stress[5,41] or the precipitation of 7-OH-MTX in the bile duct[17] in acute exposures. Factors associated with hepatotoxicity are sustained high plasma concentrations, increased cumulative dosages, chronic therapy, and host factors such as increase in age, obesity, alcoholism, and prior liver disease.[107]

Pancytopenia usually occurs within the first 2 weeks after an acute exposure. There are several reports demonstrating the occurrence of pancytopenia in individuals receiving chronic MTX therapy for rheumatoid arthritis and psoriasis.[27,54,62,80]

When used at intravenous (IV) doses of 40 to 60 mg/m², MTX is not associated with appreciable nephrotoxicity. However, at doses greater than 5,000 g/m² (approximately 130 mg/kg for an adult), several investigators report severe kidney injury, with oliguria, azotemia, and kidney failure.[13] The incidence of kidney injury (serum creatinine ≥1.5 to 3.0 × upper limit of normal) in patients with osteosarcoma and treated with high-dose MTX in conjunction with hydration, urinary alkalinization, and leucovorin is 1.8%.[109] Kidney function typically recovers over time. Patients at risk for nephrotoxicity include the elderly, those with underlying kidney disease defined as a glomerular filtration rate of less than 60 mL/min, and those who receive concurrent drug therapy that can delay MTX excretion, which includes agents that reduce renal blood flow such as NSAIDs, the nephrotoxins such as cisplatin, and the aminoglycosides, or weak organic acids such as salicylates and piperacillin which inhibit renal secretion.[46,95]

The neurologic complications associated with either high-dose systemic MTX therapy or intrathecal administration are the most consequential manifestations. The incidence of neurologic toxicity from high dose MTX therapy is approximately 5% to 15%.[49] The manifestations usually occur from hours to days after the initiation of therapy and include hemiparesis, paraparesis, quadriparesis, seizures, and dysreflexia.[49,61,96,103] These events are reversible to varying degrees.[2] Clinical findings occurring within several hours (usually within 12 hours) of therapy are attributed to chemical arachnoiditis, and they include acute onset of fever, meningismus, pleocytosis, and increased cerebrospinal fluid (CSF) protein concentration.[42] Leukoencephalopathy is associated with the onset of behavioral disorders and progressive dementia from months to years after treatment and is irreversible, although manifestations presenting soon after treatment can be reversible depending on the extent of involvement.[6,113] Patients with increased age and prior cranial radiation are at risk for this disorder.[37] Patients with leukoencephalopathy have findings consistent with edema, and demyelination or necrosis of the white matter on computed tomography (CT) and magnetic resonance imaging (MRI) of the brain.[6]

Diagnostic Testing

Plasma MTX concentrations are monitored during therapy to limit clinical toxicity. For example, patients with a plasma concentration greater than 1.0 μmol/L at 48 hours posttreatment are considered at risk for bone marrow and gastrointestinal mucosal toxicities.[95] In the former example, the MTX concentration since the time of administration is used in cancer therapy to minimize bone marrow toxicity (suppression) and maximize the efficacy of the therapeutic.[32] The drug concentration and the duration of exposure are indirect indicators of the efficacy of the drug during therapy. In patients with an unintentional exposure to MTX and not receiving MTX therapy, their exposure to MTX (concentration and duration) should be minimized because they are vulnerable to GI toxicity (mucositis). The threshold concentration of MTX for the inhibition of DNA synthesis is one order of magnitude lower for intestinal epithelial cells than hematopoietic cells.

There are several analytical methods available to measure the concentration of MTX, which is routinely conducted in blood (serum or plasma) (Table 51–1). It is important to select the appropriate analytical method to measure MTX because the performance characteristics are variable among these methods.

TABLE 51–1 Analytical Techniques Used to Measure Methotrexate and Selected Metabolites

Technique	Analyte	LOD (μM/L)	LOQ (μmol/L)	CV (MTX, μmol/L)*	AMR (μmol/L)	Matrix	Comments
FPIA[1,16]	MTX	0.02	0.03	14% (0.07) 5.9% (0.8)	0.03–1.0	Serum, plasma	Assay cross-reacts with DAMPA
EMIT[7,36]	MTX	0.02	0.04	11.7% (0.07) 6.9% (0.82)	0.04–1.2	Serum, plasma	Assay cross-reacts with DAMPA
CMIA[10,16]	MTX		0.04	4.1% (0.07)+ 4.6% (0.45)+	0.04–1.5	Plasma	Assay cross-reacts with DAMPA
HPLC-UVD[12]	MTX	0.003	0.01	12.6% (0.05)+ 5.5% (1.0)+	0.025–5.0	Serum	
LC-MS[15]	MTX		0.0025	12% (0.005) 1.7% (0.01)	0.006–1.0	Urine	
	7-OH-MTX		0.01				
LC-MS/MS[79]	MTX	0.0004		16.8% (0.0022)+, & 4.1% (0.82)+	0.002–5.5	Plasma, CSF	
	7-OH-MTX	0.0004					
	DAMPA	0.0023					

*CVs for inter- and intraday at selected MTX concentrations: +CV for interday; & for measurements made in plasma.

AMR = analytical measurement range; CSF = cerebrospinal fluid; CMIA = chemiluminescent microparticle immunoassay (Abbott); CV = coefficient of variation; DAMPA = 2,4-diamino-N(10)-methylpteroic acid; EMIT = enzyme multiplied immunoassay (ARK); FPIA = fluorescence polarization immunoassay (monoclonal antibody, Abbott); HPLC = high-performance liquid chromatography; LC = liquid chromatography; LOD = limit of detection; LOQ = limit of quantification; MS = mass spectrometry; MTX = methotrexate; 7-OH-MTX = 7-hydroxymethotrexate; UVD = ultraviolet detection.

The measurement of methotrexate concentrations in the clinical setting is routinely conducted using an immunoassay technique such as enzyme multiplied immunoassay (EMIT), chemiluminescent microparticle immunoassay (CMIA), or fluorescence polarization immunoassay (FPIA) (Table 51–1).[1,7,10,16,36] These measurements are performed on serum or plasma. The presence of the MTX metabolite DAMPA but not 7-OH-MTX diminishes the specificity of these analytical methods for MTX. The amount by which DAMPA affects the MTX concentration depends on the assay.

At low concentrations of MTX, analytical methods based on high-performance liquid chromatography with ultraviolet detection (HPLC-UVD) or mass spectrometry (LC-MS or LC-MS/MS) provide increased sensitivity and specificity compared to the immunoassays (Table 51–1). The primary advantage of the HPLC-UVD technique over the immunoassay is the ability to measure MTX independent of DAMPA.[12] The advantages of mass spectrometry are increased sensitivity and specificity compared to HPLC-UVD or immunoassays. For example, analytical methods based on mass spectrometry detect or quantify MTX at a concentration one to 2 orders of magnitude lower than methods using either one of the former 2 techniques, and they can quantify 7-OH-MTX and DAMPA in a single analytical run.[15,79] The limitations of methods using HPLC (with UVD or mass spectrometry) are their availability and turnaround time for the test result.

When patients are treated with glucarpidase (carboxypeptidase G₂) (Antidotes in Depth: A13), it is preferable to use an HPLC method to measure MTX because of the presence of DAMPA during therapy. The FPIA method with monoclonal antibodies is recommended not to be used in patients who have developed antibodies to mouse monoclonal antibodies or elevated concentrations of DAMPA.

An elevated CSF methotrexate concentration (>100 μmol/L) is indicative of an excessive intrathecal dose or delayed cerebrospinal fluid outflow obstruction.[72] Radiologic imaging of the brain, such as computed tomography and magnetic resonance imaging, are useful to evaluate for meningeal inflammation, demyelination and necrosis of the white matter, or other pathologies such as a cerebrovascular accident.

Management

The initial approach to the patient exposed to MTX is to determine whether the exposure is acute or chronic because the priorities are different for these patients. For example, a patient with chronic MTX toxicity is more likely to die from overwhelming sepsis than the patient with an acute exposure because the former patient typically presents with bone marrow suppression and severe gastroenteritis. Fluid resuscitation, stabilization, and assessment for neutropenia and kidney and liver injuries are essential steps during the evaluation of the patient with chronic MTX toxicity.

The patient with an acute exposure to MTX typically presents early after an oral exposure. The essential steps during the evaluation of this patient are limiting further gut absorption of MTX, and administering leucovorin early. Leucovorin is most effective as a competitive antidote to MTX when the intracellular concentration of MTX is still low. The time to peak blood concentration of MTX from an oral therapeutic dose of MTX is about 2 hours (1–3 hours). Using the above perspective as a framework for the management of these patients, the following discussion will review the roles of activated charcoal, urinary alkalinization, colony-stimulating factor, and antidotal therapies.

Activated charcoal adsorbs methotrexate and administration is recommended as soon as possible to limit absorption in the setting of oral exposure.[38] The administration of multiple-dose activated charcoal and cholestyramine[29,89] can significantly decrease the elimination half-life of methotrexate by interrupting the enterohepatic circulation.[34,38] This approach can increase MTX clearance but is of most benefit to patients with diminished creatinine clearance. Multiple-dose activated charcoal is recommended for patients with evidence of delayed MTX clearance, such as kidney injury or prolonged half-life (based on blood MTX concentration). Activated charcoal should be withheld in patients with gastrointestinal hemorrhage.

Adequate hydration with 0.9% sodium chloride solution as well as urinary alkalinization with IV sodium bicarbonate (to urine pH 7 to 8) (Antidotes in Depth: A5) is recommended because these modalities prevent or limit kidney injury from the precipitation of MTX and its metabolites in patients who receive inadvertent high doses of glucarpidase.[21] Serial measurements of serum creatinine and blood MTX concentration will determine the duration of urinary alkalinization.

The complete blood count (CBC) should be monitored at least as frequently as days 7, 10, and 14 to assess the impact on the cells in the bone marrow.[56] Granulocyte-macrophage colony–stimulating factor (GM-CSF)

was used in patient with a chronic MTX overdose and pancytopenia.[94] The patient had a serum MTX concentration of 1.25 μmol/L on admission and was in kidney failure. Bone marrow biopsy showed promyelocytes, but no mature white cells, and a marked reduction of megakaryocytes. Because of deteriorating conditions, GM-CSF (125 mcg/m²/d) was administered when the MTX concentration fell below the reference value for toxicity. Seven days after the initiation of GM-CSF, the white blood cell (WBC) count rose and reached expected values within 10 days. Colony-stimulating factor is recommended for patients with febrile neutropenia and who are at high risk for complications from an infection or are likely to have a poor outcome (eg, absolute neutrophil count <100 cells/μL, prolonged neutropenia {>10 days}, age 65 years or older, and hypotension with multiorgan dysfunction).[91]

Patients presenting with meningismus or altered mental status following MTX therapy should receive an initial MRI of the brain and then CSF analysis for infection.[52] Although not considered standard, it would be reasonable to measure the CSF concentration of MTX if excessive exposure to this compartment is suspected. The peak therapeutic concentration of methotrexate in CSF after the intrathecal administration of 12 mg MTX by lumbar puncture is 100 μmol/L, and the terminal half-life of MTX in the cerebrospinal compartment is 7 to 16 hours.[72] Magnetic resonance imaging of the brain can demonstrate a high signal throughout the pachymeningeal (dura mater) region, which is consistent with a chemical meningitis,[33] or a high signal of the white matter with a decreased diffusion coefficient in a diffusion-weighted image to indicate the presence of edema, which is an early finding of leukoencephalopathy.

Antidotes

The available antidotes or rescue agents (term used in cancer therapy for therapeutics that extend the use of chemotherapeutics) for methotrexate toxicity are leucovorin (folinic acid) (Antidotes in Depth: A12) and glucarpidase (carboxypeptidase G₂) (Antidotes in Depth: A13). The effectiveness of these therapies depends on both the timing of administration and the dose, which warrants the monitoring of plasma MTX concentrations during the use of these antidotes. Leucovorin rescue therapy limits the bone marrow and gastrointestinal toxicity of MTX by allowing for the continuation of essential biochemical processes that are dependent on reduced folates. The purpose of the initial dose of leucovorin is to achieve a plasma concentration equal to the MTX and subsequent doses should be adjusted according to plasma MTX concentrations at 24 and 48 hours postexposure (Fig. 51–1).[31,108] Leucovorin treatment is continued until the MTX concentration is less than 0.01 μmol/L.[20] In patients with marrow toxicity and no cancer, leucovorin therapy should be continued until marrow recovery occurs, even if plasma MTX is no longer detectable,[60] because MTX polyglutamates can still be present in the cytosol and adversely affect cellular activity. Among 36 patients undergoing MTX therapy (amount varied from 2 to 13 mg MTX per week) for rheumatoid arthritis, all of these patients had indirectly detected MTX polyglutamates in red blood cells and nondetected MTX in the plasma by FPIA and MAB.[43,44]

Glucarpidase (carboxypeptidase G₂) is a recombinant bacterial enzyme that is used as a rescue therapy to inactivate MTX by hydrolyzing it to DAMPA and glutamate. Glucarpidase is used in patients with an elevated plasma MTX concentration (>1.0 μmol/L) and delayed renal clearance of MTX.[102] Glucarpidase is not indicated for patients with a plasma MTX concentration that is consistent with the expected clearance for MTX at the dose administered (ie, a concentration that is within 2 SD of the mean MTX elimination curve for the dose administered), or for patients with no more than mild kidney injury. Following glucarpidase therapy, plasma MTX concentrations need to be monitored because residual concentrations of MTX in the blood after initial enzymatic therapy can result from the fact that the action of glucarpidase occurs solely within the vascular compartment; inadequate dose of glucarpidase occurs in patients with large MTX exposures or following redistribution of MTX from tissue stores to the blood compartment.[18,86,110] Glucarpidase can also be successfully administered intrathecally to reduce elevated MTX concentrations in the cerebrospinal space (Special Considerations: SC7).[111]

Extracorporeal Elimination

The patient with delayed renal clearance of a toxic concentration of MTX and who is not a candidate for glucarpidase therapy can benefit the most from extracorporeal elimination of MTX when the procedure is instituted early during the patient's course. Once MTX distributes into the cell and peripheral tissue compartments, the procedure cannot remove intracellular polyglutamate derivatives of MTX, and multiple sessions can be required to clear additional MTX stored at peripheral sites.[108] In addition, the procedure can be performed safely in the patient before he or she develops pancytopenia and gastrointestinal hemorrhage from MTX toxicity.

There are several reports of the use of hemodialysis or hemoperfusion (or both) for patients with MTX toxicity.[51,68,78,97,105] Although the volume of distribution (0.6–0.9 L/kg) and protein binding (50% that is not concentration dependent) suggest that MTX is cleared by hemodialysis, older clinical evidence suggests otherwise.[94] In one report, less than 10% of an initial 700 mg dose of methotrexate was cleared in 12 sessions of hemodialysis.[97] The measured clearance was only 38 mL/min, which can be compared to 5 mL/min for peritoneal dialysis,[39] 0.28 to 24 mL/min for continuous venovenous hemodiafiltration,[50,53] and 180 mL/min for normal renal clearance.[57] The ability of hemofiltration to extract MTX from the blood is also limited by the magnitude of the concentration gradient for MTX, which decreases as the concentrations of MTX decreases in the blood.[22] Plasma exchange transfusion is not recommended to remove MTX because the drug has a low degree of protein binding, which limits the efficacy of this procedure.[13,53,73,97]

Acute intermittent hemodialysis with a (F-80B Fresenius Dialyzer) high-flux dialyzer membrane yielded an effective mean plasma MTX clearance of 92 ± 10.3 mL/min in 6 patients with kidney failure that was a result of either chronic disease or high-dose MTX therapy.[105] These patients received high-dose MTX therapy and had predialysis serum MTX concentrations ranging from 1.45 to 1,813 μmol/L. The time of dialysis initiation after MTX treatment was from 1 hour to 6 days in this patient population. A serum MTX concentration of 0.3 μmol/L was used as an end point for dialysis. The reported plasma MTX clearance by this technique closely approximates normal renal MTX clearance and is indicated to enhance the clearance of MTX in patients with diminished renal clearance and a toxic plasma MTX concentration when it can be conducted safely.[83]

Charcoal hemoperfusion removed more than 50% of MTX in 4 patients with impaired renal clearance during high dose MTX therapy.[26,78] This was thought to have prevented severe skin and mucosal toxicity. Sequential hemodialysis and hemoperfusion were used for a patient with substantial MTX toxicity.[38] These procedures decreased the half-life of elimination from 45 hours to 7.6 hours. In experimental animals, hemoperfusion significantly reduced the terminal half-life of methotrexate. In surgically anephric dogs, hemoperfusion decreased the half-life from more than 20 hours to 1.3 hours.[45] Unfortunately, hemoperfusion is currently typically unavailable but modern standard hemodialysis is quite effective in MTX removal (Chap. 6).[78]

In vitro studies indicate that the toxic effects of 100 μmol/L of MTX cannot be reversed by 1,000 μmol/L of leucovorin.[76] This suggests the need for extracorporeal elimination, such as high-flux hemodialysis, or glucarpidase (or both) to lower persistent plasma MTX concentrations of greater than 100 μmol/L.[78] It is important to perform high-flux hemodialysis early, prior to distribution into tissues. Rebound of MTX concentrations from tissues can be expected with intermittent hemodialysis, which typically begins at 2 hours postdialysis and plateau at 16 hours.[35,39,105]

Patients who are at the greatest risk for developing MTX toxicity despite leucovorin treatment should receive glucarpidase (Antidotes in Depth: A13). If the patient with diminished renal clearance and a toxic MTX concentration is not a candidate for glucarpidase therapy, it is reasonable to use hemodialysis early in the patient's course. Current standard hemodialysis can offer the additional benefit of correcting fluid and electrolyte disorders resulting from kidney failure. Other treatment options to limit additional organ toxicity, including leucovorin and urinary alkalinization, should be continued during extracorporeal MTX removal. Leucovorin needs to be replaced postdialysis because it is water-soluble and will be removed by hemodialysis.[24,78,88,90]

5-FLUOROURACIL AND CAPECITABINE

Capecitabine

5-Fluorouracil (5-FU)

The fluoropyrimidines used in chemotherapy are 5-fluorouracil (5-FU), capecitabine, tegafur, and floxuridine. The fluoropyrimidines are competitive analogues to uridine and they disrupt the syntheses of DNA (during the S-phase of the cell cycle) and RNA (Chap. 50). Although floxuridine is metabolized to 5-FU, it has limited systemic toxicity because it is administered to the target organ by the arterial route. These chemotherapeutics are used to treat breast and selected GI cancers, such as colorectal. Common risk factors for toxicity from these chemotherapeutics are selected genetic polymorphisms (ie, dihydropyrimidine dehydrogenase {DPD} deficiency), and underlying liver, kidney, and coronary artery diseases.

Pharmacology

Capecitabine is an oral pro-drug of 5-FU; it is well absorbed by the gut, and then metabolized to 5-FU. In comparison, 5-FU has an erratic oral absorption in the gut and needs to be administered by the intravenous route as a bolus or a continuous infusion. Technical problems with the infusion pump or a pump programming error are reported causes of clinical toxicity from an overdose of 5-FU.[59,84]

The time to peak blood concentration for capecitabine is 1.5 to 2 hours (3.9 mg/L).[104] A median peak blood 5-FU concentration was 55.4 mg/L for a group of 18 patients receiving bolus therapy (400 mg/m² 5-FU) for colon cancer.[19] 5-Fluorouracil has an apparent volume of distribution of 8–11 L/m², distributes to third spaces or compartments, such as peritoneal and pleural fluids, and is approximately 10% protein bound. The plasma protein binding for capecitabine is 60%. The terminal half-lives for 5-FU and capecitabine in the blood compartment are about 15 and 45 minutes, respectively.

Whether a patient experiences therapeutic effects or toxic effects from the use of these chemotherapeutics depends on the balance between the enzymatic reactions involved with the formation of active metabolites and the enzymatic reaction that degrades these metabolites and the parent compound. This is important because these chemotherapeutics require enzymes that can have variable levels of potential to activate and inactivate them.

Capecitabine undergoes 3 enzymatic reactions in the liver to form 5-FU. Capecitabine is initially metabolized by carboxylesterase to 5'-deoxy-5-fluorocytidine (5-DFCB) and then to 5'-deoxy-5-fluorouridine (5'-DFUR) by cytidine deaminase (Fig. 51–2). In the liver or at the tumor site, thymidine phosphorylase converts 5'-DFUR to 5-FU. Inside the cell, 5-FU is converted to active metabolites: FdUMP, FTP, and FdUTP. Floxuridine (5-FUDR) is metabolized to 5-FU and then to FdUTP and FdUMP. Tegafur is an additional prodrug that is bioactivated by CYP2A6 to 5-FU. CYP2C9 is also capable of metabolizing tegafur, but it did not appear to significantly contribute to overall activation of tegafur in a human liver microsome system.

Hepatic metabolism by DPD inactivates approximately 80% of 5-FU to 5,6-dihydro-5-fluorouracil and alpha-fluoro-beta-alanine (FBAL), and these

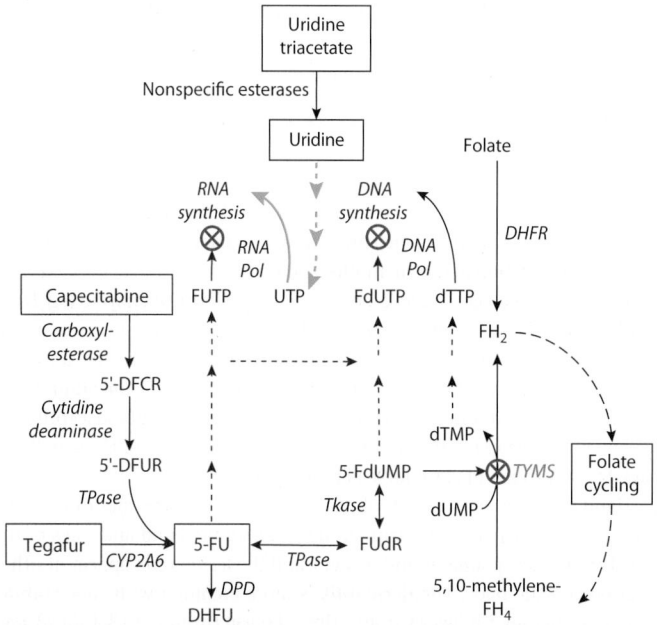

FIGURE 51–2. 5-Fluorouracil, capecitabine, and tegafur chemotherapeutic mechanisms of action and uridine triacetate antidotal rescue. 5'-DFCR = 5'-deoxy-5-fluorocytidine; 5'-DFUR = 5'-deoxy-5-fluorouridine; 5-FdUMP = fluorodeoxyuridine monophosphate; 5-FU = 5-fluorouracil; 5,10-methylene-FH4 = 5,10-methylenetetrahydrofolate; CYP2A6 = cytochrome P450, family 2, subfamily A, polypeptide 6; DHFR = dihydrofolate reductase; DHFU = 5,6-dihydrofluorouracil; DNA Pol = DNA polymerase; DPD = dihydropyrimidine dehydrogenase; dTMP = deoxythymidine monophosphate; dTTP = deoxythymidine triphosphate; dUMP = deoxyuridine monophosphate; FdUTP = fluorodeoxyuridine triphosphate; FH2 = dihydrofolate; FUdR = floxuridine; FUTP = fluorouridine triphosphate; RNA Pol = RNA polymerase; TKase = thymidine kinase; TPase = thymidine phosphorylase; TYMS = thymidylate synthase; UTP = uridine triphosphate. (Used with the permission from Silas W. Smith, MD.)

products are excreted in the urine. The enzyme DPD has nonlinear kinetics because of saturation, and its level of activity depends on the genetic variant. The frequencies of genetic variants with complete and partial DPD deficiencies in adults are 0.1% to 0.5% and 3% to 5%, respectively.[63] Patients with a significant DPD deficiency based on certain genetic variants will present with early-onset and severe manifestations of toxicity from 5-FU or capecitabine.[58,64]

Cytidine deaminase is another enzyme with a variable level of expression in the general population. Patients with a markedly elevated level of activity for this enzyme can develop capecitabine toxicity. Patients with certain genetic variants of cytidine deaminase are "ultra-metabolizers" of capecitabine, and they form higher than expected concentrations of 5-FU and present with early-onset toxicities, including severe gastroenteritis and bone marrow suppression.[25,58,65,87] Lastly, certain thymidylate synthase polymorphisms are associated with more severe toxicity.

The proportions of unchanged 5-FU that are eliminated in the urine and bile are less than 10% and approximately 2% to 3%, respectively. Capecitabine and its metabolites are eliminated primarily by the kidneys (84% in the first 24 hours).[104] Capecitabine is contraindicated when the creatinine clearance is less than 30 mL/min.

Pathophysiology

The therapeutic and toxic effects of 5-FU (and capecitabine) are based on its ability to limit DNA and RNA activities by serving as an antagonist to the pyrimidine uracil in these macromolecules (Fig. 51–2). The specific sites of action and consequence are as follows: (1) 5-FU (as FdUMP) replaces dUMP and it irreversibly inhibits thymidylate synthetase with the cofactor 5,10-methylenetetrahydrofolate (affects DNA synthesis and repair), (2) FdUTP replaces dUTP and it inhibits DNA replication (because of depleted thymidine triphosphate), and (3) fluorouridine triphosphate

(FUTP) replaces UTP and inhibits RNA and protein syntheses. Although the primary mechanism of action in chemotherapy for 5-FU is inhibition of thymidylate synthetase, the impairment of RNA synthesis causes significant toxicity to the host.

Clinical Manifestations

The clinical manifestations of toxicity from 5-FU or capecitabine are primarily gastroenteritis and bone marrow suppression.[28,66] In the setting of an overdose (5-FU), nausea and diarrhea present early (<3 days) after the completion of the administration of the chemotherapeutic.[84]

Patients with a significant genetic variant of a critical enzyme (eg, DPD, cytidine deaminase or thymidylate synthase) present with severe manifestations of toxicity that are similar to an overdose of 5-FU or capecitabine.[81] However, these clinical findings typically appear soon after the administration of the first course of treatment. For capecitabine, patients susceptible to toxicity will develop manifestations later than patients on 5-FU—usually on days 3 to 9 during a 14 day course of treatment.[25,59,65]

Hand-and-foot syndrome (palmar plantar erythrodysesthesia) presents with erythema, edema, and pain on the palms of the hand and soles of the feet. The skin desquamates and blisters, and the lesions can appear at other locations on the body. The dermatitis is more common with capecitabine than 5-FU therapy.[28] It has a variable time of onset (from 11 to 360 days), and is reversible upon discontinuation of the chemotherapeutic.[104]

Cardiac and central nervous system (CNS) manifestations of toxicity are uncommon in patients treated with these chemotherapeutics. The incidence of cardiotoxicity from 5-FU varies from 1.6% to 18%, and patents with an underlying coronary artery disease are at risk for toxicity.[82,93] Cardiac manifestations of toxicity include dysrhythmias, myocardial infarction, myocardial ischemia (from coronary artery vasospasm), heart failure, and cardiogenic shock.[59,82] In patients with documented cardiotoxicity from 5-FU, it is recommended not to resume therapy because the recurrence rate is high, varying from 82% to 100%.[93] The manifestations of CNS toxicity include confusion, encephalopathy, and coma. Although the causes of these cardiac and neurologic manifestations are unknown, toxicity from the metabolite fluoroacetate and genetic polymorphisms, such as significant DPD deficiency, are under consideration.[59,67,81]

Diagnostic Testing

Clinical laboratory tests for 5-FU or capecitabine and their metabolites (FBAL), and the type of genetic variant or level of activity for selected enzymes, such as DPD[8,63] or cytidine deaminase[25,87] are not routinely available.

Management

It is reasonable to administer activated charcoal as soon as possible to a patient presenting early after an oral overdose of capecitabine because it can limit gut absorption of the chemotherapeutic. Initiate supportive management with IV fluid hydration for dehydration and an antiemetic for vomiting (as needed) and assess for electrolyte disorders, cardiac and kidney injuries, neutropenia, and sepsis. If the patient presents with an acute coronary syndrome, conservative antianginal therapy (eg, nitrates and calcium channel blockers) should be initiated. The patient will require a cardiac monitored setting, and serial ECGs and cardiac enzymes.[82,93] Patients with a new-onset altered mental status should receive a computed tomography scan of the brain and possibly a lumbar puncture to assess for CNS infection.

Antidotes

Uridine triacetate is administered in a timely manner in an attempt to improve the survival of patients adversely affected by 5-FU or capecitabine. In an open-label, multicenter study of patients with 5-FU or capecitabine toxicity and treated with uridine triacetate, there were 117 overdoses and 18 early-onset severe symptoms. An overdose was defined as the administration of 5-FU at a dose or rate (via infusion pump) greater than the maximum tolerated dose for the patient's intended regimen of 5-FU or capecitabine. Patients with early onset of signs or symptoms were presumed susceptible

to toxicity from a genetic variant of a critical enzyme. In the study, there were 130 survivors at 30 days among the 135 patients treated with uridine triacetate.[59] By comparison, when uridine triacetate was not available in a historical reference group of patients with 5-FU or capecitabine toxicity, there were 38 deaths among 42 patients.[59] When uridine triacetate was administered within 96 hours of the last dose of the chemotherapeutic to patients with early onset of severe toxicity, all 18 patients survived. However, only 3 of 8 patients survived when uridine acetate was administered after 96 hours.[59]

Uridine triacetate is available for the emergency treatment of patients with (1) an overdose of 5-FU or capecitabine regardless of the presence of clinical toxicity, (2) an early onset (<96 hours) of severe or life-threatening manifestations of toxicity (cardiovascular, central nervous system), or (3) an early onset of an unusually severe adverse reaction, such as gastroenteritis or neutropenia, within 96 hours of the administration of 5-FU or capecitabine during the course of chemotherapy.[100] Uridine triacetate is not recommended for the treatment of patients with common or anticipated manifestations of these chemotherapeutics during therapy.[100]

Uridine triacetate is administered orally and it is deacetylated by nonspecific esterases in the gut and blood to form uridine. Upon entry into the cell, uridine is activated by phosphorylation to uridine triphosphate (UTP) (Fig. 51–2). Uridine competes with FUTP as UTP during the synthesis of RNA and serves as a source of UTP for the synthesis of new RNA. A plasma uridine concentration of at least 70 µmol/L is desired for treatment of 5-FU toxicity.[59] A single oral dose of 6 to 10 g of uridine triacetate yields a peak plasma uridine concentration of approximately 150 µmol/L at about 2 hours.[84,106] The half-life for uridine is about 3 hours.[106]

The amount of uridine triacetate indicated for 5-FU or capecitabine toxicity in adults for each single dose is 10 g administered every 6 hours for 20 doses for a total of 5 days. For children, a single dose of uridine triacetate is 6.2 g/m² of body surface area up to a maximum of 10 g per dose. The dose and schedule for uridine triacetate are not adjusted by sex, amount of 5-FU or capecitabine, or hepatic or renal clearance.[102] A common side effect from this therapy is nausea, vomiting, and diarrhea.

SUMMARY

- The number of patients with potential MTX toxicity is anticipated to increase because of the expanding therapeutic indications and available multiple formulations of this chemotherapeutic.
- Specific interventions for MTX include supportive care, monitoring plasma MTX concentration, urinary alkalinization to limit kidney toxicity, enhanced elimination, and antidotal therapy with leucovorin and enzymatic cleavage with glucarpidase.
- Patients with significant genetic variants of critical enzymes involved with 5-FU or capecitabine typically present with severe clinical toxicity soon after the administration of the first course of treatment.
- Specific interventions for 5-FU or capecitabine toxicity include supportive care and antidotal therapy with uridine triacetate.
- The early recognition of these patients and institution of these therapies can offer the patient the best outcome.

Disclaimer

The findings and conclusions in this chapter are those of the author and do not necessarily represent the official position of the Centers for Disease Control and Prevention.

REFERENCES

1. AbbottLaboratories. Methotrexate II. 2005; http://www.ilexmedical.com/files/PDF/TDX_Methotrexate.pdf. Accessed August 18, 2017.
2. Abelson HT. Methotrexate and central nervous system toxicity. *Cancer Treat Rep.* 1978;62:1999-2001.
3. Abelson HT, et al. Methotrexate-induced renal impairment: clinical studies and rescue from systemic toxicity with high-dose leucovorin and thymidine. *J Clin Oncol.* 1983;1:208-216.
4. Ahern M, et al. Methotrexate kinetics in rheumatoid arthritis: is there an interaction with nonsteroidal antiinflammatory drugs? *J Rheumatol.* 1988;15:1356-1360.

5. Akbulut S, et al. Cytoprotective effects of amifostine, ascorbic acid and *N*-acetylcysteine against methotrexate-induced hepatotoxicity in rats. *World J Gastroenterol.* 2014;20: 10158-10165.

6. Allen JC, et al. Leukoencephalopathy following high-dose IV methotrexate chemotherapy with leucovorin rescue. *Cancer Treat Rep.* 1980;64:1261-1273.

7. ARK Diagnostics Inc. Methotrexate assay. http://www.ark-tdm.com/pdfs/2017/Methotrexate/ARK_Methotrexate_Calibrator_Rev05_February_2017.pdf. Published 2017. Accessed September 8, 2017.

8. ARUP Laboratories. 5-Fluorouracil toxicity and chemotherapeutic response panel. http://ltd.aruplab.com/Tests/Pub/2007228. Published 2014. Accessed August 18, 2017.

9. Atherton LD, et al. Toxic megacolon associated with methotrexate therapy. *Gastroenterology.* 1984;86:1583-1588.

10. Aumente MD, et al. Evaluation of the novel methotrexate architect chemiluminescent inmunoassay: clinical impact on pharmacokinetic monitoring. *Ther Drug Monit.* 2017;39:492-498.

11. Barak AJ, et al. Methotrexate hepatotoxicity. *J Am Coll Nutr.* 1984;3:93-96.

12. Begas E, et al. Simple and reliable HPLC method for the monitoring of methotrexate in osteosarcoma patients. *J Chromatogr Sci.* 2014;52:590-595.

13. Benezet S, et al. Inefficacy of exchange-transfusion in case of a methotrexate poisoning [in French]. *Bull Cancer.* 1997;84:788-790.

14. Bleyer WA. The clinical pharmacology of methotrexate: new applications of an old drug. *Cancer.* 1978;41:36-51.

15. Bluett J, et al. A HPLC-SRM-MS based method for the detection and quantification of methotrexate in urine at doses used in clinical practice for patients with rheumatological disease: a potential measure of adherence. *Analyst.* 2015;140:1981-1987.

16. Bouquie R, et al. Evaluation of a methotrexate chemiluminescent microparticle immunoassay: comparison to fluorescence polarization immunoassay and liquid chromatography-tandem mass spectrometry. *Am J Clin Pathol.* 2016;146:119-124.

17. Bremnes RM, et al. Acute hepatotoxicity after high-dose methotrexate administration to rats. *Pharmacol Toxicol.* 1991;69:132-139.

18. Buchen S, et al. Carboxypeptidase G2 rescue in patients with methotrexate intoxication and renal failure. *Br J Cancer.* 2005;92:480-487.

19. Casale F, et al. Plasma concentrations of 5-fluorouracil and its metabolites in colon cancer patients. *Pharmacol Res.* 2004;50:173-179.

20. Chabner BA, Young RC. Threshold methotrexate concentration for in vivo inhibition of DNA synthesis in normal and tumorous target tissues. *J Clin Invest.* 1973;52:1804-1811.

21. Christensen ML, et al. Effect of hydration on methotrexate plasma concentrations in children with acute lymphocytic leukemia. *J Clin Oncol.* 1988;6:797-801.

22. Connors NJ, et al. Methotrexate toxicity treated with continuous venovenous hemofiltration, leucovorin and glucarpidase. *Clin Kidney J.* 2014;7:590-592.

23. Cronstein BN, et al. The antiinflammatory mechanism of methotrexate. Increased adenosine release at inflamed sites diminishes leukocyte accumulation in an in vivo model of inflammation. *J Clin Invest.* 1993;92:2675-2682.

24. Cunningham J, et al. Do patients receiving haemodialysis need folic acid supplements? *Br Med J (Clin Res Ed).* 1981;282:1582.

25. Dahan L, et al. Sudden death related to toxicity in a patient on capecitabine and irinotecan plus bevacizumab intake: pharmacogenetic implications. *J Clin Oncol.* 2012;30:e41-e44.

26. Djerassi I, et al. Removal of methotrexate by filtration-adsorption using charcoal filters or by hemodialysis. *Cancer Treat Rep.* 1977;61:751-752.

27. Doolittle GC, et al. Methotrexate-associated, early-onset pancytopenia in rheumatoid arthritis. *Arch Intern Med.* 1989;149:1430-1431.

28. Ducreux M, et al. Capecitabine plus oxaliplatin (XELOX) versus 5-fluorouracil/leucovorin plus oxaliplatin (FOLFOX-6) as first-line treatment for metastatic colorectal cancer. *Int J Cancer.* 2011;128:682-690.

29. Erttmann R, Landbeck G. Effect of oral cholestyramine on the elimination of high-dose methotrexate. *J Cancer Res Clin Oncol.* 1985;110:48-50.

30. Fong CM, Lee AC. High-dose methotrexate-associated acute renal failure may be an avoidable complication. *Pediatr Hematol Oncol.* 2006;23:51-57.

31. Frei E 3rd, et al. High dose methotrexate with leucovorin rescue. Rationale and spectrum of antitumor activity. *Am J Med.* 1980;68:370-376.

32. Frei E 3rd, et al. New approaches to cancer chemotherapy with methotrexate. *N Engl J Med.* 1975;292:846-851.

33. Fukushima T, et al. A magnetic resonance abnormality correlating with permeability of the blood-brain barrier in a child with chemical meningitis during central nervous system prophylaxis for acute leukemia. *Ann Hematol.* 1999;78:564-567.

34. Gadgil SD, et al. Effect of activated charcoal on the pharmacokinetics of high-dose methotrexate. *Cancer Treat Rep.* 1982;66:1169-1171.

35. Gibson TP, et al. Hemoperfusion for methotrexate removal. *Clin Pharmacol Ther.* 1978;23:351-355.

36. Godefroid MJ, et al. Multicenter method evaluation of the ARK Methotrexate Immunoassay. *Clin Chem Lab Med.* 2014;52:e13-e16.

37. Gowan GM, et al. Methotrexate-induced toxic leukoencephalopathy. *Pharmacotherapy.* 2002;22:1183-1187.

38. Grimes DJ, et al. Survival after unexpected high serum methotrexate concentrations in a patient with osteogenic sarcoma. *Drug Saf.* 1990;5:447-454.

39. Hande KR, et al. Methotrexate and hemodialysis. *Ann Intern Med.* 1977;87:495-496.

40. Harned TM, Mascarenhas L. Severe methotrexate toxicity precipitated by intravenous radiographic contrast. *J Pediatr Hematol Oncol.* 2007;29:496-499.

41. Hess JA, Khasawneh MK. Cancer metabolism and oxidative stress: insights into carcinogenesis and chemotherapy via the non-dihydrofolate reductase effects of methotrexate. *BBA Clin.* 2015;3:152-161.

42. Hughes PJ, Lane RJ. Acute cerebral oedema induced by methotrexate. *BMJ.* 1989; 298:1315.

43. Inoue S, et al. Erythrocyte methotrexate-polyglutamate assay using fluorescence polarization immunoassay technique: application to the monitoring of patients with rheumatoid arthritis. *Yakugaku Zasshi.* 2009;129:1001-1005.

44. Inoue S, et al. Preliminary study to identify the predictive factors for the response to methotrexate therapy in patients with rheumatoid arthritis. *Yakugaku Zasshi.* 2009;129:843-849.

45. Isacoff W. Effects of extracorporeal charcoal hemoperfusion on plasma methotrexate [abstract]. *Proc Am Assoc Cancer Res.* 1977;18:1.

46. Iven H, Brasch H. The effects of antibiotics and uricosuric drugs on the renal elimination of methotrexate and 7-hydroxymethotrexate in rabbits. *Cancer Chemother Pharmacol.* 1988;21:337-342.

47. Jackson RC, Grindley GB. The biochemical basis for methotrexate cytotoxicity. In: Sirotnak FM, et al, eds. *Folate Antagonists as Therapeutic Agents.* New York, NY: Academic Press; 1984:289-315.

48. Jacobs SA, et al. 7-Hydroxymethotrexate as a urinary metabolite in human subjects and rhesus monkeys receiving high dose methotrexate. *J Clin Invest.* 1976;57:534-538.

49. Jaffe N, et al. Transient neurologic disturbances induced by high-dose methotrexate treatment. *Cancer.* 1985;56:1356-1360.

50. Jambou P, et al. Removal of methotrexate by continuous venovenous hemodiafiltration. *Contrib Nephrol.* 1995;116:48-52.

51. Kawabata K, et al. A case of methotrexate-induced acute renal failure successfully treated with plasma perfusion and sequential hemodialysis. *Nephron.* 1995;71:233-234.

52. Kelkar R, et al. Epidemic iatrogenic *Acinetobacter* spp. meningitis following administration of intrathecal methotrexate. *J Hosp Infect.* 1989;14:233-243.

53. Kepka L, et al. Successful rescue in a patient with high dose methotrexate-induced nephrotoxicity and acute renal failure. *Leuk Lymphoma.* 1998;29:205-209.

54. Kevat SG, et al. Pancytopenia induced by low-dose methotrexate for rheumatoid arthritis. *Aust N Z J Med.* 1988;18:697-700.

55. Kremer JM, Hamilton RA. The effects of nonsteroidal antiinflammatory drugs on methotrexate (MTX) pharmacokinetics: impairment of renal clearance of MTX at weekly maintenance doses but not at 7.5 mg. *J Rheumatol.* 1995;22:2072-2077.

56. Langslow A. Nursing and the law. Deadly doses of methotrexate. *Aust Nurs J.* 1995;2: 32-34.

57. Liegler DG, et al. The effect of organic acids on renal clearance of methotrexate in man. *Clin Pharmacol Ther.* 1969;10:849-857.

58. Loganayagam A, et al. Pharmacogenetic variants in the DPYD, TYMS, CDA and MTHFR genes are clinically significant predictors of fluoropyrimidine toxicity. *Br J Cancer.* 2013;108:2505-2515.

59. Ma WW, et al. Emergency use of uridine triacetate for the prevention and treatment of life-threatening 5-fluorouracil and capecitabine toxicity. *Cancer.* 2017;123: 345-356.

60. MacKinnon SK, et al. Pancytopenia associated with low dose pulse methotrexate in the treatment of rheumatoid arthritis. *Semin Arthritis Rheum.* 1985;15:119-126.

61. Massenkeil G, et al. Transient tetraparesis after intrathecal and high-dose systemic methotrexate. *Ann Hematol.* 1998;77:239-242.

62. McIntosh S, et al. Methotrexate hepatotoxicity in children with leukemia. *J Pediatr.* 1977;90:1019-1021.

63. Mercier C, Ciccolini J. Profiling dihydropyrimidine dehydrogenase deficiency in patients with cancer undergoing 5-fluorouracil/capecitabine therapy. *Clin Colorectal Cancer.* 2006;6:288-296.

64. Mercier C, Ciccolini J. Severe or lethal toxicities upon capecitabine intake: is DPYD genetic polymorphism the ideal culprit? *Trends Pharmacol Sci.* 2007;28:597-598.

65. Mercier C, et al. Early severe toxicities after capecitabine intake: possible implication of a cytidine deaminase extensive metabolizer profile. *Cancer Chemother Pharmacol.* 2009;63:1177-1180.

66. Meulendijks D, et al. Renal function, body surface area, and age are associated with risk of early-onset fluoropyrimidine-associated toxicity in patients treated with capecitabine-based anticancer regimens in daily clinical care. *Eur J Cancer.* 2016;54:120-130.

67. Millart H, et al. The effects of 5-fluorouracil on contractility and oxygen uptake of the isolated perfused rat heart. *Anticancer Res.* 1992;12:571-576.

68. Molinari A, et al. New antineoplastic prenylhydroquinones. Synthesis and evaluation. *Bioorg Med Chem.* 2000;8:1027-1032.

69. Montesinos MC, et al. The antiinflammatory mechanism of methotrexate depends on extracellular conversion of adenine nucleotides to adenosine by ecto-5'-nucleotidase: findings in a study of ecto-5'-nucleotidase gene-deficient mice. *Arthritis Rheum.* 2007; 56:1440-1445.

70. Moriwaki Y, et al. Widespread cellular distribution of aldehyde oxidase in human tissues found by immunohistochemistry staining. *Histol Histopathol.* 2001;16:745-753.

71. Nesbit M, et al. Acute and chronic effects of methotrexate on hepatic, pulmonary, and skeletal systems. *Cancer.* 1976;37(suppl):1048-1057.

72. O'Marcaigh AS, et al. Successful treatment of intrathecal methotrexate overdose by using ventriculolumbar perfusion and intrathecal instillation of carboxypeptidase G2. *Mayo Clin Proc.* 1996;71:161-165.

73. Park ES, et al. Carboxypeptidase-G2 resuce in a patient with a high dose methotrexate-induced nephrotoxicty. *Cancer Res Treat.* 2005;37:2.

74. Peng Z, et al. Ecto-5'-nucleotidase (CD73)-mediated extracellular adenosine production plays a critical role in hepatic fibrosis. *Nucleosides Nucleotides Nucleic Acids.* 2008;27:821-824.

75. Perez-Aso M, et al. Adenosine 2A receptor promotes collagen production by human fibroblasts via pathways involving cyclic AMP and AKT but independent of Smad2/3. *FASEB J.* 2014;28:802-812.

76. Pinedo HM, et al. The reversal of methotrexate cytotoxicity to mouse bone marrow cells by leucovorin and nucleosides. *Cancer Res.* 1976;36:4418-4424.

77. Reggev A, Djerassi I. The safety of administration of massive doses of methotrexate (50 g) with equimolar citrovorum factor rescue in adult patients. *Cancer.* 1988;61:2423-2428.

78. Relling MV, et al. Removal of methotrexate, leucovorin, and their metabolites by combined hemodialysis and hemoperfusion. *Cancer.* 1988;62:884-888.

79. Roberts MS, et al. Determination of methotrexate, 7-hydroxymethotrexate, and 2,4-diamino-n10-methylpteroic acid by LC-MS/MS in plasma and cerebrospinal fluid and application in a pharmacokinetic analysis of high-dose methotrexate. *J Liq Chromatogr Relat Technol.* 2016;39:745-751.

80. Roenigk HH Jr, et al. Methotrexate therapy for psoriasis. Guideline revisions. *Arch Dermatol.* 1973;108:35.

81. Saif MW, Diasio RB. Benefit of uridine triacetate (Vistogard) in rescuing severe 5-fluorouracil toxicity in patients with dihydropyrimidine dehydrogenase (DPYD) deficiency. *Cancer Chemother Pharmacol.* 2016;78:151-156.

82. Saif MW, et al. Fluoropyrimidine-associated cardiotoxicity: revisited. *Expert Opin Drug Saf.* 2009;8:191-202.

83. Saland JM, et al. Effective removal of methotrexate by high-flux hemodialysis. *Pediatr Nephrol.* 2002;17:825-829.

84. Santos C, et al. The successful treatment of 5-fluorouracil (5-FU) overdose in a patient with malignancy and HIV/AIDS with uridine triacetate. *Am J Emerg Med.* 2017;35:802. e807-802.e808.

85. Sasaki K, et al. Theoretically required urinary flow during high-dose methotrexate infusion. *Cancer Chemother Pharmacol.* 1984;13:9-13.

86. Schwartz S, et al. Glucarpidase (carboxypeptidase G2) intervention in adult and elderly cancer patients with renal dysfunction and delayed methotrexate elimination after high-dose methotrexate therapy. *Oncologist.* 2007;12:1299-1308.

87. Serdjebi C, et al. Role of cytidine deaminase in toxicity and efficacy of nucleosidic analogs. *Expert Opin Drug Metab Toxicol.* 2015;11:665-672.

88. Sheikh-Hamad D, et al. Cisplatin-induced renal toxicity: possible reversal by N-acetylcysteine treatment. *J Am Soc Nephrol.* 1997;8:1640-1644.

89. Shinozaki T, et al. Successful rescue by oral cholestyramine of a patient with methotrexate nephrotoxicity: nonrenal excretion of serum methotrexate. *Med Pediatr Oncol.* 2000;34:226-228.

90. Skoutakis VA, et al. Folic acid dosage for chronic hemodialysis patients. *Clin Pharmacol Ther.* 1975;18:200-204.

91. Smith TJ, et al. Recommendations for the use of WBC growth factors: American Society of Clinical Oncology Clinical Practice Guideline Update. *J Clin Oncol.* 2015; 33:3199-3212.

92. Sonneveld P, et al. Pharmacokinetics of methotrexate and 7-hydroxy-methotrexate in plasma and bone marrow of children receiving low-dose oral methotrexate. *Cancer Chemother Pharmacol.* 1986;18:111-116.

93. Sorrentino MF, et al. 5-fluorouracil induced cardiotoxicity: review of the literature. *Cardiol J.* 2012;19:453-458.

94. Steger GG, et al. GM-CSF in the treatment of a patient with severe methotrexate intoxication. *J Intern Med.* 1993;233:499-502.

95. Stoller RG, et al. Use of plasma pharmacokinetics to predict and prevent methotrexate toxicity. *N Engl J Med.* 1977;297:630-634.

96. Teh HS, et al. Transverse myelopathy following intrathecal administration of chemotherapy. *Singapore Med J.* 2007;48:e46-e49.

97. Thierry FX, et al. Acute renal failure after high-dose methotrexate therapy. Role of hemodialysis and plasma exchange in methotrexate removal. *Nephron.* 1989;51: 416-417.

98. Tukova J, et al. Methotrexate bioavailability after oral and subcutaneous dministration in children with juvenile idiopathic arthritis. *Clin Exp Rheumatol.* 2009;27: 1047-1053.

99. Vakily M, et al. Coadministration of lansoprazole and naproxen does not affect the pharmacokinetic profile of methotrexate in adult patients with rheumatoid arthritis. *J Clin Pharmacol.* 2005;45:1179-1186.

100. Vistogard(TM). (uridine triacetate) [package insert]. Gaithersburg, MD: Wellstat Therapeutics Corp; 2015. https://www.accessdata.fda.gov/drugsatfda_docs/label/2015/208159s000lbl.pdf. Accessed August 18, 2017.

101. Von Hoff DD, et al. Incidence of drug-related deaths secondary to high-dose methotrexate and citrovorum factor administration. *Cancer Treat Rep.* 1977;61:745-748.

102. Voraxaze(TM). (glucaripdase) [package insert]. West Conshohocken, PA: BTG International Inc; 2012. https://www.accessdata.fda.gov/drugsatfda_docs/label/2012/125327lbl.pdf. Accessed September 8, 2017.

103. Walker RW, et al. Transient cerebral dysfunction secondary to high-dose methotrexate. *J Clin Oncol.* 1986;4:1845-1850.

104. Walko CM, Lindley C. Capecitabine: a review. *Clin Ther.* 2005;27:23-44.

105. Wall SM, et al. Effective clearance of methotrexate using high-flux hemodialysis membranes. *Am J Kidney Dis.* 1996;28:846-854.

106. Weinberg ME, et al. Enhanced uridine bioavailability following administration of a triacetyluridine-rich nutritional supplement. *PLoS One.* 2011;6:e14709.

107. Weinstein GD. Methotrexate. *Ann Intern Med.* 1977;86:199-204.

108. Widemann BC, Adamson PC. Understanding and managing methotrexate nephrotoxicity. *Oncologist.* 2006;11:694-703.

109. Widemann BC, et al. High-dose methotrexate-induced nephrotoxicity in patients with osteosarcoma. *Cancer.* 2004;100:2222-2232.

110. Widemann BC, et al. Carboxypeptidase-G2, thymidine, and leucovorin rescue in cancer patients with methotrexate-induced renal dysfunction. *J Clin Oncol.* 1997;15: 2125-2134.

111. Widemann BC, et al. Treatment of accidental intrathecal methotrexate overdose with intrathecal carboxypeptidase G2. *J Natl Cancer Inst.* 2004;96:1557-1559.

112. Widemann BC, et al. Pharmacokinetics and metabolism of the methotrexate metabolite 2, 4-diamino-N(10)-methylpteroic acid. *J Pharmacol Exp Ther.* 2000;294: 894-901.

113. Ziereisen F, et al. Reversible acute methotrexate leukoencephalopathy: atypical brain MR imaging features. *Pediatr Radiol.* 2006;36:205-212.

FOLATES: LEUCOVORIN (FOLINIC ACID) AND FOLIC ACID

Silas W. Smith and Mary Ann Howland

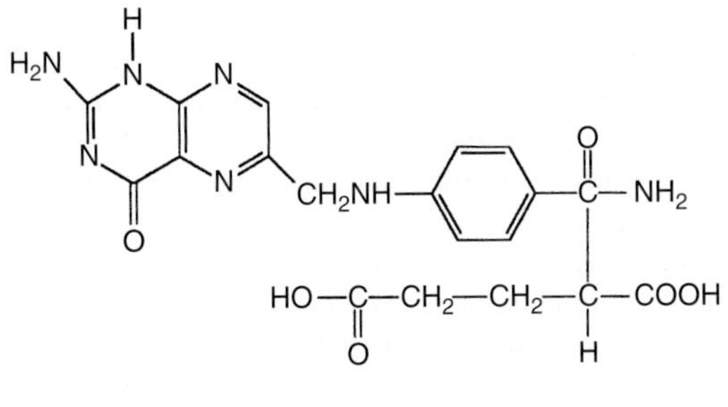

Folic Acid

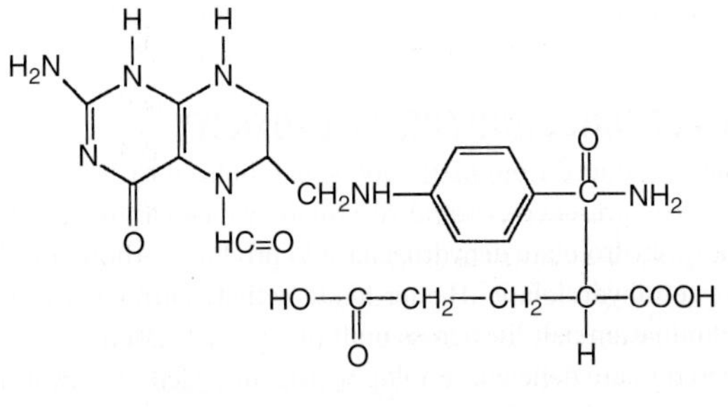

Folinic Acid

Folates refer to the metabolically active reduced forms of folic acid, including dihydrofolate and tetrahydrofolate. These folates are vital to cellular biochemistry, including the synthesis of purines and DNA. Folic acid must be reduced in vivo by dihydrofolate reductase to tetrahydrofolate. Dihydrofolate reductase inhibitors such as methotrexate (MTX), pyrimethamine and pemetrexed prevent this reduction. Leucovorin (folinic acid) and levoleucovorin, do not require dihydrofolate reductase for activation. Therefore, either leucovorin or levoleucovorin is the primary antidote for a patient who receives an overdose of MTX or another dihydrofolate reductase inhibitor.

Methanol is metabolized to the active and toxic formic acid. Folates, including folic acid and leucovorin, speed up the conversion of formic acid to nontoxic metabolites. Because methanol does not interfere with the synthesis of tetrahydrofolate, either folic acid or leucovorin is acceptable for a patient poisoned by methanol. Preliminary evidence also suggests a role for folic acid to enhance arsenic elimination.

HISTORY

In 1930–1931, Lucy Wills, while studying pregnant textile workers with macrocytic anemia in Mumbai, India, discovered that a yeast extract provided to these nutritionally deficient individuals cured and prevented their anemia.[105] Mitchell isolated the active ingredient from spinach in 1941 and named it folic acid from the Latin *folium*, meaning leaf.[35] Subsequently, the synthesis and chemical structure of folate was described in 1945–1946.[3] In 1948, the first reported clinical success in inducing temporary remission of acute leukemia by the antifolate aminopterin was reported, soon followed by success with the

less toxic amethopterin (ie, MTX).[24] That same year, in studies exploring links to anemia, a factor in the gram-positive bacteria *Leuconostoc citrovorum* was identified as required in growth media for deficient species.[79] Two years later in 1950, this "citrovorum factor"—later named leucovorin (folinic acid)—successfully reversed aminopterin and MTX toxicity, which had resisted folate therapy.[82] In the 1960s, the concept emerged of providing higher doses of MTX for improved chemotherapeutic efficacy, which was then coupled with subsequent leucovorin "rescue" to mitigate toxicity.[53] Since then, the many roles of folate and natural or induced folate deficiency continue to be studied.

PHARMACOLOGY

Folic acid (pteroylglutamic acid), an essential water-soluble vitamin, consists of a pteridine ring joined to PABA (*para*-aminobenzoic acid) and glutamic acid.[3] Folic acid is the most common of the many folate congeners that exist in nature and are essential for normal cellular metabolic functions. Folic acid is rarely called vitamin B_9. After absorption, folic acid is reduced by dihydrofolic acid reductase (DHFR) to dihydrofolic acid and then tetrahydrofolic acid (THF), which accepts one-carbon groups. Tetrahydrofolic acid serves as the precursor for several biologically active forms of folic acid, including 5-formyltetrahydrofolic acid (5-formyl THF), which is best known as folinic acid, leucovorin, and citrovorum factor. The biologically active forms of folate are enzymatically interconvertible and function as cofactors, providing the one-carbon groups necessary for many intracellular metabolic reactions, including the synthesis of thymidylate and purine nucleotides, which are essential precursors of DNA.[69,76,86,89,99] The minimum daily requirement of folic acid is normally approximately 50 mcg, but nutritionally deprived, acutely ill patients may require 100 to 200 mcg, and women who are preconception or pregnant are advised to take 400 mcg to 1,000 mcg of folic acid daily.[18,37]

Leucovorin is a mixture of the active and inactive diastereoisomers of 5-formyl-THF, of which the levo-(6S)-form is active and available as levoleucovorin.[88] Both are available as the calcium salt, with the same chemical formula. The molecular weight (MW) is 511.5 Da; levoleucovorin for injection is supplied as the calcium pentahydrate form for a total MW of 601.6.[88] Absent metabolic inhibition, folate and leucovorin are rapidly metabolized to several active folates, including 5-methyltetrahydrofolate (5-methyl-THF). The dose of levoleucovorin is half of leucovorin. Leucovorin *increases* the toxicity of 5-fluorouracil (5-FU). Leucovorin is converted to (6R)-5,10-methylene-THF, which stabilizes the ternary complex with the 5-FU metabolite, fluoro-deoxyuridine monophosphate (5-FdUMP) and thymidylate synthase, leading to thymidylate depletion.[20,80]

After a DHFR inhibitor such as MTX inhibits the formation of tetrahydrofolic acid, the intracellular machinery for the synthesis of indispensable thymidylate and purine nucleotides comes to a halt, and DNA production ceases. Leucovorin and levoleucovorin are biologically active forms of folic acid and bypass this inhibition of DHFR caused by MTX.

Folate catalyzes the formation of carbon dioxide and water from formic acid, the final metabolic step in methanol elimination. Because there is no inhibition of the formation or recycling of active folate, either folic acid or leucovorin is beneficial (Chap. 106).

Investigations suggest that folic acid aids in the methylation and subsequent elimination of arsenic. Folate supplementation in folate-deficient subjects enhanced the elimination of arsenic and potentially decreased chronic arsenic toxicity (Chap. 86).[27,70]

Related Xenobiotics

The predominant form of dietary folate, *levo*-(6*S*)-5-methyl-THF, which is required for methionine biosynthesis from homocysteine, is available commercially both as the natural form and as mefolinate, the diastereoisomeric, 1:1 mixture (6*R*,*S*)-5-methyl-THF.[20] It is also found in combination with pharmaceuticals (eg, oral contraceptive pills).[26] (6*R*)-5,10-methylene-THF also bypasses activation to produce higher (6*R*)-5,10-methylene-THF concentrations compared to leucovorin in order to enhance 5-FU efficacy.[100] It is also undergoing evaluations as an MTX rescue agent (ClinicalTrials.gov Identifier: NCT01987102).

Leucovorin Pharmacokinetics

Whereas leucovorin is naturally formed in the body as the active *levo* (*l*)-(6*S*)-isomer, the initial commercial preparation was a racemic mixture consisting of equal amounts of the inactive *dextro* (*d*)-(6*R*) and active (*l*) isomers. The pharmacokinetics of the racemic mixture of leucovorin and its active metabolite were studied after a single intravenous (IV) infusion and as a constant infusion in healthy human volunteers.[91,92] During a constant infusion of 500 mg/m^2/day, the steady-state concentration for the active (*l*) isomer was 2.33 µmol/L, the half-life was 35 minutes, and the volume of distribution (V_d) was 13.6 L. The active isomer is metabolized to an active metabolite, *l*-(6*S*)-5-methyl-THF, which achieved a steady-state concentration of 4.85 µmol/L and a half-life of 227 minutes. Similar values were achieved for half-life and V_d after single IV doses ranging from 25 to 100 mg. The inactive *d*-isomer achieved higher concentrations and had a much longer half-life with oral administration, which is saturable and stereoselective, resulting in absorption of the active isomer that is 4 to 5 times greater than that of the inactive isomer. Studies of stereospecific oral absorption demonstrate that 100% of the *l*-leucovorin is absorbed, but only 20% of the *d*-leucovorin is absorbed at this dose.[95] One study detected no adverse effects of the inactive isomer on the intracellular uptake of the active isomer and concluded that giving the active isomer provided no pharmacokinetic advantage over the racemic mixture.[81] In 5 normal subjects given 1,000 mg of leucovorin as a 2-hour intravenous infusion, peak plasma concentrations of *l*-(6*S*) leucovorin, *d*-(6*R*) leucovorin, and 5-methyl-THF were 5 9.1 ± 22 µmol/L, 148 ± 32 µmol/L, and 17.8 ± 17 µmol/L, respectively.[80] Intravenous leucovorin results in an area under the curve (AUC) for inactive (6*R*) LV that was 4.16 ± 1.4 times greater than the combined AUCs for *l*-(6*S*) leucovorin and 5-methyl-THF.[80] Two hundred milligrams of levoleucovorin was compared to 400 mg of leucovorin, each administered as a 2-hour IV infusion as a crossover study in 40 healthy volunteers; the area under the curve and the maximum serum concentrations of *l*-5-CH$_3$-THF were similar for both.[88]

The pharmacokinetics of IV leucovorin was compared with intramuscular (IM) and oral administration in male volunteers given 25 mg. At this dose, oral leucovorin was 92% bioavailable and the mean peak active *l*-5-methyl-THF concentration of 258 ng/mL (5.5 × 10^{-1} µmol/L) at 1.3 hours after IV administration, 226 ng/mL at 2.8 hours for IM, and 367 ng/mL at 2.4 hours for oral administration, respectively.[61] The pharmacokinetics of orally administered leucovorin was studied in healthy, fasted male volunteers in single doses ranging from 20 to 100 mg and 200 mg IV over 5 minutes compared with 200 mg orally.[61,74] Bioavailability decreased from 100% for the 20-mg dose to 78% for the 40-mg dose and ultimately to 31% for the 200-mg dose. A microbiologic assay was used to measure total tetrahydrofolates (reduced and active folates). Normal serum folate concentrations are approximately 0.05 µmol/L.[44] The 200-mg oral dose produced a peak serum concentration of 1.82 µmol/L compared with 0.66 µmol/L for the 20-mg oral dose and 27.1 µmol/L for the 200-mg IV dose.[61,74]

After IV administration of both leucovorin and levoleucovorin, *l*-5-methyl-THF enters the CSF. The concentration of CSF *l*-5-methyl-THF achieved was 100 to 1,000-fold less than that obtained after direct MTX intra-Ommaya reservoir administration during a period of 2 days of observation.[64] Because *l*-5-methyl-THF is cleared slowly from CSF (half-life = 85 hours), progressive accumulation occurs from chemotherapy cycle to cycle.[96] Thus, the significant reductions in *l*-5-methyl-THF that occurs with IV and intrathecal MTX

can recover with ongoing leucovorin treatment.[9,93] The limitations of oral leucovorin therapy were demonstrated in one study in which oral leucovorin (10 mg every 6 hours for 11 doses) failed to provide adequate *l*-5-methyl-THF to exceed CSF MTX concentrations in 6 of 9 patients.[2] Intrathecal administration of leucovorin and levoleucovorin is contraindicated, as it can lower seizure threshold and is associated with fatal neurotoxicity.[25,45,88,97]

ROLE IN METHOTREXATE TOXICITY

Methotrexate, an antimetabolite, is a structural analog of folic acid, differing only in the substitution of an amino group for a hydroxyl group at the number 4 position of the pteridine ring (Chap. 51). Methotrexate binds to the active site of DHFR, rendering it incapable of reducing folic acid to its biologically active forms and incapable of regenerating the necessary active forms required for the synthesis of purine nucleotides and thymidylate.[87] Under various conditions, the binding between MTX and DHFR is competitive and very tight, with an inhibition constant ranging from 0.0034 nmol/L to 0.093 ± 0.021 nmol/L.[5,19] 7-HydroxyMTX, a major MTX metabolite, more weakly inhibits DHFR (K_i = 8.9 nM).[5] This compares to a K_m of 2.7 ± 0.5 µmol/L for dihydrofolic acid.[19] Leucovorin is a reduced, active form of folate. As such, it does not require DHFR for enzymatic interconversion to the form required for purine nucleotide and thymidylate formation. Folic acid is unable to counteract MTX toxicity because after MTX therapy, DHFR is unavailable to convert folic acid to an active reduced form. High-dose MTX therapy provides chemotherapeutic benefit, although it is associated with significant toxicity. *Leucovorin rescue* describe the standard practice of limiting the toxic effects associated with high-dose MTX, by providing leucovorin after the initial MTX infusion and in cases of diminished MTX elimination, which can be due to MTX toxicity itself or other factors.[102]

ROLE IN METHANOL AND FORMATE TOXICITY

The formate produced from methanol is metabolized to 10-formyl tetrahydrofolate in the presence of tetrahydrofolate, which can be acted upon by 10-formyltetrahydrofolate dehydrogenase to produce carbon dioxide and to regenerate tetrahydrofolate.[7] Higher folate activity correlates with a faster formate elimination half-life across multiple species.[90] Monkeys experimentally rendered folate deficient develop methanol toxicity at lower methanol concentrations.[62] Folic acid supplementation (2.5 mg/kg IV) provided to dogs poisoned with 2 g/kg methanol lowered maximum formate accumulation in plasma from 3 to 1 mmol/L.[90] Similarly, administering folic acid to healthy monkeys accelerates formate metabolism.[62] Pretreatment with folic acid or leucovorin decreased both formate concentrations and the accompanying metabolic acidosis without affecting the rate of methanol elimination.[62] In monkeys given repeated injections of leucovorin, either before or concurrent with the administration of methanol, decreased formate concentrations and an absence of metabolic acidosis were observed.[4] Leucovorin remained effective in monkeys in hastening the metabolism of formate when given as late as 10 hours after methanol administration.[67]

In methanol-poisoned humans, the hepatic concentrations of total folate, leucovorin, and folate dehydrogenase (which increases leucovorin concentrations) are all diminished.[46] In a methanol-poisoned patient treated without folic acid, the formate half-life was 2.8 hours.[42] In 6 methanol-poisoned patients treated without folic acid, the mean serum formate half-life was 2.6 hours.[38] By comparison, in a single methanol-poisoned patient who was given folic acid, ethanol, and hemodialyzed, the half-life of formate was 1.1 hours during hemodialysis.[68] In another methanol-poisoned patient, the formate half-life was 3.9 hours, which decreased to 1.2 hours after leucovorin treatment.[38] In an intentional ingestion of 110 g of formic acid treated with folinic acid (1 mg/kg every 4 hours for the first 24 hours), low plasma formic acid concentrations were present during leucovorin administration, which rose significantly after leucovorin cessation.[66] In human placental ex vivo experiments, folic acid reversed the toxic effects of formic acid on the placenta of decreased maternal hCG secretion.[41] These comparative data are inadequate to draw definitive conclusions. However, the evidence supports the continued recommendation for a therapeutic role of folate or leucovorin in addition to definitive therapy with fomepizole (Antidotes in Depth: A33) and/or hemodialysis.[7]

ROLE IN ARSENIC TOXICITY

Arsenic contamination of drinking water has plagued millions, causing increased manifestations of chronic arsenic toxicity, including cancer and cardiovascular, dermatologic, and neurologic disorders.[17,60] In a folate-dependent mechanism, arsenic undergoes methylation to monomethylarsonic acid (MMA) and then to dimethylarsinic acid (DMA) via one-carbon metabolism, and this methylation facilitates urinary arsenic excretion.[28,33] Patients with higher intakes of folate-related nutrients had lower percentages of inorganic arsenic and higher MMA to inorganic arsenic ratios.[33] Folate deficiency, hyperhomocysteinemia, and low urinary creatinine, each of which is associated with decreased arsenic methylation capacity, are risk factors for arsenic-induced skin lesions.[71] In a study of arsenic's epigenetic effects on histone modification, arsenic concentration in women were associated with lower total plasma histone concentrations only among women with folate deficiency.[94] The absolute methylation amount and product probably depends on the degree of upregulation, age, and available methyl groups (Chap. 86).[31,40] In animal models, folic acid supplementation decreased arsenic embryotoxicity, malformations, and abnormal cardiac and neural development.[58] This effect appeared to be mediated by decreasing subcellular reactive oxygen species when tested in human embryonic kidney cells.[58]

These findings encouraged the study of folate supplementation, along with other nutrients, with the aim to diminish the chronic health effects of arsenic toxicity. A randomized, double-blind, placebo-controlled trial of folic acid supplementation (400 mcg daily for 12 weeks) to participants with low plasma folate concentrations demonstrated enhanced arsenic methylation.[27] In a randomized, controlled trial of 622 patients, daily folic acid of 800 mcg for 12 and 24 weeks' treatment lowered blood arsenic to a greater extent than placebo, an effect that was sustained without rebound for 12 weeks after treatment cessation.[70]

ROLE IN TOXICITY FROM DIHYDROFOLATE REDUCTASE INHIBITOR ANTIBIOTICS

Pyrimethamine is a dihydrofolate reductase competitive inhibitor used to treat infections from *Toxoplasma*, *Isospora*, and *Pneumocystis*. In a dose-dependent fashion, leucovorin significantly reduces cytogenetic aberrations associated with pyrimethamine in vitro.[21] Leucovorin is routinely added to pyrimethamine therapy for toxoplasmosis.[73,98] One large outbreak of pyrimethamine toxicity reported a 23% fatality rate in 664 cardiac patients who received isosorbide mononitrate contaminated with 50 mg of pyrimethamine.[48] Once the contaminant was determined, leucovorin was administered at a dose of 30 mg every 6 hours for 2 days and then every 12 hours until complete recovery.[48] Trimetrexate glucuronate, another dihydrofolate reductase inhibitor used in to treat *Pneumocystis*, has been discontinued in the United States. It required administration with concurrent IV leucovorin in order to preclude serious or life-threatening bone marrow suppression, oral and gastrointestinal mucosal ulceration, and renal and hepatic dysfunction (20 mg/m² over 5–10 minutes every 6 hours for a total daily dose of 80 mg/m², or orally as 4 doses of 20 mg/m² spaced equally throughout the day for 24 days).[63]

ADVERSE EFFECTS AND SAFETY ISSUES

Reports of adverse reactions to parenteral injections of folic acid, leucovorin, or levoleucovorin are uncommon. However, reported adverse reactions include allergic or anaphylactoid reactions.[95] Seizures are also rarely associated with leucovorin or levoleucovorin administration.[65] The calcium content of leucovorin and levoleucovorin warrants a slow IV infusion at a rate not faster than 160 mg/min in adults. There are 0.004 mEq of calcium per milligram of leucovorin calcium injection. Extremely large doses of leucovorin on the order of 1,000 mg every 3 hours might lead to hypercalcemia.[106] Neither leucovorin nor levoleucovorin should be administered intrathecally due to neurotoxic adverse effects.[25,45,52,77,97] As described in the pharmacology

section, leucovorin and levoleucovorin are not antidotes for 5-FU, and both enhance the chemotherapeutic and toxic effects of fluoropyrimidines including 5-FU and 5-FU prodrugs such as capecitabine and tegafur.[20,57,88,95,100]

Protocols recommend separating leucovorin and levoleucovorin from glucarpidase by 2 hours (Antidotes in Depth: A13). Otherwise, leucovorin acts as a substrate for glucarpidase, which cleaves the active *l*-(6*S*)-leucovorin approximately 50% faster than the inactive *d*-(6*R*)-form.[1,23,34,84]

There is a potential for dosing errors when interchanging leucovorin and levoleucovorin. The dose of levoleucovorin is one-half the dose of leucovorin.[88]

PREGNANCY AND LACTATION

Folic acid is a Food and Drug Administration (FDA) category A drug and is safe and essential during pregnancy and compatible with breastfeeding. Leucovorin and levoleucovorin are FDA pregnancy category C drugs.[88,95] Although definitive reproductive studies do not exist, folinic acid has successfully treated megaloblastic anemia during gestation[83] and is considered compatible with pregnancy.[13] In addition, there are case reports of maternal administration of leucovorin, in combination with 5-FU and oxaliplatin chemotherapy during pregnancy, with subsequent healthy fetal delivery.[49,59] Breast milk excretion is unstudied, but leucovorin is considered compatible with breastfeeding.[13]

DOSING AND ADMINISTRATION

After MTX overdose, a dose of leucovorin estimated to produce the same plasma concentration as the MTX dose should be given as soon as possible, preferably within one hour. One mole of MTX weighs 454.4 Da, and 1 mole of leucovorin calcium weighs 511.5 Da, with the MW of the leucovorin portion equal to 471.4 Da. Because of the safety of leucovorin and because of the toxicity of MTX, underdosing leucovorin should be avoided. Although serum MTX concentrations are often closely followed in patients on diverse oncologic regimens,[11,12] in the overdose setting, or in MTX toxicity related to treatment for tubal pregnancies, it is inappropriate to wait for a serum concentration before initiating treatment with leucovorin.[6] The toxic threshold for MTX is reported as 1×10^{-8} mol/L (0.01 µmol/L or 10 nmol/L), based on mouse studies evaluating DNA synthesis.[15] Normal serum folic acid concentrations are in the range of 13 to 43 nmol/L. Oral MTX doses as low as 2 mg in adults resulted in mean maximal MTX serum drug concentration of 0.215 µmol/L at one to 2 hours after ingestion.[85] The MTX half-life for the 2 mg dose rose from 2.4 hours to 3.2 hours when three 2-mg tablets were ingested 12 hours apart.[85] If the patient's MTX exposure is not for chemotherapeutic intent, there is no rationale to permit MTX to remain unantagonized by leucovorin. Cases and case series demonstrate that organ-level toxicity is rare, but still possible from single-adult and pediatric oral intentional and unintentional ingestions of MTX.[8,30,32,75] Even in light of the known MTX oral saturation limits, in one retrospective series of 19 cases of children and adults with MTX ingestions with subsequent MTX concentrations, all were above 0.01 µmol/L, the concentrations known to impair DNA and RNA synthesis in GI epithelium and bone marrow when present for as little as 10 hours, and several MTX concentrations were above 1 µmol/L.[16] A second poison control center review determined MTX concentrations in 15 of 103 oral ingestions, which ranged from 0.02 to 3.23 µmol/L.[32] Even when not associated with acute organ toxicity or symptoms, these MTX concentrations present a gametogenetic and stochastic carcinogenic risk.[15]

Methotrexate bioavailability decreases from 100% with oral doses less than 30 mg/m² to approximately 10% to 20% with doses greater than 80 mg/m².[10,78] A compilation of pharmacokinetic studies reported that the bioavailable dose appears to saturate at approximately 14.4 ± 1.64 mg/m², with several notable outliers.[16] As an example, if a child unintentionally ingests 100 (2.5 mg) MTX tablets for a total dose of 250 mg, only part of this dose is absorbed because MTX absorption is saturable.[30] In this case, it is reasonable to assume that a bioavailability of 50% or less would result in an absorbed dose of MTX of less than 125 mg. For this exposure, an IV dose of 125 mg of leucovorin would be reasonable to provide over 15 to 30 minutes. This dose of IV leucovorin would be expected to produce serum concentrations in excess of that of the MTX, given that the V_d of leucovorin is about 25% less than MTX and the MWs are similar. It is reasonable to repeat this dose of IV leucovorin every 3 to 6 hours until the serum MTX concentration is less than 0.01 μmol/L, preferably zero.[55,95] This differs from recommendations in patients receiving MTX therapeutically (see later discussion).

The MTX half-life varies from 5 to 45 hours, depending on the dose and the patient's kidney function. For this reason, it is reasonable to continue leucovorin therapy for 12 to 24 doses (3 days) or longer if MTX concentrations are unavailable. Patients can develop third-space storage in ascites or pleural effusions, and thus can require leucovorin dosing for an extended period of time. Patients with bone marrow toxicity require more prolonged dosing because plasma half-lives of MTX do not reflect persistent intracellular concentrations.

Therapeutic Methotrexate Therapy

The dose of leucovorin for "leucovorin rescue" after "high-dose" MTX therapy (doses of 500 mg/m² or greater) ranges from 10 to 25 mg/m² IM or IV every 6 hours for 72 hours up to 1,000 mg/m² every 6 hours in patients with renal compromise and delayed elimination.[14,39,95,101,104] If a neonate must be treated, a benzyl alcohol–free preparation must be used because of the toxicity of benzyl alcohol in neonates (Chap. 46).[29,51] For MTX overdoses, equimolar serum leucovorin concentrations theoretically provide adequate protection, but because precise determinations are invariably delayed, leucovorin administration should be initiated without delay.

As a rough guide, a single dose of 25 mg of IV leucovorin in an adult produces a peak concentration of the active *l*-5-CH₃-THF metabolite of approximately 258 ng/mL, which is 0.55 μmol/L.[95] A dosage of about 150 mg every 4 hours in an adult achieves a steady-state concentration of about 4.85 μmol/L.[91] Although the dose of leucovorin can be as high as 1,000 mg/m² every 6 hours, this is rarely warranted and cannot adequately compete with serum concentrations of MTX above 100 μmol/L.[72] Under these circumstances, it is recommended to administer glucarpidase (Antidotes in Depth: A13). An IV leucovorin dose of 150 mg/m² every 3 to 6 hours is anticipated to be effective in all but the most severe overdoses and should be administered IV as soon as possible over 15 to 30 minutes, but not faster than 160 mg/min in adults because of the calcium content. We recommend that this dose be continued a minimum of several days or until the serum MTX concentration falls below 0.01 μmol/L.[55,95] One case series of 11 patients receiving MTX over 4 hours at 10 to 12 g/m² for osteosarcoma or 3.5 g/m² for central nervous system lymphoma required high-dose leucovorin rescue for MTX concentrations at high risk for toxicity at 24, 48, or 72 hours, usually because of acute kidney injury. The dosage of leucovorin ranged from 0.24 to 10 g/day and was titrated downward as the MTX concentration fell. It took an average of 11 ± 3 days for the MTX concentration to drop below 0.1 μmol/L (Table A12–1). Table A12–2 is offered in recognition of the importance and complexity associated with switching complex methotrexate concentrations precisely.

Leucovorin rescue strategies after high-dose MTX are aligned in the leucovorin, levoleucovorin, and methotrexate package inserts, with 15 mg leucovorin (7.5 mg of levoleucovorin) provided at baseline every 6 hours for 10 doses beginning 24 hours after MTX administration, so as not to compromise chemotherapeutic efficacy.[36,88,95] In the setting of early or delayed methotrexate elimination or acute kidney injury, leucovorin dosing must be increased to counteract the persistent adverse effects of MTX (Table A12–1).[36,88,95] Other protocols call for leucovorin rescue using a 4-level tiered pharmacokinetically guided rescue strategy depending upon the MTX concentration at different time points (Fig. A12–1).[11,39,101] Healthcare facilities have also implemented leucovorin rescue stratified by multiple checkpoint MTX concentrations at 24, 36, 42, 48, and 72 hours, with multiple leucovorin dosing adjustments depending upon the MTX concentrations at these time-points.[14,39] Administration of high-dose MTX by continuous infusion over 24 hours may also invoke different leucovorin rescue protocols. Regardless of the specific rescue dosing regimen chosen, systematic protocol implementation in treatment sites reduces variance in the time to MTX concentration

TABLE A12–1 Leucovorin Dosage and Administration with Chemotherapeutic Methotrexate Use[a,b]

Clinical Situation	Laboratory Findings	Leucovorin Dosage
Normal methotrexate elimination	Serum [methotrexate] ~10 μmol/L at 24 hours after administration, 1 μmol/L at 48 hours, and <0.2 μmol/L at 72 hours	15 mg PO, IM, or IV every 6 hours for 60 hours (10 doses starting at 24 hours after the start of methotrexate infusion)
Delayed late methotrexate elimination	Serum [methotrexate] remaining >0.2 μmol/L at 72 hours and >0.05 μmol/L at 96 hours after administration	Continue 15 mg PO, IM, or IV every 6 hours until [methotrexate] is <0.05 μmol/L
Delayed early methotrexate elimination or evidence of acute kidney injury	Serum [methotrexate] of ≥50 μmol/L at 24 hours or ≥5 μmol/L at 48 hours after administration or a ≥100% increase in serum [creatinine] at 24 hours after methotrexate administration (eg, an increase from 0.5 to ≥1 mg/dL)	150 mg IV every 3 hours until [methotrexate] is <1 μmol/L; then 15 mg IV every 3 hours until [methotrexate] is <0.05 μmol/L

[a]Leucovorin should not be administered intrathecally. [b]Data from references 36, 88, and 95. IM = intramuscular; IV = intravenous; PO = oral.

measurements and time to first leucovorin rescue dose and increases appropriate leucovorin dose escalation and appropriate leucovorin at discharge.[14] A constant IV infusion of 21 mg/m²/h has been safely administered for 5 days. A transition to oral administration of leucovorin depends on the serum concentration of MTX and whether adequate serum concentrations of leucovorin can be achieved orally. In adults, a 200-mg oral dose of leucovorin produces a peak serum concentration of 1.82 μmol/L compared with 27.1 μmol/L with a 200-mg IV dose.

Levoleucovorin, the active *l*-isomer of folinic acid, is available and should be dosed at half the dose of racemic leucovorin.[88] Because of the calcium content of the levoleucovorin solution, the rate of intravenous infusion should not exceed more than 16 mL (160 mg of levoleucovorin) per minute.[88,95]

Administration of activated charcoal (AC) limits the benefit of subsequent administration of oral leucovorin. In addition to leucovorin, other modalities to treat patients with MTX overdoses include AC (Antidotes in Depth: A1), urinary alkalinization (Antidotes in Depth: A5), glucarpidase (Antidotes in Depth: A13), and extracorporeal removal (Chap. 51).

Intrathecal Methotrexate Overdose

Unintentional overdose with intrathecal MTX is potentially quite serious and is dose dependent.[45,54] In these cases, IV leucovorin and *not* intrathecal leucovorin should be administered. Intrathecal leucovorin was considered a major factor in the death of a child given a slightly higher dose of intrathecal MTX than was prescribed.[52] Although some cases have been managed with IV leucovorin with or without additional drainage procedures,

TABLE A12–2 Rapid Calculations

1 mole = 1 g molecular weight
1 molar = 1 mole/L
1×10^{-3} moles = 1 millimole = 1 mmol
1×10^{-6} moles = 1 micromole = 1 μmol
1×10^{-9} moles = 1 nanomole = 1 nmol
1 mole of methotrexate weighs 455 Da; 1 mole methotrexate = 455 g
1 molar methotrexate = 455 g/L = 455 mg/mL
0.01×10^{-6} molar methotrexate = 455×10^{-8} g/L = 455×10^{-8} mg/mL = 455×10^{-5} mcg/mL = 455×10^{-2} ng/mL = 4.55 ng/mL
To convert methotrexate concentrations in mg/L (mcg/mL) to μmol/L, multiply by 2.2
To convert methotrexate concentrations in mg/L (mcg/mL) to nmol/L, multiply by 2,200

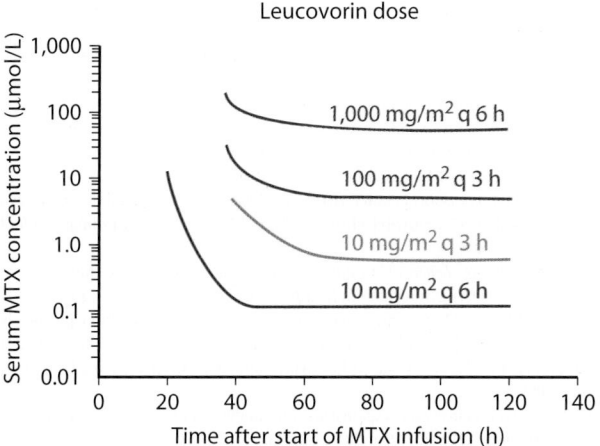

FIGURE A12–1. Example of a nomogram developed by Bleyer[10] for pharmacokinetically guided leucovorin rescue after high-dose methotrexate (MTX) administration.

it is reasonable to administer intrathecal glucarpidase in cases of significant intrathecal MTX overdose or signs of neurotoxicity.[22,43,77,103] In intrathecal MTX overdoses, consultation with experienced hematologists/oncologists and medical toxicologists is warranted (Special Considerations: SC7).[50]

Pemetrexed Toxicity

Pemetrexed toxicity is similar to that of methotrexate. Toxicity is attenuated initially with a low dose of vitamin B_{12} and leucovorin as described below. In clinical trials, leucovorin was permitted for NCI Common Terminology Criteria (CTC) Grade 4 leukopenia lasting ≥3 days, CTC Grade 4 neutropenia lasting ≥3 days, and immediately for CTC Grade 4 thrombocytopenia, bleeding associated with Grade 3 thrombocytopenia, or Grade 3 or 4 mucositis.[56] Leucovorin was administered as 100 mg/m² IV once, followed by 50 mg/m² IV every 6 hours for 8 days.[56]

Methanol Toxicity

Either folic acid or leucovorin (folinic acid) parenterally is recommended at the first suspicion of methanol poisoning. Folic acid is most commonly used. No complications were reported with the use of 50 to 70 mg of IV folic acid every 4 hours for the first 24 hours in the treatment of methanol-poisoned patients.[68] The precise dosage necessary is unknown, but 1 to 2 mg/kg every 4 to 6 hours is probably sufficient. Given that case reports demonstrate that plasma formic acid concentrations can rise after leucovorin cessation,[66] it is recommended to continue folic/folinic acid until the methanol and formate are eliminated. Because the first dose is usually administered before hemodialysis, a second dose is recommended at the completion of hemodialysis because this highly water-soluble vitamin will have been eliminated.

FORMULATION AND ACQUISITION

Leucovorin (folinic acid) powder for injection is available in 50-, 100-, 200-, and 350-mg vials. Each milligram of leucovorin contains 0.004 mEq of calcium. Reconstitution with sterile water for injection—5 mL to the 50-mg vial, 10 mL to the 100-mg vial, or 20 mL to the 200-mg vial—results in a final concentration of 10 mg/mL. Adding 17.5 mL of sterile water for injection to the 350-mg vial results in a final concentration of 20 mg/mL, where each milliliter contains 0.002 mmol of leucovorin.[95] These lyophilized products contain no preservatives. The only inactive ingredient is sodium chloride added to adjust tonicity. Reconstitute with Sterile Water for Injection, USP; when doses greater than 10 mg/m² are used (to avoid excess benzyl alcohol contained in Bacteriostatic Water for Injection, USP) and use immediately.[88] Further dilute in 100 to 1,000 mL of 0.9% sodium chloride or D_5W for infusion.[55] When protected from light, leucovorin both undiluted in glass containers and when diluted with 0.9% sodium chloride (250 mL) in polyethylene bags, has remained stable, with less than 10% degradation for at least

30 days at room and refrigerator temperatures.[47] Leucovorin is also available in a single-use vial as a solution for injection at a concentration of 10 mg/mL in a 50-mL vial. Because of the calcium content, the rate of IV administration should not be faster than 160 mg/min in adults.[95] Leucovorin is also available orally in a variety of strengths, including 5-, 10-, 15-, and 25-mg tablets.

Levoleucovorin lyophilized powder for injection is available in a single-use 50-mg vial containing the equivalent of 50 mg of levoleucovorin as the calcium pentahydrate salt and 50 mg of mannitol.[88] Reconstitution with 5.3 mL of 0.9% sodium chloride injection yields a concentration of 10 mg/mL.[88] Levoleucovorin is also available as a sterile solution in a single-use 175-mg vial that contains 17.5 mL of sterile solution in which each milliliter contains levoleucovorin calcium pentahydrate equivalent to 10 mg of levoleucovorin and 8.3 mg of sodium chloride. Because of the calcium content, the rate of IV administration should not be faster than 160 mg/min (16 mL of reconstituted solution/min).[88] Further dilution to concentrations of 0.5 mg/mL in 0.9% sodium chloride injection or 5% dextrose injection is acceptable, but should be used within 4 hours when stored at room temperature.[88]

Folic acid is available parenterally in 10-mL multidose vials with 1.5% benzyl alcohol in concentrations of 5 or 10 mg/mL from a variety of manufacturers. Once opened, the vial must be kept refrigerated.

If administration to neonates is necessary, a benzyl alcohol–free preparation must be used because of the toxicity of benzyl alcohol in neonates (Chap. 46).

SUMMARY

- Leucovorin (folinic acid) is the primary antidote for a patient who receives an overdose of methotrexate.
- Leucovorin is the biologically active, reduced form of folic acid, the synthesis of which is prevented by methotrexate.
- Only leucovorin (folinic acid) is an acceptable antidote for a patient with methotrexate toxicity, but either folic acid or leucovorin is acceptable for a patient poisoned by methanol.
- After a methanol overdose, folic acid enhances the elimination of formate.
- Leucovorin increases the toxicity of 5-FU. Uridine triacetate (Antidotes in Depth: A14) is the appropriate antidote in the case of 5-FU overdose.

REFERENCES

1. Albrecht AM, et al. Carboxypeptidase displaying differential velocity in hydrolysis of methotrexate, 5-methyltetrahydrofolic acid, and leucovorin. *J Bacteriol.* 1978;134: 506-513.
2. Allen J, et al. The inability of oral leucovorin to elevate CSF 5-methyl-tetrahydrofolate following high dose intravenous methotrexate therapy. *J Neurooncol.* 1983;1:39-44.
3. Angier RB, et al. The structure and synthesis of the liver *L. casei* factor. *Science.* 1946;103:667-669.
4. Anonymous. From the NIH: use of folate analogue in treatment of methyl alcohol toxic reactions is studied. *JAMA.* 1979;242:1961-1962.
5. Appleman JR, et al. Kinetics of the formation and isomerization of methotrexate complexes of recombinant human dihydrofolate reductase. *J Biol Chem.* 1988;263: 10304-10313.
6. Bachman EA, Barnhart K. Medical management of ectopic pregnancy: a comparison of regimens. *Clin Obstet Gynecol.* 2012;55:440-447.
7. Barceloux DG, et al. American Academy of Clinical Toxicology practice guidelines on the treatment of methanol poisoning. *J Toxicol Clin Toxicol.* 2002;40:415-446.
8. Bebarta VS, et al. Acute methotrexate ingestions in adults: a report of serious clinical effects and treatments. *J Toxicol.* 2014;2014:214574.
9. Belz S, et al. High-performance liquid chromatographic determination of methotrexate, 7-hydroxymethotrexate, 5-methyltetrahydrofolic acid and folinic acid in serum and cerebrospinal fluid. *J Chromatogr B Biomed Appl.* 1994;661:109-118.
10. Bleyer WA. The clinical pharmacology of methotrexate: new applications of an old drug. *Cancer.* 1978;41:36-51.
11. Bleyer WA. New vistas for leucovorin in cancer chemotherapy. *Cancer.* 1989;63:995-1007.
12. Booser DJ, et al. Continuous-infusion high-dose leucovorin with 5-fluorouracil and cisplatin for relapsed metastatic breast cancer: a phase II study. *Am J Clin Oncol.* 2000;23:40-41.
13. Briggs GG, et al. *Drugs in Pregnancy and Lactation.* Philadelphia, PA: Lippincott Williams & Wilkins; 2017.
14. Cerminara Z, et al. A single center retrospective analysis of a protocol for high-dose methotrexate and leucovorin rescue administration. *J Oncol Pharm Pract.* 2017 Jan 1: 1078155217729744.

15. Chabner BA, Young RC. Threshold methotrexate concentration for in vivo inhibition of DNA synthesis in normal and tumorous target tissues. *J Clin Invest*. 1973;52:1804-1811.

16. Chan BS, et al. What can clinicians learn from therapeutic studies about the treatment of acute oral methotrexate poisoning? *Clin Toxicol (Phila)*. 2017;55:88-96.

17. Chen Y, et al. Arsenic exposure from drinking water, dietary intakes of B vitamins and folate, and risk of high blood pressure in Bangladesh: a population-based, cross-sectional study. *Am J Epidemiol*. 2007;165:541-552.

18. Chitayat D, et al. Folic acid supplementation for pregnant women and those planning pregnancy: 2015 update. *J Clin Pharmacol*. 2016;56:170-175.

19. Cody V, et al. Correlations of inhibitor kinetics for *Pneumocystis jirovecii* and human dihydrofolate reductase with structural data for human active site mutant enzyme complexes. *Biochemistry*. 2009;48:1702-1711.

20. Danenberg PV, et al. Folates as adjuvants to anticancer agents: chemical rationale and mechanism of action. *Crit Rev Oncol Hematol*. 2016;106:118-131.

21. Egel C, et al. Inhibitory effects of ascorbic acid and folinic acid on chromosome aberrations induced by pyrimethamine in vitro. *Teratog Carcinog Mutagen*. 2002;22:353-362.

22. Ettinger LJ, et al. Intrathecal methotrexate overdose without neurotoxicity: case report and literature review. *Cancer*. 1978;41:1270-1273.

23. European Medicines Agency. *Pre-authorisation Evaluation of Medicines for Human Use. Withdrawal Assessment Report for Voraxaze*. London, UK: European Medicines Agency (EMEA); 2008 June 26, 2008. Report No.: EMEA/CHMP/171907/2008\.

24. Farber S, et al. Temporary remissions in acute leukemia in children produced by folic acid antagonist, 4-aminopteroyl-glutamic acid (aminopterin). *N Engl J Med*. 1948;238:787-793.

25. Finkelstein Y, et al. Intrathecal methotrexate neurotoxicity: clinical correlates and antidotal treatment. *Environ Toxicol Pharmacol*. 2005;19:721-725.

26. Food and Drug Administration Center for Drug Evaluation and Research. Application number:022532Orig1s000. Medical Review(s). Clinical Review. Daniel Davis. NDA 22-532. https://www.accessdata.fda.gov/drugsatfda_docs/nda/2010/022532orig1s000medr.pdf2011. Accessed September 2, 2017.

27. Gamble MV, et al. Folate and arsenic metabolism: a double-blind, placebo-controlled folic acid-supplementation trial in Bangladesh. *Am J Clin Nutr*. 2006;84:1093-1101.

28. Gamble MV, et al. Folate, homocysteine, and arsenic metabolism in arsenic-exposed individuals in Bangladesh. *Environ Health Perspect*. 2005;113:1683-1688.

29. Gershanik J, et al. The gasping syndrome and benzyl alcohol poisoning. *N Engl J Med*. 1982;307:1384-1388.

30. Gibbon BN, Manthey DE. Pediatric case of accidental oral overdose of methotrexate. *Ann Emerg Med*. 1999;34:98-100.

31. Hall MN, et al. Folate, cobalamin, cysteine, homocysteine, and arsenic metabolism among children in Bangladesh. *Environ Health Perspect*. 2009;117:825-831.

32. Hays H, et al. Evaluation of toxicity after acute accidental methotrexate ingestions in children under 6 years old: a 16-year multi-center review. *Clin Toxicol (Phila)*. 2018;56:120-125.

33. Heck JE, et al. Consumption of folate-related nutrients and metabolism of arsenic in Bangladesh. *Am J Clin Nutr*. 2007;85:1367-1374.

34. Hempel G, et al. Interactions of carboxypeptidase G2 with 6S-leucovorin and 6R-leucovorin in vitro: implications for the application in case of methotrexate intoxications. *Cancer Chemother Pharmacol*. 2005;55:347-353.

35. Hoffbrand AV, Weir DG. The history of folic acid. *Br J Haematol*. 2001;113:579-589.

36. Hospira I. Methotrexate Injection, USP (Contains Preservative) [presecribing information]. Lake Forest, IL: Hospira, Inc; 2014.

37. Houben PF, et al. Anticonvulsant drugs and folic acid in young mentally retarded epileptic patients. A study of serum folate, fit frequency and I.Q. *Epilepsia*. 1971;12:235-247.

38. Hovda KE, et al. Methanol and formate kinetics during treatment with fomepizole. *Clin Toxicol (Phila)*. 2005;43:221-722.

39. Howard SC, et al. Preventing and managing toxicities of high-dose methotrexate. *Oncologist*. 2016;21:1471-1482.

40. Howe CG, et al. Folate and cobalamin modify associations between *S*-adenosylmethionine and methylated arsenic metabolites in arsenic-exposed Bangladeshi adults. *J Nutr*. 2014;144:690-697.

41. Hutson JR, et al. Adverse placental effect of formic acid on hCG secretion is mitigated by folic acid. *Alcohol Alcohol*. 2013;48:283-287.

42. Jacobsen D, McMartin KE. Methanol and ethylene glycol poisonings. Mechanism of toxicity, clinical course, diagnosis and treatment. *Med Toxicol*. 1986;1:309-334.

43. Jakobson AM, et al. Cerebrospinal fluid exchange after intrathecal methotrexate overdose. A report of two cases. *Acta Paediatr*. 1992;81:359-361.

44. Janinis J, et al. Second-line chemotherapy with weekly oxaliplatin and high-dose 5-fluorouracil with folinic acid in metastatic colorectal carcinoma: a Hellenic Cooperative Oncology Group (HeCOG) phase II feasibility study. *Ann Oncol*. 2000;11:163-167.

45. Jardine LF, et al. Intrathecal leucovorin after intrathecal methotrexate overdose. *J Pediatr Hematol Oncol*. 1996;18:302-304.

46. Johlin FC, et al. Studies on the role of folic acid and folate-dependent enzymes in human methanol poisoning. *Mol Pharmacol*. 1987;31:557-561.

47. Karbownik A, et al. Stability of calcium folinate (Teva) in concentrate after re-use and in dilute infusions in 0.9% NaCl in polyethylene bags. *Acta Pol Pharm*. 2013;70:301-307.

48. Khan Assir MZ, et al. An outbreak of pyrimethamine toxicity in patients with ischaemic heart disease in Pakistan. *Basic Clin Pharmacol Toxicol*. 2014;115:291-296.

49. Kim EY, et al. Laparoscopic gastrectomy followed by chemotherapy for advanced gastric cancer diagnosed during pregnancy: a case report. *Anticancer Res*. 2016;36:4813-4816.

50. Lampkin BC, Wells R. Intrathecal leucovorin after intrathecal methotrexate. *J Pediatr Hematol Oncol*. 1996;18:249.

51. LeBel M, et al. Benzyl alcohol metabolism and elimination in neonates. *Dev Pharmacol Ther*. 1988;11:347-356.

52. Lee AC, et al. Intrathecal methotrexate overdose. *Acta Paediatr*. 1997;86:434-7.

53. Lefkowitz E, et al. Head and neck cancer. 3. Toxicity of 24-hour infusions of methotrexate (NSC-740) and protection by leucovorin (NSC-3590) in patients with epidermoid carcinomas. *Cancer Chemother Rep*. 1967;51:305-311.

54. Levitt M, et al. Transport characteristics of folates in cerebrospinal fluid; a study utilizing doubly labeled 5-methyltetrahydrofolate and 5-formyltetrahydrofolate. *J Clin Invest*. 1971;50:1301-1308.

55. Lexicomp Online. *Leucovorin Calcium*. Alphen aan den Rijn, Netherlands: Wolters Kluwer Clinical Drug Information, Inc.; 2017. Accessed September 5, 2017.

56. Lilly USA LLC. ALIMTA- pemetrexed disodium heptahydrate injection, powder, lyophilized, for solution [prescribing information]. Indianapolis, IN: Lilly USA, LLC; 2013.

57. Lonardi F, et al. Toxicity of laevo-leucovorin and dose-lowering. *Eur J Cancer*. 1992;28:1007-1008.

58. Ma Y, et al. Folic acid protects against arsenic-mediated embryo toxicity by up-regulating the expression of Dvr1. *Sci Rep*. 2015;5:16093.

59. Makoshi Z, et al. Chemotherapeutic treatment of colorectal cancer in pregnancy: case report. *J Med Case Rep*. 2015;9:140.

60. Mazumdar M, et al. Arsenic is associated with reduced effect of folic acid in myelomeningocele prevention: a case control study in Bangladesh. *Environ Health*. 2015;14:34.

61. McGuire BW, et al. Absorption kinetics of orally administered leucovorin calcium. *NCI Monogr*. 1987:47-56.

62. McMartin KE, et al. Methanol poisoning. V. Role of formate metabolism in the monkey. *J Pharmacol Exp Ther*. 1977;201:564-572.

63. MedImmune Oncology I. Neutrexin® (trimetrexate glucuronate for injection). Gaithersburg, MD: MedImmune Oncology, Inc; 2005.

64. Mehta BM, et al. Serum and cerebrospinal fluid distribution of 5-methyltetrahydrofolate after intravenous calcium leucovorin and intra-Ommaya methotrexate administration in patients with meningeal carcinomatosis. *Cancer Res*. 1983;43:435-438.

65. Meropol NJ, et al. Seizures associated with leucovorin administration in cancer patients. *J Natl Cancer Inst*. 1995;87:56-58.

66. Moore DF, et al. Folinic acid and enhanced renal elimination in formic acid intoxication. *J Toxicol Clin Toxicol*. 1994;32:199-204.

67. Noker PE, et al. Methanol toxicity: treatment with folic acid and 5-formyl tetrahydrofolic acid. *Alcohol Clin Exp Res*. 1980;4:378-383.

68. Osterloh JD, et al. Serum formate concentrations in methanol intoxication as a criterion for hemodialysis. *Ann Intern Med*. 1986;104:200-203.

69. Patel R, et al. Pharmacology and phase I trial of high-dose oral leucovorin plus 5-fluorouracil in children with refractory cancer: a report from the Children's Cancer Study Group. *Cancer Res*. 1991;51:4871-4875.

70. Peters BA, et al. Folic acid and creatine as therapeutic approaches to lower blood arsenic: a randomized controlled trial. *Environ Health Perspect*. 2015;123:1294-1301.

71. Pilsner JR, et al. Folate deficiency, hyperhomocysteinemia, low urinary creatinine, and hypomethylation of leukocyte DNA are risk factors for arsenic-induced skin lesions. *Environ Health Perspect*. 2009;117:254-260.

72. Pinedo HM, et al. The reversal of methotrexate cytotoxicity to mouse bone marrow cells by leucovorin and nucleosides. *Cancer Res*. 1976;36:4418-4424.

73. Podzamczer D, et al. Thrice-weekly sulfadiazine-pyrimethamine for maintenance therapy of toxoplasmic encephalitis in HIV-infected patients. Spanish Toxoplasmosis Study Group. *Eur J Clin Microbiol Infect Dis*. 2000;19:89-95.

74. Priest DG, et al. Pharmacokinetics of leucovorin metabolites in human plasma as a function of dose administered orally and intravenously. *J Natl Cancer Inst*. 1991;83:1806-1812.

75. Pruitt AW, et al. Accidental ingestion of methotrexate. *J Pediatr*. 1974;85:686-688.

76. Reynolds EH. Effects of folic acid on the mental state and fit-frequency of drug-treated epileptic patients. *Lancet*. 1967;1:1086-1088.

77. Riva L, et al. Successful treatment of intrathecal methotrexate overdose with folinic acid rescue: a case report. *Acta Paediatr*. 1999;88:780-782.

78. Roenigk HH Jr, et al. Methotrexate in psoriasis: consensus conference. *J Am Acad Dermatol*. 1998;38:478-485.

79. Sauberlich HE, Baumann CA. A factor required for the growth of leuconostoc citrovorum. *J Biol Chem*. 1948;176:165-173.

80. Schilsky RL, Ratain MJ. Clinical pharmacokinetics of high-dose leucovorin calcium after intravenous and oral administration. *J Natl Cancer Inst*. 1990;82:1411-1415.

81. Schleyer E, et al. Impact of the simultaneous administration of the (+)- and (−)-forms of formyl-tetrahydrofolic acid on plasma and intracellular pharmacokinetics of (−)-tetrahydrofolic acid. *Cancer Chemother Pharmacol*. 2000;45:165-171.

82. Schoenbach EB, et al. Reversal of aminopterin and amethopterin toxicity by citrovorum factor. *J Am Med Assoc*. 1950;144:1558-1560.

83. Scott JM. Folinic acid in megaloblastic anaemia of pregnancy. *Br Med J*. 1957;2:270-272.

84. Sherwood RF, et al. Purification and properties of carboxypeptidase G2 from *Pseudomonas* sp. strain RS-16. Use of a novel triazine dye affinity method. *Eur J Biochem*. 1985;148:447-453.

85. Shiozawa K, et al. Serum levels and pharmacodynamics of methotrexate and its metabolite 7-hydroxy methotrexate in Japanese patients with rheumatoid arthritis treated with 2-mg capsule of methotrexate three times per week. *Mod Rheumatol*. 2005;15:405-409.

86. Smith DB, Racusen LC. Folate metabolism and the anticonvulsant efficacy of pheno-barbital. *Arch Neurol.* 1973;28:18-22.

87. Smith SW, Nelson LS. Case files of the New York City Poison Control Center: antidotal strategies for the management of methotrexate toxicity. *J Med Toxicol.* 2008;4:132-140.

88. Spectrum Pharmaceuticals Inc. Fusilev® (levoleucovorin) [prescribing information]. Irvine, CA: Spectrum Pharmaceuticals, Inc; 2011.

89. Stover P, Schirch V. The metabolic role of leucovorin. *Trends Biochem Sci.* 1993;18:102-106.

90. Stratemann K, et al. The folate content as limiting factor for formate detoxication and methanol metabolism. *Naunyn Schmiedebergs Arch Exp Pathol Pharmakol.* 1968;260:208-209.

91. Straw JA, et al. Pharmacokinetics of leucovorin (D,L-5-formyltetrahydrofolate) after intravenous injection and constant intravenous infusion. *NCI Monogr.* 1987:41-45.

92. Straw JA, et al. Pharmacokinetics of the diastereoisomers of leucovorin after intravenous and oral administration to normal subjects. *Cancer Res.* 1984;44:3114-3119.

93. Surtees R, et al. Demyelination and single-carbon transfer pathway metabolites during the treatment of acute lymphoblastic leukemia: CSF studies. *J Clin Oncol.* 1998;16:1505-1511.

94. Tauheed J, et al. Associations between post translational histone modifications, myelomeningocele risk, environmental arsenic exposure, and folate deficiency among participants in a case control study in Bangladesh. *Epigenetics.* 2017;12:484-491.

95. Teva Parenteral Medicines Inc. Leucovorin Calcium for Injection [package insert]. Teva Parenteral Medicines, Inc. Irvine, CA; 2014.

96. Thyss A, et al. Evidence for CSF accumulation of 5-methyltetrahydrofolate during repeated courses of methotrexate plus folinic acid rescue. *Br J Cancer.* 1989;59:627-630.

97. Trinkle R, Wu JK. Intrathecal leukovorin after intrathecal methotrexate overdose. *J Pediatr Hematol Oncol.* 1997;19:267-269.

98. Van Delden C, Hirschel B. Folinic acid supplements to pyrimethamine-sulfadiazine for *Toxoplasma encephalitis* are associated with better outcome. *J Infect Dis.* 1996;173:1294-1295.

99. Weh HJ, et al. Neurotoxicity following weekly therapy with folinic acid and high-dose 5-fluorouracil 24-h infusion in patients with gastrointestinal malignancies. *Eur J Cancer.* 1993;29A:1218-1219.

100. Wettergren Y, et al. A pharmacokinetic and pharmacodynamic investigation of Modufolin(R) compared to Isovorin(R) after single dose intravenous administration to patients with colon cancer: a randomized study. *Cancer Chemother Pharmacol.* 2015;75:37-47.

101. Widemann BC, Adamson PC. Understanding and managing methotrexate nephrotoxicity. *Oncologist.* 2006;11:694-703.

102. Widemann BC, et al. High-dose methotrexate-induced nephrotoxicity in patients with osteosarcoma. *Cancer.* 2004;100:2222-2232.

103. Widemann BC, et al. Treatment of accidental intrathecal methotrexate overdose with intrathecal carboxypeptidase G2. *J Natl Cancer Inst.* 2004;96:1557-1559.

104. Widemann BC, et al. Efficacy of glucarpidase (carboxypeptidase G$_2$) in patients with acute kidney injury after high-dose methotrexate therapy. *Pharmacotherapy.* 2014;34:427-439.

105. Wills L. Treatment of "pernicious anaemia of pregnancy" and "tropical anaemia" with special reference to yeast extract as a curative agent. *Nutrition.* 1931;7:323-327; discussion 328.

106. Zoubek A, et al. Successful carboxypeptidase G$_2$ rescue in delayed methotrexate elimination due to renal failure. *Pediatr Hematol Oncol.* 1995;12:471-477.

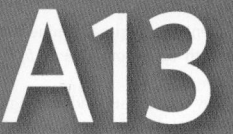

Antidotes in Depth

GLUCARPIDASE (CARBOXYPEPTIDASE G$_2$)

Silas W. Smith

INTRODUCTION

Glucarpidase (carboxypeptidase G$_2$, CPDG$_2$) is indicated for the management of methotrexate (MTX) toxicity. When given intravenously or intrathecally, it rapidly enzymatically inactivates MTX, folates, and folate analogues. It does not substitute for, and must be used in conjunction with, leucovorin (Antidotes in Depth: A12). Leucovorin should not be administered within 2 hours before or after a dose of glucarpidase.

HISTORY

Soon after the description of the structure and synthesis of folate,[6] a *Flavobacterium* species capable of removing the glutamate moiety of folate was discovered.[47] From 1955 to 1956, the inactivation of folate analogues (including chemotherapeutic aminopterin) was demonstrated in bacteria and yeasts.[61,92] Purification of "carboxypeptidase G," a pseudomonad-derived zinc-dependent enzyme responsible for MTX cleavage, was reported in 1967.[35,48] Other bacterial carboxypeptidases that differed in their substrate specificity and kinetics were isolated and purified in 1971 (*Pseudomonas stutzeri* carboxypeptidase G$_1$),[52] 1978 (*Flavobacterium* carboxypeptidase),[5] and 1992 (*Pseudomonas* sp. M-27 carboxypeptidase G$_3$).[104] By 1976, carboxypeptidase G$_1$ was scaled to pilot manufacturing production.[25] Carboxypeptidase G$_1$ (CPDG$_1$) was initially explored as a chemotherapeutic to deprive growing tumors of folate.[9,10,20,42] Human usage of CPDG$_1$ for this purpose was reported in 1974.[10] The antidotal potential of carboxypeptidase was first suggested in 1972 when it was noted that CPDG$_1$ rapidly decreased serum MTX concentrations and improved survival in mice injected with lethal MTX doses.[21] Carboxypeptidase G$_1$ was first used for rescue in a patient receiving MTX with kidney failure in 1978.[40] Carboxypeptidase G$_1$ was subsequently used to selectively eliminate systemic MTX in patients treated with high dosages targeting central nervous system (CNS) malignancies.[1,2] Unfortunately, the enzyme source of CPDG$_1$ was then lost.[4,106] The carboxypeptidase currently used in clinical practice (CPDG$_2$) was cloned from *Pseudomonas* strain R-16 and sequenced, characterized, and expressed in *Escherichia coli* in the early 1980s.[57-59,81] The preliminary crystal structure was provided in 1991, with a characterization (at 2.5 Å) and description of the active site, and biochemical mechanism of action in 1997.[49,74,89] Following the renewed availability of the recombinant CPDG$_2$ product, it underwent nonhuman primate testing for both intravenous (IV) and intrathecal (IT) rescue of MTX overdose.[3,4] Reports of successful use in human IV and IT MTX overdose rapidly emerged.[26,40,44,45,60,62,75,97,99,106] The US FDA designated glucarpidase an Orphan Product in 2003 and granted marketing approval as Voraxaze in January 2012.[16]

PHARMACOLOGY

Chemistry/Preparation

Glucarpidase is produced by recombinant DNA technology. The enzyme cloned from *Pseudomonas* strain R16 is expressed in *Escherichia coli* strain RV308.[31] The final commercial drug product is freeze-dried, and packaged in the United States.[31,39]

Mechanism of Action

Glucarpidase is a dimerized protein structure with 2 domains—a β-sheet interaction site and a zinc-dependent catalytic domain.[74] As a peptidase, the catalytic domain of glucarpidase hydrolyzes the C-terminal glutamate residues of folate and folate analogues such as MTX. Molecular modeling suggests that the 2 zinc (2$^+$) ions bind a water molecule, promoting its polarization and nucleophilic attack on the carbonyl group of the substrate (Fig. A13–1).[90] Methotrexate and its metabolite 7-OH-MTX are thus split into inactive DAMPA (2,4-diamino-*N*(10)-methylpteroic acid) and OH-DAMPA plus glutamate.[102] DAMPA undergoes subsequent hepatic metabolism. Glucarpidase similarly inactivates leucovorin and folate by cleaving their terminal glutamate residues (Fig. A13–1).[5]

Pharmacokinetics

In one study, 50 units/kg of glucarpidase was given IV to 8 volunteer subjects with normal kidney function and 4 volunteers with impaired function (calculated creatinine clearance <30 mL/min, range 9.8–27.4 mL/min).[71] Those with normal kidney function achieved a mean maximum serum concentration of glucarpidase of 3.1 mcg/mL, with a mean half-life of 9.0 hours. These values were essentially unaffected in the setting of an impaired glomerular filtration rate (GFR); therefore, renal dosing is not indicated.[16] Glucarpidase restriction to the plasma compartment was implied by a volume of distribution of 3.6 L.[71] The large protein size (83-kDa dimer) of glucarpidase precludes traversing the blood–brain barrier, crossing the cell membranes to act intracellularly, acting on MTX within the gut lumen or urinary collecting system, or treating MTX extravasation.[1,21,26,56]

Pharmacodynamics

One unit of glucarpidase activity catalyzes the hydrolysis of 1 μmol of MTX per minute at 37°C.[3] The mean enzymatic activity half-life of glucarpidase was 5.6 hours in normal volunteers and 8.2 hours in volunteers with impaired GFR.[71] Its activity is optimal at a pH between 7.0 and 7.5, compatible with human physiology. After glucarpidase administration, serum MTX concentrations rapidly declined by 71% to 99% with the original Center for Applied Microbiology and Research (CAMR) product, with the concurrent appearance of inactive DAMPA in both serum and urine.[17,45,77,82,94,95,97] DAMPA undergoes subsequent hepatic metabolism and renal elimination (~50%).[102] Commercial glucarpidase rapidly decreases serum MTX concentrations by greater than 97% within 15 minutes (Table A13–1).[16,23,32,66,82,85] In the primary efficacy study of 22 patients used as the basis for approval, glucarpidase induced MTX reductions of greater than 95% for up to 8 days, although 5 patients also received hemodialysis and 12 of 22 patients (54.5%) did not meet the primary endpoint of an MTX concentration ≤1 μmol/L in all samples, either because of a high baseline MTX concentration and/or significant MTX redistribution and rebound.[32] The ongoing glucarpidase enzymatic activity, which persists after the initial rapid MTX concentration declines, has led authors to explore glucarpidase efficacy at doses lower than the FDA-approved dose (50 units/kg). In one reported case of a patient who received late administration of approximately 8 units/kg glucarpidase, the serum MTX as measured by immunoassay declined from 1.2 to 0.5 μmol/L.[87] In 11 patients who received lower glucarpidase doses (10–31 units/kg) because of a supply shortage, there was no difference in MTX pharmacokinetics, toxicity, or survival.[77] In a retrospective evaluation of 26 patients who received glucarpidase after high-dose MTX, a multivariable analysis could not find any statistically significant relationship between glucarpidase dose and the percentage decrease in plasma MTX concentration as measured by immunoassay or high-performance liquid chromatography (HPLC).[80] Higher dosages of glucarpidase did not lead to more rapid recovery of kidney

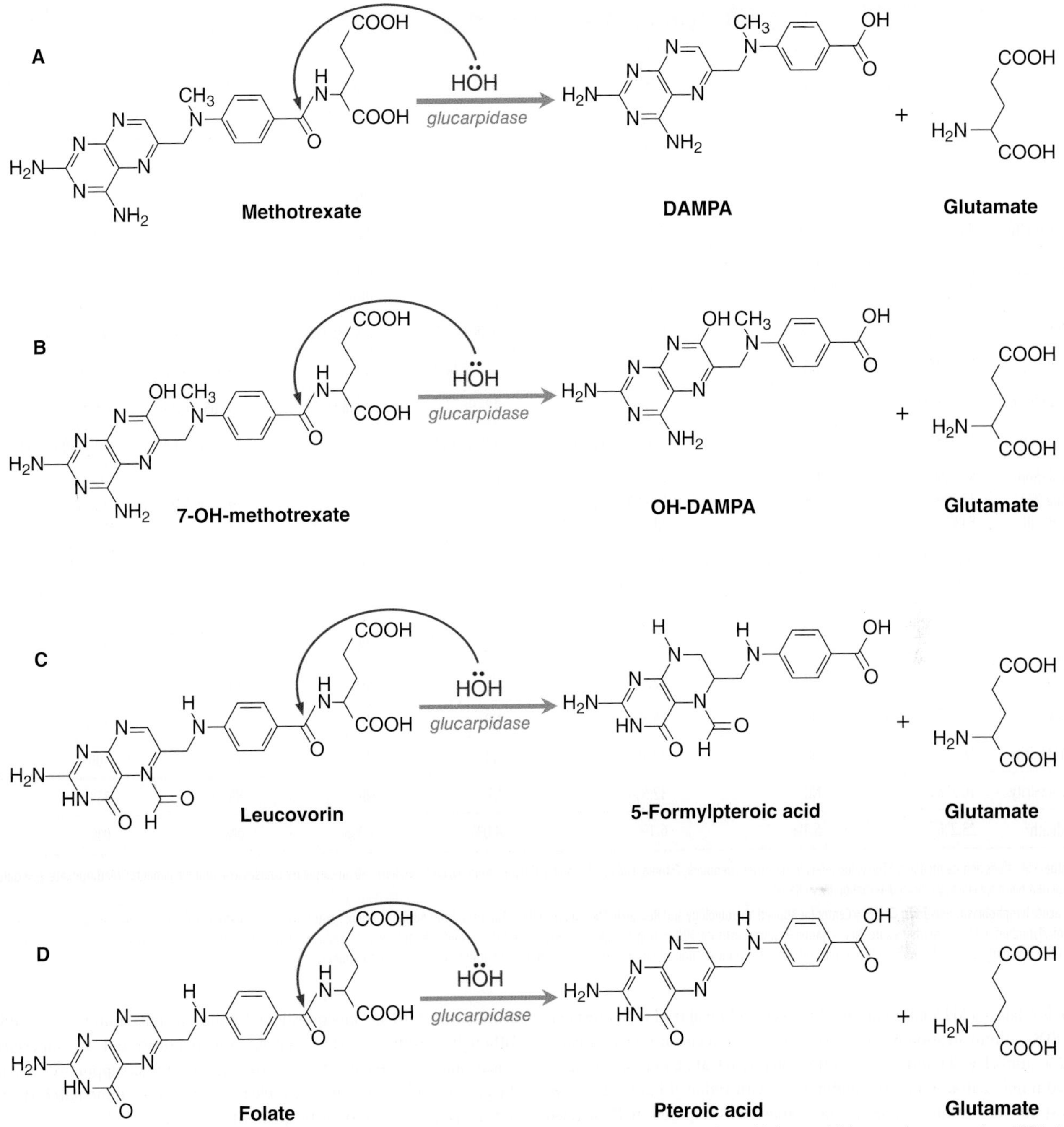

FIGURE A13–1. The catalytic domain of glucarpidase permits hydrolysis of the C-terminal glutamate residue of folate and folate analogues such as MTX via hypothesized nucleophilic attack of a zinc-bound water molecule.[90] (A, B) MTX and its metabolite 7-hydroxy-MTX are split into inactive DAMPA (2,4-diamino-N(10)-methylpteroic acid) and hydroxy-DAMPA plus glutamate. Glucarpidase similarly inactivates (C) leucovorin (folinic acid) and (D) folate by cleavage of terminal glutamate residues.

function, and lower doses (13–50 units/kg) were equally efficacious.[80] These findings were confirmed in another clinical trial in which almost half of the patients were treated with glucarpidase doses below 50 units/kg (as low as 20 units/kg), and the dose per kilogram did not correlate with the time for serum MTX concentration to decrease below 0.2 μmol/L or with the overall reduction in MTX concentration.[85]

ROLE IN METHOTREXATE TOXICITY

Patients receiving high-dose MTX therapy are routinely "rescued" with leucovorin (eg, 10–15 mg every 6 hours).[105] Treatment nomograms and institutional algorithms recommend higher leucovorin doses when MTX concentrations are excessive or the elevation of the concentration is prolonged (Antidotes in Depth: A12).[11,19,94,105] However, at MTX concentrations

above 100 μmol/L (1×10^{-4} mol/L), data suggest that adequate leucovorin concentrations cannot be achieved for competitive and complete reversal of toxicity.[17,45,50,72] Also, leucovorin administration provides 0.004 mEq calcium per milligram of leucovorin and is rarely associated with hypercalcemia in extremely high-dose therapy.[106] Necessary urine alkalinization and diuresis can also be limited by serum pH, sodium, and fluid administration ceilings once patients develop toxicity.[24,79] Thus, despite adequate leucovorin rescue, alkalization, diuresis, and supportive care, additional antidotal strategies are required in the setting of persistently elevated MTX concentrations. High-dose MTX-induced kidney dysfunction developed in 1.8% of patients with osteosarcoma enrolled in clinical trials.[95] In a 10-year retrospective review of 1,982 patients who received high-dose MTX (HDMTX) for leukemia, lymphoma, and osteosarcoma, 21 patients (1.1%) required glucarpidase

TABLE A13–1	Glucarpidase Efficacy Trials[a]						
	2000–2003	1993–2004	1997–2002	2004–2007	2007–(2010)		
	FDA Tr001[32]	FDA Tr002[32]	FDA Tr003[32]	FDA Tr006[32]	FDA Tr016[32]	2008–2010	2008–2014
Trial	"Berlin"[77]	"NCI"[65,96]	"Bonn"[17]	"NCI II"	BTG IND 11557	"St. Jude"[23]	NOPHO ALL 2008[85]
Lot	CAMR	CAMR	CAMR	Commercial	Commercial	Commercial	Commercial
Sites (n)	29	149	50	55	NR	1	7[b]
Safety data (n)	43	214	65	149	141	20	47[c]
Malignancies	ALL: 13; L: 12; +CNS: 16; others: 2	L/L: 111; OS/S: 75; others: 3	ALL: 26; NHL: 21; OS: 12; others: 6	L/L: 93; OS/S: 47; others: 9	L/L: 88; OS/S: 46; others: 7	ALL: 10; OS: 6; L:4	ALL: 47
Age (years)	18–78 (54)	0.4–82 (17)	0.9–71.8 (15.4)	0.08–85 (18)	0.5–85 (16)	4.1–20.4 (12.1)	1–17.9 (8)
TTT (hours)	27–176 (56)	NR	25–178 (52)	27–86 (48)	NR	26.3–95 (45.9)	32–82 (45)
Dose (units/kg)	10–58 (50)	NR	33–60 (50)	18–98 (49)	6–189 (50)	13–65.6 (51.6)	44.3–53.5 (50)
[MTX] (µmol/L)	1–1187	1–849 (35)	0.52–901 (11.93)	3.9–708 (38.9)	NR	1.3–590.6 (29.1)	102–200 (132)
[MTX] ↓ from baseline (%) [MTX] RSCIR	N = 24 18–99 (>97%) 83%	N = 70 NR 57%	N = 25 73–99 (97%) NR	N = 22 ≥97% 45%	NR NR NR	N = 6 99.2–99.9 (99.6) 67%	N= 8 100% NR
Leucovorin dosing	mg = [MTX] (µM) × (kg); [MTX] ≤ 5 µM: 15–75 mg/m² Q 6	1 g/m² IV Q 6 h; then 250 mg/m² Q 6 × 48 h	None 4 h prior; post 1 h @ 100 mg/m² Q 6 × 24 h	NR	NR	NR	mg = [MTX] (µM) × (kg) until MTX < 0.2 µM
Heme/myelo	60.4%	NR	4.6%	NR	NR	10%	76%
Infection	16.2%	NR	12.5%	NR	NR	20%	18%
Mucositis	34.9%	NR	15.3%	NR	NR	5%	19%
Nephrotoxicity	18.6%	NR	34.1%	NR	NR	35%	100%
Hepatotoxicity	16.2%	NR	32.5%	NR	NR	NR	35%
MTX-death[d]	23.2%	5.1%	6.1%	4.0%	2.1%	0%	0%

[a]Parenthetical values denote medians. [b]The value refers to countries (Denmark, Estonia, Finland, Iceland, Lithuania, Norway, and Sweden). [c]50 glucarpidase courses in 47 unique patients. [d]Methotrexate-associated death or death not specifically reported as malignancy related.

ALL = acute lymphoblastic leukemia; CAMR = Center for Applied Microbiology and Research (UK) lot 004; FDA = Food and Drug Administration; heme/myelo = hematological toxicity/myelosuppression; L/L = leukemia/lymphoma; MTX = methotrexate; NCI = National Cancer Institute; NHL = non-Hodgkin lymphoma; NOPHO = Nordic Organization for Pediatric Hematology and Oncology; NR = not reported in FDA summary; OS/S = osteosarcoma/sarcoma; RSCIR = rapid and sustained clinically important reduction; Tr = Trial (FDA identifier); TTT = time to treatment.

rescue for delayed MTX elimination.[22] In a recent clinical trial with prespecified $CPDG_2$ administration when the serum MTX concentration was greater than 250 µmol/L at 24 hours, greater than 30 µmol/L at 36 hours, or greater than 10 µmol/L at 42 hours in combination with reduced kidney function (at least 50% creatinine increase), glucarpidase was required in 47 of 1,286 children (3.7%).[85] This yielded a relative risk for delayed MTX elimination of approximately 0.5% per each HDMTX cycle.[85] Chemotherapeutic regimens that combine MTX with renal toxic medications such as cisplatin may also increase the risk. Thus, it is reasonable to anticipate the need for glucarpidase in approximately 1% to 4% of patients receiving HDMTX, depending on the specific indication, dose, and regimen.

Glucarpidase is labeled for patients with serum MTX concentrations greater than 1 µmol/L in the setting of impaired kidney function (as evidenced by an MTX concentration not falling within 2 standard deviations of the mean MTX excretion curve for the specific administered MTX protocol).[16] In the absence of an MTX concentration, significant mucositis, gastrointestinal distress, myelosuppression, hepatitis, or neurotoxicity should prompt administration of glucarpidase in addition to aggressive leucovorin therapy, while awaiting confirmation. The primary glucarpidase efficacy and safety studies in adults and children are summarized in Table A13–1. These trials provide data for glucarpidase use in the setting of elevated MTX concentrations and the failure of leucovorin rescue and standard care approach. The CAMR product, which was used in initial clinical trials,[17,77,96] was not

demonstrated to be bioequivalent to the current commercial product.[32] Although no fully reported trial has yet demonstrated the superiority of glucarpidase as adjuvant therapy to leucovorin and supportive care alone, the pharmacodynamic efficacy is clear: glucarpidase immediately decreases serum MTX concentrations by greater than 97%.[16,23,32,66,82,85,96]

The expansion of glucarpidase use to include routine provision at 24 hours in addition to leucovorin rescue after HDMTX was studied in a double-blind, randomized, crossover phase II clinical trial, in which HPLC plasma [MTX] were determined daily until less than 0.2 µmol/L.[68] In 16 patients, routine glucarpidase use reduced delays to subsequent chemotherapy cycles and the severity of mucositis, but it did not reduce MTX-associated nephrotoxicity or the overall total MTX area under the plasma drug concentration-time curve (AUC).[66-68] Upon further exploration, although glucarpidase decreased the MTX $AUC_{24-72\ hours}$, the overall MTX AUC was not statistically significantly changed, primarily because of the contribution of MTX exposure in the first 24 hours (prior to glucarpidase).[66-68] Clinical trials have also highlighted pharmacokinetic limitations beyond glucarpidase's impressive immediate decrease in [MTX]. In studies, a rapid and sustained clinically important reduction in MTX concentration (RSCIR, [MTX] < 1 µmol/L), occurred in only 45%,[32] 59%,[100] and 67%[23] of patients. This failure of RSCIR reflects MTX redistribution, and underscores the need for continued leucovorin therapy.[79] Patients with [MTX] of greater than or equal to 50 µmol/L were less likely to achieve RSCIR than those with of less than 50 µmol/L (although glucarpidase did lead to a higher percentage reduction in those with higher [MTX]).[100] In exploratory analysis, patients with osteosarcoma—who received higher MTX doses (eg, 8–12 g/m²)—experienced less benefit with glucarpidase.[32] Another evaluation concluded that glucarpidase was unable to prevent fatal MTX toxicity in 3% of patients.[16] However, overall, the data support the use of glucarpidase to treat those at risk for toxicity from MTX because of either persistently elevated [MTX] or kidney dysfunction.[17,36,77,95] More recent trials have demonstrated more favorable outcomes. In one trial where glucarpidase intervention was required in 50 cycles of HDMTX in 47 of a total of 1286 HDMTX-treated children, mortality was 0%.[85] The use of glucarpidase to manage MTX toxicity has also permitted earlier resumption of MTX chemotherapy.[7,23,28,68,84]

Intracellular MTX is polyglutamated, which hinders transmembrane transport and increases intracellular half-life. This MTX pool is inaccessible to glucarpidase (and hemodialysis) and can persist, causing cytotoxicity and a rebound in serum [MTX] for up to 85 hours after glucarpidase administration.[34,77,96,98] In one trial, MTX rebound was seen in 6 of 28 patients (21%) at a median of 24 hours after glucarpidase administration.[66] Delaying glucarpidase more than 96 hours after MTX initiation, once intracellular MTX is established, is associated with failure to prevent significant MTX toxicity.[77,96] This emphasizes the need for close monitoring of [MTX] to ensure early administration of glucarpidase as soon as indicated. Persistent intracellular or otherwise inaccessible MTX requires ongoing leucovorin therapy for 48 hours at the same leucovorin dose as that prior to glucarpidase, which is continued until the [MTX] is below the leucovorin treatment threshold (50–100 nmol/L, 0.05–0.1 µmol/L; 0.05–0.1 × 10⁻⁶ molar) for a minimum of 3 days.[16,17,23,32,38,43,66,77,80,85,86,94,96,100,103]

In the setting of oral MTX overdose, gastrointestinal decontamination should be performed (Chap. 51), because glucarpidase has no intraluminal activity. Leucovorin is contraindicated for IT administration, and it has rarely been associated with seizures.[30,41,55,88] Simian studies and human case reports demonstrate that IT glucarpidase provides an effective means to rapidly lower cerebrospinal fluid [MTX] in cases of overdose or prolonged CNS persistence.[3,13,62,98] Reductions in CSF [MTX] after glucarpidase administration range from 72% to 99.8%.[13,98] Intravenous leucovorin with or without steroid administration has also been employed to minimize toxicity.[46,73] Patent applications revealed experiments demonstrating glucarpidase cleavage of pemetrexed and raltitrexed.[53,54] In vitro, glucarpidase hydrolyses pemetrexed ($K_m = 25$ µM, $k_{cat} = 1,808$ s⁻¹) with a similar reaction kinetic profile to MTX ($K_m = 10$ µM, $k_{cat} = 1,039$ s⁻¹).[8] These promising kinetic data await animal and human investigations before a definitive recommendation can be made regarding glucarpidase treatment of toxicity because of other chemotherapeutic antifolates.[14]

ADVERSE EFFECTS AND SAFETY ISSUES
Antidotal Compromise
The affinity of CPDG₂ for MTX is 10- to 15-fold higher than for leucovorin; however, its affinity for the active metabolite of leucovorin, 5-methyltetrahydrofolate (5-mTHF) and folate are similar.[5,29,81] Although racemic leucovorin is commonly administered, the active enantiomer is also commercially available. Because glucarpidase cleaves active *levo*-(6S)-leucovorin approximately 50% faster than inactive *dextro*-(6R)-leucovorin,[37] glucarpidase will compromise leucovorin rescue if both antidotes are administered contemporaneously. Further, once the MTX has been rapidly cleaved, glucarpidase persistence (recalling its enzymatic activity half-life of 5.6 hours in volunteers and 8.2 hours in kidney failure) would risk compromising the endogenous folate pool and exogenously administered leucovorin. Healthy volunteers provided leucovorin 2 hours after glucarpidase had their leucovorin concentrations decreased by 50%, and activated *levo*-5-MeTHF became undetectable. When leucovorin therapy was delayed 26 hours after glucarpidase administration, enzymatic cleavage by glucarpidase still decreased leucovorin and 5-MeTHF concentrations to

80% and 75%, respectively.[29] In MTX trials within 15 minutes after administration of glucarpidase, the median leucovorin concentrations fell by 8% to 18%, with the remaining leucovorin likely being the inactive *d*-isomer.[94,96] This is of concern, as the *d*-isomer may accumulate and inhibit passive transport of the active "l"-isomer.[12] Active 5-methyltetrahydrofolate concentrations also declined precipitously by greater than 97%.[94,96] Given these concerns of antidotal leucovorin destruction, a later trial of 20 patients evaluated leucovorin and [(6S)-5-MeTHF] for a period of 3 hours after leucovorin administration in patients who had received HDMTX, glucarpidase, and leucovorin or HDMTX and leucovorin alone.[78,91] Leucovorin was not provided within 2 hours of glucarpidase (median, 2.2 hours later). The study's interpretation is limited by unbalanced trial arms. In the glucarpidase group, pretreatment [MTX] were higher; body surface areas (BSAs) and leucovorin administration were greater; and serious and other adverse events were more common. When accounting for unequal BSAs, and despite the greater than 2+-hour delay in subsequent leucovorin administration, the patients given glucarpidase experienced a decrease in dose-normalized *levo*-(6S)-leucovorin AUC$_{0-3\ hours}$, *levo*-(6S)-leucovorin C$_{max}$, active (6S)-5MeTHF AUC$_{0-3\ hours}$, and 5MeTHF C$_{max}$ by 33%, 52%, 92%, and 93%, respectively.[18] This trial and others confirmed the recommendation that leucovorin should not be administered for at least 2 hours before or after glucarpidase and that the ongoing leucovorin dose should be based on the pre-glucarpidase [MTX].[16,18,29,32,38]

Immunogenicity
Initial studies reported adverse effects in 4 of 9 patients treated with CPDG₁, including development of inactivating antibodies, "sensitization" to CPDG₁, and anaphylactoid reactions.[1,2,10,40] The current recombinant glucarpidase (CPDG₂) imparts a much lower incidence of adverse effects than the initial CPDG₁ enzyme, including paresthesias (2%), flushing (2%), nausea/vomiting (2%), hypotension (1%), headache (1%), and rash (0.3%).[16,32] However, in intentional repeated dosing of glucarpidase with HDMTX, 2 of 4 patients experienced allergic reactions.[32] In patients administered CPDG₂ fused to a murine single-chain Fv antibody, 36% (11 of 30) developed anti-CPDG₂ antibodies, but no antimurine antibodies were detected.[51] Studies using the noncommercial (CAMR) lot reported antiglucarpidase antibody (AGA) development in none of 28 patients[96] and in 3 of 7 patients,[77] respectively. In clinical trials using the commercial product, 19% (19 of 99) developed AGAs following a single glucarpidase dose and 28.5% (6 of 21) developed AGAs after 2 doses, consistent with increased antibody development with multiple exposures.[16,32] Neutralizing antibodies were found in 11 of the 25 patients who tested positive for AGA-binding antibodies, of whom 8 had received only a single dose.[16] Antiglucarpidase antibodies were found in 43% (6 of 14) of assessed patients in another trial, all of whom became positive following the second glucarpidase dose.[66] In a broader evaluation of 205 patients treated with glucarpidase from 2007 to 2012, AGAs developed in 32 of 176 (18%) patients following a single glucarpidase dose an in 11 of 29 (37.9%) after 2 or more doses; 14 of 176 (8.0%) single-dose patients had neutralizing antibodies, which increased to 8 of 29 (27.6%) after 2 or more doses.[101] Although AGAs might decrease clinical efficacy or predispose to allergic reaction upon re-exposure,[2,4,29,77] many patients have been successfully treated with more than one dose of glucarpidase for persistently elevated MTX concentrations.[17,26,45,64,70,77,83,85,99,106]

Other Considerations
Because "inactive" DAMPA has a pH-dependent urinary solubility 8 to 10 times less than MTX,[37,95] in the absence of a contraindication (eg, volume overload), alkalinization and saline diuresis should be continued to prevent DAMPA precipitation and further renal compromise.[17,94] Although the supplied product contains lactose and Tris–HCl with zinc buffer, lactose-intolerant patients can receive glucarpidase. Previous concerns of allergic reactions to lactose-containing xenobiotics and patients with rare hereditary problems of fructose intolerance, galactose intolerance, galactosemia, or glucose–galactose malabsorption, are unaddressed in prescribing guidelines.[16]

PREGNANCY AND LACTATION

Glucarpidase carries a pregnancy category C designation, although formal human and animal data are lacking. The excretion of glucarpidase in breast milk is unknown.

DOSING AND ADMINISTRATION

Glucarpidase is dosed in units per kilogram in both children and adults. After reconstituting each 1,000-unit vial with 1 mL of sterile sodium chloride (0.9%), a single dose of 50 units/kg is administered immediately by IV injection over 5 minutes. If not used immediately, reconstituted glucarpidase can be stored under refrigeration at 36° to 46°F (2°–8°C) for up to 4 hours.[16] Although clinical trials permitted additional glucarpidase doses 24 to 48 hours later in cases of persistent elevated MTX concentrations, repeat administration has not demonstrated significant efficacy and is not recommended.[16,17,65,76] The substantial cost of glucarpidase[93] and the apparent glucarpidase efficacy of lower doses[77,80,85,87] has led some authors to advocate rounding the glucarpidase doses down (eg, to the nearest vial size) or capping glucarpidase doses (eg, at 2,000 units), although this practice is not consistent with the FDA-approved dose (50 units/kg). Although this approach awaits further formal study, this approach would be reasonable in cases of glucarpidase shortage or the need to triage dosing. In cases of IT MTX overdose, a fixed dose of glucarpidase (2,000 units) reconstituted in sterile 0.9% sodium chloride has been administered intrathecally (off label) over 5 minutes and is recommended in this scenario.[13,62,98] A lack of compatibility studies precludes glucarpidase mixing with other xenobiotics.

Monitoring and Analytical Considerations

False elevations of [MTX] are reported with all of the various immunoassay techniques after glucarpidase administration.[28,37,45,70,99,106] The DAMPA metabolite significantly cross-reacts with both the MTX radioimmunoassay and competitive dihydrofolate reductase–binding assays.[27] Both MTX metabolites (7-OH-MTX and DAMPA) appreciably interfere with fluorescence polarization immunoassay (FPIA) and enzyme-multiplied immunoassay technique (EMIT) assays. For DAMPA, the cross-reactivity rates are 100% (EMIT) and 36% to 44% (FPIA).[69] The cross-reactivity of 7-OH-MTX using EMIT is 4% to 31%, and 0.6% to 3% with FPIA.[33,69] This interference persists despite newer immunoassays.[63] Clinically, the concentrations of DAMPA detected are comparable to those of MTX after administration of CPDG₂.[26] Thus, HPLC should be used to determine actual [MTX] when glucarpidase is given.[15,16]

FORMULATION AND ACQUISITION

Branded glucarpidase (Voraxaze) is available in single-use glass vials each containing lyophilized glucarpidase (1,000 units) with lactose monohydrate (10 mg), buffered to pH 6.5 to 8.0 with Tris–HCl (0.6 mg) and zinc acetate dihydrate (0.002 mg). It should be maintained at 36° to 46°F (2°–8°C), but not frozen. The manufacturer's website details acquisition information for inside and outside of the United States (http://www.btgplc.com/products/specialty-pharmaceuticals/voraxaze and http://www.btgplc.com/contact-us/contacts, respectively).

SUMMARY

- Glucarpidase is a bacterially derived enzyme used in the treatment of MTX toxicity. It cleaves MTX in the serum compartment to rapidly reduce serum [MTX].
- Glucarpidase does not substitute for leucovorin, which should be continued to counteract persistent intracellular and CNS MTX.
- Leucovorin should not be administered within 2 hours before or after a dose of glucarpidase to avoid the enzymatic destruction of leucovorin and its active metabolites.
- The measurement of [MTX] after glucarpidase administration will be unreliable unless HPLC is used.

REFERENCES

1. Abelson HT, et al. Comparative effects of citrovorum factor and carboxypeptidase G1 on cerebrospinal fluid-methotrexate pharmacokinetics. *Cancer Treat Rep.* 1978;62:1549-1552.
2. Abelson HT, et al. Treatment of central nervous system tumors with methotrexate. *Cancer Treat Rep.* 1981;65(suppl 1):137-140.
3. Adamson PC, et al. Rescue of experimental intrathecal methotrexate overdose with carboxypeptidase-G2. *J Clin Oncol.* 1991;9:670-674.
4. Adamson PC, et al. Methotrexate pharmacokinetics following administration of recombinant carboxypeptidase-G2 in rhesus monkeys. *J Clin Oncol.* 1992;10:1359-1364.
5. Albrecht AM, et al. Carboxypeptidase displaying differential velocity in hydrolysis of methotrexate, 5-methyltetrahydrofolic acid, and leucovorin. *J Bacteriol.* 1978;134:506-513.
6. Angier RB, et al. The structure and synthesis of the liver L. casei factor. *Science.* 1946;103:667-669.
7. Anoop P, et al. Methotrexate rechallenge following delayed clearance and life-threatening toxicity. *Pediatr Hematol Oncol.* 2008;25:119-121.
8. Auton T, et al. In vitro demonstration that pemetrexed is a good substrate for glucarpidase [abstract]. *Cancer Res.* 2007;67(9)(suppl):4773.
9. Bertino JR, et al. Inhibition of growth of leukemia cells by enzymic folate depletion. *Science.* 1971;172:161-162.
10. Bertino JR, et al. Initial clinical studies with carboxypeptidase G1 (CPG1), a folate depleting enzyme. *Clin Res.* 1974;22:483A.
11. Bleyer WA. Methotrexate: clinical pharmacology, current status and therapeutic guidelines. *Cancer Treat Rev.* 1977;4:87-101.
12. Bleyer WA. New vistas for leucovorin in cancer chemotherapy. *Cancer.* 1989;63:995-1007.
13. Bradley AM, et al. Successful use of intrathecal carboxypeptidase G2 for intrathecal methotrexate overdose: a case study and review of the literature. *Clin Lymphoma Myeloma Leuk.* 2013;13:166-170.
14. Brandes JC, et al. Alteration of pemetrexed excretion in the presence of acute renal failure and effusions: presentation of a case and review of the literature. *Cancer Invest.* 2006;24:283-287.
15. Brandsteterova E, et al. HPLC determination of methotrexate and its metabolite in serum. *Neoplasma.* 1990;37:395-403.
16. BTG International Inc. Prescribing Information. VORAXAZE® (glucarpidase). For injection, for intravenous use. Brentwood, TN: BTG International Inc; 2013.
17. Buchen S, et al. Carboxypeptidase G2 rescue in patients with methotrexate intoxication and renal failure. *Br J Cancer.* 2005;92:480-487.
18. Center for Drug Evaluation and Research (CDER). Application number: 125327Orig1s000. Clinical Pharmacology and Biopharmaceutics Review. Silver Spring, MD: US Food and Drug Administration; 2012. https://www.accessdata.fda.gov/drugsatfda_docs/nda/2012/125327Orig1s000ClinPharmR.pdf. Accessed October 17, 2017.
19. Cerminara Z, et al. A single center retrospective analysis of a protocol for high-dose methotrexate and leucovorin rescue administration. *J Oncol Pharm Pract.* 2017 Jan 1:1078155217729744.
20. Chabner BA, et al. Antitumor activity of a folate-cleaving enzyme, carboxypeptidase G 1. *Cancer Res.* 1972;32:2114-2119.
21. Chabner BA, Johns DG, Bertino JR. Enzymatic cleavage of methotrexate provides a method for prevention of drug toxicity. *Nature.* 1972;239:395-397.
22. Chauvin C, Touzeau C, Mahé J, et al. Evaluation of appropriate glucarpidase prescription to prevent iatrogenic incident and medical cost [abstract]. *EJOP.* 2016;10(suppl):56.
23. Christensen AM, et al. Resumption of high-dose methotrexate after acute kidney injury and glucarpidase use in pediatric oncology patients. *Cancer.* 2012;118:4321-4330.
24. Connors NJ, et al. Methotrexate toxicity treated with continuous venovenous hemofiltration, leucovorin and glucarpidase. *Clin Kidney J.* 2014;7:590-592.
25. Cornell R, Charm SE. Purification of carboxypeptidase G-1 by immunoadsorption. *Biotechnol Bioeng.* 1976;18:1171-1173.
26. DeAngelis LM, et al. Carboxypeptidase G2 rescue after high-dose methotrexate. *J Clin Oncol.* 1996;14:2145-2149.
27. Donehower RC, et al. Presence of 2,4-diamino-N10-methylpteroic acid after high-dose methotrexate. *Clin Pharmacol Ther.* 1979;26:63-72.
28. Esteve MA, et al. Severe acute toxicity associated with high-dose methotrexate (MTX) therapy: use of therapeutic drug monitoring and test-dose to guide carboxypeptidase G2 rescue and MTX continuation. *Eur J Clin Pharmacol.* 2007;63:39-42.
29. European Medicines Agency. *Pre-authorisation Evaluation of Medicines for Human Use. Withdrawal Assessment Report for Voraxaze.* London, UK: European Medicines Agency (EMEA); 2008 June 26, 2008. Report No.: EMEA/CHMP/171907/2008.
30. Finkelstein Y, et al. Intrathecal methotrexate neurotoxicity: clinical correlates and antidotal treatment. *Environ Toxicol Pharmacol.* 2005;19:721-725.
31. Food and Drug Administration Center for Drug Evaluation and Research. Application number: 125327Orig1s000. Chemistry Review(s). http://www.accessdata.fda.gov/drugsatfda_docs/nda/2012/125327Orig1s000ChemR.pdf. Published 2012. Accessed October 18, 2012.
32. Food and Drug Administration Center for Drug Evaluation and Research. Application number: 125327Orig1s000. Medical Review(s). Clinical Review. Patricia Dinndorf. BLA 125327. http://www.accessdata.fda.gov/drugsatfda_docs/nda/2012/125327Orig1s000MedR.pdf. Published 2012. Accessed August 27, 2012.

33. Fotoohi K, et al. Interference of 7-hydroxymethotrexate with the determination of methotrexate in plasma samples from children with acute lymphoblastic leukemia employing routine clinical assays. *J Chromatogr B Analyt Technol Biomed Life Sci*. 2005;817:139-144.

34. Genestier L, et al. Mechanisms of action of methotrexate. *Immunopharmacology*. 2000;47:247-257.

35. Goldman P, Levy CC. Carboxypeptidase G: purification and properties. *Proc Natl Acad Sci U S A*. 1967;58:1299-1306.

36. Green MR, Chamberlain MC. Renal dysfunction during and after high-dose methotrexate. *Cancer Chemother Pharmacol*. 2009;63:599-604.

37. Hempel G, et al. Interactions of carboxypeptidase G2 with 6S-leucovorin and 6R-leucovorin in vitro: implications for the application in case of methotrexate intoxications. *Cancer Chemother Pharmacol*. 2005;55:347-353.

38. Howard SC, et al. Preventing and managing toxicities of high-dose methotrexate. *Oncologist*. 2016;21:1471-1482.

39. Howell C. Voraxaze: a case study [presentation]. Protherics; 2008:1-53. http://www.bio-events.com/presentations/Chiron Howell.pdf. Accessed October 18, 2012.

40. Howell SB, et al. Hemodialysis and enzymatic cleavage of methotrexate in man. *Eur J Cancer*. 1978;14:787-792.

41. Jardine LF, et al. Intrathecal leucovorin after intrathecal methotrexate overdose. *J Pediatr Hematol Oncol*. 1996;18:302-304.

42. Kalghatgi KK, et al. Enhancement of antitumor activity of 2,4-diamino-5-(3',4'-dichlorophenyl)-6-methylpyrimidine and Baker's antifol (triazinate) with carboxypeptidase G1. *Cancer Res*. 1979;39:3441-3445.

43. Kamen BA, et al. Methotrexate accumulation and folate depletion in cells as a possible mechanism of chronic toxicity to the drug. *Br J Haematol*. 1981;49:355-360.

44. Krackhardt A, et al. Carboxypeptidase G2 rescue in a 79 year-old patient with cranial lymphoma after high-dose methotrexate induced acute renal failure. *Leuk Lymphoma*. 1999;35:631-635.

45. Krause AS, et al. Carboxypeptidase-G2 rescue in cancer patients with delayed methotrexate elimination after high-dose methotrexate therapy. *Leuk Lymphoma*. 2002;43:2139-2143.

46. Lee AC, et al. Intrathecal methotrexate overdose. *Acta Paediatr*. 1997;86:434-437.

47. Lemon J, et al. Conversion of pteroylglutamic acid to pteroic acid by bacterial degradation. *Arch Biochem*. 1948;19:311-316.

48. Levy CC, Goldman P. The enzymatic hydrolysis of methotrexate and folic acid. *J Biol Chem*. 1967;242:2933-2938.

49. Lloyd LF, et al. Crystallization and preliminary crystallographic analysis of carboxypeptidase G2 from *Pseudomonas* sp. strain RS-16. *J Mol Biol*. 1991;220:17-18.

50. Matherly LH, et al. Antifolate polyglutamylation and competitive drug displacement at dihydrofolate reductase as important elements in leucovorin rescue in L1210 cells. *Cancer Res*. 1986;46:588-593.

51. Mayer A, et al. A phase I study of single administration of antibody-directed enzyme prodrug therapy with the recombinant anti-carcinoembryonic antigen antibody-enzyme fusion protein MFECP1 and a bis-iodo phenol mustard prodrug. *Clin Cancer Res*. 2006;12:6509-6516.

52. McCullough JL, et al. Purification and properties of carboxypeptidase G 1. *J Biol Chem*. 1971;246:7207-7213.

53. Melton R, Atkinson A; inventors. Use of carboxypeptidase G for combating antifolate toxicity [patent application]. Publication Number WO/2005/084695. International Application Number PCT/GB2005/000751. http://patentscope.wipo.int/search/en/detail.jsf?docId=WO2005084695&recNum=1&docAn=GB2005000751&queryString=ALL:(GB2005000751)&maxRec=12005. Accessed August 29, 2017.

54. Melton R, Atkinson A; inventors. Cleavage of antifolate compounds [patent application]. Publication Number WO/2007/023243. International Application Number PCT/GB2005/003297. http://patentscope.wipo.int/search/en/detail.jsf?docId=WO20050846 95&recNum=1&docAn=GB2005000751&queryString=ALL:(GB2005000751)&maxRec=1 patent Publication number WO/2007/023243. Published 2007. Accessed August 29, 2017.

55. Meropol NJ, et al. Seizures associated with leucovorin administration in cancer patients. *J Natl Cancer Inst*. 1995;87:56-58.

56. Meyers PA. Glucarpidase for the treatment of methotrexate-induced renal dysfunction and delayed methotrexate excretion. *Pediatr Blood Cancer*. 2016;63:364.

57. Minton NP, et al. The complete nucleotide sequence of the Pseudomonas gene coding for carboxypeptidase G2. *Gene*. 1984;31:31-38.

58. Minton NP, et al. Molecular cloning of the Pseudomonas carboxypeptidase G2 gene and its expression in *Escherichia coli* and *Pseudomonas putida*. *J Bacteriol*. 1983;156:1222-1227.

59. Minton NP, Clarke LE. Identification of the promoter of the Pseudomonas gene coding for carboxypeptidase G2. *J Mol Appl Genet*. 1985;3:26-35.

60. Mohty M, et al. Carboxypeptidase G2 rescue in delayed methotrexate elimination in renal failure. *Leuk Lymphoma*. 2000;37:441-443.

61. Nickerson WJ, Webb M. Effects of folic acid analogues on growth and cell division of nonexacting microorganisms. *J Bacteriol*. 1956;71:129-139.

62. O'Marcaigh AS, et al. Successful treatment of intrathecal methotrexate overdose by using ventriculolumbar perfusion and intrathecal instillation of carboxypeptidase G2. *Mayo Clin Proc*. 1996;71:161-165.

63. Oudart JB, et al. Analytical interference in the therapeutic drug monitoring of methotrexate. *Ann Biol Clin (Paris)*. 2016;74:333-337.

64. Park ES, et al. Carboxypeptidase-G2 rescue in a patient with high dose methotrexate-induced nephrotoxicity. *Cancer Res Treat*. 2005;37:133-135.

65. Patterson DM, Lee SM. Glucarpidase following high-dose methotrexate: update on development. *Expert Opin Biol Ther*. 2010;10:105-111.

66. Perisoglou M. *Efficacy and Safety of Glucarpidase for Routine Use After High Dose Methotrexate in Patients With Bone Sarcoma* [doctoral thesis]. London, UK: University College London; 2013.

67. Perisoglou M, et al. Efficacy and safety of glucarpidase for routine use after high dose methotrexate in patients with osteosarcoma [abstract]. *Pediatr Blood Cancer*. 2012;59:1048.

68. Perisoglou M, et al. A randomized, cross-over, phase II study, to investigate the efficacy and safety of glucarpidase for routine use after high dose methotrexate in patients with bone sarcoma: interim analysis [abstract]. Chicago, IL: The Connective Tissue Oncology Society and the Musculoskeletal Tumor Society; 2011.

69. Pesce MA, Bodourian SH. Evaluation of a fluorescence polarization immunoassay procedure for quantitation of methotrexate. *Ther Drug Monit*. 1986;8:115-121.

70. Peyriere H, et al. Optimal management of methotrexate intoxication in a child with osteosarcoma. *Ann Pharmacother*. 2004;38:422-427.

71. Phillips M, et al. Pharmacokinetics of glucarpidase in subjects with normal and impaired renal function. *J Clin Pharmacol*. 2008;48:279-284.

72. Pinedo HM, et al. The reversal of methotrexate cytotoxicity to mouse bone marrow cells by leucovorin and nucleosides. *Cancer Res*. 1976;36:4418-4424.

73. Riva L, et al. Successful treatment of intrathecal methotrexate overdose with folinic acid rescue: a case report. *Acta Paediatr*. 1999;88:780-782.

74. Rowsell S, et al. Crystal structure of carboxypeptidase G2, a bacterial enzyme with applications in cancer therapy. *Structure*. 1997;5:337-347.

75. Saland JM, et al. Effective removal of methotrexate by high-flux hemodialysis. *Pediatr Nephrol*. 2002;17:825-829.

76. Schwartz S, et al. Effects of carboxypeptidase G2 (CPG2) rescue in 30 lymphoma patients with high-dose methotrexate (HD-MTX) induced renal failure abstract. *Ann Oncol*. 2005;16(suppl 5):136.

77. Schwartz S, et al. Glucarpidase (carboxypeptidase g2) intervention in adult and elderly cancer patients with renal dysfunction and delayed methotrexate elimination after high-dose methotrexate therapy. *Oncologist*. 2007;12:1299-1308.

78. Schwartz S, et al. Leucovorin (LV) pharmacokinetics in patients receiving high dose methotrexate (HDMTX), with or without glucarpidase treatment [abstract]. *J Clin Oncol*. 2013;31:e20521.

79. Scott JR, Crews KR. Reply to: glucarpidase for the treatment of methotrexate-induced renal dysfunction and delayed methotrexate excretion. *Pediatr Blood Cancer*. 2016;63:365.

80. Scott JR, et al. Comparable efficacy with varying dosages of glucarpidase in pediatric oncology patients. *Pediatr Blood Cancer*. 2015;62:1518-1522.

81. Sherwood RF, et al. Purification and properties of carboxypeptidase G2 from *Pseudomonas* sp. strain RS-16. Use of a novel triazine dye affinity method. *Eur J Biochem*. 1985;148:447-553.

82. Sieniawski M, et al. Successful carboxypeptidase G2 rescue of a high-risk elderly Hodgkin lymphoma patient with methotrexate intoxication and renal failure. *Leuk Lymphoma*. 2007;48:1641-1643.

83. Smith SW, Nelson LS. Case files of the New York City Poison Control Center: antidotal strategies for the management of methotrexate toxicity. *J Med Toxicol*. 2008;4:132-140.

84. Snyder RL. Resumption of high-dose methotrexate after methotrexate-induced nephrotoxicity and carboxypeptidase G2 use. *Am J Health Syst Pharm*. 2007;64:1163-1169.

85. Svahn T, et al. Delayed elimination of high-dose methotrexate and use of carboxypeptidase G2 in pediatric patients during treatment for acute lymphoblastic leukemia. *Pediatr Blood Cancer*. 2017;64.

86. Treon SP, Chabner BA. Concepts in use of high-dose methotrexate therapy. *Clin Chem*. 1996;42:1322-1329.

87. Trifilio S, et al. Reduced-dose carboxypeptidase-G2 successfully lowers elevated methotrexate levels in an adult with acute methotrexate-induced renal failure. *Clin Adv Hematol Oncol*. 2013;11:322-323.

88. Trinkle R, Wu JK. Intrathecal leukovorin after intrathecal methotrexate overdose. *J Pediatr Hematol Oncol*. 1997;19:267-269.

89. Tucker AD, et al. A new crystal form of carboxypeptidase G2 from *Pseudomonas* sp. strain RS-16 which is more amenable to structure determination. *Acta Crystallogr D Biol Crystallogr*. 1996;52:890-892.

90. Turra KM, et al. Molecular modeling approach to predict a binding mode for the complex methotrexate-carboxypeptidase G2. *J Mol Model*. 2012;18:1867-1875.

91. US National Library of Medicine. Sponsor: BTG International Inc. Open-label leucovorin pharmacokinetic study in patients receiving high dose methotrexate with or without Voraxaze (LVPK). ClinicalTrials.gov Identifier: NCT00634504. US National Library of Medicine, US National Institutes of Health, US Department of Health and Human Services; 2014. https://clinicaltrials.gov/ct2/show/results/NCT00634504?sect=X4370156. Accessed October 17, 2017.

92. Webb M. Inactivation of analogues of folic acid by certain non-exacting bacteria. *Biochim Biophys Acta*. 1955;17:212-225.

93. Widemann BC. Practical considerations for the administration of glucarpidase in high-dose methotrexate (HDMTX) induced renal dysfunction. *Pediatr Blood Cancer*. 2015;62:1512-1513.

94. Widemann BC, Adamson PC. Understanding and managing methotrexate nephrotoxicity. *Oncologist*. 2006;11:694-703.

95. Widemann BC, et al. High-dose methotrexate-induced nephrotoxicity in patients with osteosarcoma. *Cancer.* 2004;100:2222-2232.

96. Widemann BC, et al. Glucarpidase, leucovorin, and thymidine for high-dose methotrexate-induced renal dysfunction: clinical and pharmacologic factors affecting outcome. *J Clin Oncol.* 2010;28:3979-3986.

97. Widemann BC, et al. Carboxypeptidase-G2, thymidine, and leucovorin rescue in cancer patients with methotrexate-induced renal dysfunction. *J Clin Oncol.* 1997;15:2125-2134.

98. Widemann BC, et al. Treatment of accidental intrathecal methotrexate overdose with intrathecal carboxypeptidase G2. *J Natl Cancer Inst.* 2004;96:1557-1559.

99. Widemann BC, et al. Carboxypeptidase-G2 rescue in a patient with high dose methotrexate-induced nephrotoxicity. *Cancer.* 1995;76:521-526.

100. Widemann BC, et al. Efficacy of glucarpidase (carboxypeptidase g2) in patients with acute kidney injury after high-dose methotrexate therapy. *Pharmacotherapy.* 2014;34:427-439.

101. Widemann BC, et al. Immunogenicity and safety of glucarpidase for methotrexate toxicity [abstract]. *J Clin Oncol.* 2014;32:e20648.

102. Widemann BC, et al. Pharmacokinetics and metabolism of the methotrexate metabolite 2, 4-diamino-N(10)-methylpteroic acid. *J Pharmacol Exp Ther.* 2000;294:894-901.

103. Yamamoto T, et al. Folylpolyglutamate synthase is a major determinant of intracellular methotrexate polyglutamates in patients with rheumatoid arthritis. *Sci Rep.* 2016;6:35615.

104. Yasuda N, et al. Isolation, purification, and characterization of a new enzyme from *Pseudomonas* sp. M-27, carboxypeptidase G3. *Biosci Biotechnol Biochem.* 1992;56:1536-1540.

105. Zelcer S, et al. The Memorial Sloan Kettering Cancer Center experience with outpatient administration of high dose methotrexate with leucovorin rescue. *Pediatr Blood Cancer.* 2008;50:1176-1180.

106. Zoubek A, et al. Successful carboxypeptidase G2 rescue in delayed methotrexate elimination due to renal failure. *Pediatr Hematol Oncol.* 1995;12:471-477.

URIDINE TRIACETATE

Silas W. Smith

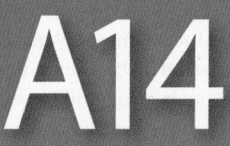

INTRODUCTION

Uridine triacetate (2′,3′,5′-tri-O-acetyluridine) is used to treat cases of toxicity from fluoropyrimidines such as fluorouracil and fluorouracil prodrugs such as capecitabine and tegafur. Uridine triacetate is a prodrug that is taken orally to provide uridine as a source for uridine triphosphate for endogenous RNA incorporation.

HISTORY

In 1950, leucovorin (folinic acid) successfully mitigated chemotherapeutic toxicity from aminopterin and methotrexate, for which folate antidotal therapy was inefficacious.[39] Fluorouracil (5-FU) synthesis and its antitumor activity were reported in 1957.[18] A decade later, the concept of leucovorin "rescue" emerged to mitigate toxicity from higher methotrexate chemotherapy doses.[27] However, in 1982 leucovorin was reported to paradoxically both increase 5-FU chemotherapeutic efficacy as well as cytotoxicity in humans by increasing inhibition of thymidylate synthase.[30] Additional studies in 1982 reported successful use of uridine to "rescue" mice from lethal 5-FU doses, as well as the ability to deliver higher 5-FU chemotherapeutic doses with concomitant uridine.[25,32] Human phase 1 uridine rescue trials soon followed in 1984.[28] Intravenous uridine was associated with severe phlebitis when administered peripherally and with cellulitis and thrombosis when given centrally.[41,42] This necessitated a shift toward oral administration. However, oral uridine was limited by poor bioavailability.[43] To prevent uridine catabolism by uridine phosphorylase and increase lipophilicity, uridine was modified to uridine triacetate in the late 1980s[45] and introduced in mice in 1996.[4] Phase 1 human studies of oral uridine, then also known as PN401, were reported soon after in 1997.[22] Meanwhile, capecitabine, which was synthesized in the early 1990s and patented abroad in 1992, underwent pilot/phase 1 studies in 1996 and received US market approval in 1998.[3,5,17] The FDA designated uridine triacetate an orphan product in 2009, and ultimately granted marketing approval in January 2015 to treat 5-FU or capecitabine overdose and early-onset, severe or life-threatening toxicity.[6]

PHARMACOLOGY

Chemistry/Preparation

Uracil (demethylated thymine) is a naturally occurring pyrimidine and one of the 4 fundamental bases of ribonucleic acid (RNA). Uracil has a molecular weight of 112.1 Da. Uridine is uracil attached by a β-N_1-glycosidic bond to a ribose ring. Uridine triacetate (or triacetyluridine) is uridine that has been triacetylated at the 2′,3′, and 5′ positions. Uridine triacetate has a molecular weight of 370.3 Da.

Mechanism of Action

Uridine as uridine triphosphate is an essential component of RNA, while uridine as uridine diphosphate glucose is an important precursor to glycogen synthesis.[48] Mechanisms of toxicity by the fluoropyrimidines (5-FU, capecitabine, tegafur, and floxuridine) are reviewed in Chap. 51 and summarized in Fig. 51–2. The 5-FU metabolite fluorouridine triphosphate (FUTP) is incorporated in RNA. Uridine triacetate, once absorbed and metabolized, supplies uridine, which can serve as a source for uridine triphosphate to compete with FUTP for RNA incorporation.[26] The enzyme thymidylate synthase generates deoxythymidine monophosphate (dTMP), which is necessary for DNA synthesis, from deoxyuridine monophosphate (dUMP). Uridine triacetate does not reverse inhibition of thymidylate synthase by the 5-FU metabolite fluorodeoxyuridine monophosphate (5-FdUMP), nor does it reverse incorporation of fluorodeoxyuridine triphosphate into DNA, as uridine is not present in DNA.

Related Agents

Various uridine formulations that are marketed as dietary supplements are available but they are not recommended to treat fluoropyrimidine toxicity because of a lack of quality control. Uridine triacetate is also packaged as branded Xuriden for treatment of hereditary orotic aciduria (HOA), at a dose that is different than for fluoropyrimidine toxicity.[47]

Pharmacokinetics and Pharmacodynamics

The pool of physiologically available uridine arises both from pyrimidine salvage pathways and through the de novo synthesis of uridine monophosphate (UMP) by the enzyme uridine monophosphate synthetase (UMPS). Uridine monophosphate synthetase catalyzes UMP generation from orotate and phosphoribosylpyrophosphate (PRPP), which is itself a product of the pentose phosphate pathway.[48] Uridine phosphorylase metabolizes uridine to uracil, and uracil is further degraded to dihydrouracil, 3-ureidopropionate, and ultimately to β-alanine by dihydropyrimidine dehydrogenase, dihydropyrimidinase, and β-ureidopropionase, respectively.[48] Unlike uracil, uridine is not a substrate for dihydropyrimidine dehydrogenase (DPD), the enzyme responsible in humans for metabolizing approximately 80% of 5-FU.[9,37]

In one of the earliest studies in a small group of 7 healthy volunteers, baseline uridine concentrations were 2.32 ± 0.58 μmol/L in plasma, and 10.44 ± 5.06 μmol/L in bone marrow.[14] Other studies found human plasma physiological uridine concentrations more typically ranging from 3 to 8 μmol/L.[28,48] When given in only trace amounts, radiolabeled uridine elimination was triphasic, with initial half-lives of 0.57±0.28 and 1.79±0.62 minutes, and a terminal half-life of 17.5±7.3 minutes.[14] This rapid elimination could be slightly altered with increasing dose. Intravenous uridine bolused at large doses of 1 to 12 g/m² cleared from the plasma in a biphasic manner with an initial half-life of 25±8 minutes and a terminal half-life of 118 minutes.[28] Uridine concentrations increased linearly with increased IV doses.[28] The volume of distribution (V_d) of uridine averaged 0.481±0.07 L/kg with trace amounts and 0.634 L/kg, with large IV doses.[14,28] The goal of sustained serum uridine concentrations higher than 70 μmol/L, which are needed to expand intestinal and bone marrow nucleotide pools and to prevent toxicity,[26,31] was explored in several pharmacokinetic evaluations. Continuous uridine infusions of 1 and 2.5 g/m²/hour increased plasma uridine concentrations to steady-state concentrations of 500 and 1,000 μmol/L, respectively.[42] Intermittent 3-hour dosing of 3 g/m² (the maximum tolerated dose) created peak and nadir concentrations of 846 to 1,306 μmol/L and 138 to 335 μmol/L, respectively.[42]

When uridine was changed to the oral route to mitigate safety concerns with the intravenous product, with single uridine doses from 0.3 to 12 g/m², bioavailability was extremely poor and ranged from only 5.8% to 9.9%.[43] At the maximum tolerated single oral dose of 8 to 12 g/m², plasma uridine concentrations reached 60 to 80 μmol/L; however, at the maximum tolerated multiple-dose regimen of 5 g/m², steady-state concentrations were only approximately 50 μmol/L.[43] Uridine's oral dosing limitations were confirmed in a separate study in which oral dosing of uridine 8 g/m² yielded mean trough concentrations of only 42.9±18 μmol/L.[40]

The significant pharmacokinetic limitations of rapid uridine plasma clearance and poor bioavailability, as well as poor oral tolerance and the safety issues surrounding intravenous administration, prompted evaluation of uridine delivery as a uridine triacetate prodrug.[4]

Uridine triacetate has several pharmacokinetic advantages. It is more lipophilic than uridine and does not require the pyrimidine transporter for absorption, which results in enhanced transport across the gastrointestinal mucosa.[19,22] Additionally, uridine triacetate is not a substrate for uridine phosphorylase, thus mitigating catabolism.[19]

Following absorption, uridine triacetate is deacetylated by nonspecific esterases to uridine and acetate. Mouse studies demonstrated that uridine triacetate had decreased first-pass effects that increased uridine bioavailability from 7% to 53% and decreased time to maximum plasma concentrations (ie, to 507 μmol/L at 0.4 hours, compared to only 20 μmol/L at one hour with uridine).[4] Subsequent human evaluations demonstrated that oral uridine triacetate doses of 3.3 g produced average uridine trough values of 37.3 μmol/L and 6.6 g doses produced average trough values of 50.8 μmol/L.[22] With intensive dosing (6 g every 2 hours for 3 doses followed by 6 g every 6 hours for 15 doses), the mean C_{max} was 259.33 μmol/L 2 hours after the third intensive dose, and this was then maintained above 100 μmol/L for more than 6 hours.[19] Following single and repeat dosing every 8 hours of a proprietary supplement that contained 0.58 g (1.61% by weight) uridine and 5.4 g uridine triacetate (15.0% by weight), the peak plasma uridine concentrations one to 2 hours later were 150.9±39.3 μmol/L with single dosing and 161.4±31.5 μmol/L with repeat dosing.[46] In clinical trials with current labeled dosing of 10 g for adults and 6 g/m² for children, the maximum uridine concentrations occurred after 2 to 3 hours, with a half-life of 2 to 2.6 hours.[21] Plasma uridine concentrations were 99 to 119 μmol/L after the first dose and rose to 153 to 160 μmol/L after the final dose.[6]

ROLE IN FLUOROPYRIMIDINE TOXICITY

Previous therapy for fluoropyrimidine toxicity was limited to supportive care, included discontinuing drugs that impaired fluoropyrimidine clearance, ECG and cardiovascular monitoring, volume resuscitation, electrolyte repletion, antiemetics and antidiarrheals, colony-stimulating factors, broad-spectrum antibiotics, glutamine enteral supplementation, and ACE inhibitors (for 5-FU-related cardiac dysfunction).[1,2,15] Despite these measures, toxicity was often severe, including bone marrow suppression (with neutropenia, infection, and sepsis), gastrointestinal toxicity (with mucositis, stomatitis, vomiting, transaminitis, and severe diarrhea), volume depletion, acute kidney injury, cardiotoxicity (dysrhythmias, congestive heart failure, and hemorrhagic pericarditis), neurotoxicity, mutisystem organ failure, and death. Uridine triacetate rescue offers a novel antidotal mechanism to mitigate fluoropyrimidine toxicity. Hematopoietic and gastrointestinal mucosal progenitors efficiently incorporate exogenous uridine by the salvage pathway, compared to solid tumors, which favor de novo synthesis, providing an explanation for the effectiveness of exogenous uridine in competing with FUTP in normal tissues.[37]

Animal Studies

In the first mice studies, intraperitoneal (IP) uridine at 1, 5, or 10 g/kg/day produced 100% survival from previously lethal doses of 5-FU (up to 800 mg/kg), although it was ineffective against higher fluorouracil doses (1,000 or 1,200 mg/kg).[25] With 2 doses of uridine 3.5 g/kg IP, the median lethal dose (LD_{50}) of fluorouracil was increased by 68% from 190 to 320 mg/kg.[32]

Furthermore, in mice with tumors given uridine rescue, the maximum tolerated dose of fluorouracil was doubled from 40 to 80 mg/kg without attendant toxicity as well as improved efficacy.[32] In another mouse study using uridine rescue with multiple doses ranging from 1.5 to 3.5 g/kg, high-dose fluorouracil 100 mg/kg/week could be extended to very-high-dose 200 or 225 mg/kg/week, with improved chemotherapeutic efficacy.[34] In mice treated with the maximum tolerated single dose of 5-FU (200 mg/kg) followed in 24 hours by a 5-day rescue uridine infusion of 5 g/kg/day, bone marrow cellularity declines were blunted and recovery was hastened significantly.[24] Mitigation of 5-FU toxicity in doses up to 800 mg/kg with this regimen was also reconfirmed.[24] In combination chemotherapy experiments of methotrexate and 5-FU in which leucovorin intended for methotrexate rescue potentially worsened 5-FU toxicity, uridine rescue permitted an increase in 5-FU doses from 100 mg/kg that was associated with a 60% mortality to 5-FU doses of 150 mg/kg with only 6% mortality.[33] Two IV uridine (3.5 g/kg) doses at 2 and 20 hours after 5-FU dose permitted 5-FU increases from 100 mg/kg to 250 and 300 mg/kg and blunted the leukocyte and erythrocyte nadirs.[35,36] In an attempt to shift to oral regimens, doses of 4 g/kg oral uridine in mice were comparable IP rescue of 5-FU at doses of 150 mg/kg as part of a multidrug chemotherapeutic regimen, which was an increase by more than 50% of the maximum tolerated weekly dose.[31] The addition of a uridine phosphorylase inhibitor in order to sustain uridine concentrations was able to further lower the oral rescue dose to 2 g/kg without compromising efficacy.[31]

The limitations of uridine alone in oral or IV formulation, including its rapid plasma clearance, led to exploration of oral prodrugs in an effort to sustain therapeutic plasma concentrations. Both immediate (at 2 hours) and delayed administration of uridine triacetate (as late as 48 hours) were evaluated, with successful doubling of the maximum tolerated 5-FU dose from 100 mg/kg/week to 200 mg/kg/week.[38] To explore the window of efficacy of uridine triacetate resuscitation, mice were given a lethal dose of 300 mg/kg of 5-FU IP followed by uridine triacetate (2 g/kg orally every 8 hours for 15 doses) at 24, 48, 72, and 96 hours after 5-FU.[9] Survival rates were 90% at 24 hours, which declined to 60%, 30%, and 20% with each subsequent day's delay in administration.[9]

Because many cases of 5-FU toxicity are associated with DPD deficiencies and delayed 5-FU clearance, an animal model was created to mimic DPD deficiency. In mice given the lethal combination of 100 mg/kg 5-FU and the DPD dehydrogenase inhibitor 5-ethynyluracil (2 mg/kg) survival was 80%, 40%, 50%, and 20% after rescue at 24, 48, 72, and 96 hours after 5-FU, respectively.[44] This demonstrated efficacy even in the setting of compromised 5-FU elimination.

Human Studies

In the first phase 1 study exploring uridine, one or 2 doses of uridine 5 to 6 g/m² as a one-hour infusion after fluorouracil administration provided insufficient uridine to eliminate 5-FU toxicity as the 5-FU dose was increased from 550 to 800 mg/m².[28] The second phase 1 uridine trial included 20 patients treated with methotrexate (250 mg/m²), 5-FU, leucovorin, and PALA, an inhibitor of the de novo pathway for the pyrimidine biosynthesis.[23] Fluorouracil doses started at 600 mg/m² (the prior maximum tolerated dose) and were escalated by 50 mg/m² until toxicity was reached. Because of high fevers with continuous uridine, uridine was given at 3 g/m² per hour for 3 hours on and then 3 hours off for a total of 72 hours of infusion. With the concomitant chemotherapy, the 5-FU dose could be increased to 750 mg/m² with uridine rescue with severe mucositis in only one patient and no decrease in functional status.[23] The oral route and additional supplementation were later explored in the last phase 1 uridine study with doses of 8 g/m² provided every 6 hours for 12 doses.[40] With this oral uridine schedule, the maximum tolerated dose of 5-FU could be increased 45% from 1.1 to 1.6 g/m² in patients also receiving methotrexate, and by 33% from 0.9 to 1.2 g/m² in patients receiving both methotrexate and doxorubicin.[40]

In the first phase 1 trial of uridine triacetate, in which 38 patients were rescued at 24 hours with 6 g as a tablet or 6.6 g as a suspension every 6 hours for 10 doses, the tolerated 5-FU dose could be increased from 0.6 to 1 g/m².[22]

In a second phase 1 trial, 6 g of uridine triacetate was given as a rescue at 8 hours after 5-FU administration and then every 8 hours for 8 doses (48 g). When 5-FU dose-limiting toxicity was reached, intensive uridine triacetate (6 g) was given every 2 hours for 3 doses, and then every 6 hours for 15 doses.[19] Fluorouracil at 1.0 g/m² was tolerated without toxicity with uridine triacetate rescue, and the 5-FU dose could be consistently elevated further to 1.25 g/m² with intensive rescue. Fluorouracil doses as high as 1.95 g/m² were possible, but with hematologic toxicity occurring at this dose.[19] In a phase 2 trial, 65 patients with gastric carcinoma were administered 1.2 g/m² of 5-FU (twice the usual dose) with leucovorin, followed by 6 g of uridine triacetate every 8 hours, with rescue at 8 hours after 5-FU, for a total of 8 doses (48 g).[16] This normally toxic 5-FU dose, which leads to 3- to 5-fold increases in 5-FU systemic exposure, was tolerated with no episodes of severe stomatitis or diarrhea, and only a 20% incidence of moderate or severe neutropenia.[16]

The pivotal efficacy trials of uridine triacetate were 2 compassionate-use studies that were summarized in 2 publications and analyses by the FDA. Those included WELL401, an open-label, single-arm, multicenter emergency use study and collection of single-patient INDs, and 401.10.001, an open-label expanded access protocol.[7,8,21,29] In these trials of 173 total patients, 142 patients had documented overdose (136 by 5-FU at 1.9 to 576 times the planned infusion rate or doses up to 10 times the intended dose and 6 by capecitabine 7,000 to 2,800 mg), an additional 26 patients had rapid onset of toxicity (severe or life-threatening toxicities within 96 hours following the end of 5-FU administration), at least one of whom was DPD deficient, and 5 were lost to follow-up.[29] There were 6 pediatric patients, of whom 3 had ingested capecitabine unintentionally. Treatment included uridine triacetate 10 g or 6.2 g/m² orally every 6 hours for 20 doses. Historical controls—albeit confounded by publication, reporting, and litigation bias—included 47 cases from the FDA (eg, the Manufacturers and User Facility Device Experience Database and Adverse Event Databases), ISMP (Institute for Safe Medication Practices), the medical and gray literature, and forensic cases, which included 25 patients with available data for 5-FU administered dose, 5-FU time and rate of administration, and the patient outcomes.[29] The primary outcome, survival to 30 days or chemotherapy resumption, was achieved overall in 158 of 168 patients (94%), with an additional 5 lost to follow-up, which included 137 of 142 patients (96%) with overdose and 21 of 26 (81%) with early-onset toxicity. Not all of these patients had expected lethality based on the infusion rate and dose. Efficacy in late administration after more than 96 hours was significantly diminished. In the 8 patients in the early toxicity cohort who had therapy initiated after 96 hours following 5-FU exposure, only 3 survived (37.5% survival).[29] Acknowledging the aforementioned limitations of historical controls, the historical cohort patients—who appeared to be comparable to the overdose patients treated with uridine triacetate as ascertained in the FDA medical review—experienced only a 16% survival (4 of 25 patients) when treated with supportive care alone.[8,21] The FDA separately reviewed the Adverse Event Reporting System for postmarketing fatal cases of fluoropyrimidine toxicity. There were 203 cases in the past 50 years (58 5-FU cases and 145 capecitabine cases), many of which were similar in their early-onset, severe, or life-threatening toxicity presentation, which ultimately all resulted in death despite supportive care.[21] In a separate phase 3 trial for which outcomes data are not yet available (NCT00024427), 2 patients with DPD deficiency were identified who had received high-dose 1.4 g/m² 5-FU followed by 8 doses of uridine triacetate every 8 hours.[37] One patient developed severe thrombocytopenia and rash and survived, whereas the other patient died with a perforated duodenal ulcer and candidemia, highlighting the risk that the DPD genetic deficiency presents to patients.[37] There are no data on uridine triacetate efficacy in overdose of tegafur, a 5-FU prodrug, although it would be reasonable to provide uridine triacetate in this circumstance.

ADVERSE EFFECTS AND SAFETY ISSUES

The most common adverse events observed in the clinical trials of uridine triacetate were vomiting (8.1%), nausea (4.6%), and diarrhea (3.5%).[29] These adverse effects are also consistent with those in patients receiving fluoropyrimidine chemotherapy both therapeutically and in overdose.[29] Of 135 patients in the pivotal studies, 3 patients had to discontinue uridine triacetate because of adverse effects within 30 days.[8] Safety data can also be gathered from use of uridine triacetate in additional patient populations. FDA reviews identified uridine triacetate use in 4 patients with hereditary orotic aciduria (HOA), 53 adults with diabetic neuropathy; 30 patients (22 children and 8 adults) with mitochondrial and metabolic disorders; 46 healthy subjects, 148 patients (6 children and 142 adults) at risk of 5-fluorouracil (5-FU) toxicity, and 288 subjects receiving high-dose 5-FU.[12,13] Providing boundaries for safe dosing regimens, the doses studied included 120 mg/kg/day for 9 months in HOA; 4 or 8 g/day for 6 to 12 months in diabetic neuropathy; 33 to 300 mg/kg/day for up to 18 years in patients with mitochondrial and metabolic disorders; and doses of 6 to 40 g/day for 5 days in 5-FU toxicity.[13] Only "non-serious" gastrointestinal adverse effects were identified, which were attributed to an undisclosed excipient that was demonstrated to be in an earlier uridine triacetate formulation.[11] No treatment discontinuations occurred in HOA clinical trials for adverse events or for any other reason. Diarrhea was reported in patients administered doses of uridine triacetate greater than 4 g/day.[11] Regarding QT interval prolongation hERG potassium channel current inhibition was reported in vitro with uridine triacetate but not with uridine, but not at physiologically relevant concentrations, and no cardiac toxicity was observed in dog or rat studies.[8,9,13] In vitro, no significant CYP450 enzyme interactions were found with uridine or uridine triacetate.[7,10] Uridine triacetate is a weak P-glycoprotein substrate and inhibitor in vitro, and the potential for local inhibition at the gut level could not be excluded.[13]

PREGNANCY AND LACTATION

There are insufficient data on the use of uridine triacetate during pregnancy to inform the risks of birth defects or miscarriage. Animal studies did not demonstrate toxicity when uridine triacetate was provided at one-half the human dose.[6] The presence of uridine triacetate in human milk is unstudied.

DOSING AND ADMINISTRATION

Uridine triacetate dosing in adults is 10 g (1 packet) orally every 6 hours for a total of 20 doses, without regard to meals.[6] The pediatric dose is 6.2 g/m² up to the adult maximum, and a table for the conversion of grams to graduated teaspoons for children is provided in the prescribing information.[6] Uridine triacetate is mixed with 3 to 4 ounces of soft foods (such as applesauce, pudding, or yogurt) and ingested within 30 minutes, along with 4 ounces of water.[6] We recommend that a 5-HT$_3$-receptor antagonist be given an antiemetic such as ondanstron, 20 to 30 minutes prior to each dose to prevent vomiting. If vomiting occurs within 2 hours of the last dose, the entire dose is given within 15 minutes of vomiting and the next dose is given at the next scheduled interval. In the event the patient cannot tolerate the oral route (eg, severe mucositis), then we recommend that uridine triacetate be given by nasogastric or gastrostomy tube. If provided via this route, then 4 ounces of a food starch–based thickening product in water should be stirred briskly until the thickener has dissolved, and the contents of one full 10-g packet of uridine triacetate granules that have been crushed to a fine powder added to the reconstituted food starch–based thickening product.[6] For pediatric patients receiving less than 10 g, the mixture should be prepared at a ratio of no greater than 1 g per 10 mL of reconstituted food starch–based thickening product and mix thoroughly.[6] The nasogastric or gastrostomy tube should be flushed with water following administration. Although uridine triacetate absorption is unaffected by food, medicines such as bismuth, cholestyramine, Kaopectolin, and sucralfate interfere with absorption.[8]

FORMULATION AND ACQUISITION

Uridine triacetate granules contain 10 g of orange-flavored, white to off-white oral granules in single-dose packets. Inactive ingredients include ethylcellulose (0.309 g), Opadry Clear (a proprietary dispersion of hydroxypropylmethylcellulose and Macrogol, 0.077 g), and natural orange juice flavor (0.131 g). Uridine triacetate is supplied as a full course of therapy with 20 single-dose packets per carton, as well as a "24-Hour Pack" containing 4 single-dose packets per carton. The manufacturer-supplied contact number for ordering uridine triacetate is 1-844-293-0007.[20]

SUMMARY

- Uridine triacetate is a uridine prodrug that is the recommended treatment for toxicity from fluoropyrimidines such as fluorouracil and its prodrugs pecitabine and Tegafur.
- Uridine triacetate should be started as early as possible after recognition of overdose or early toxicity, as efficacy declines with delay to administration.
- The antidote must be given orally or by nasogastric or gastrostomy tube.

REFERENCES

1. Alberta Health Services. Management of fluorouracil (5-Fluorouracil, 5FU) infusion overdose guideline: Alberta Health Services; 2016. http://www.albertahealthservices.ca/assets/info/hp/cancer/if-hp-cancer-guide-5fu-infusion-overdose.pdf. Accessed September 28, 2017.
2. Andreica I, et al. Fluorouracil overdose: clinical manifestations and comprehensive management during and after hospitalization. *J Hematol Oncol Pharm.* 2015;5:43-47.
3. Arasaki M, et al. *N4-(Substituted-Oxycarbonyl)-5′-Deoxy-5-Fluorocytidine Compounds, Compositions and Methods of Using Same. United States Patent Number 5,472,949.* Washington, DC: United States Patent and Trademark Office; 1995.
4. Ashour OM, et al. 5-(*m*-Benzyloxybenzyl)barbituric acid acyclonucleoside, a uridine phosphorylase inhibitor, and 2′,3′,5′-tri-*O*-acetyluridine, a prodrug of uridine, as modulators of plasma uridine concentration. Implications for chemotherapy. *Biochem Pharmacol.* 1996;51:1601-1611.
5. Bajetta E, et al. A pilot safety study of capecitabine, a new oral fluoropyrimidine, in patients with advanced neoplastic disease. *Tumori.* 1996;82:450-452.
6. BTG International Inc. VISTOGARD® (uridine triacetate) oral granules [prescribing information]. West Conshohocken, PA: BTG International Inc; 2018.
7. Center for Drug Evaluation and Research (CDER). Application Number: 208159Orig1s000. Clinical Pharmacology and Biopharmaceutics Review(s). Silver Spring, MD: US Food and Drug Administration; 2015. https://www.accessdata.fda.gov/drugsatfda_docs/nda/2015/208159Orig1s000ClinPharmR.pdf. Accessed September 28, 2017.
8. Center for Drug Evaluation and Research (CDER). Application Number: 208159Orig1s000. Medical Review(s). Silver Spring, MD: US Food and Drug Administration; 2015. https://www.accessdata.fda.gov/drugsatfda_docs/nda/2015/208159Orig1s000MedR.pdf. Accessed September 28, 2017.
9. Center for Drug Evaluation and Research (CDER). Application Number: 208159Orig1s000. Pharmacology Review(s). Silver Spring, MD: US Food and Drug Administration; 2015. https://www.accessdata.fda.gov/drugsatfda_docs/nda/2015/208159Orig1s000PharmR.pdf. Accessed September 28, 2017.
10. Center for Drug Evaluation and Research (CDER). Application Number: 208169Orig1s000. Clinical Pharmacology and Biopharmaceutics Review(s). Silver Spring, MD: US Food and Drug Administration; 2015. https://www.accessdata.fda.gov/drugsatfda_docs/nda/2015/208169Orig1s000ClinPharm.pdf. Accessed September 29, 2017.
11. Center for Drug Evaluation and Research (CDER). Application Number: 208169Orig1s000. Cross Discipline Team Leader Review. Silver Spring, MD: US Food and Drug Administration; 2015. https://www.accessdata.fda.gov/drugsatfda_docs/nda/2015/208169Orig1s000CrossR.pdf. Accessed September 28, 2017.
12. Center for Drug Evaluation and Research (CDER). Application Number: 208169Orig1s000. Medical Review(s). Silver Spring, MD: US Food and Drug Administration; 2015. https://www.accessdata.fda.gov/drugsatfda_docs/nda/2015/208169Orig1s000MedR.pdf. Accessed September 28, 2017.
13. Center for Drug Evaluation and Research (CDER). Application Number: 208169Orig1s000. Office Director Memo. Silver Spring, MD: US Food and Drug Administration; 2015. https://www.accessdata.fda.gov/drugsatfda_docs/nda/2015/208169Orig1s000ODMemo.pdf. Accessed September 28, 2017.
14. Chan TC, et al. Uridine pharmacokinetics in cancer patients. *Cancer Chemother Pharmacol.* 1988;22:83-86.
15. Daniele B, et al. Oral glutamine in the prevention of fluorouracil induced intestinal toxicity: a double blind, placebo controlled, randomised trial. *Gut.* 2001;48:28-33.
16. Doroshow JH, et al. Phase II trial of PN401, 5-FU, and leucovorin in unresectable or metastatic adenocarcinoma of the stomach: a Southwest Oncology Group study. *Invest New Drugs.* 2006;24:537-542.
17. Genentech Inc. XELODA (capecitabine) tablets, for oral use [prescribing information]. South San Francisco, CA: Genentech, Inc; 2016.
18. Heidelberger C, et al. Fluorinated pyrimidines, a new class of tumour-inhibitory compounds. *Nature.* 1957;179:663-666.
19. Hidalgo M, et al. Phase I and pharmacologic study of PN401 and fluorouracil in patients with advanced solid malignancies. *J Clin Oncol.* 2000;18:167-177.
20. BTG International Inc. Ordering Information: BTG International Inc; 2017. https://www.vistogard.com/Professional/How-to-Order. Accessed September 29, 2017.
21. Ison G, et al. FDA approval: uridine triacetate for the treatment of patients following fluorouracil or capecitabine overdose or exhibiting early-onset severe toxicities following administration of these drugs. *Clin Cancer Res.* 2016;22:4545-4549.
22. Kelsen DP, et al. Phase I trial of PN401, an oral prodrug of uridine, to prevent toxicity from fluorouracil in patients with advanced cancer. *J Clin Oncol.* 1997;15:1511-1517.
23. Kemeny NE, et al. Phase I trial of PALA, methotrexate, fluorouracil, leucovorin, and uridine rescue in patients with advanced cancer. The use of uridine to decrease fluorouracil toxicity. *Cancer Invest.* 1990;8:263-264.
24. Klubes P, Cerna I. Use of uridine rescue to enhance the antitumor selectivity of 5-fluorouracil. *Cancer Res.* 1983;43:3182-3186.
25. Klubes P, et al. Uridine rescue from the lethal toxicity of 5-fluorouracil in mice. *Cancer Chemother Pharmacol.* 1982;8:17-21.
26. Klubes P, Leyland-Jones B. Enhancement of the antitumor activity of 5-fluorouracil by uridine rescue. *Pharmacol Ther.* 1989;41:289-302.
27. Lefkowitz E, et al. Head and neck cancer. 3. Toxicity of 24-hour infusions of methotrexate (NSC-740) and protection by leucovorin (NSC-3590) in patients with epidermoid carcinomas. *Cancer Chemother Rep.* 1967;51:305-311.
28. Leyva A, et al. Phase I and pharmacokinetic studies of high-dose uridine intended for rescue from 5-fluorouracil toxicity. *Cancer Res.* 1984;44:5928-5933.
29. Ma WW, et al. Emergency use of uridine triacetate for the prevention and treatment of life-threatening 5-fluorouracil and capecitabine toxicity. *Cancer.* 2017;123:345-356.
30. Machover D, et al. Treatment of advanced colorectal and gastric adenocarcinomas with 5-FU combined with high-dose folinic acid: a pilot study. *Cancer Treat Rep.* 1982;66:1803-1807.
31. Martin DS, et al. Use of oral uridine as a substitute for parenteral uridine rescue of 5-fluorouracil therapy, with and without the uridine phosphorylase inhibitor 5-benzylacylouridine. *Cancer Chemother Pharmacol.* 1989;24:9-14.
32. Martin DS, et al. High-dose 5-fluorouracil with delayed uridine "rescue" in mice. *Cancer Res.* 1982;42:3964-3970.
33. Martin DS, et al. Improved therapeutic index with sequential *N*-phosphonacetyl-L-aspartate plus high-dose methotrexate plus high-dose 5-fluorouracil and appropriate rescue. *Cancer Res.* 1983;43:4653-4661.
34. Nord LD, et al. Biochemical modulation of 5-fluorouracil with leucovorin or delayed uridine rescue. Correlation of antitumor activity with dosage and FUra incorporation into RNA. *Biochem Pharmacol.* 1992;43:2543-2549.
35. Peters GJ, et al. In vitro biochemical and in vivo biological studies of the uridine 'rescue' of 5-fluorouracil. *Br J Cancer.* 1988;57:259-265.
36. Peters GJ, et al. Toxicity and antitumor effect of 5-fluorouracil and its rescue by uridine. *Adv Exp Med Biol.* 1986;195(pt B):121-128.
37. Saif MW, Diasio RB. Benefit of uridine triacetate (Vistogard) in rescuing severe 5-fluorouracil toxicity in patients with dihydropyrimidine dehydrogenase (DPYD) deficiency. *Cancer Chemother Pharmacol.* 2016;78:151-156.
38. Saif MW, von Borstel R. 5-Fluorouracil dose escalation enabled with PN401 (triacetyluridine): toxicity reduction and increased antitumor activity in mice. *Cancer Chemother Pharmacol.* 2006;58:136-142.
39. Schoenbach EB, et al. Reversal of aminopterin and amethopterin toxicity by citrovorum factor. *J Am Med Assoc.* 1950;144:1558.
40. Schwartz GK, et al. A phase I trial of a modified, dose intensive FAMTX regimen (high dose 5-fluorouracil+doxorubicin+high dose methotrexate+leucovorin) with oral uridine rescue. *Cancer.* 1996;78:1988-1995.
41. Seiter K, et al. Uridine allows dose escalation of 5-fluorouracil when given with *N*-phosphonacetyl-L-aspartate, methotrexate, and leucovorin. *Cancer.* 1993;71:1875-1881.
42. van Groeningen CJ, et al. Clinical and pharmacokinetic studies of prolonged administration of high-dose uridine intended for rescue from 5-FU toxicity. *Cancer Treat Rep.* 1986;70:745-750.
43. van Groeningen CJ, et al. Clinical and pharmacologic study of orally administered uridine. *J Natl Cancer Inst.* 1991;83:437-441.
44. von Borstel R, et al. Uridine triacetate as an effective antidote in preclinical models of 5-FU overdoses and impaired 5-FU clearance [abstract]. *J Clin Oncol.* 2016;34:e18232-e32.
45. Von Borstel RW, Bamat MK. Acylated uridine and cytidine and uses thereof. United States Patent number 5,583,117. Previously published as Patent number WO1989003837 A1, 1989. Washington, DC: United States Patent and Trademark Office; 1996.
46. Weinberg ME, et al. Enhanced uridine bioavailability following administration of a triacetyluridine-rich nutritional supplement. *PLoS One.* 2011;6:e14709.
47. Wellstat Therapeutics Corporation. XURIDEN (uridine triacetate) oral granules [prescribing information]. Gaithersburg, MD: Wellstat Therapeutics Corporation; 2015.
48. Yamamoto T, et al. Biochemistry of uridine in plasma. *Clin Chim Acta.* 2011;412:1712-1724.

Special Considerations

INTRATHECAL ADMINISTRATION OF XENOBIOTICS

Rama B. Rao

Cerebrospinal fluid (CSF) is produced by the choroid plexus that lines the cerebral ventricles at a rate of 15 to 30 mL/h, or approximately 500 mL/day in adults.[57] Cerebrospinal fluid flows in a rostral to caudal direction and is reabsorbed through the arachnoid villi directly into the venous circulation. The estimated total volume of CSF is 130 to 150 mL in healthy adults and 35 mL in infants.[57,74,99]

For more than 100 years, a variety of experimental and therapeutic xenobiotics have been delivered directly into the CSF[64,127] (Table SC7–1). The most common current indications for intrathecal administration include the instillation of analgesics or anesthetics and the treatment of spasticity or central nervous system (CNS) neoplasms. The clinical advantages of this route of administration include targeted delivery and lower medication dosages with fewer systemic effects. Medications are usually administered via a spinal needle or an indwelling intrathecal catheter. Catheters can be attached to either an external or subcutaneous pump. Less commonly, medications are administered into a reservoir of an intraventricular shunt. The distribution of intrathecal xenobiotics is determined by a variety of factors. Some authors speculate that the xenobiotic movement is often attributed to both diffusion and convection, and they suggest that the dilution of xenobiotics administered via a lumbar catheter is attributed to the outflow of CSF from the fourth ventricle.[92] In a radiolabeled tracer study of 5 patients with lumbar catheters, individuals received the hydrophilic radiolabeled diethylene triamine pentaacetic acid (^{111}In-DTPA) intrathecally. Neuroimaging revealed a drop in concentration of the tracer as the fluid moved rostrally.[66] The steady-state lumbar to cervical concentration for hydrophilic xenobiotics is 4:1 with marked interindividual variability.[96] Depending on the lipophilicity, the xenobiotic reaches the brain within a few minutes to 1 hour. Patient position and interindividual variations in lumbosacral CSF volume affect xenobiotic distribution and account for the differences in the level of spinal anesthesia among patients administered the same local anesthetic dosages.[55] Baricity, which is the ratio of the specific gravity of the xenobiotic to the specific gravity of CSF at 98.6°F (37°C), is also a consequential variable. Hyperbaric xenobiotics typically distribute in accordance with gravitational forces.[55] However, in overdose or administration of xenobiotics unintended for intrathecal administration, distribution, reabsorption, and clinical effects are unpredictable.

Complications occur from preparation and dosing errors or inadvertent penetration of the dura and admixture with the CSF during epidural anesthesia or analgesia.[27,54,55] Medications intended for intrathecal delivery are occasionally administered inadvertently into the wrong port of a pump delivery system, resulting in a massive overdose (see Pump Malfunction and Errors). Another potentially fatal error involves inadvertent administration of the wrong medication into the CSF.[60] This error occurs with misidentification or mislabeling of medications during pharmacy preparation or at the bedside. For patients with indwelling devices, medications intended for intravenous delivery are occasionally connected inadvertently to the intrathecal catheter, which also currently operates utilizing the same Luer lock system.

Several factors affect the clinical toxicity of intrathecal medication errors.[128] The properties of the medication are important. Ionized xenobiotics are likely to disrupt normal neurotransmission and cause toxicity, as do hyperosmolar or lipophilic xenobiotics. The site of administration is important as well. Patients administered the wrong xenobiotic into an Ommaya reservoir (an intraventricular catheter with a subcutaneous access port on the scalp) often suffer immediate alterations in mental status depending upon the xenobiotic administered. Although intrathecal administration of preservatives and excipients were investigated in animal models, the characteristics of these adjuvants in medication errors are not likely to be of value in predicting clinical effect.[56]

Patients often present with exaggerated symptoms and findings typically associated with the xenobiotic. For example, patients with intrathecal morphine overdose present with symptoms of opioid toxicity.[62] Other manifestations of intrathecal errors, regardless of the xenobiotic, include pain and paresthesias, often ascending in nature; autonomic instability, especially with extremes of blood pressure and hyperreflexic myoclonic spasms similar to those that occur in patients with tetanus. Seizures or a depressed level of consciousness also occur. The time of onset of these life-threatening symptoms is determined by the dose and characteristics of the xenobiotic. For example, a woman inadvertently administered intrathecal potassium chloride complained immediately of severe back pain.[82] Myoclonic spasms, seizures, and coma followed, and the patient died within 3 hours despite a normal serum potassium concentration. Patients with inadvertent vincristine exposures will be asymptomatic for many hours and die within a few days to a few weeks. In another example, a patient with an inadvertent intrathecal administration of aminophylline immediately developed leg cramps. He recovered and was discharged, only to return 24 hours later with leg weakness that progressed to irreversible paraplegia.[7]

TABLE SC7–1	Xenobiotics Intentionally Administered Intrathecally[a]	
Analgesics/anesthetics		Antiinflammatory
Anesthetics (local)		Corticosteroids[100]
Ketamine[53]		Antispasmodic
Morphine[70]		Baclofen[124]
Opioids[80]		Chemotherapeutics
Zinconitide[19]		Cytarabine (liposomal)[18]
Antimicrobials		Methotrexate[3]
Amikacin[15,28]		Vasoactive
Amphotericin B[48]		Epinephrine[49]
Arbekacin[42]		Papaverine[106]
Cefotiam[20]		Phenylephrine[31]
Ceftriaxone[24]		Other
Colistin[123]		Bethanecol[94]
Gentamicin[112]		Clonidine[23]
Levofloxacin[15]		Midazolam[130]
Penicillin[11]		Neostigmine[70]
Polymyxin E[14]		Octreotide[89,96]
Vancomycin[1,81]		Tetanus immunoglobulin[2]

[a]Few of these xenobiotics are approved by the US Food and Drug Administration for intrathecal administration. Most were utilized in clinical trials or as rescue therapy for refractory central nervous system disorders.

XENOBIOTIC RECOVERY FROM CEREBROSPINAL FLUID

Once a medication delivery error is identified, rapid intervention is mandatory, especially for ionized xenobiotics, chemotherapeutics, or iodinated water-soluble contrast agents because these xenobiotics usually reach the brain within an hour. In cases in which outcome is uncertain or not previously described, the exposure should be treated as potentially fatal. Any existing access to the CSF, ideally in the lumbosacral area, should be maintained.[121] Immediate withdrawal of CSF, in volumes as high as 75 mL in adults, is indicated. This can be replaced with isotonic solutions: lactated Ringer, 0.9% normal sodium chloride, or Plasma-Lyte, or a combination of these. Older cases utilized Elliot B solution, which is not readily available or advised. Some authors recommend the initial volume removal of 100 mL be performed in 20- to 30-mL aliquots. This is a reasonable initial intervention for fatal intrathecal exposures. For children, multiple aliquots of 5 to 10 mL can be removed and replaced with isotonic fluid. If the patient can tolerate an upright position, this has the potential to limit cephalad movement of xenobiotics, but positioning for any critical life support measures should take precedence.

Delays to initial CSF drainage should be minimized as the interval between the exposure and CSF drainage affects the total xenobiotic recovered (see below). In the interim, a neurosurgical consultation should be obtained to consider the placement of cerebral ventricular access for the performance of continuous CSF lavage. This procedure, also known as ventriculolumbar perfusion, involves continuous instillation of an isotonic solution into the cerebral ventricular system with CSF drainage through a lumbar site. Another intervention involves placement of an epidural catheter into the intrathecal space at a space above the lumbar drainage site so that an isotonic solution can be perfused through the catheter and drained caudally. This serves as a readily available, rapid intervention for patients awaiting placement of an emergent ventriculostomy.[84,114]

For ventriculolumbar perfusion, lavage flow rates can be as great as 150 mL/h. One author advised the addition of fresh-frozen plasma to lavage fluid after several hours to increase the CSF protein content. The ideal lavage fluid, protein components, and infusion rates are not known.[51] As multiple successful perfusions have been reported without use of this intervention, and there is unlikely to be high-quality data, the use of fresh-frozen plasma in lavage fluid is not recommended unless brain edema is already present. Some protocols previously utilized are listed in Table SC7–2. Although artificial CSF formulations exist, their role in the treatment of such medication errors is not evaluated.[86]

Depending on the xenobiotic exposure, specific antidotes or rescue xenobiotics can be employed. With most intrathecal exposures, these therapeutics will be administered via oral, intramuscular, or intravenous routes. Extreme caution should be undertaken to avoid delivery of antidotes directly into the CSF, unless specific data support their use. Immediate, aggressive CSF removal and lavage resulted in nearly 95% recovery of vincristine in the lavage fluid of a patient with inadvertent exposure. Of the published cases in which xenobiotic recovery is reported, percentages relate to both the lavage method and quantity of CSF removed. For example, withdrawal of 10 mL of CSF 45 minutes after a methotrexate overdose in a 4-year-old patient recovered 20% of the initial dose.[3] Withdrawal of 200 mL of CSF in aliquots 45 minutes after methotrexate overdose in a 9-year-old patient recovered 78% of the initial dose.[35] The specific xenobiotic affects recovery as well. For example, a patient underwent withdrawal of 30 mL of CSF 18 minutes after an overdose of simultaneously administered lidocaine, epinephrine, and fentanyl. Approximately 39% of lidocaine was recovered, whereas the recovery of fentanyl was only 7%.[113]

SPECIFIC EXPOSURES

Ionic Contrast

Several xenobiotics were utilized historically for contrast myelography. Many of these xenobiotics were abandoned because of their propensity to cause adhesive arachnoiditis chronic pain syndromes or other complications (Thorotrast). Low osmolar, nonionic contrast media are currently utilized, but unfortunately, other hyperosmolar ionic media are readily available in radiographic suites and sometimes inadvertently administered. Patients develop cranial neuropathies.[40] Exposed patients become symptomatic within 30 minutes to 6 hours after administration, with hyperreflexia and myoclonic spasms following minimal stimulation.[102,104,118] Clinical symptoms and effects typically begin in the lower extremities and move in a cephalad direction, sometimes progressing to opisthotonos. This is likely due to alterations in inhibitory neurotransmission occurring in patients with tetanus; this condition is called ascending tonic–clonic syndrome (ATCS). In one review, 3 of 7 patients with ATCS died as a result of their exposures.[102] Immediate large-volume (>100 mL) CSF drainage should be performed in 20-mL utilizing the same catheter aliquots with isotonic fluid replacement. Ventriculolumbar perfusion should be performed in severe cases.

Chemotherapeutics

Methotrexate is administered intrathecally for the prevention and treatment of leukemic meningitis or other CNS neoplasms.[9] Errors are generally dose related.[3,33-35,51,58,69,101,119] In most reported cases, aggressive drainage of as great as 250 mL of CSF in aliquots with isotonic fluid replacement was utilized without ventriculolumbar perfusion. Experimental treatment of patients with intrathecal glucarpidase was described without obvious adverse events.[87,125] The patients underwent lumbar drainage followed by intrathecal glucarpidase. Drainage removed between 32% and 58% of the methotrexate, and the antidote reduced the methotrexate concentrations by 98%. The patients received 2,000 units of intrathecal glucarpidase in 12 mL of 0.9% sodium chloride solution over 5 minutes (Antidotes in Depth: A13).

Intrathecal leucovorin is *absolutely contraindicated* as its use results in fatalities. Following intrathecal methotrexate overdose, the intravenous administration of leucovorin is appropriate[59,120] (Antidotes in Depth: A12).

Vincristine is typically administered intravenously and does not cross the blood–brain barrier. There are no therapeutic indications for intrathecal vincristine, and such errors are almost invariably fatal.[4-6,17,29,39,43,46,67] In most cases, the error is the result of confusion of either syringes or catheter access. As soon as the exposure is identified, immediate CSF drainage should be instituted, and rapid neurosurgical consultation should be obtained. The few known survivors with cognitive function underwent early neurosurgical intervention for ventriculolumbar perfusion.[5,33,84,97,134] One of the patients had an epidural catheter placed intrathecally above the drainage site for lumbolumbar perfusion while awaiting ventriculostomy. This method of intrathecal perfusion is recommended in all patients with intrathecal vincristine exposures until definitive ventriculolumbar perfusion can be established. Ideally, tubing systems should be readily available and prepared for use to prevent intrathecal medication errors.[90,116] Other rescue medications are discussed in Chaps. 34 and 51.

PUMP MALFUNCTIONS AND ERRORS

Pump malfunctions cause a sudden decrease or increase in the amount of drug delivered to the intrathecal space.

Insufficient drug delivery will result in withdrawal especially in pumps containing opioids, baclofen, or clonidine.[72] This occurs from either pump malfunction[98] or impairment of flow through the intrathecal catheter. Catheters infrequently kink, migrate, or become obstructed by an inflammatory mass.[25,26,60,91] In some devices, an impaired or reduced delivery of drug is indicated by an audible alarm.[72] Such alarms should be heeded and consultation with the implanting service is warranted to avert withdrawal.[72] Patients on chronic therapy are at highest risk of severe withdrawal signs and symptoms.[124] As intrathecal doses are 100 to 1,000 times more potent than the equivalent dose administered intravenously,[63] patients will require very high oral or intravenous doses to treat withdrawal until intrathecal delivery can be re-established. A thorough neurologic examination should be performed to evaluate for spinal cord compression symptoms that indicates a catheter-related complication.[60] An anteroposterior and lateral radiograph should be obtained to assess for kinking or fracture of the catheter.

TABLE SC7–2   Inadvertent Intrathecal Overdoses and Unintentional Exposures

Xenobiotic	Age/Sex	Mechanism	Clinical Findings/Effects	Intervention	Outcome
Aminophylline[7]	64/M	Medication error	Muscle cramps initially Paraplegia at 24 hours	Observation	Paraplegia Death in 2 years
Baclofen[132]	8/M	Probable pump malfunction	Coma, vomiting, bradycardia	20 mL CSF removed at undetermined time	Survived
Bortezomib[36,47]	Unknown	Medication error	Not reported	Not described	Three deaths
Bupivacaine[38]	34/M	Inadvertent dural puncture	Hypotension Ascending paralysis at 10 minutes	Not described	Survived
Cefotiam[20]	66/M	Catheter misconnection	Dyspnea, hypotension, myoclonic spasm, pain at 2 hours	10 mL CSF removed at 20 hours	Rhabdomyolysis Survived
Ceftriaxone[24]	74/F	Overdose	Bilateral lower extremity pain	240 mL CSF removed in 20-mL aliquots, with 0.9% NaCl replacement therapy Started at unknown time	Survived
Cytarabine[68]	4/M	Overdose	Mydriasis, delayed onset, gait impairment, tremor	50 mL CSF removed in 5-mL aliquots, with 0.9% NaCl replacement therapy Started at 65 minutes Estimated 27%–36% cytarabine recovery	Died of unknown cause
Cytarabine[77]	45/F	Overdose	Headache, vomiting	CSF removal of 54 mL from Ommaya at 2 hours	Asymptomatic at 6 hours
Dactinomycin[65]	5/F	Medication error	Hypotonia, fasciculations, hyper-reflexia at 2 hours	50 mL CSF removed with 0.9% NaCl replacement at 1 hour, then VL perfusion started at 1.5 hours using 0.9% NaCl 100 mL/h with 2.5 mg/mL hydrocortisone for 26 hours Other adjuncts	Ascending paraplegia, obstructive hydrocephalus Survived
Doxorubicin[8]	12/F	Medication error	Fever, headache, vomiting at 12 hours, seizures, hydrocephalus	No attempt at removal	Survived without sequelae at 56 days
Doxorubicin[61]	31/F	Medication error	Hypoesthesia, paraparesis, incontinence over 7 days, T8 sensory level, bowel, bladder incontinence, meningismus, adhesive arachnoiditis at 3 weeks	CSF exchange at 20 mL/h for 500 cm³ per publication; methyl prednisolone 500 mg/d and immunoglobulin 22 g/d initiated at 1 week Treatment of arachnoiditis with VP shunt placement	Lower extremity weakness 3/5 at 8 months, eventual ambulation with resolution of incontinence at 14 months
Furosemide[22]	36/M	Medication error	None	No attempt at removal	Survived
Gadolinium[9]	64/M	Medication error: gadopentetate dimeglumine	Confusion, nausea, vomiting, ataxia, nystagmus, hallucinations, blurred vision, depressed mental status	Not described	Survived
Gallamine[50]	48/M	Medication error	Hyperreflexic myoclonic spasm, onset 1 hour 45 minutes; fever, hypertension, tachycardia, miosis, coma at 3 hours	15 mL CSF drainage started at 6 hours	Survived
Iohexol[103]	52/M	Dural perforation	ATCS at 30 minutes, coma, hypoxia, fever	Not described	Survived
Ionic contrast media cases[102]	Various	Medication error	ATCS starting at 30 minutes to 6 hours	Variable	3/7 patients died; fractures, rhabdomyolysis
Iopanidol[40]	Various	Medication error	Cranial neuropathy	Not described	Survived
Ioxithalamate Contrast[122]	48/M	Medication error	ATCS, opisthotonos	Sitting position, intubation 145 mL CSF removal in 10–20-mL aliquots Other adjuncts	Survived
Labetolol[16]	32/F	Medication error	Mild drop in BP and HR	Fluid bolus	Recovered
Leucovorin[59]	11/M	Therapeutic error	Seizures	Not described	Died day 5

(Continued)

TABLE SC7–2   Inadvertent Intrathecal Overdoses and Unintentional Exposures (Continued)

Xenobiotic	Age/Sex	Mechanism	Clinical Findings/Effects	Intervention	Outcome
Lidocaine, epinephrine, fentanyl[113]					
Patient 1	28/F	Dural perforation	Hypotension, numbness at 5 minutes	20 mL CSF drained within 5 minutes; 51% lidocaine recovery, 4% fentanyl recovery	Survived
Patient 2	68/F	Dural perforation	C_5–C_6 sensory impairment at 18 minutes	30 mL CSF drained at 18 minutes; 39% lidocaine recovery; 7% fentanyl recovery	Survived
Magnesium sulfate[73]	23/F	Medication error	Backache, lower extremity weakness, intact sensation, normotension	Fowler position	Recovery within 7 hours
Mercury[115]	69/F	Inadvertent (Mercurochrome) injection into CSF fistula	Local pain, nuchal rigidity, coma at 24 hours	Lumbar drain, parenteral chelation	Sensorimotor polyneuropathy Survived
Methotrexate[34]	2/F	Overdose	Headaches	Varied	Survived
Methotrexate[41]	34/M	Overdose	Confusion, seizures, ARDS, coma at 2 hours	200 mL CSF drained and replaced with 0.9% NaCl started at 6 hours in aliquots over 48 hours, then another 150 mL CSF exchange over 36 hours (patient also inappropriately received an intrathecal leucovorin)	Cognitive and motor deficits
Methotrexate[35]	9/M	Overdose	Lower extremity numbness, seizures, flaccid paralysis, cranial neuropathy, posturing	200 mL CSF drained in 30–40-mL aliquots, replacement with Elliots B solution Started at 45 minutes 78% drug recovery	Died
Methotrexate series I[3]		Overdose			
Patient 1	12/M		Headache, vomiting at 45 minutes	30 mL CSF drained and replacement with 20-mL of Elliots B solution started at 2 hours; 28% drug recovery	Survived until relapse leukemia
Patient 2	4/M			10 mL CSF drained at 45 minutes; 20% drug recovery	Survived
Methotrexate series II[58]					
Patient 1	4/M			250 mL CSF drained in 20-mL aliquots, replacement with 0.9% NaCl started at 5 hours	Survived
Patient 2	11/M			20 mL CSF withdrawn then 210 mL CSF drained in 5-mL aliquots, replacement with 0.9% NaCl started at 3 hours; 31% drug recovery	Survived
Methotrexate[71]	3/F	Medication error: 125 mg	Seizures at 3 hours	No CSF exchange; IV leucovorin rescue and dexamethasone	Survived
Methotrexate[114]	26/M	Medication error: 625 mg	Immediate pain in leg, followed by coma and flaccid paralysis, renal failure	70 mL CSF drained at 2 hours; VL perfusion with 240 mL 0.9% NaCl over 3 hours; intrathecal administration of 1,000 units $CPDG_2$ at 8.5 hours; 32% recovery in initial drainage fluid; 58% recovery from perfusion drainage	Survived
Methotrexate[125]	Case series, n = 7	Medication errors: 155–600 mg	5/7 patients with seizures, some with headache, nausea, vomiting	Various interventions including VL perfusion started within 1 hour with 500 mL 0.9% NaCl over 4 hours	All survived
Methylene blue[37]	Case series, n = 14	Direct toxicity due to dye or pH: 10–100 mg	Pain headache, paralysis	Not described	11/14 residual paraplegia or weakness
Methylene blue[109]	59/M	6 mL 1% solution; as above	Vomiting, hypotension day 1; paralysis and urinary retention	Not described	Paraplegia and death at 5 years
Morphine[105]	45/F	Inadvertent filling of wrong port of subcutaneous infusion pump; 450 mg	Seizures, hypertension, subarachnoid hemorrhage	12 mL CSF withdrawn, then 550 mL CSF drained at 10 mL/h by gravity over 2–3 days	Survived
Morphine[62]	81/M	Inadvertent: 5 mg	Coma at 4 hours	50 mL CSF drained over 6 minutes, replacement with 50 mL 0.9% NaCl	Survived

(Continued)

TABLE SC7-2	Inadvertent Intrathecal Overdoses and Unintentional Exposures (Continued)				
Xenobiotic	**Age/Sex**	**Mechanism**	**Clinical Findings/Effects**	**Intervention**	**Outcome**
Morphine[133]	47/F	510 mg into wrong port of pump	Myoclonic spasms, coma, seizures, cranial neuropathy, hypertension then hypotension	No CSF interventions	Survived
Neostigmine[75]	26/M	Medication error	????	None	Survived
PEG asparaginase[85]	12/M	Wrong route	None	None	Survived
Penicillin[21]	22/M	Dosing error into Ommaya reservoir	Coma, hyporeflexia, tonic–clonic seizures, absence seizures, hypotension at 30 minutes	10 mL CSF withdrawal, then VL CSF drainage; replacement with LR over 30 minutes	Survived
Potassium chloride[82]	42/F	Medication error during labor	Immediate cramps, pain, seizures, normal serum potassium	None	Maternal–fetal death at 3 hours
Potassium chloride[30]	62/M	Medication error during anesthesia	Pain, cramps, hypertension, tachycardia, weakness, paresthesia, paraplegia	Removal of 50 mL CSF replaced with saline then removal of 20 mL CSF replaced with saline	Recovery beginning at 8 hours with no sequelae at 2 months
Tramadol[12]	75/F	Connection error	Diaphoresis, hypotension at 10 minutes; myoclonic spasms, opisthotonos	None	Fatal at 48 hours
Tranexamic acid[131]	49/F	Medication error, wrong route	Immediate back pain, hypertension; seizure at 2 minutes; ventricular fibrillation	None	Fatal at 1.5 hours
Vincristine[78]	5/F	Medication error: 0.9 mg	Headache at 10 hours, opisthotonos, nystagmus, flaccidity	None	Fatal on day 18
Vincristine[106]	2.5/F	Medication error: 3 mg	Opisthotonos day 2	200 mL CSF drainage in 10-mL aliquots; replacement with 0.9% NaCl	Fatal on day 3
Vincristine[69]	27/F	Medication error into Ommaya reservoir	Ascending paralysis	Detail limited: CNS "washout" FFP and "lactate solution" in undefined quantities; timing not described	Fatal on day 10
Vincristine[126]	16/M	Mislabeled	Ascending paralysis at 2 hours, fever, coma	None	Fatal
Vincristine[33]	Adult	Medication error	Ascending paralysis	CSF drainage of unreported quantity and replacement with LR immediately; VL perfusion 150 mL/h for >24 hours, then 25 mL FFP in 1 L isotonic solution at 75 mL/h for undefined time; 95% recovery of vincristine	Lower extremity neuropathy
Vincristine[39]	4/F	Medication error: 1.5 mg	Nystagmus, encephalopathy, ascending paralysis, transient improvement	Immediate drainage of 18 mL CSF in 3-mL aliquots, replacement 0.9% NaCl; an additional 30–40 mL drained over 30 minutes, starting at 10 minutes; VL perfusion using Plasma-Lyte to replace 200 mL CSF over an unknown rate, then 6 mL FFP in 250 mL Plasma-Lyte at 50 mL/h for 4 hours	Fatal on day 13
Vincristine[4]	1.25/M	Medication error: 0.7 mg	Febrile and irritable at 10 hours then lower extremity pain, nuchal rigidity, opisthotonos, ileus, hypotonia at day 2; ascending paralysis, encephalopathy by day 5; respiratory arrest at day 7	Intrathecal corticosteroids at 10 hours	Death on day 75 (withdrawal of life support)
Vincristine[5]	7/F	Medication error: 0.5 mg	Ascending weakness, pain, paraplegia	Upright position; immediate drainage 75 mL CSF within 15 min, replaced with LR; VL perfusion started within 2 hours with 150 mL/h of LR for 10 hours, then FFP 15 mL in 1 L LR as irrigant at 55 mL/h for 24 hours Other efforts	Paraplegia, neurogenic bladder Survived

(Continued)

TABLE SC7–2 Inadvertent Intrathecal Overdoses and Unintentional Exposures (*Continued*)

Xenobiotic	Age/Sex	Mechanism	Clinical Findings/Effects	Intervention	Outcome
Vincristine[6]	12/F	Medication error: 2 mg	Asymptomatic for 48 hours, then ascending paralysis, hiccups, cranial neuropathy, coma	35 mL CSF drained at 30 min, then additional drainage of 15 mL CSF replaced with LR; VL perfusion at 3 hours using FFP 15 mL in 1 L LR for total drainage of 615 mL CSF over 10 hours; 0.785 mg recovered	Death on day 83
Vincristine[17]	23/M	Medication error: 2 mg	Headache day 1; leg weakness day 2–3; ascending myeloencephalopathy with coma at day 10; seizures	Drainage of 100 mL CSF at 10 minutes, "large volume lumbar punctures" on day 2 and 3	Prolonged coma, death at 11 months
Vincristine series[29]		Medication error			
Patient 1	5/F		Ascending paralysis, opisthotonos, coma	Not described	Death on day 7
Patient 2	57/M		Ascending paralysis	"Flushing the subarachnoid space"	Death at 4 weeks
Vincristine[67]	3/M	Medication error	Day 1: leg pain; Day 2: headache, nuchal rigidity; Day 3: bladder dysfunction, fever, lower extremity paralysis, opisthotonos and coma	Not described	Death on day 6
Vincristine[83]	59/F	Medication error into Ommaya reservoir: 2 mg	Nausea, vomiting day 1; altered mental status, tremor, chills, hiccups, nystagmus, coma over 1 week	50 mL CSF drainage at 10 minutes followed by 75 mL CSF drainage at 30 minutes; VL perfusion with LR and FFP over 24 hours	Death on day 40
Vincristine[84]	10/F	Medication error	Asymptomatic for 6 days, then ascending paralysis with incontinence	Immediate drainage of CSF for 15 minutes; epidural catheter above the lumbar drainage site with lumbolumbar irrigation using 12.5 mL FFP in 500 mL LR with 96 mL drained; VL perfusion within 90 minutes for 24 hours	Survived with sensory-motor deficits of the extremities and urinary incontinence
Vincristine[110]	5.5	1.2 mg	Headache, vomiting, and backache at 3 hours, nystagmus, extremity weakness at 72 hours, autonomic instability, hiccups, encephalopathy	Drainage of 20 mL CSF at 30 minutes, repeated on day 2, intrathecal corticosteroids, 23% recovery of dose	Death on day 12
Vincristine[111]	29/F	2 mg	Headache, ascending paraplegia, cranial neuropathy, coma	Intrathecal infusion 5 mL 0.9% NaCl with drainage of 10 mL CSF, positioned upright, additional 60 mL CSF drained at 3 hours	Death on day 14, pulmonary embolus at autopsy
Ziconotide series[95]		Overtitration of therapeutic dosage in each case		Stopped medication in each case	Improved days to weeks later
Patient 1	47/M		Nystagmus, auditory and visual hallucinations, dysmetria, ataxia		Retrograde amnesia; Resolution with discontinuation of medication
Patient 2	62/M for pain of multiple sclerosis		Agitation, disorientation, waxing and waning mental status, hallucinations, allodynia, bradycardia		Resolution with discontinuation of medication; worsening multiple sclerosis at 1 year
Patient 3	45/M		Nausea, lightheadedness, nystagmus, bradycardia, agitation		Resolution with discontinuation

ATCS = ascending tonic–clonic syndrome (myoclonus, hyperreflexia on minimal stimulation, beginning in the lower extremities); CNS = central nervous system; CPDG2 = carboxypeptidase G₂; CSF = cerebrospinal fluid; FFP = fresh-frozen plasma; LR = lactated Ringer solution; VL = ventriculolumbar; VP = ventriculoperitoneal.

Pump failures also result in overinfusion. The tubing and gears can be compromised by manufacturing issues, time since implantation, or use of medications not specifically approved for the device. These unapproved drugs can leak or corrode the device and impair responsiveness of the controls on delivery rates. The combination of device age and use of drugs not specifically approved for the device substantially increased the risk of device failure from one major manufacturer.[44,76]

Intrathecal pump overdoses also occur with errors in refilling pumps that are otherwise intact. Some pumps contain 2 access sites, one of which is contiguous with the intrathecal space and allows for CSF withdrawal or injection of nonionic contrast media for imaging. The other access site is a depot port that is intermittently filled with concentrated amounts of drug (usually an opioid or baclofen) to be delivered through a programmable pump. In some patients, a template must be placed on the skin overlying subcutaneous pumps to ascertain the proper medication port. Errors occur when a concentrated bolus is inadvertently injected into the wrong port, resulting in a massive, sometimes fatal, overdose.[60,129] Massive intrathecal morphine overdose can have severe rapid symptoms, including adrenergic crisis.

When intrathecal overdose is suspected from either a refill error or pump malfunction, the clinical service that placed and manages the pump should be consulted. They can assist in device interrogation and gaining CSF access.[32] Either re-accessing the CSF port immediately or placing a spinal needle into the intrathecal space at another site is critical for the withdrawal of CSF. Large-volume drainage (>100 mL in adults in 20–30-mL aliquots) with isotonic fluid replacement is required, as well as other supportive measures such as intravenous naloxone if opioid toxicity is present. Some of these patients will require intubation and care in an intensive care unit.

If the consultant is not readily available, emptying the depot port will automatically cause the pump motor to stop. Any removed product should be carefully measured and preserved. Based on the programmed rate of delivery and time and volume of last refill, the volume expected from emptying the pump reservoir can be calculated. In suspected device failure, retrieval of a volume less than expected confirms an overinfusion into the intrathecal space. Medical care will often be specific to the xenobiotic delivered. Ideally pumps with erratic delivery or confirmed overinfusion should be replaced and the failed pump sent to the manufacturer for analysis.[44,76]

ERROR PREVENTION

All intrathecal medication errors are preventable.[47] Mechanisms for prevention are well described.[36,79] They include trained pharmacists and administering physicians, specialized packaging and handling, use of minibags for intrathecal medications whenever feasible, preadministration of any intravenous medications, removal of all syringes and other medications from the area, and a checklist and time out, with 2 persons reviewing all labels. Non-Luer lock systems are being adopted in the United Kingdom to limit connection errors, by assuring incompatibility[88] and recently FDA final guidelines has occurred on the topic in the United States. Any adopted system of prevention should include steps for intrathecal administration of required xenobiotics in all settings, including treatment wards, outpatient clinics, radiology suites, and the operating room, as well as by all intrathecal routes such as implantable pumps, Ommaya reservoirs, and lumbar or other access points.

SUMMARY

- Intrathecal medication errors can be life-threatening.
- Errors occur during preparation or administration.
- Rapid intervention with CSF drainage should be considered when a dosing or medication error occurs.
- Some intrathecal chemotherapeutic errors are fatal, and time to CSF drainage is critical to outcome.
- Pump failures precipitate either withdrawal or overdose depending on the malfunction.
- Any drug removed from a pump reservoir should be carefully measured and preserved

REFERENCES

1. Aalfs RL, Connelly JF. Comment: dilution of vancomycin for intrathecal or intraventricular administration. *Ann Pharmacother*. 1996;30:415.
2. Abrutyn E, Berlin JA. Intrathecal therapy in tetanus. A meta-analysis. *JAMA*. 1991;266: 2262-2267.
3. Addiego JE Jr, et al. The acute management of intrathecal methotrexate overdose: pharmacologic rationale and guidelines. *J Pediatr*. 1981;98:825-828.
4. al Fawaz IM. Fatal myeloencephalopathy due to intrathecal vincristine administration. *Ann Trop Paediatr*. 1992;12:339-342.
5. Al Ferayan A, et al. Cerebrospinal fluid lavage in the treatment of inadvertent intrathecal vincristine injection. *Childs Nerv Syst*. 1999;15:87-89.
6. Alcaraz A, et al. Intrathecal vincristine: fatal myeloencephalopathy despite cerebrospinal fluid perfusion. *J Toxicol Clin Toxicol*. 2002;40:557-561.
7. Amjal M. Accidental intrathecal injection of aminophylline in spinal anesthesia. *Anesthesiology*. 2011;114:998-1000.
8. Arico M, et al. Severe acute encephalopathy following inadvertent intrathecal doxorubicin administration. *Med Pediatr Oncol*. 1990;18:261-263.
9. Arlt S, et al. Gadolinium encephalopathy due to accidental intrathecal administration of gadopentetate dimeglumine. *J Neurol*. 2007;254:810-812.
10. Balis FM, et al. Methotrexate distribution within the subarachnoid space after intraventricular and intravenous administration. *Cancer Chemother Pharmacol*. 2000;45:259-264.
11. Barret GS. Treatment if pneumococcal meningitis with sulfadiazine and intrathecal penicillin G with recovery. *Ann Intern Med*. 1948;28:642-647.
12. Barrett NA, Sundaraj SR. Inadvertent intrathecal injection of tramadol. *Br J Anaesth*. 2003;91:918-920.
13. Bearer EL, et al. Squid axoplasm supports the retrograde axonal transport of herpes simplex virus. *Biol Bull*. 1999;197:257-258.
14. Benifla M, et al. Successful treatment of *Acinetobacter meningitis* with intrathecal polymyxin E. *J Antimicrob Chemother*. 2004;54:290-292.
15. Berning SE, et al. Novel treatment of meningitis caused by multidrug-resistant *Mycobacterium tuberculosis* with intrathecal levofloxacin and amikacin: case report. *Clin Infect Dis*. 2001;32:643-646.
16. Bhatia VS, Sethi SV. Inadvertent intrathecal injection of labetalol. *Saudi J Anesth*. 2016;10:345-346.
17. Bleck TP, Jacobsen J. Prolonged survival following the inadvertent intrathecal administration of vincristine: clinical and electrophysiologic analyses. *Clin Neuropharmacol*. 1991;14:457-462.
18. Bomgaars L, et al. Phase I trial of intrathecal liposomal cytarabine in children with neoplastic meningitis. *J Clin Oncol*. 2004;22:3916-3921.
19. Bonicalzi V, Canavero S. Intrathecal ziconotide for chronic pain. *JAMA*. 2004;292: 1681-1682.
20. Brossner G, et al. Accidental intrathecal infusion of cefotiam: clinical presentation and management. *Eur J Clin Pharmacol*. 2004;60:373-375.
21. Callaghan JT, et al. CSF perfusion to treat intraventricular penicillin toxicity. *Arch Neurol*. 1981;38:390-391.
22. Cardan E. Intrathecal frusemide. *Anaesthesia*. 1985;40:1025.
23. Chiari A, et al. Analgesic and hemodynamic effects of intrathecal clonidine as the sole analgesic agent during first stage of labor: a dose-response study. *Anesthesiology*. 1999;91:388-396.
24. Clara N. CSF exchange after the erroneous intrathecal injection of 800 mg ceftriaxone for pneumococcal meningitis. *J Antimicrob Chemother*. 1986;17:263-265.
25. Coffey RJ, Burchiel K. Inflammatory mass lesions associated with intrathecal drug infusion catheters: report and observations on 41 patients. *Neurosurgery*. 2002;50:78-86.
26. Coffey RJ, et al. Abrupt withdrawal from intrathecal baclofen: recognition and management of a potentially life-threatening syndrome. *Arch Phys Med Rehabil*. 2002;83:735-741.
27. Collier C. Collapse after epidural injection following inadvertent dural perforation. *Anesthesiology*. 1982;57:427-428.
28. Corpus KA, et al. Intrathecal amikacin for the treatment of pseudomonal meningitis. *Ann Pharmacother*. 2004;38:992-995.
29. Dettmeyer R, et al. Fatal myeloencephalopathy due to accidental intrathecal vincristine administration: a report of two cases. *Forensic Sci Int*. 2001;122:60-64.
30. Dias J, et al. Accidental spinal potassium chloride successfully treated with spinal lavage. *Anaesthesia*. 2014;69:72-76.
31. Dobrydnjov I, Samarutel J. Enhancement of intrathecal lidocaine by the addition of local and systemic clonidine. *Acta Anaesthesiolo Scandinavica*. 1999;43:556-562.
32. Dressnandt J, et al. Acute overdose of intrathecal baclofen. *J Neurol*. 1996;243:482-483.
33. Dyke RW. Treatment of inadvertent intrathecal injection of vincristine. *N Engl J Med*. 1989;321:1270-1271.
34. Ettinger LJ, et al. Intrathecal methotrexate overdose without neurotoxicity: case report and literature review. *Cancer*. 1978;41:1270-1273.
35. Ettinger LJ. Pharmacokinetics and biochemical effects of a fatal intrathecal methotrexate overdose. *Cancer*. 1982;50:444-450.
36. European Medicines Agency. Questions and answers: recommendations to prevent administration error with Velcade (bortezomib). http://www.ema.europa.eu/docs/en_GB/document_library/Medicine_QA/2012/01/WC500120701.pdf. Accessed January 18, 2013.
37. Evans JP, Keegan HR. Danger in the use of intrathecal methylene blue. *JAMA*. 1960; 174:856-859.
38. Evans PJ, et al. Accidental intrathecal injection of bupivacaine and dextran. *Anaesthesia*. 1981;36:685-687.
39. Fernandez CV, et al. Intrathecal vincristine: an analysis of reasons for recurrent fatal chemotherapeutic error with recommendations for prevention. *J Pediatr Hematol Oncol*. 1998;20:587-590.
40. Ferrara VL. Post myelographic nerve palsy in association with contrast agent iopamidol. *J Clin Neuroophthalmol*. 1991;11:74.
41. Finkelstein Y, et al. Emergency treatment of life-threatening intrathecal methotrexate overdose. *Neurotoxicology*. 2004;25:407-410.
42. Fujita T, et al. MRSA meningitis and intrathecal injection of arbekacin. *Surg Neurol*. 1997;48:69.
43. Gaidys WG, et al. Intrathecal vincristine. Report of a fatal case despite CNS washout. *Cancer*. 1983;52:799-801.
44. Galica R, et al. Sudden intrathecal drug delivery device motor stalls: a case series. *Reg Anesth Pain Med*. 2016;41:135-139.
45. Gilbar P. Inadvertent intrathecal administration of vincristine—has anything changed? *J Oncol Pharm Pract*. 2012;18:155-157.
46. Gilbar PJ, Carrington CV. Preventing intrathecal administration of vincristine. *Med J Aust*. 2004;181:464.
47. Gilbar PJ, Seger AC. Fatalities resulting from accidental intrathecal administration of bortezomib. Strategies for prevention. *J Clin Oncol*. 2012;30:3427-3428.

48. Goldstein EJC, et al. Intrathecal amphotericin B—a 60 year experience in treating coccoidal meningitis. *Clin Infect Dis.* 2017;64:519-526.

49. Goodman SR, et al. Epinephrine is not a useful addition to intrathecal fentanyl or fentanyl-bupivacaine for labor analgesia. *Reg Anesth Pain Med.* 2002;27:374-379.

50. Goonewardene TW, et al. Accidental subarachnoid injection of gallamine. A case report. *Br J Anaesth.* 1975;47:889-893.

51. Gopal G. Preliminary studies on cerebrospinal fluid exchange transfusion. *Indian Pediatr.* 1979;16:227-228.

52. Gosselin S, Isbister GK. Re: treatment of accidental intrathecal methotrexate overdose. *J Natl Cancer Inst.* 2005;97:609-610.

53. Govindan K, et al. Intrathecal ketamine in surgeries for lower abdomen and lower extremities. *Proc West Pharmacol Soc.* 2001;44:197-199.

54. Hew CM, et al. Avoiding inadvertent epidural injection of drugs intended for non-epidural use. *Anaesth Intensive Care.* 2003;31:44-49.

55. Hocking G, Wildsmith JA. Intrathecal drug spread. *Br J Anaesth.* 2004;93:568-578.

56. Hodgson PS, et al. The neurotoxicity of drugs given intrathecally (spinal). *Anesth Analg.* 1999;88:797-809.

57. Huang TY, et al. Supratentorial cerebrospinal fluid production rate in healthy adults: quantification with two-dimensional cine phase-contrast MR imaging with high temporal and spatial resolution. *Radiology.* 2004;233:603-608.

58. Jakobson AM, et al. Cerebrospinal fluid exchange after intrathecal methotrexate overdose. A report of two cases. *Acta Paediatr.* 1992;81:359-361.

59. Jardine LF, et al. Intrathecal leucovorin after intrathecal methotrexate overdose. *J Pediatr Hematol Oncol.* 1996;18:302-304.

60. Jones TF, et al. Neurologic complications including paralysis after a medication error involving implanted intrathecal catheters. *Am J Med.* 2002;112:31-36.

61. Jordan B, et al. Neurological improvement and rehabilitation potential following toxic myelopathy due to intrathecal injection of doxorubicin. *Spinal Cord.* 2004;42:371-373.

62. Kaiser KG, Bainton CR. Treatment of intrathecal morphine overdose by aspiration of cerebrospinal fluid. *Anesth Analg.* 1987;66:475-477.

63. Kao LW, et al. Intrathecal baclofen withdrawal mimicking sepsis. *J Emerg Med.* 2003;24:423-427.

64. Kaplan KM, Brose WG. Intrathecal methods. *Neurosurg Clin N Am.* 2004;15:289-296.

65. Kavan P, et al. Management and sequelae after misapplied intrathecal dactinomycin. *Med Pediatr Oncol.* 2001;36:339-340.

66. Kroin JS, et al. The distribution of medication along the spinal canal after chronic intrathecal administration. *Neurosurgery.* 1993;33:226-230.

67. Kwack EK, et al. Neural toxicity induced by accidental intrathecal vincristine administration. *J Korean Med Sci.* 1999;14:688-692.

68. Lafolie P, et al. Exchange of cerebrospinal fluid in accidental intrathecal overdose of cytarabine. *Med Toxicol Adverse Drug Exp.* 1988;3:248-252.

69. Lau G. Accidental intraventricular vincristine administration: an avoidable iatrogenic death. *Med Sci Law.* 1996;36:263-265.

70. Lauretti GR, et al. Dose-response study of intrathecal morphine versus intrathecal neostigmine, their combination, or placebo for postoperative analgesia in patients undergoing anterior and posterior vaginoplasty. *Anesth Analg.* 2003;82:1182-1187.

71. Lee AC, et al. Intrathecal methotrexate overdose. *Acta Paediatr.* 1997;86:434-437.

72. Lee HM, et al. Intrathecal clonidine pump failure causing acute withdrawal syndrome with stress induced cardiomyopathy. *J Med Toxicol.* 2016;12:134-138.

73. Lejuste MJ. Inadvertent intrathecal administration of magnesium sulfate. *S Afr Med J.* 1985;68:367-368.

74. Mahajan R, Gupta R. Cerebrospinal fluid physiology and cerebrospinal fluid drainage. *Anesthesiology.* 2004;100:1620.

75. Maheshwari S, et al. Accidental intrathecal injection of a very large dose of neostigmine methylsulphate. *Indian J Anaesth.* 2003;47:299-301.

76. Maino P, et al. Fentanyl overdose caused by malfunction of SynchromedII intrathecal pump. *Reg Anesth and Pain Med.* 2014;39:434-437.

77. Makar G, et al. Successful large volume cerebrospinal aspiration for an accidental overdose of cytarabine. *Med Oncol.* 2013;30:525.

78. Manelis J, et al. Accidental intrathecal vincristine administration. Report of a case. *J Neurol.* 1982;228:209-213.

79. Marliot G, et al. Securing the circuit of intrathecally administered cancer drugs: example of a collective approach. *J Oncol Pharm Pract.* 2011;17:252-259.

80. Mason N, et al. Intrathecal sufentanil and morphine for post-thoracotomy pain relief. *Br J Anaesth.* 2001;86:236-240.

81. Matsubara H, et al. Successful treatment of meningoencephalitis caused by methicillin-resistant *Staphylococcus aureus* with intrathecal vancomycin in an allogeneic peripheral blood stem cell transplant recipient. *Bone Mar Trans.* 2003;31:65-67.

82. Meel B. Inadvertent intrathecal administration of potassium chloride during routine spinal anesthesia: case report. *Am J Forens Med Pathol.* 1998;19:255-257.

83. Meggs WJ, Hoffman RS. Fatality resulting from intraventricular vincristine administration. *J Toxicol Clin Toxicol.* 1998;36:243-246.

84. Michelagnoli MP, et al. Potential salvage therapy for inadvertent intrathecal administration of vincristine. *Br J Haematol.* 1997;99:364-367.

85. Naqvi A, Fadoo Z. Inadvertent intrathecal injection of PEG-asparaginase. *J Pediatr Hematol Oncol.* 2010;32:1416.

86. Oka K, et al. The significance of artificial cerebrospinal fluid as perfusate and endoneurosurgery. *Neurosurgery.* 1996;38:733-736.

87. O'Marcaigh AS, et al. Successful treatment of intrathecal methotrexate overdose by using ventriculolumbar perfusion and intrathecal instillation of carboxypeptidase G2. *Mayo Clin Proc.* 1996;71:161-165.

88. Onia R, et al. Simulated evaluation of a non-Luer safety connector system for use in neuroaxial procedures. *Br J Anaesth.* 2012;108:134-139.

89. Paice JA, et al. Intrathecal octreotide for relief of intractable nonmalignant pain: 5-year experience with two cases. *Neurosurgery.* 1996;38:203-207.

90. Palmieri C, et al. The Vincotube System: a design solution to prevent the accidental administration of intrathecal vinca alkaloids. *J Clin Oncol.* 2004;22:965.

91. Peng P, Massicotte EM. Spinal cord compression from intrathecal catheter-tip inflammatory mass: case report and a review of etiology. *Reg Anesth Pain Med.* 2004;29:237-242.

92. Penn RD. Intrathecal medication delivery. *Neurosurg Clin N Am.* 2003;14:381-387.

93. Penn RD, Kroin JS. Treatment of intrathecal morphine overdose. *J Neurosurg.* 1995;82:147-148.

94. Penn RD, et al. Intraventricular bethanechol infusion for Alzheimer's disease: results of double-blind and escalating-dose trials. *Neurology.* 1988;38:219-222.

95. Penn RD, Paice JA. Adverse effects associated with intrathecal administration of ziconotide. *Pain.* 2000;85:291-296.

96. Penn RD, et al. Octreotide: a potent new non-opiate analgesic for intrathecal infusion. *Pain.* 1992;49:13-19.

97. Qweider M, et al. Inadvertent intrathecal vincristine administration: a neurosurgical emergency. *J Neurosurg Spine.* 2007;6:280-283.

98. Reeves RK, et al. Hyperthermia, rhabdomyolysis, and disseminated intravascular coagulation associated with baclofen pump catheter failure. *Arch Phys Med Rehabil.* 1998;79:353-356.

99. Reiber H. Flow rate of cerebrospinal fluid (CSF)—a concept common to normal blood-CSF barrier function and to dysfunction in neurological diseases. *J Neurol Sci.* 1994;122:189-203.

100. Rommer PS, et al. Long term effects of repeated cycles of intrathecal triamcinolone acetonide on spasticity in MS patients. *CNS Neuro Sci Ther.* 2016;22:74-79.

101. Root T. Accidental injection of vincristine. *J Oncol Phar Pract.* 2005;11:35.

102. Rosati G, et al. Serious or fatal complications after inadvertent administration of ionic water-soluble contrast media in myelography. *Eur J Radiol.* 1992;15:95-100.

103. Rosenberg H, Grant M. Ascending tonic-clonic syndrome secondary to intrathecal Omnipaque. *J Clin Anesth.* 2004;16:299-300.

104. Salvolini U, et al. Accidental intrathecal injection of ionic water-soluble contrast medium: report of a case, including treatment. *Neuroradiology.* 1996;38:349-351.

105. Sauter K. Correction: treatment of high dose intrathecal morphine overdose. *J Neurosurg.* 1994;81:813.

106. Schochet SS Jr, et al. Neuronal changes induced by intrathecal vincristine sulfate. *J Neuropathol Exp Neurol.* 1968;27:645-658.

107. Segal-Maurer S, et al. Successful treatment of ceftazidime-resistant *Klebsiella pneumoniae* ventriculitis with intravenous meropenem and intraventricular polymyxin B: case report and review. *Clin Infect Dis.* 1999;28:1134-1138.

108. Senbaga N, Davies EM. Inadvertent intrathecal administration of rifampicin. *Brit J Clin Pharmacol.* 2005;60:116.

109. Sharr MM, et al. Spinal cord necrosis after intrathecal injection of methylene blue. *J Neurol Neurosurg Psychiatry.* 1978;41:384-386.

110. Shepherd DA, et al. Accidental intrathecal administration of vincristine. *Med Pediatr Oncol.* 1978;5:85-88.

111. Slyter H, et al. Fatal myeloencephalopathy caused by intrathecal vincristine. *Neurology.* 1980;30:867-871.

112. Smilack J, McCloskey RV. Intrathecal gentamicin. *Ann Intern Med.* 1972;77:1002-1003.

113. Southorn P, et al. Reducing the potential morbidity of an unintentional spinal anaesthetic by aspirating cerebrospinal fluid. *Br J Anaesth.* 1996;76:467-469.

114. Spiegel RJ, et al. Treatment of massive intrathecal methotrexate overdose by ventriculolumbar perfusion. *N Engl J Med.* 1984;311:386-388.

115. Stark AM, et al. Accidental intrathecal mercury application. *Eur Spine J.* 2004;13:241-243.

116. Stefanou A, Dooley M. Simple method to eliminate risk of inadvertent intrathecal vincristine administration. *J Clin Oncol.* 2003;21:2044.

117. Svensson LG, et al. Appraisal of cerebrospinal fluid alterations during aortic surgery with intrathecal papaverine administration and cerebrospinal fluid drainage. *J Vasc Surg.* 1990;11:423-429.

118. Tartiere J, et al. Acute treatment after accidental intrathecal injection of hypertonic contrast media. *Anesthesiology.* 1989;71:169.

119. Tournel G, et al. Fatal accidental intrathecal injection of vindesine. *J Forensic Sci.* 2006;51:1166-1168.

120. Trinkle R, Wu JK. Intrathecal methotrexate overdoses. *Acta Paediatr.* 1998;87:116-117.

121. Tsui BC, et al. Reversal of an unintentional spinal anesthetic by cerebrospinal lavage. *Anesth Analg.* 2004;98:434-436.

122. van der Leede H, et al. Inadvertent intrathecal use of ionic contrast agent. *Eur Radiol.* 2002;12:S86-S93.

123. Vasen W, et al. Intrathecal use of colistin. *J Clin Microbiol.* 2000;38:3523.

124. Walker RH, et al. Intrathecal baclofen for dystonia: benefits and complications during six years of experience. *Mov Disord.* 2000;15:1242-1247.

125. Widemann BC, et al. Treatment of accidental intrathecal methotrexate overdose with intrathecal carboxypeptidase G2. *J Natl Cancer Inst.* 2004;96:1557-1559.

126. Williams ME, et al. Ascending myeloencephalopathy due to intrathecal vincristine sulfate. A fatal chemotherapeutic error. *Cancer.* 1983;51:2041-2047.

127. Wolman L. The neuropathological effects resulting from the intrathecal injection of chemical substances. *Paraplegia.* 1966;4:97-115.

128. Woods K. The prevention of intrathecal medication errors. A report to the Chief Medical Officer. Department of Health, UK: Crown Copyright; 2001.

129. Wu CL, Patt RB. Accidental overdose of systemic morphine during intended refill of intrathecal infusion device. *Anesth Analg.* 1992;75:130-132.

130. Yegin A, et al. The analgesic and sedative effects of intrathecal midazolam in perianal surgery. *Eur J Anaesthesiol.* 2004;21:658-662.

131. Yeh HM, et al. Convulsions and refractory ventricular fibrillation after intrathecal injection of a massive dose of tranexamic acid. *Anesthesiology.* 2003;98:270-272.

132. Yeh RN, et al. Baclofen toxicity in an 8-year-old with an intrathecal baclofen pump. *J Emerg Med.* 2004;26:163-167.

133. Yilmaz A, et al. Successful treatment of intrathecal morphine overdose. *Neurol India.* 2003;51:410-411.

134. Zaragoza MR, et al. Neurourologic consequences of accidental intrathecal vincristine: a case report. *Med Pediatr Oncol.* 1995;24:61-62.

EXTRAVASATION OF XENOBIOTICS

Richard Y. Wang

Extravasation injuries are among the most consequential local toxic events. When the vesicant chemotherapeutics leak into the perivascular space, significant necrosis of skin, muscles, and tendons occurs, with resultant loss of function, infection, and deformity. Typical initial manifestations include swelling, pain, and a burning sensation that can last for hours. Days later, the area becomes erythematous and indurated, followed by resolution or progression to ulceration and necrosis. These early findings are often difficult to distinguish from other forms of local drug toxicity, such as irritation and hypersensitivity, which can result from the chemotherapeutic or its vehicle (ethanol, propylene glycol) and do not progress to ulceration and necrosis. For example, fluorouracil, carmustine, cisplatin, and dacarbazine are local irritants. The local irritation and hypersensitivity manifestations are self-limiting and typified by an immediate onset of a burning sensation, pruritus, erythema, and a flare reaction of the vein receiving the infused. The extravasation of monoclonal antibodies causes minimal discomfort and inflammation.[15,37,49] When a hypersensitivity reaction or an irritation to the vessel cannot be differentiated from extravasation, it is prudent to presume extravasation and manage the situation accordingly.

The occurrence of extravasations appears to be more frequent with inexperienced clinicians.[19] Factors associated with extravasation injuries from peripheral intravenous lines include (1) poor vessel integrity and blood flow, such as those found in the elderly and in patients with numerous venipuncture attempts or who have received radiation therapy to the site; (2) limited venous and lymphatic drainage caused by either obstruction or surgical resection; and (3) the use of venous access overlying a joint, which increases the risk of dislodgments because of movement.[18,40]

In children, the use of a steel needle (butterfly) or a small catheter that easily allows blood to flow around the catheter increases the risk for an extravasation.[10] Children require frequent monitoring of the intravenous site for possible extravasation. Extravasation injuries from implanted ports in central veins occurs from inadequate placement of the needle, needle dislodgment, damaged septum, fibrin sheath formation around the catheter, perforation of the superior vena cava, and fracture of the catheter.[44] When extravasation from a central venous access device is suspected and plain radiographic studies are not diagnostic, a contrast-enhanced CT scan of the anatomic location is necessary for evaluation because the extent of the injury is often underestimated at the bedside.[1,2,37]

The factors associated with a poor outcome from extravasation injuries include (1) areas of the body with little subcutaneous tissue, such as the dorsum of the hand, volar surface of the wrist, and the antecubital fossa, where healing is poor and vital structures are more likely to be involved; (2) increased concentrations of extravasate; (3) increased volume and duration of contact with tissue; and (4) the type of chemotherapeutic.[40,41]

Vesicants, such as doxorubicin, daunorubicin, dactinomycin, epirubicin, idarubicin, mechlorethamine, mitomycin, and the vinca alkaloids produce more significant local tissue destruction than other types of chemotherapeutics, such as irritants. Mitomycin infusions cause dermal ulcerations at venipuncture sites remote from the location of administration.[36] The anthracycline antibiotics are associated with a higher incidence of significant injuries and delayed healing, which likely result from their slow release from bound tissue into surrounding viable tissue. Doxorubicin extravasation is associated with local tissue necrosis in approximately 25% of reported cases. The extravasation injuries from

taxanes appear similar to the vesicants, but are less severe in response and more delayed in presentation.[3,38]

Prevention is the best therapy for extravasation injuries. Clinicians qualified for chemotherapy administration, the development and implementation of procedures for the management of extravasations, and the safe administration of chemotherapeutics can limit the extent of these injuries.[8,32,33]

MANAGEMENT

The treatment for extravasation injuries varies by locality based on controversial practices, such as the use of selective antidotes, the use of surgical irrigation, and the timing of surgical wound debridement. This uncertainty is a result of the limited number of clinical cases available for study and the discordance between animal studies and human experience. However, the general and specific management recommendations derived from the literature and their theoretical foundations exist (Table SC8–1).[5,9,24,37,49] Clinical centers should develop and implement procedures for the management of extravasations injuries that are consistent with the current literature and guidelines.[32]

Once extravasation is suspected, the infusion should be immediately halted. A physician should be notified and the xenobiotic, its concentration, and the approximate amount infused should be noted. The venous access should be maintained to permit aspiration of as much of the infusate as possible and administration of an antidote, if indicated. The early surgical irrigation of the extravasation site is recommended by some centers for an extravasation containing more than 5 mL of a vesicant.[49] Irrigation should be initiated within 6 hours of the incident, although it has been used in patients with pain, swelling, and no ulcerations at the site when it was beyond 6 hours.[13,16,49]

The intermittent local application of a dry cold compress and elevation of the extremity is recommended for 48 to 72 hours to limit further progression of the xenobiotic and the development of dependent edema. Cooling the affected area reduces the amount of xenobiotic absorbed by the tissue and lowers the cellular metabolic rate, which limits further tissue damage and cell injury.[23,48] With just the application of a cold compress and strict elevation, only 13 (11%) of 119 patients with mild extravasations required surgical intervention for their injuries in a retrospective review of patients at one center.[28] In the past, heat was recommended to disperse the xenobiotic, but investigations with animals treated with intradermal doxorubicin demonstrated increase in the area of skin ulceration.[12,27] However, dry, warm compresses to promote systemic uptake of the vinca alkaloids (vincristine and vinblastine) and etoposide are recommended.

A warm compress is combined with the immediate local infiltration of hyaluronidase to enhance absorption of an extravasation with a vinca alkaloid or etoposide (Table SC8–1).[6] Hyaluronidase hydrolyzes the beta-1,4-glycosidic bond between N-acetyl-D-glucosamine and D-glucuronic acid in the glycosaminoglycan hyaluronate (hyaluronic acid). Hyaluronate is a natural polymer consisting of the above disaccharide unit, and it contains alternating beta-1,4-glycosidic and beta-1,3-glycosidic bonds. Hyaluronate is produced in the plasma membrane of the cell and it provides structural integrity to the extracellular matrix of soft tissues, such as connective tissue. The enzymatic hydrolysis of hyaluronate promotes the distribution of the chemotherapeutic in the soft tissue space.

Hyaluronidase is also used in the treatment of extravasations with a hyperosmotic infusate (eg, total parenteral nutrition, calcium, potassium, 10%–50% dextrose, and nafcillin).[39]

TABLE SC8–1	Management of Extravasation Injuries	
	Therapy	**Purpose/Mechanism**
General	Stop infusion and maintain intravenous cannula at the site	Decrease further extravasation
	Aspirate extravasate from the site by accessing the original intravenous cannula	Minimizes amount of chemotherapeutic localized at the site
	Apply dry cool compresses for 1 hour, every 8 hours for 3 days	Localizes area of involvement and diminishes cellular uptake of the chemotherapeutic
	Elevate extremity and administer analgesia	Promotes drainage, prevents dependent edema, and provides comfort
	For vinca alkaloids and epipodophyllotoxins, apply dry warm compresses for 1 hour, every 8 hours for 3 days (see specific management)	Promotes systemic absorption of the chemotherapeutic
Chemotherapeutic Specific		
Anthracyclines	Dexrazoxane 1,000 mg/m^2, administered daily by IV (max. 2,000 mg per day), on days 1 and 2, and 500 mg/m^2 on day 3 (max. 1,000 mg); dose is decreased for patients with kidney disease	Limits free radical formation
Mechlorethamine	Add 1.6 mL of 25% sodium thiosulfate to 8.4 mL of sterile water for injection to make a 4% solution	Prevents tissue alkylation
	Infiltrate the site of extravasation with 2 mL of 4% sodium thiosulfate per milligram of mechlorethamine at the site	
Mitomycin	Dimethyl sulfoxide (DMSO): 55%–99% (w/v) applied topically and allowed to air dry	Free radical scavenger
Vinca alkaloids and epipodophyllotoxins	Hyaluronidase: Inject subcutaneously, 150 units/mL into the site as 5 separate and equally spaced injections of 0.2 mL using a 25-gauge or smaller needle at the leading edge of the infiltrate	Degrades hyaluronic acid to enhance systemic absorption of the chemotherapeutic

Human recombinant hyaluronidase (Hylenex) is available as 150 units/mL, and recommendations are to administer it as 5 separate and equally spaced subcutaneous injections of 0.2 mL (30 units) using a 25-gauge or smaller needle at the leading edge of the infiltrate.[17,42,43] Wounds that are either cancerous or infected should not be treated with hyaluronidase. Patients treated with hyaluronidase require monitoring for allergic reactions, such as anaphylaxis, although the newer human recombinant form is less allergenic than animal-derived hyaluronidase.

The wound should be observed closely for the first 7 days, and a surgeon consulted if either pain persists or evidence of ulceration appears.[40] However, in patients with severe extravasations—where there is a high likelihood of necrosis because of the chemotherapeutic (doxorubicin), the volume or concentration, and any area where there may be significant potential for long-term morbidity such as over joints, early surgical consultation is recommended. If tissue ulceration occurs, initial management is often restricted to sterile dressings to prevent secondary infections. Once the area of necrotic skin can be clearly delineated from surviving tissue, surgical debridement is reasonable to limit secondary infection. Some patients require surgical reconstruction or skin grafts depending on the extent of the injury.

ANTIDOTES

Antidotal therapy, when available, is indicated when the extravasated xenobiotic is known to respond poorly to conservative care. The antidotal treatments are categorized by their mechanism of action. Topical steroids were used to reduce the inflammatory response, including hypersensitivity reactions, from extravasated xenobiotics.[22,49] However, this therapy remains a controversial practice for chemotherapeutics that are known to cause direct tissue necrosis, such as doxorubicin and the vinca alkaloids,[4,19,29,46] because inflammatory cells do not predominate at the wound site, and not currently recommended.[7] Sodium thiosulfate is recommended for mechlorethamine extravasation and is believed to inactivate the xenobiotic by reacting with the active ethylenimmonium ring.[18,35] The site should be infiltrated with 2 mL of a sterile 4% (isotonic) sodium thiosulfate solution for each milligram of mechlorethamine, followed by intermittent dry cold compresses for 48 to 72 hours.[6]

Finally, there are antidotes for anthracycline extravasations, such as dimethyl sulfoxide (DMSO) and dexrazoxane. Because dexrazoxane was approved by the FDA for the treatment of anthracycline extravasations in adults, the role for DMSO in the treatment of anthracycline extravasations has become secondary.[21,49] Dimethyl sulfoxide scavenges free radicals that cause tissue damage from chemotherapeutics, such as doxorubicin. Dimethyl sulfoxide was beneficial for anthracycline extravasations in both animal and human clinical trials.[6,12,29,35,45] Dimethyl sulfoxide was used at concentrations varying from 55% to 99% (w/v) and it was applied topically and then followed with intermittent cold compresses.[6,14,29,34] Additional beneficial properties of DMSO are its antiinflammatory, analgesic, and vasodilatory effects, as well as its ability to promote systemic absorption of the chemotherapeutic at local sites.[30] Dimethyl sulfoxide is also recommended for extravasations with mitomycin.

Dexrazoxane limits free radical cellular damage by chelating iron and directly acting as an antioxidant. The systemic administration of dexrazoxane limited anthracycline-induced skin lesions in a murine model[25] and was used successfully in patients following doxorubicin[11,26,47] and epirubicin[20,25] extravasations. In 2 prospective, open-label, single-arm, multicenter clinical trials, the systemic administration of dexrazoxane within 6 hours of anthracycline extravasation resulted in the need for surgical resection of the wound site in only 1 of 54 (1.8%) patients.[31] Dexrazoxane was given to these patients over 3 days intravenously at a starting dose of 1,000 mg/m^2, which was infused over 15 to 30 minutes at a site distant to that of the extravasation because of its irritating properties. Dry cold compresses at the site of the extravasation were discontinued for 15 minutes prior to therapy to promote perfusion of the antidote at the site. The dose of dexrazoxane (Table SC8–1) is decreased for patients with diminished kidney function (creatinine clearance < 40 mL/min). Patients need to be monitored with CBC and serum aminotransferases because dexrazoxane can cause reversible bone marrow suppression and result in hepatotoxicity. Additional clinical evidence needs to be gathered to better define the medical management of other chemotherapeutic extravasations. The overall incidence of extravasations with chemotherapeutics is likely small, the associated morbidity is significant.

SUMMARY

- Prevention is the best form of therapy for these injuries.
- Immediately stop the infusion following a suspected extravasation.
- Aspirate, apply dry cool compresses, elevate the extremity, and administer analgesia.

Disclaimer

The findings and conclusions in this chapter are those of the author and do not necessarily represent the official position of the Centers for Disease Control and Prevention.

REFERENCES

1. Anderson CM, et al. Mediastinitis related to probable central vinblastine extravasation in a woman undergoing adjuvant chemotherapy for early breast cancer. *Am J Clin Oncol.* 1996;19:566-568.
2. Azais H, et al. Chemotherapy drug extravasation in totally implantable venous access port systems: how effective is early surgical lavage? *J Vasc Access.* 2015;16:31-37.
3. Bailey WL, Crump RM. Taxol extravasation: a case report. *Can Oncol Nurs J.* 1997;7:96-99.
4. Barlock AL, et al. Nursing management of adriamycin extravasation. *Am J Nurs.* 1979;79:94-96.
5. Bertelli G. Prevention and management of extravasation of cytotoxic drugs. *Drug Saf.* 1995;12:245-255.
6. Bertelli G, et al. Topical dimethylsulfoxide for the prevention of soft tissue injury after extravasation of vesicant cytotoxic drugs: a prospective clinical study. *J Clin Oncol.* 1995;13:2851-2855.
7. Bhawan J, et al. Histologic changes induced in skin by extravasation of doxorubicin (adriamycin). *J Cutan Pathol.* 1989;16:158-163.
8. Boulanger J, et al. Management of the extravasation of anti-neoplastic agents. *Support Care Cancer.* 2015;23:1459-1471.
9. British Columbia Cancer Agency. Prevention and management of extravasation of chemotherapy. http://www.bccancer.bc.ca/systemic-therapy-site/Documents/Policy%20and%20Forms/III_20_ExtravasationManagement_1May2016.pdf. Published 2016. Accessed August 21, 2012.
10. Chanes DC, et al. Antineoplastic agents extravasation from peripheral intravenous line in children: a simple strategy for a safer nursing care. *Eur J Oncol Nurs.* 2012;16:17-25.
11. Conde-Estevez D, et al. Successful dexrazoxane treatment of a potentially severe extravasation of concentrated doxorubicin. *Anticancer Drugs.* 2010;21:790-794.
12. Desai MH, Teres D. Prevention of doxorubicin-induced skin ulcers in the rat and pig with dimethyl sulfoxide (DMSO). *Cancer Treat Rep.* 1982;66:1371-1374.
13. Dionyssiou D, et al. The wash-out technique in the management of delayed presentations of extravasation injuries. *J Hand Surg Eur Vol.* 2011;36:66-69.
14. Ener RA, et al. Extravasation of systemic hemato-oncological therapies. *Ann Oncol.* 2004;15:858-862.
15. Ferrari LA, et al. Cytotoxic extravasation: an issue disappearing or a problem without solution? *Tumori.* 2016;2016:290-293.
16. Giunta R. Early subcutaneous wash-out in acute extravasations. *Ann Oncol.* 2004;15:1146; author reply 1147.
17. Hylenex [TM] (recombinant hyaluronidase human injection). Halozyme Therapeutics. Halozyme[TM], Inc. http://www.hylenex.com/files/resources_docs/Infiltration-Extravasation/documentation/Hylenex%20recombinant%20and%20Infiltration-Extravasation.pdf.
18. Ignoffo RJ, Friedman MA. Therapy of local toxicities caused by extravasation of cancer chemotherapeutic drugs. *Cancer Treat Rev.* 1980;7:17-27.
19. Ignoffo RJ, Young Ly KK. Neoplastic disorders. In: *Applied Therapeutics: The Clinical Use of Drugs.* Vancouver, WA: Applied Therapeutics; 1988:1197-1201.
20. Jensen JN, et al. Dexrazoxane-a promising antidote in the treatment of accidental extravasation of anthracyclines. *Scand J Plast Reconstr Surg Hand Surg.* 2003;37:174-175.
21. Kane RC, et al. Dexrazoxane (Totect): FDA review and approval for the treatment of accidental extravasation following intravenous anthracycline chemotherapy. *Oncologist.* 2008;13:445-450.
22. Khan MS, Holmes JD. Reducing the morbidity from extravasation injuries. *Ann Plast Surg.* 2002;48:628-632.

23. Kleiter MM, et al. A tracer dose of technetium-99m-labeled liposomes can estimate the effect of hyperthermia on intratumoral doxil extravasation. *Clin Cancer Res.* 2006;12:6800-6807.
24. Kreidieh FY, et al. Overview, prevention and management of chemotherapy extravasation. *World J Clin Oncol.* 2016;7:87-97.
25. Langer SW, et al. Dexrazoxane is a potent and specific inhibitor of anthracycline induced subcutaneous lesions in mice. *Ann Oncol.* 2001;12:405-410.
26. Langer SW, et al. Dexrazoxane in anthracycline extravasation. *J Clin Oncol.* 2000;18:3064.
27. Larson DL. Treatment of tissue extravasation by antitumor agents. *Cancer.* 1982;49:1796-1799.
28. Larson DL. What is the appropriate management of tissue extravasation by antitumor agents? *Plast Reconstr Surg.* 1985;75:397-405.
29. Lawrence HJ, Goodnight SH Jr. Dimethyl sulfoxide and extravasation of anthracycline agents. *Ann Intern Med.* 1983;98:1025.
30. Lopez AM, et al. Topical DMSO treatment for pegylated liposomal doxorubicin-induced palmar-plantar erythrodysesthesia. *Cancer Chemother Pharmacol.* 1999;44:303-306.
31. Mouridsen HT, et al. Treatment of anthracycline extravasation with Savene (dexrazoxane): results from two prospective clinical multicentre studies. *Ann Oncol.* 2007;18:546-550.
32. Neuss MN, et al. 2016 Updated American Society of Clinical Oncology/Oncology Nursing Society Chemotherapy Administration Safety Standards, Including Standards for Pediatric Oncology. *J Oncol Pract.* 2016;12:1262-1271.
33. Neuss MN, et al. 2013 updated American Society of Clinical Oncology/Oncology Nursing Society chemotherapy administration safety standards including standards for the safe administration and management of oral chemotherapy. *J Oncol Pract.* 2013;9:5s-13s.
34. Olver IN, et al. A prospective study of topical dimethyl sulfoxide for treating anthracycline extravasation. *J Clin Oncol.* 1988;6:1732-1735.
35. Olver IN, Schwarz MA. Use of dimethyl sulfoxide in limiting tissue damage caused by extravasation of doxorubicin. *Cancer Treat Rep.* 1983;67:407-408.
36. Patel JS, Krusa M. Distant and delayed mitomycin C extravasation. *Pharmacotherapy.* 1999;19:1002-1005.
37. Perez Fidalgo JA, et al. Management of chemotherapy extravasation: ESMO-EONS Clinical Practice Guidelines. *Ann Oncol.* 2012;23(suppl 7):vii167-vii173.
38. Raley J, et al. Docetaxel extravasation causing significant delayed tissue injury. *Gynecol Oncol.* 2000;78:259-260.
39. Reynolds PM, et al. Management of extravasation injuries: a focused evaluation of non-cytotoxic medications. *Pharmacotherapy.* 2014;34:617-632.
40. Rudolph R, Larson DL. Etiology and treatment of chemotherapeutic agent extravasation injuries: a review. *J Clin Oncol.* 1987;5:1116-1126.
41. Rudolph R, et al. Experimental skin necrosis produced by adriamycin. *Cancer Treat Rep.* 1979;63:529-537.
42. Schulmeister L. Vesicant chemotherapy extravasation antidotes and treatments. *Clin J Oncol Nurs.* 2009;13:395-398.
43. Schulmeister L. Extravasation management: clinical update. *Semin Oncol Nurs.* 2011;27:82-90.
44. Scuderi N, Onesti MG. Antitumor agents: extravasation, management, and surgical treatment. *Ann Plast Surg.* 1994;32:39-44.
45. Svingen BA, et al. Protection against adriamycin-induced skin necrosis in the rat by dimethyl sulfoxide and alpha-tocopherol. *Cancer Res.* 1981;41:3395-3399.
46. Tsavaris NB, et al. Conservative approach to the treatment of chemotherapy-induced extravasation. *J Dermatol Surg Oncol.* 1990;16:519-522.
47. Tyson AM, Gay WE. Successful experience utilizing dexrazoxane treatment for an anthracycline extravasation. *Ann Pharmacother.* 2010;44:922-925.
48. van der Heijden AG, et al. Effect of hyperthermia on the cytotoxicity of 4 chemotherapeutic agents currently used for the treatment of transitional cell carcinoma of the bladder: an in vitro study. *J Urol.* 2005;173:1375-1380.
49. West. of Scotland Cancer Network. Cancer Nursing and Pharmacy Group. Chemotherapy extravasation guideline. 2012.

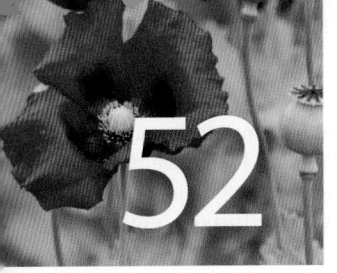

52 ANTIMIGRAINE MEDICATIONS

Jason Chu

PATHOPHYSIOLOGY OF MIGRAINE HEADACHES

A migraine headache is a neurovascular disorder often initiated by a trigger and characterized by a headache, which is preceded by an aura 20% of the time. The aura is either unilateral (40%) or bilateral (60%), reversible visual, sensory or other central nervous system symptom that gradually develops and last for minutes preceding the headache. The headache lasts 4 to 72 hours in adults and 1 to 48 hours in children and is typically a pulsatile headache of moderate to severe intensity with associated nausea, photophobia, and/or phonophobia and is typically worsened by routine physical activity. The International Headache Society establishes the diagnostic criteria for the various types of migraine, which are divided into multiple groups: migraine without aura ("common migraine"), migraine with aura ("classic migraine"), chronic migraine, complications of migraine, probable migraine, and episodic syndromes that may be associated with migraine. Further subdivisions of migraine with aura include migraine with typical aura with or without headache, migraine with brain stem aura, hemiplegic migraine, and retinal or ophthalmic migraine.[41]

The origin of migraine pain evolved from a vascular theory to a neurogenic theory but is still not fully elucidated. Migraine pain involves the trigeminovascular system as well as brain stem and diencephalic nuclei. Although the brain is insensate, the cerebral blood vessels, arteries, veins, and sinuses are innervated by C-fibers and A-δ-fibers of the trigeminal ganglion, and the dura mater is innervated by neurons from cervical dorsal root ganglia. Activation of these *first-order neurons* releases inflammatory neuropeptides such as calcitonin gene–related polypeptide (CRGP), vasoactive intestinal peptide (VIP), neurokinin A, substance P, and pituitary adenylate cyclase-activating peptide (PACAP). Pain impulses are relayed to the trigeminocervical complex composed of the trigeminal nucleus caudalis in lower medulla and the C1 and C2 region of the spinal cord. From there, nociceptive signals are relayed via *second-order neurons* via the trigeminothalamic tract to third-order neurons in the ventroposteromedial thalamus as well as the locus coeruleus, periaqueductal gray area, and hypothalamus. Thalamic *third-order neurons* in turn synapse with multiple higher and diffuse cortical areas. The trigeminocervical complex also produces retrograde parasympathetic impulses from the sphenopalatine ganglion and the superior salivatory nucleus in the pons through the sphenopalatine ganglion to the cerebral vessels.[38]

Migraine has a strong genetic component and particularly involving genetic abnormalities in the central nervous system (CNS) ion channels, namely, the P/Q calcium channels that predispose patients to specific triggers. Familial hemiplegic migraine is an autosomal dominant disorder with mutations affecting neuronal ion channels, leading to increased neuronal excitability. Four genes are known to be involved, three of these are involved in ion transport and the fourth is an axonal protein complex. Genomewide association studies have identified genes potentially involved in migraine susceptibility.[34]

Migraine auras are transient focal neurologic symptoms, which are present in about 25% to 30% of migraine patients and are typically visual although sensory, motor, speech or brain stem deficits are also described.[38] Usually auras precede the headache but can extend into the headache and postdromal phase. Visual auras are caused by a wave of neuronal depolarization, termed cortical spreading depression, at the visual cortex from a caudal to rostral fashion initially causing oligemia followed by hyperemia known as the spreading wave of oligemia. This in turn can activate the trigeminovascular system. Although cortical spreading depression accounts for migraine auras as well as the headache itself, it is still debated whether cortical spreading depression is a trigger for the initiation of migraine.[38]

Treatment of migraines encompasses a wide variety of xenobiotics that can be broadly classified either as prophylactic or abortive therapies (Table 52–1).[75] Triptans are considered the drugs of choice for abortive migraine therapy.

ERGOT ALKALOIDS

History and Epidemiology

Ergot is the product of *Claviceps purpurea*, a fungus that contaminates rye and other grains. The spores of the fungus are both windborne and transported by insects to young rye, where they germinate into hyphal filaments. When a spore germinates, it destroys the grain and hardens into a curved body called the sclerotium, which remains the major commercial source of ergot alkaloids.[11] The *C. purpurea* fungus produces diverse substances, including ergotamine, histamine, lysergic acid, tyramine, isomylamine, acetylcholine, and acetaldehyde.

In 600 B.C. an Assyrian tablet mentioned grain contamination believed to be by *C. purpurea*. In the Middle Ages, epidemics causing gangrene of the

TABLE 52–1 Xenobiotics Used in Migraine Treatment[a]	
Prophylactic	**Abortive**
β-Adrenergic antagonists	Acetaminophen
ACE inhibitors	Antiemetics: metoclopramide, prochlorperazine
Acetazolamide	
Angiotension II receptor antagonist	Aspirin
Antiepileptics: Carbamazepine, gabapentin, levetiracetam, topiramate, valproic acid, zonisamide	Butalbital
	Butyrophenones: Droperidol, haloperidol
Antipsychotics: Aripiprazole, olanzapine, quetiapine	Caffeine
	Corticosteroids
Benzodiazepines	Ergots
Butterbur root	Lidocaine (intranasal)
Calcium channel blockers	Magnesium (intravenous)
Coenzyme Q10	Nonsteroidal antiinflammatory drugs
Cyclic antidepressants	Opioids
Cyproheptadine	Oxygen
Feverfew	Sedative–hypnotics
Flunarizine	Triptans
Hormonal contraceptives	Valproic acid
Isometheptene/dichloralphenazone/acetaminophen (Midrin)	
Magnesium (oral)	
Monoamine oxidase inhibitors	
Melatonin	
Memantine	
Nefazodone	
OnabotulinumtoxinA (Botox A)	
Pizotifen	
Riboflavin	
Selective serotonin reuptake inhibitors	

[a]Prophylactic xenobiotics are usually taken to prevent triggering of migraines, and abortive xenobiotics are usually taken to stop the clinical manifestations of migraines once they are triggered. However, the separation between the two groups of xenobiotics is not strict, and some xenobiotics may be used in both roles. Triptans are currently considered the drug class of choice to abort moderate to severe migraine headache. ACE = angiotensin-converting enzyme inhibitors.

extremities, with mummification of limbs, were depicted in the literature as blackened limbs resembling the charring from fire and caused a burning sensation expressed by its victims. The disease was called *holy fire* or *St. Anthony's fire*, but the improvement that reportedly occurred when victims went to visit the shrine of St. Anthony was probably the result of a diet free of contaminated grain on the journey.[82] Abortion and seizures were also reported to result from this poisoning. On the other hand, as early as 1582, midwives used ergot to assist in the childbirth process. In 1818, Desgranges was the first physician to use ergot for obstetric care, and in 1822 Hosack reported that ergot could be used for the control of postpartum hemorrhage.[82] In the twentieth century, ergot derivatives were almost entirely limited to the treatment of vascular headaches whereas today they are rarely employed. Ergonovine, another ergot derivative, is used in obstetric care for its stimulant effect on uterine smooth muscle and was formerly used in cardiac stress tests. Methylergonovine is used for postpartum uterine atony and hemorrhage. Cabergoline is used for hyperprolactinemia. Pergolide was used for Parkinson disease but was withdrawn from the United States in 2007. Ergot derivatives were also used as "cognition enhancers,"[85] to help manage orthostatic hypotension,[77] and to prevent the secretion of prolactin.[68]

The United States, Australia, Canada, European Union, Japan, New Zealand, Switzerland, and the United Kingdom regulate the ergot level in grains, ranging from no ergots in grains in the United Kingdom to 0.03% ergot in US grain.[11] Elsewhere in the world, ergot toxicity remains a problem predominantly in poorly developed areas without ergot regulation and in animals.[11,12]

Pharmacology and Pharmacokinetics

All ergot alkaloids are derivatives of the tetracyclic compound 6-methylergoline. They are divided into 3 groups: amino acid alkaloids (ergotamine, ergotoxine), dihydrogenated amino acid alkaloids, and amine alkaloids (Fig. 52–1).

The pharmacokinetics of the ergot alkaloids are well defined by controlled human volunteer studies, whereas the toxicokinetics are essentially unknown (Table 52–2). Almost all of the ergots are poorly absorbed orally and there is considerable first-pass hepatic metabolism, resulting in highly variable bioavailability.

The pharmacologic effects of the ergot alkaloids can be subdivided into central and peripheral effects (Table 52–2). In the CNS, ergotamine stimulates serotonergic receptors, potentiates serotonergic effects, blocks

Amine alkaloids

Methylergonovine

Amino acid alkaloids

Ergotamine

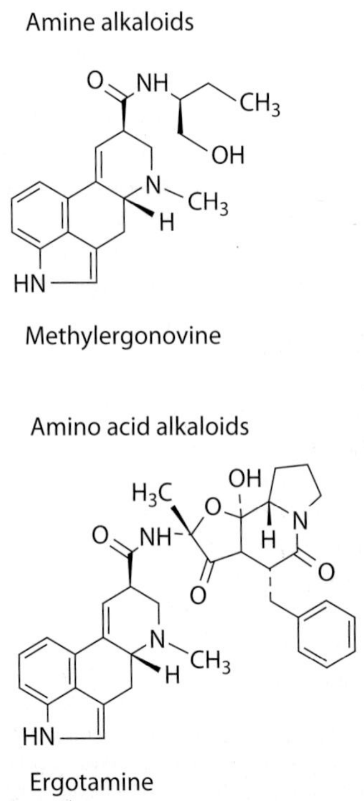

FIGURE 52–1. Chemical structures of 2 ergot derivatives representative of the amine and amino acid alkaloids.

neuronal serotonin reuptake, and has central sympatholytic actions.[19] Ergots interact with the 1A, 1B, 1D, 1F, 2A, 2C, 3, and 4 serotonin receptor subtypes, dopamine receptors and adrenergic receptors.[7] Stimulation of $5HT_{1B}$ receptors on cranial arteries causes vasoconstriction. 5-Hydroxytryptamine$_{1D}$ receptors are located presynaptically at trigeminal nerve endings and central nervous system neurons. Stimulation blocks the release of substance P and calcitonin gene–related peptide (CGRP) from trigeminal nerve endings and blocks the activation of second-order neurons of the trigeminal nucleus caudalis.[75,76] Ergotamine and dihydroergotamine decrease the neuronal firing rate and stabilize the cerebrovascular smooth musculature, which made them useful drugs for both abortive and prophylactic treatment of migraine headaches; however, newer medications with fewer adverse effects have replaced them clinically.

Peripherally, ergotamine and dihydroergotamine are α-adrenergic, 5-HT$_{2A}$ and 5-HT$_{1B}$ agonists, and vasoconstrictors.[71] The amino acid ergot alkaloids (ergotamine, ergotoxine) exhibit α-adrenergic agonism, and dehydrogenation (dihydroergotamine) of the lysergic acid nucleus increases the potency of this effect.[68] Ergotamine is a potent constrictor of peripheral arteries and veins, whereas dihydroergotamine constricts veins more than arteries.[19]

In the CNS, ergotamine and dihydroergotamine cause vasoconstriction via 5HT$_{1B}$ and α-adrenergic agonism, with both medications having similar 5-HT receptor agonist activity. As noted above, ergotamine has more peripheral arterial vasoconstriction, constricts larger cranial arteries, and possibly increases norepinephrine-induced vasoconstriction. Dihydroergotamine constricts larger cranial arteries as well but has more α-receptor antagonist activity and inhibits norepinephrine-induced vasoconstriction. Neither medication affects cranial resistance vessels nor changes cerebral blood flow.[2,69] Ergot stimulation of central 5HT$_{1A}$ receptors causes nausea and dysphoria, and stimulation of dopamine D$_2$ receptors cause nausea and vomiting.[76]

Table 52–2 summarizes the pharmacologic actions of selected ergot alkaloids currently used in clinical medicine. The spectrum of effects depends on dose, host response, and physiologic conditions. The clinical effects following overdose are an extension of the therapeutic effects. At toxic doses, extreme vasoconstriction produces the characteristic ischemic changes that occur in ergotism.

Clinical Manifestations

Ergotism, a toxicologic syndrome resulting from excessive use of ergot alkaloids, is characterized by intense burning of the extremities, hemorrhagic vesiculation, pruritus, formication, nausea, vomiting, and gangrene (Table 52–3). Headache, fixed miosis, hallucinations, delirium, cerebrovascular ischemia, and convulsions are also associated with this condition, which was called "convulsive" ergotism.[40] Chronic ergotism usually presents with peripheral ischemia of the lower extremities, although ischemia of cerebral, mesenteric, coronary, and renal vascular beds are well documented.[3,28,29,66,67] Ergotism also results from interactions of ergot derivatives with CYP3A4 inhibitors such as macrolide antibiotics and protease inhibitors, which increase bioavailability of ergots.[9,10]

The vascular effects ascribed to ergot alkaloids are complex and sometimes conflicting (Table 52–2). Subintimal and medial fibrosis, vasospasm, and arteriolar and venous thrombi (stasis related) are all reported.[55] Angiography can demonstrate distal, segmental vessel spasm with increased collateralization in patients with chronic ergotism. The coronary, renal, cerebral, ophthalmic, and mesenteric vasculature,[67] as well as the vessels of the extremities, are also affected.[72] Neuropathic changes also occur secondary to ischemia of the vasa nervorum.

Bradycardia is a characteristic effect of the ergot alkaloids and is believed to be a reflex baroreceptor–mediated phenomenon associated with vasoconstriction. However a reduction in sympathetic tone, direct myocardial depression, and increased vagal activity are also factors.[68]

Myocardial valvular abnormalities are reported with ergot alkaloids. Ergotamine, dihydroergotamine methysergide, pergolide, and cabergoline cause mitral and aortic valve leaflet thickening and immobility resulting in valvular regurgitation.[30,66,89] The mitral and aortic valves and pulmonary

TABLE 52–2   Pharmacokinetics of Ergots

Ergot Derivative	Clinical Use	t½ (hours)	Duration of Action (hours)	Bioavailability (%)	Metabolism/ Elimination	Interactions With Serotonergic Receptors	Interactions With Dopaminergic Receptors	Interactions With α-Adrenergic Receptors
Bromocriptine	Parkinsonism, amenorrhea/ prolactinemia syndrome	60 (PO)	1 week (suppression of prolactin)	28 (PO)	Liver	Weak antagonist	CNS: Partial agonist/ antagonist; inhibits prolactin secretion; emetic (high)	Vasculature: Antagonist
Dihydroergotamine	Migraine	2.4	3–4 (IM)	100 (IM) 40 (Nasal) <5 (PO)	Liver metabolism Bile excretion	Smooth muscles: Partial agonist/ antagonist CNS: Agonist lateral geniculate nucleus	CNS: Emetic (mild) Sympathetic ganglia: Antagonism	Vasculature: Partial agonist (veins); antagonist (arteries) Smooth muscles: Antagonism CNS/PNS: Antagonism
Ergonovine	Postpartum hemorrhage	1.9	3	(IV) 100	Liver	Smooth muscles: Potent antagonist Vasculature: Agonist in umbilical and placental vessels CNS: Partial antagonist/agonist	CNS: Emetic (mild); inhibits prolactin (weak); partial agonist/antagonist Vasculature: Weak antagonist	Vasculature: Partial agonist
Ergotamine	Migraine	2 (1.4–6.2)	22 (IV)	100 (IV) 47 (IM) <5 (PO)	Liver metabolism Bile excretion	Vasculature: Partial agonist Smooth muscles: Nonselective antagonist CNS: Poor agonist/ antagonist	CNS: Emetic (potent)	Vasculature: Partial agonist/antagonist Smooth muscles: Partial agonist/antagonist CNS: Antagonist PNS: Antagonist
Methylergonovine	Postpartum hemorrhage	1.4–2	3	78 (IM) 60 (PO)	Liver	Smooth muscles: Potent antagonist Vasculature: Agonist in umbilical and placental vessels CNS: Partial antagonist/agonist	CNS: Emetic (mild); inhibits prolactin (weak); partial agonist/antagonist Vasculature: Weak antagonist	Vasculature: Partial agonist
Methysergide	Migraine	2.7/10 hours (PO)	8–24	13 (PO)	Liver— metabolized to methylergonovine	Vasculature: Partial agonist CNS: Potent antagonist	None	None

IM = intramuscular; IV = intravenous; PO = oral.

arteries have high concentrations of $5HT_{2B}$ receptors. The ergot-derived medications are potent $5HT_{2B}$ receptor agonists, and stimulation activates cellular kinases leading to fibroblast proliferation and collagen synthesis.[25]

Treatment

The treatment for a patient with ergot alkaloid toxicity depends on the nature of the clinical findings. Gastric emptying is rarely used, if at all, because vomiting is a common early occurrence, and the ingestion is infrequently

TABLE 52–3   Clinical Manifestations of Ergotism

Central Effects	Peripheral Effects
Agitation	Angina
Cerebrovascular ischemia	Bradycardia
Hallucinations	Gangrene
Headaches	Hemorrhagic vesiculations and skin bullae
Miosis (fixed)	Mesenteric infarction
Nausea	Myocardial infarction
Seizures	Renal infarction
Twitching (facial)	
Vomiting	

complicated by seizures. After an acute oral overdose, 1 g/kg of oral activated charcoal is recommended. If emesis is present, antiemetics such as ondansetron or metoclopramide are reasonable to be administered intravenously to facilitate the administration of activated charcoal. In mild cases, characterized by minimal pain of the extremities, nausea, or headache, supportive measures such as hydration and analgesia are all that are needed. Immediate-release oral nifedipine is a reasonable therapy for patients with mild symptoms of vasospasm, such as dysesthesias and minimal ischemic pain of the digits.[18] With more serious cases, peripheral vasoconstriction produce ischemic changes that include angina, myocardial infarction, cerebral ischemia, intermittent claudication, and internal organ/mesenteric ischemia. Reasonable therapies include sodium nitroprusside, phentolamine, and intravenous calcium channel blockers, nicardipine, or clevidipine, titrated until resolution of vasoconstriction.[3,15,61] Although methylprednisolone at a dose of 1 mg/kg reversed ergotamine-induced lower extremity arterial vasospasm that was unresponsive to sodium nitroprusside and heparin, there is not enough data to routinely recommend this therapy.[64]

Heparin or low-molecular-weight heparins are reasonable to administer to prevent sludging and subsequent clot formation. Benzodiazepines are recommended therapies to treat ergot- or bromocriptine-associated seizures or hallucinations.[36]

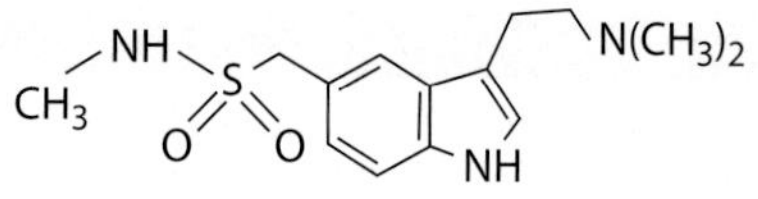

Sumatriptan

FIGURE 52–2. Representative chemical structure of the triptans.

TRIPTANS

In 1974, investigations began on a new class of compounds that produced vasoconstrictive effects via 5-HT receptors. The first compound successfully used in this way was 5-carboxamidotryptamine (5-CT). When applied to an isolated dog saphenous vein, 5-CT caused potent venoconstriction and induced significant hypotension in vivo. The next compound developed, AH25086 [(3,2-aminoethyl)-*N*-methyl-1-*H*-indole-5-acetamide], also constricted saphenous veins in dogs but had more 5-HT receptor selectivity. AH25086 was effective against acute migraine in human volunteers, but further research was stopped because it was deemed less suitable for development in humans, possibly owing to the fact that it was highly polar, lipophobic, and unsuitable for oral use.[43,70] In 1984, sumatriptan was synthesized and its clinical success led to the rapid development of 6 other triptans: almotriptan, eletriptan, frovatriptan, naratriptan, rizatriptan and zolmitriptan, and one triptan combination medication (sumatriptan/naproxen; Fig. 52–2; Table 52–4).

Pharmacology

There are numerous interrelated proposed mechanisms of action of $5HT_1$ agonists on migraine.[19] The triptans are all primarily $5\text{-}HT_{1B}$ and $5\text{-}HT_{1D}$ receptor agonists and have less activity at $5\text{-}HT_{1A}$ and $5\text{-}HT_{1F}$ receptors[31] (Chap. 13). In the CNS, $5\text{-}HT_{1B}$ receptors are located on cerebral vessels.[39] Stimulation of these receptors results in cerebral vasoconstriction,[20] reversing abnormal cerebral vasodilation. In contrast, the $5\text{-}HT_{1D}$ receptors are located presynaptically on trigeminal neurons, and act as "autoreceptors" to decrease neurotransmitter release from central trigeminal nerve terminals.[47] The triptans also inhibit dural neurogenic inflammation by preventing the release of vasoactive neuropeptides from peripheral trigeminal nerves.[57,73] Centrally, triptans stimulate $5\text{-}HT_{1B/D/F}$ receptors in the trigeminal nucleus caudalis to prevent signaling from first order trigeminal neurons to second order neurons in the trigeminal nucleus caudalis. Triptans also stimulate $5\text{-}HT_{1B/D}$ receptors to prevent signaling from second-order trigeminal nucleus caudalis neurons to third-order neurons in ventroposteromedial (VPM) thalamus. Both of the latter mechanisms block central sensitization in migraine headaches.[19] Peripherally, triptans cause vasoconstriction systemically through the $5\text{-}HT_{1B}$ receptor (Fig. 52–3).[22,51]

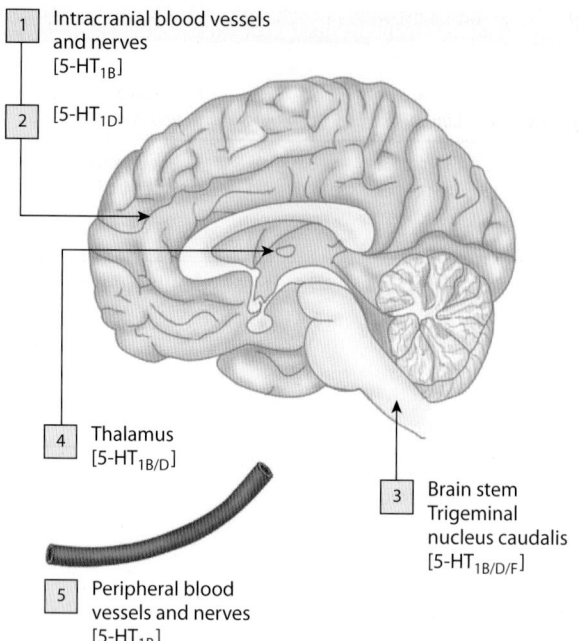

FIGURE 52–3. Some of the multiple interactive mechanisms of action of triptans. Vasoconstriction of intracranial [1] and peripheral [5] blood vessels via $5\text{-}HT_{1B}$ receptor agonism. Inhibition of vasoactive peptide release [2] from trigeminal nerve terminals at dural vessels via $5\text{-}HT_{1D}$ agonism. Modulation of nociceptive transmission to trigeminal nucleus caudalis [3] and thalamus [4].

Sumatriptan has poor oral bioavailability but good subcutaneous bioavailability (96%), and is therefore preferentially given by this route. The newer triptans differ substantially from sumatriptan with regard to oral bioavailability, plasma half-life, time to maximum effect, and recurrence rate of headaches. All triptans are pharmacodynamically similar but pharmacokinetically different (Table 52–4).

Clinical Manifestations

With appropriate therapeutic use, the common adverse effects associated with the triptans are less common and include nausea, vomiting, dyspepsia, esophageal spasm, flushing, and paresthesias.[21,68] The most consequential adverse effects are chest pressure and vasoconstriction. Chest pressure symptoms are reported in up to 15% of sumatriptan users.[14,63] Although triptans reduce coronary artery diameter by 10% to 15%, chest pressure symptoms are not believed to be secondary to cardiac ischemia. Alternate

TABLE 52–4	Pharmacokinetics of Triptans				
Triptan	$t_{1/2}$ (hours)	Duration of Action (hours)	Lipophilicity	Bioavailability O (%)	Metabolism/Elimination
Almotriptan	3.0–3.7	24	Unknown	70–80	CYP3A4, CYP2D6 MAO-A (minor)
Eletriptan	3.6–6.9	14–16	High	50	CYP3A4
Frovatriptan	25	24	Low	24–30	CYP1A2 Kidney
Naratriptan	4.5–6.6	Unknown	High	63–74	Kidney (major) P450
Rizatriptan	1.8–3.0	25	Moderate	40–45	MAO-A
Sumatriptan	2.0–2.5	4	Low	14; 96 (SC)	MAO-A
Zolmitriptan	1.5–3.6	18	Moderate	40–49	CYP1A2 MAO-A (minor)

MAO = monoamine oxidase; Oral = oral unless otherwise stated; PO = oral; SC = subcutaneous.

hypotheses for the chest pressure sensations include a generalized vasospastic disorder in migraineurs, esophageal spasm, bronchospasm, alterations of skeletal muscle energy metabolism, and central sensitization of pain pathways.[23]

Triptans can cause ischemia due to vasoconstriction. Therapeutic sumatriptan use is associated with myocardial ischemia and or infarction, dysrhythmias, renal infarction, splenic infarction, and ischemic colitis.[1,8,17,48,52,58,60,62] Cephalic vasoconstriction is the desired effect of sumatriptan, but there are reports of strokes, hemorrhages, and infarctions.[16,46,50,56] Extrapyramidal symptoms, such as akathisia and dystonia, also occur.[49] Therapeutic use of other triptans is associated with spinal cord infarction, renal infarction, myocardial infarction, ischemic colitis, and seizures.[11,33,54,83,86]

Animal studies showed a wide margin of safety with oral sumatriptan. Subcutaneous administration of 2 g/kg of sumatriptan to rats was lethal. Death was preceded by erythema, inactivity, and tremor.[44] Dogs survived 20 and 100 mg/kg subcutaneous doses, but developed hind limb paralysis, erythema, tremor, salivation, and loss of vocalization.[43] Reactions in other animals include seizures, inactivity, reduced respiratory rate, cyanosis, ptosis, ataxia, mydriasis, salivation, and lacrimation.[44,78]

Excessive triptan use is associated with vasoconstrictive adverse effects as well as tachyphylaxis. A 43-year-old man who used 23 (25 mg) tablets of sumatriptan and 32 tablets of a combination preparation of isometheptene 65 mg, dichloralphenazone 100 mg, and APAP 325 mg over 7 days for headaches developed a left occipital infarction with a right hemianopsia. Digital subtraction angiography revealed segmental narrowing in multiple cerebral vessels. The hemianopsia and vessel findings resolved after cessation of the sumatriptan and Midrin and treatment with nicardipine.[56] A 35-year-old woman who used 300 mg of sumatriptan orally and 12 mg subcutaneously developed ischemic colitis.[4] Two patients who received 4 times and 10 times the recommended dose of naratriptan developed severe hypertension.[6] However, not all triptan overdoses result in toxicity. A 36-year-old man reportedly used 66 (6 mg) doses of sumatriptan subcutaneously over 4 weeks for his cluster headaches and had no adverse effects.[80] The maximum recommended dosage of sumatriptan is 12 mg subcutaneously in a 24-hour period. Patients who took single doses of 100 to 150 mg of almotriptan had no adverse effects.[5]

In 2006, the US Food and Drug Administration (FDA) issued an alert, warning of an increased risk of serotonin toxicity with triptans used in combination with selective serotonin reuptake inhibitors (SSRIs) or selective serotonin-norepinephrine reuptake inhibitors. The alert was based on 27 cases reported to the FDA Adverse Events Reporting System between 1998 and 2002. The cases involved triptan use in conjunction with SSRIs that were coded as serotonin syndrome or symptoms indicative of serotonin toxicity.[26] A case series of serotonin toxicity from migraine medications described 3 cases associated with sumatriptan use alone, sumatriptan with sertraline, and sumatriptan with methysergide, lithium, and sertraline.[53] Other medications that might precipitate serotonin toxicity when used in conjunction with triptans include monoamine oxidase inhibitors (Chaps. 69 and 71).

Treatment
Treatment of triptan-induced vasoconstriction is dependent on the route of exposure and the organ system affected. Decontamination is not feasible after subcutaneous exposures, but can be effective following overdose of oral preparations. Gastrointestinal decontamination with activated charcoal is a reasonable approach. Because vomiting is not as prominent with triptan exposure compared to ergot alkaloids, gastric emptying procedures, such as orogastric lavage, are appropriate, but only following recent or massive ingestion. The oral forms of rizatriptan and zolmitriptan are formulated to dissolve on the tongue, limiting the effectiveness of gastrointestinal decontamination.

Many reported cases of triptan-induced vasoconstriction compromise responded to intravenous hydration and analgesia.[33,45] It is reasonable to treat triptan-associated myocardial ischemia with aspirin, heparin, and nitroglycerin.[62] Coronary angiography is recommended for transmural myocardial infarctions with ST segment elevations on electrocardiography.[52,60]

ISOMETHEPTENE
Isometheptene is a mild vasoconstrictor marketed as a combination preparation that includes dichloralphenazone, a muscle relaxant, and acetaminophen. It has indirect α- and β-adrenergic agonist effects as well as minor direct α-adrenergic agonist effects on the peripheral vasculature.[81] When administered early during a migraine exacerbation, it is as effective as sumatriptan in relieving migraine headache.[32] Cerebral vasoconstriction, intracerebral hemorrhage, and myocardial infarction are reported after therapeutic and excessive isometheptene use.[35,56,65,74] Autonomic dysreflexia, which presented as hypertension, headache, diaphoresis, and flushing, was also reported in a man with spinal cord injury who used isometheptene for treatment of a migraine headache.[87]

Isometheptene-associated vasoconstriction is rare, and reported treatments with calcium channel blockers or nitroglycerin are not routinely recommended.

CALCITONIN GENE–RELATED PEPTIDE ANTAGONISTS
During migraines, calcitonin gene–related peptide is among the many vasoactive peptides released from activated trigeminal nerves.[37] Calcitonin gene–related peptide is a potent vasodilator[13] and is involved in the transmission of nociceptive signals from cerebral vessels to the central nervous system.[24] Calcitonin gene–related peptide receptors are found in nerve fibers in cerebral and dural vessels and in multiple areas of the central nervous system postulated in migraine genesis—the cerebral cortex, periaqueductal gray, locus coeruleus, dorsal raphe nuclei, solitary tractus nucleus, spinal dorsal horn, dorsal root ganglia, and trigeminal ganglia.[79] Treatment of active migraine with sumatriptan decreased CGRP concentrations to normal.[37]

Several CGRP antagonists were developed unsuccessfully.[71,84] Erenumabaooe (Aimovig), developed for monthly subcutaneous injection, is a recently FDA-approved human immunoglobulin G2 monoclonal antibody made using recombinant DNA technology with a high affinity for the CGRP receptor and indicated for the prevention of migraines in adults. Approximately 4500 patients comprised of healthy volunteers and patients with migraines had rare adverse reactions at the injection site. Some patients develop neutralizing antibodies. The treatment was well tolerated and the benefits appear modest. No overdoses are reported. Since the xenobiotic is a monoclonal antibody, allergic reactions are a possibility.[42]

5HT$_{1F}$ Receptor Agonists
Although triptans classically exert their antimigraine effects through 5HT$_{1B}$ and 5HT$_{1D}$ agonism, naratriptan also has 5HT$_{1F}$ agonist effects. 5-Hydroxy-tryptamine$_{1F}$ receptors are found on the trigeminal ganglion and the trigeminocervical complex but not on smooth muscles, coronary arteries or cerebral vasculature.[88] Lasmiditan is a 5HT$_{1F}$ receptor agonist that decreases plasma protein extravasation at the trigeminal ganglion and inhibited nociceptive transmission from the trigeminocervical complex higher up to the CNS without vasoconstriction of vessels.[59] Reported adverse effects from oral lasmiditan include dizziness, fatigue, nausea, paresthesia, somnolence, vertigo, and sensation of heaviness.[27] Lasmiditan has undergone 2 phase II trials and is undergoing phase III trials currently.

SUMMARY
- Migraine therapies include many xenobiotics for prophylaxis as well as for abortive therapy. Triptans have supplanted ergots as the primary abortive treatment for patients with migraines.
- Ergots interact with multiple 5-HT, dopamine, and adrenergic receptors, and cause severe vasoconstriction and end organ ischemia.
- It is reasonable to treat ergot- and triptan-induced peripheral ischemia with vasodilators, calcium channel blockers, and heparin anticoagulation.
- Triptans are more selective and interact only with 5-HT$_{1B/D/F}$ receptors but also cause peripheral vasoconstriction and end organ ischemia. It is reasonable to treat triptan-induced myocardial ischemia with anticoagulation, nitrates, and coronary angiography for transmural infarctions.

■ Triptan use in conjunction with other serotonin-increasing xenobiotics is associated with increased risk of serotonin toxicity.

Acknowledgment
Neal A. Lewin, MD, contributed to this chapter in previous editions.

REFERENCES

1. Abbrescia VD, et al. Sumatriptan-associated myocardial infarction: report of case with attention to potential risk factors. *J Am Osteopath Assoc.* 1997;97:162-164.
2. Andersen AR, et al. The effect of ergotamine and dihydroergotamine on cerebral blood flow in man. *Stroke.* 1987;18:120-123.
3. Andersen PK, et al. Sodium nitroprusside and epidural blockade in the treatment of ergotism. *N Engl J Med.* 1977;296:1271-1273.
4. Andrejak M, Tribouilloy C. Drug-induced valvular heart disease: an update. *Arch Cardiovasc Dis.* 2013;106:333-339.
5. Anonymous. *Almotriptan Malate Tablets Product Information.* Toronto, Ontario, Canada: Janssen-Ortho Inc; 2003.
6. Anonymous. Naratriptan Product Information: GlaxoSmithKline, Inc; 2006.
7. Arngrim N, et al. Carbon monoxide inhalation induces headache in a human headache model [published online before print May 5, 2017]. *Cephalalgia.* doi:10.1177/0333102417708768.
8. Arora A, Arora S. Spontaneous splenic infarction associated with sumatriptan use. *J Headache Pain.* 2006;7:214-216.
9. Ausband SC, Goodman PE. An unusual case of clarithromycin associated ergotism. *J Emerg Med.* 2001;21:411-413.
10. Baldwin ZK, Ceraldi CC. Ergotism associated with HIV antiviral protease inhibitor therapy. *J Vasc Surg.* 2003;37:676-678.
11. Belser-Ehrlich S et al. Human and cattle ergotism since 1900: symptoms, outbreaks, and regulations. *Toxicol Ind Health.* 2013;29:307-316.
12. Botha CJ, et al. Gangrenous ergotism in cattle grazing fescue (*Festuca elatior* L.) in South Africa. *J S Afr Vet Assoc.* 2004;75:45-48.
13. Brain SD, et al. Calcitonin gene-related peptide is a potent vasodilator. *Nature.* 1985;313:54-56.
14. Brown EG, et al. The safety and tolerability of sumatriptan: an overview. *Eur Neurol.* 1991;31:339-344.
15. Carliner N, et al. Sodium nitroprusside treatment of ergotamine-induced peripheral ischemia. *JAMA.* 1974;227:308-309.
16. Cavazos JE, et al. Sumatriptan-induced stroke in sagittal sinus thrombosis. *Lancet.* 1994;343:1105-1106.
17. Curtin T, et al. Cardiorespiratory distress after sumatriptan given by injection. *BMJ.* 1992;305:713-714; author reply 714.
18. Dagher FJ, et al. Severe unilateral ischemia of the lower extremity caused by ergotamine: treatment with nifedipine. *Surgery.* 1985;97:369-373.
19. Dahlof C, Maassen Van Den Brink A. Dihydroergotamine, ergotamine, methysergide and sumatriptan—basic science in relation to migraine treatment. *Headache.* 2012;52:707-714.
20. Dechant KL, Clissold SP. Sumatriptan. A review of its pharmacodynamic and pharmacokinetic properties, and therapeutic efficacy in the acute treatment of migraine and cluster headache. *Drugs.* 1992;43:776-798.
21. Deleu D, Hanssens Y. Current and emerging second-generation triptans in acute migraine therapy: a comparative review. *J Clin Pharmacol.* 2000;40:687-700.
22. Dixon RM, et al. Peripheral vascular effects and pharmacokinetics of the antimigraine compound, zolmitriptan, in combination with oral ergotamine in healthy volunteers. *Cephalalgia.* 1997;17:639-646.
23. Dodick D, et al. Consensus statement: cardiovascular safety profile of triptans (5-HT agonists) in the acute treatment of migraine. *Headache.* 2004;44:414-425.
24. Durham PL. Calcitonin gene-related peptide (CGRP) and migraine. *Headache.* 2006;46(suppl 1):S3-S8.
25. Elangbam CS. Drug-induced valvulopathy: an update. *Toxicol Pathol.* 2010;38:837-848.
26. Evans RW. The FDA alert on serotonin syndrome with combined use of SSRIs or SNRIs and Triptans: an analysis of the 29 case reports. *MedGenMed.* 2007;9:48.
27. Farkkila M, et al. Efficacy and tolerability of lasmiditan, an oral 5-HT(1F) receptor agonist, for the acute treatment of migraine: a phase 2 randomised, placebo-controlled, parallel-group, dose-ranging study. *Lancet Neurol.* 2012;11:405-413.
28. Fincham RW, et al. Bilateral focal cortical atrophy and chronic ergotamine abuse. *Neurology.* 1985;35:720-722.
29. Fisher PE, et al. Ergotamine abuse and extra-hepatic portal hypertension. *Postgrad Med J.* 1985;61:461-463.
30. Flaherty KR, Bates JR. Mitral regurgitation caused by chronic ergotamine use. *Am Heart J.* 1996;131:603-606.
31. Fowler PA, et al. The clinical pharmacology, pharmacokinetics and metabolism of sumatriptan. *Eur Neurol.* 1991;31:291-294.
32. Freitag FG, et al. Comparative study of a combination of isometheptene mucate, dichloralphenazone with acetaminophen and sumatriptan succinate in the treatment of migraine. *Headache.* 2001;41:391-398.
33. Fulton JA, et al. Renal infarction during the use of rizatriptan and zolmitriptan: two case reports. *Clin Toxicol (Phila).* 2006;44:177-180.
34. Gasparini CF, et al. Genetic insights into migraine and glutamate: a protagonist driving the headache. *J Neurol Sci.* 2016;367:258-268.
35. George S, Vannozi Z. Myocardial infarction induced by migraine therapy. *Ann Emerg Med.* 1995;25:718-719.
36. Gittelman DK. Bromocriptine associated with postpartum hypertension, seizures, and pituitary hemorrhage. *Gen Hosp Psychiatry.* 1991;13:278-280.
37. Goadsby PJ, Edvinsson L. The trigeminovascular system and migraine: studies characterizing cerebrovascular and neuropeptide changes seen in humans and cats. *Ann Neurol.* 1993;33:48-56.
38. Goadsby PJ, et al. Pathophysiology of migraine: a disorder of sensory processing. *Physiol Rev.* 2017;97:553-622.
39. Hamel E. The biology of serotonin receptors: focus on migraine pathophysiology and treatment. *Can J Neurol Sci.* 1999;26(suppl 3):S2-S6.
40. Harrison TE. Ergotaminism. *J Am Coll Emerg Phys.* 1978;7:162-169.
41. Headache Classification Committee of the International Headache S. The International Classification of Headache Disorders, 3rd edition (beta version). *Cephalalgia.* 2013;33:629-808.
42. AIMOVIG™ (erenumab-aooe) injection, for subcutaneous use. Amgen Inc. (Thousand Oaks, CA 91320), and Novartis Pharmaceuticals Corporation (East Hanover, NJ 07936). Initial U.S. Approval: 2018.
43. Humphrey PP, et al. A rational approach to identifying a fundamentally new drug for the treatment of migraine. In: Saxena PR, et al., eds. *Cardiovascular Pharmacology of 5-Hydroxytryptamine.* Dordrecht: Kluwer Academic Publishers; 1990:417-431.
44. Humphrey PP, et al. Preclinical studies on the anti-migraine drug, sumatriptan. *Eur Neurol.* 1991;31:282-290.
45. Iovino M, et al. Safety, tolerability and pharmacokinetics of BIBN 4096 BS, the first selective small molecule calcitonin gene-related peptide receptor antagonist, following single intravenous administration in healthy volunteers. *Cephalalgia.* 2004;24:645-656.
46. Jayamaha JE, Street MK. Fatal cerebellar infarction in a migraine sufferer whilst receiving sumatriptan. *Intensive Care Med.* 1995;21:82-83.
47. Kaube H, et al. Inhibition by sumatriptan of central trigeminal neurones only after blood-brain barrier disruption. *Br J Pharmacol.* 1993;109:788-792.
48. Knudsen JF, et al. Ischemic colitis and sumatriptan use. *Arch Intern Med.* 1998;158:1946-1948.
49. Lopez-Alemany M et al. Akathisia and acute dystonia induced by sumatriptan. *J Neurol.* 1997;244:131-132.
50. Luman W, Gray RS. Adverse reactions associated with sumatriptan. *Lancet.* 1993;341:1091-1092.
51. MacIntyre PD, et al. Effect of subcutaneous sumatriptan, a selective 5HT1 agonist, on the systemic, pulmonary, and coronary circulation. *Circulation.* 1993;87:401-405.
52. Main ML, et al. Cardiac arrest and myocardial infarction immediately after sumatriptan injection. *Ann Intern Med.* 1998;128:874.
53. Mathew NT, et al. Serotonin syndrome complicating migraine pharmacotherapy. *Cephalalgia.* 1996;16:323-327.
54. Mazzoleni R, et al. Seizure after use of almotriptan. *Clin Neurol Neurosurg.* 2008;110:850-851.
55. Merhoff GC, Porter JM. Ergot intoxication: historical review and description of unusual clinical manifestations. *Ann Surg.* 1974;180:773-779.
56. Meschia JF, et al. Reversible segmental cerebral arterial vasospasm and cerebral infarction: possible association with excessive use of sumatriptan and Midrin. *Arch Neurol.* 1998;55:712-714.
57. Moskowitz MA. Neurogenic versus vascular mechanisms of sumatriptan and ergot alkaloids in migraine. *Trends Pharmacol Sci.* 1992;13:307-311.
58. Mueller L, et al. Vasospasm-induced myocardial infarction with sumatriptan. *Headache.* 1996;36:329-331.
59. Nelson DL, et al. Preclinical pharmacological profile of the selective 5-HT1F receptor agonist lasmiditan. *Cephalalgia.* 2010;30:1159-1169.
60. O'Connor P, Gladstone P. Oral sumatriptan-associated transmural myocardial infarction. *Neurology.* 1995;45:2274-2276.
61. O'Dell CW, et al. Sodium nitroprusside in the treatment of ergotism. *Radiology.* 1977;124:73-74.
62. Ottervanger JP, et al. Transmural myocardial infarction with sumatriptan. *Lancet.* 1993;341:861-862.
63. Ottervanger JP, et al. Postmarketing study of cardiovascular adverse reactions associated with sumatriptan. *BMJ.* 1993;307:1185.
64. Rahman A, et al. Reversal of ergotamine-induced vasospasm following methylprednisolone. *Clin Toxicol (Phila).* 2008;46:1074-1076.
65. Raroque HG Jr, et al. Postpartum cerebral angiopathy. Is there a role for sympathomimetic drugs? *Stroke.* 1993;24:2108-2110.
66. Redfield MM, et al. Valve disease associated with ergot alkaloid use: echocardiographic and pathologic correlations. *Ann Intern Med.* 1992;117:50-52.
67. Rogers DA, Mansberger JA. Gastrointestinal vascular ischemia caused by ergotamine. *South Med J.* 1989;82:1058-1059.
68. Sanders-Bush E Mayer SE. 5-Hydroxytryptamine (serotonin) receptor agonists and antagonists. In: Brunton LL, et al., eds. *Goodman and Gilman's The Pharmacological Basis of Therapeutics.* 11th ed. New York, NY: McGraw-Hill; 1992: 297-315.

69. Saper JR, Silberstein S. Pharmacology of dihydroergotamine and evidence for efficacy and safety in migraine. *Headache.* 2006;46(suppl 4):S171-S181.

70. Saxena PR, Ferrari MD. 5-HT(1)-like receptor agonists and the pathophysiology of migraine. *Trends Pharmacol Sci.* 1989;10:200-204.

71. Schytz HW, et al. Challenges in developing drugs for primary headaches. *Prog Neurobiol.* 2017;152:70-88.

72. Senter HJ, et al. Cerebral manifestations of ergotism. Report of a case and review of the literature. *Stroke.* 1976;7:88-92.

73. Shepherd SL, et al. Differential effects of 5-HT1B/1D receptor agonists on neurogenic dural plasma extravasation and vasodilation in anaesthetized rats. *Neuropharmacology.* 1997;36:525-533.

74. Shrikanth V, et al. Spontaneous intracerebral hemorrhage associated with ingestion of isometheptine containing anti-migraine medication. *Clin Neurol Neurosurg.* 2011;113:167-169.

75. Silberstein SD. Emerging target-based paradigms to prevent and treat migraine. *Clin Pharmacol Ther.* 2013;93:78-85.

76. Silberstein SD, McCrory DC. Ergotamine and dihydroergotamine: history, pharmacology, and efficacy. *Headache.* 2003;43:144-166.

77. Stumpf JL, Mitrzyk B. Management of orthostatic hypotension. *Am J Hosp Pharm.* 1994;51:648-660; quiz 697-698.

78. Sumatriptan. Product information and personal communication: Glaxo Wellcome, Inc.

79. Tepper SJ, Stillman MJ. Clinical and preclinical rationale for CGRP-receptor antagonists in the treatment of migraine. *Headache.* 2008;48:1259-1268.

80. Turhal NS. Sumatriptan overdose in episodic cluster headache: a case report of overuse without event. *Cephalalgia.* 2001;21:700.

81. Valdivia LF, et al. Pharmacological analysis of the mechanisms involved in the tachycardic and vasopressor responses to the antimigraine agent, isometheptene, in pithed rats. *Life Sci.* 2004;74:3223-3234.

82. van Dongen PW, de Groot AN. History of ergot alkaloids from ergotism to ergometrine. *Eur J Obstet Gynecol Reprod Biol.* 1995;60:109-116.

83. Vijayan N, Peacock JH. Spinal cord infarction during use of zolmitriptan: a case report. *Headache.* 2000;40:57-60.

84. Voss T, et al. A phase IIb randomized, double-blind, placebo-controlled trial of ubrogepant for the acute treatment of migraine. *Cephalalgia.* 2016;36:887-898.

85. Wadworth AN, Chrisp P. Co-dergocrine mesylate. A review of its pharmacodynamic and pharmacokinetic properties and therapeutic use in age-related cognitive decline. *Drugs Aging.* 1992;2:153-173.

86. Westgeest HM, et al. Pure naratriptan-induced ischemic colitis: a case report. *Turk J Gastroenterol.* 2010;21:42-44.

87. Wineinger MA, Basford JR. Autonomic dysreflexia due to medication: misadventure in the use of an isometheptene combination to treat migraine. *Arch Phys Med Rehabil.* 1985;66:645-646.

88. Xavier AS, et al. The journey of the non-vascular relief for migraine: from "triptans" to "ditans." *Curr Clin Pharmacol* 2017;12:36-40.

89. Zanettini R, et al. Regression of cardiac valvulopathy related to ergot-derived dopamine agonists. *Cardiovasc Ther.* 2011;29:404-410.

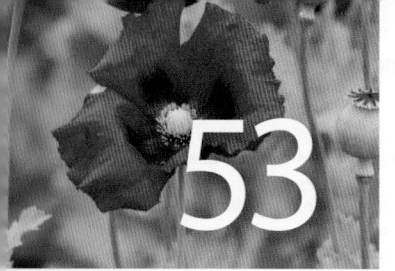

53 THYROID AND ANTITHYROID MEDICATIONS

Nicole C. Bouchard

HISTORY AND EPIDEMIOLOGY

Long before the thyroid was recognized as a functional endocrine gland, it was believed to serve a cosmetic function, especially in women. Egyptian paintings often emphasize the full and beautiful necks of women with enlarged thyroid glands. Early theories on the physiologic function of the thyroid gland included lubrication of the trachea, diversion of blood flow from the brain, and protection of women from "irritation" and "vexation" from men.[43] Although poorly defined in historical accounts, symptoms resembling hypothyroidism and myxedema that were successfully treated with ground sheep thyroid were described 500 years ago. In the 16th century, Paracelsus described the association between goiter (thyroid gland enlargement) and cretinism.[99] A syndrome of cardiac hyperactivity, goiter, and exophthalmos was first described in 1786.[99] Graves and von Basedow further detailed this syndrome and its relationship to the thyroid gland 50 years later.[43]

In 1891, injection of ground sheep thyroid extract was formally described as a treatment for myxedema.[43] Shortly afterward, oral therapy was determined to be equally effective. Seaweed, which contains large amounts of iodine, was used to treat goiter (hypothyroidism) in Chinese medicine as early as the third century A.D. In 1863, Trousseau fortuitously discovered a treatment for Graves disease when he inadvertently prescribed daily tincture of iodine instead of tincture of digitalis to a tachycardic, thyrotoxic young woman.[111]

Sir Charles R. Harington described the chemical structure and performed the first synthesis of thyroxine (tetraiodothyronine $\{T_4\}$) in 1926.[90] Triiodothyronine (T_3) was not isolated and synthesized until the 1950s.[43] Prior to this, desiccated thyroid gland from animal sources was commonly used to treat hypothyroidism. Despite becoming essentially obsolete in the modern medical community, unprocessed, desiccated thyroid is easily purchased via the Internet and in health food stores as a thyroid supplement.[104] A pharmaceutical-grade porcine-derived thyroid supplement originally produced by Armour, is still available by prescription from several manufacturers. Unfortunately, the misguided use of both organic and synthetic thyroid supplements as vitality agents, stimulants, and weight-loss aids has become increasingly common. Two epidemics of "hamburger thyrotoxicosis" that occurred in the United States in the mid-1980s secondary to consumption of ground beef contaminated with bovine thyroid gland demonstrated the potential widespread toxicologic sequelae after a community unknowingly ingested thyroid hormone.[46,60]

Today, hypothyroidism and hyperthyroidism are relatively common endocrine disorders. The global incidence of neonatal hypothyroidism is one per 3,000 to 4,500 births. It is estimated that hypothyroidism affects 1% to 5% of US adults. It is more prevalent in whites than in people of Hispanic or African American descent. In the elderly, the prevalence of hypothyroidism increases to 15% by the age of 75 years. Worldwide, iodine deficiency is the leading cause of hypothyroidism. According to US retail pharmaceutical statistics for prescription drugs, levothyroxine (both generic and brand combined; T_4) has consistently ranked in the top 5 prescription count, with an average 67 million per year. Because of widespread availability of thyroid replacement therapy, many cases of intentional and unintentional overdoses with thyroid hormone are reported.[71] However, despite the profound effects of thyroid hormones on physiologic homeostasis and the widespread use and access to exogenous thyroid hormone, morbidity and mortality from overdose is very low and clinically significant overdoses with thyroid hormone preparations are uncommon.

PHARMACOLOGY

Physiology

To properly understand the impact of thyroid supplements and antithyroid xenobiotics on the function of the human body, an understanding of thyroid physiology is required. Thyroid function is influenced by the following: (1) the hypothalamus, (2) the pituitary gland, (3) the thyroid gland, and (4) the target organs for the thyroid hormones (Fig. 53–1).

The hypothalamus, viewed by some as the "master gland," is an intermediate between cerebral centers and the pituitary gland. When the hypothalamus receives specific neurotransmitter stimulation, thyroid-releasing hormone (TRH) is produced, which is then transported through the venous sinusoids to the pituitary gland, which then releases thyroid-stimulating hormone (TSH). Thyroid-stimulating hormone enters the circulation and stimulates the production and release of the thyroid hormones T_3 and T_4 from the thyroid gland. Thyroid physiology exhibits classic autoregulation or "negative biofeedback" of hormonal function. When adequate thyroid hormones are present, they exert an inhibitory effect on the pituitary gland, diminishing production of TSH (Fig. 53–1). Suppression or upregulation of TSH production is a frequently used laboratory marker in the evaluation of hyperthyroidism and hypothyroidism, respectively.

Thyroid hormones are tyrosine molecules with iodine substitutions. Two forms of the hormone are physiologically active: T_3 and T_4 (Table 53–1). Synthesis of thyroid hormones is a multistep process. The follicles of the thyroid gland consist of an epithelial layer of thyroid cells surrounding a proteinaceous colloidal substance containing tyrosine molecules bound to thyroglobulin. After absorption, iodide (I^-) is concentrated in thyroid cells by an active transport process called *iodide trapping*. Absorbed I^- is then oxidized to iodine (I_2) by thyroid (iodide) peroxidase within the colloid matrix. Iodine rapidly iodinates tyrosine residues to form monoiodotyrosine and diiodotyrosine. These substituted tyrosine molecules then combine to form T_3 and T_4. The ratio of T_3 to T_4 in thyroglobulin is 1:5. Triiodothyronine and T_4 (thyroxine) ultimately are released into circulation from the thyroglobulin matrix.

Iodide trapping can be inhibited pharmacologically by monovalent anions such as thiocyanate (SCN^-), pertechnetate (TcO_4^-), and perchlorate (ClO_4^-). Thyroid peroxidase is inhibited by high concentrations of intrathyroidal iodide and by thioamide drugs. High intrathyroidal iodide concentrations also inhibit the release of thyroid hormone into circulation (Wolff-Chaikoff effect) (Table 53–2).

Approximately 95% of circulating or peripheral thyroid hormone is T_4; the remainder is T_3. Only 15% of the peripheral T_3 is secreted directly by the thyroid; the balance results from the peripheral (meaning outside the thyroid gland) conversion of T_4 to T_3. When circulating T_4 enters the cell, it is deiodinated to T_3. Deiodination of the T_4 molecule occurs by monodeiodination of either the outer ring or the inner ring by 5'-deiodinase or 5-deiodinase, yielding 3,5,3'-T_3 and 3,3',5-triiodothyronine (reverse T_3 $\{rT_3\}$), respectively.[11] Triiodothyronine has approximately 4 times greater hormonal activity than T_4, whereas rT_3 is metabolically inactive. Triiodothyronine exerts its effects by binding to thyroid hormone receptors inside the nucleus. This interaction with nuclear receptors regulates gene transcription and protein synthesis, which ultimately increases oxygen consumption and underlies the thermogenic effects of thyroid hormones.

Propranolol, corticosteroids, ipodate (iodinated oral contrast agent), starvation, and severe illness inhibit 5'-deiodinase, which results in decreased production of metabolically active T_3 and preferential monodeiodination to metabolically inactive rT_3, leading to a syndrome known as "sick

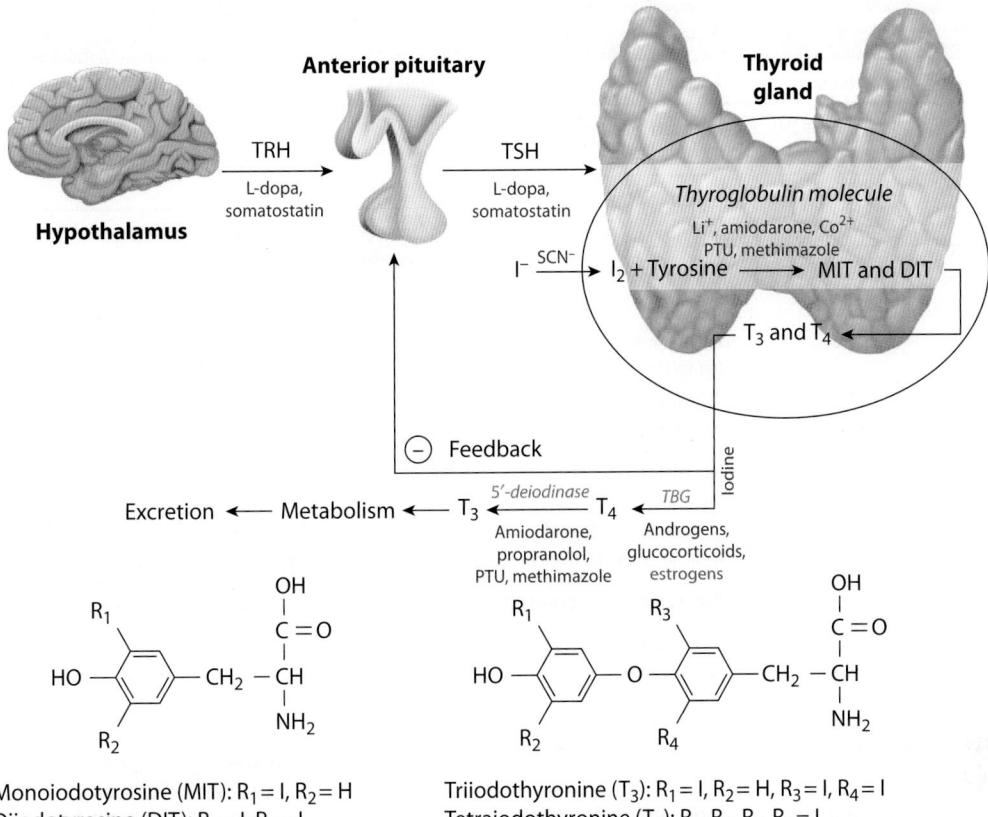

FIGURE 53–1. Thyroid hormone synthesis: its control, metabolism, and molecular structures. PTU = propylthiouracil; SCN⁻ = thiocyanate; TBG = thyroxine-binding globulin; TRH = thyrotropin-releasing hormone; TSH = thyroid-stimulating hormone; Li⁺, amiodarone, Co²⁺.

euthyroid" (Table 53–2). This energy-conserving effect allows attenuation of the thermogenic effects of thyroid hormones in times of physiologic stress.[109]

T₄ and T₃

Thyroid supplementation for treatment of hypothyroidism is in widespread use both in human and veterinary medicine. Thyroid hormones historically were derived from animal origin, but now are largely synthetically produced. Desiccated and processed porcine thyroid contains both T₃ and T₄. Because it is less pharmacologically stable and carries a risk of allergic reaction and thyrotoxicity from T₃, its use has largely been supplanted by the safer synthetic alternatives. Levothyroxine is the preparation of choice because of its low immunogenicity, 7-day half-life, and easy dosing regimen. It is also available in an intravenous (IV) formulation. Liothyronine (T₃ preparation, available in oral {PO} and IV) and combination T₃/T₄ preparations available PO. Those synthetic formulations are seldom used clinically because of their short half-lives, high cost, unique therapeutic indication, and increased risk of thyrotoxicosis.

Steady state with regard to suppression of TSH and elevation of T₄ is reached approximately 6 to 8 weeks after initiation of therapy. Doses usually are titrated in increments of 12.5 or 25 mcg/day after 6 weeks based on TSH

measurements. Typical doses for levothyroxine range from 12.5 to 300 mcg/day depending on the patient's age and body weight. Children tend to be dosed by body weight per kilogram and elderly patient dosed between 12.5 and 50 mcg/day because of enhanced sensitivity to thyroxine excess. Different sources suggest varied bioequivalence of Synthroid (T₄) to generic levothyroxine.[13,25,26,39] As a result, thyroid hormone concentrations and the patient's clinical status should be followed when transitioning between levothyroxine formulations because the switch can present a risk for an adverse drug event.

PHARMACOKINETICS AND TOXICOKINETICS

Gastrointestinal absorption of exogenous thyroid hormone occurs primarily in the duodenum and ileum. Gastrointestinal absorption is decreased by variations in intestinal flora and binding by certain xenobiotics (Table 53–2). In circulation, T₃ and T₄ both are highly but reversibly bound to plasma proteins—approximately 99.6% and 99.96%, respectively (in nonpregnant adults). Thyroxine-binding globulin binds approximately two-thirds of the circulating thyroid hormones; albumin and other proteins bind the remainder. It is estimated that only 0.4% of T₃ and 0.04% of T₄ exist in the free form. Exogenously derived thyroid hormones exhibit similar binding characteristics when dosed in a physiologic range. The amount of thyroid hormone bound to proteins varies greatly with different physiologic and pharmacologic conditions, for example, increasing in pregnancy[48] and levothyroxine overdose and decreasing in chronic disease. In pregnancy, increases in TBG binding leads to increased production of T₃ and T₄, resulting in a state of euthyroid hyperthyroxinemia. These changes in protein binding must be evaluated when measuring total thyroid hormone concentrations in the blood (see Diagnostic Testing). Table 53–1 lists some important pharmacokinetic properties of thyroid hormones.

Thyroid hormones undergo their ultimate metabolism peripherally (meaning outside the thyroid gland). Intracellular sequential deiodination accounts for approximately two-thirds of inactivation. Most of the remaining third undergoes hepatic metabolism by glucuronidation or sulfation.

TABLE 53–1	Pharmacokinetic Properties of Thyroid Hormones	
Pharmacokinetic Property	*T₃*	*T₄*
Oral bioavailability (exogenous), %	95	80
Volume of distribution (L/kg)	40	10
Half-life (days)	1	7
Protein binding (normal adult), %	99.96	99.6
Relative potency	4	1

TABLE 53–2	Xenobiotic Interactions: Effects on Thyroid Hormones and Function[8,35,40,111]	
Xenobiotic	**Interaction**	**Effect**
Dopamine, levodopa, somatostatin	Inhibit TRH and TSH synthesis	No clinical hypothyroidism
Iodides (including amiodarone), lithium, aminoglutethimide	Inhibit thyroid hormone synthesis or release	Hypothyroidism
Monovalent anions (SCN^-, TcO_4^-, ClO_4^-)	Inhibit iodide uptake to thyroid gland	Hypothyroidism
Estrogens, tamoxifen, heroin, methadone, mitotane	Increase TBG	Altered thyroid hormone transport in serum ↑ Total measured thyroid hormone (vs *free* hormone)
Androgens, glucocorticoids	Decrease TBG	Altered thyroid hormone transport in serum ↓ Total measured thyroid hormone (vs *free* hormone)
Salicylates, mefenamic acid, furosemide	Displace T_3 or T_4 from TBG	Transient hyperthyroxinemia
Thioamides (methimazole, propylthiouracil)	Inhibit thyroid peroxidase	Decrease thyroid hormone synthesis
Phenytoin, carbamazepine, phenobarbital, rifampin, rifabutin	Induction of hepatic enzymes	↓ Total thyroid hormone
Iopanoic acid, ipodate, amiodarone, propranolol, corticosteroids, propylthiouracil	Inhibition of 5'-deiodinase	Decrease peripheral conversion of T_4 ($\downarrow T_3$, $\uparrow rT_3$)
Cholestyramine, colestipol, aluminum hydroxide, sucralfate, ferrous sulfate, some calcium preparations, infant soy formula	Interfere with GI absorption of T_4	Decreased oral bioavailability of T_4
Interleukin-α, interleukin-2	Induction of autoimmune thyroid disease	Hyperthyroidism or hypothyroidism

GI = gastrointestinal; TBG = thyroid-binding globulin; TRH = thyroid-releasing hormone; TSH = thyroid-stimulating hormone. Thiocyanate (SCN^-), pertechnetate (TcO_4^-), and perchlorate (ClO_4^-).

TABLE 53–3	Common Xenobiotics That Alter Thyroid Function and Cause Clinically Important Effects[8,17,35,40,45,64,96,111,117,118]	
Xenobiotic	**Effect**	**Mechanism**
Lithium	Goiter (in 37% of patients) Hypothyroidism (in 5%–15% of patients)	Mechanism unclear
Amiodarone (37% iodine by weight)	1. Hypothyroidism (in 25% of patients) 2. Hyperthyroidism, type 1: in patients with preexisting goiters from low iodine intake 3. Hyperthyroidism, type 2: in patients with previously normal thyroid function	1. Inhibition of 5'-deiodinase 2. Type 1: iodine excess stimulates thyroid hormone production 3. Type 2: causes thyroid inflammation
Propranolol	↓Peripheral conversion of T_4 to T_3	Inhibition of 5'-deiodinase
PTU (propylthiourea) or methimazole	Decreased thyroid hormone synthesis ↓Peripheral conversion of T_4 to T_3	Inhibition of thyroid peroxidase Inhibition of 5'-deiodinase
Corticosteroids	↓Peripheral conversion of T_4 to T_3	Inhibition of 5'-deiodinase
Iodine	1. Low dose: transient or no effect 2. High doses (>10 mg/day): ↓ thyroid hormone secretion 3. Transient thyrotoxicosis (ie, Jod-Basedow effect) With rapid correction of hypothyroidism from iodine deficiency 4. Delirium 5. Caustic injury [From topical iodine]	1. Transiently stimulates thyroid hormone secretion 2. Inhibition of thyroid hormone synthesis 3. Increases thyroid hormone synthesis 4. Mechanism unclear 5. Direct cytotoxic injury to cells
Iodinated contrast material	1. Rapid ↓ peripheral conversion of T_4 to T_3 (adjunctive treatment in thyroid storm) 2. Prolonged suppression of T_4 to T_3 3. Causes thyrotoxicosis and thyroid storm 4. Iodide "mumps"	1. Inhibition of 5'-deiodinase 2. Mechanism unclear 3. Mechanism unclear 4. Idiopathic, toxic accumulation of iodide
Radioactive iodine	Treatment of hyperthyroidism, causes hypothyroidism	Uptake into thyroid follicles causes local destruction
Anion inhibitors[a]	↓Iodine uptake into thyroid follicle, used in iodide-induced hyperthyroidism	Blocks uptake of iodide into the thyroid gland by competitive inhibition

Xenobiotics that induce hepatic microsomal metabolism, such as rifampin, phenobarbital, phenytoin, and carbamazepine, increase the metabolic clearance of T_3 and T_4 (Table 53–2).

PATHOPHYSIOLOGY

Thyroid hormones are critical for optimal physiologic growth and function. Thyroid function is the most important determinant of basal metabolic rate. In addition, the thyroid exerts a permissive effect on many hormones, notably catecholamines and insulin.

Hyperthyroidism is a condition characterized by excess active thyroid hormone. Most aspects of carbohydrate, protein, and lipid metabolism are increased in the presence of thyroid hormone excess. The disorder is characterized by manifestations of increased metabolism such as hyperthermia, weight loss, diarrhea, heat intolerance, and diaphoresis, along with tachycardia, widened pulse pressure, tremor, anxiety, other behavioral changes, and sometimes tachydysrhythmias such as rapid atrial fibrillation, extrasystoles, and high output congestive heart failure.[32,61,100,101] This constellation of findings, called *thyrotoxicosis*, results from overproduction of the hormone, increased conversion from T_4 to T_3, or intake of exogenous hormone. Graves disease (diffuse toxic goiter), an autoimmune disorder, is the most common cause of excess thyroid hormone secretion. It accounts for approximately two-thirds of cases and often is accompanied by exophthalmos and diffusely enlarged, nontender thyroid gland. Toxic multinodular goiter, toxic thyroid adenoma, iodine or amiodarone exposure (which can also cause hypothyroidism; Table 53–3), thyrotoxicosis factitia, and thyroiditis (eg, postpartum, Hashimoto, DeQuervain) are some other etiologies of hyperthyroidism.[41] Severe thyrotoxicosis with significant rapid clinical decompensation is referred to as *thyroid storm* or *thyrotoxic crisis*. Thyroid storm typically occurs when untreated or undertreated hyperthyroidism occurs simultaneously with a physiologic stressor such as trauma, infection, diabetic ketoacidosis, or surgery. In early stages, patients are hyperthermic and markedly tachycardic, tremulous, agitated, or psychotic with nausea, vomiting, and diarrhea. As the disease progresses, stupor, coma, and hypotension ensue. General treatment strategies include early airway control, crystalloid fluid resuscitation, β-adrenergic antagonist administration, parenteral corticosteroids if adrenal insufficiency is suspected, and antithyroid medications such as propylthiouracil and methimazole. The β-adrenergic antagonist, propranolol, is a mainstay of treatment, as in addition to its desirable effects on tremor, heart rate, and systemic vascular resistance, it decreases peripheral conversion of T_4 to T_3.[117] Mortality in thyroid storm, even with treatment, can approach 20%.[32,97]

Because plasma catecholamine concentrations are normal or decreased in hyperthyroidism, an increase in sensitivity to catecholamines is thought to be responsible for the increased inotropy and chronotropy produced by thyroid hormones.[20,23,94] Several general mechanisms are proposed for the direct cardiac effects of thyroid hormones, although their relative contributions are uncertain.[5,21,22,55,62,113]

- T_3 increases the number of β-adrenergic receptors in various tissues, including cardiac cells.[16] This process occurs via upregulation of β-adrenergic receptor synthesis at the level of the β-adrenergic gene.[6]
- T_3 modulates myocyte intracellular signaling mechanisms that lead to increased catecholamine effects. Enhancement of intracellular signaling activity involving protein kinase A, cyclic adenosine monophosphate, G proteins, and increased phosphorylation of thyroid hormone receptor proteins all are implicated to varying degrees.[31,61,92,93,98,107,114]
- Enhancement of myocardial transmembrane and sarcoplasmic reticulum ion channel function, L-type voltage-gated Ca^{2+} channels, and accelerated Ca^{2+} entry into the sarcoplasmic reticulum also are suggested.[58,59,81,106] Whether the effects on intracellular signaling represent a direct effect of T_3 on intracellular signaling mediators or T_3 induced augmentation of the individual β-adrenergic receptor response to catecholamines with a secondary change in postreceptor signaling is unclear.[5]

In addition to these mechanisms, T_3 upregulates synthesis of cardiac thyroid hormone receptors (at TR-alpha and TR-β genes), and the thermogenic effects of thyroid hormones cause decreased systemic vascular resistance, leading to a reflex (and indirect) increase in cardiac output. Comprehensive reviews on this topic explore the more complex cellular aspects of thyroid hormones and their effects on the cardiovascular system.[21,22,61,87]

Hypothyroidism, a condition characterized by decreased basal metabolic rate and decreased catecholamine effects, is a common disorder, especially in women and the elderly. Worldwide, dietary iodine deficiency remains the leading cause of hypothyroidism. In certain parts of the world, particularly mountainous regions such as the Andes, Alps, and Himalayas, goitrous hypothyroidism remains endemic. Untreated congenital thyroid deficiency and severe dietary iodine deficiency (goitrous hypothyroidism) in young children result in profound, irreversible mental retardation and dwarfism (also referred to as cretinism). Iodine deficiency is said to be the most common cause of preventable brain damage worldwide. In developed nations, the iodization of table salt has essentially eliminated dietary iodine deficiency as a cause of hypothyroidism leaving autoimmune etiologies as the most common cause, although thyroid function diminishes significantly with age in many patients. Treatment of Graves disease with radioactive iodine typically results in hypothyroidism within one year. Thyroiditis (eg, postpartum, Hashimoto, DeQuervain) is associated with either hypothyroidism or hyperthyroidism as is exposure to certain xenobiotics such as amiodarone and lithium (Table 53–3). Myxedema and myxedema coma are potentially life-threatening emergencies that represent extremes of hypothyroidism. Hypothyroidism is not discussed in more detail in this chapter, except to note that treatment of hypothyroid emergencies, especially with T_3, can result in thyrotoxic signs and symptoms. Comprehensive reviews of hypothyroidism are available.[103]

CLINICAL MANIFESTATIONS

Signs and symptoms of toxicity from exogenous thyroid hormone resemble those of catecholamine excess. Pronounced catecholaminelike effects occur in the cardiovascular system, especially tachycardia, tachydysrhythmias (usually atrial fibrillation or flutter), thromboembolism (from both atrial fibrillation and endothelial activation), and high output cardiac failure.[32,61,100,101] Interestingly, although hyperthyroid patients typically are anxious, restless, or agitated, patients with thyroid storm sometimes present with a decreased level of consciousness or even coma.[12,52,66,95,105] Hyperthermia

occurs secondary to the thermogenic effects of thyroid hormones and psychomotor agitation. Hyperthermia can be extreme (ie, >106°F {>41°C}). The tachycardia associated with thyrotoxicosis often is disproportionately elevated when compared to the temperature elevation (Chap. 29).

Acute Toxicity

Acute overdoses with thyroid hormone preparations most commonly occur with oral levothyroxine. Significant ingestions of levothyroxine do not typically manifest clinically until 7 to 10 days after exposure, but rarely can occur as early as 1 to 3 days postingestion.[42,50,69,97,108] The delay of peripheral conversion of T_4 to the metabolically active T_3 and the time required to activate nuclear receptors and protein synthesis account for this clinical latency. By contrast, acute overdoses containing T_3 typically manifest clinically within the first 12 to 24 hours after exposure.[70]

In children, acute thyroxine overdoses almost universally are benign because the ingestions are typically unintentional and of a low dose. Most children remain asymptomatic or develop only mild signs and symptoms. No deaths are reported.[29,36,67,70,71,108,110] In a series of 15 children with unintentional ingestion, only 3 developed mild signs and symptoms within 12 to 48 hours of the exposures which resolved within 24 to 60 hours.[69] Similarly, a case series that involved 41 children (ages 1–5 years) with unintentional exposures to thyroxine (estimated doses ranged from 40 to 800 mcg) found mild signs and symptoms (hyperactive behavior, tachycardia, fever, vomiting, diarrhea, diaphoresis, and flushing) in only 27%. All children had good clinical outcomes. The degree of signs and symptoms did not correlate with the amount ingested or measured serum thyroxine concentrations (measured 1–5 hours postingestion) for most cases in that series (see Diagnostic Testing).[36] Two other series involving 78 and 92 cases of unintentional exposures in children found that mild signs and symptoms developed in only 4 and 8 patients, respectively.[108,115] A report involving an intentional exposure of 9,900 mcg in a 13-year-old boy treated empirically with activated charcoal, dexamethasone, and oral propranolol described only mild tremors and anxiety.[108] A 2.5-year-old boy exposed to an estimated 7,600 mcg and was treated with activated charcoal approximately one hour after exposure and released home. He returned approximately 24 hours later with mild tachycardia and hyperthermia and decrease in appetite. No other treatments were administered. Over the next month, he experienced desquamation of the palms and soles and irritability.[50] Very few cases of severe toxicity in children are reported: one child without a history of a seizure disorder had 2 seizures 7 days after a levothyroxine ingestion (18,000 mcg),[65] another 2-year-old developed thyroid storm with lethargy on postingestion day 5 (estimated ingestion was 6,000 mcg, no activated charcoal was administered, and she was treated with oral propranolol),[74] another child became gravely ill for a 12-hour period (blood pressure, 120/68 mm Hg; pulse, 200 beats/minute; temperature 104°F {40°C}) 6 hours after ingesting a large amount (3.2 g, or 50 grains) of a desiccated thyroid preparation containing both T_3 and T_4.[68] All of these children made a full recovery.

Exposures in adults have a wide range of toxicity. Many patients are asymptomatic or mildly symptomatic.[67,72,105] Severe sequelae occur more frequently in adults than in children. Signs and symptoms resemble thyrotoxicosis and, in extreme cases, thyroid storm. Hyperthermia,[42,67,105] dysrhythmias,[7,67,105] and severe agitation[45] are well described. Hemiparesis,[12] muscle weakness,[12,105] seizure,[2] coma,[12,67,105] respiratory failure,[34] sudden death and dysrhythmias,[10] myocardial infarction,[10] cardiac failure,[12] focal myocarditis,[10] rhabdomyolysis with muscle necrosis,[12] delayed palmar desquamation (>2 weeks postingestion),[12,105] acute kidney injury and multiorgan failure,[80] and hematuria[42] are also described. Because patients are expected to be asymptomatic shortly after ingestion and laboratory tests correlate poorly with the degree of signs and symptoms, clinical and laboratory findings early in the course of the ingestion are not reliable indicators of which patients will become ill (see Diagnostic Testing).

Chronic Toxicity

Following long-term excessive thyroid hormone ingestion, patients can present with thyrotoxicosis or have a more subtle and insidious presentation.

Classically, long-term ingestion of excess thyroid hormone occurs in patients with hypothyroidism, psychiatric disorders, and eating disorders. Persons who ingest thyroid hormones long-term can develop significant weight loss, anxiety, and accelerated osteoporosis.[83] More severe manifestations, such as cardiac dysrhythmias, sinus tachycardia, cardiac failure, and psychosis, also occur. As in patients with hyperthyroidism, intercurrent illness and physiologic stressors can trigger thyroid storm in these patients.

Numerous epidemics of hyperthyroidism and thyrotoxicosis have resulted from the consumption of ground meat containing neck muscle contaminated with thyroid gland.[27,46,60] Investigators in one of these epidemics had 3 volunteers consume a single large portion of "well-cooked" epidemic implicated ground beef that was previously frozen. Although all volunteers remained asymptomatic, the mean serum peak T_4 (8–12 hours postingestion) was elevated approximately 15 mcg/dL, and TSH remained undetectable for 4 to 17 days.[46] The practice of gullet trimming (using larynx muscles for beef) that led to these outbreaks has since been prohibited in US slaughter houses. However, the risk for sporadic cases remains, especially when laryngeal muscles are used or when farmers and hunters butcher their own meat.[88] Until an exogenous source of thyroid hormone is suspected or identified, such patients often are misdiagnosed with painless thyroiditis or thyrotoxicosis factitia.

Thyrotoxicosis factitia is a symptomatic disorder that mimics physiologic disease. It occurs with intentional long-term ingestion of exogenous thyroid hormone. The pattern of ingestion typically is surreptitious and maladaptive. Patients frequently have comorbid psychiatric disorders, such as Munchausen syndrome or eating disorders, or are taking thyroid hormone for secondary gain.[44] Patients with thyrotoxicosis factitia tend to be either health care professionals with access to medications or prescriptions or persons with access to thyroid medications prescribed for relatives, friends, or pets.[37,44,75]

Thyroid hormones remain popular among dieters and athletes who use the hormones as weight-loss aids and as stimulants. Severe consequences can occur. Sudden death was reported in 3 patients suspected of long-term ingestion of thyroid hormone for weight loss and energy enhancement (for which there is a black box warning).[10] In 2002, the heavily promoted Singaporean diet pill (Slim 10) was linked to hepatotoxicity and hyperthyroidism in numerous patients.[46] Investigators found the proprietary herbal preparation was adulterated with significant amounts of the undeclared ingredients T_4, T_3 (from thyroid gland extract), and fenfluramine (a drug banned by the US Food and Drug Administration). The medication was promptly withdrawn and the manufacturers convicted under the Singapore Poisons Act.[4] Similar cases were reported from Hong Kong, Japan, and France following ingestion of "slimming pills" containing animal thyroid extract.[57,85,91] Similarly, Redotex, a pharmaceutical Mexican diet supplement that is banned in the United States and contains T_3, norpseudoephedrine, diazepam, atropine, and a laxative was implicated in toxicity and overdose.[16,28] Unfortunately, thyroid hormone–containing supplements are promoted and are readily available to the general public without a prescription through the Internet and in stores selling nutritional supplements (Chap. 43).[104]

DIAGNOSTIC TESTING

Traditionally, thyroid testing involved combinations of measurement of total T_4 and some measurement of hormone binding (T_3 uptake). Free T_4 and T_3 are also measured by equilibrium dialysis (*free* T_4), analog assays (ie, competitive analogs of either free T_3 or free T_4 that competitively bind for spaces on the serum-binding proteins), and antibody capture assays (ie, sequential assays that capture a representative portion of the free fraction of thyroid hormone). Assessment of pituitary production of TSH has improved greatly in recent years. Because supersensitive TSH assays can readily detect suppression of TSH production, TSH is now the primary test for screening thyroid function. Suppressed or elevated concentrations of TSH should be reflexively followed up with a free T_4 assay and, if necessary, a free T_3 assay (Table 53–4).

The clinical manifestations of thyrotoxicosis and thyroid storm are well known to occur at normal, low, moderate, and high concentrations of T_3 and

TABLE 53–4 Diagnostic Tests for Thyroid Hormone and Thyroid Function

Diagnostic Test	Normal Values[a]	Comments
TSH	0.5–4.7 IU/mL	Available assays with respective detection limits: First-generation 1.0 IU/L Second-generation 0.1 IU/L Third-generation 0.01 IU/L
Total T_4 by RIA	4.5–12.5 mcg/dL (58–161 nmol/L)	↑ In pregnancy, estrogens, oral contraceptives
Total T_3 by RIA	80–200 ng/dL (0.9–2.8 nmol/L)	↑ In pregnancy, estrogens, oral contraceptives
Free T_4	8–18 pg/mL (10–23 pmol/L)	↑ In hyperthyroidism, exogenous thyroxine ingestion
Free T_3	2.3–4.2 pg/mL (3.5–6.5 pmol/L)	↑ In hyperthyroidism, exogenous thyroid hormone (T_3 or T_4)

[a]Interlaboratory and interassay variations occur.

RIA = radioimmunoassay; TSH = thyroid-stimulating hormone.

T_4.[15] This lack of correlation between signs and symptoms and serum concentrations is also true for exogenous thyroid hormone ingestion.[9,12,36,42,46,65,70,84,108,115] In a large case series of children with unintentional exposures of thyroxine estimated to be between 40 and 800 mcg, serum T_4 concentrations were drawn in 11 (1–5 hours postingestion). Serum T_4 concentrations were normal in 5 of these children and were slightly elevated in 6 (mean, 16 mcg/dL). In this series, one infant who was estimated to have ingested 4500 mcg had a significantly higher concentration (55 mcg/dL at 4.5 hours) but developed only a transient episode of diaphoresis and a "staring spell" 7 days postingestion. Another child who ingested an estimated 4,200 mcg had a concentration of 12 mcg/dL and developed significant tachycardia and hyperthermia.[38] A young child (estimated ingestion 18,000 mcg levothyroxine) had a serum T_4 concentration of 117 mcg/dL 8 hours postingestion and 38 mcg/dL on day 7, when he was symptomatic.[65] Similar trends were observed for both T_3 and T_4 in 3 other massive levothyroxine ingestions in children.[6,74,108] In an adult with a massive ingestion of levothyroxine (720,000 mcg), serum T_4 concentrations were higher than 30 mcg/dL and free T_4 was above 13 ng/dL (normal range, 0.7–1.86 ng/dL). In this case, TSH remained undetectable until postingestion day 32.[42] Overall, the observed signs and symptoms following thyroid hormone ingestion correlate poorly with the amount ingested or with measured serum T_4 concentrations. Prolonged suppression of TSH is common following ingestion of excess thyroid hormone.

Routine analysis of laboratory thyroid function tests in the setting of acute thyroid hormone overdose likely will not affect management. Analysis of thyroid hormone concentrations is indicated only if confirmation of a suspected ingestion is desired and in massive ingestions when early and severe symptoms may occur. Suppression of TSH and elevated thyroid hormone concentrations with a low serum thyroglobulin concentration help to differentiate between thyrotoxicosis factitia and true endogenous disease.[75]

MANAGEMENT

Based on the existing literature, conservative management is adequate in most cases of acute unintentional thyroxine ingestions in both adults and children. Most children with acute overdose are managed with home observation and follow-up appointments. In cases in which the acute thyroxine dose is estimated to be greater than 4,000 mcg, patient follow-up by regular telephone contact for 10 days is recommended.[36] Historically, most children with unintentional ingestions were treated with GI decontamination with activated charcoal and/or syrup of ipecac, or by gastric lavage,[36,65,69,71,108] but these procedures (especially emesis and lavage) are probably unnecessary. Based on 2 large series of unintentional exposures in children in which no toxicity was observed in the clear majority of cases, clinically significant toxicity is not expected with estimated ingestions less than 4,000 mcg.[36,51] Because children almost uniformly develop no more than minor symptoms, activated charcoal administration is recommended only if the ingestion is greater than 5,000 mcg of thyroxine. Aspiration risks are minimal in awake, alert children who are able to protect their airways and take activated charcoal orally, without nasogastric tube placement.[67,115] By extension, adults with acute ingestions greater than 5,000 mcg of thyroxine also should be treated with activated charcoal. Gastric emptying procedures such as orogastric lavage, should be reserved for early presentations with massive thyroxine ingestions (>10,000–50,000 mcg) in suicidal adults or ingestions of preparations containing large amounts of T_3.[12,42] We recommend that patients with massive ingestions (>10,000–50,000 mcg) or ingestion of T_3-containing products be admitted for observation in anticipation of developing significant symptoms.[12,42,65,68]

Treatment should be based on the development of toxicity and should include rehydration, airway protection, and control of sympathomimetic symptoms, mental status alterations, and hyperpyrexia. β-Adrenergic antagonism with propranolol is typically used for sympathomimetic symptoms in numerous cases.[9,33,65,84,108,110] Empiric treatment with β-adrenergic antagonists is not recommended. Treatment is only indicated for clinically significant tachycardia, dysrhythmias, and other signs and symptoms of catecholaminelike excess.[33,65,84,108,110]

Agitation

If sedation is required, parenteral benzodiazepines and barbiturates are recommended. Rapid-acting benzodiazepines, such as midazolam, or diazepam should be used to control severely agitated or symptomatic patients. Phenobarbital should used as an additional treatment in intubated patients or as an adjunct in patients requiring high doses of parenteral benzodiazepines for sedation because it offers the added theoretical benefit of inducing enhanced hepatic elimination of thyroxine as well as synergy with benzodiazepines (Table 53–2). Because of the general risks of sedation and the lack of evidence regarding the clinical use of enhanced hepatic elimination from phenobarbital, sedation with phenobarbital for the sole purpose of enhanced elimination is not indicated. Sedation with antipsychotics such as haloperidol and droperidol should be avoided because their significant anticholinergic properties can exacerbate thyrotoxic symptoms. In addition, the tendency for this class of drugs to prolong the QT interval and predispose to malignant dysrhythmias is of concern in the already catecholaminergic patient. Antipsychotics should be reserved for medically stable patients with psychiatric behavioral disturbances.

Catecholaminelike Excess and Cardiovascular Symptoms

The principal therapeutic role of β-adrenergic antagonists in hyperthyroidism is for their sympatholytic effects. In addition, propranolol inhibits 5′-deiodinase, thereby decreasing peripheral conversion of T_4 to T_3 (Table 53–2).[117] The clinical significance of decreased peripheral conversion in the setting of overdose is unknown. Propranolol is the most frequently used β-adrenergic antagonist in thyrotoxic patients,[36,42,65,74,84,108,110] and should be used parenterally when signs and symptoms are severe or when rapid control of heart rate is required. Starting doses of 1 to 2 mg IV propranolol every 10 to 15 minutes are recommended. Higher doses have been reported in massive thyroxine overdose, where a patient received 23 mg propranolol IV over one hour on initial presentation, then required an average of 30 mg/day IV for 5 more days.[42] Oral propranolol is recommended for persistent symptoms in patients who are both hemodynamically and medically stable and are not acutely agitated. High oral doses in the range of 20 to 120 mg every 6 hours are usually required. A 2 year-old with thyroid storm after massive levothyroixine overdose was treated with 0.8 mg/kg propanolol PO every 6 hours.[74] Other β-adrenergic antagonists, such as atenolol, nadolol, metoprolol, and esmolol, can be used for signs and symptoms of adrenergic excess, but the evidence for their inhibition of the peripheral conversion of T_4 to T_3 is not established. Continuous electrocardiographic and hemodynamic

monitoring are indicated when parenteral β-adrenergic antagonists are used or when patients require hospitalization.

When nonspecific β-adrenergic antagonists are contraindicated, as in patients with asthma or severe congestive heart failure, β_1-adrenergic receptor selective antagonists (such as atenolol or metoprolol) or calcium channel blockers are recommended. Among calcium channel blockers, diltiazem is the most studied for the management of thyrotoxicosis.[74,94] A double-blind, crossover trial that compared propranolol to diltiazem for thyrotoxic symptoms found that diltiazem was well tolerated and appeared as effective as propranolol.[79] Another study successfully used diltiazem as the sole treatment of cardiovascular signs and symptoms in 11 thyrotoxic patients.[102] Oral doses of 60 to 120 mg diltiazem 3 to 4 times daily or 5 to 10 mg/h parenterally have been used.[79,102] A possible explanation for the efficacy of calcium channel blockers in thyrotoxicosis is that thyroid hormone enhances Ca^{2+} uptake by L-type voltage-gated Ca^{2+} channels, accelerates Ca^{2+} entry into the sarcoplasmic reticulum, and increases cellular Ca^{2+} storage capacity.[58,59,81,106] The net effect of these changes is increased inotropy and chronotropy. Calcium channel blockers, particularly diltiazem and verapamil, attenuate these effects. However, the use of parenteral β-adrenergic antagonists in combination with parenteral calcium channel blockers is contraindicated because of the risk for profound hypotension and cardiovascular collapse.[86]

Hyperthermia

Antipyretics are not recommended for hyperthermia associated with catecholamine excess and thyrotoxic condition. Aspirin, particularly high doses (1.5–3 g/day), should be avoided because it carries a theoretical risk of increased thyrotoxicity from displacement of T_3 and T_4 from thyroxine-binding globulin (Table 53–2). Note, however, that hyperthermia, especially extreme hyperthermia (>106°F {>41°C}), is most likely secondary to psychomotor agitation and excess heat production from the hypermetabolic, catecholaminergic, and thyrotoxic conditions. Extreme hyperthermia is a medical emergency and should be rapidly and aggressively treated with active external cooling with ice baths or other aggressive external cooling measure and with β-adrenergic antagonism, sedation with benzodiazepines and/or barbiturates, and endotracheal intubation with paralysis if necessary (Chap. 29).

Other Therapies

Bile acid sequestrants, such as cholestyramine and colestipol, and aluminum hydroxide (antacids) and sucralfate bind to exogenous T_4 and decrease GI absorption (Table 53–2). They are used in levothyroxine overdose with possible benefit.[24] Because the evidence supporting their effectiveness is poor, they are not routinely recommended for thyroid hormone overdose.[67]

Oral iodine-containing contrast media is known to decrease peripheral conversion of T_4 to T_3. Doses of 1 to 2.5 mg/kg iodine PO daily are routinely used for thyroid storm (oral drops commonly referred to as saturated solution potassium iodide {KI or SSKI}). Thioamides, such as propylthiouracil (PTU) and methimazole, and the corticosteroids are thyroid gland inhibitors that are used for treatment of nondrug-related hyperthyroidism. In addition, thioamides inhibit peripheral conversion of T_4 to T_3. Evidence from limited case reports suggests poor efficacy of both thioamides and corticosteroids in acute overdose (see Thioamides and Iodides).[12,34,67]

Although use of antithyroid drugs such as PTU, corticosteroids, and iodine contrast media in thyroxine overdose has theoretical benefits, these xenobiotics are not validated, potentially harmful, and unlikely to offer additional benefit, or be superior to conventional therapy with activated charcoal, β-adrenergic antagonism, and sedation. These treatments are not recommended as adjunctive therapies for treatment of exogenous thyroxine overdose.

Extracorporeal Drug Removal

The use of extracorporeal drug removal procedures, such as plasma exchange or plasmapheresis, exchange transfusion (in children), and charcoal hemoperfusion, are reported in extreme cases of thyroid hormone overdose and thyroid storm.[1,12,14,34,47,54,63,67,70,77,80,82,112,116] Overall, results regarding improvement of clinical condition and plasma clearances of thyroid hormones with these methods are conflicting. The largest series of acute ingestions involved 6 patients who became critically ill after massive thyroxine ingestions of prescribed capsules containing a 1,000-fold concentration excess of thyroxine (dose range, 50,000–125,000 mcg/day for 2–12 days). Charcoal hemoperfusion and plasmapheresis were used in all patients. Plasmapheresis was found to be more effective than hemoperfusion in the extraction of thyroxine. The authors suggest this intervention shortens the duration of thyrotoxicosis. Rebound elevations in plasma concentrations occurred 24 hours later, suggesting redistribution between extravascular and intravascular compartments.[12] This redistribution is expected given the large volume of distribution for thyroid hormones (Table 53–1). It is only reasonable to perform early plasmapheresis in the exceptional situation of a known massive ingestion of thyroid hormone or critically ill patient from thyroid hormone ingestion. The outcomes from most ingestions of thyroid hormone will be favorable with good supportive care, sedation, and β-adrenergic antagonism.

XENOBIOTICS WITH ANTITHYROID EFFECTS

Thioamides

Antithyroid drugs are used to decrease the amount of thyroid hormone in hyperthyroidism, most commonly in Graves disease. Thioamides are a group of chemicals with the basic structure of R-SCN. Methimazole and propylthiouracil (PTU) are the 2 principal thioamides used for treatment of hyperthyroidism. Carbimazole, which is bioactivated methimazole, is available in Europe and China. Methimazole and PTU both inhibit the activity of thyroid peroxidase in the thyroid gland.[113] Propylthiouracil has the added effect of inactivating 5′-deiodinase, which decreases the peripheral conversion of T_4 to the metabolically more active T_3. Because thioamides act primarily by decreasing thyroid hormone synthesis (vs release), a lag time of 3 to 4 weeks may occur before T_4 is depleted. The oral bioavailability of PTU is 50% to 80%. It is rapidly absorbed from the gastrointestinal tract and may undergo first-pass effect by the liver. Although its plasma half-life is only 1.5 hours, its effects are long lasting because of accumulation in the thyroid gland. Propylthiouracil is inactivated by glucuronidation and is renally eliminated. Methimazole is completely absorbed, is concentrated in the thyroid, and is more slowly eliminated than PTU (48 vs 24 hours). We recommend a dose of PTU 100 mg orally every 8 hours. Higher doses may be required and doses in children less than 6 years old usually start at 50 mg/day. Methimazole can be given 30 mg PO daily. Although PTU is 10 times less potent than methimazole, it is more commonly used. The indications for its use are mild to moderate hyperthyroidism.

The 2 thioamides traverse the placenta (methimazole more than PTU) and should not be administered during pregnancy. However, they are minimally secreted in breast milk. Adverse effects occur in 3% to 12% of patients taking thioamides. The most common adverse effect is a maculopapular pruritic rash. Methimazole, PTU, and, to a lesser extent, carbimazole cause immune-mediated, dose-related, and age-related agranulocytosis and neutrophil dyscrasias.[73,78,89] This potentially life-threatening adverse effect is treated by administration of granulocyte colony–stimulating factor.[7] Premature withdrawal of thioamides leads to rebound symptoms and thyrotoxic states.[64]

There are little data regarding overdose with thioamides. A 12-year-old girl with a previous thyroidectomy, who was estimated to have ingested 5,000 to 13,000 mg PTU, developed only a transient decreased T_3 concentration and elevated alkaline phosphatase concentration (7350 mU/mL).[53] The absence of a functioning thyroid gland likely contributed to the benign course in this patient. No other serious sequelae are associated with acute overdose of thioamides.

Iodides

Prior to the development of thioamides, iodide salt was the principal treatment for hyperthyroidism. Iodides decrease thyroid hormone concentrations by inhibiting formation and release. In thyroid storm, high-dose iodides

(>2 g/day) decrease thyroid hormone release and produce substantial improvements by 2 to 7 days. Common sources of iodides include calcium iodide, sodium iodide, KI (pharmaceutical preparations, iopanoic acid, Lugol solution {iodine + KI solution}, oral drops {saturated solution KI}), and methyl iodide (industrial preparations).

The adverse reaction to long-term ingestion of small or excessive amounts of iodide salts, termed *iodism*, is characterized by cutaneous rash, laryngitis, bronchitis, esophagitis, conjunctivitis, drug fever, metallic taste, "mumps," salivation, headache, and bleeding diathesis. Immune-mediated hypersensitivity signs and symptoms consisting of urticaria, angioedema, eosinophilia, vasculitis, arthralgia, and lymphadenitis, and, rarely, anaphylactoid reactions may occur. Long-term iodide therapy produces goiters, hypothyroidism, and rarely hyperthyroidism. As much as 10 g sodium iodide has been administered IV without development of signs or symptoms of toxicity.

Iodide (I^-), unlike iodine (I_2), is not caustic (Chaps. 101 and 103). Potassium iodide (KI) is added to table salt to form iodized salt for prevention of goiter. It also is used prophylactically after exposure to large amounts of nuclear fallout to prevent uptake of radioactive iodine into the thyroid gland (Antidotes in Depth: A44) and is the most commonly used iodide for thyroid suppression in hyperthyroidism. "Iodide mumps" is a well-described but rare disorder characterized by severe sialadenitis (or parotitis),[56] allergic vasculitis, and/or conjunctivitis following administration of ionic and nonionic iodine-containing contrast media and oral iodide salts (Table 53–3).[18,19] Although the mechanism remains unclear, it is thought to be idiosyncratic or secondary to iodide accumulation and subsequent inflammation in the ductal systems of the salivary gland. Clinical effects tend to occur within 12 hours and resolve spontaneously within 48 to 72 hours.[18]

Iodides should be avoided in pregnancy because they readily cross the placenta. Severe fetal complications, such as cretinism and death from respiratory failure secondary to obstructive goiter, are reported.[30,48,76] Iodide salts are adsorbed to activated charcoal.

Methyl iodide is a methylating agent used in the chemical and pharmaceutical industry, as a reagent in microscopy, as a catalyst in production of organic lead compounds, as an etching agent, as a component in fire extinguishers, and formerly as a soil fumigant. Inhalational methyl iodide toxicity is associated with early pulmonary congestion, lethargy, and acute kidney injury. It also is associated with delayed cerebellar degeneration, multifocal neuropathies (cranial nerve and spinal), Parkinsonian effects, and late and persistent psychiatric symptoms (months to years).[3,49] Long-term repeated overexposures have led to misdiagnoses such as multiple sclerosis. The toxicity is similar to that of the monohalomethanes (Chap. 108).

SUMMARY

- Despite the prevalence of thyroid disorders in the general population and the widespread use of levothyroxine, remarkably little morbidity and mortality associated with overdose from thyroid hormones is reported.
- Most children with unintentional exposures can be observed as outpatients for 5 to 10 days.
- Adults with acute intentional ingestions rarely have severe symptoms that require management in an intensive care unit.
- Supportive care with sedation, cooling measures, and β-adrenergic antagonism are adequate in most cases.
- Long-term ingestions tend to produce more severe symptoms as they develop more insidiously or are complicated by thyroid storm.
- Clinicians should suspect exogenous thyroid hormone exposure in patients with thyrotoxicosis and suppressed TSH concentrations.

Acknowledgment

Christopher Keyes, MD, contributed to this chapter in previous editions.

REFERENCES

1. Aghini-Lombardi F, et al. Treatment of amiodarone iodine-induced thyrotoxicosis with plasmapheresis and methimazole. *J Endocrinol Invest.* 1993;16:823-826.

2. Allen KM, et al. Case report: clues to the diagnosis of an unsuspected massive levothyroxine overdose. *CJEM.* 2015;17:692-698.

3. Appel GB, et al. Methyl iodide intoxication. A case report. *Ann Intern Med.* 1975;82:534-536.

4. Authority HS. *Annual Report.* Singapore 2002-2003.

5. Bachman ES, et al. The metabolic and cardiovascular effects of hyperthyroidism are largely independent of beta-adrenergic stimulation. *Endocrinology.* 2004;145:2767-2774.

6. Bahouth SW, et al. Thyroid hormone induces beta1-adrenergic receptor gene transcription through a direct repeat separated by five nucleotides. *J Mol Cell Cardiol.* 1997;29:3223-3237.

7. Bartalena L, et al. Adverse effects of thyroid hormone preparations and antithyroid drugs. *Drug Saf.* 1996;15:53-63.

8. Bartalena L, et al. Treatment of amiodarone-induced thyrotoxicosis, a difficult challenge: results of a prospective study. *J Clin Endocrinol Metab.* 1996;81:2930-2933.

9. Beier C, et al. Attempted suicide with L-thyroxine in an adolescent girl [in German]. *Klin Padiatr.* 2006;218:34-37.

10. Bhasin S, et al. Sudden death associated with thyroid hormone abuse. *Am J Med.* 1981;71:887-890.

11. Bianco AC, Kim BW. Deiodinases: implications of the local control of thyroid hormone action. *J Clin Invest.* 2006;116:2571-2579.

12. Binimelis J, et al. Massive thyroxine intoxication: evaluation of plasma extraction. *Intensive Care Med.* 1987;13:33-38.

13. Bolton S. Bioequivalence studies for levothyroxine. *AAPS J.* 2005;7:E47-E53.

14. Braithwaite SS, et al. Plasmapheresis: an adjunct to medical management of severe hyperthyroidism. *J Clin Apher.* 1986;3:119-123.

15. Brooks MH, et al. Serum triiodothyronine concentration in thyroid storm. *J Clin Endocrinol Metab.* 1975;40:339-341.

16. Cantrell L. Redotex(R) revisited: intentional overdose with an illegal weight loss product. *J Emerg Med.* 2012;43:e147-e148.

17. Cappiello E, et al. Ultrastructural evidence of thyroid damage in amiodarone-induced thyrotoxicosis. *J Endocrinol Invest.* 1995;18:862-868.

18. Carter JE. Iodide "mumps." *N Engl J Med.* 1961;264:987-988.

19. Christensen J. Iodide mumps after intravascular administration of a nonionic contrast medium. Case report and review of the literature. *Acta Radiol.* 1995;36:82-84.

20. Coulombe P, et al. Plasma catecholamine concentrations in hyperthyroidism and hypothyroidism. *Metabolism.* 1976;25:973-979.

21. Danzi S, Klein I. Thyroid hormone and the cardiovascular system. *Med Clin North Am.* 2012;96:257-268.

22. Danzi S, Klein I. Thyroid disease and the cardiovascular system. *Endocrinol Metab Clin North Am.* 2014;43:517-528.

23. Das DK, et al. Thyroid hormone regulation of beta-adrenergic receptors and catecholamine sensitive adenylate cyclase in foetal heart. *Acta Endocrinol.* 1984;106:569-576.

24. de Luis DA, et al. Light symptoms following a high-dose intentional L-thyroxine ingestion treated with cholestyramine. *Horm Res.* 2002;57:61-63.

25. Dong BJ, Brown CH. Hypothyroidism resulting from generic levothyroxine failure. *J Am Board Fam Pract.* 1991;4:167-170.

26. Dong BJ, et al. Bioequivalence of generic and brand-name levothyroxine products in the treatment of hypothyroidism. *JAMA.* 1997;277:1205-1213.

27. Dymling JF, Becker DV. Occurrence of hyperthyroidism in patients receiving thyroid hormone. *J Clin Endocrinol Metab.* 1967;27:1487-1491.

28. Forrester MB. Redotex ingestions reported to Texas poison centers. *Hum Exp Toxicol.* 2010;29:789-791.

29. Funderburk SJ, Spaulding JS. Sodium levothyroxine (Synthroid R) intoxication in a child. *Pediatrics.* 1970;45:298-301.

30. Galina MP, et al. Iodides during pregnancy. An apparent cause of neonatal death. *N Engl J Med.* 1962;267:1124-1127.

31. Gardner LA, et al. Role of the cyclic AMP-dependent protein kinase in homologous resensitization of the beta1-adrenergic receptor. *J Biol Chem.* 2004;279:21135-21143.

32. Gavin LA. Thyroid crises. *Med Clin North Am.* 1991;75:179-193.

33. Geffner DL, Hershman JM. Beta-adrenergic blockade for the treatment of hyperthyroidism. *Am J Med.* 1992;93:61-68.

34. Gerard P, et al. Accidental poisoning with thyroid extract treated by exchange transfusion. *Arch Dis Child.* 1972;47:980-982.

35. Gittoes NJ, Franklyn JA. Drug-induced thyroid disorders. *Drug Saf.* 1995;13:46-55.

36. Golightly LK, et al. Clinical effects of accidental levothyroxine ingestion in children. *Am J Dis Child.* 1987;141:1025-1027.

37. Gorman CA, et al. Metabolic malingerers. Patients who deliberately induce or perpetuate a hypermetabolic or hypometabolic state. *Am J Med.* 1970;48:708-714.

38. Gorman RL, et al. Massive levothyroxine overdose: high anxiety–low toxicity. *Pediatrics.* 1988;82:666-669.

39. Green WL. New questions regarding bioequivalence of levothyroxine preparations: a clinician's response. *AAPS J.* 2005;7:E54-E58.

40. Dong BJ, Greenspan FS. Thyroid and antithyroid drugs. In: Katzung B, Trevor A, eds. *Basic and Clinical Pharmacology.* New York: McGraw Hill/Appleton Lange; 2003:644-659.

41. Guyetant S, et al. C-cell hyperplasia associated with chronic lymphocytic thyroiditis: a retrospective quantitative study of 112 cases. *Hum Pathol.* 1994;25:514-521.

42. Hack JB, et al. Severe symptoms following a massive intentional L-thyroxine ingestion. *Vet Hum Toxicol.* 1999;41:323-326.

43. Hamdy RC. The thyroid gland: a brief historical perspective. *South Med J.* 2002;95:471-473.

44. Hamolsky MW. Truth is stranger than factitious. *N Engl J Med.* 1982;307:436-437.

45. Harjai KJ, Licata AA. Effects of amiodarone on thyroid function. *Ann Intern Med.* 1997;126:63-73.

46. Hedberg CW, et al. An outbreak of thyrotoxicosis caused by the consumption of bovine thyroid gland in ground beef. *N Engl J Med.* 1987;316:993-998.

47. Henderson A, et al. Lack of efficacy of plasmapheresis in a patient overdosed with thyroxine. *Anaesth Intensive Care.* 1994;22:463-464.

48. Herbst AL, Selenkow HA. Hyperthyroidism during pregnancy. *N Engl J Med.* 1965;273:627-633.

49. Hermouet C, et al. Methyl iodide poisoning: report of two cases. *Am J Ind Med.* 1996;30:759-764.

50. Ho J, et al. Massive levothyroxine ingestion in a pediatric patient: case report and discussion. *CJEM.* 2011;13:165-168.

51. Hofe SE, Young RL. Thyrotoxicosis after a single ingestion of levothyroxine. *JAMA.* 1977;237:1361.

52. Howton JC. Thyroid storm presenting as coma. *Ann Emerg Med.* 1988;17:343-345.

53. Jackson GL, et al. Massive overdosage of propylthiouracil. *Ann Intern Med.* 1979;91:418-419.

54. Jha S, et al. Thyroid storm due to inappropriate administration of a compounded thyroid hormone preparation successfully treated with plasmapheresis. *Thyroid.* 2012;22:1283-1286.

55. Kahaly GJ, Dillmann WH. Thyroid hormone action in the heart. *Endocr Rev.* 2005;26:704-728.

56. Kalaria VG, et al. Iodide mumps: acute sialadenitis after contrast administration for angioplasty. *Circulation.* 2001;104:2384.

57. Kawata K, et al. Three cases of liver injury caused by Sennomotokounou, a Chinese dietary supplement for weight loss. *Intern Med.* 2003;42:1188-1192.

58. Kim D, Smith TW. Effects of thyroid hormone on calcium handling in cultured chick ventricular cells. *J Physiol.* 1985;364:131-149.

59. Kim D, et al. Effect of thyroid hormone on slow calcium channel function in cultured chick ventricular cells. *J Clin Invest.* 1987;80:88-94.

60. Kinney JS, et al. Community outbreak of thyrotoxicosis: epidemiology, immunogenetic characteristics, and long-term outcome. *Am J Med.* 1988;84:10-18.

61. Klein I, Ojamaa K. Thyroid hormone and the cardiovascular system. *N Engl J Med.* 2001;344:501-509.

62. Klein I, et al. Treatment of hyperthyroid disease. *Ann Intern Med.* 1994;121:281-288.

63. Kreisner E, et al. Charcoal hemoperfusion in the treatment of levothyroxine intoxication. *Thyroid.* 2010;20:209-212.

64. Kubota S, et al. Transient hyperthyroidism after withdrawal of antithyroid drugs in patients with Graves' disease. *Endocr J.* 2004;51:213-217.

65. Kulig K, et al. Levothyroxine overdose associated with seizures in a young child. *JAMA.* 1985;254:2109-2110.

66. Laman DM, et al. Thyroid crisis presenting as coma. *Clin Neurol Neurosurg.* 1984;86:295-298.

67. Lehrner LM, Weir MR. Acute ingestions of thyroid hormones. *Pediatrics.* 1984;73:313-317.

68. Levy RP, Gilger WG. Acute thyroid poisoning; report of a case. *N Engl J Med.* 1957;256:459-460.

69. Lewander WJ, et al. Acute thyroxine ingestion in pediatric patients. *Pediatrics.* 1989;84:262-265.

70. Liel Y, Weksler N. Plasmapheresis rapidly eliminates thyroid hormones from the circulation, but does not affect the speed of TSH recovery following prolonged suppression. *Horm Res.* 2003;60:252-254.

71. Litovitz TL, White JD. Levothyroxine ingestions in children: an analysis of 78 cases. *Am J Emerg Med.* 1985;3:297-300.

72. Lo DK, et al. Mild symptoms of toxicity following deliberate ingestion of thyroxine. *Vet Hum Toxicol.* 2004;46:193.

73. Luther AL, et al. Agranulocytosis secondary to methimazole therapy: report of two cases. *South Med J.* 1976;69:1356-1357.

74. Majlesi N, et al. Thyroid storm after pediatric levothyroxine ingestion. *Pediatrics.* 2010;126:e470-e473.

75. Mariotti S, et al. Low serum thyroglobulin as a clue to the diagnosis of thyrotoxicosis factitia. *N Engl J Med.* 1982;307:410-412.

76. Martin MM, Rento RD. Iodide goiter with hypothyroidism in 2 newborn infants. *J Pediatr.* 1962;61:94-99.

77. May ME, et al. Plasmapheresis in thyroxine overdose: a case report. *J Toxicol Clin Toxicol.* 1983;20:517-520.

78. Meyer-Gessner M et al. Antithyroid drug-induced agranulocytosis: clinical experience with ten patients treated at one institution and review of the literature. *J Endocrinol Invest.* 1994;17:29-36.

79. Milner MR, et al. Double-blind crossover trial of diltiazem versus propranolol in the management of thyrotoxic symptoms. *Pharmacotherapy.* 1990;10:100-106.

80. Mudoni A, et al. Multi-organ failure after massive Levothyroxine ingestion: case report [in Italian]. *G Ital Nefrol.* 2015;32.

81. Muller A, et al. Modulation of SERCA2 expression by thyroid hormone and norepinephrine in cardiocytes: role of contractility. *Am J Physiol.* 1997;272(4, pt 2):H1876-H1885.

82. Nenov VD, et al. Current applications of plasmapheresis in clinical toxicology. *Nephrol Dial Transplant.* 2003;18(suppl 5):v56-v58.

83. Nuovo J, et al. Excessive thyroid hormone replacement therapy. *J Am Board Fam Pract.* 1995;8:435-439.

84. Nystrom E, et al. Minor signs and symptoms of toxicity in a young woman in spite of massive thyroxine ingestion. *Acta Med Scand.* 1980;207:135-136.

85. Ohye H, et al. Thyrotoxicosis caused by weight-reducing herbal medicines. *Arch Intern Med.* 2005;165:831-834.

86. Packer M, et al. Hemodynamic consequences of combined beta-adrenergic and slow calcium channel blockade in man. *Circulation.* 1982;65:660-668.

87. Pantos C, et al. Thyroid hormone and phenotypes of cardioprotection. *Basic Res Cardiol.* 2004;99:101-120.

88. Parmar MS, Sturge C. Recurrent hamburger thyrotoxicosis. *CMAJ.* 2003;169:415-417.

89. Pearce SH. Spontaneous reporting of adverse reactions to carbimazole and propylthiouracil in the UK. *Clin Endocrinol.* 2004;61:589-594.

90. Pitt-Rivers R. Sir Charles Harington and the structure of thyroxine. *Mayo Clin Proc.* 1964;39:553-559.

91. Poon WT, et al. Factitious thyrotoxicosis and herbal dietary supplement for weight reduction. *Clin Toxicol (Phila).* 2008;46:290-292.

92. Pracyk JB, Slotkin TA. Thyroid hormone differentially regulates development of beta-adrenergic receptors, adenylate cyclase and ornithine decarboxylase in rat heart and kidney. *J Dev Physiol.* 1991;16:251-261.

93. Pracyk JB, Slotkin TA. Thyroid hormone regulates ontogeny of beta adrenergic receptors and adenylate cyclase in rat heart and kidney: effects of propylthiouracil-induced perinatal hypothyroidism. *J Pharmacol Exp Ther.* 1992;261:951-958.

94. Premel-Cabic A et al. Plasma noradrenaline in hyperthyroidism and hypothyroidism [in French]. *Presse Med.* 1986;15:1625-1627.

95. Pugh S, et al. Thyroid storm as a cause of loss of consciousness following anaesthesia for emergency caesarean section. *Anaesthesia.* 1994;49:35-37.

96. RC H. Chapter title. In: Gillman AG, et al., eds. *Goodman and Gilman's: The Pharmacological Basis of Therapeutics.* 8th ed. New York: McGraw-Hill; 1990:1361-1383.

97. Rennie D. Thyroid storm. *JAMA.* 1997;277:1238-1243.

98. Ririe DG, et al. Triiodothyronine increases contractility independent of beta-adrenergic receptors or stimulation of cyclic-3',5'-adenosine monophosphate. *Anesthesiology.* 1995;82:1004-1012.

99. Ralph HM. *Classic Descriptions of Disease.* Springfield, IL; 1978.

100. Roffi M, et al. Thyrotoxicosis and the cardiovascular system: subtle but serious effects. *Cleve Clin J Med.* 2003;70:57-63.

101. Roffi M, et al. Thyrotoxicosis and the cardiovascular system. *Minerva Endocrinol.* 2005;30:47-58.

102. Roti E, et al. The effect of diltiazem, a calcium channel-blocking drug, on cardiac rate and rhythm in hyperthyroid patients. *Arch Intern Med.* 1988;148:1919-1921.

103. Sawin CT. Hypothyroidism. *Med Clin North Am.* 1985;69:989-1004.

104. Sawin CT, London MH. "Natural" desiccated thyroid. A "health-food" thyroid preparation. *Arch Intern Med.* 1989;149:2117-2118.

105. Schottstaedt ES, Smoller M. "Thyroid storm" produced by acute thyroid hormone poisoning. *Ann Intern Med.* 1966;64:847-849.

106. Seppet EK, et al. Regulation of cardiac sarcolemmal Ca2+ channels and Ca2+ transporters by thyroid hormone. *Mol Cell Biochem.* 1993;129:145-159.

107. Seppet EK, et al. Mechanisms of thyroid hormone control over sensitivity and maximal contractile responsiveness to beta-adrenergic agonists in atria. *Mol Cell Biochem.* 1998;184:419-426.

108. Shilo L, et al. Massive thyroid hormone overdose: kinetics, clinical manifestations and management. *Isr Med Assoc J.* 2002;4:298-299.

109. Silva JE. The thermogenic effect of thyroid hormone and its clinical implications. *Ann Intern Med.* 2003;139:205-213.

110. Singh GK, Winterborn MH. Massive overdose with thyroxine—toxicity and treatment. *Eur J Pediatr.* 1991;150:217.

111. Surks MI, Sievert R. Drugs and thyroid function. *N Engl J Med.* 1995;333:1688-1694.

112. Tajiri J, et al. Successful treatment of thyrotoxic crisis with plasma exchange. *Crit Care Med.* 1984;12:536-537.

113. Tielens ET, et al. Acute L-triiodothyronine administration potentiates inotropic responses to beta-adrenergic stimulation in the isolated perfused rat heart. *Cardiovasc Res.* 1996;32:306-310.

114. Tse J, et al. Effects of triiodothyronine pretreatment on beta-adrenergic responses in stunned cardiac myocytes. *J Cardiothorac Vasc Anesth.* 2003;17:486-490.

115. Tunget CL, et al. Raising the decontamination level for thyroid hormone ingestions. *Am J Emerg Med.* 1995;13:9-13.

116. van Huekelom S, et al. Plasmapheresis in L-thyroxine intoxication. *Vet Hum Toxicol.* 1979;21(suppl):7.

117. Wiersinga WM. Propranolol and thyroid hormone metabolism. *Thyroid.* 1991;1:273-277.

118. Wiersinga WM. Physicochemical properties. In: Weetman AP, Grossman A, eds. *Handbook of Pharmacology.* Berlin: Springer-Verlag; 1997:225-287.

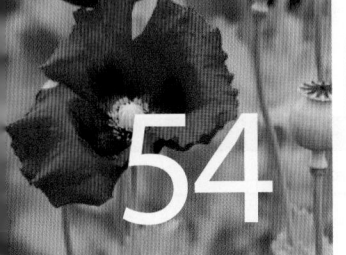

ANTIBACTERIALS, ANTIFUNGALS, AND ANTIVIRALS

Christine M. Stork

HISTORY AND EPIDEMIOLOGY

The introduction of penicillin in the 1940s revolutionized the care of patients with infectious diseases. Antimicrobials, including all categories of antibacterials, antifungals, and antivirals, significantly improve the clinical care and outcome of infected patients. Since early in their introduction, the development of antimicrobial-resistant strains of these pathogens has driven an increase in the number of antimicrobials necessary. This, in turn, continues to increase the overall potential for toxicity after use. Fortunately, with most antimicrobials, toxicity due to acute overdose is limited and chronic therapeutic doses are safe.

Most adverse drug events related to antimicrobials occur as a result of iatrogenic complications rather than intentional overdose. The diverse origins of these complications include dosing errors, route administration errors, allergic reactions, adverse drug events, and drug–drug-related interactions. Prevention, in the form of process improvements and information regarding populations at risk for adverse drug events, is continually required to minimize these untoward events. Dosing errors are prominent, particularly in neonates and infants, and those patients with compromised kidney or liver function necessitating care and constant diligence on the part of health care professionals.

Antimicrobials are more commonly associated with allergic reactions than are other pharmaceuticals. The reason is hypothesized to be either a result of their high frequency of use, repeated intermittent prescriptions, or environmental contamination. A complete allergy history is essential to minimize these adverse drug reactions in patients being considered for antimicrobial therapy.

Many adverse drug reactions attributed to antimicrobials are difficult to predict even when given patient and population specific parameters. In some cases, an excipient is found responsible for the adverse event, as is seen after the use of procaine penicillin G (Chap. 46). Antimicrobials are involved in many common and severe drug–drug interactions, primarily through the inhibition of cytochrome and other metabolic enzymes. Patients considered for antimicrobial therapy should be carefully assessed for the use of prescription and nonprescription therapies that are known to be pharmacokinetically or pharmacodynamically affected by the chosen antimicrobial.

PHARMACOLOGY AND TOXICOLOGY

Antimicrobial pharmacology is aimed at the destruction of microorganisms through the inhibition of cell cycle reproduction or the altering of a critical function within a microorganism. Table 54–1 lists antimicrobials and their associated mechanisms of activity, toxicologic effects, and related toxicologic mechanisms. Often the mechanisms for toxicologic effects following acute overdose differ from their therapeutic mechanisms.

ANTIBACTERIALS
Aminoglycosides

Aminoglycosides that are in current use in the United States include amikacin, gentamicin, kanamycin, neomycin, paromomycin, streptomycin, and tobramycin. Aminoglycosides are available in parenteral, topical, and ophthalmic forms. Overdoses, almost exclusively the result of dosing errors, are rarely life threatening, and most patients can be safely managed with

Gentamicin C_1:	$R_1 = R_2 = CH_3$
Gentamicin C_2:	$R_1 = CH_3, R_2 = H$
Gentamicin C_{1a}:	$R_1 = R_2 = H$

minimal intervention.[28,122] Adverse drug reactions, seen after aminoglycoside use, are generally class based, although subtle differences exist in the potency with which the adverse drug reactions occur (Table 54–2).

Large intravenous doses of aminoglycosides are both sufficiently safe and effective for use in single daily doses.[5] Rarely, acute aminoglycoside overdose results in nephrotoxicity, ototoxicity, or vestibular toxicity.[117,143] In one reported case, postmortem analysis confirmed a complete loss of hair cells in the inner and outer cochlear (Chap. 25).

Aminoglycosides exacerbate concomitant neuromuscular blockade, particularly at times corresponding to high peak serum aminoglycoside concentrations (Chap. 66).[173] This is caused by inhibiting presynaptic calcium channels, thereby inhibiting the release of acetylcholine from presynaptic nerve terminals. Patients at risk for enhanced neuromuscular blockade include those with abnormal neuromuscular junction function, such as occurs with myasthenia gravis or botulism.

Adverse Drug Reactions Associated With Therapeutic Use

Adverse drug reactions, including nephrotoxicity and ototoxicity, correlate most closely with elevated trough serum concentrations than with elevated peak concentrations.[109,152] Less common adverse drug reactions associated with chronic use include electrolyte abnormalities, allergic reactions, hepatotoxicity, anemia, granulocytopenia, thrombocytopenia, eosinophilia, retinal toxicity, reproductive dysfunction, tetany, and psychosis.[113,128,214,228] When aminoglycosides are administered at high doses or during once-daily dosing, sepsislike chills and malaise occur, which are likely due to excipients delivered during the infusion.[51]

Nephrotoxicity

The mechanism of nephrotoxicity and ototoxicity is incompletely understood, but involves the formation of reactive oxygen species in the presence of iron. Both the inhibition of mitochondrial respiration resulting in lipid peroxidation and the stimulation of glutamate activated N-methyl-D-aspartate

TABLE 54–1	Antimicrobial Pharmacology and Adverse Effects		
Antimicrobial	Antimicrobial Mechanism of Action	Acute Overdose	Chronic Administration
Antibacterial			
Aminoglycosides	Inhibit 30s ribosomal subunit	Neuromuscular blockade—inhibit the release of acetylcholine from presynaptic nerve terminals and acts as an antagonist at acetylcholine receptors	Nephrotoxicity/ototoxicity—form an iron complex that inhibits mitochondrial respiration and causes lipid peroxidation
Penicillins, cephalosporins, and other β-lactams	Inhibit cell wall mucopeptide synthesis	Seizures—agonist at picrotoxin-binding site, causing GABA antagonism	Hypersensitivity—immune
Chloramphenicol	Inhibits 50s ribosomal subunit and inhibits protein synthesis in rapidly dividing cells	Cardiovascular collapse	"Gray baby syndrome" Same as mechanism of action
Fluoroquinolones	Inhibit DNA topoisomerase and DNA gyrase; bind to cations (Mg^{2+})	Seizures	Not entirely known; bind to cations (Mg^{2+}), tendon rupture, hyperglycemia, or hypoglycemia
Linezolid	Inhibits bacterial protein synthesis through inhibition of N-formylmethionyl-tRNA	None clinically relevant	MAOI activity: vasopressor response to tyramine; serotonin toxicity with SSRI and possibly meperidine
Macrolides, lincosamides, and ketolides	Inhibit 50s ribosomal subunit in multiplying cells	Prolong QT interval: blocks delayed rectifier potassium channel, torsade de pointes	Not entirely known; cytotoxic effect; exacerbation of myasthenia gravis
Nitrofurantoin	Bacterial enzymatic inhibitor	Gastritis	Dermatologic, hematologic, pancreatitis, parotitis, hepatitis, crystalluria, pulmonary fibrosis
Sulfonamides	Inhibit paraaminobenzoic acid and/or paraaminoglutamic acid in the synthesis of folic acid	None clinically relevant	Hypersensitivity—metabolite acts as hapten, leading to hemolysis/methemoglobinemia; exposure to UVB causes free radical formation
Tetracycline	Inhibits 30s and 50s ribosomal subunits; binds to aminoacyl transfer RNA	None clinically relevant	Photosensitivity reaction Pregnancy: Discoloration of teeth of offspring
Vancomycin	Inhibits glycopeptidase polymerase in cell wall synthesis	"Red man syndrome"—anaphylactoid	Nephrotoxicity
Antifungal			
Amphotericin B	Binds with ergosterol on cytoplasmic membrane to create pores to facilitate organelle leak	None clinically relevant	Nephrotoxicity—vehicle deoxycholate may be involved; nephrocalcinosis
Triazoles and imidazoles	Increase permeability of cell membranes	None clinically relevant	None clinically relevant

GABA = γ-aminobutyric acid; MAOI = monoamine oxidase inhibitor; SSRI = selective serotonin reuptake inhibitor; UVB = ultraviolet light.

(NMDA) receptors are hypothesized to play a role.[98,238] The incidence of nephrotoxicity with aminoglycoside therapy is estimated at 10% to 25%.[118] Although the aminoglycosides are almost completely excreted prior to biotransformation in the kidney, a small fraction of filtered aminoglycoside is transported by absorptive endocytosis across the apical membrane of proximal tubular cells where it becomes sequestered within lysosomes. As toxicity progresses, lysosomes rupture allowing the sequestered aminoglycoside to binds to and destroy phospholipids contained on brush border membranes in the proximal renal tubule.[9]

TABLE 54–2	Predominant Manifestations of Aminoglycoside Toxicity		
Cochlear	Cochlear and Vestibular	Vestibular	Renal
Kanamycin	Amikacin	Streptomycin	Amikacin
Neomycin	Gentamicin		Gentamicin
	Tobramycin		Kanamycin
			Neomycin
			Streptomycin
			Tobramycin

In addition to tubular toxicity renal injury occurs through effects on the glomerulus and vascular system. Acute kidney injury does not generally occurs before 7 to 10 days of standard-dose therapy.[141] Because the injury occurs days prior to elevations in serum creatinine concentration, a delay in diagnosis is common.[201] Laboratory abnormalities include granular casts, proteinuria, elevated urinary sodium, and increased fractional excretion of sodium. Usually acute kidney injury (AKI) is reversible. Gentamicin and tobramycin have a higher total incidence of nephrotoxicity compared with netilmicin and amikacin.[118] Risk factors for the development of nephrotoxicity include increasing age, chronic kidney disease (CKD), female sex, previous aminoglycoside therapy, liver dysfunction, large total dose, long duration of therapy, frequent doses, high trough concentrations, the presence of other nephrotoxic xenobiotics, and shock.[9,156] Because the uptake of aminoglycosides into organs is saturable, once-daily high-dose regimens are less problematic than several lesser doses given in a single day.

Ototoxicity

Ototoxicity occurs after acute or prolonged exposure to aminoglycosides (Chap 25).[203] Both cochlear and vestibular dysfunction occur and injury is thought to result from prolonged contact time with sensory hair cells after bioaccumulation in the endolymph and perilymph spaces.[4] Vestibular toxicity, caused by destruction of sensory receptor portions of the inner ear or destruction of hair cells in the utricle and saccule, occurs in 0.4% to 10% of patients. Symptoms include vertigo or tinnitus. Table 54–2 details the relative characteristic toxicity of various aminoglycosides.

Full-tone audiometric testing first shows high-frequency hearing loss, which subsequently progress in select cases. Given the inability of cochlear hair cells to regenerate, all hearing loss that develops is permanent. After early diagnosis of vestibular dysfunction, select patients improve after discontinuation of the xenobiotic. Simultaneous administration of other ototoxic xenobiotics enhances the ototoxicity of aminoglycosides (Chap. 25).

Withdrawal of the offending xenobiotic is indicated in patients with either nephrotoxicity or ototoxicity caused by an aminoglycoside antibiotic (Chap. 27). Supportive care is the mainstay of therapy. *N*-Acetylcysteine reduced the rate of ototoxicity in patients with end-stage renal failure when given concurrently with aminoglycosides.[124] Experimental treatments in animal models include the use of deferoxamine and glutathione in an attempt to chelate and/or detoxify a reactive intermediate.[167,217] The antibiotic ticarcillin forms a renally eliminated complex with aminoglycosides; however, this is of limited value because in most instances the serum concentration of the aminoglycoside has decreased before any therapeutic measures can be used.[75]

Penicillins

$$R-\overset{\overset{\textstyle O}{\|}}{C}-NH \qquad \overset{S}{\underset{N}{\bigsqcup}} \overset{CH_3}{\underset{COOH}{<}}$$

Penicillin nucleus

Penicillin is derived from the fungus *Penicillium* and many semisynthetic derivatives have found clinical utility. Penicillins, as a class, contain a 6-aminopenicillanic acid nucleus, composed of a β-lactam ring fused to a 5-member thiazolidine ring. Classically available penicillins include penicillin G, penicillin V, and the antistaphylococcal penicillins (nafcillin, oxacillin, and dicloxacillin). Penicillins developed to enhance the spectrum of antibiotic efficacy, particularly against gram-negative bacilli, include the second-generation penicillins (ampicillin, and amoxicillin), third-generation penicillins (ticarcillin), and fourth-generation penicillins (piperacillin). Table 54–1 lists the pharmacologic mechanism of penicillins.

Acute oral overdoses of the various penicillins are usually not life threatening.[222] The most frequent complaints following acute overdose are nausea, vomiting, and diarrhea.

Seizures can occur in persons given large intravenous or cerebral intraventricular doses of penicillins.[114,125,150] More than 50 million units administered intravenously in less than 8 hours is generally required to produce seizures in adults.[206] Penicillin-induced seizures are mediated through binding to the picrotoxin-binding site on the neuronal chloride channel near the γ-aminobutyric acid (GABA)–binding site (Chap. 13).[96] Binding of the penicillin to this site produces an allosteric change in the receptor and prevents GABA from binding, resulting in a relative loss of inhibitory tone.[26] Seizures appear to be related to structure of the beta-lactam ring because penicillin analogs (such as imipenem) also cause seizures, presumably through a similar mechanism.[57]

The treatment of patients who develop penicillin-induced seizures should emphasize benzodiazepines followed by other GABA agonists, if necessary. Patients who receive an intraventricular overdose, where greater than 10,000 units or equivalent is administered, often require cerebrospinal fluid exchange or perfusion to attenuate seizure activity (Special Considerations: SC7).[46,125,154] There are rare reports of hyperkalemia resulting in electrocardiographic abnormalities after the rapid intravenous infusion of potassium penicillin G to patients with CKD and other reports of amoxicillin overdose resulting in frank hematuria and AKI.[36,88]

Adverse Drug Reactions Associated With Therapeutic Use

Penicillins are associated with a myriad of adverse drug reactions after therapeutic use, the most common of which are allergic in nature.[22]

TABLE 54–3	Classification of Anaphylactic Reactions
Grade	**Description**
I	Large local contiguous reaction (>15 cm)
II	Pruritus (urticaria) generalized
III	Asthma, angioedema, nausea, vomiting
IV	Airway (asthma, lingual edema, dysphagia, respiratory distress, laryngeal edema)
	Cardiovascular (hypotension, cardiovascular collapse)

Penicillins are commonly implicated in immune-related reactions such as bone marrow suppression, cholestasis, hemolysis, interstitial nephritis, and vasculitis.[8,86,104,216] Rare reactions include pemphigus after penicillin use and corneal damage after the use of methicillin.[19,248]

Acute Allergy

Penicillins are the pharmaceuticals most commonly implicated in the development of acute anaphylactic reactions. Anaphylactic reactions are severe, life-threatening, immunoglobulin E (IgE)–mediated immune reactions involving multiple organ systems that typically occur immediately after exposure. Table 54–3 lists the classifications of anaphylactic reactions. Anaphylaxis to penicillin occurs only after IgE antibody formation, which requires prior exposure, although that exposure could be obscure (eg, through consumption of meat from animals fed antibiotics). Life-threatening clinical manifestations include angioedema, tongue and airway edema, bronchospasm, bronchorrhea, dysrhythmias, cardiovascular collapse, and cardiac arrest.[76] The pathophysiology of systemic anaphylaxis is complex and involves multiple pathways. IgE antibodies are cross linked on the surface of mast cells and basophils, resulting in local and systemic release of preformed mediators of an immune response, including leukotrienes, C_4 and D_4, histamine, eosinophilic chemotactic factor, and other vasoactive substances, such as bradykinin, kallikrein, prostaglandin D_2, and platelet-activating factor (Fig. 54–1).

The incidence of penicillin hypersensitivity occurs in 5% of patients, with 1% of penicillin reactions manifesting as anaphylaxis. The risk for a fatal hypersensitivity after penicillin administration is 2 in 100,000 (0.002%) patient exposures.[236] All routes of penicillin administration can result in anaphylaxis; however, it occurs most commonly after intravenous administration.

Treatment is supportive with careful attention to airway, breathing, and circulation. Specific therapy for anaphylaxis is epinephrine 0.01 mg/kg in children (0.3-0.5 mg in adults) given as 1:1,000 (1 mg/mL) dilution intramuscularly (IM) every 5 to 15 minutes.[155,212] Epinephrine bronchodilates and increases cardiac output through β-adrenergic receptor stimulation. In addition, β-adrenergic receptor stimulation results in decreased peripheral vascular tone and decreased mast cell release of mediators. Oxygen, intravenous use of epinephrine (1 mcg/min of 1:100,000 or 1:250,000), intravenous crystalloid, and inhaled $β_2$-adrenergic agonists are warranted in severe cases, as are corticosteroids.[249] Refractory cases of hypotension may respond to glucagon and methylene blue administration (Antidotes in Depth: A20 and A43). H_1-receptor antagonists and H_2-receptor antagonists are useful as second-line therapeutic agents, and can be used to attenuate minor effects such as urticaria or pruritus.

Amoxicillin-Clavulanic Acid and Drug-Induced Liver Injury (DILI)

The predominant distribution of penicillin-induced hepatotoxicity is cholestatic hepatitis, which typically occurs 1 to 8 weeks after initiation of therapy.[7] The incidence of DILI is estimated at 1 per 2,300 prescriptions and is the most common cause of DILI in the United States and Europe.[25] The mechanism of hepatotoxicity is not clear, but it is hypothesized to be immunoallergic and related to clavulanate, a β-lactamase inhibitor used to prevent the bacterial destruction of β-lactam antimicrobials, or one of its metabolites. Treatment is supportive and clinical findings typically resolve after the discontinuation

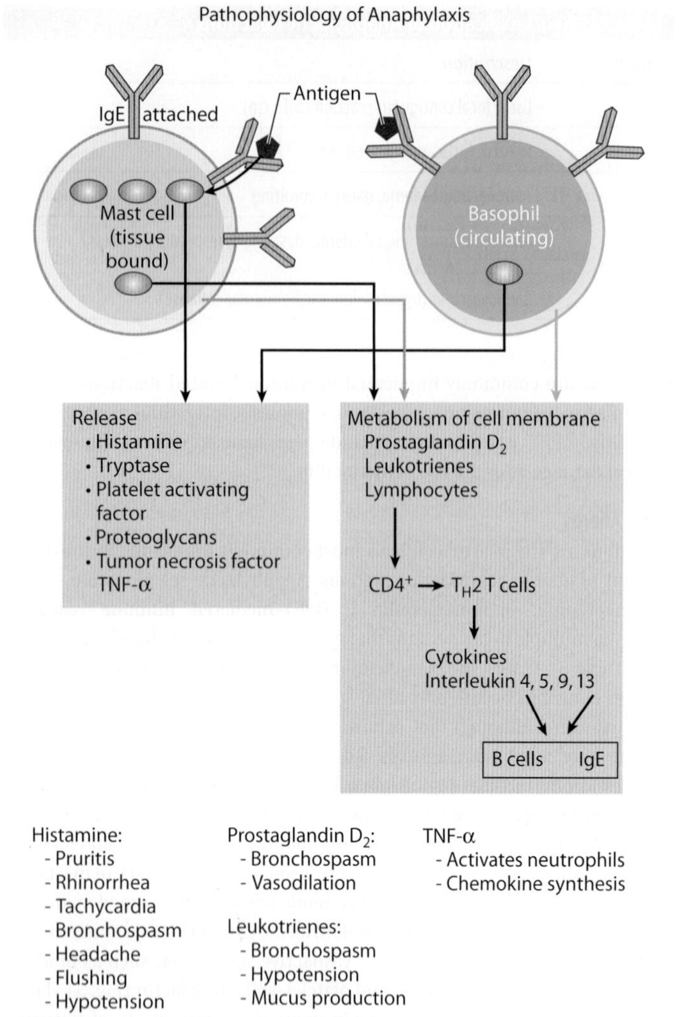

Pathophysiology of Anaphylaxis

FIGURE 54–1. Description of systemic anaphylaxis.

of therapy. However, prolonged hepatitis, ductopenia (vanishing bile duct syndrome), and pancreatitis rarely occur.[53,182] Behavioral disturbances with disorientation, agitation, and visual hallucinations temporally related to use are also reported.[16]

Hoigne Syndrome and Jarisch–Herxheimer Reaction

The most common adverse drug reactions occurring after administration of large intramuscular or intravenous doses of procaine penicillin G are the Hoigne syndrome and the Jarisch–Herxheimer reaction.[111,148] The Hoigne syndrome is characterized by extreme apprehension and fear, illusions, or hallucinations; both visual and auditory, tachycardia, systolic hypertension, and, occasionally, seizures that begin within minutes of injection.[235] These effects occur in the absence of signs or symptoms of anaphylaxis. Procaine is implicated as the etiology because of the similarity to events that occur after the administration of other local anesthetics known as the so-called caine reaction.[197,208,231] Hoigne syndrome is 6 times more common in men than in women.[211] The reason for this increased prevalence is unclear, but autosomal dominance and influences of prostaglandin and thromboxane A_2 activity occur in this population.[12]

The Jarisch–Herxheimer reaction is a self-limited reaction that develops within a few hours of antibiotic therapy for the treatment of spirochetal diseases such as syphilis or Lyme disease, leptospirosis, and in Q fever. Myalgias, chills, headache, rash, and fever spontaneously resolve within 18 to 24 hours, even with continued antibiotic therapy.[207] The pathogenesis of this reaction is likely either endotoxin induced from the lysed spirochete or cytokine elevation.[177] Antiinflammatory medications and immune modulators such as anti-TNF can be considered, but the optimal treatment is still unclear.

Cephalosporins

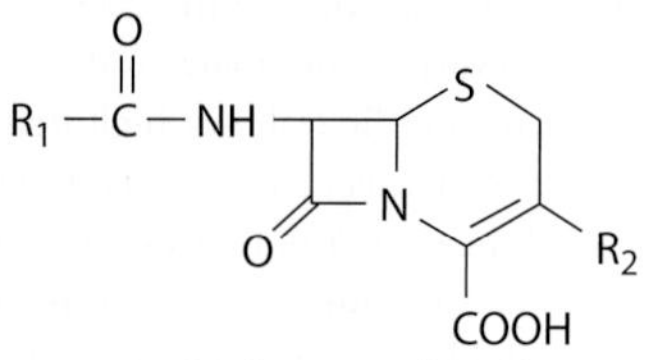

Cephem nucleus

Cephalosporins are semisynthetic derivatives of cephalosporin C produced by the fungus *Acremonium*, previously called *Cephalosporium*. Cephalosporins have a ring structure similar to that of penicillins and are generally divided into first, second, third, fourth, and fifth generations based on their antimicrobial spectrum. First-generation cephalosporins include cefadroxil, cefazolin, and cephalexin. Second-generation cephalosporins include cefaclor, cefditoren, cefotetan, cefoxitin, cefprozil, and cefuroxime. Third-generation cephalosporins include cefdinir, ceftazidime, cefixime, ceftibuten, cefotaxime, ceftriaxone, and cefpodoxime. The fourth-generation cephalosporin is cefepime, and the fifth-generation cephalosporins are ceftaroline and ceftolozane.

Effects occurring after acute overdose of cephalosporins resemble those occurring with penicillins. Some cephalosporins also have epileptogenic potential similar to penicillin.[239] Case reports demonstrate seizures after inadvertent intraventricular administration.[39,131,251] Management of cephalosporin overdose is similar to that of penicillin overdose. Table 54–1 lists the pharmacologic mechanism of cephalosporins.

Adverse Drug Reactions Associated With Therapeutic Use

Cephalosporins rarely cause an immune-mediated acute hemolytic crisis.[73] Cefaclor is the cephalosporin most commonly reported to cause systemic immune complex hypersensitivity or serum sickness, although this can occur with other cephalosporins.[119,142] Also like penicillins, first-generation cephalosporins are associated with chronic toxicity, including interstitial nephritis and hepatitis.[245] Cefepime is reported to cause reversible coma and seizures.[1,215]

Cross-Hypersensitivity

The cephalosporins contain a 6-member dihydrothiazine ring instead of the 5-member thiazolidine penicillin ring. The extent of cross-reactivity between penicillins and cephalosporins in an individual patient is largely determined by the type of penicillin allergic response experienced by the patient and the structural similarity of the beta lactam side determinants.[189] The incidence of anaphylaxis to cephalosporins is between 0.0001% and 0.1%, with a threefold increase in patients with previous penicillin allergy.[120] The overall cross-reactivity rate is approximately 1% between penicillin and a first- or second-generation cephalosporin. Cross-reactivity between penicillin and third-, fourth-, or fifth-generation cephalosporins is likely to be negligible because of a dissimilar antigenic side chain.[47] These determinants are quite distinct among cephalosporins, which cause the pattern of cross-hypersensitivity among cephalosporins to be much less well defined than among the penicillins. Caution should be used when considering first- or second-generation cephalosporins in penicillin- or cephalosporin-allergic patients; however, if a risk-to-benefit analysis demonstrates a clear benefit to the patient without equivalent alternatives, the cephalosporin should be given.

N-Methylthiotetrazole Side-Chain Effects

Cefazolin and cefotetan are the only available cephalosporins containing an *N*-methylthiotetrazole (nMTT) side chain. As these cephalosporins undergo metabolism, they release free nMTT, which (Fig. 54–2) inhibits the enzyme aldehyde dehydrogenase.[151] In conjunction with ethanol consumption, use of these medications can cause a disulfiramlike reaction (Chaps. 76 and 78).[43]

The nMTT side chain is also associated with hypoprothrombinemia, although a causal relationship is controversial.[95] It is thought that nMTT depletes vitamin K–dependent clotting factors by inhibition of vitamin K epoxide reductase.[169] In a study of children one month to one year of age who

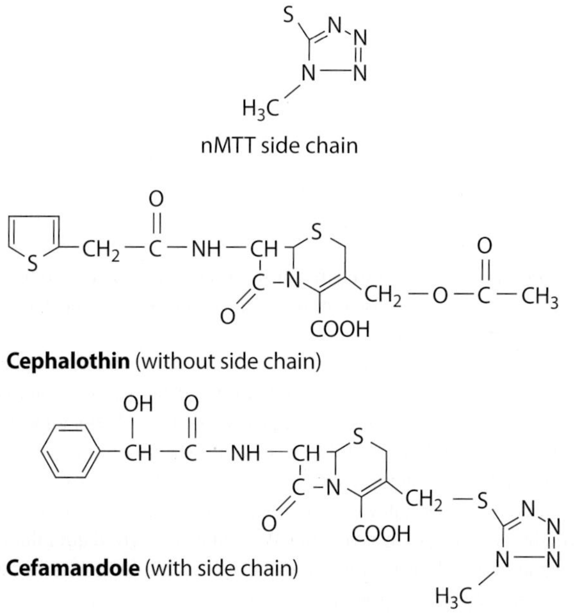

FIGURE 54–2. Characteristic structures of cephalosporins emphasizing the nMTT side chain. nMTT = *N*-methylthiotetrazole.

were maintained on a prolonged antibiotic regimen, a significant degree of vitamin K depletion was found.[21] Treatment of patients suspected of hypoprothrombinemia caused by these cephalosporins consists of clotting factor replacement, if bleeding is evident, and vitamin K_1 in doses required to reactivate vitamin K cofactors (Chap. 58 and Antidotes in Depth: A17).

Other β-Lactam Antimicrobials

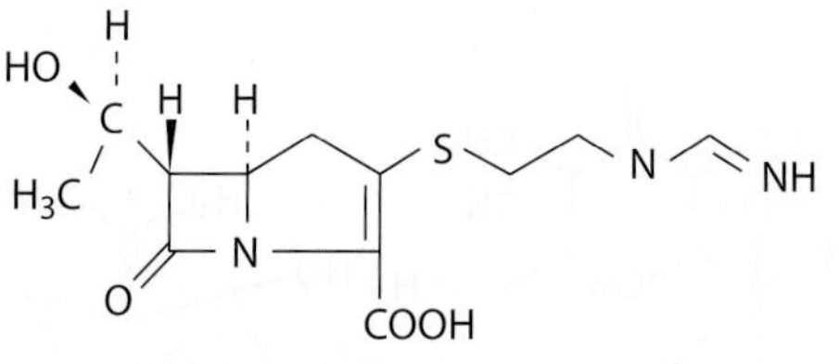

Included in this group are monobactams such as aztreonam and carbapenems such as doripenem, ertapenem, imipenem/cilastatin, and meropenem. Table 54–1 lists the pharmacologic mechanism of these xenobiotics.

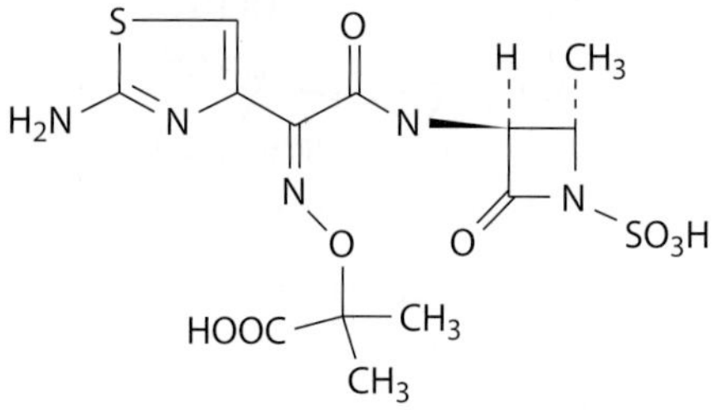

Effects occurring after acute overdose and the management of other β-lactam antimicrobials resemble those occurring after penicillin exposure. Imipenem has epileptogenic potential in both overdose and therapeutic dosing and at a higher risk than other carbapenems.[48]

Adverse Drug Reactions Associated With Therapeutic Use
The risk factors for developing imipenem-related seizures include central nervous system disease, prior seizure disorder, and abnormal kidney function.[175] The mechanism for seizures is GABA antagonism (similar to the penicillins) in conjunction with enhanced activity of excitatory amino acids.[65,220]

Cross-Hypersensitivity
Aztreonam is a monobactam that does not contain the antigenic components required for cross-allergy with penicillins, and generalized cross-allergenicity is not expected.[200] However, aztreonam cross-reacts in vitro with ceftriaxone, thought to be the result of the similarity in their side-chain structure.[174] Skin test–manifested cross-allergenicity has also been noted between imipenem and penicillin, although the clinical incidence of adverse reactions is yet to be determined.[199]

Trimethoprim–Sulfamethoxazole
Trimethoprim and sulfamethoxazole work in tandem as antibacterials effectively preventing tetrahydrofolic acid synthesis in bacterial cells. Significant toxicity after acute overdose is not expected; however, a myriad of adverse drug reactions occur after chronic therapeutic use. Hyperkalemia can result as a result of the ability of trimethoprim to competitively inhibit sodium channels in the distal nephron, causing impairment in renal potassium excretion. Clinically significant hyperkalemia is reported in patients concurrently on other xenobiotics that increase potassium and among those with CKD.[71,166] Other effects commonly reported after use of trimethoprim/sulfamethoxazole combinations include cutaneous allergic reactions, hematologic disorders, methemoglobinemia, hypoglycemia, rhabdomyolysis, neonatal kernicterus, and psychosis.[157,226]

Trimethoprim also inhibits the renal tubular secretion of creatinine, resulting in an increase in serum creatinine measurement.[66] This effect is thought to be dose related and increases in creatinine ranges from 13% to 35%. The rise in creatinine is independent of glomerular filtration rate and resolves on drug discontinuation.

Chloramphenicol

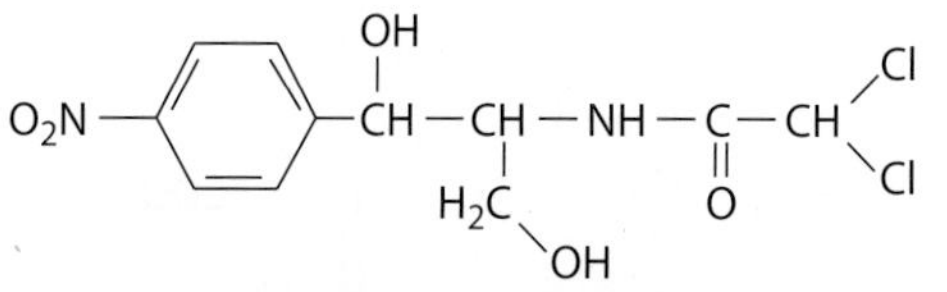

Chloramphenicol was originally derived from *Streptomyces venezuelae* and is now synthetically produced. Antimicrobial activity is demonstrated against many gram-positive and gram-negative aerobes and anaerobes.

Chloramphenicol inhibits protein synthesis in rapidly proliferating cells. Metabolic acidosis occurs as a result of the inhibition of mitochondrial enzymes, oxidative phosphorylation, and mitochondrial biogenesis.[246] Table 54–1 lists the pharmacologic mechanism of chloramphenicol.

Acute overdose of chloramphenicol commonly causes nausea and vomiting. Infrequently, sudden cardiovascular collapse can occur 5 to 12 hours after acute overdoses. Cardiovascular compromise is more frequent in patients with serum concentrations higher than 50 mcg/mL.[85,159,224] Because tissue concentration measurements are not readily available, all poisoned patients should be closely observed for at least 12 hours after exposure. Orogastric lavage should be used after recent ingestions when the patient has not vomited, and oral or nasogastric activated charcoal 1 g/kg should also be given.

Extracorporeal means of eliminating chloramphenicol are not usually required because of its rapid metabolism. However, hemodialysis, charcoal hemoperfusion, and exchange transfusion in neonates all decrease serum chloramphenicol concentrations. These extracorporeal procedures should be employed in patients presenting early after a life-threatening history of ingestion, particularly if they have severe hepatic or renal dysfunction.[83,153,213,218] Surviving patients should be closely monitored for signs of bone marrow suppression, which is dose dependent.

Adverse Drug Reactions Associated With Therapeutic Use
Chronic toxicity of chloramphenicol is similar to that which occurs following acute poisoning. The classic description of chronic chloramphenicol toxicity is the "gray baby syndrome."[159] Children with this syndrome exhibit vomiting, anorexia, respiratory distress, abdominal distension, green stools, lethargy,

cyanosis, ashen color, metabolic acidosis, hypotension, and cardiovascular collapse.

Approximately 90% of systemic chloramphenicol is metabolized via glucuronyl transferase, forming a glucuronide conjugate. The remainder is excreted renally unchanged. Infants, in particular, are predisposed to the gray baby syndrome because they have a limited capacity to form a glucuronide conjugate of chloramphenicol and, concomitantly, a limited ability to excrete chloramphenicol in the urine.[92,244]

There are 2 types of bone marrow suppression that occur after use of chloramphenicol. The most common type is dose dependent and occurs with high serum concentrations of chloramphenicol.[107,170,205] Clinical manifestations usually occur within several weeks of therapy and include anemia, thrombocytopenia, leukopenia, and, very rarely, aplastic anemia. Bone marrow suppression is generally reversible on discontinuation of therapy. A second type occurs through inhibition of protein synthesis in the mitochondria of marrow cell lines.[161] This type causes the development of aplastic anemia, which is not dose related, generally occurs in susceptible patients within 5 months of treatment and has an approximately 50% mortality rate (Chap. 20).[72,253] The dihydro and nitroso bacterial metabolites of chloramphenicol injure human bone marrow cells through inhibition of myeloid colony growth, inhibition of DNA synthesis, and inhibition of mitochondrial protein synthesis.[115]

Other adverse drug reactions associated with chloramphenicol include peripheral neuropathy, neurologic abnormalities (eg, confusion, delirium), optic neuritis, nonlymphocytic leukemia, and contact dermatitis.[61,126,136,179,210]

Fluoroquinolones

Ciprofloxacin

The fluoroquinolones are a structurally similar, synthetically derived group of antimicrobials that have diverse antimicrobial activities. They include ciprofloxacin, gatifloxacin (ophthalmic only), gemifloxacin, levofloxacin, moxifloxacin, norfloxacin, and ofloxacin. Like other antimicrobials, the fluoroquinolones rarely produce life-threatening effects following acute overdose, and most patients can be safely managed with minimal intervention.[11] Table 54–1 lists the pharmacologic mechanism of fluoroquinolones.

Rarely, acute overdose of a fluoroquinolone results in AKI or seizures.[129] The mechanism of AKI after fluoroquinolone exposure is controversial. In animals, ciprofloxacin and norfloxacin are nephrotoxic, especially in the setting of neutral or alkaline urine.[63,202] In humans, AKI is reported after both acute and chronic exposure to fluoroquinolones. A hypersensitivity reaction is postulated to explain pathologic changes consistent with interstitial nephritis.[105,185] Treatment includes discontinuation of the fluoroquinolone and supportive care. Improvement in kidney function usually occurs within several days.

Seizures are reported with ciprofloxacin and likely result from the inhibition of GABA or from elevation of neuronal glutamate.[2,58] Other authors postulate that seizures result from the ability of fluoroquinolones to bind efficiently to cations, particularly magnesium. This hypothesis is related to the inhibitory role of magnesium at the excitatory NMDA-gated ion channel (Chap. 13).[65] Treatment is supportive, using benzodiazepines and, if necessary, barbiturates to increase inhibitory tone.

Adverse Drug Reactions Associated With Therapeutic Use
Several fluoroquinolones are substrates and/or inhibitors of CYP enzymes. This can result in xenobiotic interactions, which are especially important with xenobiotics that have a narrow therapeutic index.

Serious adverse drug reactions related to fluoroquinolone use consist of central nervous system toxicity (as discussed), cardiovascular toxicity, hepatotoxicity, and notable musculoskeletal toxicity.

Fluoroquinolones prolong the QT interval, and are reported to result in torsade de pointes.[172] Prolongation is due to the ability of fluoroquinolones to block the rapid component of the delayed rectifier potassium current (I_{Kr}). Treatment of patients presenting with QT interval prolongation includes immediate discontinuation of the offending drug and supportive care (Chap. 15).

Fluoroquinolones also rarely result in potentially fatal hepatotoxicity.[138] This adverse effect was most notable with trovafloxacin, which was withdrawn from the US market.

Fluoroquinolones should be used with caution in children and pregnant women because of their potential adverse drug reactions on developing cartilage and bone.[23] There is a higher incidence of bone, joint, tendon, and muscle abnormalities in children treated with a fluoroquinolone versus alternative antibiotic therapy, which persists months after the completion of drug therapy. When followed long-term, however, it was found that these abnormalities are generally reversible. Women who received quinolones during pregnancy had larger babies and more cesarean deliveries because of fetal distress than did controls.[18]

Fluoroquinolones are implicated as a cause of tendon rupture, most commonly the Achilles, which is reported to occur for months to years after the start of treatment as well as after the discontinuation of therapy. An FDA review concluded that because of these risks, these drugs should be reserved for when there is no alternative available.[181] Risk factors include age 60 years or older, concomitant corticosteroid use, AKI or CKD, female sex, and lack of obesity.[132,247] The fluoroquinolone should be discontinued in patients, particularly athletes, who complain of symptoms consistent with painful and swollen tendons.

Macrolides and Ketolides

Erythromycin

The macrolide antimicrobials include various forms of erythromycin (base, ethylsuccinate, gluceptate, lactobionate, stearate), azithromycin, clarithromycin, and fidaxomicin. Ketolides are similar in pharmacology to macrolides; telithromycin is the only available xenobiotic at this time. Table 54–1 lists the pharmacologic mechanism of macrolides and ketolides.

Acute oral overdoses of macrolide antimicrobials are not life threatening, and symptoms, which are generally confined to the gastrointestinal tract, include nausea, vomiting, and diarrhea. Intravenous overdoses can cause dysrhythmias.[227]

Intravenous and oral therapeutic use of macrolides cause QT interval prolongation and dysrhythmias.[55] The QT interval prolongation seen occurs as a result of blockade of delayed rectifier potassium currents I_{Kr} (Chaps. 15 and 57).[186] Macrolide-associated oxidative stress to mitochondrial cells subsequently inhibited hERG potassium conductance in rat cardiomyocytes exposed to various macrolides.[195] The relative risk in a large meta-analysis for sudden cardiac death was 2.42, and ventricular tachydysrhythmia was 2.52, in patients who took macrolides versus those who did not. In children, intravenous overdoses of azithromycin resulted in similar findings.[227]

Although there are no acute overdose data regarding ketolide antimicrobials, effects are expected to be similar to macrolide antimicrobials. Therapeutic use of telithromycin is reported to result in QT interval prolongation, hepatotoxicity, toxic epidermal necrolysis, and anaphylaxis.[37,40]

Adverse Events Associated With Interactions With Xenobiotics

Erythromycin is the prototypical macrolide and, as such, has received the most attention with respect to potential and documented xenobiotic interactions. Clarithromycin, erythromycin, and troleandomycin are all potent inhibitors of CYP3A4; azithromycin does not inhibit this enzyme.[64] Erythromycin inhibits CYP enzymes after metabolism to a nitroso intermediate, which then forms an inactive complex with the iron (II) of cytochrome P450. The appendix to Chap. 11 lists substrates for CYP3A4. Clinically significant interactions occur with erythromycin and warfarin, carbamazepine, or cyclosporine.[44,100,178] Inhibition of cisapride metabolism results in increased concentrations of the parent xenobiotic, which is capable of causing prolongation of the QT interval and causing torsade de pointes.[33] Cases of carbamazepine toxicity are documented when combined with the use of erythromycin.[100] Erythromycin also inhibits CYP1A2, producing clinically significant interactions with clozapine, theophylline, and warfarin.[188]

Macrolides interact with the absorption and renal excretion of xenobiotics that are substrates for P-glycoprotein, and they also interfere with the normal gut flora responsible for metabolism. This is hypothesized to be part of the underlying mechanism of cases of macrolide-induced digoxin toxicity, for example (Chap. 62).[168]

End-Organ Effects

The most common toxic effect of macrolides after chronic use is hepatitis, which is hypothesized to be immune mediated.[49] Erythromycin estolate is the macrolide most frequently implicated in causing cholestatic hepatitis.[91,112]

Large doses (>4 g/day) of macrolides are associated with high-frequency sensorineural hearing loss that typically resolves following discontinuation of therapy.[41,135] Renal impairment is noted to be a risk factor.[193,221] Other, rare toxic effects associated with macrolides include cataracts after clarithromycin use in animals and acute pancreatitis in humans.[78,234] Allergy is rare and reported at a rate of 0.4% to 3%.[67] Telithromycin contains a carbamate side chain that is hypothesized to interfere with the normal function of neuronal cholinesterase. It should be used cautiously in patients with myasthenia gravis, particularly patients receiving pyridostigmine because of the risk of cholinergic crisis.[121]

Clindamycin is a lincosamide with structure and clinical effects similar to macrolides'. Clindamycin phosphate is commonly used topically while clindamycin hydrochloride is available intravenously and clindamycin palmitate hydrochloride is available for oral use. Data regarding acute overdose are limited. Neuromuscular blockade is reported after intravenous dosing errors.[3] The most consequential toxicity seen after therapeutic doses is esophageal ulcers, diarrhea, and *Clostridium difficile*–mediated enterocolitis.[186]

Sulfonamides

Sulfamethoxazole

Sulfonamides antagonize *para*-aminobenzoic acid or *para*-aminobenzyl glutamic acid, which are required for the biosynthesis of folic acid. Table 54–1 lists the pharmacologic mechanism of sulfonamides. Acute oral overdoses of sulfonamides are usually not life threatening, and symptoms are generally confined to nausea, although allergy and methemoglobinemia occur rarely.[82] Treatment is similar to acute oral penicillin overdoses.

Adverse Drug Reactions Associated With Therapeutic Use

The most common adverse drug reactions associated with sulfonamide therapy are nausea and cutaneous hypersensitivity reactions.[89] Hypersensitivity reactions are caused by 2 mechanisms. The first is an IgE-mediated response to the heterocyclic ring at the sulfonamide-N1 position. The more common allergic response occurs 7 to 14 days after initiation of therapy and requires an unsubstituted amine group at the N4 position of the sulfonamide. The incidence of adverse reactions to sulfonamides, including allergy, is increased in HIV-positive patients and is positively correlated to the number of previous opportunistic infections experienced by the patient.[134] This is caused by a reduction in the mechanisms available for detoxification of free radical formation, as cysteine and glutathione concentrations are low in these patients.[241]

Methemoglobinemia and hemolysis occur rarely.[70,162] The mechanism for adverse reactions is not entirely clear. However, when sulfamethoxazole is exposed to ultraviolet B radiation in vitro, free radicals are formed that can participate in the development of tissue peroxidation and hemolysis.[253] This finding is of particular importance in treating patients with glucose-6-phosphate dehydrogenase deficiency associated with decrease in reducing capabilities.[6]

The sulfonamides are associated with many chronic adverse drug reactions. Bone marrow suppression is rare, but the incidence is increased in patients with folic acid or vitamin B_{12} deficiency, and in children, pregnant women, alcoholics, dialysis patients, and immunocompromised patients, as well as in patients who are receiving other folate antagonists. Other adverse drug reactions include hypersensitivity pneumonitis, Stevens–Johnson syndrome, toxic epidermal necrolysis, stomatitis, aseptic meningitis, hepatotoxicity, renal injury, and central nervous system toxicity.[29]

Tetracyclines

Tetracycline

Tetracyclines are produced by *Streptomyces*. Currently available tetracyclines include demeclocycline, doxycycline, minocycline, and tetracycline. Table 54–1 lists the pharmacologic mechanism of tetracyclines. Significant toxicity after acute overdose of tetracyclines is unlikely. Gastrointestinal effects consisting of nausea, vomiting, and epigastric pain are reported.[42]

Adverse Drug Reactions Associated With Therapeutic Use

Tetracycline should not be used in children during the first 6 to 8 years of life or by pregnant women after the 12th week of gestation because of the risk for secondary tooth discoloration in children or fetuses.[196] Tooth discoloration can be effectively mitigated using topical application of carbamide peroxide whitening treatments.[229] Other effects associated with tetracyclines include nephrotoxicity, hepatotoxicity, skin hyperpigmentation in sun-exposed areas, and hypersensitivity reactions.[49,94,110,223] More severe hypersensitivity reactions, vertigo, xenobiotic-induced lupus, and pneumonitis are reported after minocycline use, as are cases of necrotizing vasculitis of the skin and uterine cervix, and lymphadenopathy with eosinophilia.[145,204,209] Demeclocycline rarely causes nephrogenic diabetes insipidus (Chaps. 12 and 27).[50] Degraded tetracycline is reported to result in reversible Fanconi syndrome.[84] Epi-anhydrotetracycline or anhydrotetracycline were likely the causative toxins.

Vancomycin

Vancomycin

Vancomycin is obtained from cultures of *Nocardia orientalis* and is a tricyclic glycopeptide. Vancomycin is biologically active against numerous gram-positive organisms. Table 54–1 lists the pharmacologic mechanism of vancomycin.

Acute oral overdoses of vancomycin rarely cause significant toxicity and most cases can be treated with supportive care alone. After large iatrogenic, rapidly infused intravenous overdoses, AKI can occur in patients with pre-existing kidney disease because of sustained high serum concentrations. In these patients, multiple doses of activated charcoal and hemodialysis are effective in enhancing clearance.[127,233]

Adverse Drug Reactions Associated with Therapeutic Use

Rapid infusions of intravenous vancomycin and the subsequent development of the "red man syndrome" occurs through an anaphylactoid (non–IgE-mediated) mechanism.[87] Symptoms include chest pain, dyspnea, pruritus, urticaria, flushing, and angioedema.[190] Spontaneous resolution occurs typically within 15 minutes. Other symptoms attributable to "red man syndrome" include hypotension, cardiovascular collapse, and seizures.[13,164]

The incidence of red man syndrome is approximately 14% when 1 g is given over 10 minutes, and falls dramatically to only 3.4% when given over one hour.[164,171] A trial in 11 healthy persons studied the relationship between intradermal skin hypersensitivity and the development of red man syndrome. Each of the 11 study participants underwent skin testing that was followed one week later by an intravenous dose of vancomycin 15 mg/kg over 60 minutes. Following intravenous vancomycin, all participants developed dermal flare responses and erythema, and 10 of 11 participants developed pruritus within 20 to 45 minutes. After the infusion was terminated, symptoms resolved within 60 minutes.[176]

The signs and symptoms of this syndrome are related to the rise and fall of histamine concentrations.[137,194] Tachyphylaxis occurs in patients given multiple doses of vancomycin.[99,240] Animal models demonstrated a direct myocardial depressant and vasodilatory effect of vancomycin.[62] More serious reactions result when vancomycin is given via intravenous bolus, further supporting a rate-related anaphylactoid mechanism.[20] In rare cases, oral administration of vancomycin can also result in red man syndrome.[17]

Treatment includes increasing the dilution of vancomycin and slowing intravenous administration. Antihistamines are useful as pretreatment, especially prior to the first dose.[180] A placebo-controlled trial in adult patients given 1 g of vancomycin over one hour noted a 47% incidence of reaction without diphenhydramine and a 0% incidence with diphenhydramine.[240]

Chronic use of vancomycin results in reversible nephrotoxicity, particularly in patients with prolonged excessive steady-state serum concentrations.[10,184] Concomitant administration of aminoglycoside antimicrobials increases the risk of nephrotoxicity.[191] Vancomycin also causes, though rarely, thrombocytopenia and neutropenia.[59,69]

ANTIFUNGALS

Numerous antifungals are available. Toxicity related to the use of antifungals is variable and is based generally on their mechanism of action.

Amphotericin B

Amphotericin B is a potent antifungal derived from *Streptomyces nodosus*. Amphotericin B is generally fungistatic against fungi that contain sterols in their cell membrane. Table 54–1 lists the pharmacologic mechanism of amphotericin B. Development of lipid and colloidal formulations of amphotericin B attenuate the adverse drug reactions associated with amphotericin B.[97] In these preparations, the amphotericin B is complexed with either a lipid or cholesteryl sulfate. On contact with a fungus, lipases are released to free the complexed amphotericin B, resulting in focused cell death.[102]

There are several case reports of amphotericin B overdose in infants and children. Significant clinical findings include hypokalemia, increased aspartate aminotransferase concentrations, and cardiac complications. Dysrhythmias and cardiac arrest have occurred following doses of 5 to 15 mg/kg of amphotericin B.[35,60,123] Care should be used in the doses of amphotericin B administered according to specific formulation design, as these are not interchangeable. For example, intravenous therapy for fungal infections includes a usual dose of 0.25 to 1 mg/kg/day of amphotericin B or 3 to 4 mg/kg/day of amphotericin B cholesteryl. The potential for significant dosage errors and their sequelae is readily apparent in this comparison.

Adverse Drug Reactions Associated With Therapeutic Use

Infusion of amphotericin B results in fever, rigors, headache, nausea, vomiting, hypotension, tachycardia, and dyspnea.[146] Slower rates of infusion and lower total daily doses mitigate symptoms of early infusion–related reactions as does pretreatment with diphenhydramine. In addition, acetaminophen, ibuprofen, and hydrocortisone are helpful in alleviating febrile effects.[90,232] Doses greater than 1 mg/kg/day and rapid administration in less than one hour are not recommended. Infusion concentrations of amphotericin B greater than 0.1 mg/mL can result in localized phlebitis. Slower infusion rates, hot packs, and frequent line flushing with dextrose in water is recommended help to alleviate symptoms.

Eighty percent of patients exposed to amphotericin B will sustain some degree of kidney dysfunction (Chap. 27).[45] Initial distal renal tubule damage causes renal artery vasoconstriction, ultimately resulting in azotemia.[79] Studies in animals show depressed renal blood flow and glomerular filtration rate, and increased renal vascular resistance. It is unclear why this occurs, but at this time, renal nerves, angiotensin II, and nitric oxide are excluded as etiologies.[192,198] The toxic effects associated with amphotericin B are likely caused by the deoxycholate vehicle, which accounts for differences seen with the liposomal form.[133,252] After large total doses of amphotericin B, residual decreases in glomerular filtration rate occur even after discontinuation of therapy. This is hypothesized to be the result of nephrocalcinosis. Potassium and magnesium wasting, proteinuria, decreased renal concentrating ability, renal tubular acidosis, and hematuria can also occur (Chaps. 12 and 27).[14,146] Strategies to reduce renal toxicity after amphotericin B include intravenous saline or magnesium and potassium supplementation.[32,80,101] Liposomal formulations of amphotericin B resulted in fewer patients with breakthrough fungal infections, infusion-related fever, rigors, or nephrotoxicity.[242] However, chest pain is uniquely reported after use of the liposomal preparation.[116]

Other adverse drug reactions reported after treatment with amphotericin B include normochromic, normocytic anemia secondary to decreased erythropoietin release; respiratory insufficiency with infiltrates; and, rarely, dysrhythmias, tinnitus, thrombocytopenia, peripheral neuropathy, and leukopenia.[139,144,146]

Exchange transfusion should be used in neonates and infants after large intravenous overdoses. There is a single case of the successful use of plasmapheresis concurrent with hemodialysis for evolving AKI in a 60-year-old female who had inadvertent administration of amphotericin B deoxycholate 250 mg (4.3 mg/kg) over 2 hours instead of a liposomal product.[243]

Azole Antifungals: Triazole and Imidazoles

Fluconazole

Triazole antifungals include fluconazole, isavuconazonium, itraconazole, posaconazole, terconazole, and voriconazole. Common imidazoles include butoconazole, clotrimazole, econazole, ketoconazole, miconazole, and tioconazole. Triazole antifungals treat an array of fungal pathogens, whereas imidazoles are used almost exclusively in the treatment of superficial mycoses and vaginal candidiasis. Severe toxicity is not expected in the overdose setting. Hepatotoxicity, thrombocytopenia, and neutropenia are uncommon.[30] Rare case reports implicate voriconazole in the development of toxic epidermal necrolysis.[106] Most of the toxic effects noted after the use of these xenobiotics result from their xenobiotic interactions. Fluconazole, itraconazole, ketoconazole, and miconazole competitively inhibit CYP3A4, the isoenzyme system responsible for the metabolism of many xenobiotics. Table 54–4 lists other organ system manifestations associated with antifungal agents and other antimicrobials.

ANTIPARASITICS

Antiparasitics such as mebendazole, albendazole, ivermectin, praziquantel, and pyrantel pamoate generally have limited toxicity in overdoses, although significant toxicity can be found after the use of antimalarials for the treatment of malaria (Chap. 55). Common symptoms after therapeutic use are gastrointestinal in nature and include abdominal pain, nausea, vomiting, and diarrhea. A single case of ivermectin-associated hepatic failure has been reported one month after a single dose.[237]

ANTIVIRALS

Acyclovir, famciclovir, and valacyclovir are generally well tolerated in therapeutic doses and overdoses. Neurotoxicity and, less commonly, AKI are reported after therapeutic use in humans, and similar findings are expected after overdose.[31] The most common neurotoxic complaints include lethargy, confusion, and ataxia.[108] Acute kidney injury occurs as the result of precipitation of acyclovir crystals within the renal tubules with resultant obstructive effects.[230] In 105 dogs ingesting 40 to 2,195 mg/kg, gastrointestinal symptoms were most common, with one dog developing mild creatinine increases.[183] A single case report describes a patient with AKI with crystalluria after ingestion of 30 g of valacyclovir.[187]

TABLE 54–4 Major Organ System Manifestations Associated With Antimicrobial Toxicity

Antimicrobial	System	Signs/Symptoms/Laboratory Findings
Antibacterials		
Bacitracin	Immune	Hypersensitivity reactions
Clindamycin	Immune	Hypersensitivity reactions
	Gastrointestinal	Nausea, vomiting, diarrhea
	Neurologic	Dizziness, headache, vertigo
Colistimethate (colistin sulfate)	Renal	Decreased function, acute tubular necrosis
	Neurologic	Peripheral paresthesias, confusion, coma, seizures, neuromuscular blockade
Metronidazole	Neurologic	Peripheral neuropathy, seizures
	Gastrointestinal	Nausea, vomiting
	Other	Disulfiram reactions
Nitrofurantoin	Gastrointestinal	Nausea, vomiting, diarrhea
	Hepatic	Jaundice
	Immune	Rash, acute and chronic pulmonary hypersensitivity
	Neurologic	Peripheral neuropathy
Polymyxin B sulfate	Neurologic	Muscle weakness, seizures
	Renal	Azotemia, proteinuria
Selenium sulfide	Cutaneous	Contact dermatitis, alopecia (rare)
Silver sulfadiazine	Cutaneous	Contact dermatitis
	Hematologic	Anemia, aplastic anemia
Antifungals		
Carbol-fuchsin solution (phenol/resorcinol/fuchsin)	Gastrointestinal	Nausea, vomiting, diarrhea
Gentian violet	Gastrointestinal	Nausea, vomiting, diarrhea
	Immune	Rash (rare)
Griseofulvin	Renal	Proteinuria
	Hepatic	Increased enzymes
	Gastrointestinal	Nausea, vomiting, diarrhea
	Immune	Neutropenia
	Other	Disulfiram reactions, increased porphyrins
Nystatin	Gastrointestinal	Nausea, vomiting, diarrhea
Salicylic acid	Gastrointestinal and dermal	Higher concentrations are caustic
Undecylenic acid and undecylenate salt	Gastrointestinal	Nausea, vomiting, diarrhea

ANTIMICROBIALS SPECIFIC TO THE TREATMENT OF HIV AND RELATED INFECTIONS

The evaluation and management of patients infected with HIV/AIDS continues to evolve. Medications used to manage this disorder have increased life expectancy as new, more powerful antivirals and xenobiotic combinations become available. Therapeutic for HIV commonly consists of a combination of xenobiotics from different classes. The current recommendations include highly active antiretroviral therapy (HAART), which involves the use of 2 nucleoside reverse transcriptase inhibitors (NRTI) along with a third antiretroviral drug. Options include a integrase strand transfer inhibitor (INSTI), a nonnucleoside reverse transcriptase inhibitor (NNRTI), a protease inhibitor (PI) with a pharmacokinetic enhancer (cobicistat or ritonavir), or a C-C chemokine receptor type 5 (CCR5) antagonist.[103] The unique mechanisms that each xenobiotic offers aids in inhibiting viral replication and in minimizing xenobiotic resistance. Drug and dosage errors, particularly in infants, are of significant concern and have resulted in iatrogenic overdose.[34,56,140] These drugs also have success in the antiviral treatment of hepatitis C infection.[54] Second-generation

protease inhibitors have revolutionized the care of these patients in that they can be used in combinations that exclude the need for interferon and ribavirin while achieving higher sustained virologic responses.[250] This section focuses on overdoses and major toxic effects from HIV-directed antiviral therapy, as well as from xenobiotics that are specifically used in the management of opportunistic infections. A comprehensive review of these medications and end-organ toxicities is available.[149] Several drug interactions are also possible because of these xenobiotics being substrates for both inducers and inhibitors of several CYP enzymes and P-glycoprotein–associated metabolic systems.[219] Table 54–5 lists the common antimicrobials used to treat HIV-related opportunistic infections, and their common adverse effects.

TABLE 54–5	Antimicrobials Used to Treat Common Opportunistic Infections, Overdose Effects, and Common Adverse Drug Effects		
Antimicrobial	**Opportunistic Infection**	**Overdose Effects**	**Common Adverse Drug Effects**
Albendazole	Microsporidiosis	No reported cases	Increased AST/ALT, nausea, vomiting, and diarrhea; hematologic (rare), encephalopathy, AKI, rash
Amphotericin B	Aspergillosis Candidiasis Coccidioidomycosis Cryptococcosis Histoplasmosis Leishmaniasis Paracoccidioidomycosis Penicilliosis	Hypokalemia, increased AST, dysrhythmias and cardiac arrest	Infusions related fever, rigors, headache, nausea, vomiting, hypotension, tachycardia, and dyspnea. phlebitis, AKI, potassium and magnesium wasting, proteinuria, decreased renal concentrating ability, RTA, hematuria, anemia, dysrhythmias, tinnitus, thrombocytopenia, peripheral neuropathy, leukopenia
Antimony (pentavalent)	Leishmaniasis	AKI	AKI, multiorgan system failure
Atovaquone	*Pneumocystis jiroveci* (formerly *carinii*) pneumonia (PCP)	No clinical effects	Rashes, anemia, leukopenia, increased AST/ALT
Azithromycin	*Mycobacterium avium* complex	Nausea, vomiting, diarrhea. Intravenous, dysrhythmias	QT interval prolongation, nausea, vomiting, diarrhea
Clarithromycin	*Mycobacterium avium* complex	Nausea, vomiting, diarrhea.	QT interval prolongation, nausea, vomiting, diarrhea
Caspofungin	Aspergillosis	No reported cases	Phlebitis, headache, hypokalemia, increased AST/ALT, fever
Clindamycin	*Pneumocystis jiroveci* (formerly *carinii*) pneumonia (PCP) *Toxoplasma gondii*	Intravenous, neuromuscular blockade	Esophageal ulcers, diarrhea and *Clostridium difficile* enterocolitis
Dapsone	*Pneumocystis jiroveci* (formerly *carinii*) pneumonia (PCP)	Nausea, vomiting, diarrhea, methemoglobinemia	Bone marrow suppression, hepatitis, rash
Ethambutol	*Mycobacterium avium* complex	Severe toxicity not expected	Optic neuropathy
Fluconazole	Coccidioidomycosis Histoplasmosis	Severe toxicity not expected	Hepatotoxicity, thrombocytopenia, and neutropenia
Flucytosine	Cryptococcosis	No reported cases	Bone marrow suppression, hepatotoxicity, nausea, vomiting, diarrhea, rash
Foscarnet	Cytomegalovirus	No reported cases	Azotemia, hypocalcemia, and kidney failure (common); anemia, leukopenia, thrombocytopenia, fever, headache, seizures, genital and oral ulcers, fixed-drug eruptions, nausea, vomiting, diarrhea, headaches, seizures, coma, diabetes insipidus, hypophosphatemia, hypokalemia, hypomagnesemia
Fumagillin	Microsporidiosis	No reported cases	Neutropenia, thrombocytopenia
Ganciclovir	Cytomegalovirus	Severe toxicity not expected s	Leukopenia, worsening of kidney function; can also cause nausea, vomiting, diarrhea, increased AST/ALT, anemia, thrombocytopenia, headache, dizziness, confusion, seizures
Itraconazole	Histoplasmosis	No reported cases	Hepatotoxicity, thrombocytopenia, and neutropenia
Nitazoxanide	Cryptosporidiosis Microsporidiosis	No reported cases	Hypotension, headache, abdominal pain, nausea, vomiting; may cause green-yellow urine discoloration

(Continued)

TABLE 54–5	Antimicrobials Used to Treat Common Opportunistic Infections, Overdose Effects, and Common Adverse Drug Effects (*Continued*)		
Antimicrobial	*Opportunistic Infection*	*Overdose Effects*	*Common Adverse Drug Effects*
Paromomycin	Cryptosporidiosis	No reported cases	Ototoxicity, nephrotoxicity, pancreatitis
Pentamidine	*Pneumocystis jiroveci* (formerly *carinii*) pneumonia (PCP)	40 times dosing error in a 17-month-old child resulted in cardiac arrest	Hypoglycemia (early) followed by hyperglycemia, azotemia; can cause hypotension, torsade de pointes, phlebitis, rash, Stevens Johnson syndrome, hypocalcemia, hypokalemia, anorexia, nausea, vomiting, metallic taste, leukopenia, thrombocytopenia
Primaquine	*Pneumocystis jiroveci* (formerly *carinii*) pneumonia (PCP)	No reported cases	Neutropenia, hemolytic anemia, methemoglobinemia, leukocytosis; hypertension
Pyrimethamine	*Toxoplasma gondii*	No reported cases	Agranulocytosis, aplastic anemia, thrombocytopenia, leukopenia
Rifabutin	*Mycobacterium avium* complex	High doses (>1 g daily): arthralgia/arthritis	Nausea, vomiting, diarrhea; can cause hepatotoxicity, neutropenia, thrombocytopenia, hypersensitivity reactions
Sulfadiazine	*Toxoplasma gondii*	AKI and hypoglycemia	Rash, Stevens–Johnson syndrome, toxic epidermal necrolysis, erythema multiforme; headaches, depression, hallucinations, ataxia, tremor, crystalluria, hematuria, proteinuria, and nephrolithiasis
Trimethoprim/sulfamethoxazole	*Pneumocystis jiroveci* (formerly *carinii*) pneumonia (PCP) *Toxoplasma gondii* Isosporiasis	Severe toxicity not expected	Hyperkalemia, allergy, hematologic disorders, methemoglobinemia, hypoglycemia, rhabdomyolysis, neonatal kernicterus, psychosis
Trimetrexate	*Pneumocystis jiroveci* (formerly *carinii*) pneumonia (PCP)	Severe toxicity not expected; treat similarly to methotrexate (Chap. 51)	Myelosuppression, nausea, vomiting, histaminergic reactions
Valganciclovir	Cytomegalovirus	Severe toxicity not expected; expect to be similar to ganciclovir	Anemia, neutropenia, thrombocytopenia; nausea, vomiting, headache, peripheral neuropathy
Voriconazole	Aspergillosis	Severe toxicity not expected	Hepatotoxicity, thrombocytopenia, and neutropenia, toxic epidermal necrolysis

AKI = acute kidney injury; ALT = alanine aminotransferase; AST = aspartate aminotransferase.

Specific Antiretroviral Classes

Nucleoside Analog Reverse Transcriptase Inhibitors

The nucleoside analog reverse transcriptase inhibitors inhibit the reverse transcription of viral RNA into its subsequent DNA through the use of nucleoside analogs. Currently available xenobiotics include abacavir, didanosine (ddI), emtricitabine, lamivudine, stavudine, and zidovudine.

Acute Overdose Effects

Many intentional overdoses of reverse transcriptase inhibitors occur without major toxicologic effect. The most serious adverse effect anticipated after acute overdose of an NRTI is the development of a metabolic acidosis with elevated lactate concentration, which appears to be more common in women.[52,77,147] After the incorporation of the nucleoside analog into mitochondrial DNA by viral RNA reverse transcriptase enzymes, the faulty DNA results in impaired polymerase gamma activity. This results in decreased production of mitochondrial DNA electron transport proteins, which ultimately inhibits oxidative phosphorylation (Chap. 11). Organ system toxicity follows in addition to the development of acidemia. The reported mortality in patients with NRTI-associated metabolic acidosis associated with elevated lactate is 33% to 57%.[77] Resolution of symptoms in survivors occurs within 1 to 24 weeks. Patients with NRTI-associated acidemia are reported to recover more quickly after the use of cofactors such as thiamine, riboflavin, L-carnitine, vitamin C, and antioxidants.[38] The indications for the use of these xenobiotics are unclear at this time; however, because of the relative lack of toxicity, administration is reasonable.

Chronic Effects

Development of acidemia is more commonly associated with therapeutic use of reverse transcriptase inhibitors than with acute overdose. The mechanism is likely identical to that described above. Other drug-specific adverse drug reactions include hematologic toxicity after zidovudine, pancreatitis with didanosine, hypersensitivity after abacavir, and sensory peripheral neuropathy, after stavudine and didanosine.[67,68,93,130,158]

Nonnucleoside Reverse Transcriptase Inhibitors

The nonnucleoside reverse transcriptase inhibitors bind directly to reverse transcriptase enzymes enabling allosteric inhibition of enzymatic function.[225] Delavirdine, efavirenz, etravirine, nevirapine, and rilpivirine comprise the currently available xenobiotics.

There is a paucity of acute overdose data on these xenobiotics, although they generally appear to have limited toxicity. An adult male with a reported ingestion of 6 g of nevirapine had a sustained laboratory elevation in gamma-glutamyl transferase, but no other reported effects.[74] An infant received a 40 times therapeutic dose of nevirapine with mild neutropenia and metabolic acidosis with elevated lactate concentration.[34] Finally, a 12-year-old child reported an ingestion of 3 g of efavirenz resulting in throat burning, visual impairment, peripheral nervous system abnormalities, and nightmares.[163] Treatment is entirely supportive until more information is available. The nonnucleoside reverse transcriptase inhibitors are also limited in toxicity after chronic use. Use of nevirapine and delavirdine commonly results in hypersensitivity reactions such as rash. Efavirenz is reported to result in dizziness and dysphoria. Otherwise, toxicity can result from the ability of these xenobiotics to either inhibit or enhance CYP isozymes in the metabolism of other xenobiotics.

Protease Inhibitors

Protease inhibitors inhibit the vital enzyme (protease), which is required for viral replication.[81] Currently available xenobiotics include atazanavir, darunavir, fosamprenavir, indinavir, nelfinavir, ritonavir, saquinavir, and tipranavir.

Data after protease inhibitor overdose are limited. A literature review found diarrhea and hyperlipidemia to be common findings after therapeutic use. Less common were hepatitis, rash, hyperbilirubinemia, paresthesias, and nephrolithiasis.[27] Drug interactions can occur due to almost uniform inhibition of CYP3A-enzymes, and effects on P-glycoprotein along with some having effects and/or substrates for other CYP isoenzymes.[219] A unique finding is an altered fat distribution pattern that, over time, results in lymphodystrophy central obesity, "buffalo hump," breast enlargement, cushingoid appearance, and peripheral wasting.[81]

Fusion Inhibitors

This class of xenobiotics interferes with the binding or entry of the HIV virion into the cell.[24] No acute overdose data are available for this class, but after chronic use, hypersensitivity, gastrointestinal complaints, hepatotoxicity, and infusion reactions seem to be of greatest concern.[15,160,165] The currently available drug is enfuvirtide.

Cellular Chemokine Receptor (Ccr5) Antagonist

These drugs bind to chemokine coreceptors found on CD4 cells, which then ultimately prevents the entry of the HIV virion into the cell. The currently available drug is maraviroc. There is no overdose and adverse events reported; however, maraviroc has a boxed warning due to another CCR5 inhibitor, which was halted in development because of substantial hepatotoxicity.[165]

Integrase Inhibitor

This class of xenobiotics prevents the activity of the enzyme in HIV to function normally. This enzyme is responsible for the incorporation of the virus into DNA. The currently available xenobiotics are dolutegravir, elvitegravir, and raltegravir. No information is currently available regarding its toxicity after acute overdose. It appears that these xenobiotics are well tolerated at therapeutic doses.

SUMMARY

- Adverse drug reactions attributable to antimicrobials are largely related to chronic administration, although, rarely, acute severe toxic effects occur after large exposures.
- Acute toxic effects of antimicrobials are far more common following intravenous administration, xenobiotic interactions, or after iatrogenic overdose.
- Vigilance on the part of the health care professionals will prevent the majority of acute toxic manifestations following antimicrobial use.

REFERENCES

1. Abanades S, et al. Reversible coma secondary to cefepime neurotoxicity. *Ann Pharmacother.* 2004;38:606-608.
2. Abdel-Zaher AO, et al. Involvement of glutamate, oxidative stress and inducible nitric oxide synthase in the convulsant activity of ciprofloxacin in mice. *Eur J Pharmacol.* 2012;685:30-37.
3. Ahdal OA, Bevan DR. Clindamycin-induced neuromuscular blockade. *Can J Anaesth.* 1995;42:614-617.
4. Ahmed RM, et al. Gentamicin ototoxicity: a 23-year selected case series of 103 patients. *Med J Aust.* 2012;196:701-704.
5. Ali MZ, Goetz MB. A meta-analysis of the relative efficacy and toxicity of single daily dosing versus multiple daily dosing of aminoglycosides. *Clin Infect Dis.* 1997;24: 796-809.
6. Ali NA, et al. Haemolytic potential of three chemotherapeutic agents and aspirin in glucose-6-phosphate dehydrogenase deficiency. *East Mediterr Health J Rev Santé Méditerranée Orient Al-Majallah Al-Ṣiḥḥ͟Iyah Li-Sharq Al-Mutawassiṭ.* 1999;5:457-464.
7. Amoxicillin-Clavulanate. https://livertox.nlm.nih.gov/AmoxicillinClavulanate.htm. Accessed October 31, 2016.
8. Andrade RJ, et al. Benzylpenicillin-induced prolonged cholestasis. *Ann Pharmacother.* 2001;35:783-784.
9. Appel GB. Aminoglycoside nephrotoxicity. *Am J Med.* 1990;88:16S-20S; discussion 38S-42S.
10. Appel GB, et al. Vancomycin and the kidney. *Am J Kidney Dis.* 1986;8:75-80.
11. Arcieri GM, et al. Safety of intravenous ciprofloxacin. A review. *Am J Med.* 1989;87: 92S-97S.
12. Backon J. Hoigne's syndrome: relevance of anomalous dominance and prostaglandins. *Am J Dis Child. 1960.* 1986;140:1091-1092.
13. Bailie GR, et al. Vancomycin, red neck syndrome, and fits. *Lancet Lond Engl.* 1985;2:279-280.
14. Barton CH, et al. Renal magnesium wasting associated with amphotericin B therapy. *Am J Med.* 1984;77:471-474.
15. Beilke MA. Acute hypersensitivity reaction to enfuvirtide upon re-challenge. *Scand J Infect Dis.* 2004;36:778.
16. Bell CL, et al. Acute psychosis caused by co-amoxiclav. *BMJ.* 2008;337:a2117.
17. Bergeron L, Boucher FD. Possible red-man syndrome associated with systemic absorption of oral vancomycin in a child with normal renal function. *Ann Pharmacother.* 1994;28:581-584.
18. Berkovitch M, et al. Safety of the new quinolones in pregnancy. *Obstet Gynecol.* 1994;84:535-538.
19. Berry M, et al. Toxicity of antibiotics and antifungals on cultured human corneal cells: effect of mixing, exposure and concentration. *Eye (Lond).* 1995;9:110-115.
20. Best CJ, et al. Perioperative complications following the use of vancomycin in children: a report of two cases. *Br J Anaesth.* 1989;62:576-577.
21. Bhat RV, Deshmukh CT. A study of Vitamin K status in children on prolonged antibiotic therapy. *Indian Pediatr.* 2003;40:36-40.
22. Bhattacharya S. The facts about penicillin allergy: a review. *J Adv Pharm Technol Res.* 2010;1:11-17.
23. Binz J, et al. The risk of musculoskeletal adverse events with fluoroquinolones in children what is the verdict now? *Clin Pediatr (Phila).* 2016;55:107-110.
24. Biswas P, et al. Access denied? The status of co-receptor inhibition to counter HIV entry. *Expert Opin Pharmacother.* 2007;8:923-933.
25. Björnsson ES. Drug-induced liver injury: an overview over the most critical compounds. *Arch Toxicol.* 2015;89:327-334.
26. de Boer T, et al. Effect of penicillin on transmitter release from rat cortical tissue. *Brain Res.* 1980;192:296-300.
27. Boesecke C, Cooper DA. Toxicity of HIV protease inhibitors: clinical considerations. *Curr Opin HIV AIDS.* 2008;3:653-659.
28. Bolam DL, et al. Aminoglycoside overdose in neonates. *J Pediatr.* 1982;100:835.
29. Bovino JA, Marcus DF. The mechanism of transient myopia induced by sulfonamide therapy. *Am J Ophthalmol.* 1982;94:99-102.
30. Bradbury BD, Jick SS. Itraconazole and fluconazole and certain rare, serious adverse events. *Pharmacotherapy.* 2002;22:697-700.
31. Bradley J, et al. Progressive somnolence leading to coma in a 68-year-old man. *Chest.* 1997;112:538-540.
32. Branch RA. Prevention of amphotericin B-induced renal impairment. A review on the use of sodium supplementation. *Arch Intern Med.* 1988;148:2389-2394.
33. Brandriss MW, et al. Erythromycin-induced QT prolongation and polymorphic ventricular tachycardia (torsades de pointes): case report and review. *Clin Infect Dis.* 1994;18:995-998.
34. Brasme J-F, et al. Uncomplicated outcome after an accidental overdose of nevirapine in a newborn. *Eur J Pediatr.* 2007;167:689-690.
35. Brent J, et al. Amphotericin B overdoses in infants: is there a role for exchange transfusion? *Vet Hum Toxicol.* 1990;32:124-125.
36. Bright DA, et al. Amoxicillin overdose with gross hematuria. *West J Med.* 1989;150: 698-699.
37. Brinker AD, et al. Telithromycin-associated hepatotoxicity: clinical spectrum and causality assessment of 42 cases. *Hepatology.* 2009;49:250-257.
38. Brinkman K, ter Hofstede HJM. AidsReviews. http://www.aidsreviews.com/resumen.asp?id=571&indice=199913&u=unp. Accessed May 25, 2016.
39. Brössner G, et al. Accidental intrathecal infusion of cefotiam: clinical presentation and management. *Eur J Clin Pharmacol.* 2004;60:373-375.
40. Brown SD. Benefit-risk assessment of telithromycin in the treatment of community-acquired pneumonia. *Drug Saf.* 2008;31:561-575.
41. Brummett RE. Ototoxic liability of erythromycin and analogues. *Otolaryngol Clin North Am.* 1993;26:811-819.
42. Bryant SG, et al. Increased frequency of doxycycline side effects. *Pharmacotherapy.* 1987;7:125-129.
43. Buening MK, et al. Disulfiram-like reaction to beta-lactams. *JAMA.* 1981;245:2027.
44. Bussey HI, et al. Warfarin-erythromycin interaction. *Arch Intern Med.* 1985;145:1736-1737.
45. Butler WT, et al. Electrocardiographic and electrolyte abnormalities caused by amphotericin B in dog and man. *Proc Soc Exp Biol Med.* 1964;116:857-863.
46. Callaghan JT, et al. CSF perfusion to treat intraventricular penicillin toxicity. *Arch Neurol.* 1981;38:390-391.
47. Campagna JD, et al. The use of cephalosporins in penicillin-allergic patients: a literature review. *J Emerg Med.* 2012;42:612-620.
48. Cannon JP, et al. The risk of seizures among the carbapenems: a meta-analysis. *J Antimicrob Chemother.* 2014;69:2043-2055.
49. Carson JL, et al. Acute liver disease associated with erythromycins, sulfonamides, and tetracyclines. *Ann Intern Med.* 1993;119(7, pt 1):576-583.
50. Castell DO, Sparks HA. Nephrogenic diabetes insipidus due to demethylchlortetracycline hydrochloride. *JAMA.* 1965;193:237-239.
51. Centers for Disease Control and Prevention (CDC). Endotoxin-like reactions associated with intravenous gentamicin—California, 1998. *MMWR Morb Mortal Wkly Rep.* 1998;47:877-880.

52. Chattha G, et al. Lactic acidosis complicating the acquired immunodeficiency syndrome. *Ann Intern Med*. 1993;118:37-39.

53. Chawla A, et al. Rapidly progressive cholestasis: an unusual reaction to amoxicillin/clavulanic acid therapy in a child. *J Pediatr*. 2000;136:121-123.

54. Chayama K, et al. Hepatitis C virus treatment update—a new era of all-oral HCV treatment. *Adv Dig Med*. 2016;3:153-160.

55. Cheng Y-J, et al. The role of macrolide antibiotics in increasing cardiovascular risk. *J Am Coll Cardiol*. 2015;66:2173-2184.

56. Chiappini E, et al. Preventable zidovudine overdose during postnatal prophylaxis in healthy children born to HIV-1-positive mothers. *AIDS Lond Engl*. 2008;22:316-317.

57. Chow KM, et al. Neurotoxicity induced by beta-lactam antibiotics: from bench to bedside. *Eur J Clin Microbiol Infect Dis*. 2005;24:649-653.

58. Christ W. Central nervous system toxicity of quinolones: human and animal findings. *J Antimicrob Chemother*. 1990;26(suppl B):219-225.

59. Christie DJ, et al. Vancomycin-dependent antibodies associated with thrombocytopenia and refractoriness to platelet transfusion in patients with leukemia. *Blood*. 1990;75:518-523.

60. Cleary JD, et al. Amphotericin B overdose in pediatric patients with associated cardiac arrest. *Ann Pharmacother*. 1993;27:715-719.

61. Cocke JG, et al. Optic neuritis with prolonged use of chloramphenicol. Case report and relationship to fundus changes in cystic fibrosis. *J Pediatr*. 1966;68:27-31.

62. Cohen LS, et al. Depression of cardiac function by streptomycin and other antimicrobial agents. *Am J Cardiol*. 1970;26:505-511.

63. Connor JP, et al. Acute renal failure secondary to ciprofloxacin use. *J Urol*. 1994;151:975-976.

64. Danan G, et al. Self-induction by erythromycin of its own transformation into a metabolite forming an inactive complex with reduced cytochrome P-450. *J Pharmacol Exp Ther*. 1981;218:509-514.

65. De Sarro G, et al. Effects of some excitatory amino acid antagonists and drugs enhancing gamma-aminobutyric acid neurotransmission on pefloxacin-induced seizures in DBA/2 mice. *Antimicrob Agents Chemother*. 1997;41:427-434.

66. Delanaye P, et al. Trimethoprim, creatinine and creatinine-based equations. *Nephron Clin Pract*. 2011;119:c187-c193.

67. Demoly P, et al. Allergy to macrolide antibiotics. Review of the literature [in French]. *Presse Med*. 2000;29:321-326.

68. Deray G, et al. Pharmacokinetics of zidovudine in a patient on maintenance hemodialysis. *N Engl J Med*. 1988;319:1606-1607.

69. Domen RE, Horowitz S. Vancomycin-induced neutropenia associated with anti-granulocyte antibodies. *Immunohemat Am Red Cross*. 1990;6:41-43.

70. Dunn RJ. Massive sulfasalazine and paracetamol ingestion causing acidosis, hyperglycemia, coagulopathy, and methemoglobinemia. *J Toxicol Clin Toxicol*. 1998;36:239-242.

71. Dunn RL. Exposure to trimethoprim-sulfamethoxazole is associated with hospitalisation for hyperkalaemia in older people treated with spironolactone. *Evid Based Med*. 2012;17:130-131.

72. Durosinmi MA, Ajayi AA. A prospective study of chloramphenicol induced aplastic anaemia in Nigerians. *Trop Geogr Med*. 1993;45:159-161.

73. Ehmann WC. Cephalosporin-induced hemolysis: a case report and review of the literature. *Am J Hematol*. 1992;40:121-125.

74. Elens L, et al. Acute intoxication with nevirapine in an HIV-1-infected patient: clinical and pharmacokinetic follow up. *AIDS Lond Engl*. 2009;23:1291-1293.

75. English J, et al. Attenuation of experimental tobramycin nephrotoxicity by ticarcillin. *Antimicrob Agents Chemother*. 1985;27:897-902.

76. Engrav MB, Zimmerman M. Electrocardiographic changes associated with anaphylaxis in a patient with normal coronary arteries. *West J Med*. 1994;161:602-604.

77. Falcó V, et al. Severe nucleoside-associated lactic acidosis in human immunodeficiency virus-infected patients: report of 12 cases and review of the literature. *Clin Infect Dis*. 2002;34:838-846.

78. Fang C-C, et al. Erythromycin-induced acute pancreatitis. *J Toxicol Clin Toxicol*. 1996;34:93-95.

79. Fanos V, Cataldi L. Amphotericin B-induced nephrotoxicity: a review. *J Chemother Florence Italy*. 2000;12:463-470.

80. Fisher MA, et al. Risk factors for Amphotericin B-associated nephrotoxicity. *Am J Med*. 1989;87:547-552.

81. Flexner C. HIV-protease inhibitors. *N Engl J Med*. 1998;338:1281-1292.

82. Fraser DG. Suicide attempt with Azo Gantanol resulting in methemoglobinemia. *Mil Med*. 1969;134:679-681.

83. Freundlich M, et al. Management of chloramphenicol intoxication in infancy by charcoal hemoperfusion. *J Pediatr*. 1983;103:485-487.

84. Frimpter GW, et al. Reversible Fanconi syndrome caused by degraded tetracycline. *JAMA*. 1963;184:111-113.

85. Fripp RR, et al. Cardiac function and acute chloramphenicol toxicity. *J Pediatr*. 1983;103:487-490.

86. Garratty G. Immune cytopenia associated with antibiotics. *Transfus Med Rev*. 1993;7:255-267.

87. Garrelts JC, Peterie JD. Vancomycin and the "red man's syndrome." *N Engl J Med*. 1985;312:245.

88. Geller RJ, et al. Acute amoxicillin nephrotoxicity following an overdose. *J Toxicol Clin Toxicol*. 1986;24:175-182.

89. Ghimire S, et al. An evidence-based approach for providing cautionary recommendations to sulfonamide-allergic patients and determining cross-reactivity among sulfonamide-containing medications. *J Clin Pharm Ther*. 2013;38:196-202.

90. Gigliotti F, et al. Induction of prostaglandin synthesis as the mechanism responsible for the chills and fever produced by infusing amphotericin B. *J Infect Dis*. 1987;156:784-789.

91. Gilbert FI. Cholestatic hepatitis caused by esters of erythromycin and oleandomycin. 1962. *Hawaii Med J*. 1995;54:603-605.

92. Glazko AJ. Identification of chloramphenicol metabolites and some factors affecting metabolic disposition. *Antimicrob Agents Chemother*. 1966;6:655-665.

93. Gold JW. The diagnosis and management of HIV infection. *Med Clin North Am*. 1996;80:1283-1307.

94. Gordon G, et al. Hyperpigmentation of the skin associated with minocycline therapy. *Arch Dermatol*. 1985;121:618-623.

95. Goss TF, et al. Prospective evaluation of risk factors for antibiotic-associated bleeding in critically ill patients. *Pharmacotherapy*. 1992;12:283-291.

96. Gurley D, et al. Point mutations in the M2 region of the alpha, beta, or gamma subunit of the GABAA channel that abolish block by picrotoxin. *Receptors Channels*. 1995;3:13-20.

97. Gurwith M, et al. Renal sparing by amphotericin B colloidal dispersion: clinical experience in 572 patients. *Chemotherapy*. 1999;45(suppl 1):39-47.

98. Harvey SC, et al. The antibacterial and NMDA receptor activating properties of aminoglycosides are dissociable. *Eur J Pharmacol*. 2000;387:1-7.

99. Healy DP, et al. Comparison of steady-state pharmacokinetics of two dosage regimens of vancomycin in normal volunteers. *Antimicrob Agents Chemother*. 1987;31:393-397.

100. Hedrick R, et al. Carbamazepine–erythromycin interaction leading to carbamazepine toxicity in four epileptic children. *Ther Drug Monit*. 1983;5:405-407.

101. Heidemann HT, et al. Amphotericin B nephrotoxicity in humans decreased by salt repletion. *Am J Med*. 1983;75:476-481.

102. Hiemenz JW, Walsh TJ. Lipid formulations of amphotericin B: recent progress and future directions. *Clin Infect Dis*. 1996;22(suppl 2):S133-S144.

103. HIV/AIDS treatment guidelines. AIDSinfo. https://aidsinfo.nih.gov/. Accessed November 11, 2016.

104. Ho WK, et al. Severe immune haemolysis after standard doses of penicillin. *Clin Lab Haematol*. 2004;26:153-156.

105. Hootkins R, et al. Acute renal failure secondary to oral ciprofloxacin therapy: a presentation of three cases and a review of the literature. *Clin Nephrol*. 1989;32:75-78.

106. Huang DB, et al. Toxic epidermal necrolysis as a complication of treatment with voriconazole. *South Med J*. 2004;97:1116-1117.

107. Hughes DW. Studies on chloramphenicol. 1. Assessment of haemopoietic toxicity. *Med J Aust*. 1968;2:436-438.

108. Huguenel C, et al. Case files of the Harvard Medical Toxicology Fellowship: valacyclovir neurotoxicity and unintentional overdose. *J Med Toxicol*. 2015;11:132-136.

109. Humes HD. Aminoglycoside nephrotoxicity. *Kidney Int*. 1988;33:900-911.

110. Hunt CM, Washington K. Tetracycline-induced bile duct paucity and prolonged cholestasis. *Gastroenterology*. 1994;107:1844-1847.

111. Ilechukwu ST. Acute psychotic reactions and stress response syndromes following intramuscular aqueous procaine penicillin. *Br J Psychiatry J Ment Sci*. 1990;156:554-559.

112. Inman WH, Rawson NS. Erythromycin estolate and jaundice. *Br Med J (Clin Res Ed)*. 1983;286:1954-1955.

113. Jackson TL, Williamson TH. Amikacin retinal toxicity. *Br J Ophthalmol*. 1999;83:1199-1200.

114. Jalbert EO. Seizures after penicillin administration. *Am J Dis Child. 1960*. 1985;139:1075.

115. Jimenez JJ, et al. Chloramphenicol-induced bone marrow injury: possible role of bacterial metabolites of chloramphenicol. *Blood*. 1987;70:1180-1185.

116. Johnson MD, et al. Chest discomfort associated with liposomal amphotericin B: report of three cases and review of the literature. *Pharmacother J Hum Pharmacol Drug Ther*. 1998;18:1053-1061.

117. Johnsson LG, et al. Total deafness from aminoglycoside overdosage: histopathologic case study. *Am J Otolaryngol*. 1984;5:118-126.

118. Kahlmeter G, Dahlager JI. Aminoglycoside toxicity—a review of clinical studies published between 1975 and 1982. *J Antimicrob Chemother*. 1984;13(suppl A):9-22.

119. Kearns GL, et al. Serum sickness-like reactions to cefaclor: role of hepatic metabolism and individual susceptibility. *J Pediatr*. 1994;125(5, pt 1):805-811.

120. Kelkar PS, Li JT. Cephalosporin allergy. *N Engl J Med*. 2001;345:804-809.

121. Ketek (Sanofi-aventis U.S. LLC). FDA Package Insert. MedLibrary.org. http://medlibrary.org/lib/rx/meds/ketek/. Accessed May 25, 2016.

122. Koren G, et al. Tenfold errors in administration of drug doses: a neglected iatrogenic disease in pediatrics. *Pediatrics*. 1986;77:848-849.

123. Koren G, et al. Clinical course and pharmacokinetics following a massive overdose of amphotericin B in a neonate. *J Toxicol Clin Toxicol*. 1990;28:371-378.

124. Kranzer K, et al. A systematic review and meta-analysis of the efficacy and safety of N-acetylcysteine in preventing aminoglycoside-induced ototoxicity: implications for the treatment of multidrug-resistant TB. *Thorax*. September 2015;70:1070-1077.

125. Kristof RA, et al. Treatment of accidental high dose intraventricular mezlocillin application by cerebrospinal fluid exchange. *J Neurol Neurosurg Psychiatry*. 1998;64:379-381.

126. Kubo Y, et al. Contact sensitivity to chloramphenicol. *Contact Dermatitis*. 1987;17:245-247.
127. Kucukguclu S, et al. Multiple-dose activated charcoal in an accidental vancomycin overdose. *J Toxicol Clin Toxicol*. 1996;34:83-86.
128. Kumar A, Dada T. Preretinal haemorrhages: an unusual manifestation of intravitreal amikacin toxicity. *Aust N Z J Ophthalmol*. 1999;27:435-436.
129. Kushner JM, et al. Seizures associated with fluoroquinolones. *Ann Pharmacother*. 2001;35:1194-1198.
130. Lambert JS, et al. 2′,3′-Dideoxyinosine (DDI) in patients with the acquired immunodeficiency syndrome or AIDS-related complex. A phase I trial. *N Engl J Med*. 1990;322:1333-1340.
131. Lang EW, et al. A massive intrathecal cefazoline overdose. *Eur J Anaesthesiol*. 1999;16:204-205.
132. Lang TR, et al. What tendon pathology is seen on imaging in people who have taken fluoroquinolones? A systematic review. *Fundam Clin Pharmacol*. 2017;31:4-16.
133. Laniado-Laborín R, Cabrales-Vargas MN. Amphotericin B: side effects and toxicity. *Rev Iberoam Micol*. 2009;26:223-227.
134. Lehmann DF, et al. The association of opportunistic infections with the occurrence of trimethoprim/sulfamethoxazole hypersensitivity in patients infected with human immunodeficiency virus. *J Clin Pharmacol*. 1999;39:533-537.
135. Levin G, Behrenth E. Irreversible ototoxic effect of erythromycin. *Scand Audiol*. 1986;15:41-42.
136. Levine PH, et al. Chloramphenicol-associated encephalopathy. *Clin Pharmacol Ther*. 1970;11:194-199.
137. Levy JH, Kettlekamp N, et al. Histamine release by vancomycin: a mechanism for hypotension in man. *Anesthesiology*. 1987;67:122-124.
138. Licata A, et al. Fluoroquinolone-induced liver injury: three new cases and a review of the literature. *Eur J Clin Pharmacol*. 2012;68:525-532.
139. Lin AC, et al. Amphotericin B blunts erythropoietin response to anemia. *J Infect Dis*. 1990;161:348-351.
140. Livshits Z, et al. Zidovudine (AZT) overdose in a healthy newborn receiving postnatal prophylaxis. *Clin Toxicol*. 2011;49:747-749.
141. Lopez-Novoa JM, et al. New insights into the mechanism of aminoglycoside nephrotoxicity: an integrative point of view. *Kidney Int*. 2011;79:33-45.
142. Lowery N, et al. Serum sickness-like reactions associated with cefprozil therapy. *J Pediatr*. 1994;125:325-328.
143. Lu CM, et al. Acute massive gentamicin intoxication in a patient with end-stage renal disease. *Am J Kidney Dis*. 1996;28:767-771.
144. MacGregor RR, et al. Erythropoietin concentration in amphotericin B-induced anemia. *Antimicrob Agents Chemother*. 1978;14:270-273.
145. MacNeil M, et al. Fever, lymphadenopathy, eosinophilia, lymphocytosis, hepatitis, and dermatitis: a severe adverse reaction to minocycline. *J Am Acad Dermatol*. 1997;36(2, pt 2):347-350.
146. Maddux MS, Barriere SL. A review of complications of amphotericin-B therapy: recommendations for prevention and management. *Ann Pharmacother*. 1980;14:177-181.
147. Maignen F, et al. Acute toxicity of zidovudine. Analysis of the literature and number of cases at the Paris Poison Control Center [in French]. *Therapie*. 1993;48:129-131.
148. Malone JD, et al. Procaine-induced seizures after intramuscular procaine penicillin G. *Mil Med*. 1988;153:191-192.
149. Margolis AM, et al. A review of the toxicity of HIV medications. *J Med Toxicol*. 2013;10:26-39.
150. Marks C, Cummins BH. Rescue after 2 megaunits of intrathecal penicillin. *Lancet Lond Engl*. 1981;1:658-659.
151. Matsubara T, et al. Effects of beta-lactam antibiotics and *N*-methyltetrazolethiol on the alcohol-metabolizing system in rats. *Jpn J Pharmacol*. 1987;45:303-315.
152. Mattie H, et al. Determinants of efficacy and toxicity of aminoglycosides. *J Antimicrob Chemother*. 1989;24:281-293.
153. Mauer SM, et al. Treatment of an infant with severe chloramphenicol intoxication using charcoal-column hemoperfusion. *J Pediatr*. 1980;96:136-139.
154. McCune WS, Evans JM. Intraventricular penicillin in the treatment of staphylococcic meningitis. *J Am Med Assoc*. 1944;125:705-706.
155. Moore LE, et al. Recognition, treatment, and prevention of anaphylaxis. *Immunol Allergy Clin North Am*. 2015;35:363-374.
156. Moore RD, et al. Risk factors for nephrotoxicity in patients treated with aminoglycosides. *Ann Intern Med*. 1984;100:352-357.
157. Mostafa S, Miller BJ. Antibiotic-associated psychosis during treatment of urinary tract infections: a systematic review. *J Clin Psychopharmacol*. 2014;34:483-490.
158. Moyle DGJ, Sadler M. Peripheral neuropathy with nucleoside antiretrovirals. *Drug Saf*. 2012;19:481-494.
159. Mulhall A, et al. Chloramphenicol toxicity in neonates: its incidence and prevention. *Br Med J (Clin Res Ed)*. 1983;287:1424-1427.
160. Myers SA, et al. A prospective clinical and pathological examination of injection site reactions with the HIV-1 fusion inhibitor enfuvirtide. *Antivir Ther*. 2006;11:935-939.
161. Nahata MC. Serum concentrations and adverse effects of chloramphenicol in pediatric patients. *Chemotherapy*. 1987;33:322-327.
162. Naisbitt DJ, et al. Cellular disposition of sulphamethoxazole and its metabolites: implications for hypersensitivity. *Br J Pharmacol*. 1999;126:1393-1407.
163. Nazziwa R, et al. Efavirenz poisoning in a 12 year old HIV negative African boy. *Pan Afr Med J*. 2012;12:86.
164. Newfield P, Roizen MF. Hazards of rapid administration of vancomycin. *Ann Intern Med*. 1979;91:581.
165. Nichols WG, et al. Hepatotoxicity observed in clinical trials of aplaviroc (GW873140). *Antimicrob Agents Chemother*. 2008;52:858-865.
166. Nickels LC, et al. Trimethoprim-sulfamethoxazole-induced hyperkalemia in a patient with normal renal function. *Case Rep Emerg Med*. 2012;2012:815907.
167. Nishida I, Takumida M. Attenuation of aminoglycoside ototoxicity by glutathione. *ORL J Otorhinolaryngol Relat Spec*. 1996;58:68-73.
168. Nordt SP, et al. Clarithromycin induced digoxin toxicity. *J Accid Emerg Med*. 1998;15:194-195.
169. Obata H, et al. Pathogenesis of hypoprothrombinemia induced by antibiotics. *J Nutr Sci Vitaminol (Tokyo)*. 1992;38(Special):421-424.
170. O'Gorman Hughes DW. Studies on chloramphenicol. II. Possible determinants and progress of haemopoietic toxicity during chloramphenicol therapy. *Med J Aust*. 1973;2:1142-1146.
171. O'Sullivan TL, et al. Prospective evaluation of red man syndrome in patients receiving vancomycin. *J Infect Dis*. 1993;168:773-776.
172. Owens RC, Ambrose PG. Torsades de pointes associated with fluoroquinolones. *Pharmacotherapy*. 2002;22:663-672.
173. Paradelis AG. Aminoglycoside antibiotics and neuromuscular blockade. *J Antimicrob Chemother*. 1979;5:737-738.
174. Pérez Pimiento A, et al. Aztreonam and ceftazidime: evidence of in vivo cross allergenicity. *Allergy*. 1998;53:624-625.
175. Pestotnik SL, et al. Prospective surveillance of imipenem/cilastatin use and associated seizures using a hospital information system. *Ann Pharmacother*. 1993;27:497-501.
176. Polk RE, et al. Vancomycin skin tests and prediction of "red man syndrome" in healthy volunteers. *Antimicrob Agents Chemother*. 1993;37:2139-2143.
177. Pound MW, May DB. Proposed mechanisms and preventative options of Jarisch-Herxheimer reactions. *J Clin Pharm Ther*. 2005;30:291-295.
178. Ptachcinski RJ, et al. Effect of erythromycin on cyclosporine levels. *N Engl J Med*. 1985;313:1416-1417.
179. Ramilo O, et al. Chloramphenicol neurotoxicity. *Pediatr Infect Dis J*. 1988;7:358-359.
180. Renz CL, et al. Antihistamine prophylaxis permits rapid vancomycin infusion. *Crit Care Med*. 1999;27:1732-1737.
181. Center for Drug Evaluation and Research. Drug safety and availability: FDA drug safety communication: FDA advises restricting fluoroquinolone antibiotic use for certain uncomplicated infections; warns about disabling side effects that can occur together. http://www.fda.gov/Drugs/DrugSafety/ucm500143.htm. Accessed November 10, 2016.
182. Richardet JP, et al. Prolonged cholestasis with ductopenia after administration of amoxicillin/clavulanic acid. *Dig Dis Sci*. 1999;44:1997-2000.
183. Richardson JA. Accidental ingestion of acyclovir in dogs: 105 reports. *Vet Hum Toxicol*. 2000;42:370-371.
184. Riley HD. Vancomycin and novobiocin. *Med Clin North Am*. 1970;54:1277-1289.
185. Rippelmeyer DJ, Synhavsky A. Ciprofloxacin and allergic interstitial nephritis. *Ann Intern Med*. 1988;109:170.
186. Rivera Vaquerizo PA, et al. Clindamycin-induced esophageal ulcer. *Rev Esp Enferm Dig*. 2004;96:143-145.
187. Roberts DM, et al. Acute kidney injury due to crystalluria following acute valacyclovir overdose. *Kidney Int*. 2011;79:574.
188. Rockwood RP, Embardo LS. Theophylline, ciprofloxacin, erythromycin: a potentially harmful regimen. *Ann Pharmacother*. 1993;27:651-652.
189. Romano A, et al. Cross-reactivity among beta-lactams. *Curr Allergy Asthma Rep*. 2016;16:24.
190. Rothenberg HJ. Anaphylactoid reaction to vancomycin. *J Am Med Assoc*. 1959;171:1101-1102.
191. Rybak MJ, Boike SC. Additive toxicity in patients receiving vancomycin and aminoglycosides. *Clin Pharm*. 1983;2:508.
192. Sabra R, et al. Mechanisms of amphotericin B-induced reduction of the glomerular filtration rate: a micropuncture study. *J Pharmacol Exp Ther*. 1990;253:34-37.
193. Sacristán JA, et al. Erythromycin-induced hypoacusis: 11 new cases and literature review. *Ann Pharmacother*. 1993;27:950-955.
194. Sage DJ. Management of acute anaphylactoid reactions. *Int Anesthesiol Clin*. 1985;23:175-186.
195. Salimi A, et al. Toxicity of macrolide antibiotics on isolated heart mitochondria: a justification for their cardiotoxic adverse effect. *Xenobiotica*. 2016;46:82-93.
196. Sánchez AR, et al. Tetracycline and other tetracycline-derivative staining of the teeth and oral cavity. *Int J Dermatol*. 2004;43:709-715.
197. Saravay SM, et al. "Doom anxiety" and delirium in lidocaine toxicity. *Am J Psychiatry*. 1987;144:159-163.
198. Sawaya BP, et al. Direct vasoconstriction as a possible cause for amphotericin B-induced nephrotoxicity in rats. *J Clin Invest*. 1991;87:2097-2107.
199. Saxon A, et al. Imipenem cross-reactivity with penicillin in humans. *J Allergy Clin Immunol*. 1988;82:213-217.
200. Saxon A, et al. Investigation into the immunologic cross-reactivity of aztreonam with other beta-lactam antibiotics. *Am J Med*. 1985;78:19-26.
201. Schentag JJ, Plaut ME. Patterns of urinary β2-microglobulin excretion by patients treated with aminoglycosides. *Kidney Int*. 1980;17:654-661.

202. Schluter G. Ciprofloxacin: review of potential toxicologic effects. *Am J Med*. 1987;82: 91-93.

203. Schreiber BE, et al. Sudden sensorineural hearing loss. *Lancet Lond Engl*. 2010;375: 1203-1211.

204. Schrodt BJ, et al. Necrotizing vasculitis of the skin and uterine cervix associated with minocycline therapy for acne vulgaris. *South Med J*. 1999;92:502-504.

205. Scott JL, et al. A controlled double-blind study of the hematologic toxicity of chloramphenicol. *N Engl J Med*. 1965;272:1137-1142.

206. Seamans KB, et al. Penicillin-induced seizures during cardiopulmonary bypass. A clinical and electroencephalographic study. *N Engl J Med*. 1968;278:861-868.

207. See S, et al. Penicillin-induced Jarisch-Herxheimer reaction. *Ann Pharmacother*. 2005;39:2128-2130.

208. Selden R, Sasahara AA. Central nervous system toxicity induced by lidocaine. Report of a case in a patient with liver disease. *JAMA*. 1967;202:908-909.

209. Shapiro LE, et al. Comparative safety of tetracycline, minocycline, and doxycycline. *Arch Dermatol*. 1997;133:1224-1230.

210. Shu XO, et al. Chloramphenicol use and childhood leukaemia in Shanghai. *Lancet Lond Engl*. 1987;2:934-937.

211. Silber T, D'Angelo L. Doom anxiety and Hoigne's syndrome. *Am J Psychiatry*. 1987;144: 1365.

212. Simons FER, et al. World allergy organization guidelines for the assessment and management of anaphylaxis. *World Allergy Organ J*. 2011;4:13.

213. Slaughter RL, et al. Effect of hemodialysis on total body clearance of chloramphenicol. *Am J Hosp Pharm*. 1980;37:1083-1086.

214. Slayton W, et al. Tetany in a child with AIDS receiving intravenous tobramycin. *South Med J*. 1996;89:1108-1110.

215. Smith NL, et al. Therapeutic drug monitoring when using cefepime in continuous renal replacement therapy: seizures associated with cefepime. *Crit Care Resusc*. 2012;14:312-315.

216. Somer T, Finegold SM. Vasculitides associated with infections, immunization, and antimicrobial drugs. *Clin Infect Dis*. 1995;20:1010-1036.

217. Song BB, et al. Iron chelators protect from aminoglycoside-induced cochleo- and vestibulo-toxicity. *Free Radic Biol Med*. 1998;25:189-195.

218. Stevens DC, et al. Exchange transfusion in acute chloramphenicol toxicity. *J Pediatr*. 1981;99:651-653.

219. Stolbach A, et al. A review of the toxicity of HIV medications II: interactions with drugs and complementary and alternative medicine products. *J Med Toxicol*. 2015;11:326-341.

220. Sunagawa M, et al. Structural features resulting in convulsive activity of carbapenem compounds: effect of C-2 side chain. *J Antibiot (Tokyo)*. 1995;48:408-416.

221. Swanson DJ, et al. Erythromycin ototoxicity: prospective assessment with serum concentrations and audiograms in a study of patients with pneumonia. *Am J Med*. 1992;92:61-68.

222. Swanson-Biearman B, et al. The effects of penicillin and cephalosporin ingestions in children less than six years of age. *Vet Hum Toxicol*. 1988;30:66-67.

223. Teitelbaum JE, et al. Minocycline-related autoimmune hepatitis: case series and literature review. *Arch Pediatr Adolesc Med*. 1998;152:1132-1136.

224. Thompson WL, et al. Letter: overdoses of chloramphenicol. *JAMA*. 1975;234:149-150.

225. Threlkeld SC, Hirsch MS. Antiretroviral therapy. *Med Clin North Am*. 1996;80: 1263-1282.

226. Thyagarajan B, Deshpande SS. Cotrimoxazole and neonatal kernicterus: a review. *Drug Chem Toxicol*. 2014;37:121-129.

227. Tilelli JA, et al. Life-threatening bradyarrhythmia after massive azithromycin overdose. *Pharmacotherapy*. 2006;26:147-150.

228. Timmermans L. Influence of antibiotics on spermatogenesis. *J Urol*. 1974;112:348-349.

229. Tsubura S. Clinical evaluation of three months' nightguard vital bleaching on tetracycline-stained teeth using Polanight 10% carbamide gel: 2-year follow-up study. *Odontol Soc Nippon Dent Univ*. 2010;98:134-138.

230. Tucker WE. Preclinical toxicology profile of acyclovir: an overview. *Am J Med*. 1982;73:27-30.

231. Turner WM. Lidocaine and psychotic reactions. *Ann Intern Med*. 1982;97:149-150.

232. Tynes BS, et al. Reducing amphotericin B reactions. A double-blind study. *Am Rev Respir Dis*. 1963;87:264-268.

233. Ulinski T, et al. Large-pore haemodialysis membranes: an efficient tool for rapid removal of vancomycin after accidental overdose. *Nephrol Dial Transplant*. 2005;20:1517-1518.

234. Unal M, et al. Ocular toxicity of intravitreal clarithromycin. *Retina Phila Pa*. 1999;19:442-446.

235. Utley PM, et al. Acute psychotic reactions to aqueous procaine penicillin. *South Med J*. 1966;59:1271-1274.

236. Van Arsdel PP. The risk of penicillin reactions. *Ann Intern Med*. 1968;69:1071-1073.

237. Veit O, et al. First case of ivermectin-induced severe hepatitis. *Trans R Soc Trop Med Hyg*. 2006;100:795-797.

238. Walker PD, et al. Oxidant mechanisms in gentamicin nephrotoxicity. *Ren Fail*. 1999;21:433-442.

239. Wallace KL. Antibiotic-induced convulsions. *Crit Care Clin*. 1997;13:741-762.

240. Wallace MR, et al. Red man syndrome: incidence, etiology, and prophylaxis. *J Infect Dis*. 1991;164:1180-1185.

241. Walmsley SL, et al. Oxidative stress and thiol depletion in plasma and peripheral blood lymphocytes from HIV-infected patients: toxicological and pathological implications. *AIDS Lond Engl*. 1997;11:1689-1697.

242. Walsh TJ, et al. Liposomal amphotericin B for empirical therapy in patients with persistent fever and neutropenia. National Institute of Allergy and Infectious Diseases Mycoses Study Group. *N Engl J Med*. 1999;340:764-771.

243. Wang GS, et al. Survival after amphotericin B overdose treated with plasmapheresis. *Ann Pharmacother*. 2013;47:e9.

244. Weisberger AS, et al. Mechanisms of action of chloramphenicol. *JAMA*. 1969;209:97-103.

245. Westphal JF, et al. Hepatic side-effects of antibiotics. *J Antimicrob Chemother*. 1994;33:387-401.

246. Wiest DB, et al. Chloramphenicol toxicity revisited: a 12-year-old patient with a brain abscess. *J Pediatr Pharmacol Ther JPPT*. 2012;17:182-188.

247. Wise BL, et al. Impact of age, sex, obesity, and steroid use on quinolone-associated tendon disorders. *Am J Med*. 2012;125:1228.e23-1228.e28.

248. Wolf R, Brenner S. An active amide group in the molecule of drugs that induce pemphigus: a casual or causal relationship? *Dermatology*. 1994;189:1-4.

249. Wood JP, et al. Safety of epinephrine for anaphylaxis in the emergency setting. *World J Emerg Med*. 2013;4:245-251.

250. World Health Organization, Global Hepatitis Programme. Guidelines for the Screening, Care and Treatment of Persons with Chronic Hepatitis C Infection. http://apps.who.int/iris/bitstream/10665/205035/1/9789241549615_eng.pdf. Published 2016. Accessed November 11, 2016.

251. Yoshioka DH, et al. Convulsion following intrathecal cephaloridine. *Infection*. 1975;3:123-124.

252. Zager RA, et al. Direct amphotericin B-mediated tubular toxicity: assessments of selected cytoprotective agents. *Kidney Int*. 1992;41:1588-1594.

253. Zhou W, Moore DE. Photosensitizing activity of the anti-bacterial drugs sulfamethoxazole and trimethoprim. *J Photochem Photobiol B*. 1997;39:63-72.

55 ANTIMALARIALS

James David Barry

The malaria parasite has caused untold grief throughout human history. The name originated from Italian *mal aria* (bad air) because the ancient Romans believed the disease was caused by the decay in marshes and swamps and was carried by the malodorous "foul" air emanating from these areas.[8] In the 1880s, both the *Plasmodium* protozoa and its mosquito vector were identified.[8] Today, nearly half of the world's population lives in areas where malaria is endemic. Despite markedly decreased mortality rates over the last 7 years, malaria remains a significant cause of morbidity and mortality worldwide. In 2015, there were 212 million estimated malaria cases, leading to 429,000 deaths.[119] Most of these deaths were from *Plasmodium falciparum* infections of young children and primigravid pregnant women in Africa.[15] Included among those at risk of becoming infected are 50 million travelers from industrialized countries who visit the developing countries each year. Despite using prophylactic medications, an estimated 30,000 of these travelers will acquire malaria.[96]

MALARIA OVERVIEW

Malaria is an infection of protozoan parasites in the *Plasmodium* genus with a unique life cycle involving the *Anopheles* mosquito as vector. Today malaria is primarily endemic in tropical and subtropical areas worldwide. It was once endemic in temperate areas, including Western Europe and the United States, but economic development and improvements in public health hastened its retreat.[45] Malaria was fully eradicated from the United States between 1947 and 1951 owing in large part to the powerful insecticidal effects of dichloro diphenyl trichloroethane (DDT).[45] The emergence of DDT-resistant *Anopheles* mosquitoes and chloroquine-resistant *Plasmodium* spp has impeded eradication in other parts of the world.[45]

Malaria has a unique life cycle (Fig. 55–1) beginning with inoculation of sporozoites from an infected female *Anopheles* saliva. The sporozoites travel to the liver, where they invade the host's hepatocytes and undergo asexual division (asexual exoerythrocytic cycle), ultimately causing rupture of the infected hepatocyte (tissue schizont) and release of thousands of merozoites into the bloodstream.[5] The tissue phase is complete at this point with the exception of *Plasmodium vivax* and *Plasmodium ovale*, which can remain dormant in liver cells (hypnozoites), causing recurrent infections years later. The erythrocytic cycle begins when merozoites penetrate erythrocytes (trophozoites), undergoing additional cycles of asexual division (erythrocytic schizont), leading to cell rupture and the release of a new wave of merozoites to infect additional erythrocytes. This erythrocytic cycle is responsible for the clinical manifestations of malaria. Some erythrocytic merozoites differentiate into sexual forms (macrogametocytes {female} and microgametocytes {male}). Ingestion of both sexual forms by the female *Anopheles* during a blood meal allows fertilization and zygote formation in the mosquito midgut epithelium (sporogenic cycle), ultimately leading to rupture of an oocyst and release of sporozoites that migrate to the salivary glands, awaiting injection into another victim.[115]

Six *Plasmodium* spp cause malaria in humans (Table 55–1). The majority of cases worldwide are caused by *P. falciparum* and *P. vivax*, with *P. falciparum* responsible for the overwhelming majority of deaths.[76] Traditional teaching highlights the synchronization of blood parasite cycles causing a somewhat predictable fever periodicity, described as tertian or quartan fever, depending on the causative organism. These classic periodic fevers are rarely observed in Western countries because symptomatic cases are diagnosed earlier than

in the past.[5] The routine use of antipyretics probably also contributes to atypical presentations.

Unlike the other forms of human malaria, *Plasmodium knowlesi* is a true zoonosis, the natural host being macaques (*Macaca* spp) and related monkey species. Natural transmission of a nonhuman *Plasmodium* spp to humans was thought to be rare, but increasing numbers of *P. knowlesi* malarial infections are reported in and around Malaysia, Indonesia, and Southeast Asia, causing scientists to include this parasite as a potential human pathogen.[54]

ANTIMALARIAL HISTORY

It is somewhat ironic that despite sophisticated drug development methods and advanced technologies of the 21st century, the most widely used old treatments (quinine and its derivatives) and the best new regimens (artemisinins) have both been used for centuries as ancient herbal remedies derived from plants.

The bark of the cinchona tree, the first effective remedy for malaria, was introduced to Europeans more than 350 years ago.[114] The toxicity of its active ingredient, quinine, was noted from the inception of its use. Pharmaceutical advances occurred, funded largely by the US military during World War II, yielding 4-aminoquinolines, 8-aminoquinolines, and novel antifolates. To combat emerging strains of drug-resistant *P. falciparum* that developed during the Vietnam conflict, alternate quinine derivatives (amino alcohols) were developed.[106,114] Other drugs used to treat malaria include the folate inhibitors, selected antibiotics, the sulfonamide sulfadoxine, the tetracyclines, and the macrolides (Chap. 54).

With the introduction of each new drug, resistance developed, particularly in Oceania, Southeast Asia, and Africa.[106,114] In some instances, quinine is again the first-line therapy for malaria.[118] In the past 2 decades, the search for active xenobiotics has returned to a natural product, the Chinese herb qinghaosu. The active metabolite, of which is dihydroartemisinin, is common to all the endoperoxides. These drugs are primarily used as part of an artemisinin-based combination therapy (ACT), which is recommended by the World Health Organization (WHO) as the preferred treatment of malaria in drug-resistant areas.[8,119] With increased leisure travel, a greater number of North Americans are taking prophylactic medications with potential toxicity.

This chapter highlights the toxicity of the most commonly used antimalarials using the structural and mechanistic classification outlined in Table 55–2.

AMINO ALCOHOLS
Antimalarial Mechanism

Unlike humans, who eliminate heme through the use of heme oxygenase ultimately producing the bile pigment biliverdin, *Plasmodium* spp convert heme to the nontoxic relatively inert compound hemozoin. Amino alcohols and 4-aminoquinolines concentrate in parasite food vacuoles, where they inhibit the ability of the parasite to detoxify hemozoin, leading to accumulation of toxic heme by-products and parasite death.[89,115] In resistant parasites, these antimalarials fail to concentrate in food vacuoles because of increased drug efflux. This resistance is thought to be conferred through amplification of a transmembrane pump. Interestingly, tricyclic antidepressants, phenothiazines, and calcium channel blockers reverse resistance in experimental models.[89]

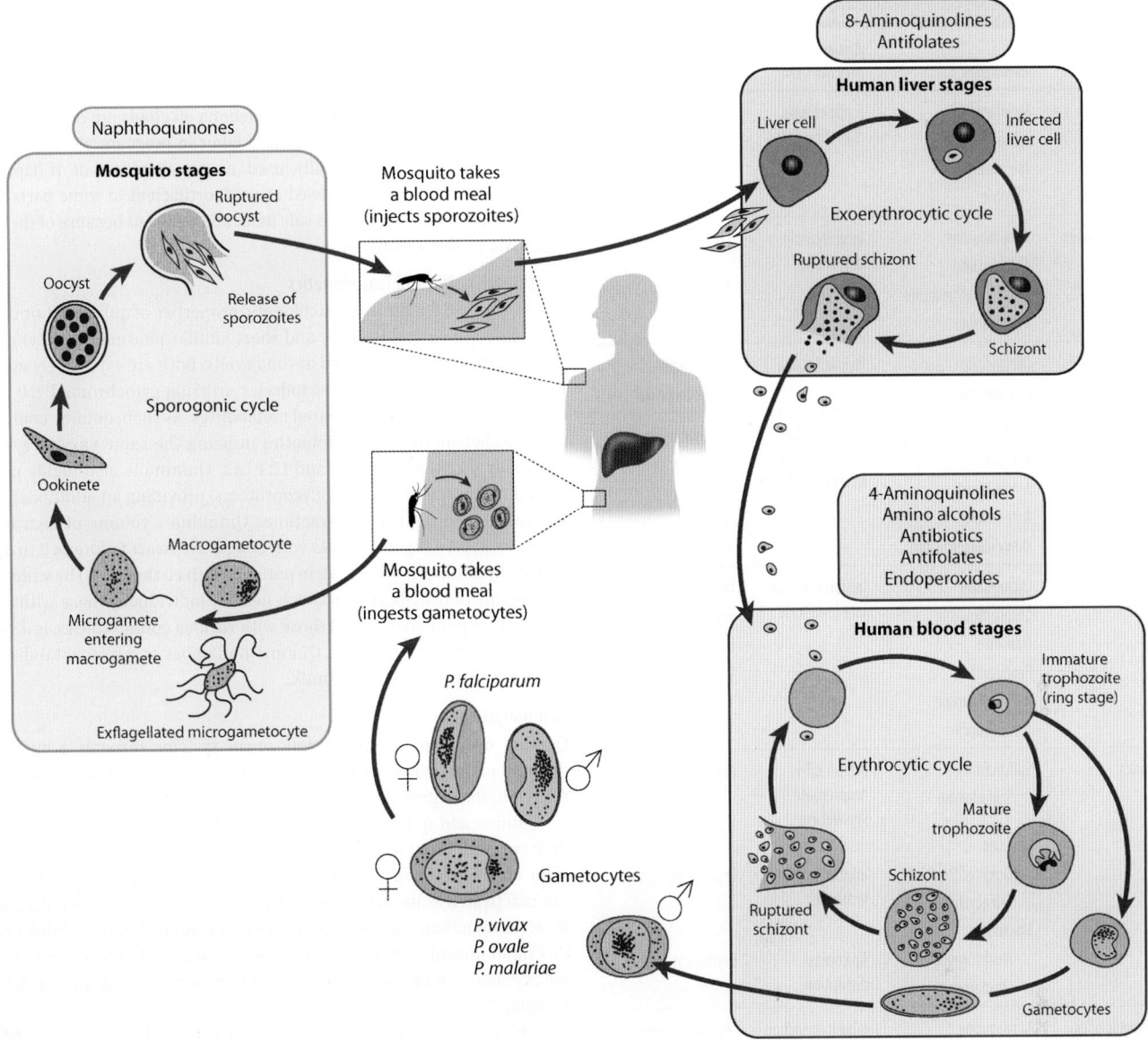

FIGURE 55–1. Life cycle stages during which antimalarials exert their effects.

TABLE 55–1	*Plasmodium* spp Affecting Humans				
Species	**Distribution**	**Fever Cycle (days)**	**RBC Preference**	**Parasitemia**	**Comments**
P. falciparum	Widespread throughout tropics	2 or less (sub-tertian)	All ages	Can be high	Most fatalities
P. knowlesi	Malaysia and neighboring countries	1	All ages	Can be high	Zoonosis (primary host Macaque monkey), severe disease in humans
P. malariae	Worldwide	3–4 (quartan)	Old	Low	Chronic infections, late recrudescence
P. ovale curtisi	Africa	2–3 (tertian)	Young	Low	Relapses/hepatic hypnozoites
P. ovale wallikeri	Africa	2–3 (tertian)	Young	Low	Relapses/hepatic hypnozoites More severe symptoms, increased parasitemia than its *R. ovale curtis*
P. vivax	Predominantly Asia	2–3 (tertian)	Young	Low	Relapses/hepatic hypnozoites

TABLE 55–2   Antimalarial Classification and Mechanisms

Class	Examples	Antimalarial Mechanism	Lifecycle Stage Effect
Amino alcohols	Halofantrine Lumefantrine Mefloquine Quinine	Inhibit heme digestion	Erythrocytic cycle[a]
4-Aminoquinolines	Amodiaquine Chloroquine Hydroxychloroquine Piperaquine	Inhibit heme digestion	Erythrocytic cycle[a]
8-Aminoquinolines	Diethylprimaquine Primaquine	Oxidant stress	Liver stages Hypnozoiticidal
Endoperoxides	Artemether Artesunate Artemisinin Artemisone Dihydroartemisinin	Unknown but oxidant stress likely contributes	Erythrocytic cycle[a]
Antifolates	Cycloguanil Chlorproguanil Dapsone Proguanil Pyrimethamine Trimethoprim	Inhibit dihydrofolate reductase	(All growing stages) Erythrocytic cycle[a] Exoerythrocytic cycle[b]
Antibiotics	Sulfonamides Sulfadoxine	Inhibit dihydropteroate synthetase	Erythrocytic cycle[a]
	Cyclines Doxycycline Tetracycline	Inhibit protein synthesis	Erythrocytic cycle[a]
	Macrolides Azithromycin Clindamycin	Apicoplast disruption	Erythrocytic cycle[a]
Naphthoquinones	Atovaquone	Inhibit mitochondrial respiration	Mosquito sporogonic cycle[c]

[a]Blood schizonticidal and blood gametocidal. [b]Liver schizonticidal but not effective against hypnozoites.
[c]Altered oocyst development.

Quinine

The therapeutic benefits of the bark of the cinchona tree have been known for centuries. As early as 1633, cinchona bark was used for its antipyretic and analgesic effects,[75] and in the 1800s, it was used for the treatment of "rebellious palpitations." Quinine, the primary alkaloid in cinchona bark, was the first effective treatment for malaria. Additionally, because of a reported

curarelike action, quinine is infrequently used as a treatment for muscle cramps. Because of its extremely bitter taste similar to that of heroin, quinine is used as an adulterant in drugs of abuse. Small quantities of quinine can be also found in some tonic waters and bitter lemon drinks.

High doses of quinine and other cinchona alkaloids are oxytocic, potentially leading to abortion or premature labor in pregnant women. Because of this, quinine is occasionally used as an abortifacient (Chap. 19).[77] Chloroquine continues to be used as an abortifacient in some parts of the developing world.[11,90] Neither is safe as an abortifacient because of their narrow toxic-to-therapeutic ratio.

Pharmacokinetics and Toxicokinetics

See Table 55–3 for the pharmacokinetic properties of quinine. Quinine and quinidine are optical isomers and share similar pharmacologic effects as class IA antidysrhythmics and antimalarials. Both are extensively metabolized in the liver, kidneys, and muscles utilizing cytochrome P450 isoenzymes to a variety of hydroxylated metabolites. As such, quinine could alter the metabolism of other xenobiotics utilizing the same enzyme systems, especially CYP3A4, CYP2D6, and CYP1A2. Quinine is also highly protein bound, primarily to α-1-acid glycoproteins, providing an additional mode for potential drug–drug interactions. Quinidine's volume of distribution varies from 0.5 L/kg in patients with congestive heart failure to 2 to 3 L/kg in healthy adults, to 3 to 5 L/kg in patients with cirrhosis.[111] The widely varied volume of distribution between healthy individuals, those with differing levels of parasitemia, and those with various comorbidities, is a shared property of all antimalarials. Quinine undergoes transplacental distribution and is secreted in breast milk.

Pathophysiology

Quinine overdose affects multiple organ systems through a number of different pathophysiologic mechanisms. Outcomes appear to be most closely related to the degree of cardiovascular dysfunction.[41]

Quinine and quinidine share anti- and prodysrhythmic effects primarily from an inhibiting effect on the cardiac sodium channels and potassium channels (Chaps. 15 and 57).[43] Blockade of the sodium channel in the inactivated state decreases inotropy, slows the rate of depolarization, slows conduction, and increases action potential duration. Inhibition of this rapid inward sodium current is increased at higher heart rates (called *use-dependent blockade*), leading to a rate-dependent widening of the QRS complex.[114,116]

Inhibition of the potassium channels suppresses the repolarizing delayed rectifier potassium current, particularly the rapidly activating component,[116] leading to prolongation of the QT interval. The resultant increase in the effective refractory period is also rate dependent, causing greater repolarization delay at slower heart rates and predisposing to torsade de pointes. As a result, syncope and sudden dysrhythmogenic death occur. This "quinidine syncope"—ventricular dysrhythmias or fibrillation—was identified more than half a century ago as a therapeutic complication.[99] An additional α-adrenergic antagonist effect contributes to the syncope and hypotension occurring in quinine toxicity. Quinidine possesses antimuscarinic activity in therapeutic dosing.[57]

Inhibition of the adenosine triphosphate (ATP)–sensitive potassium channels of pancreatic β cells results in the release of insulin, similar to the action of sulfonylureas (Chap. 47).[32] Patients at increased risk of quinine-induced hyperinsulinemia include those patients receiving high-dose intravenous (IV) quinine, intentional overdose, and patients with other metabolic stresses (eg, concurrent malaria, pregnancy, malnutrition, and ethanol consumption).[21,107]

The mechanism of quinine-induced ototoxicity appears to be multifactorial. Microstructural lengthening of the outer hair cells of the cochlea and organ of Corti occurs.[48] Additionally, vasoconstriction and local prostaglandin inhibition within the organ of Corti contributes to decreased hearing.[106] Inhibition of the potassium channel also impairs hearing and produces vertigo because it is known that the homozygous absence of gene products that form part of some potassium channels (Jervell and

TABLE 55–3 Pharmacokinetic Properties of Antimalarials

Antimalarial	Bioavailability (%)	Time to Peak (hours) (oral)	Protein Bound (%)	Volume of Distribution (L/kg)	Half-Life	Urinary Excretion (%)	Metabolism	Comments
Artemisinin	Limited	—	Large	—	2–5 h	—	CYP2B6, CYP3A4	Autoinduction of its own first-pass effect CYP2B6 inducer CYP2C19 inducer
Atovaquone	Varies	5–6	99	4.7–13	2–3 d	<1	Primarily excreted unchanged in the feces	Increased bioavailability with fatty foods Enterohepatic cycling
Dihydroartemisinin	30	1–2	—	1–35	1–2.3 h	—	—	—
Chloroquine	80–89	1.5–3	50–65	32–262	5–12 d	55	CYP2C8 CYP3A4	CYP2D6 inhibitor
Dapsone	90	2–8	70–80	0.5–2	21–30 h	20	CYP2C19	Enterohepatic circulation Genetic polymorphisms
Halofantrine	Low, varies	4–7	—	>100	1–6 d	—	CYP3A4	Active metabolite
Lumefantrine	Varies	2–66	99	0.4–8.9	3 d	—	CYP3A4	Active metabolite CYP2D6 inhibitor
Mefloquine	>85	6–24	98	15–40	15–27 d	<1	CYP3A4	Stereospecific activity Inactive metabolite
Piperaquine	Low, varies with diet	3–6	99	529–877	13–28 d	—	CYP3A4	
Primaquine	75	1–3	75	3–8	4–9 h	4	CYP2C19 CYP2D6 CYP3A4	Active metabolites primarily responsible for therapeutic and toxic effects. Genetic polymorphisms
Proguanil	60	4–5	75	13–23	12–21 h	40–60	CYP2C19 CYP3A4	Active metabolite
Pyrimethamine	>95	2–6	87	2–7	3–4 d	16–32	Hepatic	—
Quinine	76	1–3	70–90	1.8–4.6	9–15 h	20	CYP3A4 CYP2D6 CYP2C9 CYP1A2	Protein binding increased in alkaline environments CYP2D6 inhibitor

— = poorly studied or unknown.

Lange-Nielsen syndrome) causes deafness and prolonged QT intervals (Chaps. 15 and 25).[105]

Although older theories suggested that quinine caused retinal ischemia, the preponderance of evidence points to a direct toxic effect on the retina, and possibly the optic nerve fibers.[38] Quinine also antagonizes cholinergic neurotransmission in the inner synaptic layer.

Quinine has direct irritant effects on the gastrointestinal (GI) tract and stimulates the brain stem center responsible for nausea and emesis.[114]

Clinical Manifestations

Quinine overdose typically leads to GI complaints, tinnitus, and visual symptoms within hours, but the time course varies with the formulation ingested, coingestants, patient characteristics, and other case-specific details. Significant overdose is heralded by cardiovascular and central nervous system (CNS) toxicity. Death can occur within hours to days, usually from a combination of shock, ventricular dysrhythmias, respiratory arrest, or acute kidney injury (AKI).

Patients receiving even therapeutic doses often experience a syndrome known as "cinchonism," which typically includes GI complaints, headache, vasodilation, tinnitus, and decreased hearing acuity.[75,114] Vertigo, syncope, dystonia, tachycardia, diarrhea, and abdominal pain are also described.[49,63]

Quinine toxicity is correlated with total serum concentrations, but only the non–protein-bound portion is likely responsible for toxic effects. However, because free and total quinine concentrations vary widely from person to person,[37] a single quinine concentration does not always correlate with clinical toxicity. In general, serum concentrations greater than 5 mcg/mL cause cinchonism, greater than 10 mcg/mL visual impairment, greater than 15 mcg/mL cardiac dysrhythmias, and greater than 22 mcg/mL death.[4] Similar concentrations in individuals who are severely ill with malaria do not necessarily result in as severe toxicity because an increase in plasma α_1-acid glycoprotein reduces the free fraction of quinine present.[97,101]

The toxic-to-therapeutic ratio of quinine is very small. It is not surprising that patients taking therapeutic doses frequently develop toxicity because the recommended range of serum quinine concentrations for treatment of *falciparum* malaria is 5 to 15 mcg/mL, well above the concentration reported to cause cinchonism.

The average oral lethal dose of quinine is 8 g, although a dose as small as 1.5 g is reported to cause death.[39,49] Delirium, coma, and seizures are less common, usually occurring only after severe overdoses.[18]

Cardiovascular manifestations of quinine use are related to myocardial drug concentrations. They manifest on the electrocardiogram (ECG) as prolongation of the PR interval, prolongation of the QRS complex, prolongation of the QT interval, and ST depression with or without T wave inversion. Dysrhythmias and complete heart block are reported.[16] Quinine toxicity can also result in significant hypotension.

Although not commonly reported, mild hyperinsulinemia and resultant hypoglycemia occur in cases of oral quinine overdose. Hypoglycemia with elevated serum insulin concentrations was documented after therapeutic dosing in case reports complicated by severe congestive heart failure and significant ethanol consumption. Hypoglycemia is also noted in healthy patients after overdose. Hypoglycemia is fairly common in patients with severe malaria treated with quinine, occurring in up to 10% of patients and 50% of pregnant women.[107]

Eighth cranial nerve dysfunction results in tinnitus and deafness. The decreased acuity is not usually clinically apparent, although the patient recognizes tinnitus.[95] These findings usually resolve within 48 to 72 hours, and permanent hearing impairment is unlikely.

Ophthalmic presentations include blurred vision, visual field constriction, diplopia, altered color perception, mydriasis, photophobia, scotomata, and sometimes complete blindness.[18,44] The onset of blindness is invariably delayed and usually follows the onset of other manifestations by at least 6 hours. The pupillary dilation that occurs is usually nonreactive and correlates with the severity of visual loss. Funduscopic examination findings are occasionally normal but usually demonstrate extreme arteriolar constriction associated with retinal edema. Normal arteriolar caliber is commonly seen initially, but funduscopic manifestations such as vessel attenuation and disc pallor develop as clinical improvement occurs. Improvement in vision can occur rapidly but is usually slow, occurring over a period of months after a severe toxicity. Initially, improvement occurs centrally and is followed later by improvement in peripheral vision. The pupils occasionally remain dilated even after return to normal vision.[39] Patients with the greatest exposure frequently develop optic atrophy.

Hypokalemia is often described in the setting of quinine poisoning, although the mechanism is unclear. An intracellular shift of potassium rather than a true potassium deficit is the predominant theory behind the hypokalemia associated with chloroquine,[65,69] and the mechanism is assumed to be similar with quinine.

A number of immune-mediated hypersensitivity reactions are described. These are the result of antiquinine or antiquinine-hapten antibodies cross-reacting with a variety of membrane glycoproteins[19,56] dramatically increasing their binding affinity to cell-surface antigens by more than 10,000 times.[40] Asthma and dermatologic manifestations, such as urticaria, photosensitivity dermatitis, cutaneous vasculitis, lichen planus, and angioedema, also occur.[107]

Hematologic manifestations of hypersensitivity include thrombocytopenia (Chap. 20), agranulocytosis, microangiopathic hemolytic anemia, and disseminated intravascular coagulation (DIC), which can lead to jaundice, hemoglobinuria, and AKI.[49,56] Quinine is recognized as a common cause of drug-induced thrombocytopenia and the most common cause of drug-induced thrombotic microangiopathy syndrome (characteristically microangiopathic hemolytic anemia, thrombocytopenia, and acute kidney injury). Hemolysis also occurs in patients with glucose-6-phosphate dehydrogenase (G6PD) deficiency. Severe multisystem hypersensitivity reactions can occur even after minute doses of quinine, such as those in tonic drinks.[40,60] This type of interaction has previously been termed "cocktail purpura."[75,114]

A hepatitis hypersensitivity reaction, acute respiratory distress syndrome (ARDS), and a sepsislike syndrome are also reported.

Diagnostic Testing
Urine thin-layer chromatography is sensitive enough to confirm the presence of quinine even after the ingestion of tonic water.[120] Quinine immunoassay techniques are also available. Quantitative serum testing is not rapidly or widely available.

Management
Patients frequently vomit spontaneously. Emetics should not be used in the absence of vomiting because seizures, dysrhythmias, and hypotension can occur rapidly. Orogastric lavage is not routinely recommended except for patients with recent, substantial (potentially life-threatening) ingestions with no spontaneous emesis. Activated charcoal effectively adsorbs quinine and additionally decreases serum concentrations by altering enteroenteric circulation[62] but should only be administered in patients with a low risk of aspiration or protected airways.

Expectant treatment should be initiated, including oxygen, cardiac and hemodynamic monitoring, IV fluid resuscitation, and frequent ECG and blood glucose measurements. In general, patients should be monitored until vital signs normalize, mental status improves, and laboratory values stabilize. Variables including the amount ingested, patient comorbidities, and coingestions, highlight the importance of individualized care. Asymptomatic patients with suspected overdose should be monitored for 6 to 12 hours depending on variables as above, before medical clearance.

Extracorporeal membrane oxygenation was used in one case of severe quinidine poisoning with bradydysrhythmias and refractory hypotension to stabilize the cardiovascular system while a quinidine-activated charcoal bezoar was removed and the patient metabolized the remaining quinidine. A similar approach would be reasonable to consider for intractable quinine toxicity.

Cardiac. In patients with a conduction delay manifested by a QRS complex of more than 100 milliseconds (ms) we recommend treating with sodium bicarbonate alkalinization to achieve a serum pH of 7.45 to 7.50, as would be done in patients with cardiotoxicity associated with cyclic antidepressant overdoses (Antidotes in Depth: A5). Protein binding is increased in the setting of alkalemia, decreasing the cardiotoxic manifestations of quinine. Sodium bicarbonate therapy is successful in case reports[16,41,75] but has not been specifically studied. Since hypertonic sodium bicarbonate will worsen existing hypokalemia, potentially exacerbating the effect of potassium channel blockade.

Potassium supplementation for quinine-induced hypokalemia is controversial because experimental data from the 1960s suggest that hypokalemia is protective against cardiotoxicity and prolongs survival.[20,65,100] Because hypokalemia can also lead to lethal dysrhythmias, supplementation for significant hypokalemia (<3.0 mmol/L) is recommended as a reasonable intervention.

The QT interval should be carefully monitored for prolongation. If necessary, interventions for torsade de pointes, including magnesium administration, potassium supplementation, and overdrive pacing, should be initiated (Chap. 15 and Antidotes in Depth: A16).

Class IA, IC, or III antidysrhythmics and other xenobiotics with sodium channel or potassium channel blocking activity should not be used to treat quinine-overdosed patients because they would be expected to exacerbate quinine-induced conduction disturbances or dysrhythmias. The Class IB antidysrhythmics, such as lidocaine, have been used with reported success,[47] but no clinical trials have been performed (Chap. 57).

Hypotension refractory to IV crystalloid boluses should be treated with vasopressors. In controlled human studies, epinephrine infusions reverse quinidine's antidysrhythmic drug effects and prolongation of the ventricular refractory period in a dose-dependent fashion.[22,74] Although not directly studied, direct-acting vasopressors such as epinephrine, norepinephrine, and phenylephrine are recommended. An intraaortic balloon pump was successfully used for the treatment of refractory hypotension in one case report.[100]

Hypoglycemia. A low serum glucose concentration should be supported with an adequate infusion of dextrose. Serum potassium concentration and the QT interval should be monitored during correction and maintenance. Octreotide was successfully used to correct quinine-induced hyperinsulinemia in adult malaria victims.[86] In volunteers, quinine-induced hyperinsulinemia was suppressed within 15 minutes after a 100-mcg intramuscular dose of octreotide (Antidotes in Depth: A9).[85] Octreotide should be used for cases of refractory hypoglycemia in a fashion similar to that recommended in sulfonylurea toxicity, which is 50 mcg (1 mcg/kg in children) subcutaneously every 6 hours (Chap. 47).

Ophthalmic. Funduscopic examination, visual field examination, and color testing are appropriate bedside diagnostic studies. Electroretinography, electrooculography, visual-evoked potentials, and dark adaptation are helpful in assessing the injury but are not practical because they require equipment that is not portable or readily available in most clinical settings. There is no specific, effective treatment for quinine retinal toxicity.[46] Hyperbaric oxygen was used in 3 patients who recovered vision, but since its role in that recovery was not established, it cannot be routinely recommended at this time.[120]

Enhanced Elimination

The effect of multiple-dose activated charcoal (MDAC) on quinine elimination was studied in an experimental human model and in symptomatic patients.[87] In these patients, MDAC decreased the half-life of quinine from approximately 8 hours to about 4.5 hours and increased clearance by 56%.[92] Although numerous studies show that activated charcoal decreases quinine half-life,[13,62,87] evidence of clinical benefit is lacking. Nevertheless, because ophthalmic, CNS, and cardiovascular toxicity are related to serum concentration, it is prudent to reduce concentrations as quickly as practicable; thus, multiple-dose activated charcoal is recommended unless contraindications exist (Antidotes in Depth: A1).

There is conflicting evidence about a benefit of urinary acidification in enhancing clearance. But because of the increased potential for cardiotoxicity associated with acidification, this technique is never recommended.

Because quinine has a relatively large volume of distribution and is highly protein bound, hemoperfusion, hemodialysis, and exchange transfusion have only a limited effect on drug removal.[13,18,97,114] Although the blood compartment can be cleared with these techniques, total body clearance is only marginally altered. After rapid tissue distribution occurs, there is little impact on the total body burden because of the large volume of distribution and extensive protein binding; thus, extracorporeal methods of drug removal are not routinely recommended.

Mefloquine

Pharmacokinetics and Toxicodynamics

See Table 55–3 for the pharmacokinetic properties of mefloquine. Similar to its cousin quinine, mefloquine is hepatically metabolized by cytochrome P450 enzyme systems and excreted primarily in the bile and feces. Some hypothesize that the small, lipophilic structure combined with a long elimination half-life allows mefloquine to easily cross the blood–brain barrier, accumulate in the CNS, and interact with neuronal targets, leading to neurotoxic side effects.[67]

Clinical Manifestations

Common side effects with prophylactic and therapeutic dosing include nausea, vomiting, and diarrhea. These side effects are noted particularly in the extremes of age and with high therapeutic dosing. Similar findings should be expected in acute overdose.[107,117]

Mefloquine has a mild cardiodepressant effect, less than that of quinine or quinidine, which is not clinically significant in prophylactic dosing or with therapeutic administration. Bradycardia is commonly reported.[24,63,80] With prophylactic use, neither the PR interval nor the QRS complex is prolonged, but QT interval prolongation is reported.[33,63] Reports of torsade de pointes are rare, but the increase in QT interval and risk of torsade de pointes are increased when mefloquine is used concurrently with quinine, chloroquine, or most particularly, with halofantrine.[63,80,81,116] The long half-life of mefloquine means that particular care must be taken with therapeutic use of other antimalarials when breakthrough malaria occurs during mefloquine prophylaxis or within 28 days of mefloquine therapy to avoid potential drug–drug interactions. This risk would be expected to increase with acute overdose, although there is little clinical experience.

Mefloquine is commonly associated with neuropsychiatric side effects. During prophylactic use, 10% to 40% of patients experience insomnia and bizarre or vivid dreams and complain of dizziness, headache, fatigue, mood alteration, and vertigo.[98,113] Only 2% to 10% of these complications necessitate the traveler to seek medical advice or change normal activities.[24] Predisposing factors include a past history of neuropsychiatric disorders, recent prior exposure to mefloquine (within 2 months), previous mefloquine-related neuropsychiatric adverse effects, and previous treatment with psychotropics.[107] Women appear to be more likely than men to experience neuropsychiatric adverse effects.[107,113]

The risk of serious neuropsychiatric adverse effects (convulsions, altered mental status, inability to ambulate due to vertigo, ataxia, or psychosis) during prophylaxis is estimated to be one in 10,600 but is reported to be as high as one in 200 with therapeutic dosing.[31,107] Seizures occur rarely with prophylaxis and therapeutic use. In many of these cases, there is a history of previous seizures, seizures in a first-degree relative, or other seizure risk factors. Other neuropsychiatric symptoms include dysphoria, altered consciousness, encephalopathy, anxiety, depression, giddiness, and agitated delirium with psychosis. Although there is a suggestion that the severity of neuropsychiatric events is dose dependent, there does not seem to be a correlation with serum or tissue concentrations.[56]

The effect of mefloquine on the pancreatic potassium channel is much less than that of quinine, resulting in only a mild increase in insulin secretion.[32,33] Symptomatic hypoglycemia has not been reported as an effect of mefloquine alone in healthy individuals, but has occurred with concomitant use of ethanol and in a severely malnourished patient with acquired immune deficiency syndrome (AIDS).[10,33,63] In overdose, particularly when accompanied by ethanol use or starvation, hypoglycemia can be severe.

Rare events such as hypersensitivity reactions reported with prophylaxis include urticaria, alopecia, erythema multiforme, toxic epidermal necrolysis, myalgias, mouth ulcers, neutropenia, and thrombocytopenia.[81,98,103] It is unclear which, if any, would be significant after overdose. Acute respiratory distress syndrome was linked to therapeutic dosing in one case report.

In therapeutic use, mefloquine is associated with an increased incidence of stillbirth compared with quinine and a group of other antimalarials.[82] Mefloquine was not, however, linked to an increased incidence of abortion, low birth weight, mental retardation, or congenital malformations. The implications of overdose in the absence of malaria are unknown, but fetal monitoring should be instituted.

The consequences of excessive dosing and overdose are not only severe but also prolonged and potentially permanent.

Management

In overdose, treatment is primarily supportive with monitoring for potential adverse effects. Decontamination with activated charcoal is indicated if the patient presents soon after the ingestion. Specific monitoring for ECG abnormalities, hypoglycemia, and liver injury should be provided. Pregnant patients should be followed with fetal monitoring. Because of mefloquine's long half-life and potential for CNS accumulation, observation of asymptomatic patients for at least 24 hours is a reasonable approach. Central nervous system effects usually resolve within a few days, but persistent, permanent, and delayed-onset CNS effects are reported, so observation for full resolution of CNS effects would not be practical.

In 2 patients with kidney failure who received mefloquine, prophylactic hemodialysis did not remove mefloquine.[28] Given the large volume of distribution and high degree of protein binding of mefloquine, extracorporeal elimination techniques are unlikely to be effective.

In one case report, the severe neuropsychiatric manifestations of mefloquine were reversed with physostigmine, leading the authors to suggest a possible central anticholinergic mechanism. Physostigmine is not recommended as a routine treatment for mefloquine neuropsychiatric side effects.

Halofantrine

Because of erratic absorption, the potential for lethal cardiotoxicity, and concern for cross resistance with mefloquine, halofantrine is not presently recommended for malaria prophylaxis by the CDC.[6]

Pharmacokinetics and Toxicodynamics
See Table 55–3 for the pharmacokinetic properties of halofantrine.

Clinical Manifestations
The primary toxicity from therapeutic and supratherapeutic doses is prolongation of the QT interval and the risk of torsade de pointes and ventricular fibrillation.[81,109] Palpitations, hypotension, and syncope occur. First-degree atrioventricular (AV) block is common, but bradycardia is rare.[81] Dysrhythmias are also likely in the context of combined overdose or combined or serial therapeutic use with other xenobiotics that cause QT interval prolongation, particularly mefloquine.[55] Because the QT interval duration is directly related to the serum halofantrine concentration, dysrhythmias should be expected in overdose.[24,81,107] Fifty percent of children receiving a therapeutic course of halofantrine will have a QT interval greater than 440 ms.[104]

Other side effects, including nausea, vomiting, diarrhea, abdominal cramps, headache, and lightheadedness, which frequently occur in therapeutic use, are also expected in overdose.[63] Less frequently described side effects include pruritus, myalgias, and rigors. Seizures, minimal liver enzyme abnormalities, and hemolysis are described.[63,73] Whether these manifestations are related to halofantrine or to the underlying malaria is not clear.

Management
Management of patients with halofantrine overdose should focus on decontamination, supportive care, monitoring for QT interval prolongation, and treatment of any associated dysrhythmias. Based on rare case reports, non-overdose evidence, and known erratic absorption, observation of asymptomatic overdose patients for 24 hours before medical clearance would be a reasonable approach.

Lumefantrine

Lumefantrine is structurally similar to halofantrine. It is primarily used as a partner drug in the artemisinin-based combination therapy (ACT) artemether plus lumefantrine.

Little toxicity of lumefantrine alone or in combination is reported. Studies do not show QT interval prolongation or evidence of cardiac toxicity related to lumefantrine.[36] Cough and angioedema were described in one case. As in the case of all antimalarials, it is difficult to differentiate drug-related adverse events from those of malaria, comorbid diseases, or other ingested drugs, which confounds the study of potential complications.

4-AMINOQUINOLINES
The structurally related compounds chloroquine and amodiaquine were once used extensively for malaria prophylaxis. However, with the development of resistance, they are now used in fewer geographic regions. Amodiaquine is associated with a higher incidence of hepatic toxicity and agranulocytosis. In general, these xenobiotics have low toxicity when used in therapeutic doses. Because of its low toxicity, chloroquine remains the first-line drug for malaria prophylaxis and treatment in areas where *Plasmodium* spp remain sensitive.

Hydroxychloroquine is similar to chloroquine in therapeutic, pharmacokinetic, and toxicologic properties. The side effect profiles of the 2 are slightly different, favoring chloroquine use for malarial prophylaxis and hydroxychloroquine use as an antiinflammatory.[63,114] Hydroxychloroquine is used in the treatment of rheumatic diseases such as rheumatoid arthritis and lupus erythematosus. In animal studies, chloroquine is 2 to 3 times more toxic than hydroxychloroquine.[52]

Piperaquine is structurally similar to chloroquine but is primarily used in conjunction with artemisinin compounds as a component of an ACT.

Antimalarial Mechanism
The 4-aminoquinolines interfere with the digestion of heme and hemozoin formation in a manner similar to that of the amino alcohols.[34]

Chloroquine and Hydroxychloroquine

Hydroxychloroquine

Pharmacokinetics and Toxicodynamics

See Table 55–3 for the pharmacokinetic properties of chloroquine. Oral chloroquine is rapidly and completely absorbed and is ultimately sequestered in many organs, particularly the kidney, liver, lung, and erythrocytes.[17,48]

Chloroquine is slowly distributed from the blood compartment to the larger central compartment, leading to transiently high whole blood concentrations shortly after ingestion.[90,102] It is the initial high blood concentrations that are thought to be responsible for the rapid development of profound cardiorespiratory collapse typical of chloroquine toxicity. These early whole blood chloroquine concentrations correlate with death[27] and are better predictors of cardiovascular symptom severity than serum concentrations.[70] Unfortunately chloroquine concentrations are rarely rapidly available and thus unlikely to be useful for early bedside clinical decision making.

Pathophysiology

With structural similarity to quinine, the pathophysiologic mechanisms of chloroquine and hydroxychloroquine are also similar. Most notably, sodium and potassium channel blockade are the likely primary mechanisms of cardiovascular toxicity.[116]

Although less common in quinine toxicity, hypokalemia is extremely common in chloroquine overdose. The mechanism appears to be a shift of potassium from the extracellular to the intracellular space and not a true potassium deficit.[65,90,100]

Clinical Manifestations

Similar to quinine, chloroquine has a narrow toxic-to-therapeutic ratio. Severe chloroquine poisoning is usually associated with ingestions of 5 g or more in adults, systolic blood pressure less than 80 mm Hg, QRS complex duration of more than 120 ms, ventricular fibrillation, hypokalemia, and serum chloroquine concentrations exceeding 25 μmol/L (8 mcg/mL).[26,93] Not surprisingly, suspected ingested doses do not always correlate with blood concentrations,[71] but the suspected ingested dose still remains a potentially helpful historic predictor of the possibility for severe toxicity.

Symptoms usually occur within 1 to 3 hours of ingestion.[93] The range of symptoms associated with chloroquine toxicity is similar to that of quinine, but the frequencies of various manifestations differ, and other features such as cinchonism are uncommon. Nausea, vomiting, diarrhea, and abdominal pain occur less commonly than with quinine.[49,63] In contrast, respiratory depression is common, and apnea, hypotension, and cardiovascular compromise can be precipitous.[49]

The cardiovascular effects of chloroquine and hydroxychloroquine are similar to those of quinine, including QRS complex prolongation, AV block, ST and T wave depression, increased U waves, and QT interval prolongation. Hypotension is more prominent in chloroquine toxicity than with quinine.[49]

Significant hypokalemia in chloroquine toxicity is invariably associated with cardiac manifestations.[49] In fact, the extent of hypokalemia is a good indicator of the severity of chloroquine overdose[26] and mortality rate.[70]

Neurologic manifestations include CNS depression, dizziness, headache, and convulsions.[46] Rarely, dystonic reactions occur. Transient parkinsonism is also reported after excessive dosing.

Ophthalmic manifestations are infrequent in acute chloroquine toxicity and transient in nature.[49,63] More severe and irreversible vision and hearing changes are described in association with the chronic use of chloroquine and hydroxychloroquine as antiinflammatories.[63,78] Myopathy, neuropathy, and cardiomyopathy also occur when used for that purpose.[8] Dermatologic findings and hypersensitivity reactions are similar to those associated with quinine.[33] Likewise, red blood cell (RBC) oxidant stress from chloroquine results in hemolysis in patients with G6PD deficiency (Chap. 20).

Acute hydroxychloroquine toxicity is similar to chloroquine toxicity.[52] Side effects from therapeutic doses include nausea and abdominal pain; hemolysis in G6PD-deficient patients; and, rarely, retinal damage, sensorineural deafness, and hypoglycemia. Hypersensitivity reactions, including myocarditis and hepatitis, are described.

Management

Aggressive supportive care is recommended, including oxygen, cardiac and hemodynamic monitoring, and large-bore IV access, and serial blood glucose concentrations. Despite reported rapid absorption, one series reported delayed peak blood concentrations in some patients,[70] opening the possibility of a potential benefit for early GI decontamination methods. Orogastric lavage is recommended for life-threatening ingestions presenting early, but there is little evidence of efficacy. Activated charcoal adsorbs chloroquine well, binding 95% to 99% when administered within 5 minutes of ingestion.[59] The frequent development of precipitous cardiovascular and CNS toxicity should be anticipated before initiating any type of GI decontamination.

Early aggressive management of severe chloroquine toxicity decreases the mortality rate.[93] This includes early endotracheal intubation and mechanical ventilation. Evidence suggests that barbiturates are not desirable for induction in patients with chloroquine overdose. When thiopental was used to facilitate intubation, its use immediately preceded sudden cardiac arrest in 7 of 25 patients after chloroquine overdose.[27] Regardless of induction agent, an adequate FiO_2, tidal volume, and ventilatory rate should be ensured.

Although theoretically any direct-acting vasopressor would be beneficial in the setting of hypotension not responsive to fluid resuscitation, epinephrine is the vasopressor most extensively studied and is therefore the vasopressor of choice. High doses of epinephrine were used in the original studies describing the benefits of early mechanical ventilation and the administration of diazepam and epinephrine in chloroquine poisoning.[93,94] The epinephrine doses used in these studies are still recommended today.[93,94] The recommended dose is 0.25 mcg/kg/min, increasing by 0.25 mcg/kg/min until an adequate systolic blood pressure (>90 mm Hg) is achieved.[30,69,93,94] Clinicians should be mindful that high doses of epinephrine could exacerbate preexisting hypokalemia.

The use of diazepam to augment the treatment of dysrhythmias and hypotension is a unique use of this drug. Initial observations with regard to patients with mixed overdoses of chloroquine and diazepam suggested less cardiovascular toxicity and a potential benefit of high-dose diazepam.[27,65] Animal and human studies that followed also showed a potential benefit.[30,93,94] When early mechanical ventilation was combined with the administration of high-dose diazepam and epinephrine in patients severely poisoned by chloroquine, a dramatic improvement in survival compared with historical control participants (91% vs 9% survival) occurred.[93] Studies in moderately poisoned patients failed to show similar benefit,[26] and a rat model failed to show an inotropic effect. Although the definitive study has yet to be done, high-dose diazepam therapy (2 mg/kg IV over 30 minutes followed by 1–2 mg/kg/day for 2–4 days) is recommended for serious toxicity. Diazepam or an equivalent benzodiazepine should also be used to treat seizures and for sedation.

The mechanism for a potential benefit of diazepam is unclear, but multiple theories have been postulated: (1) a central antagonistic effect, (2) an anticonvulsant effect, (3) an antidysrhythmic effect by an electrophysiologic action inverse to chloroquine, (4) a pharmacokinetic interaction between diazepam and chloroquine, and (5) a decrease in chloroquine-induced vasodilation[65,90,93,94] (Antidotes in Depth: A26).

The use of sodium bicarbonate for correction of QRS complex prolongation is also controversial. Although alkalinization would be expected to counteract the effects of sodium channel blockade, it could also exacerbate preexisting hypokalemia. Although case reports describe the successful use of sodium bicarbonate in conjunction with xenobiotics for massive hydroxychloroquine overdose, no clinical trials have been performed. Before using sodium bicarbonate in the setting of chloroquine toxicity, clinicians should evaluate the overall clinical status of the patient, including the suspected degree of cardiac toxicity and severity of hypokalemia. In the setting of normal potassium, sodium bicarbonate is a reasonable intervention to counteract QRS complex prolongation.

Hypokalemia in the setting of chloroquine overdose correlates with the severity of the toxicity.[26,65] Potassium replacement in this setting is, again, controversial because it has not been shown that potassium supplementation will improve cardiac toxicity. In fact, several reports suggest a possible protective effect of hypokalemia in acute chloroquine toxicity.[26,65,90] This should be balanced against the fact that severe hypokalemia can itself result in lethal dysrhythmias and data suggesting severe hypokalemia (<1.9 mEq/L) is associated with severe, life-threatening ingestion.[24,49,65,102] Hypokalemia could not be directly attributed as the cause of death in most cases, however.[26] Based on the available evidence, potassium replacement for severe hypokalemia would be a reasonable intervention, but it is essential to anticipate rebound hyperkalemia as chloroquine toxicity resolves and redistribution of intracellular potassium occurs. Cases of hyperkalemia-related complications are reported after aggressive potassium supplementation.[52,65]

Because chloroquine and hydroxychloroquine have high volumes of distribution and significant protein binding, enhanced elimination procedures are not beneficial.[17,49] There is limited experience with lipid emulsion therapy in the setting of chloroquine poisoning; thus its use is not recommended (Antidotes in Depth: A23).

Piperaquine

See Table 55–3 for the pharmacokinetic properties of piperaquine.

Piperaquine was used extensively in China and Indonesia as an antimalarial until the development of piperaquine-resistant strains led to the use of better alternatives. Piperaquine has since undergone a rediscovery as a viable combination with artemisinin derivatives in ACT DP (dihydroartemisinin-piperaquine) therapy. Animal studies show piperaquine to be substantially less toxic than chloroquine. Cardiovascular toxicity with piperaquine requires cumulative doses 5 times higher than that of chloroquine. Hepatotoxicity occurs after chronic exposure in animals. In a human study, no significant changes in ECG or in serum glucose concentration, and no postural hypotension occurred after therapeutic doses of DP.

Patients with overdose should be managed with supportive measures and expectant observation, including cardiovascular and CNS monitoring.

Amodiaquine

Amodiaquine has pharmacologic properties similar to others in the 4-aminoquinolone family. It is rapidly absorbed from the GI tract and

hepatically metabolized by CYP2C8 into its active antimalarial metabolite, desethylamodiaquine.[118]

Amodiaquine fell out of favor as a prophylactic treatment as a result of serious and sometimes fatal liver and bone marrow toxicity,[107] but is still a component of one of 5 ACTs recommended by the WHO for treatment of active malarial infection. Hypersensitivity reactions (hepatitis and neutropenia) described in prophylactic use are uncommon with therapeutic use.[21,118] Reports of amodiaquine toxicity suggest that involuntary movements, muscle stiffness, dysarthria, syncope, and seizures can occur.[2,49] There is no overdose experience reported. Aggressive symptomatic and supportive care, expectant observation, including cardiovascular and CNS monitoring, should be provided for possible poisoning.

8-AMINOQUINOLINES
Primaquine

Primaquine and its related compounds are the only drugs licensed for the prevention of *P. ovale* and *P. vivax* relapse caused by hepatic hypnozoites (Fig. 55–1). Studies using primaquine in the early 1950s led to the discovery of G6PD deficiency after those with the disease developed hemolysis when administered the drug.[14] Glucose-6-phosphate dehydrogenase deficiency actually offers some protection against malaria because the erythrocytes of those with the disease rupture under the increased oxidative stress of the parasite's metabolism before completion of the erythrocytic cycle. Primaquine is making a resurgence in some countries for *P. falciparum* treatment as a gametocytocide to reduce transmission in campaigns to eradicate malaria from these regions.[50]

Antimalarial Mechanism
The antimalarial action of primaquine is poorly understood but thought to be related to increasing the oxidative stress of erythrocytes,[115] obstructing proper parasitic development.

Pharmacokinetics and Toxicodynamics
See Table 55–3 for the pharmacokinetic properties of primaquine. Metabolism is primarily hepatic, using multiple enzyme systems, with CYP2D6 playing a prominent role.[7] The parent compound is metabolized to reactive intermediates that are thought to mediate both its antimalarial and hemolytic effects.

Pathophysiology
Primaquine blocks sodium channels both in vitro and in animal models.[49,116] Significant cardiovascular toxicity has not been reported, although experience with primaquine overdose is limited primarily to case reports.

The predominant clinical toxicity of primaquine relates to its ability to cause RBC oxidant stress and resultant hemolysis or methemoglobinemia. Methemoglobinemia and hemolysis can occur in normal individuals given high doses as well as those with G6PD deficiency.[63,107]

The major complication of primaquine in therapeutic use is hemolysis in G6PD-deficient individuals.[32] Primaquine is contraindicated in pregnant women because of the risk of methemoglobinemia or hemolysis in the fetus. Reversible bone marrow suppression can occur.

Clinical Manifestations
Gastrointestinal irritation is common and dose related.

The extent of hemolysis in G6PD-deficient individuals depends on the extent of enzyme activity, those with greater enzyme activity having less severe hemolysis than those with less enzyme activity (Chap. 20). Other variables include the dose of primaquine and comorbid conditions, such as infection, liver disease, and administration of other drugs with hemolytic activity.

Overdose with primaquine is rarely reported, and unintentional overdoses have led to methemoglobinemia requiring IV methylene blue (Chap. 124).[107] Acute liver failure has occurred after unintentional overdose, and fatal hepatotoxicity is described in animal models.[61]

Management

Therapy should be directed at minimizing absorption with appropriate decontamination, and diagnosing then treating significant methemoglobinemia or hemolysis. Because of structural similarities with other quinolone antimalarials and animal model evidence of sodium channel blockade, cardiovascular toxicity should be anticipated with continuous monitoring and resuscitative interventions initiated as needed.

Activated charcoal is a reasonable early intervention (Antidotes in Depth: A1). Methylene blue (Chap. 124 and Antidotes in Depth: A43) is recommended for patients who are symptomatic with methemoglobinemia. Treatment of hemolysis necessitates avoiding further exposure to primaquine and possibly exchange transfusion in severe cases. Adequate hydration should be ensured to protect against hemoglobin-induced acute kidney injury. Urinary alkalinization with sodium bicarbonate is controversial in this setting but is not routinely recommended because it has not been proven to be superior to aggressive sodium chloride 0.9% hydration alone (Antidotes in Depth: A5).

Although no clinical studies have been performed, the large volume of distribution of primaquine makes it an unlikely candidate for benefit from extracorporeal removal.

ENDOPEROXIDES
Artemisinin and Derivatives

The medicinal value of natural artemisinin, the active ingredient of *Artemisia annua* (sweet wormwood or quinghao), has been known for thousands of years. Its antimalarial properties were first recognized by Chinese herbalists in A.D. 340, but the primary active component of qinghaosu, now known as artemisinin, was not isolated until 1974.[8,114] Artemisinin and its semisynthetic derivatives, artesunate, artemether, arteether, and dihydroartemisinin, are the most potent and rapidly acting of all antimalarials. They were introduced in the 1980s in China for the treatment of malaria, and since then millions of doses have been used in Asia and Africa. Because of their extremely short half-lives, the artemisinins are now used in combination with drugs with longer half-lives to delay or prevent the emergence of resistance. Artemisinin-based combination therapies are currently recommended by the WHO for the treatment of uncomplicated malaria[118] but only one has been licensed for use in the United States; artemether and lumefantrine. Five artemesin-based combination therapies (ACT) are currently recommended by the WHO. These include artemether plus lumefantrine, artesunate plus mefloquine, artesunate plus pyrimethamine–sulfadoxine, artesunate plus amodiaquine, and dihydroartemisinin and piperaquine.

Antimalarial Mechanism

The artemisinins have a unique structure containing a 1,2,4-trioxane ring. The endoperoxide linkage within this ring is cleaved when it comes into contact with ferrous iron, releasing free radicals that destroy the parasite.[1] Artemisinin is the only known natural product to contain a 1,2,4-trioxane ring, and although chemical synthesis is possible, thus far it has not been financially advantageous.

Pharmacokinetics and Toxicodynamics

See Table 55–3 for the pharmacokinetic properties of artemisinin. Artemisinin and its derivatives are rapidly metabolized to the primary active metabolite dihydroartemisinin.[68] Similar to its proposed efficacy, the toxicity of artemisinin is thought to be a result of the ability of the trioxane molecular core to form intracellular free radicals, particularly in the presence of heme. In animals, damage to brain stem nuclei is consistently produced after prolonged, high-dose, and parenteral administration.[107] Sustained CNS exposure from slowly absorbed or eliminated artemisinins is considered markedly more neurotoxic than intermittent brief exposure that occurs after oral dosing. Embryonic loss is also observed in animals.

Clinical Manifestations

In contrast to the experience with animals, the general theme throughout the literature suggests that these drugs have a very low incidence of side effects. This is consistent with the belief that long-term, rather than short-term, peak concentrations are primarily responsible for toxicity.[35] Uncommon side effects include nausea, vomiting, abdominal pain, diarrhea, and dizziness. Few large-scale trials powered to detect rare but possibly significant toxicity have been performed.

Prospective studies have failed to identify adverse neurologic outcomes.[58,107] Rare reports of adverse CNS effects during therapeutic use suggest the possibility of CNS depression, seizures, or cerebellar symptoms after intentional self-poisoning. In children with cerebral malaria, a higher incidence of seizures and a delay to recovery from coma were noted in a comparison with quinine.[112] No neurologic difference was noted in long-term follow-up. In an artemether–quinine comparative trial of adults with severe malaria, recovery from coma was also prolonged in the artemether group.[110] Rare patients receiving an artemisinin derivative in 2 other studies experienced transient dizziness or cerebellar signs.[88] Most recovered within days. One patient in each study had prolonged symptoms lasting 1 month and 4 months, respectively, but both ultimately recovered.

When serial ECGs were obtained, a small but statistically significant decrease in heart rate was noted coincident with peak drug concentrations.[72] In one therapeutic trial, 7% of adult patients receiving artemether had an asymptomatic QT interval prolongation of at least 25%.[110] Changes in the QRS complex are not reported.

Although uncommon, neutropenia, reticulocytopenia, anemia, eosinophilia, and elevated aminotransferases are reported.[107] Acute ACT overdose is rarely reported outside large population-based studies. Morbidity and mortality of overdose are frequently difficult to differentiate from those of the underlying malarial disease and coingestants.

NAPHTHOQUINONES
Atovaquone

Atovaquone is a structural analog of ubiquinone, or coenzyme Q, a mitochondrial protein involved in electron transport.[9] Atovaquone disrupts the protozoal mitochondrial membrane potential, leading to inhibition of several parasite-specific enzymes, ultimately leading to the inhibition of pyrimidine synthesis, which is necessary for protozoal survival and replication. Based on its beneficial side effect profile, the CDC recommends the combination atovaquone–proguanil for treatment of chloroquine-resistant malaria. The price of this combination as well as the variable bioavailability of atovaquone limits its use in less affluent countries.

Atovaquone alone, primarily used to treat *Pneumocystis jiroveci* in patients with AIDS, is relatively well tolerated.[84] Side effects include maculopapular rash, erythema multiforme (rarely), GI complaints, and mild aminotransferase elevations. Three cases of 3- to 42-fold overdose or excess dosing are reported.[25] No symptoms occurred in one case (at 3 times therapeutic serum concentration). Rash occurred in another, and in the third case, methemoglobinemia was attributed to a simultaneous overdose of dapsone.

When used to treat malaria, atovaquone-proguanil side effects include abdominal pain, nausea, vomiting headache, diarrhea, anorexia, and dizziness.[9] This combination is also associated with elevated aminotransferases[89] and hepatosplenomegaly.[9] Reported overdose has caused little serious toxicity.[107]

Atovaquone is reported to have extensive enterohepatic cycling, with 94% of the drug eliminated in the feces.[9,66] Although there is no evidence, multiple-dose activated charcoal is a reasonable intervention in selected overdose patients.

ANTIFOLATES AND ANTIBIOTICS

Sulfadoxine

Proguanil

Pyrimethamine

Antimalarial Mechanism

Proguanil, pyrimethamine, and the antibiotic trimethoprim interfere with malarial folate metabolism by inhibiting dihydrofolate reductase at concentrations far lower than that required to produce comparable inhibition of mammalian enzymes.[114] Dapsone and sulfonamide antibiotics also disrupt malarial folate metabolism, but by inhibiting a different enzymatic reaction—dihydropteroate synthase. Slow onset of action and concerns for the development of resistance have led to the use of these medications in synergistic combinations leading to inhibition of folate metabolism at 2 different sites.

Pharmacokinetics and Toxicodynamics

See Table 59–3 for the pharmacokinetic properties of pyrimethamine, proguanil, and dapsone.

Proguanil's active metabolite, cycloguanil, is primarily responsible for its antimalarial activity. Both the parent drug and active metabolite share substantial renal excretion, making renal insufficiency a risk factor for toxicity.[51]

Dapsone is chiefly metabolized by CYP2C19 to dapsone hydroxylamine.[108] These hydroxylamine metabolites have a long half-life, partially because of enterohepatic recirculation, and concentrate in erythrocytes leading to oxidant stress resulting in methemoglobinemia and hemolysis. Cimetidine competes for the same CYP enzymes, decreasing methemoglobin levels during therapeutic dapsone dosing[92] presumably by shunting dapsone metabolism to alternate nontoxic pathways.

Clinical Manifestations

The side effects of proguanil during prophylaxis include nausea, diarrhea, and mouth ulcers.[63] Because of the interference with folate metabolism, megaloblastic anemia is a rare but potential complication. Megaloblastic bone marrow toxicity is reported in patients with chronic kidney disease.[107] Folate supplementation is recommended in pregnancy and CKD to avoid this complication.[31] Rarely, neutropenia, thrombocytopenia, rash, and alopecia are also noted. In a single case report, hypersensitivity hepatitis was described.[31]

Overdose of pyrimethamine alone is rare. In children, it results in nausea, vomiting, a rapid onset of seizures, fever, and tachycardia.[3,49] Blindness, deafness, and developmental delay have followed. It is unclear whether the chronic neurologic deficits described in case reports are attributable to direct toxicity of pyrimethamine on the CNS or to complications of toxicity such as status epilepticus. Chronic high dose use is associated with a megaloblastic anemia and bone marrow suppression, requiring folate replacement.[3]

The sulfonamides, including the sulfone dapsone, have a long history of causing idiosyncratic reactions, including neutropenia, thrombocytopenia, eosinophilic pneumonia, aplastic anemia, neuropathy, and hepatitis.[63,107] Rare occurrence of life-threatening erythema multiforme major and toxic epidermal necrolysis, associated with pyrimethamine–sulfadoxine prophylaxis, has limited the use of this combination.

Acute ingestion of dapsone results in nausea, vomiting, and abdominal pain.[49] After overdose, dapsone produces RBC oxidant stress, leading to methemoglobinemia and, to a much lesser extent, sulfhemoglobinemia through formation of an active metabolite (Chap. 124).[23,64] Hemolysis may be either immediate or delayed. Dapsone, in particular, is known for its tendency to cause prolonged methemoglobinemia. Other symptoms, particularly tachycardia, dyspnea, dizziness, visual hallucinations, seizure, syncope, and coma resulting from end-organ hypoxia, can occur. Additional effects described in overdose include hepatitis and peripheral neuropathy.[49]

Management

Neural tube defects are associated with the use of folic acid antagonists, thus folate supplementation is reasonable in reproductive age women exposed to these agents. Folinic acid (leucovorin) would be a reasonable intervention after an overdose of proguanil or pyrimethamine (Antidotes in Depth: A12). Other efforts should include supportive care.

After dapsone ingestion, clinically significant methemoglobinemia should be treated with methylene blue (Chap. 124 and Antidotes in Depth: A43). The long half-life of dapsone and its metabolites often make repetitive doses of methylene blue necessary. The patient's clinical status is more important than a single methemoglobin level for determining treatment interventions. There is no antidote for sulfhemoglobinemia, but it constitutes an insignificant portion of total hemoglobin.

Multiple-dose activated charcoal is recommended for patients with a dapsone overdose and no contraindicators.[64] Exchange transfusion is a reasonable intervention for patients who fail to respond to methylene blue. Hemodialysis decreased methemoglobinemia concentrations in case reports but subsequent rebound dapsone concentrations were observed.[79] Continuous veno-venous hemofiltration increased dapsone clearance 3-fold in a single case report. These extracorporeal methods of removal are not routinely recommended. Hyperbaric oxygen has been used in case reports as an adjunct to methylene blue in the treatment of methemoglobinemia but is not routinely recommended (Antidotes in Depth: A43).

Cimetidine supplementation is a reasonable intervention after dapsone overdose. Other antioxidants, ascorbic acid and vitamin E, have been used to treat methemoglobinemia[12] but are not routinely recommended because their slow onset of action makes a benefit unlikely.

FUTURE DIRECTIONS

Shared cytochrome P450 metabolic pathways and genetic polymorphisms are increasingly recognized as contributing factors in drug–drug interactions and toxicity. The clarification of various antimalarial metabolic pathways has led to concern for potential toxicity due to these interactions. The clinical relevance of these interactions is unclear, however. Genetic polymorphism is described in the metabolism of proguanil and dapsone and may be a contributing factor to the hypersensitivity reactions noted with dapsone.[53,91] Table 55–3 highlights the known potentially significant metabolic interactions of antimalarials.

The development of drug resistance and search for treatments with improved efficacy, compliance and side-effect profiles fuels an ongoing pursuit for better antimalarials. Tafenoquinone (WR-238605 or etaune) is an 8-aminoquinoline with greater activity against liver-stage parasites than primaquine. It appears to have fewer side effects than primaquine, less hemolytic toxicity and a longer half-life enabling less frequent dosing that could increase compliance.[29] At the time of this writing, phase III trials of tafenoquine are ongoing. A number of new ACTs are being studied in different countries, but are not yet recommended by the WHO because of insufficient evidence. These new ACTs include combinations of artesunate and pyronaridine, arterolane and piperaquine, artemisinin and piperaquine base, artemisinin and napthoquine.[118]

Although there is no supporting evidence, one case series discussed eculizumab, a monoclonal antibody targeting the terminal portion of the complement cascade, as a potential therapy for AKI associated with quinine-induced thrombotic microangiopathy.[40] Because the role of complement in quinine-induced thrombotic microangiopathy remains unclear and it deviates from the FDA-approved indication, the use of eculizumab for quinine hypersensitivity is not presently recommended.

The complicated structure and life cycle of malaria protozoa has made the development of an effective malaria vaccine an elusive undertaking. Despite these difficulties, the Malaria Vaccine Technology Roadmap has focused strategic efforts since 2006. The most advanced vaccine in development, RTS,S/AS01, provides modest protection (26%–50%)[42] against *P. falciparum*.[83] Funding for a large-scale implementation pilot using this vaccine is established. Vaccinations in several sub-Saharan African countries began in 2018.

SUMMARY

- Malaria is a parasitic infection of human erythrocytes caused by protozoan parasites in the *Plasmodium* genus with a unique life cycle involving the *Anopheles* mosquito as the vector. It is primarily endemic in tropical and subtropical areas worldwide.
- The antimalarial properties of quinine have been known for centuries. Therapeutic dosing can result in a unique symptom complex known as "cinchonism." Significant overdose is heralded by cardiovascular and CNS toxicity.
- The development of resistance has limited the use of chloroquine to specific geographic regions harboring susceptible malarial strains. Rapid development of cardiorespiratory collapse is typical of chloroquine toxicity. Early intubation along with high-dose epinephrine and diazepam are recommended for the treatment of serious chloroquine toxicity.
- Primaquine and dapsone produce significant oxidant stress, resulting in methemoglobinemia and often hemolysis.
- Because of their extremely short half-lives, artemisinins are used in combination with drugs with longer half-lives to delay or prevent the emergence of resistance. Little is known of the acute toxicity after overdose of the newest artemisinin-based medications.

- Understanding antimalarial metabolism and toxicity, creating improved antimalarial medications, and vaccine development are among the many future research efforts under way today.

Acknowledgment

G. Randall Bond, MD, contributed to this chapter in previous editions.

REFERENCES

1. Brown D. Atremisinin and a new generation of antimalarial drugs. *Educ Chem.* 2006;43:97-99.
2. Adjei GO, et al. Amodiaquine-associated adverse effects after inadvertent overdose and after a standard therapeutic dose. *Ghana Med J.* 2009;43:135-138.
3. Akinyanju O, et al. Pyrimethamine poisoning. *Br Med J.* 1973;4:147-148.
4. AlKadi HO. Antimalarial drug toxicity: a review. *Chemotherapy.* 2007;53:385-391.
5. Antinori S, et al. Biology of human malaria plasmodia including *Plasmodium knowlesi. Mediterr J Hematol Infect Dis.* 2012;4:e2012013.
6. Arguin P, Tan K. *2016 Yellow Book, Travelers Health, Malaria.* Chap 3. https://wwwnc.cdc.gov/travel/yellowbook/2016/infectious-diseases-related-to-travel/malaria. Published 2016.
7. Ashley EA, et al. Primaquine: the risks and the benefits. *Malar J.* 2014;13:418.
8. Aweeka FT, German PI. Clinical pharmacology of artemisinin-based combination therapies. *Clin Pharmacokinet.* 2008;47:91-102.
9. Baggish AL, Hill DR. Antiparasitic agent atovaquone. *Antimicrob Agents Chemother.* 2002;46:1163-1173.
10. Baguet JP, et al. Chloroquine cardiomyopathy with conduction disorders. *Heart.* 1999;81:221-223.
11. Ball DE, et al. Chloroquine poisoning in Zimbabwe: a toxicoepidemiological study. *J Appl Toxicol.* 2002;22:311-315.
12. Barclay JA, et al. Dapsone-induced methemoglobinemia: a primer for clinicians. *Ann Pharmacother.* 2011;45:1103-1115.
13. Bateman DN, et al. Pharmacokinetics and clinical toxicity of quinine overdosage: lack of efficacy of techniques intended to enhance elimination. *Q J Med.* 1985;54:125-131.
14. Beutler E. Glucose-6-phosphate dehydrogenase deficiency: a historical perspective. *Blood.* 2008;111:16-24.
15. Birkett AJ. Status of vaccine research and development of vaccines for malaria. *Vaccine.* 2016;34:2915-2920.
16. Bodenhamer JE, Smilkstein MJ. Delayed cardiotoxicity following quinine overdose: a case report. *J Emerg Med.* 1993;11:279-285.
17. Boereboom FT, et al. Hemoperfusion is ineffectual in severe chloroquine poisoning. *Crit Care Med.* 2000;28:3346-3350.
18. Boland ME, et al. Complications of quinine poisoning. *Lancet.* 1985;1:384-385.
19. Bougie DW, et al. Patients with quinine-induced immune thrombocytopenia have both "drug-dependent" and "drug-specific" antibodies. *Blood.* 2006;108:922-927.
20. Brandfonbrener M, et al. The effect of serum potassium concentration on quinidine toxicity. *J Pharmacol Exp Ther.* 1966;154:250-254.
21. Breckenridge AM, Winstanley PA. Clinical pharmacology and malaria. *Ann Trop Med Parasitol.* 1997;91:727-733.
22. Calkins H, et al. Reversal of antiarrhythmic drug effects by epinephrine: quinidine versus amiodarone. *J Am Coll Cardiol.* 1992;19:347-352.
23. Carrazza MZ, et al. Clinical and laboratory parameters in dapsone acute intoxication. *Rev Saude Publica.* 2000;34:396-401.
24. Chattopadhyay R, et al. Assessment of safety of the major antimalarial drugs. *Expert Opin Drug Saf.* 2007;6:505-521.
25. Cheung TW. Overdose of atovaquone in a patient with AIDS. *AIDS.* 1999;13:1984-1985.
26. Clemessy JL, et al. Therapeutic trial of diazepam versus placebo in acute chloroquine intoxications of moderate gravity. *Intensive Care Med.* 1996;22:1400-1405.
27. Clemessy JL, et al. Treatment of acute chloroquine poisoning: a 5-year experience. *Crit Care Med.* 1996;24:1189-1195.
28. Crevoisier CA, et al. Influence of hemodialysis on plasma concentration-time profiles of mefloquine in two patients with end-stage renal disease: a prophylactic drug monitoring study. *Antimicrob Agents Chemother.* 1995;39:1892-1895.
29. Crockett M, Kain KC. Tafenoquine: a promising new antimalarial agent. *Expert Opin Investig Drugs.* 2007;16:705-715.
30. Crouzette J, et al. Experimental assessment of the protective activity of diazepam on the acute toxicity of chloroquine. *J Toxicol.* 1983;20:271-279.
31. Davis TM. Adverse effects of antimalarial prophylactic drugs: an important consideration in the risk-benefit equation. *Ann Pharmacother.* 1998;32:1104-1106.
32. Davis TM. Antimalarial drugs and glucose metabolism. *Br J Clin Pharmacol.* 1997;44:1-7.
33. Davis TM, et al. Neurological, cardiovascular and metabolic effects of mefloquine in healthy volunteers: a double-blind, placebo-controlled trial. *Br J Clin Pharmacol.* 1996;42:415-421.
34. de Souza NB, et al. 4-aminoquinoline analogues and its platinum (II) complexes as antimalarial agents. *Biomed Pharmacother.* 2011;65:313-316.
35. Efferth T, Kaina B. Toxicity of the antimalarial artemisinin and its derivatives. *Crit Rev Toxicol.* 2010;40:405-421.

36. Ezzet F, et al. Pharmacokinetics and pharmacodynamics of lumefantrine (benflumetol) in acute falciparum malaria. *Antimicrob Agents Chemother.* 2000;44:697-704.

37. Flanagan KL, et al. Quinine levels revisited: the value of routine drug level monitoring for those on parenteral therapy. *Acta Trop.* 2006;97:233-237.

38. Fraunfelder F, et al. Drug induced ocular side effects. In: *Clinical Ocular Toxicity: Drugs, Chemicals and Herbs.* Philadelphia, PA: Elseviers Saunders; 2008:45-287.

39. Gangitano JL, Keltner JL. Abnormalities of the pupil and visual-evoked potential in quinine amblyopia. *Am J Ophthalmol.* 1980;89:425-430.

40. George JN, et al. After the party's over. *N Engl J Med.* 2017;376:74-80.

41. Goldenberg AM, Wexler LF. Quinine overdose: review of toxicity and treatment. *Clin Cardiol.* 1988;11:716-718.

42. Goncalves BP, et al. Preparing for future efficacy trials of severe malaria vaccines. *Vaccine.* 2016;34:1865-1867.

43. Grace AA, Camm AJ. Quinidine. *N Engl J Med.* 1998;338:35-45.

44. Grant WM, Schuman JS. Quinine sulfate. In: Thomas CC, ed. *Toxicology of the Eye, Vol II: Effects on the Eyes and Visual System from Chemicals, Drugs, Metals and Minerals, Plants, Toxins and Venoms.* 4th ed. Springfield, IL: Charles C. Thomas; 1993:1225-1233.

45. Greenwood BM, et al. Malaria: progress, perils, and prospects for eradication. *J Clin Invest.* 2008;118:1266-1276.

46. Guly U, Driscoll P. The management of quinine-induced blindness. *Arch Emerg Med.* 1992;9:317-322.

47. Gunawan CA, et al. Quinine-induced arrhythmia in a patient with severe malaria. *Acta Med Indones.* 2007;39:27-32.

48. Gustafsson LL, et al. Disposition of chloroquine in man after single intravenous and oral doses. *Br J Clin Pharmacol.* 1983;15:471-479.

49. Jaeger A, et al. Clinical features and management of poisoning due to antimalarial drugs. *Med Toxicol Adverse Drug Exp.* 1987;2:242-273.

50. John CC. Primaquine plus artemisinin combination therapy for reduction of malaria transmission: promise and risk. *BMC Med.* 2016;14:65.

51. Jolink H, et al. Pancytopenia due to proguanil toxicity in a returning traveller with fever. *Eur J Clin Pharmacol.* 2010;66:811-812.

52. Jordan P, et al. Hydroxychloroquine overdose: toxicokinetics and management. *J Toxicol.* 1999;37:861-864.

53. Kaneko A, et al. Proguanil disposition and toxicity in malaria patients from Vanuatu with high frequencies of CYP2C19 mutations. *Pharmacogenetics.* 1999;9:317-326.

54. Kantele A, Jokiranta TS. Review of cases with the emerging fifth human malaria parasite, *Plasmodium knowlesi. Clin Infect Dis.* 2011;52:1356-1362.

55. Karbwang J, et al. Cardiac effect of halofantrine. *Lancet.* 1993;342:501.

56. Karbwang J, White NJ. Clinical pharmacokinetics of mefloquine. *Clin Pharmacokinet.* 1990;19:264-279.

57. Kim SY, Benowitz NL. Poisoning due to class IA antiarrhythmic drugs. Quinidine, procainamide and disopyramide. *Drug Saf.* 1990;5:393-420.

58. Kissinger E, et al. Clinical and neurophysiological study of the effects of multiple doses of artemisinin on brain-stem function in Vietnamese patients. *Am J Trop Med Hyg.* 2000;63:48-55.

59. Kivisto KT, Neuvonen PJ. Activated charcoal for chloroquine poisoning. *BMJ.* 1993; 307:1068.

60. Liles NW, et al. Diversity and severity of adverse reactions to quinine: a systematic review. *Am J Hematol.* 2016;91:461-466.

61. Lobel HO, et al. Drug overdoses with antimalarial agents: prescribing and dispensing errors. *JAMA.* 1998;280:1483.

62. Lockey D, Bateman DN. Effect of oral activated charcoal on quinine elimination. *Br J Clin Pharmacol.* 1989;27:92-94.

63. Luzzi GA, Peto TE. Adverse effects of antimalarials. An update. *Drug Saf.* 1993;8: 295-311.

64. MacDonald RD, McGuigan MA. Acute dapsone intoxication: a pediatric case report. *Pediatr Emerg Care.* 1997;13:127-129.

65. Marquardt K, Albertson TE. Treatment of hydroxychloroquine overdose. *Am J Emerg Med.* 2001;19:420-424.

66. Marra F, et al. Atovaquone-proguanil for prophylaxis and treatment of malaria. *Ann Pharmacother.* 2003;37:1266-1275.

67. McCarthy S. Malaria prevention, mefloquine neurotoxicity, neuropsychiatric illness, and risk-benefit analysis in the Australian Defence Force. *J Parasitol Res.* 2015;2015: 287651.

68. Medhi B, et al. Pharmacokinetic and toxicological profile of artemisinin compounds: an update. *Pharmacology.* 2009;84:323-332.

69. Meeran K, Jacobs MG. Chloroquine poisoning. Rapidly fatal without treatment. *BMJ.* 1993;307:49-50.

70. Megarbane B, et al. Blood concentrations are better predictors of chloroquine poisoning severity than plasma concentrations: a prospective study with modeling of the concentration/effect relationships. *Clin Toxicol (Phila).* 2010;48:904-915.

71. Megarbane B, et al. Epinephrine requirement based on the reported ingested dose in chloroquine poisoning: usefulness and limitations of dose-effect modelling. *Clin Toxicol (Phila).* 2011;49:193-194.

72. Miller LG, Panosian CB. Ataxia and slurred speech after artesunate treatment for falciparum malaria. *N Engl J Med.* 1997;336:1328.

73. Monlun E, et al. Cardiac complications of halofantrine: a prospective study of 20 patients. *Trans R Soc Trop Med Hyg.* 1995;89:430-433.

74. Morady F, et al. Antagonism of quinidine's electrophysiologic effects by epinephrine in patients with ventricular tachycardia. *J Am Coll Cardiol.* 1988;12:388-394.

75. Morrison LD, et al. Death by quinine. *Veterinary and human toxicology.* 2003;45: 303-306.

76. Nadjm B, Behrens RH. Malaria: an update for physicians. *Infect Dis Clin North Am.* 2012;26:243-259.

77. Netland KE, Martinez J. Abortifacients: toxidromes, ancient to modern—a case series and review of the literature. *Acad Emerg Med.* 2000;7:824-829.

78. Neubauer AS, et al. The multifocal pattern electroretinogram in chloroquine retinopathy. *Ophthalmic Res.* 2004;36:106-113.

79. Neuvonen PJ, et al. Acute dapsone intoxication: clinical findings and effect of oral charcoal and haemodialysis on dapsone elimination. *Acta Med Scand.* 1983;214:215-220.

80. Nosten F, Price RN. New antimalarials. A risk-benefit analysis. *Drug Saf.* 1995;12: 264-273.

81. Nosten F, et al. Cardiac effects of antimalarial treatment with halofantrine. *Lancet.* 1993;341:1054-1056.

82. Nosten F, et al. The effects of mefloquine treatment in pregnancy. *Clin Infect Dis.* 1999;28:808-815.

83. Organization WH. Questions and answers on RTS,S/ASO1 malaria vaccine. http:// www.who.int/immunization/research/development/malaria_vaccine_qa/en/. Published 2016.

84. Peters BS, et al. Adverse effects of drugs used in the management of opportunistic infections associated with HIV infection. *Drug Saf.* 1994;10:439-454.

85. Phillips RE, et al. Hypoglycaemia and counterregulatory hormone responses in severe falciparum malaria: treatment with Sandostatin. *Q J Med.* 1993;86:233-240.

86. Phillips RE, et al. Effectiveness of SMS 201-995, a synthetic, long-acting somatostatin analogue, in treatment of quinine-induced hyperinsulinaemia. *Lancet.* 1986;1: 713-716.

87. Prescott LF, et al. Treatment of quinine overdosage with repeated oral charcoal. *Br J Clin Pharmacol.* 1989;27:95-97.

88. Price R, et al. Adverse effects in patients with acute falciparum malaria treated with artemisinin derivatives. *Am J Trop Med Hyg.* 1999;60:547-555.

89. Pussard E, Verdier F. Antimalarial 4-aminoquinolines: mode of action and pharmacokinetics. *Fundam Clin Pharmacol.* 1994;8:1-17.

90. Reddy VG, Sinna S. Chloroquine poisoning: report of two cases. *Acta Anaesthesiol Scand.* 2000;44:1017-1020.

91. Reilly TP, et al. Methemoglobin formation by hydroxylamine metabolites of sulfamethoxazole and dapsone: implications for differences in adverse drug reactions. *J Pharmacol Exp Ther.* 1999;288:951-959.

92. Rhodes LE, et al. Cimetidine improves the therapeutic/toxic ratio of dapsone in patients on chronic dapsone therapy. *Br J Dermatol.* 1995;132:257-262.

93. Riou B, et al. Treatment of severe chloroquine poisoning. *N Engl J Med.* 1988;318:1-6.

94. Riou B, et al. Protective cardiovascular effects of diazepam in experimental acute chloroquine poisoning. *Intensive Care Med.* 1988;14:610-616.

95. Roche RJ, et al. Quinine induces reversible high-tone hearing loss. *Br J Clin Pharmacol.* 1990;29:780-782.

96. Ryan ET, Kain KC. Health advice and immunizations for travelers. *N Engl J Med.* 2000;342:1716-1725.

97. Sabto JK, et al. Hemodialysis, peritoneal dialysis, plasmapheresis and forced diuresis for the treatment of quinine overdose. *Clin Nephrol.* 1981;16:264-268.

98. Schlagenhauf P. Mefloquine for malaria chemoprophylaxis 1992-1998: a review. *J Travel Med.* 1999;6:122-133.

99. Selzer A, Wray HW. Quinidine syncope. Paroxysmal ventricular fibrillation occurring during treatment of chronic atrial arrhythmias. *Circulation.* 1964;30:17-26.

100. Shub C, et al. The management of acute quinidine intoxication. *Chest.* 1978;73: 173-178.

101. Silamut K, et al. Alpha 1-acid glycoprotein (orosomucoid) and plasma protein binding of quinine in falciparum malaria. *Br J Clin Pharmacol.* 1991;32:311-315.

102. Smith ER, Klein-Schwartz W. Are 1-2 dangerous? Chloroquine and hydroxychloroquine exposure in toddlers. *J Emerg Med.* 2005;28:437-443.

103. Smith HR, et al. Dermatological adverse effects with the antimalarial drug mefloquine: a review of 74 published case reports. *Clin Exp Dermatol.* 1999;24:249-254.

104. Sowunmi A, et al. Comparative cardiac effects of halofantrine and chloroquine plus chlorpheniramine in children with acute uncomplicated falciparum malaria. *Trans R Soc Trop Med Hyg.* 1999;93:78-83.

105. Splawski I, et al. Molecular basis of the long-QT syndrome associated with deafness. *N Engl J Med.* 1997;336:1562-1567.

106. Tange RA. Ototoxicity. *Adverse Drug React Toxicol Rev.* 1998;17:75-89.

107. Taylor WR, White NJ. Antimalarial drug toxicity: a review. *Drug Saf.* 2004;27: 25-61.

108. Toker I, et al. Methemoglobinemia caused by dapsone overdose: which treatment is best? *Turk J Emerg Med.* 2015;15:182-184.

109. Touze JE, et al. Electrocardiographic changes and halofantrine plasma level during acute falciparum malaria. *Am J Trop Med Hyg.* 1996;54:225-228.

110. Tran TH, et al. A controlled trial of artemether or quinine in Vietnamese adults with severe falciparum malaria. *N Engl J Med.* 1996;335:76-83.

111. Lilly, USA, LLC. Quinidine gluconate injection. USP [package insert]. Indianapolis, IN: Lilly, USA, LLC; 2012.

112. van Hensbroek MB, et al. A trial of artemether or quinine in children with cerebral malaria. *N Engl J Med.* 1996;335:69-75.

113. van Riemsdijk MM, et al. Atovaquone plus chloroguanide versus mefloquine for malaria prophylaxis: a focus on neuropsychiatric adverse events. *Clin Pharmacol Ther.* 2002;72:294-301.

114. Vinetz J, et al. Chemotherapy of malaria. In: Brunton L, et al., eds. *Goodman & Gilman's The Pharmacological Basis of Therapeutics.* 12th ed. New York: McGraw-Hill Companies; 2011.

115. Warhurst DC. Antimalarial drugs. An update. *Drugs.* 1987;33:50-65.

116. White NJ. Cardiotoxicity of antimalarial drugs. *Lancet Infect Dis.* 2007;7:549-558.

117. White NJ. The treatment of malaria. *N Engl J Med.* 1996;335:800-806.

118. WHO. Guidelines for the treatment of malaria. Third edition, April 2015. http://www.who.int/malaria/publications/atoz/9789241549127/en/. Published 2015.

119. WHO. World Health Organization: malaria fact sheet. http://www.who.int/mediacentre/factsheets/fs094/en/. Published 2016.

120. Wolf LR, et al. Cinchonism: two case reports and review of acute quinine toxicity and treatment. *J Emerg Med.* 1992;10:295-301.

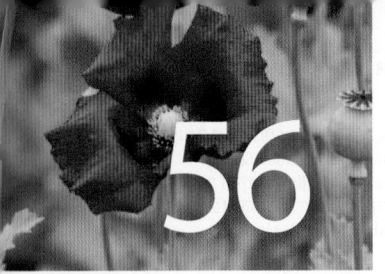

56 ANTITUBERCULOUS MEDICATIONS

Christina H. Hernon and Jeffrey T. Lai

HISTORY AND EPIDEMIOLOGY

Approximately one-third of the total population of the world, or 2 billion people, are infected with *Mycobacterium tuberculosis*. An estimated 10.4 million new cases of disease are diagnosed annually.[169] In 2010, 1.45 million deaths were reported; of which approximately 0.35 million were attributed to HIV-associated tuberculosis. In 2014, the incidence of TB in the United States was the lowest recorded (9,412 new cases) since the inception of national reporting in 1953, but in 2015, the number increased to 9557, after declining annually for more than 20 years.[25,134] The introduction of isoniazid (INH) into clinical practice in 1952 produced a steady decline in the number of TB cases in the United States over the subsequent 30 years. However, between 1985 and 1991, there was a resurgence in TB cases in the United States resulting primarily from the effects of human immunodeficiency virus (HIV), homelessness, deterioration in the health care infrastructure, and an increase in immigration. With the initiation and implementation of containment strategies, the spread of the infection slowed by aggressive case identification and patient-centered management, including directly observed therapy, social support, housing, and substance abuse treatment. These methods decreased the prevalence rate in the United States and worldwide.[115] In 2006, 20% of *Mycobacterium tuberculosis* isolates were resistant to at least isoniazid and rifampin, called multidrug-resistant tuberculosis (MDR-TB), and 2% were identified as highly resistant extensively drug-resistant tuberculosis (XDR-TB), with resistance to many additional drugs—defined as all fluoroquinolones, and at least one of 3 injectable drugs (capreomycin, kanamycin, and amikacin).[9,24] Between 1993 and 2015, 73 cases of XDR-TB were reported in the United States.[26]

At present, populations that remain at risk for TB include HIV-positive patients, homeless people, people with alcoholism, injection drug users, health care workers, prisoners, prison workers, and Native Americans. In addition, the TB rate in foreign-born persons is nearly 10 times higher than in US-born persons. In the US population, countries of birth generating the highest number of TB cases are Mexico, the Philippines, India, and Vietnam.[9]

The use of multiple drugs in regimens against MDR-TB and XDR-TB results in significant adverse drug effects, approximately 40%, and this increases to approximately 70% in treatment against coinfection with human immunodeficiency virus (HIV). These reactions include hepatotoxicity, peripheral neuropathy, arthralgias, rash, anemia, and require discontinuation of therapy if severe. These effects are greatest in the first weeks of therapy, often are irreversible, and potentially fatal.[97]

ISONIAZID
Pharmacology

Isoniazid (INH, or isonicotinic hydrazide) is structurally related to nicotinic acid (niacin, or vitamin B$_3$), nicotinamide adenosine dinucleotide (NAD), and pyridoxine (vitamin B$_6$) (Fig. 56–1). The pyridine ring is essential for

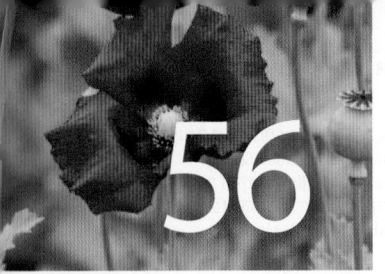

FIGURE 56–1. Isoniazid and related compounds.

antituberculous activity. Isoniazid itself does not have direct antibacterial activity. It is a prodrug that undergoes metabolic activation by KatG, a catalase peroxidase in *M. tuberculosis* that produces a highly reactive intermediate,[116,174] which in turn interacts with InhA, a mycobacterial enzyme that functions as an enoyl-acyl carrier protein (enoyl-ACP) reductase.[113,114] Enoyl-ACP reductase InhA is required for the synthesis of very long-chain lipids, mycolic acids (containing between 40 and 60 carbons) that are important components of mycobacterial cell walls.

The activated form of INH is stabilized by the pyridine ring. Enoyl-ACP reductase (InhA) catalyzes the NADH-dependent reduction of the double bonds in the growing fatty acid chain linked to acyl carrier proteins. This INH metabolite enters the binding site of InhA, where it reacts with the reduced form of nicotinamide adenine dinucleotide (NADH).[116] The covalently linked INH-NADH complex remains bound to the active site of InhA, irreversibly inhibiting the enzyme.[95,113]

Pharmacokinetics

When therapeutic doses of 300 mg are administered orally, INH is rapidly absorbed, reaching peak serum concentrations typically within 2 hours.[75,108,109] Delayed absorption of isoniazid infrequently occurs, with peak concentrations up to 6 hours after ingestion.[5] Isoniazid diffuses into all body fluids with a volume of distribution of approximately 0.6 L/kg and has negligible binding to serum proteins. After the drug penetrates infected tissue, it achieves concentrations well above those generally required for bactericidal activity.[109]

The primary metabolic pathway for INH is via *N*-acetylation via hepatic acrylamine *N*-acetyltransferase type 2 (NAT2) to acetylisoniazid, which undergoes one of the following fates: excretion by the kidney; oxidation to hydroxylamine, a hepatotoxic metabolite via CYP2E1;[171] direct hydrolyzation to hepatotoxic hydrazine; or further metabolism by NAT2 to (somewhat hepatotoxic) acetylhydrazine, which is further metabolized by NAT2 to nontoxic diacetylhydrazine. Hydrazine and (to a lesser extent) acetylhydrazine are oxidized by CYP2E1 to reactive metabolites, which induce oxidative stress or alter lipid metabolism, resulting in hepatic apoptosis or steatosis. The mechanisms and circumstances of hepatotoxicity are not yet clearly elucidated though toxicity is thought to be due to the metabolites and not to isoniazid itself.[162,171] Approximately 75% to 95% of INH is renally eliminated in the form of these hepatic metabolites within 24 hours of administration.[62] *N*-Acetyltransferase-2 (NAT2) exhibits Michaelis-Menten kinetics but is genotypically polymorphic, and the activity of an individual's enzymes is determined by an autosomal dominant inheritance pattern, with homozygous fast acetylators (FF), heterozygous fast acetylators (FS), and homozygous slow acetylators (SS). Patients are distinguishable phenotypically as fast, intermediate, and slow acetylators. Whereas the fast acetylation enzyme is found in 40% to 50% of American whites and African Americans, the fast acetylator enzyme is found in 80% to 90% of Asians and Inuits.[47] These enzymes are distinguishable by the following characteristics: (1) slow acetylators have less presystemic clearance, or first-pass effect, than do fast acetylators; (2) fast acetylators metabolize INH 5 to 6 times faster than slow acetylators; and (3) serum INH concentrations are 30% to 50% lower in fast acetylators than in slow acetylators. The elimination half-life of INH is approximately 70 minutes in fast acetylators and 180 minutes in slow acetylators. Twenty-seven percent of INH is excreted unchanged in urine by slow acetylators compared with 11% excretion in fast acetylators. Slow acetylators are at increased risk of peripheral neuropathy and dose adjustments mitigate this risk.[152] The clearance of INH averages 46 mL/min.[12,164] Additionally, a small portion of INH is directly hydrolyzed into isonicotinic acid and hydrazine, and this pathway is of greater quantitative significance in slow acetylators than in rapid acetylators. Although both hepatic microsomal oxidation by CYP2E1 of hydrazine or the acetylhydrazine intermediate into reactive intermediates are proposed as causes of INH-related hepatotoxicity, there is no significant association between variations in genetic polymorphisms and hepatotoxicity.[56,101,156,171] There is increasing evidence that hydrazine is directly linked to hepatotoxicity as well as causing hepatotoxicity via an immune-mediated, idiosyncratic mechanism.[96] Lastly, INH nonenzymatically conjugates with certain endogenous metabolites including ketone acids and vitamin B_6 (pyridoxal and pyridoxal 5-phosphate) or enzymatically with NAD^+ via human neutrophil myeloperoxidase. Interruption of homeostasis of bile acids, cholesterols, triglycerides, and free fatty acids is possible with chronic INH therapy, because of CYP2E1-dependent modulation. Fig. 56–2 illustrates the metabolism of INH.

Pathophysiology
Mechanism of Toxicity

Isoniazid induces a functional pyridoxine deficiency via 2 main mechanisms (Fig. 56–3) and culminates in refractory seizures because of a relative lack of γ-aminobutyric acid (GABA), the primary inhibitory neurotransmitter in the central nervous system, and an excess of glutamate, the primary stimulatory neurotransmitter in the central nervous system (CNS). The GABA-glutamate pathway establishes an equilibrium between the stimulatory, epileptogenic effects of glutamate against the inhibitory, sedative-hypnotic effects of GABA. Disruption of this homeostasis, with increased glutamate and insufficient GABA, is thought to be the etiology of INH-induced seizures.[73]

Pyridoxine is converted in vivo to an active form, pyridoxal-5′-phosphate, which serves as an important cofactor in many biotransformation reactions such as transamination, transketolation, and decarboxylation. Isoniazid metabolites inhibit the enzyme pyridoxine phosphokinase, which converts pyridoxine (vitamin B_6) to its active form, pyridoxal-5′-phosphate, which is a required cofactor for many pyridoxine-dependent enzyme systems in the body, including 2 enzymes that control GABA metabolism.[30,74,99] Glutamic acid decarboxylase (GAD) catalyzes GABA synthesis from glutamate, and GABA aminotransferase degrades the inhibitory neurotransmitter. The inhibitory effects are greater on GAD, which leads to both decreased GABA and elevated glutamate concentrations.[167]

Pyridoxine depletion also decreases catecholamine synthesis and interferes with the synthesis of and/or reacts with NAD^+ to form inactive hydrazine adducts, thereby disrupting cellular reduction/oxidation reactions.

Pyridoxine depletion is further compounded when INH directly reacts with pyridoxal phosphate to produce an inactive hydrazone complex that is renally excreted and thereby increases loss of this required cofactor.[99,164] Urinary excretion of pyridoxine and its metabolites increases with increasing INH dose, reflecting the effect of INH on pyridoxine metabolism.

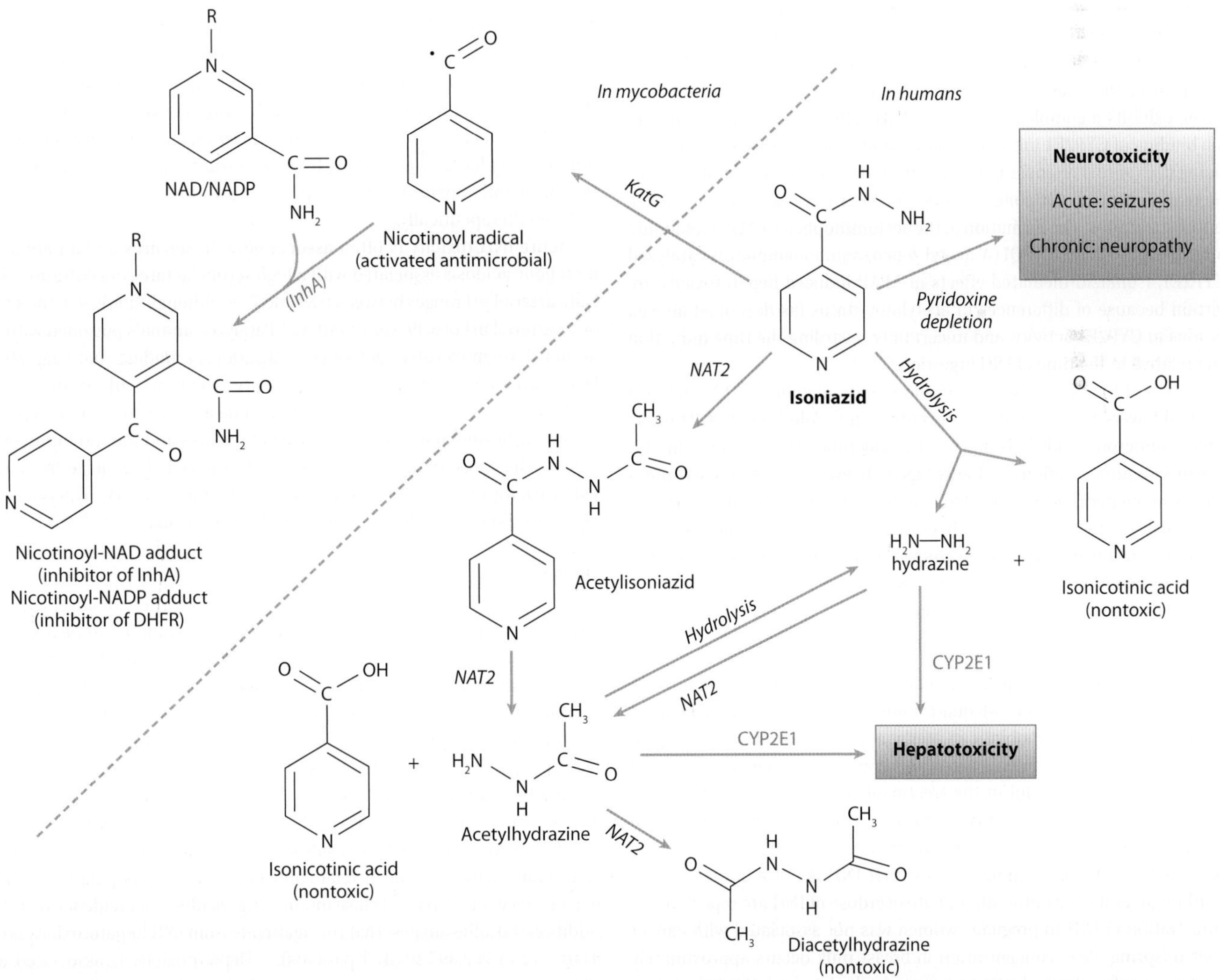

FIGURE 56–2. Metabolism of isoniazid (INH). INH metabolism occurs via enzyme N-acetyltransferase type 2 (NAT2), hydrolysis, and further oxidation via CYP2E1 into both nontoxic and hepatotoxic metabolites. Hepatotoxicity is multifactorial and occurs directly via hepatotoxic metabolites and indirectly via induced apoptosis and steatosis. DHFR = dihydrofolate reductase; InhA = mycobacterial enoyl-acyl carrier protein reductase; KatG = mycobacterial catalase peroxidase.

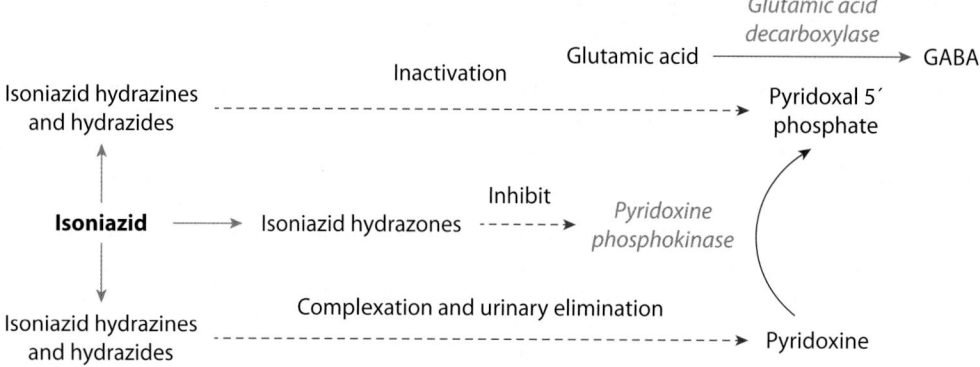

FIGURE 56–3. The effect of isoniazid on γ-aminobutyric acid (GABA) synthesis.

Structurally similar chemicals exert similar acute toxic effects. Mono-methylhydrazine, a metabolite produced from gyromitrin isolated from the *Gyromitra* spp ("false morel") mushroom, and the hydrazines used in liquid rocket fuel have a similar mechanism of action (Chap. 117).

Interactions With Other Drugs and Foods

Drug–drug interactions associated with INH are mediated through alteration of hepatic metabolism of several CYP enzymes. The majority of these interactions are inhibitory, with decreased CYP-mediated transformations, particularly demethylation, oxidation, and hydroxylation (Chap. 11). Clinically relevant adverse effects with elevated concentrations of theophylline (CYP1A2), phenytoin (CYP2C9/CYP2C19), warfarin (CYP2C9/CYP2C19), valproic acid, and carbamazepine (CYP3A4) are caused by decreased hepatic metabolism of these xenobiotics.[42,136,173] The CYP2E1 cytochrome subtype, however, exhibits a complex response to INH called ligand stabilization, in which binding of CYP2E1 initially stabilizes and inhibits its function prior to inducing it. Eventual dissociation of INH from the enzyme active site creates an increased intracellular concentration of CYP2E1 available to metabolize potential substrates. The formation of the acetaminophen (APAP) metabolite responsible for toxicity, NAPQI (*N*-acetyl-*p*-benzoquinoneimine), is catalyzed by CYP2E1. Isoniazid-mediated effects in APAP-induced hepatotoxicity are uncertain because of differences in acetylator status (as described above), variations in CYP2E1 activity, and uncertainty regarding the time induction occurs relative to the time of INH ingestion.[29,78,136]

Ingestion of food decreases the absolute bioavailability of INH and also delays and lowers maximum drug concentration.[122] Additionally, INH interacts with numerous foods.[136] Isoniazid is a weak monoamine oxidase inhibitor; both tyramine reactions to foods (aged cheeses, wines) and serotonin toxicity from meperidine are reported in patients taking INH. Clinical effects include flushing, tachycardia, and hypertension.[41,54,84,147] Furthermore, INH inhibits the enzyme histaminase, leading to exacerbated reactions after the ingestion of histamine in scombrotoxic fish.[68,98,136] Table 56–1 summarizes additional INH drug and food interactions.

Pregnancy

Isoniazid is an FDA class C drug (animal studies demonstrate an adverse effect on the fetus, with no adequate human studies; potential benefits may warrant use of the xenobiotic in pregnancy), crosses the placenta, produces umbilical cord serum concentrations comparable to maternal serum concentrations, and is useful in the treatment of tuberculosis in pregnant patients.[15,16,179] Isoniazid daily or twice weekly is the preferred regimen, and coadministration of pyridoxine is strongly recommended.[23]

Mammalian teratogen studies suggest that INH is not a human teratogen, although fetal deformities after acute overdose of INH are reported.[85,164] Administration of INH to pregnant women was not associated with cancer in their offspring. Peak concentration in breast milk occurs approximately one to 3 hours after drug administration and calculated relative infant dose is 1.2% of weight-adjusted maternal dose.[143] Although INH readily and rapidly enters breast milk, breastfeeding during therapy is acceptable.[126,164]

Clinical Manifestations of Isoniazid Toxicity
Acute Toxicity

Isoniazid produces the triad of seizures refractory to conventional therapy, severe metabolic acidosis, and coma. These clinical manifestations appear as soon as 30 minutes after ingestion.[66,72,154] The case fatality rate of a single acute ingestion classically is as high as 20%.[17,20] Vomiting, slurred speech, dizziness, and tachycardia typically represent early manifestations of toxicity, though seizures are uncommonly the initial sign of acute overdose.[88] Seizures characteristically occur after the ingestion of greater than 20 mg/kg of INH and invariably occur with ingestions greater than 35 to 40 mg/kg. Patients with underlying seizure disorders are at risk of developing seizures at lower doses, and seizures are reported with initiation of a single therapeutic dose.[17,112] Hyperreflexia or hyporeflexia are an indicator for risk of INH-induced seizures. Consciousness will return between seizures, or status epilepticus occurs.[35,104] Because GABA, the primary inhibitory neurotransmitter, is depleted in acute INH toxicity, seizure activity is often refractory to typical anticonvulsant therapy, persisting until GABA concentrations are restored therapeutically.

Acute INH toxicity is often associated with seizures and an anion gap metabolic acidosis associated with a high serum lactate concentration. Typically, arterial pH ranges between 6.80 and 7.30, although survival in the setting of an arterial pH of 6.49 was reported.[66] Paralyzed animals poisoned with INH do not develop elevated lactate concentrations, a finding that suggests the lactate arises from intense muscular activity associated with seizures.[30,105]

In acute severe INH toxicity, coma as long as 24 to 36 hours is reported, persisting beyond both the termination of seizures and the resolution of acidemia. The cause of coma is unknown.[13,66] Additional sequelae from acute INH toxicity include rhabdomyolysis, acute kidney injury, hyperglycemia, glycosuria, ketonuria, hypotension, and hyperthermia.[6,10,22,106,164,165]

Chronic Toxicity

Chronic therapeutic INH use is associated with a variety of adverse effects. Overall incidence of adverse reactions to INH is estimated to be 5.4%,[62] the most serious of which is hepatocellular necrosis.[49] Although asymptomatic elevation of aminotransferases is common in the first several months of treatment, the onset of hepatitis uncommonly presents up to one year after starting INH therapy. In 1978, after several deaths among patients receiving INH therapy, the US Public Health Service reported the incidence of clinically evident hepatitis as 1% of those taking INH; of that subgroup, 10% died, for an overall mortality rate of 0.1%.[19,80] Research performed since the resurgence of TB, however, identified a considerably lower rate of hepatotoxicity. Clinically manifest hepatitis occurred in only 11 patients in a population of 11,141 persons receiving INH and close monitoring, yielding an incidence of 0.1%.[103] Additional studies suggest that the death rate from INH hepatotoxicity is only 0.001% (2 of 202,497 treated patients).[125] Hepatotoxicity is associated with chronic overdose, increasing age, comorbid conditions such as malnutrition, and combinations of antituberculous drugs. Overt hepatic failure typically occurs when INH therapy is continued after the onset of hepatocellular

TABLE 56–1	Adverse Reactions and Drug Interactions of Antituberculous Drugs			
Drug	**Major Adverse Reactions**	**Drug Interactions Clinical Effect**	**Monitoring**	**Comments**
Isoniazid (INH)	*Acute:* seizures, acidosis, coma, hyperthermia, oliguria, anuria *Chronic:* elevation of aminotransferases, autoimmune hepatitis, arthritis, anemia, hemolysis, eosinophilia, peripheral neuropathy, optic neuritis, vitamin B$_6$ deficiency (pellagra)	Rifampin, PZA, ethanol: hepatic necrosis Warfarin: increased INR Theophylline: tachycardia, vomiting, seizures, acidosis Phenytoin: increased phenytoin concentrations Carbamazepine: altered mental status Lactose: decreased INH absorption Antacids: decreased INH absorption Red wine/soft cheese: tyramine reaction Fish (scombroid): flushing, pruritus	Hepatic aminotransferases, ANA, CBC	HIV enteropathy may decrease absorption
Rifampin	*Acute:* diarrhea, periorbital edema *Chronic:* elevation of aminotransferases, reddish discoloration of body fluids	Protease inhibitors: decreased serum concentration of protease inhibitor Delavirdine: increased HIV resistance Cyclosporine: graft rejection Warfarin: decreased INR Oral contraceptives: ineffective contraception Methadone: opioid withdrawal Phenytoin: higher frequency of seizures Theophylline: decreased theophylline concentrations Verapamil: decreased cardiovascular effect	If administered with HIV antiretrovirals, viral titers should be followed. Hepatic aminotransferases; monitor serum concentrations of drugs (ie, phenytoin, cyclosporine) or clinical markers of efficacy (ie, INR)	Interactions of rifampin with several HIV medications are very poorly described; changes in dosing or dosing interval for both rifampin and antiretroviral drugs are commonly required; teratogenic
Ethambutol	*Chronic:* optic neuritis, loss of red–green discrimination, loss of peripheral vision		Visual acuity, color discrimination	Contraindicated in children too young for formal ophthalmologic examination
Pyrazinamide (PZA)	*Chronic:* elevation of aminotransferases, decreased urate excretion	INH: increased rates of hepatotoxicity (when extended courses or high-dose pyrazinamide used)	Hepatic aminotransferases	Courses of therapy of ≤2 months are recommended
Cycloserine	*Chronic:* depression, paranoia, seizures, megaloblastic anemia	INH: increased frequency of seizures	CBC, psychiatric monitoring	
Ethionamide	*Chronic:* orthostatic hypotension, depression	Cycloserine: increases CNS effects	Blood pressure, pulse, orthostasis	
para-Aminosalicylic acid	*Chronic:* malaise, GI upset, elevation of aminotransferases, hypersensitivity reactions, thrombocytopenia		Hepatic aminotransferases, CBC	
Capreomycin	*Chronic:* hearing loss, tinnitus, proteinuria, sterile abscess at IM injection sites		Audiometry, kidney function tests	

ANA = antinuclear antibodies; CBC = complete blood count; CNS = central nervous system; HIV = human immunodeficiency virus.

injury in both adults and children.[45,46,63,91,142,170] The incidence of hepatitis is 2 to 4 times higher in pregnant women than in nonpregnant women.[52]

Isoniazid-induced hepatitis arises via 2 pathways.[45,172] The first involves an immunologic mechanism resulting in hepatic injury that is thought to be idiopathic.[131,164] The association of hepatitis with lupus erythematosus, hemolytic anemia, thrombocytopenia, arthritis, vasculitis, and polyserositis supports an immunologic process.[128,164] However, symptoms commonly found in autoimmune disorders such as fever, rash, and eosinophilia are usually absent with drug-induced lupus erythematosus, and rechallenge with INH often fails to provoke recurrence of hepatocellular injury.[45,128,172] The second, more common, mechanism involves direct hepatic injury by INH or its metabolites. The metabolites believed most responsible for hepatic injury are acetylhydrazine and hydrazine (Fig. 56–2).[56,101,155]

Peripheral neuropathy and optic neuritis are known adverse drug effects of chronic INH use. The exact pathophysiology of isoniazid-induced neurotoxicity is not known, but is believed to be caused by pyridoxine deficiency aggravated by the formation of pyridoxine-INH hydrazones.[47] Peripheral neuropathy, the most common complication of INH therapy, presents in a stocking-glove distribution that progresses proximally. Although primarily sensory in nature, myalgias and weakness are also reported.[144] Peripheral neuropathy is generally observed in severely malnourished, alcoholic, uremic, or diabetic patients; it is also associated with slow acetylator status, an effect that leads to increased INH concentrations and, consequently, increased pyridoxine depletion.[59] Optic neuritis is a central neurologic risk of isoniazid therapy which presents as decreased visual acuity, eye pain, and dyschromatopsia. Risk is greater when isoniazid is taken concurrent with other medications such as ethambutol or etanercept. Central scotomata and bitemporal hemianopsia occur on visual field testing in affected pateints.[60,72,79] Isoniazid is also associated with such findings of CNS toxicity as ataxia, psychosis, hallucinations, and coma.[2,11,58,124]

Diagnostic Testing

Acute INH toxicity is a clinical diagnosis that is inferred by history and confirmed by measuring serum INH concentrations.[135] Acute toxicity from INH correlates with serum INH concentration greater than 10 mg/L one hour after ingestion, greater than 3.2 mg/L 2 hours after ingestion, or greater than

0.2 mg/L 6 hours after the ingestion.[104] Because serum INH concentrations are not widely available, clinicians cannot rely on serum concentrations to confirm the diagnosis or initiate therapy. Because of the risk of hepatitis associated with chronic INH use, hepatic aminotransferases should be regularly monitored after therapy is started. In critically ill patients, serum should be assessed for acidemia, kidney function, creatine phosphokinase (CPK), and urine myoglobin, indicating rhabdomyolysis and possible acute kidney injury.

Management
Acute Toxicity
The antidote for INH-induced neurologic dysfunction is pyridoxine (Antidotes in Depth: A15). Pyridoxine rapidly terminates seizures, corrects metabolic acidosis, and reverses coma. The efficacy of pyridoxine is correlated with the administered dose; one study identified recurrent seizures in 60% of patients who received no pyridoxine and in 47% of those who received 10% of the ideal pyridoxine dose, and no seizures in patients who received the full dose of pyridoxine.[163] To treat acute toxicity, we recommend that the pyridoxine dose in grams should equal the amount of INH ingested in grams, with a first dose of up to 5 g intravenously in adults. Unknown quantities of ingested INH warrant initial empiric treatment with a pyridoxine dose of no more than 5 g (pediatric dose: 70 mg/kg to a maximum of 5 g). Pyridoxine should be administered at a rate of 1 g every 2 to 3 minutes. When patients have seizures that persist beyond administration of the initial dose, an additional similar dose of pyridoxine is recommended.[7]

Hospital pharmacies typically stock insufficient quantities of intravenous (IV) pyridoxine to treat even a single patient with a large INH ingestion.[127] In the event that IV formulations are unavailable in sufficient quantities, we recommend that pyridoxine tablets are crushed and administered with fluids via a nasogastric tube.[127]

Conventional antiepileptics, although generally used as first line therapy, demonstrate variable effectiveness in terminating INH-induced seizures. Benzodiazepines such as lorazepam or diazepam should be used to potentiate the antidotal efficacy of pyridoxine, particularly if optimal doses of the antidote are unavailable. The benzodiazepines act synergistically with pyridoxine, as well as possessing inherent GABA agonist activity, but they are often ineffective as the sole treatment of acute severe INH poisoning because of their reliance on GABA to exert their activity.[31,32,72,163] Phenytoin has no intrinsic GABAergic effect and is not recommended as therapy for patients with INH-induced seizures.[72,104,121] Barbiturates have potent direct and indirect GABA agonist activity and are expected to be as effective or more effective than the benzodiazepines. However, intubation may be required with use of barbiturates because of greater risk of respiratory depression with this class of antiepileptic. The efficacy of propofol in terminating INH-induced seizures is unstudied in humans, but is reasonable in cases of refractory status epilepticus.

Hemodialysis has clearance rates reported as high as 120 mL/min, but is rarely indicated for initial management of INH toxicity, unless kidney failure is present. In acute overdose, hemodialysis is not routinely recommended to enhance elimination but is reasonable following massive ingestion, when adequate supplies of pyridoxine are not available.[22,146,164]

It is recommended that asymptomatic patients who present to the emergency department within 2 hours of ingestion of toxic amounts of INH receive prophylactic administration of 5 g of oral or IV pyridoxine. This recommendation is based on the observation that INH reaches its peak serum concentration within 2 hours of ingestion of therapeutic doses. Asymptomatic patients should be observed for a 6-hour period for signs of toxicity. Acute toxicity is unlikely to manifest more than 6 hours beyond ingestion.

It is reasonable to perform early gastrointestinal (GI) decontamination by administering activated charcoal enterally by mouth to patients who are awake and able to comply with therapy or via nasogastric tube in intubated patients if no contraindications (which include absent bowel sounds, abdominal pain, abdominal distention).[141] Delayed absorption is uncommon. Late GI decontamination with activated charcoal is not reported to

increase survival or decrease toxicity and is not recommended.[133] Orogastric lavage is not routinely recommended, but is reasonable shortly after a large INH ingestion.

Chronic Toxicity
Hepatitis (defined as aminotransferase concentrations more than 2–3 times baseline) resulting from therapeutic INH administration mandates termination of therapy. After resolution of liver injury, it is appropriate to restart INH treatment, provided aminotransferase concentrations are closely monitored, with reassessment in 6 weeks or any time the patient experiences nausea, vomiting, or abdominal discomfort.[45,142] Pyridoxine does not reverse hepatic injury; consequently, surveillance for and recognition of hepatocellular injury remains essential. Cases of hepatitis refractory to medical therapy, requiring liver transplantation, are reported.[48,67,170] Research is ongoing to identify potential hepatoprotective supplements or medications to reduce INH-associated hepatotoxicity.

Isoniazid produces an axonopathy caused by pyridoxine depletion and manifests as peripheral neuropathies, cerebellar findings, and psychosis. Neurotoxicity is commonly treated with as much as 50 mg/day of oral pyridoxine, although doses as low as 6 mg/day are reportedly effective.[2,11,124,149] Because of its effectiveness in preventing neurologic toxicity, pyridoxine is often used concurrently with INH therapy. Coinfection with TB and HIV causes increased risk of pyridoxine deficiency and peripheral neuropathy with INH therapy, both before and after initiation of antiretroviral therapy, and pyridoxine supplementation should be initiated when peripheral neuropathy is evident.[158]

RIFAMYCINS

Rifampin

Pharmacology
Rifamycins are a class of macrocyclic antibiotics derived from actinomycete *Amycolatopsis mediterranei*. Xenobiotics in this class include rifampin (a semisynthetic derivative), rifabutin, and rifapentine, of which the first 2 are most commonly used.[62] Rifampin inhibits the initial steps in RNA chain polymerization through direct binding and formation of a stable drug enzyme complex with RNA polymerase. Disruption of RNA synthesis interrupts transcription and therefore inhibits protein synthesis, leading to cell death. Whereas mycobacterial RNA polymerase is susceptible to rifampin, eukaryotic RNA polymerase is not. High concentrations of rifamycin antibiotics, however, can affect mammalian mitochondrial RNA synthesis, as well as reverse transcriptases and viral DNA–dependent RNA polymerases.[62]

Pharmacokinetics and Toxicokinetics
When administered orally, rifampin reaches peak serum concentrations in 0.25 to 4 hours; foods, but not antacids, interfere with absorption.[109] Rifampin is secreted into the bile and undergoes enterohepatic recirculation. Although the recirculating antibiotic is deacetylated, the metabolite retains antimicrobial activity. The half-life of rifampin, which is normally 1.5 to 5 hours, increases in the setting of hepatic dysfunction. Additionally, rifampin autoinduces its metabolism to shorten its half-life by approximately 40%. Rifampin is distributed widely into body compartments, and imparts a reddish color

to all body fluids, including the cerebrospinal fluid,[62] and in this setting was erroneously identified as xanthochromia suggesting subarachnoid hemorrhage to the clinician.[72] Because mycobacteria rapidly develop resistance to rifampin, it should not be used as the sole therapy against TB.[62]

In large overdose, elimination half-life is observed within the normal range expected after therapeutic dosing. Transient elevation of bilirubin occurs, and is typically attributed to inhibited hepatic excretion of bilirubin or interference with the bilirubin assay because of the reddish color imparted to all body fluids, including serum.[166] Rifampin therapy carries greater teratogenic risk than other antituberculous therapies, with 4.4% incidence of malformation. Anencephaly, hydrocephalus, and congenital limb abnormality and dislocations are reported.[16,151] Rifampin is associated with hemorrhagic disease of the newborn[16] but is nevertheless compatible with breastfeeding because only minute amounts of rifampin are secreted into breast milk.[16,148]

Rifampin and rifapentine are FDA pregnancy class C, whereas rifabutin is FDA pregnancy class B (animal studies failed to demonstrate risk to the fetus, and no adequate human studies in pregnant women).

Drug–Drug Interactions

Rifamycins are potent inducers of CYP enzymes, which result in numerous drug interactions (Chap. 11). Of the rifamycins, rifampin has greater activity in inducing CYP3A4 than rifapentine; rifabutin has the least inductive activity of the class.[86] Rifampin also induces CYP1A2, CYP2C9, and CYP2C19.[173] Additionally, the ability of rifampin to induce CYP3A4 is strongly correlated with P-glycoprotein (P-gp) concentrations. P-glycoprotein is a transmembrane protein that functions as a cellular efflux pump of endogenous and exogenous xenobiotics; variations in expression of P-gp significantly affects the bioavailability of many xenobiotics and subsequent drug–drug interactions (Chaps. 9 and 11).[50] Concurrent administration of rifampin thus affects the metabolism of a wide array of drugs such as warfarin, cyclosporine, phenytoin, opioids, and oral contraceptives.[50,138,173] P-glycoprotein induction by rifampin is therefore responsible for a variety of pathophysiologic processes, including insufficient anticoagulation in patients receiving oral anticoagulants, acute graft rejection in transplant patients, graft versus host disease, difficulty controlling phenytoin concentrations, methadone withdrawal, and unplanned pregnancy. Effects arising from CYP3A4 induction begin within 5 to 6 days after rifampin is started and persist for up to 7 days after therapy is stopped.[62]

Rifamycins and HIV

Coinfection with both TB and HIV is common, causing approximately 4 million deaths per year worldwide. Approximately one-third of all patients with HIV also have TB, and concurrent highly active antiretroviral therapy (HAART) and antituberculous therapy decrease mortality.[161] However, many factors influence the efficacy and feasibility of treating these illnesses. There is decreased absorption of nearly all antituberculous medications in patients with advanced HIV caused by chronic diarrhea, intestinal pathogens, and general malabsorption. Also, there are many drug–drug interactions between antituberculous and HIV medications caused by alterations in absorption, cytochrome enzymes, P-gp transporters, and noncytochrome metabolism.[50,64,73,156] This often creates additive toxicities that compromise efficacy as well as compliance. This is particularly true when combining rifamycins and HIV medications. Toxic manifestations of individual xenobiotics are frequently additive, such as combining nevirapine and rifampin, both of which have risk of skin rash and hepatitis. Caution should be exercised when combining therapies, and individual toxicities should be reviewed to avoid cumulative effects. Table 56–1 lists common adverse effects and drug–drug interactions.

Clinical Manifestations
Acute Toxicity

The most common side effects of acute rifampin overdose are GI in nature consisting of epigastric pain, nausea, vomiting, and diarrhea.[45,62] The presence of diarrhea distinguishes rifampin ingestion from overdose of other antituberculous medications. At least 3 reported deaths are described from rifampin or rifampicin ingestion; an autopsy performed on one of these patients demonstrated the presence of pulmonary edema, although no causation was implied.[14,77,111] Other common effects include an anaphylactoid reaction manifested by flushing, urticarial rash, angioedema, and facial and periorbital edema. This occurs in both adults and children.[71] Central nervous system effects of overdose include fatigue, drowsiness, headache, dizziness, ataxia, confusion, and obtundation.[175] Anterior uveitis is occasionally observed, as are neurologic effects consisting of generalized numbness, extremity pain, ataxia, and muscular weakness.[61] Isolated rifamycin overdose infrequently produces serious acute effects.

Chronic Toxicity

When rifampin was originally introduced as an antituberculous medication, hepatitis occurred more frequently in patients taking combination therapy with INH than in those taking INH alone. These findings potentially arise from the ability of rifampin to induce cytochromes responsible for INH hepatotoxicity and not from direct hepatic injury by rifampin itself. Liver injury, when attributable to rifampin alone, is predominantly cholestatic, suggesting that clinical surveillance for hepatic injury is important as is regular biochemical monitoring.[45,102] Rifampin alters the metabolism of many other xenobiotics, including INH, pyrazinamide (PZA), and APAP, to increase their potential for hepatotoxicity.[45,102] Although some reports highlight increased compliance and typically mild and transient hepatotoxicity with combined rifampin and PZA treatment for latent TB infection, other recent studies suggest a significant risk of fatal hepatotoxicity, and the Centers for Disease Control and Prevention recommends generally avoiding this combination of drugs.[94]

A hypersensitivity reaction that is associated with rifampin therapy presents with an influenzalike syndrome. The antituberculous drug-induced hypersensitivity syndrome, formerly called DRESS syndrome (drug rash with eosinophilia and systemic symptoms), occurs in up to 20% of patients receiving high doses or intermittent (less than twice weekly) dosing and includes fever, chills, myalgias, eosinophilia, hemolytic anemia, thrombocytopenia, or interstitial nephritis (Chap. 17).[21,107] Acute kidney injury is likely related to hypersensitivity, is rarely oliguric, and is usually self-limited; patients usually recover with supportive care, although rechallenge with rifampin should be undertaken only with caution.[107]

The concomitant administration of rifampin and protease inhibitors results in increased rates of arthralgias, uveitis, leukopenia, and skin discoloration. Identical side effects occurred during the simultaneous administration of rifampin and CYP3A4 inhibitors such as clarithromycin, suggesting that toxic effects arise from elevated serum rifampin concentrations.[18] Current recommendations are that rifampin not be given with protease inhibitors, except for ritonavir in rare circumstances. In patients already taking protease inhibitors, rifabutin is recommended in place of rifampin.[110]

Diagnostic Testing and Management

Management of patients with acute rifampin overdose is primarily observational and supportive. Stabilization of vital signs is usually adequate, although clinicians should remain vigilant for toxicity from coingestants. Activated charcoal is reasonable, but not routinely recommended. For chronic toxicity, recognition of interactions between rifampin and other xenobiotics is critical. Hepatic function should be monitored because of the ability of rifampin to augment the hepatotoxicity of other xenobiotics. Treatment for hepatic injury involves withholding rifampin therapy and reassessing the appropriateness of other xenobiotics administered to the patient. Influenzalike symptoms and acute kidney injury secondary to rifampin characteristically respond to decreasing the interval between administration of the medication.[107] Although rifampin interacts with protease inhibitors, the utility of therapeutic drug monitoring is uncertain because the correlation of clinical events with serum concentrations of rifampin and antiretroviral drugs is unknown.[18]

ETHAMBUTOL

Pharmacology

Ethambutol is bacteriostatic against *Corynebacterium*, *Mycobacterium*, and *Nocardium* (CMN group) bacteria. It is most effective against mycobacteria, specifically *M. tuberculosis* and *Mycobacterium kansasii* as well as some other strains. Although it is a first-line tuberculostatic medication for TB, it is ineffective in monotherapy.[132]

Ethambutol inhibits arabinosyl transferases, interfering with biosynthesis of arabinogalactan and liparabinomannan, thus inhibiting polymerization of arabinose subunits within the arabinoglycan layer of mycobacterial cell walls.[62,77] Specifically, it blocks apical cell wall synthesis, blocking elongation growth but not cell division.[132]

Pharmacokinetics

Only the D(+) isomer is used therapeutically because the L(−) isomer is the major contributor to optic neuritis, but both enantiomers are bactericidal.[137] Ethambutol is taken up rapidly by growing cells, where bacteriostatic effects appear approximately 24 hours after incorporation by mycobacteria.[62] About 80% of an oral dose is absorbed, but both foods and antacids decrease absorption.[18,62] Maximum serum concentrations are reached within 4 hours of oral administration and are proportional to the dose. Ethambutol is approximately 20% to 30% protein bound and has a half-life of 4 to 6 hours.[62,83] Three-fourths of a standard dose is excreted unchanged in the urine by a combination of glomerular filtration and tubular secretion. Ethambutol clearance decreases with age, and this drug accumulates in patients with impaired glomerular filtration rate (GFR), making adjustments in dosing necessary in patients of advanced age or with kidney disease.[37,62] Increasingly, mutations in the *Mycobacterium embB* gene confer resistance to ethambutol, as high as 14.2%, with acquired resistance reaching nearly 40%.[77]

Ethambutol is FDA pregnancy class C, and is considered safe for use during pregnancy as a first-line medication. Although a 2.2% incidence of congenital abnormalities was identified in women receiving ethambutol therapy, no consistent pattern of abnormalities occurred in their offspring.[16] Although ethambutol is excreted into breast milk in approximately a 1:1 ratio with serum, it is considered to be compatible with breastfeeding.[16]

Clinical Manifestations and Management

Acute overdose of ethambutol is generally well tolerated, although at least one death is reported.[76] More commonly, nausea, abdominal pain, confusion, visual hallucinations, and optic neuropathy occur after acute ingestions of greater than 10 g.[44] Stabilization of vital signs is recommended, and although GI decontamination with activated charcoal was a hallmark of therapy, it is not routinely recommended. Clinicians must remain vigilant for coingestants, particularly INH. Hemodialysis is not recommended as treatment for multidrug ingestions including ethambutol.[44]

Although peripheral neuropathy and cutaneous reactions occur during chronic therapy, the most significant effect of the therapeutic use of ethambutol is unilateral or bilateral ocular toxicity presenting typically as painless blurring of vision, cecocentral scotomas (at and around the blind spot in the central field), and less commonly with decreased perception of color, and loss of peripheral vision. Ethambutol-induced optic neuropathy (EON) is largely dose and duration related and is typically reversible with drug discontinuation.[27,34,157] Optic neuritis develops in approximately 15% of patients receiving 50 mg/kg/day, 5% of patients receiving 25 mg/kg/day, and fewer than 1% of those receiving 15 mg/kg/day.[107] Patients develop ocular toxicity within 2 days of starting ethambutol and as long as 2 years after starting therapy. Age less than 60 years confers significantly greater likelihood

of full recovery with drug discontinuation.[150] The loss of peripheral vision and color discrimination that accompanies the optic neuropathy caused by ethambutol distinguishes this condition from the optic neuropathy secondary to INH.[72,107] Management of chronic toxicity from ethambutol involves cessation of therapy.

Ethambutol is a strong metal chelator, and inactivation of zinc and copper is believed to be related to its induction of retinal cell vacuoles and enlarged lysosomes. This interfere with membrane permeability, causing abnormal cell function and cell death.[34,81] The visual abnormalities induced by ethambutol are similar to those caused by a hereditary condition known as Leber optic neuropathy. Both ethambutol and Leber hereditary optic neuropathy affect oxidative phosphorylation through impairment of mitochondrial function.[33,81] Ethambutol appears to mimic this condition by binding intracellular copper, altering mitochondrial function, and producing neuronal injury.[69,81] Alternatively, alteration in zinc metabolism is believed to cause optic neuritis via progressive degeneration and irreversible neuronal destruction due to chelation of intracellular zinc, inducing vacuolar degeneration in retinal cultures.[34] The effect of this injury is a shift in the threshold for wavelength discrimination without changing the absolute sensitivity of the cone system, which leads to a loss of red–green discrimination.[145]

Diagnostic Testing and Management

All patients should receive neuroophthalmic testing before ethambutol therapy. The use of visual evoked potentials is especially useful in identifying subclinical optic nerve disease. Furthermore, patients should receive regular visual acuity examinations, and clinicians should encourage patients to report any subjective visual symptoms. The use of ethambutol is relatively contraindicated in children who are unable to comply with an ophthalmic examination.[72,107]

PYRAZINAMIDE

Pharmacology and Pharmacokinetics

Pyrazinamide is a structural analog of nicotinamide with a mechanism of action similar to that of INH. Similar to INH, PZA is a prodrug. Pyrazinamide requires deamidation to anionic pyrazinoic acid by pyrazinamidase, an endogenous cytoplasmic bacterial enzyme. In acidic conditions, PZA has enhanced antibacterial function, becoming protonated to the uncharged, active form, 5-hydroxypyrazinoic acid, which enters the cell, accumulates, and kills the bacteria by disruption of mycolic acid biosynthesis. Pyrazinamide is also active at neutral pH under certain conditions of decreased metabolism such as reduced temperature, which will facilitate drug susceptibility testing.[70] Pyrazinamide is effective against both active and dormant bacteria, and its use in antituberculous regimens shortens the course of therapy; however, resistance rapidly develops if it is used as single-agent therapy, and it should therefore only be used with other antituberculous medications.[62] After oral administration, pyrazinamide is rapidly absorbed, with maximum concentrations occurring within 1 to 2 hours of administration, and a half-life of approximately 9 hours. Hepatic metabolism to pyrazinoic acid and 5-hydroxypyrazinoic acid occurs with the metabolites subsequently renally excreted.[62] Drug clearance of PZA increases with continuing therapy, causing decreased serum pyrazinamide concentration within 1 to 2 months.[37] Pyrazinamide is synergistic with rifampin and has the greatest efficacy if administered during the first 2 months of treatment with both INH and rifampin; this regimen effectively shortens the treatment course to only 6 months.[176]

When introduced in the 1950s, PZA was administered in doses of 40 to 50 mg/kg for extended periods of time. The dosages produced clinical hepatitis, with manifestations of highly elevated aminotransferase and bilirubin concentrations. Of patients taking high-dose PZA, elevations in aminotransferases were identified in 20%, and symptomatic hepatitis was identified in 10%, with a small number of those who developed hepatitis dying from a fulminant hepatic failure. As a result of these findings, PZA was believed to be highly hepatotoxic, and its use was discouraged. The resurgence of multidrug-resistant mycobacteria, however, has forced clinicians to reconsider using PZA. Modern dosing regimens of 30 mg/kg for brief courses of 2 months infrequently produce hepatic injury, with some studies suggesting that addition of PZA to multidrug TB regimens confers no additional risk for hepatotoxicity.[45]

Pyrazinamide is FDA pregnancy class C, but is rarely used in pregnancy because the risk of poorly defined birth defects. There are examples of diagnosed patients diagnosed with tuberculosis in the first trimester (12 weeks) treated with a multidrug regimen including pyrazinamide who carried the pregnancy to term without any apparent complications.[55] Animal studies suggest that PZA has no teratogenicity at therapeutic doses.[1] Pyrazinamide is minimally excreted into breast milk and is presumed safe for breastfeeding.[16]

Diagnostic Testing

Proper dosing of PZA and short courses of therapy are the 2 most important factors in preventing toxicity. Treatment for hepatotoxicity involves cessation of PZA therapy in conjunction with supportive care.[45] Pyrazinamide inhibits the renal excretion of uric acid, and hyperuricemia results. More than 90% of children treated with short courses developed elevated uric acid concentrations.[130] Most patients, regardless of age, remain asymptomatic and do not develop symptoms of gout. Toxic effects from acute overdose of PZA have not been reported.

CYCLOSERINE

Cycloserine, previously avoided because of its adverse effects, is being used increasingly as second-line treatment with other tuberculostatic medications when treatment with primary antituberculous medications (INH, rifampin, ethambutol, and streptomycin) fail or as initial therapy when drug susceptibility testing indicates either MDR-TB or XDR-TB. Cycloserine is a structural analog of alanine and demonstrates inhibition of D-alanine racemase and D-alanine ligase, which are involved in peptidoglycan cell wall synthesis.[65] After oral doses, 70% to 90% of the drug is absorbed, and peak concentrations are reached in 3 to 8 hours. Cycloserine is distributed throughout all tissues and body fluids and easily crosses the blood–brain barrier. Less than 35% of the cycloserine is metabolized, and remaining xenobiotic is excreted unchanged in the urine.[62,178]

Toxicity is dose dependent and occurs in as many as 50% of patients taking cycloserine. Cycloserine is a partial agonist at the NMDA/glycine receptor, which contributes to neurologic effects such as somnolence, headache, tremor, dysarthria, vertigo, confusion, irritability, and seizures.[65] Psychiatric manifestations include paranoid reactions, depression, and suicidal ideation. Reversible hypersomnolence and asterixis are reported with cycloserine, suggesting reversible thalamic neurotoxicity, which is corroborated by magnetic resonance imaging.[82] Cycloserine is contraindicated in patients with a history of either seizures or depression. Whenever this drug is used, monitoring serum concentrations is recommended. Optimal treatment concentrations are between 20 and 35 mg/dL, and adverse effects are more common above 30 mg/dL. Cycloserine should be introduced slowly to avoid CNS toxicity.[72,107,178] Toxicity usually appears within the first 2 weeks of therapy and ceases upon discontinuation. Potentiation of toxicity due to ethanol consumption has been described. Because cycloserine is renally excreted, patients with impaired GFR are at increased risk of toxicity; it is removed by hemodialysis.[178] Cycloserine is FDA pregnancy class C. Although no teratogenic effects were noted in 3 women exposed to cycloserine during the first trimester of pregnancy, cycloserine is not recommended for use during pregnancy. Cord blood concentrations are approximately 70% of serum concentrations, and no adverse effects occurred in breastfed infants. Consequently, cycloserine is considered to be safe in women who are breastfeeding.[16] Reports of cycloserine overdose are scarce; however, use of peritoneal dialysis was reported in one case of intentional cycloserine ingestion in a woman

who had previously undergone a unilateral nephrectomy, with observation of improvement in CNS effects and effective decrease in serum concentrations of cycloserine.[4] In patients with evidence of CNS toxicity from cycloserine overdose and impaired renal function, it is reasonable to consider extracorporeal drug-removal.

OTHER ANTITUBERCULOUS MEDICATIONS

Ethionamide

para-Aminosalicylic acid

ETHIONAMIDE

Ethionamide, a congener of INH, is a prodrug converted to its active form, thioamide-*S*-oxide, by the bacterial cell by a flavoprotein monooxygenase enzyme. Ethionamide-*S*-oxide is believed to be further metabolized into another cytotoxic metabolite. These mycotoxic intermediary metabolites are thought to have a similar mechanism of action as INH, causing cell death from disruption of mycolic acid biosynthesis.[160] Ethionamide is rapidly absorbed, widely distributed, and crosses the blood–brain barrier. Oral doses yield peak serum concentrations within approximately 3 hours of administration. The half-life is approximately 2 hours. The most common adverse symptoms associated with ethionamide are GI irritation and anorexia. Toxic effects such as orthostatic hypotension, depression, and drowsiness are common. Rash, purpura, and gynecomastia are observed, as are tremor, paresthesias, and olfactory disturbances. It is structurally similar to methimazole, and thyroid dysfunction has occurred in several patients.[93] Approximately 5% of patients receiving ethionamide develop hepatitis. Patients using this medication should be screened intermittently for hepatic injury and thyroid function. Treatment for toxicity involves withholding ethionamide therapy.[62]

Ethionamide is FDA pregnancy class C. Birth defects were observed in 7 of 23 newborns exposed to ethionamide in utero, although a consistent pattern of anomalies was lacking. Data regarding the incidence and safety of breastfeeding while receiving ethionamide also are lacking.[16] Ethionamide is too toxic to be used as first-line therapy, but when needed, it should only be administered with another antituberculous medication because resistance develops rapidly when ethionamide is used alone.[62] Reports of ethionamide overdose are absent from the literature.

para-AMINOSALICYLIC ACID

para-Aminosalicylic acid (PAS) is a structural analog of *para*-aminobenzoic acid and appears to be a prodrug, acting as a metabolic precursor that is incorporated into the folate pathway, by dihydropteroate synthase (DHPS) and dihydrofolate synthase (DHFS) to generate a toxic hydroxyl dihydrofolate antimetabolite analog, which then inhibits dihydrofolate reductase (DHFR).[177] This inhibition occurs in mycobacteria but not in other organisms.[62] Despite common adverse effects, PAS is one of the last remaining available drugs effective against XDR-TB.[43] *para*-Aminosalicylic acid is readily absorbed from the gut and is rapidly distributed in all tissues, especially the pleural fluid and caseous material. A population based determination of volume of distribution was 79 L in a study of adult volunteers.[28] *para*-Aminosalicylic acid has a half-life of approximately one hour and is renally excreted. Adverse effects of PAS occur in 10% to 30% of patients and include anorexia, nausea, vomiting, diarrhea, sore throat, and malaise. Between 5% and 10% of patients receiving PAS develop hypersensitivity reactions characterized by high fever, rash, and arthralgias. Hematologic abnormalities of agranulocytosis, leukopenia, eosinophilia, thrombocytopenia, and acute hemolytic anemia are reported.[62] *para*-Aminosalicylic acid was removed by hemodialysis in patients with kidney failure in small amounts, but is of uncertain clinical use.[90] Adverse effects associated with chronic therapy are typically treated by termination of use. Data regarding the safety of PAS in pregnancy and breastfeeding are lacking.[16] Reports of PAS overdose are absent from the literature.

Capreomycin

Capreomycin is a cyclic polypeptide currently used more frequently because of its antibacterial activity against MDR-TB and intracellular TB bacilli. Strains of Mycoplasma that are resistant to more than one aminoglycoside are characteristically susceptible to this polypeptide. Capreomycin interferes with ribosomes and inhibits protein translation but also appears to act by other mechanisms such as alterations in topoisomerase or the glyoxylate shunt pathway.[53] Because of poor absorption after oral dosing, capreomycin must be administered intramuscularly. Toxicity associated with capreomycin use includes tinnitus, hearing loss, proteinuria, and electrolyte disturbances, although severe acute kidney injury is rare. Risk of toxicity is increased in patients with chronic kidney disease and the elderly.[117] Eosinophilia, leukocytosis, and rashes are described. Pain and sterile abscesses at the site of capreomycin injection are reported.[62] Capreomycin is FDA pregnancy class C. Data are lacking regarding the safety of capreomycin in pregnancy and breastfeeding.[16] Capreomycin overdose is not described.

BEDAQUILINE

Pharmacology and Pharmacokinetics

Bedaquiline is a diarylquinoline that received conditional approval in 2012 by the US Food and Drug Administration for the treatment of MDR-TB.[51] It exerts its antituberculous effects via inhibition of mycobacterial ATP synthase.[3] Bedaquiline is relatively slowly absorbed after oral administration, with peak plasma concentrations achieved at 4 to 6 hours.[39,119] Absorption is enhanced approximately 2-fold when bedaquiline is taken with food.[51] Bedaquiline is more than 99% protein bound and has an estimated volume of distribution of 164 L in adults.[159] Bedaquiline is metabolized primarily by CYP3A4 via demethylation to the biologically active N-desmethyl bedaquiline, which has 3- to 6-fold lower antimycobacterial activity than its parent compound; CYP2C8 and 2C19 are also implicated in bedaquiline metabolism to a lesser extent.[87] Bedaquiline is primarily excreted in the feces.[36] The terminal half-life for bedaquiline and N-desmethyl bedaquiline is estimated to be 5.5 months, likely reflecting prolonged redistribution from tissues.[38] Bedaquiline overdose has not been described. Bedaquiline is FDA pregnancy class B.

Adverse Effects

In pooled clinical trials, the most frequently reported adverse effects included nausea, vomiting, headache, arthralgias; additional adverse effects included dizziness, elevated aminotransferases, myalgias, diarrhea, and QT interval prolongation.[51] Notably, one phase 2 clinical trial (C208 Stage 2) revealed an increased number of deaths in the group receiving bedaquiline (10 of 79) as compared to the placebo group (2 of 81) when bedaquiline was added to standard antituberculous regimen.[40] However, there were no sudden deaths reported, no association between plasma concentration of bedaquiline and mortality, and no clear pattern in the causes of death; the reason for the mortality imbalance remains unclear awaiting the results of further safety trials.[40,168]

Recommended Dosing

The current recommended bedaquiline regimen for treatment of MDR-TB consists of a 2-week loading dose of 400 mg daily, then 200 mg 3 times a week to complete a 24-week course.[51]

Drug–Drug Interactions

Concomitant administration with rifamycins increases clearance of bedaquiline 5-fold, and significantly decreases serum concentration of bedaquiline; this practice should be avoided pending further evaluation of the safety profile of bedaquiline.[153,168] Similarly, the planned use of bedaquiline in patients who are taking antiretrovirals that are strong CYP3A4 inducers, such as efavirenz, will likely require alteration of the antiretroviral regimen.[168] Bedaquiline should be used with caution in patients who are also taking medications

that inhibit CYP3A4, as these are expected to lead to higher serum concentration of bedaquiline and potential resultant toxicity; there are currently no data regarding appropriate dose adjustments in these situations.[168]

Monitoring

Monitoring of serum potassium, magnesium and calcium concentrations, as well as aminotransferases (AST and ALT), is recommended at baseline and then monthly thereafter while taking bedaquiline.[168] Because of the dysrhythmogenic effects due to QT interval prolongation, an ECG should be obtained prior to initiation of treatment with bedaquiline, and at weeks 2, 4, 8, 12, and 24 after starting treatment.[168] Monthly ECGs are recommended in patients taking bedaquiline concurrently with other QT interval prolonging xenobiotics.[168]

Reports of overdose are lacking from the medical literature.

DELAMANID

Delamanid, a nitro-dihydro-imidazo-oxazole derivative, is a new antituberculous medication that received conditional approval in 2014 from the European Medicines Agency and the Japanese drug regulatory authority; it is not currently approved by the FDA.[120] Delamanid is a prodrug and requires activation by mycobacterial nitroreductase Rv 3547.[92] It exerts its effects by inhibiting synthesis of methoxymycolic and ketomycolic acids resulting in destabilization of the mycobacterial cell wall; in contrast with INH, it does not inhibit α-mycolic acid synthesis.[92]

The pharmacologic profile of delamanid has yet to be satisfactorily determined. Delamanid is administered orally, and absorption is enhanced when it is taken with food.[57] It is poorly water soluble, and more than 99% protein bound, with a large V_d over 2,000 L in adults.[89,123] Its metabolism is complex and shows significant interspecies variation: in humans, the 6-nitro-2,3-dihydro-imidazo-oxazole moiety is cleaved by plasma albumin to form the metabolite DM-6705, which is then degraded by multiple metabolic pathways, primary of which is hydroxylation and subsequent oxidation by CYP3A4.[129,139] Delamanid has a plasma half-life of 38 hours.[57]

Delamanid does not inhibit or induce CYP enzymes in vitro; its metabolites demonstrate some inhibition of CYP enzymes but only at concentrations much higher than would be encountered in clinical use.[140]

The recommended delamanid regimen is 100 mg orally twice daily for 24 weeks.[168] Adverse effects reported with delamanid therapy include nausea, vomiting, tinnitus, headache, palpitations, and QT interval prolongation.[57,168] Because of its potential dysrhythmogenic effects due to QT interval prolongation, an ECG should be obtained before initiation of treatment with delamanid, and at weeks 2, 4, 8, 12, and 24 after starting treatment.[168] Monthly ECGs are recommended in patients taking delamanid concurrently with other QT interval prolonging xenobiotics. Delamanid overdose is not described in the literature.

Many other antibiotics and immunomodulators that were overlooked or rejected for the management of TB are increasingly being used as part of multidrug regimens against resistant strains. Discussed more extensively in Chap. 54, these include fluoroquinolones such as ciprofloxacin, ofloxacin, levofloxacin, moxifloxacin, sparfloxacin; macrolides such as clarithromycin, aminoglycosides such as amikacin, streptomycin, kanamycin; interferon, amoxicillin–clavulanate, linezolid, and clofazimine.[100]

Additionally, as the prevalence of drug-resistant tuberculosis continues to increase, one novel strategy that has emerged involves the development of adjunctive therapies to enhance the effectiveness of existing medications.[118] In vitro and animal experiments have demonstrated the efficacy of a small molecule transcriptional repressor to enhance the conversion of the prodrug ethionamide to its active metabolite and to reverse acquired ethionamide resistance and clear ethionamide-resistant mycobacterial infection in mice.[8] By developing therapeutics to activate alternate mycobacterial transcription pathways and augment conversion of prodrugs within the target organism, this innovative approach may increase antimycobacterial activity without increasing risk of systemic toxicity to humans and may help to circumvent the mycobacterial enzyme mutations that underlie resistance to many antituberculous medications.

SUMMARY

- Certain antituberculous medications are potentially fatal in overdose.
- Patients acutely poisoned with INH require immediate and appropriate action to terminate seizures, with the specific antidote pyridoxine, commonly augmented by benzodiazepines.
- Although less common than previously believed, hepatocellular injury resulting from therapeutic dosing of INH requires regularly scheduled, frequent evaluations to prevent fulminant hepatic failure.
- With the increasing prevalence of MDR-TB and XDR-TB strains, antituberculous medications previously avoided or ignored are now being used typically in combination with 2 or more other antituberculous medications. Despite reduced dosages compared with those previously used, significant adverse effects remain a concern.
- Rifampin participates in numerous drug–drug interactions, some involving several antiretroviral therapies. Because antituberculous medications are commonly needed in HIV-infected patients, potential interactions between rifampin and antiretrovirals should remind clinicians to remain vigilant for unanticipated adverse effects.
- Patients receiving ethambutol, pyrazinamide, and other antituberculous medications benefit from careful surveillance for specific adverse effects such as decreased visual acuity, hepatic injury, and psychiatric manifestations. Despite the toxicity of this class of medications, rapid recognition of toxicity is typically responsive to intervention.

Acknowledgment

Edward W. Boyer, PhD, MD, contributed to this chapter in previous editions.

REFERENCES

1. Al-Hajjaj MS, et al. Evaluation of the teratogenic potential of pyrazinamide in Wistar rats. *Ups J Med Sci.* 1999;104:259-270.
2. Alao AO, Yolles JC. Isoniazid-induced psychosis. *Ann Pharmacother.* 1998;32:889-891.
3. Andries K, et al. A diarylquinoline drug active on the ATP synthase of *Mycobacterium tuberculosis. Science.* 2005;307:223-227.
4. Atkins R, et al. Acute poisoning by cycloserine. *Br Med J.* 1965;1:907-908.
5. Babalik A, et al. Therapeutic drug monitoring in the treatment of active tuberculosis. *Can Respir J.* 2011;18:225-229.
6. Bear ES, et al. Suicidal ingestion of isoniazid: an uncommon cause of metabolic acidosis and seizures. *South Med J.* 1976;69:31-32.
7. Blanchard PD, et al. Isoniazid overdose in the Cambodian population of Olmsted County, Minnesota. *JAMA.* 1986;256:3131-3133.
8. Blondiaux N, et al. Reversion of antibiotic resistance in *Mycobacterium tuberculosis* by spiroisoxazoline SMARt-420. *Science.* 2017;355:1206-1211.
9. Bloom BR, Murray CJL. Tuberculosis: commentary on a reemergent killer. *Science.* 1992;257:1055-1064.
10. Blowey DL, et al. Isoniazid-associated rhabdomyolysis. *Am J Emerg Med.* 1995;13:543-544.
11. Blumberg EA, Gil RA. Cerebellar syndrome caused by isoniazid. *DICP.* 1990;24:829-831.
12. Boxenbaum HG, Riegelman S. Pharmacokinetics of isoniazid and some metabolites in man. *J Pharmacokinet Biopharm.* 1976;4:287-325.
13. Brent J, et al. Reversal of prolonged isoniazid-induced coma by pyridoxine. *Arch Intern Med.* 1990;150:1751-1753.
14. Broadwell RO, et al. Suicide by rifampin overdose. *JAMA.* 1978;240:2283-2284.
15. Bromberg YM, et al. Placental transmission of isonicotinic acid hydrazide. *Gynecol Obstet Invest.* 1955;140:141-144.
16. Brost BC, Newman RB. The maternal and fetal effects of tuberculosis therapy. *Obstet Gynecol Clin North Am.* 1997;24:659-673.
17. Brown CV. Acute isoniazid poisoning. *Am Rev Respir Dis.* 1972;105:206-216.
18. Burman WJ, et al. Therapeutic implications of drug interactions in the treatment of human immunodeficiency virus-related tuberculosis. *Clin Infect Dis.* 1999;28:419-429, quiz 430.
19. Byrd CB. Isoniazid toxicity. A prospective study in secondary chemoprophylaxis. *JAMA.* 1972;220:1471-1473.
20. Cameron WM. Isoniazid overdose. *CMAJ.* 1978;118:1413-1415.
21. Carr DF, et al. 7th drug hypersensitivity meeting: part one. *Clin Transl Allergy.* 2016;6:1-35.
22. Cash JM, Zawada ET. Isoniazid overdose. Successful treatment with pyridoxine and hemodialysis. *West J Med.* 1991;155:644-646.
23. Centers for Disease Control and Prevention (CDC). Latent tuberculosis infection: a guide for primary health care providers. https://www.cdc.gov/tb/publications/ltbi/treatment.htm. Accessed August 4, 2017.
24. Centers for Disease Control and Prevention (CDC). Fact sheet: extensively drug-resistant tuberculosis (XDR TB). https://www.cdc.gov/tb/publications/factsheets/drtb/xdrtb.htm. Accessed May 4, 2017.
25. Centers for Disease Control and Prevention (CDC). Tuberculosis (TB). https://www.cdc.gov/tb/statistics/. Accessed May 2, 2017.
26. Centers for Disease Control and Prevention (CDC). Tuberculosis in the United States. https://www.cdc.gov/tb/statistics/surv/surv2015/default.htm. Accessed May 4, 2017.
27. Chan RYC, Kwok AKH. Ocular toxicity of ethambutol. *Hong Kong Med J.* 2006;12:56-60.
28. Chang MJ, et al. Population pharmacokinetics of moxifloxacin, cycloserine, *p*-aminosalicylic acid and kanamycin for the treatment of multi-drug-resistant tuberculosis. *Int J Antimicrob Agents.* 2017;49:677-687.
29. Chien JY, et al. Influence of polymorphic *N*-acetyltransferase phenotype on the inhibition and induction of acetaminophen bioactivation with long-term isoniazid. *Clin Pharmacol Ther.* 1997;61:24-34.
30. Chin L, et al. Convulsions as the etiology of lactic acidosis in acute isoniazid toxicity in dogs. *Toxicol Appl Pharmacol.* 1979;49:377-384.
31. Chin L, et al. Potentiation of pyridoxine by depressants and anticonvulsants in the treatment of acute isoniazid intoxication in dogs. *Toxicol Appl Pharmacol.* 1981;58:504-509.
32. Chin L, et al. Evaluation of diazepam and pyridoxine as antidotes to isoniazid intoxication in rats and dogs. *Toxicol Appl Pharmacol.* 1978;45:713-722.
33. Chowdhury D, et al. Leber's hereditary optic neuropathy masquerading as ethambutol-Induced optic neuropathy in a young male. *Ind J Ophthalmol.* 2006;54:218.
34. Chung H, et al. Ethambutol-induced toxicity is mediated by zinc and lysosomal membrane permeabilization in cultured retinal cells. *Toxicol Appl Pharmacol.* 2009;235:163-170.
35. Coyer JR, Nicholson DP. Isoniazid-induced convulsions. *South Med J.* 1976;69:294-297.
36. Cuyckens F, et al. Use of the bromine isotope ratio in HPLC-ICP-MS and HPLC-ESI-MS analysis of a new drug in development. *Anal Bioanal Chem.* 2008;390:1717-1729.
37. Denti P, et al. Pharmacokinetics of isoniazid, pyrazinamide, and ethambutol in newly diagnosed pulmonary TB patients in Tanzania. *PLoS One.* 2015;10:e0141002.
38. Diacon AH, et al. Randomized pilot trial of eight weeks of bedaquiline (TMC207) treatment for multidrug-resistant tuberculosis: long-term outcome, tolerability, and effect on emergence of drug resistance. *Antimicrob Agents Chemother.* 2012;56:3271-3276.
39. Diacon AH, et al. The diarylquinoline TMC207 for multidrug-resistant tuberculosis. *N Engl J Med.* 2009;360:2397-2405.
40. Diacon AH, et al. Multidrug-resistant tuberculosis and culture conversion with bedaquiline. *N Engl J Med.* 2014;371:723-732.
41. DiMartini A. Isoniazid, tricyclics and the "cheese reaction." *Int Clin Psychopharmacol.* 1995;10:197-198.
42. Dockweiler U. Isoniazid-induced valproic-acid toxicity, or vice versa. *Lancet.* 1987;2:152.
43. Donald PR, Diacon AH. *para*-Aminosalicylic acid: the return of an old friend. *Lancet Infect Dis.* 2015;15:1091-1099.
44. Ducobu J, et al. Acute isoniazid/ethambutol/rifampicin overdosage. *Lancet.* 1982;1:632.
45. Durand F, et al. Hepatotoxicity of antitubercular treatments. Rationale for monitoring liver status. *Drug Saf.* 1996;15:394-405.
46. Durand F, et al. Antituberculous therapy and acute liver failure. *Lancet.* 1995;345:1170.
47. Ellard GA. The potential clinical significance of the isoniazid acetylator phenotype in the treatment of pulmonary tuberculosis. *Tubercle.* 1984;65:211-227.
48. Farrell FJ, et al. Treatment of hepatic failure secondary to isoniazid hepatitis with liver transplantation. *Dig Dis Sci.* 1994;39:2255-2259.
49. Farrell GC. Drug-induced hepatic injury. *J Gastroenterol Hepatol.* 1997;12:S242-S250.
50. Finch CK, et al. Rifampin and rifabutin drug interactions: an update. *Arch Intern Med.* 2002;162:985-992.
51. Food and Drug Administration. *Anti-Infective Drugs Advisory Committee Meeting Briefing Document TMC207 (Bedaquiline) Treatment of Patients with MDR-TB NDA 204-384 28 November 2012.* Silver Spring, MD: FDA; 2012:1-253. https://www.fda.gov/downloads/advisorycommittees/committeesmeetingmaterials/drugs/anti-infectivedrugsadvisorycommittee/ucm329260.pdf.
52. Franks AL, et al. Isoniazid hepatitis among pregnant and postpartum Hispanic patients. *Public Health Rep.* 1989;104:151-155.
53. Fu LM, Shinnick TM. Genome-wide exploration of the drug action of capreomycin on *Mycobacterium tuberculosis* using Affymetrix oligonucleotide GeneChips. *J Infect.* 2007;54:277-284.
54. Gannon R, et al. Isoniazid, meperidine, and hypotension. *Ann Intern Med.* 1983;99:415.
55. Garg K, Mohapatra PR. A pregnant woman with dyspnoea, fever & decreased vision. *Indian J Med Res.* 2012;136:1062.
56. Gent WL, et al. Factors in hydrazine formation from isoniazid by paediatric and adult tuberculosis patients. *Eur J Clin Pharmacol.* 1992;43:131-136.
57. Gler MT, et al. Delamanid for multidrug-resistant pulmonary tuberculosis. *N Engl J Med.* 2012;366:2151-2160.
58. Gnam W, et al. Isoniazid-induced hallucinosis: response to pyridoxine. *Psychosomatics.* 1993;34:537-539.

59. Goel UC, et al. Isoniazid induced neuropathy in slow versus rapid acetylators: an electrophysiological study. *J Assoc Physicians India*. 1992;40:671-672.
60. González-Gay MA, et al. Optic neuritis following treatment with isoniazid in a hemodialyzed patient. *Nephron*. 1993;63:360.
61. Griffith DE, et al. Adverse events associated with high-dose rifabutin in macrolide-containing regimens for the treatment of *Mycobacterium avium* complex lung disease. *Clin Infect Dis*. 1995;21:594-598.
62. Gumbo T. Chemotherapy of tuberculosis, *Mycobacterium avium* complex disease and Leprosy. In: Brunton LL, et al., eds. *Goodman and Gilmans the Pharmcological Basis of Therapeutics*. 12th ed. New York, NY: McGraw-Hill.
63. Gurumurthy P, et al. Lack of relationship between hepatic toxicity and acetylator phenotype in three thousand South Indian patients during treatment with isoniazid for tuberculosis. *Am Rev Respir Dis*. 1984;129:58-61.
64. Gurumurthy P, et al. Decreased bioavailability of rifampin and other antituberculosis drugs in patients with advanced human immunodeficiency virus disease. *Antimicrob Agents Chemother*. 2004;48:4473-4475.
65. Halouska S, et al. Use of NMR metabolomics to analyze the targets of D-cycloserine in mycobacteria: role of D-alanine racemase. *J Proteome Res*. 2007;6:4608-4614.
66. Hankins DG, et al. Profound acidosis caused by isoniazid ingestion. *Am J Emerg Med*. 1987;5:165-166.
67. Hasagawa T, et al. Successful liver transplantation for isoniazid-induced hepatic failure—a case report. *Transplantation*. 1994;57:1274-1277.
68. Hauser MJ, Baier H. Interactions of isoniazid with foods. *Drug Intell Clin Pharm*. 1982;16:617-618.
69. Heng JE, et al. Ethambutol is toxic to retinal ganglion cells via an excitotoxic pathway. *Invest Ophthalmol Vis Sci*. 1999;40:190-196.
70. Hertog den AL, et al. Pyrazinamide is active against *Mycobacterium tuberculosis* cultures at neutral pH and low temperature. *Antimicrob Agents Chemother*. 2016;60:4956-4960.
71. Holdiness MR. A review of the Redman syndrome and rifampicin overdosage. *Med Toxicol Adverse Drug Exp*. 1989;4:444-451.
72. Holdiness MR. Neurological manifestations and toxicities of the antituberculosis drugs. A review. *Med Toxicol*. 1987;2:33-51.
73. Holland DP, et al. Therapeutic drug monitoring of antimycobacterial drugs in patients with both tuberculosis and advanced human immunodeficiency virus infection. *Pharmacotherapy*. 2009;29:503-510.
74. Holtz P, Palm D. Pharmacological aspects of vitamin B₆. *Pharmacol Rev*. 1964;16:113-178.
75. Hurwitz A, Schlozman DL. Effects of antacids on gastrointestinal absorption of isoniazid in rat and man. *Am Rev Respir Dis*. 1974;109:41-47.
76. Jack DB, et al. Fatal rifampicin-ethambutol overdosage. *Lancet*. 1978;312:1107-1108.
77. Jain A, et al. Novel mutations in emb B gene of ethambutol resistant isolates of *Mycobacterium tuberculosis*: a preliminary report. *Indian J Med Res*. 2008;128:634-639.
78. Kalsi SS, et al. Does cytochrome P450 liver isoenzyme induction increase the risk of liver toxicity after paracetamol overdose? *Open Access Emerg Med*. 2011;3:69-76.
79. Kocabay G, et al. Optic neuritis and bitemporal hemianopsia associated with isoniazid treatment in end-stage renal failure. *Int J Tuberc Lung Dis*. 2006;10:1418-1419.
80. Kopanoff DE, et al. Isoniazid-related hepatitis: a U.S. Public Health Service cooperative surveillance study. *Am Rev Respir Dis*. 1978;117:991-1001.
81. Kozak SF, et al. The role of copper on ethambutol's antimicrobial action and implications for ethambutol-induced optic neuropathy. *Diagn Microbiol Infect Dis*. 1998;30:83-87.
82. Kwon H-M, et al. Cycloserine-induced encephalopathy: evidence on brain MRI. *Eur J Neurol*. 2008;15:e60-e61.
83. Lee CS, et al. Kinetics of oral ethambutol in the normal subject. *Clin Pharmacol Ther*. 1977;22(5, pt 1):615-621.
84. Lejonc JL, et al. Paroxystic hypertension after ingestion of gruyere cheese during isoniazide treatment: a report on two cases [in French]. *Ann Med Interne (Paris)*. 1980;131:346-348.
85. Lenke RR, et al. Severe fetal deformities associated with ingestion of excessive isoniazid in early pregnancy. *Acta Obstet Gynecol Scand*. 1985;64:281-282.
86. Li AP, et al. Primary human hepatocytes as a tool for the evaluation of structure-activity relationship in cytochrome P450 induction potential of xenobiotics: evaluation of rifampin, rifapentine and rifabutin. *Chem Biol Interact*. 1997;107:17-30.
87. Liu K, et al. Bedaquiline metabolism: enzymes and novel metabolites. *Drug Metab Dispos*. 2014;42:863-866.
88. Lopez-Samblas A, Tsiligiannis T. Isoniazid intoxication in three adolescent patients. *Hosp Pharm*. 1991;26:119.
89. Szumowski J, Lynch J. Profile of delamanid for the treatment of multidrug-resistant tuberculosis. *Drug Des Devel Ther*. 2015;9:677-682.
90. Malone RS, et al. The effect of hemodialysis on cycloserine, ethionamide, para-aminosalicylate, and clofazimine. *Chest*. 1999;116:984-990.
91. Martinez-Roíg A, et al. Acetylation phenotype and hepatotoxicity in the treatment of tuberculosis in children. *Pediatrics*. 1986;77:912-915.
92. Matsumoto M, et al. OPC-67683, a nitro-dihydro-imidazooxazole derivative with promising action against tuberculosis in vitro and in mice. *PLoS Med*. 2006;3:e466.
93. McDonnell ME, et al. Hypothyroidism due to ethionamide. *N Engl J Med*. 2005;352:2757-2759.
94. McElroy PD, et al. National survey to measure rates of liver injury, hospitalization, and death associated with rifampin and pyrazinamide for latent tuberculosis infection. *Clin Infect Dis*. 2005;41:1125-1133.
95. Mdluli K, et al. Inhibition of a *Mycobacterium tuberculosis* beta-ketoacyl ACP synthase by isoniazid. *Science*. 1998;280:1607-1610.
96. Metushi IG, et al. A fresh look at the mechanism of isoniazid-induced hepatotoxicity. *Clin Pharmacol Ther*. 2011;89:911-914.
97. Michael OS, et al. Adverse events to first line anti-tuberculosis drugs in patients co-infected with HIV and tuberculosis. *Ann Ib Postgrad Med*. 2016;14:21-29.
98. Miki M, et al. An outbreak of histamine poisoning after ingestion of the ground saury paste in eight patients taking isoniazid in tuberculous ward. *Intern Med*. 2005;44:1133-1136.
99. Miller J, et al. Acute isoniazid poisoning in childhood. *Am J Dis Child*. 1980;134:290-292.
100. Mitnick CD, et al. Comprehensive treatment of extensively drug-resistant tuberculosis. *N Engl J Med*. 2008;359:563-574.
101. Nelson SD, et al. Isoniazid and iproniazid: activation of metabolites to toxic intermediates in man and rat. *Science*. 1976;193:901-903.
102. Nicod L, et al. Rifampicin and isoniazid increase acetaminophen and isoniazid cytotoxicity in human HepG2 hepatoma cells. *Hum Exp Toxicol*. 2017;16:28-34.
103. Nolan CM, et al. Hepatotoxicity associated with isoniazid preventive therapy: a 7-year survey from a public health tuberculosis clinic. *JAMA*. 1999;281:1014-1018.
104. Orlowski JP, et al. Treatment of a potentially lethal dose isoniazid ingestion. *Ann Emerg Med*. 1988;17:73-76.
105. Pahl MV, et al. Association of beta hydroxybutyric acidosis with isoniazid intoxication. *J Toxicol Clin Toxicol*. 1984;22:167-176.
106. Panganiban LR, et al. Rhabdomyolysis in isoniazid poisoning. *J Toxicol Clin Toxicol*. 2001;39:143-151.
107. Patel AM, McKeon J. Avoidance and management of adverse reactions to antituberculosis drugs. *Drug Saf*. 1995;12:1-25.
108. Paulsen O, et al. No interaction between H2 blockers and isoniazid. *Eur J Respir Dis*. 1986;68:286-290.
109. Peloquin CA, et al. Pharmacokinetics of isoniazid under fasting conditions, with food, and with antacids. *Int J Tuberc Lung Dis*. 1999;3:703-710.
110. Piscitelli SC, Gallicano KD. Interactions among drugs for HIV and opportunistic infections. http://dxdoiorg/101056/NEJM200103293441307. 2009;344:984-996.
111. Plomp TA, et al. A case of fatal poisoning by rifampicin. *Arch Toxicol*. 1981;48:245-252.
112. Puri MM, et al. Seizures with single therapeutic dose of isoniazid. *Indian J Tuberc*. 2012;59:100-102.
113. Quemard A, et al. Binding of catalase-peroxidase-activated isoniazid to wild-type and mutant *Mycobacterium tuberculosis* enoyl-ACP reductases. *J Am Chem Soc*. 1996;118:1561-1562.
114. Quémard A, et al. Enzymatic characterization of the target for isoniazid in *Mycobacterium tuberculosis*. *Biochemistry*. 1995;34:8235-8241.
115. Raviglione MC, Smith IM. XDR tuberculosis—implications for global public health. *N Engl J Med*. 2007;356:656-659.
116. Rawat R, et al. The isoniazid-NAD adduct is a slow, tight-binding inhibitor of InhA, the *Mycobacterium tuberculosis* enoyl reductase: adduct affinity and drug resistance. *Proc Natl Acad Sci U S A*. 2003;100:13881-13886.
117. Reisfeld B, et al. A physiologically based pharmacokinetic model for capreomycin. *Antimicrob Agents Chemother*. 2012;56:926-934.
118. Rubin EJ. Reviving a drug for tuberculosis? *N Engl J Med*. 2017;376:2292-2294.
119. Rustomjee R, et al. Early bactericidal activity and pharmacokinetics of the diarylquinoline TMC207 in treatment of pulmonary tuberculosis. *Antimicrob Agents Chemother*. 2008;52:2831-2835.
120. Ryan NJ, Lo JH. Delamanid: first global approval. *Drugs*. 2014;74:1041-1045.
121. Saad SF, et al. Influence of certain anticonvulsants on the concentration of γ-aminobutyric acid in the cerebral hemispheres of mice. *Eur J Pharmacol*. 1972;17:386-392.
122. Saktiawati AMI, et al. Impact of food on the pharmacokinetics of first-line anti-TB drugs in treatment-naive TB patients: a randomized cross-over trial. *J Antimicrob Chemother*. 2016;71:703-710.
123. Saliu OY, et al. Bactericidal activity of OPC-67683 against drug-tolerant *Mycobacterium tuberculosis*. *J Antimicrob Chemother*. 2007;60:994-998.
124. Salkind AR, Hewitt CC. Coma from long-term overingestion of isoniazid. *Arch Intern Med*. 1997;157:2518-2520.
125. Salpeter SR. Fatal isoniazid-induced hepatitis. Its risk during chemoprophylaxis. *West J Med*. 1993;159:560-564.
126. Sanders BM, Draper GJ. Childhood cancer and drugs in pregnancy. *BMJ*. 1979;1:717-718.
127. Santucci KA, et al. Acute isoniazid exposures and antidote availability. *Pediatr Emerg Care*. 1999;15:99-101.
128. Sarzi-Puttini P, et al. Drug-induced lupus erythematosus. *Autoimmunity*. 2005;38:507-518.
129. Sasahara K, et al. Pharmacokinetics and metabolism of delamanid, a novel anti-tuberculosis drug, in animals and humans: importance of albumin metabolism in vivo. *Drug Metab Dispos*. 2015;43:1267-1276.
130. Sánchez-Albisua I, et al. Tolerance of pyrazinamide in short course chemotherapy for pulmonary tuberculosis in children. *Pediatr Infect Dis J*. 1997;16:760-763.

131. Schreiber J, et al. Lymphocyte transformation test for the evaluation of adverse effects of antituberculous drugs. *Eur J Med Res.* 1999;4:67-71.

132. Schubert K, et al. The antituberculosis drug ethambutol selectively blocks apical growth in CMN group bacteria. *MBio.* 2017;8:e02213-e02216.

133. Scolding N, et al. Charcoal and isoniazid pharmacokinetics. *Hum Toxicol.* 1986;5:285-286.

134. Scott C, et al; Centers for Disease Control and Prevention (CDC). Tuberculosis trends—United States, 2014. *MMWR Morb Mortal Wkly Rep.* 2015;64:265-269.

135. Scott EM, Wright RC. Fluorometric determination of isonicotinic acid hydrazide in serum. *J Lab Clin Med.* 1967;70:355-360.

136. Self TH, et al. Isoniazid drug and food interactions. *Am J Med Sci.* 1999;317:304-311.

137. Sheldon R. *Chirotechnology: Industrial Synthesis of Optically Active Compounds.* New York, NY: Marcel Dekker.

138. Shenfield GM. Oral contraceptives. Are drug interactions of clinical significance? *Drug Saf.* 1993;9:21-37.

139. Shimokawa Y, et al. Metabolic mechanism of delamanid, a new anti-tuberculosis drug, in human plasma. *Drug Metab Dispos.* 2015;43:1277-1283.

140. Shimokawa Y, et al. Delamanid does not inhibit or induce cytochrome p450 enzymes in vitro. *Biol Pharm Bull.* 2014;37:1727-1735.

141. Siefkin AD, et al. Isoniazid overdose: pharmacokinetics and effects of oral charcoal in treatment. *Hum Toxicol.* 1987;6:497-501.

142. Singh J, et al. Hepatotoxicity due to antituberculosis therapy. Clinical profile and reintroduction of therapy. *J Clin Gastroenterol.* 1996;22:211-214.

143. Singh N, et al. Transfer of isoniazid from circulation to breast milk in lactating women on chronic therapy for tuberculosis. *Br J Clin Pharmacol.* 2008;65:418-422.

144. Siskind MS, et al. Isoniazid-induced neurotoxicity in chronic dialysis patients: report of three cases and a review of the literature. *Nephron.* 1993;64:303-306.

145. Sjoerdsma T, et al. Modulating wavelength discrimination in goldfish with ethambutol and stimulus intensity. *Vision Res.* 1996;36:3519-3525.

146. Skinner K, et al. Isoniazid poisoning: pharmacokinetics and effect of hemodialysis in a massive ingestion. *Hemodial Int.* 2015;19:E37-E40.

147. Smith CK, Durack DT. Isoniazid and reaction to cheese. *Ann Intern Med.* 1978;88:520-521.

148. Snider DE, Powell KE. Should women taking antituberculosis drugs breast-feed? *Arch Intern Med.* 1984;144:589-590.

149. Snider DE. Pyridoxine supplementation during isoniazid therapy. *Tubercle.* 1980;61:191-196.

150. Song W, Si S. The rare ethambutol-induced optic neuropathy: a case-report and literature review. *Medicine (Baltimore).* 2017;96:e5889.

151. Steen JS, Stainton-Ellis DM. Rifampicin in pregnancy. *Lancet.* 1977;2:604-605.

152. Steichen O, Martinez-Almoyna L, De Broucker T. Isoniazid induced neuropathy: consider prevention [in French]. *Rev Mal Respir.* 2006;23(2, pt 1):157-160.

153. Svensson EM, et al. Rifampicin and rifapentine significantly reduce concentrations of bedaquiline, a new anti-TB drug. *J Antimicrob Chemother.* 2015;70:1106-1114.

154. Terman DS, Teitelbaum DT. Isoniazid self-poisoning. *Neurology.* 1970;20:299-304.

155. Timbrell JA, et al. Isoniazid hepatotoxicity: the relationship between covalent binding and metabolism in vivo. *J Pharmacol Exp Ther.* 1980;213:364-369.

156. Toibaro JJ, Losso MH. Pharmacokinetics interaction studies between rifampicin and protease inhibitors: methodological problems. *AIDS.* 2008;22:2046-2047.

157. Tsai RK, Lee YH. Reversibility of ethambutol optic neuropathy. *J Ocul Pharmacol Ther.* 1997;13:473-477.

158. van der Watt JJ, et al. Isoniazid exposure and pyridoxine levels in human immunodeficiency virus associated distal sensory neuropathy. *Int J Tuberc Lung Dis.* 2015;19:1312-1319.

159. van Heeswijk RPG, et al. Bedaquiline: a review of human pharmacokinetics and drug-drug interactions. *J Antimicrob Chemother.* 2014;69:2310-2318.

160. Vannelli TA, et al. The antituberculosis drug ethionamide is activated by a flavoprotein monooxygenase. *J Biol Chem.* 2002;277:12824-12829.

161. Varghese GM, et al. The twin epidemics of tuberculosis and HIV. *Curr Infect Dis Rep.* 2013;15:77-84.

162. Wang P, et al. Isoniazid metabolism and hepatotoxicity. *Acta Pharm Sin B.* 2016;6:384-392.

163. Wason S, et al. Single high-dose pyridoxine treatment for isoniazid overdose. *JAMA.* 1981;246:1102-1104.

164. Weber WW, Hein DW. Clinical pharmacokinetics of isoniazid. *Clin Pharmacokinet.* 1979;4:401-422.

165. Whitefield CL, Klein RH. Isoniazid overdose: report of 40 patients, with a critical analysis of treatment and suggestions for prevention. *Am Rev Respir Dis.* 1971;103:887.

166. Wong P, et al. Acute rifampin overdose: a pharmacokinetic study and review of the literature. *J Pediatr.* 1984;104:781-783.

167. Wood JD, Peesker SJ. The effect on GABA metabolism in brain of isonicotinic acid hydrazide and pyridoxine as a function of time after administration. *J Neurochem.* 1972;19:1527-1537.

168. World Health Organization. *Companion Handbook to the WHO Guidelines for the Programmatic Management of Drug-Resistant Tuberculosis.* (Rich M, Jaramillo E, eds.). Geneva, Switzerland: WHO Document Production Services; 2014:1-464. http://apps.who.int/iris/bitstream/10665/130918/1/9789241548809_eng.pdf?ua=1&ua=1.

169. World Health Organization. Global tuberculosis report 2016. http://www.who.int/tb/publications/global_report/gtbr2016_main_text.pdf?ua=1. Published 2016.

170. Wu SS, et al. Isoniazid-related hepatic failure in children: a survey of liver transplantation centers. *Transplantation.* 2007;84:173-179.

171. Yamada S, et al. Genetic variations of NAT2 and CYP2E1 and isoniazid hepatotoxicity in a diverse population. *Pharmacogenomics.* 2009;10:1433-1445.

172. Yew WW, Leung CC. Antituberculosis drugs and hepatotoxicity. *Respirology.* 2006;11:699-707.

173. Yew WW. Clinically significant interactions with drugs used in the treatment of tuberculosis. *Drug Saf.* 2002;25:111-133.

174. Zabinski RF, Blanchard JS. The requirement for manganese and oxygen in the isoniazid-dependent inactivation of *Mycobacterium tuberculosis* enoyl reductase. *J Am Chem Soc.* 1997;119:2331-2332.

175. Zaki SA, et al. Red man syndrome due to accidental overdose of rifampicin. *Indian J Crit Care Med.* 2013;17:55-56.

176. Zhang Y, Mitchison D. The curious characteristics of pyrazinamide: a review. *Int J Tuberc Lung Dis.* 2003;7:6-21.

177. Zheng J, et al. *para*-Aminosalicylic acid is a prodrug targeting dihydrofolate reductase in *Mycobacterium tuberculosis.* *J Biol Chem.* 2013;288:23447-23456.

178. Cycloserine [package insert]. Indianapolis, IN: Eli Lilly and Company; 2005.

179. Isoniazid [package insert]. Oklahoma City, OK: PD-Rx Pharmaceuticals; Revised September 28, 2016.

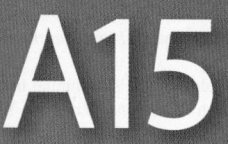

A15

PYRIDOXINE

Mary Ann Howland

INTRODUCTION

Pyridoxine (vitamin B_6), a water-soluble vitamin, is an antidote for overdoses of isonicotinic acid hydrazide (isoniazid, INH), *Gyromitra esculenta* mushrooms, hydrazine, methylated hydrazines, and ethylene glycol. With the exception of ethylene glycol, all of these xenobiotics produce seizures by the competitive inhibition of pyridoxal-5′-phosphate (PLP). Pyridoxine overcomes this inhibition. For ethylene glycol poisoning, it enhances a less toxic metabolic pathway to form benzoic and hippuric acid, instead of oxalic acid.[6] Hydrazine and methylated hydrazines (1,1-dimethylhydrazine, UDMH; monomethylhydrazine, MMH) are used as rocket fuels, and MMH is also found in *G. esculenta* mushrooms.[3]

HISTORY

Pyridoxine deficiency, which is characterized by seborrheic dermatitis, cheilosis, stomatitis, and glossitis, was first identified in 1926 but was mistakenly attributed to riboflavin (vitamin B_2) deficiency (Chap. 44).[32] Ten years later, the deficiency was fully characterized and correctly recognized as a deficiency of vitamin B_6.[32] A rare genetic abnormality that produces pyridoxine-responsive seizures in newborns was described in 1954.[5]

PHARMACOLOGY
Chemistry

The active form of pyridoxine is PLP.[32] The alcohol pyridoxine, the aldehyde pyridoxal, and the aminomethyl pyridoxamine are all naturally occurring, related compounds that are metabolized by the body to its active form PLP.[32] Pyridoxine was chosen by the Council on Pharmacy and Chemistry to represent vitamin B_6.[32] Pyridoxine hydrochloride was chosen as the commercial preparation because of its stability.[59] Pyritinol is a semi-synthetic pyridoxine analogue of 2 vitamin B_6 compounds linked by a disulfide bridge.

Mechanism of Action

Pyridoxal-5′-phosphate is an important cofactor in more than 100 enzymatic reactions, including decarboxylation and transamination of amino acids, and the metabolism of tryptophan to 5-hydroxytryptamine (serotonin) and methionine to cysteine.[24,32] In animals, iatrogenic pyridoxine deficiency produces seizures, resulting from reduced brain concentrations of PLP, glutamic acid decarboxylase, and γ-aminobutyric acid (GABA).[17]

Isoniazid and methylated hydrazines such as MMH interfere with the normal function of pyridoxine as a coenzyme. Isoniazid produces a syndrome resembling vitamin B_6 deficiency, which results in seizures.[47] Specifically, INH and other hydrazides and hydrazines inhibit the enzyme pyridoxine phosphokinase that converts pyridoxine to PLP (Fig. 56–3).[24] In addition, hydrazides directly combine with PLP, causing inactivation through the production of hydrazones that are rapidly excreted by the kidney.[24,59] Isoniazid also impairs lactate conversion to pyruvate.[16] Pyridoxal-5′-phosphate is a coenzyme for L-glutamic acid decarboxylase, which facilitates the synthesis of GABA from L-glutamic acid. Pyridoxal-5′-phosphate is also a necessary cofactor for serum glutamic-oxaloacetic transaminase (SGOT, also known as aspartate transaminase, AST), which generates L-glutamic acid from a-ketoglutarate, and for GABA transaminase, which converts GABA to succinic semialdehyde. Animal studies suggest that interference with PLP limits the formation of GABA,[24,54,55] which results in increased glutamic acid, thereby reducing cerebral inhibition and enhancing cerebral excitation, which contributes to the INH- and methylated hydrazine–induced seizures.[44,57] The administration of large doses of pyridoxine overcomes the deficiency.

Pharmacokinetics

Pyridoxine is not protein bound, has a volume of distribution of 0.6 L/kg, and easily crosses cell membranes, whereas PLP is nearly entirely plasma protein bound.[59] At extrahepatic sites, pyridoxine is rapidly metabolized to pyridoxal, PLP, and 4-pyridoxic acid, with only 7% excreted unchanged in the urine.[59] After intravenous (IV) infusion of 100 mg of pyridoxine, PLP concentration increases rapidly in serum and in erythrocytes.[59] Pyridoxal-5′-phosphate rises from 37 to 2,183 nmol/L in serum and from undetectable to 5,593 nmol/L in erythrocytes.[59] Oral pyridoxine, in doses of 600 mg, is 50% absorbed within 20 minutes of ingestion by a first-order process, with rapid achievement of peak serum concentrations of pyridoxine, PLP, and pyridoxal.[58] The concentration of PLP appears to be tightly controlled in the serum and related to alkaline phosphatase activity.[25,58] Oral doses of pyridoxine from 10 to 800 mg result in PLP concentrations of 518 to 732 nmol/L at 4 hours after ingestion.[58] Chronic alcoholic patients have lower baseline serum PLP concentrations because acetaldehyde enhances the degradation of PLP in erythrocytes through stimulation of an erythrocyte membrane–bound phosphatase that hydrolyzes phosphate-containing B_6 compounds.[31]

ROLE IN HYDRAZIDE- AND HYDRAZINE-INDUCED SEIZURES
Animal Studies

In a canine model of INH-induced toxicity, pyridoxine reduced the severity of seizures, increased the duration of seizure-free periods, and prevented death from a previously determined lethal dose of INH in a dose-dependent fashion.[13,14] Lower molar ratios prevented deaths, and higher molar ratios prevented both deaths and seizures.[14] When used as single treatments for INH-induced seizures, phenobarbital, pentobarbital, phenytoin, ethanol, and diazepam were ineffective in controlling seizures and death, but when combined with pyridoxine, each protected the animals from seizures and death.[13] Other small animal experiments document the effectiveness of pyridoxine against MMH-induced seizures when used without[24,37,50] and with diazepam.[20] Anticonvulsant efficacy is also demonstrated in feline[46] and primate[48] models.

Rat studies with intraperitoneal UDMH also demonstrate the protective effects of pyridoxine, which prevented seizures and death in a model that produced 94% mortality and 100% seizures without pyridoxine.[15] Other studies in dogs and monkeys also demonstrate the effectiveness of pyridoxine in preventing seizures and mortality, and in treating seizures.[4] Intramuscular pyridoxine protected the monkeys from death and stopped the seizures caused by IV exposure to UDMH.

Human Data

Clinical experience with pyridoxine for INH overdose in humans demonstrates favorable results.[2,11] Rapid seizure control without morbidity or mortality was achieved when the ratio in grams of pyridoxine administered to INH ingested ranged from 0.14 to 1.3, although in practice, most patients receive approximately gram-for-gram amounts. In 5 patients, the use of gram-for-gram amounts of pyridoxine resulted in the complete control of seizures and a resolution of the metabolic acidosis.[53] In 8 patients with intentional INH overdoses, basic poison management, intensive supportive care, and a mean dose of 5 g of pyridoxine IV resulted in no fatalities.[8] Seizures were controlled in a 22-month-old boy given 100 mg of IV pyridoxine after an estimated INH ingestion of 5 g.[47] Variable results are reported when lesser amounts of pyridoxine are used.[34] Seizures were reported in 2 patients after ingestion of INH–pyridoxine combination tablets, although the actual amount of pyridoxine ingested was not reported.[49] The failure to provide pyridoxine may result in persistent INH-associated seizures that do not respond to anticonvulsants.[45]

In addition to controlling seizures, administration of pyridoxine also appears to restore consciousness. Two patients, who remained obtunded for as long as 72 hours after the apparent resolution of the seizures, were reported to awaken immediately after 3 to 10 g of IV pyridoxine was administered.[10] A third patient who was lethargic awakened with IV pyridoxine. This suggests that mental status abnormalities associated with INH overdose (and possibly hydrazine overdoses) are responsive to pyridoxine and support repetitive dosing.[11,53] Patients treated with large doses of pyridoxine awaken more rapidly even after experiencing sustained seizure activity or status epilepticus.

Monomethylhydrazine poisoning is encountered in a variety of clinical situations. In the aerospace industry, where MMH is used as a rocket propellant, percutaneous or inhalational poisoning occurs. Ingestion of the false morel mushroom, *G. esculenta*, also produces toxicity when its major toxic compound, gyromitrin, is metabolized to MMH (Chap. 117).[3,19]

The neurologic effects of MMH poisoning are similar to those of INH toxicity and include seizures and respiratory failure.[17] Severe liver damage similar to INH induced hepatotoxicity is also described.[9] As in the case of INH-induced hepatotoxicity, there is no evidence that MMH-induced hepatotoxicity is treated by administration of pyridoxine.[9]

A patient who was exposed to hydrazine became comatose 14 hours later and remained comatose for 60 hours until treated with 25 mg/kg of pyridoxine.[26] A man with an altered consciousness who had ingested an unknown quantity of hydrazine improved after treatment with 10 g of pyridoxine.[23] This improvement occurred over 24 hours and may have been unrelated to pyridoxine therapy. A severe sensory peripheral neuropathy lasting for 6 months developed one week after the overdose and was most likely a result of the hydrazine ingestion and not the pyridoxine. Six patients exposed to an Aerozine-50 (1:1 mixture of hydrazine:UDMH) spill were effectively treated with pyridoxine 200 to 400 mg after developing twitching, clonic movements, hyperactivity, or gastrointestinal symptoms.[20] A patient exposed to UDMH during an explosion developed extensive burns, diverse neurologic manifestations, and electroencephalographic findings that resolved rapidly after the administration of IV pyridoxine.[18]

ROLE IN ETHYLENE GLYCOL POISONING

Pyridoxal-5′-phosphate is a cofactor in the conversion of glycolic acid to nonoxalate compounds (Chap. 106) (Fig. 106–2). We recommend that patients poisoned with ethylene glycol should receive 100 mg/day of pyridoxine IV in an attempt to shunt metabolism preferentially away from the production of oxalic acid. This approach is supported by an animal model[6] and the study of primary hyperoxaluria,[22] although there are no adequate studies of human ethylene glycol poisoning.[39]

ADVERSE EFFECTS AND SAFETY ISSUES

Pyridoxal-5′-phosphate is neurotoxic to animals and humans when administered chronically in supraphysiologic doses.[26,28,40] Delayed peripheral neurotoxicity occurred in patients taking daily doses of 200 mg to 6 g of pyridoxine for one month.[38,43,44] Healthy volunteers given 1 or 3 g/day developed a small- and large-fiber distal axonopathy, with sensory findings and quantitative

sensory threshold abnormalities occurring after 1.5 months at the high dose and 4.5 months at the low-dose exposure. When symptoms occurred, the pyridoxine was immediately stopped, but symptoms progressed for 2 to 3 weeks (Chap. 22).[7]

Pyridoxine also induces a sensory neuropathy when massive doses are administered, either as a single dose or over several days.[1,27,52] Ataxia occurred in dogs receiving 1 g/kg of pyridoxine.[52] Larger doses of pyridoxine result in loss of coordination, ataxia, seizures, and death.[48] Death after pyridoxine administration was sometimes delayed for 2 to 3 days.[52]

Two patients treated with 2 g/kg of IV pyridoxine (132 and 183 g, respectively) over 3 days developed severe and disabling sensory neuropathies.[1] One year later, both patients were still unable to walk. Inadequate information is available to determine the maximal single acute nontoxic dose in humans; however, there appears to be a wide margin of safety. Doses of pyridoxine ranging from 70 to 375 mg/kg or doses equivalent to the milligram-per-kilogram historical dose of ingested INH are routinely administered without adverse effects.[29,53]

The 0.5% chlorobutanol preservative in IV pyridoxine equates to doses of 250 to 500 mg of chlorobutanol when 5 and 10 g doses of pyridoxine are administered. Chlorobutanol is a sedative with a long elimination half-life, but doses of 600 mg were given to human volunteers without complication.[12,51] A dose of 5 g IV pyridoxine administered over 5 minutes to 5 healthy volunteers produced a transient minor increase in base deficit without any alteration in the level of consciousness.[30]

PREGNANCY AND LACTATION

Pyridoxine is Food and Drug Administration pregnancy category A. The recommended daily allowance for pyridoxine in pregnancy is 2.2 mg. Pyridoxine is routinely used in higher milligram doses (10 mg daily or up to 25 mg every 8 hours) for the treatment of hyperemesis gravidarum.[33] Although there has never been a controlled trial in pregnant women of gram doses of pyridoxine, the benefit of using pyridoxine for INH-induced seizures would clearly exceed the theoretical risk to the fetus. Pyridoxine enters breast milk and is considered compatible with breastfeeding when 10–25 mg doses are ingested. However, concentrations of pyridoxine in breast milk after maternal gram doses of pyridoxine are not known and it is reasonable to be concerned for the infant.

DOSING AND ADMINISTRATION

A safe and effective pyridoxine regimen for INH overdoses in adults is 1 g of pyridoxine for each gram of INH ingested, or 70 mg/kg in a child both to an initial maximum of 5 g.[53] The dose in children is unclear because there are so few children reported in the literature who were treated with IV pyridoxine and the history of ingested amount of INH is unreliable. Extrapolation from canine studies serve as a warning to avoid doses that approach 1 g/kg which risk pyridoxine toxicity. The gram for gram dosing of pyridoxine to INH up to 5 g in an adult or 70 mg/kg in children up to the adult dose is sufficient in the majority of patients.[35] The best way to administer pyridoxine in a patient after an INH overdose is not established. For a patient who is actively seizing, it is reasonable to give pyridoxine by slow IV infusion at approximately 0.5 g/min until the seizures stop or the maximum dose is reached. When the seizures stop, it is reasonable to infuse the remainder of the dose over 4 to 6 hours to maintain pyridoxine availability while the INH is being eliminated.[35] The dose should be repeated if seizures persist or recur or if the patient exhibits mental status depression, which could be an indication of persistent neurotoxicity, nonconvulsive status epilepticus, or a postictal phase. If IV pyridoxine is unavailable, oral pyridoxine should be administered.[42,56]

For hydrazine and methylated hydrazine (ie, MMH, UDMH) poisoning, there is no established dose.[57] Using the same dosage regimen as in the case of INH poisoning is reasonable and appropriate, although it is not tested in humans.

Benzodiazepines and barbiturates are synergistic with pyridoxine and should be used in addition to pyridoxine in rapid escalation to abort INH-induced seizures.

FORMULATION

Pyridoxine hydrochloride is available parenterally at a concentration of 100 mg/mL with a 1-mL fill in a 2-mL vial with 0.5% chlorobutanol as the preservative and 1.4 mcg/mL aluminum from Frensenius Pharmaceuticals.[41] Thus, a 5-g IV dose of pyridoxine requires fifty 100-mg/mL vials. This is an exception to the rule that appropriate doses of medications rarely require multiple vials and certainly not of this magnitude. This quantity also emphasizes the necessity of maintaining an adequate supply in the emergency department as well as in the pharmacy.[36] Oral pyridoxine is available in many tablet strengths from 10 to 500 mg depending on the manufacturer.

SUMMARY

- Pyridoxine and a benzodiazepine to achieve synergistic control of INH or MMH poisoning.
- An adequate dose of IV pyridoxine is 70 mg/kg to a maximum of 5 g. It is reasonable to treat recurrent seizures or a persistent depressed metal status with 1 to 2 additional doses and doses approaching 1 g/kg should be avoided.
- Five grams of IV pyridoxine requires administration of fifty 100-mg/mL vials.
- Adequate stocks should be ensured in the emergency department and pharmacy.
- If IV pyridoxine is unavailable, oral pyridoxine should be used.

REFERENCES

1. Albin R, et al. Acute sensory neuropathy-neuronopathy from pyridoxine overdose. *Neurology.* 1987;37:1729-1732.
2. Alvarez EG, Guntupalli KK. Isoniazid overdose: four case reports and review of the literature. *Intensive Care Med.* 1995;21:641-644.
3. Andary C, Bourrier MJ. Variations in the monomethylhydrazine content in *Gyromitra esculenta. Mycologia.* 1985;77:259-264.
4. Back KC, et al. Therapy of acute UDMH intoxication. *Aerosp Med.* 1963;34:1001-1004.
5. Baxter P. Pyridoxine-dependent seizures: a clinical and biochemical conundrum. *Biochim Biophys Acta.* 2003;1647:36-41.
6. Beasley UR, Buck WB. Acute ethylene glycol toxicosis: a review. *Vet Hum Toxicol.* 1980;22:255-263.
7. Berger AR, et al. Dose response, coasting, and differential fiber vulnerability in human toxic neuropathy: a prospective study of pyridoxine neurotoxicity. *Neurology.* 1992;42:1367-1370.
8. Blanchard P, et al. Isoniazid overdose in the Cambodian population of Olmsted County, Minnesota. *JAMA.* 1986;256:3131-3133.
9. Braun R, et al. Liver injury by the false morel poison gyromitrin. *Toxicology.* 1979;12:155-163.
10. Brent J, et al. Reversal of prolonged isoniazid-induced coma by pyridoxine. *Arch Intern Med.* 1990;150:1751-1753.
11. Brown CV. Acute isoniazid poisoning. *Am Rev Respir Dis.* 1972;105:206-216.
12. Burda A, et al. Possible adverse reactions in preservatives in high-dose pyridoxine hydrochloride IV injection. *Am J Health Syst Pharm.* 2002;59:1886-1887.
13. Chin L, et al. Potentiation of pyridoxine by depressants and anticonvulsants in the treatment of acute isoniazid intoxication in dogs. *Toxicol Appl Pharmacol.* 1981;58:504-509.
14. Chin L, et al. Evaluation of diazepam and pyridoxine as antidotes to isoniazid intoxication in rats and dogs. *Toxicol Appl Pharmacol.* 1978;45:713-722.
15. Cornish HH. The role of B$_6$ in toxicity of hydrazines. *Ann N Y Acad Sci.* 1969;166:136-145.
16. Cunningham K, et al. Pharmacometabolomic characterization of xenobiotic and endogenous metabolic phenotypes that account for inter-individual variation in isoniazid-induced toxicological response. *J Proteome Res.* 2012;11:4630-4642.
17. Dakshinamurti K, et al. Neurobiology of pyridoxine. *Ann N Y Acad Sci.* 1990;585:128-144.
18. Dhennin C, et al. Burns and the toxic effects of a derivative of hydrazine. *Burns Incl Therm Inj.* 1988;14:130-134.
19. Franke S, et al. Uber die Giftigkeit der fruhjahrslorchel *Gyromitra (Helvella) esculenta. Fr Arch Toxicol.* 1967;22:293-332.
20. Frierson WB. Use of pyridoxine HCl in acute hydrazine and UDMH intoxication. *Ind Med Surg.* 1965;34:650-651.
21. George ME, et al. Therapeutics of monomethylhydrazine intoxication. *Toxicol Appl Pharmacol.* 1982;63:201-208.
22. Gibbs DA, Watts RWE. The action of pyridoxine in primary hyperoxaluria. *Clin Sci.* 1970;38:277-286.
23. Harati Y, Niakan E. Hydrazine toxicity, pyridoxine therapy and peripheral neuropathy. *Ann Intern Med.* 1986;104:728-729.
24. Holtz P, Palm D. Pharmacological aspects of vitamin B$_6$. *Pharmacol Rev.* 1964;16:113-178.
25. Jang YM, et al. Human pyridoxal phosphatase. Molecular cloning, functional expression, and tissue distribution. *J Biol Chem.* 2003;278:50040-50046.
26. Kirlin JK. Treatment of hydrazine induced coma with pyridoxine. *N Engl J Med.* 1976;294:938-939.
27. Krinke G, et al. Pyridoxine megavitaminosis: an analysis of the early changes induced with massive doses of vitamin B$_6$ in rat primary sensory neurons. *J Neuropathol Exp Neurol.* 1985;44:117-129.
28. Krinke G, et al. Pyridoxine megavitaminosis produces degeneration of peripheral sensory neurons (sensory neuropathy) in the dog. *Neurotoxicology.* 1980;2:13-24.
29. Lheureux P, et al. Pyridoxine in clinical toxicology: a review. *Eur J Emerg Med.* 2005;12:78-85.
30. Lo Vecchio F, et al. Intravenous pyridoxine-induced metabolic acidosis. *Ann Emerg Med.* 2001;38:62-64.
31. Lumeng L, Li T. Vitamin B$_6$ metabolism in chronic alcohol abuse. *J Clin Invest.* 1974;53:693-704.
32. Marcus R, Coulston AM. Water-soluble vitamins. In: Hardman JG, et al., eds. *Goodman and Gilman's the Pharmacological Basis of Therapeutics.* 10th ed. New York, NY: McGraw-Hill; 2001:1760-1761.
33. McParlin C, et al. Treatments for hyperemesis gravidarum and nausea and vomiting in pregnancy: a systematic review. *JAMA.* 2016;316:1392-1401.
34. Miller J, et al. Acute isoniazid poisoning in childhood. *Am J Dis Child.* 1980;134:290-292.
35. Minns AB, et al. Isoniazid-induced status epilepticus in a pediatric patient after inadequate pyridoxine therapy. *Pediatr Emerg Care.* 2010;26:380-381.
36. Morrow LE, et al. Acute isoniazid toxicity and the need for adequate pyridoxine supplies. *Pharmacotherapy.* 2006;26:1529-1532.
37. O'Brien RD, et al. Poisoning of the rat by hydrazine and alkylhydrazines. *Toxicol Appl Pharmacol.* 1964;84:371-377.
38. Parry G, Bredesen D. Sensory neuropathy with low dose pyridoxine. *Neurology.* 1985;35: 1466-1468.
39. Parry MF, Wallach R. Ethylene glycol poisoning. *Am J Med.* 1974;57:143-150.
40. Perry TA, et al. Pyridoxine-induced toxicity in rats: a stereological quantification of the sensory neuropathy. *Exp Neurol.* 2004;190:133-144.
41. Pyridoxine Hydrochloride Injection, USP [package insert]. Lake Zurich, IL: Fresenius Kabi, LLC; 2015.
42. Scharman EJ, Rosencrance JG. Isoniazid toxicity: a survey of pyridoxine availability. *Am J Emerg Med.* 1994;12:386-388.
43. Schaumburg H. Sensory neuropathy from pyridoxine abuse. *N Engl J Med.* 1984;310:198.
44. Schaumburg H, et al. Sensory neuropathy from pyridoxine abuse: a new megavitamin syndrome. *N Engl J Med.* 1983;309:445-448.
45. Shah BR, et al. Acute isoniazid neurotoxicity in an urban hospital. *Pediatrics.* 1995;95: 700-704.
46. Shouse MN. Acute effects of pyridoxine hydrochloride on monomethylhydrazine seizure latency and amygdaloid kindled seizure thresholds in cats. *Exp Neurol.* 1982;75:79-88.
47. Starke H, Williams S. Acute poisoning from overdose of isoniazid: a case report. *Lancet.* 1963;83:406-408.
48. Sterman MB, Kovalesky RA. Anticonvulsant effects of restraint and pyridoxine on hydrazine seizures in the monkey. *Exp Neurol.* 1979;65:78-86.
49. Terman DS, Teitelbaum DT. Isoniazid self-poisoning. *Neurology.* 1970;20:299-304.
50. Toth B, Erickson J. Reversal of the toxicity of hydrazine an analogues by pyridoxine hydrochloride. *Toxicology.* 1977;7:31-36.
51. Tung C, et al. The pharmacokinetics of chlorbutol in man. *Biopharm Drug Dispos.* 1982;3:371-378.
52. Unna IC. Studies of the toxicity and pharmacology of vitamin B$_6$ (2-methyl, 3-hydroxy-4,5-*bis*-pyridine). *Pharmacol Exp Ther.* 1940;70:400-407.
53. Wason S, et al. Single high-dose pyridoxine treatment for isoniazid overdose. *JAMA.* 1981;246:1102-1104.
54. Wood JD, Peesker SJ. A correlation between changes in GABA metabolism and isonicotinic acid. Hydrazide-induced seizures. *Brain Res.* 1972;45:489-498.
55. Wood JD, Peesker SJ. The effect on GABA metabolism of isonicotinic acid hydrazide and pyridoxine as a function of time after administration. *J Neurochem.* 1972;19: 1527-1537.
56. Zell-Kanter M. Oral pyridoxine in the management of isoniazid poisoning. *Pediatr Emerg Care.* 2010;26:965.
57. Zelnick SD, et al. Occupational exposure to hydrazines: treatment of acute central nervous system toxicity. *Aviat Space Environ Med.* 2003;74:1285-1291.
58. Zempleni J. Pharmacokinetics of vitamin B$_6$ supplements in humans. *J Am Coll Nutr.* 1995;14:579-586.
59. Zempleni J, Kubler W. The utilization of intravenously infused pyridoxine in humans. *Clin Chim Acta.* 1994;229:27-36.

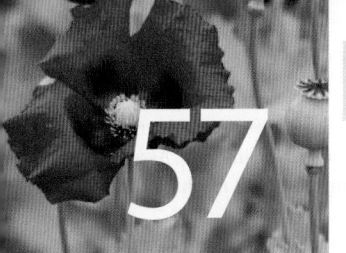

57

ANTIDYSRHYTHMICS

Maryann Mazer-Amirshahi and Lewis S. Nelson

HISTORY AND EPIDEMIOLOGY

The term *dysrhythmia* encompasses an array of abnormal cardiac rhythms that range in clinical significance from merely annoying to instantly life threatening. The word *arrhythmia* can be defined as a lack of rhythm. Some references state they are synonyms for irregular heartbeat, and others define arrhythmia as irregular heartbeat and dysrhythmia as a disturbance to an otherwise normal rhythm. Throughout the text, we have chosen the term *dysrhythmia*. Antidysrhythmics include all medications that are used to treat any of these various dysrhythmias. The importance of dysrhythmia management in the modern practice of medicine cannot be overstated because dysrhythmias are among the most common causes of preventable sudden cardiac death.[52]

For many years, antidysrhythmics were considered among the most rational of the available cardiac medications. This well-earned reputation related to their high efficacy at reducing the incidence of malignant dysrhythmias. Similarly, they are effective at controlling extrasystoles which cause patient discomfort or anxiety. However, this approach changed dramatically following publication of the Cardiac Arrhythmia Suppression Trials (CAST and CAST II)[28] and more recently with the rise of mechanical interventions, such as ablation therapy and implantable defibrillators. Cardiac Arrhythmia Suppression Trials assessed the ability of three antidysrhythmics to suppress asymptomatic ventricular dysrhythmias considered to be harbingers of sudden death. The original CAST was discontinued in 1989 before completion, when encainide and flecainide, two of the study medications, not only failed to prevent sudden death but actually increased overall mortality. The CAST II noted similar problems with moricizine.[102] It is clear that the enhanced mortality associated with many antidysrhythmics is a result of their prodysrhythmogenic effects and that virtually all medications of this group carry such risk. Because most patients with atrial fibrillation do not benefit from rhythm conversion compared with control of the ventricular response rate, the use of antidysrhythmics for this indication is less common but is still useful in some populations.[91]

In addition to the predictable, mechanism-based adverse effect of each medication, unique and often unanticipated effects also occur.[87] Experience with overdose of many of these medications is limited, and management is generally based on the underlying pharmacologic principles, existing case reports, and the experimental literature. This chapter focuses on the medications that serve primarily as antidysrhythmics and, with the exception of lidocaine (found in Chap. 64), have few other medicinal indications. Chap. 15 provides a more detailed description of the electrophysiology of dysrhythmias and a discussion of their genesis. In addition, the toxicities from β-adrenergic antagonists and Ca²⁺ channel blockers, which have indications in addition to dysrhythmia control, are discussed separately in Chaps. 59 and 60. The toxicology of cardioactive steroids such as digoxin is discussed in Chap. 62.

CLASSIFICATION OF ANTIDYSRHYTHMICS

Despite an incomplete understanding of the underlying mechanisms of dysrhythmia formation, an abundance of antidysrhythmics were developed, each attempting to alter specific electrophysiologic components of the cardiac impulse generating or conducting system.

Antidysrhythmics modify impulse generation and conduction by interacting with various membrane Na^+, K^+, and Ca^{2+} channels. Generally,

antidysrhythmics manifest electrophysiologic effects either through alteration of the channel pore or, more commonly, by modification of its gating mechanism (Fig. 57–1). Unfortunately, given their exceedingly complex mechanisms of action, the descriptive terms used to explain their molecular actions are not always completely accurate. For example, the description of an antidysrhythmic as a specific "channel blocker," although representative of the conceptual action of that medication, is inaccurate because in most cases, the molecule does not actually block the channel but rather prevents the channel from opening or closing properly. Furthermore, many of these medications are active nonspecifically at other channels or on other cells, resulting in divergent clinical actions of those similarly classified.

The Vaughan-Williams classification of antidysrhythmics by electrophysiologic properties emphasizes the connection between the basic electrophysiologic actions and the antidysrhythmic effects.[103] Although initially proposed as a descriptive model for electrophysiologic actions and not for clinical effects, the Vaughan-Williams classification is commonly invoked as a user-friendly guide to clinical therapy. A more rational classification would match the electrophysiologic effects of the antidysrhythmics with their molecular interactions on different regions of the various ion channels, such as channel gating and pore conductance.

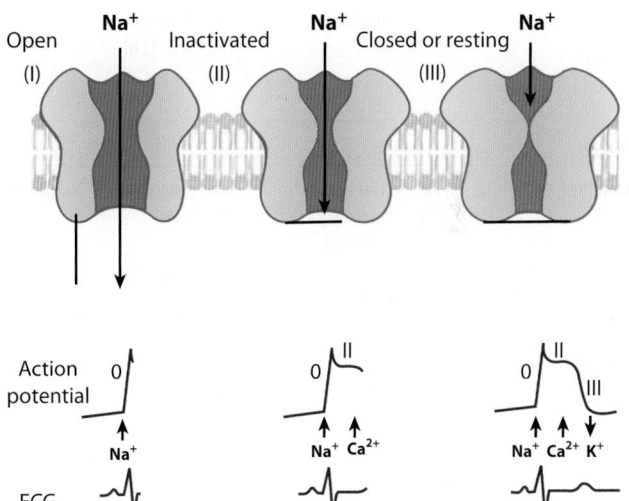

FIGURE 57–1. Sodium channel blockade. On appropriate signal, Na^+ channel activation occurs, at which time the Na^+ channel converts from the resting (III) state to the open state (I). This allows Na^+ influx to initiate phase 0 of the action potential, or cellular depolarization. The Na^+ channels subsequently assume the inactivated state by closure of an inactivation gate; this is a voltage-dependent phenomena and occurs concomitantly with, although more slowly than, channel activation. Cellular depolarization is maintained for a period of time by other ion channels that form the plateau of the action potential. Before reactivating, Na^+ channels must convert back to the resting state, which also occurs in a voltage-gated fashion. Many antidysrhythmics stabilize the inactivated state of the channel and, by slowing conversion to the resting state, prevent its reopening, reducing the excitability of the cell. Because this is a population phenomenon, there are dose-dependent effects on channel blockade; thus, more xenobiotics interfere with more channels. Interestingly, certain xenobiotics, such as ciguatoxin and aconitine, stabilize the open state of the Na^+ channel and produce persistent depolarization. ECG = electrocardiogram.

This discussion of antidysrhythmics uses the Vaughan Williams classification, recognizing its shortcomings.[109] The pharmacokinetic properties of the various medications are summarized in Table 57–1.

CLASS I ANTIDYSRHYTHMICS

All antidysrhythmics in Vaughan-Williams class I (A, B, and C) alter Na^+ conductance through cardiac voltage-gated, fast inward Na^+ channels (Table 57–1). These xenobiotics bind to the Na^+ channels and slow their recovery from the open or inactivated state to the resting state (Fig. 57–1). This conversion must occur before the channel can reopen and participate in another depolarization. Consequently, as the proportion of medication-bound Na^+ channels increases, fewer of these channels are capable of reactivation on the arrival of the next depolarizing impulse. As a result, by reducing the excitability of the myocardium, abnormal rhythms are both prevented and terminated.

Blockade of these Na^+ channels slows the rise of phase 0 of the cellular action potential, which correlates with a reduction in the rate of depolarization of the myocardial cell (or V_{max}). Similarly, conduction through the myocardium is slowed, producing a measurable prolongation of the QRS complex on the surface electrocardiogram (ECG). Correspondingly, slowed intramyocardial conduction is associated with reduced contractility, manifesting as negative inotropy. Myocardial depression also results from effects

TABLE 57–1	Antidysrhythmics: Pharmacology, Pharmacokinetics, and Adverse Effects							
Antidysrhythmic	Route	Primary Route of Elimination	Elimination Half-Life	Channel Blockade	Volume Distribution L/Kg	Protein Binding (%)	Adverse Effects and Complicating Factors	Other
Class IA								
Disopyramide	PO	Liver, kidney	Variable	Na^+, ($\tau = 9$ s), K^+, Ca^{2+}	0.59 ± 0.15	35–95 depending on plasma concentration	CHF, negative inotropic effects, anticholinergic, torsade de pointes, heart block, hypoglycemia QRS and QT prolonged	
Procainamide	IV, PO	50%–60% unchanged in kidney; active hepatic metabolite (NAPA)	PA: 3-4 h ↑ CKD NAPA: 6–10 h ↑ CKD	Na^+($\tau = 1.8$ s), K^+	1.9 ± 0.3	16 ± 9	Hypotension (ganglionic blockade), QRS and QT prolonged, fever, SLE-like syndrome, Torsade de pointes	NAPA: active metabolite, renally eliminated, K^+ channel blocker; half-life, 6–10 h A sustained-release PA preparation is available
Quinidine	PO	Liver, kidney, 10%–20% unchanged	6–8 h ↑ liver disease (to >50 h) and CKD (to 9–12 h)	Na^+($\tau = 3$ s), K^+, Ca^{2+}	2.7 ± 1.2	87 ± 3	Heart block, sinus node dysfunction QRS and QT prolonged hypotension, hypoglycemia, torsade de pointes, thrombocytopenia, ↑ [digoxin]	
Class IB								
Lidocaine	SC, IV, PO (30% BA)	Liver, active metabolite (MEGX CYP3A4)	Distribution 8 min after bolus Terminal elimination, 2 h	Na^+($\tau = 0.1$ s)	1.1 ± 0.4	70 ± 5	Fatigue, agitation, paresthesias, seizures, hallucinations, rarely bundle branch block	Metabolites: GX and MEGX are less potent as Na^+ channel blockers than lidocaine.
Mexiletine	IV, PO	Liver (CYP 2D6)	10–24 h	Na^+($\tau = 0.3$ s)	4.9 ± 0.5	63 ± 3	See lidocaine	
Phenytoin	IV, PO	Liver		Na^+($\tau = 0.2$ s)	0.64 ± 0.04	89 ± 23	Hypotension and asystole related to IV propylene glycol infusion, nystagmus, ataxia	
Tocainide	IV, PO	Kidney, liver	9-14 h	Na^+($\tau = 0.4$ s)	3.0 ± 0.2	10 ± 15	See lidocaine; aplastic anemia, interstitial pneumonia	
Class IC								
Flecainide	IV, PO	Liver (CYP2D6), 75%; kidney, 25%	20 h	Na^+($\tau = 11$ s), Ca^{2+}, K^+	4.9 ± 0.4	61 ± 10	Negative inotropic effects, bradycardia, heart block, ventricular fibrillation, ventricular tachycardia, neutropenia QT prolonged	Two major metabolites, one with minor activity, meta-O-dealkylated flecainide; and inactive meta-O-dealkylated lactam of flecainide
Moricizine	PO	Liver	2–4 h	Na^+($\tau = 10$ s)	?	95	↑ Mortality after myocardial infarction, bradycardia, CHF, ventricular fibrillation, ventricular tachycardia	

(Continued)

TABLE 57–1 Antidysrhythmics: Pharmacology, Pharmacokinetics, and Adverse Effects *(Continued)*

Antidysrhythmic	Route	Primary Route of Elimination	Elimination Half-Life	Channel Blockade	Volume Distribution L/Kg	Protein Binding (%)	Adverse Effects and Complicating Factors	Other
Propafenone	IV, PO	Liver (CYP2D6) extensive first pass	2–10 h	$Na^+(\tau = 1\,s)$, K^+	3.6 ± 2.1	85 ± 95	Asthma, congestive heart failure, hypoglycemia, AV block, QRS and QT prolonged, bradycardia, ventricular fibrillation, ventricular tachycardia	Active metabolite 5-OH-propafenone
Class II								
β-Adrenergic antagonists	IV, PO	Variable	Variable	β-Adrenergic receptor	Variable	Variable	CHF, asthma, hypoglyce-mia, Raynaud disease	
Class III								
Amiodarone	IV, PO	Liver (100%) (CYP3A4)	2 mo	Na^+, K^+, Ca^{2+}	66 ± 44	99.98 ± 0.01	Negative inotropic effects, pulmonary fibrosis, corneal microdepos-its, thyroid function abnormalities, hepatitis photosensitivity, ↑ concentrations diltiazem, quinidine, procainamide, flecainide, [digoxin] QT prolonged	Desethylamiodarone; has comparable activity to the parent compound
Dofetilide	IV, PO	Kidney	7.5 h	K^+	3.6 ± 0.8	64	Torsade de pointes QT prolonged	
Dronedarone	PO	Liver (CYP3A4)	13–19 h	Na^+, K^+, Ca^{2+}	20	>98	Contraindicated in decompensated heart failure, atrial fibrilla-tion that cannot be converted; liver, thyroid, and pulmonary toxicity QT prolonged	Active N-debutyl metabolite (10%–33% potency)
Ibutilide	IV	Kidney	2–12 h; average, 6 h	K^+, Na^+ opener	11	40	Torsade de pointes, heart block, QT prolonged	
Class IV								
Ca^{2+} channel blockers	IV, PO	Variable	Variable	Ca^{2+}	Variable	Variable	Asystole (if used IV with IV β-adrenergic recep-tor antagonists), AV block, hypotension, CNF, constipation, ↑ digoxin concentration	
Unclassified								
Adenosine	IV	All cells (intracel-lular adenosine deaminase)	Seconds	Nucleoside-specific G protein–coupled adenosine recep-tors, ↑Ca^{2+}currents activate ACh-sensitive K^+ current			Transient asystole <5 s, chest pain, dyspnea, atrial fibrillation, ↓ BP, effects potentiated by dipyridamole and in heart transplant patients, ↑ dose needed with meth-ylxanthine use	
Digoxin	IV	(Chap. 62)						
Magnesium Sulfate		(Antidotes in Depth: A16)						

$\tau_{recovery}$ describes the time it takes for the Na^+ channel to recover from blockade.

ACh = acetylcholine; AV = atrioventricular; BA = bioavailable; BP = blood pressure; CHF = congestive heart failure; CKD = chronic kidney disease; GX = glycine xylide; IV = intravenous; NAPA = N-acetylprocainamide; MEGX = monoethylglycylxylidide; PO = oral; SC = subcutaneous; PA = procainamide.

of reduced intracellular Na^+ on the Na^+-Ca^{2+} exchange mechanism.[73] This in turn reduces the intracellular Ca^{2+} concentration, which is required for adequate contractility.

The differences among class I antidysrhythmics are directly related to their pharmacologic relationships with the Na^+ channel. However, it is noteworthy that the original subdivision of class I antidysrhythmics was based on clinical observations, not current pharmacologic awareness, accounting for the somewhat illogical ordering of the class I subdivisions.[109] Type IB antidysrhythmics have their highest affinity for inactivated Na^+ channels. This occurs at the end of depolarization, during early repolarization, and during periods of myocardial ischemia, all situations in which the myocardium is partially depolarized. These xenobiotics also have rapid "on–off" binding kinetics (rapid $\tau_{recovery}$) and are thus bound only briefly, during late electrical systole, the period during which the Na^+ channels are predominantly in the inactivated form. They are almost exclusively unbound during electrical diastole, which is the major portion of the cardiac cycle at normal heart rates. However, the degree of binding increases as the heart rate accelerates because the duration of diastole decreases, and the relative proportion of time spent in systole increases; this is termed *use dependence*. Because all IB antidysrhythmics do not bind to activated Na^+ channels, in therapeutic doses they do not affect the rate of rise of phase 0 of the action potential, or V_{max}, and have no effect on the ECG. Alternatively, the class IC antidysrhythmics either act preferentially on activated Na^+ channels or they release from the Na^+ channels very slowly (slow $\tau_{recovery}$) and thus are still bound during the next cardiac cycle. This prolonged channel blockade and reduced channel reactivation results in both greater pharmacologic effects and toxicity, even at slow heart rates. These xenobiotics reduce V_{max} and prolong the QRS complex. Class IA antidysrhythmics fall between the other two subclasses.

Although in the Vaughan-Williams classification all class I antidysrhythmics are considered primarily Na^+ channel blockers, many, particularly those in class IA, have important effects on cardiac K^+ channels. These channels are critical to maintenance of the cardiac action potential and repolarization of the myocardial cell. Slowing of K^+ efflux prolongs the duration of the action potential and accounts for the persistence of refractoriness, or the time during which the cell is incapable of redepolarization. This effect produces QT interval prolongation and predisposes to the triggering of polymorphic ventricular tachycardia (torsade de pointes).[53] Because class IB antidysrhythmics have no effect on myocardial K^+ channels, they do not alter refractoriness or the QT interval. In fact, class IB antidysrhythmics often reduce the action potential duration, shortening refractoriness. Further discussion of K^+ channel blockade is found in Chap. 15 and later in the discussion of class III antidysrhythmics.

Class IA Antidysrhythmics: Procainamide, Quinidine, and Disopyramide

Procainamide (Fig. 57–2)

Procainamide is used to suppress either atrial or ventricular tachydysrhythmias. Importantly, procainamide undergoes hepatic biotransformation by acetylation to *N*-acetylprocainamide (NAPA), the rate of which is genetically determined, and rapid acetylators are prone to developing toxicity.[76] Although NAPA lacks the Na^+ channel–blocking activity of procainamide, it prolongs the action potential duration through blockade of the K^+ rectifier currents and is independently responsible for the production of cardiac dysrhythmias.[45]

Rapid intravenous (IV) dosing of procainamide is potentially dangerous because its initial volume of distribution is smaller than its final volume of distribution. Because this initial compartment includes the heart, adverse myocardial effects occur unexpectedly. In addition, procainamide exhibits ganglionic-blocking properties, which produce profound hypotension with rapid IV administration. Thus, to prevent toxicity during medication infusion, the IV loading dose is administered by slow infusion with ECG monitoring. Both procainamide and NAPA are renally eliminated and accumulate in patients with chronic kidney disease (CKD).[67]

Although the chronic use of procainamide is commonly accompanied by the development of antinuclear antibodies and infrequently progresses to

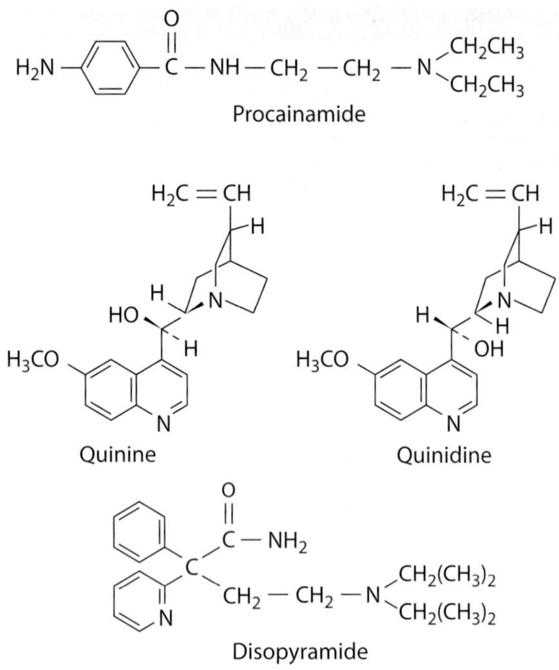

FIGURE 57–2. Structures of class IA antidysrhythmics and quinine.

drug-induced systemic lupus erythematosis,[46] this syndrome is not associated with acute poisoning. Furthermore, NAPA has less propensity than procainamide to produce this syndrome.[45] Other reported adverse effects include seizures and antimuscarinic effects with acute overdose and myopathic pain, hepatitis, thrombocytopenia, and agranulocytosis after long-term use.

Serum procainamide concentrations should be determined as part of therapeutic drug monitoring (therapeutic: 4–12 mcg/mL); NAPA concentrations should also be monitored in patients with CKD (therapeutic: 10–20 mcg/mL). In patients with procainamide overdose, both procainamide and NAPA concentrations should be obtained, although a direct prognostic role is not defined. Because the elimination half-life of procainamide is 3 to 4 hours, which is substantially shorter than that of NAPA (6–10 hours), chronic overdosing typically results in NAPA toxicity.[5] In this situation, the QT interval, a reflection of K^+ channel blockade, correlates directly and blood pressure correlates inversely with the degree of poisoning. Severe effects usually do not occur until total (procainamide plus NAPA) serum concentrations are greater than 60 mcg/mL. Because of its structural similarity with amphetamine, some patients with procainamide overdose may have a false-positive urine enzyme-multiplied immunoassay test (EMIT) for amphetamines.[110]

Quinidine

Quinidine, the *d*-isomer of quinine, is derived from the bark of the cinchona tree. Because it is a weak base, it is typically formulated as the sulfate or gluconate salt. Quinidine undergoes hydroxylation by the liver, and both active and inactive metabolites are renally eliminated.

Quinidine was once widely used for the management of atrial or ventricular dysrhythmias but has largely fallen out of favor because of its adverse effects. Quinidine has substantial cardiotoxicity that includes intraventricular conduction abnormalities and an increased QT interval. "Quinidine syncope," in which patients on therapeutic doses of quinidine experience paroxysmal, transient loss of consciousness, is almost exclusively a result of torsade de pointes.[51]

Because quinidine shares many pharmacologic properties with quinine (Chap. 55), patients occasionally have cinchonism after either chronic or acute quinidine overdose. This syndrome includes abdominal symptoms, tinnitus, and altered mental status. Quinidine also produces both peripheral and cardiac antimuscarinic effects, which enhance conduction via the atrioventricular (AV) node. Furthermore, as with quinine, quinidine-induced blockade of K⁺ channels in pancreatic islet cells causes uncontrolled insulin release, leading to hypoglycemia. Hypoglycemia occurs more commonly in patients who are critically ill because counterregulatory mechanisms are impaired in this population.[81] The antimuscarinic effects can produce classical anticholinergic findings such as dry mouth and flushed skin.[57]

Serum quinidine concentrations greater than 14 mcg/mL are associated with cardiotoxicity,[57] as evidenced by a 50% increase in either the QRS complex or QT interval. These concentrations have limited utility in clinical management.

Disopyramide

Disopyramide is more likely than other class IA antidysrhythmics to produce negative inotropy and congestive heart failure. This effect is noted both in patients receiving therapeutic dosing[98] and in those who overdose and is likely related to the blockade of myocardial Ca²⁺ channels caused by disopyramide.[48] The current use of disopyramide capitalizes on its negative inotropic effects for the treatment of patients with hypertrophic cardiomyopathy who remain symptomatic despite first-line treatment such as β-adrenergic antagonists.[30] The mono-N-dealkylated metabolite of disopyramide produces the most pronounced antimuscarinic effects of the class,[57,106] accounting for the occasional, although unproven, use of disopyramide to treat neurocardiogenic syncope.[89] Lethargy, confusion, or hallucinations are prominent in overdose.

Electrophysiologic abnormalities similar to those associated with poisoning from other class IA antidysrhythmics occur, including intraventricular conduction abnormalities, torsade de pointes, and other ventricular dysrhythmias. Disopyramide causes hyperinsulinemic hypoglycemia through its antagonism of K⁺ channels in the pancreatic islet cells.[1]

Management of Class IA Antidysrhythmic Toxicity

Management concentrates on assessment and correction of cardiovascular dysfunction. After airway evaluation and IV line placement, 12-lead ECG and continuous ECG monitoring are of paramount importance. Appropriate gastrointestinal (GI) decontamination is recommended when the patient is sufficiently stabilized. Activated charcoal is recommended for early-presenting patients with a protected airway and an ingestion of a potentially toxic amount of medication. Gastric lavage is reasonable for patients with life-threatening ingestions who present within several hours depending on the severity and probability of retained ingestant. Decontamination whole-bowel irrigation is reasonable if a sustained-release preparation is involved (Chap. 5 and Antidotes in Depth: A2).

For patients who have widening of the QRS complex duration, bolus administration of IV hypertonic sodium bicarbonate is recommended (Antidotes in Depth: A5). Depolarization is accelerated, and the QRS complex duration is reduced by enhancing rapid Na⁺ ion influx through the myocardial Na⁺ channels.[10] However, hypokalemia from the use of sodium bicarbonate may further prolong the QT interval, requiring careful monitoring of the serum K⁺ and ECG. Class IA antidysrhythmic-induced hypotension is treated primarily with rapid infusion of 0.9% NaCl to expand intravascular volume and to simultaneously increase myocardial contractility by enhancing the Starling force. Hypotension in the setting of QRS complex prolongation responds favorably to hypertonic sodium bicarbonate, which enhances inotropy by both accelerating depolarization and raising intravascular volume. In refractory cases, dobutamine or a catecholamine such as epinephrine or norepinephrine is recommended based on the assessment of the hemodynamic requirements for inotropy versus pressor effect. Epinephrine, by analogy with chloroquine and tricyclic antidepressants, may be superior to norepinephrine.[21,58] Extracorporeal life support can improve hemodynamics, but their use has not been systematically evaluated, but use in patients with standards indications, if readily available, seems reasonable. Because disopyramide also blocks Ca²⁺ channels, Ca²⁺ administration is reportedly beneficial,[2] and although evidence to support this antidotal effect is lacking, it is reasonable to administer in appropriate doses. Glucagon effectively reversed myocardial depression in canine models, but it has not been evaluated in humans because such its use remains experimental at this time.[75]

We recommend treating patients with stable ventricular dysrhythmias occurring in the setting of class IA antidysrhythmic poisoning with hypertonic sodium bicarbonate or lidocaine. Although it seem counterintuitive to administer another class I antidysrhythmic to a patient already poisoned by a class I antidysrhythmic, there is sound theoretical and experimental literature to support the use of lidocaine in this setting.[111] Because lidocaine is a class IB antidysrhythmic with rapid on–off receptor kinetics, it displaces the "slower" class IA antidysrhythmic from the binding site on the Na⁺ channel, effectively reducing channel blockade. Sodium bicarbonate enhances conduction through the myocardium, promoting spontaneous termination of the ventricular dysrhythmia.[34] Magnesium sulfate and overdrive pacing can prevent recurrent torsade de pointes after initial spontaneous resolution or defibrillation. Medications that must be avoided in treating patients with dysrhythmias associated with class IA poisoning include other class IA and IC antidysrhythmics, as well as the β-adrenergic antagonists and Ca²⁺ channel blockers, all of which exacerbate conduction abnormalities or produce hypotension.

The roles of activated charcoal hemoperfusion, hemofiltration, and continuous arteriovenous hemodiafiltration are inadequately defined, but these are reasonable and appropriate means to remove NAPA.[67] There is not sufficient clinical evidence to support the use of hemodialysis or hemoperfusion for quinidine or disopyramide poisoning.[1,43]

Class IB Antidysrhythmics: Lidocaine, Tocainide, Mexiletine, and Moricizine

Lidocaine (Fig. 57–3)

Lidocaine is an aminoacyl amide that is a synthetic derivative of cocaine. Its predominant clinical uses are as a local anesthetic and, for mechanistically

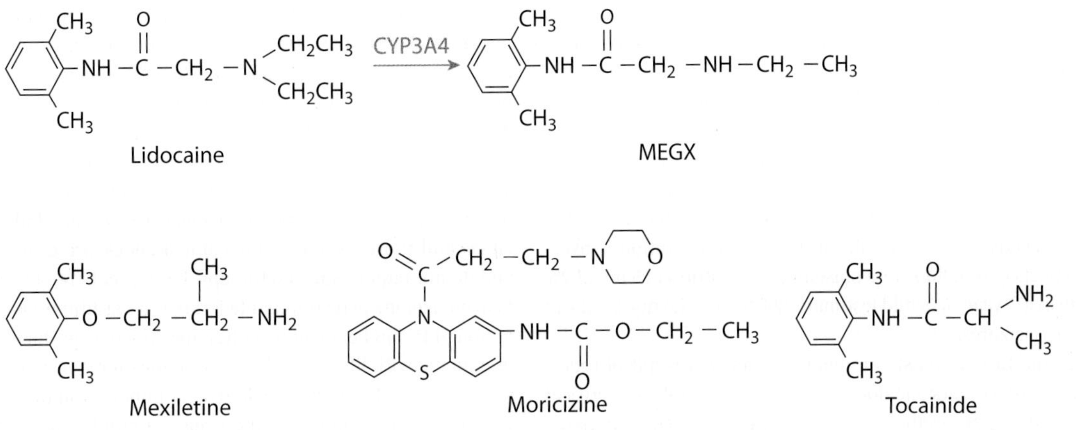

FIGURE 57–3. Structures of the class IB antidysrhythmics lidocaine (and metabolite monoethylglycylxylidide {MEGX}), tocainide, mexiletine, and moricizine.

similar reasons, to control ventricular dysrhythmias. The high frequency of lidocaine-related medication errors relates in part to its wide use in the past as well as the availability of "amps" of varying quantities, designed for specific uses such as preparation of IV infusions or for local anesthesia.[54] Many of the current cases of lidocaine toxicity result from its use in liposuction, discussed later. Lidocaine prevents myocardial reentry and subsequent dysrhythmias (Chap. 15) by preferentially suppressing conduction in compromised tissue.[99] After an IV bolus, lidocaine rapidly enters the central nervous system (CNS) but quickly redistributes into the peripheral tissue with a distribution half-life of approximately 8 minutes.[11] Lidocaine is 95% dealkylated by hepatic CYP3A4 to an active metabolite, monoethylglycylxylidide (MEGX) and, subsequently, to the inactive glycine xylidide (GX). Glycine xylidide is further metabolized to monoethylglycine and xylidide. Monoethylglycylxylidide, although less potent as a Na^+ channel blocker than lidocaine, bioaccumulates because of its substantially longer half-life.[8]

Patients with massive lidocaine exposures develop both CNS and cardiovascular effects, generally in that order. Because of its rapid entry into the CNS, acute lidocaine poisoning typically produces CNS dysfunction, with paresthesias or convulsion, as the initial manifestation.[33,86,95] Concomitant respiratory arrest generally occurs. Shortly after the CNS effects, depression in the intrinsic cardiac pacemakers leads to sinus arrest, AV block, intraventricular conduction delay, hypotension, or cardiac arrest. If the patient is supported through this period, the xenobiotics rapidly distributes away from the heart, and spontaneous cardiac function returns.

Acute lidocaine toxicity is generally related to excessive or inappropriate parenteral therapeutic dosing. Common settings include inadvertent IV or intraarterial administration instead of the intended route and excessive subcutaneous administration during laceration repair or other procedures.[105] Acute lidocaine toxicity is reported with topical tracheal application of lidocaine used for bronchoscopy,[113] during circumcision,[86] and during ureteral application during ureteroscopic stone extraction.[78] The typical CNS manifestations of submassive lidocaine poisoning include drowsiness, weakness, a sensation of "drifting away," euphoria, diplopia, decreased hearing, paresthesias, muscle fasciculations, and seizures. The more severe of these effects develop when serum lidocaine concentrations exceed 5 mcg/mL and are often preceded by paresthesias or somnolence. Any of these symptoms should, therefore, prompt the clinician to examine the patient's medication administration history or medication-infusion rate. Apnea and seizures, as well as hypotonia in neonates, are reported to result from submassive acute lidocaine toxicity.[85]

A related form of toxicity and death results from subcutaneous and adipose administration of lidocaine during tumescent liposuction.[83] In this technique, a large volume of dilute lidocaine is used to distend subcutaneous fat before liposuction.[9] Although in some reports, the cause of death was controversial,[82] postmortem lidocaine concentrations were commonly elevated, and it is likely that lidocaine metabolites were also involved in the adverse events.[55] Interestingly, proponents of this procedure suggest that lidocaine doses up to a maximum of 55 mg/kg are safe,[9] but the conventional recommended limit for subcutaneous lidocaine with epinephrine is only 5 to 7 mg/kg. Of significant concern is that the recommended doses used for liposuction procedures do not consider the ability of lidocaine to saturate the CYP3A4 enzymes. When saturation occurs, elimination lags behind absorption, and lidocaine toxicity results.

Numerous publications unequivocally demonstrate the toxicity associated with orally administered lidocaine despite its poor bioavailability.[20,115] Some of the toxicity is attributed to MEGX. Because of the relatively high concentration of viscous lidocaine (typically 4%), this preparation is overrepresented in reports of oral lidocaine poisoning.[115] As little as 15 mL of 2% viscous lidocaine in a 3-year-old child (estimate, 300 mg or 21.4 mg/kg/dose) is reported to cause seizures.

Chronic lidocaine toxicity most commonly occurs as a result of therapeutic misadventure in patients on lidocaine infusions, generally in a critical care unit. Toxicity after appropriate dosing is most likely to occur in patients with reduced hepatic blood flow as occurs with congestive heart failure,

liver disease, or concomitant therapy with CYP3A4 and CYP1A2 inhibitors (Chap. 11).[104] Adverse reactions to lidocaine also increase with advancing age, decreasing body weight, and increasing infusion rate. Chronic lidocaine toxicity occurs in 6% to 15% of patients receiving infusions at 3 mg/min for several days.[93] Partly for this reason, lidocaine is no longer routinely used to prevent dysrhythmias in the immediate postmyocardial infarction period. The clearance of lidocaine falls after approximately 24 hours of the start of an infusion, and this effect may be caused by competition for hepatic metabolism between lidocaine and its metabolites.

Mexiletine

Mexiletine, originally developed as an anorectic, was found to have antidysrhythmic, local anesthetic, and anticonvulsant activity.[17] It is currently available in oral form for the management of ventricular dysrhythmias and is used for the management of chronic neuropathic pain. Its chemical structure and electrophysiologic properties are similar to those of lidocaine. Mexiletine, a base, is absorbed in the small intestine; therefore, its absorption is increased when the gastric contents are alkalinized. Congestive heart failure and cirrhosis, as well as therapy with cimetidine or disulfiram, decrease the clearance of mexiletine.[62] Its metabolism, predominantly through CYP2D6, is accelerated by concomitant use of phenobarbital, rifampin, and phenytoin.

Adverse effects with therapeutic dosing are primarily neurologic and are similar to those that occur with lidocaine. The few reported cases of mexiletine overdose describe prominent cardiovascular effects such as complete heart block, torsade de pointes, and asystole.[23,37] Neurotoxicity resulting from overdose includes self-limited seizures, generally in the setting of cardiotoxicity. Moreover, a single case report described a patient with mexiletine poisoning who experienced status epilepticus without any hemodynamic or ECG abnormalities.[72] Mexiletine is reported to produce a false-positive result on the amphetamine immunoassay of the urine.[23,59]

Moricizine

Moricizine possesses the general qualities of class I antidysrhythmics but is difficult to specifically subclassify because it has properties that place it in both classes IB or IC.[22] Historically, it is discussed as a class IB antidysrhythmic, as it is here. The parent medication undergoes extensive and rapid metabolism. Dose-related lengthening of PR interval and QRS complex are expected, as are hemiblocks, bundle blocks, and sustained ventricular tachydysrhythmias. Experience in the setting of myocardial infarction during CAST II suggests that it is a prodysrhythmic.[102] Clinical experience with overdose is limited but is expected to be similar to that of other class I antidysrhythmics.

Management of Class IB Antidysrhythmic Toxicity

The focus of the initial management for IV lidocaine-induced cardiac arrest is continuous cardiopulmonary resuscitation to allow lidocaine to redistribute away from the heart. Apart from this setting, management of hemodynamic compromise includes fluid replacement and other conventional strategies. Catecholamine administration is recommended for the management of resistant hypotension, and if refractory toxicity persists, insertion of an intraaortic balloon assist pump or cardiac bypass.[39] Cardiopulmonary bypass, which does not directly enhance elimination, maintains hepatic perfusion, thereby allowing the lidocaine to be metabolized.[39] When bradydysrhythmias do not respond to atropine, chronotrope such as norepinephrine or isoproterenol is recommended. External pacing or insertion of a transvenous pacemaker is reportedly successful in some instances, but the myocardium is often refractory to electrical capture. Lidocaine-induced seizures, and those related to lidocaine analogs, are generally brief in nature and do not require specific therapy. For patients requiring treatment, an IV benzodiazepine is recommended; rarely, a barbiturate is required. Similarly, although IV lipid emulsion is often described as useful for the resuscitation of patients with life-threatening local anesthetic overdose (local anesthetic systemic toxicity) its use for lidocaine poisoned patients is limited to case reports and likely unnecessary given the rapid time course of recovery. As such, lipid emulsion is not recommended for lidocaine poisoning except in cases of severe and prolonged toxicity that are refractory to other therapies.[49] Lipid emulsion was used in the successful resuscitation from cardiac arrest after local infiltration of lidocaine for an incision and drainage procedure.[105] It was also used to reverse the CNS toxicity of lidocaine used for local anesthesia during procedures (Antidotes in Depth: A23).[63] Enhanced elimination techniques are limited after IV poisoning because of the rapid time course of poisoning.

After oral poisoning by a class IB antidysrhythmic, activated charcoal is recommended. Lidocaine and its metabolites are not well cleared by hemodialysis,[27] and there are no adequate data to support the use of extracorporeal removal for mexiletine or moricizine. There is one case report of a patient with a large oral mexiletine overdose who was successfully treated with hemodialysis, but how to apply this more broadly remains unclear.[4]

Class IC Antidysrhythmics: Flecainide and Propafenone
Flecainide

Flecainide, a derivative of procainamide, is orally administered to maintain sinus rhythm in patients with structurally normal hearts who have atrial fibrillation or supraventricular tachycardia.[100] Kidney disease, medication interactions, and congestive heart failure all decrease the clearance of flecainide and its active metabolite. Additionally, alkaluria reduces its clearance, presumably by enhanced tubular reuptake of nonionized flecainide. Therapeutic doses produce left ventricular dysfunction with worsening congestive heart failure. This is presumably a result of the negative inotropic effect of flecainide, which itself relates to its antagonistic effects on Ca^{2+} channels. Furthermore, sudden dysrhythmic death occurs, particularly in patients with underlying ischemic heart disease.[100]

Flecainide toxicity is associated with an increase in QRS complex duration, prolongation of the PR interval, and prolongation of the QT interval. The duration of the QRS complex has significant prognostic value: a QRS duration of 200 ms or greater is predictive of the need for mechanical circulatory support.[108] The expected consequences of these electrophysiologic disturbances include bradycardia, premature ventricular contractions, and ventricular fibrillation. Occasionally, supraventricular tachycardia can present with a bizarre axis and is often mistaken for ventricular tachycardia, which results in inappropriate treatment.[108] The combination of marked QRS complex and PR interval changes, associated with minimal QT interval prolongation, is characteristic of flecainide toxicity and contrasts with those described with other antidysrhythmics.

Propafenone

Propafenone bears a structural resemblance to propranolol,[36] as well as similar qualitative, but not quantitative, electrophysiologic properties.[32] Propafenone blocks fast inward Na^+ channels, is a weak β-adrenergic antagonist, and is an L-type Ca^{2+} channel blocker.[32] Its long half-life allows the accumulation of propafenone, particularly in patients with the slow metabolizer pharmacogenetic variant of CYP2D6 or those exposed to xenobiotics that inhibit this enzyme.[64] Propafenone overdose produces sinus bradycardia, ventricular dysrhythmias, and negative inotropy. The ECG often shows a right bundle branch block pattern, first-degree AV block, and prolongation of the QT interval. Generalized seizures have occurred.[77]

Management of Class IC Antidysrhythmic Toxicity

Management concentrates on assessment and correction of cardiovascular dysfunction. After airway evaluation and IV line placement, 12-lead ECG and continuous ECG monitoring are of paramount importance. Appropriate GI decontamination is recommended when the patient is sufficiently stabilized. Activated charcoal is recommended for early-presenting patients with a protected airway and an ingestion of a potentially toxic amount of medication. Gastric lavage is reasonable for patients with life-threatening ingestions who present within several hours depending on the severity and probability of retained ingestant. Decontamination should also include whole-bowel irrigation are recommended if a sustained-release preparation is involved (Chap. 5 and Antidotes in Depth: A2).

Standard management strategies for hypotension, such as fluid resuscitation, and for seizures, with benzodiazepines as well as careful attention to maintaining the airway as indicated. Additionally, therapy for hypotension and the ECG manifestations of class IC poisoning include IV hypertonic sodium bicarbonate to overcome the Na^+ channel blockade.[60] The utility of calcium salts for the treatment of propafenone toxicity is undefined. Several reports of overdose in humans verify QRS complex narrowing in response to hypertonic sodium bicarbonate administration on flecainide[12,50,66] and propafenone.[77] The renal elimination of flecainide is reduced by urinary alkalinization, suggesting that sodium chloride, in equimolar doses, is superior to sodium bicarbonate; however, the routine attempt to enhance urinary clearance with saline is not supported by evidence and is not recommended.[70] The administration of other class IC or IA antidysrhythmics is contraindicated because of their additive blockade of the Na^+ channel. Similarly, the administration of phenytoin to a child with propafenone poisoning was associated with a prolongation of the QRS complex, which initially responded to sodium bicarbonate, but the patient subsequently developed bradyasystolic arrest.[69] However, amiodarone was successful in the setting of flecainide-induced ventricular fibrillation refractory to other therapy.[96] As with β-adrenergic antagonists, an animal model and human case reports suggest that hyperinsulinemic euglycemic therapy is beneficial after propafenone poisoning.[7,116] In patients with refractory bradycardia, pacing should be attempted with the caveat that the efficacy of an external or internal pacemaker may be limited because of the xenobiotic-induced increased electrical pacing threshold of the ventricle. Successful therapy with cardiopulmonary bypass or extracorporeal membrane oxygenation (ECMO) is reported and is recommended in patients with severe toxicity when available.[6,13,25] Intravenous fat emulsion therapy was reportedly successful in two patients with severe flecainide poisoning[29] and in propafenone poisoning.[7,107] Although the safety and efficacy of lipid emulsion therapy in this setting remains undefined, it is reasonable for those who are seriously ill, deteriorating, and refractory to conventional therapy.

Extracorporeal removal is not expected to be beneficial for patients with flecainide poisoning. Although hemodialysis was successful in removing propafenone after overdose, additional studies are needed to determine its clinical benefit.[14] It is not recommended at this time.

CLASS III ANTIDYSRHYTHMICS
Amiodarone, Dofetilide, Dronedarone, and Ibutilide

The class III antidysrhythmics prevent and terminate reentrant dysrhythmias by prolonging the action potential duration and effective refractory period without slowing conduction velocity during phase 0 or 1 of the action potential. This effect on the action potential is generally caused by blockade of the rapidly activating component of the delayed rectifier K^+ current, which is responsible for repolarization.

The class III antidysrhythmics in use today prolong repolarization of both the atria and ventricles. Thus, common ECG effects at therapeutic doses include prolongation of the PR and QT intervals and abnormal T and U waves. Chap. 15 contains a detailed discussion of the pharmacologic mechanisms of class III antidysrhythmics. Also, Chaps. 16 and 59 discuss sotalol.

Amiodarone and Dronedarone

Amiodarone (Fig. 57–4) is an iodinated benzofuran derivative that is structurally similar to both thyroxine and procainamide. Forty percent of its molecular weight is iodine. Dronedarone is an analog of amiodarone that does not contain iodine.[60] The 2015 revision of the Advanced Cardiovascular Life Support guidelines places significant emphasis on the early IV administration of amiodarone for ventricular dysrhythmias. Both medications are used primarily to terminate or prevent atrial fibrillation, and although dronedarone is less effective and has safety issues,[24] it is not associated with many of the potentially severe adverse effects of amiodarone.[92]

Although amiodarone and dronedarone have multiple pharmacologic effects, their efficacy is primarily the result of their class III antidysrhythmic effects. They also have weak α- and β-adrenergic antagonist activity and can

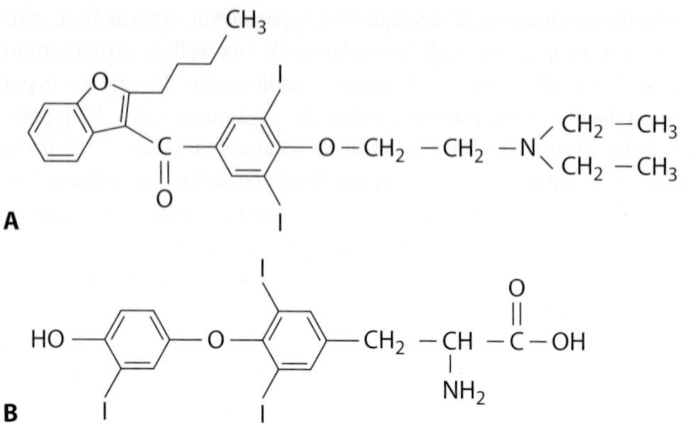

FIGURE 57–4. Structures of amiodarone (**A**) compared with triiodothyronine (**B**). Note that amiodarone is nearly 40% iodine by weight.

block both L-type Ca^{2+} channels and inactivated Na^+ channels. Amiodarone is slowly absorbed by the oral route and concentrates in the liver, lung, and adipose tissue. It has a very long elimination half-life, measured in weeks, and steady-state pharmacokinetics do not occur until after 1 month of use. Dronedarone has a half-life of about 24 hours and a smaller volume of distribution.

The ECG effects of amiodarone differ based on the route of medication administration. Therapeutic oral doses prolong the PR and QT intervals but do not alter the QRS complex. Intravenous dosing prolongs the PR interval but has few other ECG manifestations. Ventricular dysrhythmias and sinus bradycardia are the most serious cardiac complications of therapeutic doses of amiodarone. Ventricular tachycardia reported to be resistant to cardioversion and pharmacologic interventions occur[35] but are surprisingly uncommon given the frequency and extent to which the QT interval prolongation occurs. The ability of amiodarone to compete for P-glycoprotein is responsible for several drug interactions, including elevated digoxin and cyclosporin concentrations and enhanced anticoagulation effectiveness of warfarin[61] (Chap. 9).

The diverse complications associated with long-term amiodarone therapy do not occur after short-term IV use. Chronic therapy with oral amiodarone causes substantial pulmonary, thyroid, corneal, hepatic, and cutaneous toxicity caused by bioaccumulation in these organs. Dronedarone rarely causes hepatic or pulmonary toxicity.[26] Many of these effects appear to be dose related, but because of the wide range of bioavailabilities and metabolic patterns among different patients, as well as the overlap between therapeutic and toxic serum concentrations, therapeutic drug monitoring is of limited benefit.[41] Pneumonitis, the most consequential extracardiac adverse effect, occurs in up to 5% of patients taking the xenobiotic therapeutically. Amiodarone pneumonitis rarely develops within days of initiating therapy but typically occurs only after years of therapy. Its occurrence appears to be dose related: a daily dose of greater than 400 mg is a risk factor, and pneumonitis is rare in those taking less than 200 mg daily. Focusing on using the minimal effective dose has reduced the incidence of pneumonitis.[31] Oxygen supplementation speeds the development of pneumonitis, which explains the initial belief that patients with chronic lung disease are at increased risk for amiodarone pneumonitis. Manifestations of pneumonitis include dyspnea, cough, hemoptysis, crackles, hypoxia, and radiographic changes.[18] A chest computed tomography scan is the most helpful initial diagnostic test for pneumonitis but is not useful for monitoring purposes, which is often done with diffusing capacity of carbon monoxide.[41] Bronchoalveolar lavage typically reveals interstitial pneumonitis with many macrophages and a characteristic finely vacuolated foamy cytoplasm, but confirmation of the diagnosis requires open lung biopsy.

Thyroid dysfunction, either amiodarone-induced thyrotoxicosis (AIT) or amiodarone-induced hypothyroidism (AIH), occurs in approximately 4% of patients.[19] Amiodarone-induced hypothyroidism is more common than AIT when iodine intake is sufficient.[41] Amiodarone-induced hypothyroidism is likely caused by an exaggerated Wolff-Chaikoff effect, in which iodine—in this case from amiodarone—inhibits the organification and release of thyroid hormone. Amiodarone-induced thyrotoxicosis appears to exist in two distinct forms: type I AIT, which occurs in patients with abnormal thyroid glands and iodine-induced excessive thyroid hormone synthesis and release, and type II AIT, in which destructive thyroiditis leads to release of thyroid hormone from the damaged follicular cells. The relative prevalence of the two forms of AIT is unknown. Amiodarone also reduces the effect of thyroid hormone on peripheral tissue. The diagnosis is confirmed with standard thyroid function testing (thyroid-stimulating hormone, total triiodothyronine and free thyroxine[101] (Chap. 53).

Corneal microdeposits are extremely common during chronic therapy and leads to vision loss.[68] Abnormal elevation of hepatic enzymes occurs in more than 30% of those on long-term therapy, and the hepatotoxicity progresses to cirrhosis. Periodic monitoring of aminotransferases is recommended.[41] Hepatotoxicity has occurred after initial loading of amiodarone.[84] Slate-gray or bluish discoloration of the skin is common, particularly in sun-exposed portions of the body.[88]

Dofetilide

Dofetilide is approved for conversion of atrial fibrillation or atrial flutter to a normal sinus rhythm. Dofetilide increases the effective refractory period more substantially in atrial tissue than in ventricular fibers, accounting for this clinical indication.[90] Dofetilide has no known effect on Ca^{2+} or Na^+ channels, nor does it result in β-adrenergic antagonism. Dofetilide increases the QT interval but does not change either the PR interval or QRS complex in humans. Heart rate and blood pressure are also not appreciably affected.

Although limited data are available, the expected and reported adverse cardiac events include ventricular tachycardia, particularly torsade de pointes.[112] The approximate incidence of torsade de pointes in patients receiving high therapeutic doses of the medication is 3%.[3] For this reason, the US Food and Drug Administration has in place strict requirements for the use of dofetilide, such as an individualized dose initiation algorithm and mandatory hospitalization for initial therapy.[56]

Overdose data reported by the manufacturer include two cases. One patient reportedly ingested 28 capsules and experienced no events, but a second patient inadvertently received two supratherapeutic doses 1 hour apart and experienced fatal ventricular fibrillation.[80] A 33-year-old man ingested 5 mg (20 capsules) and developed QT interval prolongation within 1 hour of ingestion but had no dysrhythmia during his 4-day hospital stay.[16] One patient with a 90-fold intentional overdose experienced nonsustained ventricular tachycardia, frequent multifocal premature ventricular contractions, and ventricular bigeminy, which were successfully treated with potassium and magnesium.[47]

Ibutilide

Ibutilide is an antidysrhythmic with predominant class III activity used for the rapid conversion of atrial fibrillation and flutter to normal sinus rhythm. Because of its extensive first-pass metabolism, ibutilide can only be administered parenterally. Its metabolic pathways are not well understood but do not involve the isoenzymes CYP3A4 or CYP2D6. Pharmacokinetic data thus far do not indicate that age, sex, hepatic, or CKD necessitates adjustment of recommended dosage of ibutilide. In addition to its effects on the delayed rectifier current, ibutilide activates a slow inward Na^+ current.[71]

Ibutilide increases the QT interval and causes torsade de pointes, especially in patients with congenital long-QT syndrome and in women.[42] Although ibutilide enhances the efficacy of transthoracic cardioversion for atrial fibrillation, its use in patients with ejection fractions below 20% is associated with an increased incidence of sustained polymorphic ventricular tachycardia. Acute kidney injury, including biopsy-identified crystals, is reported in association with ibutilide cardioversion, but a causal relationship is not yet definitive.[38] Acute overdose information, only available in limited form (four patients) through the manufacturer, suggests that ventricular dysrhythmias and high-degree AV conduction abnormalities should be expected.[79]

Management of Class III Antidysrhythmic Toxicity

Treatment experience with class III antidysrhythmic overdose is limited. Isoproterenol, magnesium sulfate, and overdrive pacing can prevent recurrent torsade de pointes after initial spontaneous resolution or defibrillation. However, prolonged therapy may be required for amiadorone overdose because of the long half-life of drug.[94] Administration of class IB antidysrhythmics or propranolol for the control of monomorphic ventricular tachycardia cannot be recommended on theoretical grounds. Paradoxically, amiodarone may reduce the risk of torsade de pointes associated with the other class III antidysrhythmics.[97] This effect is likely mediated by the beneficial effects of amiodarone on the dispersion of myocardial repolarization and its Ca²⁺ channel–blocking activity.

Oral activated charcoal is recommended if patients present shortly after overdose. Hemodialysis is not expected to be beneficial in general, either because of extensive protein binding or because of large volumes of distribution (Table 57–1). A neonate survived cardiovascular collapse with the use of ECMO after an iatrogenic IV amiodarone overdose.[44] Although the benefit versus risk profile of this intervention is undefined, it is reasonable to implement ECMO if it is available or reasonably attainable through transfer. Lipid emulsion sequesters amiodarone and is demonstrated to be beneficial in swine models.[114] It is only reasonable administered to patients with severe amiodarone poisoning refractory to standard resuscitative efforts. However, when amiodarone is used as a treatment for poisoning by another xenobiotic, lipid emulsion therapy will reduce the effectiveness of the amiodarone because of subsequent sequestration.[74]

ANTIDYSRHYTHMICS-UNCLASSIFIED

Adenosine, a nucleoside found in all cells, is released from myocardial cells under physiologic and pathophysiologic conditions. It is administered as a rapid IV bolus to terminate reentrant supraventricular tachycardia. The effects of adenosine are mediated by its interaction with specific G protein–coupled adenosine (A₁) receptors that activate acetylcholine-sensitive outward K⁺ current in the atrium, sinus nodes, and AV nodes. The resultant hyperpolarization reduces the rate of cellular firing. Adenosine also reduces the Ca²⁺ currents, and its antidysrhythmic activity results from its effect in increasing AV nodal refractoriness and from inhibiting delayed afterdepolarizations elicited by sympathetic stimulation.[65]

Adverse effects of adenosine administration are very common and include transient asystole, dyspnea, chest tightness, flushing, hypotension, and atrial fibrillation. Although bronchospasm occurs after pulmonary vascular administration, it is not reported after routine IV use. Dyspnea, and probably chest tightness, is related to adenosine stimulation of the pulmonary vagal C fibers.[15] Fortunately, most of the adverse effects of adenosine are transient because of its rapid metabolism to inosine by both extracellular and intracellular deaminases. The clinical effects are potentiated by dipyridamole, an adenosine uptake inhibitor,[40] and by denervation hypersensitivity in cardiac transplant recipients. Methylxanthines block adenosine receptors (Chap. 63). In this setting, larger-than-usual doses of adenosine are required to produce an antidysrhythmic effect. Overdose of adenosine is not reported. Treatment is supportive because of the rapid elimination of the medication.

Digoxin, a cardioactive steroid, is often considered a member of this class. A complete discussion of digoxin can be found in Chap. 62.

Magnesium ion is occasionally included in this class as well because of its ability to prevent the development of recurrent torsade de pointes. A complete discussion of magnesium sulfate can be found in Antidotes in Depth: A16.

SUMMARY

- In the overdose setting, the class IA, B, and C antidysrhythmics all produce Na⁺ channel blockade, which can induce profound wide-complex cardiac dysrhythmias and morbidity if not treated judiciously.
- The class IC antidysrhythmics are considerably more toxic than the other class I antidysrhythmics, although even the class IB antidysrhythmics are lethal in overdose. Dysrhythmias are their primary toxicologic effect.

- The class III antidysrhythmics in overdose cause malignant dysrhythmias, particularly torsade de pointes. Amiodarone has many noncardiac effects, particularly pneumonitis and thyroid effects, which limit its therapeutic usefulness.
- Proper management of both adverse effects and overdose can be accomplished only by understanding the pharmacokinetics and toxicokinetics of these medications.

Acknowledgments

Neal A. Lewin, MD; Mary Ann Howland, PharmD; and Harold Osborn, MD, (deceased) contributed to this chapter in a previous edition.

REFERENCES

1. Abe M, et al. Disopyramide-induced hypoglycemia in a non-diabetic hemodialysis patient: a case report and review of the literature. *Clin Nephrol.* 2011;76:401-406.
2. Accornero F, et al. Prolonged cardiopulmonary resuscitation during acute disopyramide poisoning. *Vet Hum Toxicol.* 1993;35:231-232.
3. Aktas MK, et al. Dofetilide-induced long QT and torsades de pointes. *Ann Noninvasive Electrocardiol.* 2007;12:197-202.
4. Akıncı E, et al. Hemodialysis as an alternative treatment of mexiletine intoxication. *Am J Emerg Med.* 2011;29:1235.e5.e6.
5. Atkinson AJ, et al. Comparison of the pharmacokinetic and pharmacodynamic properties of procainamide and N-acetylprocainamide. *Angiology.* 1988;39(7 Pt 2):655-667.
6. Auzinger GM, Scheinkestel CD. Successful extracorporeal life support in a case of severe flecainide intoxication. *Crit Care Med.* 2001;29:887-890.
7. Bayram B, et al. Propafenone-induced cardiac arrest: full recovery with insulin, is it possible? *Am J Emerg Med.* 2013;31:457.e5-e7.
8. Bennett PB, et al. Competition between lidocaine and one of its metabolites, glycylxylidide, for cardiac sodium channels. *Circulation.* 1988;78:692-700.
9. Boeni R. Safety of tumescent liposuction under local anesthesia in a series of 4,380 patients. *Dermatology (Basel).* 2011;222:278-281.
10. Bou-Abboud E, Nattel S. Relative role of alkalosis and sodium ions in reversal of class I antiarrhythmic drug-induced sodium channel blockade by sodium bicarbonate. *Circulation.* 1996;94:1954-1961.
11. Boyes RN, et al. Pharmacokinetics of lidocaine in man. *Clin Pharmacol Ther.* 1971;12:105-116.
12. Brubacher J. Bicarbonate therapy for unstable propafenone-induced wide complex tachycardia. *CJEM.* 2004;6:349-356.
13. Brumfield E, et al. Life-threatening flecainide overdose treated with intralipid and extracorporeal membrane oxygenation. *Am J Emerg Med.* 2015;33:1840.e3-e5.
14. Burgess ED, Duff HJ. Hemodialysis removal of propafenone. *Pharmacotherapy.* 1989;9:331-333.
15. Burki NK, et al. Intravenous adenosine and dyspnea in humans. *J Appl Physiol.* 2005;98:180-185.
16. Campbell KB, Mando JD, Gray AL, Robinson E. Management of dofetilide overdose in a patient with known cocaine abuse. *Pharmacotherapy.* 2007;27:459-463.
17. Campbell RWF. Mexiletine. *N Engl J Med.* 2013;316:29-34.
18. Camus P, et al. Amiodarone pulmonary toxicity. *Clin Chest Med.* 2004;25:65-75.
19. Cardenas GA, et al. Amiodarone induced thyrotoxicosis: diagnostic and therapeutic strategies. *Cleve Clin J Med.* 2003;70:624-626.
20. Centini F, et al. Suicide due to oral ingestion of lidocaine: a case report and review of the literature. *Forensic Sci Int.* 2007;171:57-62.
21. Clemessy JL, et al. Treatment of acute chloroquine poisoning: a 5-year experience. *Crit Care Med.* 1996;24:1189-1195.
22. Clyne CA, et al. Moricizine. *N Engl J Med.* 1992;327:255-260.
23. Cocco G, et al. Torsades de pointes as a manifestation of mexiletine toxicity. *Am Heart J.* 1980;100(6 Pt 1):878-880.
24. Connolly SJ, et al. Dronedarone in high-risk permanent atrial fibrillation. *N Engl J Med.* 2011;365:2268-2276.
25. Corkeron MA, et al. Extracorporeal circulatory support in near-fatal flecainide overdose. *Anaesth Intensive Care.* 1999;27:405-408.
26. De Ferrari GM, Dusi V. Drug safety evaluation of dronedarone in atrial fibrillation. *Expert Opin Drug Saf.* 2012;11:1023-1045.
27. De Martin S, et al. Differential effect of chronic renal failure on the pharmacokinetics of lidocaine in patients receiving and not receiving hemodialysis. *Clin Pharmacol Ther.* 2006;80:597-606.
28. Echt DS, et al. Mortality and morbidity in patients receiving encainide, flecainide, or placebo. The Cardiac Arrhythmia Suppression Trial. *N Engl J Med.* 1991;324:781-788.
29. Ellsworth H, et al. A life-threatening flecainide overdose treated with intravenous fat emulsion. *Pacing Clin Electrophysiol.* 2013;36:e87-e89.
30. Elmariah S, Fifer MA. Medical, surgical and interventional management of hypertrophic cardiomyopathy with obstruction. *Curr Treat Options Cardiovasc Med.* 2012;14:665-678.
31. Ernawati DK, et al. Amiodarone-induced pulmonary toxicity. *Br J Clin Pharmacol.* 2008;66:82-87.

32. Faber TS, Camm AJ. The differentiation of propafenone from other class Ic agents, focusing on the effect on ventricular response rate attributable to its beta-blocking action. *Eur J Clin Pharmacol*. 1996;51:199-208.

33. Finkelstein F, Kreeft J. Massive lidocaine poisoning. *N Engl J Med*. 1979;301:50.

34. Foianini A, et al. What is the role of lidocaine or phenytoin in tricyclic antidepressant-induced cardiotoxicity? *Clin Toxicol*. 2010;48:325-330.

35. Foley P, et al. Amiodarone—Avoid the danger of Torsade de Pointes. *Resuscitation*. 2008;76:137-141.

36. Fonck K, et al. ECG changes and plasma concentrations of propafenone and its metabolites in a case of severe poisoning. *J Toxicol Clin Toxicol*. 1998;36:247-251.

37. Frank SE, Snyder JT. Survival following severe overdose with mexiletine, nifedipine, and nitroglycerine. *Am J Emerg Med*. 1991;9:43-46.

38. Franz M, et al. Acute renal failure after ibutilide. *Lancet*. 353:467-467.

39. Freed CR, Freedman MD. Lidocaine overdose and cardiac bypass support. *JAMA*. 253:3094-3095.

40. Gamboa A, et al. Role of adenosine and nitric oxide on the mechanisms of action of dipyridamole. *Stroke*. 2005;36:2170-2175.

41. Goldschlager N, et al. A practical guide for clinicians who treat patients with amiodarone: 2007. *Heart Rhythm*. 2007;4:1250-1259.

42. Gowda RM, et al. Female preponderance in ibutilide-induced torsade de pointes. *Int J Cardiol*. 2004;95:219-222.

43. Haapanen EJ, Pellinen TJ. Hemoperfusion in quinidine intoxication. *Acta Med Scand*. 1981;210:515-516.

44. Haas NA, et al. ECMO for cardiac rescue in a neonate with accidental amiodarone overdose. *Clin Res Cardiol*. 2008;97:878-881.

45. Harron DW, Brogden RN. Acecainide (N-acetylprocainamide). A review of its pharmacodynamic and pharmacokinetic properties, and therapeutic potential in cardiac arrhythmias. *Drugs*. 1990;39:720-740.

46. Heyman MR, et al. Procainamide-induced lupus anticoagulant. *South Med J*. 1988;81:934-936.

47. Hieger MA, et al. Dofetilide in overdose: a case series from poison center data. *Cardiovasc Toxicol*. 2017;17:368-374.

48. Hiraoka M, et al. New observations on the mechanisms of antiarrhythmic actions of disopyramide on cardiac membranes. *Am J Cardiol*. 1989;64:15J-19J.

49. Hoegberg LCG, et al. Systematic review of the effect of intravenous lipid emulsion therapy for local anesthetic toxicity. *Clin Toxicol*. 2016;54:167-193.

50. Jang DH, et al. A Case of Near-fatal flecainide overdose in a neonate successfully treated with sodium bicarbonate. *J Emerg Med*. 2013;44:781-783.

51. Jenzer HR, Hagemeijer F. Quinidine syncope: torsade de pointes with low quinidine plasma concentrations. *Eur J Cardiol*. 1976;4:447-451.

52. John RM, et al. Ventricular arrhythmias and sudden cardiac death. *Lancet*. 2012;380:1520-1529.

53. Kallergis EM, et al. Mechanisms, risk factors, and management of acquired long QT syndrome: a comprehensive review. *Scientific World Journal*. 2012;2012:1-8.

54. Kempen PM. Lethal/toxic injection of 20% lidocaine: a well-known complication of an unnecessary preparation? *Anesthesiology*. 1986;65:564-565.

55. Kenkel JM, et al. Pharmacokinetics and safety of lidocaine and monoethylglycinexylidide in liposuction: a microdialysis study. *Plast Reconstr Surg*. 2004;114:516-524, discussion 525-526.

56. Kim MH, et al. Cost of hospital admission for antiarrhythmic drug initiation in atrial fibrillation. *Ann Pharmacother*. 2009;43:840-848.

57. Kim SY, Benowitz NL. Poisoning due to class IA antiarrhythmic drugs. Quinidine, procainamide and disopyramide. *Drug Saf*. 1990;5:393-420.

58. Knudsen K, Abrahamsson J. Effects of epinephrine, norepinephrine, magnesium sulfate, and milrinone on survival and the occurrence of arrhythmias in amitriptyline poisoning in the rat. *Crit Care Med*. 1994;22:1851-1855.

59. Kozer E, et al. Misdiagnosis of a mexiletine overdose because of a nonspecific result of urinary toxicologic screening. *N Engl J Med*. 2000;343:1971-1972.

60. Kozlowski D, et al. Dronedarone: an overview. *Ann Med*. 2012;44:60-72. doi:10.3109/078 53890.2011.594808.

61. Kurnik D, et al. Complex drug-drug-disease interactions between amiodarone, warfarin, and the thyroid gland. *Medicine*. 2004;83:107-113.

62. Labbe L, Turgeon J. Clinical pharmacokinetics of mexiletine. *Clin Pharmacokinet*. 1999;37:361-384.

63. Lange DB, et al. Use of intravenous lipid emulsion to reverse central nervous system toxicity of an iatrogenic local anesthetic overdose in a patient on peritoneal dialysis. *Ann Pharmacother*. 2012;46:e37-e37.

64. Lee JT, et al. The role of genetically determined polymorphic drug metabolism in the beta-blockade produced by propafenone. *N Engl J Med*. 1990;322:1764-1768.

65. Lerman BB, Belardinelli L. Cardiac electrophysiology of adenosine. Basic and clinical concepts. *Circulation*. 1991;83:1499-1509.

66. Lovecchio F, et al. Hypertonic sodium bicarbonate in an acute flecainide overdose. *Am J Emerg Med*. 1998;16:534-537.

67. Low CL, et al. Relative efficacy of haemoperfusion, haemodialysis and CAPD in the removal of procainamide and NAPA in a patient with severe procainamide toxicity. *Nephrol Dial Transplant*. 1996;11:881-884.

68. Mantyjarvi M, et al. Ocular side effects of amiodarone. *Surv Ophthalmol*. 1998;42:360-366.

69. McHugh TP, Perina DG. Propafenone ingestion. *Ann Emerg Med*. 1987;16:437-440.

70. Muhiddin KA, et al. The influence of urinary pH on flecainide excretion and its serum pharmacokinetics. *Br J Clin Pharmacol*. 1984;17:447-451.

71. Murray KT. Ibutilide. *Circulation*. 1998;97:493-497.

72. Nelson LS, Hoffman RS. Mexiletine overdose producing status epilepticus without cardiovascular abnormalities. *J Toxicol Clin Toxicol*. 1994;32:731-736.

73. Nelson LS. Toxicologic myocardial sensitization. *J Toxicol Clin Toxicol*. 2002;40:867-879.

74. Niiya T, et al. Intravenous lipid emulsion sequesters amiodarone in plasma and eliminates its hypotensive action in pigs. *Ann Emerg Med*. 2010;56:402-408.e402.

75. O'Keeffe B, et al. Cardiac consequences and treatment of disopyramide intoxication: experimental evaluation in dogs. *Cardiovasc Res*. 13:630-634.

76. Okumura K, et al. Genotyping of N-acetylation polymorphism and correlation with procainamide metabolism. *Clin Pharmacol Ther*. 1997;61:509-517.

77. Ovaska H, et al. Propafenone poisoning—a case report with plasma propafenone concentrations. *J Med Toxicol*. 2010;6:37-40.

78. Pantuck AJ, et al. Seizures after ureteral stone manipulation with lidocaine. *J Urol*. 1997;157:2248.

79. Pfizer Pharmaceuticals. *Corvert (Ibutilide Fumarate) Prescribing Information*. 2009:1-12. http://labeling.pfizer.com/showlabeling.aspx?id=886.

80. Pfizer Pharmaceuticals. *Tikosyn (Dofetilide) Prescribing Information*. 2011. http://www.tikosyn.com.

81. Phillips RE, et al. Hypoglycaemia and antimalarial drugs: quinidine and release of insulin. *Br Med J (Clin Res Ed)*. 292:1319-1321.

82. Platt MS, et al. Deaths associated with liposuction: case reports and review of the literature. *J Forensic Sci*. 2002;47:205-207.

83. Rao RB, et al. Deaths related to liposuction. *N Engl J Med*. 1999;340:1471-1475.

84. Rätz Bravo AE, et al. Hepatotoxicity during rapid intravenous loading with amiodarone: description of three cases and review of the literature. *Crit Care Med*. 2005;33:128-134.

85. Resar LM, Helfaer MA. Recurrent seizures in a neonate after lidocaine administration. *J Perinatol*. 1998;18:193-195.

86. Rezvani M, et al. Generalized seizures following topical lidocaine administration during circumcision: establishing causation. *Paediatr Drugs*. 2007;9:125-127.

87. Roden DM. Risks and benefits of antiarrhythmic therapy. *N Engl J Med*. 1994;331:785-791.

88. Rogers KC, Wolfe DA. Amiodarone-induced blue-gray syndrome. *Ann Pharmacother*. 2000;34:1075-1075.

89. Romme JJ, et al. Drugs and pacemakers for vasovagal, carotid sinus and situational syncope. *Cochrane Database Syst Rev*. 2011;:CD004194.

90. Roukoz H, Saliba W. Dofetilide: a new class III antiarrhythmic agent. *Expert Rev Cardiovasc Ther*. 2007;5:9-19.

91. Roy D, et al. Rhythm control versus rate control for atrial fibrillation and heart failure. *N Engl J Med*. 2008;358:2667-2677.

92. Santangeli P, et al. Examining the safety of amiodarone. *Expert Opin Drug Saf*. 2012;11:191-214.

93. Sawyer DR, et al. Continuous infusion of lidocaine in patients with cardiac arrhythmias. Unpredictability of plasma concentrations. *Arch Intern Med*. 1981;141:43-45.

94. Sclarovsky S, et al. Amiodarone-induced polymorphous ventricular tachycardia. *Am Heart J*. 105:6-12.

95. Shimizu K, et al. The tissue distribution of lidocaine in acute death due to overdosing. *Legal Medicine*. 2000;2:101-105.

96. Siegers A, Board PN. Amiodarone used in successful resuscitation after near-fatal flecainide overdose. *Resuscitation*. 2002;53:105-108.

97. Singh BN, Wadhani N. Antiarrhythmic and proarrhythmic properties of QT-prolonging antianginal drugs. *J Cardiovasc Pharmacol Ther*. 2004;9(suppl 1 IS):85-97.

98. Takada Y, et al. Effects of antiarrhythmic agents on left ventricular function during exercise in patients with chronic left ventricular dysfunction. *Ann Nucl Med*. 2004;18:209-219.

99. Takeo S, et al. A possible involvement of sodium channel blockade of class-I-type antiarrhythmic agents in postischemic contractile recovery of isolated, perfused hearts. *J Pharmacol Exp Ther*. 1995;273:1403-1409.

100. Tamargo J, et al. Safety of flecainide. *Drug Saf*. 2012;35:273-289.

101. Tanda ML, et al. Diagnosis and management of amiodarone-induced thyrotoxicosis: similarities and differences between North American and European thyroidologists. *Clin Endocrinol (Oxf)*. 2008;69:812-818.

102. The Cardiac Arrhythmia Suppression Trial II Investigators. Effect of the antiarrhythmic agent moricizine on survival after myocardial infarction. *N Engl J Med*. 1992;327:227-233.

103. Thireau J, et al. New drugs vs. old concepts: a fresh look at antiarrhythmics. *Pharmacol Ther*. 2011;132:125-145.

104. Thomson PD, et al. Lidocaine pharmacokinetics in advanced heart failure, liver disease, and renal failure in humans. *Ann Intern Med*. 1973;78:499-508.

105. Tierney KJ, et al. Lidocaine-induced cardiac arrest in the emergency department: effectiveness of lipid therapy. *J Emerg Med*. 2016;50:47-50.

106. Tsuchishita Y, et al. Effects of serum concentrations of disopyramide and its metabolite mono-N-dealkyldisopyramide on the anticholinergic side effects associated with disopyramide. *Biol Pharm Bull*. 2008;31:1368-1370.

107. Tusscher ten BL, et al. Intravenous fat emulsion therapy for intentional propafenone intoxication. *Clin Toxicol.* 2011;49:701.

108. Valentino MA, et al. Flecainide toxicity: a case report and systematic review of its electrocardiographic patterns and management. *Cardiovasc Toxicol.* 2016:1-7.

109. Vaughan-Williams EM. Classifying antiarrhythmic actions: by facts or speculation. *J Clin Pharmacol.* 1992;32:964-977.

110. White SR, et al. The case of the slandered Halloween cupcake: survival after massive pediatric procainamide overdose. *Pediatr Emerg Care.* 2002;18:185-188.

111. Winecoff AP, et al. Reversal of the electrocardiographic effects of cocaine by lidocaine. Part 1. Comparison with sodium bicarbonate and quinidine. *Pharmacotherapy.* 1994;14:698-703.

112. Wolbrette DL. Risk of proarrhythmia with class III antiarrhythmic agents: sex-based differences and other issues. *Am J Cardiol.* 2003;91(6A SP -):44.

113. Wu FL, et al. Seizure after lidocaine for bronchoscopy: case report and review of the use of lidocaine in airway anesthesia. *Pharmacotherapy.* 1993;13:72-78.

114. Xanthos T, et al. Intralipid™ administration attenuates the hypotensive effects of acute intravenous amiodarone overdose in a swine model. *Am J Emerg Med.* 2016;34:1389-1393.

115. Yamashita S, et al. Lidocaine toxicity during frequent viscous lidocaine use for painful tongue ulcer. *J Pain Symptom Manage.* 2002;24:543-545.

116. Yi H-Y, et al. Cardioprotective effect of glucose-insulin on acute propafenone toxicity in rat. *Am J Emerg Med.* 2012;30:680-689.

Silas W. Smith

INTRODUCTION

Although magnesium is a divalent cation like other metals, we will refer to it as magnesium in this text. It is an essential cofactor in more than 350 enzyme reactions in cardiac, neurologic, neuromuscular, and endocrine processes, as well as in basic energy, structural, nucleic acid, and signal transduction pathways.[107,136] Hypomagnesemia results in nausea, vomiting, weakness, muscle spasms, neurologic and muscular excitation (tremor, hyperreflexia, and tetany), and cardiac dysrhythmias. Hypermagnesemia produces cardiovascular effects, including conduction disturbances, hypotension, and cardiac arrest; respiratory depression; gastrointestinal (GI) complaints of nausea, vomiting, and thirst; and neuromuscular sequelae, including weakness, paralysis, and central nervous system (CNS) depression.[4,77,131] Magnesium as chloride, citrate, hydroxide, oxide or sulfate is used to repair xenobiotic-associated hypomagnesemia and as an adjunctive treatment for cardiovascular toxins, fluoride toxicity, pesticide poisoning, and alcohol use disorders.

HISTORY

In 1679, Nehemiah Grew described the process of obtaining the eponymous salts in the springs of Epsom through evaporation, which he later published in 1695 to be magnesium sulfate ($MgSO_4$).[105] Later as an antidote, $MgSO_4$ was used as a therapy for tetanus in 1906.[63] In 1923, $MgSO_4$ was introduced to treat the convulsions of nephritis in children, which was later extended to the advanced chronic nephritis in adults.[131] On the basis of reports in 1925 and 1926, $MgSO_4$ came into common practice for the prevention and control of seizures in severe toxemia of pregnancy; its use for this indication was "grandfathered" by the US Food and Drug Administration (FDA).[20] The cardiac utility of $MgSO_4$ was demonstrated in 1935 and 1943 as therapy to suppress "paroxysmal tachycardia."[13,139] Magnesium sulfate also continues in use as a uterine tocolytic, a bronchodilator a migraine therapy and as a nutritional adjunct to prevent hypomagnesemia in hyperalimentation.

PHARMACOLOGY

Chemistry and Preparation

Magnesium has the atomic number 12, with a molecular weight of 24.3 Da. Despite having a smaller atomic radius than calcium, magnesium binds water tighter, with two hydration shells, leading to a radius 400 times larger than its dehydrated form.[64] This property underlies its calcium antagonism, despite similar chemical reactivity and charge.[64] For clinical use, magnesium is prepared as a salt, typically in combination with chloride, citrate, hydroxide oxide, or sulfate. Magnesium as $MgSO_4$ is typically formulated in its heptahydrate form $MgSO_4 \cdot 7H_2O$, with a molecular weight of 120.38 Da alone and 246.47 when accounting for water. It occurs as colorless crystals or white powder, which is freely soluble in water.

Related Agents

The use of magnesium as an oral saline cathartic (eg, magnesium citrate, magnesium hydroxide, and $MgSO_4$) is discussed in Antidotes in Depth: A2.

Pharmacokinetics

Magnesium is the fourth most common plasma cation after sodium, potassium, and calcium but follows potassium as the second most prevalent intracellular cation.[37] Adults contain approximately 1 mole (21–28 g)

of magnesium; homeostasis balances intestinal absorption and renal excretion.[107] A normal serum magnesium concentration is 1.5 to 2.0 mEq/L (1.7–2.4 mg/dL; 0.7–1 mmol/L).[16] Magnesium is approximately 30% to 40% protein bound.[16,82] Extracellular magnesium represents only 1% of the body's total stores, with the remaining magnesium found in bone (~60%), muscle (~20%), and soft tissues (~19%). Serum values do not always accurately reflect tissue concentrations and can be normal despite intracellular deficiency.[37] This discrepancy was assessed by determining retained magnesium in response to an intravenous (IV) load: those retaining more than 30% of an 800-mg load of IV magnesium were considered magnesium depleted; those retaining less than 20% were replete.[120] Magnesium is not metabolized, but only ionized magnesium is physiologically active. After being absorbed, magnesium is eliminated by the kidney and occurs at a rate proportional to the plasma concentration and glomerular filtration. As kidney function declines, compensatory decreases in tubular resorption occur; however, in end-stage kidney disease, limited magnesium excretion can lead to hypermagnesemia.[136]

Pharmacokinetic studies of $MgSO_4$ typically have involved pregnant women with preeclampsia. After a 4-g loading dose followed by a 1-g/h continuous maintenance infusion, serum magnesium concentrations approximately doubled from 0.74 to 0.85 mmol/L to 1.48 to 1.70 mmol/L at 30 minutes and remained constant for at least 24 hours.[91] When a 4-g loading dose is followed by a 2-g/h continuous maintenance infusion, magnesium concentrations reach 1.73 to 2.25 mmol/L.[91] After IV $MgSO_4$ administration, the apparent volume of distribution (V_d) increases rapidly and becomes constant within 2 hours in healthy nonpregnant individuals but may not become constant for up to 4 hours in pregnant women.[21] Given intramuscularly, [$MgSO_4$] does not peak until 90 to 120 minutes followed by a slow decline back to baseline concentrations over 4 to 8 hours, unless repeated intramuscular (IM) magnesium is provided at 4 hours.[21,82,91]

Pharmacodynamics and Mechanisms of Action

The critical roles and functions of magnesium are more completely reviewed in Chap. 12. Selected key magnesium actions provide the physiologic basis for antidotal strategies. Adenosine triphosphate (ATP) avidly binds and requires magnesium to participate in enzymatic reactions.[103] Separately, magnesium acts as a calcium channel blocker. In the heart, this produces negative inotropy in isolated preparations. However it results in positive inotropy in healthy human volunteers, presumably because of decreased systemic and pulmonary arterial vascular resistance.[37,103] Additionally, limiting calcium outflow from the sarcoplasmic reticulum and restricting outward potassium movement appear to underlie the role of magnesium in reduction of sinus node rate firing, increased atrioventricular (AV) node refractoriness, and suppression of ectopy.[37,103] The role of magnesium in calcium channel blocker, activation of adenylate cyclase, and increased production of endothelial vasodilator prostacyclin and cyclic adenosine monophosphate (cAMP) lead to vascular relaxation in peripheral and intracranial blood vessels.[6,12,128] In the pulmonary system, the inhibitory actions of magnesium on smooth muscle lead to a weak bronchodilating effect.[58]

In the nervous system, the glutamate N-methyl-D-aspartate (NMDA) receptor mediates excitatory neurotransmission. The NMDA receptor undergoes voltage-dependent blockade following magnesium administration with a high permeability for calcium in those receptors expressing

NR1 and NR2 although not NR3 subunits.[18] Magnesium used as an NMDA antagonist has demonstrated neuroprotective and antinociceptive effects in clinical trials.[3,133] Magnesium competitively blocks presynaptic calcium entry to decrease or abolish acetylcholine release at motor endplates and postsynaptically decreases sensitivity to acetylcholine.[48,77] Magnesium similarly blocks N- (and L-) type calcium channels to inhibit catecholamine release from adrenergic nerves.[110] Effective serum concentrations for the prevention or treatment of eclamptic seizures range from 4 to 7 mEq/L (2.0–3.5 mmol/L).[91]

ROLE IN XENOBIOTIC-INDUCED HYPOMAGNESEMIA

Table 12–10 lists common xenobiotic causes of hypomagnesemia. These include xenobiotics that cause GI or renal losses (laxatives, alcohol, and diuretics), chemotherapeutics (cisplatin, human epidermal growth factor receptor antagonists), antimicrobials (aminoglycosides, amphotericin B, pentamidine), immunosuppressants (cyclosporine and tacrolimus), and proton pump inhibitors. In animal models, magnesium administration is additionally protective against cisplatin-induced nephrotoxicity while improving chemotherapeutic efficacy.[78,104] Receptor activator of nuclear factor κ-B ligand (RANKL) inhibitors used to treat osteoporosis and bone metastases also place patients at risk for hypomagnesemia.[79] The choice of oral or IV repletion should depend on the degree of hypomagnesemia and the clinical scenario, with IV treatment used for severe cases.

ROLE IN POISONING BY CARDIAC TOXINS

Digoxin inhibits the magnesium-dependent sodium-potassium adenosine triphosphatase (Na^+-K^+-ATPase). Antidotal use of $MgSO_4$ in cardiovascular poisoning dates back to 1935, when it was used to mitigate digoxin-associated dysrhythmias in 15 patients.[139] In 1950, Szekely reported that 3 to 4 g of $MgSO_4$ interrupted digoxin-associated bidirectional tachycardia or extrasystolic bigeminy in six patients.[115] In controlled studies of cardioactive steroids toxicity in dogs[71,126] and monkeys,[127] cardiotoxicity (ie, ventricular dysrhythmias and death) was significantly more pronounced and occurred at lower concentrations in magnesium-deficient animals. In another dog experiment, $MgSO_4$ reversed cardioactive steroids–induced myocardial potassium egress (a measure of sodium-Na^+,K^+-ATPase inhibition).[89] In humans, $MgSO_4$ abolished digoxin-associated extrasystoles in all but 1 of 14 patients.[42] Magnesium sulfate eliminated digoxin-associated tachydysrhythmias in all 7 patients who were also determined to have decreased intracellular [magnesium] despite normal serum [magnesium] and [digoxin].[25]

In seven patients taking digoxin for chronic Chagasic cardiomyopathy, all of those with magnesium deficiency as determined by muscle biopsy had cardiac dysrhythmias (eg, ventricular tachycardia {VT}, AV dissociation), some despite normal serum magnesium.[17] Twenty-one hospitalized patients with low intracellular magnesium concentrations as determined by monocyte analysis or serum hypomagnesemia, experienced classic digoxin toxicity (eg, ventricular tachycardia, multiple premature or multifocal ventricular beats, supraventricular tachycardia with AV nodal block) at relatively low serum digoxin concentrations (three of 2 nmol/L).[135] Three of 21 patients with digoxin toxicity had low intracellular magnesium concentrations but normal serum concentrations. In human case reports, magnesium has stabilized refractory digoxin-associated ventricular dysrhythmias when digoxin-specific antibody fragments were unavailable.[46,68] Magnesium augmented the efficacy of Digifab in reversing marinobufagenin-induced Na^+,K^+-ATPase inhibition in humans with pregnancy-induced hypertension and elevated marinobufagenin concentrations, providing an experimental link for magnesium efficacy in preeclampsia.[137] On the basis of these data, it is reasonable to administer magnesium to patients with tachydysrhythmias evidence of digoxin poisoning, even in the setting of normal digoxin concentrations.

Magnesium sulfate has been used sporadically to treat patients with other specific cardiovascular poisonings. In murine models of amitriptyline poisoning, $MgSO_4$ was effective and superior to lidocaine in converting VTs and synergistic with norepinephrine in reducing occurrence of dysrhythmias.[72,73]

Case reports demonstrate similar benefit of magnesium in converting refractory ventricular dysrhythmias in cyclic antidepressant overdose.[23,49,74,108] In one randomized trial of 72 patients with cyclic antidepressant poisoning, $MgSO_4$ 1 g every 6 hours in addition to standard care with bicarbonate infusion decreased intensive care unit (ICU) duration and decreased the mortality rate from 33% to 14%.[41] In a review of ventricular dysrhythmias associated with aconite poisoning, $MgSO_4$ terminated dysrhythmias in two of nine patients, although its precise role was unclear.[29]

Magnesium use in patients with cardiac dysrhythmias has demonstrated efficacy and safety. Large doses of $MgSO_4$ (7–12 g) were initially explored to suppress multifocal atrial tachycardia.[62] As an adjunct, $MgSO_4$ improved rate control and rhythm conversion in patients with atrial fibrillation primarily treated with digoxin.[32] A separate study found that twice as much IV digoxin was required for rate control of atrial fibrillation in hypomagnesemic patients (<1.5 mEq/L).[34] Intravenous $MgSO_4$ (3±2 g initially) enhanced the efficacy of dofetilide to chemically cardiovert 160 patients with atrial fibrillation and flutter, a 107% increased odd of success.[26] From a safety perspective, in 20 patients who received ibutilide for atrial fibrillation and flutter, 2 g of $MgSO_4$ eliminated the 29% increase in QT interval induced by ibutilide.[57] In a trial of 476 patients with atrial fibrillation and flutter, IV infusion of 5 g of $MgSO_4$ for 1 hour before the ibutilide administration followed by an additional IV infusion of 5 g of magnesium increased the rate of conversion to sinus rhythm from 67.3% to 76.5% and decreased the incidence of ventricular dysrhythmias (including torsade de pointes) from 7.4% to 1.2%.[95] In a separate trial of 229 consecutive patients who received ibutilide, $MgSO_4$ (1–4 g) was associated with a dose-responsive 78% increased odds of successful chemical conversion.[117] Magnesium sulfate (0.037 g/kg body weight followed by 0.025 g/kg/h) eliminated the need to administer amiodarone (for heart rate >110 or non–sinus rhythm) in 16 of 29 patients critically ill patients with new-onset atrial fibrillation who would have otherwise received it per protocol.[113] An oral dose of only 250 to 500 mg/day $MgSO_4$ did not improve the efficacy of conversion of atrial fibrillation with sotalol.[47] However, in a study of 34 patients, oral magnesium (500 mg) reduced the QTc interval prolongation induced by sotalol and dofetilid.[86] Although one meta-analysis was unable to demonstrate a benefit of prophylactic $MgSO_4$ in preventing postoperative atrial fibrillation in cardiac surgery,[27] subsequent evaluations have found a distinct dose–response benefit when magnesium was added to cardioplegic solutions.[50] These data suggest a benefit of magnesium as a primary antidysrhythmic and the ability of magnesium to mitigate cardiotoxicity from other antidysrhythmics.

Torsade de pointes is a subset of polymorphic VT that often self-terminates and occurs in the setting of a prolonged QT interval.[14] Not all polymorphic VT is torsade de pointes. This is a critical distinction in interpreting the literature. Previously unrecognized blockade of the cardiac rapidly activating delayed potassium rectifier current (hERG/KCNH2 gene) has led to multiple drug withdrawals and led the FDA to mandate hERG assays and electrocardiogram trials since 2005 to evaluate "QT liability" and the prodysrhythmic cardiovascular risk of new chemical entities.[80] Many drugs possess QT liability, which can be exacerbated in overdose or occur with coingestants that modify metabolism. The QT interval has limitations as a surrogate marker for torsade de pointes, and toxins may be torsadogenic through mechanisms other than directly blocking hERG, such as by interfering with channel synthesis or surface expression (eg, pentamidine).[80] Furthermore, QT interval prolongation in poisoning is likely multifactorial.

The 2015 American Heart Association (AHA) guidelines update for emergency cardiovascular care did not readdress the use of magnesium in cardiac arrest with polymorphic VT.[81] These guidelines noted that routine use of magnesium for ventricular fibrillation (VF) or polymorphic VT was not recommended in adult patients on the basis of randomized trials showing no benefit of magnesium in patients with out-of-hospital cardiac arrest receiving cardiopulmonary resuscitation,[43] in-hospital cardiac arrest,[118] and refractory or recurrent VF.[5,55,81] These guidelines apply to a different population than those encountered in poisoning. The prehospital trial[43] did not mention polymorphic VT (or torsade de pointes); the in-hospital cardiac arrest trial[118] specifically excluded patients with clinical indications for magnesium and torsade de pointes, the remaining trials[5,55,81] evaluated patients with VF (not with torsade de pointes or polymorphic ventricular tachycardia), and all failed to ascribe or associate a case of dysrhythmia or arrest to a toxicologic cause. The guidelines acknowledged that the most common cause of polymorphic VT in these cases was myocardial ischemia.[81] The importance of this distinction between ischemic versus xenobiotic-induced QT interval prolongation was highlighted by a study in which IV $MgSO_4$ (3.75 g over 3 minutes) in nine patients shortened QTc interval prolongation induced by amiodarone and quinidine (despite normal electrolytes and magnesium concentrations) but did not do so in those with a prolonged QTc interval because of ischemic coronary disease.[53] Low serum magnesium is associated with an increased risk of sudden cardiac death.[67] The AHA guidelines recommend "consideration of" IV $MgSO_4$ when polymorphic VT was secondary to a long QT interval (ie, torsade de pointes).[81]

Magnesium sulfate was first reported to treat three patients with torsade de pointes induced by quinidine and amiodarone, procainamide, and imipramine in 1984.[123] A subsequent case series of 6 and 12 patients demonstrated similar benefit for torsade de pointes, as well as a benefit in patients with intractable ventricular tachydysrhythmias despite normomagnesemia.[62,97,122] $MgSO_4$ also eliminated torsade de pointes in pediatric patients with congenital and acquired long QT syndrome.[59,60] Case reports variously describe the success of $MgSO_4$ in resolving QRS complex and QTc interval abnormalities in poisonings by escitalopram,[109] flecainide,[129] antipsychotics,[90] and arsenic trioxide.[38] There is significant divergence of opinion among toxicologists about what constitutes a prolonged or corrected QT interval, QT interval thresholds that require intervention (if any), and magnesium dosing (if any) in cases of drug-induced QT interval prolongation.[92] Other than where described in the clinical trials earlier, magnesium does not typically affect the QT interval, making ascertainment of efficacy difficult. Based on the limited available data, it is reasonable to ensure eumagnesemia in patients with prolonged QT interval and administer magnesium in patients with progressive QT interval prolongation due to poisoning. After an episode of torsade de pointes, it is recommended to administer IV $MgSO_4$.[81,119]

ROLE IN ETHANOL DISORDERS AND THIAMINE DEFICIENCY

Chronic alcohol use is associated with hypomagnesemia. In one series of 105 patients with heavy alcohol use, magnesium deficiency was present in 48%.[36] Magnesium deficiency correlated with worse cognitive test scores, even in the setting of normal thiamine pyrophosphate concentrations.[36] A smaller study found magnesium deficiency in 53% of patients admitted for detoxification.[35] In another study of 62 active drinkers, hypomagnesemia was present in 23% and directly correlated with QT interval prolongation.[87] Magnesium is an essential cofactor of the thiamine-dependent enzymes transketolase and pyruvate dehydrogenase, and magnesium increases the activity of a third critical thiamine-dependent enzyme α-ketoglutarate dehydrogenase.[94] In people with alcoholism and nutritionally deficient patients, Wernicke's encephalopathy and thiamine deficiency remained refractory despite thiamine repletion until magnesium deficiency was addressed.[28,39,121] More than 4 decades ago, murine studies confirmed early human observations of the critical role of adequate magnesium in thiamine efficacy. Magnesium deficiency results in a loss of thiamine from tissues and limits the response to exogenous thiamine; magnesium supplementation augments the response to thiamine repletion in thiamine-deficient rats.[138] Furthermore, thiamine pyrophosphokinase, the enzyme that activates thiamine to thiamine pyrophosphate (thiamine diphosphate), requires magnesium as a cofactor.[106] In a controlled trial of 36 patients with chronic alcohol use disorders, those given $MgSO_4$ in addition to thiamine demonstrated significantly greater transketolase activity.[96]

Separately, magnesium was evaluated for its role in mitigating the consequences of alcohol withdrawal and neuronal hyperactivity. Hypomagnesemia is associated with higher structured scores of alcohol withdrawal.[101] The degree of hypomagnesemia in patients with alcoholism correlates with stroboscopic-inducible seizure (photoconvulsion) thresholds, which itself

correlates with incidence of spontaneous seizures and delirium tremens.[132] Unfortunately, there are few appropriately designed studies, and they are often limited in their clinical scope. In a randomized, parallel group, double-blind trial of 119 patients with mild to moderate alcohol withdrawal designed to evaluate biochemical parameters, 8 weeks of oral daily magnesium (500 mg) sped recovery of aspartate aminotransferase (AST).[100] In a randomized, placebo-controlled trial of 59 consecutive patients with alcoholic liver disease, 2 days of 729 mg (30 mmol)/day of IV $MgSO_4$ followed by 6 to 7 weeks of 304 mg (12.5 mmol)/day of oral magnesium (as magnesium oxide) did not improve muscle mass or strength beyond placebo but did improve serum magnesium concentrations and was associated with higher muscle magnesium concentrations in subsequent analysis.[1] The study was confounded by a failure to control for spironolactone treatment, which is magnesium-sparing. In 49 patients with alcoholism randomized in a double-blind fashion to receive either 364 mg (15 mmol) oral magnesium daily (as magnesium-lactate-citrate tablets) or matching placebo for 6 weeks, magnesium supplementation improved aminotransferases, maximal muscle hand grip strength, and sense of general well-being.[52] An early review of treatment of delirium tremens before the routine use of benzodiazepines found that $MgSO_4$ administration decreased the duration of tremor and visual hallucinations.[45] However, in one of the few studies evaluating acute withdrawal, a double-blind, placebo-controlled trial of 100 patients, four doses of IM $MgSO_4$ (2 g every 6 hours) did not alter chlordiazepoxide use or the incidence of diaphoresis, tremor, vomiting, hallucinations, or withdrawal severity.[130] The study was underpowered to detect a difference in grand mal seizures and delirium tremens. This is in contrast to the findings of a retrospective review of 781 patients with alcoholism being treated for detoxification, which documented a lower seizure incidence in the patients treated with magnesium.[31] In a separate controlled study of eight patients with acute withdrawal, magnesium repletion either completely abolished inducible photoconvulsive responses or raised photoconvulsion thresholds.[132] Given the significant prevalence of magnesium and thiamine deficiency in individuals with alcoholism and magnesium's critical role for thiamine efficacy and its alteration of seizure thresholds in controlled human experimental studies, it is reasonable to actively screen for magnesium deficiency and administer magnesium to patients with hypomagnesemia, those with moderate to severe alcoholic withdrawal (including withdrawal seizures or associated with elevated aminotransferases), and those at risk for Wernicke's encephalopathy.

The importance of magnesium to thiamine pyrophosphate function is also reflected in the guidance to administer magnesium and thiamine as adjunctive treatments for ethylene glycol poisoning.[10] Metabolism of the ethylene glycol metabolite glyoxylic acid to 2-hydroxy-3-oxoadipate requires thiamine pyrophosphate and is facilitated by magnesium administration.[88] In one in vitro study, the lack of magnesium decreased glyoxylic acid metabolism to 2-hydroxy-3-oxoadipate by 60%.[66] Separately, glyoxylic acid covalently inactivates thiamine pyrophosphate, and thus the pyruvate decarboxylase complex, making ensuring sufficient thiamine of critical importance.[44] As a relatively benign intervention, it is reasonable to administer magnesium as adjunctive therapy to ethylene glycol–poisoned patients with normal kidney function while pursuing definitive management (eg, hemodialysis, fomepizole) as reviewed in Chap. 106.

ROLE IN PESTICIDE POISONING

Because magnesium diminishes calcium channel mediated synaptic acetylcholine release, it was hypothesized that $MgSO_4$ might ameliorate organic phosphorus (OP) effects at the neuromuscular junction and elsewhere.[40] Magnesium sulfate blunted paraoxon-induced tachycardia, hypertension, and hemoconcentration in mini pigs.[98,99] In four OP-poisoned patients, $MgSO_4$ administration produced no appreciable clinical or electrophysiological change when given 9 days into poisoning; when given 2 to 3 days into care, electrophysiological alterations consistent with conversion of an OP depolarizing blockade to a presynaptic blockade occurred, with no clinical change.[112] A rat model of sarin poisoning highlighted the distinct importance of distinguishing tonic-clonic convulsions from ongoing seizure. Although magnesium attenuated visible convulsions, sustained seizure activity and brain injury continued to occur.[65] In a small controlled trial of 11 patients given 4 g/day of IV MgSO₄ compared with 34 patients given usual care (multiple-dose activated charcoal, atropine, and oximes) the requirement for atropine and oximes did not differ, but the duration of hospitalization decreased, and the mortality rate decreased from 15% to 0%.[93] In a subsequent phase 2 trial, 40 patients received MgSO₄ 4, 8,12, or 16 g in a 4:1 treatment:control pseudorandomization.[11] Compared with six patients (60%) who died in the total control group, 3 of 16 (19%), 2 of 8 (25%), 1 of 8 (13%), and 0 of 8 (0%) patients died in the 4-g, 8-g, 12-g, and 16-g groups, respectively. A double-blind, prospective randomized clinical trial of 100 patients with OP poisoning found that 4 g of MgSO₄ IV reduced atropine requirements over 30 minutes and reduced the need for intubation and ICU stay but did not alter the mortality rate.[125] Separately, the cardiovascular complications of organophosphorus compounds are well described. Severe rhythm and conductivity disorders resulted in cardiac arrest and death in 29 patients poisoned with organic phosphorus compounds.[85] In a review of 168 organ, QT interval prolongation, ST segment and T wave anomalies were present in 134 (80%), and frequent dysrhythmias appeared in 56 patients (33%).[69,70] A separate study confirmed these findings and reported QT interval prolongation in 14 of 15 patients (93%) and malignant dysrhythmias in 6 of 15 (40%).[83] Magnesium sulfate (dose unspecified) was used to suppress ventricular ectopy is these cases.[70] Given the available data, it would be reasonable to provide MgSO₄ in organic phosphorus compound poisoning.

Metal phosphides (eg, aluminum and zinc), used as rodenticides and fumigants, have become a common cause of self-poisoning in certain countries (Chap. 108). For example, phosphine was found in 619 of 674 cases (92%) of suicidal poisonings in Tehran.[75] Magnesium concentrations in the setting of poisoning are quite variable. The lack of specific antidotes and the significant toxicity of phosphides led to the search for other interventions. Administration of magnesium in the form of the novel pharmacophore porphylleren–MC16 reversed aluminum phosphide–induced bradycardia, hypotension, energy depletion, and lipid peroxidation in mice.[9] One human trial found decreased markers of oxidative stress in aluminum phosphide–poisoned patients given MgSO₄.[22] Human studies conflict as to the efficacy of magnesium administration; some demonstrate efficacy and other no benefit, leaving magnesium's role unclear.[8,102] Given the absence of any meaningful alternatives to supportive care in phosphide poisoning, it is reasonable to administer MgSO₄. In barium poisoning, oral MgSO₄ is administered to precipitate insoluble barium sulfate to preclude absorption and is reviewed in Chap. 107.

ROLE IN HYDROFLUORIC ACID AND FLUORIDE-RELEASING XENOBIOTICS

In addition to binding calcium, fluoride (Chap. 104) also binds to potassium and magnesium. Calcium administration (Antidotes in Depth: 32) remains a mainstay of treatment for hydrofluoric acid (HF) exposures. In murine studies, oral MgCl₂ administration for decontamination successfully increased the LD₅₀ of sodium fluoride, but oral MgSO₄ was unsuccessful in increasing survival in another pretreatment HF ingestion model.[56,76,84] Intravenous MgCl₂ increased the lethal dose and delayed death in a porcine HF ingestion model.[24] Clinical experience has demonstrated that relatively small skin surface HF burns (3.5% or less of concentration HF) in humans can lead to profound hypomagnesemia (in addition to hypocalcemia), which, if left unaddressed and not aggressively reversed (in addition to calcium administration), can contribute to death.[30,116,134] Survival and mitigation of lethal dysrhythmias in HF or sodium fluoride ingestion both typically require large amounts of magnesium and calcium.[2,114] It is reasonable to administer magnesium in cases of systemic toxicity from fluoride-releasing xenobiotics.

ADVERSE EFFECTS AND SAFETY ISSUES

The side effects of MgSO₄ administration were all well described in a series of 100 parenteral administrations in 1941. These included cardiovascular effects of cutaneous vasodilation; conduction disturbances such as bradycardia,

hypotension, and cardiac arrest; respiratory depression; GI complaints of nausea, vomiting, and thirst; and neurologic sequelae of restlessness, confusion, a sense of impending doom, CNS depression, and paralysis.[131] The usefulness of surveillance of patellar reflexes in anticipating respiratory depression was also recognized.[131] Hypocalcemia and hyperkalemia are also reported with MgSO₄ treatment for preeclampsia.[61] Patients with acute or chronic kidney disease or low urine flow rates are at increased risk for hypermagnesemia.[82,136] Frequent serum magnesium concentrations should be obtained. Magnesium sulfate inhibits platelet function in vitro and in vivo, which is reported to prolong bleeding times.[51,54]

Case series and reports abound of iatrogenic hypermagnesemia through a variety of mechanisms. These include free-flowing ("runaway") or misprogrammed pump infusions; confounding with IV bags of other infusing solutions (eg, oxytocin, lactated ringers); mislabeled infusions; 10-fold administration errors; and concentration, dilution, and admixture errors.[19,111] In the event of hypermagnesemia or hypocalcemia leading to significant symptoms (eg, respiratory muscle paralysis, hypotension, or dysrhythmia), IV calcium (Antidotes in Depth: 32) is used to counteract the effects.

PREGNANCY AND LACTATION

In 2013, the status of magnesium was changed from Pregnancy Class A to D (positive evidence of human fetal risk, but the potential benefits are acceptable in certain situations despite its risks). An FDA safety alert cautioned that continuous MgSO₄ administration to pregnant women for longer than 5 to 7 days was associated with fetal hypocalcemia, osteopenia, skeletal abnormalities, and fractures.[124] Magnesium sulfate was associated with neonatal cord serum concentrations of 70% to 100% of maternal concentrations but did not lower neonatal Apgar scores.[15] Magnesium sulfate was not associated with congenital malformations.[15]

Magnesium distributes into breast milk during parenteral magnesium administration. Breast milk values in patients with preeclampsia given MgSO₄ were similar to those of control participants by 48 hours.[15] Although caution should be exercised when MgSO₄ is administered to a nursing mother, the American Academy of Pediatrics considers MgSO₄ to be compatible with breastfeeding.[7]

DOSING AND ADMINISTRATION

Magnesium dosing varies significantly. In the setting of magnesium deficiency, several grams of MgSO₄ provided over the first day in divided doses of 1 to 2 g are often required for repletion, with frequent serum determinations to guide therapy. For torsade de pointes in adults, 2 g (25–50 mg/kg in children up to 2 g) of MgSO₄ intravenously is recommended.[119] The caveat for the potential need for repeated doses may be missed. In perspective, 2 to 5 g or more of MgSO₄ was typically used in the cardiac conversion and dysrhythmia trials. A dose of 2 g in adults followed by an infusion or intermittent doses of 0.5 to 1 g/h to sustain serum (and intracellular) concentrations appears more rational. Again by comparison, 4 g of IV MgSO₄ is recommended to initiate therapy for severe preeclampsia or eclampsia for maternal and fetal neuroprotection, with maintenance doses typically of 1 to 2 g/h.[33,82,91] Empiric IV MgSO₄ administration for a prolonged QT interval is controversial; approximately 50% of toxicologists use a QTc threshold of 500 ms, although this was scenario dependent.[92] Eumagnesemia (and normal potassium) should be ensured in patients with prolonged QT interval, and given the lack of consensus, it would be reasonable to administer magnesium in patients with progressive QT interval prolongation from poisoning. The recommended dose mirrors that for torsade de pointes: 2 g of MgSO₄ in adults followed by infusion or intermittent doses of 0.5 to 1 g/h with endpoints guided by the specific clinical circumstances. The rate of administration depends on the clinical scenario. For example, in a seizing patient with eclampsia, a dose of 4 g MgSO₄ is rapidly provided over 5 minutes.[82] Use in life-threatening ventricular dysrhythmia would predispose to a similar rapid rate, recalling that care should prioritize electrical therapy (cardioversion or defibrillation) in unstable rhythms. In nonemergent scenarios, MgSO₄ is administered at a rate not to exceed 150 mg/min. If used in organic phosphorus compound poisoning, $MgSO_4$ doses mirroring the clinical trials (at least 4 g/day) are recommended. Magnesium requirements in fluoride poisoning are significant and guided by serum and clinical assessment. Magnesium sulfate should be diluted to a less than or equal to 20% concentration for IV administration.

FORMULATION AND ACQUISITION

A variety of $MgSO_4$ formulations are available for parenteral administration: 4% (40 mg/mL) or 8% (80 mg/mL) in sterile water volumes ranging from 100 mL to 1 L. Magnesium sulfate injection, 50% in water (500 mg/mL), is typically supplied as 2 or 10 mL. Magnesium sulfate is also formulated in 5% dextrose in concentrations ranging from 1% (10 mg/mL) to 2% (20 mg/mL) and in similar volume ranges.

Magnesium in much smaller concentrations (eg, 0.3 mg/mL) is found as a component of multiple or mixed electrolyte or parenteral nutritional infusion formulations (eg, in combination with acetate, chloride, potassium, and sodium). These would not be anticipated to be sufficient for antidotal purposes. Of note, dialysate solutions containing magnesium present the potential for medication error and should not be confused with those intended for IV infusion.

SUMMARY

- Magnesium sulfate is used to treat xenobiotic-associated hypomagnesemia and as an adjunctive therapy to treat cardiovascular toxins, fluoride toxicity, and pesticide poisoning.
- Ectopy in patients taking cardioactive steroids can be mitigated by $MgSO_4$ while awaiting definitive therapy (digoxin Fab fragments).
- Magnesium sulfate therapy and correction of electrolytes are mainstays of therapy to preclude recurrent torsade de pointes, although optimal dosing remains to be defined.
- The decision to intervene with $MgSO_4$ in isolated QT interval prolongation is complex. Repletion of hypomagnesemia should occur. An initial dose followed by an infusion is reasonable because cellular exchange of magnesium is slow compared with more rapid kidney excretion.
- Hypomagnesemia should be assessed and treated in patients with alcohol use disorders.

REFERENCES

1. Aagaard NK, et al. Magnesium supplementation and muscle function in patients with alcoholic liver disease: a randomized, placebo-controlled trial. *Scand J Gastroenterol.* 2005;40:972-979.
2. Abukurah AR, et al. Acute sodium fluoride poisoning. *JAMA.* 1972;222:816-817.
3. Afshari D, et al. Evaluation of the intravenous magnesium sulfate effect in clinical improvement of patients with acute ischemic stroke. *Clin Neurol Neurosurg.* 2013;115:400-404.
4. Alhosaini M, Leehey DJ. Magnesium and dialysis: the neglected cation. *Am J Kidney Dis.* 2015;66:523-531.
5. Allegra J, et al. Magnesium sulfate in the treatment of refractory ventricular fibrillation in the prehospital setting. *Resuscitation.* 2001;49:245-249.
6. Altura BM, et al. Mg2+-Ca2+ interaction in contractility of vascular smooth muscle: Mg2+ versus organic calcium channel blockers on myogenic tone and agonist-induced responsiveness of blood vessels. *Can J Physiol Pharmacol.* 1987;65:729-745.
7. American Academy of Pediatrics Committee on Drugs. Transfer of drugs and other chemicals into human milk. *Pediatrics.* 2001;108:776-789.
8. Anand R, et al. Aluminum phosphide poisoning: an unsolved riddle. *J Appl Toxicol.* 2011;31:499-505.
9. Baeeri M, et al. On the benefit of magnetic magnesium nanocarrier in cardiovascular toxicity of aluminum phosphide. *Toxicol Indust Health.* 2013;29:126-135.
10. Barceloux DG, et al. American Academy of Clinical Toxicology practice guidelines on the treatment of ethylene glycol poisoning. Ad Hoc Committee. *J Toxicol Clin Toxicol.* 1999;37:537-560.
11. Basher A, et al. Phase II study of magnesium sulfate in acute organophosphate pesticide poisoning. *Clin Toxicol (Phila).* 2013;51:35-40.
12. Belfort MA, Moise KJ Jr. Effect of magnesium sulfate on maternal brain blood flow in preeclampsia: a randomized, placebo-controlled study. *Am J Obstet Gynecol.* 1992;167:661-666.
13. Boyd LJ, Scherf D. Magnesium sulfate in paroxysmal tachycardia. *Am J Med Sci.* 1943;206:43.
14. Bradfield JS, et al. Ventricular arrhythmias. In: Fuster V, et al., eds: *Hurst's The Heart.* 14th ed. New York, NY: McGraw-Hill Education; 2017.
15. Briggs GG, et al. *Drugs in Pregnancy and Lactation.* Philadelphia, PA: Lippincott Williams & Wilkins; 2017.
16. Bringhurst F, et al. Bone and mineral metabolism in health and disease. In: Kasper D, et al., eds: *Harrison's Principles of Internal Medicine.* 19th ed. New York, NY: McGraw-Hill; 2014.
17. Camara EJ, et al. Muscle magnesium content and cardiac arrhythmias during treatment of congestive heart failure due to chronic Chagasic cardiomyopathy. *Braz J Med Biol Res.* 1986;19:49-58.
18. Cavara NA, et al. Residues at the tip of the pore loop of NR3B-containing NMDA receptors determine Ca2+ permeability and Mg2+ block. *BMC Neurosci.* 2010;11:133.
19. Cavell GF, et al. Iatrogenic magnesium toxicity following intravenous infusion of magnesium sulfate: risks and strategies for prevention. *BMJ Case Rep.* 2015;2015.
20. Center for Drug Evaluation and Research (CDER). Approval Package for Application Number: 20-488. Magnesium sulfate in 5% dextrose injection in plastic container, 10 mg/mL and 20 mg/mL. Rockville, MD: US Food and Drug Administration; 1995.
21. Chesley LC. Parenteral magnesium sulfate and the distribution, plasma levels, and excretion of magnesium. *Am J Obstet Gynecol.* 1979;133:1-7.
22. Chugh SN, et al. A critical evaluation of anti-peroxidant effect of intravenous magnesium in acute aluminium phosphide poisoning. *Magnes Res.* 1997;10:225-230.
23. Citak A, et al. Efficacy of long duration resuscitation and magnesium sulphate treatment in amitriptyline poisoning. *Eur J Emerg Med.* 2002;9:63-66.
24. Coffey JA, et al. Limited efficacy of calcium and magnesium in a porcine model of hydrofluoric acid ingestion. *J Med Toxicol.* 2007;3:45-51.
25. Cohen L, Kitzes R. Magnesium sulfate and digitalis-toxic arrhythmias. *JAMA.* 1983;249:2808-2810.
26. Coleman CI, et al. Intravenous magnesium sulfate enhances the ability of dofetilide to successfully cardiovert atrial fibrillation or flutter: results of the Dofetilide and Intravenous Magnesium Evaluation. *Europace.* 2009;11:892-895.
27. Cook RC, et al. Prophylactic magnesium does not prevent atrial fibrillation after cardiac surgery: a meta-analysis. *Ann Thorac Surg.* 2013;95:533-541.
28. Coughlan JJ, et al. Thiamine refractory Wernickes encephalopathy reversed with magnesium therapy. *BMJ Case Rep.* 2016;2016.
29. Coulson JM, et al. The management of ventricular dysrhythmia in aconite poisoning. *Clin Toxicol (Phila).* 2017;55:313-321.
30. Dalamaga M, et al. Hypocalcemia, hypomagnesemia, and hypokalemia following hydrofluoric acid chemical injury. *J Burn Care Res.* 2008;29:541-543.
31. Daus AT, et al. Clinical experience with 781 cases of alcoholism evaluated and treated on an inpatient basis by various methods. *Int J Addict.* 1985;20:643-650.
32. Davey MJ, Teubner D. A randomized controlled trial of magnesium sulfate, in addition to usual care, for rate control in atrial fibrillation. *Ann Emerg Med.* 2005;45:347-353.
33. De Silva DA, et al. Magnesium sulphate for eclampsia and fetal neuroprotection: a comparative analysis of protocols across Canadian tertiary perinatal centres. *J Obstet Gynaecol Can.* 2015;37:975-987.
34. DeCarli C, et al. Serum magnesium levels in symptomatic atrial fibrillation and their relation to rhythm control by intravenous digoxin. *Am J Cardiol.* 1986;57:956-959.
35. Denison H, et al. Influence of increased adrenergic activity and magnesium depletion on cardiac rhythm in alcohol withdrawal. *Br Heart J.* 1994;72:554-560.
36. Dingwall KM, et al. Hypomagnesaemia and its potential impact on thiamine utilisation in patients with alcohol misuse at the Alice Springs Hospital. *Drug Alcohol Rev.* 2015;34:323-328.
37. Dube L, Granry JC. The therapeutic use of magnesium in anesthesiology, intensive care and emergency medicine: a review. *Can J Anaesth.* 2003;50:732-746.
38. Ducas RA, et al. Monomorphic ventricular tachycardia caused by arsenic trioxide therapy for acute promyelocytic leukaemia. *J R Coll Physicians Edinb.* 2011;41:117-118.
39. Dyckner T, et al. Aggravation of thiamine deficiency by magnesium depletion. A case report. *Acta Med Scand.* 1985;218:129-131.
40. Eddleston M, Chowdhury FR. Pharmacological treatment of organophosphorus insecticide poisoning: the old and the (possible) new. *Br J Clin Pharmacol.* 2016;81:462-470.
41. Emamhadi M, et al. Tricyclic antidepressant poisoning treated by magnesium sulfate: a randomized, clinical trial. *Drug Chem Toxicol.* 2012;35:300-303.
42. Enselberg CD, et al. The effects of magnesium upon cardiac arrhythmias. *Am Heart J.* 1950;39:703-712.
43. Fatovich DM, et al. Magnesium in cardiac arrest (the magic trial). *Resuscitation.* 1997;35:237-241.
44. Flatau S, et al. 31P NMR investigations on free and enzyme bound thiamine pyrophosphate. *FEBS Lett.* 1988;233:379-382.
45. Flink EB. Magnesium deficiency syndrome in man. *JAMA.* 1956;160:1406-1409.
46. French JH, et al. Magnesium therapy in massive digoxin intoxication. *Ann Emerg Med.* 1984;13:562-566.
47. Frick M, et al. The effect of oral magnesium, alone or as an adjuvant to sotalol, after cardioversion in patients with persistent atrial fibrillation. *Eur Heart J.* 2000;21:1177-1185.
48. Fuchs-Buder T, Tassonyi E. Magnesium sulphate enhances residual neuromuscular block induced by vecuronium. *Br J Anaesth.* 1996;76:565-566.
49. Fukushima N, et al. A neonatal prolonged QT syndrome due to maternal use of oral tricyclic antidepressants. *Eur J Pediatr.* 2016;175:1129-1132.
50. Gholipour Baradari A, et al. A double-blind randomized clinical trial comparing different doses of magnesium in cardioplegic solution for prevention of atrial fibrillation after coronary artery bypass graft surgery. *Cardiovasc Ther.* 2016;34:276-282.

51. Gries A, et al. The effect of intravenously administered magnesium on platelet function in patients after cardiac surgery. *Anesth Analg*. 1999;88:1213-1219.

52. Gullestad L, et al. Oral magnesium supplementation improves metabolic variables and muscle strength in alcoholics. *Alcohol Clin Exp Res*. 1992;16:986-990.

53. Gurfinkel E, et al. Abnormal QT intervals associated with negative T waves induced by antiarrhythmic drugs are rapidly reduced using magnesium sulfate as an antidote. *Clin Cardiol*. 1993;16:35-38.

54. Guzin K, et al. The effect of magnesium sulfate treatment on blood biochemistry and bleeding time in patients with severe preeclampsia. *J Matern Fetal Neonatal Med*. 2010;23:399-402.

55. Hassan TB, et al. A randomised trial to investigate the efficacy of magnesium sulphate for refractory ventricular fibrillation. *Emerg Med J*. 2002;19:57-62.

56. Heard K, Delgado J. Oral decontamination with calcium or magnesium salts does not improve survival following hydrofluoric acid ingestion. *J Toxicol Clin Toxicol*. 2003;41:789-792.

57. Henyan N, White CM. Adjunctive intravenous magnesium to reduce toxicity and enhance efficacy of class III antiarrhythmic agents. *Conn Med*. 2004;68:627-629.

58. Hill JM, Britton J. Effect of intravenous magnesium sulphate on airway calibre and airway reactivity to histamine in asthmatic subjects. *Br J Clin Pharmacol*. 1996;42:629-631.

59. Hoshino K, et al. Optimal administration dosage of magnesium sulfate for torsades de pointes in children with long QT syndrome. *J Am Coll Nutr*. 2004;23(suppl):497S-500S.

60. Hoshino K, et al. Successful uses of magnesium sulfate for torsades de pointes in children with long QT syndrome. *Pediatr Int*. 2006;48:112-117.

61. Hudali T, Takkar C. Hypocalcemia and hyperkalemia during magnesium infusion therapy in a pre-eclamptic patient. *Clin Case Rep*. 2015;3:827-831.

62. Iseri LT, et al. Magnesium and potassium therapy in multifocal atrial tachycardia. *Am Heart J*. 1985;110:789-794.

63. Blake JA. The use of magnesium sulfate in the production of anesthesia and in the treatment of tetanus. *Surg Gynecol Obstet*. 1906;2:541-550.

64. Jahnen-Dechent W, Ketteler M. Magnesium basics. *Clin Kidney J*. 2012;5:i3-i14.

65. Katalan S, et al. Magnesium sulfate treatment against sarin poisoning: dissociation between overt convulsions and recorded cortical seizure activity. *Arch Toxicol*. 2013;87:347-360.

66. Kawasaki H, et al. Alpha-ketoglutarate-dependent oxidation of glyoxylic acid in rat-liver mitochondria. *J Biochem*. 1966;59:419-421.

67. Kieboom BC, et al. Serum magnesium and the risk of death from coronary heart disease and sudden cardiac death. *J Am Heart Assoc*. 2016;5.

68. Kinlay S, Buckley NA. Magnesium sulfate in the treatment of ventricular arrhythmias due to digoxin toxicity. *J Toxicol Clin Toxicol*. 1995;33:55-59.

69. Kiss Z, Fazekas T. Arrhythmias in organophosphate poisonings. *Acta Cardiol*. 1979;34:323-330.

70. Kiss Z, Fazekas T. Organophosphates and torsade de pointes ventricular tachycardia. *J R Soc Med*. 1983;76:984-985.

71. Kleiger RE, et al. Effects of chronic depletion of potassium and magnesium upon the action of acetylstrophanthidin on the heart. *Am J Cardiol*. 1966;17:520-527.

72. Knudsen K, Abrahamsson J. Effects of epinephrine, norepinephrine, magnesium sulfate, and milrinone on survival and the occurrence of arrhythmias in amitriptyline poisoning in the rat. *Crit Care Med*. 1994;22:1851-1855.

73. Knudsen K, Abrahamsson J. Effects of magnesium sulfate and lidocaine in the treatment of ventricular arrhythmias in experimental amitriptyline poisoning in the rat. *Crit Care Med*. 1994;22:494-498.

74. Knudsen K, Abrahamsson J. Magnesium sulphate in the treatment of ventricular fibrillation in amitriptyline poisoning. *Eur Heart J*. 1997;18:881-882.

75. Kordrostami R, et al. Forensic toxicology analysis of self-poisoning suicidal deaths in Tehran, Iran; trends between 2011-2015. *Daru*. 2017;25:15.

76. Koskinen-Kainulainen M, et al. The LD50, excretion and serum and bone levels of F after a high single F and F + Mg dose in rats with findings on cardiac Ca and Mg. *Magnes Trace Elem*. 1990;9:15-27.

77. Krendel DA. Hypermagnesemia and neuromuscular transmission. *Semin Neurol*. 1990;10:42-45.

78. Kumar G, et al. Magnesium improves cisplatin-mediated tumor killing while protecting against cisplatin-induced nephrotoxicity. *Am J Physiol Renal Physiol*. 2017;313:F339-F350.

79. Laskowski LK, et al. A RANKL Wrinkle: denosumab-induced hypocalcemia. *J Med Toxicol*. 2016;12:305-308.

80. Lester RM, Olbertz J. Early drug development: assessment of proarrhythmic risk and cardiovascular safety. *Expert Rev Clin Pharmacol*. 2016;9:1611-1618.

81. Link MS, et al. Part 7: adult advanced cardiovascular life support: 2015 American Heart Association guidelines update for cardiopulmonary resuscitation and emergency cardiovascular care. *Circulation*. 2015;132(suppl):S444-S464.

82. Lu JF, Nightingale CH. Magnesium sulfate in eclampsia and pre-eclampsia: pharmacokinetic principles. *Clin Pharmacokinet*. 2000;38:305-314.

83. Ludomirsky A, et al. Q-T prolongation and polymorphous ("torsade de pointes") ventricular arrhythmias associated with organophosphorus insecticide poisoning. *Am J Cardiol*. 1982;49:1654-1658.

84. Luoma H, et al. Reduction of the lethality and the nephrocalcinotic effect of single fluoride doses by magnesium in rats. *Magnesium*. 1984;3:81-87.

85. Lyzhnikov EA, et al. [Pathogenesis of disorders of cardiac rhythm and conductivity in acute organophasphate insecticide poisoning]. *Kardiologiia*. 1975;15:126-129.

86. McBride BF, et al. An evaluation of the impact of oral magnesium lactate on the corrected QT interval of patients receiving sotalol or dofetilide to prevent atrial or ventricular tachyarrhythmia recurrence. *Ann Noninvasive Electrocardiol*. 2006;11:163-169.

87. Moulin SR, et al. QT interval prolongation associated with low magnesium in chronic alcoholics. *Drug Alcohol Depend*. 2015;155:195-201.

88. Nakada HI, Sund LP. Glyoxylic acid oxidation by rat liver. *J Biol Chem*. 1958;233:8-13.

89. Neff MS, et al. Magnesium sulfate in digitalis toxicity. *Am J Cardiol*. 1972;29:377-382.

90. Nelson S, Leung JG. Torsades de pointes after administration of low-dose aripiprazole. *Ann Pharmacother*. 2013;47:e11.

91. Okusanya BO, et al. Clinical pharmacokinetic properties of magnesium sulphate in women with pre-eclampsia and eclampsia. *BJOG*. 2016;123:356-366.

92. Othong R, et al. Medical toxicologists' practice patterns regarding drug-induced QT prolongation in overdose patients: a survey in the United States of America, Europe, and Asia Pacific region. *Clin Toxicol (Phila)*. 2015;53:204-209.

93. Pajoumand A, et al. Benefits of magnesium sulfate in the management of acute human poisoning by organophosphorus insecticides. *Hum Exp Toxicol*. 2004;23:565-569.

94. Panov A, Scarpa A. Independent modulation of the activity of alpha-ketoglutarate dehydrogenase complex by Ca2+ and Mg2+. *Biochemistry*. 1996;35:427-432.

95. Patsilinakos S, et al. Effect of high doses of magnesium on converting ibutilide to a safe and more effective agent. *Am J Cardiol*. 2010;106:673-676.

96. Peake RW, et al. The effect of magnesium administration on erythrocyte transketolase activity in alcoholic patients treated with thiamine. *Scott Med J*. 2013;58:139-142.

97. Perticone F, et al. Efficacy of magnesium sulfate in the treatment of torsade de pointes. *Am Heart J*. 1986;112:847-849.

98. Petroianu G, Ruefer R. Beta-blockade or magnesium in organophosphorus insecticide poisoning (OPIP). *Anaesth Intensive Care*. 1992;20:538-589.

99. Petroianu G, et al. Control of blood pressure, heart rate and haematocrit during high-dose intravenous paraoxon exposure in mini pigs. *J Appl Toxicol*. 1998;18:293-298.

100. Poikolainen K, Alho H. Magnesium treatment in alcoholics: a randomized clinical trial. *Subst Abuse Treat Prev Policy*. 2008;3:1.

101. Prior PL, et al. Influence of microelement concentration on the intensity of alcohol withdrawal syndrome. *Alcohol*. 2015;50:152-156.

102. Proudfoot AT. Aluminium and zinc phosphide poisoning. *Clin Toxicol (Phila)*. 2009;47:89-100.

103. Reinhart RA. Clinical correlates of the molecular and cellular actions of magnesium on the cardiovascular system. *Am Heart J*. 1991;121:1513-1521.

104. Saito Y, et al. Magnesium co-administration decreases cisplatin-induced nephrotoxicity in the multiple cisplatin administration. *Life Sci*. 2017;189:18-22.

105. Sakula A. Doctor Nehemiah Grew (1641-1712) and the Epsom salts. *Clio Med*. 1984;19:1-21.

106. Santini S, et al. Structural characterization of CA1462, the Candida albicans thiamine pyrophosphokinase. *BMC Struct Biol*. 2008;8:33.

107. Saris NE, et al. Magnesium. An update on physiological, clinical and analytical aspects. *Clin Chim Acta*. 2000;294:1-26.

108. Sarisoy O, et al. Efficacy of magnesium sulfate for treatment of ventricular tachycardia in amitriptyline intoxication. *Pediatr Emerg Care*. 2007;23:646-648.

109. Schreffler SM, et al. Sodium channel blockade with QRS widening after an escitalopram overdose. *Pediatr Emerg Care*. 2013;29:998-1001.

110. Shimosawa T, et al. Magnesium inhibits norepinephrine release by blocking N-type calcium channels at peripheral sympathetic nerve endings. *Hypertension*. 2004;44:897-902.

111. Simpson KR, Knox GE. Obstetrical accidents involving intravenous magnesium sulfate: recommendations to promote patient safety. *MCN Am J Matern Child Nurs*. 2004;29:161-169; quiz 170-171.

112. Singh G, et al. Neurophysiological monitoring of pharmacological manipulation in acute organophosphate (OP) poisoning. The effects of pralidoxime, magnesium sulphate and pancuronium. *Electroencephalogr Clin Neurophysiol*. 1998;107:140-148.

113. Sleeswijk ME, et al. Efficacy of magnesium-amiodarone step-up scheme in critically ill patients with new-onset atrial fibrillation: a prospective observational study. *J Intensive Care Med*. 2008;23:61-66.

114. Stremski ES, et al. Survival following hydrofluoric acid ingestion. *Ann Emerg Med*. 1992;21:1396-1369.

115. Szekely P, Wynne NA. The effects of magnesium on cardiac arrhythmias caused by digitalis. *Clin Sci*. 1951;10:241-253.

116. Tepperman PB. Fatality due to acute systemic fluoride poisoning following a hydrofluoric acid skin burn. *J Occup Med*. 1980;22:691-692.

117. Tercius AJ, et al. Intravenous magnesium sulfate enhances the ability of intravenous ibutilide to successfully convert atrial fibrillation or flutter. *Pacing Clin Electrophysiol*. 2007;30:1331-1335.

118. Thel MC, et al. Randomised trial of magnesium in in-hospital cardiac arrest. Duke Internal Medicine Housestaff. *Lancet*. 1997;350:1272-1276.

119. Thomas SH, Behr ER. Pharmacological treatment of acquired QT prolongation and torsades de pointes. *Br J Clin Pharmacol*. 2016;81:420-427.

120. Topf JM, Murray PT. Hypomagnesemia and hypermagnesemia. *Rev Endocr Metab Disord*. 2003;4:195-206.

121. Traviesa DC. Magnesium deficiency: a possible cause of thiamine refractoriness in Wernicke-Korsakoff encephalopathy. *J Neurol Neurosurg Psychiatry*. 1974;37:959-962.

122. Tzivoni D, et al. Treatment of torsade de pointes with magnesium sulfate. *Circulation*. 1988;77:392-397.

123. Tzivoni D, et al. Magnesium therapy for torsades de pointes. *Am J Cardiol*. 1984; 53:528-530.

124. US Food and Drug Administration. FDA Drug Safety Communication: FDA recommends against prolonged use of magnesium sulfate to stop pre-term labor due to bone changes in exposed babies. https://www.fda.gov/drugs/drugsafety/ucm353333.htm. Accessed April 27, 2017.

125. Vijayakumar HN, et al. Study of effect of magnesium sulphate in management of acute organophosphorous pesticide poisoning. *Anesth Essays Res*. 2017;11:192-196.

126. Vitale JJ, et al. Effects of magnesium-deficient diet upon puppies. *Circ Res*. 1961; 9:387-394.

127. Vitale JJ, et al. Magnesium deficiency in the Cebus monkey. *Circ Res*. 1963;12:642-650.

128. Watson KV, Moldow CF, Ogburn PL, et al. Magnesium sulfate: rationale for its use in preeclampsia. *Proc Natl Acad Sci U S A*. 1986;83:1075-8.

129. Williamson DG, et al. Management of persistent wide QRS in flecainide overdose with magnesium sulphate. *Emerg Med J*. 2010;27:487-488.

130. Wilson A, Vulcano B. A double-blind, placebo-controlled trial of magnesium sulfate in the ethanol withdrawal syndrome. *Alcohol Clin Exp Res*. 1984;8:542-545.

131. Winkler AW, et al. Intravenous magnesium sulfate in the treatment of nephritic convulsions in adults. *J Clin Invest*. 1942;21:207-216.

132. Wolfe SM, Victor M. The relationship of hypomagnesemia and alkalosis to alcohol withdrawal symptoms. *Ann N Y Acad Sci*. 1969;162:973-984.

133. Wu L, et al. The efficacy of N-methyl-D-aspartate receptor antagonists on improving the postoperative pain intensity and satisfaction after remifentanil-based anesthesia in adults: a meta-analysis. *J Clin Anesthes*. 2015;27:311-324.

134. Wu ML, et al. Survival after hypocalcemia, hypomagnesemia, hypokalemia and cardiac arrest following mild hydrofluoric acid burn. *Clin Toxicol (Phila)*. 2010;48:953-955.

135. Young IS, et al. Magnesium status and digoxin toxicity. *Br J Clin Pharmacol*. 1991; 32:717-721.

136. Yu L, et al. Serum magnesium and mortality in maintenance hemodialysis patients. *Blood Purif*. 2017;43:31-36.

137. Zazerskaya IE, et al. Magnesium sulfate potentiates effect of DigiFab on marinobufagenin-induced Na/K-ATPase inhibition. *Am J Hypertens*. 2013;26:1269-1272.

138. Zieve L. Influence of magnesium deficiency on the utilization of thiamine. *Ann N Y Acad Sci*. 1969;162:732-743.

139. Zwillinger L. Uber die Magnesiumwirkung auf das Herz. *Klinische Wochenschrift*. 1935;14:1429-1433.

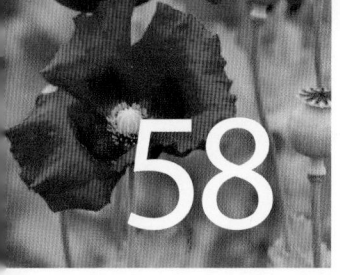

58 ANTITHROMBOTICS

Betty C. Chen and Mark K. Su

HISTORY AND EPIDEMIOLOGY

Antithrombotics have numerous clinical applications, including in the treatment of coronary artery disease, cerebrovascular events, hypercoagulable states, deep vein thrombosis (DVT), and pulmonary embolism (PE). The antithrombotics are a diverse group of xenobiotics that are widely studied and constantly in the process of therapeutic evolution.

The origins and discovery of antithrombotics are extraordinary.[6,29,156,259] The discovery of modern-day oral anticoagulants originated after investigations of a hemorrhagic disorder in Wisconsin cattle in the early 20th century that resulted from the ingestion of spoiled sweet clover silage. The hemorrhagic agent, eventually identified as bishydroxycoumarin, would be the precursor to its synthetic congener warfarin (named after the *Wisconsin Alumni Research Foundation*). Warfarin was rapidly marketed as both a medicine and a rodenticide. "Superwarfarins" were subsequently developed for the rat population that had developed increasing genetic resistance to warfarin.

The origins of the anticoagulant heparin are equally fascinating. A medical student initially attempting to study ether soluble procoagulants derived from porcine intestines serendipitously found that, over time, these apparent "procoagulants" actually prevented normal blood coagulation. The phospholipid anticoagulant responsible for this effect would later be identified as a variant form of heparin. Shortly thereafter, the water-soluble mucopolysaccharide termed *heparin* (because of its abundance in the liver) was discovered. *Unfractionated* heparin (UFH) is a mixture of polysaccharide chains with varying molecular weights. After the identification of the active pentasaccharide segment of heparin in the 1970s, multiple *low-molecular-weight* heparins (LMWHs) were isolated, and synthetic forms were created.

Hirudin, a 65–amino acid polypeptide, was produced by the salivary glands of the medicinal leech (*Hirudo medicinalis*).[256] Antistasin and antistasinlike proteins are naturally secreted by the Mexican leech, *Haementeria officinalis*, and the earthworm.[106,370] These xenobiotics have not been used therapeutically; however, they inspired the development of the synthetic factor inhibitors, such as direct thrombin inhibitors (DTIs) and factor Xa inhibitors.

In the late 19th century, human urine was noted to have proteolytic activity with specificity for fibrin. A substance found to be an activator of endogenous plasminogen leading to the consumption of fibrin, fibrinogen, and other coagulation proteins was isolated and purified and given the name *urokinase*. Streptokinase, a protein produced by β-hemolytic streptococci, tissue plasminogen activator (t-PA), and other synthetic thrombolytics were later discovered. Although known to exist for many years, ancrod, a purified derivative of Malayan pit viper, only recently gained therapeutic attention as a naturally occurring antithrombotic.

In the early 20th century, the antithrombotic properties of aspirin were noted in anecdotal reports of patients having a predisposition to bleeding while taking aspirin. Clinicians also noted lower rates of myocardial infarction (MI), and studies to elucidate the effects of aspirin on coagulation soon followed with further research exposing the role of platelet aggregation in thrombosis.[251] These discoveries led to the development of the antiplatelet xenobiotics.

The diversity of these antithrombotics led to ever-increasing use in many fields of medicine. Although warfarin is the most common oral anticoagulant in use today because of its utility in patients with cerebrovascular disease, cardiac dysrhythmias, and thromboembolic disease, the emergence of newly developed oral antithrombotics has changed the landscape of modern anticoagulation. During the period from 2011 to 2015, the American Association of Poison Control Centers has listed anticoagulants in the top 25 categories associated with the largest number of fatalities (Chap. 130).

The total number of cases of reported antithrombotic exposures to the American Association of Poison Control Centers was 96,498 with 130 deaths during that 5-year period (Chap. 130). During that time period, new antithrombotics such as apixaban, edoxaban, and ticagrelor joined the market. In 2011, dabigatran and warfarin led the US Food and Drug Administration (FDA) Safety Information and Adverse Event Reporting Program's list of adverse drug events, with 3,781 reports of serious adverse events associated with dabigatran, including 542 patient deaths. By comparison, warfarin alone accounted for 1,106 reports with 72 deaths.[255] Since then, the FDA is continually reviewing dabigatran and initiated its own study that demonstrated lower risks of death, stroke, and intracranial hemorrhage but higher risks of gastrointestinal (GI) bleeding in patients anticoagulated with dabigatran compared with warfarin.[371]

PHYSIOLOGY

Balance Between Coagulation and Anticoagulation

An understanding of the normal function of the coagulation pathways is essential to appreciate the etiology of a coagulopathy. This section summarizes the critical steps of the coagulation cascade. For additional details, readers are referred to Chap. 20 and several reviews.[135,252,257,304]

Coagulation consists of a series of events that prevent blood loss and assist in the restoration of blood vessel integrity. Although the traditional understanding of the events that occur in the coagulation cascade,[91,231] as discussed later, adequately describe in vitro events, the current understanding emphasizes some distinct differences that occur in vivo.[135,257,304] Despite these differences, an understanding of the traditional model is most useful for interpreting the results of diagnostic tests of coagulation.

Within the cascade, coagulation factors exist as inert precursors and are transformed into enzymes when activated. Activation of the cascade occurs through one of two distinct pathways, the *intrinsic* and *extrinsic* systems (Fig. 58–1).[91,231] After being activated, these enzymes catalyze a series of reactions that ultimately converge to generate thrombin with the subsequent formation of a fibrin clot.

The *intrinsic* pathway is activated by the complexation of factor XII (Hageman factor) with high-molecular-weight kininogen (HMWK) and prekallikrein or vascular subendothelial collagen. This results in sequential activation of factor XII, active kallikrein, active factors IX to XI, and prothrombin (factor II) (Fig. 58–1). Prothrombin is converted to thrombin in the presence of factor V, calcium, and phospholipid. The integrity of this system is usually evaluated by determining the partial thromboplastin time (PTT).

In the *extrinsic* or tissue factor–dependent pathway, a complex is formed between factor VII, calcium, and tissue factor, which is released after injury. A calcium- and lipid-dependent complex is then created between factors VII and X. The factor VII–X complex subsequently converts prothrombin to thrombin, which promotes the formation of fibrin from fibrinogen (Fig. 58–1). The integrity of this pathway is usually assessed by determining the prothrombin time (PT or international normalized ratio {INR}[120]). The distinction between PT and INR is discussed in Chap. 20.

Activation of factor X provides the important link between the intrinsic and extrinsic coagulation pathways. Additional evidence that tissue factors can activate both factors IX and X suggests that there are more interrelations between the two pathways.[275] Furthermore, cell surfaces facilitate the process of clotting. Platelets are also known to interact with proteins of the coagulation cascade through surface receptors for factors V, VIII, IX, and X.[142,265,339] As a final step, factor XIII assists in the cross-linking of fibrin to form a stable thrombus.

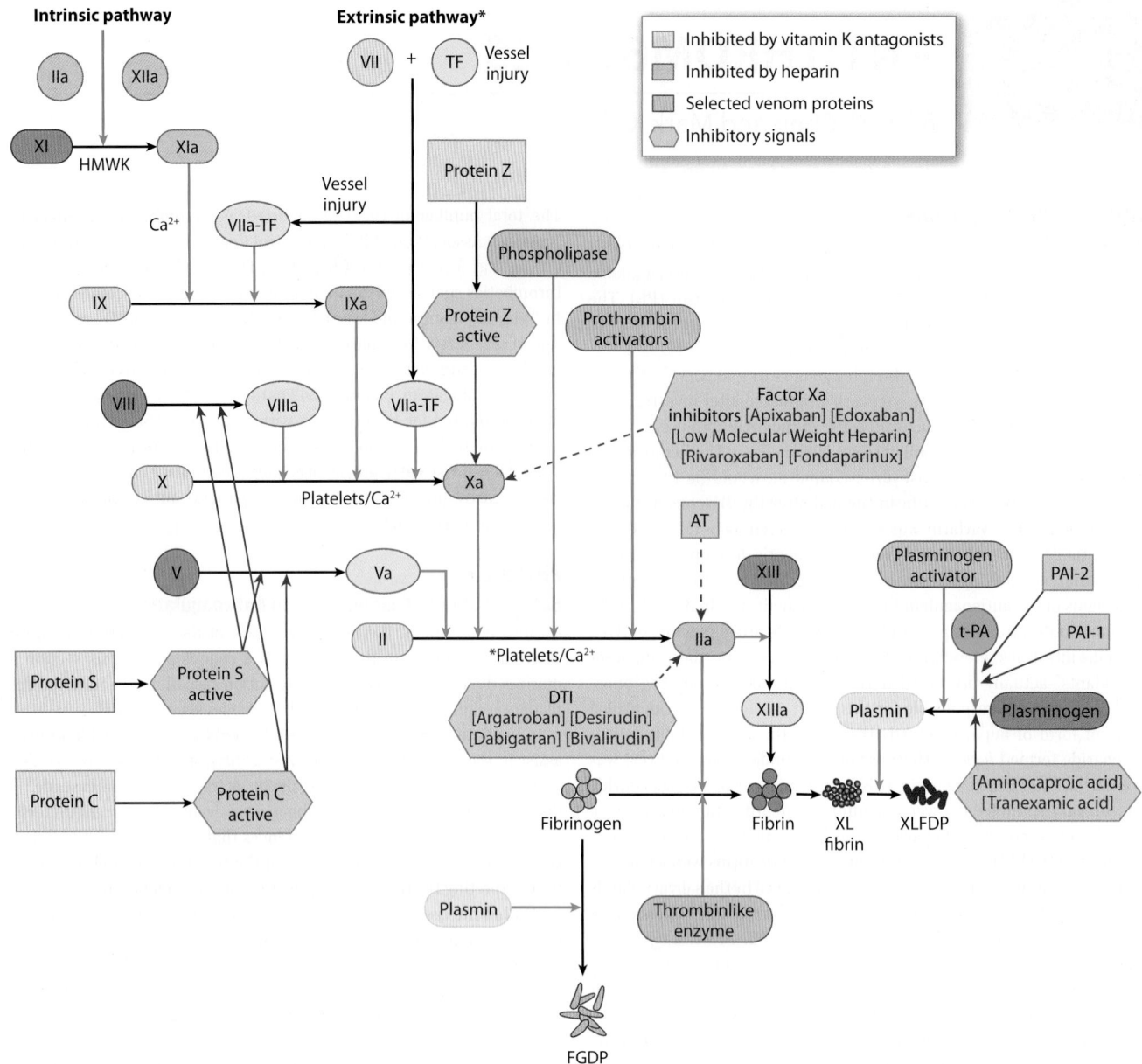

FIGURE 58–1. A schematic overview of the coagulation, platelet activation, and fibrinolytic pathways indicating where phospholipids on the platelet surface interact with the coagulation pathway intermediates. Arrows are not shown from platelets to phospholipids involved in the tissue factor VIIa and the factor IX to VIIIa interactions to avoid confusion. Interactions of selected venom proteins are indicated in the purple boxes. The diagram is not complete with reference to the multiple sites of interaction of the serine protease inhibitors (SERPINs) to avoid overcrowding. Solid red lines indicate inhibition of a reaction effect. Black arrows refer to chemical conversion of coagulation factors. Green arrows represent activation of the chemical conversion pathway. Dashed red lines indicate inhibition of a specific clotting factor. *Refer to Figs. 58–4 and 58–5 for the platelet activation pathway. DTI = direct thrombin inhibitor; FDP = fibrin degradation products; FGDP = fibrinogen degradation product; HMWK = high-molecular-weight kininogen; TF = tissue factor; t-PA = tissue plasminogen activator; XL = cross-linked.

Antithrombin (AT), and proteins C, S, and Z serve as inhibitors, maintaining the homeostasis that is required to prevent spontaneous clotting and keep blood fluid. Protein C, when aided by protein S, inactivates two plasma factors, V and VIII.[46,73,135] Protein Z is a glycoprotein (GP) molecule that forms a complex with the protein Z–dependent protease inhibitor (ZPI) which, in turn, inhibits the activated factor X (Xa).[380] Antithrombin complexes with all the serine protease coagulation factors (factor Xa, factor IXa, and contact factors, including XIIa, kallikrein, and HMWK), except factor VII.[46,135,304]

Thrombolytics such as streptokinase, urokinase, anistreplase, and recombinant tissue plasminogen activator (rt-PA) enhance the normal processes that lead to clot degradation.[257]

Thrombosis is initiated when exposed endothelium or released tissue factors lead to platelet adherence and aggregation, the formation of thrombin, and cross-linking of fibrinogen to form fibrin strands.[135,257,304]

This results in a hemostatic plug or thrombus formation. Thrombus formation, in turn, leads to generation of plasmin from plasminogen, which causes fibrinolysis and eventual dissolution of the hemostatic plug.[74,75] Thus, the fibrinolytic system is a natural balance against unregulated coagulation. Thrombolytic therapy increases fibrinolytic activity by accelerating the conversion of plasminogen to plasmin, which actively degrades fibrin.[74,75] After the administration of thrombolytics, a drug-induced coagulopathy ensues, and fibrin degradation products (FDPs) are elevated secondary to the rapid turnover of clot.

DEVELOPMENT OF COAGULOPATHY

Impaired coagulation results from decreased production or enhanced consumption of coagulation factors, the presence of inhibitors of coagulation, activation of the fibrinolytic system, or abnormalities in platelet number or function. Platelets are involved in the initial phases of clotting after blood vessel injury by assisting in the formation of the fibrin plug.

Decreased production of coagulation factors results from congenital and acquired etiologies. Although congenital disorders of factor VIII (hemophilia A), factor IX (Christmas factor Hemophilia B), factor XI, and factor XII (Hageman factor) are all reported, their overall incidence is still quite low. Clinical conditions that result in acquired factor deficiencies are much more common and result from either a decrease in synthesis or activation. Factors II, V, VII, and X are entirely synthesized in the liver,[135,257,304] making hepatic dysfunction a common cause of acquired coagulopathy. In addition, factors II, VII, IX, and X also require postsynthetic modification by an enzyme that uses vitamin K as a cofactor,[353,358,359] such that vitamin K deficiency (from malnutrition, changes in gut flora secondary to xenobiotics, or malabsorption), and inhibition of vitamin K cycling (from warfarin) are capable of impairing coagulation.

Excessive consumption of coagulation factors usually results from massive activation of the coagulation cascade. Massive activation occurs during severe bleeding or disseminated intravascular coagulation (DIC). The latter results from infection, such as sepsis, and from conditions that introduce tissue factor into the blood, such as neoplasms, snake envenomations, stagnant blood flow, diffuse endothelial injury secondary to hyperthermia, ruptured aortic aneurysm, or aortic dissection. The hallmark of a consumptive coagulopathy is a depressed concentration of fibrinogen with an elevation of FDPs. This combination suggests the rapid turnover of fibrin in the coagulation process. In the other coagulopathic conditions, the failure to activate the coagulation cascade is associated with normal or high fibrin concentrations and low FDPs because of limited clot formation.

Hypothermia is a well-known cause of DIC leading to death.[365] Canine studies show decreased fibrinogen, factor II, and factor VII concentrations when cooled to 68°F (20°C) while a simultaneous rise in factor V concentration occurs.[140] In vitro studies show increased coagulation time, clot formation time, and maximum clot strength in hypothermic whole-blood samples from healthy volunteers.[103,311] In addition, thrombocytopenia occurs secondary to sequestration in the spleen, liver, and splanchnic circulation.[301,355] Infants with hypothermia have an increased risk for intracranial and pulmonary hemorrhage.[62]

Inhibitors of the coagulation cascade (circulating anticoagulants) are of two types: immunoglobulins to coagulation factors or antibodies to phospholipid membrane surfaces. Immunoglobulins develop without obvious cause, are part of a systemic autoimmune disorder, or result from repeated transfusions with exogenous factors (as occurs in patients with hemophilia).[162,209,330] Antibodies to factors V, VII to XI, and XIII are described.[35,330] The clinical syndromes associated with antibody inhibitors are similar to those associated with deficiencies of the particular coagulation factors involved. Antiphospholipid antibodies are directed against phospholipid membrane surfaces and β_2-GP I, also known as apolipoprotein H. This protein is essential in preventing hemostasis by inhibiting adenosine diphosphate (ADP)–induced platelet aggregation, inhibiting activation of the intrinsic pathway of the coagulation cascade, and inhibiting both platelet-mediated factor Xa and factor VII activation. Therefore, destroying β_2-GP I creates a prothrombotic clinical status.[324,325,334] Paradoxically, this antibody creates a prolonged PTT because the antibody also binds to most phospholipid-containing PTT reagents. This reduction in amount of active reagent results in a falsely elevated PTT.[162,209]

GENERAL MANAGEMENT

Gastrointestinal decontamination should be performed on patients who are believed to have potentially significant life-threatening ingestions unless they already present with significant bleeding. For patients who present after a few hours of ingestion, gastric emptying is not indicated (Chap. 5). In general, a single dose of activated charcoal (AC) decreases absorption of some anthrombotics and should be given unless contraindicated.[272,377,391] Oral cholestyramine enhances warfarin elimination,[299] but no studies are available that compare these two therapies or evaluate the role of combined AC and

cholestyramine therapy. Therefore, early administration of AC after ingestion is the preferred form of GI decontamination, even for patients who overdose on warfarin. In addition to general supportive measures, the patient should be placed in a supervised medical and psychiatric environment that offers protection against external or self-induced trauma and permits observation for the onset of coagulopathy.

Blood transfusion is required for any patient with a history of blood loss or active bleeding who is hemodynamically unstable, has impaired oxygen transport, or is expected to become unstable. Although a transfusion of packed red blood cells (PRBCs) is ideal for replacing lost blood, it cannot correct a coagulopathy, so patients will continue to bleed. Massive transfusion protocols (MTPs) aim to correct coagulopathy with an array of blood products, electrolytes, and antifibrinolytics. If available, it is reasonable to use an MTP for unstable patients. If an MTP is not available, whole blood is reasonable in severe cases because it contains many components, including platelets, white blood cells, and non–vitamin K–dependent factors.

VITAMIN K ANTAGONISTS
Warfarin and "Warfarinlike" Anticoagulants

The vitamin K antagonist (VKA) anticoagulants can be divided into two groups: (1) hydroxycoumarins, including warfarin, difenacoum, coumafuryl, fumasol, prolin, ethyl biscoumacetate, phenprocoumon, dicumarol, bishydroxycoumarin, and acenocoumarin, and (2) indanediones, including chlorphacinone, diphacinone, diphenadione, phenindione, and anisindione. Regardless of the classification, their mechanism of action involves inhibition of the vitamin K cycle. Vitamin K is a cofactor in the postribosomal synthesis of clotting factors II, VII, IX, and X (Fig. 58–2). The vitamin K–sensitive enzymatic step that occurs in the liver involves the γ-carboxylation of 10 or more glutamic acid residues at the amino terminal end of the precursor proteins to form a unique amino acid γ-carboxyglutamate.[104,353,358,359] These

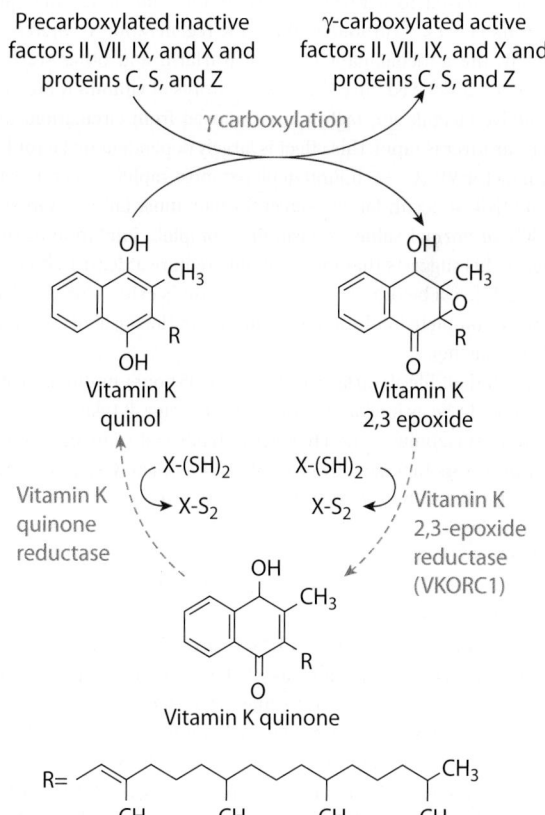

FIGURE 58–2. The vitamin K cycle. Dotted lines represent pathways that can be blocked with warfarin and warfarinlike anticoagulants. The aliphatic side chain (R) of vitamin K is shown below the metabolic pathway. VKORC1 = vitamin K reductase complex 1.

amino acids chelate calcium in vivo, which allows the binding of the four vitamin K–dependent clotting factors to phospholipid membranes during activation of the coagulation cascade.[400]

Vitamin K is inactive until it is reduced from its quinone form to a quinol (or hydroquinone) form in hepatic microsomes. This reduction of vitamin K must precede the carboxylation of the precursor factors. The carboxylation activity is coupled to an epoxidase activity for vitamin K, whereby vitamin K is oxidized simultaneously to vitamin K 2,3-epoxide (Fig. 58–2).[358,399] This inactive form of the vitamin is converted back to the active form by two successive reductions.[104,233,277,395] In the first step, an epoxide reductase (known as vitamin K 2,3-epoxide reductase) uses reduced nicotinamide adenine dinucleotide (NADH) as a cofactor to convert vitamin K 2,3-epoxide to a quinone form.[270,271,358] Subsequently, the quinone is reduced to the active vitamin K quinol form (Antidotes in Depth: A18).

Warfarin is a racemic mixture of R warfarin and S warfarin enantiomers. In humans, S warfarin is approximately 2.7 to 3.8 times more potent than R warfarin.[37] Warfarin and all warfarinlike compounds inhibit the activity of vitamin K 2,3-epoxide reductase, as is demonstrated by the observation of elevated concentrations of vitamin K 2,3-epoxide.[69,403] Vitamin K quinone reductase is also inhibited by warfarin and its related compounds (Fig. 58–2).[104,121] This reduction in the cyclic activation of vitamin K subsequently inhibits the formation of activated clotting factors.

Pharmacology of Vitamin K Antagonists

Oral warfarin is well absorbed, and peak serum concentrations occur approximately 3 hours after administration.[357] Because only the free warfarin is therapeutically active, concurrent administration of xenobiotics that alter the concentration of free warfarin, either by competing for binding to albumin or by inhibiting warfarin metabolism, markedly influences the anticoagulant effect.[24,126,357] The pharmacologic response to warfarin is a polygenic trait with approximately 30 genes contributing to its therapeutic effects.[195] Readers are referred to a review of xenobiotics and foods that potentiate warfarin's effects.[398] Although vitamin K regeneration is altered almost immediately, the anticoagulant effect of warfarin and other warfarinlike anticoagulants is delayed until the existing stores of vitamin K are depleted and the active coagulation factors are removed from circulation. Because vitamin K turnover is rapid, this effect is largely dependent on factor half-life ($t_{1/2}$), with factor VII ($t_{1/2}$ ~5 hours) depleted most rapidly.[126] For a prolongation of the INR to occur, factor concentrations must fall to approximately 25% to 30% of normal values.[72] Assuming complete inhibition of the vitamin K cycle, this suggests that most patients require at least 15 hours (three factor VII half-lives) before the effect of warfarin is evident on the INR.[123] In fact, because complete inhibition does not occur, the onset of coagulation is delayed even further.

Because the half-life of warfarin in humans is 35 hours, its duration of action is documented to be as long as 5 days.[50,357] On average, it takes approximately 6 days of warfarin administration to reach a steady-state anticoagulant effect.

R warfarin is metabolized by enzymes CYP1A2 and CYP3A4, and S warfarin is metabolized by CYP2C9. Whereas R warfarin is metabolized by side-chain reduction to secondary alcohols that are subsequently excreted by the kidney, S warfarin is metabolized by hydroxylation to 7-hydroxy warfarin, which is excreted into the bile.[357] The elimination of S warfarin is more rapid than that of R warfarin.[49]

Dosing of warfarin and other VKAs is problematic in many patients. In one study, genetic polymorphisms of the vitamin K epoxide reductase complex 1 (VKORC1) and CYP2C9 genes were the strongest predictors of interindividual variability in the anticoagulant effect of warfarin.[195] Pharmacogenomic research with complex xenobiotics, such as warfarin, improves safety of treatment and predicts or prevents interactions with other xenobiotics. Although the FDA has approved a commercially available test to identify variants within these genes,[193] current guidelines do not advocate genetic testing to guide VKA dosing.[154]

Within the coumarin group are two 4-hydroxycoumarin derivatives, difenacoum and brodifacoum, that differ from warfarin by their longer, higher molecular weight polycyclic hydrocarbon side chains. Together with chlorophacinone, an indandione derivative, they are known as *superwarfarins* or long-acting VKAs.

Long-acting VKAs were designed to be effective rodenticides in warfarin-resistant rodents.[230] Their mechanism of action is identical to that of the traditional warfarinlike anticoagulants, as demonstrated by increased concentrations of vitamin K 2,3-epoxide after administration.[48,51,56,210,277] The ability of these xenobiotics to perform as superior rodenticides is attributed to their high lipid solubility and concentration in the liver.[210,230,277] They also saturate hepatic enzymes at very low concentrations, as demonstrated by zero-order elimination after overdose.[56] These factors make them about 100 times more potent than warfarin on a molar basis.[210,230,277] In addition, they have a longer duration of action than the traditional warfarins.[210,230,277] For example, to obtain 100% lethality in a mouse, more than 21 days of feeding with a warfarin-containing rodenticide (0.025% anticoagulant by weight of bait) is required.[230] Similar efficacy is achieved with a single ingestion of brodifacoum (0.005% anticoagulant by weight of bait).[230] Furthermore, more concentrated liquid formulations, such as brodifacoum (0.5% anticoagulant), are available through illegal vendors and are implicated in prolonged coagulopathy in humans.[138] It should also be noted that although ingestion of these xenobiotics is the most common route of exposure and subsequent cause of toxicity, dermal absorption of liquid preparations occurs, also resulting in a coagulopathy.[344]

Clinical Manifestations

Although intentional ingestions of warfarin-containing products are uncommon, adverse drug events resulting in excessive anticoagulation and bleeding frequently occur. The risk of bleeding during VKA therapy depends on a myriad of factors, including the intensity of anticoagulation, patient characteristics, and comorbid conditions. Clearly, the most serious complication of excessive anticoagulation is intracranial bleeding, which is reported to occur in as many as 2% of patients on long term therapy, which is an 8- to 10-fold increase in risk compared with patients who are not anticoagulated.[125,126,405] The overall risk of major bleeding in patients can be estimated using tools such as the Hypertension, Abnormal Renal/Liver Function, Stroke, Bleeding History or Predisposition, Labile INR, Elderly, Drugs/Alcohol Concomitantly (HAS-BLED) score, which was prospectively validated in patients with atrial fibrillation.[225,285] Bleeding ranges between 1 and 12.5 episodes per 100 patient-years, with a higher risk in patients with multiple risk factors.[285] Another study showed that patients older than the age of 80 years have a cumulative incidence of major bleeding at 13.1 per 100 person-years with major bleeding defined as bleeding at serious sites (eg, intracranial, retroperitoneal, intraspinal, or pericardial) or bleeding that results in blood transfusion or death. Patients between the ages of 65 and 80 years have a lower risk of 4.7 major episodes of bleeding per 100 person-years.[176] Major bleeding complications are associated with a fatality rate as high as 77%.[239] In patients with intracranial bleeding a decreased level of consciousness and an increased size of hematoma are predictors of poor prognosis.[419] Somewhat surprisingly, the degree of INR elevation was not associated with worse outcome.[419]

Many cases of intentional overdose of long-acting VKAs in humans are reported. The clinical courses of these patients are characterized by a severe coagulopathy that last weeks to months, often accompanied by consequential blood loss. Most patients do not seek medical care until bruising or bleeding is evident,[19,56,57,119,170,194] which often occurs many days after ingestion. The most common sites of bleeding are the GI and genitourinary tracts. In one study describing 12 patients with surreptitious ingestion of oral anticoagulants, nine were health care professionals.[271] These patients presented with bruising, hematuria, hematochezia, and menorrhagia. Bleeding into the neck with resultant airway compromise is a rare but life-threatening complication.[43]

Patients with unintentional ingestions must be distinguished from those with intentional ingestions because the former demonstrate a low likelihood of developing a coagulopathy and have rare morbidity or mortality. Most patients (usually children) are entirely asymptomatic and have a normal coagulation profile after an acute unintentional exposure. Typical warfarin-like rodenticides contain only small concentrations of anticoagulant, 0.005% (or 5 mg of brodifacoum per 100 g of product). A 10-kg child would require an initial dose of 10 g of rodenticide (8 pellets, each of which is approximately 25 mm in size). These quantities are far greater than those that occur in typical "tastes." Thus, single small unintentional ingestions of warfarin-containing rodenticides pose a minimal threat to normal patients.[190] Prolongation of the INR is unlikely with a single small ingestion of a long-acting VKA rodenticide. Clinically significant anticoagulation is even rarer. In a combined pediatric case series, prolongation of the INR occurred in only 8 of 142 children (5.6%) reported with single small ingestions of long-acting VKAs.[28,189,190,342] Only one child in this group was reported to have "abnormal prolonged bleeding," but this required no medical attention.[342] In a single case report, a 36-month-old child developed a coagulopathy manifested by epistaxis and hematuria, with anticoagulation persisting for more than 100 days after a presumed, but unwitnessed, single unintentional ingestion of brodifacoum.[366] Clinically significant coagulopathy can result, however, after small repeated ingestions. Two children reportedly became poisoned by repeated ingestions of a long-acting anticoagulant. One child presented with a neck hematoma that compromised his airway and the other with a hemarthrosis.[151] Similarly, a 7-year-old girl required multiple hospitalizations over a 20-month period after repeated unintentional ingestions of brodifacoum.[32] Finally, a 24-month-old child who presented with unexplained bruising and a PT greater than 125 seconds was the victim of brodifacoum poisoning secondary to Munchausen syndrome by proxy, which is currently called *pediatric condition falsification* (Chap. 31).[15]

Laboratory Assessment

Although warfarin concentrations are useful to confirm the diagnosis in unknown cases and to study drug kinetics,[155,268] the routine use of simple and inexpensive measures such as INR determination seems more appropriate (Table 58–1). When blood loss is evident, serial determinations of hemoglobin concentration are indicated.

For patients with an acute and significant long acting VKA overdose, daily INR evaluations for 2 days are adequate to identify most patients at risk for coagulopathy. Earlier detection through direct coagulation factor analysis is available but is typically reserved to trend patients with known coagulopathy for treatment purposes.[155,170] Concentrations of long-acting VKAs can now be measured, although they are usually only performed in reference laboratories.[199,268] We recommend that children with possibly significant exposures be followed up with at least a single INR at least 48 hours after the exposure. Even though significant toxicity from long-acting VKAs is rare, it should be recognized that the reported benign courses of exposures in children are somewhat misleading. Multiple retrospective studies suggest that children with unintentional acute exposures do not require any follow-up coagulation studies.[256,260,279,332] However, this conclusion and approach to management is an unjustified attempt to decrease the cost of "unnecessary" coagulation studies. There are clearly insufficient data to justify this conclusion because many of these "exposed" children were never documented to have ingested long-acting VKAs (Chap. 130). We recommend that clinicians continue to manage these children as possibly significant exposures and that all children be followed up with at least a single INR at a minimum of 2 days after the exposure. A baseline INR is usually unnecessary but is reasonable if there is a suspicion of an antecedent ingestion. A baseline INR is also helpful when chronic exposure is suspected.

Treatment of Vitamin K Antagonist–Induced Coagulopathy

Life-threatening bleeding secondary to VKA toxicity should be immediately reversed with factor replacement followed by vitamin K_1 (Table 58–1). The American College of Chest Physicians (ACCP) and the FDA recommend factor replacement with four-factor prothrombin complex concentrate (PCC) as a first-line treatment for major bleeding in the setting of VKA-induced coagulopathy.[172] This recommendation is reasonable given the ease of administration as compared with fresh-frozen plasma (FFP). Most countries use traditional four-factor PCC, which contains concentrated factors II, VII,

IX, X, C, and S. Dosing of PCC is based on INR and body weight. The typical doses range between 25 and 50 units/kg with the largest dose based on a maximum weight of 100 kg. The PCC is contained in both 500-unit and 1,000-unit vials. However, the factor IX content of each vial is variable: 500-unit vial may contain between 400 to 620 units/vial, and a 1,000-unit vial may contain between 800 and 1,240 units/vial. Each individual vial states the actual factor IX content in each bottle, and the dosage should be based on the actual factor IX content in each vial.[88] Most forms of PCC, contain small amounts of heparin. These heparin-containing PCCs are contraindicated in patients with a history of heparin-induced thrombocytopenia (HIT) and heparin-induced thrombocytopenia and thrombosis syndrome (HITT). In those cases, factor eight inhibitor bypassing activity (FEIBA), an activated prothrombin complex concentrate (aPCC), is recommended. Activated aPCCs contain factors II, VII, IX, and X in inactive and activated forms. Factor eight inhibitor bypassing activity is typically used to treat patients with hemophilia A and B. Unfortunately, FEIBA has not been studied extensively in the setting of VKA-induced coagulopathy. Therefore, there is no standard dose for coagulopathy reversal. Typical doses for treating bleeding or for perioperative management range between 50 and 100 units/kg with the dose based on the amount of factor VIII inhibitor bypass activity.[23] Despite its increased cost, the rationale for using PCC instead of FFP includes less risk of infection transmission.[172] In addition, small-volume factor replacement is preferable in patients at risk of volume overload, such as patients with heart failure, chronic kidney disease (CKD), or intracranial bleeding.[2] Unfortunately, there are only a few studies comparing PCC with FFP in reversing coagulopathy. These studies show that PCC safely produces complete INR reversal faster than FFP with more consistent factor IX replacement.[95,185,234] However, unequal factor replacement in these small studies favors more factor replacement in patients receiving PCC.[315] Fresh-frozen plasma is rich in active vitamin K–dependent coagulation factors and will reverse oral anticoagulant-induced coagulopathy in most patients. In general, approximately 15 mL/kg of FFP should be adequate to reverse any VKA-induced coagulopathy.[87] However, the specific factor quantities and volume of each unit may be varied, leading to an unpredictable response.[234] In addition, delay to FFP administration is accentuated by requirements for blood type matching and thawing. Therefore, we recommend in acute major bleeding in the setting of VKA-induced coagulopathy the use of PCC as the preferred reversal agent.

Activated recombinant factor VII (rFVIIa) is approved for patients with hemophilia or various factor inhibitors and has successfully reversed warfarin toxicity.[284] The safety of off-label rFVIIa to reverse VKA coagulopathy is unclear. Preliminary data using rFVIIa suggested its utility for bleeding secondary to warfarin-induced excessive anticoagulation and a case series showing beneficial effects in four patients with long acting VKA toxicity.[420] However, adverse outcomes, such as arterial thrombotic events, occur at higher than acceptable rates. Initial concerns for thromboembolic adverse events were raised when review of the FDA's Adverse Event Reporting System database found that the majority of these complications arose in patients who received rFVIIa for off-label purposes. Cerebrovascular accident, acute MI, PE, venous thrombosis, and clotted devices all occurred at higher rates in off-label applications.[269] The Factor Seven for Acute Hemorrhagic Stroke Trial (FAST) showed that arterial thromboembolic adverse events increased in a dose-dependent fashion with the administration of rFVIIa.[102] A subsequent meta-analysis confirmed that an increased rate of arterial thrombosis occurs in patients who receive rFVIIa.[219] The risk of continued bleeding versus the benefit of rapid reversal of coagulopathy with rFVIIa is unknown, and further experience with rFVIIa is necessary to determine its safety and efficacy in anticoagulant-induced bleeding. We do not recommend routine use of rFVIIa for reversing VKA-associated coagulopathy. If FFP, PCC, and FEIBA are not available, then it is reasonable that rFVIIa be given in life-threatening situations.[1] It should also be noted that if rFVIIa is used, assays based on PT are inaccurate and should be avoided when administering rFVIIa.[191]

Treatment with vitamin K_1 takes several hours to activate enough factors to reverse a patient's coagulopathy,[234,278] and this delay is potentially fatal. Repetitive, large doses of vitamin K_1 (on the order of 60 mg/d or greater) are

TABLE 58–1   Antithrombotics: Laboratory Testing, Antidotes, and Treatment Strategies

	Laboratory Testing Results (Expected)	Antidotes and Treatment Strategies
Antiplatelet Agents Cyclooxygenase inhibitors Phosphodiesterase inhibitors Adenosine reuptake inhibitors Adenosine diphosphate receptor inhibitors Glycoprotein IIb/IIIa inhibitors	Bleeding time prolonged; platelet function assays abnormal	Desmopressin 0.3 mcg/kg IV over 15–30 min for life-threatening bleeding; platelet administration is controversial but is recommended in life-threatening situations.

Antithrombin Agonists
Unfractionated heparin
	PTT prolonged; TT abnormal; ACT elevated; fibrinogen normal, anti–factor Xa activity increased	1 mg of protamine per 100 units of heparin[a]. In overdose, if unknown quantity of heparin administered, treat based on ACT:[b]
		    ACT <150 s: no protamine needed
		    ACT 200–300 s: 0.6 mg/kg protamine
		    ACT 300–400 s: 1.2 mg/kg protamine
		Alternatively, empiric treatment with 25–50 mg of protamine
		Ciraparantag (in clinical trials)

Low-molecular-weight heparin (eg, enoxaparin, dalteparin)	Anti–factor Xa activity increased; PTT is insensitive	1 mg of protamine per 100 antifactor Xa units (or 1 mg of enoxaparin) given in the previous 8 h. Administer an additional 0.5 mg protamine per 100 anti–factor Xa units if bleeding continues. Protamine does not completely neutralize LMWHs.

Direct Thrombin Inhibitors
 	
Dabigatran
	PTT prolonged; TT prolonged; ECT prolonged; anti–factor Xa activity elevated (at low concentrations, PT and PTT may be normal); dTT prolonged[d,351]	
		
		Activated charcoal in overdose
		Idarucizumab 5 g IV
		If idarucizumab is unavailable:
		    4F-PCC administration with up to 100 units/kg in repeated 50 units/kg doses as needed. If bleeding continues 30 min after PCC[c], give FEIBA ©.[237,376]
		    Hemodialysis
		FFP 15 mL/kg

Bivalirudin		Stop the infusion
Argatroban		FFP 15 mL/kg
Direct Factor Xa Inhibitors Rivaroxaban Apixaban Edoxaban	PT and PTT can be normal or prolonged (varies with reagents); anti–factor Xa activity elevated with specific modified chromogenic antifactor Xa assay[d]	AC in overdose PCC[c] administration with up to 50 units/kg in repeated 25 units/kg doses as needed Andexanet alfa[e] Low dose: 400 mg IV High dose: 800 mg IV Ciraparantag (in clinical trials)
Fibrinolytics	PT and PTT prolonged; TT abnormal; fibrinogen abnormal	Cryoprecipitate Factor replacement with 15 mL/kg of FFP or 50 units/kg of PCC[c] For life-threatening hemorrhage, give tranexamic acid at 1 g intravenously over 10 minutes followed by 1 g over 8 h. If tranexamic acid is unavailable, IV aminocaproic acid is recommended as a loading dose of 5 g over 1 h followed by an infusion at 1 g/h for 23 h. Stop infusion if bleeding ceases.
Pentasaccharide Fondaparinux	Fondaparinux-specific anti-Xa assay PTT does not reflect degree of anticoagulation	PCC administration with up to 50 units/kg in repeated 25 units/kg doses as needed to maximum of 100 units/kg.
Vitamin K Antagonist Warfarin	*Early* (PT prolonged; PTT normal) *Late* (PT and PTT prolonged; TT and fibrinogen normal)	Vitamin K Factor replacement with 4F-PCC[c] or if not available FFP (15 mL/Kg) 4F-PCC for major or life-threatening hemorrhage See Table 58–2 for detailed management recommendations.

[a]May need to repeat in 2–8 h because of potential heparin rebound. [b]Use of activated clotting time (ACT) is only validated in the operative setting after cardiopulmonary bypass. [c]In patients with a history of heparin-induced thrombocytopenia, avoid prothrombin complex concentrate (PCC) (except Profilnine) and use factor eight inhibitor bypassing activity (FEIBA) or recombinant factor VII (rFVIIA). [d]No readily available method to assess extent of anticoagulation at this time. [e]FDA approved for rivaroxaban and apixaban (but should also be effective for edoxaban) and low dose vs high dose is based on timing and amount of last dose of Anti-Xa inhbitor.

AC = activated charcoal; ECT = ecarin clotting time; dTT= dilute thrombin time; FFP = fresh-frozen plasma; 4F-PCC = four-factor prothrombin complex concentrate; LMWH = low molecular weight heparin; PCC = prothrombin complex concentrate; PT = prothrombin time; PTT = partial thromboplastin time; TT = thrombin time.

reported in some patients with massive ingestion.[155,271] If complete reversal of INR prolongation occurs or is desirable (as in most cases of life-threatening bleeding) and the underlying medical condition of the patient still requires some degree of anticoagulation, the patient can then receive anticoagulation with heparin after the bleeding is controlled and clinical stability restored. Heparin anticoagulation was used without apparent bleeding complications in 25% of patients in one cross-sectional study.[402]

Vitamin K$_1$ is preferable over the other forms of vitamin K; the other forms are ineffective[183,262,270,373] are potentially toxic,[17] and are unavailable in the United States. Parenteral administration of vitamin K$_1$ (phytonadione) is traditionally preferred as initial therapy by many authors, but success can also be achieved with early oral therapy, especially when the coagulopathy is not severe.[56] In most cases, the patient can be switched to oral vitamin K$_1$ for long-term care. Vitamin K$_1$ can be administered intramuscularly, subcutaneously, intradermally, or intravenously. Although intravenous (IV) therapy has the most rapid onset of action of all routes of delivery, its use as the sole therapeutic is still associated with a delay of several hours[278,395] and carries the added risk of anaphylactoid reactions.[302] The use of low doses and slow rate of administration reduces this risk[335] (Antidotes in Depth: A18). In cases in which oral administration is undesirable, for example, with significant GI bleeding the subcutaneous (SC) route should not be used because absorption is erratic. In this case, we recommend the IV route of administration of vitamin K$_1$ because the benefits outweigh the risks.

For patients with non–life-threatening bleeding, the clinician must evaluate whether anticoagulation is required for long-term care. In patients not requiring chronic anticoagulation we recommend treating even small elevations of the INR with vitamin K$_1$ alone to prevent deterioration in coagulation status and reduce the risk of bleeding. In contrast to ingestions of warfarin, we recommend not to give prophylactic vitamin K$_1$ to asymptomatic patients with unintentional ingestions of long-acting warfarinlike anticoagulants because (1) if the patient develops a coagulopathy, it will last for weeks, and the one or two doses of vitamin K$_1$ given will not prevent complications; (2) a gradual decline in coagulation factors occurs over the first day of anticoagulation, so an individual would not be expected to develop a life-threatening coagulopathy in 1 or 2 days; and (3) after vitamin K$_1$ is administered, the onset of an INR abnormality will be delayed, which could impair the ability of the clinician to recognize a coagulation abnormality, possibly requiring the patient to undergo an unnecessarily prolonged observation period.

For patients requiring chronic anticoagulation we agree with the ACCP guidelines for the management of patients with elevated INRs (Table 58-2). It should also be noted that low-dose vitamin K is safe to administer to patients with mildly elevated INRs (4–10) to decrease the INR more rapidly; however, one study did not demonstrate decreased bleeding in the treatment group.[86] Furthermore, simply omitting warfarin

doses is usually adequate for a patient without active bleeding who has an INR between 4 and 9.[86]

It is often unclear why patients with consistent therapeutic dosing have seemingly random elevations in their INR. A case-control study identified the following risk factors associated with overanticoagulation from VKAs: previous medical history of increased INR, antibiotic therapy, fever, and concomitant use of amiodarone and proton pump inhibitors.[60] Clinicians should pay particular attention to patients with these conditions, and close monitoring of coagulation profiles should be performed.[60]

Treatment of Long-Acting Vitamin K Antagonist Overdoses
In patients with unintentional, small ingestions of long-acting VKAs, the risk of coagulopathy is low. However, it takes days to develop coagulopathy. Administration of AC is recommended to prevent absorption in acute ingestions if no contraindication exists.[190,342]

Treatment of a patient with a coagulopathy resulting from a long-acting anticoagulant overdose is essentially the same as the treatment of oral anticoagulant toxicity with certain exceptions. Although initial parenteral vitamin K$_1$ doses as high as 400 mg have been required for reversal,[57] daily oral vitamin K$_1$ requirements are often in the range of 50 to 200 mg. Recent experience in both animals and humans suggests that parenteral vitamin K$_1$ therapy is not required after initial stabilization (Antidotes in Depth: A18).[56,411]

In one case report, a 2-year-old child with confirmed brodifacoum-associated coagulopathy developed anemia, epistaxis, ecchymosis and GI bleeding. She developed an anaphylactoid reaction after several doses of IV vitamin K$_1$. Patients typically tolerate IV vitamin K$_1$ well as long as it is administered appropriately. In stable patients, oral vitamin K is recommended. However, because oral vitamin K was not available at this hospital, the patient received five plasma exchange treatments, which resulted in normalization of her coagulation studies. In addition, repeat brodifacoum concentrations were undetectable after her third plasma exchange treatment.[94] Because there are other less invasive methods of correcting VKA-induced coagulopathy and lack of established experience with plasma exchange beyond this case report, we do not recommend plasma exchange therapy for VKA-induced coagulopathy.

Long-acting VKAs are metabolized by the cytochrome P450 system.[16,270] In a rat model, the duration of coagulopathy was shortened by administering phenobarbital, a CYP3A4 inducer.[16] Although phenobarbital has never been systematically studied in humans, this approach was used by several authors in isolated human cases of long-acting anticoagulant toxicity.[57,183,226,366,393] These anecdotal reports suggest some improvement with phenobarbital therapy, but the risk of sedation in a patient who might be prone to bleeding complications outweighs any purported benefit.

Patients with long-acting VKA overdose should be followed until their coagulation studies remain normal without treatment for several days. This usually requires daily or even twice-daily INR measurements until the INR is at the lower limit of the therapeutic range. Monitoring of serial INR measurements should allow for a gradual decrease in vitamin K$_1$ requirement over time. Periodic coagulation factor analysis (particularly factor VII), however, provides an early marker of toxicity resolution.[170] An anticoagulated patient will require weeks to months of close observation for both psychiatric and medical management. A critical superwarfarin concentration below which anticoagulation does not occur is not defined.[57] In one case report, brodifacoum was observed to follow zero-order elimination kinetics.[56]

Nonbleeding Complications of Vitamin K Antagonists
Warfarin therapy is associated with three nonhemorrhagic lesions of the skin: urticaria,[323] purple toe syndrome,[122] and warfarin skin necrosis.[77,193,202,242,384] Although warfarin skin necrosis was once thought to be a rare and idiosyncratic reaction,[193,202] more recent evidence suggests a link between this disorder and protein C deficiency.[202,384] Protein C synthesis is also dependent on vitamin K.[73] Patients who are homozygotes for protein C deficiency have an increased incidence of thrombosis and embolic events, such that they often require long-term anticoagulant therapy.[73] Because the half-life of

TABLE 58–2 Recommendations for Management of Elevated International Normalized Ratio or Bleeding in Patients Receiving Vitamin K Antagonists[154]

International Normalized Ratio	Recommendation[a]
<4.5; no significant bleeding	Lower or omit the next dose of warfarin.
≥4.5–10; no significant bleeding	Omit warfarin for the next one or two doses.
>10; no evidence of bleeding	Give oral vitamin K$_1$ (1–2.5 mg). If more rapid reversal is necessary, give oral vitamin K$_1$ (≤5 mg) and wait 24 h. Give additional vitamin K$_1$ orally (1–2 mg) as needed.
Serious bleeding at any INR value or life-threatening bleeding	Hold warfarin therapy and give 4F-PCC supplemented with vitamin K$_1$ (5–10 mg by slow IV[a] infusion). Vitamin K$_1$ administration often needs to be repeated every 12 h.

[a]Intravenous (IV) infusion of vitamin K$_1$ rarely may cause severe anaphylactoid reactions
FFP = fresh-frozen plasma; 4F-PCC = four-factor prothrombin complex concentrate; INR = international normalized ratio; PCC = prothrombin complex concentrate.

protein C is shorter than that of many of the vitamin K–dependent coagulation factors, protein C concentrations fall rapidly during the first hours of warfarin therapy. This results in an imbalance that actually favors coagulation, and skin necrosis results because of microvascular thrombosis in dermal vessels.[242,384] Although warfarin skin necrosis is more common in patients with protein C deficiency, this disorder is also described in patients with protein S and AT deficiencies.[77] Unfortunately, these deficiencies are neither necessary nor sufficient to account for the incidence of warfarin necrosis.[77] If necrosis occurs, warfarin should be discontinued, and heparin should be initiated to decrease thrombosis of postcapillary venules. Some patients also require surgical debridement.[314]

The purple toe syndrome, in contrast to warfarin-induced skin necrosis, is presumed to result from small atheroemboli that are no longer adherent to their plaques by clot (Fig. 17–13).

Warfarin-related nephropathy (WRN) is a well-recognized form of non-hemorrhagic warfarin toxicity. In patients with CKD, an acute increase in the INR above 3 was associated with an increase in serum creatinine and accelerated reduction in kidney function. The etiology of the WRN is attributed to acute tubular injury and glomerular bleeding, demonstrated by the finding of red blood cell (RBCs) filling Bowman's capsule and RBCs casts obstructing glomeruli on specimens from kidney biopsies.[54,55] Further studies that retrospectively reviewed kidney function in patients on long-term warfarin anticoagulation showed 33% of patients with CKD and 16.5% of patients without CKD developed WRN. Warfarin-related nephropathy is associated with a mortality rate of 31.1%, a significant increase in risk compared with 18.9% in patients without WRN.[54]

An additional major nonhemorrhagic complication of warfarin therapy is warfarin embryopathy. Most warfarin-induced fetal abnormalities occur during weeks 6 to 12 of gestation, but central nervous system (CNS) and ocular abnormalities can develop at any time during gestation (Chap. 30).[158,354]

ANTITHROMBIN AGONISTS

Heparin

Conventional heparin also known as unfractionated heparin C or unfractionated heparin (UFH) is a heterogeneous group of molecules within the class of glycosaminoglycans.[180] The heparin precursor molecule is composed of long chains of mucopolysaccharides, a polypeptide, and carbohydrates. The main carbohydrate components of heparin molecules include uronic acids and amino sugars in polysaccharide chains. Heparin for pharmaceutical use is extracted from bovine lung tissue and porcine intestines.[328]

Heparin inhibits thrombosis by accelerating the binding of AT to thrombin (activated factor II) and other serine proteases involved in coagulation.[232,308] Thus, factors IX to XII, kallikrein, and thrombin are inhibited. Heparin also affects plasminogen activator inhibitor, protein C inhibitor, and other components of coagulation. The therapeutic effect of heparin is usually measured through the activated PTT. The activated clotting time (ACT) is more useful for monitoring large therapeutic doses or in the overdose situation.[201]

Low-molecular-weight heparins are 4,000- to 6,000-Da fractions obtained from conventional heparin.[128] As such, they share many of the pharmacologic and toxicologic properties of conventional heparin.[45] The various LMWHs (eg, nadroparin, enoxaparin, dalteparin) are prepared by different methods of depolymerization of heparin; consequently, they each differ to a certain extent regarding their pharmacokinetic properties and anticoagulant profiles. The major differences between LMWHs and conventional heparin are greater bioavailability, longer half-life, more predictable anticoagulation with fixed dosing, targeted activity against activated factor X, and less targeted activity against thrombin.[45,128] As a result of this targeted factor X activity, LMWHs have minimal effect on the activated PTT, thereby eliminating either the need for, or the usefulness of monitoring. They are therefore administered on a fixed dose schedule. However, in certain instances (eg, patients with CKD, pregnancy), monitoring of anti–factor Xa activity is performed to assess adequacy of anticoagulation and to prevent the risk of bleeding.[159] Controversy exists as to whether such testing is clinically necessary,[44] but

studies have not shown significant benefit in determining risk of thromboembolic recurrence or consistent risk of major bleeding. We do not recommend the routine testing of anti–factor Xa activity.

Studies investigating LMWHs for the prevention of thromboembolic disease after hip surgery and trauma, in patients with stroke or DVT, in pregnancy, and in other conditions where anticoagulation with heparin would otherwise be indicated (eg, at the onset of oral anticoagulation therapy) are numerous. Low-molecular-weight heparins have a minimal risk in pregnancy[246] because they do not cross the placenta,[124,356] and they are therefore preferred for the treatment or prophylaxis of thromboembolic disease in pregnancy.[306] Most studies demonstrate a lower incidence of embolization; however, there is still a trend toward increased bleeding.[30,152,220] The PROTECT trial, which compared dalteparin and UFH in terms of rates of proximal leg DVT, PE, and major bleeding in critically ill patients, found that patients randomized to the dalteparin group had statistically fewer PE. This study found no statistically significant differences in proximal DVT and major bleeding rates.[153]

Pharmacology

Because of the large size of heparin and negative charge, the molecule is unable to cross cellular membranes. These factors prevent oral administration, and heparin must be administered parenterally. After parenteral administration, heparin remains in the intravascular compartment, in part bound to globulins, fibrinogen, and low-density lipoproteins, resulting in a volume of distribution of 0.06 L/kg in humans.[118,273] Because of its rapid metabolism in the liver by a heparinase, heparin has a short duration of effect.[232] Although the half-life of elimination is dose dependent and ranges from 1 to 2.5 hours,[232,241,273] the duration of anticoagulant effect is usually reported as 1 to 3 hours.[232] Dosing errors or drug interactions with thrombolytics, antiplatelet drugs, or nonsteroidal antiinflammatory drugs increase the risk of bleeding.[161] Low-molecular-weight heparins are nearly 90% bioavailable after SC administration and have an elimination half-life of 3 to 6 hours.[137] Anti–factor Xa activity peaks between 3 and 5 hours after dosing.[137] Low-molecular-weight heparins are renally eliminated and patients with stage 4 or 5 CKD are at increased risk of toxicity.[386] Although there are insufficient data guiding therapeutic LMWH dosing in patients with severe CKD, some advocate dose reduction to decrease the risk of bleeding. However, no dosage regimens are provided.[154]

Clinical Manifestations

Intentional overdoses with heparin are rare.[238] Most reported cases involve iatrogenic toxicity in hospitalized patients.[136,145,238,276,326] These cases involved the administration of large amounts of heparin as a consequence of misidentification of heparin vials, during the process of flushing IV lines, and secondary to IV pump malfunction. Significant bleeding complications occurred in several cases, including at least one fatality.[136] However, intentional overdoses of LMWHs are reported, although none of them were fatal.[58,254]

Similar adverse effects to UFH are also reported with LMWHs and include epidural or spinal hematoma, intrahepatic bleeding,[173] abdominal wall hematomas,[13] psoas hematoma after lumbar plexus block,[192] and intracranial bleeding in patients with CNS malignancy.[98] Although these complications were all reported in patients who received the LMWH enoxaparin, there are no data to suggest differing toxicities among LMWHs.

Diagnostic Testing

For therapeutic anticoagulation, the effect of heparin is usually monitored with activated partial thromboplastin time (aPTT). Most hospitals have heparin nomograms that recommend heparin dose alterations based on aPTT, although these nomograms need to be individualized by each hospital because of the variation expected from the particular aPTT reagent and laboratory technology used. For patients undergoing cardiovascular procedures, the ACT is used to monitor them because they require higher dose heparin.[137] More recently, an anti-Xa assay specific for heparin was FDA approved. Heparin dosing is titrated based on the anti-Xa assay results, with therapeutic ranges higher than prophylactic ranges. Goal ranges also differ depending on whether LMWH or UFH is being used.

In patients with heparin resistance, in whom extremely high doses of heparin are required to accomplish a therapeutic aPTT, anti-Xa activity is recommended to guide heparin dosing. Despite lower heparin dosing and subtherapeutic aPTTs, patients monitored with anti-Xa activity had similar rates of recurrent thromboembolism and bleeding compared with the patients who were given high-dose heparin to maintain therapeutic aPTTs in a prospectively collected randomized control trial.[221]

Low-molecular-weight heparins are usually administered at fixed doses for venous thromboembolism (VTE) prophylaxis or at weight-based doses for VTE treatment. Laboratory monitoring is not done unless patients are pregnant, have CKD, or are obese. In these cases, anti-Xa activity is measured, with target ranges varying based on agent and dosing regimen.[137] In patients without the aforementioned risk factors, monitoring and dose adjustment are of no benefit compared with fixed-dose regimens of LMWH.[5] In addition, several studies show no correlation between anti-Xa activity and bleeding propensity.[18,215,389]

Treatment

After stabilization of the airway and breathing and circulation is ensured, the physician should be prepared to replace blood loss and reverse the coagulopathy, if indicated. Because of the relatively short duration of action of heparin, observation alone is indicated if significant bleeding has not occurred. For a patient requiring anticoagulation, serial aPTT determinations will indicate when it is safe to resume therapy. If significant bleeding occurs, either removal of the heparin or reversal of its anticoagulant effect is indicated. Because heparin has a very small volume of distribution, it can be effectively removed by exchange transfusion.[326] Although this technique has been used successfully in neonates, protamine has also safely been given to neonates without a history of fish allergy or previous exposure to protamine or protamine-containing insulin.[253] Exchange transfusion to remove heparin should be performed in neonates with significant bleeding if protamine is contraindicated.

When severe bleeding occurs, protamine sulfate partially neutralizes UFH[7] (Table 58–1). Protamine is a low-molecular-weight protein found in the sperm and testes of salmon, which forms ionic bonds with heparin and renders it devoid of anticoagulant activity.[232] One milligram of protamine sulfate injected intravenously neutralizes 100 units of UFH.[232] The dose of protamine should be calculated from the dose of heparin administered if known and assuming the approximate half-life of heparin to be 60 to 90 minutes; the amount of protamine should not exceed the amount of heparin expected to be found intravascularly at the time of infusion. As with other foreign proteins, protamine administration is associated with numerous adverse effects such as hypotension, bradycardia, and allergic reactions. Because approximately 0.2% of patients receiving protamine experience anaphylaxis, a complication that carries a 30% mortality rate, we recommend that protamine be reserved for patients with life-threatening bleeding (Antidotes in Depth: A19).[173] Clinicians should be aware that excess protamine administration does result in paradoxical anticoagulation, but this should not deter clinicians from administering protamine in life-threatening situations.

Because of the severe adverse effects associated with protamine, research has focused on safer methods to reverse heparin anticoagulation. These agents include heparinase,[248] synthetic protamine variants,[387,388] and platelet factor 4 (PF4). These therapies are not widely available, and their efficacy and safety are not established.

If life-threatening bleeding occurs after LMWH administration we also recommend treating patients with protamine. Several studies show that protamine partially reverses LMWHs such as enoxaparin, dalteparin, and tinzaparin. In one case report of a 10-fold dosing error of enoxaparin, protamine effectively reversed the anticoagulant effects.[404] In a series of 14 bleeding patients given protamine to reverse LMWH, bleeding ceased in two-thirds of the patients. These data, however, are complicated by repeat dosing of protamine as well as administration of other procoagulant antidotes such as clotting factors and vitamin K in a subset of patients. In addition, patients received protamine between 30 minutes and 48 hours after their last dose of LMWH.[379] Approximately 1 mg protamine will neutralize 100 anti–factor Xa units, and 1 mg of enoxaparin will neutralize 100 anti–factor Xa units for up to 8 hours after LMWH administration.[137] A second dose of 0.5 mg protamine per 100 anti–factor Xa units is reasonable if bleeding continues. If more than 8 hours has elapsed, a smaller dose of protamine should be administered. The maximum dose of 50 mg should not be exceeded.[137] The appropriate dosages for protamine are described in detail in the Antidotes in Depth: A19. The newer experimental protamine variants appear to be effective against LMWHs but are not yet clinically available.[387,388] Interestingly, there is one case report of recombinant activated factor VII (rFVIIa) reversing the effects of LMWH in the setting of postoperative acute kidney injury (AKI),[96,249,264] and there is also a single case report demonstrating efficacy at reversing severe bleeding caused by enoxaparin.[175] Based on this limited reported experience, we do not recommend rFVIIA for LMWH-associated bleeding.

NONBLEEDING COMPLICATIONS

Postoperative thrombocytopenia that occurs in the first 1 or 2 days after surgery usually results from platelet consumption. This early fall in platelet count tends to cause concern for a drug-induced thrombocytopenia called HIT because postoperative VTE prophylaxis with heparin is usually started simultaneously.[392] However, postoperative thrombocytopenia usually improves by the third postoperative day, distinguishing itself from HIT, which typically occurs between days 5 and 10 after heparin initiation. In patients who were previously treated with heparin, HIT-related events sometimes occur within 24 hours after reexposure.[223]

Heparin-induced thrombocytopenia affects up to 5% of patients receiving heparin.[223,392] Heparin stimulates platelets to release PF4, which subsequently complexes with heparin to provoke an IgG response, causing platelet aggregation and thrombocytopenia.[14,416] A more severe form of thrombocytopenia, HITT (formerly known as HIT-2 or the white clot syndrome), occurs in up to 55% of patients with untreated HIT.[223] The antibodies against the heparin–PF4 complex activate platelets, which leads to platelet–fibrin thrombotic events.[14,416]

Patients present with either hemorrhagic or thromboembolic complications. Low-molecular-weight heparin is also associated with thrombocytopenia (isolated HIT) and less frequently with HITT.[223] Consequently, when HITT occurs, LMWH is contraindicated.[223] Treatment of patients with HIT includes discontinuation of heparin or LMWH and immediate use of alternative anticoagulant such as lepirudin, argatroban, or danaparoid.[68,223] In addition to HIT and HITT, necrotizing skin lesions[286] and hyperkalemia from aldosterone suppression[274] also rarely occur in patients receiving heparin therapy. These patients should not receive heparin or LMWH again, not even in low doses to maintain venous patency.

Some additional complications of heparin use include osteoporosis, which mostly occurs in patients on long-term therapy with UFH.[174] A small percentage of these patients develop bone fractures if treated continuously for more than 3 months. Data for LMWHs are limited, and the incidence of osteoporosis is less compared with UFH.[174] In 2008, an outbreak of adverse events was linked to heparin contaminated with oversulfated chondroitin sulfate.[227] The contaminated heparin, which was found in at least 10 countries, originated in China.[38] Many patients developed anaphylactoid-type reactions with at least 100 reported deaths.[227]

DIRECT THROMBIN INHIBITORS

Hirudin and its congeners (lepirudin and desirudin) are used in patients with acute coronary syndromes, the prevention of thromboembolic disease, and in patients with HITT.[36,322,329] Desirudin is at least as effective as UFH and without an increased risk of bleeding or thrombocytopenia. However, in the Global Use of Strategies to Open Occluded Coronary Arteries (GUSTO) IIb study of patients with unstable angina or non–Q wave MI, there was an increase in the number of blood transfusions in patients who received desirudin compared with those who received heparin.[338] This increased risk of bleeding compared with heparin has caused desirudin to fall out of favor. Instead bivalirudin and argatroban tend to be used more often, especially in the setting of HITT. In fact, initial studies using bivalirudin during coronary artery angioplasty for unstable or postinfarction angina showed that it is a safe substitute for heparin with lower bleeding rates.[36] Unfortunately, all of these DTIs are short acting and require parenteral administration.

Because of the potential therapeutic limitations of warfarin (eg, dosing, risk of bleeding, narrow therapeutic window), direct oral anticoagulants were developed with directed activity against specific clotting factors. The proposed benefits of these medications include the convenience of fixed dosing and avoidance of close therapeutic monitoring. Ximelagatran was one of the first DTIs that was as effective as warfarin in the treatment of stroke prevention, nonvalvular atrial fibrillation, and DVT.[168] Ximelagatran had many advantages over warfarin, including rapidity of onset, fixed dosing, stable absorption, decreased risk of drug interactions, and lack of necessity for therapeutic monitoring.[168] However, in 2006, drug manufacturers abandoned ximelagatran after noticing a high rate of hepatic failure. Countries that had approved ximelagatran withdrew the medication from the market.

Subsequently, dabigatran was approved for systemic anticoagulation in patients with nonvalvular atrial fibrillation in the United States and many other countries. Later it was approved for the treatment and prophylaxis of VTE. The Randomized Evaluation of Long Term Anticoagulant Therapy (RE-LY) trial demonstrated that dabigatran administration was associated with lower rates of systemic embolic events, with similar rates of bleeding, compared with anticoagulation with warfarin.[81] However, subsequent evaluation of the data acquired from the RE-LY trial demonstrates that patients 75 years of age and older an increased risk of extracranial bleeding when compared with those taking warfarin.[110] In multiple noninferiority trials, dabigatran demonstrated similar efficacy to enoxaparin in reducing VTE without increasing bleeding risk after hip joint replacement.[114,115]

Pharmacology

Thrombin has four separate binding sites, each of which is specific for substrate, inhibitor, or cofactors.[368] Whereas bivalent DTIs, such as hirudin and bivalirudin, bind the active site and one of two exosites (binding sites outside of the active site), univalent DTIs, such as dabigatran, bind just the active site[97] (Fig. 58–3). By directly inhibiting thrombin, anticoagulation is possible without the need for AT.[329] In addition, inhibiting thrombin also inhibits platelet activation because thrombin is a potent and direct-acting platelet activator. Unlike heparin, DTIs are able to enter clots and inhibit clot-bound thrombin because of their small size, offering the distinct advantage of restricting further thrombus formation.

Desirudin, bivalirudin, and argatroban are all administered parenterally. Desirudin is given as SC injections for VTE prophylaxis. Although the dosing for desirudin is 15 mg as a subcutaneous injection every 12 hours, this dose should be decreased or stopped in patients with stage 3 or greater CKD. In addition, patients previously treated with the hirudins develop antibodies, creating the potential for anaphylaxis with repeat dosing.[137] Bivalirudin is also an analogue of hirudin. It is used in patients with HITT who require cardiac catheterization or cardiopulmonary bypass surgery.[137] Argatroban binds noncovalently to the active site of thrombin to function as a competitive inhibitor.[137] It is metabolized by CYP3A4/5 in the liver and is particularly useful in patients with CKD.[137]

Dabigatran is orally administered as dabigatran etexilate. This prodrug has no anticoagulant properties, and serum esterase coverts it to dabigatran, the active drug.[347] At therapeutic doses, peak concentrations occur in 2 hours (Table 58–3). Approximately 35% of dabigatran is protein bound; 85% is eliminated renally, with 78% of it is eliminated within the first 24 hours. Its mean terminal half-life is approximately 8 to 12 hours.[37] Contraindications to dabigatran are active hemorrhage or a hypersensitivity reaction to dabigatran. The manufacturer recommends either dose adjustment or avoidance

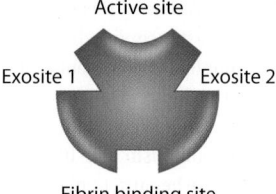

Thrombin binding sites
Active site

Exosite 1   Exosite 2

Fibrin binding site

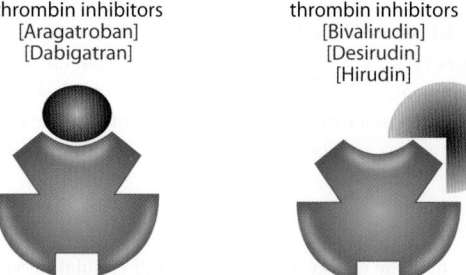

Direct thrombin inhibitors

Univalent direct
thrombin inhibitors
[Aragatroban]
[Dabigatran]

Bivalent direct
thrombin inhibitors
[Bivalirudin]
[Desirudin]
[Hirudin]

FIGURE 58–3. Thrombin has four separate binding sites. Each site is specific for substrate, inhibitor, or cofactors. Bivalent direct thrombin inhibitors, such as hirudin and bivalirudin, bind the active site and one of two exosites. Univalent direct thrombin inhibitors, such as dabigatran, bind only the active site.

of concomitant administration of P-glycoprotein inhibitors in patients with renal insufficiency. It also recommended to avoid coadministration of rifampin, a P-glycoprotein inducer.[39] P-glycoprotein activity prevents enteric absorption of dabigatran, and rifampin augments this activity, resulting in subtherapeutic dabigatran serum concentrations.

Clinical Manifestations

Intentional overdoses with the DTIs are rare events. Although there are reports of patients who develop significant coagulopathy after unintentional ingestion of excess dabigatran,[64,261,409] the more common scenario is that patients become overanticoagulated because of improper dosing in patients with CKD or failure to adjust dosing in patients who develop AKI. In general, the parenterally administered medications have short elimination half-lives, and iatrogenic medication administration errors, if recognized, are often less risky than those that are longer acting.

Dabigatran, the newest of the DTIs, is orally administered with a longer duration of action. Since its approval in 2010, bleeding was rapidly recognized as a complication of therapy. Only recently has a specific monoclonal antibody reversal xenobiotic, idarucizumab (Praxbind), been approved by the FDA. In 2011, the FDA released an advisory announcing that a review of postmarketing reports of serious bleeding associated with dabigatran use was initiated. In addition, dabigatran leads the list of fatalities reported to the MedWatch system. There are many published case reports of patients bleeding while anticoagulated with dabigatran. Patients may have been subjected to increased risk of bleeding because of risk factors such as increased age or CKD. In New Zealand and Australia, a significant number of bleeding events, including intracranial bleeding, GI bleeding, hematuria, and hemoptysis, were reported in the period immediately after the approval of the medication. Up to 25% of the reports in this series involved errors in prescribing practices.[160] In particular, off-label use of dabigatran for anticoagulation in the setting of mechanical heart valves led to valve thrombosis.[70,293] Cardiac tamponade from hemopericardium, fatal epistaxis, serious GI bleeding, postoperative bleeding complications, and intracranial bleeding are all reported.[26,65,107,340,367] In addition, clinicians have expressed difficulties in treating hemorrhage in trauma victims while anticoagulated with dabigatran.[85]

Furthermore, several questions regarding other adverse effects related to dabigatran use have been raised. A meta-analysis comparing patients

TABLE 58–3	Pharmacology of Oral Antithrombotics[a]				
	Warfarin	Dabigatran (Pradaxa)	Rivaroxaban (Xarelto)	Apixaban (Eliquis)	Edoxaban (Savayasa)
T_{max} (h)	3	2	3	1–3	1-2
$t_{1/2}$ (h)[a]	35	8–12	5–13	8–15	10–15
Protein binding (%)	97	35	>90	87	55
Metabolism and elimination	Hepatic metabolites (primarily CYP1A2, CYP3A4, and CYP2C9) excreted via renal and biliary systems	80%–85% renal; 15%–20% biliary	33% renal (unchanged); 33% renal metabolite; 33% hepatic metabolite	25% renal; 55% fecal, 15% hepatic metabolite	35% renal; 49% fecal; 16% hepatic metabolism
Drug interactions	Many interactions[357]	P-gp inducers; rifampin	Combined P-gp and strong CYP3A4 inhibitors and inducers	Strong dual inhibitors of CYP3A4 and P-gp; Combined CYP3A4 and P-gp inducers	Rifampin

[a]Antithrombotic metabolism and plasma half-life ($t_{1/2}$) may be altered by a number of factors such as diet, genetic polymorphisms, and kidney disease.
P-gp = P-glycoprotein; T_{max} = time to maximum blood concentration.

anticoagulated with dabigatran versus warfarin, enoxaparin, or placebo showed higher rates of MI or acute coronary syndrome.[372] Additionally, though clinical trials implied that discontinuation of dabigatran does not cause rebound thrombosis, the authors of anecdotal reports of thrombotic events after cessation of dabigatran anticoagulation have questioned whether thrombosis is caused by rebound or just sequelae from underlying hypercoagulability or illness.[364]

Laboratory Assessment
Monitoring the anticoagulant effect in the setting of DTI use is complex. For bivalirudin and argatroban, serial aPTT measurements are commonly used to estimate the degree of anticoagulation.[137] Admittedly, the aPTT is not a good test because the degree of anticoagulation does not follow a linear relationship. This is particularly emphasized with dabigatran, the most recently developed DTI. For example, the aPTT increases at higher dabigatran concentrations, but the relationship is nonlinear, with the aPTT plateauing at dabigatran concentrations greater than 200 ng/mL.[346,378] Furthermore, the PT and INR are usually elevated, but they do not correlate with the anticoagulant effect of dabigatran.[349,378] Dilute thrombin time (dTT) and ecarin clotting time (ECT) are proposed as more accurate reflections of the anticoagulation effect.[378] Several assays are used to measure serum dabigatran effect using the dTT assay. In these assays, standards with known dabigatran concentrations are used. Unfortunately, none of these modalities are FDA approved.[105,317,348] Ecarin clotting time is a laboratory assay that uses ecarin, a derivative of sawscaled viper venom, as the reagent to activate prothrombin. Although some hospitals are able to obtain a thrombin time (TT) in a clinically relevant time, the dTT and the ECT are usually unavailable.

Treatment of Direct Thrombin Inhibitor–Induced Coagulopathy
In the event of an acute ingestion of dabigatran, AC is indicated based on data from an in vitro model.[377] It should be noted that there have been at least two cases of intentional dabigatran overdose that were managed via orogastric lavage and AC. The initial dabigatran concentrations were later found to be 970 ng/mL and 4,170 ng/mL, respectively.[261,410] Based on a small prospective study with dabigatran assays, the average peak concentration in patients receiving therapeutic dosing of dabigatran was 112.7 ± 66.6 ng/mL.[317] However, because both patients after intentional dabigatran overdoses cases did not have bleeding complications, they were observed until the resolution of coagulopathy. One patient was given FFP for an aPTT of 79s (normal, 23–37 s) and an INR of 3.3. The other patient was noted to have a mild coagulopathy with an aPTT of 48.8 s and an INR of 1.3.[261,410] An overdose of argatroban was successfully treated with FFP in a case report.[415] With the widespread dabigatran use, the first of the novel oral anticoagulants, the absence of a reversal agent became a potentially deadly complication. The manufacturer fast-tracked the development of idarucizumab (Praxbind), a monoclonal antibody targeting dabigatran.[374,375] In murine and human studies, idarucizumab

administration results in normalization of a battery of functional clotting assays, including clotting time, aPTT, and TT.[321] In a prospective study containing 90 patients who received 5 g of IV idarucizumab for urgent reversal of dabigatran-induced coagulopathy, reversal of coagulopathy occurred in 100% of patients despite 18 deaths in the study population. Study investigators noted that hemostasis in bleeding patients was restored at a median of 11.4 hours after administration of idarucizumab. In addition, antidotal therapy restored ECT and dTT in 88% to 98% of the patients. In patients undergoing an emergent procedure, normal intraoperative hemostasis was noted in 85% of cases. There are a significant number of limitations with this particular study. It should be noted that in addition to idarucizumab, 56% of patients received some type of blood products, including PRBCs, FFP, platelets, cryoprecipitate, PCCs, or whole blood. Thrombotic events were noted in five patients. One thrombotic event (simultaneous DVT and PE) occurred within 72 hours of idarucizumab administration in a single patient. Other complications noted were left atrial thrombus at 9 days, DVT at 7 days, MI at 13 days, and ischemic stroke at 26 days. Unfortunately, there was no control group to determine if morbidity or mortality outcomes were changed by administration of idarucizumab. In addition, dabigatran concentrations in enrolled patients ranged between 5 and 3,600 ng/mL with a median of 132 and 114 ng/mL in the two study groups.[287] Although the majority of patients in the RE-LY trial had dabigatran concentrations less than 1,000 ng/mL, the literature reports exceedingly high dabigatran concentrations in many patients, particularly in patients who have kidney injury or in patients who have intentionally overdosed on dabigatran. The standard dose of idarucizumab, 5 g, will be insufficient in reversing coagulopathy in patients with these extremely high dabigatran concentrations.

There are many case reports describing the use of idarucizumab in various clinical scenarios. It has been used in life-threatening bleeding, intentional overdose, and therapeutic accumulation secondary to kidney injury and in the preoperative or preprocedural setting.[47,140,165,166,235,282,303,307,319,331,351,363] At least one case report showed continuation of life-threatening GI bleeding despite receiving recommended dosing of idarucizumab.[4] One report described using idarucizumab in conjunction with hemodialysis to achieve normal coagulation function.[235] It should be noted that several case reports demonstrated a rebound drug effect after administration of idarucizumab. One case described a patient with a massive dabigatran overdose with an initial dabigatran concentration of 3,337 ng/mL. After receiving idarucizumab, the patient's dabigatran concentration fell to 513 ng/mL, with improvement in his coagulopathy. However, 7 hours after receiving idarucizumab, the patient's[294] dabigatran concentration rebounded to 1,126 ng/mL with corresponding increases in INR, PT, and aPTT.[309] Dabigatran rebound after idarucizumab treatment is noted in other case reports.[169] Some advocate for idarucizumab administration before thrombolytic therapy for acute ischemic cerebrovascular accidents in patients anticoagulated with dabigatran.

In these case reports, patients received 5 g of idarucizumab followed by t-PA without adverse consequence.[31,139,187,263,320,327] Some clinicians routinely recommend idarucizumab treatment before thrombolytic therapy for acute ischemic stroke.[100,139] However, given the paucity of data and lack of a formal clinical trial, this should not be the standard of care as case reports cannot determine the efficacy and safety of this practice.

Before the FDA approval of idarucizumab in 2015, the manufacturer suggested several strategies to treat patients with significant bleeding while anticoagulated with dabigatran. Transfusion of RBCs and FFP in addition to supportive care were the mainstays of treatment (Table 58–1). Recombinant factor FVIIa, PCCs, and hemodialysis were also used, but these interventions are incompletely studied. In a murine study of dabigatran, collagenase-induced intracranial hematoma expansion was inhibited in a dose-dependent fashion by PCC with the best results at 100 units/kg, the equivalent of 200% factor replacement. In the same study, high-dose PCC decreased but did not normalize the tail vein bleeding time. Recombinant factor VIIa was ineffective in limiting intracranial hematoma volume, and FFP limited intracranial hematoma size in the mice given a lower dose of dabigatran.[418]

However, conclusions based on data obtained from murine studies should be interpreted with caution when treating humans. First, the hemostatic therapies used in these murine experiments are human derived, and cross-species effects cannot be predicted. Second, these mice had prolongation of their tail vein bleeding times, but dabigatran at therapeutic doses does not change bleeding time in humans.[186] Another study done in healthy humans found that aPTT, endogenous thrombin potential lag time, TT, and ECT did not decrease with the administration of four-factor PCC.[108]

One ex-vivo study showed that after a single dose of dabigatran in healthy volunteers, FEIBA decreased endogenous thrombin potential and lag time, and thrombin generation increased in a dose dependent fashion.[237] In a murine study, aPCC reduced bleeding time at low doses. Unfortunately, at high doses, this effect was reduced.[376]

Hemodialysis for dabigatran removal remains a controversial intervention. A single study showed that after a subtherapeutic dose of dabigatran in patients with stage 5 CKD, the extraction ratios were up to 68% at 4 hours after the initiation of hemodialysis.[350] Although this suggests that dabigatran is effectively removed from the serum, the greater implication of this finding is unknown. This study did not address the safety of hemodialysis in bleeding patients who are actively bleeding or the possibility of rebound concentrations after hemodialysis.[349,350] Several published case reports demonstrated significant drug rebound after hemodialysis in bleeding patients, up to 87% of the initial dabigatran concentration within 2 hours after the cessation of hemodialysis.[63,64,340] In one case, hemodialysis was not effective in stopping bleeding, and despite massive transfusion of RBCs, FFP, and platelets, deaths from exsanguination occurred. In some cases, a repeat hemodialysis session or continuous venovenous hemodiafiltration (CVVHD) was performed in anticipation of posthemodialysis rebound. Although they were successful in decreasing serum dabigatran concentrations, they did not normalize the aPTT or the TT.[340]

Although the safety and efficacy of these adjunctive therapies are unknown, they are reasonable in patients with serious bleeding if idarucizumab is not available or if a patient continues to have life-threatening hemorrhage despite idarucizumab administration. Repletion of blood volume and coagulation factors with PCC is reasonable. If maximal efforts at repletion of blood volume and coagulation factors are ineffective, then hemodialysis followed by CVVHD is reasonable if the patient can tolerate the procedure hemodynamically.

Ciraparantag is a "universal antidote" being developed to reverse the activity of a number of anticoagulants, including the oral DTIs, the factor Xa inhibitors, and the heparins.[9-11] Clinical trial results have yet to be published.

FACTOR Xa INHIBITORS

Rivaroxaban was the first orally active direct factor Xa inhibitor approved for VTE and stroke prophylaxis and treatment. Development of this class of drugs started in the 1980s after the discovery of antistasin, a naturally occurring factor Xa inhibitor found in leeches. After screening a library of more than 200,000 compounds, a pharmaceutical company was able to identify structures that inhibit factor Xa. After structure optimization, rivaroxaban was created for clinical trials.[283]

Numerous clinical trials investigated the efficacy and safety of rivaroxaban.[22,113,114,188,203,369] Compared with warfarin, rivaroxaban prevented more strokes or systemic thromboembolic events and significantly reduced the number of intracranial hemorrhages in patients with nonvalvular atrial fibrillation.[281] The most recent published trial compared the use of rivaroxaban compared with placebo in patients with acute coronary syndrome. There was a significant risk reduction in death attributed to any cardiac cause or stroke. However, rivaroxaban-treated patients had statistically significant increased rates of major and intracranial hemorrhages.[243]

Apixaban is another oral factor Xa inhibitor that is approved by the FDA for VTE prophylaxis in patients with atrial fibrillation. Numerous studies showed benefit of apixaban in preventing VTE in specific populations while simultaneously lowering mortality or specific types of bleeding, such as intracranial hemorrhage.[80,147,150,203-206]

In trials investigating the use of apixaban in patients with recent acute coronary syndrome, excess bleeding caused early cessation of trials; however, most patients were concurrently treated with dual antiplatelet therapy.[3,76]

Edoxaban is the newest of the approved factor Xa inhibitors based on studies for VTE prophylaxis in patients with atrial fibrillation and for the treatment of VTE disease.[66,71,111,143,144,171,296,396,414] Studies with edoxaban demonstrated promising results compared with enoxaparin in post–orthopedic surgery VTE prophylaxis, although it is not currently FDA approved for this indication.[129-132,297] The risk of hemorrhage compared with enoxaparin varies among the many studies.[52,66,71,129-132,414] Compared with warfarin in patients with nonvavular atrial fibrillation, the ENGAGE AF-TIMI 48 trial demonstrated a lower risk of cardiovascular death and hemorrhage, including intracranial hemorrhages and fatal bleeding.[111,143,144,396] However, a study demonstrated the addition of an antiplatelet agent, such as aspirin, to edoxaban therapy in patients with atrial fibrillation resulted in a higher risk of hemorrhage compared with patients who received warfarin in conjunction with a single antiplatelet agent.[412]

Factor Xa inhibitor development continues. Betrixaban is undergoing clinical trials to determine its efficacy and safety in VTE prophylaxis.[79]

Pharmacology

The factor Xa inhibitors are ideal anticoagulants because their site of action is the intersection of the intrinsic and extrinsic pathways, preventing thrombin activation.[59] These synthetic drugs reversibly inhibit factor Xa without any cofactor requirements. Theoretically, this class of anticoagulants is safer than the DTIs because they do not completely neutralize thrombin.

Rivaroxaban and apixaban selectively bind free and clot-bound factor Xa without inhibiting related serine proteases, including thrombin, trypsin, plasmin, or other activated clotting factors.[116] In addition, rivaroxaban and apixaban inhibit tissue factor or collagen-induced thrombin formation. In vitro, the factor Xa inhibitors hinder tissue factor–induced platelet aggregation.[116,408] Rivaroxaban does not directly inhibit platelet aggregation, and concomitant aspirin use does not affect the pharmacokinetics or safety of rivaroxaban in studies of healthy humans.[59,116,196]

Rivaroxaban has an oral bioavailability of approximately 80%.[397] Inhibition of factor Xa peaks approximately 3 hours after administration of the rivaroxaban. This inhibition lasts for approximately 12 hours.[198] However, kidney or liver disease lengthens its duration of action (Table 58–3). Dosing varies by indication and kidney function. The manufacturer provides recommended dose adjustments for each indication based on kidney function.

Approximately one-third of rivaroxaban is eliminated unchanged by the kidneys, and one-third is metabolized to an inactive form and excreted by the kidney. The remaining one-third is metabolized by the CYP3A4-dependent and -independent pathways in the liver and then excreted fecally. Concomitant use of CYP3A4 inhibitors or P-glycoprotein inhibitors is contraindicated because of increased risk of drug accumulation of up to 160%.[164,397]

In the future, rivaroxaban could be a suitable anticoagulant alternative in patients with HITT because in vitro studies do not show platelet aggregation or activation in the presence of HITT antibodies or release of PF4 from platelets.[390] Future studies proving efficacy and safety are needed before these xenobiotics can be recommended for use in patients with HITT.

In preclinical studies, the oral bioavailability of apixaban is approximately 66%. Apixaban is primarily distributed to the blood compartment and is approximately 87% protein bound.[116] Peak serum concentrations occur between 1 and 3 hours postingestion. There are multiple elimination pathways, suggesting that patients with either renal or hepatic impairment should be able to tolerate apixaban well. Approximately 25% of apixaban is excreted in the urine, and the majority of apixaban is excreted fecally between 24 to 48 hours after ingestion.[116,295] Simultaneous administration of strong CYP3A4 inhibitors is contraindicated with apixaban.

Apixaban is approved in the United States for stroke prevention in patients with nonvalvular atrial fibrillation, for VTE prophylaxis, and for VTE treatment.[80,150] Dosing is based on indication. The manufacturer recommends either decreasing the dose or avoiding coadministration of apixaban if strong inhibitors of CYP3A4 and P-glycoprotein are administered.[53]

Edoxaban is approved for the treatment of nonvalvular atrial fibrillation and for the treatment of DVT and PE. The dosage varies by indication. For patients with atrial fibrillation, the dosage also depends on creatinine clearance. Edoxaban is not recommended for patients with creatinine clearance less than 95 mL/min. Patients with VTE disease should receive edoxaban after 5 to 10 days of treatment with a parenteral anticoagulant.[89,310] The manufacturer also notes that coadministration of rifampin, due to CYP3A4 induction, and coadministration of other anticoagulants are contraindicated.[89,247] The prescribing information provided by the manufacturers of edoxaban also recommend a maximum dose of 30 mg/day for patients with body weight less than 60 kg.[89]

Edoxaban is orally administered and has a bioavailability of 61.8%.[240,250] P-glycoprotein appears to be the key factor as a transporter of edoxaban. Edoxaban metabolism is minor, and the compound is largely excreted in the urine and feces.[250] Approximately 35% of an oral dose is eliminated renally, and 49% of the oral dose is excreted in the feces.[240] Peak edoxaban concentrations occur 1 to 2 hours after ingestion, and the terminal half-life is 10 to 14 hours.[89]

Clinical Manifestations

Hemorrhage is the most concerning consequence of the factor Xa inhibitors, even at therapeutic doses. However, hemorrhage does not always occur in overdose. There are reports of no hemorrhage despite acute overdoses of both rivaroxaban and apixaban. In a multi–poison control center study involving 223 rivaroxaban or apixaban exposures, 12 patients involved suicide attempts, and none of these patients developed hemorrhage, although confirmation of ingestion was not verified in all cases.[345] A case report describes a 21-month-old girl who developed an INR of 3.5 approximately 12 hours after ingesting an unknown quantity of rivaroxaban. She did not have any hemorrhagic consequences.[245] Another case report describes a 71-year-old man who intentionally ingested 1,940 mg of rivaroxaban, resulting in an INR of 7.2 drawn 2 hours after ingestion and rivaroxaban concentration of 160 ng/mL drawn 3 days after ingestion. He never developed bleeding, and he was monitored until his coagulopathy resolved. He did not receive any blood products or reversal agents.[300] In another case, a 42-year-old man intentionally ingested multiple pharmaceuticals, including 1,400 mg of rivaroxaban. He never developed any bleeding, but given his INR of 2.4 drawn 5 hours after ingestion, he was given 1 g of tranexamic acid and 3,000 units of PCC. He was discharged 1 day after this ingestion without any bleeding or adverse events.[224] There are many other cases reporting massive intentional factor Xa inhibitor overdose, resulting in abnormal coagulation studies or supratherapeutic concentrations.[20,212,213] More predictably, bleeding occurs at therapeutic doses. In the previously mentioned multi–poison control center study, all bleeding events occurred in patients on long-term anticoagulant therapy.[345] Another case report describes a 58-year-old man taking

10 mg of rivaroxaban per day who developed prolonged rectal bleeding 31 days after initiating treatment for prophylaxis after hip replacement.[40]

Diagnostic Testing

Some studies done in healthy volunteers show that rivaroxaban inhibits factor Xa activity and prolongs PT, aPTT, and LMWH activity in a dose-dependent fashion.[197,198] Unfortunately, PT and aPTT are not reliable measures of the anticoagulant effect of rivaroxaban because results vary widely depending on the reagent used. Thrombin generation assays are prolonged, and endogenous thrombin potential is decreased. Unfortunately, these assays are not readily available in most medical centers. Chromogenic anti–factor Xa activity reliably measures rivaroxaban effect over a large range of concentrations.[316]

Studies investigating the effect of apixaban on hematologic laboratory studies are limited, but multiple in vitro studies show that aPTT and PT increase in a dose-dependent fashion. The Heptest, a newly developed clotting assay that measures anti-Xa and anti-IIa activity, correlates best with the antithrombotic effect of apixaban. Unfortunately, it is not widely available because it is not yet FDA approved.[105,116,407]

Treatment of Factor Xa Inhibitor–Induced Coagulopathy

A study in healthy volunteers demonstrated that rivaroxaban absorption, as defined by area under the concentration–time curve, is decreased after AC administration up to 8 hours after a single oral dose of rivaroxaban. Absorption is decreased by 43% if AC is administered within 2 hours of a rivaroxaban ingestion. Activated charcoal given 8 hours after rivaroxaban ingestion resulted in a 29% decrease in absorption.[272] Another study showed that AC at 2 hours and 6 hours after single-dose apixaban ingestion also reduced apixaban absorption by 50% and 28%, respectively. In this study, the half-life of apixaban decreased from 13 hours to 5 hours after AC was administered at either 2 hours or 6 hours after apixaban ingestion.[391] The administration of AC after an acute overdose is therefore recommended (Table 58–1). A single human study evaluated the use of four-factor PCC in reversing patients given rivaroxaban 20 mg twice daily for 2.5 days. The PT and endogenous thrombin time rapidly normalized after administration of 50 units/kg of PCC.[108] Rivaroxaban anticoagulated rabbits showed improvements in coagulation assays after treatment with PCC and rFVIIa. However, these agents were clinically ineffective in achieving hemostasis.[146] Because of its high protein binding, hemodialysis is unlikely to be an effective adjunct method to accelerate rivaroxaban removal.

Preliminary in vitro studies show that four-factor PCC may improve thrombin generation and coagulation parameters in blood aliquots treated with apixaban.[117] However, there are no human studies with clinically relevant outcomes to support the use of PCC in factor Xa-associated bleeding.

Although edoxaban is the newest of the factor Xa inhibitors, hemorrhage remains a concern. There is a report of diffuse alveolar hemorrhage in addition to the bleeding complications mentioned in the numerous clinical trials.[267] There are few studies evaluating reversal methods. There is one human study evaluating four-factor PCC in the reversal after a single dose of edoxaban. In this study, participants received 10, 25, or 50 units/kg of 4 factor PCC after a single dose of edoxaban. Participants then underwent punch biopsy, and coagulation studies and clinical bleeding were evaluated. After 50 units/kg of 4 factor PCC the bleeding duration and endogenous thrombin potential normalized. However, the PT and bleeding volume were only partially reversed.[417] There are two animal studies showing that rFVIIa and FEIBA are effective in reversing edoxaban-induced coagulopathy.[133,167] However, given that these agents have not been studied in for this indication in humans, neither rFVIIa nor FEIBA are recommended as treatment for edoxaban-induced coagulopathy.

Although the half-lives of the factor Xa inhibitors are substantially shorter than that of warfarin, normalization of hemostasis because of drug clearance often requires more than 24 hours without intervention. During this time, supportive measures such as restoration of intravascular volume are helpful but do not correct the xenobiotic-induced coagulopathy. Prothrombin complex concentrates at a starting dose of 25 units/kg appears to be the only antidote that improves laboratory parameters immediately after infusion, but their effect on hemostasis is unknown. Regardless, in the case of life-threatening bleeding, PCC is reasonable to attempt to achieve hemostasis. Their peak coagulation effect should occur immediately after administration. In severe cases, repeat doses may need to be administered. The risk of thrombosis is unknown, and providers should be aware of this adverse effect when administering PCC. If PCC is unavailable, FEIBA should be used as a second-line agent. If both PCC and FEIBA are unavailable, it is reasonable to use rFVIIa with the caveat that the risk of thrombosis is higher with this drug compared with PCC and FEIBA.

Andexanet alfa (Andexxa) is a recombinant protein recently FDA approved for reversal of anticoagulation caused by factor Xa inhibitors. This antidote was developed by altering the structure of factor X. Although the drug still binds factor Xa inhibitors, it has been altered to inhibit the catalytic activation of thrombin, and the factor Va binding site, which is necessary for anticoagulation, is no longer present.[229] Studies in healthy elderly volunteers demonstrated that andexanet alfa administration given to patients who had achieved a steady-state concentration of either apixaban or rivaroxaban resulted in rapid reduction in plasma-free inhibitor concentrations and increased thrombin formation. Antifactor Xa activity decreased by more than 90% immediately after andexanet alfa infusion but rebounded to placebo concentrations within 1 to 2 hours.[337] In an open-label single-group study, andexanet alfa was given to patients who had ingested a factor Xa inhibitor within 18 hours of acute major bleeding onset. After infusion of andexanet alfa, 79% of patients achieved hemostasis and antifactor Xa activity decreased 12 hours after andexanet alfa infusion. Thrombotic events occurred in 6% of patients within 3 days of andexanet alfa infusion, and 15% of the patients died. An unclear number of patients received blood products such as PRBCs, FFP, or PCC. There was no control group to determine if there were any changes in patient outcomes such as morbidity or mortality resulting from andexanet alfa adminstration (Antidotes in Depth: A17).[82]

PENTASACCHARIDES

Pentasaccharides are synthetic anticoagulants that possess activity against factor Xa and are used for the prevention and treatment of VTE. Fondaparinux is the only pentasaccharide currently available for clinical use.[217] The pentasaccharide binds to AT with an affinity higher than that of heparin facilitating the formation of the AT–factor Xa complex. After this complex forms, fondaparinux dissociates from the AT–factor Xa complex and can bind and activate additional AT.[137] Routine measurements of coagulation are not generally performed. When the degree of anticoagulation needs to be assessed, the fondaparinux-specific anti-Xa assay is the most helpful. The pentasaccharides have long half-lives and have no reliable reversal agent if bleeding occurs; they do not bind to protamine.[137] Patients with stage 3 CKD should have their dose reduced 50%; fondaparinux is contraindicated in patients with stages 4 and 5 CKD.[137] No controlled trials are available yet. However, normalization of coagulation studies and thrombin generation occurred after healthy volunteers received fondaparinux followed by rFVIIa.[34] In a case series of eight patients who received 90 mcg/kg of rFVIIa for hemorrhage, only 50% of patients had favorable outcomes. Anti-Xa activity remained unchanged, and none of the patients had any thrombotic complications. However, many of these patients were on other antithrombotics, including antiplatelet drugs. With respect to PCCs, a single trial investigated the use of PCC and aPCC to reverse fondaparinux-induced anticoagulation. In this study, the effect of PCC could not be assessed because the coagulation assay was incompatible with the formulation of PCC used. However, the addition of aPCC to plasma samples from fondaparinux-treated volunteers reversed thrombin generation time. This study was an ex vivo study, and further studies are required before PCC can be routinely recommended for the purpose of reversing fondaparinux-induced coagulopathy.[112] If a patient develops significant bleeding from fondaparinux, based on opinion only, it is reasonable to administer 25 to 50 units of PCC in addition to standard supportive measures.

ANTICOAGULANT APTAMERS

Aptamer anticoagulants are small nucleic acid molecules that are currently under development to target specific blood coagulation proteins.[266] They are direct protein inhibitors and function similarly to monoclonal antibodies.[266] Specific aptamers that are currently being studied include the anti–factor IX aptamer, the anti–activated protein C aptamer, and the anti–factor VIIa aptamer.[149] These xenobiotics may have future clinical utility because their anticoagulant effects appear to be easier to control, and consequently safer, compared with the most commonly used anticoagulants.

Although not yet approved, pegnivacogin is an RNA aptamer that inhibits factor IX and is undergoing human trials to evaluate its efficacy and safety. Several clinical trials are being conducted in healthy volunteers and patients with coronary artery disease.[289,291] The effects of pegnivacogin mimic hemophilia B, also known as Christmas disease. By inhibiting factor IX, the conversion of factor X to factor Xa is inhibited.[382] Studies show that approximately 1 mg/kg of pegnivacogin inhibits more than 99% of factor IX. Pharmacokinetic studies demonstrate a half-life of pegnivacogin to be approximately 100 hours with stable antithrombotic effects lasting for 30 hours.[288,289] Similar to the heparins, pegnivacogin anticoagulation should be monitored with aPTT because previous studies have demonstrated that the degree of factor IX inhibition correlates well with aPTT.[289] Unfortunately, despite its theoretical benefits, an unexpectedly high number of participants in the most recent clinical trial developed severe allergic reactions after pegnivacogin administration, causing the trial to be terminated early. In this study, pegnivacogin was being compared with bivalirudin in patients undergoing percutaneous coronary intervention (PCI). At the point of the trial's termination, there was no obvious difference in reduction of bleeding compared with the bivalirudin group.[222] Further studies demonstrated that these allergic reactions are the result of anti–polyethylene glycol antibodies.[290] Because this aptamer is a synthetically tailored nucleic acid sequence, its antidote is easily manufactured. By creating a complementary aptamer that possesses a nucleic acid sequence that binds to pegnivacogin through Watson-Crick base pairing, it can effectively neutralize the original xenobiotic by creating an inactive complex. In fact, pegnivacogin is being studied in conjunction with anivamersen, the complementary aptamer to pegnivacogin.[381]

FIBRINOLYTICS

The fibrinolytic system is designed to remove unwanted clots while leaving those clots protecting sites of vascular injury intact. Plasminogen exists as a proenzyme that is converted to the active form, plasmin, by plasminogen activators.[74,75] The actions of plasmin are nonspecific in that it degrades fibrin clots and some plasma proteins and coagulation factors.[395] Inhibition of plasmin occurs through α_2-antiplasmin.[395] Tissue plasminogen activator is released from the endothelium and is under the inhibitory control of two inactivators known as tissue plasminogen activator inhibitors 1 and 2 (t-PAI-1 and t-PAI-2).[74,75,257,395] Under physiological conditions, endogenous t-PA does not induce a fibrinolytic state because there is no fibrin to initiate the conversion of plasminogen to plasmin. However, exogenous t-PA administration results in supraphysiological concentrations that promote a fibrinolytic state.[395]

With their diverse indications in acute MI, unstable angina, arterial and venous thrombosis and embolism, and cerebrovascular disease, the thrombolytics are commonly used.[27] Readers are referred to a number of reviews for specific indications and dosing regimens.[84,208,280,341,395,401] Although all fibrinolytics enhance fibrinolysis, they differ in their specific sites of action and duration of effect. Tissue plasminogen activator is produced by recombinant DNA technology, and it is clot specific (ie, it does not increase fibrinolysis in the absence of a thrombus). Newer thrombolytics such as reteplase and tenecteplase possess longer half-lives that facilitate administration via bolus dosing rather than infusion.[395] On the other hand, streptokinase, urokinase, and anistreplase are not clot specific. Tissue plasminogen activator has the shortest half-life and duration of effect (5 minutes and 2 hours, respectively) and anistreplase the longest (90 minutes and 18 hours, respectively).[280,341] Streptokinase has the additional risk of potential severe allergic reaction on rechallenge, limiting its use to once in a lifetime. In fact, streptokinase is no longer used in the United States.

Thrombolytics such as monteplase, lanoteplase, pamiteplase, and desmoteplase are used in other countries or are currently being evaluated for therapeutic use.[228] These fibrinolytics have longer half-lives and are administered via single or repeated bolus injections. They also have increased fibrin selectivity but no apparent improvement in mortality compared with t-PA.[184]

A number of contraindications preclude the use of fibrinolytics. Undesired bleeding occurs because of clot destruction at vascular compromised sites and destruction of coagulation factors from plasmin generation.[395] Risk factors for bleeding, such as recent surgery or bleeding, known vascular lesions, malignancy, or prior intracranial hemorrhage, are contraindications for fibrinolytic administration.

Clinical Manifestations

Although the incidence of bleeding requiring transfusion is as high as 7.7% after high-dose (150 mg) t-PA and 4.4% after low-dose t-PA,[84] the incidence of intracranial hemorrhage with t-PA appears to be similar to the newer fibrinolytics (monteplase, tenecteplase, reteplase, and lanoteplase).[383] The addition of heparin to thrombolytic therapy increases the risk of bleeding. Reviews of multiple trials suggest that life-threatening events such as intracranial hemorrhage occur in 0.30% to 0.58% of patients receiving anistreplase, 0.42% to 0.73% of patients receiving alteplase, and 0.08% to 0.30% of patients receiving streptokinase.[401] Regardless of the thrombolytic used, the frequency of bleeding events is similar, with the exception that lanoteplase has a decreased incidence of significant hemorrhage.[93]

Treatment

Patients with minor hemorrhage complications caused by the fibrinolytic agents should receive supportive care as necessary, with focus on volume replacement and attempts to control the bleeding if possible. However, for patients with significant bleeding such as intracranial hemorrhage, it is reasonable to administer fibrinogen and coagulation factor replacement with cryoprecipitate, FFP, or PCC.[318] One study showed that after thrombolytic-induced intracranial hemorrhage, coagulopathy went untreated in 45% of cases.[148] A recent study of 3,894 patients showed that the mortality rate associated with postfibrinolytic intracranial hemorrhage is up to 52%, and the rate of intracranial hematoma expansion is 26.8%. When studied, postfibrinolytic patients with expanding intracranial hematomas tended to have severe hypofibrinogenemia, highlighting the need for cryoprecipitate repletion.[413] If fibrinogen and factor replacement are ineffective, then antifibrinolytics such as aminocaproic acid and tranexamic acid are recommended (Table 58–1). These fibrinolytics prevent activation of plasmin by competing with fibrin to bind to plasminogen and plasmin. Although a significant amount of fibrinolysis has already occurred, competitive inhibition of further plasmin-activated fibrinolysis is theoretically helpful in cases of life-threatening bleeding despite no clinical evidence available to show improved morbidity or mortality. Aminocaproic acid is also able to prevent the binding of t-PA to fibrin. Not only can these antifibrinolytics prevent fibrinolysis, but they can also reverse excessive fibrinolysis,[318,395] although it is not well studied in the setting of fibrinolytic therapy.

Aminocaproic acid is administered orally or intravenously. When administered intravenously, a loading dose of 4 to 5 g over 1 hour is followed by an infusion of 1 to 1.25 g/h with a maximum of 30 g given in 24 hours. The infusion should be stopped before 24 hours if the bleeding has ceased. Aminocaproic acid should not be given to patients with hematuria. These patients are at risk for developing obstructive AKI from ureteral clots that cannot be lysed. There are also rare reports of myopathy and muscle necrosis.[395] Although theoretically, aminocaproic acid could reverse hemorrhage after fibrinolytic therapy, there are no case reports or studies supporting its use in this situation.

Tranexamic acid is also reasonable to administer orally or intravenously. It is currently approved for the treatment of menorrhagia and is dosed at 1 g orally four times a day for four days.[395] It is also used in hemophiliac patients undergoing cardiac surgery. However, recent studies received significant attention for the use of tranexamic acid in patients with traumatic hemorrhage. The CRASH-2 study, a multicentered randomized controlled trial evaluating outcomes of patients receiving tranexamic acid with traumatic bleeding found that infusion of 1 g over 10 minutes, followed by 1 g over 8 hours, resulted in a significant reduction in mortality rate. In addition, the risk of arterial thrombosis, as well as fatal and nonfatal thrombosis, was significantly reduced compared with control participants who received placebo.[305] A case report describes the successful use of tranexamic acid in a patient who developed an intracranial hemorrhage after thrombolytic therapy. After receiving 1.675 g of IV tranexamic acid, repeat computed tomography and magnetic resonance imaging of the brain revealed no hematoma expansion, and the patient did not develop any thrombotic complications.[127] In the Japanese Observational Study for Coagulation and Thrombolysis in Early Trauma (J-OCTET) study, early administration of tranexamic acid resulted in lower rates of mortality, including in the subset of patients with primary brain injury.[336] An additional study demonstrates that tranexamic acid also has a protective effect on gut barrier function, particularly in ischemia-reperfusion injuries.[99]

Unfortunately, aminocaproic acid and tranexamic acid are associated with generalized tonic-clonic seizures in up to 7.6% of patients. The precise mechanism of seizures is not known. In murine studies, competitive antagonism of glycine receptors is suggested. When the mice were treated with isoflurane and propofol, seizure activity ceased.[211]

In summary, patients with severe bleeding, such as intracranial hemorrhage, after t-PA administration, replacement of coagulation factors and fibrinogen is recommended as soon as possible. While there are no significant studies using tranexamic acid or aminocaproic acid in factor and fibrinogen replacement failure, in patients who are gravely ill, tranexamic acid and aminocaproic acid could theoretically help decrease bleeding if all other measures fail. Because mortality rates in this population are so high, it is reasonable to recommend this intervention despite the lack of evidence.

ANTIPLATELET DRUGS

Under normal conditions, vascular endothelium provides thromboregulators that prevent thrombus formation. When the endothelium becomes compromised, exposed collagen triggers two cascades of events to promote platelet aggregation. First, a tissue factor–mediated pathway indirectly activates platelets. Tissue factor, either from the damaged vessel wall or carried in the blood, complexes with factor VIIa and activates factor IX and the extrinsic pathway of the coagulation cascade. Thrombin then directly stimulates further platelet adhesion.[134] Second, when von Willebrand factor (vWF) adheres to the exposed endothelium, platelet GP Ib-V-IX binds to the vWF and anchors platelets to the site of vascular injury. In addition, platelet GP VI and Ia tether the platelets to exposed collagen[90,134,200] (Fig. 58–4).

After platelet adhesion, modulators such as ADP and thromboxane A_2 (TXA_2) maintain platelet activation.[90,134,395] Intracellular signaling results in the release of arachidonic acid (AA) via phospholipase A2. Next, AA is converted into prostacyclin via cyclooxygenase-1 (COX-1) or cyclooxygenase-2 (COX-2). This stimulates the production of TXA_2, which further propagates platelet activation and aggregation[90,182] (Fig. 58–5).

These mediators recruit more platelets to the area of vessel injury. Glycoprotein IIb/IIIa is expressed on the surface of the platelets and allows platelet cross-linking via this receptor with vWF acting as a bridge.[90,134]

Thrombus formation perpetuates platelet aggregation and adhesion to the vessel wall. Platelet GP IIb/IIIa activation results in further thrombus formation by binding fibrinogen and vWF, essential to the linking of platelets.[90]

Antiplatelet therapies aim to decrease platelet activation or aggregation by inhibiting one of the steps in the many pathways, leading to GP IIb/IIIa activation of platelets.

CYCLOOXYGENASE INHIBITORS

Widespread use of aspirin as an antiplatelet drug is associated with significantly decreased vascular events. Aspirin acetylates the COX-1 enzyme, prevents substrate binding to the enzyme, and results in irreversible inhibition

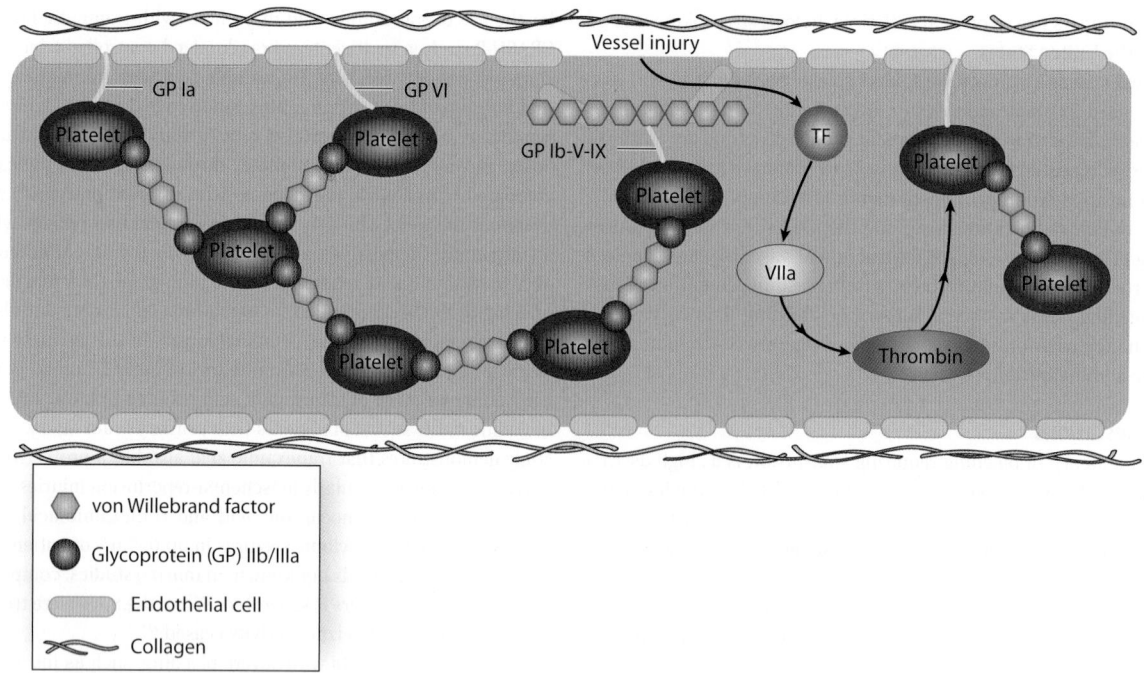

FIGURE 58–4. A schematic diagram of platelet aggregation. An injury to the endothelium results in initial platelet tethering by means of von Willebrand factor (vWF) and glycoprotein (GP) Ib-V-IX. Platelet GP VI and Ia tether the platelets to exposed collagen. GP IIb-IIIa is expressed on the surface of the platelets and allows platelet cross-linking with vWF bridging. TF = tissue factor.

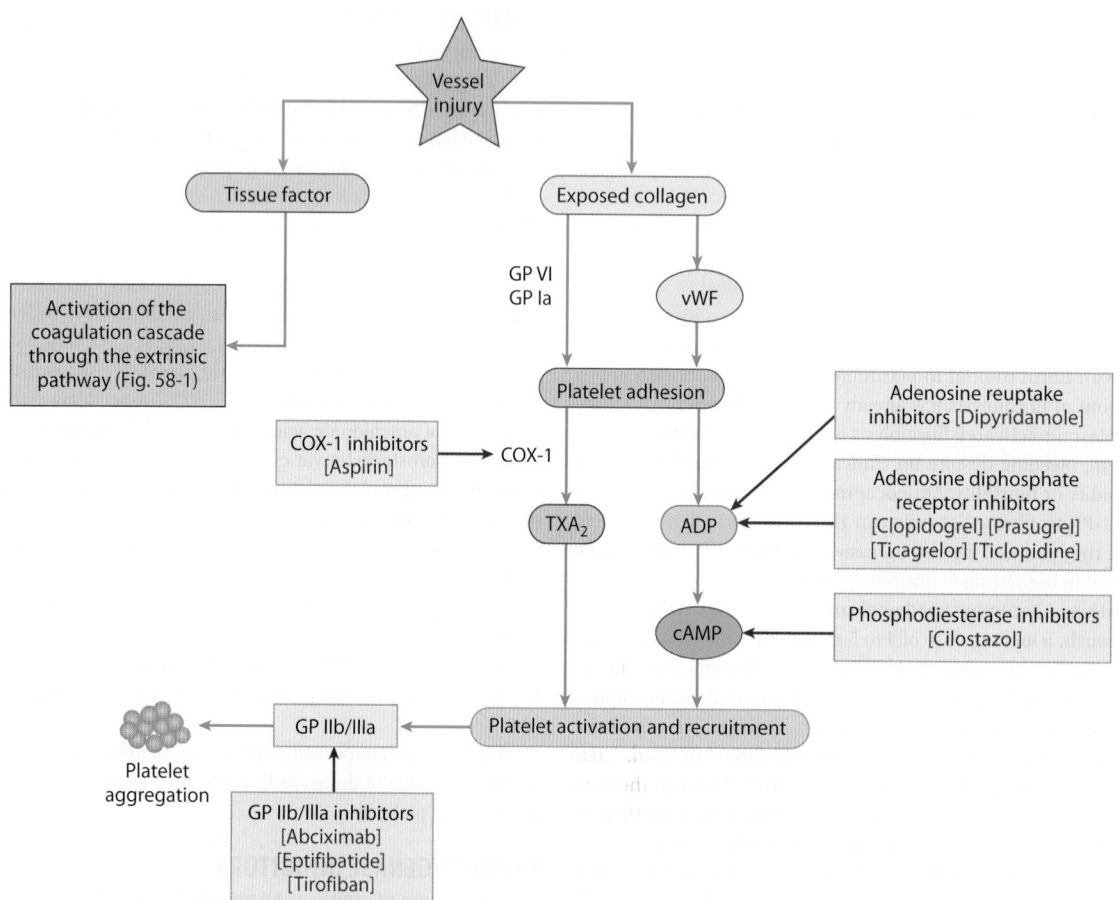

FIGURE 58–5. The antiplatelet drugs act in various stages of platelet aggregation. ADP = adenosine diphosphate; cAMP = cyclic adenosine monophosphate; COX-1 = cyclooxygenase 1; GP = glycoprotein; TXA_2 = thromboxane A_2; vWF = von Willebrand factor.

of TXA$_2$ generation. Daily low-dose aspirin fully inhibits COX-1 function and subsequent platelet aggregation because platelets are unable to regenerate COX-1.[109] However, although aspirin irreversibly inhibits COX-2, larger doses of aspirin are required to decrease COX-2–mediated processes because of rapid synthesis of new COX-2.[109]

Aspirin dosed between 75 and 150 mg showed the best odds reduction in preventing MI and stroke compared with other doses.[12,109] In fact, high-dose aspirin causes inhibition of other downregulators of platelet adhesion such as endothelium-derived prostacyclin. Although effective in preventing vascular events, the risks of bleeding and GI irritation are real. In a randomized trial comparing low dose (70–150 mg/d) and standard-dose (300–325 mg/d) aspirin in patients with acute coronary syndrome, standard-dose aspirin conferred an increased risk of GI bleeding without significant additional cardiovascular benefit.[177] However, even daily low-dose aspirin resulted in a significantly increased risk of GI bleeding compared with nonaspirin use, but this risk is outweighed by the benefits of cardiovascular disease and stroke prevention.[394]

CYCLIC ADENOSINE MONOPHOSPHATE MODULATORS

Phosphodiesterase Inhibitors

Cilostazol is a phosphodiesterase inhibitor marketed for the treatment of intermittent claudication secondary to peripheral vascular disease (PVD). By increasing cyclic adenosine monophosphate (cAMP), vasodilation is achieved by inhibiting myosin light-chain kinase, essential for smooth muscle contraction. Additionally, cAMP inhibits platelet aggregation. Small trials demonstrate that cilostazol improves walking distances, decreases arterial thrombosis, and improves rethrombosis rates in patients with PVD. In the Cilostazol for Prevention of Secondary Stroke (CSPS) study, cilostazol was not inferior to aspirin in preventing secondary stroke. However, because of its common GI adverse effects and headache, a high rate of discontinuation precludes this xenobiotic from being more widely used.[109]

Adenosine Reuptake Inhibitors

Dipyridamole has antiplatelet properties, although its mechanism of action is not completely known. Evidence suggests that by inhibiting degradation of cAMP and by blocking adenosine reuptake, intracellular cAMP accumulates and inhibits platelet aggregation.[109,395] Dipyridamole also has antiinflammatory properties by decreasing monocyte gene expression of chemokines.[400] Dipyridamole 200 mg is marketed alone or in combination with 25 mg of aspirin (Aggrenox).

Randomized studies demonstrate a significant reduction in stroke in high-risk patients taking dipyridamole with aspirin compared with patients taking aspirin alone. However, many patients discontinue dipyridamole because of headache.[101,157] Unfortunately, compared with clopidogrel, dipyridamole and aspirin offer no improvement in stroke prevention and an increase in the risk of major bleeding.[313]

ADENOSINE DIPHOSPHATE RECEPTOR INHIBITORS

Platelets require stimulation of P2Y1 and P2Y12, ADP receptors, to inhibit adenyl cyclase. Cyclic AMP formation decreases as a result of the inhibition of adenyl cyclase, and the platelet loses its ability to activate. Clopidogrel, prasugrel, ticagrelor, cangrelor, and ticlopidine are ADP receptor inhibitors. By increasing cAMP concentrations through inhibition of the P2Y12 receptor, these xenobiotics are able to inhibit platelet activation.[109,395]

Ticlopidine is a first-generation ADP receptor inhibitor. It is typically taken orally at 250 mg twice daily. Despite its rapid absorption with peak plasma concentrations between 1 and 3 hours, peak platelet inhibition occurs 1 week after initiation. Two of the many metabolites are noted to have significantly stronger ADP receptor inhibitor activity than the parent drug. Ticlopidine does not confer an overall reduction of cardiovascular death, stroke, or MI risk,[141] but coadministration with aspirin decreases stent thrombosis in some situations.[216]

The relatively high risk of neutropenia and the risks of agranulocytosis, thrombocytopenia, and thrombotic thrombocytopenic purpura–hemolytic

uremic syndrome and the development of newer generation ADP receptor inhibitors have rendered the use of ticlopidine nearly obsolete.[109,395]

Clopidogrel irreversibly binds and inhibits ADP receptors. Maximal platelet inhibition is achieved between day 4 and 7 after initiation of maintenance doses but occurs 2 to 4 hours after a 600-mg loading dose.[109] Clopidogrel requires conversion via CYP2C19 to form its active metabolite. Up to one-third of patients are resistant to clopidogrel. Many of these patients possess a CYP2C19 genetic polymorphism that results in loss of function, and these patients have an increased risk of major cardiovascular adverse events, especially after coronary artery stenting.[109,244] Similarly, concomitant administration of medications that inhibit numerous CYP enzymes may result in decreased efficacy. Further studies are required to determine if dosing modification may improve efficacy in preventing adverse vascular events. [109]

Clopidogrel is dosed at 75 mg/day. It is commonly administered with aspirin as numerous studies, such as the CREDO, COMMIT, and CLARITY trials, demonstrate that dual antiplatelet therapy to be beneficial in the reduction of vascular events.[67,312,352] However, in the ACTIVE trials, warfarin was superior to dual antiplatelet therapy with aspirin and clopidogrel in preventing major vascular events.[78] The risk of bleeding remains a major concern associated with the use of clopidogrel, particularly in dual antiplatelet regimens.[67,83]

Another ADP receptor inhibitor, prasugrel, similarly requires conversion to an active metabolite, which occurs within 30 minutes of dosing. CYP2C19 inhibition or concomitant proton pump inhibitor administration does not alter efficacy. A head-to-head comparison of prasugrel and clopidogrel in patients undergoing coronary artery intervention found a decreased incidence of overall vascular adverse outcomes and death and stent thrombosis in patients on prasugrel but no improvement in overall morbidity, mortality, or bleeding events.[109,406]

Cangrelor, approved in 2015, is another ADP receptor inhibitor with rapid onset of action. It has a short half-life, between 2.6 to 3.3 minutes.[8] Rates of adverse events such as severe bleeding are favorable compared with clopidogrel when used during PCI.[33]

Ticagrelor is the newest of the ADP receptor inhibitors that exerts its effects by allosterically and reversibly inhibiting the ADP receptor. Absorption is rapid with peak plasma concentrations in approximately 2.5 hours.[362] Dosing of ticagrelor includes a loading dose of 180 mg followed by a maintenance dose of 90 mg twice daily. The mortality and morbidity associated with ticagrelor has been compared with many other antiplatelet agents. Numerous studies delineate the risks of bleeding, in particular, based on antiplatelet therapy.[41,42,258,385]

GLYCOPROTEIN IIb/IIIa INHIBITORS

Three GP IIb/IIIa inhibitors are available for use with patients with acute coronary syndromes. Abciximab is a monoclonal Fab antibody that binds the GP IIb/IIIa receptor. When administered with heparin and aspirin in patients undergoing coronary artery intervention, stent thrombosis, MI, and mortality all decrease. Abciximab is administered as an IV bolus dose of 0.25 mg/kg is followed by an infusion of 0.125 mg/kg/min. The plasma half-life is short, with plasma concentrations becoming negligible approximately 30 minutes after cessation of the infusion. However, the Fab fragments bind to the platelets and inhibit platelet function for up to 24 hours.[395]

Eptifibatide is a synthetic GP IIb/IIIa inhibitor used in patients with acute coronary syndrome undergoing coronary artery interventions. Its molecular structure is based on snake venom disintegrin. An IV loading dose of 180 mcg/kg is followed by an infusion of 2 mcg/kg/min.[395] Dosing in patients with CKD is unstudied, but there is a demonstrable increase in rates of bleeding in patients with a creatinine clearance less than 60 mL/min.[298] Tirofiban also inhibits the GP IIb/IIIa receptor and has similar clinical efficacy compared with eptifibatide.[395]

Up to 10% of patients treated with GP IIb/IIIa inhibitors have major bleeding events. Thrombocytopenia can also occur as a result of antigenic recognition of the xenobiotic-bound platelets.[109]

A number of trials examining the efficacy and safety of the GP IIb/IIIa inhibitors describe positive trends in decreasing predefined endpoints such as 30-day mortality, stent rethrombosis, and MI. After evaluation of the combined data from multiple trials, the benefits of GP IIb/IIIa inhibitor therapy without early coronary artery revascularization are unclear when weighing the risks of bleeding. However, with early coronary artery revascularization, adding a GP IIb/IIIa inhibitor is beneficial, although the benefit of treatment in the highest risk patients is uncertain.[92,109]

DEVELOPMENT OF NOVEL RECEPTOR AND ENZYME INHIBITORS

Recent pharmaceutical development has focused on inhibition of several key enzymes or receptors in platelet activation and aggregation. Thromboxane A_2 function is inhibited by TXA_2 synthase inhibitors or by antagonizing the TXA_2 receptor. Clinical trials are currently underway to evaluate the efficacy of inhibiting protease-activated receptors, also called thrombin receptors.[361]

Laboratory Assessment

Bleeding time is traditionally the most useful and widely available used to assess platelet function. However, its popularity has decreased because of its insensitivity, invasiveness, scarring, and high degree of variability. A variety of platelet function assays exist, but few are widely available. The gold standard assay, light transmission aggregometry, is commonly used in specialty laboratories, but it does not reflect physiologic platelet adhesion or aggregation. Furthermore, this test is time consuming and expensive. Several widely used tests to assess platelet function, such as flow cytometry and serum TXA_2 assay, are available. Each of these tests has significant disadvantages such as being artifact prone, expensive, nonspecific, or insensitive to select antiplatelet agents. In addition, extrapolating these results to determine a patient's risk of bleeding or thrombosis is not possible.[163]

Management

When managing bleeding in patients taking antiplatelet xenobiotics, blood transfusion should be used in patients with significant blood loss. However, transfusion of PRBCs will not increase platelet adhesion or aggregation. Unfortunately, the published literature that assesses interventions on bleeding patients maintained on antiplatelet xenobiotics is conflicting, and there is no clear consensus on appropriate reversal strategies and agents. The most widely evaluated intervention is platelet transfusion. The existing studies are small and mostly retrospective. Prospective studies are biased by nonrandomization, specifically by the clinician ultimately deciding whether to transfuse the platelets. Many of these studies show that platelet transfusion is potentially harmful and independently predict increased mortality and bleeding (Table 58–1).[21,61] Although transfusing platelets is associated with worse outcomes, it is important to notice that these studies only demonstrate association and not causation. Therefore, blood transfusion to replace lost volume and coagulation factors is reasonable. It is also reasonable to administer platelets to patients in extremis, such as those requiring massive transfusion caused by extensive blood loss.

Desmopressin is approved for the treatment of inherited defects of hemostasis and potentiates thrombosis by releasing vWF and factor VIII from the endothelium into the plasma. In these patients, complications such as arterial thrombosis and MI are reported after desmopressin administration.[207,218] However, some proposed protocols for reversing antiplatelet xenobiotics in the setting of life-threatening bleeding include desmopressin. Most of these protocols are based on case reports because the majority of the studies evaluated prophylactic desmopressin before surgery to prevent blood loss. A single study evaluated the administration of desmopressin on platelet aggregation and platelet activity in healthy volunteers given a single dose of clopidogrel. They found that platelet reactivity and platelet aggregation increased after desmopressin administration. There was no mention of adverse outcomes in any of the study participants.[214] The risk of desmopressin-induced thrombosis in patients taking antiplatelet xenobiotics is unknown; in patients taking antiplatelet medications for atherosclerosis, the risk of thrombosis is greater.[214] There is not enough information to routinely recommend the use of desmopressin in this setting at this time.

In the case of abciximab, cessation of the infusion results in a rapid decrease in circulating antibodies. If severe bleeding occurs, platelet transfusion after discontinuation of the infusion is effective in restoring platelet activation and aggregation.[395] In most cases, discontinuation of eptifibatide and tirofiban results in restoration of normal platelet function within hours. However, patients with renal dysfunction have prolonged platelet inhibition. Both of these xenobiotics are renally cleared, and some have suggested hemodialysis as a means to enhance clearance.[360] Although not formally studied, case reports of patients with protracted platelet inhibition in the setting of eptifibatide use and end-stage CKD suggest that hemodialysis restores platelet aggregation capacity.[343] However, there are insufficient data at this time to routinely recommend this intervention, especially because initiating hemodialysis typically takes several hours, during which time platelet function typically improves. Unlike abciximab platelet toxicity, transfusion of platelets to patients receiving eptifibatide is believed to be ineffective in restoring platelet function. At therapeutic concentrations, the concentration of these xenobiotics far outnumbers the inhibited GP IIb/IIIa receptors by several orders of magnitude.[360] Further studies are required to produce recommendations or guidelines for emergent reversal of antiplatelet xenobiotics to determine if any interventions are effective and offer a favorable risk-to-benefit profile. In the meantime, clinicians should volume resuscitate accordingly with fluids and blood products as necessary.

SNAKE VENOMS

A detailed discussion of snake envenomations is found in Chap. 119 and Special Considerations: SC10; only a few specific issues are discussed here. Snake venoms are composed of a vast number of complex proteins and peptides that interact with components of the human hemostatic system. In general, their functions may be thought of as being procoagulant, anticoagulant, fibrinolytic, vessel wall interactive, platelet active, or as protein inactivators. Additionally, they are more specifically classified based on their specific biologic activity; some of the various mechanisms include individual factor activation, inhibition of protein C and thrombin, fibrinogen degradation, platelet aggregation, and inhibition of serine protease inhibitors (SERPINS). Currently, more than 100 different snake venoms affect the hemostatic system.[178,179]

Figure 58–1 is an overview of their multiple interactions with the coagulation and fibrinolytic systems.[236]

Some of these venom proteins are being used as therapeutically for human diseases. Ancrod, a purified derivative of the Malayan pit viper, *Calloselasma rhodostoma* (formerly known as *Agkistrodon rhodostoma*), is therapeutically used because of its defibrinogenating property.[25] The mechanism of action of ancrod and other similar xenobiotics is to link fibrinogen end to end and subsequently prevent cross-linking. It is under investigation for the treatment of DVT, MI, PE, acute cerebrovascular thrombosis, HITT, and warfarin-related vascular complications. In a multicenter study of 500 patients with acute or progressing ischemic neurologic events, ancrod showed a favorable benefit-to-risk ratio compared with placebo.[333] As expected, an increased risk of bleeding is observed; however, the risk is less than that with thrombolytics.[333] Monitoring of fibrinogen concentrations is essential to avoid potential complications because no specific antidote exists. Following envenomation, snakes such as those of the Crotalinae family that induce bleeding, antivenin treatment is indicated.

SUMMARY

- The development of new antithrombotics and the increasing frequency of antithrombotic therapeutic use are associated with complications and adverse outcomes.
- A complete understanding of the normal mechanisms of coagulation, anticoagulation, and thrombolysis combined with an understanding of the pharmacology of the xenobiotic and the clinical needs of the patient will allow clinicians to better choose among the complex therapies currently available.
- Complications of the antithrombotics should be managed with supportive care, starting with volume resuscitation and blood replacement.

■ More aggressive interventions and specific reversal therapeutics are necessary depending if the patient is experiencing severe, life-threatening hemorrhage. In these instances, clinical studies do not always ensure a favorable risk-to-benefit profile because further studies are required.

■ Ongoing development of new antithrombotics will raise new challenges for clinicians as adverse outcomes and bleeding complications arise, and new antidotes will be developed to address these issues.

Acknowledgments

Theresa Kierenia, MD (deceased), and Robert S. Hoffman, MD, contributed to this chapter in previous editions.

REFERENCES

1. Ageno W, et al. Oral anticoagulant therapy: antithrombotic therapy and prevention of thrombosis, 9th ed: American College of Chest Physicians Evidence-Based Clinical Practice Guidelines. *Chest.* 2012;141(2 suppl):e44S-88S.
2. Aiyagari V, Testai FD. Correction of coagulopathy in warfarin associated cerebral hemorrhage. *Curr Opin Crit Care.* 2009;15:87-92.
3. Alexander JH, et al. Apixaban with antiplatelet therapy after acute coronary syndrome. *N Engl J Med.* 2011;365:699-708.
4. Alhashem HM, et al. Persistent life-threatening hemorrhage after administration of idarucizumab. *Am J Emerg Med.* 2017;35:193 e193-193 e195.
5. Alhenc-Gelas M, et al. Adjusted versus fixed doses of the low-molecular-weight heparin Fragmin in the treatment of deep vein thrombosis. Fragmin-Study Group. *Thromb Haemost.* 1994;71:698-702.
6. Ancalmo N, Ochsner J. Heparin, the Miracle Drug: A Brief History of Its Discovery. *J La State Med Soc.* 1990;142:22-24.
7. Andersen MN, et al. Experimental studies of heparin-protamine activity with special reference to protamine inhibition of clotting. *Surgery.* 1959;46:1060.
8. Angiolillo DJ, Capranzano P. Pharmacology of emerging novel platelet inhibitors. *Am Heart J.* 2008;156(2 suppl):S10-15.
9. Ansell JE, et al. Use of PER977 to reverse the anticoagulant effect of edoxaban. *N Engl J Med.* 2014;371:2141-2142.
10. Ansell JE, et al. Single-dose ciraparantag safely and completely reverses anticoagulant effects of edoxaban. *Thromb Haemost.* 2017;117:238-245.
11. Ansell JE, et al. Ciraparantag safely and completely reverses the anticoagulant effects of low molecular weight heparin. *Thromb Res.* 2016;146:113-118.
12. Antithrombotic Trialists Collaboration. Collaborative meta-analysis of randomised trials of antiplatelet therapy for prevention of death, myocardial infarction, and stroke in high risk patients. *BMJ.* 2002;324:71-86.
13. Antonelli D, et al. Enoxaparin associated with high abdominal wall hematomas: a report of two cases. *Am Surg.* 2000;66:797-800.
14. Aster RH. Heparin-induced thrombocytopenia and thrombosis. *N Engl J Med.* 1995;332:1374-1376.
15. Babcock J, et al. Rodenticide-induced coagulopathy in a young child. A case of Munchausen syndrome by proxy. *Am J Pediatr Hematol Oncol.* 1993;15:126-130.
16. Bachmann KA, Sullivan TJ. Dispositional and pharmacodynamic characteristics of brodifacoum in warfarin-sensitive rats. *Pharmacology.* 1983;27:281-288.
17. Badr M, et al. Menadione causes selective toxicity to periportal regions of the liver lobule. *Toxicol Lett.* 1987;35:241-246.
18. Bara L, et al. Occurrence of thrombosis and haemorrhage, relationship with anti-Xa, anti-IIa activities, and D-dimer plasma levels in patients receiving a low molecular weight heparin, enoxaparin or tinzaparin, to prevent deep vein thrombosis after hip surgery. *Br J Haematol.* 1999;104:230-240.
19. Barlow AM, et al. Difenacoum (Neosorexa) poisoning. *Br Med J (Clin Res Ed).* 1982;285:541-541.
20. Barton J, et al. Anti-Xa activity in apixaban overdose: a case report. *Clin Toxicol (Phila).* 2016;54:871-873.
21. Batchelor JS, Grayson A. A meta-analysis to determine the effect on survival of platelet transfusions in patients with either spontaneous or traumatic antiplatelet medication-associated intracranial haemorrhage. *BMJ Open.* 2012;2.
22. Bauersachs R, et al. Oral rivaroxaban for symptomatic venous thromboembolism. *N Engl J Med.* 2010;363:2499-2510.
23. Baxalta US Inc. FEIBA (Anti-Inhibitor Coagulant Complex). http://www.shirecontent.com/PI/PDFs/FEIBA_USA_ENG.pdf. Accessed April 30, 2017.
24. Becker RC. Seminars in thrombosis, thrombolysis, and vascular biology. Part 2: coagulation and thrombosis. *Cardiology.* 1991;78:257-266.
25. Bell WR. Defibrinogenating enzymes. *Drugs.* 1997;54(suppl 3):18-30, discussion 30-31.
26. Bene J, et al. Rectal bleeding and hemostatic disorders induced by dabigatran etexilate in 2 elderly patients. *Ann Pharmacother.* 2012;46:e14.
27. Benedict CR, et al. Thrombolytic therapy: a state of the art review. *Hosp Pract (Off Ed).* 1992;27:61-72.
28. Bennett DL, et al. Long-acting anticoagulant ingestion: a prospective study. *Vet Hum Toxicol.* 1987;29:472-473.
29. Beretz A, Cazenave JP. Old and new natural products as the source of modern antithrombotic drugs. *Planta Med.* 1991;57:S68-72.
30. Bergqvist D, et al. Low-molecular-weight heparin (enoxaparin) as prophylaxis against venous thromboembolism after total hip replacement. *N Engl J Med.* 1996;335: 696-700.
31. Berrouschot J, et al. Intravenous thrombolysis with recombinant tissue-type plasminogen activator in a stroke patient receiving dabigatran anticoagulant after antagonization with idarucizumab. *Stroke.* 2016;47:1936-1938.
32. Berry RG, et al. Surreptitious superwarfarin ingestion with brodifacoum. *South Med J.* 2000;93:74-75.
33. Bhatt DL, et al. Effect of platelet inhibition with cangrelor during PCI on ischemic events. *N Engl J Med.* 2013;368:1303-1313.
34. Bijsterveld NR, et al. Ability of recombinant factor VIIa to reverse the anticoagulant effect of the pentasaccharide fondaparinux in healthy volunteers. *Circulation.* 2002;106:2550-2554.
35. Bithell T. Acquired coagulation disorders. In: Lee G, Bet al eds. *Wintrobe's Clinical Hematology.* 9th ed. Philadelphia: Lea & Febiger; 1993:1473-1503.
36. Bittl JA, et al. Treatment with bivalirudin (Hirulog) as compared with heparin during coronary angioplasty for unstable or postinfarction angina. *N Engl J Med.* 1995;333:764-769.
37. Blech S, et al. The metabolism and disposition of the oral direct thrombin inhibitor, dabigatran, in humans. *Drug Metab Dispos.* 2008;36:386-399.
38. Blossom DB, et al. Outbreak of adverse reactions associated with contaminated heparin. *N Engl J Med.* 2008;359:2674-2684.
39. Boehringer Ingelheim Pharmaceuticals Inc. 2015. http://docs.boehringer-ingelheim.com/Prescribing Information/PIs/Pradaxa/Pradaxa.pdf. Accessed September 28, 2017.
40. Boland M, et al. Acute-onset severe gastrointestinal tract hemorrhage in a postoperative patient taking rivaroxaban after total hip arthroplasty: a case report. *J Med Case Rep.* 2012;6:129-129.
41. Bonaca MP, et al. Long-term use of ticagrelor in patients with prior myocardial infarction. *N Engl J Med.* 2015;372:1791-1800.
42. Bonaca MP, et al. Prevention of stroke with ticagrelor in patients with prior myocardial infarction: insights from PEGASUS-TIMI 54 (Prevention of Cardiovascular Events in Patients With Prior Heart Attack Using Ticagrelor Compared to Placebo on a Background of Aspirin-Thrombolysis in Myocardial Infarction 54). *Circulation.* 2016;134:861-871.
43. Boster SR, Bergin JJ. Upper airway obstruction complicating warfarin therapy—with a note on reversal of warfarin toxicity. *Annals of emergency medicine.* 1983;12:711-715.
44. Bounameaux H, de Moerloose P. Is laboratory monitoring of low-molecular-weight heparin therapy necessary? No. *J Thromb Haemost.* 2004;2:551-554.
45. Bounameaux H, Goldhaber SZ. Uses of low-molecular-weight heparin. *Blood Rev.* 1995;9:213-219.
46. Bowen KJ, Vukelja SJ. Hypercoagulable states. Their causes and management. *Postgrad Med.* 1992;91:117-118, 123-115-128 passim.
47. Braemswig TB, et al. Emergency LP in a patient receiving dabigatran after antagonization with idarucizumab. *Am J Emerg Med.* 2017;35:662 e663-662 e664.
48. Braithwaite GB. Vitamin K and brodifacoum. *J Am Vet Med Assoc.* 1982;181:531, 534.
49. Breckenridge A, et al. Pharmacokinetics and pharmacodynamics of the enantiomers of warfarin in man. *Clin Pharmacol Ther.* 1974;15:424-430.
50. Breckenridge A, Orme ML. The plasma half lives and the pharmacological effect of the enantiomers of warfarin in rats. *Life Sci II.* 1972;11:337-345.
51. Breckenridge AM, et al. Mechanisms of action of the anticoagulants warfarin, 2-chloro-3-phytylnaphthoquinone (Cl-K), acenocoumarol, brodifacoum and difenacoum in the rabbit [proceedings]. *Br J Pharmacol.* 1978;64:399P.
52. Brekelmans MP, et al. Clinical impact and course of major bleeding with edoxaban versus vitamin K antagonists. *Thromb Haemost.* 2016;116:155-161.
53. Bristol-Myers Squibb Company. Eliquis package insert. http://packageinserts.bms.com/pi/pi_eliquis.pdf. Accessed February 19, 2018.
54. Brodsky SV, et al. Warfarin-related nephropathy occurs in patients with and without chronic kidney disease and is associated with an increased mortality rate. *Kidney Int.* 2011;80:181-189.
55. Brodsky SV, et al. Acute kidney injury during warfarin therapy associated with obstructive tubular red blood cell casts: a report of 9 cases. *Am J Kidney Dis.* 2009;54:1121-1126.
56. Bruno GR, et al. Long-acting anticoagulant overdose: brodifacoum kinetics and optimal vitamin K dosing. *Ann Emerg Med.* 2000;36:262-267.
57. Burucoa C, et al. Chlorophacinone intoxication. A biological and toxicological study. *J Toxicol Clin Toxicol.* 1989;27:79-89.
58. Byrne M, Zumberg M. Intentional low-molecular-weight heparin overdose: a case report and review. *Blood Coagul Fibrinolysis.* 2012;23:772-774.
59. Cabral KP, Ansell J. Oral direct factor Xa inhibitors for stroke prevention in atrial fibrillation. *Nat Rev Cardiol.* 2012;9:385-391.
60. Cadiou G, et al. Risk factors of vitamin K antagonist overcoagulation. A case-control study in unselected patients referred to an emergency department. *Thromb Haemost.* 2008;100:685-692.
61. Campbell PG, et al. Emergency reversal of antiplatelet agents in patients presenting with an intracranial hemorrhage: a clinical review. *World Neurosurg.* 2010;74:279-285.
62. Chadd MA, Gray OP. Hypothermia and coagulation defects in the newborn. *Arch Dis Child.* 1972;47:819-821.

63. Chang DN, et al. Removal of dabigatran by hemodialysis. *Am J Kidney Dis.* 2013;61: 487-489.

64. Chen BC, et al. Hemodialysis for the treatment of pulmonary hemorrhage from dabigatran overdose. *Am J Kidney Dis.* 2013;62:591-594.

65. Chen BC, et al. Hemorrhagic complications associated with dabigatran use. *Clin Toxicol (Phila).* 2012;50:854-857.

66. Chen J, et al. Efficacy and safety of edoxaban in nonvalvular atrial fibrillation: a meta-analysis of randomized controlled trials. *J Stroke Cerebrovasc Dis.* 2015;24:2710-2719.

67. Chen ZM, et al. Addition of clopidogrel to aspirin in 45,852 patients with acute myocardial infarction: randomised placebo-controlled trial. *Lancet.* 2005;366:1607-1621.

68. Chong BH, Isaacs A. Heparin-induced thrombocytopenia: what clinicians need to know. *Thromb Haemost.* 2009;101:279-283.

69. Choonara IA, et al. Vitamin K1 metabolism in relation to pharmacodynamic response in anticoagulated patients. *Br J Clin Pharmacol.* 1985;20:643-648.

70. Chu JW, et al. Thrombosis of a mechanical heart valve despite dabigatran. *Ann Intern Med.* 2012;157:304.

71. Chung N, et al. Safety of edoxaban, an oral factor Xa inhibitor, in Asian patients with non-valvular atrial fibrillation. *Thromb Haemost.* 2011;105:535-544.

72. Ciavarella D, et al. Clotting factor levels and the risk of diffuse microvascular bleeding in the massively transfused patient. *Br J Haematol.* 1987;67:365-368.

73. Clouse LH, Comp PC. The regulation of hemostasis: the protein C system. *N Engl J Med.* 1986;314:1298-1304.

74. Collen D. On the regulation and control of fibrinolysis. Edward Kowalski Memorial Lecture. *Thromb Haemost.* 1980;43:77-89.

75. Collen D, Lijnen HR. Basic and clinical aspects of fibrinolysis and thrombolysis. *Blood.* 1991;78:3114-3124.

76. APPRAISE Steering Committee and Investigators; Alexander JH, et al. Apixaban, an oral, direct, selective factor Xa inhibitor, in combination with antiplatelet therapy after acute coronary syndrome: results of the Apixaban for Prevention of Acute Ischemic and Safety Events (APPRAISE) trial. *Circulation.* 2009;119:2877-2885.

77. Comp PC. Coumarin-induced skin necrosis. Incidence, mechanisms, management and avoidance. *Drug Saf.* 1993;8:128.

78. Connolly S, et al. Clopidogrel plus aspirin versus oral anticoagulation for atrial fibrillation in the Atrial Fibrillation Clopidogrel Trial with Irbesartan for prevention of Vascular Events (ACTIVE W): a randomised controlled trial. *Lancet.* 2006;367:1903-1912.

79. Connolly SJ, et al. Betrixaban compared with warfarin in patients with atrial fibrillation: results of a phase 2, randomized, dose-ranging study (Explore-Xa) *Eur Heart J.* 2013;34:1498-1505.

80. Connolly SJ, et al. Apixaban in patients with atrial fibrillation. *N Engl J Med.* 2011;364:806-817.

81. Connolly SJ, et al. Dabigatran versus warfarin in patients with atrial fibrillation. *N Engl J Med.* 2009;361:1139-1151.

82. Connolly SJ, et al. Andexanet alfa for acute major bleeding associated with factor xa inhibitors. *N Engl J Med.* 2016;375:1131-1141.

83. Connolly SJ, et al. Effect of clopidogrel added to aspirin in patients with atrial fibrillation. *N Engl J Med.* 2009;360:2066-2078.

84. Conti CR. Brief overview of the end points of thrombolytic therapy. *Am J Cardiol.* 1991;68:8E-10E.

85. Cotton BA, et al. Acutely injured patients on dabigatran. *N Engl J Med.* 2011;365: 2039-2040.

86. Crowther MA, et al. Oral vitamin K versus placebo to correct excessive anticoagulation in patients receiving warfarin: a randomized trial. *Ann Intern Med.* 2009;150:293-300.

87. Cruickshank J, et al. Warfarin toxicity in the emergency department: recommendations for management. *Emerg Med (Fremantle).* 2001;13:91-97.

88. CSL Behring LLC. Kcentra prescribing information. http://labeling.cslbehring.com/PI/US/Kcentra/EN/Kcentra-Prescribing-Information.pdf. Accessed April 30, 2017.

89. Daiichi Sankyo Co. LTD. Savaysa prescribing information. http://dsi.com/prescribing-information-portlet/getPIContent?productName=Savaysa&inline=true. Accessed April 29, 2017.

90. Davì G, Patrono C. Platelet activation and atherothrombosis. *N Engl J Med.* 2007;357: 2482-2494.

91. Davie EW, Ratnoff OD. Waterfall sequence for intrinsic blood clotting. *Science.* 1964;145:1310-1312.

92. De Luca G, et al. Risk profile and benefits from Gp IIb-IIIa inhibitors among patients with ST-segment elevation myocardial infarction treated with primary angioplasty: a meta-regression analysis of randomized trials. *Eur Heart J.* 2009;30:2705-2713.

93. den Heijer P, et al. Evaluation of a weight-adjusted single-bolus plasminogen activator in patients with myocardial infarction: a double-blind, randomized angiographic trial of lanoteplase versus alteplase. *Circulation.* 1998;98:2117-2125.

94. Deng Y, Qiu L. Therapeutic plasma exchange as a second-line treatment for brodifacoum poisoning following an anaphylactoid reaction to vitamin K. *Clin Case Rep.* 2017;5:35-38.

95. Dentali F, Crowther MA. Management of excessive anticoagulant effect due to vitamin K antagonists. *Hematology.* 2008:266-270.

96. Deveras RAE, Kessler CM. Reversal of warfarin-induced excessive anticoagulation with recombinant human factor VIIa concentrate. *Ann Intern Med.* 2002;137: 884-888.

97. Di Nisio M, et al. Direct thrombin inhibitors. *N Engl J Med.* 2005;353:1028-1040.

98. Dickinson LD, et al. Enoxaparin increases the incidence of postoperative intracranial hemorrhage when initiated preoperatively for deep venous thrombosis prophylaxis in patients with brain tumors. *Neurosurgery.* 1998;43:1074-1081.

99. Diebel ME, et al. Early tranexamic acid administration: a protective effect on gut barrier function following ischemia/reperfusion injury. *J Trauma Acute Care Surg.* 2015;79:1015-1022.

100. Diener HC, et al. Thrombolysis and thrombectomy in patients treated with dabigatran with acute ischemic stroke: expert opinion. *Int J Stroke.* 2017;12:9-12.

101. Diener HC, et al. European stroke prevention study. 2. Dipyridamole and acetylsalicylic acid in the secondary prevention of stroke. *J Neurol Sci.* 1996;143:1-13.

102. Diringer MN, et al. Thromboembolic Events with recombinant activated factor vii in spontaneous intracerebral hemorrhage: results from the Factor Seven for Acute Hemorrhagic Stroke (FAST) trial. *Stroke.* 2010;41:48-53.

103. Dirkmann D, et al. Hypothermia and acidosis synergistically impair coagulation in human whole blood. *Anesthes Analges.* 2008;106:1627-1632.

104. Dowd P, et al. The mechanism of action of vitamin K. *Ann Rev Nutr.* 1995;15:419-440.

105. Du S, et al. Measurement of non-vitamin K antagonist oral anticoagulants in patient plasma using Heptest-STAT coagulation method. *Ther Drug Monit.* 2015;37:375-380.

106. Dunwiddie CT, et al. Purification and characterization of recombinant antistasin—a leech-derived inhibitor of coagulation Factor-Xa. *Arteriosclerosis.* 1990;10:A913-A913.

107. Dy EA, Shiltz DL. Hemopericardium and cardiac tamponade associated with dabigatran use. *Ann Pharmacother.* 2012;46:e18.

108. Eerenberg ES, et al. Reversal of rivaroxaban and dabigatran by prothrombin complex concentrate: a randomized, placebo-controlled, crossover study in healthy subjects. *Circulation.* 2011;124:1573-1579.

109. Eikelboom JW, et al. Antiplatelet drugs: antithrombotic therapy and prevention of thrombosis, 9th ed: American College of Chest Physicians Evidence-Based Clinical Practice Guidelines. *Chest.* 2012;141(2 suppl):e89S-e119S.

110. Eikelboom JW, et al. Risk of bleeding with 2 doses of dabigatran compared with warfarin in older and younger patients with atrial fibrillation: an analysis of the Randomized Evaluation of Long-Term Anticoagulant Therapy (RE-LY) trial. *Circulation.* 2011;123:2363-2372.

111. Eisen A, et al. Edoxaban vs warfarin in patients with nonvalvular atrial fibrillation in the US Food and Drug Administration approval population: an analysis from the Effective Anticoagulation with Factor Xa Next Generation in Atrial Fibrillation-Thrombolysis in Myocardial Infarction 48 (ENGAGE AF-TIMI 48) trial. *Am Heart J.* 2016;172:144-151.

112. Elmer J, Wittels KA. Emergency reversal of pentasaccharide anticoagulants: a systematic review of the literature. *Transfus Med.* 2012;22:108-115.

113. Eriksson BI, et al. A once-daily, oral, direct factor Xa inhibitor, rivaroxaban (BAY 59-7939), for thromboprophylaxis after total hip replacement. *Circulation.* 2006;114: 2374-2381.

114. Eriksson BI, et al. Oral dabigatran versus enoxaparin for thromboprophylaxis after primary total hip arthroplasty (RE-NOVATE II®). A randomised, double-blind, non-inferiority trial. *Thromb Haemost.* 2011;105:721-729.

115. Eriksson BI, et al. Dabigatran etexilate versus enoxaparin for prevention of venous thromboembolism after total hip replacement: a randomised, double-blind, non-inferiority trial. *Lancet.* 2007;370:949-956.

116. Eriksson BI, et al. Comparative pharmacodynamics and pharmacokinetics of oral direct thrombin and factor Xa inhibitors in development. *Clin Pharmacokinet.* 2009;48:1-22.

117. Escolar G, et al. Effects of apixaban on hemostasis and reversal of its anticoagulant action by different coagulation factor concentrates: studies in vitro with circulating human blood. *PLoS One.* 2012;130:S113-S113.

118. Estes JW, Poulin PF. Pharmacokinetics of heparin. Distribution and elimination. *Thromb Diath Haemorrh.* 1975;33:26.

119. Exner DV, et al. Superwarfarin ingestion. *CMAJ.* 1992;146:34-35.

120. Farrell M, et al. Response of life threatening dimenhydrinate intoxication to sodium bicarbonate administration. *J Toxicol Clin Toxicol.* 1991;29:527-535.

121. Fasco MJ, et al. Evidence that warfarin anticoagulant action involves two distinct reductase activities. *J Biol Chem.* 1982;257:11210-11212.

122. Feder W, Auerbach R. "Purple toes": an uncommon sequela of oral coumarin drug therapy. *Ann Intern Med.* 1961;55:911-917.

123. Fihn SD, et al. The risk for and severity of bleeding complications in elderly patients treated with warfarin. *Ann Intern Med.* 1996;124:970-979.

124. Forestier F, et al. Low molecular weight heparin (PK 10169) does not cross the placenta during the second trimester of pregnancy study by direct fetal blood sampling under ultrasound. *Thromb Res.* 1984;34:557.

125. Franke CL, et al. Intracerebral hematomas during anticoagulant treatment. *Stroke.* 1990;21:726-730.

126. Freedman MD, Olatidoye AG. Clinically significant drug interactions with the oral anticoagulants. *Drug Saf.* 1994;10:381-394.

127. French KF, et al. Treatment of intracerebral hemorrhage with tranexamic acid after thrombolysis with tissue plasminogen activator. *Neurocrit Care.* 2012;17:107-111.

128. Frydman A. Low-molecular-weight heparins: an overview of their pharmacodynamics, pharmacokinetics and metabolism in humans. *Haemostasis.* 1996;26(suppl 2):24-38.

129. Fuji T, et al. A randomized, open-label trial of edoxaban in Japanese patients with severe renal impairment undergoing lower-limb orthopedic surgery. *Thromb J.* 2015;13:6.

130. Fuji T, et al. Efficacy and safety of edoxaban versus enoxaparin for the prevention of venous thromboembolism following total hip arthroplasty: STARS J-V. *Thromb J.* 2015;13:27.

131. Fuji T, et al. Safety and efficacy of edoxaban in patients undergoing hip fracture surgery. *Thromb Res*. 2014;133:1016-1022.

132. Fuji T, et al. A dose-ranging study evaluating the oral factor Xa inhibitor edoxaban for the prevention of venous thromboembolism in patients undergoing total knee arthroplasty. *J Thromb Haemost*. 2010;8:2458-2468.

133. Fukuda T, et al. Reversal of anticoagulant effects of edoxaban, an oral, direct factor Xa inhibitor, with haemostatic agents. *Thromb Haemost*. 2012;107:253-259.

134. Furie B, Furie BC. Mechanisms of thrombus formation. *N Engl J Med*. 2008;359:938-949.

135. Furie B, Furie BC. Molecular and cellular biology of blood coagulation. *N Engl J Med*. 1992;326:800-806.

136. Galant SP. Accidental heparinization of a newborn infant. *Am J Dis Child*. 1967;114:313-319.

137. Garcia DA, et al. Parenteral anticoagulants: antithrombotic therapy and prevention of thrombosis, 9th ed: American College of Chest Physicians Evidence-Based Clinical Practice Guidelines. *Chest*. 2012;141(2 suppl):e24S-e43S.

138. Garlich FM, et al. Public health response following poisoning with illegal brodifacoum (0.5%) rodenticide. *Clin Toxicol*. 2012;50:357-357.

139. Gawehn A, et al. Successful thrombolysis with recombinant tissue plasminogen activator after antagonizing dabigatran by idarucizumab: a case report. *J Med Case Rep*. 2016;10:269.

140. Gendron N, et al. Real-world use of idarucizumab for dabigatran reversal in three cases of serious bleeding. *Clin Case Rep*. 2017;5:346-350.

141. Gent M, et al. The Canadian American Ticlopidine Study (Cats) in thromboembolic stroke. *Lancet*. 1989;1:1215-1220.

142. Gilbert GE, et al. Platelet-derived microparticles express high affinity receptors for factor VIII. *J Biol Chem*. 1991;266:17261-17268.

143. Giugliano RP, et al. Edoxaban versus warfarin in patients with atrial fibrillation. *N Engl J Med*. 2013;369:2093-2104.

144. Giugliano RP, et al. Cerebrovascular events in 21 105 patients with atrial fibrillation randomized to edoxaban versus warfarin: effective anticoagulation with factor Xa next generation in atrial fibrillation-thrombolysis in myocardial infarction 48. *Stroke*. 2014;45:2372-2378.

145. Glueck HI, et al. Inadvertent sodium heparin administration to a newborn infant. *JAMA*. 1965;191:1031-1032.

146. Godier A, et al. Evaluation of prothrombin complex concentrate and recombinant activated factor VII to reverse rivaroxaban in a rabbit model. *Anesthesiology*. 2012;116:94-102.

147. Goldhaber SZ, et al. Apixaban versus enoxaparin for thromboprophylaxis in medically ill patients. *N Engl J Med*. 2011;365:2167-2177.

148. Goldstein JN, et al. Management of thrombolysis-associated symptomatic intracerebral hemorrhage. *Arch Neurol*. 2010;67:965-969.

149. Gopinath SC. Anti-coagulant aptamers. *Thromb Res*. 2008;122:838-847.

150. Granger CB, et al. Apixaban versus warfarin in patients with atrial fibrillation. *N Engl J Med*. 2011;365:981-992.

151. Greeff MC, et al. "Superwarfarin" (bromadiolone) poisoning in two children resulting in prolonged anticoagulation. *Lancet*. 1987;2:1269.

152. Green D, et al. Low molecular weight heparin: a critical analysis of clinical trials. *Pharmacol Rev*. 1994;46:89-109.

153. PROTECT Investigators for the Canadian Critical Care Trials Group and the Australian and New Zealand Intensive Care Society Clinical Trials Group; Cook D, et al. Dalteparin versus unfractionated heparin in critically ill patients. *N Engl J Med*. 2011;364:1305-1314.

154. Guyatt GH, et al. Executive summary: antithrombotic therapy and prevention of thrombosis, 9th ed: American College of Chest Physicians Evidence-Based Clinical Practice Guidelines. *Chest*. 2012;141(2 suppl):7S-47S.

155. Hackett LP, et al. Plasma warfarin concentrations after a massive overdose. *Me J Aust*. 1985;142:642-643.

156. Haines ST, Bussey HI. Thrombosis and the pharmacology of antithrombotic agents. *Ann Pharmacother*. 1995;29:892-905.

157. Halkes PHA, et al. Aspirin plus dipyridamole versus aspirin alone after cerebral ischaemia of arterial origin (ESPRIT): randomised controlled trial. *Lancet*. 2006;367:1665-1673.

158. Hall JG, et al. Maternal and fetal sequelae of anticoagulation during pregnancy. *Am J Med*. 1980;68:122-140.

159. Harenberg J. Is laboratory monitoring of low-molecular-weight heparin therapy necessary? Yes. *J Thromb Haemost*. 2004;2:547-550.

160. Harper P, et al. Bleeding risk with dabigatran in the frail elderly. *N Engl J Med*. 2012;366:864-866.

161. Harrington R, Ansell J. Risk-benefit assessment of anticoagulant therapy. *Drug Saf*. 1991;6:54-69.

162. Harris EN, et al. Antiphospholipid antibodies: a review. *Eur J Rheumatol Inflamm*. 1984;7:5-8.

163. Harrison P, et al. Measuring antiplatelet drug effects in the laboratory. *Thromb Res*. 2007;120:323-336.

164. Heidbuchel H, et al. European Heart Rhythm Association Practical Guide on the use of new oral anticoagulants in patients with non-valvular atrial fibrillation. *Europace*. 2013;15:625-651.

165. Held V, et al. Idarucizumab as antidote to intracerebral hemorrhage under treatment with dabigatran. *Case Rep Neurol*. 2016;8:224-228.

166. Henderson RS Jr, et al. Idarucizumab for dabigatran reversal in emergency type-A aortic dissection. *J Cardiothorac Vasc Anesth*. 2017;31:e80-e81.

167. Herzog E, et al. Effective reversal of edoxaban-associated bleeding with four-factor prothrombin complex concentrate in a rabbit model of acute hemorrhage. *Anesthesiology*. 2015;122:387-398.

168. Ho S-J, Brighton TA. Ximelagatran: direct thrombin inhibitor. *Vasc Health Risk Manag*. 2006;2:49-58.

169. Hofer S, et al. Reversal of anticoagulation with dabigatran in an 82-year-old patient with traumatic retroperitoneal arterial bleeding using the new antidote idarucizumab: a case report. *A A Case Rep*. 2016;7:227-231.

170. Hoffman RS, et al. Evaluation of coagulation factor abnormalities in long-acting anticoagulant overdose. *J Toxicol Clin Toxicol*. 1988;26:233-248.

171. Hokusai VTEI, et al. Edoxaban versus warfarin for the treatment of symptomatic venous thromboembolism. *N Engl J Med*. 2013;369:1406-1415.

172. Holbrook A, et al. Evidence-based management of anticoagulant therapy: antithrombotic therapy and prevention of thrombosis, 9th ed: American College of Chest Physicians Evidence-Based Clinical Practice Guidelines. *Chest*. 2012;141(2 suppl):e152S-e184S.

173. Houde JP, Steinberg G. Intrahepatic hemorrhage after use of low-molecular-weight heparin for total hip arthroplasty. *The Journal of arthroplasty*. 1999;14:372-374.

174. Hovanessian HC. New-generation anticoagulants: the low molecular weight heparins. *Ann Emerg Med*. 2012;34:768-779.

175. Hu Q, Brady JO. Recombinant activated factor VII for treatment of enoxaparin-induced bleeding. *Mayo Clin Proc*. 2004;79:827.

176. Hylek EM, et al. Major hemorrhage and tolerability of warfarin in the first year of therapy among elderly patients with atrial fibrillation. *Circulation*. 2007;115:2689-2696.

177. CURRENT-OASIS 7 Investigators; Mehta SR, et al. Dose comparisons of clopidogrel and aspirin in acute coronary syndromes. *N Engl J Med*. 2010;363:930-942.

178. Iyaniwura TT. Snake venom constituents: biochemistry and toxicology (Part 1). *Vet Hum Toxicol*. 1991;33:468-474.

179. Iyaniwura TT. Snake venom constituents: biochemistry and toxicology (Part 2). *Vet Hum Toxicol*. 1991;33:475-480.

180. Jacques LB. Heparin: an old drug with a new paradigm. *Science*. 1979;206:528-533.

181. Janssen Pharmaceuticals Inc. Xarelto prescribing information. https://www.xareltohcp.com/shared/product/xarelto/prescribing-information.pdf. Accessed September 21, 2017.

182. Jin RC, et al. Endogenous mechanisms of inhibition of platelet function. *Microcirculation*. 2005;12:247-258.

183. Jones EC, et al. Prolonged anticoagulation in rat poisoning. *JAMA*. 1984;252:3005-3007.

184. Jones JB, Docherty A. Non-invasive treatment of ST elevation myocardial infarction. *Postgrad Med J*. 2007;83:725-730.

185. Junagade P, et al. Fixed dose prothrombin complex concentrate for the reversal of oral anticoagulation therapy. *Hematology*. 2007;12:439-440.

186. Kaatz S, et al. Guidance on the emergent reversal of oral thrombin and factor Xa inhibitors. *Am J Hematol*. 2012;(87 suppl 1):S141-S145.

187. Kafke W, Kraft P. Intravenous thrombolysis after reversal of dabigatran by idarucizumab: a case report. *Case Rep Neurol*. 2016;8:140-144.

188. Kakkar AK, et al. Extended duration rivaroxaban versus short-term enoxaparin for the prevention of venous thromboembolism after total hip arthroplasty: a double-blind, randomised controlled trial. *Lancet*. 2008;372:31-39.

189. Katona B, et al. Anticoagulant rodenticide poisoning. *Vet Hum Toxicol*. 1986;28:478-478.

190. Katona B, Wason S. Superwarfarin poisoning. *J Emerg Med*. 1989;7:627-631.

191. Keeney M, et al. Effect of activated recombinant human factor 7 (Niastase) on laboratory testing of inhibitors of factors VIII and IX. *Lab Hematol*. 2005;11:118-123.

192. Klein SM, et al. Enoxaparin associated with psoas hematoma and lumbar plexopathy after lumbar plexus block. *Anesthesiology*. 1997;87:1576-1579.

193. Koch-Weser J. Coumarin necrosis. *Ann Intern Med*. 1968;68:1365-1367.

194. Kruse JA, Carlson RW. Fatal rodenticide poisoning with brodifacoum. *Ann Emerg Med*. 1992;21:331-336.

195. Krynetskiy E, McDonnell P. Building individualized medicine: prevention of adverse reactions to warfarin therapy. *J Pharmacol Exp Ther*. 2007;322:427-434.

196. Kubitza D, et al. Safety, tolerability, pharmacodynamics, and pharmacokinetics of rivaroxaban—an oral, direct Factor Xa inhibitor—are not affected by aspirin. *J Clin Pharmacol*. 2006;46:981-990.

197. Kubitza D, et al. Safety, pharmacodynamics, and pharmacokinetics of single doses of BAY 59-7939, an oral, direct factor Xa inhibitor. *Clin Pharmacol Ther*. 2005;78:412-421.

198. Kubitza D, et al. Safety, pharmacodynamics, and pharmacokinetics of BAY 59-7939—an oral, direct Factor Xa inhibitor—after multiple dosing in healthy male subjects. *Eur J Clin Pharmacol*. 2005;61:873-880.

199. Kuijpers EA, et al. A method for the simultaneous identification and quantitation of five superwarfarin rodenticides in human serum. *J Anal Toxicol*. 1995;19:557-562.

200. Kulkarni S, et al. A revised model of platelet aggregation. *J Clin Investig*. 2000;105:783-791.

201. Kunert M, et al. Value of activated blood coagulation time in monitoring anticoagulation during coronary angioplasty. *Z Kardiol*. 1996;85:118-124.

202. Lacy JP, Goodin RR. Letter: warfarin-induced necrosis of skin. *Ann Intern Med*. 1975;82:381-382.

203. Lassen MR, et al. Rivaroxaban versus enoxaparin for thromboprophylaxis after total knee arthroplasty. *N Engl J Med*. 2008;358:2776-2786.

204. Lassen MR, et al. The efficacy and safety of apixaban, an oral, direct factor Xa inhibitor, as thromboprophylaxis in patients following total knee replacement. *J Thromb Haemost*. 2007;5:2368-2375.

205. Lassen MR, et al. Apixaban versus Enoxaparin for thromboprophylaxis after hip replacement. *N Engl J Med*. 2010;363:2487-2498.

206. Lassen MR, et al. Apixaban versus enoxaparin for thromboprophylaxis after knee replacement (ADVANCE-2): a randomised double-blind trial. *Lancet*. 2010;375: 807-815.

207. Laupacis A, Fergusson D. Drugs to minimize perioperative blood loss in cardiac surgery: meta-analyses using perioperative blood transfusion as the outcome. The International Study of Peri-operative Transfusion (ISPOT) Investigators. *Anesthes Analg*. 1997;85:1258-1267.

208. Lawrence PF, Goodman GR. Thrombolytic therapy. *Surg Clin North Am*. 1992;72: 899-918.

209. Lechner K, Pabinger-Fasching I. Lupus anticoagulants and thrombosis. A study of 25 cases and review of the literature. *Haemostasis*. 1985;15:254-262.

210. Leck JB, Park BK. A comparative study of the effects of warfarin and brodifacoum on the relationship between vitamin K1 metabolism and clotting factor activity in warfarin-susceptible and warfarin-resistant rats. *Biochem Pharmacol*. 1981;30:123-128.

211. Lecker I, et al. Tranexamic acid concentrations associated with human seizures inhibit glycine receptors. *J Clin Investig*. 2012;122:4654-4666.

212. Lehmann T, et al. Massive human rivaroxaban overdose. *Thromb Haemost*. 2014;112: 834-836.

213. Leikin SM, et al. The X factor: lack of bleeding after an acute apixaban overdose. *Am J Emerg Med*. 2016.

214. Leithauser B, et al. Effects of desmopressin on platelet membrane glycoproteins and platelet aggregation in volunteers on clopidogrel. *Clinical Hemorheol Microcirc*. 2008;39:293-302.

215. Leizorovicz A, et al. Factor Xa inhibition: correlation between the plasma levels of anti-Xa activity and occurrence of thrombosis and haemorrhage. *Haemostasis*. 1993;23(suppl 1):89-98.

216. Leon MB, et al. A clinical trial comparing three antithrombotic drug regimens after coronary-artery stenting. *N Engl J Med*. 1998;339:1665-1671.

217. Levi M. Emergency reversal of antithrombotic treatment. *Intern Emerg Med*. 2009;4: 137-145.

218. Levi M, et al. Pharmacological strategies to decrease excessive blood loss in cardiac surgery: a meta-analysis of clinically relevant endpoints. *Lancet*. 1999;354:1940-1947.

219. Levi M, et al. Safety of recombinant activated factor VII in randomized clinical trials. *N Engl J Med*. 2010;363:1791-1800.

220. Levine M, et al. A comparison of low-molecular-weight heparin administered primarily at home with unfractionated heparin administered in the hospital for proximal deep-vein thrombosis. *N Engl J Med*. 1996;334:677-681.

221. Levine MN, et al. A randomized trial comparing activated thromboplastin time with heparin assay in patients with acute venous thromboembolism requiring large daily doses of heparin. *Arch Intern Med*. 1994;154:49-56.

222. Lincoff AM, et al. Effect of the REG1 anticoagulation system versus bivalirudin on outcomes after percutaneous coronary intervention (REGULATE-PCI): a randomised clinical trial. *Lancet*. 2016;387:349-356.

223. Linkins L-A, et al. Treatment and prevention of heparin-induced thrombocytopenia: antithrombotic therapy and prevention of thrombosis, 9th ed: American College of Chest Physicians Evidence-Based Clinical Practice Guidelines. *Chest*. 2012;141(2 suppl): e495S-530S.

224. Linkins LA, Moffat K. Monitoring the anticoagulant effect after a massive rivaroxaban overdose. *J Thromb Haemost*. 2014;12:1570-1571.

225. Lip GY, et al. Comparative validation of a novel risk score for predicting bleeding risk in anticoagulated patients with atrial fibrillation: the HAS-BLED (Hypertension, Abnormal Renal/Liver Function, Stroke, Bleeding History or Predisposition, Labile INR, Elderly, Drugs/Alcohol Concomitantly) score. *J Am Coll Cardiol*. 2011;57:173-180.

226. Lipton RA, Klass EM. Human ingestion of a "superwarfarin" rodenticide resulting in a prolonged anticoagulant effect. *JAMA*. 1984;252:3004-3005.

227. Liu H, et al. Lessons learned from the contamination of heparin. *Natural Prod Rep*. 2009;26:313-321.

228. Longstaff C, et al. Fibrin binding and the regulation of plasminogen activators during thrombolytic therapy. *Cardiovasc Hematol Agents Med Chem*. 2008;6:212-223.

229. Lu G, et al. A specific antidote for reversal of anticoagulation by direct and indirect inhibitors of coagulation factor Xa. *Nat Med*. 2013;19:446-451.

230. Lund M. Comparative effect of the three rodenticides warfarin, difenacoum and brodifacoum on eight rodent species in short feeding periods. *J Hygiene*. 1981;87:101-107.

231. Macfarlane RG. An enzyme cascade in the blood clotting mechanism, and its function as a biochemical amplifier. *Nature*. 1964;202:498-499.

232. MacLean JA, et al. Adverse reactions to heparin. *Ann Allergy*. 1990;65:254-259.

233. Majerus P, et al. Anticoagulant, thrombolytic, and antiplatelet drugs. In: Hardiman J, et al., eds. *Goodman and Gilman's The Pharmacologic Basis of Therapeutics*. 9th ed. New York, NY: McGraw-Hill; 1996:1341-1359.

234. Makris M, et al. Emergency oral anticoagulant reversal: the relative efficacy of infusions of fresh frozen plasma and clotting factor concentrate on correction of the coagulopathy. *Thromb Haemost*. 1997;77:477.

235. Marino KK, et al. Management of dabigatran-associated bleeding with two doses of idarucizumab plus hemodialysis. *Pharmacotherapy*. 2016;36:e160-e165.

236. Markland FS. Snake venoms and the hemostatic system. *Toxicon*. 1998;36:1749-1800.

237. Marlu R, et al. Effect of non-specific reversal agents on anticoagulant activity of dabigatran and rivaroxaban. A randomised crossover ex vivo study in healthy volunteers. *Thromb Haemost*. 2012;108:217-224.

238. Martin CM, et al. Surreptitious self-administration of heparin. *JAMA*. 1970;212:475-476.

239. Mathiesen T, et al. Intracranial traumatic and non-traumatic haemorrhagic complications of warfarin treatment. *Acta Neurol Scand*. 1995;91:208-214.

240. Matsushima N, et al. Bioavailability and safety of the factor Xa inhibitor edoxaban and the effects of quinidine in healthy subjects. *Clin Pharmacol Drug Dev*. 2013;2:358-366.

241. McAvoy TJ. Pharmacokinetic modeling of heparin and its clinical implications. *J Pharmacokinet Biopharm*. 1979;7:331-354.

242. McGehee WG, et al. Coumarin necrosis associated with hereditary protein C deficiency. *Ann Intern Med*. 1984;101:59-60.

243. Mega JL, et al. Rivaroxaban in patients with a recent acute coronary syndrome. *N Engl J Med*. 2012;366:9-19.

244. Mega JL, et al. Reduced-function cyp2c19 genotype and risk of adverse clinical outcomes among patients treated with clopidogrel predominantly for PCI: a meta-analysis. *JAMA*. 2010;304:1821-1830.

245. Mehta PD, et al. Coagulopathy after accidental pediatric rivaroxaban ingestion. *Clin Toxicol*. 2012;50:602-603.

246. Melissari E, et al. Use of low molecular weight heparin in pregnancy. *Thromb Haemost*. 1992;68:652-656.

247. Mendell J, et al. The effect of rifampin on the pharmacokinetics of edoxaban in healthy adults. *Clin Drug Investig*. 2015;35:447-453.

248. Michelsen LG, et al. Heparinase I (neutralase) reversal of systemic anticoagulation. *Anesthesiology*. 1996;85:339-346.

249. Midathada MV, et al. Recombinant factor VIIa in the treatment of bleeding. *Am J Clin Pathol*. 2004;121:124-137.

250. Mikkaichi T, et al. Edoxaban transport via *P*-glycoprotein is a key factor for the drug's disposition. *Drug Metab Dispos*. 2014;42:520-528.

251. Miner J, Hoffhines A. The discovery of aspirin's antithrombotic effects. *Texas Heart Inst J*. 2007;34:179-186.

252. Monagle P, et al. Antithrombotic therapy in children: the Seventh ACCP Conference on Antithrombotic and Thrombolytic Therapy. *Chest*. 2004;126(3 suppl):645S-687S.

253. Monagle P, et al. Antithrombotic therapy in neonates and children: antithrombotic therapy and prevention of thrombosis, 9th ed: American College of Chest Physicians Evidence-Based Clinical Practice Guidelines. *Chest*. 2012;141(2 suppl):e737S-e801S.

254. Monte AA, et al. Low-molecular-weight heparin overdose: management by observation. *Ann Pharmacother*. 2010;44:1836-1839.

255. Moore T, et al. Monitoring FDA MedWatch Reports: anticoagulants the, leading reported drug risk in 2011. http://www.ismp.org/QuarterWatch/pdfs/2011Q4.pdf. Accessed September 28, 2017.

256. Morrissey B, et al. Washington's experience and recommendations re: anticoagulant rodenticides. *Vet Hum Toxicol*. 1995;37:362-363.

257. Mosher DF. Blood coagulation and fibrinolysis: an overview. *Clin Cardiol*. 1990;13 (4 suppl 6): VI5-11.

258. Motovska Z, et al. Prasugrel versus ticagrelor in patients with acute myocardial infarction treated with primary percutaneous coronary intervention: multicenter Randomized PRAGUE-18 Study. *Circulation*. 2016;134:1603-1612.

259. Mueller RL, Scheidt S. History of drugs for thrombotic disease. Discovery, development, and directions for the future. *Circulation*. 1994;89:432-449.

260. Mullins ME, et al. Unintentional pediatric superwarfarin exposures: do we really need a prothrombin time? *Pediatrics*. 2000;105:402-404.

261. Mumoli N, et al. Conservative management of intentional massive dabigatran overdose. *J Am Geriatr Soc*. 2015;63:2205-2207.

262. Murdoch DA. Prolonged anticoagulation in chlorphacinone poisoning. *Lancet*. 1983;1:355-356.

263. Mutzenbach JS, et al. Intravenous thrombolysis in acute ischemic stroke after dabigatran reversal with idarucizumab - a case report. *Ann Clin Transl Neurol*. 2016;3: 889-892.

264. Ng HJ, et al. Successful control of postsurgical bleeding by recombinant factor VIIa in a renal failure patient given low molecular weight heparin and aspirin. *Ann Hematol*. 2003;82:257-258.

265. Nichols WL. Von Willebrand disease and hemorrhagic abnormalities of platelet and vascular function. In: Lee Goldman AIS, ed. *Goldman-Cecil Medicine*. 25th ed. New York, NY: Elsevier Saunders; 2015.

266. Nimjee SM, et al. The potential of aptamers as anticoagulants. *Trends Cardiovasc Med*. 2005;15:41-45.

267. Nitta K, et al. Diffuse alveolar hemorrhage associated with edoxaban therapy. *Case Rep Crit Care*. 2016;2016:7938062.

268. O'Bryan SM, Constable DJ. Quantification of brodifacoum in plasma and liver tissue by HPLC. *J Anal Toxicol*. 1991;15:144-147.

269. O'Connell KA, et al. Thromboembolic adverse events after use of recombinant human coagulation factor VIIa. *JAMA*. 2006;295:293-298.

270. O'Reilly RA. Vitamin K antagonists. In: Colman RW, et al., eds. *Hemostasis and Thrombosis*. Philadelphia, PA: Lippincott; 1987.

271. O'Reilly RA, Aggeler PM. Surreptitious ingestion of coumarin anticoagulant drugs. *Ann Intern Med.* 1966;64:1034-1041.

272. Ollier E, et al. Effect of activated charcoal on rivaroxaban complex absorption. *Clin Pharmacokinet.* 2017;56:793-801.

273. Olsson P, et al. The elimination from plasma of intravenous heparin. An experimental study on dogs and humans. *Acta Med Scand.* 1963;173:619-630.

274. Oster JR, et al. Heparin-induced aldosterone suppression and hyperkalemia. *Am J Med.* 1995;98:575-586.

275. Osterud B, Rapaport SI. Activation of factor IX by the reaction product of tissue factor and factor VII: additional pathway for initiating blood coagulation. *Proc Nat Acad Sci U S A.* 1977;74:5260-5264.

276. Pachman DJ. Accidental heparin poisoning in an infant. *Am J Dis Child.* 1965;110:210-212.

277. Park BK, Leck JB. A comparison of vitamin K antagonism by warfarin, difenacoum and brodifacoum in the rabbit. *Biochem Pharmacol.* 1982;31:3635-3639.

278. Park BK, et al. Plasma disposition of vitamin K1 in relation to anticoagulant poisoning. *Br J Clin Pharmacol.* 1984;18:655-662.

279. Parsons BJ, et al. Rodenticide poisoning among children. *Aust N Z J Public Health.* 1996;20:488-492.

280. Paspa PA, Movahed A. Thrombolytic therapy in acute myocardial infarction. *Am Fam Phys.* 1992;45:640-648.

281. Patel MR, et al. Rivaroxaban versus warfarin in nonvalvular atrial fibrillation. *N Engl J Med.* 2011;365:883-891.

282. Peetermans M, et al. Idarucizumab for dabigatran overdose. *Clin Toxicol (Phila).* 2016;54:644-646.

283. Perzborn E, et al. The discovery and development of rivaroxaban, an oral, direct factor Xa inhibitor. *Nat Rev Drug Discov.* 2011;10:61-75.

284. Pinner NA, et al. Treatment of warfarin-related intracranial hemorrhage: a comparison of prothrombin complex concentrate and recombinant activated factor VII. *World Neurosurg.* 2010;74:631-635.

285. Pisters R, et al. A novel user-friendly score (HAS-BLED) to assess 1-year risk of major bleeding in patients with atrial fibrillation: the Euro Heart Survey. *Chest.* 2010;138:1093-1100.

286. Platell CF, Tan EG. Hypersensitivity reactions to heparin: delayed onset thrombocytopenia and necrotizing skin lesions. *Aust N Z J Surg.* 1986;56:621-623.

287. Pollack CV Jr, et al. Idarucizumab for dabigatran reversal. *N Engl J Med.* 2015;373:511-520.

288. Povsic TJ, et al. Dose selection for a direct and selective factor ixa inhibitor and its complementary reversal agent: translating pharmacokinetic and pharmacodynamic properties of the REG1 system to clinical trial design. *J Thromb Thrombolysis.* 2011;32:21-31.

289. Povsic TJ, et al. A randomized, partially blinded, multicenter, active-controlled, dose-ranging study assessing the safety, efficacy, and pharmacodynamics of the REG1 anticoagulation system in patients with acute coronary syndromes: design and rationale of the RADAR Phase IIb trial. *Am Heart J.* 2011;161:261-268.e262.

290. Povsic TJ, et al. Pre-existing anti-PEG antibodies are associated with severe immediate allergic reactions to pegnivacogin, a PEGylated aptamer. *J Allergy Clin Immunol.* 2016;138:1712-1715.

291. Povsic TJ, et al; RADAR Investigators. A phase 2, randomized, partially blinded, active-controlled study assessing the efficacy and safety of variable anticoagulation reversal using the REG1 system in patients with acute coronary syndromes: results of the RADAR trial. *Eur Heart J.* 2013;34:2481-2489.

293. Price J, et al. Mechanical valve thrombosis with dabigatran. *J Am Coll Cardiol.* 2012;60:1710-1711.

294. Quintard H, et al. Idarucizumab administration for reversing dabigatran effect in an acute kidney injured patient with bleeding. *Thromb Haemost.* 2017;117:196-197.

295. Raghavan N, et al. Apixaban metabolism and pharmacokinetics after oral administration to humans. *Drug Metab Dispos.* 2009;37:74-81.

296. Raskob G, et al. Extended duration of anticoagulation with edoxaban in patients with venous thromboembolism: a post-hoc analysis of the Hokusai-VTE study. *Lancet Haematol.* 2016;3:e228-236.

297. Raskob G, et al. Oral direct factor Xa inhibition with edoxaban for thromboprophylaxis after elective total hip replacement. A randomised double-blind dose-response study. *Thromb Haemost.* 2010;104:642-649.

298. Reddan DN, et al. Treatment effects of eptifibatide in planned coronary stent implantation in patients with chronic kidney disease (ESPRIT Trial). *Am J Cardiol.* 2003;91:17-21.

299. Renowden S, et al. Oral cholestyramine increases elimination of warfarin after overdose. *BMJ.* 1985;291:513-514.

300. Repplinger DJ, et al. Lack of significant bleeding despite large acute rivaroxaban overdose confirmed with whole blood concentrations. *Clin Toxicol (Phila).* 2016;54:647-649.

301. Reuler JB. Hypothermia: pathophysiology, clinical settings, and management. *Ann Intern Med.* 1978;89:519-527.

302. Rich EC, Drage CW. Severe complications of intravenous phytonadione therapy. Two cases, with one fatality. *Postgrad Med.* 1982;72:303-306.

303. Rimsans J, et al. Idarucizumab for urgent reversal of dabigatran for heart transplant: a case report. *Am J Hematol.* 2017;92:E34-E35.

304. Roberts HR, Lozier JN. New perspectives on the coagulation cascade. *Hosp Pract (Off Ed).* 1992;27:97-105, 109-112.

305. Roberts I, et al. Effect of tranexamic acid on mortality in patients with traumatic bleeding: prespecified analysis of data from randomised controlled trial. *BMJ.* 2012;345:e5839.

306. Romualdi E, et al. Anticoagulant therapy for venous thromboembolism during pregnancy: a systematic review and a meta-analysis of the literature. *J Thromb Haemost.* 2013;11:270-281.

307. Rosenberg L, et al. Idarucizumab for reversal of dabigatran prior to acute surgery: a schematic approach based on a case report. *Basic Clin Pharmacol Toxicol.* 2017;120:407-410.

308. Rosenberg RD. Actions and interactions of antithrombin and heparin. *N Engl J Med.* 1975;292:146-151.

309. Rottenstreich A, et al. Idarucizumab for dabigatran reversal—does one dose fit all? *Thromb Res.* 2016;146:103-104.

310. Ruff CT, al. Association between edoxaban dose, concentration, anti-Factor Xa activity, and outcomes: an analysis of data from the randomised, double-blind ENGAGE AF-TIMI 48 trial. *Lancet.* 2015;385:2288-2295.

311. Rundgren M, Engstrom M. A thromboelastometric evaluation of the effects of hypothermia on the coagulation system. *Anesthes Analg.* 2008;107:1465-1468.

312. Sabatine MS, et al. Addition of clopidogrel to aspirin and fibrinolytic therapy for myocardial infarction with ST-segment elevation. *N Engl J Med.* 2005;352:1179-1189.

313. Sacco RL, et al. Aspirin and extended-release dipyridamole versus clopidogrel for recurrent stroke. *N Engl J Med.* 2008;359:1238-1251.

314. Sallah S, et al. Warfarin and heparin-induced skin necrosis and the purple toe syndrome: infrequent complications of anticoagulant treatment. *Thromb Haemost.* 1997;78:785-790.

315. Samama CM. Prothrombin complex concentrates: a brief review. *Eur J Anaesthesiol.* 2008;25:784-789.

316. Samama MM, et al. Laboratory assessment of rivaroxaban: a review. *Thromb J.* 2013;11:11.

317. Samos M, et al. Monitoring of dabigatran therapy using Hemoclot((R)) Thrombin Inhibitor assay in patients with atrial fibrillation. *J Thromb Thrombolysis.* 2015;39:95-100.

318. Sane DC, et al. Bleeding during thrombolytic therapy for acute myocardial infarction: mechanisms and management. *Ann Intern Med.* 1989;111:1010-1022.

319. Sauter TC, et al. Reversal of dabigatran using idarucizumab in a septic patient with impaired kidney function in real-life practice. *Case Rep Emerg Med.* 2016;2016:1393057.

320. Schafer N, et al. Systemic thrombolysis for ischemic stroke after antagonizing dabigatran with idarucizumab—a case report. *J Stroke Cerebrovasc Dis.* 2016;25:e126-127.

321. Schiele F, et al. A specific antidote for dabigatran: functional and structural characterization. *Blood.* 2013;121:3554-3562.

322. Schiele F, et al. [Anticoagulant therapy with recombinant hirudin in patients with thrombopenia induced by heparin]. *Presse Med.* 1996;25:757-760.

323. Schiff BL, Kern AB. Cutaneous reactions to anticoagulants. *Arch Dermatol.* 1968;98:136-137.

324. Schousboe I. beta 2-Glycoprotein I: a plasma inhibitor of the contact activation of the intrinsic blood coagulation pathway. *Blood.* 1985;66:1086-1091.

325. Schousboe I, Rasmussen MS. Synchronized inhibition of the phospholipid mediated autoactivation of factor XII in plasma by beta 2-glycoprotein I and anti-beta 2-glycoprotein I. *Thromb Haemost.* 1995;73:798-804.

326. Schreiner RL, et al. Accidental heparin toxicity in the newborn intensive care unit. *J Pediatr.* 1978;92:115-116.

327. Schulz JG, Kreps B. Idarucizumab elimination of dabigatran minutes before systemic thrombolysis in acute ischemic stroke. *J Neurol Sci.* 2016;370:44.

328. Schwartz BS. Heparin: what is it? How does it work? *Clin Cardiol.* 1990;13(4 suppl 6):VI12-15.

329. Serruys PW, et al. A comparison of hirudin with heparin in the prevention of restenosis after coronary angioplasty. Helvetica Investigators. *N Engl J Med.* 1995;333:757-763.

330. Shapiro S. Acquired anticoagulants. In: Williams W, et al., eds. *Hematology.* 2nd ed. New York, NY: McGraw-Hill; 1973:1447-1454.

331. Shapiro S, et al. Idarucizumab for dabigatran overdose in a child. *Br J Haematol.* 2018;180:457-459.

332. Shepherd G, et al. Acute, unintentional pediatric brodifacoum ingestions. *Pediatr Emerg Care.* 2002;18:174-178.

333. Sherman DG, Atkinson RP. Intravenous ancrod for treatment of acute ischemic stroke: the STAT study: a randomized controlled trial. Stroke Treatment with Ancrod Trial. *JAMA.* 2000;283:2395-2403.

334. Shi W, et al. Anticardiolipin antibodies block the inhibition by beta 2-glycoprotein I of the factor Xa generating activity of platelets. *Thromb Haemost.* 1993;70:342-345.

335. Shields RC, et al. Efficacy and safety of intravenous phytonadione (vitamin K1) in patients on long-term oral anticoagulant therapy. *Mayo Clin Proc.* 2001;76:260-266.

336. Shiraishi A, et al. Effectiveness of early administration of tranexamic acid in patients with severe trauma. *Br J Surg.* 2017;104:710-717.

337. Siegal DM, et al. Andexanet alfa for the reversal of factor Xa inhibitor activity. *N Engl J Med.* 2015;373:2413-2424.

338. Simoons ML. A comparison of recombinant Hirudin with heparin for the treatment of acute coronary syndromes. The Global Use of Strategies to Open Occluded Coronary Arteries (GUSTO) IIb Investigators. *N Engl J Med.* 1996;335:775-782.

339. Sims PJ, et al. Complement proteins C5b-9 cause release of membrane vesicles from the platelet surface that are enriched in the membrane receptor for coagulation factor Va and express prothrombinase activity. *J Biol Chem.* 1988;263:18205-18212.

340. Singh T, et al. Extracorporeal therapy for dabigatran removal in the treatment of acute bleeding: a single center experience. *Clin J Am Soc Nephrol.* 2013;8:1533-1539.

341. Smitherman TC. Considerations affecting selection of thrombolytic agents. *Mol Biol Med.* 1991;8:207-218.

342. Smolinske SC, et al. Superwarfarin poisoning in children: a prospective study. *Pediatrics.* 1989;84:490-494.

343. Sperling RT, et al. Platelet glycoprotein IIb/IIIa inhibition with eptifibatide: prolongation of inhibition of aggregation in acute renal failure and reversal with hemodialysis. Ca4theter *Cardiovasc Interv.* 2003;59:459-462.

344. Spiller HA, et al. Dermal absorption of a liquid diphacinone rodenticide causing coagulopathy. *Vet Hum Toxicol.* 2003;45:313-314.

345. Spiller HA, et al. An observational study of the factor Xa inhibitors rivaroxaban and apixaban as reported to eight poison centers. *Ann Emerg Med.* 2016;67:189-195.

346. Stangier J. Clinical pharmacokinetics and pharmacodynamics of the oral direct thrombin inhibitor dabigatran etexilate. *Clin Pharmacokinet.* 2008;47:285-295.

347. Stangier J, et al. Pharmacokinetic profile of the oral direct thrombin inhibitor dabigatran etexilate in healthy volunteers and patients undergoing total hip replacement. *J Clin Pharmacol.* 2005;45:555-563.

348. Stangier J, Feuring M. Using the HEMOCLOT direct thrombin inhibitor assay to determine plasma concentrations of dabigatran. *Blood Coagul Fibrinolysis.* 2012;23:138-143.

349. Stangier J, et al. The pharmacokinetics, pharmacodynamics and tolerability of dabigatran etexilate, a new oral direct thrombin inhibitor, in healthy male subjects. *Br J Clin Pharmacol.* 2007;64:292-303.

350. Stangier J, et al. Influence of renal impairment on the pharmacokinetics and pharmacodynamics of oral dabigatran etexilate: an open-label, parallel-group, single-centre study. *Clin Pharmacokinet.* 2010;49:259-268.

351. Starke RM, et al. A prospective cohort study of idarucizumab for reversal of dabigatran-associated hemorrhage. *Neurosurgery.* 2015;77:N11-13.

352. Steinhubl SR, et al. Early and sustained dual oral antiplatelet therapy following percutaneous coronary intervention—a randomized controlled trial. *JAMA.* 2002;288:2411-2420.

353. Stenflo J, Suttie JW. Vitamin K-dependent formation of gamma-carboxyglutamic acid. *Ann Rev Biochem.* 1977;46:157-172.

354. Stevenson RE, et al. Hazards of oral anticoagulants during pregnancy. *JAMA.* 1980;243:1549-1551.

355. Stine RJ. Accidental hypothermia. *J Am Coll Emerg Phys.* 1977;6:413-416.

356. Sturridge F, et al. The use of low molecular weight heparin for thromboprophylaxis in pregnancy. *British J Obstet Gynaecol.* 1994;101:69-71.

357. Sutcliffe FA, et al. Aspects of anticoagulant action: a review of the pharmacology, metabolism and toxicology of warfarin and congeners. *Rev Drug Metab Drug Interact.* 1987;5:225-272.

358. Suttie JW. Warfarin and vitamin K. *Clin Cardiol.* 1990;13(4 suppl 6):VI16-18.

359. Suttie JW, Jackson CM. Prothrombin structure, activation, and biosynthesis. *Physiol Rev.* 1977;57:1-70.

360. Tcheng JE. Clinical challenges of platelet glycoprotein IIb/IIIa receptor inhibitor therapy: bleeding, reversal, thrombocytopenia, and retreatment. *Am Heart J.* 2000;139(2 suppl):s38-s45.

361. Tello-Montoliu A, et al. Antiplatelet therapy: thrombin receptor antagonists. *Br J Clin Pharmacol.* 2011;72:658-671.

362. Teng R, et al. Absorption, distribution, metabolism, and excretion of ticagrelor in healthy subjects. *Drug Metab Dispos.* 2010;38:1514-1521.

363. Thorborg C, et al. Reversal by the specific antidote, idarucizumab, of elevated dabigatran exposure in a patient with rectal perforation and paralytic ileus. *Br J Anaesth.* 2016;117:407-409.

364. Thorne KM, et al. Thrombotic events after discontinuing dabigatran: rebound or resumption? *BMJ.* 2012;345:e4469.

365. Tolman KG, Cohen A. Accidental hypothermia. *Can Med Assoc J.* 1970;103:1357-1361.

366. Travis SF, et al. Spontaneous hemorrhage associated with accidental brodifacoum poisoning in a child. *J Pediatr.* 1993;122:982-984.

367. Truumees E, et al. Epidural hematoma and intraoperative hemorrhage in a spine trauma patient on Pradaxa (dabigatran). *Spine.* 2012;37:E863-E865.

368. Tulinsky A. Molecular interactions of thrombin. *Semin Thromb Hemost.* 1996;22:117-124.

369. Turpie AGG, et al. Rivaroxaban versus enoxaparin for thromboprophylaxis after total knee arthroplasty (RECORD4): a randomised trial. *Lancet.* 2009;373:1673-1680.

370. Tuszynski GP, et al. Isolation and characterization of antistasin- an inhibitor of metastasis and coagulation. *J Biol Chem.* 1987;262:9718-9723.

371. US Food and Drug Administration. FDA Drug Safety Communication: FDA study of Medicare patients finds risks lower for stroke and death but higher for gastrointestinal bleeding with Pradaxa (dabigatran) compared to warfarin. https://www.fda.gov/downloads/Drugs/DrugSafety/UCM397606.pdf. Accessed August 25, 2017.

372. Uchino K, Hernandez AV. Dabigatran association with higher risk of acute coronary events: meta-analysis of noninferiority randomized controlled trials. *Arch Intern Med.* 2012;172:397-402.

373. Udall JA. Don't use the wrong vitamin K. *Calif Med.* 1970;112:65-67.

374. Van Ryn J, et al. An antibody selective to dabigatran safely neutralizes both dabigatran-induced anticoagulant and bleeding activity in in vitro and in vivo models. *J Thromb Haemost.* 2011;9:110-110.

375. van Ryn J, et al. Dabigatran anticoagulant activity is neutralized by an antibody selective to dabigatran in in vitro and in vivo models. *J Am Coll Cardiol.* 2011;57:E1130-E1130.

376. van Ryn J, et al. Reversibility of the anticoagulant effect of high doses of the direct thrombin inhibitor dabigatran, by recombinant factor VIIa or activated prothrombin complex concentrate. *Haematologica.* 2008;93(suppl 1):148.

377. van Ryn J, et al. Adsorption of dabigatran etexilate in water or dabigatran in pooled human plasma by activated charcoal in vitro. *Blood.* 2009;114:440-440.

378. van Ryn J, et al. Dabigatran etexilate—a novel, reversible, oral direct thrombin inhibitor: interpretation of coagulation assays and reversal of anticoagulant activity. *Thromb Haemost.* 2010;103:1116-1127.

379. van Veen JJ, et al. Protamine reversal of low molecular weight heparin: clinically effective? *Blood Coagul Fibrinolysis.* 2011;22:565-570.

380. Vasse M. Protein Z, a protein seeking a pathology. *Thromb Haemost.* 2008;100:548-556.

381. Vavalle JP, Cohen MG. The REG1 anticoagulation system: a novel actively controlled factor IX inhibitor using RNA aptamer technology for treatment of acute coronary syndrome. *Future Cardiol.* 2012;8:371-382.

382. Vavalle JP, et al. A phase 1 ascending dose study of a subcutaneously administered factor IXa inhibitor and its active control agent. *J Thromb Haemost.* 2012;10:1303-1311.

383. Verstraete M. Third-generation thrombolytic drugs. *Am J Med.* 2000;109:52-58.

384. Vigano S, et al. Decrease in protein C antigen and formation of an abnormal protein soon after starting oral anticoagulant therapy. *Br J Haematol.* 1984;57:213-220.

385. Vilahur G, et al. Protective effects of ticagrelor on myocardial injury after infarction. *Circulation.* 2016;134:1708-1719.

386. Von Visger J, Magee C. Low molecular weight heparins in renal failure. *J Nephrol.* 2003;16:914-916.

387. Wakefield TW, et al. Effective and less toxic reversal of low-molecular weight heparin anticoagulation by a designer variant of protamine. *J Vasc Surg.* 1995;21:839-849; discussion 849-850.

388. Wakefield TW, et al. A [+18RGD] protamine variant for nontoxic and effective reversal of conventional heparin and low-molecular-weight heparin anticoagulation. *J Surg Res.* 1996;63:280-286.

389. Walenga JM, et al. Laboratory monitoring of the clinical effects of low molecular weight heparins. *Thromb Res Suppl.* 1991;14:49-62.

390. Walenga JM, et al. Rivaroxaban—an oral, direct factor Xa inhibitor—has potential for the management of patients with heparin-induced thrombocytopenia. *Br J Haematol.* 2008;143:92-99.

391. Wang X, et al. Effect of activated charcoal on apixaban pharmacokinetics in healthy subjects. *Am J Cardiovasc Drugs.* 2014;14:147-154.

392. Warkentin TE, et al. Heparin-induced thrombocytopenia in patients treated with low-molecular-weight heparin or unfractionated heparin. *N Engl J Med.* 1995;332:1330-1335.

393. Watts RG, et al. Accidental poisoning with a superwarfarin compound (brodifacoum) in a child. *Pediatrics.* 1990;86:883-887.

394. Weil J, et al. Prophylactic aspirin and risk of peptic ulcer bleeding. *BMJ.* 1995;310:827-830.

395. Weitz JI. Blood coagulation and anticoagulant, fibrinolytic, and antiplatelet drugs. In: Brunton LL, et al., eds. *Goodman & Gilman's The Pharmacological Basis of Therapeutics* 12th ed. New York, NY: McGraw-Hill; 2012.

396. Weitz JI, et al. Randomised, parallel-group, multicentre, multinational phase 2 study comparing edoxaban, an oral factor Xa inhibitor, with warfarin for stroke prevention in patients with atrial fibrillation. *Thromb Haemost.* 2010;104:633-641.

397. Weitz JI, et al. New antithrombotic drugs: antithrombotic therapy and prevention of thrombosis, 9th ed: American College of Chest Physicians Evidence-Based Clinical Practice Guidelines. *Chest.* 2012;141(2 suppl):e120S-e151S.

398. Wells PS, et al. Interactions of warfarin with drugs and food. *Ann Intern Med.* 1994;121:676-683.

399. Wessler S, Gitel SN. Warfarin. From bedside to bench. *N Engl J Med.* 1984;311:645-652.

400. Weyrich AS, et al. Dipyridamole selectively inhibits inflammatory gene expression in platelet-monocyte aggregates. *Circulation.* 2005;111:633-642.

401. White HD. Comparative safety of thrombolytic agents. *Am J Cardiol.* 1991;68:30E-37E.

402. White RH, et al. Management and prognosis of life-threatening bleeding during warfarin therapy. National Consortium of Anticoagulation Clinics. *Arch Intern Med.* 1996;156:1197-1201.

403. Whitlon DS, et al. Mechanism of coumarin action: significance of vitamin K epoxide reductase inhibition. *Biochemistry.* 1978;17:1371-1377.

404. Wiernikowski JT, et al. Reversal of anti-thrombin activity using protamine sulfate. experience in a neonate with a 10-fold overdose of enoxaparin. *Thromb Res.* 2007;120:303-305.

405. Wintzen AR, et al. The risk of intracerebral hemorrhage during oral anticoagulant treatment: a population study. *Ann Neurol.* 1984;16:553-558.

406. Wiviott SD, et al. Prasugrel versus clopidogrel in patients with acute coronary syndromes. *N Engl J Med.* 2007;357:2001-2015.

407. Wong PC, et al. Apixaban, an oral, direct and highly selective factor Xa inhibitor: in vitro, antithrombotic and antihemostatic studies. *J Thromb Haemost*. 2008;6:820-829.

408. Wong PC, Jiang X. Apixaban, a direct factor Xa inhibitor, inhibits tissue-factor induced human platelet aggregation in vitro: comparison with direct inhibitors of factor VIIa, XIa and thrombin. *Thromb Haemost*. 2010;104:302-310.

409. Woo J, et al. Positive outcome after intentional overdose of dabigatran. *J Med Toxicol*. 2012:1-4.

410. Woo JS, et al. Positive outcome after intentional overdose of dabigatran. *J Med Toxicol*. 2013;9:192-195.

411. Woody BJ, et al. Coagulopathic effects and therapy of brodifacoum toxicosis in dogs. *J Vet Intern Med*. 1992;6:23-28.

412. Xu H, et al. Concomitant use of single antiplatelet therapy with edoxaban or warfarin in patients with atrial fibrillation: analysis from the ENGAGE AF-TIMI48 Trial. *J Am Heart Assoc*. 2016;5.

413. Yaghi S, et al. Treatment and outcome of thrombolysis-related hemorrhage: a multi-center retrospective study. *JAMA Neurol*. 2015;72:1451-1457.

414. Yamashita T, et al. Randomized, multicenter, warfarin-controlled phase II study of edoxaban in Japanese patients with non-valvular atrial fibrillation. *Circ J*. 2012;76: 1840-1847.

415. Yee AJ, Kuter DJ. Successful recovery after an overdose of argatroban. *Ann Pharmacother*. 2006;40:336-339.

416. Young MA, et al. Heparin-associated thrombocytopenia and thrombosis syndrome in a rehabilitation patient. *Arch Phys Med Rehabil*. 1989;70:468-470.

417. Zahir H, et al. Edoxaban effects on bleeding following punch biopsy and reversal by a 4-factor prothrombin complex concentrate. *Circulation*. 2015;131:82-90.

418. Zhou W, et al. Hemostatic therapy in experimental intracerebral hemorrhage associated with the direct thrombin inhibitor dabigatran. *Stroke*. 2011;42:3594-3599.

419. Zubkov AY, et al. Predictors of outcome in warfarin-related intracerebral hemorrhage. *Arch Neurol*. 2008;65:1320-1325.

420. Zupancic-Salek S, et al. Successful reversal of anticoagulant effect of superwarfarin poisoning with recombinant activated factor VII. *Blood Coagul Fibrinolysis*. 2005;16: 239-244.

A17

PROTHROMBIN COMPLEX CONCENTRATES AND DIRECT ORAL ANTICOAGULANT ANTIDOTES

Betty C. Chen and Mark K. Su

INTRODUCTION

Prothrombin complex concentrate (PCC) is a lyophilized powder that consists of coagulation factors II, VII, IX, and X in addition to other factors and additives. Prothrombin complex concentrates come in two forms, activated and nonactivated. Activated PCCs (aPCCs) are typically used to treat hemophilia, and formulations consist of a mixture of nonactivated and activated factors. Nonactivated factors require activation by the other cofactors to function in the coagulation cascade. In the United States, nonactivated PCCs are available in both four-factor and three-factor formulations (4F-PCC and 3F-PCC, respectively). Prothrombin complex concentrates are also widely available in Europe, Asia, and Australia. In addition to clotting factors, 4F-PCC contains heparin and antithrombotic factors C and S.[13] Three-factor PCC contains only small amounts of factor VII and heparin.[16] Although some direct oral anticoagulants (DOACs) now have a reversal agent, PCCs are still used to attempt rapid reversal of DOAC-induced coagulopathy.

With dabigatran, the first of the DOACs, the need for a definitive reversal agent became apparent after adverse effects and fatalities were reported. The manufacturer of dabigatran developed idarucizumab, a monoclonal antibody, as a result.[83,84] Similarly, with the rising use of the oral Xa inhibitors, andexanet alfa (Andexxa), a recombinant modified human Factor Xa was recently approved.

PROTHROMBIN COMPLEX CONCENTRATES

History

Prothrombin complex concentrates were initially used for the treatment of patients with hemophilia A. This iteration of PCC is referred to as 3F-PCC because it contains a lower concentration of factor VII compared with 4F-PCC to limit thrombogenic complications. 3F-PCC is approved for the treatment of hemophilia A, but it was used off label to reverse warfarin-induced coagulopathy before the approval of 4F-PCC in the United States. The use of 4F-PCC became routine when consensus guidelines recommended their use to reverse warfarin-associated coagulopathy. Four Factor-PCC was approved for use in the United States in 2013 solely for the purpose of reversing warfarin-associated coagulopathy, but it is routinely used for other indications.

Pharmacology

Prothrombin complex concentrates contain the coagulation factors that are inhibited by vitamin K antagonists (VKAs) such as warfarin. These factors include factors II, VII, IX, and X. They also include proteins C and S. Kcentra (a 4F-PCC) is manufactured from pooled United States sourced plasma. Other countries used pooled regionally sourced plasma. It is then purified, heat treated, nanofiltered, and lyophilized to produce concentrated factors II, VII, IX, and X and proteins C and S (Table A17–1). Nonactivated PCCs also contain antithrombin, albumin, heparin, sodium chloride, and sodium citrate.[44] Three Factor-PCCs contain factors II, IX, and X. In addition, a small amount of factor VII is included. This decreased dose of factor VII is thought to limit thrombogenic complications in patients with hemophilia. The manufacturing process is similar to that of 4F-PCC and therefore contains factors C and S and heparins. Activated prothrombin complex concentrates do not contain heparins, but they do contain some factors of the kinin-generating system.[6]

Mechanism of Action

Vitamin K antagonists impair the synthesis of gamma-carboyxlated factors II, VII, IX, and X in the coagulation cascade. Prothrombin complex concentrates correct warfarin-associated coagulopathy by direct replacement of factors whose synthesis was inhibited.

Pharmacokinetics and Pharmacodynamics

Because PCC products are administered intravenously, their bioavailability is 100%. In a study of 15 healthy volunteers receiving 50 IU/kg of 4F-PCC, maximal concentration of factors and proteins C and S occurred at the earliest sampling point, at 5 minutes postinfusion. These concentrations remained stable the first hour after infusion. Terminal half-lives of factors II, VII, IX, and X were calculated and are shown in Table A17–2.[66] In a prospective study, patients with an international normalized ratio (INR) greater than 2 and requiring emergency reversal of warfarin were treated with 25 to 50 IU/kg of 4F-PCC. The mean infusion rate of 4F-PCC was 7.5 mL/min or 188 IU/min, resulting in normalization of INR (<1.3) in 935 of patients within 30 minutes after completion of 4F-PCC infusion. In addition, the INR remained less than 1.3 for 48 hours after the infusion.[67] In another randomized controlled trial, the INR was reduced to less than 1.3 in 62% of participants at 30 minutes after 4F-PCC infusion.[76]

Adverse Effects and Safety Issues

Most forms of PCC contain small amounts of heparin. These heparin-containing PCCs are contraindicated in patients with a history of heparin-induced thrombocytopenia (HIT) and heparin-induced thrombocytopenia and thrombosis syndrome (HITT). Prothrombin complex concentrates are also contraindicated in patients with disseminated intravascular coagulation (DIC) or with known anaphylactic or severe allergic reactions to any of its components.[16]

Because PCCs are made from human blood, they can theoretically transmit infectious diseases such as viruses, Creutzfeldt-Jakob disease agent, or the variant Creutzfeldt-Jakob disease agent. The manufacturing

TABLE A17–1	Factor and Protein Content in Prothrombin Complex Concentrates[44]					
	Factor II	*Factor VII*	*Factor IX*	*Factor X*	*Protein C*	*Protein S*
Four-factor prothrombin complex concentrate (Kcentra) (IU)	380–800	200–500	400–620	500–1,020	420–820	240–680
Three-factor prothrombin complex concentrate (Bebulin)	120 IU/100 IU of factor IX	13 IU/100 IU of factor IX	100 IU/100 IU of factor IX	100 IU/100 IU of factor IX	NA	NA

NA = not available.

TABLE A17–2	Coagulation Factor and Protein Pharmacokinetics After Four-Factor Prothrombin Complex Concentrate in Healthy Volunteers[66]					
	Factor II	*Factor VII*	*Factor IX*	*Factor X*	*Protein C*	*Protein S*
Terminal half-life (h)	59.7 (45.5–65.9)	4.2 (3.9–6.6)	16.7 (14.2–67.7)	30.7 (23.7–41.1)	47.2 (28.4–65.1)	49.1 (39–59.7)
Volume of distribution (mL/kg)	71 (61.2–78.9)	41.8 (39.3–52.5)	92.4 (76.2–182.2)	56.1 (52.9–60.1)	62.9 (50.1–65)	76.6 (69.8–85.8)

process has minimized the likelihood of disease transmission by screening plasma via a polymerase chain reaction and including pasteurization and nanofiltration, two virus reduction steps. Although the risk of virus transmission is still theoretically possible, it is exceedingly low. Although there are cases of suspected hepatitis and HIV transmission in patients who have received PCCs, these patients also received other blood products, which could have been the source of infection. There are no proven virus transmission cases from 4F-PCC because the virus processing step was introduced in 1996.[6,7,16,30,66]

Fatal and nonfatal thrombotic events are reported with 4F-PCC use. These complications include myocardial infarction (MI), arterial thrombosis, venous thrombosis, pulmonary embolism (PE), cerebrovascular accident, and DIC.[25,48] The risk of developing a thrombotic complication is approximately 1.6% to 2.5% based on a review and meta-analysis that used PCC for reversing warfarin anticoagulation. Data from one publication cited a less than 1% rate of thrombosis based on 4F-PCC administration internationally.[30] Some study investigators have postulated that the rate of thrombotic complications is related to a patient's underlying risk of thrombosis and the original indication for systemic anticoagulation rather than as a result of the PCC.[12,48] This explanation is reasonable considering patients who received 4F-PCC for other indications had a lower rate of thrombosis at 0.9%.[68]

In one study of healthy volunteers receiving 4F-PCC, thrombogenicity was assessed via serial measurements of prothrombin fragment 1+2 (F_{1+2}) and D-dimer. After 4F-PCC infusion, maximal F_{1+2} concentrations occurred 5 minutes postinfusion, the first sampling point.[68] However, many thrombogenic complications are reported to occur long after the first 5 minutes after PCC administration. Therefore, the risk of thrombosis does not seem to be related to thrombogenicity from PCCs alone. Other risk factors such as underlying thrombosis risk and prolonged immobilization also play a large role in risk of thrombogenic complications.

Further studies are required to assess the risk of thrombosis after 4F-PCC administration for the treatment of non-VKA antagonist factor deficiencies. The use of 4F-PCC should be used cautiously because the risk of thrombosis is likely higher than in patients requiring reversal of VKA antagonist coagulopathy. Several studies suggest that patients with liver disease who receive 4F-PCC are at a higher risk of thrombosis because of rebalanced hemostasis via intact thrombin generation and decreased fibrinolytic ability despite abnormal coagulation test results.[50-52,82]

Finally, hypersensitivity to 4F-PCC is reported to have an incidence of 3%. Other side effects include headache, gastrointestinal disturbances, arthralgias, and hypotension.[16] Other formulations of PCC such as 3F-PCC and aPCC also warn of possible hypersensitivity reaction. However, rates of these occurrences are not reported.[6,7]

Pregnancy and Lactation
There are no studies or data available to elucidate the risks of 4F-PCC, 3F-PCC, or aPCC use in pregnancy or breastfeeding. Four Factor-PCC has not been evaluated in pregnant animals and therefore has the potential to cause harm to fetuses.[16] Warfarin is contraindicated in pregnancy because of its teratogenic potential. Therefore, PCCs have no current indication in pregnant women. However, if a pregnant woman is anticoagulated with warfarin and requires emergent reversal, fresh-frozen plasma (FFP) should be used. If the volume associated with FFP is a concern because of the risk of volume overload, then providers can use PCCs but with the caveat that the effects on the pregnancy and fetus are unknown.

There are also no available data regarding excretion of PCC in breast milk, and there is potential for PCC to be excreted in milk. There are also no data

on the effects of PCC on nursing infants or the ability of PCC on the reproductive system. Therefore, PCC should only be used in nursing mothers under severe circumstances, and babies should not be permitted to nurse from mothers who recently received PCC.

Dosing and Administration
Most countries use 4F-PCC for the reversal of VKA-induced anticoagulation. The only brand of 4F-PCC currently available in the United States is Kcentra, although Octaplex is under review by the US Food and Drug Administration (FDA). Dosing of Kcentra is based on INR and actual body weight. The doses are based on factor IX concentration and range between 25 and 50 units/kg with a maximum weight of 100 kg (Table A17–3). The contents of each vial are variable and range between 400 and 620 IU of factor IX. Each individual vial states the actual factor IX content in each bottle, and the individual dosage should be based on the actual factor IX content in each vial.[16,44]

Kcentra must be administered within 4 hours of reconstitution. Reconstitution requires the use of the included Mix2 Vial and diluent vial. Kcentra must be stored at temperatures between 20° and 25°C prior to administration in a separate infusion line. The rate of administration should be started at a rate of 0.12 mL/kg/min (~3 units/kg/min) up to a maximum of 8.4 mL/min (~210 units/min).[16]

All US studies evaluating the safety and efficacy of 4F-PCC have enrolled adults. However, PCC has been used to correct warfarin-associated coagulopathy in a severely ill child with a favorable outcome.[1] Prothrombin complex concentrates have been increasingly used in pediatric patients undergoing cardiac surgery. However, these patients are given PCCs to correct coagulopathy associated with operative complications and not warfarin-associated coagulopathy.[4]

Although current PCC dosing is based on a patient's weight and INR, there has been at least one study evaluating the use of fixed dosing of PCC for the reversal of warfarin-associated coagulopathy. This study noted that this technique was not associated with any thromboembolic complications. Furthermore, the authors postulated that the main benefit of this method of PCC administration minimizes the time to administration of PCC.[45] Unfortunately, this study did not include a control group, and mortality and morbidity were not evaluated or discussed. There are insufficient data to recommend this dosing approach at this time.

Four-Factor Versus Three-Factor Prothrombin Complex Concentrates
Numerous studies have evaluated the efficacy and safety of 4F-PCC versus 3F-PCC. Several retrospective studies indicate faster reversal, high rates of reversal, or lower mortality rates in patients receiving 4F-PCC compared with 3F-PCC.[3,17,57,86] One investigator concluded that the cost effectiveness of 4F-PCC was better than 3F-PCC because of its improved efficacy at reversing coagulopathy.[57] However, not all studies were resoundingly in favor of 4F-PCC over 3F-PCC. In several retrospective studies, the efficacy of reversing INR

TABLE A17–3	Kcentra Dosing Recommendations from the Manufacturer[16]		
Pretreatment INR	2–<4	4–6	>6
Dose of Kcentra (units of factor IX)/kg body weight	25	35	50
Maximum dose (units of factor IX)	Not to exceed 2,500 IU	Not to exceed 3,500 IU	Not to exceed 5,000 IU

INR = international normalized ratio.

Table from manufacturer's prescribing insert.

was about equal regardless of which formulation of PCC was used. Although the rates of thromboembolic complications were similar between the groups in one study, thrombosis complications were higher if 4F-PCC was given.[38,46]

One study evaluated the use of 4F-PCC versus 3F-PCC combined with recombinant factor VIIa (rFVIIa). Although the 3F-PCC with rFVIIa combination resulted in a lower INR, 4F-PCC alone resulted in both decreased deep vein thrombosis (DVT) rates and mortality.[60]

Four-Factor Prothrombin Complex Concentrates Versus Plasma

Numerous studies have evaluated the safety and efficacy of 4F-PCC compared with fresh frozen plasma (FFP) infusion for warfarin reversal.[19,41,56,76] The conclusions from many of these studies show that PCCs leads to more rapid correction of INR compared with plasma. However, it must be noted that the amount of factor replacement between the PCC groups versus the plasma groups was unequal. Typically, the patients in the PCC groups received a dose of 25 to 50 IU/kg, but patients in the plasma group received 10 to 15 mL/kg. These represent factor replacements at ranges of 50% to 100% versus 20% to 30%, respectively.[43,56,75,76] Mortality data have therefore been exceedingly difficult to quantify because of this disparity in factor replacement when comparing PCC versus plasma. A recently published meta-analysis claimed that the odds ratio of mortality for receiving 4F-PCC versus FFP was 0.64 showing an improved mortality rate with 4F-PCC.[12] However, the odds ratio was not statistically significant. Furthermore, when comparing the complications of 4F-PCC to FFP, the rate of thrombosis or thromboembolic disease was higher in patients who received FFP (6.4% versus 2.5%).[12] Despite the potential favorable risk-to-benefit ratio of PCC compared with FFP, it should be noted that these authors were compensated by the manufacturers of PCC. Additionally, there is one other study, included in the aforementioned meta-analysis, that demonstrated no difference in mortality in patients with intracranial hemorrhages.[55] There do appear to be several theoretical advantages of PCCs over FFP, including a smaller volume of infusion, bypassing blood type matching, avoidance of delay for thawing of plasma, and predictable dosing of factors. Despite its significantly increased cost, PCC possesses a lower risk of infection transmission compared with FFP.[33] Aside from four cases of parvovirus B19 transmission associated with Octaplex, there are very few reports of virus transmission associated with PCC administration, and risk is further minimized by additional protective steps added in the manufacturing process.[16,44]

Other Uses for Prothrombin Complex Concentrates

Prothrombin Complex Concentrates for Direct Oral Anticoagulants

Prothrombin complex concentrations can be used to treat coagulopathy from the DOACs. The manufacturers of dabigatran have suggested that PCC can be used to partially reverse the anticoagulant effect of dabigatran, but they admit that its efficacy and safety have not be evaluated in any clinical trials. They now recommended the use of a monoclonal antibody idarucizumab.[11] The manufacturers of rivaroxaban have noted that PCC can be used to partially reverse its anticoagulant activity, but this information is derived from healthy volunteers.[23,37] In theory, PCC can reverse anticoagulation from these DOACs if the amount of factor replacement overwhelms the amount of available DOAC. However, it is very difficult to determine what dose of PCC can establish normal hemostatic conditions, and clinical evidence is scant on their efficacy in this setting. For patients requiring emergent reversal of dabigatran-induced anticoagulation, PCC is a reasonable second-line agent for achieving reversal of anticoagulation after idarucizumab administration. For patients requiring emergent reversal of factor Xa inhibitor–induced anticoagulation, PCC is also a reasonable second line therapy after andexanet alfa administration.

Prothrombin Complex Concentrates in Liver Disease

There are studies evaluating the use of PCC to reverse coagulopathy associated with liver disease. Unfortunately, the rate of INR reversal in patients with liver disease treated with 4F-PCC seems to be significantly less than elevated INRs for other reasons such as warfarin-associated coagulopathy. In one study, INR less than 1.5 was achieved in only 19% of patients who

received 4F-PCC for elevated INR related to liver disease. On the other hand, 81.5% of non–liver disease patients had successful decreases in INR below 1.5 with 4F-PCC.[36] In another study evaluating the use of 3F-PCC or 4F-PCC for elevated INR, patients with nonwarfarin elevation of their INR, in general, had less success (27.7%) of INR reversal to less than 1.3.[63] However, in this study, the patients with liver disease and elevated INR had the most consistent correction to an INR below 1.3.[63] There has been one study comparing the use of FFP versus PCC versus rFVIIa to facilitate procedures in critically ill patients with liver disease. Although bleeding rates were similar among the groups, patients receiving PCC and rFVIIa experienced expedited procedures and fewer blood products compared with those receiving FFP.[47] At this time, there is currently insufficient information to routinely recommend PCC administration to patients with liver disease for the sole purpose of INR correction. For patients with the collective criteria of liver disease, elevated INR, and life-threatening hemorrhage, it would be reasonable to give PCC.

Prothrombin Complex Concentrates in Trauma

There have not been any high-quality studies evaluating the use of 4F-PCC in the setting of coagulopathy from trauma. There are some small studies that have evaluated the use of 3F-PCC in trauma, which have had varying results. There is no overall consensus of whether or not 3F-PCC resulted in a decreased requirement for red blood cell transfusion.[39,61,71,73] Therefore, there is not enough evidence to recommend routine use of PCC to correct coagulopathy from trauma at this time.

Availability

The only brand of 4F-PCC currently available in the United States is Kcentra. Another brand of 4F-PCC, Octaplex, is being evaluated for FDA approval. 3F-PCCs is available as Bebulin. Outside of the United States, the PCCs are available as Beriplex, Confidex, Cofact, OcPlex, Octaplex, Octaplex 1000, Octaplex 500, PPSB S.D., PPSB-HT Nichiyaku Profilnine, Profilnine SD, ProthoRAAS, Prothrombin Complex Octapharm, Prothrombinex-HT, Prothromblex, Prothromplex Immuno Tim 4, Prothromblex NF, Prothromblex Total, Prothromblex Total NF, Protromplex TIM3, Pushu Laishi, TachoSil, Uman Complex, and Uman-Complex D.I.

Activated Prothrombin Complex Concentrates

Similar to 4F-PCCs, aPCCs contain factors II, VII IX, and X. However, the difference between the two PCCs is that aPCCs contain *activated* factor VII instead of nonactivated factor VII. The other clotting factors are nonactivated in both concentrates. The only aPCC product currently available in the United States is factor eight inhibitor bypassing activity (FEIBA). Factor eight inhibitor bypassing activity is traditionally used for the treatment of hemophilia A or B, and it is not FDA approved for warfarin reversal. However, because FEIBA does not contain heparin, it is the recommended therapy to reverse warfarin-associated coagulopathy in critically ill patients with HIT or HITT.

Unfortunately, aPCC has not been studied extensively in the setting of VKA-induced coagulopathy. In one study comparing the aPCC FEIBA versus FFP for reversing warfarin-associated coagulopathy, aPCC was superior to FFP in time to reversal of anticoagulation. However, it should be noted that patients in the aPCC group received more overall factor replacement than the patients in the FFP group. Whereas dosing of the aPCC was either 500 or 1,000 units, the median dose of FFP given was 400 mL. This study did note that successful hemostasis was similar in both arms, and there was no significant difference in hospital length of stay.[5,87] For reversal of DOACs, studies have been limited to small studies, animal studies, or healthy volunteers.[5] In one small study, patients with intracranial hemorrhages who received aPCC did not have intracranial hematoma expansion or thrombotic complications.[20] However, another small study evaluating the use of aPCC in patients with intracranial hemorrhage found that patients receiving aPCC resulted in stable repeat head imaging without hematoma expansion 55% of the time, and 18% of patients experienced thromboembolic complications.[58] In a porcine model, dabigatran-treated study participants had less blood loss after polytrauma after receiving 50 U/kg of aPCC.[34] In the laboratory, both PCC and aPCC corrected thromboelastography and rotational thromboelastometry (laboratory measures of thrombin generation) in patients receiving dabigatran or rivaroxaban.[31] One ex vivo study showed that after a single dose of dabigatran in healthy volunteers, aPCC decreased endogenous thrombin potential and lag time, and thrombin generation increased in a dose-dependent fashion.[59] In a murine study, aPCC reduced bleeding time from dabigatran at low doses. Unfortunately, at high doses, this effect was reduced.[85]

There is no standard dose of aPCC for coagulopathy reversal. Providers should weigh the risks and benefits of aPCC use in anticoagulated patients. If a patient is critically ill and FFP is not rapidly available to reverse warfarin coagulopathy, aPCC is a reasonable intervention. Typical doses for treating bleeding or for perioperative management range between 50 and 100 units/kg with the units measuring the amount of factor VIII inhibitor bypass activity.[6] However, one study evaluated fixed doses of aPCC in adult patients because lower doses which resulted in cessation of bleeding in 93% patients. In this study, patients with an INR of less than 5 received 500 units of aPCC. Patients with INR of greater than 5 received 1,000 units of aPCC; 87% of patients survived to discharge, and no thrombotic complications were noted.[81] Given the thrombogenic potential of FEIBA, this lower dose recommendation is reasonable if FFP is unavailable in warfarin-anticoagulated patients. In patients requiring reversal of direct factor Xa–induced anticoagulation, there are very little data on ideal dosing. Small studies have reported dosages of a PCC between 25 and 100 units/kg to reverse DOAC coagulopathy. If Andexanet alpha or another antidote is unavailable, it is reasonable to administer aPCC to patients with a contraindication to nonactivated PCC in aliquots of 25 units/kg up to a maximum of 100 units/kg. This therapy should be reserved for critically ill patients who need emergent reversal of their anticoagulation.

Recombinant Factor VIIa

Recombinant factor VIIa is approved for patients with hemophilia or various factor inhibitors and has been successfully used to reverse VKA toxicity. However, the safety of off-label use of rFVIIa to reverse VKA coagulopathy is generally unfavorable. Despite weak evidence showing beneficial effects in four patients with long-acting VKA toxicity, there are several studies that consider rFVIIa inferior to PCC in terms of hospital length of stay, blood product transfusion requirements, or mortality.[18,40,88] These studies include both warfarin and other VKA antagonists, which needs to be considered when evaluating the specific effect of rFVIIa on warfarin reversal.

There is also concern that arterial thrombotic events may occur at higher than acceptable rates when factor rFVIIa is administered. Reviewing the data from the FDA's Adverse Event Reporting System database, thromboembolic adverse events were frequent in patients who received rFVIIa for off-label purposes.[65] The Factor Seven for Acute Hemorrhagic Stroke Trial (FAST) showed that arterial thromboembolic complications rose in a dose-dependent fashion with rfVIIa administration.[22] These findings were confirmed in subsequent studies and a meta-analysis.[49] The risk of continued bleeding versus the benefit of rapid reversal of coagulopathy with rFVIIa is unknown, but studies suggest the risk for complications is higher than that of other reversal agents such as PCC. The use of rFVIIa for reversing VKA-associated coagulopathy is generally not recommended given the availability of safer agents. However, if FFP and PCC (activated or nonactivated) cannot be administered or are unavailable, then it is reasonable to administer rFVIIa in life-threatening situations.[2]

IDARUCIZUMAB
History

Idarucizumab was approved by the FDA in 2015. It was designed specifically to reverse the effects of dabigatran, the first of the DOACs. It was approved through the FDA's accelerated approval program because there were no other definitive antidotes or reversal agents for dabigatran before idarucizumab's creation. Idarucizumab is recommended for reversal of dabigatran-associated coagulopathy in the setting of either emergency or urgent surgery (or procedures) and in uncontrolled or life-threatening bleeding.[10]

Pharmacology and Chemistry

Idarucizumab is a humanized monoclonal antibody fragment to dabigatran. To create idarucizumab, mice are immunized with dabigatran-derived haptens, resulting in the production of antibodies targeted against dabigatran. Antibodies with the highest affinity for dabigatran are then chosen and processed to retain the Fab fragment, the antigen binding section of the antibody. Murine protein sequences are then replaced with human protein sequences and then further refined with recombinant DNA processing. The end result is a monoclonal antibody with lower immunogenicity.[78]

Mechanism of Action

Idarucizumab binds directly to dabigatran at an affinity of approximately 350 times higher to the affinity of dabigatran to thrombin. When dabigatran is bound to idarucizumab, its anticoagulant effect is deactivated via normalization of various coagulation parameters.[24,35,78]

Pharmacokinetics and Pharmacodynamics

The bioavailability of idarucizumab is 100% because it is administered intravenously. Peak plasma concentrations occur immediately after infusion.[27] Manufacturers state that the binding of idarucizumab is irreversible given its high affinity for dabigatran.

The volume of distribution of idarucizumab is approximately 0.06 L/kg.[27] Because idarucizumab is primarily located in plasma, it is able to bind plasma dabigatran and encourage extravascular unbound dabigatran to move into the vascular space to reequilibrate. If there is excess or unbound intravascular idarucizumab available, it will be able to bind any newly arriving dabigatran to further neutralize dabigatran and its anticoagulant effects.[9,24,28]

Idarucizumab possesses two half-lives. After peak concentrations are reached, the initial half-life of idarucizumab is approximately 45 minutes. Four hours after administration, only 4% of the peak idarucizumab concentration is detectable in plasma. At that point, the half-life ranges between 4.5 to 8.1 hours.[28] In one study, healthy volunteers were given 220 mg of dabigatran twice daily for 3 days. Then they were given 1 to 7.5 g of idarucizumab. After infusion of idarucizumab, thrombin time, ecarin clotting time, and activated partial thromboplastin time (aPTT) immediately normalized in a dose-dependent fashion. Thirty minutes after idarucizumab infusion, investigators noted that endogenous thrombin potential and thrombin lag time significantly trended toward baseline in a dose-dependent fashion for 4 hours.[28,78]

In a prospective study of patients taking dabigatran and requiring rapid reversal of anticoagulation for either life-threatening hemorrhage or for emergent surgery or procedures, patients who received 5 g of intravenous (IV) idarucizumab had a reversal rate of 100% of patients. However, despite this apparent success, there was a total of 18 deaths in the both study groups (9 in each group). Only 5 of the deaths appeared to be related to bleeding events, and 9 of the deaths occurred within the first 96 hours after idarucizumab administration. Causes of death included septic shock, intracranial hemorrhage, multiorgan failure, hemodynamic collapse, respiratory failure, and cardiac arrest. It is unclear whether the cause of death was related to poor hemostasis but in bleeding patients; hemostasis was restored at a median of 11.4 hours after administration of idarucizumab. In patients undergoing an emergent procedure, normal intraoperative hemostasis was noted in 85% of cases.[70]

Idarucizumab is renally eliminated. The proximal renal tubules are able to reuptake or degrade idarucizumab. However, this process is saturable. The remaining amount of idarucizumab is excreted in the urine unchanged.[14,28,62] There is a dose-dependent increase in the amount of idarucizumab that is recovered in urine. At a dose of 1 mg, 10% of idarucizumab is received in the urine. At 4 g, 40% of idarucizumab is recovered in the urine.[24,27] Dabigatran-bound idarucizumab is also processed in the renal tubules. If the renal tubules process the idarucizumab portion of the complex, then the free dabigatran may be renally excreted.[29,69]

In murine and human studies, idarucizumab administration results in normalization of a battery of functional clotting assays, such as clotting time, aPTT, and thrombin time.[78]

Several case reports suggest that a rebound drug effect occurs after idarucizumab administration. A patient with a massive dabigatran overdose with an initial dabigatran concentration of 3,337.3 ng/mL (the average peak concentration in patients receiving therapeutic dosing of dabigatran is 112.7 ± 66.6 ng/mL[74]) received idarucizumab, resulting in a dabigatran concentration of 513 ng/mL and improvement in coagulopathy. However, 7 hours after receiving idarucizumab, the dabigatran concentration rebounded to 1,126 ng/mL with corresponding increases in INR, PT, and aPTT.[72] Dabigatran rebound after idarucizumab treatment was noted in other case reports.[32] Despite the apparent rapid reversal of anticoagulation by idarucizumab in most cases, some patients experience a recurrent coagulopathy between 12 and 24 hours after receiving idarucizumab, perhaps caused by dabigatran redistribution.[10]

Adverse Effects and Safety Issues

Before approval of idarucizumab, it was tested in over 200 volunteers and well tolerated in doses up to 8 g. No hypersensitivity reactions were reported in any of the volunteers. In addition, no severe antibody reactions were reported in any of the volunteers.[24]

However, patients with hereditary fructose intolerance are at risk for serious adverse effects because the medication contains sorbitol.[10]

Thrombotic events such as DVT, PE, MI, or ischemic stroke are reported after idarucizumab use.[24,70] The true incidence of these thromboembolic complications is unknow, and neither idarucizumab nor its complex with dabigatran is believed to directly cause platelet aggregation or clot formation.[24,78]

Other Uses of Idarucizumab

There are several case reports describing the use of idarucizumab to reverse dabigatran's anticoagulant effect before thrombolytic therapy in patients with acute ischemic strokes. Luckily, the patients in these handful of cases did not have adverse consequences as a result of this practice.[8,26,42,64,77,79] Because of these reports, some clinicians now routinely recommend idarucizumab treatment before thrombolytic therapy for acute ischemic stroke.[21,26] However, there are no quality clinical studies that accurately describes the safety of this practice; therefore, we cannot recommend this practice until better evidence of safety and efficacy is available.

Pregnancy and Lactation

There are no studies or data available to elucidate the risks of idarucizumab use in pregnancy or while breastfeeding. Reproductive and developmental studies have not been performed in animals, and idarucizumab has the potential to cause harm to fetuses.[10]

There are also no available data regarding excretion of idarucizumab in breast milk. There is potential for idarucizumab to be excreted in milk, and its effects on nursing infants or the reproductive system are unknown.[10]

Dosing and Administration

Idarucizumab is dosed at 5 g. Each package of idarucizumab contains two vials, each containing 50 mL of fluid and 2.5 g of idarucizumab. The medication is ready to be infused without the need to be reconstituted in a separate diluent. Vials must be stored between 2° and 8°C. Before drug administration, the IV line should be flushed with saline. The medication can then be administered in two fashions. One option is to infuse each vial as two consecutive infusions of 2.5 g as was done in phase III clinical trials. The second option is to use a syringe to bolus inject both vials intravenously. There is no evidence that one approach is better than the other. If the medication is withdrawn from the vial, it must be given within 1 hour.[10,70]

There is a small subset of patients who have recurrent coagulopathy between 12 and 24 hours after receiving idarucizumab.[70] For patients who have this rebound effect in conjunction with clinically significant bleeding or need for repeat surgery or procedure, it is reasonable to administer a second dose of idarucizumab at 5 g.[10] However, there have been no studies to evaluate the efficacy or safety of this practice.

Availability

Idarucizumab is available as a parenteral solution with each vial containing 2.5 g of idarucizumab in 50 mL of fluid for injection. If idarucizumab is not immediately available, an online directory of available doses of idarucizumab is accessible on the manufacturer's website at www.praxbind.com.

ANDEXANET ALFA

History

Given the increasing use of oral factor Xa inhibitors for systemic anticoagulation, there was motivation to find a safe and efficacious reversal agent. Andexanet alfa "Andexxa" is a recombinant protein that reverses anticoagulation caused by factor Xa inhibitors. It is currently FDA approved.

Pharmacology and Mechanism of Action

Andexanet alfa was created by altering the structure of factor X. Andexanet alfa binds factor Xa inhibitors, but its structure was modified to inhibit the catalytic activation of thrombin. In addition, the factor V_a binding site on factor X, which is necessary for anticoagulation, is no longer present.[53]

Pharmacokinetics and Pharmacodynamics

A study in healthy elderly volunteers demonstrated that andexanet alfa administration given to participants with a steady-state concentration of either apixaban or rivaroxaban resulted in rapid reduction in plasma free inhibitor concentrations and increased thrombin formation. Immediately after andexanet alfa infusion, antifactor Xa activity decreased by more than 90%. However, within 1 to 2 hours, concentrations rebounded to concentrations comparable to those of the placebo group.[80] In a multicenter, prospective, open-label, single-group study, andexanet alfa was given to patients who had ingested a factor Xa inhibitor within 18 hours of onset of acute hemorrhage. After infusion of andexanet alfa, anti factor Xa activity decreased 12 hours after andexanet alfa infusion, and 79% of patients achieved hemostasis.[15]

Adverse Effects and Safety Issues

In the study in healthy volunteers, there were no serious or thrombotic complications in any of the participants.[80] However, in the aforementioned prospective study, thrombotic complications occurred in 18% of patients during the 30-day follow-up period. One-third of these events occurred in the first 72 hours after infusion. Documented thrombotic events included MI, stroke, DVT, and PE. Some patients had more than one thrombotic complication. Only 27% of patients were restarted on their anticoagulation during the 30-day follow-up period. In this study, 15% of patients died. The only reported details regarding these deaths were that 60% of them were related to cardiovascular events, and 40% of deaths were related to noncardiac events. There was no control group to determine if there were any changes in patient outcomes such as morbidity or mortality resulting from andexanet alfa administration.[15]

There have been no reports of anaphylaxis in human or animal studies.[15,54,80]

Pregnancy and Lactation

There are no data available to elucidate the risks of andexanet alfa use in pregnancy or while breastfeeding. Reproductive and developmental studies were not performed in animals, and andexanet alfa has the potential to cause harm to fetuses.

Dosing and Administration

Andexanet alfa is administered intravenously in a low dose/high dose protocol based on the timing and amount of the last dose of rivaroxaban and apixaban. All patients receive a loading dose administered over 15 to 30 minutes. A 2-hour infusion dose is then given immediately after the loading dose. For patients who received a factor Xa inhibitor more than 7 hours before AnXa administration, the loading dose is 400 mg, and the infusion dose is 480 mg. For patients who received a factor Xa inhibitor within 7 hours of AnXa administration, the loading dose is 800 mg, and the infusion dose is 960 mg.[15]

Availability

Andexanet alfa received FDA approval in May 2018 for the reversal of rivaroxaban and apixiban-associated hemorrhage. It is avaialble as a lyophylized powder in single use vials of 100 mg of recombinant coagulation factor Xa (recombinant-inactivated-zhzo).

SUMMARY

- Patients with life-threatening bleeding secondary to anticoagulants should be treated with appropriate antidotal therapy.
- VKA coagulopathy is reversed with factor replacement in bleeding patients. If bleeding is severe or life threatening or if the patient requires emergent surgical intervention, 4F-PCC is recommended as first-line treatment. It is recommended that IV vitamin K_1 be administered to γ-carboxylate factors II, VII, IX and X when the effects of 4F-PCC have disappeared.
- Alternatives to 4F-PCC include FFP, 3F-PCC, rFVIIa, and aPCCs. However, in the absence of 4F-PCC, 3F-PCC, rFVIIa and aPCC are all reasonable alternatives despite their less favorable risk profiles.
- For dabigatran-induced anticoagulation, we recommend reversal with idarucizumab for patients requiring emergent interventions or for patients who have life-threatening bleeding.
- For patients with hemorrhage from rivaroxaban or apixaban we recommend andexanet alfa.

REFERENCES

1. Adams CB, et al. Emergent pediatric anticoagulation reversal using a 4-factor prothrombin complex concentrate. *Am J Emerg Med.* 2016;34:1182 e1181-1182.
2. Ageno W, et al. Oral anticoagulant therapy: antithrombotic therapy and prevention of thrombosis, 9th ed: American College of Chest Physicians Evidence-Based Clinical Practice Guidelines. *Chest.* 2012;141(2 suppl):e44S-88S.
3. Al-Majzoub O, et al. Evaluation of warfarin reversal with 4-factor prothrombin complex concentrate compared to 3-factor prothrombin complex concentrate at a tertiary academic medical center. *J Emerg Med.* 2016;50:7-13.
4. Ashikhmina E, et al. Prothrombin complex concentrates in pediatric cardiac surgery: the current state and the future. *Ann Thorac Surg.* 2017;104:1423-1431.
5. Awad NI, Cocchio C. Activated prothrombin complex concentrates for the reversal of anticoagulant-associated coagulopathy. *P T.* 2013;38:696-701.
6. Baxalta US Inc. FEIBA (Anti-Inhibitor Coagulant Complex). http://www.shirecontent .com/PI/PDFs/FEIBA_USA_ENG.pdf. Accessed April 30, 2017.
7. Baxter Healthcare Corporation. Bebulin. http://www.baxter.com.sg/downloads/healthcare_professionals/products/bebulin-vh_pi.pdf. Accessed October 13, 2017.
8. Berrouschot J, et al. Intravenous thrombolysis with recombinant tissue-type plasminogen activator in a stroke patient receiving dabigatran anticoagulant after antagonization with idarucizumab. *Stroke.* 2016;47:1936-1938.
9. Blech S, et al. The metabolism and disposition of the oral direct thrombin inhibitor, dabigatran, in humans. *Drug Metab Dispos.* 2008;36:386-399.
10. Boehringer Ingelheim Pharmaceuticals Inc. http://docs.boehringer-ingelheim.com/Prescribing%20Information/PIs/Praxbind/Praxbind.pdf. Accessed September 21, 2017.
11. Boehringer Ingelheim Pharmaceuticals Inc. http://docs.boehringer-ingelheim.com/Prescribing%20Information/PIs/Pradaxa/Pradaxa.pdf. Accessed September 21, 2017.
12. Brekelmans MPA, et al. Benefits and harms of 4-factor prothrombin complex concentrate for reversal of vitamin K antagonist associated bleeding: a systematic review and meta-analysis. *J Thromb Thrombolysis.* 2017;44:118-129.
13. Chai P, Babu K. Toxin-induced coagulopathy. *Emerg Med Clin North Am.* 2014;32:53-78.
14. Christensen EI, et al. Endocytic receptors in the renal proximal tubule. *Physiology (Bethesda).* 2012;27:223-236.
15. Connolly SJ, et al. Andexanet alfa for acute major bleeding associated with factor Xa inhibitors. *N Engl J Med.* 2016;375:1131-1141.
16. CSL Behring LLC. http://labeling.cslbehring.com/PI/US/Kcentra/EN/Kcentra-Prescribing-Information.pdf. Accessed April 30, 2017.
17. DeAngelo J, et al. Comparison of 3-factor versus 4-factor prothrombin complex concentrate with regard to warfarin reversal, blood product use, and costs. *Am J Ther.* July 26, 2017. [Epub ahead of print].
18. DeLoughery EP, DeLoughery TG. Use of three procoagulants in improving bleeding outcomes in the warfarin patient with intracranial hemorrhage. *Blood Coagul Fibrinolysis.* 2017;28:612-616.
19. Dentali F, Crowther MA. Management of excessive anticoagulant effect due to vitamin K antagonists. Hematology/the Education Program of the American Society of Hematology. American Society of Hematology. Education Program. 2008:266-270.
20. Dibu JR, et al. The role of FEIBA in reversing novel oral anticoagulants in intracerebral hemorrhage. *Neurocrit Care.* 2016;24:413-419.

21. Diener HC, et al. Thrombolysis and thrombectomy in patients treated with dabigatran with acute ischemic stroke: expert opinion. *Int J Stroke.* 2017;12:9-12.
22. Diringer MN, et al. thromboembolic events with recombinant activated factor vii in spontaneous intracerebral hemorrhage: results from the Factor Seven for Acute Hemorrhagic Stroke (FAST) Trial. *Stroke.* 2010;41:48-53.
23. Eerenberg ES, et al. Reversal of rivaroxaban and dabigatran by prothrombin complex concentrate: a randomized, placebo-controlled, crossover study in healthy subjects. *Circulation.* 2011;124:1573-1579.
24. Eikelboom JW, et al. Idarucizumab: the antidote for reversal of dabigatran. *Circulation.* 2015;132:2412-2422.
25. Franchini M, Lippi G. Prothrombin complex concentrates: an update. *Blood Transfus.* 2010;8:149-154.
26. Gawehn A, et al. Successful thrombolysis with recombinant tissue plasminogen activator after antagonizing dabigatran by idarucizumab: a case report. *J Med Case Rep.* 2016;10:269.
27. Glund S, et al. A randomised study in healthy volunteers to investigate the safety, tolerability and pharmacokinetics of idarucizumab, a specific antidote to dabigatran. *Thromb Haemost.* 2015;113:943-951.
28. Glund S, et al. Safety, tolerability, and efficacy of idarucizumab for the reversal of the anticoagulant effect of dabigatran in healthy male volunteers: a randomised, placebo-controlled, double-blind phase 1 trial. *Lancet.* 2015;386:680-690.
29. Greinacher A, et al. Reversal of anticoagulants: an overview of current developments. *Thromb Haemost.* 2015;113:931-942.
30. Hanke AA, et al. Long-term safety and efficacy of a pasteurized nanofiltrated prothrombin complex concentrate (Beriplex P/N): a pharmacovigilance study. *Br J Anaesth.* 2013;110:764-772.
31. Herrmann R, et al. Thrombin generation using the calibrated automated thrombinoscope to assess reversibility of dabigatran and rivaroxaban. *Thromb Haemost.* 2014;111:989-995.
32. Hofer S, et al. Reversal of anticoagulation with dabigatran in an 82-year-old patient with traumatic retroperitoneal arterial bleeding using the new antidote idarucizumab: a case report. *A A Case Rep.* 2016;7:227-231.
33. Holbrook A, et al. Evidence-based management of anticoagulant therapy: antithrombotic therapy and prevention of thrombosis, 9th ed: American College of Chest Physicians Evidence-Based Clinical Practice Guidelines. *Chest.* 2012;141(2 suppl):e152S-e184S.
34. Honickel M, et al. Therapy with activated prothrombin complex concentrate is effective in reducing dabigatran-associated blood loss in a porcine polytrauma model. *Thromb Haemost.* 2016;115:271-284.
35. Honickel M, et al. Reversal of dabigatran anticoagulation ex vivo: porcine study comparing prothrombin complex concentrates and idarucizumab. *Thromb Haemost.* 2015;113:728-740.
36. Huang WT, et al. Four-factor prothrombin complex concentrate for coagulopathy reversal in patients with liver disease. *Clin Appl Thromb Hemost.* 2016:1076029616668406.
37. Janssen Pharmaceuticals Inc. https://www.xareltohcp.com/shared/product/xarelto/prescribing-information.pdf. Accessed September 21, 2017.
38. Jones GM, et al. 3-factor versus 4-factor prothrombin complex concentrate for warfarin reversal in severe bleeding: a multicenter, retrospective, propensity-matched pilot study. *J Thromb Thrombolysis.* 2016;42:19-26.
39. Joseph B, et al. Factor IX complex for the correction of traumatic coagulopathy. *J Trauma Acute Care Surg.* 2012;72:828-834.
40. Joseph B, et al. Prothrombin complex concentrate: an effective therapy in reversing the coagulopathy of traumatic brain injury. *J Trauma Acute Care Surg.* 2013;74:248-253.
41. Junagade P, et al. Fixed dose prothrombin complex concentrate for the reversal of oral anticoagulation therapy. *Hematology.* 2007;12:439-440.
42. Kafke W, Kraft P. Intravenous thrombolysis after reversal of dabigatran by idarucizumab: a case report. *Case Rep Neurol.* 2016;8:140-144.
43. Karaca MA, et al. Use and effectiveness of prothrombin complex concentrates vs fresh frozen plasma in gastrointestinal hemorrhage due to warfarin usage in the ED. *Am J Emerg Med.* 2014;32:660-664.
44. Kinard TN, Sarode R. Four factor prothrombin complex concentrate (human): review of the pharmacology and clinical application for vitamin K antagonist reversal. *Expert Rev Cardiovasc Ther.* 2014;12:417-427.
45. Klein L, et al. Evaluation of fixed dose 4-factor prothrombin complex concentrate for emergent warfarin reversal. *Am J Emerg Med.* 2015;33:1213-1218.
46. Kuroski JE, Young S. Comparison of the safety and efficacy between 3-factor and 4-factor prothrombin complex concentrates for the reversal of warfarin. *Am J Emerg Med.* 2017;35:871-874.
47. Kwon JO, MacLaren R. Comparison of fresh-frozen plasma, four-factor prothrombin complex concentrates, and recombinant factor VIIa to facilitate procedures in critically ill patients with coagulopathy from liver disease: a retrospective cohort study. *Pharmacotherapy.* 2016;36:1047-1054.
48. Leissinger CA, et al. Role of prothrombin complex concentrates in reversing warfarin anticoagulation: a review of the literature. *Am J Hematol.* 2008;83:137-143.
49. Levi M, et al. Safety of recombinant activated factor VII in randomized clinical trials. *N Engl J Med.* 2010;363:1791-1800.
50. Lisman T, et al. Intact thrombin generation and decreased fibrinolytic capacity in patients with acute liver injury or acute liver failure. *J Thromb Haemost.* 2012;10:1312-1319.
51. Lisman T, et al. Haemostatic abnormalities in patients with liver disease. *J Hepatol.* 2002;37:280-287.

52. Lisman T, Porte RJ. Rebalanced hemostasis in patients with liver disease: evidence and clinical consequences. *Blood.* 2010;116:878-885.
53. Lu G, et al. A specific antidote for reversal of anticoagulation by direct and indirect inhibitors of coagulation factor Xa. *Nat Med.* 2013;19:446-451.
54. Lu G, et al. Preclinical safety and efficacy of andexanet alfa in animal models. *J Thromb Haemost.* 2017;15:1747-1756.
55. Majeed A, et al. Mortality in vitamin K antagonist-related intracerebral bleeding treated with plasma or 4-factor prothrombin complex concentrate. *Thromb Haemost.* 2014;111:233-239.
56. Makris M, et al. Emergency oral anticoagulant reversal: the relative efficacy of infusions of fresh frozen plasma and clotting factor concentrate on correction of the coagulopathy. *Thromb Haemost.* 1997;77:477.
57. Mangram A, et al. Is there a difference in efficacy, safety, and cost-effectiveness between 3-factor and 4-factor prothrombin complex concentrates among trauma patients on oral anticoagulants? *J Crit Care.* 2016;33:252-256.
58. Mao G, et al. Factor eight inhibitor bypassing agent (FEIBA) for reversal of target-specific oral anticoagulants in life-threatening intracranial bleeding. *J Emerg Med.* 2017;52:731-737.
59. Marlu R, et al. Effect of non-specific reversal agents on anticoagulant activity of dabigatran and rivaroxaban. A randomised crossover ex vivo study in healthy volunteers. *Thromb Haemost.* 2012;108:217-224.
60. Martin DT, et al. Emergent reversal of vitamin K antagonists: addressing all the factors. *Am J Surg.* 2016;211:919-925.
61. Matsushima K, et al. Prothrombin complex concentrate in trauma patients. *Am J Surg.* 2015;209:413-417.
62. Meibohm B, Zhou H. Characterizing the impact of renal impairment on the clinical pharmacology of biologics. *J Clin Pharmacol.* 2012;52(1 suppl):54S-62S.
63. Mohan S, et al. The use of 3- and 4-factor prothrombin complex concentrate in patients with elevated INR. *J Pharm Pract.* 2017;897190017707119.
64. Mutzenbach JS, et al. Intravenous thrombolysis in acute ischemic stroke after dabigatran reversal with idarucizumab—a case report. *Ann Clin Transl Neurol.* 2016;3:889-892.
65. O'Connell KA, et al. Thromboembolic adverse events after use of recombinant human coagulation factor VIIa. *JAMA.* 2006;295:293-298.
66. Ostermann H, et al. Pharmacokinetics of Beriplex P/N prothrombin complex concentrate in healthy volunteers. *Thromb Haemost.* 2007;98:790-797.
67. Pabinger I, et al. Prothrombin complex concentrate (Beriplex P/N) for emergency anticoagulation reversal: a prospective multinational clinical trial. *J Thromb.* 2008;6:622-631.
68. Pabinger I, et al. Impact of infusion speed on the safety and effectiveness of prothrombin complex concentrate: a prospective clinical trial of emergency anticoagulation reversal. *Ann Hematol.* 2010;89:309-316.
69. Pollack CV Jr, et al. Design and rationale for RE-VERSE AD: a phase 3 study of idarucizumab, a specific reversal agent for dabigatran. *Thromb Haemost.* 2015;114:198-205.
70. Pollack CV Jr, et al. Idarucizumab for Dabigatran Reversal. *N Engl J Med.* 2015;373:511-520.
71. Quick JA, et al. Experience with prothrombin complex for the emergent reversal of anticoagulation in rural geriatric trauma patients. *Surgery.* 2012;152:722-726; discussion 726-728.
72. Rottenstreich A, et al. Idarucizumab for dabigatran reversal—does one dose fit all? *Thromb Res.* 2016;146:103-104.
73. Safaoui MN, et al. A promising new alternative for the rapid reversal of warfarin coagulopathy in traumatic intracranial hemorrhage. *Am J Surg.* 2009;197:785-790.
74. Samos M, et al. Monitoring of dabigatran therapy using Hemoclot((R)) Thrombin Inhibitor assay in patients with atrial fibrillation. *J Thromb Thrombolysis.* 2015;39:95-100.
75. Sarode R. Four-factor prothrombin complex concentrate versus plasma for urgent vitamin K antagonist reversal: new evidence. *Clin Lab Med.* 2014;34:613-621.
76. Sarode R, et al. Efficacy and safety of a 4-factor prothrombin complex concentrate in patients on vitamin K antagonists presenting with major bleeding: a randomized, plasma-controlled, phase IIIb study. *Circulation.* 2013;128:1234-1243.
77. Schafer N, et al. Systemic thrombolysis for ischemic stroke after antagonizing dabigatran with idarucizumab—a case report. *J Stroke Cerebrovasc Dis.* 2016;25:e126-127.
78. Schiele F, et al. A specific antidote for dabigatran: functional and structural characterization. *Blood.* 2013;121:3554-3562.
79. Schulz JG, Kreps B. Idarucizumab elimination of dabigatran minutes before systemic thrombolysis in acute ischemic stroke. *J Neurol Sci.* 2016;370:44.
80. Siegal DM, et al. Andexanet alfa for the reversal of factor Xa inhibitor activity. *N Engl J Med.* 2015;373:2413-2424.
81. Stewart WS, Pettit H. Experiences with an activated 4-factor prothrombin complex concentrate (FEIBA) for reversal of warfarin-related bleeding. *Am J Emerg Med.* 2013;31:1251-1254.
82. Tripodi A, et al. Evidence of normal thrombin generation in cirrhosis despite abnormal conventional coagulation tests. *Hepatology.* 2005;41:553-558.
83. Van Ryn J, et al. An antibody selective to dabigatran safely neutralizes both dabigatran-induced anticoagulant and bleeding activity in in vitro and in vivo models. *J Thromb Haemost.* 2011;9:110-110.
84. van Ryn J, et al. Dabigatran anticoagulant activity is neutralized by an antibody selective to dabigatran in in vitro and in vivo models. *J Am Coll Cardiol.* 2011;57:E1130-E1130.
85. van Ryn J, et al. Reversibility of the anticoagulant effect of high doses of the direct thrombin inhibitor dabigatran, by recombinant factor VIIa or activated prothrombin complex concentrate. *Haematologica.* 2008;93(suppl 1):148.
86. Voils SA, et al. Comparative effectiveness of 3- versus 4-factor prothrombin complex concentrate for emergent warfarin reversal. *Thromb Res.* 2015;136:595-598.
87. Wojcik C, et al. Activated prothrombin complex concentrate factor VIII inhibitor bypassing activity (FEIBA) for the reversal of warfarin-induced coagulopathy. *Int J Emerg Med.* 2009;2:217-225.
88. Zupancic-Salek S, et al. Successful reversal of anticoagulant effect of superwarfarin poisoning with recombinant activated factor VII. *Blood Coagul Fibrinolysis.* 2005;16:239-244.

A18

VITAMIN K$_1$

Mary Ann Howland

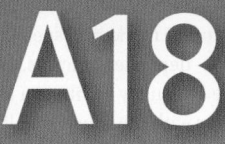

Vitamin K$_1$ (phytonadione) is the commercial preparation of the natural form of vitamin K (phylloquinone) that is indicated for the reversal of an elevated prothrombin time (PT) or an international normalized ratio (INR) in patients with vitamin K deficiency. Acquired vitamin K deficiency most commonly results from the therapeutic administration of warfarin or after an overdose of warfarin or a long-acting anticoagulant rodenticide (LAARs), such as brodifacoum. The optimal dosage regimen of vitamin K$_1$ to treat patients who develop an elevated INR while receiving warfarin was given in the 2012 American College of Chest Physicians consensus guidelines.[1] Oral administration of vitamin K$_1$ is safe and effective. Because intravenous (IV) administration of vitamin K$_1$ is associated with anaphylactoid reactions, its use is not recommended unless serious or life-threatening hemorrhage is present. Subcutaneous (SC) administration should only be used when a patient is unable to tolerate oral vitamin K therapy and is not clinically compromised enough to necessitate IV vitamin K$_1$.[10]

HISTORY

It was noted in 1929 that chickens fed a poor diet developed spontaneous bleeding. In 1935, Dam and coworkers discovered that incorporating a fat-soluble substance, defined as a "koagulation factor," into the diet could correct the bleeding, leading to the name vitamin K.[23,40,45]

PHARMACOLOGY

Chemistry

Vitamin K is an essential fat-soluble vitamin that encompasses at least two distinct natural forms. Vitamin K$_1$ (phytonadione, phylloquinone) is the only form synthesized by plants and algae. Vitamin K$_2$ (menaquinones) is actually a series of compounds with the same 2-methyl-1, 4-naphthoquinone ring structure as phylloquinone but with a variable number (1–13) of repeating five-carbon units on the side chain. Bacteria synthesize vitamin K$_2$ (menaquinones). Most of the vitamin K ingested in the diet is phylloquinone (vitamin K$_1$).

Related Vitamin K Compounds

Vitamin K$_1$ (phytonadione) is the only vitamin K preparation that should be used to reverse anticoagulant-induced vitamin K deficiency or to treat infants or pregnant women. Vitamin K$_1$ is superior to the other previously commercially available vitamin K preparations because it is more active, requires smaller doses, and has fewer associated risks.[19,42] In addition, patients with glucose-6-phosphate dehydrogenase (G6PD) deficiency have an increased risk of hemolysis with other vitamin K preparations.

Vitamins K$_3$ (menadione) and K$_4$ (menadiol sodium diphosphate) are no longer approved by the US Food and Drug Administration (FDA) because they produce hemolysis, hyperbilirubinemia, and kernicterus in neonates, as well as hemolysis in G6PD-deficient patients. The only advantage that menadione and menadiol sodium diphosphate have is their direct absorption from the intestine by a passive process that does not require the presence of bile salts. However, even for patients with cholestasis or severe pancreatic insufficiency, they are neither interchangeable with vitamin K$_1$ nor a substitute for vitamin K$_1$ when anticoagulants such as warfarin or a LAAR are responsible for coagulation deficits. Therefore, for a patient deficient in bile salts who requires vitamin K$_1$, exogenous bile salts, such as ox bile extract 300 mg or dehydrocholic acid 500 mg, are recommended with each dose of oral vitamin K$_1$.[32]

Mechanism of Action

A postsynthetic modification of coagulation factors II, VII, IX, and X and proteins S, C and Z requires γ-carboxylation of the glutamate residues in a vitamin K–dependent process. Only the reduced (K$_1$H$_2$, hydroquinone) form of vitamin K manifests biologic activity. During the carboxylation step, the active reduced vitamin K$_1$ is converted to an epoxide. This 2,3-epoxide is reduced and recycled to the active K$_1$H$_2$ in a process that is inhibited by warfarin (Fig. 58–2). For further details, readers are referred to an in-depth model of the chemical basis of this reaction.[13,51] The phytonadione form of vitamin K is activated to the reduced, vitamin K$_1$H$_2$ form directly by nicotinamide adenine dinucleotide (phosphate) (NAD(P)H)-dehydrogenase (DT-diaphorase) enzymes that use both NADH and NADPH in a pathway that is relatively insensitive to warfarin; the vitamin K 2,3-epoxide form cannot be activated through this pathway.[38,40,44,45,47] Exogenous phytonadione allows γ-carboxylation of clotting factors that are present and does not rely on recycling.[11,38]

Daily Requirement

The human daily requirement for vitamin K is small; the Food and Nutrition Board set the recommended daily allowance at 1 mcg/kg/d of phylloquinone for adults, although 10 times that amount is required for infants to maintain normal hemostasis.[39] Vitamin K–dependent extrahepatic enzymatic reactions relate to carboxylation of proteins in the bone, kidney, placenta, lung, pancreas, and spleen and include the synthesis of osteocalcin, matrix Gla protein, plaque Gla protein, and one or more renal Gla proteins.[39,40,44] Variations in dietary vitamin K intake while receiving therapeutic oral anticoagulation with warfarin can result in significant over- or underanticoagulation.[1,18] One study measured vitamin K concentrations before and after treatment with warfarin, and as expected, the concentrations fell from 1.72 ng/mL to 0.59 ng/mL. Patients taking warfarin exhibited large inter- and intravariability in vitamin K concentrations (0.2–4.2 ng/mL).[24]

Pharmacokinetics of Dietary Vitamin K

Dietary vitamin K in the forms of phylloquinone and menaquinones is solubilized in the presence of the bile salts, free fatty acids, and monoglycerides, which enhance absorption. Vitamin K is incorporated into chylomicrons, entering the circulation through the lymphatic system in transit to the liver.[40] In the plasma, vitamin K is primarily in the phylloquinone form, but liver stores are 90% menaquinones and 10% phylloquinone.[40] Within 3 days of a diet low in vitamin K, a group of surgical patients showed a fourfold decrease of liver vitamin K concentrations without an effect on their PTs.[43] Rats given a vitamin K–deficient diet develop severe bleeding within 2 to 3 weeks.

Pharmacokinetics of Administered Vitamin K$_1$

There are only a limited number of pharmacokinetic studies of vitamin K$_1$.[8,20,31,52] One study evaluated the pharmacokinetics of vitamin K$_1$ in healthy volunteers, brodifacoum-anticoagulated rabbits, and a patient poisoned with brodifacoum.[31] In the volunteers and the poisoned patient, a 10-mg IV dose of vitamin K_1 had a half-life of 1.7 hours. After oral administration of doses of 10 and 50 mg of vitamin K_1, peak concentrations of 100 to 400 ng/mL and 200 to 2,000 ng/mL, respectively, occurred at 3 to 5 hours. Bioavailability varied significantly among patients (10%–65%) for both doses and in individual patients with the 50-mg dose. Oral vitamin K_1 is absorbed in an energy-dependent saturable process in the proximal small intestine, which contributes to the variability.[31] In maximally brodifacoum-anticoagulated rabbits, IV vitamin K_1 (10 mg/kg) increased prothrombin complex activity from 14% to 50% by 4 hours and to 100% by 9 hours, after which it declined with a half-life of 6 hours.[31] High doses of oral vitamin K_1 were effectively used to treat a patient anticoagulated with brodifacoum.[8]

The pharmacokinetics of oral and intramuscular (IM) vitamin K_1 were compared in eight healthy female volunteers. Baseline serum vitamin K_1 concentrations were 0.23 ng/mL. After the oral administration of 5 mg of vitamin K_1, peak serum concentrations of 90 ng/mL were achieved between 4 and 6 hours. These concentrations dropped to a steady state of 3.8 ng/mL and exhibited a half-life of about 4 hours.

The pharmacokinetics were distinctly different and quite variable after IM administration. Intramuscular administration of 5 mg of vitamin K resulted in peak serum concentrations of only 50 ng/mL, with delays from 2 to 30 hours after administration and with the maintenance of a plateau for about 30 hours.[20] Consequently, IM administration is not recommended; either oral or IV administration is more appropriate, and the route will be defined by the severity of bleeding. Only in the case of acute gastrointestinal disease in a patient without serious life-threatening hemorrhage is the SC route an appropriate alternative to the oral route (Table 58–2).

Pharmacodynamics of Administered Vitamin K_1

The time necessary for the INR to return to a safe or normal range is variable and dependent on the rate of absorption of vitamin K_1, the serum concentration achieved, and the time necessary for the synthesis of activated clotting factors. A decrease in the INR often occurs within several hours, although it often takes 8 to 24 hours to reach target values.[1,7,16,28,35] Maintenance of a normal INR depends on the half-life of the vitamin K_1, maintenance of an effective serum concentration, and the half-life of the anticoagulant involved. The IV route is unpredictably faster than the oral route in restoring the INR to the chosen target range.[1,20,26] However, the onset of action for the IV route is faster.[26,48] A comparison of oral versus IV vitamin K_1 therapy for excessive anticoagulation, without major hemorrhage, demonstrated that individuals with INRs of 6 to 10 had similarly improved INRs at 24 hours.[26] The onset of action began at 2 hours with IV compared with 6 hours with oral.[26] The IV group more often overcorrected to an INR of less than 2.[26] In a retrospective analysis of 64 patients requiring vitamin K for nonurgent reversal of anticoagulation before a procedure, the IV route corrected more patients to an INR less than 4 at 4 hours than the oral route.[48] In a randomized controlled trial in asymptomatic patients on warfarin with an INR between 4.5 and 10, the administration of 1 mg of vitamin K orally was associated with a faster return to a therapeutic INR than with 1 mg administered subcutaneously.[10]

Vitamin K Deficiency and Monitoring

Vitamin K deficiency results from inadequate intake, malabsorption, or interference with the vitamin K cycle. Malnourishment and any condition in which bile salts or fatty acids are inadequate, such as extrahepatic cholestasis or severe pancreatic insufficiency, often leads to vitamin K deficiency. Multifactorial etiologies place newborns at risk for hemorrhage. Phylloquinone does not readily cross the placenta, and breast milk contains less phylloquinone than vitamin K–fortified formula. Fetal hepatic stores of phylloquinone are low, and treatments such as maternal antiepileptic therapy lead to increased vitamin K metabolism.[40,44] Although menaquinones are produced in the colon by bacteria, it is unlikely that enteric production contributes significantly to vitamin K stores or that eradication of the bacteria with antibiotics, without a coexistent dietary deficiency of vitamin K, results in deficiency.[40] Determination of vitamin K deficiency is usually established

on the basis of a prolonged PT or INR, which are surrogate markers of specific coagulation factors. Measurement of the vitamin K–dependent factors, II, VII, IX, and X, is an effective way to determine the adequacy of vitamin K_1 dosing.[21] Serial measurements of factor VII, the factor with the shortest half-life, allow for the early detection of inadequate vitamin K in the diet or a therapeutic regimen.[8] Direct measurement of serum vitamin K concentrations is done by high-performance liquid chromatography analysis. The human serum vitamin K concentration required for adequate production of activated clotting factors in the presence of long-acting vitamin K antagonists (LAARs) is still unclear. A single study in a patient who overdosed on brodifacoum suggested that a serum vitamin K concentration of 200 to 400 ng/mL was sufficient to achieve a normal coagulation profile. Prior studies suggested 1,000 ng/mL was necessary in rabbits.[8,31]

ROLE IN XENOBIOTIC-INDUCED VITAMIN K DEFICIENCY

Warfarin and LAARs are vitamin K antagonists that interfere with the vitamin K cycle, causing the accumulation of vitamin K 2,3-epoxide, an inactive metabolite. Warfarin is a strong irreversible inhibitor of the vitamin K 2,3-epoxide reductase, which regenerates vitamin K into its active (K_1H_2, hydroquinone) form.[3] The superwarfarins are even more potent vitamin K reductase inhibitors. Under ideal nutritional circumstances in a healthy individual, vitamin K is recycled, and only 1 mcg/kg/d is required in adults to maintain adequate coagulation. DT-diaphorases are warfarin-insensitive enzymes capable of reducing vitamin K_1 to its active hydroquinone form, but they are incapable of regenerating vitamin K from vitamin K 2,3-epoxide after carboxylation of the coagulation factor (Fig. 58–2).[3] Thus, in the presence of warfarin or superwarfarins, additional vitamin K_1 must be administered to supply this active cofactor for each and every carboxylation step because it can no longer be recycled.[8,15] The minimum vitamin K_1 requirement in the presence of a LAAR is unknown. Other compounds including the N-methyl-thiotetrazole side chain–containing antibiotics such as moxalactam and cefamandole (Chap. 54), as well as salicylates have varying degrees of vitamin K antagonistic activity (Chap. 37).[9,40]

ADVERSE EFFECTS AND SAFETY ISSUES

Although vitamin K_1 can be administered orally, subcutaneously, intramuscularly, or intravenously, the oral route is preferred for maintenance therapy. When administered orally, vitamin K_1 is virtually free of adverse effects, except for overcorrection of the INR for a patient requiring maintenance anticoagulation. The preparations available for IV administration are rarely associated with anaphylactoid reactions. Because of the lipid solubility of vitamin K, these preparations are not available in solution but rather as an aqueous colloidal suspension of a polyoxyethylated castor oil derivative, dextrose, and benzyl alcohol. Intravenous administration has resulted in death secondary to anaphylactoid reactions, probably as a result of the colloidal formulation of the preparation.[4,12,27] Numerous anaphylactoid reactions are reported, even when the preparation is properly diluted and administered slowly.[17,30,36,50] In a 5-year retrospective study, two patients experienced presumed anaphylactoid reactions shortly after initiation of 0.5 to 1 mg of IV vitamin K_1 diluted in 50 mL of dextrose 5% in water to be infused over 1 hour. Based on the total number of 6,572 administered doses of vitamin K_1 infused according to this protocol, the estimated incidence of presumed anaphylactoid reactions was 3 in 10,000.[6,17] Rarely, the SC and IM routes of administration also result in anaphylactoid reactions.[17] Liposomal preparations, which may become safer alternatives, are in development.

PREGNANCY AND LACTATION

Vitamin K_1 is listed as FDA pregnancy Category C. There are no reproductive studies in animals. Vitamin K is the treatment of choice for vitamin K deficiency during pregnancy and for prevention of hemorrhagic disease in newborns.[5] A standard textbook on drugs in pregnancy also states that vitamin K is compatible with breastfeeding. However, the amount of vitamin K transferred in mother's milk is not usually adequate to prevent hemorrhagic disease in a newborn without supplementing the newborn directly.[5]

DOSING AND ADMINISTRATION

The optimal regimen for vitamin K₁ remains unclear. Variables include the vitamin K₁ pharmacokinetics and the amount and type of anticoagulant ingested.[37] Reported cases of LAAR poisoning have required as much as 50 to 250 mg of vitamin K₁ daily for weeks to months.[2,8,14,15,22,25,41,49] A recommended initial regimen starting approach for a patient who has overdosed on LAAR is 25 to 50 mg of vitamin K₁ orally three to four times a day for 1 to 2 days. For unusually large oral vitamin K doses, the IV formulation can be given orally.[10] The INR should be monitored, and the vitamin K₁ dose adjusted accordingly. When the INR is less than 2, a downward titration in the dose of vitamin K₁ should be made on the basis of factor VII analysis. For an ingestion of brodifacoum, serial serum concentrations of brodifacoum are recommended in determining the ultimate duration of treatment, although the effect of brodifacoum is demonstrated to persist at very low or undetectable blood concentrations.[8,29]

The management of patients with elevated INRs secondary to excessive warfarin is described in Table 58–2. Intravenous administration of vitamin K₁ should be reserved for serious or life-threatening hemorrhage at any elevation of INR.[1] Under these circumstances, supplementation with prothrombin complex concentrate (PCC) and fresh-frozen plasma (FFP) is recommended, based on a risk-to-benefit analysis. A starting dose of 10 mg of vitamin K₁ is recommended. To minimize the risk of an anaphylactoid reaction, the preparation should be diluted with preservative-free 5% dextrose, 0.9% sodium chloride, or 5% dextrose in 0.9% sodium chloride and administered slowly, using an infusion pump, over a minimum of 20 minutes.[1] The administration recommended rate is not to exceed 1 mg/min in adults.[46] Precautions should be anticipated in the event of an anaphylactoid reaction.

Because the duration of action of vitamin K₁ is short lived, the dose is recommended for administration two to four times daily. The onset of the effect of vitamin K₁ is not immediate regardless of the route of administration.

FORMULATION AND ACQUISITION

Vitamin K₁ is available for IV and SC administration as phytonadione injection emulsion in 2 mg/mL (0.5-mL ampule and vial or prefilled drug delivery system) and 10-mg/mL (1-mL ampule) concentrations.by different manufacturers. Each 1 mL of the 10-mg/mL preparations contain benzyl alcohol (0.9%) as a preservative and 70 mg of polyoxyethylated fatty acid derivative (polyoxyl 35 castor oil).[33] Many of the 2-mg/mL (0.5-mL) preparations also contain these excipients, and one manufacturer offers a 2-mg/mL (0.5-mL) preparation that is free of the polyoxyl 35 castor oil and instead contains 1 mg of phytonadione, 10 mg of polysorbate 80, 10.4 mg of propylene glycol, 0.17 mg of sodium acetate anhydrous, and 0.00002 mL of glacial acetic acid.[34] Oral vitamin K₁ is available as Mephyton in 5-mg tablets.

SUMMARY

- Vitamin K₁ (phytonadione) is recommended for the reversal of an elevated PT or INR in patients with xenobiotic-induced vitamin K deficiency.
- Intravenous administration is reserved for patients with serious or life-threatening hemorrhage. The IV route is rarely associated with serious anaphylactoid reactions.
- Vitamin K₁ is administered with other therapies such as PCC and FFP that have rapid onsets of action.
- The onset of action of vitamin K₁ is delayed for several hours with the IV route and even longer delays occur with the oral route.
- Patients with LAAR poisoning usually require large doses of oral vitamin K₁ for weeks to months.

REFERENCES

1. Ageno W, et al. Oral anticoagulant therapy: antithrombotic therapy and prevention of thrombosis, 9th ed: American College of Chest Physicians Evidence-Based Clinical Practice Guidelines. *Chest.* 2012;41(2 suppl):e44S-e88S.
2. Babcock J, et al. Rodenticide induced coagulopathy in a young child. *Am J Pediatr Hematol Oncol.* 1993;15:126-130.
3. Baglin T. Management of warfarin (Coumadin) overdose. *Blood Rev.* 1998;12:91-98.
4. Barash P, et al. Acute cardiovascular collapse after intravenous phytonadione. *Anesth Analg.* 1976;55:304-306.
5. Briggs' Drugs in Pregnancy and Lactation. Phytonadione. Facts & Comparisons Searchable Drug Information Databases. http://www.wolterskluwercdi.com/facts-comparisons-online/databases. Accessed July 28, 2017.
6. Britt RB, Brown JN. Characterizing the severe reactions of parenteral vitamin K1. *Clin Appl Thromb Hemost.* 2018;24:5-12.
7. Brophy M, et al. Low-dose vitamin K therapy in excessively anticoagulated patients: a dose finding study. *J Thromb Thrombolysis.* 1997;4:289-292.
8. Bruno GR, et al. Long-acting anticoagulant overdose: brodifacoum kinetics and optimal vitamin K₁ dosing. *Ann Emerg Med.* 2000;36:262-267.
9. Chen LJ, et al. Use of hypoprothrombinemia-inducing cephalosporins and the risk of hemorrhagic events: a nationwide nested case-control study. *PLoS One.* 2016;11:e0158407.
10. Crowther MA, et al. Oral vitamin K reversed warfarin-associated coagulopathy faster than subcutaneous vitamin K. *Ann Intern Med.* 2002;137:251-254.
11. Curtis R, et al. Reversal of warfarin anticoagulation for urgent surgical procedures. *Can J Anaesth.* 2015;62:634-649.
12. De la Rubia J, et al. Anaphylactic shock and vitamin K₁. *Ann Intern Med.* 1989;110:943.
13. Dowd P, et al. The mechanism of action of vitamin K. *Annu Rev Nutr.* 1995;15:419-440.
14. Exner DV, et al. Superwarfarin ingestion. *CMAJ.* 1992;146:34-35.
15. Feinstein DL, et al. The emerging threat of superwarfarins: history, detection, mechanisms, and countermeasures. *Ann N Y Acad Sci.* 2016;1374:111-122.
16. Fetrow CW, et al. Antagonism of warfarin induced hypoprothrombinemia with use of low-dose subcutaneous vitamin K₁. *J Clin Pharmacol.* 1997;37:751-757.
17. Fiore L, et al. Anaphylactoid reactions to vitamin K. *J Thromb Thrombolysis.* 2001; 11:175-183.
18. Franco V, et al. Role of dietary vitamin K intake in chronic oral anticoagulation: prospective evidence from observational and randomized protocols. *Am J Med.* 2004;116: 651-656.
19. Gamble JR, et al. Clinical comparison of vitamin K₁ and water-soluble vitamin K. *Arch Intern Med.* 1955;5:52-58.
20. Hagstrom JN, et al. The pharmacokinetics and lipoprotein fraction distribution of intramuscular versus oral vitamin K₁ supplementation in women of childbearing age: effects on hemostasis. *Thromb Haemost.* 1995;74:1486-1490.
21. Hoffman R, et al. Evaluation of coagulation factor abnormalities in long-acting anticoagulant overdose. *J Toxicol Clin Toxicol.* 1998;26:233-248.
22. Hollinger B, Pastoor T. Case management and plasma half-life in a case of brodifacoum poisoning. *Arch Intern Med.* 1993;153:1925-1928.
23. Kaushansky K, Kipps TJ. Hematopoietic agents: growth factors, minerals, and vitamins. In: Brunton LL, et al., eds. *Goodman & Gilman's The Pharmacological Basis of Therapeutics.* 12th ed. New York, NY: McGraw-Hill; 2011.
24. Kim YE, et al. High intra- and inter-individual variability of plasma vitamin K concentrations in patients with atrial fibrillation under warfarin therapy. *Eur J Clin Nutr.* 2015;69:703-706.
25. La Rosa F, et al. Brodifacoum intoxication with marijuana smoking. *Arch Pathol Lab Med.* 1997;121:67-69.
26. Lubetsky A, et al. Comparison of oral vs intravenous phytonadione (vitamin K₁) in patients with excessive anticoagulation: a prospective randomized controlled study. *Arch Intern Med.* 2003;163:2469-2473.
27. Mattea E, Quinn K. Adverse reactions after intravenous phytonadione administration. *Hosp Pharm.* 1981;16:230-235.
28. Nee R, et al. Intravenous versus subcutaneous vitamin K₁ in reversing excessive oral anticoagulation. *Am J Cardiol.* 1999;83:286-288.
29. Olmos V, Lopez C. Brodifacoum poisoning with toxicokinetic data. *Clin Toxicol.* 2007; 45:487-489.
30. O'Reilly R, Kearns P. Intravenous vitamin K injections: dangerous prophylaxis. *Arch Intern Med.* 1995;155:2127-2128.
31. Park BK, et al. Plasma disposition of vitamin K₁ in relation to anticoagulant poisoning. *Br J Clin Pharmacol.* 1984;18:655-662.
32. Phytonadione. In: McEvoy GK, ed. *AHFS Drug Information.* Bethesda, MD: American Society of Health System Pharmacists; 2004:3525-3527.
33. Phytonadione Injection, Emulsion Hospira (repackaged by both Cardinal Health and General Injectables & Vaccines, Inc.). Lake Forest, IL; 2017.
34. Phytonadione Injection Emulsion International Medication Systems, Limited So. El Monte, CA; 2016.
35. Raj G, et al. Time course of reversal of anticoagulant effect of warfarin by intravenous and subcutaneous phytonadione. *Arch Intern Med.* 1999;159:2721-2724.
36. Riegert-Johnson DL, Volcheck GW. The incidence of anaphylaxis following intra-venous phytonadione (vitamin K1): a 5-year retrospective review. *Ann Allergy Asthma Immunol.* 2002;89:400-406.
37. Routh CR, et al. Superwarfarin ingestion and detection. *Am J Hematol.* 1991;36:50-54.
38. Schulman S, Furie B. How I treat poisoning with vitamin K antagonists. *Blood.* 2015;125: 438-442.
39. Shearer MJ. Vitamin K. *Lancet.* 1995;345:229-233.
40. Shearer MJ. Vitamin K metabolism and nutrition. *Blood Rev.* 1992;6:92-104.
41. Sheen S, Spiller H. Symptomatic brodifacoum ingestion requiring high-dose phytonadione therapy. *Vet Hum Toxicol.* 1994;36:216-217.

42. Udall JA. Don't use the wrong vitamin K. *West J Med*. 1970;112:65-67.

43. Usuri Y, et al. Vitamin K concentrations in the plasma and liver of surgical patients. *Am J Clin Nutr*. 1990;51:846-852.

44. Vermeer C, Hamulyak K. Pathophysiology of vitamin K deficiency and oral anticoagulants. *Thromb Haemost*. 1991;66:153-159.

45. Vermeer C, Schurgers L. A comprehensive review of vitamin K and vitamin K antagonists. *Hematol Oncol Clin North Am*. 2000;15:339-353.

46. Vitamin K1 phytonadione injectable emulsion USP [package insert]: Lake Forest, IL: Hospira; 2017.

47. Wallin R, Hutson S. Warfarin and the vitamin K dependent γ-carboxylation system. *Trends Molec Med*. 2004;10:299-302.

48. Watson HG, et al. A comparison of the efficacy and rate of response to oral and intravenous Vitamin K in reversal of over-anticoagulation with warfarin. *Br J Haematol*. 2001 Oct;115:145-149.

49. Weitzel J, et al. Surreptitious ingestion of a long-acting vitamin K antagonist/rodenticide, brodifacoum: clinical and metabolic studies of three cases. *Blood*. 1990;76:2555-2559.

50. Wjasow C, McNamara R. Anaphylaxis after low dose intravenous vitamin K. *J Emerg Med*. 2003;24:169-172.

51. Wilson CR, et al. Species comparison of vitamin K_1 2,3-epoxide reductase activity in vitro: kinetics and warfarin inhibition. *Toxicology*. 2003;189:191-198.

52. Winn MJ, et al. An investigation of the pharmacological response to vitamin K_1 in the rabbit. *Br J Pharmacol*. 1988;94:1077-1084.

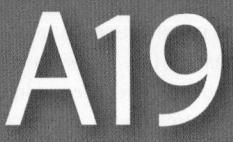

PROTAMINE

Mary Ann Howland

Protamine is a rapidly acting antidote that physically complexes unfraction-ated heparin (UFH) and reverses its anticoagulant effects. Protamine neu-tralizes the anti-IIa activity of low-molecular-weight heparin (LMWH) and incompletely neutralizes the anti-Xa activity of LMWH, which often normal-izes the activated partial thromboplastin time (aPTT) and the thrombin time but minimally affects the anti–factor Xa activity and cannot be expected to limit hemmorhage. Protamine has no effect on heparin pentasaccharide fragments or analogs such as fondaparinux.

HISTORY

In 1868, Friedric Miescher discovered and named the basic protein that resides in the sperm of salmon as protamine.[91] The antidotal properties of protamine were recognized in the late 1930s, leading to its approval as an antidote for heparin overdose in 1968.[30] However, the largest body of litera-ture pertaining to protamine originates from its use in neutralizing heparin after cardiopulmonary bypass and dialysis procedures.

PHARMACOLOGY
Chemistry

The protamines are a group of simple basic cationic proteins found in fish sperm that bind to heparin to form a stable neutral salt. The effects of prot-amine sulfate and protamine chloride are comparable.[62] The binding of heparin to protamine is stronger than the binding of heparin to antithrom-bin (AT), consequently protamine rapidly inactivates heparin and reverses its anticoagulant effects.[45,86] Commercially available protamine sulfate is derived from the sperm of mature testes of salmon and related species. Upon hydrolysis, protamine yields basic amino acids, particularly arginine, pro-line, serine, and valine, but not tyrosine and tryptophan.

Related Protamine Variants

In animal studies, synthetic protamine variants, not available for clinical use, were effective in reversing the anticoagulant effects of LMWH, and are reported to be less toxic than protamine.[13,49,98,99]

Mechanism of Action

Heparins are large electronegative xenobiotics that are rapidly complexed by the electropositive protamine, forming an inactive salt. Heparin is an indirect anticoagulant, requiring a cofactor. This cofactor, AT, was formerly called AT III. Heparin alters the stereochemistry of AT, thereby catalyzing the subsequent inactivation of thrombin and other clotting factors.[38] Only about one-third of an administered dose of UFH binds to AT, and this frac-tion is responsible for most of its anticoagulant effect.[4,64] Low-molecular-weight heparin has a reduced ability to inactivate thrombin as a result of lesser AT binding, but the smaller fragments of LMWH inactivate factor Xa almost as well as the larger molecules of UFH, allowing for equivalent efficacy. Immunoelectrophoretic studies demonstrate that because of the net positive charge of protamine, it has a greater affinity for heparin than heparin for AT, producing a dissociation of the heparin–AT complex and favoring a protamine–heparin complex.[83] This complex is removed by the reticuloendothelial system.[3] The ability of protamine to bind to LMWH is limited by the smaller chain length and molecular weight (MW) and the lesser sulfate charge density.[32,45]

PHARMACOKINETICS AND PHARMACODYNAMICS

Normal volunteers, free from cardiovascular disease and heparin free, received 0.5 mg/kg of protamine intravenously over 10 min. In this study, the protamine plasma half-life was 7.4 minutes, and it was undetectable within 20 minutes. Pharmacokinetic modeling did not fit a typical pattern.[10] When the same investigators administered 250 mg of protamine intravenously over 5 minutes at the end of cardiopulmonary bypass for heparin reversal, the total protamine half-life (free plus bound to heparin) was 4.5 minutes, and a two-compartment model best explained the data. Protamine has a very rapid onset of action and can neutralize the effects of heparin within 5 min.[86]

ROLE IN REVERSING HEPARIN

Protamine is indicated to reverse anticoagulant effects of heparin.[34] It is commonly used during coronary artery bypass graft (CABG) and car-diac valve surgeries, during abdominal aortic aneurysm and other open abdominal surgeries, in fistula placement and noncardiac vascular surger-ies, during catheterization for cardiac or electrophysiologic procedures, and in hemodialysis.[11,43,70,105] Multiple controlled human trials substantiate the effectiveness of protamine in terminating the effects of heparin.[39,43,105] Protamine should be used in patients with consequential bleeding from excessive heparin.[29,34,47]

ROLE IN REVERSING LOW-MOLECULAR-WEIGHT HEPARIN

In contrast to heparin, there is no proven method for completely neutraliz-ing LMWH. Protamine neutralizes the anti-IIa activity of LMWH and a vari-able portion of the anti-Xa activity of LMWH.[34] Because the interaction of protamine and heparin is dependent on the MW of heparin, LMWH (mean MW, 4,500 Da) has reduced protamine binding. The protamine-resistant fraction in LMWH is an ultra–low-molecular-weight fraction with a low sul-fate charge.[21] No human studies offer strong evidence for or against a ben-eficial effect of protamine as treatment for hemorrhage after LMWH use.[34] Case studies and case reviews report both success and failure of protamine administration to reverse LMWH-associated bleeding.[7,12,13,18,49,71,73,75,96-99,108] Not all LMWHs are the same and tinzaparin, a highly sulfated LMWH, is more responsive to protamine than enoxaparin and dalteparin but still incomplete.[5,32,45] Protamine is reasonable therapy for LMWH excess associ-ated with hemorrhage, but complete reversal should not be expected, and caution should limit the protamine dose.

ADVERSE EFFECTS AND SAFETY ISSUES

Protamine is routinely used in the neutralization of heparin at the com-pletion of CABG surgery. More than 1 million coronary revascularizations are performed each year in the United States. However, unlike previous years, only one-fourth of these cases are now CABGs and routinely expose patients to protamine. Since the advent of CABG surgery, there have been approximately 100 deaths reported in total associated with the use of prot-amine. It is largely in this setting that the adverse effects of protamine are also documented and studied.[44,46,60,68,82] It is often difficult to separate the adverse effects caused by protamine from those of the protamine–heparin complex or those actually related to heparin. Adverse effects associated with protamine include both administration rate- and non–rate-related hypotension,[20,27-31,35,37,51,54,90,93] anaphylaxis,[50,67] anaphylactoid reactions,[53,76,78] bradycardia,[2] thrombocytopenia,[103] thrombogenicity,[22] leukopenia, decreased oxygen consumption,[100,102] acute respiratory distress syndrome (ARDS),[9,95] pulmonary hypertension and pulmonary vasoconstriction,[15,41] cardiovascular collapse,[65,88] and dose-dependent paradoxical anticoagulation with protamine excess.[3,8,55,60,80,81]

Mechanisms for these adverse effects are multifactorial.[91] Some contribution results from the significant electropositivity of protamine.[87] The protamine–heparin complex activates the arachidonic acid pathway, and the production of thromboxane A_2 is at least partly responsible for some of the hemodynamic changes, including pulmonary hypertension.[15,21,42,77,104] Pretreatment with indomethacin limits these effects.[21,42,77,104] Free protamine or protamine complexed with heparin converts L-arginine to nitric oxide (formerly called endothelium-derived relaxing factor), which in turn causes vasodilation and inhibits platelet aggregation and adhesion, potentially increasing bleeding risks.[84] Methylene blue, via reduction in the amount and effect of nitric oxide, was used with success to treat the vasoplegia secondary to a severe protamine reaction.[1,24,69,97] Protamine in excess of heparin enters the myocardium and decreases cyclic adenosine monophosphate (cAMP), causing myocardial depression.[15,92] Protamine and protamine–heparin complexes activate the complement pathway and contribute to vasoactive events.[15,85] Mast cells in the human heart and skin to are stimulated by protamine to release histamine.[15,69] In the absence of heparin or in an amount exceeding that necessary for heparin neutralization protamine acts as an anticoagulant through several mechanisms. Protamine impairs adenosine diphosphate–induced platelet aggregation, clot initiation, clot kinetics, and platelet function, resulting in weaker clot formation.[52,55,100] Additionally, protamine reduces factor V activation by both thrombin and factor Xa, decreases factor VII[8,80,81] activation by tissue factor, and enhances tissue-type plasminogen activator mediated fibrinolysis. A study in patients undergoing CABG reported higher rates of microvascular bleeding and coagulation factor replacement in those receiving excess protamine.[60]

Risk factors for protamine-induced adverse reactions include prior exposure to protamine in insulin, exposure during previous surgery with protamine reversal, vasectomy, fish allergy, or a rapid protamine infusion rate.[65,85] A prospective study reported a 0.06% incidence of anaphylactic reactions to protamine in all patients undergoing CABG, but a 2% incidence in diabetics using neutral protamine Hagedorn (NPH) insulin.[14] Patients with diabetes receiving daily subcutaneous injections of a protamine containing insulin (NPH) have a 40% to 50% increased risk of immune-mediated adverse reactions, including anaphylaxis.[34,36,40,50,59,93] A systematic review of the literature revealed an anaphylaxis incidence of 1%, but the authors were cautious in interpreting the results because of study heterogeneity.[82] Histamine concentrations; the activation of complement; and elevated IgE, IgA, and IgG concentrations are mechanisms for the immune-mediated adverse effects.[63,94,106,107]

Occasionally, patients manifesting a protamine allergy are incorrectly presumed to have an insulin allergy.[58] In patients with diabetes receiving protamine insulin injections, the presence of serum antiprotamine IgE antibody is a significant risk factor for acute protamine reactions. Only patients with previous exposure to protamine insulin injections had serum antiprotamine IgE antibodies. However, in the group without previous protamine insulin exposure, antiprotamine IgG antibody was noted as a risk factor for protamine reactions.[107] Either naturally occurring cross-reacting antibodies or perhaps previously unrecognized protamine exposure was responsible for the generation of these IgG antibodies.

ALTERNATIVES TO PROTAMINE IN PATIENTS AT RISK FOR ADVERSE DRUG REACTIONS

There are limited options to replace protamine for the reversal of heparin in patients who have previously experienced anaphylaxis after protamine therapy or in patients who are suspected of being at high risk. Recommended strategies usually depend on local preferences and include clotting factor replenishment, exchange transfusion in neonates, protamine avoidance, protamine administration with expectant management of anaphylaxis, or

heparin avoidance and use of bivalrudin.[61] Several investigational alternatives include heparin removal devices in the coronary artery bypass extracorporeal circuit, as well as the use of hexadimethrine, methylene blue, platelet factor-4, and heparinase antidotes.[14,57] Pretreatment with antihistamines and corticosteroids is often sufficient for immune-mediated mechanisms but will probably not be beneficial for pulmonary vasoconstriction and non–immune-mediated anaphylactoid reactions.[48]

PREGNANCY AND LACTATION

Protamine is FDA Pregnancy Category C. No animal studies have been done on reproduction. Taking into consideration the benefit-to-risk assessment, protamine is reasonable to reverse or partially reverse the bleeding in a pregnant woman considered secondary to UFH or LMWH, respectively.[6] Protamine excretion in breast milk is unknown.

DOSING AND ADMINISTRATION

Dosing in Cardiopulmonary Bypass

Protamine is most frequently used at the conclusion of cardiopulmonary bypass operations to reverse the effects of heparin. Many regimens are used for protamine dosing. These include using arbitrary amounts of protamine and dosing on the basis of the total amount of heparin used. We recommend the most commonly used approach using a ratio of 0.3 to 1 mg of protamine to 100 units of heparin and subsequently titrating based on activating clotting time (ACT) point-of-care testing.[25,39,52,66,109]

Heparin Rebound

A heparin anticoagulant rebound effect is noted after cardiopulmonary bypass and is attributed to the presence of detectable circulating heparin several hours after apparently adequate heparin neutralization with protamine. It is likely that the rapid clearance of protamine and redistribution of heparin from reservoirs in plasma proteins and vascular cytology contributes to this finding. The incidence of heparin rebound and the need for additional protamine range from 4% to 42%, depending on the neutralization protocol.[38,72,89] It is probable that larger heparin doses prolong the heparin clearance, contributing to higher than expected heparin concentrations.[89] When 300 units/kg of body weight doses of heparin were reversed with 3 mg/kg of protamine at the conclusion of cardiopulmonary bypass, a 14% incidence of small but detectable concentrations of circulating heparin was noted at 2 hours, which lasted less than 1 hour in all but one case.[72] A prolonged prothrombin time (PT) and thrombocytopenia occurred without increase in hemorrhage.

Dosing for Heparin and Low-Molecular-Weight Heparin

Approximately 1 mg of protamine will neutralize about 100 units (1 mg) of heparin (UFH). In the case of unintentional overdose, the half-life of heparin should be used to calculate the remaining quantity of heparin because half of the administered dose of heparin is eliminated within 60 to 90 minutes under normal dosing conditions. This means that if bleeding occurs 2 hours after a single dose, only half of that initial dose will require reversal with protamine.[34] We recommend this kinetic dosing, which is slightly more conservative than the package insert, which states that if protamine is administered 30 minutes after heparin, half of the usual dose of protamine is likely sufficient.[86] In the case of an unintentional overdose without hemorrhage, the short half-life of heparin and the potential risks of protamine diminish the benefit from protamine administration. If protamine is necessary to reverse active hemorrhage, it must be administered very slowly intravenously either undiluted or diluted in dextrose 5% in water or 0.9% sodium chloride over 10 to 15 minutes to limit the incidence of rate-related hypotension.[56,86,101] The dose of protamine should not exceed 50 mg intravenously.[32,34,86] In the absence of hemorrhage, repeat doses should be guided by the severity of the clinical status of the patient and the level of abnormality of the aPTT, thrombin time and antifactor Xa (anti-FXa) heparin concentrations.[32,86] The package insert has a specific warning: "Hyperheparinemia or bleeding has been reported in experimental animals and in some patients 30 minutes to 18 hours after cardiac surgery (under cardiopulmonary bypass) in spite of complete neutralization of heparin by adequate doses of protamine sulfate at the end of the operation. It is important to keep the patient under close observation after cardiac surgery. Additional doses of protamine sulfate should be administered if indicated by coagulation studies, such as the heparin titration test with protamine and the determination of plasma thrombin time."

Most studies demonstrate incomplete protamine neutralization of the LMWHs enoxaparin, dalteparin, and tinzaparin. We recommend administering 1 mg of protamine per 100 anti–factor Xa units, in which 1 mg of enoxaparin equals 100 anti–factor Xa units if administered within 8 hours of the LMWH. A second dose of 0.5 of mg protamine should be administered per 100 anti–factor Xa units if bleeding continues.[26,34,86] If more than 8 hours has elapsed, then a smaller fractional dose of protamine should be administered based on the actual time from the initiation of therapy.

A number of tests directly measure heparin concentrations or indirectly measure the effect of heparin on the clotting cascade.[16,19,25] These tests are helpful in determining the appropriate protamine dosing. Because excessive protamine acts as an anticoagulant, the dose chosen should be an underestimation of that which is needed.

The dosing of protamine in children for the reversal of heparin is similar to that of adults if the dose of heparin was given within 30 minutes and is 1 mg of protamine/100 units heparin received.[74] However if the dose of heparin has been 30 to 60 minutes earlier, then the dose of protamine should be 0.5 to 0.75 mg/100 units of heparin received. For 60 to 120 minutes after the heparin dose, the protamine dose is 0.375 to 0.5 mg/100 units heparin received, and for longer than 120 minutes, the protamine dose is 0.25 mg to 0.375 mg/100 units of heparin received. The maximum dose in each of these circumstances is 50 mg.[74]

DOSING IN THE OVERDOSE SETTING

When a patient is believed to have received an overdose of an unknown quantity of heparin, the decision to use protamine should be determined by the presence of a prolonged aPTT and thrombin time (TT) and antifactor Xa heparin concentration or the presence of persistent hemorrhage. The risks of protamine use, especially in those who have had a prior life-threatening reaction to protamine, as well as in a patient with diabetes receiving protamine-containing insulin, and the risks of continued heparin anticoagulation are essential to determine the appropriate use. A baseline ACT, TT, heparin-neutralized TT, heparin activity, platelets, PT, partial thromboplastin time, hemoglobin, and hematocrit ideally should be obtained. Because of the routine nature of heparin reversal after cardiopulmonary bypass, consultation with members of the bypass team would be reasonable. An empiric dose of protamine is determined by the baseline ACT: (1) an ACT of less than 200 seconds necessitates no protamine, (2) an ACT of 200 to 300 seconds necessitates 0.6 mg/kg, and (3) an ACT of 300 to 400 seconds necessitates 1.2 mg/kg. These doses should be given up to a single maximum dose of 50 mg. The dose can be repeated if dictated by persistent bleeding and an elevated aPTT, TT, and ACT. These doses have not been validated outside of the operating room. The ACT should be repeated 5 to 15 minutes after protamine administration and in 2 to 8 hours to evaluate for potential heparin rebound. Further dosing should be based on these values and the patient's clinical condition.[33]

When an ACT is unavailable, protamine 25 mg to a maximum of 50 mg should be administered to an adult and adjusted accordingly.[86] Repeat dosing in several hours will be necessary with heparin rebound if bleeding or ACT is prolonged. The dose should be administered slowly intravenously over 15 minutes with resuscitative equipment immediately available. Neonates should not receive protamine that has been diluted with bacteriostatic water containing benzyl alcohol.

AVAILABILITY

Protamine is available as a parenteral solution ready for injection in a concentration of 10 mg/mL in either a 5-mL or 25-mL vial containing totals of 50 mg and 250 mg, respectively, with and without preservatives.[86]

SUMMARY

- Protamine effectively and rapidly reverses the anticoagulant effect of UFH.
- Protamine variably reverses the anticoagulant effects of LMWH and cannot be expected to limit hemorrhage.
- Protamine has no effect on heparin pentasaccharide fragments or analogs.
- Protamine should only be used for a prolonged aPTT in the presence of active hemorrhage, given the risks of hypotension, anaphylaxis, anaphylactoid reactions, dysrhythmias, leukopenia, thrombocytopenia, and ARDS.
- Protamine must be given intravenously over 10 to 15 min because faster administration is likely to produce hypotension.
- In most circumstances outside of the operating room, the maximum single dose of protamine is 50 mg.

REFERENCES

1. Albuquerque AA, et al. Methylene blue to treat protamine-induced anaphylaxis reactions. An experimental study in pigs. *Braz J Cardiovasc Surg*. 2016;31:226-231.
2. Alvarez J, et al. Sinus node function and protamine sulfate. *J Cardiothorac Anesth*. 1989;3:44-51.
3. Andersen MN, et al. Experimental studies of heparin-protamine activity with special reference to protamine inhibition of clotting. *Surgery*. 1959;46:1060-1068.
4. Andersson LO, et al. Anticoagulant properties of heparin fractionated by affinity chromatography on matrix-bound antithrombin III and by gel filtration. *Thromb Res*. 1976;6:575-583.
5. Balla I, et al. Intentional overdose with tinzaparin: management dilemmas. *J Emerg Med*. 2014;46:197-201.
6. Bates SM, et al. VTE, thrombophilia, antithrombotic therapy, and pregnancy: antithrombotic therapy and prevention of thrombosis, 9th ed: American College of Chest Physicians Evidence-Based Clinical Practice Guidelines. *Chest*. 2012;141(2 suppl): e691S-e736S.
7. Bjornaas MA, et al. Nonfatal self-poisoning with LMW heparin and the use of antidote. *Thromb Res*. 2010;126:e403-e405.
8. Bolliger D, et al. The anticoagulant effect of protamine sulfate is attenuated in the presence of platelets or elevated factor VIII concentrations. *Anesth Analg*. 2010;111: 601-608.
9. Brooks JC. Noncardiogenic pulmonary edema immediately following rapid protamine administration. *Ann Pharmacother*. 1999;33:927-930.
10. Butterworth J, et al. The pharmacokinetics and cardiovascular effects of a single intravenous dose of protamine in normal volunteers. *Anesth Analg*. 2002;94:514-522.
11. Butterworth J, et al. Rapid disappearance of protamine in adults undergoing cardiac operation with cardiopulmonary bypass. *Ann Thorac Surg*. 2002;74:1589-1595.
12. Byrne M, Zumberg M. Intentional low-molecular-weight heparin overdose: a case report and review. *Blood Coagul Fibrinolysis*. 2012;23:772-774.
13. Byun Y, et al. Low molecular weight protamine: a potential nontoxic heparin antagonist. *Thromb Res*. 1999;94:53-61.
14. Carr JA, Silverman N. The heparin-protamine interaction. A review. *J Cardiovasc Surg (Torino)*. 1999;40:659-666.
15. Carr ME, Carr, SL. At high heparin concentrations, protamine concentrations which reverse heparin anticoagulant effects are insufficient to reverse heparin antiplatelet effects. *Thromb Res*. 1994;75:617-630.
16. Castellani WJ, et al. Effect of protamine sulfate on the ACA heparin assay. *Clin Chem*. 1991;37:1119-1120.
17. Chang SW, et al. Pulmonary vascular injury by polycations in perfused rat lungs. *J Appl Physiol*. 1987;62:1932-1943.
18. Chawla L, et al. Incomplete reversal of enoxaparin toxicity by protamine: implications of renal insufficiency, obesity and low molecular weight heparin sulfate content. *Obesity Surg*. 2004;14:695-698.
19. Chen W, Yang V. Versatile non-clotting based heparin assay requiring no instrumentation. *Clin Chem*. 1991;37:832-837.
20. Chilukuri K, et al. Incidence and outcomes of protamine reactions in patients undergoing catheter ablation of atrial fibrillation. *J Interv Card Electrophysiol*. 2009;25: 175-181.
21. Conzen PF, et al. Thromboxane mediation of pulmonary hemodynamic responses after neutralization of heparin by protamine in pigs. *Anesth Analg*. 1989;68:25-31.
22. Cosgrove J, et al. Protamine usage following implantation of drug-eluting stents: a word of caution. *Cath Cardiovas Interv*. 2008;71:913-914.
23. Crowther MA, et al. Mechanisms responsible for the failure of protamine to inactivate low-molecular-weight heparin. *Br J Haematol*. 2002;116:178-186.
24. Del Duca D, et al. Use of methylene blue for catecholamine-refractory vasoplegia from protamine and aprotinin. *Ann Thorac Surg*. 2009;87:640-642.
25. Despotis GJ, et al. Anticoagulation monitoring during cardiac surgery: a review of current and emerging techniques. *Anesthesiology*. 1999;91:1122-1151.

26. Dietrich CP, et al. Structural features and bleeding activity of commercial low-molecular-weight heparins: neutralization by ATP and protamine. *Semin Thromb Hemost.* 1999;3:43-50.

27. Fadali MA, et al. Mechanism responsible for the cardiovascular depressant effect of protamine sulfate. *Ann Surg.* 1974;180:232-235.

28. Fadali MA, et al. Cardiovascular depressant effect of protamine sulfate. *Thorax.* 1976; 31:320-323.

29. Figueiredo S, et al. Emergency reversal of heparin overdose in a neurosurgical patient guided by thromboelastography. *Br J Anaesth.* 2013;111:303-304.

30. Food and Drug Administration. New drug application: Washington, DC: Food and Drug Administration; 1968:6460, log 775.

31. Frater RMW, et al. Protamine-induced circulatory changes. *J Thorac Cardiovasc Surg.* 1984;87:687-692.

32. Frontera JA, et al. Guideline for reversal of antithrombotics in intracranial hemorrhage: a statement for healthcare professionals from the Neurocritical Care Society and Society of Critical Care Medicine. *Neurocrit Care.* 2016;24:6-46.

33. Galeone A, et al. Monitoring incomplete heparin reversal and heparin rebound after cardiac surgery. *J Cardiothorac Vasc Anesth.* 2013;27:853-858.

34. Garcia DA, et al. Parenteral anticoagulants: antithrombotic therapy and prevention of thrombosis, 9th ed: American College of Chest Physicians Evidence-Based Clinical Practice Guidelines. *Chest.* 2012;141(2 suppl):e24S-43S.

35. Goldman BS, et al. Cardiovascular effects of protamine sulfate. *Ann Thorac Cardiovasc Surg.* 1969;7:459-471.

36. Gottschlich GM, et al. Adverse reactions to protamine sulfate during cardiac surgery in diabetic and nondiabetic patients. *Ann Allergy.* 1988;61:277-281.

37. Gourin A, et al. Protamine sulfate administration and the cardiovascular system. *J Thorac Cardiovasc Surg.* 1971;62:193-204.

38. Gundry SR, et al. Postoperative bleeding in cardiovascular surgery: does heparin rebound really exist? *Am Surg.* 1989;55:162-165.

39. Guo Y, et al. Protamine dosage based on two titrations reduces blood loss after valve replacement surgery: a prospective, double-blinded, randomized study. *Can J Cardiol.* 2012;28:547-552.

40. Gupta SK, et al. Anaphylactoid reactions to protamine: an often lethal complication in insulin-dependent diabetic patients undergoing vascular surgery. *J Vasc Surg.* 1989; 9:342-350.

41. Hiong Y, et al. A case of catastrophic pulmonary vasoconstriction after protamine administration in cardiac surgery: role of intraoperative transesophageal echocardiography. *J Cardiothorac Vascular Anesth.* 2008;22:727-731.

42. Hobbhahn J, et al. Beneficial effect of cyclooxygenase inhibition on adverse hemodynamic responses after protamine. *Anesth Analg.* 1988;67:253-260.

43. Hofmann B, et al. Immediate effects of individualized heparin and protamine management on hemostatic activation and platelet function in adult patients undergoing cardiac surgery with tranexamic acid antifibrinolytic therapy. *Perfusion.* 2013;28: 412-418.

44. Holland CL, et al. Adverse reactions to protamine sulfate following cardiac surgery. *Clin Cardiol.* 1984;7:157-162.

45. Holst J, et al. Protamine neutralization of intravenous and subcutaneous low-molecular-weight heparin (tinzaparin, Logiparin). An experimental investigation in healthy volunteers. *Blood Coagul Fibrinolysis.* 1994;5:795-803.

46. Horrow JC. Protamine: a review of its toxicity. *Anesth Analg.* 1985;64:348-361.

47. Hudcova J, Talmor D. Life-threatening hemorrhage following subcutaneous heparin therapy. *Ther Clin Risk Manag.* 2009;5:51-54.

48. Hughes C, Haddock M. Protamine reaction in a patient undergoing coronary artery bypass grafting. *CRNA.* 1995;6:172-176.

49. Hulin MS, et al. Comparison of the hemodynamic and hematologic toxicity of a protamine variant after reversal of low-molecular-weight heparin anticoagulation in a canine model. *Lab Anim Sci.* 1997;47:153-160.

50. Jackson DR. Sustained hypotension secondary to protamine sulfate. *Angiology.* 1970; 21:295-298.

51. Jastrebski MK, et al. Cardiorespiratory effects of protamine after cardiopulmonary bypass in man. *Thorax.* 1974;20:534-538.

52. Jobes DR, et al. Increased accuracy and precision of heparin and protamine dosing reduces blood loss and transfusion in patients undergoing primary cardiac operations. *J Thorac Cardiovasc Surg.* 1995;110:36-45.

53. Kambam JR, et al. Histamine$_2$ receptor blocker in the treatment of protamine-related anaphylactoid reactions: two case reports. *Can J Anaesth.* 1989;36:463-465.

54. Katz NM, et al. Hemodynamics of protamine administration. *J Thorac Cardiovasc Surg.* 1987;94:881-886.

55. Khan NU, et al. The effects of protamine overdose on coagulation parameters as measured by the thrombelastograph. *Eur J Anaesthes.* 2010;27:624-627.

56. Kien ND, et al. Mechanism of hypotension following rapid infusion of protamine sulfate in anesthetized dogs. *J Cardiothorac Vasc Anesth.* 1992;6:143-147.

57. Kikura M, et al. Heparin neutralization with methylene blue, hexadimethrine, or vancomycin after cardiopulmonary bypass. *Anesth Analg.* 1996;83:223-227.

58. Kim R. Anaphylaxis to protamine masquerading as an insulin allergy. *Del Med J.* 1993;65:17-23.

59. Kimmel SE, et al. Risk factors for clinically important adverse events after protamine administration following cardiopulmonary bypass. *J Am Coll Cardiol.* 1998;32:1916-1922.

60. Koster A, et al. Protamine overdose and its impact on coagulation, bleeding, and transfusions after cardiopulmonary bypass: results of a randomized double-blind controlled pilot study. *Clin Appl Thromb Hemost.* 2014; 20:290-295.

61. Koster A, et al. Management of protamine allergy with bivalirudin during coronary artery revascularization. *Ann Thorac Surg.* 2010;90:276-277.

62. Kuitunen AH, et al. Heparin rebound: a comparative study of protamine chloride and protamine sulfate in patients undergoing coronary artery bypass surgery. *J Cardiothorac Vasc Anesth.* 1991;5:221-226.

63. Lakin JD, et al. Anaphylaxis to protamine sulfate mediated by a complement dependent IgG antibody. *J Allergy Clin Immunol.* 1978;61:102-107.

64. Lam LH, et al. The separation of active and inactive forms of heparin. *Biochem Biophys Res Commun.* 1976;69:570-577.

65. Levy J, Adkinson N. Anaphylaxis during cardiac surgery: implications for clinicians. *Anesth Analg.* 2008;106:392-403.

66. Levy J, Tanaka K. Anticoagulation and reversal paradigms: is too much of a good thing bad? *Anesth Analg.* 2009;108:692-694.

67. Lieberman P, et al. The diagnosis and amanagement of anaphylaxis: an updated practice parameter. *J Allergy Clin Immunol.* 2005;115(suppl):S483-S523.

68. Lindblad B. Protamine sulphate: a review of its effects—hypersensitivity and toxicity. *Eur J Vasc Surg.* 1989;3:195-201.

69. Lutjen DL, Arndt KL. Methylene blue to treat vasoplegia due to a severe protamine reaction: a case report. *AANA J.* 2012;80:170-173.

70. Mahan CE. A 1-year drug utilization evaluation of protamine in hospitalized patients to identify possible future roles of heparin and low molecular weight heparin reversal agents. *J Thromb Thrombolysis.* 2014;37:271-278.

71. Makris M, et al. Poor reversal of low molecular weight heparin by protamine. *Br J Hematol.* 2000;108:884-885.

72. Martin P, et al. Heparin rebound phenomenon: much ado about nothing. *Blood Coagul Fibrinolysis.* 1992;3:187-191.

73. Massonnet-Castel S, et al. Partial reversal of low molecular weight heparin (PK 10169) anti-Xa activity by protamine sulfate: in vitro and in vivo study during cardiac surgery with extracorporeal circulation. *Hemostasis.* 1986;16:139-146.

74. Monagle P, et al. Antithrombotic therapy in neonates and children: antithrombotic therapy and prevention of thrombosis, 9th ed: American College of Chest Physicians Evidence-Based Clinical Practice Guidelines. *Chest.* 2012;141(2 suppl):e737S-e801S. Erratum in: *Chest.* 2014;146:1422. *Chest.* 2014 Dec;146:1694. Dosage error in article text.

75. Monte AA, et al. Low-molecular-weight heparin overdose: management by observation. *Ann Pharmacother.* 2010;44:1836-1839.

76. Moorthy SS, et al. Severe circulatory shock following protamine (an anaphylactoid reaction). *Anesth Analg.* 1980;59:77-78.

77. Morel DR, et al. C5a and thromboxane generation associated with pulmonary vaso- and broncho-constriction during protamine reversal of heparin. *Anesthesiology.* 1987;66:597-604.

78. Neidhart PP, et al. Fatal anaphylactoid response to protamine after percutaneous transluminal coronary angioplasty. *Eur Heart J.* 1992;13:856-858.

79. Ng HJ, et al. Successful control of postsurgical bleeding by recombinant factor VIIa in a renal failure patient given low molecular weight heparin and aspirin. *Ann Hematol.* 2003;82:257-258.

80. Ni Ainle F, et al. Protamine sulfate down-regulates thrombin generation by inhibiting factor V activation. *Blood.* 2009;114:1658-1665.

81. Nielsen VG, Malayaman SN. Protamine sulfate: crouching clot or hidden hemorrhage? *Anesth Analg.* 2010;111:593-594.

82. Nybo M, Madsen S. Serious anaphylaxis reactions to protamine sulfate: a systematic literature review. *Basic Clin Pharmacol Toxicol.* 2008;103:192-196.

83. Okajirna Y, et al. Studies on the neutralizing mechanism of antithrombin activity of heparin by protamine. *Thromb Res.* 1981;24:21-29.

84. Pearson PJ, et al. Protamine releases endothelium-derived relaxing factor from systemic arteries. *Anesth Prog.* 1991;38:99-100.

85. Porsche R, Brenner ZR. Allergy to protamine sulfate. *Heart Lung.* 1999;28:418-428.

86. Protamine sulfate injection, USP [package insert]: Lake Zurich, IL: Frensenius Kabi; 2017.

87. Pugsley MK, et al. Charge is an important determinant of hemodynamic and adverse cardiovascular effects of cationic drugs. *Pharmacol Res.* 2015;102:46-52.

88. Pugsley MK, et al. Protamine is a low molecular weight polycationic amine that produces actions on cardiac muscle. *Life Sci.* 2002;72:293-305.

89. Raul TK, et al. Heparin administration during extracorporeal circulation: heparin rebound and postoperative bleeding. *J Thorac Cardiovasc Surg.* 1979;78:95-102.

90. Shapira N, et al. Cardiovascular effects of protamine sulfate in man. *J Thorac Cardiovasc Surg.* 1982;84:505-514.

91. Sokolowska E, et al. The toxicology of heparin reversal with protamine: past, present and future. *Expert Opin Drug Metab Toxicol.* 2016;12:897-909.

92. Stefaniszyn HJ, et al. Toward a better understanding of the hemodynamic effects of protamine and heparin interaction. *J Thorac Cardiovasc Surg.* 1984;87:678-686.

93. Stewart WJ, et al. Increased risk of severe protamine reactions in NPH insulin-dependent diabetics undergoing cardiac catheterization. *Circulation.* 1984;70:788-792.

94. Stoelting RK, et al. Hemodynamic changes and circulating histamine concentrations following protamine administration to patients and dogs. *Can Anaesth Soc J.* 1984;31:534-540.

95. Urdaneta F, et al. Noncardiogenic pulmonary edema associated with protamine administration during coronary artery bypass graft surgery. *J Clin Anesth.* 1999;11:675-681.

96. van Veen JJ, et al. Protamine reversal of low molecular weight heparin: clinically effective? *Blood Coagul Fibrinolysis.* 2011;22:565-570.

97. Viaro F, et al. Catastrophic cardiovascular adverse reactions to protamine are nitric oxide/cyclic guanosine monophosphate dependent and endothelium mediated: should methylene blue be the treatment of choice? *Chest.* 2002;122:1061-1066.

98. Wakefield TW, et al. A [18RGD] protamine variant for nontoxic and effective reversal of conventional heparin and low-molecular-weight anticoagulation. *J Surg Res.* 1996;63:280-296.

99. Wakefield TW, et al. Effective and less toxic reversal of low-molecular weight heparin anticoagulation by a designer variant of protamine. *J Vasc Surg.* 1995;21:839-849.

100. Wakefield TW, et al. Impaired myocardial function and oxygen utilization due to protamine sulfate in an isolated rabbit heart preparation. *Ann Surg.* 1990;212:387-393.

101. Wakefield TW, et al. Effects of differing rates of protamine reversal of heparin anticoagulation. *Surgery.* 1996;119:123-128.

102. Wakefield TW, et al. Decreased oxygen consumption as a toxic manifestation of protamine sulfate reversal of heparin anticoagulation. *J Vasc Surg.* 1989;9:772-777.

103. Wakefield TW, et al. Heparin-mediated reduction of the toxic effects of protamine sulfate on rabbit myocardium. *J Vasc Surg.* 1992;16:47-53.

104. Wakefield TW, et al. Increased prostacyclin and adverse hemodynamic responses to protamine sulfate in an experimental canine model. *J Surg Res.* 1991;50:449-456.

105. Wang J, Ma et al. Blood loss after cardiopulmonary bypass, standard vs titrated protamine: a meta-analysis. *Neth J Med.* 2013;71:123-127.

106. Weiss ME, et al. Serial immunologic investigations in a patient who had a life-threatening reaction to intravenous protamine. *Clin Exp Allergy.* 1990;20:713-720.

107. Weiss ME, et al. Association of protamine IgE and IgG antibodies with life-threatening reactions to intravenous protamine. *N Engl J Med.* 1989;320:886-892.

108. Wiernikowski J, et al. Reversal of anti-thrombin activity using protamine sulfate. Experience in a neonate with a 10-fold overdose of enoxaparin. *Thromb Res.* 2007;120:303-305.

109. Wright SJ, et al. Calculating the protamine-heparin reversal ratio: a pilot study investigating a new method. *J Cardiothorac Vasc Anesth.* 1993;7:416-421.

History A 48-year-old woman was transported to the hospital by emergency medical services (EMS). According to the paramedics, they were called to the house after the patient sent a text message to a friend saying that she no longer wanted to live. The friend went to the patient's house, and when no one answered, she called 911 to have the police break down the door. The patient was found on her bed with a suicide note. The friend related that the patient had migraine headaches but did not know what medications she used.

Emergency medical services personnel reported that at the scene the patient was lethargic with the following vital signs: blood pressure, 70/40 mm Hg; pulse, 25 beats/min; and respiratory rate, 8 breaths/min. Emergency medical services administered oxygen via nasal cannula at 4L/min inserted an intravenous (IV) catheter, infused 0.9% sodium chloride running wide open, and administered 0.5 mg of atropine IV before arrival to the hospital.

Physical Examination On arrival to the hospital, the patient had the following vital signs: blood pressure, 76/42 mm Hg; pulse, 35 beats/min; respiratory rate, 10 breaths/min; temperature, 98.3°F; O_2 saturation, 99% on room air; end-tidal CO_2, 38 mm Hg; and rapid reagent bedside glucose, 58 mg/dL. Physical examination was notable for pupils that were 2 to 3 mm and sluggishly reactive to light. Gag reflex was intact, and there were no secretions, pills, or blood in the mouth. The patient's chest was clear to auscultation, and other than bradycardia, her cardiac examination was normal. The abdomen was soft with normal bowel sounds, and her skin was normal. The patient responded to sternal rub by opening her eyes but mumbled incoherently. She moved all four extremities to pain and was able to localize the source of the pain.

Initial Management Dextrose (50 g IV) and naloxone (0.04 mg followed by 0.08 mg and 0.4 mg IV) were given with no clinical response. Blood samples were sent for a complete blood count, electrolytes, ethanol, and acetaminophen (APAP), and an electrocardiogram (ECG) was ordered.

What Is the Differential Diagnosis?
Many xenobiotics cause bradycardia (Chap. 15), but this patient has the combined features of hypotension and bradycardia. Here, the differential diagnosis is narrower, with the most common causes listed in Table CS8–1.

What Clinical and Laboratory Analyses Help Exclude Life-Threatening Causes of This Patient's Presentation? Often, the physical examination provides significant insight into the diagnosis. Patients who overdose with either opioids or α_2-adrenergic agonists may present with the classic opioid toxic syndrome (Chaps. 3, 36, and 61 and Table 3–2) that is manifested by miosis and depression of both the central nervous system and the respiratory drive. Although this patient has many features consistent with that toxic syndrome, the normal oxygen saturation on room air, normal end-tidal CO_2, and failure to respond to naloxone essentially exclude the diagnosis of an opioid overdose. Also, most other causes of hypotension and bradycardia routinely decrease the level of consciousness except for nondihydropyridine calcium channel blockers, which tend to preserve the level of consciousness (Chap. 60).

An ECG should be evaluated (Fig. CS8–1). Although patients with all of the causes listed in Table CS8–1 can present with sinus bradycardia, certain features may be suggestive of the etiology. When bradycardia is associated with traditional class I antidysrhythmics, the QRS complex is usually significantly widened as a result of sodium channel blockade (Chap. 57). Patients prescribed

TABLE CS8–1	Differential Diagnosis

Most Common Toxicologic Causes of Combined Hypotension and Bradycardia

α_2-Adrenergic agonists	Calcium channel blockers
β-Adrenergic antagonists	Cardioactive steroids
Antidysrhythmics (Class I)	Opioids
Baclofen	

cardioactive steroids often have underlying atrial fibrillation or demonstrate a "digoxin effect" (Chap. 62). In overdose, they may have ventricular premature beats, high degrees of atrioventricular blockade, or delayed after depolarizations on their ECGs (Chap. 15). Finally, although a prolongation of the QT interval is nonspecific, it is expected with class IA and IC antidysrhythmics and some opioids, most notably methadone (Chap. 36).

Rapid laboratory testing may also be of some utility. With acute toxicity from cardioactive steroids, the serum potassium concentration rises, and this increase has prognostic implications (Chap. 62). Less dramatic rises occur with β-adrenergic antagonist overdose but have unclear prognostic value. This patient's serum potassium concentration was 5.2 mEq/L. β-Adrenergic antagonists also tend to cause hypoglycemia. In contradistinction, hyperglycemia, although not only common with calcium channel blockers, has prognostic implications.

Further Diagnosis and Treatment
A clinical decision was made to forgo attempts at gastrointestinal decontamination given the patient's mental status. She was infused a second liter of 0.9% sodium chloride intravenously and administered glucagon for a presumed β-adrenergic antagonist overdose (Antidotes in Depth: A20). This diagnosis was suspected given the history of migraines (because this class of medication is commonly prescribed prophylactically for migraine headache), the ECG, the serum potassium concentration, and the blood glucose concentration. After 3 mg of glucagon IV, the patient's blood pressure rose to 102/62 mm Hg with a pulse of 60 beats/min, and this dose was repeated in 15 minutes when her blood pressure fell again. Her anion gap was normal, and both APAP and ethanol concentrations were negative. By the next day, she was awake, and her vital signs remained normal. During a subsequent psychiatric evaluation, she admitted to taking an unspecified amount of propranolol. She was voluntarily admitted for psychiatric care.

CASE STUDY 8 (CONTINUED)

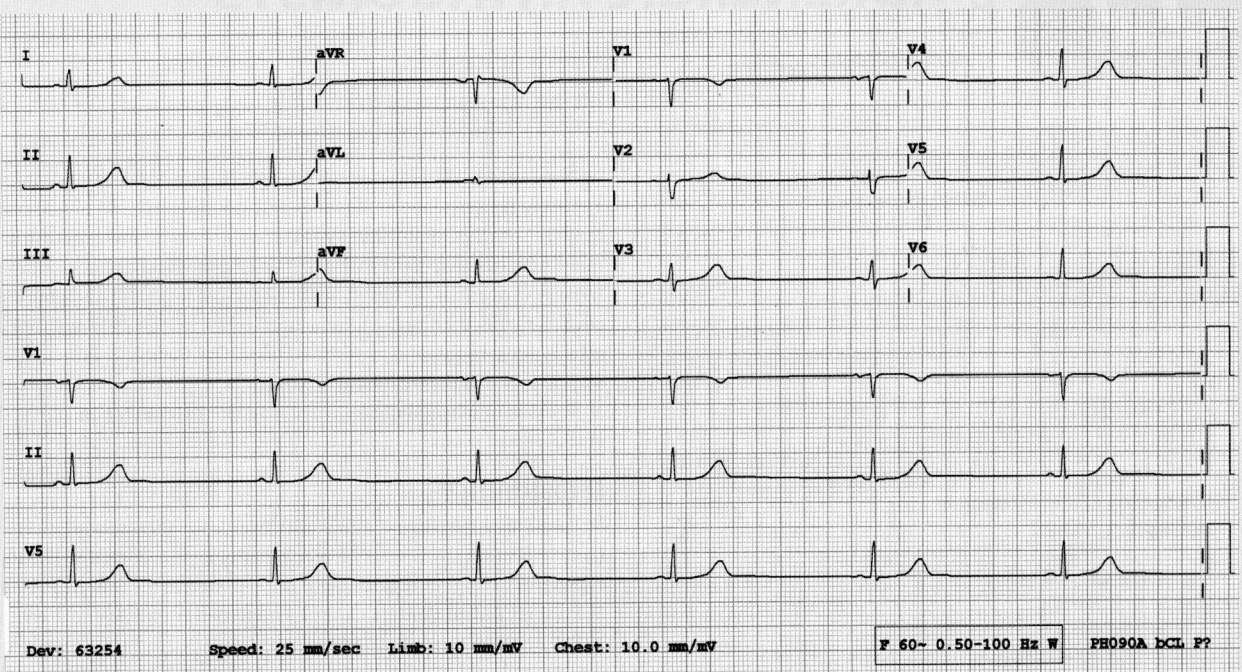

FIGURE CS8–1. Electrocardiogram on presentation showing profound sinus bradycardia with a heart rate of 36 beats/min. The axis is normal, as are the PR interval of 120 ms and the QRS complex duration of 80 ms. The QT interval is slightly prolonged at 510 ms, and there is no evidence of ischemia or infarction.

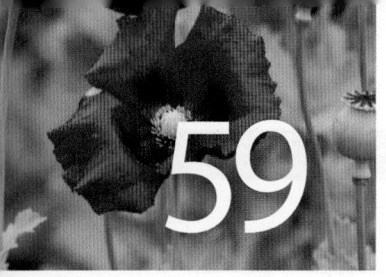

59 β-ADRENERGIC ANTAGONISTS

Jeffrey R. Brubacher

O—CH₂–CH—CH₂–NH—CH(CH₃)₂
|
OH

Atenolol

CH₂–C—NH₂

O—CH₂–CH—CH₂–NH—CH(CH₃)₂
|
OH

Metoprolol

CH₂–CH₂–O–CH₃

O—CH₂–CH—CH₂–NH—CH(CH₃)₂
|
OH

Pindolol

N
|
H

O—CH₂–CH—CH₂–NH—CH(CH₃)₂
|
OH

Propranolol

HISTORY

In 1948, Raymond Alquist postulated that epinephrine's cardiovascular actions of hypertension and tachycardia were best explained by the existence of two distinct sets of receptors that he generically named α and β receptors. At that time, the contemporary "antiepinephrine" agents such as phenoxybenzamine reversed the hypertension but not the tachycardia associated with epinephrine. According to Alquist's theory, these xenobiotics acted at the α receptors. The β receptors, in his schema, mediated catecholamine-induced tachycardia. British pharmacist Sir James Black was influenced by Alquist's work and recognized the potential clinical benefit of a β-adrenergic antagonist. In 1958, Black synthesized the first β-adrenergic antagonist, pronethalol. Pronethalol was briefly marketed as "Alderlin," named after Alderly Park, the research headquarters of ICI Pharmaceuticals. Pronethalol was discontinued because it produced thymic tumors in mice. Propranolol was soon developed and marketed as "Inderal" (an incomplete anagram of Alderlin) in the United Kingdom in 1964[31,235] and in the United States in 1973. Before the introduction of β-adrenergic antagonists, the management of angina was limited to xenobiotics such as nitrates, which reduced preload through dilation of the venous capacitance vessels and increased myocardial oxygen delivery by vasodilation of the coronary arteries. Propranolol gave clinicians the ability to decrease myocardial oxygen utilization. This new approach decreased morbidity and mortality in patients with ischemic heart disease.[134] New medications soon followed, and by 1979, there were 10 β-adrenergic antagonists available in the United States.[74] Unfortunately, it soon became apparent that these xenobiotics were dangerous when taken in overdose, and by 1979, severe toxicity and death from β-adrenergic overdose

were reported.[74] There are currently 20 US Food and Drug Administration–approved β-adrenergic antagonists with additional β-adrenergic antagonists available worldwide (Table 59–1). They are commonly used in the treatment of cardiovascular disease: hypertension, coronary artery disease, and tachydysrhythmias. Other indications for β-adrenergic antagonists include congestive heart failure, migraine headaches, benign essential tremor, panic attack, stage fright, and hyperthyroidism. Ophthalmic β-adrenergic antagonists are used in the treatment of glaucoma.[101] The pharmacology, toxicology, and poison management issues discussed in this chapter are applicable to all of these indications.

EPIDEMIOLOGY

Intentional β-adrenergic antagonist overdose, although relatively uncommon, continues to account for a number of deaths annually. The number of exposures to β-adrenergic antagonists reported to the American Association of Poison Control Centers (AAPCC) increased from 9,500 in 1999 to almost 25,000 in 2014. During the 5-year period from 2010 to 2014, there were 120,409 β-adrenergic antagonist exposures reported to the AAPCC (Chap. 130). These exposures resulted in 326 deaths of which β adrenergic antagonists were the first listed cause of death in 216 cases. Children younger than the age of 6 years accounted for 15,623 exposures and no fatalities. The youngest fatality attributed to β-adrenergic antagonists in this period was aged 14 years. Just under half of these exposures (52,347) were single-substance exposures. Each year since 2010, single-substance exposures to β-adrenergic antagonists resulted in 70 to 110 cases with major morbidity and 5 to 14 fatalities (Chap. 130).[39,184,186]

Compared with the other β-adrenergic antagonists, propranolol accounts for a disproportionate number of reported cases of self-poisoning[50,204] and deaths.[130,156] This may be explained by the fact that propranolol is frequently prescribed to patients with diagnoses such as anxiety, stress, and migraine who may be more prone to suicide attempts. Propranolol is more lethal because of its lipophilic and membrane-stabilizing properties.[96,204]

PHARMACOLOGY

The Cardiac Cycle

Normal cardiac electrical activity involves a complex series of ion fluxes that result in myocyte depolarization and repolarization. Cardiac electrical activity is coupled to myocyte contraction and relaxation, respectively, by increases and decreases in intracellular calcium concentrations. Cardiac electrical and mechanical activity is closely regulated by the autonomic nervous system.

Under normal conditions, heart rate is determined by the rate of spontaneous discharge of specialized pacemaker cells that comprise the sinoatrial (SA) node (Fig. 59–1). Pacemaker cells are also found in the atrioventricular (AV) node and in Purkinje fibers. Spontaneous pacemaker cell depolarization was once attributed to inward cation current through "pacemaker channels."[2,60] More recent research suggests that spontaneous depolarization of pacemaker cells involves several mechanisms, including a "membrane clock," consisting of "pacemaker channels" and other inward cation channels located on the cell membrane, and a "calcium clock," which is driven by rhythmic release of calcium from the sarcoplasmic reticulum (SR).[47,133,139,164,167,267] β-Adrenergic stimulation significantly increases the rate of pacemaker cell depolarization by phosphorylating proteins within the SR, thereby increasing the rate of the "calcium clock." There is also a direct, phosphorylation-independent action of cyclic adenosine monophosphate (cAMP) at the pacemaker channels, which increases the rate of the "membrane clock."[47] Depolarization of cells in the SA

TABLE 59–1	Pharmacologic Properties of the β-Adrenergic Antagonists								
	Adrenergic Blocking Activity	Partial Agonist Activity (ISA)	Membrane-Stabilizing Activity	Vasodilating Property	Log D[b]	Protein Binding (%)	Oral Bioavailability (%)	Half-Life (h)	Metabolism	Volume of Distribution (L/kg)
Acebutolol	β_1	Yes	Yes	No	0.52	25	40	2–4	Hepatic or renal	1.2
Atenolol	β_1	No	No	No	-2.03	<5	40–50	5–9	Renal	1
Betaxolol (tablets and ophthalmic)	β_1	No	Yes	Yes (calcium channel blockade)	0.56	50	80–90	14–22	Hepatic or renal	4.9–8.8
Bisoprolol	β_1	No	No	No	0.11	30	80	9–12	Hepatic or renal	3.2
Bucindolol[a]	β_1, β_2	β_2	NA	Yes (β_2 agonism and α_1 blockade)	NA	NA	30	8 +/− 4.5	Hepatic	NA
Carteolol (ophthalmic)	β_1, β_2	Yes	No	Yes (β_2 agonism and nitric oxide mediated)	-0.42	30	85	5–6	Renal	NA
Carvedilol (long acting form available)	$\alpha_1, \beta_1, \beta_2$	No	Yes	Yes (α_1 blockade, calcium channel blockade)	3.16	~98	25–35	6–10	Hepatic	2
Celiprolol	α_2, β_1	β_2	NA	Yes (β_2 agonism, nitric oxide mediated)	NA	22–24	30–70	5	Hepatic	NA
Esmolol	β_1	No	No	No	-0.22	50	NA	~8 min	RBC esterases	2
Labetalol	$\alpha_1, \beta_1, \beta_2$	β_2	Low	Yes (α_1 blockade, β_2 agonism)	0.99	50	20–33	4–8	Hepatic	9
Levobunolol (ophthalmic)	β_1, β_2	No	No	No	0.56	NA	NA	6	NA	NA
Metipranolol (ophthalmic)	β_1, β_2	No	No	No	0.53	NA	NA	3–4	NA	NA
Metoprolol (long-acting form available)	β_1	No	Low	No	-0.34	10	40–50	3–4	Hepatic	4
Nadolol	β_1, β_2	No	No	No	-0.84	20–30	30–35	10–24	Renal	2
Nebivolol	β_1	No	NA	Yes (nitric oxide mediated)	NA	98	12–96	8–32	Hepatic	10–40
Oxprenolol	β_1, β_2	Yes	Yes	No	NA	80	20%–70%	1–3	Hepatic	1.3
Penbutolol	β_1, β_2	Yes	No	No	2.05	90	~100	5	Hepatic or renal	NA
Pindolol	β_1, β_2	Yes	Low	No	-0.19	50	75–90	3–4	Hepatic or renal	2
Propranolol (long-acting form available)	β_1, β_2	No	Yes	No	0.99	90	30–70	3–5	hepatic	4
Sotalol	β_1, β_2	No	No	No	-1.82	0	90	9–12	Renal	2
Timolol (tablets and ophthalmic)	β_1, β_2	No	No	No	-1.99	60	75	3–5	Hepatic or renal	2

[a]Xenobiotics in italics are not approved by the Food and Drug Administration. [b]Log D is the octanol/water partition coefficient at a pH of 7.

ISA = intrinsic sympathomimetic activity; NA = information not available; RBC = red blood cell; NA = not available.

Information from references 75, 77, 96, 169, 172, 175, 191, 251, and 268.

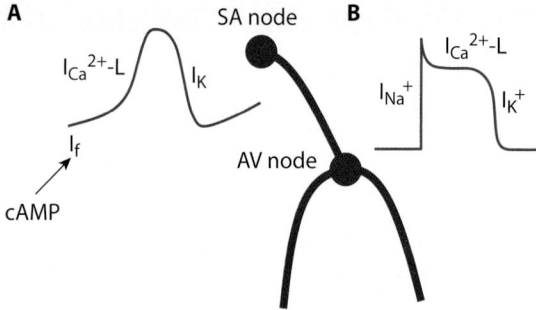

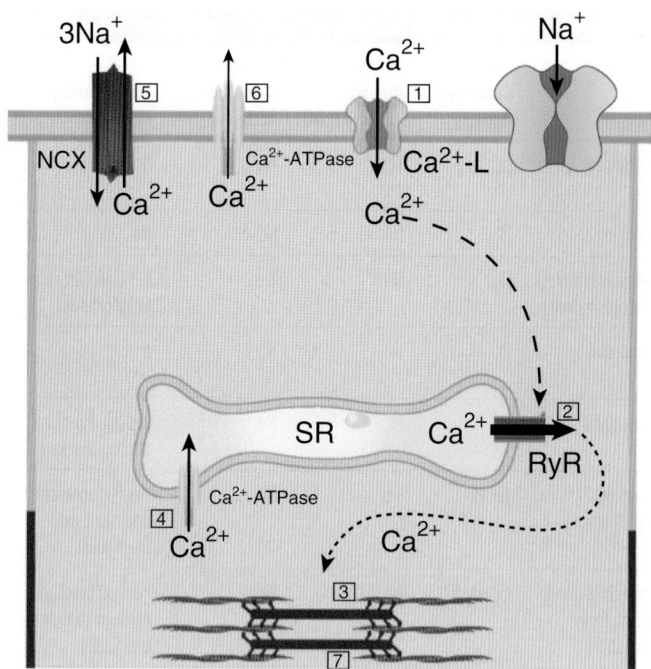

FIGURE 59–1. The cardiac conduction system. (**A**) The cardiac cycle begins when pacemaker cells in the sinoatrial (SA) node depolarize spontaneously. Traditionally, this depolarization was attributed to inward "pacemaker" currents (I_f). There is now evidence that pacemaker cell depolarization may also be driven by cyclical calcium release from a "calcium clock" in the sarcoplasmic reticulum (SR). β-Adrenergic stimulation increases both the frequency of the "calcium clock" by a phosphokinase A (PKA)–mediated effect and the magnitude of the pacemaker current secondary to a direct effect of cyclic adenosine monophosphate (cAMP). These effects both increase the heart rate. Cholinergic stimulation has the opposite effects and results in bradycardia. Pacemaker cells lack fast Na^+ channels. Pacemaker cell depolarization triggers the opening of voltage-gated type calcium channels ($I_{Ca^{2+}}$-L), and the impulse is transmitted to surrounding cells. (**B**) Coordinated SA nodal depolarization generates an impulse sufficient to open fast Na^+ channels in surrounding atrial tissue, and the impulse spreads along specialized pathways to depolarize the atria and ventricles. AV = atrioventricular.

FIGURE 59–2. Fluctuations in Ca^{2+} concentrations couple myocyte depolarization with contraction and myocyte repolarization with relaxation. (1) Depolarization, driven by Na^+ influx through Na^+ channels, causes voltage-gated Ca^{2+} channels to open and calcium to flow down its concentration gradient into the myocyte. (2) This Ca^{2+} current triggers the opening of Ca^{2+} release channels in the sarcoplasmic reticulum (SR), and calcium pours out of the SR. The amount of Ca^{2+} released from the SR is proportional to the initial inward Ca^{2+} current and to the amount of calcium stored in the SR. (3) At rest, actin–myosin interaction is prevented by troponin. When Ca^{2+} binds to troponin, this inhibition is removed, actin and myosin slide relative to each other, and the cell contracts.

After contraction, calcium is actively removed from the myocyte to allow relaxation. (4) Most Ca^{2+} is actively pumped into the SR, where it is bound to calsequestrin. Calcium stored in the SR is thus available for release during subsequent depolarizations. The sarcoplasmic Ca^{2+} ATPase is inhibited by phospholamban (Fig. 59–3). (5) NCX, the Ca^{2+}, Na^+ antiporter, couples the flow of three molecules of Na^+ flow in one direction to that of a single molecule of Ca^{2+} in the opposite direction. This transporter is passively driven by electrochemical gradients, which usually favor the inward flow of sodium coupled to the extrusion of calcium. Extrusion of Ca^{2+} is inhibited by high intracellular sodium or extracellular Ca^{2+} concentrations and by cell depolarization. Under these conditions, the pump may "run in reverse." (6) Some calcium is actively pumped from the cell by a Ca^{2+} ATPase. (7) As myocyte Ca^{2+} concentrations fall, Ca^{2+} is released from troponin, and the myocyte relaxes.

node spreads to surrounding atrial cells, where it triggers the opening of fast sodium channels. This initiates an electric current that spreads from cell to cell along specialized pathways to depolarize the entire heart. This depolarization, referred to as cardiac excitation, is linked to mechanical activity of the heart by the process of electrical–mechanical coupling (Chap. 15).

Myocyte Calcium Flow and Contractility

During systole, voltage-gated slow Ca^{2+} channels (L-type channels) on the myocyte membrane open in response to cell depolarization, allowing Ca^{2+} to flow down its concentration gradient into the myocyte (Fig. 59–2). Invaginations of the myocyte membrane known as T-tubules place L-type Ca^{2+} channels in close approximation to Ca^{2+} release channels (ryanodine receptors: RyR) on the SR. The local increase in calcium concentration that follows the opening of a single L-type Ca^{2+} channel on the cell membrane triggers the opening of the associated RyR channels, resulting in a large release of calcium from the SR, a phenomenon known as calcium-induced calcium release.[87,269] Myocytes contain tens of thousands of *couplons*, clusters of L-type calcium channels and RyR channels. The Ca^{2+} released from one *couplon* is not sufficient to trigger firing of neighboring couplons.[41] Organized myocyte contraction requires synchronized release of calcium from numerous couplons throughout the myocyte. This process depends on membrane depolarization to synchronize opening of L-type channels and subsequent calcium release. This occurs rapidly throughout an extensive network of T-tubules that spans the myocyte.[106] After release from the SR, cytostolic calcium binds to troponin C and allows actin myosin interaction and subsequent myocyte contraction. The strength of contraction is proportional to the amount of calcium release from the SR during depolarization, which depends, in part, on the magnitude of SR calcium stores. Actin–myosin interaction is also modulated by β-adrenergic–mediated troponin phosphorylation, ischemia, intracellular pH, and myofilament stretch.[13,27,28,247]

During diastole, several ion pumps actively remove calcium from the cytoplasm (Fig. 59–2). The most important of these are the SR Ca^{2+} ATPase (SERCA2a) that pumps cytosolic Ca^{2+} into the SR, and the calcium–sodium transporter (NCX) that exchanges one intracellular Ca^{2+} ion for three sodium ions from extracellular fluid. The SR Ca^{2+} ATPase is important for maintaining SR Ca^{2+} stores and is modulated by β-adrenergic stimulation (see later). When

calcium concentrations drop during diastole, calcium dissociates from troponin, and relaxation occurs.[21,26,28,223]

β-Adrenergic Receptors and the Heart

β-Adrenergic receptors are divided into $β_1$, $β_2$, and $β_3$ subtypes. In the healthy heart, approximately 80% of human cardiac β-adrenergic receptors are $β_1$, and 20% are $β_2$. Human hearts also contain a small number of $β_3$-adrenergic receptors.[24,81,177] The relative density of cardiac $β_2$-adrenergic receptors increases with heart failure.[38,236] $β_1$-Adrenergic receptors mediate increased inotropy by a well-described pathway involving cAMP, which acts as a second messenger to activate protein kinases (Fig. 59–3). $β_1$-Adrenergic receptors are coupled to G_s proteins that activate adenylate cyclase when the receptor is stimulated. This increases intracellular production of cAMP, which binds to and activates protein kinase A (PKA) and other cAMP-dependent protein kinases.[145] Protein kinase A (PKA), in turn, phosphorylates important myocyte proteins, including phospholamban, the voltage-sensitive calcium channels, the calcium release (RyR) channels, and troponin.[28,223] Phosphorylation of the L-type calcium channel increases contractility by increasing the influx of calcium during each cell depolarization triggering

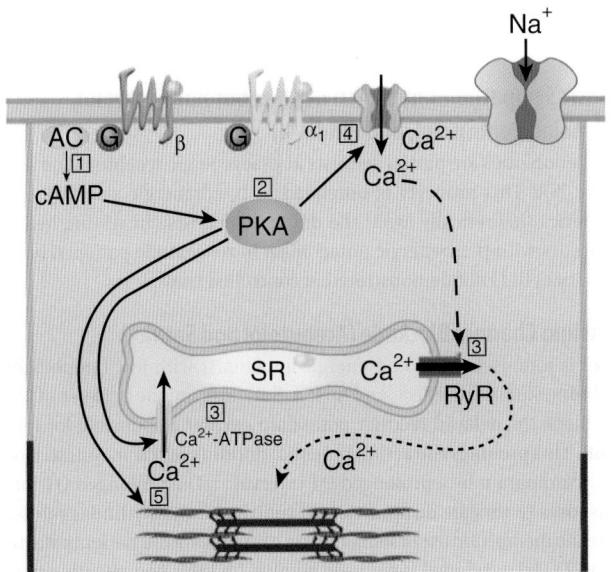

FIGURE 59–3. $β_1$-Adrenergic agonists are positive inotropes by virtue of their ability to activate protein kinase A (PKA). (1) $β_1$-adrenergic receptors are coupled to G_s proteins, which activate adenylate cyclase when catecholamines bind to the receptor. This causes increased formation of cyclic adenosine monophosphate (cAMP) from adenosine triphosphate (ATP). (2) Increased cAMP concentrations activate PKA, which mediates the ultimate effects of β-adrenergic receptor stimulation by phosphorylating key intracellular proteins. (3) Phosphorylation of phospholamban disinhibits the sarcoplasmic reticulum (SR) Ca^{2+} ATPase, resulting in increased SR calcium stores available for release during subsequent depolarizations, and phosphorylation of SR calcium release channels enhances Ca^{2+} release from SR stores during contraction. (4) Phosphorylation of voltage-gated Ca^{2+} channels increases Ca^{2+} influx through these channels during systole. (5) Troponin phosphorylation improves cardiac performance by facilitating Ca^{2+} unbinding during diastole. $β_2$ adrenergic receptors are also coupled to G_s proteins and mediate positive inotropy through a cAMP mechanism (see text). Increased cAMP directly increases heart rate (**Fig. 59–1A**).

greater release of calcium from the SR.[206,226,233] Phospholamban inhibits SER-CA2a. Phosphorylation of phospholamban by PKA at Ser16 and at Thr17 by Ca^{2+}/calmodulin-dependent protein kinase removes this inhibition[46,170] and increases the activity of SERCA2a, resulting in increased "reloading" of SR calcium stores and hence enhanced subsequent contractility.[55,241] Improved activity of the SR Ca^{2+} ATPase also results in more rapid removal of cytoplasmic Ca^{2+} during diastole and aids in myocyte relaxation (ie, lusitropy). Phosphorylation of the RyR channels results in more rapid release of Ca^{2+} from SR stores.[28,223,247] Troponin phosphorylation facilitates Ca^{2+} unbinding and thus improves cardiac performance by enhancing myocyte relaxation.[3,21,146,241] $β_1$-Adrenergic receptors increase chronotropy by an incompletely understood mechanism that is hypothesized to involve phosphorylation of SR proteins, resulting in an increased rate of Ca^{2+} discharge from the SR,[164,166] in addition to direct cAMP interaction with membrane-bound pacemaker channels.[2,35] Although β-adrenergic stimulation acutely improves cardiac function, chronic β-adrenergic stimulation, acting through $β_1$-adrenergic receptors, results in a number of detrimental effects including calcium overload, increased risk of dysrhythmias, impaired excitation–contraction coupling, takotsubo stress cardiomyopathy, and myocyte apoptosis.[28,38,275,248]

Cardiac $β_2$-adrenergic receptors are dually linked to both excitatory G_s proteins and inhibitory G_i proteins.[122,212,276] Under normal conditions, the G_s pathway predominates in human cardiac $β_2$-adrenergic receptors, and $β_2$-adrenergic stimulation increases contractility, relaxation, and chronotropy through the PKA pathway described earlier. However, in a failing heart, the inhibitory G_i protein pathway becomes dominant, and $β_2$-adrenergic stimulation inhibits cardiac function.[38,94,223] Chronic $β_2$-adrenergic stimulation reportedly prevents myocyte apoptosis.[275] The $β_3$-adrenergic receptors are best understood as metabolic regulators in adipose tissue.[64] The role of

cardiac $β_3$-adrenergic receptors is poorly understood, but evidence suggests that they prevent the maladaptive myocardial remodeling that occurs with chronic sympathetic overstimulation.[17,18,24]

Noncardiac Effects of β-Adrenergic Receptor Activation

β-Adrenergic agonists have important noncardiac effects. β-Adrenergic receptors mediate smooth muscle relaxation in several organs. Relaxation of arteriolar smooth muscle, predominately by $β_2$-adrenergic stimulation, reduces peripheral vascular resistance and decreases blood pressure. This counteracts α-adrenergic–mediated arteriolar constriction. In the lungs, $β_2$-adrenergic receptors mediate bronchodilation. Unfortunately, chronic β-adrenergic stimulation causes adverse pulmonary effects, including mucous cell proliferation, hyperreactive airways, and inflammation.[52] Third trimester uterine tone and contractions are inhibited by $β_2$-adrenergic agonists, and gut motility is decreased by both $β_1$- and $β_2$-adrenergic stimulation. Chronic, high-dose $β_2$-adrenergic stimulation causes skeletal muscle hypertrophy.[125]

β-Adrenergic receptors play a role in the immune system. Mast cell degranulation is inhibited by $β_2$-adrenergic stimulation, explaining the role of epinephrine in aborting and treating anaphylaxis. Polymorphonuclear leukocytes demarginate in response to β-adrenergic stimulation, resulting in the increased white blood cell counts with catecholamine infusions or with increased endogenous release of epinephrine the occurs with pain or physiological stress.

β-Adrenergic agonists also have important metabolic effects. Insulin secretion is increased by $β_2$-adrenergic receptor stimulation. Despite increased insulin concentrations, the net effect of $β_2$-adrenergic receptor stimulation is to increase glucose because of increased skeletal muscle glycogenolysis and hepatic gluconeogenesis and glycogenolysis. $β_2$-Adrenergic receptors also cause glucagon secretion from pancreatic α cells.[132] β-Adrenergic agonists act at fat cells to cause lipolysis and thermogenesis. Stimulation of adipocyte β-adrenergic receptors results in breakdown of triglycerides and release of free fatty acids. Skeletal muscle potassium uptake is increased by $β_2$-adrenergic stimulation, resulting in hypokalemia, explaining the role of $β_2$-adrenergic agonists in the treatment of hyperkalemia. Finally, renin secretion is increased by $β_1$-adrenergic stimulation, resulting in increased blood pressure.[268]

Action of β-Adrenergic Antagonists

β-Adrenergic antagonists competitively antagonize the effects of catecholamines at β-adrenergic receptors and blunt the chronotropic and inotropic response to catecholamines. Severe bradycardia and hypotension often results in patients who take additional medications that impair cardiac conduction or contractility or in those with underlying cardiac or medical conditions that make them reliant on sympathetic stimulation. In addition to slowing the rate of SA node discharge, β-adrenergic antagonists inhibit ectopic pacemakers and slow conduction through atrial and AV nodal tissue. β-Adrenergic antagonists limit the detrimental effects of chronic adrenergic overstimulation and have become standard of care for patients with all stages of compensated chronic heart failure, including patients with stable New York Heart Association class III or IV disease.[1,86,271] β-Adrenergic antagonism occasionally exacerbates symptoms in patients with decompensated congestive heart failure, but in the absence of cardiogenic shock or symptomatic bradycardia, β-adrenergic antagonists should not be routinely discontinued in heart failure patients admitted to hospital.[274] β-Adrenergic antagonists reduce the number of adverse cardiac events in patients with recent myocardial infarctions (MIs) but not in patients with prior myocardial infarct, stable coronary artery disease, or risk factors for coronary artery disease.[19]

The antihypertensive effect of β-adrenergic antagonists is counteracted by a reflex increase in peripheral vascular resistance. This effect is augmented by the $β_2$-adrenergic antagonism of nonselective β-adrenergic antagonists. By causing increased peripheral vascular resistance, $β_2$-adrenergic antagonists rarely worsen peripheral vascular disease.

Some patients with reactive airways disease experience severe bronchospasm after using β-adrenergic antagonists because of loss of

β_2-adrenergic–mediated bronchodilation. Catecholamines inhibit mast cell degranulation through a β_2-adrenergic mechanism. Interference with this can predispose to life-threatening effects after anaphylactic reactions in atopic individuals.[109] β_2-Adrenergic antagonists impair the ability to recover from hypoglycemia and sometimes mask the sympathetic discharge that serves to warn of hypoglycemia. This combination of effects is dangerous for patients with diabetes at risk for hypoglycemic episodes.[268]

β-Adrenergic antagonism inhibits catecholamine-mediated potassium uptake at skeletal muscle. This causes slight elevations in serum [potassium], especially after exercise,[48,245] and in rare cases is associated with severe hyperkalemia.[23,80,88,89,168] Although β_2-adrenergic stimulation augments insulin release, β-adrenergic antagonists seldom lower insulin concentrations. In fact, they occasionally cause hypoglycemia, especially in children, by interference with glycogenolysis and gluconeogenesis.[200] These effects are important in people with diabetes, who are at risk for hypoglycemia. β-Adrenergic antagonists also alter lipid metabolism. Although the release of free fatty acids from adipose tissue is inhibited, patients taking nonselective β-adrenergic antagonists typically have increased plasma concentrations of triglycerides and decreases in high-density lipoproteins.[268] There are reports of cardiac arrest, believed secondary to reduced cardiac output, when propranolol was used in patients with thyrotoxic cardiomyopathy.[51,190]

PHARMACOKINETICS

The pharmacokinetic properties of the β-adrenergic antagonists depend in large part on their lipophilicity. Propranolol is the most lipid soluble of the β-adrenergic antagonists, and atenolol is the most water soluble. The oral bioavailability of the β-adrenergic antagonists ranges from approximately 25% for propranolol to almost 100% for pindolol and penbutolol.

The highly lipid-soluble β-adrenergic antagonists cross lipid membranes rapidly and concentrate in adipose tissue. These properties allow rapid entry into the central nervous system (CNS) and typically result in large volumes of distribution. In contrast, highly water-soluble medications, cross lipid membranes slowly, distribute in total body water, and tend to have less CNS toxicity. Volumes of distribution range from about 1 L/kg for atenolol to more than 100 L/kg for carvedilol.

The highly lipid-soluble β-adrenergic antagonists are highly protein bound and poorly excreted by the kidneys. They require hepatic biotransformation before they can be eliminated and accumulate in patients with liver failure. In contrast, the water-soluble β-adrenergic antagonists tend to be slowly absorbed, poorly protein bound, and renally eliminated. They accumulate in patients with kidney failure. Esmolol, although water soluble, is rapidly metabolized by red blood cell esterases and does not accumulate in patients with renal failure. The half-life of esmolol is about 8 minutes. Half-lives of the other β-adrenergic antagonists range from about 2 hours for oxprenolol to as long as 32 hours for nebivolol. The β-adrenergic antagonists also differ in their β_1-adrenergic selectivity, intrinsic sympathomimetic activity (ISA), and vasodilatory properties[191,202,207,243,268] (Table 59–1 and later discussion).

β_1 Selectivity (Acebutolol, Atenolol, Betaxolol, Bisoprolol, Celiprolol, Esmolol, Metoprolol, and Nebivolol)

β_1-Selective antagonists avoid some of the adverse effects of the nonselective antagonists. Short-term use of β_1-adrenergic selective antagonists appears to be safe in patients with mild to moderately severe reactive airways.[217] These medications are safer for patients with diabetes mellitus or peripheral vascular disease. Their β_1-adrenergic selectivity, however, is incomplete, and adverse reactions secondary to β_2-adrenergic antagonism occur with therapeutic dosage as well as in overdose.[147,268]

Membrane-Stabilizing Effects (Acebutolol, Betaxolol, Carvedilol, Oxprenolol, and Propranolol)

β-Adrenergic antagonists that inhibit fast sodium channels (also known as type I antidysrhythmic activity) are said to possess "membrane-stabilizing activity." No significant membrane stabilization occurs with therapeutic

use of β-adrenergic antagonists, but this property contributes to toxicity in overdose.

Intrinsic Sympathomimetic Activity (Acebutolol, Carteolol, Oxprenolol, Penbutolol, and Pindolol)

These xenobiotics are partial agonists at β-adrenergic receptors and are said to have ISA. This property is unrelated to β_1-adrenergic selectivity. These xenobiotics theoretically avoid the dramatic decrease in resting heart rate that occurs with β-adrenergic antagonism in susceptible patients, but their clinical benefit is not demonstrated in controlled trials.[70,77]

Potassium Channel Blockade (Acebutolol and Sotalol)

Sotalol is a nonselective β-adrenergic antagonist with low lipophilicity, no membrane stabilizing effect, and no ISA. Sotalol is unique because of its ability to block the delayed rectifier potassium current responsible for repolarization. This prolongs the action potential duration and is manifested on the electrocardiogram by a prolonged QT interval.[102] The prolonged QT interval predisposes to torsade de pointes, and ventricular dysrhythmias rarely complicate the therapeutic use of sotalol.[129] In a case series of 672 patients started on sotalol, 7 (1%) developed torsade de pointes, and this complication typically occurred within the first days of starting the xenobiotic.[262] In patients taking sotalol therapeutically, torsade de pointes is most common in those who have kidney failure; use other medications that prolong the QT interval; or have predisposing factors for QT interval prolongation such as hypokalemia, hypomagnesemia, bradycardia, or congenital QT interval prolongation.[53,102] QT interval prolongation is relatively easy to monitor; it is a poor indicator of risk of torsade de pointes. Other ECG findings such as changes in T wave morphology are better indicators of torsade de pointes risk, but identifying these changes requires sophisticated analysis that is not readily available in the clinical setting.[180,240] Sotalol was associated with increased mortality in the SWORD trial, a randomized trial comparing sotalol with placebo for patients with recent MI or remote MI with symptomatic heart failure.[259] The cause of excess mortality in the SWORD trial was assumed to be from dysrhythmias, but that assumption is unproven and has been challenged.[61] Acebutolol also prolongs the QT interval presumably secondary to blockade of outward potassium channels.[149]

Vasodilation (Betaxolol, Bucindolol, Carteolol, Carvedilol, Celiprolol, Labetalol, and Nebivolol)

Labetalol and some newer β-adrenergic antagonists (betaxolol, bucindolol, carteolol, carvedilol, celiprolol, nebivolol) are also vasodilators. Labetalol and carvedilol are nonselective β-adrenergic antagonists that also possess α-adrenergic antagonist activity. Nebivolol is a selective β_1-adrenergic antagonist that causes vasodilation by release of nitric oxide.[169] Bucindolol, carteolol, and celiprolol vasodilate because they are agonists at β_2-adrenergic receptors. Celiprolol and carteolol also vasodilate because of nitric oxide–mediated effects. Bucindolol was recently approved while celiprolol are not yet FDA approved. Carteolol is currently available as an ocular preparation. Betaxolol and carvedilol also have calcium channel blocking properties that result in vasodilation (Table 59–1). Despite theoretical advantages, β-adrenergic antagonists with vasodilating properties have not been proven to be more beneficial than other β-adrenergic antagonists for patients with congestive heart failure.[36,203] These xenobiotics also have a theoretical advantage over other β_2-adrenergic agonists for managing hypertension in patients with peripheral vascular disease, but there is very little research on this topic.[194] Xenobiotics with β_2-adrenergic agonist activity are likely safer in patients with reactive airways.

β-Adrenergic antagonists should not be given without appropriate α-adrenergic blockade in situations of catecholamine excess such as pheochromocytoma. In these conditions, β_2-adrenergic–mediated vasodilation is essential to counteract α-adrenergic–mediated vasoconstriction, and β-adrenergic antagonists result in "unopposed α-adrenergic effect, causing dangerous increases in vascular resistance.[67,268] Even xenobiotics with combined α- and β-adrenergic antagonist properties, such as labetalol, can cause this problem.[69,131] Labetalol, for example, is 5- to 10-fold more potent as a β-adrenergic antagonist than as an α-adrenergic antagonist.[83] Medications with β2-adrenergic agonist properties might avoid the "unopposed α adrenergic" effect, but their use in this situation has not been investigated.

Other Preparations (Ophthalmic Preparations and Combined Products)

Therapeutic use of ophthalmic solutions containing β-adrenergic antagonists rarely causes systemic adverse effects such as bradycardia, high-grade AV block, heart failure, and bronchospasm.[33,76,179,225,227,258,268]

Several combination tablets containing both β-adrenergic antagonists and thiazide diuretics are available to treat hypertension in the United States. These include atenolol–chlorthalidone, bisoprolol–hydrochlorothiazide, metoprolol–chlorthalidone, metoprolol–hydrochlorothiazide, nadolol–bendroflumethiazide, and propranolol–hydrochlorothiazide.[9] Internationally, products containing β-adrenergic antagonists in combination with calcium channel antagonists are available. These include amlodipine in combination with atenolol, bisoprolol, or metoprolol and nifedipine in combination with acebutolol, atenolol, or metoprolol. None of these products are FDA approved.[8]

PATHOPHYSIOLOGY

Most of the toxicity of β-adrenergic antagonists is due to their ability to competitively antagonize the action of catecholamines at cardiac β-adrenergic receptors. The peripheral vascular effects of β-adrenergic antagonism are less prominent in overdose. β-Adrenergic antagonists also appear to have toxic effects independent of their action at catecholamine receptors. In catecholamine-depleted, spontaneously beating isolated rat hearts, propranolol, timolol, and sotalol all decreased heart rate and contractility.[58] Surprisingly, these effects were similar in catecholamine-depleted and non-depleted hearts.[137] A membrane-depressant effect likely contributes to the negative inotropic effects of propranolol but not to that of timolol or sotalol. Hence, β-adrenergic antagonists appear to possess myocardial depressant properties that are independent of catecholamine antagonism or membrane depressant activity, possibly because of interference with calcium handling at the level of the SR.[137]

β-Adrenergic antagonists also interfere with calcium uptake into intracellular organelles. Interference with cytosolic calcium handling stimulates calcium-sensitive outward potassium channels, resulting in myocyte hyperpolarization and subsequent refractory bradycardia. Lowering extracellular potassium or raising extracellular sodium concentrations was conjectured to counteract this effect and, in fact, partially reversed propranolol and atenolol toxicity in isolated rat hearts.[118] In another series of experiments with isolated rat hearts, calcium improved the function of rat hearts poisoned with β-adrenergic antagonists.[137]

Although cardiovascular effects are most prominent in overdose, β-adrenergic antagonists also cause respiratory depression.[136] This effect is centrally mediated and is an important cause of death in spontaneously breathing animal models of β-adrenergic antagonism toxicity.[138] There is evidence that propranolol is concentrated in synaptic vessels and impairs synaptic function by inhibition of membrane ion pumps, including the Na^+, K^+-ATPase, the Ca^{2+} ATPase, and the Mg^{2+} ATPase pumps. These actions likely explain some of the CNS effects noted in propranolol overdose.[84]

CLINICAL MANIFESTATIONS

The clinical findings of toxicity generally occur within hours after β-adrenergic antagonist overdose. Propranolol overdose, in particular, is often complicated by the rapid development of hypoglycemia, seizures, coma, and dysrhythmias. In a retrospective review of published report of adult β-adrenergic antagonist overdose, there were 39 symptomatic patients with well-documented times from ingestion to symptom onset. Only 1 patient had ingested a sustained-release product. Thirty-one patients (80%) displayed signs and symptoms of toxicity at 2 hours, all but one (97%) at

4 hours, and everyone within the first 6 hours. The authors conclude that there are no well-documented reports of immediate release β-adrenergic antagonist overdose resulting in toxicity delayed more than 6 hours after ingestion.[148] The authors of an Australian series also noted that in their 58 patients with β-adrenergic antagonist overdose, all major clinical findings of poisoning began within 6 hours of ingestion.[204] These observations do not apply to sotalol, which is well known to cause delayed toxicity in overdose, or to sustained-release preparations of any of the β-adrenergic antagonists.

Isolated β-adrenergic antagonist overdose in healthy people is often benign. In several series, one-third or more of patients reporting a β-adrenergic overdose remained asymptomatic.[63,71,150,243] This is partially explained by the fact that β-adrenergic antagonism is often well tolerated in healthy persons who do not rely on sympathetic stimulation to maintain cardiac output. In particular, unintentional ingestions in children rarely result in significant toxicity.[25] In fact, a review of published cases found a few reports of hypoglycemia but no deaths or serious cardiovascular morbidity after β-adrenergic antagonist ingestion in children younger than the age of 6 years.[158]

β-Adrenergic antagonists severely impair the ability of the heart to respond to peripheral vasodilation, bradycardia, or decreased contractility caused by other xenobiotics. Therefore, even relatively benign vasoactive xenobiotics cause catastrophic toxicity when coingested with β-adrenergic antagonists.[78] The most important predictor of toxicity in patients with β-adrenergic antagonist overdose is likely the presence of a cardioactive coingestant.[152] Isolated β-adrenergic antagonist overdose is most likely to cause clinical abnormalities in persons with congestive heart failure, sick sinus syndrome, or impaired AV conduction who rely on sympathetic stimulation to maintain heart rate or cardiac output. Nevertheless, severe toxicity and death occur in healthy persons who have ingested β-adrenergic antagonists alone.[74,204,234] This is explained by an increased susceptibility of certain persons to β-adrenergic antagonism or by special properties that increase the toxicity of certain β-adrenergic antagonists (see later). In patients without a coingestant, toxicity is most likely to occur in those who ingest a β-adrenergic antagonist with membrane-stabilizing activity.[152]

Patients with symptomatic β-adrenergic antagonist overdose are most often hypotensive and bradycardic. Decreased SA node function results in sinus bradycardia, sinus pauses, or sinus arrest. Impaired AV conduction manifested as prolonged PR interval or high-grade AV block occurs rarely. Prolonged QRS complex duration and QT interval duration occur, and severe poisoning results in asystole. Congestive heart failure often complicates β-adrenergic antagonist overdose. Delirium, coma, and seizures occur most commonly in the setting of severe hypotension but also occur with normal blood pressure, especially with exposure to the more lipophilic medications such as propranolol.[74,204] Respiratory depression and apnea may have an additional role in toxicity.[7] In a review of reported cases, 18% of patients with propranolol toxicity and 6% of those with atenolol toxicity had a respiratory rate less than 12 breaths/min.[204] Respiratory depression after β-adrenergic antagonist overdose typically occurs in patients who are hypotensive and comatose but is reported in awake patients.[182] Hypoglycemia often complicates β-adrenergic antagonist poisoning in children[98,158] but is uncommon in acutely poisoned adults. In a series of 15 cases of β-adrenergic antagonist overdose, none of the 13 adults were hypoglycemic, but both of the 2 children had symptomatic hypoglycemia.[74] Bronchospasm is relatively uncommon after β-adrenergic antagonist overdose and appears to occur only in susceptible patients. In the series mentioned, only 2 of the 15 patients developed bronchospasm,[74] and in a review of 39 cases of symptomatic adults with β-adrenergic antagonist overdose, only 1 patient developed bronchospasm.[148] Clinical use of β-adrenergic antagonists slightly increases serum potassium,[159] but significant hyperkalemia is rare.

β1 Selectivity (Acebutolol, Atenolol, Betaxolol, Bisoprolol, Esmolol, Metoprolol, and Nebivolol)

In overdose, cardioselectivity is largely lost, and deaths caused by the β1-adrenergic selective antagonists, including acebutolol,[96] atenolol,[156] betaxolol,[29] and metoprolol,[209,234] are reported. There are reports of minor toxicity after acute overdose with bisoprolol[253] and with nebivolol.[95] There is also one report of death after an iatrogenic overdose of bisoprolol in an older adult patient with impaired bisoprolol metabolism.[93]

Membrane-Stabilizing Effects (Acebutolol, Betaxolol, Carvedilol, Oxprenolol, and Propranolol)

Propranolol possesses the most membrane-stabilizing activity of this class, and propranolol poisoning is characterized by coma, seizures, hypotension, bradycardia, impaired AV conduction, and a widened QRS interval. Ventricular tachydysrhythmias can occur.[5,156] A Brugada pattern on the ECG caused by Na⁺ channel blockade or by revealing underlying Brugada syndrome is reported after propranolol overdose.[10,205] Hypotension is often out of proportion to bradycardia, and deaths from propranolol overdose are well reported.[74,96,156] Acebutolol, betaxolol, and oxprenolol also possess significant membrane-stabilizing activity and have caused fatalities when taken in overdose.[29,96,121,191,201]

Lipid Solubility

In overdose, the more lipophilic β-adrenergic antagonists more often cause delirium, coma, and seizures even in the absence of hypotension.[74,204] Atenolol, the least lipid soluble of β-adrenergic antagonists, appears to be one of the safer β-adrenergic antagonists when taken in overdose.[96] In fact, in one series of β-adrenergic antagonist overdoses, none of the 18 patients with atenolol overdose had seizures compared with 8 of 28 patients with propranolol overdose.[204] Nevertheless, atenolol overdose is reported to result in severe toxicity and cardiovascular death.[156,197,238]

Intrinsic Sympathomimetic Activity (Acebutolol, Carteolol, Oxprenolol, Penbutolol, and Pindolol)

There is little experience with overdose of these xenobiotics, but ISA would theoretically make these xenobiotics safer than the other β-adrenergic antagonists. Sympathetic stimulation with mild tachycardia or hypertension often predominates in pindolol overdose, and this class of xenobiotics appears to be relatively safe in overdose.[74,130,202] In addition to ISA, acebutolol and oxprenolol have significant membrane-stabilizing activity, making them dangerous in overdose, and deaths due to acute toxicity from these xenobiotics are reported.[74,96,149,201] Overdose with carteolol or penbutolol has not been reported.

Potassium Channel Blockade (Acebutolol and Sotalol)

In six patients with sotalol overdose, the average QT interval was 172% of normal, and five patients had ventricular dysrhythmias, including multifocal ventricular extrasystoles, ventricular tachycardia, and ventricular fibrillation.[189] Sotalol overdose is also be complicated by hypotension, bradycardia, and asystole,[6,189] and fatalities are well documented.[181,196]

Sotalol overdose often causes delayed and prolonged toxicity, although ECG changes appear to occur early. In a series of six patients with sotalol overdose, all had prolonged QT intervals noted on the initial ECG taken 30 minutes to 4.5 hours after ingestion. It is not clear whether these patients were taking sotalol therapeutically before their overdoses, so it is possible that the prolonged QT interval on the initial ECG was present before the overdoses. The greatest QT interval prolongation occurred 4 to 15 hours after ingestion, and the risk of ventricular dysrhythmias was highest between 4 and 20 hours. All four patients who developed ventricular tachycardia did so after 4 hours, and in two patients, ventricular dysrhythmias first occurred 9 hours after ingestion. One patient continued to have ventricular dysrhythmias at 48 hours, and abnormally prolonged QT intervals were noted as long as 100 hours after ingestion. In this series, the average sotalol half-life was 13 hours, and the average time until normalization of the QT interval was 82 hours.[189] Acebutolol-induced QT interval prolongation likely contributes to the ventricular tachydysrhythmias that occur in patients with severe acebutolol toxicity.[62,149,156]

Vasodilation (Betaxolol, Bucindolol, Carteolol, Carvedilol, Celiprolol, Labetalol, and Nebivolol)

The vasodilatory properties of these xenobiotics should theoretically act in synergy with β-adrenergic antagonism to increase toxicity. Conversely, the low membrane-stabilizing effect of these xenobiotics would be expected to make them relatively safe in overdose. Betaxolol is the sole medication in this class with membrane-stabilizing properties. Overdose with labetalol appears to be similar to that of other β-adrenergic antagonists with hypotension and bradycardia as prominent features.[124,126,230] Experience with overdose of the newer vasodilating β-adrenergic antagonists is limited. Similar to conventional β-adrenergic antagonists, carvedilol overdose causes hypotension and bradycardia.[32,90,242] In a case report from Germany, nebivolol overdose was complicated by bradycardia, lethargy, and hypoglycemia. The patient received standard treatment and had a benign outcome.[95] Another patient who overdosed on nebivolol became hypotensive and bradycardic and then had a cardiac arrest. That person was successfully resuscitated with lipid emulsion and high-dose insulin.[237] Severe toxicity and death have occurred after betaxolol[29,30] and celiprolol[213] poisoning. Overdoses with bucindolol or carteolol have not been reported.

Other Preparations (Ophthalmic Preparations, Sustained Release, and Combined Products)

There is very little published experience with overdoses of the sustained-release β-adrenergic antagonists, but it is reasonable to expect that overdose with these xenobiotics will result in both a delayed onset and prolonged duration of toxicity. Acute overdose of ophthalmic β-adrenergic antagonists has not been reported. Patients who take mixed overdoses with calcium channel antagonists and β-adrenergic antagonists are difficult to manage because of synergistic toxicity.[59,216,224,231,249] Overdoses with combined β-adrenergic antagonist and calcium channel blocker preparations such as felodipine and metoprolol or atenolol and nifedipine have not been reported, but these combinations would be expected to be quite dangerous in overdose.

DIAGNOSTIC TESTING

All patients with an intentional overdose of a β-adrenergic antagonist require a 12-lead ECG and continuous cardiac monitoring. Serum glucose should be measured regardless of mental status because β-adrenergic antagonists can cause hypoglycemia. A chest radiograph and assessment of oxygen saturation should be obtained if the patient is at risk for or has symptoms of congestive heart failure. Patients with bradycardia of uncertain etiology should have thyroid function, potassium, renal function, and cardiac enzymes measured. Digoxin concentration should be measured for bradycardic patients who have access to digoxin or who have a clinical presentation suggestive of cardioactive steroid poisoning (Chap. 62). Serum concentrations of β-adrenergic antagonists are not readily available for routine clinical use but may prove helpful in making a retrospective diagnosis in selected cases. Lactate concentration should be measured in patients who are symptomatic after a β-adrenergic antagonist overdose. Elevated lactate is associated with increased likelihood of fatality in these patients. However, because β-adrenergic antagonists inhibit the development of hyperlactatemia in the presence of shock, lactate is a poor predictor of survival, and fatalities are reported in β-adrenergic antagonist–poisoned patients with normal or modestly elevated lactate concentrations.[174]

MANAGEMENT

Airway and ventilation should be maintained with endotracheal intubation if necessary. Because laryngoscopy sometimes induces a vagal response, it is reasonable to give atropine before intubation of patients with bradycardia. This is particularly true for children, who are more susceptible to this complication. The initial treatment of patients with bradycardia and hypotension consists of atropine and intravenous (IV) fluids. These measures will likely be insufficient in patients with severe toxicity but often suffice in patients with mild poisoning or other causes of bradycardia.

Gastrointestinal (GI) decontamination is warranted for all persons who have ingested significant amounts of a β-adrenergic antagonist. Induction of emesis is contraindicated because of the potential for catastrophic deterioration of mental status and vital signs in these patients and because vomiting increases vagal stimulation that could potentially worsen bradycardia.[232]

Orogastric lavage is recommended for patients with significant toxic effects such as seizures, hypotension, or bradycardia if the patient presents in a time frame when the medication is still expected to be in the stomach. Orogastric lavage is also recommended for all patients who present shortly after ingestion of large (gram amount) ingestions of propranolol or one of the other more toxic β-adrenergic antagonists (ie, acebutolol, betaxolol, metoprolol, oxprenolol, sotalol). Orogastric lavage causes vagal stimulation and carries the risk of worsening bradycardia, so it is reasonable to pretreat patients with standard doses of atropine or, at a minimum, be prepared to treat if it develops. Activated charcoal alone is recommended for persons with minor effects after an overdose with one of the more water-soluble β-adrenergic antagonists who present within several hours after ingestion (Antidotes in Depth: A1). Whole-bowel irrigation with polyethylene glycol is reasonable in patients who have ingested sustained-release preparations (Antidotes in Depth: A2).

Seizures or coma associated with cardiovascular collapse is treated by attempting to restore circulation. Seizures in the patient with relatively normal vital signs should be treated with an adequate trial of benzodiazepines followed by barbiturates if benzodiazepines fail. Refractory seizures are rare in patients with isolated β-adrenergic antagonist overdose.

Specific Management
Patients who fail to respond to atropine and fluids require management with the inotropic agents discussed later (Fig. 59–4). When time permits, it is

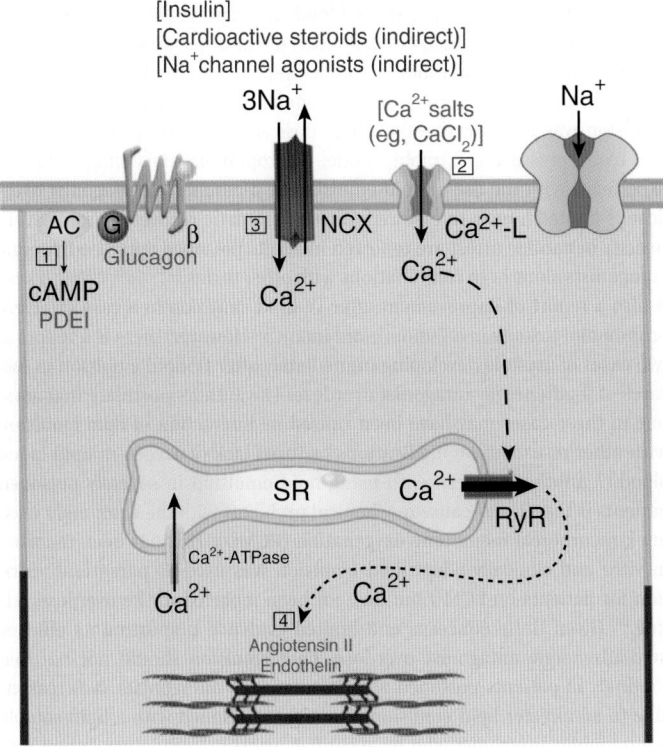

FIGURE 59–4. Positive inotropes improve cardiac function by a number of mechanisms, which usually result in increased intracellular Ca^{2+}. (1) Xenobiotics that increase cyclic adenosine monophosphate (cAMP). Glucagon receptors and β-adrenergic receptors are coupled to G_s proteins so that receptor binding increases cAMP by activation of adenylate cyclase. Phosphodiesterase inhibitors increase cAMP by inhibiting its breakdown. (2) Xenobiotics that increase calcium influx. Calcium salts increase calcium influx through L-type Ca^{2+} channels by a direct mass effect. (3) Xenobiotics that inhibit extrusion of calcium via the Na^+, Ca^{2+} exchange pump: Xenobiotics that increase intracellular sodium such as digoxin and Na^+ channel agonists (eg, aconitine) and those such as 4-aminopyridine that prolong the action potential duration alter the electrochemical gradients in a way that hinders the extrusion of calcium. (4) Xenobiotics that increase the sensitivity of the contractile elements to calcium. Angiotensin II and endothelin do this by inducing an intracellular alkalosis. The calcium sensitizers levosimendan and pimobendan are used to treat heart failure in some countries. NCX = the calcium sodium antiporter

preferable to introduce new medications sequentially so that the effects of each may be assessed. The author recommends glucagon followed by calcium and high-dose insulin euglycemia therapy. In critically ill patients, there may not be enough time for this stepwise approach, and multiple treatments may be started simultaneously. If these therapies fail, the author suggests starting a catecholamine pressor. Advanced hemodynamic monitoring, when available, is advisable to guide therapy for all patients receiving catecholamine pressors or phosphodiesterase inhibitors. Lipid emulsion therapy is reasonable in β-adrenergic antagonist–poisoned patients who have cardiovascular collapse unresponsive to other interventions, but caution is warranted given reports of sudden asystole after lipid emulsion in this situation.[49] Mechanical life support with intraaortic balloon pump (IABP) or extracorporeal circulation is recommended when medical management fails.

Glucagon
Cardiac glucagon receptors, like β-adrenergic receptors, are coupled to G_s proteins.[264] Glucagon binding increases adenylate cyclase activity independent of β-adrenergic receptor binding.[272] Glucagon's inotropic effect is enhanced by its ability to inhibit phosphodiesterase and thereby prevent cAMP breakdown.[176]

There have been no controlled trials of glucagon in human cases of β-adrenergic antagonist poisoning.[16,34] Nevertheless, with more than 45 years of clinical use,[128,260] glucagon is still recognized as a useful treatment of choice for severe β-adrenergic antagonist toxicity.[117,199,243,266] This is supported by animal models[82,127,155] and a case series suggesting that glucagon is also effective in correcting symptomatic bradycardia and hypotension secondary to therapeutic β-adrenergic antagonist use.[157] Glucagon is a vasodilator, and in animal models of propranolol poisoning, it is more effective in restoring contractility, cardiac output, and heart rate than in restoring blood pressure.[16,155]

The initial adult dose of glucagon for β-adrenergic antagonist toxicity is 3 to 5 mg given slowly over 1 to 2 minutes. The initial pediatric dose is 50 mcg/kg. If there is no response to the initial dose, titrated doses, up to a cumulative dose of approximately 10 mg, is recommended. When a response occurs, a glucagon infusion is started. It is reasonable to start the glucagon infusion at the "response dose" per hour. Thus, for example, if the patient receives 7 mg of glucagon before a response occurs, the glucagon infusion should be started at 7 mg/h. When a full 10-mg dose of glucagon fails to restore blood pressure and heart rate and the diagnosis of β-adrenergic antagonist toxicity is probable, we still recommends starting an infusion of glucagon at 10 mg/h because glucagon will have synergistic effects with subsequent antidotes. Glucagon sometimes causes vomiting with risk of aspiration, and it is reasonable to pretreat with an antiemetic but to remain cognizant of the fact that many antiemetics cause QT interval prolongation. Other side effects of glucagon in this setting include hyperglycemia and mild hypocalcemia,[107] and these should be treated appropriately if they develop. Patients also develop rapid tachyphylaxis to glucagon, and the need for increasing doses and additional therapies should be expected even when patients initially respond (Antidotes in Depth: A20).

Calcium
Calcium salts effectively treat hypotension but not heart rate in animal models of β-adrenergic antagonist toxicity.[137,151] Calcium chloride successfully reverses hypotension in patients with β-adrenergic antagonist overdose[37,197] and in combined calcium channel blocker and β-adrenergic antagonist toxicity.[97] The adult starting dose of calcium gluconate is 3 g of the 10% solution given intravenously. For patients with persistent hypotension, the author recommends repeat at this same dose of calcium gluconate every 10 to 20 minutes up to a total of 9 g. The initial dose of calcium gluconate in children is 60 mg/kg up to 3 g followed by repeat boluses every 10 to 20 minutes, as needed for persistent hypotension, up to a total of 180 mg/kg (Antidotes in Depth: A32).

Insulin and Glucose
High-dose insulin improves cardiac function after cardiac surgery[85] and survival after MI.[68,161,163] There is evidence that high-dose insulin combined with sufficient glucose to maintain euglycemia is beneficial in β-adrenergic

antagonist poisoning. In a canine model of propranolol toxicity, all six animals treated with insulin and glucose survived compared with four of six in the glucagon group along with one of six in the epinephrine group and no survivors in the sham treatment group.[120] Insulin plus glucose was markedly more effective than vasopressin plus epinephrine in a porcine model of propranolol toxicity. In that experiment, all five animals in the insulin group survived the 4-hour protocol, and all five in the vasopressin plus epinephrine group died within 90 minutes.[103] In a rabbit model of severe propranolol toxicity, high-dose insulin was more effective than lipid emulsion in restoring blood pressure and heart rate, but there was no difference in survival rate.[91] Clinical experience with high dose insulin for β-adrenergic antagonist poisoning is increasing but still limited to case reports and case series.[65] Improvements in heart rate and blood pressure after high-dose insulin are reported in patients with isolated overdoses of metoprolol, nebivolol, and propranolol.[105,193,237] High-dose insulin was also effective in combined poisoning with β-adrenergic antagonists and calcium channel blockers.[105,273]

High-dose insulin is simple to use and safe (with appropriate monitoring of glucose and potassium) and does not require invasive monitoring. For these reasons, we recommend using high-dose insulin and glucose infusions for patients with β-adrenergic antagonist toxicity who have not responded to fluids, atropine, and glucagon. Although the dose of insulin is not definitively established, therapy typically begins with a bolus of 1 unit/kg of regular human insulin along with 0.5 gm/kg of dextrose. If blood glucose is greater than 300 mg/dL (16.7 mmol/L), the dextrose bolus is not necessary. An infusion of regular insulin should follow the bolus starting at 1 unit/kg/h. A continuous dextrose infusion, beginning at 0.5 gm/kg/h, should also be started. Glucose should be monitored every 15 to 30 minutes until stable and then every 1 to 2 hours and titrated to maintain the blood glucose between 100 and 250 mg/dL. Cardiac function should also be reassessed every 10 to 15 minutes, and if it remains depressed, the insulin infusion should be increased up to 10 units/kg/h as required (rarely higher). The goal of therapy is improved organ perfusion with improvements in cardiac output, mental status, urine output, and acid–base abnormalities. The response to insulin is typically delayed for 15 to 60 minutes, so it will usually be necessary to start a catecholamine infusion before the full effects of insulin are apparent. It is important to continue monitoring glucose and electrolytes for several hours after insulin is discontinued (Antidotes in Depth: A21).

Catecholamines

Patients who do not respond to the preceding therapies usually require a catecholamine infusion. The choice of catecholamine is somewhat controversial. Theoretically, the pure β-adrenergic agonist isoproterenol would seem to be the ideal agent because it can overcome β-adrenergic blockade without causing any α-adrenergic effects. Unfortunately, this therapy has several potential drawbacks that limit its efficacy. In the presence of β-adrenergic antagonism, extraordinarily high doses of isoproterenol and other catecholamines are frequently required.[50,201,208,243,256] Individual case reports document isoproterenol infusions as high as 800 mcg/min.[202] At these high doses, the β₂-adrenergic effects of isoproterenol cause peripheral vasodilation and can result in lower blood pressure.[208] Nevertheless, in some animal models, isoproterenol is the most effective catecholamine and is even more effective than glucagon in reversing β-adrenergic antagonist toxicity.[239,263] Clinical experience, however, has not shown this to be the case. In a review of reported cases, glucagon increased heart rate 67% of the time and blood pressure 50% of the time. In contrast, isoproterenol was effective in increasing heart rate only 11% of the time and blood pressure only 22% of the time. Epinephrine was more effective than isoproterenol.[266] The selective β₁-adrenergic agonist prenalterol, which is not FDA approved, may avoid some of the problems associated with isoproterenol and was used successfully to treat β-adrenergic antagonist overdose.[72,130] Prenalterol would be expected to be especially effective after overdose of the cardioselective β-adrenergic antagonists.[72] Prenalterol therapy is limited by its relatively long half-life (~2 hours), which makes titration difficult.[210] Dobutamine is a β₁-adrenergic agonist with relatively little effect on vascular resistance that might be useful in this setting. However,

experience is limited and dobutamine is not always effective in patients with β-adrenergic antagonist overdose.[201,229] In the setting of β-adrenergic antagonism, catecholamines with substantial α-adrenergic agonist properties can increase peripheral vascular resistance without improving contractility, resulting in acute cardiac failure. Severe hypertension caused by a lack of β₂-adrenergic–mediated vasodilation is another potential adverse reaction from this so-called unopposed α-adrenergic effect.[79] Because of these potential problems, it is recommended that catecholamine use be guided by hemodynamic monitoring either using noninvasive techniques such as bioimpedance or echocardiographic monitoring or by direct invasive measures of determining cardiac performance. Catecholamine infusions should be started at the usual rates and then increased rapidly until a clinical effect is obtained. If advanced monitoring is impossible and the diagnosis of β-adrenergic antagonist overdose is fairly certain, it is reasonable to begin an isoproterenol or epinephrine infusion with careful monitoring of the patient's blood pressure and clinical status. The infusion should be stopped immediately if the patient becomes more hypotensive or develops congestive heart failure.

Lipid Emulsion

Lipid emulsion is intravenous has a potential role in selected cases of severe β-adrenergic antagonist overdose. Intravenous administration of lipid emulsion is hypothesized to reduce the toxicity of lipid-soluble xenobiotics by lowering free serum concentrations of these compounds as they partition into the lipemic component of blood and improve the bioenergetics of the heart. Intravenous lipid emulsion was effective in some animal models of poisoning with propranolol, a highly lipid-soluble β-adrenergic antagonist, but not with the water-soluble atenolol or metoprolol.[40,42,43,45,160] Lipid emulsion was less effective than high-dose insulin in restoring heart rate and blood pressure in a rabbit model of propranolol poisoning.[91] Human experience with the use of lipid emulsion in β-adrenergic antagonist overdose is limited largely to case reports, but dramatic recoveries from severe toxicity or cardiac arrest are reported in adults poisoned with β-adrenergic antagonists alone or in combinations with other toxins.[22,44,111,218,237,242,257] There is also a report of improvement after IV lipid emulsion in a case of severe propranolol toxicity in a 7-month-old infant.[250] However, there is a report of two cases of asystole developing immediately after IV lipid emulsion in two cases of β-adrenergic antagonist overdose. The authors postulate that asystole in these cases may have been caused by interaction of lipid emulsion with other resuscitation medications or "brief lack of oxygen in lipid-laden blood."[49] Another concern with using lipid emulsion in severely poisoned patients is that it may cause mechanical problems with the equipment used in extracorporeal membrane oxygenation (ECMO). This has been reported in vitro and clinically when lipid emulsion was used as parenteral nutrition for patients on ECMO but has not been reported in the overdose setting.[140] Given these concerns and limited evidence supporting its efficacy in β-adrenergic antagonist overdose, lipid emulsion should not be used routinely in patients poisoned with β-adrenergic antagonists. It is reasonable to administer lipid emulsion in patients poisoned with a lipid-soluble β-adrenergic antagonist who have cardiac arrest or circulatory failure that does not respond to usual therapy,[45,92] especially if mechanical life support is not promptly available (see later). The optimal dose and formulation of lipid emulsion for this purpose is unknown. One protocol calls for a 1.5 mL/kg of 20% lipid emulsion followed by an infusion of 0.25 mL/kg/min. The bolus can be repeated in 3 to 5 minutes if necessary. The total dose should be less than 8 mL/kg[265] (Antidotes in Depth: A23).

Phosphodiesterase Inhibitors

The phosphodiesterase inhibitors amrinone, milrinone, and enoximone are theoretically beneficial in β-adrenergic antagonist overdose because they inhibit the breakdown of cAMP by phosphodiesterase and hence increase cAMP independently of β-adrenergic receptor stimulation. Phosphodiesterase inhibitors increase inotropy in the presence of β-adrenergic antagonism in both animal models[141] and in humans.[254] Although these xenobiotics appear to be as effective as glucagon in animal models of β-adrenergic antagonist toxicity,[155,221] controlled dog models were unable to demonstrate an additional benefit over glucagon.[154,222] Phosphodiesterase inhibitors have been used clinically to treat β-adrenergic antagonist–poisoned patients, but experience is limited.[100,124,219,220] Therapy with phosphodiesterase inhibitors is often limited by hypotension secondary to peripheral vasodilation. Furthermore, these xenobiotics are difficult to titrate because of relatively long half-lives (30–60 minutes for milrinone, 2–4 hours for amrinone, and ~2 hours for enoximone).[115,183] For these reasons, they are not routinely recommended in β-adrenergic antagonist–poisoned patients, especially in patients without arterial and pulmonary artery pressure monitoring.

Ventricular Pacing

Ventricular pacing is not a particularly useful intervention in patients with β-adrenergic antagonist toxicity, but it will increase the heart rate in some patients.[116] Unfortunately, there will frequently be failure to capture or pacing increases the heart rate with no increase in cardiac output or blood pressure.[5,130,135,243] In fact, some authors have noticed that ventricular pacing occasionally decreases blood pressure perhaps secondary to loss of organized atrial contraction or because of impaired ventricular relaxation.[243] For these reasons, ventricular pacing is not recommended for management of β-adrenergic antagonist toxicity except for heart rate control in patients with an IABP.

Extracorporeal Removal

Extracorporeal removal is not routinely recommended in patients with β-adrenergic antagonist overdose. It is ineffective for the lipid-soluble β-adrenergic antagonists because of their large volumes of distribution. Hemodialysis does remove water-soluble renally eliminated β-adrenergic antagonists such as atenolol[215] and acebutolol[211] but is often technically difficult in β-adrenergic antagonist–poisoned patients because of hypotension and bradycardia. Extracorporeal removal is reasonable in certain circumstances such as patients with severe toxicity from a water-soluble β-adrenergic antagonist whose blood pressure is maintained with mechanical life support.

Mechanical Life Support

It is important to remember that a patient with circulatory failure from an acute overdose will typically recover without sequelae if ventilation and circulation are maintained until the xenobiotic is eliminated. When the preceding medical treatment fails, it is recommended to use extracorporeal life support (ECLS). Extracorporeal life support includes venoarterial extracorporeal membrane oxygenation (VA-ECMO), emergency cardiac bypass, IABP, or left ventricular assist devices. Several case reports describe remarkable recoveries after the use of these therapies for refractory β-adrenergic antagonist toxicity[30,66,135,173] or combined β-adrenergic antagonist and calcium channel blocker overdose.[73,108,123,198,214,270] In one report, a neonate who developed refractory circulatory collapse from an iatrogenic overdose of propranolol was supported with VA-ECMO for 5 days and survived neurologically intact.[57] A case series documents experience with ECLS for patients with cardiac arrest caused by cardiovascular medication poisoning. In this series of 6 patients, 2 deaths were attributed to delayed institution of ECLS. The other 4 patients survived without sequelae.[15] In another series, ECLS was used in 17 patients with circulatory failure after an overdose. Eight patients had taken β-adrenergic antagonists either alone or in combination with other cardiovascular toxins. A total of 13 of the 17 patients had long-term survival. The authors conclude that ECLS is efficient and relatively safe as a last resort treatment for patients with cardiac arrest or refractory shock after an overdose.[54] More recently, researchers studied 62 poisoned patients with persistent cardiac arrest or circulatory failure and compared survival in 14 patients treated with ECLS versus 48 managed with conventional therapy. Six patients in the ECLS group and 10 in the conventional therapy group had ingested β-adrenergic antagonists. In this series, 12 of 14 (86%) of the ECLS patients survived compared with 23 of 48 (48%) in the conventional therapy

group. None of the patients with persistent cardiac arrest survived without ECLS. The outcome of the patients poisoned with β-adrenergic antagonists was not reported separately, but the authors commented that these patients had a lower mortality rate and that ECLS was associated with a lower mortality rate after adjusting for β-adrenergic antagonist intoxication.[171] Consistent with several recent reviews of ECLS in poisoned patients,[56,110,192] we recommend that ECLS be used, in centers where it is available, in β-adrenergic antagonist–poisoned patients with persistent cardiac arrest or circulatory failure unresponsive to standard therapy. Given the high risk of complications, including severe bleeding, stroke, and intracranial hemorrhage, ECLS should be reserved for severely poisoned patients who are failing medical therapy. Because there is evidence that lipid emulsion can cause mechanical problems with VA-ECMO circuits,[140] the author suggests that lipid emulsion be withheld and the patient supported with cardiopulmonary resuscitation if ECLS can be initiated promptly.

Experimental Treatment

Vasopressin is a hypothalamic hormone that acts at G protein–coupled receptors to mediate vasoconstriction (at V_1 receptors), water retention (at V_2 receptors), and corticotropin secretion (at V_3 receptors) and to increase the response to catecholamines. Vasopressin analogues have been used as vasopressors clinically in shock states and for patients in cardiopulmonary arrest.[20,255] Vasopressin was as effective as glucagon but less effective than high-dose insulin in a porcine model of propranolol toxicity.[103,104] Clinical experience with vasopressin in β-adrenergic antagonist poisoning is limited. Vasopressin was used without effect in a patient in cardiac arrest after metoprolol poisoning who subsequently survived after initiation of mechanical life support.[66] The American Heart Association has removed vasopressin from its most recent Adult Cardiac Arrest Algorithm.[188] Methylene blue inhibits guanylate cyclase and acts as a vasoconstrictor. It is reported to reverse refractory vasodilatory shock after cardiac surgery.[178] Methylene blue was used in a patient who had overdosed on atenolol and amlodipine. In that case, calcium, glucagon, high-dose insulin, and three other pressors (dopamine, norepinephrine, and vasopressin) failed to reverse hypotension (mean arterial pressure in the low 40s), but there was a marked improvement in blood pressure 20 minutes after 1 mg/kg of methylene blue was infused over 10 minutes.[4] The routine use of either vasopressin or methylene blue is not recommended in patients with β-adrenergic antagonist poisoning.

The calcium sensitizers levosimendan and pimobendan interact with the contractile proteins to improve cardiac function and are used clinically to treat heart failure.[11,142,143,195] Levosimendan is both a positive inotrope and a vasodilator and has a better safety profile than pimobendan. It is approved in Europe for use in heart failure patients and is as effective as dobutamine in increasing contractility. Levosimendan infusions allow uptitration of β-adrenergic antagonists in patients with severe heart failure.[274] Levosimendan improved survival in a porcine model of propranolol toxicity[144] and improved cardiac output in a murine model of metoprolol toxicity[114] but was not beneficial in a murine model of propranolol toxicity.[113] Calcium sensitizers are not available in the United States or Canada. They may eventually prove to have a role in managing patients poisoned with β-adrenergic antagonists.

Fructose 1, 6-diphosphate (FDP) is an intermediate in the glycolytic pathway. Fructose 1, 6-diphosphate is able to cross cell membranes, and it increases cardiac contractility.[187,246] Compared with glucose infusion, FDP infusion resulted in improved survival in murine models of propranolol toxicity and verapamil toxicity.[112] Fructose 1, 6-diphosphate may eventually prove to have a role in the management of β-adrenergic antagonist poisoning but cannot be recommended at this time.

Special Circumstances

The preceding discussion applies to the generic management of patients with β-adrenergic antagonists. Certain β-adrenergic antagonists have unique properties that modify their toxicity. The management considerations for these unique agents are discussed next.

Sotalol

In addition to bradycardia and hypotension, sotalol toxicity results in a prolonged QT interval and ventricular dysrhythmias, including torsade de pointes. Sotalol-induced bradycardia and hypotension should be managed as with other β-adrenergic antagonists. Specific management of patients with sotalol overdose includes correction of hypokalemia and hypomagnesemia. Overdrive pacing and magnesium infusions are recommended for prevention of recurrent episodes in patients who have developed sotalol induced torsade de pointes.[12,252] Lidocaine is also reportedly effective for sotalol-induced torsade de pointes.[14] In the future, potassium channel openers such as the cardioprotective medication nicorandil may prove effective for sotalol-induced torsade de pointes.[228,244,261]

Peripheral Vasodilation (Betaxolol, Bucindolol, Carteolol, Carvedilol, Celiprolol, Labetalol, and Nebivolol)

Treatment of patients who have overdosed with one of the vasodilating β-adrenergic antagonists is similar to that for patients who ingest other β-adrenergic antagonists. Decisions about the need for vasopressors should be guided by clinical findings. If vasodilation is a prominent feature, then high doses of pressors with α-adrenergic agonist properties (eg, norepinephrine or phenylephrine) would be reasonable.[99] Conversely, if β-adrenergic antagonism is prominent, glucagon is recommended to increase intracellular cAMP.[95,124]

Membrane-Stabilizing Effects (Acebutolol, Betaxolol, Carvedilol, Oxprenolol, and Propranolol)

It might be expected that hypertonic sodium bicarbonate would be beneficial in treating the ventricular dysrhythmias that occur with these xenobiotics. Unfortunately, there is limited experience with the use of sodium bicarbonate in this situation, and the experimental data are mixed. Sodium bicarbonate was not beneficial in a canine model of propranolol toxicity, although there was a trend toward QRS complex duration narrowing in the sodium bicarbonate group.[153] In models with propranolol-poisoned isolated rat hearts, however, hypertonic sodium chloride proved beneficial.[118,119] Perhaps most compelling is the fact that sodium bicarbonate appeared to reverse ventricular tachycardia in a human case of acebutolol poisoning.[62] Because sodium bicarbonate is a relatively safe and simple intervention, we recommend that it be used in addition to standard therapy for β-adrenergic antagonist–poisoned patients with QRS duration prolongation, ventricular dysrhythmias, or severe hypotension. Sodium bicarbonate would not be expected to be beneficial in sotalol-induced ventricular dysrhythmias and, by causing hypokalemia, may actually increase the risk of torsade de pointes. The usual dose of hypertonic sodium bicarbonate is 1 to 2 mEq/kg given as an IV bolus. This should either be followed by an infusion or by repeated boluses as needed. Care should be taken to avoid severe alkalosis or hypokalemia (Antidotes in Depth: A5).

Observation

All patients who have bradycardia, hypotension, abnormal ECGs, or CNS toxicity after β-adrenergic antagonist overdose should be observed in a critical care setting until these findings resolve. Toxicity from regular release β-adrenergic antagonist poisoning other than with sotalol almost always occurs within the first 6 hours.[148,152,204] Therefore, patients without any findings of toxicity after an overdose of a regular release β-adrenergic antagonist other than sotalol can safely be discharged from medical care after an observation time of 6 to 8 hours if they remain asymptomatic with normal vital signs and a normal ECG and have had GI decontamination with activated charcoal. Because ingestion of extended-release preparations is associated with delayed toxicity, these patients should be observed for 24 hours in an intensive care unit. It would also be reasonable to extend the observation period for patients at risk for delayed absorption because of a mixed overdose or underlying GI disease. Sotalol toxicity is sometimes delayed with ventricular dysrhythmias first occurring as late as 9 hours after ingestion.[189] We recommend that all patients with sotalol overdose be monitored for at least 12 hours. Patients who remain stable without QT interval prolongation can then be discharged from a monitored setting.

SUMMARY

- β-Adrenergic antagonists are commonly used to treat hypertension, angina, tachydysrhythmias, tremor, migraine, and panic attacks.
- Overdoses of β-adrenergic antagonists are relatively uncommon but continue to cause deaths worldwide.
- Patients who develop clinical findings after ingesting regular release β-adrenergic antagonists do so within the first 6 hours. Patients with sotalol ingestions are an exception to this in that sotalol causes delayed and prolonged toxicity. Extended-release formulations also result in delayed toxicity and require 24-hour observation.
- Patients with consequential β-adrenergic antagonist overdose typically develop bradycardia and hypotension.
- Propranolol and other β-adrenergic antagonists with membrane-stabilizing properties and high lipid solubility are the most toxic in overdose. They cause prolongation of the QRS complex, severe hypotension, coma, seizures, and apnea.
- Sotalol and acebutolol are unique in their ability to prolong the QT interval, and sotalol toxicity often results in refractory ventricular dysrhythmias, which should be treated by cardioversion followed by overdrive pacing or magnesium infusion.
- In addition to supportive and symptomatic care, the most important initial therapies for patients with β-adrenergic antagonist toxicity are calcium salts and glucagon if available. High doses of insulin together with glucose is recommended early in the course of treatment if the response to the initial therapy is not rapid and complete. Catecholamine infusions should be closely monitored and large doses are typically required. Patients who fail treatment with glucagon, insulin, and catecholamines are critically ill and may respond to IV lipid emulsion therapy, phosphodiesterase inhibitors, or mechanical support of circulation. Fortunately, most patients respond to simpler measures, and this aggressive therapy is rarely required.

REFERENCES

1. Abraham WT. Beta-blockers: the new standard of therapy for mild heart failure. *Arch Intern Med.* 2000;160:1237-1247.
2. Accili EA, et al. From funny current to HCN channels: 20 years of excitation. *News Physiol Sci.* 2002;17:32-37.
3. Adelstein RS, Eisenberg E. Regulation and kinetics of the actin-myosin-ATP interaction. *Annu Rev Biochem.* 1980;49:921-956.
4. Aggarwal N, et al. Methylene blue reverses recalcitrant shock in beta-blocker and calcium channel blocker overdose. *BMJ Case Rep.* 2013;2013.
5. Agura ED, et al. Massive propranolol overdose: successful treatment with high-dose isoproterenol and glucagon. *Am J Med.* 1986;80:755-757.
6. Alderfliegel F, et al. Sotalol poisoning associated with asystole. *Intensive Care Med.* 1993;19:57-58.
7. Annane D. Beta-adrenergic mediation of the central control of respiration: myth or reality. *J Toxicol Clin Exp.* 1991;11:325-336.
8. Anonymous. https://www.drugs.com/drug-class/beta-blockers-with-calcium-channel-blockers.html. Last accessed June 6, 2018.
9. Anonymous. *Approved Drug Products with Therapeutic Equivalence Evaluations.* 36th edition. Silver Spring, MD, U.S. Department of Health and Human Services, Food and Drug Administration; 2016.
10. Aouate P, et al. Propranolol intoxication revealing a Brugada syndrome. *J Cardiovasc Electrophysiol.* 2005;16:348-351.
11. Archan S, Toller W. Levosimendan: current status and future prospects. *Curr Opin Anaesthesiol.* 2008;21:78-84.
12. Arstall MA, et al. Sotalol-induced torsade de pointes: management with magnesium infusion. *Postgrad Med J.* 1992;68:289-290.
13. Asghari P, et al. The structure and functioning of the couplon in the mammalian cardiomyocyte. *Protoplasma.* 2012;249(suppl 1):S31-S38.
14. Assimes TL, Malcolm I. Torsade de pointes with sotalol overdose treated successfully with lidocaine. *Can J Cardiol.* 1998;14:753-756.
15. Babatasi G, et al. Severe intoxication with cardiotoxic drugs: value of emergency percutaneous cardiocirculatory assistance. *Arch Mal Coeur Vaiss.* 2001;94:1386-1392.
16. Bailey B. Glucagon in beta-blocker and calcium channel blocker overdoses: a systematic review. *J Toxicol Clin Toxicol.* 2003;41:595-602.

17. Balligand JL. Beta3-adrenoreceptors in cardiovascular diseases: new roles for an "old" receptor. *Curr Drug Delivery.* 2013;10:64-66.

18. Balligand JL. Cardiac salvage by tweaking with beta-3-adrenergic receptors. *Cardiovasc Res.* 2016;111:128-133.

19. Bangalore S, et al; REACH Registry Investigators. B-blocker use and clinical outcomes in stable outpatients with and without coronary artery disease. *JAMA.* 2012;308: 1340-1349.

20. Barrett LK, et al. Vasopressin: mechanisms of action on the vasculature in health and in septic shock. *Crit Care Med.* 2007;35:33-40.

21. Barry WH, Bridge JH. Intracellular calcium homeostasis in cardiac myocytes. *Circulation.* 1993;87:1806-1815.

22. Barton CA, et al. Successful treatment of a massive metoprolol overdose using intravenous lipid emulsion and hyperinsulinemia/euglycemia therapy. *Pharmacotherapy.* 2015;35:e56-60.

23. Belen B, et al. A complication to be aware of: hyperkalaemia following propranolol therapy for an infant with intestinal haemangiomatozis. *BMJ Case Rep.* 2014;pii: bcr2014203746.

24. Belge C, et al. Enhanced expression of beta3-adrenoceptors in cardiac myocytes attenuates neurohormone-induced hypertrophic remodeling through nitric oxide synthase. *Circulation.* 2014;129:451-462.

25. Belson MG, et al. Beta-adrenergic antagonist exposures in children. *Vet Hum Toxicol.* 2001;43:361-365.

26. Bers DM. Calcium fluxes involved in control of cardiac myocyte contraction. *Circ Res.* 2000;87:275-281.

27. Bers DM. Cardiac excitation-contraction coupling. *Nature.* 2002;415:198-205.

28. Bers DM. Calcium cycling and signaling in cardiac myocytes. *Annu Rev Physiol.* 2008;70:23-49.

29. Berthault F, et al. A fatal case of betaxolol poisoning. *J Anal Toxicol.* 1997;21:228-231.

30. Bilbault P, et al. Near-fatal betaxolol self-poisoning treated with percutaneous extracorporeal life support. *Eur J Emerg Med.* 2007;14:120-122.

31. Black JW, et al. Comparison of some properties of pronethalol and propranolol. 1965. *Br J Pharmacol.* 1997;120:285-299.

32. Bouchard NC, et al. Carvedilol overdose with quantitative confirmation. *Basic Clin Pharmacol Toxicol.* 2008;103:102-103.

33. Bourgeois JA. Depression and topical ophthalmic beta adrenergic blockade. *J Am Optom Assoc.* 1991;62:403-406.

34. Boyd R, Ghosh A. Towards evidence based emergency medicine: best bets from the Manchester Royal Infirmary. Glucagon for the treatment of symptomatic beta blocker overdose. *Emerg Med J.* 2003;20:266-267.

35. Boyett MR, et al. The sinoatrial node, a heterogeneous pacemaker structure. *Cardiovasc Res.* 2000;47:658-687.

36. Briasoulis A, et al. Meta-analysis of the effects of carvedilol versus metoprolol on all-cause mortality and hospitalizations in patients with heart failure. *Am J Cardiol.* 2015;115:1111-1115.

37. Brimacombe JR, et al. Propranolol overdose—a dramatic response to calcium chloride. *Med J Aust.* 1991;155:267-268.

38. Brodde O-E, et al. Cardiac adrenoceptors: physiological and pathophysiological relevance. *J Pharmacol Sci.* 2006;100:323-337.

39. Bronstein AC, et al. 2010 Annual Report of the American Association of Poison Control Centers' National Poison Data System (NPDS): 28th Annual Report. *Clin Toxicol.* 2011;49:910-941.

40. Browne A, et al. Intravenous lipid emulsion does not augment blood pressure recovery in a rabbit model of metoprolol toxicity. *J Med Toxicol.* 2010;6:373-378.

41. Cannell MB, Kong CHT. Local control in cardiac E-C coupling. *J Mol Cell Cardiol.* 2012;52:298-303.

42. Cave G Harvey, M. Intravenous lipid emulsion as antidote beyond local anesthetic toxicity: a systematic review. *Acad Emerg Med.* 2009;16:815-824.

43. Cave G, Harvey M. Lipid emulsion may augment early blood pressure recovery in a rabbit model of atenolol toxicity. *J Med Toxicol.* 2009;5:50-51.

44. Cave G, et al. Intravenous lipid emulsion as antidote: a summary of published human experience. *Emerg Med Australas.* 2011;23:123-141.

45. Cave G, et al. The role of fat emulsion therapy in a rodent model of propranolol toxicity: a preliminary study. *J Med Toxicol.* 2006;2:4-7.

46. Cerra MC, Imbrogno S. Phospholamban and cardiac function: a comparative perspective in vertebrates. *Acta Physiologica.* 2012;205:9-25.

47. Chen P-S, et al. The initiation of the heart beat. *Circ J.* 2010;74:221-225.

48. Cleroux J, et al. Exercise-induced hyperkalaemia: effects of beta-adrenoceptor blocker vs diuretic. *Br J Clin Pharmacol.* 1987;24:225-229.

49. Cole JB, et al. Asystole immediately following intravenous fat emulsion for overdose. *J Med Toxicol.* 2014;10:307-310.

50. Critchley JA, Ungar A. The management of acute poisoning due to beta-adrenoceptor antagonists. *Med Toxicol Adverse Drug Exp.* 1989;4:32-45.

51. Dalan R, Leow MK. Cardiovascular collapse associated with beta blockade in thyroid storm. *Exp Clin Endocrinol Diabetes.* 2007;115:392-396.

52. Dal, CJ, McGrath JC. Previously unsuspected widespread cellular and tissue distribution of beta-adrenoceptors and its relevance to drug action. *Trends Pharmacol Sci.* 2011;32:219-226.

53. Dancey D, et al. Sotalol-induced torsades de pointes in patients with renal failure. *Can J Cardiol.* 1997;13:55-58.

54. Daubin C, et al. Extracorporeal life support in severe drug intoxication: a retrospective cohort study of seventeen cases. *Crit Care.* 2009;13:R138.

55. Davis BA, et al. The role of phospholamban in the regulation of calcium transport by cardiac sarcoplasmic reticulum. *Mol Cell Biochem.* 1990;99:83-88.

56. de Lange DW, et al. Extracorporeal membrane oxygenation in the treatment of poisoned patients. *Clin Toxicol.* 2013;51:385-393.

57. De Rita F, et al. Rescue extracorporeal life support for acute verapamil and propranolol toxicity in a neonate. *Artif Organs.* 2011;35:416-420.

58. de Wildt D, et al. Different toxicological profiles for various beta-blocking agents on cardiac function in isolated rat hearts. *J Toxicol Clin Toxicol.* 1984;22:115-132.

59. Deniel A, et al. Fatal cardiac arrest associated with concomitant bisoprolol and verapamil overdose. *J Am Geriatr Soc.* 2016;64:451-452.

60. DiFrancesco D, Borer JS. The funny current: cellular basis for the control of heart rate. *Drugs.* 2007;67(suppl 2):15-24.

61. Doggrell SA, Brown L. D-sotalol: death by the sword or deserving of further consideration for clinical use [review]? *Exp Opin Investig Drugs.* 2000;9:1625-1634.

62. Donovan KD, et al. Acebutolol-induced ventricular tachycardia reversed with sodium bicarbonate. *J Toxicol Clin Toxicol.* 1999;37:481-484.

63. Elkharrat D, et al. Beta adrenergic receptor blockade: a self-limited phenomenon explaining the benignancy of acute poisoning with beta adrenergic inhibitors. Report of a series of 40 patients seen at the Fernand-Widal toxicology center, with a 0% mortality rate. *Semin Hop.* 1982;58:1073-1076.

64. Emorine LJ, et al. Molecular characterization of the human beta 3-adrenergic receptor. *Science.* 1989;245:1118-1121.

65. Engebretsen KM, et al. High-dose insulin therapy in beta-blocker and calcium channel-blocker poisoning. *Clin Toxicol.* 2011;49:277-283.

66. Escajeda JT, et al. Successful treatment of metoprolol-induced cardiac arrest with high-dose insulin, lipid emulsion, and ECMO. *Am J Emerg Med.* 2015;33:1111.e1111-1114.

67. Fareed FN, et al. Death temporally related to the use of a beta adrenergic receptor antagonist in cocaine associated myocardial infarction. *J Med Toxicol.* 2007;3:169-172.

68. Fath-Ordoubadi F, Beatt KJ. Glucose-insulin-potassium therapy for treatment of acute myocardial infarction: an overview of randomized placebo-controlled trials. *Circulation.* 1997;96:1152-1156.

69. Feek CM, Earnshaw PM. Hypertensive response to labetalol in phaeochromocytoma. *Br Med J.* 1980;281:387.

70. Fitzgerald JD. Do partial agonist beta-blockers have improved clinical utility? *Cardiovasc Drugs Ther.* 1993;7:303-310.

71. Forrester MB. Pediatric carvedilol ingestions reported to Texas poison centers, 2000 to 2008. *Pediatr Emerg Care.* 2010;26:730-732.

72. Freestone S, et al. Severe atenolol poisoning: treatment with prenalterol. *Hum Toxicol.* 1986;5:343-345.

73. Frierson J, et al. Refractory cardiogenic shock and complete heart block after unsuspected verapamil-SR and atenolol overdose. *Clin Cardiol.* 1991;14:933-935.

74. Frishman W, et al. Clinical pharmacology of the new beta-adrenergic blocking drugs. Part 8. Self-poisoning with beta-adrenoceptor blocking agents: recognition and management. *Am Heart J.* 1979;98:798-811.

75. Frishman WH, Alwarshetty M. Beta-adrenergic blockers in systemic hypertension: pharmacokinetic considerations related to the current guidelines. *Clin Pharmacokinet.* 2002;41:505-516.

76. Frishman WH, et al. Cardiovascular considerations in using topical, oral, and intravenous drugs for the treatment of glaucoma and ocular hypertension: focus on beta-adrenergic blockade. *Heart Dis.* 2001;3:386-397.

77. Frishman WH, Saunders E. beta-Adrenergic blockers. *J Clin Hypertens.* 2011;13: 649-653.

78. Frithz G. Letter: toxic effects of propranolol on the heart. *Br Med J.* 1976;1:769-770.

79. Gandy W. Severe epinephrine-propranolol interaction. *Ann Emerg Med.* 1989;18:98-99.

80. Ganigara A, et al. Fatal hyperkalemia following succinylcholine administration in a child on oral propranolol. *Drug Metab Pers Ther.* 2015;30:69-71.

81. Gauthier C, et al. Beta 3-adrenoceptors in the cardiovascular system. *Clin Hemorheol Microcirc.* 2007;37:193-204.

82. Glick G, et al. Glucagon. Its enhancement of cardiac performance in the cat and dog and persistence of its inotropic action despite beta-receptor blockade with propranolol. *Circ Res.* 1968;22:789-799.

83. Gold EH, et al. Synthesis and comparison of some cardiovascular properties of the stereoisomers of labetalol. *J Med Chem.* 1982;25:1363-1370.

84. Gopalaswamy UV, et al. Effect of propranolol on rat brain synaptosomal Na(+)-K(+)-ATPase, Mg(2+)-ATPase and Ca(2+)-ATPase. *Chem Biol Interact.* 1997;103:51-58.

85. Gradinac S, et al. Improved cardiac function with glucose-insulin-potassium after aortocoronary bypass grafting. *Ann Thorac Surg.* 1989;48:484-489.

86. Guyatt GH, Devereaux PJ. A review of heart failure treatment. *Mt Sinai J Med.* 2004;71:47-54.

87. Gyorke I, Gyorke S. Regulation of the cardiac ryanodine receptor channel by luminal Ca2+ involves luminal Ca2+ sensing sites. *Biophys J.* 1998;75:2801-2810.

88. Hahn, L, Hahn M. Carvedilol-induced hyperkalemia in a patient with chronic kidney disease. *J Pharm Pract.* 2015;28:107-111.

89. Hamad A, al. Life-threatening hyperkalemia after intravenous labetalol injection for hypertensive emergency in a hemodialysis patient. *Am J Nephrol.* 2001;21:241-244.

90. Hantson P, et al. Carvedilol overdose. *Acta Cardiol.* 1997;52:369-371.

91. Harvey M, et al. Insulin versus lipid emulsion in a rabbit model of severe propranolol toxicity: a pilot study. *Crit Care Res Pract*. 2011;2011:361737.

92. Harvey MG, Cave G. Intralipid infusion ameliorates propranolol-induced hypotension in rabbits. *J Med Toxicol*. 2008;4:71-76.

93. Hashiyada M, et al. Unexpectedly high blood concentration of bisoprolol after an incorrect prescription: a case report. *Leg Med*. 2013;15:103-105.

94. He J-Q, et al. Crosstalk of beta-adrenergic receptor subtypes through Gi blunts beta-adrenergic stimulation of L-type Ca2+ channels in canine heart failure. *Circ Res*. 2005;97:566-573.

95. Heinroth KM, et al. Acute beta 1-selective beta-receptor blocker nebivolol poisoning in attempted suicide. *Dtsch Med Wochenschr*. 1999;124:1230-1234.

96. Henry JA, Cassidy SL. Membrane stabilising activity: a major cause of fatal poisoning. *Lancet*. 1986;1:1414-1417.

97. Henry M, et al. Cardiogenic shock associated with calcium-channel and beta blockers: reversal with intravenous calcium chloride. *Am J Emerg Med*. 1985;3:334-336.

98. Hesse B, Pedersen JT. Hypoglycaemia after propranolol in children. *Acta Med Scand*. 1973;193:551-552.

99. Hicks PR, Rankin AP. Massive adrenaline doses in labetalol overdose. *Anaesth Intensive Care*. 1991;19:447-449.

100. Hoeper MM, Boeker KH. Overdose of metoprolol treated with enoximone. *N Engl J Med*. 1996;335:1538.

101. Hoffman BB, et al. Catecholamines, sympathomimetic drugs, and adrenergic receptor antagonists. *Goodman and Gilman's*. New York, NY: McGraw-Hill; 2001: 215-268.

102. Hohnloser SH, Woosley RL. Sotalol. *N Engl J Med*. 1994;331:31-38.

103. Holger JS, et al. Insulin versus vasopressin and epinephrine to treat beta-blocker toxicity. *Clin Toxicol*. 2007;45:396-401.

104. Holger JS, et al. A comparison of vasopressin and glucagon in beta-blocker induced toxicity. *Clin Toxicol*. 2006;44:45-51.

105. Holger JS, et al. High-dose insulin: a consecutive case series in toxin-induced cardiogenic shock. *Clin Toxicol*. 2011;49:653-658.

106. Ibrahim M, et al. The structure and function of cardiac t-tubules in health and disease. *Proc Biol Sci*. 2011;278:2714-2723.

107. Illingworth RN. Glucagon for beta-blocker poisoning. *Lancet*. 1980;2:86.

108. Janion M, et al. Is the intra-aortic balloon pump a method of brain protection during cardiogenic shock after drug intoxication? *J Emerg Med*. 2010;38:162-167.

109. Javeed N, et al. Refractory anaphylactoid shock potentiated by beta-blockers. *Cathet Cardiovasc Diagn*. 1996;39:383-384.

110. Johnson NJ, et al. A review of emergency cardiopulmonary bypass for severe poisoning by cardiotoxic drugs. *J Med Toxicol*. 2013;9:54-60.

111. Jovic-Stosic J, et al. Severe propranolol and ethanol overdose with wide complex tachycardia treated with intravenous lipid emulsion: a case report. *Clin Toxicol*. 2011;49:426-430.

112. Kalam Y, Graudins A. The effects of fructose-1,6-diphosphate on haemodynamic parameters and survival in a rodent model of propranolol and verapamil poisoning. *Clin Toxicol*. 2012;50:546-554.

113. Kalam Y, Graudin, A. Levosimendan does not improve cardiac output or blood pressure in a rodent model of propranolol toxicity when administered using various dosing regimens. *Int J Toxicol*. 2012;31:166-174.

114. Kalam Y, Graudins A. Levosimendan infusion improves cardiac output but not blood pressure in a rodent model of severe metoprolol toxicity. *Hum Exp Toxicol*. 2012;31:955-963.

115. Kelly RA, et al. *Pharmacologic Treatment of Heart Failure*. New York, NY: McGraw-Hill; 1996:809-838.

116. Kenyon CJ, et al. Successful resuscitation using external cardiac pacing in beta adrenergic antagonist-induced bradyasystolic arrest. *Ann Emerg Med*. 1988;17:711-713.

117. Kerns W 2nd. Management of beta-adrenergic blocker and calcium channel antagonist toxicity. *Emerg Med Clin North Am*. 2007;25:309-331; abstract viii.

118. Kerns W 2nd, et al. The effects of extracellular ions on beta-blocker cardiotoxicity. *Toxicol Appl Pharmacol*. 1996;137:1-7.

119. Kerns W 2nd, et al. The effect of hypertonic sodium and dantrolene on propranolol cardiotoxicity. *Acad Emerg Med*. 1997;4:545-551.

120. Kerns W 2nd, etal. Insulin improves survival in a canine model of acute beta-blocker toxicity. *Ann Emerg Med*. 1997;29:748-757.

121. Khan, A, Muscat-Baron JM. Fatal oxprenolol poisoning. *Br Med J*. 1977;1:552.

122. Kobilka BK. Structural insights into adrenergic receptor function and pharmacology. *Trends Pharmacol Sci*. 2011;32:213-218.

123. Kolcz J, et al. Extracorporeal life support in severe propranolol and verapamil intoxication. *J Intensive Care Med*. 2007;22:381-385.

124. Kollef MH. Labetalol overdose successfully treated with amrinone and alpha-adrenergic receptor agonists. *Chest*. 1994;105:626-627.

125. Koopman R, et al. The role of beta-adrenoceptor signaling in skeletal muscle: therapeutic implications for muscle wasting disorders. *Curr Opin Clin Nutr Metab Care*. 2009;12:601-606.

126. Korzets A, et al. Acute renal failure associated with a labetalol overdose. *Postgrad Med J*. 1990;66:66-67.

127. Kosinski EJ, Malindzak GS Jr. Glucagon and isoproterenol in reversing propranolol toxicity. *Arch Intern Med*. 1973;132:840-843.

128. Kosinski EJ, et al. Glucogan and propranolol (inderal) toxicity. *N Engl J Med*. 1971;285:1325.

129. Krapf R, Gertsch M. Torsade de pointes induced by sotalol despite therapeutic plasma sotalol concentrations. *Br Med J*. 1985;290:1784-1785.

130. Kulling P, et al. Beta-adrenoceptor blocker intoxication: epidemiological data. Prenalterol as an alternative in the treatment of cardiac dysfunction. *Hum Toxicol*. 1983;2:175-181.

131. Kuok CH, et al. Cardiovascular collapse after labetalol for hypertensive crisis in an undiagnosed pheochromocytoma during cesarean section. *Acta Anaesthesiol Taiwan*. 2011;49:69-71.

132. Lacey RJ, et al. Selective stimulation of glucagon secretion by beta 2-adrenoceptors in isolated islets of Langerhans of the rat. *Br J Pharmacol*. 1991;103:1824-1828.

133. Lakatta EG, DiFrancesco D. What keeps us ticking: a funny current, a calcium clock, or both? *J Mol Cell Cardiol*. 2009;47:157-170.

134. Lambert DM. Effect of propranolol on mortality in patients with angina. *Postgrad Med J*. 1976;52(suppl 4):57-60.

135. Lane AS, et al. Massive propranolol overdose poorly responsive to pharmacologic therapy: use of the intra-aortic balloon pump. *Ann Emerg Med*. 1987;16:1381-1383.

136. Langemeijer J, et al. Respiratory arrest as main determinant of toxicity due to overdose with different beta-blockers in rats. *Acta Pharmacol Toxicol (Copenh)*. 1985;57:352-356.

137. Langemeijer J, et al. Calcium interferes with the cardiodepressive effects of beta-blocker overdose in isolated rat hearts. *J Toxicol Clin Toxicol*. 1986;24:111-133.

138. Langemeijer JJ, et al. Centrally induced respiratory arrest: main cause of death in beta-adrenoceptor antagonist intoxication. *Hum Toxicol*. 1986;5:65.

139. Lau DH, et al. Sinus node revisited. *Curr Opin Cardiol*. 2011;26:55-59.

140. Lee HM, et al. What are the adverse effects associated with the combined use of intravenous lipid emulsion and extracorporeal membrane oxygenation in the poisoned patient? *Clin Toxicol*. 2015;53:145-150.

141. Lee KC, et al. Cardiovascular and renal effects of milrinone in beta-adrenoreceptor blocked and non-blocked anaesthetized dogs. *Drugs Exp Clin Res*. 1991;17:145-158.

142. Lehmann A, et al. The role of Ca++-sensitizers for the treatment of heart failure. *Curr Opin Crit Care*. 2003;9:337-344.

143. Lehtonen L, Poder P. The utility of levosimendan in the treatment of heart failure. *Ann Med*. 2007;39:2-17.

144. Leppikangas H, et al. Levosimendan as a rescue drug in experimental propranolol-induced myocardial depression: a randomized study. *Ann Emerg Med*. 2009;54:811-817. e811-813.

145. Levitzki A, et al. The signal transduction between beta-receptors and adenylyl cyclase. *Life Sci*. 1993;52:2093-2100.

146. Li L, et al. Phosphorylation of phospholamban and troponin I in beta-adrenergic-induced acceleration of cardiac relaxation. *Am J Physiol Heart Circ Physiol*. 2000;278:H769-H779.

147. Lofdahl CG, Svedmyr N. Cardioselectivity of atenolol and metoprolol. A study in asthmatic patients. *Eur J Respir Dis*. 1981;62:396-404.

148. Love JN. Beta blocker toxicity after overdose: when do symptoms develop in adults? *J Emerg Med*. 1994;12:799-802.

149. Love JN. Acebutolol overdose resulting in fatalities. *J Emerg Med*. 2000;18:341-344.

150. Love JN, et al. Electrocardiographic changes associated with beta-blocker toxicity. *Ann Emerg Med*. 2002;40:603-610.

151. Love JN, et al. Hemodynamic effects of calcium chloride in a canine model of acute propranolol intoxication. *Ann Emerg Med*. 1996;28:1-6.

152. Love JN, et al. Acute beta blocker overdose: factors associated with the development of cardiovascular morbidity. *J Toxicol Clin Toxicol*. 2000;38:275-281.

153. Love JN, et al. The effect of sodium bicarbonate on propranolol-induced cardiovascular toxicity in a canine model. *J Toxicol Clin Toxicol*. 2000;38:421-428.

154. Love JN, et al. A comparison of combined amrinone and glucagon therapy to glucagon alone for cardiovascular depression associated with propranolol toxicity in a canine model. *Am J Emerg Med*. 1993;11:360-363.

155. Love JN, et al. A comparison of amrinone and glucagon therapy for cardiovascular depression associated with propranolol toxicity in a canine model. *J Toxicol Clin Toxicol*. 1992;30:399-412.

156. Love JN, et al. Characterization of fatal beta blocker ingestion: a review of the American Association of Poison Control Centers data from 1985 to 1995. *J Toxicol Clin Toxicol*. 1997;35:353-359.

157. Love JN, et al. A potential role for glucagon in the treatment of drug-induced symptomatic bradycardia. *Chest*. 1998;114:323-326.

158. Love JN, Sikka N. Are 1-2 tablets dangerous? Beta-blocker exposure in toddlers. *J Emerg Med*. 2004;26:309-314.

159. Lundborg, P. The effect of adrenergic blockade on potassium concentrations in different conditions. *Acta Med Scand Suppl*. 1983;672:121-126.

160. Macala K, Tabrizchi R. The effect of fat emulsion on hemodynamics following treatment with propranolol and clonidine in anesthetized rats. *Acad Emerg Med*. 2014;21:1220-1225.

161. Malmberg K. Prospective randomised study of intensive insulin treatment on long term survival after acute myocardial infarction in patients with diabetes mellitus. Digami (diabetes mellitus, insulin glucose infusion in acute myocardial infarction) study group. *BMJ*. 1997;314:1512-1515.

162. Malmberg K. Role of insulin-glucose infusion in outcomes after acute myocardial infarction: the diabetes and insulin-glucose infusion in acute myocardial infarction (DIGAMI) study. *Endocr Pract*. 2004;10(suppl 2):13-16.

163. Malmberg K, et al. Randomized trial of insulin-glucose infusion followed by subcutaneous insulin treatment in diabetic patients with acute myocardial infarction (DIGAMI study): effects on mortality at 1 year. *J Am Coll Cardiol.* 1995;26:57-65.
164. Maltsev AV, et al. Synchronization of stochastic Ca2(+) release units creates a rhythmic Ca2(+) clock in cardiac pacemaker cells. *Biophys J.* 2011;100:271-283.
165. Maltsev VA, Lakatta EG. Normal heart rhythm is initiated and regulated by an intracellular calcium clock within pacemaker cells. *Heart Lung Circ.* 2007;16:335-348.
166. Maltsev VA, et al. The emergence of a general theory of the initiation and strength of the heartbeat. *J Pharmacol Sci.* 2006;100:338-369.
167. Maltsev VA, et al. Modern perspectives on numerical modeling of cardiac pacemaker cell. *J Pharmacol Sci.* 2014;125:6-38.
168. Mandic D, et al. Severe hyperkalemia induced by propranolol. *Med Pregl.* 2014;67:181-184.
169. Mangrella M, et al. Pharmacology of nebivolol. *Pharmacol Res.* 1998;38:419-431.
170. Marks AR. Calcium cycling proteins and heart failure: mechanisms and therapeutics. *J Clin Invest.* 2013;123:46-52.
171. Masson R, et al. A comparison of survival with and without extracorporeal life support treatment for severe poisoning due to drug intoxication. *Resuscitation.* 2012;83:1413-1417.
172. McDevitt DG. Comparison of pharmacokinetic properties of beta-adrenoceptor blocking drugs. *Eur Heart J.* 1987;8(suppl M):9-14.
173. McVey FK, Corke CF. Extracorporeal circulation in the management of massive propranolol overdose. *Anaesthesia.* 1991;46:744-746.
174. Megarbane B, et al. Usefulness of the serum lactate concentration for predicting mortality in acute beta-blocker poisoning. *Clin Toxicol.* 2010;48:974-978.
175. Meredith PA, et al. The pharmacokinetics of bucindolol and its major metabolite in essential hypertension. *Xenobiotica.* 1985;15:979-985.
176. Mery PF, et al. Glucagon stimulates the cardiac Ca2+ current by activation of adenylyl cyclase and inhibition of phosphodiesterase. *Nature.* 1990;345:158-161.
177. Michel MC, et al. Are there functional beta3-adrenoceptors in the human heart? *Br J Pharmacol.* 2011;162:817-822.
178. Michel S, et al. Use of methylene blue in the treatment of refractory vasodilatory shock after cardiac assist device implantation: report of four consecutive cases. *J Clin Med Res.* 2012;4:212-215.
179. Miki A, et al. Betaxolol-induced deterioration of asthma and a pharmacodynamic analysis based on beta-receptor occupancy. *Int J Clin Pharmacol Ther.* 2003;41:358-364.
180. Minchole A, et al. ECG-based estimation of dispersion of APD restitution as a tool to stratify sotalol-induced arrhythmic risk. *J Electrocardiol.* 2015;48:867-873.
181. Montagna M, Groppi A. Fatal sotalol poisoning. *Arch Toxicol.* 1980;43:221-226.
182. Montgomery AB, et al. Marked suppression of ventilation while awake following massive ingestion of atenolol. *Chest.* 1985;88:920-921.
183. Morita S, et al. Pharmacokinetics of enoximone after various intravenous administrations to healthy volunteers. *J Pharm Sci.* 1995;84:152-157.
184. Mowry JB, et al. 2014 Annual Report of the American Association of Poison Control Centers' National Poison Data System (NPDS): 32nd Annual Report. *Clin Toxicol (Phila).* 2015;53:962-1147.
185. Mowry JB, et al. 2012 Annual Report of the American Association of Poison Control Centers' National Poison Data System (NPDS): 30th Annual Report. *Clin Toxicol (Phila).* 2013;51:949-1229.
186. Mowry JB, et al. 2013 Annual Report of the American Association of Poison Control Centers' National Poison Data System (NPDS): 31st Annual Report. *Clin Toxicol (Phila).* 2014;52:1032-1283.
187. Munger MA, et al. Effect of intravenous fructose-1,6-diphosphate on myocardial contractility in patients with left ventricular dysfunction. *Pharmacotherapy.* 1994;14:522-528.
188. Neumar RW, et al. Part 1: executive summary: 2015 American Heart Association Guidelines Update for Cardiopulmonary Resuscitation and Emergency Cardiovascular Care. *Circulation.* 2015;132:S315-367.
189. Neuvonen PJ, et al. Prolonged QT interval and severe tachyarrhythmias, common features of sotalol intoxication. *Eur J Clin Pharmacol.* 1981;20:85-89.
190. Ngo AS, Lung Tan DC. Thyrotoxic heart disease. *Resuscitation.* 2006;70:287-290.
191. Olin BR, et al. Beta-adrenergic blocking agents. St. Louis, MO: Wolters Kluwer; 2000:467-486.
192. Ouellet G, et al. Available extracorporeal treatments for poisoning: overview and limitations. *Semin Dial.* 2014;27:342-349.
193. Page C, et al. The use of high-dose insulin-glucose euglycemia in beta-blocker overdose: a case report. *J Med Toxicol.* 2009;5:139-143.
194. Paravastu SC, et al. Beta blockers for peripheral arterial disease. *Cochrane Database Syst Rev.* 2013:Cd005508.
195. Perrone SV, Kaplinsky EJ. Calcium sensitizer agents: a new class of inotropic agents in the treatment of decompensated heart failure. *Int J Cardiol.* 2005;103:248-255.
196. Perrot D, et al. A case of sotalol poisoning with fatal outcome. *J Toxicol Clin Toxicol.* 1988;26:389-396.
197. Pertoldi F, et al. Electromechanical dissociation 48 hours after atenolol overdose: usefulness of calcium chloride. *Ann Emerg Med.* 1998;31:777-781.
198. Pfaender M, et al. Successful treatment of a massive atenolol and nifedipine overdose with CVVHDF. *Minerva Anestesiol.* 2008;74:97-100.
199. Pollack CV Jr. Utility of glucagon in the emergency department. *J Emerg Med.* 1993;11:195-205.
200. Poterucha JT, et al. Frequency and severity of hypoglycemia in children with beta-blocker-treated long QT syndrome. *Heart Rhythm.* 2015;12:1815-1819.
201. Prichard BN, et al. Overdosage with beta-adrenergic blocking agents. *Adverse Drug React Acute Poisoning Rev.* 1984;3:91-111.
202. Pritchard BN, Thorpe, P. Pindolol in hypertension. *Med J Aust.* 1971;58:1242.
203. Reed BN, Sueta CA. A practical guide for the treatment of symptomatic heart failure with reduced ejection fraction (HFrEF). *Curr Cardiol Rev.* 2015;11:23-32.
204. Reith DM, et al. Relative toxicity of beta blockers in overdose. *J Toxicol Clin Toxicol.* 1996;34:273-278.
205. Rennyson SL, Littmann L. Brugada-pattern electrocardiogram in propranolol intoxication. *Am J Emerg Med.* 2010;28:256.e257-258.
206. Reute, H, Porzig H. Beta-adrenergic actions on cardiac cell membranes. *Adv Myocardiol.* 1982;3:87-93.
207. Reynolds RD, et al. Pharmacology and pharmacokinetics of esmolol. *J Clin Pharmacol.* 1986;26(suppl A):A3-A14.
208. Richards DA, Prichard BN. Self-poisoning with beta-blockers. *Br Med J.* 1978;1:1623-1624.
209. Riker CD, et al. Massive metoprolol ingestion associated with a fatality—a case report. *J Forensic Sci.* 1987;32:1447-1452.
210. Ronn O, et al. Haemodynamic effects and pharmacokinetics of a new selective beta1-adrenoceptor agonist, prenalterol, and its interaction with metoprolol in man. *Eur J Clin Pharmacol.* 1979;15:9-13.
211. Rooney M, et al. Acebutolol overdose treated with hemodialysis and extracorporeal membrane oxygenation. *J Clin Pharmacol.* 1996;36:760-763.
212. Rosenbaum DM, et al. The structure and function of G-protein-coupled receptors. *Nature.* 2009;459:356-363.
213. Roussel O, et al. Celiprolol poisoning: two case reports. *Therapie.* 2005;60:81-84.
214. Rygnestad T, et al. Severe poisoning with sotalol and verapamil. Recovery after 4 h of normothermic CPR followed by extra corporeal heart lung assist. *Acta Anaesthesiol Scand.* 2005;49:1378-1380.
215. Saitz R, et al. Atenolol-induced cardiovascular collapse treated with hemodialysis. *Crit Care Med.* 1991;19:116-118.
216. Sakurai H, et al. Cardiogenic shock triggered by verapamil and atenolol: a case report of therapeutic experience with intravenous calcium. *Jpn Circ J.* 2000;64:893-896.
217. Salpeter S, et al. Cardioselective beta-blockers for reversible airway disease. *Cochrane Database Syst Rev.* 2002:CD002992.
218. Samuels TL, et al. Intravenous lipid emulsion treatment for propranolol toxicity: another piece in the lipid sink jigsaw fits. *Clin Toxicol.* 2011;49:769.
219. Sandroni C, et al. Successful treatment with enoximone for severe poisoning with atenolol and verapamil: a case report. *Acta Anaesthesiol Scand.* 2004;48:790-792.
220. Sandron C, et al. Enoximone in cardiac arrest caused by propranolol: two case reports. *Acta Anaesthesiol Scand.* 2006;50:759-761.
221. Sato S, et al. Milrinone versus glucagon: comparative hemodynamic effects in canine propranolol poisoning. *J Toxicol Clin Toxicol.* 1994;32:277-289.
222. Sato S, et al. Combined use of glucagon and milrinone may not be preferable for severe propranolol poisoning in the canine model. *J Toxicol Clin Toxicol.* 1995;33:337-342.
223. Schaub MC, et al. Integration of calcium with the signaling network in cardiac myocytes. *J Mol Cell Cardiol.* 2006;41:183-214.
224. Schier JG, et al. Fatality from administration of labetalol and crushed extended-release nifedipine. *Ann Pharmacother.* 2003;37:1420-1423.
225. Schweitzer I, et al. Antiglaucoma medication and clinical depression. *Aust N Z J Psychiatry.* 2001;35:569-571.
226. Scoote M, et al. The therapeutic potential of new insights into myocardial excitation-contraction coupling. *Heart.* 2003;89:371-376.
227. Sharifi M, et al. Third degree AV block due to ophthalmic timilol solution. *Int J Cardiol.* 2001;80:257-259.
228. Shimizu W, Antzelevitch C. Effects of a K(+) channel opener to reduce transmural dispersion of repolarization and prevent torsade de pointes in LQT1, LQT2, and LQT3 models of the long-QT syndrome. *Circulation.* 2000;102:706-712.
229. Shore ET, et al. Metoprolol overdose. *Ann Emerg Med.* 1981;10:524-527.
230. Smit AJ, et al. Acute renal failure after overdose of labetalol. *Br Med J.* 1986;293:1142-1143.
231. Snook CP, et al. Severe atenolol and diltiazem overdose. *J Toxicol Clin Toxicol.* 2000;38:661-665.
232. Soni N, et al. Cardiovascular collapse and propranolol overdose. *Med J Aust.* 1983;2:629-630.
233. Sperelakis N. Regulation of calcium slow channels of cardiac muscle by cyclic nucleotides and phosphorylation. *J Mol Cell Cardiol.* 1988;20(suppl 2):75-105.
234. Stajic M, et al. Fatal metoprolol overdose. *J Anal Toxicol.* 1984;8:228-230.
235. Stapleton MP. Sir James Black and propranolol. The role of the basic sciences in the history of cardiovascular pharmacology. *Tex Heart Inst J.* 1997;24:336-342.
236. Steinberg SF. The molecular basis for distinct beta-adrenergic receptor subtype actions in cardiomyocytes. *Circ Res.* 1999;85:1101-1111.
237. Stellpflug SJ, et al. Intentional overdose with cardiac arrest treated with intravenous fat emulsion and high-dose insulin. *Clin Toxicol.* 2010;48:227-229.
238. Stinson J, et al. Ventricular asystole and overdose with atenolol. *BMJ.* 1992;305:693.
239. Strubelt O. Evaluation of antidotes against the acute cardiovascular toxicity of propranolol. *Toxicology.* 1984;31:261-270.

240. Sugrue A, et al. Electrocardiographic predictors of torsadogenic risk during dofetilide or sotalol initiation: utility of a novel T wave analysis program. *Cardiovasc Drugs Ther.* 2015;29:433-441.

241. Sulakhe PV, Vo XT. Regulation of phospholamban and troponin-I phosphorylation in the intact rat cardiomyocytes by adrenergic and cholinergic stimuli: roles of cyclic nucleotides, calcium, protein kinases and phosphatases and depolarization. *Mol Cell Biochem.* 1995;149-150:103-126.

242. Tabone D, Ferguson C. Bet 2: intralipid/lipid emulsion in beta-blocker overdose. *Emerg Med J.* 2011;28:991-993.

243. Taboulet P, et al. Pathophysiology and management of self-poisoning with beta-blockers. *J Toxicol Clin Toxicol.* 1993;31:531-551.

244. Takahashi N, et al. Clinical suppression of bradycardia dependent premature ventricular contractions by the potassium channel opener nicorandil. *Heart.* 1998;79:64-68.

245. Takaichi K, et al. of factors causing hyperkalemia. *Intern Med.* 2007;46:823-829.

246. Takeuchi K, et al. Administration of fructose 1,6-diphosphate during early reperfusion significantly improves recovery of contractile function in the postischemic heart. *J Thorac Cardiovasc Surg.* 1998;116:335-343.

247. Taur Y, Frishman WH. The cardiac ryanodine receptor (RyR2) and its role in heart disease. *Cardiol Rev.* 2005;13:142-146.

248. Templin C, et al. Clinical features and outcomes of takotsubo (stress) cardiomyopathy. *N Engl J Med.* 2015;373:929-938.

249. Thakrar R, et al. Management of a mixed overdose of calcium channel blockers, beta-blockers and statins. *BMJ Case Rep.* 2014;pii: bcr2014204732.

250. Thompson AM, et al. Intravenous lipid emulsion and high-dose insulin as adjunctive therapy for propranolol toxicity in a pediatric patient. *Am J Health Syst Pharm.* 2016;73:880-885.

251. Toda N. Vasodilating beta-adrenoceptor blockers as cardiovascular therapeutics. *Pharmacol Ther.* 2003;100:215-234.

252. Totterman KJ, et al. Overdrive pacing as treatment of sotalol-induced ventricular tachyarrhythmias (torsade de pointes). *Acta Med Scand Suppl.* 1982;668:28-33.

253. Tracqui A, et al. Self-poisoning with the beta-blocker bisoprolol. *Hum Exp Toxicol.* 1990;9:255-256.

254. Travill CM, et al. The inotropic and hemodynamic effects of intravenous milrinone when reflex adrenergic stimulation is suppressed by beta-adrenergic blockade. *Clin Ther.* 1994;16:783-792.

255. Treschan TA, Peters J. The vasopressin system: physiology and clinical strategies. *Anesthesiology.* 2006;105:599-612; quiz 639-540.

256. Tynan RF, et al. Self-poisoning with propranolol. *Med J Aust.* 1981;1:82-83.

257. van den Berg MJ, Bosch FH. Case report: hemodynamic instability following severe metoprolol and imipramine intoxication successfully treated with intravenous fat emulsion. *Am J Ther.* 2016;23:e246-248.

258. Vinti H, et al. Systemic complications of beta-blocking eyedrops. Apropos of 6 cases. *Rev Med Intern.* 1989;10:41-44.

259. Waldo AL, et al. Effect of d-sotalol on mortality in patients with left ventricular dysfunction after recent and remote myocardial infarction. The SWORD Investigators. Survival With Oral d-Sotalol. [Erratum appears in *Lancet.* 1996 Aug 10;348(9024):416]. *Lancet.* 1996;348:7-12.

260. Ward DE, Jones B. Glucagon and beta-blocker toxicity. *Br Med J.* 1976;2:151.

261. Watanabe O, et al. Nicorandil, a potassium channel opener, abolished torsades de pointes in a patient with complete atrioventricular block. *Pacing Clin Electrophysiol.* 1999;22:686-688.

262. Weeke P, et al. QT variability during initial exposure to sotalol: experience based on a large electronic medical record. *Europace.* 2013;15:1791-1797.

263. Wei J, et al. Pharmacologic antagonism of propranolol in dogs. Effects of dopamine-isoproterenol and glucagon on hemodynamics and myocardial oxygen consumption in ischemic hearts during chronic propranolol administration. *J Thorac Cardiovasc Surg.* 1984;87:732-742.

264. Wei Y, Mojsov S. Tissue-specific expression of the human receptor for glucagon-like peptide-I: brain, heart and pancreatic forms have the same deduced amino acid sequences. *FEBS Lett.* 1995;358:219-224.

265. Weinberg G. (2007). LipidRescue™ resuscitation for cardiac toxicity. Treatment Regimens. http://lipidrescue.org.

266. Weinstein RS. Recognition and management of poisoning with beta-adrenergic blocking agents. *Ann Emerg Med.* 1984;13:1123-1131.

267. Weisbrod D, et al. Mechanisms underlying the cardiac pacemaker: the role of SK4 calcium-activated potassium channels. *Acta Pharmacol Sin.* 2016;37:82-97.

268. Westfall TC, Westfall DP. Adrenergic agonists and antagonists. In: Brunton L, ed. *Goodman and Gilman's The Pharmacological Basis of Therapeutics* (electronic edition). New York, NY: McGrawHill; 2006.

269. Wier WG, Balke CW. Ca(2+) release mechanisms, Ca(2+) sparks, and local control of excitation-contraction coupling in normal heart muscle. *Circ Res.* 1999;85:770-776.

270. Wnek W. The use of intra-aortic balloon counterpulsation in the treatment of severe hemodynamic instability from myocardial depressant drug overdose. *Przegl Lek.* 2003;60:274-276.

271. Wu AH, Cody RJ. Medical and surgical treatment of chronic heart failure. *Curr Probl Cardiol.* 2003;28:229-260.

272. Yagami T. Differential coupling of glucagon and beta-adrenergic receptors with the small and large forms of the stimulatory G protein. *Mol Pharmacol.* 1995;48:849-854.

273. Yuan TH, et al. Insulin-glucose as adjunctive therapy for severe calcium channel antagonist poisoning. *J Toxicol Clin Toxicol.* 1999;37:463-474.

274. Zafrir B, Amir O. Beta blocker therapy, decompensated heart failure, and inotropic interactions: current perspectives. *Isr Med Assoc J.* 2012;14:184-189.

275. Zhu W, et al. beta-adrenergic receptor subtype signaling in the heart: from bench to the bedside. *Curr Top Membr.* 2011;67:191-204.

276. Zhu W, et al. The enigma of beta2-adrenergic receptor Gi signaling in the heart: the good, the bad, and the ugly. *Circ Res.* 2005;97:507-509.

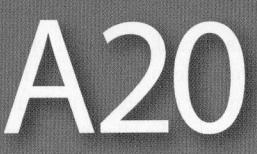

A20

Antidotes in Depth

GLUCAGON

Mary Ann Howland and Silas W. Smith

INTRODUCTION

The traditional role of glucagon was to reverse life-threatening hypoglycemia in patients with diabetes unable to receive dextrose in the outpatient setting. However, in clinical toxicology, glucagon is used early in the management of β-adrenergic antagonist and calcium channel blocker toxicity to increase heart rate, contractility, and blood pressure by increasing myocardial cyclic adenosine monophosphate (cAMP) via a non–β-adrenergic receptor mechanism of action. The use of glucagon is based primarily on animal studies as well as human case series and case reports. The effects of glucagon are often transient.

HISTORY

Glucagon was discovered in 1922, the year after insulin's discovery, when acetone precipitates of pancreatic extracts were found to produce "a distinctly hyperglycemic effect" in animals.[34] Originally viewed as a mere contaminant in insulin products, glucagon was eventually attributed to pancreatic α-cells and sequenced in 1957.[7,22] The positive inotropic and chronotropic effects of glucagon were recognized in the 1960s.[18,20] Clinical use in human poisonings began in 1971.[39]

PHARMACOLOGY
Chemistry and Preparation

Glucagon is a single-chain polypeptide counterregulatory hormone with a molecular weight of 3,500 Da that is secreted by the α-cells of the pancreas. The previously animal-derived product was possibly contaminated with insulin; the form approved in 1998 by the US Food and Drug Administration (FDA) is synthesized by recombinant DNA technology and thus is free of insulin and the prior phenol preservative.[31,57]

Mechanism of Action

In both animals and humans, glucagon receptors are found in the heart, brain, and pancreas.[26,42,90] Binding of glucagon to cardiac receptors is closely correlated with activation of cardiac adenylate cyclase.[68] A large number of glucagon binding sites are demonstrated, and as little as 10% occupancy produces near maximal stimulation of adenylate cyclase. Binding of glucagon to its receptor results in coupling with two isoforms of the G_s protein and catalyzes the exchange of guanosine triphosphate (GTP) for guanosine diphosphate on the α subunit of the G_s protein.[25,67,95] One isoform is coupled to β-adrenergic agonists, and both isoforms are coupled to glucagon.[95] The GTP-G_s units stimulate adenylate cyclase to convert adenosine triphosphate (ATP) to cAMP.[41,51] In animal hearts, glucagon inhibits the phosphodiesterase PDE_3.[6,56] Selective inhibition of PDE_4 potentiated the cAMP response to glucagon in adult rat ventricular myocytes.[66] Glucagon, along with $β_2$-adrenergic agonists (not $β_1$-adrenergic agonists), histamine, and serotonin, also activates G_i, which inhibits cAMP formation in human atrial heart tissue.[33]

Evidence suggests an additional mechanism of action for glucagon independent of cAMP and dependent on arachidonic acid.[76] Cardiac tissue metabolizes glucagon, liberating mini-glucagon, an active smaller terminal fragment.[76,92] Mini-glucagon stimulates phospholipase A_2, releasing arachidonic acid. Arachidonic acid acts to increase cardiac contractility through an effect on calcium. The effect of arachidonic acid—and therefore of mini-glucagon—is synergistic with the effect of glucagon and cAMP.[61,75] Stimulation of glucagon receptors in the liver and adipose tissue increases cAMP synthesis, resulting in glycogenolysis, gluconeogenesis, and ketogenesis.[41] Other properties of glucagon include relaxation of smooth muscle in the lower esophageal sphincter, stomach, small and large intestines, common bile duct, and ureters.[21,25,64]

Cardiovascular Effects

Investigations of the mechanism of action of glucagon on the heart were performed on cardiac tissue obtained from patients during surgical procedures and in a variety of in vivo and ex vivo animal studies. The results are often species specific and are affected by the presence or absence of congestive heart failure. The inotropic action of glucagon is related to an increase in cardiac cAMP concentrations.[18,41,51] Glucagon increases cAMP to augment the sarcoplasmic reticulum calcium pool.[16] Glucagon improves chronotropy at both the sinus node and the atrioventricular (AV) junctional region, even in the presence of escape rhythms.[87] Both the positive inotropic and chronotropic actions of glucagon are very similar to those of the β-adrenergic agonists, except that they are not blocked by β-adrenergic antagonists.[5,16,18,20,36,49,51,59,64,93,95] Glucagon also improves coronary blood flow.[3] Although in some canine experiments, glucagon caused ventricular tachycardia, glucagon is not dysrhythmogenic in patients with severe chronic congestive heart failure or myocardial infarction–related acute congestive heart failure or in postoperative patients with myocardial depression.[31,44,50,53] The effects of glucagon diminish markedly as the severity and chronicity of congestive heart failure increases.[59]

Pharmacokinetics and Pharmacodynamics

The volume of distribution of glucagon is 0.25 L/kg.[57] The plasma, liver, and kidney extensively metabolize glucagon with an elimination half-life of 8-18 minutes.[57] In human volunteers, after a single IV bolus, the cardiac effects of glucagon begin within 1 to 3 minutes is maximal within 5 to 7 minutes, and persists for 10 to 15 minutes.[59] The time to maximal glucose concentration is 5 to 20 minutes, with a duration of action of 60 to 90 minutes.[57] Smooth muscle relaxation begins within one minute and lasts 10 to 20 minutes.[57] The onset of action after intramuscular and subcutaneous administration occurs in about 10 minutes, with a peak at about 30 minutes.[57] Activation of adenylate cyclase in adipose, myocardial, and hepatic tissue and myocardial contractility requires pharmacologic concentrations of glucagon greater than 0.1 nM.[68] At physiologic concentrations of glucagon of less than 0.1 nM, glucagon enhances the cardiac metabolic effects of insulin by activating a phosphatidylinositol-3 kinase (PI3K)–dependent signal without stimulating adenylate cyclase.[68] Tachyphylaxis (desensitization of receptors) may occur with repetitive dosing. Experimental heart preparations exposed to glucagon for varying lengths of time demonstrated a decrease in the amount of generated cAMP.[28,96] Possible explanations for tachyphylaxis include uncoupling from the glucagon receptor, increased PDE hydrolysis of cAMP, or both.[28,92,96,99] Other experiments demonstrated a limited effect of glucagon on contractility and hyperglycemia, suggesting tachyphylaxis.[24,32]

Volunteer Studies

Cardiovascular effects were extensively studied in 21 patients with heart failure who were given varied doses and durations of glucagon therapy.[60] Eleven patients who received 3 to 5 mg via intravenous (IV) bolus had increases in the force of contraction, as measured by maximum dP/dT (upstroke pattern on apex echocardiogram), heart rate, cardiac index, blood pressure, and stroke

941

work. There were no changes in systemic vascular resistance, left ventricular end-diastolic pressure, or stroke index. Additionally, glucose concentrations increased by 50%, and the potassium concentrations fell. A study of nine patients demonstrated a 30% increase in coronary blood flow after a 50-mcg/kg IV dose.[53] Patients who received 1 mg via IV bolus also had an increase in cardiac index, but systemic vascular resistance fell, probably secondary to splanchnic and hepatic vascular smooth muscle relaxation.[60] Patients who received an infusion of 2 to 3 mg/min for 10 to 15 minutes responded similarly to those who received the 3- to 5-mg IV boluses, but patients receiving boluses experienced significant dose-limiting nausea and vomiting.[60]

ROLE IN THE MANAGEMENT OF β-ADRENERGIC ANTAGONIST TOXICITY

β-adrenergic antagonist toxicity is manifested by hypotension, bradycardia, prolonged AV conduction times, depressed cardiac output, and cardiac failure. Other noncardiovascular effects include alterations in consciousness; seizures; and, rarely, hypoglycemia.[1,19,23,91] Original management of β-adrenergic antagonist toxicity included provision of large doses of competitive β-agonists such as isoproterenol.[38] Glucagon was found superior to this approach in animal evaluations and human cases.[14,38,39,62,94] Animal studies document the ability of glucagon to increase contractility, restore the sinus node function after sinus node arrest, increase AV conduction, and rarely improve survival.[4,46,59,74] Glucagon successfully reversed bradydysrhythmias and hypotension in patients unresponsive to the aforementioned traditional xenobiotics and is recommended for administration early in the management of patients with severe toxicity.[72,89] By increasing myocardial cAMP concentrations independent of the β receptor, glucagon is able to increase both inotropy and chronotropy.[5,20,46,49,58,59,93]

Glucagon successfully reversed the bradycardia, low-output heart failure, and hypotension that developed in a premature newborn, presumably as a result of an inappropriately large prenatal dose of labetalol given to the mother. This neonate, delivered at 32 weeks' gestation and weighing 1.8 kg, received 0.3 mg/kg of glucagon IV initially and five additional doses of 0.3 to 0.6 mg/kg over the next 5 hours, with improvement in heart rate, blood pressure, and perfusion. Epinephrine and diuretics were also used.[81] Other case reports, case series, and reviews document full or partial beneficial hemodynamic response to glucagon administration in β-adrenergic antagonist toxicity, although at times, it has yielded no effect.[47,54,80] Because the management of β-adrenergic antagonist toxicity is often complicated, many other therapies, including atropine, epinephrine, norepinephrine, dopamine, dobutamine, and various combinations are used with variable success.[19,37] High-dose insulin (HDI) (Antidotes in Depth: A21) and lipid emulsion (Antidotes in Depth: A23) were added to the available therapeutic interventions. In canine studies, HDI therapy has a more sustained effect on hemodynamic parameters and an improved survival rate compared with glucagon.[26] We recommend HDI early in the resuscitation of severe β-adrenergic antagonist overdoses with myocardial depression.

Glucagon was used to improve blood pressure in cases of anaphylactic shock refractory to epinephrine in patients on β-adrenergic antagonists.[85] A small pretreatment study demonstrated a survival advantage of glucagon over epinephrine in anaphylaxis induced in guinea pigs that were pretreated with propranolol.[79] In addition to previously described mechanisms of action, glucagon decreases histamine release and concentrations, increases nitric oxide release, and prevents the increased release of free radicals during ex vivo animal models of anaphylaxis.[2,43,69] We recommend glucagon use in refractory anaphylaxis in patients taking β-adrenergic antagonists.[8,30]

Combined Effects with Phosphodiesterase Inhibitors and Calcium

Previous strategies for enhancing the effects of glucagon have involved combining it with the PDE$_3$ inhibitor amrinone (inamrinone), its derivative milrinone, and the now discontinued selective PDE$_4$ inhibitor rolipram. In a canine model of propranolol toxicity, both amrinone and milrinone alone were comparable to glucagon,[46,73] but the combination of amrinone and glucagon

resulted in a decrease in mean arterial pressure.[45] Tachycardia occurred when milrinone was used with glucagon.[74] In an ex vivo model using strips of rat ventricular heart, rolipram enhanced the inotropic effect of glucagon and limited glucagon tachyphylaxis.[28] Although the evidence for the effectiveness of combining glucagon with a PDE inhibitor was demonstrated in animal models and human case reports, we recommend against the use of this approach. The relationship between calcium and the chronotropic effects of glucagon was demonstrated in rats.[11] Maximal chronotropic effects of glucagon are dependent on a normal circulating ionized calcium. Both hypocalcemia and hypercalcemia blunt the maximal chronotropic response.[10,11]

ROLE IN CALCIUM CHANNEL BLOCKER TOXICITY

Calcium channel blocker toxicity produces a constellation of clinical findings similar to those recognized with β-adrenergic antagonist toxicity, including hypotension, bradycardia, conduction block, and myocardial depression. Animal studies demonstrate the ability of glucagon to improve heart rate and AV conduction and reverse the myocardial depression produced by nifedipine, diltiazem, and verapamil.[4,27,71,82,83,86,97,98] However, there was no survival benefit attributed to glucagon in these studies, and a canine model of verapamil toxicity comparing glucagon to HDI only revealed a survival benefit for HDI.[4,35] Human case reports demonstrate improved hemodynamics, including in cases refractory to other standard measures. Therefore, it is reasonable to continue glucagon therapy while preparing for HDI utilization.[13,17,52,58,80,88]

ROLE IN OTHER CARDIOVASCULAR TOXINS

A bolus of glucagon followed by infusion significantly increased the mean arterial pressure and decreased the QRS complex duration in amitriptyline-poisoned rats.[29] In human pediatric and adult cases of cyclic antidepressant overdoses refractory to multiple measures, glucagon produced immediate hemodynamic improvement.[70,77,78,80] Sodium bicarbonate (Antidotes in Depth: A5) remains the treatment of choice for cyclic antidepressant poisoning followed by other treatment strategies outlined in Chap. 68. Glucagon should be a reasonable therapeutic option if appropriate therapeutic use of sodium bicarbonate fails to improve the hemodynamic status.

ROLE IN REVERSAL OF HYPOGLYCEMIA

Glucagon was once proposed as part of the initial treatment for all comatose patients because it stimulates glycogenolysis in the liver.[65] The theoretical rationale for this approach is only partially sound in that glucagon requires time to act and will often be ineffective in a patient with depleted glycogen stores, such as in patients with prolonged fasting, severe liver disease, alcoholism, starvation, adrenal insufficiency, or chronic hypoglycemia.[15,57] Patients with type 2 diabetes are more likely to respond than are patients with type 1 diabetes. The IV administration of 0.5 to 1.0 g/kg of 50% dextrose in adults rapidly reverses hypoglycemia and does not rely on glycogen stores for its effect. Therefore, IV dextrose is preferred over glucagon as the initial substrate to be given to all patients with an altered mental status presumed to be related to hypoglycemia (Antidotes in Depth: A8). Glucagon is reasonable as a temporizing measure, until medical help can be obtained, in the home where IV dextrose is not an option or when IV access is not rapidly available. In patients with an insulinoma, after an initial hyperglycemic response to glucagon, an increase in insulin will exacerbate the hypoglycemia.[55]

ADVERSE EFFECTS AND SAFETY ISSUES

Side effects associated with glucagon include dose-dependent nausea, vomiting, hyperglycemia, hypoglycemia, and hypokalemia; relaxation of the smooth muscle of the stomach, duodenum, small bowel, and colon; and, rarely, urticaria, respiratory distress, and hypotension.[50,57] Hypotension is reported up to 2 hours after administration in patients receiving glucagon as premedication for upper gastrointestinal (GI) endoscopy procedures.[57] Hyperglycemia is followed by an immediate rise in insulin, which causes an intracellular shift in potassium, resulting in hypokalemia.[24,50,59] It is unclear whether stimulation of the Na$^+$,K$^+$-ATPase in skeletal muscle also contributes to the hypokalemia as occurs with β-adrenergic agonists.[35,40,63] Glucagon increases the anticoagulant effect of warfarin.[57]

Glucagon also increases the release of catecholamines in a patient with a pheochromocytoma, resulting in a hypertensive crisis,[24] which is treated with phentolamine.[57] Continuous prolonged exposure to glucagon in a patient with a glucagonoma led to a reversible dilated cardiomyopathy.[9] The smooth muscle relaxation associated with a continuous infusion might impede attempts at GI decontamination with multiple-dose activated charcoal or whole-bowel irrigation.

PREGNANCY AND LACTATION

Glucagon is FDA Pregnancy Category B. It is presumed that benefit exceeds risk. There are no reports of glucagon use during lactation. However, the size and peptide nature of glucagon suggest that the exposure to a lactating infant would be limited.

DOSAGE AND ADMINSTRATION

The dosing regimen for glucagon administration in toxicologic emergencies has never been formally studied and is based on case reports. Intravenous infusion of an initial dose of 50 mcg/kg (3-5 mg in a 70 kg adult) over 3 to 10 min is recommended and likely minimizes nausea and vomiting. If the initial dose is inadequate, a higher dose (up to 10 mg) is recommended.[26] Using too small a dose can potentially decrease systemic vascular resistance.[60] the effect of glucagon is often transient. We recommend either repeat doses of 3 to 5 mg as needed or a continuous infusion of 2 to 5 mg/h (10 mg/h or less) in 5% dextrose in water to be tapered as the patient improves and allows time for HDI to become effective.[1,21,22,47,54,65] Experimental heart preparations clearly demonstrate tachyphylaxis with continuous infusion, but whether this occurs in humans is unclear.[28,96]

FORMULATION AND ACQUISITION

Glucagon (rDNA origin) for injection is available as a sterile, lyophilized white powder in a vial alone or accompanied by sterile water for reconstitution, also in a vial. It is also supplied in the form of a kit for treatment of hypoglycemia with one vial containing 1 mg (1 unit) of glucagon (rDNA origin) for injection with a disposable prefilled syringe containing sterile water for reconstitution, as well as a "10-pack" with 10 vials, each containing 1 mg (1 unit of glucagon {rDNA origin} for injection). The glucagon powder should be reconstituted with 1 mL of sterile water for injection, after which the vial should be shaken gently until the powder completely dissolves. The final solution should be clear, without visible particles.[57] The reconstituted glucagon should be used immediately after reconstitution and any unused part discarded. Concentrations greater than 1 mg/mL should not be used. An adequate supply of glucagon in the emergency department is at least 20 (1-mg) vials, with assurance of another 90 mg for up to 8 hours of therapy (Special Considerations: SC1).[12,48] Severe cases requiring prolonged infusions have exhausted local supplies.[84] The use of HDI has reduced the need for prolonged glucagon administration.

SUMMARY

- Glucagon produces positive inotropic and chronotropic effects despite β-adrenergic antagonism and calcium channel blockade.
- Glucagon is often beneficial in the treatment of patients with severe β-adrenergic antagonist and calcium channel blocker toxicity.
- The effects of glucagon are not persistent, and other therapies, such as HDI, are recommended (Chaps. 59 and 60 and Antidotes in Depth: A21).
- The relatively benign character of an IV bolus of glucagon in the patient with a serious β-adrenergic antagonist or calcium channel blocker toxicity should lead the clinician to use glucagon early in patient management.
- Rapid administration of glucagon results in nausea and vomiting will limit the adverse effects. Diminishing the initial dose, rate of infusion, or both will limit the adverse effects.

REFERENCES

1. Agura E, et al. Massive propranolol overdose. Successful treatment with high-dose isoproterenol and glucagon. *Am J Med.* 1986;80:755-757.
2. Andjelkovic I, Zlokovic B. Protective effects of glucagon during the anaphylactic response in guinea-pig isolated heart. *Br J Pharmacol.* 1982;76:483-489.
3. Bache RJ, et al. Coronary and systemic hemodynamic effects of glucagon in the intact unanesthetized dog. *J Appl Physiol.* 1970;29:769-774.
4. Bailey B. Glucagon in beta-blocker and calcium channel blocker overdoses: a systematic review. *J Toxicol Clin Toxicol.* 2003;41:595-602.
5. Benvenisty AI, et al. Antagonism of chronic canine beta-adrenergic blockade with dopamine-isoproterenol, dobutamine, and glucagon. *Surg Forum.* 1979;30:187-188.
6. Brechler V, et al. Inhibition by glucagon of the cGMP-inhibited low-Km cAMP phosphodiesterase in heart is mediated by a pertussis toxin-sensitive G-protein. *JBiolChem.* 1992;267:15496-15501.
7. Bromer WW, et al. The amino acid sequence of glucagon. *Diabetes.* 1957;6:234-238.
8. Campbell RL, et al. Emergency department diagnosis and treatment of anaphylaxis: a practice parameter. *Ann Allergy Asthma Immunol.* 2014;113:599-608.
9. Chang-Chretien K, et al. Reversible dilated cardiomyopathy associated with glucagonoma. *Heart.* 2004;90:e44.
10. Chernow B, et al. Glucagon: endocrine effects and calcium involvement in cardiovascular actions in dogs. *Circ Shock.* 1986;19:393-407.
11. Chernow B, et al. Glucagon's chronotropic action is calcium dependent. *J Pharmacol Exp Ther.* 1987;241:833-837.
12. Dart RC, et al. Expert consensus guidelines for stocking of antidotes in hospitals that provide emergency care. *Ann Emerg Med.* 2017;Jun 29. pii: S0196-0644(17)30657-1.
13. Doyon S, Roberts JR. The use of glucagon in a case of calcium channel blocker overdose. *Ann Emerg Med.* 1993;22:1229-3123.
14. Ehgartner GR, Zelinka MA. Hemodynamic instability following intentional nadolol overdose. *Arch Intern Med.* 1988;148:801-802.
15. Eli Lilly and Company. Glucagon for Injection (rDNA origin). Indianapolis, IN: Eli Lilly and Company; 2012.
16. Entman ML, et al. Mechanism of action of epinephrine and glucagon on the canine heart. Evidence for increase in sarcotubular calcium stores mediated by cyclic 3',5'-AMP. *Circ Res.* 1969;25:429-438.
17. Fant JS, et al. The use of glucagon in nifedipine poisoning complicated by clonidine ingestion. *Pediatr Emerg Care.* 1997;13:417-419.
18. Farah AE. Glucagon and the circulation. *Pharmacol Rev.* 1983;35:181-217.
19. Frishman W, et al. Clinical pharmacology of the new beta-adrenergic blocking drugs. Part 8. Self-poisoning with beta-adrenoceptor blocking agents: recognition and management. *Am Heart J.* 1979;98:798-811.
20. Glick G, et al. Glucagon. Its enhancement of cardiac performance in the cat and dog and persistence of its inotropic action despite beta-receptor blockade with propranolol. *Circ Res.* 1968;22:789-799.
21. Hall-Boyer K, et al. Glucagon: hormone or therapeutic agent? *Crit Care Med.* 1984;12:584-589.
22. Heard RD, et al. An alpha-cell hormone of the islets of Langerhans. *JBiolChem.* 1948;172:857.
23. Heath A. Beta-adrenoceptor blocker toxicity: clinical features and therapy. *Am J Emerg Med.* 1984;2:518-525.
24. Hendy GN, et al. Impaired responsiveness to the effect of glucagon on plasma adenosine 3':5'-cyclic monophosphate in normal man. *Eur J Clin Invest.* 1977;7:155-160.
25. Homcy CJ. The beta-adrenergic signaling pathway in the heart. *Hosp Pract (Off Ed).* 1991;26:43-50.
26. Illingworth RN. Glucagon for beta-blocker poisoning. *Practitioner.* 1979;223:683-685.
27. Jolly SR, et al. Cardiovascular depression by verapamil: reversal by glucagon and interactions with propranolol. *Pharmacology.* 1987;35:249-255.
28. Juan-Fita MJ, et al. Rolipram reduces the inotropic tachyphylaxis of glucagon in rat ventricular myocardium. *Naunyn Schmiedebergs Arch Pharmacol.* 2004;370:324-329.
29. Kaplan YC. Effect of glucagon on amitriptyline-induced cardiovascular toxicity in rats. *Hum Exp Toxicol.* 2008;27:321-325.
30. Kemp AM, Kemp SF. Pharmacotherapy in refractory anaphylaxis: when intramuscular epinephrine fails. *Curr Opin Allergy Clin Immunol.* 2014;14:371-378.
31. Kerns W 2nd. Management of beta-adrenergic blocker and calcium channel antagonist toxicity. *Emerg Med Clin North Am.* 2007;25:309-331; abstract viii.
32. Kerns W 2nd, et al. Insulin improves survival in a canine model of acute beta-blocker toxicity. *Ann Emerg Med.* 1997;29:748-757.
33. Kilts JD, et al. Beta(2)-adrenergic and several other G protein-coupled receptors in human atrial membranes activate both G(s) and G(i). *Circ Res.* 2000;87:705-709.
34. Kimball CP, Murlin JR. Aqueous extracts of pancreas III. Some precipitation reactions of insulin. *JBiolChem.* 1923;58:337-348.
35. Kline JA, et al. Insulin is a superior antidote for cardiovascular toxicity induced by verapamil in the anesthetized canine. *J Pharmacol Exp Ther.* 1993;267:744-750.
36. Kobayashi T, et al. Effects of glucagon, prostaglandin E 1 and dibutyryl cyclic 3',5'-AMP upon the transmembrane action potential of guinea pig ventricular fiber and myocardial contractile force. *Jpn Circ J.* 1971;35:807-819.
37. Koch-Weser J, Frishman WH. beta-Adrenoceptor antagonists: new drugs and new indications. *N Engl J Med.* 1981;305:500-506.

38. Kosinski EJ, Malindzak GS Jr. Glucagon and isoproterenol in reversing propranolol toxicity. Arch Intern Med. 1973;132:840-843.

39. Kosinski EJ, et al. Glucagon and propranolol (Inderal) toxicity. *N Engl J Med.* 1971;285:1325.

40. Kraus-Friedmann N, et al. Glucagon stimulation of hepatic Na+, K+-ATPase. *Mol Cell Biochem.* 1982;44:173-180.

41. Levey GS, Epstein SE. Activation of adenyl cyclase by glucagon in cat and human heart. *Circ Res.* 1969;24:151-156.

42. Levey GS, et al. Characterization of 125I-glucagon binding in a solubilized preparation of cat myocardial adenylate cyclase. Further evidence for a dissociable receptor site. *JBiolChem.* 1974;249:2665-2673.

43. Levi R. Hypersensitivity reactions of the heart: reduction of anaphylactic crisis by theophylline or glucagon. *Bull N Y Acad Med.* 1971;47:1229.

44. Lipski JI, et al. Electrophysiological effects of glucagon on the normal canine heart. *Am J Physiol.* 1972;222:1107-1112.

45. Love JN, et al. A comparison of combined amrinone and glucagon therapy to glucagon alone for cardiovascular depression associated with propranolol toxicity in a canine model. *Am J Emerg Med.* 1993;11:360-363.

46. Love JN, et al. A comparison of amrinone and glucagon therapy for cardiovascular depression associated with propranolol toxicity in a canine model. *J Toxicol Clin Toxicol.* 1992;30:399-412.

47. Love JN, et al. A potential role for glucagon in the treatment of drug-induced symptomatic bradycardia. *Chest.* 1998;114:323-326.

48. Love JN, Tandy TK. Beta-adrenoceptor antagonist toxicity: a survey of glucagon availability. *Ann Emerg Med.* 1993;22:267-268.

49. Lucchesi BR. Cardiac actions of glucagon. *Circ Res.* 1968;22:777-787.

50. Lvoff R, Wilcken DE. Glucagon in heart failure and in cardiogenic shock. Experience in 50 patients. *Circulation.* 1972;45:534-542.

51. MacLeod KM, et al. Characterization of glucagon-induced changes in rate, contractility and cyclic AMP levels in isolated cardiac preparations of the rat and guinea pig. *J Pharmacol Exp Ther.* 1981;217:798-804.

52. Mahr NC, et al. Use of glucagon for acute intravenous diltiazem toxicity. *Am J Cardiol.* 1997;79:1570-1571.

53. Manchester JH, et al. Effects of glucagon on myocardial oxygen consumption and coronary blood flow in man and in dog. *Circulation.* 1970;41:579-588.

54. Mansell PI. Glucagon in the management of deliberate self-poisoning with propranolol. *Arch Emerg Med.* 1990;7:238-240.

55. Marks V, Samols E. Glucagon test for insulinoma: a chemical study in 25 cases. *J Clin Pathol.* 1968;21:346-352.

56. Mery PF, et al. Glucagon stimulates the cardiac Ca2+ current by activation of adenylyl cyclase and inhibition of phosphodiesterase. *Nature.* 1990;345:158-161.

57. Novo Nordisk Inc. GlucaGen® (glucagon [rDNA origin] for injection) [prescribing information]. Plainsboro, NJ: Novo Nordisk A/S; 2015.

58. Papadopoulos J, O'Neil MG. Utilization of a glucagon infusion in the management of a massive nifedipine overdose. *J Emerg Med.* 2000;18:453-455.

59. Parmley WW. The role of glucagon in cardiac therapy. *N Engl J Med.* 1971;285:801-802.

60. Parmley WW, et al. Cardiovascular effects of glucagon in man. *N Engl J Med.* 1968;279:12-17.

61. Pavoine C, et al. Miniglucagon [glucagon-(19-29)] is a component of the positive inotropic effect of glucagon. *Am J Physiol.* 1991;260:C993-C999.

62. Peterson CD, et al. Glucagon therapy for beta-blocker overdose. *Drug Intell Clin Pharm.* 1984;18:394-398.

63. Pettit GW, et al. The contribution of renal and extrarenal mechanisms to hypokalemia induced by glucagon. *Eur J Pharmacol.* 1977;41:437-441.

64. Powers AC, D'Alessio D. Endocrine pancreas and pharmacotherapy of diabetes mellitus and hypoglycemia. In: Brunton LL, et al., eds. *Goodman & Gilman's The Pharmacological Basis of Therapeutics.* 12th ed. New York, NY: McGraw-Hill; 2011.

65. Rappolt RT Sr, et al. NAGD regime [naloxone (Narcan), activated charcoal, glucagon, doxapram (Dopram)] for the coma of drug-related overdoses. *Clin Toxicol.* 1980;16:395-396.

66. Rochais F, et al. A specific pattern of phosphodiesterases controls the cAMP signals generated by different Gs-coupled receptors in adult rat ventricular myocytes. *Circ Res.* 2006;98:1081-1088.

67. Rodbell M. The role of hormone receptors and GTP-regulatory proteins in membrane transduction. *Nature.* 1980;284:17-22.

68. Rodgers RL. Glucagon and cyclic AMP: time to turn the page? *Curr Diabetes Rev.* 2012;8:362-381.

69. Rosic M, et al. Glucagon effects on 3H-histamine uptake by the isolated guinea-pig heart during anaphylaxis. *Biomed Res Int.* 2014;2014:782709.

70. Ruddy JM, et al. Management of tricyclic antidepressant ingestion in children with special reference to the use of glucagon. *Med J Aust.* 1972;1:630-633.

71. Sabatier J, et al. Antagonistic effects of epinephrine, glucagon and methylatropine but not calcium chloride against atrio-ventricular conduction disturbances produced by high doses of diltiazem, in conscious dogs. *Fundam Clin Pharmacol.* 1991;5:93-106.

72. Salzberg MR, Gallagher EJ. Propranolol overdose. *Ann Emerg Med.* 1980;9:26-27.

73. Sato S, et al. Milrinone versus glucagon: comparative hemodynamic effects in canine propranolol poisoning. *J Toxicol Clin Toxicol.* 1994;32:277-289.

74. Sato S, et al. Combined use of glucagon and milrinone may not be preferable for severe propranolol poisoning in the canine model. *J Toxicol Clin Toxicol.* 1995;33:337-342.

75. Sauvadet A, et al. Synergistic actions of glucagon and miniglucagon on Ca2+ mobilization in cardiac cells. *Circ Res.* 1996;78:102-109.

76. Sauvadet A, et al. Arachidonic acid drives mini-glucagon action in cardiac cells. *JBiolChem.* 1997;272:12437-12345.

77. Sener EK, et al. Response to glucagon in imipramine overdose. *J Toxicol Clin Toxicol.* 1995;33:51-53.

78. Sensky PR, Olczak SA. High-dose intravenous glucagon in severe tricyclic poisoning. *Postgrad Med J.* 1999;75:611-612.

79. Serwonska MH, Frick OL. Anti-anaphylactic activity of glucagon in guinea pigs (gp) with beta-adrenergic blockade [abstract]. *J Allergy Clin Immunol.* 1988;81:238.

80. Skoog CA, Engebretsen KM. Are vasopressors useful in toxin-induced cardiogenic shock? *Clin Toxicol (Phila).* 2017;55:285-304.

81. Stevens TP, Guillet R. Use of glucagon to treat neonatal low-output congestive heart failure after maternal labetalol therapy. *J Pediatr.* 1995;127:151-153.

82. Stone CK, et al. Treatment of verapamil overdose with glucagon in dogs. *Ann Emerg Med.* 1995;25:369-374.

83. Stone CK, et al. Glucagon and phenylephrine combination vs glucagon alone in experimental verapamil overdose. *Acad Emerg Med.* 1996;3:120-125.

84. Thakrar R, et al. Management of a mixed overdose of calcium channel blockers, beta-blockers and statins. *BMJ Case Rep.* 2014;2014.

85. Thomas M, Crawford I. Best evidence topic report. Glucagon infusion in refractory anaphylactic shock in patients on beta-blockers. *Emerg Med J.* 2005;22:272-273.

86. Tuncok Y, et al. The effects of amrinone and glucagon on verapamil-induced cardiovascular toxicity in anaesthetized rats. *Int J Exp Pathol.* 1996;77:207-212.

87. Urthaler F, et al. Comparative effects of glucagon on automaticity of the sinus node and atrioventricular junction. *Am J Physiol.* 1974;227:1415-1421.

88. Walter FG, et al. Amelioration of nifedipine poisoning associated with glucagon therapy. *Ann Emerg Med.* 1993;22:1234-1237.

89. Ward DE, Jones B. Glucagon and beta-blocker toxicity. *Br Med J.* 1976;2:151.

90. Wei Y, Mojsov S. Tissue-specific expression of the human receptor for glucagon-like peptide-I: brain, heart and pancreatic forms have the same deduced amino acid sequences. *FEBS Lett.* 1995;358:219-224.

91. Weinstein RS. Recognition and management of poisoning with beta-adrenergic blocking agents. *Ann Emerg Med.* 1984;13:1123-1131.

92. White CM. A review of potential cardiovascular uses of intravenous glucagon administration. *J Clin Pharmacol.* 1999;39:442-447.

93. Whitehouse FW, James TN. Chronotropic action of glucagon on the sinus node. *Proc Soc Exp Biol Med.* 1966;122:823-826.

94. Whitsitt LS, Lucchesi BR. Effects of beta-receptor blockade and glucagon on the atrioventricular transmission system in the dog. *Circ Res.* 1968;23:585-595.

95. Yagami T. Differential coupling of glucagon and beta-adrenergic receptors with the small and large forms of the stimulatory G protein. *Mol Pharmacol.* 1995;48:849-854.

96. Yao LF, et al. Glucagon-induced densensitization: correlation between cyclic AMP levels and contractile force. *Eur J Pharmacol.* 1982;79:147-150.

97. Zaloga GP, et al. Glucagon reverses the hypotension and bradycardia of verapamil overdose in rats. *Crit Care Med.* 1985;13:273.

98. Zaritsky AL, et al. Glucagon antagonism of calcium channel blocker-induced myocardial dysfunction. *Crit Care Med.* 1988;16:246-251.

99. Zeiders JL, et al. Ontogeny of cardiac beta-adrenoceptor desensitization mechanisms: agonist treatment enhances receptor/G-protein transduction rather than eliciting uncoupling. *J Mol Cell Cardiol.* 1999;31:413-423.

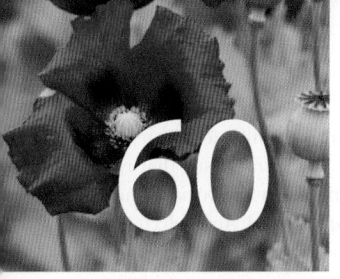

60 CALCIUM CHANNEL BLOCKERS

David H. Jang

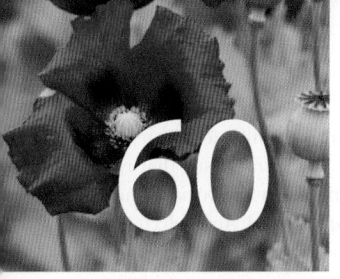

Amlodipine

Diltiazem

Verapamil

HISTORY AND EPIDEMIOLOGY

In 1964, Albretch Fleckenstein described an inhibitory action of verapamil and prenylamine on excitation–contraction coupling that was similar to calcium depletion.[3] By the late 1970s, the clinical use of calcium channel blockers (CCBs) was widely accepted for a variety of cardiovascular indications, including hypertension, dysrhythmias, and angina. Later indications for the use of CCBs include Raynaud phenomenon and disease, migraine and cluster headaches and subarachnoid hemorrhage.[1] There are currently 10 individual CCBs marketed in the United States that are available as immediate- or sustained-release formulations and as combination products with other antihypertensives.[31]

The cardiovascular drug class is one of the leading classes of drugs associated with poisoning fatality. Over the past 5 years of available data, there were more than 12 million poisonings with more than 7,000 poisoning-related deaths reported to the American Association of Poison Control Centers National Poisons Data System (NPDS). Cardiovascular drugs were involved in more than 400,000 of the reported poisonings and accounted for nearly 15% of the overall poisoning fatalities. Within this class, CCBs were the most common cardiovascular drugs involved in poisoning fatalities. Calcium channel blockers accounted for more than 50,000 cases reported over the past 5 years, with more than 300 cases resulting in major effects and more than 100 deaths (Chap. 130).[15,16,77,78] There is a bimodal distribution within the pediatric population that involves unintentional exposures in young infants and toddlers with intentional ingestions in teenagers.[40]

PHARMACOLOGY

Calcium (Ca^{2+}) ion channels exist as either voltage-dependent or ligand-gated channels. There are many types of voltage-gated Ca^{2+} channels that include P-, N-, R-, T-, Q-, and L-type channels (Table 60–1). Ligand-gated Ca^{2+} channels include IP_3 and ryanodine receptors, which are found intracellularly and play a critical role in cell signaling. Voltage-gated Ca^{2+} channels are located throughout the body in the heart, nervous system, pancreas, and muscles.[106] Voltage-gated Ca^{2+} channels are composed of several components, including α_2, β, δ, and the ion-conducting α_1-subunit. The α_1-subunit is the most important component of the Ca^{2+} channel because it contains the actual pore through which Ca^{2+} ions pass, and it also serves as the binding site of all CCBs. The other subunits such as β and δ act to modulate the function of the α_1-subunit.[79,122]

The primary action of all CCBs available in the United States is antagonism of the L-type or "long-acting" voltage-gated Ca^{2+} channels. Calcium channel blockers are often classified into three groups based on their chemical structure (Table 60–2).[41,71,79] A fourth class, the diarylaminopropylamines included mibefradil, but this drug was withdrawn because of significant adverse drug interactions.[114] Each group binds a slightly different region of the α_{1c} subunit of the Ca^{2+} channel and thus has different affinities for the various L-type Ca^{2+} channels, both in the myocardium and the vascular smooth muscle.[18] It is often more logical to classify them as nondihydropyridine versus dihydropyridine CCBs. Whereas the former includes verapamil and diltiazem, the latter includes many drugs, the chemical names of which all currently end in –pine, such as nifedipine and amlodipine. Verapamil and diltiazem have inhibitory effects on both the sinoatrial (SA) and atrioventricular (AV) nodal tissue and thus are commonly used for the treatment of hypertension, to reduce myocardial oxygen demand, and to achieve rate control in a variety of tachydysrhythmias. In contrast, the dihydropyridines have very little direct effect on the myocardium at therapeutic doses and act primarily as peripheral vasodilators.[122] They are therefore commonly used as vasodilators for conditions with increased vascular tone such as hypertension, migraine headaches, and postintracranial hemorrhage–associated vasospasm. Dihydropyridines bind to a site that is formed by amino acid residues in two adjacent S6 segments plus the S5 segment between them, and in some cases, enantiomeric pairs are activators or inhibitors, respectively, indicating that very subtle changes in the drug–receptor interaction are sufficient to convert from agonist to antagonist action.[64]

Experimental studies suggest an additional vasodilatory effect of some CCBs caused by stimulation of nitric oxide release. Amlodipine and other dihydropyridine CCBs release nitric oxide in a dose-dependent fashion from canine coronary microvessels.[127-129] Although the exact mechanism is uncertain, it is hypothesized that this amlodipine-induced nitric oxide production results from increasing endothelial nitric oxide synthase activity through phosphorylation of this enzyme. Bradykinin B_2 receptors also contribute to vasodilation. Bradykinin is a vasodilator that exerts its action by causing endothelial release of prostacyclin, nitric oxide, and endothelium-derived hyperpolarizing factor.[128]

TABLE 60–1	Voltage-Gated Calcium Channel Subtypes		
Type	**Distribution**	**Function**	**Blocked By**
T (transient)	Polysynaptic nerve terminals and cardiac nodal tissue	Pacemaker activity	Mibefradil
R	Neural tissue	Neurotransmitter release	Cadmium
Q	Presynaptic nerve terminals	Neurotransmitter release	Agatoxin
P (Purkinje)	Cerebellar Purkinje neurons	Neurotransmitter release	Agatoxin
N (neuronal)	Presynaptic nerve terminals	Catecholamine release	ω-Conotoxin
L (long-acting)	Myocardium and smooth muscle	Muscular contraction	Verapamil, diltiazem, dihydropyridines

TABLE 60–2	Classification[38] of Calcium Channel Blockers Available in the United States		
Class	Specific Compounds	Volume of Distribution (L/kg)	Time to Peak* Concentrations (h)
Phenylalkylamine	Verapamil	3–5	1–2
Benzothiazepine	Diltiazem	5.3	2–4
Dihydropyridines	Amlodipine	21	6–12
	Clevidipine	0.17	<1
	Felodipine	10	2.5–5
	Isradipine	3	1–2
	Nicardipine	8.3	1–4
	Nifedipine	0.75	2.5–5
	Nimodipine	2	1–2
	Nisoldipine	1.6	>6

*All are oral ingestion of an immediate release formulation: at therapeutic doses.

PHARMACOKINETICS AND TOXICOKINETICS

Absorption

All CCBs are well absorbed orally, but many exhibit low bioavailability because of extensive hepatic first-pass metabolism. When the CCBs reach the liver, they undergo hepatic oxidative metabolism predominantly via the CYP3A4 subgroup of the enzyme system.[76]

Distribution

All CCBs are highly protein bound which limits the role of extracorporeal removal. Volumes of distribution are large for amlodipine (21 L/kg), verapamil (3–5 L/kg), and diltiazem (5.3 L/kg) and somewhat smaller for nifedipine (0.75 L/kg).[47,84]

Metabolism

Norverapamil, formed by N-demethylation of verapamil, is the only active metabolite and retains 20% of the activity of the parent compound. Diltiazem is predominantly deacetylated into minimally active deacetyldiltiazem, which is then eliminated via the biliary tract.[48,57] After repeated doses, as well as after overdose, these hepatic enzymes become saturated, reducing the potential of the first-pass effect and increasing the quantity of active drug absorbed systemically.[124] Saturation of metabolism as well as the modified-release dosage form contribute to the prolongation of the apparent half-lives reported after overdose of various CCBs.[95]

Excretion

The CCBs undergo a significant, but variable, amount of renal excretion after metabolism with a small percentage eliminated in the urine unchanged. For example, amlodipine undergoes 60% renal excretion after metabolism to inactive metabolites compared with 70% for verapamil (3.4% as unchanged drug) and 90% for nifedipine as inactive metabolites.[34,80]

One interesting aspect of the pharmacology of CCBs is their potential for drug–drug interactions. CYP3A4, which metabolizes most CCBs, is also responsible for the initial oxidation of numerous other xenobiotics. Verapamil and diltiazem specifically compete for this enzyme and can decrease the clearance of many drugs, including carbamazepine, cisapride, quinidine, various β-hydroxy-β-methylglutaryl-coenzyme A (HMG-CoA) reductase inhibitors, cyclosporine, tacrolimus, most human immunodeficiency virus–protease inhibitors, and theophylline (Chap. 11 and Appendix).[39,92] In June 1998, mibefradil, a structurally unique CCB, was voluntarily withdrawn after several reports of serious adverse xenobiotic interactions caused in part by its potent inhibition of CYP3A4.[66] Other inhibitors of CYP3A4, such as cimetidine, fluoxetine, some antifungals, macrolide antibiotics, and even the flavonoids in grapefruit juice, raise serum concentrations of several CCBs, which results in toxicity.[38,102]

In addition to affecting CYP3A4, verapamil and diltiazem also inhibit P-glycoprotein–mediated drug transport into peripheral tissue that results in elevated serum concentrations of xenobiotics such as cyclosporine and digoxin that use this transport system (Chap. 11 and Appendix). Unlike diltiazem and verapamil, nifedipine and the other dihydropyridines do not appear to affect the clearance of other xenobiotics via CYP3A4 or P-glycoprotein–mediated transport. Similarly, inhibition of P-glycoprotein–mediated transport by certain xenobiotics such as statins result in increased oral bioavailability of CCBs, which requires closer outpatient follow-up for the development of bradycardia or hypotension.

PHYSIOLOGY AND PATHOPHYSIOLOGY

Calcium plays an essential role in many cellular processes throughout the body, and many types of cells depend on the maintenance of a Ca^{2+} concentration gradient across cell membranes in order to function. The extracellular Ca^{2+} concentration is approximately 10,000 times greater than the intracellular concentration. This concentration gradient is important for contraction and relaxation of muscle cells (Fig. 60–1). Ca^{2+} channels and various exchange pumps located on the cell membrane play a key role in maintaining this concentration gradient within muscle cells.[59,81]

Calcium is driven down a large electrical and concentration gradient through L-type Ca^{2+} channels located in all muscle cell types (cardiac, striated, and smooth). This influx of Ca^{2+} is critical for the function of both cardiac and smooth muscle cells; however, skeletal muscle depends primarily on intracellular Ca^{2+} stores for excitation–contraction coupling and not the intracellular influx of Ca^{2+}. In smooth muscle, the rapid influx of Ca^{2+} binds calmodulin, and the resulting complex stimulates myosin light chain kinase activity. The myosin light chain kinase phosphorylates, and thus activates, myosin, which subsequently binds actin, causing contraction.[74]

Calcium plays a similarly important role in myocardial contractility. In myocardial cells, Ca^{2+} influx is slower relative to the initial Na^+ influx that

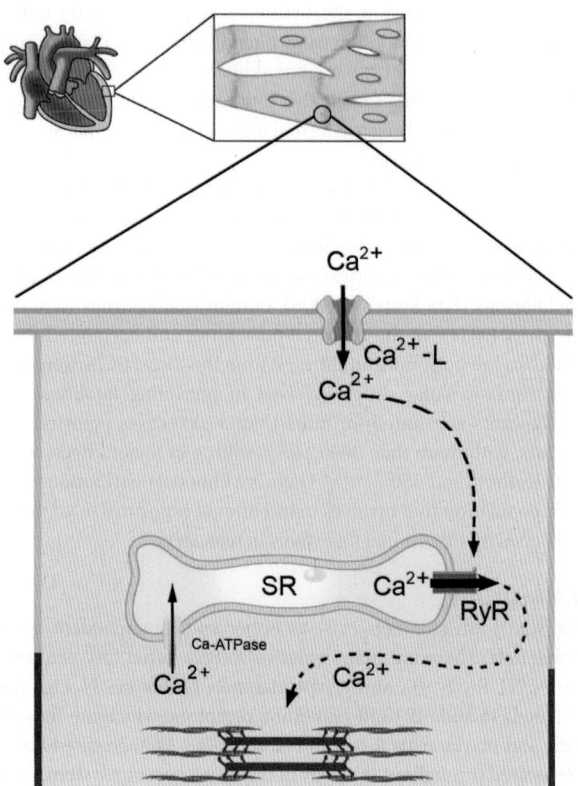

FIGURE 60–1. Normal contraction of myocardial cells. The L-type voltage-gated Ca^{2+} channels (Cav-L) open to allow Ca^{2+} ion influx during myocyte depolarization. This causes the concentration-dependent release of more Ca^{2+} ions from the ryanodine receptor (RyR) of the sarcoplasmic reticulum (SR).

initiates cellular depolarization and prolongs this depolarization, creating the plateau phase (phase 2) of the action potential (Chap. 15 and Fig. 15–2). The Ca^{2+} subsequently stimulates a receptor-operated Ca^{2+} channel on the sarcoplasmic reticulum (SR), known as the ryanodine receptor, releasing Ca^{2+} from the vast stores of the SR into the cytosol.[87] This is often termed *Ca²⁺-induced Ca²⁺ release*. Calcium then binds troponin C, which causes a conformational change that displaces troponin and tropomyosin from actin, allowing actin and myosin to bind, resulting in a contraction.[19,28] Calcium influx is also plays important in the spontaneous depolarization (phase 4) of the action potential in the SA node. This Ca^{2+} influx also allows normal propagation of electrical impulses via the specialized myocardial conduction tissues, particularly the AV node. After opening, the rates of recovery of these slow Ca^{2+} channels, in both the SA and AV nodal tissue, determine the rate of conduction.

The nondihydropyridine CCBs such as verapamil and diltiazem have the greatest affinity for the myocardium, with verapamil considered the most potent. In addition, not only do verapamil and, to a lesser extent, diltiazem impede Ca^{2+} influx and channel recovery in the myocardium, but their blockade is also potentiated as the frequency of channel opening increases. Dihydropyridines are modulated by the membrane potential and calcium channel blockade is more pronounced when current is measured from depolarized holding potentials as opposed to verapamil; where this voltage-dependent block occurs in the absence of repetitive depolarizations.[44,89] Therefore, in frequently contracting tissue, such as myocardium, the blockade of verapamil and diltiazem is augmented. Verapamil and diltiazem are therefore commonly used for controlling the ventricular rate in patients with atrial tachydysrhythmia.

At therapeutic doses, the dihydropyridine CCBs such as nifedipine have little effect at the myocardium and have most of their effect at the peripheral vascular tissue; thus, they have the most potent vasodilatory effects compared with the nondihydropyridine CCBs. Dihydropyridines bind the Ca^{2+} channel best at less-negative membrane potentials. Because the resting potential for myocardial muscle (–90 mV) is lower than that of vascular smooth muscle (–70 mV), dihydropyridines bind preferentially in the peripheral vascular tissue.[89]

The toxicity of CCBs is largely an extension of their therapeutic effects within the cardiovascular system. Inhibition of the L-type Ca^{2+} channels within both the myocardium and peripheral vascular smooth muscle results in a combination of decreased inotropy and heart rate, as well as arterial vasodilation. Because dihydropyridines have limited myocardial effect at therapeutic concentrations, the baroreceptor reflex remains intact, and slight increases in heart rate and cardiac output often occur. Isradipine is the only dihydropyridine whose inhibitory effect on the SA node is significant enough to blunt any reflex tachycardia. Calcium channel blocker poisoning also results in blockade of L-type Ca^{2+} channels located in the pancreas. This results in decreased insulin release, resulting in hyperglycemia.

CLINICAL MANIFESTATIONS

The hallmarks of CCB poisoning are hypotension and bradycardia, which result from depression of myocardial contraction and peripheral vasodilation.[100] Myocardial conduction is impaired, producing AV conduction abnormalities, idioventricular rhythms, and complete heart block, most commonly with nondihydropyridine poisoning. Junctional escape rhythms occur in patients with significant poisonings.[13,45,51,91,125] The negative inotropic effects are often so profound, particularly with verapamil, that ventricular contraction is completely ablated.[5,9,11,23]

Hypotension is the most common and life-threatening finding in acute CCB poisoning, caused by a combination of decreased inotropy, bradycardia, and peripheral vasodilation.[93] Patients can present asymptomatically early after ingestion and subsequently deteriorate rapidly to severe cardiogenic shock.[5,9,54] The associated clinical findings reflect the degree of cardiovascular compromise and hypoperfusion, particularly to the central nervous system. Early symptoms include fatigue, dizziness, and lightheadedness. Alteration in mentation in the absence of hypotension should

prompt the clinician to evaluate for other causes and ingestions. Severely poisoned patients manifest syncope, altered mental status, coma, and sudden death.[97,101] Gastrointestinal (GI) effects, such as nausea and vomiting, are not a typical feature of CCB poisoning. Acute respiratory distress syndrome (ARDS) is also described with severe CCB poisoning. This is due to precapillary vasodilation with a subsequent increase in transcapillary pressure. The elevated pressure gradient results in increased capillary transudates and possible interstitial edema.[33,53]

In mild to moderate overdose of dihydropyridine CCBs, the predominantly peripheral effect induces a reflex tachycardia. However, severe poisoning with any CCBs can result in loss of receptor selectivity, resulting in bradycardia. A prospective poison control center study noted AV nodal block to occur more frequently with verapamil poisoning.[94] Although deaths are attributed mainly to the nondihydropyridines, a significant number of dihydropyridine-related deaths are also reported, which likely reflects the wider use of dihydropyridine CCBs.[94,107]

Several factors ultimately determine CCB toxicity. These include medication formulation, dose, and coingestion with other cardioactive medications such as β-adrenergic antagonists, underlying comorbidities, and age. Older adult patients and those with underlying cardiovascular disease such as congestive heart failure are more sensitive to CCBs.[75] Even at therapeutic doses, these patients are more susceptible to the cardioactive effects of these medications and develop symptomatic hypotension.

Pediatric cases of CCB overdose commonly result from medication errors or unwitnessed ingestions of pills found at home.[12,40] Children with CCB poisoning can develop nonspecific clinical effects such as lethargy, emesis, and confusion. Although CCB poisoning in children is uncommon, there are reported cases of severe poisoning and death.[107]

DIAGNOSTIC TESTING

All patients with suspected CCB poisoning should be considered at risk for cardiovascular collapse and be evaluated with a 12-lead electrocardiogram (ECG) followed by continuous cardiac and hemodynamic monitoring. A chest radiograph, pulse oximetry, end-tidal carbon dioxide ($EtCO_2$), and serum chemistry should also be obtained if any degree of hypoperfusion is suspected. Assessment of electrolytes, including magnesium, and a serum digoxin concentration in a bradycardic patient with unknown exposure history are indicated, although a careful history, if possible, may narrow down the etiology. Cardioactive steroids should be a consideration in a patient with undifferentiated bradycardia with hyperkalemia but are less likely in the setting of hypotension. Assays for CCB serum concentrations are not routinely available and therefore have no role in the management of patients poisoned with CCBs.

Hyperglycemia is considered a prognostic sign in cases of severe CCB poisoning. The release of insulin from the β-islet cells in the pancreas is dependent on Ca^{2+} influx through the L-type Ca^{2+} channel. Calcium channel blocker poisoning reduces insulin release with resultant hyperglycemia. An additional mechanism also includes dysregulation of the insulin-dependent phosphatidylinositol-3 kinase (PI3K) pathway.[11] It should be noted that hyperglycemia might also be the result of diabetes or the administration of glucagon for suspected β-adrenergic antagonist poisoning. A retrospective study suggests that serum glucose concentration correlated with the severity of nondihydropyridine CCB poisoning. The initial mean serum glucose concentration was 188 mg/dL in patients who met a composite endpoint of requiring vasopressors, a pacemaker, or death versus 122 mg/dL in those not requiring intervention. Peak serum glucose concentrations were also significantly different.[69] This finding is interpreted to be an early sign of severity and an indicator for when to initiate high dose insulin (HDI) (Antidotes in Depth: A21) therapy.

MANAGEMENT
Overview
All patients with suspected CCB poisoning should undergo prompt evaluation even when the initial vital signs are normal. This urgency is due to the

potential to initiate early GI decontamination and pharmacologic therapies before patients manifest severe poisoning. This is particularly important with ingestions involving sustained-release formulations. Intravenous (IV) access should be obtained, and initial treatment should be directed toward aggressive GI decontamination of patients with large recent ingestions. All patients who become hypotensive should initially receive a fluid bolus of 10 to 20 mL/kg of crystalloid. This is repeated as needed with constant monitoring of volume status with repeat serial examinations for volume overload. Caution is required because aggressive fluid resuscitation should not be given to patients with congestive heart failure, evidence of ARDS, or chronic kidney disease. Although there are currently both outpatient and inpatient consensus guidelines in the management of CCB poisoning, there is still no clear pathway for treatment, and the inpatient guidelines are too ambiguous for clinicians unfamiliar with this type of poisoning to be useful.[82,108]

Pharmacotherapy should focus on maintenance or improvement of both cardiac output and peripheral vascular tone. Although atropine, calcium, insulin, glucagon, isoproterenol, dopamine, epinephrine, norepinephrine, and phosphodiesterase (PDE) inhibitors have been used with reported success in CCB-poisoned patients, no single intervention has consistently demonstrated efficacy. It is also important to be aware that certain treatments such as vasopressors are detrimental with long-term use, so these should be avoided when there are more effective and safer treatment options.

Although therapy for hypotension and bradycardia should begin with crystalloids and atropine, most critically poisoned patients do not respond to these initial efforts and require further pharmacotherapy. Although it would be ideal to initiate each therapy individually and monitor the patient's hemodynamic response, in the most critically ill patients, multiple therapies are administered simultaneously. A reasonable treatment sequence based on existing data and clinical experience should initially consist of isotonic fluids, atropine, calcium, and glucagon (Antidotes in Depth: A20). If the patient does not respond to these initial treatments, HDI therapy should be initiated. Because the onset of effect of HDI is delayed for 15 to 40 minutes and given the relative safety of its use, earlier initiation is preferable. The use of vasopressors such as norepinephrine or dopamine can result in tissue ischemia with long-term use and thus should be avoided, when possible, in favor of HDI therapy. Phosphodiesterase inhibitors such as inamrinone, milrinone, and enoximone have been used to treat patients with CCB poisoning.[65,98,121] These xenobiotics inhibit the breakdown of cyclic adenosine diphosphate (cAMP) by PDE inhibition, thereby increasing intracellular cAMP concentrations, resulting in increased cardiac output. Despite some reported success, PDE inhibitors are not readily available, other xenobiotics are more effective and easier to use and we do not recommend routine use (Fig. 60–2).

Gastrointestinal Decontamination

Because CCB poisoning is a leading cause of poisoning fatality, attempts to prevent absorption from the GI tract are recommended, assuming there are no contraindications for the described techniques in this chapter. This is particularly important if sustained-release CCBs are suspected. Patients who present early with minimal or no symptoms can have delayed cardiovascular toxicity, which can be profound and refractory to conventional treatment, making early GI decontamination a cornerstone in CCB management.

We recommend that all patients with CCB ingestions should receive 1 g/kg of activated charcoal (AC) orally or via nasogastric tube as long as the airway is stable or protected. Multiple-dose activated charcoal (MDAC) (0.5 g/kg every 4–6 hours) without a cathartic is reasonable for nearly all patients with either sustained-release pill ingestions or signs of continuing absorption. Although data are limited, there is no evidence that MDAC increases CCB clearance from the serum.[95] Rather, its efficacy is a result of the continuous presence of AC throughout the GI tract, which adsorbs any active xenobiotic from its slow-release formulation. Multiple-dose activated charcoal should not be administered to a patient with inadequate GI function (eg, hypotension, diminished peristalsis sounds (Antidotes in Depth: A1).

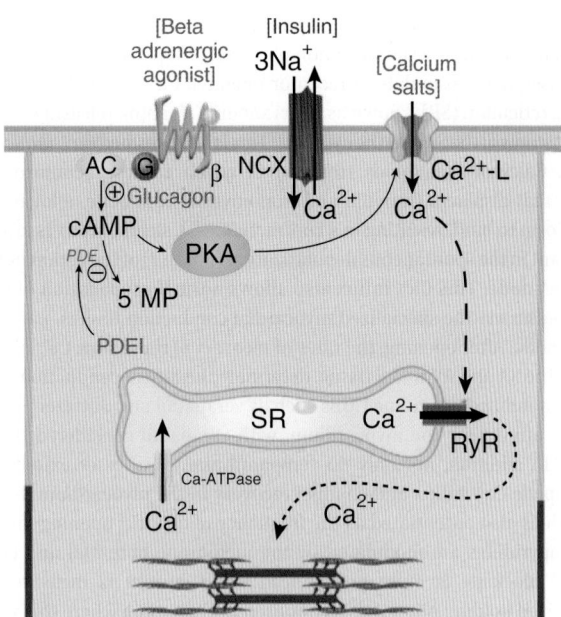

FIGURE 60–2. Myocardial toxicity of calcium channel blockers (CCBs) and use of antidotal therapies. Calcium channel blockers reduce calcium ion influx through the L-type Ca^{2+} channel (Ca^{2+}-L) and thus reduce contractility. The entry of calcium via voltage-gated channels (Ca^{2+}-L) initiates a cascade of events that result in actin–myosin coupling and contractions. Mechanisms to increase intracellular Ca^{2+} include recruitment of new or dormant Ca^{2+} channels by increasing cyclic adenosine monophosphate (cAMP) by stimulating its formation by adenylate cyclase (AC) with glucagon (see text). The use of calcium salts may increase the $[Ca^{2+}]$ gradient across the cellular membrane to further its influx and improve contractility. The mechanism by which insulin therapy enhances inotropy is not fully known. 5'MP = 5'-monophosphate; NCX = Ca^{2+}, Na^+ antiporter; PDEI = phosphodiesterase inhibitor; PKA = protein kinase A; RyR = ryanodine receptor; SR = sarcoplasmic reticulum.

Orogastric lavage is recommended for all patients who present early (1–2 hours postingestion) after large ingestions and for those who are critically ill and require immediate endotracheal intubation, although the effects of orogastric lavage after overdose of a sustained-release CCB are not specifically studied. When performing orogastric lavage in a CCB-poisoned patient, it is important to remember that lavage increases vagal tone and potentially exacerbates any bradydysrhythmias; we routinely pretreat with atropine.[111] It is important to note that although AC is less invasive than lavage, orogastric lavage followed by AC may be more practical in critically ill patients who are intubated[68,110]

Whole-bowel irrigation (WBI) with polyethylene glycol solution (1–2 L/h orally or via nasogastric tube in adults, up to 500 mL/h in children) is recommended for patients who ingest sustained-release products and for whom there are no contraindications. Although the benefit is uncertain, in patients with severe poisoning. The risk of WBI is limited in these cases. It should be continued until the rectal effluent is clear (Antidotes in Depth: A2).[17,24]

Atropine

Atropine is often first-line therapy for patients with symptomatic bradycardia from xenobiotic poisoning such as organic phosphorus compounds, β-adrenergic antagonists, and CCBs. Although the use of atropine improved both heart rate and cardiac output in an early dog model of verapamil poisoning and a few patients with bradycardia from CCB poisoning,[37,94] reports of patients with severe CCB poisoning demonstrate atropine to be largely ineffective.[56,90,105] The decreased effectiveness is largely due to the negative inotropic effects or peripheral vasodilation of CCBs. Given its availability, familiarity, efficacy in mild poisonings, and safety profile, atropine is recommended as initial therapy in patients with symptomatic bradycardia.

Dose

The dosing of atropine for xenobiotic induced bradycardia is similar to the dose used for Advanced Cardiac Life Support. Dosing should begin with 0.5 to 1.0 mg (minimum of 0.1 mg in children >5 kg; 0.02 mg/kg in children) intravenously every 2 or 3 minutes up to a maximum dose of 3 mg in all patients with symptomatic bradycardia. However, treatment failures should be anticipated in severely poisoned patients and other therapies such as calcium and glucagon should be administered. In patients in whom WBI or MDAC will be used, the use of atropine should also be administered particularly if increased vagal tone is apparent.

Calcium

Calcium is another treatment often used for CCB poisoning to increase extracellular Ca^{2+} concentration with an increase in transmembrane concentration gradient. Pretreatment with IV Ca^{2+} prevents hypotension without diminishing the antidysrhythmic efficacy before therapeutic verapamil use in reentrant supraventricular tachydysrhythmias.[29,104] This also is observed with CCB poisoning in which Ca^{2+} tends to improve blood pressure more than heart rate. Experimental models demonstrate the utility of Ca^{2+} salts with CCB poisoning. In verapamil-poisoned dogs, improvement in inotropy and blood pressure was demonstrated after increasing the serum Ca^{2+} concentration by 2 mEq/L with an IV infusion of 10% calcium chloride ($CaCl_2$) at 3 mg/kg/min.[37,45]

Clinical experience demonstrates that Ca^{2+} reverses the negative inotropy, impaired conduction, and hypotension in many humans poisoned by CCBs.[67,72,95] Unfortunately, this effect is often short lived, and more severely poisoned patients do not improve significantly with Ca^{2+} administration alone.[22,56,99] Although some authors believe that these failures might represent inadequate dosing, optimal effective dosing of Ca^{2+} is unclear, and they recommend repeat doses of Ca^{2+} to markedly increase the serum ionized Ca^{2+} concentrations.[51,67] The excessive use of Ca^{2+} can result in significant complications such as vasoconstriction and renal failure, particularly if a Ca^{2+} infusion is used.[103] Caution should be exercised in the administration of Ca^{2+} in patients suspected of an acute cardioactive steroid poisoning as a cause of their bradycardia.[14] The use of Ca^{2+} in the setting of cardioactive steroid poisoning is reported to result in cardiac complications such as dysrhythmia (Chap. 62).

Dose

For poisoned adults, an initial IV infusion of approximately 13 to 25 mEq of Ca^{2+} (10–20 mL of 10% $CaCl_2$ or 30–60 mL of 10% Ca^{2+} gluconate) is given over 10 minutes followed by repeat doses every 10 minutes up to two doses then every 20 to 60 minutes as needed. It is important to monitor [Ca^{2+}] every 30 to 60 minutes (Antidotes in Depth: A32). Careful selection and attention to the type of Ca^{2+} used is critical for dosing. Although there is no difference in efficacy of $CaCl_2$ or calcium gluconate, 1 g of $CaCl_2$ contains 13.4 mEq of Ca^{2+}, which is about three times the 4.65 mEq found in 1 g of calcium gluconate. Thus, to administer equal doses of Ca^{2+}, three times the volume of calcium gluconate compared with that of $CaCl_2$ is required. The main limitation of using $CaCl_2$, however, is that it has significant potential for causing tissue injury if extravasated we recommend administration through a central venous line, intraosseous line or peripheral line if no other route is accessible. Adverse effects of IV Ca^{2+} include nausea, vomiting, flushing, constipation, confusion, hypercalcemia, and hypophosphatemia.

Glucagon

Glucagon is an endogenous polypeptide hormone secreted by the pancreatic α cells in response to hypoglycemia and catecholamines. In addition, it has significant inotropic and chronotropic effects (Antidotes in Depth: A20).[20,21,109,126] Glucagon is a therapy of choice for β-adrenergic antagonist poisoning (Chap. 59) because of its ability to bypass the β-adrenergic receptor and activate adenylate cyclase via a G_s protein in the myocardium.[123] Thus, glucagon is unique in that it is functionally a "pure" β_1 agonist, with no peripheral vasodilatory effects (Fig. 60–2). Although there are reports of both successes and failures of glucagon in CCB-poisoned patients who failed

to respond to fluids, Ca^{2+}, or dopamine and dobutamine, the authors recommend a trial of glucagon.[23,30,46,56]

Dose

Dosing for glucagon is not well established.[6] An initial dose of 3 to 5 mg IV, slowly over 3 to 5 minutes and if there is no hemodynamic improvement within 5 minutes, and retreatment with a dose of 4 to 10 mg is effective. The initial pediatric dose is 50 mcg/kg. Because of the short half-life of glucagon, repeat doses are often required. A maintenance infusion should be initiated after a desired effect is achieved. Adverse effects include vomiting and hyperglycemia, particularly in patients with diabetes or during continuous infusion. In other models repeat administration leads to tachyphylaxis, which is an acute decrease in response to a drug after repeated administration.

High-Dose Insulin Therapy

High-dose insulin (HDI) therapy is the treatment of choice for patients who are severely poisoned by CCBs. The mechanisms of action for HDI are varied and include utilization of free fatty acids for myocardial metabolic needs; CCB poisoning forces the myocardium to become more carbohydrate dependent.[60,61,63] At the same time, CCBs inhibit Ca^{2+}-mediated insulin secretion from the β-islet cells in the pancreas, making glucose uptake in myocardial cells dependent on passive diffusion down a concentration gradient rather than insulin-mediated active transport.[27] In addition, there is evidence that the CCB-poisoned myocardium also becomes insulin resistant, possibly by dysregulation of the PI3K pathway (Antidotes in Depth: A21). This prevents normal recruitment of insulin-responsive glucose transporter proteins. The combination of inhibited insulin secretion and impaired glucose utilization may explain why severe CCB toxicity often produces significant hyperglycemia.[61,62] However, the current accepted mechanism is that insulin impairs the Na^+-Ca^{2+} antiporter, resulting in an increase in the intracellular [Ca^{2+}]. This increase of calcium results in an increase in the Ca^{2+} load from the SR, leading to increased cardiac contractility.[52,113]

Many CCB-poisoned patients have been successfully treated with HIE therapy as demonstrated by improved hemodynamic function, mainly resulting from improved contractility, with little effect on heart rate. There are also reports of the failure of this treatment, but this represents initiation of therapy in terminally ill patients with multiple organ failure and delayed initiation of treatment.[35]

Dose

We recommend to begin therapy with a bolus of 1 unit/kg of regular human insulin along with 0.5 g/kg of dextrose. If blood glucose is greater than 300 mg/dL (16.65 mmol/L), the dextrose bolus is unnecessary. An infusion of regular insulin should follow the bolus starting at 1 units/kg/h titrated up to 2 units/kg/h if there is no improvement after 30 minutes. Even higher doses (10 units/kg h) of insulin have been successfully reported, and we recommend escalating to this dose if 1 to 2 units/kg/h is not successful.[32] A continuous dextrose infusion, beginning at 0.5 g/kg/h, should also be started. Glucose should be monitored every 30 minutes for the first 4 hours and titrated to maintain euglycemia. The response to insulin is typically delayed for 15 to 40 minutes, so early use of HDI should be initiated very early in the patient's course if severe CCB poisoning is suspected. Primary complications of HDI include hypoglycemia and hypokalemia from intracellular shifting of potassium. It is essential to note that the development of hypoglycemia is an indication to increase glucose delivery rather than decrease the insulin infusion rate. The blood glucose should be monitored every 15 to 30 minutes until stable and then every 1 to 2 hours. Kidney failure will alter the pharmacokinetics of insulin elimination and we recommend closer glucose monitoring and to use the dosing of insulin as recommended. Concentrating the insulin infusion to 10 units/mL prevents fluid overload from large doses of insulin.

Intravenous Lipid Emulsion

The use of intravenous lipid emulsion (ILE) as an antidote is best studied for the treatment of local anesthetic systemic toxicity with expanded use for the treatment of nonlocal anesthetic overdose such as with CCBs. Xenobiotics that are highly lipophilic may benefit more from the use of ILE in severe poisoning (Antidotes in Depth: A23).

There is controversy whether ILE is a valuable treatment for CCB poisoning because of inconsistent reported outcomes.[43] Existing experimental evidence supports that ILE decreases the toxicity of several intravenously administered lipid-soluble drugs, most notably bupivacaine.[117,118] Pretreatment with ILE also increased the dose of certain medications to cause toxicity, but its generalizability to CCBs in debatable.[119]

Intravenous lipid emulsion was used on a patient with severe verapamil poisoning who failed Ca[2+] and HDI but when given ILE showed improvement and survival. Serum verapamil concentrations were measured before and after ILE treatment. There was a decrease in verapamil after ILE administration after the lipid was removed from the samples, which demonstrate sequestration of verapamil.[35] However, there are also reports that ILE enhances intestinal absorption of other xenobiotics and lacks clinical benefit.[85,86] Intravenous lipid emulsion has the potential for interfering with the circuitry of extracorporeal membrane oxygenation (ECMO), and it is not clear what interaction ILE has on other medications being used as treatment. The Lipid Emulsion Workgroup is composed of representatives of all major toxicology associations' published evidence-based recommendations in which ILE was recommended for cardiac arrest from bupivacaine toxicity. At this time, the Workgroup's evidence-based recommendation on the use of ILE in CCB poisoning state that in the setting of life-threatening and non–life-threatening CCB poisoning, ILE should not be used as first-line therapy. The use of ILE is reasonable for CCB induced severe cardiovascular toxicity that persists despite maximal treatment with standard resuscitative measures (including GI decontamination) and ECMO and other ECLS are not available.[42,43]

Adjunctive Pharmacologic Treatment

Other pharmacotherapies are studied in the setting of CCB poisoning. There are limited data with these therapies, and therefore we do not recommend routine use. Digoxin was evaluated experimentally in CCB poisoning because it raises the intracellular Ca[2+] concentration.[8] In a canine model of verapamil poisoning, digoxin, in conjunction with atropine or Ca[2+], improved both systolic blood pressure and myocardial inotropy.[7] However, because digoxin requires a significant amount of time to distribute into tissue and because limited efficacy data and no safety data have yet been collected, we do not recommend use of digoxin in CCB poisoning. Another xenobiotic that was used as a treatment for CCB poisoning is levosimendan. Levosimendan is a Ca[2+] sensitizer used in the management of acutely decompensated congestive heart failure. Although there are reported cases of success with the use of this drug, there is also existing experimental evidence that does not support its use.[2,83,112]

Methylene blue (Antidotes in Depth: A43) was reported in a confirmed ingestion of amlodipine poisoning in a patient who failed conventional therapy, including HIE treatment. A Swan-Ganz catheter confirmed pure vasodilatory shock, which responded to methylene blue (2 mg/kg).[56] Methylene blue is also reported with success in a case of a mixed β-adrenergic antagonist and CCB overdose,[4] and it is used in other causes of refractory vasodilatory shock such as anaphylaxis and sepsis caused by inhibition of methylene blue along the nitric oxide–cyclic guanosine monophosphate pathway and contributes electrons to mitochondrial glycerophosphate dehydrogenase to improve mitochondrial respiration. Experimental evidence also shows improvement in hemodynamics with no change in mortality rate.[55] Some evidence suggests that certain dihydropyridines, such as amlodipine mediate, their vasodilatory effects via nitric oxide, but the importance of this pathway in acute poisoning is unclear. Further investigation is required before methylene blue can routinely be recommended in patients with CCB poisoning.[115]

Inotropes and Vasopressors

Catecholamines are often administered after first-line therapy such as atropine, Ca[2+], glucagon, and isotonic fluids fail. There are numerous cases that describe either success or failure with various inotropes and vasopressors, including epinephrine, norepinephrine, dopamine, isoproterenol,

dobutamine, and vasopressin.[22,46,50,73] Based on experimental and clinical data, no single inotrope or vasopressor is consistently effective. The variability in response is from the differences of CCB involved, coingestants with other cardioactive medications, and patient response. Calcium channel blocker poisoning often involve the myocardium (verapamil and diltiazem) resulting in negative chronotropy or inotropy or peripheral smooth muscle relaxation (dihydropyridines) with vasodilation mediated by α_1-adrenergic receptors. In a retrospective study in a series of patients with nondihydropyridine poisoning, they were managed with the use of multiple vasopressors and without HDI in all but three cases. Despite high doses of vasopressors, ischemic complications were uncommon and were attributed to the hypotension related to the poisoning. In this study, the use of vasopressors after nondihydropyridine poisoning was associated with good clinical outcomes.[70] Despite variable success in CCB poisoning, the existing data described previously show that all vasopressors are generally inferior with significantly more adverse effects such as tissue ischemia with long-term use. The authors therefore recommend avoiding their use if possible or using as a bridge to HDI.

Adjunctive Hemodynamic Support

The most severely CCB-poisoned patients will not respond to any pharmacologic intervention. Transthoracic or IV cardiac pacing is reasonable to improve heart rate, as several case reports demonstrate.[105,116] However, in a prospective cohort of CCB poisonings, two of four patients with significant bradycardia requiring electrical pacing had no electrical capture.[93] In addition, even if electrical pacing is effective in increasing the heart rate, blood pressure often remains unchanged.[49,50]

Intraaortic balloon pump (IABP) is another invasive supportive option that is reasonable to attempt in CCB poisoning refractory to pharmacologic therapy.[58] Because IABPs are ECG gated, in patients with very low heart rates, IABP is often not effective with increasing cardiac output with counterpulsation. Insertion of an IABP successfully improved cardiac output and blood pressure in a patient with a mixed verapamil and atenolol overdose.[36]

Severely CCB-poisoned patients have also been supported for days and subsequently recovered fully with much more invasive and technologically demanding ECMO and emergent open and percutaneous cardiopulmonary bypass.[49,96] Extracorporeal membrane oxygenation has been increasingly used in pharmacology-refractory CCB poisoning.[26,120] The advantage of ECMO over IABP is that it is independent of cardiac electrical and mechanical activity. There are currently two ECMO modalities available, which include venovenous EMCO (VV-EMCO) and venoarterial ECMO (VA-ECMO). Venovenous-extracorporeal membrane oxygenation is used primarily for patients with refractory respiratory failure and is not adequate in shock from severe CCB poisoning. Venoarterial-extracorporeal membrane oxygenation is recommended in severe circulatory shock. Reported complications of VA-ECMO include bleeding at the cannulation site, leg ischemia, and clotting of the machine circuitry, especially if ILE is given.[10,25]

Molecular adsorbents recirculating system (MARS) therapy is a specific extracorporeal albumin dialysis that is reported in the treatment of patients with severe CCB poisoning. Molecular adsorbents recirculating system therapy has the unique ability to selectively remove from circulation protein-bound xenobiotics that are not cleared by conventional hemodialysis. The use of MARS therapy is under current investigation with *Amanita* poisoning but reportedly was successfully used in three patients with severe nondihydropyridine CCB poisoning.[88] Despite potential application, we recommend the use of VA-ECMO or some other form of ECLS. The major limitation of all these technologies, however, is that they are available only at tertiary care facilities.

DISPOSITION

Patients who manifest signs or symptoms of toxicity should be admitted to an intensive care setting. Because of the potential for delayed toxicity, patients who ingest sustained-release products should be admitted for

24 hours to a monitored setting even if they are asymptomatic. This precautionary approach is particularly important for toddlers and small children in whom even one or a few tablets may produce significant toxicity. Criteria for safe discharge or medical stability apply only to patients with a reliable history of an ingestion of an "immediate-release" preparation who have received adequate GI decontamination, had serial ECGs over 6 to 8 hours that have remained unchanged, and are asymptomatic.

SUMMARY

- The hallmarks of CCB toxicity include bradydysrhythmias and hypotension, which are an extension of their pharmacologic effects.
- Although most patients develop symptoms and clinical findings of hypoperfusion, such as lightheadedness, nausea, or fatigue, within hours of a significant ingestion, ingestion of sustained-release formulations result in significant delays in any hemodynamic consequences with prolonged toxicity.
- Aggressive decontamination of patients with exposures to sustained-release products should begin as soon as possible and should not be delayed while awaiting signs of toxicity.
- Because HDI therapy has a delay to onset on action, it should be instituted early in the clinical course in an attempt to avoid the use of vasopressors.
- Patients who fail to respond to all pharmaceutical interventions should be considered for lipid emulsion adjunctive hemodynamic support, such as VA-ECMO, whenever available.

REFERENCES

1. Abernethy DR, Schwartz JB. Calcium-antagonist drugs. *N Engl J Med.* 1999;341: 1447-1457.
2. Abraham MK et al. Levosimendan does not improve survival time in a rat model of verapamil toxicity. *J Med Toxicol.* 2009;5:3-7.
3. Acierno LJ, Worrell LT. Albrecht Fleckenstein: father of calcium antagonism. *Clin Cardiol.* 2004;27:710-711.
4. Aggarwal N, et al. Methylene blue reverses recalcitrant shock in beta-blocker and calcium channel blocker overdose. *BMJ Case Rep.* 2013;pii: bcr2012007402.
5. Ashraf M, et al. Massive overdose of sustained-release verapamil: a case report and review of literature. *Am J Med Sci.* 1995;310:258-263.
6. Bailey B. Glucagon in beta-blocker and calcium channel blocker overdoses: a systematic review. *J Toxicol Clin Toxicol.* 2003;41:595-602.
7. Bania TC, et al. Calcium and digoxin vs. calcium alone for severe verapamil toxicity. *Acad Emerg Med.* 2000;7:1089-1096.
8. Bania TC, et al. Dose-dependent hemodynamic effect of digoxin therapy in severe verapamil toxicity. *Acad Emerg Med.* 2004;11:221-227.
9. Barrow PM, et al. Overdose of sustained-release verapamil. *Br J Anaesth.* 1994;72:361-365.
10. Baud FJ, et al. Clinical review: aggressive management and extracorporeal support for drug-induced cardiotoxicity. *Crit Care.* 2007;11:207.
11. Bechtel LK, et al. Verapamil toxicity dysregulates the phosphatidylinositol 3-kinase pathway. *Acad Emerg Med.* 2008;15:368-374.
12. Belson MG, et al. Calcium channel blocker ingestions in children. *Am J Emerg Med.* 2000;18:581-586.
13. Benaim ME. Asystole after verapamil. *Br Med J.* 1972;2:169-170.
14. Bower JO, Mengle H. The additive effects of calcium and digitalis: a warning with a report of two deaths. 1936;106:1151-1153.
15. Bronstein AC, et al. 2009 Annual Report of the American Association of Poison Control Centers' National Poison Data System (NPDS): 27th Annual Report. *Clin Toxicol.* 2010;48:979-1178.
16. Bronstein AC, et al. 2011 Annual report of the American Association of Poison Control Centers' National Poison Data System (NPDS): 29th Annual Report. *Clin Toxicol (Phila).* 2012;50:911-1164.
17. Buckley N, et al. Slow-release verapamil poisoning. Use of polyethylene glycol whole-bowel lavage and high-dose calcium. *Med J Aust.* 1993;158:202-204.
18. Catterall WA, Swanson TM. Structural basis for pharmacology of voltage-gated sodium and calcium channels. *Mol Pharmacol.* 2015;88:141-150.
19. Chakraborti S, et al. Calcium signaling phenomena in heart diseases: a perspective. *Molecular and cellular biochemistry.* 2007;298:1-40.
20. Chernow B. Glucagon: a potentially important hormone in circulatory shock. *Progress Clin Biol Res.* 1988;264:285-293.
21. Chernow B, et al. Glucagon: endocrine effects and calcium involvement in cardiovascular actions in dogs. *Circ Shock.* 1986;19:393-407.
22. Chimienti M, et al. Acute verapamil poisoning: successful treatment with epinephrine. *Clin Cardiol.* 1982;5:219-222.
23. Connolly DL, et al. Massive diltiazem overdose. *Am J Cardiol.* 1993;72:742-743.
24. Cumpston KL, et al. Whole bowel irrigation and the hemodynamically unstable calcium channel blocker overdose: primum non nocere. *J Emerg Med.* 2010;38:171-174.
25. de Lange DW, et al. Extracorporeal membrane oxygenation in the treatment of poisoned patients. *Clin Toxicol (Phila).* 2013;51:385-393.
26. De Rita F, et al. Rescue extracorporeal life support for acute verapamil and propranolol toxicity in a neonate. *Artifi Organs.* 2011;35:416-420.
27. Devis G, et al. Calcium antagonists and islet function. I. Inhibition of insulin release by verapamil. *Diabetes.* 1975;24:247-251.
28. Dibb KM, et al. Analysis of cellular calcium fluxes in cardiac muscle to understand calcium homeostasis in the heart. *Cell Calcium.* 2007;42:503-512.
29. Dolan DL. Intravenous calcium before verapamil to prevent hypotension. *Ann Emerg Med.* 1991;20:588-589.
30. Doyon S, Roberts JR. The use of glucagon in a case of calcium channel blocker overdose. *Ann Emerg Med.* 1993;22:1229-1233.
31. Eisenberg MJ, et al. Calcium channel blockers: an update. *Am J Med.* 2004;116:35-43.
32. Engebretsen KM, et al. High-dose insulin therapy in beta-blocker and calcium channel-blocker poisoning. *Clin Toxicol.* 2011;49:277-283.
33. Fauville JP, et al. Severe diltiazem poisoning with intestinal pseudo-obstruction: case report and toxicological data. *J Toxicol Clin Toxicol.* 1995;33:273-277.
34. Foster TS, et al. Nifedipine kinetics and bioavailability after single intravenous and oral doses in normal subjects. *J Clin Pharmacol.* 1983;23:161-170.
35. French D, et al. Serum verapamil concentrations before and after Intralipid(R) therapy during treatment of an overdose. *Clin Toxicol.* 2011;49:340-344.
36. Frierson J, et al. Refractory cardiogenic shock and complete heart block after unsuspected verapamil-SR and atenolol overdose. *Clin Cardiol.* 1991;14:933-935.
37. Gay R, et al. Treatment of verapamil toxicity in intact dogs. *J Clin Invest.* 1986;77:1805-1811.
38. Geronimo-Pardo M, et al. Clarithromycin-nifedipine interaction as possible cause of vasodilatory shock. *Ann Pharmacother.* 2005;39:538-542.
39. Gladding P, et al. Potentially fatal interaction between diltiazem and statins. *Ann Intern Med.* 2004;140:W31.
40. Gleyzer A, et al. Calcium channel blocker ingestions in children. *Am J Emerg Med.* 2001;19:456-457.
41. Godfraind T. Pharmacological basis of the classification of calcium antagonists. *Acta Otolaryngol Suppl.* 1988;460:33-41.
42. Gosselin S, et al. Evidence-based recommendations on the use of intravenous lipid emulsion therapy in poisoning. *Clin Toxicol (Phila).* 2016;54:899-923.
43. Gosselin S, et al. Methodology for AACT evidence-based recommendations on the use of intravenous lipid emulsion therapy in poisoning. *Clin Toxicol (Phila).* 2015;53:557-564.
44. Grace AA, Camm AJ. Voltage-gated calcium-channels and antiarrhythmic drug action. *Cardiovasc Res.* 2000;45:43-51.
45. Hariman RJ, et al. Reversal of the cardiovascular effects of verapamil by calcium and sodium: differences between electrophysiologic and hemodynamic responses. *Circulation.* 1979;59:797-804.
46. Hendren WG, et al. Extracorporeal bypass for the treatment of verapamil poisoning. *Ann Emerg Med.* 1989;18:984-987.
47. Hermann P, Morselli PL. Pharmacokinetics of diltiazem and other calcium entry blockers. *Acta Pharmacol Toxicol.* 1985;57(suppl 2):10-20.
48. Hermann P, et al. Pharmacokinetics of diltiazem after intravenous and oral administration. *Eur J Clin Pharmacol.* 1983;24:349-352.
49. Holzer M, et al. Successful resuscitation of a verapamil-intoxicated patient with percutaneous cardiopulmonary bypass. *Crit Care Med.* 1999;27:2818-2823.
50. Horowitz BZ, Rhee KJ. Massive verapamil ingestion: a report of two cases and a review of the literature. *Am J Emerg Med.* 1989;7:624-631.
51. Howarth DM, et al. Calcium channel blocking drug overdose: an Australian series. *Hum Exp Toxicol.* 1994;13:161-166.
52. Hsu CH, et al. Cellular mechanisms responsible for the inotropic action of insulin on failing human myocardium. *J Heart Lung Transplant.* 2006;25:1126-1134.
53. Humbert VH Jr, et al. Noncardiogenic pulmonary edema complicating massive diltiazem overdose. *Chest.* 1991;99:258-259.
54. Ishikawa T, et al. Atrioventricular dissociation and sinus arrest induced by oral diltiazem. *N Engl J Med.* 1983;309:1124-1125.
55. Jang DH, et al. Efficacy of methylene blue in an experimental model of calcium channel blocker-induced shock. *Ann Emerg Med.* 2015;65:410-415.
56. Jang DH, et al. Methylene blue in the treatment of refractory shock from an amlodipine overdose. *Ann Emerg Med.* 2011;58:565-567.
57. Johnson KE, et al. Electrophysiologic effects of verapamil metabolites in the isolated heart. *J Cardiovasc Pharmacol.* 1991;17:830-837.
58. Johnson NJ, et al. A review of emergency cardiopulmonary bypass for severe poisoning by cardiotoxic drugs. *J Med Toxicol.* 2013;9:54-60.
59. Katz AM. Molecular biology of calcium channels in the cardiovascular system. *Am J Cardiol.* 1997;80:17I-22I.
60. Kline JA, et al. Beneficial myocardial metabolic effects of insulin during verapamil toxicity in the anesthetized canine. *Crit Care Med.* 1995;23:1251-1263.
61. Kline JA, et al. Insulin improves heart function and metabolism during non-ischemic cardiogenic shock in awake canines. *Cardiovasc Res.* 1997;34:289-298.

62. Kline JA, et al. The diabetogenic effects of acute verapamil poisoning. *Toxicol Appl Pharmacol.* 1997;145:357-362.

63. Kline JA, et al. Insulin is a superior antidote for cardiovascular toxicity induced by verapamil in the anesthetized canine. *J Pharmacol Exp Ther.* 1993;267:744-750.

64. Kokubun S, et al. The voltage-dependent effect of 1,4-dihydropyridine enantiomers on Ca channels in cardiac cells. *Jpn Heart J.* 1986;27(suppl 1):57-63.

65. Koury SI, et al. Amrinone as an antidote in experimental verapamil overdose. *Acad Emerg Med.* 1996;3:762-767.

66. Krayenbuhl JC, et al. Drug-drug interactions of new active substances: mibefradil example. *European J Clin Pharmacol.* 1999;55:559-565.

67. Lam YM, et al. Continuous calcium chloride infusion for massive nifedipine overdose. *Chest.* 2001;119:1280-1282.

68. Lapatto-Reiniluoto O, et al. Activated charcoal alone and followed by whole-bowel irrigation in preventing the absorption of sustained-release drugs. *Clin Pharmacol Ther.* 2001;70:255-260.

69. Levine M, et al. Assessment of hyperglycemia after calcium channel blocker overdoses involving diltiazem or verapamil. *Crit Care Med.* 2007;35:2071-2075.

70. Levine M, et al. Critical care management of verapamil and diltiazem overdose with a focus on vasopressors: a 25-year experience at a single center. *Ann Emerg Med.* 2013; 62:252-258.

71. Luscher TF, Cosentino F. The classification of calcium antagonists and their selection in the treatment of hypertension. A reappraisal. *Drugs.* 1998;55:509-517.

72. Luscher TF, et al. Calcium gluconate in severe verapamil intoxication. *N Engl J Med.* 1994;330:718-720.

73. MacDonald D, Alguire PC. Case report: fatal overdose with sustained-release verapamil. *Am J Med Sci.* 1992;303:115-117.

74. Marston S, El-Mezgueldi M. Role of tropomyosin in the regulation of contraction in smooth muscle. *Adv Exp Med Biol.* 2008;644:110-123.

75. Materne P, et al. Hemodynamic effects of intravenous diltiazem with impaired left ventricular function. *Am J Cardiol.* 1984;54:733-737.

76. McAllister RG Jr, et al. Pharmacokinetics of calcium-entry blockers. *Am J Cardiol.* 1985;55:30B-40B.

77. Mowry JB, et al. 2014 Annual Report of the American Association of Poison Control Centers' National Poison Data System (NPDS): 32nd Annual Report. *Clin Toxicol (Phila).* 2015;53:962-1147.

78. Mowry JB, et al. 2015 Annual Report of the American Association of Poison Control Centers' National Poison Data System (NPDS): 33rd Annual Report. *Clin Toxicol (Phila).* 2016;54:924-1109.

79. Nargeot J, et al. Molecular basis of the diversity of calcium channels in cardiovascular tissues. *Eur Heart J.* 1997;18(suppl A):A15-26.

80. Nawrath H, Wegener JW. Kinetics and state-dependent effects of verapamil on cardiac L-type calcium channels. *Naunyn Schmiedebergs Arch Pharmacol.* 1997;355:79-86.

81. Nilsson H. Interactions between membrane potential and intracellular calcium concentration in vascular smooth muscle. *Acta Physiol Scand.* 1998;164:559-566.

82. Olson KR, et al. Calcium channel blocker ingestion: an evidence-based consensus guideline for out-of-hospital management. *Clin Toxicol (Phila).* 2005;43:797-822.

83. Osthoff M, et al. Levosimendan as treatment option in severe verapamil intoxication: a case report and review of the literature. *Case Rep Med.* 2010;2010.

84. Padrini R, et al. Physiological, pharmacological and pathological factors affecting the pharmacokinetics of calcium entry blockers. *G Ital Cardiol.* 1987;17:786-790.

85. Perez E, et al. Determining the optimal dose of intravenous fat emulsion for the treatment of severe verapamil toxicity in a rodent model. *Acad Emerg Med.* 2008; 15:1284-1289.

86. Perichon D, et al. An assessment of the in vivo effects of intravenous lipid emulsion on blood drug concentration and haemodynamics following oro-gastric amitriptyline overdose. *Clin Toxicol (Phila).* 2013;51:208-215.

87. Petrovic MM, et al. Ryanodine receptors, voltage-gated calcium channels and their relationship with protein kinase A in the myocardium. *Physiol Res.* 2008;57:141-149.

88. Pichon N, et al. Extracorporeal albumin dialysis in three cases of acute calcium channel blocker poisoning with life-threatening refractory cardiogenic shock. *Ann Emerg Med.* 2012;59:540-544.

89. Pitt B. Diversity of calcium antagonists. *Clin Ther.* 1997;19(suppl A):3-17.

90. Proano L, et al. Calcium channel blocker overdose. *Am J Emerg Med.* 1995;13:444-450.

91. Quezado Z, et al. Severe cardiac, respiratory, and metabolic complications of massive verapamil overdose. *Crit Care Med.* 1991;19:436-438.

92. Quinn DI, Day RO. Drug interactions of clinical importance. An updated guide. *Drug Saf.* 1995;12:393-452.

93. Ramoska EA, et al. Calcium channel blocker toxicity. *Ann Emerg Med.* 1990;19:649-653.

94. Ramoska EA, et al. A one-year evaluation of calcium channel blocker overdoses: toxicity and treatment. *Ann Emerg Med.* 1993;22:196-200.

95. Roberts D, et al. Diltiazem overdose: pharmacokinetics of diltiazem and its metabolites and effect of multiple dose charcoal therapy. *J Toxicol Clin Toxicol.* 1991;29:45-52.

96. Rosansky SJ. Verapamil toxicity—treatment with hemoperfusion. *Ann Intern Med.* 1991;114:340-341.

97. Samniah N, Schlaeffer F. Cerebral infarction associated with oral verapamil overdose. *J Toxicol Clin Toxicol.* 1988;26:365-369.

98. Sandroni C, et al. Successful treatment with enoximone for severe poisoning with atenolol and verapamil: a case report. *Acta Anaesthesiol Scand.* 2004;48:790-792.

99. Schiffl H, et al. Clinical features and management of nifedipine overdosage in a patient with renal insufficiency. *J Toxicol Clin Toxicol.* 1984;22:387-395.

100. Schoffstall JM, et al. Effects of calcium channel blocker overdose-induced toxicity in the conscious dog. *Ann Emerg Med.* 1991;20:1104-1108.

101. Shah AR, Passalacqua BR. Case report: sustained-release verapamil overdose causing stroke: an unusual complication. *Am J Med Sci.* 1992;304:357-359.

102. Sica DA. Interaction of grapefruit juice and calcium channel blockers. *Am J Hypertens.* 2006;19:768-773.

103. Sim MT, Stevenson FT. A fatal case of iatrogenic hypercalcemia after calcium channel blocker overdose. *J Med Toxicol.* 2008;4:25-29.

104. Singh NA. Intravenous calcium and verapamil—when the combination may be indicated. *Int J Cardiol.* 1983;4:281-284.

105. Snover SW, Bocchino V. Massive diltiazem overdose. *Ann Emerg Med.* 1986;15: 1221-1224.

106. Spedding M, Paoletti R. Classification of calcium channels and the sites of action of drugs modifying channel function. *Pharmacol Rev.* 1992;44:363-376.

107. Spiller HA, et al. Amlodipine fatality in an infant with postmortem blood levels. *J Med Toxicol.* 2012;8:179-182.

108. St-Onge M, et al. Experts consensus recommendations for the management of calcium channel blocker poisoning in adults. *Crit Care Med.* 2017;45:e306-e315.

109. Stone CK, et al. Treatment of verapamil overdose with glucagon in dogs. *Ann Emerg Med.* 1995;25:369-374.

110. Thanacoody R, et al. Position paper update: whole bowel irrigation for gastrointestinal decontamination of overdose patients. *Clin Toxicol (Phila).* 2015;53:5-12.

111. Thompson AM, et al. Changes in cardiorespiratory function during gastric lavage for drug overdose. *Hum Toxicol.* 1987;6:215-218.

112. Varpula T, et al. Treatment of serious calcium channel blocker overdose with levosimendan, a calcium sensitizer. *Anesthes Analg.* 2009;108:790-792.

113. von Lewinski D, et al. Insulin causes [Ca2+]i-dependent and [Ca2+]i-independent positive inotropic effects in failing human myocardium. *Circulation.* 2005;111:2588-2595.

114. Wandel C, et al. Mibefradil is a P-glycoprotein substrate and a potent inhibitor of both P-glycoprotein and CYP3A in vitro. *Drug Metab Dispos.* 2000;28:895-898.

115. Warrick BJ, et al. A systematic analysis of methylene blue for drug-induced shock. *Clin Toxicol (Phila).* 2016;54:547-555.

116. Watling SM, et al. Verapamil overdose: case report and review of the literature. *Ann Pharmacother.* 1992;26:1373-1378.

117. Weinberg G, et al. Lipid emulsion infusion rescues dogs from bupivacaine-induced cardiac toxicity. *Reg Anesthesia Pain Med.* 2003;28:198-202.

118. Weinberg GL, et al. Lipid infusion accelerates removal of bupivacaine and recovery from bupivacaine toxicity in the isolated rat heart. *Reg Anesthesia Pain Med.* 2006;31:296-303.

119. Weinberg GL, et al. Pretreatment or resuscitation with a lipid infusion shifts the dose-response to bupivacaine-induced asystole in rats. *Anesthesiology.* 1998;88:1071-1075.

120. Weinberg RL, et al. Venoarterial extracorporeal membrane oxygenation for the management of massive amlodipine overdose. *Perfusion.* 2014;29:53-56.

121. Wolf LR, et al. Use of amrinone and glucagon in a case of calcium channel blocker overdose. *Ann Emerg Med.* 1993;22:1225-1228.

122. Woscholski R, Marme D. Dihydropyridine binding of the calcium channel complex from skeletal muscle is modulated by subunit interaction. *Cell Signal.* 1992;4:209-218.

123. Yagami T. Differential coupling of glucagon and beta-adrenergic receptors with the small and large forms of the stimulatory G protein. *Mol Pharmacol.* 1995;48: 849-854.

124. Yeung PK, et al. Pharmacokinetics and metabolism of diltiazem in rats: comparing single vs repeated subcutaneous injections in vivo. *Biopharm Drug Dispos.* 2007; 28:403-407.

125. Yust I, et al. Life-threatening bradycardic reactions due to beta blocker-diltiazem interactions. *Isr J Med Sci.* 1992;28:292-294.

126. Zaritsky AL, et al. Glucagon antagonism of calcium channel blocker-induced myocardial dysfunction. *Crit Care Med.* 1988;16:246-251.

127. Zhang X, Hintze TH. Amlodipine releases nitric oxide from canine coronary microvessels: an unexpected mechanism of action of a calcium channel-blocking agent. *Circulation.* 1998;97:576-580.

128. Zhang X, et al. Amlodipine enhances NO production induced by an ACE inhibitor through a kinin-mediated mechanism in canine coronary microvessels. *J Cardiovasc Pharmacol.* 2000;35:195-202.

129. Zhang XP, et al. Paradoxical release of nitric oxide by an L-type calcium channel antagonist, the R+ enantiomer of amlodipine. *J Cardiovasc Pharmacol.* 2002;39: 208-214.

HIGH-DOSE INSULIN

Samuel J. Stellpflug and William Kerns II

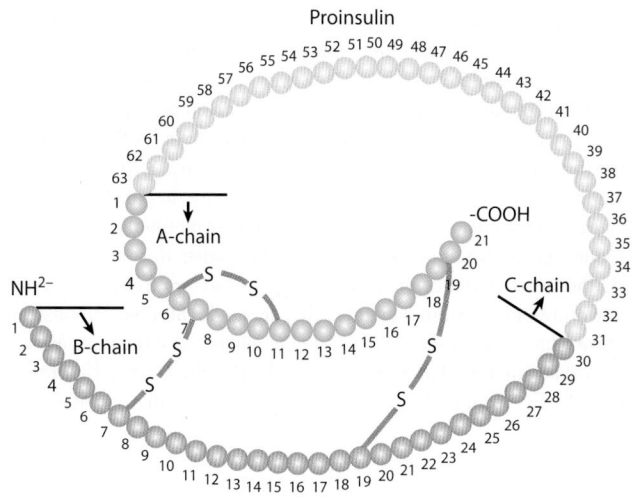

Proinsulin

HISTORY

Insulin was discovered and named in 1922, although its existence had been previously surmised. Clinicians at Toronto General Hospital successfully achieved glycemic control in a 14-year-old boy with diabetes by injecting him with pancreatic extract, culminating more than 30 years of research.[76] In the past 2 decades, insulin has gained increased attention and importance in the management of a spectrum of critical illnesses, including sepsis, heart failure, and cardiovascular drug toxicity. The benefits of insulin go well beyond simple glucose control. In xenobiotic-induced myocardial depression, the use of high-dose insulin (HDI) along with sufficient dextrose can restore normal hemodynamic status.

PHARMACOLOGY

Chemistry and Physiology

To understand the role of insulin specifically for resuscitating patients with cardiac drug toxicity, the altered myocardial physiology that occurs during drug-induced shock is briefly reviewed. The hallmarks of severe β-adrenergic antagonist (BAA) and calcium channel blocker (CCB) toxicity are bradycardia and decreased inotropy that compromise cardiac output and produce cardiogenic shock.[17] This is caused by direct β-adrenergic receptor antagonism and calcium channel blockade. In some cases, peripheral vasodilation also occurs, especially in the context of dihydropyridine CCB ingestions.[22,75] In addition to direct receptor and ion channel effects, metabolic derangements occur that closely resemble diabetes with hyperglycemia, insulin deficiency, insulin resistance, and acidemia.

In the nonstressed state, the heart primarily catabolizes free fatty acids for its energy needs. On the other hand, the stressed myocardium switches its preferred energy substrate to carbohydrates, as demonstrated in models of both BAA and CCB toxicity.[21,42,70] The greater the degree of shock, the greater the carbohydrate demand.[43] The liver responds to stress by making more glucose available via glycogenolysis. As a result, blood glucose concentrations increase. Hyperglycemia is noted both in animal models and in human cases of some cardiac drug overdoses; it can be especially

evident with CCB toxicity.[10,23,45,71] The degree of hyperglycemia can correlate directly with the severity of shock for cases involving verapamil and diltiazem.[48] Calcium channel blockers interfere with carbohydrate processing by inhibiting pancreatic insulin release, which is necessary to transport glucose across cell membranes. Insulin release from islet cells requires functioning L-type or voltage-gated calcium channels similar to those found in myocardial and vascular tissue. Calcium channel blockers directly inhibit pancreatic calcium channels (Fig. A21–1).[16] In vitro models of verapamil infusion confirm this toxicity; circulating glucose concentrations increase without an associated increase in insulin.[43] Calcium channel blockers also create a state of insulin resistance by interfering with glucose transporter 1 (GLUT-1) and phosphatidylinositol 3-kinase (PI3K) glucose transport (Fig. A21–2).[5,50] As a result of diminished circulating insulin and inhibited enzymatic glucose uptake, glucose movement into

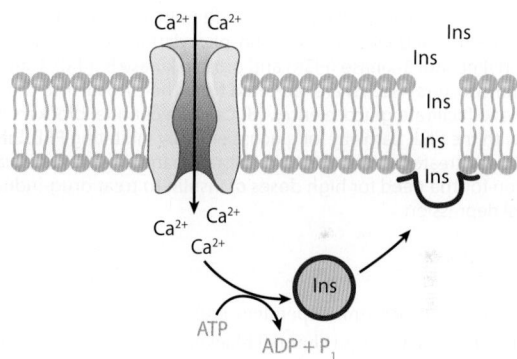

L-type calcium channel

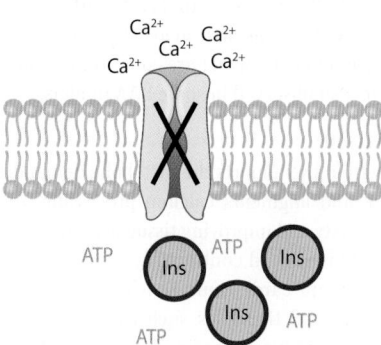

L-type calcium channel

FIGURE A21–1. (A) Insulin (Ins) release from the β-pancreatic islet cell is mediated via influx of calcium through voltage-gated (L-type) calcium channels and requires adenosine triphosphate (ATP). **(B)** Ca^{2+} channel blockers (CCBs) inhibit pancreatic insulin release by antagonizing calcium entry via L-type calcium channel. This results in insufficient insulin to support the glucose demands of the stressed heart and contributes to hyperglycemia that occurs with CCB toxicity. ADP = adenosine diphosphate.

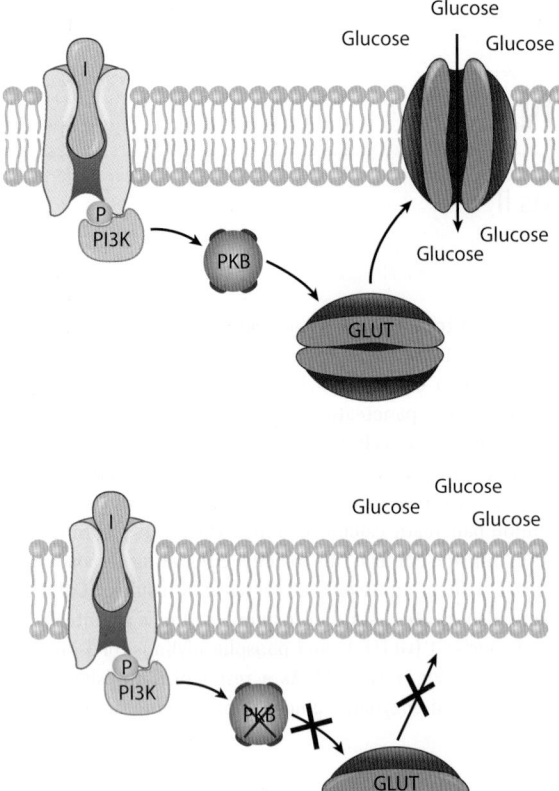

FIGURE A21–2. (**A**) The binding of insulin (I) to its receptor stimulates glucose entry into cells via a series of phosphorylation reactions involving phosphatidylinositol 3-kinase (PI3K) and protein kinase B (PKB). Ultimately, glucose transporters (GLUTs) are recruited from the cytosol into the cell membrane to facilitate glucose entry. (**B**) Calcium channel blockers (CCBs) interfere with the PI3K pathway for glucose entry by inhibiting PKB. Inhibition of this pathway creates a state of insulin resistance and provides one plausible explanation for the need for high doses of insulin to treat drug-induced myocardial depression.

cells becomes concentration dependent and may not sufficiently support myocardial demand. Calcium channel blockers further contribute to metabolic abnormalities by inhibiting lactate oxidation.[42,46] This likely occurs through inhibition of pyruvate dehydrogenase, the enzyme responsible for conversion of pyruvate to acetylcoenzyme A (acetyl-CoA). As a result, pyruvate is preferentially converted to lactate rather than the acetyl-CoA that would ordinarily enter the citric acid cycle; lactate then accumulates. Lactate accumulation and acidemia are consistent manifestations of CCB toxicity[17,46] and are also observed in some BAA models.[12]

Mechanism of Action

High-dose insulin therapy supports the metabolic demands associated with cardiogenic shock and augments calcium processing, thereby increasing myocardial contractility and improving tissue perfusion.

Insulin-mediated improved contractility appears to be a critical factor leading to survival from cardiogenic shock. In studies comparing insulin with more traditional therapies such as epinephrine and glucagon, insulin improves drug-induced cardiac function and work efficiency.[32,44] Epinephrine and glucagon performed less well, possibly because they promote free fatty acid utilization. As such, epinephrine and glucagon afforded limited increases in contractility at the expense of less efficient work, increased oxygen demand, and ultimately a higher mortality rate. Similar observations were noted when HDI was studied in cardiothoracic surgery postoperative care: improved myocardial function with economy

of oxygen demand and work.[24,30,81] Interestingly, in BAA and CCB studies using HDI, survival occurs without dramatic improvement in hypotension or bradycardia.[22,32,42,46] The lack of effect on drug-induced hypotension in animal studies and human cases may be due to the vasodilatory properties of insulin.[19] These vasodilatory effects occur in the systemic, coronary, and pulmonary vasculature; this vasodilation contradicts the occasionally published idea that insulin is a vasopressor. The mechanism is likely due to activation of the PI3K pathway enhancing endothelial nitric oxide synthase (eNOS) activity (Fig. A21–3).[5,33] Vasodilation in concert with improved cardiac contractility allows for improved tissue perfusion. Improved tissue perfusion explains why insulin is associated with superior survival effect compared with vasopressor adrenergic xenobiotics such as epinephrine.[32]

Initially, the ability of insulin to improve cardiac function was attributed to increased catecholamine release. However, evidence does not support this explanation. For example, β-receptor antagonism did not prevent improved contractility that followed insulin administration.[51,70] In a CCB toxic model, insulin therapy improved cardiac function and survival without increasing circulating catecholamine concentrations.[45] Evidence demonstrates that the positive inotropic effects of insulin occur because of metabolic support of the heart during hypodynamic shock. As alluded to earlier, during drug-induced shock, the heart switches preferred energy precursors from fatty acids to carbohydrates, and insulin facilitates this demand.[42] Studies demonstrate a direct correlation between carbohydrate metabolism and the improved indices of cardiac function that occur with insulin therapy. Despite β-adrenergic antagonism by propranolol, insulin increased myocardial glucose uptake

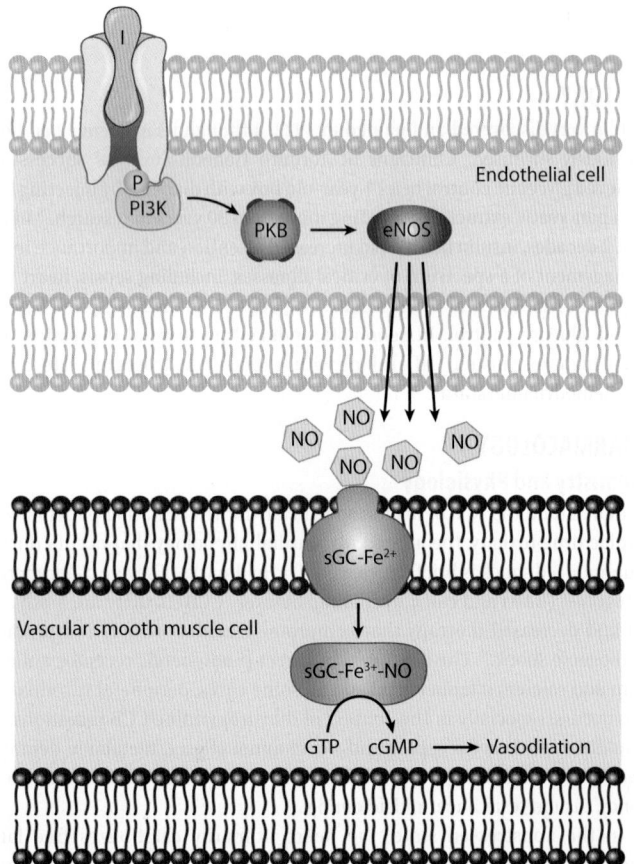

FIGURE A21–3. Nitric oxide (NO) is released from endothelial cells in response to insulin. This process involves two kinases: phosphatidylinositol 3-kinase (PI3K) and protein kinase B (PKB). NO diffuses into adjoining vascular smooth muscle cells and binds at a ferric site on the enzyme soluble guanylate cyclase (sGC). Activation of sGC produces cyclic guanosine monophosphate (cGMP) a signaler of cell relaxation, ultimately leading to vasodilation. GTP = guanosine triphosphate.

with subsequent increased contractility.[70] In a model of verapamil toxicity, insulin increased glucose uptake with resultant improved contractility.[42] Insulin therapy also increased lactate uptake by restoring pyruvate dehydrogenase activity.[44] In this way, lactate serves as a carbohydrate energy source after conversion to pyruvate and ultimately acetyl-CoA, which can then enter the citric acid cycle.

There is also evidence that insulin exerts an effect beyond enhanced carbohydrate usage via direct effects on calcium and, to a lesser extent, potassium and sodium ion homeostasis.[19,51] Insulin increases available intracellular calcium by enhancing reverse mode sodium–calcium exchange, with a resultant increase in the sarcoplasmic reticulum (SR) calcium load, thus causing increased contractility.[35,86] Furthermore, insulin-mediated increase in SR calcium availability seems to result from further activation of sodium/hydrogen exchange (Fig. 60–2).[35] An additional and unexplored mechanism is insulin's effect on protein kinase B (PKB or Akt), a kinase that influences contractile function and glucose uptake. Insulin stimulates PKB/Akt[3] and in turn PKB/Akt phosphorylates phospholamban, a protein that regulates calcium cycling in the SR.[11]

Pharmacokinetics and Pharmacodynamics

Regular insulin administered as HDI therapy is given intravenously, so gastrointestinal absorption is not an issue. The peak plasma concentration is essentially immediate. The onset and peak of the cardiovascular effect of insulin is roughly 15 to 40 minutes.[12,32,33,44,46] Insulin is slightly soluble in water, has a volume of distribution of roughly 21 L in an adult human, and demonstrates protein binding of roughly 5%, which can increase in a patient with diabetes with insulin antibodies.[55,72] More than half of insulin metabolism occurs in the liver, but there is also a sizable degree that occurs in adipose tissue, muscle, and the kidneys.[66] The elimination half-life of intravenously administered insulin is roughly 5 to 10 minutes, and it is partially eliminated in both the kidneys and the bile.[69,72]

ROLE IN DRUG-INDUCED CARDIOVASCULAR TOXICITY

As mentioned earlier, the positive inotropic effects of insulin were recognized in 1927; however, HDI therapy for drug-induced shock in humans was first reported in 1999.[84,87] This case series included four patients who overdosed on verapamil and one with a combined amlodipine–atenolol overdose. All patients failed traditional antidote therapy but responded to rescue insulin therapy. Since this initial case series, more than 90 cases have been published reporting use of insulin therapy for treatment of isolated or mixed drug-induced cardiac drug toxicity.[1,2,4,6-9,13-15,18,20,25-29,31,38,52,53,56-59,61,62,64,65,67,68,71,74,77-79,82,83] The vast majority of cases involved primary ingestion of β-adrenergic antagonists or calcium channel blockers. High-dose insulin was also used for poison-induced shock resulting from amiodarone,[18] amitriptyline, citalopram,[31] and morphine.[49] In one case of digoxin and insulin overdose, the coingested insulin was thought to be protective.[4] Various regimens of classic antidotes were used before insulin therapy in many of these cases. No direct outcome comparisons can be made between insulin and these other therapies once thought to be standard care. That being said and recognizing the inherent reporting bias, overall survival was very good when insulin was included in resuscitation. Further review of these cases and animal models yields important clinical information that can be used to guide HDI therapy.

Experimental models suggest that large doses of regular insulin (2.5–10 units/kg/h) are necessary to provide inotropic support.[5,12,41,44,46] The most recent human case series used 10 units/kg/h as the standard dose.[34] In one case, 22 units/kg/h was used with survival after cardiac arrest from nebivolol.[78] However, humans respond to less insulin. Most patients in the early reports were treated with HDI ranging between 0.5 and 2 units/kg/h. Many of the literature reported patients received an initial insulin bolus (between 0.1 and 1 unit/kg) before continuous infusion. The theoretical advantage to giving an initial insulin bolus is to rapidly saturate insulin receptors to speed the physiological response. Interestingly, one report noted that patients receiving an insulin bolus before the infusion showed a better blood pressure response than patients

who received only a continuous infusion.[25] Three patients received bolus insulin without continuous infusion, including a patient who inadvertently received 1,000 units.[68] In this case, hemodynamics improved, and there were no adverse events related to the extreme insulin dose. The typical reported duration of insulin infusion is 24 to 48 hours, with a range of 0.75 to 96 hours. The need for prolonged infusion likely reflects prolonged drug toxicokinetics often observed after overdose.

The predominant clinical effect of insulin is increased cardiac contractility with subsequent improvement in perfusion, often without initial increase in blood pressure. Contractility typically increased within 15 to 40 minutes after initiating insulin and often allowed a decrease in concurrent vasopressor use, sparing the toxicity of these xenobiotics. The timing of increased contractility is consistent with the observed response times in animal models.[12,32,33,41,46] Although prior studies did not find a survival benefit for vasopressors compared with insulin, a recent investigation demonstrated synergy between HDI and vasopressors regarding cerebral perfusion when norepinephrine was added after reaching severe malperfusion despite maximal HDI therapy.[39] In this swine model of severe propranolol shock, combined HDI and norepinephrine increased cerebral perfusion compared with HDI alone or vasopressors alone.

Other salutary effects were observed during insulin therapy. In one case of a combined amlodipine and valsartan overdose, blood pressure increased directly because of increased vascular resistance rather than increased cardiac function.[77] Two patients converted from third-degree heart block to normal sinus rhythm with an increased pulse in temporal relationship to insulin.[87] Except for these two patients, insulin therapy did not significantly affect heart rate in other reports. One reported case, technically a HDI failure, strongly supports the idea of insulin as an inotrope.[79] A patient with baseline hypertrophic cardiomyopathy but no baseline obstructive pathophysiology ingested diltiazem, metoprolol, and amiodarone. With insulin dosing quickly escalating to 10 units/kg/h, there was increased cardiac contractility documented by ultrasonography to the point of inducing hemodynamically significant obstructive outflow. The patient's clinical course ultimately improved after intravenous lipid emulsion administration. There are cases in which authors reported a lack of response to insulin. Reasons for no response in three of these reports include inadequate dosing and excessive delay to insulin therapy.[14]

Based on the sum of experimental and clinical experience, we recommend using HDI (bolus of regular insulin 1 unit/kg {total body weight} followed by 1 to 10 units/kg/h continuous infusion) early in the resuscitation of severe BAA- and CCB-induced myocardial depression. This recommendation is supported by multidisciplinary consensus guidelines.[80] It is also reasonable to use HDI for other xenobiotic-induced cardiogenic shock that is failing resuscitation with inotropes and vasopressors.

ADVERSE EVENTS AND SAFETY ISSUES

The major anticipated adverse event associated with the use of large amounts of insulin, especially in patients naïve to insulin, is hypoglycemia, defined as blood glucose less than 60 mg/dL (3.3 mmol/L) regardless of the presence or absence of symptoms. Because of potential hypoglycemia, all experimental animals received sufficient dextrose during insulin infusion to maintain euglycemia. In the aggregate human cases, patients typically received empiric supplemental dextrose based on frequent glucose monitoring. The typical dextrose dose was 25 g/h, but requirements varied widely from 0.5 to 75 g/h. The duration of exogenous dextrose supplementation was roughly 2 days, but it varied significantly from 9 to 100 hours. Dextrose supplementation was necessary beyond cessation of insulin for most cases. Despite empiric dextrose and blood glucose monitoring (albeit with no standard frequency of testing), hypoglycemia was observed in some patients. In one retrospective series, hypoglycemia occurred in 5 of 37 patients and resulted in HDI cessation.[57] In a prospective evaluation of seven separate CCB overdoses, there was one clinically insignificant episode.[25] In another retrospective 12-patient case series, there were 6 patients with a total of 19 hypoglycemic events (8 in one patient), all of uncertain but unlikely clinical significance.[34] Of note, dextrose requirement does not directly correlate well with insulin dose or severity of shock. Patients with severe shock and marked hyperglycemia often do not need any supplemental dextrose during the initial hours of insulin therapy because of insulin deficiency and insulin resistance. Additionally, there is likely a ceiling requirement for dextrose as glucose transport is saturable. One animal model demonstrated that dextrose need was greater for animals treated with 5 versus 1 unit/kg/h of insulin but not between groups treated with 5 versus 10 units/kg/h.[12] There is other evidence that glucose requirements are not predictable.[54] Overall, hypoglycemia is a potential consequence of HDI therapy, but clinically significant hypoglycemia is rare. A combination of rigorous glucose monitoring and dextrose administration can prevent hypoglycemia and avoid unnecessary cessation of insulin treatment.

Another anticipated consequence of insulin treatment is hypokalemia. Although serum potassium concentrations often falls below normal laboratory ranges, HDI does not typically cause profound hypokalemia. The observed decrease reflects a shifting of potassium from the extracellular to intracellular space that occurs as a result of the action of insulin. Patients maintain normal total body potassium stores and do not experience true deficiency unless they have other reasons for potassium loss. In the initial case series, three patients had a nadir of potassium ranging from 2.2 to 2.8 mEq/L without sequelae.[85] In two case series of 7 and 12 patients, there were 2 of 7 and 7 of 12 patients, respectively, who demonstrated clinically insignificant hypokalemia.[25,34] There is a theoretical risk of excessive potassium replacement in the instance of lowered serum potassium but normal total body stores. Hyperkalemia is also reported to worsen verapamil-induced myocardial depression.[37,60]

Other observed ion changes during insulin therapy include hypomagnesemia and hypophosphatemia. Similar to action on potassium, insulin causes an intracellular shift of both phosphorus and magnesium.[40,63] In the initial series of drug-induced shock treated with insulin, four patients had lowered magnesium (0.4–0.6 mmol/L; normal, 0.8–1.2 mmol/L) and phosphorus (0.2–0.5 mmol/L; normal, 1–1.4 mmol/L) concentrations. No symptoms were attributed to these lowered serum concentrations, but three patients received supplementation of both electrolytes. No other insulin-treated CCB cases address these two electrolytes. Insulin (0.1 units/kg/h) for diabetic ketoacidosis is likewise associated with similar effects on magnesium and phosphorus, so it is unlikely that alterations of magnesium and phosphorus are dose related.[36]

PREGNANCY AND LACTATION

Regular insulin is Pregnancy Category B and is compatible with breastfeeding.

DOSING AND ADMINISTRATION

Based on the experimental studies and aggregate human cases, HDI will most likely benefit patients with cardiac drug-induced myocardial depression. High-dose insulin is recommended for patients with malperfusion refractory to large doses of vasopressors even when there is no associated poor contractility. The experimental evidence and human case experience are strongest for CCB toxicity. Animal studies and growing human experience also support its use for BAA toxicity.

Myocardial function should be measured or estimated. Options include cardiac ultrasonography or through machine-estimated cardiac output using pulse contour analysis attached to a standard arterial catheter. This can be done more invasively via placement of a pulmonary artery catheter. When myocardial function is decreased, insulin therapy is initiated by first administering a 1-unit/kg bolus of regular human insulin along with 0.5-g/kg bolus of dextrose; if blood glucose is greater than 300 mg/dL (16.7 mmol/L), the dextrose bolus is not necessary. An infusion of regular insulin should immediately follow the bolus starting at 1 unit/kg/h. Ideally, this insulin infusion should be concentrated to prevent fluid overload that would occur with large doses. We typically concentrate the infusion at 10 unit/mL compared with the typical insulin infusion concentration of 1 unit/mL used for diabetic ketoacidosis. This unusual pharmacy formulation requires close collaboration with hospital pharmacists. Concentrated insulin solutions are stable for 14 days.[47] A continuous dextrose infusion, beginning at 0.5 g/kg/h, is concurrently recommended when necessary. Dextrose can be started as D_{10}, especially without central venous access and while determining the dextrose need, but it is ultimately best delivered as D_{25} or D_{50} via central venous access, also with the intent to lessen large fluid volumes that would otherwise be necessary with administration of more dilute dextrose solutions. Recently, more concentrated dextrose (D_{70}) was safely used in two patients with BAA shock to support HDI therapy while minimizing total fluid infusion.[73]

If possible, cardiac function should be reassessed every 10 to 15 minutes after starting HDI therapy. If cardiac function remains depressed, then the insulin dose should be increased. This assessment can be done with complex cardiac output measurement or simply as a gross bedside ultrasound interpretation, depending on availability. Although we typically recommend dosing up to 10 units/kg/h, doses up to 22 units/kg/h have been used, and the maximum dose is not established.[12,78] The blood glucose should be monitored every 15 to 30 minutes until stable and then every 1 to 2 hours. The dextrose infusion should be increased to maintain blood glucose concentrations between 100 and 250 mg/dL (5.5–14 mmol/L) rather than reducing the insulin.

The serum potassium concentration should be measured during HDI therapy. If it is low, especially when potassium loss is suspected, then supplementation is indicated to maintain the concentration in the "mildly hypokalemic" range (2.8–3.2 mEq/L). A reasonable time frame is to evaluate serum potassium hourly while actively titrating the insulin infusion and every 6 hours after the infusion rate is stabilized. Magnesium and phosphorus should also be measured and supplemented as indicated. However, unless there is reason for loss of these three electrolytes, lowered serum concentrations likely reflect compartmental shifts, not depletion.

The ultimate goal of HDI is improvement in organ perfusion as demonstrated by increased cardiac output, improved mental status, adequate urine output, and reversal of metabolic abnormalities, as indicated by serum lactate, bicarbonate, pH, and base excess. This improvement is often, but not always, accompanied by an improvement in mean arterial blood pressure. Because insulin improves both cardiac function and perfusion while slightly vasodilating, treatment goals should focus more on organ perfusion and outcome as opposed to simply the numerical blood pressure. An increase in the rate of dextrose infusion to maintain euglycemia often accompanies hemodynamic and metabolic improvements. This increase in dextrose demand is due, in part, to increased CCB or BAA metabolism and loss of the CCB-induced diabetogenic influences, and it can be regarded as a favorable prognostic indicator.

The typical duration of therapy is 1 to 2 days, although HDI has been used for up to 4 days. We recommend reducing the insulin infusion rate by 1 unit/kg/h after the patient has stabilized and reassessing hourly for additional infusion reduction while maintaining adequate perfusion. In many patients, the dextrose infusion will continue to be necessary after the insulin is reduced and ultimately eliminated. The reduction of insulin and dextrose will cause potassium shifting, which should also be monitored.

SUMMARY

- High-dose insulin is recommended to augment cardiac function and perfusion in the context of cardiogenic shock caused by CCBs and BAAs.
- This therapy supports the metabolic demands associated with the cardiogenic shock and augments calcium processing, thereby increasing myocardial contractility and improving tissue perfusion.
- High doses of concentrated regular insulin are given intravenously, along with appropriate amounts of dextrose, and specific monitoring is required of serum glucose and potassium, in addition to surrogate markers of tissue perfusion, such as cardiac output, urine output, bicarbonate, pH, and lactate.

REFERENCES

1. Aaronson PM, et al. Hyperinsulinemia euglycemia, continuous veno-venous hemofiltration, and extracorporeal life support for severe verapamil poisoning: case report. *Clin Toxicol.* 2009;47:742.

2. Armenian P, et al. Prolonged absorption from a sustained-release verapamil preparation with documentation of serum levels and their response to intralipid. *Clin Toxicol.* 2010;48:646.

3. Bertrand L, et al. Insulin signaling in the heart. *Cardiovasc Res.* 2008;79:238-248.

4. Bilbault P, et al. Is digoxin poisoning improved by insulin? A case report. *Clin Toxicol.* 2005;43:510.

5. Bechtel LK, et al. Verapamil toxicity dysregulates the phosphatidylinositol 3-kinase pathway. *Acad Emerg Med.* 2008;15:368-374.

6. Boyer EW, et al. Hyperinsulinemia/euglycemia therapy for calcium channel blocker poisoning. *Pediatr Emerg Care.* 2002;18:36-37.

7. Boyer EW, Shannon M. Treatment of calcium-channel-blocker intoxication with insulin infusion. *N Engl J Med.* 2001;344:1721-1722.

8. Bryant SM, et al. Seven years of high dose insulin therapy for calcium channel antagonist poisoning. *Clin Toxicol.* 2009;27:751.

9. Bouchard NC, et al. Prolonged resuscitation for massive amlodipine overdose with maximal vasopressors, intralipids and veno arterial-extracorporeal membrane oxygenation (VA ECMO). *Clin Toxicol.* 2010;48:613.

10. Buiumsohn A, et al. Seizures and intraventricular conduction defect in propranolol poisoning. A report of two cases. *Ann Intern Med.* 1979;91:860-862.

11. Catalucci D, et al. Akt increases sarcoplasmic reticulum Ca2+ cycling by direct phosphorylation of phopholamban at Thr 17. *J Biol Chem.* 2009;284:28180-28187.

12. Cole JB, et al. A blinded, randomized, controlled trial of three doses of high-dose insulin in poison-induced cardiogenic shock. *Clin Toxicol.* 2013;51:201-207.

13. Cole JB, et al. Failure of high dose insulin and intravenous fat emulsion in 2 patients with poison-induced cardiogenic shock. *Clin Toxicol.* 2011;49:537-538.

14. Cumpston K, et al. Failure of hyperinsulinemia/euglycemia therapy in severe diltiazem overdose. *J Toxicol Clin Toxicol.* 2002;40:618.

15. Cumpston KL, Rose SR. Titration of hyperinsulinemia euglycemia therapy for the treatment of acute diltiazem toxicity. *Clin Toxicol.* 2009;47:724.

16. Devis G, et al. Calcium antagonists and islet function. I. Inhibition of insulin release by verapamil. *Diabetes.* 1975;24:247-251.

17. DeWitt CR, Waksman JC. Pharmacology, pathophysiology, and management of calcium channel blocker and beta-blocker toxicity. *Toxicol Rev.* 2004;23:223-238.

18. Dolcourt BA, Hedge MW. Hyperinsulinemia euglycemic therapy for symptomatic amiodarone ingestion. *Clin Toxicol.* 2009;47:717.

19. Draznin B. Intracellular calcium, insulin secretion, and action. *Am J Med.* 1988;85:44-58.

20. Engebretsen KM, et al. Therapeutic misadventure of high dose insulin without adverse effects. *Clin Toxicol.* 2008;26:604.

21. Engebretsen KM, et al. High-dose insulin therapy in beta-blocker and calcium channel-blocker poisoning. *Clin Toxicol.* 2011;49:277-283.

22. Engebretsen KM, et al. Addition of phenylephrine to high-dose insulin in dihydropyridine overdose does not improve outcome. *Clin Toxicol.* 2010;48:806-812.

23. Enyeart JJ, et al. Profound hyperglycemia and metabolic acidosis after verapamil overdose. *J Am Coll Cardiol.* 1983;2:1228-1231.

24. Gradinac S, et al. Improved cardiac function with glucose-insulin-potassium after aorto-coronary bypass grafting. *Ann Thorac Surg.* 1989;48:484-489.

25. Greene SL, et al. Relative safety of hyperinsulinaemia/euglycaemia in the management of calcium channel blocker overdose: a prospective observational study. *Intensive Care Med.* 2007;33:2019-2024.

26. Goldberg RJ, et al. Glucagon treatment of combined beta-blocker and calcium channel blocker toxicity. *Clin Toxicol.* 2002;40:351.

27. Harris NS. Case records of the Massachusetts General Hospital. Case 24-2006. A 40-year-old woman with hypotension after an overdose of amlodipine. *N Engl J Med.* 2006;355:602-611.

28. Hasin T, et al. The use of low-dose insulin in cardiogenic shock due to combined overdose of verapamil, enalapril and metoprolol. *Cardiology.* 2006;106:233-236.

29. Herbert JX, et al. Verapamil overdosage unresponsive to dextrose/insulin therapy. *J Toxicol Clin Toxicol.* 2001;39:293-294.

30. Hiesmayr M, et al. Effects of dobutamine versus insulin on cardiac performance, myocardial oxygen demand, and total body metabolism after coronary artery bypass grafting. *J Cardiothoracic Vasc Anesth.* 1995;9:653-658.

31. Holger JS, et al. High dose insulin in toxic cardiogenic shock. *Clin Toxicol.* 2009;47:303-307.

32. Holger JS, et al. Insulin versus vasopressin and epinephrine to treat beta-blocker toxicity. *Clin Toxicol.* 2007;45:396-401.

33. Holger JS, et al. Cardiovascular and metabolic effects of high-dose insulin in a porcine septic shock model. *Acad Emerg Med.* 2010;17:429-435.

34. Holger JS, et al. High-dose insulin: a consecutive case series in toxin-induced cardiogenic shock. *Clin Toxicol.* 2011;49:653-658.

35. Hsu CH, et al. Cellular mechanisms responsible for the inotropic action of insulin on failing human myocardium. *J Heart Lung Transplant.* 2006;25:1126-1134.

36. Ionescu-Tirgoviste C, et al. Plasma phosphorus and magnesium values during treatment of severe diabetic ketoacidosis. *Med Intern.* 1981;19:66-68.

37. Jolly SR, et al. Effect of hyperkalemia on experimental myocardial depression by verapamil. *Am Heart J.* 1991;121:517-523.

38. Kanagarajan K, et al. The use of vasopressin in the setting of recalcitrant hypotension due to calcium channel blocker overdose. *Clin Toxicol.* 2007;45:56-59.

39. Katzung KG, et al. Randomized controlled trial comparing high-dose insulin (HDI) to vasopressors or combination therapy in refractory toxin-induced shock [abstract]. *J Med Toxicol.* 2016;12:3.

40. Kebler R, et al. Dynamic changes in serum phosphorus levels in diabetic ketoacidosis. *Am J Med.* 1985;79:571-576.

41. Kerns W, et al. Insulin improves survival in a canine model of acute beta-blocker toxicity. *Ann Emerg Med.* 1997;29:748-757.

42. Kline J, et al. Beneficial myocardial metabolic effects of insulin during verapamil toxicity in the anesthetized canine. *Crit Care Med.* 1995;23:1251-1263.

43. Kline J, et al. Myocardial metabolism during graded intraportal verapamil infusion in awake dogs. *J Cardiovasc Pharmacol.* 1996; 27:719-726.

44. Kline JA, et al. Insulin improves heart function and metabolism during non-ischemic cardiogenic shock in awake canines. *Cardiovasc Res.* 1997;34:289-298.

45. Kline JA, et al. The diabetogenic effects of acute verapamil poisoning. *Toxicol Appl Pharmacol.* 1997;145:357-362.

46. Kline JA, et al. Insulin is a superior antidote for cardiovascular toxicity induced by verapamil in the anesthetized canine. *J Pharmacol Exp Ther.* 1993;267:744-750.

47. Laskey D, et al. Stability of high-dose insulin in normal saline bags for treatment of calcium channel blocker and beta blocker overdose. *Clin Toxicol.* 2016;54:829-832.

48. Levine M, et al. Assessment of hyperglycemia after calcium channel blocker overdoses including diltiazem or verapamil. *Crit Care Med.* 2007;35:2071-2075.

49. Lookabill SK, et al. Undifferentiated toxin-induced cardiogenic shock treated with high dose insulin [abstract]. *J Med Toxicol.* 2016;12:23-24.

50. Louters LL, et al. Verapamil inhibits the glucose transport activity of GLUT-1. *J Med Toxicol.* 2010;6:100-105.

51. Lucchesi BR, et al. The positive inotropic actions of insulin in the canine heart. *Eur J Pharmacol.* 1972;18:107-115.

52. Marques M, et al. Treatment of calcium channel blocker intoxication with insulin infusion: case report and literature review. *Resuscitation.* 2003;57:211-213.

53. Masters TN, Glaviano VV. Effects of d,l-propranolol on myocardial free fatty acid and carbohydrate metabolism. *J Pharmacol Exp Ther.* 1969;167:187-193.

54. Mégarbane B, et al. Intentional overdose with insulin: prognostic factors and toxicokinetic/toxicodynamic profiles. *Crit Care.* 2007;11:R115.

55. Merimee TJ. The relationship of insulin I131 to serum protein fractions. *Bull Johns Hopkins Hosp.* 1965;116:191.

56. Meyer M, et al. Verapamil-induced hypotension reversed with dextrose-insulin. *J Toxicol Clin Toxicol.* 2001;39:500.

57. Miller AD, et al. Hypoglycemia in patients treated with high-dose insulin for calcium channel blocker poisoning. *J Toxicol Clin Toxicol.* 2006;44:782-783.

58. Min L, DeshPande K. Diltiazem overdose haemodynamic response to hyperinsulinaemia-euglycaemia therapy: a case report. *Crit Care Resusc.* 2004;6:28-30.

59. Montiel V, et al. Diltiazem poisoning treated with hyperinsulinemic euglycemia therapy and intravenous lipid emulsion. *Eur J Emerg Med.* 2011;18:121-123.

60. Morris-Kukoski CL, et al. Insulin "euglycemia" therapy for accidental nifedipine overdose. *J Toxicol Clin Toxicol.* 2000;38:577.

61. Nickson CP, Little M. Early use of high-dose insulin euglycaemic therapy for verapamil toxicity. *Med J Aust.* 2009;191:350-352.

62. Nugent M, et al. Verapamil worsens rate of development and hemodynamic effects of acute hyperkalemia in halothane-anesthetized dogs: effects of calcium therapy. *Anesthesiology.* 1984;60:435-439.

63. Ortiz-Munoz L, et al. Hyperinsulinemia-euglycemia therapy for intoxication with calcium channel blockers. *Boletin Associacion Medica de Puerto Rico.* 2005;97:182-189.

64. Page CB, et al. The use of high-dose insulin glucose euglycemia in beta-blocker overdose: a case report. *J Med Toxicol.* 2009;5:139-142.

65. Paolisso G, et al. Insulin induces opposite changes in plasma and erythrocyte magnesium concentrations in man. *Diabetologia.* 1986;29:644-647.

66. Patterson KR, et al. Undesired effects of insulin therapy. *Adverse Drug React Acute Poisoning Rev.* 1983;2:219-234.

67. Pizon AF, et al. Calcium channel blocker overdose: one center's experience. *Clin Toxicol.* 2005;43:679-680.

68. Place R, et al. Hyperinsulin therapy in the treatment of verapamil overdose. *J Toxicol Clin Toxicol.* 2000;38:576-577.

69. Rabkin R, et al. Effects of renal disease on renal uptake and excretion of insulin in man. *N Engl J Med.* 1970;282:182-187.

70. Rasmussen L, et al. Severe intoxication after an intentional overdose of amlodipine. *Acta Anaesthesiol Scand.* 2003;47:1038-1040.

71. Reikeras O, et al. Metabolic effects of high doses of insulin during acute left ventricular failure in dogs. *Eur Heart J.* 1985;6:451-457.

72. Robinson DM, Wellington K. Insulin glulisine. *Drugs.* 2006;66:861-869.

73. Robinson H, et al. Infusion of 70% Dextrose to minimize risk of fluid overload in high dose insulin therapy: a case series [abstract]. *J Med Toxicol.* 2017;13:26-27.

74. Saely S, et al. Case series of severe calcium channel blocker toxicity treated with high concentration of high dose insulin therapy. *Clin Toxicol.* 2011;49:593.

75. Schoffstall JM, et al. Effects of calcium channel blocker overdose-induced toxicity in the conscious dog. *Ann Emerg Med.* 1991;20:1104-1108.

76. Shah SN, et al. History of insulin. *J Assoc Physicians Ind.* 1997;45(suppl 1):4-9.

77. Smith SW, et al. Prolonged severe hypotension following combined amlodipine and valsartan ingestion. *Clin Toxicol.* 2008;46:470-474.

78. Stellpflug SJ, et al. Intentional overdose with cardiac arrest treated with intravenous fat emulsion and high-dose insulin. *Clin Toxicol.* 2010;48:227-229.

79. Stellpflug SJ, et al. Cardiotoxic overdose treated with intravenous fat emulsion and high dose insulin in the setting of hypertrophic cardiomyopathy. *J Med Toxicol.* 2011;7:151-153.

80. St-Onge M, et al. Recommendations for the treatment of calcium channel blocker poisoning. *Crit Care Med.* 2017;45:e306-e315.

81. Svedjeholm R, et al. High-dose insulin improves the efficacy of dopamine early after cardiac surgery. A study of myocardial performance and oxygen consumption. *Scand J Thorac Cardiovasc Surg.* 1991;25:215-221.

82. Weibrecht KW, Rhyee SH. Delayed hyperglycemia following verapamil overdose. *Clin Toxicol.* 2010;48:656.

83. Verbrugge LB, van Wezel HB. Pathophysiology of verapamil overdose: new insights in the role of insulin. *J Cardiothorac Vasc Anesth.* 2007;21:406-409.

84. Visscher MB, Muller EA. The influence of insulin upon the mammalian heart. *J Physiol.* 1927;62:341-348.

85. Vogt S, et al. Survival of severe amlodipine intoxication due to medical intensive care. *Forensic Sci Int.* 2006;161:216-220.

86. von Lewinsk D, et al. Insulin causes $[Ca^{2+}]_i$-dependent and $[Ca^{2+}]_i$-independent positive inotropic effects in failing human myocardium. *Circulation.* 2005;111:2588-2595.

87. Yuan TH, et al. Insulin-glucose as adjunctive therapy for severe calcium channel antagonist poisoning. *J Toxicol Clin Toxicol.* 1999;37:463-467.

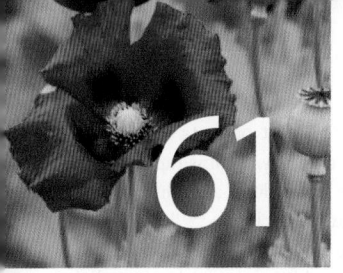

61 MISCELLANEOUS ANTIHYPERTENSIVES AND PHARMACOLOGICALLY RELATED AGENTS

Hallam Melville Gugelmann and Francis Jerome DeRoos

Hypertension is one of the most prevalent chronic medical problems and one of the most readily amenable to pharmacotherapy. Antihypertensive pharamacotherapeutics were first used in the 1960s after two studies independently linked asymptomatic hypertension to significant adverse effects such as stroke, myocardial infarction (MI), and sudden death.[74,92] The first antihypertensives used included centrally acting sympatholytics, direct vasodilators, sodium nitroprusside, and diuretics. Unfortunately, these often had significant adverse events, leading to the development of β-adrenergic antagonists, calcium channel blockers (CCBs), angiotensin-converting enzyme inhibitors (ACEIs), angiotensin receptor blockers (ARBs), and direct renin inhibitors (DRIs) (Table 61-1). This chapter reviews early antihypertensives, as well ACEIs, ARBs, and DRIs. In general, the majority of antihypertensives manifest clinical signs and symptoms in terms of the degree of hypotension produced. Particular attention will be placed on mechanisms of action and unique toxicologic considerations for each of these xenobiotics.

CLONIDINE AND OTHER CENTRALLY ACTING ANTIHYPERTENSIVES

Clonidine is an imidazoline compound synthesized in the early 1960s. Because of its potent peripheral α_2-adrenergic agonist effects, it was initially studied as a topical nasal decongestant.[218] However, hypotension

TABLE 61–1 Antihypertensives and Pharmacologically Related Xenobiotics

β-Adrenergic antagonists (Chap. 59)
Calcium channel blockers (Chap. 60)
Sympatholytics (antagonize α-adrenergic vasoconstriction)
   Central α_2-adrenergic agonists
      Clonidine, dexmedetomidine, guanabenz,[a] guanfacine,[a] methyldopa,[a] tizanidine
   Central imidazoline agonists
      Moxonidine, rilmenidine
   Ganglionic blockers
      Trimethaphan[a]
   Peripheral adrenergic neuron antagonists
      Guanadrel,[a] metyrosine,[a] reserpine[a]
   Peripheral α_1-adrenergic antagonists
      Doxazosin, prazosin, silodosin, terazosin
Diuretics
   Thiazides
      Bendroflumethiazide,[a] chlorthalidone,[a] chlorothiazide, hydrochlorothiazide, hydroflumethiazide,[a] indapamide, methyclothiazide,[a] metolazone, polythiazide,[a] trichlormethiazide[a]
   Loop diuretics
      Bumetanide, ethacrynic acid, furosemide, torsemide
   Potassium-sparing diuretics
      Amiloride, eplerenone, spironolactone, triamterene
Vasodilators
   Diazoxide,[a] hydralazine, minoxidil,[a] nitroprusside
Angiotensin-converting enzyme inhibitor
   Benazepril, captopril, enalapril, fosinopril, lisinopril, moexipril, perindopril, quinapril, ramipril, spirapril, trandolapril
Angiotensin II receptor blockers
   Azilsartan, candesartan, eprosartan, irbesartan, losartan, olmesartan, telmisartan, valsartan
Direct renin inhibitors
   Aliskiren

[a]Included for historical reference; use as an antihypertensive is limited in the United States.

was a common adverse event, which redirected its consideration for other therapeutic applications.[101] Clonidine is the most commonly used of all the centrally acting antihypertensives, a group that includes methyldopa, guanfacine, and guanabenz. Although these drugs differ chemically and structurally, they all decrease blood pressure in a similar manner. The imidazoline compounds oxymetazoline and tetrahydrozoline, which are used as ophthalmic topical vasoconstrictors and nasal decongestants (Chap. 49), produce similar systemic effects when ingested.[101]

Although the increased efficacy and improved adverse event profiles of newer antihypertensives diminished the use of the α_2-adrenergic agonists in routine hypertension management, use of these xenobiotics is increasing as a result of a wide variety of applications, including attention deficit hyperactivity disorder, peripheral nerve and spinal anesthesia, and compounded skin creams[181] and as an adjunct in the management of opioid, ethanol, and nicotine withdrawal.[117,122] In addition, abuse of clonidine remains a problem in opioid-dependent patients and is reportedly used in criminal acts of chemical submission.[21,137]

Ingestion of centrally acting imidazolines can cause significant toxicity, particularly in children. One report from two large pediatric hospitals identified 47 children requiring hospitalization for unintentional clonidine ingestions over a 5-year period.[239] Significant clonidine poisoning also results from formulation and dosing errors in children[193,221] and after imidazolines used as ocular vasoconstrictors, especially if ingested.[129,141,184]

Pharmacology

Clonidine and the other centrally acting antihypertensives exert their hypotensive effects primarily by stimulating two sets of receptors: presynaptic α_2-adrenergic receptors[22,75] and imidazoline receptors.[135,187] Central α_2-adrenergic receptor agonism enhances the activity of inhibitory neurons in the vasoregulatory regions of the central nervous system (CNS), including the locus ceruleus, the nucleus tractus solitarii in the medulla, and—possibly most prominently—in the rostral ventrolateral medulla,[35] resulting in decreased norepinephrine release.[200] Central agonism by imidazolines results in decreased sympathetic outflow from the intermediolateral cell columns of the thoracolumbar spinal tracts into the periphery and reduces the heart rate' vascular tone' and, ultimately, arterial blood pressure.[231] This centrally mediated sympatholytic effect is partially modulated by nitric oxide and γ-aminobutyric acid (GABA), which explains some of the clinical variability that occurs among patients who overdose with clonidine.[33,84,233] Imidazolines also have profound effects at imidazoline receptors, one of their primary sites of action. There are three recognized classes of imidazoline receptors. Imidazoline-1 (I_1) receptors mediate hypotensive effects of imidazolines by functioning upstream from presynaptic α_2-adrenergic receptors, likely in addition to other physiologic effects. Imidazoline-2 (I_2) receptors are involved in pain perception modulation and interact with monoamine oxidases A and B. Imidazoline-3 (I_3) receptors have effects on glucose homeostasis within pancreatic β-islet cells.[135] In addition to α- and imidazoline receptor–mediated effects, clonidine has opioidlike effects that are mediated through I_2 receptors[22] and through the release of β-endorphin, which directly stimulates opioid receptors.[242]

Pharmacokinetics

Clonidine is well absorbed from the gastrointestinal (GI) tract (~75%) with an onset of action within 30 to 60 minutes. The peak serum concentration occurs at 2 to 3 hours and lasts as long as 8 hours.[54] Clonidine has 20% to 40% protein binding (primarily to albumin) and an apparent volume of distribution of 3.2 to 5.6 L/kg.[130] The majority of clonidine is eliminated unchanged via the kidneys.[134]

Clonidine is available in both oral and transdermal ("patch") forms. Transdermal systems allow slow, continuous delivery of drug over a prolonged period of time, ranging from 72 hours to 1 week (Special Considerations: SC3). This formulation, however, offers unique clinical challenges. Each patch contains significantly more drug than is typically delivered during the prescribed duration of use. For example, a patch that delivers 0.1 mg/day of clonidine contains a total of 2.5 mg, the product that delivers 0.3 mg/day contains a total of 7.5 mg.[32] Even after 1 week of use, between 35% and 50% and, in some instances, as much as 70% of the drug remains in the patch.[32,95] Puncturing the outer membrane layer or backing opens the drug reservoir and allows a significant amount of the drug to be released rapidly. In addition, patients do not perceive this delivery system as a medication and thus do not always exercise appropriate precautions when disposing of used patches. For example, numerous reports of toxicity in both adults and children have resulted from dermal exposure of discarded patches, mouthing, or ingesting a clonidine patch.[32,45,185] Compounding creams, often inadvertently containing massive amounts of clonidine, have caused significant toxicity.[193]

Guanfacine and guanabenz are structurally and pharmacologically very similar to each other. They are well absorbed orally, achieving peak concentrations within 3 to 5 hours, and both have large volumes of distribution (4–6 L/kg for guanfacine and 7–17 L/kg for guanabenz).[104,216] Whereas guanabenz is metabolized predominantly in the liver and undergoes extensive first-pass effect, guanfacine is eliminated equally by the liver and kidney.[104,216] The metabolism of neither drug results in the production of significant active metabolites. Guanabenz is infrequently used.[145]

Whereas clonidine, guanabenz, and guanfacine are all active drugs with direct α_2-adrenergic agonist effects, methyldopa is a prodrug. It enters the CNS, probably by an active transport mechanism, before it is converted into its pharmacologically active degradation products.[24] α-Methylnorepinephrine is the most significant of its metabolites, although α-methyldopamine and α-methylepinephrine also are active.[71,97,191] These metabolites are direct α_2-adrenergic agonists and have similar effects and mechanism as the other centrally acting antihypertensives. Approximately 50% of an oral dose of methyldopa is absorbed, and peak serum concentrations are achieved in 2 to 3 hours.[158] However, because methyldopa requires metabolism into its active form, these concentrations have little correlation with its clinical effects. Methyldopa has a small volume of distribution (0.24 L/kg) and little protein binding (15%).[158] It is eliminated in the urine, both as parent compound and after hepatic sulfation.[165] Methyldopa is still used for the management of postpartum hypertension.[87]

Pathophysiology

In therapeutic oral dosing, clonidine and the other centrally acting antihypertensives have little effect on the peripheral α_2 receptors, the peripheral sympathetic nervous system, or the normal circulatory responses that occur with exercise or the Valsalva maneuver.[157,169] However, when serum concentrations increase above 2 ng/mL, as in the setting of intravenous (IV) administration or oral overdose, peripheral postsynaptic α_1-adrenergic stimulation occurs, producing temporary vasoconstriction and hypertension.[42,54] Shortly afterward, however, potent centrally mediated sympathetic inhibition becomes the predominant effect, and bradycardia with hypotension ensues.[5,156,191]

Clinical Manifestations

Although the majority of the published cases involve clonidine, the signs and symptoms of poisoning with any centrally acting antihypertensive are similar. The CNS and cardiovascular toxicity reflect an exaggeration of their pharmacologic action. In the context of large overdoses, initial α_1 agonism results in hypertension and tachycardia, typically transient,[113] followed by the more predominant signs of imidazoline toxicity, including CNS depression, bradycardia,

hypotension, and occasionally hypothermia.[7,208,229] Most patients who ingest clonidine or the other similarly acting drugs manifest symptoms rapidly, typically within 30 to 90 minutes.[239] The exception is methyldopa, a prodrug, which requires metabolism to be activated, delaying toxicity for hours.[208,241]

Central nervous system depression is the most frequent clinical finding, ranging from mild lethargy to coma.[147] In addition, severely obtunded patients often experience decreased ventilatory effort and hypoxia.[5] Respirations are often slow and shallow, with intermittent deep, sighing breaths. Various other terms are used to describe this phenomenon, including gasping, Cheyne-Stokes respirations, and periodic apnea.[7,11,147] This hypoventilation is characteristically responsive to tactile stimuli in children, although mechanical ventilation is required in severe cases.[5,98] The associated CNS depression typically resolves over 12 to 36 hours.[11,168] Other manifestations of this CNS depression include hypotonia, hyporeflexia, and irritability.[42,147,220] The cranial nerve examination often demonstrates miotic pupils, typically reactive to light.[5,7,223] Two unusual case reports describe seizures in the setting of clonidine poisoning,[42,176] the mechanism of which is unclear.

Hypothermia is associated with overdoses involving centrally acting antihypertensives.[7,147,176,191] This is thought to be a consequence of α-adrenergic effects within the thermoregulatory center, although some authors suggest that these drugs activate central serotonergic pathways that alter normal thermoregulation.[130,151] Although this phenomenon sometimes lasts for several hours, it rarely requires treatment and typically responds well to passive rewarming.[42,176] Sinus bradycardia occurs in up to 50% of patients who ingest clonidine, resulting from the combination of an exaggerated centrally mediated sympatholytic effect, a centrally mediated increase in vagal tone or a direct stimulation of α_2-adrenergic receptors on the myocardium.[33,50,127,220,239]

Other conduction abnormalities, including first-degree heart block, type 1 and 2 Mobitz atrioventricular block, and complete heart block, are described both in overdose and after therapeutic dosing.[119,168,202] It appears that very young patients and patients who have underlying sinus node dysfunction, concurrent sympatholytic drug therapy, or chronic kidney disease (CKD) are at particular risk of developing bradydysrhythmia after central antihypertensive ingestion.[28,220,224] Hypotension is the major cardiovascular manifestation of central antihypertensive toxicity.[7,32] Although studies suggest a dose–response relationship between the estimated quantity of the centrally acting antihypertensive ingested and the severity of the clinical manifestations, clonidine ingestions as small as 0.2 mg can cause clinically severe poisoning, mandating the necessity to individually assess each exposure. The presence of any symptoms should prompt immediate medical evaluation,[19,168] especially in pediatric patients and exposures to compounding creams.[34] Fatalities from any of these xenobiotics are rare.[109]

After deaths of four children who were prescribed clonidine were reported, concerns that there was a causal association between combination clonidine–methylphenidate therapy and sudden death were raised.[67] Closer scrutiny of these cases revealed significant confounders, however, and a formal investigation by the US Food and Drug Administration concluded that there was inadequate evidence to confirm this association.[222]

Diagnostic Testing

Clonidine and other centrally acting antihypertensives are not routinely included in rapidly accessible serum or urine toxicologic assays. Consequently, management decisions should be based on clinical parameters. No electrolyte or hematologic abnormalities are associated with this exposure. Because of the potential for bradydysrhythmia and hypoventilation, 12-lead electrocardiography (ECG), end-tidal CO_2, and continuous cardiac and pulse oximetry monitoring are recommended.

Management

Appropriate therapy begins with particular focus on the patient's respiratory and hemodynamic status. Administration of activated charcoal (AC) is the primary mode of GI decontamination in most cases of ingestion; however, altered mental status and severe respiratory depression typically limit the ability to administer AC. Patients often present after the onset of symptoms rather than immediately after ingestion, and patients respond well to supportive care. In cases involving clonidine patch ingestions, whole-bowel irrigation (WBI) appears to be an effective intervention and is reasonable only if the airway status is stable or secure.[99,106]

All patients with CNS depression should be evaluated for hypoxia and hypoglycemia. Those with respiratory compromise, including apnea, often respond well to simple auditory or tactile stimulation.[5,7,98] Significant arousal during preparation for intubation often precludes the need for mechanical ventilation.[5] Endotracheal intubation should be performed in patients who fail to arouse to stimuli or those with evidence of airway compromise.

Patients with isolated hypotension should initially be treated with IV boluses of crystalloid: 20 mL/kg in children and 500 to 1,000 mL in adults. Bradycardia is typically mild and usually does not require any therapy if adequate peripheral perfusion exists. If symptomatic bradycardia occurs, then atropine is recommended but, frequently requires multiple doses.[5,7,140]

It is likely that naloxone was first used in clonidine-poisoned patients because the clinical findings of CNS and respiratory depression and miosis are similar to opioid-poisoned patients.[163] Clonidine-poisoned patients, particularly children, often show increased arousal, respiratory effort, heart rate, and blood pressure after naloxone administration.[11,125,163,223] Although unclear mechanistically, this effect is likely related to modulation of CNS sympathetic outflow by endogenous CNS opioids.[25,66] This concept is supported by a clinical study in which clonidine administration to hypertensive patients for 3 days resulted in a significant decrease in blood pressure. Subsequent administration of 0.4 mg of parenteral naloxone reversed the decrease in blood pressure and heart rate in almost 60% of the patients.[65] Because of the short duration of effects of naloxone (20–60 minutes), redosing or continuous infusions are often required. As with some synthetic opioids, such as propoxyphene and fentanyl, clinical improvement sometimes occurs only after high doses (4–10 mg) of naloxone,[70,144] and some patients have no response regardless of dose used.[140,239] Hypertension can occur after administration of naloxone in pediatric clonidine overdoses.[86]

Early-onset hypertension in imidazoline toxicity is typically self-limited, and therapy should be cautiously undertaken. Treatment with esmolol theoretically can exacerbate this paradoxical hypertension in a manner similar to that which occurs when β-adrenergic antagonists are used in cocaine toxicity, namely by inducing unopposed α_1-receptor stimulation (Chap. 75). Although oral nifedipine has been used,[53] it cannot be titrated and has unpredictable efficacy. If hypertension is severe or prolonged, treatment with a short-acting and titratable antihypertensive such as IV nicardipine and sodium nitroprusside is reasonable.[147]

Withdrawal

Abrupt cessation of central antihypertensive therapy results in withdrawal, typically characterized by excessive sympathetic activity. Symptoms include agitation, insomnia, tremor, palpitations, tachycardia, and hypertension that begin between 16 and 48 hours after cessation of therapy.[29,186,197] Complications of clonidine withdrawal can include ventricular tachycardia and MI.[20,160,177] The frequency and severity of symptoms appear to be greater in patients treated with higher doses for several months and in those with the most severe pretreatment hypertension.[186] Shorter acting xenobiotics such as clonidine and guanabenz are more frequently associated with withdrawal.[79,183] In addition, because of prolonged and continuous exposures, children being treated with extended-release guanfacine formulations and transdermal patches are at greater risk of developing withdrawal upon cessation. The mechanism for this hyperadrenergic phenomenon involves an increase in CNS noradrenergic activity in the setting of decreased α_2-receptor sensitivity.[61] Animal and human data suggest that β-adrenergic antagonists, including labetalol, are contraindicated in clonidine withdrawal.[10,114] As noted earlier, esmolol can, in theory, exacerbate this paradoxical hypertension in a manner similar to that which is proposed when these xenobiotics are used for patients manifesting cocaine toxicity (ie, by inducing unopposed α_1-receptor stimulation) (Chap. 75). Reasonable treatment strategies include administering clonidine

or benzodiazepines, via either the oral or IV route, followed by a closely monitored tapering of the dosing over several weeks.

CENTRAL IMIDAZOLINE AGONISTS

Moxonidine and related rilmenidine are known as second-generation centrally acting oral antihypertensives.[58] They are structurally similar to clonidine but selectively attach at I_1 imidazoline binding sites (found predominantly in the rostral ventrolateral medulla), with much less affinity for the α_2-adrenergic receptor.[62] As noted earlier, I_1 binding ultimately leads to decreased sympathetic outflow from the medulla, vasodilation, and reduction in blood pressure. Although nitric oxide or GABA mechanisms are also contributory,[174,175] animal studies suggest that α_2-adrenergic receptor effects predominantly mediate central effects with these xenobiotics.[41] Therapeutically, moxonidine is used both as monotherapy or in combination with other antihypertensives. Patients with diabetes or metabolic syndrome benefit from moxonidine because of its positive effects on insulin resistance, impaired glucose tolerance, and hyperlipidemia.[58,68] Case reports of seizures (resolving with benzodiazepines) without development of hypotension suggest that weak α_2-adrenergic receptor affinity is overwhelmed in overdose.[139]

Dexmedetomidine is a newer centrally acting imidazoline agonist used for sedation in intensive care settings. In contrast to moxonidine and rilmenidine, dexmedetomidine is highly selective for the α_2-adrenergic receptor and has profound sedating, analgesic-sparing, and sympatholytic effects. Side effects include bradycardia and hypotension.[118] Withdrawal from this xenobiotic can result in tachycardia, agitation, and hypertension.[124]

OTHER SYMPATHOLYTIC ANTIHYPERTENSIVES

Several other xenobiotics also exert their antihypertensive effect by decreasing the effects of the sympathetic nervous system. Often termed *sympatholytics*, they can be classified as ganglionic blockers (eg, trimetaphan), presynaptic adrenergic blockers (eg, reserpine), or α_1-adrenergic antagonists (eg, prazosin), depending on their mechanism of action. Of these xenobiotics, the ganglionic blockers are rarely used clinically, and little is known about their effects in overdose; the presynaptic adrenergic blockers and α_1-adrenergic antagonists are reviewed briefly next.

Presynaptic Adrenergic Antagonists

Guanethidine

These xenobiotics exert their sympatholytic action by decreasing norepinephrine release from presynaptic nerve terminals. Whereas guanethidine and guanadrel interfere with the action potential that triggers norepinephrine release,[205] reserpine depletes norepinephrine, serotonin, and other catecholamines from the presynaptic nerve terminals by direct binding and inactivation of catecholamine storage vesicles.[80] Adverse events limit their clinical usefulness. These effects include a high incidence of orthostatic and exercise-induced hypotension, diarrhea, increased gastric secretions, and impotence;[161] hypotensive effects have lasted for as long as 1 week.[116,206] Likely because of its ability to cross the blood–brain barrier, reserpine depletes central catecholamines and produces drowsiness, extrapyramidal symptoms, hallucinations, migraine headaches, or depression.[133] In overdose, an extension of their pharmacologic effects is expected. Patients with severe orthostatic hypotension are treated with IV crystalloid boluses and a direct-acting vasopressor. If reserpine is involved, significant CNS depression should also be anticipated.[133]

Peripheral α₁-Adrenergic Antagonists

The selective α_1-adrenergic antagonists include prazosin, terazosin, and doxazosin. The α_1 receptor is a postsynaptic receptor primarily located on vascular smooth muscle, although they are also found in the eye and in the GI and genitourinary tracts.[46,103] These xenobiotics are used to treat urinary dysfunction secondary to benign prostatic hyperplasia.[18] They produce arterial smooth muscle relaxation, vasodilation, and a reduction of the blood pressure. Although better tolerated than ganglionic blockers and peripheral adrenergic neuron blockers, these medications are associated with significant symptoms of postural hypotension, including lightheadedness, syncope, or palpitations, particularly after the first dose or if the dosing is rapidly increased.[18] Hypotension and CNS depression ranging from lethargy to coma are reported in overdose.[128,131,199] Their use has also resulted in priapism.[189] Treatment of peripheral α_1–adrenergic agonist includes supportive care, IV crystalloid boluses, and a vasopressor, with phenylephrine being a logical initial choice.

DIRECT VASODILATORS

Hydralazine, Minoxidil, and Diazoxide

These xenobiotics produce vascular smooth muscle relaxation independent of innervation or known pharmacologic receptors.[56,115,121] This vasodilatory effect is attributed to stimulation of nitric oxide release from vascular endothelial cells. The nitric oxide then diffuses into the underlying smooth muscle cells, stimulating guanylate cyclase to produce cyclic guanosine monophosphate (cGMP). This second messenger indirectly inhibits calcium entry into the smooth muscle cells, producing vasodilation.[198] Minoxidil, however, also has direct potassium channel activation effects;[123,161] the opening of these adenosine triphosphate-linked potassium channels results in potassium influx and cell depolarization, thereby reducing calcium influx and ultimately relaxing vascular smooth muscle.[30] As this vasodilation occurs, the baroreceptor reflexes, which remain intact, produce an increased sympathetic outflow to the myocardium, resulting in an increase in heart rate and contractile force. Historically, these xenobiotics were used therapeutically in patients with severe, refractory hypertension and in conjunction with a β-adrenergic antagonist to diminish reflex tachycardia. Hydralazine continues to be used for the management of severe postpartum hypertension.[234] Hydralazine, minoxidil, and diazoxide are effective orally, but sodium nitroprusside is only used intravenously. Minoxidil is also used topically in a 2% solution to promote hair growth, and ingestion can cause significant poisoning.[64,150] Diazoxide, although previously used to rapidly reduce blood pressure in hypertensive emergencies, is rarely used for this indication now, given that it is not easily titrated and causes a variable, occasionally profound, hypotensive effect.[120] Adverse effects associated with daily hydralazine use include several immunologic phenomena such as hemolytic anemia, vasculitis, acute glomerulonephritis, and most notably a lupuslike syndrome.[178] Minoxidil is associated with changes on ECG, both in therapeutic doses and in overdose. Sinus tachycardia, ST-segment depression, and T-wave inversion are all reported.[91,180,213] There also appears to be an association with supratherapeutic doses of minoxidil and left ventricular multifocal, subacute necrosis, and subsequent fibrosis.[93,94] The significance of either of these changes is unknown; they typically resolve with either continued therapy or as other toxic manifestations resolve.[91,94] The common toxic manifestations of these xenobiotics in overdose are an extension of their pharmacologic action. Symptoms include lightheadedness, syncope, palpitations, and nausea.[3,138] Signs include tachycardia alone[180] or with flushing or alterations in mental status, typically related to the degree of hypotension.[150]

In the case of hydralazine, minoxidil, or diazoxide overdose, GI decontamination—including AC and, possibly, WBI—is reasonable followed by routine supportive care, with special consideration to maintaining adequate mean arterial pressure. If intravenous crystalloid boluses are insufficient, then a peripherally acting α-adrenergic agonist, such as norepinephrine or phenylephrine, is reasonable as the next therapy. Dopamine and epinephrine should be avoided to prevent an exaggerated myocardial response and tachycardia from β-adrenergic stimulation.

Nitroprusside

Nitroprusside

Sodium nitroprusside is effectively a prodrug, exerting its vasodilatory effects only after its breakdown and the release of nitric oxide. The nitroprusside molecule also contains five cyanide radicals that, although gradually released, occasionally produce cyanide or thiocyanate toxicity.[164,203] Methemoglobin binds small amounts of liberated cyanide, which are also cleared by interacting with various sulfhydryl groups and enzymatically in the liver by rhodanese, which couples them to thiosulfate-producing thiocyanate.[73] This cyanide detoxification process in healthy adults occurs at a rate of about 1 mcg/kg/min, which corresponds to a sodium nitroprusside infusion rate of 2 mcg/kg/min.[48,203] A variety of factors—including poor nutrition, critical illness, surgery, diuretic use, and young age—place patients at risk for developing cyanide toxicity.[37,48] The hemolysis associated with cardiopulmonary bypass (CPB) places patients at particular risk because the elevated free hemoglobin accelerates the release of cyanide from the sodium nitroprusside moiety.[37] Therefore, depending on the balance of cyanide release (eg, rate of sodium nitroprusside infusion) and the rate of cyanide detoxification (eg, sulfur donor stores), cyanide toxicity can develop within hours. Infusion rates greater than 4 mcg/kg/min of nitroprusside for longer than 12 hours are expected to overwhelm the capacity of rhodanese for detoxifying cyanide.[188] Signs and symptoms of cyanide toxicity include alteration in mental status; anion gap metabolic acidosis; elevated lactate concentration; and in late stages, hemodynamic instability. If cyanide poisoning does occur, hydroxycobalamin is the current treatment of choice (Chap. 123).

One method of preventing cyanide toxicity from sodium nitroprusside is to expand the thiosulfate pool available for detoxification by the concomitant administration of sodium thiosulfate.[48,89,153] Dosing of 1 g of sodium thiosulfate for every 100 mg of nitroprusside is typically sufficient to prevent cyanide accumulation.[188] Thiocyanate thus formed accumulates, particularly in patients with CKD or acute kidney injury (AKI), and produces thiocyanate toxicity.[73,203] Simultaneous infusion of thiosulfate does not interfere with the vasodilatory effects of sodium nitroprusside (Antidotes in Depth: A42).[100]

Thiocyanate is almost exclusively renally eliminated, with an elimination half-life of 3 to 7 days. It is postulated that a continuous sodium nitroprusside infusion of 2.5 mcg/kg/min in patients with normal renal function could produce thiocyanate toxicity within 7 to 14 days, although it may be as short as 3 to 6 days or as little as 1 mcg/kg/min in patients with CKD who are not receiving hemodialysis.[203] The signs and symptoms of thiocyanate toxicity begin to appear at serum concentrations of 60 mcg/mL (1 mmol/L) and are very nonspecific, ranging from nausea, vomiting, fatigue, and dizziness to confusion, delirium, and seizures.[73] Severe thiocyanate toxicity causes life-threatening effects, such as hypotension with intracranial pressure elevation, when serum concentrations are above 200 mcg/mL.[48,73,89] Anion gap metabolic acidosis and hemodynamic instability do not occur with thiocyanate toxicity. Although cyanide or thiocyanate concentrations are not typically useful in the management of patients with cyanide toxicity, they should be considered for monitoring critically ill patients who are at risk of thiocyanate poisoning. Hemodialysis clears thiocyanate from the serum; patients with significant clinical manifestations of thiocyanate toxicity benefit from hemodialysis.[60,146,154]

Another therapy used to prevent cyanide toxicity from sodium nitroprusside is a simultaneous infusion of hydroxocobalamin.[123] Dosing of 25 mg/h has successfully reduced cyanide poisoning in humans.[146] As with thiosulfate, simultaneous infusion of hydroxocobalamin does not interfere with the vasodilatory effects of sodium nitroprusside.[100] Because of the relative higher cost of hydroxocobalamin as well its interactions with some laboratory tests, thiosulfate should remain the mainstay of prophylaxis against sodium nitroprusside-induced cyanide toxicity (Antidotes in Depth: A41 and A42).

DIURETICS

Diuretics are divided into three main groups: (1) the thiazides and related compounds, including hydrochlorothiazide and chlorthalidone; (2) the loop diuretics, including furosemide, bumetanide, and ethacrynic acid; and (3) the potassium-sparing diuretics, including amiloride, triamterene, and spironolactone. Two other groups of diuretics—the carbonic anhydrase inhibitors, such as acetazolamide, and osmotic diuretics (eg, mannitol)—are not used in the treatment of hypertension.

The thiazides produce their diuretic effect by inhibition of sodium and chloride reabsorption in the distal convoluted tubule. Loop diuretics, in contrast, inhibit the coupled transport of sodium, potassium, and chloride in the thick ascending limb of the loop of Henle. Although their exact antihypertensive mechanism is unclear, an increased urinary excretion of sodium, potassium, and magnesium results from the use of loop diuretics. Potassium-sparing diuretics act either as aldosterone antagonists, such as spironolactone, or as renal epithelial sodium channel antagonists, such as triamterene, in the late distal tubule and collecting duct.[111]

The majority of toxicity associated with diuretics is metabolic and occurs during chronic therapy or overuse.[237] Hyponatremia develops within the first 2 weeks of initiation of diuretic therapy in more than 67% of susceptible patients, and female sex, old age, and malnourishment are the greatest risk factors.[9,215] Manifestations of severe hyponatremia ($[Na^+] <120$ mEq/L) include headache, nausea, vomiting, confusion, seizures, or coma (Chap. 12). The osmotic demyelination syndrome, formally known as central pontine myelinolysis, is reported during rapid correction of severe hyponatremia secondary to diuretic abuse.[44]

Diuretic use is associated with hypokalemia and hypomagnesemia and can thus precipitate ventricular dysrhythmias such as torsade de pointes and sudden death.[23,72,209,211] Although it is unclear how great a risk, if any, diuretic use poses, it remains prudent to monitor and correct potassium and magnesium concentrations.[27,209] This is particularly important in older adult patients and for patients who concomitantly use digoxin, in which setting hypokalemia is clearly associated with dysrhythmias (Chap. 62).[27] Potassium-sparing diuretics can cause hyperkalemia, particularly in the setting of CKD or AKI or when combined with other hyperkalemia-producing drugs such as ACEIs.[115]

Thiazide diuretics can causes hyperglycemia, particularly in patients with diabetes mellitus, through depletion of total-body potassium stores. Because insulin secretion is dependent on transmembrane potassium fluxes, an overall decrease in potassium concentration reduces the amount of insulin secreted.[136] This effect is dose dependent and reversible either by potassium supplementation or discontinuation of the thiazide diuretic.[36,96] Thiazide diuretics are also associated with inducing hyperuricemia, renal calculi, and gout.[31,88,90] This is because the renal elimination of uric acid is extremely dependent on intravascular and urinary volume, so diuretic-induced volume depletion reduces uric acid filtration and increases its proximal tubule resorption.[207,219] Several unusual reactions are associated with thiazide diuretic use, including pancreatitis; cholecystitis; and hematologic abnormalities, such as hypercoagulability, thrombocytopenia, and hemolytic anemia.[57,59,194,196,228,235]

Despite the widespread use of these xenobiotics, isolated acute overdoses are distinctly rare. Major signs and symptoms include GI distress, brisk diuresis, possible hypovolemia and electrolyte abnormalities, and altered mental status.[132] Typically, the diuresis is short lived because of the limited duration of effect and the rapid clearance of the majority of diuretics. Assessment should focus on fluid and electrolyte status, which should be corrected as needed. If hyperkalemia is unexpectedly discovered, it could be due to either the ingestion of a potassium-sparing xenobiotic or, more likely, an overdose of potassium supplements, which are frequently prescribed in conjunction with thiazide and loop diuretics.[107,108] Diuretic overdose can cause altered mental status, including coma, without evidence of any fluid or electrolyte abnormalities.[132,195] Postulated mechanisms include a direct drug effect and induction of transient cerebral ischemia caused by hypotension.[166]

ANGIOTENSIN-CONVERTING ENZYME INHIBITORS

Angiotensin-converting enzyme inhibitors are among the most widely prescribed antihypertensives (Table 61-1). In general, they are well absorbed from the GI tract, reaching peak serum concentrations within 1 to 4 hours. Enalapril and ramipril are prodrugs and require hepatic metabolism to produce their active forms. Elimination is primarily via the kidneys.

All ACEIs have a common core structure of a 2-methylpropanolol-L-proline moiety.[78] This structural element binds directly to the active site of ACE, which is found in the lung and vascular endothelium, preventing the conversion of angiotensin I to angiotensin II. Because angiotensin II is a potent vasoconstrictor and stimulant of aldosterone secretion, it causes vasodilation; decreased peripheral vascular resistance; decreased blood pressure; increased cardiac output; and a relative increase in renal, cerebral, and coronary blood flow.[78] This hypotensive response can be severe in select patients after their initial dose, resulting in syncope and cardiac ischemia.[39,102] Patients with renovascular-induced hypertension and patients who are hypovolemic from concomitant diuretic use appear to be at greatest risk.[102] Overall, however, these drugs are well tolerated and have a very low incidence of side effects. Some reported adverse effects include rash, dysgeusia, neutropenia, hyperkalemia, chronic cough, and angioedema.[15,52,78] Because of their interference with the renin–angiotensin system, ACEIs are potential teratogens and should never be used by pregnant women or women of childbearing age.[15]

Angiotensin-Converting Enzyme Inhibitor–Induced Angioedema

Angioedema is an inflammatory reaction in which there is increased capillary blood flow and permeability, resulting in an increase in interstitial fluid. If this process is confined to the superficial dermis, urticaria develops; if the deeper layers of the dermis or subcutaneous tissue are involved, angioedema results. Angioedema most commonly involves the periorbital, perioral, or oropharyngeal tissues.[190] This swelling can progress rapidly over minutes and result in complete airway obstruction and death.[77,81]

The pathogenesis of acquired angioedema involves multiple vasoactive substances, including histamine, prostaglandin D_2, leukotrienes, and bradykinin.[105] Because ACE also inactivates bradykinin and substance P, ACE inhibition results in elevations in bradykinin concentrations that appear to be the primary cause of both ACEI angioedema and cough (Fig. 61-1).[4,110] Unlike anaphylaxis, there is no evidence that the ACEI angioedema phenomenon is immunoglobulin E (IgE) mediated,[4] although these two entities can be difficult to differentiate clinically.

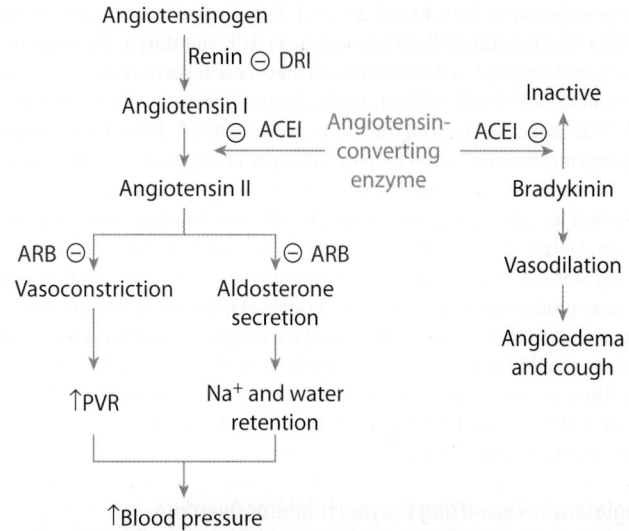

FIGURE 61-1. An overview of the normal function of the renin–angiotensin–aldosterone system (RAAS) and the mechanisms of action of angiotensin-converting enzyme inhibitors (ACEIs), angiotensin II receptor blockers (ARBs), and direct renin inhibitors (DRIs) on that system. PVR = peripheral vascular resistance.

Although the literature is replete with reports of ACEI angioedema, the overall incidence is only approximately 0.1%, and it is idiosyncratic.[69,110,212]

One-third of these reactions occur within hours of the first dose, and another third occurs within the first week.[143,212] It is important to remember that the remaining third of cases occur at any time during therapy, even after years.[38] Women, African Americans, and patients with a history of idiopathic angioedema appear to be at greater risk.[143,170] In addition, there is evidence that patients who develop ACEI angioedema are at increased subsequent risk of developing angioedema from any etiology.[17]

Treatment varies depending on the severity and rapidity of the swelling. Because of its propensity to involve the tongue, face, and oropharynx, the airway must remain the primary focus of management. A nasopharyngeal airway is often helpful. If there is any potential for or suggestion of airway compromise, then early endotracheal intubation should be performed. Severe tongue and oropharyngeal swelling make orotracheal or nasotracheal intubation extremely difficult, if not impossible. If this is a concern, then fiberoptic nasal intubation is a viable solution, if available. Other potential intubation techniques include retrograde intubation over a guidewire passed through the cricothyroid membrane and emergent cricothyrotomy.[82] However, the most important aspect of airway management in patients experiencing ACEI angioedema is early risk assessment for airway obstruction and rapid intervention before the development of severe and obstructive swelling.[2]

Because ACEI angioedema is not an IgE-mediated phenomenon, pharmacologic therapy targeting an allergic cascade—such as epinephrine, diphenhydramine, and corticosteroids—should not be expected to be effective. However, when the history is unclear, these medications should not be withheld to ensure providing life-saving therapy to someone having a severe IgE-mediated allergic reaction.

Newer potential treatment modalities target various points along the cascade of events associated with hereditary angioedema. Hereditary angioedema results from a genetically mediated defect in C_1 esterase inhibitor, resulting in limited activity of this enzyme and an increase in kallikrein concentrations. Kallikrein is a protease that cleaves kininogen into bradykinin. The end result is very similar to the cause of ACEI angioedema, namely an activation of vascular bradykinin B_2 receptors.[15] Additional treatments include the C_1 esterase inhibitor Berinert, the kallikrein inhibitor ecallantide, and the bradykinin B_2 receptor antagonist icatibant. Some case reports of successful treatment of ACEI angioedema with these xenobiotics exist,[16,76,162] and a review summarized clinical trials (phase II for icatibant and phases II and III for ecallantide).[201] Significant costs associated with these treatment modalities should limit their use to patients with rapidly progressive or severe angioedema.

Fresh-frozen plasma (FFP) is described in case reports to reverse or slow the progression of both hereditary and ACEI angioedema.[227] Fresh-frozen plasma contains kinase II, which acts as an ACE and thus leads to the degradation of accumulated bradykinin. In these case reports, doses range from 1 to 5 units of FFP (200–250 mL/unit) with most using an infusion of 2 units of FFP as initial, and typically definitive, treatment.[182,227] Fresh-frozen plasma is a reasonable intervention for patients experiencing severe angioedema.

All patients with mild or rapidly resolving angioedema should be observed for several hours to ensure that the swelling does not progress or return. Outpatient therapy with a short course of oral antihistamines and corticosteroids is reasonable if there is any question as to whether ACEI therapy produced the angioedema because allergic-mediated angioedema will benefit from this treatment. Patients developing angioedema from ACEI therapy should be instructed to discontinue them permanently and to consult their primary care physicians about other antihypertensive options. Because this is a mechanistic and not allergic adverse effect, the use of any other ACEIs is contraindicated.

Angiotensin-Converting Enzyme Inhibitor Overdose

The toxicity of ACEIs in overdose appears to be limited.[40,132] Although several reports of overdoses involving ACEIs have been published, the majority of the cases reported manifested toxicity of a coingestant.[49,85,236] Although hypotension is reported,[12,13,126] deaths are rarely related to isolated ACEI

ingestions.[172] Other patients remain asymptomatic despite high serum drug concentrations.[126]

Treatment should focus on supportive care and on identifying any potentially toxic coingestants, particularly other antihypertensives such as β-adrenergic antagonists and CCBs. In most cases, AC alone is adequate GI decontamination. Intravenous crystalloid boluses are often effective in correcting hypotension, although catecholamines are often required.[12] Naloxone is another potential treatment option. Angiotensin-converting enzyme inhibitors inhibit the metabolism of enkephalins and potentiate their opioid effects, which include lowering blood pressure.[51,155] In a controlled human volunteer study, continuous naloxone infusion effectively blunted the hypotensive response of captopril.[1] In one case report, naloxone appeared to be effective in reversing symptomatic hypotension secondary to a captopril overdose;[232] in another published case, naloxone was ineffective.[12] Although its role in the setting of ACEI overdose remains unclear, a trial of naloxone is reasonable in opioid-naïve patients.

ANGIOTENSIN II RECEPTOR BLOCKERS

Angiotensin II receptor blockers (ARBs) were first introduced in 1995. These xenobiotics are rapidly absorbed from the GI tract, reaching peak serum concentrations in 1 to 4 hours, and then are eliminated either unchanged in the feces or, after undergoing hepatic metabolism predominantly CYP 3A4 and 2C9,[14] eliminated in the bile.[167]

Although these xenobiotics are similar to ACEIs in that they decrease the effects of angiotensin, they may have similar effects on blood pressure. The ARBs block whereas the ACEIs decrease the formation of angiotensin II, they act by antagonizing angiotensin II at the type 1 angiotensin (AT-1) receptor (Fig. 61–1).[226] This inhibits the vasoconstrictive- and aldosterone-promoting effects of angiotensin II and reduces blood pressor by blunting both the sympathetic as well as the renin–angiotensin systems.[149] Despite the mechanistic evidence that ARBs do not affect bradykinin degradation and therefore have a much lower incidence of angioedema compared with ACEIs, serious cases of angioedema associated with ARB therapy are reported.[143,230] In addition, there is a significantly higher incidence of angioedema associated with ARBs compared with other antihypertensives, such as β-adrenergic antagonists.[225] One meta-analysis found that the incidence of angioedema with ARBs was less than half that with ACEIs and not significantly different from placebo.[142] Similar to ACEIs, ARBs should never be used by pregnant patient because of their teratogenic potential.[15,210] In addition, when initiating ARB therapy, up to 1% develop of patients first-dose orthostatic hypotension.[83]

There are few published reports of isolated overdoses involving ARBs. Adverse signs and symptoms reflect orthostatic or absolute hypotension and include palpitations, diaphoresis, dizziness, lethargy, or confusion.[26,152,214] Hypotension should be treated with crystalloid boluses and catecholamine therapy.[152,214] Significant hypotension can occur during the induction of general anesthesia in patients who chronically taking ARBs. Hypotension in this case is reportedly refractory to traditional vasoconstrictor therapy, such as norepinephrine, ephedrine, and phenylephrine but appear to respond to vasopressin.[63]

One promising treatment for hypotension produced by ARBs and ACEIs is methylene blue[148,159] (Antidotes in Depth: A43), This treatment was first explored in patients placed on cardiopulmonary bypass (CPB).[171,217] During CPB, systemic blood pressure and peripheral vascular resistance decrease because of a number of factors, including acute hemodilution, citrate use during cardioplegia, a poorly defined inflammatory response that results in nitric oxide release, and an increase in circulating bradykinin.[43,47,240] This increase in bradykinin, which also mediates its vasodilatory effects via nitric oxide, occurs because bradykinin metabolism is primarily in pulmonary tissue and CPB mechanically bypasses the pulmonary system.[43,47] Angiotensin-converting enzyme inhibitors and ARBs exacerbate this vasodilation by further inhibiting bradykinin metabolism.[179] In a double-blind, placebo-controlled study of 30 patients taking ACEIs who were undergoing elective cardiac surgery requiring CPB, administration of methylene blue at the onset of CPB resulted in an increase in mean arterial pressure and systemic vascular resistance and less use of phenylephrine and norepinephrine.[148] A reasonable starting dose of methylene blue, when used as a vasopressor, is 2 mg/kg with subsequent intermittent boluses or possibly continuous infusions starting at 0.5 mg/kg/h.[112,148]

DIRECT RENIN INHIBITORS

Direct renin inhibitors such as aliskiren exert their antihypertensive effects by directly inhibiting circulating renin in the renin–angiotensin–aldosterone system (RAAS).[238] Unfortunately, all RAAS acting antihypertensives such as ACEIs, ARBs, and DRIs induce a compensatory increase in serum renin concentrations; however, only DRIs are able to blunt the physiologic effects of this rise.[204,238] Aliskiren is well tolerated and is an effective antihypertensive both as monotherapy and in combination with other antihypertensives, including hydrochlorothiazide, CCBs, and β-adrenergic antagonists.[136] However, significant controversy surrounds aliskiren use when combined ARBs or ACEIs after a clinical trial was halted because of an increased incidence of ischemic stroke, AKI, hyperkalemia, and hypotension was noted in patients with diabetes and CKD.[173] Currently, aliskiren is contraindicated in patients receiving ARBs or ACEIs.[6] There are no reported cases of poisoning or overdose; however, hypotension should be anticipated and treatment that includes supportive care, including IV crystalloid and catecholamines, seems reasonable.

SUMMARY

- These xenobiotics are not often associated with severe poisonings, either because of limited use, as with most of the sympatholytics and direct vasodilators, or because of limited toxicity, as is the case of diuretics, ACEIs, ARBs, and DRIs.
- Severe clonidine poisoning classically presents as the opioid toxidrome producing profound CNS depression and bradycardia.
- Clonidine withdrawal manifests as agitation, tachycardia, and hypertension and should be treated with clonidine or benzodiazepines.
- Nitroprusside infusions greater than 4 mcg/kg/min result in cyanide poisoning, which can be prevented with coadministration of thiosulfate or hydroxycobalamin.
- Because of the pathogenesis of ACEI-induced angioedema, it is unlikely to respond to "typical" allergic treatment such as antihistamines, epinephrine, and corticosteroids. Rather, focus should be on definitive airway management in patients with rapidly progressing swelling or symptoms.

REFERENCES

1. Ajayi AA, et al. Effect of naloxone on the actions of captopril. *Clin Pharmacol Ther.* 1985;38:560-565.
2. Al-Khudari S, et al. Management of angiotensin-converting enzyme inhibitor-induced angioedema. *Laryngoscope.* 2011;121:2327-2334.
3. Allon M, et al. Prolonged hypotension after initial minoxidil dose. *Arch Intern Med.* 1986;146:2075-2076.
4. Anderson MW, deShazo RD. Studies of the mechanism of angiotensin-converting enzyme (ACE) inhibitor-associated angioedema: the effect of an ACE inhibitor on cutaneous responses to bradykinin, codeine, and histamine. *J Allergy Clin Immunol.* 1990;85:856-858.
5. Anderson RJ, et al. Clonidine overdose: report of six cases and review of the literature. *Ann Emerg Med.* 1981;10:107-112.
6. Angeli F, et al. Efficacy and safety profile of aliskiren: practical implications for clinicians. *Curr Drug Saf.* 2014;9:106-117.
7. Artman M, Boerth RC. Clonidine poisoning. A complex problem. *Am J Dis Child.* 1983;137:171-174.
9. Baglin A, et al. Metabolic adverse reactions to diuretics. Clinical relevance to elderly patients. *Drug Saf.* 1995;12:161-167.
10. Bailey RR, Neale TJ. Rapid clonidine withdrawal with blood pressure overshoot exaggerated by beta-blockade. *Br Med J.* 1976;1:942-943.
11. Bamshad MJ, Wasserman GS. Pediatric clonidine intoxications. *Vet Hum Toxicol.* 1990;32:220-223.
12. Barr CS, et al. Profound prolonged hypotension following captopril overdose. *Postgrad Med J.* 1991;67:953-954.
13. Barr M. Teratogen update: angiotensin-converting enzyme inhibitors. *Teratology.* 1994;50:399-409.
14. Barreras A, Gurk-Turner C. Angiotensin II receptor blockers. *Proc (Bayl Univ Med Cent).* 2003;16:123-126.
15. Bas M, et al. Nonallergic angioedema: role of bradykinin. *Allergy.* 2007;62:842-856.
16. Bas M, et al. Therapeutic efficacy of icatibant in angioedema induced by angiotensin-converting enzyme inhibitors: a case series. *Ann Emerg Med.* 2010;56:278-282.
17. Beltrami L, et al. Long-term follow-up of 111 patients with angiotensin-converting enzyme inhibitor-related angioedema. *J Hypertens.* 2011;29:2273-2277.
18. Bendall MJ, et al. Side effects due to treatment of hypertension with prazosin. *Br Med J.* 1975;2:727-728.
19. Benson BE, et al. TESS-based dose-response using pediatric clonidine exposures. *Toxicol Appl Pharmacol.* 2006;213:145-151.
20. Berge KH, Lanier WL. Myocardial infarction accompanying acute clonidine withdrawal in a patient without a history of ischemic coronary artery disease. *Anesth Analg.* 1991;72:259-261.
21. Beuger M, et al. Clonidine use and abuse among methadone program applicants and patients. *J Subst Abuse Treat.* 1998;15:589-593.
22. Bhalla S, et al. Determination of α(2)-adrenoceptor and imidazoline receptor involvement in augmentation of morphine and oxycodone analgesia by agmatine and BMS182874. *Eur J Pharmacol.* 2011;651:109-121.
23. Bigger JT. Diuretic therapy, hypertension, and cardiac arrest. *N Engl J Med.* 1994;330:1899-1900.
24. Bobik A, et al. Evidence for a predominantly central hypotensive effect of alpha-methyldopa in humans. *Hypertension.* 1986;8:16-23.
25. Boxwalla M, et al. Involvement of imidazoline and opioid receptors in the enhancement of clonidine-induced analgesia by sulfisoxazole. *Can J Physiol Pharmacol.* 2010;88:541-552.
26. Brabant SM, et al. Refractory hypotension after induction of anesthesia in a patient chronically treated with angiotensin receptor antagonists. *Anesth Analg.* 1999;89:887-888.
27. Brater DC, Morrelli HF. Digoxin toxicity in patients with normokalemic potassium depletion. *Clin Pharmacol Ther.* 1977;22:21-33.
28. Byrd BF, et al. Risk factors for severe bradycardia during oral clonidine therapy for hypertension. *Arch Intern Med.* 1988;148:729-733.
29. Campbell BC, Reid JL. Regimen for the control of blood pressure and symptoms during clonidine withdrawal. *Int J Clin Pharmacol Res.* 1985;5:215-222.
30. Campese VM. Minoxidil: a review of its pharmacological properties and therapeutic use. *Drugs.* 1981;22:257-278.
31. Campion EW, et al. Asymptomatic hyperuricemia. Risks and consequences in the normative aging study. *Am J Med.* 1987;82:421-426.
32. Caravati EM, Bennett DL. Clonidine transdermal patch poisoning. *Ann Emerg Med.* 1988;17:175-176.
33. Castro JL, et al. Central benzodiazepine involvement in clonidine cardiovascular actions. *Can J Physiol Pharmacol.* 1999;77:844-851.
34. Cates AL, et al. Clonidine overdose in a toddler due to accidental ingestion of a compounding cream. *Pediatr Emerg Care.* 2016.
35. Chan CKS, et al. Contribution of imidazoline receptors and alpha2-adrenoceptors in the rostral ventrolateral medulla to sympathetic baroreflex inhibition by systemic rilmenidine. *J Hypertens.* 2007;25:147-155.
36. Chan JC, et al. Drug-induced disorders of glucose metabolism. Mechanisms and management. *Drug Saf.* 1996;15:135-157.
37. Cheung AT, et al. Cardiopulmonary bypass, hemolysis, and nitroprusside-induced cyanide production. *Anesth Analg.* 2007;105:29-33.
38. Chin HL, Buchan DA. Severe angioedema after long-term use of an angiotensin-converting enzyme inhibitor. *Ann Intern Med.* 1990;112:312-313.
39. Cleland JG, et al. Severe hypotension after first dose of enalapril in heart failure. *Br Med J (Clin Res Ed).* 1985;291:1309-1312.
40. Cobaugh D, et al. Angiotensin converting enzyme inhibitor overdoses: a multi-centre study. *Vet Hum Toxicol.* 1990;32:352.
41. Cobos-Puc LE, et al. α2A-adrenoceptors, but not nitric oxide, mediate the peripheral cardiac sympatho-inhibition of moxonidine. *Eur J Pharmacol.* 2016;782:35-43.
42. Conner CS, Watanabe AS. Clonidine overdose: a review. *Am J Hosp Pharm.* 1979;36:906-911.
43. Conti VR, McQuitty C. Vasodilation and cardiopulmonary bypass: the role of bradykinin and the pulmonary vascular endothelium. *Chest.* 2001;120:1759-1761.
44. Copeland PM. Diuretic abuse and central pontine myelinolysis. *Psychother Psychosom.* 1989;52:101-105.
45. Corneli HM, et al. Toddler eats clonidine patch and nearly quits smoking for life. *JAMA.* 1989;261:42.
46. Cubeddu LX. New alpha 1-adrenergic receptor antagonists for the treatment of hypertension: role of vascular alpha receptors in the control of peripheral resistance. *Am Heart J.* 1988;116(1 Pt 1):133-162.
47. Cugno M, et al. Increase of bradykinin in plasma of patients undergoing cardiopulmonary bypass: the importance of lung exclusion. *Chest.* 2001;120:1776-1782.
48. Curry SC, Arnold-Capell P. Toxic effects of drugs used in the ICU. Nitroprusside, nitroglycerin, and angiotensin-converting enzyme inhibitors. *Crit Care Clin.* 1991;7:555-581.
49. Dawson AH, et al. Lisinopril overdose. *Lancet.* 1990;335:487-488.
50. de Jonge A, et al. Quantitative aspects of alpha adrenergic effects induced by clonidine-like imidazolidines. II. Central and peripheral bradycardic activities. *J Pharmacol Exp Ther.* 1982;222:712-719.

51. Di Nicolantonio R, et al. Captopril potentiates the vasodepressor action of met-enkephalin in the anaesthetized rat. *Br J Pharmacol*. 1983;80:405-408.

52. DiBianco R. Adverse reactions with angiotensin converting enzyme (ACE) inhibitors. *Med Toxicol*. 1986;1:122-141.

53. Dire DJ, Kuhns DW. The use of sublingual nifedipine in a patient with a clonidine overdose. *J Emerg Med*. 1988;6:125-128.

54. Dollery CT, et al. Clinical pharmacology and pharmacokinetics of clonidine. *Clin Pharmacol Ther*. 1976;19:11-17.

56. DuCharme DW, et al. Pharmacologic properties of minoxidil: a new hypotensive agent. *J Pharmacol Exp Ther*. 1973;184:662-670.

57. Eckhauser ML, et al. Diuretic-associated pancreatitis: a collective review and illustrative cases. *Am J Gastroenterol*. 1987;82:865-870.

58. Edwards LP, et al. Pharmacological properties of the central antihypertensive agent, moxonidine. *Cardiovasc Ther*. 2012;30:199-208.

59. Eisner EV, Crowell EB. Hydrochlorothiazide-dependent thrombocytopenia due to IgM antibody. *JAMA*. 1971;215:480-482.

60. Elberg AJ, et al. Prolonged nitroprusside and intermittent hemodialysis as therapy for intractable hypertension. *Am J Dis Child*. 1978;132:988-989.

61. Engberg G, et al. Clonidine withdrawal: activation of brain noradrenergic neurons with specifically reduced alpha 2-receptor sensitivity. *Life Sci*. 1982;30:235-243.

62. Ernsberger P, et al. Role of imidazole receptors in the vasodepressor response to clonidine analogs in the rostral ventrolateral medulla. *J Pharmacol Exp Ther*. 1990;253:408-418.

63. Eyraud D, et al. Treatment of intraoperative refractory hypotension with terlipressin in patients chronically treated with an antagonist of the renin-angiotensin system. *Anesth Analg*. 1999;88:980-984.

64. Farrell SE, Epstein SK. Overdose of Rogaine extra strength for men topical minoxidil preparation. *J Toxicol Clin Toxicol*. 1999;37:781-783.

65. Farsang C, et al. Reversal by naloxone of the antihypertensive action of clonidine: involvement of the sympathetic nervous system. *Circulation*. 1984;69:461-467.

66. Farsang C, et al. Possible role of an endogenous opiate in the cardiovascular effects of central alpha adrenoceptor stimulation in spontaneously hypertensive rats. *J Pharmacol Exp Ther*. 1980;214:203-208.

67. Fenichel R. Combining methylphenidate and clonidine: the role of post-marketing surveillance. *J Child and Adolesc Psychopharmacol*. 2009;5:155-156.

68. Fenton C, et al. Moxonidine: a review of its use in essential hypertension. *Drugs*. 2006;66:477-496.

69. Finley CJ, et al. Angiotensin-converting enzyme inhibitor-induced angioedema: still unrecognized. *Am J Emerg Med*. 1992;10:550-552.

70. Fowler MA, et al. Case 01-1995: A two-year-old female with alteration of consciousness. *Pediatr Emerg Care*. 1995;11:62-65.

71. Freed CR, et al. Hypotension and hypothalamic amine metabolism after long-term alpha-methyldopa infusions. *Life Sci*. 1978;23:313-322.

72. Freis ED. Adverse effects of diuretics. *Drug Saf*. 1992;7:364-373.

73. Friederich JA, Butterworth JF. Sodium nitroprusside: twenty years and counting. *Anesth Analg*. 1995;81:152-162.

74. Fries E, et al. Effects of treatment on morbidity in hypertension. Results in patients with diastolic blood pressures averaging 115 through 129 mm hg. *JAMA*. 1967;202:1028-1034.

75. Frohlich ED, et al. Hemodynamic and cardiac effects of centrally acting antihypertensive drugs. *Hypertension*. 1984;6(5 Pt 2):81.

76. Gallitelli M, Alzetta M. Icatibant: a novel approach to the treatment of angioedema related to the use of angiotensin-converting enzyme inhibitors. *Am J Emerg Med*. 2012;30:2.

77. Gannon TH, Eby TL. Angioedema from angiotensin converting enzyme inhibitors: a cause of upper airway obstruction. *Laryngoscope*. 1990;100:1156-1160.

78. Gavras H, Gavras I. Angiotensin converting enzyme inhibitors. Properties and side effects. *Hypertension*. 1988;11(3 Pt 2):41.

79. Geyskes GG, et al. Clonidine withdrawal. Mechanism and frequency of rebound hypertension. *Br J Clin Pharmacol*. 1979;7:55-62.

80. Giachetti A, Shore PA. The reserpine receptor. *Life Sci*. 1978;23:89-92.

81. Giannoccaro PJ, et al. Fatal angioedema associated with enalapril. *Can J Cardiol*. 1989;5:335-336.

82. Gill M, et al. Retrograde endotracheal intubation: an investigation of indications, complications, and patient outcomes. *Am J Emerg Med*. 2005;23:123-126.

83. Goldberg AI, et al. Safety and tolerability of losartan potassium, an angiotensin II receptor antagonist, compared with hydrochlorothiazide, atenolol, felodipine ER, and angiotensin-converting enzyme inhibitors for the treatment of systemic hypertension. *Am J Cardiol*. 1995;75:793-795.

84. Gozlinska B, et al. Clonidine action in spontaneously hypertensive rats (SHR) depends on the GABAergic system function. *Amino Acids*. 1999;17:131-138.

85. Graham SR, et al. Captopril overdose. *Med J Aust*. 1989;151:111.

86. Gremse DA, et al. Hypertension associated with naloxone treatment for clonidine poisoning. *J Pediatr*. 1986;108(5 Pt 1):776-778.

87. Griffis KR Jr, et al. Utilization of hydralazine or alpha-methyldopa for the management of early puerperal hypertension. *Am J Perinatol*. 1989;6:437-441.

88. Gurwitz JH, et al. Thiazide diuretics and the initiation of anti-gout therapy. *J Clin Epidemiol*. 1997;50:953-959.

89. Hall AH, Rumack BH. Hydroxycobalamin/sodium thiosulfate as a cyanide antidote. *J Emerg Med*. 1987;5:115-121.

90. Hall AP, et al. Epidemiology of gout and hyperuricemia. A long-term population study. *Am J Med*. 1967;42:27-37.

91. Hall D, et al. ECG changes during long-term minoxidil therapy for severe hypertension. *Arch Intern Med*. 1979;139:790-794.

92. Hamilton M, et al. The role of blood-pressure control in preventing complications of hypertension. *Lancet*. 1964;1:235-238.

93. Hanton G, et al. Use of M-mode and doppler echocardiography to investigate the cardiotoxicity of minoxidil in beagle dogs. *Arch Toxicol*. 2004;78:40-48.

94. Hanton G, et al. Cardiovascular toxicity of minoxidil in the marmoset. *Toxicol Lett*. 2008;180:157-165.

95. Head GA, et al. Relationship between imidazoline and alpha2-adrenoceptors involved in the sympatho-inhibitory actions of centrally acting antihypertensive agents. *J Auton Nerv Syst*. 1998;72:163-169.

96. Helderman JH, et al. Prevention of the glucose intolerance of thiazide diuretics by maintenance of body potassium. *Diabetes*. 1983;32:106-111.

97. Henning M, Rubenson A. Evidence that the hypotensive action of methyldopa is mediated by central actions of methylnoradrenaline. *J Pharm Pharmacol*. 1971;23:407-411.

98. Henretig F. Clonidine and centrally acting antihypertensives. In: Ford M, et al., eds. *Clinical Toxicology*. Philadelphia, PA: Saunders; 2001:391-396.

99. Henretig F, et al. Clonidine patch toxicity: the proof is in the poop. *J Toxicol Clin Toxicol*. 1995;33:520.

100. Hewick DS, et al. Sodium nitroprusside: pharmacological aspects of its interaction with hydroxocobalamin and thiosulphate. *J Pharm Pharmacol*. 1987;39:113-117.

101. Higgins GL, et al. Pediatric poisoning from over-the-counter imidazoline-containing products. *Ann Emerg Med*. 1991;20:655-658.

102. Hodsman GP, et al. Factors related to first dose hypotensive effect of captopril: prediction and treatment. *Br Med J (Clin Res Ed)*. 1983;286:832-834.

103. Hoffman B, Lefkowitz R. Catecholamines, sympathomimetic drugs, and adrenoceptor antagonists. In: Hardman J, et al., eds. *Goodman and Gilman's The Pharmacological Basis of Therapeutics*. 9th ed. New York, NY: McGraw-Hill; 1996:199-248.

104. Holmes B, et al. A review of its pharmacodynamic properties and therapeutic efficacy in hypertension. *Drugs*. 1983;26:212-229.

105. Hoover T, et al. Angiotensin converting enzyme inhibitor induced angio-oedema: a review of the pathophysiology and risk factors. *Clin Exp Allergy*. 2010;40:50-61.

106. Horowitz R, et al. Accidental clonidine patch ingestion in a child. *Am J Ther*. 2005;12:272-274.

107. Hume L, Forfar JC. Hyperkalaemia and overdose of antihypertensive agents. *Lancet*. 1977;2:1182.

108. Illingworth RN, Proudfoot AT. Rapid poisoning with slow-release potassium. *Br Med J*. 1980;281:485-486.

109. Isbister GK, et al. Adult clonidine overdose: prolonged bradycardia and central nervous system depression, but not severe toxicity. *Clin Toxicol (Phila)*. 2017;55:187-192.

110. Israili ZH, Hall WD. Cough and angioneurotic edema associated with angiotensin-converting enzyme inhibitor therapy. A review of the literature and pathophysiology. *Ann Intern Med*. 1992;117:234-242.

111. Jackson E. Diuretics. In: Hardman J, Limbird L, eds. *Goodman and Gilman's The Pharmacological Basis of Therapeutics*. 10th ed. New York, NY: McGraw-Hill; 2001:757-787.

112. Jang DH, et al. Methylene blue in the treatment of refractory shock from an amlodipine overdose. *Ann Emerg Med*. 2011;58:565-567.

113. Johnson ML, et al. Massive clonidine overdose during refill of an implanted drug delivery device for intrathecal analgesia: a review of inadvertent soft-tissue injection during implantable drug delivery device refills and its management. *Pain Med*. 2011;12:1032-1040.

114. Jonkman FA, et al. Beta 2-adrenoceptor antagonists intensify clonidine withdrawal syndrome in conscious rats. *J Cardiovasc Pharmacol*. 1989;14:886-891.

115. Juurlink DN, et al. Rates of hyperkalemia after publication of the randomized Aldactone evaluation study. *N Engl J Med*. 2004;351:543-551.

116. Kalmanovitch DV, Hardwick PB. Hypotension after guanethidine block. *Anaesthesia*. 1988;43:256.

117. Kamibayashi T, Maze M. Clinical uses of alpha2-adrenergic agonists. *Anesthesiology*. 2000;93:1345-1349.

118. Keating GM. Dexmedetomidine: a review of its use for sedation in the intensive care setting. *Drugs*. 2015;75:1119-1130.

119. Kibler LE, Gazes PC. Effect of clonidine on atrioventricular conduction. *JAMA*. 1977;238:1930-1932.

120. Koch-Weser J. Diazoxide. *N Engl J Med*. 1976;294:1271-1273.

121. Koch-Weser J. Hydralazine. *N Engl J Med*. 1976;295:320-323.

122. Kosten TR, O'Connor PG. Management of drug and alcohol withdrawal. *N Engl J Med*. 2003;348:1786-1795.

123. Krapez JR, et al. Effects of cyanide antidotes used with sodium nitroprusside infusions: sodium thiosulphate and hydroxocobalamin given prophylactically to dogs. *Br J Anaesth*. 1981;53:793-804.

124. Kukoyi A, et al. Two cases of acute dexmedetomidine withdrawal syndrome following prolonged infusion in the intensive care unit: report of cases and review of the literature. *Hum Exp Toxicol*. 2013;32:107-110.

125. Kulig K, et al. Naloxone for treatment of clonidine overdose. *JAMA*. 1982;247:1697.

126. Lau CP. Attempted suicide with enalapril. *N Engl J Med*. 1986;315:197.

127. Laubie M, et al. Action of clonidine on the baroreceptor pathway and medullary sites mediating vagal bradycardia. *Eur J Pharmacol*. 1976;38:293-303.

128. Lenz K, et al. Acute intoxication with prazosin: case report. *Hum Toxicol*. 1985; 4:53-56.

129. Lev R, Clark RF. Visine overdose: case report of an adult with hemodynamic compromise. *J Emerg Med*. 1995;13:649-652.

130. Lin MT, et al. Serotonergic mechanisms of clonidine-induced hypothermia in rats. *Neuropharmacology*. 1981;20:15-21.

131. Lip GY, Ferner RE. Poisoning with anti-hypertensive drugs: angiotensin converting enzyme inhibitors. *J Hum Hypertens*. 1995;9:711-715.

132. Lip GY, Ferner RE. Poisoning with antihypertensive drugs: diuretics and potassium supplements. *J Hum Hypertens*. 1995;9:295-301.

133. Loggie JM, et al. Accidental reserpine poisoning: clinical and metabolic effects. *Clin Pharmacol Ther*. 1967;8:692-695.

134. Lowenthal DT. Pharmacokinetics of clonidine. *J Cardiovasc Pharmacol*. 1980;2(suppl 1):29.

135. Lowry JA, Brown JT. Significance of the imidazoline receptors in toxicology. *Clin Toxicol (Phila)*. 2014;52:454-469.

136. Luna B, Feinglos MN. Drug-induced hyperglycemia. *JAMA*. 2001;286:1945-1948.

137. Lusthof KJ, et al. Use of clonidine for chemical submission. *J Toxicol Clin Toxicol*. 2000;38:329-332.

138. MacMillan AR, et al. Minoxidil overdose. *Chest*. 1993;103:1290-1291.

139. Magdalan J, et al. Acute poisoning with moxonidine? A case report. *Clin Toxicol (Phila)*. 2008;46:921-922.

140. Maggi JC, et al. Severe clonidine overdose in children requiring critical care. *Clin Pediatr (Phila)*. 1986;25:453-455.

141. Mahieu LM, et al. Imidazoline intoxication in children. *Eur J Pediatr*. 1993;152:944-946.

142. Makani H, et al. Meta-analysis of randomized trials of angioedema as an adverse event of renin-angiotensin system inhibitors. *Am J Cardiol*. 2012;110:383-391.

143. Malde B, et al. Investigation of angioedema associated with the use of angiotensin-converting enzyme inhibitors and angiotensin receptor blockers. *Ann Allergy Asthma Immunol*. 2007;98:57-63.

144. Mannelli M, et al. Naloxone administration releases catecholamines. *N Engl J Med*. 1983;308:654-655.

145. Manolio TA, et al. Trends in pharmacologic management of hypertension in the United States. *Arch Intern Med*. 1995;155:829-837.

146. Marbury TC, et al. Combined antidotal and hemodialysis treatments for nitroprusside-induced cyanide toxicity. *J Toxicol Clin Toxicol*. 1982;19:475-482.

147. Marruecos L, et al. Clonidine overdose. *Crit Care Med*. 1983;11:959-960.

148. Maslow AD, et al. The hemodynamic effects of methylene blue when administered at the onset of cardiopulmonary bypass. *Anesth Analg*. 2006;103:8, table of contents.

149. Mazzolai L, Burnier M. Comparative safety and tolerability of angiotensin II receptor antagonists. *Drug Saf*. 1999;21:23-33.

150. McCormick MA, et al. Severe toxicity from ingestion of a topical minoxidil preparation. *Am J Emerg Med*. 1989;7:419-421.

151. McLennan PL. The hypothermic effect of clonidine and other imidazolidines in relation to their ability to enter the central nervous system in mice. *Eur J Pharmacol*. 1981;69:477-482.

152. McNamee JJ, et al. Terlipressin for refractory hypotension following angiotensin-II receptor antagonist overdose. *Anaesthesia*. 2006;61:408-409.

153. Mégarbane B, et al. Antidotal treatment of cyanide poisoning. *J Chin Med Assoc*. 2003;66:193-203.

154. Messerli FH, et al. Risk/benefit assessment of beta-blockers and diuretics precludes their use for first-line therapy in hypertension. *Circulation*. 2008;117:2715; discussion 2715.

155. Millar JA, et al. Attenuation of the antihypertensive effect of captopril by the opioid receptor antagonist naloxone. *Clin Exp Pharmacol Physiol*. 1983;10:253-259.

156. Minns AB, et al. Guanfacine overdose resulting in initial hypertension and subsequent delayed, persistent orthostatic hypotension. *Clin Toxicol (Phila)*. 2010;48:146-148.

157. Muir AL, et al. Circulatory effects at rest and exercise of clonidine, an imidazoline derivative with hypotensive properties. *Lancet*. 1969;2:181-184.

158. Myhre E, et al. Clinical pharmacokinetics of methyldopa. *Clin Pharmacokinet*. 1982;7:221-233.

159. Nabbi R, et al. Angiotensin-receptor-blocker-induced refractory hypotension responds to methylene blue. *Acta Anaesthesiol Scand*. 2012;56:933-934.

160. Nakagawa S, et al. Ventricular tachycardia induced by clonidine withdrawal. *Br Heart J*. 1985;53:654-658.

161. Newgreen DT, et al. The action of diazoxide and minoxidil sulphate on rat blood vessels: a comparison with cromakalim. *Br J Pharmacol*. 1990;100:605-613.

162. Nielsen EW, Gramstad S. Angioedema from angiotensin-converting enzyme (ACE) inhibitor treated with complement 1 (C1) inhibitor concentrate. *Acta Anaesthesiol Scand*. 2006;50:120-122.

163. Niemann JT, et al. Reversal of clonidine toxicity by naloxone. *Ann Emerg Med*. 1986;15:1229-1231.

164. Norris JC, Hume AS. In vivo release of cyanide from sodium nitroprusside. *Br J Anaesth*. 1987;59:236-239.

165. Oates J, Brown N. Antihypertensive agents and the drug therapy of hypertension. In: Hardman J, et al., eds. *Goodman and Gilman's The Pharmacological Basis of Therapeutics*. 10th ed. New York, NY: McGraw-Hill; 2001:871-900.

166. O'Doherty NJ. Thiazides and cerebral ischaemia. *Lancet*. 1965;2:1297.

167. Ohtawa M, et al. Pharmacokinetics and biochemical efficacy after single and multiple oral administration of losartan, an orally active nonpeptide angiotensin II receptor antagonist, in humans. *Br J Clin Pharmacol*. 1993;35:290-297.

168. Olsson JM, Pruitt AW. Management of clonidine ingestion in children. *J Pediatr*. 1983;103:646-650.

169. Onesti G, et al. Pharmacodynamic effects of a new antihypertensive drug, Catapres (ST-155). *Circulation*. 1969;39:219-228.

170. Orfan N, et al. Severe angioedema related to ACE inhibitors in patients with a history of idiopathic angioedema. *JAMA*. 1990;264:1287-1289.

171. Pappalardo F, et al. Prolonged refractory hypotension in cardiac surgery after institution of cardiopulmonary bypass. *J Cardiothorac Vasc Anesth*. 2002;16:477-479.

172. Park H, et al. Suicide by captopril overdose. *J Toxicol Clin Toxicol*. 1990;28:379-382.

173. Parving H, et al. Cardiorenal end points in a trial of aliskiren for type 2 diabetes. *N Engl J Med*. 2012;367:2204-2213.

174. Peng J, et al. Sympathoinhibitory mechanism of moxonidine: role of the inducible nitric oxide synthase in the rostral ventrolateral medulla. *Cardiovasc Res*. 2009; 84:283-291.

175. Peng J, et al. GABAergic mechanism in the rostral ventrolateral medulla contributes to the hypotension of moxonidine. *Cardiovasc Res*. 2011;89:473-481.

176. Perrone J, et al. Guanabenz induced hypothermia in a poisoned elderly female. *J Toxicol Clin Toxicol*. 1994;32:445-449.

177. Peters RW, et al. Cardiac arrhythmias after abrupt clonidine withdrawal. *Clin Pharmacol Ther*. 1983;34:435-439.

178. Pettinger WA, Mitchell HC. Side effects of vasodilator therapy. *Hypertension*. 1988; 11(3 Pt 2):36.

179. Pigott DW, et al. Effect of omitting regular ACE inhibitor medication before cardiac surgery on haemodynamic variables and vasoactive drug requirements. *Br J Anaesth*. 1999;83:715-720.

180. Poff SW, Rose SR. Minoxidil overdose with ECG changes: case report and review. *J Emerg Med*. 1992;10:53-57.

181. Pomerleau AC, et al. Dermal exposure to a compounded pain cream resulting in severely elevated clonidine concentration. *J Med Toxicol*. 2014;10:61-64.

182. Prematta M, et al. Fresh frozen plasma for the treatment of hereditary angioedema. *Ann Allergy Asthma Immunol*. 2007;98:383-388.

183. Ram CV, et al. Withdrawal syndrome following cessation of guanabenz therapy. *J Clin Pharmacol*. 1979;19:148-150.

184. Rangan C, et al. Central alpha-2 adrenergic eye drops: case series of 3 pediatric systemic poisonings. *Pediatr Emerg Care*. 2008;24:167-169.

185. Rapko DA, Rastegar DA. Intentional clonidine patch ingestion by 3 adults in a detoxification unit. *Arch Intern Med*. 2003;163:367-368.

186. Reid JL, et al. Withdrawal reactions following cessation of central alpha-adrenergic receptor agonists. *Hypertension*. 1984;6(5 Pt 2):75.

187. Reis DJ, Piletz JE. The imidazoline receptor in control of blood pressure by clonidine and allied drugs. *Am J Physiol*. 1997;273(5 Pt 2):1569.

188. Rindone JP, Sloane EP. Cyanide toxicity from sodium nitroprusside: risks and management. *Ann Pharmacother*. 1992;26:515-519.

189. Robbins DN, et al. Priapism secondary to prazosin overdose. *J Urol*. 1983;130:975.

190. Roberts JR, Wuerz RC. Clinical characteristics of angiotensin-converting enzyme inhibitor-induced angioedema. *Ann Emerg Med*. 1991;20:555-558.

191. Robertson D, et al. Antihypertensive metabolites of alpha-methyldopa. *Hypertension*. 1984;6(5 Pt 2):50.

192. Romano MJ, Dinh A. A 1000-fold overdose of clonidine caused by a compounding error in a 5-year-old child with attention-deficit/hyperactivity disorder. *Pediatrics*. 2001;108:471-472.

194. Rosenberg L, et al. Thiazides and acute cholecystitis. *N Engl J Med*. 1980;303:546-548.

195. Rougraff ME. Chlorothiazide overdosage effects in two-year-old child. *Pa Med J*. 1959;62:694.

196. Rubinstein I. Fatal thrombosis of left internal carotid artery following diuretic abuse. *Ann Emerg Med*. 1985;14:275.

197. Rupp H, et al. Drug withdrawal and rebound hypertension: differential action of the central antihypertensive drugs moxonidine and clonidine. *Cardiovasc Drugs Ther*. 1996;10(suppl 1):251-262.

198. Rybalkin SD, et al. Cyclic GMP phosphodiesterases and regulation of smooth muscle function. *Circ Res*. 2003;93:280-291.

199. Rygnestad TK, Dale O. Self-poisoning with prazosin. *Acta Med Scand*. 1983; 213:157-158.

200. Saunders C, Limbird LE. Localization and trafficking of alpha2-adrenergic receptor subtypes in cells and tissues. *Pharmacol Ther*. 1999;84:193-205.

201. Scalese MJ, Reinaker TS. Pharmacologic management of angioedema induced by angiotensin-converting enzyme inhibitors. *Am J Health Syst Pharm*. 2016;73:873-879.

202. Scheinman MM, et al. Adverse effects of sympatholytic agents in patients with hypertension and sinus node dysfunction. *Am J Med*. 1978;64:1013-1020.

203. Schulz V. Clinical pharmacokinetics of nitroprusside, cyanide, thiosulphate and thiocyanate. *Clin Pharmacokinet*. 1984;9:239-251.

204. Sealey JE, Laragh JH. Aliskiren, the first renin inhibitor for treating hypertension: reactive renin secretion may limit its effectiveness. *Am J Hypertens.* 2007;20:587-597.

205. Shand DG, et al. The release of guanethidine and bethanidine by splenic nerve stimulation: a quantitative evaluation showing dissociation from adrenergic blockade. *J Pharmacol Exp Ther.* 1973;184:73-80.

206. Sharpe E, et al. A case of prolonged hypotension following intravenous guanethidine block. *Anaesthesia.* 1987;42:1081-1084.

207. Shekarriz B, Stoller ML. Uric acid nephrolithiasis: current concepts and controversies. *J Urol.* 2002;168(4 Pt 1):1307-1314.

208. Shnaps Y, et al. Methyldopa poisoning. *J Toxicol Clin Toxicol.* 1982;19:501-503.

209. Siegel D, et al. Diuretics, serum and intracellular electrolyte levels, and ventricular arrhythmias in hypertensive men. *JAMA.* 1992;267:1083-1089.

210. Simonetti GD, et al. Non-lethal fetal toxicity of the angiotensin receptor blocker candesartan. *Pediatr Nephrol.* 2006;21:1329-1330.

211. Siscovick DS, et al. Diuretic therapy for hypertension and the risk of primary cardiac arrest. *N Engl J Med.* 1994;330:1852-1857.

212. Slater EE, et al. Clinical profile of angioedema associated with angiotensin converting-enzyme inhibition. *JAMA.* 1988;260:967-970.

213. Smith BA, et al. Acute hydralazine overdose: marked ECG abnormalities in a young adult. *Ann Emerg Med.* 1992;21:326-330.

214. Smith SW, et al. Prolonged severe hypotension following combined amlodipine and valsartan ingestion. *Clin Toxicol (Phila).* 2008;46:470-474.

215. Sonnenblick M, et al. Diuretic-induced severe hyponatremia. review and analysis of 129 reported patients. *Chest.* 1993;103:601-606.

216. Sorkin EM, Heel RC. Guanfacine. A review of its pharmacodynamic and pharmacokinetic properties, and therapeutic efficacy in the treatment of hypertension. *Drugs.* 1986;31:301-336.

217. Sparicio D, et al. Angiotensin-converting enzyme inhibitors predispose to hypotension refractory to norepinephrine but responsive to methylene blue. *J Thorac Cardiovasc Surg.* 2004;127:608.

218. Stähle H. A historical perspective: development of clonidine. *Best Pract Res Clin Anaesthesiol.* 2000;14:237-246.

219. Steele TH, Oppenheimer S. Factors affecting urate excretion following diuretic administration in man. *Am J Med.* 1969;47:564-574.

220. Stein B, Volans GN. Dixarit overdose: the problem of attractive tablets. *Br Med J.* 1978;2:667-668.

221. Suchard JR, Graeme KA. Pediatric clonidine poisoning as a result of pharmacy compounding error. *Pediatr Emerg Care.* 2002;18:295-296.

222. Swanson J, et al. Clonidine in the treatment of ADHD: questions about safety and efficacy. *J Child Adolesc Psychopharmacol.* 2009;5:301-304.

223. Tenenbein M. Naloxone in clonidine toxicity. *Am J Dis Child.* 1984;138:1084-1085.

224. Thormann J, et al. Effects of clonidine on sinus node function in man. *Chest.* 1981; 80:201-206.

225. Toh S, et al. Comparative risk for angioedema associated with the use of drugs that target the renin-angiotensin-aldosterone system. *Arch Intern Med.* 2012;172: 1582-1589.

226. Unger T, Sandmann S. Angiotensin receptor blocker selectivity at the AT1- and AT2-receptors: conceptual and clinical effects. *J Renin Angiotensin Aldosterone Syst.* 2000; 1(2 suppl):6.

227. van den Elzen M, et al. Efficacy of treatment of non-hereditary angioedema. *Clin Rev Allergy Immunol.* 2016.

228. Van der Linden W, et al. Acute cholecystitis and thiazides. *Br Med J (Clin Res Ed).* 1984;289:654-655.

229. Van Dyke MW, et al. Guanfacine overdose in a pediatric patient. *Vet Hum Toxicol.* 1990;32:46-47.

230. van Rijnsoever EW, et al. Angioneurotic edema attributed to the use of losartan. *Arch Intern Med.* 1998;158:2063-2065.

231. van Zwieten PA. Pharmacology of centrally acting hypotensive drugs. *Br J Clin Pharmacol.* 1980;10 Suppl 1:20S.

232. Varon J, Duncan SR. Naloxone reversal of hypotension due to captopril overdose. *Ann Emerg Med.* 1991;20:1125-1127.

233. Venturini G, et al. Selective inhibition of nitric oxide synthase type I by clonidine, an anti-hypertensive drug. *Biochem Pharmacol.* 2000;60:539-544.

234. Vigil-De Gracia P, et al. Management of severe hypertension in the postpartum period with intravenous hydralazine or labetalol: a randomized clinical trial. *Hypertens Pregnancy.* 2007;26:163-171.

235. Vila JM, et al. Thiazide-induced immune hemolytic anemia. *JAMA.* 1976;236: 1723-1724.

236. Waeber B, et al. Self poisoning with enalapril. *Br Med J (Clin Res Ed).* 1984; 288:287-288.

237. Weinberger MH. Diuretics and their side effects. Dilemma in the treatment of hypertension. *Hypertension.* 1988;11(3 Pt 2):20.

238. Weintraub HS, et al. benefits of aliskiren beyond blood pressure reduction. *Cardiol Rev.* 2011;19:90-94.

239. Wiley JF, et al. Clonidine poisoning in young children. *J Pediatr.* 1990;116: 654-658.

240. Yiu P, et al. Reversal of refractory hypotension with single-dose methylene blue after coronary artery bypass surgery. *J Thorac Cardiovasc Surg.* 1999;118:195-196.

241. Zarifis J, et al. Poisoning with anti-hypertensive drugs: methyldopa and clonidine. *J Hum Hypertens.* 1995;9:787-790.

242. Zheng X, et al. Plasma levels of beta-endorphin, leucine enkephalin and arginine vasopressin in patients with essential hypertension and the effects of clonidine. *Int J Cardiol.* 1995;51:233-244.

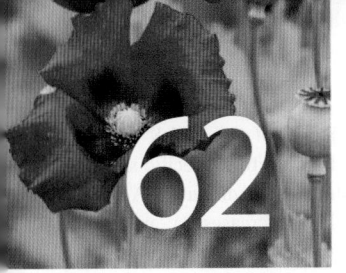

62 CARDIOACTIVE STEROIDS

Jason B. Hack

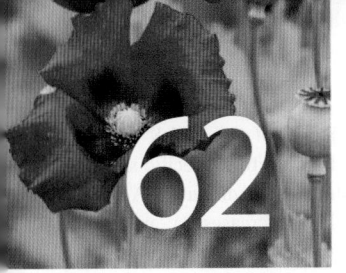

Digoxin
MW: = 780 Da

Unsaturated
lactone ring

Digitoxoses

Steroid nucleus
(cyclopentanoperhydrophenanthrene)

Aglycones, genin
(basic cardenolide structure)

HISTORY AND EPIDEMIOLOGY

The *Ebers Papyrus* provides evidence that the Egyptians used plants containing cardioactive steroids (CASs) at least 3,000 years ago. However, it was not until 1785, when William Withering wrote the first systematic account about the effects of the foxglove plant, that the use of CASs was more widely accepted into the Western apothecary. Foxglove, the most common source of plant CASs, was initially used as a diuretic and for the treatment of "dropsy" (edema), and Withering eloquently described its "power over the motion of the heart, to a degree yet unobserved in any other medicine."[123]

In the past, CASs were the primary treatment for congestive heart failure and control of ventricular response rate in atrial tachydysrhythmias. Because of their narrow therapeutic index, acute and chronic toxicities remain important problems.[84] According to the American Association of Poison Control Centers data, between the years 2011 and 2015, there were more than 7,000 exposures to CAS-containing plants with five attributable deaths and about 12,00 exposures to CAS-containing xenobiotics resulting in more than 120 deaths (Chap. 130).

Most cases of pharmaceutically induced CAS toxicity encountered in the United States result from digoxin; other internationally available but much less commonly used preparations are digitoxin, ouabain, lanatoside C, deslanoside, and gitalin. Digoxin toxicity most commonly occurs in patients at the extremes of age or those with chronic kidney disease (CKD). In children, most acute overdoses are unintentional, either by mistakenly ingesting an adult's medication or iatrogenically resulting from decimal point dosing errors. (Digoxin is prescribed in microgram doses, inviting 10-fold calculation errors.) In older adults, digoxin toxicity most commonly occurs either from interactions with another medication in their chronic regimen or indirectly as a consequence of an alteration in the absorption or elimination kinetics. These drug–drug interactions result from an adult's chronic polypharmacy or from the addition of a new xenobiotic that changes CAS clearance in the liver or kidney or alters protein binding resulting in increased bioavailability.

Cardioactive steroid toxicity also results from exposure to certain plants or animals, including oleander (*Nerium oleander*); yellow oleander (*Thevetia peruviana*), which are implicated in the suicidal deaths of thousands of patients in Southeast Asia;[25,26] foxglove (*Digitalis* spp); lily of the valley (*Convallaria majalis*); common milkweed (*Asclepias syriaca*);[104] sea mango (*Cerbera manghas*);[89] dogbane (*Apocynum cannabinum*); and red

squill (*Urginea maritima*). Cardioactive steroid poisoning results from teas containing seeds of these plants and herbal products contaminated with plant CASs (Chaps. 43 and 118).[16,19,53,77,89,91,97,104,115] Toxicity has resulted from ingestion, instead of the intended topical application, of a purported aphrodisiac derived from the dried secretion of toads from the *Bufo* species, which contains a bufadienolide-class CAS.[10-12] Although there have been no reported human exposures, fireflies of the *Photinus* species (*P. ignitus*, *P. marginellu*, and *P. pyralis)* contain the CAS lucibufagin that is structurally a bufadienolides (see Chemistry).[28,63]

CHEMISTRY

Cardioactive steroids contain an aglycone or "genin" nucleus structure with a steroid core and an unsaturated lactone ring attached at C-17. Cardioactive glycosides contain additional sugar groups attached to C-3. The sugar residues confer increased water solubility and enhance the ability of the molecule to enter cells. Cardenolides are primarily plant-derived aglycones with a five-membered unsaturated lactone ring. The bufadienolide and lucibufagin groups of CAS molecules are mainly animal derived and contain a six-membered unsaturated lactone ring (a plant derived exception is scillaren from red squill). Thus, when the aglycone digoxigenin is linked to one or more hydrophilic sugar (digitoxoses) moieties at C-3, it forms digoxin, a cardiac glycoside. The aglycone of digitoxin differs from that of digoxin by the absence of a hydroxyl group on C-12, and ouabain differs from digoxin by both the absence of a hydroxyl group on C-12 and the addition of hydroxyl groups on C-1, C-5, C-10, and C-11. The cardioactive components in toad secretions are genins and lack sugar moieties.

PHARMACOKINETICS

The correlation between clinical effects and serum concentrations is based on steady-state concentrations, which is dependent on absorption, distribution, and elimination (Table 62–1). Although not proven,

TABLE 62–1	Pharmacology of Selected Cardioactive Steroids	
Pharmacology	**Digoxin**	**Digitoxin**
Onset of action		
PO	1.5–6 h	3–6 h
IV	5–30 min	30 min–2 h
Maximal effect (h)		
PO	4–6	6–12
IV	1.5–3	4–8
Intestinal absorption (%)	40–90 (mean, 75)	>95
Plasma protein binding (%)	25	97
Volume of distribution (L/kg)	5–7 (adults)	0.6 (adults)
	16 (infants)	
	10 (neonates)	
	4–5 (adults with kidney failure)	
Elimination half-life (days)	1.6	6–7
Route of elimination (%)	Renal (60%–80%), with limited hepatic metabolism	Hepatic metabolism (80%)
Enterohepatic circulation (%)	7	26

IV = intravenous; PO = oral.

nonpharmaceutical CASs likely follow the absorption and distribution pattern of digoxin or digitoxin, therefore obtaining a serum concentration before 6 hours after ingestion (when tissue concentrations ultimately reach steady state) will give a misleadingly high (predistribution) serum concentration. After therapeutic dosing, the intravascular distribution of digoxin from the plasma is best described using a two-compartment model. The distribution or α phase represents the decrease in intravascular drug concentration and is dependent on whether the route of exposure was intravenous (IV) or oral (PO). Blood concentrations decline exponentially with a distribution half-life of 30 minutes as the drug moves from the blood to the peripheral tissues. Most of the intravascular CAS leaves the blood and distributes to the tissues, resulting in a large volume of distribution (V_d) (eg, the V_d of digoxin is 5–7 L/kg with therapeutic use). The β or elimination phase for digoxin has a half-life of approximately 36 hours and represents the total-body clearance of the drug, which is achieved primarily by the kidneys (70% of its clearance in a person with normal kidney function).[18,47]

After a massive acute digoxin overdose, the apparent half-life shortens to as little as 13 to 15 hours because elevated serum concentrations result in greater renal clearance before distribution to the tissues.[51,111] Even with therapeutic administration of CAS, adjustments to the dosing regimen must be made to avoid toxicity caused by the physiologic changes associated with aging, including hypothyroidism, chronic hypoxemia with alkalosis, and decreased glomerular filtration rate. Physiologic changes in CAS kinetics occur with functional decline of the liver, kidney, and heart and dynamics with electrolyte abnormalities, including hypomagnesemia, hypercalcemia, hypernatremia, and commonly hypokalemia. Therefore, serum concentrations of CAS should be monitored to avoid inadvertent toxicity. Hypokalemia resulting from a variety of mechanisms (eg, loop diuretics, poor dietary intake, diarrhea, and administration of potassium-binding resins) enhances the effects of CASs on the myocardium and is associated with toxicity at lower serum CAS concentrations. Chronic hypokalemia reduces the number of Na^+,K^+ adenosine triphosphatase (ATPase) units in skeletal muscle, which also alters drug effects.[15]

Drug interactions between digoxin and quinidine, verapamil, diltiazem, carvedilol, amiodarone, and spironolactone are common.[20,23,46,66,93] For example, quinidine decreases CAS tissue binding, which causes a reduction in the volume of distribution of the CAS, increasing its serum concentration; a reduction in excretion as a consequence of a decrease in renal perfusion; or, as a result of interference with secretion by the kidneys and intestines, because of inactivation of P-glycoproteins. Also, in approximately 10% to 15% of patients receiving digoxin, a significant amount of digoxin is inactivated in the gastrointestinal (GI) tract by enteric bacterium, primarily *Eubacterium lentum*. Inhibition of this inactivation by the alteration of the GI flora by many antibiotics, particularly macrolides, results in increased bioavailability[71] and increased serum CAS concentrations.[92]

MECHANISMS OF ACTION AND PATHOPHYSIOLOGY

Electrophysiologic Effects on Inotropy

Cardioactive steroids increase the force of contraction of the heart (positive inotropic effect) by increasing cytosolic Ca^{2+} during systole. Both Na^+ and Ca^{2+} ions enter and exit cardiac muscle cells during each cycle of depolarization–contraction and repolarization–relaxation. During depolarization–contraction, sodium entry heralds the start of the action potential (phase 0) and carries the inward, depolarizing positive charge. Calcium subsequently enters the cardiac myocyte through L-type calcium channels during late phase 0 and the plateau phase of the action potential. This extracellular Ca^{2+} entry into the cell triggers the release of additional Ca^{2+} into the cytosol from the sarcoplasmic reticulum (SR). During repolarization–relaxation (diastole), Ca^{2+} removed from the cytosol by two mechanisms—it is sequestered back into the SR by a local Ca^{2+}-ATPase and is moved out of the cell by an Ca^{2+}, Na^+-antiporter (Fig. 62–1 and Chap. 15).[76]

Cardioactive steroids inhibit active transport of Na^+ and K^+ across the cell membrane during repolarization by binding to a specific site on the extracellular face of the alpha-subunit of the membrane Na^+,K^+-ATPase. This inhibits the cellular Na^+ pump activity, which decreases Na^+ extrusion and increases Na^+ in the cytosol, thereby decreasing the transmembrane Na^+ gradient. Because the Ca^{2+}, Na^+-antiporter is not driven by adenosine triphosphate (ATP) but rather from the Na^+ gradient generated by the Na^+,K^+ transport mechanism (the antiporter extrudes one calcium ion from the cell in exchange for three sodium ions moving into the cell down a concentration gradient),[27] the dysfunction of the Na^+,K^+-ATPase pump reduces Ca^{2+} extrusion from the cell. The accumulation of cytoplasmic Ca^{2+} enhances the Ca^{2+} release from the SR during systole,[7] which increases the force of contraction of the cardiac muscle. Additional mechanisms of action are being explored and include creation of transmembrane calcium channels by cardioactive glycosides.[1]

Effects on Cardiac Electrophysiology

At therapeutic serum concentrations, CASs increase automaticity and shorten the repolarization intervals of the atria and ventricles (Table 62–2). There is a concurrent decrease in the rate of depolarization and conduction through the sinoatrial (SA) and atrioventricular (AV) nodes, respectively. This is mediated directly by depression of myocardial tissue and indirectly via an enhancement in vagally mediated parasympathetic tone. These changes in nodal conduction are reflected on the electrocardiogram (ECG) by a decrease in ventricular response rate to suprajunctional rhythms and by PR interval prolongation. The effects of CASs on ventricular repolarization are related to the elevated intracellular resting potential caused by accumulated cytosolic Ca^{2+} that manifests on the ECG as QT interval shortening and ST-segment and T-wave forces opposite in direction to the major QRS forces. The last effect results in the characteristic scooping of the ST segments (referred to as the *digitalis effect*; Fig. 62–2).

Excessive increases in intracellular Ca^{2+} caused by CAS toxicity result in delayed afterdepolarizations (DADs). Delayed afterdepolarizations are fluxes in membrane potential caused by Ca^{2+} release from the SR, which is caused by excess cytosolic Ca^{2+} and appear on the ECG as U waves. Occasionally, DADs initiate a cellular depolarization that manifests as a premature ventricular contraction (Chap. 16).[27,58]

Hypokalemia reduces Na^+,K^+-ATPase activity and enhances pump inhibition induced by CASs. This enhances myocardial automaticity and increases myocardial susceptibility to CAS-related dysrhythmias, partly as a result of decreased competitive inhibition between the CAS and potassium at the Na^+,K^+-ATPase exchange.[95] Severe hypokalemia (<2.5 mEq/L) reduces the efficacy of sodium–potassium pump function, slowing the pump and exacerbating concomitant Na^+–K^+ ATPase exchange inhibition by CASs.[58] Magnesium is a cofactor of the Na^+,K^+-ATPase exchange.[29] Hypomagnesemia reduces the Na^+,K^+-ATPase exchange activity, enhancing the inhibition affects and increasing the sensitivity to CASs.[95] Cardioactive steroid toxicity, evidenced by increased dysrhythmias and myocardial irritability, is closely associated with magnesium deficiency.[118,125]

Effects of Cardioactive Steroids on the Autonomic Nervous System

The parasympathetic system is affected by CASs by an increase in release of acetylcholine from vagal fibers,[72,114] possibly through augmentation of intracellular Ca^{2+}.

The sympathetic system is affected by CASs by an increase in efferent sympathetic discharge,[85,109] which exacerbates dysrhythmias.

MANIFESTATIONS OF CARDIOACTIVE STEROID TOXICITY

Detection of CAS toxicity is based on an accurate history of CAS exposure, high clinical suspicion based on subtle symptoms, and ECG and electrolyte abnormalities, coupled with a detectable CAS concentration. Although there are differences in the signs and symptoms of acute versus chronic CAS poisoning, adults and children have similar manifestations when poisoned.

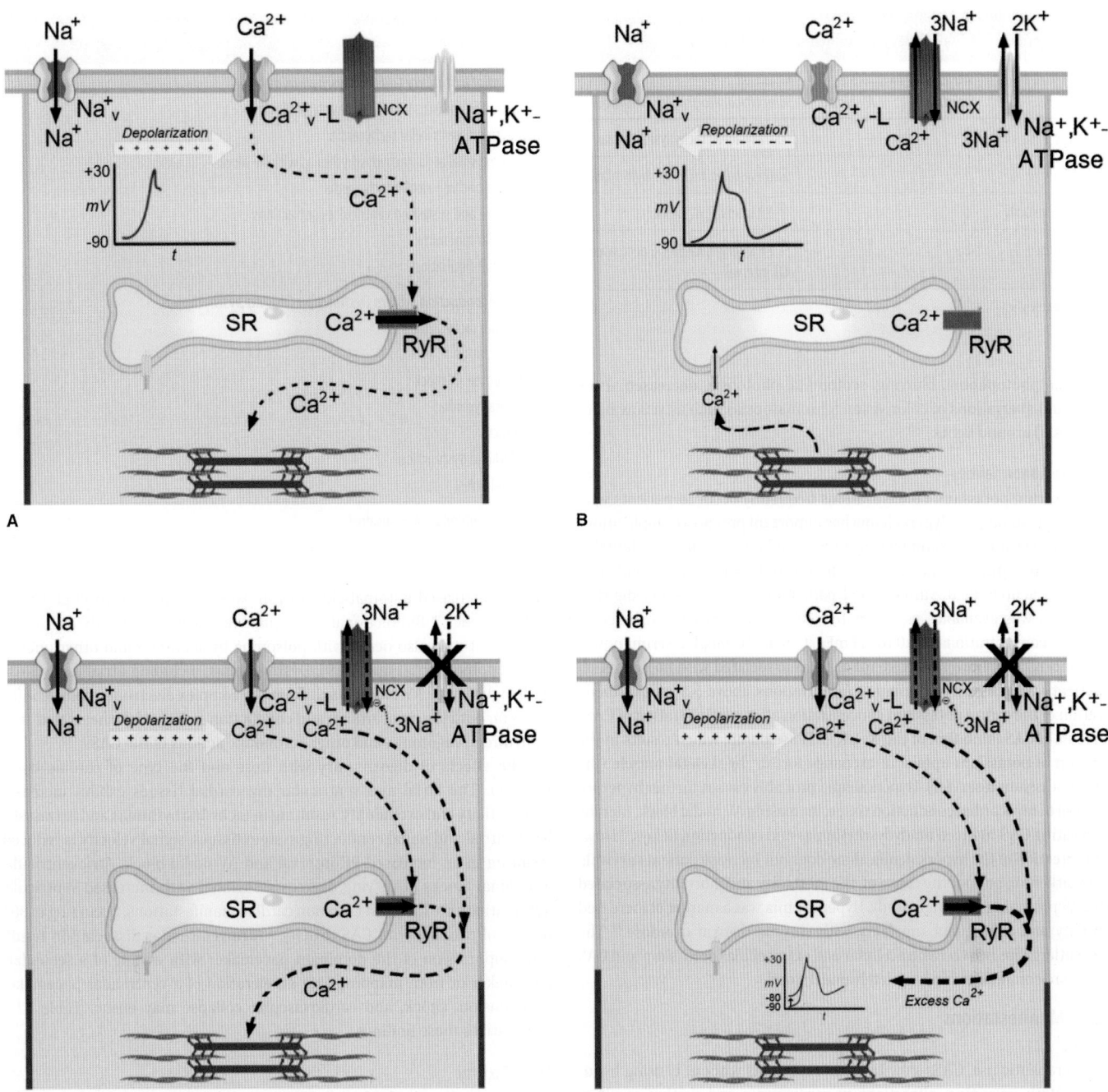

FIGURE 62–1. Pharmacology and toxicology of the cardioactive steroids (CASs). (**A**) Normal depolarization. Depolarization occurs after the opening of fast Na$^+$ channels; the increase in intracellular potential opens voltage-dependent Ca^{2+} channels, and the influx of Ca^{2+} induces the massive release of Ca^{2+} from the sarcoplasmic reticulum (SR), producing contraction. (**B**) Normal repolarization. Repolarization begins with active expulsion of 3Na$^+$ ions in exchange for 2K$^+$ ions using an ATPase. This electrogenic (3Na$^+$ for 2K$^+$) pump creates a Na$^+$ gradient used to expel Ca^{2+} via an antiporter (NCX). The SR sequesters its Ca^{2+} load via a separate ATPase. (**C**) Pharmacologic CAS. Digitalis inhibition of the Na$^+$,K$^+$-ATPase raises the intracellular Na$^+$ content, preventing the antiporter from expelling 1Ca^{2+} in exchange for 3Na$^+$. The net result is an elevated intracellular Ca^{2+}, resulting in enhanced inotropy through enhanced SR calcium release. (**D**) Toxicologic CAS. Excessive elevation of the intracellular Ca^{2+} elevates the resting potential, producing myocardial sensitization and predisposing to dysrhythmias. RyR = ryanodine receptor.

Noncardiac Manifestations

Acute Toxicity

An asymptomatic period of several minutes to several hours often follows a single administered toxic dose of CAS. The first clinical effects are typically nausea, vomiting, or abdominal pain. Central nervous system effects of acute toxicity include lethargy, confusion, and weakness that are not caused by hemodynamic changes.[3,16] The absence of nausea and vomiting within several hours after exposure makes severe acute CAS poisoning unlikely.

Chronic Toxicity

Chronic toxicity is often difficult to diagnose as a result of its insidious development and protean manifestations, including weakness, anhedonia, and loss of appetite.[84] Symptoms also include those that occur with acute poisonings; however, they are often less obvious. Gastrointestinal findings include anorexia, nausea, vomiting, abdominal pain, and weight loss. Neuropsychiatric disorders include delirium, confusion, drowsiness, headache, hallucinations, and, rarely, seizures.[16,39,41] Visual disturbances include transient

TABLE 62–2	Electrophysiologic Effects of Cardioactive Steroids on the Myocardium		
	Atria and Ventricles	AV Node	Electrocardiography Findings
Excitability	↑	—	Extrasystoles, tachydysrhythmias
Automaticity	↑	—	Extrasystoles, tachydysrhythmias
Conduction velocity	↓	↓	↑ PR interval, AV block
Refractoriness	↓	↑	↑ PR interval, AV block, decreased QT interval

AV = atrioventricular.

TABLE 62–3	Cardiac Dysrhythmias Associated With Cardioactive Steroid Poisoning

Myocardial Irritability Causing Dysrhythmias
Atrial flutter and atrial fibrillation with AV block
Bidirectional ventricular tachycardia
Nonparoxysmal atrial tachydysrhythmias with AV block
Nonsustained ventricular tachycardia
Premature and sustained ventricular contractions
Ventricular bigeminy
Ventricular fibrillation

Primary Conduction System Dysfunction Causing Dysrhythmias
Junctional tachycardia
AV dissociation
High-degree AV block
Sinus bradycardia
Exit blocks
His-Purkinje dysfunction
SA nodal arrest

AV = atrioventricular; SA = sinoatrial.

amblyopia, photophobia, blurring, scotomata, photopsia, decreased visual activity, and aberrations of color vision (chromatopsia) such as yellow halos (xanthopsia) around lights.[67,68]

Electrolyte Abnormalities

Elevated serum potassium concentrations frequently occur in patients with acute CAS poisoning.[15,58] Hyperkalemia has important prognostic implications because the serum potassium concentration is a better predictor of lethality than either the initial ECG changes or the serum CAS concentration.[5,6] In a study of 91 acutely digitoxin-poisoned patients conducted before digoxin-specific Fab was available, approximately 50% of the patients with serum potassium concentrations of 5.0 to 5.5 mEq/L died. Although a serum potassium concentration lower than 5.0 mEq/L was associated with no deaths, all 10 patients with serum potassium concentrations above 5.5 mEq/L died.[5] Elevation of the serum potassium concentration after administration of CASs is a result of CAS inhibition of the Na$^+$,K$^+$-ATPase pump, which results in the inhibition of potassium uptake in exchange for Na$^+$ by skeletal muscle (the largest potassium reservoir). Hyperkalemia probably causes further hyperpolarization of myocardial conduction tissue, increasing AV nodal block, thereby exacerbating CAS-induced bradydysrhythmias and conduction delays.[58] However, correction of the hyperkalemia alone does not increase patient survival;[5] it is a marker for, but not the cause of, the morbidity and mortality associated with CAS poisoning in a single study. Hyperkalemia was a marker of increased morbidity and subsequent mortality with chronic digoxin overdose.[74] The interrelationships between intracellular and extracellular potassium and CAS therapy are complex and incompletely understood.

Cardiac Manifestations
General

With therapeutic use, CASs slow tachydysrhythmias without causing hypotension. With poisoning, alterations in cardiac rate and rhythm result in nearly any dysrhythmia with the exception of a rapidly conducted supraventricular tachydysrhythmia because of the prominent AV nodal depressive effect of CASs. In 10% to 15% of cases, the first sign of toxicity is the appearance of an ectopic ventricular rhythm.[95] Although no single dysrhythmia is pathognomonic of CAS toxicity, toxicity should be suspected when

there is increased automaticity with impaired conduction through the SA and AV nodes.[58] Bidirectional ventricular tachycardia is nearly diagnostic, although it may also occur with poisoning by aconitine and other uncommon xenobiotics[106] (Fig. 15–19). Dysrhythmias, including atrial tachycardia with high-degree AV block, result from the complex electrophysiologic influences on both the myocardium and conduction system of the heart that stem from direct, vagotonic, and other autonomic actions of the CASs.

The effects of digoxin vary with dose and the type of cardiac tissue involved. The atrial and ventricular myocardial tissues exhibit increased automaticity and excitability, resulting in tachydysrhythmias and extrasystoles. In atrial and nodal conducting system tissues, signal velocity is reduced, resulting in an increased PR interval and AV nodal block. Atrioventricular junctional blocks of varying degrees associated with increased ventricular automaticity are the most common cardiac manifestations, occurring in 30% to 40% of patients with CAS toxicity.[73] Atrioventricular dissociation results from suppression of the dominant pacemaker with escape of a secondary pacemaker or from inappropriate acceleration of a ventricular pacemaker. Hypotension, shock, and cardiovascular collapse may ensue. Table 62–3 summarizes these findings.

Acute Toxicity

A variety cardiac dysrhythmias are associated with CAS toxicity. These dysrhythmias are unified by the presence of a sensitized myocardium and a depressed AV node (Table 62–3). Early bradydysrhythmias result from increased vagal tone at the SA and AV nodes and are often responsive to atropine.[37,80]

Chronic Toxicity

Later appearing bradydysrhythmias in both acute and chronic CAS toxicity occur by direct actions on the heart and often are minimally responsive to atropine.[37] Ventricular tachydysrhythmias are more common in patients with chronic or later in acute poisoning.

DIAGNOSTIC TESTING

Properly obtained and interpreted serum digoxin concentrations aid significantly in the management of patients with suspected digoxin toxicity, as well as in the management of patients poisoned by other CASs. Although most institutions report a therapeutic range for serum digoxin concentration from 0.5 to 2.0 ng/mL (SI units, 1.0–2.6 nmol/mL), current understanding suggests an upper limit of 1.0 ng/mL to maintain benefit while decreasing

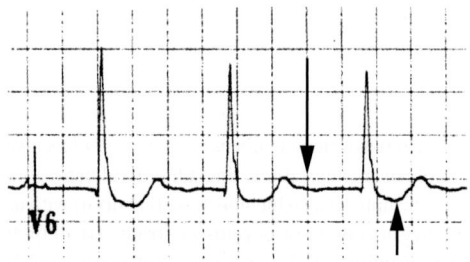

FIGURE 62–2. Digitalis effect noted in the lateral precordial lead, V6. Note the prolonged PR interval (long arrow) and the repolarization abnormality (scooping of the ST segment) (short arrow).

the risk of toxicity.[98,107] In addition to determining a serum CAS concentration, care must be taken to interpret the concentration as a correlate with other factors—the clinical condition of the patient; the interval between the last dose and the time the blood sample was taken; the presence of other metabolic abnormalities, including hypokalemia, hypomagnesemia, hypercalcemia, hypernatremia, alkalosis, hypothyroidism, and hypoxemia; and the use of xenobiotics such as amiodarone, calcium channel blockers, catecholamines, quinidine, and diuretics.

Cardioactive steroid poisoning is multifactorial, and using the upper limit of the therapeutic range of digoxin as the sole indicator of toxicity is misleading[101] because there is an overlap in serum digoxin concentrations between toxic and nontoxic patients. In general, a patient's clinical condition and serum concentration correlate well; the significance of a serum concentration depends on when the value is obtained after an acute ingestion to account for the distribution phase of the drug. Asymptomatic patients with CAS concentrations obtained before completion of the α distribution, found to be above the therapeutic range, are less often toxic but require close observation and retesting. Patients with mean pharmaceutical CAS serum concentrations above 2 ng/mL for digoxin and above 40 ng/mL for digitoxin measured 6 hours after the last dose often are clinically toxic.[59] A patient with a markedly elevated CAS concentration at any point after ingestion (eg, 15 ng/mL or greater for digoxin) requires definitive therapy.

In most hospitals, "digoxin levels" are the only estimation available to physicians in the acute setting when evaluating a patient for presumed nondigoxin CAS poisoning. The assays typically used in most institutions frequently, but unpredictably, cross-react with other plant- or animal-derived CASs. Although a monoclonal digoxin immunoassay accurately only quantifies the serum digoxin concentration, an elevated digoxin concentration in the correct clinical setting will qualitatively assist in making a presumptive diagnosis of nonpharmaceutical CAS exposure (Chaps. 43 and 118).[13,88] For example, using various techniques, including high-performance liquid chromatography and monoclonal and polyclonal antibody analysis, "digoxin" concentrations were determined from serum to which oleandrin and oleandrigenin from *Nerium oleander* was added or from patients exposed to *Thevetia peruviana* (yellow oleander) or toad-secreted bufadienolides.[11,25,55] Patients with CAS poisoning from plant- or animal-derived CASs may have a positive detection of CAS when using a polyclonal digoxin assay and a low or negative finding when using a monoclonal assay (Chaps. 43 and 118).

Serum concentrations of digoxin are measured in one of two ways: free digoxin and total digoxin. The most common method of quantifying total digoxin in the serum is by fluorescence polarization immunoassay. Under normal circumstances, 6 hours after the last dose, measuring total digoxin in the serum accurately predicts cardiac concentrations.[13,24] However, after the administration of digoxin-specific Fab (which remains almost entirely within the intravascular space (V_d, 0.40 L/kg), there is a large elevation in blood CAS concentrations because the CAS is drawn from the tissues and complexes with the antibody fragment. A large increase in total serum digoxin concentrations occurs, representing free CAS plus bound (inactivated) CAS. In this situation, requesting a "free digoxin level" will avoid this spurious increase and reflect clinically relevant unbound digoxin concentration. Paradoxically, excess digoxin Fab may itself cause a false elevation in digoxin concentration (Chap. 7).

ENDOGENOUS DIGOXINLIKE IMMUNOREACTIVE SUBSTANCE

Some patients have a positive digoxin assay resulting from an endogenous digoxinlike immunoreactive substance (EDLIS) that is structurally and functionally similar to prescribed CASs.[45,46] This substance is found in patients with increased inotropic need or reduced renal clearance, including neonates;[116] patients with end-stage kidney disease,[17,42,54] liver disease,[79] subarachnoid hemorrhage,[122] congestive heart failure,[40,102] insulin-dependent diabetes,[35] stress,[41,117] or hypothermia;[52] after strenuous exercise;[117] and in pregnancy.[31,43,50] An endogenous Na+,K+-ATPase–inhibiting dihydropyrone-substituted bufadienolide CAS was isolated from human placenta.[32] It differs from the toad bufadienolides by a single double-bond pyrone ring. Because

bufadienolides are not normally found in either healthy humans or edible plants, a synthetic pathway to produce dihydropyrone-substituted steroids in humans is thought to be responsible for EDLIS. Further research is necessary to confirm this pathway.[50] A clinician suspecting this problem should consult the clinical laboratory.[34] Clinical observations indicate that the serum digoxin concentration contributed by EDLIS is usually less than 2 ng/mL.

Other endogenous substances that can cross-react with the digoxin assay to produce a false-positive result include bilirubin[79] and xenobiotics, such as spironolactone.[103]

THERAPY
Acute Management Overview
Initial treatment of a patient with acute CAS poisoning includes providing general care (eg, GI decontamination, monitoring for dysrhythmias, measuring electrolyte and digoxin concentrations) and definitive care (eg, administering digoxin-specific antibody fragments {DSFab}). Secondary care includes treating complications such as dysrhythmias and electrolyte abnormalities.

Gastrointestinal Decontamination
The initial treatment should be directed toward prevention of further GI absorption. Rarely, if ever, is emesis or lavage recommended because efficacy is limited because of rapid absorption from the gut and to the emetic effects of the drug itself. Because many CASs, such as digitoxin and digoxin, are recirculated enterohepatically, both late and repeated activated charcoal (AC) administration (1 g/kg of body weight every 2–4 hours for up to four doses) are beneficial in reducing serum concentrations.[18,21,65,69,86,120] Activated charcoal prevents reabsorption of CAS from the GI tract and reduces the serum half-life. Activated charcoal is recommended in CAS-toxic patients if definitive therapy with digoxin-specific Fab is not immediately available or when kidney function is impaired.[21]

Advanced Management
Digoxin-Specific Antibody Fragments
Definitive therapy for patients with life-threatening dysrhythmias from CAS toxicity (in descending order of associated mortality: ventricular tachycardia, AV junctional tachycardia, and AV block[33]) is to administer DSFab.[2,34,36,87,91,97,108,112,124] Purified digoxin-specific Fab administration causes an immediate sharp decrease in free serum digoxin concentrations; a concomitant, but clinically unimportant, massive increase in total serum digoxin concentration; an increase in renal clearance of inactivated bound CAS; and a decrease in serum potassium concentration.[2] In addition, the administration of digoxin-specific Fab is pharmacoeconomically advantageous in economically developed countries.[22] Although the antidote itself is expensive, its expense is far outweighed by obviating the need, risk, and expense of long-term intensive care unit stays and of repetitive evaluation of potassium and digoxin concentrations. Table 62–4 lists the indications for administering digoxin-specific Fab. Extensive discussion is found in Antidotes in Depth: A22.

Other Cardiac Therapeutics
Secondary treatments used in patients with symptomatic CAS poisoning include the use of atropine for supraventricular bradydysrhythmias or high degrees of AV block. Atropine dosing is 0.5 mg administered IV to an adult or 0.02 mg/kg with a minimum of 0.1 mg to a child. Atropine should be titrated to block the vagotonic effects of CASs. The dose should be repeated at 5-minute intervals if necessary. Therapeutic success is unpredictable because the depressant actions of CASs are mediated only partly through the vagus nerve.

Phenytoin and lidocaine were used to manage CAS-induced ventricular tachydysrhythmias and ventricular irritability. These xenobiotics depress the enhanced ventricular automaticity without significantly slowing, and perhaps enhancing, AV nodal conduction.[96] In fact, phenytoin reverses digitalis-induced prolongation of AV nodal conduction while suppressing digitalis-induced ectopic tachydysrhythmia without diminishing myocardial contractile forces.[49] In addition, phenytoin terminates supraventricular dysrhythmias induced by digitalis more effectively than lidocaine.[96]

TABLE 62–4	Indications for Administration of Digoxin-Specific Antibody Fragments

Any digoxin related life-threatening dysrhythmias, regardless of SDC

—Includes ventricular tachycardia or ventricular fibrillation or progressive bradydysrhythmias such as atropine-resistant symptomatic sinus bradycardia or second or third-degree heart block

Potassium concentration >5 mEq/L in the setting of acute digoxin poisoning

Chronic elevation of SDC associated with dysrhythmias, significant GI symptoms, or altered mental status

SDC ≥15 ng/mL at any time or ≥10 ng/mL 6 h postingestion, regardless of clinical effects

Acute ingestion of 10 mg of digoxin in an adult

Acute ingestion of 4 mg of digoxin in a child

Poisoning with a nondigoxin cardioactive steroid

Digoxin-specific Fab dosing (round up to number of whole vials in calculation)

$$\text{No. of vials} = \frac{\text{SDC (ng/mL)} \times \text{Patient weight (kg)}}{100}$$

$$\text{No. of vials} = \frac{\text{Amount ingested (mg)}}{0.5 \,(\text{mg/vial})} \times 80\% \text{ bioavailability}$$

Empiric therapy for acute poisoning:

10–20 vials (adult or pediatric {must watch for volume overload})

Empiric therapy for chronic poisoning:

Adults: 3–6 vials

Children: 1–2 vials

GI = gastrointestinal; SDC = serum digoxin concentration.

Underlying atrial fibrillation and flutter typically do not convert to a normal sinus rhythm with administration of phenytoin or lidocaine. When used, phenytoin should be slowly IV infused (~50 mg/min) or in boluses of 100 mg repeated every 5 minutes until control of the dysrhythmias is achieved or a maximum of 1,000 mg has been given in adults or 15 to 20 mg/kg in children.[9,78] Fosphenytoin has not been evaluated in this setting. Maintenance PO doses of phenytoin (300–400 mg/day in adults and 6–10 mg/kg/day in children) should be continued until digoxin toxicity is resolved. Lidocaine is given as a 1- to 1.5-mg/kg IV bolus followed by continuous infusion at 1 to 4 mg/min in adults or as a 1- to 1.5-mg/kg IV bolus followed by 30 to 50 mcg/kg/min in children as required to control the rhythm disturbance (Chap. 57). Indications for the use of phenytoin and lidocaine in the setting of CAS toxicity are rare because of the effectiveness and definitiveness of Fab fragments, which has obviated their utility.

Class IA antidysrhythmics (eg, quinidine, procainamide, disopyramide) are contraindicated in the setting of CAS poisoning because they may induce or worsen AV nodal block by increasing vagal tone and decreasing His-Purkinje conduction by blocking fast Na⁺ channel opening and because their α-adrenergic receptor blockade and vagal inhibition may induce significant hypotension and tachycardia[37,83] Class IA antidysrhythmics are also prodysrhythmogenic, and their safety in the setting of CAS poisoning is unstudied. Additionally, quinidine reduces renal clearance of digoxin and digitoxin.[23] The use of isoproterenol should be avoided in CAS-induced conduction disturbances because there may be an increased incidence of ventricular ectopic activity in the presence of toxic concentrations of CAS.

Pacemakers and Cardioversion

External or transvenous pacemakers have had limited indications in the management of patients with CAS poisoning. In one retrospective study of 92 digitalis-poisoned patients, 51 patients were treated with cardiac pacing, digoxin-specific Fab, or both; the overall mortality rate was 13%.[113] Prevention of life-threatening dysrhythmias failed in 8% of

patients treated with immunotherapy and 23% of patients treated with internal pacemakers. The main reasons for failure of digoxin-specific Fab were pacing-induced dysrhythmias and delayed or insufficient doses of digoxin-specific Fab. Iatrogenic complications of pacing occurred in 36% of patients. Thus, overdrive suppression with a temporary transvenous pacemaker would only be reasonable in the scenario of unavailability or failure of digoxin-specific Fab in the presence of CAS poisoning.[6,113] In the setting of digoxin poisoning, administration of transthoracic electrical cardioversion for atrial tachydysrhythmias is associated with the development of potentially lethal ventricular dysrhythmias. The dysrhythmias were related to the degree of toxicity and the amount of administered current in cardioversion.[99] It is reasonable to attempt transthoracic pacing for atropine unresponsive bradydysrhythmias in settings when definitive care (digoxin-specific Fab fragments) is delayed or unavailable. In CAS-poisoned patients with unstable rhythms, such as unstable ventricular tachycardia or ventricular fibrillation, cardioversion, and defibrillation, respectively, are indicated.

Electrolyte Therapy

Potassium

Hypokalemia and hyperkalemia exacerbate CAS cardiotoxicity even at "therapeutic" digoxin concentrations. When hypokalemia is noted in conjunction with tachydysrhythmias or bradydysrhythmias, potassium replacement should be administered with serial monitoring of the serum potassium concentration. Digoxin-specific Fab administration generally should be withheld until the hypokalemia is corrected because the life-threatening manifestations of CAS cardiotoxicity often resolves.

In hyperkalemic patients, reduction in potassium concentrations should be judiciously initiated with care to avoid hypokalemia prior to initiating DsFab. Any exacerbation of CAS cardiotoxicity despite this correction should be treated immediately with Fab fragments.

In acute CAS toxicity, if potassium is at least 5 mEq/L, DSFab are recommended. If digoxin-specific Fab is not available immediately and ECG evidence of a dysrhythmia suggestions of hyperkalemia is present, an attempt should be made to lower the serum potassium with IV insulin, dextrose, sodium bicarbonate and PO administration of an ion-exchange substrate (eg, resin sodium polystyrene sulfonate) as indicated. Caution should be applied to the subsequent administration of digoxin-specific Fab because of concern for profound hypokalemia.

Although calcium is beneficial in most hyperkalemic patients, in the setting of CAS poisoning, administration of calcium salts is considered to be potentially dangerous. A number of experimental studies cite the additive or synergistic actions of calcium and CAS₍ₛ₎ on the heart (because intracellular hypercalcemia is already present), resulting in dysrhythmias,[38,82,105] cardiac dysfunction[60] (eg, hypercontractility, so-called stone heart hypocontractility), and cardiac arrest.[70,105,118] Although a 2004 study was unable to show an adverse effect,[44] there exist three case reports[8,62] of CAS-poisoned patients who died at various intervals after calcium administration, which supports the withholding of calcium administration in the setting of hyperkalemia induced by CAS poisoning.

Although rate of administration of Ca²⁺ may play a role in exaggerating CAS cardiac toxicity,[70,82] calcium administration should be avoided because better, safer, alternative treatments, such as digoxin-specific Fab, insulin, and sodium bicarbonate, are available for CAS-induced hyperkalemia.[14,58,87,108,112,124] The purported mechanism of exaggerated cardiac effects in CAS-toxic patients with the administration of Ca²⁺ is attributed to the preexisting CAS augmented intracellular cytoplasmic Ca²⁺. Exogenous Ca²⁺ is thought to increase Ca²⁺ transmembrane concentration gradient that further inhibits calcium extrusion through the Na⁺-Ca²⁺ exchange or increased intracytoplasmic stores.[59] This additional cytoplasmic calcium results in altered contraction of myofibril organelles,[60] less negative intracellular resting potential that allows delayed afterdepolarizations to reach firing threshold,[48,59,82] altered function of the SR,[60,94] or increased calcium interfering with myocardial mitochondrial function (Chaps. 15 and 16).[60]

Magnesium

Hypomagnesemia also occurs in CAS-poisoned patients secondary to the contributory factors mentioned with hypokalemia, such as long-term diuretic use to treat congestive heart failure. The theoretical benefits of magnesium therapy in the setting of hypomagnesemia include blockade of the transient inward calcium current, antagonism of calcium at intracellular binding sites, decreased CAS-related ventricular irritability,[61] and blockade of potassium egress from CAS-poisoned cells.[4,30,56,90,100,110,121] Although hypomagnesemia increases myocardial digoxin uptake and decreases cellular Na^+,K^+-ATPase activity, there is conflicting evidence as whether magnesium "reactivates" the CAS-bound Na^+,K^+-ATPase activity.[81,100,110]

Cardioactive steroid–toxic patients found to be hypomagnesemic should have magnesium repleted. A common regimen uses 2 g of magnesium sulfate IV over 20 minutes in adults (25–50 mg/kg/dose to a maximum of 2 g in children). After stabilization, adult patients with severe hypomagnesemia require a magnesium infusion of 1 to 2 g/h (25–50 mg/kg/h to a maximum of 2 g in children), with serial monitoring of serum magnesium concentrations, telemetry, respiratory rate (observing for bradypnea), deep tendon reflexes (observing for hyporeflexia), and monitoring of blood pressure.

Extracorporal Removal of Cardioactive Steroids

Forced diuresis,[64] hemoperfusion,[75,119] and hemodialysis[119] are ineffective in enhancing the elimination of digoxin because of its large volume of distribution (4–10 L/kg), which makes it relatively inaccessible to these techniques. Because of its high affinity for tissue proteins, only approximately 10% of the amount of the total body digoxin is found in the serum, and of that amount, approximately 20% to 40% is protein bound.[57]

SUMMARY

- Digoxin and digitoxin are the most commonly prescribed members of the drugs classified as CASs, and they have a narrow therapeutic index.
- Both cardiac and noncardiac effects occur after CAS poisoning, including nausea, vomiting, headache, weakness, altered mental status bradycardia, atrial and ventricular ectopy with block, or hyperkalemia.
- Dysrhythmias in patients with therapeutic cardioactive steroid concentrations often occur from hypokalemia and hypomagnesemia and these dysrhythmias will only be resolved with electrolyte repletion.
- Definitive therapy for acute CAS poisoning is the early administration of digoxin-specific Fab immunotherapy coupled with decontamination techniques, including AC and supportive therapy.

REFERENCES

1. Arispe N, et al. Heart failure drug digitoxin induces calcium uptake into cells by forming transmembrane calcium channels. *Proc Natl Acad Sci U S A.* 2008;105:2610-2615.
2. Banner W Jr, et al. Influence of assay methods on serum concentrations of digoxin during FAB fragment treatment. *J Toxicol Clin Toxicol.* 1992;30:259-267.
3. Bayer MJ. Recognition and management of digitalis intoxication: implications for emergency medicine. *Am J Emerg Med.* 1991;9:29-32.
4. Beller GA, et al. Correlation of serum magnesium levels and cardiac digitalis intoxication. *Am J Cardiol.* 1974;33:225-229.
5. Bismuth C, et al. Hyperkalemia in acute digitalis poisoning: prognostic significance and therapeutic implications. *Clin Toxicol.* 1973;6:153-162.
6. Bismuth C, et al. Acute digitoxin intoxication treated by intracardiac pacemaker: experience in sixty-eight patients. *Clin Toxicol.* 1977;10:443-456.
7. Blaustein MP. Physiological effects of endogenous ouabain: control of intracellular Ca2+ stores and cell responsiveness. *Am J Physiol.* 1993;264(6 Pt 1):C1367-1387.
8. Bower J, Mengle H. The additive effect of calcium and digitalis: a warning, with a report of two deaths. *JAMA.* 1936;106:1151-1153.
9. Bristow MR, et al. Treatment of heart failure: pharmacologic methods. In: Braunwald E, et al., eds. *Heart Disease: A Textbook of Cardiovascular Medicine.* 6th ed. Philadelphia, PA: Saunders; 2001:573-575.
10. Centers for Disease Control and Prevention (CDC). Deaths associated with a purported aphrodisiac—New York City, February 1993-May 1995. *MMWR Morb Mortal Wkly Rep.* 1995;44:853-855, 861.
11. Brubacher JR, et al. Treatment of toad venom poisoning with digoxin-specific Fab fragments. *Chest.* 1996;110:1282-1288.
12. Chern MS, et al. Biologic intoxication due to digitalis-like substance after ingestion of cooked toad soup. *Am J Cardiol.* 1991;67:443-444.
13. Cheung K, et al. Detection of poisoning by plant-origin cardiac glycoside with the Abbott TDx analyzer. *Clin Chem.* 1989;35:295-297.
14. Chillet P, et al. Digoxin poisoning and anuric acute renal failure: efficiency of the treatment associating digoxin-specific antibodies (Fab) and plasma exchanges. *Int J Artif Organs.* 2002;25:538-541.
15. Clausen T, et al. Effects of denervation on sodium, potassium and [3H] ouabain binding in muscles of normal and potassium-depleted rats. *J Physiol.* 1983;345:123.
16. Cooke DM. The use of central nervous system manifestations in the early detection of digitalis toxicity. *Heart Lung.* 1993;22:477-481.
17. Craver JL, Valdes R Jr. Anomalous serum digoxin concentrations in uremia. *Ann Intern Med.* 1983;98:483-484.
18. Critchley JA, Critchley LA. Digoxin toxicity in chronic renal failure: treatment by multiple dose activated charcoal intestinal dialysis. *Hum Exp Toxicol.* 1997;16:733-735.
19. Dasgupta A, et al. Effect of Asian and Siberian ginseng on serum digoxin measurement by five digoxin immunoassays. Significant variation in digoxin-like immunoreactivity among commercial ginsengs. *Am J Clin Pathol.* 2003;119:298-303.
20. De Mey C, et al. Carvedilol increases the systemic bioavailability of oral digoxin. *Br J Clin Pharmacol.* 1990;29:486-490.
21. de Silva HA, et al. Multiple-dose activated charcoal for treatment of yellow oleander poisoning: a single-blind, randomised, placebo-controlled trial. *Lancet.* 2003;361:1935-1938.
22. DiDomenico RJ, et al. Analysis of the use of digoxin immune fab for the treatment of non-life-threatening digoxin toxicity. *J Cardiovasc Pharmacol Ther.* 2000;5:77-85.
23. Doering W. Quinidine-digoxin interaction: pharmacokinetics, underlying mechanism and clinical implications. *The New England journal of medicine.* 1979;301:400-404.
24. Doherty JE, et al. The distribution and concentration of tritiated digoxin in human tissues. *Ann Intern Med.* 1967;66:116-124.
25. Eddleston M, et al. Acute yellow oleander (Thevetia peruviana) poisoning: cardiac arrhythmias, electrolyte disturbances, and serum cardiac glycoside concentrations on presentation to hospital. *Heart.* 2000;83:301-306.
26. Eddleston M, et al. Deliberate self harm in Sri Lanka: an overlooked tragedy in the developing world. *BMJ.* 1998;317:133-135.
27. Eisner DA, Smith TW. The Na-K pump and its effect in cardiac muscle. In: Fozzard HA, ed. *The Heart and Cardiovascular System: Scientific Foundations.* 2nd ed. New York, NY: Raven Press; 1991:863-902.
28. Eisner T, et al. Lucibufagins: defensive steroids from the fireflies Photinus ignitus and P. marginellus (Coleoptera: Lampyridae). *Proc Natl Acad Sci U S A.* 1978;75:905-908.
29. Fawcett WJ, et al. Magnesium: physiology and pharmacology. *Br J Anaesth.* 1999;83:302-320.
30. French JH, et al. Magnesium therapy in massive digoxin intoxication. *Ann Emerg Med.* 1984;13:562-566.
31. Friedman HS, et al. Urinary digoxin-like immunoreactive substance in pregnancy. Relation to urinary electrolytes. *Am J Med.* 1987;83:261-264.
32. Gao S, et al. [The source of endogenous digitalis-like substance in normal pregnancy]. *Zhonghua Fu Chan Ke Za Zhi.* 1998;33:539-541.
33. Gaultier M, et al. [Acute digitalis poisoning (70 cases)]. *Bull Mem Soc Med Hop Paris.* 1968;119:247-274.
34. George S, et al. Digoxin measurements following plasma ultrafiltration in two patients with digoxin toxicity treated with specific Fab fragments. *Anna Clin Biochem.* 1994;31(Pt 4):380-382.
35. Giampietro O, et al. Increased urinary excretion of digoxin-like immunoreactive substance by insulin-dependent diabetic patients: a linkage with hypertension? *Clin Chem.* 1988;34:2418-2422.
36. Gibb I, et al. Plasma digoxin: assay anomalies in Fab-treated patients. *Br J Clin Pharmacol.* 1983;16:445-447.
37. Gold H. Pharmacologic basis of cardiac therapy. *J Am Med Assoc.* 1946;132:547-554.
38. Gold H, Edwards DJ. The effects of ouabain on the heart in the presence of hypercalcemia. *Am Heart J.* 1927;3:45-50.
39. Gorelick DA, et al. Paranoid delusions and auditory hallucinations associated with digoxin intoxication. *J Nerv Ment Dis.* 1978;166:817-819.
40. Graves SW. Endogenous digitalis-like factors. *Crit Rev Clin Lab Sci.* 1986;23:177-200.
41. Graves SW, et al. Increases in plasma digitalis-like factor activity during insulin-induced hypoglycemia. *Neuroendocrinology.* 1989;49:586-591.
42. Graves SW, et al. An endogenous digoxin-like substance in patients with renal impairment. *Ann Intern Med.* 1983;99:604-608.
43. Graves SW, et al. Endogenous digoxin-immunoreactive substance in human pregnancies. *J Clin Endocrinol Metab.* 1984;58:748-751.
44. Hack JB, et al. The effect of calcium chloride in treating hyperkalemia due to acute digoxin toxicity in a porcine model. *J Toxicol Clin Toxicol.* 2004;42:337-342.
45. Haddy FJ. Endogenous digitalis-like factor or factors. *N Engl J Med.* 1987;316:621-623.
46. Hager WD, et al. Digoxin-quinidine interaction Pharmacokinetic evaluation. *N Engl J Med.* 1979;300:1238-1241.
47. Hastreiter AR, et al. Digitalis, digitalis antibodies, digitalis-like immunoreactive substances, and sodium homeostasis: a review. *Clin Perinatol.* 1988;15:491-522.
48. Hauptman PJ, Kelly RA. Digitalis. *Circulation.* 1999;99:1265-1270.
49. Helfant RH, et al. Protection from digitalis toxicity with the prophylactic use of diphenylhydantoin sodium. An arrhythmic-inotropic dissociation. *Circulation.* 1967;36:119-124.

50. Hilton PJ, et al. An inhibitor of the sodium pump obtained from human placenta. *Lancet.* 1996;348:303-305.

51. Hobson JD, Zettner A. Digoxin serum half-life following suicidal digoxin poisoning. *JAMA.* 1973;223:147-149.

52. Hoffman RS, et al. Endogenous digitalis-like factors in hypothermic patients. *Gen Int Med Clin Innov.* 2016;1(4).

53. Hollman A. Plants and cardiac glycosides. *Br Heart J.* 1985;54:258-261.

54. Isensee L, et al. Digoxin levels in dialysis patients. *Hosp Physician.* 1988;24:50-52.

55. Jortani SA, et al. Inhibition of Na,K-ATPase by oleandrin and oleandrigenin, and their detection by digoxin immunoassays. *Clin Chem.* 1996;42:1654-1658.

56. Kaneko T, et al. Successful treatment of digoxin intoxication by haemoperfusion with specific columns for beta2-microgloblin-adsorption (Lixelle) in a maintenance haemodialysis patient. *Nephrol Dial Transplant.* 2001;16:195-196.

57. Katzung BG, Parmley WM. Cardiac glycosides & other drugs used in congestive heart failure. In: Katzung BG, ed. *Basic & Clinical Pharmacology.* 7th ed. Stamford, CT: Appleton & Lange; 1998:197-215.

58. Kelly RA, Smith TW. Recognition and management of digitalis toxicity. *Am J Cardiol.* 1992;69:108G-118G; disc. 118G-119G.

59. Kelly RA, Smith TW. Pharmacological treatment of heart failure. In: Goodman LS, et al., eds. *Goodman & Gilman's The Pharmacological basis of Therapeutics.* 9th ed. New York, NY: McGraw-Hill, Health Professions Division; 1996:809-838.

60. Khatter JC, et al. Digitalis cardiotoxicity: cellular calcium overload a possible mechanism. *Basic Res Cardiol.* 1989;84:553-563.

61. Kinlay S, Buckley NA. Magnesium sulfate in the treatment of ventricular arrhythmias due to digoxin toxicity. *J Toxicol Clin Toxicol.* 1995;33:55-59.

62. Kne T, et al. Fatality from calcium chloride in a chronic digoxin toxic patient. *J Toxicol Clin Toxicol.* 1997;5:505.

63. Knight M, et al. Firefly toxicosis in lizards. *J Chem Ecol.* 1999;25:1981-1986.

64. Koren G, Klein J. Enhancement of digoxin clearance by mannitol diuresis: in vivo studies and their clinical implications. *Vet Hum Toxicol.* 1988;30:25-27.

65. Lalonde RL, et al. Acceleration of digoxin clearance by activated charcoal. *Clin Pharmacol Ther.* 1985;37:367-371.

66. Leahey EB Jr, et al. Interaction between quinidine and digoxin. *JAMA.* 1978;240:533-534.

67. Lee TC. Van Gogh's vision. Digitalis intoxication? *JAMA.* 1981;245:727-729.

68. Lely AH, van Enter CH. Large-scale digitoxin intoxication. *Br Med J.* 1970;3:737-740.

69. Levy G. Gastrointestinal clearance of drugs with activated charcoal. *N Engl J Med.* 1982;307:676-678.

70. Lieberman AL. Studies on calcium VI. Some inter-relationships of the cardiac activities of calcium gluconate and scillaren-B. *J Pharmacol Exp Ther.* 1933;47:183-192.

71. Lindenbaum J, et al. Inactivation of digoxin by the gut flora: reversal by antibiotic therapy. *N Engl J Med.* 1981;305:789-794.

72. Madan BR, et al. Effect of some arrhythmogenic agents upon the acetylcholine content of the rabbit atria. *J Pharm Pharmacol.* 1970;22:621-622.

73. Mahdyoon H, et al. The evolving pattern of digoxin intoxication: observations at a large urban hospital from 1980 to 1988. *Am Heart J.* 1990;120:1189-1194.

74. Manini AF, et al. Prognostic utility of serum potassium in chronic digoxin toxicity: a case-control study. *Am J Cardiovasc Drugs.* 2011;11:173-178.

75. Marbury T, et al. Advanced digoxin toxicity in renal failure: treatment with charcoal hemoperfusion. *South Med J.* 1979;72:279-281.

76. McGarry SJ, Williams AJ. Digoxin activates sarcoplasmic reticulum Ca(2+)-release channels: a possible role in cardiac inotropy. *Br J Pharmacol.* 1993;108:1043-1050.

77. McRae S. Elevated serum digoxin levels in a patient taking digoxin and Siberian ginseng. *CMAJ.* 1996;155:293-295.

78. Miller JM, Zipes DP. Management of the patient with cardiac arrhythmias. In: Braunwald E, et al., eds. *Heart Disease: A Textbook of Cardiovascular Medicine.* 6th ed. Philadelphia, PA: Saunders; 2001:726-727.

79. Nanji AA, Greenway DC. Falsely raised plasma digoxin concentrations in liver disease. *Br Med J (Clin Res Ed).* 1985;290:432-433.

80. Navab F, Honey M. Self-poisoning with digoxin: successful treatment with atropine. *Br Med J.* 1967;3:660-661.

81. Neff MS, et al. Magnesium sulfate in digitalis toxicity. *Am J Cardiol.* 1972;29:377-382.

82. Nola GT, et al. Assessment of the synergistic relationship between serum calcium and digitalis. *Am Heart J.* 1970;79:499-507.

83. Opie LH. Adverse cardiovascular drug interactions. *Curr Probl Cardiol.* 2000;25:621-676.

84. Ordog GJ, et al. Serum digoxin levels and mortality in 5,100 patients. *Ann Emerg Med.* 1987;16:32-39.

85. Pace DG, Gillis RA. Neuroexcitatory effects of digoxin in the cat. *J Pharmacology Exp Ther.* 1976;199:583-600.

86. Pond S, et al. Treatment of digitoxin overdose with oral activated charcoal. *Lancet.* 1981;2:1177-1178.

87. Rabetoy GM, et al. Treatment of digoxin intoxication in a renal failure patient with digoxin-specific antibody fragments and plasmapheresis. *Am J Nephrol.* 1990;10:518-521.

88. Radford DJ, et al. Immunological detection of cardiac glycosides in plants. *Aust Vet J.* 1994;71:236-238.

89. Radford DJ, et al. Naturally occurring cardiac glycosides. *Med J Aust.* 1986;144:540-544.

90. Reisdorff EJ, et al. Acute digitalis poisoning: the role of intravenous magnesium sulfate. *J Emerg Med.* 1986;4:463-469.

91. Rich SA, et al. Treatment of foxglove extract poisoning with digoxin-specific Fab fragments. *Ann Emerg Med.* 1993;22:1904-1907.

92. Rodin SM, Johnson BF. Pharmacokinetic interactions with digoxin. *Clin Pharmacokinet.* 1988;15:227-244.

93. Rose AM, Valdes R Jr. Understanding the sodium pump and its relevance to disease. *Clin Chem.* 1994;40:1674-1685.

94. Rosen MR. Cellular electrophysiology of digitalis toxicity. *J Am Coll Cardiol.* 1985;5 (5 suppl A):22a-34a.

95. Rosen MR, et al. Electrophysiology and pharmacology of cardiac arrhythmias. IV. Cardiac antiarrhythmic and toxic effects of digitalis. *Am Heart J.* 1975;89:391-399.

96. Rumack BH, et al. Phenytoin (diphenylhydantoin) treatment of massive digoxin overdose. *Br Heart J.* 1974;36:405-408.

97. Safadi R, et al. Beneficial effect of digoxin-specific Fab antibody fragments in oleander intoxication. *Arch Intern Med.* 1995;155:2121-2125.

98. Sameri RM, et al. Lower serum digoxin concentrations in heart failure and reassessment of laboratory report forms. *Am J Med Sci.* 2002;324:10-13.

99. Sarubbi B, et al. Atrial fibrillation: what are the effects of drug therapy on the effectiveness and complications of electrical cardioversion? *Can J Cardiol.* 1998;14:1267-1273.

100. Seller RH. The role of magnesium in digitalis toxicity. *Am Heart J.* 1971;82:551-556.

101. Selzer A. Role of serum digoxin assay in patient management. *J Am Coll Cardiol.* 1985;5(5 suppl A):106a-110a.

102. Shilo L, et al. Endogenous digoxin-like immunoreactivity in congestive heart failure. *Br Med J (Clin Res Ed).* 1987;295:415-416.

103. Silber B, et al. Spironolactone-associated digoxin radioimmunoassay interference. *Clin Chem.* 1979;25:48-50.

104. Simpson NS, et al. What toxicity may result from ingestion of the plant pictured below? Answer: cardioactive steroid toxicity from common milkweed. *J Med Toxicol.* 2013;9:287-288.

105. Smith PK, et al. Calcium and digitalis synergism: the toxicity of calcium salts injected intravenously into digitalized animals. *Arch Intern Med.* 1939;64:322-329.

106. Smith SW, et al. Bidirectional ventricular tachycardia resulting from herbal aconite poisoning. *Ann Emerg Med.* 2005;45:100-101.

107. Smith TW. Pharmacokinetics, bioavailability and serum levels of cardiac glycosides. *J Am Coll Cardiol.* 1985;5(5 suppl A):43a-50a.

108. Smith TW, et al. Reversal of advanced digoxin intoxication with Fab fragments of digoxin-specific antibodies. *N Engl J Med.* 1976;294:797-800.

109. Somberg JC, et al. The antiarrhythmic effects of quinidine and propranolol in the ouabain-intoxicated spinally transected cat. *Eur J Pharmacol.* 1979;54:161-166.

110. Specter MJ, et al. Studies on magnesium's mechanism of action in digitalis-induced arrhythmias. *Circulation.* 1975;52:1001-1005.

111. Springer M, et al. Acute massive digoxin overdose: survival without use of digitalis-specific antibodies. *Am J Emerg Med.* 1986;4:364-368.

112. Sullivan JB Jr. Immunotherapy in the poisoned patient. Overview of present applications and future trends. *Med Toxicol.* 1986;1:47-60.

113. Taboulet P, et al. Acute digitalis intoxication—is pacing still appropriate? *J Toxicol Clin Toxicol.* 1993;31:261-273.

114. Torsti P. The acetylcholine content and cholinesterase activities in the rabbit heart in experimental heart failure and the effect of g-strophanthin treatment upon them. *Ann Med Exp Biol Fenn.* 1959;37(suppl 4):1-71.

115. Tuncok Y, et al. Urginea maritima (squill) toxicity. *J Toxicol Clin Toxicol.* 1995;33:83-86.

116. Valdes R Jr, et al. Endogenous substance in newborn infants causing false positive digoxin measurements. *J Pediatr.* 1983;102:947-950.

117. Valdes R Jr, et al. Endogenous digoxin-like immunoreactivity in blood is increased during prolonged strenuous exercise. *Life Sci.* 1988;42:103-110.

118. Wagner J, Salzer WW. Calcium-dependent toxic effects of digoxin in isolated myocardial preparations. *Arch Int Pharmacodyn Ther.* 1976;223:4-14.

119. Warren SE, Fanestil DD. Digoxin overdose. Limitations of hemoperfusion-hemodialysis treatment. *JAMA.* 1979;242:2100-2101.

120. Watson WA. Factors influencing the clinical efficacy of activated charcoal. *Drug Intell Clin Pharm.* 1987;21:160-166.

121. Whang R, Aikawa JK. Magnesium deficiency and refractoriness to potassium repletion. *J Chronic Dis.* 1977;30:65-68.

122. Wijdicks EF, et al. Digoxin-like immunoreactive substance in patients with aneurysmal subarachnoid haemorrhage. *Br Med J (Clin Res Ed).* 1987;294:729-732.

123. Withering W. An account of the foxglove and some of its medical uses: with practical remarks on dropsy and other diseases. In: Kelly EC, ed. *Medical Classics.* Baltimore, MD: Williams & Wilkins; 1936:295-443.

124. Woolf AD, et al. The use of digoxin-specific Fab fragments for severe digitalis intoxication in children. *N Engl J Med.* 1992;326:1739-1744.

125. Young IS, et al. Magnesium status and digoxin toxicity. *Br J Clin Pharmacol.* 1991;32:717-721.

A22

DIGOXIN-SPECIFIC ANTIBODY FRAGMENTS

Silas W. Smith and Mary Ann Howland

INTRODUCTION

Digoxin-specific antibody fragments (DSFab) are indicated for the management of patients with digoxin and digitoxin toxicity, as well as toxicity from other pharmaceutical, plant, and animal cardioactive steroids (CASs, eg, ouabain, dogbane, oleander, squill, and *Bufo* and *Birgus* species). Digoxin-specific antibody fragments have an excellent record of efficacy and safety, and they should be administered early in both established and suspected CAS poisoning.

HISTORY

The production of antibody fragments to treat patients poisoned with digoxin followed the development of digoxin antibodies for measuring serum digoxin concentrations by radioimmunoassay (RIA).[21] This RIA technique permitted the correlation between serum digoxin concentrations and clinical digoxin toxicity.[10,31,38,91] In 1967, Butler and Chen suggested that purified antidigoxin antibodies with a high affinity and specificity should be developed to treat digoxin toxicity in humans.[21] The digoxin molecule alone, with a molecular weight of 780 Da, was too small to be immunogenic. But digoxin could function as a hapten when joined to an immunogenic protein carrier such as albumin. These investigators immunized sheep with this conjugate to generate antibodies.[115,117] The immunized sheep subsequently produced a mixture of antibodies that included antialbumin antibodies and antidigoxin antibodies. The antibodies were separated and highly purified to retain the digoxin antibodies while removing the antibodies to the albumin and all other extraneous proteins. The antibodies that were developed had a high affinity for digoxin and sufficient cross-reactivity with digitoxin and other CASs to be clinically useful for the treatment of all CAS poisonings.[23,106,107]

Intact IgG antidigoxin antibodies reversed digoxin toxicity in dogs.[22] Unfortunately, the urinary excretion of digoxin was delayed, and free digoxin was released after antibody degradation occurred. Furthermore, there was significant concern with regard to the development of hypersensitivity reactions. To make such antibodies both safer and effective in humans, whole IgG antidigoxin antibodies were cleaved with papain, yielding two antigen-binding fragments (Fab) and one (discarded) Fc fragment.[22] Affinity chromatography was used to isolate and purify the DSFab after papain digestion. Because the Fc fragment does not bind antigen and increases the potential for hypersensitivity reactions, it was eliminated. When compared with whole IgG antibodies, the advantages of DSFab included a larger volume of distribution (V_d) and distribution to the extravascular space, more rapid onset of action, diminished risk of adverse immunologic effects, and more rapid elimination.[22,76,79,83,117] In 1976, Digibind was used with clinical success,[116] and it became commercially available in 1986, before being discontinued in 2011.[59] Another commercial product, DigiFab, approved by the US Food and Drug Administration (FDA) in 2001, is currently available.[20]

PHARMACOLOGY

Chemistry and Preparation

DigiFab is prepared from the blood of healthy sheep that were immunized with a digoxin derivative, digoxin-dicarboxymethoxylamine (DDMA).[20] Digoxin-dicarboxymethoxylamine contains a functionally essential cyclopentaperhydrophenanthrene:lactone ring moiety coupled to keyhole limpet hemocyanin (KLH), a metalloprotein found in the hemolymph of the great keyhole limpet (*Megathura crenulata*) that functions as the hapten instead of the previously used albumin. Papain digestion yields digoxin-specific Fab fragments, which are isolated by affinity chromatography.[20] The molecular weight of each fragment is approximately 46,200 Da.

Mechanism of Action

Immediately after intravenous (IV) administration, the antigen-binding fragments bind intravascular free digoxin (or digitoxin). Uncomplexed antibody fragments then diffuse into the interstitial space, where they bind free digoxin. A concentration gradient is then established, which facilitates movement into the interstitial or intravascular spaces of both the free intracellular digoxin and digoxin that is dissociated from its binding sites on the external surface of Na$^+$,K$^+$-adenosine triphosphatase (ATPase) enzyme in the heart and in skeletal muscles.[84,105] The dissociation rate constant of digoxin for Na$^+$,K$^+$-ATPase, therefore, affects the time course for binding to DSFab and, consequently, the onset of action.[62,86,109] The binding affinities of DSFab for digoxin and digitoxin are about 10^9 to 10^{10} M^{-1} and 10^8 to 10^9 M^{-1}, respectively. They are greater than the affinities of digoxin or digitoxin for the Na$^+$,K$^+$-ATPase enzyme.[20]

Pharmacokinetics

The pharmacokinetics of Digibind and DigiFab (previously named DigiTAb) were compared in human volunteers.[129] Sixteen participants received 1 mg of digoxin intravenously as a 5-minute bolus followed 2 hours later by a 30-minute IV infusion of 76 mg (an equimolar neutralizing dose) of either Digibind or DigiFab. Free and total digoxin (free plus DSFab bound) were assayed using an ultrafiltration method over 48 hours. At 30 minutes after infusion of either DSFab, the serum free digoxin concentration was below the level of assay detection and remained so for several hours. A few patients in both groups had free digoxin concentrations rebound to 0.5 ng/mL at approximately 18 hours, and the area under the serum drug concentration versus time curve (AUC) for 2 to 48 hours for free digoxin was similar for both treatment groups. The elimination half-life of total digoxin averaged 18 hours for DigiFab and 21 hours for Digibind, and the distribution half-life was 1 hour for each. In another study, the elimination half-life of the DSFab-glycoside complex was 20 to 30 hours, with free digoxin concentrations rising between 8 and 12 hours.[118] The volumes of distribution were 0.3 L/kg for DigiFab versus 0.4 L/kg for Digibind.[25,20] Systemic clearance of DigiFab was higher than for Digibind, accounting for the shorter elimination half-life of DigiFab (15 hours versus 23 hours).[129] Urine sampling over the first 24 hours demonstrated mostly free digoxin and very little free DSFab for both groups. The authors postulated that during renal excretion, the DSFab digoxin complex is metabolized in the kidney by the proximal tubular cells, releasing free digoxin and unmeasured DSFab metabolites.[129]

Similar findings were described after the first clinical use of Digibind in a patient who gave a history of ingesting 90 (0.25 mg) digoxin tablets.[116] The total serum digoxin concentration, which was 17.6 ng/mL at the time Digibind infusion was initiated, rose to 226 ng/mL at 1 hour and remained there for 11 hours, before falling off the next 44 hours, with a half-life of 20 hours.[116] Digibind concentrations peaked at the end of the infusion and then apparently exhibited a biphasic or triphasic decline, probably reflecting distribution into different compartments, as well as excretion and catabolism. Free serum digoxin concentrations were undetectable for the first 9 hours; rose to a peak of 2 ng/mL at 16 hours; and fell to 1.5 ng/mL at both 36 hours and 56 hours, at which time sampling stopped. An analysis of

977

renal elimination based on an incomplete collection suggested that digoxin was excreted only in the bound form during the first 6 hours, but by 30 hours after Fab administration, all digoxin in the urine was free digoxin.

A study designed to measure efficacy of DSFab delivery compared a loading dose of DSFab followed by an infusion of the DSFab dose infused over a short amount of time.[105] The former strategy increased the ratio of digoxin bound to uncomplexed DSFab in the serum from 50% to 70%.[105] The authors hypothesized that a very rapid infusion regimen would result in the elimination of DSFab before the fragments could optimally bind the digoxin redistributing from tissue sites.[105]

Digoxin takes several hours to distribute from the blood to the tissue compartment. As expected, a rodent model demonstrated that DSFab was more effective when administered before complete distribution of digoxin.[101] When distribution was complete, increasing the dose of DSFab significantly improved efficacy, as measured by comparing the AUC of digoxin with that of the Fab–digoxin complex.[101]

Pharmacokinetic studies in patients with kidney failure demonstrate that the half-life of DSFab is prolonged 10-fold, with no change in the apparent DSFab V_d. In this situation, serum DSFab concentrations can remain detectable for 2 to 3 weeks or more.[87] Total serum digoxin concentrations generally follow DSFab serum concentrations. Case reports and series demonstrate that free digoxin concentrations can persist and reappear up to 10 days after administration of DSFab to patients end-stage kidney disease compared with 12 to 24 hours in patients with normal kidney function.[39,43,68,87,88,111,113,121-123,133] In one series of patients with end-stage kidney disease, the maximum average concentration of free digoxin was 1.30 ± 0.7 ng/mL and occurred at 127 ± 40 hours.[122] After the peak, there is a slow decline that parallels the elimination of DSFab.

In an attempt to hasten digoxin elimination with and without DSFab treatment, various extracorporal modalities were explored, with predictably disappointing results given digoxin's V_d and the digoxin–antibody complex's size. The inability of extracorporeal elimination has been demonstrated in several experimental models and case reports. Continuous arteriovenous hemofiltration was ineffective in removing the digoxin–Fab fragment complex in a piglet model.[96] Low concentrations of total digoxin were measured in peritoneal dialysate of a 3-day-old child with digoxin overdose.[11] Plasmapheresis was capable of clearing DSFab-bound digoxin and preventing rebound in one case.[97] In another case, a 4-hour session was used to reverse persistent cardiotoxicity from recrudescence at 18 hours after a massive digoxin ingestion (serum concentration 35.6 ng/mL > 20 hours after overdose).[100] In another patient, plasma exchange was capable of removing DSFab–digoxin complexes and precluding rebound, but it was without significant impact in improving total digoxin clearance (< 1% of the total amount of ingested drug) because of digoxin's large apparent V_d.[139] Last, plasma exchange closely after DSFab administration in a patient with junctional rhythm, hemodynamic instability, and a digoxin concentration of 16.7 ng/mL was associated with gradual recovery of consciousness and sinus rhythm, although discerning the effect of plasma exchange from antidotal administration was unclear.[104] A multispecialty-working group, which reviewed the available literature, recommended against performing extracorporeal treatments in severe digoxin poisoning when DSFab is administered.[85] Provision of additional DSFab is recommended as a more rational approach.

Pharmacodynamics

At the tissue level, in ex vivo isolated human ventricular myocardium with a 1.5-fold higher molar DSFab dosing, digoxin toxicity was reversed within 30 minutes.[86] A key finding from this study and an additional investigation in human postmortem left ventricles was that the maximal rate of digoxin removal from Na^+,K^+-ATPase was limited by the dissociation rate of digoxin from Na^+,K^+-ATPase, with a half-life for this decay ranging from 46 to 54 minutes.[86,109] Later pharmacokinetic and pharmacodynamic studies inferred two digoxin receptor subtypes, (1) a high-affinity, low-capacity binding site that constituted 11% of receptors and mediates digoxin-induced positive inotropic effect and (2) a low-affinity, high-capacity binding site that

constituted 89% of total receptors.[62,131] The effects of the low-affinity receptor increased as dose increased, and its dissociation time constant was 18 times lower than high-affinity, low-capacity receptor, implying kinetic limits to DSFab efficacy even in the setting of sufficient molar administration.[62,85] At the blood compartment level, in six patients in whom free digoxin or digitoxin concentrations were measured in a clinical toxicity scenario, free serum concentrations decreased to zero or near zero within 1 to 2 minutes after administration of the antibody fragments.[134] In a later study in 36 patients with chronic digoxin poisoning who received one, two, or three or more DSFab vials, free digoxin concentrations decreased to almost zero after administration, regardless of dose.[27]

Clinically, in the multicenter study of 150 patients, the mean time to initial response from the completion of the Digibind infusion (accomplished over 15 minutes to 2 hours) was 19 minutes (range, 0–60 minutes), and the time to complete response was 88 minutes (range, 30–360 minutes). Time to response was not affected by age, concurrent cardiac disease, or presence of chronic or acute ingestion.[5] In another study of 63 adult and pediatric patients, therapeutic response generally occurred by 30 minutes, although some pediatric patients responded within minutes, and complete response sometimes took hours.[134] Dysrhythmia reversal occurred within an average of 3.2 hours (range, 0.5–13 hours) in 34 patients with life threatening dysrhythmias.[118] In another series, 15 of 19 pediatric patients had complete resolution within 180 minutes, with a median time to initial response of 25 minutes.[135]

ROLE IN DIGOXIN TOXICITY

A large study evaluating adults and pediatric patients with acute and chronic digoxin toxicity established the efficacy of Digibind.[5] Of the 150 patients treated, 148 were evaluated for cardiovascular manifestations of toxicity before treatment: 79 patients (55%) had high-grade atrioventricular (AV) block, 68 (46%) had refractory ventricular tachycardia, 49 (33%) had ventricular fibrillation, and 56 (37%) had hyperkalemia. Complete resolution of all signs and symptoms of digoxin toxicity occurred in 80% of cases. Partial response was observed in 10% of patients, and of the 15 patients who did not respond, 14 were moribund before initiation of therapy or later found to not be digoxin toxic. The success of Digibind was demonstrated by the fact that of the 56 patients who had cardiac arrest caused by digoxin, 54% survived to discharge compared with 100% mortality before the availability of DSFab.[5] In 34 patients (27 with suicidal intent) with life-threatening dysrhythmias and a mean serum digoxin concentration of 12.2 ng/mL (range, 3.4–29 ng/mL), 32 (94%) made a full recovery after administration of DSFab (as Digitalis Antidote BM).[118] In a prospective study of suicidal, acute, and chronic patients poisoned by digoxin and digitoxin, in which 22 required cardiopulmonary resuscitation (ie, chest compressions), 53 of 56 (95%) patients responded to DSFab.[134] The three deaths were associated with nonequimolar DSFab administration, concomitant cyclic antidepressant overdose, and severe underlying cardiac disease. In a postmarketing observational surveillance study of 717 patients, 50% of patients had a complete response to treatment, 24% had a partial response, and 12% had no response.[54] In the 89 patients with no response, digoxin was deemed contributory in only 14 patients. Four of these patients had unexplained treatment failure; 2 received inadequate Digibind dosing; and 8 were moribund, unevaluable, or of questionable toxicity.[54] A later single-center, retrospective review of 66 patients used equimolar therapy in cases of lethal dysrhythmia, arrest, bradycardia less than 40 beats/min, potassium greater than 5 mEq/L, cardiogenic shock, and half-molar reversal in patients at risk for deterioration; DSFab treatment reversed poisoning in 91%.[75] In the 5 patients who ultimately died, 3 had successful responses to DSFab but died of other complications, 1 had iatrogenic digoxin administration for dysrhythmia associated with septic shock, and 1 had a combined verapamil poisoning. Repeat therapy was required in 11 of 66 (16.7%) patients initially treated with a median dose of three vials.[75] In a large retrospective, multicenter review of 838 patients, the mortality rate was significantly decreased with DSFab use from 15% (117 of 770 patients) to 6% (4 of 67 patients).[74] A prospective study of 36 patients was confounded by patients' use of multiple cardiac medications, potential spironolactone interference with the digoxin assay, digoxin clearance, potassium elimination, and digoxin concentrations with unclear relationship to the distributional phase.[32,89,126] The administration of DSFab eliminated gastrointestinal (GI) symptoms suggestive of toxicity, increased heart rate in a dose-dependent fashion when one, two, or three or more vials were provided by 4.5, 10, and 17.3 beats/min, respectively, and decreased potassium by 0.3 mmol/L in an apparent dose-independent fashion.[27] As was demonstrated by multiple studies, DSFab is efficacious in reversing digoxin-associated cardiac arrest.[5,75,94,134] Newborns, infants, and children have all been successfully treated with DSFab.[11,44,65,110,111] In a large series of 29 pediatric patients poisoned with digoxin or digitoxin, DSFab at doses of 0.30 to 0.96 mg/kg reversed severe cardiac manifestations or hyperkalemia in 27 (93%).[135]

ROLE OF DIGOXIN-SPECIFIC ANTIBODY FRAGMENTS WITH OTHER CARDIOACTIVE STEROIDS

Digoxin-specific antibody fragments were designed to have high-affinity binding for digoxin and digitoxin. There are structural similarities, however, among the CASs. In fact, detectable "digoxin concentrations" using immunoassays were reported with some, but not all, nondigoxin CASs.[17,34,35,46,64,92] This interference suggested a potential for cross-reactivity between DSFab and other CASs. Thus, DSFab can have variable efficacy for multiple natural CAS poisonings, including those unique CASs in common and yellow oleander (*Nerium oleander* and *Thevetia peruviana*), dogbane (*Apocynum cannabinum*), lily of the valley (*Convallaria majalis*), the ordeal bean (*Tanghinia venenifera*), (red) squill (sea onion, *Urginea maritima*), sea mango (*Cerbera manghas*), *Bufo* toad species, coconut crab (*Birgus latro L.*).[8,18,19,29,40,51,67,81,103]

In vitro studies also suggested the remarkable diagnostic importance and clinical efficacy of the binding affinity of DSFab for CASs such as bufalin, convallatoxin, cinobufotalin, oleandrin, oleandrigenin, and oubain and those in the balloon plant (*Gomphocarpus physocarpus* and *fruticosus*), bushman's poison (*Carissa acokanthera*), conkerberry (*Carissa laxiflora*), frangipani (*Plumeria rubra*), king's crown (*Calotropis procera*), mother of millions (*Bryophyllum tubiflorum*), pheasants eye (*Adonis microcarpa*), sea mango (*Cerbera manghas*), redheaded cotton-bush (*Asclepias curassavica*), rubber vine (*Cryptostegia grandifolia*), and wintersweet (*Carissa spectabilis*).[29,33,35,95,98,132] Distinctions between assay detection and DSFab efficacy are critical. One in vitro study demonstrated cross-reactivity of steroidal alkaloidal compounds in *Veratrum viride* (false hellebore) with the digoxin assay but no binding to DigiFab.[9] Conversely, DSFab binds the cardioactive steroid cerberin, although serum cerberin did not react with a clinical digoxin assay.[64] Highlighting the heterogeneity of DSFab antibodies, only a fraction of the total Digibind and DigiFab antibodies bound to ouabain with high affinity in vitro, and the ouabain-binding capacity of Digibind was approximately twice that of DigiFab.[95] Both older and newer immunoassays were capable of detecting oleandrin (from *N. oleander*) in human serum, with the Digoxin III assay being highly sensitive.[34]

Several animal studies explored DSFab use in atypical CAS poisoning. In mice poisoned with an LD_{90} of Chan Su extract containing bufalin, cinobufotalin, and cinobufagin, Digibind at doses of 1,600 mg/kg followed by 800 mg/kg decreased the mortality rate from 100% to 47%.[18] A placebo-controlled canine study of experimentally induced *N. oleander* poisoning used 60 mg/kg of DSFab to prevent death and normalize dysrhythmias.[30] Larger doses may be required in cases of poisoning by other CAS because of the lower affinity binding of DSFab for these toxins. DigiFab is expected to have similar affinity binding toward CASs as Digibind. Both products are polyclonal, contributing to their broad spectrum of affinity for nondigoxin CASs. Several case reports discuss successful use of DSFab to reverse cardiotoxicity resulting from ingestion of *N. oleander* and *T. peruviana* at dose up to 480 mg of Digibind.[24,103,112] A double-blind study in patients with severe poisoning from yellow oleander provided 1,200 mg of DigiTAb to reverse serious dysrhythmias.[40] An observational study confirmed a threefold rise in oleander fatalities when DSFab was unavailable.[41] Twenty vials and more of Digibind have been required in cases of Chan Su poisoning.[19] A case of toad egg poisoning was successfully reversed with three vials

of brand-unspecified DSFab.[70] Twenty vials of brand-unspecified DSFab successfully reversed cardiotoxicity from suicidal ingestion of seeds from the pong-pong ("suicide") tree (*Cerbera odollam*), which contains the CAS cerberin.[64] Similarly, 20 vials (760 mg) of Digibind were required to reverse life-threatening coconut crab poisoning, from the CAS neriifolin.[81] Complicating the diagnosis and therapeutic decision-making, *Digitalis* species lanatosides have contaminated botanical dietary supplements not otherwise anticipated to contain CASs.[8,114] On the basis of the common and yellow oleander poisonings studies, a minimum of 20 vials (800 mg) DSFab is recommended.[7] We recommend that treatment decisions be based on clinical and diagnostic findings such as ECG or electrolyte abnormalities (eg, life-threatening dysrhythmias, shock or hemodynamic instability, potassium concentrations > 5 mEq/L and those provided in Table 62–4), with initial therapy consisting of 10 to 20 vials in cases of nonpharmaceutical cardiac glycoside poisonings. Subsequent doses should be based on clinical response. Gastrointestinal decontamination is recommended because of the potential ongoing absorption of ingested products.

In humans, DSFab were also used to mitigate preeclampsia (toxemia of pregnancy) associated with endogenous digitalis-like substances (EDLIS) such as marinobufagenin.[2,45,50] DigiFab neutralizes EDLIS and reverses preeclampsia-induced Na⁺,K⁺-ATPase inhibition in a manner similar to Digibind.[58] The effects of EDLIS are mitigated, and DSFab effectiveness is potentiated in the presence of magnesium, providing an experimental link for magnesium efficacy in preeclampsia.[138] In a randomized, double-blind trial of women with severe preeclampsia, DSFab administration was associated with prevention of maternal renal impairment, lowered rates of maternal pulmonary edema, and prevention of neonatal intraventricular hemorrhage.[3,72] Definitive therapy in preeclampsia remains delivery.

INDICATIONS FOR DIGOXIN-SPECIFIC ANTIBODY FRAGMENTS

Life-threatening, or potentially life-threatening, toxicity from any CAS should prompt DSFab treatment.[20] Patients with known or suggestive CAS exposure with progressive bradydysrhythmias, including symptomatic sinus bradycardia or second- or third-degree heart block unresponsive to atropine, and patients with severe ventricular dysrhythmias, such as ventricular tachycardia or ventricular fibrillation, should also be treated with DSFab.[75] Ventricular tachycardia with a fascicular block is likely to be a digoxin-toxic rhythm.[82] We recommend treating with DsFab patient with a potassium concentration exceeding 5 mEq/L that is attributable to a CAS in the presence of other manifestations of acute or chronic digoxin toxicity.[13] Digoxin-specific antibody fragments is recommended for acute ingestions greater than 4 mg in a healthy child (or > 0.1 mg/kg) or 10 mg in a healthy adult, with a lower threshold in compromised patients. Serum digoxin concentrations do not correlate with myocardial concentrations until 4 to 6 hours after ingestion, when an equilibrium from the serum to the myocardium is achieved. Serum concentrations of greater than or equal to 10 ng/mL soon after an acute ingestion may predict the need for treatment with DSFab. Because older adults are at greatest risk of lethality with digoxin poisoning,[14] the treatment threshold for patients older than 60 years of age is recommended to be lower. Some authors decrease this age threshold to 55 years.[75] This approach is reasonable in the setting of other comorbidities. Before the advent of DSFab, the mortality rate in patients older than 60 years of age was 58% compared with 8% in patients younger than 40 years of age and 34% in patients between 40 and 50 years of age.[14] A rapid progression of clinical signs and symptoms, such as cardiac and GI toxicity and an elevated or rising potassium concentration, in the presence of an acute overdose, suggests a potentially life-threatening exposure and the need for DSFab.

Cardioactive steroid toxicity causes an increase in intracellular calcium, and the administration of exogenous calcium may further exacerbate conduction abnormalities and potentially result in cardiac arrest, unresponsive to further resuscitation. Thus, in a patient with an unknown exposure who is clinically ill with characteristics suggestive of poisoning by a CAS, DSFab should be administered early in the management and always before administration of calcium gluconate or chloride. The CAS effects can be reversed, obviating the risk associated with the administration of calcium. It also can be difficult to distinguish clinically between digoxin poisoning and intrinsic cardiac disease, which the administration of DSFab can resolve.

A computer-based simulation model compared the treatment of non–life-threatening digoxin toxicity with standard therapy. The authors concluded that treatment with DSFab could decrease length of hospitalization by 1.5 days, a major cost containment benefit.[37] In a 2016, US national hospital database study of 24,547 patients, in patients treated with DSFab for digoxin toxicity, the length of stay was significantly shorter than the remainder of the cohort (7.2 days versus 11.6 days), and even after adjusting for disease and severity variables, DSFab reduced the mean length of stay by 0.3 to 0.7 days.[53] The sometimes rapidly changing pharmaceutical, personnel, and facility costs likely will modify local pharmacoeconomic considerations for DSFab administration.

ADVERSE EFFECTS AND SAFETY ISSUES

Digoxin-specific antibody fragments are generally safe and effective. Reported adverse effects include hypokalemia as a consequence of reactivation of the Na^+,K^+-ATPase; withdrawal of the inotropic or AV nodal blocking effects of digoxin, leading to congestive heart failure or a rapid ventricular rate in patients with atrial fibrillation; and, rarely, allergic reactions.[25,20] Hypokalemia with associated cardiac dysrhythmia requiring potassium repletion was reported in one of 29 children in a multicenter study.[135] Serum potassium should be monitored after DSFAb administration because potassium can rapidly shift intracellularly.[20] In a multicenter study of 150 patients treated with Digibind, hypokalemia was reported in 6 patients (4%), worsening of congestive heart failure occurred in 4 patients (3%), and transient apnea was reported in a neonate who was several hours old.[5] There were no other reactions reported in any of the patients in this series. In a postmarketing surveillance study of Digibind that included 717 patients, 6 patients (0.8%) had an allergic reaction to DSFab, of whom 3 of the 6 had a prior history of allergy to antibiotic drugs.[54] One of these patients developed a total-body rash, facial swelling, and a flush during the infusion. Two others experienced a pruritic rash. Three other reported adverse reactions were thrombocytopenia and rigors, and there were two episodes of wheezing and dyspnea that appeared to be unrelated to Digibind use.[54] One patient received Digibind on three separate occasions over the course of 1 year for multiple suicide attempts, with no adverse effects.[15] During the clinical trials with DigiFab, one patient developed pulmonary edema, bilateral pleural effusions, and kidney failure, most likely caused by the loss of the inotropic and chronotropic digoxin effects.[20] Phlebitis and postural hypotension were related to the infusion of DigiFab in two healthy volunteers.[20]

Patients with allergies to papain, chymopapain, or other papaya extracts or the pineapple enzyme bromelain may be at risk for allergic reactions because trace residues of papaya may remain in the DSFab.[20] Patients with an allergy to sheep protein or those who have previously received ovine antibodies or ovine Fab may also be at risk for allergic reactions, although this is not reported.

PREGNANCY AND LACTATION

Digoxin-specific antibody fragments are FDA Pregnancy Category C. Reproduction studies have not been done, and human case reports are limited. However, considering the maternal benefit of DSFab, it should be used as clinically indicated to protect the maternal–fetal dyad. At least one randomized trial used DSFab for up to eight total doses therapeutically in pregnancy.[3,72] Digoxin-specific antibody fragments use should not be withheld in maternal poisoning because of pregnancy. It is unknown whether DSFab is excreted into breast milk, but it is considered compatible with breastfeeding.[16]

DOSING AND ADMINISTRATION

The dose of DSFab depends on the total body load (TBL) of digoxin. This amount varies depending on the size of the patient and the V_d. Adults and children receiving digoxin therapeutically who develop chronic digoxin toxicity require small doses of DSFab because their total body burden of digoxin is usually small. Tolerance to digoxin does not appear to develop in

patients.[108] Children with acute overdoses require DSFab doses based on the amount of digoxin ingested and their subsequent total body load, as in adults.

Estimates of digoxin TBL can be made in three ways: (1) estimate the quantity of digoxin acutely ingested and assume 80% bioavailability (milligrams ingested × 0.8 equals TBL), which is on the higher end of the value incorporated into successful treatment regimens;[5,75,118] (2) obtain a serum digoxin concentration and, using a pharmacokinetic formula, incorporate the apparent V_d of digoxin and the patient's body weight (in kilograms); or (3) use an empiric dose based on the average requirements for an acute or chronic overdose in an adult or child.

Each of these methods of estimating the dose of DSFab has limitations. The history of ingestion is often unreliable, and empiric doses based on averages can overestimate or underestimate DSFab requirements. Additionally, bioavailability varies by P-glycoprotein (MDR1) genotype and the gut microbiome.[71,80] Using the pharmacokinetic formula assumes a steady-state V_d of 5 L/kg.[5] In studies reviewing efficacy, a value of 5.6 L/kg has been used previously.[5,75] Although the value of 5 L/kg achieves mathematical simplicity in equations (because each vial binds 0.5 mg of digoxin), this V_d is not accurate in the acute setting and can change with comorbid disease. In addition, the V_d of 5 L/kg is a population average that varies with the individual, lean body mass, kidney disease, thyroid disease, and pharmacokinetic model and is lower than a more typical V_d of 7 L/kg.[26,28,42,102,137] Acknowledging these limitations, sample calculations for each of these methods are shown in Tables A22–1 to A22–3. Each vial contains 40 mg (DigiFab) of purified DSFab that will bind approximately 0.5 mg of digoxin or digitoxin. The number of vials is rounded up to the next whole vial, which provides some margin when not incorporating higher values for V_d or bioavailability. If the quantity of ingestion cannot be reliably estimated, it is safest to use the largest calculated estimate. The clinician should always be prepared to increase or repeat the dose if symptoms fail to resolve.

Because of the increasing cost of DSFab and availability concerns, several authors have suggested partial or non-neutralization in various scenarios, particularly in cases of chronic toxicity. We do not recommend this approach. Part of the difficulty lies within heterogeneity of clinically meaningful endpoints and determining the contribution of digoxin to the overall clinical presentation or outcome. In a study of 20 patients with severe digoxin poisoning, 30% failed a strategy of providing only two DSFab vials and waiting for ECG signs of digoxin toxicity to abate, with a mortality rate of 5%.[12] Repeat DSFab therapy was required in 3 of 21 patients (14%) with equimolar dosing compared to 8 of 45 patients (18%) treated with half-molar reversal, despite the full reversal patients having more severe clinical presentations.[75] A significant mortality rate of 15% is associated with therapeutic nihilism (failure to administer DSFab) in acute and chronic toxicity.[74]

Given that studies demonstrate a mean Na^+,K^+-ATPase occupancy of 24% in digitalized patients, poisoned patients are anticipated to have an even higher occupancy, risking clinical and pharmaceutical recrudescence (rebound toxicity).[108] In 717 patients, recrudescence was seen in 2.8%, which

TABLE A22–1	Sample Calculation Based on History of Acute Digoxin Ingestion	
Adult	**Child**
Weight: 70 kg	Weight: 10 kg
Ingestion: 50 (0.25 mg) digoxin tablets	Ingestion: 50 (0.25 mg) digoxin tablets
Calculation:	Calculation: Same as for adult. Child will require 20 vials.
0.25 mg × 50 = 12.5 mg ingested dose	
12.5 mg × 0.80 (assume 80% bioavailability) = 10 mg (absorbed dose)	
$\dfrac{10 \text{ mg}}{0.5 \text{ mg/vial}} = 20$ vials	

TABLE A22–2	Sample Calculations Based on the Serum Digoxin Concentration[a]	
Adult	**Child**	**Quick Estimation (for Adults and Children)**

Adult

Weight: 70 kg
SDC: 10 ng/mL
V_d: 5 L/kg
Calculation:[b]

$$\text{No. of vials}^c = \frac{\text{Total body load (mg)}}{0.5\,\text{mg/vial}}$$

$$= \frac{\text{SDC} \times V_d \times \text{Patient wt (kg)}}{1,000 \times 0.5\ \text{mg/vial}}$$

$$\text{No. of vials}^c = \frac{10\,\text{ng/mL} \times 5\,\text{L/kg} \times 70\,\text{kg}}{1,000 \times 0.5\,\text{mg/vial}}$$

No. of vials = 7

Child

Weight: 10 kg
SDC: 10 ng/mL
V_d: 5 L/kg
Calculation:[b]

$$\text{No. of vials}^c = \frac{10\,\text{ng/mL} \times 5\,\text{L/kg} \times 10\,\text{kg}}{1,000 \times 0.5\,\text{mg/vial}}$$

No. of vials = 1

Quick Estimation (for Adults and Children)

$$\text{No. of vials}^c = \frac{\text{SDC (ng/mL)} \times \text{Patient wt (kg)}}{100}$$

[a]If the serum digoxin concentration (SDC) is provided in units of nmol/L, a factor of 0.78 is used to convert to ng/mL. [b]1,000 is a conversion factor to change ng/mL to mg/L. [c]Round up to the nearest whole vial to determine the number of vials indicated.

V_d = volume of distribution.

was correlated with less than equimolar DSFab dosing.[54] In a pediatric series, 3 of 29 (10%) received retreatment with DSFab; 1 case was associated with half molar dosing, 1 had concomitant quinidine poisoning, and 1 had it provided empirically after initial reversal of cardiac toxicity.[135] In a kinetic evaluation, continuous infusion of DSFab at 0.5 mg/min was sufficient to absorb digoxin rediffusing into the serum during the first 8 hours, suggesting a requirement for sufficient ongoing DSFab.[105] Lower DSFab doses were less efficacious in increasing heart rate in a prospective observational study, and rebound was frequent (25 of 36 patients), with 9 patients achieving a rebound of greater than 2 nmol/L (1.56 ng/mL).[27] Such a rate of recrudescence would require ongoing monitoring, and studies advocating partial reversal have not completely accounted for the attendant facility, monitoring, and personnel costs in the event that a full equimolar reversal is not provided, which might mitigate any pharmaceutical cost saving. Given the known inherent rate limitations of digoxin removal from Na+, K+-ATPase(s),[62,86,109] the need to create sufficient gradient for redistribution to serum for this to occur, the efficacy seen with higher than equimolar dosing,[25,101,120] and inadequate free DSFab monitoring at most institutions, until pharmacokinetic arguments for partial dosing are rigorously tested in sufficiently powered clinical trials, the authors believe that equimolar DSFab dosing should be employed. Slower or ongoing administration of DSFab[105] has a rational basis to preclude antidotal elimination but awaits further definitive study.

Each 40-mg vial of DigiFab (which binds 0.5 mg of digoxin) should be reconstituted with 4 mL of sterile water for IV injection and gently mixed to provide a solution containing 10 mg/mL of DSFab.[20] The reconstituted product should be used promptly, or if refrigerated, it should be used within 4 hours. This preparation can be further diluted with sterile isotonic saline for injection. DigiFab should be administered slowly as an IV infusion over at least 30 minutes unless the patient is critically ill, in which case the DigiFab can be given by IV bolus. If a rate-related infusion reaction occurs, the infusion should be stopped, the patient stabilized, and the infusion restarted at a slower rate. For infants and small children, the manufacturer recommends diluting the 40-mg vial with 4 mL of sterile water for IV injection and

TABLE A22–3	Empiric Dosing Recommendations	
Acute Ingestion		**Chronic Toxicity**
Adult: 10–20 vials		Adult: 3–6 vials
Child:[a] 10–20 vials		Child:[b] 1–2 vials

[a]Monitor for volume overload in very small children. [b]The prescribing information contains a table for infants and children, with corresponding serum concentrations.

administering the dose undiluted using a tuberculin syringe. For very small doses, this preparation can be further diluted with an additional 36 mL of sterile 0.9% sodium chloride for injection (for a total of 40 mL) to achieve a 1-mg/mL concentration.

MEASUREMENT OF SERUM DIGOXIN CONCENTRATION AFTER DIGOXIN-SPECIFIC ANTIBODY FRAGMENT ADMINISTRATION

Most laboratories are not equipped to determine free serum digoxin concentrations within a clinically reasonable timeframe. This is relevant because after DSFab administration, total serum digoxin concentrations are clinically meaningless because they represent both free and bound digoxin and may rise up to 10- to 20-fold compared with pretreatment values.[6,49,57,77,84,119,134] The type of test for total digoxin concentrations used can either result in falsely high or falsely low serum concentrations, depending on which phase (solid or supernatant) is sampled.[56,83] Free serum digoxin concentrations should be near zero after initial DSFab administration.[26,27,133] Free digoxin concentrations begin to reappear 5 to 24 hours or longer after Fab administration, depending on the antibody dose, infusion technique, and the patient's renal function. Newer commercial methods, using ultrafiltration or immunoassays, make free digoxin concentration measurements easier to perform and therefore more clinically useful, but they remain associated with errors in the underestimation or overestimation of the free digoxin concentration.[48,61,90,99,121,124] Free digoxin concentrations are particularly useful in patients with end-stage kidney disease. Independent of the availability of these data, serum digoxin values represent only an imperfect marker of target (cardiac) organ toxicity and only approximate the need for ongoing therapy. As such, and given the experimental data demonstrating that digoxin Na+,K+-ATPase is rate limited, the patient's cardiac status must be carefully clinically and electrocardiographically monitored for signs of persistent or recurrent toxicity and need for additional DSFab.

Additional pitfalls in the measurement and utility of serum digoxin concentrations include endogenous and exogenous factors. Spironolactone, eplerenone, canrenone, and canrenone's prodrug potassium canrenoate can positively or negatively interfere with serum digoxin measurements, depending on the analytical method.[32,136] Endogenous digitalis-like substances are described in infants, women in the third trimester of pregnancy, high altitude exposure, hypothermia, acute respiratory distress syndrome, essential hypertension, congestive heart failure, right ventricular dysfunction, hypertrophic cardiomyopathy, kidney and liver failure, kidney and liver transplant recipients, and critically ill patients without liver or kidney disease.[1,32,36,47,52,55,63,66,125,127,130] Exogenous measurement factors relate primarily to EDLIS measurement techniques and interpretation.[69] When EDLISs are free or weakly bound, as in these circumstances, they are measurable by the typical RIA and can account for factitiously high reported serum digoxin concentrations in the absence of digoxin treatment, although the degree of interference, if any, depends on the assay and can vary significantly between assays.[60,73] The role of EDLIS is incompletely elucidated; however, sympathetic stimulation of adrenal cortex leads to endogenous marinobufagenin production, which causes decreased sodium reabsorption, arterial constriction, and salt-sensitive hypertension.[4] Endogenous digoxinlike immunoreactive substances are thus implicated as a causative factor in cardiac and kidney disease, including kidney and cardiac fibrosis and preeclampsia.[93] Additionally, digoxin metabolites have varying degrees of cardioactivity.[78] Some metabolites cross-react and are measured by RIA, but others do not. The in vivo production of these metabolites varies in patients and may depend on intestinal metabolism by gut flora as well as renal and liver clearance.[128]

FORMULATION AND ACQUISITION

Digoxin-specific antibody fragments are available as DigiFab. Vials contain 40 mg of purified lyophilized digoxin-immune ovine immunoglobulin fragments, approximately 75 mg of mannitol USP, and approximately 2 mg of sodium acetate USP as a buffer. The diluent is not included. The product contains no preservatives and is intended for IV administration after reconstitution with 4 mL of sterile water for injection USP. Each vial binds approximately 0.5 mg of digoxin.

SUMMARY

- Digoxin-specific antibody fragments have dramatically advanced the care and are lifesaving in patients poisoned with CASs.
- In the more than 40 years since the release of DSFab, a potentially lethal overdose of a CAS has become manageable, allowing clinicians to treat patients with minimal risks.
- Recrudescence after therapy is reported, particularly in cases of kidney failure, and patients should be monitored for recurrence of symptoms in these cases. Rarely, additional dosing of DSFab is needed.
- Nonpharmaceutical CAS poisoning often requires large doses for reversal.

REFERENCES

1. Abbas MMK, et al. Involvement of the bufadienolides in the detection and therapy of the acute respiratory distress syndrome. *Lung.* 2017;195:323-332.
2. Adair CD, et al. Elevated endoxin-like factor complicating a multifetal second trimester pregnancy: treatment with digoxin-binding immunoglobulin. *Am J Nephrol.* 1996;16:529-531.
3. Adair CD, et al. Digoxin immune fab treatment for severe preeclampsia. *Am J Perinatol.* 2010;27:655-662.
4. AlGhatrif M, et al. The pressure of aging. *Med Clin North Am.* 2017;101:81-101.
5. Antman EM, et al. Treatment of 150 cases of life-threatening digitalis intoxication with digoxin-specific Fab antibody fragments. Final report of a multicenter study. *Circulation.* 1990;81:1744-1752.
6. Argyle JC. Effect of digoxin antibodies on TDx digoxin assay. *Clin Chem.* 1986;32:1616-1617.
7. Bandara V, et al. A review of the natural history, toxinology, diagnosis and clinical management of Nerium oleander (common oleander) and Thevetia peruviana (yellow oleander) poisoning. *Toxicon.* 2010;56:273-281.
8. Barrueto F Jr, et al. Cardioactive steroid poisoning from an herbal cleansing preparation. *Ann Emerg Med.* 2003;41:396-399.
9. Bechtel LK, et al. Ingestion of false hellebore plants can cross-react with a digoxin clinical chemistry assay. *Clin Toxicol (Phila).* 2010;48:435-442.
10. Beller GA, et al. Digitalis intoxication. A prospective clinical study with serum level correlations. *N Engl J Med.* 1971;284:989-997.
11. Berkovitch M, et al. Acute digoxin overdose in a newborn with renal failure: use of digoxin immune Fab and peritoneal dialysis. *Ther Drug Monit.* 1994;16:531-533.
12. Bilbault P, et al. Emergency step-by-step specific immunotherapy in severe digoxin poisoning: an observational cohort study. *Eur J Emerg Med.* 2009;16:145-149.
13. Bismuth C, et al. Hyperkalemia in acute digitalis poisoning: prognostic significance and therapeutic implications. *Clin Toxicol.* 1973;6:153-162.
14. Borron SW, et al. Advances in the management of digoxin toxicity in the older patient. *Drugs Aging.* 1997;10:18-33.
15. Bosse GM, Pope TM. Recurrent digoxin overdose and treatment with digoxin-specific Fab antibody fragments. *J Emerg Med.* 1994;12:179-185.
16. Briggs GG, et al. *Drugs in Pregnancy and Lactation.* Philadelphia, PA: Lippincott Williams & Wilkins; 2017.
17. Brubacher JR, et al. Toad venom poisoning: failure of a monoclonal digoxin immunoassay to cross-react with the cardioactive steroids. *J Toxicol Clin Toxicol.* 1996;34:529-530.
18. Brubacher JR, et al. Efficacy of digoxin specific Fab fragments (Digibind) in the treatment of toad venom poisoning. *Toxicon.* 1999;37:931-492.
19. Brubacher JR, et al. Treatment of toad venom poisoning with digoxin-specific Fab fragments. *Chest.* 1996;110:1282-1288.
20. BTG International Inc.: DigiFab, Digoxin Immune Fab (Ovine) [prescribing information]. West Conshohocken, PA: BTG International Inc.; 2014.
21. Butler VP Jr, Chen JP. Digoxin-specific antibodies. *Proc Natl Acad Sci U S A.* 1967;57:71-78.
22. Butler VP Jr, et al. Effects of sheep digoxin-specific antibodies and their Fab fragments on digoxin pharmacokinetics in dogs. *J Clin Invest.* 1977;59:345-359.
23. Butler VP Jr, et al. Immunological reversal of the effects of digoxin. *Fed Proc.* 1977;36:2235-2241.
24. Camphausen C, et al. Successful treatment of oleander intoxication (cardiac glycosides) with digoxin-specific Fab antibody fragments in a 7-year-old child: case report and review of literature. *Z Kardiol.* 2005;94:817-823.
25. Cano NJ, et al. Affinity and dose-dependent digoxin Na+K+ATPase dissociation by monoclonal digoxin-specific antibodies. *Biochem Pharmacol.* 1995;50:1867-1872.
26. Chan BS, Buckley NA. Digoxin-specific antibody fragments in the treatment of digoxin toxicity. *Clin Toxicol (Phila).* 2014;52:824-836.
27. Chan BS, et al. Efficacy and effectiveness of anti-digoxin antibodies in chronic digoxin poisonings from the DORA study (ATOM-1). *Clin Toxicol (Phila).* 2016;54:488-494.
28. Cheng JW, et al. Is the volume of distribution of digoxin reduced in patients with renal dysfunction? Determining digoxin pharmacokinetics by fluorescence polarization immunoassay. *Pharmacotherapy.* 1997;17:584-590.
29. Cheung K, et al. Plant cardiac glycosides and digoxin Fab antibody. *J Paediatr Child Health.* 1991;27:312-313.
30. Clark RF, et al. Digoxin-specific Fab fragments in the treatment of oleander toxicity in a canine model. *Ann Emerg Med.* 1991;20:1073-1077.
31. D'Angio RG, et al. Therapeutic drug monitoring: improved performance through educational intervention. *Ther Drug Monit.* 1990;12:173-181.
32. Dasgupta A. Therapeutic drug monitoring of digoxin: impact of endogenous and exogenous digoxin-like immunoreactive substances. *Toxicol Rev.* 2006;25:273-281.
33. Dasgupta A, et al. The Fab fragment of anti-digoxin antibody (digibind) binds digitoxin-like immunoreactive components of Chinese medicine Chan Su: monitoring the effect by measuring free digitoxin. *Clin Chim Acta.* 2001;309:91-95.
34. Dasgupta A, et al. Rapid detection of oleander poisoning by Digoxin III, a new Digoxin assay: impact on serum Digoxin measurement. *Am J Clin Pathol.* 2008;129:548-553.
35. Dasgupta A, Scott J. Unexpected suppression of total digoxin concentrations by cross-reactants in the microparticle enzyme immunoassay: elimination of interference by monitoring free digoxin concentration. *Am J Clin Pathol.* 1998;110:78-82.
36. De Angelis C, et al. Effects of high altitude exposure on plasma and urinary digoxin-like immunoreactive substance. *Am J Hypertens.* 1992;5:600-607.
37. DiDomenico RJ, et al. Analysis of the use of digoxin immune fab for the treatment of non-life-threatening digoxin toxicity. *J Cardiovasc Pharmacol Ther.* 2000;5:77-85.
38. Duhme DW, et al. Reduction of digoxin toxicity associated with measurement of serum levels. A report from the Boston Collaborative Drug Surveillance Program. *Ann Intern Med.* 1974;80:516-519.
39. Dunham G, Califf RM. Digoxin toxicity in renal insufficiency treated with digoxin immune fab: case summaries of two patients. *Prim Cardiol.* 1988;15:31-34.
40. Eddleston M, et al. Anti-digoxin Fab fragments in cardiotoxicity induced by ingestion of yellow oleander: a randomised controlled trial. *Lancet.* 2000;355:967-972.
41. Eddleston M, et al. Deaths due to absence of an affordable antitoxin for plant poisoning. *Lancet.* 2003;362:1041-1044.
42. el-Desoky ES, et al. Application of two-point assay of digoxin serum concentration in studying population pharmacokinetics in Egyptian pediatric patients with heart failure: does it make sense? *Am J Ther.* 2005;12:320-327.
43. Erdmann E, et al. Digitalis intoxication and treatment with digoxin antibody fragments in renal failure. *Klin Wochenschr.* 1989;67:16-19.
44. Eyal D, et al. Digoxin toxicity: pediatric survival after asystolic arrest. *Clin Toxicol (Phila).* 2005;43:51-54.
45. Fedorova OV, et al. Interaction of Digibind with endogenous cardiotonic steroids from preeclamptic placentae. *J Hypertens.* 2010;28:361-366.
46. Fink SL, et al. Rapid detection of convallatoxin using five digoxin immunoassays. *Clin Toxicol (Phila).* 2014;52:659-663.
47. Frisolone J, et al. False-positive serum digoxin concentrations determined by three digoxin assays in patients with liver disease. *Clin Pharm.* 1988;7:444-449.
48. George S, et al. Digoxin measurements following plasma ultrafiltration in two patients with digoxin toxicity treated with specific Fab fragments. *Ann Clin Biochem.* 1994;31(Pt 4):380-382.
49. Gibb I, et al. Plasma digoxin: assay anomalies in Fab-treated patients. *Br J Clin Pharmacol.* 1983;16:445-447.
50. Goodlin RC. Antidigoxin antibodies in eclampsia. *N Engl J Med.* 1988;318:518-519.
51. Graham JC. The Pharmacology of Apocynum Cannabinum. *Biochem J.* 1909;4:385-404.
52. Graves SW, et al. An endogenous digoxin-like substance in patients with renal impairment. *Ann Intern Med.* 1983;99:604-608.
53. Hauptman PJ, et al. Digoxin toxicity and use of digoxin immune fab: insights from a national hospital database. *JACC Heart Fail.* 2016;4:357-364.

54. Hickey AR, et al. Digoxin Immune Fab therapy in the management of digitalis intoxication: safety and efficacy results of an observational surveillance study. *J Am Coll Cardiol*. 1991;17:590-598.

55. Hoffman RS, et al. Endogenous digitalis-like factors in hypothermic patients. *Gen Int Med Clin Innov*. 2016;1:67-70.

56. Honda SA, et al. Problems in determining levels of free digoxin in patients treated with digoxin immune FAb. *J Clin Lab Anal*. 1995;9:407-412.

57. Hursting MJ, et al. Determination of free digoxin concentrations in serum for monitoring Fab treatment of digoxin overdose. *Clin Chem*. 1987;33:1652-1655.

58. Ishkaraeva-Yakovleva VV, et al. DigiFab interacts with endogenous cardiotonic steroids and reverses preeclampsia-induced Na/K-ATPase inhibition. *Reprod Sci*. 2012;19:1260-1267.

59. Johnson AR, et al. Discrepancies in reported US pricing information for digoxin-Fab. *Clin Toxicol (Phila)*. 2015;53:71.

60. Jones TE, Morris RG. Discordant results from "real-world" patient samples assayed for digoxin. *Ann Pharmacother*. 2008;42:1797-1803.

61. Jortani SA, et al. Validity of unbound digoxin measurements by immunoassays in presence of antidote (Digibind). *Clin Chim Acta*. 1999;283:159-169.

62. Kang W, Weiss M. Digoxin uptake, receptor heterogeneity, and inotropic response in the isolated rat heart: a comprehensive kinetic model. *J Pharmacol Exp Ther*. 2002;302:577-583.

63. Karboski JA, et al. Marked digoxin-like immunoreactive factor interference with an enzyme immunoassay. *Drug Intell Clin Pharm*. 1988;22:703-705.

64. Kassop D, et al. An unusual case of cardiac glycoside toxicity. *Int J Cardiol*. 2014; 170:434-437.

65. Kaufman J, et al. Use of digoxin Fab immune fragments in a seven-day-old infant. *Pediatr Emerg Care*. 1990;6:118-121.

66. Kelly RA, et al. Characterization of digitalis-like factors in human plasma. Interactions with NaK-ATPase and cross-reactivity with cardiac glycoside-specific antibodies. *J Biol Chem*. 1985;260:11396-11405.

67. Kolliker A, Pelikan E. Some remarks on the physiological action of the Tanghinia venenifera. *Proc R Soc Lond*. 1857;9:173-174.

68. Koren G, et al. Agonal elevation in serum digoxin concentrations in infants and children long after cessation of therapy. *Crit Care Med*. 1988;16:793-795.

69. Koren G, Parker R. Interpretation of excessive serum concentrations of digoxin in children. *Am J Cardiol*. 1985;55:1210-1214.

70. Kuo HY, et al. Life-threatening episode after ingestion of toad eggs: a case report with literature review. *Emerg Med J*. 2007;24:215-216.

71. Kurata Y, et al. Role of human MDR1 gene polymorphism in bioavailability and interaction of digoxin, a substrate of P-glycoprotein. *Clin Pharmacol Ther*. 2002;72:209-219.

72. Lam GK, et al. Digoxin antibody fragment, antigen binding (Fab), treatment of preeclampsia in women with endogenous digitalis-like factor: a secondary analysis of the DEEP Trial. *Am J Obstet Gynecol*. 2013;209:119 e1-6.

73. Lampon N, et al. Investigation of possible interference by digoxin-like immunoreactive substances on the Architect iDigoxin CMIA in serum samples from pregnant women, and patients with liver disease, renal insufficiency, critical illness, and kidney and liver transplant. *Clin Lab*. 2012;58:1301-1304.

74. Lapostolle F, et al. Assessment of digoxin antibody use in patients with elevated serum digoxin following chronic or acute exposure. *Intensive Care Med*. 2008;34:1448-1453.

75. Lapostolle F, et al. Digoxin-specific Fab fragments as single first-line therapy in digitalis poisoning. *Crit Care Med*. 2008;36:3014-3308.

76. Lechat P, et al. Reversal of lethal digoxin toxicity in guinea pigs using monoclonal antibodies and Fab fragments. *J Pharmacol Exp Ther*. 1984;229:210-213.

77. Lemon M, et al. Concentrations of free serum digoxin after treatment with antibody fragments. *Br Med J (Clin Res Ed)*. 1987;295:1520-1521.

78. Lindenbaum J, et al. Inactivation of digoxin by the gut flora: reversal by antibiotic therapy. *N Engl J Med*. 1981;305:789-794.

79. Lloyd BL, Smith TW. Contrasting rates of reversal of digoxin toxicity by digoxin-specific IgG and Fab fragments. *Circulation*. 1978;58:280-283.

80. Lu L, et al. Intestinal microbiome and digoxin inactivation: meal plan for digoxin users? *World J Microbiol Biotechnol*. 2014;30:791-799.

81. Maillaud C, et al. First successful curative use of digoxin-specific Fab antibody fragments in a life-threatening coconut crab (Birgus latro L.) poisoning. *Toxicon*. 2012;60:1013-1017.

82. Marchlinski FE, et al. Which cardiac disturbances should be treated with digoxin immune Fab (ovine) antibody? *Am J Emerg Med*. 1991;9:24-28; discussion 33-34.

83. Marcus L, et al. Therapy of digoxin intoxication in dogs by specific hemoperfusion through agarose polyacrolein microsphere beads-antidigoxin antibodies. *Am Heart J*. 1985;110:30-39.

84. McMillin GA, et al. Comparable effects of DIGIBIND and DigiFab in thirteen digoxin immunoassays. *Clin Chem*. 2002;48:1580-1584.

85. Mowry JB, et al. Extracorporeal treatment for digoxin poisoning: systematic review and recommendations from the EXTRIP Workgroup. *Clin Toxicol (Phila)*. 2016;54:103-114.

86. Nabauer M, Erdmann E. Reversal of toxic and non-toxic effects of digoxin by digoxin-specific Fab fragments in isolated human ventricular myocardium. *Klin Wochenschr*. 1987;65:558-561.

87. Nollet H, et al. Delayed elimination of digoxin antidotum determined by radioimmunoassay. *J Clin Pharmacol*. 1989;29:41-45.

88. Nuwayhid NF, Johnson GF. Digoxin elimination in a functionally anephric patient after digoxin-specific Fab fragment therapy. *Ther Drug Monit*. 1989;11:680-685.

89. O'Brien MS, et al. Effect of spironolactone on the renal clearance of digoxin in dogs. *J Pharmacol Exp Ther*. 1985;234:190-194.

90. Ocal IT, Green TR. Serum digoxin in the presence of digibind: determination of digoxin by the Abbott AxSYM and Baxter Stratus II immunoassays by direct analysis without pretreatment of serum samples. *Clin Chem*. 1998;44:1947-1950.

91. Ordog GJ, et al. Serum digoxin levels and mortality in 5,100 patients. *Ann Emerg Med*. 1987;16:32-39.

92. Osterloh J, et al. Oleander interference in the digoxin radioimmunoassay in a fatal ingestion. *JAMA*. 1982;247:1596-1597.

93. Paczula A, et al. The role of endogenous cardiotonic steroids in pathogenesis of cardiovascular and renal complications of arterial hypertension. *Postepy Hig Med Dosw*. 2016;70:243-250.

94. Patel SH, et al. Successful treatment of prolonged digoxin-induced cardiac arrest with mechanical chest compressions and digoxin-specific antibody fragments. *Resuscitation*. 2017;115:e7-e8.

95. Pullen MA, et al. Comparison of non-digitalis binding properties of digoxin-specific Fabs using direct binding methods. *J Immunol Methods*. 2008;336:235-241.

96. Quaife EJ, et al. Failure of CAVH to remove digoxin-Fab complex in piglets. *J Toxicol Clin Toxicol*. 1990;28:61-68.

97. Rabetoy GM, et al. Treatment of digoxin intoxication in a renal failure patient with digoxin-specific antibody fragments and plasmapheresis. *Am J Nephrol*. 1990;10: 518-521.

98. Radford DJ, et al. Naturally occurring cardiac glycosides. *Med J Aust*. 1986;144:540-544.

99. Rainey P. Digibind and free digoxin. *Clin Chem*. 1999;45:719-721.

100. Rajpal S, et al. Recrudescent digoxin toxicity treated with plasma exchange: a case report and review of literature. *Cardiovasc Toxicol*. 2012;12:363-368.

101. Renard C, et al. Time- and dose-dependent digoxin redistribution by digoxin-specific antigen binding fragments in a rat model. *Toxicology*. 1999;137:117-127.

102. Reuning RH, et al. Role of pharmacokinetics in drug dosage adjustment. I. Pharmacologic effect kinetics and apparent volume of distribution of digoxin. *J Clin Pharmacol New Drugs*. 1973;13:127-141.

103. Safadi R, et al. Beneficial effect of digoxin-specific Fab antibody fragments in oleander intoxication. *Arch Intern Med*. 1995;155:2121-2125.

104. Santos-Araujo C, et al. Combined use of plasmapheresis and antidigoxin antibodies in a patient with severe digoxin intoxication and acute renal failure. *Nephrol Dial Transplant*. 2007;22:257-258.

105. Schaumann W, et al. Kinetics of the Fab fragments of digoxin antibodies and of bound digoxin in patients with severe digoxin intoxication. *Eur J Clin Pharmacol*. 1986;30:527-533.

106. Schmidt DH, Butler VP Jr. Immunological protecion against digoxin toxicity. *J Clin Invest*. 1971;50:866-871.

107. Schmidt DH, Butler VP Jr. Reversal of digoxin toxicity with specific antibodies. *J Clin Invest*. 1971;50:1738-1744.

108. Schmidt TA, et al. No adaptation to digitalization as evaluated by digitalis receptor (Na,K-ATPase) quantification in explanted hearts from donors without heart disease and from digitalized recipients with end-stage heart failure. *Am J Cardiol*. 1993; 71:110-114.

109. Schmidt TA, Kjeldsen K. Enhanced clearance of specifically bound digoxin from human myocardial and skeletal muscle samples by specific digoxin antibody fragments: subsequent complete digitalis glycoside receptor (Na,K-ATPase) quantification. *J Cardiovasc Pharmacol*. 1991;17:670-677.

110. Schmitt K, et al. Massive digitoxin intoxication treated with digoxin-specific antibodies in a child. *Pediatr Cardiol*. 1994;15:48-49.

111. Sherron PA, Gelband H. Case study: reversal of digoxin toxicity with Fab fragments in a pediatric patient with acute renal failure. Management of digitalis toxicity: the role of DIGIBIND. Research Triangle Park, NC: Burroughs Wellcome Co.; 1986:50-54.

112. Shumaik GM, et al. Oleander poisoning: treatment with digoxin-specific Fab antibody fragments. *Ann Emerg Med*. 1988;17:732-735.

113. Sinclair AJ, et al. Kinetics of digoxin and anti-digoxin antibody fragments during treatment of digoxin toxicity. *Br J Clin Pharmacol*. 1989;28:352-356.

114. Slifman NR, et al. Contamination of botanical dietary supplements by Digitalis lanata. *N Engl J Med*. 1998;339:806-811.

115. Smith TW. New advances in the assessment and treatment of digitalis toxicity. *J Clin Pharmacol*. 1985;25:522-528.

116. Smith TW, et al. Reversal of advanced digoxin intoxication with Fab fragments of digoxin-specific antibodies. *N Engl J Med*. 1976;294:797-800.

117. Smith TW, et al. Immunogenicity and kinetics of distribution and elimination of sheep digoxin-specific IgG and Fab fragments in the rabbit and baboon. *Clin Exp Immunol*. 1979;36:384-396.

118. Smolarz A, et al. Digoxin specific antibody (Fab) fragments in 34 cases of severe digitalis intoxication. *J Toxicol Clin Toxicol*. 1985;23:327-340.

119. Soldin SJ. Digoxin—issues and controversies. *Clin Chem*. 1986;32:5-12.

120. Timsina MP, Hewick DS. The plasma kinetics of digoxin-specific Fab fragments and digoxin in the rabbit. *J Pharm Pharmacol*. 1991;43:807-810.

121. Ujhelyi MR, et al. Monitoring serum digoxin concentrations during digoxin immune Fab therapy. *DICP*. 1991;25:1047-1049.

122. Ujhelyi MR, et al. Influence of digoxin immune Fab therapy and renal dysfunction on the disposition of total and free digoxin. *Ann Intern Med*. 1993;119:273-277.

123. Ujhelyi MR, et al. Disposition of digoxin immune Fab in patients with kidney failure. *Clin Pharmacol Ther*. 1993;54:388-394.

124. Valdes R Jr, Jortani SA. Monitoring of unbound digoxin in patients treated with anti-digoxin antigen-binding fragments: a model for the future? *Clin Chem*. 1998;44:1883-1885.

125. Vasdev S, et al. Plasma endogenous digitalis-like factors in healthy individuals and in dialysis-dependent and kidney transplant patients. *Clin Nephrol*. 1987;27:169-174.

126. Velazquez H, Wright FS. Control by drugs of renal potassium handling. *Annu Rev Pharmacol Toxicol*. 1986;26:293-309.

127. Vinge E, Ekman R. Partial characterization of endogenous digoxinlike substance in human urine. *Ther Drug Monit*. 1988;10:8-15.

128. Vlasses PH, et al. False-positive digoxin measurements due to conjugated metabolite accumulation in combined renal and hepatic dysfunction. *Am J Nephrol*. 1987;7:355-359.

129. Ward SB, et al. Comparison of the pharmacokinetics and in vivo bioaffinity of DigiTAb versus Digibind. *Ther Drug Monit*. 2000;22:599-607.

130. Weinberg U, et al. Digoxinlike immunoreactive factor isolated from human pleural fluid is structurally similar to digoxin. *Am J Med Sci*. 1997;314:28-30.

131. Weiss M, et al. Systems analysis of digoxin kinetics and inotropic response in the rat heart: effects of calcium and KB-R7943. *Am J Physiol Heart Circ Physiol*. 2004;287:H1857-H1867.

132. Welsh KJ, et al. Rapid detection of the active cardiac glycoside convallatoxin of lily of the valley using LOCI digoxin assay. *Am J Clin Pathol*. 2014;142:307-312.

133. Wenger TL. Experience with digoxin immune Fab (ovine) in patients with renal impairment. *Am J Emerg Med*. 1991;9:21-3; discussion 33-34.

134. Wenger TL, et al. Treatment of 63 severely digitalis-toxic patients with digoxin-specific antibody fragments. *J Am Coll Cardiol*. 1985;5:118A-23A.

135. Woolf AD, et al. The use of digoxin-specific Fab fragments for severe digitalis intoxication in children. *N Engl J Med*. 1992;326:1739-1744.

136. Yamada T, et al. Interference between eplerenone and digoxin in fluorescence polarization immunoassay, microparticle enzyme immunoassay, and affinity column-mediated immunoassay. *Ther Drug Monit*. 2010;32:774-777.

137. Yukawa E, et al. Population pharmacokinetics of digoxin in Japanese patients: a 2-compartment pharmacokinetic model. *Clin Pharmacokinet*. 2001;40:773-781.

138. Zazerskaya IE, et al. Magnesium sulfate potentiates effect of DigiFab on marinobufagenin-induced Na/K-ATPase inhibition. *Am J Hypertens*. 2013;26:1269-1272.

139. Zdunek M, et al. Plasma exchange for the removal of digoxin-specific antibody fragments in renal failure: timing is important for maximizing clearance. *Am J Kidney Dis*. 2000;36:177-183.

63

METHYLXANTHINES AND SELECTIVE β₂-ADRENERGIC AGONISTS

Robert J. Hoffman

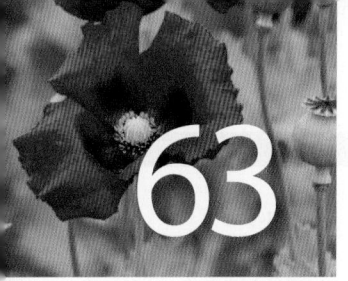

Caffeine
(1,3,7-trimethylxanthine)

Theophylline
(1,3-dimethylxanthine)

Theobromine
(3,7-dimethylxanthine)

Caffeine
Molecular weight = 194.19 Da
Therapeutic serum concentration = 1–10 mcg/mL

Theophylline
Molecular Weight = 180.17 Da
Therapeutic serum concentration = 5–15 mcg/mL
= 28–83 µmol/L

Theobromine
Molecular weight = 180.17 Da

HISTORY AND EPIDEMIOLOGY

Methylated derivatives of xanthine, or methylxanthines, are plant-derived alkaloids that include caffeine (1,3,7-trimethylxanthine), theobromine (3,7-dimethylxanthine), and theophylline (1,3-dimethylxanthine). Members of this group share pharmacologic properties and clinical effects. The naturally occurring methylxanthines caffeine and theobromine are used ubiquitously throughout the world. Caffeine is most commonly contained in beverages imbibed for their stimulant, mood-elevating, and fatigue-abating effects. The plant *Coffea arabica* and related species are used to make coffee, a beverage rich in caffeine. Cocoa and chocolate are derived from the seeds of *Theobroma cacao*, which contains theobromine and to a lesser extent caffeine. *Thea sinensis*, a shrub native to China but now cultivated worldwide, produces leaves from which various teas, rich in caffeine and containing small amounts of theophylline and theobromine, are brewed. *Paullinia* spp, commonly known as guarana, is a South American plant that produces berries with caffeine content much greater than that of coffee beans.

Selective β₂-adrenergic agonists were developed for the treatment of bronchoconstriction. Their receptor selectivity improved therapy for patients with reversible airways disease, allowing avoidance of the adverse effects of the previously used therapies: epinephrine, an α and β-adrenergic agonist, as well as isoproterenol, a β₁ and β₂-adrenergic agonist. Most selective β₂-adrenergic agonists are pharmacodynamically similar, with similar clinical effects; the principal differences are their pharmacokinetics. Clenbuterol and ritodrine have unique toxicities distinct from other β₂-adrenergic agonists. This chapter does not examine each β₂-adrenergic agonist individually but instead discusses them as a class, with a separate discussion of the unique toxicities of clenbuterol and ritodrine. The β₂-adrenergic agonists in the United States include arformoterol, albuterol, clenbuterol, bitolterol, formoterol, levalbuterol, metaproterenol, pirbuterol, ritodrine, salmeterol, terbutaline, although numerous others are used outside the United States.

The American Association of Poison Control Centers (AAPCC) follows trends in methylxanthine and β₂-adrenergic agonists exposures in National Poisoning Data System (NPDS). Theophylline exposures, which previously caused thousands of poisonings and dozens of deaths annually, have remained uncommon and are continuing to decrease in frequency. From 2012 to 2015, there were approximately 200 exposures annually, consistent with how infrequently theophylline is now used therapeutically. Caffeine exposures continue to slowly decrease. In 1998, there were 7,390 reported caffeine exposures, with a steady decline: from 2007 with 5,448 exposures, to 2011 with 3,667 exposures, and to 2015 with 3,598 exposures. Caffeine is an important component of many energy drinks, and these have only been included as a subcategory of poisoning in NPDS since 2010, when there were 308 reported exposures. In 2015, the number of reported exposures to caffeine-containing energy drinks increased to 1,161, and exposures to caffeine-containing alcoholic beverages was 150.

The number of selective β₂-adrenergic agonist exposures is decreasing, with approximately 6,500 cases annually from 2012 to 2015, which is a decrease from the past 5 years, which had approximately 8,000 to 9,000 reported in 2007 to 2011 reports annually. There are no reported deaths from these substances (Chap. 130).

Most caffeine consumed is in beverages, with a lesser but concerning portion of caffeine consumed as in concentrated form as powders of liquids.[6] With limited scientific evidence demonstrating benefit, caffeine use is advocated for various beneficial health effects, as well as to improve athletic performance and concentration.[16,53,77] Products with high caffeine content are widely available as dietary supplements, which are generally not regulated by the Food and Drug Administration (FDA). These include powder, tablets, concentrated liquid, and liquid energy "shots" all for oral (PO) consumption as well as newer topical and transdermal caffeine products (Table 63–1).[64]

Energy drinks, which are FDA regulated, typically containing caffeine and other stimulant ingredients are increasingly popular, particularly with adolescents and athletes. A surge in poisoning from pure caffeine powder prompted the FDA to issue warning letters to manufacturers in 2015,[32] and the FDA also issued a safety alerts advising consumers to avoid use of these powdered caffeine products because of the potential for severe illness or death.[34] These drinks also have significant adverse side effects.[61,42] Although these do not routinely result in severe toxicity, major morbidity and mortality result from their use and misuse. Between 30% and 50% of adolescents and young adults in the United States regularly consume energy drinks.[79] Surveys of parents in the United States reveal that children as young as 5 years of age drink caffeinated beverages daily.[97]

Beverages that combine alcohol with relatively large doses of caffeine are commonly used, particularly among young adults and underage drinkers. Toxicity from use of such drinks became apparent very soon after they were introduced in the United States.[21] In some instances, the incidence of toxicity and adverse events associated with such drinks was so significant that some were banned because they are considered exceptionally dangerous. Caffeine is a very common ingredient as well as adulterant in illicit stimulants sold by Internet vendors.[28]

Caffeine, theophylline, and aminophylline are used in neonates to treat the apnea and bradycardia syndrome of prematurity. The result of such treatment is an increased respiratory rate, decreased apnea, increased cardiac chronotropy and inotropy, and increased cardiac output.[13] Caffeine is also used as an analgesic adjuvant, particularly when combined acetaminophen, aspirin, and ibuprofen or ergots.[30]

Theophylline or its water-soluble salt, aminophylline, is used to treat varied respiratory conditions, primarily reversible bronchospastic airway disease, particularly asthma. Theophylline was once the mainstay of therapy for such diseases, but inhaled selective β₂-adrenergic agonists with fewer adverse effects have almost completely replaced theophylline.

TABLE 63–1	Caffeine and Stimulant Content of Commonly Used Products			
Product	Caffeine Content in Typical Single Serving (mg)	Volume of Typical Single Serving (mL)	Other Relevant Beverage Ingredients	Category
Arizona AZ RX Energy Shot	110	240	Niacin, vitamin B_{12}	Dietary supplement
Caffeine pill (Vivarin, No-Doz)	200	—	—	Medication
Chocolate (Hershey Kiss)	1	—	—	Food
Chocolate milk	10–15	240	Theobromine	Beverage
Coffee (regular)	115–175	330		Beverage
Cola	30	330		Beverage
Espresso	55	30		Beverage
Five-Hour Energy	207	60	Niacin, taurine, vitamin B_6, vitamin B_{12}	Dietary supplement
Hot chocolate	8	240	Theobromine	Beverage
Red Bull	110	250	Taurine	Beverage
Tea (black)	40–100	240	Theobromine, theophylline	Beverage

Spectrum of Toxicity

Methylxanthine toxicity is generally classified as acute, acute on chronic, or chronic in nature. In neonates receiving methylxanthine therapy, both acute and chronic toxicities are reported, and acute-on-chronic toxicity occurs in acute overdose in adults already being treated with theophylline therapeutically.

Chronic toxicity from caffeine most typically results from frequent self-administration of excessive caffeine. The *Diagnostic and Statistical Manual of Mental Disorders*, 5th edition, notes five distinct caffeine-related disorders: caffeine toxicity, caffeine withdrawal, caffeine use disorder, other caffeine-induced disorders, and unspecified caffeine-related disorder.[1] *Caffeinism* is the classical syndrome associated with chronic caffeine use, consisting of headache, palpitations, tachycardia, insomnia, and delirium.

Theobromine poisoning is reported in veterinary literature and typically results from dogs or other small animals ingesting cocoa or chocolate. In 2015, the death of four wild bears after they ingested of chocolate used as bait demonstrated the potential for theobromine lethality in large and animals.[22] Because of its greater thermogenic and ergogenic activity relative to caffeine, theobromine is now an ingredient of numerous energy and sports drinks used for stimulation and athletic enhancement, but human toxicity is unreported.

Use of selective β_2-adrenergic agonists is widespread. Adverse effects are associated with both therapeutic dosing and overdose. Excessive use of β_2-adrenergic agonists results in tachyphylaxis, a phenomenon in which downregulation of receptors occurs and the effects of the xenobiotic diminish as a result of excessive use.[52] Consequently, patients require higher doses to achieve the same clinical effects previously experienced at lower doses, resulting in consequential adverse effects. The most common acute selective β_2-adrenergic agonist toxicity results from children ingesting albuterol syrup. Toxicity associated with terbutaline and ritodrine is infrequently reported. Clenbuterol, a long-acting β_2 adrenergic agonist used in countries outside the United States for treating bronchoconstriction in countries outside the United States, emerged as an abused anabolic xenobiotic as well as additive in street drugs.[45] Epidemic clenbuterol toxicity occurs as a result of both its admixture with illicit drugs and its intentional use for bodybuilding purposes in the United States.[27] These outbreaks demonstrate that, for reasons incompletely understood, clenbuterol has unique toxicities relative to other β_2-adrenergic agonists. Food poisoning by consumption of animal meat from livestock treated with clenbuterol occurs in Europe.[5] Ritodrine, removed from the US market in 2013 but still used in other countries, was used in parenteral and PO formulations as a tocolytic. Besides typical adverse effects

of other β_2-adrenergic agonists, it is associated with acute development of pulmonary edema, rhabdomyolysis, and agranulocytosis.[56,105]

PHARMACOLOGY
Methylxanthines

Methylxanthines cause the release of endogenous catecholamines, resulting in stimulation of β_1 and β_2 receptors. Endogenous catecholamine concentrations are extremely elevated in patients with methylxanthine poisoning.[7] Methylxanthines are structural analogs of adenosine and function pharmacologically as adenosine antagonists. Adenosine modulates histamine release and causes bronchoconstriction. This is a putative mechanism explaining the primary therapeutic efficacy of adenosine antagonists in the treatment of bronchospasm. Additionally, adenosine antagonism results in release of norepinephrine, and to a lesser extent epinephrine, through blockade of presynaptic A_2 receptors. The additional methyl group possessed by caffeine (1,3,7-trimethylxanthine) permits greater central nervous system (CNS) penetration relative to theophylline and theobromine, which are dimethylxanthines. Caffeine is an effective analgesic adjuvant, possibly because of its stimulant properties.

Methylxanthines also inhibit phosphodiesterase, the enzyme responsible for degradation of intracellular cyclic adenosine monophosphate (cAMP), which has many effects, including an increase in intracellular calcium concentrations. Phosphodiesterase inhibition was long considered to be the primary therapeutic mechanism of the methylxanthines, but clinically significant elevations in cAMP concentrations are not achieved until serum methylxanthine concentrations are well above the therapeutic range. This likely occurs as a result of the structural similarity of the adenosine moiety of cAMP and the methylxanthines. Cyclic AMP is involved in the postsynaptic second messenger system of β-adrenergic stimulation. Thus, elevated cAMP concentrations cause clinical effects similar to adrenergic stimulation, including smooth muscle relaxation, peripheral vasodilation, myocardial stimulation, skeletal muscle contractility, and CNS excitation.

Selective β_2-Adrenergic Agonists

Selective β_2-adrenergic agonists act very specifically at β_2-adrenergic receptors, resulting in an increase in intracellular cAMP. Effects of β_2 agonism include relaxation of vascular, bronchial, and uterine smooth muscle; glycogenolysis in skeletal muscle; and hepatic glycogenolysis and gluconeogenesis. Selective β_2-adrenergic agonists are characterized as directly activating the β_2 receptor, such as albuterol; being taken up into a membrane depot, such as formoterol; or interacting with a receptor-specific auxiliary binding site, such as salmeterol. These differences do not appear to be relevant in acute toxicity. However, emerging evidence suggests that chronic use of long-acting β_2-adrenergic agonists is associated with increased incidence of intubation as well as fatalities with future exacerbations of asthma.[77]

PHARMACOKINETICS AND TOXICOKINETICS

Caffeine Pharmacokinetics

Caffeine is bioavailable by all routes of administration. Oral administration, which is by far the most common route of exposure, results in nearly 100% bioavailability. Peak concentration of caffeine occurs 30 to 60 minutes after oral intake, and food in the gastrointestinal (GI) tract delays the time to peak concentration. Caffeine rapidly diffuses into the total body water and all tissues and readily crosses the blood–brain barrier and into the placenta. The volume of distribution (V_d) is 0.6 L/kg, and 36% is protein bound. Caffeine is secreted in breast milk with concentrations of 2 to 4 mcg/mL in breast milk after 100 mg PO dosing in a breastfeeding mother. Consumption of caffeine does not result in clinically relevant breast milk caffeine concentrations in lactating women or toxicity in their breastfeeding children. Breast milk caffeine concentrations are much lower than maternal serum caffeine concentrations, with breast milk having 0.006% to 1.5% of the quantity of maternal serum.[8]

When taken in amounts that produce serum caffeine concentrations exceeding a therapeutic range, or approximately 20 mg/kg, caffeine exhibits Michaelis-Menten kinetics and is metabolized, primarily by CYP1A2. The major pathway involves demethylation to 1,7-dimethylxanthine (paraxanthine) followed by hydroxylation or repeated demethylation followed by hydroxylation. To a lesser extent, caffeine is also metabolized to theobromine and theophylline. Neonates demethylate caffeine, producing theophylline, and possess the unique ability to convert theophylline to caffeine by methylation.[39] By 4 to 7 months of age, infants metabolize and eliminate caffeine in a manner similar to adults. All patients demethylate some quantity of caffeine to active metabolites, including theophylline and theobromine. The degree to which this occurs depends on the patient's age, CYP1A2 induction status, and other factors.

Less than 5% of caffeine is excreted in the urine unchanged. The half-life of caffeine is highly variable and dependent on several factors. In a healthy, nonsmoking, adult patient, the half-life is 4.5 hours; in smokers, the half-life shortened by up to 50%. Younger patients, particularly infants, and patients with CYP1A2 inhibition, such as pregnant patients or patients with cirrhosis, have longer caffeine half-lives.

Caffeine Toxicokinetics

Caffeine toxicity is a dose-dependent phenomenon. The range of toxic concentrations reported in different references varies greatly, suggesting there is a wide range of clinical effects at any given serum concentration. Therapeutic dosing in neonates is typically consists of a loading dose of 20 mg/kg, with daily maintenance dosing of 5 mg/kg. Based on case reports and series, a lethal dose in adults is estimated at 150 to 200 mg/kg, and death is reported with serum concentrations above 80 mcg/mL. Numerous fatalities are reported with serum concentrations under 200 mcg/mL, and survival is reported of a patient with an acute caffeine overdose and a serum concentration over 400 mcg/mL.[93] Infants tolerate greater serum concentrations of caffeine than do children and adults.

Theophylline Pharmacokinetics

Theophylline is nearly 100% orally bioavailable. Many of the available PO preparations are sustained-release ones designed to provide stable serum concentrations over a prolonged period of time with less frequent dosing. Peak absorption for immediate-release preparations is 60 to 90 minutes; peak absorption of sustained-release preparations generally occurs 6 to 10 hours after ingestion. Theophylline rapidly diffuses into the total body water and all tissues, readily crosses the blood–brain barrier, and crosses into the placenta and breast milk. The V_d of theophylline is 0.5 L/kg, and 56% of it is protein bound at therapeutic concentrations.

Theophylline is metabolized primarily by CYP1A2. The major pathway is demethylation to 3-methylxanthine in addition to being demethylated or oxidized to other metabolites. Less than 10% of theophylline is excreted in the urine unchanged. The half-life of theophylline is highly variable and depends on several factors. In healthy, adult, nonsmoking patients, the half-life is 4.5 hours. Infants and older adults as well as patients with CYP1A2 inhibition, pregnant patients, and those with cirrhosis have theophylline half-lives twice as long as healthy children and nonsmoking adults.[24] Factors that induce CYP1A2, such as cigarette smoking, decrease methylxanthine half-life and increase clearance, but others that inhibit CYP1A2, such as exposure to cimetidine, macrolides, and oral contraceptives can significantly decrease theophylline clearance.[95] Cessation of smoking, such as when a patient with chronic obstructive pulmonary disease develops bronchitis, leads to a reversal of CYP1A2 induction and predisposes to the development of chronic toxicity.

Theophylline Toxicokinetics

As in the case of caffeine, theophylline exhibits Michaelis-Menten kinetics, presumably when greater than a single therapeutic dose is taken. At higher doses and in overdose, it undergoes zero-order elimination, and only a fixed amount of the xenobiotic is eliminated in a given time because of saturation of metabolic enzymes.[43]

Therapeutic serum concentrations of theophylline are 5 to 15 mcg/mL. Although morbidity and mortality are not always predictable based on serum concentrations, life-threatening toxicity is associated with serum concentrations of 80 to 100 mcg/mL in acute overdoses and of 40 to 60 mcg/mL in chronic overdoses.[82,84]

Theobromine Toxicokinetics and Pharmacokinetics

Theobromine is well absorbed from the GI tract and taken as food, such as in chocolate, is 77% bioavailable.[90] Theobromine has 21% protein binding, a V_d of 0.62 L/kg, and a serum half-life of 6 to 10 hours.[74] Theobromine undergoes hepatic metabolism by CYP1A2 and CYP2E1. Theobromine is excreted in breast milk. Toxic concentrations of theobromine in animals are known, but comparable human data are lacking.

Selective β₂-Adrenergic Agonist Pharmacokinetics

The β_2-adrenergic agonists are bioavailable by both inhalation and ingestion, and much of "inhaled" β_2-adrenergic agonists may actually be swallowed and absorbed from the GI tract. Absorption, distribution, and elimination are quite variable. The half-life of albuterol is approximately 4 hours, and less than 5% crosses the blood–brain barrier. It is metabolized extensively in the liver, and it is excreted in urine and feces as albuterol and metabolites.

Terbutaline is partially metabolized in the liver, mainly to inactive conjugates. With parenteral administration, 60% of a given dose is excreted in the urine unchanged.

Clenbuterol has a terminal half-life of approximately 22 hours and a prolonged duration of action. It is more potent than other β_2-adrenergic agonist, with a typical therapeutic dose of 20 to 40 mcg, as opposed to milligram doses for other β_2-adrenergic agonists. Clenbuterol has lipolytic and anabolic effects desired by athletes and others who use the drug.

Selective β₂-Adrenergic Agonist Toxicokinetics

Overdose of albuterol, which happens predominantly in young children treated with PO albuterol preparations, uncommonly causes significant effects. For PO albuterol poisoning, 1 mg/kg appears to be the dose threshold for developing clinically significant toxicity.[101] Clenbuterol toxicity occurs after illicit drug use by ingestion, intranasal, and IV use of clenbuterol or clenbuterol-tainted street drugs.[49]

METHYLXANTHINE AND β₂-ADRENERGIC AGONIST TOXICITY

Caffeine, theobromine, and theophylline affect the same organ systems and cause qualitatively similar effects. Toxicity affects the GI, cardiovascular, central nervous, and musculoskeletal systems in addition to causing a constellation of metabolic derangements. A putative cause for toxicity involves the increase in metabolism that occurs with methylxanthine toxicity, particularly in the setting of a decreased tissue perfusion. Concomitant poisoning with other xenobiotics that result in adrenergic stimulation, such as pseudoephedrine, ephedrine, amphetamines, or cocaine, may be particularly severe.[29]

Gastrointestinal

In overdose, methylxanthines cause nausea, and most significant acute overdoses result in severe and protracted emesis. Whereas emesis occurs in 75% of cases of acute theophylline poisoning, only 30% of cases of chronically poisoned patients experience emesis.[85] When it occurs, the emesis is usually severe and requires use of potent antiemetics. This is especially evident with sustained-release theophylline preparations.[2] Emesis is less common and less severe with selective β_2-adrenergic agonist toxicity.

Methylxanthines increase gastric acid secretion and relax smooth muscle. These factors contribute to the gastritis and esophagitis reported in chronic methylxanthine users. Gastritis is noted in drinkers of decaffeinated coffee, and therefore some adverse gastric effects associated with coffee drinking are caused by ingredients other than caffeine such as the pH of the beverage.

Cardiovascular

Methylxanthines are cardiac stimulants and result in positive inotropy and chronotropy even with therapeutic dosing. Dysrhythmias, particularly tachydysrhythmias, are common in patients with methylxanthine overdose. Tachydysrhythmias, particularly ventricular extrasystoles, are more common after methylxanthine overdose.[19,82] Cardiac dysrhythmias, although described with selective β_2-adrenergic agonist poisoning, are most frequently supraventricular in origin and clinically inconsequential. Dysrhythmias other than sinus tachycardia associated with β_2-adrenergic agonist toxicity are not routinely noted with toxicity from other β_2-adrenergic agonists, but clenbuterol is known to cause atrial fibrillation.[27] Palpitations, tachycardia, and chest pain are common presenting complaints for patients with clenbuterol toxicity.

In the setting of acute poisoning, generally benign sinus tachycardia is nearly universal in patients without antecedent cardiac disease. In any patient, particularly those with underlying cardiac disease, sinus tachycardia degenerates to a more severe rhythm disturbance, and these represent the most common causes of fatality associated with methylxanthine poisoning. Both atrial and ventricular dysrhythmias, including supraventricular tachycardia (SVT), multifocal atrial tachycardia, atrial fibrillation, premature ventricular contractions, and ventricular tachycardia, result from methylxanthine toxicity.[9] Concomitant electrolyte disturbances, particularly hypokalemia, contribute to the development of dysrhythmias. Dysrhythmias occur more commonly and at lower serum concentrations in cases of chronic poisoning with methylxanthines. Consequential dysrhythmias occur in 35% of patients with chronic theophylline poisoning but in only 10% of patients with acute poisoning.[84] Ventricular dysrhythmias occur at serum concentrations of 40 to 80 mcg/mL in patients with chronic theophylline overdoses and most commonly at serum concentrations greater than 80 mcg/mL in patients with acute overdoses. Neonates born to mothers who consumed more than 500 mg/day of caffeine are more likely to have dysrhythmias compared with cohorts born to mothers consuming less than 250 mg/day of caffeine. See Table 63–1 for the caffeine content of popular products.

Myocardial ischemia and myocardial infarction (MI) are associated from acute caffeine or theophylline poisoning. Myocardial infarction is also associated with albuterol and more recently clenbuterol overdose. Isoproterenol, once a common asthma therapy before widespread use of selective β_2-adrenergic agonists, has both β_1 and β_2-adrenergic agonist activity and is a well-reported cause of MI. Given the frequency of use of selective β_2-adrenergic agonists and in light of the well-known safety and toxicity profile, MI is very unlikely to occur from selective β_2-adrenergic agonists other than clenbuterol. Clenbuterol is clearly capable of causing myocardial ischemia and MI in young otherwise healthy patients without coronary artery disease.[72]

Elevation of troponin, muscle creatine phosphokinase (CK-MM) and cardiac (CK-MB) fractions are described and expected after large doses of β_2-adrenergic agonists, particularly terbutaline infusions and continuous albuterol nebulization.[23,91] In the absence of electrocardiographic (ECG) changes suggestive of ischemia, the clinical significance of increased CK-MB and cardiac troponin concentrations in patients receiving terbutaline infusions, particularly children, is unclear and does not correlate with clinically adverse effects.[20]

In therapeutic doses, methylxanthines cause cerebral vasoconstriction. In overdose, this effect likely exacerbates CNS toxicity by diminishing cerebral perfusion. Tolerance to the vasopressor effects of methylxanthines develops after several days of use and rapidly disappears after relatively brief periods of abstinence.

Dietary caffeine increases blood pressure, which is believed to contribute to population levels of morbidity and mortality.[51] At elevated serum concentrations, patients with methylxanthine or selective β_2-adrenergic agonist poisoning often develop a characteristic widened pulse pressure. This is caused by enhanced inotropy (β_1) that increases in systolic blood pressure combined with peripheral vasodilation (β_2), which causes diastolic hypotension. In cases of acute theophylline overdose, serum concentrations greater than 100 mcg/mL are usually associated with severe toxicity, and the associated shock involves significant hypotension rather than simply widened pulse pressure. Methylxanthines cause renal vasodilation that, in addition to the increased cardiac output, results in a mild diuresis.

Pulmonary

Methylxanthines stimulate the CNS respiratory center, causing an increase in respiratory rate. For this reason, caffeine and theophylline are used to treat neonatal apnea syndromes. Severe caffeine and theophylline overdoses cause hyperventilation, respiratory alkalosis, respiratory failure, respiratory arrest, and acute respiratory distress syndrome.

Neuropsychiatric

The stimulant and psychoactive properties of methylxanthines, particularly caffeine, elevate mood and improve performance of manual tasks. The CNS stimulation associated with use is an effect sought by users of coffee, tea, cocoa, and chocolate. Central nervous system stimulation resulting from therapeutic use of theophylline is generally considered to be an undesirable side effect. Although at low doses, methylxanthines have beneficial effects, with increasing doses, they result in adverse effects. Headache, anxiety, agitation, insomnia, tremor, irritability, hallucinations, and seizures occur from caffeine or theophylline poisoning. In adults, caffeine doses of 50 to 200 mg result in increased alertness, decreased drowsiness, and lessened fatigue, and caffeine doses of 200 to 500 mg produce adverse effects such as tremor, anxiety, diaphoresis, and palpitations. Children tend to develop CNS symptoms at lower serum theophylline concentrations than adults, and such excitation is a significant clinical disadvantage of theophylline use.

Seizures are a major complication of methylxanthine poisoning. The ability of caffeine to both promote and prolong seizures is well recognized, and caffeine was once used to prolong therapeutically induced seizures in electroconvulsive therapy.[26] Seizures resulting from methylxanthine overdose tend to be severe and recurrent and refractory to conventional treatment. Antagonism of adenosine, the endogenous neurotransmitter responsible for halting seizures, contributes to the profound seizures associated with methylxanthine overdose.[31,87] When studied prospectively, chronic theophylline toxicity results in seizures in 14% of patients, but 5% of acutely poisoned patients experience seizures. In cases of chronic and acute-on-chronic toxicity, seizures are more likely to occur, and they occur at lower serum concentrations.[68] Patients at extremes of age—those younger than age 3 years and older than age 60 years—are more likely to experience seizures with overdose.

Musculoskeletal

Methylxanthines increase striated muscle contractility, secondarily decreasing muscle fatigue. They also increase muscle oxygen consumption and increase the basal metabolic rate. These effects are sought by users to enhance or improve athletic performance or weight loss. All methylxanthines cause smooth muscle relaxation.

Tremor is the most common adverse effect of methylxanthines. Skeletal muscle excitation associated with methylxanthine overdose includes fasciculation, hypertonicity, myoclonus, or even rhabdomyolysis.[63] Mechanisms for rhabdomyolysis include increased muscle activity, particularly from seizures, and direct cytotoxicity from excessive sequestered intracytoplasmic calcium. The mechanism of injury is unknown, but multiple case reports associate a nontraumatic compartment syndrome with rhabdomyolysis with theophylline overdose.[62,94]

Metabolic

Numerous metabolic derangements result from acute methylxanthine toxicity and are similar to those in other hyperadrenergic situations.[43] Methylxanthines result in adrenal release of endogenous catecholamines,[89] which contribute to the metabolic effects associated with methylxanthine exposure. Severe hypokalemia from β₂-adrenergic stimulation is well reported.[96] This results from influx of extracellular potassium into the intracellular compartment despite normal total body potassium content. Both ECG and neuromuscular complications secondary to hypokalemia are possible. Other metabolic effects of methylxanthine and selective β₂-adrenergic agonist poisoning include hypomagnesemia and hypophosphatemia.[12]

Transient hypokalemia resulting from β-adrenergic agonism occurs in 85% of patients with acute theophylline overdose, and typically the serum potassium decreases to approximately 3 mEq/L.[2,86] Stimulation of Na^+,K^+-ATPase results in a shift of serum potassium to the intracellular compartment of skeletal muscle. Total body potassium stores are unchanged. The significance of hypokalemia in patients with methylxanthine overdose or in patients with hypokalemia secondary to selective β₂-adrenergic agonists, is unclear. Hyperkalemia secondary to rhabdomyolysis or overly aggressive repletion of potassium is a rare but potential adverse effect of methylxanthine poisoning.

Metabolic acidosis with an increased serum lactate concentration is commonly noted as a complication of theophylline overdose and is also described as a result of clenbuterol overdose and with therapeutic albuterol use.[9,49,76] Tachypnea and respiratory alkalosis secondary to stimulation of the respiratory center are also common with methylxanthine toxicity, but this does not result from selective β₂-adrenergic agonists.

Hyperglycemia with serum glucose of approximately 200 mg/dL in those without diabetes is common and occurs in 75% of patients with acute theophylline overdose. Rebound hypoglycemia after albuterol overdose is reported in children,[98] but this is probably an extraordinarily rare occurrence. Hyperthermia caused by increased metabolic activity and increased muscle activity occurs after caffeine and theophylline overdose. Leukocytosis, probably secondary to the high concentrations of circulating catecholamines, results from acute methylxanthine overdose and lacks clinical significance. In the absence of seizures or protracted emesis, chronic methylxanthine poisoning does not typically lead to metabolic derangements other than mild hypokalemia because such toxicity is an ongoing, compensated process.

CHRONIC METHYLXANTHINE TOXICITY

The distinction between acute and chronic toxicity is based on the duration of exposure. Signs and symptoms of chronic toxicity are usually more subtle or nonspecific, such as anorexia, nausea, palpitations, or emesis, but chronic toxicity also presents as seizures or dysrhythmias. Patients chronically receiving theophylline or caffeine have higher total body stores of these xenobiotics and often underlying medical disorders and thus develop toxicity with a smaller amount of additional theophylline or caffeine. Chronic methylxanthine poisoning typically occurs in the setting of therapeutic use of theophylline or caffeine, as well as from frequent, chronic consumption of caffeinated products. Patients often manifest subtle signs of illness, such as anorexia, nausea, palpitations, or emesis. However, the initial presentation in these patients, even with serum concentrations in the 40- to 60-mcg/mL

range, can be a seizure. Children chronically overdosed with theophylline often have peak serum theophylline concentrations in the high end of the normal range, and thus this laboratory testing fails to identify some who will progress to life-threatening toxicity. In the absence of protracted emesis or seizures, the initial electrolytes other than potassium and blood gases are expected to be normal in patients with chronic methylxanthine toxicity.

CHRONIC METHYLXANTHINE USE

Data on the effect of caffeine on many chronic health issues are mixed and highly contradictory. Studies show inconclusive links to Alzheimer's disease, depression, cancer, heart disease, osteoporosis, hyperlipidemia, and hypercholesterolemia associated with caffeine use.[17,41,99,102,103] Hypokalemia secondary to excessive consumption of caffeine-containing beverages is reported.

CAFFEINE WITHDRAWAL

Caffeine induces tolerance, and a withdrawal syndrome, including headache, yawning, nausea, drowsiness, rhinorrhea, lethargy, irritability, nervousness, a disinclination to work, and depression, occurs on abstinence in tolerant users. Use of caffeinated analgesics to treat headache causes rebound headaches upon cessation. Caffeine withdrawal symptoms are described in neonates born to mothers with consequential caffeine use.[65] The onset of caffeine withdrawal symptoms begins 12 to 24 hours after cessation and lasts up to 1 week. In a double-blind trial, 52% of adults with low to moderate caffeine intake, defined as 2.5 cups of coffee daily, developed a withdrawal syndrome on caffeine abstinence.[91]

REPRODUCTION

Massive doses of methylxanthines are teratogenic, but the doses of typical use are not associated with birth defects. Decreased fecundity and adverse fetal outcome are noted in animals with chronic exposure to methylxanthines. Human studies of fertility, fetal loss, and fetal outcome produce divergent results, and the effects of methylxanthine use during gestation are unclear.[15]

DIAGNOSTIC TESTING

An ECG, serum electrolytes, and serum caffeine or theophylline concentrations are indicated in cases of suspected methylxanthine toxicity. Because toxicity is dose related in acute overdose, serum concentrations of caffeine and theophylline correlate with toxicity, but for caffeine, there is a much wider range of severity associated with a given serum concentration.

Hospitals that use caffeine therapeutically can typically assay serum caffeine concentration within the institution, and likewise hospitals using theophylline therapeutically typically can assay serum theophylline concentrations. Overdose of caffeine causes a spuriously elevated serum theophylline concentration.[35]

Theophylline concentrations—and to a lesser extent, caffeine concentrations—are used prognostically to guide management of poisoning. Proper interpretation requires knowledge of whether the poisoning is acute, chronic, or acute on chronic. In the setting of toxicity, serum caffeine or theophylline concentrations should be obtained immediately and then serially every 1 to 2 hours until a downward trend is evident.

Likewise, serum electrolytes, particularly potassium, should be monitored serially as long as the poisoned patient remains symptomatic and significantly abnormal values warrant treatment. Cardiac monitoring should continue until the patient is free of dysrhythmias other than sinus tachycardia, has a falling serum methylxanthine concentration, and is clinically stable. In patients with systemic illness, hyperthermia, or increased muscle tone, assessing serum CK and urinalysis to detect rhabdomyolysis is also indicated.

MANAGEMENT

General Principles and Gastrointestinal Decontamination

After assuring adequacy of airway, breathing, and circulation, supportive care and maintenance of vital signs within acceptable limits are the mainstays of therapy for patients with methylxanthine and selective β₂-adrenergic agonist toxicity. Decisions regarding GI decontamination, including orogastric lavage, administration of activated charcoal (AC), or whole-bowel irrigation (WBI), depend on the dosage and type of preparation involved, the time since exposure, and the patient's physical condition. Activated charcoal is the only GI decontamination that is routinely recommended for selective β_2-adrenergic agonist ingestion.

Orogastric Lavage

Orogastric lavage is an acceptable option for patients with methylxanthine ingestions capable of causing severe toxicity or fatality given an appropriate time frame (Chap. 5) and who are not already experiencing spontaneous emesis. If orogastric lavage can be performed safely by a skilled clinician, an approximated dose of ingestion of 50 mg/kg of theophylline tablets is a reasonable threshold. Most patients with caffeine ingestion are unlikely to be appropriate for orogastric lavage because concentrated caffeine is most commonly in powder, liquid, or rapidly disintegrating tablets, and caffeine is very rapidly absorbed from the stomach. Therefore, we recommend orogastric lavage for caffeine tablet ingestions of 50 mg/kg or greater that have occurred 60 minutes or less from the time orogastric lavage can be started. Lavage after ingestion of caffeine powder or liquid would preferably be performed with a nasogastric tube rather than an orogastric tube. Caffeine powder or liquid could be readily retrieved through a nasogastric tube. Because of the much greater ease, greater safety, and lesser need for clinician experience to safely perform, nasogastric lavage is reasonable after recent ingestion of 50 mg/kg or more caffeine liquid or powder. If the patient has ingested an unknown but likely greater than 1 tsp of concentrated powder, which would contain nearly 5 g, it should be presumed this is a massive mg/kg dose, and similarly nasogastric lavage is reasonable. At the completion of orogastric or nasogastric lavage, the lavage tube should be used to deliver an appropriate dose of AC. If a nasogastric tube is used, it may be left in place for delivery of multiple-dose activated charcoal (MDAC).

Likewise, for patients with recent ingestion of large quantities of selective β_2-adrenergic agonist in liquid form who have not already had spontaneous emesis, aspiration of gastric contents with a small nasogastric tube is reasonable followed by administration of AC.

Activated Charcoal

Activated charcoal is essential for the treatment of methylxanthine poisoning. Activated charcoal can adsorb methylxanthines and selective β_2-adrenergic agonist present in the GI tract and limit their absorption. Multiple-dose activated charcoal is helpful to enhance the elimination of methylxanthines but is not indicated for selective β_2-adrenergic agonist ingestion. Multiple-dose activated charcoal is recommended for any significant methylxanthine ingestion. Multiple-dose activated charcoal enhances elimination of theophylline, and probably caffeine and theobromine, by "gut dialysis" (Antidotes in Depth: A1). Although MDAC's utility is only proven for theophylline, the pharmacologic similarity of the methylxanthines and the relative safety of MDAC therapy warrant the use of such treatment for patients with any methylxanthine toxicity.

Whole-Bowel Irrigation

Whole-bowel irrigation for the xenobiotics covered in this chapter is reasonable for sustained-release pills, with very specific limitations. Ingestion of sustained-release theophylline tablets is associated with the formation of bezoars that are difficult to remove or dislodge and require endoscopic removal.[18] Use of a brief period of initial WBI for patients with ingestion of sustained-release theophylline tablets is reasonable to prevent bezoar formation (Antidotes in Depth: A2). Polyethylene glycol electrolyte lavage solution used for WBI can displace theophylline already bound to AC.[47] This is a concern in patients who have taken several doses of AC before WBI, in which desorption of methylxanthine from AC will result in some additional methylxanthine available for GI absorption. Also, WBI is experimentally demonstrated to provide no additional benefit to AC in treatment of sustained-released theophylline ingestion.[14] Thus if orogastric lavage was not used, MDAC, possibly preceded by an initial period of WBI to prevent bezoar formation, is reasonable treatment of a patient with ingestion of sustained-release theophylline.

Specific Treatment
Gastrointestinal Toxicity

Use of a highly effective antiemetic, such as ondansetron or granisetron, sometimes in doses used for chemotherapy, plays a role in management of methylxanthine-induced vomiting, which is usually severe and prolonged. However, ondansetron is capable of resulting in QT interval prolongation,[33] particularly in the setting of likely hypokalemia and hypomagnesemia, both common with methylxanthine toxicity. We recommend confirmation of a normal QT interval before ondansetron use. Phenothiazine antiemetics are contraindicated in methylxanthine poisoning because they are typically ineffective, and they lower the seizure threshold. Less effective antiemetics such as metoclopramide are reasonable if ondansetron or granisetron is unavailable or if the maximal ondansetron or granisetron dose has been reached or if the QT interval is already prolonged.[75] Histamine (H_2) blockers and proton pump inhibitors are reasonable in any patient with hematemesis. Cimetidine is contraindicated because it inhibits multiple CYP enzymes, delaying clearance of methylxanthines.

Cardiovascular Toxicity

Patients with hypotension should initially be treated by administration of isotonic intravenous (IV) fluid, such as 0.9% sodium chloride or lactated Ringer solution, in bolus volumes of 20 mL/kg. If acceptable blood pressure cannot be maintained despite several fluid boluses or if there are contraindications to fluid bolus, additional therapy using vasopressors or β-adrenergic antagonists such as esmolol is recommended. There are less available data on use of esmolol for this purpose, but animal models[36] and human case reports confirm its efficacy.[80]

Methylxanthine and selective β_2-adrenergic agonist toxicity cause hypotension via β-adrenergic agonism; therefore, administration of vasopressors with β-adrenergic agonist effects, such as epinephrine, dobutamine, or isoproterenol, is suboptimal. An α-adrenergic agonist such as phenylephrine is the first-line pressor of choice in such a situation, although norepinephrine is also acceptable.

In cases of refractory hypotension, the administration of a β-adrenergic antagonist is recommended. Administration of a β-adrenergic antagonist to a hypotensive patient is counterintuitive, but it can reverse β_2-adrenergic–mediated vasodilation. In addition, β_1-adrenergic blockade treats tachycardia and any associated decreased cardiac output. In dogs with aminophylline-induced tachycardia and hypotension, administration of esmolol results in a return to normal heart rate and blood pressure, and it does not exacerbate hypotension.[36] Propranolol, esmolol, and metoprolol were used successfully to treat methylxanthine-induced hypotension and dysrhythmias in humans.[10,71] It is most appropriate to use a β-adrenergic antagonist with a brief duration of action, such as esmolol, at least initially, in such circumstances. In the event of an adverse reaction or side effect such as hypotension or bronchospasm were to occur, the duration of such will be relatively brief. Any β-adrenergic antagonist therapy should ideally be preceded and accompanied by assessment of cardiac output and central venous pressure, either directly or noninvasively.[55] Because of its long half-life and possibly potency, toxicity from clenbuterol exposure appears more likely to require treatment with β-adrenergic antagonist medications.[48]

When xenobiotic toxicity is not causal, adenosine or electrical cardioversion is the preferred treatment for SVT. This is not so for SVT resulting from methylxanthine toxicity. Because of the antagonist effects at the adenosine receptor, administration of adenosine is not expected to convert a methylxanthine-induced SVT. Even if adenosine is successfully used to convert an SVT, the effect is likely to be transient. Because methylxanthine toxicity has a global effect on the myocardium and methylxanthine concentrations do not change rapidly, cardioversion, which is effective in electrically "reorganizing" depolarization, is unlikely to result is a sustained normal rhythm.

The primary treatment for methylxanthine-induced SVT includes administration of benzodiazepines, and focused pharmacologic therapy to treat SVT would be use of a β-adrenergic antagonist such as esmolol, of if that were not possible, we recommend cautious administration of a conduction-attenuating calcium channel blocker such as diltiazem or verapamil. Pharmacologic treatment of methylxanthine-induced ventricular dysrhythmias would involve, in addition to typical Advanced Cardiovascular Life Support resuscitation medications, use of esmolol.[58]

In animal models, treatment of patients with acute theophylline toxicity with the calcium channel blockers diltiazem, verapamil, and nifedipine each results in decreased cardiac-related deaths and prevention of dysrhythmias, hypotension, myocardial necrosis, and seizures.[100] In addition to the cardiovascular benefit of calcium channel blockers, they also afford neurologic protection and prevention of seizure.

Central Nervous System Toxicity

Administration of a benzodiazepine, such as diazepam, lorazepam, or midazolam, is the recommended treatment for anxiety, agitation, or seizure. Because of the long duration of effect of methylxanthines, lorazepam is preferable, and if diazepam or midazolam is used, the need for multiple doses should be expected. Seizures associated with methylxanthine toxicity are severe and often refractory to treatment. In patients with seizures not controlled with one or two therapeutic doses of a benzodiazepine we recommend treatment with a barbiturate such as phenobarbital or pentobarbital or another suitable sedative–hypnotic such as propofol. No delay should occur before escalating management to include more potent medications. Unsuccessful antiepileptic therapy of methylxanthine-induced seizures should quickly be escalated to use a more potent antiepileptic. The administration of barbiturates or propofol may result in, or exacerbate hypotension. Treatment of agitation or seizure with benzodiazepines, barbiturates, propofol, or other sedative–hypnotic requires repeated dosing until clinical effect is achieved.

Administration of phenobarbital to prevent seizures in theophylline-poisoned rabbits and mice increases survival by decreasing the incidence of seizures.[25,40] Although historically phenobarbital was the recommended medication for such prophylaxis, use of a benzodiazepine such as lorazepam seems preferable based on pharmacokinetic and practical considerations. Patients at risk for seizure include those identified earlier in this chapter—patients older than age 60 years or younger than age 3 years, those with chronic overdose and a serum concentration above 40 mcg/mL, and acutely overdosed patients with serum concentrations greater than 100 mcg/mL.

Phenytoin and fosphenytoin are contraindicated to treat methylxanthine-induced seizures. Phenytoin and fosphenytoin are of no benefit in controlling methylxanthine-induced seizures. Phenytoin shortens the time to seizure and increases the mortality rate when administered to theophylline-poisoned animals.[11,46] Retrospective review of human cases demonstrated phenytoin to be ineffective in treating seizures in nearly all cases.[70]

Metabolic Abnormalities

Patients with symptomatic hypokalemia should be treated with electrolyte repletion. Most cases of hypokalemia are well tolerated and do not require potassium supplementation, but any patient with symptomatic hypokalemia, particularly those associated with ECG changes of abnormal T waves or QT interval prolongation, should be treated. The frequency of ventricular dysrhythmias in methylxanthine poisoning is exacerbated by hypokalemia coupled with increased intrinsic catecholamine release. Correction of hypokalemia is crucial in methylxanthine poisoning associated with ventricular dysrhythmias.

There is no specific degree of hypokalemia that absolutely necessitates treatment, and potassium supplementation should not be routinely used. In the absence of associated dysrhythmias or prolonged QT interval, the clinical significance of such hypokalemia is unclear. When potassium correction is needed, it is generally performed with the administration of IV or PO potassium, but hypokalemia experimentally responds to treatment with β-adrenergic antagonists.

If administration of potassium to treat symptomatic hypokalemia is indicated, it is in lesser quantities than that needed for total body potassium repletion. Methylxanthine and β₂-adrenergic agonists result in a potassium shift rather than potassium loss. In cases of hypokalemia secondary to β-adrenergic

agonism, after the β-adrenergic agonism resolves, an efflux of potassium from the intracellular compartment occurs with a concomitant increase in the serum potassium concentration. Aggressive attempts to correct hypokalemia result in hyperkalemia after the β-adrenergic agonist effects abate.

Experimentally, administration of propranolol to theophylline-poisoned dogs prevented or partially reversed hypokalemia, hypophosphatemia, hyperglycemia, and metabolic acidosis as well as hypotension.[54] Prevention or correction of the metabolic derangements associated with theophylline toxicity by administration of β-adrenergic antagonists is congruent with the fact that these derangements, particularly hypokalemia, are the consequence of β-adrenergic agonism. Indications to treat hypomagnesemia, hypophosphatemia, or hypocalcemia include ECG abnormalities such as prolongation of the QT interval or dysrhythmia.

Hyperglycemia, likely resulting from increased circulating catecholamines, is common. This hyperglycemia does not necessitate treatment, both because it is a transient effect and because in other situations of hyperglycemia resulting from adrenergic agonism, rebound hypoglycemia is a risk.

Musculoskeletal Toxicity

The use of benzodiazepines is a reasonable treatment for fasciculations, hypertonicity, myoclonus, and rhabdomyolysis. Rhabdomyolysis necessitates aggressive therapy with IV fluid and sodium bicarbonate (Antidotes in Depth: A5).

Enhanced Elimination

Fortunately, methylxanthine toxicity lends itself well to several methods of enhanced elimination, including disrupting enterohepatic or enteroenteric recirculation with MDAC or hemodialysis as well as increasingly used methods such as continuous arteriovenous and continuous venovenous hemoperfusion.[50,60]

Although intermittent hemodialysis has a long record of efficacy in treating methylxanthine toxicity, in some settings when hemodialysis is not an option, continuous renal replacement therapy (CRRT) is an alternative treatment. Particularly in infants, MDAC, CRRT, and exchange blood transfusion are effective methods of enhanced elimination, and these may be used concurrently, particularly if hemodialysis is not feasible.[69,86,88]

Enhanced elimination of methylxanthines by use of MDAC is recommended for toxicity with elevated serum methylxanthine concentrations unless there is a specific contraindication. Such MDAC use allows elimination of theophylline limiting enteroenteric or enteroenteric recirculation.[4] Multiple-dose activated charcoal is extremely effective at enhancing elimination of theophylline.[37,59,67] Experimentally in animals and human volunteers, AC administered after IV aminophylline administration results in increased systemic clearance and decreased half-life of theophylline.[57,66,73] The pharmacologic similarity of the methylxanthines suggests that MDAC is probably effective in caffeine or theobromine poisoning, and MDAC certainly is effective in eliminating theophylline generated from metabolism of caffeine or theobromine. The efficacy of MDAC combined with the safety and ease with which this therapy can be administered makes MDAC the mainstay of enhanced elimination in methylxanthine toxicity. Severe emesis associated with methylxanthine poisoning results in intolerance of MDAC (Antidotes in Depth: A1).[81]

Charcoal hemoperfusion was once considered the most effective method of enhanced elimination of methylxanthines, decreasing theophylline's half-life to 2 hours and increasing its clearance up to sixfold.[104] Variations of charcoal hemoperfusion, including albumin colloid hemoperfusion, resin hemoperfusion, and charcoal hemoperfusion in series with hemodialysis, are reported. Because of widespread availability and efficiency, hemodialysis is the recommended first-line method of extracorporeal treatment (ECTR) for methylxanthine poisoning.[38] In addition to the extracorporeal removal of methylxanthines, hemodialysis can also correct fluid and electrolyte imbalances, is more widely available,[83] is technically easier, with lower complication rates.

Consensus guidelines give specific indications for extracorporeal removal of theophylline,[38] which should also be applied to caffeine

TABLE 63–2	Methylxanthine Poisoning: Indications for Hemodialysis or Charcoal Hemoperfusion

1. Extracorporeal xenobiotic removal is recommended if:
   a. Serum theophylline or caffeine concentration >100 mg/L (555 mmol/L).
   b. Seizures are present.
   c. Life-threatening dysrhythmias are present.
   d. Shock is present.
   e. Theophylline or caffeine concentration is rising despite optimal treatment.
   f. Clinical deterioration occurs despite optimal therapy.
2. Extracorporeal xenobiotic removal is suggested if:
   a. Theophylline or caffeine >60 mg/L (333 mmol/L) in chronic exposure.
   b. The patient is <6 months or >60 years of age and the theophylline or caffeine >50 mg/mL (278 mmol/L in chronic exposure.
   c. Gastrointestinal decontamination cannot be performed.

poisoning. These include theophylline concentration greater than 100 mg/L (555 μmol/L); presence of seizures; life-threatening dysrhythmias, or shock; a rising serum concentration despite optimal GI decontamination; and clinical deterioration despite optimal care. In patients with chronic poisoning, extracorporeal removal is suggested if the theophylline serum concentration is greater than 60 mg/L (333 μmol/L) or a lower cutoff of concentration greater than 50 mg/L (278 μmol/L) for patients younger than 6 months of age or older than 60 years of age. Another suggested indication for extracorporeal removal is inability to administer GI decontamination. Extracorporeal treatment should be continued until clinical improvement is apparent or the concentration is less than 15 mg/L (83 μmol/L). Intermittent hemodialysis is the preferred method of extracorporeal removal but hemoperfusion or CRRT are reasonable if hemodialysis is not feasible. Exchange transfusion is an adequate alternative to hemodialysis in neonates. Multiple-dose activated charcoal should be continued during extracorporeal treatment. Although CRRT is less effective than intermittent hemodialysis, it is more widely available and easier to perform, particularly in children (Table 63–2).

SUMMARY

- Caffeine is one of the most commonly consumed xenobiotics worldwide, and as a result of novel products such as pure caffeine in powder or tablet form, energy drinks and caffeinated alcoholic beverages, poisoning from these products is a continuing problem.
- There are significant differences in the clinical presentation and management of patients with acute and chronic methylxanthine poisoning. Supportive care and treatment of GI, cardiovascular, CNS, metabolic, and musculoskeletal effects are the mainstay of therapy. The unique properties of methylxanthines necessitate specific therapies for the GI, cardiovascular, and CNS toxicities of methylxanthines.
- Methylxanthines result in much more severe poisoning than selective β_2-adrenergic agonists. Cardiotoxicity with dysrhythmias and neurotoxicity with severe seizures and status epilepticus are the most significant results of methylxanthine poisoning.
- Clenbuterol is unique among β_2-adrenergic agonists. It has a long half-life and results in cardiotoxicity as well as metabolic toxicity with metabolic acidosis with elevated lactate concentration. Treatment includes supportive care and use of β-adrenergic antagonists.
- Methods of enhanced elimination, particularly extracorporeal elimination by hemodialysis, and gut dialysis with MDAC, are effective treatments for patients with methylxanthine toxicity.

REFERENCES

1. American Psychiatric Association. *Diagnostic and Statistical Manual of Mental Disorders.* 5th ed. Washington, DC: American Psychiatric Association; 2013:280.
2. Amitai Y, Lovejoy FH. Characteristics of vomiting associated with acute sustained release theophylline poisoning: implications for management with oral activated charcoal. *J Toxicol Clin Toxicol.* 1987;25:539-554.
3. Amitai Y, Lovejoy FH. Hypokalemia in acute theophylline poisoning. *Am J Emerg Med.* 1988;6:214-218.
4. Arimori K, Nakano M. Transport of theophylline from blood to the intestinal lumen following i.v. administration to rats. *J Pharmacobiodyn.* 1985;8:324-327.
5. Barbosa J, et al. Food poisoning by clenbuterol in Portugal. *Food Addit Contam.* 2005;22:563-566.
6. Beauchamp GA, et al. A retrospective study of clinical effects of powdered caffeine exposures reported to three US poison control centers. *J Med Toxicol.* 2016;12:295-300.
7. Benowitz NL, et al. Massive catecholamine release from caffeine poisoning. *JAMA.* 1982;248:1097-1098.
8. Berlin CM, et al. Disposition of dietary caffeine in milk, saliva, and plasma of lactating women. *Pediatrics.* 1984;73:59-63.
9. Bernard S. Severe lactic acidosis following theophylline overdose. *Ann Emerg Med.* 1991;20:1135-1137.
10. Biberstein MP, et al. Use of beta-blockade and hemoperfusion for acute theophylline poisoning. *West J Med.* 1984;141:485-490.
11. Blake KV, et al. Relative efficacy of phenytoin and phenobarbital for the prevention of theophylline-induced seizures in mice. *Ann Emerg Med.* 1988;17:1024-1028.
12. Bodenhamer J, et al. Frequently nebulized beta-agonists for asthma: effects on serum electrolytes. *Ann Emerg Med.* 1992;21:1337-1342.
13. Brouard C, et al. Comparative efficacy of theophylline and caffeine in the treatment of idiopathic apnea in premature infants. *Am J Dis Child.* 1985;139:698-700.
14. Burkhart KK, et al. Whole-bowel irrigation as adjunctive treatment for sustained-release theophylline overdose. *Ann Emerg Med.* 1992;21:1316-1320.
15. Cao H, et al. Is caffeine intake a risk factor leading to infertility? A protocol of an epidemiological systematic review of controlled clinical studies. *Syst Rev.* 2016;5:45.
16. Cappelletti S, et al. Caffeine: cognitive and physical performance enhancer or psychoactive drug? *Curr Neuropharmacol.* 2015;13:71-88.
17. Carman AJ, et al. Current evidence for the use of coffee and caffeine to prevent age-related cognitive decline and Alzheimer's disease. *J Nutr Heal Aging.* 2014;18:383-392.
18. Cereda JM, et al. Endoscopic removal of pharmacobezoar of slow release theophylline. *Br Med J (Clin Res Ed).* 1986;293:1143.
19. Chazan R, et al. Cardiac arrhythmias as a result of intravenous infusions of theophylline in patients with airway obstruction. *Int J Clin Pharmacol Ther.* 1995;33:170-175.
20. Chiang VW, et al. Cardiac toxicity of intravenous terbutaline for the treatment of severe asthma in children: a prospective assessment. *J Pediatr.* 2000;137:73-77.
21. Cleary K, et al. Adolescents and young adults presenting to the emergency department intoxicated from a caffeinated alcoholic beverage: a case series. *Ann Emerg Med.* 2012;59:67-69.
22. CNN. *Bears Overdose on Chocolate Bait.* 2015. http://www.cnn.com/2015/01/23/us/bears-overdose-on-chocolate-irpt/.
23. Craig VL, et al. Efficacy and safety of continuous albuterol nebulization in children with severe status asthmaticus. *Pediatr Emerg Care.* 1996;12:1-5.
24. Cusack B, et al. Theophylline kinetics in relation to age: the importance of smoking. *Br J Clin Pharmacol.* 1980;10:109-114.
25. Czuczwar SJ, et al. Inhibition of aminophylline-induced convulsions in mice by antiepileptic drugs and other agents. *Eur J Pharmacol.* 1987;144:309-315.
26. Datto C, et al. Augmentation of seizure induction in electroconvulsive therapy: a clinical reappraisal. *J ECT.* 2002;18:118-125.
27. Daubert GP, et al. Acute clenbuterol overdose resulting in supraventricular tachycardia and atrial fibrillation. *J Med Toxicol.* 2007;3:56-60.
28. Davies S, et al. Risk of caffeine toxicity associated with the use of "legal highs" (novel psychoactive substances). *Eur J Clin Pharmacol.* 2012;68:435-439.
29. Derlet RW, et al. Potentiation of cocaine and d-amphetamine toxicity with caffeine. *Am J Emerg Med.* 1992;10:211-216.
30. Derry CJ, et al. Caffeine as an analgesic adjuvant for acute pain in adults. *Cochrane Database Syst Rev.* 2014;12:CD009281.
31. Eldridge FL, et al. Role of endogenous adenosine in recurrent generalized seizures. *Exp Neurol.* 1989;103:179-185.
32. US Food and Drug Administration. FDA takes action bulk pure powdered caffeine prod. https://www.fda.gov/Food/NewsEvents/ConstituentUpdates/ucm460097.htm.
33. US Food and Drug Administration. FDA drug safety communication: abnormal heart rhythms may be associated with use of Zofran (ondansetron). https://www.fda.gov/Drugs/DrugSafety/ucm271913.htm.
34. US Food and Drug Administration. FDA consumer advice on pure powdered caffeine. https://www.fda.gov/Food/RecallsOutbreaksEmergencies/SafetyAlertsAdvisories/ucm405787.htm.
35. Fligner CL, Opheim KE. Caffeine and its dimethylxanthine metabolites in two cases of caffeine overdose: a cause of falsely elevated theophylline concentrations in serum. *J Anal Toxicol.* 1988;12:339-343.
36. Gaar GG, et al. The effects of esmolol on the hemodynamics of acute theophylline toxicity. *Ann Emerg Med.* 1987;16:1334-1339.
37. Gal P, et al. Oral activated charcoal to enhance theophylline elimination in an acute overdose. *JAMA.* 1984;251:3130-3131.
38. Ghannoum M, et al. Extracorporeal treatment for theophylline poisoning: systematic review and recommendations from the EXTRIP workgroup. *Clin Toxicol.* 2015;53:215-229.

39. Giacoia G, et al. Theophylline pharmacokinetics in premature infants with apnea. *J Pediatr.* 1976;89:829-832.

40. Goldberg MJ, et al. Phenobarbital improves survival in theophylline-intoxicated rabbits. *J Toxicol Clin Toxicol.* 1986;24:203-211.

41. Grobbee DE, et al. Coffee, caffeine, and cardiovascular disease in men. *N Engl J Med.* 1990;323:1026-1032.

42. Gunja N, Brown JA. Energy drinks: health risks and toxicity. *Med J Aust.* 2012;196:46-49.

43. Hall KW, et al. Metabolic abnormalities associated with intentional theophylline overdose. *Ann Intern Med.* 1984;101:457-462.

44. Heath A, Knudsen K. Role of extracorporeal drug removal in acute theophylline poisoning. A review. *Med Toxicol Advers Drug Exp.* 1987;2:294-308.

45. Hieger MA, et al. A case series of clenbuterol toxicity caused by adulterated heroin. *J Emerg Med.* 2016;51:259-261.

46. Hoffman A, et al. Effect of pretreatment with anticonvulsants on theophylline-induced seizures in the rat. *J Crit Care.* 1993;8:198-202.

47. Hoffman RS, et al. Theophylline desorption from activated charcoal caused by whole bowel irrigation solution. *J Toxicol Clin Toxicol.* 1991;29:191-201.

48. Hoffman RJ, et al. Clenbuterol ingestion causing prolonged tachycardia, hypokalemia, and hypophosphatemia with confirmation by quantitative levels. *J Toxicol Clin Toxicol.* 2001;39:339-344.

49. Hoffman RS, et al. A descriptive study of an outbreak of clenbuterol-containing heroin. *Ann Emerg Med.* 2008;52:548-553.

50. Jacobi J. Use of plasmapheresis in acute theophylline toxicity. *Crit Care Med.* 1992; 20:151.

51. James JE. Critical review of dietary caffeine and blood pressure: a relationship that should be taken more seriously. *Psychosom Med.* 2004;66:63-71.

52. January B, et al. β2-Adrenergic receptor desensitization, internalization, and phosphorylation in response to full and partial agonists. *J Biol Chem.* 1997;272: 23871-23879.

53. Kamimori GH, et al. Effect of three caffeine doses on plasma catecholamines and alertness during prolonged wakefulness. *Eur J Clin Pharmacol.* 2000;56:537-544.

54. Kearney TE, et al. Theophylline toxicity and the beta-adrenergic system. *Ann Intern Med.* 1985;102:766-769.

55. Kempf J, et al. Haemodynamic study as guideline for the use of beta blockers in acute theophylline poisoning. *Intensive Care Med.* 1996;22:585-587.

56. Kimura M, et al. Pulmonary edema complicating ritodrine infusion in a patient with premature labor. *Intern Med.* 2013;52:155.

57. Kulig KW, et al. Intravenous theophylline poisoning and multiple-dose charcoal in an animal model. *Ann Emerg Med.* 1987;16:842-846.

58. Laskowski LK, et al. Start me up! Recurrent ventricular tachydysrhythmias following intentional. *Clin Toxicol.* 2015;53:830-833.

59. Lim DT, et al. Absorption inhibition and enhancement of elimination of sustained-release theophylline tablets by oral activated charcoal. *Ann Emerg Med.* 1986; 15:1303-1307.

60. Lin JL, Jeng LB. Critical, acutely poisoned patients treated with continuous arteriovenous hemoperfusion in the emergency department. *Ann Emerg Med.* 1995;25:75-80.

61. Lippi G, et al. Energy drinks and myocardial ischemia: a review of case reports. *Cardiovasc Toxicol.* 2016;16:207-212.

62. Lloyd D, et al. Acute compartment syndrome secondary to theophylline overdose. *Lancet.* 1990;336:312.

63. MacDonald JB, et al. Rhabdomyolysis and acute renal failure after theophylline overdose. *Lancet.* 1985;325:932-933.

64. Malinauskas BM, et al. A survey of energy drink consumption patterns among college students. *Nutr J.* 2007;6:35.

65. McGowan JD, et al. Neonatal withdrawal symptoms after chronic maternal ingestion of caffeine. *South Med J.* 1988;81:1092-1094.

66. Mckinnon RS, et al. Studies on the mechanisms of action of activated charcoal on theophylline pharmacokinetics. *J Pharm Pharmacol.* 1987;39:522-525.

67. Nobel PA, Light GS. Theophylline-induced diuresis in the neonate. *J Pediatr.* 1977; 90:825-826.

68. Olson KR, et al. Theophylline overdose: acute single ingestion versus chronic repeated overmedication. *Am J Emerg Med.* 1985;3:386-394.

69. Osborn HH, et al. Theophylline toxicity in a premature neonate—elimination kinetics of exchange transfusion. *J Toxicol Clin Toxicol.* 1993;31:639-644.

70. Paloucek FP, Rodvold KA. Evaluation of theophylline overdoses and toxicities. *Ann Emerg Med.* 1988;17:135-144.

71. Price KR, Fligner DJ. Treatment of caffeine toxicity with esmolol. *Ann Emerg Med.* 1990;19:44-46.

72. Quinley KE, et al. Clenbuterol causing non–ST-segment elevation myocardial infarction in a teenage female desiring to lose weight: case and brief literature review. *Am J Emerg Med.* 2016;34:1739-e5.

73. Radomski L, et al. Model for theophylline overdose treatment with oral activated charcoal. *Clin Pharmacol Ther.* 1984;35:402-408.

74. Resman BH, et al. Breast milk distribution of theobromine from chocolate. *J Pediatr.* 1977;91:477-480.

75. Roberts JR, et al. Ondansetron quells drug-resistant emesis in theophylline poisoning. *Am J Emerg Med.* 1993;11:609-610.

76. Rodrigo GJ, Rodrigo C. Elevated plasma lactate level associated with high dose inhaled albuterol therapy in acute severe asthma. *Emerg Med J.* 2005;22:404-408.

77. Salpeter SR, et al. Meta-analysis: effect of long-acting β-agonists on severe asthma exacerbations and asthma-related deaths. *Ann Intern Med.* 2006;144:904-912.

78. Schubert MM, Astorino T. A systematic review of the efficacy of ergogenic aids for improving running performance. *J Strength Cond Res.* 2013;27:1699-1707.

79. Seifert SM, et al. Health effects of energy drinks on children, adolescents, and young adults. *Pediatrics.* 2011;127:511-528.

80. Seneff M, et al. Acute theophylline toxicity and the use of esmolol to reverse cardiovascular instability. *Ann Emerg Med.* 1990;19:671-673.

81. Sessler CN. Poor tolerance of oral activated charcoal with theophylline overdose. *Am J Emerg Med.* 1987;5:492-495.

82. Sessler CN, Cohen MD. Cardiac arrhythmias during theophylline toxicity. A prospective continuous electrocardiographic study. *Chest.* 1990;98:672-678.

83. Shalkham AS, et al. The availability and use of charcoal hemoperfusion in the treatment of poisoned patients. *Am J Kidney Dis.* 2006;48:239-241.

84. Shannon M. Life-threatening events after theophylline overdose: a 10-year prospective analysis. *Arch Intern Med.* 1999;159:989-994.

85. Shannon M. Predictors of major toxicity after theophylline overdose. *Ann Intern Med.* 1993;119:1161-1167.

86. Shannon M, et al. Multiple dose activated charcoal for theophylline poisoning in young infants. *Pediatrics.* 1987;80:368-370.

87. Shannon M, Maher T. Anticonvulsant effects of intracerebroventricular adenocard in theophylline-induced seizures. *Ann Emerg Med.* 1995;26:65-68.

88. Shannon M, et al. Exchange transfusion in the treatment of severe theophylline poisoning. *Pediatrics.* 1992;89:145-147.

89. Shannon M. Hypokalemia, hyperglycemia and plasma catecholamine activity after severe theophylline intoxication. *J Toxicol Clin Toxicol.* 1994;32:41-47.

90. Shively CA, et al. High levels of methylxanthines in chocolate do not alter theobromine disposition. *Clin Pharmacol Ther.* 1985;37:415-424.

91. Silverman K, et al. Withdrawal syndrome after the double-blind cessation of caffeine consumption. *N Engl J Med.* 1992;327:1109-1114.

92. Sykes AP, et al. Creatine kinase activity in patients with brittle asthma treated with long term subcutaneous terbutaline. *Thorax.* 1991;46:580-583.

93. Tisdell R, et al. Caffeine poisoning in an adult-survival with a serum concentration of 400 mg/L and need for adenosine agonist antidotes. *Vet Hum Toxicol.* 1986;28:492.

94. Titley OG, Williams N. Theophylline toxicity causing rhabdomyolysis and acute compartment syndrome. *Intensive Care Med.* 1992;18:129-130.

95. Tjia JF, et al. Theophylline metabolism in human liver microsomes: inhibition studies. *J Pharmacol Exp Ther.* 1996;276:912-917.

96. Udezue E, et al. Hypokalemia after normal doses of nebulized albuterol (salbutamol). *Am J Emerg Med.* 1995;13:168-171.

97. Warzak WJ, et al. Caffeine consumption in young children. *J Pediatr.* 2011;158:508-509.

98. Wasserman D, Amitai Y. Hypoglycemia following albuterol overdose in a child. *Am J Emerg Med.* 1992;10:556-557.

99. Whayne TF. Coffee: a selected overview of beneficial or harmful effects on the cardiovascular system? *Curr Vasc Pharmacol.* 2015;13:637-648.

100. Whitehurst VE, et al. Reversal of acute theophylline toxicity by calcium channel blockers in dogs and rats. *Toxicology.* 1996;110:113-121.

101. Wiley JF, et al. Unintentional albuterol ingestion in children. *Pediatr Emerg Care.* 1994;10:193-196.

102. Willett WC, et al. Coffee consumption and coronary heart disease in women. A ten-year follow-up. *JAMA.* 1996;275:458-462.

103. Wilson PWF, Bloom HL. Caffeine consumption and cardiovascular risks: little cause for concern. *J Am Heart Assoc.* 2016;5:e003089.

104. Woo OF, et al. Benefit of hemoperfusion in acute theophylline intoxication. *J Toxicol Clin Toxicol.* 1984;22:411-424.

105. Zhang L, et al. Ritodrine-induced agranulocytosis in pregnancy. *J Obstet Gynaecol.* 2014;34:533-534.

64

LOCAL ANESTHETICS

Matthew D. Sztajnkrycer

HISTORY AND EPIDEMIOLOGY

Local anesthetics block excitation of and transmission along a nerve axon in a predictable and reversible manner. In contrast to the nonselective effects of a general anesthetic, the anesthesia produced is selective to the chosen body part. Because local anesthetics do not require the circulation as an intermediate carrier and usually are not transported to distant organs, their actions are largely confined to the structures with which they come into direct contact. Local anesthetics are used to provide analgesia in various parts of the body by topical application, injection in the vicinity of peripheral nerve endings and major nerve trunks, or via instillation within the ophthalmic, epidural or subarachnoid spaces. The various local anesthetics differ with regard to their potency, duration of action, and degree of effects on sensory and motor nerve fibers. Toxicity is either local or systemic. With systemic toxicity, central nervous system (CNS) and cardiovascular effects are of greatest concern.

Until the 1880s, the only available analgesics were centrally acting depressants such as alcohol and opioids, which blunted the perception of pain rather than addressing the underlying cause. In 1860, the chemist Albert Niemann extracted the active alkaloid *cocaine* (Chap. 75) from the leaves of the coca shrub (*Erythroxylon coca*). Over the next 2 decades, the local anesthetic properties of the drug were identified. In 1884, Koller performed glaucoma surgery with only topical cocaine anesthesia.[54]

Although the clinical benefits of cocaine anesthesia were significant, so were its toxic and addictive potential. At least 13 deaths were reported in the first 7 years after the introduction of cocaine in Europe, and within 10 years after the introduction of cocaine as a regional anesthetic, reviews of "cocaine poisoning" appeared in the literature.[89,111] The toxicity of cocaine, coupled with the tremendous advantages it provided for surgery, led to a search for less toxic substitutes.

After the elucidation of the chemical structure of cocaine (the benzoic acid methyl ester of the alkaloid ecgonine) in 1895, other amino esters were examined. Synthetic compounds with local anesthetic activity were introduced but were highly toxic or irritating or had an impractically brief clinical effect. In 1904, Einhorn synthesized procaine, but its short duration of action limited its clinical utility. Research turned to focus on synthesis of local anesthetics with more prolonged durations of action.

The potent, long-acting local anesthetics dibucaine and tetracaine were synthesized in 1925 and 1928, respectively, and were introduced into clinical practice shortly thereafter. These anesthetics were not safe for regional anesthetic techniques because of potential systemic toxicity secondary to the combination of high potency, delayed metabolism, and the larger volumes of drug required for regional anesthesia compared with local anesthesia. On the other hand, these anesthetics were very useful for spinal anesthesia, which required much smaller volumes.

Lofgren synthesized lidocaine in 1943 from a series of aniline derivatives. This amino amide combined high tissue penetration and a moderate duration of action with acceptably low systemic toxicity. Additionally, unlike amino ester anesthetics, the metabolites of lidocaine did not include *para*-aminobenzoic acid (PABA), responsible for allergic reactions. Subsequent to the release of lidocaine in 1944, several other amino amide compounds were introduced into clinical practice including mepivacaine (1956), prilocaine (1959), bupivacaine (1963), etidocaine (1971), and ropivacaine (1996).

Considering the frequency of local anesthetic use, both within and outside health care facilities, clinically significant toxic reactions are relatively uncommon. In reports of fatalities resulting from toxic exposures reported to US poison control centers, local anesthetics are rarely implicated, representing fewer than 0.5% of cases (Chap. 130). Iatrogenic poisonings result from inadvertent injection of a therapeutic dose into a blood vessel, repeated use of a therapeutic dose, or unintentional administration of a toxic dose. The amide local anesthetics have largely replaced the esters in clinical use because of their increased stability and relative absence of hypersensitivity reactions (see Pharmacology later). Poisoning from topical benzocaine is relatively common because of the large number of nonprescription products available for treatment of teething and hemorrhoids. With nonprescription use, toxic effects after exposure are typically mild, and death rarely occurs. Toxicity usually occurs as a therapeutic misadventure, the potential for child abuse or neglect should be evaluated if the patient is younger than 2 years, and potential suicide should be evaluated in older children and adults.

Benzocaine spray is the most important cause of severe acquired methemoglobinemia in the hospital setting (Chap. 124).[33] Between November 1997 and March 2002, the US Food and Drug Administration (FDA) received 198 reported adverse events secondary to benzocaine products. A total of 132 cases (66.7%) involved definite or probable methemoglobinemia; most were serious adverse events, and 2 deaths occurred.[98] In these cases, a single spray of unspecified duration of 20% benzocaine was the dose most commonly reported. In 2003 and again in 2006, the FDA issued advisories regarding the use of benzocaine spray for topical mucosal anesthesia before intubation, upper endoscopy, and transesophageal echocardiography. In 2006, the US Veterans Health Administration halted the use of benzocaine spray for topical anesthesia. At this point in time, any continued use of topical benzocaine spray should be undertaken with extreme caution after careful assessment of risks, benefits, and alternatives, with antidotal therapy readily available.

PHARMACOLOGY

Local anesthetics fall into one of two chemically distinct groups: amino esters and amino amides (Fig. 64–1). The basic structure of all local anesthetics consists of three major components: a lipophilic, aromatic ring connected by an ester or amide linkage to a short alkyl intermediate chain that in turn is bound to a hydrophilic tertiary (or less commonly, secondary) amine. The amine group acts as a base, accepting protons and becoming charged at a higher pH. The proportion of charged molecules is dependent upon the pKa of the specific local anesthetic.

All local anesthetics function primarily by reversibly binding to specific receptor proteins within the membrane-bound sodium channels of conducting tissues. These receptors are reached only via the cytoplasmic (intracellular) side of the cell membrane. Blockade of ion conductance through the sodium channel eventually leads to failure to initiate and propagate action potentials (Fig. 64–2). The analgesic effect results from inhibiting axonal transmission of the nerve impulse in small-diameter myelinated Aδ ("fast pain") and unmyelinated C ("slow pain") nerve fibers carrying pain and temperature sensation. Conduction block of these fibers occurs at lower local anesthetic concentrations than required for the larger fibers responsible for touch, motor function, and proprioception.[30] This likely occurs in myelinated nerves because smaller fibers have closer spacing of the nodes of Ranvier. Given that a fixed number of nodes must be blocked for conduction failure to occur, the shorter critical length of nerve is reached sooner by

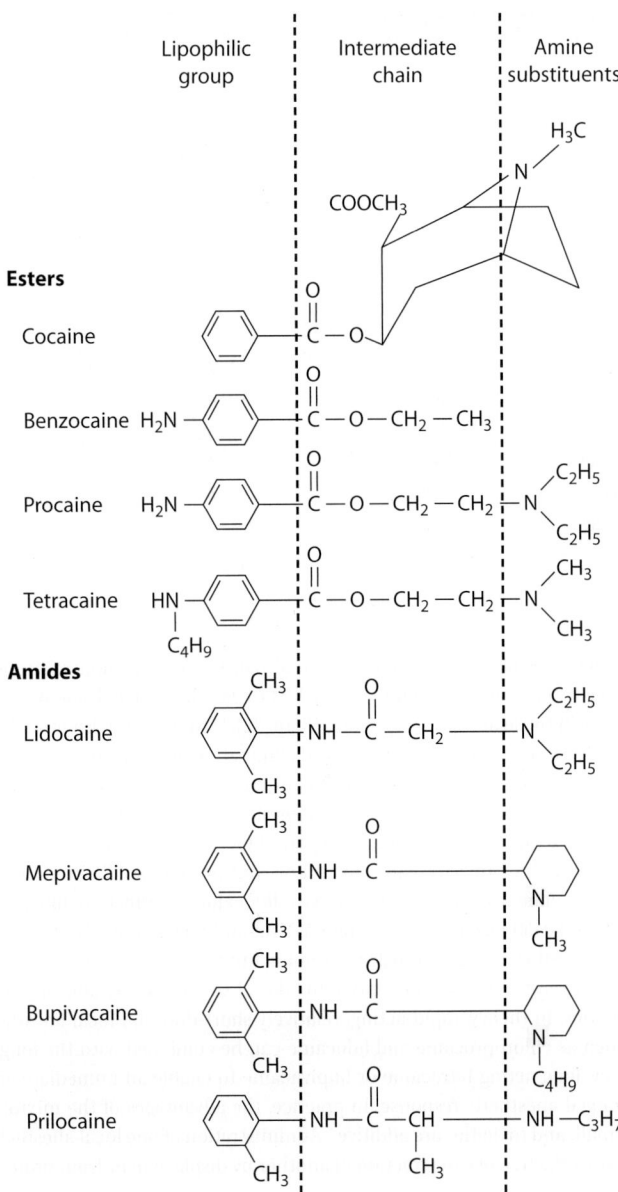

FIGURE 64–1. Representative local anesthetics.

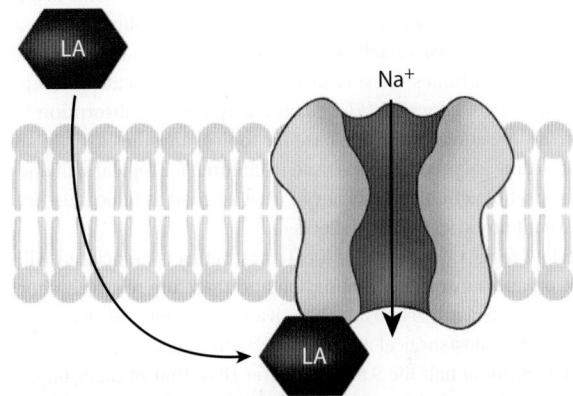

FIGURE 64–2. The multi-unit sodium channel is embedded in the nerve cell membrane. Local anesthetics (LAs) enter the nerve cell at the exposed membranes of the nodes of Ranvier and bind to the cytoplasmic side of the sodium channel (also located at the node of Ranvier) and alter sodium conductance.

the locally placed anesthetic in small fibers.[46] For unmyelinated fibers, the smaller diameter limits the distance that such fibers can passively propagate the electrical impulse. Differential nerve blockade is also related to voltage- and time-dependent affinity of local anesthetics to the sodium channels.

The sodium channel exists in three classes (Chap. 15 and Fig. 15–2). At resting membrane potential or in the hyperpolarized membrane, the channel is closed to sodium conductance. With an appropriate activating stimulus, the channel opens, allowing rapid sodium influx and membrane depolarization. Milliseconds later, the channel is inactivated, terminating the fast sodium current. Local anesthetic blockade is much stronger for channels that are activated (open) or inactivated than for channels that are resting. Analogous to the use-dependent kinetics of class I antidysrhythmics, pain fibers have a higher firing rate and longer action potential (ie, more time with the sodium channel open or inactivated) than other fiber types and therefore are more susceptible to local anesthetic action.[62]

These effects also occur in conductive tissues in the heart and brain that rely on sodium current. Although sodium channel blockade initially was believed to be the sole cause of systemic toxicity, mechanisms are more complex, especially in the heart, and occur at systemic concentrations lower than previously thought.[91] Recent proteomics analyses suggest that phosphatidyl-3-kinase (PI3K) plays a central role in pathways associated with bupivacaine-associated neurotoxicity.[145]

Growing evidence indicates that local anesthetics directly affect many other organ systems and functions such as the coagulation, immune, and respiratory systems, all at concentrations much lower than those required to achieve sodium channel blockade.[20,61,62] For example, lidocaine inhibited muscarinic signaling in *Xenopus* oocytes at less than 50% of the concentration required for sodium channel blockade.[62] Study of these less well-described effects may help elucidate both therapeutic and toxic phenomena that are incompletely explained.

The primary determinant of the onset of action of a local anesthetic is its pK$_a$, which affects its lipophilicity (Table 64–1). All local anesthetics are weak bases, with a pK$_a$ between 7.8 and 9.3. At physiologic pH (7.4), xenobiotics with a lower pK$_a$ have more uncharged molecules capable of crossing nerve cell membranes, producing a faster onset of action than xenobiotics with a higher pK$_a$. The onset of action also is influenced by the total dose of local anesthetic administered, which effects the concentration responsible for diffusion.

Local anesthetic potency is highly correlated with the lipid solubility of the xenobiotic. Therefore, the aromatic side of the anesthetic is the primary determinant of potency. The hydrophilic amine is important in occupying the sodium channel, which involves an ionic interaction with the charged form of the tertiary amine. The length of the intermediate chain is another determinant of local anesthetic activity, with three to seven carbon equivalents providing maximal activity.[30] Shorter or longer intermediate chain lengths are associated with rapid loss of local anesthetic action, suggesting that a critical length of physical separation between the aromatic group and the tertiary amine is required for sodium channel blockade to occur.

The degree of protein binding influences the duration of action of a local anesthetic. Anesthetics with greater protein binding remain associated with the neural membrane for a longer time interval and therefore have longer durations of action.[30] When high serum concentrations are achieved, a higher degree of protein binding increases the risk for cardiac toxicity.

PHARMACOKINETICS

A distinction must be made between local disposition (distribution and elimination) and systemic disposition of the anesthetic. Local distribution is influenced by several factors, including spread of local anesthetic by bulk flow, diffusion, transport via adjacent blood vessels, and binding to proximate tissues. Local elimination occurs through systemic absorption, transfer into the general circulation, and local hydrolysis of amino ester anesthetics. Systemic absorption decreases the amount of local anesthetic that is available for anesthetic effect, thereby limiting the duration of the block. Systemic absorption depends on the avidity of binding of local anesthetics to tissues

TABLE 64–1	Pharmacologic Properties of Local Anesthetics[48,100]					
	pK_a	Protein Binding (%)	Log D[a]	Relative Potency	Duration of Action	Approximate Maximum Allowable Subcutaneous Dose (mg/kg)
Esters						
Chloroprocaine	9.3	Unknown	1.17	Intermediate	Short	10
Cocaine	8.7	92	1.14	Low	Medium	3
Procaine	9.1	5	0.72	Low	Short	10
Tetracaine	8.4	76	2.23	High	Long	3
Amides						
Bupivacaine	8.1	95	2.45	High	Long	2
Etidocaine	7.9	95	3.16[b]	High	Long	4
Lidocaine	7.8	70	2.36	Low	Medium	4.5
Mepivacaine	7.9	75	0.93	Intermediate	Medium	4.5
Prilocaine	8.0	40	0.75	Intermediate	Medium	8
Ropivacaine	8.2	95	1.92	Intermediate	Long	2–3

[a]Log D is the octanol/water partition coefficient at a pH of 7. [b]Log D for etidocaine is at a pH of 7.4.

near the site of injection and on local perfusion. Both these factors vary with the site of injection. In general, areas with greater blood flow will have more rapid and complete systemic uptake of local anesthetic; for example, intravenous (IV) > tracheal > intercostal > paracervical > epidural > brachial plexus > sciatic > subcutaneous.

Because of their lipophilicity, local anesthetics readily cross cell membranes, the blood–brain barrier, and the placenta. After being absorbed, systemic tissue distribution is highly dependent on tissue perfusion. After local anesthetics enter the venous circulation, they pass through the lungs, where significant uptake occurs, thereby lowering peak arterial concentrations. Thus, the lungs serve as a buffer against systemic toxicity, but the capacity of the lungs to accumulate drug is saturable.[80] Part of the reason why most local anesthetic–induced seizures result from unintentional intravascular bolus injection rather than absorptive uptake is that lung uptake of these drugs exceeds 90%. The very high peak venous concentrations produced by rapid injection usually are necessary to produce toxic arterial concentrations.

All local anesthetics, except cocaine, cause peripheral vasodilation by direct relaxation of vascular smooth muscle. Vasodilation enhances vascular absorption of the local anesthetic. Addition of epinephrine (5 mcg/mL or 1:200,000) to the local anesthetic solution decreases the rate of vascular absorption, thereby improving the depth and prolonging the duration of local action, and mitigating risk of systemic toxicity. Local anesthetic mixed with epinephrine also decreases bleeding into the surgical field and serves as a marker for inadvertent intravascular injection (by producing tachycardia) when a test dose of the mixture is injected through a needle or catheter.[95] Significant drawbacks to epinephrine use include uncomfortable side effects such as palpitations and tremors, local tissue ischemia, and life-threatening systemic adverse reactions in susceptible patients (eg, myocardial ischemia and hypertensive crises). Inadvertent intravascular injection of local anesthetics mixed with epinephrine can be fatal, although generally the epinephrine in these mixtures is very dilute.[86]

The two classes of local anesthetics undergo metabolism by different routes (Chap. 75). The amino esters are rapidly metabolized by plasma cholinesterase to the major metabolite, PABA. The amino amides are metabolized more slowly in the liver to a variety of metabolites that do not include PABA.[29] Patients with enzymatic mutations or low or absent concentrations of plasma cholinesterase (pseudocholinesterase) are at increased risk for systemic toxicity from amino ester local anesthetics. Factors that decrease hepatic blood flow or impair hepatic function increase the risk for toxic reactions to the amino amides and make management of serious reactions more difficult. Patient age, as it relates to liver enzyme activity and plasma protein binding, influences the rate of metabolism of local

anesthetics. Whereas lidocaine's terminal half-life after IV administration averaged 80 minutes in volunteers aged 22 to 26 years, the half-life was 138 minutes in those aged 61 to 71 years (Chap. 32).[103] Newborns with immature hepatic enzyme systems have prolonged elimination of amino amides, which is associated with seizures when high continuous infusion rates are used.[1,92] Lidocaine elimination is reduced by congestive heart failure or coadministration of xenobiotics that reduce hepatic blood flow, thus explaining the increased risk of toxicity with cimetidine and propranolol.[117] Propranolol and cimetidine also potentially decrease lidocaine clearance by inhibiting hepatic CYP450 enzymes, including CYP1A2 and CYP3A4 involved in lidocaine N-deethylation and 3-hydroxylation in humans.[137]

Local anesthetics are often mixed to take advantage of desirable pharmacokinetics. In theory, rapid-acting, relatively short-duration local anesthetics such as chloroprocaine and lidocaine can be combined with the longer latency, long-acting tetracaine or bupivacaine to enable an immediate and prolonged anesthetic response. In practice, the advantages of the mixtures are small, and toxicities are additive.[6] Administration of one local anesthetic increases the free plasma fraction of another by displacement from protein-binding sites.[67]

Local anesthetics usually cannot penetrate intact skin in sufficient quantities to produce reliable anesthesia.[14] Efficient skin penetration requires the combination of a high water content and a high concentration of the water-insoluble base form of the local anesthetic. This combination of properties is achieved by mixing lidocaine and prilocaine in their base forms in a 1:1 ratio (eutectic mixture of local anesthetics {EMLA}).[18] Application for at least 45 minutes is required to achieve adequate dermal analgesia. Local anesthetic uptake continues for several hours during application. A liposomal formulation of 4% lidocaine (ELA-Max) facilitates skin absorption.[49] It is as effective as lidocaine–prilocaine base for topical anesthesia.[40,71] In addition, a 4% tetracaine gel preparation is used in children for topical skin anesthesia with an onset of action and efficacy at least as good as lidocaine–prilocaine base without any systemic side effects

The low molecular weight of local anesthetics is associated with rapid absorption and subsequent elimination and therefore relatively short duration of action. Recently, a liposomal bupivacaine formulation was introduced as a long acting postsurgical anesthetic.[22,85] After local infiltration, the product has a terminal half-life 9.8-fold greater than that of plain bupivacaine. Significantly elevated plasma bupivacaine concentrations were observed for 96 hours after local infiltration of the liposomal formulation but do not correlate with local efficacy.[3,64] Current manufacturer recommendations warn against use of all local anesthetics within 96 hours of liposomal bupivacaine administration because local infiltration has the potential to precipitate an immediate release of local anesthetic from the liposomal formulation, with subsequent systemic toxicity.

CLINICAL MANIFESTATIONS OF TOXICITY

Although the most common adverse reactions to local anesthetics are vasopressor syncopal events associated with injection, the following sections focus on their local and systemic toxicity.[134]

Toxic Reactions

Regional Side Effects and Tissue Toxicity

At a sufficient concentration, all local anesthetics are directly cytotoxic to nerve cells. However, in clinically relevant doses, they rarely produce localized nerve damage.[73,102] Significant direct neurotoxicity results from intrathecal injection or infusion of local anesthetics for spinal anesthesia. In this setting, lidocaine has an increased risk for both persistent lumbosacral neuropathy and a syndrome of painful but self-limited postanesthesia buttock and leg pain or dysesthesia referred to as *transient neurologic symptoms*.[66] Nerve damage often is attributed to the use of excessively concentrated solutions or inappropriate formulations. Several reports of cauda equina syndrome are associated with use of hyperbaric 5% lidocaine solutions for spinal anesthesia. Hyperbaric solutions are denser than cerebrospinal fluid. This neurotoxicity appears to be a phenomenon that occurs when the anesthetic is injected through narrow-bore needles or through continuous spinal catheters. This process results in very high local concentrations of the anesthetic that might pool around the sacral roots because of inadequate mixing.[118] The mechanism of this neurotoxicity is unknown but is believed to be independent of sodium channel blockade.[66] Because an equally effective block can be achieved with injection of larger volumes of lower concentration, 5% lidocaine is generally avoided and bupivacaine used instead. There is a significant (up to 10-fold) increase in the development of new neurologic dysfunction after receiving a neuraxial block in patients with preexisting peripheral neuropathy, a fact emphasizing the importance of informed consent and risk communication.[57]

Similar severe neurotoxic reactions occur after massive subarachnoid injection of chloroprocaine during attempted epidural anesthesia.[115] The neurotoxicity initially was attributed to use of the antioxidant sodium bisulfite and the low pH of the commercial solution rather than use of the anesthetic itself.[136] Despite reformulation without bisulfite, subsequent animal data suggest that chloroprocaine itself is responsible for the neurotoxicity.[131] Skeletal muscle changes are observed after intramuscular injection of local anesthetics, especially the more potent, longer acting local anesthetics. The effect is reversible, and muscle regeneration is complete within 2 weeks after injection of local anesthetics.[10]

Although rare, after peripheral nerve or plexus block, transient or prolonged postoperative neuropathy is well recognized. Likely mechanisms include direct injury of the nerve related to intraneuronal injection and local anesthetic neurotoxicity. The frequency of peripheral neuropathies reported after peripheral nerve blockade varies from 0% to more than 5%.[15] Direct visualization of peripheral nerves via ultrasonography reduces this complication, avoiding traumatic injury and allowing for injection of less local anesthetic to produce adequate nerve block.[80,126] In one study, intraneural injection occurred in 17% of supraclavicular or interscalene blocks, but ultrasonographic identification prevented further injection.[8] Analysis of 12,668 ultrasound-guided nerve blocks for peripheral regional anesthesia found that the incidences of postoperative neurologic symptoms lasting longer than 5 days and 6 months were 0.18% and 0.008%, respectively.[126] Visualization of the target site via ultrasound guidance also decreases local anesthetic systemic toxicity, likely because of reduced incidence of inadvertent vascular puncture.[8]

Systemic Side Effects and Toxicity

Allergic Reactions

Allergic reactions to local anesthetics are extremely rare. Fewer than 1% of all adverse drug reactions caused by local anesthetics are immunoglobulin (Ig) E mediated.[49] In one study designed to determine the prevalence of true local anesthetic allergy in patients referred to an allergy clinic for suspected hypersensitivity, skin prick and intradermal testing results were negative for all 236 participants tested.[11] As noted, the amino esters are responsible for the majority of true allergic reactions. When hydrolyzed, the amino ester local anesthetics produce PABA, a known allergen (Chap. 46). Cross-sensitivity to other amino ester anesthetics is common. Some multidose commercial preparations of amino amides contain the preservative methylparabens (Chap. 46), chemically related to PABA, and most likely the cause of the much rarer allergic reactions attributed to amino amides. Preservative-free amino amides, including lidocaine, are appropriate for use in patients who have reactions to drug preparations containing methylparabens unless the patient is specifically sensitive to lidocaine. If the patient with a history of allergic reaction to a particular anesthetic requires a local anesthetic, a paraben preservative-free drug from the opposite class can be chosen because there is no cross-reactivity between the amides and esters.

Methemoglobinemia

Methemoglobinemia is a frequent adverse effect of topical and oropharyngeal benzocaine and is occasionally reported with lidocaine, tetracaine, or prilocaine use. Most reports of methemoglobinemia associated with local anesthetics are the result of an excessive dose or a break in the normal mucosal barrier for topical anesthetics (Chap. 124).

Benzocaine is initially metabolized to aniline and then further metabolized to phenylhydroxylamine and nitrobenzene, which are both potent oxidizing agents (Chap. 124). Although reports describe methemoglobinemia resulting from standard doses of benzocaine topical oropharyngeal spray given for laryngoscopy or gastrointestinal upper endoscopy, affected patients commonly have abnormal mucosal integrity as occurs with thrush or mucositis.[38,98] Prilocaine is an amino ester local anesthetic primarily used in obstetric anesthesia because of its rapid onset of action and low systemic toxicity in both the mother and fetus. Use of large doses of prilocaine lead to the development of methemoglobinemia.[59,82] An aniline derivative, prilocaine undergoes hepatic metabolism to produce *ortho*-toluidine, another oxidizing agent.[59] A direct relationship exists between the amount of epidural prilocaine administered and the incidence of methemoglobinemia. A dose greater than approximately 8 mg/kg is generally necessary to produce effects and symptoms, which are often not apparent until several hours after epidural administration of the drug. Lidocaine–prilocaine cream, often used in the outpatient setting for minor dermal procedures, is associated with significant methemoglobinemia, more commonly in children than in adults.[53] Standard doses of lidocaine–prilocaine cream used for circumcision in term neonates are associated with minimal production of methemoglobin, but risks may be increased in neonates with metabolic disorders.[129] The diagnosis of methemoglobinemia is suggested by cyanosis unresponsive to oxygen in individuals with normal cardiopulmonary examinations and known oxidant exposure and presence of chocolate brown blood. It is confirmed by direct measurement of methemoglobin with a cooximeter. When clinically indicated, we recommend treating affected patients with symptomatic methemoglobinemia with IV methylene blue (Chap. 124 and Antidotes in Depth: A43).

Local Anesthetic Systemic Toxicity

Systemic toxicity for all local anesthetics correlates with serum concentrations. Factors that determine the concentration include dose; rate of administration; site of injection (absorption occurs more rapidly and completely from vascular areas, such as with neck and intercostal blocks); the presence or absence of a vasoconstrictor; and the degree of tissue–protein binding, fat solubility, and pK_a of the local anesthetic.[97] The brain and heart are the primary target organs for systemic toxicity because of their rich perfusion, moderate tissue–blood partition coefficients, lack of diffusion limitations, and presence of cells that rely on voltage-gated sodium channels to produce an action potential.

Recommendations for maximal local anesthetic doses designed to minimize the risk for systemic toxic reactions were developed but remain controversial.[127] These maximal recommended doses aim to prevent

TABLE 64–2	Toxic Intravenous (IV) Doses of Local Anesthetics
Local Anesthetic	Minimum IV Toxic Dose of Local Anesthetic in Humans (mg/kg)
Bupivacaine	1.6
Chloroprocaine	22.8
Etidocaine	3.4
Lidocaine	6.4
Mepivacaine	9.8
Procaine	19.2
Tetracaine	2.5

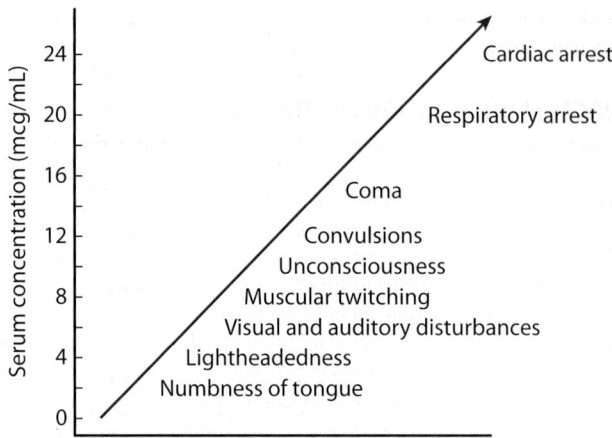

FIGURE 64–3. Relationship of signs and symptoms of toxicity to serum lidocaine concentrations.

infiltration of excessive drug. However, because most episodes of systemic toxicity from local anesthetics, with the exception of methemoglobinemia from topical drug, occur secondary to unintentional intravascular injection rather than from overdosage, limiting the maximal dose will not prevent most toxic systemic reactions.[123]

Toxicity is also related to the metabolism of a given local anesthetic. The rapidity of elimination from the plasma influences the total dose delivered to the CNS or heart. The amino esters are rapidly hydrolyzed in the plasma and eliminated, explaining their relatively low potential for systemic toxicity. The amino amides have a much greater potential for producing systemic toxicity because termination of the therapeutic effect of these drugs is achieved through redistribution and slower metabolic inactivation.[45] Another factor that creates difficulty in specifying the minimal toxic plasma concentration of lidocaine results from the fact that its N-dealkylated metabolites are pharmacologically active and monoethylglycylxylide has a prolonged half life (Chap. 57 and Fig. 57-3). Although these factors make it difficult to establish safe doses of local anesthetics, Table 64–2 summarizes the estimates of minimal toxic IV doses of various local anesthetics.

Central Nervous System Toxicity

Systemic toxicity in humans usually presents initially with CNS abnormalities. Intravenous infusion studies in volunteers demonstrate an inverse relationship between anesthetic potency and dose required to induce signs of CNS toxicity.[125] A similar relationship exists between the convulsive concentration and the relative anesthetic potency. In humans, seizures are reported at serum concentrations of approximately 2 to 4 mcg/mL for bupivacaine and etidocaine. Concentrations in excess of 10 mcg/mL are usually required for production of seizures when less potent drugs such as lidocaine are administered. Despite the strong relationship between local anesthetic potency and CNS toxicity, several other factors influence the CNS effects, including the rate of injection, drug interactions, and acid–base status.[32]

The rapidity with which a particular serum concentration is achieved influences anesthetic toxicity. Volunteers tolerated an average dose of 236 mg of etidocaine and a serum concentration of 3 mcg/mL before onset of CNS effects and symptoms when the anesthetic was infused at a rate of 10 mg/min. However, when the infusion rate was increased to 20 mg/min, the same individuals only tolerated an average of 161 mg which produced a serum concentration of approximately 2 mcg/mL.[124]

Both metabolic and respiratory acidoses increase local anesthetic induced CNS toxicity. Acidemia decreases plasma protein binding, increasing the amount of free drug available for CNS diffusion despite promoting the charged form of the amine group. The convulsive threshold of various local anesthetics is inversely related to arterial PCO_2.[34,41,42] Hypercarbia lowers the seizure threshold by several mechanisms: (1) increased cerebral blood flow, which increases drug delivery to the CNS; (2) increased conversion of the drug base to the active cation in the presence of decreased intracellular pH; and (3) decreased plasma protein binding, which increases the amount of free drug available for diffusion into the brain.[19,34,41,42] In general, CNS depressants

minimize the signs and symptoms of CNS excitation and increase the threshold for local anesthetic–induced seizures. Flumazenil increases the sensitivity of the CNS to the amino amide anesthetics.[17]

A gradually increasing serum lidocaine concentration usually produces a stereotypical pattern of signs and symptoms (Fig. 64-3). In an awake patient, the initial effects include tinnitus, lightheadedness, circumoral numbness, disorientation, confusion, auditory and visual disturbances, and lethargy. Subjective side effects occur at serum concentrations between 3 and 6 mcg/mL. Significant psychological effects of local anesthetics are also reported. Near-death experiences and delusions of actual death are described as specific symptoms of local anesthetic toxicity.[87] Thus, the appearance of psychological symptoms during administration of local anesthetics should not be disregarded as unrelated nervous reactions or effects of sedatives given as premedication but rather as a possible early sign of CNS toxicity.

Clinical signs, usually excitatory, then develop, and include shivering, tremors, and ultimately generalized tonic–clonic seizures.[106] Objective CNS toxicity usually is evident at lidocaine concentrations between 5 and 9 mcg/mL. Seizures typically occur at concentrations above 10 mcg/mL, with higher concentrations producing coma, apnea, and cardiovascular collapse. The excitatory phase has a wide range of intensity and duration, depending on the chemical properties of the local anesthetic. With the highly lipophilic, highly protein-bound local anesthetics, the excitement phase is brief and mild. Toxicity from large IV boluses of bupivacaine often present without CNS excitement, with bradycardia, cyanosis, and coma as the first signs.[120] Rapid intravascular injection of lidocaine produces a brief excitatory phase followed by generalized CNS depression with respiratory arrest. Seizures are reported after even small doses injected into the vertebral or carotid artery (as rarely occurs during stellate ganglion block).[72] A relative overdose produces a slower onset of effects (usually within 5–15 minutes of drug injection), with irritability progressing to seizures.

The mechanism of the initial CNS excitation involves selective sodium channel blockade of cerebral cortical inhibitory pathways in the amygdala.[130,135] The resulting increase in unopposed excitatory activity leads to seizures. As the concentration increases further, both inhibitory and excitatory neurons are blocked, and generalized CNS depression ensues. Levobupivacaine causes increased neuronal excitation and neurotoxicity by inhibition of KCNQ2/3 channels, an effect reversed by the channel activator retigabine.[25]

Cardiovascular Toxicity

Cardiovascular side effects are the most feared manifestations of local anesthetic toxicity. Shock and cardiovascular collapse are related to effects on vascular tone, inotropy, and dysrhythmias related to indirect CNS and direct cardiac and vascular effects of the local anesthetic. Animal studies and clinical observations clearly demonstrate that for most local anesthetics, CNS toxicity develops at significantly lower serum concentrations than those needed to produce cardiac toxicity. With the exception of bupivacaine, local anesthetics have a high cardiovascular: CNS toxicity ratio.[72,100,101,120]

Some of the discrepancy between the incidence of CNS and cardiac toxicity result from a detection bias. Not only can the treating physicians fail to recognize cardiac effects because of preoccupation with CNS manifestations of toxicity, but early cardiac toxicity is often quite subtle. An experimental study attempting to identify early warning signs of bupivacaine-induced cardiac toxicity in pigs evaluated bupivacaine induced changes in cardiac output, heart rate, blood pressure, and electrocardiogram (ECG).[108] A 40% reduction in cardiac output was not associated with significant change in heart rate or blood pressure, the latter secondary to a direct vasoconstrictive effect of bupivacaine at the concentrations produced.[23] If cardiac toxicity develops, management is exceedingly difficult.

Changes in systemic vascular tone induced by local anesthetics are mediated by direct effect on vascular smooth muscle or indirectly via effects on spinal cord sympathetic outflow. Predictably, sympathetic blockade after spinal anesthesia or epidural anesthesia above the T5 dermatome results in peripheral venodilation and arterial dilation. Shock results when high doses of anesthetic are used in hypovolemic patients. Local anesthetics have a biphasic effect on peripheral vascular smooth muscle. Whereas lower doses produce direct vasoconstriction, higher doses are associated with severe cardiovascular toxicity and cause vasodilation, contributing to cardiovascular collapse.

All local anesthetics directly produce a dose dependent decrease in cardiac contractility, with the effects roughly proportional to their peripheral anesthetic effect. Although the classic anesthetic action of sodium channel blockade in heart muscle accounts in large part for the negative inotropy by affecting excitation–contraction coupling, it does not explain the entire difference in myocardial depression produced by different anesthetics.[36] Poorly understood effects on calcium handling or effects of the intracellular drug directly on contractile proteins or mitochondrial function underlie these effects.[36,43] Bupivacaine impairs regulation of glucose homeostasis through inhibition of protein kinase B (Akt) and activation of 5′-adenosine monophosphate activated protein kinase (AMPK) activities: interacts with peripheral δ- and κ-opioid receptors; and inhibits myosin phosphatase target subunit I (MYPTI), protein kinase C (PKC), and phosphorylation-dependent inhibitory protein of myosin phosphatase (CPI-17).[27,109]

Blockade of the fast sodium channels of cardiac myocytes decreases maximum upstroke velocity (V_{max}) of the action potential (Chaps. 15 and 16 and Fig. 15–2). This effect slows impulse conduction in the sinoatrial and atrioventricular (AV) nodes, the His-Purkinje system, and atrial and ventricular muscle.[28] These changes are reflected on ECG by increases in PR interval and QRS complex duration. At progressively higher anesthetic concentrations, hypotension, sinus arrest with junctional rhythm, and eventually cardiac arrest occur.[5] Asystole is described in patients who received unintentional IV bolus injections of 800 to 1,000 mg of lidocaine.[5,44] Cardiovascular toxicity of local anesthetics usually occurs after a sudden increase in serum concentration, as in unintentional intravascular injection. Cardiovascular toxicity is rare in other circumstances because high serum concentrations are necessary to produce this effect and because CNS toxicity precedes cardiovascular events, providing a warning. Cardiac toxicity usually is not observed with lidocaine use in humans until the serum lidocaine concentration greatly exceeds 10 mcg/mL unless the patient is also receiving xenobiotics that depress sinus and AV nodal conduction such as calcium channel blockers, β-adrenergic antagonists, or cardioactive steroids. Intravascular lidocaine injection used to diminish pain associated with IV propofol injection was associated with episodes of bradycardia (heart rate <30 beats/min) and sinus arrest in a 69-year-old man later diagnosed with sick sinus syndrome.[69]

Animal studies compared the dose or serum concentrations of local anesthetics required to produce irreversible circulatory collapse with those necessary to produce seizures.[33,100,101] The cardiovascular collapse:CNS toxicity (CC:CNS) ratio for lidocaine is approximately 7; therefore, CNS toxicity should become evident well before potentially cardiotoxic concentrations are reached. In contrast, bupivacaine is significantly more cardiotoxic than most other local anesthetics commonly used, with a CC:CNS ratio of 3:7.

Inadvertent intravascular injection produces near simultaneous signs of CNS and cardiovascular toxicity. Bupivacaine produces myocardial depression out of proportion to its anesthetic potency and, more importantly, causes refractory ventricular dysrhythmias.[122] The enhanced cardiovascular toxicity of bupivacaine relates to enhanced CNS effects at cardiovascular centers, direct effects on myocyte metabolism, and important differences related to sodium channel blockade.[132] Although lidocaine and bupivacaine both block sodium channels in the open or inactivated states, lidocaine quickly dissociates from the channel at diastolic potentials, allowing rapid recovery from block during diastole (known as fast on–fast off kinetics). Therefore, sodium channel blockade with lidocaine is much more pronounced at rapid heart rates (accounting for the antidysrhythmic effects for ventricular tachycardia).[86] In contrast, at high concentrations, bupivacaine rapidly binds to and slowly dissociates from sodium channels (fast on–slow off kinetics), with significant block accumulating at all physiologic heart rates.[28] Accordingly, at heart rates of 60 to 150 beats/min, approximately 70 times more lidocaine is needed than bupivacaine to produce an equal effect on V_{max} of the action potential. Enhanced conduction block in Purkinje fibers and ventricular muscle cells sets up a reentrant circuit responsible for the ventricular tachydysrhythmias induced by bupivacaine.[93]

Bupivacaine is problematic both in terms of having the highest potential for cardiovascular toxicity and for the refractoriness of its toxicity to conventional therapy. Bupivacaine has an asymmetrically substituted carbon, and the kinetics of sodium channel binding are stereospecific.[75] The S (levo)-enantiomer levobupivacaine is significantly less cardiotoxic than the R (dextro)-enantiomer despite having similar anesthetic properties.[7,91] Consequently, bupivacaine, the racemic mixture of both enantiomers, is more cardiotoxic than levobupivacaine, which contains only the levo-enantiomer.[52] The stereospecific effect on sodium channels seems to differ between the heart and the peripheral nerves because the local anesthetic potency of levobupivacaine is the same as, or perhaps even greater than, that of bupivacaine.[39,104] Ropivacaine is a pure enantiomer and is less cardiotoxic than bupivacaine, but it is also slightly less potent as an anesthetic.[112,113]

Effects other than sodium channel blockade contribute to cardiotoxicity. Lipophilic local anesthetics such as bupivacaine directly impair mitochondrial energy transduction via two mechanisms: (1) uncoupling of oxygen consumption and adenosine triphosphate (ATP) synthesis and (2) inhibition of complex I in the respiratory chain.[122] These effects are related to the lipophilic properties of the drug rather than to stereospecific effects on ion channels. Lidocaine has no effect on mitochondrial respiration, and ropivacaine has less effect than bupivacaine.[142] There is no difference between the two bupivacaine enantiomers. These effects occur with higher concentrations of the local anesthetic, as occur after unintentional intravascular injection.

Low-dose bupivacaine-induced cardiotoxic effects are described in humans under certain circumstances and at concentrations that are not associated with seizures in pigs.[68,140] Severe cardiac toxicity is described after injection of a small subcutaneous dose of bupivacaine in a patient with secondary carnitine deficiency.[140] Myocytes are highly dependent on oxidation of free fatty acids for energy. Interference with this mechanism via bupivacaine-induced inhibition of carnitine–acylcarnitine translocase contributes to the cardiotoxicity of lipophilic local anesthetics (Chap. 48, Fig. 48–3, and Antidotes in Depth: A10).[141] Bupivacaine produce dysrhythmias by blocking GABAergic neurons that tonically inhibit the autonomic nervous system.[59] In addition to its other effects on the heart, bupivacaine induces a marked decrease in cardiac contractility by altering Ca^{2+} release from sarcoplasmic reticulum.[84]

In a large series of patients receiving bupivacaine, systemic toxicity occurred in only 15 of 11,080 nerve blocks.[96] Of these patients, 80% manifested seizures; the other 20% had milder symptoms. Bupivacaine use, particularly at 0.75% concentration, is associated with severe cardiovascular depression, ventricular dysrhythmias, and even death.[116] Pregnant women were disproportionately affected. Some of these patients required prolonged resuscitation, and restoration of adequate spontaneous circulation proved exceedingly difficult.[116] In 1983, 49 incidents of cardiac arrest or ventricular tachycardia occurring over a 10-year period were presented to the

TABLE 64–3	Types of Local Anesthetic Reactions
Cause	**Major Clinical Features**
Local anesthetic toxicity (intravascular injection)	Immediate seizure or dysrhythmias
Reaction to adjuvant catecholamine	Tachycardia, hypertension, headache
Vasodepressor syncope	Bradycardia, hypotension, pallor rapid onset and recovery, loss of conscientiousness
Allergic reaction	Anaphylaxis
High spinal or epidural block	Bradycardia, hypotension, respiratory distress, respiratory arrest

FDA Anesthetic and Life Support Advisory Committee. Among these cases, 0.75% bupivacaine was used in 27 obstetric patients with 10 deaths, and 0.5% bupivacaine was used in 8 obstetric patients with 6 deaths. Among the 14 nonobstetric patients, 5 died. The overall mortality rate was 43% (21 of 49). Partly as a result of these reports, in 1984, the FDA withdrew approval of bupivacaine 0.75% for use as obstetric anesthesia.[116]

Acid–base and electrolyte status influence the cardiac toxicity of a given drug because all depressant properties are potentiated by acidosis, hypoxia, or hypercarbia.[16] Table 64–3 outlines the spectrum of acute local anesthetic reactions.

DIAGNOSTIC TESTING

In cases of possible local anesthetic toxicity, the patient should be attached to continuous cardiac monitoring, and an ECG should be obtained to detect dysrhythmias and conduction disturbances. Serum electrolytes, blood urea nitrogen, creatinine, and blood gas analysis should be obtained to help assess the cause of cardiac dysrhythmias. Cooximetry should be obtained in patients in whom methemoglobinemia is suspected clinically. Rapid, sensitive assays are available for measuring concentrations of lidocaine and its monoethylglycinexylidide (MEGX) metabolite. When properly interpreted, the results of these assays are used to prevent lidocaine toxicity and to identify lidocaine toxicity in the nontherapeutic setting (Chap. 57, Fig. 57-3). Assays for determining serum concentrations of other local anesthetics are not routinely available. Treatment should never be delayed while waiting for results of xenobiotic concentration determinations.

TREATMENT

If toxicity results from ingestion of liquid medications, it is reasonable to give oral activated charcoal within 1 to 2 hours of ingestion, provided airway protective reflexes are intact. Contaminated mucous membranes should be washed off. Neither hemodialysis nor hemoperfusion has proven utility.

Treatment of Local Anesthetic Central Nervous System Toxicity

At the first sign of possible CNS toxicity, administration of the drug must be discontinued. One hundred percent oxygen should be supplied immediately, and ventilation should be supported if necessary. Patients with minor symptoms usually do not require treatment, provided adequate respiratory and cardiovascular functions are maintained. The patient must be followed closely so that progression to more severe effects can be detected.

Although most seizures caused by local anesthetics are self-limited, they should be treated quickly because the hypoxia and acidemia produced by prolonged seizures increase both CNS and cardiovascular toxicity.[99,101] Intubation is not mandatory, and the decision to intubate must be individualized. Maintaining adequate ventilation is of proven value. Modest hyperventilation extracorporeal life support (ECLS) is reasonable to produce respiratory alkalemia. By decreasing CNS extraction of drug, lowering extracellular potassium, and hyperpolarizing the neuronal cell membrane, normalizing (lowering) PCO_2 decreases the affinity for, or accelerates separation of, the local anesthetic from the sodium channel. Ultra-short-acting

barbiturates and benzodiazepines are recommended for treatment of local anesthetic–induced seizures, but either of these medication groups can also exacerbate circulatory and respiratory depression.[32,94] Propofol 1 mg/kg IV was as effective as thiopental 2 mg/kg IV in stopping bupivacaine induced seizures in rats and was used successfully in a patient with uncontrolled muscle twitching secondary to local anesthetic toxicity.[13,55] However, propofol causes significant bradydysrhythmias and even asystole, especially when used with other xenobiotics that cause bradycardia. Based on currently available data, benzodiazepines are recommended as the first-line treatment for local anesthetic CNS toxicity. Neuromuscular blockers are proposed as adjunctive treatment for local anesthetic–induced seizures. They block muscular activity, decreasing oxygen demand and lactic acid production. However, neuromuscular blockers should never be used to treat seizures per se because they have no anticonvulsant effect and can make clinical diagnosis of ongoing seizures problematic by abolishing muscle contractions. To avoid this potentially lethal complication, chemical paralysis should be used only to facilitate endotracheal intubation if needed, unless continuous electroencephalography is also used. If used, short-acting neuromuscular blockers are desirable, facilitating subsequent repeated neurologic assessments. Succinylcholine is not routinely recommended because of significant side effects, including hyperkalemia and dysrhythmias. Given less potential for adverse cardiac effects, nondepolarizing neuromuscular blockers such as rocuronium are preferentially recommended (Chap. 66).

When severe systemic toxicity occurs, the cardiovascular system must be monitored closely because cardiovascular depression often goes unnoticed while seizures are being treated. Because local anesthetic–induced myocardial depression occurs even with preserved blood pressure, it is important to be aware of early signs of cardiac toxicity, including ECG changes.

Treatment of Local Anesthetic Cardiovascular Toxicity

Treatment of cardiovascular toxicity is complicated by the complex effects of local anesthetics on the heart. Initial therapy should focus on correcting the physiologic derangements that potentiate the cardiac toxicity of local anesthetics, including hypoxemia, acidemia, and hyperkalemia.[16,119] Prompt support of ventilation and circulation limits hypoxia and acidemia. Early recognition of potential cardiac toxicity is critical to achieving a good outcome because patients with cardiac toxicity that goes unrecognized for any interval are more difficult to resuscitate.[9] If a potentially massive intravascular local anesthetic injection is suspected, maximizing oxygenation of the patient before cardiovascular collapse occurs is critical.

Standard Advanced Cardiac Life Support (ACLS) protocols should be followed when dealing with most local anesthetic cardiac toxicity. Bupivacaine-induced dysrhythmias often are refractory to cardioversion, defibrillation, and pharmacologic treatment. Lidocaine, phenytoin, magnesium, bretylium, amiodarone, calcium channel blockers, and combined therapy with clonidine and dobutamine were all used in animal models with variable results.[37,88,90] Lidocaine competes with bupivacaine for cardiac sodium channels and at high doses may displace it. Anecdotal reports suggest that lidocaine has occasionally helped in this application.[31] However, concern exists about additive CNS effects when lidocaine is used to treat bupivacaine cardiac toxicity, and its use in this manner cannot be routinely recommended.

With toxicity from the longer acting, highly lipid-soluble, protein-bound amide local anesthetics (bupivacaine and etidocaine), if the patient does not respond promptly to therapy, cardiopulmonary resuscitation is expected to be difficult and prolonged (1–2 hours) before depression of the cardiac conduction system spontaneously reverses as a result of redistribution and metabolism of the drugs.[2,114] Vital organ perfusion is seriously compromised during CPR despite optimal chest compression. The significance of this problem increases with the duration of resuscitation; therefore, rapid initiation of is recommended when practical. Cardiopulmonary bypass resulted in successful outcomes in some cases of lidocaine and bupivacaine overdose.[47,81] Cardiopulmonary bypass provides circulatory support that is far superior to that provided by closed-chest cardiac massage. The improved perfusion prevents tissue hypoxia and the development of metabolic acidosis, which in turn decreases the binding of local anesthetics to myocardial sodium channel receptors. Hepatic blood flow is better maintained, enhancing local anesthetic metabolism, and increased myocardial blood flow helps redistribute local anesthetics out of the myocardium.[81] Increasingly, ECLS using venoarterial extracorporeal membrane oxygenation (VA-ECMO) is being used in the management of critically ill overdose patients in both the emergency department and intensive care unit environments.[35]

Atropine supplemented with electrical pacing is reasonable to treat bradycardia. Cardiac pacing was used successfully for treatment of cardiac arrest after unintentional administration of a 2-g bolus of lidocaine into a cardiopulmonary bypass circuit as the patient was being removed from bypass.[107] Pharmacologic therapy was unsuccessful, and resumption of bypass was necessary. Forty-five minutes after the injection, AV pacing restored perfusion and permitted discontinuation of bypass.

Use of sodium bicarbonate early in resuscitation to prevent acidemia-mediated potentiation of cardiac toxicity is reasonable.[31] Although a canine model of bupivacaine-induced cardiotoxicity demonstrated utility of high dose insulin compared with saline or dextrose, its use cannot be routinely recommended at this time (Antidotes in Depth: A21).[26]

Intravenous Lipid Emulsion

While investigating the relationship between lipid metabolism and bupivacaine toxicity, a rat study of bupivacaine induced asystolic arrest showed that pretreatment with IV lipid emulsion (ILE) increased the toxic dose of bupivacaine by 50%.[143] In addition, a dose of bupivacaine that was uniformly fatal in control rats resulted in universal survival in animals that also received fat emulsion.[143] Subsequent studies of local anesthetic toxicity demonstrated accelerated return of cardiac function and systemic vascular resistance after ILE both in isolated hearts and in intact animals.[21,58,139,140]

Numerous case reports describe successful use of ILE (in various formulations) to treat patients (including pregnant and pediatric patients) in cardiac arrest after regional anesthesia with various local anesthetics, including bupivacaine, ropivacaine, and levobupivacaine (Antidotes in Depth: A23).[12,60]

The most recent guidelines by the American Society of Regional Anesthesia and Pain Medicine (ASRA) suggest dosing for a patient in cardiac arrest is a 1.5-mL/kg bolus of 20% ILE over 1 minute while continuing chest compressions followed by continuous infusion of 0.25 mL/kg/min.[105] For persistent cardiovascular collapse, it is reasonable to repeat the bolus once or twice and double the infusion rate. If there is evidence of recovery, it is reasonable to continue the infusion for at least 10 minutes after stability. After initiating standard ACLS protocols, including ensuring adequate oxygenation and ventilation, we recommend that ILE be given as soon as possible after signs of significant local anesthetic toxicity become manifest (Antidotes in Depth: A23).[143] Initiation of VA-ECMO in association with ILE use is associated with fat deposition in the VA-ECMO circuit and increased blood clot formation within the circuit.[74] However, given that ILE administration can be accomplished more readily than initiation of VA-ECMO, it is reasonable to administer ILE to the severely intoxicated patient even if the patient eventually is transitioned to VA-ECMO.

Prevention of Systemic Toxicity of Local Anesthetics

Despite the development of new, relatively less toxic amino amide local anesthetics such as levobupivacaine and ropivacaine, severe CNS and cardiovascular effects remain a risk. Several cases of ropivacaine-induced cardiac arrest are reported.[24,70] In these cases, patients with both asystolic arrest and ventricular fibrillation–associated arrest were successfully resuscitated. Nonetheless, it is clear that prevention is more prudent and effective than treatment of toxicity. The keys to prevention are to use the lowest possible anesthetic concentration and volume consistent with effective anesthesia and to avoid a significant intravascular injection. The latter is accomplished by ensuring extravascular placement demonstrated repetitively by ultrasonographic guidance and by careful, slow aspiration of a needle or catheter before injection; injection of a small test dose of anesthetic mixed with epinephrine to assess a cardiovascular response if injection is intravascular; and use of slow, fractional dosing of large-volume injections with vigilance for early signs of CNS and cardiac toxicity.

SUMMARY

- Local anesthetics are frequently used xenobiotics that provide surgical analgesia and acute and chronic pain relief.
- The analgesic effect of local anesthetics is primarily caused by inhibition of neural conductance secondary to sodium channel blockade.
- Systemic toxicity, which primarily affects the heart and brain, is also largely related to sodium channel blockade.
- Severe systemic toxicity usually occurs secondary to inadvertent intravascular injection.
- If cardiovascular collapse and cardiac arrest occur, especially in the setting of bupivacaine toxicity, resuscitation is difficult and prolonged. In addition to standard ACLS protocols emphasizing maintenance of oxygenation and ventilation, ILE is recommended.
- Cardiopulmonary bypass is useful because it provides cardiovascular support, limits exacerbating factors such as tissue hypoxia and acidemia, and improves hepatic blood flow, thereby increasing local anesthetic metabolism, but it is difficult to initiate in a timely manner. Although increasingly available, extracorporeal life support will be limited by the use of ILE, which has been noted to clog the VA-ECMO circuit.

Acknowledgment

Brian Kaufman, MD; Staffan Wahlander, MD; and David R. Schwartz, MD, contributed to this chapter in previous editions.

REFERENCES

1. Agarwal R, et al. Seizures occurring in pediatric patients receiving continuous infusion of bupivacaine. *Anesth Analg.* 1992;75:284-286.
2. Albright G. Cardiac arrest following regional anesthesia with etidocaine or bupivacaine. *Anesthesiology.* 1979;51:285-287.
3. Anonymous. Exparel bupivacaine liposome injectable suspension. Prescribing information. San Diego, CA: Pacira Pharmaceuticals, Inc; 2015.
4. Ash-Bernal R, et al. Acquired methemoglobinemia—a retrospective series of 138 cases at 2 teaching hospitals. *Medicine.* 2004;83:265-273.
5. Babui E, et al. Inadvertent massive lidocaine overdose causing temporary complete heart block in myocardial infarction. *Am Heart J.* 1981;102:801-803.
6. Badgwell J. Cardiovascular and central nervous system effects of co-administered lidocaine and bupivacaine in piglets. *Reg Anesth.* 1991;16:89-94.
7. Bardsley H, et al. A comparison of the cardiovascular effects of levobupivacaine and rac-bupivacaine following intravenous administration to healthy volunteers. *Br J Clin Pharmacol.* 1998;46:245-249.
8. Barrington MJ, Kluger R. Ultrasound guidance reduces the risk of local anesthetic systemic toxicity following peripheral nerve blockade. *Reg Anesth Pain Med.* 2013;38:289-299.
9. Batra MS, et al. Bupivacaine cardiotoxicity in a pregnant patient with mitral valve prolapse: an example of an improperly administered epidural block. *Anesthesiology.* 1984;60:170-171.
10. Benoit P, Belt WD. Some effects of local anesthetic agents on skeletal muscle. *Exp Neurol.* 1972;34:264–278.
11. Berkun Y, et al. Evaluation of adverse reactions to local anesthetics: experience with 236 patients. *Ann Allergy Asthma Immunol.* 2003;91:342-345.
12. Bern S, Weinberg G. Local anesthetic toxicity and lipid resuscitation in pregnancy. *Curr Opin Anaesthesiol.* 2011;24:262-267.
13. Bishop D, Johnstone R. Lidocaine toxicity treated with low-dose propofol. *Anesthesiology.* 1993;78:788-789.
14. Bonadio W. TAC: a review. *Pediatr Emerg Care.* 1989;5:128-130.
15. Borgeat A, et al. Acute and nonacute complications associated with interscalene block and shoulder surgery: a prospective study. *Anesthesiology.* 2001; 85:875-880.
16. Bosnjak Z, et al. Comparison of lidocaine and bupivacaine depression of sinoatrial node activity during hypoxia and acidosis in adult and neonatal guinea pigs. *Anesth Analg.* 1986;65:911-917.
17. Bruguerolle B, Emperaire N. Local anesthetic-induced toxicity may be modified by low-dose flumazenil. *Life Sci.* 1992;50:185-187.
18. Buckley MM, Benfield P. Eutectic lidocaine/prilocaine cream: a review of the topical anaesthetic/analgesic efficacy of a eutectic mixture of local anaesthetics (EMLA). *Drugs.* 1993;46:126-151.
19. Burney R, et al. Effects of pH on protein binding of lidocaine. *Anesth Analg.* 1978;57:478–480.

20. Butterworth JF, Strichartz G. Molecular mechanisms of local anesthesia: a review. *Anesthesiology*. 1990;72:711-734.

21. Candela D, et al. Reversal of bupivacaine-induced cardiac electrophysiologic changes by two lipid emulsions in anesthetized and mechanically ventilated piglets. *Anesth Analg*. 2010;110:1473-1479.

22. Chahar P, Cummings KC III. Liposomal bupivacaine: a review of a new bupivacaine formulation. *J Pain Res*. 2012;5:257-264.

23. Chang KS, et al. Bupivacaine inhibits baroreflex control of heart rate in conscious rats. *Anesthesiology*. 2000;92:197-207.

24. Chazalon P, et al. Ropivacaine-induced cardiac arrest after peripheral nerve block: successful resuscitation. *Anesthesiology*. 2003;99:1253-1254.

25. Cheng Y, et al. Effectiveness of retigabine against levobupivacaine-induced central nervous system toxicity: a prospective, randomized animal study. *J Anesth*. 2016;30:109-115.

26. Cho H, et al. Insulin reverses bupivacaine-induced cardiac depression in dogs. *Anesth Analg*. 2000;91:1096-1102.

27. Cho H, et al. Lipid emulsion inhibits vasodilation induced by a toxic dose of bupivacaine by suppressing bupivacaine-induced PKC and CPI-17 dephosphorylation but has no effect on vasodilation induced by a toxic dose of mepivacaine. *Korean J Pain*. 2016;29:229-238.

28. Clarkson C, Hondeghem LM. Mechanism for bupivacaine depression of cardiac conduction: fast block of sodium channels during the action potential with slow recovery from block during diastole. *Anesthesiology*. 1985;62:396-405.

29. Covino BG. New developments in the field of local anesthetics and the scientific basis for their clinical use. *Acta Anaesth Scand*. 1982;26:242-249.

30. Covino BG. Pharmacology of local anesthetic agents. *Br J Anaesth*. 1986;58:701-716.

31. Davis N, de Jong R. Successful resuscitation following massive bupivacaine overdose. *Anesth Analg*. 1982;61:62-64.

32. de Jong R, Heavner J. Local anesthetic seizure prevention: diazepam versus pentobarbital. *Anesthesiology*. 1972;36:449-457.

33. de Jong R, et al. Cardiovascular effects of convulsant and supraconvulsant doses of amide local anesthetics. *Anesth Analg*. 1982;61:3-9.

34. de Jong R, et al. Effect of carbon dioxide on the cortical seizure threshold to lidocaine. *Exp Neurol*. 1967;17:221-232.

35. de Lange DW, et al. Extracorporeal membrane oxygenation in the treatment of poisoned patients. *Clin Toxicol*. 2013;51:385-393.

36. de la Coussaye J, et al. Experimental evidence in favor of role of intracellular actions of bupivacaine in myocardial depression. *Anesth Analg*. 1992;74:698-702.

37. de la Coussaye J, et al. Reversal of electrophysiologic and hemodynamic effects induced by high-dose of bupivacaine by the combination of clonidine and dobutamine in anesthetized dogs. *Anesth Analg*. 1992;74:703-711.

38. Dinneen S, et al. Methemoglobinemia from topically applied anesthetic spray. *Mayo Clin Proc*. 1994;69:886-888.

39. Dyhre H, et al. The duration of action of bupivacaine, levobupivacaine, ropivacaine, and pethidine in peripheral nerve block in the rat. *Acta Anaesthesiol Scand*. 1997;41:1345-1352.

40. Eichenfeld LA. Clinical study to evaluate the efficacy of ELA-Max (4% liposomal lidocaine) as compared with eutectic mixture of local anesthetics cream for pain reduction of venipuncture in children. *Pediatrics*. 2002;109:1093-1099.

41. Englesson S. The influence of acid-base changes on central nervous system toxicity of local anesthetic agents. I. An experimental study in cats. *Acta Anaesthesiol Scand*. 1974;18:79-87.

42. Englesson S. The influence of acid-base changes on central nervous system toxicity of local anesthetic agents: II. *Acta Anaesthesiol Scand*. 1974;18:88-103.

43. Fettiplace MR, et al. Insulin signaling in bupivacaine-induced cardiac toxicity: sensitization during recovery and potentiation by limited emulsion. *Anesthesiology*. 2016;124:428-442.

44. Finkelstein F, Kreeft J. Massive lidocaine poisoning. *N Engl J Med*. 1979;301:50.

45. Foldes FF, et al. The intravenous toxicity of local anesthetic agents in man. *Clin Pharm Ther*. 1965;6:328-335.

46. Franz D, Perry R. Mechanisms for differential block among single myelinated and nonmyelinated axons by procaine. *J Physiol*. 1974;236:193-210.

47. Freedman M, et al. Extracorporeal pump assistance—novel treatment for acute lidocaine poisoning. *Eur J Clin Pharmacol*. 1982;22:129-135.

48. Fujita Y. Amrinone reverses bupivacaine-induced regional myocardial dysfunction. *Acta Anaesthesiol Scand*. 1996;40:47-52.

49. Giovannitti JA, Bennett CR. Assessment of allergy to local anesthetics. *J Am Dent Assoc*. 1979;98:701-706.

50. Goldman RD. ELA-max: a new topical lidocaine formulation. *Ann Pharmacother*. 2004;38:892-894.

51. Gosselin S, et al. Evidence-based recommendations on the use of intravenous lipid emulsion therapy in poisoning. *Clin Toxicol*. 2016;54:899-923.

52. Graf BM, et al. Stereospecific effect of bupivacaine isomers on atrioventricular conduction in the isolated perfused guinea pig heart. *Anesthesiology*. 1997;86:410-419.

53. Hahn I, et al. EMLA-induced methemoglobinemia (metHb) and systemic topical anesthetic toxicity. *J Emerg Med*. 2004;26:85-88.

54. Halsted WS. Practical comments on the use and abuse of cocaine suggested by its invariably successful employment in more than a thousand minor surgical operations. *N Y Med J*. 1885;42:294.

55. Heavner J, et al. Comparison of propofol with thiopentone for treatment of bupivacaine-induced seizures in rats. *Br J Anaesth*. 1993;71:715-719.

56. Heavner JE. Cardiac dysrhythmias induced by infusion of local anesthetics into the lateral ventricle of cats. *Anesth Analg*. 1986;65:133-138.

57. Hebl JR, et al. Neurologic complications after neuraxial anesthesia or analgesia in patients with preexisting peripheral sensorimotor neuropathy or diabetic polyneuropathy. *Anesth Analg*. 2006;103:1294-1299.

58. Heinonen JA, et al. The effects of intravenous lipid emulsion on hemodynamic recovery and myocardial cell mitochondrial function after bupivacaine toxicity in anesthetized pigs. *Human Exp Toxicol*. 2016;1:1-11.

59. Hjelm M, Holmdahl M. Biochemical effects of aromatic amines II. Cyanosis methemoglobinemia and Heinz-body formation induced by a local anaesthetic agent (prilocaine). *Acta Anaesthesiol Scand*. 1965;2:99-120.

60. Hoegberg LCG, et al. Systematic review of the effect of intravenous lipid emulsion therapy for local anesthetic toxicity. *Clin Toxicol*. 2016;54:167-193.

61. Hollmann MW, Durieux ME. Local anesthetics and the inflammatory response: a new therapeutic indication? *Anesthesiology*. 2000;93:858-875.

62. Hollmann MW, et al. Local anesthetic inhibition of m1 muscarinic acetylcholine signaling. *Anesthesiology*. 2000;93:497-509.

63. Hondeghem L, Miller R. *Local Anesthetics, Basic and Clinical Pharmacology*. 4th ed. Stamford, CT: Appleton and Lange; 1989:315-322.

64. Hu D, et al. Pharmacokinetic profile of liposome Bupivacaine injection following a single administration at the surgical site. *Clin Drug Invest*. 2013;33:109-115.

65. Jin Z, et al. Epinephrine administration in lipid-based resuscitation in a rat model of bupivacaine-induced cardiac arrest. Optimal timing. *Reg Anesth Pain Med*. 2015;40:222-231.

66. Johnson M. Potential neurotoxicity of spinal anesthesia with lidocaine. *Mayo Clin Proc*. 2000;75:921-932.

67. Jorfeldt L, et al. Lung uptake of lidocaine in man as influenced by anaesthesia, mepivacaine infusion or lung insufficiency. *Acta Anaesth Scand*. 1983;27:5-9.

68. Kasten G, Martin S. Successful cardiovascular resuscitation after massive intravenous bupivacaine overdosage in anesthetized dogs. *Anesth Analg*. 1985;64:491-497.

69. Kim KO, et al. Profound bradycardia with lidocaine during anesthesia induction in a silent sick sinus syndrome patient. *J Clin Anesth*. 2011;23:227-230.

70. Klein S, et al. Successful resuscitation after ropivacaine-induced ventricular fibrillation. *Anesth Analg*. 2004;97:901-903.

71. Koh JL, et al. A randomized, double-blind comparison study of EMLA and ELA-Max for topical anesthesia in children undergoing intravenous insertion. *Paediatr Anaesth*. 2004;14:977-982.

72. Kozody R, et al. Dose requirements of local anesthetic to produce grand mal seizure during stellate ganglion block. *Can Anaesth Soc J*. 1982;29:489-491.

73. Lambert L, et al. Irreversible conduction block in isolated nerve by high concentrations of local anesthetics. *Anesthesiology*. 1994;80:1082-1093.

74. Lee HMD, et al. What are the adverse effects associated with the combined use of intravenous lipid emulsion and extracorporeal membrane oxygenation in the poisoned patient? *Clin Toxicol*. 2015;53:145-150.

75. Lee-Son S, et al. Stereoselective inhibition of neuronal sodium channels by local anesthetics: evidence for two sites of action? *Anesthesiology*. 1992;77:324-335.

76. Li B, et al. Association of sustained cardiac recovery with epinephrine in the delayed lipid-based resuscitation from cardiac arrest induced by bupivacaine overdose in rats. *Br J Anaesth*. 2012;108:857-863.

77. Lindgren L, et al. The effect of amrinone on recovery from severe bupivacaine intoxication in pigs. *Anesthesiology*. 1992;77:309-315.

78. Liu F, et al. Epinephrine reversed high-concentration bupivacaine-induced inhibition of calcium channels and transient outward potassium current channels, but not on sodium channel in ventricular myocytes of rats. *BMC Anesth*. 2015;15:66.

79. Liu SS, et al. Incidence of unintentional intraneural injection and postoperative neurological complications with ultrasound-guided interscalene and supraclavicular nerve blocks. *Anesthesia*. 2011;66:168-174.

80. Lofstrom JB. Physiologic disposition of local anesthetics. *Reg Anesth*. 1982;7:33-38.

81. Long W, et al. Successful resuscitation of bupivacaine-induced cardiac arrest using cardiopulmonary bypass. *Anesth Analg*. 1989;69:403-406.

82. Lund P, Cwik J. Propitocaine (Citanest) and methemoglobinemia. *Anesthesiology*. 1965;26:569-571.

83. Luo M, et al. Giving priority to lipid administration can reduce lung injury caused by epinephrine in bupivacaine-induced cardiac depression. *Reg Anesth Pain Med*. 2016;41:469-476.

84. Lynch C III. Depression of myocardial contractility in vitro by bupivacaine, etidocaine, and lidocaine. *Anesth Analg*. 1986;65:551-559.

85. Ma P, et al. Local anesthetic effects of bupivacaine loaded lipid-polymer hybrid nanoparticles: in vitro and in vivo evaluation. *Biomed Pharmacother*. 2017;89:689-695.

86. Mallampati SR, et al. Convulsions and ventricular tachycardia from bupivacaine with epinephrine: successful resuscitation. *Anesth Analg*. 1984;63:856-859.

87. Marsch SCU, et al. Unusual psychological manifestation of systemic local anesthetic toxicity. *Anesthesiology*. 1998;88:531-533.

88. Matsuda F, et al. Nicardipine reduces the cardio-respiratory toxicity of intravenously administered bupivacaine in rats. *Can J Anaesth*. 1990;37:920-923.

89. Mattison JB. Cocaine poisoning. *Med Surg Rep*. 1891;60:645-650.

90. Maxwell L, et al. Bupivacaine-induced cardiac toxicity in neonates: successful treatment with intravenous phenytoin. *Anesthesiology*. 1994;80:682-686.

91. Mazoit JX, et al. Comparative ventricular electrophysiologic effect of racemic bupivacaine, levobupivacaine, and ropivacaine on the isolated rabbit heart. *Anesthesiology*. 2000;92:784-792.

92. McCloskey J, et al. Bupivacaine toxicity secondary to continuous caudal epidural infusion in children. *Anesth Analg*. 1992;75:287-290.

93. Moller R, Covino B. Cardiac electrophysiologic effects of lidocaine and bupivacaine. *Anesth Analg*. 1988;67:107-114.

94. Moore D, et al. Convulsive arterial plasma levels of bupivacaine and the response to diazepam therapy. *Anesthesiology*. 1979;50:454-456.

95. Moore DC, Batra M. The components of an effective test dose prior to epidural block. *Anesthesiology*. 1981;55:693-696.

96. Moore DC, et al. Bupivacaine: a review of 11,080 cases. *Anesth Analg*. 1978;57:42-53.

97. Moore DC, et al. Factors determining dosages of amide-type local anesthetic drugs. *Anesthesiology*. 1977;47:263-268.

98. Moore T, et al. Reported adverse event cases of methemoglobinemia associated with benzocaine products. *Arch Intern Med*. 2004;164:1192-1196.

99. Morishima H, Corvino B. Toxicity and distribution of lidocaine in nonasphyxiated and asphyxiated baboon fetuses. *Anesthesiology*. 1981;54:182-186.

100. Morishima H, et al. Bupivacaine toxicity in pregnant and nonpregnant ewes. *Anesthesiology*. 1985;63:134-139.

101. Morishima H, et al. Toxicity of lidocaine in adult, newborn, and fetal sheep. *Anesthesiology*. 1981;55:57-61.

102. Myers RR, et al. Neurotoxicity of local anesthetics: altered perineural permeability, edema, and nerve fiber injury. *Anesthesiology*. 1986;64:29-35.

103. Nation R, et al. Lignocaine kinetics in cardiac and aged subjects. *Br J Clin Pharmacol*. 1977;4:439-445.

104. Nau C, et al. Stereoselectivity of bupivacaine in local anesthetic-sensitive ion channels of peripheral nerve. *Anesthesiology*. 1999;91:786-795.

105. Neal JM, et al. American Society of Regional Anesthesia and Pain Medicine checklist for managing local anesthetic systemic toxicity: 2012 version. *Reg Anesthes Pain Med*. 2012;37:16-18.

106. Nicholas E, Thornton MD. Lidocaine toxicity during attempted epistaxis cautery. *J Emerg Med*. 2016;51:303-304.

107. Noble J, et al. Massive lignocaine overdose during cardiopulmonary bypass: successful treatment with cardiac pacing. *Br J Anaesth*. 1984;56:1439-1441.

108. Nystrom EUM, et al. Blood pressure is maintained despite profound myocardial depression during acute bupivacaine overdose in pigs. *Anesth Analg*. 1999;88:1143-1148.

109. Ok S-H, et al. Lipid emulsion inhibits vasodilation induced by a toxic dose of bupivacaine via attenuated dephosphorylation of myosin phosphatase of myosin phosphatase target subunit I in isolated rat aorta. *Int J Med Sci*. 2015;12:958-967.

110. Ozcan M, Weinberg G. Intravenous lipid emulsion for the treatment of drug toxicity. *J Intensive Care Med*. 2014;29:59-70.

111. Peterson RC. History of cocaine. *NIDA Res Monogr*. 1977;13:17-34.

112. Pitkanen M, et al. Chronotropic and inotropic effects of ropivacaine, bupivacaine, and lidocaine in the spontaneously beating and electrically paced isolated perfused rabbit heart. *Reg Anesth Pain Med*. 1992;17:183-192.

113. Polley LS, et al. Relative analgesic potencies of ropivacaine and bupivacaine for epidural analgesia in labor: implications for therapeutic indexes. *Anesthesiology*. 1999;90:944-950.

114. Prentiss J. Cardiac arrest following caudal anesthesia. *Anesthesiology*. 1979;50:51-53.

115. Reisner LS, et al. Persistent neurologic deficit and adhesive arachnoiditis following intrathecal 2-chloroprocaine injection. *Anesth Analg*. 1980;59:452-454.

116. Reiz S, Nath S. Cardiotoxicity of local anesthetic agents. *Br J Anaesth*. 1986;58:736-746.

117. Reynolds F. Adverse effects of local anaesthetics. *Br J Anaesth*. 1987;59:78-95.

118. Rigler M, et al. Cauda equina syndrome after continuous spinal anesthesia. *Anesth Analg*. 1991;72:275-281.

119. Rosen M, et al. Bupivacaine-induced cardiotoxicity in hypoxic and acidotic sheep. *Anesth Analg*. 1985;64:1089-1096.

120. Rosenberg PH, et al. Acute bupivacaine toxicity as a result of venous leakage under the tourniquet cuff during a bier block. *Anesthesiology*. 1983;58:95-98.

121. Rosenberg PH, et al. Maximum recommended doses of local anesthetics: a multifactorial concept. *Reg Anesth Pain Med*. 2004;29:564-575.

122. Rosenblatt MA, et al. Successful use of a 20% lipid emulsion to resuscitate a patient after a presumed bupivacaine-related cardiac arrest. *Anesthesiology*. 2006;105:217-218.

123. Scott DB. "Maximal recommended doses" of local anaesthetic drugs. *Br J Anaesth*. 1989;63:373-374.

124. Scott DB. Evaluation of the toxicity of local anaesthetic agents in man. *Br J Anaesth*. 1975;47:56-61.

125. Scott DB.: Toxicity caused by local anaesthetic drugs. *Br J Anaesth*. 1981;53:553-554.

126. Sites BD, et al. Incidence of local anesthetic systemic toxicity and postoperative neurologic symptoms associated with 12,668 ultrasound-guided nerve blocks: an analysis from a prospective clinical registry. *Reg Anesth Pain Med*. 2012; 37:478482.

127. Strichartz GR, Berde CB. Local anesthetics. In: Miller RD, ed. *Anesthesia*. 4th ed. New York, NY: Churchill Livingstone; 1994:489-521.

128. Sztark F, et al. Comparison of the effects of bupivacaine and ropivacaine on heart cell mitochondrial bioenergetics. *Anesthesiology*. 1998;88:1340-1349.

129. Taddio A, et al. Efficacy and safety of lidocaine prilocaine cream for pain during circumcision. *N Engl J Med*. 1997;336:1197-1201.

130. Tanaka K, Yamasaki M. Blocking of cortical inhibitory synapses by intravenous lidocaine. *Nature*. 1966;209:207-208.

131. Taniguchi M, et al. Sodium bisulfite: scapegoat for chloroprocaine neurotoxicity? *Anesthesiology*. 2004;100:85-91.

132. Thomas R, et al. Cardiovascular toxicity of local anesthetics: an alternative hypothesis. *Anesth Analg*. 1986;65:444-450.

133. Tong YCI, et al. Liposomal bupivacaine and clinical outcomes. *Best Practice Res Clin Anaesth*. 2014;28:15-27.

134. Verrill PJ. Adverse reactions to local anesthetics and vasoconstrictor drugs. *Practitioner*. 1975;214:380-387.

135. Wagman IH, et al. Effects of lidocaine on the central nervous system. *Anesthesiology*. 1967;28:155-172.

136. Wang BC, et al. Chronic neurologic deficits and Nesacaine: an effect of the anesthetic 2-chloroprocaine or the antioxidant sodium bisulfite? *Anesth Analg*. 1984;63:445-447.

137. Wang JS, et al. Involvement of CYP1A2 and CYP3A4 in lidocaine N-deethylation and 3-hydroxylation in humans. *Drug Metab Dispos*. 2000;28:959-965.

138. Weinberg G, et al. Lipid emulsion infusion rescues dogs from bupivacaine-induced cardiac toxicity. *Reg Anesth Pain Med*. 2003;28:198-202.

139. Weinberg G, et al. Lipid infusion accelerates removal of bupivacaine and recovery from bupivacaine toxicity in the isolated rat heart. *Reg Anesth Pain Med*. 2006;31:296-303.

140. Weinberg GL, et al. Resuscitation with lipid versus epinephrine in a rat model of bupivacaine overdose. *Anesthesiology*. 2008;108:907-913.

141. Weinberg GL, et al. Bupivacaine inhibits acylcarnitine exchange in cardiac mitochondria. *Anesthesiology*. 2000;92:523-528.

142. Weinberg GL, et al. Pretreatment or resuscitation with a lipid infusion shifts the dose-response to bupivacaine-induced asystole in rats. *Anesthesiology*. 1998:88:1071-1075.

143. Weinberg GL. Lipid infusion therapy. Translation to clinical practice. *Anesth Analg*. 2008;106:1340-1342.

144. Weinberg GL. Lipid rescue—caveats and recommendations for the "Silver Bullet" [letter]. *Reg Anesth Pain Med*. 2004;29:74-75.

145. Zhao W, et al. iTRAQ proteomics analysis reveals that PI3K is highly associated with bupivacaine-induced neurotoxicity pathways. *Proteomics*. 2016;16:564-575.

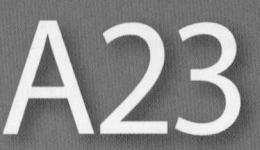
LIPID EMULSION

Sophie Gosselin and Theodore C. Bania

INTRODUCTION

The use of intravenous lipid emulsion (ILE) as an antidote is best studied for the treatment of local anesthetic systemic toxicity. However, it is also used for the treatment of overdose from other lipophilic xenobiotics such as calcium channel blockers, cyclic antidepressants, insecticides, and β-adrenergic antagonists, among many others.

HISTORY

Lipid emulsion was used as one component of parenteral nutrition for more than 40 years and is also used as a diluent for intravenous (IV) drug delivery of highly lipophilic xenobiotics such as amphotericin and propofol. More recently, liposomal suspensions containing local anesthetics such as bupivacaine were formulated that slowly release xenobiotics to increase their duration of anesthetic effect.

Bupivacaine toxicity is uncommon and sometimes refractory to Advanced Cardiac Life Support measures (Chap. 64). In the setting of local anesthetic–induced cardiovascular collapse, fatalities occur. Previously, cardiopulmonary bypass was essentially the only effective treatment for these patients.[4] Intravenous lipid emulsion (ILE) was initially evaluated in animal models of bupivacaine toxicity with some reported efficacy. Because of the success in animal models and the limitations of other therapies, ILE was attempted in humans with local anaesthetic toxicity. Multiple reports are published that suggest benefit.[34,41] Intravenous lipid emulsion was subsequently recommended by several anesthesia and medical toxicology specialty societies for the treatment of local anesthetic toxicity, especially bupivacaine.[56] The most commonly proposed mechanism of action is the entrapment of local anesthetic in the serum lipid phase thus, likely decreasing the amount of xenobiotic at the site of toxicity.

In 2008, the first case of nonlocal anaesthetic toxicity treated with ILE was published. After this report, ILE was evaluated in animal models of toxicity from a multitude of lipid-soluble xenobiotics. Based on these studies, ILE was used in many cases of human and animal clinical poisoning.[41]

PHARMACOLOGY

Chemistry and Preparation

Lipid emulsion is composed of two types of lipids, triglycerides and phospholipids. Triglycerides are hydrophobic molecules that are formed when three fatty acids are linked to one glycerol. The fatty acid chain lengths vary, producing different triglycerides. The primary triglycerides in lipid emulsions are linoleic, linolenic, oleic, palmitic, and stearic acids; their concentrations vary slightly in the different commercially available formulations. These long-chain triglycerides (12 or more carbons) are extracted from safflower oil or soybean oil (or both), depending on the brand.[25] Newer lipid emulsions containing long-chain triglycerides in addition to medium-chain triglycerides (6–12 carbons) are derived from coconut, olive, and fish oils, and their availability and cost vary.[51]

Phospholipids contain two fatty acids bound to glycerol and a phosphoric acid moiety that is located at the third hydroxyl group. Phospholipids are amphipathic; the nonpolar fatty acids are hydrophobic, and the polar phosphate head is hydrophilic. This imparts important pharmacologic properties to this carrier molecule, allowing it to solubilize nonpolar xenobiotics in aqueous serum.

The lipids are dispersed in the serum by forming an emulsion of small lipid droplets, in which the phospholipids form a layer around a triglyceride core. The hydrophobic fatty acid component of the phospholipid molecule is directed toward the triglycerides while the hydrophilic glycerol component is directed outward away from the triglyceride core. The presence of small amounts of glycerol, which is hydrophilic, allows the lipid droplets to be suspended as an emulsion in water and serum.

The lipid emulsion per se is a white, milky liquid. It is sterile and nonpyrogenic with an average pH of 8 (range, 6–9). Lipid emulsions are isoosmotic solutions (260–310 mOsm/L) made for parenteral use and thus are easily delivered through a peripheral or central vein[49] and intraosseously.[16]

Lipid emulsions have different globule sizes depending on their uses.[13] Microemulsions containing droplet sizes less than 0.1 μm are used for drug delivery. Miniemulsions containing droplet sizes greater than 0.1 μm but less than 1.0 μm are used for parenteral nutrition and are the ones used off label in clinical toxicology. Droplet sizes in commercially available nutritional lipid emulsions range from 0.4 to 0.5 μm. Phospholipid emulsifiers such as egg phosphatide are added and prevent droplet coalescence. After IV administration, lipid emulsions are found in the serum as lipid droplets that resemble chylomicrons and turn the serum turbid or milky.[10] Macroemulsions containing droplet sizes greater than 1.0 μm are used for chemoembolization. These macroemulsions contain chemotherapeutics that are delivered intraarterially directly into the tumor blood supply. The lipid droplets occlude the artery and slowly release the chemotherapeutic.

Related Lipid Formulations

Most case reports that support the treatment of local anesthetic toxicity with ILE use branded Intralipid or standard long-chain triglyceride mixtures. Other lipid emulsions, that contain mixtures of long-chain and medium-chain triglycerides, are also reportedly successful in clinical cases of poisoning.[29,81] However, formulations containing oleic acid are theoretically problematic at high doses because IV sodium oleate is used in animal models to induce acute respiratory distress syndrome (ARDS) and ingestion of sodium oleate was reported to produce severe respiratory distress.[58,68]

Controversy exists as to whether or not lipid emulsions containing both long- and medium-chain triglyceride mixtures are more effective at partitioning xenobiotics than are long-chain triglycerides.[43] In one rodent model of bupivacaine toxicity, although the rate of return to spontaneous circulation was identical in both groups, asystole recurred 15 to 45 minutes after ILE administration, and serum and cardiac bupivacaine concentrations were lower in the group treated with the long-chain mixtures.[43] In human serum, a mixture of long- and medium-chain triglycerides increased the extraction of bupivacaine, ropivacaine, and mepivacaine compared with long-chain triglyceride mixtures alone.[66] However, in a rodent model of bupivacaine toxicity, long- and medium-chain mixtures were equally effective in reversing bupivacaine toxicity, but the long-chain mixture resulted in fewer recurrences of asystole and lower myocardial bupivacaine concentrations.[44]

Mechanism of Action

The mechanisms of action of parenteral lipid emulsion in toxicology are not clearly understood. The three proposed mechanisms of action of ILE are modulation of intracellular metabolism; a lipid sink, sponge, or conduit mechanism; and activation of ion channels.

Modulation of Intracellular Metabolism

In experimental models of poisoning from xenobiotics that alter intracellular energy metabolism, toxicity was successfully treated with ILE, suggesting that repairing or circumventing this dysfunction is involved. Bupivacaine blocks carnitine-dependent mitochondrial lipid transport and inhibits adenosine triphosphatase (ATPase) synthetase in the electron transport chain.[9,85] Verapamil inhibits intracellular processing of fatty acids,[38,39] but it also inhibits insulin release and produces insulin resistance.[39] This reduces the consumption of free fatty acid during shock, perhaps caused by the high oxygen demand required of fatty acid oxidation.[26] The cyclic antidepressant amitriptyline depresses human myocardial contraction independent of an effect on conduction[29] and inhibits medium- and short-chain fatty acid metabolism.[81] Propranolol changes intracellular energy from primarily fatty acid to carbohydrate-dependent metabolism.[46]

Theoretically, the addition of excess fatty acids overcomes blocked or inhibited enzymes by mass action, providing energy to an energy "starved" heart, reversing toxicity. Some support for this mechanism comes from the ability of ILE to reverse myocardial depression resulting from myocardial ischemia.[76] In a canine model using 10 minutes of regional myocardial ischemia, treatment with ILE after ischemia resulted in improved systolic wall contraction. In the same canine model, pretreatment with oxfenicine, which blocks carnitine palmitoyltransferase-1, blocked the beneficial effect of lipid emulsion.[39] This finding suggests that the effects of ILE on myocardial contraction after ischemia are mediated by mitochondrial metabolism. However, other authors reported increased myocardial free fatty acid (FFA) uptake and increased oxygen consumption in dogs given an infusion of ILE without any change in left ventricular pressure, heart rate, or cardiac output.[53] Moreover, in a human septic shock model studying the various substrates used by the myocardium, the contribution of FFAs as a myocardial energy source was markedly diminished (12% versus 54% in the control group), but that of lactate was increased (36% versus 12%). The observed shift in myocardial substrate extraction was associated with a discrepancy between measured myocardial oxygen consumption: 41% of myocardial oxygen consumption was not explained by the utilization of commonly available substrates extracted from coronary circulation.[12] This raises the question as to whether or not an exogenous source of FFAs such as provided by lipid emulsion, is actually useful in a xenobiotic induced shock state.

Unfortunately, there is limited experimental evidence to support a modulation of intracellular energy metabolism as the mechanism of action of the ILE. Some evidence comes from experimental studies in bupivacaine toxicity. In an isolated rat heart model of bupivacaine-induced cardiotoxicity, doses of lipid emulsion in the perfusate that were thought to be too low to significantly decrease bupivacaine concentrations reversed bupivacaine-induced cardiac dysfunction.[73] Similarly, in an in vivo model of bupivacaine-induced toxicity rodents pretreated with a single dose of a fatty acid oxidation inhibitor (CVT-4325) were unable to be rescued by ILE, suggesting that lipid emulsion works by providing energy in the form of FFAs.[60] Although these results suggest that lipid emulsion works by a mechanism other than binding bupivacaine and suggest a metabolic effect, other studies support the theory that lipid emulsion works by a nonmetabolic mechanism. In one study, verapamil toxicity was induced in rodents that were pretreated with the fatty acid oxidation inhibitor oxfenicine or control solution. Both groups were then resuscitated with ILE.[2] There were no significant differences in survival time and mean arterial pressure between the oxfenicine-treated and control groups. Analogous to some models of bupivacaine toxicity, this study suggests that in verapamil toxicity, ILE works by a mechanism other than mitochondrial energy supply.

Lipid Sink, Sponge, or Conduit Mechanism

This mechanism theorizes that lipid emulsion "soaks up" lipid-soluble xenobiotic, removing it from the site of toxicity. In a variation of this proposed mechanism, ILE sequesters the xenobiotic out of the aqueous plasma, which bathes the tissue, and within a nonaqueous part of the plasma that is not in contact with the site of toxicity. Intravenous lipid emulsion is also thought to alter the distribution of lipid-soluble xenobiotics and redistribute them away from the site of toxicity into an area with high lipid content (ie, create a "lipid conduit"). Some experimental support comes from studies of bupivacaine toxicity.

Stronger evidence for the lipid sink or sponge mechanism is seen in the effect of lipid emulsion on the pharmacokinetics and tissue distribution of bupivacaine in rats. Lipid emulsion decreased the distribution of bupivacaine into tissue, resulting in decreased concentrations in the brain and myocardium.[69] Similarly, in a pharmacokinetic study of clomipramine toxicity, after infusion of lipid emulsion into the peritoneal cavity, concentrations of clomipramine increased and volume of distribution decreased in addition to an increase in blood pressure.[27] In a pharmacokinetic study of amiodarone toxicity, ILE pretreatment resulted in higher concentrations of amiodarone and higher blood pressures compared with pretreatment with saline.[57] In a well-perfused swine model, ILE decreased amitriptyline concentrations in the brain by 25% and decreased the heart-to-plasma amitriptyline ratio.[29] In a successful resuscitation from bupropion overdose, bupropion concentrations increased dramatically after ILE administration.[77] Concentrations also increased after successful treatment of verapamil.[18] These findings in experimental models and case reports are used to support the lipid sink or sponge model, in which ILE removes a xenobiotic away from the compartment of toxicity, although the increased concentrations is also explained by an increased perfusion of tissues and release of the drug.

Additional indirect evidence supports the lipid sink or sponge and a nonmetabolic mechanism. Although the myocardium can utilize fatty acids for metabolism, the central nervous system (CNS) does not use fatty acids to a substantial degree, implying that the reversal of sedation results from xenobiotic removal from the CNS as opposed to an altered metabolism. This reversal of CNS effects was demonstrated in two animal models of thiopental sedation,[8,67] but in another animal model of thiopental anesthesia, ILE increased the CNS effects. These findings are also used to support the lipid sink or sponge mechanism because in this model, it was proposed that the lipid emulsion maintained a high serum thiopental concentration, permitting subsequent thiopental diffusion into the CNS.[37]

The degree of lipid solubility of a xenobiotic is measured using the partition coefficients log P or log D. Both measure the xenobiotic distribution between a lipophilic organic phase (usually octanol) and a polar aqueous phase (usually water) and report the logarithm of the ratio of concentration of the xenobiotic between the two phases. Whereas log P measures the partition of the nonionized form of the xenobiotic between the two phases, log D measures the partition of both the nonionized and the ionized form of the xenobiotic and varies based on pH. Whereas log P is reported across a range of often unspecified pH values, the log D at pH of 7 is considered by the editors of this text as an acceptable evaluation of lipid solubility in normal plasma. Conditions that vary the lipid solubility are likely clinically important because they will alter the amount of xenobiotic partitioning into the serum lipid. In an in vitro model, the distribution of bupivacaine and ropivacaine in lipid emulsion decreased at lower pH.[48]

Activation of Ion Channels

Lipid emulsion was also hypothesized to activate either or both Ca^{2+} and Na^+ channels. Linolenic and stearic acids decreased bupivacaine-induced Na^+ channel blockade in an experimental model of human embryonic kidney cell expression of human cardiac Na^+ channels bathed in lipid emulsion.[54] Fatty acids directly activated myocardial Ca^{2+} channels and induced a dose-dependent increase in the Ca^{2+} current, promoting dysrhythmias. Oleic, linoleic, and linolenic acids act directly on the Ca^{2+} channel to increase Ca^{2+} current.[31] None of these studies are representative of the administration of ILE in humans or animals, and the amount of ILE used in this setting cannot be converted to a meaningful dosing regimen.

Mechanism of Action: Conclusion

Despite the lack of definitive studies on mechanisms of action, the lipid sink, conduit, and sponge model is the most compelling because beneficial effects from ILE are most frequently noted for lipid-soluble xenobiotics independent of their mechanisms of toxicity.[19] Multiple consequential mechanisms of action may exist, and depending on the xenobiotic, the mechanisms of action likely vary and are multifactorial.

Pharmacokinetics

Lipid droplets that are smaller than 1 μm are primarily removed from circulation as they move through the capillaries of adipose and hepatic tissue. The capillary endothelium in these tissues contains lipoprotein lipase, which hydrolyzes triglycerides, releasing fatty acids and glycerol that then diffuses into the cells. Fatty acids enter the cardiac myocyte either by passive diffusion or protein-mediated transport.[72]

The half-life of intravenously administered lipid emulsion is 30 to 60 minutes and can vary substantially depending on the patient's clinical status, lipid emulsion dose, and droplet size.[17] More than 2.5 g of lipid/kg/d (12.5 mL/kg of 20% ILE or 875 mL in a 70-kg person) overwhelms lipoprotein lipase activity, resulting in decreased clearance.[59] Mean droplet sizes vary across lipid emulsion formulations and the number of fat globules per milliliter of lipid emulsion solution are affected by the time to expiration date, storage temperature, and possibly plastic bag versus glass containers.[13] Larger droplet sizes have slower clearances and are removed by reticuloendothelial phagocytosis. Solutions containing larger than recommended droplets are considered unstable and increase the risk of triglyceride accumulation in various target organs. These larger droplets are more likely to induce an inflammatory response, obstruct the microvasculature, and produce capillary fat emboli. The liver is the organ most commonly involved in accumulation of larger lipid emulsion droplets.[13]

Pharmacodynamics

When inside the cells, fatty acids are used as energy or resynthesized into triglycerides and stored. For use as energy, triglycerides are transported into the mitochondria by carnitine palmitoyltransferase, where they undergo β oxidation sequentially releasing acetylcoenzyme A (acetyl-CoA) as the fatty acid chain is reduced in length. These acetyl-CoA molecules enter the citric acid cycle, where they ultimately generate adenosine triphosphate (ATP) (Figs. 11–3 and 11–9). Although glucose, lactate, and fatty acid metabolism all are used in the production of acetyl-CoA, fatty acid metabolism produces the largest amount of energy. For example, whereas 1 mole of glucose produces 36 moles of ATP, 1 mole of stearic acid produces 146 moles of ATPs;[86] the metabolism of longer fatty acid chains may produce even more ATP.

ROLE IN LOCAL ANESTHETIC TOXICITY

The swine model appropriateness to evaluate lipid resuscitation therapy was questioned. Certain species of swine develop complement activation-related pseudoallergy (CARPA), an acute hypersensitivity reaction to liposomes. Complement activation-related pseudoallergy is characterized by mottling, hypoxia, and cardiovascular instability, which might compromise ILE resuscitation. This was thought to explain the incongruous effect of ILE in these swine models and hypotension when ILE is administered in some swine models.[29,83] However, subsequent adequately powered studies reported no difference in the hemodynamic parameters of swine treated with ILE and a veterinary literature review on the use of ILE in pets does not mention this rare pseudoallergy as a contraindication.[11,24]

Based on the experimental evidence in bupivacaine toxicity, ILE was reportedly successfully used in several reported human cases of cardiovascular collapse from local anesthetic overdose. The first human case occurred after the inadvertent IV administration of bupivacaine and mepivacaine during an interscalene block.[64] The patient developed cardiac arrest and was treated with cardiopulmonary resuscitation (CPR) and Advanced Cardiac Life Support (ACLS) for 20 minutes but only had return of spontaneous circulation after administration of the first dose of ILE (100 mL of 20% ILE followed by 0.5 mL/kg/min for 2 hours). Of note, cardiac catheterization revealed total occlusion of the right coronary artery, and the patient was discharged with an implantable cardiac defibrillator.

In addition to its use during resuscitation, ILE was used to treat milder clinical scenarios of local anesthetic toxicity such as altered consciousness and cardiac dysrhythmias without loss of pulse. A recent review of 76 human case reports documented using ILE for resuscitation for local anesthetic toxicity, and the majority report some improvement, especially with bupivacaine toxicity.[34] The nature of the clinical findings as well as the dose and the duration of ILE administration reported were heterogenous. The absence of a control group and publication bias inherent to case reporting remains significant confounders in interpretation.[34] A randomized trial with healthy volunteers and subtoxic doses of local anesthetics given to reach the threshold of early neurotoxicity gave 120 mL of ILE 20% and could not find a difference between its groups.[15] Another study used 1.5 mL/kg of 20% ILE in pretreatment for a dose of 1 mL/kg of lidocaine and found no difference in the lipid phase entrapment of lidocaine or in patient electroencephalographic patterns.[30]

For local anesthetic poisoning, earlier recommendations limited use of ILE to situations after the failure of standard resuscitative measures. As a result of the experimental evidence and many successful case reports, some authors recommend adding ILE at the first signs of local anesthetic toxicity, but others suggest using it only in the setting of cardiovascular collapse. In the latter setting, ILE should be used concomitantly with CPR and ACLS, and high doses of epinephrine should be avoided.[84]

We recommend administering ILE when there is rapid progression of bupivacaine toxicity affecting the CNS (agitation, confusion, seizures) or cardiovascular system (hypertension, tachycardia, ventricular dysrhythmias, hypotension, conduction blocks). In the setting of cardiovascular collapse, ILE is recommended with CPR and standard ACLS. Lipid emulsion should be stored for easy and rapid access in operating rooms or in areas where local anesthetics are frequently used.

ROLE IN NON–LOCAL ANESTHETIC TOXICITY

After the experience with bupivacaine toxicity, ILE was evaluated for toxicity of calcium channel blockers, cyclic antidepressant, β-adrenergic antagonists, organic phosphorus compounds, amiodarone, cocaine, and many other xenobiotics, with conflicting results.[41]

Based on some positive experimental evidence, ILE use was expanded to non–local anesthetic toxicity. Intravenous lipid emulsion was successfully used to resuscitate a 17-year-old patient with prolonged cardiovascular collapse after bupropion and lamotrigine overdose. In this case, the patient experienced seizures and received ACLS and CPR for 70 minutes, with return of spontaneous circulation after ILE administration (a bolus of 100 mL of 20%). Asystole recurred 90 minutes after ILE administration and resolved with epinephrine.[70]

To date, the latest and most exhaustive systematic review[41] found more than 159 case reports, 137 of which are in humans, three low-quality randomized control trials,[20,36,42,74] and one observational study of ILE for resuscitation in non–local anesthetic toxicity.[20]

The first randomized trial explored the efficacy of 10 mL/kg of 10% ILE on 30 patients with various sedative-hypnotic poisonings. The trial unfortunately suffers from serious methodological flaws in the authors' selection bias, lack of blinding, and outcome measurement in which the statistically significant outcome represents a change of 1 point on the pre- and postintubation Glasgow Coma Scale.[74] The other two studies on tricyclic antidepressant overdoses did not show a difference in mortality rate.[36] An isoflurane study gave 2 mL/kg of 30% ILE to patients receiving anesthesia for various procedures. It reported a benefit of 4 and 5 minutes in time to eye opening and time to exit of the operating room, respectively, between the groups but no difference on time to extubation.[42] Other case studies report improvement with varied amounts of ILE for poisonings with diverse amounts of amlodipine, diltiazem, verapamil, atenolol, nebivolol, propranolol, carvedilol, flecainide, haloperidol, amitriptyline, dosulepin, doxepin, imipramine, quetiapine, venlafaxine, carbamazepine, lamotrigine, phenobarbital, diphenhydramine, bupropion, hydroxychloroquine, cocaine, and bromadiolone.

Subsequently, the largest case series of ILE was published reporting an overall survival rate of 69% in 25 of 36 patients poisoned with various non–local anesthetics such as calcium channel blockers and β-adrenergic antagonists (10 of 36), cyclic antidepressant (5 of 36), or bupropion (3 of 36).[52] This study failed to demonstrate a meaningful increase in mean arterial pressure (MAP) a priori defined as a sustained increase of 10 mm Hg for 1 hour even in the survivor-only group. Wide variability in the dosing regimen, total lipid emulsion amount, and additional treatment received was noted. Despite successful reports, data on the efficacy of ILE are severely limited by reporting biases, therapeutic effects resulting from additional coadministered therapies, and coingestant xenobiotic toxicity. A study on fatality cases of the US National Poison Database system from 2006 to 2016 reported more than 450 cases of unsuccessful use of ILE for various overdoses, attesting to the fact that this therapy requires controlled studies to determine its effectiveness and adverse effect profile when used for poisonings.[71a]

The Lipid Emulsion Workgroup, composed of representative of all major toxicology associations, published evidence-based recommendations in which ILE was recommended for cardiac arrest from bupivacaine toxicity and after failure of other modalities in amitriptyline, bupropion, and toxicity from other local anesthetics. The workgroup could not find evidence to recommend ILE in other situations because of a lack of data or balance between risks and possible benefits.[21] Based on the current data available from animal models and clinical case reports, the Lipid Emulsion Workgroup published recommendations that ILE is a reasonable consideration in cardiac arrest from bupivacaine toxicity and serious hemodynamic instability from a bupropion, amitriptyline, and other local anaesthetics after conventional treatments failed.[21] However, given the lack of data, which yield overall neutral opinions from the Lipid Emulsion workgroup, the authors of this textbook provide the following recommendation pending new available evidence. Lipid emulsion can be administered for patients with hemodynamic instability refractory to standard resuscitation measures when the risk-to-benefit ratio of interaction with other pharmacological or specific antidotal therapies or extracorporeal life support (ECLS) measures such as extracorporeal membrane oxygenation (ECMO) is carefully evaluated. Thus it is reasonable that lipid emulsion be used in the setting of severe toxicity (prolonged cardiovascular instability with nonperfusion or poor perfusion caused by hypotension, or dysrhythmias or seizures) resulting from a lipid soluble xenobiotic(s) despite maximal treatment with standard resuscitation measures even if the current available evidence for the efficacy of this therapy is of very low grade. Standard antidotal therapy and resuscitative measures are shown to be superior or equivalent to lipid emulsion and should not be abandoned in a rush to administer ILE.

ADVERSE EFFECTS AND SAFETY ISSUES

The adverse effects attributed to ILE administration are infrequently reported in the poisoning literature.[7] A systematic review evaluated all possible adverse effects with ILE given for parenteral nutrition or poisoning up to 14 days. Potential complications of ILE include acute kidney injury, cardiac arrest, ventilation perfusion mismatch, ARDS, venous thromboembolism, hypersensitivity, fat embolism, fat overload syndrome, pancreatitis, extracorporeal circulation machine circuit obstruction, allergic reaction, and increased susceptibility to infection.[28]

Because of the limited number of case reports, complications or toxicity from ILE at dosages exceeding the daily recommended amount for parenteral nutrition remains a concern. Pulmonary toxicity is reported when ILE is used as a source of parenteral nutrition. In patients with ARDS, 500 mL of 20% ILE administered over 8 hours resulted in increased pulmonary artery pressures, pulmonary shunting, increased pulmonary vascular resistance, and decreased partial pressures of oxygen in the alveoli/fraction of inspired oxygen ratio (PaO_2/FIO_2).[79] Similar results were found in patients with ARDS administered 500 mL of 10% ILE over 4 hours, resulting in an increase in pulmonary shunting and a decrease in the fraction of PaO_2/FIO_2.[35] The pulmonary effect of ILE in ARDS may be related to infusion rate. In patients with ARDS, 500 mL of 20% ILE infused over 5 hours resulted in an increase

in pulmonary pressures, but a slower infusion over 10 hours left pulmonary pressures unchanged.[47]

In these studies, when pulmonary effects occurred, they were mild and resolved after the ILE infusion was stopped or within 3 to 4 hours. Larger doses may result in clinically significant toxicity and more prolonged effects. However, studies using lipid emulsions with medium-chain triglycerides have shown less pulmonary toxicity.[17,71]

Intravenous lipid emulsion causes pulmonary toxicity by at least two mechanisms. Intravenous lipid emulsion may occlude the pulmonary vasculature with microfat emboli. Macrophages containing lipid droplets are demonstrated in the bronchioalveolar lavage fluid of ARDS patients treated with ILE.[40] Experimental evidence also suggests that a substantial amount of the high concentrations of linoleic acid in ILE is converted to arachidonic acid and then into vasoactive prostaglandins. Indomethacin, an inhibitor of prostaglandin synthesis, prevented any pulmonary vascular effect caused by ILE in one sheep model.[50]

Elevated triglycerides and pancreatitis are reported when ILE is used for parenteral nutrition. The precise mechanism of ILE-induced pancreatitis is unknown but may be the result from the large concentration of triglycerides forming large lipid droplets that obstruct the small vessels of the pancreas, leading to ischemia. Lipase then degrades the triglycerides, releasing cytotoxic FFAs. Laboratory assays differ in how they measure triglycerides.

Hyperamylasemia and pancreatitis were reported in two cases of ILE use in treatment of xenobiotic toxicity. After successful resuscitation with ILE from bupivacaine-induced cardiac arrest, an elevated amylase concentration without associated elevated lipase or associated symptoms was reported.[77] Elevated lipase concentrations were reported after administering ILE to a 13-year-old girl who developed delayed seizures and cardiac arrest after amitriptyline ingestion. Lipase concentrations peaked at 1,849 IU/L 5 days after ILE and were associated with elevated triglycerides and abdominal pain.[40]

Large doses or rapid infusions of ILE have the potential to induce a fat overload syndrome. Fat overload syndrome is characterized by hyperlipemia, fever, fat infiltration, hepatomegaly, jaundice, splenomegaly, anemia, leukopenia, thrombocytopenia, coagulation disturbances, seizures, and coma. Multiple end-organ dysfunction is attributed to inadequate clearance of lipids and sludging in the lungs, brain, kidney, retina, and liver. Because of the rapid redistribution of most local anesthetics, prolonged ILE infusion should not be required (Chap. 64). However, many other lipid-soluble xenobiotics have a long duration of toxicity, and prolonged and repeated ILE infusions, if given, increase the risk of fat overload syndrome.

Particularly when administered early in the clinical course of an oral overdose, ILE has the potential to increase gastrointestinal absorption or facilitate distribution of lipid-soluble xenobiotics, resulting in increased toxicity. In an orogastric model of amitriptyline and verapamil overdose, ILE increased amitriptyline concentrations and resultant toxicity.[62,63] Gastric decontamination should be performed under these circumstances.

Intravenous lipid emulsions also have the potential to interact with other essential antidotes and especially epinephrine and vasopressin.[5,31,33] If an antidote is lipid soluble, it may be incorporated by the ILE and result in decreased effectiveness. Intravenous lipid emulsion was also used with several other medications during resuscitation for toxicity, including atropine, amiodarone, sodium bicarbonate, magnesium sulfate, calcium chloride, naloxone, and metaraminol.[6,37,65,80]

The addition of ILE to high dose insulin (HDI) therapy was evaluated in a model of severe verapamil toxicity, and there were no improvements in hemodynamics, metabolic parameters, or survival.[3] Also, ILE did not improve hypotension in a swine model of amitriptyline-induced toxicity[78] Therefore, although other resuscitative xenobiotics should be used as indicated, there is no evidence yet to support or refute the simultaneous use of ILE and bicarbonate or HDI therapy.

Hyperlipidemia after using ILE interferes with many laboratory studies, making them uninterpretable.[23] This interference lasts for several hours and is dependent in part on the type of laboratory system used. Intravenous lipid emulsion variably alters analytical test results and results in erroneous measurement, no significant effect, or the inability to perform a laboratory test. In vitro testing of ILE demonstrated that colorimetric methods were more prone to the effects of ILE than potentiometric methods. In the setting of ILE, glucose measurement by colorimetric method did not accurately report hypoglycemia. For example, a glucose concentration of 48.6 mg/dL (2.7 mmol/L) may be falsely reported as 223.2 mg/dL (12.4 mmol/L). Centrifugation at 140,000 g for 10 minutes minimized most interference. Troponin-I, sodium, potassium, chloride, calcium, bicarbonate, or urea assays had the least interference. Albumin and magnesium assays demonstrated significant interference. Amylase, lipase, phosphate, creatinine, total protein, alanine aminotransferase, creatine kinase, and bilirubin became unmeasurable.[22] The effect of ILE on toxic drug concentrations assays is largely unknown. Ideally, analytic testing should be performed before ILE administration.[23]

DOSING AND ADMINISTRATION

Although the optimal dosing regimen for human poisonings remains undefined, several animal models evaluate the effects of high-dose ILE. In both rodent and canine models of verapamil toxicity, 12.4- and 7-mL/kg boluses of 20% ILE were given,[3,75] and in a rabbit model of clomipramine, 12 mL/kg of 20% ILE was used.[49] In a small rodent model, the median lethal dose of ILE 20% was reported at 67 mL/kg,[32] which is much higher than the current recommended clinical doses, but an LD_{50} cannot be use to guide safety. In a model of IV verapamil toxicity in which ILE was administrated 5 minutes after the start of the verapamil infusion, higher doses up to a maximum of 18.6 mL/kg of 20% ILE were more effective in improving blood pressure, acidemia, and mean time survival than lower doses. Higher doses than 18.6 mL/kg improved hemodynamic parameters transiently but resulted in overall decreased survival times than the 18.6-mL/kg dose but twice the time than the 12.4-mL/kg dose.[61] These animal models used large doses of xenobiotic and were designed to produce a rapid onset of toxicity; it is difficult to extrapolate their findings to typical human overdose cases. One controlled human study used as much as 10 mL/kg of 10% ILE with questionable clinical results and did not report on adverse effects.[74]

Dosing was initially arbitrarily defined for local anesthetic toxicity, specifically bupivacaine, with generalization of this dosing regimen to poisoning by other local anesthetics and other xenobiotics. The American Society of Regional Anesthesia and Pain Management, the Association of Anesthetists of Great Britain and Ireland, and the American Heart Association[55] accepted similar guidelines and recommendations on the use of ILE in local anesthetic toxicity.

These societies recommend a dose of 1.5 mL/kg bolus of 20% ILE followed by 0.25 mL/kg/min or 15 mL/kg/h to run for 30 to 60 minutes.[55] They suggest repeating this bolus several times for persistent dysrhythmias and that the infusion rate can be increased if blood pressure decreases.

The precise dose of ILE for non–local anesthetics has not been studied, and it is not known if boluses or infusion are more effective. The reasonable safe total dose is also unknown but would depend on the degree of toxicity and response to previous doses of ILE.

The most common route of administration is IV either peripherally or via central catheters. The intraosseous route was also, albeit seldom, reported as successful.[16]

The American College of Medical Toxicology published interim guidance on the use of ILE in lipophilic xenobiotic toxicity.[1] When ILE is used, they recommend a bolus dose of 1.5 mL/kg of 20% ILE. They also recommend that repeat boluses of ILE can be administered for persistent severe symptoms and that that the bolus "may" be followed by an infusion for 30 to 60 minutes of 0.25 mL/kg/min or to a maximum total dose of 10 mL/kg. To date, no experimental, animal, or human clinical studies exist to inform on what benefit, if any, could be expected from any infusion of ILE. We agree on a maximum total dose of 10 mL/kg.

Propofol is formulated as a 10% lipid emulsion, but it is not recommended for use in ILE therapy because of the adverse effect of the propofol from the dose needed to achieve the doses of lipid typically used in ILE therapy.[82] A 1.5-mL/kg bolus of 20% ILE equates to 3 mL/kg of the 10% lipid emulsion in the propofol solution. A normal dose of propofol (1%) for general anesthesia is 2.5 mg/kg or 0.25 mL/kg.[68] If propofol is used as a ILE therapy, it would deliver a bolus of 12 times the recommended dose of propofol. This would exacerbate any drug-induced hypotension and bradycardia and therefore is not recommended.

Pregnancy and Lactation

Intravenous lipid emulsion is a Pregnancy Category C pharmaceutical. It is not known whether ILE can cause fetal harm when administered to gravid patients. Few cases of ILE resuscitation have been published in pregnant patients.[14,45] Potentially, large doses can result in elevated triglyceride concentrations, and lipid globules may occlude placental vasculature. The risk of potential toxicity should be weighed against potential benefit to the pregnant woman and fetus. There is no reported risk of ILE on breastfeeding infants.

FORMULATION AND ACQUISITION

Lipid emulsion is available in parenteral formulation of 5%, 10%, 20%, and 30% solutions. The 20% solution is the formulation we recommend and the one used most often. The 30% solution is a pharmacy bulk admixture and is used to prepare dilute concentrations. The 30% solution should be diluted before administration and has not been used clinically for xenobiotic toxicity.

SUMMARY

- Lipid emulsion is recommended for the treatment of local anesthetic systemic toxicity, particularly bupivacaine, in the case of rapidly progressive toxicity or cardiac arrest.
- In local anesthetic systemic toxicity, a bolus of ILE is recommended if still needed after standard resuscitation medications and should be stored where local anesthetics are administered.
- Lipid emulsion use for other xenobiotics is only reasonable when severe toxicity resulting from a lipid-soluble xenobiotic persists despite maximal treatment with standard resuscitation measures.
- When used for either local anesthetic or non–local anesthetic toxicity, we recommend a bolus dose of 1.5 mL/kg of 20% ILE. Repeat boluses of ILE are reasonable for persistent severe signs and symptoms to a maximum total dose of 10 mL/kg.
- The IV route is preferred although in absence of IV access, the intraosseous route can be used.

REFERENCES

1. American College of Medical Toxicology. ACMT Position Statement: Guidance for the Use of Intravenous Lipid Emulsion. *J Med Toxicol.* 2017;13:124-125.
2. Bania T, et al. The role of cardiac free fatty acid metabolism in verapamil toxicity treated with intravenous fat emulsions. 2007 Society for Academic Emergency Medicine Annual Meeting. *Acad Emerg Med.* 2007;14(suppl 5):S196-S197.
3. Bania TC, et al. Hemodynamic effects of intravenous fat emulsion in an animal model of severe verapamil toxicity resuscitated with atropine, calcium, and saline. *Acad Emerg Med.* 2007;14:105-111.
4. Barrington MJ, Kluger R. Ultrasound guidance reduces the risk of local anesthetic systemic toxicity following peripheral nerve blockade. *Reg Anesth Pain Med.* 2013;38:289-299.
5. Carreiro S, et al. Intravenous lipid emulsion alters the hemodynamic response to epinephrine in a rat model. *J Med Toxicol.* 2013;9:220-225.
6. Cave G, et al. Intravenous lipid emulsion as antidote: a summary of published human experience. *Emerg Med Australas.* 2011;23:123-141.
7. Cave G, Harvey MG. Should we consider the infusion of lipid emulsion in the resuscitation of poisoned patients? *Crit Care.* 2014;18:457.
8. Cave G, et al. Intralipid ameliorates thiopentone induced respiratory depression in rats: investigative pilot study. *Emerg Med Australas.* 2005;17:180-181.
9. Chazotte B, Vanderkooi G. Multiple sites of inhibition of mitochondrial electron transport by local anesthetics. *Biochim Biophys Acta.* 1981;636:153-161.
10. Corwin DJ, et al. Adverse events associated with a large dose of intravenous lipid emulsion for suspected local anesthetic toxicity. *Clin Toxicol (Phila).* 2017;55:603-607.
11. Crane C, et al. Utilization of a swine (Sus scrofa) model for lipid emulsion resuscitation studies. *ISRN Anesthesiology.* 2012;2012:1-5.
12. Dhainaut JF, et al. Coronary hemodynamics and myocardial metabolism of lactate, free fatty acids, glucose, and ketones in patients with septic shock. *Circulation.* 1987;75:533-541.
13. Driscoll DF. Lipid injectable emulsions: pharmacopeial and safety issues. *Pharm Res.* 2006;23:1959-1969.

14. Dun-Chi Lin J, et al. Two for one: a case report of intravenous lipid emulsion to treat local anesthetic systemic toxicity in term pregnancy. *A A Case Rep.* 2017; 8: 235-237.

15. Dureau P, et al. Effect of Intralipid(R) on the dose of ropivacaine or levobupivacaine tolerated by volunteers: a clinical and pharmacokinetic study. *Anesthesiology.* 2016; 125:474-483.

16. Elliott A, et al. Intraosseous administration of antidotes - a systematic review. *Clin Toxicol (Phila).* 2017:1-30.

17. Faucher M, et al. Cardiopulmonary effects of lipid emulsions in patients with ARDS. *Chest.* 2003;124:285-291.

18. French D, et al. Serum verapamil concentrations before and after Intralipid® therapy during treatment of an overdose. *Clin Toxicol.* 2011;49:340-344.

19. French D, et al. Partition constant and volume of distribution as predictors of clinical efficacy of lipid rescue for toxicological emergencies. *Clin Toxicol (Phila).* 2011;49:801-809.

20. Gil HW, et al. Effect of intravenous lipid emulsion in patients with acute glyphosate intoxication. *Clin Toxicol.* 2013;51:767-771.

21. Gosselin S, et al. Evidence-based recommendations on the use of intravenous lipid emulsion therapy in poisoning. *Clin Toxicol (Phila).* 2016;54:899-923.

22. Grunbaum AM, et al. Analytical interferences resulting from intravenous lipid emulsion. *Clin Toxicol.* 2012;50:812-817.

23. Grunbaum AM, et al. Review of the effect of intravenous lipid emulsion on laboratory analyses. *Clin Toxicol (Phila).* 2016;54:92-102.

24. Gwaltney- et al. Use of intravenous lipid emulsions for treating certain poisoning cases in small animals. *Vet Clin North Am Small Anim Pract.* 2012;42:251-262, vi.

25. Haber LM, et al. Fat overload syndrome. An autopsy study with evaluation of the coagulopathy. *Am J Clin Pathol.* 1988;90:223-227.

26. Hantson P, Beauloye C. Myocardial metabolism in toxin-induced heart failure and therapeutic implications. *Clin Toxicol (Phila).* 2012;50:166-171.

27. Harvey M, et al. Correlation of plasma and peritoneal diasylate clomipramine concentration with hemodynamic recovery after intralipid infusion in rabbits. *Acad Emerg Med.* 2009;16:151-156.

28. Hayes BD, et al. Systematic review of clinical adverse events reported after acute intravenous lipid emulsion administration. *Clin Toxicol (Phila).* 2016;54:365-404.

29. Heinonen JA, et al. Intravenous lipid emulsion entraps amitriptyline into plasma and can lower its brain concentration--an experimental intoxication study in pigs. *Basic Clin Pharmacol Toxicol.* 2013;113:193-200.

30. Heinonen JA, et al. Intravenous lipid emulsion given to volunteers does not affect symptoms of lidocaine brain toxicity. *Basic Clin Pharmacol Toxicol.* 2015;116:378-383.

31. Hicks SD, et al. Lipid emulsion combined with epinephrine and vasopressin does not improve survival in a swine model of bupivacaine-induced cardiac arrest. *Anesthesiology.* 2009;111:138-146.

32. Hiller DB, et al. Safety of high volume lipid emulsion infusion: a first approximation of LD50 in rats. *Reg Anesth Pain Med.* 2010;35:140-144.

33. Hiller DB, et al. Epinephrine impairs lipid resuscitation from bupivacaine overdose: a threshold effect. *Anesthesiology.* 2009;111:498-505.

34. Hoegberg LC, et al. Systematic review of the effect of intravenous lipid emulsion therapy for local anesthetic toxicity. *Clin Toxicol (Phila).* 2016;54:167-193.

35. Hwang TL, et al. Effects of intravenous fat emulsion on respiratory failure. *Chest.* 1990;97:934-938.

36. Kasnavieh SMH. Intravenous lipid emulsion for the treatment of tricyclic antidepressant toxicity a randomized controlled trial. Paper presented at the VIIth Mediterranean Emergency Medicine Congress, September 8 to 11, 2013, Marseille, France.

37. Kazemi A, et al. The effect of lipid emulsion on depth of anaesthesia following thiopental administration to rabbits. *Anaesthesia.* 2011;66:373-378.

38. Kline JA, et al. Myocardial metabolism during graded intraportal verapamil infusion in awake dogs. *J Cardiovasc Pharmacol.* 1996;27:719-726.

39. Kline JA, et al. The diabetogenic effects of acute verapamil poisoning. *Toxicol Appl Pharmacol.* 1997;145:357-362.

40. Levine M, et al. Delayed-onset seizure and cardiac arrest after amitriptyline overdose, treated with intravenous lipid emulsion therapy. *Pediatrics.* 2012;130:e432-438.

41. Levine M, et al. Systematic review of the effect of intravenous lipid emulsion therapy for non-local anesthetics toxicity. *Clin Toxicol (Phila).* 2016;54:194-221.

42. Li Q, et al. Intravenous lipid emulsion improves recovery time and quality from isoflurane anaesthesia: a double-blind clinical trial. *Basic Clin Pharmacol Toxicol.* 2014;115:222-228.

43. Li Z, et al. Lipid resuscitation of bupivacaine toxicity: long-chain triglyceride emulsion provides benefits over long- and medium-chain triglyceride emulsion. *Anesthesiology.* 2011;115:1219-1228.

44. Litonius ES, et al. Intravenous lipid emulsion only minimally influences bupivacaine and mepivacaine distribution in plasma and does not enhance recovery from intoxication in pigs. *Anesth Analg.* 2012;114:901-906.

45. Lynch W, et al. Lipid Emulsion rescue of amniotic fluid embolism-induced cardiac arrest: a case report. *A A Case Rep.* 2017;8:64-66.

46. Masters TN, Glaviano VV. Effects of dl-propranolol on myocardial free fatty acid and carbohydrate metabolism. *J Pharmacol Exp Ther.* 1969;167:187-193.

47. Mathru M, et al. Effect of fast vs slow intralipid infusion on gas exchange, pulmonary hemodynamics, and prostaglandin metabolism. *Chest.* 1991;99:426-429.

48. Mazoit JX, et al. Binding of long-lasting local anesthetics to lipid emulsions. *Anesthesiology.* 2009;110:380-386.

49. McEvoy GK, American Society of Health-System P. *Handbook on Injectable Drugs.* 2015.

50. McKeen CR, et al. Pulmonary vascular effects of fat emulsion infusion in unanesthetized sheep. Prevention by indomethacin. *J Clin Invest.* 1978;61:1291-1297.

51. Mirtallo JM, et al. State of the art review: intravenous fat emulsions: Current applications, safety profile, and clinical implications. *Ann Pharmacother.* 2010;44:688-700.

52. Mithani S, et al. A cohort study of unstable overdose patients treated with intravenous lipid emulsion therapy. *CJEM.* 2016;19:256-264.

53. Mjos OD, Akre S. Effect of catecholamines on blood flow, oxygen consumption, and release-uptake of free fatty acids in adipose tissue. *Scand J Clin Lab Invest.* 1971; 27:221-225.

54. Mottram AR, et al. Fatty acids antagonize bupivacaine-induced INa blockade. *Clin Toxicol.* 2011;49:729-733.

55. Neal JM, et al. ASRA practice advisory on local anesthetic systemic toxicity. *Reg Anesth Pain Med.* 2010;35:152-161.

56. Neal JM, et al. American Society of Regional Anesthesia and Pain Medicine checklist for managing local anesthetic systemic toxicity: 2012 version. *Reg Anesth Pain Med.* 2012;37:16-18.

57. Niiya T, et al. Intravenous lipid emulsion sequesters amiodarone in plasma and eliminates its hypotensive action in pigs. *Ann Emerg Med.* 2010;56:402-408.e402.

58. Okumura T, et al. Severe respiratory distress following sodium oleate ingestion. *J Toxicol Clin Toxicol.* 1998;36:587-589.

59. Palmblad J. Intravenous lipid emulsions and host defense - a critical review. *Clin Nutr.* 1991;10:303-308.

60. Partownavid P, et al. Fatty-acid oxidation and calcium homeostasis are involved in the rescue of bupivacaine-induced cardiotoxicity by lipid emulsion in rats. *Crit Care Med.* 2012;40:2431-2437.

61. Perez E, et al. Determining the optimal dose of intravenous fat emulsion for the treatment of severe verapamil toxicity in a rodent model. *Acad Emerg Med.* 2008;15:1284-1289.

62. Perichon D, et al. An assessment of the in vivo effects of intravenous lipid emulsion on blood drug concentration and haemodynamics following oro-gastric amitriptyline overdose. *Clin Toxicol.* 2013;51:208-215.

63. Perichon D, et al. Intravenous lipid emulsion does not improve hemodynamics or survival in a rodent model of oral verapamil poisoning. *Clin Toxicol.* 2013;51:277.

64. Rosenblatt MA, et al. Successful use of a 20% lipid emulsion to resuscitate a patient after a presumed bupivacaine-related cardiac arrest. *Anesthesiology.* 2006;105:217-218.

65. Rothschild L, et al. Intravenous lipid emulsion in clinical toxicology. *Scand J Trauma Resusc Emerg Med.* 2010;18:51.

66. Ruan W, et al. A mixed (long- and medium-chain) triglyceride lipid emulsion extracts local anesthetic from human serum in vitro more effectively than a long-chain emulsion. *Anesthesiology.* 2012;116:334-339.

67. Russell RL, Westfall BA. Alleviation of barbiturate depression. *Anesth Analg.* 1962; 41:582-585.

68. Schuster DP. ARDS: clinical lessons from the oleic acid model of acute lung injury. *Am J Respir Crit Care Med.* 1994;149:245-260.

69. Shi K, et al. The effect of lipid emulsion on pharmacokinetics and tissue distribution of bupivacaine in rats. *Anesth Analg.* 2013;116:804-809.

70. Sirianni AJ, et al. Use of lipid emulsion in the resuscitation of a patient with prolonged cardiovascular collapse after overdose of bupropion and lamotrigine. *Ann Emerg Med.* 2008;51:412-415, 415.e411.

71. Smiseth OA, Mjos OD. Haemodynamic and metabolic consequences of elevated plasma free fatty acids during acute ischaemic left ventricular failure in dogs. *Scand J Clin Lab Invest.* 1985;45:515-520.

71a. Smolinske S, Hoffman RS, Villeneuve E, et al. When lipid rescue is not the magic bullet. *Clin Toxicol.* 2017;55:694-695.

72. Stanley WC, et al. Myocardial substrate metabolism in the normal and failing heart. *Physiol Rev.* 2005;85:1093-1129.

73. Stehr SN, et al. The effects of lipid infusion on myocardial function and bioenergetics in l-bupivacaine toxicity in the isolated rat heart. *Anesth Analg.* 2007;104:186-192.

74. Taftachi F, et al. Lipid emulsion improves Glasgow coma scale and decreases blood glucose level in the setting of acute non-local anesthetic drug poisoning—a randomized controlled trial. *Eur Rev Med Pharmacol Sci.* 2012;16(suppl 1):38-42.

75. Tebbutt S, et al. Intralipid prolongs survival in a rat model of verapamil toxicity. *Acad Emerg Med.* 2006;13:134-139.

76. Van de Velde M, et al. Long-chain triglycerides improve recovery from myocardial stunning in conscious dogs. *Cardiovasc Res.* 1996;32:1008-1015.

77. Vanden Hoek TL, et al. Part 12: cardiac arrest in special situations: 2010 American Heart Association Guidelines for Cardiopulmonary Resuscitation and Emergency Cardiovascular Care. *Circulation.* 2010;122(18 suppl 3):S829-S861.

78. Varney SM, et al. Intravenous lipid emulsion therapy does not improve hypotension compared to sodium bicarbonate for tricyclic antidepressant toxicity: a randomized, controlled pilot study in a swine model. *Acad Emerg Med.* 2014;21:1212-1219.

79. Venus B, et al. Cardiopulmonary effects of Intralipid infusion in critically ill patients. *Crit Care Med.* 1988;16:587-590.

80. Waring WS. Intravenous lipid administration for drug-induced toxicity: a critical review of the existing data. *Expert Rev Clin Pharmacol.* 2012;5:437-444.

81. Weinbach EC, et al. Effects of tricyclic antidepressant drugs on energy-linked reactions in mitochondria. *Biochem Pharmacol.* 1986;35:1445-1451.

82. Weinberg G, et al. Lipid, not propofol, treats bupivacaine overdose. *Anesth Analg.* 2004;99:1875-1876; author reply 1876.

83. Weinberg G, Rubinstein I. Pig in a poke: species specificity in modeling lipid resuscitation. *Anesth Analg.* 2012;114:907-909.

84. Weinberg GL. Lipid infusion therapy: translation to clinical practice. *Anesth Analg.* 2008;106:1340-1342.

85. Weinberg GL, et al. Bupivacaine inhibits acylcarnitine exchange in cardiac mitochondria. *Anesthesiology.* 2000;92:523-528.

86. Yudkin M, et al. *A Guidebook to Biochemistry.* 4th ed. Cambridge, UK: Cambridge University Press; 1980.

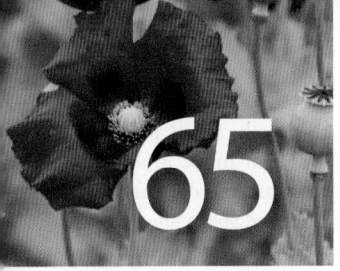

65 INHALATIONAL ANESTHETICS

Caitlin J. Guo and Brian S. Kaufman

HISTORY AND EPIDEMIOLOGY

Paracelsus, a Swiss physician and alchemist, is credited with the earliest use of an inhalational anesthetic when he prepared a mixture of diethyl ether, alcohol, and water called sweet oil of vitriol. He described the administration of this preparation to hens that fell into what appeared to be a deep sleep from which they recovered unharmed. In 1735, Wilhelm Froben gave this substance its modern name of "ether." Ether was used topically, particularly via the intranasal route, as a treatment of headache, nervous diseases, and fits.

Modern anesthetic practice began in 1846 at the Massachusetts General Hospital, when the dentist William Morton gave the first public demonstration of the ability of inhaled ether vapor to alleviate the pain of surgery. Oliver Wendell Holmes chose the Greek-related noun *anesthesia* (without feeling) to characterize the process.

Observations on circulatory and respiratory physiology eventually led to an understanding of the effects of inhalation gases and vapors. In the last decade of the 18th century, centers for the "pneumatic treatment" of disease were established in Birmingham and Bristol, England. Experiments with ether that was inhaled via a funnel and with nitrous oxide were conducted at these institutions. After Humphry Davy described his own pleasurable and exhilarating experience when he inhaled the "laughing" gas, many of his colleagues and friends inhaled nitrous oxide to experience its inebriating effects. Davy also described how inhalation of nitrous oxide relieved headache and the pain of an erupting molar tooth. Although Davy recognized the analgesic properties of nitrous oxide and its possible application for surgery, he failed to pursue the idea.

The public soon took up the use of nitrous oxide in the form of nitrous oxide frolics. Audience members at itinerant medicine shows volunteered to experience the exhilarating effects of nitrous oxide inhalation. At one such show in 1844 in Hartford, Connecticut, a man under the influence of nitrous oxide injured his leg but felt no pain. Dr. Horace Wells, a dentist in the audience that day, inhaled nitrous oxide the following day and had his partner painlessly remove a troublesome tooth. A subsequent public demonstration of the use of nitrous oxide for dental extraction had limited success, leaving his colleagues doubtful regarding its efficacy and safety and thereby impeding its general acceptance as a surgical anesthetic.

In Great Britain in 1847, James Simpson, an obstetrician, first used ether to relieve the pain of labor. He subsequently adopted chloroform for this purpose because of its more pleasant odor and more rapid induction and emergence. The clergy and other physicians opposed the concept of relieving pain during childbirth, but the method ultimately was accepted after Queen Victoria gave birth to Prince Leopold while receiving chloroform administered by John Snow.

Over the next century, several "volatile" anesthetics were introduced, including ethyl chloride in 1848, divinyl ether in 1933, trichloroethylene in 1934, and ethyl vinyl ether in 1947. All of these inhalational anesthetics had significant safety problems associated with their use, including combustibility and direct organ toxicity.

Advances in fluorine chemistry led to the cost-effective incorporation of fluorine into molecules used in the development of modern anesthetics. Fluroxene was the first of the new fluorinated anesthetics to be widely used clinically. However, this anesthetic was flammable and hepatotoxic. It was largely replaced by the nonflammable halothane, which was synthesized in 1951 and introduced into clinical practice in 1956. Methoxyflurane was evaluated in humans in 1960 but is no longer used because of nephrotoxicity (Chap. 27) and hepatotoxicity. Other halogenated hydrocarbons with improved clinical properties were introduced, including enflurane, isoflurane, desflurane, and sevoflurane (Fig. 65–1). The inert gas xenon holds promise as a useful anesthetic and is both cardio- and neuroprotective in experimental studies.[47] The clinical use of xenon is limited both by its cost and difficulty to manufacture. Although xenon is environmentally friendly compared with presently used anesthetic gases, its toxicity is relatively unknown but is believed to be minimal.

PHARMACOLOGY

Inhalational anesthetics remain the most popular anesthetics used for maintenance of anesthesia primarily because they are easily and safely administered by modern anesthesia machines and are rapidly titratable to effect. Inhalational anesthetics used in current clinical practice are available as either volatile liquids (halothane, isoflurane, sevoflurane, and desflurane) or as compressed gases (nitrous oxide).

Because a wide range of chemically distinct xenobiotics can produce anesthesia, a unique receptor for the inhaled anesthetics is improbable. More likely, the volatile anesthetics cause general anesthesia by modulating synaptic function from within cell membranes. The most likely, but not yet proven, targets for the inhalational anesthetics are the ion channels that control ion flow across the cytoplasmic membrane.[13] An in-depth discussion is beyond the scope of this chapter, but several concepts are important to consider. First, more than 20 different ion channels are identified, each controlling various anion and cation flows. The results of these ion channel effects include release of inhibitory neurotransmitters and inhibition of excitatory neurotransmitters. In fact, each anesthetic type has variable actions. The receptor for γ-aminobutyric acid type A (GABA$_A$) is the best studied and is important because GABA$_A$ is an inhibitory neurotransmitter. The interaction of all of these receptor effects produces the condition we refer to as general anesthesia. Many of the adverse effects of the inhalational anesthetics result directly from ion channel effects in non-neural tissue, primarily cardiac cell membranes.

FIGURE 65–1. The inhalational anesthetics.

Reversible changes in neurologic function cause loss of perception and reaction to pain, unawareness of immediate events, and loss of memory of those events. The common pharmacologic mechanisms for general anesthesia include the physical–chemical behavior of volatile hydrocarbons with lipids and proteins within the hydrophobic regions of biologic membrane.

The potency of the various inhaled anesthetics correlates with their physicochemical properties. The dominant theories of the molecular mechanisms by which volatile anesthetics affect membrane function are based on the lipid solubility of the anesthetic and experimental demonstration of pressure reversal of anesthesia. Anesthetic potency correlates directly with the relative lipid solubility of each gaseous anesthetic, suggesting that the primary molecular actions occur in the lipid portion of cell membranes. This mechanism described by the Meyer-Overton lipid solubility theory.[37] Potential membrane regions for anesthetic action include the hydrophobic areas of proteins and protein–lipid interface regions, as well as the phospholipid matrix. High atmospheric pressures can reverse the effects of several anesthetics, suggesting that anesthesia results from increasing membrane volume at normal atmospheric pressure, an effect described by the volume expansion theory.[33]

PHARMACOKINETICS

The route of exposure of inhaled anesthetics are the lungs. Factors that influence their absorption by blood and distribution to other tissues, particularly the brain, include anesthetic solubility, pulmonary pathology, lung and tissue blood flow, and tissue solubility. The goal of inhalational anesthesia is to develop and maintain a satisfactory partial pressure of anesthetic in the brain, the primary site of action.

The pharmacokinetics of anesthetics are linked to their pharmacodynamic effects through the concept of anesthetic potency. The linkage exists because anesthesia strives to achieve and maintain a desired alveolar concentration. For the inhaled anesthetics, potency is commonly designated by the minimum alveolar concentration (MAC) of the anesthetic. The MAC is the alveolar concentration at 1 atm that prevents movement in 50% of participants in response to a painful stimulus (ie, it is the analgesic median effective concentration $\{EC_{50}\}$). Minimum alveolar concentration is used when comparing the effects of equipotent doses of anesthetics on various organ functions.

NITROUS OXIDE

Nitrous oxide (N_2O), a compresses gas, is the most commonly used inhalational anesthetic in the world, but its safety is debated.[30] Its advantages include a mild odor, absence of airway irritation, rapid induction and emergence, potent analgesia, and minimal respiratory and circulatory effects. When administered in a modern operating room (OR) using current standards of monitoring to prevent unintentional hypoxia, nitrous oxide is remarkably safe. Unfortunately, nitrous oxide also has a potential for abuse because of its euphoric effects, particularly among hospital and dental personnel.[29] Death and permanent brain injury are reported but do not generally result from direct toxic effects; instead, they are secondary to hypoxia as a result of simple asphyxiation (Chap. 121).[17]

Nitrous oxide is also used as a food additive to generate foam, a property exploited to produce whipped cream. Sold in supermarkets as "bulbs," death has occurred secondary to asphyxiation, when homemade mouthpieces failed to separate from the user after unconsciousness occurred during use.[46] Recreational abuse of nitrous oxide among teenagers and adults of all ages is on the rise. In 2015, the National Institute on Drug Abuse reported that 527,000 people aged 12 years or older reported using inhalants, and many of them used whippets. This is most assuredly an underestimate of true usage.

Death also occurred when patients received commercially prepared nitrous oxide from tanks contaminated with impurities such as nitric oxide or nitrogen dioxide. Pulmonary toxicity resulting from similar contaminants was reported after illicit preparation of nitrous oxide from the combustion of ammonium nitrate fertilizer.[36]

Injury results from the physical properties of this anesthetic. Nitrous oxide is 35 times more soluble in blood than is nitrogen. When nitrous oxide is inhaled, any compliant air-containing space, such as the bowel, increases in size; noncompliant spaces, such as the Eustachian tubes, exhibit an increase in pressure. These effects occur because nitrous oxide diffuses along the concentration gradient from the blood into a closed space much more rapidly than nitrogen can be transferred in the opposite direction. Clinical consequences include rapid progression of a pneumothorax to a tension pneumothorax, tympanic membrane rupture with hearing loss, bowel distension, and tracheal or laryngeal trauma caused by increased endotracheal cuff pressure resulting from replacement of air by a larger volume of nitrous oxide. Nitrous oxide is particularly dangerous in patients who have suffered air emboli, and its use should be immediately discontinued upon recognition of these events. When intracranial or neuraxial air is injected during placement of an epidural catheter, it also can theoretically expand upon subsequent exposure to nitrous oxide.

Hematologic Effects

Bone marrow suppression was first recognized as a complication of long-term nitrous oxide exposure in the 1950s, when the gas was used to sedate intubated patients who had severe tetanus.[28] Leukopenia with hypoplastic bone marrow and megaloblastic erythropoiesis typically developed 3 to 5 days after initial exposure and was followed by thrombocytopenia. Recovery usually occurred within 4 days after discontinuation of the anesthetic. Healthy patients undergoing routine surgical procedures demonstrate mild megaloblastic bone marrow changes within 12 hours of exposure to 50% nitrous oxide and marked changes within 24 hours of exposure.[44] Critically ill patients appear to be more sensitive to the effects of nitrous oxide on the bone marrow, with megaloblastic changes described after only one hour of exposure, but changes are unlikely in individuals with less than 6 hours of exposure in the absence of preexistent folate or vitamin B_{12} deficiencies.[3]

The hematologic effects of exposure to nitrous oxide strongly resemble the biochemical characteristics of pernicious anemia.[2,42,43] Vitamin B_{12}, or cyanocobalamin, is a bound coenzyme of cytoplasmic methionine synthase. The cobalt moiety in the enzyme functions as a methyl carrier in its transfer from 5-methyltetrahydrofolate to homocysteine to form methionine (Fig. 65–2). Nitrous oxide oxidizes the cobalt ion, converting vitamin B_{12} from the active monovalent form (Co^+) to the inactive divalent form (Co^{2+}), which irreversibly inhibits methionine synthase.[42] The metabolic consequences of this inhibition are significant because methionine and tetrahydrofolate are required for both DNA synthesis and myelin production. This interference is responsible for the development of bone marrow depression and polyneuropathy resembling the characteristic findings that occur in pernicious anemia.[43]

Neurologic Effects

Disabling polyneuropathy in health care workers who habitually abused nitrous oxide was first described in 1978.[29] This neurologic disorder improved slowly when the patients abstained from further nitrous oxide abuse. This neuropathy is clinically indistinguishable from subacute combined degeneration of the spinal cord associated with pernicious anemia.[48] The syndrome of nitrous oxide neuropathy is characterized by sensorimotor polyneuropathy, often combined with signs of posterior and lateral spinal cord involvement. Signs and symptoms include numbness and paresthesias in the extremities, weakness, and truncal ataxia. Magnetic resonance imaging (MRI) findings typically show abnormal signal involving in the posterior and anterior spinal cord columns (Fig. 65–3).[24]

Neurologic changes usually develop after several months of frequent exposure to nitrous oxide, although neurologic manifestations may develop within days of use in patients with subclinical vitamin B_{12} deficiency. Those at risk include individuals who chronically abuse the gas and those who are occupationally exposed for prolonged periods to environments contaminated with high concentrations of nitrous oxide.[6] Animal studies demonstrate that methionine synthase is inactivated by exposure to greater than 1,000 per million (ppm) of nitrous oxide. This scenario is highly unlikely in modern ORs, where inhalational anesthetics are scavenged, but it may occur

SH
|
CH₂ Homocysteine
|
CH₂
|
H₂N—C—H
|
COOH

5-Methyltetrahydrofolate

Methionine
synthase

N₂O
B₁₂
S-Adenosylmethionine (SAM)

CH₃
|
S
|
CH₂
|
CH₂ Methionine
|
H₂N—C—H
|
COOH

Tetrahydrofolate

FIGURE 65–2. Hematologic effects of exposure to nitrous oxide (N₂O) resemble those characteristic of pernicious anemia and are related to oxidation and inactivation of vitamin B₁₂. The irreversible blockade of methionine synthase impairs DNA synthesis and myelin production.

in poorly ventilated dental offices. This problem probably is underdiagnosed because the neurologic changes that occur in mild cases mimic other more common neurologic conditions.[11]

Immunologic Effects

Concern has been raised regarding detrimental effects of nitrous oxide on immune function. Nitrous oxide is associated with varied effects on immune function with evidence of decreased proliferation of human peripheral blood mononuclear cells and decreased neutrophil chemotaxis. The ENIGMA trial evaluated patients undergoing major surgery comparing nitrous oxide–based and nitrous oxide–free anesthesia, and showed an increase in secondary outcomes including wound infection, pneumonia, and atelectasis.[38] However, ENIGMA-II, the follow-up trial with a much larger sample size of

7,112 patients, did not demonstrate any differences in any of the previous reported results.[40]

Cardiovascular Effects

Concern over nitrous oxide and increased risk of cardiovascular complications is mostly theoretical. Nitrous oxide increases postoperative homocysteine concentrations and impairs endothelial function by inhibiting an enzyme that converts homocysteine to methionine.[39] Chronic homocysteinemia is associated with cardiovascular disease. Although the initial ENIGMA trial[38] showed an increase of long-term myocardial infarctions, the most recent ENIGMA-II, with a much larger sample size and a study design that specifically evaluated cardiovascular complications, did not demonstrate any difference (8% versus 8%; $P = 0.64$).[40]

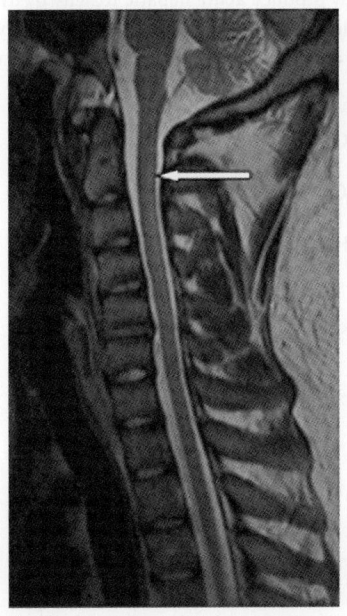
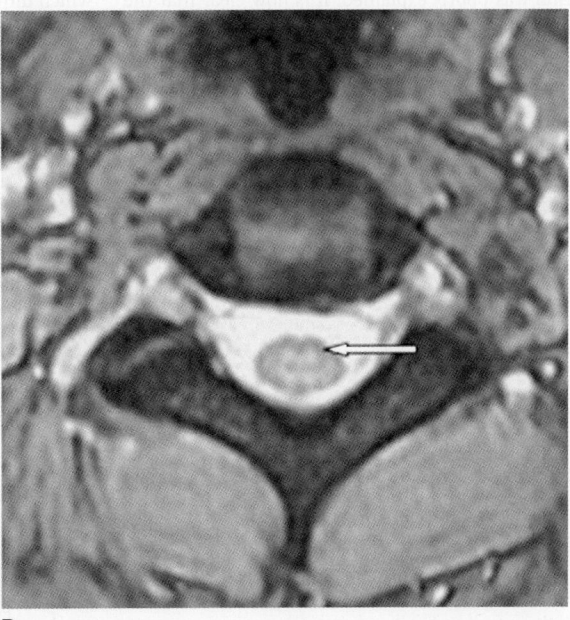

A **B**

FIGURE 65–3. Magnetic resonance imaging findings in a 19 year-old man with a 4-month history of nitrous oxide abuse who presented with gait imbalance, limb weakness, and numbness from the nipples to the toes. (**A**) T₂-weighted (4,000/120) sagittal image shows increased signal intensity (arrow) in the cervical spinal cord. (**B**) T₂-weighted (4,000/120) axial image shows (arrow) abnormal signal involvement in the posterior and anterior spinal cord columns.[24]

Treatment

General

Removal of the acutely affected person from the toxic environment should be the initial intervention in addition to ensuring adequate oxygenation and ventilation. Individuals who have developed toxicity from occupational exposure or abuse of the gas should be educated about the relationship between their activities and their clinical findings.

Specific

Acute overdose of nitrous oxide can lead to life-threatening hypoxia. Patients admitted with respiratory compromise should be administered supplemental oxygen and monitored for 24 hours. Supportive treatment such as intensive care unit (ICU) care and mechanical ventilation is warranted in the presence of severe respiratory failure.

The treatment regimen for the neurologic sequelae of vitamin B_{12} deficiency from nitrous oxide toxicity includes parenteral vitamin B_{12} and oral methionine. Vitamin B_{12} is recommended in a manner similar to that used in the treatment of pernicious anemia by either (1) intramuscular injection of 1,000 mcg vitamin B_{12} daily for 1 week followed by weekly injection of 1,000 mcg for 4 to 9 weeks and then monthly injection of 1,000 mcg until clinical resolution or (2) daily oral administration of 1,000 to 2,000 mcg of vitamin B_{12} until clinical resolution.[50]

Up to 20% of the population may have unrecognized vitamin B_{12} deficiency from dietary restriction, malabsorption, or autoimmune gastritis, which is exacerbated when exposed to nitrous oxide.[50] It is worth noting that in some of the early case reports, before recognition of vitamin B_{12} deficiency in nitrous oxide toxicity, many had improvement of symptoms simply after cessation. Methionine was also successfully used when vitamin B_{12} treatment alone failed to improve neurologic effects. There is no guideline for dosing vitamin B_{12} for patients with nitrous oxide toxicity, although case reports have used a 3-g daily oral regimen.[51]

The bone marrow abnormalities associated with nitrous oxide toxicity should be treated with a single 30-mg intravenous (IV) dose of folinic acid (Antidotes in Depth: A12).

HALOGENATED HYDROCARBONS

The volatile anesthetics which are liquids under standard conditions with a very high vapor pressure, were initially considered biochemically inert. Toxicity after administration was poorly explained. It is now clear that the metabolites of the inhalational anesthetics are responsible for acute and chronic toxicities, which are predictable and dose related.

Halothane Hepatitis

Two distinct types of hepatotoxicity are associated with halothane use. The first is a mild dysfunction that develops in approximately 20% of exposed patients. Patients often are asymptomatic but exhibit mild elevated serum aminotransferase concentrations within a few days after anesthetic exposure. Recovery is usually complete.[25] In contrast, appearance of serum aminotransferase concentrations above 10 times the upper normal limits indicates a life-threatening hepatitis that occurs in approximately 1 in 10,000 exposed patients and produces fatal massive hepatic necrosis in 1 in 35,000 patients.[4] Because the histologic findings of massive hepatocellular necrosis are indistinguishable from many of the causes of viral hepatitis,[55] differentiating halothane hepatitis from other causes of hepatitis in the postoperative period is difficult. Jaundice, which is common after anesthesia and surgery, can result from many factors such as preexisting liver disease, perioperative hypotension, blood transfusion, sepsis, or other causes of hepatitis. Thus, halothane hepatitis is a diagnosis of exclusion or inclusion based on the clinical history and time course.

Several studies report an association between multiple exposures to halothane and subsequent development of hepatitis.[48,54,59] In one study, 95% of cases of halothane hepatitis occurred after repeated exposures, 55% of which involve reexposure within 4 weeks.[59] Under these circumstances, hepatic dysfunction usually is more severe, and the latency before clinical presentation usually is shorter compared with the initial exposure.[54]

Obesity is a risk factor commonly implicated in halothane hepatotoxicity.[1,56] Increased fat stores act as a reservoir for halothane, with slow and prolonged release into the circulation and subsequent increase in production of potentially hepatotoxic metabolites.

Most cases of halothane hepatitis occur in middle-aged patients; with women having twice the risk.[25] Genetic factors likely play an important role in some patients, as indicated by a case report of this syndrome in three pairs of related Mexican women.[23]

Mechanism of Toxicity

Halothane is the most extensively metabolized inhalational anesthetic. Approximately 20% of the absorbed anesthetic undergoes oxidative metabolism, principally by CYP2E1 in the liver, to trifluoroacetic acid. Reduction to trifluorochloroethane and difluorochloroethylene is a minor route of halothane metabolism that requires the absence of oxygen and the presence of an electron donor (Fig. 65–4). These volatile metabolites are free radicals, which directly produce acute hepatic toxicity by irreversibly binding to and destroying hepatocellular structures. Alternatively, by acting as haptens, they trigger an immune-mediated hypersensitivity response.[45,57] The high

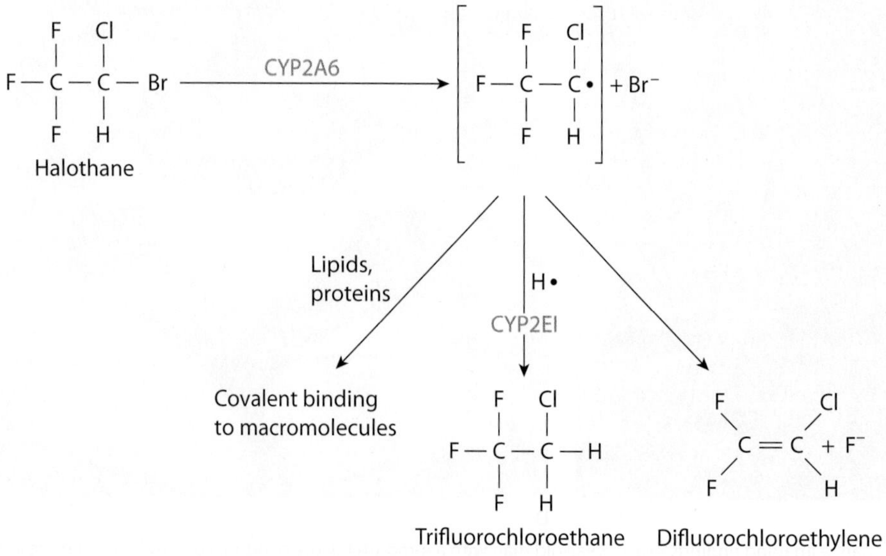

FIGURE 65–4. Reductive metabolism of halothane results in the formation of a reactive metabolite that may directly bind macromolecules and create neoantigens or undergo further metabolism to trifluorochloroethane and difluorochloroethylene. CYP = cytochrome P450.

percentage of patients with halothane hepatitis who had recent reexposure is most consistent with the latter mechanism in which the first exposure primes the development of antibodies to a haptenized protein.[25]

The use of halothane for inhalational anesthesia has markedly decreased in North America with the widespread availability of newer, safer halogenated anesthetics. Halothane is still widely used in some countries because it is inexpensive and provides a smooth induction of anesthesia.

Isoflurane and desflurane are pungent gases that can be airway irritants. Isoflurane, desflurane, and sevoflurane all appear to have low hepatotoxic potential. Rare case reports of hepatitis are still reported with all anesthetics but at a much lower incidence compared to halothane. Cross-sensitivity may exist, such that prior exposure to one anesthetic triggers hepatotoxicity upon subsequent exposure to a different anesthetic.

Nephrotoxicity

The kidneys are at risk for toxicity from modern inhalational anesthetics. Methoxyflurane is an anesthetic that was introduced in 1962. By 1966, this anesthetic was linked to the development of vasopressin-resistant polyuric renal insufficiency (nephrogenic diabetes insipidus) in 16 of 94 patients receiving prolonged methoxyflurane anesthesia for abdominal surgery (Chap. 27).[15] Polyuria was associated with a negative fluid balance, elevations of serum sodium and urea nitrogen concentrations, osmolality, and a fixed urinary osmolality approximating that of serum. Kidney abnormalities lasted from 10 to 20 days in most patients but persisted for more than one year in 3 of the 17 patients.[15] Subsequent studies demonstrated that kidney toxicity was caused by inorganic fluoride released during biotransformation of methoxyflurane.[53] The risk of toxicity was highly correlated with both the total dose of methoxyflurane (concentration times duration) and the peak serum fluoride concentration.[14] The nephrotoxic serum fluoride concentration is 50 to 60 μmol/L.[14] The factors that enhance biotransformation such as obesity and enzyme induction also increase the risk of toxicity. Although the precise mechanism by which fluoride produces its toxic effect in the kidneys is not clear, one hypothesis is that fluoride inhibits adenylate cyclase, thereby interfering with the normal action of antidiuretic hormone on the distal convoluted tubules.

Although methoxyflurane is no longer used, lessons learned regarding its toxicity are applicable when evaluating the nephrotoxic potential of other fluorinated anesthetics. Of the currently used anesthetics (halothane, isoflurane, desflurane, sevoflurane), only sevoflurane undergoes biotransformation by defluorination.

Approximately 5% of sevoflurane is metabolized by defluorination, occasionally resulting in sufficient serum fluoride concentrations to produce transient decreases in urine-concentrating ability.[27] However, clinically evident renal impairment almost never occurs with use of sevoflurane.[20] In volunteer studies, exposure to sevoflurane that resulted in high serum fluoride concentrations did not result in any urine concentrating defects. In patients with chronic kidney disease (CKD), the risk of postoperative kidney dysfunction is believed to be worse with exposure to inhalational anesthetics. However, studies demonstrate that deterioration of kidney function does not occur after exposure to desflurane and isoflurane,[32] possibly because intrarenal fluoride concentrations are more important than serum fluoride concentrations in the development of nephrotoxicity.

Sevoflurane reacts with the alkali within carbon dioxide absorbers to produce several degradation products, including a vinyl ether called compound A ($CF_2C(CF_3)OCH_2F$). Compound A causes renal tubular necrosis in rats, especially at the corticomedullary junction.[26,58] The extent of nephrotoxicity is determined by both the concentration of compound A and the duration of exposure. Compound A is also conjugated, and its breakdown products are nephrotoxic.

Technical Issues

Extensive clinical experience with several million patients who were exposed to sevoflurane and 4,000 closely studied volunteers failed to demonstrate

nephrotoxicity.[34] Higher concentrations of compound A are generated during low-flow anesthesia, use of high concentrations of sevoflurane, and increased temperature conditions. A high fresh-gas flow rate dilutes the concentration of compound A. Concern that higher compound A concentrations are generated when a low fresh-gas flow rate (eg, <2 L/min) is used in a closed circuit led to the current sevoflurane package labeling, which warns against fresh-gas flow rates below 2 L/min in a circle absorber system.[18]

Some controversy exists regarding the safety of low-flow sevoflurane anesthesia. Although there have been no clinical reports of sevoflurane- induced nephrotoxicity as measured by changes in blood urea nitrogen (BUN), serum creatinine, or creatinine clearance, clinical data demonstrate transient nephrotoxicity when more subtle measurements of glomerular and tubular function are used.[18,20,22] For example, when young, healthy patients without underlying kidney disease were anesthetized with low-flow sevoflurane for a mean of 6.7 hours, transient but statistically significant increases in urinary glucose and protein excretion were documented without any changes in BUN, creatinine, or creatinine clearance.[22] The clinical significance of such transient abnormalities in kidney function is uncertain. Regardless, it seems prudent to avoid the practice of low-flow sevoflurane in patients with CKD until clinical data document safety. Newer carbon dioxide absorbents that are free of strong alkali are now available to decrease compound A generation.

INHALATION ANESTHETIC–RELATED CARBON MONOXIDE POISONING
Pharmacology

Desflurane and isoflurane contain a difluoromethoxy moiety that can be degraded to carbon monoxide (CO). This process occasionally results in toxic exposure to patients. Carboxyhemoglobin levels as high as 36% were reported from intraoperative desflurane degradation.[8] Although there was no evidence of patient harm in this case, morbidity or mortality could occur at this level in patients (Chap. 122). The true incidence of carbon monoxide exposure during clinical anesthesia is unknown. Routine detection of intraoperative carbon monoxide exposure is now possible using multiwavelength pulse cooximeters, but these devices are not widely adopted, and conventional pulse oximeters used in ORs cannot detect carbon monoxide (Chaps. 28 and 122).[9]

Carbon monoxide production is inversely proportional to the water content of CO_2 absorbents. Soda lime (a granular mixture of calcium, sodium, and potassium hydroxide) is the most frequently used CO_2 absorbent. It is sold wet (13%–15% water by weight) but may dry with high gas-inflow rates, reducing its effectiveness at removing CO. Higher concentrations of carbon monoxide are most apt to be present during the first case after a weekend because of drying of CO_2 absorbent from a continuous inflow of dry oxygen if the anesthesia machine was not in use.[19]

Other factors influence the concentration of carbon monoxide resulting from anesthetic degradation, including temperature (higher temperature increases carbon monoxide formation), type of absorbent, choice of anesthetic, and concentration of anesthetic. Strong alkalis, such as potassium and sodium hydroxide, initiate the reaction that forms carbon monoxide.

Mass spectrometry (available in some ORs) cannot directly detect carbon monoxide because its molecular weight is equivalent to that of nitrogen, a gas usually present in much greater amounts. In addition, detection of carbon monoxide by fragmentation products is not possible by mass spectrometry because CO_2 is present in greater amounts and has similar fragmentation products.

Unfortunately, the diagnosis of carbon monoxide poisoning during anesthesia is difficult because the main clinical features of toxicity are masked by anesthesia, and no routinely available means can identify carbon monoxide within the breathing circuit or detect when the CO_2 absorbent is desiccated. Delayed neurologic sequelae from intraoperative carbon monoxide poisoning are typically missed on the anesthesiologist's postoperative patient evaluation because the delayed manifestations may develop days following the procedure.[61]

The product label of desflurane and isoflurane advises that the CO_2 absorbent should be replaced when a practitioner suspects the absorbent is desiccated. However, this warning fails to account for the lack of a reliable method of actionable data to determine when the absorbent is fully or partially desiccated.

If an anesthetic machine is found with the fresh-gas flow on at the beginning of the day, a reasonable practice is to replace the absorbent. Newer CO_2 absorbents that are less likely to degrade anesthetics are now available. These newer absorbents have decreased amounts of strong bases.

LONG-TERM USE OF HALOGENATED ANESTHETICS IN INTENSIVE CARE UNITS

Halogenated anesthetics have been used since the 1990s in ICUs for long-term sedation of patients receiving mechanical ventilation and more recently as part of the treatment for patients with refractory status epilepticus. Use is limited by concerns regarding atmospheric pollution, but also ambient ICU air, and high costs (because of a lack of rebreathing systems in the ICU). The development of anesthetic-conserving devices for use with ICU ventilators has addressed these issues. Potential advantages include more rapid wakeup and shorter times to extubation with minimal risk of toxicity.[35]

Clinical studies report the use of isoflurane and sevoflurane for ICU sedation. In one study, 19 patients were mechanically for more than 24 hours in the ICU with sevoflurane used for sedation.[35] Toxic effects of sevoflurane were not found even though serum fluoride concentrations often exceeded 50 μmol/L (the concentration suggested to be the nephrotoxic threshold).[14]

Isoflurane is being used as a first-choice for long-term sedation during mechanical ventilation in some ICUs. Experimental models demonstrate that isoflurane is potentially neurotoxic, primarily through induction of neuronal apoptosis. In rats, isoflurane substantially decreases local glucose utilization in various brain regions, including the thalamus. Reversible psychomotor dysfunction was reported in 3.6% of 335 patients who received isoflurane for more than 12 hours as a primary sedative during mechanical ventilation in a general ICU.[5] Psychomotor dysfunction occurred in 42% of patients aged 4 years or younger but in only 1.3% of patients older than 4 years.

Isoflurane is an alternate treatment for patients with refractory status epilepticus. Reversible MRI abnormalities developed in two patients who received inhaled isoflurane for a prolonged time (35 and 85 days).[21] Serial MRIs demonstrated the development of hyperintense T2 signals involving the medulla, cerebellar cortex, deep cerebellar nuclei, thalamus, and hypothalamus bilaterally. These abnormalities improved after discontinuation of the isoflurane.

CHRONIC EXPOSURE TO WASTE ANESTHETIC GASES

Waste anesthetic gases are defined as inhalation gases and vapors that are released into work areas associated with or adjacent to the administration of a gas or volatile liquid for anesthetic purposes. Because anesthesia machines are not airtight and consist of hundreds of parts, it is inevitable that clinical personnel will be exposed to waste anesthetic gases. Exposure to waste anesthetic gas produces short- and long-term effects. Common short-term effects are lethargy and fatigue in staff members who are exposed to significant quantities of waste anesthetic gas. Chronic long-term effects correlate with the concentration of gas and duration of exposure. Animal studies demonstrate that exposure to high concentrations of nitrous oxide and halogenated xenobiotics can cause cellular, mutagenic, carcinogenic, and teratogenic effects.

The US government has been involved with the regulation and management of waste anesthetic gas since 1970. The OR environment in the United States is highly regulated and monitored, but exposure limits vary in other countries and can exceed the concentrations permitted in the United States. Even in a modern working environment with low-leakage anesthesia machines, scavenging systems, and high room ventilation exchange rates, exposure to inhalational anesthetics could not be kept below acceptable threshold concentrations in all cases. However, a cause-and-effect relationship between human exposure to waste anesthetic gases and poor reproductive outcomes could not be identified in an analysis requested by the American Society of Anesthesiologists.[12]

Dentists and dental assistants are often exposed to greater concentrations of waste anesthetic gases than are individuals working in well-vented ORs. An epidemiologic survey compared 15,000 dentists who used nitrous oxide in their practices with 15,000 dentists who did not.[11] A 1.2- to 1.8-fold increase in hepatic, kidney, and neurologic disease was found in the dentists and their chair-side assistants who were chronically exposed to trace concentrations of nitrous oxide. For those with heavy office use of nitrous oxide, a fourfold increase in the incidence of neurologic complaints compared with the nonexposed group was observed. Female dental assistants who were exposed to nitrous oxide had a two- to threefold increase in spontaneous abortion rates, reduced fertility, and a higher rate of congenital abnormalities in their offspring.[11]

ABUSE OF HALOGENATED VOLATILE ANESTHETICS

Fatal or life-threatening complications occur when halogenated inhalational anesthetics are used for nonanesthetic purposes such as suicide attempts, mood elevation, and topical treatment of herpes simplex labialis.

When ingested, halothane, a volatile liquid, usually produces gastroenteritis with vomiting followed by depressed levels of consciousness, hypotension, hypothermia, shallow breathing, respiratory failure, and bradycardia with varying degrees of heart block and extrasystoles. A depressed level of consciousness is attributed to large amount halothane that is absorbed from gastric mucosa, which also causes systemic vasodilation resulting in hypotension and hypothermia.[16,60] The diagnosis should be suspected when these features occur in a patient with the sweet or fruity odor of halothane on the breath. If suspected, nasogastric lavage is recommended to remove the reminder of halothane that is still in the stomach. Case reports have used ice-cold saline for hourly gastric lavage with success. The gastric aspirate also smelled of halothane.[60] Supportive care, including mechanical ventilation, fluid and electrolyte resuscitation, inotropic support, electrolytes correction, antidysrhythmics, normothermia, and antibiotics, should be provided. Full recovery can occur without permanent organ injury.

Intravenous injections of halothane may occur as a suicide attempt or unintentionally during anesthesia induction. A young patient who was found unconscious and hypotensive with ARDS after self-administered IV injection of halothane was unable to be resuscitated.[7] A 16-year-old girl received an unintentional IV injection of 2.5 mL of halothane during anesthesia induction.[52] She became unconscious and apneic within 30 seconds but began to awaken within 2 to 3 minutes. Four hours later, she developed ARDS but subsequently made a full recovery.

Transient coma and apnea probably are secondary to a halothane bolus reaching the brain on its first pass through the bloodstream. Redistribution then occurs, explaining the rapid awakening. The ARDS that develops after injection of halothane most likely results from a direct toxic effect of high concentrations of the hydrocarbon on the pulmonary vasculature. After injection, the anesthetic likely travels as a bolus during the first passage through the pulmonary circulation because of its poor solubility in blood.

Hospital personnel are involved in most reported cases of halothane abuse by inhalation.[49] Inhalation of halothane produces a pleasurable sensation similar to that described with other inhaled hydrocarbons, such as the solvents in glue and paint (Chap. 81). Death may result from upper airway obstruction after loss of consciousness or from dysrhythmias. Death occurred in a student nurse anesthetist suggested to have applied a full 250-mL bottle of enflurane over 3 hours to "cold sores" on her lower lip.[31]

SUMMARY

- Inhalational anesthetics remain a popular choice for maintenance of anesthesia due to their safety profile and titratability. Toxicity is uncommon when properly administered and monitored.
- Health care practitioners who use inhaled anesthetics should be knowledgeable about their pharmacology and potential toxicity.

- Nitrous oxide abuse, typically in the form of "whippets," is common and can lead acutely to life-threatening hypoxia. It causes bone marrow suppression and disabling polyneuropathy with chronic abuse. Treatment is supportive in acute setting, and patients with long-term hematologic and neurologic sequelae are treated with vitamin B_{12}, methionine, and folinic acid.

- Halothane, an older halogenated hydrocarbon, is no longer used in North America but is still in widespread use around the world and is associated with fulminant hepatitis.

- Sevoflurane is associated with production of compound A, which can cause renal tubular necrosis; however, it is not shown to cause acute kidney injury in vivo.

- Abuse of halogenated volatile anesthetics is rare; treatment is supportive.

Acknowledgment

Martin Griffel, MD, contributed to this chapter in previous editions.

REFERENCES

1. Abernethy DR, Greenblatt DJ. Pharmacokinetics of drugs in obesity. *Clin Pharmacokinet.* 1982;7:108-124.
2. Amess JA, et al. Megaloblastic haemopoiesis in patients receiving nitrous oxide. *Lancet.* 1978;2:339-342.
3. Amos RJ, et al. Incidence and pathogenesis of acute megaloblastic bone-marrow change in patients receiving intensive care. *Lancet.* 1982;2:835-838.
4. Anonymous. Summary of the national Halothane Study. Possible association between halothane anesthesia and postoperative hepatic necrosis. *JAMA.* 1966;197:775-88.
5. Ariyama J, et al. Risk factors for the development of reversible psychomotor dysfunction following prolonged isoflurane inhalation in the general intensive care unit. *J Clin Anesth.* 2009;21:567-573.
6. Baird PA. Occupational exposure to nitrous oxide--not a laughing matter. *N Engl J Med.* 1992;327:1026-1027.
7. Berman P, Tattersall M. Self-poisoning with intravenous halothane. *Lancet.* 1982;1:340.
8. Berry PD, et al. Severe carbon monoxide poisoning during desflurane anesthesia. *Anesthesiology.* 1999;90:613-616.
9. Bledsoe BE, et al. Use of pulse co-oximetry as a screening and monitoring tool in mass carbon monoxide poisoning. *Prehosp Emerg Care.* 2010;14:131-133.
10. Bouche MP, et al. No compound a formation with Superia during minimal-flow sevoflurane anesthesia: a comparison with Sofnolime. *Anesth Analg.* 2002;95:1680-1685, table of contents.
11. Brodsky JB, et al. Exposure to nitrous oxide and neurologic disease among dental professionals. *Anesth Analg.* 1981;60:297-301.
12. Buring JE, et al. Health experiences of operating room personnel. *Anesthesiology.* 1985;62:325-330.
13. Campagna JA, et al. Mechanisms of actions of inhaled anesthetics. *N Engl J Med.* 2003;348:2110-2124.
14. Cousins MJ, Mazze RI. Methoxyflurane nephrotoxicity. A study of dose response in man. *JAMA.* 1973;225:1611-1616.
15. Crandell WB, et al. Nephrotoxicity associated with methoxyflurane anesthesia. *Anesthesiology.* 1966;27:591-607.
16. Curelaru I, et al. A case of recovery from coma produced by the ingestion of 250 ml of halothane. *Br J Anaesth.* 1968;40:283-288.
17. DiMaio VJ, Garriott JC. Four deaths resulting from abuse of nitrous oxide. *J Forensic Sci.* 1978;23:169-172.
18. Eger EI 2nd, et al. Dose-related biochemical markers of renal injury after sevoflurane versus desflurane anesthesia in volunteers. *Anesth Analg.* 1997;85:1154-1163.
19. Fang ZX, et al. Carbon monoxide production from degradation of desflurane, enflurane, isoflurane, halothane, and sevoflurane by soda lime and Baralyme. *Anesth Analg.* 1995;80:1187-1193.
20. Frink EJ Jr, et al. Renal concentrating function with prolonged sevoflurane or enflurane anesthesia in volunteers. *Anesthesiology.* 1994;80:1019-1025.
21. Fugate JE, et al. Prolonged high-dose isoflurane for refractory status epilepticus: is it safe? *Anesth Analg.* 2010;111:1520-1524.
22. Higuchi H, et al. Effects of sevoflurane and isoflurane on renal function and on possible markers of nephrotoxicity. *Anesthesiology.* 1998;89:307-322.
23. Hoft RH, et al. Halothane hepatitis in three pairs of closely related women. *N Engl J Med.* 1981;304:1023-1024.
24. Hsu CK, et al. Myelopathy and polyneuropathy caused by nitrous oxide toxicity: a case report. *Am J Emerg Med.* 2012;30:1016 e3-6.
25. Inman WH, Mushin WW. Jaundice after repeated exposure to halothane: a further analysis of reports to the Committee on Safety of Medicines. *Br Med J.* 1978;2:1455-1456.
26. Kandel L, et al. Nephrotoxicity in rats undergoing a one-hour exposure to compound A. *Anesth Analg.* 1995;81:559-563.
27. Kobayashi Y, et al. Serum and urinary inorganic fluoride concentrations after prolonged inhalation of sevoflurane in humans. *Anesth Analg.* 1992;74:753-757.
28. Lassen HC, et al. Treatment of tetanus; severe bone-marrow depression after prolonged nitrous-oxide anaesthesia. *Lancet.* 1956;270:527-530.
29. Layzer RB, et al. Neuropathy following abuse of nitrous oxide. *Neurology.* 1978;28:504-506.
30. Leslie K, et al. Nitrous oxide and long-term morbidity and mortality in the ENIGMA trial. *Anesth Analg.* 2011;112:387-393.
31. Lingenfelter RW. Fatal misuse of enflurane. *Anesthesiology.* 1981;55:603.
32. Litz RJ, et al. Renal responses to desflurane and isoflurane in patients with renal insufficiency. *Anesthesiology.* 2002;97:1133-1136.
33. Lugli AK, et al. Anaesthetic mechanisms: update on the challenge of unravelling the mystery of anaesthesia. *Eur J Anaesthesiol.* 2009;26:807-820.
34. Mazze RI, Jamison R. Renal effects of sevoflurane. *Anesthesiology.* 1995;83:443-445.
35. Mesnil M, et al. Long-term sedation in intensive care unit: a randomized comparison between inhaled sevoflurane and intravenous propofol or midazolam. *Intensive Care Med.* 2011;37:933-941.
36. Messina FV, Wynne JW. Homemade nitrous oxide: no laughing matter. *Ann Intern Med.* 1982;96:333-334.
37. Meyer KH. Contributions to the theory of narcosis. *Trans Faraday Soc.* 1937;33:1062-1063.
38. Myles PS, et al. Avoidance of nitrous oxide for patients undergoing major surgery: a randomized controlled trial. *Anesthesiology.* 2007;107:221-231.
39. Myles PS, et al. Effect of nitrous oxide on plasma homocysteine and folate in patients undergoing major surgery. *Br J Anaesth.* 2008;100:780-786.
40. Myles PS, et al. The safety of addition of nitrous oxide to general anaesthesia in at-risk patients having major non-cardiac surgery (ENIGMA-II): a randomised, single-blind trial. *Lancet.* 2014; 384:1446-1454.
41. Neuberger J, Williams R. Halothane hepatitis. *Dig Dis.* 1988;6:52-64.
42. Nunn JF. Clinical aspects of the interaction between nitrous oxide and vitamin B12. *Br J Anaesth.* 1987;59:3-13..
43. Nunn JF, et al. Megaloblastic bone marrow changes after repeated nitrous oxide anaesthesia. Reversal with folinic acid. *Br J Anaesth.* 1986;58:1469-1470.
44. O'Sullivan H, et al. Human bone marrow biochemical function and megaloblastic hematopoiesis after nitrous oxide anesthesia. *Anesthesiology.* 1981;55:645-649.
45. Pohl LR, Gillette JR. A perspective on halothane-induced hepatotoxicity. *Anesth Analg.* 1982;61:809-811.
46. Potocka-Banas B, et al. Death caused by addictive inhalation of nitrous oxide. *Hum Exp Toxicol.* 2011;30:1875-1877.
47. Preckel B, et al. Molecular mechanisms transducing the anesthetic, analgesic, and organ-protective actions of xenon. *Anesthesiology.* 2006;105:187-197.
48. Scott JM, et al. Pathogenesis of subacute combined degeneration: a result of methyl group deficiency. *Lancet.* 1981;2:334-337.
49. Spencer JD, et al. Halothane abuse in hospital personnel. *JAMA.* 1976;235:1034-1035.
50. Stabler, S.P., Clinical practice. Vitamin B12 deficiency. *N Engl J Med.* 2013;368:149-160.
51. Stacy CB, et al. Methionine in the treatment of nitrous-oxide-induced neuropathy and myeloneuropathy. *J Neurol.* 1992;239:401-403.
52. Sutton J, et al. Accidental intravenous injection of halothane. Case report. *Br J Anaesth.* 1971;43:513-520.
53. Taves DR, et al. Toxicity following methoxyflurane anesthesia. II. Fluoride concentrations in nephrotoxicity. *JAMA.* 1970;214:91-95.
54. Touloukian J, Kaplowitz N. Halothane-induced hepatic disease. *Semin Liver Dis.* 1981;1:134-142.
55. Uzunalimoglu B, et al. The liver in mild halothane hepatitis. Light and electron microscopic findings with special reference to the mononuclear cell infiltrate. *Am J Pathol.* 1970;61:457-478.
56. Vaughan RW. Biochemical and biotransformation alterations in obesity. *Contemp Anesth Pract.* 1982;5:55-70.
57. Vergani D, et al. Sensitisation to halothane-altered liver components in severe hepatic necrosis after halothane anaesthesia. *Lancet.* 1978;2:801-803.
58. Versichelen LF, et al. Only carbon dioxide absorbents free of both NaOH and KOH do not generate compound A during in vitro closed-system sevoflurane: evaluation of five absorbents. *Anesthesiology.* 2001;95:750-755.
59. Walton B, et al. Unexplained hepatitis following halothane. *Br Med J.* 1976;1:1171-1176.
60. Wig J, et al. Coma following ingestion of halothane. Its successful management. *Anaesthesia.* 1983;38:552-555.
61. Woehlck HJ, et al. Reduction in the incidence of carbon monoxide exposures in humans undergoing general anesthesia. *Anesthesiology.* 1997;87:228-234.

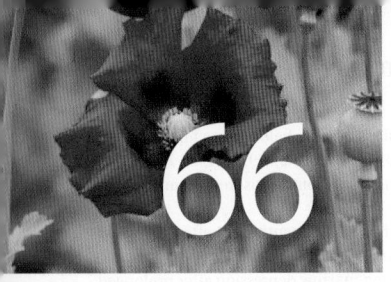

66 NEUROMUSCULAR BLOCKERS

Caitlin J. Guo and Kenneth M. Sutin

HISTORY AND EPIDEMIOLOGY

Curare is the generic term for the resinous arrowhead poisons used to paralyze hunted animals.[116] The curare alkaloids are derived from the bark of the *Strychnos* vine, and the most potent alkaloids, the toxiferines, are derived from *Strychnos toxifera*. Fortunately for the hunters who used curare, ingestion of their prey did not cause paralysis. Sir Walter Raleigh discovered the use of curare in Guyana in 1595, and he was the first person to bring curare to Europe. Curare played a pivotal role in the discovery of the mechanism of neuromuscular transmission. In 1844, Claude Bernard placed a small piece of dry curare under the skin of a live frog and observed that the frog became limp and died.[8] He performed an immediate autopsy and discovered that the heart was beating. Because direct muscle stimulation produced contraction but nerve stimulation did not, Bernard concluded that curare paralyzed the motor nerves. He later observed, however, that bathing the isolated nerve did not affect neuromuscular transmission, leading him to conclude: "Curare must act on the terminal plates of motor nerves."[18] Curare was used by Nobel Laureate physiologists Charles Sherrington, John Eccles, and Bernard Katz to further elucidate neuromuscular physiology. Its first clinical use was described in 1878 when Hunter used curare to treat patients with tetanus and seizures.[116] In 1932, Raynard West used curare to reduce the muscular rigidity of hemiplegia.[116]

Curare (d-tubocurarine) was introduced into clinical anesthesia in 1943 by Harold Griffith and Enid Johnson.[43] Endotracheal intubation during general anesthesia was not common those days, so d-tubocurarine was administered in a dose that spared the diaphragm and maintained spontaneous ventilation. It was not until 1954 when Henry Beecher found that patients receiving d-tubocurarine had a sixfold increase in respiratory-related anesthesia mortality that artificial ventilation and reversal of residual d-tubocurarine became a routine practice.[9] Use of d-tubocurarine spanned almost 40 years until it was replaced by superior nondepolarizing neuromuscular blockers that caused less histamine release and hypotension.

Around the same time in the 1950s that curare gained popularity in the operating room, succinylcholine also came to clinical use to facilitate orotracheal intubation.[9] In the nonmedical world, succinylcholine carried a reputation of being the "person poison."[3] This came to media attention when a high-profile killing case involving an anesthesiologist Dr. Carl Coppolino and his mistress were accused of murdering his wife and the mistress's husband in 1966 and 1967, respectively, by injecting succinylcholine.[77] In 1983, shortly after Dr. Michael Swango began his internship at Ohio State University Hospital, patients began dying inexplicably, and he was relieved of his duties.[109] Following switching residencies and jobs for 14 years, prosecutors secured Swango's guilty plea for the murder of three victims. The toxicological analysis of the 7-year-old remains of Thomas Sammarco revealed succinylcholine in the liver and gallbladder and its metabolite succinylmonocholine in multiple organs, which assisted in the conviction.

With the advent of new modalities of drug delivery, toxicologists must be attuned to possible malicious intent. Emergency personnel responding to a 911 call observed the widow removing an insulin pump reservoir from her dead husband's body with the stated intent to donate the costly equipment.[5] A natural cause of death was presumed, yet surprisingly, forensic analysis revealed etomidate and laudanosine (a metabolite of atracurium) in the victim's liver.

Understanding the pharmacokinetics and pharmacodynamics of the depolarizing and nondepolarizing neuromuscular blockers (NDNMBs) is critical to maximizing benefit while minimizing toxicity.

MECHANISM OF NEUROMUSCULAR TRANSMISSION AND BLOCK

The purpose of a NMB is to selectively and reversibly inhibit signal transmission at the skeletal neuromuscular junction (NMJ). All NMBs possess at least one positively charged quaternary ammonium moiety that binds to the postsynaptic nicotinic acetylcholine (nACh) receptor at the NMJ, inhibiting its normal activation by acetylcholine (ACh). The nACh receptor is a ligand-gated ion channel that consists of 4 different protein subunits in a pentameric structure surrounding a central channel. The nACh receptor found in human skeletal muscle is present in 2 primary forms: a mature type found at the NMJ ($\alpha 1_2 \beta \epsilon \delta$) or as a fetal (immature) type found on muscle at extrajunctional regions of the muscle fiber ($\alpha 1_2 \beta \gamma \delta$). Figure 66–1 provides an overview normal neuromuscular transmission and excitation–contraction coupling.

Skeletal muscle paralysis can occur by several mechanisms. For example, tetrodotoxin blocks voltage-sensitive sodium channels, preventing action potential conduction in the motor neuron (Chap. 39). On the other hand, botulinum toxin blocks ACh release from the presynaptic neuron by inhibiting the binding of ACh-containing vesicles to the neuronal membrane in the region of the synaptic cleft (Chap. 38). Modulation of postsynaptic ACh receptor activity at the NMJ may produce paralysis by one of two mechanisms: depolarizing (phase I block) and nondepolarizing (phase II block). Succinylcholine is the only depolarizing neuromuscular blocker (DNMB) in current clinical use. High doses of nicotine also cause a depolarizing block. All other drugs discussed are NDNMBs.

The process of DNMB requires several steps. First, two molecules of succinylcholine must bind to each α site of the nACh receptor. This action causes a prolonged open state of the nACh receptor ion channel. The initial depolarization generates a muscle action potential and usually causes brief contractions (fasciculations). In contrast to ACh, succinylcholine is not hydrolyzed efficiently by acetylcholinesterase (AChE) located in the synaptic cleft. Thus, the effect of succinylcholine lasts much longer than ACh. Succinylcholine persistence at the ACh receptor causes a sustained local muscle endplate depolarization that, in turn, causes the voltage-gated sodium channel in the perijunctional region to remain in a prolonged inactive state, inducing a desensitization block. The muscle is temporarily refractory to presynaptic release of further ACh (phase I block).

The NDNMBs cause skeletal muscle paralysis by competitively inhibiting the effects of ACh and thus preventing muscle depolarization. One molecule of an NDNMB bound to a single nACh receptor (also on the α site) is sufficient to competitively inhibit normal channel activation. Because the NDNMBs do not block voltage-gated sodium channels on the skeletal muscle membrane, direct electrical stimulation with a current sufficient to cause membrane depolarization will still elicit a muscular contraction. The NDNMBs are classified by duration of action as ultra-short, short, intermediate, and long. They are also classified by chemical structure as either a synthetic benzylisoquinolinium or an aminosteroid (Table 66–1).

The NDNMBs also block nACh receptors on the prejunctional nerve terminal and inhibit ACh-stimulated ACh production and release by blocking local autoregulation of available ACh.[98] This effect reduces the available pool of ACh and augments the extent of neuromuscular block.[11]

PHARMACOKINETICS

The NMBs are highly water soluble and relatively insoluble in lipids. Thus, they are rapidly distributed in the extracellular space and very slowly permeate lipid membranes such as the gut, placenta, and the normal blood–brain

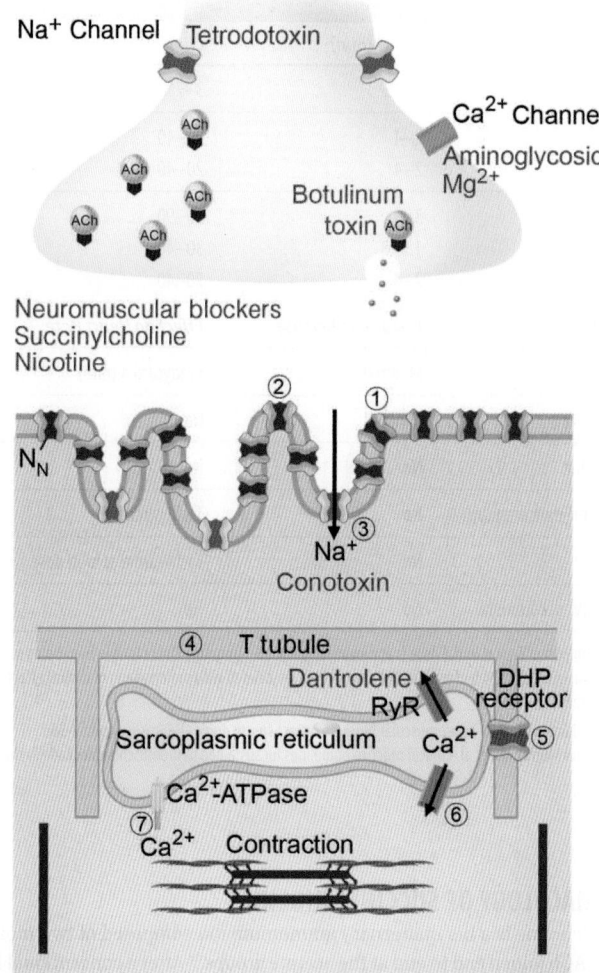

FIGURE 66–1. Excitation–contraction coupling in skeletal muscle. At the neuromuscular junction, acetylcholine (2) released from the presynaptic nerve terminal crosses the 50-nm synaptic cleft to reach the nicotinic acetylcholine (nACh) receptor (1). When an agonist simultaneously occupies both receptor sites, this ion channel opens, becoming nonselectively permeable to monovalent cations, resulting in an influx of Na^+ and an efflux of K^+. This produces local membrane depolarization (endplate potential), which in turn opens voltage-gated Na^+ channels (3). A depolarization of sufficient amplitude generates a propagated muscle action potential (MAP), which is conducted along the muscle membrane and down the transverse (T) tubules (4). In the T tubule, the MAP triggers a voltage-gated calcium channel (7) and the dihydropyridine receptor (5), which then activates the skeletal muscle ryanodine receptor/channel (6). To allow the fastest activation of mammalian skeletal muscle, calcium diffusion is not necessary for activation of the type 1 ryanodine receptor (RyR-1); instead, there is a direct electrical (protein) linkage between the dihydropyridine (DHP) receptor and the ryanodine receptor.[33] Active ATPase-driven calcium reuptake terminates muscle contraction. Many factors influence the activity of the RyR-1 channel, including Ca^{2+}, Mg^{2+}, and xenobiotics such as inhalational anesthetics that accelerate Ca^{2+} release in persons susceptible to malignant hyperthermia. Antagonists such as conotoxin are red and agonists such as nicotine are green.

barrier. For this reason, they are devoid of central nervous system (CNS) effects. Because these drugs distribute in the extracellular space, their dose is based on ideal body mass. Thus, in obese patients, estimation of drug requirement based on total body mass results in the administration of an excessive dose.

The speed of onset of an NMB is inversely related to its molar potency (ie, ED_{95} expressed as moles NMB drug per kilogram body weight).[59,60] Stated differently, the greater the affinity of the NDNMB for the ACh receptor, the fewer molecules per kilogram of tissue are required to produce a given degree of ACh receptor occupancy. Atracurium is the only NDNMB that does not

follow this generalization because it is a mixture of 10 isomers, each having a unique receptor affinity (cisatracurium consists of only one isomer).

In general, small, fast-contracting muscles such as the extraocular muscles are more susceptible to neuromuscular block than are larger, slower muscles such as the diaphragm. This is the so-called *respiratory-sparing effect*. After an intravenous (IV) bolus of NDNMB, paralysis of the diaphragm is coincident with paralysis of laryngeal muscles because high tissue perfusion results in rapid drug distribution and diffusion into the NMJ of all tissues.[25] However, recovery from NMB is fastest for the diaphragm and intercostal muscles; intermediate for the large muscles of the trunk and extremities; and slowest for the adductor pollicis, larynx, pharynx, and extraocular muscles.[25]

COMPLICATIONS OF NEUROMUSCULAR BLOCKERS

Complications associated with the use of NMBs include (1) problems associated with the care of a paralyzed patient (eg, inability to secure a definitive airway, undetected hypoventilation resulting from ventilator or airway problems, impaired ability to monitor neurologic function, unintentional patient awareness, peripheral nerve injury, deep vein thrombosis, and skin breakdown); (2) immediate side effects; and (3) delayed effects occurring after prolonged drug exposure.[85,86]

Consciousness

Even though NMBs do not affect consciousness, misconceptions about these drugs persist.[73] The pupillary light reflex, an important indicator of midbrain function, is preserved in healthy subjects who receive NDNMBs because pupillary function is mediated by muscarinic cholinergic receptors, for which the NMBs have no affinity.[42]

Histamine Release

Neuromuscular blockers may elicit dose- and injection rate–related nonimmunologic (non–IgE-mediated) histamine release from tissue mast cells by an uncertain mechanism (Table 66–1). The NMBs most commonly associated with histamine release are atracurium and succinylcholine.[81]

Anaphylaxis

Anaphylactic reactions are rare, with an incidence of 1 in 3,500 to 1 in 20,000 and up to 60% are related to NMBs.[81] Part of this variability is due to difficulty in determining the exact exposures in the operative setting when numerous xenobiotics and, blood products NMBs are administered simultaneously. Rocuronium and succinylcholine are the two most cited offenders among all NMB-associated anaphylaxis.[66,115]

Control of Respiration

At subparalyzing doses, NDNMBs blunt the peripheral hypoxic ventilatory response (HVR) but not the ventilatory response to hypercapnia.[30,31] Hypoxic ventilatory response returns to normal when chemical paralysis is completely reversed. Hypoventilation resulting from blunting of the HVR, especially when combined with the residual effects of other xenobiotics used during anesthesia such as opioids or inhalational anesthetics, causes delayed respiratory failure after general anesthesia.

Autonomic Side Effects

Nicotinic ACh receptors found in autonomic ganglia, similar to those at the NMJ, are pentamers composed of α and β subunits. In general, they are less susceptible to block by NMBs.[74] There is one notable exception. At the same dose that produces neuromuscular block, tubocurarine also blocks nACh receptors at the parasympathetic ganglia, causing tachycardia, and at the sympathetic ganglia, blunting the sympathetic response.[102] In combination with tubocurarine-related histamine release, the sympathetic block causes significant hypotension, particularly in patients with heart failure or hypovolemia.[11] This is an important reason why tubocurarine is no longer available in the United States.

The muscarinic receptors (M_1–M_5) are members of the seven-transmembrane G-protein–coupled receptor family. As such, they are structurally unique and mostly unaffected by NMBs. At clinical doses, pancuronium

TABLE 66–1	Pharmacology of Selected Neuromuscular Blockers					
Generic Name	Class	Duration	Initial Dose (mg/kg)[a,b]	Onset (min)[c]	Clinical Duration (min)[d]	
Succinylcholine	Depolarizer	Ultrashort	0.6–1	1–1.5	3–7	
Atracurium	Nondepolarizer, benzylisoquinolinium	Intermediate	0.4	2–4	20–40	
Cisatracurium		Intermediate	0.1	2–4	20–40	
Pancuronium	Nondepolarizer, aminosteroid	Long	0.1	3–6	60–90	
Rocuronium		Intermediate	0.6	1.5–3	30–40	
Vecuronium		Intermediate	0.1	2–4	20–40	
	Renal Excretion (%)[e]	Biliary Excretion (%)[f]	Metabolite	Histamine Release	Effect on Heart Rate	
Succinylcholine	<10	Minimal	Succinic acid	Minimal	Bradycardia (rare)	
Atracurium	5–10	Minimal	Laudanosine	Minimal	No	
Cisatracurium	10–20	Minimal	Laudanosine	No	No	
Pancuronium	40–60	10–20	3-Desacetyl-pancuronium[g]	No	Tachycardia	
Rocuronium	10–20	50–70	No	No	Tachycardia at high dose	
Vecuronium	15–25	40–70	3-Desacetyl-vecuronium[c]	No	No	

[a]Cisatracurium is labeled as milligram of base per milliliter. Other drugs are labeled and packaged as milligram of salt per milliliter. [b]Typical initial dose is approximately $2 \times ED_{95}$ (mg/kg). [c]Onset is time from bolus to 100% block. [d]Clinical duration is time from drug injection until 25% recovery of single twitch height. [e]Percent renal excretion in the first 24 h of unchanged drug; if high, associated with prolongation of clinical effect. [f]Percent biliary excretion in first 24 h of unchanged drug; if high, associated with prolongation of clinical effect. [g]Active metabolite.

Data from Donati F. Neuromuscular blocking drugs for the new millennium: current practice, future trends—comparative pharmacology of neuromuscular blocking drugs. *Anesth Analg.* 2000;90(suppl):S2-S6; McManus MC. Neuromuscular blockers in surgery and intensive care, part 1. *Am J Health Syst Pharm.* 2001;58:2287-2299; and Murray MJ, et al. Clinical practice guidelines for sustained neuromuscular blockade in the adult critically ill patient. *Crit Care Med.* 2002;30:142-156.

elicits dose- and injection rate–related increases in heart rate, blood pressure, cardiac output, and sympathetic tone.[26,103,110] This is attributed to a selective block of parasympathetic transmission at the cardiac muscarinic receptors, an atropine-like effect,[103] block of presynaptic (feedback) muscarinic receptors at sympathetic nerve terminals, and perhaps an indirect norepinephrine-releasing effect at postganglionic fibers.[26]

Dysrhythmias such as bradycardia, junctional rhythms, ventricular dysrhythmias, and asystole occur rarely after use of succinylcholine. Dysrhythmias most likely result from stimulation of the cardiac muscarinic receptors and can be prevented by pretreatment with 15 to 20 mcg/kg of IV atropine. Bradycardia is uncommon, but it may be especially severe in children during anesthetic induction when large or repeated doses of succinylcholine are given.

INTERACTIONS OF NEUROMUSCULAR BLOCKERS WITH OTHER XENOBIOTICS AND PATHOLOGIC CONDITIONS

The NMBs have significant interactions with many xenobiotics and coexisting medical conditions. These interactions affect the neuromuscular system at any level from the CNS to the muscle itself (Table 66–2).[94,114]

In most neuromuscular diseases, such as muscular dystrophy, Guillain-Barré syndrome, myasthenia gravis, and postpolio syndrome, the sensitivity to NDNMB is increased, so a small dose of NMB produces a profound degree of block.[2,13,45] However, persons with myasthenia gravis typically demonstrate resistance to the effects of succinylcholine.[2,13] In individuals with myopathy in whom the specific cause is not yet known, succinylcholine should be avoided because of the possible sensitivity to malignant hyperthermia (MH), hyperkalemia, or rhabdomyolysis. In place of succinylcholine, a short-acting NDNMB can be used to lessen the chance of prolonged weakness.

Many pathologic conditions potentiate the duration or intensity of NDNMB, such as respiratory acidosis, hypokalemia, hypocalcemia, hypermagnesemia, hypophosphatemia, hypothermia, shock, and liver or kidney failure.[97] Alternatively, acute sepsis and inflammatory conditions are associated with mild resistance to the effect of NDNMB.[88]

PHARMACOLOGY OF SUCCINYLCHOLINE

Succinylcholine is a bis-quaternary ammonium ion composed of two molecules of ACh joined end to end at the acetate groups.[28] After a conventional IV induction dose of 1 mg/kg, typical plasma concentrations are approximately 62 mcg/mL.[90]

Succinylcholine is hydrolyzed primarily by plasma cholinesterase (PChE, also known as pseudocholinesterase or butyrylcholinesterase; BChE, EC 3.1.1.8) and to a slight extent by alkaline hydrolysis. Hydrolysis is a two-step reaction; first succinylmonocholine and choline are formed, and then succinic acid and choline are formed. The latter two are normal products of intermediary metabolism. The first reaction is approximately six times faster than the second reaction. Less than 3% of the administered dose is excreted unchanged in the urine.[40] After an IV bolus, the plasma succinylcholine concentration increases abruptly, and there is a rapid onset of NMJ block. Later, the plasma succinylcholine concentration undergoes a rapid decline as a result of drug redistribution to extravascular tissues and hydrolysis in plasma. Finally, succinylcholine leaves the NMJ to reenter the plasma as a result of reversal of the concentration gradient.[39,55]

At an induction dose of 1 mg/kg IV, succinylcholine theoretically increases cerebral blood flow, cortical electrical activity, intracranial pressure (ICP),[61] and intraocular pressure, but the clinical implication is unclear. Most data come from small nonrandomized studies involving ICP, and results are mixed. In addition, there has not been sufficient evidence that supports routine use of NDMBs as a pretreatment for succinylcholine.

TOXICITY OF SUCCINYLCHOLINE

The important adverse drug reactions associated with succinylcholine include anaphylaxis, prolonged drug effect, hyperkalemia, acute rhabdomyolysis in patients with muscular dystrophy, MH in susceptible patients, masseter spasms or trismus in patients with congenital myopathies, and cardiac dysrhythmias. This is especially relevant for children who present with undiagnosed or a cyclically subtle myopathy.

TABLE 66–2 Effect of Prior Administration of Xenobiotics on Subsequent Response to Succinylcholine or Nondepolarizing Neuromuscular Blockers

Xenobiotic	Response to Succinylcholine	Response to Nondepolarizer	Comments
Aminoglycosides (eg, amikacin, gentamicin)	Potentiates	Potentiates	Dose-related decrease in presynaptic ACh release. Decrease postjunctional response to ACh. Partially reversible with calcium administration. The ability of neostigmine to reverse this effect is unpredictable.
Anticholinesterase, peripherally acting: neostigmine, edrophonium	Prolongs succinylcholine (except edrophonium)	No effect	Neostigmine, pyridostigmine, and physostigmine inhibit plasma AChE and prolong succinylcholine block. Edrophonium does not inhibit plasma cholinesterase.
Anticholinesterase, centrally acting: donepezil	Potentiates	No effect	Inhibits AChE (junctional ≫ plasma); long half-life (70 h).
β-Adrenergic antagonist: propranolol	Potentiates in cats, effects in humans uncertain	Potentiates	When given alone, unmasks myasthenic syndrome. Blocks ACh binding at postsynaptic membrane. Reversal of block with neostigmine causes severe bradycardia.
β-Adrenergic antagonist: esmolol	? Mild prolongation	Slows onset of rocuronium	Competes for PChE or red blood cell cholinesterase.
Botulinum toxin	?	Early potentiation, delayed resistance	Subclinical systemic denervation leads to hypersensitivity.
Calcium channel blockers	Potentiates	Potentiates	Causes calcium channel block pre- and postjunctionally. Verapamil has local cholinesterase inhibitor effect on nerve. Inhibits block reversal of NDNMBs by cholinesterase inhibitors.
Carbamazepine	?	Inhibits, shortened duration	Chronic therapy causes resistance to NDNMB, except for atracurium.
Cardioactive steroids	More prone to cardiac dysrhythmias	Pancuronium increases catecholamines and causes dysrhythmias	
Dantrolene	?	Potentiates	Blocks excitation–contraction coupling by blocking ryanodine receptor channel in sarcoplasmic reticulum of skeletal muscle.
Furosemide <10 mcg/kg 1–4 mg/kg	Potentiates or inhibits	Potentiates or inhibits	Biphasic dose response in cats; protein kinase inhibition at low doses and phosphodiesterase inhibition at high doses. Diuretic-related hypokalemia potentiates pancuronium in cats.
Glucocorticoids	?	Inhibits	Chronic steroid use induces resistance to pancuronium and decrease plasma cholinesterase activity by 50%. Steroids ± NDNMB associated with myopathies.
Inhalational anesthetics: isoflurane	Potentiates	Potentiates	Decrease CNS activity and potentiates NMB in anesthetic doses: dependent fashion (postsynaptic and muscle effects). Halothane causes less muscle relaxation than isoflurane.
Lidocaine	Potentiates	Low dose potentiates block; high dose inhibits nerve terminals and blocks ACh binding site at postsynaptic membrane.	The fast Na+ channel blockers decrease action potential propagation, ACh release, postsynaptic membrane sensitivity, and muscle excitability. Weak inhibitor of PChE. This potentially is observed with all local anesthetic, but practically lidocaine one that is intravenously administered.
Lithium	Prolongs onset and duration	Prolongs effect of pancuronium	Inhibits synthesis and release of ACh. Lithium alone causes myasthenic reaction.
Magnesium	Potentiates; blocks fasciculations	Potentiates or prolongs blocks	Decreases prejunctional ACh release, postjunctional membrane sensitivity, and muscle excitability.
NDNMB: pancuronium, vecuronium, rocuronium	"Precurarization" with NDNMB shortens the onset and decreases side effects of succinylcholine; pancuronium increases block duration.	Chronic NDNMB induces resistance to their effect; mixing different NDNMBs causes greater than additive effects, especially combining pancuronium with tubocurarine or metocurine.	Prior NDNMB inhibits plasma PChE and prolongs mivacurium and succinylcholine block. Rank order: pancuronium > vecuronium > atracurium. Heterozygote for atypical PChE develops phase II block when given succinylcholine and pancuronium.
Organic phosphorus compounds	Potentiates	?	Irreversible PChE inhibitor. Which totally blocks enzyme activity.
Phenelzine (MAOI)	Prolongs	?	Decreases PChE activity.
Phenytoin	?	Resistant, shortened duration	Acutely, potentiates NDNMB paralysis. With chronic use (except for atracurium), phenytoin induces resistance to NDNMB and increases metabolism. This increases the initial dose and decreases the repeat dosing interval.
Polypeptide antibiotics: polymyxin	Potentiates	Potentiates	Causes severe weakness and induces postsynaptic neuromuscular block. Neostigmine increases block.

(Continued)

TABLE 66–2	Effect of Prior Administration of Xenobiotics on Subsequent Response to Succinylcholine or Nondepolarizing Neuromuscular Blockers (Continued)		
Xenobiotic	Response to Succinylcholine	Response to Nondepolarizer	Comments
Succinylcholine	Small initial dose of succinylcholine are used to limit muscular fasciculations.	Pancuronium and vecuronium slightly prolonged by prior succinylcholine.	
Theophylline		Inhibits	The combination of pancuronium and theophylline increases cardiac dysrhythmias.
Cyclic antidepressants (CA)			The combination of pancuronium and CA cause cardiac dysrhythmias due to sympathetic effects.

ACh = acetylcholine; AChE = acetylcholinesterase; CNS = central nervous system; MAOI = monoamine oxidase inhibitor; NDNMB = nondepolarizing neuromuscular blocker; NMB = neuromuscular blocker; NMJ = neuromuscular junction; PChE = plasma cholinesterase.

Data from Crowe S, Collins L. Suxamethonium and donepezil: a cause of prolonged paralysis. *Anesthesiology.* 2003;98:574-575; Flacchino F, et al. Sensitivity to vecuronium after botulinum toxin administration. *J Neurosurg Anesthesiol.* 1997;9:1491153; Fleming NW, et al. Neuromuscular blocking action of suxamethonium after antagonism of vecuronium by edrophonium, pyridostigmine or neostigmine. *Br J Anaesth.* 1996;77:492-495; Kaeser HE. Drug-induced myasthenic syndromes. *Acta Neurol Scand Suppl.* 1984;100:39-47; Kato M, et al. Inhibition of human plasma cholinesterase and erythrocyte acetylcholinesterase by nondepolarizing neuromuscular blocking agents. *J Anesth.* 2000;14:30-34; Ostergaard D, et al. Adverse reactions and interactions of the neuromuscular blocking drugs. *Med Toxicol Adverse Drug Exp.* 1989; 4:351-368; and Viby-Mogensen J. Interaction of other drugs with muscle relaxants. In: Katz RL, ed. *Muscle Relaxants: Basic and Clinical Aspects.* New York, NY: Grune & Stratton; 1985:233-256.

PROLONGED EFFECT

The effects of succinylcholine last for several hours if metabolism is significantly slowed because of decreased PChE concentration, abnormal PChE activity (genetic variant or drug inhibition), or a phase II block.[20] Acquired PChE deficiency is caused by hepatic disease, malnutrition, plasmapheresis, or pregnancy.[20] Inactivation of PChE results from fluoride poisoning, organic phosphorus compounds, or carbamates. However, even with only 20% to 30% of normal PChE activity, the clinical duration of succinylcholine is less than doubled.[35]

Many genetic variants of PChE are known. The most common atypical PChE (atypical type, homozygous; incidence 1:3,000) can be assayed by its resistance to inhibition by the local anesthetic dibucaine.[95] A history of uneventful exposure to succinylcholine *excludes* the possibility of atypical PChE except in the case of hepatic transplantation. Dibucaine inhibits the ability of normal PChE to hydrolyze benzoylcholine by more than 70% (ie, dibucaine number >70), heterozygous atypical PChE by 40% to 60%, and homozygous atypical PChE by 30% or less. Dibucaine number is an effective method of identifying patients at increased risk for prolonged neuromuscular blockade from succinylcholine. The lower the number, the greater likelihood there will be prolonged neuromuscular blockade from atypical reasonable PChE activity. Fresh-frozen plasma or PChE concentrates are infused to hasten recovery in the case of a genetic enzyme defect or an acquired PChE deficiency. However, to avoid the risks of transfusion, it is best to provide supportive care, simply keep the patient sedated, intubated, and ventilated until the drug is metabolized. In this setting, spontaneous reversal usually occurs within 3 to 4 hours, although in rare cases, full recovery requires up to 12 hours.[20] When the duration of succinylcholine is very prolonged, blood samples should be drawn for measurement of PChE concentration and activity.

Prolonged nondepolarizing block also occurs when unusually large IV doses of succinylcholine (3–5 mg/kg) are given over minutes.[68] This is called *phase II block*, and it can be partially reversed by neostigmine.

Interestingly, pseudocholinesterase is also involved in metabolism of cocaine. Plasma cholinesterase catalyzes the hydrolysis of cocaine, and low PChE concentrations are associated with increased risk of cocaine toxicity.[24,51,92] There have been few small studies demonstrating that exogenously administered PChE degrades cocaine more quickly and is theoretically able to treat cocaine-induced toxicity.[16,75,78,105]

HYPERKALEMIA

Succinylcholine 1 mg/kg IV typically causes a transient serum K^+ concentration increase of approximately 0.5 mEq/L within minutes of administration both in normal individuals and in persons with kidney failure. The acute hyperkalemic response to succinylcholine is greatly exaggerated with coexisting myopathy or proliferation of extrajunctional muscle ACh receptors. However, the mortality rate is highest (approaching 30%) when rhabdomyolysis is present.[44] Severe, precipitous, potentially life-threatening hyperkalemia also occurs after succinylcholine administration in several conditions associated with proliferation of ACh receptors. These conditions include denervation caused by head or spinal cord injury, stroke, neuropathy, prolonged use of NDNMBs because of muscle pathology direct trauma, crush or compartment syndrome, or muscular dystrophy; critical illness due to hemorrhagic shock, neuropathy, myopathy, or prolonged immobility; thermal burn or cold injury; and sepsis lasting several days. After a neurologic injury, susceptibility to hyperkalemia begins within 4 to 7 days and persist for an extended period of time. In patients who have been in the intensive care unit (ICU) for more than 1 week, succinylcholine should be avoided altogether because of the risk of hyperkalemic cardiac arrest, which is associated with a mortality rate of at least 19%.[7,10,44] Severe hyperkalemia can be mitigated, but not prevented, by a small dose of an NDNMB (10%–30% ED_{95} of the NDNMB or 5%–15% of the intubation dose). This dose should be sufficient to prevent succinylcholine-induced muscle fasciculations.[106]

Severe or even fatal hyperkalemia is reported in a few patients who received succinylcholine immediately after exsanguinating hemorrhage or massive trauma. The mechanism for this condition differs from that after neurologic injury because of inadequate time for proliferation of extrajunctional ACh receptors. Succinic acid, a tricarboxylic acid cycle intermediate that is also a metabolite of succinylcholine, facilitates activation of voltage-gated sodium channels in a dose-dependent fashion, increasing skeletal muscle excitability.[46] In hemorrhagic shock, accumulation of succinic acid as a result of cell breakdown and anaerobic metabolism possibly augments the potassium-releasing effect of succinylcholine.

RHABDOMYOLYSIS

Severe hyperkalemia rarely occurs in the absence of a clinical history that readily discloses an obvious risk factor, with one important exception. Acute or delayed onset of rhabdomyolysis, hyperkalemia, ventricular dysrhythmias, cardiac arrest, and death are reported in apparently healthy children who were subsequently found to have an undiagnosed myopathy.[64] Since March 1995, a black box warning on the package insert has stated that succinylcholine should be avoided in elective surgery in children, particularly in children younger than 8 years of age, because of the risk of a previously undiagnosed skeletal myopathy, especially Duchenne muscular dystrophy. Sudden cardiac arrest occurring immediately after succinylcholine administration should always be assumed to be caused by hyperkalemia. If fever, muscle rigidity, and elevated lactate concentration or metabolic and respiratory acidosis are also present, the presumptive diagnosis of MH should prompt immediate therapy with dantrolene.

MALIGNANT HYPERTHERMIA

Malignant hyperthermia is a syndrome characterized by extreme skeletal muscle hypermetabolism. It is most often initiated after exposure to an anesthetic that triggers a cycle of abnormal calcium release from the skeletal muscle sarcoplasmic reticulum and can have a variable presentation.[100] Malignant hyperthermia is observed in patients with underlying muscle diseases, such as muscular dystrophy and myotonia. It is also strongly linked to three rare genetic myopathies, central core disease, King Denborough syndrome, and multiminicore disease.

Although MH is linked with rare congenital myopathies, it typically affects individuals who are otherwise healthy.[63] It is inherited as an autosomal dominant trait with variable penetrance.[76] Triggering xenobiotics that can precipitate an attack of MH include succinylcholine and volatile inhalational anesthetics (the prototypical xenobiotic is halothane). In individuals considered MH susceptible, xenobiotics that can be administered safely include NDNMBs, nitrous oxide, propofol, ketamine, etomidate, benzodiazepines, barbiturates, opioids, and local anesthetics.

In human MH, there is a causal association with several unique defects involving a skeletal muscle receptor or regulatory protein, especially defects involving the voltage sensitive calcium release channel found in skeletal muscle; the type 1 ryanodine receptor (or RYR1, chromosome 19q13.1). Mutations of the RYR1 receptor are detected in 50% to 70% of patients with MH, and more than 200 different mutations are described[12,50] (Fig. 66–1). The structurally distinct type 2 ryanodine receptor (RYR2) is the primary type expressed in cardiac muscle, and this could explain why the myocardium is relatively spared in the early phase of MH (with the exception of an acute hyperdynamic response).[99] The existence of multiple mutations across multiple alleles means that genetic testing is not likely to prove useful in detecting all individuals who are MH susceptible or to exclude the risk of MH.

Although the prevalence of a genetic disorder associated with MH is between 1 in 3,000 and 1 in 8,500, the observed incidence of fulminant MH in patients exposed to general anesthesia when triggering anesthetic agents are used is 1 in 62,000 and 1 in 84,000.[93,100] Each year in the United States, there are an estimated 700 cases of MH.[62] Even in those who are MH susceptible after exposure to anesthesia with known triggers, clinical manifestations develop less than half the time. For this reason, a previous uneventful anesthetic exposure does not preclude development of MH on a subsequent exposure.[4] In the operating room, MH most often presents abruptly soon after initial exposure to a triggering anesthetic, although the onset of MH may be delayed several hours during the anesthesia[84] or occur as long as 12 hours after surgery. In addition, recrudescence of MH occurs within 24 to 36 hours after an initial episode in up to 25% of patients.

The immediate systemic manifestations of MH result from extreme skeletal muscle hypermetabolism. The uncontrolled release of calcium from the terminal cisternae of the sarcoplasmic reticulum causes skeletal muscle contraction. Although generalized muscular rigidity is a specific sign of MH, it is only observed in 40%; masseter spasm is a finding observed in 27% of MH patients.[63] Futile calcium cycling by sarcoplasmic Ca^{2+}-ATPase rapidly depletes intracellular adenosine triphosphate and leads to anaerobic metabolism. Clinically, MH presents as skeletal muscle hypermetabolism with an increase in cardiac output and sinus tachycardia; increased CO_2 production causes hypercapnia; increased O_2 consumption can cause: mixed venous O_2 desaturation (below the normal value of 75%), arterial hypoxemia, anaerobic metabolism, metabolic acidosis, elevated lactate concentration, cyanosis, and skin mottling; and excess heat production that leads to a rapid increase in core temperature with hyperthermia.[47] Other clinical findings include tachycardia, cardiac dysrhythmias, hyperkalemia, rhabdomyolysis, and disseminated intravascular coagulopathy.

The earliest signs of MH include an early and rapid increase in CO_2 production, causing an increase in arterial, venous, and end-tidal CO_2, followed

by or associated with tachycardia; tachypnea; hypertension or labile blood pressure; and skeletal and jaw muscle rigidity. Despite the name of the syndrome, hyperthermia is not a universal finding in MH, and moreover, it may be a late sign.[113] Acute potassium release from skeletal muscle cells produce life-threatening hyperkalemia. Subsequent rhabdomyolysis exacerbates the elevation of potassium by causing acute kidney injury. In late-stage MH, cardiac decompensation results from hyperkalemia, heart failure, vascular collapse, or myocardial ischemia (especially with coexisting coronary artery disease).

The differential diagnosis of MH includes antipsychotic malignant syndrome, propofol infusion syndrome, serotonin toxicity, thyroid storm, pheochromocytoma, baclofen withdrawal, tetanus, meningitis, poisoning by salicylates, amphetamines, cocaine, or antimuscarinics, unintentional intraoperative hyperthermia, environmental heat stroke, and transfusion reactions (Chap. 29). Of note, early septic shock is also associated with hypermetabolism, increased cardiac output, and fever; however, in contrast to MH, early septic shock is associated with an elevated mixed venous O_2 saturation (typically >75%).

Rarely, MH is triggered by severe exercise in a hot climate, IV potassium (which depolarizes the muscle membrane), antipsychotics, or infection.[23,54] There is of a possible link between MH and exertional heat illness (EHI) or exertional rhabdomyolysis (eg, a patient with exertional rhabdomyolysis who at a later time develops MH).[14,15] There is no evidence that patients with heat-related illness have MH, even if, on occasion, some patients appear to improve following many interventions including dantrolene. Furthermore, a presumptive diagnosis of heat-related illness does not necessarily exclude the diagnosis of MH, and one must maintain clinical suspicion for possible MH, especially because environmental factors can be a sole precipitating factor in the absence of anesthetics.[50]

One theory of the pathogenesis of MH suggests that MH-triggering xenobiotics interact with an abnormal RYR1 channel, causing it to stay in a prolonged open state and leading to rapid efflux of calcium from the skeletal muscle sarcoplasmic reticulum into the myoplasm. Succinylcholine prolongs muscle depolarization, leading to an elevated myoplasmic calcium concentration. This action initiates the voltage sensitive calcium release channel of the sarcoplasmic reticulum.[44] However, not all cases of MH can be explained by an RYR1 mutation.[36] For example, MH is also associated with defects in the CACNA1S protein that encodes a subunit of the skeletal muscle L-type calcium channel (known as the dihydropyridine receptor) and possibly with certain disorders of sodium channels (observed in the myotonic disorders).[36,83]

The antidote for MH is dantrolene, and the key aspects of MH therapy are rapid initial diagnosis, discontinuation of triggering anesthetics, active cooling, and immediate therapy with dantrolene (within minutes). By partially blocking calcium release from skeletal muscle sarcoplasmic reticulum, dantrolene rapidly reverses the signs and symptoms of hypermetabolism (Antidotes in Depth: A24). The precise mechanism of dantrolene activity is not known, but it modulates several calcium pathways.[50] Before the introduction of dantrolene, the mortality rate of MH was 64%.[62] When patients with acute MH are treated immediately with dantrolene, removal of triggering agents, and supportive measures (volume resuscitation, active cooling, control of hyperkalemia), the mortality rate is less than 5%.[62] Factors associated with an increase in mortality rate are a muscular body habitus, development of disseminated intravascular coagulation, and a longer duration of anesthesia before the peak in end-tidal carbon dioxide.[62] Even if administration is delayed for hours or days, dantrolene still improves survival after an acute episode of MH. Patients with significant dysrhythmias can be treated with standard antidysrhythmics; however, calcium channel blockers must *not* be given with dantrolene because they precipitate hyperkalemia and severe hypotension[101] (Table 66–3).

Persons who have experienced a possible episode of MH or have a positive family history should be referred to the Malignant Hyperthermia Registry and may be considered for muscle biopsy or genetic sequencing of the *RYR1* gene. The muscle biopsy is considered to be the gold standard, but patients must

TABLE 66–3	Therapy for Malignant Hyperthermia (MH)[a]

Acute Phase Treatment of MH

1. Call for help. Immediately summon experienced help when MH is suspected. Call MH hotline, 800-644-9737.

2. Discontinue triggers: volatile inhalational anesthetics and succinylcholine.

3. Hyperventilate with 100% O_2 with flow ≥10 L/min and monitor end-tidal CO_2.

4. Halt procedure as soon as possible and continue sedation and analgesia with nontriggering agents: opioids and benzodiazepines.

5. Administer dantrolene, initial IV bolus of 2.5 mg/kg followed by additional boluses (every 15 minutes), until signs of MH are controlled (tachycardia, rigidity, increased end-tidal CO_2, hyperthermia). Typically, a total dose of 10 mg/kg IV controls symptoms, but occasionally 30 mg/kg is required.
   - Dantrium/Revonto:[b] Each 20-mg vial is reconstituted by adding 60 mL of sterile water.
   - Ryanodex: Each 250-mg vial is reconstituted by adding 5 mL of sterile water.

6. Monitor core temperature closely (tympanic membrane, nasopharynx, esophagus, rectal, or pulmonary artery) and actively cool the patient with core temperature >39°C (immersion in ice-water slurry is preferred, cooling by peritoneal or gastric lavage, surface cool or surface cooling techniques are also reasonable).

7. Hyperkalemia is common and should be treated aggressively with hyperventilation, IV calcium gluconate (30 mg/kg up to 3 g) or chloride (10 mg/kg up to 1 g), sodium bicarbonate, IV dextrose, and insulin. Hypokalemia should be treated with caution because of the potential for rhabdomyolysis induced hyperkalemia.[c]

8. Sodium bicarbonate. 1–2 mEq/kg (up to 50 mEq/kg) is reasonable if blood gas values have not yet been obtained or if clinically indicated.

9. Monitor continuously: ECG, pulse oximetry, end-tidal CO_2, core temperature, CVP, urine output; and serially measure: arterial and mixed venous blood gases, metabolic profile (especially potassium), calcium, CBC, coagulation indices, and creatine kinase.

10. Dysrhythmias usually respond to dantrolene, cooling, and correction of acidosis and hyperkalemia. If dysrhythmias persist or are life threatening, standard antidysrhythmics are indicated, including amiodarone, magnesium, and procainamide.
   - Calcium channel blockers (verapamil or diltiazem) should not be used to treat dysrhythmias because they may cause hyperkalemia and cardiac arrest.

11. Ensure adequate urine output by restoration of intravascular volume followed by administration of mannitol or furosemide. Insert a urinary bladder catheter and consider central venous or pulmonary artery catheterization.

12. For emergency consultation, refer to the MHAUS at http://www.mhaus.org/. Call the MH Emergency Hotline:
   - Inside the United States or Canada, call 800-MH-HYPER (800-644-9737).
   - Outside the United States and Canada, call 001 315-464-7079.

Postacute Phase Treatment of MH

1. Observe the patient in an ICU setting for at least 24 h because recrudescence of MH occurs in 25% of cases, particularly after a fulminant case resistant to treatment. Observe for pulmonary edema, kidney failure, and compartment syndrome.

2. Administer dantrolene 1 mg/kg IV q4–6h or 0.25 mg/kg/h by infusion for at least 24 h after the episode.

3. Serially monitor arterial blood gases, metabolic profile, CBC, creatine kinase, calcium, phosphorus, coagulation indices, urine and serum myoglobin, and core body temperature until they return to normal values.

4. Counsel the patient and family regarding MH and further precautions.
   - For nonemergency patient referrals, contact the MHAUS at 800-644-9737, 1 North Main Street, PO Box 1069, Sherburne, NY 13460.
   - Report patients who have had an acute MH episode to the North American MH Registry of MHAUS at 888-274-7899.
   - Alert family members to the possible dangers of MH and anesthesia.

5. Recommend an MH medical identification tag or bracelet for the patient, which should be worn at all times.

[a]The guidelines may not apply to every patient and of necessity must be altered according to specific patient needs. [b]There are two formulation of dantrolene, Dantrium/Revonto and Ryanodex. [c]Sudden unexpected cardiac arrest in children: Children younger than about 10 years of age who experience sudden cardiac arrest after succinylcholine administration in the absence of hypoxemia and anesthetic overdose should be treated for acute hyperkalemia first. In this situation, calcium chloride should be administered along with means to reduce serum potassium. They should be presumed to have subclinical muscular dystrophy, and a pediatric neurologist should be consulted.

CBC = complete blood count; CVP = central venous pressure; ECG = electrocardiogram; ICU = intensive care unit; IV = intravenous; MHAUS = Malignant Hyperthermia Association of the United States.

Modified with permission from Malignant Hyperthermia Association of the United States (mhaus.org).

travel to an authorized testing center for biopsy. There are currently four centers in the United States and one center in Canada. A fresh tissue specimen is placed in a tissue bath perfused with Krebs solution, and halothane or caffeine is added. According to the North America Malignant Hyperthermia Group, an MH-susceptible individual is one who demonstrates a positive muscle contraction in response to either halothane or caffeine. On the other hand, genetic testing can be performed. Additional information regarding testing options can be found on the website of the Malignant Hyperthermia Association of the United States (www.mhaus.org).

MUSCLE SPASMS

Masseter muscle rigidity was observed in 0.3% to 1.0% of children when general anesthesia was induced with succinylcholine and halothane (a technique now obsolete) and currently is much less frequently encountered. Masseter muscle rigidity is clinically significant because it will complicate airway management and herald the onset of MH.[91]

When administered to persons genetically predisposed to myotonia, succinylcholine precipitates tonic muscular contractions, ranging from trismus (which prevents orotracheal intubation) to severe generalized myoclonus and chest wall rigidity (which prevent ventilation).[32] Because the myotonic contractions are independent of neural activity, they cannot be aborted by an NDNMB. Usually the contractions are self-limited, but occasionally they will be life threatening if an airway cannot be established and hypoxemia ensues.

PHARMACOLOGY OF NONDEPOLARIZING NEUROMUSCULAR BLOCKERS

Table 66–1 summarizes the pharmacology and toxicity of the NDNMBs.[53,79,80,86] Whereas atracurium is composed of 10 different isomers, each having its unique pharmacokinetic and pharmacodynamic profile, cisatracurium contains only the 1R-*cis* and 1'R-*cis* isomers. Both atracurium and cisatracurium exhibit organ-independent elimination and are rapidly metabolized by spontaneous (nonenzymatic) temperature- and pH-dependent Hoffmann degradation and, to a lesser extent, by ester hydrolysis. The latter is catalyzed by nonspecific plasma esterases distinct from the PChE that hydrolyzes succinylcholine. In addition, significant drug metabolism or elimination occurs in the liver and kidney.[34]

TOXICITY OF NONDEPOLARIZING NEUROMUSCULAR BLOCKERS

The most important toxic effects of the NDNMBs are accumulation of laudanosine and persistent weakness. In general, limiting the drug dose and monitoring the drug effect with a portable nerve stimulator reduce the incidence of prolonged weakness.

Laudanosine

Metabolism of atracurium and cisatracurium generates laudanosine, which crosses the blood–brain and placental barriers and may cause neuroexcitation but lacks any neuromuscular blocking activity.[29] Metabolism of each atracurium molecule generates one molecule of laudanosine.[89] Cisatracurium is an improvement over atracurium because it produces one-third as much laudanosine (and is three times more potent).[38,58]

In the CNS, laudanosine has an inhibitory effect at the γ-aminobutyric acid, nACh, and opioid receptors. At high serum concentrations in experimental animals, laudanosine causes dose-related neuroexcitation, myoclonic activity (>14 mcg/mL), and generalized seizures (>17 mcg/mL).[17,38] In humans, the toxic serum laudanosine concentration is unknown, and seizures directly attributable to atracurium are not reported even after prolonged infusion in the ICU.[38,117] In ICU patients who received a 72-hour infusion of atracurium (1 mg/kg/h), the highest serum laudanosine concentrations (10–20 mcg/mL) were observed in patients with impaired glomerular filtration rate.[69] Laudanosine is excreted primarily in the bile, and its elimination is prolonged in patients with liver disease, biliary obstruction, and kidney disease.[96]

Persistent Weakness Associated with Nondepolarizing Neuromuscular Blockers

Short-term blockade with a NDNMB usually resolves promptly upon discontinuation. When an NDNMB is administered for more than 48 hours, there is a risk that weakness will persist longer than anticipated based on the kinetics of drug elimination. In addition, critical illness is associated with dysfunction of the peripheral nerve, NMJ, and muscle (Table 66–4). For instance, in the ICU, persistent weakness is observed in 68% to 100% of patients with sepsis or multiorgan failure[22,37,112] and in 20% to 30% of patients who receive NDNMB for only 48 to 72 hours.[71] Persistent weakness is multifactorial and associated with illness severity; sepsis; acute respiratory distress syndrome; multiorgan failure; hyperglycemia; NDNMB; use of systemic corticosteroids;

muscle injury; thermal injury, and electrolyte, endocrine, and nutritional disorders.[21,27,49,70] Many xenobiotics given to patients in the ICU can cause weakness by themselves or potentiate the effects of NDNMB.[52,94] Progressive weakness and acute respiratory failure are even described after discharge from the ICU and will be life threatening if not immediately recognized.[65] Patients who develop persistent weakness have a 2.5- to 3.5-fold increase in ICU mortality and ICU stay.[71]

PHARMACOLOGIC REVERSAL OF NEUROMUSCULAR BLOCKADE

Acetylcholinesterase Inhibitors

Termination of NMB effect initially results from drug redistribution and later from drug elimination, metabolism, or chemical antagonism. Pharmacologic antagonism of a partial NDNMB is achieved by giving a reversal agent that inhibits junctional AChE and thereby increases ACh at the NMJ. This increase in ACh can overcome the competitive inhibition caused by residual NDNMB. The commonly used anti-ChEs are polar molecules that possess a quaternary ammonium (Table 66–5). Neostigmine and pyridostigmine are hydrolyzed by ChE and form short-lived carbamyl complexes (half-life, 15–20 minutes) with the esteratic site of the enzyme.[6] In contrast, edrophonium is not hydrolyzed by ChE; rather, it forms an electrostatic interaction and a hydrogen bond with the cationic site of ChE that is both competitive and reversible. Neostigmine and pyridostigmine, but not edrophonium, inhibit PChE and thus prolong the effects of xenobiotics metabolized by this enzyme, such as succinylcholine.[35]

The most common and troublesome clinical side effect of ChE inhibition is bradycardia, which usually is prevented by coadministration of an antimuscarinic such as atropine.[19] Bradydysrhythmias are severe and lead to nodal or idioventricular rhythm, complete heart block, or even asystole.[72] These side effects occur more frequently in patients with preexisting bradycardia and those receiving chronic β-adrenergic antagonist therapy. They are not necessarily prevented by prior administration of atropine.[108] Other problems that result from excess ChE inhibition are hypersalivation, lacrimation, bronchospasm, increased bronchial secretions, abdominal cramping from intestinal hyperperistalsis, and increased bladder tone. After general anesthesia, use of anti-ChE pharmacologic reversal increases the incidence of nausea, vomiting, and abdominal cramps.[57] Because atropine crosses the blood–brain barrier, it may produce central anticholinergic syndrome.

Sugammadex

Sugammadex (Bridion) is a selective NDNMB binder that was developed specifically for rapid and complete reversal of neuromuscular blockage induced by rocuronium and vecuronium (Fig. 66–2). Approved by the European Union in 2008 for use, the US Food and Drug Administration initially rejected

TABLE 66–4	Acute Neuromuscular Pathology Associated With Critical Illness or Nondepolarizing Neuromuscular Blockers			
	Critical Illness Polyneuropathy	**Residual Neuromuscular Block**	**Disuse (Cachectic) Myopathy**	**Critical Illness Myopathy**
Sensory	Moderate to severe, distal > proximal	Normal	Normal	Normal
Motor	Symmetric weakness, lower > upper extremity, proximal > distal or diffuse, respiratory failure	Diffuse symmetric weakness, respiratory failure	Diffuse weakness, proximal > distal	Symmetric weakness, proximal > distal or diffuse, respiratory failure
Creatine phosphokinase	Normal	Normal	Normal	Elevated in ≤50%
Electrodiagnostic studies (EMG, NCV)	Axonal degeneration of motor > sensory, reduced sensory and motor compound action potentials, normal NCV	Fatigue at NMJ assessed by fade on repetitive nerve stimulation	Normal EMG and NCV	Myopathic changes, muscle membrane inexcitability, normal NCV
Muscle biopsy	Denervation atrophy	Normal	Atrophy of type 2 fibers, no myosin loss, no necrosis	Atrophy of type 2 fibers, myosin loss, mild myonecrosis, no inflammatory infiltration

EMG = electromyography; NCV = nerve conduction velocity; NMJ = neuromuscular junction.

Data from Bolton CF. Critical illness polyneuropathy and myopathy. *Crit Care Med.* 2001;29:2388-2390; Lacomis D. Critical illness myopathy. *Curr Rheumatol Rep.* 2002;4:403-408; Lacomis D, Campellone JV. Critical illness neuromyopathies. *Adv Neurol.* 2002;88:325-335; and Leijten FSS, de Weerd AW. Critical illness polyneuropathy: a review the literature, definition and pathophysiology. *Clin Neurol Neurosurg.* 1994;96:10-19.

TABLE 66–5   Pharmacology of Intravenous Neuromuscular Blockade Reversal Drugs and Coadministered Antimuscarinics

	Anticholinesterases		
	Neostigmine	**Pyridostigmine**	**Edrophonium**
Initial dose (mg/kg)	0.04–0.08	0.2–0.4	0.5–1.0
Onset (min)	7–11	10–16	1–2
Duration (min)	60–120	60–120	60–120
Recommended antimuscarinic	Glycopyrrolate	Glycopyrrolate	Atropine (preferred because of time of onset is better paired with edrophonium)

	Antimuscarinics	
	Glycopyrrolate	**Atropine**
Structure	Quaternary ammonium	Tertiary amine
Initial dose (mg/kg)	0.01–0.02	0.02–0.03
Onset (min)	2–3	1
Duration (min)	30–60	30–60
Elimination	Renal	Renal
Crosses blood–brain barrier	No	Yes

sugammadex because of concerns of hypersensitivity and allergic reactions but it was approved in December 2015.

Sugammadex reverses the effect of steroidal NMBs by directly binding to the steroidal NMB at 1:1 ratio to form sugammadex–NMB complex, thus preventing the binding of NMBs to the nicotinic receptors. Although sugammadex can bind to all steroidal NMBs, its affinity is greatest for rocuronium followed by vecuronium and least with pancuronium.[87] Administration of IV sugammadex results in rapid removal of NMB from plasma, which facilitates the movement of NMBs from the NMJ into plasma through a concentration gradient effect, where they bind to any free remaining sugammadex. Thus, sugammadex can reverse any depth of neuromuscular blockade in a dose-dependent fashion. After the sugammadex–NMB complex is formed, it is eliminated through biliary (75%) and renal (25%) clearance and excreted via the urine (65%–97%).[48] In addition, the sugammadex–NMB complex is inert and does not cause any muscarinic effect. There are some concerns over hypersensitivity and allergic reactions, which occurred in 0.3% of healthy volunteers, which delayed its approval in the United States. A particular precaution for sugammadex exists on utilizing women on hormonal

contraceptives. In vitro studies indicate sugammadex binds to progesterone and decreases the concentration. Administration of sugammadex is considered to be equivalent to missing a dose (or doses) of an oral contraceptive. Therefore, patients must be counseled regarding the use additional non-hormonal or back-up method of contraception for the subsequent 7 days if they received the sugammadex and are receiving hormonal contraceptives.

The doses of sugammadex based on actual body weight are:[1]

- 2 mg/kg for shallow blockade: if spontaneous recovery has been reached up to the reappearance of the second twitch to train-of-four stimulation after rocuronium and vecuronium blockage
- 4 mg/kg for profound blockage: if 1 or 2 posttetanic counts and response to train-of-four stimulation after rocuronium and vecuronium blockade
- 16 mg/kg for immediate reversal: 3 minutes after administration of 1.2 mg/kg of rocuronium. Immediate reversal of vecuronium is unstudied.

Sugammadex is not effective for nonsteroidal NMBS such as mivacurium, atracurium, and cisatracurium. Therefore, if neuromuscular blockage needs to be reestablished after sugammadex, succinylcholine or one of the nonsteroidal neuromuscular blockers should be used. In the meantime, supportive management is continued with establishing a definitive airway and mechanical ventilation.

CHOICE OF REVERSAL

Choice of reversal between sugammadex versus acetylcholinesterase inhibitor is complex. Although sugammadex has been available in Europe since 2008, experience has been limited in the United States due to availability and cost, largely because of its very recent approval.

Sugammadex offers two major advantages: rapid reversal and lack of cholinergic side effects. Its disadvantages include a lack of affinity for nonsteroidal NDNMB and a variable affinity for steroidal NMB (rocuronium > vecuronium >> pancuronium). Thus, it is unlikely to replace acetylcholinesterase inhibitors completely. In routine anesthesia care, rapid reversal of NDNMB is rarely needed, and the anticholinergic effects are well tolerated when administered with an antimuscarinic. However, there are clearly situations when rapid reversal of an NDNMB with sugammadex can be beneficial such as difficult airway management, brief surgical procedures that require deep neuromuscular blockade, patients with cardiac comorbidities who do not tolerate dysrhythmias from AChE inhibition, and pediatric patients in whom neuromuscular blockage have been avoided because of unknown myopathy.

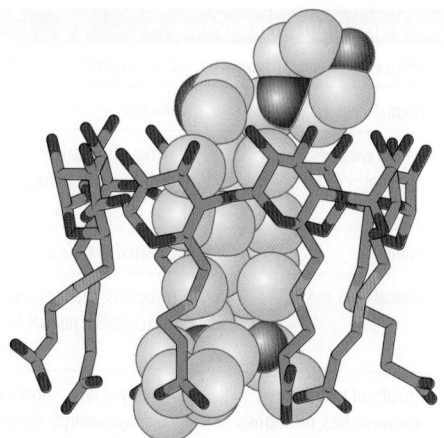

FIGURE 66–2. Sugammadex encapsulating a molecule of rocuronium. *(Reproduced with permission from Hemmerling TM, Zaouter C, Geldner G, et al. Sugammadex—a short review and clinical recommendations for the cardiac anesthesiologist. Ann Card Anaesth. 2010;Sep-Dec;13(3):206-216.)*

DIAGNOSTIC TESTING

Quantitative methods for analysis of blood and tissue NDNMB and metabolite concentrations using high-performance liquid chromatography and mass spectrometry are described.[56,104]

Succinylcholine and succinylmonocholine can be assayed by gas chromatography and mass spectrometry in blood, urine, or the site of intramuscular injection.[90,107] Less than 3% of administered succinylcholine and 10% of its metabolite succinylmonocholine are excreted in the urine. However, both the parent drug and the metabolite undergo spontaneous hydrolysis, especially in alkaline conditions.[111] Historically, detection of succinylcholine was difficult because of its rapid hydrolysis. However, techniques for detecting this parent compound in tissues even after embalming are described.[41] Because succinic acid is also a product of normal intermediary metabolism, assay of this metabolite is not useful for positive identification of prior succinylcholine exposure.[82] Surprisingly, the presence of succinylmonocholine in forensic samples also cannot prove prior exposure to succinylcholine. Succinylmonocholine in concentrations of 0.01 to 0.20 mcg/g has been detected in tissues of six autopsy cases with no history of succinylcholine exposure.[67]

SUMMARY

- Succinylcholine is the only DNMB in current clinical use. Its immediate adverse effects include dose- and rate-related histamine release and modulation of autonomic tone.
- Acute and potentially fatal hyperkalemia occurs after succinylcholine administration; in patients with certain myopathies such as Duchenne muscular dystrophy; or after stroke, spinal cord injury, neuropathy, prolonged immobility, or crush syndrome.
- In MH, acute onset of severe hypermetabolism causing acidosis, rhabdomyolysis, hyperkalemia, and death occurs if treatment with dantrolene and aggressive cooling is not rapidly administered. One vial of Ryanodex, the newer formulation of dantrolene, contains the initial 2.5 mg/kg dose for patients up to 100 kg, whereas the older formulation requires mixing of 12.5 vials to provide the same dose.
- The most important complications associated with use of NDNMBs are undetected hypoventilation and prolonged drug effect.
- In most neuromuscular diseases, sensitivity to NDNMB is increased and fatal hyperkalemia is a potential result.
- Reversal of nonsteroidal NDNMB can be achieved with acetylcholinesterase inhibitors, and steroidal NDNMB can be achieved with acetylcholinesterase inhibitors or sugammadex.
- Choice of reversal depends on availability, cost, and indications. The main advantage of sugammadex is rapid reversal of selected steroidal NDNMB without cholinergic effects.

REFERENCES

1. Abrishami A, et al. Sugammadex, a selective reversal medication for preventing postoperative residual neuromuscular blockade. *Cochrane Database Syst Rev.* 2009;:CD007362.
2. Azar I. The response of patients with neuromuscular disorders to muscle relaxants: a review. *Anesthesiology.* 1984;61:173-187.
3. Bailey FL. *The Defense Never Rests.* New York, NY: Signet Books; 1972.
4. Bendixen D, et al. Analysis of anaesthesia in patients suspected to be susceptible to malignant hyperthermia before diagnostic in vitro contracture test. *Acta Anaesthesiol Scand.* 1997;41:480-484.
5. Benedict B, et al. The insulin pump as murder weapon: a case report. *Am J Forensic Med Pathol.* 2004;25:159-160.
6. Bevan DR, et al. Reversal of neuromuscular blockade. *Anesthesiology.* 1992;77:785-805.
7. Biccard BM, Hughes M. Succinylcholine in the intensive care unit. *Anesthesiology.* 2002;96:253-254.
8. Black J. Claude Bernard on the action of curare. *BMJ.* 1999;319:622.
9. Booij LH. The history of neuromuscular blocking agents. *Curr Anaesth Crit Care.* 2000;11:7.
10. Booij LH. Is succinylcholine appropriate or obsolete in the intensive care unit? *Crit Care.* 2001;5:245-246.
11. Bowman WC. Non-relaxant properties of neuromuscular blocking drugs. *Br J Anaesth.* 1982;54:147-160.
12. Brandom BW. Genetics of malignant hyperthermia. *ScientificWorldJournal.* 2006;6: 1722-1730.
13. Briggs ED, Kirsch JR. Anesthetic implications of neuromuscular disease. *J Anesth.* 2003;17:177-185.
14. Capacchione JF, Muldoon SM. The relationship between exertional heat illness, exertional rhabdomyolysis, and malignant hyperthermia. *Anesth Analg.* 2009;109: 1065-1069.
15. Capacchione JF, et al. Exertional rhabdomyolysis and malignant hyperthermia in a patient with ryanodine receptor type 1 gene, L-type calcium channel alpha-1 subunit gene, and calsequestrin-1 gene polymorphisms. *Anesthesiology.* 2010;112:239-244.
16. Carmona GN, et al. Intravenous butyrylcholinesterase administration and plasma and brain levels of cocaine and metabolites in rats. *Eur J Pharmacol.* 2005;517: 186-190.
17. Chapple DJ, et al. Cardiovascular and neurological effects of laudanosine. Studies in mice and rats, and in conscious and anaesthetized dogs. *Br J Anaesth.* 1987;59: 218-225.
18. Conti, F. Claude Bernard's Des Fonctions du Cerveau: an ante litteram manifesto of the neurosciences? *Nat Rev Neurosci.* 2002;3:979-985.
19. Cronnelly R, Morris RB. Antagonism of neuromuscular blockade. *Br J Anaesth.* 1982; 54:183-194.
20. Davis L, et al. Cholinesterase. Its significance in anaesthetic practice. *Anaesthesia.* 1997;52:244-260.
21. de Letter MA, et al. Risk factors for the development of polyneuropathy and myopathy in critically ill patients. *Crit Care Med.* 2001;29:2281-2286.
22. Deem S, et al. Acquired neuromuscular disorders in the intensive care unit. *Am J Respir Crit Care Med.* 2003;168:735-739.
23. Denborough M. Malignant hyperthermia. *Lancet.* 1998;352:1131-1136.
24. Devenyi P. Cocaine complications and pseudocholinesterase. *Ann Intern Med.* 1989; 110:167-168.
25. Dhonneur G, et al. Effects of an intubating dose of succinylcholine and rocuronium on the larynx and diaphragm: an electromyographic study in humans. *Anesthesiology.* 1999;90:951-955.
26. Domenech JS, et al. Pancuronium bromide: an indirect sympathomimetic agent. *Br J Anaesth.* 1976;48:1143-1148.
27. Douglass JA, et al. Myopathy in severe asthma. *Am Rev Respir Dis.* 1992;146:517-519.
28. Durant NN, Katz RL. Suxamethonium. *Br J Anaesth.* 1982;54:195-208.
29. Eddleston JM, et al. Concentrations of atracurium and laudanosine in cerebrospinal fluid and plasma during intracranial surgery. *Br J Anaesth.* 1989;63:525-530.
30. Eriksson LI. The effects of residual neuromuscular blockade and volatile anesthetics on the control of ventilation. *Anesth Analg.* 1999;89:243-251.
31. Eriksson LI. Reduced hypoxic chemosensitivity in partially paralysed man. A new property of muscle relaxants? *Acta Anaesthesiol Scand.* 1996;40:520-523.
32. Farbu E, et al. Anaesthetic complications associated with myotonia congenita: case study and comparison with other myotonic disorders. *Acta Anaesthesiol Scand.* 2003;47:630-634.
33. Fill M, Copello JA. Ryanodine receptor calcium release channels. *Physiol Rev.* 2002;82: 893-922.
34. Fisher DM, et al. Elimination of atracurium in humans: contribution of Hofmann elimination and ester hydrolysis versus organ-based elimination. *Anesthesiology.* 1986;65:6-12.
35. Fleming NW, et al. Neuromuscular blocking action of suxamethonium after antagonism of vecuronium by edrophonium, pyridostigmine or neostigmine. *Br J Anaesth.* 1996;77:492-495.
36. Fletcher JE, et al. Sodium channel in human malignant hyperthermia. *Anesthesiology.* 1997;86:1023-1032.
37. Fletcher SN, et al. Persistent neuromuscular and neurophysiologic abnormalities in long-term survivors of prolonged critical illness. *Crit Care Med.* 2003;31:1012-1016.
38. Fodale V, Santamaria LB. Laudanosine, an atracurium and cisatracurium metabolite. *Eur J Anaesthesiol.* 2002;19:466-473.
39. Foldes FF. Distribution and biotransformation of succinylcholine. *Int Anesthesiol Clin.* 1975;13:101-115.
40. Foldes FF, Norton S. The urinary excretion of succinyldicholine and succinylmonocholine in man. *Br J Pharmacol Chemother.* 1954;9:385-388.
41. Forney RB Jr, et al. Extraction, identification and quantitation of succinylcholine in embalmed tissue. *J Anal Toxicol.* 1982;6:115-119.
42. Gray AT, et al. Neuromuscular blocking drugs do not alter the pupillary light reflex of anesthetized humans. *Arch Neurol.* 1997;54:579-584.
43. Griffith HR, Johnson GE. The use of curare in general anesthesia. *Anesthesiology.* 1943;3:3.
44. Gronert GA, et al. Aetiology of malignant hyperthermia. *Br J Anaesth.* 1988;60:253-267.
45. Gyermek L. Increased potency of nondepolarizing relaxants after poliomyelitis. *J Clin Pharmacol.* 1990;30:170-173.
46. Haeseler G, et al. Succinylcholine metabolite succinic acid alters steady state activation in muscle sodium channels. *Anesthesiology.* 2000;92:1385-1391.
47. Heffron JJ. Malignant hyperthermia: biochemical aspects of the acute episode. *Br J Anaesth.* 1988;60:274-278.
48. Hemmerling TM, et al. Sugammadex—a short review and clinical recommendations for the cardiac anesthesiologist. *Ann Card Anaesth.* 2010;13:206-216.
49. Herridge MS, et al. One-year outcomes in survivors of the acute respiratory distress syndrome. *N Engl J Med.* 2003;348:683-693.

50. Hirshey Dirksen SJ, et al. Special article: future directions in malignant hyperthermia research and patient care. *Anesth Analg.* 2011;113:1108-1119.

51. Hoffman RS, et al. Association between life-threatening cocaine toxicity and plasma cholinesterase activity. *Ann Emerg Med.* 1992;21:247-253.

52. Kaeser H E. Drug-induced myasthenic syndromes. *Acta Neurol Scand Suppl.* 1984;100:39-47.

53. Kampe SJ, et al. Muscle relaxants. *Best Pract Res Clin Anaesthesiol.* 2003;17:137-146.

54. Kasamatsu Y, et al. Rhabdomyolysis after infection and taking a cold medicine in a patient who was susceptible to malignant hyperthermia. *Intern Med.* 1998;37:169-173.

55. Kato M, et al. Comparison between in vivo and in vitro pharmacokinetics of succinylcholine in humans. *J Anesth.* 1999;13:189-192.

56. Kerskes CH, et al. The detection and identification of quaternary nitrogen muscle relaxants in biological fluids and tissues by ion-trap LC-ESI-MS. *J Anal Toxicol.* 2002;26:29-34.

57. King MJ, et al. Influence of neostigmine on postoperative vomiting. *Br J Anaesth.* 1988;61:403-406.

58. Kisor DF, Schmith VD. Clinical pharmacokinetics of cisatracurium besilate. *Clin Pharmacokinet.* 1999;36:27-40.

59. Kopman AF, et al. Molar potency is predictive of the speed of onset of neuromuscular block for agents of intermediate, short, and ultrashort duration. *Anesthesiology.* 1999;90:425-431.

60. Kopman AF, et al. Molar potency is not predictive of the speed of onset of atracurium. *Anesth Analg.* 1999;89:1046-1049.

61. Kovarik WD, et al. Succinylcholine does not change intracranial pressure, cerebral blood flow velocity, or the electroencephalogram in patients with neurologic injury. *Anesth Analg.* 1994;78:469-473.

62. Larach MG, et al. Cardiac arrests and deaths associated with malignant hyperthermia in North America from 1987 to 2006: a report from the North American Malignant Hyperthermia Registry of the malignant hyperthermia association of the United States. *Anesthesiology.* 2008;108:603-611.

63. Larach MG, et al. Clinical presentation, treatment, and complications of malignant hyperthermia in North America from 1987 to 2006. *Anesth Analg.* 2010;110:498-507.

64. Larach MG, et al. Hyperkalemic cardiac arrest during anesthesia in infants and children with occult myopathies. *Clin Pediatr (Phila).* 1997;36:9-16.

65. Latronico N, et al. Acute neuromuscular respiratory failure after ICU discharge. Report of five patients. *Intensive Care Med.* 1999;25:1302-1306.

66. Laxenaire MC. Neuromuscular blocking drugs and allergic risk. *Can J Anaesth.* 2003;50:429-433.

67. LeBeau M, Quenzer C. Succinylmonocholine identified in negative control tissues. *J Anal Toxicol.* 2003;27:600-601.

68. Lee C. Dose relationships of phase II, tachyphylaxis and train-of-four fade in suxamethonium-induced dual neuromuscular block in man. *Br J Anaesth.* 1975;47:841-845.

69. Lefrant JY, et al. Pharmacodynamics and atracurium and laudanosine concentrations during a fixed continuous infusion of atracurium in mechanically ventilated patients with acute respiratory distress syndrome. *Anaesth Intensive Care.* 2002;30:422-427.

70. Leijten FS, et al. Critical illness polyneuropathy in multiple organ dysfunction syndrome and weaning from the ventilator. *Intensive Care Med.* 1996;22:856-861.

71. Leijten FS, et al. The role of polyneuropathy in motor convalescence after prolonged mechanical ventilation. *JAMA.* 1995;274:1221-1225.

72. Lonsdale M, Stuart J. Complete heart block following glycopyrronium/neostigmine mixture. *Anaesthesia.* 1989;44:448-449.

73. Loper KA, et al. Paralyzed with pain: the need for education. *Pain.* 1989;37:315-316.

74. Lukas RJ, et al. International Union of Pharmacology. XX. Current status of the nomenclature for nicotinic acetylcholine receptors and their subunits. *Pharmacol Rev.* 1999;51:397-401.

75. Lynch TJ, et al. Cocaine detoxification by human plasma butyrylcholinesterase. *Toxicol Appl Pharmacol.* 1997;145:363-371.

76. MacLennan DH, Phillips MS. Malignant hyperthermia. *Science.* 1992;256:789-794.

77. Maltby JR. Criminal poisoning with anaesthetic drugs: murder, manslaughter, or not guilty. *Forensic Sci.* 1975;6:91-108.

78. Mattes CE, et al. Therapeutic use of butyrylcholinesterase for cocaine intoxication. *Toxicol Appl Pharmacol.* 1997;145:372-380.

79. McManus MC. Neuromuscular blockers in surgery and intensive care, Part 1. *Am J Health Syst Pharm.* 2001;58:2287-2299.

80. McManus MC. Neuromuscular blockers in surgery and intensive care, Part 2. *Am J Health Syst Pharm.* 2001;58:2381-2395.

81. Mertes PM, Laxenaire MC. Adverse reactions to neuromuscular blocking agents. *Curr Allergy Asthma Rep.* 2004;4:7-16.

82. Meyer E, et al. Succinic acid is not a suitable indicator of suxamethonium exposure in forensic blood samples. *J Anal Toxicol.* 1997;21:170-171.

83. Monnier N, et al. Correlations between genotype and pharmacological, histological, functional, and clinical phenotypes in malignant hyperthermia susceptibility. *Hum Mutat.* 2005;26:413-425.

84. Morrison AG, Serpell MG. Malignant hyperthermia during prolonged surgery for tumour resection. *Eur J Anaesthesiol.* 1998;15:114-117.

85. Murphy GS, Vender JS. Neuromuscular-blocking drugs. Use and misuse in the intensive care unit. *Crit Care Clin.* 2001;17:925-942.

86. Murray MJ, et al. Clinical practice guidelines for sustained neuromuscular blockade in the adult critically ill patient. *Crit Care Med.* 2002;30:142-156.

87. Naguib M. Sugammadex: another milestone in clinical neuromuscular pharmacology. *Anesth Analg.* 2007;104:575-581.

88. Narimatsu E, et al. Sepsis attenuates the intensity of the neuromuscular blocking effect of d-tubocurarine and the antagonistic actions of neostigmine and edrophonium accompanying depression of muscle contractility of the diaphragm. *Acta Anaesthesiol Scand.* 1999;43:196-201.

89. Nigrovic V, Fox JL. Atracurium decay and the formation of laudanosine in humans. *Anesthesiology.* 1991;74:446-454.

90. Nordgren IK, et al. Analysis of succinylcholine in tissues and body fluids by ion-pair extraction and gas chromatography-mass spectrometry. *Arch Toxicol Suppl.* 1983;6:339-350.

91. O'Flynn RP, et al. Masseter muscle rigidity and malignant hyperthermia susceptibility in pediatric patients. An update on management and diagnosis. *Anesthesiology.* 1994;80:1228-1233.

92. Om A, et al. Medical complications of cocaine: possible relationship to low plasma cholinesterase enzyme. *Am Heart J.* 1993;125:1114-1117.

93. Ording H. Incidence of malignant hyperthermia in Denmark. *Anesth Analg.* 1985;64:700-704.

94. Ostergaard DJ, et al. Adverse reactions and interactions of the neuromuscular blocking drugs. *Med Toxicol Adverse Drug Exp.* 1989;4:351-368.

95. Pantuck EJ. Plasma cholinesterase: gene and variations. *Anesth Analg.* 1993;77:380-386.

96. Parker CJ, et al. Disposition of infusions of atracurium and its metabolite, laudanosine, in patients in renal and respiratory failure in an ITU. *Br J Anaesth.* 1988;61:531-540.

97. Prielipp RC, Coursin DB. Applied pharmacology of common neuromuscular blocking agents in critical care. *New Horiz.* 1994;2:34-47.

98. Rike W. Pre-junctional effects of neuromuscular blocking and facilitatory drugs. In: Katz R, ed. *Muscle Relaxants.* Amsterdam, Netherlands: North-Holland Publishing Co.; 1975:59-102.

99. Roewer N, et al. Cardiovascular and metabolic responses to anesthetic-induced malignant hyperthermia in swine. *Anesthesiology.* 1995;83:141-159.

100. Rosenberg H, et al. Malignant hyperthermia. *Orphanet J Rare Dis.* 2007;2:21.

101. Saltzman LS, et al. Hyperkalemia and cardiovascular collapse after verapamil and dantrolene administration in swine. *Anesth Analg.* 1984;63:473-478.

102. Savarese JJ. The autonomic margins of safety of metocurine and d-tubocurarine in the cat. *Anesthesiology.* 1979;50:40-46.

103. Saxena PR, Bonta IL. Mechanism of selective cardiac vagolytic action of pancuronium bromide. Specific blockade of cardiac muscarinic receptors. *Eur J Pharmacol.* 1970;11:332-341.

104. Sayer H, et al. Identification and quantitation of six non-depolarizing neuromuscular blocking agents by LC-MS in biological fluids. *J Anal Toxicol.* 2004;28:105-110.

105. Schindler CW, Goldberg SR. Accelerating cocaine metabolism as an approach to the treatment of cocaine abuse and toxicity. *Future Med Chem.* 2012;4:163-175.

106. Schreiber JU, et al. Prevention of succinylcholine-induced fasciculation and myalgia: a meta-analysis of randomized trials. *Anesthesiology.* 2005;103:877-884.

107. Somogyi G, et al. Drug identification problems in two suicides with neuromuscular blocking agents. *Forensic Sci Int.* 1989;43:257-266.

108. Sprague DH. Severe bradycardia after neostigmine in a patient taking propranolol to control paroxysmal atrial tachycardia. *Anesthesiology.* 1975;42:208-210.

109. Stewart JB. *Blind Eye: How the Medical Establishment Let a Doctor Get Away with Murder.* New York, NY: Simon & Schuster; 1999:336.

110. Stoelting RK. The hemodynamic effects of pancuronium and d-tubocurarine in anesthetized patients. *Anesthesiology.* 1972;36:612-615.

111. Tsutsumi H, et al. Adsorption and stability of suxamethonium and its major hydrolysis product succinylmonocholine using liquid chromatography-electrospray ionization mass spectrometry. *J Health Sci.* 2003;49:285-291.

112. van Mook WN, Hulsewe-Evers RP. Critical illness polyneuropathy. *Curr Opin Crit Care.* 2002;8:302-310.

113. Verburg MP, et al. In vivo induced malignant hyperthermia in pigs. I. Physiological and biochemical changes and the influence of dantrolene sodium. *Acta Anaesthesiol Scand.* 1984;28:1-8.

114. Viby-Mogensen J. Interaction of other drugs with muscle relaxants. In: Katz R, ed. *Muscle Relaxants: Basic and Clinical Aspects.* New York, NY: Grune & Stratton; 1985:233-256.

115. Watkins J. Adverse reaction to neuromuscular blockers: frequency, investigation, and epidemiology. *Acta Anaesthesiol Scand Suppl.* 1994;102:6-10.

116. West R. Curare in man. *Proc Royal Soc Med.* 1932;25:1107-1116.

117. Yate PM, et al. Clinical experience and plasma laudanosine concentrations during the infusion of atracurium in the intensive therapy unit. *Br J Anaesth.* 1987;59:211-217.

DANTROLENE SODIUM

Caitlin J. Guo and Kenneth M. Sutin

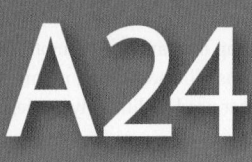

Dantrolene

INTRODUCTION

Dantrolene produces relaxation of skeletal muscle without causing complete paralysis. It is the only therapy proven to be effective for both treatment and prophylaxis of malignant hyperthermia (MH).[8] Malignant hyperthermia is a rare life-threatening condition that is triggered by the use of either an inhalational anesthetic or succinylcholine. It is a syndrome of hypermetabolism involving the skeletal muscle, which overwhelms the ability of the body to supply oxygen, remove carbon dioxide, and regulate body temperature and can quickly lead to circulatory collapse if untreated. Typical signs include severe hyperthermia, increased CO_2 production and oxygen consumption, hemodynamic instability, mixed respiratory and metabolic acidosis, hyperkalemia, muscle rigidity, and rhabdomyolysis.

HISTORY

Dantrolene was first synthesized in 1967.[33] Four years later, it was used in oral form to treat skeletal muscle spasticity secondary to neurologic disorders.[6] The ability of intravenous (IV) dantrolene to rapidly reverse MH was first reported in swine in 1975[11] and subsequently in humans in 1982.[16] The delay from dantrolene discovery to clinical use was in part due to the difficulty encountered in formulating a parenteral (water-soluble) solution of the lipid-soluble drug.

PHARMACOLOGY

Dantrolene is a hydantoin derivative that is structurally similar to local anesthetics and anticonvulsants but possess neither property.[17,37] It is highly lipophilic and relatively insoluble in water. Widespread use had to wait until a there was a suitable IV preparation. Today mannitol is added to the lyophilized dantrolene to improve solubility. In plasma, dantrolene is bound to plasma proteins, especially albumin. Oral dantrolene exhibits variable absorption by the small intestine, bioavailability is up to 70%, and peak blood concentrations are achieved 3 to 6 hours after ingestion.[17]

Quantitative analysis of dantrolene and its metabolites were performed using reverse-phase, high-performance liquid chromatography.[1] After a 2.4-mg/kg IV dose, the mean serum dantrolene concentration was 4.2 mcg/mL.[8] This concentration produced a 75% reduction in twitch contraction of skeletal muscle.[8] The therapeutic plasma concentration in humans is estimated at 2.8 to 4.2 mcg/mL.[8]

Dantrolene is metabolized in the liver by 5-hydroxylation of the hydantoin ring or by reduction of the nitro group to an amine.[37] Up to 20% of administered dantrolene is excreted in the urine as the 5-hydroxydantrolene, which is an active metabolite that is half as potent as the parent drug.[37] In adults, the elimination half-lives are 6 to 9 hours for dantrolene and 15.5 hours for the 5-hydroxydantrolene metabolite.[37] In one study of children ages 2 to 7 years, the dantrolene elimination half-life was 10 hours, and that for 5-hydroxydantrolene was 9 hours.[18]

At therapeutic concentrations, dantrolene inhibits binding of [^{3}H]ryanodine to the ryanodine receptor type 1 (RYR-1) receptor on sarcoplasmic reticulum membrane of skeletal muscle,[24] causing a dose-dependent inhibition of both the steady and peak components of calcium release.[34] This reduces the free myoplasmic calcium concentration and thereby directly inhibits excitation–contraction coupling.[20] Dantrolene causes skeletal muscle weakness but not complete paralysis, which may be related to its low water solubility. This plateau effect (achieved at a plasma concentration of 4.2 mcg/mL) produces a 75% reduction of skeletal muscle twitch contraction and a 42% reduction in hand grip strength.[8] Dantrolene does not change the electrical properties or excitation of nerve excitation–contraction coupling at the neuromuscular junction (NMJ), or skeletal muscle, and it does not alter sarcoplasmic calcium reuptake. Dantrolene does not bind to the cardiac ryanodine receptor (RYR-2) and thus does not have any direct cardiac effects.[10,36,39] In animal models, the combination with verapamil use is associated with a significant decrease in cardiac function, although this has not been described in humans.[21,30] Dantrolene also stabilizes adverse ventricular electrophysiological characteristics and ventricular dysrhythmias in rat models of chronic β-adrenergic receptor activation.[19]

ROLE IN MALIGNANT HYPERTHERMIA AND OTHER HYPERTHERMIAS

Dantrolene is indicated for treatment of skeletal muscle hypermetabolism characteristic of MH after an acute episode of MH to prevent recrudescence. Long-term oral dantrolene therapy is used rarely to treat chronic spasticity.[15] Historically, dantrolene was used prophylactically in MH-susceptible individuals; however, current practice is simply to avoid exposure to triggers of MH during anesthesia in potentially susceptible patients.

It is reasonable to administer dantrolene for patients with severe hypermetabolism when the diagnosis of MH cannot be excluded with certainty, especially when there is coexisting respiratory and metabolic acidosis, coagulopathy, hyperthermia, or rhabdomyolysis.[7] In typical fulminant MH, the diagnosis is not subtle, and the course of treatment is obvious once the diagnosis is considered. This is not true when the clinical presentation is atypical. Atypical clinical presentations of MH in the presence or absence of triggering anesthetics are reported, especially in MH-susceptible individuals.

Dantrolene use is reported in hyperthermic syndromes other than MH, including antipsychotic malignant syndrome,[25] heat stroke,[2] serotonin toxicity,[12] monoamine oxidase inhibitor interaction or overdose,[13] methylenedioxymethamphetamine ("ecstasy") overdose,[22,27] intrathecal baclofen withdrawal,[14] and thyroid storm.[5] Given the lack of evidence-based support for these conditions, dantrolene therapy is not recommended for indications other than MH. However, given that (1) the differential diagnosis of a hyperthermic syndrome does not necessarily exclude (and often includes) that of MH, (2) the definitive diagnosis of a hyperthermic syndrome may be subtle or delayed, and (3) MH may occur simultaneously with another hyperthermic syndrome,[23] it is reasonable to give dantrolene when MH cannot be specifically excluded because its use may be lifesaving and response to standard cooling measure is not rapidly effective. It bears emphasis that dantrolene provided for hyperthermia does not substitute for aggressive cooling and resuscitation.

ADVERSE EFFECTS AND SAFETY ISSUES

The alkaline pH of the reconstituted dantrolene causes pain at the injection site and thrombophlebitis in 9% of patients.[3] Unintended extravasation can cause tissue necrosis, highlighting that dantrolene should only be given through a central vein or a large peripheral vein. There is no evidence to suggest allergic cross-reactivity with dantrolene in patients with prior phenytoin allergy.

When given to healthy persons or for MH prophylaxis or treatment, dantrolene causes skeletal muscle weakness in 15% to 22%, and diaphragm weakness (dyspnea) is noted.[3,38] In healthy volunteers, dantrolene 2.5 mg/kg does not reduce respiratory rate, vital capacity, or peak expiratory flow rate.[8] However, in patients with diminished respiratory reserve (eg, end stage pulmonary disease, preexisting neuromuscular disease), dantrolene is reported to precipitate respiratory failure.[3,17] Dantrolene also causes gastrointestinal distress, nausea, and vomiting. Other reported side effects include dizziness, somnolence, disorientation, ptosis, blurred vision, and dysphagia.[3,8,38] Uncommonly, compartment syndrome is observed, and even though likely secondary to MH or trauma, it is associated with dantrolene administration.[3]

Dantrolene and verapamil should not be used in combination because of the risk of hyperkalemia and hypotension; however, the mechanistic details of this drug interaction remain unclear.[17,26,30] Intravenous calcium salts are safe to administer with dantrolene if needed, such as for the treatment of cardiac dysrhythmias or hyperkalemia (during an episode of MH).

When dantrolene is given orally for more than 2 months to treat skeletal muscle spasticity, there is a 1.8% risk of dose- and duration-related chronic hepatitis, including elevated aminotransferase concentrations and hyperbilirubinemia[35] that it is not always fully reversible after dantrolene is discontinued.[4]

PREGNANCY AND LACTATION

Dosing during pregnancy is based on total body weight. Dantrolene rapidly crosses the placenta and is slowly excreted in breast milk.[32] The elimination half-life in neonates is about 20 hours.[32] At the concentrations achieved in serum or breast milk, there are no reports of significant adverse neonatal effects, although there is a potential for neonatal respiratory depression. However, it is suggested that breastfeeding only resume 48 hours after the last dose of dantrolene.[9] Dantrolene carries a Pregnancy Category C designation because embryo lethality in rabbits and decreased pup survival in rats were observed at doses seven times the human oral dose.[28]

FORMULATION

There are currently two formulations of dantrolene, Dantrium or Revonto, and Ryanodex. Approved by the US Food and Drug Administration in 2014, Ryanodex[29,31] offers significant advantages over the older formulations.

Dantrium and Revonto are long-standing formulations of dantrolene, they are supplied as a sterile lyophilized powder in a 70-mL vial that contains 20 mg of dantrolene sodium and 3,000 mg of mannitol. After addition of 60 mL of sterile water to each vial, each vial is shaken for approximately 20 seconds and until the solution becomes clear. The final solution is isotonic and has a pH of approximately 9.5. Caution must be taken to avoid extravasation. The extreme alkalinity of the reconstituted solution also can corrode glass and thus must not be transferred into a glass bottle for prophylactic infusion.

Ryanodex is supplied as a sterile nanocrystalline powder suspension containing 250 mg of dantrolene sodium (or 12.5 times more dantrolene per vial than the older formulations) and 125 mg of mannitol. Each vial of Ryanodex is reconstituted with 5 mL of preservative-free sterile water. It is not compatible with dextrose-containing solutions nor 0.9% sodium chloride because they may cause precipitation. The reconstituted vial is shaken for 10 seconds until a uniform orange color suspension forms. Ryanodex can be administered by IV bolus into a free running infusion line of either 0.9% sodium chloride or 5% dextrose solution. Because of the extreme alkalinity of the reconstituted solution (pH of 10.5), care must be taken to prevent extravasation into surrounding tissue and possible tissue necrosis.

A single vial of Ryanodex is sufficient to provide a loading dose for a patient weighing up to 100 kg, and it can be mixed and administered in less than 1 minute. For the older dantrolene formulations, a 100-kg patient requires 12.5 vials to be prepared and in a much larger volume of sterile water, a process that could take 15 to 20 minutes and multiple providers to mix and administer.

Of note, each vial of Ryanodex contains 125 mg of mannitol compared with 3,000 mg of mannitol in the older formulations. The additional mannitol may not be required because the volume of water used to dilute Ryanodex is much less than for the older formulations.

DOSING AND ADMINISTRATION

The initial dose of dantrolene for treatment of acute MH is an IV bolus of 2.5 mg/kg in the adults and children.[18] Depending on the formulation, for a typical adult, the initial dose may require multiple bottles of dantrolene to be simultaneously reconstituted. The newer formulation provides 250 mg dantrolene per vial, and the older formulation provides 20 mg per vial. Initial dosing probably should be determined by total body weight given that dantrolene is lipophilic; however, its pharmacokinetics in obesity are not determined.[8] Redosing of 2.5 mg/kg IV is recommended every 15 minutes until the signs of hypermetabolism are reversed or until a total dose of approximately 10 mg/kg has been administered. Occasionally, doses in excess of 10 mg/kg are required; however, alternative diagnosis should be considered in such cases. The key point is that the total dose of dantrolene is determined by titration to a metabolic endpoint and resolution of skeletal muscle hypermetabolism. When an effective dose of dantrolene is given, signs of muscle hypermetabolism usually start to normalize within 30 minutes.[16]

After successful termination of the acute episode of hypermetabolism, it is recommended that dantrolene therapy be continued for at least 24 hours to prevent reoccurrences, with bolus dosing at 1 mg/kg IV every 4 to 6 hours or 0.25 mg/kg/h IV as a continuous infusion. After 24 hours, dantrolene can be discontinued or the interval doses increased to every 8 or 12 hours if the patient has achieved metabolic stability and is clinically improving. The Malignant Hyperthermia Association of the United States (MHAUS) has similar recommendations for postexposure.

SUMMARY

- Dantrolene is the only specific antidote to treat malignant hyperthermia.
- Dantrolene should be stocked whenever MH-triggering xenobiotics are used.
- Dantrolene is primarily eliminated by the liver and about 20% is excreted in the urine as an active metabolite, that is half potent as the parent drug.
- Dantrolene is lipophilic, crosses the placenta and is excreted in breast milk.
- The initial dose of dantrolene for treatment of acute MH is an IV bolus of 2.5 mg/kg in adults and children, which is repeated every 15 minutes until clinical signs of hypermetabolism are corrected.
- The Malignant Hyperthermia Association of the United States maintains a website, www.mhaus.org; a toll-free hotline for MH emergencies, 800-MH-HYPER (644-9737); and a national MH registry.

REFERENCES

1. Allen GC, et al. Plasma levels of dantrolene following oral administration in malignant hyperthermia-susceptible patients. *Anesthesiology.* 1988;69 Comp/PM: Remove the issue number during revisions:900-904.
2. Bouchama A, et al. Cooling and hemodynamic management in heatstroke: practical recommendations. *Crit Care.* 2007;11:R54.
3. Brandom BW, et al. Complications associated with the administration of dantrolene 1987 to 2006: a report from the North American Malignant Hyperthermia Registry of the Malignant Hyperthermia Association of the United States. *Anesth Analg.* 2011;112:1115-1123.
4. Chan CH. Dantrolene sodium and hepatic injury. *Neurology.* 1990;40:1427-1432.
5. Christensen PA, Nissen LR. Treatment of thyroid storm in a child with dantrolene. *Br J Anaesth.* 1987;59:523.
6. Chyatte SB, et al. The effects of dantrolene sodium on spasticity and motor performance in hemiplegia. *South Med J.* 1971;64:180-185.
7. Denborough M. Malignant hyperthermia. *Lancet.* 1998;352:1131-1136.
8. Flewellen EH, et al. Dantrolene dose response in awake man: implications for management of malignant hyperthermia. *Anesthesiology.* 1983;59:275-280.
9. Fricker RM, et al. Secretion of dantrolene into breast milk after acute therapy of a suspected malignant hyperthermia crisis during cesarean section. *Anesthesiology.* 1998;89:1023-1025.

10. Fruen BR, et al. Dantrolene inhibition of sarcoplasmic reticulum Ca2+ release by direct and specific action at skeletal muscle ryanodine receptors. *J Biol Chem.* 1997;272:26965-26971.
11. Harrison GG. Control of the malignant hyperpyrexic syndrome in MHS swine by dantrolene sodium. *Br J Anaesth.* 1975;47:62-65.
12. John L, et al. Serotonin syndrome associated with nefazodone and paroxetine. *Ann Emerg Med.* 1997;29:287-289.
13. Kaplan RF, et al. Phenelzine overdose treated with dantrolene sodium. *JAMA.* 1986;255:642-644.
14. Khorasani A, Peruzzi WT. Dantrolene treatment for abrupt intrathecal baclofen withdrawal. *Anesth Analg.* 1995;80:1054-1056.
15. Kita M, Goodkin DE. Drugs used to treat spasticity. *Drugs.* 2000;59:487-495.
16. Kolb ME, et al. Dantrolene in human malignant hyperthermia. *Anesthesiology.* 1982;56:254-262.
17. Krause T, et al. Dantrolene—a review of its pharmacology, therapeutic use and new developments. *Anaesthesia.* 2004;59:364-373.
18. Lerman J, et al. Pharmacokinetics of intravenous dantrolene in children. *Anesthesiology.* 1989;70:625-629.
19. Liu T, et al. Effects of dantrolene treatment on ventricular electrophysiology and arrhythmogenesis in rats with chronic beta-adrenergic receptor activation. *J Cardiovasc Pharmacol Ther.* 2015;20:414-427.
20. Lopez JR, et al. Effects of dantrolene on myoplasmic free [Ca2+] measured in vivo in patients susceptible to malignant hyperthermia. *Anesthesiology.* 1992;76:711-719.
21. Lynch C 3rd, et al. Effects of dantrolene and verapamil on atrioventricular conduction and cardiovascular performance in dogs. *Anesth Analg.* 1986. 65:252-258.
22. Moon J, Cros J. Role of dantrolene in the management of the acute toxic effects of Ecstasy (MDMA). *Br J Anaesth.* 2007;99:146.
23. Nishiyama K, et al. Malignant hyperthermia in a patient with Graves' disease during subtotal thyroidectomy. *Endocr J.* 2001;48:227-232.
24. Paul-Pletzer K, et al. Identification of a dantrolene-binding sequence on the skeletal muscle ryanodine receptor. *J Biol Chem.* 2002;277:34918-34923.
25. Reulbach U, et al. Managing an effective treatment for neuroleptic malignant syndrome. *Crit Care.* 2007;11:R4.
26. Rubin AS, Zablocki AD. Hyperkalemia, verapamil, and dantrolene. *Anesthesiology.* 1987;66:246-249.
27. Rusyniak DE, et al. Dantrolene use in 3,4-methylenedioxymethamphetamine (ecstasy)-mediated hyperthermia. *Anesthesiology.* 2004;101:263; author reply 264.
28. Eagle Pharmaceuticals. Ryanodex (dantrolene sodium) for injectable suspension, for intravenous use [prescribing information]. Woodcliff Lake, NJ: Eagle Pharmaceuticals; 2014.
29. Anonymous. Ryanodex—a new dantrolene formulation for malignant hyperthermia. *Med Lett Drugs Ther.* 2015;57:100.
30. Saltzman LS, et al. Hyperkalemia and cardiovascular collapse after verapamil and dantrolene administration in swine. *Anesth Analg.* 1984;63:473-478.
31. Schutte JK, et al. Comparison of the therapeutic effectiveness of a dantrolene sodium solution and a novel nanocrystalline suspension of dantrolene sodium in malignant hyperthermia normal and susceptible pigs. *Eur J Anaesthesiol.* 2011;28:256-264.
32. Shime J, et al. Dantrolene in pregnancy: lack of adverse effects on the fetus and newborn infant. *Am J Obstet Gynecol.* 1988;159:831-834.
33. Snyder HR Jr, et al. 1-[(5-arylfurfurylidene)amino]hydantoins. A new class of muscle relaxants. *J Med Chem.* 1967;10:807-810.
34. Szentesi P, et al. Effects of dantrolene on steps of excitation-contraction coupling in mammalian skeletal muscle fibers. *J Gen Physiol.* 2001;118:355-375.
35. Utili R, et al. Dantrolene-associated hepatic injury. Incidence and character. *Gastroenterology.* 1977;72(4 Pt 1):610-616.
36. Van Winkle WB. Calcium release from skeletal muscle sarcoplasmic reticulum: site of action of dantrolene sodium. *Science.* 1976;193:1130-1131.
37. Ward A, et al. Dantrolene. A review of its pharmacodynamic and pharmacokinetic properties and therapeutic use in malignant hyperthermia, the neuroleptic malignant syndrome and an update of its use in muscle spasticity. *Drugs.* 1986;32:130-168.
38. Wedel DJ, et al. Clinical effects of intravenously administered dantrolene. *Mayo Clin Proc.* 1995;70:241-246.
39. Zhao F, et al. Dantrolene inhibition of ryanodine receptor Ca2+ release channels. Molecular mechanism and isoform selectivity. *J Biol Chem.* 2001;276:13810-13816.

67

ANTIPSYCHOTICS

David N. Juurlink

HISTORY AND EPIDEMIOLOGY

The development of antipsychotic drugs dramatically altered the practice of psychiatry and eventually, medical care in general. Before the introduction of chlorpromazine in 1950, patients with schizophrenia were treated with nonspecific sedatives such as barbiturates or chloral hydrate. Agitated patients were housed in large "mental institutions" and often placed in physical restraints, and thousands underwent surgical disruption of the connections between the frontal cortices and other areas of the brain (leucotomy). By 1955, approximately 500,000 patients with mental health disorders were institutionalized in the United States. The advent of antipsychotic drugs in the 1950s revolutionized the care of these patients. These drugs, originally termed *major tranquilizers* and subsequently *neuroleptics,* dramatically reduced the characteristic hallucinations, delusions, thought disorders and paranoia—the "positive" symptoms of schizophrenia.

Shortly after the introduction of these drugs, it became apparent that they were capable of causing significant toxicity after overdose, a common occurrence in patients with mental illness. Moreover, they were also associated with a host of adverse effects during routine therapeutic use, particularly involving the endocrine and nervous systems. The latter includes the extrapyramidal syndromes (EPS), a constellation of disorders that are relatively common, sometimes irreversible, and occasionally life threatening.

The search for new drugs led to the development of multiple antipsychotics in several distinct chemical classes. These drugs exhibited varying potencies and markedly different adverse effect profiles. The novel antipsychotic clozapine was first synthesized in 1959 but did not enter widespread clinical use until the early 1970s. Clozapine was unusual because it conferred a relatively low risk of EPS and was often effective in patients who had not responded well to other antipsychotics. Moreover, unlike other antipsychotic drugs available at the time, it often improved the "negative" symptoms of schizophrenia, such as avolition, alogia, and social withdrawal, symptoms that, although often less outwardly apparent than the positive symptoms, result in significant disability. Reports of life-threatening agranulocytosis led to the withdrawal of clozapine from the market in 1974, although it was reintroduced in 1990 with stringent monitoring requirements.[8,56] However, clozapine's unique therapeutic and pharmacologic properties led to its characterization as an *atypical* antipsychotic, the forerunner and prototype of many other second-generation antipsychotics that have now largely supplanted the earlier drugs in clinical practice.

Most antipsychotic toxicity occurs through one of two mechanisms. After overdose, antipsychotic toxicity is dose dependent and reflects an extension of the drug's effects on neurotransmitter systems and other biologic processes. The features of antipsychotic overdose are therefore generally predictable based on an understanding of the drug's pharmacology. Unpredictable (idiosyncratic) adverse effects also occur in the context of therapeutic use. These toxicities result from individual susceptibility, which may in part have a genetic basis, and are less reliably correlated with the antipsychotic dose. In both types of toxicity, the severity of illness ranges from minor to life threatening, depending on variety of other factors, including concomitant drug exposures, comorbidity, and access to medical care.

The true incidences of antipsychotic overdose and adverse effects are not known with certainty. Some patients never seek medical attention, and others are misdiagnosed. Even among those who seek medical attention and are correctly diagnosed, notification of poison control centers or other adverse event reporting systems is discretionary and incomplete (Chap. 130). With these limitations in mind, a few observations can be made.

In 2015, poison control centers in the United States were contacted about more than 2.17 million human exposures involving potential poisons.[92] Antipsychotic exposures are reported together with sedative–hypnotics, but these collectively represented 151,433 exposures (5.84% of all exposures). The vast majority of poison control center calls involving antipsychotic drugs pertain to intentional overdoses in patients 20 years or older, most of whom have a good outcome. However, these drugs were associated with more fatalities than any other group ($n = 401$ deaths), although the extent to which they played a causal role in death is unclear. Importantly, poison control center data underestimate the annual incidence of poisoning and mortality associated with antipsychotic drugs and likely identify only a small minority of adverse drug reactions involving these drugs (Chap. 130).

Although all antipsychotics exhibit significant toxicity in overdose, a substantial body of clinical experience and some observational data suggest that the low-potency, first-generation antipsychotics such as thioridazine, chlorpromazine, and mesoridazine are associated with greater toxicity than other antipsychotics.[18,20] Inferences regarding the relative toxicity of the antipsychotics derived from aggregated data should be extrapolated to individual patients with caution.[18,42]

PHARMACOLOGY

Classification

Antipsychotics are classified in several ways, according to their chemical structures, their receptor binding profiles, or as *typical* or *atypical* antipsychotics. Table 67–1 outlines the taxonomy of some of the more commonly used antipsychotics. Classification by chemical structure was most useful before the 1970s, when phenothiazines and butyrophenones constituted most of the antipsychotics in clinical use. At present, however, the spectrum of available antipsychotics and their structural heterogeneity renders this scheme of little use to clinicians. It is worth noting, however, that the phenothiazines exhibit a high degree of structural similarity to the tricyclic antidepressants (TCAs) (Fig. 67–1) and share many of their manifestations in overdose. The phenothiazines are further classified according to the nature of the substituent on the nitrogen atom at position 10 of the center ring as aliphatic, piperazine, or piperidine compounds.

Of greater clinical utility is the classification of antipsychotics according to their binding affinities for various receptors (Table 67–2). However, by far the most widely used classification system categorizes antipsychotics as either *typical* or *atypical*. Typical (also called *traditional*; *conventional*; or, increasingly, *first-generation*) antipsychotics dominated the first 40 years of antipsychotic therapy. They were subcategorized according to their affinity for the D_2 receptor as either low potency (exemplified by thioridazine and chlorpromazine) or high potency (exemplified by haloperidol).

The concept of atypicality has evolved over time with the introduction of new antipsychoticss[110,130] and connotes different features to pharmacologists and clinicians. From a clinical perspective, atypical (*second-generation*) antipsychotics treat both the positive and negative symptoms of schizophrenia, are less likely than traditional drugs to produce EPS at clinically effective doses, and cause little or no elevation of the serum prolactin concentration.[66] From a pharmacologic perspective, many atypical antipsychotics also inhibit the activity of serotonin at the 5-HT$_{2A}$ receptor. Some antipsychotics are

TABLE 67–1 Classification of Commonly Used Antipsychotics

Classification	Antipsychotic	Usual Daily Adult Dose (mg)	Volume of Distribution (L/kg)	Half-Life (Range, h)	Protein Binding (%)	Active Metabolite
Typicals						
Butyrophenones	Droperidol	1.25–30	2–3	2–10	85–90	N
	Haloperidol	1–20	18–30	14–41	90	Y
Diphenylbutylpiperidines	Pimozide	1–20	11–62	28–214	99	Y
Phenothiazines						
Aliphatic	Chlorpromazine	100–800	10–35	18–30	98	Y
	Methotrimeprazine	2–50	23–42	17–78	NR	Y
	Promazine	50–1,000	30–40	8–12	98	N
	Promethazine	25–150	9–25	9–16	93	Y
Piperazine	Fluphenazine	0.5–20	220	13–58[b]	99	NR
	Perphenazine	8–64	10–35	8–12	>90	NR
	Prochlorperazine	10–150	13–32	17–27	>90	NR
	Trifluoperazine	4–50	NR	7–18	>90	Y
Piperidine	Mesoridazine	100–400	3–6	2–9	98	Y
	Thioridazine	200–800	18	26–36	96	Y
	Pipotiazine	25–250 (monthly IM depot)	7.5	3–11	NR	N
Thioxanthenes	Chlorprothixene	30–300	11–23	8–12	NR	NR
	Flupentixol	3–6	7–8	7–36	NR	NR
	Thiothixene	5–30	NR	12–36	>90	NR
	Zuclopenthixol	20–100	10	20	NR	NR
Atypicals						
Benzamides	Amisulpride	50–1,200	5.8	12	16	N
	Raclopride	3–6	1.5	12–24	NR	N
	Remoxipride	150–600	0.7	3–7	80	Y
	Sulpiride	200–1,200	0.6–2.7	4–11	14–40	N
Benzepines						
Dibenzodiazepine	Clozapine	50–900	15–30	6–17	95	Y
Dibenzoxazepine	Loxapine[a]	20–250	NR	2–8	90–99	Y
Thienobenzodiazepine	Olanzapine	5–20	10–20	21–54	93	N
Dibenzothiazepine	Quetiapine	150–750	10	3–9	83	N
Indoles						
Benzisoxazole	Risperidone	2–16	0.7–2.1	3–20	90	Y
	Paliperidone	1–12 mg (IM 25–150 monthly)	7	23	74	N
	Iloperidone	12–14	30–36	18–33	96	Y
Imidazolidinone	Sertindole	12–24	20–40	24–200	99	Y
Benzisothiazole	Ziprasidone	40–160	2	4–10	99	N
	Lurasidone	20–160	80–90	29–37	99	Y
Dibenzo-oxepino pyrroles	Asenapine	5–20	20–25	13–39	95	N
Quinolinones	Aripiprazole	10–30	5	47–68	99	Y

[a]Loxapine's atypical profile is lost at doses >50 mg/d; it is sometimes therefore categorized as a typical antipsychotic. [b]For hydrochloride salt; enanthate and decanoate have ranges of 3–4 days and 5–12 days, respectively.

IM = intramuscular; N = no; NR = not reported; Y = yes.

Data from references 9, 11, 14, 39, 62, 70, and 86.

classified as third generation, reflecting the property of antagonism (or partial antagonism) of D_2 receptors with agonist at 5-HT$_{1A}$ receptors.[96]

More than two dozen atypical antipsychotics are now in clinical use or under development. Despite their considerably higher cost, they have largely supplanted traditional antipsychotics because of their effectiveness in treating the negative symptoms of schizophrenia and their somewhat more favorable adverse effect profile in addition to the perception that they cause fewer long-term adverse effects than conventional antipsychotics—a belief that may result, in part, from the use of higher doses of older drugs in studies comparing the tolerability of typical and atypical antipsychotics.[55] Controversy exists regarding the superiority of these drugs over first-generation antipsychotics, and it is worth noting that the use of the newer antipsychotics for indications other than schizophrenia is extremely common, including their use as adjunctive treatment for depression, eating disorders, attention

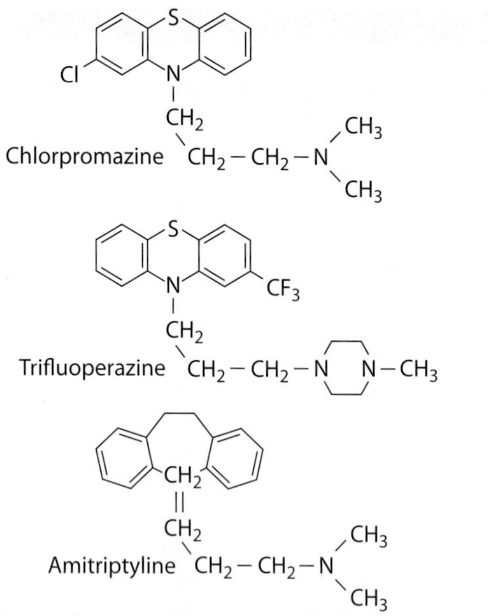

FIGURE 67–1. Structural similarity between phenothiazines and cyclic antidepressants.

deficit hyperactivity disorder, insomnia, posttraumatic stress disorder, personality disorders, and Tourette syndrome.[81] However, the most extensive off-label use of atypical antipsychotics is for the management of agitation association with cognitive impairment in older adults.

Mechanisms of Antipsychotic Action

Of the many contemporary theories of schizophrenia, the most enduring has been the *dopamine hypothesis*.[123] First advanced in 1967 and supported by in vivo data,[1] this theory posits that the "positive symptoms" of schizophrenia result from excessive dopaminergic signaling in the mesolimbic and mesocortical pathways.[88] This hypothesis arose in part from the observation that hallucinations and delusions could be produced in otherwise normal individuals by drugs that augment dopaminergic transmission, such as cocaine and amphetamine, and that these effects could be blunted by dopamine antagonists.

There are at least five subtypes of dopamine receptors (D_1 through D_5), but schizophrenia principally involves excess signaling at the D_2 subtype,[123] and antagonism of D_2 neurotransmission is the *sine qua non* of antipsychotic activity. Antipsychotics have different binding profiles at this receptor, reflected by the dissociation constant (K_d), which in turn reflects release of the drug from the receptor. For example, the receptor releases clozapine and quetiapine more rapidly than it does any other drugs.[121,123]

Dopamine receptors are present in many other areas of the central nervous system (CNS), including the nigrostriatal pathway (substantia nigra, caudate and putamen, which collectively govern the coordination of movement), tuberoinfundibular pathway, hypothalamus and pituitary, and area postrema of the medulla, which contains the chemoreceptor trigger zone (CTZ). Antipsychotic-related blockade of D_2 neurotransmission in these areas is associated with many of the beneficial and adverse effects of these drugs. For example, whereas D_2 antagonism in the CTZ alleviates nausea and vomiting, blockade of hypothalamic D_2 receptors increases pituitary prolactin release, resulting in gynecomastia and galactorrhea. Blockade of nigrostriatal D_2 receptors underlies many of the movement disorders associated with antipsychotic therapy.[136,150]

TABLE 67–2	Clinical and Toxicologic Manifestations of Selected Antipsychotics			
	α_1-Adrenergic Antagonism	Muscarinic Antagonism	Fast Sodium Channel (I_{Na}) Blockade	Delayed Rectifier (I_{Kr}) Blockade
Clinical effect	Hypotension	Central and peripheral anticholinergic effects	QRS complex widening; myocardial depression	QT interval prolongation; torsade de pointes
Typical				
Chlorpromazine	+++	++	++	++
Fluphenazine	−	−	+	+
Haloperidol	−	−	+	++
Loxapine	+++	++	++	+
Mesoridazine	+++	+++	+++	++
Perphenazine	+	−	+	++
Pimozide	+	−	+	++
Thioridazine	+++	+++	+++	+++
Trifluoperazine	+	−	+	++
Atypical				
Amisulpride	−	−	−	++
Asenapine	++	−	−	−
Aripiprazole	++	−	−	−
Clozapine	+++	+++	−	+
Iloperidone	+++	−	−	++
Lurasidone	−	−	−	−
Olanzapine	++	+++	−	−
Paliperidone	++	−	−	+
Quetiapine	+++	+++	+	− to +
Remoxipride	−	−	−	−
Risperidone	++	−	−	−
Sertindole	+	−	−	++
Ziprasidone	++	−	−	+++

+ to ++ = effect present in increasing degree; − − = effect is absent; − to + = presence of effect minimal or absent.
Data from references 19, 22, 51, 80, 112, and 114.

Antipsychotics interfere with signaling at other receptors to varying degrees, including muscarinic receptors, H_1 histamine receptors, and α-adrenergic receptors. The extent to which these receptors are blocked at therapeutic doses can be used to predict the adverse effect of each antipsychotic profile.[22] For example, those that antagonize muscarinic receptors at clinically effective doses (most notably the aliphatic and piperidine phenothiazines as well as clozapine, loxapine, olanzapine, and quetiapine) often produce anticholinergic effects during routine use and can produce pronounced anticholinergic manifestations after overdose (Table 67–2). Similarly, blockade of peripheral α_1-adrenergic receptors by the aliphatic and piperidine phenothiazines, clozapine, risperidone, paliperidone, iloperidone, and others increases the risk of postural hypotension during therapy and clinically important hypotension after overdose. In contrast, haloperidol overdose, for example, is characterized by neither antimuscarinic effects nor hypotension.

Several antipsychotics also block voltage-gated fast sodium channels (I_{Na}). Although this effect is of little consequence during therapy, in the setting of overdose this can slow cardiac conduction (phase 0 depolarization) and impair myocardial contractility. This effect, most notable with the phenothiazines, is both rate and voltage dependent and is therefore more pronounced at faster heart rates and less negative transmembrane potentials.[19] Blockade of the delayed rectifier potassium current (I_{Kr}) can produce prolongation of the QT interval, creating a substrate for development of torsade de pointes.[94] Prolongation of the QT interval is sometimes evident during maintenance therapy, particularly in patients with previously unrecognized repolarization abnormalities or additional risk factors for QT interval prolongation. This effect may partially explain the dose-dependent increase in risk of sudden cardiac death among patients treated with typical and atypical antipsychotic drugs.[108,109]

Several antipsychotics exhibit a relatively high degree of antagonism at the $5-HT_{2A}$ receptor, which imparts two important therapeutic properties: (1) greater effectiveness for the treatment of the negative symptoms of schizophrenia and (2) a significantly lower incidence of extrapyramidal side effects. Some antipsychotics produce unique effects through effects at other receptors. For example, loxapine and clozapine inhibit the presynaptic reuptake of catecholamines and antagonize γ-aminobutyric acid (GABA)$_A$ receptors,[129] which may explain the apparent increase in the occurrence of seizures with overdose of these antipsychotics.[105] A more detailed description of the pharmacology of the most commonly used second-generation antipsychotics is warranted in light of their increasing role in therapy.

Clozapine, a dibenzodiazepine, binds to dopamine receptors (D_1–D_5) and serotonin receptors ($5-HT_{1A/1C}$, $5-HT_{2A/2C}$, $5-HT_3$, and $5-HT_6$) with moderate to high affinity.[8,106,114] It also antagonizes α_1-adrenergic, α_2-adrenergic, and H_1 histamine receptors. It has the highest binding affinity of any atypical antipsychotic at M_1 muscarinic receptors.[113] Despite this feature, clozapine paradoxically activates the M_4 genetic subtype of the muscarinic receptor and frequently produces sialorrhea during therapy.[112]

Olanzapine, a thienobenzodiazepine, binds with high affinity to serotonin ($5-HT_{2A/2C}$, $5-HT_3$, and $5-HT_6$) and dopamine receptors (D_1, D_2, and D_4), although its potency at D_2 receptors is lower than that of most traditional antipsychotics.[70,114] It is an exceptionally potent H_1 antagonist, binding more avidly than pyrilamine, which is a widely used antihistamine. It is also has a high affinity for M_1 receptors and is a relatively weak α_1 antagonist.

Risperidone, a benzisoxazole derivative, has high affinity for several receptors, including serotonin receptors ($5-HT_{2A/2C}$), D_2 receptors, and α_1 and H_1 receptors.[70,112,114] It has no appreciable activity at M_1 receptors. Its primary metabolite (9-hydroxyrisperidone) is nearly equipotent as the parent compound at D_2 and $5-HT_{2A}$ receptors.[70] Paliperidone is the major active metabolite of risperidone and is available orally and as a long-acting parenteral preparation that exhibits a similar receptor binding profile.[86]

Quetiapine, a dibenzothiazepine, is a weak antagonist at D_2, M_1, and $5-HT_{1A}$ receptors, but it is a potent antagonist of α_1-adrenergic and H_1 receptors.[70] At least 2 of its 11 metabolites are pharmacologically active, but they circulate at low concentrations and likely contribute little to the quetiapine's

clinical effects. A considerable proportion of fatalities involving antipsychotics reported to North American Poison Control Centers involve quetiapine, usually in combination with other drugs.[16]

Ziprasidone, a benzothiazole derivative, is an antagonist at D_2 and several serotonin ($5-HT_{2A/2C}$, $5-HT_{1D}$, and $5-HT_7$) receptors, but it also displays agonist activity at $5-HT_{1A}$ receptors.[70,71,114] Its α_1 antagonist activity is particularly strong, with a binding affinity approximately one 10th that of prazosin. In addition, it is a strong inhibitor of the delayed rectifier channel (I_{Kr}) and can significantly prolong repolarization.[71,83]

Lurasidone is an active metabolite of risperidone. It exhibits high affinity for D_2 and $5-HT_{2A}$ receptors, as well as for $5-HT_{1A}$ and $5-HT_7$, but low affinity α_1 adrenergic receptors and no appreciable affinity for muscarinic or H_1 receptors.[86]

Aripiprazole, a quinolinone derivative, is a novel antipsychotic that binds avidly to D_2 and D_3 receptors as well as $5-HT_{1A}$, $5-HT_{2A}$, and $5-HT_{2B}$ receptors.[93,114] Some evidence suggests that its efficacy in the treatment of schizophrenia and its lower propensity for EPS relates to partial agonist activity at dopamine D_2 receptors.[91] Aripiprazole acts as a partial agonist at $5-HT_{1A}$ receptors but is an antagonist at $5-HT_{2A}$ receptors. Its principal active metabolite, dehydroaripiprazole, has affinity for D_2 receptors and thus has pharmacologic activity similar to that of the parent compound.[93]

Like aripiprazole, bifeprunox is a partial agonist at D_2 and $5-HT_{1A}$ receptors. It is characterized as a third-generation antipsychotic and has no appreciable affinity for serotonin $5-HT_{2A}$ and $5-HT_{2C}$, muscarinic, or H_1 receptors.[31,96,122]

Amisulpride is a substituted benzamide derivative that preferentially blocks dopamine receptors in limbic rather than striatal structures. At low doses, it blocks presynaptic D_2 and D_3 receptors with high affinity, thereby accentuating dopamine release, and at high doses, it blocks postsynaptic D_2 and D_3 receptors. It has no appreciable affinity for serotonergic, histaminergic, adrenergic, and cholinergic receptors.[86]

Sertindole is a second-generation antipsychotic recently reintroduced into the market after being voluntarily withdrawn in 1998 over concerns about its effects on the QT interval. It binds to striatal D_2 receptors, although less avidly than olanzapine, and exhibits antagonism at $5-HT_{2A}$ and α_1 adrenergic receptors.[68,102,128] It is estimated that between 3.1% and 7.8% of patients receiving sertindole develop QT intervals greater than 500 ms.[148]

Asenapine is a second-generation antipsychotic administered sublingually because of its high first-pass metabolism. It acts as an antagonist at multiple dopamine, 5-HT, histamine, and α-adrenergic receptors but has no appreciable activity at muscarinic receptors or on the QT interval.[28,29]

PHARMACOKINETICS AND TOXICOKINETICS

With a few exceptions, the antipsychotics have similar pharmacokinetic characteristics regardless of their chemical classification. Most are lipophilic; have a large volume of distribution; and with the exception of asenapine, are generally well absorbed, although some antipsychotics with prominent anticholinergic effects are likely to exhibit delayed absorption. Plasma concentrations generally peak within 2 to 3 hours after a therapeutic dose but can be delayed after overdose.

Most antipsychotics are substrates for one or more isoforms of the hepatic cytochrome (CYP) enzyme system. For example, haloperidol, perphenazine, thioridazine, sertindole, and risperidone are extensively metabolized by the CYP2D6 system, which is functionally absent in approximately 7% of white patients and overexpressed in 1% to 25% of patients, depending on ethnicity.[53] These polymorphisms influence the tolerability and efficacy of treatment with these antipsychotics during therapeutic use[15,32,33,65,142] but are unlikely to significantly alter the severity of acute antipsychotic overdose.

Drugs that inhibit CYP2D6 (eg, paroxetine, fluoxetine, and bupropion) can increase concentrations of these antipsychotics, increasing the risk of adverse effects. In contrast, metabolism of clozapine and asenapine is primarily mediated by CYP1A2, and increased clozapine concentrations follow exposure to CYP1A2 inhibitors such as fluvoxamine, macrolide, or fluoroquinolone antibiotics or upon smoking cessation because the polycyclic aromatic hydrocarbons in cigarette smoke induce CYP1A2.[38] The kidneys play a relatively small role in the elimination of antipsychotics, and dose adjustment is generally not necessary for patients with chronic kidney disease.

PATHOPHYSIOLOGY AND CLINICAL MANIFESTATIONS

Table 67–3 lists the adverse effects of antipsychotics. Some of these effects develop primarily following overdose, but others occur during the course of therapeutic use.

Adverse Effects During Therapeutic Use

The Extrapyramidal Syndromes. The EPSs (Table 67–4) are a group of disorders that share the common feature of abnormal muscular activity. Among the typical antipsychotics, the incidence of EPS appears to be highest with the more potent antipsychotics such as haloperidol and flupenthixol and lower with less potent antipsychotics such as chlorpromazine and thioridazine. Atypical antipsychotics are associated with an even lower incidence of EPS. Although the physiologic mechanisms for this observation are not fully understood, several hypotheses have been put forth, including 5-HT$_{2A}$ antagonism, rapid dissociation from the D$_2$ receptor, and a lower degree of nigrostriatal dopaminergic hypersensitivity during chronic use.[66,67,84] However, it is important to note that EPS occur during treatment with any antipsychotic, regardless of typicality or potency.

Acute Dystonia. Acute dystonia is a movement disorder characterized by sustained involuntary muscle contractions, often involving the muscles of the head and neck, including the extraocular muscles and the tongue, but occasionally involving the extremities. These contractions are sometimes referred to as *limited reactions,* reflecting their transient nature rather than

their severity. All of the currently available antipsychotics are associated with the development of acute dystonic reactions.[136] Spasmodic torticollis, facial grimacing, protrusion of the tongue, and oculogyric crisis are among the more common manifestations. Laryngeal dystonia is a rare but potentially life-threatening variant that is easily misdiagnosed because it presents with throat pain, dyspnea, stridor, and dysphonia rather than the more characteristic features of dystonia.[40]

Acute dystonia typically develops within a few hours of starting of treatment but may be delayed in onset for several days. Left untreated, dystonia resolves slowly over several days after the offending antipsychotic is withdrawn. Risk factors for acute dystonia include male gender, young age (children are particularly susceptible), a previous episode of acute dystonia, and recent cocaine use.[137,150] Although the reaction often appears dramatic and sometimes is mistaken for seizure activity, it is rarely life threatening. Of note, xenobiotics other than antipsychotics sometimes cause acute dystonia, particularly metoclopramide, the antidepressants, some antimalarials, histamine H$_2$ receptor antagonists, anticonvulsants, and cocaine.[137]

Treatment of Acute Dystonia. Acute dystonia is generally more distressing than serious, but rare cases compromise respiration, necessitating supplemental oxygen and, occasionally, assisted ventilation.[40,137] The response to parenteral anticholinergics is generally rapid and dramatic, and benztropine is recommended as the first-line treatment (2 mg intravenously or intramuscularly in adults or 0.05 mg/kg in children). Diphenhydramine is often more readily available, and it is also reasonable to use (50 mg intravenously or intramuscularly in adults, or 1 mg/kg in children). Parenteral benzodiazepines such as lorazepam (0.05–0.10 mg/kg intravenously or intramuscularly) or diazepam (0.1 mg/kg intravenously) can be used for patients who do not respond to anticholinergics but can also be effective as initial therapy. It is important to recognize that additional doses of anticholinergics are often necessary because the duration of action of most antipsychotics exceeds that of either benztropine or diphenhydramine.[30] We recommend that patients in whom acute dystonia jeopardizes respiration be observed for at least 12 to 24 hours after initial resolution.

Akathisia. Akathisia (from the Greek phrase "not to sit") is characterized by a feeling of restlessness, anxiety, or sense of unease, often in conjunction with the objective finding of an inability to remain still. Patients with akathisia frequently appear uncomfortable or fidgety. They typically rock back and forth while standing or repeatedly cross and uncross their legs while seated. Akathisia is sometimes misinterpreted as a manifestation of the underlying psychiatric disorder rather than an adverse effect of drug therapy.

Akathisia is common and often reduces adherence to therapy. Like acute dystonia, akathisia tends to occur relatively early in the course of treatment and coincides with peak antipsychotic concentrations in plasma.[150] The incidence appears highest with typical, high-potency antipsychotics and lowest with atypical antipsychotics. Although most cases develop within days to weeks after initiation of treatment or an increase in dose, a delayed-onset (tardive) variant is also recognized.

The pathophysiology of akathisia is incompletely understood but appears to involve antagonism of postsynaptic D$_2$ receptors in the mesocortical pathways.[84,136] Interestingly, a similar phenomenon is described in patients after the initiation of treatment with antidepressants, particularly the selective serotonin reuptake inhibitors.[7,78]

Treatment of Akathisia. Akathisia can be difficult to treat. A reduction in the antipsychotic dose is a reasonable initial intervention. If this fails or is impractical, substitution of another (generally atypical) antipsychotic drug or treatment with lipophilic β-adrenergic antagonists such as propranolol lessen akathisia. In the absence of good data, the choice of intervention should be guided by individual patient considerations.[76,104] Benzodiazepines produce short-term relief, and anticholinergics such as benztropine or procyclidine lessen akathisia in some patients but are more likely to be effective for akathisia induced by antipsychotics with little or no intrinsic anticholinergic activity.[21,77]

TABLE 67–3	Adverse Effects of Antipsychotics
Central nervous system	Somnolence, progressing to coma
	Respiratory depression with loss of airway reflexes
	Hyperthermia
	Seizures
	Extrapyramidal syndromes
	Central anticholinergic syndrome
Cardiovascular	
Clinical	Tachycardia
	Hypotension (orthostatic or resting)
	Myocardial depression
Electrocardiographic	QRS complex prolongation
	Right deviation of terminal 40 ms of frontal plane axis
	QT interval prolongation
	Torsade de pointes
	Nonspecific repolarization changes
Endocrine	Amenorrhea, oligomenorrhea, or metrorrhagia
	Breast tenderness and galactorrhea
Gastrointestinal	Impaired peristalsis
	Dry mouth[a]
Genitourinary	Urinary retention
	Ejaculatory dysfunction
	Priapism
Ophthalmic	Mydriasis or miosis; visual blurring
Dermatologic	Impaired sweat production
	Cutaneous vasodilation

[a]An exception is clozapine, which can cause sialorrhea.

TABLE 67–4	The Extrapyramidal Syndromes			
Disorder	Time of Maximal Risk	Features	Postulated Mechanism	Suggested Treatments
Akathisia	Hours to days	Restlessness and general unease; inability to sit still	Mesocortical D_2 antagonism	Dose reduction, trial of alternate drug, propranolol, benzodiazepines, anticholinergics
Dystonia	Hours to days	Sustained, involuntary muscle contraction, including torticollis, blepharospasm, oculogyric crisis	Imbalance of dopaminergic or cholinergic transmission	Anticholinergics, benzodiazepines
Neuroleptic malignant syndrome	2–10 days	Many (Table 67–5): altered mental status, motor symptoms, hyperthermia, autonomic instability, catatonia, mutism	D_2 antagonism in striatum, hypothalamus, and mesocortex	Cooling, benzodiazepines, supportive care, bromocriptine, amantadine, or other direct-acting dopamine agonist
Parkinsonism	Weeks	Bradykinesia, rigidity, shuffling gait, masklike facies, resting tremor	Postsynaptic striatal D_2 antagonism	Dose reduction, anticholinergics, dopamine agonists
Tardive dyskinesia	3 months to years	Late-onset involuntary choreiform movements, buccolinguomasticatory movements	Excess dopaminergic activity	Recognize early and stop offending drug; addition of other antipsychotic; cholinergics

Data from references 104 and 136.

Parkinsonism. Antipsychotics occasionally produce a parkinsonian syndrome characterized by rigidity, akinesia or bradykinesia, and postural instability. It is similar to idiopathic Parkinson disease, although the classic "pill-rolling" tremor is often less pronounced.[104] The syndrome typically develops during the first few months of therapy, particularly with high-potency antipsychotics. It is more common among older women, and in some patients, it represents iatrogenic unmasking of latent Parkinson disease. Parkinsonism results from antagonism of postsynaptic D_2 receptors in the striatum.[136]

Treatment of Drug-Induced Parkinsonism. The risk of drug-induced parkinsonism is minimized by using the lowest effective dose of antipsychotic. The addition of an anticholinergic often attenuates symptoms at the expense of additional side effects. This strategy is often effective in younger patients, although the routine use of prophylactic anticholinergics is not recommended. A dopamine agonist such as amantadine is sometimes added, particularly in older patients who may be less tolerant of anticholinergics, but this may aggravate the underlying psychiatric disturbance and is not generally recommended.[82]

Tardive Dyskinesias. The term *tardive dyskinesia* was coined in 1952 to describe the delayed onset of persistent orobuccal masticatory movements occurring in a three women after several months of antipsychotic therapy.[136] The adjective *tardive,* meaning delayed, was used to distinguish these movement disorders from the Parkinsonian movements described earlier. The incidence of tardive dyskinesia in younger patients is approximately 3% to 5% per year but rises considerably with age. A prospective study of older patients treated with high-potency typical antipsychotics identified a 60% cumulative incidence of tardive dyskinesia after 3 years of treatment.[61] Potential risk factors for tardive dyskinesia include alcohol use, affective disorder, prior electroconvulsive therapy, diabetes mellitus, and various genetic factors.[136]

Several distinct tardive syndromes are recognized, including the classic orobuccal lingual masticatory stereotypy, chorea, dystonia, myoclonus, blepharospasm, and tics. It is generally accepted that the atypical antipsychotics are associated with a lower incidence of tardive dyskinesia and other drug-related movement disorders. However, whether this is true of all atypical antipsychotics is unclear. Among the atypical antipsychotics, clozapine is associated with the lowest incidence of tardive dyskinesia and risperidone with the highest incidence (when higher doses are used), but the reasons for this are uncertain.[132,133,136]

Treatment of Tardive Dyskinesia. Tardive dyskinesia is highly resistant to the usual pharmacologic treatments for movement disorders. A recent systematic review of various treatment options concluded that none was supported by good evidence, including dose reduction, switching between antipsychotics, anticholinergics, benzodiazepines, β-adrenergic antagonists, buspirone,

calcium channel blockers, or vitamin E.[12] Consequently, no firm guidance can be offered regarding the management of tardive dyskinesia, which should be guided by individual patient considerations. Despite the absence of good data, a recent review proposed strategies for management of tardive dyskinesia, beginning with primary prevention (avoidance of antipsychotic therapy where possible and use of the lowest effective dose).[141] Tetrabenazine, an inhibitor of vesicular monoamine transporter type 2 (VMAT2), was suggested as the first-line treatment, although it is expensive and may cause somnolence, depression, or parkinsonism.[4] Valbenazine, a recently approved VMAT2 inhibitor with a longer half-life, appears to be better tolerated than tetrabenazine.[59] For focal tardive dyskinesia (cervical or oromandibular, for example), the same review suggested botulinum toxin injections.

Neuroleptic Malignant Syndrome. Neuroleptic malignant syndrome (NMS) is a potentially life-threatening emergency. First described in 1960 in patients treated with haloperidol, this syndrome is now associated with virtually every antipsychotic.[35] The reported incidence of NMS ranges from 0.2% to 1.4% of patients receiving antipsychotics,[2,24,131] but less severe episodes may go undiagnosed or unreported. As a result, much of what is known about the epidemiology and treatment of NMS is speculative and based on case reports and case series. Most cases of NMS are diagnosed in young adulthood, with the frequency of diagnosis diminishing gradually thereafter.[46]

The pathophysiology of NMS is incompletely understood but involves abrupt reductions in central dopaminergic neurotransmission in the striatum and hypothalamus, altering the core temperature "set point"[48] and leading to impaired thermoregulation and other manifestations of autonomic dysfunction. Blockade of striatal D_2 receptors contributes to muscle rigidity and tremor.[13,26,138] In some cases, a direct effect on skeletal muscle may play a role in the pathogenesis of hyperthermia, but the thermodysregulation of NMS is principally a centrally mediated phenomenon.[48] Altered mental status is multifactorial and reflects one or more of hypothalamic and spinal dopamine receptor antagonism, a genetic predisposition, or the direct effects of hyperthermia and other drugs.[50] Although NMS most often occurs during treatment with a D_2 receptor antagonist, withdrawal of dopamine agonists sometimes produces an indistinguishable syndrome. The latter typically occurs in patients with long-standing Parkinson disease who abruptly change or discontinue treatment with dopamine agonists such as levodopa/carbidopa, amantadine,[43] or bromocriptine.[13] The resulting disorder is sometimes referred to as the Parkinsonian-hyperpyrexia syndrome, and mortality rates of up to 4% are reported.[95] Hospitalization for aspiration pneumonia, a common occurrence in older patients with Parkinson disease, is a particularly high-risk setting for this complication and is particularly dangerous because the cardinal manifestations of NMS are easily misattributed to the combined effects of pneumonia and the underlying movement disorder.

The vast majority of NMS cases occur in the context of therapeutic use of antipsychotics rather than after overdose. Postulated risk factors for the development of NMS include young age, male gender, extracellular fluid volume contraction, use of high-potency antipsychotics, depot preparations, cotreatment with lithium, multiple drugs in combination, and rapid dose escalation.[2,25,75,97] One large observational study[97] suggests that treatment with high-potency first-generation antipsychotics is associated with a more than 20-fold increase in the risk of NMS, although this may partly reflect heightened suspicion of the disorder in patients receiving those drugs. The mortality rate of NMS associated with first-generation antipsychotics is estimated at approximately 16%, and the rate associated with second-generation antipsychotics is estimated at 3%.[135]

The manifestations of NMS include the tetrad of altered mental status, muscular rigidity (classically described as "lead pipe"), hyperthermia, and autonomic dysfunction. These findings appear in any sequence, although a review of 340 NMS cases found that mental status changes and rigidity usually preceded the development hyperthermia and autonomic instability.[139] Occasionally, rigidity is not present when creatine kinase concentrations are elevated but emerges thereafter.[98] Signs typically evolve over a period of several days, with the majority occurring within 2 weeks of antipsychotic initiation. However, it is important to recognize that NMS occurs even after prolonged use of an antipsychotic, particularly after a dose increase, the addition of another antipsychotic, or the development of intercurrent illness. It is also worth noting that the clinical course of NMS often fluctuates, sometimes waxing and waning dramatically over a few hours.

There are no universally accepted criteria for the diagnosis of NMS, and more than a dozen sets of criteria have been proposed.[3,24,37,75] The operating characteristics of these criteria have not been formally evaluated, in part because of the absence of a gold standard. An international group published the results of a Delphi consensus panel regarding the diagnosis of NMS (Table 67–5).[47] A recent validation exercise suggested that an aggregate cutoff score of 74 (of a possible 100) was associated with the highest degree of agreement between expert-generated criteria and *Diagnostic and Statistical Manual of Mental Disorders*, fourth edition, text revision, criteria (sensitivity,

69.6%; specificity, 90.7%).[49] However, the authors caution that in the absence of a biological reference standard, this scoring system should be used adjunctively with current clinical standards for the diagnosis of NMS.

It may be difficult to distinguish NMS from other toxin-induced hyperthermia syndromes, such as those associated with anticholinergics (antimuscarinics) (Chap. 49) and the serotonergics (Chap. 69), all of which share common features of elevated temperature, altered mental status, and neuromuscular abnormalities. The most important differentiating feature is the medication history, with dopamine antagonists, antimuscarinic drugs, and direct or indirect serotonin agonists (often in combination) as the most likely etiologies, respectively. The time course of the illness also helps to differentiate among the disorders. Whereas serotonin toxicity and the antimuscarinic syndrome tend to develop rapidly after exposure to causative xenobiotics, NMS typically develops more gradually, often waxing and waning over several days or more. Occasionally, clinicians must attempt to differentiate NMS from other disorders in the absence of a reliable medication history. The physical examination is of some utility in this regard.[103] Although NMS is classically characterized by "lead-pipe" rigidity, the presence of ocular or generalized clonus is more suggestive of serotonin toxicity, particularly when accompanied by shivering and hyperreflexia, findings not typical of NMS. Because skeletal muscle contraction occurs through nicotinic rather than muscarinic transmission, patients with the antimuscarinic syndrome generally have few muscular abnormalities. However, such patients are sometimes resistant to physical restraint, giving the appearance of increased muscle tone.

Treatment of Neuroleptic Malignant Syndrome: General Measures. Treatment recommendations are largely based on general physiologic principles, case reports, and case series. Therapy should be individualized according to the severity and duration of illness and the modifying influences of comorbidity.[13,111,140] The provision of good supportive care is the cornerstone for treatment of NMS. It is essential to recognize the condition as an emergency and to withdraw the offending xenobiotic immediately. When NMS ensues after abrupt discontinuation of a dopamine agonist such as levodopa, the drug should be reinstituted promptly. Most patients with suspected NMS should be admitted to an intensive care unit. Supplemental oxygen should be administered, and assisted ventilation is necessary in cases of respiratory failure, which result from one or more of central hypoventilation, loss of protective airway reflexes, rigidity of the chest wall muscles or oversedation.

The hyperthermia associated with NMS is multifactorial in origin and, when present, warrants aggressive treatment. Antipyretics are not effective. Immersion of patients with severe drug-induced hyperthermia (>106°F) in an ice-water bath has been shown to rapidly lower body temperature (Chaps. 29 and 75).[74] Despite the absence of good data in patients with NMS, we recommend ice-water immersion in patients with severe hyperthermia given the urgency with which it should be corrected. Other strategies include active cooling blankets; the placement of ice packs in the groin and axillae; or evaporative cooling, which can be accomplished by removing the patient's clothing and exposing the patient to cooled water or towels immersed in ice water while maintaining continuous air circulation with the use of fans. Although often used,[145] these approaches are inferior to ice water immersion and are not recommended unless immersion is impractical or unsafe.

Hypotension should be treated initially with isotonic crystalloid followed by vasopressors if necessary. Maintenance of intravascular volume and adequate renal perfusion are recommended to reduce the incidence of myoglobinuric acute kidney injury in patients with high creatine kinase concentrations. Tachycardia does not require specific treatment, but hemodynamically significant bradycardia necessitates transcutaneous or transvenous pacing. Venous thromboembolism is a major cause of morbidity and mortality in patients with NMS, and prophylactic doses of low-molecular-weight heparin are reasonable in patients who likely will be immobilized for more than 12 to 24 hours.

Pharmacologic Treatment of Neuroleptic Malignant Syndrome. Benzodiazepines are the most widely used pharmacologic adjuncts for treatment of

TABLE 67–5	Suggested Diagnostic Criteria for the Neuroleptic Malignant Syndrome	
Criterion		*Priority Score*
Exposure to a dopamine antagonist or withdrawal of a dopamine agonist in previous 72 hours		20
Hyperthermia (>100.4°F or 38.0°C on at least two occasions, measured orally		18
Rigidity		17
Mental status alteration (reduced or fluctuating level of consciousness)		13
Creatine kinase elevation (at least four times the upper limit of normal)		10
Sympathetic nervous system lability, defined as at least two of: Blood pressure elevation (SBP or DBP ≥25% above baseline) Blood pressure fluctuation (≥20% DBP change or ≥25% SBP change in 24 hours) Diaphoresis Urinary incontinence		10
Hypermetabolic state (defined as heart rate increase ≥25% above baseline *and* respiratory rate increase ≥50% above baseline)		5
Negative workup for other toxic, metabolic, infectious, or neurologic causes		7

DBP = diastolic blood pressure; SBP = systolic blood pressure.

Data from Fryml L, Williams KR, Pelic CG, et al. The role of amantadine withdrawal in 3 cases of treatment-refractory altered mental status. *J Psychiatr Pract.* 2017 May;23(3):191-199.

NMS and are recommended as first line-therapy. Dantrolene and bromocriptine are not well studied, and their incremental benefit over good supportive care is debated.[111,116] Benzodiazepines are frequently used in the management of NMS because of their rapid onset of action, which is particularly important when patients are agitated or restless. They attenuate the sympathetic hyperactivity that characterizes NMS by facilitating GABA-mediated chloride transport and producing neuronal hyperpolarization, in a fashion analogous to their beneficial effects in cocaine toxicity.[50] The primary disadvantage of benzodiazepines is that they will cloud the assessment of the patient's mental status.

Dantrolene reduces skeletal muscle activity by inhibiting ryanodine receptor type 1 calcium release channels, interfering with calcium release from the sarcoplasmic reticulum.[69] In theory, this should reduce body temperature and total oxygen consumption and lessen the risk of myoglobinuric acute kidney injury. The role of dantrolene in NMS is controversial because the available literature is limited to case reports and case series with varying conclusions. Moreover, unlike malignant hyperthermia (in which the use of dantrolene is unquestioned), the muscle rigidity of NMS is principally a centrally mediated process. Nevertheless, several reports describe rapid, dramatic reductions in rigidity and temperature after its administration.[17,53,72] Dantrolene is not recommended as a routine treatment in patients with NMS but is reasonable in those with prominent muscular rigidity or rhabdomyolysis, in light of its potential benefits and relative safety.[13] It can be given by mouth or nasogastric tube (50–100 mg/d) or by intravenous (IV) infusion (2–3 mg/kg/d, or up to 10 mg/kg/d in severe cases). Bromocriptine is a centrally acting dopamine agonist given orally or by nasogastric tube at dosages of 2.5 to 10 mg three or four times daily. The rationale for its use rests in the belief that reversal of antipsychotic-related striatal D_2 antagonism will ameliorate the manifestations of NMS. It is recommended in patients with moderate to severe NMS, but other dopamine agonists anecdotally associated with success may be used instead, including ropinirole, levodopa,[100,127] and amantadine.[44,60,131] Of note, dopaminergics are associated with exacerbation of underlying psychiatric illness.

When these medications are used, they should be tapered slowly after the patient improves to minimize the likelihood of recrudescent NMS. In severe cases with prominent rigidity it is reasonable to use dantrolene and a dopamine agonist should be used in combination with benzodiazepines.

Electroconvulsive Therapy. Electroconvulsive therapy (ECT) is reported to dramatically improve the manifestations of NMS, presumably by enhancing central dopaminergic transmission. In one report, five patients received an average of 10 ECT treatments, and resolution generally occurred after the third or fourth session.[99] Whether this result represents a true effect of ECT or simply the natural course of NMS with good supportive care alone is not clear. As with drug therapies for NMS, the effectiveness of ECT remains unproven, but its use seems reasonable in patients with severe, persistent, or treatment-resistant NMS as well as those with residual catatonia or psychosis after resolution of other manifestations.[13,100]

Adverse Effects on Other Organ Systems. Sedation, dry mouth, and urinary retention occur commonly with antipsychotics, particularly during the initial period of therapy. These effects occur most commonly with antipsychotics that exhibit antihistaminic and antimuscarinic activity. All antipsychotics lower the seizure threshold, but seizures are uncommon during therapeutic use. Because hypothalamic dopamine inhibits hypophyseal prolactin release, hyperprolactinemia and galactorrhea can occur. All antipsychotics are associated with a host of metabolic derangements, including weight gain, dyslipidemia, and steatohepatitis. The metabolic syndrome appears most commonly in association with clozapine, olanzapine, and chlorpromazine therapy.[34] Rare but dramatic instances of glucose intolerance, including fatal cases of diabetic ketoacidosis, are also described.[6,54,107,134] The mechanism of this is incompletely understood, but it is not adequately explained by the weight gain associated with antipsychotic therapy because glucose disturbances often develop shortly after therapy is instituted. The risk of hyperglycemia appears greatest during the initial weeks of antipsychotic therapy.[79] Other idiosyncratic reactions reported with use of antipsychotics include photosensitivity, skin pigmentation and cholestatic hepatitis (particularly with the phenothiazines), myocarditis, and agranulocytosis (the latter occurs with many antipsychotics, most notably clozapine, occurring in up to 2% of patients).[90] Most of these conditions result from an immunologically based hypersensitivity reaction and develop during the first month of therapy. Finally, an increasing number of reports associate antipsychotic drugs with venous thromboembolism.[52,63] This may partially explain the high incidence of thromboembolic disease found in patients with NMS (see later).

Acute Overdose

Antipsychotic overdose produces a spectrum of toxic manifestations involving multiple organ systems, but the most serious toxicity involves the CNS and cardiovascular system. Some of these manifestations are present to a minor degree during therapeutic use, although they tend to be most pronounced during the early period of therapy and dissipate with continued use.

Depressed level of consciousness is a common and dose-dependent feature of antipsychotic overdose, ranging from somnolence to coma. It may be associated with impaired airway reflexes, but significant respiratory depression is uncommon in the absence of other factors. Many antipsychotics, including several of the atypicals, are potent muscarinic antagonists and produce anticholinergic features in overdose.[10,22,27] Peripheral manifestations include tachycardia, decreased production of sweat and saliva, flushed skin, urinary retention, diminished bowel sounds, and mydriasis, although miosis also occurs. These findings may be present in isolation or coexist with central manifestations, including agitation, delirium, psychosis, hallucinations, and coma, some of which may be mistakenly attributed to the underlying psychiatric illness.

Mild elevations in body temperature are common and reflect impaired heat dissipation as a result of impaired sweating, as well as increased heat production in agitated patients. Hyperthermia should always prompt a search for other features of NMS. Tachycardia is a common finding in patients with antipsychotic overdose and reflects reduced vagal tone and, with some antipsychotics, a compensatory response to hypotension. Bradycardia is distinctly uncommon, and although it may be a preterminal finding, its presence should prompt a search for alternative causes, including in ingestion of negative chronotropic drugs such as β-adrenergic antagonists, calcium channel blockers, cardioactive steroids, and opioids. Hypotension is a common feature of antipsychotic overdose and is generally caused by peripheral α_1-adrenergic blockade and, particularly with the phenothiazines, reduced myocardial contractility.

The electrocardiographic (ECG) manifestations of antipsychotic overdoses vary, sometimes exhibiting similarities to those of cyclic antidepressant toxicity (Chaps 15 and 68). These include prolongation of the QRS complex and a rightward deflection of the terminal 40 ms of the QRS complex, typically manifesting as a tall, broad terminal positive deflection of the QRS complex in lead aVR. These changes reflect blockade of the inward sodium current (I_{Na}). Prolongation of the QT interval results from blockade of the delayed rectifier potassium current (I_{Kr}), creating a substrate for development of torsade de pointes and other ventricular dysrhythmias.[94] This situation is sometimes evident during maintenance therapy and may underlie the apparent increase in sudden cardiac death among users of antipsychotic drugs.[108,109]

DIAGNOSTIC TESTS

The diagnosis of antipsychotic poisoning is supported by the clinical history, the physical examination, and a limited number of adjunctive tests. Both the clinical and ECG findings are nonspecific and shared by other drug classes, including TCAs, skeletal muscle relaxants, carbamazepine, and first-generation antihistamines such as diphenhydramine. Moreover, the absence of typical ECG changes does not exclude a significant antipsychotic ingestion, particularly early after overdose, and at least one additional ECG is recommended in the following 2 to 3 hours.

Abdominal radiography sometimes reveals densities in the gastrointestinal tract because some solid dosage forms of phenothiazines are radiopaque. However, these tests are neither sensitive nor specific, and they are not recommended in the absence of another indication.

Plasma concentrations of antipsychotics are not widely available, do not correlate well with clinical signs and symptoms, and do not help guide therapy. Comprehensive urine drug screens using high-performance liquid chromatography, gas chromatography–mass spectrometry, or tandem mass spectrometry can detect antipsychotics, but these tests are available at only a few hospitals and in most instances provide only a qualitative result and are not recommended. Urine immunoassays for TCAs occasionally produce a false-positive result in the presence of phenothiazines.[5,115]

MANAGEMENT

The care of a patient with an antipsychotic overdose should proceed with the recognition that other drugs, particularly other psychotropics, may have been coingested and can confound both the clinical presentation and management. Regularly encountered coingestants include other psychotropic drugs such as antidepressants, sedative–hypnotics, opioids, anticholinergic agents, valproic acid, and lithium, as well as ethanol and nonprescription analgesics such as acetaminophen and aspirin.

Supportive care is the cornerstone of treatment for patients with antipsychotic overdose. Supplemental oxygen should be administered if hypoxia is present. Intubation and ventilation are rarely required for patients with single xenobiotic ingestions but may be necessary for patients with very large overdoses of antipsychotics or coingestion of other CNS depressants. Patients with altered mental status should receive thiamine, as well as parenteral dextrose if hypoglycemia is present. Naloxone is recommended based on clinical grounds (Antidotes in Depth: A4). All symptomatic patients should undergo continuous cardiac monitoring. An ECG should be recorded upon presentation and reliable venous access obtained. Asymptomatic patients with a normal ECG 6 hours after overdose are at exceedingly low risk of complications and generally do not require ongoing cardiac monitoring. Symptomatic patients and those with an abnormal ECG should have continuous monitoring for a minimum of 24 hours.

Gastrointestinal Decontamination

Gastrointestinal decontamination with activated charcoal (1 g/kg by mouth or nasogastric tube) is recommended for patients who present within a few hours of a large or multidrug overdose and have no contraindications. Although this intervention is time sensitive, many antipsychotics exhibit significant antimuscarinic activity and slow gastric emptying, thereby increasing the likelihood that activated charcoal will be beneficial. Although it is unknown whether activated charcoal improves clinically important outcomes,[64] a Bayesian analysis of pharmacokinetic data from a series of quetiapine overdoses concluded that activated charcoal use led to a 35% reduction in the fraction of quetiapine absorbed.[57] Orogastric lavage and whole-bowel irrigation likely will not improve clinical outcomes and should be used rarely in the management of patients with antipsychotic overdose.

Treatment of Cardiovascular Complications

Vital signs should be monitored closely. Hypotension most often results from peripheral α-adrenergic blockade and is most likely to occur with older, low-potency antipsychotics such as thioridazine.[91] Hypotension should be treated initially with appropriate titration of 0.9% sodium chloride. If vasopressors are required, direct-acting agonists such as norepinephrine or phenylephrine are recommended over dopamine, which is an indirect agonist and likely will be ineffective. Vasopressin or its analogs should be used with great caution in patients who have coingested a negative inotropic drug such as a β-adrenergic antagonist or calcium channel blocker. Continuous blood pressure monitoring may be warranted in such cases.

Progressive prolongation of the QRS complex is uncommon and reflects sodium channel blockade and slowing of phase 0 depolarization in the His-Purkinje system. This is usually associated with reduced cardiac output

and malignant ventricular dysrhythmias. Much of what is known about the treatment of sodium channel blocker toxicity derives from the cyclic antidepressant literature, with treatment recommendations extended to sodium channel blocking antipsychotic drugs by analogy. Sodium bicarbonate (1–2 mEq/kg) is the first-line therapy for ventricular dysrhythmias and is recommended for patients with dysrhythmias or QRS complex greater than 0.12 seconds (Antidotes in Depth: A5 and Chap. 68). At least two mechanisms underlie the beneficial effects of sodium bicarbonate, sodium channel blockade is partially overcome by an increase in extracellular sodium, and the binding of antipsychotics to the sodium channel is less extensive binding at higher pH values.

Repeated boluses of bicarbonate are recommended to achieve a target blood pH of no greater than 7.5, although we recommend continuous infusions.[125] If the patient is intubated, hyperventilation is recommended only if sodium bicarbonate is unavailable. If significant conduction abnormalities or ventricular dysrhythmias persist despite the use of sodium bicarbonate, lidocaine (1–2 mg/kg, followed by continuous infusion) is a reasonable second-line antidysrhythmic. Although lidocaine is also a sodium channel blocker, it exhibits rapid on/off sodium channel binding with preferential binding in the inactivated state and reportedly lessens the cardiotoxicity associated with antipsychotic drug overdose.[124] Class IA antidysrhythmics (procainamide, disopyramide, and quinidine), class IC antidysrhythmics (propafenone, encainide, and flecainide), and class III antidysrhythmics (amiodarone, sotalol, and bretylium) can aggravate cardiotoxicity and are contraindicated. When administering sodium bicarbonate to patients with antipsychotic overdose, caution must be taken to avoid hypokalemia because many of these antipsychotics block cardiac potassium channels, thereby prolonging the QT interval. Hypokalemia and hypomagnesemia exacerbate this blockade, potentially leading to torsade de pointes and other lethal dysrhythmias, particularly in patients with overdoses involving amisulpride or ziprasidone.

Sinus tachycardia related to anticholinergic activity should not be treated unless it is associated with active ischemia, which, although uncommon, may complicate antipsychotic overdose in patients with existing coronary disease. If symptomatic sinus tachycardia requires emergent treatment, a short-acting β-adrenergic antagonist such as esmolol is recommended. Prolongation of the QT interval requires no specific treatment other than monitoring and correction of potential contributing causes such as hypokalemia and hypomagnesemia. After torsade de pointes has resolved spontaneously resolved or after cardioversion, intravenous magnesium sulfate is recommended to lessen the likelihood of recurrence, taking care to prevent hypotension, which is dose and rate dependent. Overdrive pacing with isoproterenol or transcutaneous or transvenous pacing is recommended if the patient does not respond to magnesium; however, magnesium is preferred because pacing may worsen rate-dependent sodium channel blockade.

Most antipsychotics exhibit a high degree of lipophilicity in addition to significant cardiovascular toxicity. Considerable enthusiasm has emerged for the use of intravenous lipid emulsion (ILE) therapy for patients with significant cardiac toxicity from lipophilic drugs (Antidotes in Depth: A23). The rationale for this therapy rests, in part, in the concept that highly lipophilic drugs selectively partition into the exogenous lipid, minimizing toxicity at the biophase. This treatment has been extensively studied in animal models of bupivacaine toxicity,[36,143,144] but published experience with antipsychotic drugs is limited to a handful of case reports.[41,85,87,151] Recently published evidence-based recommendations on the use of ILE in acute poisoning note the very low quality of evidence supporting the intervention for most poisonings.[45] As a result, it is reasonable to give ILE only in cases of not rapidly treatable cardiovascular collapse after antipsychotic overdose. Dosing for ILE is not well established, but a reasonable protocol begins with 20% lipid emulsion given as a bolus of 1.5 mL/kg (Antidotes in Depth: A23). Extracorporeal circulatory support is associated with survival in severe quetiapine overdose; however, this is only an option in selected centers. This intervention, when available, in critically ill patients unresponsive to other therapies is reasonable but therefore not routinely recommended at this time.[73]

Treatment of Seizures

Seizures associated with antipsychotic overdose are generally short-lived and often require no pharmacologic treatment. Multiple or refractory seizures should prompt a search for other causes, including hypoglycemia and ingestion of other proconvulsant xenobiotics. When treatment is necessary, benzodiazepines such as lorazepam or diazepam generally suffice, although phenobarbital is a reasonable second-line therapy. Although phenytoin is part of the standard algorithm for status epilepticus, it is of limited effectiveness for xenobiotic-induced seizures.[126] Patients with refractory seizures should respond to propofol infusion or general anesthesia. Finally, seizures abruptly lower serum pH and thereby increase the cardiotoxicity of antipsychotics by enhancing binding to the sodium channel; therefore, an ECG should be obtained after resolution of seizure activity.

Treatment of the Central Antimuscarinic Syndrome

Many of the older and newer generation antipsychotics have pronounced anticholinergic properties. Case reports and observational studies suggest that the cholinesterase inhibitor physostigmine (Antidotes in Depth: A11) can safely and effectively ameliorate the agitated delirium associated with the central antimuscarinic (anticholinergic) syndrome by indirectly increasing synaptic acetylcholine levels.[26,118-120] Although benzodiazepines control agitation, they further impair alertness, obfuscating the assessment of mental status and increasing the risk of complications.[23]

Physostigmine has been used successfully in patients with antipsychotic overdose,[23,117,120,146,147] but it should be used with caution. It should not be used in patients with ventricular dysrhythmias, any degree of heart block, or prolongation of the QRS complex. If physostigmine is used, it is recommended to be given in 0.5-mg increments every 3 to 5 minutes, with close observation. If bradycardia, bronchospasm, or bronchorrhea develops, these can be treated with glycopyrrolate 0.2 to 0.4 mg IV. Atropine is often more widely available and is a reasonable alternative to glycopyrrolate but it crosses the blood–brain barrier and is likely to aggravate delirium. The effects of physostigmine are transient, typically ranging in duration from 30 to 90 minutes, and additional doses are often necessary. Of note, physostigmine does not prevent other complications of antipsychotic overdose, particularly those involving the cardiovascular system.

Other commonly used cholinesterase inhibitors, such as edrophonium, neostigmine, and pyridostigmine, should not be used to treat anticholinergic delirium because they do not cross the blood–brain barrier. Case reports involving other anticholinergics suggest that cholinesterase inhibitors used for treatment of dementia (eg, tacrine, donepezil, and galantamine) are reasonable alternatives to physostigmine for patients able to take medications orally.[58,89,101]

Enhanced Elimination

No pharmacologic rationale supports the use of multiple-dose charcoal or manipulation of urinary pH to increase the clearance of antipsychotics. One volunteer study found that urinary acidification may increase remoxipride elimination,[149] but this practice is impractical and possibly dangerous. Because most antipsychotics exhibit large volumes of distribution and extensive protein binding (Table 67–1), extracorporeal removal is unwarranted and should be performed only if the patient has coingested other xenobiotics amenable to extracorporeal removal.

SUMMARY

- Over the past decade, the atypical antipsychotics have largely supplanted traditional antipsychotics, which were associated with greater toxicity in overdose and a higher incidence of extrapyramidal reactions. Consequently, atypical antipsychotics are now implicated in the majority of overdoses.
- With both typical and atypical antipsychotics, significant toxicity can occur either during the course of therapy or after overdose. Of the various toxicities that arise during therapeutic use, NMS is the most dangerous. Its manifestations are protean, and it may be difficult to recognize. Altered mental status, muscle rigidity, hyperthermia, and autonomic instability are its hallmarks, but the diagnosis should be considered in any unwell patient treated with antipsychotics, particularly in the 2 weeks after a change in therapy or in a patient with another stressor such as severe intercurrent illness or general anesthesia. Treatment of NMS is largely supportive and often involves the use of benzodiazepines. Dopamine agonists such as bromocriptine and ropinirole are recommended in patients with moderate to severe NMS, while dantrolene is recommended only in those with severe muscle rigidity or rhabdomyolysis. Electroconvulsive therapy is anecdotally associated with dramatic clinical improvement.
- The principal manifestations of antipsychotic overdose involve the CNS and cardiovascular system. Depressed mental status, hypotension, and anticholinergic signs are nonspecific features that support the diagnosis of, particularly in conjunction with typical ECG findings of sodium channel blockade and QT interval prolongation, although these vary considerably among the available antipsychotic drugs.
- Most fatalities after antipsychotic overdose occur in cases involving coingestion of other CNS depressants or cardiotoxic medications.
- Supportive care is the mainstay of therapy for patients with antipsychotic overdose, although selective use of nonspecific antidotes, such as activated charcoal, sodium bicarbonate, or physostigmine, may improve outcomes in selected patients. Particularly severe or refractory cardiovascular toxicity may warrant a trial of ILE or extracorporeal life support, although these interventions are not well studied in the context of antipsychotic drug overdose.

Acknowledgments

Frank LoVecchio and Neal Lewin contributed to this chapter in a previous edition.

REFERENCES

1. Abi-Dargham A, et al. Increased baseline occupancy of D2 receptors by dopamine in schizophrenia. *Proc Natl Acad Sci U S A.* 2000;97:8104-8109.
2. Addonizio G, et al. Neuroleptic malignant syndrome: review and analysis of 115 cases. *Biol Psychiatry.* 1987;22:1004-1020.
3. Adnet P, et al. Neuroleptic malignant syndrome. *Br J Anaesth.* 2000;85:129-135.
4. Aia PG, et al. Tardive dyskinesia. *Curr Treat Options Neurol.* 2011;13:231-241.
5. Asselin WM, Leslie JM. Use of the EMITtox serum tricyclic antidepressant assay for the analysis of urine samples. *J Anal Toxicol.* 1990;14:168-171.
6. Avella J, et al. Fatal olanzapine-induced hyperglycemic ketoacidosis. *Am J Forensic Med Pathol.* 2004;25:172-175.
7. Baldassano CF, et al. Akathisia: a review and case report following paroxetine treatment. *Compr Psychiatry.* 1996;37:122-124.
8. Baldessarini RJ, et al. A novel antipsychotic agent. *N Engl J Med.* 1991;324:746-754.
9. Baldessarini RJ, Tarazi FI. Drugs and the treatment of psychiatric disorders: psychosis and mania. 2001:10:485-520.
10. Balit CR, et al. Quetiapine poisoning: a case series. *Ann Emerg Med.* 2003;42:751-758.
11. Baselt RC. Disposition of toxic drugs and chemicals in man. 2004;7.
12. Bergman H, et al. Systematic review of interventions for treating or preventing antipsychotic-induced tardive dyskinesia. *Health Technol Assess.* 2017;21:1-218.
13. Bhanushali MJ, Tuite, PJ. The evaluation and management of patients with neuroleptic malignant syndrome. *Neurol Clin.* 2004;22:389-411.
14. Borison RL. Recent advances in the pharmacotherapy of schizophrenia. *Harv Rev Psychiatry.* 1997;4:255-271.
15. Brockmoller J, et al. The impact of the CYP2D6 polymorphism on haloperidol pharmacokinetics and on the outcome of haloperidol treatment. *Clin Pharmacol Ther.* 2002;72:438-452.
16. Bronstein AC, et al. 2011 Annual report of the American Association of Poison Control Centers' National Poison Data System (NPDS): 29th Annual Report. *Clin Toxicol (Phila).* 2012;50:911-1164.
17. Brvar M, Bunc M. Video of dantrolene effectiveness on neuroleptic malignant syndrome associated muscular rigidity and tremor. *Crit Care.* 2007;11:415.
18. Buckley N, McManus P. Fatal toxicity of drugs used in the treatment of psychotic illnesses. *Br J Psychiatry.* 1998;172:461-464.
19. Buckley NA, Sanders P. Cardiovascular adverse effects of antipsychotic drugs. *Drug Saf.* 2000;23:215-228.
20. Buckley NA, et al. Cardiotoxicity more common in thioridazine overdose than with other neuroleptics. *J Toxicol Clin Toxicol.* 1995;33:199-204.
21. Burgyone K, et al. The use of antiparkinsonian agents in the management of drug-induced extrapyramidal symptoms. *Curr Pharm Des.* 2004;10:2239-2248.

22. Burns MJ. The pharmacology and toxicology of atypical antipsychotic agents. *J Toxicol Clin Toxicol*. 2001;39:1-14.

23. Burns MJ, et al. A comparison of physostigmine and benzodiazepines for the treatment of anticholinergic poisoning. *Ann Emerg Med*. 2000;35:374-381.

24. Caroff SN, Mann SC. Neuroleptic malignant syndrome. *Med Clin North Am*. 1993;77:185-202.

25. Caroff SN, Mann SC. Neuroleptic malignant syndrome and malignant hyperthermia. *Anaesth Intensive Care*. 1993;21:477-478.

26. Caroff SN, et al. Movement disorders associated with atypical antipsychotic drugs. *J Clin Psychiatry*. 2002;63(suppl 4):12-19.

27. Chue P, Singer P. A review of olanzapine-associated toxicity and fatality in overdose. *J Psychiatry Neurosci*. 2003;28:253-261.

28. Citrome L. Asenapine review, part I: chemistry, receptor affinity profile, pharmacokinetics and metabolism. *Expert Opin Drug Metab Toxicol*. 2014;10:893-903.

29. Citrome L. Asenapine review, part II: clinical efficacy, safety and tolerability. *Expert Opin Drug Saf*. 2014;13:803-830.

30. Corre KA, et al. Extended therapy for acute dystonic reactions. *Ann Emerg Med*. 1984;13:194-197.

31. Dahan L, et al. Effects of bifeprunox and aripiprazole on rat serotonin and dopamine neuronal activity and anxiolytic behaviour. *J Psychopharmacol*. 2009;23:177-189.

32. Dahl ML. Cytochrome p450 phenotyping/genotyping in patients receiving antipsychotics: useful aid to prescribing? *Clin Pharmacokinet*. 2002;41:453-470.

33. Dahl-Puustinen ML, et al. Disposition of perphenazine is related to polymorphic debrisoquin hydroxylation in human beings. *Clin Pharmacol Ther*. 1989;46:78-81.

34. De HM, et al. Metabolic and cardiovascular adverse effects associated with antipsychotic drugs. *Nat Rev Endocrinol*. 2012;8:114-126.

35. Delay J, et al. [A non-phenothiazine and non-reserpine major neuroleptic, haloperidol, in the treatment of psychoses.]. *Ann Med Psychol (Paris)*. 1960;118:145-152.

36. Di Gregorio G, et al. Lipid emulsion is superior to vasopressin in a rodent model of resuscitation from toxin-induced cardiac arrest. *Crit Care Med*. 2009;37:993-999.

37. American Psychiatric Association. *Diagnostic and Statistical Manual of Mental Disorders* (DSM-IV). Washington, DC: American Psychiatric Association; 1994;4:739-742.

38. Dresser GK, Bailey DG. A basic conceptual and practical overview of interactions with highly prescribed drugs. *Can J Clin Pharmacol*. 2002;9:191-198.

39. Ereshefsky L. Pharmacologic and pharmacokinetic considerations in choosing an antipsychotic. *J Clin Psychiatry*. 1999;60(suppl 10):20-30.

40. Fines RE, et al. Acute laryngeal dystonia related to neuroleptic agents. *Am J Emerg Med*. 1999;17:319-320.

41. Finn SD, et al. Early treatment of a quetiapine and sertraline overdose with Intralipid. *Anaesthesia*. 2009;64:191-194.

42. Frey R, et al. [Fatal poisonings with antidepressive drugs and neuroleptics. Analysis of a correlation with prescriptions in Vienna 1991 to 1997]. *Nervenarzt*. 2002;73:629-636.

43. Fryml L, et al. The role of amantadine withdrawal in 3 cases of treatment-refractory altered mental status. *J Psychiatr Pract*. 2017;23:191-199.

44. Gangadhar BN, et al. Amantadine in the neuroleptic malignant syndrome. *J Clin Psychiatry*. 1984;45:526.

45. Gosselin S, et al. Evidence-based recommendations on the use of intravenous lipid emulsion therapy in poisoning. *Clin Toxicol (Phila)*. 2016;54:899-923.

46. Gurrera RJ. A systematic review of sex and age factors in neuroleptic malignant syndrome diagnosis frequency. *Acta Psychiatr Scand*. 2017;135:398-408.

47. Gurrera RJ, et al. An international consensus study of neuroleptic malignant syndrome diagnostic criteria using the Delphi method. *J Clin Psychiatry*. 2011;72:1222-1228.

48. Gurrera RJ, Chang, SS. Thermoregulatory dysfunction in neuroleptic malignant syndrome. *Biol Psychiatry*. 1996;39:207-212.

49. Gurrera RJ, et al. A Validation Study of the International Consensus Diagnostic Criteria for Neuroleptic Malignant Syndrome. *J Clin Psychopharmacol*. 2017;37:67-71.

50. Gurrera RJ, Romero, JA. Sympathoadrenomedullary activity in the neuroleptic malignant syndrome. *Biol Psychiatry*. 1992;32:334-343.

51. Haddad PM, Anderson IM. Antipsychotic-related QTc prolongation, torsade de pointes and sudden death. *Drugs*. 2002;62:1649-1671.

52. Hagg S, Spigset O. Antipsychotic-induced venous thromboembolism: a review of the evidence. *CNS Drugs*. 2002;16:765-776.

53. Henderson A, Longdon P. Fulminant metoclopramide induced neuroleptic malignant syndrome rapidly responsive to intravenous dantrolene. *Aust N Z J Med*. 1991;21:742-743.

54. Henderson DC. Atypical antipsychotic-induced diabetes mellitus; how strong is the evidence? *CNS Drugs*. 2002;16:77-89.

55. Hugenholtz GW, et al. Haloperidol dose when used as active comparator in randomized controlled trials with atypical antipsychotics in schizophrenia: comparison with officially recommended doses. *J Clin Psychiatry*. 2006;67:897-903.

56. Iqbal MM, et al. Clozapine: a clinical review of adverse effects and management. *Ann Clin Psychiatry*. 2003;15:33-48.

57. Isbister GK, et al. Pharmacokinetics of quetiapine in overdose and the effect of activated charcoal. *Clin Pharmacol Ther*. 2007;81:821-827.

58. Isbister GK, et al. Presumed Angel's trumpet (Brugmansia) poisoning: clinical effects and epidemiology. *Emerg Med (Fremantle)*. 2003;15:376-382.

59. Jankovic J. Dopamine depleters in the treatment of hyperkinetic movement disorders. *Expert Opin Pharmacother*. 2016;17:2461-2470.

60. Jee A. Amantadine in neuroleptic malignant syndrome. *Postgrad Med J*. 1987;63:508-509.

61. Jeste DV, et al. Risk of tardive dyskinesia in older patients. A prospective longitudinal study of 266 outpatients. *Arch Gen Psychiatry*. 1995;52:756-765.

62. Jibson MD, Tandon R. New atypical antipsychotic medications. *J Psychiatr Res*. 1998;32:215-228.

63. Jonsson AK, et al. Venous thromboembolism in recipients of antipsychotics: incidence, mechanisms and management. *CNS Drugs*. 2012;26:649-662.

64. Juurlink DN. Activated charcoal for acute overdose: a reappraisal. *Br J Clin Pharmacol*. 2016;81:482-487.

65. Kakihara S, et al. Prediction of response to risperidone treatment with respect to plasma concentrations of risperidone, catecholamine metabolites, and polymorphism of cytochrome P450 2D6. *Int Clin Psychopharmacol*. 2005;20:71-78.

66. Kapur S, Mamo D. Half a century of antipsychotics and still a central role for dopamine D2 receptors. *Prog Neuropsychopharmacol Biol Psychiatry*. 2003;27:1081-1090.

67. Kapur S, Seeman P. Does fast dissociation from the dopamine d(2) receptor explain the action of atypical antipsychotics? A new hypothesis. *Am J Psychiatry*. 2001;158:360-369.

68. Kasper S, et al. Sertindole and dopamine D2 receptor occupancy in comparison to risperidone, clozapine and haloperidol—a 123I-IBZM SPECT study. *Psychopharmacology (Berl)*. 1998;136:367-373.

69. Katus LE, Frucht SJ. Management of serotonin syndrome and neuroleptic malignant syndrome. *Curr Treat Options Neurol*. 2016;18:39.

70. Keck PE Jr, McElroy SL. Clinical pharmacodynamics and pharmacokinetics of antimanic and mood-stabilizing medications. *J Clin Psychiatry*. 2002;63(suppl 4):3-11.

71. Keck PE Jr, et al. Ziprasidone: a new atypical antipsychotic. *Expert Opin Pharmacother*. 2001;2:1033-1042.

72. Kouparanis A, et al. Neuroleptic malignant syndrome in a patient on long-term olanzapine treatment at a stable dose: successful treatment with dantrolene. *Brain Inj*. 2015;29:658-660.

73. Lannemyr L, Knudsen K. Severe overdose of quetiapine treated successfully with extracorporeal life support. *Clin Toxicol (Phila)*. 2012;50:258-261.

74. Laskowski LK, et al. Ice water submersion for rapid cooling in severe drug-induced hyperthermia. *Clin Toxicol (Phila)*. 2015;53:181-184.

75. Levenson JL. Neuroleptic malignant syndrome. *Am J Psychiatry*. 1985;142:1137-1145.

76. Lima AR, et al. Central action beta-blockers versus placebo for neuroleptic-induced acute akathisia. *Cochrane Database Syst Rev*. 2004;CD001946.

77. Lima AR, et al. Anticholinergics for neuroleptic-induced acute akathisia. *Cochrane Database Syst Rev*. 2004;CD003727.

78. Lipinski JF Jr, et al. Fluoxetine-induced akathisia: clinical and theoretical implications. *J Clin Psychiatry*. 1989;50:339-342.

79. Lipscombe LL, et al. Antipsychotic drugs and hyperglycemia in older patients with diabetes. *Arch Intern Med*. 2009;169:1282-1289.

80. Luchini F, et al. Catatonia and neuroleptic malignant syndrome: two disorders on a same spectrum? Four case reports. *J Nerv Ment Dis*. 2013;201:36-42.

81. Maher AR, Theodore G. Summary of the comparative effectiveness review on off-label use of atypical antipsychotics. *J Manag Care Pharm*. 2012;18:S1-20.

82. Mamo DC, et al. Managing antipsychotic-induced parkinsonism. *Drug Saf*. 1999;20:269-275.

83. Manini AF, et al. QT prolongation and Torsades de Pointes following overdose of ziprasidone and amantadine. *J Med Toxicol*. 2007;3:178-181.

84. Marsden CD, Jenner P. The pathophysiology of extrapyramidal side-effects of neuroleptic drugs. *Psychol Med*. 1980;10:55-72.

85. Matsumoto H, et al. Effect of lipid emulsion during resuscitation of a patient with cardiac arrest after overdose of chlorpromazine and mirtazapine. *Am J Emerg Med*. 2015;33:1541-1542.

86. Mauri MC, et al. Clinical pharmacology of atypical antipsychotics: an update. *EXCLI J*. 2014;13:1163-1191.

87. McAllister RK, et al. Lipid 20% emulsion ameliorates the symptoms of olanzapine toxicity in a 4-year-old. *Am J Emerg Med*. 2012;30:1012-1012.

88. Meltzer HY, Stahl SM. The dopamine hypothesis of schizophrenia: a review. *Schizophr Bull*. 1976;2:19-76.

89. Mendelson G. Pheniramine aminosalicylate overdosage. Reversal of delirium and choreiform movements with tacrine treatment. *Arch Neurol*. 1977;34:313

90. Miller DD. Review and management of clozapine side effects. *J Clin Psychiatry*. 2000;61(suppl 8):14-17, discussion 18-19.

91. Minns AB, Clark RF. Toxicology and overdose of atypical antipsychotics. *J Emerg Med*. 2012;43:906-913.

92. Mowry JB, et al. 2015 Annual Report of the American Association of Poison Control Centers' National Poison Data System (NPDS): 33rd Annual Report. *Clin Toxicol (Phila)*. 2016;54:924-1109.

93. Naber D, Lambert M. Aripiprazole: a new atypical antipsychotic with a different pharmacological mechanism. *Prog Neuropsychopharmacol Biol Psychiatry*. 2004;28:1213-1219.

94. Nelson LS. Toxicologic myocardial sensitization. *J Toxicol Clin Toxicol*. 2002;40:867-879.

95. Newman EJ, et al. The parkinsonism-hyperpyrexia syndrome. *Neurocrit Care*. 2009;10:136-140.

96. Newman-Tancredi A, et al. Neuropharmacological profile of bifeprunox: merits and limitations in comparison with other third-generation antipsychotics. *Curr Opin Investig Drugs*. 2007;8:539-554.

97. Nielsen RE, et al. Neuroleptic malignant syndrome-an 11-year longitudinal case-control study. *Can J Psychiatry*. 2012;57:512-518.
98. Nisijima K. Elevated creatine kinase does not necessarily correspond temporally with onset of muscle rigidity in neuroleptic malignant syndrome: a report of two cases. *Neuropsychiatr Dis Treat*. 2012;8:615-618.
99. Nisijima K, Ishiguro T. Electroconvulsive therapy for the treatment of neuroleptic malignant syndrome with psychotic symptoms: a report of five cases. *J ECT*. 1999;15:158-163.
100. Nisijima K, et al. Intravenous injection of levodopa is more effective than dantrolene as therapy for neuroleptic malignant syndrome. *Biol Psychiatry*. 1997;41:913-914.
101. Noyan MA, et al. Donepezil for anticholinergic drug intoxication: a case report. *Prog Neuropsychopharmacol Biol Psychiatry*. 2003;27:885-887.
102. Perquin L, Steinert T. A review of the efficacy, tolerability and safety of sertindole in clinical trials. *CNS Drugs*. 2004;18(suppl 2):19-30, discussion 41-43.
103. Perry PJ, Wilborn CA. Serotonin syndrome vs neuroleptic malignant syndrome: a contrast of causes, diagnoses, and management. *Ann Clin Psychiatry*. 2012;24:155-162.
104. Pierre JM. Extrapyramidal symptoms with atypical antipsychotics: incidence, prevention and management. *Drug Saf*. 2005;28:191-208.
105. Pisani F, et al. Effects of psychotropic drugs on seizure threshold. *Drug Saf*. 2002;25:91-110.
106. Pope HG Jr, et al. Frequency and presentation of neuroleptic malignant syndrome in a large psychiatric hospital. *Am J Psychiatry*. 1986;143:1227-1233.
107. Ragucci KR, Wells BJ. Olanzapine-induced diabetic ketoacidosis. *Ann Pharmacother*. 2001;35:1556-1558.
108. Ray WA, et al. Atypical antipsychotic drugs and the risk of sudden cardiac death. *N Engl J Med*. 2009;360:225-235.
109. Ray WA, et al. Antipsychotics and the risk of sudden cardiac death. *Arch Gen Psychiatry*. 2001;58:1161-1167.
110. Remington G. Understanding antipsychotic "atypicality": a clinical and pharmacological moving target. *J Psychiatry Neurosci*. 2003;28:275-284.
111. Reulbach U, et al. Managing an effective treatment for neuroleptic malignant syndrome. *Crit Care*. 2007;11:R4.
112. Richelson E. Receptor pharmacology of neuroleptics: relation to clinical effects. *J Clin Psychiatry*. 1999;60(suppl 10):5-14.
113. Richelson E, Nelson A. Antagonism by antidepressants of neurotransmitter receptors of normal human brain in vitro. *J Pharmacol Exp Ther*. 1984;230:94-102.
114. Richelson E, Souder T. Binding of antipsychotic drugs to human brain receptors focus on newer generation compounds. *Life Sci*. 2000;68:29-39.
115. Robinson K, Smith RN. Radioimmunoassay of tricyclic antidepressant and some phenothiazine drugs in forensic toxicology. *J Immunoassay*. 1985;6:11-22.
116. Rosebush PI, et al. The treatment of neuroleptic malignant syndrome. Are dantrolene and bromocriptine useful adjuncts to supportive care? *Br J Psychiatry*. 1991;159:709-712.
117. Ross SR, Rodgers SR. Physostigmine in amoxapine overdose. *Am J Hosp Pharm*. 1981;38:1121-1122.
118. Schneir AB, et al. Complications of diagnostic physostigmine administration to emergency department patients. *Ann Emerg Med*. 2003;42:14-19.
119. Schuster MA, et al. A national survey of stress reactions after the September 11, 2001, terrorist attacks. *N Engl J Med*. 2001;345:1507-1512.
120. Schuster P, et al. Reversal by physostigmine of clozapine-induced delirium. *Clin Toxicol*. 1977;10:437-441.
121. Seeman P. Atypical antipsychotics: mechanism of action. *Can J Psychiatry*. 2002;47:27-38.
122. Seeman P. Dopamine D2 High receptors moderately elevated by bifeprunox and aripiprazole. *Synapse*. 2008;62:902-908.
123. Seeman P, Kapur S. Schizophrenia: more dopamine, more D2 receptors. *Proc Natl Acad Sci U S A*. 2000;97:7673-7675.
124. Seger DL. A critical reconsideration of the clinical effects and treatment recommendations for sodium channel blocking drug cardiotoxicity. *Toxicol Rev*. 2006;25:283-296.
125. Seger DL, et al. Variability of recommendations for serum alkalinization in tricyclic antidepressant overdose: a survey of U.S. Poison Center medical directors. *J Toxicol Clin Toxicol*. 2003;41:331-338.
126. Shah AS, Eddleston M. Should phenytoin or barbiturates be used as second-line anticonvulsant therapy for toxicological seizures? *Clin Toxicol (Phila)*. 2010;48:800-805.
127. Shoop SA, Cernek PK. Carbidopa/levodopa in the treatment of neuroleptic malignant syndrome. *Ann Pharmacother*. 1997;31:119.
128. Spina E, Zoccali R. Sertindole: pharmacological and clinical profile and role in the treatment of schizophrenia. *Expert Opin Drug Metab Toxicol*. 2008;4:629-638.
129. Squires RF, Saederup E. Mono N-aryl ethylenediamine and piperazine derivatives are GABAA receptor blockers: implications for psychiatry. *Neurochem Res*. 1993;18:787-793.
130. Stahl SM. Introduction: what makes an antipsychotic atypical? *J Clin Psychiatry*. 1999;60(suppl 10):3-4.
131. Strawn JR, et al. Neuroleptic malignant syndrome. *Am J Psychiatry*. 2007;164:870-876.
132. Tarsy D. Movement disorders with neuroleptic drug treatment. *Psychiatr Clin North Am*. 1984;7:453-471.
133. Tarsy D, et al. Effects of newer antipsychotics on extrapyramidal function. *CNS Drugs*. 2002;16:23-45.
134. Torrey EF, Swalwell CI. Fatal olanzapine-induced ketoacidosis. *Am J Psychiatry*. 2003;160:2241.
135. Trollor JN, et al. Comparison of neuroleptic malignant syndrome induced by first- and second-generation antipsychotics. *Br J Psychiatry*. 2012;201:52-56.
136. Trosch RM. Neuroleptic-induced movement disorders: deconstructing extrapyramidal symptoms. *J Am Geriatr Soc*. 2004;52:S266-S271.
137. van Harten PN, et al. Acute dystonia induced by drug treatment. *BMJ*. 1999;319:623-626.
138. Velamoor VR. Neuroleptic malignant syndrome. Recognition, prevention and management. *Drug Saf*. 1998;19:73-82.
139. Velamoor VR, et al. Progression of symptoms in neuroleptic malignant syndrome. *J Nerv Ment Dis*. 1994;182:168-173.
140. Velamoor VR, et al. Management of suspected neuroleptic malignant syndrome. *Can J Psychiatry*. 1995;40:545-550.
141. Vijayakumar D, Jankovic J. Drug-induced dyskinesia, part 2: treatment of tardive dyskinesia. *Drugs*. 2016;76:779-787.
142. von Bahr C, et al. Plasma levels of thioridazine and metabolites are influenced by the debrisoquin hydroxylation phenotype. *Clin Pharmacol Ther*. 1991;49:234-240.
143. Weinberg G, et al. Lipid, not propofol, treats bupivacaine overdose. *Anesth Analg*. 2004;99:1875-1876.
144. Weinberg G, et al. Lipid emulsion infusion rescues dogs from bupivacaine-induced cardiac toxicity. *Reg Anesth Pain Med*. 2003;28:198-202.
145. Weiner JS, Khogali M. A physiological body-cooling unit for treatment of heat stroke. *Lancet*. 1980;1:507-509.
146. Weisdorf D, et al. Physostigmine for cardiac and neurologic manifestations of phenothiazine poisoning. *Clin Pharmacol Ther*. 1978;24:663-667.
147. Weizberg M, et al. Altered mental status from olanzapine overdose treated with physostigmine. *Clin Toxicol (Phila)*. 2006;44:319-325.
148. Wenzel-Seifert K, et al. QTc prolongation by psychotropic drugs and the risk of Torsade de Pointes. *Dtsch Arztebl Int*. 2011;108:687-693.
149. Widerlov E, et al. Effect of urinary pH on the plasma and urinary kinetics of remoxipride in man. *Eur J Clin Pharmacol*. 1989;37:359-363.
150. Wirshing WC. Movement disorders associated with neuroleptic treatment. *J Clin Psychiatry*. 2001;62(suppl 21):15-18.
151. Yurtlu BS, et al. Intravenous lipid infusion restores consciousness associated with olanzapine overdose. *Anesth Analg*. 2012;114:914-915.

68 CYCLIC ANTIDEPRESSANTS

Matthew Valento and Erica L. Liebelt

HISTORY AND EPIDEMIOLOGY

The term *cyclic antidepressant* (CA) refers to a group of pharmacologically related xenobiotics used for treatment of depression, neuralgic pain, migraines, enuresis, and attention deficit hyperactivity disorder (ADHD). Most CAs have at least three rings in their chemical structure. They include the traditional tricyclic antidepressants (TCAs) imipramine, desipramine, amitriptyline, nortriptyline, doxepin, trimipramine, protriptyline, and clomipramine, as well as other cyclic compounds such as the tetracyclic, maprotiline and the dibenzoxapine amoxapine, antidepressants.

Imipramine was the first TCA used for treatment of depression in the late 1950s. However, the synthesis of iminodibenzyl, the "tricyclic" core of imipramine, and the description of its chemical characteristics date back to 1889. Structurally related to the phenothiazines, imipramine was originally developed as a hypnotic for agitated or psychotic patients and was serendipitously found to alleviate depression. From the 1960s until the late 1980s, the TCAs were the major pharmacologic treatment for depression in the United States. However, by the early 1960s, cardiovascular and central nervous system (CNS) toxicities were recognized as major complications in patients with TCA overdoses. The newer CAs developed in the 1980s and 1990s were designed to decrease some of the adverse effects of older TCAs, improve the therapeutic index, and reduce the incidence of serious toxicity. The epidemiology of CA poisoning has evolved significantly in the past 30 years, resulting in great part from the introduction of the selective serotonin reuptake inhibitors (SSRIs and SSNRIs) and other newer antidepressants for the treatment of depression. Although the use of CAs for depression has decreased, other medical indications, including chronic pain, sleep disorders, obsessive-compulsive disorder, and, particularly in children, enuresis and ADHD, have emerged, resulting in their continued use.[19,87] The antidepressants are a leading cause of drug-related self-poisonings in the developed world, primarily because of their ready availability to people with depression or chronic pain who by virtue of their diseases are at high risk for overdose. However, despite the increase in SSRI use and overdose, patients with TCA overdoses continue to have a higher incidence of hospitalization and fatality than do those with SSRI overdose and continue to be among the leading xenobiotics associated with fatality reported to poison control centers (Chap. 130).

Despite the emergence of the SSRIs in the early 1990s, TCAs are still frequently prescribed by pediatric office-based practices for many of the conditions noted earlier. Since the October 2004 US Food and Drug Administration boxed warning about the increased risk of suicidal behavior associated with antidepressant use, several reports describe significant declines in antidepressant dispensing in children compared with historical trends.[25] Nevertheless, CA poisoning likely will continue to be among the most lethal unintentional drug ingestions in younger children because only one or two adult-strength pills can produce serious clinical effects in young children.

PHARMACOLOGY

The TCAs are classified into tertiary and secondary amines based on the presence of a methyl group on the propylamine side chain (Table 68–1). The tertiary amines amitriptyline and imipramine are metabolized to the secondary amines nortriptyline and desipramine, respectively, which themselves are marketed as antidepressants. In therapeutic doses, the CAs produce similar pharmacologic effects on the autonomic system, CNS, and cardiovascular system. However, they can be distinguished from each other by their relative potencies and side effect profiles.[124]

At therapeutic doses, CAs inhibit presynaptic reuptake of norepinephrine or serotonin, functionally increasing the amount of these neurotransmitters at CNS receptors. Whereas the tertiary amines, especially clomipramine, are more potent inhibitors of serotonin reuptake, the secondary amines are more potent inhibitors of norepinephrine reuptake. Although these pharmacologic actions formed the basis of the monoamine hypothesis of depression in the 1960s, antidepressant actions of these drugs appear to be much more complex.

The "receptor sensitivity hypothesis of antidepressant drug action" postulates that after chronic CA administration, alterations in the sensitivity of various receptors are responsible for antidepressant effects. Chronic CA administration alters the number or function of central β-adrenergic and serotonin receptors. In addition, CAs modulate glucocorticoid receptor gene expression and cause alterations at the genomic level of other receptors.[8] All of these actions likely play a role in the antidepressant effects of CAs.

Additional pharmacologic mechanisms of CAs are responsible for their side effects with therapeutic dosing and clinical effects after overdose. All of the CAs are competitive antagonists of the muscarinic acetylcholine receptors, although they have different affinities. The CAs also antagonize peripheral α_1-adrenergic receptors. The most prominent effects of CA overdose result from binding to the cardiac sodium channels, which is also described as a membrane-stabilizing effect (Fig. 68–1) (Chap. 15). The TCAs are potent inhibitors of both peripheral and central postsynaptic histamine receptors.

TABLE 68–1	Cyclic Antidepressants—Classification by Chemical Structure
Tertiary Amines	
Amitriptyline Clomipramine Doxepin Imipramine Trimipramine	Imipramine
Secondary Amines	
Desipramine Nortriptyline Protriptyline	Nortriptyline
Amoxapine	
Maprotiline	

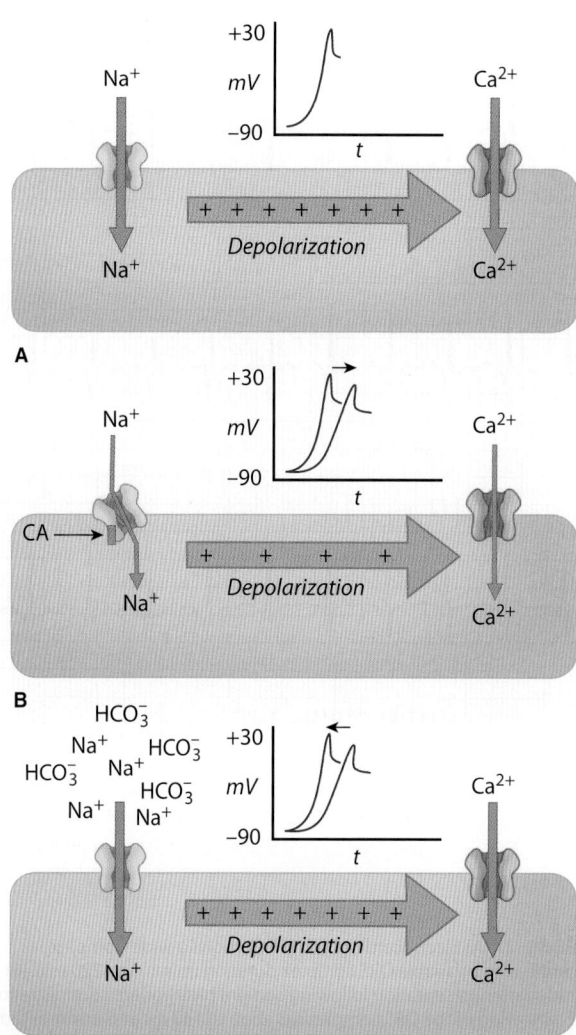

FIGURE 68–1. Effects of cyclic antidepressants (CAs) on the fast sodium channel. (**A**) Sodium depolarizes the cell, which both propagates conduction, allowing complete cardiac depolarization, and opens voltage-dependent Ca²⁺ channels, producing contraction. (**B**) CAs and other sodium channel blockers alter the conformation of the sodium channel, slowing the rate of rise of the action potential, which produces both negative dromotropic and inotropic effects. (**C**) Raising the Na⁺ gradient across the affected sodium channel speeds the rate of rise of the action potential, counteracting the drug-induced effects. Raising the pH removes the CA from the binding site on the Na⁺ channel. See Fig. 68–3 for the effects noted on the electrocardiograph.

Finally, the CAs interfere with chloride conductance by binding to the picro-toxin site on the γ-aminobutyric acid (GABA)–chloride complex.[112]

Amoxapine is a dibenzoxazepine CA derived from the active antipsychotic loxapine. Although it has a three-ringed structure, this drug has little similarity to the other tricyclics. It is a potent norepinephrine reuptake inhibitor, has no effect on serotonin reuptake, and blocks dopamine receptors. Maprotiline is a tetracyclic antidepressant that predominantly blocks norepinephrine reuptake. Both of these CAs have a slightly different toxic profile than the traditional TCAs.[59,61,124]

PHARMACOKINETICS AND TOXICOKINETICS

In therapeutic dosing, the CAs are rapidly and almost completely absorbed from the gastrointestinal (GI) tract, with peak concentrations 2 to 8 hours after administration of a therapeutic dose. They are weak bases (high pK$_a$). In overdose, the decreased GI motility caused by anticholinergic effects and ionization in gastric acid delay CA absorption. Because of extensive first-pass metabolism by the liver, the oral bioavailability of CAs is low and variable, although metabolism saturates in overdose, increasing bioavailability.

The CAs are highly lipophilic and possess large and variable volumes of distribution (15–40 L/kg). They are rapidly distributed to the heart, brain, liver, and kidney, in which the tissue to plasma ratio generally exceeds 10:1. The octanol/water partition coefficient (log P) is an often cited measure of lipid-solubility with the log D representing Log P at physiological pH—a more representative measure. Some examples of log D values for CAs are amitriptyline, 3.96; nortriptyline, 2.86; imipramine, 2.06; desipramine, 1.05; and doxepin, 2.93.

Less than 2% of the ingested dose is present in blood several hours after overdose, and serum CA concentrations decline biexponentially. The CAs are extensively bound to α$_1$-acid glycoprotein (AAG) in the plasma, although differential binding among the specific CAs is observed.[2] Changes in AAG concentration or pH can alter binding and the percentage of free or unbound drug.[94,106] Specifically, a low blood pH (which often occurs in a severely poisoned patient) increases the amount of free drug, making it more available to exert its effects. This property serves as one basis for alkalinization therapy (see later).

The CAs undergo demethylation, aromatic hydroxylation, and glucuronide conjugation of the hydroxy metabolites. The tertiary amines imipramine and amitriptyline are demethylated to desipramine and nortriptyline, respectively. The hydroxy metabolites of both tertiary and secondary amines are pharmacologically active and contribute to toxicity. The glucuronide metabolites are inactive.

Genetically based differences in the activity of the CYP2D6, which are responsible for hydroxylation of imipramine and desipramine, account for wide interindividual variability in metabolism and steady-state serum concentrations.[18] "Poor metabolizers" are reported to recover more slowly from an overdose or demonstrate toxicity with therapeutic dosing, which is a major risk factor for attaining high serum CA concentrations.[47,116] The metabolism of CAs is also influenced by concomitant ingestion of ethanol and other xenobiotics that induce or inhibit CYP2D6 (Chap. 11 and Appendix). Increased plasma CA concentrations in older adult patients are likely because of decreased renal clearance.[100]

Elimination half-lives for therapeutic doses of CAs vary from 7 to 58 hours (54–92 hours for protriptyline), with even longer half-lives in older adults. The half-lives are also be prolonged following overdose as a result of saturable metabolism. A small fraction (15%–30%) of CA elimination occurs through biliary and gastric secretion. The metabolites are then reabsorbed in the systemic circulation, resulting in enterohepatic and enterogastric recirculation and reducing their fecal excretion. Finally, less than 5% of CAs are excreted unchanged by the kidney.

PATHOPHYSIOLOGY

The CAs slow the recovery from inactivation of the fast sodium channel, slowing phase 0 depolarization of the action potential in the distal His-Purkinje system and the ventricular myocardium (Figs. 68–1 and 15–2 and Chap. 15). Impaired depolarization within the ventricular conduction system slows the propagation of ventricular depolarization, which manifests as prolongation of the QRS complex on the electrocardiogram (ECG) (Figs. 68–2 and 68-3). The right bundle branch has a relatively longer refractory period, and it is affected disproportionately by xenobiotics that slow intraventricular conduction. This slowing of depolarization results in a rightward shift of the terminal 40 ms (T40-ms) of the QRS axis and the right bundle branch block pattern that is noted on the ECG of patients who are exposed to or overdose with a CA.[126]

Because CAs are weakly basic, they are increasingly ionized as the ambient pH falls and less ionized as the pH rises. Changing the ambient pH therefore alters their binding to the sodium channel. This probably occurs because 90% of the binding of CA to the sodium channel occurs in the ionized state, alkalinizing the blood facilitates the movement of the CA away from the hydrophilic sodium channel and into the lipid membrane (Antidotes in Depth: A5).

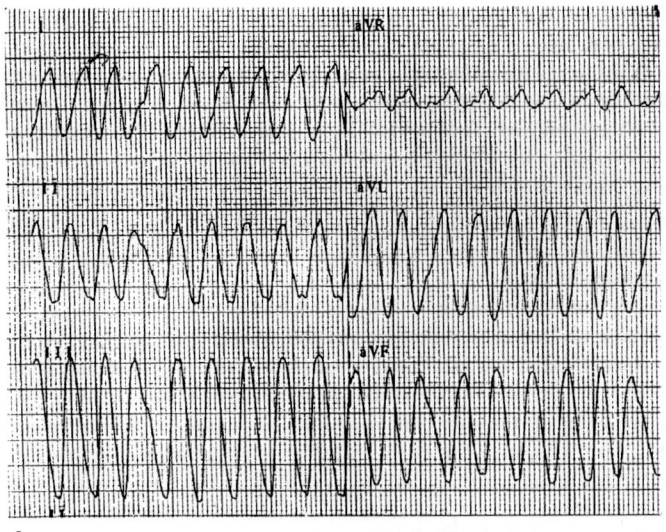

A

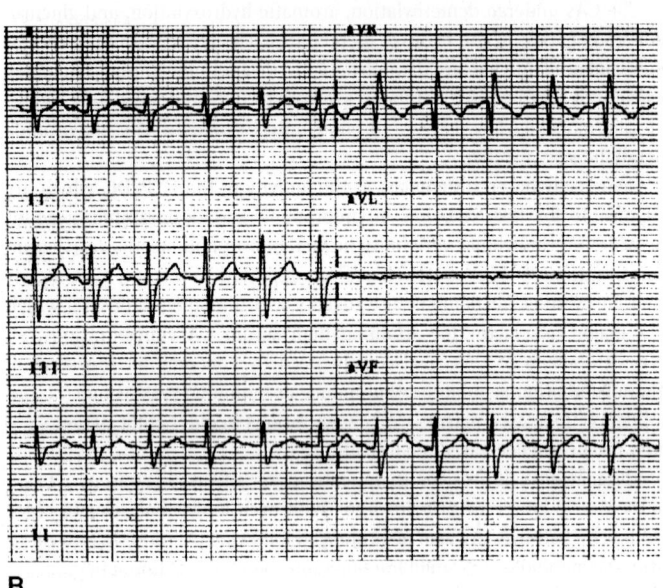

B

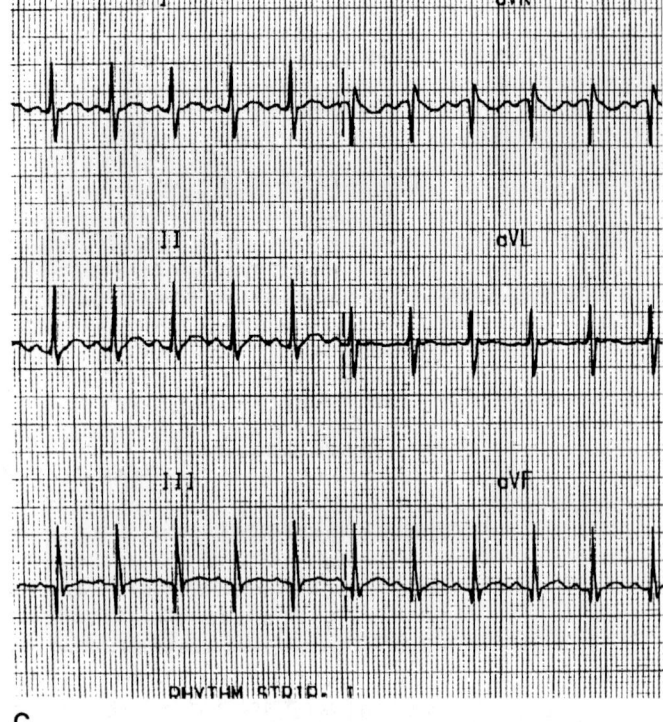

C

FIGURE 68–2. (A) Electrocardiograph (ECG) shows a wide-complex tachycardia with a variable QRS complex duration (minimum, 220 ms). **(B)** ECG 30 minutes after presentation following sodium bicarbonate administration shows narrowing of the QRS complex duration to 140 ms and an amplitude of the R in aV$_R$ of 6.0 mm. **(C)** ECG 9 hours after presentation shows further narrowing of the QRS complex to 80 ms and decrease in the amplitude of the R in aV$_R$ to 4.5 mm. *(Reproduced with permission from Liebelt EL. Targeted management strategies for cardiovascular toxicity from tricyclic antidepressant overdose: the pivotal role for alkalinization and sodium loading. Pediatr Emerg Care. 1998 Aug;14(4):293-298.)*

Sinus tachycardia is caused by the antimuscarinic, vasodilatory (reflex tachycardia), and sympathomimetic effects of the CAs. Wide-complex tachycardia most commonly represents aberrantly conducted sinus tachycardia rather than ventricular tachycardia. However, by prolonging anterograde conduction, nonuniform ventricular conduction can result, leading to reentrant ventricular dysrhythmias.

Electrophysiologic studies in a canine model demonstrate that prolongation of the QRS complex duration is rate dependent, a characteristic effect of the Vaughn Williams class IA antidysrhythmics (Chap. 57). Furthermore, pharmacologic induction of bradycardia prevents or narrows wide-complex tachycardia by allowing time for recovery of the sodium channel from inactivation.[4,103] However, because bradycardia adversely affects cardiac output, induction of bradycardia is not recommended.

A Brugada ECG pattern, specifically type 1 or "coved" pattern, is rarely associated with CA overdose. The Brugada syndrome originates from a structural change in the myocardial sodium channel that results in functional sodium channel alterations similar to those caused by the CAs.[11,83] It is possible that this small cohort of patients have subclinical Brugada syndrome that was uncovered by the CA (Chap. 15).

Prolongation of the QT interval also occurs in the setting of both therapeutic use and overdose of CAs. This apparent prolongation of repolarization results primarily from slowed depolarization (ie, QRS complex prolongation) rather than altered repolarization.[99] Although QT interval prolongation predisposes to the development of torsade de pointes, this dysrhythmia is uncommon in patients with CA poisoning where tachycardia is prominent.

Hypotension is caused by direct myocardial depression secondary to altered sodium channel function, which disrupts the subsequent excitation-contraction coupling of myocytes and impairs cardiac contractility. Peripheral vasodilation from α-adrenergic blockade by CAs also contributes prominently to postural hypotension. In addition, downregulation of adrenergic receptors blunts the physiologic response to catecholamines.[82]

Agitation, delirium, and depressed sensorium are primarily caused by central anticholinergic and antihistaminic effects. Details regarding the exact mechanism of CA-induced seizures remain elusive. Cyclic antidepressant-induced seizures may result from a combination of an increased concentration of monoamines (particularly norepinephrine), muscarinic antagonism, neuronal sodium channel alteration, and GABA inhibition.[84]

Acute respiratory distress syndrome (ARDS) occurs in the setting of CA overdose. In one study, amitriptyline exposure caused dose-related vasoconstriction and bronchoconstriction in isolated rat lungs.[115] Many substances implicated in ARDS, such as platelet-activating factor and protein kinase activation, were important in mediating amitriptyline-induced impairment of lung function in this experimental model. Another animal model demonstrated that acute amitriptyline poisoning causes dose-dependent rises in

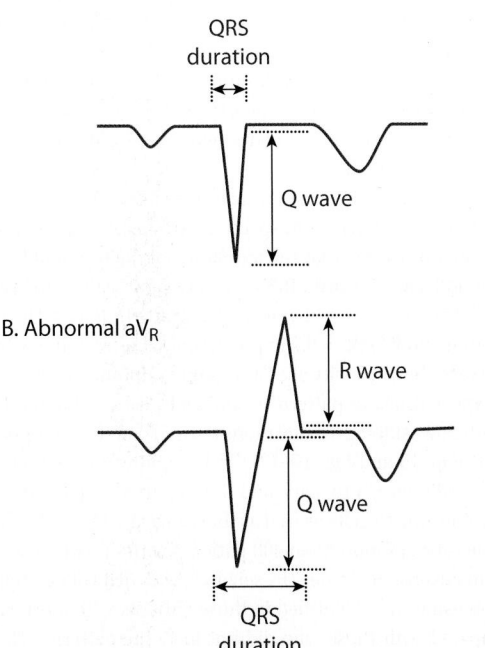

A. Normal aV$_R$

QRS duration

Q wave

B. Abnormal aV$_R$

R wave

Q wave

QRS duration

FIGURE 68–3. (**A**) Normal QRS complex in lead aVR. (**B**) Abnormal QRS complex in a patient with cyclic antidepressant (CA) poisoning. The R wave in lead aV$_R$ is measured as the maximal height in millimeters of the terminal upward deflection in the QRS complex. In this example, the QRS complex duration is prolonged, indicating significant CA poisoning.

pulmonary artery pressure, pulmonary edema, and sustained vasoconstriction that could be attenuated by either calcium channel inhibition or a nitric oxide donor.[72]

CLINICAL MANIFESTATIONS

The toxic profile is qualitatively the same for all of the first-generation TCAs but is slightly different for some of the other CAs.[124] The progression of clinical toxicity is unpredictable and often rapid. Patients commonly present to the emergency department (ED) with minimal apparent clinical abnormalities, only to develop life-threatening cardiovascular and CNS toxicity within hours.

The CAs have a narrow therapeutic index, meaning that a small increase in serum concentration over the therapeutic range results in toxicity. Acute ingestion of 10 to 20 mg/kg of most CAs causes significant cardiovascular and CNS manifestations (therapeutic dose, 2–4 mg/kg/d). Thus, in adults, ingestions of more than 1 g of a CA is usually associated with life-threatening effects. In a series of children with unintentional TCA exposure, all patients with reported ingestions of more than 5 mg/kg manifested clinical toxicity.[78]

Acute Toxicity

Most of the reported toxicity from CAs derives from patients with acute ingestions, especially in patients who are chronically taking the medication. Clinical manifestations of these two cohorts do not appear to be different, and most studies do not distinguish between them.

Acute Cardiovascular Toxicity

Cardiovascular toxicity is primarily responsible for the morbidity and mortality attributed to CAs. Refractory hypotension caused by myocardial depression is the most common cause of death from CA overdose.[20,114] Hypoxia, acidosis, volume depletion, seizures, or concomitant ingestion of other cardiodepressant or vasodilating drugs exacerbate hypotension and predispose to ventricular dysrhythmia.[69,118]

The most common dysrhythmia observed after CA overdose is sinus tachycardia (rate, 120–160 beats/min in an adult), and this finding is present in most patients with clinically significant TCA poisoning. The ECG typically

demonstrates intraventricular conduction delay that manifests as a rightward shift of the T40-ms QRS complex axis and a prolongation of the QRS complex duration. These findings can be used to identify and risk stratify patients with CA poisoning (see Diagnostic Testing). Prolongation of the PR interval, QRS complex, and QT interval can occur in the setting of both therapeutic and toxic amounts of TCAs.[74]

Wide-complex tachycardia is the characteristic potentially life-threatening dysrhythmia observed in patients with severe toxicity (Fig. 68–2). Ventricular tachycardia is often difficult to distinguish from the aberrantly conducted sinus tachycardia that occurs more commonly. In the former cases, the preceding P wave may not be apparent because of prolonged atrioventricular conduction, widened QRS interval, or both. Ventricular tachycardia occurs most often in patients with prolonged QRS complex duration or hypotension.[69,118] Fatal dysrhythmias are rare because ventricular tachycardia and fibrillation occur in only approximately 4% of all cases.[41,92] Both the Brugada type I ECG pattern and torsade de pointes are uncommon with acute TCA overdose.

Acute Central Nervous System Toxicity

Altered mental status and seizures are the primary manifestations of CNS toxicity. Delirium, agitation, or psychotic behavior with hallucinations most likely result from antagonism of muscarinic and histaminergic receptors. These alterations in consciousness usually are followed by lethargy, which is followed by rapid progression to coma. The duration of coma is variable and does not necessarily correlate with or occur concomitantly with ECG abnormalities.[61]

Seizures usually are generalized and brief, most often occurring within 1 to 2 hours of ingestion.[28] The incidence of seizures is similar to ventricular tachycardia and occurs in an estimated 4% of patients presenting with overdose and 13% of fatal cases.[128] Status epilepticus is uncommon. Abrupt deterioration in hemodynamic status, namely hypotension and ventricular dysrhythmias, often develops during or within minutes after a seizure.[28,69,118] This rapid cardiovascular deterioration likely results from seizure-induced acidemia that exacerbates cardiovascular toxicity. The risk of seizures in patients with CA overdoses is increased in those undergoing long-term therapy or who have other risk factors such as history of seizures, head trauma, or concomitant drug withdrawal.[110] Myoclonus and extrapyramidal symptoms also occur in CA-poisoned patients, and cerebellitis is reported.[119]

Cessation of CAs produces a drug discontinuation syndrome in some patients, which is typified by GI and somatic distress, sleep disturbances, movement disorders, and mania.[37]

Other Clinical Effects

Anticholinergic effects can occur early or late in the course of CA toxicity. Pupils are dilated and poorly reactive to light. Other anticholinergic effects include dry mouth, dry flushed skin, urinary retention, and ileus. Although prominent, these findings are typically inconsequential.

Reported pulmonary complications include ARDS, aspiration pneumonitis, and multisystem organ failure. Acute respiratory distress syndrome results from aspiration, hypotension, pulmonary infection, and excessive fluid administration, along with the primary toxic effects of CAs.[107,109] Bowel ischemia, pseudoobstruction, and pancreatitis are reported in patients with CA overdose.[80]

Death directly caused by CA toxicity usually occurs in the first several hours after presentation and is secondary to refractory hypotension in patients who reach health care facilities. Late deaths (>1–2 days after presentation) usually are secondary to other factors such as aspiration pneumonitis, ARDS from refractory hypotension, or infection.[21]

Chronic Toxicity

Chronic CA toxicity usually manifests as exaggerated side effects, such as sedation and sinus tachycardia or is identified by supratherapeutic drug concentrations in the blood in the absence of an acute overdose.[39] Unlike patients with chronic theophylline and aspirin poisoning, chronic CA toxicity does not appear to cause life-threatening effects.

A sparse literature describes the clinical course of this cohort. However, a case report described chronic amitriptyline overdose in a child (15 mg/kg a day for 1 month) that resulted in status epilepticus and significant cardiac conduction abnormalities but normal neurologic outcome.[26] Genetic analysis showed two copies of wild-type alleles for the genes responsible for CYP2D6 activity, concluding the patient was not a "rapid metabolizer." Several possible protective mechanisms are presented by the authors that further illustrate the complexity of this drug, its metabolism, and toxicity. These include a unique pharmacogenomics profile that yields an abnormal receptor profile or metabolic pathway (eg, polymorphism in the gene for myocardial fast sodium channels), another xenobiotic causing a beneficial drug–drug interaction, and the protective effect from other drugs the patient was taking—guanfacine and clonidine—adrenergic medications that may have offered some protective effect from the α-adrenergic blockade caused by amitriptyline.

Several reports describe sudden death in children taking therapeutic doses of CAs.[96,98,117] Prolongation of the QT interval with resultant torsade de pointes, advanced atrioventricular conduction delays, blood pressure fluctuations, and ventricular tachycardia are postulated mechanisms, although whether any of these effects contributed to the deaths is unknown. Prospective studies using 12-lead ECG, 24-hour ECG recording, and Doppler echocardiography in children receiving therapeutic doses of CAs have failed to find any significant cardiac abnormalities when compared to children not taking CAs.[14,31] However, it is recommend that CAs not be initiated or continued in any child with a resting QT interval greater than 450 ms or with a bundle branch block.[34] This is an ongoing area of research because it becomes problematic in making decisions about pharmacotherapy interventions.

Unique Toxicity from "Atypical" Cyclic Antidepressants

Although the incidence of serious cardiovascular toxicity is lower in patients with amoxapine overdoses, the incidence of seizures is significantly greater than with the traditional CAs.[61,71] Moreover, seizures are more frequent, or status epilepticus occurs.[83] Similarly, the incidences of seizures, cardiac dysrhythmias, and duration of coma are greater with maprotiline toxicity compared with the CAs.[59]

DIAGNOSTIC TESTING

Diagnostic testing for patients with CA poisoning primarily relies on indirect bedside tests (ECG) and other qualitative laboratory analyses. Quantification of CA concentration provides little help in the acute management of patients with CA overdose but provides adjunctive information to support the diagnosis.

Electrocardiography

The ECG provides important diagnostic information and predicts clinical toxicity after a CA overdose. Toxicity results in distinctive and diagnostic ECG changes that allows early diagnosis and targeted therapy even when the clinical history and physical examination are unreliable.

A rightward T40-ms axis shift is a sensitive indicator of drug presence.[22,86,126] A terminal QRS complex vector between 130 degrees and 270 degrees discriminated between 11 patients with positive toxicology screens for CAs and 14 patients with negative toxicology screen results.[86] In one report, the positive and negative predictive values of this ECG parameter for CA ingestions were 66% and 100%, respectively, in a population of 299 general overdose patients. A retrospective study reported that a CA-poisoned patient was 8.6 times more likely to have a T40-ms axis greater than 120 degrees than was a non–CA-poisoned patient.[126] This parameter was a more sensitive indicator of CA-induced altered mental status but not necessarily of seizure or dysrhythmia. An abnormal terminal rightward axis is easily estimated by observing a negative deflection (terminal S wave) in leads I and aV_L and a positive deflection (terminal R wave) in lead aV_R (Fig. 68–3).

The maximal limb lead QRS complex duration is an easily measured ECG parameter that is a sensitive indicator of toxicity. A landmark investigation reported that 33% of patients with a limb lead QRS complex duration greater than or equal to 100 ms developed seizures, and 14% developed ventricular dysrhythmias.[16] No seizures or dysrhythmias occurred in those patients whose QRS complex duration remained less than 100 ms. There was a 50% incidence of ventricular dysrhythmias among patients with a QRS complex duration greater than or equal to 160 ms. No ventricular dysrhythmias occurred in patients with a QRS complex duration less than 160 ms. Subsequent studies confirmed that a QRS complex duration greater than 100 ms is associated with an increased incidence of serious toxicity, including coma, need for intubation, hypotension, seizures, and dysrhythmias, making this ECG parameter a useful indicator of toxicity.[22,66]

Evaluation of lead aV_R on a routine ECG is also reported to predict toxicity (Figs. 68–2 and 68–3). When prospectively studied, 79 patients with acute CA overdoses demonstrated that the amplitude of the terminal R wave and R/S wave ratio in lead aV_R (RaV_R, R/SaV_R) were significantly greater in patients who developed seizures and ventricular dysrhythmias.[66] The sensitivity of $RaV_R = 3$ mm and $R/SaV_R = 0.7$ in predicting seizures and dysrhythmias was comparable to the sensitivity of a QRS complex duration greater than 100 ms.

The type 1 Brugada pattern is similar to a right bundle branch block (rSR′), with downsloping ST elevations ("coved") in the right precordial leads (V1–V3) (Chap. 15 and Fig. 15–12).[11,83] This pattern is neither highly sensitive nor specific for CA toxicity, and it is reported in patients with cocaine and phenothiazine toxicity as well as those on class IA antidysrhythmic therapy. In one series of more than 400 patients with CA overdose, a significant increase in adverse outcomes (ie, seizures, widened QRS complex duration, and hypotension) was identified in those patients with a Brugada ECG pattern compared with those who did not have the pattern.[11] However, there were no deaths or dysrhythmias in the nine patients with this pattern.

Serial ECGs are recommended because the ECG changes are dynamic. Electrocardiograph parameters should always be interpreted in conjunction with the clinical presentation, history, and course during the first several hours to assist in decision making regarding interventions and disposition.[67]

Laboratory Tests

Determination of serum CA concentrations has limited utility in the immediate evaluation and management of patients with acute overdoses. In one study, serum drug concentrations failed to accurately predict the development of seizures or ventricular dysrhythmias.[16] The pharmacologic properties of CAs—namely, large volumes of distributions, prolonged absorption phase, long distribution half-lives, pH-dependent protein binding, and the wide interpatient variability of terminal elimination half-lives—explain the limited value of serum concentrations in this situation. Any concentration above the therapeutic range (50–300 ng/mL, including active metabolites) is associated with adverse effects and is an indication to decrease or discontinue the medication.

Although CA concentrations greater than 1,000 ng/mL usually are associated with significant clinical toxicity such as coma, seizures, and dysrhythmias, life-threatening toxicity occurs in patients with serum concentrations of less than 1,000 ng/mL.[16,62] Serious toxicity at lower concentrations probably results from a number of factors, including the timing of the specimen in relation to the ingestion and the limitations of measuring the concentration in blood and not the affected tissue. Quantitative concentrations usually cannot be readily obtained in most hospital laboratories. However, qualitative screens for CAs using an enzyme-multiplied immunoassay test are available at many hospitals. Unfortunately, false-positive results occur with many drugs such as carbamazepine, cyclobenzaprine, thioridazine, diphenhydramine, quetiapine, and cyproheptadine (Chap. 7). Thus, the presence of a CA on a qualitative assay should not be relied on to confirm the diagnosis of CA poisoning in the absence of corroborating historical or clinical evidence, and obtaining these laboratory results is not recommended.

An ultra-pressure liquid chromatography tandem mass spectrometry (UPLC-MS) assay capable of quantifying nine CA drugs in less than 5 minutes was recently validated, although its clinical application is limited because it is not currently widely available.[68]

Quantitative concentrations are helpful in determining the cause of death in suspected overdose patients. Concentrations reported in lethal overdoses typically range from 1,100 to 21,800 ng/mL. However, it should be noted that CA concentrations increase more than fivefold because of postmortem redistribution (Chap. 140).[5] Measurement of liver CA concentration or the parent-to-metabolite drug ratio provide additional information in the post-mortem setting.

MANAGEMENT

Any person with a suspected or known ingestion of a CA requires immediate evaluation and treatment (Table 68–2). The patient should be attached to a cardiac monitor, and intravenous access should be secured. Early intubation is recommended for patients with CNS depression or hemodynamic instability because of the potential for rapid clinical deterioration. A 12-lead ECG should be obtained for all patients. Laboratory tests, including concentrations of glucose and electrolytes, should be performed for all patients with altered mental status, as well as blood gas analysis to both assess the degree of acidemia and guide alkalinization therapy. Aggressive interventions for maintenance of blood pressure and peripheral perfusion must be performed early to avoid irreversible damage. Both children and adults receiving cardiopulmonary resuscitation have recovered successfully despite periods of asystole exceeding 90 minutes.[24,27,86,111] The options for GI decontamination are discussed in the following section.

TABLE 68–2 Treatment of Cyclic Antidepressant (CA) Toxicity

Toxic Effect	Treatment
Sinus rhythm with a QRS complex >100 ms	Sodium bicarbonate: 1–2 mEq/kg IV boluses at 3- to 5-min intervals to reverse the abnormality or to a target serum pH ≤7.55
	Sodium bicarbonate: 150 mEq in 1 L of D_5W continuous infusion at twice maintenance rate up to target serum pH ≤7.55
	Controlled ventilation (if clinically indicated for hypoventilation)
Wide-complex tachycardia or ventricular tachycardia	Sodium bicarbonate: 1–2 mEq/kg IV boluses at 3- to 5-min intervals to reverse the abnormality or to a target serum pH ≤7.55
	Sodium bicarbonate: 150 mEq in 1 L of D_5W continuous infusion at twice maintenance rate up to target serum pH ≤7.55
	Correct hypoxia, acidemia, hypotension
	Lidocaine for refractory dysrhythmias despite sodium bicarbonate administration: 1 mg/kg slow IV bolus followed by infusion of 20–50 mcg/kg/min
	Hypertonic saline (3% sodium chloride): 1-2 mEq/kg bolus
	Magnesium sulfate 25–50 mg/kg (maximum 2 g) IV over 2 min
Torsade de pointes	DC cardioversion followed by
	Magnesium sulfate or
	Overdrive pacing (caution because of rate dependence of CA)
Hypotension	0.9% sodium chloride boluses (up to 30 mL/kg)
	Correct hypoxia, acidemia
	Sodium bicarbonate: 1–2 mEq/kg IV boluses at 3- to 5-min intervals to reverse the abnormality or to a target serum pH ≤7.55
	Sodium bicarbonate: 150 mEq in 1 L of D_5W continuous infusion at twice maintenance rate up to target serum pH ≤7.55
	Norepinephrine in standard titrated doses
Seizures	Benzodiazepines
	Secure airway with intubation if necessary
	Correct hypoxia, acidemia
	Continuous infusion of midazolam or propofol if benzodiazepines fail
	Neuromuscular paralysis or general anesthesia with EEG monitoring if all other measures fail
Refractory poisoning	If standard therapies fail, ILE for cardiac arrest
	Extracorporeal mechanical circulation (ECMO, cardiopulmonary bypass); no evidence to support hemodialysis or hemoperfusion

DC = direct current; D_5W = dextrose 5% in water; ECMO = extracorporeal membrane oxygenation; EEG = electroencephalography; ILE = intravenous lipid emulsion; IV = intravenous.

Gastrointestinal Decontamination

The benefits of orogastric lavage for CA toxicity are not substantiated by controlled trials. The potential benefits of removing significant quantities of a highly toxic drug must be weighed against the risks of the procedure (Chap. 5).[17] The anticholinergic actions of some CAs decrease spontaneous gastric emptying, allowing unabsorbed drug to remain in the stomach for several hours. However, because of the potential for rapid deterioration of mental status and seizures, orogastric lavage should not be performed on patients without a protected airway. As such, this procedure should be limited to patients presenting shortly after ingestion (within 2 hours) who have already undergone endotracheal intubation for depressed mental status or other clinical toxicity. Endotracheal intubation should not be performed for the sole purpose of GI decontamination. Orogastric lavage in young children with unintentional ingestions of CAs may be associated with more risk and impracticalities, such as the inadequate hole size of pediatric tubes, and less benefit given the amount of drug usually ingested.

Activated charcoal (AC) is recommended in all patients presenting within 2 hours of ingestion with a normal mental status, and in patients with altered mental status and a protected airway. Irrespective of age, an additional dose of AC several hours later is reasonable in a seriously poisoned patient in whom unabsorbed drug may still be present in the GI tract or in the case of desorption of CAs from AC. It is important to monitor for the development of an ileus to prevent abdominal complications from additional doses of AC.[80]

Wide-Complex Dysrhythmias, Conduction Delays, and Hypotension

The mainstay of therapy for treating wide-complex dysrhythmias and for reversing conduction delays and hypotension is the combination of serum alkalinization and sodium loading. Increasing the extracellular concentration of sodium, or sodium loading, overwhelms the effective blockade of sodium channels, presumably through gradient effects (Fig. 68–1). Controlled in vitro and in vivo studies in various animal models demonstrate that hypertonic sodium bicarbonate effectively reduces QRS complex prolongation, increases blood pressure, and reverses or suppresses ventricular dysrhythmias caused by CAs.[89,102-104] These studies showed a clear benefit of hypertonic sodium bicarbonate compared with hyperventilation, hypertonic sodium chloride, or nonsodium buffer solutions. A systematic review of all animal and human studies revealed that alkalinization therapy was the most beneficial therapy for consequential dysrhythmias and shock[15] (Antidotes in Depth: A5).

The optimal dosing and mode of administration of hypertonic sodium bicarbonate and the indications for initiating and terminating this treatment are unsupported by controlled clinical studies. Instead, the information is extrapolated from animal studies, clinical experience, and an understanding of the pathophysiologic mechanisms of CA toxicity. A bolus, or rapid infusion over several minutes, of hypertonic sodium bicarbonate (1–2 mEq/kg) is recommended initially.[76,108] Additional boluses every 3 to 5 minutes are recommended until the QRS complex duration narrows and the hypotension improves (Fig. 68–2). Blood pH should be carefully monitored after several bicarbonate boluses, aiming for a target pH of no greater than 7.50 or 7.55. Because CAs redistribute from the tissues into the blood over several hours, it is reasonable to begin a continuous sodium bicarbonate infusion to maintain the pH in this range. Although diluting sodium bicarbonate in 5% dextrose in water and infusing it slowly renders it less able to increase the sodium gradient across the cell, the beneficial effects of pH elevation still warrant its use after the patient is stabilized. No evidence supports prophylactic alkalinization in the absence of cardiovascular toxicity (eg, QRS complex duration < 100 ms). In addition, alkalinization inevitably decreases in potassium and ionized calcium, which result in QT interval prolongation and potentially contribute to other dysrhythmias. Hypertonic sodium chloride (3% NaCl) reverses cardiotoxicity in several animal studies,[49,77,89] and numerous reports and extensive clinical experience support its efficacy in humans.[15,50,51,79] However, the dose of hypertonic saline for CA poisoning has never been evaluated in humans for safety or efficacy, and the dose suggested by animal studies (up to 15 mEq/kg) exceeds the amount that most clinicians would consider safe (1–2 mEq/kg). Hypertonic sodium chloride is associated with a hyperchloremic metabolic acidosis, an undesired effect that highlights one benefit of hypertonic sodium bicarbonate. However, it is reasonable to administer hypertonic saline in situations in which alkalinization with sodium bicarbonate is not possible. Sodium acetate is a possible alternative treatment if sodium bicarbonate is unavailable, although this cannot be given as a rapid bolus because high acetate concentrations result in hypotension.[85]

Hyperventilation of an intubated patient is a more rapid and easily titratable method of serum alkalinization but is not as effective as sodium bicarbonate in reversing cardiotoxicity.[55,76] Simultaneous hyperventilation and sodium bicarbonate administration may result in profound alkalemia and should be performed only with extreme caution and careful monitoring of serum pH. Hyperventilation without bicarbonate administration is a reasonable alternative in patients with ARDS or congestive heart failure in whom administration of large quantities of sodium is contraindicated.

Alkalinization and sodium loading with hypertonic sodium bicarbonate and or hypertonic saline along with controlled ventilation (if clinically indicated) should be administered to all CA overdose patients presenting with major cardiovascular toxicity. Indications include conduction delays (QRS complex >100 ms) and hypotension. It is imperative to initiate treatment until CA toxicity is excluded because of the risk of rapid and precipitous deterioration. Although commonly assumed, it is unclear whether the failure of the QRS complex to narrow with sodium bicarbonate treatment excludes CA toxicity.

It is also unclear whether alkalinization and sodium loading are effective for reversing the Brugada pattern. The sparse available literature is equivocal.[12,83] It is prudent to administer sodium bicarbonate in the presence of a presumed CA-induced Brugada pattern, especially with concomitant signs of other CA toxicity.

Alkalinization should be continued for at least 12 to 24 hours after the ECG has normalized because of the redistribution of the drug from the tissue. However, the time observed for resolution or normalization of conduction abnormalities is extremely variable, ranging from several hours to several days, despite continuous bicarbonate infusion.[67] We recommend stopping alkalinization when the patient's mental status improves and there is improvement, but not necessarily normalization, of abnormal ECG findings.

Antidysrhythmic Therapy

Lidocaine is the antidysrhythmic most commonly advocated for treatment of CA-induced dysrhythmias, although no controlled human studies demonstrate its efficacy.[93] Because lidocaine has sodium channel blocking properties, some investigators argue against its use in CA poisoning.[1] These theoretical concerns are not well supported in the literature, and the class IB antidysrhythmic channel binding kinetics may prove favorable. Lidocaine should be used for ventricular dysrhythmias not responsive to sodium bicarbonate therapy. Although limited data also suggest that the IB antidysrhythmic phenytoin prevents or reverses conduction abnormalities,[44,75] these data were poorly controlled for other confounding factors, such as blood pH and sodium bicarbonate administration; they had very small numbers; and, in some, the cardiotoxicity was not severe. Because phenytoin exacerbates ventricular dysrhythmias in animals and fails to protect against seizures, its use is no longer recommended.[10,21]

The use of class IA (quinidine, procainamide, disopyramide, and moricizine) and class IC (flecainide, propafenone) antidysrhythmics is absolutely contraindicated because they have similar pharmacologic actions to CAs and thus will worsen the sodium channel inhibition and exacerbate cardiotoxicity. Class III antidysrhythmics (amiodarone, bretylium, and sotalol) prolong the QT interval and, although unstudied, are contraindicated as well (Chap. 57).

Because magnesium sulfate has antidysrhythmic properties, it may be beneficial in the treatment of ventricular dysrhythmias. Animal studies of the effects of magnesium on CA-induced dysrhythmias yield conflicting results.[56,57] However, successful use of magnesium sulfate in the treatment of refractory ventricular fibrillation after TCA overdose is reported.[24,27,58,101] A case control study suggested that magnesium sulfate and sodium bicarbonate

resulted in lower fatality incidence and shorter intensive care unit (ICU) stay compared to sodium bicarbonate alone.[29] When dysrhythmias fail to reverse after alkalinization, sodium loading, and a trial of lidocaine and then magnesium sulfate is reasonable.

Slowing the heart rate in the presence of CAs allows more time during diastole for CA unbinding from sodium channels and results in an improvement in ventricular conduction.[3,4,104] This abolishes the reentry mechanism for dysrhythmias and was one rationale for the past use of physostigmine and propranolol. However, results from animal studies and limited clinical reports fail to show a clear benefit from these interventions. Propranolol terminated ventricular tachycardia in an animal model but also caused significant hypotension and death.[103] In one case series, patients developed severe hypotension or had a cardiac arrest shortly after receiving a β-adrenergic antagonist.[36] The combined negative inotropic effects of β-adrenergic antagonists and CAs, along with the significant cardiac and CNS effects reported with physostigmine use, do not support their use in the management of CA-induced tachydysrhythmias.

Hypotension

Standard initial treatment for hypotension should include volume expansion with isotonic saline or sodium bicarbonate. Hypotension unresponsive to these therapeutic interventions necessitates the use of inotropic or vasopressor support and possibly extracorporeal cardiovascular support.

No controlled human trials are available to guide the use of vasopressor therapy. The pharmacologic properties of CAs complicate the choice of a specific agent. Specifically, CA blockade of neurotransmitter reuptake theoretically could result in depletion of intracellular catecholamines, blunting the effect of dopamine, which is dependent on the release of endogenous norepinephrine for its inotropic activity. This pharmacologic effect and limited clinical data suggest that a direct-acting vasopressor such as norepinephrine is more efficacious than an indirect-acting catecholamine such as dopamine.[32,120,121,123]

Based on the available data, pharmacologic effects, theoretical concerns, and experience, norepinephrine (0.1–0.2 mcg/kg/min) is recommended for hypotension that is unresponsive to volume expansion and hypertonic sodium bicarbonate therapy. Central venous pressure measurement can guide the choice of additional vasopressor or inotropic agents, especially in the presence of other cardiodepressant drugs.

If these measures fail to correct hypotension, extracorporeal life support measures are reasonable, if available. Extracorporeal membrane oxygenation, extracorporeal circulation, and cardiopulmonary bypass are successful adjuncts for refractory hypotension and life support when maximum therapeutic interventions fail.[42,52,60,111,125] These modalities can provide critical perfusion to the heart and brain and maintain metabolic function while giving the body time to redistribute and eliminate the CA by maintaining hepatorenal blood flow.

Additional Therapies

Intravenous lipid emulsion (ILE) is reported to be effective in reversing cardiovascular toxicity caused by several lipophilic drugs, including amitriptyline and clomipramine. Its utilization and effectiveness appear logical given their pharmacological properties—log D and log P—octanol/water partition coefficient discussed previously.

Several controlled animal studies have demonstrated improved survival in clomipramine-induced cardiovascular collapse when ILE is given either as pretreatment or resuscitation in comparison with saline controls and sodium bicarbonate infusion.[45,46] Other animal studies failed to demonstrate any benefit or have shown poor results compared with standard therapies.[7,70,95,122] Case series and case reports demonstrate clinical improvement when ILE was administered for cardiovascular collapse or instability refractory to other therapies.[38,45,54,63,105] The dosing and timing of administration are variable as well as other concomitant therapies, making it difficult to reach any definitive conclusions regarding its effectiveness. In addition, significant adverse reactions and complications are noted, including ARDS, pancreatitis, and interference with laboratory assays. A recent extensive review by the Lipid

Emulsion Workgroup found only one randomized control trial of ILE utilization on CA-poisoned patients, which found no difference in time to ECG improvement, mortality, or hospitalization length compared with standard therapy.[53,64] There is no evidence to promote ILE use for non–life-threatening toxicity.[43] Given the current available data, ILE is reasonable for cardiac arrest after CA poisoning and for refractory hypotension or cardiac dysrhythmias if other interventions fail but should not be used as a first-line therapy and should not delay efforts to achieve sodium loading and serum alkalinization in patients with cardiovascular toxicity (Antidotes in Depth: A23).[97]

Successful use of vasopressin for intractable hypotension caused by CA toxicity, unresponsive to α-receptor agonists and pH manipulation, is described.[9] The vasoconstrictive effects of this drug may provide benefit in the setting of vasodilatory shock. Data are insufficient to recommend vasopressin as a first-line therapy for CA toxicity, and its use should be restricted to hypotension refractory to other treatments.

Central Nervous System Toxicity

Seizures caused by CAs usually are brief and often stop before treatment can be initiated. Recurrent seizures, prolonged seizures (>2 minutes), and status epilepticus require prompt treatment to prevent worsening acidosis, hypoxia, and development of hyperthermia and rhabdomyolysis. Benzodiazepines are effective as first-line therapy for seizures. If this therapy fails, either a barbiturate or propofol is recommended. Propofol controls refractory seizures resulting from amoxapine toxicity.[81] Failure to respond to barbiturates or propofol should prompt the use of neuromuscular paralysis and general anesthesia with continuous electroencephalographic monitoring. Phenytoin is contraindicated for seizures because data not only demonstrate a failure to terminate seizures but also suggest enhanced cardiovascular toxicity.[9,21]

Use of flumazenil in a patient with known or suspected CA ingestion is contraindicated. Several case reports of patients with CA overdoses describe seizures after administration of flumazenil (Antidotes in Depth: A25).[65] Physostigmine was used in the past to reverse the acute CNS toxicity (Antidotes in Depth: A11). However, physostigmine is contraindicated because it precipitates seizures in acutely CA-poisoned patients increasing the risk of cardiac toxicity, causing bradycardia and asystole.[91]

Enhanced Elimination

No specific treatment modalities have demonstrated clinical significant efficacy in enhancing the elimination of CAs. Some investigators propose multiple doses of AC to enhance CA elimination because of their small enterohepatic and enterogastric circulation.[73] Human volunteer studies and case series of patients with CA overdoses suggest that the half-life of CAs is be decreased by multiple-dose activated charcoal (MDAC). Activated charcoal reduced the apparent half-life of amitriptyline to 4 to 40 hours in overdose patients compared with previously published values of 30 to more than 60 hours.[117] Changes in the severity or duration of clinical toxicity, however, were not reported. Other investigators showed that in human volunteers, MDAC reduced the half-life of therapeutic doses of amitriptyline approximately 20% compared with no AC administration. However, the methodologic flaws and equivocal findings of these studies and the lack of any positive outcome data for this intervention from additional studies do not provide evidence supporting its use in this setting.[23,40] Pharmacokinetic properties of CAs (large volumes of distribution, high plasma protein binding) weighed against the small increases in clearance and the potential complications of MDAC, such as impaction, intestinal infarction, and perforation, do not warrant its routine use.[23,80] One additional dose of AC is reasonable to decrease GI absorption in patients with evidence of significant CNS and cardiovascular toxicity if bowel sounds are present.

Measures to enhance urinary CA excretion have a minimal effect on total clearance. Urinary alkalinization does not enhance, and may reduce, urinary clearance because of passive reabsorption of the nonionized CA from an alkaline urine.[127] Hemodialysis is ineffective in enhancing the elimination of CAs because of their large volumes of distribution, high lipid solubility, and extensive protein binding.[48] Redistribution of drug to the plasma and a rebound effect would be expected after this procedure. Although several uncontrolled case reports and a case series described improvement in cardiotoxicity during hemoperfusion, this finding is likely coincidental.[13,24,35] Given these limitations, hemodialysis or hemoperfusion should not be performed for patients with CA toxicity.

Hospital Admission Criteria

All patients who present with known or suspected CA ingestion should undergo continuous cardiac monitoring and serial ECG for a minimum of 6 hours. Recommendations in the older literature for 48 to 72 hours of ICU monitoring even for patients with minor CA ingestions stem from isolated case reports of late-onset dysrhythmias, CNS effects, and sudden deaths.[90] However, review of these cases shows inadequate GI decontamination, inadequate therapeutic interventions, and significant ongoing complications of overdose. Several retrospective studies demonstrate that late, unexpected complications in CA overdoses such as seizures, dysrhythmias, and death did not occur in patients who had few or no major signs of toxicity at presentation or a normal level of consciousness and a normal ECG for 24 hours.[20,27,30,92] The following previously proposed disposition algorithm, based on clinical signs and symptoms, is reasonable: If the patient is asymptomatic at presentation, undergoes GI decontamination, has normal ECGs, or has sinus tachycardia (with normal QRS complexes) that resolves and the patient remains asymptomatic in the health care facility for a minimum of 6 hours without any treatment interventions, the patient may be medically cleared for psychiatric evaluation or discharged home, as appropriate.[6,118]

A prospective study of 67 patients used the Antidepressant Overdose Risk Assessment (ADORA) criteria to identify patients who were at high risk for developing serious toxicity and proposed criteria for hospitalization.[33] In this study, the presence of QRS complex duration greater than 100 ms, cardiac dysrhythmias, altered mental status, seizures, respiratory depression, or hypotension on presentation to the ED (or within 6 hours of ingestion, if the time was known) was 100% sensitive in identifying patients with significant toxicity and subsequent complications. Criteria specific for ICU admission (other than patients requiring ventilatory and or blood pressure support), versus an inpatient bed with continuous cardiac monitoring, are less clear and probably are institution dependent.[113]

The disposition of patients with persistent isolated sinus tachycardia, prolonged QT interval with no concomitant altered mental status, or blood pressure changes is not clearly defined. Previous studies demonstrate that these two parameters alone are not predictive of subsequent clinical toxicity or complications.[33,34] In addition, the sinus tachycardia may persist for up to 1 week after ingestion. However, a study of isolated CA overdose patients reported that a heart rate greater than 120 beats/min and a QT interval greater than 480 ms were associated with an increased likelihood of major toxicity.[22] These patients are candidates for observation with continuous ECG monitoring and serial ECGs for 24 hours.

Inpatient Cardiac Monitoring

The duration of cardiac monitoring in any patient initially exhibiting signs of major clinical toxicity depends on many factors. Certainly, the duration of CA cardiotoxicity and neurotoxicity may be prolonged, and using normalization of ECG abnormalities as an endpoint for therapy and discharge is problematic. Some studies document the variable resolution and normalization of QRS prolongation and T40-ms axis rotation.[88,109] Based on the available literature, patients admitted to the hospital for significant poisoning should be monitored for another 24 hours after termination of CA therapy, including alkalinization, antidysrhythmics, and inotropics or vasopressors, after resolution of clinical toxicity.

SUMMARY

- Cyclic antidepressant poisoning continues to be a cause of serious morbidity and mortality worldwide.
- The distinctive characteristics of these drugs cause significant CNS and cardiovascular toxicity, the latter being responsible for mortality as a result of overdose of these drugs. Cardiovascular toxicity ranges from

mild conduction abnormalities and sinus tachycardia to wide-complex tachycardia, hypotension, and asystole. Central nervous system toxicity includes delirium, lethargy, seizures, and coma.

■ The ECG is a simple, readily available diagnostic test that can predict the development of significant toxicity, particularly seizures and dysrhythmias.

■ Management strategies are based primarily on the pathophysiology of these drugs, namely, sodium channel blockade in the myocardium. Alkalinization and sodium loading with hypertonic sodium bicarbonate is the principal therapy for cardiovascular toxicity.

■ Guidelines for observing or admitting patients to the hospital are based on initial clinical presentation or development of clinical effects and ECG changes.

REFERENCES

1. Ahmad S. Management of cardiac complications in tricyclic antidepressant poisoning. *J R Soc Med.* 1980;73:79.

2. Amitai Y, et al. Distribution of amitriptyline and nortriptyline in blood: role of alpha-1-glycoprotein. *Ther Drug Monit.* 1993;15:267-273.

3. Ansel GM, et al. Mechanisms of ventricular arrhythmia during amitriptyline toxicity. *J Cardiovasc Pharmacol.* 1993;22:798-803.

4. Ansel GM, et al. Prevention of tricyclic antidepressant-induced ventricular tachyarrhythmia by a specific bradycardic agent in a canine model. *J Cardiovasc Pharmacol.* 1994;24:256-260.

5. Apple FS. Postmortem tricyclic antidepressant concentrations: assessing cause of death using parent drug to metabolite ratio. *J Anal Toxicol.* 1989;13:197-198.

6. Banahan BF Jr, Schelkun PH. Tricyclic antidepressant overdose: conservative management in a community hospital with cost-saving implications. *J Emerg Med.* 1990;8:451-454.

7. Bania TC, Chu J. Hemodynamic effect of intralipid prolongs survival in amitriptyline toxicity. *Acad Emerg Med.* 2006;13:S1777.

8. Barden N. Modulation of glucocorticoid receptor gene expression by antidepressant drugs. *Pharmacopsychiatry.* 1996;29:12-22.

9. Barry JD, et al. Vasopressin treatment for cyclic antidepressant overdose. *J Emerg Med.* 2006;31:65-68.

10. Beaubien AR, et al. Antagonism of imipramine poisoning by anticonvulsants in the rat. *Toxicol Appl Pharmacol.* 1976;38:1-6.

11. Bebarta VS, et al. Incidence of Brugada electrocardiographic pattern and outcomes of these patients after intentional tricyclic antidepressant ingestion. *Am J Cardiol.* 2007;100:656-660.

12. Bebarta VS, Waksman JC. Amitriptyline-induced Brugada pattern fails to respond to sodium bicarbonate. *Clin Toxicol (Phila).* 2007;45:186-188.

13. Bek K, et al. Charcoal haemoperfusion in amitriptyline poisoning: experience in 20 children. *Nephrology (Carlton).* 2008;13:193-197.

14. Biederman J, et al. A naturalistic study of 24-hour electrocardiographic recordings and echocardiographic findings in children and adolescents treated with desipramine. *J Am Acad Child Adolesc Psychiatry.* 1993;32:805-813.

15. Blackman K, et al. Plasma alkalinization for tricyclic antidepressant toxicity: a systematic review. *Emerg Med (Fremantle).* 2001;13:204-210.

16. Boehnert MT, Lovejoy FH Jr. Value of the QRS duration versus the serum drug level in predicting seizures and ventricular arrhythmias after an acute overdose of tricyclic antidepressants. *N Engl J Med.* 1985;313:474-479.

17. Bosse GM, et al. Comparison of three methods of gut decontamination in tricyclic antidepressant overdose. *J Emerg Med.* 1995;13:203-209.

18. Brosen K, et al. Role of P450IID6, the target of the sparteine-debrisoquin oxidation polymorphism, in the metabolism of imipramine. *Clin Pharmacol Ther.* 1991;49:609-617.

19. Caldwell PH, et al. Tricyclic and related drugs for nocturnal enuresis in children. *Cochrane Database Syst Rev.* 2016:CD002117.

20. Callaham M, Kassel D. Epidemiology of fatal tricyclic antidepressant ingestion: implications for management. *Ann Emerg Med.* 1985;14:1-9.

21. Callaham M, et al. Phenytoin prophylaxis of cardiotoxicity in experimental amitriptyline poisoning. *J Pharmacol Exp Ther.* 1988;245:216-220.

22. Caravati EM, Bossart PJ. Demographic and electrocardiographic factors associated with severe tricyclic antidepressant toxicity. *J Toxicol Clin Toxicol.* 1991;29:31-43.

23. Chyka PA. Multiple-dose activated charcoal and enhancement of systemic drug clearance: summary of studies in animals and human volunteers. *J Toxicol Clin Toxicol.* 1995;33:399-405.

24. Citak A, et al. Efficacy of long duration resuscitation and magnesium sulphate treatment in amitriptyline poisoning. *Eur J Emerg Med.* 2002;9:63-66.

25. Clarke G, et al. Trends in youth antidepressant dispensing and refill limits, 2000 through 2009. *J Child Adolesc Psychopharmacol.* 2012;22:11-20.

26. Clement A, et al. Chronic amitriptyline overdose in a child. *Clin Toxicol (Phila).* 2012;50:431-434.

27. Deegan C, O'Brien K. Amitriptyline poisoning in a 2-year old. *Paediatr Anaesth.* 2006;16:174-177.

28. Ellison DW, Pentel PR. Clinical features and consequences of seizures due to cyclic antidepressant overdose. *Am J Emerg Med.* 1989;7:5-10.

29. Emamhadi M, et al. Tricyclic antidepressant poisoning treated by magnesium sulfate: a randomized, clinical trial. *Drug Chem Toxicol.* 2012;35:300-303.

30. Fasoli RA, Glauser FL. Cardiac arrhythmias and ECG abnormalities in tricyclic antidepressant overdose. *Clin Toxicol.* 1981;18:155-163.

31. Fletcher SE, et al. Prospective study of the electrocardiographic effects of imipramine in children. *J Pediatr.* 1993;122:652-654.

32. Follmer CH, Lum BK. Protective action of diazepam and of sympathomimetic amines against amitriptyline-induced toxicity. *J Pharmacol Exp Ther.* 1982;222:424-429.

33. Foulke GE. Identifying toxicity risk early after antidepressant overdose. *Am J Emerg Med.* 1995;13:123-126.

34. Foulke GE, et al. Tricyclic antidepressant overdose: emergency department findings as predictors of clinical course. *Am J Emerg Med.* 1986;4:496-500.

35. Frank RD, Kierdorf HP. Is there a role for hemoperfusion/hemodialysis as a treatment option in severe tricyclic antidepressant intoxication? *Int J Artif Organs.* 2000;23:618-623.

36. Freeman JW, Loughhead MG. Beta blockade in the treatment of tricyclic antidepressant overdosage. *Med J Aust.* 1973;1:1233-1235.

37. Garner EM, et al. Tricyclic antidepressant withdrawal syndrome. *Ann Pharmacother.* 1993;27:1068-1072.

38. Geib AJ, et al; Toxicology Investigators' Consortium (ToxIC). Clinical experience with intravenous lipid emulsion for drug-induced cardiovascular collapse. *J Med Toxicol.* 2012;8:10-14.

39. Giller EL Jr, et al. Chronic amitriptyline toxicity. *Am J Psychiatry.* 1979;136(4A):458-459.

40. Goldberg MJ, et al. Lack of effect of oral activated charcoal on imipramine clearance. *Clin Pharmacol Ther.* 1985;38:350-353.

41. Goldberg RJ, et al. Cardiac complications following tricyclic antidepressant overdose. Issues for monitoring policy. *JAMA.* 1985;254:1772-1775.

42. Goodwin DA, et al. Extracorporeal membrane oxygenation support for cardiac dysfunction from tricyclic antidepressant overdose. *Crit Care Med.* 1993;21:625-627.

43. Gosselin S, et al. Evidence-based recommendations on the use of intravenous lipid emulsion therapy in poisoning. *Clin Toxicol (Phila).* 2016;54:899-923.

44. Hagerman GA, Hanashiro PK. Reversal of tricyclic-antidepressant-induced cardiac conduction abnormalities by phenytoin. *Ann Emerg Med.* 1981;10:82-86.

45. Harvey M, Cave G. Intralipid outperforms sodium bicarbonate in a rabbit model of clomipramine toxicity. *Ann Emerg Med.* 2007;49:178-185, 185 e171-174.

46. Harvey M, et al. Intravenous lipid emulsion-augmented plasma exchange in a rabbit model of clomipramine toxicity; survival, but no sink. *Clin Toxicol (Phila).* 2014;52:13-19.

47. Haufroid V, Hantson P. CYP2D6 genetic polymorphisms and their relevance for poisoning due to amphetamines, opioid analgesics and antidepressants. *Clin Toxicol (Phila).* 2015;53:501-510.

48. Heath A, et al. Treatment of antidepressant poisoning with resin hemoperfusion. *Hum Toxicol.* 1982;1:361-371.

49. Hoegholm A, Clementsen P. Hypertonic sodium chloride in severe antidepressant overdosage. *J Toxicol Clin Toxicol.* 1991;29:297-298.

50. Hoffman JR, McElroy CR. Bicarbonate therapy for dysrhythmia and hypotension in tricyclic antidepressant overdose. *West J Med.* 1981;134:60-64.

51. Hoffman JR, et al. Effect of hypertonic sodium bicarbonate in the treatment of moderate-to-severe cyclic antidepressant overdose. *Am J Emerg Med.* 1993;11:336-341.

52. Johnson NJ, et al. A review of emergency cardiopulmonary bypass for severe poisoning by cardiotoxic drugs. *J Med Toxicol.* 2013;9:54-60.

53. Kasnavieh FH KM, et al. Intravenous lipid emulsion for the treatment of tricyclic antidepressant toxicity: a randomized controlled trial. VIIth Mediterranean Emergency Medicine Conference, Marseille, France; 2013.

54. Kiberd MB, Minor SF. Lipid therapy for the treatment of a refractory amitriptyline overdose. *CJEM.* 2012;14:193-197.

55. Kingston ME. Hyperventilation in tricyclic antidepressant poisoning. *Crit Care Med.* 1979;7:550-551.

56. Kline JA, et al. Magnesium potentiates imipramine toxicity in the isolated rat heart. *Ann Emerg Med.* 1994;24:224-232.

57. Knudsen K, Abrahamsson J. Effects of magnesium sulfate and lidocaine in the treatment of ventricular arrhythmias in experimental amitriptyline poisoning in the rat. *Crit Care Med.* 1994;22:494-498.

58. Knudsen K, Abrahamsson J. Magnesium sulphate in the treatment of ventricular fibrillation in amitriptyline poisoning. *Eur Heart J.* 1997;18:881-882.

59. Knudsen K, Heath A. Effects of self poisoning with maprotiline. *Br Med J (Clin Res Ed).* 1984;288:601-603.

60. Kochert E PK, Kaczorowski D. Extracorporeal membrane oxygenation for TCA poisoning refractory to lipid emulsion therapy. *Vis J Emerg Med.* 2016:42-44.

61. Kulig K, et al. Amoxapine overdose. Coma and seizures without cardiotoxic effects. *JAMA.* 1982;248:1092-1094.

62. Lavoie FW, et al. Value of initial ECG findings and plasma drug levels in cyclic antidepressant overdose. *Ann Emerg Med.* 1990;19:696-700.

63. Levine M, et al. Delayed-onset seizure and cardiac arrest after amitriptyline overdose, treated with intravenous lipid emulsion therapy. *Pediatrics.* 2012;130:e432-438.

64. Levine M, et al. Systematic review of the effect of intravenous lipid emulsion therapy for non-local anesthetics toxicity. *Clin Toxicol (Phila).* 2016;54:194-221.

65. Lheureux P, et al. Flumazenil in mixed benzodiazepine/tricyclic antidepressant overdose: a placebo-controlled study in the dog. *Am J Emerg Med.* 1992;10:184-188.

66. Liebelt EL, et al. ECG lead aVR versus QRS interval in predicting seizures and arrhythmias in acute tricyclic antidepressant toxicity. *Ann Emerg Med.* 1995;26:195-201.

67. Liebelt EL, et al. Serial electrocardiogram changes in acute tricyclic antidepressant overdoses. *Crit Care Med.* 1997;25:1721-1726.

68. Lin CN, et al. Method validation of a tricyclic antidepressant drug panel in urine by UPLC-MS/MS. *Ann Clin Lab Sci.* 2014;44:431-436.

69. Lipper B, et al. Recurrent hypotension immediately after seizures in nortriptyline overdose. *Am J Emerg Med.* 1994;12:452-453.

70. Litonius E, et al. No antidotal effect of intravenous lipid emulsion in experimental amitriptyline intoxication despite significant entrapment of amitriptyline. *Basic Clin Pharmacol Toxicol.* 2012;110:378-383.

71. Litovitz TL, Troutman WG. Amoxapine overdose. Seizures and fatalities. *JAMA.* 1983;250:1069-1071.

72. Liu X, et al. Adverse pulmonary vascular effects of high dose tricyclic antidepressants: acute and chronic animal studies. *Eur Respir J.* 2002;20:344-352.

73. Manoguerra AS. Poisoning with tricyclic antidepressant drugs. *Clin Toxicol.* 1977;10:149-158.

74. Marshall JB, Forker AD. Cardiovascular effects of tricyclic antidepressant drugs: therapeutic usage, overdose, and management of complications. *Am Heart J.* 1982;103:401-414.

75. Mayron R, Ruiz E. Phenytoin: does it reverse tricyclic-antidepressant-induced cardiac conduction abnormalities? *Ann Emerg Med.* 1986;15:876-880.

76. McCabe JL, et al. Experimental tricyclic antidepressant toxicity: a randomized, controlled comparison of hypertonic saline solution, sodium bicarbonate, and hyperventilation. *Ann Emerg Med.* 1998;32(3 Pt 1):329-333.

77. McCabe JL, et al. Recovery from severe cyclic antidepressant overdose with hypertonic saline/dextran in a swine model. *Acad Emerg Med.* 1994;1:111-115.

78. McFee RB, et al. Selected tricyclic antidepressant ingestions involving children 6 years old or less. *Acad Emerg Med.* 2001;8:139-144.

79. McKinney PE, Rasmussen R. Reversal of severe tricyclic antidepressant-induced cardiotoxicity with intravenous hypertonic saline solution. *Ann Emerg Med.* 2003;42:20-24.

80. McMahon AJ. Amitriptyline overdose complicated by intestinal pseudo-obstruction and caecal perforation. *Postgrad Med J.* 1989;65:948-949.

81. Merigian KS, et al. Successful treatment of amoxapine-induced refractory status epilepticus with propofol (Diprivan). *Acad Emerg Med.* 1995;2:128-133.

82. Merigian KS, et al. Plasma catecholamine levels in cyclic antidepressant overdose. *J Toxicol Clin Toxicol.* 1991;29:177-190.

83. Monteban-Kooistra WE, et al. Brugada electrocardiographic pattern elicited by cyclic antidepressants overdose. *Intensive Care Med.* 2006;32:281-285.

84. Nakashita M, et al. Effects of tricyclic and tetracyclic antidepressants on the three subtypes of GABA transporter. *Neurosci Res.* 1997;29:87-91.

85. Neavyn MJ, et al. Sodium acetate as a replacement for sodium bicarbonate in medical toxicology: a review. *J Med Toxicol.* 2013;9:250-254.

86. Niemann JT, et al. Electrocardiographic criteria for tricyclic antidepressant cardiotoxicity. *Am J Cardiol.* 1986;57:1154-1159.

87. Otasowie J, et al. Tricyclic antidepressants for attention deficit hyperactivity disorder (ADHD) in children and adolescents. *Cochrane Database Syst Rev.* 2014:CD006997.

88. Pellinen TJ, et al. Electrocardiographic and clinical features of tricyclic antidepressant intoxication. A survey of 88 cases and outlines of therapy. *Ann Clin Res.* 1987;19:12-17.

89. Pentel P, Benowitz N. Efficacy and mechanism of action of sodium bicarbonate in the treatment of desipramine toxicity in rats. *J Pharmacol Exp Ther.* 1984;230:12-19.

90. Pentel P, et al. Late complications of tricyclic antidepressant overdose. *West J Med.* 1983;138:423-424.

91. Pentel P, Peterson CD. Asystole complicating physostigmine treatment of tricyclic antidepressant overdose. *Ann Emerg Med.* 1980;9:588-590.

92. Pentel P, Sioris L. Incidence of late arrhythmias following tricyclic antidepressant overdose. *Clin Toxicol.* 1981;18:543-548.

93. Pentel PR, Benowitz NL. Tricyclic antidepressant poisoning. Management of arrhythmias. *Med Toxicol.* 1986;1:101-121.

94. Pentel PR, Keyler DE. Effects of high dose alpha-1-acid glycoprotein on desipramine toxicity in rats. *J Pharmacol Exp Ther.* 1988;246:1061-1066.

95. Perichon D, et al. An assessment of the in vivo effects of intravenous lipid emulsion on blood drug concentration and haemodynamics following oro-gastric amitriptyline overdose. *Clin Toxicol (Phila).* 2013;51:208-215.

96. Popper CW, ZB. Sudden death putatively related to desipramine treatment in youth: a fifth case and a review of speculative mechanisms. *J Child Adolesc Psychopharmacol.* 1995;5:283-300.

97. Ramasubbu B, et al. Serum alkalinisation is the cornerstone of treatment for amitriptyline poisoning. *BMJ Case Rep.* 2016;2016:10 1136/bcr-2016-214685.

98. Riddle MA, et al. Sudden death in children receiving Norpramin: a review of three reported cases and commentary. *J Am Acad Child Adolesc Psychiatry.* 1991;30:104-108.

99. Rodriguez S, Tamargo J. Electrophysiological effects of imipramine on bovine ventricular muscle and Purkinje fibres. *Br J Pharmacol.* 1980;70:15-23.

100. Rudorfer MV, Potter WZ. Metabolism of tricyclic antidepressants. *Cell Mol Neurobiol.* 1999;19:373-409.

101. Sarisoy O, et al. Efficacy of magnesium sulfate for treatment of ventricular tachycardia in amitriptyline intoxication. *Pediatr Emerg Care.* 2007;23:646-648.

102. Sasyniuk BI, Jhamandas V. Mechanism of reversal of toxic effects of amitriptyline on cardiac Purkinje fibers by sodium bicarbonate. *J Pharmacol Exp Ther.* 1984;231:387-394.

103. Sasyniuk BI, et al. Experimental amitriptyline intoxication: treatment of cardiac toxicity with sodium bicarbonate. *Ann Emerg Med.* 1986;15:1052-1059.

104. Sasyniuk BI, Jhamandas V. Frequency-dependent effects of amitriptyline on Vmax in canine Purkinje fibers and its alteration by alkalosis. *Proc West Pharmacol Soc.* 1986;29:73-75.

105. Scholten HJ, et al. Intralipid as antidote for tricyclic antidepressants and SSRIs: a case report. *Anaesth Intensive Care.* 2012;40:1076-1077.

106. Seaberg DC, et al. Effects of alpha-1-acid glycoprotein on the cardiovascular toxicity of nortriptyline in a swine model. *Vet Hum Toxicol.* 1991;33:226-230.

107. Shannon M, Lovejoy FH Jr. Pulmonary consequences of severe tricyclic antidepressant ingestion. *J Toxicol Clin Toxicol.* 1987;25:443-461.

108. Shannon M, et al. Hypotension in severe tricyclic antidepressant overdose. *Am J Emerg Med.* 1988;6:439-442.

109. Shannon MW. Duration of QRS disturbances after severe tricyclic antidepressant intoxication. *J Toxicol Clin Toxicol.* 1992;30:377-386.

110. Skowron DM, Stimmel GL. Antidepressants and the risk of seizures. *Pharmacotherapy.* 1992;12:18-22.

111. Southall DP, Kilpatrick SM. Imipramine poisoning: survival of a child after prolonged cardiac massage. *Br Med J.* 1974;4:508.

112. Squires RF, Saederup E. Antidepressants and metabolites that block GABAA receptors coupled to 35S-t-butylbicyclophosphorothionate binding sites in rat brain. *Brain Res.* 1988;441:15-22.

113. Stern TA, et al. Complications after overdose with tricyclic antidepressants. *Crit Care Med.* 1985;13:672-674.

114. Strom J, et al. Acute self-poisoning with tricyclic antidepressants in 295 consecutive patients treated in an ICU. *Acta Anaesthiol Scand.* 1984;28:666-670.

115. Svens K, Ryrfeldt A. A study of mechanisms underlying amitriptyline-induced acute lung function impairment. *Toxicol Appl Pharmacol.* 2001;177:179-187.

116. Swanson JR, et al. Death of two subjects due to imipramine and desipramine metabolite accumulation during chronic therapy: a review of the literature and possible mechanisms. *J Forensic Sci.* 1997;42:335-339.

117. Swartz CM, Sherman A. The treatment of tricyclic antidepressant overdose with repeated charcoal. *J Clin Psychopharmacol.* 1984;4:336-340.

118. Taboulet P, et al. Cardiovascular repercussions of seizures during cyclic antidepressant poisoning. *J Toxicol Clin Toxicol.* 1995;33:205-211.

119. Tatli O, et al. Cerebellitis developing after tricyclic antidepressant poisoning. *Am J Emerg Med.* 2013;31:1419 e1413-1415.

120. Teba L, et al. Beneficial effect of norepinephrine in the treatment of circulatory shock caused by tricyclic antidepressant overdose. *Am J Emerg Med.* 1988;6:566-568.

121. Tran TP, et al. Response to dopamine vs norepinephrine in tricyclic antidepressant-induced hypotension. *Acad Emerg Med.* 1997;4:864-868.

122. Varney SM, et al. Intravenous lipid emulsion therapy does not improve hypotension compared to sodium bicarbonate for tricyclic antidepressant toxicity: a randomized, controlled pilot study in a swine model. *Acad Emerg Med.* 2014;21:1212-1219.

123. Vernon DD, et al. Efficacy of dopamine and norepinephrine for treatment of hemodynamic compromise in amitriptyline intoxication. *Crit Care Med.* 1991;19:544-549.

124. Wedin GP, et al. Relative toxicity of cyclic antidepressants. *Ann Emerg Med.* 1986;15:797-804.

125. Williams JM, et al. Extracorporeal circulation in the management of severe tricyclic antidepressant overdose. *Am J Emerg Med.* 1994;12:456-458.

126. Wolfe TR, et al. Terminal 40-ms frontal plane QRS axis as a marker for tricyclic antidepressant overdose. *Ann Emerg Med.* 1989;18:348-351.

127. Yates C, et al. Extracorporeal treatment for tricyclic antidepressant poisoning: recommendations from the EXTRIP Workgroup. *Semin Dial.* 2014;27:381-389.

128. Zaccara G, et al. Clinical features, pathogenesis and management of drug-induced seizures. *Drug Saf.* 1990;5:109-151.

69 SEROTONIN REUPTAKE INHIBITORS AND ATYPICAL ANTIDEPRESSANTS

Christine M. Stork

INTRODUCTION

In the United States, major depressive disorder is a leading cause of disability and affects 15.7 million American adults; representing 6.7% of all US adults in 2015.[97] Although major depressive disorder can develop at any age, a higher percentage of 15- to 25-year-old adults are found to have depression, and women are affected nearly twice as often as men. The exact etiology of depression and the mechanism by which increased serotonergic and norepinephrine neurotransmission modulates mood remain unclear. A complex interaction of genetics and altered serotonin neurotransmission along with alterations in brain-derived neurotrophic factor, neurotrophin-3, dopamine, norepinephrine, and excitatory neuronal pathways likely have a role in depressive disorders.[119] Although termed *selective serotonin reuptake inhibitors* (SSRIs), these antidepressants have complex pharmacologic effects and interact with a number of other receptors and neurotransmitters. The class of SSRIs includes citalopram, escitalopram (citalopram's active enantiomer), fluoxetine, fluvoxamine, paroxetine, and sertraline (Fig. 69–1). Atypical antidepressants extend the pharmacologic principles of SSRIs to achieve beneficial effects for patients with depression. The SSRIs and atypical antidepressants comprise the current standard for the treatment of depression.[70] The SSRIs also are used to treat anxiety disorders, insomnia, chronic pain, panic disorders, social phobia, fibromyalgia, migraine, obsessive–compulsive disorders, bipolar disorders, premenstrual syndrome, menopausal symptoms, nicotine dependence, attention deficit hyperactivity disorder (ADHD), posttraumatic stress disorder, sexual dysfunction, digestive system disorders, urinary system disorders, and bulimia nervosa.[10,110,116,125] They have excellent safety profiles compared with previous antidepressants such as monoamine oxidase inhibitors (MAOIs) and the cyclic antidepressants (Cas) (Chaps. 68 and 71). Similar to many xenobiotics, the appropriateness of their use, their effectiveness, and the associated morbidity and mortality have made their use increasingly controversial as the patient population, especially those at the extremes of age, and the comorbidity profiles of those using the SSRIs are expanding.

HISTORY AND EPIDEMIOLOGY

Serotonin (5-hydroxytryptamine) got its name after its initial discovery as a vasoconstrictor. The SSRIs were initially marketed in the United States in the early 1980s and are today considered one of the first-line therapies for treatment of major depressive disorders.[54] The SSRIs are as effective as the CAs and MAOIs for the treatment of major depression, have fewer significant adverse events associated with their therapeutic use, and are less problematic in overdose (Chaps. 68 and 71) An increased risk of suicidal behavior is reported with the use of many antidepressants compared with herbals or counseling alone in children and adults.[65,92] This may be related to delayed onset of therapeutic efficacy coupled with increased energy associated with the initiation of therapy.

PATHOPHYSIOLOGY

Table 69–1 lists the pharmacology, therapeutic doses, and metabolism of the available SSRIs and atypical antidepressants. Modulation of serotonin and norepinephrine neurotransmission has a significant role in the treatment of depression.[131] There are seven widely known classes of serotonin receptors, with many containing subtype classifications (Chap. 13). The SSRIs selectively inhibit serotonin reuptake via the serotonin transporter (SERT) caused by p-trifluoromethyl or p-fluoro substitution present in many of these xenobiotics.[161] Serotonin transporter functions through conformational changes as it moves serotonin across the membranes. An increase in transport and in the related conformational change is also associated with an increase in cyclic guanosine monophosphate (cGMP) phosphorylation within the neuron. Serotonergic neurons are located almost exclusively in the median raphe nucleus of the brainstem, where they extend into and are in close proximity to norepinephrine neurons that are located primarily in the locus ceruleus[9] (Fig. 69–2). The interplay between norepinephrine and serotonin likely explains the effectiveness of antidepressants that do not directly modulate serotonin neurotransmission.

PHARMACOKINETICS AND TOXICOKINETICS

The SSRIs display diverse elimination patterns and have numerous active metabolites, which substantially increase both the duration of therapeutic effectiveness and the duration during which drug interactions and adverse drug effects occur. These latter effects often persist even after the medication is discontinued (Table 69–1). Important pharmacokinetic and pharmacodynamic drug interactions are reported with therapeutic dosing (see Serotonin Toxicity). The SSRIs and their active metabolites are substrates

FIGURE 69–1. Structures of common selective serotonin reuptake inhibitors. Citalopram is shown as the *S*-enantiomer (escitalopram).

TABLE 69–1 Drug Mechanism and Pharmacokinetic Data for Available Selective Serotonin Reuptake Inhibitors and Atypical Antidepressants[a]

Drug	Typical Daily Dose Range (mg)	$t_{1/2}$ (h)	Major Metabolic Mechanism	Major Active Metabolites	Major Active Metabolite $t_{1/2}$	Drug (d) or Metabolite (m) Inhibits CYP
SSRIs						
Citalopram	20–60	33–37	2C19, 3A4, 2D6	Monodesmethylcitalopram, didesmethylcitalopram	59 h	None or unknown
Escitalopram	10–20	22–32	2C19, 3A4, 2D6	S(+)-Desmethylcitalopram	59 h	None
Fluoxetine	10–80	24–144	2C9, 2D6	Norfluoxetine	4–16 d	2D6 (d,m), 2C19 (d,m), 2D6 (d,m), 3A4 (m)
Fluvoxamine	100–300	15–23	1A2, 2D6	None	N/A	1A2, 2C9, 2C19, 3A4
Paroxetine	10–50	2.9–44	2D6	None	N/A	2D6
Sertraline	50–200	24	2C9, 2B6, 2C19, 2D6, 3A4	Desmethylsertraline	62–104 h	2C19 (d,m)
SPARIs						
Vilazodone	10–40	25	3A4, 2C19, 2D6	None	NA	None or unknown
Vortioxetine	5–20	66	2D6, 3A4	None	NA	None or unknown
SARIs						
Trazodone	50–600	3–9	2D6, 3A4 inhibitors may increase concentration	m-Chlorophenylpiperazine	?	None or unknown
Nefazodone	300–600	3.5	3A4	Triazoledione, hydroxynefazodone	10 hours	(m)3A4
SMRIs						
Desvenlafaxine	50	11	Conjugation, 2D6	None or unknown	N/A	None or unknown
Duloxetine	40–60	8–17	2D6, 1A2	None	N/A	2D6
Levomilnacipran	40–120	12	3A4, P-glycoprotein Minor: 2C19, 2C8 and 2D6	None	N/A	None or unknown
Milnacipran	25–200	6–8	Glucuronidation	None	N/A	None
Venlafaxine	75–375	3–4	2D6	0-desmethylvenlafaxine, depends on 3A4 and 2C19 for metabolism	10 h	None or unknown
PSNR						
Mirtazapine	15–45	20–40	3A4	Desmethylmirtazapine	Unknown	3A4 induction
NDRI						
Bupropion	150–450	9.6–20.9	2D6	Hydroxybupropion, erythrohydrobupropion, threohydrobupropion	24–37 h	2D6

[a]The volume of distribution for all these xenobiotics is large except for trazodone.

N/A = not applicable; NDRI = norepinephrine/dopamine reuptake inhibitor; PSNR = presynaptic serotonin and norepinephrine releaser; SARI = serotonin antagonist/partial agonist/reuptake inhibitor; SNRI = serotonin/norepinephrine reuptake inhibitor; SPARI = serotonin reuptake inhibitors/partial receptor agonists; SSRI = selective serotonin reuptake inhibitor.

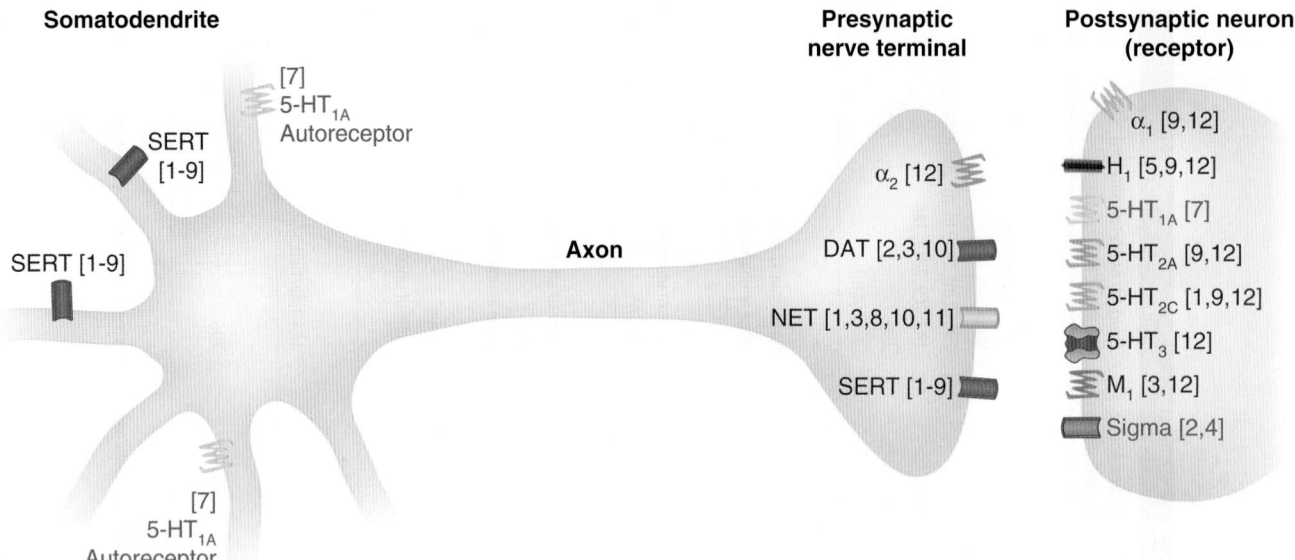

FIGURE 69–2. Simplified sites of action of select serotonin and noradrenergic antidepressants. Xenobiotics in green numbers are agonists, and those in red numbers are antagonists. (**A**) All of the following inhibit the serotonin transporter (SERT) and affect other receptors: (1) fluoxetine blocks norepinephrine reuptake transporter (NET) (weak) and 5-HT$_{2C}$; (2) sertraline blocks the dopamine reuptake transporter (DAT) (weak) and binds to the sigma receptor; (3) paroxetine blocks NET (weak) and the muscarinic receptor (M$_1$) and inhibits nitric oxide synthase (NOS); (4) fluvoxamine binds to the sigma receptor; (5) citalopram has mild histamine receptor (H$_1$) receptor inhibition and increases QTc prolongation at high doses; (6) escitalopram is a pure selective serotonin reuptake inhibitor (SSRI); (7) serotonin reuptake inhibitors/partial receptor agonists (SPARIs) include the partial 5-HT$_{1A}$ agonist vilazodone (buspirone; not a SERT); (8) serotonin/norepinephrine reuptake inhibitors (SNRIs), including venlafaxine, deslafaxine, and duloxetine, indirectly increase dopamine in the prefrontal cortex); and (9) serotonin antagonist/partial agonist/reuptake inhibitors (SARIs; trazodone) block 5-HT$_{2A}$, 5-HT$_{2C}$, H$_1$, and α$_1$ receptor (dose dependent). (**B**) All of the following have no SERT inhibition but exhibit other effects: (10) norepinephrine/dopamine reuptake inhibitors (NDRIs; bupropion); (11) norepinephrine reuptake inhibitors (NRIs; atomoxetine); and (12) noradrenergic and specific serotonergic antidepressants (NASSAs; mirtazapine), which blocks central α$_2$ presynaptic receptors, 5-HT$_{2A}$, 5-HT$_{2C}$, 5-HT$_3$, H$_1$, M$_1$ (weak) and peripheral α$_1$ receptor (weak). The xenobiotics listed next to the receptors affect the receptors to varying degrees of potency.

for and potent inhibitors of CYP2D6 and other cytochrome P-450 metabolizing enzymes (CYPs).[63] For example, whereas fluoxetine, fluvoxamine, citalopram, venlafaxine, mirtazapine, paroxetine, sertraline, and vortioxetine are substrates for CYP2D6, paroxetine, norfluoxetine, and fluoxetine inhibit the same enzyme (Table 69–1). Fluvoxamine inhibits CYP1A2 and CYP2C19, nefazodone inhibits CYP3A4, and mirtazapine induces CPY3A4. The metabolism of trazodone, vilazodone, and vortioxetine is decreased after this same enzyme is inhibited.[146] The consequences of these interactions manifest when the metabolism of xenobiotics that rely on these enzymes for metabolic transformation is altered (Chap. 11).

PATHOPHYSIOLOGY

The causes of depression and the mechanisms by which antidepressants ameliorate depressive symptoms are not well understood. Population-based studies demonstrate heritability in major depression, and a unique genotype was identified in the 5HT$_{2A}$ receptor in patients with seasonal affective disorder.[42] Mutations in the serotonin transporter are known to cause conformational changes as serotonin moves across the membrane.[163] These mutations also affect the regulation of cGMP-dependent signaling processes and are found to be associated with psychiatric disorders. The current postulated causes of depression include a disruption in function in the signal transduction cascade or events that occur thereafter that influences the regulation of neuronal ion channels, receptor modulation, neurotransmitter release, synaptic potentiation, and neuronal survival.[23] Multiple neurotransmitters are likely involved, including serotonin, norepinephrine, and dopamine. Further research evaluating the lesser known influences of γ-aminobutyric acid (GABA), excitatory amino acids, substance P antagonists, and antimuscarinic xenobiotics is ongoing. In addition to the direct pharmacologic effect of increasing synaptic concentrations of serotonin, antidepressants increase neurogenesis in the prefrontal cortex and glia in oligodendrocytes and activate complementary factors such as brain-derived neurotrophic factor and mitogen-activated protein kinase. The secondary effects, including conformational changes occurring

after exposure to these endogenous mediators, may explain previous research finding no difference in the concentration of serotonin-binding sites or serotonin receptor activity between depressed patients who respond to SSRIs and those who do not respond.[24,134] Unlike the CAs and other atypical antidepressants, the SSRIs have little direct interaction with cholinergic receptors, GABA receptors, sodium channels, or adrenergic reuptake (Table 69–2).

CLINICAL MANIFESTATIONS

Most of the effects that occur after overdose are direct extensions of the pharmacologic activity of the SSRIs in therapeutic doses. Excess serotonergic stimulation is prominent and nonselective. Common signs and symptoms include drowsiness, tremor, nausea, and vomiting. Less commonly, central nervous system (CNS) depression and sinus tachycardia occur.[13] Seizures and changes on electrocardiography (ECG), including prolongation of the QRS complex and QT interval duration, are reported, but they rarely occur with most SSRIs, even after large overdoses (Table 69–3). Infrequently, SSRI overdose results in life-threatening effects with fatalities often associated with coadministration of other xenobiotics.

Citalopram

Citalopram and its S(+)-enantiomer, escitalopram, cause QT interval prolongation in therapeutic doses in a linear, dose-related, and delayed manner.[74,90] In healthy adults, an increase of 8.5 ms occurred at a dose of 20 mg/day and 18.5 ms with a dose of 60 mg/day. The development of torsade de pointes is reported in therapeutic doses but only when concurrent xenobiotics are used or when there are electrolyte abnormalities. In large case series, patients are at risk for seizures and QT interval prolongation after ingestions exceeding 600 mg of citalopram or with serum concentrations more than 40 times the expected therapeutic concentrations.[27,122,123] Seizures were an early finding, occurring within 2 hours of ingestion, but the development of abnormalities on ECG were delayed for as long as 24 hours after ingestion.[123] Other case series report survival with seizures and significant QT interval prolongation

TABLE 69–2	Receptor Activity of Selective Serotonin Reuptake Inhibitors and Related Antidepressants				
Drug	Mechanism	Degree of Norepinephrine Reuptake Inhibition	Degree of Serotonin Reuptake Inhibition	Degree of Dopamine Reuptake Inhibition	Degree of Peripheral α-Adrenergic Effects
SSRIs					
Citalopram	SSRI, antimuscarinic	0	++++	0	0
Escitalopram	SSRI	0	++++	0	0
Fluoxetine	SSRI, inhibition of 5-HT$_{2C}$	0	++++	0	0
Fluvoxamine	SSRI	0	++++	0	0
Paroxetine	SSRI, antimuscarinic	+	++++	+	0
Sertraline	SSRI, weak reuptake norepinephrine and dopamine inhibitor	0	++++	+	+
Other					
Bupropion	Inhibits reuptake of biogenic amines	++	0	+	++
Duloxetine	SRI, norepinephrine reuptake inhibitor	++	++++	0	++
Desvenlafaxine	SRI, norepinephrine reuptake inhibitor	++	++++	0	++
Levomilnacipran	SRI, norepinephrine reuptake inhibitor	++	++++	0	0
Milnacipran	SRI, norepinephrine reuptake inhibitor	++	++++	0	+
Mirtazapine	α$_2$-Adrenergic antagonism, 5-HT$_2$/5-HT$_3$ antagonism	0	++++	0	+
Nefazodone	SRI, α$_1$-adrenergic antagonist	0	+	0	+
Trazodone	SRI, α$_1$-adrenergic antagonist	0	+	0	+
Venlafaxine	SRI, norepinephrine reuptake inhibitor	++	++++	0	++
Vilazodone	SSRI, 5-HT$_{1A}$ agonist	0	++++	0	0
Vortioxetine	SSRI, 5-HT$_{1A}$, 5-HT$_3$ agonist	0	++++	0	0

+ = weak if any agonism; ++ = weak agonism; +++ = strong agonism; ++++ = very strong agonism; 0 = no effect; SRI = serotonin reuptake inhibitor; SSRI = selective serotonin reuptake inhibitor.

TABLE 69–3	Predictive Analysis of the Relative Potential for Seizures and Abnormalities on Electrocardiography of Selective Serotonin Reuptake Inhibitors and Related Antidepressants		
Drug	Seizures	QT Interval Prolongation	QRS Complex Prolongation
Classic SSRIs			
Citalopram	+++	+++	+
Escitalopram	+++	+++	+
Fluoxetine	+	0	0
Fluvoxamine	+	0	0
Paroxetine	+	0	0
Sertraline	+	0	0
Atypical Antidepressants			
Bupropion	++++	+	+
Desvenlafaxine	+++	+	+++
Duloxetine	++++	Unknown	Unknown
Levomilnacipran	Unknown	Unknown	Unknown
Milnacipran	Unknown	Unknown	Unknown
Mirtazapine	Unknown	Unknown	++
Nefazodone	0	0	0
Trazodone	+	+	0
Venlafaxine	+++	+	+++
Vilazodone	+	Unknown	Unknown
Vortioxetine	Unknown	Unknown	Unknown

0 = does not cause; + = very rarely causes; ++ = rarely causes; +++ = causes; ++++ = very commonly causes; SSRI = selective serotonin reuptake inhibitor.

after a reported ingestion of 2.0 to 5.2 g of citalopram.[13,64] In 50 forensic cases, femoral blood citalopram concentrations were between 1.5 and 27 mcg/mL. Therapeutic concentrations identified at postmortem are reported to be up to 0.4 mcg/mL.[129]

Although the mechanisms are unclear, experimental models suggest that the didesmethylcitalopram metabolite of citalopram prolongs the QT interval by blocking I$_{Kr}$, but high concentrations of both the parent drug and this metabolite result in seizures (Chaps. 15 and 57).[19,160] The elimination half-life of the *R*-enantiomer of citalopram exceeds that of the *S*-enantomer.[104]

MANAGEMENT

Treatment of patients with acute SSRI overdose is largely supportive. Dextrose and thiamine should be given when clinically indicated for patients who present with altered mental status. Although cardiac manifestations after SSRI overdose are rare, a 12-lead ECG should be obtained to identify other cardiotoxic drugs, such as the CAs, to which the patient might access (Chaps. 15, 67, and 68). We recommend that patients suspected of overdose with citalopram or escitalopram be attached to a cardiac monitor to exclude the possibility of delayed QT interval prolongation and subsequent risk for ventricular dysrhythmias.[152] After the patient is initially stabilized, oral activated charcoal (AC) (1 g/kg) is recommended to adsorb drug remaining in the gastrointestinal (GI) tract. Lowering of blood concentrations and reduction in risk for QT interval prolongation are demonstrated when AC is given within the first 4 hours after escitalopram and citalopram ingestion.[49,50,59] Patients with small unintentional overdoses of SSRIs other than citalopram and escitalopram are not expected to develop significant signs and symptoms of poisoning. Adults with well-defined unintentional ingestions of up to 100 mg of citalopram and 50 mg of escitalopram can be managed safely at home with close observation.[112] The dose at which children can be safely managed in the home is less well defined. Fatalities resulting from SSRIs are rare and most commonly occur after ingestions of multiple xenobiotics or are manifestations of drug interactions resulting from excess serotonergic effects (see Serotonin Toxicity).[57] Forensic analysis of femoral blood samples is useful as corroborative data regarding death caused by SSRIs. In a forensic case study, blood concentrations in fatalities were higher concentrations than those found after purported therapeutic use of SSRIs.[129]

ADVERSE EVENTS AFTER THERAPEUTIC DOSES

Adverse events commonly associated with therapeutic doses of SSRIs as well as with overdose include GI (anorexia, nausea, vomiting, diarrhea), sexual dysfunction, weight gain, sleep disturbance, and discontinuation reactions.[44] Less common adverse events include sedation, particularly after citalopram and paroxetine, which result from their weak antimuscarinic activity, and anxiety after fluoxetine treatment.[93] Serotonin activity inhibits platelet secretory response, platelet aggregation, and platelet plug formation.[16] Although the effect increases in SSRIs with increased potency, clinically consequential bleeding is rare and is significant only in patients concurrently taking other antiplatelet medications.[1,87] This effect is of potential benefit in patients at risk for cardiovascular events.[6] Other rarely reported adverse events include new-onset panic disorder, priapism, bradycardia, hepatotoxicity, and urinary incontinence.[44] Movement disorders, most commonly akathisia, parkinsonism, myoclonus, and dystonia, also occur after SSRI use.[136,147] These extrapyramidal adverse events appear to be related to the complex interplay between serotonergic and dopaminergic activity. Predisposing factors for the development of movement disorders include concomitant use of dopamine antagonists such as the antipsychotics.[88]

The use of SSRIs is associated with the syndrome of inappropriate antidiuretic hormone secretion (SIADH; Chap. 12), in which severe hyponatremia occurs rapidly. The effect appears to be serotonin mediated in animal models, with increased concentrations of serum cortisol, adrenocorticotropin, and vasopressin noted.[51] Rat studies demonstrate that stimulation of 5-HT_{1C} and 5-HT_2 receptors increases antidiuretic hormone secretion.[144,145] However, human case control studies using water-loading tests have not confirmed defects in osmoregulated release of vasopressin through measurement of vasopressin concentrations after 3 to 11 months of paroxetine use.[99] A review of the literature identified increasing age, female sex, concurrent medications known to cause hyponatremia, low body weight, a previous history of hyponatremia, and excessive fluid intake as risk factors for hyponatremia.[76,83,84] Although reported to occur from 3 days to 4 months after initiation of therapy, a case-matched control study of 203 patients identified that SIADH occurs most frequently within the first 2 weeks of therapy.[106] Hyponatremia is also reported when switching from one SSRI to another.[8] Neither CYP2D6 genotype metabolizer status nor high serum concentrations predicts risk of hyponatremia.[149] Patients older than 40 years of age using SSRIs are at increased risk for bone fracture, presumably caused by a serotonergic effect on osteoblasts and osteoclasts.[140]

Serotonin Toxicity

The most common severe adverse event associated with SSRIs is the development of serotonin toxicity. This was formerly referred to in life-threatening cases as *serotonin syndrome* and *serotonin behavioral* or *hyperactivity syndrome*. It was first described in patients treated with MAOIs who were given other xenobiotics that enhance serotonergic activity.[30,115,143] However, ingestion of an MAOI is not required for serotonin toxicity to develop, and its occurrence is unpredictable (Table 69–4).

Pathophysiology

The pathophysiologic mechanism of serotonin toxicity is not completely understood but likely involves excessive selective stimulation and genetic variation of serotonin 5-HT_{2A} and perhaps 5-HT_{1A} receptors.[32,109,113] Initial animal models demonstrate that specific stimulation of 5-HT_{1A} receptors results in serotonin toxicity even when 5-HT_{2A} receptors were inactivated using a specific antagonist.[35,113] However, a subsequent animal study and a human retrospective case series showed that the potency of 5-HT_{2A} agonist therapy was directly related to the development of the findings attributed to serotonin toxicity.[56] 5-HT_{1D} receptors are not implicated in cases of serotonin toxicity.

TABLE 69–4	Potential Causes of Serotonin Toxicity[21]

Inhibitors of Serotonin Metabolism

Linezolid

Methylene blue

Monoamine oxidase inhibitors (nonselective)
  Phenelzine, moclobemide, clorgyline, isocarboxazid

Harmine and harmaline from Ayahuasca preparations, psychoactive beverage used for religious purposes in the Amazon and Orinoco River basins

St. John's wort *(Hypericum perforatum)*

Syrian rue *(Peganum harmala)*

Blockers of Serotonin Reuptake

Bupropion

Clomipramine, imipramine

Cocaine

Dextromethorphan

Fentanyl

Meperidine

Pentazocine

SSRIs: all

Milnacipran

Tramadol

Trazodone, nefazodone

Venlafaxine

Serotonin Precursors or Agonists

L–Tryptophan

Lysergic acid diethylamide (LSD)

Triptans (sumatriptan)

Enhancers of Serotonin Release

Substituted amphetamines and analogs: phenylethylamines, especially MDMA, cathinones, aminoindanes

Methylone

Buspirone

Butylone

Cocaine

Lithium

Mirtazapine

Other

Ginseng

Lithium

Ondansetron, granisetron, and metoclopramide

Sibutramine

Ritonavir

Valproic acid

MDMA = 3,4-methylenedioxymethamphetamine; SSRI = selective serotonin reuptake inhibitor.

Serotonin toxicity occurs most frequently after use of combinations of serotonergic xenobiotics (Table 69–4) but also occurs after high therapeutic dosing or overdoses of isolated serotonergic xenobiotics.[34,68,81,117] Interactions resulting in serotonin toxicity also occur while alternating serotonergic xenobiotic regimens, particularly when an insufficient time lag occurs before initiating the alternative therapy.[95] Residual pharmacologic effects, receptor downregulation or upregulation, and the presence of active metabolites are likely causative in these circumstances. For example, fluoxetine metabolism results in the active metabolite norfluoxetine, which has comparable pharmacologic effects and a half-life substantially longer than fluoxetine. The clearance of norfluoxetine takes approximately 2 weeks.

TABLE 69–5	Diagnostic Criteria for Serotonin Toxicity

After Introduction of a Serotonergic Xenobiotic:

Spontaneous clonus alone

Inducible or ocular clonus *plus* agitation *or* diaphoresis or hypertonicity with temperature >38°C (100.4°F)

Tremor with hyperreflexia

Other Common Manifestations

Diaphoresis and shivering

Diarrhea

Hyperthermia

Incoordination

Mental status changes

Myoclonus

Although sporadic reports occur, selective MAO subtype B (MAO-B) inhibitor xenobiotic combinations and triptans (5-HT$_{1B/1D}$ receptor agonists) can result in serotonin toxicity at therapeutic doses.[43,45]

Manifestations

Signs of serotonin toxicity include altered mental status, agitation, tachycardia, myoclonus, hyperreflexia, diaphoresis, tremor, diarrhea, incoordination, muscle rigidity, and hyperthermia (Table 69–5). The neuromuscular effects are often more prominent in the lower extremities. The clinical manifestations of serotonin toxicity are diverse, and minor manifestations are common after initiation of SSRI and atypical antidepressant therapy. In fact, a prospective study of depressed inpatients given clomipramine demonstrated that 16 of the 38 patients experienced manifestations consistent with serotonin toxicity, with 14 having spontaneous resolution within 1 week without discontinuation of therapy.[91] Life-threatening effects invariably result from hyperthermia caused by excessive muscle activity that is more prominent in the lower extremities. Sustained severe hyperthermia can lead to death through denaturation of essential protein and enzymatic function that ultimately results in an elevated lactate concentration and metabolic acidosis, rhabdomyolysis, renal and hepatic dysfunction, disseminated intravascular coagulation, or acute respiratory distress syndrome (Chap. 29).[103,150]

Diagnosis

Although fulminant life-threatening cases are easy to recognize, mild cases of serotonin toxicity are more difficult to distinguish from similarly appearing disorders from other causes. In an effort to determine diagnostic criteria, a study that included 38 cases of presumed serotonin toxicity suggested diagnostic criteria to include three of the following signs and symptoms—altered level of consciousness, agitation, myoclonus, hyperreflexia, diaphoresis, tremor, diarrhea, and incoordination—when other causes were excluded.[150] A modification, the Hunter Serotonin Toxicity Criteria, which included the variables of myoclonus, agitation, diaphoresis, hyperreflexia, hypertonicity, and fever, was validated in 473 patients and found to correlate best with a clinical toxicologic diagnosis of serotonin toxicity (Table 69–5).[41] Currently, no diagnostic test capable of determining whether a patient is experiencing serotonin toxicity is available. A single case report demonstrated increased urinary serotonin concentrations associated with serotonin toxicity.[25] There are likely genetic alterations of SERT or 5-HT$_{2A}$ receptors or polymorphisms of drug metabolism via CYP2D6 involved.[47] Mice with *SERT* gene deficiency showed increased serotonergic response when given serotoninergic drugs. A T102C single-nucleotide polymorphism of the 5-HT$_{2A}$ was associated with SSRI adverse event–related drug discontinuation after initiation of paroxetine therapy, although this was unable to be validated after acute overdose.[32,108]

Management

Treatment of patients with serotonin toxicity begins with supportive care and focuses on decreasing core body temperature and muscle activity. Because muscular rigidity is thought to be primarily responsible for hyperthermia and death, rapid, aggressive external cooling using ice water immersion if severe in conjunction with sedative hypnotics such as benzodiazepines are recommended to limit complications and mortality (Chap. 29). In severe cases, neuromuscular blockade with a definitive airway is a recommended approach to achieve rapid muscle relaxation. The time course of serotonin toxicity is variable and related to the time required to eliminate the offending xenobiotics. In most patients, the manifestations of serotonin toxicity resolve within 24 hours after the offending xenobiotic is removed. However, serotonin toxicity can be prolonged when it is caused by xenobiotics with long half-lives, protracted duration of effects, or active metabolites.

Animal models indicate that pretreatment with serotonin antagonists can prevent development of serotonin toxicity.[113] Several case reports suggest success after use of 4 mg of oral cyproheptadine, an antihistamine with nonspecific serotonin antagonist effects, including 5-HT$_{1A}$ and 5-HT$_{2A}$ receptors.[62,89] Patients who responded typically had no hyperthermia and only mild to moderate manifestations of serotonin toxicity. Evidence supports the use of cyproheptadine in this patient group. We currently recommend doses of 8 to 16 mg orally repeated hourly, as needed, to achieve muscle relaxation in more severe cases. Further research is warranted to determine the success of higher doses given to gain sufficient 5-HT$_{2A}$ antagonistic effects in more severely affected patients.[56] Other xenobiotics, such as methysergide, chlorpromazine, atypical antipsychotics, and propranolol, are anecdotally reported to be successful for the treatment of serotonin toxicity.[21,56,66,133] These therapies are not currently recommended.

Differentiating Serotonin Toxicity from Neuroleptic Malignant Syndrome

Many features overlap between serotonin toxicity and the neuroleptic malignant syndrome (NMS; Chap. 67). Although altered mental status, autonomic instability, and changes in neuromuscular tone that result in hyperthermia are common to both disorders: many differences are apparent. It is also clear that the implicated xenobiotics, time course, pathophysiology, and manifestations are distinct (Table 69–6).[56] Signs and symptoms of serotonin toxicity develop within minutes to hours after exposure to the offending xenobiotics, but NMS typically develops days to weeks after daily exposure.[124] In addition, after syndrome onset, even with the offending xenobiotics discontinued, NMS can persist for as long as 2 weeks. However, serotonin toxicity usually resolves

TABLE 69–6	Comparison of Neuroleptic Malignant Syndrome (NMS) and Serotonin Toxicity	
	NMS	**Serotonin Toxicity**
Historical Diagnostic Clue		
Inciting drug pharmacology	Dopamine antagonist	Serotonin agonist
Time course of initiation of symptoms after exposure	Days to weeks	Hours
Duration of symptoms	Days to 2 wk	Usually 24 h
Symptoms		
Altered mental status (depressed or confusion)	+++	+++
Altered mental status (agitation or hyperactivity)	+++	+++
Autonomic instability	+++	+++
Bradykinesia	+++	–
Gastrointestinal findings (diarrhea)	–	+++
Hyperthermia	+++	+++
Lead pipe rigidity	+++	+
Shivering	–	+++
Tremor, hyperreflexia, myoclonus	+	+++

− = not found; + = rare finding; +++ = common finding.

within 24 hours and is directly correlated with the pharmacokinetic metabolic profile of the offending xenobiotic. A review of the literature indicates that patients presenting with serotonin toxicity are more likely to exhibit agitation, hyperactivity, clonus, myoclonus, ocular oscillations (opsoclonus), shivering, tremors, and lower limb hyperreflexia, but patients presenting with NMS were more likely to exhibit bradykinesia and lead pipe rigidity.[56,121]

ATYPICAL ANTIDEPRESSANTS

Atypical antidepressants are defined as not belonging strictly within a class of antidepressants. They are not SSRIs, CAs, or MAOIs. Most are derivatives of SSRIs and have additional pharmacologic effects that were selected in an attempt to decrease the undesirable side effects of traditional antidepressants.

Serotonin/Norepinephrine Reuptake Inhibitors: Venlafaxine, Desvenlafaxine, Duloxetine, Milnacipran, and Levomilnacipran

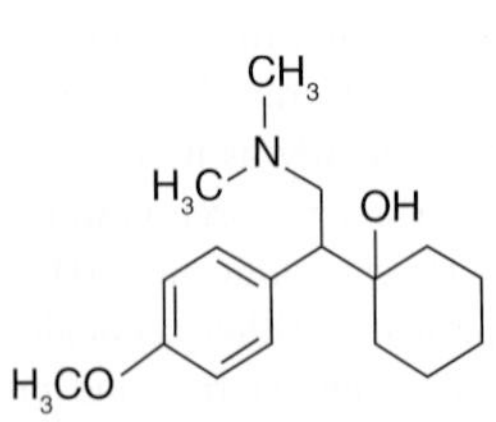

Venlafaxine

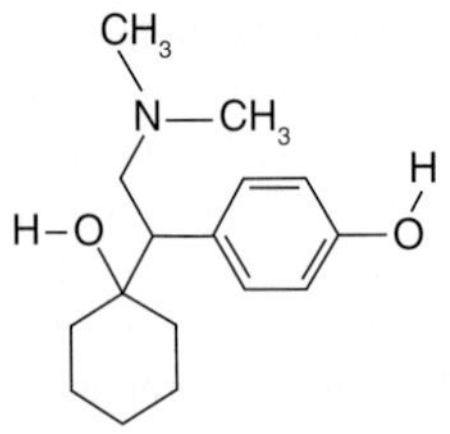

Desvenlafaxine

In addition to inhibiting serotonin reuptake, venlafaxine inhibits norepinephrine reuptake. Venlafaxine produces rapid downregulation of central β-adrenergic receptors, which results in a faster onset of antidepressant effect.[137] Patients with acute venlafaxine overdose present with nausea, vomiting, dizziness, tachycardia, CNS depression, hypotension, hypoglycemia, hyperthermia, hepatic toxicity (including zone 3 necrosis), rhabdomyolysis, and seizures.[48,100,118,139] Sodium and potassium channel blocking effects are rarely clinically apparent; however, prolongation of the QRS complex and QT interval can lead to ventricular tachycardia and death.[18,132,156] One report indicated a positive incremental association of clinical toxicity with a maximum measured serum venlafaxine concentration of 25.8 μmol/L.[102] Although no clinical data regarding efficacy are available, we recommend sodium bicarbonate to attenuate the sodium channel blocking effects that lead to QRS complex prolongation (Antidotes in Depth: A5). In addition, GI decontamination with AC with or without whole-bowel irrigation (WBI) decreases serum concentrations and decreases the incidence of seizures in select patients, particularly after the ingestion of extended-release formulations.[85,86] Adverse events associated with chronic therapeutic doses of venlafaxine include alopecia, yawning, focal myositis, facial flushing, and dose-related increases in blood pressure.[79,120] Although limited information is available, venlafaxine appears to be more dangerous than SSRIs, and the other serotonin/norepinephrine reuptake inhibitors (SNRIs)—desvenlafaxine, duloxetine, milnacipran, and levomilnacipran—after overdose.[31,77,156]

Serotonin Reuptake Inhibitors/Partial Receptor Agonists: Vilazodone and Vortioxetine

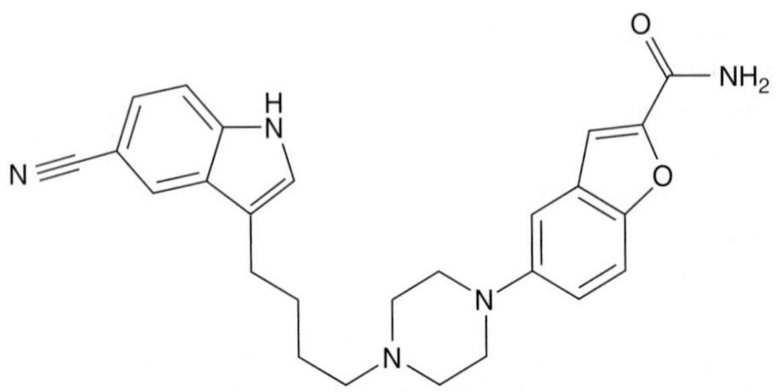

Vilazodone

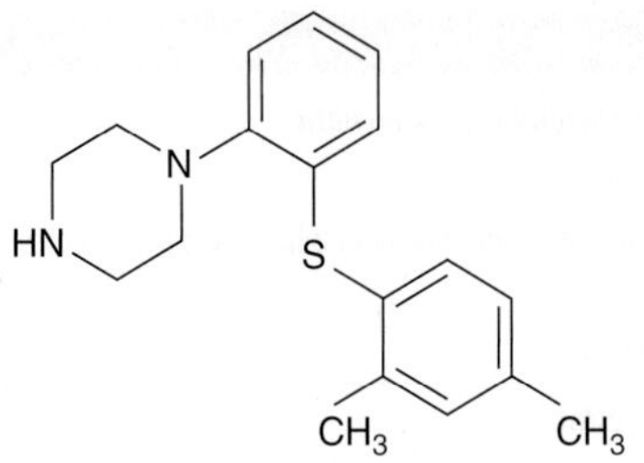

Vortioxetine

Vilazodone is an SSRI with additional 5-HT$_{1A}$ receptor agonism. Little information is available about vilazodone after overdose. After therapeutic doses, a case report suggested that vilazodone resulted in breakthrough seizures shortly after dose escalation in a patient with a seizure disorder who had been seizure free for 8 years.[101] However, in an analysis of published literature regarding therapeutic doses, only GI side effects occurred in more than 2,000 patients taking therapeutic doses.[162] A single report of a child with a reported ingestion of 37 mg/kg of vilazodone exhibited altered mental status, signs of serotonin toxicity, and a seizure.[2] Similarly, there is little information available regarding vortioxetine overdose, but it is anticipated to have effects similar to other SSRIs.

Serotonin Antagonist/Partial Agonist/Reuptake Inhibitors: Trazodone and Nefazodone

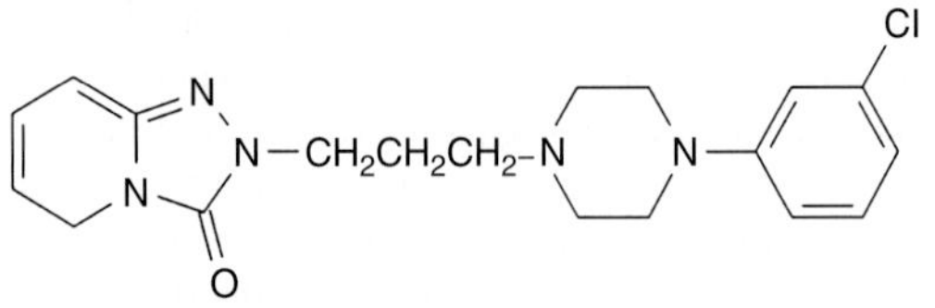

Trazodone is an antagonist at 5-HT$_{2A}$ and 5-HT$_{2C}$ receptors, a partial agonist at 5-HT$_1$ receptors, and a weak serotonin reuptake inhibitor. In addition, trazodone has α-adrenergic antagonist activity and weak H$_1$ receptor antagonism. Central nervous system depression and orthostatic hypotension are the most common complications after acute overdose of trazodone.[53] Less common, seizures and cardiac conduction delays, such as QT interval prolongation and ventricular dysrhythmias, and death.[29,39,126,138] Trazodone is rarely reported to cause SIADH and cholestatic hepatitis.[46,155,26,115,126] Priapism, reported with therapeutic doses of trazodone, occurs occasionally after overdose.[69] Treatment is supportive and includes monitoring the ECG for conduction delays and the administration of fluids and vasopressors for hypotension if necessary.

Nefazodone is an antagonist at 5-HT$_{2A}$ receptors and α-adrenergic receptors in addition to moderate inhibition of serotonin and norepinephrine reuptake.[38] Nefazodone is rarely used because of concerns of severe hepatic toxicity, including jaundice, hepatitis, and hepatocellular necrosis.[28] The most common manifestations seen after acute overdose include drowsiness, nausea, dizziness, and hypotension.[15] Treatment is similar to trazodone overdose.

Presynaptic Serotonin and Norepinephrine Releaser: Mirtazapine

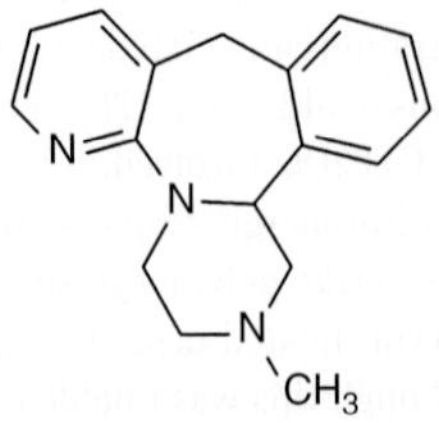

The mechanism of action of mirtazapine is unique. It is a central presynaptic α$_2$-adrenergic inhibitor which increases neuronal norepinephrine and serotonin release.[20] Mirtazapine also blocks some subtypes of 5-HT receptors, including 5-HT$_{2A}$, 5-HT$_{2C}$, and 5-HT$_3$. Finally, mirtazapine blocks H$_2$ receptors, peripheral α_1 receptors, and muscarinic acetylcholine receptors.[114] The main effects that occur after acute mirtazapine overdoses include altered mental status, tachycardia, and hypothermia.[96,157] Large overdoses cause respiratory depression and prolongation of the QT interval.[22,130] Rare adverse reactions associated with the therapeutic use of mirtazapine causing serotonin toxicity, hepatitis, and reversible agranulocytosis are reported.[71,75,111]

Norepinephrine/Dopamine Reuptake Inhibitor: Bupropion

The use of bupropion, especially extended-release formulations, is common for the treatment of depression. Bupropion is also frequently used in the treatment of smoking cessation therapy, weight loss, ADHD, and, occasionally, in compulsive eating disorders.[4,52,98] The pharmacologic mechanism of action of bupropion, a substituted cathinone (β-keto amphetamine) and its active metabolite, hydroxybupropion, include inhibition of reuptake of dopamine and, to a lesser extent, norepinephrine.[7] Chronic doses above 450 mg/day place patients at risk for seizures.[37,80] Frequent effects that occur after overdose include tachycardia, hypertension, GI symptoms, and agitation.[12,14] Large acute overdoses result in seizures (infrequently status epilepticus), QRS complex prolongation, and occasionally QT interval prolongation.[12,77,78,153] In some cases, effects were delayed for up to 10 hours, and seizures up to 24 hours, particularly after the ingestion of sustained-release preparations.[148] Effects can continue for up to 48 hours. Euphoria, hallucinations, and seizures are reported after nasal insufflation.[72,128] This is caused by extensive mucosal absorption, effectively bypassing first-pass hepatic metabolism.

It remains unclear whether seizures are caused by bupropion or its metabolite hydroxybupropion.[37,141] Elevated bupropion and hydroxybupropion concentrations are documented after seizures. The exact mechanism for seizures caused by hydroxybupropion is unclear at this time. Treatment, when required for seizures, should be supportive and includes judicious use of benzodiazepines. Significant cardiotoxicity and QRS complex prolongation are likely because of delayed and sustained elevation of serum bupropion serum concentration.[3] As assessed in animal studies, the mechanism is a deficiency in intracellular communication via gap junctions and therefore may not be responsive to sodium bicarbonate (Antidotes in Depth: A5).[26] Research is warranted to define the role of intravenous lipid emulsion (ILE) in life-threatening cases. Evidence-based recommendations suggest the use of ILE for life-threatening bupropion overdose after other therapies fail.[60,142] Intravenous lipid emulsion is not recommended in the situation of bupropion overdose without life-threatening cardiac toxicity. When a patient presents shortly after an overdose or the patient has taken a massive overdose, we recommend the use of multiple doses of AC with the addition of WBI if the airway is protected.

Other serious adverse events reported after chronic bupropion use include cholestatic and hepatocellular dysfunction and rhabdomyolysis, with isolated reports of chest pain, dystonia, trigeminal nerve dysfunction, mania, generalized erythrodermic psoriasis, erythema multiforme, dyskinesia, altered vestibular and sensory function, and serum sickness.[5,33,36,58,61,82,94,154]

DRUG DISCONTINUATION SYNDROME

The term *drug discontinuation syndrome* is used to describe the physiologic manifestations that occur after abrupt antidepressant cessation. The distinction between a withdrawal syndrome and drug discontinuation syndrome is unclear, but it likely distinguishes the manifestations occurring after therapeutic use versus misuse, that is, alcohol or heroin withdrawal and SSRI discontinuation syndrome. Drug discontinuation syndromes are commonly reported after abrupt discontinuation of all antidepressants, including SSRIs and atypical antidepressants.[158] Selective serotonin reuptake inhibitors cause a discontinuation syndrome that usually begins within 5 days after drug discontinuation and continues up to 3 weeks.[67] The most frequently reported symptoms include dizziness, lethargy, paresthesias, nausea, vivid dreams, irritability, and depressed mood.[135] The risk factors associated with development of a discontinuation syndrome are not fully clarified; however, in a given individual, a genetic polymorphism of the 5-HT$_{1A}$ receptor is hypothesized to play a role.[107] The syndrome is more common with SSRIs with shorter elimination half-lives (paroxetine > fluvoxamine > sertraline > fluoxetine). Of published cases, approximately 65% were attributed to paroxetine, approximately 20% to sertraline, and only 10% to fluoxetine and fluvoxamine.[11,17] Fluoxetine discontinuation syndrome occurs less frequently, at only 2 cases per 1 million prescriptions.[127] The long elimination half-life of fluoxetine and its active metabolite norfluoxetine probably decrease the incidence of discontinuation syndrome by providing a tapered effect after cessation. The discontinuation symptoms found with paroxetine were classified as mild to moderate in 20% to 40% of patients receiving 20 mg/day.[11]

Because of difficulty in distinguishing symptoms of discontinuation syndrome from underlying disease, some authors have proposed diagnostic criteria for the SSRI discontinuation syndrome.[17] All proposed criteria include discontinuation of the SSRI in concordance with CNS effects, GI distress, or anxiety.[151] The prominent CNS findings include dizziness; ataxia; vertigo; sensory abnormalities, including electric shocklike sensations and paresthesias; and behavior abnormalities, including aggression and impulsivity.

The biochemical basis of the discontinuation syndrome appears to be similar to tryptophan depletion, which results in an acute decrease in synaptic serotonin.[40] In fact, abrupt discontinuation versus drug taper was a noted risk factor for the discontinuation syndrome in paroxetine cases compared with drug taper.[73]

Treatment of patients exhibiting the discontinuation syndrome should include supportive care and resumption of the discontinued drug or administration of another SSRI if the implicated drug is contraindicated.[159] The drug then should be tapered at a rate that allows for improved patient tolerance. Many of the other antidepressants discussed in this chapter also result in discontinuation reactions. Symptoms appear similar to those reported after discontinuation of the SSRIs and are treated in a similar manner.[159]

Drug discontinuation syndrome is also identified to occur in neonates.[55] It is commonly referred to as the neonatal (serotonin) abstinence syndrome (NSAS). Neonatal (serotonin) abstinence syndrome is reported to occur after in utero exposure to SSRIs and other atypical antidepressants. The incidence of NSAS was reported to be as high as 30% in a cohort of neonates whose mothers were taking SSRIs.[93] Another literature review found an overall relative risk of 3 compared with those without exposure. In these cases, symptoms were generally confined to the CNS, respiratory system, and GI system and resolved over a 2-week period.[105]

SUMMARY

- Acute overdose with SSRIs or atypical antidepressants are not usually life threatening, although seizures or cardiac toxicity occur.
- Monitoring is recommended for 24 hours for the delayed cardiotoxicity with citalopram or escitalopram.
- Monitoring is also recommended for 24 hours for delayed seizures after extended-release bupropion ingestion.
- Drug interactions and adverse drug events are associated with serotonin reuptake inhibitors and lead to acute life-threatening events, including serotonin toxicity.
- Serotonin toxicity can produce life-threatening hyperthermia and should be treated with aggressive cooling and sedation. Cyproheptadine is recommended for symptomatic patients and neuromuscular blockade is recommended for those with refractory hyperthermia.

REFERENCES

1. Aarts N, et al. Inhibition of serotonin reuptake by antidepressants and cerebral microbleeds in the general population. *Stroke*. 2014;45:1951-1957.

2. Acker EC, et al. Acute vilazodone toxicity in a pediatric patient. *J Emerg Med*. 2015;49:284-286.

3. Al-Abri SA, et al. Delayed bupropion cardiotoxicity associated with elevated serum concentrations of bupropion but not hydroxybupropion. *Clin Toxicol*. 2013;51:1230-1234.

4. Alberg AJ, Carpenter MJ. Enhancing the effectiveness of smoking cessation interventions: a cancer prevention imperative. *J Natl Cancer Inst*. 2012;104:260-262.

5. Amann B, et al. Bupropion-induced isolated impairment of sensory trigeminal nerve function. *Int Clin Psychopharmacol*. 2000;15:115-116.

6. Andrade C, et al. Serotonin reuptake inhibitor antidepressants and abnormal bleeding: a review for clinicians and a reconsideration of mechanisms. *J Clin Psychiatry*. 2010;71:1565-1575.

7. Arias HR, et al. Pharmacological and neurotoxicological actions mediated by bupropion and diethylpropion. *Int Rev Neurobiol*. 2009;88:223-255.

8. Arinzon ZH, et al. Delayed recurrent SIADH associated with SSRIs. *Ann Pharmacother*. 2002;36:1175-1177.

9. Asnis GM, et al. Functional interrelationship of serotonin and norepinephrine: cortisol response to MCPP and DMI in patients with panic disorder, patients with depression, and normal control subjects. *Psychiatry Res*. 1992;43:65-76.

10. Atkinson JH, et al. Effects of noradrenergic and serotonergic antidepressants on chronic low back pain intensity. *Pain*. 1999;83:137-145.

11. Baldwin DS, et al. Discontinuation symptoms in depression and anxiety disorders. *Int J Neuropsychopharmacol*. 2007;10:73-84.

12. Balit CR, et al. Bupropion poisoning: a case series. *Med J Aust*. 2003;178:61-63.

13. Barbey JT, Roose SP. SSRI Safety in overdose. *J Clin Psychiatry*. 1998;59(suppl 15):42-48.

14. Belson MG, Kelley TR. Bupropion exposures: clinical manifestations and medical outcome. *J Emerg Med*. 2002;23:223-230.

15. Benson BE, et al. Toxicities and outcomes associated with nefazodone poisoning: an analysis of 1,338 exposures. *Am J Emerg Med*. 2000;18:587-592.

16. Bismuth-Evanzal Y, et al. Decreased serotonin content and reduced agonist-induced aggregation in platelets of patients chronically medicated with SSRI drugs. *J Affect Disord*. 2012;136:99-103.

17. Black K, et al. Selective serotonin reuptake inhibitor discontinuation syndrome: proposed diagnostic criteria. *J Psychiatry Neurosci*. 2000;25:255-261.

18. Blythe D, Hackett LP. Cardiovascular and neurological toxicity of venlafaxine. *Hum Exp Toxicol*. 1999;18:309-313.

19. Boeck V, et al. Studies on acute toxicity and drug levels of citalopram in the dog. *Acta Pharmacol Toxicol (Copenh)*. 1982;50:169-174.

20. de Boer T. The pharmacologic profile of mirtazapine. *J Clin Psychiatry*. 1996;57(suppl 4):19-25.

21. Boyer EW, Shannon M. The serotonin syndrome. *N Engl J Med*. 2005;352:1112-1120.

22. Bremner JD, et al. Safety of mirtazapine in overdose. *J Clin Psychiatry*. 1998;59:233-235.

23. Brigitta B. Pathophysiology of depression and mechanisms of treatment. *Dialogues Clin Neurosci*. 2002;4:7-20.

24. Briley M, Moret C. Neurobiological mechanisms involved in antidepressant therapies. *Clin Neuropharmacol*. 1993;16:387-400.

25. Brvar M, et al. Urinary serotonin level is associated with serotonin syndrome after moclobemide, sertraline, and citalopram overdose. *Clin Toxicol (Phila)*. 2007;45:458-460.

26. Caillier B, et al. QRS widening and QT prolongation under bupropion: a unique cardiac electrophysiological profile. *Fundam Clin Pharmacol*. 2012;26:599-608.

27. Catalano G, et al. QTc interval prolongation associated with citalopram overdose: a case report and literature review. *Clin Neuropharmacol*. 2001;24:158-162.

28. Choi S. Nefazodone (Serzone) withdrawn because of hepatotoxicity. *CMAJ*. 2003;169:1187.

29. Chung KJ, et al. Management of ventricular dysrhythmia secondary to trazodone overdose. *J Emerg Med*. 2008;35:171-174.

30. Cohen RM, et al. Myoclonus-associated hypomania during MAO-inhibitor treatment. *Am J Psychiatry*. 1980;137:105-106.

31. Cooper JM, et al. Desvenlafaxine overdose and the occurrence of serotonin toxicity, seizures and cardiovascular effects. *Clin Toxicol (Phila)*. 2016:1-7.

32. Cooper JM, et al. Serotonin toxicity from antidepressant overdose and its association with the T102C polymorphism of the 5-HT2A receptor. *Pharmacogenomics J*. 2014;14:390-394.

33. Cox NH, et al. Generalized pustular and erythrodermic psoriasis associated with bupropion treatment. *Br J Dermatol*. 2002;146:1061-1063.

34. Daniels RJ. Serotonin syndrome due to venlafaxine overdose. *J Accid Emerg Med*. 1998;15:333-334.

35. Darmani NA, Zhao W. Production of serotonin syndrome by 8-OH DPAT in Cryptotis parva. *Physiol Behav*. 1998;65:327-331.

36. David D, Esquenazi J. Rhabdomyolysis associated with bupropion treatment. *J Clin Psychopharmacol*. 1999;19:185-186.

37. Davidson J. Seizures and bupropion: a review. *J Clin Psychiatry*. 1989;50:256-261.

38. Davis R, et al. A review of its pharmacology and clinical efficacy in the management of major depression. *Drugs*. 1997;53:608-636.

39. De Meester A, et al. Fatal overdose with trazodone: case report and literature review. *Acta Clin Belg*. 2001;56:258-261.

40. Delgado PL. Monoamine depletion studies: implications for antidepressant discontinuation syndrome. *J Clin Psychiatry*. 2006;67(suppl 4):22-26.

41. Dunkley EJC, et al. The Hunter Serotonin Toxicity Criteria: simple and accurate diagnostic decision rules for serotonin toxicity. *QJM*. 2003;96:635-642.

42. Enoch MA, et al. Association between seasonal affective disorder and the 5-HT2A promoter polymorphism, -1438G/A. *Mol Psychiatry*. 1999;4:89-92.

43. Evans RW, et al. The FDA alert on serotonin syndrome with use of triptans combined with selective serotonin reuptake inhibitors or selective serotonin-norepinephrine reuptake inhibitors: American Headache Society position paper. *Headache*. 2010;50:1089-1099.

44. Ferguson JM. SSRI antidepressant medications: adverse effects and tolerability. *Prim Care Companion J Clin Psychiatry*. 2001;3:22-27.

45. Fernandes C, et al. Rasagiline-induced serotonin syndrome. *Mov Disord*. 2011;26:766-767.

46. Fernandes NF, et al. Trazodone-induced hepatotoxicity: a case report with comments on drug-induced hepatotoxicity. *Am J Gastroenterol*. 2000;95:532-535.

47. Fox MA, et al. Receptor mediation of exaggerated responses to serotonin-enhancing drugs in serotonin transporter (SERT)-deficient mice. *Neuropharmacology*. 2007;53:643-656.

48. Francino M-C, et al. Hypoglycaemia: a little known effect of Venlafaxine overdose. *Clin Toxicol (Phila)*. 2012;50:215-217.

49. Friberg LE, et al. Pharmacokinetic–pharmacodynamic modelling of QT interval prolongation following citalopram overdoses. *Br J Clin Pharmacol*. 2006;61:177-190.

50. Friberg LE, et al. The population pharmacokinetics of citalopram after deliberate self-poisoning: a Bayesian approach. *J Pharmacokinet Pharmacodyn*. 2005;32:571-605.

51. Fuller RW. Serotonergic stimulation of pituitary-adrenocortical function in rats. *Neuroendocrinology*. 1981;32:118-127.

52. Gadde KM, et al. Bupropion for weight loss: an investigation of efficacy and tolerability in overweight and obese women. *Obes Res*. 2001;9:544-551.

53. Gamble DE, Peterson LG. Trazodone overdose: four years of experience from voluntary reports. *J Clin Psychiatry*. 1986;47:544-546.

54. Gartlehner G, et al. Comparative benefits and harms of antidepressant, psychological, complementary, and exercise treatments for major depression: an evidence report for a clinical practice guideline from the American college of physicians. *Ann Intern Med*. 2016;164:331-341.

55. Gentile S. Serotonin reuptake inhibitor-induced perinatal complications. *Paediatr Drugs*. 2007;9:97-106.

56. Gillman PK. The serotonin syndrome and its treatment. *J Psychopharmacol (Oxf)*. 1999;13:100–109.

57. Goeringer KE, et al. Postmortem forensic toxicology of selective serotonin reuptake inhibitors: a review of pharmacology and report of 168 cases. *J Forensic Sci*. 2000;45:633-648.

58. Goren JL, Levin GM. Mania with bupropion: a dose-related phenomenon? *Ann Pharmacother*. 2000;34:619-621.

59. van Gorp F, et al. Population pharmacokinetics and pharmacodynamics of escitalopram in overdose and the effect of activated charcoal. *Br J Clin Pharmacol*. 2012;73:402-410.

60. Gosselin S, et al. Evidence-based recommendations on the use of intravenous lipid emulsion therapy in poisoning. *Clin Toxicol*. 2016.

61. de Graaf L, Diemont WL. Chest pain during use of bupropion as an aid in smoking cessation. *Br J Clin Pharmacol*. 2003;56:451-452.

62. Graudins A, et al. Treatment of the serotonin syndrome with cyproheptadine. *J Emerg Med*. 1998;16:615-619.

63. Greenblatt DJ, et al. Human cytochromes and some newer antidepressants: kinetics, metabolism, and drug interactions. *J Clin Psychopharmacol*. 1999;19(5 suppl 1):23S-35S.

64. Grundemar L, et al. Symptoms and signs of severe citalopram overdose. *The Lancet*. 1997;349:1602.

65. Gunnell D. Selective serotonin reuptake inhibitors (SSRIs) and suicide in adults: meta-analysis of drug company data from placebo controlled, randomised controlled trials submitted to the MHRA's safety review. *BMJ*. 2005;330:385-0.

66. Guzé BH, Baxter LR. The serotonin syndrome: case responsive to propranolol. *J Clin Psychopharmacol*. 1986;6:119-120.

67. Haddad P. Newer antidepressants and the discontinuation syndrome. *J Clin Psychiatry*. 1997;58(suppl 7):17-21; discussion 22.

68. Hanekamp BB, et al. Serotonin syndrome and rhabdomyolysis in venlafaxine poisoning: a case report. *Neth J Med*. 2005;63:316-318.

69. Hanno PM, et al. Trazodone-induced priapism. *Br J Urol*. 1988;61:94.

70. Hawton K, et al. Toxicity of antidepressants: rates of suicide relative to prescribing and non-fatal overdose. *Br J Psychiatry*. 2010;196:354-358.

71. Hernández JL, et al. Severe serotonin syndrome induced by mirtazapine monotherapy. *Ann Pharmacother*. 2002;36:641-643.

72. Hill S, et al. A case report of seizure induced by bupropion nasal insufflation. *Prim Care Companion J Clin Psychiatry*. 2007;9:67-69.

73. Himei A, Okamura T. Discontinuation syndrome associated with paroxetine in depressed patients: a retrospective analysis of factors involved in the occurrence of the syndrome. *CNS Drugs.* 2006;20:665-672.

74. Howland RH. A critical evaluation of the cardiac toxicity of citalopram: part 1. *J Psychosoc Nurs Ment Health Serv.* 2011;49:13-16.

75. Hui C-K, et al. Mirtazapine-induced hepatotoxicity. *J Clin Gastroenterol.* 2002;35: 270-271.

76. Jacob S, Spinler SA. Hyponatremia associated with selective serotonin-reuptake inhibitors in older adults. *Ann Pharmacother.* 2006;40:1618-1622.

77. Jasiak NM, Bostwick JR. Risk of QT/QTc prolongation among newer non-SSRI antidepressants. *Ann Pharmacother.* 2014;48:1620-1628.

78. Jepsen F, et al. Sustained release bupropion overdose: an important cause of prolonged symptoms after an overdose. *Emerg Med J.* 2003;20:560-561.

79. Jewell DPA, et al. Reversible focal myositis in a patient taking venlafaxine. *Rheumatol Oxf Engl.* 2004;43:1590-1593.

80. Johnston JA, et al. A 102-center prospective study of seizure in association with bupropion. *J Clin Psychiatry.* 1991;52:450-456.

81. Keltner NL, Hall S. Neonatal serotonin syndrome. *Perspect Psychiatr Care.* 2005;41: 88-91.

82. Khoo A-L, et al. Acute liver failure with concurrent bupropion and carbimazole therapy. *Ann Pharmacother.* 2003;37:220-223.

83. Kirby D, Ames D. Hyponatraemia and selective serotonin re-uptake inhibitors in elderly patients. *Int J Geriatr Psychiatry.* 2001;16:484-493.

84. Kirby D, et al. Hyponatraemia in elderly psychiatric patients treated with Selective Serotonin Reuptake Inhibitors and venlafaxine: a retrospective controlled study in an inpatient unit. *Int J Geriatr Psychiatry.* 2002;17:231-237.

85. Kumar VVP, et al. The effect of decontamination procedures on the pharmacodynamics of venlafaxine in overdose. *Br J Clin Pharmacol.* 2011;72:125-132.

86. Kumar VVP, et al. The effect of decontamination procedures on the pharmacokinetics of venlafaxine in overdose. *Clin Pharmacol Ther.* 2009;86:403-410.

87. Labos C, et al. Risk of bleeding associated with combined use of selective serotonin reuptake inhibitors and antiplatelet therapy following acute myocardial infarction. *CMAJ.* 2011;183:1835-1843.

88. Lane RM. SSRI-induced extrapyramidal side-effects and akathisia: implications for treatment. *J Psychopharmacol Oxf Engl.* 1998;12:192-214.

89. Lappin RI, Auchincloss EL. Treatment of the serotonin syndrome with cyproheptadine. *N Engl J Med.* 1994;331:1021-1022.

90. Le Bloc'h Y, et al. Routine therapeutic drug monitoring in patients treated with 10-360 mg/day citalopram. *Ther Drug Monit.* 2003;25:600-608.

91. Lejoyeux M, et al. Prospective evaluation of the serotonin syndrome in depressed inpatients treated with clomipramine. *Acta Psychiatr Scand.* 1993;88:369-371.

92. Lenzer J. Secret US report surfaces on antidepressants in children. *BMJ.* 2004; 329:307.

93. Levinson ML, et al. Adverse effects and drug interactions associated with fluoxetine therapy. *DICP Ann Pharmacother.* 1991;25:657-661.

94. Lineberry TW, et al. Bupropion-induced erythema multiforme. *Mayo Clin Proc.* 2001;76:664-666.

95. Liu P-T, et al. Serotonin syndrome in an octogenarian after switch from fluoxetine to duloxetine. *J Am Geriatr Soc.* 2009;57:2384.

96. LoVecchio F, et al. Outcomes after isolated mirtazapine (Remeron) supratherapeutic ingestions. *J Emerg Med.* 2008;34:77-78.

97. National Institutes of Mental Health. Major Depression Among Adults. http:// www.nimh.nih.gov/health/statistics/prevalence/major-depression-among-adults .shtml.

98. Makowski CT, et al. Naltrexone/bupropion: an investigational combination for weight loss and maintenance. *Obes Facts.* 2011;4:489-494.

99. Marar IE, et al. Effect of paroxetine on plasma vasopressin and water load testing in elderly individuals. *J Geriatr Psychiatry Neurol.* 2000;13:212-216.

100. Mazur JE, et al. Fatality related to a 30-g venlafaxine overdose. *Pharmacotherapy.* 2003;23:1668-1672.

101. McKean J, et al. Breakthrough seizures after starting vilazodone for depression. *Pharmacotherapy.* 2015;35:e6-8.

102. Mégarbane B, et al. Pharmacokinetic/pharmacodynamic modelling of cardiac toxicity in venlafaxine overdose. *Intensive Care Med.* 2007;33:195-196; author reply 197.

103. Miller F, et al. Disseminated intravascular coagulation and acute myoglobinuric renal failure: a consequence of the serotonergic syndrome. *J Clin Psychopharmacol.* 1991;11:277-279.

104. von Moltke LL, et al. Escitalopram (S-citalopram) and its metabolites in vitro: cytochromes mediating biotransformation, inhibitory effects, and comparison to R-citalopram. *Drug Metab Dispos Biol Fate Chem.* 2001;29:1102-1109.

105. Moses-Kolko EL, et al. Neonatal signs after late in utero exposure to serotonin reuptake inhibitors: literature review and implications for clinical applications. *JAMA.* 2005;293:2372-2383.

106. Movig KLL, et al. Serotonergic antidepressants associated with an increased risk for hyponatraemia in the elderly. *Eur J Clin Pharmacol.* 2002;58:143-148.

107. Murata Y, et al. Effects of the serotonin 1A, 2A, 2C, 3A, and 3B and serotonin transporter gene polymorphisms on the occurrence of paroxetine discontinuation syndrome. *J Clin Psychopharmacol.* 2010;30:11-17.

108. Murphy GM, et al. Pharmacogenetics of antidepressant medication intolerance. *Am J Psychiatry.* 2003;160:1830-1835.

109. Nakayama H, et al. Two cases of mild serotonin toxicity via 5-hydroxytryptamine 1A receptor stimulation. *Neuropsychiatr Dis Treat.* 2014;10:283-287.

110. Naranjo CA, Knoke DM. The role of selective serotonin reuptake inhibitors in reducing alcohol consumption. *J Clin Psychiatry.* 2001;62(suppl 20):18-25.

111. Nelson JC. Safety and tolerability of the new antidepressants. *J Clin Psychiatry.* 1997;58(suppl 6):26-31.

112. Nelson LS, et al. Selective serotonin reuptake inhibitor poisoning: an evidence-based consensus guideline for out-of-hospital management. *Clin Toxicol (Phila).* 2007;45:315-332.

113. Nisijima K, et al. Potent serotonin (5-HT)(2A) receptor antagonists completely prevent the development of hyperthermia in an animal model of the 5-HT syndrome. *Brain Res.* 2001;890:23-31.

114. Nutt D. Mirtazapine: pharmacology in relation to adverse effects. *Acta Psychiatr Scand Suppl.* 1997;391:31-37.

115. Oates JA, Sjoerdsma A. Neurologic effects of tryptophan in patients receiving a monoamine oxidase inhibitor. *Neurology.* 1960;10:1076-1078.

116. O'Reardon JP, et al. A randomized, placebo-controlled trial of sertraline in the treatment of night eating syndrome. *Am J Psychiatry.* 2006;163:893-898.

117. Paruchuri P, et al. Rare case of serotonin syndrome with therapeutic doses of paroxetine. *Am J Ther.* 2006;13:550-552.

118. Pascale P, et al. Severe rhabdomyolysis following venlafaxine overdose. *Ther Drug Monit.* 2005;27:562-564.

119. Peng G, et al. Research on the pathological mechanism and drug treatment mechanism of depression. *Curr Neuropharmacol.* 2015;13:514-523.

120. Pereira CE, Goldman-Levine JD. Extended-release venlafaxine-induced alopecia. *Ann Pharmacother.* 2007;41:1084.

121. Perry PJ, Wilborn CA. Serotonin syndrome vs neuroleptic malignant syndrome: a contrast of causes, diagnoses, and management. *Ann Clin Psychiatry.* 2012;24:155-162.

122. Personne M, et al. Citalopram toxicity. *Lancet.* 1997;350:518-519.

123. Personne M, et al. Citalopram overdose—review of cases treated in Swedish hospitals. *J Toxicol Clin Toxicol.* 1997;35:237-240.

124. Pileggi DJ, Cook AM. Neuroleptic malignant syndrome review: focus on treatment and rechallenge. *Ann Pharmacother.* 2016;50:973-981.

125. Pilkinton P, et al. An open label pilot study of adjunctive asenapine for the treatment of posttraumatic stress disorder. *Psychopharmacol Bull.* 2016;46:8-17.

126. Pisani F, et al. Effects of psychotropic drugs on seizure threshold. *Drug Saf.* 2002;25: 91-110.

127. Price JS, et al. A comparison of the post-marketing safety of four selective serotonin re-uptake inhibitors including the investigation of symptoms occurring on withdrawal. *Br J Clin Pharmacol.* 1996;42:757-763.

128. Reeves RR, Ladner ME. Additional evidence of the abuse potential of bupropion. *J Clin Psychopharmacol.* 2013;33:584-585.

129. Reis M, et al. Reference concentrations of antidepressants. A compilation of postmortem and therapeutic levels. *J Anal Toxicol.* 2007;31:254-264.

130. Retz W, et al. Non-fatal mirtazapine overdose. *Int Clin Psychopharmacol.* 1998;13: 277-279.

131. Richelson E. Pharmacology of antidepressants. *Mayo Clin Proc.* 2001;76:511-527.

132. Rudolph RL, Derivan AT. The safety and tolerability of venlafaxine hydrochloride: analysis of the clinical trials database. *J Clin Psychopharmacol.* 1996;16(3 suppl 2):54S-59S; discussion 59S-61S.

133. Sandyk R. L-dopa induced "serotonin syndrome" in a parkinsonian patient on bromocriptine. *J Clin Psychopharmacol.* 1986;6:194-195.

134. Sargent PA, et al. Brain serotonin1A receptor binding measured by positron emission tomography with [11C]WAY-100635: effects of depression and antidepressant treatment. *Arch Gen Psychiatry.* 2000;57:174-180.

135. Schatzberg AF, et al. Serotonin reuptake inhibitor discontinuation syndrome: a hypothetical definition. Discontinuation Consensus panel. *J Clin Psychiatry.* 1997;58(suppl 7): 5-10.

136. Schillevoort I, et al. Extrapyramidal syndromes associated with selective serotonin reuptake inhibitors: a case-control study using spontaneous reports. *Int Clin Psychopharmacol.* 2002;17:75-79.

137. Schweizer E, et al. Placebo-controlled trial of venlafaxine for the treatment of major depression. *J Clin Psychopharmacol.* 1991;11:233-236.

138. Service JA, Waring WS. QT Prolongation and delayed atrioventricular conduction caused by acute ingestion of trazodone. *Clin Toxicol (Phila).* 2008;46:71-73.

139. Shaw MW, Sheard JDH. Fatal venlafaxine overdose with acinar zone 3 liver cell necrosis. *Am J Forensic Med Pathol.* 2005;26:367-368.

140. Sheu Y, et al. SSRI use and risk of fractures among perimenopausal women without mental disorders. *Inj Prev.* 2015;21:397-403.

141. Silverstone PH, et al. Convulsive liability of bupropion hydrochloride metabolites in Swiss albino mice. *Ann Gen Psychiatry.* 2008;7:19.

142. Sirianni AJ, et al. Use of lipid emulsion in the resuscitation of a patient with prolonged cardiovascular collapse after overdose of bupropion and lamotrigine. *Ann Emerg Med.* 2008;51:412-415, 415.e1.

143. Smith B, Prockop DJ. Central-nervous-system effects of ingestin of L-tryptophan by normal subjects. *N Engl J Med.* 1962;267:1338-1341.

144. Spigset O, Hedenmalm K. Hyponatremia in relation to treatment with antidepressants: a survey of reports in the world health organization data base for spontaneous reporting of adverse drug reactions. *Pharmacotherapy*. 1997;17:348-352.

145. Spigset O, Mjorndal T. The effect of fluvoxamine on serum prolactin and serum sodium concentrations: relation to platelet 5-HT2A receptor status. *J Clin Psychopharmacol*. 1997;17:292-297.

146. Spina E, et al. Clinically relevant pharmacokinetic drug interactions with second-generation antidepressants: an update. *Clin Ther*. 2008;30:1206-1227.

147. SSRI antidepressants: extrapyramidal reactions. *Prescrire Int*. 2016;25:100.

148. Starr P, et al. Incidence and onset of delayed seizures after overdoses of extended-release bupropion. *Am J Emerg Med*. 2009;27:911-915.

149. Stedman CAM, et al. Cytochrome P450 2D6 genotype does not predict SSRI (fluoxetine or paroxetine) induced hyponatraemia. *Hum Psychopharmacol*. 2002;17:187-190.

150. Sternbach H. The serotonin syndrome. *Am J Psychiatry*. 1991;148:705-713.

151. Tamam L, Ozpoyraz N. Selective serotonin reuptake inhibitor discontinuation syndrome: a review. *Adv Ther*. 2002;19:17-26.

152. Tarabar AF, et al. Citalopram overdose: late presentation of torsades de pointes (TdP) with cardiac arrest. *J Med Toxicol*. 2008;4:101-105.

153. Thundiyil JG, et al. Evolving epidemiology of drug-induced seizures reported to a Poison Control Center System. *J Med Toxicol*. 2007;3:15-19.

154. Tripathi A, Greenberger PA. Bupropion hydrochloride induced serum sickness-like reaction. *Ann Allergy Asthma Immunol*. 1999;83:165-166.

155. Vanpee D, et al. Seizure and hyponatraemia after overdose of trazadone. *Am J Emerg Med*. 1999;17:430-431.

156. Venlafaxine: more dangerous than most "selective" serotonergic antidepressants. *Prescrire Int*. 2016;25:96-99.

157. Waring WS, et al. Lack of significant toxicity after mirtazapine overdose: a five-year review of cases admitted to a regional toxicology unit. *Clin Toxicol (Phila)*. 2007;45:45-50.

158. Warner CH, et al. Antidepressant discontinuation syndrome. *Am Fam Physician*. 2006;74(3).

159. Wilson E, Lader M. A review of the management of antidepressant discontinuation symptoms. *Ther Adv Psychopharmacol*. 2015;5:357-368.

160. Witchel HJ, et al. Inhibitory actions of the selective serotonin re-uptake inhibitor citalopram on HERG and ventricular L-type calcium currents. *FEBS Lett*. 2002;512:59-66.

161. Wong DT, et al. A new selective inhibitor for uptake of serotonin into synaptosomes of rat brain: 3-(p-trifluoromethylphenoxy). N-methyl-3-phenylpropylamine. *J Pharmacol Exp Ther*. 1975;193:804-811.

162. Yu S-Y, et al. Evaluation of the efficacy and safety of vilazodone for treating major depressive disorder. *Neuropsychiatr Dis Treat*. 2015;11:1957-1965.

163. Zhang Y-W, et al. Control of serotonin transporter phosphorylation by conformational state. *Proc Natl Acad Sci U S A*. 2016;113:E2776-2783.

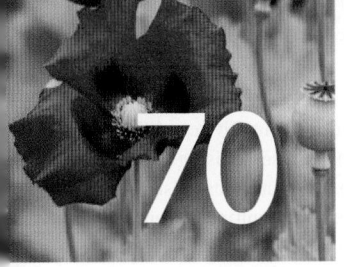

70 LITHIUM

Howard A. Greller

MW	= 6.94 Da
Lithium concentration (serum):	
Therapeutic concentration for	
bipolar depression	= 0.6–1.2 mEq/L (mmol/L)

HISTORY AND EPIDEMIOLOGY

Lithium derives its name from *lithos*, the Greek word for stone, conferred to the element on its discovery in 1817 by the Swedish chemistry student Arfwedson. Lithium is a metal with no charge; lithium salts that are used therapeutically are monovalent cations. By the mid 19th century, lithium salts were used therapeutically for the treatment of gout, as well as mania and depression. The soft drink 7-Up originally contained lithium as its "active ingredient," and during the 1930s and 1940s, it was used as a salt substitute ("Westal") for patients with congestive heart failure until several cases of poisoning led to its discontinuation.[7,17,61] In 1949, Cade "rediscovered" the calming effects of lithium by initially injecting a combination of lithium carbonate and urea (believed a source of mania) into normally "frenetic" guinea pigs and noting the resulting sedation. He subsequently tested it on 10 patients with mania.[46,59] In 1954, Mogens Schou performed a randomized placebo controlled trial of lithium for mania, with promising results.[59,204] However, for 20 years, until reapproved in 1974, lithium was banned by the US Food and Drug Administration in response to multiple reports of toxicity.[7,59]

Lithium is considered the most effective long-term therapy for treatment and prevention of relapse of bipolar affective disorders.[58,80,86,97,207,212] It has a demonstrated antisuicidal effect[57] and the ability to improve both the manic and the depressive symptoms, as well as augment the therapeutic efficacy of other approaches that have failed to achieve symptom remission.[17,51,60,86,92,97,130,135,142,159] Lithium is also effective for compulsive gambling[112,178] and has shown promise for use in neurodegenerative disorders such as Alzheimer disease, ischemic stroke, amyotrophic lateral sclerosis, Huntington disease, multiple sclerosis, and traumatic brain injury.[53,139,152,172,202,240,241]

PHARMACOLOGY

Lithium is the chemically simplest xenobiotic in the modern pharmacopeia. It has a complex mechanism of action that eludes complete explication after more than 50 years of clinical use and study. The exploration of the mechanism of action of lithium is tied to the understanding of the physiology of mood disorders. In the classic model of psychopharmacology, xenobiotics exert their effects through interaction with monoamine neurotransmission, primarily dopamine, norepinephrine, and serotonin, in addition to their secondary signaling systems, primarily G protein–coupled receptors.[28] Clinically, the therapeutic effects of lithium and similar mood-stabilizing pharmaceuticals become evident only after chronic administration, so their mechanism of action is unlikely solely the result of acute biochemical interactions.

One of the central processes involved in the pathogenesis of mood disorders and schizophrenia, as well as the therapeutic effects of lithium, is interaction with the β form of the multifunctional enzyme glycogen synthase kinase 3 (GSK-3β). Glycogen synthase kinase 3 is a serine/threonine kinase at the nexus of multiple signaling pathways. It is the central kinase involved in both neuronal cell survival (through interaction with Akt, a GSK-3β–modifying enzyme) as well as neurogenesis (through interaction with Wnt/β-catenin),[161] in addition to a number of significant processes, including gene transcription, neuronal function, synaptic plasticity, and the circadian cycle, as well as cellular structure, apoptosis, and cell death.[30,52,120,132] In fact, GSK-3β phosphorylates more than 100 substrates, with a suggestion of many more.[30,52,187]

Postmortem tissue from the ventral prefrontal cortex of patients with major depressive disorder showed elevated GSK-3β activity as well as decreased activity in Akt.[121,122] Glycogen synthase kinase 3 is inadequately inhibited in association with mood disorders and is inhibited in humans treated with lithium.[120] Overactivity of GSK-3β is associated with neuronal degeneration and sensitivity to apoptotic stimulation. Dysregulation of GSK-3β is implicated in tumor growth and the neurofibrillary tangles of Alzheimer disease.[65,235] It also is a key regulator of neuronal cell fate, with a proapoptotic effect in many settings.[4,24,26,29,120,144,159,194] It is involved in regulating the activity of Wnt/β-catenin, Jun, and cyclic adenosine monophosphate (cAMP) response element–binding protein (CREB), transcription factors important in embryonic patterning, cell proliferation, neuronal modeling and plasticity, neuronal signal transduction, memory consolidation, and cytoskeletal remodeling. Its other targets include transcription factors such as c-Jun, nuclear factor activated T cells, proteins bound to microtubules (Tau, microtubule-associated protein 1B, kinesin light chain), cell cycle mediators (cyclin D), and metabolic regulators (glycogen synthase, pyruvate dehydrogenase).[161,185,187,197,224] Hypoxia contributes to increased GSK-3β activity, which is counteracted or inhibited with mood-stabilizing drugs. Vascular depression, or depression after stroke, is an organic model of major depression.[113,162] The finding that this form of depression responds similarly to intervention with mood stabilizers lends further support to the GSK-3β hypothesis.[82,94,109,182,234]

Many older generation antipsychotics are known to affect GSK-3β signaling in mice.[145] Glucogen synthase kinase (GSK-3β) activity is regulated not only by first- and second-generation antipsychotics but also through serotonin (5-hydroxytriptamine or 5-HT) neurotransmission and activation of 5-HT$_{2A}$ receptors as well as through monoamine-affecting antidepressants that modify these neurotransmitters.[23,24,26,27,29-31,143] Atypical antipsychotics and antagonists of D$_2$ dopamine receptors, as well as antagonism of 5-HT$_{2A}$ serotonin receptors, exert some of their utility through inhibition of GSK-3β activity.[29,30] Lithium modulates dopamine neurotransmission both pre- and postsynaptically, reducing the functional output of the mesolimbic system. Abnormal functioning of this pathway results in mania in animal models.[28,49]

The link between neuropsychiatric illness and these centrally placed mediators of signaling comes from exploration of dopamine neurotransmission (Fig. 70–1). Scaffolding proteins, the β-arrestins, are traditionally associated with the termination of G protein–coupled receptor (GPCR) signaling and desensitization. After a receptor is stimulated, GPCRs are phosphorylated, leading to the β-arrestin recruitment that uncouples the receptor from the G protein and leads to GPCR internalization. β-Arrestins also act as scaffolds for the formation of a protein complex that allows for GPCRs to signal independently from G proteins.[24,26,28,29,49] Dopaminergic neurotransmission through GPCRs is mediated through a complex that involves Akt, β-arrestin2 (βArr2) and protein phosphatase 2A (PP2A). Akt is a serine/threonine kinase that is additionally regulated through phosphatidylinositol-mediated signaling.[30] Akt activity results from an equilibrium between phosphorylation (activation) and dephosphorylation (inactivation).[27] Regulation of GSK-3β activity is achieved through phosphorylation of its *N*-terminal serine residue, leading to inhibition.[144] The Akt–βArr2–PP2A complex, when activated, dephosphorylates (deactivates) Akt, which leads to the activation of GSK-3β through loss of inhibition (loss of phosphorylation).[25,27,30,67,82]

Lithium is a direct inhibitor of GSK-3β that can also inhibit its activity indirectly through a mechanism involving Akt activation.[26,27,54,120] Lithium activates Akt by disrupting assembly of the Akt–βArr2–PP2A complex through displacement of the magnesium cofactor required for assembly.[23,26,27,224]

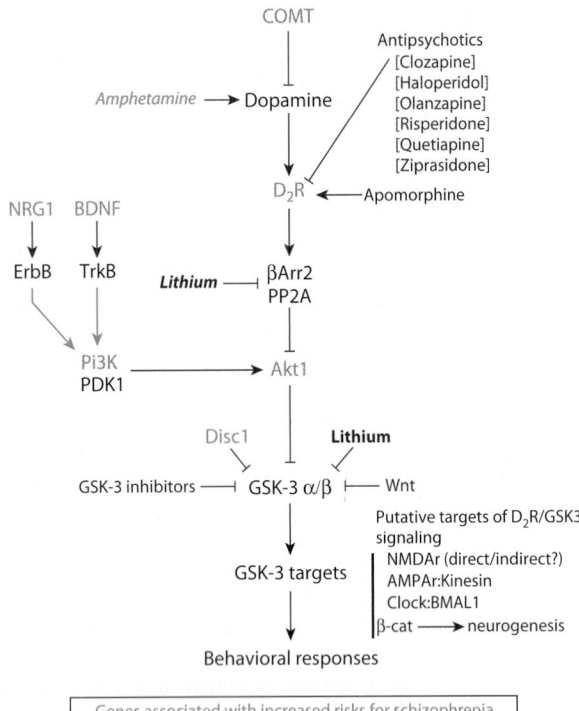

FIGURE 70–1. Regulation of GSK-3 (glycogen synthase kinase 3) and Akt (GSK-3β–modifying enzyme) signaling by psychoactive drugs and related network of gene products associated with mental disorders. Proteins labeled in orange are the product of genes associated with an increased risk of developing schizophrenia or bipolar disorders. Blue arrows indicate activation, and the red T arrows indicate inhibition. Black arrows indicate actions that can either activate or inhibit the function of specific substrates. Behavioral changes in dopaminergic responses have been reported in Akt1 and β-arrestin 2 knock out mice and in GSK-3β–HET mice. Growth factors, including neurotrophins, activate Akt, which phosphorylates, and inhibits GSK-3, allowing activation of downstream effectors to promote cell survival. Wnt (wingless-related integration site) inhibits GSK-3, stabilizing β-catenin, which activates Wnt target genes, and promotes neurogenesis.[224] β-cat = β-catenin; COMT = catechol-O-methyltransferase; D₂R = D₂ dopamine receptor; Disc1 = disrupted-in-schizophrenia 1; NRG1 = neuregulin 1; PDK1 = phosphatidylinositol-dependent kinase 1; Pi3K = phosphatidylinositol 3-kinase. *(Reproduced with permission from Beaulieu JM, Gainetdinov RR. The physiology, signaling, and pharmacology of dopamine receptors. Pharmacol Rev. 2011 Mar;63(1):182-217.)*

Through disruption of this complex, which normally inactivates Akt, lithium promotes Akt activation, leading to increased phosphorylation and subsequent inactivation of GSK-3β. This is demonstrated in β-arrestin knockout mice, which, unable to create this complex, are resistant to the behavioral effects of lithium.[27,30,82,120] Thus, lithium demonstrates both direct and indirect mechanisms of GSK-3β inhibition.

Identification of the Akt–βArr2–PP2A signaling complex as a target of lithium lends credence to the use of lithium as an adjunct to enhance the action of atypical antipsychotics and antidepressants in poorly responsive subjects by acting through Akt–GSK-3β signaling.[26,27,120]

Inhibition of GSK-3β by lithium is thought to be neuroprotective by modifying the downstream targets and effectors of GSK-3β activity.[4,23,27,82,109,182,196] Lithium is implicated in the neuroprotective modulation of the bcl-2 gene, which is known for its role in preventing apoptosis and in downregulation of the proapoptotic protein p53. Lithium increases bcl-2 concentrations in cultured nervous tissue of both rats and humans.[55,157] Additional support comes from patients undergoing long-term therapy with either lithium or valproic acid (VPA) whose prefrontal cortex volumes are significantly greater than in untreated patients, suggesting a protective effect in humans.[53,196] Further evidence points toward a neuroprotective and neurotrophic effect of lithium with

evidence to support benefit in such diverse neurodegenerative conditions as Parkinson disease (in a mice model of Parkinson disease using N-methyl-4-pheynyl-1,2,3,6-tetrahydropyridine {MPTP}),[239] Huntington disease,[152,202] amyotrophic lateral sclerosis (ALS),[79] stroke and multiple sclerosis,[23,53] traumatic brain injury,[139,240,241] and Alzheimer disease.[4,20,29,30,47,159,166]

The interplay among lithium, GSK-3β, and the Akt pathway and all of its downstream targets is one major link between mood disorder and the effects of lithium. The other is the interaction between lithium and the Wnt pathway, also mediated through the interaction of lithium and GSK-3β (Fig. 70–1). Glucogen synthase kinase (GSK-3β) constitutively antagonizes Wnt signaling and must be inhibited for the pathway to function. Wnt modulates transcription through β-catenin signaling in the nucleus. β-Catenin is involved in a cycle of synthesis and destruction mediated through the β-catenin destruction complex, composed of scaffolding proteins, including axin and tumor suppressor adenomatous polyposis coli (APC). Wnt inhibits GSK-3β, stabilizing and promoting β-catenin signaling. Lithium, through its effects on GSK-3β does the same, enhancing cell survival. Wnt signaling removes APC from the complex and relocalizes the other components to the plasma membrane, leading to stabilization of β-catenin, allowing it to enter the nucleus and modulate transcription.[197,224]

It is unlikely that lithium has a single mechanism of action. Other mechanisms, such as the inhibition of inositol monophosphatases, contribute to its pleiotropic effects on behavior. Evidence has bridged the current molecular targets and downstream regulators of the effects of lithium with the classic proposed mechanism of action, the inositol-depletion hypothesis, one of the first proposed mechanisms of action of lithium.[109] Inositol is a six-carbon sugar that forms the backbone of a number of cellular signaling mechanisms. Lithium treatment results in a decreased myoinositol (the most biologically active stereoisomer of inositol) concentration in the cerebral cortex.[36,109,159] Abnormalities in regional brain myoinositol concentrations are found in patients with bipolar disorder. This theory is partially supported by experimental magnetic resonance spectroscopy data.[213,238] Myoinositol is phosphorylated to form phosphatidyl inositol (PIP), which is further phosphorylated and combined with diacylglycerol (DAG) to form phosphatidyl 4,5-bisphosphate (PIP-2). Upon stimulation of a cell, GPCRs activate phospholipase C (PLC), which hydrolyzes PIP-2 to release the secondary messengers DAG and inositol 1,4,5-trisphosphate (IP3).[37,108] Each of these secondary messengers in turn initiates a cascade of events, including activation of protein kinase C, which is important for calcium homeostasis and neurotransmitter release,[159,213] as well as independent mobilization and regulation of intracellular calcium.[181,196,213] Many extracellular signals, including some serotonin receptor subtypes, neurotrophin signaling pathways, receptor tyrosine kinase pathways, and G protein–mediated signaling, activate PLC to exert their actions.[96,186,187]

Serial dephosphorylation of IP3 leads to regeneration of myoinositol and recycling of the inositol pool. Two enzymes involved in this pathway are inhibited by lithium. The first enzyme, inositol 1,4-bisphosphate 1-phosphatase (IPPase), dephosphorylates the bisphosphate to inositol monophosphate (IMP). The second enzyme, inositol 1-monophosphatase (IMPase), dephosphorylates IMP to myoinositol[4] (Fig. 70–2).

Lithium inhibits IMPase in an uncompetitive fashion by binding to the enzyme–substrate complex and preventing the release of phosphate. It performs this function by displacing a magnesium ion from the active site after hydrolysis similar to its effects on GSK-3β.[54] Uncompetitive inhibitors only bind to the enzyme–substrate complex, inhibiting the reaction at that point; the higher the concentration of the substrate, the more the enzyme is inhibited.[82,102,154] Uncompetitive inhibitor kinetics are related proportionally to the concentration of the enzyme–substrate complex and cannot be overcome by increasing the concentration of the substrate, unlike a competitive inhibitor.[82,102,154] The nature of the action of lithium serves as a regulator to preferentially block pathologic signaling caused by excessive myoinositol while leaving the normal signaling intact. As described, IMPase is an important step in the cellular recycling of the inositol pool and is inhibited by lithium.

Myoinositol is also generated de novo from glucose-6-phosphate by inositol synthase, which forms IMP. The inhibition of IMPase by lithium

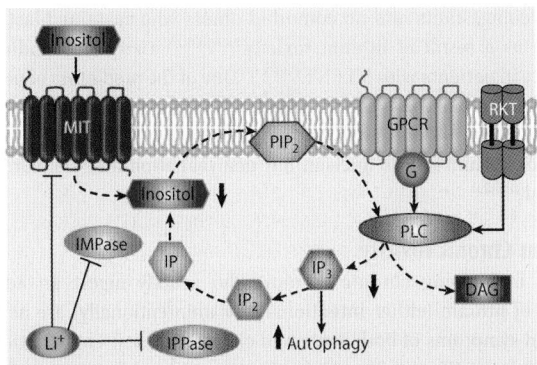

FIGURE 70–2. The actions of lithium on inositol depletion and autophagy induction. Extracellular signal binding to its cell surface receptor, either G protein–coupled receptor (GPCR) or RTK, activates phospholipase C (PLC), which hydrolyzes the phospholipid phosphatidyl bisphosphate (PIP$_2$) to yield second messengers inositol triphosphate (IP$_3$) and diacylglycerol (DAG). Inositol triphosphate is recycled by enzymes inositol bisphosphate phosphatase (IPPase) and inositol monophosphatase (IMPase) and converted to inositol (mainly myoinositol), which is required for PIP$_2$ resynthesis. Lithium decreases intracellular inositol concentrations by directly inhibiting IPPase, IMPase, and myoinositol transporter (MIT) that uptakes extracellular inositol. Decreased intracellular inositol concentrations are expected to subsequently reduce PIP$_2$ and prevent the formation of IP$_3$ and DAG, thus blocking transmembrane signaling and triggering the induction of autophagy. Lines with solid arrows represent stimulatory connections; lines with flattened ends represent inhibitory connections. Dashed lines represent pathways with reduced activity as a result of lithium treatment. IP = inositol monophosphate; IP$_2$ = inositol bisphosphate. *(Reproduced with permission from Chiu CT, Chuang DM. Molecular actions and therapeutic potential of lithium in preclinical and clinical studies of CNS disorders. Pharmacol Ther. 2010 Nov;128(2):281-304.)*

subsequently leads to myoinositol depletion by preventing the conversion of the newly synthesized IMP to myoinositol. Valproic acid also inhibits inositol synthase, illustrating a potential mechanism for the synergy of these complementary mood stabilizers.[71,141] A third mechanism of intracellular diminution of inositol by lithium (as well as VPA and carbamazepine) is by reducing the activity and transcription of the sodium myoinositol transporter, preventing the uptake of exogenous myoinositol by the cell.[109]

The result of these effects is depletion of the inositol pool available to the cell, causing a series of events at different points in the signal transduction cascade that leads to differential gene transcription and expression. This sequence ultimately is responsible for some of the observed clinical effects of lithium on the central nervous system (CNS).[209] Experimental data using dextroamphetamine as a model for clinical mania demonstrate increased regional inositol signaling in the human brain that is attenuated by pretreatment with lithium, lending support to the hypothesis.[34,95]

The inositol depletion hypothesis, an original attempt to explain in molecular terms the therapeutic effects of lithium, does not fully elucidate nor replicate clinical disease or response to therapy. In vivo studies with more drastic inositol depletion than that which occurs from lithium therapy fail to replicate predicted behavioral patterns. Studies in knockout mice lacking various isoforms of inositol monophosphatase fail to replicate the antidepressant or antimanic effects of lithium. However, the model remains attractive, and the flaws may represent species variation with validity more in humans with bipolar disorder than the mouse model illustrates.[23,159,209] There is a synergy with the other proposed mechanisms of the effects of lithium. In a yeast model, GSK-3β is required for de novo inositol synthesis, and the loss of GSK-3β activity leads to inositol depletion. This finding links two of the targets of not only lithium but other mood stabilizers as well.[11,64]

In summary, although the precise mechanism of action is unknown, some common features of investigation have emerged. The potential targets, widely found and disparate in function, all seem to be inhibited by lithium in an uncompetitive fashion, most commonly through displacement of a divalent cation, usually Mg^{2+}. The systems affected by this inhibition vary widely. Downstream targets modulate secondary cell messengers and intracellular

signal transduction, transcription factors and gene expression, and neuronal plasticity and cellular differentiation. Further study is needed to elucidate the complex interaction of these pathways with the action of lithium to form an integrated hypothesis, along with the disruption that occurs in cases of lithium toxicity.

PHARMACOKINETICS AND TOXICOKINETICS

Lithium has a volume of distribution of between 0.6 and 0.9 L/kg. It has no discernible protein binding and distributes freely in total body water, with the exception of the cerebrospinal fluid (CSF), from which it is actively extruded.[72,98,198] The extrusion is believed to occur through active transport mechanism involving sodium–lithium exchange at the arachnoid processes.[70] Immediate-release preparations of lithium are rapidly absorbed from the gastrointestinal (GI) tract, and peak serum concentrations are achieved within 1 to 2 hours. Sustained-release products demonstrate variable absorption, with a delay to peak of 4 to 5 hours.[98,223] In overdose, a longer delay to peak concentrations and multiple peaks are reported.[69,98] Chronic therapy prolongs the elimination of lithium, as does advancing age.[98] Although lithium is rapidly absorbed, tissue distribution is a complex phenomenon, with a significant delay to achieve steady state, similar to digoxin. Lithium exhibits preferential uptake into the kidney, thyroid, bone, and other organs and tissues such as the liver and muscle. Lithium distribution into the brain can take up to 24 hours to reach equilibrium. Lithium is concentrated in red blood cells (RBCs) by both passive diffusion and active transport. Although the RBC concentration correlates closely with the brain concentration, this does not appear to be clinically useful.[48] The pharmacokinetic profile of lithium is described as an open, two-compartment model.[72,98]

Each 300-mg lithium carbonate tablet contains 8.12 mEq of lithium.[98] Ingestion of a single 300-mg tablet is expected to increase the serum lithium concentration by approximately 0.1 to 0.3 mEq/L (assuming a volume of distribution of approximately 0.6–0.9 L/kg and a patient weight of 50–100 kg).

Lithium is not metabolized and is eliminated almost entirely (95%) by the kidneys, with a small amount eliminated in the feces.[72] Lithium is also be found in sweat, saliva, and breast milk.[68,228] In an adult with normal kidney function, lithium clearance varies from 10 to 40 mL/min.[98,222] Given the elimination of lithium being primarily renal, when at steady state, total body clearance equals renal clearance.

Lithium is handled by the kidneys much in the same way as sodium. Lithium is freely filtered, and more than 80% is reabsorbed by the proximal tubule. There is also a small amount reabsorbed in the loop of Henle and distal tubule.[39,81,136,222] Lithium excretion is therefore dependent on factors that affect the glomerular filtration rate (GFR) or decrease serum sodium concentration. Any condition that makes the kidney sodium avid, such as volume depletion or salt restriction, increases lithium reabsorption in the proximal tubule.[98,222] Thus, risk factors for accumulation of lithium and subsequent development of toxicity include advanced age (decrease in GFR); use of thiazide diuretics, nonsteroidal antiinflammatory drugs (NSAIDs), or angiotensin-converting enzyme (ACE) inhibitors and angiotensin-receptor blockers (ARBs); decreased sodium intake; and low-output heart failure.[16,163,229]

The therapeutic index of lithium is narrow. The generally accepted steady-state therapeutic range of serum lithium concentrations is 0.6 to 1.0 mmol/L, although much disagreement exists about whether this serum concentration truly reflects therapeutic efficacy.[80,98,147] A detailed review of 246 studies examining long-term treatment of mood disorders found that although the target concentration should be individualized, tighter control (0.6–0.8 mmol/L) was associated with the best efficacy with the most tolerated side effect profile.[208] Both in therapeutic and overdose situations, clinical signs and symptoms seem to be a more valuable indicator of brain lithium concentrations than serum measurements.[18,169]

CLINICAL MANIFESTATIONS

Similar to other xenobiotics having prolonged redistributive phases and tissue burdens, lithium toxicity is characteristically divided into three main categories: acute, acute on chronic, and chronic. In acute lithium toxicity, the patient has no body burden of lithium present at the time of ingestion. The toxicity that develops depends on the amount ingested, along with rates of absorption, distribution, and elimination. In chronic toxicity, the patient has a stable body burden of lithium as the serum concentration is maintained in the therapeutic range, and then some factor disturbs this balance, either by enhancing absorption, or more commonly, decreasing elimination. For chronic users of lithium, small perturbations in the equilibrium between intake and elimination often leads to toxicity. In acute-on-chronic toxicity, the patient ingests an increased amount of lithium (intentionally or unintentionally) in the setting of a stable body burden. With tissue saturation, any additional lithium leads to signs and symptoms of toxicity.

Acute Toxicity

Acute ingestions of lithium salts produce clinical findings similar to that of ingestions of other metal salts, with predominant early GI effects. Nausea, vomiting, and diarrhea are prevalent. Significant volume losses may result, leading patients to complain of lightheadedness, dizziness, and orthostasis. Neurologic manifestations occur several hours after ingestion in acute toxicity because the lithium redistributes slowly into the CNS from the serum.

Chronic Toxicity

Lithium is primarily a neurotoxin. The earliest case reports of lithium toxicity described predominantly neurologic symptoms.[215,231] Most important, neurotoxicity does not precisely correlate with serum concentrations.[73,195] The initial clinical condition of the patient and the duration of exposure to an elevated concentration are more closely predictive of outcome than the initial serum lithium concentration.[1,8,104,106,206]

Approximately 27% of patients using lithium develop tremor, making this one of the most common movement disorders encountered in clinical practice.[165] Tremor is positively correlated with age, male sex, and concomitant use of neuroleptics and other antidepressants.[12,227] It may also be the most common drug-induced tremor encountered clinically, although it is typically mild.[170] The tremor is classified as a postural tremor and subcategorized as an exaggerated physiologic tremor, with a frequency of 8 to 12 Hz most commonly seen in the hands.[12] Drug-induced Parkinsonism also rarely occurs.[110] The mechanism that leads to development of the tremor is unknown.

The tremor diminishes over time with continued therapy but increases with toxicity. Other findings of chronic toxicity include fasciculations, hyperreflexia, choreoathetoid movements, clonus, dysarthria, nystagmus, and ataxia.[165,223] The mental status is often altered and progresses from confusion to stupor, coma, and seizures.[147,163] Electroencephalographic (EEG) changes are most frequently reported as "slowing."[105,210] The progression of these symptoms follows no order, and any patient undergoing chronic therapy can have one or any combination of these features. In rats, lithium overdose consistently induced encephalopathy with increasing severity as per the pattern of exposure. The occurrence of seizures and fatality paralleled the severity of the encephalopathy. The neurotoxic effects of lithium, as evidenced by EEG abnormalities and clinical signs and symptoms outlast the normalization of serum lithium concentrations.[73,105]

The syndrome of irreversible lithium-effectuated neurotoxicity (SILENT) is a descriptive syndrome of the irreversible neurologic and neuropsychiatric sequelae of lithium toxicity.[1,103,116,183] The syndrome of irreversible lithium-effectuated neurotoxicity is defined as neurologic dysfunction that is caused by lithium in the absence of prior neurologic illness and persists for at least 2 months after cessation of the drug. Case reports support these findings and this definition. However, as is true in most case reports, confounders make wide applicability of the findings difficult. Because of the polypharmacy prevalent in psychiatry, long-term neurologic sequelae attributed to lithium are frequently described in patients using lithium in combination with other xenobiotics, such as haloperidol, chlorpromazine, carbamazepine, phenytoin, aspirin, VPA, amitriptyline, β-adrenergic antagonists, calcium channel blockers, angiotensin-converting enzyme inhibitors, diuretics, and NSAIDs.[1,76,103,107,156,168] However, there exist reports of patients using lithium

without coingestants and no comorbid illness who sustained lasting dysfunction as a result of lithium toxicity.[2,8,127,175,206] Cerebellar findings predominate in patients with SILENT.[1-3,158,183] One of the predictors of persistent neurologic dysfunction is the concomitant finding of hyperpyrexia, an ominous finding in patients with lithium toxicity.[99,158] The mechanism of the persistent dysfunction is unclear, but demyelination and cellular loss are proposed.[1,158,203]

Acute-on-Chronic Toxicity

Patients undergoing chronic therapy who acutely ingest an additional amount of lithium (either intentionally or unintentionally) are at risk for signs and symptoms of both acute and chronic toxicity. These patients display prominent GI and neurologic effects, which adds some confusion to diagnosis and management. Serum lithium concentrations in cases of acute or chronic toxicity are often difficult to interpret.

Other Systemic Manifestations of Chronic Lithium Therapy

The most common adverse effect of chronic lithium therapy is nephrogenic diabetes insipidus (NDI), which can develop within weeks of the initiation of therapy and affects up to 40% of patients (Chap. 12).[100,174]

Lithium inhibits the transport of sodium through the amiloride-sensitive epithelial sodium channel (ENaC), which is also the main route of entry for lithium. Lithium has a twofold higher affinity than sodium for entry through this channel, without a corresponding means of extrusion and thus becomes concentrated intracellularly.[100,174] Lithium inhibits magnesium-dependent G proteins that activate vasopressin-sensitive adenylate cyclase, leading to decreased generation of cAMP in the cell membranes of distal tubular cells.[38,56,221,230] Decreased cAMP leads to reduced expression and translocation of the vasopressin-regulated water channel aquaporin-2 (AQP2), making the distal tubules resistant to the action of vasopressin, and thus unable to concentrate urine.[5,38,146,232] There is a potential mechanistic overlap with GSK-3β. With GSK-3β inhibition by lithium, the tonic inhibition of cyclooxygenase-2 (COX-2) is removed, and increased COX-2 activity leads to increased prostaglandin expression in the renal medulla. Increased prostaglandin expression is important in NDI through regulation of glomerular blood flow,[188,189] as well as increasing the degradation of AQP2, further decreasing the ability to form a concentrated urine.[128,129,188,189]

Chronic lithium therapy is associated with chronic tubulointerstitial nephropathy, as manifested by the development of acute kidney injury (AKI) and chronic kidney disease (CKD) with little or no proteinuria and biopsy findings of tubular cysts. This association was demonstrated in a biopsy-based study of 24 chronically treated patients, although the overall prevalence of this condition is low.[100] Long-term treatment (> 10 years) is associated with the development of CKD, including a small percentage of chronic kidney failure.[6,125]

Lithium causes a number of endocrine disorders. The most prevalent endocrine manifestation of chronic lithium therapy is hypothyroidism, which has a multifactorial etiology.[44] Lithium is selectively concentrated in the thyroid gland and competes for iodide transport, synthesis of triiodothyronine (T_3), responsiveness of the gland to thyroid-stimulating hormone (TSH), release of T_3 and tetraiodothyronine (T_4), and peripheral conversion of T_4 to T_3.[44,85] Lithium decreases the responsiveness of peripheral tissues to T_3 and increases antithyroglobulin antibodies if already present, although it does not induce development de novo (Fig. 53–1).[13,134,173] Although hypothyroidism is most common, hyperthyroidism and thyrotoxicosis are also reported.[33,41,110,220] Hyperthyroidism, by altering proximal tubule function, leads to decreased lithium excretion.[21] Thus, hyperthyroidism leads to chronic lithium toxicity through impaired elimination, and the elevated lithium concentrations often can mask the manifestations of hyperthyroidism.[19,173] Interestingly, because lithium inhibits the release of thyroid hormone, it has been used as an adjunctive therapy for hyperthyroidism.[101,134]

The combination of hyperparathyroidism and hypercalcemia is frequently reported in patients receiving chronic lithium therapy, most commonly in older women. The mechanism is thought to be modification of calcium feedback on parathyroid hormone release through alteration of a calcium-sensing receptor that prevents suppression of parathyroid hormone release in response to elevated calcium,[191] although stimulation of parathyroid hormone release, parathyroid gland hyperplasia, and adenomas are alternative suggested mechanisms.[10,140,160,218]

Lithium is associated with a number of electrocardiographic (ECG) abnormalities, although the evidence for significant toxicity is lacking. Most reports are uncontrolled case reports without corroborating experimental data or biologic plausibility. The most commonly reported manifestation is T-wave flattening or inversion, primarily in the precordial leads,[177] although prolongation of the QT interval is also noted.[131,226] One study associated elevated serum lithium concentrations with QT interval prolongation above 440 ms, although the number of patients studied was small.[115] Associations exist between lithium and sinoatrial dysfunction, with resultant bradycardia.[9,91,176,211,219] However, many of these cases had either electrolyte disturbances or multiple other cardioactive xenobiotics involved that would be more likely causative.[50,155,171,211,219,233] Numerous case reports link lithium with an ECG pattern that is consistent with a myocardial infarction, without biochemical markers of injury.[123,124,184] Additional case reports link lithium to ventricular dysrhythmias.[42] Lithium blocks cardiac sodium channels in a transfected Chinese hamster ovary cell, which is the putative link between lithium therapy and the unmasking of a Brugada pattern and cardiomyopathy.[50,62,89,211,219,233] For the most part, lithium has few consequential effects on cardiac function, even in overdose, and malignant dysrhythmias or significant dysfunction are very uncommon.

Developmentally, in utero exposure to lithium increases the incidence of congenital heart defects (approximately 1 additional case per 100 live births), specifically right ventricular outflow obstructions (including Ebstein abnormality), in a dose-dependent fashion.[68,179,237] Additionally, many effects similar to those that occur in patients undergoing chronic therapy are found in infants exposed in utero, including thyroid disease and neurotoxicity.[88]

Lithium causes a leukocytosis and an increase in neutrophils. It was proposed as an adjunct to chemotherapy-induced neutropenia, other marrow suppressive therapies, and acquired immunodeficiency syndrome (AIDS).[63] Although lithium increases the total neutrophil count, no improved clinical outcomes are documented, and its use is now superseded by recombinant colony-stimulating factors.[77,182,193]

DIAGNOSTIC TESTING

Because of the prevalence of lithium use, therapeutic drug monitoring is readily available in most settings, and serum concentrations are usually readily obtainable.[236] A lithium concentration should be determined upon patient presentation and serial measurements obtained in most instances in which overdose or toxicity is likely, especially after ingestion of sustained-release preparations. Emphasis should be placed on the lithium concentration as a marker of exposure and response to therapy but not necessarily as a determinant of toxicity or treatment. The history, symptoms, and clinical signs, rather than the absolute lithium concentration, should guide therapy. The sample must be sent in an appropriate lithium-free tube because use of lithiated-heparin tubes will lead to false-positive results, up to an additional 4 mEq/L.[137] Serum electrolyte concentrations and kidney function should be assessed because kidney function is important in determining the need for more aggressive therapy, such as hemodialysis. If the patient is hypernatremic, NDI should be suspected, and determinations of serum and urine osmolarity and electrolytes help confirm the diagnosis (Chap. 12). If thyroid disease is suspected, thyroid function tests should be obtained. If a deliberate ingestion has occurred, a serum acetaminophen concentration should be obtained. An ECG is also indicated. The complete blood count may indicate a leukocytosis as a stress response or caused by the hematologic effects of lithium.

MANAGEMENT

The initial management and stabilization should begin with assessment and, if necessary, support of airway, breathing, and circulation. Lithium rarely, if ever, affects the patient's airway or breathing, although coingestants may.

Emesis, which occurs with significant frequency after acute exposure, may lead to aspiration and respiratory compromise. After the patient is stable, the characteristics of the exposure should be determined while the physical examination and laboratory assessment commence. The formulation and nature of the product should be ascertained and, most important, identified as immediate- or sustained-release. Whether or not lithium is part of the patient's medication regimen is helpful to determine whether the ingestion is acute, acute on chronic, or chronic.

Gastrointestinal Decontamination

For patients who present after an acute overdose or an acute-on-chronic overdose, a risk benefit analysis of GI decontamination must be undertaken. Two factors should be considered. With an acute overdose and predominance of early GI symptoms, including emesis, self-decontamination may already have occurred. Second, immediate-release preparations are often rapidly absorbed and may not lend themselves to GI evacuation.

Gastrointestinal decontamination options are limited. Lithium salts are monovalent do not bind readily to activated charcoal.[149] Because of the danger of a depressed level of consciousness, potential loss of protective airway reflexes, and emesis, no beneficial effect from activated charcoal is expected unless indicated for treatment of a coingestant. Orogastric lavage has a limited role in the acute management of a patient with a lithium overdose but remains of reasonable benefit early in the clinical course after a substantial ingestion. Immediate-release preparations of lithium are rapidly absorbed and typically produce emesis, obviating the role of lavage, and sustained-release formulations of lithium (ie, controlled-release tablets) are compounded in a slowly dissolving film-coated formulation, often making the tablet too large to fit through even the largest lavage tube.

Sodium polystyrene sulfonate (SPS) is a cationic exchange resin often used for the treatment of severe hyperkalemia. It binds potassium in exchange for sodium, allowing elimination of excess potassium in the feces. Because of the ionic similarity between potassium and lithium, use of SPS has been proposed for decontamination of patients being treated for lithium toxicity. A number of models have examined the effectiveness of this technique.[149-151] Use of SPS has many theoretical benefits, including demonstrated effectiveness of lithium binding in vitro compared with activated charcoal and the ability of orally administered SPS to reduce serum concentrations of intravenously administered lithium in mice.[149] Unfortunately, the finding that doses used to increase lithium elimination also lead to significant hypokalemia in human participants limits the application of this technique.[201] In a murine model, potassium supplementation with SPS was found to mitigate this process but only at the expense of elevating lithium concentrations.[151] Two reports in the literature demonstrate increased lithium elimination with SPS, one in a healthy volunteer and another in a patient with an acute overdose. However, the serum potassium concentration was not reported in either case.[87] In a retrospective cohort review of 12 chronically poisoned patients, it was suggested that SPS reduced the elimination half-life of lithium by 50%. However, many of the patients had altered kidney function that was corrected at the same time as the intervention (which was not standardized), and no clinical outcomes were reported.[90] We therefore recommend against the routine use of SPS in the management of the lithium-poisoned patients.

Whole-bowel irrigation (WBI) is the only GI decontamination that has some demonstrated efficacy in eliminating lithium from volunteers. In one of the few clinical trials of WBI, the serum lithium concentrations of 10 normal volunteers who ingested sustained-release lithium carbonate were plotted against time over a 72-hour period. In the second phase of the trial, when the volunteers received 2 L/h of polyethylene glycol solution 1 hour after the ingestion, there was a significant reduction (67%) in the serum concentration, even as early as 1 hour after the therapeutic intervention.[214] Whole-bowel irrigation is recommended for patients manifesting significant toxicity (ie, neurologic dysfunction) and who have ingested sustained-release lithium preparations and have no contraindications (eg, protected airway, no obstruction or ileus) (Antidotes in Depth: A2).

Fluid and Electrolytes

The critical initial management of the lithium-poisoned patient should focus on restoration of intravascular volume, both in those with acute poisonings with GI losses and in chronic poisonings with toxic effects that are often the result of disturbances of kidney function and lithium elimination. Many patients with lithium toxicity have volume-responsive decreases in kidney function,[190] which we recommend to manage with infusion of 0.9% sodium chloride solution at 1.5 to 2 times the maintenance rate.[40,138] This therapy increases renal perfusion, and GFR, which will increase lithium elimination. When the kidney is sodium avid (as in volume depletion) it will retain lithium. Increased intravascular volume will reduce this retention and increase the elimination of lithium. Urine output must be closely monitored and any electrolyte abnormalities corrected. Caution must be used in patients with prerenal AKI, CKD, and congestive heart failure. Monitoring for the development of hypernatremia in patients suspected of having NDI is critical because this occurs in approximately 55% of patients on long-term therapy.[146,199,222]

Lithium-induced NDI is sometimes reversed by discontinuation of the drug and repletion of electrolytes and water, although it may be permanent.[128,222] Use of amiloride, as well as acetazolamide, to mitigate lithium-induced polyuria is described, although the potential for volume contraction and stimulation of lithium reabsorption prevents recommendation of this drug as a routine adjunct to acute care.[33,75,93,128,190] A novel proposed therapeutic, the direct renin inhibitor aliskiren, improved the urinary concentrating defect in lithium-treated mice. Aliskiren upregulated AQP2 protein expression in inner medullary collecting duct principal cells and prevented lithium-induced NDI.[148]

We recommend against any attempt to enhance elimination of lithium by forced diuresis using loop diuretics (furosemide), osmotic agents (mannitol), carbonic anhydrase inhibitors (acetazolamide), or phosphodiesterase inhibitors (aminophylline). An initial small increase in elimination may be achieved, but typically salt and water depletion subsequently developed followed by increased lithium retention.[39] We also recommend against sodium bicarbonate administration for urinary alkalinization because it does not significantly increase elimination over volume expansion with sodium chloride and may lead to hypokalemia, alkalemia, and fluid overload.

Extracorporeal Drug Removal

Lithium has pharmacokinetic properties that make it amenable to extracorporeal removal,[22,74,114,118,136] and with these characteristics, it would seem to be an ideal candidate for hemodialysis. In fact, hemodialysis is often recommended for treatment of acute, acute-on-chronic, and chronic lithium toxicity.[14,74,117,180,223] The original criteria for hemodialysis originated from a case series of 23 patients and a review of 100 other patients published in 1978, which was before the introduction of sustained-release products.[106] Those recommendations were never prospectively evaluated or subsequently reevaluated.[15,74,84]

Some characteristics of lithium make impactful extracorporeal elimination difficult. Lithium is predominantly localized intracellularly and diffuses slowly across cell membranes.[74] When traditional intermittent hemodialysis is used for patients with chronic exposures, clearance of the blood compartment is often followed by a rebound phenomenon of redistribution from tissue stores, leading to recurrent increased serum concentrations. The clinical significance of this rebound is uncertain, but without additional elimination, this can redistribute back into target tissues.[43] There have only been three cases reported of clinical deterioration after rebound from an extracorporeal elimination method, likely as a result of failed decontamination in an extended-release ingestion and ongoing absorption.[41,45,83] An additional complicating factor is that the brain, the "target organ" of toxicity, is not directly amenable to a rapid artificial elimination process. Attempts have been made to correlate the serum concentration with the lithium concentration in the CSF and brain. But in the few studies in which CSF concentrations were obtained, although serum and CSF lithium concentrations correlated, brain concentrations and clinical effects did not.[111,119] Magnetic resonance spectroscopy studies of bipolar patients with steady-state lithium concentrations demonstrated a significant

variability between brain and serum concentrations, especially within the therapeutic range.[78,192] In addition, because of the toxicokinetic profile of lithium, serum concentrations do not correlate well with toxicity.[73,97,119,223]

Consensus exists regarding when to perform an extracorporeal elimination technique (extracorporeal treatment {ECTR}). The Extracorporeal Treatments in Poisoning Workgroup (ExTRIP) performed an extensive analysis of the data available regarding lithium. Their consensus provides the following analysis: "ECTR is recommended in severe lithium poisoning," graded (1, D). The "1" indicates that more than 85% of the members strongly recommend, and the D that there is a very low level of evidence (no observational studies or randomized controlled trials).[66] In the statement, there is a movement away from absolute values and serum concentrations with simple thresholds combined with clinical symptoms as guidelines for intervention.

Extracorporeal treatment is recommended if kidney function is impaired and the lithium concentration is greater than 4.0 mEq/L or in the presence of a decreased level of consciousness, seizures, or life-threatening dysrhythmias regardless of the lithium concentration[66] (Table 70–1).

Extracorporeal treatment is suggested if the concentration is greater than 5.0 mEq/L, if confusion is present or if the expected time to obtain a concentration less than 1.0 mEq/L with optimal management is more than 36 hours.[66]

Whether hemodialysis diminishes or enhances the risk of permanent neurologic sequelae is the subject of ongoing debate.[216,217] Although no controlled studies have analyzed this important management question, a preponderance of evidence suggests a reduced risk.[1,8,14,74,114,119,167,180,183,205,223] A Cochrane systematic review was methodologically flawed because there have been no randomized controlled trials of hemodialysis for lithium poisoning, and thus was inconclusive regarding the benefits of hemodialysis in lithium poisoning.[133]

The choice of ECTR should be guided by the availability of the equipment and the clinical status of the patient. The recommended methodology is intermittent hemodialysis (IHD), although continuous methods are acceptable if IHD is not available. After the technique is complete, serial measurements should be obtained over 12 hours to determine if the ECTR should be repeated. After the initial treatment, both continuous and intermittent methods are equally acceptable.[66]

Continuous venovenous hemodialysis and continuous venovenous hemodiafiltration are two continuous renal replacement therapies (CRRTs) commonly used in the treatment of patients with AKI or volume overload and for elimination of xenobiotics.[14,32,225] Both techniques are effective in patients who are hemodynamically unstable because they are not dependent on arterial blood pressure.[84,164,225] Traditional IHD offers clearance rates that vary between 50 and 170 mL/min with blood flows of 250 mL/min or more.[74,126,153,180,225] Although CRRT techniques offer lower clearance per hour than does IHD, their overall daily clearances are similar.[74] With continued improvements in techniques, use of high volumes, and high dialysate flow rates, clearances are improving, approaching more than half the clearance per hour achieved by IHD in some studies.[84] One case of a rebound concentration was reported in a patient treated with continuous arteriovenous hemodiafiltration,[35] and one case with use of combined renal replacement therapies, including veno-venous techniques, showed no rebound.[14]

TABLE 70–1   Consensus Recommendations for Hemodialysis[a]

Strength of Recommendation	Concentration	OR Clinical Features
Recommended	>4.0 mEq/L with ↓GFR	Decreased level of consciousness, seizures, or life-threatening dysrhythmias
Reasonable	>5.0 mEq/L	Confusion or [Li⁺] not expected to fall to <1.0 mEq/L with optimal management in 36 h

[a]↓ GFR = glomerular filtration rate <60 mL/min.

Data from Decker BS, Goldfarb DS, Dargan PI, et al. Extracorporeal Treatment for Lithium Poisoning: Systematic Review and Recommendations from the EXTRIP Workgroup. *Clin J Am Soc Nephrol.* 2015 May 7;10(5):875-887.

These techniques are most likely to be after IHD to prevent redistribution of lithium and rebound of serum concentrations (Chap. 6).

After an initial session of an ECTR such as IHD, a second session or more are recommended until serum lithium concentrations fall consistently below 1.0 mEq/L; clinical improvement is apparent; or as per the ExTrip consensus, after a minimum of 6 hours of therapy when a concentration is not readily available.[66]

Peritoneal dialysis offers no increased efficacy of clearance of lithium over the natural clearance of normal kidneys.[14,74] Although recommended in the past, given its lack of efficacy coupled with its infrequent use and potential for serious complications such as bowel perforation, peritoneal dialysis has no role in the management of lithium-poisoned patients.

SUMMARY

- Lithium is a simple ion with extensive current usage and extremely varied and complex clinical and pathophysiologic effects.
- Lithium is available in multiple formulations, both immediate release and sustained release, and has an essential role in clinical psychiatry.
- Because of the complexity of the pharmacokinetic profile of lithium, toxicity develops in a wide range of conditions and is precipitated by both intentional overdose and therapeutic misadventure.
- The care of lithium-poisoned patients should be predicated on rapid clinical evaluation of the condition of the patient coupled with identification of the type of poisoning.
- Management includes the use of volume resuscitation and WBI and or another extracorporeal treatment, when indicated, to prevent or treat severe neurologic morbidity and to prevent death.
- Syndrome of irreversible lithium-effectuated neurotoxicity is a persistent neuropsychiatric consequence of lithium toxicity with predominant cerebellar findings that continue at least 2 months after cessation of lithium.

REFERENCES

1. Adityanjee, et al. The syndrome of irreversible lithium-effectuated neurotoxicity. *Clin Neuropharmacol.* 2005;28:38-49.
2. Adityanjee. The syndrome of irreversible lithium effectuated neurotoxicity. *J Neurol Neurosurg Psychiatr.* 1987;50:1246-1247.
3. Adityanjee. The syndrome of irreversible lithium-effectuated neurotoxicity (SILENT). *Pharmacopsychiatry.* 1989;22:81-83.
4. Aghdam SY, Barger SW. Glycogen synthase kinase-3 in neurodegeneration and neuroprotection: lessons from lithium. *Curr Alzheimer Res.* 2007;4:21-31.
5. Agre P, et al. Aquaporin water channels—from atomic structure to clinical medicine. *J Physiol (Lond).* 2002;542(Pt 1):3-16.
6. Aiff H, et al. Effects of 10 to 30 years of lithium treatment on kidney function. *J Psychopharmacol.* 2015;29:608-614.
7. Aita JF, et al. 7-Up anti-acid lithiated lemon soda or early medicinal use of lithium. *Nebr Med J.* 1990;75:277-279; discussion 280.
8. Apte SN, Langston JW. Permanent neurological deficits due to lithium toxicity. *Ann Neurol.* 1983;13:453-455.
9. Armstrong EJ, et al. Lithium-associated Mobitz II block: case series and review of the literature. *Pacing Clin Electrophysiol.* 2011;34:e47-e51.
10. Awad SS, et al. Parathyroid adenomas versus four-gland hyperplasia as the cause of primary hyperparathyroidism in patients with prolonged lithium therapy. *World J Surg.* 2003;27:486-488.
11. Azab AN, et al. Glycogen synthase kinase-3 is required for optimal de novo synthesis of inositol. *Mol Microbiol.* 2007;63:1248-1258.
12. Baek JH, et al. Lithium tremor revisited: pathophysiology and treatment. *Acta Psychiatr Scand.* 2014;129:17-23.
13. Baethge C, et al. Long-term lithium treatment and thyroid antibodies: a controlled study. *J Psychiatry Neurosci.* 2005;30:423-427.
14. Bailey AR, et al. Comparison of intermittent haemodialysis, prolonged intermittent renal replacement therapy and continuous renal replacement haemofiltration for lithium toxicity: a case report. *Crit Care Resusc.* 2011;13:120-122.
15. Bailey B, McGuigan M. Comparison of patients hemodialyzed for lithium poisoning and those for whom dialysis was recommended by PCC but not done: what lesson can we learn? *Clin Nephrol.* 2000;54:388-392.
16. Baird-Gunning J, et al. Lithium Poisoning. *J Intensive Care Med.* 2016;32:249-263.
17. Baldessarini RJ, Tondo L. Suicidal risks during treatment of bipolar disorder patients with lithium versus anticonvulsants. *Pharmacopsychiatry.* 2009;42:72-75.
18. Balkhi El S, et al. Lithium poisoning: is determination of the red blood cell lithium concentration useful? *Clin Toxicol (Phila).* 2009;47:8-13.
19. Bandyopadhyay D, Nielsen C. Lithium-induced hyperthyroidism, thyrotoxicosis and mania: a case report. *QJM.* 2012;105:83-85.
20. Bartzokis G. Neuroglial pharmacology: myelination as a shared mechanism of action of psychotropic treatments. *Neuropharmacology.* 2012;62:2137-2153.
21. Baum M, et al. Effects of thyroid hormone on the neonatal renal cortical Na+/H+ antiporter. *Kidney Int.* 1998;53:1254-1258.
22. Bayliss G. Dialysis in the poisoned patient. *Hemodial Int.* 2010;14:158-167.
23. Beaulieu J-M, Caron MG. Looking at lithium: molecular moods and complex behaviour. *Mol Interv.* 2008;8:230-241.
24. Beaulieu J-M, et al. Beyond cAMP: the regulation of Akt and GSK3 by dopamine receptors. *Front Mol Neurosci.* 2011;4:38.
25. Beaulieu J-M, et al. Dopamine receptors—IUPHAR Review 13. *Br J Pharmacol.* 2015;172:1-23.
26. Beaulieu J-M, et al. Akt/GSK3 signaling in the action of psychotropic drugs. *Annu Rev Pharmacol Toxicol.* 2009;49:327-347.
27. Beaulieu J-M, et al. A β-arrestin 2 signaling complex mediates lithium action on behavior. *Cell.* 2008;132:125-136.
28. Beaulieu J-M. Converging evidence for regulation of dopamine neurotransmission by lithium: an editorial highlight for "Chronic lithium treatment rectifies maladaptive dopamine release in the nucleus accumbens." *J Neurochem.* 2016;139:520-522.
29. Beaulieu J-M. Not only lithium: regulation of glycogen synthase kinase-3 by antipsychotics and serotonergic drugs. *Int J Neuropsychopharmacol.* 2007;10:3-6.
30. Beaulieu JM, Gainetdinov RR. The physiology, signaling, and pharmacology of dopamine receptors. *Pharmacol Rev.* 2011;63:182-217.
31. Beaulieu JM, et al. Role of GSK3 beta in behavioral abnormalities induced by serotonin deficiency. *Proc Natl Acad Sci U S A.* 2008;105:1333-1338.
32. Beckmann U, et al. Efficacy of continuous venovenous hemodialysis in the treatment of severe lithium toxicity. *J Toxicol Clin Toxicol.* 2001;39:393-397.
33. Bedford JJ, et al. Amiloride restores renal medullary osmolytes in lithium-induced nephrogenic diabetes insipidus. *Am J Physiol Renal Physiol.* 2008;294:F812-F820.
34. Bell EC, et al. Lithium and valproate attenuate dextroamphetamine-induced changes in brain activation. *Hum Psychopharmacol Clin Exp.* 2005;20:87-96.
35. Bellomo R, et al. Treatment of life-threatening lithium toxicity with continuous arteriovenous hemodiafiltration. *Crit Care Med.* 1991;19:836-837.
36. Bersudsky Y, et al. Homozygote inositol transporter knockout mice show a lithium-like phenotype. *Bipolar Disord.* 2008;10:453-459.
37. Bersudsky Y, et al. Glycogen synthase kinase-3beta heterozygote knockout mice as a model of findings in postmortem schizophrenia brain or as a model of behaviors mimicking lithium action: negative results. *Behav Pharmacol.* 2008;19:217-224.
38. Blount MA, et al. Expression of transporters involved in urine concentration recovers differently after cessation of lithium treatment. *Am J Physiol Renal Physiol.* 2010;298:F601-F608.
39. Boer WH, et al. Evaluation of the lithium clearance method: direct analysis of tubular lithium handling by micropuncture. *Kidney Int.* 1995;47:1023-1030.
40. Boltan DD, Fenves AZ. Effectiveness of normal saline diuresis in treating lithium overdose. *Proc (Bayl Univ Med Cent).* 2008;21:261-263.
41. Borras-Blasco J, et al. Unrecognized delayed toxic lithium peak concentration in an acute intoxication with sustained release lithium product. *South Med J.* 2007;100:321-323.
42. Bosak AR, et al. Hemodialysis treatment of monomorphic ventricular tachycardia associated with chronic lithium toxicity. *J Med Toxicol.* 2014;10:303-306.
43. Bosinski T, et al. Massive and extended rebound of serum lithium concentrations following hemodialysis in two chronic overdose cases. *Am J Emerg Med.* 1998;16:98-100.
44. Bou Khalil R, Richa S. Thyroid adverse effects of psychotropic drugs: a review. *Clin Neuropharmacol.* 2011;34:248-255.
45. Branger B, et al. Voluntary lithium salt poisoning: risks of slow release forms. *Nephrologie.* 2000;21:291-293.
46. Cade JF. Lithium salts in the treatment of psychotic excitement. *Med J Aust.* 1949;2:349-352.
47. Cai Z, et al. Roles of glycogen synthase kinase 3 in Alzheimer's disease. *Curr Alzheimer Res.* 2012;9:864-879.
48. Camus M, et al. Comparison of lithium concentrations in red blood cells and plasma in samples collected for TDM, acute toxicity, or acute-on-chronic toxicity. *Eur J Clin Pharmacol.* 2003;59(8-9):583-587.
49. Can A, et al. Chronic lithium treatment rectifies maladaptive dopamine release in the nucleus accumbens. *J Neurochem.* 2016;139:576-585.
50. Canan F, et al. Lithium intoxication related multiple temporary ECG changes: a case report. *Cases J.* 2008;1:156.
51. Cantor C. The impact of lithium long-term medication on suicidal behavior and mortality of bipolar patients. *Arch Suicide Res.* 2006;10:303-304.
52. Chen G, et al. Looking ahead: electroretinographic anomalies, glycogen synthase kinase-3, and biomarkers for neuropsychiatric disorders. *Biol Psychiatry.* 2014;76:86-88.
53. Chiu C-T, Chuang D-M. Molecular actions and therapeutic potential of lithium in preclinical and clinical studies of CNS disorders. *Pharmacol Ther.* 2010;128:281-304.
54. Chiu C-T, et al. Therapeutic potential of mood stabilizers lithium and valproic acid: beyond bipolar disorder. *Pharmacol Rev.* 2013;65:105-142.
55. Chou C-H, et al. GSK3β regulates Bcl2L12 and Bcl2L12A anti-apoptosis signaling in glioblastoma and is inhibited by LiCl. *Cell Cycle.* 2012;11:532-542.

56. Christensen S, et al. Pathogenesis of nephrogenic diabetes insipidus due to chronic administration of lithium in rats. *J Clin Invest.* 1985;75:1869-1879.

57. Cipriani A, et al. Lithium in the prevention of suicidal behavior and all-cause mortality in patients with mood disorders: a systematic review of randomized trials. *Am J Psychiatry.* 2005;162:1805-1819.

58. Cipriani A, et al. Lithium versus antidepressants in the long-term treatment of unipolar affective disorder. *Cochrane Database Syst Rev.* 2006;:CD003492.

59. Cole N, Parker G. Cade's identification of lithium for manic-depressive illness—the prospector who found a gold nugget. *J Nerv Ment Dis.* 2012;200:1101-1104.

60. Collins JC, McFarland BH. Divalproex, lithium and suicide among Medicaid patients with bipolar disorder. *J Affect Disord.* 2008;107:23-28.

61. Corcoran AC, et al. Lithium poisoning from the use of salt substitutes. *JAMA.* 1949;139:685-688.

62. Crawford RR, et al. Multiple lithium-dependent Brugada syndrome unmasking events in a bipolar patient. *Clin Case Rep.* 2015;3:14-18.

63. Crews L, et al. Molecular pathology of neuro-AIDS (CNS-HIV). *Int J Mol Sci.* 2009;10:1045-1063.

64. Damri O, et al. Molecular effects of lithium are partially mimicked by inositol-monophosphatase (IMPA)1 knockout mice in a brain region-dependent manner. *Eur Neuropsychopharmacol.* 2015;25:425-434.

65. De Strooper B, Woodgett J. Alzheimer's disease: mental plaque removal. *Nature.* 2003;423:392-393.

66. Decker BS, et al. Extracorporeal treatment for lithium poisoning: systematic review and recommendations from the EXTRIP Workgroup. *Clin J Am Soc Nephrol.* 2015;10:875-887.

67. Del Guidice T, Beaulieu J-M. Selective disruption of dopamine D2-receptors/beta-arrestin2 signaling by mood stabilizers. *J Recept Signal Transduct Res.* 2015;35:224-232.

68. Dodd S, Berk M. The pharmacology of bipolar disorder during pregnancy and breast-feeding. *Expert Opin Drug Saf.* 2004;3:221-229.

69. Dupuis RE, et al. Multiple delayed peak lithium concentrations following acute intoxication with an extended-release product. *Ann Pharmacother.* 1996;30:356-360.

70. Ehrlich BE, Wright EM. Choline and PAH transport across blood-CSF barriers: the effect of lithium. *Brain Res.* 1982;250:245-249.

71. Eickholt BJ, et al. Effects of valproic acid derivatives on inositol trisphosphate depletion, teratogenicity, glycogen synthase kinase-3beta inhibition, and viral replication: a screening approach for new bipolar disorder drugs derived from the valproic acid core structure. *Mol Pharmacol.* 2005;67:1426-1433.

72. Eyer F, et al. Lithium poisoning: pharmacokinetics and clearance during different therapeutic measures. *J Clin Psychopharmacol.* 2006;26:325-330.

73. Fernández-Torre JL, et al. Creutzfeldt-Jakob-like syndrome secondary to severe lithium intoxication: a detailed follow-up electroencephalographic study. *Clin Neurophysiol.* 2014;125:2315-2317.

74. Fertel BS, et al. Extracorporeal removal techniques for the poisoned patient: a review for the intensivist. *J Intensive Care Med.* 2010;25:139-148.

75. Finch CK, et al. Treatment of lithium-induced diabetes insipidus with amiloride. *Pharmacotherapy.* 2003;23:546-550.

76. Finley PR, et al. Clinical relevance of drug interactions with lithium. *Clin Pharmacokinet.* 1995;29:172-191.

77. Focosi D, et al. Lithium and hematology: established and proposed uses. *J Leukoc Biol.* 2009;85:20-28.

78. Forester BP, et al. Brain lithium levels and effects on cognition and mood in geriatric bipolar disorder: a lithium-7 magnetic resonance spectroscopy study. *Am J Geriatr Psychiatry.* 2009;17:13-23.

79. Fornai F, et al. Lithium delays progression of amyotrophic lateral sclerosis. *Proc Natl Acad Sci U S A.* 2008;105:2052-2057.

80. Fountoulakis KN, et al. The International College of Neuro-Psychopharmacology (CINP) treatment guidelines for bipolar disorder in adults (CINP-BD-2017), part 3: the clinical guidelines. *Int J Neuropsychopharm.* 2017;20:180-195.

81. Fransen R, et al. Effects of furosemide or acetazolamide infusion on renal handling of lithium: a micropuncture study in rats. *Am J Physiol.* 1993;264(1 Pt 2):R129-R134.

82. Freland L, Beaulieu J-M. Inhibition of GSK3 by lithium, from single molecules to signaling networks. *Front Mol Neurosci.* 2012;5:14.

83. Friedberg RC, et al. Massive overdoses with sustained-release lithium carbonate preparations: pharmacokinetic model based on two case studies. *Clin Chem.* 1991;37:1205-1209.

84. Garlich FM, Goldfarb DS. Have advances in extracorporeal removal techniques changed the indications for their use in poisonings? *Adv Chronic Kidney Dis.* 2011;18:172-179.

85. Gau C-S, et al. Association between mood stabilizers and hypothyroidism in patients with bipolar disorders: a nested, matched case-control study. *Bipolar Disord.* 2010;12:253-263.

86. Geddes JR, Miklowitz DJ. Treatment of bipolar disorder. *Lancet.* 2013;381:1672-1682.

87. Gehrke JC, et al. In-vivo binding of lithium using the cation exchange resin sodium polystyrene sulfonate. *Am J Emerg Med.* 1996;14:37-38.

88. Gentile S. Lithium in pregnancy: the need to treat, the duty to ensure safety. *Expert Opin Drug Saf.* 2012;11:425-437.

89. Gentille-Lorente DI, Lechuga-Durán I. Brugada type 1 pattern and lithium therapy. *Actas Esp Psiquiatr.* 2015;43:235-236.

90. Ghannoum M, et al. Successful treatment of lithium toxicity with sodium polystyrene sulfonate: a retrospective cohort study. *Clin Toxicol.* 2010;48:34-41.

91. Goldberger ZD. Sinoatrial block in lithium toxicity. *Am J Psychiatry.* 2007;164:831-832.

92. Gonzalez-Pinto A, et al. Suicidal risk in bipolar I disorder patients and adherence to long-term lithium treatment. *Bipolar Disord.* 2006;8(5 Pt 2):618-624.

93. Gordon CE, et al. Acetazolamide in Lithium-Induced Nephrogenic Diabetes Insipidus. *N Engl J Med.* 2016;375:2008-2009.

94. Gould TD, et al. Beta-catenin overexpression in the mouse brain phenocopies lithium-sensitive behaviors. *Neuropsychopharmacology.* 2007;32:2173-2183.

95. Gould TD, et al. Strain differences in lithium attenuation of d-amphetamine-induced hyperlocomotion: a mouse model for the genetics of clinical response to lithium. *Neuropsychopharmacology.* 2007;32:1321-1333.

96. Gould TD, et al. Emerging experimental therapeutics for bipolar disorder: insights from the molecular and cellular actions of current mood stabilizers. *Mol Psychiatry.* 2004;9:734-755.

97. Grandjean EM, Aubry J-M. Lithium: updated human knowledge using an evidence-based approach. *CNS Drugs.* 2009;23:397-418.

98. Grandjean EM, Aubry J-M. Lithium: updated human knowledge using an evidence-based approach. Part II: clinical pharmacology and therapeutic monitoring. *CNS Drugs.* 2009;23:331-349.

99. Grignon S, Bruguerolle B. Cerebellar lithium toxicity: a review of recent literature and tentative pathophysiology. *Therapie.* 1996;51:101-106.

100. Grünfeld J-P, Rossier BC. Lithium nephrotoxicity revisited. *Nat Rev Nephrol.* 2009;5:270-276.

101. Gupta Y, et al. Development of Graves' disease after long-standing hypothyroidism on treatment, with acute toxicity to thionamides and lithium. *Case Rep.* 2012;2012(jul31 1):bcr2012006433-bcr2012006433.

102. Haimovich A, et al. Determination of the lithium binding site in inositol monophosphatase, the putative target for lithium therapy, by magic-angle-spinning solid-state NMR. *J Am Chem Soc.* 2012;134:5647-5651.

103. Hallab B, et al. [Syndrome of irreversible lithium-effectuated neurotoxicity or SILENT: a case report]. *Therapie.* 2017;72:403-407.

104. Hanak A-S, et al. Neurobehavioral effects of lithium in the rat: investigation of the effect/concentration relationships and the contribution of the poisoning pattern. *Prog Neuropsychopharmacol Biol Psychiatry.* 2017;76:1-22.

105. Hanak A-S, et al. Electroencephalographic patterns of lithium poisoning: a study of the effect/concentration relationships in the rat. *Bipolar Disord.* 2017;19:135-145.

106. Hansen HE, Amdisen A. Lithium intoxication. (Report of 23 cases and review of 100 cases from the literature). *Q J Med.* 1978;47:123-144.

107. Harvey NS, Merriman S. Review of clinically important drug interactions with lithium. *Drug Saf.* 1994;10:455-463.

108. Harwood AJ, Agam G. Search for a common mechanism of mood stabilizers. *Biochem Pharmacol.* 2003;66:179-189.

109. Harwood AJ. Lithium and bipolar mood disorder: the inositol-depletion hypothesis revisited. *Mol Psychiatry.* 2005;10:117-126.

110. Hermida AP, et al. A case of lithium-induced parkinsonism presenting with typical motor symptoms of Parkinson's disease in a bipolar patient. *Int Psychogeriatr.* 2016;28:2101-2104.

111. Hillert M, et al. Uptake of lithium into rat brain after acute and chronic administration. *Neurosci Lett.* 2012;521:62-66.

112. Hollander E, et al. FDG-PET study in pathological gamblers. 1. Lithium increases orbitofrontal, dorsolateral and cingulate metabolism. *Neuropsychobiology.* 2008;58:37-47.

113. Holley CK, Mast BT. The effects of widowhood and vascular risk factors on late-life depression. *Am J Geriatr Psychiatry.* 2007;15:690-698.

114. Holubek WJ, et al. Use of hemodialysis and hemoperfusion in poisoned patients. *Kidney Int.* 2008;74:1327-1334.

115. Hsu C-H, et al. Electrocardiographic abnormalities as predictors for over-range lithium levels. *Cardiology.* 2005;103:101-106.

116. Ikeda Y, et al. Total and regional brain volume reductions due to the Syndrome of Irreversible Lithium-Effectuated Neurotoxicity (SILENT): a voxel-based morphometric study. *Prog Neuropsychopharmacol Biol Psychiatry.* 2010;34:244-246.

117. Jacobsen D, et al. Lithium intoxication: pharmacokinetics during and after terminated hemodialysis in acute intoxications. *J Toxicol Clin Toxicol.* 1987;25:81-94.

118. Jaeger A, et al. Toxicokinetics of lithium intoxication treated by hemodialysis. *J Toxicol Clin Toxicol.* 1985;23(7-8):501-517.

119. Jaeger A, et al. When should dialysis be performed in lithium poisoning? A kinetic study in 14 cases of lithium poisoning. *J Toxicol Clin Toxicol.* 1993;31:429-447.

120. Jope RS. Glycogen synthase kinase-3 in the etiology and treatment of mood disorders. *Front Mol Neurosci.* 2011;4:16.

121. Karege F, et al. Alteration in kinase activity but not in protein levels of protein kinase B and glycogen synthase kinase-3beta in ventral prefrontal cortex of depressed suicide victims. *Biol Psychiatry.* 2007;61:240-245.

122. Karege F, et al. Alterations in phosphatidylinositol 3-kinase activity and PTEN phosphatase in the prefrontal cortex of depressed suicide victims. *Neuropsychobiology.* 2011;63:224-231.

123. Kayrak M, et al. Lithium intoxication causing ST segment elevation and wandering atrial rhythms in an elderly patient. *Cardiology J.* 2010;17:404-407.

124. Kayrak M, et al. A bizarre electrocardiographic pattern due to chronic lithium therapy. *Ann Noninvasive Electrocardiol.* 2010;15:289-292.

125. Kessing LV, et al. Use of Lithium and anticonvulsants and the rate of chronic kidney disease: a nationwide population-based study. *JAMA Psychiatry.* 2015;72:1182-1191.

126. Komaru Y, et al. Use of the anion gap and intermittent hemodialysis following continuous hemodiafiltration in extremely high dose acute-on-chronic lithium poisoning: a case report. *Hemodial Int.* 2017;10:666.

127. Kores B, Lader MH. Irreversible lithium neurotoxicity: an overview. *Clin Neuropharmacol.* 1997;20:283-299.

128. Kortenoeven MLA, et al. Amiloride blocks lithium entry through the sodium channel thereby attenuating the resultant nephrogenic diabetes insipidus. *Kidney Int.* 2009;76:44-53.

129. Kortenoeven MLA, et al. Lithium reduces aquaporin-2 transcription independent of prostaglandins. *Am J Physiol Cell Physiol.* 2012;302:C131-C140.

130. Kovacsics CE, et al. Lithium's antisuicidal efficacy: elucidation of neurobiological targets using endophenotype strategies. *Annu Rev Pharmacol Toxicol.* 2009;49:175-198.

131. La Rocca R, et al. QT interval prolongation and bradycardia in lithium-induced nephrogenic diabetes insipidus. *Int J Cardiol.* 2012;162:e1-e2.

132. Lavoie J, et al. Glycogen synthase kinase-3β haploinsufficiency lengthens the circadian locomotor activity period in mice. *Behavioural Brain Research.* 2013;253:262-265.

133. Lavonas EJ, Buchanan J. Hemodialysis for lithium poisoning. *Cochrane Database Syst Rev.* 2015;9:CD007951.

134. Lazarus JH. Lithium and thyroid. *Best Pract Res Clin Endocrinol Metab.* 2009;23:723-733.

135. Leary OFO, et al. Lithium augmentation of the effects of desipramine in a mouse model of treatment-resistant depression: a role for hippocampal cell proliferation. *Neuroscience.* 2013;228(C):36-46.

136. Leblanc M, et al. Lithium poisoning treated by high-performance continuous arteriovenous and venovenous hemodiafiltration. *Am J Kidney Dis.* 1996;27:365-372.

137. Lee DC, Klachko MN. Falsely elevated lithium levels in plasma samples obtained in lithium containing tubes. *J Toxicol Clin Toxicol.* 1996;34:467-469.

138. Lee Y-C, et al. Outcome of patients with lithium poisoning at a far-east poison center. *Hum Exp Toxicol.* 2011;30:528-534.

139. Leeds PR, et al. A new avenue for lithium: intervention in traumatic brain injury. *ACS Chem Neurosci.* 2014;5:422-433.

140. Lehmann SW, Lee J. Lithium-associated hypercalcemia and hyperparathyroidism in the elderly What do we know? *J Affect Disord.* 2012:1-7.

141. Leng Y, et al. Synergistic neuroprotective effects of lithium and valproic acid or other histone deacetylase inhibitors in neurons: roles of glycogen synthase kinase-3 inhibition. *J Neurosci.* 2008;28:2576-2588.

142. Lewitzka U, et al. The suicide prevention effect of lithium: more than 20 years of evidence-a narrative review. International *J Bipolar Disord.* 2014 2:1. 2015;3:32.

143. Li X, et al. Lithium regulates glycogen synthase kinase-3beta in human peripheral blood mononuclear cells: implication in the treatment of bipolar disorder. *Biol Psychiatry.* 2007;61:216-222.

144. Li X, Jope RS. Is glycogen synthase kinase-3 a central modulator in mood regulation? *Neuropsychopharmacology.* 2010;35:2143-2154.

145. Li X, et al. Regulation of mouse brain glycogen synthase kinase-3 by atypical antipsychotics. *Int J Neuropsychopharmacol.* 2007;10:7-19.

146. Li Y, et al. Development of lithium-induced nephrogenic diabetes insipidus is dissociated from adenylyl cyclase activity. *J Am Soc Nephrol.* 2006;17:1063-1072.

147. Licht RW. Lithium: still a major option in the management of bipolar disorder. *CNS Neurosci Ther.* 2012;18:219-226.

148. Lin Y, et al. Aliskiren increases aquaporin-2 expression and attenuates lithium-induced nephrogenic diabetes insipidus. *Am J Physiol Renal Physiol.* 2017;313:F914-F925.

149. Linakis JG, et al. Administration of activated charcoal or sodium polystyrene sulfonate (Kayexalate) as gastric decontamination for lithium intoxication: an animal model. *Pharmacol Toxicol.* 1989;65:387-389.

150. Linakis JG, et al. Potassium repletion fails to interfere with reduction of serum lithium by sodium polystyrene sulfonate in mice. *Acad Emerg Med.* 2001;8:956-960.

151. Linakis JG, et al. Use of sodium polystyrene sulfonate for reduction of plasma lithium concentrations after chronic lithium dosing in mice. *J Toxicol Clin Toxicol.* 1998;36:309-313.

152. Linares GR, et al. Preconditioning mesenchymal stem cells with the mood stabilizers lithium and valproic acid enhances therapeutic efficacy in a mouse model of Huntington's disease. *Exp Neurol.* 2016;281:81-92.

153. Lopez JC, et al. Higher requirements of dialysis in severe lithium intoxication. *Hemodial Int.* 2012;16:407-413.

154. Lu S, et al. Insights into the role of magnesium triad in myo-inositol monophosphatase: metal mechanism, substrate binding, and lithium therapy. *J Chem Inf Model.* 2012;52:2398-2409.

155. Maddala RNM, et al. Chronic lithium intoxication: varying electrocardiogram manifestations. *Indian J Pharmacol.* 2017;49:127-129.

156. Mani J, et al. Prolonged neurological sequelae after combination treatment with lithium and antipsychotic drugs. *J Neurol Neurosurg Psychiatr.* 1996;60:350-351.

157. Manji HK, Chen G. PKC, MAP kinases and the bcl-2 family of proteins as long-term targets for mood stabilizers. *Mol Psychiatry.* 2002;7(suppl 1):S46-S56.

158. Manto M, et al. Analysis of cerebellar dysmetria associated with lithium intoxication. *Neurol Res.* 1996;18:416-424.

159. Marmol F. Lithium: bipolar disorder and neurodegenerative diseases Possible cellular mechanisms of the therapeutic effects of lithium. *Prog Neuropsychopharmacol Biol Psychiatry.* 2008;32:1761-1771.

160. Marti JL, et al. Surgical approach and outcomes in patients with lithium-associated hyperparathyroidism. *Ann Surg Oncol.* 2012;19:3465-3471.

161. Martin P-M, et al. DIXDC1 contributes to psychiatric susceptibility by regulating dendritic spine and glutamatergic synapse density via GSK3 and Wnt-catenin signaling. *Mol Psychiatry.* 2016;468:1-9.

162. Mast BT. Cerebrovascular disease and late-life depression: a latent-variable analysis of depressive symptoms after stroke. *Am J Geriatr Psychiatry.* 2004;12:315-322.

163. McKnight RF, et al. Lithium toxicity profile: a systematic review and meta-analysis. *Lancet.* 2012;379:721-728.

164. Meertens JHJM, et al. Haemodialysis followed by continuous veno-venous haemodiafiltration in lithium intoxication; a model and a case. *Eur J Intern Med.* 2009;20:e70-e73.

165. Mehta SH, et al. Drug-induced movement disorders. *Neurol Clin.* 2015;33:153-174.

166. Mendes CT, et al. Lithium reduces Gsk3b mRNA levels: implications for Alzheimer disease. *Eur Arch Psychiatry Clin Neurosci.* 2009;259:16-22.

167. Meyer RJ, et al. Hemodialysis followed by continuous hemofiltration for treatment of lithium intoxication in children. *Am J Kidney Dis.* 2001;37:1044-1047.

168. Mignat C, Unger T. ACE inhibitors. Drug interactions of clinical significance. *Drug Saf.* 1995;12:334-347.

169. Moore CM, et al. Brain-to-serum lithium ratio and age: an in vivo magnetic resonance spectroscopy study. *Am J Psychiatry.* 2002;159:1240-1242.

170. Morgan JC, Sethi KD. Drug-induced tremors. *Lancet Neurol.* 2005;4:866-876.

171. Newland KD, Mycyk MB. Hemodialysis reversal of lithium overdose cardiotoxicity. *Am J Emerg Med.* 2002;20:67-68.

172. Nunes MA, et al. Microdose lithium treatment stabilized cognitive impairment in patients with Alzheimer's disease. *Curr Alzheimer Res.* 2013;10:104-107.

173. Oakley PW, et al. Lithium: thyroid effects and altered renal handling. *J Toxicol Clin Toxicol.* 2000;38:333-337.

174. Oliveira JL de, et al. Lithium nephrotoxicity. *Rev Assoc Med Bras.* 2010;56:600-606.

175. Omata N, et al. A patient with lithium intoxication developing at therapeutic serum lithium levels and persistent delirium after discontinuation of its administration. *Gen Hosp Psychiatry.* 2003;25:53-55.

176. Oudit GY, et al. Lithium-induced sinus node disease at therapeutic concentrations: linking lithium-induced blockade of sodium channels to impaired pacemaker activity. *Can J Cardiol.* 2007;23:229-232.

177. Paclt I, et al. Electrocardiographic dose-dependent changes in prophylactic doses of dosulepine, lithium and citalopram. *Physiol Res.* 2003;52:311-317.

178. Pallanti S, et al. Lithium and valproate treatment of pathological gambling: a randomized single-blind study. *J Clin Psychiatry.* 2002;63:559-564.

179. Patorno E, et al. Lithium use in pregnancy and the risk of cardiac malformations. *N Engl J Med.* 2017;376:2245-2254.

180. Peces R, Pobes A. Effectiveness of haemodialysis with high-flux membranes in the extracorporeal therapy of life-threatening acute lithium intoxication. *Nephrol Dial Transplant.* 2001;16:1301-1303.

181. Pedrosa E, et al. β-catenin promoter ChIP—ChIP reveals potential schizophrenia and bipolar disorder gene network. *J Neurogenet.* 2010;24:182-193.

182. Phiel CJ, Klein PS. Molecular targets of lithium action. *Annu Rev Pharmacol Toxicol.* 2001;41:789-813.

183. Porto FHG, et al. The Syndrome of Irreversible Lithium-Effectuated Neurotoxicity (SILENT): one-year follow-up of a single case. *J Neurol Sci.* 2009;277:172-173.

184. Puhr J, et al. Lithium overdose with electrocardiogram changes suggesting ischemia. *J Med Toxicol.* 2008;4:170-172.

185. Qu Z, et al. Lithium promotes neural precursor cell proliferation: evidence for the involvement of the non-canonical GSK-3β-NF-AT signaling. *Cell Biosci.* 2011;1:18.

186. Quiroz JA, et al. Molecular effects of lithium. *Mol Interv.* 2004;4:259-272.

187. Quiroz JA, et al. Novel insights into lithium's mechanism of action: neurotrophic and neuroprotective effects. *Neuropsychobiology.* 2010;62:50-60.

188. Rao R, et al. GSK3beta mediates renal response to vasopressin by modulating adenylate cyclase activity. *J Am Soc Nephrol.* 2010;21:428-437.

189. Rao R. Glycogen synthase kinase-3 regulation of urinary concentrating ability. *Cur Opin Nephrol Hypertens.* 2012;21:541-546.

190. Rej S, et al. The effects of lithium on renal function in older adults—a systematic review. *J Geriatr Psychiatry Neurol.* 2012;25:51-61.

191. Riccardi D, Brown EM. Physiology and pathophysiology of the calcium-sensing receptor in the kidney. *Am J Physiol Renal Physiol.* 2010;298:F485-F499.

192. Riedl U, et al. Duration of lithium treatment and brain lithium concentration in patients with unipolar and schizoaffective disorder--a study with magnetic resonance spectroscopy. *Biol Psychiatry.* 1997;41:844-850.

193. Roberts DE, et al. Effect of lithium carbonate on zidovudine-associated neutropenia in the acquired immunodeficiency syndrome. *Am J Med.* 1988;85:428-431.

194. Roh M-S, et al. Hypoxia activates glycogen synthase kinase-3 in mouse brain in vivo: protection by mood stabilizers and imipramine. *Biol Psychiatry.* 2005;57:278-286.

195. Rossi FH, et al. Permanent cerebellar degeneration after acute hyperthermia with nontoxic lithium levels: a case report and review of literature. *Cerebellum.* 2017;351:1-6.

196. Rowe MK, Chuang DM. Lithium neuroprotection: molecular mechanisms and clinical implications. *Expert Rev Mol Med*. 2004;6:1-18.

197. Saito-Diaz K, et al. The way Wnt works: components and mechanism. *Growth Factors*. 2012;31:1-31.

198. Sakae R, et al. Decreased lithium disposition to cerebrospinal fluid in rats with glycerol-induced acute renal failure. *Pharm Res*. 2008;25:2243-2249.

199. Sands JM, Bichet DG; American College of Physicians, American Physiological Society. Nephrogenic diabetes insipidus. *Ann Intern Med*. 2006;144:186-194.

200. Sato Y, et al. Lithium toxicity precipitated by thyrotoxicosis due to silent thyroiditis: cardiac arrest, quadriplegia, and coma. *Thyroid*. 2013;23:766-770.

201. Scharman EJ. Methods used to decrease lithium absorption or enhance elimination. *J Toxicol Clin Toxicol*. 1997;35:601-608.

202. Scheuing L, et al. Preclinical and clinical investigations of mood stabilizers for Huntington's disease: what have we learned? *Int J Biol Sci*. 2014;10:1024-1038.

203. Schneider JA, Mirra SS. Neuropathologic correlates of persistent neurologic deficit in lithium intoxication. *Ann Neurol*. 1994;36:928-931.

204. Schou M, et al. The treatment of manic psychoses by the administration of lithium salts. *J Neurol Neurosurg Psychiatr*. 1954;17:250-260.

205. Schou M. Lithium treatment at 52. *J Affect Disord*. 2001;67:21-32.

206. Schou M. Long-lasting neurological sequelae after lithium intoxication. *Acta Psychiatr Scand*. 1984;70:594-602.

207. Severus E, et al. Lithium for prevention of mood episodes in bipolar disorders: systematic review and meta-analysis. *Int J Bipolar Disord*. 2014;2:15.

208. Severus WE, et al. What is the optimal serum lithium level in the long-term treatment of bipolar disorder—a review? *Bipolar Disord*. 2008;10:231-237.

209. Shaldubina A, et al. Behavioural phenotyping of sodium-myo-inositol cotransporter heterozygous knockout mice with reduced brain inositol. *Genes Brain Behav*. 2007;6:253-259.

210. Sheean GL. Lithium neurotoxicity. *Clin Exp Neurol*. 1991;28:112-127.

211. Shiraki T, et al. Complete atrioventricular block secondary to lithium therapy. *Circ J*. 2008;72:847-849.

212. Shorter E. The history of lithium therapy. *Bipolar Disord*. 2009;11(s2):4-9.

213. Silverstone PH, et al. Bipolar disorder and myo-inositol: a review of the magnetic resonance spectroscopy findings. *Bipolar Disord*. 2005;7:1-10.

214. Smith SW, et al. Whole-bowel irrigation as a treatment for acute lithium overdose. *Ann Emerg Med*. 1991;20:536-539.

215. Stern RL. Severe lithium chloride poisoning with complete recovery. *JAMA*. 1949;139:710.

216. Swartz CM, Dolinar LJ. Encephalopathy associated with rapid decrease of high levels of lithium. *Ann Clin Psychiatry*. 1995;7:207-209.

217. Swartz CM, Jones P. Hyperlithemia correction and persistent delirium. *J Clin Pharmacol*. 1994;34:865-870.

218. Szalat A, et al. Lithium-associated hyperparathyroidism: report of four cases and review of the literature. *Eur J Endocrinol*. 2009;160:317-323.

219. Talati SN, et al. Sinus node dysfunction in association with chronic lithium therapy: a case report and review of literature. *Am J Ther*. 2009;16:274-278.

220. Tan LH, et al. Lithium-associated silent thyroiditis: clinical implications. *Aust NZ J Psychiatry*. 2013;47:965-966.

221. Thomsen K, et al. Chronic lithium treatment inhibits amiloride-sensitive sodium transport in the rat distal nephron. *J Pharmacol Exp Ther*. 1999;289:443-447.

222. Thomsen K, Shirley DG. A hypothesis linking sodium and lithium reabsorption in the distal nephron. *Nephrol Dial Transplant*. 2006;21:869-880.

223. Timmer RT, Sands JM. Lithium intoxication. *J Am Soc Nephrol*. 1999;10:666-674.

224. Valvezan AJ, Klein PS. GSK-3 and Wnt signaling in neurogenesis and bipolar disorder. *Front Mol Neurosci*. 2012;5:1.

225. van Bommel EF, et al. Treatment of life-threatening lithium toxicity with high-volume continuous venovenous hemofiltration. *Am J Nephrol*. 2000;20:408-411.

226. van Noord C, et al. Psychotropic drugs associated with corrected QT interval prolongation. *J Clin Psychopharmacol*. 2009;29:9-15.

227. Vestergaard P, et al. Prospective studies on a lithium cohort. 3. Tremor, weight gain, diarrhea, psychological complaints. *Acta Psychiatr Scand*. 1988;78:434-441.

228. Viguera AC, et al. Lithium in breast milk and nursing infants: clinical implications. *Am J Psychiatry*. 2007;164:342-345.

229. Vodovar D, et al. Lithium poisoning in the intensive care unit: predictive factors of severity and indications for extracorporeal toxin removal to improve outcome. *Clin Toxicol*. 2016;54:615-623.

230. Waise A, Fisken RA. Unsuspected nephrogenic diabetes insipidus. *BMJ*. 2001;323:96-97.

231. Waldron AM. Lithium intoxication occurring with the use of a table salt substitute in the low sodium dietary treatment of hypertension and congestive heart failure. *Univ Hosp Bull*. 1949;15:9.

232. Walker RJ, et al. Lithium-induced reduction in urinary concentrating ability and urinary aquaporin 2 (AQP2) excretion in healthy volunteers. *Kidney Int*. 2005;67:291-294.

233. White B, et al. Protracted presyncope and profound bradycardia due to lithium toxicity. *Int J Cardiol*. 2008;125:e48-e50.

234. Williams RSB. Employing multiple models, methods and mechanisms in bipolar disorder research. *Biochem Soc Trans*. 2009;37(Pt 5):1077-1079.

235. Woodgett JR. Physiological roles of glycogen synthase kinase-3: potential as a therapeutic target for diabetes and other disorders. *Curr Drug Targets Immune Endocr Metabol Disord*. 2003;3:281-290.

236. Wu AHB, et al. National academy of clinical biochemistry laboratory medicine practice guidelines: recommendations for the use of laboratory tests to support poisoned patients who present to the emergency department. *Clin Chem*. 2003;49:357-379.

237. Yacobi S, Ornoy A. Is lithium a real teratogen? What can we conclude from the prospective versus retrospective studies? A review. *Isr J Psychiatry Relat Sci*. 2008;45:95-106.

238. Yildiz A, et al. Lithium-induced alterations in nucleoside triphosphate levels in human brain: a proton-decoupled 31P magnetic resonance spectroscopy study. *Psychiatry Res*. 2005;138:51-59.

239. Youdim MB, Arraf Z. Prevention of MPTP (*N*-methyl-4-phenyl-1,2,3,6-tetrahydropyridine) dopaminergic neurotoxicity in mice by chronic lithium: involvements of Bcl-2 and Bax. *Neuropharmacology*. 2004;46:1130-1140.

240. Yu F, et al. Posttrauma cotreatment with lithium and valproate: reduction of lesion volume, attenuation of blood-brain barrier disruption, and improvement in motor coordination in mice with traumatic brain injury. *J Neurosurg*. 2013;119:766-773.

241. Yu F, et al. Lithium ameliorates neurodegeneration, suppresses neuroinflammation, and improves behavioral performance in a mouse model of traumatic brain injury. *J Neurotrauma*. 2012;29:362-374.

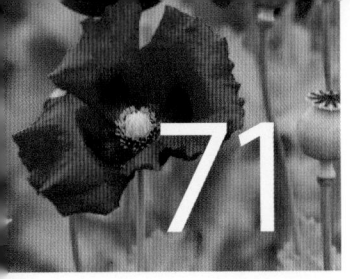

71 MONOAMINE OXIDASE INHIBITORS

Alex F. Manini

HISTORY AND EPIDEMIOLOGY

Monoamine oxidase inhibitors (MAOIs) have a unique history, pharmacology, and toxic syndrome. Although toxicity from MAOI ingestion is becoming less common because of more limited clinical usage of the traditional nonselective MAOIs, an understanding of MAOI toxicity is fundamental to any clinician who cares for patients with acute poisoning.

Monoamine oxidase (MAO) was discovered in 1928 and named by Zeller when the enzyme was recognized to metabolize primary, secondary, and tertiary amines such as tyramine and norepinephrine.[132] Subsequently, the "monoamine hypothesis" postulated depression as a condition of monoamine deficiency, and MAOIs targeted monoamine metabolism for therapeutic benefit. In the early 1950s, iproniazid, a drug previously used to treat tuberculosis, was found to produce favorable behavioral effects. By the mid-1950s, it was demonstrated that iproniazid inhibited MAO, and it then became the first antidepressant used clinically.[22]

In the late 1960s, two MAO isoforms were identified, each with substrate and inhibitor specificity. This determination led to the development of selective MAOIs in attempts to minimize the many food and drug interactions that occur with the traditional nonselective MAOIs. Nonselective MAOIs proved to be potent and efficient antidepressants and became the first-line therapy for depression. In the 1970s, alternative therapies for depression, such as the tricyclic antidepressants, were developed and achieved clinical success without as many food and drug interactions.

Intentional MAOI overdose is relatively uncommon and accounts for a dwindling number of annual exposures reported to the American Association of Poison Control Centers. From 2011 to 2015, there was a decreasing trend in the number of exposures with fewer than 100 exposures reported in 2015 (Chap. 130), representing less than 1% of all antidepressant exposures. Of the reported exposures in 2010, there were only five cases of "major toxic effect" (defined as life-threatening signs or symptoms), and no deaths were reported. Over the past 2 decades, annual reported MAOI exposures have decreased 34% since 1985 (Chap. 130). Global MAOI exposure rates declined in proportion with the United States, with the possible exception of exposures to moclobemide, a drug not approved by the US Food and Drug Administration (FDA).[33]

Many authors recommend the prescription of nonselective MAOIs only for resistant or atypical depression with prominent neurovegetative symptoms.[30] However, selective and reversible MAOIs are the subject of renewed clinical applicability and basic science research interest. Monoamine oxidase-B selective xenobiotics, such as selegiline, are widely used for the treatment of Parkinson disease. Reversible inhibitors of MAO, such as moclobemide, are used in Europe for depression, phobias, anxiety, and other select indications.[130] Current applicability of a new generation of experimental MAOIs is being investigated as neuroprotective xenobiotics for a variety of neurodegenerative diseases.[132]

PHARMACOLOGY

Chemistry

Monoamines, also known as biogenic amines, include the catecholamines (epinephrine, norepinephrine, dopamine, tyrosine), indolamines (serotonin, melatonin), and some naturally occurring amines (eg, tyramine, benzylamine). They share the presence of a single amine group and the ability to be metabolized by MAO, a flavin-containing enzyme present on the outer mitochondrial membrane of central nervous system (CNS) neurons, hepatocytes, and platelets. In a two-step reaction, MAO catalyzes the oxidative deamination of its various substrates. The reaction liberates H_2O_2, a reactive oxygen

species. Deamination by MAO is one of two major routes of elimination of monoamines, the other being extracellular degradation by catechol-O-methyltransferase (COMT). Serotonin and tyramine, which are not metabolized by COMT, are the exceptions to this rule.

Monoamine Neurotransmitter Stores

Monoamine neurotransmitter synthesis, vesicle transport, vesicle storage, uptake, and degradation are described in detail in Chap. 13. In the neuron, MAO functions as a "safety valve" to metabolize and inactivate excess monoamine neurotransmitter molecules. After monoamines reenter the cytoplasm from the synaptic cleft, they can either reenter vesicles for further storage and release or can be rapidly enzymatically degraded by MAO.

Monoamine Oxidase Isoforms

There are two MAO isoforms, each with its own substrate and inhibitor specificity (Table 71–1). Whereas MAO-A preferentially metabolizes norepinephrine and serotonin, MAO-B preferentially metabolizes phenylethylamine. Both isoforms metabolize tyramine and dopamine with comparable efficiency, but they are localized to different anatomic regions. Monoamine oxidase-A is concentrated in the intestine and liver, and MAO-B is concentrated in the basal ganglia of the brain.[20]

Mechanism of Action

Monoamine oxidase inhibitors are transported into the neuron by the Na^+-dependent membrane norepinephrine-reuptake transporter.[72] Inhibition of MAO prevents presynaptic degradation of monoamines, thus increasing the concentration of monoamine neurotransmitters available for synaptic storage and subsequent release (Fig. 71–1). Inhibition of MAO also results in indirect release of norepinephrine into the synapse via displacement from presynaptic vesicles in a manner similar to amphetamines (Chap. 73).[116]

Elevated synaptic concentrations of serotonin are best correlated with the antidepressant therapeutic effects of MAOIs. The enzymatic inhibition produced by MAOIs precedes the clinical effects by as long as 2 weeks. This finding, which is similar to other antidepressants, most likely relates to the relatively slow downregulation of postsynaptic CNS serotonin receptors.[93]

In overdose, MAOIs also impair norepinephrine synthesis caused by dopamine-β-hydroxylase inhibition. Impaired norepinephrine synthesis

TABLE 71–1 Monoamine Oxidase (MAO) Isoforms: Substrate Affinities and Localization

	MAO Isoforms	
	MAO-A	**MAO-B**
Substrate Affinity		
Dopamine	Moderate	Moderate
Epinephrine	Moderate	Moderate
Norepinephrine	High	Low
Serotonin	High	Low
Tyramine	Moderate	Moderate
Localization		
Brain	Low	High
Intestine	Moderate	Low
Liver	Moderate	Moderate
Placenta	High	Absent
Platelets	Absent	High

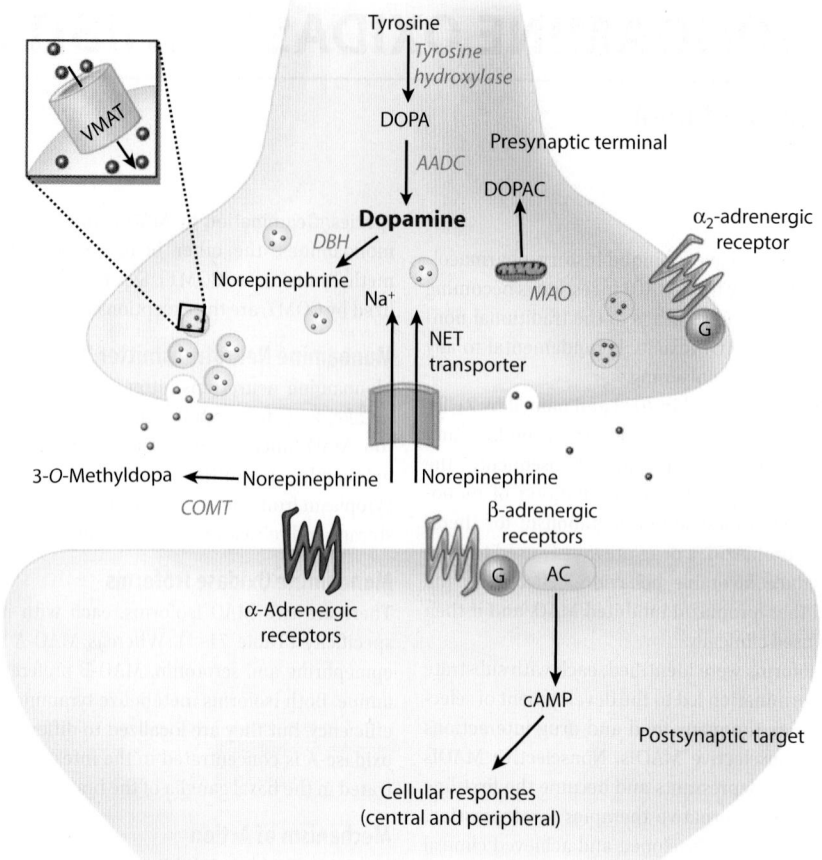

FIGURE 71–1. Sympathetic nerve terminal. Dopamine is synthesized in the sympathetic nerve cell and transported into vesicles, where it is converted to norepinephrine (NE) and stored in vesicles (⊙). An action potential causes the vesicles to migrate to and fuse with the presynaptic membrane. Norepinephrine diffuses across the synaptic cleft and binds with and activates postsynaptic α- and β-adrenergic receptors. Neuronal NE reuptake occurs via the monoamine transporter. Norepinephrine is transported back into vesicles by the vesicular monoamine transporter (VMAT; inset) or metabolized to 3,4 dihydroxyphenyl acetic acid (DOPAC) by mitochondrial monoamine oxidase (MAO). Norepinephrine that diffuses away from the synaptic cleft is inactivated by catechol-O-methyl transferase (COMT). AADC = aromatic ʟ-amino acid decarboxylase; cAMP = cyclic adenosine monophosphate; DBH = dopamine β-hydroxylase; NET = Membrane NE reuptake transporter.

leads to eventual depletion of norepinephrine stores. Additionally, indirect dopamine agonism occurs via elevated synaptic concentrations of dopamine. Dopamine agonism results in β-adrenergic stimulation, peripheral vasodilation, and direct α-adrenergic stimulation at high doses.

The hydrazide MAOIs (eg, phenelzine, isocarboxazid) are thought to be cleaved to liberate pharmacologically active products (eg, hydrazides), which are metabolized by acetylation in the liver.

First-Generation Monoamine Oxidase Inhibitors: Nonselective and Irreversible

Monoamine oxidase inhibitors are a chemically heterogeneous group of xenobiotics (Fig. 71–2). First-generation MAOIs (ie, irreversible and nonselective) in clinical use worldwide include the reactive hydrazide derivatives (phenelzine, isocarboxazid) and an amphetamine derivative (tranylcypromine).[45] First-generation MAOIs bind covalently to MAO and irreversibly inhibit the function of the enzyme. Thus, patients taking these MAOIs are depleted of the enzyme until new MAO is synthesized, a process that typically takes up to 3 weeks, resulting in short half-lives but long durations of effect. Patients taking first-generation MAOIs remain at risk for food and xenobiotic interactions during much of this period. Because nonselective MAOIs inhibit both isoforms of MAO (ie, MAO-A and MAO-B), inhibition of intestinal and hepatic degradation of biogenic amines occurs.

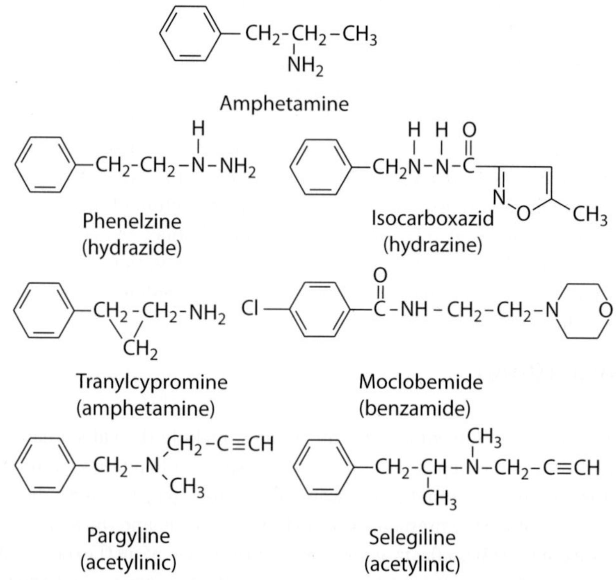

FIGURE 71–2. Structural similarities between amphetamine and the monoamine oxidase inhibitors (MAOIs). The words in parentheses are the chemical classes of the MAOI.

As a result, patients who receive these MAOIs must be placed on a restrictive diet to prevent adverse events resulting from the absorption of undigested tyramine from the gut.

Phenelzine, isocarboxazid, and tranylcypromine are currently FDA approved for treatment of refractory depression.[57,76] Other enzyme systems inhibited by first-generation MAOIs include amine oxidases such as diamine oxidase and semicarbazide-sensitive oxidases, arylamine N-acetyltransferase (by tranylcypromine), ceruloplasmin, alcohol dehydrogenase (by tranylcypromine), dopa decarboxylase, L-glutamic acid decarboxylase, γ-aminobutyric acid (GABA) decarboxylase and GABA transaminase (by hydrazide MAOIs), alanine aminotransferase (by phenelzine), and other pyridoxine (B_6)-containing enzyme systems.[48] The clinical implications of inhibiting these diverse enzyme systems, other than alcohol dehydrogenase and cytochrome P450 enzymes,[104] are poorly understood.

Second-Generation Monoamine Oxidase Inhibitors: Selective and Irreversible

Selective MAOIs preferentially inhibit one of the two MAO isoforms, although isoform selectivity is dose dependent.

MAO-A Inhibitors

Clorgyline is an MAO-A inhibitor structurally related to pargyline. Once thought to be useful for treatment of depression, it has not found widespread use in psychiatry because of disappointing results from clinical trials.

MAO-B Inhibitors

Selegiline is a selective MAO-B inhibitor that is FDA approved for the treatment of Parkinson disease.[57,67] Monoamine oxidase-B selectivity may be last in large overdoses. Selegiline transdermal system is FDA approved for treatment of major depressive disorder in adults as an alternative to the traditional oral delivery system.[1,2,57] Rasagiline is another MAO-B selective MAOI that is FDA approved to treat Parkinson disease.[19]

Third-Generation Monoamine Oxidase Inhibitors: Selective and Reversible

Reversible inhibitors of monoamine oxidase-A (RIMAs) are a class of drugs that selectively and reversibly inhibit MAO-A.[57] These xenobiotics were developed in an effort to compensate for the limitations of first- and second-generation MAOIs (see Clinical Manifestations). Reversible inhibitors of monoamine oxidase-A can be displaced by tyramine from the active site of the enzyme MAO-B, thereby enabling peripheral metabolism of the amine. Because tyramine is not present in high concentrations in the brain, MAO-A continues to be inhibited, and the antidepressant effects are achieved.[57] Moclobemide is the most widely studied RIMA and is approved as an antidepressant in Europe and other parts of the world but not the United States.[33]

Naturally Occurring Monoamine Oxidase Inhibitors

The extract of the plant St. John's wort (*Hypericum perforatum*) is licensed in Germany for use as an antidepressant. Although the major constituents, hypericin and hyperforin, have weak MAOI activity, it is uncertain whether this activity is responsible for its antidepressant effect. However, MAOI activity explains sporadic reports of hypertensive crises, cardiovascular collapse during anesthesia, and the development of serotonin toxicity associated with use of St. John's wort.[51,84]

Ayahuasca, a hallucinogenic beverage used by South American natives, is an ethnobotanical mixture of dimethyltryptamine and harmala alkaloids that circumvents gastrointestinal (GI) MAO. Dimethyltryptamine, which is a potent hallucinogen, is derived from several local plant species[26] but is not normally orally bioavailable because of its first-pass metabolism by MAO.[75] When *Banisteriopsis caapi*, a plant containing the MAO-inhibiting harmala alkaloids, is mixed with dimethyltryptamine-containing plants, the bioavailability of this hallucinogenic amine is increased.[73,74] Cortical activation occurs in the anterior and posterior cingulate cortex, parietal and occipital cortex, and other areas. 5-HT_{2A} mediated reductions in α oscillations in the parietal and occipital cortex correlate with visual imagery intensity.[23] Ayahuasca has been evaluated in preclinical studies for its potential antidepressant, anxiolytic, and antiaddictive properties, with limited success. Ayahuasca is currently being used as an alternative medicine approach to drug detoxification at many centers in North and Central America, although data on efficacy are lacking. Toxicity includes visual hallucinations, perceptual modifications, blurred vision, euphoria, intense "emotional modification," panic, cerebellar signs (incoordination, ataxia), anxiety, listlessness, CNS depression, seizures, tachycardia, hypertension, tachypnea, nausea, vomiting, and in some instances prolonged psychotic disorders. Similarly, Syrian rue (*Peganum harmala*) contains harmine and harmaline alkaloids, short-acting inhibitors of MAO_A. It has been used alone or in combination with *Acacia confusa*, which contains dimethyltryptamine (DMT) for similar hallucinogenic intent.

Monoamine oxidase-B activity in tobacco plants has prompted studies to find a link between the lower platelet MAO-B activity of smokers and their lower rate of Parkinson disease.[15] This finding has led to interest in studying other MAO-B inhibitors for potential applications as neuroprotective xenobiotics.[132]

Miscellaneous and Experimental Monoamine Oxidase Inhibitors

Other xenobiotics with nonselective MAO inhibitory properties are used for purposes unrelated to MAO inhibition. Furazolidone is an antimicrobial used to treat protozoan-related diarrhea and bacterial enteritis. Procarbazine is a hydrazide derivative indicated as a chemotherapeutic for stage III and IV Hodgkin disease as part of the MOPP (nitrogen mustard, vincristine, procarbazine, prednisone) regimen. Linezolid is an antibiotic that produces weak, nonselective MAO inhibition in Parkinson disease.[29,113,120] Azure B, a metabolite of methylene blue, is a high-potency reversible inhibitor of MAO.[85]

Research is active for novel MAO combination xenobiotics that target multiple mechanistic approaches for the treatment of dementia and parkinsonism.[27] Ladostigil combines the cholinergic effects of a carbamate with the aminergic effects of MAO-B inhibition.[103] M30 is an actively researched xenobiotic that combines iron chelation and radical scavenger effects with irreversible, nonselective MAO inhibition.[35] Neither xenobiotic has been approved by the FDA.

PHARMACOKINETICS AND TOXICOKINETICS

Monoamine oxidase inhibitors are absorbed readily when given by mouth, and peak plasma concentrations are reached within 2 to 3 hours. Similar to other antidepressants, these xenobiotics are lipophilic and readily cross the blood–brain barrier. Monoamine oxidase inhibitors are hepatically metabolized by both oxidation (various CYP enzymes, including CYP2D6 and CYP2C19) and acetylation (N-acetyltransferase), to metabolites that are excreted in the urine.[4]

Similar to the original MAOI, iproniazid, phenelzine and isocarboxazid are metabolized to hydrazides. The rate of metabolism of the hydrazide MAOIs is dependent on the N-acetyltransferase phenotype (ie, "acetylator status") of the patient (ie, fast or slow). About half of the US population, but as low as 10% of Native Americans, have a recessive single gene trait that effects the N-acetyltransferase enzyme to cause slow acetylator status in the liver, contributing to exaggerated clinical effects despite standard therapeutic dosing or even mild overdose.

The clinical effects of MAOI inhibition occur rapidly and are usually maximal within a few days. First-generation, irreversible MAOIs have durations of effect that far surpass their pharmacologic half-lives, as discussed earlier.[117] Thus, when switching from one MAOI to another serotonergic drug such as a selective serotonin reuptake inhibitor (SSRI) or cyclic antidepressant, a sufficient time period of 2 to 3 weeks must be allowed to prevent an adverse drug interaction. It should be noted that the reverse is not true (ie, switching from SSRI to MAOI), except in the case of fluoxetine, whose active metabolite, norfluoxetine, has a long half-life; therefore, a time period of 5 weeks is recommended when switching from fluoxetine to an MAOI.

PATHOPHYSIOLOGY

As discussed earlier (see Mechanism of Action), MAOIs contribute to adrenergic stimulation via release of norepinephrine from sympathetic nerve terminals.[63] This leads to hyperadrenergic crises particularly in the presence of xenobiotics that serve as substrates for, or enhancers of, monoamine formation, such as tyramine.[62] In addition, norepinephrine release combined with MAO inhibition results in so-called "autopotentiation," or synergistic sympathomimetic effects. Autopotentiation is responsible for paradoxical or hypertensive reactions sometimes observed after therapeutic doses of MAOIs.[21,96]

Hydrazide MAOIs such as phenelzine inactivate pyridoxal 5′ phosphate, the cofactor necessary for neuronal decarboxylation of glutamic acid to the inhibitory neurotransmitter GABA. In addition, hydrazides complex with pyridoxine, the precursor of pyridoxal 5′ phosphate, thus enhancing its urinary elimination and further inhibiting the formation of neuronal GABA.[83] Decreased availability of neuronal GABA leads to CNS excitation after overdose of hydrazide MAOIs (Chaps. 56 and 117).[60]

Impaired $GABA_A$ activity contributes to symptoms of CNS excitation such as seizures, which occur in MAOI overdose. In animal models, isocarboxazid and tranylcypromine directly inhibit GABA-mediated Cl⁻ influx at $GABA_A$ receptors (Chap. 13).[113] The exact binding site of MAOIs on the $GABA_A$ receptor complex is unknown. γ-Aminobutyric acid effects appear to be most localized in the caudate putamen and nucleus accumbens areas in one animal model.[83] Elevated neuronal glutamate concentrations caused by MAOI effects also synergistically enhance CNS excitation.[106]

ADVERSE EFFECTS

Overdose

Monoamine oxidase inhibitor overdose results in severe and life-threatening clinical manifestations, especially if the MAOI is a first-generation drug such as phenelzine. Classically, the clinical course involves a biphasic response characterized by initial CNS excitation and peripheral sympathetic stimulation that terminates in coma and cardiovascular collapse.[65] This biphasic model is hypothesized to result from an initial adrenergic crisis followed by inhibition of norepinephrine release[134] and is supported by animal studies.[37,41] Additionally, depletion of norepinephrine stores is responsible for delayed hypotension observed over the course of an MAOI overdose. Toxic dose–response relationships in humans are unclear, but an overdose of 5 mg/kg of a first-generation MAOI is potentially life threatening.[8,65] Clinical manifestations of MAOI overdose are summarized in Table 71–2.

Patients with MAOI overdose are initially asymptomatic for several hours. Delays in clinical toxicity are well described.[69,71,95] Hypotheses that might explain this phenomenon include all of the following: initial reversible binding to MAO, cumulative effects, time-dependent alterations to MAO

substrate stores, individual acetylator status, and hydrolysis of the hydrazide MAOIs. Although clinical toxicity should generally be apparent within the first several hours (initially with neuromuscular and sympathetic effects),[65] maximal toxicity is reportedly delayed up to 24 hours after overdose.[65,71,95]

Neurologic effects can be considered neuropsychiatric, neuromuscular, mental status alteration, seizures, and chronic effects. Neuropsychiatric effects include agitation, akathisia, and hallucinations. Neuromuscular effects include flailing and tremor of the extremities, nystagmus, opsoclonus, fasciculation, myoclonus, hypertonia, hyperreflexia, muscular irritability, and muscular rigidity, the latter of which leads to secondary effects such as hyperthermia and rhabdomyolysis. Effects on mental status include a variable spectrum from confusion to coma, the latter of which is a typically endstage finding.

Severe hyperthermia (>106°F) caused by MAOI toxicity has a multifactorial etiology and is an ominous sign.[107] Temperature dysregulation is caused by adrenergic crisis, muscular hypertonia, or CNS effects. Secondary effects from severe hyperthermia include disseminated intravascular coagulation and metabolic acidosis.[71]

Cardiovascular effects follow the previously described initial hyperadrenergic crisis followed by cardiovascular collapse. Thus, initially, hypertension, tachycardia, palpitations, and tachydysrhythmias are to be expected.[54] In severe poisoning, late toxicity includes development of hypotension, reflex tachycardia or bradycardia, bradydysrhythmias, and sudden death.[69,97] Alterations in myocardial supply–demand dynamics lead to myocardial injury with possible elevations of serum cardiac biomarkers (eg, troponin I). Myonecrosis[87] and myocarditis[126] are also attributed to MAOI overdose.

Abnormalities on electrocardiography (ECG) include ischemic changes on ECG (contiguous lead findings of T-wave inversion or ST-segment depression or elevation). Peaked T waves, in the presence[65] or absence[90] of hyperkalemia, are also noted. Myocardial manifestations associated with catastrophic CNS processes (eg, intracranial hemorrhage) can also lead to T-wave inversions.

In addition to the effects mentioned above and listed in Table 71–2, reported complications of MAOI overdose include acute kidney injury,[65,69,87,97] fetal demise,[97] and hemolysis.[65,71]

Selegiline Overdose

Selegiline is metabolized to L-methamphetamine, which results in hypertension and tachycardia, even at therapeutic doses.[6,3,101] Postmarketing surveillance safety data on the selegiline transdermal system demonstrated that only 13 (< 1%) of 1,516 patients studied reported a hypertensive event, none of which were objectively confirmed.[80] Selegiline overdose produces hallucinations and convulsions and is associated with elevated urinary concentrations of L-methamphetamine and L-amphetamine.[32,56]

TABLE 71–2	Comparison of the Clinical Manifestations of Monoamine Oxidase Inhibitor (MAOI) Toxicity		
Clinical Category	**Hyperadrenergic Crisis**	**Serotonin Toxicity**	**MAOI Overdose**
Onset	Minutes to hours	Minutes to hours	≤24 h
Duration	Hours	Hours	Days
Temperature	Normal	Elevated	Elevated
Neurologic	Headache, hemorrhagic stroke Neuromuscular excitation	Akathisia, hyperreflexia, shivering, tremor, seizures, autonomic instability, coma Myoclonus, "wet dog shakes," muscular rigidity	Neuropsychiatric effects, neuromuscular effects, headache, seizures Myoclonus, muscular rigidity
Cardiovascular	Hypertension, dysrhythmias, myocardial injury	Hypertension, hypotension, tachycardia, palpitations, dysrhythmias	Hypertension (early), hypotension (late), tachycardia, palpitations, dysrhythmias, myocardial injury
Gastrointestinal	Nausea	Hyperactive bowel sounds	Nausea, vomiting, diarrhea
Dermatologic	Flushing, diaphoresis	Diaphoresis	Flushing, piloerection, diaphoresis
Ophthalmologic	Mydriasis	Mydriasis	Mydriasis, ocular clonus

Moclobemide Overdose

Moclobemide overdose typically produces mild to moderate CNS depression (drowsiness, disorientation), GI effects (nausea), and cardiovascular effects (tachycardia and mild hypertension).[33,75] Serotonin toxicity caused by the ingestion of moclobemide, alone[49] and in combination with other serotonergics[77,86,124,129] is well described. In massive overdose, fatalities attributed solely to the toxic effects of moclobemide are reported.[14,34,40]

Hyperadrenergic Crisis

Hyperadrenergic crisis occurs in patients with MAO-A inhibition in the setting of exposure to other sympathomimetic drugs such as cocaine, epinephrine, or amphetamines or when tyramine-containing foods such as aged cheeses and fermented drinks are eaten (Table 71–3).[132] Tyramine is an indirect-acting sympathomimetic amine with an amphetaminelike mechanism of action.[134] The MAO-A present in the intestinal wall and liver extensively metabolizes dietary amines preventing them from entering the circulation, but in the presence of irreversible MAO-A inhibition, this protective mechanism is lost, allowing tyramine and other dietary monoamines to enter the circulation.[9] This enzymatic failure results in an amphetaminelike release of norepinephrine from peripheral adrenergic neurons and provocation of hyperadrenergic crisis. A meal that contains 6 to 8 mg of tyramine per serving can potentially precipitate this reaction, and ingestion of a total of 25 to 50 mg can produce a severe and possibly life-threatening reaction.[28,118,125] A European study of biogenic amines contained in retail meat products (eg, sausage, cold cuts) found that such products contained up to 50 mg/kg of tyramine, which would pose a high risk for individuals receiving first-generation MAOI therapy.[82] Additionally, despite compliance with diet, chronically elevated cytoplasmic and synaptic concentrations of norepinephrine caused by therapeutic MAOI administration leads to adrenergic crises in some patients. Dietary restrictions and recommendations for patients prescribed first-generation MAOIs are summarized in Table 71–3.[28,118,125] As detailed earlier, a period of 3 weeks is sufficient to allow a normal diet to be resumed.[119]

The clinical syndrome of tyramine-related hyperadrenergic crisis is characterized by hypertension, headache, flushing, diaphoresis, mydriasis, neuromuscular excitation, and potential cardiac dysrhythmias.[121] This reaction is subjectively reported in up to 10% of patients taking MAOIs chronically.[91] Monoamine oxidase inhibitors specific for the MAO-B isoform are less likely to predispose to food or drug interactions by maintaining significant hepatic MAO-A activity; however, isoform specificity is lost as dose is increased.

Serotonin Toxicity

Any xenobiotic with serotonin-potentiating activity can interact with the MAOIs to produce serotonin toxicity[10] (Chap. 69). Combinations of xenobiotics commonly implicated in this reaction are involved with serotonin synthesis (eg, L-tryptophan), release (eg, amphetamines), agonism (eg, triptans metabolized by MAO), neuromodulation (eg, lithium), or reuptake inhibition (eg, selective serotonin reuptake inhibitors, serotonin–norepinephrine reuptake inhibitors, meperidine, tramadol, dextromethorphan). Animal studies demonstrate that both meperidine[108] and dextromethorphan[109] administration can lead to fatal serotonin toxicity. Serotonin toxicity most commonly occurs in patients receiving combination therapy with two or more serotonergic xenobiotics; however, it rarely occurs with just one serotonergic xenobiotic such as venlafaxine.[81]

Clinically, serotonin toxicity runs a spectrum of severity[10] and is described in detail in Chap. 69. Minor findings can include akathisia, myoclonus, hyperreflexia, diaphoresis, penile erection, shivering, hyperactive bowel sounds, and tremor. Tremor and hyperreflexia are typically greater in the lower extremities. Shivering is classically described as similar to "wet dog shakes"[43] and can occur at a range of body temperatures.[79] Severe signs and symptoms include life-threatening autonomic instability, muscular rigidity, and hyperthermia.

Several diagnostic schemes for serotonin toxicity exist.[10,24,46,92,114] However, the key diagnostic criterion is exposure to a serotonergic. Because no diagnostic test is yet available, the diagnosis of serotonin toxicity must be established on clinical grounds. The onset of clinical symptoms typically occurs within minutes after a change in medication or self-poisoning.[68] Most patients with serotonin toxicity develop symptoms within 6 hours. Key clinical features of MAOI-induced serotonin toxicity are summarized in Table 71–2.

Other Adverse Drug Reactions

Clinically significant drug interactions with MAOIs can be caused by serotonergic effects (see Serotonin Toxicity) and alterations to drug metabolism. Chronic use of phenelzine is also associated with an isoniazidlike peripheral neuropathy,[42] possibly explained by pyridoxine deficiency.[115] Administration of opioids with serotonergic properties (eg, meperidine, dextromethorphan) is absolutely contraindicated because of the risk of precipitating the serotonin toxicity.[10,39,100,108,109] Adverse drug reactions are expected with other coadministered drugs that are metabolized by cytochrome P450 enzymes because first-generation MAOIs have an extensive inhibitory effect on CYP2C9, CYP2C19, and CYP2D6.[4,104] Thus, prolonged sedation and respiratory depression is reported when barbiturates (eg, phenobarbital) and benzodiazepines (eg, diazepam, lorazepam), which are both metabolized by hepatic cytochrome P450 enzymes, are coadministered. Table 71–4 summarizes analgesic safety in combination with MAOI drugs.[39]

TABLE 71–3	Dietary Restrictions for Patients Taking Monoamine Oxidase Inhibitors[a]	
Low Tyramine Content (0–4 mg/serving)	Moderate Tyramine Content (4–8 mg/serving)	High Tyramine Content (> 8 mg/serving)
Chocolate	Avocado or guacamole	Aged, mature cheeses
Cottage cheese, cream cheese, yogurt, sour cream	Banana peels or stewed whole bananas	Broad beans or fava beans
Distilled alcohol	Meat extracts	Fermented sausage
Non-overripe fruit	Overripe fruit or figs	Liver
Soy sauce	Pasteurized light and pale beers	Red wines, selected beers
		Smoked, pickled, aged, putrefying meats or fish, caviar
		Yeast and meat extracts

[a]Recommendation: Foods with *high* tyramine content should be avoided, those with *moderate* content should be consumed in restricted moderation, and those with *low* content can be cautiously consumed.

TABLE 71–4	Analgesics/Anesthetics/Sedatives Safety When Combined with Monoamine Oxidase Inhibitors (MAOIs)		
Analgesic Class	Safe	Monitor Closely or Use Alternative if Medically Appropriate	Avoid Combination (Contraindicated)
Nonprescription	Acetaminophen Aspirin Nonsteroidal antiinflammatory drugs		Dextromethorphan
Opioids	Buprenorphine Codeine Morphine Oxycodone	Propoxyphene	Meperidine Pentazocine Tramadol Tapentadol
Nonopioids	Inhalational anesthetics Nitroglycerin	Barbiturates[a] Benzodiazepines[a] Ketamine	
Local anesthetics	Lidocaine		Cocaine

[a]Drugs metabolized by hepatic cytochrome P450 may produce prolonged sedation and respiratory depression when combined with MAOIs.

Drug Discontinuation Syndrome

Monamine oxidase inhibitor drug discontinuation syndrome typically begins 24 to 72 hours after discontinuation. Classically, sudden discontinuation of MAOI produces symptoms that are the worst after high therapeutic doses of tranylcypromine and isocarboxazid.[5] Symptoms range from nausea, vomiting, and malaise to CNS symptoms such as agitation, psychosis, and convulsions. Treatment is generally supportive and typically involves a benzodiazepine such as diazepam or lorazepam and restarting the medication if clinically indicated.

DIAGNOSTIC TESTING

The clinical utility of therapeutic drug monitoring in the routine use of MAOIs is limited. Evaluation of MAO activity is not routinely available, requires a fresh specimen (preferably jejunal biopsy),[64] and is therefore not recommended. Experimental evidence suggests that inhibition of human platelet MAO-B activity by at least 85% is associated with a favorable clinical antidepressant response to phenelzine.[31,36]

Evaluation of MAOI toxicity remains a clinical diagnosis. Serum concentrations of MAOIs that correlate meaningfully with clinical effects are not well established. In addition, serum concentrations of any antidepressant, in general, can be misleading when obtained postmortem for forensic purposes.[89,99] Hyperglycemia and leukocytosis are reported but likely are nonspecific findings. Elevations in serum lactate concentrations and metabolic acidosis result from seizures, muscular hypertonia, or hyperthermia.

Measurement of blood and urinary concentrations of MAO substrates provides indirect evidence of MAOI effects. Monoamine oxidase inhibitors increase serum serotonin, increase or decrease serum norepinephrine, increase urinary epinephrine and norepinephrine, and decrease urinary serotonin metabolites. Because of the indirect nature of this testing and the fact that its interpretation is fraught with confounding factors (eg, if the patient is receiving vasopressors), the routine measurement of serum and urinary MAO substrates is not recommended in the assessment of MAOI toxicity. Of note, patients taking selegiline[105] and tranylcypromine[132] occasionally test positive for amphetamines on drug screens because of their metabolites.

MANAGEMENT

Out of Hospital

Decisions regarding referral to the emergency department (ED) must take into account factors such as patient age, intent of exposure, and symptoms, as well as timing of exposure. All patients with MAOI exposures who display suicidal intent should be referred to an ED for evaluation. Children with exposure to even one adult formulation MAOI tablet or selegiline patch should be referred to the ED because of the potential for late-onset significant toxicity.[3] Patients who exhibit more than mild headache or minimal diaphoresis after an acute therapeutic error involving MAOI ingestion should be referred to an ED. Observation at home is warranted in patients who are asymptomatic and more than 24 hours have elapsed since the time of ingestion. Because of the paucity of data at this time, patients with selegiline patch ingestion should be referred to the ED for observation, even if suicidal intent is absent.

Prehospital

Activated charcoal is reasonable to be administered to asymptomatic patients who have ingested overdoses of MAOI if no contraindications are present.[17] Transportation to the hospital should not be delayed to administer activated charcoal. Use of intravenous (IV) benzodiazepines for seizures and external cooling measures for severe hyperthermia (>106°F {>41.1°C})[107] is recommended in consultation or authorization with medical direction from emergency medical services, by a written treatment protocol or policy, or with direct medical oversight.

Initial Approach in the Emergency Department

As with any serious ingestion, initial stabilization must include rapid assessment of the airway, breathing, and circulation as well as establishment of IV access, supplemental oxygen, and continuous cardiac monitoring. Hyperthermia or hemodynamic instability after MAOI ingestion is a manifestation of significant toxicity. Intravenous volume repletion should begin while focusing on stabilization of hyperthermia, seizures, and muscular rigidity. In any patient with altered mental status who will likely deteriorate, early endotracheal intubation not only protects the airway but also facilitates safe gastric decontamination measures.

Gastrointestinal Decontamination

Patients who overdose with MAOIs are more likely to benefit from GI decontamination than most other overdose patients because of their high potential for morbidity and mortality.[58,88] Orogastric lavage with a large bore orogastric tube (36–40 Fr) is recommended if a life-threatening ingestion is suspected to have occurred within several hours before presentation.[39,58,88] Single-dose activated charcoal is recommended orally (or via nasogastric tube) for patients who present within several hours of ingestion unless contraindications are present. Whole-bowel irrigation with oral polyethylene glycol electrolyte solution likely has limited utility unless there are coingestions with other sustained-release preparation medications and therefore not routinely recommended. The lack of early clinical findings of poisoning should not dissuade the use of GI decontamination given the potential for delayed clinical deterioration.

Cooling Measures

Severe hyperthermia must be treated with aggressive cooling. Ice baths (first choice for life-threatening hyperthermia),[110] cold water, and fans are the mainstays of treatment (Chap. 29). There is no available evidence to support use of invasive cooling devices either catheter based or noninvasive devices such as cooling blankets. Indications for ice bath immersion to treat MAOI toxicity include a rectal temperature greater than 106°F (41.1°C),[107] rigidity, and altered mental status. Benzodiazepines help to control muscular rigidity, seizures, and agitation and to contribute to amelioration of hyperthermia and tachycardia. Patients with refractory hyperthermia despite the above measures require neuromuscular blockade, using nondepolarizing paralytics, in conjunction with endotracheal intubation and ventilation. The depolarizing paralytic succinylcholine should be avoided in severe MAOI toxicity because of the risk of precipitating lethal dysrhythmia caused by hyperkalemia in the setting of rhabdomyolysis. Neuromuscular blockade eliminates hyperthermia that results from muscular rigidity and is recommended if first-line treatments are unsuccessful. Antipyretics such as acetaminophen and nonsteroidal antiinflammatory drugs should not be administered because the hyperthermia is not caused by alterations in the hypothalamic temperature set point (Chap. 29).[105]

Blood Pressure Control

Because there is characteristic fluctuation in vital signs associated with MAOI overdose, hemodynamic monitoring should be instituted even for patients who initially are stable. When supporting the patient's blood pressure, preference should be given to titratable drugs with a rapid onset and termination of action because of the potential for rapid hemodynamic changes. Use of β-adrenergic antagonists is contraindicated for control of hypertension in MAOI-related toxicity because the action of monoamines (eg, norepinephrine) at the neuronal synapse in the autonomic nervous system could result in refractory hypertension caused by unopposed α-adrenergic agonism.[94]

Patients who are normotensive at baseline and who experience MAOI-related severe hypertension can be preferably treated with phentolamine for effective control (2–5 mg IV).[9] Alternatively, nicardipine, nitroprusside, and nitroglycerin all allow for titratable blood pressure control.[19] Tyramine-related mild hypertensive crises can theoretically be controlled with the dihydropyridine calcium channel blockers such as nifedipine and possibly the oral α-adrenergic antagonists such as terazosin but should be used with caution.[18,47] Particular caution must be exercised in patients with baseline hypertension because overly aggressive blood pressure lowering will reduce cerebral perfusion pressure, potentially causing cerebral ischemia.

Patients who are hypotensive require aggressive support with IV fluid resuscitation and vasopressors. The direct-acting sympathetic vasopressors epinephrine and norepinephrine can be used safely in patients taking MAOIs.[11] Rather than causing release of a stored pool of norepinephrine, they bind directly with postsynaptic α- and β-adrenergic receptors, unlike dopamine.

Dopamine is contraindicated in hypotensive patients who have overdosed on MAOIs for several reasons. The indirect action of dopamine administration may produce a synergistic effect with MAOI, resulting in excessive adrenergic activity and exaggerated rises in blood pressure. In addition, most of the α-adrenergic receptor mediated vasoconstriction of dopamine is secondary to norepinephrine release; in the presence of MAOIs, norepinephrine synthesis is likely impaired from concomitant dopamine-β-hydroxylase inhibition, and dopamine will not reliably raise blood pressure if cytoplasmic and vesicular neuronal stores have been depleted. Finally, in the presence of impaired norepinephrine release or α-adrenergic blockade by any cause, unopposed dopamine-induced vasodilation from action on peripheral dopamine and β adrenoceptors may paradoxically lower blood pressure further.

Dysrhythmias

Because of the unique pharmacologic and toxicokinetic considerations of MAOI toxicity, Advanced Cardiac Life Support protocols should be slightly tailored to the patient.[122] Removal of the offending xenobiotic as well as correction of hypoxia, hypokalemia, and hypomagnesemia, if present, is the recommended initial step.

Patients with immediately life-threatening dysrhythmias require rapid cardioversion. In the presence of the nonperfusing dysrhythmias such as ventricular fibrillation, pulseless ventricular tachycardia, and torsade de pointes, unsynchronized electrical defibrillation is the treatment of choice.

In patients with stable ventricular tachycardia, a trial of an antidysrhythmic such as procainamide or amiodarone is recommended. High-quality studies evaluating the use of these xenobiotics in the setting of MAOI overdose are not available.

Hemodynamically significant supraventricular tachycardia from MAOI toxicity should be corrected to prevent myocardial ischemia or infarction, ventricular dysrhythmia, and high-output heart failure. Benzodiazepines are safe and effective to treat sinus tachycardia as long as respiratory status remains monitored. Adenosine and synchronized cardioversion are unlikely to be useful in the setting of ongoing presence of the MAOI, but are reasonable in rare cases that are unresponsive to benzodiazepines. In patients with borderline hypotension, nondihydropyridine calcium channel antagonists such as diltiazem and verapamil are relatively contraindicated because they may further lower blood pressure due to bradycardia and heart block.

Hemodynamically significant bradycardia from MAOI toxicity includes management of IV fluid and atropine as first-line therapy to temporize the patient with bradycardia and hypotension. Epinephrine and isoproterenol are recommended second choices while a pacemaker (transcutaneous or transvenous) is prepared.

Management of Central Nervous System Manifestations

In any patient with acute altered mental status, hypoglycemia should be rapidly excluded.[12,102] For patients with mild to moderate CNS excitation with small incremental doses of parenteral diazepam or midazolam are recommended. Patients with seizures should be treated with benzodiazepines in standard incremental doses. Empiric administration of pyridoxine (vitamin B₆), intravenously at 70 mg/kg, up to 5 g in adults, is reasonable in patients with status epilepticus, particularly after massive ingestions of hydrazide-derived MAOIs such as phenelzine because of its ability to deplete endogenous pyridoxine stores (Antidotes in Depth: A15).[115] Phenytoin should not be used for treatment of MAOI-induced seizures because there is no distinct seizure focus but rather generalized neuronal dysfunction in the presence of MAOI (and metabolites) in the CNS.

Cyproheptadine

Cyproheptadine is a nonselective serotonin antagonist (with additional anticholinergic, histaminic, and some serotonin agonism) that is recommended as third-line therapy (after benzodiazepine administration and cooling measures) for serotonin toxicity.[10] Cyproheptadine prevents lethality in animal models of serotonin toxicity[78] and reportedly is beneficial in humans, although its efficacy has not been rigorously established.[38,44] It is suggested when the diagnosis of serotonin toxicity is likely, especially if incomplete response has been achieved with aggressive cooling and benzodiazepine therapy.[61] In addition, its use to treat neuromuscular rigidity and hyperthermia associated with MAOI overdose is reported.[7,25]

The recommended initial dose in adults is 12 mg orally followed by 2 mg every 2 hours while symptoms continue.[10] A dose of 12 to 32 mg will bind 85% to 95% of serotonin receptors.[55] The dose of cyproheptadine used to treat the serotonin toxicity may cause sedation, but this effect is a goal of therapy and should not deter clinicians from using the drug. Relative contraindications to its use include acute asthma exacerbation, GI obstruction, and age younger than 2 years (because of a lack of safety information for this age group).

Dantrolene

Use of dantrolene in patients with serotonin toxicity is not recommended (Antidotes in Depth: A24). Case reports citing its utility with off-label usage probably involved misdiagnosis.[10,52] Malignant hyperthermia, for which dantrolene is indicated, is a disease that is completely unrelated to serotonin toxicity. In animal models of serotonin toxicity, dantrolene administration has no effect on survival.[50,78] In addition, dantrolene is implicated in the fatality of one case of serotonin toxicity.[55]

Extracorporeal Elimination

The utility of extracorporeal measures, such as hemodialysis, to treat MAOI toxicity remains to be demonstrated. There is limited rationale to perform hemodialysis because toxicity persists long after the xenobiotic is gone. Additionally, the data regarding protein binding and volumes of distribution of the first-generation MAOI drugs such as isocarboxazid are not well characterized. Use of peritoneal dialysis[66] and hemodialysis[72] to treat MAOI overdose has been reported in the literature. However, time to resolution of symptoms for all cases did not differ (~24 hours) from those in which hemodialysis was not used. Therefore, extracorporeal elimination is not recommended in the management of MAOI overdose unless other indications are present such as severe acidemia or life-threatening hyperkalemia or the need to eliminate dialyzable toxic coingestions.

Disposition

Recommendations for the ideal time frame for observation of patients with suspected MAOI overdose are limited by a paucity of relevant studies in the clinical toxicology literature. For patients with presumed MAOI (selective or nonselective) overdose, it is reasonable to observe them with telemetry monitoring, preferably in an intensive care unit, for at least 24 hours regardless of the initial clinical findings. This recommendation takes into account the potential for delayed-onset of clinical toxicity as well as the potential for severe morbidity and mortality.[69,71,95] However, patients with MAOI–food or MAOI–xenobiotic interactions often do not require hospital admission if the interaction is mild and resolution of symptoms is complete.

SUMMARY

- Toxicity from MAOI exposures is becoming less common because of more limited clinical usage of the traditional nonselective MAOIs; however, clinical and research use of selective MAOIs and RIMAs is increasing.
- Inhibition of MAO has effects on myriad neuronal neurotransmitters, which are responsible for the majority of the therapeutic and toxic effects of MAOIs.
- The clinical effects of MAOI overdose include neurotoxicity and cardiovascular collapse; this overdose is potentially life threatening and should be managed aggressively.
- Aside from overdose, other consequential manifestations of MAOI toxicity include hyperadrenergic crisis and the serotonin toxicity.

REFERENCES

1. American Academy of Pediatrics Committee on Injury, Violence, and Poison Prevention. Poison Treatment in the Home. *Pediatrics.* 2003;112:1182-1185.
2. Amsterdam JD. A double-blind, placebo-controlled trial of the safety and efficacy of selegiline transdermal system without dietary restrictions in patients with major depressive disorder. *J Clin Psychiatry.* 2003;64:208-214.
3. Azzaro AJ, et al. Evaluation of the potential for pharmacodynamic and pharmacokinetic drug interactions between selegiline transdermal system and two sympathomimetic agents (pseudoephedrine and phenylpropanolamine) in healthy volunteers. *J Clin Pharmacol.* 2007;47:978-990.
4. Baker GB, et al. Metabolism of monoamine oxidase inhibitors. *Cell Mol Neurobiol.* 1999;19:411-426.
5. Baldessarini RJ, et al. Discontinuing psychotropic agents. *J Psychopharmacol.* 1999;13:292-293; discussion 299.
6. Bar Am O, et al. Contrasting neuroprotective and neurotoxic actions of respective metabolites of anti-Parkinson drugs rasagiline and selegiline. *Neurosci Lett.* 2004;355:169-172.
7. Beasley CM Jr, et al. Possible monoamine oxidase inhibitor-serotonin uptake inhibitor interaction: fluoxetine clinical data and preclinical findings. *J Clin Psychopharmacol.* 1993;13:312-320.
8. Bell DB 2nd, Scaff J. Fatal reaction to tranylcypromine (Parnate). *Hawaii Med J.* 1963;22:440-441.
9. Bieck PR, Antonin KH. Oral tyramine pressor test and the safety of monoamine oxidase inhibitor drugs: comparison of brofaromine and tranylcypromine in healthy subjects. *J Clin Psychopharmacol.* 1988;8:237-245.
10. Boyer EW, Shannon M. The serotonin syndrome. *N Engl J Med.* 2005;352:1112-1120.
11. Braverman B, et al. Vasopressor challenges during chronic MAOI or TCA treatment in anesthetized dogs. *Life Sci.* 1987;40:2587-2595.
12. Bressler R, et al. Tranylcypromine: a potent insulin secretagogue and hypoglycemic agent. *Diabetes.* 1968;17:617-624.
13. Bronstein AC, et al. 2010 Annual Report of the American Association of Poison Control Centers' National Poison Data System (NPDS): 28th annual report. *Clin Toxicol (Phila).* 2011;49:910-941.
14. Camaris C, Little D. A fatality due to moclobemide. *J Forens Sci.* 1997;42:954-955.
15. Castagnoli K, Murugesan T. Tobacco leaf, smoke and smoking, MAO inhibitors, Parkinson's disease and neuroprotection; are there links? *Neurotoxicology.* 2004;25:279-291.
16. Chen JJ, et al. Comprehensive review of rasagiline, a second-generation monoamine oxidase inhibitor, for the treatment of Parkinson's disease. *Clin Ther.* 2007;29:1825-1849.
17. Chyka PA, et al. Position paper: single-dose activated charcoal. *Clin Toxicol (Phila).* 2005;43:61-87.
18. Clary C, Schweizer E. Treatment of MAOI hypertensive crisis with sublingual nifedipine. *J Clin Psychiatry.* 1987;48:249-250.
19. Cockhill LA, Remick RA. Blood pressure effects of monoamine oxidase inhibitors—the highs and lows. *Can J Psychiatry.* 1987;32:803-808.
20. Collins GGS, et al. Multiple forms of human brain mitochondrial monoamine oxidase. *Nature.* 1970;225:817-820.
21. Cooper AJ, et al. A hypertensive syndrome with tranylcypromine medication. *Lancet.* 1964;1:527-529.
22. Healy D. *The Antidepressant Era.* Cambridge, MA: Harvard University Press; 1997.
23. Dos Santos RG, et al. Antidepressive, anxiolytic, and antiaddictive effects of ayahuasca, psilocybin and lysergic acid diethylamide (LSD): a systematic review of clinical trials published in the last 25 years. *Ther Adv Psychopharmacol.* 2016;6:193-213.
24. Dunkley EJ, et al. The Hunter Serotonin Toxicity Criteria: simple and accurate diagnostic decision rules for serotonin toxicity. *QJM.* 2003;96:635-642.
25. Erich JL, et al. "Ping-pong" gaze in severe monoamine oxidase inhibitor toxicity. *J Emerg Med.* 1995;13:653-655.
26. Erowid. The vaults of N.N-DMT. http://www.erowid.org/chemicals/dmt.
27. Fernandez HH, Chen JJ. Monoamine oxidase inhibitors: current and emerging agents for Parkinson disease. *Clin Neuropharmacol.* 2007;30:150-168.
28. Folks DG. Monoamine oxidase inhibitors: reappraisal of dietary considerations. *J Clin Psychopharmacol.* 1983;3:249-252.
29. French G. Safety and tolerability of linezolid. *J Antimicrob Chemother.* 2003;51(suppl 2):ii45-53.
30. Frieling H, Bleich S. Tranylcypromine: new perspectives on an "old" drug. *Eur Arch Psychiatry Clin Neurosci.* 2006;256:268-273.
31. Fritz RR, et al. Tranylcypromine lowers human platelet MAO B activity but not concentration. *Biol Psychiatry.* 1983;18:685-694.
32. Fujita Y, et al. Detection of levorotatory methamphetamine and levorotatory amphetamine in urine after ingestion of an overdose of selegiline. *Yakugaku Zasshi.* 2008;128:1507-1512.
33. Fulton B, Benfield P. Moclobemide. An update of its pharmacological properties and therapeutic use. *Drugs.* 1996;52:450-474.
34. Gaillard Y, Pepin G. Moclobemide fatalities: report of two cases and analytical determinations by GC-MS and HPLC-PDA after solid-phase extraction. *Forens Sci Int.* 1997;87:239-248.
35. Gal S, et al. M30, a novel multifunctional neuroprotective drug with potent iron chelating and brain selective monoamine oxidase-ab inhibitory activity for Parkinson's disease. *J Neural Transm Suppl.* 2006:447-456.
36. Georgotas A, et al. Prediction of response to nortriptyline and phenelzine by platelet MAO activity. *Am J Psychiatry.* 1987;144:338-340.
37. Gessa GL, et al. On the mechanism of hypotensive effects of MAO inhibitors. *Ann N Y Acad Sci.* 1963;107:935-944.
38. Gillman PK. The serotonin syndrome and its treatment. *J Psychopharmacol.* 1999;13:100-109.
39. Gillman PK. Monoamine oxidase inhibitors, opioid analgesics and serotonin toxicity. *Br J Anaesth.* 2005;95:434-441.
40. Giroud C, et al. Death following acute poisoning by moclobemide. *Forens Sci Int.* 2004;140:101-107.
41. Goldberg ND, Shideman FE. Species differences in the cardiac effects of a monoamine oxidase inhibitor. *J Pharmacol Exp Ther.* 1962;136:142-151.
42. Goodheart RS, et al. Phenelzine associated peripheral neuropathy—clinical and electrophysiologic findings. *Aust N Z J Med.* 1991;21:339-340.
43. Gorzalka BB, Hanson LA. Sexual behavior and wet dog shakes in the male rat: regulation by corticosterone. *Behav Brain Res.* 1998;97:143-151.
44. Graudins A, et al. Treatment of the serotonin syndrome with cyproheptadine. *J Emerg Med.* 1998;16:615-619.
45. Haefely W, et al. Biochemistry and pharmacology of moclobemide, a prototype RIMA. *Psychopharmacology.* 1992;106(suppl):S6-S14.
46. Hegerl U, et al. The serotonin syndrome scale: first results on validity. *Eur Arch Psychiatry Clin Neurosci.* 1998;248:96-103.
47. Hesselink JM. Safer use of MAOIs with nifedipine to counteract potential hypertensive crisis. *Am J Psychiatry.* 1991;148:1616.
48. Holt A, et al. On the binding of monoamine oxidase inhibitors to some sites distinct from the MAO active site, and effects thereby elicited. *Neurotoxicology.* 2004;25:251-266.
49. Isbister GK, et al. Moclobemide poisoning: toxicokinetics and occurrence of serotonin toxicity. *Br J Clin Pharmacol.* 2003;56:441-450.
50. Isbister GK, Whyte IM. Serotonin toxicity and malignant hyperthermia: role of 5-HT2 receptors. *Br J Anaesth.* 2002;88:603; author reply 603-604.
51. Izzo AA. Drug interactions with St. John's Wort (Hypericum perforatum): a review of the clinical evidence. *Int J Clin Pharmacol Ther.* 2004;42:139-148.
52. Kaplan RF, et al. Phenelzine overdose treated with dantrolene sodium. *JAMA.* 1986;255:642-644.
53. Kapur S, et al. Cyproheptadine: a potent in vivo serotonin antagonist. *Am J Psychiatry.* 1997;154:884.
54. Keck PE Jr, et al. Acute cardiovascular response to monoamine oxidase inhibitors: a prospective assessment. *J Clin Psychopharmacol.* 1989;9:203-206.
55. Kline SS, et al. Serotonin syndrome versus neuroleptic malignant syndrome as a cause of death. *Clin Pharm.* 1989;8:510-514.
56. Kobayashi T, et al. Pharmacoresistant convulsions and visual hallucinations around two weeks after selegiline overdose: a case report. *Pharmacopsychiatry.* 2011;44:346-347.
57. Krishnan KR. Revisiting monoamine oxidase inhibitors. *J Clin Psychiatry.* 2007;68 (suppl 8):35-41.
58. Kulig K, et al. Management of acutely poisoned patients without gastric emptying. *Ann Emerg Med.* 1985;14:562-567.
59. Lancranjan I. The endocrine profile of bromocriptine: its application in endocrine diseases. *J Neural Transm.* 1981;51:61-82.
60. Landolt HP, Gillin JC. Different effects of phenelzine treatment on EEG topography in waking and sleep in depressed patients. *Neuropsychopharmacology.* 2002;27:462-469.
61. Lappin RI, Auchincloss EL. Treatment of the serotonin syndrome with cyproheptadine. *N Engl J Med.* 1994;331:1021-1022.
62. Lavin MR, et al. Spontaneous hypertensive reactions with monoamine oxidase inhibitors. *Biol Psychiatry.* 1993;34:146-151.
63. Lee WC, et al. Cardiac activities of several monoamine oxidase inhibitors. *J Pharmacol Exp Ther.* 1961;133:180.
64. Levine RJ, Sjoerdsma A. Estimation of monamine oxidase activity in man: techniques and applications. *Ann N Y Acad Sci.* 1963;107:966-974.
65. Linden CH, et al. Monoamine oxidase inhibitor overdose. *Ann Emerg Med.* 1984;13:1137-1144.
66. Lipkin D, Kushnick T. Pargyline hydrochloride poisoning in a child. *JAMA.* 1967;201:135-136.
67. Mann JJ, et al. Studies of selective and reversible monoamine oxidase inhibitors. *J Clin Psychiatry.* 1984;45(7 Pt 2):62-66.
68. Mason PJ, et al. Serotonin syndrome. Presentation of 2 cases and review of the literature. *Medicine.* 2000;79:201-209.
69. Matell G, Thorstrand C. A case of fatal nialamide poisoning. *Acta Med Scand.* 1967;181:79-82.
70. Matter BJ, et al. Tranylcypromine sulfate poisoning; successful treatment by hemodialysis. *Arch Intern Med.* 1965;116:18-20.
71. Mawdsley JA. "Parstelin." A case of fatal overdose. *Med J Aust.* 1968;2:292.
72. McDaniel KD. Clinical pharmacology of monoamine oxidase inhibitors. *Clin Neuropharmacol.* 1986;9:207-234.
73. McKenna DJ. Clinical investigations of the therapeutic potential of ayahuasca: rationale and regulatory challenges. *Pharmacol Ther.* 2004;102:111-129.

74. McKenna DJ, et al. Monoamine oxidase inhibitors in South American hallucinogenic plants: tryptamine and beta-carboline constituents of ayahuasca. *J Ethnopharmacol.* 1984;10:195-223.

75. Myrenfors PG, et al. Moclobemide overdose. *J Intern Med.* 1993;233:113-115.

76. Nelson SD, et al. Isoniazid and iproniazid: activation of metabolites to toxic intermediates in man and rat. *Science.* 1976;193:901-903.

77. Neuvonen PJ, et al. Five fatal cases of serotonin syndrome after moclobemide-citalopram or moclobemide-clomipramine overdoses. *Lancet.* 1993;342:1419.

78. Nisijima K, et al. Potent serotonin (5-HT)(2A) receptor antagonists completely prevent the development of hyperthermia in an animal model of the 5-HT syndrome. *Brain Res.* 2001;890:23-31.

79. Okada F, Okajima K. Abnormalities of thermoregulation induced by fluvoxamine. *J Clin Psychopharmacol.* 2001;21:619-621.

80. Pae CU, et al. Safety of selegiline transdermal system in clinical practice: analysis of adverse events from postmarketing exposures. *J Clin Psychiatry.* 2012;73:661-668.

81. Pan JJ, Shen WW. Serotonin syndrome induced by low-dose venlafaxine. *Ann Pharmacother.* 2003;37:209-211.

82. Papavergou EJ, et al. Levels of biogenic amines in retail market fermented meat products. *Food Chem.* 2012;135:2750-2755.

83. Parent MB, et al. Effects of the antidepressant/antipanic drug phenelzine and its putative metabolite phenylethylidenehydrazine on extracellular gamma-aminobutyric acid levels in the striatum. *Biochem Pharmacol.* 2002;63:57-64.

84. Patel S, et al. Hypertensive crisis associated with St. John's Wort. *Am J Med.* 2002;112:507-508.

85. Petzer A, et al. Azure B, a metabolite of methylene blue, is a high-potency, reversible inhibitor of monoamine oxidase. *Toxicol Appl Pharmacol.* 2012;258:403-409.

86. Pilgrim JL, et al. Serotonin toxicity involving MDMA (ecstasy) and moclobemide. *Forens Sci Int.* 2012;215:184-188.

87. Platts MM, et al. Phenelzine and trifluoperazine poisoning. *Lancet.* 1965;2:738.

88. Pond SM, et al. Gastric emptying in acute overdose: a prospective randomised controlled trial. *Med J Aust.* 1995;163:345-349.

89. Prouty RW, Anderson WH. The forensic science implications of site and temporal influences on postmortem blood-drug concentrations. *J Forens Sci.* 1990;35:243-270.

90. Quill TE. Peaked "T" waves with tranylcypromine (Parnate) overdose. *Int J Psychiatry Med.* 1981;11:155-160.

91. Rabkin JG, et al. Adverse reactions to monoamine oxidase inhibitors. Part II. Treatment correlates and clinical management. *J Clin Psychopharmacol.* 1985;5:2-9.

92. Radomski JW, et al. An exploratory approach to the serotonin syndrome: an update of clinical phenomenology and revised diagnostic criteria. *Med Hypotheses.* 2000;55:218-224.

93. Raft D, et al. Relationship between response to phenelzine and MAO inhibition in a clinical trial of phenelzine, amitriptyline and placebo. *Neuropsychobiology.* 1981;7:122-126.

94. Ramoska E, Sacchetti AD. Propranolol-induced hypertension in treatment of cocaine intoxication. *Ann Emerg Med.* 1985;14:1112-1113.

95. Reid DD, Kerr WC. Phenelzine poisoning responding to phenothiazine. *Med J Aust.* 1969;2:1214-1215.

96. Richards DW. Paradoxical hypertension from tranylcypromine sulfate. *JAMA.* 1963;186:854.

97. Robertson JC. Recovery after massive MAOI overdose complicated by malignant hyperpyrexia, treated with chlorpromazine. *Postgrad Med J.* 1972;48:64-65.

98. Robinson DS, Amsterdam JD. The selegiline transdermal system in major depressive disorder: a systematic review of safety and tolerability. *J Affect Disord.* 2008;105:15-23.

99. Rogde S, et al. Fatal combined intoxication with new antidepressants. Human cases and an experimental study of postmortem moclobemide redistribution. *Forens Sci Int.* 1999;100:109-116.

100. Rogers KJ, Thornton JA. The interaction between monoamine oxidase inhibitors and narcotic analgesics in mice. *Br J Pharmacol.* 1969;36:470-480.

101. Rose LM, et al. A hypertensive reaction induced by concurrent use of selegiline and dopamine. *Ann Pharmacother.* 2000;34:1020-1024.

102. Rowland MJ, et al. Hypoglycemia caused by selegiline, an antiparkinsonian drug: can such side effects be predicted? *J Clin Pharmacol.* 1994;34:80-85.

103. Sagi Y, et al. The neurochemical and behavioral effects of the novel cholinesterase-monoamine oxidase inhibitor, ladostigil, in response to L-dopa and L-tryptophan, in rats. *Br J Pharmacol.* 2005;146:553-560.

104. Salsali M, et al. Inhibitory effects of the monoamine oxidase inhibitor tranylcypromine on the cytochrome P450 enzymes CYP2C19, CYP2C9, and CYP2D6. *Cell Mol Neurobiol.* 2004;24:63-76.

105. Shin HS. Metabolism of selegiline in humans. Identification, excretion, and stereochemistry of urine metabolites. *Drug Metab Dispos.* 1997;25:657-662.

106. Shioda K, et al. Extracellular serotonin, dopamine and glutamate levels are elevated in the hypothalamus in a serotonin syndrome animal model induced by tranylcypromine and fluoxetine. *Prog Neuropsychopharmacol Biol Psychiatry.* 2004;28:633-640.

107. Simon HB. Hyperthermia. *N Engl J Med.* 1993;329:483-487.

108. Sinclair JG. The effects of meperidine and morphine in rabbits pretreated with phenelzine. *Toxicol Appl Pharmacol.* 1972;22:231-240.

109. Sinclair JG. Dextromethorphan-monoamine oxidase inhibitor interaction in rabbits. *J Pharm Pharmacol.* 1973;25:803-808.

110. Smith J, Wallis L. Cooling methods used in the treatment of exertional heat illness. *Br J Sports Med.* 2005;39:503-507.

111. Snider SR, et al. Increase in brain serotonin produced by bromocriptine. *Neurosci Lett.* 1975;1:237-241.

112. Sola CL, et al. Anticipating potential linezolid-SSRI interactions in the general hospital setting: an MAOI in disguise. *Mayo Clin Proc.* 2006;81:330-334.

113. Squires RF, Saederup E. Antidepressants and metabolites that block GABA$_A$ receptors coupled to 35S-t-butylbicyclophosphorothionate binding sites in rat brain. *Brain Res.* 1988;441:15-22.

114. Sternbach H. The serotonin syndrome. *Am J Psychiatry.* 1991;148:705-713.

115. Stewart JW, et al. Phenelzine-induced pyridoxine deficiency. *J Clin Psychopharmacol.* 1984;4:225-226.

116. Sulzer D, Rayport S. Amphetamine and other psychostimulants reduce pH gradients in midbrain dopaminergic neurons and chromaffin granules: a mechanism of action. *Neuron.* 1990;5:797-808.

117. Szuba MP, et al. Rapid conversion from one monoamine oxidase inhibitor to another. *J Clin Psychiatry.* 1997;58:307-310.

118. Tailor SA, et al. Hypertensive episode associated with phenelzine and tap beer—a reanalysis of the role of pressor amines in beer. *J Clin Psychopharmacol.* 1994;14:5-14.

119. Thase ME, et al. MAOIs in the contemporary treatment of depression. *Neuropsychopharmacology.* 1995;12:185-219.

120. Thomas CR, et al. Serotonin syndrome and linezolid. *J Am Acad Child Adolesc Psychiatry.* 2004;43:790.

121. Tollefson GD. Monoamine oxidase inhibitors: a review. *J Clin Psychiatry.* 1983;44:280-288.

122. Ulus IH, et al. Characterization of phentermine and related compounds as monoamine oxidase (MAO) inhibitors. *Biochem Pharmacol.* 2000;59:1611-1621.

123. Vanden Hoek TL, et al. Part 12: cardiac arrest in special situations: 2010 American Heart Association Guidelines for Cardiopulmonary Resuscitation and Emergency Cardiovascular Care. *Circulation.* 2010;122(18 suppl 3):S829-861.

124. Vuori E, et al. Death following ingestion of MDMA (ecstasy) and moclobemide. *Addiction.* 2003;98:365-368.

125. Walker SE, et al. Tyramine content of previously restricted foods in monoamine oxidase inhibitor diets. *J Clin Psychopharmacol.* 1996;16:383-388.

126. Waring WS, Wallace WA. Acute myocarditis after massive phenelzine overdose. *Eur J Clin Pharmacol.* 2007;63:1007-1009.

127. Wells DG, Bjorksten AR. Monoamine oxidase inhibitors revisited. *Can J Anaesth.* 1989;36:64-74.

128. White K, et al. Combined monoamine oxidase inhibitor-tricyclic antidepressant treatment: a pilot study. *Am J Psychiatry.* 1980;137:1422-1425.

129. Wu ML, Deng JF. Fatal serotonin toxicity caused by moclobemide and fluoxetine overdose. *Chang Gung Med J.* 2011;34:644-649.

130. Yamada M, Yasuhara H. Clinical pharmacology of MAO inhibitors: safety and future. *Neurotoxicology.* 2004;25:215-221.

131. Youdim MB, et al. Tranylcypromine ("Parnate") overdose: measurement of tranylcypromine concentrations and MAO inhibitory activity and identification of amphetamines in plasma. *Psychol Med.* 1979;9:377-382.

132. Youdim MB, Bakhle YS. Monoamine oxidase: isoforms and inhibitors in Parkinson's disease and depressive illness. *Br J Pharmacol.* 2006;147(suppl 1):S287-S296.

133. Youdim MB, Riederer PF. A review of the mechanisms and role of monoamine oxidase inhibitors in Parkinson's disease. *Neurology.* 2004;63(7 suppl 2):S32-S35.

134. Youdim MB, Weinstock M. Therapeutic applications of selective and non-selective inhibitors of monoamine oxidase A and B that do not cause significant tyramine potentiation. *Neurotoxicology.* 2004;25:243-250.

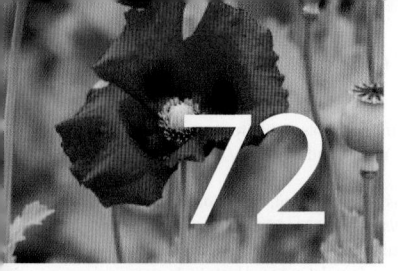

72 SEDATIVE–HYPNOTICS

Payal Sud and David C. Lee

HISTORY AND EPIDEMIOLOGY

Sedative–hypnotics are xenobiotics that limit excitability (sedation) and or induce drowsiness and sleep (hypnosis). *Anxiolytics* (formerly known as *minor tranquilizers*) are medications prescribed for their sedative–hypnotic properties. Mythology of ancient cultures is replete with stories of xenobiotics that cause sleep or unconsciousness (Chap. 1). Sedative–hypnotic overdoses were described in the medical literature soon after the commercial introduction of bromide preparations in 1853. Other commercial xenobiotics that subsequently were developed include chloral hydrate, paraldehyde, sulfonyl, and urethane.

Barbiturates were introduced in 1903 and quickly supplanted older xenobiotics. Barbiturates dominated the sedative–hypnotic market for the first half of the 20th century. Because of their narrow therapeutic index and substantial potential for abuse, they quickly became a major health problem. By the 1950s, barbiturates were frequently implicated in overdoses and were responsible for the majority of drug-related suicides. As fatalities from barbiturates increased, attention shifted toward preventing their abuse and finding less toxic alternatives.[19] After their introduction in the early 1960s, benzodiazepines quickly became the most commonly used sedatives in the United States.

Intentional and unintentional overdoses with sedative–hypnotics occur frequently. According to the American Association of Poison Control Centers, sedative–hypnotics is consistently one of the top five classes of xenobiotics associated with overdose fatalities (Chap. 130). With the ubiquitous worldwide use of sedative–hypnotics, they may be associated with a substantially higher number of overdoses and deaths than are officially reported. Compared with barbiturate overdoses, overdoses of benzodiazepines alone account for relatively few deaths.[29,36,43] Most deaths associated with benzodiazepines result from mixed overdoses with other respiratory depressants.[36,112]

Chlordiazepoxide, the first commercially available benzodiazepine, was initially marketed in 1960. Since then, more than 50 benzodiazepines have been marketed, and more are being developed. Although the benzodiazepines remain the most popular prescribed anxiolytics, several benzodiazepine-receptor agonists were developed in 1989 in an attempt to circumvent some of the side effects of benzodiazepines. These drugs include zolpidem, as zaleplon, zopiclone, and eszopiclone.[6,107] Newer formulations of zolpidem tartrate such as Intermezzo are now available, which is a low-dose sublingual tablet form (1.75 mg and 3.5 mg compared with 5 mg and 10 mg). Ramelteon and tasimelteon are newer sleep aids that function as melatonin receptor (MT$_1$ and MT$_2$) agonists rather than benzodiazepine-receptor agonists.[112,134] Dexmedetomidine, a central α_2-adrenergic agonist, is now increasingly used in the hospital setting for short-term sedation.[143] An additional medication is suvorexant, a dual orexin receptor antagonist that inhibits the action of orexin, a neuropeptide that promotes wakefulness.[30]

This chapter focuses primarily on pharmaceuticals prescribed for their sedative–hypnotic effects, many of which interact with the γ-aminobutyric acid-A (GABA$_A$) receptor (Table 72–1). Specific sedative–hypnotics such as ethanol and γ-hydroxybutyric acid (GHB) are discussed in more depth in their respective chapters (Chaps. 76 and 80).

PHARMACODYNAMICS AND TOXICODYNAMICS

All sedative–hypnotics induce central nervous system (CNS) depression. Most clinically effective sedative–hypnotics produce their physiologic effects by enhancing the function of GABA-mediated chloride channels via agonism at the GABA$_A$ receptor. These receptors are the primary mediators of inhibitory neurotransmission in the brain (Chap. 13). The GABA$_A$ receptor is a pentameric structure composed of varying polypeptide subunits associated with a chloride on the postsynaptic membrane. These subunits are classified into families (eg, α, β, γ). Variations in the five subunits of the GABA receptor confer drug selectivity and clinical effects such as sedation, anxiolysis, hypnosis, amnesia, and muscle relaxation.[133] The most common GABA$_A$ receptor in the brain is composed of $\alpha_1\beta_2\gamma_2$ subunits. Almost all sedative–hypnotics bind to GABA$_A$ receptors containing the α_1 subunit. One exception may be etomidate, which produces sedation at the β_2 unit and anesthesia at the β_3 subunit.[24,94] Benzodiazepines are effective only at GABA$_A$ receptors with the γ_2 subunit. Even within classes of sedative–hypnotics, there are varying affinities and actions for differing subunits of the GABA receptor.[33,78] The α_1 subunit is responsible for sedation and amnesia, the α_2 subunit is responsible for anxiolysis, and the α_4 and α_6 subunits are completely insensitive to benzodiazepines. Nonbenzodiazepine sedative–hypnotics such as zolpidem, zaleplon, and zopiclone selectively bind the α_1 subunit and thus cause primarily sedation and not anxiolysis at therapeutic doses.

The role of GABA receptors in the peripheral nervous system has been increasingly recognized, especially in the gastrointestinal (GI) tract. γ-Aminobutyric acid agonism is involved in modulation of GI visceral pain processing.[7] Furthermore, GABA$_B$ agonism by baclofen was found to reduce duodenal ulcer formation.[64]

Many sedative–hypnotics also act at receptors other than the GABA$_A$ receptor. Trichloroethanol and propofol also inhibit glutamate-mediated *N*-methyl-D-aspartate (NMDA) receptors, thereby inhibiting excitatory neurotransmission.[26,102,121] Certain benzodiazepines inhibit adenosine metabolism and reuptake, thereby potentiating both A$_1$-adenosine (negative dromotropy) and A$_2$-adenosine (coronary vasodilation) receptor-mediated effects.[90,131] Benzodiazepines can also interact with serotonergic pathways. The anxiolytic effects of clonazepam can be partially explained by upregulation of serotonergic receptors, specifically 5-HT$_1$ and 5-HT$_2$.[9] Sleep aids such as melatonin, ramelteon, and tasimelteon are agonists at melatonin receptor subtypes MT$_1$ and MT$_2$ in the suprachiasmatic nucleus of the brain.[116,134,140,146] Dexmedetomidine is a central α_2-adrenergic agonist similar to clonidine.[143]

PHARMACOKINETICS AND TOXICOKINETICS

Most orally administered sedative–hypnotics are rapidly absorbed via the GI tract, with the rate-limiting step consisting of dissolution and dispersion of the xenobiotic. Barbiturates and benzodiazepines are primarily absorbed in the small intestine. Clinical effects are determined by their relative ability to penetrate the blood–brain barrier. Xenobiotics that are highly lipophilic penetrate most rapidly. The ultrashort-acting barbiturates are clinically active in the most vascular parts of the brain (gray matter first), with sleep occurring within 30 seconds of administration. Table 72–1 lists individual sedative–hypnotics and some of their pharmacokinetic properties.

After initial distribution, many of the sedative–hypnotics undergo a redistribution phase as they are dispersed to other body tissues, specifically adipose tissue. Xenobiotics that are extensively redistributed, such as the lipophilic (ultrashort-acting) barbiturates, have a brief clinical effect as the early peak concentrations in the brain rapidly decline.

Many of the sedative–hypnotics are metabolized to pharmacologically active intermediates. This is particularly true for chloral hydrate and some of the benzodiazepines. The benzodiazepines can be demethylated, hydroxylated, or conjugated with glucuronide in the liver. Glucuronidation results in the production of inactive metabolites. Benzodiazepines such as diazepam and chlordiazepoxide are demethylated, which produces active intermediates with a more prolonged half-lives than the parent compound

TABLE 72–1	Sedative-Hypnotics: Duration of Action and Active Metabolites	
	Duration of Action[a]	Active Metabolite Important
Benzodiazepines		
Alprazolam	S	No
Chlordiazepoxide	I	Yes
Clonazepam	L	Yes
Clorazepate	L	Yes
Diazepam	Single dose: S Multiple doses: L	Yes
Estazolam	I	No
Flunitrazepam	L	Yes
Flurazepam	L	Yes
Lorazepam	I	No
Midazolam	S	Yes
Oxazepam	I	No
Temazepam	I	No
Triazolam	S	No
Eszopiclone	S	No
Zaleplon	S	No
Zolpidem	S	No
Barbiturates		
Amobarbital	I	Yes
Butabarbital	I	Unknown
Mephobarbital	S	Yes
Methohexital	S	No
Pentobarbital	Single dose: S Multiple doses: I	No
Phenobarbital	L	No
Primidone	I	Yes
Secobarbital	I	Unknown
Other		
Chloral hydrate	I	Yes
Dexmedetomidine	S	No
Etomidate	US	Unclear
Propofol	US	No
Ramelteon	S	Yes
Tasimelteon	S	No
Suvorexant	I	No

[a]The duration of action usually approximates the half-life (t½); some lipophilic xenobiotics have a short duration of action with a single dose because of redistribution from the central nervous system but with multiple doses become longer acting.

I = intermediate acting t½ = 6–24 h; L = long acting t½ >24 h (a long-acting metabolite may contribute to a long duration of action); S = short acting t½ <6 h; US = ultrashort acting t½ <1 h.

(Table 72-1). Because of the individual pharmacokinetics of sedative–hypnotics and the production of active metabolites, there is often little correlation between the duration of effect and biologic half-lives.

Most sedative–hypnotics, such as the highly lipid-soluble barbiturates and the benzodiazepines, are highly protein bound. These drugs are poorly filtered by the kidneys. Elimination occurs principally by hepatic metabolism. Chloral hydrate and meprobamate are notable exceptions. Xenobiotics with a low lipophilicity and limited protein binding are more subject to renal excretion.

Overdoses as well concomitant therapeutic usage of combinations of sedative–hypnotics enhance toxicity through additive and synergistic effects. For example, both barbiturates and benzodiazepines act on the GABA$_A$ receptor, but barbiturates prolong the opening of the chloride ionophore,

and benzodiazepines increase the frequency of ionophore opening.[135] Various sedative–hypnotics increase the affinity of another xenobiotic at its respective binding site. For example, pentobarbital increases the affinity of γ-hydroxybutyric acid (GHB) for its non–GABA binding site.[137] Propofol potentiates the effect of pentobarbital on chloride influx at the GABA$_A$ receptor.[111] Propofol also increases the affinity and decreases the rate of dissociation of benzodiazepines from their site on the GABA$_A$ receptor.[18,150] These actions increase the clinical effect of each xenobiotic and lead to deeper CNS and respiratory depression when they are used concomitantly.

Another mechanism of synergistic toxicity occurs via alteration of metabolism. The combination of ethanol and chloral hydrate, historically known as a "Mickey Finn," has synergistic CNS depressant effects. Chloral hydrate competes for alcohol and aldehyde dehydrogenases, thereby prolonging the half-life of ethanol. The metabolism of ethanol generates the reduced form of nicotinamide adenine dinucleotide (NADH), which is a cofactor for the metabolism of choral hydrate to trichloroethanol, an active metabolite. Finally, ethanol inhibits the conjugation of trichloroethanol, which in turn inhibits the oxidation of ethanol (Fig. 72–1).[1,80,128,129] The end result of these synergistic pharmacokinetic interactions is enhanced CNS depression.

Multiple drug–drug interactions prolong the half-life of sedative–hypnotics and significantly increase their potency or duration of action (Chap. 9). The half-life of midazolam, which undergoes hepatic metabolism via cytochrome CYP3A4, can change dramatically in the presence of

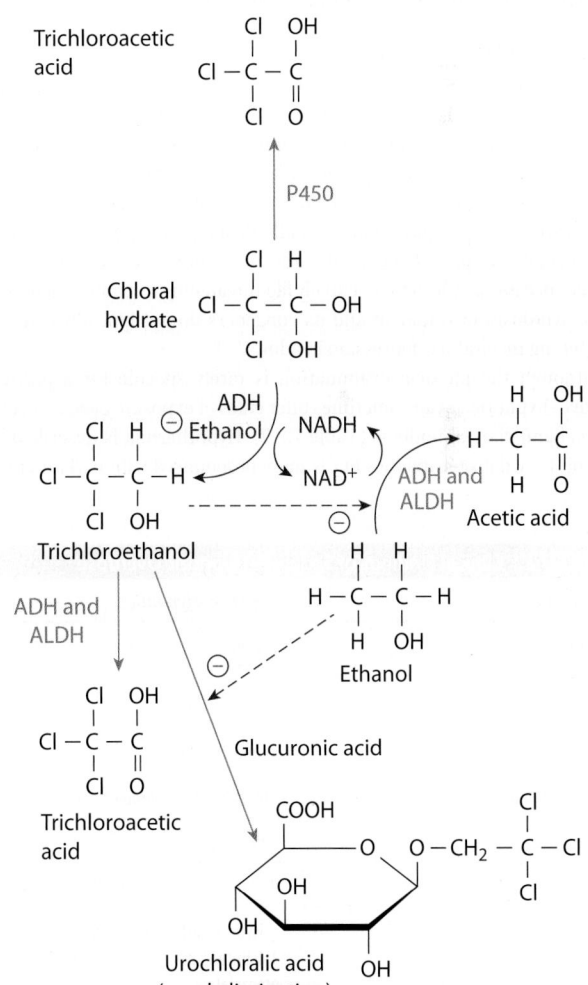

FIGURE 72–1. Metabolism of chloral hydrate and ethanol demonstrating the interactions between chloral hydrate and ethanol metabolism. Note the inhibitory effects (dotted lines) of ethanol on trichloroethanol metabolism and the converse. ADH = alcohol dehydrogenase; ALDH = aldehyde dehydrogenase; NAD$^+$ = Nicotinamide adenine dinucleotide; NADH = nicotinamide adenine dinucleotide.

certain xenobiotics that compete for its metabolism or that induce or inhibit CYP3A4 (Table 11–2).[96,153] For example, the half-life of midazolam rises 400-fold when coadministered with itraconazole.[8,136]

TOLERANCE AND WITHDRAWAL

Ingestions of typical doses of sedative–hypnotics have less predictable effects in patients who chronically use them. This is due to *tolerance,* defined as the progressive diminution of effect of a particular drug with repeated administrations that results in a need for greater doses to achieve the same effect. Tolerance occurs when adaptive neural and receptor changes (plasticity) occur after repeated exposures. These changes include a decrease in the number of receptors (downregulation), reduction of firing of receptors (receptor desensitization), structural changes in receptors (receptor shift), or reduction of coupling of sedative–hypnotics and their respective GABA$_A$-related receptor site (Chap. 14). Tolerance can also be secondary to pharmacokinetic factors, such as increased metabolism after repetitive doses. However, in most cases, tolerance to sedative–hypnotics is caused by pharmacodynamic changes such as receptor downregulation.[136]

Cross-tolerance readily exists among the sedative–hypnotics. For example, chronic use of benzodiazepines not only decreases the activity of the benzodiazepine site on the GABA receptor but also decreases the binding affinity of the barbiturate sites.[2,54] Many sedative–hypnotics are also associated with drug dependence after chronic exposure. Some of these—classically, the barbiturates, benzodiazepines, and ethanol—are also associated with life-threatening withdrawal syndromes.

CLINICAL MANIFESTATIONS

Patients with sedative–hypnotic overdoses exhibit slurred speech, ataxia, and incoordination. Larger doses result in stupor or coma. In most instances, respiratory depression parallels CNS depression. However, not all sedative–hypnotics cause significant hypoventilation. Although oral overdoses of benzodiazepines alone produce sedation and hypnosis, they rarely produce life-threatening hypoventilation. Typically, the patient appears comatose but with normal vital signs. In contrast, large intravenous (IV) doses of benzodiazepines occasionally lead to potentially life-threatening respiratory depression. Single overdoses of zolpidem and its congeners do not typically cause life-threatening respiratory depression in adults.[127,162]

Although the physical examination is rarely specific for a particular sedative–hypnotic, it can sometimes offer clues of exposure based on certain physical and clinical findings (Table 72–2). Hypothermia is described with most of the sedative–hypnotics but is more pronounced with barbiturates.[55,119]

TABLE 72–2	Clinical Findings of Sedative–Hypnotic Overdose
Clinical Signs	**Sedative–Hypnotics**
Acneiform rash	Bromides
Cardiotoxicity	
Hypotension from myocardial depression	Meprobamate
Dysrhythmias	Chloral hydrate
Coma (fluctuating)	Glutethimide, meprobamate
GI hemorrhage	Chloral hydrate
Hypothermia	Barbiturates, bromides, ethchlorvynol
Muscular twitching	γ-Hydroxybutyric acid, γ-butyrolactone, 1,4-butanediol, γ-valerolactone, propofol, etomidate
Odors (Unique)	Chloral hydrate (pear), ethchlorvynol (new vinyl shower curtain)
Urine (discolored)	Propofol (green/pink)

GI = gastrointestinal.

Fixed drug eruptions that are often bullous can appear over pressure-point areas. Although classically referred to as "barbiturate blisters," this phenomenon is not specific to barbiturates because other CNS xenobiotics, including carbon monoxide, methadone, imipramine, benzodiazepines, and several others, can lead to the same finding.

Large single doses or prolonged duration of IV dosing of sedative–hypnotics can also cause toxicities due to their diluents. Propylene glycol accumulates with prolonged infusions of certain medications such as lorazepam. Rapid infusions of propylene glycol induce hypotension. Accumulated amounts of propylene glycol lead to metabolic acidosis and a hyperosmolar state with elevated lactate concentrations.[101,110,152,154] In one study, two-thirds of critical care patients given high doses of lorazepam (0.16 mg/kg/h) for more than 48 hours had significant accumulations of propylene glycol as manifested by hyperosmolarity and an anion gap metabolic acidosis[5] (Chap. 46).

DIAGNOSTIC TESTING

When overdose is a primary concern in an undifferentiated comatose patient without a clear history, laboratory testing is useful to exclude metabolic abnormalities. This includes electrolytes, liver function tests, thyroid function tests, blood urea nitrogen, creatinine, glucose, venous blood gas analysis, and cerebrospinal fluid analysis as clinically indicated. With any suspected intentional overdose, a serum acetaminophen concentration should be obtained. Diagnostic imaging studies, such as neuroimaging of the head, are warranted on a case-by-case basis.

Routine laboratory screening for "drugs of abuse" generally is not helpful in the management of undifferentiated comatose adult patients. However, screening may be useful for epidemiologic purposes in a particular community or in psychiatric patients. These tests vary in type, sensitivity, and specificity. Furthermore, many sedative–hypnotics are not included on standard screening tests for drugs of abuse. For example, a typical benzodiazepine urine screen identifies metabolites of 1,4-benzodiazepines, such as oxazepam or nordiazepam (desmethyldiazepam). Many benzodiazepines, including the commonly used lorazepam and clonazepam, are metabolized to alternative compounds and remain undetected, thus exhibiting a false-negative result on the benzodiazepine-screening assay. Alprazolam and triazolam are not detected because they undergo minimal metabolism.[34]

Specific concentrations of xenobiotics such as ethanol or phenobarbital, although readily available at most hospitals, are rarely crucial in clinical decision making. Concentrations of most other sedative–hypnotics are not routinely performed in hospital laboratories. Because of its radiopacity, large ingestions of chloral hydrate are evident on abdominal radiography (Chap. 8). Although immediate identification of a particular sedative–hypnotic may be helpful in predicting the length of toxicity, it rarely affects the acute management of the patient. One exception is phenobarbital, for which urinary alkalinization and multiple-dose activated charcoal (MDAC) enhance elimination.[38,73,106,117] The EXtracorporeal TReatments in Poisoning (EXTRIP) workgroup recommends intermittent hemodialysis for severe barbiturate poisoning, and hemoperfusion and continuous renal replacement therapy are viable alternatives.[74]

MANAGEMENT

Death secondary to sedative–hypnotic overdose usually results from cardiorespiratory collapse. Careful attention should focus on monitoring and maintaining adequate airway, oxygenation, and hemodynamic support. Supplemental oxygen, respiratory support, and prevention of aspiration are the cornerstones of treatment. Hemodynamic instability should be treated initially with volume expansion. With proper supportive care and adequate airway and respiratory support as needed, patients with sedative–hypnotic overdoses should eventually recover. Patients with meprobamate and chloral hydrate overdoses occasionally present with both respiratory depression and cardiac toxicity. In 40% of cases, meprobamate toxicity was found to be associated with myocardial depression and significant hypotension, often resistant to IV fluid resuscitation.[21] The cardiotoxic effects of chloral hydrate include lethal ventricular dysrhythmias resulting from its active halogenated metabolite trichloroethanol causing myocardial sensitization to catecholamines. In the setting of cardiac dysrhythmias from chloral hydrate, use of β-adrenergic antagonists such as propranolol is reported to cause resolution of the dysrhythmia.[15,17,166,175] We recommend administering IV β-adrenergic antagonists in patients with chloral hydrate–induced dysrhythmias resistant to standard therapy.

The use of GI decontamination should be decided on a case-by-case basis. The benefits of activated charcoal (AC) must be balanced with the risks of its aspiration and subsequent potential for pulmonary toxicity. The use of AC should be determined based on the current mental status of the patient, the potential for further deterioration, the xenobiotic(s) ingested, and the expected clinical course. Phenobarbital overdose is one particular scenario in which MDAC increases elimination by 50% to 80%.[10,11,14] In a prospective study of 10 comatose patients after phenobarbital overdose, the serum half-life of phenobarbital was significantly decreased after multiple dose activated charcoal (MDAC) administration (36 ± 13 hours) compared with the group treated with single dose activated charcoal (SDAC) (93 ± 52 hours) (Antidotes in Depth: A1).[105]

Although the efficacy of orogastric lavage is controversial, orogastric lavage is reasonable in overdoses with xenobiotics that slow GI motility or that are known to develop concretions, specifically phenobarbital and meprobamate.[21,59,125] Orogastric lavage in the setting of oral benzodiazepine overdoses alone is not recommended because the benefits of lavage are minimal compared with the significant risks of aspiration (Chap. 5). No antidote counteracts all sedative–hypnotic overdoses. Flumazenil, a competitive benzodiazepine antagonist, rapidly reverses the sedative effects of benzodiazepines as well as zolpidem and its congeners.[71,123,165,172] However, flumazenil can precipitate life-threatening benzodiazepine withdrawal in benzodiazepine-dependent patients. Flumazenil use is also associated with seizures, especially in patients who have overdosed on tricyclic antidepressants (Antidotes in Depth: A25).[56,139] Because the lethality of sedative–hypnotics is associated with their ability to cause respiratory depression, asymptomatic patients can be downgraded to a lower level of care after a period of observation when there are no signs of respiratory depression. The exact length of the observation period will vary based on the patient's clinical presentation, age, and the type and amount of xenobiotic(s) ingested. Patients with symptomatic overdoses of long-acting sedative–hypnotics, such as meprobamate and clonazepam, or drugs that have significant enterohepatic circulation may require 24 hours of observation in the intensive care unit. Patients with mixed overdoses of various sedative–hypnotics and CNS depressants also warrant closer observation for respiratory depression because of synergistic respiratory depressant effects.

SPECIFIC SEDATIVE–HYPNOTICS

Barbiturates

The general structure of barbiturates is shown above. Barbital became the first commercially available barbiturate in 1903. Although many other barbiturates were subsequently developed, their popularity has greatly waned since the introduction of benzodiazepines. Barbiturates are derivatives of barbituric acid (2,4,6-trioxo-hexa-hydropyrimidine), which itself has no CNS depressant properties. The addition of various side chains influences the pharmacologic properties. Barbiturates with long side chains tend to have increased lipophilicity and potency and slower rates of elimination. However, the observed clinical effects also depend on absorption, redistribution, and the presence of active metabolites. For this reason, the duration of action of barbiturates (like those of benzodiazepines) does not correlate well with their biologic half-lives.

Oral barbiturates are preferentially absorbed in the small intestine and are eliminated by both hepatic and renal mechanisms. Shorter acting barbiturates tend to be more lipid soluble, more protein bound, have a higher pK_a, and are metabolized almost completely by the liver. Longer acting barbiturates such as phenobarbital accumulate less extensively in tissues and are excreted renally as the parent drug. An example of this is phenobarbital, with a relatively low pK_a (7.24). Alkalinizing the urine with sodium bicarbonate to a urinary pH of 7.5 to 8.0 can increase the elimination of phenobarbital by 5- to 10-fold. This procedure is not effective for the short-acting barbiturates because they have higher pK_a values, are more protein bound, and are primarily metabolized by the liver with very little unchanged drug excreted by the kidneys (Antidotes in Depth: A5 and Chap. 6). Urinary alkalinization is utilized to decrease the serum half-life of phenobarbital. The clinical benefits are supported in a prospective controlled trial and few case reports.[117] Given the pharmacokinetic properties of barbiturates, the EXTRIP Workgroup recommends dialysis for cases of severe long-acting barbiturate poisoning presenting with prolonged coma, respiratory depression requiring mechanical ventilation, shock, persistent toxicity or persistently elevated or rising serum concentrations despite MDAC. Intermittent hemodialysis and continuation of MDAC during dialysis is recommended.[74]

Barbiturates (especially the shorter acting barbiturates) can accelerate their own hepatic metabolism by cytochrome P450 enzyme autoinduction. Phenobarbital is a nonselective inducer of hepatic cytochromes, the greatest effects being on CYP2B1, CYP2B2, and CYP2B10, although CYP3A4 is also affected.[120,151] Not surprisingly, a variety of interactions are reported after the use of barbiturates. Clinically significant interactions as a result of enzyme induction lead to increased metabolism of β-adrenergic antagonists, corticosteroids, doxycycline, estrogens, phenothiazines, quinidine, theophylline, and many other xenobiotics.

Early deaths caused by barbiturate ingestions result from respiratory arrest and cardiovascular collapse. Delayed deaths result from acute kidney failure, pneumonia, acute respiratory distress syndrome, cerebral edema, and multiorgan system failure as a result of prolonged cardiorespiratory depression.[3,42]

Benzodiazepines

The general structure of benzodiazepines is shown above. The commercial use of benzodiazepines began with the introduction of chlordiazepoxide for anxiety in 1961 and diazepam for seizures in 1963. Benzodiazepines are used principally as sedatives and anxiolytics. Clonazepam is the only benzodiazepine approved for use as a chronic anticonvulsant. Benzodiazepines rarely cause paradoxical psychological effects, including nightmares, delirium, psychosis, and transient global amnesia.[83,86,176] The incidence and intensity of CNS adverse events increase with age.[81]

Similar to barbiturates, variations of the benzodiazepine side chains influence potency, duration of action, metabolites, and rate of elimination. Most benzodiazepines are highly protein bound and lipophilic. They passively diffuse into the CNS, their main site of action. Because of their lipophilicity, benzodiazepines are extensively metabolized via oxidation and conjugation in the liver before their renal elimination.

Benzodiazepines bind nonselectively to "central" benzodiazepine sites located throughout the brain. These sites contain the $GABA_A$ α and γ subunits.[33,161] The binding of the benzodiazepine to its particular site changes the GABA receptor to "lock" into a position that promotes GABA binding to the GABA receptor. Whereas benzodiazepines that are active at the α_1 subunit affect anxiety, sleep, and amnesia, those that are active in the α_2 and α_3 subunits tend to have greater anxiolytic properties. "Peripheral" benzodiazepine sites are found throughout the body, with the greatest concentrations in steroid-producing cells in the adrenal gland, anterior pituitary gland, and reproductive organs. These sites are not affiliated with the GABA receptor (Antidotes in Depth: A26).

One unique property of the benzodiazepines is their relative safety even after substantial ingestion, which probably results from their GABA receptor properties.[33,97] Unlike many other sedative–hypnotics, benzodiazepines do not open GABA channels independently at high concentrations. Benzodiazepines do not cause any specific systemic injury, and their long-term use is not associated with specific organ toxicity. Most often deaths are secondary to a combination of alcohol or other sedative–hypnotics.[130,168,170] Supportive care is the mainstay of treatment.

Flumazenil is a competitive benzodiazepine receptor antagonist that is ideal for either benzodiazepine-naïve patients with a sole benzodiazepine overdose or benzodiazepine-naïve patients who develop respiratory depression after IV administration of benzodiazepines (Antidotes in Depth: A25). Caution should be exercised if flumazenil is administered to patients with an unknown overdose because seizures and dysrhythmias are reported to occur from the effects of the coingestant after the effect of the benzodiazepine has been reversed. Similarly, chronic benzodiazepine users are at risk of developing withdrawal symptoms, including seizures, after receiving flumazenil. The duration of effect of flumazenil is shorter than that of most benzodiazepines, and resedation can occur.[118]

Tolerance to the sedative effects of benzodiazepines occurs more rapidly than does tolerance to the antianxiety effects.[73,115] Abrupt discontinuation after long-term use of benzodiazepines precipitates benzodiazepine withdrawal, characterized by autonomic instability, changes in perception, paresthesias, headaches, tremors, and seizures.[13] Withdrawal from benzodiazepines is common, manifested by almost one-third of chronic users.[66] Alprazolam and lorazepam are associated with more severe withdrawal syndromes compared with chlordiazepoxide and diazepam.[66,67] This is likely because both chlordiazepoxide and diazepam have active metabolites, accumulation of which prolongs the clinical effect of the drug and results in a gradual tapering effect. This leads to delayed presentation of withdrawal from benzodiazepines with active metabolites. Withdrawal may also occur when a chronic user of a particular benzodiazepine is switched to another benzodiazepine with a greater affinity for different receptor subunits.[76]

Chloral Hydrate

First introduced in 1832, chloral hydrate belongs to one of the oldest classes of pharmaceutical hypnotics, the chloral derivatives. Although still used sporadically in children, its use has substantially decreased.[1,75,93,103] Chloral hydrate is well absorbed but is irritating to the GI tract. It has extensive tissue distribution, rapid onset of action, and rapid hepatic metabolism by alcohol and aldehyde dehydrogenases. Trichloroethanol is a lipid-soluble, active metabolite that is responsible for the hypnotic effects of chloral hydrate. It has a serum half-life of 4 to 12 hours and is metabolized to inactive trichloroacetic acid by alcohol dehydrogenases. It is also conjugated with glucuronide and excreted by the kidney as urochloralic acid. Less than 10% of trichloroethanol is excreted unchanged.

Metabolic rates in children vary widely because of variable development and function of hepatic enzymes, in particular those achieving glucuronidation.[16,80] The elimination half-life of chloral hydrate and trichloroethanol is markedly increased in children younger than 2 years. This is especially concern in neonates and in infants exposed to repetitive doses.

Acute chloral hydrate poisoning is unique compared with that of other sedative–hypnotics because of the production of toxic metabolites. Cardiac dysrhythmias are the major cause of death.[41] Chloral hydrate and its metabolites reduce myocardial contractility, shorten the refractory period, and increase myocardial sensitivity to catecholamines. Persistent cardiac dysrhythmias (ventricular fibrillation, ventricular tachycardia, torsade de pointes) are common terminal events.[79] β-Adrenergic antagonists such as propranolol mitigate this myocardial sensitivity and are recommended in patients with chloral hydrate–induced dysrhythmias resistant to standard therapy.[15,17,166,175]

In addition to cardiotoxicity, chloral hydrate toxicity causes vomiting, hemorrhagic gastritis, and rarely gastric and intestinal necrosis, leading to perforation and esophagitis with stricture formation.[69,157] Although large ingestions of chloral hydrate are evident on abdominal radiographs because of its radiopacity, a normal radiograph should not be used to exclude chloral hydrate ingestion. Few hospital-based laboratories have the ability to rapidly detect chloral hydrate or its metabolites.

Bromides

Bromides were used in the past as "nerve tonics," headache remedies, and anticonvulsants. Although medicinal bromides have largely disappeared from the US pharmaceutical market, bromide toxicity still occurs through the availability of bromide salts of common drugs, such as dextromethorphan hydrobromine, in large overdoses.[91] There is also documentation of bromism from excessive consumption of cola with brominated vegetable oils.[52] Poisoning may also occur in immigrants and travelers from other countries where bromides are still therapeutically used.[37] An epidemic of more than 400 cases of mass bromide poisoning occurred in the Cacuaco municipality of Luanda Province, Angola, in 2007. According to a World Health Organization report, the etiology of the bromide exposure in these cases was believed to be table salt contaminated with sodium bromide. Although the majority of persons affected were children, no actual deaths were attributed to bromide poisoning in this epidemic.[167]

Bromides tend to have long half-lives, and toxicity typically occurs over-time as concentrations accumulate in tissue. Bromide and chloride ions have a similar distribution pattern in the extracellular fluid. It is postulated that because the bromide ion moves across membranes slightly more rapidly than the chloride ion, it is more quickly reabsorbed in the tubules from the glomerular filtrate than the chloride ion. Although osmolar equilibrium persists, CNS function is progressively impaired by a poorly understood mechanism, with resulting inappropriateness of behavior, headache, apathy, irritability, confusion, muscle weakness, anorexia, weight loss, thickened speech, psychotic behavior, tremulousness, ataxia, and eventually, coma. Delusions and hallucinations occur. Bromides lead to hypertension, increased intracranial pressure, and papilledema.[20,37,149] Chronic use of bromides also produces dermatologic changes called bromoderma, with the hallmark characteristic of a facial acneiform rash.[49,149] Toxicity with bromides during pregnancy causes accumulation of bromide in the fetus and resultant CNS depression.[104] A spurious laboratory result of hyperchloremia with decreased or negative anion gap results from the interference of bromide with the chloride assay on some analyzers[109,171] (Chap. 12). Thus, an isolated elevated serum chloride concentration with neurologic symptoms should raise suspicion of possible bromide poisoning.

Carisoprodol and Meprobamate

Meprobamate was introduced in 1950 and was used for its muscle-relaxant and anxiolytic characteristics. Carisoprodol, which was introduced in 1955, is metabolized to meprobamate. Both drugs have pharmacologic effects on the GABA$_A$ receptor similar to those of the barbiturates. Similar to the barbiturates, meprobamate can directly open the GABA-mediated chloride channel and inhibits NMDA receptor currents.[113] Both are rapidly absorbed from the GI tract. Meprobamate is metabolized in the liver to inactive hydroxyl and glucuronide metabolites that are excreted almost exclusively by the kidney. Of all the nonbarbiturate tranquilizers, meprobamate is most likely to produce euphoria; the exact mechanism of this is unknown.[57,58] Unlike most sedative–hypnotics, meprobamate causes profound hypotension from direct myocardial depression.[21] Adherent masses or bezoars of pills are reported in the stomach at autopsy after large meprobamate ingestions.[125] Orogastric lavage with a large-bore tube and MDAC is reasonable for patients with a significant meprobamate ingestion while keeping in mind the risk of aspiration. Whole-bowel irrigation is also reasonable if multiple pills or small concretions are suspected. Patients can experience recurrent toxic manifestations as a result of concretion formation with delayed drug release and absorption. Careful monitoring of the clinical course is essential even after the patient shows initial improvement because recurrent and cyclical CNS depression can occur.[125]

Zolpidem, Zaleplon, Zopiclone, and Eszopiclone

Zolpidem   Zaleplon

These oral hypnotics have supplanted benzodiazepines as the most commonly prescribed sleep aid medications.[35] Although they are structurally unrelated to the benzodiazepines, they bind preferentially to the benzodiazepine site subtype in the brain that contains the $GABA_A$ α_1 subunit.[33] They have a lower affinity for benzodiazepine sites that contain the other α isoforms; therefore, they have potent hypnotic effects with less potential for dependence and antiepileptics properties.[48] Each of these xenobiotics has a relatively short half-life (6 hours or less), with zaleplon exhibiting the shortest half-life (1 hour). Unlike benzodiazepines that prolong the first two stages of sleep and shorten stages 3 and 4 of rapid eye movement sleep, zolpidem and its congeners all decrease sleep latency with little effect on sleep architecture. Because of their receptor selectivity, they appear to have minimal effect at other sites on the $GABA_A$ receptor that mediate anxiolytic, antiepileptic, or muscle-relaxant effects.[68,158] A low-dose sublingual tablet of zolpidem tartrate (Intermezzo) was recently approved for middle of the night awakenings. An unusual side effect of these drugs, even during therapeutic dosing, is somnambulism, transient anterograde global amnesia, with the majority of these reports involving zolpidem.[45]

They are hepatically metabolized by various CYP450 enzymes. Zolpidem is mainly metabolized by CYP3A4. Zaleplon is primarily metabolized by aldehyde oxidase, but CYP3A4 is also involved in parent compound oxidation. Whereas zopiclone is primarily metabolized by CYP3A4 and CYP2C8, eszopiclone is metabolized mainly by CYP3A4 and CYP2E1. Various pharmacokinetic interactions with inhibitors or inducers of CYP450 enzymes and these medications are reported.[47]

In isolated overdoses, drowsiness and CNS depression are common. However, prolonged coma with respiratory depression is exceptionally rare. Isolated overdoses usually manifest with depressed level of consciousness without respiratory depression. For example, even at 40 times the therapeutic dose of zolpidem, no biologic or electrocardiographic abnormalities were reported.[40] Zopiclone overdoses are rarely associated with methemoglobinemia.[39] Tolerance to zolpidem and its congeners occurs, and as expected, withdrawal follows abrupt discontinuation of chronic use.

The withdrawal syndrome is typically mild.[46,164] Flumazenil reverses the hypnotic and cognitive effects of these xenobiotics, and given the lack of antiepileptic effects of these xenobiotics, flumazenil reversal may be safer here than in the case of benzodiazepines (Antidotes in Depth: A25).[71,172] Because of increasing prevalence of these xenobiotics, they have been associated with increasing hospitalizations especially when ingested with other sedative-hypnotics.[179] Deaths result when zolpidem is taken in large amounts with other CNS depressants.[40]

Propofol

Propofol is a rapidly acting IV sedative–hypnotic that is both a postsynaptic $GABA_A$ agonist and induces presynaptic release of GABA.[95,150] Propofol is also an antagonist at NMDA receptors.[63,138,177] In addition, propofol interacts with dopamine, promotes nigral dopamine release possibly via $GABA_B$ receptors,[98,126] and has partial agonist properties at dopamine (D_2) receptors.[124] Propofol is used for procedural sedation and either induction or maintenance of general anesthesia, as well as an antiepileptic to manage status epilepticus. It is highly lipid soluble, so it crosses the blood–brain barrier rapidly. The onset of anesthesia usually occurs in less than 1 minute. The duration of action after short-term dosing is usually less than 8 minutes because of its rapid redistribution from the CNS.

Propofol use is associated with various adverse events. Acutely, propofol causes dose-related respiratory depression. Propofol decreases systemic arterial pressure and causes myocardial depression. Although short-term use of propofol does not typically cause dysrhythmias or myocardial ischemia, atropine-sensitive bradydysrhythmias are noted, specifically sinus bradycardia and Mobitz type 1 atrioventricular block.[148,163,174] Short-term use of propofol in the perioperative setting is associated with a myoclonic syndrome manifesting as opisthotonus, myoclonus, and sometimes myoclonic seizure–like activity.[84,92]

Prolonged propofol infusions, typically more than 48 hours at rates of 4 to 5 mg/kg/h or greater, are associated with a life-threatening propofol-infusion syndrome involving metabolic acidosis, cardiac dysrhythmias, and skeletal muscle injury.[60,61] The clinical signs of propofol infusion syndrome often begin with the development of a new right bundle branch block and ST-segment convex elevations in the electrocardiogram precordial leads.[60] Predisposing factors to the development include young age, severe brain injury (especially in the setting of trauma), respiratory compromise, concurrent exogenous administration of catecholamines or glucocorticoids, inadequate carbohydrate intake, and undiagnosed mitochondrial myopathy. Some authors propose a "priming" and "triggering" mechanism for propofol infusion syndrome with endogenous glucocorticoids, catecholamines, and possibly cytokines as "priming" agents and exogenous catecholamines and glucocorticoids in the setting of high-dose propofol infusion as "triggering" stimuli.[155] Propofol disrupts mitochondrial free fatty acid utilization and metabolism, causing a syndrome of energy imbalance and myonecrosis similar to mitochondrial myopathies.[22,132,156] Most case reports associate propofol with metabolic acidosis, elevated lactate concentration, and fatal myocardial failure in both children and young adults. However, this syndrome is also reported in older adults.[100] Some cases of metabolic acidosis are associated with an inborn disorder of acylcarnitine metabolism.[169] Prolonged propofol infusions unmask previously undiagnosed myopathy that would cause them to be at increased risk for propofol infusion syndrome, especially in children.

The unique nature of the carrier base of propofol, a milky soybean emulsion formulation, is associated with multiple adverse drug events such as impairment of macrophage function,[22] hypertriglyceridemia,[65,72,156] histamine-mediated anaphylactoid reactions,[33,62,156] and impairment of platelet and coagulation function.[3,31] Additionally, the carrier base is a fertile medium for many organisms, such as enterococcal, pseudomonal, staphylococcal, streptococcal, and candidal species. In 1990, the US Centers for Disease Control and Prevention first reported an outbreak of *Staphylococcus aureus* associated with contaminated propofol.[87] Since then, 20 propofol-related outbreaks have been reported, which have affected 144 patients and caused 10 deaths.[178]

Etomidate

Etomidate is an IV nonbarbiturate, hypnotic primarily used for an anesthesia induction. It is active at the $GABA_A$ receptor, specifically the β_2 and β_3 subunits.[24,94] Only the IV formulation is available in the United States. The onset of action is less than 1 minute, and its duration of action is less than 5 minutes.

Etomidate is commercially available as a 2-mg/mL solution in a 35% propylene glycol solution. Propylene glycol toxicity from prolonged etomidate infusions is implicated in the development of hyperosmolar metabolic acidosis (Chap. 46).[70,152,154] Etomidate has minimal effect on cardiac function, but rare cases of hypotension are reported because of adrenal suppression.[142] Etomidate has both proconvulsant and antiepileptic properties.[25,108] Involuntary muscle movements are common during induction and are caused by etomidate interaction with glycine receptors at the spinal cord level.[28,88,89]

Etomidate depresses adrenal production of cortisol and aldosterone; therefore, it is associated with adrenocortical suppression, usually after prolonged infusions.[122,159,160] Etomidate is associated with increased morbidity and mortality in critically ill and trauma patients.[27,50] However, the clinical significance of adrenal suppression from etomidate administration is disputed.[51,144,145] In the appropriate setting, etomidate does not appear to have any greater risk of significant adverse events compared with its counterparts.

Dexmedetomidine

Dexmedetomidine is a central α_2-adrenergic agonist that decreases central presynaptic catecholamine release, primarily in the locus ceruleus. When dexmedetomidine is used to help wean patients from ventilators, sedation is achieved with less associated delirium compared with other agents.[99,143] It is also used for procedural sedation in certain settings such as interventional radiology procedures and awake fiberoptic intubations. Compared with propofol, dexmedetomidine sedation lessens opioid requirements in postoperative patients.

Dexmedetomidine has minimal effect at the $GABA_A$ receptor. Unlike other sedative–hypnotics, it is not associated with significant respiratory depression. Although mechanistically similar to clonidine, dexmedetomidine does not appear to cause as much respiratory depression as clonidine. Dexmedetomidine is said to induce a state of "cooperative sedation" in which a patient is sedated but yet able to interact with health care providers. Dexmedetomidine also has analgesic effects.[23]

Dexmedetomidine is currently only approved for use for less than 24 hours. Extensive safety trials have not yet explored its use beyond 24 hours. Unlike clonidine, rebound hypertension and tachycardia have not been described upon cessation. Because dexmedetomidine decreases central sympathetic outflow, its use should probably be avoided in patients whose clinical stability is dependent on high resting sympathetic tone. The most common adverse effects from its use are nausea, dry mouth, bradycardia, and varying effects on blood pressure (usually hypertension followed by hypotension). Slowing of the continuous infusion may help to prevent or lessen the hypotensive effects.[23] In one case, a 60-fold overdose in a child was associated with hypoglycemia.[12]

Melatonin, Ramelteon, and Tasimelteon

Melatonin (*N*-acetyl-5-methoxytryptamine) and melatonin-containing products are sold as dietary supplements. Melatonin is naturally synthesized from tryptophan by the enzyme 5-hydroxyindole-O-methyltransferase, primarily within the pineal gland in humans. Ramelteon is a synthetic melatonin-analog that is FDA approved for the treatment of chronic insomnia. Ramelteon is thought to decrease both latency to sleep induction and length of persistent sleep.[134] Tasimelteon, the newest melatonin receptor agonist, is the only FDA-approved drug used to treat non–24-hour sleep–wake disorder that occurs in blind individuals in whom light cues do not reach the suprachiasmatic nucleus of the brain to allow for a normal sleep–wake cycle.[53] Melatonin, ramelteon, and tasimelteon act as agonists at MT_1 and MT_2 receptors, which are G protein–coupled receptors mainly located in the suprachiasmatic nucleus of the brain.[127] Whereas MT_1 receptors are involved in sleep induction, MT_2 receptors are involved in regulation of the circadian sleep–wake cycle in humans.[140]

Ramelteon administered orally is rapidly absorbed but undergoes significant first-pass metabolism primarily by CYP1A2.

Adverse effects of ramelteon are mild and usually include drowsiness, dizziness, fatigue, and headache. The endocrine effects of long-term exposure to ramelteon seem to be limited to subclinical increases in serum prolactin concentration in women and do not appear to affect adrenal or thyroid function.[114] In addition, ramelteon appears to have a low abuse potential and does not appear to be associated with a withdrawal syndrome or rebound insomnia.[44,77,85] A retrospective review of 222 poison control center calls of ramelteon overdose reported no significant clinical effect in 88.3% of cases. Isolated cases of bradycardia, hypotension, and seizures did occur.[147] There are no published reports of tasimelteon toxicity from overdose.

Suvorexant

Suvorexant is a newly approved dual orexin receptor antagonist. Orexin (also known as hypocretin) promotes wakefulness; as an orexin antagonist, suvorexant induces and maintains sleep. This is the first drug in this class of sedative–hypnotics.[141,173] Preliminary studies have shown that patients taking this drug have a shorter sleep latency and stayed asleep longer than the control group taking placebo. There are no reports of physical dependence on this drug or withdrawal upon its cessation. There are no trials comparing suvorexant with other drugs for noninferiority or efficacy. The most commonly reported side effect with overdose is somnolence after awakening.[82]

SUMMARY

- Sedative–hypnotics encompass a wide range of xenobiotics that predominantly interact with the $GABA_A$ receptor but can also have varying mechanisms of action.
- Patients with sedative–hypnotic overdoses often present with the primary manifestation of CNS depression; however, death typically results from respiratory depression and subsequent cardiovascular collapse in the setting of concurrent coingestion of other CNS depressants.
- Treatment is largely supportive, including careful monitoring, airway protection, and proper supportive care, with a rare need for GI decontamination in select severe cases.
- Specific antidotes such as flumazenil and hemodialysis are rarely indicated.

Acknowledgment

Kathy Lynn Ferguson, DO, contributed to this chapter in previous editions.

REFERENCES

1. American Academy of Pediatrics Committee on Drugs and Committee on Environmental Health. Use of chloral hydrate for sedation in children. *Pediatrics*. 1993;92:471-473.
2. Allan AM, et al. Barbiturate tolerance: effects on GABA-operated chloride channel function. *Brain Res*. 1992;588:255-260.
3. Aoki H, et al. In vivo and in vitro studies of the inhibitory effect of propofol on human platelet aggregation. *Anesthesiology*. 1998;88:362-370.
4. Armstrong D, Schep L. Comparing bromism with methyl bromide toxicity. *Clin Toxicol*. 2009;47:371-372.

5. Arroliga AC, et al. Relationship of continuous infusion lorazepam to serum propylene glycol concentration in critically ill adults. *Crit Care Med.* 2004;32:1709-1714.

6. Asnis GM, et al. Pharmacotherapy treatment options for insomnia: a primer for clinicians. *Int J Mol Sci.* 2016;17:50.

7. Auteri M, et al. The GABAergic system and the gastrointestinal physiopathology. *Curr Pharm Des.* 2015;21:4996-5016

8. Backman JT, et al. The area under the plasma concentration-time curve for oral midazolam is 400-fold larger during treatment with itraconazole than with rifampicin. *Eur J Clin Pharmacol.* 1998;54:53-58.

9. Bailey SJ, Toth M. Variability in the benzodiazepine response of serotonin 5-HT1A receptor null mice displaying anxiety-like phenotype: evidence for genetic modifiers in the 5-HT-mediated regulation of GABA(A) receptors. *J Neurosci.* 2004;24: 6343-6351.

10. Berg MJ, et al. Acceleration of the body clearance of phenobarbital by oral activated charcoal. *N Engl J Med.* 1982;307:642-644.

11. Berg MJ, et al. Effect of charcoal and sorbitol-charcoal suspension on the elimination of intravenous phenobarbital. *Ther Drug Monit.* 1987;9:41-47.

12. Bernard PA, et al. Hypoglycemia associated with dexmedetomidine overdose in a child? *J Clin Anesth.* 2009;21:50-53.

13. Blais D, Petit L. Benzodiazepines: dependence and a therapeutic approach to gradual withdrawal. *Can Fam Physician.* 1990;36:1779-1782.

14. Boldy DA, et al. Treatment of phenobarbitone poisoning with repeated oral administration of activated charcoal. *Q J Med.* 1986;61:997-1002.

15. Bowyer K, Glasser SP. Chloral hydrate overdose and cardiac arrhythmias. *Chest.* 1980; 77:232-235.

16. Bronley-DeLancey A, et al. Application of cryopreserved human hepatocytes in trichloroethylene risk assessment: relative disposition of chloral hydrate to trichloroacetate and trichloroethanol. *Environ Health Perspect.* 2006;114:1237-1242.

17. Brown AM, Cade JF. Cardiac arrhythmias after chloral hydrate overdose. *Med J Aust.* 1980;1:28-29.

18. Bruner KR, Reynolds JN. Propofol modulation of [3H]flunitrazepam binding to GABAA receptors in guinea pig cerebral cortex. *Brain Res.* 1998;806:122-125.

19. Buckley NA, et al. Correlations between prescriptions and drugs taken in self-poisoning. Implications for prescribers and drug regulation. *Med J Aust.* 1995;162:194-197.

20. Carney MW. Five cases of bromism. *Lancet.* 1971;2:523-524.

21. Charron C, et al. Incidence, causes and prognosis of hypotension related to meprobamate poisoning. *Intensive Care Med.* 2005;31:1582-1586.

22. Chen RM, et al. Propofol suppresses macrophage functions and modulates mitochondrial membrane potential and cellular adenosine triphosphate synthesis. *Anesthesiology.* 2003;98:1178-1185.

23. Chrysostomou C, Schmitt CG. Dexmedetomidine: sedation, analgesia and beyond. *Expert Opin Drug Metab Toxicol.* 2008;4:619-627.

24. Cirone J, et al. Gamma-aminobutyric acid type A receptor beta 2 subunit mediates the hypothermic effect of etomidate in mice. *Anesthesiology.* 2004;100:1438-1445.

25. Conca A, et al. Etomidate vs. thiopentone in electroconvulsive therapy. An interdisciplinary challenge for anesthesiology and psychiatry. *Pharmacopsychiatry.* 2003;36: 94-97.

26. Criswell HE, et al. Macrokinetic analysis of blockade of NMDA-gated currents by substituted alcohols, alkanes and ethers. *Brain Res.* 2004;1015:107-113.

27. Cuthbertson BH, et al. The effects of etomidate on adrenal responsiveness and mortality in patients with septic shock. *Intensive Care Med.* 2009;35:1868-1876.

28. Daniels S, Roberts RJ. Post-synaptic inhibitory mechanisms of anaesthesia; glycine receptors. *Toxicol Lett.* 1998;100-101:71-76.

29. Darrouj J, et al. Dexmedetomidine infusion as adjunctive therapy to benzodiazepines for acute alcohol withdrawal. *Ann Pharmacother.* 2008;42:1703-1705.

30. Davis JF, et al. Orexigenic hypothalamic peptides behavior and feeding. In: Preedy VR, et al, eds. *Handbook of Behavior, Food and Nutrition.* New York: Springer; 2011:361-362.

31. De La Cruz JP, et al. Antiplatelet effect of the anaesthetic drug propofol: influence of red blood cells and leucocytes. *Br J Pharmacol.* 1999;128:1538-1544.

32. Doble A. New insights into the mechanism of action of hypnotics. *J Psychopharmacol.* 1999;13:S11-S20.

33. Ducart AR, et al. Propofol-induced anaphylactoid reaction during anesthesia for cardiac surgery. *J Cardiothorac Vasc Anesth.* 2000;14:200-201.

34. Dunn W. Various laboratory methods screen and confirm benzodiazepines. *Emerg Med News.* 2000;21-24.

35. Elie R, et al. Sleep latency is shortened during 4 weeks of treatment with zaleplon, a novel nonbenzodiazepine hypnotic. Zaleplon Clinical Study Group. *J Clin Psychiatry.* 1999;60:536-544.

36. Finkle BS, et al. Diazepam and drug-associated deaths. A survey in the United States and Canada. *JAMA.* 1979;242:429-434.

37. Frances C, et al. Bromism from daily over intake of bromide salt. *J Toxicol Clin Toxicol.* 2003;41:181-183.

38. Fukunaga K, et al. Effects of urine pH modification on pharmacokinetics of phenobarbital in healthy dogs. *J Vet Pharmacol Ther.* 2008;31:431-436.

39. Fung HT, et al. Two cases of methemoglobinemia following zopiclone ingestion. *Clin Toxicol.* 2008;46:167-170.

40. Garnier R, et al. Acute zolpidem poisoning—analysis of 344 cases. *J Toxicol Clin Toxicol.* 1994;32:391-404.

41. Graham SR, et al. Overdose with chloral hydrate: a pharmacological and therapeutic review. *Med J Aust.* 1988;149:686-688.

42. Greenblatt DJ, et al. Overdosage with pentobarbital and secobarbital: assessment of factors related to outcome. *J Clin Pharmacol.* 1979;19:758-768.

43. Greenblatt DJ, et al. Acute overdosage with benzodiazepine derivatives. *Clin Pharmacol Ther.* 1977;21:497-514.

44. Griffiths RR, Johnson MW. Relative abuse liability of hypnotic drugs: a conceptual framework and algorithm for differentiating among compounds. *J Clin Psychiatry.* 2005;66(suppl 9):31-41.

45. Gunja N. In the zzz zone: the effects of z-drugs on human performance and driving. *J Med Toxicol.* 2013;9:163-171.

46. Hajak G, et al. Abuse and dependence potential for the non-benzodiazepine hypnotics zolpidem and zopiclone: a review of case reports and epidemiological data. *Addiction.* 2003;98:1371-1378.

47. Hesse LM, et al. Clinically important drug interactions with zopiclone, zolpidem and zaleplon. *CNS Drugs.* 2003;17:513-532.

48. Heydorn WE. Zaleplon a review of a novel sedative hypnotic used in the treatment of insomnia. *Expert Opin Investig Drugs.* 2000;9:841-858.

49. Hezemans-Boer M, et al. Skin lesions due to exposure to methyl bromide. *Arch Dermatol.* 1988;124:917-921.

50. Hildreth AN, et al. Adrenal suppression following a single dose of etomidate for rapid sequence induction: a prospective randomized study. *J Trauma.* 2008;65:573-579.

51. Hohl CM, et al. The effect of a bolus dose of etomidate on cortisol levels, mortality, and health services utilization: a systematic review. *Ann Emerg Med.* 2010;56:105-113.e105.

52. Horowitz BZ. Bromism from excessive cola consumption. *J Toxicol Clin Toxicol.* 1997;35:315-20.

53. US Food and Drug Administration. https://www.accessdata.fda.gov/drugsatfda_docs/label/2014/205677s000lbl.pdf

54. Hu XJ, Ticku MK. Chronic benzodiazepine agonist treatment produces functional uncoupling of the gamma-aminobutyric acid-benzodiazepine receptor ionophore complex in cortical neurons. *Mol Pharmacol.* 1994;45:618-625.

55. Ivnitsky JJ, et al. Intermediates of Krebs cycle correct the depression of the whole body oxygen consumption and lethal cooling in barbiturate poisoning in rat. *Toxicology.* 2004;202:165-172.

56. Jacobsen D. The relative efficacy of antidotes. *J Toxicol Clin Toxicol.* 1995;33:705-708.

57. Jacobsen D, et al. Clinical course in acute self-poisonings: a prospective study of 1125 consecutively hospitalised adults. *Hum Toxicol.* 1984;3:107-116.

58. Jacobsen D, et al. A prospective study of 1212 cases of acute poisoning: general epidemiology. *Hum Toxicol.* 1984;3:93-106.

59. Johanson WG Jr. Massive phenobarbital ingestion with survival. *JAMA.* 1967;202: 1106-1107.

60. Kam PC, Cardone D. Propofol infusion syndrome. *Anaesthesia.* 2007;62:690-701.

61. Kang TM. Propofol infusion syndrome in critically ill patients. *Ann Pharmacother.* 2002;36:1453-1456.

62. Kimura K, et al. Histamine release during the induction of anesthesia with propofol in allergic patients: a comparison with the induction of anesthesia using midazolam-ketamine. *Inflamm Res.* 1999;48:582-587.

63. Kingston S, et al. Propofol inhibits phosphorylation of N-methyl-D-aspartate receptor NR1 subunits in neurons. *Anesthesiology.* 2006;104:763-769.

64. Krantis A, McKay A. Cysteine interacts with enteric GABAergic mechanisms: effects on experimental duodenal ulceration. In: Szabo S, ed. *Hans Selye Symposia on Neuroendocrinology and Stress.* Berlin, Germany: Springer Verlag, 1990.

65. Kunst G, Bohrer H. Serum triglyceride levels and propofol infusion. *Anaesthesia.* 1995;50:1101.

66. Lader M. Anxiolytic drugs: dependence, addiction and abuse. *Eur Neuropsychopharmacol.* 1994;4:85-91.

67. Lader M. Biological processes in benzodiazepine dependence. *Addiction.* 1994;89: 1413-1418.

68. Langtry HD, Benfield P. Zolpidem. A review of its pharmacodynamic and pharmacokinetic properties and therapeutic potential. *Drugs.* 1990;40:291-313.

69. Lee DC, Vassalluzzo C. Acute gastric perforation in a chloral hydrate overdose. *Am J Emerg Med.* 1998;16:545-546.

70. Levy ML, et al. Propylene glycol toxicity following continuous etomidate infusion for the control of refractory cerebral edema. *Neurosurgery.* 1995;37:363-371.

71. Lheureux P, et al. Zolpidem intoxication mimicking narcotic overdose: response to flumazenil. *Hum Exp Toxicol.* 1990;9:105-107.

72. Lindholm M. Critically ill patients and fat emulsions. *Minerva Anestesiol.* 1992;58: 875-879.

73. Linton AL, et al. Methods of forced diuresis and its application in barbiturate poisoning. *Lancet.* 1967;2:377-379.

74. Mactier R, et al. Extracorporeal treatment for barbiturate poisoning: recommendations from the EXTRIP Workgroup. *Am J Kidney Dis.* 2014;64:347-358.

75. Malis DJ, Burton DM. Safe pediatric outpatient sedation: the chloral hydrate debate revisited. *Otolaryngol Head Neck Surg.* 1997;116:53-57.

76. Marks J. Techniques of benzodiazepine withdrawal in clinical practice. A consensus workshop report. *Med Toxicol Adverse Drug Exp.* 1988;3:324-333.

77. Mayer G, et al. Efficacy and safety of 6-month nightly ramelteon administration in adults with chronic primary insomnia. *Sleep.* 2009;32:351-360.

78. Mehta AK, Ticku MK. An update on GABAA receptors. *Brain Res Brain Res Rev.* 1999;29:196-217.

79. Mercer AE, et al. Functional and toxicological consequences of metabolic bioactivation of methapyrilene via thiophene S-oxidation: induction of cell defence, apoptosis and hepatic necrosis. *Toxicol Appl Pharmacol.* 2009;239:297-305.

80. Merdink JL, et al. Kinetics of chloral hydrate and its metabolites in male human volunteers. *Toxicology.* 2008;245:130-140.

81. Meyer BR. Benzodiazepines in the elderly. *Med Clin North Am.* 1982;66:1017-1035.

82. Michelson D, et al. Safety and efficacy of suvorexant during 1-year treatment of insomnia with subsequent abrupt treatment discontinuation: a phase 3 randomised, double-blind placebo-controlled trial. *Lancet Neurol.* 2014;13:461-471.

83. Miller NS, Gold MS. Benzodiazepines: reconsidered. *Adv Alcohol Subst Abuse.* 1990;8:67-84.

84. Miner JR, et al. Randomized clinical trial of etomidate versus propofol for procedural sedation in the emergency department. *Ann Emerg Med.* 2007;49:15-22.

85. Mini L, et al. Ramelteon 8 mg/d versus placebo in patients with chronic insomnia: post hoc analysis of a 5-week trial using 50% or greater reduction in latency to persistent sleep as a measure of treatment effect. *Clin Ther.* 2008;30:1316-1323.

86. Mitler MM. Nonselective and selective benzodiazepine receptor agonists—where are we today? *Sleep.* 2000;23(suppl 1):S39-S47.

87. Centers for Disease Control (CDC). Postsurgical infections associated with an extrinsically contaminated intravenous anesthetic Agent—California, Illinois, Maine, and Michigan, 1990. *MMWR Morb Mortal Wkly Rep.* 1990;39:426-427, 433.

88. Modica PA, et al. Pro- and anticonvulsant effects of anesthetics (Part I). *Anesth Analg.* 1990;70:303-315.

89. Modica PA, et al. Pro- and anticonvulsant effects of anesthetics (Part II). *Anesth Analg.* 1990;70:433-444.

90. Narimatsu E, Aoki M. Involvement of the adenosine neuromodulatory system in the benzodiazepine-induced depression of excitatory synaptic transmissions in rat hippocampal neurons in vitro. *Neurosci Res.* 1999;33:57-64.

91. Ng YY, et al. Spurious hyperchloremia and decreased anion gap in a patient with dextromethorphan bromide. *Am J Nephrol.* 1992;12:268-270.

92. Nimmaanrat S. Myoclonic movements following induction of anesthesia with propofol: a case report. *J Med Assoc Thai.* 2005;88:1955-1957.

93. Nordt SP, et al. Pediatric chloral hydrate poisonings and death following outpatient procedural sedation. *J. Med. Toxicol.* 2013;10:219-222

94. O'Meara GF, et al. The GABA-A beta3 subunit mediates anaesthesia induced by etomidate. *Neuroreport.* 2004;15:1653-1656.

95. O'Shea SM, et al. Propofol increases agonist efficacy at the GABA(A) receptor. *Brain Res.* 2000;852:344-348.

96. Olkkola KT, et al. Midazolam should be avoided in patients receiving the systemic antimycotics ketoconazole or itraconazole. *Clin Pharmacol Ther.* 1994;55:481-485.

97. Orser BA, et al. General anaesthetics and their effects on GABA(A) receptor desensitization. *Toxicol Lett.* 1998;100-101:217-224.

98. Pain L, et al. In vivo dopamine measurements in the nucleus accumbens after nonanesthetic and anesthetic doses of propofol in rats. *Anesth Analg.* 2002;95:915-919.

99. Pandharipande PP, et al. Effect of sedation with dexmedetomidine vs lorazepam on acute brain dysfunction in mechanically ventilated patients: the MENDS randomized controlled trial. *JAMA.* 2007;298:2644-2653.

100. Parke TJ, et al. Metabolic acidosis and fatal myocardial failure after propofol infusion in children: five case reports. *BMJ.* 1992;305:613-616.

101. Parker MG, et al. Removal of propylene glycol and correction of increased osmolar gap by hemodialysis in a patient on high dose lorazepam infusion therapy. *Intensive Care Med.* 2002;28:81-84.

102. Peoples RW, Weight FF. Trichloroethanol potentiation of gamma-aminobutyric acid-activated chloride current in mouse hippocampal neurones. *Br J Pharmacol.* 1994;113:555-563.

103. Pershad J, et al. Chloral hydrate: the good and the bad. *Pediatr Emerg Care.* 1999; 15:432-435.

104. Pleasure JR, Blackburn MG. Neonatal bromide intoxication: prenatal ingestion of a large quantity of bromides with transplacental accumulation in the fetus. *Pediatrics.* 1975;55:503-506.

105. Pond SM, et al. Randomized study of the treatment of phenobarbital overdose with repeated doses of activated charcoal. *JAMA.* 1984;251:3104-3108.

106. Proudfoot AT, et al. Position paper on urine alkalinization. *J Toxicol Clin Toxicol.* 2004;42:1-26.

107. Qasim A, et al. Management of chronic insomnia disorder in adults: a clinical practice guideline from the American College of Physicians. *Ann Intern Med.* 2016;165:125-133.

108. Reddy RV, et al. Excitatory effects and electroencephalographic correlation of etomidate, thiopental, methohexital, and propofol. *Anesth Analg.* 1993;77:1008-1011.

109. Repplinger D, Nelson LS. Mind the gap. *Emerg Med.* 2015:47:216-220.

110. Reynolds HN, et al. Hyperlactatemia, increased osmolar gap, and renal dysfunction during continuous lorazepam infusion. *Crit Care Med.* 2000;28:1631-1634.

111. Reynolds JN, Maitra R. Propofol and flurazepam act synergistically to potentiate GABAA receptor activation in human recombinant receptors. *Eur J Pharmacol.* 1996;314:151-156.

112. Reynoldson JN, et al. Ramelteon: a novel approach in the treatment of insomnia. *Ann Pharmacother.* 2008;42:1262-1271.

113. Rho JM, et al. Barbiturate-like actions of the propanediol dicarbamates felbamate and meprobamate. *J Pharmacol Exp Ther.* 1997;280:1383-1391.

114. Richardson G, Wang-Weigand S. Effects of long-term exposure to ramelteon, a melatonin receptor agonist, on endocrine function in adults with chronic insomnia. *Hum Psychopharmacol.* 2009;24:103-111.

115. Rickels K, et al. Long-term treatment of anxiety and risk of withdrawal. Prospective comparison of clorazepate and buspirone. *Arch Gen Psychiatry.* 1988;45:444-450.

116. Rivara S, et al. Melatonin receptor agonists: SAR and applications to the treatment of sleep-wake disorders. *Curr Top Med Chem.* 2008;8:954-968.

117. Roberts DM, Buckley NA. Enhanced elimination in acute barbiturate poisoning a systematic review. *Clin Toxicol.* 2011;49:2-12.

118. Romazicon [package insert]. Nutley, NJ: Roche Laboratories, Inc.; April 2010.

119. Rosenberg J, et al. Pharmacokinetics of drug overdose. *Clin Pharmacokinet.* 1981;6:161-192.

120. Sahi J, et al. Regulation of cytochrome P450 2C9 expression in primary cultures of human hepatocytes. *J Biochem Mol Toxicol.* 2009;23:43-58.

121. Scheibler P, et al. Trichloroethanol impairs NMDA receptor function in rat mesencephalic and cortical neurones. *Eur J Pharmacol.* 1999;366:R1-R2.

122. Schenarts CL, et al. Adrenocortical dysfunction following etomidate induction in emergency department patients. *Acad Emerg Med.* 2001;8:1-7.

123. Schmidt-Mutter C, et al. The anxiolytic effect of gamma-hydroxybutyrate in the elevated plus maze is reversed by the benzodiazepine receptor antagonist, flumazenil. *Eur J Pharmacol.* 1998;342:21-27.

124. Schulte D, et al. Propofol decreases stimulated dopamine release in the rat nucleus accumbens by a mechanism independent of dopamine D2, GABAA and NMDA receptors. *Br J Anaesth.* 2000;84:250-253.

125. Schwartz HS. Acute meprobamate poisoning with gastrotomy and removal of a drug-containing mass. *N Engl J Med.* 1976;295:1177-1178.

126. Schwieler L, et al. The anaesthetic agent propofol interacts with GABA(B)-receptors: an electrophysiological study in rat. *Life Sci.* 2003;72:2793-2801.

127. Seay RE, et al. Comment: possible toxicity from propylene glycol in lorazepam infusion. *Ann Pharmacother.* 1997;31:647-648.

128. Sellers EM, et al. Interaction of chloral hydrate and ethanol in man. II. Hemodynamics and performance. *Clin Pharmacol Ther.* 1972;13:50-58.

129. Sellers EM, et al. Interaction of chloral hydrate and ethanol in man. I. Metabolism. *Clin Pharmacol Ther.* 1972;13:37-49.

130. Serfaty M, Masterton G. Fatal poisonings attributed to benzodiazepines in Britain during the 1980s. *Br J Psychiatry.* 1993;163:386-393.

131. Seubert CN, et al. Midazolam selectively potentiates the A(2A) but not A1-receptor–mediated effects of adenosine: role of nucleoside transport inhibition and clinical implications. *Anesthesiology.* 2000;92:567-577.

132. Short TG, Young Y. Toxicity of intravenous anaesthetics. *Best Pract Res Clin Anaesthesiol.* 2003;17:77-89.

133. Sigel E, Steinmann ME. Structure, function, and modulation of GABA$_A$ receptors. *J. Biol. Chem.* 2012;287(402224-40231).

134. Simpson D, Curran MP. Ramelteon: a review of its use in insomnia. *Drugs.* 2008;68: 1901-1919.

135. Sivilotti L, Nistri A. GABA receptor mechanisms in the central nervous system. *Prog Neurobiol.* 1991;36:35-92.

136. Smith PF, Darlington CL. The behavioural effects of long-term use of benzodiazepine sedative and hypnotic drugs: what can be learned from animal studies? *N Z J Psychol.* 1994;23:48-63.

137. Snead OC 3rd, et al. Gamma-hydroxybutyric acid binding sites: interaction with the GABA-benzodiazepine-picrotoxin receptor complex. *Neurochem Res.* 1992;17:201-204.

138. Snyder GL, et al. General anesthetics selectively modulate glutamatergic and dopaminergic signaling via site-specific phosphorylation in vivo. *Neuropharmacology.* 2007;53: 619-630.

139. Spivey WH. Flumazenil and seizures: analysis of 43 cases. *Clin Ther.* 1992;14:292-305.

140. Srinivasan V, et al. Melatonin and melatonergic drugs on sleep: possible mechanisms of action. *Int J Neurosci.* 2009;119:821-846.

141. Stahl SM. Mechanism of action of suvorexant. *CNS Spectrums.* 2016;21:215-218.

142. Stowe DF, et al. Comparison of etomidate, ketamine, midazolam, propofol, and thiopental on function and metabolism of isolated hearts. *Anesth Analg.* 1992;74:547-558.

143. Szumita PM, et al. Sedation and analgesia in the intensive care unit: evaluating the role of dexmedetomidine. *Am J Health Syst Pharm.* 2007;64:37-44.

144. Tekwani KL, et al. The effect of single-bolus etomidate on septic patient mortality: a retrospective review. *West J Emerg Med.* 2008;9:195-200.

145. Tekwani KL, et al. A prospective observational study of the effect of etomidate on septic patient mortality and length of stay. *Acad Emerg Med.* 2009;16:11-14.

146. Tibbitts GM. Sleep disorders: causes, effects, and solutions. *Prim Care.* 2008;35:817-837.

147. Todd CM, Forrester MB. Ramelteon ingestions reported to Texas poison centers, 2005-2009. *J Emerg Med.* 2012:43:189-193.

148. Tramer MR, et al. Propofol and bradycardia: causation, frequency and severity. *Br J Anaesth.* 1997;78:642-651.

149. Trump DL, Hochberg MC. Bromide intoxication. *Johns Hopkins Med J.* 1976;138:119-123.

150. Uchida I, et al. The role of the GABA(A) receptor alpha1 subunit N-terminal extracellular domain in propofol potentiation of chloride current. *Neuro-pharmacology.* 1997;36:1611-1621.

151. van de Kerkhof EG, et al. Induction of metabolism and transport in human intestine: validation of precision-cut slices as a tool to study induction of drug metabolism in human intestine in vitro. *Drug Metab Dispos.* 2008;36:604-613.

152. Van de Wiele B, et al. Propylene glycol toxicity caused by prolonged infusion of etomidate. *J Neurosurg Anesthesiol.* 1995;7:259-262.

153. van Herwaarden AE, et al. Midazolam and cyclosporin a metabolism in transgenic mice with liver-specific expression of human CYP3A4. *Drug Metab Dispos.* 2005;33:892-895.

154. Varon J, Marik P. Etomidate and propylene glycol toxicity. *J Emerg Med.* 1998;16:485.

155. Vasile B, et al. The pathophysiology of propofol infusion syndrome: a simple name for a complex syndrome. *Intensive Care Med.* 2003;29:1417-1425.

156. Vasileiou I, et al. Propofol: a review of its non-anaesthetic effects. *Eur J Pharmacol.* 2009;605:1-8.

157. Veller ID, et al. Gastric necrosis: a rare complication of chloral hydrate intoxication. *Br J Surg.* 1972;59:317-319.

158. Wagner J, et al. Beyond benzodiazepines: alternative pharmacologic agents for the treatment of insomnia. *Ann Pharmacother.* 1998;32:680-691.

159. Wagner RL, White PF. Etomidate inhibits adrenocortical function in surgical patients. *Anesthesiology.* 1984;61:647-651.

160. Wagner RL, et al. Inhibition of adrenal steroidogenesis by the anesthetic etomidate. *N Engl J Med.* 1984;310:1415-1421.

161. Wala EP, et al. Substantia nigra: the involvement of central and peripheral benzodiazepine receptors in physical dependence on diazepam as evidenced by behavioral and EEG effects. *Pharmacol Biochem Behav.* 1999;64:611-623.

162. Walsh JK, et al. Efficacy and safety of zolpidem extended release in elderly primary insomnia patients. *Am J Geriatr Psychiatry.* 2008;16:44-57.

163. Warden JC, Pickford DR. Fatal cardiovascular collapse following propofol induction in high-risk patients and dilemmas in the selection of a short-acting induction agent. *Anaesth Intensive Care.* 1995;23:485-487.

164. Watsky E. Management of zolpidem withdrawal. *J Clin Psychopharmacol.* 1996;16:459.

165. Wesensten NJ, et al. Reversal of triazolam- and zolpidem-induced memory impairment by flumazenil. *Psychopharmacology (Berl).* 1995;121:242-249.

166. White JF, Carlson GP. Epinephrine-induced cardiac arrhythmias in rabbits exposed to trichloroethylene: role of trichloroethylene metabolites. *Toxicol Appl Pharmacol.* 1981;60:458-465.

167. World Health Organization. Outbreak of neurological illness of unknown etiology in Cacuaco Municipality, Angola: WHO rapid assessment and cause finding mission, 2 November—23 November 2007: executive summary http://www.who.int/environmental_health_emergencies/events/Angola%20cause%20finding%20mission%20report%20Exeutive%20Summary%20for%20Web%20V190308.pdf.

168. Wiley CC, Wiley JF 2nd. Pediatric benzodiazepine ingestion resulting in hospitalization. *J Toxicol Clin Toxicol.* 1998;36:227-231.

169. Withington DE, et al. A case of propofol toxicity: further evidence for a causal mechanism. *Paediatr Anaesth.* 2004;14:505-508.

170. Wolf BC, et al. Alprazolam-related deaths in Palm Beach County. *Am J Forensic Med Pathol.* 2005;26:24-27.

171. Yamamoto K, et al. False hyperchloremia in bromism. *J Anesth.* 1991;5:88-91.

172. Yang CC, Deng JF. Utility of flumazenil in zopiclone overdose. *Clin Toxicol.* 2008;46:920-921.

173. Yin J, et al. Structure and ligand-binding mechanism of the human OX1 and OX2 receptors. *Nat Struct Mol Biol.* 2016;23:293-299

174. Zaballos M, et al. Comparative effects of thiopental and propofol on atrial vulnerability: electrophysiological study in a porcine model including acute alcoholic intoxication. *Br J Anaesth.* 2004;93:414-421.

175. Zahedi A, et al. Successful treatment of chloral hydrate cardiac toxicity with propranolol. *Am J Emerg Med.* 1999;17:490-491.

176. Zavala F. Benzodiazepines, anxiety, and immunity. *Pharmacol Ther.* 1997;75:199-216.

177. Zhu H, et al. The effect of thiopental and propofol on NMDA- and AMPA-mediated glutamate excitotoxicity. *Anesthesiology.* 1997;87:944-951.

178. Zorilla-Vaca A, et al. Infectious disease risk associated with contaminated propofol anesthesia, 1989-2014. *Emerg Infect Dis.* 2016;22:981-992

179. Zosel A, et al. Zolpidem misuse with other medications or alcohol frequently results in intensive care unit admission. *Am J Ther.* 2011;18:305-308.

FLUMAZENIL

Mary Ann Howland

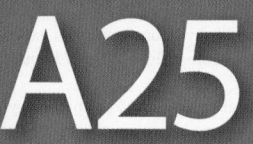

Flumazenil

Diazepam

Midazolam

INTRODUCTION

Flumazenil is a competitive benzodiazepine receptor antagonist. Its role in patients with an unknown overdose is limited because seizures and dysrhythmias may develop when the effects of a benzodiazepine are reversed if the patient has taken a mixed overdose of a benzodiazepine and a proconvulsant. Flumazenil also has the potential to induce benzodiazepine withdrawal symptoms, including seizures in patients who are benzodiazepine dependent. Flumazenil does not reliably reverse the respiratory depression induced by intravenous (IV) benzodiazepines.[24] Flumazenil is the ideal antidote for the relatively few patients who are both naïve to benzodiazepines and who overdose solely on a benzodiazepine as well as benzodiazepine-naïve patients whose benzodiazepines must be reversed during or after procedural sedation. Because the duration of effect of flumazenil is shorter than that of most benzodiazepines, repeat doses may be necessary and vigilance is warranted. Flumazenil has no role in the management of ethanol intoxication. In patients with hepatic encephalopathy, further study is necessary before it can be recommended.[4] Case reports raise the possibility of a role for flumazenil in patients with paradoxical reactions to therapeutic doses of benzodiazepines.[78,86] Flumazenil is neither rational nor effective in patients who overdose with baclofen.[15] Flumazenil is effective for overdoses of zolpidem and zaleplon, nonbenzodiazepines that interact with ω_1 receptors, a subclass of central benzodiazepine receptors.[50,62,65,79]

HISTORY

The initial work of Haefely and Hunkeler[42,82] on chlordiazepoxide synthesis led to an attempt to develop benzodiazepine derivatives that would act as antagonists.[37] This endeavor was initially unsuccessful but led to the promising γ-aminobutyric acid (GABA) hypothesis as the benzodiazepine mechanism of action. Radioligand binding identified specific high-affinity benzodiazepine binding sites and others isolated a product produced by a *Streptomyces* species that had the basic 1,4-benzodiazepine structure.

Synthetic derivatives of this molecule led to the creation of benzodiazepines with potent anxiolytic and anticonvulsant activity and diminished sedative and muscle-relaxing properties. Testing revealed these derivatives had high in vitro binding affinities but lacked in vivo agonist activity. An inability to enter the central nervous system (CNS) was considered an explanation for the discordance. During an experiment that attempted to demonstrate CNS penetration of these derivatives, diazepam given to incapacitate the animals had a surprisingly weak effect. This lack of efficacy of diazepam led to the discovery of a benzodiazepine antagonist. Further modifications led to the synthesis of flumazenil.[23,68]

PHARMACOLOGY
Mechanism of Action

The benzodiazepine receptor modulates the effect of GABA on the GABA$_A$ receptor by increasing the frequency of Cl$^-$ channel opening, leading to hyperpolarization. Agonists such as diazepam stimulate the benzodiazepine receptor to produce anxiolytic, anticonvulsant, sedative–hypnotic, amnestic, and muscle relaxant effects.[38] Flumazenil is a water-soluble benzodiazepine analog with a molecular weight of 303 Da. It acts as a competitive antagonist at the α_1 subtype of GABA$_A$ benzodiazepine receptors with very weak partial agonist properties at the α_2, α_3, and α_5 subtypes of the GABA$_A$ benzodiazepine receptors in animal models and possibly in humans.[21,52] Inverse agonists bind the benzodiazepine receptor and result in the opposite effects of anxiety, agitation, and seizures. Antagonists, such as flumazenil, competitively occupy the benzodiazepine receptor without causing any functional change and without allowing an agonist or inverse agonist access to the receptor. The zero setpoint of intrinsic activity may be influenced by the activity of the GABA system or by chronic treatment with benzodiazepines.[27] Positron emission tomography investigations in adult humans revealed that 1.5 mg of flumazenil led to an initial receptor occupancy of 55%, but 15 mg caused almost total blockade of benzodiazepine receptor sites.[72]

PHARMACOKINETICS AND PHARMACODYNAMICS

Table A25–1 summarizes the physicochemical and pharmacologic properties of flumazenil.[24,42] Volunteer studies demonstrate that the ability of flumazenil to reverse the effects of sedating doses of IV benzodiazepines (eg, 30 mg diazepam, 3 mg lorazepam, 10 mg midazolam) is dose dependent and begins within minutes.[21] Peak effects occur within 6 to 10 minutes.[24] Most individuals achieve complete reversal of benzodiazepine effect with a total IV dose of 1 mg, titrated in 0.2-mg aliquots.[5,14] A 3-mg IV dose produces similar effects that last approximately twice as long as the 1-mg dose. A study in monkeys reports the pharmacodynamic half-life of flumazenil as similar to the pharmacokinetic half-life.[91]

ROLE IN CONSCIOUS SEDATION

A number of studies evaluated patients who received midazolam or diazepam (average doses of 10 and 30 mg, respectively) as conscious sedation for endoscopy or cardioversion.[6,13,14,18,45,47] When a benzodiazepine is given for conscious sedation during a procedure, flumazenil appears safe and effective for reversal of prolonged sedation and partial reversal of amnesia and cognitive impairment.[30,40,46] The practitioner performing conscious sedation is able to obtain a more reliable history of whether contraindications to flumazenil exist. Most patients respond to total doses of 0.4 to 1 mg.[24]

TABLE A25–1	Physicochemical and Pharmacologic Properties of Flumazenil
pK$_a$	Weak base
LogD	1.15 (octanol/aqueous PO$_4$ buffer)
Volume of distribution (SS)	1.06 L/kg
Distribution half-life (min)	4–11
Metabolism	Hepatic: three inactive metabolites Clearance dependent on hepatic blood flow
Elimination	First order
Protein binding (%)	54–64
Elimination half-life (min)	54
Onset of action (min)	1–2
Duration of action	Dependent on dose and elimination of benzodiazepine, time interval, dose of flumazenil, and hepatic function

Administering flumazenil slowly at a rate of 0.1 mg/min minimizes the disconcerting symptoms associated with rapid arousal, such as confusion, agitation, and emotional lability. Persistent or recurrent sedation becomes evident within 20 to 120 minutes, depending on the dose and pharmacokinetics of the specific chosen benzodiazepine and the dose of flumazenil.[30] One study evaluated 887 patients who received 5 mg of midazolam for endoscopy followed by a median reversal dose of 0.2 mg of flumazenil. Most procedures lasted 30 minutes, and flumazenil was administered 5 minutes after arrival in the recovery room. Patients left for home 65 minutes after the last dose of midazolam with only 83% of the patients fully alert. Of concern is that 3 patients fainted, fell or had a near fall, although without harm demonstrating the risks of incomplete or transient reversal.[57] Flumazenil does not alter the clinical course of most patients who receive it and provides a false sense of effectiveness to the clinician. Therefore, patients must be carefully monitored and subsequent doses of flumazenil titrated to clinical response. Because the amnestic effect of benzodiazepines and the cognitive and psychomotor effects are not fully reversed, posttreatment instructions should be reinforced in writing and given to a responsible caregiver accompanying the patient.[21,30]

Two patients undergoing endoscopy who developed seizures after benzodiazepine reversal are reported.[77] One patient had a history of seizures, and the other had no obvious etiology. Both patients recovered uneventfully.

ROLE IN PARADOXICAL REACTIONS

Paradoxical reactions to benzodiazepines are unpredictable and documented in as many as 10% of adults and in 3.4% of children.[16,34,55,56,78] Common features include worsening restlessness, agitation, disorientation, irrational talking, flailing and excessive movements, hostile behavior, and dysphoria.[29,32,63,78,86] The mechanism is unclear and is attributed to disinhibition.[26] These reactions are reported to occur from several minutes to 210 minutes after initiation of sedation.[32,86] One study of 98 pediatric patients found that administering a flumazenil dose of 0.1 mg/kg as a 0.1% solution at 0.2 mL/s compared with 1 mL/s significantly reduced the occurrence of paradoxical reactions.[58] Management strategies include administering higher doses of the benzodiazepines, adding other drugs such as opioids or droperidol, stopping the procedure, and using flumazenil.[20,26,29,43,56,63,86] Intravenous flumazenil was administered to six adults with paradoxical reactions to midazolam in 0.1-mg aliquots. Doses of 0.2 to 0.5 mg were effective in all the patients with a response occurring within 30 seconds.[86] Attention to other causes of unexpected behavior such as hypoxia or hypoglycemia must be addressed and corrected.

ROLE IN THE OVERDOSE SETTING

Although the flumazenil package insert prescribing information carries an indication for the management of benzodiazepine overdose, the role of flumazenil in the overdose setting is controversial.[24,48,83] The first argument against flumazenil use is the rare morbidity and mortality associated with benzodiazepine use. An analysis of 702 patients who had taken benzodiazepines alone or in combination with ethanol or other xenobiotics and were subsequently admitted to a medical intensive care unit over a 14-year period revealed a 0.7% fatality rate (five deaths) and 9.8% complication rate (69 patients).[41] In comparison, the fatality rate for patients with nonbenzodiazepine-related overdoses was 1.6% (55 of 3,430 patients). In the benzodiazepine group, two patients died, and 18 (12.5%) of 144 patients had complications, mostly aspiration pneumonitis and decubitus ulcers. Proponents of flumazenil therapy suggest that some of the 29 diagnostic procedures used in the patients were unnecessary, and some of the complications could have been prevented by the use of flumazenil. We and others suggest that many of the cases of aspiration pneumonitis occurred before hospital admission and that the patients also suffered from trauma and infectious diseases, making most diagnostic procedures necessary.

In an effort to develop indications for safe and effective use of flumazenil, overdosed comatose patients were retrospectively assigned to either a low-risk or non–low-risk group.[35] Low-risk patients had CNS depression with normal vital signs, no other neurologic findings, no evidence of ingestion of a tricyclic antidepressant by history or electrocardiography, no seizure history, and absence of an available history of chronic benzodiazepine use. All other patients fell into the non–low-risk category. Of 35 consecutive comatose patients, 4 were assigned to the low-risk group. Flumazenil resulted in complete awakening in three patients and partial awakening in the fourth patient in the low-risk group, with no adverse events. In the non–low-risk group of 31 patients, flumazenil caused complete awakening in 4 patients and partial awakening in 5 patients. Seizures occurred in 5 patients, of whom only 1 had a history of seizures, 5 were long-term benzodiazepine users, 4 had abnormal vital signs before reversal, and 3 had evidence of hyperreflexia or myoclonus. Therefore, although flumazenil use probably was safe and effective in the low-risk group, few patients could be considered low risk. The risk of seizures appears substantial in non–low-risk patients.

A systematic review with an analysis of randomized controlled trials of the use of flumazenil compared to placebo in emergency department patients with coma and a suspicion of benzodiazepine overdose included a total of 994 patients divided equally between flumazenil and placebo.[66] More serious adverse events (supraventricular dysrhythmias and seizures) and more adverse events in general (eg, aggressive behavior, nausea, vomiting, and abdominal cramps, sweating, shivering, and anxiety) occurred in the flumazenil group than placebo.[75]

The risks of flumazenil usually outweigh the benefits in patients with overdoses.[66,67,73,75] When non–benzodiazepine-dependent patients solely ingest benzodiazepines in overdose, as rarely occurs in adults but might be expected in children, the risks associated with flumazenil are limited.[49,88] Table A25–2 summarizes the indications for flumazenil use in the overdose setting.

ROLE IN NONBENZODIAZEPINE TOXICITY
Hepatic Encephalopathy

Hepatic encephalopathy is considered a reversible metabolic encephalopathy characterized by a spectrum of CNS effects. Symptoms may progress

TABLE A25–2	Indications for Flumazenil Use in the Overdose Setting

Pure benzodiazepine overdose in a nontolerant individual who has
- CNS depression
- Normal vital signs, including SaO$_2$
- Normal ECG findings
- Otherwise normal neurologic examination

CNS = central nervous system; ECG = electrocardiogram.

from confusion and somnolence to coma. One current hypothesis implicates an increase in GABAergic tone in the development of encephalopathy.[7,76]

Animal studies of hepatic encephalopathy secondary to galactosamine or thioacetamide (hepatotoxins) demonstrate an increase in GABA effect, which is antagonized by flumazenil, bicuculline (a GABA receptor antagonist), and isopropylbiclophosphate chloride (a calcium channel blocker).[7] Cerebrospinal fluid (CSF) from these animals contained a benzodiazepine receptor ligand with agonist activity. Rat studies involving hepatic encephalopathy resulting from acute liver ischemia showed only a slight response to flumazenil but significant improvement after administration of a partial inverse agonist.[12,84]

Human studies have detected benzodiazepine binding activity in the CSF and serum of patients with hepatic encephalopathy. One group identified four to 19 peaks representing benzodiazepine binding ligands from the frontal cortex of 11 patients who died of hepatic encephalopathy.[10] Two of the peaks were further characterized as diazepam and N-desmethyldiazepam. Brain concentrations of these substances were 2 to 10 times higher than normal in 6 of the patients and were normal in 5 patients. Patients with idiopathic recurring stupor have measurable "endozepines" (endogenous benzodiazepine ligands) in serum and CSF.[69,81]

Flumazenil improves the clinical and electrophysiologic responses of patients with hepatic encephalopathy and idiopathic recurring stupor.[4,8,22,69,81] Some patients with encephalopathy have improved from stage IV to stage II encephalopathy after IV flumazenil. Maximal improvement after flumazenil lasts approximately 1 to 2 hours and gradually dissipates within 6 hours. The response rate in a meta-analysis averaged approximately 30%.[33] The proposed explanations for the unresponsiveness include cerebral edema, hypoxia, other systemic diseases or complications, and irreversible CNS damage.

Animal and human data convincingly support the concept that increased GABAergic tone is responsible for hepatic encephalopathy. Evidence for endogenous benzodiazepine ligands that enhance GABA action also are demonstrated but controversial.[1,3] The source of these benzodiazepine receptor agonists is unclear, but diet or production by gut bacteria (or both) is postulated.[7] Some authorities believe endogenous de novo synthesis is unlikely and propose prior benzodiazepine exposure and persistence of clinical effects as an explanation. Hyperammonemia, neurosteroids, and hemoglobin metabolites are also implicated in the pathophysiology of hepatic encephalopathy.[3,11,19,71]

Flumazenil can lead to short-term improvement of the clinical condition of a subgroup of patients with hepatic encephalopathy and may prove useful as an addition to conventional therapy.[2,4,9] Existing guidelines recommend that use be reserved for patients with acute hepatic encephalopathy and a history of benzodiazepine use.[11,25] Additional research is necessary to prospectively identify responders, provide dosing considerations, and evaluate adverse events. There is no known survival benefit, and we do not currently recommend flumazenil utilization.[31]

Ethanol Intoxication

Animal studies indicate that many of the actions of ethanol are mediated through GABA neurotransmission.[80] Acute ethanol administration appears to enhance GABA transmission and inhibit N-methyl-D-aspartate excitation. Chronic ethanol administration leads to downregulation of the GABA system. Ethanol enhances $GABA_A$-induced chloride influx in a dose-dependent fashion without a direct effect on chloride. Flumazenil does not influence this action of GABA. Chronic ethanol use selectively increases the sensitivity to inverse benzodiazepine agonists, invoking a change in coupling or conformation of the receptor. These changes may explain the development of tolerance as well as the kindling effect and production of seizures that occur during ethanol withdrawal.

A randomized, double-blind, crossover study was conducted in eight male volunteers given IV ethanol to achieve a constant serum ethanol concentration of 160 mg/dL.[17] After being stabilized, the volunteers were given either placebo or 5 mg of flumazenil. Subjective and objective psychomotor tests were conducted, with no differences noted between groups. Thus, the probability of ethanol reversal at the doses achieved appears unlikely.[76]

Based on this information, flumazenil likely does not have a significant effect on ethanol intoxication, and low doses (< 1 mg) of flumazenil have no effect.[51,54] The 5-mg doses reportedly produce favorable changes in sensorium, but these findings may be the result of confounding factors. Flumazenil should not be administered in this dose range in the overdose setting. Therefore, to avoid the increased risk of adverse effects, flumazenil cannot be recommended for reversal of ethanol intoxication.

ADVERSE EFFECTS AND SAFETY ISSUES

More than 3,500 patients worldwide received flumazenil, including healthy volunteers and overdosed patients, or patients who had undergone conscious sedation. The safety of flumazenil in healthy volunteers is well established without discernible objective or subjective effects. However, seizures in benzodiazepine-dependent patients, dysrhythmias in patients who coingest a benzodiazepine and a prodysrhythmic xenobiotic, and resedation within 20 to 120 minutes in patients receiving benzodiazepines for conscious sedation are recognized adverse events associated with flumazenil administration.

The ability of flumazenil to precipitate acute benzodiazepine withdrawal seizures in a more controlled environment than the overdose setting was demonstrated by reversal of long-term benzodiazepine sedation in the intensive care unit. A study of 1,700 patients revealed that 14 patients developed adverse drug reactions; probably half of these reactions were related to abrupt arousal.[6] Two patients with a history of epilepsy developed tonic–clonic seizures, and one patient developed myoclonic seizures.[6] Dose-dependent induction of withdrawal reactions is therefore suggested. Small total doses (< 1 mg) of titrated flumazenil are suggest to allow sufficient occupation of the benzodiazepine receptor sites by benzodiazepines to limit the occurrence of withdrawal seizures.

In a study of 12 patients receiving midazolam sedation for 4 ± 3 days, 0.5 mg of flumazenil was administered as a rapid bolus. Serum norepinephrine and epinephrine concentrations rose within 10 minutes, returned to baseline within 30 minutes, and correlated with increased heart rate, blood pressure, and myocardial oxygen consumption.[44] Flumazenil causes a significant overshoot in cerebral blood flow and risks causing a large increase in intracranial pressure in patients who have received midazolam for severe head injury.[90]

Thirty published case series involving 758 patients with benzodiazepine overdoses were reviewed.[28] In total, 387 patients participated in double-blind study protocols and 371 patients in open-label studies.[28] Fifty percent of cases were associated with mixed benzodiazepine overdoses. The doses of flumazenil ranged from 0.2 to 5 mg. Five cases of seizures were temporally related to flumazenil administration, all followed large bolus doses. In three of the five patients, high concentrations of TCAs were present in the blood. The seizures resolved either without treatment or after administration of a small dose of a benzodiazepine. Dysrhythmias developed in two patients given small doses of flumazenil, both presumably associated with the presence of a TCA. Of 497 patients enrolled in two clinical US studies sponsored by the manufacturer,[28] 6 patients developed seizures (5 had coingested TCAs), and 1 patient who had taken a TCA and carbamazepine had a junctional tachycardia, which normalized after several minutes. Thus, in reviewing 1,255 patients, 11 patients had seizures, and 3 developed dysrhythmias, for an incidence of approximately 0.9%. We agree with the consensus report, which stated that (1) flumazenil is not a substitute for primary emergency care; (2) hypoxia and hypotension should be corrected before flumazenil is used; (3) when used, small titrated doses of flumazenil should be given; (4) flumazenil should not be used in patients with a history of seizures, evidence of seizures or jerking movements, or evidence of a TCA overdose; and (5) flumazenil should not be used by inexperienced clinicians.

An analysis was published of all seizures associated with flumazenil gathered from previously published cases or reports to the manufacturer.[77] Forty-three patients had seizures, and six patients died, but the author believed that none of the deaths were attributable to flumazenil.[77] Four patients developed status epilepticus; two were presumed to be caused by concomitant TCA exposure, and the other two patients had received benzodiazepines

TABLE A25-3	Contraindications to Flumazenil Use
History	**Clinical**
Seizure history or current treatment of seizures	Potential ECG evidence of cyclic antidepressant use: terminal rightward 40-ms axis, QRS or QT interval prolongation
Ingestion of a xenobiotic capable of provoking seizures or cardiac dysrhythmias	Hypoxia or hypoventilation[a]
	Hypotension
	Head trauma
Long-term use of benzodiazepines	

[a]Do not rely on flumazenil to reverse benzodiazepine-induced respiratory depression.

ECG = electrocardiogram.

to treat status epilepticus before flumazenil therapy. In six of 43 seizure episodes, the relationship to flumazenil use was believed to be inadequately defined. The remaining 37 patients were stratified into five categories. In category 1, seven patients were given flumazenil after they had received a benzodiazepine for treatment of a seizure disorder. Six of these seven patients received greater than 1 mg flumazenil. In category 2, 20 patients received flumazenil for reversal of a benzodiazepine in a mixed drug overdose. Many of these patients had coingested TCAs. Thirteen of these patients received more than 1 mg of flumazenil. Two of the patients in this group developed status epilepticus and died, possibly secondary to a severe TCA overdose. Category 3 included five patients who received benzodiazepines for suppression of non–drug-induced seizures. Two of these five patients received more than 1 mg of flumazenil. Category 4 included three patients with acute benzodiazepine overdoses in the presence of chronic benzodiazepine dependence. Category 5 included two patients who received a benzodiazepine for conscious sedation. Therefore, flumazenil use places the patient at risk for seizures by unmasking a toxic effect in mixed overdose, by removing the protective anticonvulsant effect in a patient with non–drug-induced seizures, or by precipitating acute benzodiazepine withdrawal. Table A25-3 summarizes the contraindications and precautions essential to evaluate before flumazenil use.

Flumazenil does not consistently reverse benzodiazepine-induced respiratory depression and is not suggested as the initial intervention if respiratory depression occurs.[24,53,59,74] Interestingly, in one preliminary observational study of 13 patients being mechanically ventilated for more than 4 days who were receiving midazolam, the administration of flumazenil increased diaphragm electrical activity.[70] It is likely that after oral overdose, benzodiazepine-induced respiratory insufficiency is related to smooth muscle relaxation, resulting in a mechanical effect with an increase in upper airway resistance and obstructive apnea rather than a central effect.[36] Although flumazenil might improve the clinical situation,[36,64] other standard procedures such as airway repositioning, supplemental oxygen, bag-valve-mask ventilation, and endotracheal intubation, if indicated, should be used either before or during reversal.

PREGNANCY AND LACTATION

Flumazenil is US Food and Drug Administration (FDA) Pregnancy Category C. There are no adequate studies done in pregnant women.[24] It is not known whether flumazenil is excreted in breast milk.[24]

DOSING AND ADMINISTRATION

Slow IV titration (0.1 mg/min) and waiting 1 minute between doses, to a total dose no higher than 1 mg, seems most reasonable in adults. In pediatric patients, for the reversal of conscious sedation, the package insert recommends an initial dose of 0.01 mg/kg (up to 0.2 mg). We think it is prudent to administer the flumazenil slowly as described for adults. Administration into a large freely running vein minimizes the potential for pain at the injection site. Resedation should be anticipated to occur between 20 and 120 minutes, and readministration of flumazenil may be necessary. Flumazenil

is compatible with 5% dextrose in water, lactated Ringer's solution, and normal saline.[24] Although not approved by the FDA, continuous IV infusion of flumazenil 0.1 to 1.0 mg/h in 0.9% sodium chloride solution or 5% dextrose in water is used by some authors after the loading dose, although we do not consider this approach of well-defined value or appropriate.[50,87,89]

FORMULATION

Flumazenil is available by many manufacturers in a concentration of 0.1 mg/mL with parabens in 5- and 10-mL vials.

SUMMARY

- The risks of flumazenil greatly outweigh the potential benefits of reversal when benzodiazepines are used chronically or acutely to treat a seizure disorder.
- We believe that flumazenil can be safely administered to patients naïve to benzodiazepines for the reversal of CNS sedation.
- We recommend that flumazenil be avoided in the overdose setting when evidence indicates coingestion of a drug capable of causing seizures or dysrhythmias.
- Flumazenil should not be used when involvement of a TCA is strongly suggested based on history, clinical findings, or findings on electrocardiography (prolonged QRS complex).[39,52,60,85]
- We recommend that flumazenil be avoided in any patients where theophylline, carbamazepine, chloral hydrate, chloroquine, and or chlorinated hydrocarbons are a part of the overdose history.[85]
- We believe that in the event of a seizure induced by a therapeutic dose of flumazenil, a benzodiazepine such as diazepam or lorazepam should be effective; however, because of the competitive nature of flumazenil, higher doses are necessary to reverse higher doses of flumazenil.

REFERENCES

1. Ahboucha S, Butterworth RF. Pathophysiology of hepatic encephalopathy: a new look at GABA from the molecular standpoint. *Metab Brain Dis.* 2004;19:331-343.
2. Ahboucha S, Butterworth RF. Role of endogenous benzodiazepine ligands and their GABA-A–associated receptors in hepatic encephalopathy. *Metab Brain Dis.* 2005;20:425-437.
3. Ahboucha S, et al. Increased brain concentrations of endogenous (non-benzodiazepine) GABA-a receptor ligands in human hepatic encephalopathy. *Metab Brain Dis.* 2004;19:241-251.
4. Als-Nielsen B, et al. Benzodiazepine receptor antagonists for acute and chronic hepatic encephalopathy. *Cochrane Database Syst Rev.* 2004;2:CD002798.
5. Amrein R, et al. Clinical pharmacology of flumazenil. *Eur J Anaesth.* 1988;2:65-80.
6. Amrein R, et al. Flumazenil in benzodiazepine antagonism: actions and clinical use in intoxications and anaesthesiology. *Med Toxicol.* 1987;2:411-429.
7. Anonymous. Benzodiazepine compounds and hepatic encephalopathy. *N Engl J Med.* 1991;325:509-510.
8. Anonymous. Flumazenil in the treatment of hepatic encephalopathy. *Ann Pharmacother.* 1993;27:46-47.
9. Barbaro G, et al. Flumazenil for hepatic encephalopathy grade III and IVa in patients with cirrhosis: an Italian multicenter double-blind, placebo-controlled, cross-over study. *Hepatology.* 1998;28:374-378.
10. Basile AS, et al. Elevated brain concentrations of 1,4-benzodiazepines in fulminant hepatic failure. *N Engl J Med.* 1991;325:473-478.
11. Blei AT, Córdoba J. Hepatic encephalopathy: Practice Parameters Committee of the American College of Gastroenterology. *Am J Gastroenterol.* 2001;96:1968-1976.
12. Bosman DK, et al. The effects of benzodiazepine-receptor antagonists and partial inverse agonists on acute hepatic encephalopathy in the rat. *Gastroenterology.* 1991;101:772-781.
13. Breheny FX. Reversal of midazolam sedation with flumazenil. *Crit Care Med.* 1991;20:736-739.
14. Brogden RN, Goa KL. Flumazenil: a reappraisal of its pharmacological properties and therapeutic efficacy as a benzodiazepine antagonist. *Drugs.* 1991;42:1061-1089.
15. Byrnes SMA, et al. Flumazenil: an unreliable antagonist in baclofen overdose. *Anaesthesiology.* 1996;51:481-482.
16. Chung HJ, et al. Delayed flumazenil injection after endoscopic sedation increases patient satisfaction compared with immediate flumazenil injection. *Gut Liver.* 2014;8:7-12.
17. Clausen TG, et al. The effect of the benzodiazepine antagonist, flumazenil, on psychometric performance in acute ethanol intoxication in man. *Eur J Clin Pharmacol.* 1990;38:233-236.
18. Coll-Vincent B, et al. Sedation of cardioversion in the emergency department: analysis of effectiveness in four protocols. *Ann Emerg Med.* 2003;42:767-772.

19. Cordoba J. Hepatic encephalopathy: from the pathogenesis to the new treatments. *ISRN Hepatol.* 2014;1-16.

20. Drobish JK, et al. Emergence delirium with transient associative agnosia and expressive aphasia reversed by flumazenil in a pediatric patient. *A A Case Rep.* 2015;4:148-150.

21. Dunton AW, et al. Flumazenil: US clinical pharmacology studies. *Eur J Anaesth.* 1988;2:81-95; discussion *Eur J Anaest.* 1988;2(suppl):233-235.

22. Ferenci P, et al. Successful long-term treatment of portal—systemic encephalopathy by the benzodiazepine antagonist flumazenil. *Gastroenterology.* 1989;96:240-243.

23. File SE, Pellow S. Intrinsic actions of the benzodiazepine receptor antagonist Ro 15-1788. *Psychopharmacology.* 1986;88:1-11.

24. Flumazenil injection [package insert]. Princeton NJ: Sandoz Canada Inc for Sandoz Inc; 2012.

25. Foster K, et al. Current and emerging strategies for treating hepatic encephalopathy. *Crit Care Nurs Clin North Am.* 2010;22:341-350.

26. Fulton SA, Mullen KD. Completion of upper endoscopic procedures despite paradoxical reaction to midazolam: a role for flumazenil? *Arch J Gastroenterol.* 2000;95:809-811.

27. Gardner CR. Functional in vivo correlates of the benzodiazepine agonist-inverse agonist continuum. *Prog Neurobiol.* 1988;31:425-476.

28. Geller E, et al. Risks and benefits of therapy with flumazenil (Anexate) in mixed drug intoxications. *Eur Neurol.* 1991;31:241-250.

29. George M, Sury M. Reversal of paradoxical excitement to diazepam sedation. *Pediatr Anesth.* 2008;18:546-547.

30. Girdler NM, et al. A randomised crossover trial of post-operative cognitive and psychomotor recovery from benzodiazepine sedation: effects of reversal with flumazenil over a prolonged recovery period. *Br Dent J.* 2002;192:335-339.

31. Goh ET, et al. Flumazenil versus placebo or no intervention for people with cirrhosis and hepatic encephalopathy. *Cochrane Database Syst Rev.* 2017;8:CD002798.

32. Golparvar M, et al. Paradoxical reaction following intravenous midazolam premedication in pediatric patients—a randomized placebo controlled trial of ketamine for rapid tranquilization. *Pediatr Anesth.* 2004;14:924-930.

33. Goulenok C, et al. Flumazenil vs. placebo in hepatic encephalopathy in patients with cirrhosis: a meta-analysis. *Aliment Pharmacol Ther.* 2002;16:361-372.

34. Greenblatt DJ, Shader RI. Benzodiazepines (first of two parts). *N Engl J Med.* 1974;291:1011-1015.

35. Gueye PN, et al. Empiric use of flumazenil in comatose patients: limited applicability of criteria to define low risk. *Ann Emerg Med.* 1996;27:730-735.

36. Gueye P, et al. Mechanism of respiratory insufficiency in pure or mixed drug-induced coma involving benzodiazepines. *J Toxicol Clin Toxicol.* 2002;40:35-47.

37. Haefely W, Hunkeler W. The story of flumazenil. *Eur J Anaesth.* 1988;2:3-14.

38. Hart YM, et al. The effect of intravenous flumazenil on interictal electroencephalographic epileptic activity: results of a placebo-controlled study. *J Neurol Neurosurg Psychiatry.* 1991;54:305-309.

39. Haverkos GP, et al. Fatal seizures after flumazenil administration in a patient with mixed overdose. *Ann Pharmacother.* 1994;28:1347-1349.

40. Henthorn KM, Dickinson C. The use of flumazenil after midazolam-induced conscious sedation. *Br Dent J.* 2010;209:E18.

41. Höjer J, Baehrendtz S. The effect of flumazenil (Ro 15-1788) in the management of self-induced benzodiazepine poisoning: a double-blind controlled study. *Acta Med Scand.* 1988;224:357-365.

42. Hunkeler W. Preclinical research findings with flumazenil (Ro 15-1788, Anexate): chemistry. *Eur J Anaesth.* 1988;2(suppl):37-62.

43. Jackson BF, et al. Successful flumazenil reversal of paradoxical reaction to midazolam in a child. *J Emerg Med.* 2015;48:e67-72.

44. Kamijo Y, et al. Cardiovascular response and stress reaction to flumazenil injection in patients under infusion with midazolam. *Crit Care Med.* 2000;28:318-323.

45. Katz JA, et al. Flumazenil reversal of midazolam sedation of the elderly. *Reg Anesth Pain Med.* 1991;16:247-252.

46. Kim SI, et al. Conscious sedation using midazolam and sequential flumazenil in cirrhotic patients for prophylactic endoscopic variceal ligation. *Digestion.* 2015;92:220-226.

47. Kirkegaard L, et al. Benzodiazepine antagonist Ro 15-1788. *Anaesthesia.* 1986;41:1184-1188.

48. Kreshak A, et al. A poison center's 10 year experience with flumazenil administration to acutely poisoned adults. *J Emerg Med.* 2012;43:677-682.

49. Kreshak A, et al. Flumazenil administration to poisoned pediatric patients. *Ped Emerg Care.* 2012;28:448-450.

50. L'heureux P. Continuous flumazenil for zolpidem toxicity—commentary. *J Toxicol Clin Toxicol.* 1998;36:745-746.

51. L'heureux P, Askenasi R. Efficacy of flumazenil in acute alcohol intoxication: double-blind placebo controlled evaluation. *Hum Exp Toxicol.* 1991;10:235-239.

52. L'heureux P, et al. Flumazenil in mixed benzodiazepine/tricyclic antidepressant overdose: a placebo-controlled study in the dog. *Am J Emerg Med.* 1992;10:184-188.

53. Lim AG. Death after flumazenil. *BMJ.* 1989;299:858-859.

54. Linowiecki K, et al. Reversal of ethanol-induced respiratory depression by flumazenil. *Vet Hum Toxicol.* 1992; 34:417-419.

55. Litchfield NB. Complications of intravenous diazepam. Adverse psychological reactions. *Anesth Prog.* 1980;27:175-183.

56. Mancuso C, Tanzi M. Paradoxical reactions to benzodiazepines: literature review and treatment options. *Pharmacotherapy.* 2004;24:1177-1185.

57. Mathus-Vliegen EM, et al. Significant and safe shortening of the recovery time after flumazenil-reversed midazolam sedation. *Dig Dis Sci.* 2014;59:1717-1725.

58. Moallemy A, et al. The injection rate of intravenous midazolam significantly influences the occurrence of paradoxical reaction in pediatric patients. *J Res Med Sci.* 2014;19:965-969.

59. Mora CT, et al. Effects of diazepam and flumazenil on sedation and hypoxic ventilatory response. *Anesth Analg.* 1989;68:473-478.

60. Mordel A, et al. Seizures after flumazenil administration in a case of combined benzodiazepine and tricyclic antidepressant overdose. *Crit Care Med.* 1992;20:1733-1734.

61. Neave N, et al. Dose-dependent effects of flumazenil on cognition, mood, and cardiorespiratory physiology in healthy volunteers. *Br Dent J.* 2000;189:668-674.

62. Noguchi H, et al. Binding and neuropharmacological profile of zaleplon, a novel nonbenzodiazepine sedative/hypnotic. *Eur J Pharmacol.* 2002;434:21-28.

63. Olshaker J, Flanigan J. Flumazenil reversal of lorazepam induced acute delirium. *J Emerg Med.* 2003;24:181-183.

64. Oshima T, et al. Flumazenil antagonizes midazolam-induced airway narrowing during nasal breathing in humans. *Br J Anaesthesia.* 1999;82:698-702.

65. Patat A, et al. Flumazenil antagonizes the central effects of zolpidem, an imidazopyridine hypnotic. *Clin Pharmacol Ther.* 1994;56:430-436.

66. Penninga E, et al. Adverse events associated with flumazenil treatment for the management of suspected benzodiazepine intoxication—a systematic review with meta-analyses of randomised trials. *Basic Clin Pharmacol Toxicol.* 2016;118:37-44.

67. Penninga E, et al. Reply to Pajoumand A, Hassanian-Moghaddam H, Zamani N's Letter to the Editor regarding our article "Adverse events associated with flumazenil treatment for the management of suspected benzodiazepine intoxication—a systematic review with meta-analyses of randomised trials." *Basic Clin Pharmacol Toxicol.* 2016;118:325-326.

68. Persson A, et al. Saturation analysis of specific[11] C Ro 15-1788 binding to the human neocortex using positron emission tomography. *Hum Psychopharmacol.* 1989;4:21-31.

69. Rothstein JD, et al. Endogenous benzodiazepine receptor ligands in idiopathic recurring stupor. *Lancet.* 1992;340:1002-1004.

70. Rozé H, et al. Effect of flumazenil on diaphragm electrical activation during weaning from mechanical ventilation after acute respiratory distress syndrome. *Br J Anaesth.* 2015;114:269-275.

71. Ruscito BJ, Harrison NL. Hemoglobin metabolites mimic benzodiazepines and are possible mediators of hepatic encephalopathy. *Blood.* 2003;102:1525-1528.

72. Savic I, et al. Feasibility of reversing benzodiazepine tolerance with flumazenil. *Lancet.* 1991;337:133-137.

73. Seger DL. Flumazenil—treatment or toxin. *J Toxicol Clin Toxicol.* 2004;42:209-216.

74. Shalansky SJ, et al. Therapy update: effect of flumazenil on benzodiazepine-induced respiratory depression. *Clin Pharm.* 1993;12:483-487.

75. Sivilotti ML. Flumazenil, naloxone and the "coma cocktail." *Br J Clin Pharmacol.* 2016;81:428-436.

76. Jones EA, et al. NIH conference. The gamma-aminobutyric acid A (GABAA) receptor complex and hepatic encephalopathy. Some recent advances. *Ann Intern Med.* 1989;100:532-546.

77. Spivey WH. Flumazenil and seizures: analysis of 43 cases. *Clin Ther.* 1992;14:292-305.

78. Tae CH, et al. Paradoxical reaction to midazolam in patients undergoing endoscopy under sedation: incidence, risk factors and the effect of flumazenil. *Dig Liver Dis.* 2014;46:710-715.

79. Thornton SL, et al. Pediatric zolpidem ingestion demonstrating zero-order kinetics treated with flumazenil. *Pediatr Emerg Care.* 2013;29:1204-1206.

80. Ticku MK, et al. Modulation of GABAergic transmission by ethanol. In: Biggio G, Costa E, eds. *GABAergic Synaptic Transmission.* New York, NY: Raven; 1992:255-268.

81. Tinuper P, et al. Idiopathic recurring stupor: a case with possible involvement of the gamma-aminobutyric acid (GABA)ergic system. *Ann Neurol.* 1992;31:503-506.

82. Tobin JM, Lewis N. New psychotherapeutic agent chlordiazepoxide. *JAMA.* 1960;174:1242-1249.

83. Tote S, Mulleague L. The role of flumazenil in self-harm with benzodiazepines: to give or not to give? *Hosp Med.* 2005;66:308.

84. Van der Rijt CC, et al. Flumazenil does not improve hepatic encephalopathy associated with acute ischemic liver failure in the rabbit. *Metab Brain Dis.* 1990;3:131-141.

85. Weinbroum A, et al. The use of flumazenil in the management of acute drug poisoning: a review. *Intensive Care Med.* 1991;17:S32-S38.

86. Weinbroum A, et al. The midazolam-induced paradox phenomenon is reversible by flumazenil. Epidemiology, patient characteristics and review of the literature. *Eur J Anaesthesiol.* 2001;18:789-797.

87. Weinbroum MD, et al. Use of flumazenil in the treatment of drug overdose: a double-blind and open clinical study in 110 patients. *Crit Care Med.* 1996;24:199-206.

88. Wiley CC, Wiley JF II. Pediatric benzodiazepine ingestion resulting in hospitalization. *J Toxicol Clin Toxicol.* 1998;36:227-231.

89. Winkler E, et al. Use of flumazenil in the diagnosis and treatment of patients with coma of unknown etiology. *Crit Care Med.* 1993;21:538-542.

90. Whitwan G, Amrein R. Pharmacology of flumazenil. *Acta Anaesthesiol Scand.* 1995; 39(suppl 108):3-14.

91. Zanettini C, et al. Quantitative pharmacological analyses of the interaction between flumazenil and midazolam in monkeys discriminating midazolam: determination of the functional half life of flumazenil. *Eur J Pharmacol.* 2014;723:405-409.

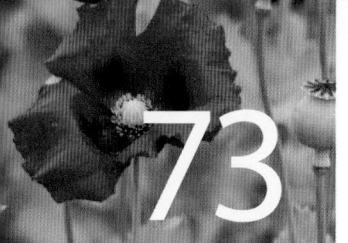

73

AMPHETAMINES

Meghan B. Spyres and David H. Jang

Methylenedioxymethamphetamine

Methamphetamine Epinephrine

HISTORY AND EPIDEMIOLOGY

Amphetamine was first synthesized in 1887 but was essentially lost until the 1920s, when concerns arose regarding the supply of ephedrine for asthma therapy.[67] The attempt to synthesize ephedrine lead to the rediscovery of dextroamphetamine in the United States and methamphetamine (*d*-phenylisopropylmethylamine hydrochloride) in Japan. Amphetamine was first marketed by Smith, Kline, and French in 1932 as the nasal decongestant Benzedrine. Both amphetamine and methamphetamine were supplied as stimulants for soldiers and prisoners of war during World War II. Amphetamine tablets were later available in 1935 for the treatment of narcolepsy and were advocated as anorexiants in 1938.[17]

The stimulant and euphoric effects of amphetamine were immediately recognized, with abuse reported as early as 1940.[74] As a result, Benzedrine inhalers were banned by the US Food and Drug Administration (FDA) in 1959. From 1950 to the 1970s, there were sporadic periods of widespread amphetamine use and abuse in the United States. In the 1960s and early 1970s, various amphetamines such as methylenedioxyamphetamine (MDA), *para*-methoxyamphetamine (PMA), and *para*-methoxymethamphetamine (PMMA) were popularized as hallucinogens.[97,127] The Controlled Substance Act of 1970 placed amphetamines in Schedule II to prevent the diversion of pharmaceutical amphetamines for nonmedicinal uses. Abuse of amphetamines subsequently declined.[136]

In the 1980s, use of methylenedioxy derivatives of amphetamine and methamphetamine surfaced and circumvented existing regulations. The best known of these derivatives were 3,4-methylenedioxymethamphetamine (MDMA) and 3,4-methylenedioxyethamphetamine (MDEA).[6] Since the late 1980s, a dramatic resurgence of methamphetamine abuse has spread throughout much of the United States. A high-purity preparation of methamphetamine hydrochloride was illegally marketed in a large crystalline form termed "ice" by abusers.[46] Methamphetamine-related deaths in the United States increased through the 1990s, initially at several hundred per year. From 2010 to 2014, deaths involving methamphetamine doubled from 1,388 to 3,728 per year.[171] Men who have sex with men in New York City (and perhaps elsewhere) remain a specific population at risk, with a persistently high prevalence of methamphetamine use.[72] The ease and low cost of methamphetamine synthesis encourage establishment of illegal clandestine laboratories in the United States.[72] Since the

mid-1990s, MDMA has been widely used by college students and teenagers in large gatherings, known as "rave" or "techno" parties, in Europe and the United States.[134] Methcathinone (a khat-derived substance) and 4-bromo-2,5-methoxyphenylethylamine (2CB) were popular in dance clubs in the Midwestern United States in the 1990s, but use was not widespread.[59,62] Synthetic cathinones are currently sold as "bath salts" or "legal highs" to circumvent existing laws, resulting in serious toxicity and deaths.[31] Recently, older amphetamines such as PMA and PMMA made a resurgence, with new reports of toxicity and deaths.[102]

PHARMACOLOGY

Amphetamine is the acronym for racemic β-phenylisopropylamine. Amphetamine is representative of a broader group of compounds with a shared phenylethylamine structure, which is a more accurate term. Numerous substitutions on the phenylethylamine backbone are possible, resulting in a variety of xenobiotics, some with unique properties. For the purposes of this chapter, all phenylethylamines, even those that are not actually amphetamines, will be called *amphetamines* for simplicity, and the name *amphetamine* specifically refers to β-phenylisopropylamine.

The pharmacologic effects of amphetamines are complex, but their primary mechanism of action is the release of biogenic amines. Release of catecholamines from the presynaptic terminals, particularly dopamine and norepinephrine, leads to a hyperadrenergic condition, but release of serotonin favors a serotonergic condition. Although there are conflicting mechanistic models of amphetamine induction of catecholamine release, these variable results are directly correlated with the different concentrations of amphetamine used in experimental models. Our understanding of the mechanism of action of amphetamines is based on dopaminergic neurons; similar mechanisms occur with norepinephrine and serotonin. Two storage pools exist for dopamine in the presynaptic terminals: the vesicular pool and the cytoplasmic pool. The vesicular storage of dopamine and other biogenic amines is maintained by the acidic environment within the vesicles and the persistence of a stabilizing electrical gradient within the cytoplasm. This environment is maintained by an adenosine triphosphate–dependent active proton transport system.[115,145]

Amphetamines enter the nerve cell either by passive diffusion or by exchange diffusion through a reuptake transporter that is partially dose dependent. At low concentrations, amphetamines enter the cell by exchange diffusion at the dopamine reuptake transporter and cause the release of dopamine from the cytoplasmic pool. At moderate concentrations, amphetamines passively diffuse through the presynaptic terminal membrane and interact with the neurotransmitter transporter on the vesicular membrane to cause exchange release of dopamine into the cytoplasm. Dopamine is subsequently released into the synapse by reverse transport at the dopamine reuptake site.[145,170] At high concentrations, an additional mechanism is invoked as amphetamines diffuse through the cellular and vesicular membranes. Because amphetamines are bases, they alkalinize the vesicles, reducing the pH gradient necessary for vesicle integrity, resulting in dopamine release from the vesicles and delivery into the synapse by reverse transport (Chap. 13 and Fig. 73–1).[161,162] Amphetamines also block the reuptake of biogenic amines by competitive inhibition.[68,181] However, the contribution of this to the ultimate clinical effects are likely minor. Amphetamine's structural

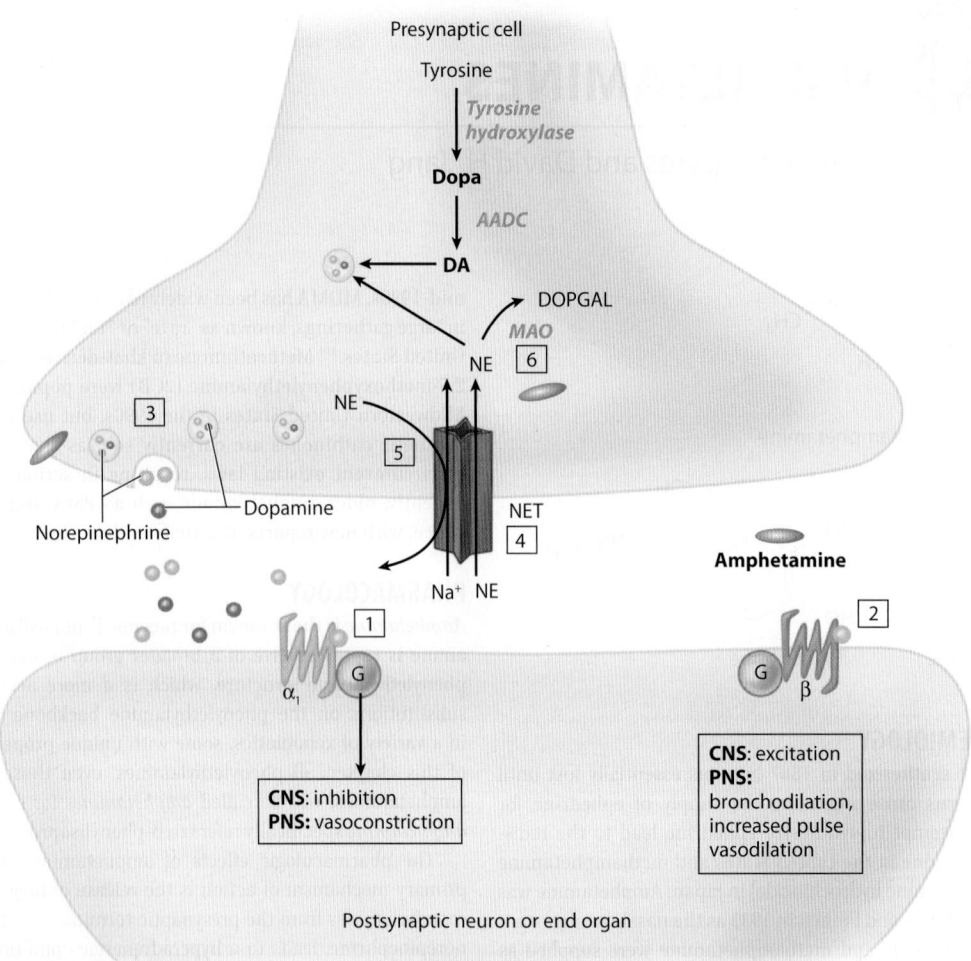

FIGURE 73–1. Noradrenergic nerve ending. The postsynaptic membrane represents an end organ or another neuron in the central nervous system (CNS). The primary mechanism of action of amphetamine is the release of catecholamines, particularly dopamine (DA) and norepinephrine (NE), from the presynaptic terminals. Two storage pools exist for DA in the presynaptic terminals: the vesicular pool and the cytoplasmic pool. The vesicular storage of DA and other biogenic amines is maintained by the acidic environment within the vesicles and the persistence of a stabilizing electrical gradient with respect to the cytoplasm. (1, 2) Activating or antagonizing postsynaptic α- and β-adrenoceptors. (3) Amphetamines release DA or NE from the cytoplasmic pool by exchange diffusion at the DA uptake transporter site in the membrane. (4) Amphetamines diffuse through the presynaptic terminal membrane and interact with the neurotransmitter transporter on the vesicular membrane to cause exchange release of DA or NE into the cytoplasm. DA is subsequently released into the synapse by reverse transport at the DA uptake site. (5) Amphetamine diffuses through the cellular and vesicular membranes, alkalinizing the vesicles, and permitting dopamine release from the vesicles and delivery into the synapse by reverse transport. (6) Inhibiting monoamine oxidase (MAO) to prevent NE degradation; or inhibiting catechol-O-methyltransferase (COMT) to prevent NE degradation. AADC = aromatic L-amino acid decarboxylase; DOPGAL = 3,4-dihydroxyphenylglycoaldehyde; G = G protein; NET = membrane norepinephrine uptake transporter; NME = normetanephrine; PNS = peripheral nervous system.

similarity to amphetamine derived monoamine oxidase inhibitors (MAOIs) such as tranylcypromine explains their weak MAOI effect, the clinical significance of which is unclear.[131]

Binding selectivity to the neurotransmitter transporters largely determines the range of pharmacologic effects for a particular amphetamine. The affinity of MDMA for serotonin transporters, for example, is 10 times greater than that for dopamine and norepinephrine transporters. With this high affinity for serotonin transporters, MDMA produces primarily serotonergic effects.[64] Other predominantly serotonergic amphetamines include *para*-methoxyamphetamine and bromo-dragonFLY (Table 73–1).

The most identifiable effects of amphetamines are those caused by excessive biogenic amine release and the resultant stimulation of various receptors including α-adrenergic, β-adrenergic, dopamine, and serotonin receptors. The majority of serotonergic neurons in the central nervous system (CNS) are located in the raphe nuclei, which connects the brainstem to the rest of the CNS via serotonergic projections. Within the CNS,

serotonin regulates a wide variety of functions, including, but not limited to, mood, memory, temperature regulation, sleep, and pain.[67] Serotonin is also involved in the release of antidiuretic hormone, the excessive release of which leads to hyponatremia. This is particularly associated with amphetamines with potent serotonergic effects such as MDMA.[73] Additional effects of serotonin include regulation of fluid secretion and peristalsis, as well as regulation of many vascular beds, predominantly via vasoconstriction. Peripherally, serotonergic actions of amphetamines can result in carcinoidlike effects.[103,144]

Norepinephrine is another important neurotransmitter central to the action of amphetamines. Norepinephrine is found in the CNS and is also released peripherally from postganglionic sympathetic fibers. The main noradrenergic nucleus in the CNS is the locus ceruleus. Amphetamine induced excessive release of norepinephrine within the CNS results in decreased fatigue and increased attentiveness. Peripherally, norepinephrine acts on the adrenergic receptors (α and β), which mediate

TABLE 73–1   Examples of Amphetamines

Xenobiotic	Clinical Manifestations	Structure
4-Bromo-2,5-dimethoxyamphetamine (DOB)	Marked psychoactive effect, potency > mescaline Fantasy, mood altering Agitation, sympathetic excess Sold as impregnated paper, like LSD	
4-Bromo-2,5-methoxyphenylethylamine (2CB, MFT)	Relaxation Sensory distortion Agitation Hallucination Potency > mescaline	
Methcathinone (cat, Jeff, khat, ephedrone)	Hallucinations Sympathetic excess	
4-Methyl-2,5-dimethoxyamphetamine (DOM/STP) (serenity, tranquility, peace)	Narrow therapeutic index Euphoria, perceptual distortion Hallucinations, sympathetic excess	
3,4-Methylenedioxyamphetamine (MDA, love drug)	Empathy, euphoria Agitation, delirium, hallucinations, death associated with sympathetic excess	
3,4-Methylenedioxyethamphetamine (MDEA, Eve)	Comparable to MDMA Sympathetic excess	
3,4-Methylenedioxymethamphetamine (MDMA, Adam, molly, ecstasy, XTC)	Psychotherapy "facilitator" Euphoria, empathy nausea, anorexia, anxiety, insomnia Sympathetic excess	
para-Methoxyamphetamine (PMA)	Potent hallucinogen Sympathetic excess	
2,4,5-Trimethoxyamphetamine	Similar to mescaline	

LSD = lysergic acid diethylamide.

vasoconstriction and increased cardiac activity, resulting in hypertension and tachycardia.

The increase in CNS dopamine, particularly in the neostriatum, mediates stereotypical behavior and other locomotor activities as well as reward pathways.[36] The activity of dopamine in the neostriatum appears to be linked to glutamate release and inhibition of γ-aminobutyric acid (GABA) efferent neurons.[86] Stimulation of the glutamatergic system contributes significantly to the stereotypical behavior, locomotor activity, and neurotoxicity of amphetamines.[86,152,153] The effects of serotonin and dopamine on the mesolimbic system alter perception, cause psychotic behavior and anorexia.[76,160]

Structure Modification

Phenylethylamines are chemical structures with an ethyl group backbone that has an aromatic group and a terminal amine. Specific substitutions made to the phenylethylamine backbone have led to the wide variety of novel drugs, described later. Substitutions at different positions of the phenylethylamine molecule alter the general pharmacology and clinical effects of amphetamines, as demonstrated by both animal and human observations. Large-group substitution at the α carbon reduces the stimulant and cardiovascular effects of the amphetamine but allows retention of the anorectic properties (such as phentermine). Substitution at the *para* position of the phenyl ring enhances the hallucinogenic or serotonergic effects of amphetamines (such as in *para*-chloroamphetamine and MDMA).[60] Although these generalizations enable an understanding of the effects of amphetamines, there are many exceptions, and such generalizations do not necessarily apply after exposure to large doses of a particular molecule. There is a broad spectrum of clinical effects that derive from the various amphetamines: methamphetamine results in the most potent cardiovascular effects, and 2,5-dimethoxy-4-bromoamphetamine (DOB) results in the most consequential hallucinogenic and serotonergic effects.[60,117] Table 73–2 further describes the pharmacology of specific substitutions.

Other specific substitutions are worth noting. The addition of an extra methyl group to the terminal amine in amphetamine produces methamphetamine, greatly increasing CNS activity. This extra methyl group also makes methamphetamine more lipid soluble, allowing faster penetration across the blood–brain barrier and more resistance to degradation by monoamine oxidase. The addition of an α-methyl group results in strong stimulant, cardiovascular, and anorectic properties.[60,117] This is largely due to resistance to metabolism by monoamine oxidase conferred by the addition of this group. These characteristics permit better oral bioavailability and longer duration of effect. The α-methyl group in the amphetamine structure also introduces chirality to the molecule. With few notable exceptions including MDMA, the *d*-enantiomer is typically 4 to 10 times more potent than the *l* form of amphetamine. Addition of a methoxy group to either the 2 or 5 position of the aromatic ring on the amphetamine or methamphetamine compound increases serotonergic activity. Another important substitution to the phenylethylamine backbone is the addition of a halogen group (eg, iodine or bromine), which increases the potency and neurotoxicity of the compound compared to nonhalogenated compounds. Neurotoxicity is thought to be due to significant serotonin depletion, leading to irreversible neuron damage.[76] The ability of amphetamines to directly interact with neurotransmitter transporters enable minor modifications of the molecule to significantly alter its pharmacologic profile.[80] The addition of a ketone group at the β position results in a group of compounds

known as the synthetic cathinones. Specifically, the addition of this group to amphetamine results in cathinone. The β-ketone group is responsible for increased polarity, which decreases penetration of the blood–brain barrier.

PHARMACOKINETICS AND TOXICOKINETICS
Absorption
Amphetamines can be absorbed by intravenous, oral, intranasal, and inhalational routes. Amphetamines are rapidly absorbed, with bioavailability that ranges between 60% and 90% depending on the route of administration. Peak serum concentrations are variable and are substance and route dependent. Methamphetamine has peak serum concentrations in less than 15 minutes when used via an intravenous (IV) or intranasal route and up to 180 minutes when taken orally.

Distribution
After absorption, amphetamines are distributed to most compartments of the body. Most amphetamines are also relatively lipophilic and readily cross the blood–brain barrier. Amphetamines have large volumes of distribution, varying from 3 to 5 L/kg for amphetamine, 3 to 4 L/kg for methamphetamine and phentermine, and to 11 to 33 L/kg for methylphenidate. Some amphetamines such as pemoline have a small volume of distribution (0.2–0.6 L/kg).

Metabolism
Amphetamines are eliminated via multiple pathways, including diverse routes of hepatic transformation and renal elimination. For MDMA and its analogs, *N*-dealkylation, hydroxylation, and demethylation are the dominant hepatic pathways. Depending on the particular amphetamines, active metabolites of amphetamines and ephedrine derivatives are formed. *N*-demethylation of methamphetamine and MDMA result in the formation of amphetamine and MDA, respectively.[108] Dealkylation and demethylation are mainly performed by CYP1A2, CYP2D6, and CYP3A4, as well as flavin monooxygenase. Polymorphism of CYP2D6 in humans was recognized because of the diversity of rates of *p*-hydroxylation of amphetamines. Since its discovery, CYP2D6 polymorphism has been implicated in drug toxicity, substance use and abuse, and lack of drug efficacy in selected individuals.[146] Increased toxicity of amphetamines is a potential concern in patients with decreased CYP2D6 activity. Although animals with CYP2D6 deficiency are more susceptible to MDMA toxicity, limited studies in humans do not demonstrate an association between mortality and CYP2D6 polymorphism.[121] In general, because multiple enzymes and elimination pathways (including renal) are involved in amphetamine metabolism, it is less likely that CYP2D6 polymorphism or drug interactions with CYP3A4 alone will significantly increase toxicity. However, it is unclear if toxicity is enhanced when multiple mechanisms for altering drug metabolism and kidney dysfunction are present simultaneously.

Elimination
Renal elimination of the parent compound is substantial for amphetamine (30%), methamphetamine (40%–50%), MDMA (65%), and phentermine (80%). Amphetamines are bases with a typical pK_a range of 9 to 10, and renal elimination varies depending on the urine pH, with elimination increasing as pH decreases.[14] The half-life of amphetamines varies significantly: amphetamine, 8 to 30 hours; methamphetamine, 12 to 34 hours; MDMA, 5 to 10 hours; methylphenidate, 2.5 to 4 hours; and phentermine, 19 to 24 hours. Repetitive administration, which occurs typically during binge use, leads to drug accumulation and prolongation of the apparent half-life and duration of effect.[13,108]

PATHOPHYSIOLOGY
Most complications associated with amphetamines are a result of an uncontrolled hyperadrenergic condition similar to that which occurs with other sympathomimetics such as cocaine, except the duration of effect is typically longer (Table 73–3). Most patients with acute amphetamine toxicity manifest effects in the CNS and cardiovascular system. The majority of the specific

TABLE 73–2	Specific Substitutions on Phenylethylamine

Substitution	Pharmacological Effect
α-Carbon	Indirect acting; resists oxidation by monoamine oxidase
β-Carbon	Decreases central nervous system penetration Whereas hydroxyl (–OH): increases adrenergic activity
Amino group	No substitution: α-adrenergic > β-adrenergic effects Larger group: β-adrenergic > α-adrenergic effects t-Butyl group: β₂-adrenergic selective Methyl (–CH₃) group: maximum α- and β-adrenergic effects
3-, 4- of aromatic ring	Hydroxylation at 3- and 4-: increased α- and β-adrenergic effects Absence of hydroxylation (at one or both positions) prevents degradation by catechol-O-methyltransferase.
Halogenation	Enhances potency of neurotoxic properties of amphetamines by selective action on the serotonin system

TABLE 73–3	Clinical Manifestations of Amphetamine Toxicity

Acute

Cardiovascular System
- Aortic dissection
- Dysrhythmias
- Hypertension
- Myocardial ischemia
- Tachycardia
- Vasospasm

Central Nervous System
- Agitation
- Anorexia
- Bruxism
- Choreoathetoid movements
- Euphoria
- Headache
- Hyperreflexia
- Hyperthermia
- Intracerebral hemorrhage
- Paranoid psychosis
- Seizures

Other Sympathomimetic Symptoms
- Diaphoresis
- Mydriasis
- Nausea
- Tachypnea
- Tremor

Other Organ System Manifestations
- Acute respiratory distress syndrome
- Ischemic colitis
- Muscle rigidity
- Rhabdomyolysis

Laboratory Abnormalities
- Creatine phosphokinase elevated
- Hyperglycemia
- Hyponatremia
- Leukocytosis
- Liver enzymes elevated
- Myoglobinuria

Chronic
- Aortic and mitral regurgitation
- Cardiomyopathy
- Dopaminergic and serotonergic neuron damage
- Pulmonary hypertension
- Vasculitis

effects are from excessive catecholamine release as opposed to direct effects from the amphetamines themselves. Additional organ-specific pathophysiologic effects are described later.

Central Nervous System

Anxiety, agitation, and hallucinations are typical CNS findings that result from adrenergic stimulation. Choreoathetoid movements, often described as irregular jerking or twisting movements, are related to increased dopaminergic stimulation in the striatal area.[88,101,107] Seizures are the direct result of amphetamine or occur secondarily to hyponatremia as reported with MDMA and certain synthetic cathinones.[19] Psychosis, often a finding with acute use, is likely to recur with subsequent use, even after periods of prolonged

abstinence. This phenomenon of recurrent psychosis on reexposure is likely related to a kindling phenomenon.[112]

Cardiac

Cardiomyopathy is reported in chronic amphetamine users. Excessive catecholamine exposure is likely responsible for their associated cardiomyopathies, similar to that occurring in patients with pheochromocytomas or chronic cocaine use.[85,177] Some postulate that polymorphisms in CYP2D6 activity influences the risk of developing cardiomyopathy; however, a clear association is not demonstrated.[164] Valvular heart disease and pulmonary hypertension are associated with amphetamines taken for diet suppression. The mechanism of toxicity is incompletely understood but is likely do to serotonergic activity occurs in carcinoid pathology. Specifically, alterations in serotonin reuptake transporter (SERT) activity is thought to play a significant role in the pathophysiology of both diseases, and drug effect at the $5HT_{2B}$ receptor is implicated in the development of valvular heart disease.[103,144]

Vascular

Necrotizing vasculitis of small- and medium-sized arteries occurs in association with amphetamine use and affects multiple organ systems as described later. The etiology of the arteritis remains unclear. Although various contaminants associated with injection drug use are postulated as potential etiologies, in animal models, oral and IV amphetamine administration is also associated with vasculitis, suggesting that this is a direct amphetamine effect.[18,32,165]

Chronic Central Nervous System Toxicity

Chronic administration of certain amphetamines to animals alters dopamine and serotonin transporter functions, depletes dopamine and serotonin in the neuronal synapses, and produces irreversible destruction of those neurons.[16,56,139,140,145,180] The cause of neuronal toxicity is related to the generation of oxygen free radicals, resulting in the generation of toxic dopamine and serotonin metabolites as well as neuronal destruction. Based on animal models, dose, frequency and duration of exposure, and ambient temperature affect toxicity. Intact dopamine or serotonin transporters are necessary to produce neurologic injury. Xenobiotics that inhibit transporter function appear to prevent neurologic injuries in animals.[64] Although not as well studied as MDMA, studies of former methamphetamine users demonstrate impaired memory and psychomotor functions, as well as corresponding dopamine transporter dysfunction and abnormal glucose metabolism on positron emission tomography scans. However, species-specific susceptibility to neurologic injuries, the duration of effects in primates and humans, and functional consequences of neurotoxicity in humans remain unclear and require further study.

CLINICAL MANIFESTATIONS

Acute and chronic toxicity of amphetamines are described next. Refer to the section Individual Amphetamines for effects specific to each individual molecule.

Acute Toxicity

Central nervous system effects from acute amphetamine use include anxiety, agitation, hallucinations, seizures, mydriasis, diaphoresis, and hyperthermia.[47,48,143] The pathophysiology of amphetamine-induced hyperthermia is multifactorial and includes increased catecholamine release, increased metabolic and psychomotor activity, and vasoconstriction-mediated impaired heat dissipation.[106] Psychosis appears to be a more prominent feature after amphetamine than after cocaine use.[2] Intracerebral hemorrhage and cerebral infarction are also reported with amphetamine use.[49,84,110,129]

Cardiovascular toxicity from acute amphetamine use involves hypertension, tachycardia, and dysrhythmias. Reported dysrhythmias range from premature ventricular complexes to ventricular tachycardia and ventricular fibrillation.[78] Other vascular complications reported with acute use include myocardial ischemia or infarction,[113,173] aortic dissection,[176] acute respiratory distress syndrome,[166,175] obstetric complications, fetal death,[63,99] and ischemic colitis.[77,82] Additional acute complications include metabolic acidosis, rhabdomyolysis,[50] acute kidney injury (AKI); acute tubular necrosis), and coagulopathy, often from uncontrolled agitation and hyperthermia.[39,70,170] Unless these systemic signs and symptoms are rapidly reversed, multiorgan failure and death ensue.

Chronic Toxicity

Amphetamine users seeking intense "highs" go on "speed runs" for days to weeks. Because of the development of tolerance, they use increasing amounts of amphetamine during these periods, usually without much nutritional sustenance or sleep, while attempting to achieve their desired euphoria.[150] Acute psychosis resembling paranoid schizophrenia occurs during these binges and has contributed to both amphetamine-related suicides and homicides.[51] A normal sensorium usually returns within a few days after discontinuation of the drug. Typically, after such binges, patients sleep for prolonged periods of time, feel hungry and depressed when awake, and often have amphetamine cravings.[89,93]

Compulsive repetitive behavior patterns from the use of amphetamines are reported in humans and animals. Individuals pick at their skin, grind their teeth (bruxism), or perform repetitive tasks, such as constantly cleaning the house or car. 3,4-Methylenedioxymethamphetamine users often carry pacifiers to relieve bruxism and prevent tooth damage. Choreoathetoid movements, although uncommon, are reported with acute and chronic amphetamine use.[88,101,107]

Necrotizing vasculitis is associated with amphetamine abuse. Angiography typically demonstrates beading and narrowing of the small- and medium-sized arteries (Fig. 8–29). Progressive necrotizing arteritis involves multiple organ systems, including the brain, heart, gut, and kidney.[18,32,92,165] Complications include cerebral infarction and hemorrhage, coronary artery disease, pancreatitis, and AKI. Cardiomyopathy is also reported with acute and chronic amphetamine abuse.[156,182] Valvular disease and pulmonary hypertension are reported when amphetamines such as fenfluramine, dexfenfluramine, and phentermine are used for dieting.[144,163]

Finally, complications can result from IV drug use and from the associated contaminants. Contamination with microbials leads to human immunodeficiency virus infection, hepatitis, and malaria. Bacterial and foreign body contamination results in endocarditis, tetanus, wound botulism, osteomyelitis, and pulmonary and soft tissue abscesses.[100]

DIAGNOSTIC TESTING

The choice and extent of diagnostic tests should be guided by the history and physical examination. In all patients with altered mental status, blood specimens should be sent for glucose, blood urea nitrogen, and electrolyte assays. An electrocardiogram should be obtained in all patients to screen for tachydysrhythmias and coingestants, and continuous cardiac monitoring should be initiated. A complete blood count, urinalysis, coagulation profile, creatine phosphokinase, chest radiograph, computed tomography scan of the head, echocardiogram of the heart, and lumbar puncture will be necessary, depending on the clinical presentation.

Qualitative urine immunoassays are available for amphetamines, but several considerations limit their utility in the management of acutely poisoned patients. Although point-of-care urine tests are available, these tests rarely contribute to management in the acute setting. A major limitation is the high rate of false-positive and false-negative results common to the amphetamine immunoassay. For example, many cold preparations contain pseudoephedrine, which is structurally similar and cross-reacts with the immunoassay.[33,53] Likewise, selegiline, a selective monoamine oxidase type B inhibitor used for the treatment of parkinsonism, is metabolized to amphetamine and methamphetamine. Other common drugs that produce false-positive results include bupropion, trazodone, amantadine, and certain antihistamines.[21,119,123] Even a true-positive result only means that the patient has used certain amphetamines within the past several days and does not distinguish remote from acute use. False-negative results may occur with certain amphetamines such as MDMA and cathinones, which are not recognized on standard

urinary drug testing.[33,155] Utilization of such tests is often misleading and rarely directly contributes to the acute management of patients. The gold standard for drug testing, gas chromatography–mass spectrometry analysis, can misidentify isomeric substances such as *l*-methamphetamine, which is present in nasal inhalers, with *d*-methamphetamine, if performed by inexperienced personnel.[10] In summary, the use of urine immunoassays should not guide clinical management of patients who present with suspected toxicity from amphetamines.

MANAGEMENT

The initial medical assessment of the agitated patient must include vital signs, a rapid glucose determination, and a complete physical examination. Determination of core body temperature is essential to diagnose the presence and degree of hyperthermia, which is a frequent and rapidly fatal manifestation in patients with drug-induced delirium. Significant hyperthermia necessitates immediate interventions to achieve rapid cooling[24,58] (Chap. 29). Some patients require temporary physical restraint to gain pharmacologic control and prevent personal harm to themselves or others. Physical restraints should be discontinued as soon as possible; prolonged restraints result in rhabdomyolysis and continued heat generation. IV access should be obtained so that IV sedation can be initiated. If IV access cannot be obtained, it is necessary to attempt to administer intramuscular benzodiazepines such as midazolam until definitive access is accomplished.

The most appropriate choice of chemical sedation is a benzodiazepine because of the characteristic high therapeutic index, good antiepileptic activity, and predictable pharmacokinetic properties. Benzodiazepines are effective not only for the treatment of delirium induced by acute overdose of cocaine, amphetamines, and other xenobiotics but also the delirium associated with ethanol and sedative–hypnotic withdrawal (Antidotes in Depth: A26).[44,61,122] Sedation should be titrated rapidly until the patient is calm. In our clinical experience, cumulative benzodiazepine doses required in the initial 30 minutes to achieve adequate sedation will periodically exceed 100 mg of diazepam or its equivalent (Table 73–4).

Antipsychotics, particularly potent dopamine antagonists such as haloperidol and droperidol, are frequently recommended as adjuncts for amphetamine-induced delirium. Potent blockade of dopamine receptors functions

---

TABLE 73–4 | **Management of Patients with Amphetamine Toxicity**

Agitation

Benzodiazepines (usually adequate for the cardiovascular manifestations)

Diazepam 10 mg (or equivalent) intravenously; repeat rapidly until the patient is calm (cumulative dose periodically be as high as 100 mg of diazepam). An equivalent dose of IM midazolam is recommended if IV access is not available.

Seizures

Benzodiazepines

Barbiturates

Propofol for status epilepticus (typically will require endotracheal intubation)

Hyperthermia

External cooling

Control agitation rapidly

Gastric Decontamination and Elimination

Activated charcoal for recent ingestions

Hypertension

Control agitation first

α-Adrenergic antagonist (phentolamine)[a]

Vasodilators (nitroglycerin, or nicardipine)

Delirium or Hallucinations with Abnormal Vital Signs

If agitated: benzodiazepines

[a]Avoid β-adrenergic antagonists, especially with suspected cocaine toxicity.

IM = intramuscular; IV = intravenous.

to antagonize the psychiatric and psychomotor effects of amphetamines. In experimental models, antipsychotics are not always as effective as benzodiazepines in treatment of amphetamine toxicity; however, results are mixed regarding their safety and efficacy.[40,45,61] Very little clinical data are available evaluating antipsychotics in the management of amphetamine toxicity, but at least one study in children demonstrates safety when antipsychotics are used adjunctively with benzodiazepines.[40,142] In our clinical experience, antipsychotics are very effective for benzodiazepine-resistant methamphetamine toxicity in children, particularly for symptoms of psychomotor agitation. However, antipsychotics have several negative effects that must be taken into consideration. Antipsychotics lower the seizure threshold, alter temperature regulation, cause acute dystonia, and precipitate cardiac dysrhythmias. Hyperthermia and seizures are potential life-threatening complications of amphetamine toxicity, and the use of antipsychotics could worsen these outcomes. Additionally, they do not interact with the benzodiazepine–GABA–chloride channel receptor complex, which could aggravate the clinical outcomes related to occult or concomitant cocaine toxicity and ethanol withdrawal.[61,65,122] Based on these concerns, benzodiazepines are recommended as first-line treatments in the management of acute toxicity from amphetamines. In a patient without hyperthermia or seizure activity, in whom psychomotor or psychiatric agitation is a predominant feature, adjunctive use of antipsychotics after benzodiazepine administration is reasonable, particularly in children.

Rhabdomyolysis from amphetamines usually results from psychomotor agitation and hyperthermia.[141] Sedation, typically with benzodiazepines, prevents further muscle contraction and heat production. External cooling should be instituted for hyperthermia.[95] Although some promote dantrolene as potential treatment option for amphetamine-induced hyperthermia, evidence is limited to case reports, predominantly involving MDMA.[69] Strong evidence to support the use of dantrolene is limited to cases of malignant hyperthermia, and side effects, including significant respiratory muscle weakness, are reported.[90] Given the potential harms of dantrolene and limited supportive evidence, in contrast to known efficacy of supportive measures, we do not currently recommended its use for amphetamine-induced hyperthermia. Adequate IV hydration and cardiovascular support should maintain urine output of at least 1 to 2 mL/kg/h. Although urinary acidification can significantly increase amphetamine elimination and decrease the half-lives of amphetamine and methamphetamine,[13,14] urinary pH manipulation does not decrease toxicity and instead increases the risk of AKI from rhabdomyolysis by precipitating ferrihemate in the renal tubules.[37] Some patients with AKI, acidemia, and hyperkalemia require urgent hemodialysis.

Amphetamine body packers, although uncommon, should be treated similarly to those who transport cocaine (Special Considerations: SC5). Any sympathomimetic symptom suggesting leakage of the packets requires surgical intervention.[172] Intravenous fluids, benzodiazepines, intubation, and external cooling are often necessary to stabilize these patients.

INDIVIDUAL AMPHETAMINES
Methamphetamine

Amphetamine

Phenylethylamine

Methamphetamine

Methamphetamine is known by many names, including, but not limited to, "yaba," "speed," "go," "crack," "uppers," and "dexies." The terms "crystal," "shard," and "ice" refer to the crystalline form of methamphetamine. Methamphetamine was first synthesized from ephedrine in Japan in 1893, soon after the synthesis of amphetamine in 1887. Crystallized methamphetamine was synthesized in 1919 through the reduction of ephedrine using red phosphorus. From the 1950s to the 1970s, there were multiple epidemics of methamphetamine abuse in the United States.[135] Methamphetamine is approved by the FDA for the short-term treatment of attention deficit hyperactivity disorder and obesity, and it is sold under the trade name Desoxyn as a Schedule II drug. It is also prescribed for off-label use for refractory depression and narcolepsy.

The production of methamphetamine is relatively simple, requiring minimal equipment and chemicals. There are many methods of methamphetamine production that initially use pseudoephedrine, ephedrine, or phenyl-2-propanone (P2P). The primary ingredient of methamphetamine synthesis is ephedrine, which can be hydrogenated into methamphetamine. The ephedrine method, using pharmaceutical grade L-ephedrine, produces a product with few contaminants that is stereochemically pure.[46,132] Phenyl-2-propanone, as an alternative ingredient, can be methylated into ephedrine and then transformed into methamphetamine.[23] Because of the strict control of ephedrine and P2P, illicit chemists use phenylacetic acid to synthesize P2P.[23,38] Lead acetate, which is used as a substrate for the reaction, resulted in an epidemic of lead poisoning associated with methamphetamine abuse in Oregon.[3,120] Mercury contamination was also documented, although clinical mercury toxicity has not been reported.[23] Methamphetamine laboratories use many potentially toxic xenobiotics, including phosphine gas, methylamine gas, chloroform, and hydrochloric acid.[4,79] These laboratories therefore pose a significant health risk to law enforcement officers and the general public, causing respiratory and ophthalmic irritation, headaches, and burns.[29,154] Currently, the sale of other potential amphetamine synthetic ingredients, such as hydrochloric acid, hydrogen chloride, anhydrous ammonia, red phosphorus, and iodine, is also monitored and restricted in the United States.[23,30]

Methamphetamine exists as a chiral molecule with two isomers that include levomethamphetamine and dextromethamphetamine. Although the levorotatory form is devoid of CNS stimulatory properties, it retains its vasoactive effects and is used in nonprescription nasal decongestant inhalers. In the racemic mixture, the dextrorotatory form is solely responsible for the stimulant effects observed with methamphetamines. Methamphetamine undergoes metabolism in the liver mainly to amphetamine and 4-hydroxymethamphetamine and has prolonged half-life of 19 to 34 hours, although the duration of its acute effects can be greater than 24 hours.[46]

3,4-Methylenedioxymethamphetamine

Methamphetamine   Methylenedioxymethamphetamine

3,4-Methylenedioxymethamphetamine, also known as MDMA, was first synthesized in 1912 and was rediscovered in 1965 by Shulgin. 3,4-Methylenedioxymethamphetamine is known as "ecstasy," "E," "Adam," "XTC," "Molly," and "MDM," and it is commonly abused.[128,174,178] Other amphetamines similar to MDMA include MDEA ("Eve") and MDA ("love drug"). With similar clinical effects, these xenobiotics are also used or distributed as MDMA in areas of MDMA popularity. Amphetamines sold as MDMA include 2CB, 2,4-dimethoxy-4-(n)-propylthiophenylethylamine (2C-T7), and N-methyl-1-(3,4-methylenedioxyphenyl)-2-butanamine (MBDB).[28,59] Typically, MDMA is available in 50- to 200-mg colorful and branded tablets.

3,4-Methylenedioxymethamphetamine and similar analogs are so-called *entactogens* (meaning "touching within"), capable of producing euphoria, inner peace, and a desire to socialize.[151] In addition, some psychologists used MDMA to enhance psychotherapy until the Controlled Substances Act of 1986 placed MDMA in Schedule I, thereby eliminating its medical use.[127] People who use MDMA report that it enhances pleasure, heightens sexuality, and expands consciousness without the loss of control.[66] Negative effects reported with acute use included ataxia, restlessness, confusion, poor concentration, and impaired memory.[151] 3,4-Methylenedioxymethamphetamine has about one-tenth the CNS stimulant effect of amphetamine. Unlike amphetamine and methamphetamine, MDMA is a potent stimulus for the release of serotonin.[25,41,68] The concentration of MDMA required to stimulate the release of serotonin is 10 times less than that required for the release of dopamine or norepinephrine. In animal models, the stereotypic and discriminatory effects of MDMA, and its congeners can be distinguished from those of other amphetamines.[25]

The sympathetic effects of MDMA are mild in low doses. However, when a large amount of MDMA is taken, the clinical presentation is similar to that of other amphetamines. Dysrhythmias, hyperthermia, rhabdomyolysis, disseminated intravascular coagulation (DIC), and deaths are reported.[57,87,137] Significant hyponatremia is also reported with MDMA use.[1,22,73] 3,4-Methylenedioxymethamphetamine and its metabolites increase the release of vasopressin (antidiuretic hormone), and this is thought to be related to the serotonergic effects.[52] Furthermore, substantial free water intake combined with sodium loss from physical exertion in dance clubs increases the risk of the development of hyponatremia.

Molly is a purified or crystallized form of MDMA that is typically sold as a powder rather than a pill and is taken orally. It gained popularity because of what was perceived as a more rapid onset of symptoms and a subtler offset or "come-down" period. Molly is also commonly viewed as a safer form of MDMA because it is erroneously believed by users to contain no adulterants. The use of Molly is associated with typical amphetamine adverse effects.[83] Although Molly is often sold on the street as pure MDMA, Molly may contain various compounds including members of the 2C series, amphetamines that have two methoxy groups and a halogen such as iodine (2C-I) or bromide (2C-B).

A major concern with MDMA is its long-term effects on the brain. In numerous animal models, acute administration of MDMA leads to the decrease in SERT function and number. Recovery of SERT function takes several weeks. Repetitive administration of MDMA ultimately results in permanent damage to serotonergic neurons, typically causing injury to the axons and the terminals while sparing the cell bodies.[109,139] Some regeneration of synaptic terminals occurs even with neuronal damage, but functional recovery is incomplete. Intact SERT function is necessary for MDMA-induced neurotoxicity. Xenobiotics that inhibit the reuptake of serotonin prevent MDMA-induced neurotoxicity in animals. Animal data suggest that MDMA induces hydroxyl free radical generation and decreases antioxidants in serotonergic neurons.[147] 3,4-Methylenedioxymethamphetamine itself is not the ultimate neurotoxin; rather, its metabolites 3-methyldopamine and N-methyl-α-methyldopamine appear to be responsible in animals.[114] When antioxidants are depleted, neuronal damage occurs.

Para-methoxyamphetamine and Para-methoxymethamphetamine-Monomethoxy Derivatives

Amphetamine

Para-methoxy-N-methylamphetamine (PMA)

Methamphetamine

Para-methoxy-N-methylamphetamine (PMMA)

Para-methoxyamphetamine (PMA) is the 4-methoxylated analog of amphetamine, and *para*-methoxy-*N*-methylamphetamine (PMMA; methyl-MA) is the 4-methoxy analog of methamphetamine. *Para*-methoxyamphetamine was first produced in 1973 and sold as a hallucinogen for a short period of time and then reemerged in the 1990s. *Para*-methoxy-*N*-methylamphetamine soon appeared after PMA, with multiple reports of death also emerging during that time.[12,81,91] *Para*-methoxyamphetamine and PMMA are commonly found as tablets or capsules sold as MDMA or "ecstasy." Although the effects of PMA and PMMA mimic some aspects of MDMA and methamphetamine, unique properties of PMA and PMMA make them considerably more lethal, earning the street name "death." More than 100 fatalities and severe poisonings attributed to PMMA and PMA are reported in North America, Australia, and Europe.[94,98,102,105]

Methoxy ring substitution of amphetamine or methamphetamine at the 3 or 4 positions (*para* substitution is the most common) yields PMA and PMMA derivatives that have significantly less sympathomimetic activity than amphetamine but very potent serotonergic activity.[35,158] Both PMA and PMMA inhibit reuptake of serotonin and inhibit monoamine oxidase A found centrally and peripherally. The methoxy ring substitution is also responsible for poor penetration of the blood–brain barrier.[8,54]

Para-methoxyamphetamine and PMMA poisoning results in autonomic hyperactivity similar to that observed with other amphetamines, namely, hypertension, tachycardia, and agitation. Poor blood–brain barrier penetration results in a delayed onset of CNS effects and overall a comparatively weak euphoric effect. These properties often lead users to repeat doses, resulting in severe toxicity and the seemingly high mortality rate.

Cathinones (Methcathinone, Methylenedioxypyrovalerone, and Mephedrone)—"Bath Salts"

Methamphetamine

Methcathinone

Cathinone (2-amino-1-phenyl-1-propanone) is a naturally occurring substance found in the leaves of the *Catha edulis* (khat) plant. Also known as guat and gat, the fresh leaves and stems are commonly used as a stimulant in Africa and the Middle East. The plant form contains numerous amphetamines in minute quantities, but the primary active ingredient is cathinone. As the leaves age, cathinone is degraded to cathine, which has about one-tenth the stimulant effect of D-amphetamine. Imported fresh khat must be consumed within a week, or much of its potency is lost. The primary effects of khat are increased alertness, insomnia, euphoria, anxiety, and hyperactivity. Khat chewing is linked to cardiac and gastrointestinal (GI) disease.[124,125]

The syntheses of cathinone derivatives were reported in the early 1920s, with the production of methcathinone in 1928 and mephedrone in 1929. Methcathinone, the methyl derivative of cathinone, was used in Russia as an antidepressant in the 1930s and 1940s. Also known as "Cat" and "Jeff," cathinone was used recreationally, historically most often in countries formerly part of the Soviet Union. Various synthetic cathinones, including mephedrone and methylenedioxypyrovalerone (MDPV), have gained popularity in both the United States and Europe in recent years.[7] Increased popularity of synthetic cathinones is likely be due to a combination of media attention and widespread Internet availability.[133,149] Many other synthetic cathinones produced include methylone, mephedrone, butylone, MDPV, dimethylcathinone, ethcathinone, ethylone, 3-,4-fluoromethcathinone, and α-pyrrolidinovalerophenone. α-Pyrrolidinovalerophenone (1-phenyl-2-(pyrrolidin-1)-ylpentan-1-one), sold on the street as "flakka," in particular is a popular drug of abuse.[168] Bupropion, a popular pharmaceutical licensed for treatment of depression and smoking cessation, is the only medicinally used cathinone.[111] Sustained-release bupropion overdoses are associated with delayed toxicity. Serious toxicity in overdose, including seizures and refractory dysrhythmias requiring extracorporeal membrane oxygenation as well as fatalities, are reported.[75,157]

The synthetic cathinones differ structurally from other amphetamines by the addition of a ketone at the β position. The β-ketone group is responsible for increased polarity, which decreases penetration of the blood–brain barrier. Cathinones possess amphetamine-like properties and have sympathomimetic effects, although as a group, they are considered less potent. Both the US Poison Control Centers and the Toxicology Investigator's Consortium Registry (ToxIC) data report common adverse effects to include agitation, tachycardia, hallucinations, and a general sympathomimetic toxidrome.[55,155] Some synthetic cathinones cause hyponatremia, although the mechanism is not clear and may differ from that of MDMA.[11,26,27,104,130] Reported complications include compartment syndrome, DIC, AKI, cardiomyopathy, myocardial infarction, seizures, and sudden cardiac death.[55,96,116,138,148,183] An irreversible Parkinson syndrome was also described in chronic users of IV methcathinone that was manufactured with the use of potassium permanganate as an oxidizing agent. In one case series, T1-weighted magnetic resonance imaging showed symmetric hyperintensity in the globus pallidus, substantia nigra, and innominata in all active methcathinone users, characteristic of manganese poisoning. These cases were also confirmed with elevated whole-blood manganese concentrations.[159]

Synthetic cathinones are often sold as "bath salts" or "plant food" and labeled as "not for human consumption" to circumvent controlled substances legislation. The legal status differs among countries and changes over time. In the United States, the synthetic cathinones were initially unscheduled but were made illegal for human consumption under the Federal Analogue Act of 1986. In 2011, the Drug Enforcement Administration used its emergency scheduling authority to enact temporary control, making possession or sale of methylenedioxypyrovalerone, methylone, and mephedrone illegal. This was later written into permanent law. In 2014, an additional 10 synthetic cathinones were given temporary Schedule I status.

Bromo-dragonFLY

Amphetamine   Bromo-dragonFLY

1-(8-Bromobenzo[1,2-b;4,5-b]difuran-4-yl)-2-aminopropane, also known as Bromo-dragonFLY (BDF), was first synthesized in 1998. Bromo-dragonFLY was named after its superficial structural resemblance to a dragonfly, similar to its less potent predecessor, the dihydrofuran series nicknamed FLY. Bromo-dragonFLY is a member of a new class of benzodifurans, which were used as potent tools for investigation of the serotonin receptor family. Benzodifurans were also briefly investigated as potential antidepressants.[179]

Structurally, BDF is closely related to other phenylethylamines such as DOB and 2C-B but contains two furan rings on either side of the benzene ring, creating a fully aromatic tricyclic structure. There are several similar compounds to BDF, differing by substitution of the bromine atom with other entities. Bromo-dragonFLY exists as R- and S-enantiomers, which are both biologically active. The R-enantiomer is considered more potent, with a significant hallucinogenic effect mediated primarily through the 5-HT$_{2A}$ serotonin receptor (also with affinity for the 5-HT$_{2B}$ and 5-HT$_{2C}$ serotonin receptors).[126]

Bromo-dragonFLY use is associated with deaths in Europe and the United States. Reports demonstrate delayed complications owing to severe peripheral vasoconstriction and limb ischemia. Such complications likely result from BDF's potent serotonergic properties.[5,34,41,167,179]

2,5-Dimethoxy-4-Methylamphetamine and 2,5-Dimethoxy-4-Iodoamphetamine

Amphetamine   2,5-Dimethoxy-4-methylamphetamine

2,5-Dimethoxy-4-methylamphetamine (DOM), also known as STP, which stands for "serenity, tranquility, and peace," emerged in the 1960s as a hallucinogen. It was noted for its delayed onset of action and duration of effect, which resulted in a short-lived appearance. 2,5-Dimethoxy-4-iodoamphetamine (DOI) is another potent hallucinogen, previously sold as a substitute for lysergic acid diethylamide, or LSD.

Dimethoxy amphetamine derivatives are structurally characterized by methoxy ring substitution at the 2 and 5 positions on the aromatic ring, with varying substitution of hydrophobic moieties at the 4 position. 2,5-Dimethoxy-4-methylamphetamine and DOI are both serotonin receptor agonists with selectivity at the 5-HT$_{2A}$, 5-HT$_{2B}$, and 5-HT$_{2C}$ receptor subtypes. Because of this selectivity, DOM and DOI are often used in scientific research involving study of the 5-HT$_2$ receptor subfamily. 2,5-Dimethoxy-4-methylamphetamine exists as a chiral molecule, with the R-(-)-enantiomer considered the more potent.[15]

Potent hallucinogenic effects and dysphoria characterize the use of DOB and DOI, with minimal sympathomimetic effects. These symptoms can often be delayed with a prolonged duration of effect, sometimes refractory to the use of benzodiazepines. Reversible vasospasm with the use of dimethoxy amphetamine derivatives is reported.[9,20]

The 2C-Series and N-2-methoxybenzylphenylethylamines

The 2C-series and its derivatives are similar in structure and function DOM and DOI as all are dimethoxy phenylethylamine derivatives with potent hallucinogenic properties. The 2C series differs in that they lack an α-carbon methyl group and are thus not true amphetamines in structure.

The first of this series 2C-B was initially intended for psychotherapy, however, it fell out of favor because of GI side effects and limited entactogenic effects. Multiple other 2C compounds have been developed by altering substitutions at positions 2,4 and 5 on the phenyl ring. The compound 2C-I is an iodo-substituted dimethoxy phenylethylamine popularized in recent years as "smiles." Reported clinical effects of this series include sympathomimetic effects, delirium, hallucinations, and psychosis.[42]

2-(4-Iodo-2,5-dimethoxyphenyl)-N-[(2-methoxyphenyl)methyl]ethanamine (2C-I-NBOMe, N-Bomb) was discovered in 2003, along with other similar NBOMe compounds. It possesses strong 5-HT$_{2A}$ agonism and was initially used as a pharmacologic tool to study 5-HT$_{2A}$ receptors. 2C-I-NBOMe is synthesized by N-benzyl substitution of 2C-I and is currently used recreationally as an LSD alternative. The high potency of NBOMe compounds compared with 2C-I allow efficacy in microgram doses, with subsequent potential for accidental overdose. NBOMes are used by all routes, but poor oral bioavailability limits oral use.[71,118] Reported clinical effects include euphoria, hallucinations, and sympathomimetic effects. Deaths are reported.[118,169]

SUMMARY

■ Novel amphetamines, often created to evade designer drug laws, continue to increase dramatically throughout the United States.

■ The extensive knowledge of the modifications to the existing phenylethylamine backbone allows clinicians to predict the effects of the amphetamines. These effects are attributed to variable degrees of selectivity affecting dopamine, norepinephrine, and serotonin.

■ Many complications associated with amphetamines are similar to those of cocaine, such as agitation, hyperthermia, rhabdomyolysis, myocardial ischemia, and cerebral infarction.

■ The management of patients with acute toxicity of any of the amphetamines includes supportive care, with the judicious use of benzodiazepines and anticipation of complications of adrenergic and serotonergic toxicity such as hyperthermia and rhabdomyolysis.

Acknowledgment
William K. Chiang, MD, contributed to this chapter in previous editions.

REFERENCES

1. Aitchison KJ, et al. Ecstasy (MDMA)-induced hyponatraemia is associated with genetic variants in CYP2D6 and COMT. *J Psychopharmacol.* 2012;26:408-418.
2. Alexander PD, et al. A comparison of psychotic symptoms in subjects with methamphetamine versus cocaine dependence. *Psychopharmacology (Berl).* 2017;234:1535-1547.
3. Allcott JV 3rd, et al. Acute lead poisoning in two users of illicit methamphetamine. *JAMA.* 1987;258:510-511.
4. Allen A, Cantrell T. Synthetic reductions in clandestine amphetamine and methamphetamine labs. *J Forensic Sci.* 1989;42:183-199.
5. Andreasen MF, et al. A fatal poisoning involving Bromo-Dragonfly. *Forensic Sci Int.* 2009;183:91-96.
6. Anonymous. Clinical aspects of amphetamine abuse. *JAMA.* 1978;240:2317-2319.
7. Anonymous. *United Nations Office on Drugs and Crime World Drug Report.* United Nations Publication, New York; 2015.
8. Ask AL, et al. Selective inhibition of monoamine oxidase in monoaminergic neurons in the rat brain. *Naunyn Schmiedebergs Arch Pharmacol.* 1983;324:79-87.
9. Balikova M. Nonfatal and fatal DOB (2,5-dimethoxy-4-bromoamphetamine) overdose. *Forensic Sci Int.* 2005;153:85-91.
10. Barron RP, et al. Identification of impurities in illicit methamphetamine samples. *J Assoc Off Anal Chem.* 1974;57:1147-1158.
11. Baumann MH, et al. Powerful cocaine-like actions of 3,4-methylenedioxypyrovalerone (MDPV), a principal constituent of psychoactive "bath salts" products. *Neuropsychopharmacology.* 2013;38:552-562.
12. Becker J, et al. A fatal paramethoxymethamphetamine intoxication. *Leg Med (Tokyo).* 2003;5(suppl 1):S138-141.
13. Beckett AH, Rowland M. Urinary excretion kinetics of amphetamine in man. *J Pharm Pharmacol.* 1965;17:628-639.
14. Beckett AH, et al. Influence of urinary pH on excretion of amphetamine. *Lancet.* 1965;1:303.
15. Berankova K, et al. Distribution profile of 2,5-dimethoxy-4-bromoamphetamine (DOB) in rats after oral and subcutaneous doses. *Forensic Sci Int.* 2007;170:94-99.
16. Berger UV, et al. Depletion of serotonin using p-chlorophenylalanine (PCPA) and reserpine protects against the neurotoxic effects of p-chloroamphetamine (PCA) in the brain. *Exp Neurol.* 1989;103:111-115.
17. Bett WR. Benzedrine sulphate in clinical medicine; a survey of the literature. *Postgrad Med J.* 1946;22:205-218.
18. Bostwick DG. Amphetamine induced cerebral vasculitis. *Hum Pathol.* 1981;12:1031-1033.
19. Boulanger-Gobeil C, et al. Seizures and hyponatremia related to ethcathinone and methylone poisoning. *J Med Toxicol.* 2012;8:59-61.
20. Bowen JS, et al. Diffuse vascular spasm associated with 4-bromo-2,5-dimethoxyamphetamine ingestion. *JAMA.* 1983;249:1477-1479.
21. Brahm NC, et al. Commonly prescribed medications and potential false-positive urine drug screens. *Am J Health Syst Pharm.* 2010;67:1344-1350.
22. Budisavljevic MN, et al. Hyponatremia associated with 3,4-methylenedioxymethylamphetamine ("Ecstasy") abuse. *Am J Med Sci.* 2003;326:89-93.
23. Burton BT. Heavy metal and organic contaminants associated with illicit methamphetamine production. *NIDA Res Monogr.* 1991;115:47-59.
24. Callaway CW, Clark RF. Hyperthermia in psychostimulant overdose. *Ann Emerg Med.* 1994;24:68-76.
25. Callaway CW, et al. Amphetamine derivatives induce locomotor hyperactivity by acting as indirect serotonin agonists. *Psychopharmacology (Berl).* 1991;104:293-301.
26. Cameron K, et al. Mephedrone and methylenedioxypyrovalerone (MDPV), major constituents of "bath salts," produce opposite effects at the human dopamine transporter. *Psychopharmacology (Berl).* 2013;227:493-499.
27. Cameron KN, et al. Bath salts components mephedrone and methylenedioxypyrovalerone (MDPV) act synergistically at the human dopamine transporter. *Br J Pharmacol.* 2013;168:1750-1757.
28. Carter N, et al. Deaths associated with MBDB misuse. *Int J Legal Med.* 2000;113:168-170.
29. Centers for Disease Control and Prevention. Acute public health consequences of methamphetamine laboratories—16 states, January 2000–June 2004. *MMWR Morb Mortal Wkly Rep.* 2005;54:356-359.
30. Centers for Disease Control and Prevention. Anhydrous ammonia thefts and releases associated with illicit methamphetamine production—16 states, January 2000–June 2004. *MMWR Morb Mortal Wkly Rep.* 2005;54:359-361.
31. Centers for Disease Control and Prevention. Emergency department visits after use of a drug sold as "bath salts"–Michigan, November 13, 2010–March 31, 2011. *MMWR Morb Mortal Wkly Rep.* 2011;60:624-627.
32. Citron BP, et al. Necrotizing angiitis associated with drug abuse. *N Engl J Med.* 1970;283:1003-1011.
33. Cody JT, Schwarzhoff R. Fluorescence polarization immunoassay detection of amphetamine, methamphetamine, and illicit amphetamine analogues. *J Anal Toxicol.* 1993;17:23-33.
34. Corazza O, et al. Designer drugs on the internet: a phenomenon out-of-control? The emergence of hallucinogenic drug Bromo-Dragonfly. *Curr Clin Pharmacol.* 2011;6:125-129.
35. Corrigall WA, et al. The reinforcing and discriminative stimulus properties of para-ethoxy- and para-methoxyamphetamine. *Pharmacol Biochem Behav.* 1992;41:165-169.
36. Costall B, Naylor RJ. Extrapyramidal and mesolimbic involvement with the stereotypic activity of D- and L-amphetamine. *Eur J Pharmacol.* 1974;25:121-129.
37. Curry SC, et al. Drug- and toxin-induced rhabdomyolysis. *Ann Emerg Med.* 1989;18:1068-1084.
38. Dal Carson TA, et al. A clandestine approach to the synthesis of phenyl-2-propanone from phenylpropenes. *J Forensic Sci.* 1984;29:1187-1208.
39. Dar KJ, McBrien ME. MDMA induced hyperthermia: report of a fatality and review of current therapy. *Intensive Care Med.* 1996;22:995-996.
40. Davis WM, et al. Antagonism of acute amphetamine intoxication by haloperidol and propranolol. *Toxicol Appl Pharmacol.* 1974;29:397-403.
41. De Souza EB, Battaglia G. Effects of MDMA and MDA on brain serotonin neurons: evidence from neurochemical and autoradiographic studies. *NIDA Res Monogr.* 1989;94:196-222.
42. Dean BV, et al. 2C or not 2C: phenethylamine designer drug review. *J Med Toxicol.* 2013;9:172-178.
43. Delliou D. Bromo-DMA: new hallucinogenic drug. *Med J Aust.* 1980;1:83.
44. Derlet RW, et al. Antagonism of cocaine, amphetamine, and methamphetamine toxicity. *Pharmacol Biochem Behav.* 1990;36:745-749.
45. Derlet RW, et al. Protection against d-amphetamine toxicity. *Am J Emerg Med.* 1990;8:105-108.
46. Derlet RW, Heischober B. Methamphetamine. Stimulant of the 1990s? *West J Med.* 1990;153:625-628.
47. Derlet RW, et al. Amphetamine toxicity: experience with 127 cases. *J Emerg Med.* 1989;7:157-161.
48. Devan GS. Phentermine and psychosis. *Br J Psychiatry.* 1990;156:442-443.
49. Edwards M, et al. Cerebral infarction with a single oral dose of phenylpropanolamine. *Am J Emerg Med.* 1987;5:163-164.
50. Eilert RJ, Kliewer ML. Methamphetamine-induced rhabdomyolysis. *Int Anesthesiol Clin.* 2011;49:52-56.
51. Ellinwood EH Jr. Assault and homicide associated with amphetamine abuse. *Am J Psychiatry.* 1971;127:1170-1175.
52. Fallon JK, et al. Action of MDMA (ecstasy) and its metabolites on arginine vasopressin release. *Ann N Y Acad Sci.* 2002;965:399-409.
53. Fitzgerald RL, et al. Resolution of methamphetamine stereoisomers in urine drug testing: urinary excretion of R(-)-methamphetamine following use of nasal inhalers. *J Anal Toxicol.* 1988;12:255-259.
54. Freezer A, et al. Effects of 3,4-methylenedioxymethamphetamine (MDMA, 'Ecstasy') and para-methoxyamphetamine on striatal 5-HT when co-administered with moclobemide. *Brain Res.* 2005;1041:48-55.
55. Froberg BA, et al. Acute methylenedioxypyrovalerone Toxicity. *J Med Toxicol.* 2015;11:185-194.
56. Gibb JW, et al. Neurotoxicity of amphetamines and their metabolites. *NIDA Res Monogr.* 1997;173:128-145.
57. Gill JR, et al. Ecstasy (MDMA) deaths in New York City: a case series and review of the literature. *J Forensic Sci.* 2002;47:121-126.
58. Ginsberg MD, et al. Amphetamine intoxication with coagulopathy, hyperthermia, and reversible renal failure. A syndrome resembling heatstroke. *Ann Intern Med.* 1970;73:81-85.
59. Giroud C, et al. 2C-B: a new psychoactive phenylethylamine recently discovered in Ecstasy tablets sold on the Swiss black market. *J Anal Toxicol.* 1998;22:345-354.
60. Glennon RA. Stimulus properties of hallucinogenic phenalkylamines and related designer drugs: formulation of structure-activity relationships. *NIDA Res Monogr.* 1989;94:43-67.
61. Goldfrank LR, Hoffman RS. The cardiovascular effects of cocaine. *Ann Emerg Med.* 1991;20:165-175.
62. Goldstone MS. "Cat": methcathinone—a new drug of abuse. *JAMA.* 1993;269:2508.
63. Gorman MC, et al. Outcomes in pregnancies complicated by methamphetamine use. *Am J Obstet Gynecol.* 2014;211:429 e421-427.
64. Green AR, et al. The pharmacology and clinical pharmacology of 3,4-methylenedioxymethamphetamine (MDMA, "ecstasy"). *Pharmacol Rev.* 2003;55:463-508.
65. Greenblatt DJ, et al. Fatal hyperthermia following haloperidol therapy of sedative-hypnotic withdrawal. *J Clin Psychiatry.* 1978;39:673-675.
66. Greer G, Tolbert R. Subjective reports of the effects of MDMA in a clinical setting. *J Psychoactive Drugs.* 1986;18:319-327.

67. Grinspoon L, Bakalar JB. *Amphetamines: Medical and Health Hazards.* Boston, MA: CK Hall; 1979.

68. Groves PM, et al. Neuronal actions of amphetamine in the rat brain. *NIDA Res Monogr.* 1989;94:127-145.

69. Grunau BE, et al. Dantrolene in the treatment of MDMA-related hyperpyrexia: a systematic review. *CJEM.* 2010;12:435-442.

70. Hahn L. Consumption coagulopathy after amphetamine abuse in pregnancy. *Acta Obstet Gynecol Scand.* 1995;74:652-654.

71. Halberstadt AL, Geyer MA. Effects of the hallucinogen 2,5-dimethoxy-4-iodophenethylamine (2C-I) and superpotent N-benzyl derivatives on the head twitch response. *Neuropharmacology.* 2014;77:200-207.

72. Halkitis PN, et al. Longitudinal investigation of methamphetamine use among gay and bisexual men in New York City: findings from Project BUMPS. *J Urban Health.* 2005;82(1(suppl 1)):i18-25.

73. Hartung TK, et al. Hyponatraemic states following 3,4-methylenedioxymethamphetamine (MDMA, "ecstasy") ingestion. *QJM.* 2002;95:431-437.

74. Heal DJ, et al. Amphetamine, past and present—a pharmacological and clinical perspective. *J Psychopharmacol.* 2013;27:479-496.

75. Heise CW, et al. Two cases of refractory cardiogenic shock secondary to bupropion successfully treated with veno-arterial extracorporeal membrane oxygenation. *J Med Toxicol.* 2016;12:301-304.

76. Hirata H, et al. Methamphetamine-induced serotonin neurotoxicity is mediated by superoxide radicals. *Brain Res.* 1995;677:345-347.

77. Holubar SD, et al. Methamphetamine colitis: a rare case of ischemic colitis in a young patient. *Arch Surg.* 2009;144:780-782.

78. Hung YM, Chang JC. Weight-reducing regimen associated with polymorphic ventricular tachycardia. *Am J Emerg Med.* 2006;24:714-716.

79. Irvine GD, Chin L. The environmental impact and adverse health effects of the clandestine manufacture of methamphetamine. *NIDA Res Monogr.* 1991;115:33-46.

80. Iversen L. Neurotransmitter transporters: fruitful targets for CNS drug discovery. *Mol Psychiatry.* 2000;5:357-362.

81. Johansen SS, et al. Three fatal cases of PMA and PMMA poisoning in Denmark. *J Anal Toxicol.* 2003;27:253-256.

82. Johnson TD, Berenson MM. Methamphetamine-induced ischemic colitis. *J Clin Gastroenterol.* 1991;13:687-689.

83. Kahn DE, et al. 3 cases of primary intracranial hemorrhage associated with "Molly", a purified form of 3,4-methylenedioxymethamphetamine (MDMA). *J Neurol Sci.* 2012;323:257-260.

84. Kaku DA, Lowenstein DH. Emergence of recreational drug abuse as a major risk factor for stroke in young adults. *Ann Intern Med.* 1990;113:821-827.

85. Karch SB, Billingham ME. The pathology and etiology of cocaine-induced heart disease. *Arch Pathol Lab Med.* 1988;112:225-230.

86. Karler R, et al. The dopaminergic, glutamatergic, GABAergic bases for the action of amphetamine and cocaine. *Brain Res.* 1995;671:100-104.

87. Karlovsek MZ, et al. Our experiences with fatal ecstasy abuse (two case reports). *Forensic Sci Int.* 2005;147(suppl):S77-S80.

88. Klawans HL, Weiner WJ. The effect of d-amphetamine on choreiform movement disorders. *Neurology.* 1974;24:312-318.

89. Kokkinidis L, et al. Amphetamine withdrawal: a behavioral evaluation. *Life Sci.* 1986;38:1617-1623.

90. Kolb ME, et al. Dantrolene in human malignant hyperthermia. *Anesthesiology.* 1982;56:254-262.

91. Kraner JC, et al. Fatalities caused by the MDMA-related drug parameioxyamphetamine (PMA). *J Anal Toxicol.* 2001;25:645-648.

92. Kwon C, et al. Transient proximal tubular renal injury following Ecstasy ingestion. *Pediatr Nephrol.* 2003;18:820-822.

93. Lago JA, Kosten TR. Stimulant withdrawal. *Addiction.* 1994;89:1477-1481.

94. Lamberth PG, et al. Fatal parametoxy-amphetamine (PMA) poisoning in the Australian Capital Territory. *Med J Aust.* 2008;188:426.

95. Laskowski LK, et al. Ice water submersion for rapid cooling in severe drug-induced hyperthermia. *Clin Toxicol (Phila).* 2015;53:181-184.

96. Levine M, et al. Compartment syndrome after "bath salts" use: a case series. *Ann Emerg Med.* 2013;61:480-483.

97. Lin DL, et al. Recent parameioxymethamphetamine (PMMA) deaths in Taiwan. *J Anal Toxicol.* 2007;31:109-113.

98. Ling LH, et al. Poisoning with the recreational drug parameioxyamphetamine ("death"). *Med J Aust.* 2001;174:453-455.

99. Little BB, et al. Methamphetamine abuse during pregnancy: outcome and fetal effects. *Obstet Gynecol.* 1988;72:541-544.

100. Louria DB, et al. The major medical complications of heroin addiction. *Ann Intern Med.* 1967;67:1-22.

101. Lundh H, Tunving K. An extrapyramidal choreiform syndrome caused by amphetamine addiction. *J Neurol Neurosurg Psychiatry.* 1981;44:728-730.

102. Lurie Y, et al. Severe parameioxymethamphetamine (PMMA) and parameioxyamphetamine (PMA) outbreak in Israel. *Clin Toxicol (Phila).* 2012;50:39-43.

103. MacLean MR, Dempsie Y. Serotonin and pulmonary hypertension—from bench to bedside? *Curr Opin Pharmacol.* 2009;9:281-286.

104. Marinetti LJ, Antonides HM. Analysis of synthetic cathinones commonly found in bath salts in human performance and postmortem toxicology: method development, drug distribution and interpretation of results. *J Anal Toxicol.* 2013;37:135-146.

105. Martin TL. Three cases of fatal parameioxyamphetamine overdose. *J Anal Toxicol.* 2001;25:649-651.

106. Matsumoto RR, et al. Methamphetamine-induced toxicity: an updated review on issues related to hyperthermia. *Pharmacol Ther.* 2014;144:28-40.

107. Mattson RH, Calverley JR. Dextroamphetamine-sulfate-induced dyskinesias. *JAMA.* 1968;204:400-402.

108. Maurer HH, et al. Toxicokinetics and analytical toxicology of amphetamine-derived designer drugs ('Ecstasy'). *Toxicol Lett.* 2000;112-113:133-142.

109. McCann UD, et al. Positron emission tomographic evidence of toxic effect of MDMA ("Ecstasy") on brain serotonin neurons in human beings. *Lancet.* 1998;352:1433-1437.

110. McGee SM, et al. Spontaneous intracerebral hemorrhage related to methamphetamine abuse: autopsy findings and clinical correlation. *Am J Forensic Med Pathol.* 2004;25:334-337.

111. Meltzer PC, et al. 1-(4-Methylphenyl)-2-pyrrolidin-1-yl-pentan-1-one (Pyrovalerone) analogues: a promising class of monoamine uptake inhibitors. *J Med Chem.* 2006;49:1420-1432.

112. Minabe Y, Emori K. Two types of neuroplasticities in the kindling phenomenon: effects of chronic MK-801 and methamphetamine. *Brain Res.* 1992;585:237-242.

113. Moller M, et al. Ecstasy-induced myocardial infarction in a teenager: rare complication of a widely used illicit drug. *Clin Res Cardiol.* 2010;99:849-851.

114. Monks TJ, et al. The role of metabolism in 3,4-(+)-methylenedioxyamphetamine and 3,4-(+)-methylenedioxymethamphetamine (ecstasy) toxicity. *Ther Drug Monit.* 2004;26:132-136.

115. Morgan JP. Amphetamine and methamphetamine during the 1990s. *Pediatr Rev.* 1992;13:330-333.

116. Murray BL, et al. Death following recreational use of designer drug "bath salts" containing 3,4-methylenedioxypyrovalerone (MDPV). *J Med Toxicol.* 2012;8:69-75.

117. Nichols DE, Oberlender R. Structure-activity relationships of MDMA-like substances. *NIDA Res Monogr.* 1989;94:1-29.

118. Nikolaou P, et al. 2C-I-NBOMe, an "N-bomb" that kills with "Smiles." Toxicological and legislative aspects. *Drug Chem Toxicol.* 2015;38:113-119.

119. Nixon AL, et al. Bupropion metabolites produce false-positive urine amphetamine results. *Clin Chem.* 1995;41(6 Pt 1):955-956.

120. Norton RL, et al. Blood lead of intravenous drug users. *J Toxicol Clin Toxicol.* 1996;34:425-430.

121. O'Donohoe A, et al. MDMA toxicity: no evidence for a major influence of metabolic genotype at CYP2D6. *Addict Biol.* 1998;3:309-314.

122. Olmedo R, Hoffman RS. Withdrawal syndromes. *Emerg Med Clin North Am.* 2000;18:273-288.

123. Olsen KM, et al. Metabolites of chlorpromazine and brompheniramine may cause false-positive urine amphetamine results with monoclonal EMIT d.a.u. immunoassay. *Clin Chem.* 1992;38:611-612.

124. Pantelis C, et al. Khat, toxic reactions to this substance, its similarities to amphetamine, and the implications of treatment for such patients. *J Subst Abuse Treat.* 1989;6:205-206.

125. Pantelis C, et al. Use and abuse of khat (Catha edulis): a review of the distribution, pharmacology, side effects and a description of psychosis attributed to khat chewing. *Psychol Med.* 1989;19:657-668.

126. Parker MA, et al. A novel (benzodifuranyl)aminoalkane with extremely potent activity at the 5-HT2A receptor. *J Med Chem.* 1998;41:5148-5149.

127. Passie T, Benzenhofer U. The History of MDMA as an Underground Drug in the United States, 1960-1979. *J Psychoactive Drugs.* 2016;48:67-75.

128. Pedersen W, Skrondal A. Ecstasy and new patterns of drug use: a normal population study. *Addiction.* 1999;94:1695-1706.

129. Perez JA Jr, et al. Methamphetamine-related stroke: four cases. *J Emerg Med.* 1999;17:469-471.

130. Petrie M, et al. Cross-reactivity studies and predictive modeling of "Bath Salts" and other amphetamine-type stimulants with amphetamine screening immunoassays. *Clin Toxicol (Phila).* 2013;51:83-91.

131. Pitts DK, Marwah J. Cocaine and central monoaminergic neurotransmission: a review of electrophysiological studies and comparison to amphetamine and antidepressants. *Life Sci.* 1988;42:949-968.

132. Puder KS, et al. Illicit methamphetamine: analysis, synthesis, and availability. *Am J Drug Alcohol Abuse.* 1988;14:463-473.

133. Ramsey J, et al. Buying 'legal' recreational drugs does not mean that you are not breaking the law. *QJM.* 2010;103:777-783.

134. Randall T. Ecstasy-fueled 'rave' parties become dances of death for English youths. *JAMA.* 1992;268:1505-1506.

135. Rasmussen N. America's first amphetamine epidemic 1929-1971: a quantitative and qualitative retrospective with implications for the present. *Am J Public Health.* 2008;98:974-985.

136. Rasmussen N. Medical science and the military: the Allies' use of amphetamine during World War II. *J Interdiscip Hist.* 2011;42:205-233.

137. Ravina P, et al. Hyperkalemia in fatal MDMA ('ecstasy') toxicity. *Int J Cardiol.* 2004;93:307-308.

138. Regunath H, et al. Bath salt intoxication causing acute kidney injury requiring hemodialysis. *Hemodial Int.* 2012;16(suppl 1):S47-S49.

139. Ricaurte GA, et al. 3,4-Methylenedioxyethylamphetamine (MDE), a novel analogue of MDMA, produces long-lasting depletion of serotonin in the rat brain. *Eur J Pharmacol.* 1987;137:265-268.

140. Ricaurte GA, et al. Further evidence that amphetamines produce long-lasting dopamine neurochemical deficits by destroying dopamine nerve fibers. *Brain Res.* 1984;303:359-364.

141. Richards JR, et al. Methamphetamine abuse and rhabdomyolysis in the ED: a 5-year study. *Am J Emerg Med.* 1999;17:681-685.

142. Ruha AM, Yarema MC. Pharmacologic treatment of acute pediatric methamphetamine toxicity. *Pediatr Emerg Care.* 2006;22:782-785.

143. Rusyniak DE. Neurologic manifestations of chronic methamphetamine abuse. *Psychiatr Clin North Am.* 2013;36:261-275.

144. Seghatol FF, Rigolin VH. Appetite suppressants and valvular heart disease. *Curr Opin Cardiol.* 2002;17:486-492.

145. Seiden LS, Kleven MS. Methamphetamine and related drugs: toxicity and resulting behavioral changes in response to pharmacological probes. *NIDA Res Monogr.* 1989;94:146-160.

146. Sellers EM, et al. The potential role of the cytochrome P-450 2D6 pharmacogenetic polymorphism in drug abuse. *NIDA Res Monogr.* 1997;173:6-26.

147. Shankaran M, et al. Ascorbic acid prevents 3,4-methylenedioxymethamphetamine (MDMA)-induced hydroxyl radical formation and the behavioral and neurochemical consequences of the depletion of brain 5-HT. *Synapse.* 2001;40:55-64.

148. Sivagnanam K, et al. "Bath salts" induced severe reversible cardiomyopathy. *Am J Case Rep.* 2013;14:288-291.

149. Slomski A. A trip on "bath salts" is cheaper than meth or cocaine but much more dangerous. *JAMA.* 2012;308:2445-2447.

150. Smith DE, Fischer CM. An analysis of 310 cases of acute high-dose methamphetamine toxicity in Haight-Ashbury. *Clin Toxicol.* 1970;3:117-124.

151. Solowij N, et al. Recreational MDMA use in Sydney: a profile of 'Ecstasy' users and their experiences with the drug. *Br J Addict.* 1992;87:1161-1172.

152. Sonsalla PK. The role of N-methyl-D-aspartate receptors in dopaminergic neuropathology produced by the amphetamines. *Drug Alcohol Depend.* 1995;37:101-105.

153. Sonsalla PK, et al. Role for excitatory amino acids in methamphetamine-induced nigrostriatal dopaminergic toxicity. *Science.* 1989;243:398-400.

154. Spann MD, et al. Characteristics of burn patients injured in methamphetamine laboratory explosions. *J Burn Care Res.* 2006;27:496-501.

155. Spiller HA, et al. Clinical experience with and analytical confirmation of "bath salts" and "legal highs" (synthetic cathinones) in the United States. *Clin Toxicol (Phila).* 2011;49:499-505.

156. Srikanth S, et al. Methamphetamine-associated acute left ventricular dysfunction: a variant of stress-induced cardiomyopathy. *Cardiology.* 2008;109:188-192.

157. Starr P, et al. Incidence and onset of delayed seizures after overdoses of extended-release bupropion. *Am J Emerg Med.* 2009;27:911-915.

158. Steele TD, et al. Evaluation of the neurotoxicity of N-methyl-1-(4-methoxyphenyl)-2-aminopropane (para-methoxymethamphetamine, PMMA). *Brain Res.* 1992;589:349-352.

159. Stepens A, et al. A Parkinsonian syndrome in methcathinone users and the role of manganese. *N Engl J Med.* 2008;358:1009-1017.

160. Sudilovsky A. Disruption of behavior in cats by chronic amphetamine intoxication. *Int J Neurol.* 1975;10:259-275.

161. Sulzer D, et al. Amphetamine redistributes dopamine from synaptic vesicles to the cytosol and promotes reverse transport. *J Neurosci.* 1995;15(5 Pt 2):4102-4108.

162. Sulzer D, et al. Weak base model of amphetamine action. *Ann N Y Acad Sci.* 1992;654:525-528.

163. Surapaneni P, et al. Valvular heart disease with the use of fenfluramine-phentermine. *Tex Heart Inst J.* 2011;38:581-583.

164. Sutter ME, et al. Polymorphisms in CYP2D6 may predict methamphetamine related heart failure. *Clin Toxicol (Phila).* 2013;51:540-544.

165. Syed RH, Moore TL. Methylphenidate and dextroamphetamine-induced peripheral vasculopathy. *J Clin Rheumatol.* 2008;14:30-33.

166. Tashkin DP. Airway effects of marijuana, cocaine, and other inhaled illicit agents. *Curr Opin Pulm Med.* 2001;7:43-61.

167. Thorlacius K, et al. [Bromo-dragon fly—life-threatening drug. Can cause tissue necrosis as demonstrated by the first described case]. *Lakartidningen.* 2008;105:1199-1200.

168. Umebachi R, et al. Clinical characteristics of alpha-pyrrolidinovalerophenone (alpha-PVP) poisoning. *Clin Toxicol (Phila).* 2016;54:563-567.

169. Walterscheid JP, et al. Pathological findings in 2 cases of fatal 25I-NBOMe toxicity. *Am J Forensic Med Pathol.* 2014;35:20-25.

170. Walubo A, Seger D. Fatal multi-organ failure after suicidal overdose with MDMA, 'ecstasy': case report and review of the literature. *Hum Exp Toxicol.* 1999;18:119-125.

171. Warner M, et al. Drugs most frequently involved in drug overdose deaths: United States, 2010-2014. *Natl Vital Stat Rep.* 2016;65:1-15.

172. Watson CJ, et al. Body-packing with amphetamines—an indication for surgery. *J R Soc Med.* 1991;84:311-312.

173. Watts DJ, McCollester L. Methamphetamine-induced myocardial infarction with elevated troponin I. *Am J Emerg Med.* 2006;24:132-134.

174. Weir E. Raves: a review of the culture, the drugs and the prevention of harm. *CMAJ.* 2000;162:1843-1848.

175. Wells SM, et al. Acute inhalation exposure to vaporized methamphetamine causes lung injury in mice. *Inhal Toxicol.* 2008;20:829-838.

176. Westover AN, Nakonezny PA. Aortic dissection in young adults who abuse amphetamines. *Am Heart J.* 2010;160:315-321.

177. Wiener RS, et al. Dilated cardiomyopathy and cocaine abuse. Report of two cases. *Am J Med.* 1986;81:699-701.

178. Williams H, et al. "Saturday night fever": ecstasy related problems in a London accident and emergency department. *J Accid Emerg Med.* 1998;15:322-326.

179. Wood DM, et al. Delayed onset of seizures and toxicity associated with recreational use of Bromo-dragonFLY. *J Med Toxicol.* 2009;5:226-229.

180. Wrona MZ, et al. Potential new insights into the molecular mechanisms of methamphetamine-induced neurodegeneration. *NIDA Res Monogr.* 1997;173:146-174.

181. Yamamoto BK, Zhu W. The effects of methamphetamine on the production of free radicals and oxidative stress. *J Pharmacol Exp Ther.* 1998;287:107-114.

182. Yeo KK, et al. The association of methamphetamine use and cardiomyopathy in young patients. *Am J Med.* 2007;120:165-171.

183. Young AC, et al. Two cases of disseminated intravascular coagulation due to "bath salts" resulting in fatalities, with laboratory confirmation. *Am J Emerg Med.* 2013;31:445 e443-445.

74 CANNABINOIDS

Jeff M. Lapoint

HISTORY AND EPIDEMIOLOGY

Cannabis has been used for more than 4,000 years. The earliest documentation of the therapeutic use of marijuana is the fourth century B.C. in China.[172] Cannabis use spread from China to India to North Africa, reaching Europe around A.D. 500.[138] In colonial North America, cannabis was cultivated as a source of fiber. Similar to cocaine and morphine, cannabis was the focus of research efforts in the 19th century. Although the active chemical constituents of the former were isolated during this time, that of cannabis remained elusive.[97] This was because the active compounds of opium poppy and coca leaf are both alkaloids and were possible to extract with the technological means of the time, whereas the methods to isolate the active terpenes in cannabis were not available to researchers until several decades later.

The first pure phytocannabinoid to be isolated was cannabinol, in 1898. Synthesis of its structural isomers yielded the first synthetic cannabinoid (SC) years later—Δ^9-tetrahydrocannabinol (THC). Cannabinol was previously shown to lack psychoactive effects, but this new compound demonstrated similar effects to cannabis in a model of ataxia in dogs. Pure Δ^9-THC was subsequently isolated from hashish extract in 1964, and the structure was elucidated in 1967.[98]

Cannabis was used in the United States as a substance of abuse from the 1850s until the 1930s when the US Federal Bureau of Narcotics began to portray marijuana as a powerful, addictive substance. Despite this, marijuana was listed in the US Pharmacopoeia from 1850 to 1942. In 1970, the Controlled Substances Act classified marijuana as a Schedule I drug.

In all populations, cannabis use by men exceeds use by women. Currently, marijuana is the most commonly used illicit xenobiotic in the United States; however, it is legal for recreational use in an increasing number of states, including at the time of this writing Colorado, Washington, California, Oregon, and Alaska. In 2015 in the United States, 8.2% (22 million persons) 12 years of age or older used marijuana in the month before the survey; this prevalence is increased from 6% in previous years. The prevalence of past-month users aged 12 to 17 years was 7% (increased from 6.8% in 2006). The number of first-time users was estimated to be 2.1 million, with 63.3% younger than 18 years of age.[128]

Interest in SCs as potential therapeutics increased after the progress of the late 1960s, and several SCs similar in structure to THC were created. These semisynthetic compounds were based on the dibenzopyran ring structure of THC and had varying cannabinoid receptor binding affinities relative to THC. The search for a nonopioid analgesic sparked research and development efforts by pharmaceutical companies, most notably Pfizer, from the 1960s to 1980s.[67] Despite its efforts, no medications came to market; new analgesics retained unwanted psychoactive side effects. During this period, an extensive understanding of structure activity relationships for cannabinoids developed.[66]

Subsequent synthetic compounds were developed as cannabinoid research tools and were important in the discovery of central and peripheral cannabinoid receptors (CB_1 and CB_2) in the 1980s.[34] Many of these did not retain structural similarity to THC but remained potent and efficacious agonists at CB_1 and CB_2.[66] In the 1990s, the endogenous cannabinoids were discovered and were subsequently synthesized.[84] These free fatty acids are quickly hydrolyzed in vivo, a fact that previously limited potential for pharmaceutical development. Researchers have since synthesized stable versions of endocannabinoids (Fig. 74-1).

In 2004, SC-laced herbal incense blends became available over the Internet and through smoke shops in Western Europe.[88] Popular use and subsequent publicity increased, resulting in several users presenting to emergency departments in Germany. As the result of efforts by the German government and THC Pharma, JWH-018 was isolated as the psychoactive ingredient present in these early incense blends. The discovery led to legislative action and subsequent ban of herbal incense containing JWH-018 in Germany, but almost as soon as the ban took effect, manufacturers substituted a different SC—JWH-073. Since that time, many Western European countries have legislated further control of SCs.

The incidence of SC exposure in the United States increased, and in November 2010, the Drug Enforcement Administration (DEA) began the process of listing selected SCs as Schedule I drugs on a temporary basis. By March 2011, the DEA listed several nonclassical SCs as Schedule I, but as was the case in Germany, manufacturers of herbal incense blends in the United States switched to other unscheduled SCs. Second- and third-generation SCs, such as AM-2201, XLR-11, and the indazole derivatives, have since emerged and further complicate the clinical, regulatory, and public health efforts.

Toxicologists face a new era in the field of cannabinoids: Research continues to advance understanding of the cannabinoid system, a myriad of new and discrete SCs emerge ever year, and even the familiar marijuana is found with higher potency and changing phytocannabinoid ratios that may affect patients in unanticipated ways.

MEDICAL USES

Cannabis has been used medicinally for thousands of years to treat a seemingly endless array of conditions. However, modern medicine is supported by an evidence-based system rather than the belief-based medicine of the past. Therefore, potential medicinals must be proven through rigorous investigation to be not only safe but effective in the treatment of a targeted malady. Although smoked marijuana and THC preparations have not typically proven acutely dangerous, efficacy is questionable. Several issues must be considered when examining the body of evidence both for and against the medical use of cannabinoids. Marijuana is not the same entity as, nor is interchangeable with, Δ^9-THC. Although the latter is the chief psychoactive constituent of marijuana, the multiple additional cannabinoids present in marijuana are biologically active and must be considered. Second, significant study design flaws limit the conclusions that can be drawn from existing studies. Finally, poor overall understanding of cannabinoid physiology may hamper future study design. Proposed uses for medical cannabis and the available evidence supporting that use are reviewed next.

Pain

Acute Pain

Studies examining the efficacy of cannabis in the setting of induced acute pain showed no improvement. These studies were limited by the lack of a positive control and examined only extremes of induced pain.[30] Smoked marijuana failed to attenuate thermal pain in volunteers, and an oral THC analog had no effect on postsurgical pain.[73]

Chronic Pain

When used for the treatment of chronic and neuropathic pain, cannabinoids have had some favorable outcomes, although design flaws severely limit the quality of medical evidence.[118] Initial trials of combined cannabinoid and opioid therapy are encouraging, and the principle may have mechanistic merit based on the knowledge that opioid and cannabinoid receptors can form heterodimers,[131] but lack of proper controls and the presence of confounders limit the clinical applicability of cannabinoids as analgesics at this time.

Cannabinoids

Endocannabinoids

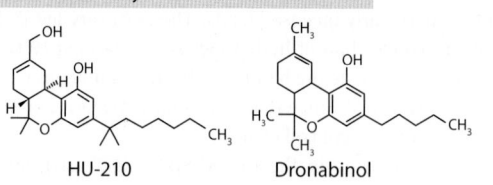

Anandamide

2-Arachidonoylglycerol
(2AG)

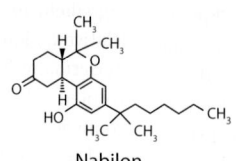

2-Arachidonyl glyceryl
ether

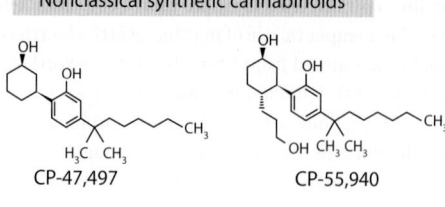

N-Arachidonoyl dopamine

Classical synthetic cannabinoids

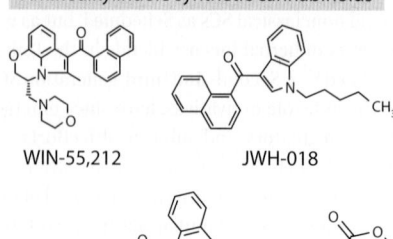

HU-210

Dronabinol

Nabilon

Nonclassical synthetic cannabinoids

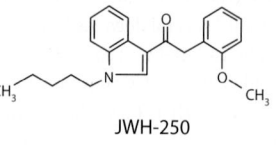

CP-47,497

CP-55,940

Aminoalkylindole synthetic cannabinoids

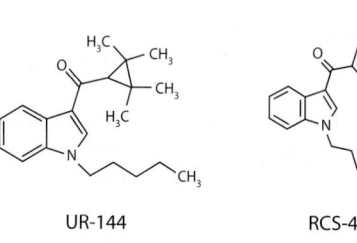

WIN-55,212   JWH-018

JWH-073

JWH-250

JWH-200

AM-2201   BB-22   XLR-11   UR-144   RCS-4

Phytocannabinoids

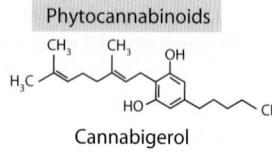

Cannabigerol

Cannabidiol

Tetrahydrocannabinol

Cannabinoid antagonists

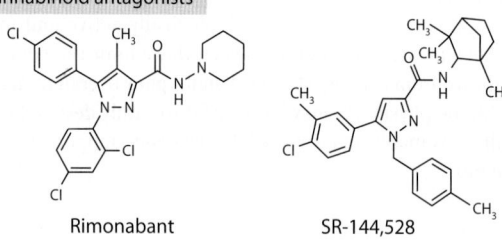

Rimonabant

SR-144,528

Fatty acid amide hydrolase inhibitor

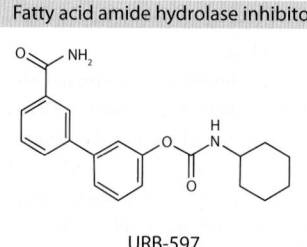

URB-597

Indole and indazole synthetic cannabinoids

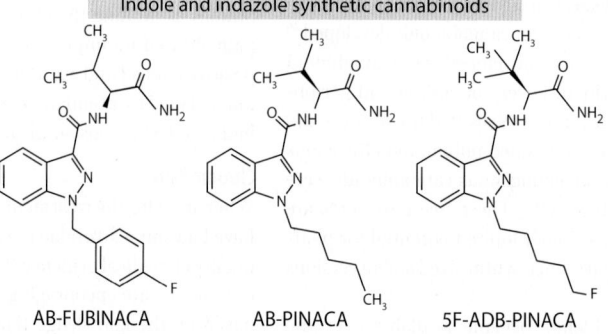

AB-FUBINACA   AB-PINACA   5F-ADB-PINACA

FIGURE 74–1. Cannabinoid structural classes.

Nausea and Vomiting

Trials of cannabinoids for treatment of chemotherapy-induced nausea and vomiting demonstrate superiority over placebo but compared with serotonin and dopamine antagonists, this difference is not statistically significant.[17,38,90,100,169] Dronabinol is currently FDA approved for this indication.

Glaucoma

Trials investigating the efficacy of cannabinoids for the treatment of glaucoma demonstrate the inferiority to longer acting traditional therapeutics, which have more significant effects on intraocular pressure (IOP) and longer durations of effect. One small trial found no difference between the effect of cannabinoids and placebo on IOP.[162]

Summary of Medical Use

In 2003, the Institute of Medicine undertook an extensive review of the evidence supporting the medical use of marijuana. It concluded that in some circumstances, cannabinoids show promise for use as therapeutics, but the quality of current studies necessitated further research specifically for the treatment of chronic pain. In addition, smoking marijuana provides a crude and unpredictable delivery mechanism, and safer, more precise methods of administration are needed.[167]

Similarly, a meta-analysis in 2015 composed of randomized clinical trials (RCTs) showed only moderate evidence to support the efficacy of cannabinoids in treating chronic pain and spasticity related to multiple sclerosis.[169] A Cochrane review of 23 RCTs found that pharmaceutical cannabinoids for use in the management of many clinical conditions but are only currently FDA approved for the control of chemotherapy-related nausea and vomiting that are resistant to conventional antiemetics, for breakthrough postoperative nausea and vomiting, and for appetite stimulation in patients with human immunodeficiency virus (HIV) patients with anorexia-cachexia syndrome.[59] The claims of benefit in the other medical conditions are not clearly supported by evidence.[6,170]

PHARMACOLOGY AND PATHOPHYSIOLOGY

The term *cannabinoid* refers to compounds that bind to the cannabinoid receptors regardless of whether they are derived from plants (phytocannabinoids), synthetic processes (SCs), or endogenous sources (endocannabinoids). At one time, the term may have been used to delineate a structural similarity to Δ^9-THC, but this naming convention was largely abandoned during the past 30 years of cannabinoid research as new compounds were discovered and synthesized. The structural diversity of cannabinoid receptor ligands and the absence of a true pharmacophore make nomenclature based purely on structure cumbersome and inconsistent. It is preferable then to use the term *cannabinoid* to denote receptor binding and subclassify cannabinoids further based on origin and structure (Fig. 74–1). The *terms cannabinoid, cannabinometic,* and *cannabinoid receptor agonist* are interchangeable.

Cannabis is a collective term referring to the bioactive substances from the cannabis plant. The *Cannabis* genus (species *sativa* and *indica*) produces more than 60 chemicals (C21 group) called cannabinoids. The major cannabinoids are cannabinol, cannabidiol (CBD), and tetrahydrocannabinol. The principal psychoactive cannabinoid is THC, also known as Δ^9-tetrahydrocannabinol. *Marijuana* is the common name for a mixture of dried leaves and flowers of the *C. sativa* plant. Hashish and hashish oil are the pressed resin and the oil expressed from the pressed resin, respectively. The concentration of THC varies from 1% in low-potency marijuana up to 50% in hash oil. Δ^9-Tetrahydrocannabinol extracted from marijuana using butane (butane hash oil or BHO) approaches THC concentrations of 100%. Pure THC and several pharmaceutical SCs are available by prescription with the generic names of dronabinol and nabilone, respectively. Nabiximol is the generic name for an oral mucosal spray containing THC and cannabidiol, which is approved for medical use in Canada, the United Kingdom, and parts of Europe. Unregulated SCs originally designed as research chemicals have emerged as designer drugs of abuse over the past several years.

Cannabinoid receptors are G protein–linked neuromodulators that inhibit adenyl cyclase in a dose-dependent and stereospecific manner. Although historically the cannabinoid receptor system is described as having a central CB_1 and a peripheral CB_2 receptor, the available evidence points to the central nervous system (CNS) presence of CB_2 receptors.[147] The two currently identified cannabinoid receptors are labeled CB_1 and CB_2 and are distinguished largely by their anatomic distribution and mechanisms of cellular messaging (Fig. 74–2).

CB_1 Receptors and the Psychogenic Effects of Cannabis

The CB_1 receptors are structurally composed of seven transmembrane protein units coupled to pertussis-sensitive (decrease adenyl cyclase) G proteins. They exhibit genetic variation via splice variants and are found as heterodimers with a multitude of other receptor types.[67]

Isolated agonism of CB_2 receptors was the target for novel pharmaceutical candidates as antiinflammatory agents with minimal success as the psychoactive effects of CB_1 agonism persisted.

The CB_1 receptors are the most numerous G protein–coupled receptors in the mammalian brain, accounting for the multiple and varied effects of cannabinoids on behavior, learning, and mood as well as suggesting the enormous complexity of the endocannabinoid system.[58] The highest concentration of CB_1 receptors is located in areas of the brain associated with movement and higher functions of cognition and emotions. A relative lack of CB_1 receptors in the brainstem also explains lack of coma and respiratory depression that occurs with *Cannabis* use.

Mechanism of Cellular Signaling

Cannabinoid receptors both in the CNS and in the periphery exist on the presynaptic terminus of various neurons. Depolarization in the postsynaptic portion of the neuron and subsequent increase in intracellular Ca^{2+} leads to on-demand synthesis and release of endocannabioids.[117] These free fatty acid–based messengers diffuse into the synapse and bind to the presynaptic cannabinoid receptor. Ligand binding causes conformational change in the G protein subunits and inhibition of adenyl cyclase, resulting in decreased intracellular cyclic adenosine monophosphate (cAMP) concentrations, decreased activity of voltage-gated Ca^{2+} channels, and ultimately decreased neurotransmitter release (Fig. 74–2). Exogenous cannabinoids act similarly to endogenous cannabinoids upon receptor binding, except that binding affinity will vary among exogenous ligands and endogenous cannabinoids, which are rapidly metabolized by fatty acid amide hydrolases.[84] Interestingly, some online chemical suppliers offer fatty acid amide hydrolase inhibitors for sale, along with various SCs, perhaps providing a glimpse into future products more closely related to endocannabinoids coming to market.

Both receptors inhibit adenyl cyclase and stimulate K^+ channel conductance.[121] CB_1 receptors are located either presynaptically or postsynaptically, and their activation can inhibit or enhance the release of acetylcholine, L-glutamate, γ-aminobutyric acid, noradrenaline, dopamine, and 5-hydroxytryptamine.[71,77,140]

The neuropharmacologic mechanisms by which cannabinoids produce their psychoactive effects are not fully elucidated.[60,71,121] Nevertheless, activity at the CB_1 receptors is believed to be responsible for the clinical effects of cannabinoids,[12,40,71,153] including the regulation of cognition, memory, motor activities, nociception, nausea, and vomiting. Chronic administration of a cannabinoid agonist reduces CB_1 receptor density in several regions of the rat brain.[13]

PHARMACOKINETICS AND TOXICOKINETICS

Absorption

The pharmacokinetics of phytocannabinoids was extensively reviewed.[50] The rate and completeness of absorption of cannabinoids depend on the route of administration and the type of cannabis product.

Inhalation of smoke containing THC results in the onset of psychoactive effects within minutes typically reaching peak serum concentration before

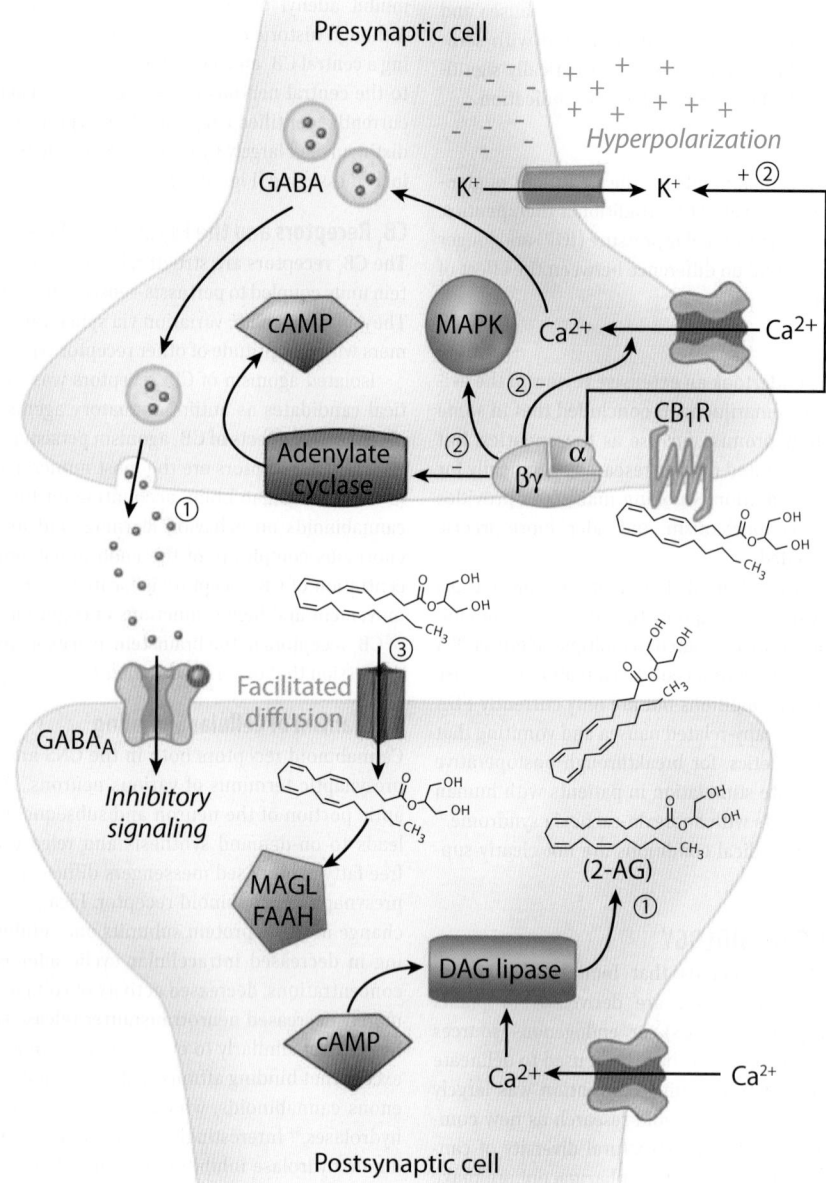

FIGURE 74–2. Endocannabinoids act as allosteric cellular messengers. ① In response to presynaptic γ-aminobutyric acid (GABA) release and postsynaptic binding resulting in increased cyclic adenosine monophosphate (cAMP), endocannabinoids are synthesized on demand and bind to presynaptic cannabinoid receptors. ② Activation of these G protein receptors results in decreased presynaptic adenylate cyclase, decreased cAMP, decreased calcium ion influx, and increased potassium efflux. The net results are hyperpolarization of the presynaptic cell and decreased neurotransmitter release. ③ After binding, endocannabinoids diffuse back to the postsynaptic area, where they undergo degradation by monoacylglycerol lipase (MAGL) and fatty acid amide hydrolase (FAAH). CB₁R = cannabinoid type ₁ receptor; DAG lipase = diacylglycerol lipase; MAPK = mitogen-activated protein kinase. 2-AG=2-arachidonoylglycerol. *(Adapted with permission from Seely KA, Prather PL, James LP, et al. Marijuana-based drugs: innovative therapeutics or designer drugs of abuse? Mol Interv. 2011 Feb;11(1):36-51.)*

finishing the cigarette. From 10% to 35% of available THC is absorbed during smoking, and peak serum. Peak serum concentrations depend on the dose. A marijuana cigarette containing 1.75% THC produces a peak serum THC concentration of approximately 85 ng/mL.[63]

Ingestion of cannabis results in an unpredictable onset of psychoactive effects in 1 to 3 hours. Only 5% to 20% of available THC reaches the systemic circulation after ingestion. Peak serum THC concentrations usually occur 2 to 4 hours after ingestion, but delays up to 6 hours are described.[86] Dronabinol has an oral bioavailability of approximately 10% with high interindividual variability.[47,111] Nabilone has an oral bioavailability estimated to be greater than 90% and reaches peak serum concentrations 2 hours after ingestion.[137]

Distribution

Δ⁹-Tetrahydrocannabinol has a steady-state volume of distribution of approximately 2.5 to 3.5 L/kg.[47] Cannabinoids are lipid soluble and accumulate in fatty tissue in a biphasic pattern. Initially, THC is distributed to highly vascularized tissues such as the liver, kidneys, heart, and muscle. After smoking or intravenous (IV) administration, the distribution half-life is less than 10 minutes.[64] After the initial distribution phase, THC accumulates more slowly in less vascularized tissues and body fat. Repeated administration of Δ⁸-THC (an isomer of Δ⁹-THC) to rats over 2 weeks resulted in steadily increasing concentrations of Δ⁸-THC in body fat and liver but not in brain tissue. After administration of Δ⁸-THC stopped, the cannabinoids are slowly released from fat stores during adipose tissue turnover.[116]

Δ^9-Tetrahydrocannabinol crosses the placenta and enters the breast milk. Concentrations in fetal serum are 10% to 30% of maternal concentrations. Daily cannabis smoking by a nursing mother resulted in concentrations of THC in breast milk eightfold higher than concomitant maternal serum concentrations; THC metabolites do not accumulate in breast milk.[123]

Metabolism

Δ^9-Tetrahydrocannabinol is nearly completely metabolized by hepatic microsomal hydroxylation and oxidation (primarily CYP2C9 and CYP3A4).[50] The primary metabolite (11-hydroxy-Δ^9-THC or 11-OH-THC) is active and is subsequently oxidized to the inactive 11-nor-Δ^9-THC carboxylic acid metabolite (THC-COOH) and many other inactive metabolites.[1,4,127]

In six volunteers, peak serum THC concentrations occurred at 8 minutes (range, 6–10 minutes) after the onset of smoking, peak 11-OH-THC at 13 minutes (range, 9–23 minutes), and peak THC-COOH at 120 minutes (range, 48–240 minutes) (Fig. 74–3).[63] Approximately 1 hour after beginning to smoke a marijuana cigarette, the THC to 11-OH-THC ratio is 3:1, and the THC to THC-COOH ratio is 1:2; at approximately 2 hours, the ratios are 2.5:1 and 1:8, respectively; and at 3 hours, the ratios are 2:1 and 1:16, respectively.[63] Ingestion of cannabis results in much more variable concentrations and time courses of THC and metabolites (Fig. 74–3). Nonetheless, at 2 to 3 hours after ingestion, the ratios are similar to those after smoking: THC to 11-OH-THC is 2:1, and THC to THC-COOH ranges from 1:7 to 1:14.[165] Δ^9-Tetrahydrocannabinol is detectable in serum 1.5 to 4.5 hours after ingestion of dronabinol.[46]

Of the many aminoalkylindole (AAI) SCs isolated in "Spice" incense blends, human metabolic analyses are only published for JWH-018, JWH-073, and AM 2201.[14,15] In contrast to THC, these cannabinoids are metabolized largely through hydroxylation and oxidation by CYP2C9 and CYP1A2 (with minor contributions of CYP2D6) to active metabolites that retain affinity for and in most are agonists at both CB_1 and CB_2 receptors.[27,28] These metabolites undergo glucuronic acid conjugation in phase II metabolism.

Excretion

Reported elimination half-lives of THC and its major metabolites vary considerably. After IV doses of THC, the mean elimination half-life ranges from 1.6 to 57 hours.[50] Elimination half-lives are expected to be similar after inhalation.[50,63] The elimination half-life of 11-OH-THC is 12 to 36 hours, and that of THC-COOH ranges from 1 to 6 days.[79,165]

Δ^9-Tetrahydrocannabinol and its metabolites are excreted in the urine and the feces. In the 72 hours after ingestion, approximately 15% of a THC dose is excreted in the urine, and roughly 50% is excreted in the feces.[1,21,168] After IV administration, approximately 15% of a THC dose is excreted in the urine, and only 25% to 35% is excreted in the feces.[165] Inhalation is expected to produce results similar to IV administration.[50,63] Within 5 days, 80% to 90% of a THC dose is excreted from the body.[55,68]

Cannabinoids were measured in the urine after smoking a marijuana cigarette containing 27 mg of THC (Fig. 74–3).[94] After smoking THC, urine concentrations peaked at 2 hours (mean, 21.5 ng/mL; range, 3.2–53.3 ng/mL) and were undetectable (<1.5 ng/mL) in five of the eight participants by 6 hours. Urine concentrations of 11-OH-THC peaked at 3 hours (77.3 ± 29.7 ng/mL). The primary urinary metabolite is the glucuronide conjugate of THC-COOH.[170] The urine concentration of THC-COOH peaks at 4 hours (179.4 ± 146.9 ng/mL),[95] and it has an average urinary excretion half-life of 2 to 3 days (range, 0.9–9.8 days).[50] Both 11-OH-THC and THC-COOH remained detectable in the urine of all eight participants for the 8 hours of the study.[94]

After discontinuation of use, metabolites are often detected in the urine of chronic users for several weeks.[39,74] Factors such as age, weight, and frequency of use only partially explained the long excretion period.[39] Primary urinary metabolites of nonclassical SCs are summarized in Fig. 74–4.

CLINICAL MANIFESTATIONS

The clinical effects of THC use, including time of onset and duration of effect, vary with the dose, the route of administration (ingestion is slower in onset than inhalation), the experience of the user, the vulnerability of the user to psychoactive effects, and the setting in which the THC is used. The concomitant use of CNS depressants such as ethanol or stimulants such as cocaine alters the psychological and physiological effects of marijuana. The therapeutic serum THC concentration for the treatment of nausea and vomiting is greater than 10 ng/mL.[23]

Psychological Effects

Use of marijuana produces variable psychological effects.[40] The variation, which occurs both between and within users, is likely the result of drug tolerance, phase of clinical effects, strain of cannabis, physical and social settings, or user expectations or cognitive capacity. The most commonly self-reported effect is relaxation. Other commonly reported effects are perceptual alterations (heightened sensory awareness, slowing of time), a feeling of well-being (including giddiness or laughter), and increased appetite.[49]

Physiological Effects

Use of cannabis is associated with physiologic effects on cerebral blood flow, the heart, the lungs, and the eyes. In a controlled, double-blind positron emission tomography study,[95] Intravenous THC increased cerebral blood flow, particularly in the frontal cortex, insula, cingulate gyrus, and subcortical regions. These increases in cerebral blood flow occurred 30 to 60 minutes after use and were still elevated at 120 minutes.[96] Similar blood flow changes result from smoking marijuana.[120]

Common acute cardiovascular effects of cannabis use include increases in heart rate and decreases in vascular resistance.[75,148] Cannabis produces dose-dependent increases in heart rate within 15 minutes of using a marijuana cigarette (from a baseline mean of 66 beats/min to a mean of 89 beats/min) that reach a maximum (mean, 92 beats/min) 10 to 15 minutes after peak serum THC concentrations. These changes last for 2 to 3 hours.[8] Increases in blood pressure occur with cannabis use. In a study of six participants, an increase in blood pressure from a baseline mean of 119/74 mm Hg to a mean of 129/81 mm Hg occurred but was not statistically significant.[8] In a double-blind, controlled study of men being investigated for angina pectoris, smoking a marijuana cigarette resulted in statistically significant changes in blood pressure from a baseline mean of 123/79 mm Hg to a peak mean of 132/84 mm Hg.[129] In contrast, in one study, repeated THC use resulted in significant slowing of heart rate (from a mean of 68 beats/min to a low of 62 beats/min) and lowering of blood pressure (from a mean of 116/62 mm Hg to a low of 108/53 mm Hg).[10] Decreased vascular tone causes postural hypotension accompanied by dizziness and syncope.

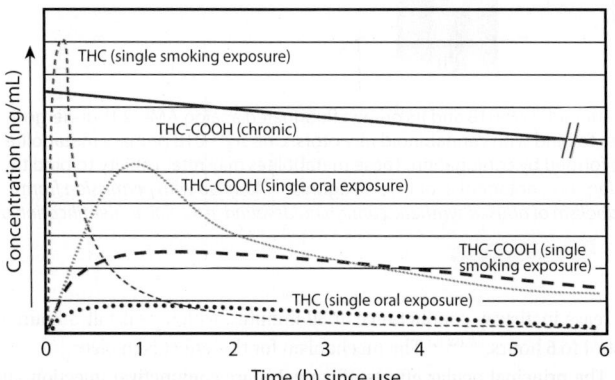

FIGURE 74–3. Estimated relative time course of Δ^9 tetrahydrocannabinol (THC) and its major metabolite in the urine based on the route of exposure. THC-COOH = Δ^9 THC carboxylic acid.

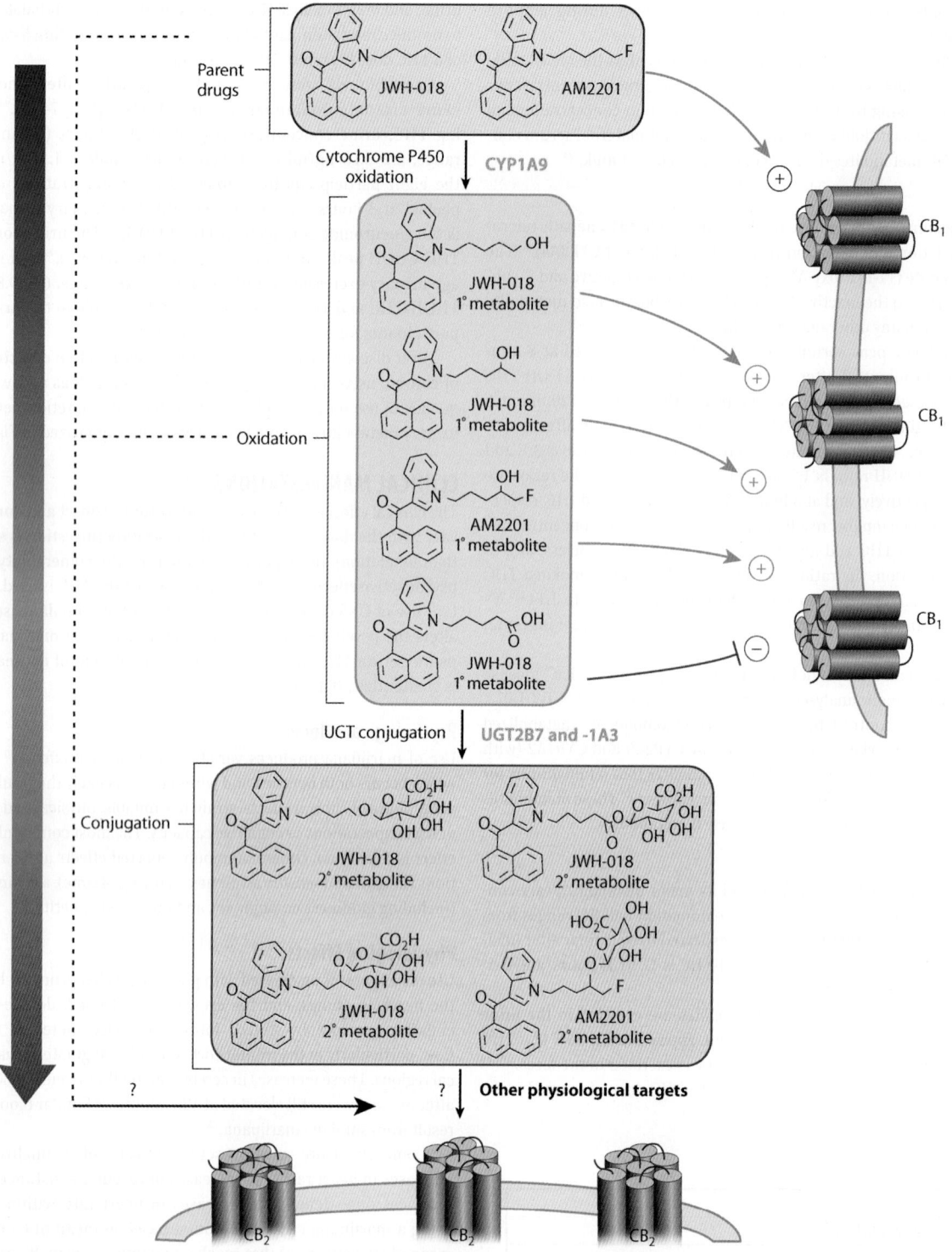

FIGURE 74–4. JWH-018 and AM-2201 metabolism. Aminoalkylindole synthetic cannabinoid JWH-018 and its omega fluorinated analog AM-2201 undergo oxidation by CYP2C9 and CYP1A9 to primary metabolites that retain affinity and ability to bind with cannabinoid receptors. One JWH-018 primary metabolite acts as an antagonist at cannabinoid type 1 receptor (CB₁). Secondary metabolites are formed by conjugation. These metabolites may retain ability to bind to cannabinoid receptors, but at this time it is unclear which do so and in what capacity (agonist, antagonist, or inverse agonist). *(Adapted with permission from Chimalakonda KC, Seely KA, Bratton SM, et al. Cytochrome P450-mediated oxidative metabolism of abused synthetic cannabinoids found in K2/Spice: identification of novel cannabinoid receptor ligands. Drug Metab Dispos. 2012 Nov;40(11):2174-2184.)*

Inhalation or ingestion of THC produces a dose-related short-term decrease in airway resistance and an increase in airway conductance in both normal individuals and individuals with asthma.[156] Smoking marijuana results in an immediate increase in airway conductance, which peaks at 15 minutes and lasts 60 minutes. Ingestion of cannabis produces a significant increase in airway conductance at 30 minutes, which peaks at 3 hours and lasts 4 to 6 hours.[157,158,161] The mechanism for this effect is unclear.

The principal ocular effects of cannabis are conjunctival injection and a transient decrease in IOP. Cannabinoids, applied topically to a rabbit eye, resulted in hyperemia of the conjunctival blood vessels for 2 hours after application.[103] Regardless of route of administration, cannabis causes a fall in IOP in 60% of users[48] by acting on CB_1 receptors in the ciliary body.[126] The mean reduction in IOP is 25% and lasts 3 to 4 hours.

Physiological effects of novel SCs are not yet studied in any controlled settings.

ACUTE TOXICITY

In addition to the physiological and psychological effects described, acute toxicity includes decreases in coordination, muscle strength, and hand steadiness. Lethargy, sedation, postural hypotension, inability to concentrate, decreased psychomotor activity, slurred speech, and slow reaction time also occur.[115,168]

In young children, the acute ingestion of cannabis is potentially consequential.[93] Ingestion of estimated amounts of 250 to 1,000 mg of hashish resulted in obtundation in 30 to 75 minutes. Tachycardia (>150 beats/min) was found in one-third of the children. Less commonly reported findings include apnea, cyanosis, bradycardia, hypotonia, and opisthotonus.

The acute toxicity profile of nonclassical SCs stands in stark contrast to the relatively mild effects of smoked or ingested phytocannabinoid products. Given the general similarity in receptor binding, both users and clinicians initially expected the effects to be largely identical to marijuana and hashish. The significant differences are likely a result of AAI cannabinoids found in "incense blends" being more potent and efficacious at cannabinoid receptors as well as having active metabolites. Moreover, these products are unregulated, and the presence of additional xenobiotics, such as cathinones, methylxanthines, and long-acting β-adrenergic agonists such as clenbuterol must be considered.

The recent published reports of presumed SC toxicity are challenging to interpret because many lack laboratory confirmation of exposure. In addition, in cases involving "spice" blends, adverse effects may result from the plant matter or adulterants. Finally, the concentration of SCs varies by incense package, even of the same brand and lot, making dose estimation difficult if not impossible.

Agitation[142] and seizures are reported.[85,141] In one report with laboratory confirmation, a patient experienced multiple seizures within 30 minutes after ingesting JWH-018 in powder form.[85] The sample was confirmed as pure JWH-018.

Psychosis (new onset, acute exacerbation of existing psychiatric disorders, and increased risk of psychosis relapse) and anxiety have resulted after a single dose.[57,69,124]

Tachycardia was a common finding detailed in one series, and tachydysrhythmias requiring cardioversion are reported.[85] Chest pain and increased troponin concentrations were observed in three patients who claimed to have smoked spice several days before presenting to the hospital, but laboratory confirmation of SC exposure was not performed.[104]

Diffuse pulmonary infiltrates and dyspnea requiring intubation and mechanical ventilation were reported in a habitual spice user. Laboratory confirmation revealed three parent SCs (AM-2201, JWH-122, and JWH-210).[2]

Accounts of acute kidney injury are described in a case series of 16 previously healthy participants. All patients reported smoking spice incense blends before presentation. The patients had flank pain, nausea, and vomiting with elevated serum creatinine concentrations. Laboratory confirmation was achieved in eight of the patients, and a previously unreported SC was isolated (XLR-11). Several of the patients required hemodialysis, but all eventually recovered.[1]

Cerebral ischemia was reported in a patient using a product confirmed to contain XLR-11. The patient presented after smoking SC with right-sided weakness and later had CT of the brain confirming a left insular stroke. Forensic testing of the product revealed XLR-11, but neither the parent or metabolites could not be identified in the patient's urine, suggesting rapid metabolism.[155]

The fourth-generation indazole derivative SCs were likely responsible for several recent outbreaks of somnolence and bradycardia in suspected users.

This stands in contrast to earlier generations of SCs users who presented with sympathomimetic-like symptoms. Patients using nonclassical SCs respond to supportive care.[106]

ADVERSE REACTIONS
Acute Use

Cannabis users occasionally experience distrust, dysphoria, fear, panic reactions, or transient psychoses. Commonly reported adverse reactions at the prescribed dose of dronabinol or nabilone include postural hypotension, dizziness, sedation, xerostomia, abdominal discomfort, nausea, and vomiting. Acute pancreatitis (serum amylase concentration up to 3,200 IU/mL) after a period of heavy cannabis use is reported, but the causal relationship is unclear.[47]

Life-threatening ventricular tachycardia is reported.[132] In six individuals with acute cardiovascular deaths, postmortem whole-blood THC concentrations ranged from 2 to 22 ng/mL (mean, 7.2 ng/mL; median, 5 ng/mL).[5] Although the temporal association is clear, causality is less clear because three of the six people had significant preexisting cardiac pathology. The risk of myocardial infarction is increased five times over baseline in the 60 minutes after marijuana use, but subsequently declines rapidly to baseline risk levels.[105] Atrial fibrillation with palpitations, nausea, and dizziness was temporally associated with smoking marijuana in four patients.[41,83,151]

Chronic Use

Long-term use of cannabis is associated with a number of adverse effects.

Immune System

Cannabinoids affect host resistance to infection by modulating the secondary immune response (macrophages, T and B lymphocytes, acute phase and immune cytokines). However, an immune-mediated health risk from using cannabis was not documented.[81]

Respiratory System

Chronic use of smoked marijuana is associated with clinical findings compatible with obstructive lung disease.[161] Smoking marijuana delivers more particulates to the lower respiratory tract than does smoking tobacco,[171] and marijuana smoke contains carcinogens similar to tobacco smoke. Case reports and a hospital-based case control study suggest that cancers of the respiratory tract (mouth, larynx, sinuses, lung) are associated with daily or near daily smoking of marijuana, although exposure to tobacco smoke and ethanol may be confounding factors.[22,156,159] By contrast a systematic review and a cohort study with 8 years of follow-up demonstrated no association between marijuana smoking and smoking-related cancers,[53,99] and a population-based case-control study found that marijuana use was not associated with an increased risk of developing oral squamous cell carcinoma.[136]

Cardiovascular System

Marijuana use is a risk for individuals with coronary artery disease. An exploratory prospective study of self-reported marijuana use among patients admitted for myocardial infarction found that patients who used marijuana were at significantly increased risk for cardiovascular and noncardiovascular mortality compared with nonusers.[105,111]

Reproductive System

Reduced fertility in chronic users is a result of oligospermia, abnormal menstruation, and decreased ovulation.[18] Cannabis is probably the most common illicit drug of abuse during the reproductive age. No definitive patterns of malformations are recognized.[16] Statistically significant reductions in birth weight (mean, 79 g less than nonusers) and length (mean, 0.5 cm shorter than nonusers) are reported in women who had urine assays positive for cannabis during pregnancy.[163] The results of three other studies are difficult to interpret because marijuana use in pregnancy was poorly documented.[54,173] Epidemiologic studies based on self-reporting of cannabis use do not support an association between the use of cannabis during pregnancy and teratogenesis.[82,89,173]

The effect of maternal use of cannabis during pregnancy on neurobehavioral development in the offspring was studied. No detrimental effects were reported in children born to women who smoked marijuana daily (more than 21 cigarettes per week) in rural Jamaica.[36] Tremors and increased startling were reported in infants younger than 1 week of age whose mothers used cannabis during pregnancy.[43] These findings, which persisted beyond 3 days, were not associated with other signs of a withdrawal syndrome. There were no abnormalities in the children of parents who used more than five marijuana cigarettes per week in Ottawa, Canada, at 12, 24, and 36 months of age, but lower scores in verbal and memory domains at 48 months of age are reported.[42,44,55] The results of studies evaluating the effect of in utero exposure to cannabis on postnatal neurobehavioral development are equivocal because of methodologic concerns regarding exposure assessment and control of covariates,[33] including the continued parental use of cannabis during the postnatal and early childhood periods. The role of secondhand exposure to cannabis on postnatal and early childhood development of neurobehavioral problems remains unstudied.

Endocrine System

In experimental animals, cannabis exposure is associated with suppression of gonadal steroids, growth hormone, prolactin, and thyroid hormone. In addition, cannabis alters the activity of the hypothalamic-pituitary-adrenal axis.[18] In human studies, the results are inconsistent, long term effects are not demonstrated, and clinical consequences are undefined.[18]

Neurobehavioral Effects

There is a concern that chronic cannabis use results in deficits in cognition and learning that last well after cannabis use has stopped. Neuropsychological tests were administered to 27 adolescents:10 cannabis abusers, 8 infrequent cannabis abusers, and 9 who used no psychoactive substances showed significant differences that persisted for the duration of the study (6 weeks of abstinence) between the cannabis group and the other groups in a visual retention test and a memory test.[145] In a study of three experienced marijuana smokers, arithmetic and recall tasks were impaired for up to 24 hours after smoking.[56] Adults who used cannabis more than seven times per week had impairments in math skills, verbal expression, and memory retrieval processes; people who used cannabis one to six times per week showed no impairments.[11] After 1 day of abstinence, 65 heavy marijuana users (median, use on 29 of past 30 days) showed greater impairment on neuropsychological tests of attention and executive functions than light marijuana users (median, use on 1 day of past 30 days).[125] The authors were uncertain whether this difference was caused by residual THC in the brain, a withdrawal effect from the drug, or a direct neurotoxic effect of cannabis.

There is little evidence that adverse cognitive effects persist after stopping the use of cannabis[72] or that cannabis use causes psychosocial harm to the user.[92] Patients using cannabinoids at younger ages, those using potent cannabinoids such as SCs, and those who have underlying psychiatric disorders are more likely to exhibit psychotic features after cannabinoid exposure.[9,130] An "amotivational syndrome" is attributed to cannabis use. The syndrome is a poorly defined complex of characteristics such as apathy, underachievement, and lack of energy.[26,144] The association of the syndrome with cannabis use is based primarily on anecdotal, uncontrolled observations.[60] Anthropologic field studies, evaluations of US college students, and controlled laboratory experiments have failed to identify a causal relationship between cannabis use and the amotivational syndrome.[60] A study evaluating the role of depression in the amotivational syndrome found significantly lower scores on "need for achievement" scales in heavy users (median, daily use for 6 years) with depressive symptoms compared with heavy users without depressive symptoms and light users (median, several times per month for 4.5 years) with or without depressive symptoms.[113] These data suggest that symptoms attributed to an amotivational syndrome are caused by depression, not cannabis.

Another study found that behavior that could be interpreted as amotivation was inversely related to the perceived size of the reward.[26]

Abuse, Dependence, and Withdrawal

The *Diagnostic and Statistical Manual of Mental Disorders*, 5th edition, defines marijuana abuse as repeated instances of use under hazardous conditions; repeated, clinically meaningful impairment in social, occupational, or educational functioning; or legal problems related to marijuana use. The amount, frequency, and duration of cannabis use required to develop dependence are not well established.[25,154] Much of the support for cannabis dependence is based on the existence of a withdrawal syndrome. In animals repeatedly given cannabis, the administration of a CB$_1$ receptor antagonist produced signs of withdrawal.[87,152] In humans, chronic users experience unpleasant effects when abstaining from cannabis.[19] The time of onset of withdrawal symptoms is not well characterized.[18] The most reliably reported effects are irritability, restlessness, and nervousness as well as appetite and sleep disturbances.[152] Other reported acute withdrawal manifestations include tremor, diaphoresis, fever, and nausea. These symptoms and signs are reversed by the oral administration of THC.[9,51] The duration of withdrawal manifestations, without treatment, is not clearly established.[20,152] There are reports of a withdrawal syndrome observed after heavy and prolonged nonclassical SC use.[32,91,114,139]

Cannabinoid Hyperemesis Syndrome

Chronic, heavy marijuana use is associated with a clinical syndrome (CHS) composed of abdominal discomfort, nausea, and hyperemesis. Symptoms are often refractory to opioids and antiemetics.[166] Patients typically have multiple visits to the emergency department and are subjected to a host of diagnostic and therapeutic modalities ranging from CT scans and endoscopy to cholecystectomy. The hallmark of the syndrome is almost immediate relief of symptoms with bathing or showering in hot water, and a major diagnostic feature is compulsive bathing. The pathophysiology of this syndrome is unclear. In animal models, excessive cannabinoid administration results in downregulation of CB$_1$ receptors. Endogenous cannabinoids, such as anandamide, demonstrate increased binding affinity for other G protein receptors such as transient receptor potential cation channel subfamily V member 1 (TPRV1).

Relief with hot water may indicate dysfunction of pain perception, excess substance P release, and involvement of TRPV1 which these factors may assist in elucidating the mechanism for this syndrome as well as providing new treatment modalities.[133] This hypothesis is supported by reports of successful treatment of CHS treatment with topical capsaicin. Ultimately, resolution of this syndrome depends on cessation of marijuana use.[3,24,35,45,149,150,166]

Reports also exist of successful CHS treatment with, benzodiazepines, dopamine antagonists, and substance P inhibitors. Opioids are not shown to be effective and are not indicated. Upon discharge, patients should be educated that the syndrome will likely return if the individual continues to use exogenous cannabinoids, and full resolution of symptoms should take place in 10 to 14 days.

CANNABIS AND DRIVING

The perceptual alterations caused by cannabis suggest that its recent use could be associated with automobile crashes. Experimental and epidemiologic studies have provided limited evidence with regard to the effects of cannabis use on driving ability. The published analytical studies of the relationship between cannabis and driving behavior and motor vehicle crashes were reviewed elsewhere.[7] In experimental driving studies, cannabis impairs driving ability, but cannabis using drivers recognize their impairment and compensate for it by driving at slower speeds and increasing following distance. However, the slower reaction time caused by cannabis results in impaired emergency response behavior.

The epidemiologic studies evaluating the association of cannabis use and traffic crashes provide no evidence that cannabis alone increases the risk of causing fatal crashes or serious injuries.[7,119] Regardless, cannabis use decreases reaction times and results in significant driving impairment.[52] One study comparing past driving records of subjects entering a drug treatment center with control participants found that a self-reported history of cannabis use was associated with a statistically significant increase in adjusted relative risk for all crashes (relative risk, 1.49; 95% confidence interval {CI}, 1.17–1.89) and for "at fault" crashes (relative risk, 1.68; 95%CI, 1.21–2.34).[29]

DIAGNOSTIC TESTING

Cannabinoids can be detected in plasma or urine. Immunoassays are routinely available; gas chromatography–mass spectrometry (GC-MS) is the most specific assay and is considered the reference method.

Enzyme-multiplied immunoassay technique (EMIT) is a qualitative urine test that is often used for screening purposes. Enzyme-multiplied immunoassay technique identifies the metabolites of THC. In these tests, the concentrations of all metabolites present are additive. For the EMIT II Cannabinoid Assay, the cutoff concentration for distinguishing positive from negative samples is 20 ng/mL. A positive test result means that the total concentration of all the assayed metabolites present in the urine is at least 20 ng/mL. A positive urine test result for cannabis only indicates the presence of cannabinoids, and it does not identify which metabolites are present or at what concentrations. Qualitative urine test results do not indicate or measure toxicity or degree of exposure. The National Institute on Drug Abuse guidelines for urine testing specify test cutoff concentrations of 50 ng/mL for screening and 15 ng/mL for confirmation.

Variables affecting the duration of detection of urinary metabolites include dose, duration of use, acute versus chronic use, route of exposure, and sensitivity of the method. In addition, factors affecting the quantitative values of urine THC and metabolites include urine volume, concentration, and pH. Using GC/MS, metabolites are typically detected in the urine up to 7 days after the use of single marijuana cigarette.[64,65]

The length of time between stopping cannabis use and a negative EMIT urine test result (<20 ng/mL) depends on the extent of use. Release of THC from adipose tissue is important in drug test interpretation because many chronic users release cannabinoids in quantities sufficient to result in positive urine test results for several weeks. In addition, vigorous exercise stimulates the release of cannabinoids from fat depots. In light users being tested daily under observed abstinence, the mean time to the first negative urine test result is 8.5 days (range, 3–18 days), and the mean time to the last positive urine is 18.2 days (range, 7–34 days).[39] In heavy users (mean, 9 years of using at least once a day) being tested under the same conditions, the mean time to the first negative urine test result (EMIT assay less than 20 ng/mL) was 19.1 days (range, 3–46 days), and the mean time to the last positive urine sample was 31.5 days (range, 4–77 days).[39]

Standard laboratory analyses identify THC and its metabolites but cannot identify the source of the THC (eg, marijuana, hashish, dronabinol). Immunoassays for THC will not identify nabilone because it is not THC; however, nabilone can be specifically identified using high-performance liquid chromatography–tandem mass spectrometry.[146]

Immunoassays give false-negative and false-positive test results (Table 74–1). To help identify evidence tampering, negative urine immunoassays should be accompanied by examining the urine for clarity and measuring urinary specific gravity, pH, temperature, and creatinine[146,163] (Chap. 7).

Immunoassays for THC will not detect nonclassical SCs or their metabolites. Commercial urine immunoassays are available but need to be directed toward a specific nonclassical SCs. High-performance liquid chromatography–tandem mass spectrometry or gas chromatography mass spectrometry are currently the gold standard for laboratory confirmation for SCs, but their clinical utility is limited retrospective confirmation. Further challenges are presented by the multitude of known nonclassical SCs and the rate at which new illicit SCs are introduced to the illegal high market.[49,70,76,78,107,108,135,160,164]

TABLE 74–1	Xenobiotics or Conditions Reported to Produce Inaccurate Screening Test Results for Tetrahydrocannabinol
False Negative[a]	**False Positive**
Bleach (NaOCl)	Dronabinol
Citric acid	Efavirenz
Detergent additives	Ethacrynic acid
Dettol	Hemp seed oil
Dilution	Nonsteroidal antiinflammatory drugs
Glutaraldehyde	Promethazine
Lemon juice	Riboflavin
Niacin	
Potassium nitrite (KNO$_2$)	
Table salt (NaCl)	
Tetrahydrozoline	
Vinegar (acetic acid)	
Water	

[a]Xenobiotics "possibly" producing false-negative urine test results are usually added to a urine sample, not ingested.

Passive Inhalation

Studies of passive exposure to marijuana smoke and the urinary excretion of cannabinoids have used enclosed spaces with nonsmokers present during and after active smoking by others.[31,86,110,119,122] In an unventilated room (12,225.8 L of air), five adult volunteers were exposed to the side stream smoke of 4 or 16 marijuana cigarettes (THC, 25 mg/cigarette) smoked simultaneously over 1 hour on each of 6 consecutive days.[33] After being exposed to four marijuana cigarettes, four of the volunteers had at least one positive urine by EMIT assay (cutoff, 20 ng/mL) at some unspecified time during the six study days; exposure to 16 marijuana cigarettes resulted in positive EMIT assays only after the second day of exposure.

In a car (1,650 L of air), three adult volunteers were exposed to the smoke from 12 marijuana cigarettes smoked by two people over 30 minutes.[110] Enzyme-multiplied immunoassay technique analyses of urine samples from one passive inhaler were positive at time 0 to 4 hours and on days 2 and 3; a second passive inhaler had one positive urine test result at time 4 to 24 hours after exposure.

Three adult volunteers in an unventilated room (21,600 L of air) were exposed to the side stream smoke of four marijuana cigarettes (THC, 27 mg/cigarette) smoked simultaneously over 1 hour.[112] The concentrations of cannabinoids in urine samples taken 20 to 24 hours after exposure were less than 6 ng/mL when analyzed using radioimmunoassay (RIA) methodology. Another study used an unventilated room (total volume of 27,950 L) containing three desks and a filing cabinet.[86] Over 10 to 34 minutes, each of six volunteers smoked a marijuana cigarette (THC, 17.1 mg/cigarette) and left the room. Four nonsmoking men were in the study room for 3 hours from the start of smoking. The door was opened and closed 18 times during the study. The maximum urine cannabinoid concentration (measured by RIA) in the nonsmokers was 6.8 ng/mL at 6 hours after the start of smoking.

Another study used a closed room (15,500 L of air) with each of four participants smoking two marijuana cigarettes containing 2.5% THC on one occasion and 2.8% THC on a second occasion.[122] On each occasion, two nonsmoking participants were in the room for 1 hour from the onset of smoking. None of the nonsmokers' urine samples (0–24 hours) from either exposure period tested positive on an EMIT assay with a cutoff of 20 ng/mL. An identical experiment in a closed car (~3,500 L of air) resulted in 1 of 23 urine specimens testing positive at 6 hours.

Therefore, passive inhalation of marijuana smoke is unlikely to result in positive urine test results unless the exposure is substantial.

Saliva

Saliva samples are used to establish the presence of cannabinoids and time of cannabis consumption. Cannabinoids (THC, THC-COOH, 11-OH-THC) in saliva are derived from either the smoke of the marijuana or hashish or from a preliminary metabolism in the mouth.[143] Saliva THC concentrations above 10 ng/mL are consistent with recent use and correlate with subjective toxicity and heart rate changes.[101]

Hair

Hair sample analysis is not useful in identifying THC or its metabolites. Only small quantities of non–nitrogen-containing substances, such as cannabinoids, are found in hair pigments.[37,80,102]

Sweat

Perspiration deposits drug metabolites on the skin, and these are renewed even after the skin is washed. Detection threshold is reported to be 10 ng/mL, but forensic confirmation by alternative means is required.[80]

Estimating Time of Exposure

A measurable serum concentration of THC is consistent with recent exposure and toxicity, but there is poor correlation between serum THC concentrations and actual clinical effects.[61] The ratio of THC to THC-COOH is used to estimate time of smoking marijuana. Similar concentrations of each indicate cannabis use within 20 to 40 minutes and imply toxicity. In naïve users, a concentration of THC-COOH that is greater than THC indicates that use probably occurred more than 30 minutes ago. The high background concentrations of THC-COOH in habitual users make estimations of time of exposure unreliable in this population.

Serum concentrations of THC and THC-COOH were used in a logarithmic equation to predict the time since smoking a marijuana cigarette.[94] The ratio provided acceptable results up to 3 hours after smoking (predicted time of exposure averaged 27 minutes longer than actual exposure time), but more than 3 hours after smoking, the predicted exposure time was overestimated by 3 hours. Mean overestimations of predicted exposure time of 2.5 to 4.2 hours for smoking and of 1.6 hours for ingestions are reported when serum samples are taken more than 4 hours after exposure.[63]

Chronic use or oral administration of cannabis increases the concentration of 11-OH-THC relative to the concentrations of THC or THC-COOH. In these cases, estimating time of exposure based on relative concentrations is problematic.[62] In four participants, ingestion of cannabis produced total serum metabolite concentrations less than 20 times the serum THC concentration for 3 hours after ingestion, suggesting that a ratio of this magnitude is consistent with recent oral consumption.[86]

MANAGEMENT

Gastrointestinal (GI) decontamination is not recommended for patients who ingest cannabis products, nabilone, dronabinol, or nonclassical SCs because clinical toxicity is rarely serious and responds to supportive care. In addition, a patient with a significantly altered mental status, such as somnolence, agitation, or anxiety, has risks associated with GI decontamination that outweigh the potential benefits of the intervention.

We recommend that agitation, anxiety seizures or transient psychotic episodes be treated with quiet reassurance and benzodiazepines (midazolam 1–2 mg intramuscularly or diazepam 5–10 mg intravenously) as needed. The management of patients exposed to SCs should not be expected to mirror that of THC or prescription THC-based cannabinoids. Symptomatic and supportive care is often necessary.

Laboratory evaluation should be initiated for signs of electrolyte disturbances and direct toxicity of the CNS, cardiovascular, renal, and musculoskeletal systems. Appropriate crystalloid fluid resuscitation should be given for rhabdomyolysis and acute kidney injury.

Antipsychotics are not recommended at this time during any phase of undifferentiated agitated delirium. If psychotic features persist after the resolution of sympathomimetic features, a quiet space with close observation

is indicated, and antipsychotic medications are reasonable if resolution is prolonged. Patients should be observed until asymptomatic.

If available, drug samples in addition to the patient's blood and urine, although not clinically useful, may aid in unknown designer SC identification and understanding of clinical effects.

There are no specific antidotes for cannabis or SC toxicity. Coingestants, such as cocaine, ethanol, designer amphetamines, methylxanthines, and long-acting β-adrenergic agonists, should be identified and their effects anticipated and treated as indicated.

SUMMARY

- Phytocannabinoids were used for centuries both as medicinal substances and as intoxicants.
- Despite the collective human history with cannabinoids, we are only beginning to understand the endocannabinoid system and the consequences of alterations to that system.
- Medical use of THC and smoked marijuana have long existed, and although the safety profile of these xenobiotics is established, evidence of the efficacy of medical marijuana over the gamut of currently prescribed maladies is sparse. Still, the cannabinoid system provides an attractive target for treatment of chronic pain and appetite modulation, but more rigorous and properly designed investigations are needed.
- The toxicity profile of traditional cannabinoids and designer SCs used as drugs of abuse and research chemicals are as different as their chemical structures. Clinicians, users, and public health policy makers alike would do well to separate these groups of cannabinoids in both thought and practice.

Acknowledgment

Michael A. McGuigan, MD, contributed to this chapter in previous editions.

REFERENCES

1. Agurell S, et al. Pharmacokinetics and metabolism of delta 1-tetrahydrocannabinol and other cannabinoids with emphasis on man. *Pharmacol Rev.* 1986;38:21-43.
2. Alhadi S, et al. High times, low sats: diffuse pulmonary infiltrates associated with chronic synthetic cannabinoid use. *J Med Toxicol.* 2013;9:199-206.
3. Allen JH, et al. Cannabinoid hyperemesis: cyclical hyperemesis in association with chronic cannabis abuse. *Gut.* 2004;53:1566-1570.
4. Anderson PO, McGuire GG. Delta-9-tetrahydrocannabinol as an antiemetic. *Am J Hosp Pharm.* 1981;38:639-646.
5. Bachs L, Morland H. Acute cardiovascular fatalities following cannabis use. *Forensic Sci Int.* 2001;124:200-203.
6. Bagshaw SM, Hagen NA. Medical efficacy of cannabinoids and marijuana: a comprehensive review of the literature. *J Palliat Care.* 2002;18:111-122.
7. Bates MN, Blakely TA. Role of cannabis in motor vehicle crashes. *Epidemiol Rev.* 1999;21:222-232.
8. Beaconsfield P, et al. Marihuana smoking. Cardiovascular effects in man and possible mechanisms. *N Engl J Med.* 1972;287:209-212.
9. Ben AM, Potvin S. Cannabis and psychosis: what is the link? *J Psychoactive Drugs.* 2007;39:131-142.
10. Benowitz NL, Jones RT. Cardiovascular effects of prolonged delta-9-tetrahydrocannabinol ingestion. *Clin Pharmacol Ther.* 1975;18:287-297.
11. Block RI, Ghoneim MM. Effects of chronic marijuana use on human cognition. *Psychopharmacology (Berl).* 1993;110:219-228.
12. Breivogel CS, Childers SR. The functional neuroanatomy of brain cannabinoid receptors. *Neurobiol Dis.* 1998;5:417-431.
13. Breivogel CS, et al. Chronic delta9-tetrahydrocannabinol treatment produces a time-dependent loss of cannabinoid receptors and cannabinoid receptor-activated G proteins in rat brain. *J Neurochem.* 1999;73:2447-2459.
14. Brents LK, et al. Monohydroxylated metabolites of the K2 synthetic cannabinoid JWH-073 retain intermediate to high cannabinoid 1 receptor (CB1R) affinity and exhibit neutral antagonist to partial agonist activity. *Biochem Pharmacol.* 2012;83:952-961.
15. Brents LK, et al. Phase I hydroxylated metabolites of the K2 synthetic cannabinoid JWH-018 retain in vitro and in vivo cannabinoid 1 receptor affinity and activity. *PLoS One.* 2011;6:e21917.
16. Briggs GG, et al. *Drugs in Pregnancy and Lactation: A Reference Guide to Fetal and Neonatal Risk.* Philadelphia, PA: Lippincott Williams & Wilkins; 2012.
17. Broder LE, et al. A randomized blinded clinical trial comparing delta-9-tetrahydrocannabinol (THC) and hydroxizine (HZ) as antiemetics (AE) for cancer chemotherapy (CT). *Proc Am Assoc Cancer Res.* 1982;23:514.
18. Brown TT, Dobs AS. Endocrine effects of marijuana. *J Clin Pharmacol.* 2002;42:90S-96S.

19. Budney AJ, Hughes JR. The cannabis withdrawal syndrome. *Curr Opin Psychiatry.* 2006;19:233-238.
20. Budney AJ, Moore BA. Development and consequences of cannabis dependence. *J Clin Pharmacol.* 2002;42:28S-33S.
21. Busto U, et al. Clinical pharmacokinetics of non-opiate abused drugs. *Clin Pharmacokinet.* 1989;16:1-26.
22. Caplan GA. Marihuana and mouth cancer. *J Royal Soc Med.* 1991;84:386.
23. Chang AE, et al. Delata-9-tetrahydrocannabinol as an antiemetic in cancer patients receiving high-dose methotrexate. A prospective, randomized evaluation. *Ann Intern Med.* 1979;91:819-824.
24. Chang YH, Windish DM. Cannabinoid hyperemesis relieved by compulsive bathing. *Mayo Clin Proc.* 2009;84:76-78.
25. Chen K, et al. Relationships between frequency and quantity of marijuana use and last year proxy dependence among adolescents and adults in the United States. *Drug Alcohol Depend.* 1997;46:53-67.
26. Cherek DR, et al. Possible amotivational effects following marijuana smoking under laboratory conditions. *Exp Clin Psychopharmacol.* 2002;10:26-38.
27. Chimalakonda KC, et al. Conjugation of synthetic cannabinoids JWH-018 and JWH-073, metabolites by human UDP-glucuronosyltransferases. *Drug Metab Dispos.* 2011;39:1967-1976.
28. Chimalakonda KC, et al. Cytochrome P450-mediated oxidative metabolism of abused synthetic cannabinoids found in K2/spice: identification of novel cannabinoid receptor ligands. *Drug Metab Dispos.* 2012;40:2174-2184.
29. Chipman ML, et al. Being "at fault" in traffic crashes: does alcohol, cannabis, cocaine, or polydrug abuse make a difference? *Inj Prev.* 2003;9:343-348.
30. Clark WC, et al. Effects of moderate and high doses of marihuana on thermal pain: a sensory decision theory analysis. *J Clin Pharmacol.* 1981;21:299S-310S.
31. Cone EJ, et al. Passive inhalation of marijuana smoke: urinalysis and room air levels of delta-9-tetrahydrocannabinol. *J Anal Toxicol.* 1987;11:89-96.
32. Cooper ZD. Adverse effects of synthetic cannabinoids: management of acute toxicity and withdrawal. *Curr Psychiatry Rep.* 2016;18:52.
33. Day NL, Richardson GA. Prenatal marijuana use: epidemiology, methodologic issues, and infant outcome. *Clin Perinatol.* 1991;18:77-91.
34. Devane WA, et al. Determination and characterization of a cannabinoid receptor in rat brain. *Mol Pharmacol.* 1988;34:605-613.
35. Donnino MW, et al. Cannabinoid hyperemesis: a case series. *J Emerg Med.* 2011;40:e63-e66.
36. Dreher MC, et al. Prenatal marijuana exposure and neonatal outcomes in Jamaica: an ethnographic study. *Pediatrics.* 1994;93:254-260.
37. DuPont RL, Baumgartner WA. Drug testing by urine and hair analysis: complementary features and scientific issues. *Forensic Sci Int.* 1995;70:63-76.
38. Duran M, et al. Preliminary efficacy and safety of an oromucosal standardized cannabis extract in chemotherapy-induced nausea and vomiting. *Br J Clin Pharmacol.* 2010;70:656-663.
39. Ellis GJ, et al. Excretion patterns of cannabinoid metabolites after last use in a group of chronic users. *Clin Pharmacol Ther.* 1985;38:572-578.
40. Felder CC, Glass M. Cannabinoid receptors and their endogenous agonists. *Annu Rev Pharmacol Toxicol.* 1998;38:179-200.
41. Fisher B, et al. Cardiovascular complications induced by cannabis smoking: a case report and review of the literature. *Emerg Med J.* 2005;22:679-680.
42. Fried PA. Behavioral outcomes in preschool and school-age children exposed prenatally to marijuana: a review and speculative interpretation. *NIDA Res Monogr.* 1996;164:242-260.
43. Fried PA, Makin JE. Neonatal behavioural correlates of prenatal exposure to marihuana, cigarettes and alcohol in a low risk population. *Neurotoxicol Teratol.* 1987;9:1-7.
44. Fried PA, Watkinson B. 36- and 48-month neurobehavioral follow-up of children prenatally exposed to marijuana, cigarettes, and alcohol. *J Dev Behav Pediatr.* 1990;11:49-58.
45. Galli JA, et al. Cannabinoid hyperemesis syndrome. *Curr Drug Abuse Rev.* 2011;4:241.
46. Goodwin RS, et al. Delta(9)-tetrahydrocannabinol, 11-hydroxy-delta(9)-tetrahydrocannabinol and 11-nor-9-carboxy-delta(9)-tetrahydrocannabinol in human plasma after controlled oral administration of cannabinoids. *Ther Drug Monit.* 2006;28:545-551.
47. Grant P, Gandhi P. A case of Cannabis-induced pancreatitis. *JOP.* 2004;5:41-43.
48. Green K. Marijuana smoking vs cannabinoids for glaucoma therapy. *Arch Ophthalmol.* 1998;116:1433-1437.
49. Grigoryev A, et al. Chromatography-mass spectrometry studies on the metabolism of synthetic cannabinoids JWH-018 and JWH-073, psychoactive components of smoking mixtures. *J Chromatography B.* 2011;879:1126-1136.
50. Grotenhermen F. Pharmacokinetics and pharmacodynamics of cannabinoids. *Clin Pharmacokinet.* 2003;42:327-360.
51. Haney M, et al. Marijuana withdrawal in humans: effects of oral THC or divalproex. *Neuropsychopharmacology.* 2004;29:158-170.
52. Hartman RL, Huestis MA. Cannabis effects on driving skills. *Clin Chem.* 2013;59:478-492.
53. Hashibe M, et al. Marijuana smoking and head and neck cancer. *J Clin Pharmacol.* 2002;42:103S-107S.
54. Hatch EE, Bracken MB. Effect of marijuana use in pregnancy on fetal growth. *Am J Epidemiol.* 1986;124:986-993.
55. Hawks RL. The constituents of cannabis and the disposition and metabolism of cannabinoids. *NIDA Res Monogr.* 1982;42:125-137.
56. Heishman SJ, et al. Acute and residual effects of marijuana: profiles of plasma THC levels, physiological, subjective, and performance measures. *Pharmacol Biochem Behav.* 1990;37:561-565.
57. Helmer DA, Kosten TR. Psychosis associated with synthetic cannabinoid agonists: a case series. *Am J Psychiatry.* 2011;168:10.
58. Herkenham M, et al. Characterization and localization of cannabinoid receptors in rat brain: a quantitative in vitro autoradiographic study. *J Neurosci.* 1991;11:563-583.
59. Hirst RA, et al. Pharmacology and potential therapeutic uses of Cannabis. *Br J Anaesth.* 1998;81:77-84.
60. Hollister LE. Health aspects of Cannabis. *Pharmacol Rev.* 1986;38:1-20.
61. Hollister LE, et al. Do plasma concentrations of delta 9-tetrahydrocannabinol reflect the degree of intoxication? *J Clin Pharmacol.* 1981;21:171S-177S.
62. Huestis MA, et al. Estimating time of last oral ingestion of cannabis from plasma THC and THCCOOH concentrations. *Ther Drug Monit.* 2006;28:540-544.
63. Huestis MA, et al. Blood cannabinoids. II. Models for the prediction of time of marijuana exposure from plasma concentrations of Δ9-tetrahydrocannabinol (THC) and 11-nor-9-carboxy-Δ9-tetrahydrocannabinol (THCCOOH). *J Anal Toxicol.* 1992;16:283-290.
64. Huestis MA, et al. Detection times of marijuana metabolites in urine by immunoassay and GC-MS. *J Anal Toxicol.* 1995;19:443-449.
65. Huestis MA, et al. Urinary excretion profiles of 11-nor-9-carboxy-delta 9-tetrahydrocannabinol in humans after single smoked doses of marijuana. *J Anal Toxicol.* 1996;20:441-452.
66. Huffman JW. Cannabimimetic indoles, pyrroles and indenes. *Curr Med Chem.* 1999;6:705-720.
67. Huffman JW, Padgett LW. Recent developments in the medicinal chemistry of cannabimimetic indoles, pyrroles and indenes. *Curr Med Chem.* 2005;12:1395-1411.
68. Hunt CA, Jones RT. Tolerance and disposition of tetrahydrocannabinol in man. *J Pharmacol Exp Ther.* 1980;215:35-44.
69. Hurst D, et al. Psychosis associated with synthetic cannabinoid agonists: a case series. *Am J Psychiatry.* 2011;168:1119.
70. Hutter M, et al. Identification of the major urinary metabolites in man of seven synthetic cannabinoids of the aminoalkylindole type present as adulterants in "herbal mixtures" using LC-MS/MS techniques. *J Mass Spectrom.* 2012;47:54-65.
71. Iversen L. Cannabis and the brain. *Brain.* 2003;126:1252-1270.
72. Iversen L. Long-term effects of exposure to Cannabis. *Curr Opin Pharmacol.* 2005;5:69-72.
73. Jain AK, et al. Evaluation of intramuscular levonantradol and placebo in acute postoperative pain. *J Clin Pharmacol.* 1981;21:320S-326S.
74. Johansson E, Halldin MM. Urinary excretion half-life of delta 1-tetrahydrocannabinol-7-oic acid in heavy marijuana users after smoking. *J Anal Toxicol.* 1989;13:218-223.
75. Jones RT. Cardiovascular system effects of marijuana. *J Clin Pharmacol.* 2002;42:58S-63S.
76. Kacinko SL, et al. Development and validation of a liquid chromatography-tandem mass spectrometry method for the identification and quantification of JWH-018, JWH-073, JWH-019, and JWH-250 in human whole blood. *J Anal Toxicol.* 2011;35:386-393.
77. Katona I, et al. GABAergic interneurons are the targets of cannabinoid actions in the human hippocampus. *Neuroscience.* 2000;100:797-804.
78. Kavanagh P, et al. The Identification of the urinary metabolites of 3-(4-Methoxybenzoyl)-1-Pentylindole (RCS-4), a novel cannabimimetic, by gas chromatography–mass spectrometry. *J Anal Toxicol.* 2012;36:303-311.
79. Kelly P, Jones RT. Metabolism of tetrahydrocannabinol in frequent and infrequent marijuana users. *J Anal Toxicol.* 1992;16:228-235.
80. Kidwell DA, et al. Testing for drugs of abuse in saliva and sweat. *J Chromatogr B Biomed Sci Appl.* 1998;713:111-135.
81. Klein TW. Marijuana, immunity and infection. *J Neuroimmunol.* 1998;83:102-115.
82. Kline J, et al. Marijuana and spontaneous abortion of known karyotype. *Paediatr Perinat Epidemiol.* 1991;5:320-332.
83. Kosior DA, et al. Paroxysmal atrial fibrillation following marijuana intoxication: a two-case report of possible association. *Int J Cardiol.* 2001;78:183-184.
84. Lambert DM, Fowler CJ. The endocannabinoid system: drug targets, lead compounds, and potential therapeutic applications. *J Med Chem.* 2005;48:5059-5087.
85. Lapoint J, et al. Severe toxicity following synthetic cannabinoid ingestion. *Clin Toxicol.* 2011;49:760-764.
86. Law B, et al. Passive inhalation of cannabis smoke. *J Pharm Pharmacol.* 1984;36:578-581.
87. Lichtman AH, Martin BR. Marijuana withdrawal syndrome in the animal model. *J Clin Pharmacol.* 2002;42:20S-27S.
88. Lindigkeit R, et al. Spice: a never ending story? *Forensic Sci Int.* 2009;191:58-63.
89. Linn S, et al. The association of marijuana use with outcome of pregnancy. *Am J Public Health.* 1983;73:1161-1164.
90. Long A, et al. A randomized double-blind cross-over comparison of the antiemetic activity of levonantradol and prochlorperazine. *Proc Am Soc Clin Oncol.* 1982;1: C-220.
91. Macfarlane V, Christie G. Synthetic cannabinoid withdrawal: a new demand on detoxification services. *Drug Alcohol Rev.* 2015;34:147-153.
92. Macleod J, et al. Psychological and social sequelae of cannabis and other illicit drug use by young people: a systematic review of longitudinal, general population studies. *Lancet.* 2004;363:1579-1588.

93. Macnab A, et al. Ingestion of cannabis: a cause of coma in children. *Pediatr Emerg Care.* 1989;5:238-239.

94. Manno JE, et al. Temporal indication of marijuana use can be estimated from plasma and urine concentrations of delta9-tetrahydrocannabinol, 11-hydroxy-delta9-tetra-hydrocannabinol, and 11-nor-delta9-tetrahydrocannabinol-9-carboxylic acid. *J Anal Toxicol.* 2001;25:538-549.

95. Mathew RJ, et al. Marijuana intoxication and brain activation in marijuana smokers. *Life Sci.* 1997;60:2075-2089.

96. Mathew RJ, et al. Time course of tetrahydrocannabinol-induced changes in regional cerebral blood flow measured with positron emission tomography. *Psychiatry Res.* 2002;116:173-185.

97. Mechoulam R. A historical overview of chemical research on cannabinoids. *Chem Physics Lipids.* 2000;108:1-13.

98. Mechoulam R, Gaoni Y. The absolute configuration of delta-1-tetrahydrocannabinol, the major active constituent of hashish. *Tetrahedron Lett.* 1967;12:1109-1111.

99. Mehra R, et al. The association between marijuana smoking and lung cancer: a systematic review. *Arch Intern Med.* 2006;166:1359-1367.

100. Meiri E, et al. Efficacy of dronabinol alone and in combination with ondansetron versus ondansetron alone for delayed chemotherapy-induced nausea and vomiting. *Curr Med Res Opin.* 2007;23:533-543.

101. Menkes DB, et al. Salivary THC following cannabis smoking correlates with subjective intoxication and heart rate. *Psychopharmacology.* 1991;103:277-279.

102. Mieczkowski T. A research note: the outcome of GC/MS/MS confirmation of hair assays on 93 cannabinoid (+) cases. *Forensic Sci Int.* 1995;70:83-91.

103. Mikawa Y, et al. Ocular activity of topically administered anandamide in the rabbit. *Jap J Ophthalmol.* 1997;41:217-220.

104. Mir A, et al. Myocardial infarction associated with use of the synthetic cannabinoid K2. *Pediatrics.* 2011;128:e1622-e1627.

105. Mittleman MA, et al. Triggering myocardial infarction by marijuana. *Circulation.* 2001;103:2805-2809.

106. Monte AA, et al. An outbreak of exposure to a novel synthetic cannabinoid. *N Engl J Med.* 2014;370:389-390.

107. Moosmann B, et al. A fast and inexpensive procedure for the isolation of synthetic cannabinoids from "Spice" products using a flash chromatography system. *Anal Bioanal Chem.* 2012:1-7.

108. Moran CL, et al. Quantitative measurement of JWH-018 and JWH-073 metabolites excreted in human urine. *Anal Chem.* 2011;83:4228-4236.

109. Centers for Disease Control and Prevention (CDC). Acute kidney injury associated with synthetic cannabinoid use—multiple states, 2012. *MMWR Morb Mortal Wkly Rep.* 2013;62:93-98.

110. Morland J, et al. Cannabinoids in blood and urine after passive inhalation of cannabis smoke. *J Forensic Sci.* 1985;30:997-1002.

111. Mukamal KJ, et al. An exploratory prospective study of marijuana use and mortality following acute myocardial infarction. *Am Heart J.* 2008;155:465-470.

112. Mule SJ, et al. Active and realistic passive marijuana exposure tested by three immunoassays and GC/MS in urine. *J Anal Toxicol.* 1988;12:113-116.

113. Musty RE, Kaback L. Relationships between motivation and depression in chronic marijuana users. *Life Sci.* 1995;56:2151-2158.

114. Nacca N, et al. The synthetic cannabinoid withdrawal syndrome. *J Addict Med.* 2013; 7:296-298.

115. Nahas G, et al. The kinetics of cannabinoid distribution and storage with special reference to the brain and testis. *J Clin Pharmacol.* 1981;21:208S-214S.

116. Nahas GG. Lethal cannabis intoxication. *N Engl J Med.* 1971;284:792.

117. Nocerino E, et al. Cannabis and cannabinoid receptors. *Fitoterapia.* 2000;71(suppl 1): S6-S12.

118. Noyes RJ, et al. The analgesic properties of delta-9-tetrahydrocannabinol and codeine. *Clin Pharmacol Ther.* 1975;18:84-89.

119. O'Kane CJ, et al. Cannabis and driving: a new perspective. *Emerg Med (Fremantle).* 2002;14:296-303.

120. O'Leary DS, et al. Effects of smoking marijuana on brain perfusion and cognition. *Neuropsychopharmacology.* 2002;26:802-816.

121. Onaivi ES, et al. Endocannabinoids and cannabinoid receptor genetics. *Prog Neurobiol.* 2002;66:307-344.

122. Perez-Reyes M, et al. Passive inhalation of marihuana smoke and urinary excretion of cannabinoids. *Clin Pharmacol Ther.* 1983;34:36-41.

123. Perez-Reyes M, Wall ME. Presence of delta9-tetrahydrocannabinol in human milk. *N Engl J Med.* 1982;307:819-820.

124. Pierre JM. Cannabis, synthetic cannabinoids, and psychosis risk: what the evidence says. *Curr Psychiatry.* 2011;10.

125. Pope HJ, Yurgelun-Todd D. The residual cognitive effects of heavy marijuana use in college students. *JAMA.* 1996;275:521-527.

126. Porcella A, et al. The synthetic cannabinoid WIN55212-2 decreases the intraocular pressure in human glaucoma resistant to conventional therapies. *Eur J Neurosci.* 2001;13:409-412.

127. Poster DS, et al. delta 9-tetrahydrocannabinol in clinical oncology. *JAMA.* 1981;245: 2047-2051.

128. Poznyak V. Global epidemiology of cannabis use and implications for public health [abstract]. *Alcohol and Alcoholism.* 2014;49:i14.

129. Prakash R, et al. Effects of marihuana and placebo marihuana smoking on hemodynamics in coronary disease. *Clin Pharmacol Ther.* 1975;18:90-95.

130. Rabin R, George T. Understanding the link between cannabinoids and psychosis. *Clin Pharmacol Ther.* 2017;101:197-199.

131. Ramesh D, et al. Blockade of endocannabinoid hydrolytic enzymes attenuates precipitated opioid withdrawal symptoms in mice. *J Pharmacol Exp Ther.* 2011;339: 173-185.

132. Rezkalla SH, et al. Coronary no-flow and ventricular tachycardia associated with habitual marijuana use. *Ann Emerg Med.* 2003;42:365-369.

133. Richards JR, et al. Cannabinoid hyperemesis syndrome: potential mechanisms for the benefit of capsaicin and hot water hydrotherapy in treatment. *Clin Toxicol.* 2017;1-10.

134. Romolo FS, et al. Determination of nabilone in bulk powders and capsules by high-performance liquid chromatography/tandem mass spectrometry. *Rapid Commun Mass Spectrom.* 2004;18:128-130.

135. Rosenbaum CD, et al. Here today, gone tomorrow... and back again? A review of herbal marijuana alternatives (K2, Spice), synthetic cathinones (bath salts), kratom, Salvia divinorum, methoxetamine, and piperazines. *J Med Toxicol.* 2012;8:15-32.

136. Rosenblatt KA, et al. Marijuana use and risk of oral squamous cell carcinoma. *Cancer Res.* 2004;64:4049-4054.

137. Rubin A, et al. Physiologic disposition of nabilone, a cannabinol derivative, in man. *Clin Pharmacol Ther.* 1977;22:85-91.

138. Russo EB. History of cannabis and its preparations in saga, science, and sobriquet. *Chem Biodivers.* 2007;4:1614-1648.

139. Sampson CS, et al. Withdrawal seizures seen in the setting of synthetic cannabinoid abuse. *Am J Emerg Med.* 2015 Nov;33:1712.e3.

140. Schlicker E, Kathmann M. Modulation of transmitter release via presynaptic cannabinoid receptors. *Trends Pharmacol Sci.* 2001;22:565-572.

141. Schneir AB, Baumbacher T. Convulsions associated with the use of a synthetic cannabinoid product. *J Med Toxicol.* 2012;8:62-64.

142. Schneir AB, et al. "Spice" girls: synthetic cannabinoid intoxication. *J Emerg Med.* 2011;40:296-299.

143. Schramm W, et al. Drugs of abuse in saliva: a review. *J Anal Toxicol.* 1992;16:1-9.

144. Schwartz RH. Marijuana: an overview. *Pediatr Clin North Am.* 1987;34:305-317.

145. Schwartz RH, et al. Short-term memory impairment in Cannabis-dependent adolescents. *Am J Dis Child.* 1989;143:1214-1219.

146. Schwartz RH, Hawks RL. Laboratory detection of marijuana use. *JAMA.* 1985;254: 788-792.

147. Seely KA, et al. Marijuana-based drugs: innovative therapeutics or designer drugs of abuse? *Mol Interv.* 2011;11:36-51.

148. Sidney S. Cardiovascular consequences of marijuana use. *J Clin Pharmacol.* 2002;42: 64S-70S.

149. Simonetto DA, et al. Cannabinoid hyperemesis: a case series of 98 patients. *Mayo Clin Proc.* 2012;87:114-119.

150. Singh E, Coyle W. Cannabinoid hyperemesis. *Am J Gastroenterol.* 2008;103:1048-1049.

151. Singh GK. Atrial fibrillation associated with marijuana use. *Pediatr Cardiol.* 2000;21:284.

152. Smith NT. A review of the published literature into cannabis withdrawal symptoms in human users. *Addiction.* 2002;97:621-632.

153. Sugiura T, Waku K. Cannabinoid receptors and their endogenous ligands. *J Biochem.* 2002;132:7-12.

154. Swift W, et al. One year follow-up of cannabis dependence among long-term users in Sydney, Australia. *Drug Alcohol Depend.* 2000;59:309-318.

155. Takematsu M, et al. A case of acute cerebral ischemia following inhalation of a synthetic cannabinoid." *Clin Toxicol.* 2014;52:973-975.

156. Tashkin DP. Airway effects of marijuana, cocaine, and other inhaled illicit agents. *Curr Opin Pulm Med.* 2001;7:43-61.

157. Tashkin DP, et al. Acute effects of smoked marijuana and oral delta9-tetrahydrocannabinol on specific airway conductance in asthmatic subjects. *Am Rev Respir Dis.* 1974;109:420-428.

158. Tashkin DP, et al. Acute pulmonary physiologic effects of smoked marijuana and oral 9-tetrahydrocannabinol in healthy young men. *N Engl J Med.* 1973;289:336-341.

159. Taylor F. Marijuana as a potential respiratory tract carcinogen: a retrospective analysis of a community hospital population. *South Med J.* 1988;81:1213-1216.

160. Teske J, et al. Sensitive and rapid quantification of the cannabinoid receptor agonist naphthalen-1-yl-(1-pentylindol-3-yl) methanone (JWH-018) in human serum by liquid chromatography-tandem mass spectrometry. *J Chromatogr B.* 2010;878: 2659-2663.

161. Tetrault JM, et al. Effects of marijuana smoking on pulmonary function and respiratory complications: a systematic review. *Arch Intern Med.* 2007;167:221-228.

162. Tomida I, et al. Effect of sublingual application of cannabinoids on intraocular pressure: a pilot study. *J Glaucoma.* 2006;15:349-353.

163. Uebel RA, Wium CA. Toxicological screening for drugs of abuse in samples adulterated with household chemicals. *S Afr Med J.* 2002;92:547-549.

164. Vardakou I, et al. Spice drugs as a new trend: mode of action, identification and legislation. *Toxicol Lett.* 2010;197:157-162.

165. Wall ME, et al. Metabolism, disposition, and kinetics of delta-9-tetrahydrocannabinol in men and women. *Clin Pharmacol Ther.* 1983;34:352-363.

166. Wallace EA, et al. Cannabinoid hyperemesis syndrome: literature review and proposed diagnosis and treatment algorithm. *South Med J.* 2011;104:659-664.

167. Watson SJ, et al. Marijuana and medicine: assessing the science base: a summary of the 1999 Institute of Medicine report. *Arch Gen Psychiatry.* 2000;57:547-552.

168. Weil AT. Adverse reactions to marihuana. Classification and suggested treatment. *N Engl J Med.* 1970;282:997-1000.

169. Whiting PF, et al. Cannabinoids for medical use: a systematic review and meta-analysis. *JAMA.* 2015;313:2456-2473.

170. Williamson EM, Evans FJ. Cannabinoids in clinical practice. *Drugs.* 2000;60:1303-1314.

171. Wu TC, et al. Pulmonary hazards of smoking marijuana as compared with tobacco. *N Engl J Med.* 1988;318:347-351.

172. Zuardi AW. History of Cannabis as a medicine: a review. *Rev Bras Psiquiatr.* 2006;28:153-157.

173. Zuckerman B, et al. Effects of maternal marijuana and cocaine use on fetal growth. *N Engl J Med.* 1989;320:762-768.

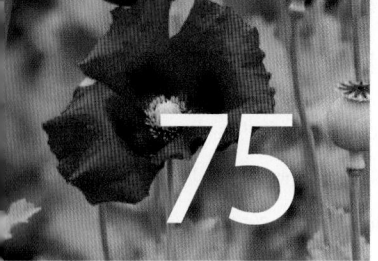

75 COCAINE

Craig G. Smollin and Robert S. Hoffman

HISTORY AND EPIDEMIOLOGY

Cocaine is contained in the leaves of *Erythroxylum coca* (coca plant), a shrub that grows abundantly in Colombia, Peru, Bolivia, the West Indies, and Indonesia. As early as the sixth century, the inhabitants of Peru chewed or sucked on the leaves for social and religious reasons. In the 1100s, the Incas used cocaine-filled saliva as local anesthesia for ritual trephinations of the skull.[78]

In 1859, Albert Niemann isolated cocaine as the active ingredient of the plant. By 1879, Vassili von Anrep demonstrated that cocaine could numb the tongue.[118] However, Europeans knew little about cocaine until 1884, when the Austrian ophthalmologist Karl Koller introduced cocaine as an effective local anesthetic for eye surgery and Koller's colleague, Sigmund Freud, wrote extensively on the psychoactive properties of cocaine.[63] Following these revelations, Merck, the main cocaine producer in Europe, increased production from less than 0.75 pounds in 1883 to more than 150,000 pounds in 1886.[114]

Simultaneously, reports of complications from the therapeutic use of cocaine began to appear. In 1886, a 25-year-old man had a "pulseless" syncope after cocaine was applied to his eye to remove a foreign body.[229] By 1887, more than 30 cases of severe toxicity were reported,[198] and by 1895, at least eight fatalities resulting from a variety of doses and routes of administration were summarized in one article.[66] Recreational cocaine use was legal in the United States until the passage of the Harrison Narcotics Act of 1914, when cocaine was restricted to medicinal use. Not until 1982, however, was the first cocaine-associated myocardial infarction (MI) reported in the United States.[36]

Currently, cocaine is an approved pharmaceutical. It is used primarily for topical anesthesia of cutaneous lacerations or during otolaryngology procedures as a vasoconstrictor and topical anesthetic. Although multiple factors fostered a decline in the medicinal use of cocaine,[24,73,142] the recreational use of cocaine remains a significant problem.

The United Nations office on Drugs and Crime estimates that there are 19 million cocaine users worldwide.[233] In the United States, it was estimated that in 2015, there were 1.9 million cocaine users,[51] and in 2011, cocaine was the most common illicit xenobiotic resulting in emergency department (ED) visits.[52] The dramatic evolution of the cannabinoid and opioid epidemics will probably change the profile of the ED patients using illicit xenobiotics (Chaps. 36 and 74).

PHARMACOLOGY

The alkaloid form of cocaine, benzoylmethylecgonine, is a weak base that is relatively insoluble in water. It is extracted from the leaf by mechanical degradation in the presence of a hydrocarbon. The resulting product is converted into a hydrochloride salt to yield a white powder, cocaine hydrochloride, which is very water soluble. Cocaine hydrochloride is used by insufflation, application topically to mucous membranes, injection after dissolution in water, or ingestion; however, it degrades rapidly when pyrolyzed. Smokable cocaine (crack) is formed by dissolving cocaine hydrochloride in water and adding a strong base. A hydrocarbon solvent is added, the cocaine base is extracted into the organic phase, and then evaporated. The term "free-base" refers to the use of cocaine base in solution.

Cocaine is rapidly absorbed after all routes of exposure; however, when applied to mucous membranes or ingested, its vasoconstrictive properties slow the rate of absorption and delay the peak effect. Bioavailability when smoking cocaine exceeds 90% and is approximately 80% after nasal application.[110] Data for ingested cocaine and application to other mucous membranes such as the urethra, vagina, or rectum are inadequately documented. Table 75–1 lists the typical onsets and durations of action for various routes of cocaine use.

After absorption, cocaine is approximately 90% bound to plasma proteins, primarily α_1-acid glycoprotein.[178] Based on human volunteer studies with small doses of cocaine, the volume of distribution is reported to range from 1.6 to 2.7 L/kg,[11,32,110] but it is unclear if the volume of distribution changes with overdose.

The metabolism of cocaine is complex and dependent on both genetic and acquired factors. Three major pathways of cocaine metabolism are well described (Fig. 75–1). Cocaine undergoes *N*-demethylation in the liver to form norcocaine, a minor metabolite that rarely accounts for more than 5% of drug.[106,223] However, norcocaine readily crosses the blood–brain barrier and produces clinical effects in animals that are quite similar to cocaine.[17,113,210] Nearly half of a dose of cocaine is both nonenzymatically[222] and enzymatically hydrolyzed[48] to form benzoylecgonine (BE). When BE is injected into animals, some reports suggest that it is virtually inactive,[115,218] but other studies demonstrate cerebral vasoconstriction[41] and seizures.[122,160] When either injected directly into the cerebral ventricles[161,210] or applied to the surface of cerebral arteries,[145] BE is a potent vasoconstrictor. Although BE traverses the blood–brain barrier poorly,[162] the potential effects are of concern as some BE is probably formed from cocaine that has already entered the central nervous system (CNS). In vitro, BE has little or no effect on cardiac sodium or potassium channels.[41,58] Finally, plasma cholinesterase (PChE) and other esterases metabolize cocaine to ecgonine methyl ester (EME). In normal individuals, between 32% and 49% of cocaine is metabolized to EME.[4,106] Similar to BE, EME crosses the blood–brain barrier poorly.[161] Although many authors state that EME has little or no pharmacologic activity,[160,161,207] diverse animal models demonstrate contradictory results, concluding that EME is a vasodilator,[145,176,208] sedative, anticonvulsant,[210] and protective metabolite against lethal doses of cocaine.[90]

Genetic or acquired alterations in PChE activity modulate the effects of cocaine. Early in vitro studies showed that cocaine was poorly metabolized in serum from patients with succinylcholine sensitivity (low PChE activity). In subsequent studies and case series, patients with low PChE activity

TABLE 75–1	Pharmacology of Cocaine by Various Routes of Administration			
Route of Exposure	Onset of Action (min)	Peak Action (min)	Duration of Action (min)	Relative Peak Concentrations (ng/mL)
Intravenous	<1	3–5	30–60	180 ± 56
Nasal insufflation	1–5	20–30	60–120	220 ± 39
Smoking	<1	3–5	30–60	203 ± 88
Gastrointestinal	30–60	60–90	30–140	210 ± 58

Data from Jeffcoat AR, Perez-Reyes M, Hill JM, et al. Cocaine disposition in humans after intravenous injection, nasal insufflation (snorting), or smoking. *Drug Metab Dispos.* 1989 Mar-Apr;17(2):153-159 and Van Dyke C, Jatlow P, Ungerer J, et al. Oral cocaine: plasma concentrations and central effects. *Science.* 1978 Apr 14;200(4338):211-213.

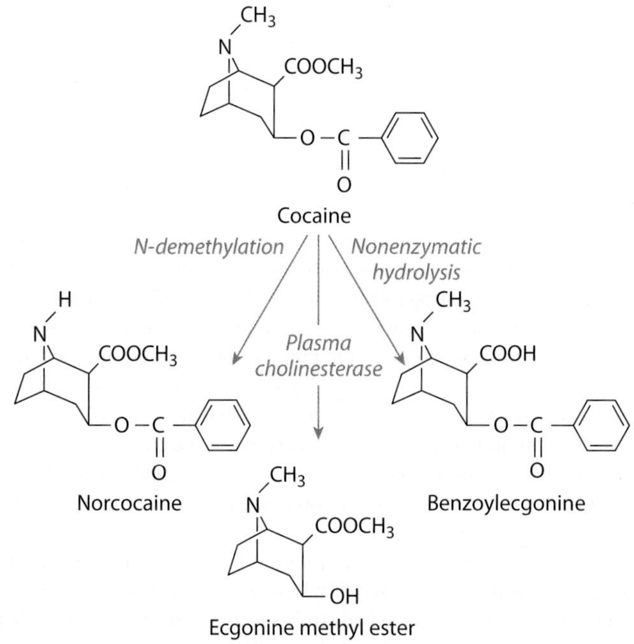

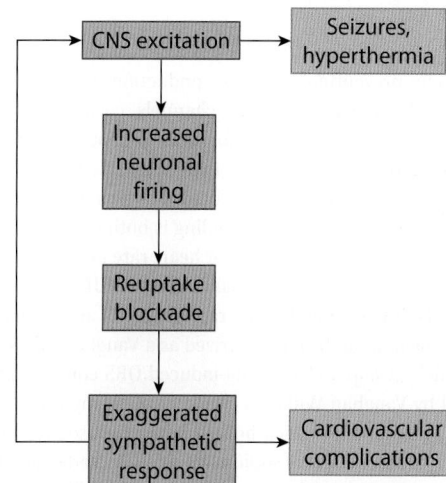

FIGURE 75-1.
Metabolism of cocaine. The three principal metabolic pathways of cocaine are depicted.

FIGURE 75-2. Cocaine-induced central nervous (CNS) system effects modulate peripheral events.

demonstrate increased sensitivity to cocaine,[89,174] findings that are corroborated in multiple animal models.[26,90,143]

Multiple other metabolites of cocaine are well characterized.[39] Several have clinical or diagnostic importance. In 1990, a unique metabolite was identified in patients who smoke cocaine, now known either as anhydroecgonine methyl ester (AEME) or methylecgonide.[108] The presence of this compound and its metabolite, ecgonidine, are useful to help determine the route of administration in cocaine users.[206] Additionally, AEME has demonstrable agonism and antagonism at various muscarinic receptor subtypes, which has important clinical implications.[65,250] Animal models also suggest that AEME has greater neurotoxic potential compared with cocaine.[65]

Ethanol has a unique pharmacologic interaction with cocaine. A transesterification reaction between the two drugs produces ethylbenzoylecognine, which is also called "ethyl cocaine" or "cocaethylene" (CE).[17] In human volunteers given cocaine and ethanol, CE accounted for approximately 17% of the metabolites, producing a decrease in the amount of BE and an increase in the amount of EME formed.[82,83] Cocaethylene has a longer duration of action than cocaine and similar neurotoxic and cardiotoxic effects.

PATHOPHYSIOLOGY

Neurotransmitter Effects

Cocaine blocks the reuptake of biogenic amines. Specifically, these effects are described on serotonin and the catecholamines dopamine, norepinephrine, and epinephrine. Several animal investigations elucidated the particular roles of each neurotransmitter. Mice lacking the dopamine transporter are relatively insensitive to the locomotor effects of cocaine.[68] Whereas tachycardia emanates from adrenally derived epinephrine, hypertension results from neuronally derived norepinephrine.[227,228] Serotonin is an important modulator of dopamine and has a role in cocaine addiction, reward, and seizures.[80,133,153]

Although much emphasis is placed on the reuptake blockade of these biogenic amines, it is clear that this effect is insufficient to account for the clinical manifestations of cocaine toxicity. Other xenobiotics that block the reuptake of biogenic amines, such as cyclic antidepressants, produce quite distinct clinical manifestations[230] (Chap. 68). Xenobiotics that block the effects of dopamine, epinephrine, and norepinephrine not only fail to protect against cocaine toxicity but actually exacerbate toxicity.[29,75,142,201] Although this results in part from an unopposed α-adrenergic effect, hypertension and vasospasm fail to explain the increase in psychomotor agitation, seizures, and

hyperthermia that result.[29,75] These effects most likely result from an interaction between cocaine and excitatory amino acids. Cocaine increases excitatory amino acid concentrations in the brain,[217] and excitatory amino acid antagonists prevent both seizures and death in experimental animals.[18,192] Finally, because experimental evidence in animals[28,75,211] and clinical experience in humans demonstrate that sedation treats both the central effects of cocaine and the peripheral effects of biogenic amines, a newer model was proposed (Fig. 75–2). This model emphasizes the necessity of diffuse CNS excitation as a prerequisite for cocaine toxicity, explains experimental and clinical observations, and provides insight into the treatment of acute toxicity.

Cardiovascular Effects

Cocaine use is associated with myocardial ischemia and MI. The increased risk of MI results from several different mechanisms, including hypertension and tachycardia with resultant increase in myocardial oxygen demand, vasospasm resulting in decrease coronary artery blood flow, accelerated atherogenesis, and hypercoagulability. In addition, chronic exposure to high concentrations of catecholamines results in mitochondrial disruption and oxidative stress on a cellular level with direct myocardial injury.[138]

Vasospasm

Although increased myocardial oxygen demand is sufficient to cause ischemia in some individuals, it is clear that cocaine also produces profound vasoconstriction. Evidence suggests that cocaine-induced vasoconstriction is mediated through both neuronal norepinephrine and BE.[127,144] Benzoylecgonine has a direct effect on vessels that is calcium mediated.[144] Additionally nicotine, which is simultaneously used by many substance users, has additive, if not synergistic, effects with cocaine.[166]

Oxidative Stress

Chronic exposure to elevated concentrations of catecholamines in the context of repetitive cocaine use results in the formation of reactive oxygen species and oxidation products known as "aminochromes" that directly damage myocardial cells. Evidence suggests that this pathophysiologic pathway is important in the development of cocaine-induced cardiomyopathy.[138]

Atherogenesis

Cocaine use accelerates atherosclerosis. Rabbits fed a normal diet supplemented with cholesterol do not develop atherosclerotic vascular disease. However, when that diet includes cocaine, rabbits develop classic atherosclerotic lesions.[120,129,130] Experiments with human endothelial cells demonstrate that cocaine directly increases the permeability to lipids by altering tight junctions.[121] This probably promotes the formation of subendothelial atherosclerotic plaques.

Dysrhythmias

Like other local anesthetics (Chap. 64), cocaine blocks neuronal sodium channels, thereby preventing saltatory conduction. Because of homology between neuronal and cardiac sodium channels, cocaine also inhibits the rapid inward Na^+ current responsible for phase 0 depolarization of the cardiac action potential (Chaps. 15 and 68). Experimental evidence suggests that cocaine enters the sodium channel and binds on the inner membrane.[42,119,183] Like many sodium channel blockers, binding is both pH and use dependent such that binding increases as pH falls or heart rate increase (Chap. 68).[43,242] Furthermore, although norcocaine has a greater affinity for inactivated sodium channels, it has a much more rapid offset of action than cocaine.[42] Consequently, cocaine can be characterized as a Vaughan-Williams class 1C antidysrhythmic[249] (Chap. 57). Cocaine-induced QRS complex prolongation is exacerbated by Vaughan-Williams class IA antidysrhythmics[247] and ameliorated by hypertonic sodium bicarbonate, hypertonic sodium chloride, and lidocaine.[13,73,177] Another effect of sodium channel blockade, the Brugada pattern, is also associated with cocaine use (Fig. 15–12).[141,171]

In addition to its sodium channel-blocking properties, cocaine also blocks cardiac potassium channels (Chap. 15). This results in QT interval prolongation[181,226,242] and increases the risk of torsade de pointes.[209] Cocaethylene also has dysrhythmogenic effects.[172] In vivo experiments demonstrated inhibition of the myocardial hERG potassium channels, which helps to explain this phenomenon.[58] In animal studies, CE is associated with increased incidence of dysrhythmias, prolonged myocardial depression, and increased lethality.[115,246]

Hematologic Effects

Enhanced coagulation and impaired thrombolysis compound the effects of accelerated atherogenesis and vasospasm. Cocaine activates human platelets and causes α-granule release, resulting in platelet aggregation.[85,126] Thus, even in the absence of endothelial injury, cocaine initiates a thrombotic cascade while simultaneously enhancing the activity of plasminogen activator inhibitor type 1 (PAI-1), thereby impairing clot lysis.[165]

Pulmonary Effects

Bronchospasm

The association between cocaine use and asthma[195] was not recognized until smoked cocaine became prevalent.[56] Furthermore, experiments in human volunteers demonstrate that only smoked cocaine (not intravenous {IV} cocaine) produces bronchospasm.[225] Although it is possible that bronchospasm results from direct administration of cocaine to the airways, inhaled contaminants of cocaine, or thermal insult, and the unique pyrolytic metabolite of cocaine that acts as a muscarinic agonist (AEME) produces bronchospasm in experimental animals.[31]

CLINICAL MANIFESTATIONS

Many clinical manifestations of toxicity develop immediately after cocaine use. These are typically associated with the sympathetic overactivity, and their duration of effect is predictable based on the pharmacokinetics of cocaine use. Other manifestations, such as those associated with tissue ischemia, often present in a delayed fashion, with a clinical latency of hours to even days after last cocaine use. The reasons for this delay are not clear but may relate to the presence of an altered sensorium associated with acute cocaine use and its anesthetic effects (see the later section Cessation of Use).

Vital sign abnormalities that develop during cocaine toxicity are characteristic of the sympathomimetic toxidrome. Thus, varying degrees of hypertension, tachycardia, tachypnea, and hyperthermia occur. Although any of these vital sign abnormalities can be life threatening, experimental and clinical evidence suggests that hyperthermia is the most critical.[29,75,150] Initially, with typically used doses, and at any time with a massive dose, apnea, hypotension, and bradycardia can result, all from direct suppression (anesthesia) of brainstem centers.[127,142,158] These effects are fleeting and rarely noted when patients present a health care facility when either the sympathetic overdrive rapidly ensues or sudden death results. Additional sympathomimetic findings include mydriasis, diaphoresis, and neuropsychiatric manifestations.

Cocaine produces end-organ toxicity in virtually every organ system in the body. These events result from vasospasm, hemorrhage secondary to increased vascular shear force (dP/dT), or enhanced coagulation. Each organ system is discussed separately in the following sections.

Central Nervous System

Seizures, coma, headache, focal neurologic signs or symptoms, or behavioral abnormalities that persist longer than the predicted duration of effect of cocaine should alert the clinician to a potential catastrophic CNS event. Hemorrhage occurs at any anatomic site in the CNS. Subarachnoid, intraventricular, and intraparenchymal bleeding are all well described in association with cocaine use.[2,46,136,148,185,212] Early discussions suggested an underlying predisposition due to the presence of arteriovenous malformations or congenital aneurysms,[248] but subsequent larger studies failed to support this analysis, suggesting that effects occur independently of preexisting disease.[2,170,237] Ruptured intracerebral aneurysms in cocaine users are almost exclusively in the carotid artery circulation.[2,170,237] Presumably, CNS bleeding is a manifestation of abnormal shear force. Spontaneous extraaxial bleeding is also associated with cocaine use.[200]

Both vasospastic infarction and transient ischemic attack are reported in association with cocaine use.[46,47,136] In one epidemiologic study, women younger than age 45 years who had strokes were seven times more likely to report cocaine use than control participants.[182] Patients can present with any of the classic physical findings associated with thrombotic or embolic stroke. Additionally, paralysis is reported after cocaine-associated vasospasm of an anterior spinal artery.[46,164]

Seizures are commonly provoked by cocaine use.[92,167] Typically, they are discrete and occur within minutes after exposure; however, in some cases, they occur after as long as 24 hours after last use.[191] Although cocaine use serves as a trigger in some patients with epilepsy, an underlying focus is not necessary for seizures to occur.[123]

Headache is also well described in cocaine users. Although the exact mechanism is unclear, hypertension or dysregulation of neurotransmitters are likely contributory. In addition to typical tension headache, classic migraine and cluster headaches are also reported.[180,202]

Eyes, Nose, and Throat

Sympathetic excess produces mydriasis through stimulation of the dilator fibers of the iris with characteristic retention of the ability to respond to light. Like other mydriatics, cocaine produces acute narrow angle-closure glaucoma.[81] Vasospasm of the retinal vessels causes both unilateral and bilateral loss of vision.[91,139] Additionally, although cocaine produces excellent corneal anesthesia, it is highly toxic to the corneal epithelium. After application of cocaine to the eye, the superficial corneal layer is shed, resulting in pain and decreased acuity.[186] The loss of eyebrow and eyelash hair from thermal injury associated with smoking crack cocaine is called madarosis.[224]

Chronic intranasal insufflation of cocaine produces perforation of the nasal septum. This finding most likely results from repeated ischemic injury with resultant cartilage loss. This ischemia is usually asymptomatic, and necrotic tissue is sloughed. At least one reported case of wound botulism (Chap. 38) was associated with intranasal insufflation. Presumably, this resulted from accumulation of necrotic tissue in the nose, serving as a culture medium for *Clostridium botulinum*.[125]

Angioedema and oropharyngeal burns, located as far distally as the esophagus, are associated with smoking crack cocaine.[27,33,117,159] These effects are probably the result of inhalation or ingestion of superheated fumes and hot liquid (from the smoking apparatus) rather than direct toxicity from cocaine.

Pulmonary

Pneumothorax, pneumomediastinum, and pneumopericardium are reported after both smoked and intranasal cocaine use.[146,187,204,230,234] These findings do not result directly from cocaine toxicity but rather are epiphenomena related to the mechanism of drug use. After insufflation or inhalation, the user commonly performs a Valsalva maneuver in an attempt to retain the drug. Bearing down against a closed epiglottis increases intrathoracic pressure, and an alveolar bleb ruptures against the pleural, mediastinal, or pericardial surfaces.

Cocaine use exacerbates reversible airways disease, and it is common for patients to present with shortness of breath and wheezing.[56,135,176,194] Like so many manifestations of cocaine toxicity, it is unclear whether this is a direct effect of cocaine or related to inhalation of some contaminant of the drug. However, as discussed earlier, the muscarinic agonist effects of the pyrolysis metabolite AEME might be contributory.

"Crack lung" is the term given to an acute pulmonary syndrome that occurs after inhalational use of crack cocaine. The syndrome is a poorly defined constellation of symptoms, including fever, hemoptysis, hypoxia, acute respiratory distress syndrome, and respiratory failure. It is associated with diffuse alveolar and interstitial infiltrates on chest radiography.[187] Histopathology shows diffuse alveolar damage and hemorrhage with inflammatory cell infiltration and hemosiderin-laden macrophages. Eosinophilia was noted in several cases.[62] The syndrome is variously attributed to impurities mixed with the crack, carbonaceous material generated from pyrolysis, and direct cocaine toxicity.

Vasospasm and subsequent thrombosis of the pulmonary artery or its branches can produce pulmonary infarction.[49] Patients present with shortness of breath and pleuritic chest pain characteristic of a pulmonary embolus. Clinical signs and symptoms of ventilation–perfusion (V/Q) mismatch (Chap. 28), as well as abnormalities on arterial blood gas analysis, are noted.

Cardiovascular

Chest pain or discomfort is a common ED complaint in cocaine users.[21] Cocaine use is associated with cardiac ischemia and infarction in young people and reportedly accounts for as much as 25% of MIs in patients younger than 45 years of age.[184] Although MI is of concern, only approximately 6% of patients with complaints referable to the heart manifest biochemical evidence of myocardial injury.[96,243] Many others have an ischemic cardiac event, but for the remainder, the differential diagnosis is broad.[128] Entities to consider include the pulmonary and esophageal etiologies described previously, referred abdominal symptoms (see Abdominal), chest wall injury,[44,72,104,137,140] aortic dissection, coronary artery dissection,[203,221] and dysrhythmias. No single sign or symptom or combination of signs and symptoms reliably identifies cardiovascular injury from among the discussed differential diagnosis.[96]

Catecholamine-induced direct myocardial toxicity contributes to both acute and chronic cardiac disease. Takotsubo cardiomyopathy is a reversible form of left ventricular apical ballooning associated with myocardial ischemia in the absence of atherosclerotic lesions. It is thought to result from catecholamine toxicity on the myocardium during high levels of stress and is also reported after cocaine use.[7] Chronic cocaine use is associated with a dilated cardiomyopathy,[86,128] the etiology of which is presumed to be the result of repeated subclinical ischemic events. Patients typically present with signs and symptoms of congestive heart failure or pulmonary edema. The pathologic finding of contraction band necrosis is indicative of some direct catecholamine-induced oxidative damage to cardiac myocytes because this finding only commonly occurs with cocaine and amphetamine use, pheochromocytoma, and in patients receiving high-dose vasopressors.[60,239]

Abdominal

Abdominal pain or other gastrointestinal (GI) complaints suggest a broad differential diagnosis. Cocaine users have a disproportionate incidence of perforated ulcers.[134,179,215] The etiology is not elucidated but is hypothesized to be related to local ischemia of the GI tract or increased acid production associated with sympathetic activity. Vasospasm produces ischemic colitis that presents with abdominal pain or bloody stools.[140,169] More severe vasospasm, with or without thrombosis, leads to intestinal infarction[64,87,101,175] with associated hypotension and metabolic acidosis. Signs and symptoms of bowel obstruction, such as vomiting or distension, might suggest body packing (GI drug smuggling). Although less common, splenic[171] and renal infarctions[53,163,199] also occur, and splenic rupture with

associated hemoperitoneum and hemodynamic instability is reported.[8,10,100] Spontaneous hemoperitoneum without identifiable organ injury is also described, although occult trauma could not be definitively excluded.[14]

Animals frequently develop hepatotoxicity after cocaine administration. In human cocaine users, minor elevations of liver enzyme concentrations are common and rarely associated with symptoms.[25,124] When more severe liver injury occurs, it is usually associated with multisystem organ dysfunction from hyperthermia or another type of hepatic injury.[9] Isolated hepatic injury from cocaine is distinctly uncommon because of differences in metabolic pathways because animals are known to make a hepatotoxic metabolite of cocaine that is not described in humans.[236]

Musculoskeletal

Rhabdomyolysis is common in all conditions that produce an agitated delirium and or hyperthermia; cocaine is no exception.[40,103,196] Unlike most other toxicologic disorders, however, psychomotor agitation is not a prerequisite for cocaine-associated rhabdomyolysis.[251] Muscle injury also results from either vasospasm or direct muscle toxicity; however, the exact mechanism remains unclear. Patients with cocaine toxicity present with a spectrum of illness that ranges from asymptomatic enzyme and electrolyte abnormalities characteristic of rhabdomyolysis, to localized or diffuse muscle pain, to frank compartment syndrome and acute kidney injury.[54]

Limb ischemia associated with cocaine use is reported.[37,50,76,155,157] Although vasospasm, accelerated atherogenesis, and increased thrombogenesis (see Pathophysiology) place users at increased risk, the majority of the cases reported above appear to result from vasospasm.

Traumatic injury is also fairly common in the setting of cocaine use.[152] Clinicians should be aware of the possibilities of occult fractures or other injuries that are masked by the anesthetic properties of cocaine or the patient's altered level of consciousness.[142,151]

Neuropsychiatric

The neuropsychiatric effects of cocaine are most likely dose dependent. Low-dose administration produces alertness, exhilaration, hypersexual behavior, and other "desired" effects. These effects rarely bring users to health care facilities. As the cocaine dose increases, agitation, aggressive behavior, confusion, disorientation, and hallucinations develop.

Other possible manifestations include a variety of movement disorders that most likely result from dysregulation of dopamine. Some patients develop acute dystonias[28,59,235] or choreoathetoid movements that are referred to as "crack dancing."[45,77]

Obstetric

The majority of obstetric findings associated with cocaine use involve developmental problems in the fetus and neonate and are probably a result of a combination of chronic vascular insufficiency from cocaine-induced spasm of the uterine artery or distal vessels and other risk factors, such as poor maternal nutrition, cigarette smoking, and a lack of prenatal care (Chap. 30). These events are extensively reviewed elsewhere.[30,57,214] Acute cocaine use during pregnancy is associated with abruptio placentae, causing patients to present with abdominal pain and vaginal bleeding.[1,61] The remaining maternal and fetal complications comprise every possible complication described in nonpregnant patients.

DIAGNOSTIC TESTING

Cocaine and BE, its principal metabolite, can be detected in blood, urine, saliva, hair, and meconium. Routine drug of abuse testing relies on urine testing using a variety of immunologic techniques (Chap. 7) Although cocaine is rapidly eliminated within just a few hours of use, BE is easily detected in the urine for 2 to 3 days after last use.[4] When more sophisticated testing methodology is applied to chronic users, cocaine metabolites are identified for several weeks after the last use.[245]

Urine testing, even using rapid point-of-care assays, offers little to clinicians managing patients with presumed cocaine toxicity because it cannot distinguish recent from remote cocaine use. In addition, false-negative testing results when there is a large quantity of urine in the bladder with very recent cocaine use or when the urine is intentionally diluted by increased fluid intake,[38] leading to a urine cocaine concentration below the cutoff value and interpretation of the test result as negative. Under these circumstances, repeat testing is almost always positive. False-positive test results are extremely unlikely.

Although false-positive test results do occur, they are more common with hair testing than urine or blood because of the increased risk of external contamination.[38,193] Because of the very low rate of false-positive results, confirmation of a positive urine is unnecessary for medical indications (Chap. 7).

The greatest benefit for cocaine testing is in cases of unintentional poisoning or suspected child abuse and neglect. Here confirmation of a clinical suspicion is essential to support a legal argument. In addition, there is a role for urine testing of body packers, especially when the concealed xenobiotic is unknown.[232] Although many body packers have negative urine throughout their hospitalizations, a positive urine test result is suggestive of the concealed drug but obviously not confirmatory. More important, a conversion from a negative study on admission to a positive study not only confirms the substance ingested but also suggests packet leakage, which could be a harbinger of life-threatening toxicity (Special Considerations: SC5). Another indication for urine testing for cocaine occurs in young patients with chest pain syndromes in whom the history of drug use, specifically cocaine, is not forthcoming.[93] Routine diagnostic tests such as a bedside rapid reagent glucose, electrolytes, renal function tests, and markers of skeletal muscle and cardiac muscle injury are more likely to be useful than urine drug screening. Occasionally, the electrocardiogram (ECG) will show signs of ischemia or infarction, or dysrhythmias that require specific therapy. Unfortunately, in the setting of cocaine-associated chest pain, the ECG has neither the sensitivity nor the specificity necessary to permit exclusion or confirmation of cardiac injury.[98] Cardiac markers are therefore always required adjuncts when considering myocardial ischemia or MI. Because cocaine use is associated with diffuse muscle injury, assays for troponin are preferred over myoglobin or myocardial band enzymes of creatine phosphokinase (CPKMB).[97] Additionally, computed tomography (CT) angiography of the coronary arteries is reported by some to be a useful tool to exclude MI after cocaine use (CPKMB).[241] This test exposes the patient to high levels of radiation, and the relative risk versus benefit has not been studied, especially given the likelihood of repeated episodes of chest pain and inconsistent follow-up. For these reasons, we believe the data are insufficient to routinely recommend coronary CT at this time. Chest radiography is useful to exclude certain causes in patients with chest discomfort or to identify free air under the diaphragm when GI perforation is suspected. Supplemental diagnostic studies, such as CT scans of the head, chest, or abdomen and functional cardiac imaging, should be guided by the clinical condition of the patient.[40,55,79]

CESSATION OF USE

A cocaine withdrawal syndrome is not reported. After binge use of cocaine, a "washed-out" syndrome occurs that is best described by dopamine depletion.[220,231] Patients complain of anhedonia and lethargy, and they have trouble initiating and sustaining movement. However, they are arousable with minimal stimulation and usually remain cognitively intact.

Symptoms typically associated with cocaine toxicity sometimes present in a delayed fashion after cessation of cocaine use. The reasons for this delay are multifactorial and not entirely apparent but are presumed to be related to prolonged elimination of metabolites such as CE; changes in receptor regulation;[168] or effects on platelets, coagulation, and thrombolysis that stimulate a slow cascade, leading to thrombosis.

MANAGEMENT
General Supportive Care
As in the case of all poisoned patients, the initial emphasis should be on stabilization and control of the patient's airway, breathing, and circulation. If

tracheal intubation is required, it is important to recognize that cocaine toxicity is a relative contraindication to the use of succinylcholine.[154] Specifically, in the setting of rhabdomyolysis, hyperkalemia will be exacerbated by succinylcholine administration, and life-threatening dysrhythmias may result (Chap. 66). Additionally, it is essential to recognize that PChE metabolizes both cocaine and succinylcholine.[109] Thus, their simultaneous use will either prolong cocaine toxicity, paralysis, or both. Human data are insufficient to predict which interaction is more likely to occur. If hypotension is present, the initial approach should be intravenous (IV) infusion of 0.9% sodium chloride solution because many patients are volume depleted as a result of poor oral intake and excessive fluid losses from uncontrolled agitation, diaphoresis, and hyperthermia. Administration of IV fluids is also important in patients with rhabdomyolysis secondary to cocaine-associated agitation and hyperthermia.

In the setting of cocaine toxicity, it is important to recognize that both animal[29,75] and human[150] experience suggests that elevated temperature represents the most critical vital sign abnormality. Determination of the core temperature is an essential element of the initial evaluation, even when patients are severely agitated. When hyperthermia is present, rapid cooling with ice water immersion is required to normalize core body temperature (Chap. 29).[132] Sedation or paralysis and intubation are often necessary to facilitate the rapid cooling process. We recommend not to use antipyretics, drugs that prevent shivering (chlorpromazine or meperidine), and dantrolene[62] because they are ineffective and have the potential for adverse drug interactions such as serotonin toxicity (meperidine) (Chap. 36) or seizures (chlorpromazine).

Sedation remains the mainstay of therapy in patients with cocaine-associated agitation. It is important to remember that cocaine use is associated with hypoglycemia caused by catecholamine discharge.[19,163] Clinical findings of hypoglycemia and increased catecholamines are similar; consequently, a rapid bedside glucose should be obtained, or hypertonic dextrose should be empirically administered if indicated before or while simultaneously achieving sedation.

Both animal models[29,75] and extensive clinical experience in humans support the central role of benzodiazepines. Antipsychotics have also been used in the treatment of acute cocaine toxicity. A meta-analysis evaluating benzodiazepines and antipsychotics in animal models of cocaine toxicity found that both reduced mortality rates. However, benzodiazepine treatment reduced the mortality rate by 52% compared with only 29% for antipsychotics.[84] Although the choice among individual benzodiazepines is not well studied, an understanding of the pharmacology of these drugs allows for rational decision making. The goal is to use parenteral therapy with a drug that has a rapid onset and a rapid peak of action, making titration easy. Using this rationale, we recommend midazolam and diazepam over lorazepam because significant delay to peak effect for lorazepam often results in oversedation when it is dosed rapidly or in prolonged agitation when the appropriate dosing interval is used. Drugs should be administered in initial doses that are consistent with routine practices and increased incrementally based on an appropriate understanding of their pharmacology. For example, if using diazepam, the starting dose should be 5 to 10 mg IV, which can be repeated every 3 to 5 minutes and increased if necessary. Large doses of benzodiazepines are often necessary (on the order of 1 mg/kg of diazepam). This may result from cocaine-induced alterations in benzodiazepine receptor function (Antidotes in Depth: A26).[69,70,112]

On the rare occasion when benzodiazepines fail to achieve an adequate level of sedation, it is reasonable to administer either a rapidly acting barbiturate or propofol. There is recent interest in the use of ketamine to control patients with acute agitation,[35,99,173,190,205] but there is insufficient evidence demonstrating safety and efficacy to support its use in patients with cocaine-associated behavioral disorders. Controlled animal studies clearly show that the use of phenothiazines or butyrophenones as monotherapy is contraindicated.[29,75,139] In animal models, these drugs enhance toxicity (seizures), lethality, or both. Additional concerns about these drugs include interference with heat dissipation, exacerbation of tachycardia, prolongation of the QT interval, induction of torsade de pointes, and precipitation of dystonic reactions.

After sedation is accomplished, often no additional therapy is required. Specifically, patients with hypertension and tachycardia usually respond to sedation and volume resuscitation. In the uncommon event that hypertension or tachycardia persists, a direct-acting vasodilator such as nitroglycerin, nicardipine, or an α-adrenergic antagonist (eg, phentolamine) is recommended. The use of a β-adrenergic antagonist or a mixed α- and β-adrenergic antagonists in patients with acute cocaine toxicity is contraindicated. In both animal models and human reports, these drugs increase lethality and fail to treat the underlying CNS excitation[16,29,75,201,231] (see Specific Management later.) Severe and life-threatening hypertension or vasospasm will result from an unopposed α-adrenergic effect.

Decontamination

The majority of patients who present to the hospital after cocaine use do not require GI decontamination because the most popular methods of cocaine use are smoking and IV and intranasal administration. If the nares contain residual white powder presumed to be cocaine, gentle irrigation with 0.9% sodium chloride solution will help remove adherent material. Less commonly, patients ingest cocaine unintentionally or in an attempt to conceal evidence during an arrest (body stuffing)[88,111,147,219] or transport large quantities of drug across international borders (body packing).[67,73] These patients often require intensive decontamination and possibly surgical removal (Special Considerations: SC5).

Specific Management

In patients with end-organ manifestations of vasospasm that do not resolve with sedation, cooling, and volume resuscitation we recommend treatment with vasodilators (eg, phentolamine). When possible, direct delivery via intra-arterial administration to the affected vascular bed is preferable. Because this approach is not always feasible, systemic therapy is typically indicated. Phentolamine is dosed IV in increments of 1 to 2.5 mg and repeated as necessary until symptoms resolve or systemic hypotension develops.

Acute Coronary Syndrome

A significant amount of animal, in vitro, and in vivo human experimentation has been directed at defining the appropriate approach to patients with presumed cardiac ischemia or infarction. In some instances, an approach that is similar to the treatment of coronary artery disease (CAD) is indicated, although there are certain notable exceptions. An overall approach to care is available in the American Heart Association (AHA) guidelines and a number of reviews.[3,5,6,93,127,156]

In the setting of hypoxia, high-flow oxygen therapy is clearly indicated because it will help overcome some of the supply–demand mismatch that occurs with coronary insufficiency. Aspirin is likely safe in patients with cocaine-associated chest pain and is recommended for routine use.[156] In addition, administration of morphine is likely to be effective because it relieves cocaine-induced vasoconstriction.[198] Morphine also offers the same theoretical benefits of preload reduction and reduction of catecholamine release associated with pain.

Nitroglycerin is recommended because it reduces cocaine-associated coronary constriction of both normal and diseased vessels and relieves chest pain and associated symptoms.[89] Interestingly, in several clinical trials of cocaine-associated chest pain, benzodiazepines are at least as effective or superior to nitroglycerin.[12,102] Although the reasons for this are unclear, possible etiologies include blunting of central catecholamines or direct effects on cardiac benzodiazepine receptors. Either or both drugs are recommended in standard dosing (Antidotes in Depth: A26).

Although the benefits of β-adrenergic antagonism are demonstrated in patients with CAD, there is controversy surrounding their use in patients with cocaine-associated chest pain. In determining the risks and benefits of β-adrenergic antagonist administration, the established safety of their use should be compared with the magnitude of the benefit achieved in relation to other available therapies.

Several studies in both animals and humans underscore the potential risks of β-adrenergic antagonism in the setting of acute cocaine toxicity. β-Adrenergic antagonism increases lethality in cocaine-poisoned animals[29,75] and in humans exacerbates cocaine-induced coronary vasoconstriction.[127] In one study, the administration of esmolol to patients with acute cocaine poisoning produced severe paradoxical hypertension.[201] Mixed α- and β-adrenergic antagonists do not appear to offer any advantage in the treatment of patients with cocaine-associated coronary artery vasospasm. Labetalol was no better than placebo in this regard,[16] likely due in part to the relative ratios of receptor blockade. Intravenous labetalol has a relative β:α receptor blockage of 7:1.[188] Carvedilol has a ratio of 2.4:1.[20]

Despite these studies, β-adrenergic antagonists are frequently administered in the context of cocaine-associated chest pain for a variety of reasons, and several authors have argued in favor of their safety.[189] They often fail to distinguish acute toxicity from chronic or remote use, suggest that the aforementioned adverse events are extremely rare compared with the overall number of patients receiving β-adrenergic antagonists[189] and point to the absence of any documented cases of severe adverse events with the administration of combined α- and β-adrenergic antagonists.[189]

Even if the frequency of severe adverse events is rare, no quality data currently support the efficacy of β-adrenergic antagonism in the context of acute cocaine use. Studies in this area produce variable and conflicting results and are based on case reports and retrospective reviews using inconsistent outcome measures.

Thus, in the setting of acute cocaine toxicity, β-adrenergic antagonism is contraindicated. The 2008 AHA guidelines for the treatment of cocaine-associated chest pain and MI state that use of β-adrenergic antagonists should be avoided in the acute setting.[156] The 2014 AHA guidelines on the management of non–ST-segment elevation MI list β-adrenergic antagonists as class III (harm) because of the risk of potentiating coronary artery vasospasm.[5] If, after the measures mentioned previously are initiated, hypertension or vasospasm is still present and treatment is indicated, phentolamine is recommended based on its demonstrable experimental and clinical results.[95,127] If tachycardia does not respond to these accepted therapies, then diltiazem administration is reasonable.[15] Before the administration of any negative inotrope, it is essential to confirm that the tachycardia is not compensatory for a low cardiac output resulting from global myocardial dysfunction. Noninvasive methods of assessment of cardiac function have been used successfully in patients with cocaine-associated acute coronary syndromes and are recommended.[12]

There are no data on the use of unfractionated heparin (UFH) or low-molecular-weight heparins (LMWHs), glycoprotein IIb/IIIa inhibitors, or clopidogrel. The recent AHA guidelines recommend the administration of UFH or LMWH in patients with cocaine-associated MI.[156] The decision to use any of these medications should be based on a risk-to-benefit analysis. The possibility of underlying atherosclerotic heart disease should be evaluated. When acute thrombosis is likely, thrombolytic therapy is reasonable. Mechanistically, cocaine inhibits endogenous thrombolysis through augmentation of the inhibitor of tissue plasminogen activator. Additionally, there is sufficient clinical evidence to support the safety of thrombolytic therapy in patients with cocaine-associated MI.[89,94] Even though the number of patients treated with thrombolytic therapy is insufficient to demonstrate efficacy in terms of mortality, evidence of revascularization is encouraging. If available, cardiac catheterization with revascularization is preferable to thrombolysis.[213,216] A high rate of stent thrombosis after MI is reported in cocaine users. Thrombolysis would not be expected to be useful in treating ischemia caused by vasospasm. Because of the high incidence of coexisting atherosclerotic disease and an increased hypercoagulable state in cocaine-associated MI, thrombolysis is an acceptable alternative when catheterization is unavailable. Standard contraindications such as persistent hypertension, aortic dissection, trauma, and altered mental status must be considered before thrombolysis.

Dysrhythmias

Most patients present with sinus tachycardia that resolves after sedation, cooling, rehydration, and time to metabolize the drug. Other stable dysrhythmias should be treated similarly and often spontaneously revert because of the short duration of effect of cocaine. However, cocaine use is associated with atrial, supraventricular, and ventricular dysrhythmias, including torsade de pointes.[107,128,209] Most notably, wide complex tachycardias result from sodium channel blockade.

When approaching patients with cocaine-associated dysrhythmias, there are several important points to consider. The first is that β-adrenergic antagonism is contraindicated. Furthermore, class IA and IC antidysrhythmics are also contraindicated because of their ability to exacerbate cocaine induced sodium and potassium channel blockade.[128,247] Additionally, although popular in many advanced cardiac life support dysrhythmia algorithms, the effects of amiodarone are largely unknown in the setting of cocaine toxicity. Because of the lack of data demonstrating a benefit for amiodarone and because of concerns about its β-adrenergic antagonist effects, the use of this drug is not recommended at this time. Finally, although adenosine and synchronized cardioversion transiently help convert narrow complex tachycardias, if a substantial amount of cocaine is unmetabolized, the patient will likely revert back to the original dysrhythmia as these therapeutic interventions have short durations of effect. Thus, for rapid atrial fibrillation and narrow complex reentrant tachycardias, a calcium channel blocker such as diltiazem is reasonable. For wide-complex dysrhythmias, a trial of hypertonic sodium bicarbonate is recommended and has demonstrable usefulness analogous to treating patients with cyclic antidepressant overdose (Antidotes in Depth: A5).[116,126,177,198,242,247] When the use of hypertonic sodium bicarbonate fails to treat the dysrhythmia, lidocaine is recommended. Although lidocaine blocks sodium channels, its fast-on, fast-off properties allow it to antagonize the effects of cocaine. The benefits and safety of lidocaine were demonstrated in multiple animal models[74,79,85,90,247] and in humans with cocaine-associated MI.[115,234]

Ischemic Stroke

The safety of thrombolysis in cocaine-associated ischemic stroke is uncertain. Cocaine use can increase the risk of both ischemic stroke and intracerebral hemorrhage. One study found no increase in intracerebral hemorrhage after administration of tissue plasminogen activator in patients who had recently used cocaine, although acute cocaine intoxication was not specifically investigated.[149] Mechanical intervention with stent placement for ischemic stroke secondary to vasospasm was used, but data are insufficient to recommend routine use at this time.[238]

Limb and Bowel Ischemia

Only limited case reports address the management of patients with limb and bowel ischemia. Imaging is essential because it is important to try to distinguish thrombosis or embolus from vasospasm. If a discrete lesion is found, either angioplasty[50] or thrombolysis is reasonable depending on institutional resources. Because embolectomy or bypass may be required, a consultation with either interventional radiology or vascular surgery should be obtained. Vasodilators such as phentolamine, nitroglycerin,[76,157] and nicardipine and anticoagulation are also reasonable in an attempt to improve the low flow state and prevent clot.[37,155,157] Interestingly, continuous infusion of iloprost (an analog of the vasodilatory prostacyclin PGI_2) was reportedly beneficial in several cases.[37,155,157] If the patient is hemodynamically unstable, there is a theoretical role for direct intraarterial administration of vasodilators in an attempt to minimize the systemic effects.

ADULTERANTS

A variety of adulterants, contaminants, and diluents, collectively called "cutting agents," are present in cocaine. Adulterants are pharmacologically active substances intentionally added to enhance or mimic the effects of a drug. Diluents describe inert substances added to increase bulk, and contaminants describe unintentional byproducts present as a result of impure

manufacturing processes or drug storage. Historically, common cocaine adulterants included starches, sympathomimetics, and other local anesthetics.[34] Currently, the main adulterants of cocaine supplies include caffeine, diltiazem, hydroxyzine, levamisole, and phenacetin.[22]

The adulterant levamisole is worth special mention. First identified in cocaine in 2003, levamisole is an antihelminthic and immunomodulator. It was withdrawn from the US market in 2000 primarily because of agranulocytosis. By 2009, the US Drug Enforcement Administration estimated that 69% of cocaine contained levamisole.[131] Levamisole is metabolized to aminorex, a drug with potent amphetaminelike effects at dopamine and norepinephrine transporters. It is postulated that the addition of levamisole acts to both enhance and potentially lengthen the duration of effects of cocaine.[23] Two primary categories of levamisole toxicity are identified. The first is hematologic effects, including neutropenia and agranulocytosis. The second is dermatologic effects, including vasculitis and purpura. Reexposure to cocaine with levamisole is associated with recurrence of these symptoms. A multifocal inflammatory leukoencephalopathy characterized by cerebral demyelination and white matter lesions is also reported after use of cocaine adulterated with levamisole.[71,240]

DISPOSITION

Patients who present to health care facilities with classic sympathomimetic signs and symptoms that resolve spontaneously in the absence of signs of end-organ damage can be safely discharged after short periods of observation. When hyperthermia, rhabdomyolysis, or other signs of end-organ damage are evident, hospital admission is usually required. Patients who use cocaine are at increased risk for sudden death likely related in part to dysrhythmias and myocardial ischemia. In one series, patients with cardiac arrest after smoking crack cocaine were younger, more likely to survive, and less likely to have neurologic sequelae than case controls.[105]

For patients with chest pain, a specific management algorithm was derived based on substantial clinical experience. Those patients with clearly diagnostic or evolving ECGs suggestive of ischemia or infarction, positive cardiac biomarkers, dysrhythmias other than sinus tachycardia, congestive heart failure, or persistent pain require admission. Patients who become pain free and whose ECGs are stable are candidates for discharge if a single cardiac marker obtained at least 8 hours after the onset of chest pain is normal.[244] Although the AHA guidelines recommend 9 to 12 hours of observation for low-and intermediate-risk patients with cocaine-associated chest pain,[156] it is unclear whether the few extra hours offers additional benefit.

For all patients, it is essential to provide a referral for detoxification. Repeated cocaine use is the greatest risk factor for future cardiovascular complications.[96,197,245] Additionally, cocaine use in patients treated for traumatic injury is a risk factor for subsequent death from unintentional injury.

SUMMARY

- A sympathomimetic toxidrome is the typical clinical presentation.
- Hyperthermia is the most life-threatening vital sign abnormality and should be rapidly treated with ice water immersion.
- Treatment of agitation should focus on rapid sedation with a benzodiazepine and cooling if indicated.
- Myocardial infarction and dysrhythmias occur via diverse mechanisms.
- Both ischemic and hemorrhagic stroke also occur.

REFERENCES

1. Addis A, et al. Fetal effects of cocaine: an updated meta-analysis. *Reprod Toxicol.* 2001;15:341-369.
2. Aggarwal SK, et al. Cocaine-associated intracranial hemorrhage: absence of vasculitis in 14 cases. *Neurology.* 1996;46:1741-1743.
3. Albertson TE, et al. TOX-ACLS: toxicologic-oriented advanced cardiac life support. *Ann Emerg Med.* 2001;37(4 suppl):S78-S90.
4. Ambre J, et al. Urinary excretion of ecgonine methyl ester, a major metabolite of cocaine in humans. *J Anal Toxicol.* 1984;8:23-25.
5. Amsterdam EA, et al. 2014 AHA/ACC guideline for the management of patients with non-ST-elevation acute coronary syndromes: executive summary: a report of the

American College of Cardiology/American Heart Association Task Force on Practice Guidelines. *Circulation.* 2014;130:2354-2394.

6. Anderson JL, et al. 2012 ACCF/AHA focused update incorporated into the ACCF/AHA 2007 guidelines for the management of patients with unstable angina/non-ST-elevation myocardial infarction: a report of the American College of Cardiology Foundation/American Heart Association Task Force on Practice Guidelines. *J Am Coll Cardiol.* 2013;61:e179-347.

7. Arora S, et al. Transient left ventricular apical ballooning after cocaine use: is catecholamine cardiotoxicity the pathologic link? *Mayo Clin Proc.* 2006;81:829-832.

8. Azar F, et al. Cocaine-associated hemoperitoneum following atraumatic splenic rupture: a case report and literature review. *World J Emerg Surg.* 2013;8:33.

9. Balaguer F, et al. Cocaine-induced acute hepatitis and thrombotic microangiopathy. *JAMA.* 2005;293:797-798.

10. Ballard DH, et al. Atraumatic splenic rupture and ileal volvulus following cocaine abuse. *Clin Imaging.* 2015;39:1112-1114.

11. Barnett G, et al. Cocaine pharmacokinetics in humans. *J Ethnopharmacol.* 1981;3:353-366.

12. Baumann BM, et al. Cardiac and hemodynamic assessment of patients with cocaine-associated chest pain syndromes. *J Toxicol Clin Toxicol.* 2000;38:283-290.

13. Beckman KJ, et al. Hemodynamic and electrophysiological actions of cocaine. Effects of sodium bicarbonate as an antidote in dogs. *Circulation.* 1991;83:1799-1807.

14. Bellows CF, Raafat AM. The surgical abdomen associated with cocaine abuse. *J Emerg Med.* 2002;23:383-386.

15. Billman GE. Effect of calcium channel antagonists on cocaine-induced malignant arrhythmias: protection against ventricular fibrillation. *J Pharmacol Exp Ther.* 1993;266:407-416.

16. Boehrer JD, et al. Influence of labetalol on cocaine-induced coronary vasoconstriction in humans. *Am J Med.* 1993;94:608-610.

17. Borne RF, et al. Biological effects of cocaine derivatives I: improved synthesis and pharmacological evaluation of norcocaine. *J Pharm Sci.* 1977;66:119-120.

18. Brackett RL, et al. Prevention of cocaine-induced convulsions and lethality in mice: effectiveness of targeting different sites on the NMDA receptor complex. *Neuropharmacology.* 2000;39:407-418.

19. Brady WJ Jr, Duncan CW. Hypoglycemia masquerading as acute psychosis and acute cocaine intoxication. *Am J Emerg Med.* 1999;17:318-319.

20. Bristow MR. Beta-adrenergic receptor blockade in chronic heart failure. *Circulation.* 2000;101:558-569.

21. Brody SL, et al. Cocaine-related medical problems: consecutive series of 233 patients. *Am J Med.* 1990;88:325-331.

22. Broseus J, et al. The cutting of cocaine and heroin: a critical review. *Forensic Sci Int.* 2016;262:73-83.

23. Brunt TM, et al. Adverse effects of levamisole in cocaine users: a review and risk assessment. *Arch Toxicol.* 2017;91:2303-2313.

24. Bush S. Is cocaine needed in topical anaesthesia? *Emerg Med J.* 2002;19:418-422.

25. Cantilena LR, et al. Prevalence of abnormal liver-associated enzymes in cocaine experienced adults versus healthy volunteers during phase 1 clinical trials. *Contemp Clin Trials.* 2007;28:695-704.

26. Carmona GN, et al. Butyrylcholinesterase accelerates cocaine metabolism: in vitro and in vivo effects in nonhuman primates and humans. *Drug Metab Dispos.* 2000;28:367-371.

27. Castro-Villamor MA, et al. Cocaine-induced severe angioedema and urticaria. *Ann Emerg Med.* 1999;34:296-297.

28. Catalano G, et al. Dystonia associated with crack cocaine use. *South Med J.* 1997;90:1050-1052.

29. Catravas JD, Waters IW. Acute cocaine intoxication in the conscious dog: studies on the mechanism of lethality. *J Pharmacol Exp Ther.* 1981;217:350-356.

30. Chasnoff IJ, et al. Cocaine use in pregnancy. *N Engl J Med.* 1985;313:666-669.

31. Chen LC, et al. Pulmonary effects of the cocaine pyrolysis product, methylecgonidine, in guinea pigs. *Life Sci.* 1995;56:PL7-12.

32. Chow MJ, et al. Kinetics of cocaine distribution, elimination, and chronotropic effects. *Clin Pharmacol Ther.* 1985;38:318-324.

33. Cohen ME, Kegel JG. Candy cocaine esophagus. *Chest.* 2002;121:1701-1703.

34. Cole C, et al. Adulterants in illicit drugs: a review of empirical evidence. *Drug Test Anal.* 2011;3:89-96.

35. Cole JB, et al. A prospective study of ketamine versus haloperidol for severe prehospital agitation. *Clin Toxicol (Phila).* 2016;54:556-562.

36. Coleman DL, et al. Myocardial ischemia and infarction related to recreational cocaine use. *West J Med.* 1982;136:444-446.

37. Collins CG, et al. Cocaine-associated lower limb ischemia. *Vascular.* 2008;16:297-299.

38. Cone EJ, et al. Urine testing for cocaine abuse: metabolic and excretion patterns following different routes of administration and methods for detection of false-negative results. *J Anal Toxicol.* 2003;27:386-401.

39. Cone EJ, et al. Cocaine metabolism and urinary excretion after different routes of administration. *Ther Drug Monit.* 1998;20:556-560.

40. Counselman FL, et al. Creatine phosphokinase elevation in patients presenting to the emergency department with cocaine-related complaints. *Am J Emerg Med.* 1997;15:221-223.

41. Covert RF, et al. Hemodynamic and cerebral blood flow effects of cocaine, cocaethylene and benzoylecgonine in conscious and anesthetized fetal lambs. *J Pharmacol Exp Ther.* 1994;270:118-126.

42. Crumb WJ Jr, Clarkson CW. Characterization of the sodium channel blocking properties of the major metabolites of cocaine in single cardiac myocytes. *J Pharmacol Exp Ther.* 1992;261:910-917.

43. Crumb WJ Jr, Clarkson CW. The pH dependence of cocaine interaction with cardiac sodium channels. *J Pharmacol Exp Ther.* 1995;274:1228-1237.

44. Daniel JC, et al. Acute aortic dissection associated with use of cocaine. *J Vasc Surg.* 2007;46:427-433.

45. Daras M, et al. Cocaine-induced choreoathetoid movements ('crack dancing'). *Neurology.* 1994;44:751-752.

46. Daras M, et al. Central nervous system infarction related to cocaine abuse. *Stroke.* 1991;22:1320-1325.

47. Daras MD, et al. Bilateral symmetrical basal ganglia infarction after intravenous use of cocaine and heroin. *Clin Imaging.* 2001;25:12-14.

48. Dean RA, et al. Human liver cocaine esterases: ethanol-mediated formation of ethylcocaine. *FASEB J.* 1991;5:2735-2739.

49. Delaney K, Hoffman RS. Pulmonary infarction associated with crack cocaine use in a previously healthy 23-year-old woman. *Am J Med.* 1991;91:92-94.

50. Denegri A, et al. Lower limb ischemia due to long-term abuse of cocaine. *J Cardiovasc Med (Hagerstown).* 2016;17(suppl 2):e176-e177.

51. Department of Health and Human Services SAaMHS. *Results from 2015 National Survey on Drug Use and Health*; 2015.

52. Department of Health and Human Services SAMHSA. *Results from the Drug Abuse Warning Network.* National Estimates of Drug-Related Emergency Department Visits; Rockville, MD 2011.

53. Edmondson DA, et al. Cocaine-induced renal artery dissection and thrombosis leading to renal infarction. *WMJ.* 2004;103:66-69.

54. el-Hayek BM, et al. [Rhabdomyolysis, compartment syndrome and acute kidney failure related to cocaine consume]. *Nefrologia.* 2003;23:469-470.

55. Eng JG, et al. False-negative abdominal CT scan in a cocaine body stuffer. *Am J Emerg Med.* 1999;17:702-704.

56. Ettinger NA, Albin RJ. A review of the respiratory effects of smoking cocaine. *Am J Med.* 1989;87:664-668.

57. Fajemirokun-Odudeyi O, Lindow SW. Obstetric implications of cocaine use in pregnancy: a literature review. *Eur J Obstet Gynecol Reprod Biol.* 2004;112:2-8.

58. Ferreira S, et al. Effects of cocaine and its major metabolites on the HERG-encoded potassium channel. *J Pharmacol Exp Ther.* 2001;299:220-226.

59. Fines RE, et al. Cocaine-associated dystonic reaction. *Am J Emerg Med.* 1997;15:513-515.

60. Fineschi V, et al. Myocardial necrosis and cocaine. A quantitative morphologic study in 26 cocaine-associated deaths. *Int J Legal Med.* 1997;110:193-198.

61. Flowers D, et al. Cocaine intoxication associated with abruptio placentae. *J Natl Med Assoc.* 1991;83:230-232.

62. Fox AW. More on rhabdomyolysis associated with cocaine intoxication. *N Engl J Med.* 1989;321:1271.

63. Freud S. Uber coca. *Wein Centralbl Ther.* 1884;2:289-314.

64. Freudenberger RS, et al. Intestinal infarction after intravenous cocaine administration. *Ann Intern Med.* 1990;113:715-716.

65. Garcia RC, et al. Anhydroecgonine methyl ester, a cocaine pyrolysis product, may contribute to cocaine behavioral sensitization. *Toxicology.* 2017;376:44-50.

66. Garland O. Fatal acute poisoning by cocaine. *Lancet.* 1895;1:1104-1105.

67. Gill JR, Graham SM. Ten years of "body packers" in New York City: 50 deaths. *J Forensic Sci.* 2002;47:843-846.

68. Giros B, et al. Hyperlocomotion and indifference to cocaine and amphetamine in mice lacking the dopamine transporter. *Nature.* 1996;379:606-612.

69. Goeders NE. Cocaine differentially affects benzodiazepine receptors in discrete regions of the rat brain: persistence and potential mechanisms mediating these effects. *J Pharmacol Exp Ther.* 1991;259:574-581.

70. Goeders NE, et al. Tolerance and sensitization to the behavioral effects of cocaine in rats: relationship to benzodiazepine receptors. *Pharmacol Biochem Behav.* 1997;57:43-56.

71. Gonzalez-Duarte A, Williams R. Cocaine-induced recurrent leukoencephalopathy. *Neuroradiol J.* 2013;26:511-513.

72. Gotway MB, et al. Thoracic complications of illicit drug use: an organ system approach. *Radiographics.* 2002;22(Spec No):S119-135.

73. Grant SA, et al. Tetracaine protects against cocaine lethality in mice. *Ann Emerg Med.* 1993;22:1799-1803.

74. Grawe JJ, et al. Reversal of the electrocardiographic effects of cocaine by lidocaine. Part 2. Concentration-effect relationships. *Pharmacotherapy.* 1994;14:704-711.

75. Guinn MM, et al. of intravenous cocaine lethality in nonhuman primates. *Clin Toxicol.* 1980;16:499-508.

76. Gutierrez A, et al. Cocaine-induced peripheral vascular occlusive disease—a case report. *Angiology.* 1998;49:221-224.

77. Habal R, et al. Cocaine and chorea. *Am J Emerg Med.* 1991;9:618-620.

78. Haddad LM. 1978: Cocaine in perspective. *JACEP.* 1979;8:374-376.

79. Hahn IH, et al. Contrast CT scan fails to detect the last heroin packet. *J Emerg Med.* 2004;27:279-283.

80. Hall FS, et al. Molecular mechanisms underlying the rewarding effects of cocaine. *Ann N Y Acad Sci.* 2004;1025:47-56.

81. Hari CK, et al. Acute angle closure glaucoma precipitated by intranasal application of cocaine. *J Laryngol Otol.* 1999;113:250-251.

82. Harris DS, et al. The pharmacology of cocaethylene in humans following cocaine and ethanol administration. *Drug Alcohol Depend.* 2003;72:169-182.

83. Hart CL, et al. Comparison of intravenous cocaethylene and cocaine in humans. *Psychopharmacology (Berl).* 2000;149:153-162.

84. Heard K, et al. Benzodiazepines and antipsychotic medications for treatment of acute cocaine toxicity in animal models–a systematic review and meta-analysis. *Hum Exp Toxicol.* 2011;30:1849-1854.

85. Heit J, et al. The effects of lidocaine pretreatment on cocaine neurotoxicity and lethality in mice. *Acad Emerg Med.* 1994;1:438-442.

86. Henzlova MJ, et al. Apparent reversibility of cocaine-induced congestive cardiomyopathy. *Am Heart J.* 1991;122:577-579.

87. Hoang MP, et al. Histologic spectrum of arterial and arteriolar lesions in acute and chronic cocaine-induced mesenteric ischemia: report of three cases and literature review. *Am J Surg Pathol.* 1998;22:1404-1410.

88. Hoffman RS, et al. Prospective evaluation of "crack-vial" ingestions. *Vet Hum Toxicol.* 1990;32:164-167.

89. Hoffman RS, Hollander JE. Thrombolytic therapy and cocaine-induced myocardial infarction. *Am J Emerg Med.* 1996;14:693-695.

90. Hoffman RS, et al. Ecgonine methyl ester protects against cocaine lethality in mice. *J Toxicol Clin Toxicol.* 2004;42:349-354.

91. Hoffman RS, Reimer BI. "Crack" cocaine-induced bilateral amblyopia. *Am J Emerg Med.* 1993;11:35-37.

92. Holland RW 3rd, et al. Grand mal seizures temporally related to cocaine use: clinical and diagnostic features. *Ann Emerg Med.* 1992;21:772-776.

93. Hollander JE. The management of cocaine-associated myocardial ischemia. *N Engl J Med.* 1995;333:1267-1272.

94. Hollander JE, et al. Cocaine-associated myocardial infarction. Clinical safety of thrombolytic therapy. Cocaine Associated Myocardial Infarction (CAMI) Study Group. *Chest.* 1995;107:1237-1241.

95. Hollander JE, et al. Nitroglycerin in the treatment of cocaine associated chest pain—clinical safety and efficacy. *J Toxicol Clin Toxicol.* 1994;32:243-256.

96. Hollander JE, et al. Prospective multicenter evaluation of cocaine-associated chest pain. Cocaine Associated Chest Pain (COCHPA) Study Group. *Acad Emerg Med.* 1994;1:330-339.

97. Hollander JE, et al. Effect of recent cocaine use on the specificity of cardiac markers for diagnosis of acute myocardial infarction. *Am Heart J.* 1998;135(2 Pt 1):245-252.

98. Hollander JE, et al. "Abnormal" electrocardiograms in patients with cocaine-associated chest pain are due to "normal" variants. *J Emerg Med.* 1994;12:199-205.

99. Hollis GJ, et al. Prehospital ketamine use by paramedics in the Australian Capital Territory: a 12 month retrospective analysis. *Emerg Med Australas.* 2017;29:89-95.

100. Homler HJ. Nontraumatic splenic hematoma related to cocaine abuse. *West J Med.* 1995;163:160-162.

101. Hon DC, et al. Crack-induced enteric ischemia. *N J Med.* 1990;87:1001-1002.

102. Honderick T, et al. A prospective, randomized, controlled trial of benzodiazepines and nitroglycerine or nitroglycerine alone in the treatment of cocaine-associated acute coronary syndromes. *Am J Emerg Med.* 2003;21:39-42.

103. Horowitz BZ, et al. Severe rhabdomyolysis with renal failure after intranasal cocaine use. *J Emerg Med.* 1997;15:833-837.

104. Hsue PY, et al. Cardiac arrest in patients who smoke crack cocaine. *Am J Cardiol.* 2007;99:822-824.

105. Hsue PY, et al. Acute aortic dissection related to crack cocaine. *Circulation.* 2002;105:1592-1595.

106. Inaba T, et al. Metabolism of cocaine in man. *Clin Pharmacol Ther.* 1978;23:547-552.

107. Isner JM, et al. Acute cardiac events temporally related to cocaine abuse. *N Engl J Med.* 1986;315:1438-1443.

108. Jacob P 3rd, et al. Cocaine smokers excrete a pyrolysis product, anhydroecgonine methyl ester. *J Toxicol Clin Toxicol.* 1990;28:121-125.

109. Jatlow P, et al. Cocaine and succinylcholine sensitivity: a new caution. *Anesth Analg.* 1979;58:235-238.

110. Jeffcoat AR, et al. Cocaine disposition in humans after intravenous injection, nasal insufflation (snorting), or smoking. *Drug Metab Dispos.* 1989;17:153-159.

111. June R, et al. Medical outcome of cocaine bodystuffers. *J Emerg Med.* 2000;18:221-224.

112. Jung ME, et al. Cocaine increases benzodiazepine receptors labeled in the mouse brain in vivo with [3H]Ro 15-1788. *NIDA Res Monogr.* 1989;95:512-513.

113. Just WW, Hoyer J. The local anesthetic potency of norcocaine, a metabolite of cocaine. *Experientia.* 1977;33:70-71.

114. Karch SB. Cocaine: history, use, abuse. *J R Soc Med.* 1999;92:393-397.

115. Katz JL, et al. Comparative behavioral pharmacology and toxicology of cocaine and its ethanol-derived metabolite, cocaine ethyl-ester (cocaethylene). *Life Sci.* 1992;50:1351-1361.

116. Kerns W 2nd, et al. Cocaine-induced wide complex dysrhythmia. *J Emerg Med.* 1997;15:321-329.

117. Kestler A, Keyes L. Images in clinical medicine. Uvular angioedema (Quincke's disease). *N Engl J Med.* 2003;349:867.

118. Knuepfer MM. Cardiovascular disorders associated with cocaine use: myths and truths. *Pharmacol Ther.* 2003;97:181-222.

119. Knuepfer MM, Branch CA. Cardiovascular responses to cocaine are initially mediated by the central nervous system in rats. *J Pharmacol Exp Ther.* 1992;263:734-741.

120. Kolodgie FD, et al. Increased prevalence of aortic fatty streaks in cholesterol-fed rabbits administered intravenous cocaine: the role of vascular endothelium. *Toxicol Pathol.* 1993;21:425-435.

121. Kolodgie FD, et al. Cocaine-induced increase in the permeability function of human vascular endothelial cell monolayers. *Exp Mol Pathol.* 1999;66:109-122.

122. Konkol RJ, et al. Seizures induced by the cocaine metabolite benzoylecgonine in rats. *Epilepsia.* 1992;33:420-427.

123. Koppel BS, et al. Relation of cocaine use to seizures and epilepsy. *Epilepsia.* 1996;37:875-878.

124. Kothur R, et al. Liver function tests in nonparenteral cocaine users. *Arch Intern Med.* 1991;151:1126-1128.

125. Kudrow DB, et al. Botulism associated with Clostridium botulinum sinusitis after intranasal cocaine abuse. *Ann Intern Med.* 1988;109:984-985.

126. Kugelmass AD, et al. Activation of human platelets by cocaine. *Circulation.* 1993;88:876-883.

127. Lange RA, et al. Cocaine-induced coronary-artery vasoconstriction. *N Engl J Med.* 1989;321:1557-1562.

128. Lange RA, Hillis LD. Cardiovascular complications of cocaine use. *N Engl J Med.* 2001;345:351-358.

129. Langner RO, Bement CL. Cocaine-induced changes in the biochemistry and morphology of rabbit aorta. *NIDA Res Monogr.* 1991;108:154-166.

130. Langner RO, et al. Arteriosclerotic toxicity of cocaine. *NIDA Res Monogr.* 1988;88:325-336.

131. Larocque A, Hoffman RS. Levamisole in cocaine: unexpected news from an old acquaintance. *Clin Toxicol (Phila).* 2012;50:231-241.

132. Laskowski LK, et al. Ice water submersion for rapid cooling in severe drug-induced hyperthermia. *Clin Toxicol (Phila).* 2015;53:181-184.

133. Lason W. Neurochemical and pharmacological aspects of cocaine-induced seizures. *Pol J Pharmacol.* 2001;53:57-60.

134. Lee HS, et al. Acute gastroduodenal perforations associated with use of crack. *Ann Surg.* 1990;211:15-17.

135. Levine M, et al. The effects of cocaine and heroin use on intubation rates and hospital utilization in patients with acute asthma exacerbations. *Chest.* 2005;128:1951-1957.

136. Levine SR, et al. Cerebrovascular complications of the use of the "crack" form of alkaloidal cocaine. *N Engl J Med.* 1990;323:699-704.

137. Li W, et al. Cocaine-induced relaxation of isolated rat aortic rings and mechanisms of action: possible relation to cocaine-induced aortic dissection and hypotension. *Eur J Pharmacol.* 2004;496:151-158.

138. Liaudet L, et al. Pathophysiological mechanisms of catecholamine and cocaine-mediated cardiotoxicity. *Heart Fail Rev.* 2014;19:815-824.

139. Libman RB, et al. Transient monocular blindness associated with cocaine abuse. *Neurology.* 1993;43:228-229.

140. Linder JD, et al. Cyclooxygenase-2 inhibitor celecoxib: a possible cause of gastropathy and hypoprothrombinemia. *South Med J.* 2000;93:930-932.

141. Littmann L, et al. Brugada-type electrocardiographic pattern induced by cocaine. *Mayo Clin Proc.* 2000;75:845-849.

142. Long H, et al. Medicinal use of cocaine: a shifting paradigm over 25 years. *Laryngoscope.* 2004;114:1625-1629.

143. Lynch TJ, et al. Cocaine detoxification by human plasma butyrylcholinesterase. *Toxicol Appl Pharmacol.* 1997;145:363-371.

144. Madden JA, et al. Cocaine and benzoylecgonine constrict cerebral arteries by different mechanisms. *Life Sci.* 1995;56:679-686.

145. Madden JA, Powers RH. Effect of cocaine and cocaine metabolites on cerebral arteries in vitro. *Life Sci.* 1990;47:1109-1114.

146. Maeder M, Ullmer E. Pneumomediastinum and bilateral pneumothorax as a complication of cocaine smoking. *Respiration.* 2003;70:407.

147. Malbrain ML, et al. A massive, near-fatal cocaine intoxication in a body-stuffer. Case report and review of the literature. *Acta Clin Belg.* 1994;49:12-18.

148. Mangiardi JR, et al. Cocaine-related intracranial hemorrhage. Report of nine cases and review. *Acta Neurol Scand.* 1988;77:177-180.

149. Martin-Schild S, et al. Intravenous tissue plasminogen activator in patients with cocaine-associated acute ischemic stroke. *Stroke.* 2009;40:3635-3637.

150. Marzuk PM, et al. Ambient temperature and mortality from unintentional cocaine overdose. *JAMA.* 1998;279:1795-1800.

151. Marzuk PM, et al. Fatal injuries after cocaine use as a leading cause of death among young adults in New York City. *N Engl J Med.* 1995;332:1753-1757.

152. Marzuk PM, et al. Prevalence of recent cocaine use among motor vehicle fatalities in New York City. *JAMA.* 1990;263:250-256.

153. Mateo Y, et al. Role of serotonin in cocaine effects in mice with reduced dopamine transporter function. *Proc Natl Acad Sci U S A.* 2004;101:372-377.

154. Matsuo S, et al. Interaction of muscle relaxants and local anesthetics at the neuromuscular junction. *Anesth Analg.* 1978;57:580-587.

155. Mazzone A, et al. Cocaine-related peripheral vascular occlusive disease treated with iloprost in addition to anticoagulants and antibiotics. *Clin Toxicol (Phila).* 2007;45:65-66.

156. McCord J, et al. Management of cocaine-associated chest pain and myocardial infarction: a scientific statement from the American Heart Association Acute Cardiac Care Committee of the Council on Clinical Cardiology. *Circulation.* 2008;117:1897-1907.

157. McMullin CM, et al. Profound acute limb ischemia affecting all four limbs following cocaine inhalation. *J Vasc Surg.* 2015;61:504-506.

158. Mehta A, et al. Electrocardiographic effects of intravenous cocaine: an experimental study in a canine model. *J Cardiovasc Pharmacol.* 2003;41:25-30.

159. Meleca RJ, et al. Mucosal injuries of the upper aerodigestive tract after smoking crack or freebase cocaine. *Laryngoscope.* 1997;107:620-625.

160. Mets B, Virag L. Lethal toxicity from equimolar infusions of cocaine and cocaine metabolites in conscious and anesthetized rats. *Anesth Analg.* 1995;81:1033-1038.

161. Misra AL, et al. Estimation and disposition of [3H]benzoylecgonine and pharmacological activity of some cocaine metabolites. *J Pharm Pharmacol.* 1975;27:784-786.

162. Mochizuki Y, et al. Acute aortic thrombosis and renal infarction in acute cocaine intoxication: a case report and review of literature. *Clin Nephrol.* 2003;60:130-133.

163. Mochson CM, et al. Hypoglycemia in cocaine-intoxicated mice. *Acad Emerg Med.* 2001;8:768.

164. Mody CK, et al. Neurologic complications of cocaine abuse. *Neurology.* 1988;38: 1189-1193.

165. Moliterno DJ, et al. Influence of intranasal cocaine on plasma constituents associated with endogenous thrombosis and thrombolysis. *Am J Med.* 1994;96:492-496.

166. Moliterno DJ, et al. Coronary-artery vasoconstriction induced by cocaine, cigarette smoking, or both. *N Engl J Med.* 1994;330:454-459.

167. Mott SH, et al. Neurologic manifestations of cocaine exposure in childhood. *Pediatrics.* 1994;93:557-560.

168. Nademanee K, et al. Myocardial ischemia during cocaine withdrawal. *Ann Intern Med.* 1989;111:876-880.

169. Niazi M, et al. Spectrum of ischemic colitis in cocaine users. *Dig Dis Sci.* 1997;42: 1537-1541.

170. Nolte KB, et al. Intracranial hemorrhage associated with cocaine abuse: a prospective autopsy study. *Neurology.* 1996;46:1291-1296.

171. Novielli KD, Chambers CV. Splenic infarction after cocaine use. *Ann Intern Med.* 1991;114:251-252.

172. O'Leary ME. Inhibition of HERG potassium channels by cocaethylene: a metabolite of cocaine and ethanol. *Cardiovasc Res.* 2002;53:59-67.

173. Olives TD, et al. intubation of profoundly agitated patients treated with prehospital ketamine. *Prehosp Disaster Med.* 2016;31:593-602.

174. Om A, et al. Medical complications of cocaine: possible relationship to low plasma cholinesterase enzyme. *Am Heart J.* 1993;125:1114-1117.

175. Osorio J, et al. Cocaine-induced mesenteric ischaemia. *Dig Surg.* 2000;17:648-651.

176. Pane MA, et al. Ecgonine methyl ester, a major cocaine metabolite, causes cerebral vasodilation in neonatal sheep. *Pediatr Res.* 1997;41:815-821.

177. Parker RB, et al. Comparative effects of sodium bicarbonate and sodium chloride on reversing cocaine-induced changes in the electrocardiogram. *J Cardiovasc Pharmacol.* 1999;34:864-869.

178. Parker RB, et al. Factors affecting serum protein binding of cocaine in humans. *J Pharmacol Exp Ther.* 1995;275:605-610.

179. Pecha RE, et al. Association of cocaine and methamphetamine use with giant gastro-duodenal ulcers. *Am J Gastroenterol.* 1996;91:2523-2527.

180. Penarrocha M, et al. Cluster headache and cocaine use. *Oral Surg Oral Med Oral Pathol Oral Radiol Endod.* 2000;90:271-274.

181. Perera R, et al. Prolonged QT interval and cocaine use. *J Electrocardiol.* 1997;30: 337-339.

182. Petitti DB, et al. Stroke and cocaine or amphetamine use. *Epidemiology.* 1998;9: 596-600.

183. Przywara DA, Dambach GE. Direct actions of cocaine on cardiac cellular electrical activity. *Circ Res.* 1989;65:185-192.

184. Qureshi AI, et al. Cocaine use and the likelihood of nonfatal myocardial infarction and stroke: data from the Third National Health and Nutrition Examination Survey. *Circulation.* 2001;103:502-506.

185. Ramadan NM, et al. Scintillating scotomata associated with internal carotid artery dissection: report of three cases. *Neurology.* 1991;41:1084-1087.

186. Ravin JG, Ravin LC. Blindness due to illicit use of topical cocaine. *Ann Ophthalmol.* 1979;11:863-864.

187. Restrepo CS, et al. Pulmonary complications from cocaine and cocaine-based substances: imaging manifestations. *Radiographics.* 2007;27:941-956.

188. Richards DA, et al. Pharmacological basis for antihypertensive effects of intravenous labetalol. *Br Heart J.* 1977;39:99-106.

189. Richards JR, et al. beta-Blockers, cocaine, and the unopposed alpha-stimulation phenomenon. *J Cardiovasc Pharmacol Ther.* 2017;22:239-249.

190. Riddell J, et al. Ketamine as a first-line treatment for severely agitated emergency department patients. *Am J Emerg Med.* 2017.

191. Riezzo I, et al. Side effects of cocaine abuse: multiorgan toxicity and pathological consequences. *Curr Med Chem.* 2012;19:5624-5646.

192. Rockhold RW, et al. Glutamate receptor antagonists block cocaine-induced convulsions and death. *Brain Res Bull.* 1991;27:721-723.

193. Romano G, et al. Hair testing for drugs of abuse: evaluation of external cocaine contamination and risk of false positives. *Forensic Sci Int.* 2001;123:119-129.

194. Rome LA, et al. Prevalence of cocaine use and its impact on asthma exacerbation in an urban population. *Chest.* 2000;117:1324-1329.

195. Ruetsch YA, et al. From cocaine to ropivacaine: the history of local anesthetic drugs. *Curr Top Med Chem.* 2001;1:175-182.

196. Ruttenber AJ, et al. Cocaine-associated rhabdomyolysis and excited delirium: different stages of the same syndrome. *Am J Forensic Med Pathol.* 1999;20:120-127.

197. Ryb GE, et al. Suicides, homicides, and unintentional injury deaths after trauma center discharge: cocaine use as a risk factor. *J Trauma.* 2009;67:490-496; discussion 497.

198. Saland KE, et al. Influence of morphine sulfate on cocaine-induced coronary vasoconstriction. *Am J Cardiol.* 2002;90:810-811.

199. Saleem TM, et al. Renal infarction: a rare complication of cocaine abuse. *Am J Emerg Med.* 2001;19:528-529.

200. Samkoff LM, et al. Spontaneous spinal epidural hematoma. Another neurologic complication of cocaine? *Arch Neurol.* 1996;53:819-821.

201. Sand IC, et al. Experience with esmolol for the treatment of cocaine-associated cardiovascular complications. *Am J Emerg Med.* 1991;9:161-163.

202. Satel SL, Gawin FH. Migrainelike headache and cocaine use. *JAMA.* 1989;261: 2995-2996.

203. Satran A, et al. Increased prevalence of coronary artery aneurysms among cocaine users. *Circulation.* 2005;111:2424-2429.

204. Savader SJ, et al. Pneumothorax, pneumomediastinum, and pneumopericardium: complications of cocaine smoking. *J Fla Med Assoc.* 1988;75:151-152.

205. Scaggs TR, et al. prehospital ketamine is a safe and effective treatment for excited delirium in a community hospital based EMS system. *Prehosp Disaster Med.* 2016;31:563-569.

206. Scheidweiler KB, et al. Pharmacokinetics and pharmacodynamics of methylecgonidine, a crack cocaine pyrolyzate. *J Pharmacol Exp Ther.* 2003;307:1179-1187.

207. Schindler CW, et al. Effects of cocaine and cocaine metabolites on cardiovascular function in squirrel monkeys. *Eur J Pharmacol.* 2001;431:53-59.

208. Schreiber MD, et al. Effects of cocaine, benzoylecgonine, and cocaine metabolites in cannulated pressurized fetal sheep cerebral arteries. *J Appl Physiol.* (1985) 1994;77:834-839.

209. Schrem SS, et al. Cocaine-induced torsades de pointes in a patient with the idiopathic long QT syndrome. *Am Heart J.* 1990;120:980-984.

210. Schuelke GS, et al. Effect of cocaine metabolites on behavior: possible neuroendocrine mechanisms. *Brain Res Bull.* 1996;39:43-48.

211. Schwartz AB, et al. Electrocardiographic and hemodynamic effects of intravenous cocaine in awake and anesthetized dogs. *J Electrocardiol.* 1989;22:159-166.

212. Schwartz KA, Cohen JA. Subarachnoid hemorrhage precipitated by cocaine snorting. *Arch Neurol.* 1984;41:705.

213. Shah DM, et al. Percutaneous transluminal coronary angioplasty and stenting for cocaine-induced acute myocardial infarction: a case report and review. *Catheter Cardiovasc Interv.* 2000;49:447-451.

214. Shankaran S, et al. Impact of maternal substance use during pregnancy on childhood outcome. *Semin Fetal Neonatal Med.* 2007;12:143-150.

215. Sharma R, et al. Clinical observation of the temporal association between crack cocaine and duodenal ulcer perforation. *Am J Surg.* 1997;174:629-632; discussion 632-633.

216. Singh S, et al. Increased incidence of in-stent thrombosis related to cocaine use: case series and review of literature. *J Cardiovasc Pharmacol Ther.* 2007;12:298-303.

217. Smith JA, et al. Cocaine increases extraneuronal levels of aspartate and glutamate in the nucleus accumbens. *Brain Res.* 1995;683:264-269.

218. Spealman RD, et al. Effects of cocaine and related drugs in nonhuman primates. II. Stimulant effects on schedule-controlled behavior. *J Pharmacol Exp Ther.* 1989;251:142-149.

219. Sporer KA, Firestone J. Clinical course of crack cocaine body stuffers. *Ann Emerg Med.* 1997;29:596-601.

220. Sporer KA, Lesser SH. Cocaine washed-out syndrome. *Ann Emerg Med.* 1992;21:112.

221. Steinhauer JR, Caulfield JB. Spontaneous coronary artery dissection associated with cocaine use: a case report and brief review. *Cardiovasc Pathol.* 2001;10:141-145.

222. Stewart DJ, et al. Cocaine metabolism: cocaine and norcocaine hydrolysis by liver and serum esterases. *Clin Pharmacol Ther.* 1979;25:464-468.

223. Stewart DJ, et al. Hydrolysis of cocaine in human plasma by cholinesterase. *Life Sci.* 1977;20:1557-1563.

224. Tames SM, Goldenring JM. Madarosis from cocaine use. *N Engl J Med.* 1986;314:1324.

225. Tashkin DP, et al. Acute effects of inhaled and i.v. cocaine on airway dynamics. *Chest.* 1996;110:904-910.

226. Taylor D, et al. Cocaine induced prolongation of the QT interval. *Emerg Med J.* 2004;21:252-253.

227. Tella SR, et al. Pathophysiological and pharmacological mechanisms of acute cocaine toxicity in conscious rats. *J Pharmacol Exp Ther.* 1992;262:936-946.

228. Tella SR, et al. Cocaine: cardiovascular effects in relation to inhibition of peripheral neuronal monoamine uptake and central stimulation of the sympathoadrenal system. *J Pharmacol Exp Ther.* 1993;267:153-162.

229. Thompson A. Toxic action of cocaine. *Br Med J.* 1886;1:67.

230. Torre M, Barberis M. Spontaneous pneumothorax in cocaine sniffers. *Am J Emerg Med.* 1998;16:546-549.

231. Trabulsy ME. Cocaine washed out syndrome in a patient with acute myocardial infarction. *Am J Emerg Med.* 1995;13:538-539.

232. Traub SJ, et al. Body packing—the internal concealment of illicit drugs. *N Engl J Med.* 2003;349:2519-2526.

233. United Nations Office on Drugs and Crime. *World Drug Report.* United Nations Publication, New York 2016.

234. Uva JL. Spontaneous pneumothoraces, pneumomediastinum, and pneumoperitoneum: consequences of smoking crack cocaine. *Pediatr Emerg Care.* 1997;13:24-26.

235. van Harten PN, et al. Cocaine as a risk factor for neuroleptic-induced acute dystonia. *J Clin Psychiatry.* 1998;59:128-130.

236. Van Thiel DH, Perper JA. Hepatotoxicity associated with cocaine abuse. *Recent Dev Alcohol.* 1992;10:335-341.

237. Vannemreddy P, et al. Influence of cocaine on ruptured intracranial aneurysms: a case control study of poor prognostic indicators. *J Neurosurg.* 2008;108:470-476.

238. Vidale S, et al. Intra-arterial thrombolysis in a young patient with cocaine-associated stroke. *Neurol Sci.* 2014;35:1465-1466.

239. Virmani R, et al. Cardiovascular effects of cocaine: an autopsy study of 40 patients. *Am Heart J.* 1988;115:1068-1076.

240. Vitt JR, et al. Confirmed case of levamisole-associated multifocal inflammatory leukoencephalopathy in a cocaine user. *J Neuroimmunol.* 2017;305:128-130.

241. Walsh K, et al. Coronary computerized tomography angiography for rapid discharge of low-risk patients with cocaine-associated chest pain. *J Med Toxicol.* 2009;5:111-119.

242. Wang RY. pH-dependent cocaine-induced cardiotoxicity. *Am J Emerg Med.* 1999;17:364-369.

243. Weber JE, et al. Cocaine-associated chest pain: how common is myocardial infarction? *Acad Emerg Med.* 2000;7:873-877.

244. Weber JE, et al. Validation of a brief observation period for patients with cocaine-associated chest pain. *N Engl J Med.* 2003;348:510-517.

245. Willens HJ, et al. Cardiovascular manifestations of cocaine abuse. A case of recurrent dilated cardiomyopathy. *Chest.* 1994;106:594-600.

246. Wilson LD, et al. Cocaine, ethanol, and cocaethylene cardiotoxicity in an animal model of cocaine and ethanol abuse. *Acad Emerg Med.* 2001;8:211-222.

247. Winecoff AP, et al. Reversal of the electrocardiographic effects of cocaine by lidocaine. Part 1. Comparison with sodium bicarbonate and quinidine. *Pharmacotherapy.* 1994;14:698-703.

248. Wojak JC, Flamm ES. Intracranial hemorrhage and cocaine use. *Stroke.* 1987;18:712-715.

249. Wood DM, et al. Management of cocaine-induced cardiac arrhythmias due to cardiac ion channel dysfunction. *Clin Toxicol (Phila).* 2009;47:14-23.

250. Yang Y, et al. Evidence for cocaine and methylecgonidine stimulation of M(2) muscarinic receptors in cultured human embryonic lung cells. *Br J Pharmacol.* 2001;132:451-460.

251. Zamora-Quezada JC, et al. Muscle and skin infarction after free-basing cocaine (crack). *Ann Intern Med.* 1988;108:564-566.

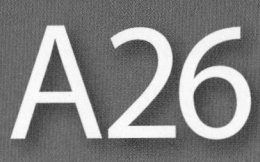
A26

BENZODIAZEPINES

Fiona Garlich Horner, Robert S. Hoffman, Lewis S. Nelson, and Mary Ann Howland

Benzodiazepines are a class of sedative–hypnotics that share similar chemical structures, receptor physiology, and clinical effects. Benzodiazepines are used broadly for a range of clinical indications, including xenobiotic-induced seizures, xenobiotic-induced psychomotor agitation, withdrawal from ethanol and other sedative–hypnotics, cocaine-associated myocardial ischemia, chloroquine overdose, and to induce muscle relaxation in serotonin toxicity, neuroleptic malignant syndrome, strychnine poisoning, and black widow spider envenomation. This Antidotes in Depth provides a summary of the clinical pharmacology of benzodiazepines and a review of their use in specific clinical scenarios, with an emphasis on specific drug selection and safe administration. A discussion of the manifestations and treatment of overdose of benzodiazepines and similar xenobiotics is found in Chap. 72.

HISTORY

The first benzodiazepine, chlordiazepoxide, was discovered serendipitously in 1957 as part of a quest to develop safer and more marketable sedatives.[70] Before this, the most commonly prescribed sedative–hypnotics were the barbiturates, which by the 1920s had largely supplanted chloral hydrate, bromides, and opium as the sedatives of choice.[71] Although safer than their predecessors, barbiturates were associated with dependence, abuse, and numerous overdose deaths, limiting their therapeutic use. Meprobamate, marketed in the 1950s as the first anxiolytic, was soon withdrawn from the market because of similar problems. The introduction of chlordiazepoxide in 1960 represented a major breakthrough in the field of psychopharmacology and ushered in an era of rapid development and widespread use of numerous other benzodiazepines. The improved safety profile of benzodiazepines as a class allowed them to become, for a time, the most widely prescribed drugs in the world.[70]

CHEMISTRY

All benzodiazepines share a common chemical structure, shown in Fig. A26–1. This structure links a benzene ring with a diazepine ring and gives rise to the name used to describe the drug class. The additional phenyl ring is present in all clinically important benzodiazepines and serves as a site of substitution that modulates certain pharmacologic characteristics. Modification of side chains of the ring structures leads to differences in lipophilicity, central nervous system (CNS) penetration, duration of action, potency, and rate of elimination. The majority of benzodiazepines are highly protein bound and lipophilic, entering the CNS via passive diffusion.[48] The nonbenzodiazepine hypnotics (zolpidem, zopiclone, and zaleplon) lack the typical benzodiazepine structure but have similar pharmacologic effects.[40] A discussion of the manifestations and treatment of overdose of benzodiazepines and other sedative–hypnotics is found in Chap. 72.

FIGURE A26–1. Generic structure of benzodiazepines.

γ-AMINOBUTYRIC ACID TYPE A RECEPTORS

Benzodiazepines bind to a specific site on the postsynaptic γ-aminobutyric acid type A (GABA$_A$) receptor. The GABA$_A$ receptor is a ligand-gated chloride channel that, when bound by the inhibitory neurotransmitter GABA, opens to allow an inward flux of negatively charged chloride ions. This results in membrane hyperpolarization and subsequent inhibition of neuronal excitability. When benzodiazepines bind to the GABA$_A$ receptor, the frequency of channel opening is increased in the presence of GABA, resulting in increased chloride ion influx and enhanced neuronal inhibition.[112] In the absence of GABA, the benzodiazepines have no effect on chloride conductance.

The GABA$_A$ receptor is formed by five polypeptide subunits that span the cell membrane in a circular fashion to create the chloride channel. These subunits are coded as α, β, γ, δ, ε, θ, λ, or ρ, and at least 19 isoforms of these subunits (eg, α_{1-5}) are identified.[106,114] Numerous subunit configurations are possible, but the most common pentamer is composed of two α subunits; two β subunits; and an additional subunit, most commonly γ_2.[100,114] Different GABA$_A$ receptor subunit isoforms predominate in different areas of the CNS and confer distinct functional effects and pharmacologic properties.[100] Benzodiazepines have no appreciable binding to GABA$_B$ receptors.

BENZODIAZEPINE RECEPTORS

Rapidly evolving neuroscience has resulted in an exponential expansion in the understanding of benzodiazepine receptors. As a result, significant evolution in nomenclature has occurred. Older, imprecise terminology was replaced by more specific characterization of binding sites defined by molecular structure and function.[100]

Central

The term "central benzodiazepine receptors" is used to refer to benzodiazepine binding sites on GABAergic neurons of the nervous system. The benzodiazepine binding site is located at the interface of an α and a γ subunit; most commonly an α_1 and a γ_2 subunit.[106,114] Anatomical variations in the α isoforms of GABA$_A$ receptors confer distinct pharmacologic response to benzodiazepine binding.[80] The α_1 isoform, located in the sensory and motor areas of the brain, mediates sedative and hypnotic effects. The α_2, α_3, and α_5 isoforms are dispersed throughout the subcortical and limbic areas of the brain and mediate anxiolytic and anticonvulsant effects. γ-aminobutyric acid type A receptors that contain α_4 and α_6 subunits are insensitive to benzodiazepines and are of low prevalence in the brain.[100]

In older nomenclature, GABA$_A$ receptors with primarily α_1 isoforms were termed benzodiazepine type 1 (BZ$_1$) receptors or ω_1 receptors, and those with predominance of α_2, α_3, and α_5 isoforms were called benzodiazepine type 2 (BZ$_2$) receptors or ω_2 receptors.[81] Most typical benzodiazepines have substantial affinity for the α_1, α_2, α_3, and α_5 isoforms, which explains their combined sedative–hypnotic, anxiolytic, and anticonvulsant effects. In contrast, the nonbenzodiazepine hypnotics (eg, zolpidem) have high affinity for α_1, intermediate affinity for α_2 and α_3, and low affinity for α_5 isoforms, which explains their lack of antiepileptic effects.[40] γ-Aminobutyric acid type A receptors are now more simply classified as having high-, low-, or intermediate-affinity benzodiazepine binding sites.[100]

Opposite the benzodiazepine binding site, situated at the α–β subunit interface, is the binding site for neurosteroids such as pregnenolone (Fig. A26–2).[53] These neurosteroids are potent modulators of GABA$_A$ receptor function and

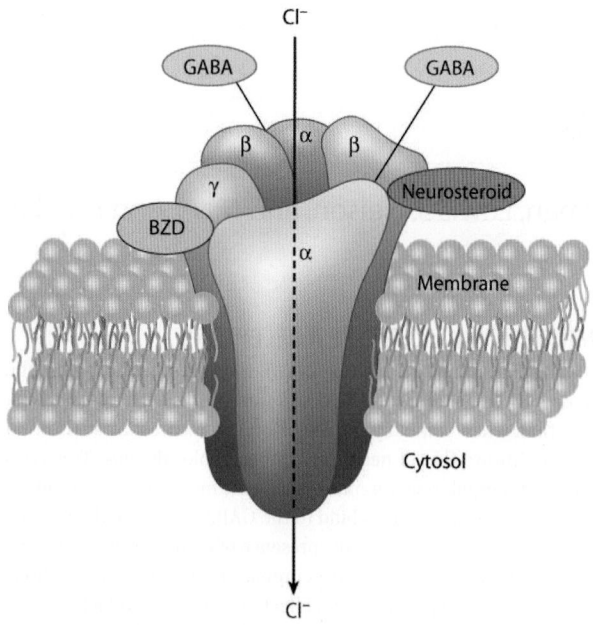

FIGURE A26–2. The γ-aminobutyric acid type A (GABA_A) chloride (Cl⁻) channel. The figure demonstrates a typical configuration of the GABA_A Cl⁻ channel, which consists of two α, two β, and one γ isoforms. The benzodiazepine (BZD) receptor is located between an α and a γ subunit. Neurosteroid binding at the opposite side of the α isoform is a positive allosteric modulator.

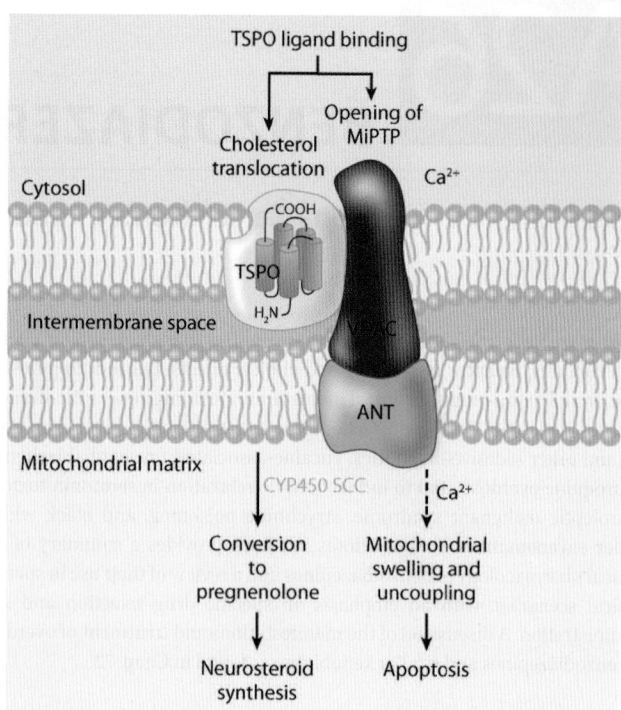

FIGURE A26–3. The "peripheral benzodiazepine receptor" has three main components: the tryptophan-rich sensory protein (TSPO; 18-kDa translocator protein), a voltage-dependent anion channel (VDAC), and an adenine nucleotide transporter (ANT), which are shown on the mitochondrial membrane. Stimulation of the TSPO can trigger influx of Ca²⁺ or cholesterol across the mitochondrial membrane. MiPTP = mitochondrial permeability transition pore; SCC = side chain cleavage.

are important products of the tryptophan-rich sensory protein receptor (see below).

Peripheral (Tryptophan-Rich Sensory Protein)

The term "peripheral benzodiazepine receptor" (PBR) was originally used in the 1970s to define any benzodiazepine binding sites outside of the nervous system.[18] They were also termed BZ₃ or ω₃ receptors to distinguish them from the "central receptors" described earlier.[63] However, it was subsequently discovered that this receptor was also expressed in CNS tissues, that it was the binding site for numerous other nonbenzodiazepine ligands, and that its structure and function were immensely complex and vastly dissimilar from that expressed in GABAergic neurons.[91] The PBR was determined to be an 18-kDa translocator protein located primarily on the outer mitochondrial membrane, and a member of a family of proteins involved in transmembrane signaling as part of host defense, stress response, and regulatory mechanisms in many species.[22,35,37,91] This protein is termed tryptophan-rich sensory protein and abbreviated as TSPO. Although the term PBR remains attractive, for simplicity and consistency, the current term TSPO will be used in the remainder of this discussion.

The TSPO has a heterotrimer structure that is composed of an isoquinoline binding protein, which is the actual receptor (TSPO); a voltage-dependent anion channel (VDAC); and an adenine nucleotide transporter (ANT).[91] The TSPO protein and the VDAC span the outer mitochondrial membrane, and the ANT bridges the outer and inner membranes (Fig. A26–3). Sequencing of TSPOs demonstrates that they are of ancient evolutionary origin with DNA from bacteria and fungi having a nearly 50% homology of the isoquinoline binding domain with human DNA.[35,38] This finding suggests that the TSPO performs a "housekeeping function," that is, they are involved in a process or processes that are essential for life. In higher life forms, TSPOs are found in the brain, adrenal glands, heart, and kidney and are especially concentrated in tissues in which steroids are synthesized.[91] Tryptophan-rich sensory proteins are implicated in cholesterol and protoporphyrin transport required for the synthesis of neurosteroids, heme, and bile salts; ischemia and reperfusion; regulation of calcium channels; mitochondrial respiration; apoptosis; microglial activation; and the immune response.[38,91,113] More recently, TSPO ligands were investigated as potential targets for a variety of disorders, including

anxiety, cancer, ischemia, and others.[24,30,57,59,86,92,107,122] It is hypothesized that the TSPO has two major roles: opening of the mitochondrial permeability transition pore, leading to calcium influx and apoptosis,[11,37,69] and, as noted earlier, in synthesis of neurosteroids that modulate GABA_A function.[90,101]

PHARMACOKINETICS AND PHARMACODYNAMICS

In the hospital setting, benzodiazepines are usually administered to treat seizures, psychomotor agitation, or sedative–hypnotic withdrawal. This Antidotes in Depth focuses on the most commonly used parenteral benzodiazepines: diazepam, lorazepam, and midazolam. Clinically important pharmacologic parameters of these three benzodiazepines are listed in Table A26–1. Of note, although they are often used interchangeably for a variety of indications, the onsets and peak effects of sedative and antiepileptic activity are distinctly different for each benzodiazepine. Thus, an understanding of pharmacology is crucial in selecting the optimal benzodiazepine, dose, route, and interval to ensure adequate response and limit adverse reactions.

The intravenous (IV) route is preferred in critically ill patients because it guarantees immediate and complete absorption with a relatively rapid onset of action. Intraosseous delivery of benzodiazepines is equivalent to IV administration and thus should be used in critically ill patients when IV access cannot be rapidly established.[64] When IV or intraosseous access is unavailable, intramuscular (IM) lorazepam or midazolam is recommended because they both have good absorptive profiles.[43,54,105,118] In contrast, the absorption after IM diazepam is best described as slow, incomplete, erratic, and dependent on the site of administration and the skill of the person administering it.[33,54,61] We therefore recommend not to use IM injection of diazepam unless no other alternatives exist.

Intranasal and rectal administration is occasionally used for benzodiazepine delivery when IV access is not available, especially in children with seizures. However, both routes are inferior to IV administration. When rectal diazepam was compared with IV diazepam in children with seizures, the

TABLE A26–1   Pharmacologic Properties of Select Benzodiazepines

Parameter	Diazepam	Midazolam	Lorazepam
Molecular weight (g/mol)	284.7	325.78	321.2
Oral bioavailability	>90%	40%	>90%
Volume of distribution (healthy adults) (L/kg)	0.89 ± 0.18	0.80 ± 0.19	1.28 ± 0.34
Protein binding (%)	97–99	96	85
Lipid solubility (LogD; octanol/water at pH 7)	3.86	3.68	2.48
Hepatic metabolism	Phase 1	Phase 1	Phase 2
Active metabolites	Yes (desmethyldiazepam and others)	Yes: α-hydroxymidazolam (10% of parent, but accumulates with chronic dosing)	No
Average dose (mg) in a 70-kg adult[a] Sedation	10 mg IV over 2 min Wait 2 min before redosing	2 mg IV over >2 min (maximum, 1.5 mg over >2 min in older adult or debilitated patients), or 5–10 mg IM Wait 2 min before IV redosing	2 mg IV over one minute (dilute with equal volume of NS or D$_5$W before injection) Wait 15 min before redosing
Status epilepticus (initial dose)	10 mg IV	10 mg IM	4 mg IV
Diluent(s)	Alcohol 10% Benzyl alcohol 1.5% Propylene glycol 40%	Benzyl alcohol 1% Sodium edetate 1%	Benzyl alcohol 2% Propylene glycol 80%
Formulations	5 mg/mL 5 mg/mL (Rectal gel)	1 mg/mL 5 mg/mL	2 mg/mL 4 mg/mL

[a]Avoid intraarterial administration because severe spasm may occur with resulting ischemia or gangrene. Also avoid extravasation.

D$_5$W = 5% dextrose in water; IV = intravenous; NS = 0.9% NaCl.

peak concentration was more variable, was delayed by about 20 minutes, and resulted in higher failure rates.[88,96] Similarly, although midazolam is more rapidly absorbed than diazepam after both nasal and rectal administration, the kinetic profile of nasal or rectal midazolam is still inferior to IV administration of either diazepam or midazolam (Table A26–2).[50,75,96]

TABLE A26–2   Relative Pharmacodynamic Properties of Benzodiazepines in Humans

	Diazepam	Midazolam	Lorazepam
Anticonvulsant			
Onset of action			
IV	Rapid (minutes)	Rapid (minutes)	Rapid (minutes)
IM	Not advisable	~3 min	9 min
IN	3–5 min	5 min	~10 min
PR	5–10 min	10–20 min	20 min
Duration of action			
IV	1–2 h	30–80 min	Many hours
IM	Unpredictable	1–2 h	Many hours
Sedative			
Onset of action			
IV	1–2 min	1–2 min	5–20 min
IM	Unpredictable	5–10 min	20–30 min
IN	3–5 min	5–10 min	~10 min
Relative duration of action			
Single dose	Short	Short	Long
Repeated doses	Long (secondary to active metabolites)	Intermediate (secondary to active metabolites)	Long

IM = intramuscular; IN = intranasal; IV = intravenous; PR = per rectum.

After being absorbed, benzodiazepines distribute into the CNS to produce their sedative and antiepileptic effects. The differences among individual drugs are evaluated in terms of their pharmacokinetics, such as plasma or cerebral drug concentrations, or their onset and pharmacodynamics, such as changes in either consciousness or electroencephalographic (EEG) findings. In animal and human studies, whereas diazepam demonstrates the most rapid onset and time to peak clinical effects, lorazepam is associated with significant pharmacodynamic delays.[10,44,45] In a cat model, intravenously administered diazepam, midazolam, and lorazepam all appeared rapidly in the cerebrospinal fluid (CSF), but lorazepam exhibited a slower time to peak concentration, a slower onset of EEG effect, and a longer duration of EEG activity.[10]

In similar human studies, volunteers were given a 1-minute IV infusion of diazepam (0.15 mg/kg), midazolam (0.1 mg/kg), or lorazepam (low dose, 0.0225 mg/kg; high dose, 0.045 mg/kg).[44,45] Electroencephalographic analysis was used as a surrogate for the pharmacodynamic effects of sedation. Peak EEG effects were present immediately at the end of the diazepam infusion but were delayed for 5 to 10 minutes after midazolam administration[45] and 30 minutes after lorazepam administration (Table A26–3).[44] The delay to peak effect after lorazepam administration is due to its decreased lipophilicity compared with diazepam and midazolam, whose greater lipophilicity allows them to rapidly cross the blood–brain barrier.[46]

Benzodiazepines, like many centrally acting xenobiotics, undergo a two-phase elimination in which they redistribute from the central to the peripheral compartment (represented by the alpha half-life) and then are eliminated from the body via metabolism and excretion (represented by the β half-life).[110] Benzodiazepines are classically categorized as long acting (diazepam and chlordiazepoxide), intermediate acting (lorazepam, alprazolam, clonazepam), and short acting (midazolam) based on their terminal beta elimination half-lives.[47] However, this does not necessarily correlate accurately with their clinical duration of action, which is more dependent on α redistribution. For example, because of rapid peripheral redistribution,

TABLE A26–3	Selected Pharmacokinetic and Pharmacodynamic Properties of Intravenous Benzodiazepines [44,45]		
Parameter	Diazepam (0.15 mg/kg)	Midazolam (0.1 mg/kg)	Lorazepam (0.045 mg/kg)
Onset of EEG effect	Immediate	Immediate	Slow
Time to peak EEG effect (min)	1	5–10	30
Duration of EEG effect (h)	5–6	2	8
Elimination half-life (h)	33 ± 5	2.8 ± 0.5	12 ± 2

EEG = electroencephalographic; IV = intravenous.

a single dose of diazepam has a relatively short duration of action despite its long elimination half-life of 20 to 70 hours. Lorazepam has a much shorter elimination half-life of 10 to 20 hours, but the duration of action after a single dose is relatively long.[47] These characteristics change after repeated dosing.

The presence of pharmacologically active metabolites prolongs the duration of action of select benzodiazepines, especially when repeated doses are administered. All benzodiazepines undergo hepatic metabolism, either by oxidation (phase I) or by conjugation with glucuronide (phase II).[93] Drugs that undergo phase I oxidation, such as diazepam, midazolam, and chlordiazepoxide, produce active metabolites. Diazepam is metabolized to nordiazepam (desmethyldiazepam, half-life, 48–72 hours) and temazepam (half-life, 8–22 hours), which are both subsequently metabolized to oxazepam (half-life, 4–15 hours).[47,121] These long-acting active metabolites effectively prolong the clinical effect of diazepam, though because of redistribution out of the CNS, the duration of clinical effect is significantly less than the elimination half-life. Glucuronidation, as in the case of lorazepam, results in the production of pharmacologically inactive metabolites. Older adult patients and those with hepatic failure have decreased clearance of drugs that undergo phase I oxidative metabolism.[93] As such, administration of diazepam, midazolam, or chlordiazepoxide in these patients often results in excessive accumulation of parent drug, a prolonged half-life, and increased adverse effects. Lorazepam is often recommended in patients with cirrhosis for this reason. The relative pharmacodynamic properties of diazepam, lorazepam, and midazolam are shown in Table A26–2.

ROLE OF BENZODIAZEPINES IN SELECT CLINICAL SCENARIOS

Many chapters in this text discuss the use of benzodiazepines as $GABA_A$ agonists in the management of poisoned patients (Chaps. 13, 14, 69, 73, 75, 77, 79, and 83). A few commonly encountered clinical scenarios deserve brief discussion here: xenobiotic-induced seizures, sedative–hypnotic withdrawal, and psychomotor agitation. There is extensive pharmacologic and clinical evidence supporting the use of $GABA_A$ agonists in these settings, although the choice of agonist is based on many variables. In contrast, the use of benzodiazepines as modulators of TSPOs for the treatment of poisoned patients is a more speculative but evolving field. As such, focused discussions of two additional xenobiotics, chloroquine (Chap. 55) and cocaine (Chap. 75), are warranted.

Xenobiotic-Induced Seizures

Benzodiazepines are well-established as the initial treatment of choice for xenobiotic-induced seizures.[25,31,72,103,104,123,124] Unlike in traumatic or epileptic seizure disorders which arise from a localized seizure focus, the initiation and propagation of xenobiotic-induced seizures result from a global decrease in seizure threshold, either from a decrease in GABAergic tone or an increase in excitatory amino acid neurotransmission.[25] Therefore, non–sedative–hypnotic antiepileptics such as phenytoin are likely to be ineffective in treating xenobiotic-induced seizures and should be avoided.[5,103] Furthermore, there is evidence that use of non–sedative–hypnotic antiepileptics result in increased toxicity, as occurs with the enhanced cardiotoxicity of phenytoin in tricyclic antidepressant poisoning.[21,103]

The selection of a specific benzodiazepine is informed by pharmacokinetic data and clinical studies of patients with epileptic seizures and status epilepticus. Current data and clinical guidelines indicate that IV lorazepam

or IM midazolam is preferred for rapid seizure cessation. Clinical trials demonstrate that despite its slower CNS penetration, IV lorazepam is more effective than other IV benzodiazepines in the cessation of status epilepticus, with a lower risk of seizure recurrence.[2,8,68,94,111] Intravenous midazolam may be as effective as IV lorazepam, but it is not as well studied.[94] A large multicenter, randomized, double-blind trial demonstrated that a large dose of IM midazolam (10 mg) was at least, if not more, effective than IV lorazepam (4 mg) for seizure cessation in the prehospital setting.[105,117] Another study suggests that IM or intranasal benzodiazepines are superior to the IV route if IV access is not already established.[3] Thus, IV lorazepam and IM midazolam are the recommended first-line antiepileptics for seizures or status epilepticus in the absence of withdrawal.[20,117]

If seizure control is not achieved promptly with rapidly escalating doses of benzodiazepines, second-line sedative–hypnotics such as phenobarbital or propofol are recommended along with appropriate management of airway, ventilation, and circulation.[25] If overdose of isoniazid or other hydrazine-containing compound is suspected, high-dose pyridoxine should be administered (Chaps. 56 and Antidotes in Depth: A15).[115] Benzodiazepines potentiate the effect of pyridoxine by acting synergistically[28] but are often ineffective as sole treatment for hydrazine-induced seizures because of their upstream blockade of GABA synthesis.

Sedative–Hypnotic Withdrawal

Benzodiazepines were established almost 50 years ago as the first-line treatment of alcohol withdrawal in a landmark study in which patients treated with chlordiazepoxide had significantly lower incidence of seizures and delirium tremens.[58] Since then, the benzodiazepines have also been used as the primary management of withdrawal from benzodiazepines,[89] γ-hydroxybutyric acid (GHB)[16,109] and GHB precursors 1,4-butanediol and gamma-butyrolactone,[102,120] as well as important adjuncts in the treatment of withdrawal from baclofen,[99,125] gabapentin,[14] and the nonbenzodiazepine hypnotics (eg, zolpidem, zopiclone).[9,26]

Numerous trials have investigated various benzodiazepines, routes, doses, and treatment strategies. Diazepam has favorable properties that make it a desirable first-line treatment for moderate to severe sedative–hypnotic withdrawal, in which prolonged agitation is expected. It has the most rapid time to onset and peak clinical effect, which limits oversedation when repeated dosing is required. The presence of active diazepam metabolites also confers a longer duration of therapeutic effect and an autotapering effect at the end of therapy.[121] The delay of lorazepam to onset and peak clinical effect frequently results in oversedation when serial doses are administered in rapid succession ("dose stacking"). The relatively short duration of action of midazolam limits its utility in xenobiotic withdrawal. Oral chlordiazepoxide is commonly used in early uncomplicated alcohol withdrawal because of its long duration of action and active metabolites (Chap. 77).

Psychomotor Agitation

In patients with extreme psychomotor agitation caused by sympathomimetic or other xenobiotic toxicity, IV diazepam or midazolam is recommended because of their rapid onset and rapid peak effects. The relatively slow onset and delayed peak of lorazepam often leads to the administration of several doses before the full effect of the first dose is appreciated, with resultant oversedation. When a short duration of sedation is anticipated, such as when treating a patient with toxicity after IV or inhaled use of cocaine, midazolam is recommended over diazepam or lorazepam in that the duration of the effects of midazolam better matches the duration of effects of cocaine, thereby limiting oversedation when cocaine is rapidly metabolized. In some patients with severe psychomotor agitation, obtaining IV access can be difficult or impractical and can place staff at undue risk. In such cases, we recommend IM midazolam for the treatment of undifferentiated agitation.[56,60,77] This should be followed, when conditions permit, by IV diazepam or midazolam if agitation persists (Chaps. 73 and 75).

Chloroquine

Although chloroquine overdose is uncommon, case fatality rates are extremely high, and ingestion of 5 g or more was once considered universally fatal. However, in 1988, a case series of patients with chloroquine overdose who survived with the use of an aggressive new regimen was described.[97] The protocol, consisting of early endotracheal intubation, high-dose epinephrine infusion, and IV diazepam (2 mg/kg over 30 min), resulted in the survival of 10 of 11 patients who ingested at least 5 g of chloroquine. This treatment strategy was based on observations that patients with mixed chloroquine and diazepam overdoses experienced less cardiovascular toxicity.[29] Subsequent animal studies demonstrated that diazepam mitigated the convulsant effect[4] as well as the hemodynamic and electrocardiographic manifestations[98] of chloroquine poisoning.

The mechanism of the beneficial cardiovascular effect of diazepam in chloroquine toxicity is unclear, but peripheral TSPO agonism appears to play a role. In isolated perfused hearts, high-dose diazepam has positive inotropic effects that are suppressed by a TSPO antagonist.[67] Benzodiazepines, chloroquine, and experimental TSPO agonists share some structural elements, suggesting a receptor-based mechanism (Fig. A26–4). Functional similarity is also suggested by evidence that both flurazepam and PK 11195 (a TSPO agonist) have antimalarial activity.[34] Thus, despite the limitations in translating laboratory data to human poisoning, one could speculate that the beneficial effects of high-dose diazepam result from competitive inhibition between chloroquine and TSPOs. Although the ideal regimen has not been defined, for patients with severe chloroquine toxicity it is reasonable to administer high-dose diazepam at a dose of 2 mg/kg IV over 30 minutes followed by 1 to 2 mg/kg/d for 2 to 4 days. Seizures should be treated with diazepam or another IV benzodiazepine.

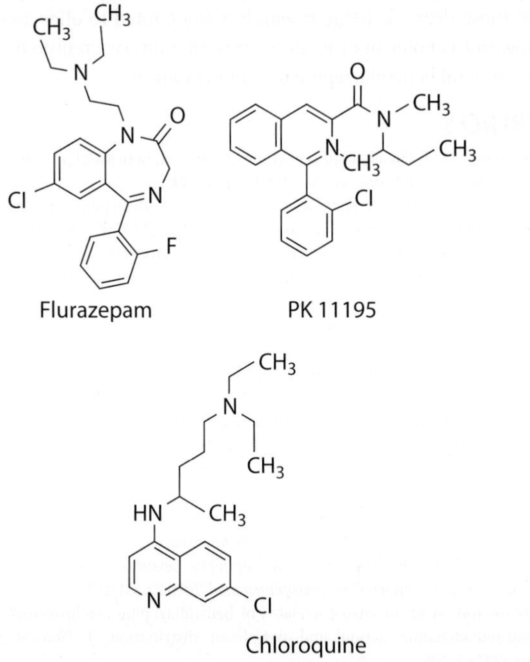

FIGURE A26–4. Comparative structures of flurazepam, PK 11195 (a PBR agonist), and chloroquine. Note the similarity and particularly the shared isoquinoline rings of chloroquine and PK 11195.

Cocaine-Associated Chest Pain

Patients who use cocaine frequently present to emergency departments with chest pain or signs or symptoms that could represent myocardial ischemia or infarction.[19] Unlike most patients with acute cocaine toxicity, however, these patients often present hours after their last drug use and without the classic sympathomimetic findings of acute cocaine toxicity.[51] Although the pathophysiology of cocaine-induced myocardial ischemia is complex and multifactorial (Chap. 75), one component of delayed myocardial ischemia likely results from the vasoconstrictive actions of benzoylecgonine, the principal metabolite of cocaine.[74] Benzoylecgonine is distinct from cocaine in that it has a much longer half-life,[6,7] does not produce CNS stimulation,[83,84] and is a direct constrictor vasoconstricts or through modulation of calcium channels.[73]

Limited research suggests that chronic cocaine use is associated with an increased number of TSPOs on human platelets.[27] Also in humans, cocaine withdrawal is associated with a decrease in TSPOs on neutrophils. In the myocardium, TSPOs are either present on mitochondria or coupled to calcium channels.[82] Specifically, TSPO ligands have inhibitory effects on myocardial L-type calcium channels.[23] Also in experimental models of cardiac ischemia and reperfusion injury, TSPO agonists limit myocardial infarction size and improve cardiac function.[65,122] This effect most likely occurs through inhibition of the opening of the mitochondrial permeability transition pore,[87] the opening of which is a common final mechanism of cell death. Additionally, although the exact mechanism is unclear, TSPO agonists directly antagonize the vasoconstrictive effects of norepinephrine in rat aortic tissue.[41]

Benzodiazepines are commonly used to treat the agitation associated with sympathomimetic overdose (Chaps. 73 and 75). Although it is assumed that the normalization of vital signs results from a decrease in CNS stimulation and psychomotor agitation, it is reasonable to believe that the effects on TSPOs are contributory. In the same isolated perfused hearts described earlier, low-dose diazepam has a negative inotropic effect that results from an interaction with calcium currents.[66]

Two randomized controlled studies evaluated the use of benzodiazepines in patients with cocaine-associated chest pain.[15,52] In the first study, patients were randomized to receive nitroglycerin, diazepam, or combined therapy.[15] Diazepam was equivalent to nitroglycerin in improving chest pain, and combined therapy appeared to offer no additional benefit. The second study randomized patients to nitroglycerin or combined nitroglycerin with lorazepam therapy.[52] In this trial, combined therapy was better than nitroglycerin alone. Thus, it is reasonable to administer IV lorazepam or diazepam as an adjunct to nitroglycerin therapy in patients with chest pain in the setting of recent cocaine use.

ADVERSE EFFECTS AND SAFETY ISSUES

The most common adverse effects of benzodiazepines are CNS and respiratory depression. Although this is unavoidable in some cases, it is limited by selecting the optimal drug and the proper dose and dosing interval. Extra caution is advised in older adult patients because they are more sensitive, particularly to the sedative and respiratory depressant effects of midazolam.[1] Additionally, patients with hepatic failure are at increased risk of adverse effects with diazepam or midazolam because of decreased drug clearance. For this reason, we recommend lorazepam in patients with cirrhosis. In contrast, paradoxical reactions rarely occur in which some patients become more agitated after benzodiazepine administration, particularly children.[76,78,116] These infrequent reactions probably result from disinhibition and typically respond to larger doses of benzodiazepines. Although paradoxical agitation also responds to flumazenil (Antidotes in Depth: A25), we recommend against reversal when benzodiazepines are used for most toxicologic indications.

Intravenous benzodiazepines produce a mild reduction in heart rate and both systolic and diastolic blood pressure. The effects of midazolam are reportedly greater than diazepam,[95] but this may merely be based on an inability to determine an equivalent dosing regimen. Although these reductions result in part from diminished sympathetic tone, direct myocardial effects are rarely severe and are often considered desirable in the overdose setting.

Whereas respiratory depression is generally not a concern with oral benzodiazepines, parenteral administration is documented to impair ventilation. Early investigations demonstrated that IM diazepam (10 mg) blunted the hypoxic ventilatory drive in normal subjects.[62] Intravenous diazepam impaired the ventilatory response to a rising PCO_2 in normal volunteers.[12] The impaired response to a rising PCO_2 was evident almost immediately and lasted for at least 25 minutes after injection of 0.4 mg/kg of diazepam in healthy volunteers.[49] Studies with midazolam demonstrate similar alterations in respiratory physiology[36] that are comparable in magnitude to those reported with diazepam.[17] Apnea is reported after IV midazolam and is dose and rate related, with doses greater than or equal to 0.15 mg/kg being of particular concern.[65] Individuals with preexisting pulmonary disorders, extremes of age, or exposure to other CNS or respiratory depressants are more susceptible. When IM midazolam is used for the treatment of agitation, some transient respiratory depression is noted, but the need for ventilatory support is uncommon.[56,60,62]

Pregnancy and Lactation

Diazepam, lorazepam, and midazolam all cross the placenta and are labeled as US Food and Drug Administration Pregnancy Category D because of the risk of adverse effects with chronic use or at the time of delivery.[55,79] Administration of benzodiazepines late in pregnancy or during labor can result in neonatal flaccidity, respiratory difficulties, and hypothermia, termed the "floppy infant syndrome." Chronic use late in pregnancy can result in neonatal withdrawal symptoms. Additionally, an association with congenital anomalies is suggested with use of prescription benzodiazepines in early pregnancy,[32,79] although the bulk of evidence suggests risk of teratogenicity is very low, if not nonexistent.[39,55,119] The risk to a fetus is likely negligible from short-term benzodiazepine administration in emergent situations, in which the risk of harm from untreated xenobiotic poisoning vastly outweighs any potential adverse medication effects. Thus, we recommend that benzodiazepines not be withheld in critically ill poisoned patients because of pregnancy status. If delivery is imminent, it is reasonable to select a short-acting benzodiazepine such as midazolam.

Benzodiazepines are excreted into breast milk in very small quantities.[55,79] Although single standard doses typically do not result in adverse effects, high doses, repeated administration, or prolonged use may result in accumulation in the serum of breastfed infants, with a resultant risk of sedation.[108] It is thus reasonable to forgo breastfeeding (by discarding pumped breast milk, ie, "pumping and dumping") for several hours after a single IV dose or for 24 hours after repeated benzodiazepine dosing (Chaps. 30 and 31).[85]

DOSING AND ADMINISTRATION

When selecting a benzodiazepine for a given clinical scenario, the pharmacokinetic and pharmacodynamic parameters presented in Tables A26–1 and A26–3 should be considered, along with existing clinical data. Onset of effect, peak effect, and duration of effect should be weighed in the context of the anticipated clinical course. It is worth noting that each of the three benzodiazepines discussed will likely have some efficacy in all clinical scenarios for which a benzodiazepine is indicated. Although selection of a specific benzodiazepine is often based on availability within the hospital and regional historic preferences, some general recommendations can be made.

Intravenous dosing is recommended for critically ill patients, although other routes such as IM, intranasal, or intraosseous are effective when IV access is unavailable or impractical. Benzodiazepines with rapid onset of action, such as diazepam or midazolam, are recommended when rapid symptom control is necessary. A long-acting benzodiazepine with active metabolites, such as diazepam, is recommended in cases of sedative–hypnotic withdrawal and ethanol withdrawal when prolonged symptoms are anticipated. Lorazepam is reasonable in patients with hepatic failure because of its relatively preserved clearance and lack of active metabolites. Intravenous lorazepam or IM midazolam is recommended for seizure cessation.

Common equivalent initial IV doses in adults are: lorazepam 1 mg, diazepam 5 mg, and midazolam 2 mg.[13,42] When repeated administration is

necessary, appropriate spacing between doses is crucial to avoid oversedation and respiratory depression. Intravenous diazepam and midazolam can be safely administered every 2 to 5 minutes, but we recommend delays prior to repeating lorazepam doses of at least 15 minutes to account for the slower time to peak effect. It is important to note that switching from one benzodiazepine to another is rarely indicated and increases the risk of an adverse drug event from unpredictable peak effects or improper therapeutic doses or dosing intervals (Chaps. 14, 73, 75, and 77).

FORMULATION AND ACQUISITION

Parenteral benzodiazepines are available from multiple manufacturers in varying concentrations. It is essential to recognize that some formulations contain several significant and varied diluents, most notably propylene glycol (Table A26–1). Large doses or prolonged continuous infusions of benzodiazepines may result in toxicity from these excipients (Chap. 46).

SUMMARY

- Although benzodiazepines are commonly used in a variety of medical settings, subtle differences exist in their pharmacokinetics and pharmacodynamics. Optimal use of these drugs requires a thorough understanding of these differences.
- When choosing among different benzodiazepines, the desired onset of action, peak effect, and duration of action aid in selecting the preferred therapy.
- In general, IV administration is preferred in an emergency because of rapid and reliable absorption.
- Because of rapid onset of action and short time to peak effect, expedient sedation is best achieved with midazolam when a short duration of action is desirable or diazepam for a longer duration of action.
- When IV access is not available, pharmacokinetic and pharmacodynamic parameters favor the use of IM midazolam for sedation.
- When used for control of the agitated patient, the delayed peak effect of lorazepam (regardless of route of administration) is undesirable.
- Intravenous lorazepam is highly effective for seizure cessation, with a longer duration of antiepileptic effect than IV diazepam or midazolam. Large doses of IM midazolam are effective for status epilepticus in the prehospital setting.
- Although the use of benzodiazepines as TSPO (peripheral benzodiazepine receptor) agonists may explain some unique therapeutic effects of these drugs, existing research is too limited to offer guidance with regard to choice of drug, dose, or dosing interval required to optimize peripheral benzodiazepine receptor response.

REFERENCES

1. Albrecht S, et al. The effect of age on the pharmacokinetics and pharmacodynamics of midazolam. *Clin Pharmacol Ther.* 1999;65:630-639.
2. Alldredge BK, et al. A comparison of lorazepam, diazepam, and placebo for the treatment of out-of-hospital status epilepticus. *N Engl J Med.* 2001;345:631-637.
3. Alshehri A, et al. Intravenous versus nonintravenous benzodiazepines for the cessation of seizures: a systematic review and meta-analysis of randomized controlled trials. *Acad Emerg Med.* 2017;24:875-883.
4. Amabeoku G. Involvement of GABAergic mechanisms in chloroquine-induced seizures in mice. *Gen Pharmacol.* 1992;23:225-229.
5. Amabeoku GJ, Chikuni O. Effects of some GABAergic agents on quinine-induced seizures in mice. *Experientia.* 1992;48:659-662.
6. Ambre J. The urinary excretion of cocaine and metabolites in humans: a kinetic analysis of published data. *J Anal Toxicol.* 1985;9:241-245.
7. Ambre J, et al. Urinary excretion of ecgonine methyl ester, a major metabolite of cocaine in humans. *J Anal Toxicol.* 1984;8:23-25.
8. Appleton R, et al. Lorazepam versus diazepam in the acute treatment of epileptic seizures and status epilepticus. *Dev Med Child Neurol.* 1995;37:682-688.
9. Aragona M. Abuse, dependence, and epileptic seizures after zolpidem withdrawal: review and case report. *Clin Neuropharmacol.* 2000;23:281-283.
10. Arendt RM, et al. In vitro correlates of benzodiazepine cerebrospinal fluid uptake, pharmacodynamic action and peripheral distribution. *J Pharmacol Exp Ther.* 1983;227:98-106.
11. Azarashvili T, et al. The peripheral-type benzodiazepine receptor is involved in control of Ca2+-induced permeability transition pore opening in rat brain mitochondria. *Cell Calcium.* 2007;42:27-39.

12. Bailey PL, et al. Variability of the respiratory response to diazepam. *Anesthesiology*. 1986;64:460-465.

13. Barr J, et al. A double-blind, randomized comparison of i.v. lorazepam versus midazolam for sedation of ICU patients via a pharmacologic model. *Anesthesiology*. 2001;95:286-298.

14. Barrueto F, et al. Gabapentin withdrawal presenting as status epilepticus. *J Toxicol Clin Toxicol*. 2002;40:925-928.

15. Baumann BM, et al. Randomized, double-blind, placebo-controlled trial of diazepam, nitroglycerin, or both for treatment of patients with potential cocaine-associated acute coronary syndromes. *Acad Emerg Med*. 2000;7:878-885.

16. Bennett WRM, et al. Gamma-hydroxybutyric acid (GHB) withdrawal: a case report. *J Psychoactive Drugs*. 2007;39:293-296.

17. Berggren L, et al. Changes in respiratory pattern after repeated doses of diazepam and midazolam in healthy subjects. *Acta Anaesthesiol Scand*. 1987;31:667-672.

18. Braestrup C, Squires RF. Specific benzodiazepine receptors in rat brain characterized by high-affinity (3H) diazepam binding. *Proc Natl Acad Sci U S A*. 1977;74:3805-3809.

19. Brody SL, et al. Cocaine-related medical problems: consecutive series of 233 patients. *Am J Med*. 1990;88:325-331.

20. Brophy GM, et al. Guidelines for the evaluation and management of status epilepticus. *Neurocrit Care*. 2012;17:3-23.

21. Callaham M, et al. Phenytoin prophylaxis of cardiotoxicity in experimental amitriptyline poisoning. *J Pharmacol Exp Ther*. 1988;245:216-220.

22. Campanella M, Turkheimer FE. TSPO: functions and applications of a mitochondrial stress response pathway. *Biochem Soc Trans*. 2015;43:593-594.

23. Campiani G, et al. Synthesis, biological activity, and SARs of pyrrolobenzoxazepine derivatives, a new class of specific "peripheral-type" benzodiazepine receptor ligands. *J Med Chem*. 1996;39:3435-3450.

24. Cappelli A, et al. Synthesis and structure-activity relationship studies in peripheral benzodiazepine receptor ligands related to alpidem. *Bioorg Med Chem*. 2008;16: 3428-3437.

25. Chen H-Y, et al. Treatment of drug-induced seizures. *Br J Clin Pharmacol*. 2016;81: 412-419.

26. Chen S-C, et al. Detoxification of high-dose zolpidem using cross-titration with an adequate equivalent dose of diazepam. *Gen Hosp Psychiatry*. 2012;34:210.e5-210.e7.

27. Chesley SF, et al. Cocaine augments peripheral benzodiazepine binding in humans. *J Clin Psychiatry*. 1990;51:404-406.

28. Chin L, et al. Potentiation of pyridoxine by depressants and anticonvulsants in the treatment of acute isoniazid intoxication in dogs. *Toxicol Appl Pharmacol*. 1981;58: 504-509.

29. Clemessy JL, et al. Therapeutic trial of diazepam versus placebo in acute chloroquine intoxications of moderate gravity. *Intensive Care Med*. 1996;22:1400-1405.

30. Danovich L, et al. The influence of clozapine treatment and other antipsychotics on the 18 kDa translocator protein, formerly named the peripheral-type benzodiazepine receptor, and steroid production. *Eur Neuropsychopharmacol*. 2008;18:24-33.

31. Derlet RW, et al. Antagonism of cocaine, amphetamine, and methamphetamine toxicity. *Pharmacol Biochem Behav*. 1990;36:745-749.

32. Dolovich LR, et al. Benzodiazepine use in pregnancy and major malformations or oral cleft: meta-analysis of cohort and case-control studies. *BMJ*. 1998;317:839-843.

33. Dundee JW, et al. Letter: plasma-diazepam levels following intramuscular injection by nurses and doctors. *Lancet*. 1974;2:1461.

34. Dzierszinski F, et al. Ligands of the peripheral benzodiazepine receptor are potent inhibitors of Plasmodium falciparum and Toxoplasma gondii in vitro. *Antimicrob Agents Chemother*. 2002;46:3197-3207.

35. Fan J, et al. Structural and functional evolution of the translocator protein (18 kDa). *Curr Mol Med*. 2012;12:369-386.

36. Forster A, et al. Respiratory depressant effects of different doses of midazolam and lack of reversal with naloxone—a double-blind randomized study. *Anesth Analg*. 1983;62:920-924.

37. Gatliff J, Campanella M. The 18 kDa translocator protein (TSPO): a new perspective in mitochondrial biology. *Curr Mol Med*. 2012;12:356-368.

38. Gavish M, et al. Enigma of the peripheral benzodiazepine receptor. *Pharmacol Rev*. 1999;51:629-650.

39. Gedzelman E, Meador KJ. Antiepileptic drugs in women with epilepsy during pregnancy. *Ther Adv Drug Saf*. 2012;3:71-87.

40. George CF. Pyrazolopyrimidines. *Lancet*. 2001;358:1623-1626.

41. Gimeno M, et al. The role of cyclic nucleotides in the action of peripheral-type benzodiazepine receptor ligands in rat aorta. *Gen Pharmacol*. 1994;25:1553-1561.

42. Gold JA, et al. A strategy of escalating doses of benzodiazepines and phenobarbital administration reduces the need for mechanical ventilation in delirium tremens. *Crit Care Med*. 2007;35:724-730.

43. Greenblatt DJ, et al. Clinical pharmacokinetics of lorazepam. III. Intravenous injection. Preliminary results. *J Clin Pharmacol*. 17:490-494.

44. Greenblatt DJ, et al. Kinetic and dynamic study of intravenous lorazepam: comparison with intravenous diazepam. *J Pharmacol Exp Ther*. 1989;250:134-140.

45. Greenblatt DJ, et al. Pharmacokinetic and electroencephalographic study of intravenous diazepam, midazolam, and placebo. *Clin Pharmacol Ther*. 1989;45:356-365.

46. Greenblatt DJ, Sethy VH. Benzodiazepine concentrations in brain directly reflect receptor occupancy: studies of diazepam, lorazepam, and oxazepam. *Psychopharmacology (Berl)*. 1990;102:373-378.

47. Greenblatt DJ, et al. Benzodiazepines: a summary of pharmacokinetic properties. *Br J Clin Pharmacol*. 1981;11(suppl 1):11S-16S.

48. Griffin CE, et al. Benzodiazepine pharmacology and central nervous system-mediated effects. *Ochsner J*. 2013;13:214-223.

49. Gross JB, et al. Time course of ventilatory response to carbon dioxide after intravenous diazepam. *Anesthesiology*. 1982;57:18-21.

50. Hardmeier M, et al. Intranasal midazolam: pharmacokinetics and pharmacodynamics assessed by quantitative EEG in healthy volunteers. *Clin Pharmacol Ther*. 2012;91:856-862.

51. Hollander JE, et al. Prospective multicenter evaluation of cocaine-associated chest pain. Cocaine Associated Chest Pain (COCHPA) Study Group. *Acad Emerg Med*. 1:330-339.

52. Honderick T, et al. A prospective, randomized, controlled trial of benzodiazepines and nitroglycerine or nitroglycerine alone in the treatment of cocaine-associated acute coronary syndromes. *Am J Emerg Med*. 2003;21:39-42.

53. Hosie AM, et al. Endogenous neurosteroids regulate GABAA receptors through two discrete transmembrane sites. *Nature*. 2006;444:486-489.

54. Hung OR, et al. Comparative absorption kinetics of intramuscular midazolam and diazepam. *Can J Anaesth*. 1996;43(5 Pt 1):450-455.

55. Iqbal MM, et al. Effects of commonly used benzodiazepines on the fetus, the neonate, and the nursing infant. *Psychiatr Serv*. 2002;53:39-49.

56. Isbister GK, et al. Randomized controlled trial of intramuscular droperidol versus midazolam for violence and acute behavioral disturbance: the DORM study. *Ann Emerg Med*. 2010;56:392-401.e1.

57. Jaiswal A, et al. Peripheral benzodiazepine receptor ligand Ro5-4864 inhibits isoprenaline-induced cardiac hypertrophy in rats. *Eur J Pharmacol*. 2010;644: 146-153.

58. Kaim SC, et al. Treatment of the acute alcohol withdrawal state: a comparison of four drugs. *Am J Psychiatry*. 1969;125:1640-1646.

59. Kaynar G, et al. Effects of peripheral benzodiazepine receptor ligand Ro5-4864 in four animal models of acute lung injury. *J Surg Res*. 2013;182:277-284.

60. Knott JC, et al. Randomized clinical trial comparing intravenous midazolam and droperidol for sedation of the acutely agitated patient in the emergency department. *Ann Emerg Med*. 2006;47:61-67.

61. Korttila K, Linnoila M. Absorption and sedative effects of diazepam after oral administration and intramuscular administration into the vastus lateralis muscle and the deltoid muscle. *Br J Anaesth*. 1975;47:857-862.

62. Lakshminarayan S, et al. Effect of diazepam on ventilatory responses. *Clin Pharmacol Ther*. 1976;20:178-183.

63. Langer SZ, Arbilla S. Imidazopyridines as a tool for the characterization of benzodiazepine receptors: a proposal for a pharmacological classification as omega receptor subtypes. *Pharmacol Biochem Behav*. 1988;29:763-766.

64. Lathers CM, et al. A comparison of intraosseous and intravenous routes of administration for antiseizure agents. *Epilepsia*. 1989;30:472-479.

65. Leducq N, et al. Role of peripheral benzodiazepine receptors in mitochondrial, cellular, and cardiac damage induced by oxidative stress and ischemia-reperfusion. *J Pharmacol Exp Ther*. 2003;306:828-837.

66. Leeuwin RS, et al. Flunarizine but not theophylline modulates inotropic responses of the isolated rat heart to diazepam. *Eur J Pharmacol*. 1996;315:153-157.

67. Leeuwin RS, et al. PK 11195 antagonizes the positive inotropic response of the isolated rat heart to diazepam but not the negative inotropic response. *Eur J Pharmacol*. 1996;299:149-152.

68. Leppik IE, et al. Double-blind study of lorazepam and diazepam in status epilepticus. *JAMA*. 1983;249:1452-1454.

69. Li J, et al. Peripheral benzodiazepine receptor ligand, PK11195 induces mitochondria cytochrome c release and dissipation of mitochondria potential via induction of mitochondria permeability transition. *Eur J Pharmacol*. 2007;560:117-122.

70. Lopez-Munoz F, et al. The discovery of chlordiazepoxide and the clinical introduction of benzodiazepines: half a century of anxiolytic drugs. *J Anxiety Disord*. 2011;25: 554-562.

71. López-Muñoz F, et al. The history of barbiturates a century after their clinical introduction. *Neuropsychiatr Dis Treat*. 2005;1:329-343.

72. Luongo R, et al. Diazepam and pentobarbital protect against scorpion venom toxin-induced epilepsy. *Brain Res Bull*. 2009;79:296-302.

73. Madden JA, et al. Cocaine and benzoylecgonine constrict cerebral arteries by different mechanisms. *Life Sci*. 1995;56:679-686.

74. Madden JA, Powers RH. Effect of cocaine and cocaine metabolites on cerebral arteries in vitro. *Life Sci*. 1990;47:1109-1114.

75. Malinovsky JM, et al. Plasma concentrations of midazolam after i.v., nasal or rectal administration in children. *Br J Anaesth*. 1993;70:617-620.

76. Mancuso CE, et al. Paradoxical reactions to benzodiazepines: literature review and treatment options. *Pharmacotherapy*. 2004;24:1177-1185.

77. Martel M, et al. Management of acute undifferentiated agitation in the emergency department: a randomized double-blind trial of droperidol, ziprasidone, and midazolam. *Acad Emerg Med*. 2005;12:1167-1172.

78. Massanari M, et al. Paradoxical reactions in children associated with midazolam use during endoscopy. *Clin Pediatr (Phila)*. 1997;36:681-684.

79. McElhatton PR. The effects of benzodiazepine use during pregnancy and lactation. *Reprod Toxicol*. 8:461-475.

80. McLeod M, et al. The heterogeneity of central benzodiazepine receptor subtypes in the human hippocampal formation, frontal cortex and cerebellum using [3H]flumazenil and zolpidem. *Brain Res Mol Brain Res.* 2002;104:203-209.
81. Meldrum BS, Chapman AG. Benzodiazepine receptors and their relationship to the treatment of epilepsy. *Epilepsia.* 1986;27(suppl 1):S3-S13.
82. Mestre M, et al. Electrophysiological and pharmacological evidence that peripheral type benzodiazepine receptors are coupled to calcium channels in the heart. *Life Sci.* 1985;36:391-400.
83. Mets B, Virag L. Lethal toxicity from equimolar infusions of cocaine and cocaine metabolites in conscious and anesthetized rats. *Anesth Analg.* 1995;81:1033-1038.
84. Misra AL, et al. Estimation and disposition of [3H]benzoylecgonine and pharmacological activity of some cocaine metabolites. *J Pharm Pharmacol.* 1975;27:784-786.
85. Nitsun M, et al. Pharmacokinetics of midazolam, propofol, and fentanyl transfer to human breast milk. *Clin Pharmacol Ther.* 2006;79:549-557.
86. Nothdurfter C, et al. Translocator protein (18 kDa) (TSPO) as a therapeutic target for anxiety and neurologic disorders. *Eur Arch Psychiatry Clin Neurosci.* 2012;262(suppl 2):S107-S112.
87. Obame FN, et al. Peripheral benzodiazepine receptor-induced myocardial protection is mediated by inhibition of mitochondrial membrane permeabilization. *J Pharmacol Exp Ther.* 2007;323:336-345.
88. Ogutu BR, et al. Pharmacokinetics and anticonvulsant effects of diazepam in children with severe falciparum malaria and convulsions. *Br J Clin Pharmacol.* 2002;53:49-57.
89. Onyett SR. The benzodiazepine withdrawal syndrome and its management. *J R Coll Gen Pract.* 1989;39:160-163.
90. Owen DRJ, et al. Variation in binding affinity of the novel anxiolytic XBD173 for the 18 kDa translocator protein in human brain. *Synapse.* 2011;65:257-259.
91. Papadopoulos V, et al. Translocator protein (18kDa): new nomenclature for the peripheral-type benzodiazepine receptor based on its structure and molecular function. *Trends Pharmacol Sci.* 2006;27:402-409.
92. Papadopoulos V, Lecanu L. Translocator protein (18 kDa) TSPO: an emerging therapeutic target in neurotrauma. *Exp Neurol.* 2009;219:53-57.
93. Peppers MP. Benzodiazepines for alcohol withdrawal in the elderly and in patients with liver disease. *Pharmacotherapy.* 1996;16:49-57.
94. Prasad M, et al. Anticonvulsant therapy for status epilepticus. *Cochrane Database Syst Rev.* 2014:CD003723.
95. Reves JG, et al. Midazolam: pharmacology and uses. *Anesthesiology.* 1985;62:310-324.
96. Rey E, et al. Pharmacokinetic optimization of benzodiazepine therapy for acute seizures. Focus on delivery routes. *Clin Pharmacokinet.* 1999;36:409-424.
97. Riou B, et al. Treatment of severe chloroquine poisoning. *N Engl J Med.* 1988;318:1-6.
98. Riou B, et al. Protective cardiovascular effects of diazepam in experimental acute chloroquine poisoning. *Intensive Care Med.* 1988;14:610-616.
99. Ross JC, et al. Acute Intrathecal baclofen withdrawal: a brief review of treatment options. *Neurocrit Care.* 2011;14:103-108.
100. Sankar R. GABA(A) receptor physiology and its relationship to the mechanism of action of the 1,5-benzodiazepine clobazam. *CNS Drugs.* 2012;26:229-244.
101. Scarf AM, et al. The translocator protein (18 kDa): central nervous system disease and drug design. *J Med Chem.* 2009;52:581-592.
102. Schneir AB, et al. A case of withdrawal from the GHB precursors gamma-butyrolactone and 1,4-butanediol. *J Emerg Med.* 2001;21:31-33.
103. Sharma AN, Hoffman RJ. Toxin-related seizures. *Emerg Med Clin North Am.* 2011;29:125-139.
104. Shih T-M, et al. Control of nerve agent-induced seizures is critical for neuroprotection and survival. *Toxicol Appl Pharmacol.* 2003;188:69-80.
105. Silbergleit R, et al. Intramuscular versus intravenous therapy for prehospital status epilepticus. *N Engl J Med.* 2012;366:591-600.
106. Smith TA. Type A gamma-aminobutyric acid (GABAA) receptor subunits and benzodiazepine binding: significance to clinical syndromes and their treatment. *Br J Biomed Sci.* 2001;58:111-121.
107. Soustiel JF, et al. The effect of oxygenation level on cerebral post-traumatic apoptosis is modulated by the 18-kDa translocator protein (also known as peripheral-type benzodiazepine receptor) in a rat model of cortical contusion. *Neuropathol Appl Neurobiol.* 2008;34:412-423.
108. Spigset O. Anaesthetic agents and excretion in breast milk. *Acta Anaesthesiol Scand.* 1994;38:94-103.
109. Tarabar AF, Nelson LS. The gamma-hydroxybutyrate withdrawal syndrome. *Toxicol Rev.* 2004;23:45-49.
110. Teboul E, Chouinard G. A guide to benzodiazepine selection. Part I: pharmacological aspects. *Can J Psychiatry.* 1990;35:700-710.
111. Treiman DM, et al. A comparison of four treatments for generalized convulsive status epilepticus. Veterans Affairs Status Epilepticus Cooperative Study Group. *N Engl J Med.* 1998;339:792-798.
112. Twyman RE, et al. Differential regulation of GABA acid receptor channels by diazepam and phenobarbital. *Ann Neurol.* 1988;25:213-220.
113. Venneti S, et al. The peripheral benzodiazepine receptor (translocator protein 18kDa) in microglia: from pathology to imaging. *Prog Neurobiol.* 2006;80:308-322.
114. Wafford KA. GABAA receptor subtypes: any clues to the mechanism of benzodiazepine dependence? *Curr Opin Pharmacol.* 2005;5:47-52.
115. Wason S, et al. Single high-dose pyridoxine treatment for isoniazid overdose. *JAMA.* 1981;246:1102-1104.
116. Weinbroum AA, et al. The midazolam-induced paradox phenomenon is reversible by flumazenil. Epidemiology, patient characteristics and review of the literature. *Eur J Anaesthesiol.* 2001;18:789-797.
117. Welch RD, et al. Intramuscular midazolam versus intravenous lorazepam for the prehospital treatment of status epilepticus in the pediatric population. *Epilepsia.* 2015;56:254-262.
118. Wermeling DP, et al. Bioavailability and pharmacokinetics of lorazepam after intranasal, intravenous, and intramuscular administration. *J Clin Pharmacol.* 2001;41:1225-1231.
119. Wikner BN, et al. Use of benzodiazepines and benzodiazepine receptor agonists during pregnancy: neonatal outcome and congenital malformations. *Pharmacoepidemiol Drug Saf.* 2007;16:1203-1210.
120. Wojtowicz JM, et al. Withdrawal from gamma-hydroxybutyrate, 1,4-butanediol and gamma-butyrolactone: a case report and systematic review. *CJEM.* 2008;10:69-74.
121. Wretlind M, et al. Disposition of three benzodiazepines after single oral administration in man. *Acta Pharmacol Toxicol (Copenh).* 1977;40(suppl 1):28-39.
122. Xiao J, et al. 4'-Chlorodiazepam, a translocator protein (18 kDa) antagonist, improves cardiac functional recovery during postischemia reperfusion in rats. *Exp Biol Med (Maywood).* 2010;235:478-486.
123. Yokoyama M, et al. Effects of flumazenil on intravenous lidocaine-induced convulsions and anticonvulsant property of diazepam in rats. *Anesth Analg.* 1992;75:87-90.
124. Yoshikawa H. First-line therapy for theophylline-associated seizures. *Acta Neurol Scand.* 2007;115(s186):57-61.
125. Zuckerbraun NS, et al. Intrathecal baclofen withdrawal: emergent recognition and management. *Pediatr Emerg Care.* 2004;20:759-764.

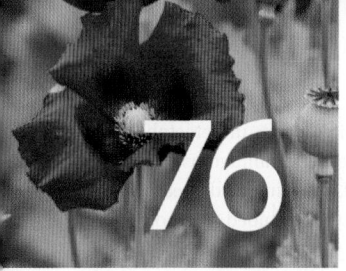

76 ETHANOL

Luke Yip

HISTORY AND EPIDEMIOLOGY

Ethanol, or ethyl alcohol, is commonly referred to as "alcohol." This term is somewhat misleading because there are numerous other alcohols. However, ethanol is one of the most commonly used and abused xenobiotics in the world. Its use is pervasive among adolescents and adults of all ages and socioeconomic groups and represents a tremendous financial and social cost.[3,228] The ethanol content of alcoholic beverages is expressed by volume percent or by proof. Proof is a measure of the absolute ethanol content of distilled liquor, made by determining its specific gravity at an index temperature. In the United Kingdom, the Customs and Excise Act of 1952 declared proof spirits (100 proof) as those in which the weight of the spirits is 12/13 the weight of an equal volume of distilled water at 11°C (51°F). Thus, 100-proof spirits are 48.24% ethanol by weight or 57.06% by volume. Other spirits are designated over or under proof, with the percentage of variance noted. In the United States, a proof spirit (100 proof) is one containing 50% ethanol by volume.

The derivation of proof comes from the days when sailors in the British Navy suspected that the officers were diluting their rum (grog) ration and demanded "proof" that this was not the case. They achieved this by pouring a sample of grog on black granular gunpowder. If the gunpowder ignited by match or spark, the rum was up to standard, 100% proof that the liquor was at least 50% ethanol. This became shortened to 100 proof (Table 76–1).

In addition to beverages, ethanol is present in hundreds of medicinal preparations used as a diluent or solvent in concentrations ranging from 0.3% to 75%.[36,52,61,169,173,227] Mouthwashes have up to 75% ethanol (150 proof), and colognes typically contain 40% to 60% ethanol (80–120 proof).[17,107,173,192] These products occasionally cause inebriation, especially when unintentionally ingested by children.[39,58,94,229] Other sources in which significant amounts of ethanol are found include alcohol-based hand sanitizers and food extracts or flavorings for baking and cooking. Alcohol-based hand sanitizers are widely available as low-viscosity rinses, gels, or foams. They contain 60% to 95% ethanol, isopropanol, or both. Ingestion of these products for their ethanol content is reported in adults and children with an intention to be inebriated and results in serious consequences.[56,100,183,195] Vanilla extract is required by US Food and Drug Administration to have an ethanol content not less than 35% by volume, and inebriation after vanilla extract ingestion is reported.[139]

Veisalgia, "alcohol hangover," comes from the Norwegian kveis, "uneasiness following debauchery" and the Greek algia, "pain." The "hangover" syndrome is attributable to congeners that appear in alcoholic beverages in addition to ethanol and water.[33,41,42] Congeners contribute to the special characteristics of taste, flavor, aroma, and color of a beverage. The combinations and exact amounts of congeners vary with the type of beverage, ranging from 33 mg/L in vodka, to averages of 500 mg/L in some whiskies and as much as 29,000 mg/L in specially aged whiskies or brandies.[33,41,42] The conventional listing of congeners includes fusel oil (a mixture containing amyl, butyl, propyl, and methyl alcohol), aldehydes, furfural, esters, low-molecular-weight organic acids, phenols, and other carbonyl compounds, tannins, solids, and a relatively large number of additional organic and inorganic compounds, usually in trace amounts.[33,42]

Consumption of illicitly produced ethanol ("moonshine") results in methanol, lead or arsenic poisoning, and botulism.[21,54,74,104,125,131,149,170] Incidental lead contamination is also reported in draught beers or wine contained in lead-capped bottles.[202,203] Of historic interest is that the addition of cobalt salts to beer to stabilize the "head" (foam) led to outbreaks of congestive cardiomyopathy among heavy beer drinkers in the United States, Canada, and Belgium in the 1960s (Chap. 91). The clinical-pathological pattern of this disease is distinct from the classical alcoholic cardiomyopathy.[142,144]

Alcoholism is the leading cause of morbidity and mortality in the United States. The prevalence of ethanol dependence in the United States is relatively stable, at around 6% for men and 2% for women.[29] The overall estimated annual cost of excessive drinking in the United States for 2010 was $249 billion with binge drinking representing 76.7% of the total costs.[188] More than 70% of this cost was attributed to lost productivity, most of which resulted from ethanol-related impaired productivity at work or death. Most of the remaining estimated costs were expenditures for health care services to treat ethanol-induced disorders (11.4%), criminal justice system costs of ethanol-related crime (10.0%), and ethanol-related motor vehicle crashes (5.4%). Excessive ethanol use is the fourth leading cause of preventable

TABLE 76–1	Basic Information and Calculations

Ethanol MW: 46 Da

$$mmol = \frac{mg}{MW} = \frac{mg}{46}$$

$$mmol/L = \frac{mg/dL}{4.6}$$

Specific gravity:[a] 0.7939 (~0.8) g/mL

Volume of distribution (V_d): 0.6 L/kg

$$\text{Serum ethanol concentration (mg/dL)}^{b} = \frac{\text{Dose (mg)}}{V_d \text{ (L/kg)} \times \text{Body weight (kg)} \times 10}$$

Average reduction in serum ethanol concentration (elimination phase):

Nontolerant adults: 3.26–4.35 mmol/L/h (15–20 mg/dL/h, 100–125 mg/kg/h)

Tolerant adults: 6.52–8.70 mmol/L/h (30–40 mg/dL/h, 175 mg/kg/h)

For a 70-kg individual:

Dose of Ethanol	Serum Ethanol Concentration[b]
10 mL/kg of 10% (20 proof)	153 mg/dL (36.30 mmol/L)
3 mL/kg of 10% (20 proof)	46 mg/dL (10.87 mmol/L)
1.5 mL/kg of 10% (20 proof)	23 mg/dL (5.43 mmol/L)
150 mL (5 "shots") of 40% (80 proof)	125 mg/dL (31.09 mmol/L)
30 mL (1 "shot") of 40% (80 proof)	25 mg/dL (5.87 mmol/L)
One "standard drink" (~0.6 fluid (fl) oz or 14 grams of "pure" ethanol): 1.5 fl oz of 80-proof distilled spirits or "hard liquor" (eg, whiskey, gin, rum, vodka, and tequila), 2–3 fl oz of cordial, liqueur, or aperitif (24% ethanol), 3–4 fl oz of fortified wine (eg, sherry or port, 14% ethanol), 5 fl oz of table wine (12% ethanol), 8–9 fl oz of malt liquor (7% ethanol), or 12 fl oz of regular beer (5% ethanol)[158]	25 mg/dL (9.11 mmol/L)

[a]Specific gravity of ethanol is dependent on its water content and temperature. The specific gravity of 100% ethanol at temperature between 20° and 35°C ranges from 0.78934 to 0.77641 (~0.8) g/mL.
[b]This is the theoretical maximum concentration, based on instantaneous and complete ethanol absorption and no distribution or metabolism. Principle 1 and Principle 2 concentration consistent with legal intoxication = 10.87–17.39 mmol/L (50–80 mg/dL or 0.05–0.08 g/dL %). The legal breath ethanol concentration to serum ethanol concentration ratio has been set at 1:2100; the amount of ethanol in 1 mL of blood is the same amount in 2,100 mL of exhaled air: Measured breath ethanol concentration (mmol/L) × 2,100 = (Calculated) serum ethanol concentration (mmol/L).

death[148] and accounted for an average of 88,129 American deaths per year from 2006 through 2010; 1 in 10 deaths among working-age adults age 20 to 64 years.[32] In 2015, there were 10,265 ethanol-related traffic fatalities in the United States that accounted for 29% of total traffic fatalities; 63% of ethanol-impaired driving fatalities were drivers with serum ethanol concentration 80 mg/dL or higher.[155] Drivers age 21 to 34 years accounted for 27%, and drivers between 16 and 20 years accounted for 16% of all ethanol-impaired drivers in fatal crashes. Among 16- to 20-year-old male drivers, an increase of 20 mg/dL in serum ethanol concentration was estimated to more than double the relative risk of fatal single vehicle crash injury compared with sober drivers of the same age and gender.[240] When the serum ethanol concentration was between 80 and 100 mg/dL (17–22 mmol/L), 100 and 150 mg/dL (22–33 mmol/L), and greater than 150 mg/dL (33 mmol/L), the relative risks of fatal single-vehicle crash injury were 52, 241, and 15,560 respectively.

The Global Burden of Disease Study identified 3 effects of ethanol: harmful effects in relation to injuries, harmful effects in relation to disease, and the protective effect in relation to ischemic heart disease.[157] Overall, ethanol accounted for 3.5% of mortality and disability, 1.5% of all deaths, 2.1% of all life years lost, and 6% of all the years lived with disability.[157] In the United States, according to National Highway Traffic Safety Administration (NHTSA) information, all jurisdictions have enacted per se serum ethanol concentration for adults operating noncommercial motor vehicles.[156] The term "illegal per se" refers to state laws that make it a criminal offense to operate a motor vehicle at or above a specified ethanol concentration in the blood, breath, or urine, which is independent of any determination of clinical impairment (Special Considerations: SC11). For example, although some ethanol-tolerant individuals will not exhibit impairment even at serum ethanol concentrations greater than 300 mg/dL (65 mmol/L), they are still considered impaired with regard to the laws that governs motor vehicle operation.[1]

There is a dose–response relationship between ethanol consumption and risk of death in men age 16 to 34 years and in women age 16 to 54 years. Meta-analysis of aggregate data from epidemiologic dose–response ethanol and mortality cohort studies suggests that the amount of ethanol consumption at which all-cause risk is lowest is approximately 5 g/day and that ethanol exerts a protective effect (J-shaped dose response curve) up to a daily intake of approximately 45 g.[11] "Sensible" or "responsible" drinking of ethanol (not drinking alcohol to excess) for men is 8 to 10 g/d up to age 34 years, 16 to 20 g/d between 34 and 44 years of age, 24 to 30 g/d between 44 and 54 years of age, 32 to 40 g/d up between 54 and 84 years of age, and 40 to 50 g/d over age 85 years. Women are advised to limit their drinking to 8 to 10 g/d up to age 44 years, 16 to 20 g/d between 44 and 74 years of age, and 24 to 30 g/d over age 75 years.[232] However, no safe amount of prenatal ethanol exposure is established. The combination of a national tolerance of drinking and heavy advertising of ethanol makes it especially appealing to young people. In a society increasingly concerned with drug abuse, the excessive use of ethanol constitutes a serious and pervasive problem as well as a major health issue.

PHARMACOKINETICS AND TOXICOKINETICS

Ethanol is rapidly absorbed from the gastrointestinal (GI) tract, with approximately 20% absorbed from the stomach and the remainder from the small intestine.[162] Factors that enhance absorption include rapid gastric emptying, ethanol intake without food, the absence of congeners, dilution of ethanol (maximum absorption occurs at a concentration of 20%), and carbonation. Under optimal conditions for absorption, 80% to 90% of an ingested dose is fully absorbed within 60 minutes. Factors that delay or decrease ethanol absorption include high concentrations of ethanol (by causing pylorospasm), the presence of food, the coexistence of GI disease, coingestion of xenobiotics such as aspirin and anticholinergics,[105,167] time taken to ingest the drink, and individual variation. When any of these factors is present, absorption may be delayed for 2 to 6 hours. The relative amount of ethanol that is absorbed from the stomach is determined by the presence of an alcohol dehydrogenase (ADH) enzyme in the gastric mucosa, which oxidizes a proportion of the ingested ethanol, thus reducing the amount available for absorption. This effect is more pronounced in men than in women and in nonalcoholics

than in alcoholics.[13,67] However, this gender difference is undetectable after age 50 years.[197] Although histamine$_2$ (H$_2$) receptor antagonists such as cimetidine and ranitidine inhibit gastric ADH, resulting in decreased first-pass metabolism and increased bioavailability of imbibed ethanol,[28,48,60,198] the clinical significance of this effect after a moderate ethanol dose is unclear.[7,24,66,124,218]

After complete distribution, ethanol is present in body tissues in a concentration proportional to that of the tissue water content. Ethanol freely passes through the placenta, exposing the fetus to ethanol concentrations comparable to those achieved in the mother.

Ethanol is primarily eliminated by the liver, with 2% to 5% excreted unchanged by the kidneys, lungs, and sweat.[98] Ethanol is metabolized via at least 3 different pathways: the aforementioned ADH pathway located in the cytosol of the hepatocytes, cytochrome P450 2E1 (CYP2E1) located on the endoplasmic reticulum, and the peroxidase-catalase system associated with the hepatic peroxisomes (Fig. 76–1).[162]

For a given ethanol dose, 95% to 98% is metabolized in the liver, first to acetaldehyde by ADH and then further to acetic acid by aldehyde dehydrogenase (ALDH).[98] The end products of ethanol oxidation are carbon dioxide and water. The remaining 2% to 5% is excreted unchanged in urine, sweat, and expired air. In addition, less than 0.1% undergoes nonoxidative biotransformation, the products of which include fatty acid ethyl esters (FAEEs), ethyl glucuronide, and ethyl sulfate. Fatty acid ethyl esters are formed by esterification of ethanol with endogenous fatty acids and acyl-CoA fatty acids and is catalyzed by cytosolic FAEE synthases. Whereas ethyl glucuronide is formed by the conjugation of ethanol with glucuronic acid catalyzed by uridine diphosphate-glucuronosyltransferase, ethyl sulfate is formed by the transfer of a sulfur group from 3′-phosphoadenosine-5′-phosphosulfate to ethanol mediated by mitochondrial sulfotransferases.[10,40,84,194]

The ADH system is the main pathway for ethanol metabolism and is also the rate-limiting step. Alcohol dehydrogenase is a zinc metalloenzyme that uses oxidized nicotinamide adenine dinucleotide (NAD$^+$) as a hydrogen ion acceptor to oxidize ethanol to acetaldehyde. In this process, a hydrogen ion is transferred from ethanol to NAD$^+$, converting it to its reduced form, NADH. Subsequently, hydrogen ion is transferred from acetaldehyde to NAD$^+$. Under normal conditions, acetate is converted to acetylcoenzyme A (acetyl-CoA), which enters the citric acid cycle—also historically known as the Krebs cycle—and is metabolized to carbon dioxide and water. The entry of acetyl-CoA into the citric acid cycle is thiamine dependent (Antidotes in Depth: A27). When thiamine is deficient, acetyl-CoA accumulates, and high acetyl-CoA concentration favors formation of acetoacetate and its subsequent reduction to β-hydroxybutyrate in the setting of a high redox state defined by NADH excess.

The *ADH* gene family encodes enzymes that metabolize a wide variety of substrates. There are at least 7 genetic loci that code for human ADH arising from the association of different subunits, and there are more than 20 ADH enzymes.[2] These ADH forms are divided into 5 major classes (I–V) according to their subunit, enzyme composition, and physicochemical properties.[99] Two of these gene loci exhibit polymorphism, and they both involve class I *ADH* genes; 3 alleles exist for ADH2 (*ADH1B*) *ADH2*1* (*ADH1B*1*), *ADH2*2* (*ADH1B*2*), and *ADH2*3* (*ADH1B*3*) and 3 for ADH3 (*ADH1C*) *ADH3*1* (*ADH1C*1*), *ADH3*2* (*ADH1C*2*), and *ADH3*3* (*ADH1C*3*).[38] Class I enzymes are inducible intracellular hepatic enzymes and play a major role in ethanol metabolism.[128] Class IV ADH6 (σ-ADH) is the major ADH expressed in human gastric mucosa.[13,67] Alcohol dehydrogenase is usually present in non-Asians, but in a majority of Pacific Rim Asians, the enzyme activity is either low or not detectable.[13,14,50] The *ADH1B*2* allele is present in 90% of Pacific Rim Asians but occurs infrequently in most whites, except for people of Jewish and perhaps Hispanic descent.[233] This allele is responsible for the unusually rapid conversion of ethanol to acetaldehyde. People carrying *ADH1B*2* alleles are about one-third as likely to be alcoholic compared with people without this allele.[233]

In the liver, ADH metabolizes ethanol to acetaldehyde, which is then converted to acetate by mitochondrial NAD$^+$-dependent ALDH. Human ALDH

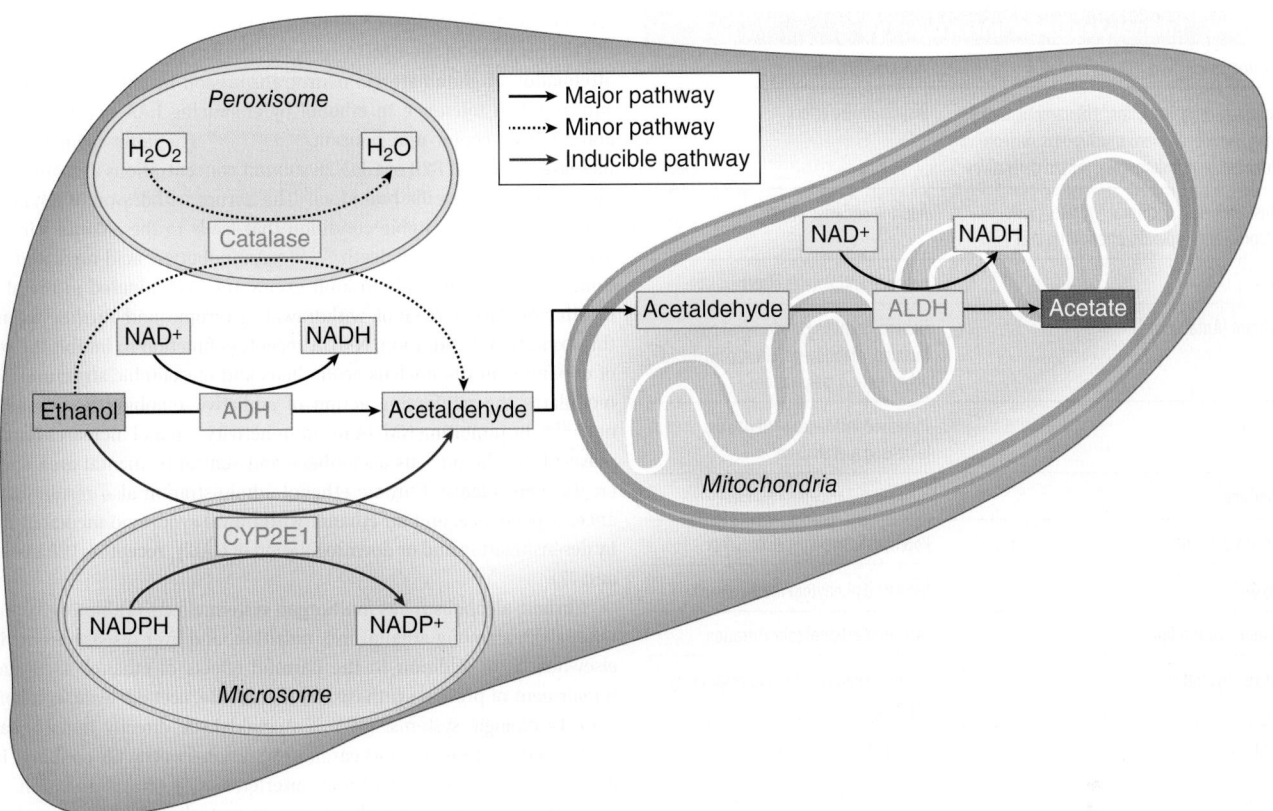

FIGURE 76–1. Ethanol is metabolized in the cytoplasm of hepatocytes to acetaldehyde through major, minor, and inducible pathways. Acetaldehyde is metabolized in the mitochondria to acetic acid.

is divided into 9 major gene families. There is a functional polymorphism of the mitochondrial *ALDH2* gene and expression of an inactive form of the ALDH2, glutamate to lysine substitution at position 487 (E487K), results in impaired acetaldehyde metabolizing capacity. The variant allele *ALDH2*2* encodes a protein subunit that confers low activity to the enzyme, resulting in marked differences in the steady-state kinetic constants, which appears to be most prevalent in Pacific Rim Asians.[2,38,76,212,213] These metabolic polymorphisms contribute to differences in ethanol and acetaldehyde elimination rates; high-activity ADH variants are predicted to increase the rate of acetaldehyde generation, but the low-activity ALDH2 variant is associated with limited capacity to metabolize this compound and contributes to differences in ethanol-related behavior. Asians possessing an atypical *ALDH2* gene are more sensitive to acute adverse responses to ethanol, which tends to discourage ethanol consumption. Homozygous *ALDH2*2* individuals are strikingly sensitive to a small dose of ethanol (0.2 g/kg), as evidenced by the intense flushing, pronounced cardiovascular and hemodynamic effects as well as subjective perception of general discomfort.[57,76,171,217,222] This effect is also associated with the *ADH2*2* and *ADH3*1* allele and is similar to that induced by disulfiram (Chap. 78). The ethanol flushing response involves prostaglandin and histamine release. Both prostaglandin antagonists (aspirin)[219] and antihistamines (H_1 and H_2)[145,208,215] attenuate this response.

Cytochrome P450 2E1 is responsible for very little ethanol metabolism in the nontolerant drinker but becomes more important as the ethanol concentration rises or as ethanol use becomes chronic (Fig. 76–1). Cytochrome P450 2E1 uses reduced nicotinamide adenine dinucleotide phosphate (NADPH) as an electron acceptor to oxidize ethanol to acetaldehyde.[117] In this process, electrons are transferred from ethanol to NADPH, converting it to its oxidized form, NADP⁺. Subsequently, acetaldehyde is further oxidized to acetate as hydrogen ion is transferred from acetaldehyde to NAD. The ability of ethanol to induce the CYP2E1 forms the basis for the well-established interactions between ethanol and a host of other xenobiotics metabolized by

this system.[49,65] In alcoholics and those with higher ethanol concentrations, cimetidine also delays ethanol clearance by inhibiting CYP2E1.[80] However, the increase in serum ethanol concentration from such an interaction is of questionable clinical significance.[6,7,24,27]

Alcohol dehydrogenase is saturated at relatively low serum ethanol concentrations; class I ADH is not inducible.[31] As the system is saturated, ethanol elimination changes from first-order to zero-order kinetics (Chap. 9). In adults, the average rate of ethanol metabolism is 100 to 125 mg/kg/h in occasional drinkers and up to 175 mg/kg/h in habitual drinkers.[20,75] As a result, the average-sized adult metabolizes 7 to 10 g/h, and the serum ethanol concentration falls 15 to 20 mg/dL/h (3.26–4.35 mmol/L/h). Tolerant drinkers, by recruiting CYP2E1, increase their clearance of ethanol to 30 mg/dL/h (6.52 mmol/L/h) or even higher.[20,75] Studies of inebriated patients indicate that although the average ethanol clearance rate is about 20 mg/dL/h (4.35 mmol/L/h), there is considerable individual variation (standard deviation of about 6 mg/dL/h (1.30 mmol/L/h).[20,75]

XENOBIOTIC INTERACTIONS

Ethanol interacts with a variety of xenobiotics (Table 76–2).[103,227] The most frequent ethanol–drug interactions occur as a result of ethanol-induced increase in hepatic enzyme activity. By contrast, acute ethanol use inhibits metabolism of other xenobiotics due to competitive inhibition of hepatic enzyme activity or a reduction in hepatic blood flow. The interaction between ethanol and disulfiram (Antabuse) is well described and it can be life threatening (Chap. 78).

Concomitant use of cocaine and ethanol leads to the formation of an active metabolite, ethylbenzoylecgnine, through transesterification of cocaine by the liver.[178] Cocaethylene has a longer half-life than cocaine itself (2 hours versus 48 minutes), and this explains some of the delayed cardiovascular effects attributed to cocaine use.[9,234] Both ethanol and cocaethylene inhibit the metabolism of cocaine, thereby prolonging the elimination of cocaine and enhancing its effect (Chap. 75).[168]

TABLE 76–2	Ethanol–Xenobiotic Interactions
Xenobiotics	**Adverse Effects**
Carbamates, cephalosporins,[a] chloramphenicol, chlorpropamide, *Coprinus* mushrooms, griseofulvin, metronidazole, nitrofurantoin, thiram derivatives	Disulfiramlike effect
Antihistamines (H₁), chloral hydrate, cyclic antidepressants, opioids, phenothiazines	Additive sedative effect
Aspirin	Enhance antiplatelet effect
Disulfiram (Antabuse)	Nausea, vomiting, abdominal pain, flushing, diaphoresis, chest pain, headache, vertigo, palpitations
Isoniazid	Increased incidence of hepatitis; increased metabolism[b]
Methadone	Increased methadone metabolism[b]
Oral hypoglycemics	Potentiates hypoglycemic effect
Phenytoin	Increased phenytoin metabolism[b]
Ranitidine, cimetidine	Increased ethanol concentration
Sedative–hypnotics	Additive sedative effect or respiratory depression
Vasodilators	Potentiates vasodilator effect
Warfarin	Increased warfarin metabolism[b]

[a]Those containing a *N*-methylthiotetrazole side chain. [b]Effect possibly associated with chronic ethanol consumption.

The combination of ethanol and chloral hydrate (ie, "Mickey Finn") has additive central nervous system (CNS) depressant effects. Chloral hydrate competes for ADH, thereby prolonging the half-life of ethanol.[199] The metabolism of ethanol generates NADH, which is a necessary cofactor for choral hydrate metabolism to trichloroethanol, an active metabolite. In addition, ethanol inhibits the conjugation of trichloroethanol, which in turn inhibits ethanol oxidation.

Case reports and retrospective case series suggest that chronic ethanol consumption predisposes a person to acetaminophen (APAP) hepatotoxicity (Chap. 33)[55,133,141,193,244] even when APAP is taken according to the manufacturer's recommended dosage.[243] Because ethanol induces CYP2E1, the enzyme involved in the metabolism of APAP to its hepatotoxic intermediate, NAPQI, a theoretical basis for this association exists. However, in randomized, placebo-controlled trials in which people with confirmed alcoholism were given APAP 4 g/day or placebo, there were no differences between the 2 groups with regard to liver enzymes or to their coagulation profile.[187] Recent fasting, common in people with alcoholism, was also associated with a predisposition to APAP hepatotoxicity, likely because of depletion of glutathione (Chap. 33).[231] However, in a retrospective study, heavy drinkers did not develop more severe hepatoxicity after APAP overdose than nondrinkers.[134]

PATHOPHYSIOLOGY

Despite the long history of ethanol use and study, no specific receptor for ethanol is identified, and the mechanism of action leading to inebriation remains the subject of debate.[172] Ethanol affects a large number of membrane proteins that participate in signaling pathways such as neurotransmitter receptors, enzymes, and ion channels,[154,224] and there is extensive evidence that ethanol interacts with a variety of neurotransmitters.[59,220,221] The major actions of ethanol involve enhancing the inhibitory effects of γ-aminobutyric acid (GABA) at GABA_A receptors and blockade of the *N*-methyl-*D*-aspartate (NMDA) subtype of glutamate, an excitatory amino acid (EAA) receptor.[45,115,116,224] Animal studies indicate that the acute effects of ethanol result from competitive inhibition of glycine binding to the NMDA

receptor and disruption of glutamatergic neurotransmission by inhibiting the response of the NMDA receptor. Persistent glycine antagonism and attenuation of glutamatergic neurotransmission by chronic ethanol exposure result in tolerance to ethanol by enhancing EAA neurotransmission and NMDA receptor upregulation.[25,92,95,153,220,221] The latter involves selective increases in NMDA R2B or GluN2B subunit concentrations and other molecular changes in specific brain loci.[4] The abrupt withdrawal of ethanol thus produces a hyperexcitable condition that leads to the alcohol withdrawal and excitotoxic neuronal death.[18,45,221] γ-Aminobutyric acid-mediated inhibition, which normally acts to limit excitation, is eliminated in the absence of ethanol during ethanol withdrawal syndrome and further intensifies this excitation. In addition, NMDA receptors function to inhibit the release of dopamine in the nucleus accumbens and mesolimbic structures, which modulates the reinforcing action of addictive xenobiotics such as ethanol.[22,23,207] By inhibiting NMDA receptor activity, ethanol increases dopamine release from the nucleus accumbens and ventral tegmental area and thus creates dependence. Chronic ethanol administration also results in tolerance, dependence, and an ethanol withdrawal syndrome mediated in part by desensitization and or downregulation of GABA_A receptors (Chaps. 13, 14, and 77).

Chronic alcoholism has multiorgan system effects (Table 76–3), and the relationships among ethanol use, nutrition, and liver disease are reviewed elsewhere.[127] In addition to the harmful effects of ethanol itself such as impairment of protein synthesis, its metabolite, acetaldehyde, is inherently toxic to biologic systems.[121,129,223,242] Acetaldehyde directly impairs cardiac contractile function, disrupts cardiac excitation–contractile coupling, inhibits myocardial protein synthesis, interferes with phosphorylation, cause structural and functional alterations in mitochondria and hepatocytes, and inactivates acetyl-coenzyme A. Acetaldehyde also reacts with intracellular proteins to generate adducts. Acetaldehyde-protein and DNA adducts promote oxidative stress, lipid peroxidation, hepatic stellae cell activation-associated inflammation and fibrosis, and mutagenesis. Acetaldehyde adducts are believed to be important in the early phase of alcoholic liver disease, and in advanced liver disease, they contribute to the development of hepatic fibrosis as well as hepatocellular carcinoma.[200]

Ethanol metabolism through the CYP2E1 pathway generates highly reactive oxygen radicals, including the hydroxyethyl radical (HER) molecule. Elevated oxygen radical concentrations generate a state of oxidative stress, which leads to cell damage. Oxygen radicals also initiate lipid peroxidation, resulting in reactive molecules such as malondialdehyde (MDA) and 4-hydroxy-2-nonenal (HNE). These molecules react with proteins or acetaldehyde to form adducts, which contribute to the development of alcoholic liver injury.[46]

Oxidation of ethanol generates an excess of acetyl-CoA and reducing potential in the cytosol in the form of NADH with the ratio of NADH to NAD⁺ being dramatically increased. This ratio, also known as the redox potential, determines the ability of the cell to carry on various oxidative processes. The excess acetyl-CoA and the unfavorable change in redox potential caused by ethanol metabolism contribute to the development of metabolic disorders such as impaired gluconeogenesis, alterations in fatty acid metabolism, fatty liver, hyperlipidemia, hypoglycemia, elevated lactate concentration, hyperuricemia (gouty attacks), increased collagen and scar tissue formation, and alcoholic ketoacidosis (AKA) (Fig. 76–2).

Studies in alcoholic liver disease focused on Kupffer cell activation by endotoxin that is released by intestinal bacteria. When Kupffer cells are activated, they produce regulatory nuclear factor κB (NFκB) and generation of significant amounts of superoxide radicals (O_2^-) and cytokines (tumor necrosis factor and interleukin-8), which is an essential factor in the injury to hepatocytes associated with alcoholic liver disease.[140,230]

ACUTE CLINICAL FEATURES

Ethanol is a selective CNS depressant at low doses and a general depressant at high doses. Initially, it depresses the areas of the brain involved with highly integrated functions. Cortical release leads to animated behavior and the

TABLE 76–3	Systemic Effects Associated With Alcoholism

Cardiovascular
   Cardiomyopathy
   "Holiday heart" (dysrhythmias)
   "Wet" beriberi or high-output heart failure (thiamine deficiency)

Endocrine and Metabolic
   Hypoglycemia
   Hypokalemia
   Hypomagnesemia
   Hypophosphatemia
   Hypothermia
   Hypertriglyceridemia
   Hyperuricemia
   Metabolic acidosis
   Malnutrition

Gastrointestinal
   Mouth
      Cancer of the mouth, pharynx, larynx
      Cheilosis
      Stomatitis (nutritional)
   Esophagus
      Boerhaave syndrome
      Cancer of the esophagus
      Esophageal spasm (diffuse)
      Esophagitis
      Mallory-Weiss tear
   Stomach and duodenum
      Diarrhea
      Gastritis (Acute)
      Gastritis (chronic hypertrophic)
      Hematemesis
      Malabsorption
      Peptic ulcer
   Liver
      Cirrhosis
      Hepatitis
      Steatosis
   Pancreas
      Pancreatitis (acute or chronic)

Genitourinary
   Hypogonadism
   Impotence
   Infertility

Hematologic
   Coagulopathy
   Folate, B_{12}, iron-deficiency anemias
   Hemolysis (Zieve syndrome, stomatocytosis, spur-cell anemia)
   Leukopenia
   Thrombocytopenia

Neurologic
   Alcohol amnestic syndrome
   Alcoholic hallucinosis
   Alcohol withdrawal
   Cerebellar degeneration
   Cerebral atrophy (dementia)
   Cerebrovascular accident (hemorrhage, infarction)
   Inebriation
   Korsakoff psychosis
   Marchiafava-Bignami disease
   Myopathy
   Osmotic demyelination syndrome
   Pellagra
   Polyneuropathy
   Subdural hematoma
   Wernicke encephalopathy

Ophthalmic
   Tobacco—ethanol amblyopia

Psychiatric
   Animated behavior
   Loss of self-restraint
   Manic-depressive illness
   Suicide and depression

Respiratory
   Atelectasis
   Pneumonia
   Respiratory acidosis
   Respiratory depression

loss of restraint. This paradoxical CNS stimulation is due to disinhibition. The signs of inebriation are quite variable. The patients are energized and loquacious, expansive, emotionally labile, increasingly gregarious or appear to have lost self-control, exhibit antisocial behavior, and are ill tempered. As the degree of inebriation increases, there are successive inhibition and impairment of neuronal activity. Patients become irritable, abusive, aggressive, violent, dysarthric, confused, disoriented, or lethargic. With severe inebriation, there is loss of airway protective reflexes, coma, and increasing risk of death from respiratory depression. An ethanol-naïve adult with a serum ethanol concentration of greater than 250 mg/dL (54 mmol/L) is usually comatose.[1]

However, the acute effects of ethanol ingestion also depend on the habituation of the drinker. This is mainly because of the development of tolerance, which has both a metabolic (pharmacokinetic) and a functional (pharmacodynamic) component.[211] Metabolic tolerance to ethanol is based on enhanced elimination by CYP2E1. Functional tolerance (resistance to the effects of ethanol at the cellular level) is a more important determinant of

habituation and is mediated through alterations in $GABA_A$ receptor subunits (eg, decrease in α_{-1} and α_{-2} subunit, increase in α_{-6} subunit, glycine antagonism, and glutamatergic neurotransmission attenuation) and upregulation of NMDA receptors (eg, NMDA R2B or GluN2B subunit) as well as interaction between serotonergic (eg, $5HT_{1A}$) and adrenergic (eg, norepinephrine and dopamine) neurons.[25,92,95,108,109,150,153,176,210,221] Acute ethanol tolerance is demonstrated by the Mellanby effect, which involves the comparison of physiologic responses or behavioral effects at the same serum ethanol concentration on the ascending and descending limbs of the serum ethanol vs time curve. Impairment is greater at a given serum ethanol concentration when it is increasing than for the same serum ethanol concentration when it is falling.[160,226] Although individuals who are acutely inebriated move through a progressive sequence of events, the association of a particular aspect of inebriation with a specific serum ethanol concentration is not usually possible without knowing the pattern of ethanol use of the patient. Acute inebriation occurs in habitual drinkers when they raise their ethanol concentration an equivalent amount above baseline and specific clinical manifestations of

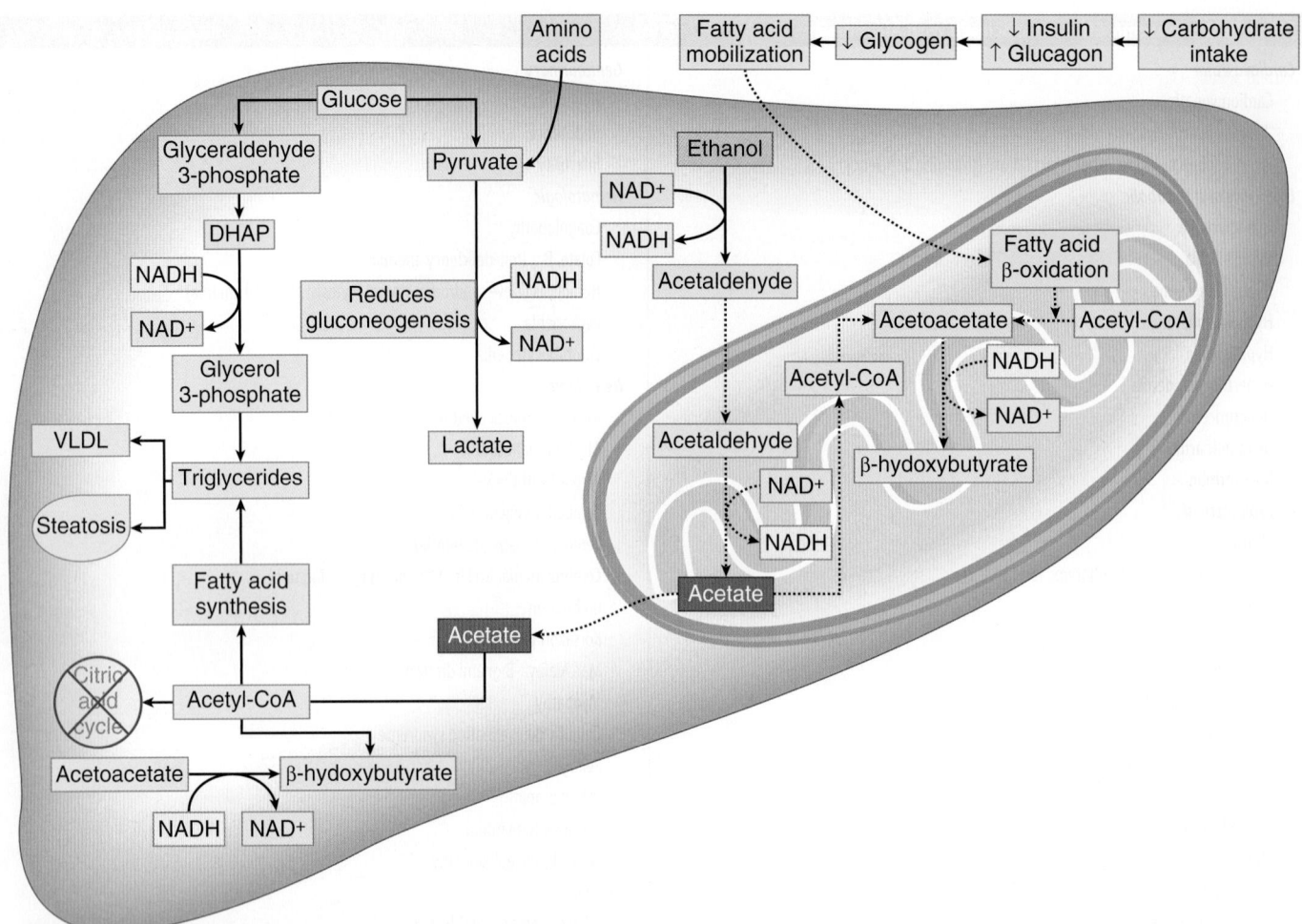

FIGURE 76–2. Ethanol metabolism drives reactions towards NADH and acetate. The high cytoplasmic redox state favors the reduction of pyruvate to lactate and diverts pyruvate from being a substrate for gluconeogenesis, favors the reduction of dihydroxyacetone phosphate (DHAP) to glycerol 3-phosphate, and serves as substrate for triglycerides formation. The high cytoplasmic redox state and acetate load limits the citric acid cycle, thus decreasing the supply of NADH for oxidative phosphorylation, resulting in a decrease in adenosine triphosphate (ATP) production and favoring conversion of acetyl-CoA to ketone bodies and fatty acid synthesis. Abrupt discontinuation of ethanol and starvation results in mobilization and oxidation of fatty acids. Fatty acid metabolism results in the formation of acetyl-CoA, which combines with the excess acetate, in the form of acetyl-CoA, that is generated from ethanol metabolism to form acetoacetate. Most of the acetoacetate is reduced to β-hydroxybutyrate because of the high cellular redox state.

inebriation typically occur with significantly higher serum ethanol concentration than nontolerant individuals. Regardless, the absolute change above baseline is an important factor.

Many patients present with obvious signs and symptoms consistent with inebriation that include flushed facies, diaphoresis, tachycardia, hypotension, hypothermia, hypoventilation, mydriasis, nystagmus, vomiting, dysarthria, muscular incoordination, ataxia, altered consciousness, and coma. However, an inebriated patient presenting to an emergency department (ED) has a broad range of diagnostic possibilities and should prompt a careful evaluation for a variety of occult clinical and metabolic disorders. A meticulous and systematic approach to the evaluation and management of an inebriated patient will help avoid the potential pitfalls in such a situation.[69] The presence or absence of an odor of ethanol on the breath is an unreliable means of ascertaining whether a person is inebriated or whether ethanol was recently consumed.[152] Diplopia, visual disturbances, and nystagmus are caused by either the toxic effects of ethanol or represent Wernicke encephalopathy. Hypothermia is exacerbated by environmental exposure, from malnutrition and loss of carbohydrate or energy substrate, and ethanol-induced vasodilation; conversely heat-related illness is exacerbated during a heat wave. Inebriation impairs cardiac output in patients with preexisting cardiac disease[77] and induces dysrhythmias such as atrial fibrillation, atrioventricular block, and nonsustained ventricular tachycardia.[53,78,79] The association between ethanol use and cardiac dysrhythmias, particularly supraventricular tachydysrhythmias, in apparently healthy people is called "holiday heart

syndrome."[110,118,143] The syndrome was first described in people with consequential ethanol consumption, who typically presented on weekends or after holidays, and it also occurs in patients who binge but who usually drink little ethanol. The most common dysrhythmia is atrial fibrillation, which usually reverts to normal sinus rhythm within 24 hours. Although the syndrome recurs, the clinical course is benign in patients without anatomic cardiac pathology, and specific antidysrhythmic therapy is usually not warranted.[68,79] Acute consequential ethanol drinking precipitates silent myocardial ischemia in patients with stable angina pectoris.[186] A variant form of angina pectoris, or Prinzmetal angina, occurs at rest but not usually with exertion and is associated with transient ST-segment elevation caused by focal spasm of an epicardial coronary artery and is reported to occur in patients after ethanol ingestion at a time when the serum ethanol concentration has decreased almost to zero.[62,102,137,146,166,190,214] Ethanol-related seizures occur as a consequence of ethanol dependence. Most commonly these seizures are caused by alcohol withdrawal and are classically characterized by generalized tonic-clonic activity followed by a brief postictal period. However, a significant percentage of patients with ethanol-related seizures have other identifiable causes, and they include head trauma (eg, intracranial hemorrhage or contusion), idiopathic generalized epilepsy, cerebrovascular accident, intracranial lesions (eg, tumors, infection, and gliosis), and toxic-metabolic (eg, hypoglycemia).[159,179,180] Patients presenting with acute inebriation commonly have decreased serum ionized magnesium concentrations while their total serum magnesium concentration is within the normal range.[239] However, total-body magnesium depletion occurs because of poor dietary intake, decreased GI absorption secondary to ethanol, and renal wasting caused by ethanol-related diuresis.[63,101,182,201,209]

DIAGNOSTIC TESTS

There are numerous qualitative and quantitative assays for ethanol in biological fluids and exhaled breath. Immunoassay or gas chromatography is commonly used for determination of ethanol in liquid specimens in most hospitals. Hospital laboratory analysis of blood samples for ethanol content is usually based on serum (liquid portion of whole blood after the cellular components and clotting factors are removed) or rarely plasma (acellular liquid portion of whole blood). By contrast, forensic casework expresses ethanol concentration in terms of ethanol concentration in whole blood (Special Considerations: SC11).

Ethanol saliva testing is a promising alternative to breath ethanol analysis in the rapid assessment of serum ethanol concentrations in patients regardless of their mental status.[43,204] Fatty acid ethyl esters are a highly sensitive and specific test for recent ethanol use.[16,51,205] Because FAEEs remain in the system for at least 24 hours, they have a role as a marker of recent ethanol use even after ethanol is completely metabolized. The presence of FAEEs in meconium and hair is currently the most used tool to detect prenatal ethanol exposure.[10]

Ethyl glucuronide and ethyl sulfate are nonoxidative direct ethanol metabolites and are excreted for considerably longer time than ethanol.[19,40,83,189,194] Testing for these metabolites in urine has gained popularity as a sensitive method to detect recent ethanol intake and is favored over tests such as γ-glutamyl transferase (GGT) or carbohydrate-deficient transferrin, particularly by agencies concerned with monitoring an individual for recent ethanol consumption or relapse, confirm abstinence in treatment programs, workplaces, and schools, and provide legal proof of drinking.[82,175] The presence of ethyl glucuronide and ethyl sulfate provides a strong indication of recent drinking even when ethanol is no longer detectable.[83] However, caution should be applied in the interpretation of ethyl glucuronide testing results. Ethyl glucuronide is sensitive to degradation or is synthesized by bacteria (eg, *Escherichia coli*) such that infected urine results in either a false-negative or false-positive test result, particularly when specimens are improperly stored; ethyl sulfate degradation or formation is not detected under similar conditions.[85,87] Detection windows for ethyl glucuronide and ethyl sulfate after drinking are limited and dependent on the amount of ethanol consumed. For example, these metabolites are detectable in urine for 24 hours or less after intake of 0.25 g/kg ethanol and 48 hours or less after intake of 0.50 g/kg ethanol.[40,81,83,90,91,237] Depending on the analytical cut-off limit, unintentional exposure to ethanol including mouthwash and hand sanitizers results in a urine positive for ethyl glucuronide or ethyl sulfate.[37,185] There appears to be a marked interindividual variation in the concentration–time profiles for both metabolites. When the times for ethanol intake and urine specimen collection between drinking and sampling are uncertain, it is not possible to link a single ethyl glucuronide and sulfate result to a specific ethanol dose taken at a specific time.[86] A common cut-off or reporting limit has yet to be determined for urinary ethyl glucuronide and ethyl sulfate when used as ethanol biomarkers.

Laboratory investigations that are recommended for inebriated patients include a rapid reagent glucose test, complete blood count, electrolytes, blood urea nitrogen, creatinine urine, ketones, acetone, lipase, liver enzymes, ammonia, calcium, and magnesium. Patients with an anion gap metabolic acidosis should have urine ketones and a serum lactate concentration determined (Chaps. 12 and 106). Whereas high serum acetone concentrations are indicative of isopropanol toxicity or accelerated fatty acid metabolism, elevated serum or urinary ketones are indicative of AKA, starvation ketosis, or diabetic ketoacidosis (DKA). Because the laboratory nitroprusside reaction detects only ketones (acetoacetate and acetone) and not β-hydroxybutyrate, the assay for urinary ketones is only mildly positive in many patients with AKA.

A serum ethanol concentration will be infrequently necessary in the initial laboratory studies of patients who appear inebriated or have an altered mental status.[93] When performed if the serum ethanol concentration is inconsistent with the patient's clinical condition, prompt reevaluation of the patient is indicated to elucidate the etiology of the altered mental status, including toxic-metabolic (eg, hypoglycemia, electrolyte or acid–base disorder, toxic alcohols, therapeutic or illicit drug overdose, ethanol withdrawal, hepatic encephalopathy, and Wernicke-Korsakoff syndrome), trauma-related, neurologic (eg, postictal condition), and infectious (eg, CNS infections) etiologies. The threshold for head computed tomography (CT) imaging should be low in comatose patients with concentrations below 300 mg/dL (65 mmol/L) and those with values in excess of 300 mg/dL (65 mmol/L) who fail to improve clinically during a limited period of close observation followed by a lumbar puncture if warranted. There should also be a low threshold for head CT imaging in chronically ethanol-tolerant patients because they are prone to trauma and coagulopathies, both of which cause intracranial bleeding.

If the osmol gap, the difference between the measured osmolality and the calculated osmolarity, is to be used as a tool to assist in the diagnosis of toxic alcohol ingestion, the presence of ethanol in patients needs to be included in the calculation.[89] Ethanol increases the calculated osmolarity, making the osmol gap smaller or even possibly negative. Small osmol gaps cannot be safely used to exclude the possibility of toxic alcohol ingestions, but very large osmol gaps are suggestive of toxic alcohol ingestions.

MANAGEMENT OF POSSIBLY INEBRIATED PATIENTS

Ethanol is rapidly absorbed from the GI tract. Occasionally, an extremely inebriated or comatose patient will have severe respiratory depression, necessitating endotracheal intubation and ventilatory support. Any patient with an acute altered mental status mandates immediate investigation and treatment of reversible causes such as hypoxia, hypoglycemia, and opioid toxicity. In addition, treatment for presumed thiamine depletion is recommended. Supplemental oxygen should be administered if the patient is hypoxic; intravenous (IV) dextrose (0.5–1.0 g/kg) and naloxone 0.04 mg should be administered as clinically indicated. Abnormal vital signs should be addressed and stabilized. Patients who are combative and violent should be both physically restrained and then chemically sedated (Special Considerations: SC4). Randomized clinical trials suggest both benzodiazepines (ie, midazolam) and antipsychotics (ie, droperidol and haloperidol) are effective as chemical sedation in the ED setting.[96,111,136,161] Midazolam has a more rapid onset of action and a shorter duration of effect than droperidol.[96,111,136,161] Patients receiving midazolam required more additional sedation and required airway management compared with patients receiving droperidol.[96,111,136] Although the efficacy of midazolam and various antipsychotics are confirmed in multiple studies,[96,111,136,161] these studies were not designed to inform about the safety, equivalence, or superiority of midazolam and droperidol. Caution should be taken because of additive effects of ethanol and benzodiazepine on respiratory depression. Attempts by those who are clinically inebriated to sign out against medical advice or attempt to leave should also be prevented. Under these circumstances reevaluation, observation and additional laboratory studies will enhance the assessment to ensure the patient is safe for discharge (Chap. 138 and Special Considerations: SC11). It is reasonable to reassess patient's fluid and electrolyte status and abnormalities corrected. It is reasonable to add multivitamins with folate, thiamine, and magnesium to the maintenance IV solution.

A variety of therapies are advocated either to reverse the intoxicating effects of ethanol or to enhance its elimination. Those proven to be either ineffective or unreliable include caffeine, naloxone, flumazenil, and rapid IV saline loading.[64,126,163,164,184] Hemodialysis is an effective means of enhancing the systemic elimination of ethanol because of the small volume of distribution and low molecular weight of ethanol. In severe ethanol poisoning resulting in respiratory failure or coma, hemodialysis is a reasonable adjunct treatment to supportive care. However, the risks of hemodialysis usually exceed its benefit.

INDICATIONS FOR HOSPITALIZATION

A patient with uncomplicated inebriation can be safely discharged after a careful observation with social service or psychiatric counseling. An individual should not be discharged while impairment of cognitive and motor function persists. However, it is reasonable to discharge a mildly intoxicated patient to a protected environment under the supervision of a responsible, not intoxicated adult. In all cases except allowing a person to drive, the clinical assessment of the patient is more important than the serum ethanol concentration. Indications for hospital admission include persistently abnormal vital signs, persistently abnormal mental status with or without an obvious cause, an overdose with intended self-harm, concomitant serious trauma, consequential ethanol withdrawal, and those with an associated serious disease process such as pancreatitis or GI hemorrhage.

Chronic alcoholism leads to an organic brain syndrome that is irreversible. The patient's socioeconomic condition, capacity, and lack of ability to comply with a treatment plan are critical in making a disposition. Patients with alcoholism requesting ethanol detoxification should be assisted in finding an appropriate rehabilitation site. Inpatient detoxification programs differ substantially from outpatient programs, but their most consequential advantages are that they enforce abstinence, provide more support and structure, and separate the patient from the social surroundings associated with drinking.[157,225] For patients who are not admitted, a referral should be offered to Alcoholics Anonymous or another suitable ethanol rehabilitation program.

Ethanol-Associated Hypoglycemia

Hypoglycemia associated with ethanol consumption occurs when ethanol metabolism increases the cellular redox ratio. The higher redox state favors the conversion of pyruvate to lactate, diverting pyruvate from being a substrate for gluconeogenesis (Fig. 76–2).[113,241] Hypoglycemia typically occurs when there is a reduced caloric intake and only after the hepatic glycogen stores are depleted, as in an overnight fast. The mechanism by which hypoglycemia is associated with ethanol consumption in the well-nourished individual is less well defined.

Although the conditions associated with hypoglycemia in adults are also present in infants and children, children with their smaller livers have less glycogen stores than adults and are more likely to develop hypoglycemia. Hypoglycemia associated with ethanol consumption usually occurs in malnourished chronic alcoholics and children (Chap. 47). Hypoglycemia also occurs in binge drinkers who do not have adequate caloric intake. A 22% incidence of hypoglycemia was reported in one retrospective study of children with documented ethanol ingestion.[128] In another retrospective study of children and adolescents, there was a 3.4% incidence of hypoglycemia (serum glucose concentration <67 mg/dL or 3.7 mmol/L);[58] children age younger than 5 years have an increased risk of developing hypoglycemia, and it is the most common reported clinical abnormality related to ethanol ingestion in this age group.[119,120]

Clinical Features

Patients with ethanol associated hypoglycemia usually present with an altered consciousness 2 to 10 hours after ethanol ingestion. Other physical findings include hypothermia and tachypnea. Laboratory findings, in addition to hypoglycemia, usually include a positive serum ethanol concentration, ketonuria without glucosuria, and mild metabolic acidosis.

Management

Acute treatment of ethanol-associated hypoglycemia is similar to other causes of hypoglycemia (Chap. 47 and Antidotes in Depth: A8) and should prompt a systematic evaluation for coexisting clinical and metabolic disorders. Hospital admission is reasonable in severe or resistant cases. Because this represents serious metabolic impairment that cannot be rapidly rectified.

Alcoholic Ketoacidosis

The development of AKA requires a combination of physical (eg, abrupt discontinuation of ethanol and starvation) and physiologic events to occur. The normal response to starvation and depletion of hepatic glycogen stores is for amino acids to be converted to pyruvate. Pyruvate serves as a substrate for gluconeogenesis and is converted to acetyl-CoA, which can enter the citric acid cycle or is used in various biosynthetic pathways (eg, fatty acids, ketone bodies, cholesterol, and acetylcholine). As described earlier, ethanol metabolism generates an excess of acetate and a high cellular redox potential. This excess acetate is converted to acetyl-CoA by cytoplasmic and mitochondrial adenosine triphosphate (ATP)–dependent acetyl-CoA synthetases (Fig. 76–2). The consequences of increased cellular acetyl-CoA and cellular redox potential include inhibition of pyruvate dehydrogenase complex thus entry of pyruvate into the citric acid cycle, inhibition of the citric acid cycle, and favors formation of the ketone bodies (ie, acetoacetate, beta-hydroxybutyrate, and acetone). The high redox state also favors the conversion of pyruvate to lactate, diverting pyruvate from being a substrate for gluconeogenesis. To compensate for the lack of normal metabolic substrates, the body mobilizes fat from adipose tissue and increases fatty acid metabolism as an alternative source of energy. This response is mediated by a decrease in insulin and an increase in glucagon, catecholamines, growth hormone, and cortisol. Fatty acid metabolism results in the formation of acetyl-CoA. Two molecules of acetyl-CoA condense to form acetoacetyl-CoA, which is metabolized to acetoacetate via the 3-hydroxy-3-methylglutaryl CoA (HMG-CoA) pathway.[30] Similarly, the high acetyl-CoA concentration that is generated from excess acetate favors condensation to acetoacetyl-CoA and metabolism to acetoacetate, both in the mitochondria as well as in the cytoplasm. Most of the acetoacetate is reduced to β-hydroxybutyrate because of the excess reducing potential or high redox state of the cell. Volume depletion interferes with the renal elimination of acetoacetate and β-hydroxybutyrate and contributes to the metabolic acidosis. An elevated lactate concentration results from shunting from pyruvate or from hypoperfusion or infection that may coexist with the underlying ketoacidosis.

Clinical Features

Patients with AKA are typically chronic ethanol users, presenting after a few days of "binge" drinking, who become acutely starved because of cessation in oral intake due to binging itself or because of nausea, vomiting, abdominal pain from gastritis, hepatitis, pancreatitis, or a concurrent acute illness.[69,70,72] The patient usually appears acutely ill with salt and water depletion, tachypnea, tachycardia, and hypotension. Medical conditions such as sepsis, meningitis, pyelonephritis, or pneumonia occur simultaneously, and ethanol withdrawal subsequently develops.

The serum ethanol concentration is usually low or undetectable because ethanol intake substantially decreased earlier in the clinical course. In one report of 23 episodes of AKA, serum ethanol was undetectable in 13 and above 50 mg/dL in only 5.[70] The hallmarks of AKA include an elevated anion gap metabolic acidosis with an elevated serum lactate concentration. However, some patients will have a normal arterial pH or be even alkalemic because of an associated primary metabolic alkalosis because of vomiting and a compensatory respiratory alkalosis (Chap. 12).[70,72,206] When patients with AKA were compared with patients with DKA, those with AKA tended to have a higher blood pH, lower serum potassium and chloride concentrations, and a higher serum bicarbonate concentration.[71] The etiology of anion gaps in patients with AKA and DKA are very similar with β-hydroxybutyrate being the primary anion in AKA and acetoacetate in DKA.[71]

The nitroprusside test used to detect the presence of ketones in serum and urine is negative or mildly positive in patients with AKA because the nitroprusside reaction only detects molecules containing ketone moieties. This includes acetoacetate and acetone but not β-hydroxybutyrate. Reliance on the nitroprusside test alone underestimates the severity of ketoacidosis. Specific assays for β-hydroxybutyrate are performed in some hospital laboratories and are available as point-of-care testing at bedside. The blood glucose concentration is typically low or mildly elevated. It is postulated that ethanol induced hypoglycemia occurs first, causing increased cortisol, growth hormone, glucagon, and epinephrine concentrations, which mobilizes fatty acids that are then converted to ketone bodies.[44] Therefore, alcoholic hypoglycemia and AKA frequently are sequential events of the same process depending on the point in this process at which the patient is evaluated.

Management

Treatment should begin with adequate crystalloid fluid replacement, dextrose, thiamine and folic acid. Supplemental multivitamins, potassium, and magnesium are recommended on an individual basis. The administration of dextrose will stimulate the release of insulin, decrease the release of glucagon, and reduce the oxidation of fatty acids. Exogenous glucose also facilitates the synthesis of ATP, which reverses the pyruvate-to-lactate and NAD$^+$/NADH ratios. The provision of thiamine facilitates pyruvate entry into the citric acid cycle, thus increasing ATP production. Volume replacement restores glomerular filtration and improves excretion of ketones and organic acids. Administration of either insulin or sodium bicarbonate in the management of AKA is usually unnecessary.[72]

During the recovery phase of AKA, β-hydroxybutyrate is converted back to acetoacetate. As this process occurs, the nitroprusside test becomes more positive because of higher concentrations of acetoacetate resulting in a hyperketonemia and ketonuria, which represents improvement of the metabolic status.

Patients presenting with AKA are manifesting serious metabolic impairment and frequently require hospital admission. They often succumb to other precipitating or coexisting medical or surgical disorders[69] such as occult trauma, pancreatitis, GI hemorrhage or hepatorenal dysfunction, and infections. However, death is rare from ethanol-induced ketoacidosis.

ALCOHOLISM

Alcoholism is traditionally defined as a chronic, progressive disease characterized by tolerance and physical dependence to ethanol and pathologic organ changes and is recognized to be a multifactorial, genetically influenced disorder.[38,88,157,171,181,196,216] The most recent edition of the American Psychiatric Association's *Diagnostic and Statistical Manual of Mental Disorders* (*DSM-5*) integrated alcohol abuse and alcohol dependence into a single disorder called *alcohol use disorder* (AUD) with mild, moderate, and severe subclassifications.[5] The presence of at least 2 of the symptoms (Table 76–4) within 12 months indicates an AUD. The severity of AUD is defined by the number of symptoms present (ie, mild, 2 or 3 symptoms; moderate, 4 or 5 symptoms; and severe, 6 or more symptoms).

Although many people drink in an attempt to ameliorate their depression, all available evidence suggests that alcoholism adversely affects mood and cognitive ability. Research suggests alcoholism is partly under genetic control.[12,106,112,130] Chromosomal linkage analysis has implicated chromosomes 9, 15, and 16 in the genetic predisposition to alcoholism.[15,47,132] Polymorphism in *ADH* and *ALDH* genes appears to be a marker for risk of alcoholism.[34,38,57,216,217] The *ADH1B*2*, *ADH1C*1*, and *ALDH2*2* alleles are associated with reduced risk of alcoholism. Genetic epidemiologic studies

TABLE 76–4 *DSM-5* Alcohol Use Disorder

Drinking more or longer than intended?

Desire or unsuccessful efforts to control alcohol use?

A lot of time drinking or to recover from alcohol effects?

Craving to use alcohol?

Drinking or sick from drinking interfering with obligations at work, home, or school?

Continued drinking even though it is causing social or interpersonal problems?

Alcohol use reducing social, occupational, or recreational activities?

Recurrent alcohol use in situations where it is physically hazardous?

Continued drinking in spite of physical or psychological problems?

Need for increased drinking to achieve desired effect?

Drinking to relieve or avoid withdrawal symptoms?

Data from American Psychiatric Association: Diagnostic and Statistical Manual of Mental Disorders, 5th ed. Arlington, VA: American Psychiatric Association; 2013.

TABLE 76–5 The Brief Michigan Alcoholism Screening Test

Question	Circle Correct Answer		Points
1. Do you feel you are a normal drinker?	Yes	No	N2
2. Do friends or relatives think you are a normal drinker?	Yes	No	N2
3. Have you ever attended a meeting of Alcoholics Anonymous?	Yes	No	Y5
4. Have you ever lost friends or girlfriends/boyfriends because of drinking?	Yes	No	Y2
5. Have you ever gotten into trouble at work because of drinking?	Yes	No	Y2
6. Have you ever neglected your obligations, your family, or your work for 2 or more days in a row because you were drinking?	Yes	No	Y2
7. Have you ever had delirium tremens (DTs) or severe shaking, or heard voices, or seen things that weren't there after heavy drinking?	Yes	No	Y2
8. Have you ever gone to anyone for help about your drinking?	Yes	No	Y5
9. Have you ever been in a hospital because of drinking?	Yes	No	Y5
10. Have you ever been arrested for drunk driving after drinking?	Yes	No	Y2

Score 6 = Probable diagnosis of alcoholism.

Reproduced with permission from Pokorny AD, Miller BA, Kaplan HB. The brief MAST: a shortened version of the Michigan Alcoholism Screening Test. *Am J Psychiatry*. 1972 Sep;129(3):342-345.

strongly correlate Asians with homozygous *ADH1B*2* and *ALDH2*2* alleles with reduced ethanol consumption and incidence of alcoholism.[38,171,233] The incidence of both homozygous *ADH1B*1* and *ALDH2*1* alleles was significantly higher in patients with ethanol dependence and in patients with alcoholic liver disease.

Screening is a preliminary procedure to assess the likelihood that an individual has a substance use disorder or is at risk of negative consequences from alcohol or other xenobiotics use. Whereas screening tools, such as the Brief Michigan Alcoholism Screening Test (MAST)[174] and the CAGE questions[138] (Tables 76–5 and 76–6), were initially developed to identify people with active alcohol dependence for referral to treatment, the screening, brief intervention, and referral to treatment (SBIRT) was developed as a public health model designed to provide universal screening, secondary prevention in detecting risky or hazardous substance use before the onset of abuse or dependence, early intervention, and treatment for people who have problematic or hazardous alcohol problems within health care settings.[8] Based on the Substance Abuse and Mental Health Services Administration (SAMHSA) model, SBIRT allows for universal screening of all patients regardless of an identified disorder, allowing health care professionals to address the spectrum of such behavioral health problems even when the patient is not actively seeking intervention or treatment.

The Alcohol Use Disorders Identification Test (AUDIT) was developed from a 6-country World Health Organization collaborative project as a screening instrument to identify heavy drinkers and explicitly

TABLE 76–6 The CAGE Questions[138]

1. Have you ever felt you should **c**ut down on your drinking?
2. Have people **a**nnoyed you by criticizing your drinking?
3. Have you ever felt bad or **g**uilty about your drinking?
4. Have you ever had a drink first thing in the morning to steady your nerves or to get rid of a hangover (**e**ye opener)?

Two or more affirmatives = probable diagnosis of alcoholism.

TABLE 76–7   AUDIT-C Alcohol Use Disorders Identification Test-Dealing With Alcohol Consumption

Questions	Scoring[a]				
	0	1	2	3	4
How often do you have a drink containing alcohol?	Never	≤Monthly	2–4 times/mo	2–3 times/wk	≥4 times/k
How many alcohol units do you drink on a typical day when you are drinking?	0–2	3–4	5–6	7–9	≥10
How often have you had ≥6 units if female, or ≥8 units if male, on a single occasion in the past year?	Never	<Monthly	Monthly	Weekly	Daily (almost)

[a]One alcohol unit (10 mL or 8 g of "pure" ethanol) is equal 25 mL of whisky (alcohol by volume 40%), a third of a pint of beer (alcohol by volume, 5%–6%), or a 175-mL glass of red wine (alcohol by volume, 12%).

addresses alcohol-related problems and symptoms of dependence over the past year.[191] It is a 10-item questionnaire that covers the domains of alcohol consumption, drinking behavior, and alcohol-related problems. The AUDIT screen provides a simple method of early detection of hazardous and harmful alcohol use in primary health care settings. A modified version of the AUDIT instrument, the first 3 questions of AUDIT dealing with alcohol consumption (AUDIT-C), is used to help identify patients who are hazardous drinkers or have active alcohol use disorders and performed better than AUDIT for identification of heavy drinkers who might benefit from brief primary care interventions (Table 76–7).[26,114] In addition, there was no significant difference between these screening questionnaires for identification of patients with heavy drinking or active alcohol abuse or dependence. However, AUDIT performed better than AUDIT-C in identifying active alcohol abuse or dependence. The AUDIT-C is scored on a scale of 0 to 12 points; 0 reflect no alcohol use in the past year. In men, a score of 4 points or more is considered positive for alcohol misuse; in women, a score of 3 points or more is considered positive. Generally, the higher the AUDIT-C score, the more likely it is that the drinking is affecting the patient's health and safety.

The presence of tolerance or dependence is not essential for a diagnosis of alcoholism. Emphasis instead is placed on the social and behavioral concomitants of heavy drinking.[151] In the ED setting, questions concerning the patient's ability to function physically and psychologically are just as appropriate as quantifying the amount of ethanol consumed per day.

Alcoholism is commonly associated with affective disorders, especially depression.[147,177] There is a higher rate of alcoholism among patients with bipolar disorder than in the general population, and there is evidence for a genetic relationship between alcoholism and depression.[106,165,235,236] Ethanol affects mood, judgment, and self-control and creates a clinical condition conducive to violence directed at self and others and is an important risk factor for suicide.

Various strategies are used to treat alcoholism, including psychosocial interventions, pharmacologic interventions, or both. One psychosocial experiment is the "project-based Housing First" model, the so-called wet houses, in which chronically homeless individuals with alcohol problems are provided food and permanent housing, but unlike other housing agencies or shelters, wet houses do not require participants to observe curfews or abstain from drinking, and they can elect to receive onsite case management and other supportive services.[35,122] Contrary to the enabling hypothesis that provision of non–abstinence-based Housing First would result in stable or increasing levels of alcohol use and alcohol-related problems, residence of project-based Housing First reduced their alcohol use on typical and peak drinking days by 7% and 8%, respectively, for every 3 months of their stay; increased their avoidance in drinking to inebriation at least 1 day in the previous month by 19% at the end of a 2-year stay; and reported a decrease in delirium tremens occurrence by 42% during at the end of 2-year residence. Pharmacologic treatment of ethanol dependence that is of potential collateral toxicologic consequence include opioid antagonists such as naltrexone and nalmefene, disulfiram, serotonergic agents, and topiramate.[73,97]

Although it is a serious disease with important health and economic consequences, alcoholism remains underdiagnosed and remains a treatment challenge.[135,238]

SUMMARY

- Ethanol is widely used in our society and ethanol use problems impose a staggering personal, social, and economic burden on our society.
- Domestic violence, motor vehicle crashes, child abuse, fires, falls, rape, and other crimes such as robbery and assault and medical consequences such as cancer, liver disease, and heart disease are all associated with ethanol misuse.
- One interesting area in ethanol research is the finding that genetics are an important determinant in vulnerability to ethanol dependence. This finding suggests the biological basis of alcoholism.
- Acute inebriation and alcoholism are among the most common and complex toxicologic and societal problems.
- Patients with acute inebriation or alcoholism present with a diversity of clinical problems (eg, hypoglycemia, AKA, and ethanol withdrawal) that challenge the clinicians to be meticulous and systematic in their evaluation and management of these patients.

REFERENCES

1. Adinoff B, et al. Acute ethanol poisoning and the ethanol withdrawal syndrome. *Med Toxicol Adverse Drug Exp.* 1988;3:172-196.
2. Agarwal DP. Genetic polymorphisms of alcohol metabolizing enzymes. *Pathol Biol.* 2001;49:703-709.
3. Alcohol Epidemiologic Data Directory, June 2012. http://pubs.niaaa.nih.gov/publications/2012DataDirectory/2012DataDirectory.pdf.
4. Allgaier C. Ethanol sensitivity of NMDA receptors. *Neurochem Int.* 2002;41:377-382.
5. American Psychiatric Association. *Diagnostic and Statistical Manual of Mental Disorders.* 5th ed. Washington, DC: American Psychiatric Association; 2013.
6. Amir I, et al. Ranitidine increases the bioavailability of imbibed alcohol by accelerating gastric emptying. *Life Sci.* 1996;58:511-518.
7. Arora S, et al. Alcohol levels are increased in social drinkers receiving ranitidine. *Am J Gastroenterol.* 2000;95:208-213.
8. Babor TF, et al. Screening, Brief Intervention, and Referral to Treatment (SBIRT): toward a public health approach to the management of substance abuse. *Subst Abus.* 2007;28:7-30.
9. Bailey DN, et al. Cocaine and cocaethylene-creatinine clearance ratios in humans. *J Anal Toxicol.* 1997;21:41-43.
10. Bager H, et al. Biomarkers for the detection of prenatal alcohol exposure: a review. *Alcohol Clin Exp Res.* 2017;41:251-261.
11. Bagnardi V, et al. Flexible meta-regression functions for modeling aggregate dose-response data, with an application to alcohol and mortality. *Am J Epidemiol.* 2004;159:1077-1086.
12. Ball DM, Murray RM. Genetics of alcohol misuse. *Br Med J.* 1994;50:18-35.
13. Baraona E, et al. Gender differences in pharmacokinetics of alcohol. *Alcohol Clin Exp Res.* 2001;25:502-507.
14. Baraona E, et al. Lack of alcohol dehydrogenase isoenzyme activities in the stomach of Japanese subjects. *Life Sci.* 1991;49:1929-1934.
15. Bergen AW, et al. Framingham Heart Study: genomic regions linked to alcohol consumption in the Framingham Heart Study. *BMC Genet.* 2003;4(suppl 1):S101.
16. Best CA, Laposata M. Fatty acid ethyl esters: toxic non-oxidative metabolites of ethanol and markers of ethanol intake. *Front Biosci.* 2003;8:e202-217.

17. Bhatti SA, et al. Ethanol and pH levels of proprietary mouthrinses. *Community Dent Health.* 1994;11:71-74.

18. Bleich S, et al. Homocysteine as a neurotoxin in chronic alcoholism. *Prog Neuropsychopharmacol Biol Psychiatry.* 2004;28:453-464.

19. Borucki K, et al. Detection of recent ethanol intake with new markers: comparison of fatty acid ethyl esters in serum and of ethyl glucuronide and the ratio of 5-hydroxytryptophol to 5-hydroxyindole acetic acid in urine. *Alcohol Clin Exp Res.* 2005;29:781-787.

20. Brennan DF, et al. Ethanol elimination rates in an ED population. *Am J Emerg Med.* 1995;13:276-280.

21. Briggs G, et al. Notes from the field: botulism from drinking prison-made illicit alcohol—Arizona, 2012. *MMWR Morb Mortal Wkly Rep.* 2013;62:88.

22. Brodie MS. Increased ethanol excitation of dopaminergic neurons of the ventral tegmental area after chronic ethanol treatment. *Alcohol Clin Exp Res.* 2002;26:1024-1030.

23. Brodie MS, et al. Ethanol directly excites dopaminergic ventral tegmental area reward neurons. *Alcohol Clin Exp Res.* 1999;23:1848-1852.

24. Brown AS, James OF. Omeprazole, ranitidine, and cimetidine have no effect on peak blood ethanol concentrations, first pass metabolism or area under the time-ethanol curve under "real-life" drinking conditions. *Aliment Pharmacol Ther.* 1998;12:141-145.

25. Burnett EJ, et al. Glutamatergic plasticity and alcohol dependence-induced alterations in reward, affect and cognition. *Prog Neuropsychopharmacol Biol Psychiatry.* 2016;65:309-320.

26. Bush K, et al. The AUDIT alcohol consumption questions (AUDIT-C): an effective brief screening test for problem drinking. Ambulatory Care Quality Improvement Project (ACQUIP). Alcohol Use Disorders Identification Test. *Arch Intern Med.* 1998;158:1789-1795.

27. Bye A, et al. Effect of ranitidine hydrochloride (150 mg twice daily) on the pharmacokinetics of increasing doses of ethanol (0.15, 0.3, 0.6 g kg-1). *Br J Clin Pharmacol.* 1996;41:129-133.

28. Caballeria J, et al. Effects of cimetidine on gastric alcohol dehydrogenase activity and blood ethanol levels. *Gastroenterology.* 1989;96:388-392.

29. Caetano R, Cunradi C. Alcohol dependence: a public health perspective. *Addiction.* 2002;97:633-645.

30. Caldwell IC, Drummond GI. Synthesis of acetoacetate by liver enzymes. *J Biol Chem.* 1963;238:64-68.

31. Cederbaum AI. Alcohol metabolism. *Clin Liver Dis.* 2012;16:667-685.

32. Centers for Disease Control and Prevention. Alcohol Related Disease Impact (ARDI) application, 2013. http://www.cdc.gov/ARDI.

33. Chapman LF. Experimental induction of hangover. *Q J Stud Alcohol.* 1970;31:67-86.

34. Chen YC, et al. Alcohol metabolism and cardiovascular response in an alcoholic patient homozygous for the ALDH2*2 variant gene allele. *Alcohol Clin Exp Res.* 1999;23:1853-1860.

35. Collins SE, et al. Project-based Housing First for chronically homeless individuals with alcohol problems: within-subjects analyses of 2-year alcohol trajectories. *Am J Public Health.* 2012;102:511-519.

36. Committee on Drugs. 1983–1984, American Academy of Pediatrics: ethanol in liquid preparations intended for children. *Pediatrics.* 1984;73:405-407.

37. Costantino A, et al. The effect of the use of mouthwash on ethylglucuronide concentrations in urine. *J Anal Toxicol.* 2006;30:659-662.

38. Crabb DW, et al. Overview of the role of alcohol dehydrogenase and aldehyde dehydrogenase and their variants in the genesis of alcohol-related pathology. *Proc Nutr Soc.* 2004;63:49-63.

39. Cummins LH. Hypoglycemia and convulsions in children following alcohol ingestion. *J Pediatr.* 1961;58:23-26.

40. Dahl H, et al. Comparison of urinary excretion characteristics of ethanol and ethyl glucuronide. *J Anal Toxicol.* 2002;26:201-204.

41. Damrau F, Liddy E. Hangovers and whisky congeners: comparison of whisky with vodka. *J Nat Med Assoc.* 1960;52:262-264.

42. Damrau F, Goldberg AH. Adsorption of whisky congeners by activated charcoal. *Southwest Med.* 1971;53:175-182.

43. Degutis LC, et al. The saliva strip test is an accurate method to determine blood alcohol concentration in trauma patients. *Acad Emerg Med.* 2004;11:885-887.

44. Devenyi P. Alcoholic hypoglycemia and alcoholic ketoacidosis: sequential events of the same process? *Can Med Assoc J.* 1982;127:513.

45. De Witte P. Imbalance between neuroexcitatory and neuroinhibitory amino acids causing craving for ethanol. *Addict Behav.* 2004;29:1325-1339.

46. Dey A, Cederbaum AI. Alcohol and oxidative liver injury. *Hepatology.* 2006;43:S63-S74.

47. Dick DM, et al. Association of GABRG3 with alcohol dependence. *Alcohol Clin Exp Res.* 2004;28:4-9.

48. Di Padova C, et al. Effects of ranitidine on blood alcohol levels after ethanol ingestion. *JAMA.* 1992;267:83-86.

49. Djordjevic D, et al. Ethanol interactions with other cytochrome P450 substrates including drugs, xenobiotics, and carcinogens. *Pathol Biol.* 1998;46:760-770.

50. Dohmen K, et al. Ethnic differences in gastric-alcohol dehydrogenase activity and ethanol first-pass metabolism. *Alcohol Clin Exp Res.* 1996;20:1569-1576.

51. Doyle KM, et al. Fatty acid ethyl esters in the blood as markers of ethanol intake. *JAMA.* 1996;276:1152-1156.

52. Dukes GE, et al. Alcohol in pharmaceutical products. *Am Fam Physician.* 1977;16:97-103.

53. Eilam O, Heyman SN. Wenckebach-type atrioventricular block in severe alcohol intoxication. *Am J Emerg Med.* 1991;9:1170.

54. Ellis T, Lacy R. Illicit alcohol (moonshine) consumption in West Alabama revisited. *South Med J.* 1998;91:858-860.

55. Embly DI, Fraser BN. Hepatotoxicity of paracetamol enhanced by ingestion of alcohol. *S Afr Med J.* 1977;51:208-209.

56. Engel JS, Spiller HA. Acute ethanol poisoning in a 4-year-old as a result of ethanol-based hand-sanitizer ingestion. *Pediatr Emerg Care.* 2010;26:508-509.

57. Eriksson CJ, et al. Functional relevance of human ADH polymorphism. *Alcohol Clin Exp Res.* 2001;25(5 suppl ISBRA):157S-163S.

58. Ernst AA, et al. Ethanol ingestion and related hypoglycemia in a pediatric and adolescent emergency department population. *Acad Emerg Med.* 1996;3:46-49.

59. Faingold CL, et al. Ethanol and neurotransmitter interactions—from molecular to integrative effects. *Prog Neurobiol.* 1998;55:509-535.

60. Feely J, Wood AJ. Effects of cimetidine on the elimination and actions of ethanol. *JAMA.* 1982;247:2819-2821.

61. Feldstein TJ. Carbohydrate and alcohol content of 200 oral liquid medications for use in patients receiving ketogenic diets. *Pediatrics.* 1996;97:506-511.

62. Fernandez D, et al. Alcohol-induced Prinzmetal variant angina. *Am J Cardiol.* 1973;32:238-239.

63. Flink EB. Magnesium deficiency in alcoholism. *Alcohol Clin Exp Res.* 1986;10:590-594.

64. Fluckiger A, et al. Lack of effect of the benzodiazepine antagonist flumazenil and the performance of healthy subjects during experimentally induced ethanol intoxication. *Eur J Clin Pharmacol.* 1988;34:273-276.

65. Fraser AG. Pharmacokinetic interactions between alcohol and other drugs. *Clin Pharmacokinet.* 1997;33:79-90.

66. Fraser AG, et al. Ranitidine has no effect on postbreakfast ethanol absorption. *Am J Gastroenterol.* 1993;88:217-221.

67. Frezza M, et al. High blood alcohol levels in women: the role of decreased gastric alcohol dehydrogenase activity and first pass metabolism. *N Engl J Med.* 1990;322:95-110.

68. Fuenmayor AJ, Fuenmayor AM. Cardiac arrest following holiday heart syndrome. *Int J Cardiol.* 1997;59:101-103.

69. Fulop M. Alcoholism, ketoacidosis, and lactic acidosis. *Diabetes Metab Rev.* 1989;5:365-378.

70. Fulop M, et al. Alcoholic ketosis. *Alcohol Clin Exp Res.* 1986;10:610-615.

71. Fulop M, Hoberman HD. Diabetic ketoacidosis and alcoholic ketosis. *Ann Intern Med.* 1979;91:796-797.

72. Fulop M, Hoberman HD. Alcoholic ketosis. *Diabetes.* 1975;24:785-790.

73. Garbutt JC, et al. Pharmacological treatment of alcohol dependence, a review of the evidence. *JAMA.* 1999;281:1318-1325.

74. Gerhardt RE, et al. Moonshine-related arsenic poisoning. *Arch Intern Med.* 1980;140:211-213.

75. Gershman H, Steper J. Rate of clearance of ethanol from the blood of intoxicated patients in the emergency department. *J Emerg Med.* 1991;9:307-311.

76. Goedde HW, et al. Distribution of ADH2 and ALDH2 genotypes in different populations. *Hum Genet.* 1992;88:344-346.

77. Gould L. Hemodynamic effects of ethanol in patients with cardiac disease. *Q J Stud Alcohol.* 1972;33:714-722.

78. Greenspon AJ. Provocation of ventricular tachycardia after consumption of alcohol. *N Engl J Med.* 1979;301:1049-1156.

79. Greenspon AJ, Schaal SF. The "holiday heart": electrophysiological studies of alcohol effects in alcoholics. *Ann Intern Med.* 1983;98:135-140.

80. Haber PS, et al. Metabolism of alcohol by human gastric cells: relation to first-pass metabolism. *Gastroenterology.* 1996;111:863-870.

81. Halter CC, et al. Kinetics in serum and urinary excretion of ethyl sulfate and ethyl glucuronide after medium dose ethanol intake. *Int J Legal Med.* 2008;122:123-128.

82. Helander A. Biological markers in alcoholism. *J Neural Transm Suppl.* 2003:15-32.

83. Helander A, Beck O. Ethyl sulfate: a metabolite of ethanol in humans and a potential biomarker of acute alcohol intake. *J Anal Toxicol.* 2005;29:270-274.

84. Helander A, Beck O. Mass spectrometric identification of ethyl sulfate as an ethanol metabolite in humans. *Clin Chem.* 2004;50:936-937.

85. Helander A, Dahl H. Urinary tract infection: a risk factor for false-negative urinary ethyl glucuronide but not ethyl sulfate in the detection of recent alcohol consumption. *Clin Chem.* 2005;51:1728-1730.

86. Helander A, et al. Detection times for urinary ethyl glucuronide and ethyl sulfate in heavy drinkers during alcohol detoxification. *Alcohol Alcohol.* 2009;44:55-61.

87. Helander A, et al. Postcollection synthesis of ethyl glucuronide by bacteria in urine may cause false identification of alcohol consumption. *Clin Chem.* 2007;53:1855-1857.

88. Higuchi S, et al. Alcohol and aldehyde dehydrogenase genotypes and drinking behavior in Japanese. *Alcohol Clin Exp Res.* 1996;20:493-497.

89. Hoffman RS, et al. Osmol gaps revisited: normal values and limitations. *J Toxicol Clin Toxicol.* 1993;31:81-93.

90. Høiseth G, et al. A pharmacokinetic study of ethyl glucuronide in blood and urine: applications to forensic toxicology. *Forensic Sci Int*. 2007;172:119-124.

91. Høiseth G, et al. Comparison between the urinary alcohol markers EtG, EtS, and GTOL/5-HIAA in controlled drinking experiment. *Alcohol Alcohol*. 2008;43:187-191.

92. Holmes A, et al. Glutamatergic targets for new alcohol medications. *Psychopharmacology*. 2013;229:539-554.

93. Holt S, et al. Alcohol and the emergency service patient. *Br Med J*. 1980;281:638-640.

94. Hornfeldt CS. A report of acute ethanol poisoning in a child. *J Toxicol Clin Toxicol*. 1992;30:115-121.

95. Hu XJ, et al. Chronic ethanol treatment produces a selective upregulation of the NMDA receptor subunit gene expression in mammalian cultured cortical neurons. *Brain Res Mol Brain Res*. 1996;36:211-218.

96. Isbister GK, et al. Randomized controlled trial of intramuscular droperidol versus midazolam for violence and acute behavioral disturbance: the DORM study. *Ann Emerg Med*. 2010;56:392-401.

97. Johnson RA. Progress in the development of topiramate for treating alcohol dependence: from a hypothesis to a proof-of-concept study. *Alcohol Clin Exp Res*. 2004;28:1137-1144.

98. Jones AW. Excretion of alcohol in urine and diuresis in healthy men in relation to their age, the dose administered and the time after drinking. *Forensic Sci Int*. 1990;45:217-224.

99. Jornvall H, Hoog JO. Nomenclature of alcohol dehydrogenases. *Alcohol Alcohol*. 1995;30:153-161.

100. Joseph MM, et al. Acute ethanol poisoning in a 6-year-old girl following ingestion of alcohol-based hand sanitizer at school. *World J Emerg Med*. 2011;2:232-233.

101. Kalbfleisch JM, et al. Effects of ethanol administration on urinary excretion of magnesium and other electrolytes in alcoholic and normal subjects. *J Clin Invest*. 1963;42:1471-1475.

102. Kashima T, et al. Variant angina induced by alcohol ingestion. *Angiology*. 1982;33:137-139.

103. Kater RM, et al. Increased rate of clearance of drugs from the circulation of alcoholics. *Am J Med Sci*. 1969;258:35-39.

104. Kaufmann RB, et al. Deaths related to lead poisoning in the United States, 1979-1998. *Environ Res*. 2003;91:78-84.

105. Kechagias S, et al. Low-dose aspirin decreases blood alcohol concentrations by delaying gastric emptying. *Eur J Clin Pharmacol*. 1997;53:241-246.

106. Kendler KS, et al. Alcoholism and major depression in women. A twin study of the causes of comorbidity. *Arch Gen Psychiatry*. 1993;50:690-698.

107. Khan F, et al. Overlooked sources of ethanol. *J Emerg Med*. 1999;17:985-988.

108. Khanna JM, et al. Role of serotonergic and adrenergic systems in alcohol tolerance. *Prog Neuropsychopharmacol*. 1981;5:459-465.

109. Khanna JM, et al. Effect of NMDA antagonists, an NMDA agonist, and serotonin depletion on acute tolerance to ethanol. *Pharmacol Biochem Behav*. 2002;72:291-298.

110. Klatsky AL. Alcohol and cardiovascular diseases: a historical overview. *Novartis Found Symp*. 1998;216:2-12.

111. Knott JC, et al. Randomized clinical trial comparing intravenous midazolam and droperidol for sedation of the acutely agitated patient in the Emergency Department. *Ann Emerg Med*. 2006;47:61-67.

112. Koopmans JR, Boomsma DI. Familial resemblance in alcohol use: genetic or cultural transmission? *J Stud Alcohol*. 1996;57:19-28.

113. Krebs HA, et al. Inhibition of hepatic gluconeogenesis by ethanol. *Biochem J*. 1969;112:117-124.

114. Kriston L, et al. Meta-analysis: are 3 questions enough to detect unhealthy alcohol use? *Ann Intern Med*. 2008;149:879-888.

115. Krystal JH, et al. NMDA receptor antagonism and the ethanol intoxication signal: from alcoholism risk to pharmacotherapy. *Ann N Y Acad Sci*. 2003;1003:176-184.

116. Krystal JH, et al. N-methyl-D-aspartate glutamate receptors and alcoholism: reward, dependence, treatment, and vulnerability. *Pharmacol Ther*. 2003;99:79-94.

117. Kunitoh S, et al. Acetaldehyde as well as ethanol is metabolized by human CYP2E1. *J Pharmacol Exp Ther*. 1997;280:527-532.

118. Kupari M, Koskinen P. Time of onset of supraventricular tachyarrhythmia in relation to alcohol consumption. *Am J Cardiol*. 1991;67:718-722.

119. Lamminpaa A. Alcohol intoxication in childhood and adolescence. *Alcohol Alcohol*. 1995;30:5-12.

120. Lamminpaa A, Vilska J. Acute alcohol intoxications in children treated in hospital. *Acta Paediatr Scand*. 1990;79:847-854.

121. Lang CH, et al. Alcohol myopathy: impairment of protein synthesis and translation initiation. *Int J Biochem Cell Biol*. 2001;33:457-473.

122. Larimer ME, et al. Health care and public service use and costs before and after provision of housing for chronically homeless persons with severe alcohol problems. *JAMA*. 2009;301:1349-1357.

123. Levitt MD. Review article: lack of clinical significance of the interaction between H2-receptor antagonists and ethanol. *Aliment Pharmacol Ther*. 1993;7:131-138.

124. Leung AK. Ethyl alcohol ingestion in children. A 15-year review. *Clin Pediatr (Phila)*. 1986;25:617-619.

125. Levy P, et al. Methanol contamination of Romanian home-distilled alcohol. *J Toxicol Clin Toxicol*. 2003;41:23-28.

126. Li J, et al. Intravenous saline has no effect on blood ethanol clearance. *J Emerg Med*. 1999;17:1-5.

127. Lieber CS. Relationships between nutrition, alcohol use, and liver disease. *Alcohol Res Health*. 2003;27:220-231.

128. Lieber CS. Ethnic and gender differences in ethanol metabolism. *Alcohol Clin Exp Res*. 2000;24:417-418.

129. Lieber CS. Biochemical and molecular basis of alcohol-induced injury to the liver and other tissues. *N Engl J Med*. 1988;319:1639-1644.

130. Liu IC, et al. Genetic and environmental contributions to the development of alcohol dependence in male twins. *Arch Gen Psychiatry*. 2004;61:897-903.

131. Liu JJ, et al. Methanol-related deaths in Ontario. *J Toxicol Clin Toxicol*. 1999;37:69-73.

132. Ma JZ, et al. Mapping susceptibility loci for alcohol consumption using number of grams of alcohol consumed per day as a phenotype measure. *BMC Genet*. 2003;4(suppl 1):S104.

133. Maddrey WC. Hepatic effects of acetaminophen—Enhanced toxicity in alcoholics. *J Clin Gastroenterol*. 1987;9:180-185.

134. Makin A, Williams R. Paracetamol hepatotoxicity and alcohol consumption in deliberate and accidental overdose. *QJM*. 2000;93:341-349.

135. Mann K, et al. One hundred years of alcoholism: the twentieth century. *Alcohol Alcohol*. 2000;35:10-15.

136. Martel M, et al. Management of acute undifferentiated agitation in the emergency department: e randomized double-blind trial of droperidol, ziprasidone, and midazolam. *Acad Emerg Med*. 2005;12:1167-1172.

137. Matsuguchi T, et al. Provocation of variant angina by alcohol ingestion. *Eur Heart J*. 1984;5:906-912.

138. Mayfield D, et al. The CAGE questionnaire: validation of a new alcoholism screening instrument. *Am J Psychiatry*. 1974;131:1121-1126.

139. Mazor C, et al. Adolescent ethanol intoxication from vanilla extract ingestion: a case report. *Internet J Family Pract*. 2004;4.

140. McClain CJ, et al. Monocyte activation in alcoholic liver disease. *Alcohol*. 2002;27:53-61.

141. McClain CJ, et al. Potentiation of acetaminophen hepatotoxicity. *JAMA*. 1980;244:251-253.

142. McDermott PH, et al. Myocarditis and cardiac failure in men. *JAMA*. 1966;198:253-256.

143. Menz V, et al. Alcohol and rhythm disturbance: the holiday heart syndrome. *Herz*. 1996;21:227-231.

144. Mercier G, Patry G. Quebec beer-drinkers' cardiomyopathy: clinical signs and symptoms. *Can Med Assoc J*. 1967;97:884-888.

145. Miller NS, et al. Antihistamine blockade of alcohol-induced flushing in orientals. *J Stud Alcohol*. 1988;49:16-20.

146. Miwa K, et al. Importance of magnesium deficiency in alcohol-induced variant angina. *Am J Cardiol*. 1994;73:813-816.

147. Modesto-Lowe V, Kranzler HR. Diagnosis and treatment of alcohol-dependent patients with comorbid psychiatric disorders. *Alcohol Res Health*. 1999;23:144-149.

148. Mokdad AH, et al. Actual causes of death in the United States, 2000. *JAMA*. 2004;291:1238-1245.

149. Morgan BW, et al. Lead contaminated moonshine: a report of Bureau of Alcohol, Tobacco and Firearms analyzed samples. *Vet Hum Toxicol*. 2004;46:89-90.

150. Morrow AL, et al. GABAA and NMDA receptor subunit mRNA expression in ethanol dependent rats. *Alcohol Alcohol* Suppl. 1994;2:89-95.

151. Morse RM, Flarin DK. The definition of alcoholism. *JAMA*. 1992;268:1012-1014.

152. Moskowitz H, et al. Police officers' detection of breath odors from alcohol ingestion. *Accid Anal Prev*. 1999;31:175-180.

153. Nagy J. The NR2B subtype of NMDA receptor: a potential target for the treatment of alcohol dependence. *Curr Drug Targets CNS Neurol Disord*. 2004;3:169-179.

154. Narahashi T, et al. Neuroreceptors and ion channels as targets of alcohol. *Alcohol Clin Exp Res*. 2001;25(5 suppl ISBRA):182S-188S.

155. National Highway Traffic Safety Administration. *Traffic Safety Facts 2015 Data: Alcohol-Impaired Driving*. December 2016, DOT HS 812 350. https://crashstats.nhtsa.dot.gov/Api/Public/ViewPublication/812350.

156. National Highway Traffic Safety Administration. *Traffic Safety Facts 2012 Data: Alcohol-Impaired Driving*. December 2013, DOT HS 811 870. https://crashstats.nhtsa.dot.gov/Api/Public/ViewPublication/811870.

157. National Institute on Alcohol Abuse and Alcoholism. Congressional Report to Congress. Tenth Special Report to the U.S. Congress on Alcohol and Health. https://pubs.niaaa.nih.gov/publications/10report/10thspecialreport.pdf.

158. National Institute on Alcohol Abuse and Alcoholism. What is a standard drink? https://www.niaaa.nih.gov/alcohol-health/overview-alcohol-consumption/what-standard-drink.

159. Ng SK, et al. Alcohol consumption and withdrawal in new-onset seizures. *N Engl J Med*. 1988;319:666-673.

160. Nicholson ME, et al. Variability in behavioral impairment involved in the rising and falling BAC curve. *J Stud Alcohol*. 1992;53:349-356.

161. Nobay F, et al. A prospective, double-blind, randomized trial of midazolam versus haloperidol versus lorazepam in the chemical restraint of violent and severely agitated patients. *Acad Emerg Med*. 2004;11:744-749.

162. Norberg A, et al. Role of variability in explaining ethanol pharmacokinetics: research and forensic applications. *Clin Pharmacokinet*. 2003;42:1-31.

163. Nuotto E. Coffee and caffeine and alcohol effects on psychomotor function. *Clin Pharmacol Ther.* 1982;31:68-72.

164. Nuotto E, Palva ES. Naloxone fails to counteract heavy alcohol intoxication. *Lancet.* 1983;2:167-170.

165. Nurnberger JI Jr, et al. Is there a genetic relationship between alcoholism and depression? *Alcohol Res Health.* 2002;26:233-240.

166. Oda H, et al. Alcohol and coronary spasm. *Angiology.* 1994;45:187-197.

167. Oneta CM, et al. First pass metabolism of ethanol is strikingly influenced by the speed of gastric emptying. *Gut.* 1998;43:612-619.

168. Parker RB, et al. Effects of ethanol and cocaethylene on cocaine pharmacokinetics in conscious dogs. *Drug Metab Dispos.* 1996;24:850-853.

169. Parker WA. Alcohol-containing pharmaceuticals. *Am J Drug Alcohol Abuse.* 1982;9:195-209.

170. Pegues DA, et al. Elevated blood lead levels associated with illegally distilled alcohol. *Arch Intern Med.* 1993;153:1501-1504.

171. Peng GS, et al. Involvement of acetaldehyde for full protection against alcoholism by homozygosity of the variant allele of mitochondrial aldehyde dehydrogenase gene in Asians. *Pharmacogenetics.* 1999;9:463-476.

172. Peoples RW, et al. Lipid vs. protein theories of alcohol action in the nervous system. *Annu Rev Pharmacol Toxicol.* 1996;36:185-201.

173. Petroni NC, Cardoni AA. Alcohol content of liquid medicinals. *Clin Toxicol.* 1979;14:407-432.

174. Pokorny AD, et al. The brief MAST. *Am J Psychiatry.* 1972;129:342-350.

175. Politi L, et al. Bioanalytical procedures for determination of conjugates or fatty acid esters of ethanol as markers of ethanol consumption: a review. *Anal Biochem.* 2007;368:1-16.

176. Popova NK, Ivanova EA. 5-HT(1A) receptor antagonist p-MPPI attenuates acute ethanol effects in mice and rats. *Neurosci Lett.* 2002;322:1-4.

177. Raimo EB, Schuckit MA. Alcohol dependence and mood disorders. *Addict Behav.* 1998;23:933-946.

178. Randall T. Cocaine alcohol mix in body to form even longer lasting, more lethal drug. *JAMA.* 1992;267:1043-1044.

179. Rathlev NK, et al. Alcohol-related seizures. *J Emerg Med.* 2006;31:157-163.

180. Rathlev NK, et al. Etiology and weekly occurrence of alcohol-related seizures. *Acad Emerg Med.* 2002;9:824-828.

181. Reich T, et al. Genome-wide search for genes affecting the risk for alcohol dependence. *Am J Med Genet.* 1998;81:207-215.

182. Rivlin RS. Magnesium deficiency and alcohol intake: mechanisms, clinical significance and possible relation to cancer development. *J Am Coll Nutr.* 1994;13:416-423.

183. Roberts HS, et al. An unusual complication of hand hygiene. *Anaesthesia.* 2005;60:100-101.

184. Roberts JR, Greenberg MI. Fluid loading: neither safe nor efficacious in the treatment of the alcohol-intoxicated patient in the ED. *Am J Emerg Med.* 2000;18:121.

185. Rohrig TP, et al. Detection of ethylglucuronide in urine following the application of Germ-X. *J Anal Toxicol.* 2006;30:703-704.

186. Rossinen J, et al. Acute heavy alcohol intake increases silent myocardial ischaemia in patients with stable angina pectoris. *Heart.* 1996;75:563-567.

187. Rumack B, et al. Effect of therapeutic doses of acetaminophen (up to 4 g/day) on serum alanine aminotransferase levels in subjects consuming ethanol: systematic review and meta-analysis of randomized controlled trials. *Pharmacotherapy.* 2012;32:784-791.

188. Sacks JJ, et al. 2010 national and state costs of excessive alcohol consumption. *Am J Prev Med.* 2015;49:e73-e79.

189. Sarkola T, et al. Urinary ethyl glucuronide and 5-hydroxytryptophol levels during repeated ethanol ingestion in healthy human subjects. *Alcohol Alcohol.* 2003;38:347-351.

190. Sato A, et al. Prinzmetal's variant angina induced only by alcohol ingestion. *Clin Cardiol.* 1981;4:193-195.

191. Saunders JB, et al. Development of the Alcohol Use Disorders Identification Test (AUDIT): WHO Collaborative Project on Early Detection of Persons with Harmful Alcohol Consumption—II. *Addiction.* 1993;88:791-804.

192. Scherger DL, et al. Ethyl alcohol (ethanol)-containing cologne, perfume, and after-shave ingestions in children. *Am J Dis Child.* 1988;142:630-632.

193. Schiodt FV, et al. Acetaminophen toxicity in an urban county hospital. *N Engl J Med.* 1997;337:1112-1117.

194. Schmitt G, et al. Ethyl glucuronide: an unusual ethanol metabolite in humans. Synthesis, analytical data, and determination in serum and urine. *J Anal Toxicol.* 1995;19:91-94.

195. Schneir AB, Clark RF. Death caused by ingestion of an ethanol-based hand sanitizer. *J Emerg Med.* 2013;45:358-360.

196. Schuckit MA. Biological, psychological, and environmental predictors of alcoholism risk: a longitudinal study. *J Stud Alcohol.* 1998;59:485-494.

197. Seitz HK, et al. Human gastric alcohol dehydrogenase activity: effect of age, sex, and alcoholism. *Gut.* 1993;34:1433-1437.

198. Seitz HK, et al. In vivo interactions between H2-receptor antagonists and ethanol metabolism in man and in rats. *Hepatology.* 1984;4:1231-1234.

199. Sellers EM, et al. Interaction of chloral hydrate and ethanol in man. I. Metabolism. *Clin Pharmacol Ther.* 1972;13:37-49.

200. Setshedi M, et al. Acetaldehyde adducts in alcoholic liver disease. *Oxid Med Cell Longev.* 2010;3:178-185.

201. Shane SR, Flink EB. Magnesium deficiency in alcohol addiction and withdrawal. *Magnes Trace Elem.* 1991-1992;10:263-268.

202. Sherlock JC, et al. Lead in alcoholic beverages. *Food Addit Contam.* 1986;3:347-354.

203. Smart GA, et al. Lead in alcoholic beverages: a second survey. *Food Addit Contam.* 1990;7:93-99.

204. Smolle KH, et al. Q.E.D. Alcohol test: a simple and quick method to detect ethanol in saliva of patients in emergency departments. Comparison with the conventional determination in blood. *Intensive Care Med.* 1999;25:492-495.

205. Soderberg BL, et al. Fatty acid ethyl esters. Ethanol metabolites that reflect ethanol intake. *Am J Clin Pathol.* 2003;119(suppl):S94-S99.

206. Soffer A, Hamburger S. Alcoholic ketoacidosis: a review of 30 cases. *J Am Med Womens Assoc.* 1982;37:106-110.

207. Stobbs SH, et al. Ethanol suppression of ventral tegmental area GABA neuron electrical transmission involves N-methyl-D-aspartate receptors. *J Pharmacol Exp Ther.* 2004;311:282-289.

208. Stowell A, et al. Diphenhydramine and the calcium carbimide-ethanol reaction: a placebo-controlled clinical study. *Clin Pharmacol Ther.* 1986;39:521-525.

209. Sullivan JF, et al. Serum magnesium in chronic alcoholism. *Ann NY Acad Sci.* 1969;162:947-955.

210. Suwaki H, et al. Recent research on alcohol tolerance and dependence. *Alcohol Clin Exp Res.* 2001;25(5 suppl ISBRA):189S-196S.

211. Tabakoff B, et al. Alcohol tolerance. *Ann Emerg Med.* 1986;15:1005-1012.

212. Takeshita T, et al. The contribution of polymorphism in the alcohol dehydrogenase beta subunit to alcohol sensitivity in a Japanese population. *Hum Genet.* 1996;97:409-413.

213. Takeshita T, et al. Characterization of the three genotypes of low Km aldehyde dehydrogenase in a Japanese population. *Hum Genet.* 1994;94:217-223.

214. Takizawa A, et al. Variant angina induced by alcohol ingestion. *Am Heart J.* 1984;107:25-27.

215. Tan OT, et al. Suppression of alcohol-induced flushing by a combination of H1 and H2 histamine antagonists. *Br J Dermatol.* 1982;107:647-652.

216. Tanaka F, et al. High incidence of ADH2*1/ALDH2*1 genes among Japanese alcohol dependents and patients with alcoholic liver disease. *Hepatology.* 1996;23:234-239.

217. Thomasson HR, et al. Alcohol and aldehyde dehydrogenase polymorphisms and alcoholism. *Behav Genet.* 1993;23:131-136.

218. Toon S, et al. Absence of effect of ranitidine on blood alcohol concentrations when taken morning, midday, or evening with or without food. *Clin Pharmacol Ther.* 1994;55:385-391.

219. Truitt EB Jr, et al. Aspirin attenuation of alcohol-induced flushing and intoxication in Oriental and Occidental subjects. *Alcohol Alcohol.* 1987;Suppl 1:595-599.

220. Tsai GE, et al. Increased glutamatergic neurotransmission and oxidative stress after alcohol withdrawal. *Am J Psychiatry.* 1998;155:726-732.

221. Tsai GE, Coyle JT. The role of glutamatergic neurotransmission in the pathophysiology of alcoholism. *Annu Rev Med.* 1998;49:173-184.

222. Tsutaya S, et al. Analysis of aldehyde dehydrogenase 2 gene polymorphism and ethanol patch test as a screening method for alcohol sensitivity. *Tohoku J Exp Med.* 1999;187:305-310.

223. Tuma DJ, Casey CA. Dangerous byproducts of alcohol breakdown-focus on addicts. *Alcohol Res Health.* 2003;27:285-290.

224. Ueno S, et al. Alcohol actions on GABA(A) receptors: from protein structure to mouse behavior. *Alcohol Clin Exp Res.* 2001;25(5 suppl ISBRA):76S-81S.

225. Walsh DC, et al. A randomized trial of treatment options for alcohol abusing workers. *N Engl J Med.* 1991;325:775-782.

226. Wang MQ, et al. Proprioceptive responses under rising and falling BACs: a test of the Mellanby effect. *Percept Mot Skills.* 1993;77:83-88.

227. Weathermon R, Crabb DW. Alcohol and medication interactions. *Alcohol Res Health.* 1999;23:40-45.

228. Welch C, et al. The increasing burden of alcoholic liver disease on United Kingdom critical care units: secondary analysis of a high quality clinical database. *J Health Serv Res Policy.* 2008;13(suppl 2):40-44.

229. Weller-Fahy ER, et al. Mouthwash: a source of acute ethanol intoxication. *Pediatrics.* 1980;66:302-305.

230. Wheeler MD. Endotoxin and Kupffer cell activation in alcoholic liver disease. *Alcohol Res Health.* 2003;27:300-306.

231. Whitcomb DC, Block GD. Association of acetaminophen hepatotoxicity with fasting and ethanol use. *JAMA.* 1994;272:1845-1850.

232. White IR, et al. Alcohol consumption and mortality: modelling risks for men and women at different ages. *BMJ.* 2002;325:191-197.

233. Whitfield JB. Meta-analysis of the effects of alcohol dehydrogenase genotype on alcohol dependence and alcoholic liver disease. *Alcohol Alcohol.* 1997;32:613-619.

234. Wilson LD, et al. Cocaethylene causes dose-dependent reductions in cardiac function in anesthetized dogs. *J Cardiovasc Pharmacol.* 1995;26:965-973.

235. Winokur G, et al. Alcoholism and drug abuse in three groups--bipolar I, unipolars and their acquaintances. *J Affect Disord.* 1998;50:81-89.

236. Winokur G, et al. Familial alcoholism in manic-depressive (bipolar) disease. *Am J Med Genet*. 1996;67:197-201.

237. Wojcik MH, Hawthorne JS. Sensitivity of commercial ethyl glucuronide testing in screening for alcohol abstinence. *Alcohol Alcohol*. 2007;42:317-320.

238. Wright C. Physician interventions in alcoholism—past and present. *Md Med J*. 1995;44:447-452.

239. Wu C, Kenny MA. Circulating total and ionized magnesium after ethanol ingestion. *Clin Chem*. 1996;42:625-629.

240. Zador PL, et al. Alcohol-related relative risk of driver fatalities and driver involvement in fatal crashes in relation to driver age and gender: an update using 1996 data. *J Stud Alcohol*. 2000;61:387-395.

241. Zaleski J, Bryła J. Ethanol-induced impairment of gluconeogenesis from lactate in rabbit hepatocytes: correlation with an increased reduction of mitochondrial NAD pool. *Int J Biochem*. 1980;11:237-242.

242. Zhang X, et al. Ethanol and acetaldehyde in alcoholic cardiomyopathy: from bad to ugly en route to oxidative stress. *Alcohol*. 2004;32:175-186.

243. Zimmerman HJ, Maddrey WC. Acetaminophen (paracetamol) hepatotoxicity with regular intake of alcohol: analysis of instances of therapeutic misadventure. *Hepatology*. 1995;22:767-773.

244. Zimmerman HJ. Effects of alcohol on other hepatotoxins. *Alcoholism*. 1986;10:3-15.

A27

THIAMINE HYDROCHLORIDE

Robert S. Hoffman

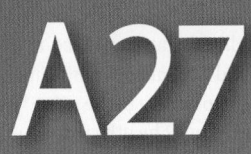

INTRODUCTION

Thiamine (vitamin B_1) is a water-soluble vitamin found in organ meats, yeast, eggs, and green leafy vegetables that is essential in the creation and utilization of cellular energy. Although there is no toxicity associated with thiamine excess, thiamine deficiency is responsible for "wet" beriberi high output (congestive heart failure) and "dry" beriberi (Wernicke encephalopathy and the Wernicke-Korsakoff syndrome). Patients at risk include those with malnutrition (HIV/AIDS, cancer, end-stage kidney disease, fad diets, anorexia nervosa, bulimia, cyclic vomiting, hyperemesis gravidarum, and after bariatric surgery), those with impaired absorption (alcoholism, sepsis, bariatric surgery, inflammatory bowel disease), and those with enhanced elimination (high-dose loop diuretic therapy). Typical signs of Wernicke encephalopathy include ataxia, altered mental status, and ophthalmoplegia. Although administration of 100 mg of parenteral thiamine hydrochloride protects against thiamine deficiency for more than 1 week, patients with clinical deficiencies require larger doses for a longer period of time.

HISTORY

Kanehiro Takaki, a physician in the Japanese navy, first established the relationship between a nutritional deficiency and beriberi in 1884. It was not until 1901 that Gerrit Grijns determined that the nutrient, as yet unnamed, was contained in the outer coat of rice and was lost during the polishing process. Ten years later, Casimir Funk isolated thiamine, and Williams finally determined its structure in 1934. Originally thiamine was called aneurin for "antineuritic vitamin"[22] and was ultimately synthesized by Cline, Williams, and Finkelstein.[28] In 1936, Peters demonstrated that thiamine could reverse neurologic disease in nutritionally deprived pigeons and that improvement was coupled to an enhanced ability to metabolize pyruvate.[109]

In 1881, Carl Wernicke reported 3 patients with alcoholism who died after developing confusion, ataxia, and ophthalmoplegia.[149] Autopsies showed characteristic hemorrhages surrounding the third and fourth cerebral ventricles. A few years later, Sergei Korsakoff reported amnesia and confabulation in 30 individuals with alcoholism and 16 without alcoholism that was preceded in many by the clinical findings reported by Wernicke.[157] Today, these 2 neurologic disorders are often combined and called the Wernicke-Korsakoff syndrome in recognition that they are a spectrum of the same disease.

PHARMACOLOGY
Biochemistry

As a coenzyme in the pyruvate dehydrogenase complex, thiamine diphosphate (thiamine pyrophosphate), the active form of thiamine, facilitates the conversion (with bound lipoamide and magnesium as cofactors) of pyruvate to acetylcoenzyme A (acetyl-CoA). This reaction occurs at the C2 atom

of thiamine, which is located between the nitrogen and sulfur atoms on the thiazolium ring.[53] In the protein-rich environment of the enzyme complex, this C2 atom is deprotonated to form a carbanion that rapidly attaches to the carbonyl group of pyruvate, thereby stabilizing it for decarboxylation.[73] In a series of subsequent reactions, the hydroxyethyl group that remains bound to thiamine diphosphate is transferred to lipoamide, where an acetyl group is later broken off and attached to coenzyme A (CoA). This overall process links pyruvate production from anaerobic glycolysis to the citric acid cycle, in which the sum of anaerobic and aerobic metabolism produces the equivalent of 36 moles of adenosine triphosphate (ATP) from each mole of glucose (Fig. A27–1). When pyruvate cannot be converted to acetyl-CoA

FIGURE A27–1. Thiamine links anaerobic glycolysis to the citric acid cycle. Anaerobic glycolysis only yields 2 moles of adenosine triphosphate (ATP) as each mole of glucose is metabolized to 2 moles of pyruvate. To obtain the 34 additional ATP equivalents that can be derived as the citric acid converts pyruvate to CO_2 and H_2O, pyruvate must first be combined with coenzyme A (CoA) to form acetylcoenzyme A (acetyl-CoA) and CO_2. This process is dependent on the thiamine-requiring enzyme system known as pyruvate dehydrogenase complex.

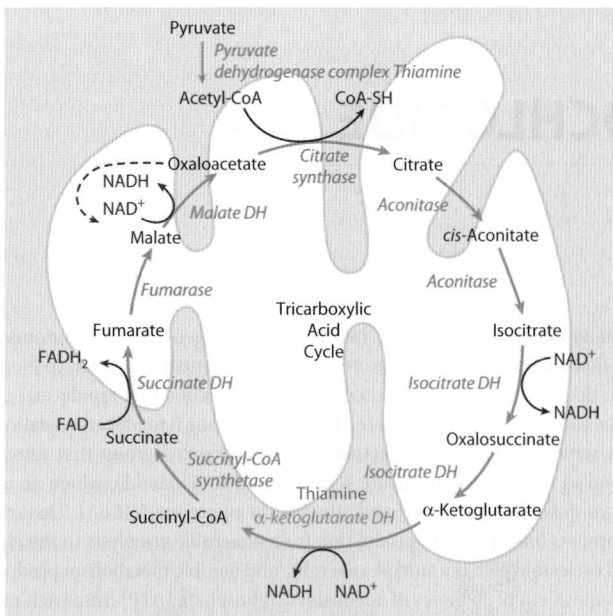

FIGURE A27–2. Thiamine is essential for α-ketoglutarate dehydrogenase activity, which is a rate-limiting step within the citric acid cycle. Thiamine deficiency leads to an accumulation of α-ketoglutarate, which is shunted to glutamate and causes excitatory neurotoxicity.

because of thiamine deficiency, for example, only 2 moles of ATP are generated by anaerobic metabolism from each mole of glucose. Within the citric acid cycle, thiamine is also required as a cofactor for the α-ketoglutarate dehydrogenase complex to catalyze the reaction of α-ketoglutarate to succinyl-CoA (Fig. A27–2), and in the pentose phosphate pathway for transketolase, an enzyme in which nicotinamide adenine dinucleotide phosphate (NADPH) is formed for subsequent use in reductive biosynthesis.[15,172] In addition to its metabolic effects, thiamine also has a role as a neuromodulator, influencing acetylcholine release.[64]

Naturally occurring thiamine is a base composed of a substituted pyrimidine ring and a substituted thiazole ring connected by a methylene bridge. This connection between the 2 rings is weak, and the molecule is unstable in both an alkaline milieu and in a high-temperature environment. In addition, thiamine is highly water soluble, allowing it to leach out of foods following prolonged washing or cooking in water. However, thiamine, which is synthesized as a hydrochloride salt, is usually quite stable. Thiamine requirements are determined by total caloric intake and energy demand, with 0.33 mg of thiamine required for every 4,400 kJ (1,000 kcal) of energy.[132] The recommended daily consumption is 0.5 mg/1,000 kcal to provide a margin of safety.[131]

Pharmacokinetics

Thiamine is well absorbed from the human gastrointestinal (GI) tract by a complex process.[81,116] At low concentrations, thiamine absorption occurs through a saturable mechanism that is most effective in the duodenum, with absorption occurring to a lesser degree in the large bowel and stomach.[81] As thiamine concentrations increase, however, the majority of absorption occurs through simple passive diffusion. A placebo-controlled human volunteer study evaluated the kinetics of oral administration of 100, 500, and 1,500 mg in healthy participants.[132] After the oral 100-mg dose, peak concentrations occurred in whole blood in 3.43 hours. Although higher doses produced higher peak concentrations with a delay in time, the lack of linearity of the dose–response relationship confirmed complex absorption kinetics.[132] The kinetics of oral and intravenous (IV) thiamine were compared in 6 healthy volunteers after a 50-mg dose.[144] Intravenous administration peaked rapidly and had an apparent elimination half-life of 96 minutes but showed restricted distribution with 53% recovered in the

urine over the next 24 hours. By contrast, oral administration peaked in a mean of 53 minutes, was only 5.3% bioavailable, and had an apparent elimination half-life of 154 minutes, and only 2.5% was recoverable in the urine.[144] The effects of varied rates of infusion were compared in 12 healthy individuals when 150 mg of thiamine was given IV over either 1 hour or 24 hours in a controlled trial.[41] As expected, although the rapid infusion produced a higher peak concentration. However, the slower infusion increased the AUC of thiamine pyrophosphate and decreased the urinary elimination from 83.6% of the dose to 57.6%, suggesting a benefit for slower administration rates.[41] Synthesized analogs such as thiamine propyl disulfide, benfotiamine, and fursultiamine have enhanced bioavailability, but their use remains largely experimental.[53,151,168] Chronic liver disease, folate deficiency, steatorrhea, and other forms of malabsorption all significantly decrease the absorption of thiamine.[33,133] Bariatric surgery also predisposes patients to thiamine deficiency.[1,5,48,125,126] Malabsorption has even greater clinical relevance in patients with alcoholism.[9,148] In experimental studies, when healthy volunteers were given small amounts of ethanol, a 50% reduction in GI thiamine absorption resulted.[148] A rat model confirmed that the simple presence of ethanol in the gut impairs thiamine absorption.[65]

Two genes are involved in the cellular transport of thiamine: a high-affinity thiamine transporter known as THTR1 (SLC19A2) and a low-affinity thiamine transporter known as THTR2 (SLC19A3).[54,55] Variations or mutations in these genes predispose to thiamine deficiency causing thiamine-responsive megaloblastic anemia syndrome. Homozygous or compound heterozygous mutations in THTR2 manifest as 2 distinct clinical phenotypes, thiamine-biotin-responsive basal ganglia disease and Wernicke-like encephalopathy.[169] Experimental evidence suggests that ethanol intake directly alters gene transcription, further increasing risk.[152] These models demonstrate that ethanol reduces the expression of intestinal and pancreatic acinar thiamine transporters at the protein, mRNA, and transcriptional (promoter activity) levels.[140]

Thiamine is eliminated from the body largely by renal clearance, which consists of a combination of glomerular filtration, flow-dependent tubular secretion, and saturable tubular reabsorption.[161] In an animal model, furosemide, acetazolamide, chlorothiazide, amiloride, mannitol, and salt loading all significantly increased urinary elimination of thiamine.[69] This nonspecific flow-dependent elimination was confirmed in humans given small doses of furosemide.[115] Interestingly, spironolactone use is associated with higher thiamine concentrations.[117] Additionally, both furosemide and digoxin appear to inhibit thiamine uptake into myocardial cells.[171]

THIAMINE DEFICIENCY
Pathophysiology

Mice develop signs of encephalopathy 10 days after being rendered thiamine deficient. Immunohistochemistry in these animals demonstrates destruction of the blood–brain barrier with resultant extravasation of albumin.[59] Similarly, rats develop symptoms after 10 days of thiamine deficiency and subsequently demonstrate deterioration of the blood–brain barrier with hemorrhage into the mammillary bodies and other areas of the brain.[20] This pattern is similar to findings described in humans with Wernicke encephalopathy (Fig. A27-3).[56,111] Although there are no controlled trials of thiamine deprivation in humans, several unfortunate events support this time course. One report describes 3 patients who were given total parenteral nutrition (TPN) without multivitamins; signs and symptoms developed in 7, 10, and 14 days, respectively.[155] Similar reports confirm this time course with some variability based on the nutritional status of the patients.[6,80,99,105] Infants aged 2 to 12 months given a soy-based formula that lacked thiamine also developed findings consistent with Wernicke encephalopathy, irritability, vomiting, nystagmus, ophthalmoplegia and metabolic acidosis with elevated lactate.[45]

The proximate cause of Wernicke encephalopathy is unclear. In human autopsy studies, brain samples from alcoholic patients with Wernicke-Korsakoff syndrome demonstrate decreased function of pyruvate dehydrogenase, α-ketoglutarate dehydrogenase, and transketolase compared with control participants.[18] However, a similar decrease in enzyme activity of neuronal

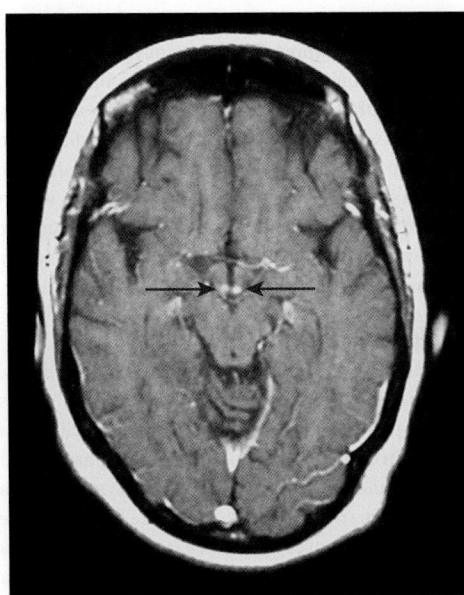

FIGURE A27–3. Postgadolinium axial and coronal T1-weighted magnetic resonance image of a patient with Wernicke encephalopathy showing pronounced enhancement of the mammillary bodies (arrows). *(Used with permission from Dr. Alexander Baxter, Department of Radiology, New York University School of Medicine.)*

tissue was demonstrated in alcoholics who died from hepatic coma without ever manifesting signs of Wernicke encephalopathy.[85] This finding is understandable given that high concentrations of ammonia inhibit α-ketoglutarate dehydrogenase.[15] Likewise, the activity of thiamine-requiring citric acid cycle enzymes is reduced in thiamine-replete patients with neurodegenerative diseases.[14] Thus, although thiamine deficiency produces deficits in critical enzymes in humans, many have argued that it is unclear whether these deficits are either necessary or sufficient to produce clinical disease.

Animal models offer insight into the mechanisms involved in developing thiamine-deficient neurologic injury. Although the exact chain of events leading to these structural abnormalities is unclear, several models demonstrate key portions of the pathway. Thiamine deficiency in rats produces 200% to 640% increases in concentrations of glutamate,[83,84] which presumably results from blockade of α-ketoglutarate dehydrogenase. Excess α-ketoglutarate is shunted away from the citric acid cycle to form glutamate. Astrocytes seem uniquely sensitive to these effects with decreases in both glutamate and glutamate-aspartate transporters noted, which further increase interstitial glutamate concentrations.[2,3] Rats subsequently develop increases in lactate in vulnerable regions of the brain marked by the induction of the protooncogene c-fos. Both the histochemical lesions and the gene induction are blocked by the administration of the calcium channel blocker nicardipine.[98] This suggests a strong role for excitatory amino acid–induced alterations in calcium transport in the genesis of thiamine-deficient encephalopathy.[70] In other animal models of thiamine deficiency, neuronal tissues are also directly injured by oxidative stress and lipid peroxidation.[21,61,62,70] Additional investigations demonstrate roles for triggered mast cell degranulation,[46] histamine,[83] and nitric oxide[51,77] in the generation of neuronal injury. The final common pathway is localized cerebral edema, which appears to result from altered expression of aquaporin.[26]

In what may be the most important finding since Wernicke's original report described 2 healthy nonalcoholic brothers who developed signs, symptoms, and neuroimaging findings consistent with Wernicke encephalopathy despite normal serum thiamine concentrations.[76] Both brothers were confirmed to have compound mutations of the *SLC19A3* gene (K44E and E320Q) encoding for low-affinity thiamine transporter (THTR2). High-dose thiamine (up to 600 mg) was clinically effective. The more severe E320Q homozygous THTR2 mutation manifests as impaired thiamine uptake, progressive brain atrophy, bilateral thalamic and basal ganglia lesions, and epileptic spasms

beginning early in infancy.[169] Several other mutations (including G23V and T422A and those inducing premature termination codons) produce loss of thiamine THTR2 transport function and a spectrum of generalized dystonia; epilepsy; and bilateral striatal, caudate, putamen, and cortical lesions.[35,128,139] Patients may respond to high-dose thiamine (150–300 mg/every 8 hours in adults or 10–40 mg/kg/day in children) or biotin (or both).[128] As demonstrated by magnetic resonance imaging, vasogenic edema is a characteristic finding during the acute crises.[142] When added to the cases in which thiamine was excluded from TPN or infant formula, these findings definitively relate intracellular thiamine concentrations to clinical and anatomical manifestations of Wernicke encephalopathy and thiamine deficiency.

In addition, several human cases and case series suggest an important role for insufficient magnesium (a cofactor) in Wernicke pathogenesis.[37,93,120] The adversely synergistic effects of magnesium and thiamine codeficiency mirrors detrimental effects observed in animal species.[86] Chronic alcoholic patients supplemented with magnesium in addition to thiamine recover their erythrocyte transketolase activity to a greater extent compared with those receiving thiamine alone.[108] Patients with Wernicke encephalopathy may be clinically unresponsive to thiamine treatment in the setting of untreated hypomagnesemia.[47]

Clinical Manifestations

When thiamine is completely removed from the human diet, tachycardia is often the first sign of deficiency. The clinical symptoms of thiamine deficiency present as 2 distinct patterns: "wet" beriberi or cardiovascular disease and "dry" beriberi, the neurologic disease known as Wernicke-Korsakoff syndrome. Although some patients display symptoms consistent with both disorders, usually either the cardiovascular or the neurologic manifestations predominate. A genetic variant of transketolase activity, combined with low physical activity and low-carbohydrate diet, predisposes to neurologic symptoms, but high-carbohydrate diets and increased physical activity lead to cardiovascular symptoms.[13,165] Thus, cardiovascular disease is more common in the Asian population, and neurologic disease predominates in the northern European population.

Wet beriberi results from high-output cardiac failure induced by peripheral vasodilation and the formation of arteriovenous fistulae secondary to thiamine deficiency. These patients complain of fatigue, decreased exercise tolerance, shortness of breath, and peripheral edema. Myocardial edema is reported.[43] Patients with congestive heart failure seem to have an analogous worsening cardiac function caused by diuretic-associated thiamine use, which improves with thiamine supplementation.[39,146] Fulminant cardiovascular beriberi (Shoshin beriberi) presents as shock and cardiovascular collapse.[32,95] The classic triad of oculomotor abnormalities, ataxia, and global confusion defines dry beriberi or Wernicke encephalopathy. Other manifestations include hypothermia and the absence of deep-tendon reflexes.[44,160] Vomiting and anorexia are common[45,155] and are presumed to be related to increases in intracranial pressure. Additionally, patients develop a peripheral neuropathy with paresthesias, hypesthesias, and an associated myopathy, all related to axonal degeneration.[131] Laboratory studies may reflect a metabolic acidosis with elevated lactate concentration brought on by excessive anaerobic glycolysis resulting from blocked entry of substrate into the Krebs cycle.[25,27,74,75,82,106,118,160] Interestingly, a primary respiratory alkalosis of unclear etiology seems to be simultaneously present.[40] Korsakoff psychosis, a frequently irreversible disorder of learning and processing of new information characterized by a deficit in short-term memory and confabulation, often occurs together with Wernicke encephalopathy.[157] A 10% to 20% mortality rate is associated with Wernicke encephalopathy, with survivors having an 80% risk of developing Korsakoff psychosis.[114] Only about 21% of patients with Korsakoff psychosis will have a complete recovery, with others having variable degrees of improvement that typically take months.[156]

A clinical tool for identifying patients with Wernicke encephalopathy used 4 signs: dietary deficiencies, oculomotor abnormalities, cerebellar dysfunction, and either an altered mental status or mild memory impairment. When 2 or more signs were present, the tool was highly sensitive and specific.[19] Despite this tool, autopsy studies suggest that Wernicke encephalopathy remains underrecognized in the critically ill patients.[47]

Epidemiology: Populations at Risk

In the United States, a healthy diet and mandatory thiamine supplementation of numerous food products protect most people from the manifestations of thiamine deficiency. Despite this, the prevalence of Wernicke encephalopathy in the general US population is estimated to be between 0.2% and 2.2%, although only 20% of these cases are estimated to be diagnosed during their lifetime.[90,138] This is, unfortunately, not true in other countries. A survey of the 17 major public hospitals in the Sydney, Australia, area identified more than 1,000 cases of either acute Wernicke encephalopathy or Korsakoff psychosis between 1978 and 1993.[91] Similarly, a single Australian hospital identified 32 cases of Wernicke encephalopathy during a 33-month period.[166] In Australia, mandatory supplementation of flour with thiamine in 1991 resulted in a dramatic reduction in hospitalized cases during 1992 and 1993,[91] as well as of the percentage of cases diagnosed by postmortem studies.[60] Other countries at risk include Ireland and New Zealand, where lack of a mandatory thiamine supplementation program is correlated with a high prevalence of biochemical evidence of thiamine deficiency.[102,103] In countries where bread is not a major dietary staple, alternative supplemental strategies such as adding thiamine to fish sauce seem promising.[163]

Alcoholic patients, whose consumption of ethanol is their major source of calories, are the best described and most easily recognized patients at risk for thiamine deficiency.[114] In Scotland, 21% of alcoholics requiring emergency admission to the hospital were thiamine deficient, as determined by erythrocyte transketolase activity.[68] The prevalence in US alcoholics is estimated to be 12.5%.[138] In patients with sepsis, thiamine deficiency rates are between 20% and 70%.[30] Likewise, in patients with congestive heart failure, thiamine deficiency is reported to range from just a few percent to over 90% depending on the population studied and the use of diuretics.[39,146]

Consequential thiamine deficiency is also described in the following settings: incarceration,[69] drug rehabilitation,[49] hemodialysis,[36] hyperemesis gravidarum or anorexia nervosa,[147] parenteral nutrition,[6,23,24,27,80,82,105,106,141,155,158] acquired immunodeficiency syndrome (AIDS),[7,16,17,124] malignancies,[11,66,78,119,135,153] institutionalized older adults,[79,102-104] critically ill children,[72,88] sepsis,[40] congestive heart failure on furosemide therapy,[79] malabsorption secondary to diarrhea,[33,170] eating disorders,[113,159] the refeeding syndrome,[92] and patients who had undergone bariatric surgery.[1,5,48,52,96,125] Thus, despite routine dietary supplementation, many people are still at risk because of dietary limitations, alcohol abuse, or underlying medical or surgical conditions. Additionally there is some evidence to suggest that the use of metformin is associated with thiamine deficiency which contributes to neuropathies in patients with diabetes.[87]

ROLE IN PREVENTION AND TREATMENT OF WERNICKE ENCEPHALOPATHY

Thiamine hydrochloride is included in the initial therapy for any patient with an altered mental status, potentially acting as both treatment and prevention of Wernicke encephalopathy. Many patients with altered levels of consciousness have had or will have a poor nutritional status or will be hospitalized and deprived of oral intake for a number of days because of GI disorders or altered mental status. Although thiamine concentrations can be either directly measured or functionally assessed by measuring erythrocyte transketolase activity at baseline and in response to thiamine diphosphate administration,[63] these determinations are unavailable for clinical use and do not correlate with disease severity.[90] Likewise, although clinical prediction models exist, they are cumbersome and unvalidated.[129] Glucose loading increases thiamine requirements, which can exacerbate marginal thiamine deficiencies, elevate lactate concentrations,[101] or precipitate coma in the absence of parenteral thiamine supplementation.[114] Although it is commonly believed that acute glucose loading, in the form of a bolus of hypertonic dextrose, can precipitate Wernicke encephalopathy over several hours in normal individuals, there is evidence to support this effect only in patients

who already have grave manifestations of thiamine deficiency or exaggerated delay in the provision of thiamine.[94,121,160] Previously healthy patients require prolonged dextrose administration in the absence of thiamine to develop Wernicke encephalopathy. Because the morbidity and mortality associated with Wernicke encephalopathy are so severe and underdiagnosed and treatment is both benign and inexpensive, parenteral thiamine hydrochloride should be included in the initial therapy for all patients who receive dextrose, all patients with altered consciousness, and every potential alcoholic or nutritionally deprived individual who presents to the emergency department or other clinical setting.

ROLE IN THE TREATMENT OF OTHER DISORDERS

A supplementary indication for the administration of thiamine hydrochloride occurs in patients with ethylene glycol poisoning. As shown in Fig. 106–2, a minor pathway for the elimination of glyoxylic acid involves its conversion to α-hydroxy-β-ketoadipate by α-ketoglutarate: glyoxylate carboligase, a thiamine and magnesium-requiring enzyme. There are no data to support an increase in α-hydroxy-β-ketoadipate formation after thiamine administration in ethylene glycol–poisoned animals or humans. However, animal models of primary hyperoxaluria show increases in urinary oxalate during thiamine deficiency, suggesting at least a potential importance of this pathway.[58,143] Because therapy is benign and inexpensive, it is reasonable to administer standard doses of thiamine to patients with suspected or confirmed ethylene glycol poisoning.

Standard doses of thiamine are also recommended for patients with alcoholic ketoacidosis (AKA) and starvation ketoacidosis. Glucose is required to stimulate insulin secretion, which subsequently terminates ketogenesis. Because by definition, AKA occurs in malnourished alcoholics who are at risk for Wernicke encephalopathy, parenteral thiamine administration is recommended (Chap. 76).[10]

It is also reasonable to include routine thiamine administration in patients with congestive heart failure treated with long-term use of loop diuretics. Diuretics enhance renal thiamine elimination.[127] In one randomized trial, 200 mg of daily IV thiamine was able to increase cardiac ejection fraction by 22% at 7 weeks.[130] Another study showed that a daily oral dose of 300 mg of thiamine in patients with chronic heart failure was able to increase left ventricular ejection fraction by 10% over placebo.[123] Repletion of thiamine and other water soluble vitamin repletion is common practice in clinical dialysis centers.

ADVERSE EFFECTS

Very few complications are associated with the parenteral administration of thiamine. A single case of repeated angioedema was reported with oral thiamine.[107] The older literature emphasized intramuscular (IM) administration because of numerous reports of anaphylactoid reactions associated with IV thiamine delivery.[42,112,122,137,162] It is generally believed that these reactions resulted from responses to contaminants rather than thiamine itself. Despite the availability of purer, aqueous preparations of thiamine, rare adverse reports still occur.[8,71,97,110,136] Although the IM route is theoretically comparably efficacious in a healthy individual, many patients requiring thiamine have diminished muscle mass or a coagulopathy, exacerbating the potential for pain and unpredictable absorption. The safety of thiamine use was evaluated in a large case series in which nearly 1,000 patients received parenteral doses of up to 500 mg of thiamine without significant complications.[167] This study suggests that if anaphylaxis to thiamine exists, its occurrence is exceedingly rare, permitting the safe IV administration of thiamine to most patients.

PREGNANCY AND LACTATION

Thiamine hydrochloride is listed in Pregnancy Category A and is also considered safe for use in lactating mothers. When the use of oral thiamine supplementation was studied in thiamine-deficient Cambodian mothers, a significant increase in breast milk concentrations was noted, but these concentrations were insufficient to correct deficiencies in their children over the 5-day study period.[29] Over the course of study, the median breast milk thiamine concentration increased from 180 nmol/L to 503 nmol/L (360–808 nmol/L) on day 6, which is within the reported values of American breast milk. Although the infants' thiamine concentration increased from 3.0 nmol/L to 5.6 nmol/L, these values still qualified as deficient.

DOSING AND ADMINISTRATION

For prevention of Wernicke encephalopathy, initial therapy usually consists of the immediate parenteral administration of 100 mg of thiamine hydrochloride. This can be given either intramuscularly or intravenously, but the oral route should be avoided because of its unpredictable absorption. In countries where thiamine propyl disulfide (a lipid-soluble thiamine preparation) is available, the oral route is equally efficacious for the replacement of serious thiamine deficiencies.[9,151] Although there are no dose finding studies, some authorities recommend daily doses as high as 250 mg/day in high-risk patients without signs and symptoms of Wernicke encephalopathy.[150] Current recommendations also exist for patients on TPN (3–3.5 mg/d), enteral feeding (2.2–2.9 mg/1,500 kcal), and renal replacement therapy (100 mg/d).[134] Unfortunately, despite consensus statements and guidelines, evidence suggests that clinicians uniformly fail to protect their patients appropriately[34,67] and that there will likely be public health benefits to increasing the duration of parenteral thiamine administration to patients at risk.[164]

The practice of requiring the administration of parenteral thiamine before hypertonic dextrose in patients with altered consciousness is illogical.[57] Besides the fact that the first dose of dextrose is unlikely to cause thiamine deficiency, thiamine uptake into cells and activation of enzyme systems is slower than that of glucose uptake, which suggests that even pretreatment with thiamine offers little benefit over posttreatment.[145] Despite these limitations, it is prudent to administer at least 100 mg of parenteral thiamine at the time of initial dextrose administration. The biochemical link between dextrose and thiamine is obvious, which demonstrates to the clinician the scientific basis for the administration of thiamine. Although thiamine is unlikely to offer immediate benefits for patients with altered consciousness, it will offer some long-term protection for these individuals at risk and initiate therapy for a serious, insidious, and easily overlooked disorder.

For treatment of Wernicke encephalopathy, in some patients, symptoms such as ophthalmoplegia are reported to respond rapidly to as little as 2 mg of thiamine; however, the other neurologic and cardiovascular manifestations of thiamine deprivation necessitate higher doses and generally respond more slowly, if at all. Although many sources recommend that daily doses of 100 mg of thiamine are sufficient as in preventive therapy, others recommend initial doses of at least 200 or 250 mg[4,153] based on limited data. We agree with current guidelines recommended by the British National Formulary and the Royal College of Physicians, British Association for Psychopharmacology, the European Federation of Neurological Societies (EFNS), and the National Institute for Health and Clinical Excellence (NICE) guidelines, all of which suggest that the initial thiamine regimen for patients with Wernicke encephalopathy is 500 mg intravenously 3 times daily for 2 to 3 days and 250 mg intravenously daily for the next 3 to 5 days.[50,89] This increase over formerly recommended regimens is reflective of reports of patients failing standard therapy and the safety of parenteral thiamine.[31] As stated earlier, because there is pharmacokinetic evidence favoring slow infusions over bolus therapy, this practice is reasonable after the first dose.[41] Additionally, because data suggest that transketolase activity is improved when magnesium supplementation is routinely added to thiamine administration,[108] we recommend administering 2 g of magnesium sulfate IV to patients with normal kidney function.

Because of the safety of thiamine hydrochloride and the urgency to correct the manifestations of thiamine deficiency, up to 1,000 mg of thiamine hydrochloride is reasonable for use in the first 12 hours if a patient demonstrates persistent neurologic abnormalities.[100]

Dosing in other disorders is less well defined. In patients with congestive heart failure, regimens have varied from 100 mg twice per week to 300 mg/day,[38,39] but for sepsis, single doses of 200 mg were given.[12] For ethylene glycol poisoning and AKA, we recommend a dose of 100 mg intravenously.

For all these disorders, strong evidence to favor one regimen over alternatives is lacking.

FORMULATION AND ACQUISITION

Multiple manufacturers formulate thiamine hydrochloride for IV or IM administration. Typical concentrations are either 50 or 100 mg/mL. Although more concentrated solutions are available, their use is usually reserved for preparation of TPN solutions. Thiamine available in the United States is formulated in 0.5% (5 mg/mL) chlorobutanol as a preservative. In the United Kingdom, the formulation Pabrinex is chlorobutanol free. Chlorobutanol is a sedative with a long elimination half-life, but doses of 600 mg were given to human volunteers without complication.[154] Thus, following UK and EFNS recommendations of 1,500 mg/day of thiamine would only deliver 75 to 150 mg of chlorobutanol depending on which preparation was used. Even with the long elimination half-life, many days of high dose thiamine could be administered without delivering a single sedating dose.

SUMMARY

- Thiamine is an essential water-soluble vitamin for cellular energy.
- Thiamine deficiency can present as either Wernicke encephalopathy or high output cardiac failure (wet beriberi).
- Wernicke encephalopathy manifests as ataxia, ophthalmoplegia, altered mental status, decreased deep tendon reflexes, metabolic acidosis with elevated lactate, and hypothermia.
- Parenteral administration of 100 mg of thiamine is required to protect an individual at risk for 1 to 2 weeks.
- When Wernicke encephalopathy is present or suspected, higher doses of thiamine are recommended. The exact dose and speed of administration of thiamine has yet to be established for these patients, but we favor the higher dosing regimens that are proposed.
- Although thiamine requirements are based on caloric intake, there is no evidence that thiamine must be given before dextrose administration.

REFERENCES

1. Aasheim ET. Wernicke encephalopathy after bariatric surgery: a systematic review. *Ann Surg.* 2008;248:714-720.
2. Abdou E, Hazell AS. Thiamine deficiency: an update of pathophysiologic mechanisms and future therapeutic considerations. *Neurochem Res.* 2015;40:353-361.
3. Afadlal S, et al. Role of astrocytes in thiamine deficiency. *Metab Brain Dis.* 2014;29:1061-1068.
4. Ambrose ML, et al. Thiamin treatment and working memory function of alcohol-dependent people: preliminary findings. *Alcohol Clin Exp Res.* 2001;25:112-116.
5. Angstadt JD, Bodziner RA. Peripheral polyneuropathy from thiamine deficiency following laparoscopic Roux-en-Y gastric bypass. *Obesity Surg.* 2005;15:890-892.
6. Anon. Beriberi can complicate TPN. *Nutr Rev.* 1987;45:239-243.
7. Arici C, et al. Severe lactic acidosis and thiamine administration in an HIV-infected patient on HAART. *Int J STD AIDS.* 2001;12:407-409.
8. Assem ESK. Anaphylactic reaction to thiamine. *Practitioner.* 1973;322:565.
9. Baker H, Frank O. Absorption, utilization and clinical effectiveness of allithiamines compared to water-soluble thiamines. *Journal of nutritional science and vitaminology.* 1976;22(suppl):63-68.
10. Bakker SJ, et al. Protection against cardiovascular collapse in an alcoholic patient with thiamine deficiency by concomitant alcoholic ketoacidosis. *J Intern Med.* 1997;242:179-183.
11. Barbato M, Rodriguez PJ. Thiamine deficiency in patients admitted to a palliative care unit. *Palliat Med.* 1994;8:320-324.
12. Berg KM, et al. Intravenous thiamine is associated with increased oxygen consumption in critically ill patients with preserved cardiac index. *Ann Am Thorac Soc.* 2014;11:1597-1601.
13. Blass JP, Gibson GE. Abnormality of a thiamine-requiring enzyme in patients with Wernicke-Korsakoff syndrome. *N Engl J Med.* 1977;297:1367-1370.
14. Bubber P, et al. Tricarboxylic acid cycle enzymes following thiamine deficiency. *Neurochem Int.* 2004;45:1021-1028.
15. Butterworth RF. Thiamine deficiency-related brain dysfunction in chronic liver failure. *Metab Brain Dis.* 2009;24:189-196.
16. Butterworth RF, et al. Thiamine deficiency and Wernicke's encephalopathy in AIDS. *Metab Brain Dis.* 1991;6:207.
17. Butterworth RF, et al. Thiamine deficiency in AIDS. *Lancet.* 1991;338:1086.
18. Butterworth RF, et al. Thiamine-dependent enzyme changes in the brains of alcoholics: relationship to the Wernicke-Korsakoff syndrome. *Alcohol Clin Exp Res.* 1993;17:1084-1088.

19. Caine D, et al. Operational criteria for the classification of chronic alcoholics: identification of Wernicke's encephalopathy. *J Neurol Neurosurg Psychiatry.* 1997;62:51-60.

20. Calingasan NY, et al. Blood-brain barrier abnormalities in vulnerable brain regions during thiamine deficiency. *Exp Neurol.* 1995;134:64-72.

21. Calingasan NY, et al. Oxidative stress is associated with region-specific neuronal death during thiamine deficiency. *J Neuropathol Exp Neurol.* 1999;58:946-958.

22. Carpenter KJ. *Beriberi, White Rice, and Vitamin B: A Disease, a Cause, and a Cure.* Berkeley, CA: University of California Press; 2000:xiv, 282.

23. Centers for Disease Control. Deaths associated with thiamine-deficient total parenteral nutrition. Erratum appears in *MMWR Morb Mortal Wkly Rep.* 1989;38:79.

24. Centers for Disease Control. Lactic acidosis traced to thiamine deficiency related to nationwide shortage of multivitamins for total parenteral nutrition—United States, 1997. *MMWR Morb Mortal Wkly Rep.* 1997;46:523.

25. Chadda K, et al. Acute lactic acidosis with Wernicke's encephalopathy due to acute thiamine deficiency. *Intensive Care Med.* 2002;28:1499.

26. Chan H, et al. Primary cultures of rat astrocytes respond to thiamine deficiency-induced swelling by downregulating aquaporin-4 levels. *Neurosci Lett.* 2004;366:231-234.

27. Cho YP, et al. Severe lactic acidosis and thiamine deficiency during total parenteral nutrition—case report. *Hepatogastroenterology.* 2004;51:253-255.

28. Cline JK, et al. Nutrition classics. *J Am Chem Soc.* 1937;59:1052-1054.

28a. Synthesis of vitamin B1. By Joseph K. Cline, Robert R. Williams, and Jacob Finkeltstein. *Nutr Rev.* 1977;35:238-240.

29. Coats D, et al. Thiamine pharmacokinetics in Cambodian mothers and their breastfed infants. *Am J Clin Nutr.* 2013;98:839-844.

30. Costa NA, et al. Thiamine as a metabolic resuscitator in septic shock: one size does not fit all. *J Thorac Dis.* 2016;8:E471-E472.

31. Cresce ND, et al. Encephalopathy despite thiamine repletion during alcohol withdrawal. *Cleve Clin J Med.* 2014;81:350-352.

32. Dabar G, et al. Shoshin beriberi in critically-Ill patients: case series. *Nutr J.* 2015; 14:51.

33. Davies SB, et al. Wernicke's encephalopathy in a non-alcoholic patient with a normal blood thiamine level. *Med J Aust.* 2011;194:483-484.

34. Day GS, et al. Thiamine prescribing practices within university-affiliated hospitals: a multicenter retrospective review. *J Hosp Med.* 2015;10:246-253.

35. Debs R, et al. Biotin-responsive basal ganglia disease in ethnic Europeans with novel SLC19A3 mutations. *Arch Neurol.* 2010;67:126-130.

36. Descombes E, et al. Acute encephalopathy due to thiamine deficiency (Wernicke's encephalopathy) in a chronic hemodialyzed patient: a case report. *Clin Nephrol.* 1991;35:171-175.

37. Dingwall KM, et al. Hypomagnesaemia and its potential impact on thiamine utilisation in patients with alcohol misuse at the Alice Springs Hospital. *Drug Alcohol Rev.* 2015;34:323-328.

38. Dinicolantonio JJ, et al. Effects of thiamine on cardiac function in patients with systolic heart failure: systematic review and metaanalysis of randomized, double-blind, placebo-controlled trials. *Ochsner J.* 2013;13:495-499.

39. DiNicolantonio JJ, et al. Thiamine supplementation for the treatment of heart failure: a review of the literature. *Congest Heart Fail.* 2013;19:214-222.

40. Donnino MW, et al. Thiamine deficiency in critically ill patients with sepsis. *J Crit Care.* 2010;25:576-581.

41. Drewe J, et al. Effect of intravenous infusions of thiamine on the disposition kinetics of thiamine and its pyrophosphate. *J Clin Pharm Ther.* 2003;28:47-51.

42. Eisenstadt WS. Hypersensitivity to thiamine hydrochloride. *Minn Med.* 1942;85: 861-863.

43. Essa E, et al. Cardiovascular magnetic resonance in wet beriberi. *J Cardiovasc Magn Reson.* 2011;13:41.

44. Faigle R, et al. Dry beriberi mimicking Guillain-Barre syndrome as the first presenting sign of thiamine deficiency. *Eur J Neurol.* 2012;19:e14-e15.

45. Fattal-Valevski A, et al. Outbreak of life-threatening thiamine deficiency in infants in Israel caused by a defective soy-based formula. *Pediatrics.* 2005;115:e233-e238.

46. Ferguson M, et al. Increased mast cell degranulation within thalamus in early prelesion stages of an experimental model of Wernicke's encephalopathy. *J Neuropathol Exp Neurol.* 1999;58:773-783.

47. Flannery AH, et al. Unpeeling the evidence for the banana bag: evidence-based recommendations for the management of alcohol-associated vitamin and electrolyte deficiencies in the ICU. *Crit Care Med.* 2016;44:1545-1552.

48. Foster D, et al. Wernicke encephalopathy after bariatric surgery: losing more than just weight. *Neurology.* 2005;65:1987.

49. Fozi K, et al. Prevalence of thiamine deficiency at a drug rehabilitation centre in Malaysia. *Med J Malaysia.* 2006;61:519-525.

50. Galvin R, et al. EFNS guidelines for diagnosis, therapy and prevention of Wernicke encephalopathy. *Eur J Neurol.* 2010;17:1408-1418.

51. Gioda CR, et al. Thiamine deficiency leads to reduced nitric oxide production and vascular dysfunction in rats. *Nutr Metab Cardiovasc Dis.* 2014;24:183-188.

52. Grao Castellote C, et al. [Carencial neuropathy by thiamine deficiency secondary bariatric surgery]. *Med Clin (Barc).* 2008;131:437-438.

53. Greb A, Bitsch R. Comparative bioavailability of various thiamine derivatives after oral administration. *Int J Clin Pharmacol Ther.* 1998;36:216-221.

54. Guerrini I, et al. Direct genomic PCR sequencing of the high affinity thiamine transporter (SLC19A2) gene identifies three genetic variants in Wernicke Korsakoff syndrome (WKS). *Am J Med Genet B Neuropsychiatr Genet.* 2005;137B:17-19.

55. Guerrini I, et al. Molecular genetics of alcohol-related brain damage. *Alcohol Alcohol.* 2009;44:166-170.

56. Gupta RK, et al. Thiamine deficiency related microstructural brain changes in acute and acute-on-chronic liver failure of non-alcoholic etiology. *Clin Nutr.* 2012;31:422-428.

57. Hack JB, Hoffman RS. Thiamine before glucose to prevent Wernicke encephalopathy: examining the conventional wisdom. *JAMA.* 1998;279:583-584.

58. Hannett B, et al. Formation of oxalate in pyridoxine or thiamin deficient rats during intravenous xylitol infusions. *J Nutr.* 1977;107:458-465.

59. Harata N, Iwasaki Y. Evidence for early blood-brain barrier breakdown in experimental thiamine deficiency in the mouse. *Metab Brain Dis.* 1995;10:159-174.

60. Harper CG, et al. Prevalence of Wernicke-Korsakoff syndrome in Australia: has thiamine fortification made a difference? *Med J Aust.* 1998;168:542-545.

61. Hazell AS. Astrocytes are a major target in thiamine deficiency and Wernicke's encephalopathy. *Neurochem Int.* 2009;55:129-135.

62. Hazell AS, Butterworth RF. Update of cell damage mechanisms in thiamine deficiency: focus on oxidative stress, excitotoxicity and inflammation. *Alcohol Alcohol.* 2009;44:141-147.

63. Herve C, et al. Comparison of erythrocyte transketolase activity with thiamine and thiamine phosphate ester levels in chronic alcoholic patients. *Clin Chim Acta.* 1995;234:91-100.

64. Hirsch JA, Parrott J. New considerations on the neuromodulatory role of thiamine. *Pharmacology.* 2012;89:111-116.

65. Hoyumpa AM Jr, et al. Intestinal thiamin transport: effect of chronic ethanol administration in rats. *Am J Clin Nutr.* 1978;31:938-945.

66. Isenberg-Grzeda E, et al. Nonalcoholic thiamine-related encephalopathy (Wernicke-Korsakoff syndrome) among inpatients with cancer: a series of 18 cases. *Psychosomatics.* 2016;57:71-81.

67. Isenberg-Grzeda E, et al. Prescribing thiamine to inpatients with alcohol use disorders: how well are we doing? *J Addict Med.* 2014;8:1-5.

68. Jamieson CP, et al. The thiamin, riboflavin and pyridoxine status of patients on emergency admission to hospital. *Clin Nutr.* 1999;18:87-91.

69. Jeyakumar D. Thiamine responsive ankle oedema in detention centre inmates. *Med J Malaysia.* 1995;50:17-20.

70. Jhala SS, Hazell AS. Modeling neurodegenerative disease pathophysiology in thiamine deficiency: consequences of impaired oxidative metabolism. *Neurochem Int.* 2011;58:248-260.

71. Juel J, et al. Anaphylactic shock and cardiac arrest caused by thiamine infusion. *BMJ Case Rep.* 2013;2013.

72. Kauffman G, et al. Thiamine deficiency in ill children. *Am J Clin Nutr.* 2011;94:616-617.

73. Kern D, et al. How thiamine diphosphate is activated in enzymes. *Science.* 1997;275:67-70.

74. Kitamura K, et al. Two cases of thiamine deficiency-induced lactic acidosis during total parenteral nutrition. *Tohoku J Exp Med.* 1993;171:129-133.

75. Klein M, et al. Fatal metabolic acidosis caused by thiamine deficiency. *J Emerg Med.* 2004;26:301-303.

76. Kono S, et al. Mutations in a thiamine-transporter gene and Wernicke's-like encephalopathy. *N Engl J Med.* 2009;360:1792-1794.

77. Kruse M, et al. Increased brain endothelial nitric oxide synthase expression in thiamine deficiency: relationship to selective vulnerability. *Neurochem Int.* 2004;45:49-56.

78. Kuba H, et al. Thiamine-deficient lactic acidosis with brain tumor treatment. Report of three cases. *J Neurosurg.* 1998;89:1025-1028.

79. Kwok T, et al. Thiamine status of elderly patients with cardiac failure. *Age Ageing.* 1992;21:67-71.

80. La Selve P, et al. Shoshin beriberi: an unusual complication of prolonged parenteral nutrition. *JPEN J Parenter Enteral Nutr.* 1986;10:102-103.

81. Laforenza U, et al. Thiamine uptake in human intestinal biopsy specimens, including observations from a patient with acute thiamine deficiency. *Am J Clin Nutr.* 1997;66:320-326.

82. Lange R, et al. Lactic acidosis from thiamine deficiency during parenteral nutrition in a two-year-old boy. *Eur J Pediatr Surg.* 1992;2:241-244.

83. Langlais PJ, et al. Depletion of brain histamine produces regionally selective protection against thiamine deficiency-induced lesions in the rat. *Metab Brain Dis.* 2002;17:199-210.

84. Langlais PJ, Zhang SX. Extracellular glutamate is increased in thalamus during thiamine deficiency-induced lesions and is blocked by MK-801. *J Neurochem.* 1993;61:2175-2182.

85. Lavoie J, Butterworth RF. Reduced activities of thiamine-dependent enzymes in brains of alcoholics in the absence of Wernicke's encephalopathy. *Alcohol Clin Exp Res.* 1995;19:1073-1077.

86. Lee BJ, et al. Effects of dietary vitamin B(1) (thiamine) and magnesium on the survival, growth and histological indicators in lake trout (Salvelinus namaycush) juveniles. *Comp Biochem Physiol A Mol Integr Physiol.* 2012;162:219-226.

87. Liang X, et al. Metformin is a substrate and inhibitor of the human thiamine transporter, THTR-2 (SLC19A3). *Mol Pharm.* 2015;12:4301-4310.

88. Lima LF, et al. Low blood thiamine concentrations in children upon admission to the intensive care unit: risk factors and prognostic significance. *Am J Clin Nutr.* 2011;93:57-61.

89. Lingford-Hughes AR, et al. BAP updated guidelines: evidence-based guidelines for the pharmacological management of substance abuse, harmful use, addiction and comorbidity: recommendations from BAP. *J Psychopharmacol.* 2012;26:899-952.

90. Lough ME. Wernicke's encephalopathy: expanding the diagnostic toolbox. *Neuropsychol Rev.* 2012;22:181-194.

91. Ma JJ, Truswell AS. Wernicke-Korsakoff syndrome in Sydney hospitals: before and after thiamine enrichment of flour. *Med J Aust.* 1995;163:531-534.

92. Maiorana A, et al. Acute thiamine deficiency and refeeding syndrome: similar findings but different pathogenesis. *Nutrition.* 2014;30:948-952.

93. McLean J, Manchip S. Wernicke's encephalopathy induced by magnesium depletion. *Lancet.* 1999;353:1768.

94. Merola JF, et al. Clinical problem-solving. At a loss. *N Engl J Med.* 2012;367:67-72.

95. Misumida N, et al. Shoshin beriberi induced by long-term administration of diuretics: a case report. *Case Rep Cardiol.* 2014;2014:878915.

96. Moize V, et al. Nystagmus: an uncommon neurological manifestation of thiamine deficiency as a serious complication of sleeve gastrectomy. *Nutr Clin Pract.* 2012;27:788-792.

97. Morinville V, et al. Anaphylaxis to parenteral thiamine (vitamin B1). *Schweiz Med Wochenschr.* 1998;128:1743-1744.

98. Munujos P, et al. Proto-oncogene c-fos induction in thiamine-deficient encephalopathy. Protective effects of nicardipine on pyrithiamine-induced lesions. *J Neurol Sci.* 1993;118:175-180.

99. Naidoo DP, et al. Acute pernicious beriberi in a patient receiving parenteral nutrition. A case report. *South Afr Med J.* 1989;75:546-548.

100. Nakada T, Knight RT. Alcohol and the central nervous system. *Med Clin North Am.* 1984;68:121-131.

101. Navarro D, et al. Glucose loading precipitates focal lactic acidosis in the vulnerable medial thalamus of thiamine-deficient rats. *Metab Brain Dis.* 2008;23:115-122.

102. O'Keeffe ST. Thiamine deficiency in elderly people. *Age Ageing.* 2000;29:99-101.

103. O'Keeffe ST, et al. Thiamine deficiency in hospitalized elderly patients. *Gerontology.* 1994;40:18-24.

104. O'Rourke NP, et al. Thiamine status of healthy and institutionalized elderly subjects: analysis of dietary intake and biochemical indices. *Age Ageing.* 1990;19:325-329.

105. Oguz SS, et al. A rare case of severe lactic acidosis in a preterm infant: lack of thiamine during total parenteral nutrition. *J Pediatr Endocrinol Metab.* 2011;24:843-845.

106. Oriot D, et al. Severe lactic acidosis related to acute thiamine deficiency. *JPEN J Parenter Enteral Nutr.* 1991;15:105-109.

107. Osman M, Casey P. Angioneurotic oedema secondary to oral thiamine. *BMJ Case Rep.* 2013;2013.

108. Peake RW, et al. The effect of magnesium administration on erythrocyte transketolase activity in alcoholic patients treated with thiamine. *Scott Med J.* 2013;58:139-142.

109. Peters R. The biochemical lesion in vitamin B1 deficiency. *Lancet.* 1936;227:1161-1165.

110. Proebstle TM, et al. Specific IgE and IgG serum antibodies to thiamine associated with anaphylactic reaction. *J Allergy Clin Immunol.* 1995;95(5 Pt 1):1059-1060.

111. Rao VL, Butterworth RF. Thiamine phosphatases in human brain: regional alterations in patients with alcoholic cirrhosis. *Alcohol Clin Exp Res.* 1995;19:523-526.

112. Reingold IM, Webb FR. Sudden death following intravenous injection of thiamine hydrochloride. *JAMA.* 1946;130:491-492.

113. Renthal W, et al. Thiamine deficiency secondary to anorexia nervosa: an uncommon cause of peripheral neuropathy and Wernicke encephalopathy in adolescence. *Pediatr Neurol.* 2014;51:100-103.

114. Reuler JB, et al. Current concepts. Wernicke's encephalopathy. *N Engl J Med.* 1985;312:1035-1039.

115. Rieck J, et al. Urinary loss of thiamine is increased by low doses of furosemide in healthy volunteers. *J Lab Clin Med.* 1999;134:238-243.

116. Rindi G, Laforenza U. Thiamine intestinal transport and related issues: recent aspects. *Proc Soc Exp Biol Med.* 2000;224:246-255.

117. Rocha RM, et al. Influence of spironolactone therapy on thiamine blood levels in patients with heart failure. *Arq Bras Cardiol.* 2008;90:324-328.

118. Romanski SA, McMahon MM. Metabolic acidosis and thiamine deficiency. *Mayo Clin Proc.* 1999;74:259-263.

119. Rovelli A, et al. Severe lactic acidosis due to thiamine deficiency after bone marrow transplantation in a child with acute monocytic leukemia. *Haematologica.* 1990;75:579-581.

120. Sanchez-Larsen A, et al. Cerebral vasospasm and Wernicke encephalopathy secondary to adult cyclic vomiting syndrome: the role of magnesium. *BMC Neurol.* 2016;16:135.

121. Schabelman E, Kuo D. Glucose before thiamine for Wernicke encephalopathy: a literature review. *J Emerg Med.* 2012;42:488-494.

122. Schiff L. Collapse following parenteral administration of solution of thiamine hydrochloride. *JAMA.* 1941;117:609.

123. Schoenenberger AW, et al. Thiamine supplementation in symptomatic chronic heart failure: a randomized, double-blind, placebo-controlled, cross-over pilot study. *Clin Res Cardiol.* 2012;101:159-164.

124. Schramm C, et al. Thiamine for the treatment of nucleoside analogue-induced severe lactic acidosis. *Eur J Anaesthesiol.* 1999;16:733-735.

125. Sebastian JL, et al. Thiamine deficiency in a gastric bypass patient leading to acute neurologic compromise after plastic surgery. *Surg Obes Relat Dis.* 2010;6:105-106.

126. Sekiyama S, et al. Peripheral neuropathy due to thiamine deficiency after inappropriate diet and total gastrectomy. *Tokai J Exp Clin Med.* 2005;30:137-140.

127. Seligmann H, et al. Thiamine deficiency in patients with congestive heart failure receiving long-term furosemide therapy: a pilot study. *Am J Med.* 1991;91:151-155.

128. Serrano M, et al. Reversible generalized dystonia and encephalopathy from thiamine transporter 2 deficiency. *Mov Disord.* 2012;27:1295-1298.

129. Sgouros X, et al. Evaluation of a clinical screening instrument to identify states of thiamine deficiency in inpatients with severe alcohol dependence syndrome. *Alcohol Alcohol.* 2004;39:227-232.

130. Shimon I, et al. Improved left ventricular function after thiamine supplementation in patients with congestive heart failure receiving long-term furosemide therapy. *Am J Med.* 1995;98:485-490.

131. Skelton WP 3rd, Skelton NK. Thiamine deficiency neuropathy. It's still common today. *Postgrad Med.* 1989;85:301-306.

132. Smithline HA, et al. Pharmacokinetics of high-dose oral thiamine hydrochloride in healthy subjects. *BMC Clin Pharmacol.* 2012;12:4.

133. Spinazzi M, et al. Subacute sensory ataxia and optic neuropathy with thiamine deficiency. *Nat Rev Neurol.* 2010;6:288-293.

134. Sriram K, et al. Thiamine in nutrition therapy. *Nutr Clin Pract.* 2012;27:41-50.

135. Steinberg A, et al. Thiamine deficiency in stem cell transplant patients: a case series with an accompanying review of the literature. *Clin Lymphoma Myeloma Leuk.* 2014;14(suppl):S111-S113.

136. Stephen JM, et al. Anaphylaxis from administration of intravenous thiamine. *Am J Emerg Med.* 1992;10:61-63.

137. Stiles MH. Hypersensitivity to thiamine chloride with a note on sensitivity to pyridoxine hydrochloride. *J Allergy.* 1941;12:507-509.

138. Strain J, Kling C. Thiamine dosing for Wernicke's encephalopathy in alcoholics: is traditional dosing inadequate? *S D Med.* 2010;63:316-317.

139. Subramanian VS, et al. Biotin-responsive basal ganglia disease-linked mutations inhibit thiamine transport via hTHTR2: biotin is not a substrate for hTHTR2. *Am J Physiol Cell Physiol.* 2006;291:C851-C859.

140. Subramanya SB, et al. Chronic alcohol consumption and intestinal thiamin absorption: effects on physiological and molecular parameters of the uptake process. *Am J Physiol Gastrointest Liver Physiol.* 2010;299:G23-G31.

141. Svahn J, et al. Severe lactic acidosis due to thiamine deficiency in a patient with B-cell leukemia/lymphoma on total parenteral nutrition during high-dose methotrexate therapy. *J Pediatr Hematol Oncol.* 2003;25:965-968.

142. Tabarki B, et al. Biotin-responsive basal ganglia disease revisited: clinical, radiologic, and genetic findings. *Neurology.* 2013;80:261-267.

143. Takasaki E. The urinary excretion of oxalic acid in vitamin B1 deficient rats. *Invest Urol.* 1969;7:150-153.

144. Tallaksen CM, et al. Kinetics of thiamin and thiamin phosphate esters in human blood, plasma and urine after 50 mg intravenously or orally. *Eur J Clin Pharmacol.* 1993;44:73-78.

145. Tate JR, Nixon PF. Measurement of Michaelis constant for human erythrocyte transketolase and thiamin diphosphate. *Anal Biochem.* 1987;160:78-87.

146. Teigen LM, et al. Prevalence of thiamine deficiency in a stable heart failure outpatient cohort on standard loop diuretic therapy. *Clin Nutr.* 2016;35:1323-1327.

147. Tesfaye S, et al. Pregnant, vomiting, and going blind. *Lancet.* 1998;352:1594.

148. Thomson AD, et al. Patterns of 35S-thiamine hydrochloride absorption in the malnourished alcoholic patient. *J Lab Clin Med.* 1970;76:34-45.

149. Thomson AD, et al. Wernicke's encephalopathy revisited. Translation of the case history section of the original manuscript by Carl Wernicke "Lehrbuch der Gehirnkrankheiten fur Aerzte und Studirende" (1881) with a commentary. *Alcohol Alcohol.* 2008;43:174-179.

150. Thomson AD, et al. The Royal College of Physicians report on alcohol: guidelines for managing Wernicke's encephalopathy in the accident and Emergency Department. *Alcohol Alcohol.* 2002;37:513-521.

151. Thomson AD, et al. Thiamine propyl disulfide: absorption and utilization. *Ann Intern Med.* 1971;74:529-534.

152. Thomson AD, et al. The evolution and treatment of Korsakoff's syndrome: out of sight, out of mind? *Neuropsychol Rev.* 2012;22:81-92.

153. Thomson AD, Marshall EJ. The treatment of patients at risk of developing Wernicke's encephalopathy in the community. *Alcohol Alcohol.* 2006;41:159-167.

154. Tung C, et al. The pharmacokinetics of chlorbutol in man. *Biopharm Drug Dispos.* 1982;3:371-378.

155. Velez RJ, et al. Severe acute metabolic acidosis (acute beriberi): an avoidable complication of total parenteral nutrition. *JPEN J Parenter Enteral Nutr.* 1985;9:216-219.

156. Victor M, et al. The Wernicke-Korsakoff syndrome. A clinical and pathological study of 245 patients, 82 with post-mortem examinations. *Contemp Neurol Ser.* 1971;7:1-206.

157. Victor M, Yakovlev PI. S.S. Korsakoff's psychic disorhic disorder in conjunction with peripheral neuritis; a translation of Korsakoff's original article with comments on the author and his contribution to clinical medicine. *Neurology.* 1955;5:394-406.

158. Vortmeyer AO, et al. Haemorrhagic thiamine deficient encephalopathy following prolonged parenteral nutrition. *J Neurol Neurosurg Psychiatry*. 1992;55:826-829.

159. Ward KE, Happel KI. An eating disorder leading to wet beriberi heart failure in a 30-year-old woman. *Am J Emerg Med*. 2013;31:460 e5-6.

160. Watson AJ, et al. Acute Wernickes encephalopathy precipitated by glucose loading. *Ir J Med Sci*. 1981;150:301-303.

161. Weber W, et al. Nonlinear kinetics of the thiamine cation in humans: saturation of nonrenal clearance and tubular reabsorption. *J Pharmacokinet Biopharm*. 1990;18:501-523.

162. Weigand CG. Reactions attributed to administration of thiamine chloride. *Geriatrics*. 1950;5:274-279.

163. Whitfield KC, et al. Perinatal consumption of thiamine-fortified fish sauce in rural Cambodia: a randomized clinical trial. *JAMA Pediatr*. 2016:e162065.

164. Wilson EC, et al. The long-term cost to the UK NHS and Social Services of different durations of IV thiamine (vitamin B1) for chronic alcohol misusers with symptoms of Wernicke's encephalopathy presenting at the emergency department. *Appl Health Econ Health Policy*. 2016;14:205-215.

165. Wilson JD, Madison LL. Deficiency of thiamine (beriberi), pyridoxine, and riboflavin. In: Isaselbacher KJ, et al., eds. *Harrison's Principles of Internal Medicine*, 9th ed. New York, NY: McGraw-Hill; 1980:425-429.

166. Wood B, Currie J. Presentation of acute Wernicke's encephalopathy and treatment with thiamine. *Metab Brain Dis*. 1995;10:57-72.

167. Wrenn KD, et al. A toxicity study of parenteral thiamine hydrochloride. *Ann Emerg Med*. 1989;18:867-870.

168. Xie F, et al. Pharmacokinetic study of benfotiamine and the bioavailability assessment compared to thiamine hydrochloride. *J Clin Pharmacol*. 2014;54:688-695.

169. Yamada K, et al. A wide spectrum of clinical and brain MRI findings in patients with SLC19A3 mutations. *BMC Med Genet*. 2010;11:171.

170. Yeh WY, et al. Thiamine-deficient optic neuropathy associated with Wernicke's encephalopathy in patients with chronic diarrhea. *J Formos Med Assoc*. 2013;112:165-170.

171. Zangen A, et al. Furosemide and digoxin inhibit thiamine uptake in cardiac cells. *Eur J Pharmacol*. 1998;361:151-155.

172. Zhao Y, et al. Decreased transketolase activity contributes to impaired hippocampal neurogenesis induced by thiamine deficiency. *J Neurochem*. 2009;111:537-546.

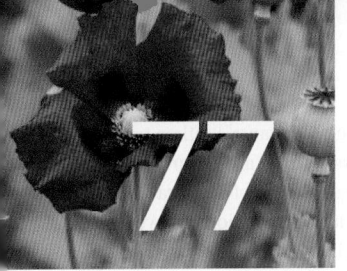

77 ALCOHOL WITHDRAWAL

Jeffrey A. Gold and Lewis S. Nelson

HISTORY AND EPIDEMIOLOGY

The medical problems associated with alcoholism and alcohol withdrawal were initially described by Pliny the Elder in the first century B.C. In his work *Naturalis Historia*, the alcoholic and alcohol withdrawal were described as follows: "drunkenness brings pallor and sagging cheeks, sore eyes, and trembling hands that spill a full cup, of which the immediate punishment is a haunted sleep and unrestful nights."[74] Initial treatments as described by Osler at the turn of the 20th century were focused on supportive care, including confinement to bed, cold baths to reduce fever, and judicious use of potassium bromide, chloral hydrate, hyoscine, and possibly opium.[18]

Some of the initial large series of alcohol related complications in the early 20th century describe alcohol use as a major public health concern. At Bellevue Hospital in New York City, there were 7,000 to 10,000 admissions per year for alcohol-related problems from 1902 to 1935, with an estimated rate of 2.5 to 5 admissions per 1,000 New York City residents.[45] Many of these patients were described as having "alcoholomania" or "acute alcoholic delirium."

A similar number of admissions to Boston City Hospital was also reported, with up to 10% of people with alcoholism admitted with evidence of delirium tremens (DTs).[69] The mortality rate at the beginning of the study among patients with DTs was 52% (1912), and DTs was the leading cause of death among admitted people with alcoholism. Over the ensuing 20 years, this rate declined to approximately 10% to 12%, a decrease believed to be secondary to improved supportive care and nursing.

Although people with alcoholism were widely recognized as having a high incidence of delirium and psychomotor agitation, whether this was caused by ethanol use, ethanol abstinence, or coexisting psychological disorders was debated. Isbell and colleagues performed a highly controversial study in 1955, proving that abstinence from alcohol was responsible for DTs when they subjected 9 male prisoners to chronic alcohol ingestion for a period of 6 to 12 weeks followed by 2 weeks of abstinence.[43] During the abstinence phase, 6 of the 9 men developed tremor, elevations in blood pressure and heart rate, diaphoresis, and varying degrees of either auditory or visual hallucinations, consistent with the diagnosis of DTs. In addition, 2 of the 9 men developed convulsions, further linking alcohol abstinence to seizures. However, it should be noted that the high rate of development of DTs (67%) is atypical and does not represent the true prevalence found in later epidemiologic studies.[16]

Alcoholism and the various manifestations of the alcohol withdrawal syndrome (AWS) still represent major problems in both the inpatient and outpatient setting. Ethanol is responsible for approximately 3.8% of all deaths worldwide (6.3% of men and 1.1% of women) and accounts for 4.6% of the global burden of disease (7.6% of men and 1.4% of women).[79] The lifetime risk of alcohol use disorders in men is more than 20%, with a risk of about 15% for alcohol abuse and 10% for alcohol dependence.[88]

Alcohol-related complications accounted for 21% of all medical intensive care unit (ICU) admissions, with alcohol withdrawal being the most common alcohol-related diagnosis.[61] Further, the presence of any alcohol use disorder (alcohol abuse, dependence or harmful alcohol use) was associated with a 2-fold increase in mortality amongst ICU patients with organ failure.[66] In other studies, 8% of all general hospital admissions, 16% of all postsurgical patients, and 31% of all trauma patients developed alcohol withdrawal.[29] The development of alcohol withdrawal in postsurgical and trauma patients is associated nearly threefold increase in mortality in this population.[5]

PATHOPHYSIOLOGY

Intensive research over the past 2 decades provides valuable insight into the mechanism of alcohol withdrawal, allowing for better understanding of both the clinical spectrum of the disorder and potential therapeutic interventions (Chap. 14). Alcohol withdrawal syndrome is a neurologic disorder with a continuum of progressively worsening effects caused by the reduction or discontinuation of ethanol in a person who has developed ethanol dependence following chronic and heavy ethanol use. Alcohol withdrawal syndrome is often exacerbated by the clinical manifestations of heavy alcohol intake (eg, nutritional depletion, impaired immunity, anemia, cirrhosis, and head trauma).

The effects of chronic alcohol consumption on neurotransmitter function best explains the clinical findings. Persistent stimulation of the inhibitory γ-aminobutyric acid (GABA) receptor chloride channel complex by ethanol leads to downregulation.[14] This allows the alcohol user to maintain a relatively normal level of consciousness, as well as cognitive and motor function despite the presence of sedative concentrations of ethanol in the brain. A continued escalation of the steady-state serum ethanol concentration is required to achieve euphoria due to the development of tolerance, which results from progressive desensitization of the GABA receptor chloride channel complex.[53] The exact mechanism by which this adaptive change occurs is incompletely understood but involves in part substitution of an α_4 for an α_1 receptor subunit on the $GABA_A$ receptor (Chaps. 13 and 14). A converse series of events occurs at the N-methyl-D-aspartate (NMDA) subtype of glutamate receptor. Binding of ethanol to the glycine binding site of this receptor inhibits the NMDA receptor function, resulting in compensatory quantitative upregulation of these excitatory receptors (as opposed to a subunit component change in the GABA receptors).[36] Thus withdrawal of alcohol is associated with both a decrease in GABAergic activity and an increase in glutamatergic activity.[14] This phenomenon of a concomitant loss of inhibition and increased excitation results in the clinical manifestations of autonomic excitability and psychomotor agitation associated with alcohol withdrawal (Figs. 14-1 and 14-2).[73]

Repeated episodes of alcohol withdrawal lead to permanent alterations in neurotransmitters and their receptors. In rats, repeated episodes of alcohol withdrawal leads to persistent and progressive electroencephalographic abnormalities, with subsequent episodes of withdrawal becoming increasingly resistant to benzodiazepines. Both clinical observation and in vitro data also suggest permanent dysregulation of GABA receptors, and thiamine and other nutritional deficiencies are implicated in structural brain changes in animal models.[70] These effects are proposed explanation for both the "kindling phenomenon," which is the clinical observation of an increasing severity of alcohol withdrawal among individual subjects, and the development of benzodiazepine-resistant alcohol withdrawal.[106]

CLINICAL MANIFESTATIONS

Alcohol withdrawal is defined in the *Diagnostic and Statistical Manual of Mental Disorders*, 5th edition (*DSM-V*) as the cessation of heavy or prolonged alcohol use resulting, within a period of a few hours to several days, in the development of 2 or more of the clinical findings listed in Table 77–1. Alcohol withdrawal can be qualitatively classified both by timing (eg, early versus late) and severity (eg, mild, moderate, severe). However, despite the availability of scoring systems (see next paragraph), there are no adequate or fully accepted criteria by which to define these categorizations, and many of the components require subjective interpretation. Furthermore, the clinical

TABLE 77–1	Diagnostic Criteria for Alcohol Withdrawal Syndrome[4]

A. Cessation of or reduction in alcohol intake, which has previously been prolonged or heavy.

B. Criterion A, plus any 2 of the following symptoms developing within several hours to a few days:

Anxiety

Autonomic hyperactivity

Hallucinations

Insomnia

Nausea and vomiting

Psychomotor agitation

Seizures (generalized tonic–clonic)

Tremor (worsening)

C. The above symptoms cause clinically significant distress or impairment in social, occupational, or other important areas of functioning.

D. The above symptoms are not attributable to other causes; for example, another mental disorder, intoxication, or withdrawal from another substance.

Specify if hallucinations (usually visual or tactile) occur with intact reality testing, or if auditory, visual, or tactile illusions occur in the absence of a delirium.

course of alcohol withdrawal varies widely among patients, and progression of individual patients through these different stages is also highly variable.[100] In fact, some extensive alcohol users experience no significant withdrawal after the cessation of alcohol consumption. Recognizing these limitations, this conceptual framework still proves helpful in the clinical management of patients with alcohol withdrawal.

One of the more commonly used means for accurately assessing the severity of alcohol withdrawal is the Clinical Institute Withdrawal Assessment of Alcohol Scale, Revised (CIWA-Ar) score.[95] This scoring system contains 10 clinical categories and requires less than 5 minutes to complete. In an attempt to improve the specificity and simplicity of the score, the Glasgow Modified Alcohol Withdrawal Scale (GMAWS) was developed and validated, demonstrating clinical comparability to the CIWA-Ar.[15] However, use of either CIWA or GNWAS is limited by the requirement of subjective assessments by the patient; they cannot be adequately performed in highly agitated or sedated patients and are difficult to use in situations with language barriers. For these reasons, we prefer the use of general alertness scales such as the Richmond Agitation Sedation Scale (RASS) or Riker Sedation Anesthesia Scale (SAS), which are observer based.[81,90] In one study, use of the SAS was associated with a reduction in intensive care unit (ICU) length of stay and reduction in sedative use compared with use of the CIWA.[89] Scoring systems are essential not only for symptom-triggered therapy, but they also provide a basis for comparative analysis of clinical trials in ethanol withdrawal. Greater use of semiobjective CIWA-Ar, GMWAS, RASS, SAS, or a comparable validated scale remain essential for interpretation of both genetic and treatment trials.

Early Uncomplicated Withdrawal

Alcohol withdrawal begins as early as 6 hours after the cessation of drinking. Early withdrawal is characterized by autonomic hyperactivity, including tachycardia, hypertension, fine tremor, and diaphoresis, as well as psychological changes such as emotional lability, anxiety, insomnia, and psychomotor agitation. This constellation of findings is sometimes called *alcoholic tremulousness.*[98] Although these clinical effects are uncomfortable, they are not generally harmful. Most patients who ultimately develop severe manifestations of AWS initially develop these findings, but this is not universal. At this "stage" of AWS, the clinical effects are still readily amenable to treatment with ethanol, as is done daily by many patients with alcohol use disorder when they take an "eye opener."

Alcoholic Hallucinosis

Nearly 25% of patients with alcohol withdrawal will develop transient hallucinations, and a subset of these patients will develop alcoholic hallucinosis, which is characterized by vivid hallucinations that are generally transient but do infrequently last several weeks.[31,99] Although classically

these hallucinations are tactile or visual ("pink elephants"), other types of hallucinations, particularly auditory and persecutory, are described. Tactile hallucinations include formication, or the sensation of ants crawling on the skin, which can result in repeated itching and excoriations. However, as opposed to DTs, patients with alcoholic hallucinosis have a clear sensorium. The presence of alcoholic hallucinosis is neither a positive nor a negative predictor of the subsequent development of DTs.[32]

Alcohol Withdrawal Seizures

Approximately 10% of patients with alcohol withdrawal develop seizures, or "rum fits." For many patients, a generalized seizure is the first manifestation of the alcohol withdrawal.[98] Approximately 40% of patients with alcohol withdrawal seizures have isolated seizures, and 3% develop status epilepticus.[100] Alcohol withdrawal seizures often occur in the absence of other signs of alcohol withdrawal and are characteristically brief, generalized, tonic–clonic events with a short postictal period. However, for approximately one-third of patients with DTs, the sentinel event is an isolated alcohol withdrawal seizure.[65] Rapid recovery and normal mental status initially minimize the seriousness of an alcohol withdrawal seizures.[100] Finally, clinicians should be cognizant that many people with alcoholism are prescribed antiepileptics because they have a preexisting seizure disorder, often related to repetitive brain trauma.[42] Conversely, the use of antiepileptics does not unequivocally indicate the presence of a preexisting seizure disorder because of the difficulty in differentiating these seizures from those of alcohol withdrawal.

Delirium Tremens

Delirium tremens is the most serious manifestation of alcohol withdrawal and generally occurs between 48 and 96 hours after the cessation of drinking.[98] Many of the clinical characteristics of DTs are similar to those of uncomplicated early alcohol withdrawal, differing only in severity, and include tremors, autonomic instability (hypertension and tachycardia), and psychomotor agitation. However, unlike the other forms of alcohol withdrawal, DTs is defined by either (1) disturbance of consciousness (eg, reduced clarity of awareness of the environment) with reduced ability to focus, sustain, or shift attention, delirium, confusion, and frank psychosis, or (2) a change in cognition (eg, memory deficit, disorientation, and language disturbance) or the development of a perceptual disturbance that is not better accounted for by a preexisting, established, or evolving dementia.[4] Unlike the early manifestations of alcohol withdrawal, which typically last for 3 to 5 days, DTs often lasts for up to 2 weeks.

RISK FACTORS FOR THE DEVELOPMENT OF ALCOHOL WITHDRAWAL

Factors determining whether an individual will develop withdrawal and to what severity are not well identified. As already mentioned, the development of alcohol dependence is a prerequisite, and this requires several days or longer of nearly continuous consumption of alcohol. The strongest predictor for the development of alcohol withdrawal is a history of prior episodes of withdrawal or DTs or a family history of alcoholic withdrawal.[34,49] These factors, in addition to a select number of clinical and biochemical variables, were combined to create the Prediction of Alcohol Withdrawal Severity Scale (PAWSS), which demonstrated a 93% sensitivity for predicting complicated alcohol withdrawal among hospitalized patients.[60]

The influence of family history on the development of withdrawal suggests a strong role for genetic factors. A growing number of studies have identified associated polymorphisms, including genes involved in dopaminergic neurotransmission, glutamate signaling, cannabinoid receptors, serotonin signaling, and neuropeptide Y.[97] However, these findings must be interpreted with caution. First, whether these findings represent a predisposition to greater ethanol consumption because of an enhanced mesolimbic reward system or some other underlying pathophysiologic effect is unclear. Second, many of the studies do not systematically discriminate among alcoholic tremulousness, alcoholic hallucinosis, withdrawal seizures, and DTs, all of which are potentially regulated by different pathways. Finally, almost uniformly these studies are small (fewer than 200 participants) and are racially homogenous, making it imperative that these be replicated on a larger scale and among different racial groups. Larger and more varied patient cohorts that include both women and nonwhite ethnic groups are required before any definitive conclusions can be drawn. Racial predisposition to the development or severity of alcohol withdrawal is not definitive, but the experience at our institution suggests that African American patients are at lower risk of developing severe DTs than whites.[19]

DIAGNOSTIC TESTING
Clinical and Biochemical Predictors
Numerous attempts have been made to develop biochemical predictors for the presence or severity of alcohol withdrawal. Although consistent abnormalities in readily obtained laboratory values are observed in patients with alcohol withdrawal (eg, aminotransferases, magnesium, mean corpuscular volume), their role in predicting the severity is poorly understood. In one study, an alanine aminotransferase of greater than 50 U/L, a serum chloride less than 96 mEq/L, and a serum potassium less than 3.6 mEq/L were all associated with the development of alcohol withdrawal in patients admitted to a detoxification center.[104] Another study noted that risk factors for DTs included a significant hypokalemia, thrombocytopenia, and prevalence of structural brain lesions.[27] However, the varied and generally low specificity of these derangements makes it difficult to assess their predictive value, especially when accounting for other clinical characteristics such as prior history, initial ethanol concentration, and admission CIWA-Ar or RASS score. In addition, there is a negative association between the presence of severe alcohol withdrawal and histopathologic cirrhosis, further clouding the usefulness of routine laboratory testing for prognostication.[6]

Other investigators have focused specifically on blood ethanol concentration as a predictor for the severity of alcohol withdrawal in at-risk subjects. In one study of patients entering a detoxification program, an admission blood ethanol concentration of greater than 150 mg/dL had a 100% sensitivity and a 57% specificity for the need for treatment of alcohol withdrawal.[101] At a different treatment facility, an ethanol concentration of greater than 150 mg/dL had an 81% positive predictive value for the need to use more than a single dose of chlordiazepoxide.[101] In a third study, an ethanol concentration of greater than 200 mg/dL was a factor in predicting complicated alcohol withdrawal.[60] In addition, admission blood ethanol concentrations in patients with alcohol withdrawal seizures were twofold higher than in those without seizures, irrespective of whether or not they had a history of prior withdrawal seizures. However, these results should be interpreted with caution and in the context of the clinical presentation because other studies yield conflicting results. For example, in one study, an admission ethanol concentration of lower than 100 mg/dL was associated with an increased risk of recurrent alcohol withdrawal seizures, and in another study, admission ethanol concentrations failed to predict the development of DTs.[20,77] There are many potential explanations, including differences in patient population, differences in cohort size, and the late onset of DTs, at a time when ethanol concentrations would be extremely low or nonexistent.

Homocysteine and B vitamin concentrations as well as hepatic function tests are associated with the development of alcohol withdrawal, although there are several contradictory study results.[38,49] Because many studies are based on small numbers of often highly selected subjects and some are promising but not prospectively validated, their generalizability is typically poor.[104] Numerous reports document hyperhomocysteinemia in alcoholism, presumably caused by a deficiency of dietary folic acid. Furthermore, homocysteine and its metabolites act as excitatory neurotransmitters at the NMDA receptor and cause seizures and excitatory neuronal death. In one study, serum homocysteine concentrations were predictive of the development of alcohol withdrawal seizures.[11] However, in this study, there was very strong correlation ($r^2 = 0.7666$; $P <0.001$) between admission blood ethanol concentrations and homocysteine concentrations and the development of seizures, raising doubts as to whether the determination of homocysteine concentration holds any advantage over blood ethanol concentrations.

MANAGEMENT
Alcohol Withdrawal Seizures
Alcohol withdrawal seizures are perhaps the most rigorously studied complication of alcohol withdrawal. They are generally self-limited, and if treatment is needed, benzodiazepines are preferred. In a randomized, placebo-controlled trial of 229 participants with alcohol withdrawal seizures, 2 mg of intramuscular lorazepam reduced the risk of recurrent seizure from 24% to 3% ($P <0.001$) at 6 hours and the need for hospital admission from 42% to 29% ($P = 0.02$).[23] However, whether this interrupts the natural history of progression to DTs is not known. There is no role for phenytoin in either treatment or prevention of alcohol withdrawal seizures. In multiple trials, phenytoin was ineffective in preventing recurrent seizures.[2,76] The most likely explanation for the failure of phenytoin is its inability to regulate γ-aminobutyric acid (GABA) or N-methyl-D-aspartate (NMDA) receptors, the principal mediators of seizures in alcohol withdrawal. One exception to this lack of usefulness occurs in alcoholic patients with a non–alcohol withdrawal–mediated seizure (eg, traumatic injury) or a history of underlying seizure disorders.

Alcohol Withdrawal
In the early stages of alcohol withdrawal, many patients are able to self-medicate with additional ethanol consumption. Among those who seek medical attention, many patients with alcohol withdrawal can be safely managed as outpatients. Outpatient management has significant cost savings with little effect on treatment outcome.[92] In one study, patients who were not clinically intoxicated, had no history of either DTs or alcohol withdrawal seizures, had no comorbid psychiatric or medical disorders, and had a CIWA-Ar score of less than 8 were safely managed as outpatients.[3] Patients not meeting these criteria were referred to inpatient detoxification centers or medical units, depending on the severity of withdrawal and other comorbid conditions.

For all patients with alcohol withdrawal, the initial stages of therapy remain the same and should include a thorough assessment to identify a coexisting medical, psychiatric, or toxicologic disorder. In particular, an assessment for CNS trauma and infection should include the use of computed tomography and lumbar puncture as indicated. Patients with altered cognition and an elevated body temperature should receive antibiotics, pending the results of a lumbar puncture. In concert with this approach, adequate supportive care should be instituted, including maneuvers to address any abnormal vital signs such as body temperature.

Chronic ethanol consumption leads to severe vitamin and nutritional deficiencies and electrolyte disturbances that should be corrected. Specifically, thiamine is recommended for all patients to prevent the development of Wernicke encephalopathy.[25] It was historically suggested that thiamine should be given before the administration of dextrose to prevent precipitation of Wernicke encephalopathy.[64,102] This is a highly unlikely event, and it will suffice to administer the thiamine simultaneously or shortly after the dextrose.

A systematic review of all articles related to nutritional and electrolyte deficiencies in patients with alcohol use disorders and not specific to alcohol withdrawal suggests that the typical "banana bag" be abandoned in lieu of specific nutritional supplementation.[28] The recommendations, which are not subsequently validated, suggest that there is strong support for the administration of thiamine, 200 to 500 mg intravenously every 8 hours in the first day. In addition, the authors suggest that there is reasonable support for the administration of magnesium sulfate, 64 mg/kg intravenously and folic acid, 400 to 1,000 mcg intravenously over this same time period. We believe that these higher doses of thiamine are appropriate in the range of therapy for Wernicke–Korsakoff syndrome. We recommend an initial dose of parenteral thiamine of 100 mg in the management of the patient with alcohol withdrawal.

In addition, there is a high incidence of intravascular volume depletion among people with alcoholism, volume resuscitation is recommended in patients with clinically significant alcohol withdrawal. Of 39 deaths between 1915 and 1936 attributed to DTs in which volume status was recorded, all participants were volume depleted.[69] Finally, for patients with AWS, prevention of nosocomial complications is paramount for reducing hospital stays. Currently, in addition to adequate volume replacement, we recommend that all patients (1) be kept with the head of the bed elevated to prevent aspiration and (2) that deep vein thrombosis prophylaxis be given if the patient is bed bound for an extended period.

The association of alcohol withdrawal with severe psychomotor agitation led to early use of sedative–hypnotics. In a landmark study, 547 patients were randomized to one of 4 drugs (chlordiazepoxide, chlorpromazine, hydroxyzine, or thiamine) or to placebo for the treatment of alcohol withdrawal.[46] Patients receiving chlordiazepoxide had the lowest incidence of both alcohol withdrawal seizures and DTs, establishing benzodiazepines as a first-line agent for treatment of alcohol withdrawal. Of note, use of chlorpromazine, an antipsychotic, is associated with a significant increase in the incidence of seizures in both humans and animal models.[13,46]

Since this study, numerous trials have compared different routes of administration among various sedative–hypnotics, both to each other and to placebo. Because of the historical use noted earlier, chlordiazepoxide remains widely used in outpatient clinics and inpatient detoxification services. Oral benzodiazepine administration is generally effective in patients with early or mild alcohol withdrawal, although initial rapid titration with an intravenous (IV) regimen may be more efficient. Benzodiazepines administered intravenously have a rapid onset of action and among the benzodiazepines, IV diazepam offers the most rapid time to peak clinical effects, which limits the oversedation that may occur after the administration of lorazepam, which has a slower onset to the peak drug effect. Because of the delayed peak clinical effect of lorazepam of approximately 10 to 20 minutes, several doses may be administered in rapid succession with little clinical effect followed by the appearance of the sedative effect of the cumulative doses. Midazolam may be administered intramuscularly if IV access is not available.[91] Although no significant differences are observed among benzodiazepines and barbiturates in terms of mortality or the duration of delirium, the improved pharmacokinetic and safety profile as well as the ease of administration favor benzodiazepines over barbiturates when an IV medication is required.[3,50]

Other pharmacokinetic factors and experience confirm that diazepam is the preferred benzodiazepine for initial IV use in patients with moderate to severe alcohol withdrawal. Diazepam has a long half-life and 2 active metabolites (desmethyldiazepam and oxazepam). The prolonged half-life (48–72 hours) of desmethyldiazepam further extends the effective duration of action of the initial dose of diazepam.[111] A study comparing oral diazepam with oral lorazepam found that the former was associated with a more comfortable recovery, likely because of the active metabolites.[82] A retrospective review reported that the use of a single benzodiazepine rather than multiple benzodiazepines was a marker for treatment success in surgical patients experiencing alcohol withdrawal during surgical admission.[72] These data suggest that it is more important to sedate the patient rapidly with adequate doses of a single benzodiazepine than to use multiple treatments in hopes of finding an effective regimen. Finally, it should be noted that in patients with advanced liver disease, the use of diazepam may result in a very prolonged period of sedation because of impaired clearance of the parent compound and its metabolites. Consequently, in these patients, a benzodiazepine without active metabolites, such as lorazepam, is recommended.

The initial management of patients with AWS should include rapid titration with a benzodiazepine to achieve sedation.[71] An oral benzodiazepine, such as chlordiazepoxide or diazepam, should be sufficient, but certain patients require IV medication. The goal of therapy is to have the patient sedated but breathing spontaneously, with normal vital signs. Although normalization of vital signs is not a mandatory therapeutic endpoint, abnormal vital signs despite adequate sedation should prompt a search for comorbidities. In many patients, attaining complete sedation using a loading protocol allows for autotitration; that is, as alcohol withdrawal resolves, the blood concentrations of the benzodiazepine decrease, allowing gradual clinical recovery.[59] In practicality, most patients need periodic symptom triggered redosing with benzodiazepines to maintain adequate sedation. This

is particularly important in patients develop withdrawal with alcohol withdrawal a concomitantly elevated blood alcohol concentration. Their benzodiazepine requirements using symptom-triggered therapy typically parallel the decline in their blood alcohol concentration.

Multiple studies suggest that if additional doses are required, they should be administered based on symptoms ("symptom triggered") as opposed to on a fixed dosing schedule.[17] In 2 randomized controlled trials, administration of benzodiazepine in a symptom-triggered fashion reduced both the total amount of benzodiazepine and the duration of treatment.[24,85] In these trials, benzodiazepines were administered every hour as long as the CIWA-Ar score remained greater than 8 to 10. In both trials, symptom-triggered therapy resulted in a 4- to 6-fold reduction in the duration of therapy and a 4- to 5-fold reduction in the total amount of benzodiazepine administered, with no increase in withdrawal seizures or adverse events. Symptom-triggered doses in patients with moderate or severe alcohol withdrawal using IV diazepam 10 to 20 mg or lorazepam 2 to 4 mg. For less symptomatic patients, oral chlordiazepoxide 50 to 100 mg is recommended. However, it is important to note that the decision to treat in the symptom-triggered group was made based on CIWA-Ar score (usually >8), which demonstrates the usefulness of standardized scoring and evaluation tools. It should also be noted that in both these trials, patients had very mild withdrawal symptoms, with mean CIWA-Ar scores of 9 to 11. Although experience suggests that this same regimen is also effective in patients with more severe withdrawal or DTs, it has not been validated in this population. Furthermore, it must be emphasized that protocolized use of the CIWA-Ar score depends on a significant history of recent heavy drinking and a communicative subject. A prospective analysis of complex medical-surgical patients enrolled in a CIWA-Ar protocol suggested that more than 50% of the patients failed to have recent alcohol use and could not communicate, leading to unnecessary treatment.[37] Consequently, we agree with studies that use generalized sedation or agitation scales such as the SAS or RASS in these populations. Using the SAS was associated with reduced ICU length of stay compared with CIWA in ICU admitted patients with withdrawal/DTs.[89]

Resistant Alcohol Withdrawal and Delirium Tremens

There is a subgroup of patients with alcohol withdrawal who require very large doses of diazepam or another comparable drug to achieve initial sedation.[35] This same group often has exceedingly high benzodiazepine requirements to maintain this degree of sedation. Patients with resistant alcohol withdrawal and DTs are often have benzodiazepine requirements that exceed 2,600 mg of diazepam within the first 24 hours and generally require admission to an ICU or step-down unit.[86,106] Patients admitted to the Bellevue hospital medical ICU for resistant alcohol withdrawal had very high diazepam requirements, with a mean of 234 mg (range, 10–1,490 mg) required in the first 24 hours and individual doses of diazepam that often exceeded 100 mg to control their agitation. These patients comprised approximately 5% of all ICU admissions, with nearly 40% of patients requiring mechanical ventilation and a mean ICU length of stay of 5.7 days.[33]

The approach to the management of patients with resistant alcohol withdrawal depends on several factors, including the availability of an ICU bed. In the ICU, despite the perception of failure of high benzodiazepine requirements, we recommend administration of benzodiazepines in a symptom-triggered fashion. This approach was confirmed in a study of patients who developed AWS postoperatively in the ICU.[93] In this study, a symptom-triggered strategy resulted in a shorter length of stay and a lower incidence of mechanical ventilation than did continuous infusion of midazolam. Patients who receive this therapy generally respond to doses of diazepam, which results in a brief period of sedation followed by recrudescence of their symptoms. However, the dose range and other sedative–hypnotics required to achieve this may be dramatically different than that which is observed in subjects with nonresistant alcohol withdrawal. In another study, use of escalating doses of diazepam, up to 200 mg as an individual dose, combined with phenobarbital in participants with continued benzodiazepine resistance (defined as the requirement for bolus doses more frequently than every hour), reduced the need for mechanical ventilation by nearly 50%.[33] In non-ICU settings, the ability to administer frequent IV doses of diazepam is limited.

In instances of extreme benzodiazepine resistance, patients often receive a second GABAergic drug because of "failure" of benzodiazepine therapy. Phenobarbital, given in combination with a benzodiazepine, in IV doses of up to 260 mg, is recommended.[33] Caution is required to avoid stacking doses of phenobarbital because the onset of clinical effect takes approximately 20 to 40 minutes.[37] With the growing use of phenobarbital in resistant cases, a number of studies have now documented its safety and efficacy, even as a first-line therapy.[62] Furthermore, when administered in a symptom-triggered fashion, administration of a single loading dose of 10 mg/kg of phenobarbital, compared with administration of lorazepam according to a CIWA protocol, reduced the need for ICU admission for alcohol withdrawal from 25 to 8%.[39,50,83] Combined, these data suggest that phenobarbital is the preferred adjunct to benzodiazepines for cases of resistant alcohol withdrawal.[68] Although studies and reviews suggest its use as initial therapy,[62] additional prospective studies are needed before it can be routinely recommended as primary therapy (as opposed to benzodiazepines) for routine management.

Alternatively, propofol, either as individual bolus or as an infusion (in standard ICU dosing regimens, 10–50 mcg/kg/min), can serve as an adjunct to benzodiazepines for patients with resistant alcohol withdrawal. Although propofol has a rapid onset, it is difficult to titrate, and high-dose or long-term use is associated with profound metabolic consequences.[21] However, in an observational study, propofol was safely administered to 21 patients intubated for severe benzodiazepine-resistant DTs.[33] The main drawback to the use of propofol and barbiturates are their narrow therapeutic indices, with the potential for profound respiratory depression. This is especially true for propofol, which should generally only be used in the setting of mechanical ventilation. Both of these sedative–hypnotics can act synergistically with benzodiazepines to enhance GABA-induced chloride channel opening. In addition, propofol antagonizes NMDA receptors, thus reducing the excitatory component of alcohol withdrawal. The safety concerns with propofol were highlighted in a recent retrospective study that compared patients treated with escalating doses of benzodiazepine with or without propofol, The addition of propofol led to longer ICU length of stay and need for mechanical ventilation.[108] Given the uncontrolled nature of the data, it is difficult to make definitive safety claims based on this study, but given the known adverse effects of intubation and mechanical ventilation, relegating propofol to patients with RAW is judicious.[33,94] Therefore, based on best available data we recommend against using propofol as a primary therapeutic and only recommend using it after patients have failed escalating doses of oral or IV benzodiazepines.

Ethanol

Ethanol consumption is a common and effective means by which people with alcoholism can self-medicate to treat or prevent mild alcohol withdrawal. Consequently, some hospitals still administer ethanol for either prophylaxis or treatment of alcohol withdrawal. In one survey, 72% of 122 hospitals surveyed had administered either IV or oral ethanol for these indications; in another, 25% of Veterans Administration Hospitals allowed consumption of alcoholic beverages.[12,87] Despite its widespread use, little randomized controlled data supports its use. In one trial, 39 trauma patients without hepatic or CNS disease were successfully treated with 10% ethanol infusion for treatment of presumed alcohol withdrawal.[17,22] Conversely, IV ethanol was no more effective than flunitrazepam in one trial and inferior to diazepam in another in the prevention of alcohol withdrawal in postoperative surgical patients.[26,103] Although the authors did not report any adverse effects in these trials, the necessity for frequent blood alcohol monitoring, unpredictable elimination kinetics, potential for significant hepatic complications, postulated adverse effects of ethanol on wound healing, and difficulty in safely administering this therapy make it inappropriate to recommend the use of ethanol for the medical treatment of alcohol withdrawal.[40]

Adrenergic Antagonists

Numerous studies have investigated the use of sympatholytics to control the autonomic symptoms of alcohol withdrawal. Both β-adrenergic antagonists and clonidine reduced blood pressure and heart rate in randomized, placebo-controlled trials.[8,51] However, the inability of these xenobiotics to address the underlying pathophysiologic mechanism of alcohol withdrawal and subsequently control the neurologic manifestations makes them suboptimal as the sole therapeutic. Additionally, by altering the physiologic parameters that serve as classic markers for the severity of withdrawal, there is a risk of under administering necessary amounts of benzodiazepines.[110] This was observed in a randomized controlled trial of the central α_2-agonist lofexidine, and it is particularly complicated if using the peripheral manifestations to assess alcohol withdrawal severity as is done with CIWA.[47] There are a growing number of reports documenting the use of the central α-adrenergic agonist dexmedetomidine as an adjuvant to benzodiazepines for treatment of alcohol withdrawal.[9,10,57,78] The majority of observational studies document an improvement in CIWA or RASS score with dexmedetomidine administration and with a subsequent reduction in the amount of benzodiazepine administered.[109] This is also associated with a reduction in global adrenergic tone, manifest by reductions in heart rate and blood pressure.[78] However, the impact on global outcomes remains mixed, with studies reporting increased or decreased duration of hospitalization with dexmedetomidine use.[9,10] Consequently, with the high cost of dexmedetomidine, the unclear efficacy, and the potential for bradycardia, we recommend not to use it for the routine primary treatment of alcohol withdrawal. In the setting in which standard therapies, such as escalating doses of benzodiazepines and barbiturates, fail to provide adequate sedation (eg, RASS) or control of the alcohol withdrawal (eg, CIWA), a trial of dexmedetomidine seems reasonable whole continuing the therapies.

Magnesium

The theoretical benefits of magnesium supplementation are based both on the high prevalence of magnesium deficiency in people with alcoholism, its ability to block NMDA receptors, and its usefulness in preventing seizures in other disorders, including eclampsia.[41,44,84] Furthermore, magnesium deficiency has many clinical similarities to alcohol withdrawal, clouding the differential diagnosis. Numerous studies have evaluated the efficacy of magnesium supplementation.[75] However, in a randomized, placebo-controlled trial, magnesium had no effect on either the incidence of withdrawal seizures or severity of alcohol withdrawal.[105] Consequently, aside from repletion of electrolyte abnormalities as part of routine patient care, we recommend against the routine administration of magnesium for the treatment of alcohol withdrawal.

Antiepileptics

Carbamazepine has been used in multiple trials for treatment of mild alcohol withdrawal, more commonly in Europe, where an IV preparation is available. In animal studies, carbamazepine increases both the CNS GABA concentrations and the seizure threshold in alcohol withdrawal models. However, there are insufficient data to recommend the use of carbamazepine in lieu of benzodiazepines in patients with either alcohol withdrawal or DTs.[7,67] Valproic acid appears to have a benzodiazepine-sparing effect in patients with mild withdrawal, but the true clinical benefit is unclear.[2] In contrast, a recent randomized placebo-controlled study of the newer epileptic, oxcarbazepine, showed no difference between this xenobiotic and placebo in inpatient detoxification.[48] Consequently, although this class of drugs may be reasonably recommended as an adjunct to benzodiazepines, we recommend against using antiepileptics as monotherapy or primary therapy for treatment of patients with moderate or severe alcohol withdrawal.

Gabapentin

Gabapentin, originally introduced as an antiepileptic, has been used extensively for treatment of neuropathic pain and delirium. Contrary to its name, its primary mechanism of action appears to be inhibition of the voltage-gated calcium channel, which inhibits the activity of stimulatory neurotransmitters, such as glutamate.[52] An extensive literature demonstrates that gabapentin, administered in doses up to 2,400 mg/day is extremely effective in treatment of alcohol dependence, reducing alcohol cravings in people with alcoholism, and promoting abstinence.[63] However, literature related to its use for the treatment of established alcohol withdrawal remains mixed. Currently, the only studies have focused on its outpatient use for mild alcohol withdrawal. When pooled, these studies confirm a reduction in alcohol use when the withdrawal has resolved but also suggest a potential increase in the rate of seizures (6%) and potential worsening of delirium in patients with severe alcohol withdrawal. Therefore, although it may be appropriate for mild alcohol withdrawal, its use, especially as monotherapy, cannot be recommended for patients with severe alcohol withdrawal, DTs, or a history of seizures.[55]

Other Therapeutics

Recently there has been growing attention toward the use of baclofen, a GABA$_B$ receptor agonist, because of its purported ability to reduce alcohol cravings and treat alcohol withdrawal. However, data from 3 randomized controlled clinical studies have failed to demonstrate clinical benefit. In one study, baclofen was found to be equivalent to placebo, but in another, no difference was found between baclofen and benzodiazepines, with one of the studies demonstrating inferiority to chlordiazepoxide.[1,30,58] Based on these data and a recent Cochrane review we recommend against using baclofen for monotherapy at this time, although its use as an adjunctive therapy deserves further study.[56]

Ketamine is also proposed as an adjunct for treatment of severe alcohol withdrawal or DTs. Ketamine is an NMDA receptor antagonist, already used in the emergency department and ICU for procedural sedation and more recently as a continuous infusion for sedation, particularly in mechanically ventilated patients.[54,80,96] A recent retrospective study of the use of ketamine in 23 ICU patients with alcohol withdrawal[107] found that it was associated with a reduction in the need for diazepam. However, the uncontrolled use of multiple other adjuncts combined with a lack of a controlled comparator group makes it difficult to assess the true clinical benefit. Psychological adverse effects are common, and their effects on an inadequately sedated patient with alcohol withdrawal are unknown. Therefore, pending more controlled clinical data, ketamine is only reasonable in cases of severe benzodiazepine-resistant alcohol withdrawal for whom other more established adjuncts, including phenobarbital and possibly propofol, have either failed or are unable to be tolerated.[107]

SUMMARY

- Ethanol withdrawal is a complex physiologic process involving both enhanced neuronal excitation and reduced inhibition.
- The manifestations of greatest concern are neurologic and include altered mental status and seizures, but the autonomic excess is always of great concern.
- Treatment includes supportive care and sedation with benzodiazepines in escalating doses in a symptom-triggered fashion.
- When benzodiazepines cannot produce adequate sedation, sedative–hypnotics such as phenobarbital or propofol are recommended.

REFERENCES

1. Addolorato G, et al. Baclofen in the treatment of alcohol withdrawal syndrome: a comparative study vs diazepam. *Am J Med.* 2006;119:276 e213-278.
2. Alldredge BK, et al. Placebo-controlled trial of intravenous diphenylhydantoin for short-term treatment of alcohol withdrawal seizures. *Am J Med.* 1989;87:645-648.
3. Asplund CA, et al. 3 regimens for alcohol withdrawal and detoxification. *J Fam Pract.* 2004;53:545-554.
4. Association AP. *Diagnostic and Statistical Manual of Mental Disorders.* 5th ed. Washington, DC: American Psychiatric Association; 2013.
5. Bard MR, et al. Alcohol withdrawal syndrome: turning minor injuries into a major problem. *J Trauma.* 2006;61:1441-1445; discussion 1445-1446.
6. Barrio E, et al. Liver disease in heavy drinkers with and without alcohol withdrawal syndrome. *Alcohol Clin Exp Res.* 2004;28:131-136.
7. Barrons R, Roberts N. The role of carbamazepine and oxcarbazepine in alcohol withdrawal syndrome. *J Clin Pharm Ther.* 2010;35:153-167.
8. Baumgartner GR, Rowen RC. Clonidine vs chlordiazepoxide in the management of acute alcohol withdrawal syndrome. *Arch Intern Med.* 1987;147:1223-1226.
9. Beg M, et al. Treatment of alcohol withdrawal syndrome with and without dexmedetomidine. *Perm J.* 2016;20:49-53.
10. Bielka K, et al. Addition of dexmedetomidine to benzodiazepines for patients with alcohol withdrawal syndrome in the intensive care unit: a randomized controlled study. *Ann Intensive Care.* 2015;5:33.
11. Bleich S, et al. Elevated homocysteine levels in alcohol withdrawal. *Alcohol Alcohol.* 2000;35:351-354.
12. Blondell RD, et al. Ethanol in formularies of US teaching hospitals. *JAMA.* 2003;289:552.
13. Blum K, et al. Enhancement of alcohol withdrawal convulsions in mice by haloperidol. *Clin Toxicol.* 1976;9:427-434.
14. Brousse G, et al. Alteration of glutamate/GABA balance during acute alcohol withdrawal in emergency department: a prospective analysis. *Alcohol Alcohol.* 2012;47:501-508.
15. Brown J, et al. An overview and evaluation of combining an addiction liaison nurse outpatient service with hepatitis C outpatient clinics in Glasgow, Scotland. *Gastroenterol Nurs.* 2013;36:98-104.
16. Caetano R, et al. Prevalence, trends, and incidence of alcohol withdrawal symptoms: analysis of general population and clinical samples. *Alcohol Health Res World.* 1998;22:73-79.
17. Cassidy EM, et al. Symptom-triggered benzodiazepine therapy for alcohol withdrawal syndrome in the emergency department: a comparison with the standard fixed dose benzodiazepine regimen. *Emerg Med J.* 2012;29:802-804.
18. de Medilis CE. *Sajous's Analytical Cyclopædia of Practical Medicine.* Philadelphia: F. A. Davis Company; 1905.
19. Chan GM, et al. Racial variations in the incidence of severe alcohol withdrawal. *J Med Toxicol.* 2009;5:8-14.
20. Clothier J, et al. Varying rates of alcohol metabolism in relation to detoxification medication. *Alcohol.* 1985;2:443-445.
21. Corbett SM, et al. Propofol-related infusion syndrome in intensive care patients. *Pharmacotherapy.* 2008;28:250-258.
22. Craft PP, et al. Intravenous ethanol for alcohol detoxification in trauma patients. *South Med J.* 1994;87:47-54.
23. D'Onofrio G, et al. Lorazepam for the prevention of recurrent seizures related to alcohol. *N Engl J Med.* 1999;340:915-919.
24. Daeppen JB, et al. Symptom-triggered vs fixed-schedule doses of benzodiazepine for alcohol withdrawal: a randomized treatment trial. *Arch Intern Med.* 2002;162:1117-1121.
25. Donnino MW, et al. Myths and misconceptions of Wernicke's encephalopathy: what every emergency physician should know. *Ann Emerg Med.* 2007;50:715-721.
26. Eggers V, et al. Blood alcohol concentration for monitoring ethanol treatment to prevent alcohol withdrawal in the intensive care unit. *Intensive Care Med.* 2002;28:1475-1482.
27. Eyer F, et al. Risk assessment of moderate to severe alcohol withdrawal—predictors for seizures and delirium tremens in the course of withdrawal. *Alcohol Alcohol.* 2011;46:427-433.
28. Flannery AH, et al. Unpeeling the evidence for the banana bag: evidence-based recommendations for the management of alcohol-associated vitamin and electrolyte deficiencies in the ICU. *Crit Care Med.* 2016;44:1545-1552.
29. Foy A, et al. The course of alcohol withdrawal in a general hospital. *QJM.* 1997;90:253-261.
30. Girish K, et al. A randomized, open-label, standard controlled, parallel group study of efficacy and safety of baclofen, and chlordiazepoxide in uncomplicated alcohol withdrawal syndrome. *Biomed J.* 2016;39:72-80.
31. Glass IB. Alcoholic hallucinosis: a psychiatric enigma—2. Follow-up studies. *Br J Addict.* 1989;84:151-164.
32. Glass IB. Alcoholic hallucinosis: a psychiatric enigma—1. The development of an idea. *Br J Addict.* 1989;84:29-41.
33. Gold JA, et al. A strategy of escalating doses of benzodiazepines and phenobarbital administration reduces the need for mechanical ventilation in delirium tremens. *Crit Care Med.* 2007;35:724-730.
34. Goodson CM, et al. Predictors of severe alcohol withdrawal syndrome: a systematic review and meta-analysis. *Alcohol Clin Exp Res.* 2014;38:2664-2677.
35. Hack JB, et al. Resistant alcohol withdrawal: does an unexpectedly large sedative requirement identify these patients early? *J Med Toxicol.* 2006;2:55-60.
36. Haugbol SR, et al. Upregulation of glutamate receptor subtypes during alcohol withdrawal in rats. *Alcohol Alcohol.* 2005;40:89-95.
37. Hecksel KA, et al. Inappropriate use of symptom-triggered therapy for alcohol withdrawal in the general hospital. *Mayo Clin Proc.* 2008;83:274-279.
38. Heese P, et al. Alterations of homocysteine serum levels during alcohol withdrawal are influenced by folate and riboflavin: results from the German Investigation on Neurobiology in Alcoholism (GINA). *Alcohol Alcohol.* 2012;47:497-500.
39. Hendey GW, et al. A prospective, randomized, trial of phenobarbital versus benzodiazepines for acute alcohol withdrawal. *Am J Emerg Med.* 2011;29:382-385.
40. Hodges B, Mazur JE. Intravenous ethanol for the treatment of alcohol withdrawal syndrome in critically ill patients. *Pharmacotherapy.* 2004;24:1578-1585.
41. Hoes MJ. Plasma concentrations of magnesium and vitamin B-1 in alcoholism and delirium tremens. Pathogenic and prognostic implications. *Acta Psychiatr Belg.* 1981; 81:72-84.

42. Hughes JR. Alcohol withdrawal seizures. *Epilepsy Behav.* 2009;15:92-97.
43. Isbell H, et al. An experimental study of the etiology of "rum fits" and delirium tremens. *Q J Stud Alcohol.* 1955;16:1-33.
44. Jin C, et al. Enhanced ethanol inhibition of recombinant *N*-methyl-D-aspartate receptors by magnesium: role of NR3A subunits. *Alcohol Clin Exp Res.* 2008;32:1059-1066.
45. Jolliffe N. The alcoholic admissions to Bellevue Hospital. *Science.* 1936;83:306-309.
46. Kaim SC, et al. Treatment of the acute alcohol withdrawal state: a comparison of four drugs. *Am J Psychiatry.* 1969;125:1640-1646.
47. Keaney F, et al. A double-blind randomized placebo-controlled trial of lofexidine in alcohol withdrawal: lofexidine is not a useful adjunct to chlordiazepoxide. *Alcohol Alcohol.* 2001;36:426-430.
48. Koethe D, et al. Oxcarbazepine—efficacy and tolerability during treatment of alcohol withdrawal: a double-blind, randomized, placebo-controlled multicenter pilot study. *Alcohol Clin Exp Res.* 2007;31:1188-1194.
49. Kraemer KL, et al. Independent clinical correlates of severe alcohol withdrawal. *Subst Abus.* 2003;24:197-209.
50. Kramp P, Rafaelsen OJ. Delirium tremens: a double-blind comparison of diazepam and barbital treatment. *Acta Psychiatr Scand.* 1978;58:174-190.
51. Kraus ML, et al. Randomized clinical trial of atenolol in patients with alcohol withdrawal. *N Engl J Med.* 1985;313:905-909.
52. Kukkar A, et al. Implications and mechanism of action of gabapentin in neuropathic pain. *Arch Pharm Res.* 2013;36:237-251.
53. Kumar S, et al. Ethanol and xylitol production from glucose and xylose at high temperature by Kluyveromyces sp. IIPE453. *J Ind Microbiol Biotechnol.* 2009;36:1483-1489.
54. Kurdi MS, et al. Ketamine: current applications in anesthesia, pain, and critical care. *Anesth Essays Res.* 2014;8:283-290.
55. Leung JG, et al. The role of gabapentin in the management of alcohol withdrawal and dependence. *Ann Pharmacother.* 2015;49:897-906.
56. Liu J, Wang LN. Baclofen for alcohol withdrawal. *Cochrane Database Syst Rev.* 2015:CD008502.
57. Ludtke KA, et al. Retrospective review of critically ill patients experiencing alcohol withdrawal: dexmedetomidine versus propofol and/or lorazepam continuous infusions. *Hosp Pharm.* 2015;50:208-213.
58. Lyon JE, et al. Treating alcohol withdrawal with oral baclofen: a randomized, double-blind, placebo-controlled trial. *J Hosp Med.* 2011;6:469-474.
59. Maldonado JR, et al. Benzodiazepine loading versus symptom-triggered treatment of alcohol withdrawal: a prospective, randomized clinical trial. *Gen Hosp Psychiatry.* 2012;34:611-617.
60. Maldonado JR, et al. Prospective Validation Study of the Prediction of Alcohol Withdrawal Severity Scale (PAWSS) in medically ill inpatients: a new scale for the prediction of complicated alcohol withdrawal syndrome. *Alcohol Alcohol.* 2015;50:509-518.
61. Marik P, Mohedin B. Alcohol-related admissions to an inner city hospital intensive care unit. *Alcohol Alcohol.* 1996;31:393-396.
62. Martin K, Katz A. The role of barbiturates for alcohol withdrawal syndrome. *Psychosomatics.* 2016;57:341-347.
63. Mason BJ, et al. Gabapentin treatment for alcohol dependence: a randomized clinical trial. *JAMA Intern Med.* 2014;174:70-77.
64. Mayo-Smith MF, et al. Management of alcohol withdrawal delirium. An evidence-based practice guideline. *Arch Intern Med.* 2004;164:1405-1412.
65. McMicken D, Liss JL. Alcohol-related seizures. *Emerg Med Clin North Am.* 2011;29:117-124.
66. McPeake JM, et al. Do alcohol use disorders impact on long term outcomes from intensive care? *Crit Care.* 2015;19:185.
67. Minozzi S, et al. Anticonvulsants for alcohol withdrawal. *Cochrane Database Syst Rev.* 2010:CD005064.
68. Mo Y, et al. Barbiturates for the treatment of alcohol withdrawal syndrome: a systematic review of clinical trials. *J Crit Care.* 2016;32:101-107.
69. Moore M, Gray MG. Delerium tremens: a study of cases at the Boston City Hospital, 1915-1936. *N Engl J Med.* 1939;220:953-956.
70. Mulholland PJ, et al. Thiamine deficiency in the pathogenesis of chronic ethanol-associated cerebellar damage in vitro. *Neuroscience.* 2005;135:1129-1139.
71. Muzyk AJ, et al. The role of diazepam loading for the treatment of alcohol withdrawal syndrome in hospitalized patients. *Am J Addict.* 2013;22:113-118.
72. Newman JP, et al. Trends in the management of alcohol withdrawal syndrome. *Laryngoscope.* 1995;105:1-7.
73. Ozsoy S, et al. Expression of glutamate transporters in alcohol withdrawal. *Pharmacopsychiatry.* 2016;49:14-17.
74. Picciotto MR. Common aspects of the action of nicotine and other drugs of abuse. *Drug Alcohol Depend.* 1998;51:165-172.
75. Prior PL, et al. Influence of microelement concentration on the intensity of alcohol withdrawal syndrome. *Alcohol Alcohol.* 2015;50:152-156.
76. Rathlev NK, et al. The lack of efficacy of phenytoin in the prevention of recurrent alcohol-related seizures. *Ann Emerg Med.* 1994;23:513-518.
77. Rathlev NK, et al. Clinical characteristics as predictors of recurrent alcohol-related seizures. *Acad Emerg Med.* 2000;7:886-891.
78. Rayner SG, et al. Dexmedetomidine as adjunct treatment for severe alcohol withdrawal in the ICU. *Ann Intensive Care.* 2012;2:12.
79. Rehm J, et al. Global burden of disease and injury and economic cost attributable to alcohol use and alcohol-use disorders. *Lancet.* 2009;373:2223-2233.
80. Riddell J, et al. Ketamine as a first-line treatment for severely agitated emergency department patients. *Am J Emerg Med.* 2017;35:1000-1004.
81. Riker RR, et al. Prospective evaluation of the Sedation-Agitation Scale for adult critically ill patients. *Crit Care Med.* 1999;27:1325-1329.
82. Ritson B, Chick J. Comparison of two benzodiazepines in the treatment of alcohol withdrawal: effects on symptoms and cognitive recovery. *Drug Alcohol Depend.* 1986;18:329-334.
83. Rosenson J, et al. Phenobarbital for acute alcohol withdrawal: a prospective randomized double-blind placebo-controlled study. *J Emerg Med.* 2013;44:592-598 e592.
84. Ruppersberg JP, et al. The mechanism of magnesium block of NMDA receptors. *Semin Neurosci.* 1994;6:87-96.
85. Saitz R, et al. Individualized treatment for alcohol withdrawal. A randomized double-blind controlled trial. *JAMA.* 1994;272:519-523.
86. Sarff M, Gold JA. Alcohol withdrawal syndromes in the intensive care unit. *Crit Care Med.* 2010;38:S494-501.
87. Sattar SP, et al. Use of alcoholic beverages in VA medical centers. *Subst Abuse Treat Prev Policy.* 2006;1:30.
88. Schuckit MA. Alcohol-use disorders. *Lancet.* 2009;373:492-501.
89. Sen S, et al. Evaluation of a symptom-triggered benzodiazepine protocol utilizing SAS and CIWA-Ar scoring for the treatment of alcohol withdrawal syndrome in the critically ill. *Ann Pharmacother.* 2017;51:101-110.
90. Sessler CN, et al. The Richmond Agitation-Sedation Scale: validity and reliability in adult intensive care unit patients. *Am J Respir Crit Care Med.* 2002;166:1338-1344.
91. Silbergleit R, et al. Intramuscular versus intravenous therapy for prehospital status epilepticus. *N Engl J Med.* 2012;366:591-600.
92. Soyka M, Horak M. Outpatient alcohol detoxification: implementation efficacy and outcome effectiveness of a model project. *Eur Addict Res.* 2004;10:180-187.
93. Spies CD, et al. Alcohol withdrawal severity is decreased by symptom-orientated adjusted bolus therapy in the ICU. *Intensive Care Med.* 2003;29:2230-2238.
94. Stewart R, et al. Outcomes of patients with alcohol withdrawal syndrome treated with high-dose sedatives and deferred intubation. *Ann Am Thorac Soc.* 2016;13:248-252.
95. Sullivan JT, et al. Assessment of alcohol withdrawal: the revised clinical institute withdrawal assessment for alcohol scale (CIWA-Ar). *Br J Addict.* 1989;84:1353-1357.
96. Umunna BP, et al. Ketamine for continuous sedation of mechanically ventilated patients. *J Emerg Trauma Shock.* 2015;8:11-15.
97. van Munster BC, et al. Genetic polymorphisms related to delirium tremens: a systematic review. *Alcohol Clin Exp Res.* 2007;31:177-184.
98. Victor M, Adams RD. The effect of alcohol on the nervous system. *Res Publ Assoc Res Nerv Ment Dis.* 1953;32:526-573.
99. Victor M, et al. Auditory hallucinations in the alcoholic patient. *Trans Am Neurol Assoc.* 1953;3:273-275.
100. Victor M, Brausch C. The role of abstinence in the genesis of alcoholic epilepsy. *Epilepsia.* 1967;8:1-20.
101. Vinson DC, Menezes M. Admission alcohol level: a predictor of the course of alcohol withdrawal. *J Fam Pract.* 1991;33:161-167.
102. Watson AJ, et al. Acute Wernickes encephalopathy precipitated by glucose loading. *Ir J Med Sci.* 1981;150:301-303.
103. Weinberg JA, et al. Comparison of intravenous ethanol versus diazepam for alcohol withdrawal prophylaxis in the trauma ICU: results of a randomized trial. *J Trauma.* 2008;64:99-104.
104. Wetterling T, et al. Clinical predictors of alcohol withdrawal delirium. *Alcohol Clin Exp Res.* 1994;18:1100-1102.
105. Wilson A, Vulcano B. A double-blind, placebo-controlled trial of magnesium sulfate in the ethanol withdrawal syndrome. *Alcohol Clin Exp Res.* 1984;8:542-545.
106. Wojnar M, et al. Differences in the course of alcohol withdrawal in women and men: a Polish sample. *Alcohol Clin Exp Res.* 1997;21:1351-1355.
107. Wong A, et al. Evaluation of adjunctive ketamine to benzodiazepines for management of alcohol withdrawal syndrome. *Ann Pharmacother.* 2015;49:14-19.
108. Wong A, et al. Management of benzodiazepine-resistant alcohol withdrawal across a healthcare system: benzodiazepine dose-escalation with or without propofol. *Drug Alcohol Depend.* 2015;154:296-299.
109. Woods AD, et al. The use of dexmedetomidine as an adjuvant to benzodiazepine-based therapy to decrease the severity of delirium in alcohol withdrawal in adult intensive care unit patients: a systematic review. *JBI Database System Rev Implement Rep.* 2015;13:224-252.
110. Worner TM. Propranolol versus diazepam in the management of the alcohol withdrawal syndrome: double-blind controlled trial. *Am J Drug Alcohol Abuse.* 1994;20:115-124.
111. Wretlind M, et al. Disposition of three benzodiazepines after single oral administration in man. *Acta Pharmacol Toxicol (Copenh).* 1977;40(suppl 1):28-39.

DISULFIRAM AND DISULFIRAMLIKE REACTIONS

Amit K. Gupta

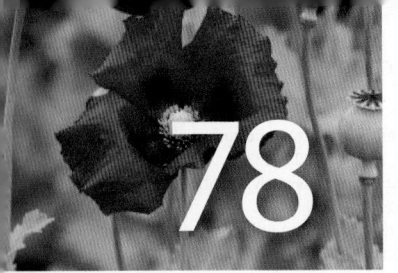

Disulfiram

HISTORY AND EPIDEMIOLOGY

Disulfiram, tetraethylthiuram disulfide (TETD), was synthesized from thiocarbamide in the 1880s to accelerate the vulcanization (stabilization) of rubber by the addition of sulfur.[108] Sixty years later, it was the first Western medication used to treat alcohol dependence. By the turn of the 20th century, most rubber factory workers exposed to disulfiram found that they were intolerant to alcohol.[3,34] E.E Williams, a rubber factory occupational physician, wrote, "If the chemical compound disulfiram is not harmful to man, one wonders if one has discovered a cure for alcoholism." Apart from its use in the rubber industry, beginning in the early 1940s, disulfiram was also used in medicine as a scabicide. Two scientists, Hald and Jacobsen, were exploring the antiparasitic effects of disulfiram when they made the rediscovery that ingesting alcohol after loading doses of disulfiram was "quite unpleasant."[39] Subsequently, in 1951, the US Food and Drug Administration approved disulfiram for the treatment for alcoholism. Disulfiram is typically prescribed at an initial dose of 500 mg/day for 1 to 2 weeks followed by a maintenance dose of 125 to 500 mg/day.

Disulfiram was never widely used clinically, and its use further declined after several studies revealed no significant difference in drinking outcomes between unsupervised disulfiram administration and placebo.[33] Studies evaluating the efficacy of disulfiram that span nearly 60 years yield mixed results, with many studies having small sample sizes, nonrandomization, unblinded conditions, short follow-up periods, and no measurement of treatment adherence. With the worldwide approval of naltrexone in 1993 and later acamprosate, the clinical use of disulfiram declined. More recent interest in disulfiram for treating cocaine and other stimulant dependence has provided some renewed clinical interest.[35,82,85] Disulfiram is being studied for its possible antineoplastic properties, which include the induction of oxidative stress, leading to cooper-dependent cytotoxicity, proteasome inhibition, and nuclear factor-kB inhibition.[15,38] Oxidative stress is enhanced by the presence of the disulfiram–copper chelation complex, and copper-binding drugs inhibit proteasome activity and generate reactive oxygen species.[90] Disulfiram is undergoing clinical trials for the treatment of various cancers, including melanoma and liver, lung, and prostate cancers.

In considering disulfiram toxicity, a distinction must be made between the clinical manifestations of a disulfiram–ethanol reaction and the toxic effects of disulfiram itself. Direct disulfiram toxicity can be further classified as acute or chronic poisoning. Although life-threatening effects associated with disulfiram are rare, clinicians should be aware of proper diagnosis and management of patients with disulfiram-associated toxicity.

Specific epidemiologic information about the 3 different forms of disulfiram toxicity is difficult to elucidate, even from an analysis of the American Association of Poison Control Centers (AAPCC). Data from the National Poison Data System from 2015 revealed 221 exposures to disulfiram, with the majority of cases being in adults and classified as unintentional. No deaths and only one major adverse outcome was reported. Since 1982, 14 deaths associated with disulfiram were reported to the AAPCC, most involving a disulfiram–ethanol reaction (Chap. 130). Serious adverse effects associated

with both therapeutic use of disulfiram and with disulfiram overdose continue to be reported mostly in case reports and case series. As such, these reports are difficult to interpret because of complications and comorbidities associated with alcohol use; the potential effects of polypharmacy; and the difficulty in relating the adverse effect to disulfiram, alcohol, or a disulfiram–ethanol reaction.

PHARMACOLOGY AND PHARMACOKINETICS OF DISULFIRAM

Approximately 70% to 90% of disulfiram is absorbed from the gastrointestinal (GI) tract after oral administration.[13] Upon absorption, disulfiram is immediately converted to diethyldithiocarbamate (DDC) followed by rapid conversion to carbon disulfide and diethylamine.[24] Diethyldithiocarbamate also chelates copper to form a bis(DDC)–copper complex.[13] Bis(DDC)–copper is absorbed from the small intestine. Peak serum concentrations of disulfiram and DDC are achieved 8 to 10 hours after a 250-mg dose, and that for carbon disulfide occurs 5 to 6 hours.[24] In one study, the mean serum disulfiram concentration in humans after a 250-mg dose was reported to be 0.38 ± 0.03 mcg/mL.[24]

Within 5 to 10 minutes after absorption, disulfiram is rapidly reduced to DDC via glutathione reductase, which then can undergo nonenzymatic degradation to diethylamine and carbon disulfide or chelate copper to form a bis(DDC)–copper complex (Fig. 78–1).[13] As such, it is difficult to detect the parent drug blood concentrations. Metabolism of disulfiram occurs primarily in the liver and the erythrocyte. The oxidation of DDC in the liver is catalyzed by at least 4 enzymes of cytochrome P450 (CYP3A4, CYP1A2, CYP2A6, CYP 2D6) and to a minor extent by human flavin monooxygenase.[63] Diethyldithiocarbamate is also metabolized by glucuronidation, methylation, and oxidation. Methylation of DDC produces diethyldithiomethylcarbamate (MeDDC).[17] Diethyldithiomethylcarbamate is oxidized primarily to the intermediate metabolite MeDDC sulfine, which is ultimately converted to MeDDC sulfoxide.[63] Genetic differences in various enzymatic activity among

FIGURE 78–1. Disulfiram metabolism occurs in the liver and in the erythrocyte. The most consequential metabolites are diethyldithiocarbamate and carbon disulfide.

individuals lead to variable concentrations of the individual metabolites.[24] Carbon disulfide undergoes oxidation to carbonyl sulfide and further oxidation to carbon dioxide.

Disulfiram is highly lipid soluble and approximately 80% protein bound.[46] The hepatic metabolites of disulfiram are mostly excreted renally, and an estimated 5% to 20% is not metabolized and is excreted unchanged in the feces.[24] The volume of distribution is not described.

Disulfiram has a half-life estimated at 60 to 120 hours. Diethyldithiocarbamate is estimated to have a half-life of 13.9 hours and carbon disulfide 8.9 hours.[46] With chronic dosing of disulfiram, carbon disulfide also is excreted through the lungs, and this explains the side effects of metallic taste and halitosis.[23] Because of the long half-lives of disulfiram and its metabolites, 1 or 2 weeks is often needed before disulfiram is totally eliminated from the body after the last dose.[3]

Disulfiram and DDC are selective mechanism-based inhibitors of CYP2E1.[52] One study in normal healthy volunteers demonstrated that a single 500-mg dose of disulfiram markedly reduced (by 93%) the 6-hydroxylation of chlorzoxazone, a putative index of CYP2E1 activity.[53] Drugs metabolized by the cytochrome oxidase systems, specifically CYP2E1 (eg, amitriptyline, warfarin, phenytoin, chlordiazepoxide, and diazepam), have increased serum concentrations and prolonged half-lives in patients taking disulfiram.[32] Using probe drugs selectively metabolized by individual CYP enzymes, 500 mg of disulfiram had no effect on the metabolism of coumarin (CYP2A6), tolbutamide (CYP2C9), mephenytoin (CYP2C19), dextromethorphan (CYP2D6), or intravenously administered midazolam (CYP3A).[51] Disulfiram does not significantly alter the metabolism of a therapeutic dose of acetaminophen in either healthy patients or those with alcoholic liver disease.[87]

OTHER ENZYMES INHIBITED BY DISULFIRAM

Disulfiram and its active metabolites have many other targets besides aldehyde dehydrogenase (ALDH). Diethyldithiocarbamate is a potent metal chelator, which explains interest in the treatment of nickel (Chap. 96) and its effects on the activity of copper-dependent enzymes such as microsomal carboxylesterases, plasma cholinesterases, and cytochrome oxidase.[66] Inhibition of microsomal carboxylesterases and plasma cholinesterases is theorized to play a role in the pharmacokinetic increases in plasma cocaine concentrations caused by disulfiram.[68]

Diethyldithiocarbamate also inhibits dopamine β-hydroxylose (DBH), which converts dopamine to norepinephrine.[36,75] Inhibition of DBH leads to increased concentrations of dopamine in the brain and periphery and decreased concentrations of norepinephrine and epinephrine.[36] The increased concentrations of dopamine associated with disulfiram is supportive of the possible therapeutic benefit in cocaine dependence and the potentiation of psychosis in psychotic individuals. Decreased urinary concentrations of vanillylmandelic acid, the metabolite of epinephrine and norepinephrine, are noted in individuals taking disulfiram, and this offer an explanation explain the hypotension that occurs in patients with the disulfiram–ethanol reaction.[40]

DISULFIRAM–ETHANOL REACTION
Pharmacology and Pharmacokinetics
The primary indication for disulfiram is as an avoidant and aversive treatment for alcohol dependence. Either the fear of having a disulfiram–ethanol reaction or the memory of having one is a form of conditioned avoidance meant to deter the patient from using alcohol. Disulfiram inhibits both cytosolic and mitochondrial hepatic aldehyde–nicotinamide adenine dinucleotide (NAD) oxidoreductase, which is more commonly known as ALDH. This enzyme catalyzes the oxidation of acetaldehyde to acetate, the inhibition of which results in an accumulation of acetaldehyde in the blood and tissues after ethanol ingestion (Fig. 78–2).[3] The increased concentration of acetaldehyde is responsible for the symptoms produced by the disulfiram–ethanol reaction.

Elevations of blood acetaldehyde are largely determined by the extent of ALDH inhibition produced as well as the ethanol dose ingested.[83] After

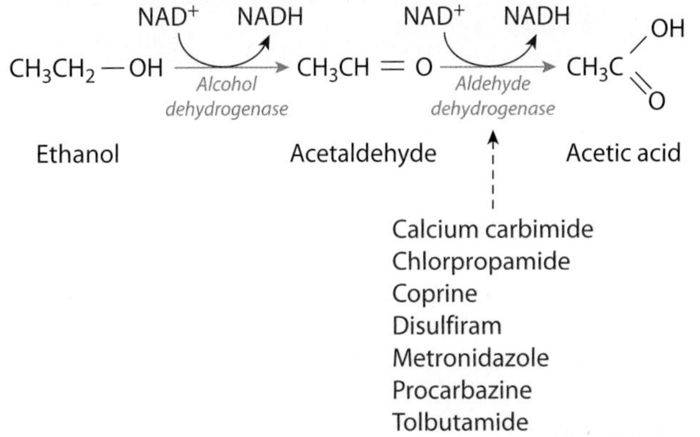

FIGURE 78–2. The site of action of disulfiram and other xenobiotics. The irreversible inactivation of aldehyde dehydrogenase results in an increased acetaldehyde concentration after ethanol is administered. NAD$^+$ = nicotinamide adenine dinucleotide (oxidized); NADH = nicotinamide adenine dinucleotide (reduced).

oral disulfiram administration, low-Km ALDH is inhibited with doses greater than 150 mg/kg, but disulfiram does not inhibit high-Km ALDH even in high doses (eg, 600 mg/kg).[67] Thus, ALDH is inhibited by disulfiram at a more or less constant first-order kinetic rate regardless of variations in the concentration of ALDH. Aldehyde dehydrogenase inhibition with disulfiram develops over 12 hours and is mainly irreversible.[46] Recovery of enzymatic activity depends on de novo ALDH synthesis that takes place in 6 or more days.[53] The exact mechanism by which disulfiram and its metabolites inhibit ALDH is still unknown but may be due to oxidizing sulfhydryl groups or competition for NAD.[91] The metabolites of disulfiram, including DDC and its sulfoxide and sulfone metabolites, also inhibit ALDH.[39]

The disulfiram–ethanol reaction occurs up to 3 weeks after the cessation of disulfiram therapy. There are also sustained-release and depot disulfiram preparations, but none is available in the United States. One patient developed a reaction 3 weeks after the subcutaneous injection of 2 g of disulfiram.[86]

Disulfiram–ethanol reactions occur after exposure to the ethanol contained in many household products. Table 78–1 lists some of these products.

Clinical Manifestations
Symptoms of the disulfiram–ethanol reaction often begin within 15 minutes of ethanol ingestion, peak at 30 to 60 minutes, and gradually resolve over the next several hours. Symptoms are diverse and include flushing, pruritus, diaphoresis, lightheadedness, headache, nausea, vomiting, and abdominal pain. Esophageal rupture caused by forceful vomiting is reported.[26] Electrocardiographic (ECG) changes, including ST-segment depressions and flattening of T waves, occur as well as dysrhythmias and myocardial infarction.[70,73] Other rare complications include methemoglobinemia, hypertension, bronchospasm, and myoclonus.[106,109,123] Severe shock and hypotension requiring vasopressor support are reported.[11,74] Deaths attributed to the disulfiram–ethanol reaction are extremely rare and are associated with disulfiram doses in excess of current recommendations.[5,47]

TABLE 78–1	Common Household Products That Contain Ethanol and May Cause a Reaction with Disulfiram[22,58,84,86,94]

Adhesives

Alcohols: denatured alcohol, rubbing alcohol

Detergents

Foods: liquor-containing desserts, fermented vinegar, some sauces

Nonprescription xenobiotics: analgesics, antacids, antidiarrheals, cough and cold preparations, topical anesthetics, vitamins

Personal hygiene products: aftershave lotions, colognes, contact lens solutions, deodorants, liquid soaps, mouthwashes, perfumes, shampoos, skin liniments, and lotions

Solvents

TABLE 78–2	Xenobiotics Reported to Cause a Disulfiramlike Reaction With Ethanol[8,14,23,41,55,56,72,76,99,113,119,122]

Antimicrobials

Cephalosporins, especially those that contain an nMTT side chain, such as cefotetan, cefoperazone, cefamandole, and cefmenoxime

Metronidazole

Moxalactam

Trimethoprim–sulfamethoxazole

Possible reactions with chloramphenicol, furazolidone, griseofulvin, nitrofurantoin, procarbazine quinacrine, sulfonamides

Calcium carbimide (citrated)

Carbon disulfide

Carbon tetrachloride

Chloral hydrate

Dimethylformamide

Mushrooms

Coprinus mushrooms, including *C. atramentaria, C. insignis, C. variegatus,* and *C. quadrifidus, Boletus luridus, Clitocybe clavipes, Polyporus sulphureus, Pholiota squarosa, Tricholoma aurantum, Verpa bohemica*

Nitrefazole

Phentolamine

Procarbazine

Sulfonylurea oral hypoglycemics

Chlorpropamide

Tolbutamide

Tacrolimus

Thiram analogs (fungicides)

Copper, mercuric, and sodium diethyldithiocarbamate

Zinc and ferric dimethyldithiocarbamate

Zinc and disodium ethylenebis (dithiocarbamate)

Thiuram analogs

Tetraethylthiuram monosulfide and disulfide (disulfiram)

Tetramethylthiuram disulfide (thiram)

Tolazoline

Trichloroethylene

nMTT = *N*-methylthiotetrazole.

Disulfiram-like reactions occur when ethanol is ingested with xenobiotics other than disulfiram. Symptoms are similar to those of disulfiram–ethanol reactions. Health care providers should warn patients of such reactions when prescribing certain medications that cause this adverse effect. Unfortunately, these reactions are idiosyncratic and are not been studied extensively.[116] Table 78–2 lists xenobiotics reported to cause disulfiramlike reactions.

MANAGEMENT OF DISULFIRAM–ETHANOL REACTIONS

The duration of the disulfiram–alcohol reaction varies from 30 to 60 minutes in mild cases to several hours and is largely dependent on the amount of alcohol absorbed and its metabolism. Because of vomiting and volume depletion, serum glucose, electrolytes, and kidney function should be evaluated. Because only small amounts of ethanol precipitate a disulfiram–ethanol reaction, it is useful to quantify the presence of ethanol with a blood concentration. Patients with cardiovascular instability should have an ECG and attached to continue cardiac monitoring. Symptomatic and supportive care is the mainstay of treatment. Most patients with hypotension respond to intravenous (IV) 0.9% sodium chloride. Refractory hypotension is rare, but if necessary, a vasopressor should be administered. A direct-acting adrenergic agonist such as norepinephrine is recommended because disulfiram inhibits DBH, an enzyme necessary for norepinephrine synthesis. As such, indirect vasopressors, such as dopamine, that require functioning norepinephrine synthesis are less effective.

For further symptomatic care, antiemetics are reasonable, and for cutaneous flushing, a histamine (H_1) receptor antagonist, such as diphenhydramine, is useful.[105] Most patients with a disulfiram–ethanol reaction have mild symptoms, are hemodynamically stable, and should safely discharged after resolution of symptoms.

Fomepizole halts the accumulation of acetaldehyde and thus halts the severity of disulfiram–ethanol reactions. Fomepizole, an inhibitor of alcohol dehydrogenase, limits the progression of the disulfiram reaction by blocking ethanol metabolism to acetaldehyde (Antidotes in Depth: A33). In a study of patients with alcoholism, fomepizole decreased acetaldehyde concentrations and improved clinical symptoms in those experiencing a disulfiram–ethanol reaction.[62] A case series reported 2 patients who developed severe disulfiram–ethanol reactions with hypotension and tachycardia unresponsive to fluids who were treated successfully with a single dose of fomepizole.[101] One patient improved clinically 90 minutes after administration of fomepizole and the other within 30 minutes. Fomepizole is only be recommended for patients experiencing a severe disulfiram–ethanol reaction leading to cardiogenic or distributive shock.

CLINICAL MANIFESTATIONS OF DISULFIRAM TOXICITY
Acute Disulfiram Toxicity

Reported cases of acute disulfiram overdose are infrequent and typically do not cause life-threatening toxicity. Most patients rapidly develop GI symptoms within 1 to 2 hours that include nausea, vomiting, and abdominal pain. Neurologic symptoms are present after acute disulfiram overdose, including lethargy and coma.[61] Dysarthria and movement disorders, including myoclonus, ataxia, dystonia, and akinesia, usually take 3 or more days to develop, occur rarely, and are related to direct effects of carbon disulfide on the basal ganglia.[59,60,64] Hypotonia is present in children.[6] Persistent neurologic abnormalities, such as paresis, myoclonus, and neuropathy, lasting weeks to months, are reported in both children and adults but are rare.[95,124]

Chronic Disulfiram Toxicity

The disulfiram–ethanol reaction, characterized by tachycardia, hypotension, diaphoresis, and facial erythema, is familiar to most physicians. However, the toxic effects of disulfiram alone, including depression, lethargy, loss of libido, psychosis, delirium, meningeal signs, unilateral weakness, optic neuritis, and peripheral neuropathy, are not well recognized by most clinicians, perhaps because the behavioral symptoms confused with manic-depressive or schizophrenic psychoses and the neurologic findings with the sequelae of alcoholism.[19,23,27,57,81,91,100]

The only significant adverse event reported in a placebo-controlled trial of abstinent individuals with oral disulfiram 250 mg/day versus placebo was drowsiness.[33] Over a 23-year period (1968–1991), 155 adverse drug events (ADEs) were reported for disulfiram, giving it an ADR rate of 1 per 200 to 2,000 patients per year (categorized as an "intermediate" rate of ADRs for a medication). Hepatic reactions were the most frequent ADR (34%) followed by neurologic (21%), cutaneous (15%), psychiatric (4%), and other (26%).[23]

Disulfiram-induced hepatitis was first reported in 1974.[50] In 1977, 6 additional cases were reported; 5 of the patients died.[92] Incidence of disulfiram-induced fatal hepatitis is reportedly 1 in 30,000 patients treated per year.[16] The onset of symptoms of hepatotoxicity caused by disulfiram occurs within 4 to 6 weeks (range, 2–24 weeks) after initiating treatment.[16,29,92] Signs and symptoms include fatigue, headache, fever, pruritus, rash, myalgias, malaise, anorexia, nausea, vomiting, abdominal pain, jaundice, light stools, dark urine, and hepatomegaly. Symptoms usually resolve within 2 weeks of stopping disulfiram, but liver function requires up to 12 weeks to normalize.[16,29,92] Liver biopsy demonstrates a predominantly hepatocellular degeneration with focal or extensive hepatocellular necrosis as well as portal and periportal eosinophilic infiltration.[16,29] Although the exact mechanism of disulfiram-induced liver damage is unclear, most reports suggest an idiosyncratic hypersensitivity reaction as the primary mechanism involved.[16,29,92] Alternatively, a carbon disulfide–induced hepatic injury resulting from covalent binding of electrophilic oxides or carbene derivatives of these oxides to macromolecules is considered responsible.[30]

Asymptomatic elevations in aminotransferase concentrations, up to 3 times the upper limits of normal, associated with disulfiram therapy are reported to range from 6% to 30% in alcoholics.[37,110,121] Although hepatic effects are most commonly reported with oral dosage forms, they also occur with implantable depot disulfiram.[69]

Liver transplantation for disulfiram-induced liver failure was first reported in 1989.[114] Since then, several case reports of liver transplantation for disulfiram-induced liver failure are noted[71]; the first North American case was performed in 1998.[89] A 5-year review from a hospital in Denmark revealed that disulfiram was the most common cause of idiosyncratic drug-induced liver failure, accounting for 13 of the 43 cases (30%).[2]

Disulfiram induces a peripheral neuropathy characterized by distal sensory impairment with loss of coordination, painful paresthesias, and distal weakness with foot drop.[1,31] The severity of the neuropathy is directly related to dose and duration of exposure.[81,118] If disulfiram is not discontinued, sensory and motor impairment progresses proximally.[7,98] Wallerian-type axonal degeneration, intermediate filament accumulation, and marked loss of larger myelinated fibers are the pathological hallmarks of disulfiram toxicity.[10,79] Experiments in animals showed that disulfiram causes Schwann cell damage and demyelination of peripheral nerves.[111,112] In addition, isolated descriptions of both axonal and myelin involvement are reported.[78]

The mechanisms underlying disulfiram-induced parkinsonism and catatonia are still controversial. One of the main hypotheses is that the lesions result from the toxicity of the disulfiram metabolite, carbon disulfide.[49,91] Histopathologic lesions of the globus pallidus and substantia nigra are observed after chronic exposure to carbon disulfide in animals.[97] Other research suggest involvement of brain dopaminergic transmission in disulfiram neurotoxicity.[17,44] This is supported by an experiment in mice, in which the toxic effects of 1-methyl-4-phenyl-1,2,3,6-tetrahydropyridine on nigrostriatal dopaminergic systems were enhanced by pretreatment with disulfiram.[18]

The exact mechanism of disulfiram-mediated encephalopathy is not known. However, both DDC and carbon disulfide are implicated, and both inhibit the activity of DBH, leading to the accumulation of dopamine, producing a relative deficiency of adrenaline and noradrenaline in the area of the basal ganglia.[42] Dopamine-mediated cellular injury is related to its ability to induce excitatory toxic effects of glutamate and calcium-mediated cell death and to impair the cellular ability to eliminate free oxygen radicals.[98]

Disulfiram and Carbon Disulfide

Carbon disulfide is a colorless volatile liquid and a commonly used nonpolar chemical solvent. The principal industrial use of carbon disulfide is the manufacture of viscose rayon. In addition, carbon disulfide is used as an insecticide for the fumigation of grains, nursery stock, in fresh fruit conservation, and as a soil pesticide against insects and nematodes.[21] The clinical, biochemical, and pathological neurotoxic effects of disulfiram are similar to those of carbon disulfide. Both are associated with depression, lethargy, loss of libido, psychosis, ataxia, incoordination, and peripheral neuropathy.[91] Both inhibit DBH in vitro and produce increased brain dopamine and decreased brain norepinephrine, demyelination, and denervation in vivo.[104] Acute exposure to carbon disulfide causes a rapid onset of headache, confusion, nausea, hallucinations, delirium, seizures, coma, and death.[4] Chronic carbon disulfide exposure causes pyridoxine deficiency and interacts with pyridoxal-5-phosphate, a cofactor in the production of γ-aminobutyric acid (GABA) from glutamate, thereby depleting GABA concentrations in the brain and leading to benzodiazepine-resistant seizures.[88] These findings suggest that disulfiram induced seizures are similar to that of carbon disulfide. However, there is no evidence that administering pyridoxine to a patient with disulfiram-induced seizure is of any benefit.

Although patients with occupational exposure to carbon disulfide have an increased risk of atherosclerosis and ischemic heart disease, this has not been proven for patients using disulfiram.[108] Disulfiram therapy increases serum cholesterol concentration.[65]

Disulfiram and Pediatrics

The presence of this drug in the household makes it a potential xenobiotic encountered in unintentional poisonings; however, reports of significant toxicity are rare. One case report details a 5-year-old girl with exposure to 19 tablets of disulfiram, who subsequently developed dystonia, complete loss of developmental milestones, and spastic tetraparesis over a 2-year follow-up period.[64] A 2-year-old child who developed an encephalopathy and dystonia after exposure to disulfiram brain magnetic resonance imaging showed edema and symmetrical hyperintense signal changes involving the globus pallidus and substantia nigra.[117]

Disulfiram and Pregnancy

There is a paucity of information regarding the teratogenic effects, if any, of disulfiram in humans or animals. Case reports suggest congenital defects, and one spontaneous miscarriage occurred.[25,43,77] A confounder could be the combination of disulfiram and alcohol itself, which enhances the incidence of birth defects. The embryotoxic properties of disulfiram could be related because of its lead- and copper-chelating properties.[20]

DIAGNOSTIC TESTING

Acute Disulfiram Toxicity

Serum concentrations of disulfiram and its metabolites, including diethyldithiomethylcarbamate acid and diethyldithiomethylcarbamate acid, can be measured but are not useful when managing most patients with suspected acute or chronic disulfiram overdose, disulfiram toxicity, or a disulfiram–ethanol reaction. Other markers of ingestion include carbon disulfide in the breath and diethylamine in the urine.[28] Because of rapid metabolism, only a small proportion of ingested disulfiram reaches the blood as the parent drug.[46] Leukocyte ALDH correlates most closely with hepatic mitochondrial ALDH. Decreased erythrocyte ALDH1 and leukocyte ALDH2 activity are markers of disulfiram exposure, but neither enzyme assay is commonly available. Elevated acetaldehyde concentrations in the blood will occur but are not readily available and thus also not clinically useful in managing patients.

Chronic Disulfiram Toxicity

The development of hepatotoxicity is a concern with chronic disulfiram administration. Two common strategies used for detecting and preventing severe hepatotoxicity include routine clinical monitoring for signs or symptoms of hepatic injury as well as periodic monitoring of biomarkers, including alanine aminotransferase, aspartate aminotransferase, alkaline phosphatase, and total bilirubin.[120,121]

There is no agreement on when disulfiram therapy should be modified or discontinued based on the finding of mildly elevated aminotransferase concentrations. There is much greater agreement that the development of an aminotransferase concentration greater than 3 times the upper limit of the reference range in combination with evidence of impaired hepatic synthetic function, elevated total bilirubin greater than 2 times the upper limit of the reference range, or international normalized ratio greater than 1.5 is suggestive of more severe drug-induced liver injury. In such situations, the mortality rate may be 16% or higher and necessitate discontinuing disulfiram.[9,102]

MANAGEMENT OF DISULFIRAM TOXICITY

Acute Disulfiram Toxicity

There is no antidote for acute disulfiram overdose. No specific studies have evaluated GI decontamination for acute overdose. Unless otherwise contraindicated, activated charcoal at a dose of 1 g/kg is recommended. Induced emesis is not indicated, and orogastric lavage or whole-bowel irrigation is not required.

Chronic Disulfiram Toxicity

Most patients receiving disulfiram will not develop hepatotoxicity, but those who develop mild increase in their aminotransferases will likely normalize with continued disulfiram therapy.[102] Continued periodic monitoring of liver function tests should be performed, and therapy should be discontinued with symptoms of hepatic injury such as jaundice, abdominal pain, nausea, vomiting, or fever.

Treatment of hepatotoxicity is supportive and usually resolves after discontinuation of disulfiram therapy. Liver transplantation was successfully performed for disulfiram-induced hepatic failure in both adults and children.[71,89]

DISULFIRAM AS AN ANTIDOTE

Disulfiram is used for the treatment of nickel dermatitis. However, a small double-blind, placebo-controlled study of patients with hand eczema and nickel allergy did not find a clinically significant difference between those treated with disulfiram and those treated with placebo.[48] In fact, the conditions of some patients worsened after disulfiram therapy.[54]

Diethyldithiocarbamate is available as the chelator dithiocarb. Although animal studies suggest that DDC is effective for nickel-carbonyl poisoning, there are no human studies to confirm this[12,107] (Chap. 96).

SUMMARY

- Although the role of disulfiram in treating alcoholism is diminishing, its use for the treatment of cocaine dependence is gaining interest.
- It is critical to understand the distinction among the different forms of disulfiram toxicity, including toxicity from an acute overdose, from chronic therapy, and from a disulfiram–ethanol reaction.
- Disulfiram and its metabolites both irreversibly inhibit ALDH. This leads to accumulation of acetaldehyde and is responsible for many of the symptoms produced by the disulfiram–ethanol reaction. Symptoms are typically self-limiting and include facial and generalized body warmth and flushing, pruritus, urticaria, diaphoresis, lightheadedness, vertigo, headache, nausea, vomiting, and abdominal pain.
- Treatment for the disulfiram–ethanol reaction is mostly supportive and includes IV crystalloid administration, antiemetics, and histamine receptor antagonists. Fomepizole, an alcohol dehydrogenase inhibitor, is appropriate for more serious reactions when the serum ethanol concentration remains elevated.
- Disulfiram toxicity after an acute overdose is unlikely to be life threatening. Early symptoms are mostly GI. Rarely, persistent neurologic symptoms occur and include myopathy, movement disorders, ataxia, parkinsonism, and psychosis.
- Hepatotoxicity is the most common ADE associated with chronic disulfiram therapy. Neurotoxicity is also reported with chronic disulfiram toxicity, and symptoms are similar to those of acute disulfiram toxicity.

Acknowledgment

Edwin K. Kuffner, MD, contributed to this chapter in previous editions.

REFERENCES

1. Ansbacher LE, et al. Disulfiram neuropathy: a neurofilamentous distal axonopathy. *Neurology*. 1982;32:424-428.
2. Baekdal M, et al. Drug-induced liver injury: a cohort study on patients referred to the Danish transplant center over a five year period. *Scand J Gastroenterol*. 2017;52:450-454.
3. Barth KS, Malcolm RJ. Disulfiram: an old therapeutic with new applications. *CNS Neurol Disord Drug Targets*. 2010;9:5-12.
4. Beauchamp RO Jr, et al. A critical review of the literature on carbon disulfide toxicity. *Crit Rev Toxicol*. 1983;11:169-278.
5. Becker MC, Sugarman G. Death following "test drink" of alcohol in patients receiving Antabuse. *JAMA*. 1952;149:568-571.
6. Benitz WE, Tatro DS. Disulfiram intoxication in a child. *J Pediatr*. 1984;105:487-489.
7. Bevilacqua JA, et al. [Disulfiram neuropathy. Report of 3 cases]. *Rev Med Chil*. 2002;130:1037-1042.
8. Billstein SA, Sudol TE. Disulfiram-like reactions rare with ceftriaxone. *Geriatrics*. 1992;47:70.
9. Bjornsson E, et al. Clinical characteristics and prognostic markers in disulfiram-induced liver injury. *J Hepatol*. 2006;44:791-797.
10. Bouldin TW, et al. Pathology of disulfiram neuropathy. *Neuropathol Appl Neurobiol*. 1980;6:155-160.
11. Bourcier S, et al. Disulfiram ethanol reaction mimicking anaphylactic, cardiogenic, and septic shock. *Am J Emerg Med*. 2013;31:270; e271-e273.
12. Bradberry SM, Vale JA. Therapeutic review: do diethyldithiocarbamate and disulfiram have a role in acute nickel carbonyl poisoning? *J Toxicol Clin Toxicol*. 1999;37:259-264.
13. Brien JF, Loomis CW. Disposition and pharmacokinetics of disulfiram and calcium carbimide (calcium cyanamide). *Drug Metab Rev*. 1983;14:113-126.
14. Brown KR, et al. Theophylline elixir, moxalactam, and a disulfiram reaction. *Ann Intern Med*. 1982;97:621-622.
15. Chen D, et al. Disulfiram, a clinically used anti-alcoholism drug and copper-binding agent, induces apoptotic cell death in breast cancer cultures and xenografts via inhibition of the proteasome activity. *Cancer Res*. 2006;66:10425-10433.
16. Chick J. Safety issues concerning the use of disulfiram in treating alcohol dependence. *Drug Saf*. 1999;20:427-435.
17. Cobby J, et al. Methyl diethyldithiocarbamate, a metabolite of disulfiram in man. *Life Sci*. 1977;21:937-942.
18. Corsini GU, et al. 1-Methyl-4-phenyl-1,2,3,6-tetrahydropyridine (MPTP) neurotoxicity in mice is enhanced by pretreatment with diethyldithiocarbamate. *Eur J Pharmacol*. 1985;119:127-128.
19. Daniel DG, et al. Capgras delusion and seizures in association with therapeutic dosages of disulfiram. *South Med J*. 1987;80:1577-1579.
20. Danielsson BR, et al. Placental transfer and fetal distribution of lead in mice after treatment with dithiocarbamates. *Arch Toxicol*. 1984;55:27-33.
21. Davidson M, Feinleib M. Carbon disulfide poisoning: a review. *Am Heart J*. 1972;83:100-114.
22. Ehrlich RI, et al. Disulfiram reaction in an artist exposed to solvents. *Occup Med (Lond)*. 2012;62:64-66.
23. Enghusen Poulsen H, et al. Disulfiram therapy—adverse drug reactions and interactions. *Acta Psychiatr Scand Suppl*. 1992;369:59-65; discussion 65-56.
24. Faiman MD, et al. Elimination kinetics of disulfiram in alcoholics after single and repeated doses. *Clin Pharmacol Ther*. 1984;36:520-526.
25. Favre-Tissort M, Delatour P. [Psychopharmacology and teratogenesis a propos of disulfiram: experimental trial]. *Ann Med Psychol (Paris)*. 1965;123:735-740.
26. Fernandez D. Another esophageal rupture after alcohol and disulfiram. *N Engl J Med*. 1972;286:610.
27. Fisher CM. "Catatonia" due to disulfiram toxicity. *Arch Neurol*. 1989;46:798-804.
28. Fletcher K, et al. A breath test to assess compliance with disulfiram. *Addiction*. 2006;101:1705-1710.
29. Forns X, et al. Disulfiram-induced hepatitis. Report of four cases and review of the literature. *J Hepatol*. 1994;21:853-857.
30. Friis H, Andreasen PB. Drug-induced hepatic injury: an analysis of 1100 cases reported to the Danish Committee on Adverse Drug Reactions between 1978 and 1987. *J Intern Med*. 1992;232:133-138.
31. Frisoni GB, Di Monda V. Disulfiram neuropathy: a review (1971–1988) and report of a case. *Alcohol Alcohol*. 1989;24:429-437.
32. Frye RF, Branch RA. Effect of chronic disulfiram administration on the activities of CYP1A2, CYP2C19, CYP2D6, CYP2E1, and N-acetyltransferase in healthy human subjects. *Br J Clin Pharmacol*. 2002;53:155-162.
33. Fuller RK, et al. Disulfiram treatment of alcoholism. A Veterans Administration cooperative study. *JAMA*. 1986;256:1449-1455.
34. Garbutt JC, et al. Pharmacological treatment of alcohol dependence: a review of the evidence. *JAMA*. 1999;281:1318-1325.
35. Gaval-Cruz M, Weinshenker D. Mechanisms of disulfiram-induced cocaine abstinence: Antabuse and cocaine relapse. *Mol Interv*. 2009;9:175-187.
36. Goldstein M, et al. Inhibition of dopamine-beta-hydroxylase by disulfiram. *Life Sci*. 1964;3:763-767.
37. Goyer PF, Major LF. Hepatotoxicity in disulfiram-treated patients. *J Stud Alcohol*. 1979;40:133-137.
38. Gui X, et al. Disulfiram/copper complex inhibiting NF-$_k$B activity and potentiating cytotoxic effect of gemcitabine on colon and breast cancer cel lines. *Cancer Lett*. 2010;290:104-113.
39. Hald J, et al. Formation of acetaldehyde in the organism in relation to dosage of Antabuse (tetraethylthiuramdisulfide) and to alcohol-concentration in blood. *Acta Pharmacol Toxicol (Copenh)*. 1949;5:179-188.
40. Heath RG, et al. Behavioral and metabolic changes associated with administration of tetraethylthiuram disulfide (Antabuse). *Dis Nerv Syst*. 1965;26:99-105.
41. Heelon MW, White M. Disulfiram-cotrimoxazole reaction. *Pharmacotherapy*. 1998;18:869-870.
42. Heikkila RE, et al. In vivo inhibition of superoxide dismutase in mice by diethyldithiocarbamate. *J Biol Chem*. 1976;251:2182-2185.
43. Helmbrecht GD, Hoskins IA. First trimester disulfiram exposure: report of two cases. *Am J Perinatol*. 1993;10:5-7.
44. Hotson JR, Langston JW. Disulfiram-induced encephalopathy. *Arch Neurol*. 1976;33:141-142.
45. Jensen JC, et al. Elimination characteristics of disulfiram over time in five alcoholic volunteers: a preliminary study. *Am J Psychiatry*. 1982;139:1596-1598.
46. Johansson B. A review of the pharmacokinetics and pharmacodynamics of disulfiram and its metabolites. *Acta Psychiatr Scand Suppl*. 1992;369:15-26.
47. Jones RO. Death following the ingestion of alcohol in an Antabuse treated patient. *Can Med Assoc J*. 1949;60:609-612.
48. Kaaber K, et al. Treatment of nickel dermatitis with Antabuse; a double blind study. *Contact Dermatitis*. 1983;9:297-299.

49. Kane FJ Jr. Carbon disulfide intoxication from overdosage of disulfiram. *Am J Psychiatry*. 1970;127:690-694.

50. Keeffe EB, Smith FW. Disulfiram hypersensitivity hepatitis. *JAMA*. 1974;230:435-436.

51. Kharasch ED, et al. Lack of single-dose disulfiram effects on cytochrome P-450 2C9, 2C19, 2D6, and 3A4 activities: evidence for specificity toward P-450 2E1. *Drug Metab Dispos*. 1999;27:717-723.

52. Kharasch ED, et al. Single-dose disulfiram inhibition of chlorzoxazone metabolism: a clinical probe for P450 2E1. *Clin Pharmacol Ther*. 1993;53:643-650.

53. Kitson TM, Crow KE. Studies on possible mechanisms for the interaction between cyanamide and aldehyde dehydrogenase. *Biochem Pharmacol*. 1979;28:2551-2556.

54. Klein LR, Fowler JF Jr. Nickel dermatitis recall during disulfiram therapy for alcohol abuse. *J Am Acad Dermatol*. 1992;26:645-646.

55. Kline SS, et al. Cefotetan-induced disulfiram-type reactions and hypoprothrombinemia. *Antimicrob Agents Chemother*. 1987;31:1328-1331.

56. Klink DD, et al. Disulfiram-like reaction to chlorpropamide (Diabinese). *Wis Med J*. 1969;68:134-136.

57. Knee ST, Razani J. Acute organic brain syndrome: a complication of disulfiram therapy. *Am J Psychiatry*. 1974;131:1281-1282.

58. Koff RS, et al. Alcohol in cough medicines hazard to disulfiram user. *JAMA*. 1971;215:1988-1989.

59. Krauss JK, et al. Dystonia and akinesia due to pallidoputaminal lesions after disulfiram intoxication. *Mov Disord*. 1991;6:166-170.

60. Laplane D, et al. Lesions of basal ganglia due to disulfiram neurotoxicity. *J Neurol Neurosurg Psychiatry*. 1992;55:925-929.

61. Lemoyne S, et al. Delayed and prolonged coma after acute disulfiram overdose. *Acta Neurol Belg*. 2009;109:231-234.

62. Lindros KO, et al. The disulfiram (Antabuse)-alcohol reaction in male alcoholics: its efficient management by 4-methylpyrazole. *Alcohol Clin Exp Res*. 1981;5:528-530.

63. Madan A, et al. Identification of the human P-450 enzymes responsible for the sulfoxidation and thiono-oxidation of diethyldithiocarbamate methyl ester: role of P-450 enzymes in disulfiram bioactivation. *Alcohol Clin Exp Res*. 1998;22:1212-1219.

64. Mahajan P, et al. Basal ganglia infarction in a child with disulfiram poisoning. *Pediatrics*. 1997;99:605-608.

65. Major LF, Goyer PF. Effects of disulfiram and pyridoxine on serum cholesterol. *Ann Intern Med*. 1978;88:53-56.

66. Malcolm R, et al. The safety of disulfiram for the treatment of alcohol and cocaine dependence in randomized clinical trials: guidance for clinical practice. *Expert Opin Drug Saf*. 2008;7:459-472.

67. Marchner H, Tottmar O. A comparative study on the effects of disulfiram, cyanamide and 1-aminocyclopropanol on the acetaldehyde metabolism in rats. *Acta Pharmacol Toxicol (Copenh)*. 1978;43:219-232.

68. McCance-Katz EF, et al. Disulfiram effects on acute cocaine administration. *Drug Alcohol Depend*. 1998;52:27-39.

69. Meier M, et al. Acute liver failure: a message found under the skin. *Postgrad Med J*. 2005;81:269-270.

70. Milne HJ, Parke TR. Hypotension and ST depression as a result of disulfiram ethanol reaction. *Eur J Emerg Med*. 2007;14:228-229.

71. Mohanty SR, et al. Liver transplantation for disulfiram-induced fulminant hepatic failure. *J Clin Gastroenterol*. 2004;38:292-295.

72. Morales-Molina JA, et al. Alcohol ingestion and topical tacrolimus: a disulfiram-like interaction? *Ann Pharmacother*. 2005;39:772-773.

73. Moreels S, et al. Intractable hypotension and myocardial ischaemia induced by co-ingestion of ethanol and disulfiram. *Acta Cardiol*. 2012;67:491-493.

74. Motte S, et al. Refractory hyperdynamic shock associated with alcohol and disulfiram. *Am J Emerg Med*. 1986;4:323-325.

75. Musacchio JM, et al. Inhibition of dopamine-beta-hydroxylase by disulfiram in vivo. *J Pharmacol Exp Ther*. 1966;152:56-61.

76. Neu HC, Prince AS. Interaction between moxalactam and alcohol. *Lancet*. 1980;1:1422.

77. Nora AH, et al. Limb-reduction anomalies in infants born to disulfiram-treated alcoholic mothers. *Lancet*. 1977;2:664.

78. Nukada H, Pollock M. Disulfiram neuropathy. A morphometric study of sural nerve. *J Neurol Sci*. 1981;51:51-67.

79. Olney RK, Miller RG. Peripheral neuropathy associated with disulfiram administration. *Muscle Nerve*. 1980;3:172-175.

80. Orakzai A, et al. Disulfiram-induced transient optic and peripheral neuropathy: a case report. *Ir J Med Sci*. 2007;176:319-321.

81. Palliyath SK, et al. Peripheral nerve functions in chronic alcoholic patients on disulfiram: a six month follow up. *J Neurol Neurosurg Psychiatry*. 1990;53:227-230.

82. Pani PP, et al. Disulfiram for the treatment of cocaine dependence. *Cochrane Database Syst Rev*. 2010:CD007024.

83. Peachey JE, et al. Cardiovascular changes during the calcium carbimide-ethanol interaction. *Clin Pharmacol Ther*. 1981;29:40-46.

84. Petroni NC, Cardoni AA. Alcohol content of liquid medicinals. *Clin Toxicol*. 1979;14:407-432.

85. Pettinati HM, et al. A double blind, placebo-controlled trial that combines disulfiram and naltrexone for treating co-occurring cocaine and alcohol dependence. *Addict Behav*. 2008;33:651-667.

86. Phillips M. Persistent sensitivity to ethanol following a single dose of parenteral sustained-release disulfiram. *Adv Alcohol Subst Abuse*. 1987;7:51-61.

87. Poulsen HE, et al. The influence of disulfiram on acetaminophen metabolism in man. *Xenobiotica*. 1991;21:243-249.

88. Price TR, Silberfarb PM. Disulfiram-induced convulsions without challenge by alcohol. *J Stud Alcohol*. 1976;37:980-982.

89. Rabkin JM, et al. Liver transplantation for disulfiram-induced hepatic failure. *Am J Gastroenterol*. 1998;93:830-831.

90. Rae C, et al. The role of copper in disulfiram-induced cytotoxicity and raadiosensitization of cancer cells. *J Nucl Med*. 2013;54:953-960.

91. Rainey JM Jr. Disulfiram toxicity and carbon disulfide poisoning. *Am J Psychiatry*. 1977;134:371-378.

92. Ranek L, et al. Disulfiram hepatotoxicity. *Br Med J*. 1977;2:94-96.

93. Rathod NH. Toxic effects of disulfiram therapy; with two case reports. *Q J Stud Alcohol*. 1958;19:418-427.

94. Refojo MF. Disulfiram-alcohol reaction caused by contact lens wetting solution. *Contact Intraocul Lens Med J*. 1981;7:172.

95. Reichelderfer TE. Acute disulfiram poisoning in a child. *Q J Stud Alcohol*. 1969;30:724-728.

96. Reynolds WA, Lowe FH. Mushrooms and a toxic reaction to alcohol: report of four cases. *N Engl J Med*. 1965;272:630-631.

97. Richter R. Degeneration of the basal ganglia in monkeys from chronic carbon disulfide poisoning. *J Neuropathol Exp Neurol*. 1945;4:324-353.

98. Rothman SM, Olney JW. Glutamate and the pathophysiology of hypoxic-ischemic brain damage. *Ann Neurol*. 1986;19:105-111.

99. Rothstein E, Clancy DD. Toxicity of disulfiram combined with metronidazole. *N Engl J Med*. 1969;280:1006-1007.

100. Ryan TV, et al. Chronic neuropsychological impairment resulting from disulfiram overdose. *J Stud Alcohol*. 1993;54:389-392.

101. Sande M, et al. Fomepizole for severe disulfiram-ethanol reactions. *Am J Emerg Med*. 2012;30:262 e263-265.

102. Senior JR. Monitoring for hepatotoxicity: what is the predictive value of liver "function" tests? *Clin Pharmacol Ther*. 2009;85:331-334.

103. Shorter D, Kosten TR. Novel pharmacotherapeutic treatments for cocaine addiction. *BMC Med*. 2011;9:119.

104. Stanosz S, et al. Concentration of dopamine in plasma, activity of dopamine beta-hydroxylase in serum and urinary excretion of free catecholamines and vanillylmandelic acid in women chronically exposed to carbon disulphide. *Int J Occup Med Environ Health*. 1994;7:257-261.

105. Stowell A, et al. Diphenhydramine and the calcium carbimide-ethanol reaction: a placebo-controlled clinical study. *Clin Pharmacol Ther*. 1986;39:521-525.

106. Stransky G, et al. Methemoglobinemia in a fatal case of disulfiram-ethanol reaction. *J Anal Toxicol*. 1997;21:178-179.

107. Sunderman FW Sr. The treatment of acute nickel carbonyl poisoning with sodium diethyldithiocarbamate. *Ann Clin Res*. 1971;3:182-185.

108. Sweetnam PM, et al. Exposure to carbon disulphide and ischaemic heart disease in a viscose rayon factory. *Br J Ind Med*. 1987;44:220-227.

109. Syed J, Moarefi G. An unusual presentation of a disulfiram-alcohol reaction. *Del Med J*. 1995;67:183.

110. Tamai H, et al. Comparison of cyanamide and disulfiram in effects on liver function. *Alcohol Clin Exp Res*. 2000;24:97S-99S.

111. Tonkin EG, et al. Disulfiram produces a non-carbon disulfide-dependent schwannopathy in the rat. *J Neuropathol Exp Neurol*. 2000;59:786-797.

112. Tonkin EG, et al. N,N-diethyldithiocarbamate produces copper accumulation, lipid peroxidation, and myelin injury in rat peripheral nerve. *Toxicol Sci*. 2004;81:160-171.

113. Truitt EB Jr, et al. Disulfiramlike actions produced by hypoglycemic sulfonylurea compounds. *Q J Stud Alcohol*. 1962;23:197-207.

114. Vanjak D, et al. [Fulminant hepatitis induced by disulfiram in a patient with alcoholic cirrhosis. Survival after liver transplantation]. *Gastroenterol Clin Biol*. 1989;13:1075-1078.

115. Vasak V, Kopecky J. On the role of pyridoxamine in the mechanism of the toxic action of carbon disulphide. Toxicology of carbon disulphide. *Excerpta Medica*; 1967:35-41.

116. Visapaa JP, et al. Lack of disulfiram-like reaction with metronidazole and ethanol. *Ann Pharmacother*. 2002;36:971-974.

117. Vykuntaraju KN, Ramalingaiah AH. Disulfiram poisoning causing acute encephalopathy. *Indian Pediatr*. 2013;50:887-888.

118. Watson CP, et al. Disulfiram neuropathy. *Can Med Assoc J*. 1980;123:123-126.

119. Wier JK, Tyler VE Jr. An investigation of Coprinus atramentarius for the presence of disulfiram. *J Am Pharm Assoc Am Pharm Assoc*. 1960;49:426-429.

120. Wilson H. Side-effects of disulfiram. *Br Med J*. 1962;2:1610-1611.

121. Wright CT, et al. Disulfiram-induced fulminating hepatitis: guidelines for liver-panel monitoring. *J Clin Psychiatry*. 1988;49:430-434.

122. Yodaiken RE. Ethylene dibromide and disulfiram—a lethal combination. *JAMA*. 1978;239:2783.

123. Zapata E, Orwin A. Severe hypertension and bronchospasm during disulfiram-ethanol test reaction. *BMJ*. 1992;305:870.

124. Zorzon M, et al. Acute encephalopathy and polyneuropathy after disulfiram intoxication. *Alcohol Alcohol*. 1995;30:629-631.

79 HALLUCINOGENS

Mark J. Neavyn and Jennifer L. Carey

HISTORY

A "hallucination" is defined as a false perception that has no basis in the external environment. The term is derived from the Latin "to wander in mind." Hallucinations differ from illusions, which are distorted perceptions of objects based in reality. Although the term *psychedelic* has been used for years to refer to the recreational and nonmedical effects of hallucinogens, other terms, such as *entheogen* and *entactogen*, frequently appear in discussions. Entheogens are "substances that generate the god or spirit within," and entactogens create an awareness of "the touch within."[50] These terms all refer to the same xenobiotics, used with differing intent or in varying settings.

Hallucinogens are a diverse group of xenobiotics that alter and distort perception, thought, and mood without clouding the sensorium. Hallucinogens are categorized by their chemical structures and are further divided into natural and synthetic members of each family. The major structural classes of hallucinogens include the lysergamides, tryptamines (indolealkylamines), amphetamines (phenylethylamines), arylhexamines, cannabinoids, harmine alkaloids, belladonna alkaloids, and tropane alkaloids. In addition, there are several unclassified hallucinogens, such as *Salvia divinorum*, nutmeg (*Myristica fragrans*), kratom (*Mitragyna speciose*), and kava kava (*Piper methysticum*). This chapter focuses on lysergamides, tryptamines, phenylethylamines, and the aforementioned "unclassified" hallucinogens. The other classes are found in Chaps. 71, 73, 74, and 83 (Table 79-1).

Hallucinogens have been used for thousands of years by many different cultures, largely during religious ceremonies. The ancient Indian holy book, *Rig-Veda*, written more than 3,500 years ago, describes a sacramental substance called Soma both as a god and as an intoxicating substance. Although debated for many years, the source of Soma is now believed to be an extract of the mushroom *Amanita muscaria*.[121,129] The Aztecs used the psilocybin-containing mushroom *Psilocybe mexicana*, termed "teonanacatl" (flesh of the gods), and the lysergic acid amide-containing morning glory plant, *Turbina corymbosa*, known as "Ololiuqui" in their religious ceremonies. The Native American Church in the United States uses peyote in religious ceremonies.[28,31,116] In South America, ayahuasca, a tea made of dimethyltryptamine-containing plants (eg, *Psychotria viridis*), is famous for its use in shamanistic rituals.[94]

From medieval times through recent years, several large-scale epidemics of vasospastic ischemia, gangrene and hallucinations (collectively called ergotism) resulted from *Claviceps purpurea* contamination of cereal crops.[164] The hallucinations from Claviceps ingestion is attributed to the ergot alkaloid lysergic acid amide from which lysergic acid diethylamide (LSD) was chemically synthesized. *Claviceps purpurea* has been suggested, but subsequently disproved, as the cause of the mass hysteria leading up to the Salem witch trials. Many of these adverse effects after ingestion of *C. purpurea* are attributed to the serotonergic agonist effects of the ergot alkaloids (Chap. 52).[47]

Synthetic hallucinogen use is often said to have begun in 1938 when Albert Hofmann, a Swiss chemist, synthesized LSD while performing extensive research on the medicinal uses of ergot alkaloids derived from the fungus, *Claviceps purpurea*. Five years later, LSD was "tested" when Hofmann exposed himself in his laboratory and subsequently developed hallucinations.[76,141] Soon thereafter, Sandoz laboratories began marketing LSD under the trademark *Delysidas* as an adjunct for analytic psychotherapy. In the 1950s, a small number of psychiatrists began using LSD to release the repressed memories of patients and as an experimental model for schizophrenia.[149] The Central Intelligence Agency experimented with the use of LSD as a tool for interrogating suspected communists and as a mind-control agent.[27,141]

Lysergic acid diethylamide (also called acid) became a fashionable recreational drug. In the 1960s, the concept of the "fifth freedom" emerged as

the "right" for individuals to alter their consciousness as they saw fit. In one of the most famous slogans of the 1960s, Timothy Leary popularized LSD as a way to "tune in, turn on, drop out."[141] By 1966, federal law banned the use of LSD.[112] Initial reports of LSD-induced chromosomal damage appeared in the 1960s, including fetuses in utero.[36,78,90] However, further studies of pregnant women who had taken LSD did not demonstrate an increased risk of abortions or birth defects.[53,87] Lysergic acid diethylamide use diminished in the late 1970s and early 1980s, perhaps because of users' concerns regarding potential health risks of brain damage, "bad trips," and flashbacks.[120] Recurrent visual hallucinations after LSD are known to cause significant anxiety in some users, and this phenomenon is now recognized as "hallucinogen persisting perception disorder" (HPPD).[72]

In the meantime, there was a rise in the use of the "designer" hallucinogens. Exploiting a loophole in drug enforcement laws, these designer synthetic tryptamine and amphetamine hallucinogens are chemically similar to, but legally distinct from, their outlawed counterparts and therefore not subjected to legislative drug control. These are often referred to as "legal highs." A bill sponsored by Rep. Charles Dent of Pennsylvania in 2016 aimed to place additional synthetic hallucinogens, opioids, and cannabinoids in Schedule I status, but it has yet to pass in the US Senate.[37]

The Internet is now a vehicle for the rapid and facile sharing of information on the synthesis of emerging drugs, user experiences, and adverse effects. Encyclopedic content on recreational drug use is found on Erowid.org, and additional crowd-sourcing information is found on drug forums hosted on Bluelight.org, Reddit.com, and many others. Additionally, many "herbal" hallucinogens are widely available for purchase via unregulated websites.[41] Hidden "cryptomarkets" are found on the dark web, content on the Internet that requires encryption software or prior authorization to access and is not searchable through common Internet search engines.[156,157] A search on one such cryptomarket Alphabay found 120 vendors selling novel psychoactive substances to users.[157] All-night dance clubs host "rave parties" at which emerging hallucinogens are popular.[16] Although the impact of these parties on the growth of hallucinogens in the United States is unclear, many of the newer hallucinogens are christened "club drugs" because of this association.[64] A survey of dance club patrons in South London suggests that novel psychoactive substances supplement established recreational drugs like 3,4-methylenedioxymethamphetamine (MDMA).[107]

Although much of the research involving psychedelic drugs was halted in the 1960s, clinical investigations for the treatment of various psychiatric disorders, with emphasis on treatment of anxiety and addictions is reemerging. Currently, psilocybin is being evaluated for the treatment of the existential anxiety associated with end-stage cancer and obsessive-compulsive disorders, and MDMA is studied as an adjunct to psychotherapy for treatment-resistant posttraumatic stress disorder.[69,106,108,123] This clinical or research use of psychedelic drugs remains highly controversial.

EPIDEMIOLOGY

Resurgence in LSD use was reported among high school teens in the late 1990s, with more prevalent use in the suburbs than the cities.[113,130] In 1997, 2 studies of adolescents showed a lifetime prevalence of LSD use at 13% and 14%.[80,120] In 2000, Drug Enforcement Administration (DEA) agents seized an LSD-production lab and apprehended 2 men involved in massive production of LSD in Kansas. The seizure of more than 40 kg of LSD in this case was considered the largest LSD lab seizure in DEA history.[3] Their incarceration resulted in a 95% decrease in LSD availability nationwide.[4]

From 2006 to 2015, the National Survey on Drug Use and Health (NSDUH) reported the following trends in hallucinogen use: lifetime LSD use among

TABLE 79–1	Structural Classifications of Hallucinogens

Lysergamides
- D-Lysergic acid diethylamide (LSD)
- Lysergic acid hydroxyethylamide
  - Morning glory (*Ipomoea violacea*)
  - South American morning glory (*Ololiuqui*)
- Ergine
  - Woodrose (*Argyreia nervosa*)

Indolealkylamines and Tryptamines
- 5-Methoxy-*N,N*-dimethyltryptamine (5-MeO-DiPT, Foxy Methoxy)
- *N,N*-Dimethyltryptamine (DMT)
- Psilocin α-methyltryptamine (AMT)
- Psilocybin

Phenylethylamines
- Mescaline
- 3,4-Methylenedioxymethamphetamine (MDMA)
- 2C-B
- 2C-T-7

Tetrahydrocannabinoids
- Marijuana
- Hashish

Belladonna Alkaloids
- Jimsonweed (*Datura stramonium*)
- Henbane (*Hyoscyamus niger*)
- Deadly nightshade (*Atropa belladonna*)
- *Brugmansia* spp

Miscellaneous
- Kava Kava (*Piper methysticum*)
- Kratom (*Mitragyna speciose korth*)
- Nutmeg (*Myristica fragrans*)-myristicin, elemicin, safrole
- Phencyclidine (PCP), ketamine
- *Salvia divinorum*

Americans over the age of 12 years increased from 23 to 25 million, lifetime phencyclidine (PCP) use decreased from 6.6 to 6.3 million, and lifetime MDMA use increased from 12 million to 18 million. Additionally, lifetime ketamine use increased from 2.3 to 3 million people, and lifetime reported use of α-methyltryptamine (AMT), dimethyltryptamine (DMT), or 5-methoxydimethyl tryptamine (5-MeO-DMT) tripled from 700,000 to 2.1 million. About 1.8 million people reported use of *S. divinorum* during their lifetime in 2006, and 5.1 million people reported lifetime use in 2015.[117] In the reported results, the 18- to 25-year-old age group was most likely to report use of any of these hallucinogens within the previous year.[143] In 2010, the

NSDUH reported that 1.2 million Americans older than the age of 12 years were current users of hallucinogens.[152]

LYSERGAMIDES

Lysergamides are derivatives of lysergic acid, a substituted tetracyclic amine based on an indole nucleus (Fig. 79–1). Naturally occurring lysergamides are found in several species of morning glory (*Rivea corymbosa, Ipomoea violacea*) and Hawaiian baby woodrose (*Argyreia nervosa*).[71] Morning glory seeds contain multiple alkaloids, including lysergic acid hydroxyethylamide and ergonovine. Morning glory seeds were called *ololiuqui* in ancient Mexico, where Aztecs and other indigenous populations used them in religious rites.[145] However, in one volunteer study, ololiuqui caused sedation rather than hallucinations.[77] Hawaiian baby woodrose seeds contain the alkaloid ergine (D-lysergic acid amide).[7] Both morning glory and Hawaiian baby woodrose seeds are legally purchased for planting in garden stores and on the Internet.

The synthetic lysergamide, LSD, is derived from an ergot alkaloid of the fungus, *Claviceps purpurea*. Although 4 LSD isomers exist, only the D-isomer is active. Lysergic acid diethylamide is a water-soluble, colorless, tasteless, and odorless powder. Lysergic acid diethylamide is typically sold as liquid-impregnated blotter paper, microdots, tiny tablets, "window pane" gelatin squares, liquid, powder, or tablets.[130] Of note, the traditional "blotter paper" associated with LSD is commonly found to have other synthetic hallucinogens, particularly *N*-benzly-oxy-methyl (NBOME).[44,59] Lysergic acid diethylamide users typically experience heightened awareness of auditory and visual stimuli with size, shape, and color distortions. Auditory and visual hallucinations occur, as well as synesthesia, a confusion of the senses, in which users report "hearing colors" or "seeing sounds." Other more complex perceptual effects include depersonalization and a sensation of enhanced insight or awareness. A "bad trip" or dysphoric reaction is said to occur when LSD use produces anxiety, bizarre behaviors, and combativeness.

Lysergic acid diethylamide is classified by the DEA as a Schedule I drug, which is defined as having a high abuse potential, lack of established safety even under medical supervision, and no known use in medical treatment.

INDOLEALKYLAMINES (TRYPTAMINES)

Indolealkylamines, or tryptamines, represent a class of natural and synthetic compounds that structurally share a substituted monoamine group (Fig. 79–2). Endogenous tryptamines include serotonin and melatonin. Naturally occurring exogenous tryptamines include psilocybin, bufotenine and N,N-dimethyltryptamine (DMT). Psilocybin is found in three major genera of mushrooms: *Psilocyba, Panaelous,* and *Conocybe*.[129] Other psychoactive mushrooms include *Amanita muscaria* and *Amanita pantherina*, which contain ibotenic acid, muscimol, and muscazone, which are unrelated to the tryptamines.[71] Hallucinogenic mushrooms are discussed at length in Chap. 117. Psilocybin-containing mushrooms, or "magic mushrooms," are indigenous to the Pacific Northwest and southern United States, usually

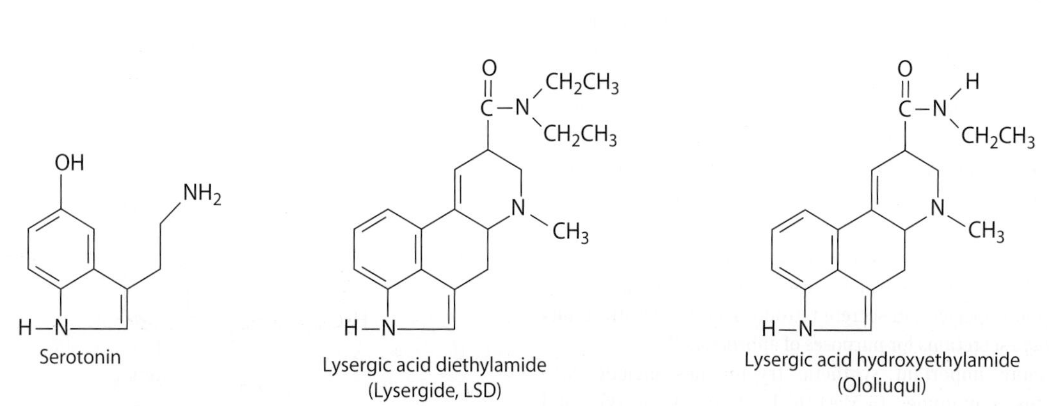

FIGURE 79–1. Hallucinogens of the lysergamide chemical class and their chemical similarity to serotonin.

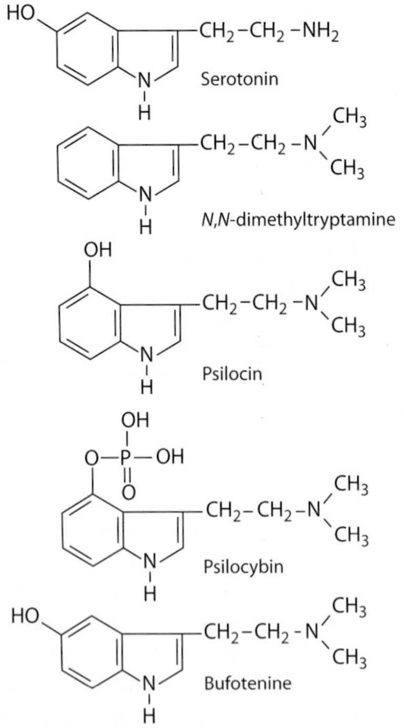

FIGURE 79–2. Hallucinogens of the indolealkylamine chemical class and their chemical similarity to serotonin.

found in cow pastures. The mushroom is recognizable by a green-blue color that it assumes after bruising, but misidentification is common.[14]

N,N-dimethyltryptamine a $5\text{-}HT_{2A}$, $5\text{-}HT_{2C}$ and $5\text{-}HT_{1A}$ receptor agonist, is a potent short-acting hallucinogen found naturally in the bark of the Yakee plant (*Virola calophylla*), a species of the Myristicaceae family, which grows in the Amazon basin. It is used by shamans as a hallucinogenic snuff to "communicate with the spirits."[129] *N,N*-dimethyltryptamine is also found in the hallucinogenic tea ayahuasca, which originates in the Amazon Basin and used by indigenous healers during religious ceremonies.[94] In ayahuasca, DMT-containing plants (eg, *Psychotria viridis*) are combined with plants containing harmine alkaloids (eg, *Banisteriopsis caapi*), which inhibit hepatic monoamine oxidases to increase the oral bioavailability of DMT (Chap. 71).[102]

The use of toads in religious ceremonies and witchcraft dates back thousands of years. All species of the toad genus Bufo have parotid glands on their backs that produce a variety of xenobiotics, including dopamine, epinephrine, and serotonin.[93] Many of these toads produce bufotenine, a tryptamine, which causes hypertension but does not cross the blood–brain barrier. Interest in bufotenine grew out of reports of a toad-licking fad in the 1980s, in which individuals would reportedly lick toads for recreational purposes.[92] However, further review suggests that bufotenine is not the hallucinogenic substance found in toad secretions. Instead, 5-methoxydimethyl tryptamine (5-MeO-DMT), was identified as the psychoactive substance.[162] 5-Methoxydimethyl tryptamine is only found in one species of toad, *Bufo alvarius* (Sonoran Desert toad or Colorado River toad).[92] Although bufotenine was classified as a Schedule I drug by the DEA for many years, 5-MeO-DMT was not scheduled until 2009.[109] Like DMT, 5-MeO-DMT is rapidly metabolized by intestinal monoamine oxidase enzymes; oral ingestion of toad venom or skins would thus have limited potential as a route of recreational use.[25] Methods for extracting and drying *B. alvarius* secretions for smoking and insufflation are available on the Internet. The toad venom glands also produce cardioactive steroids, called bufadienolides, which cause digoxinlike cardiac toxicity (Chap. 62) and in some species can secrete tetrodotoxin.[104,167] Death results from ingestion of *Bufo* secretions for purposes of aphrodisia.[34,67]

Two of the more important synthetic tryptamines include N,N-diisopropyl-5-methoxytryptamine (5-MeO-DiPT, Foxy Methoxy), and α-methyltryptamine (AMT, IT-290). Since 2001, law enforcement authorities

in more than ten states seized large amounts of 5-MeO-DiPT and AMT. These xenobiotics are often sold surreptitiously as MDMA. 5-MeO-DiPT was listed as Schedule I in 2004.[154] α-Methyltryptamine (AMT or IT-290) is a monoamine oxidase inhibitor that was sold as an antidepressant in the former Soviet Union.[135] α-Methyltryptamine was listed as Schedule I by the DEA in 2004.[154] Since 2011, AMT exposures reported to the United Kingdom Poisons Information Service are increasing.[81] This mirrors the experience in the United States as reported by the NSDUH data documenting tripling of reported lifetime use to 2.1 million people in 2015.[117]

PHENYLETHYLAMINES (AMPHETAMINES)

Dopamine, norepinephrine, and tyrosine are endogenous phenylethylamines. Exogenous phenylethylamines stimulate catecholamine release and cause a variety of physiologic and psychiatric effects, including hallucinations. Substitution on the phenylalkylamine structure has important effects on both the hallucinogenic and stimulant potential of the drug. The presence of a methyl group in the side chain of the phenylethylamines is associated with a higher degree of hallucinogenic effect (Fig. 79–3).[83] 3,4-Methylenedioxymethamphetamine, amphetamine, and methamphetamine are well-known members of this family and are discussed in detail in Chap. 73.

The best recognized of the naturally occurring psychoactive phenylethylamines is mescaline. Mescaline is found in Peyote (*Lophophora williamsii*), a small blue-green spineless cactus that grows in dry and rocky slopes throughout the southwestern United States and northern Mexico. Peyote buttons are the round, fleshy tops of the cactus that are sliced off and dried. The legal use of peyote in the United States is restricted to members of the Native American Church, for whom peyote buttons are used for both religious ceremonies and medical treatment for physical and psychological ailments.[28,31,116]

Other nonindigenous cactus species containing significant amounts of mescaline include the San Pedro cactus (*Trichocereus pachanoi*) and Peruvian torch cactus (*Trichocereus peruvianus*). These plants can be purchased for ornamental purposes in garden stores and on the Internet.[71]

The synthesis and effects of hundreds of other hallucinogenic amphetamines are well described, including 4-bromo-2,5-dimethoxyphenethylamine (2C-B, Nexus, Bromo, Spectrum) and 2,5-dimethoxy-4-N-propylthiopheneethylamine (2C-T-7, Blue Mystic).[134] During the 1980s, 2C-B gained popularity as a legal alternative to MDMA. When 2C-B became a Schedule I drug in 1995, 2C-T-7 emerged as another legal designer amphetamine.[12] In 2004, 2C-T-7 became a Schedule I drug.[39] 5-Methoxydimethyl tryptamine is a

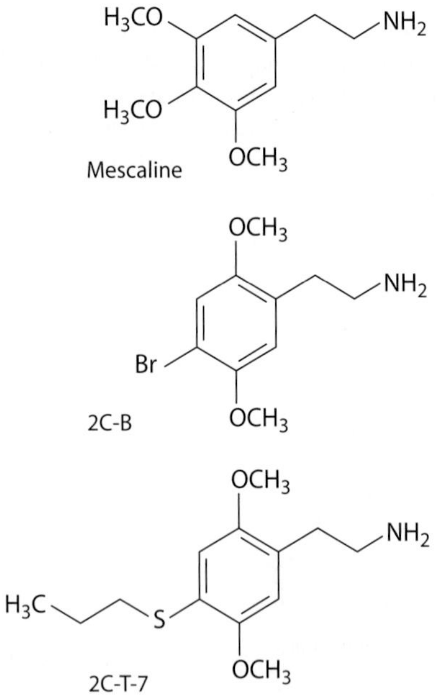

FIGURE 79–3. Hallucinogens of the phenylethylamine chemical class.

Schedule I controlled drug since 2011. Under Food and Drug Administration Safety and Innovation Act of 2012, the compounds 2C-D, 2C-C, 2C-E, 2C-I, 2C-T-2, 2C-T-4, and 2C-P are all now Schedule I drugs.[66]

SALVIA DIVINORUM

Salvia divinorum is a perennial herbaceous member of the mint family. Although there are more than 500 species of Salvia, *S. divinorum* is most recognized for its hallucinogenic properties.[155] *Salvia divinorum* is a native to areas of Oaxaca, Mexico, and grows well in sunny, temperate climates. Plants, leaves, and extracts are typically purchased online, and advice for cultivation of plants is easily accessible.

Since the 16th century, the Mazatec Indians have used *S. divinorum* as a hallucinogen in religious rites as a means of producing "visions."[155] The Mazatecs continue to revere *S. divinorum* as an incarnation of the Virgin Mary, referring to the plant as "ska Maria." Currently, although the federal Controlled Substances Act does not prohibit use of *S. divinorum* or its psychoactive extracts, the possession and sale of *S. divinorum* is illegal in several states, including Louisiana,[151] Missouri,[43] Delaware,[150] and Florida.[42] The United States is limited to local regulation in certain municipalities where *S. divinorum* use among teenagers is rampant.[153] There is wide variability among state laws against *S. divinorum*, and there continues to be widespread marketing of this hallucinogen on the Internet as a "legal hallucinogen."

KRATOM

Kratom, or *Mitragyna speciosa Korth*, is derived from the leaves of a tree native to Asia and Africa.[133] Kratom has dual properties, producing stimulant effects and opioidlike analgesic effects. It was used in Southeast Asia to enhance productivity in manual laborers. The kratom alkaloids mitragynine and 7-hydroxymitragynine are reported to activate μ-, δ-, and κ-opioid receptors. It is used as a substitute for opium; although hallucinogenic effects are uncommon, they are reported after heavy use.[144] Kratom has been illegal in Thailand since 1946 and Australia since 2005. Although there are import bans on kratom as an adulterant because it was not approved as a supplement before 1994, it is currently legal to possess and use in the United States, where it is adopted by some patients for self-treatment of chronic pain and to modulate opioid withdrawal symptoms.

NUTMEG

Nutmeg is derived from *Myristica fragrans*, an evergreen tree native to the Spice Islands. The fruits of the tree contain a central kernel called the nutmeg; the surrounding red aril is used to produce a spice called mace.[119]

Although nutmeg is commonly available as a cooking spice, it has been used medicinally for centuries as an antidiarrheal and abortifacient.[70] It is a recreational herbal that is used to produce euphoria and hallucinations; it is more likely to be abused by adolescents because of its low cost and accessibility.[40,119,126]

BELLADONNA ALKALOIDS

The belladonna alkaloids, including the tropane alkaloids atropine, hyoscyamine, and scopolamine, are isolated from a number of plants. Deadly nightshade (*Atropa belladonna*), a perennial plant, grows throughout the United States, areas of Europe, and Africa. Belladonna alkaloids are isolated from both the leaves and berries of this perennial plant. Jimson weed (*Datura stramonium*), also called locoweed, grows throughout warm and moist areas of the world. This bush contains pods full of small black seeds that are ingested or brewed as a tea for their hallucinogenic properties. The common name Angel's trumpet is used for plants of the Solanaceae family with large trumpet-shaped white flowers (*Brugmansia* or *Datura*) (Chap. 118). Given their wide availability, in the wild and over the Internet, these plants are frequently used as hallucinogens by adolescents.[65] Unfortunately, they produce significant morbidity from anticholinergic toxicity in unwary users.[61] Moonflower, a common name given to several plants, including *Datura inoxia*, was responsible for anticholinergic poisoning of more than a dozen adolescents in one series.[35] Additionally, epidemics of unintentional poisoning were reported among drug users who received heroin adulterated with scopolamine[74] (Antidotes in Depth: A11).

TOXICOKINETICS

Lysergic acid diethylamide (LSD) is the most studied hallucinogen for which there is extensive information about its pharmacokinetic data (Table 79–2). Ingestion is the most common route of exposure, and the gastrointestinal (GI) tract rapidly absorbs LSD. Other reported routes of administration include intravenous, intramuscular, intranasal, parenteral, sublingual, smoking, and conjunctival instillation. Plasma protein binding is over 80% and the volume of distribution is 0.28 L/kg. It is concentrated within the visual cortex, as well as the limbic and reticular activating systems. Metabolism takes place in the liver via hydroxylation and glucuronidation and LSD is excreted predominantly as a pharmacologically inactive compound. Lysergic acid diethylamide has an elimination half-life of about 2.5 hours. Only small amounts are eliminated unchanged in the urine. The minimum effective oral dose is 25 mcg.[84] The onset of effects generally occurs 30 to 60 minutes after exposure, with a duration of 10 to 12 hours.

TABLE 79–2	Pharmacology of Selected Hallucinogens			
Drug Name or Source	**Psychoactive Component (if Different)**	**Typical Oral Dose**	**Onset**	**Duration**
Bufo species toads	5-MeO-DMT	5–15 mg (smoked)	Immediate (smoked)	5–20 min (smoked)
DMT	—	15–60 mg	5–20 min	30–60 min
"Foxy Methoxy"	5-MeO-DiPT	6–10 mg	20–30 min	3–6 h
Woodrose (*Argyreia nervosa*)	Ergine	5–10 seeds	minutes	6–8 h
Jimson weed (*Datura stramonium*)	Atropine, hyoscyamine, scopolamine	10 seeds	20–30 min	2–3 h
Kratom (*Mitragyna speciosa Korth*)	Mitragynine, 7-hydroxy-mitragynine	2–6 g (stimulant); >7 g (sedative)	10–15 min	4–6 h
LSD	Lysergic acid diethylamide	50–100 mcg	30–60 min	10–12 h
"Magic mushrooms" (*Psilocybe* spp)	Psilocybin, psilocin	5 g mushrooms	30 min–2 h	4 h
Nutmeg (*Myristica fragrans*)	Myristicin, elemicin	20 g	1 h	24 h
Peyote (*Lophophora williamsii*)	Mescaline	6–12 buttons, 270–540 mg mescaline	1–3 h	10–12 h
Salvia divinorum	Salvinorin A	—	30 min (inhaled); 1 h (PO)	15–20 min (inhaled); 2 h (PO)
2C-B	—	16–30 mg	1 h	6–10 h

PO = oral.

Ingestion of 200 to 300 morning glory seeds is required to achieve hallucinogenic effects. Only 5 to 10 seeds of Hawaiian baby woodrose are required to produce hallucinations. After ingestion of woodrose seeds, the effects typically last for 6 to 8 hours and produce tranquility without marked euphoria.[7]

Peyote buttons are very bitter and are eaten whole or dried and crushed into a powder, which is reconstituted as tea.[71] Nausea, vomiting, and diaphoresis often precede the onset of hallucinations, which begin at 1 to 3 hours after ingestion and last for up to 12 hours.[119] About 6 to 12 peyote buttons, or 270 to 540 mg of mescaline, are commonly required to produce hallucinogenic effects.[128] Ingestion of up to 5 g of psilocybin-containing mushrooms is typically required to produce hallucinogenic effects.

After ingestion of *Psilocybe* spp mushrooms, psilocybin is converted to psilocin, the active hallucinogen in the GI tract.[68] The effects of psilocin are similar to LSD but have a shorter duration of action of about 4 hours.

For recreational purposes, DMT is typically smoked, insufflated, or injected. Hallucinogenic effects peak in 5 to 20 minutes, with a duration of 30 to 60 minutes. 5-Methoxy-*N,N*-dimethyltryptamine (5-MeO-DiPT) is usually ingested by mouth and less commonly smoked or insufflated. Effects begin 20 to 30 minutes after ingestion and include disinhibition and relaxation. There is a dose-dependent response, and at higher ranges, symptoms include mydriasis, euphoria, auditory and visual hallucinations, nausea, diarrhea, and jaw clenching.[111,136] The hallucinogenic effects last from 3 to 6 hours.[103,136] Other substances such as sildenafil, γ-hydroxybutyrate, benzodiazepines, and marijuana are used to heighten or prolong the hallucinogenic effects of 5-MeO-DiPT. α-Methyltryptamine is available as a white powder, which is ingested, smoked, or insufflated. Hallucinations typically occur within 30 minutes and last from 12 to 16 hours.[89]

Amphetamine, methamphetamine, and MDMA are well absorbed through the GI tract. The elimination half-life ranges from 8 to 30 hours for members of this class and is dependent on urine pH.[15,38] Amphetamines are weak bases and undergo more rapid elimination in acidic urine.[131] The volume of distribution ranges from 3 to 5 L/kg for amphetamine, 3 to 4 L/kg for methamphetamine, and likely more than 5 L/kg for MDMA.[15,38,88,131] Elimination of other amphetamines occurs through multiple mechanisms, including aromatic hydroxylation, aliphatic hydroxylation, and N-dealkylation.[88] Tolerance occurs with chronic amphetamine use.[85] There is little information about 2C-B and 2C-T-7 in the medical literature. Both drugs are used via oral, intranasal, and rectal routes. Both 2C-B and 2C-T-7 exert their hallucinogenic effects within 1 hour of use, and physiologic and psychologic effects persist for 6 to 10 hours. Additional information on the kinetics of amphetamine and congeners can be found in Chap. 73.

Salvia divinorum is chewed, smoked, or ingested as tea. Hallucinations occur rapidly after exposure and are typically quite vivid. Synesthesia is reported among Salvia users. Hallucinogenic effects after *S. divinorum* use are typically brief, lasting only 1 to 2 hours. Pharmacokinetic data for *S. divinorum* and its primary psychoactive, salvinorin A, were described in a volunteer study.[137] Psychoactive effects were typically experienced 5 to 10 minutes after absorption of salvinorin A via the buccal mucosa, reaching a plateau during the first hour after exposure and resolving within 2 hours. Vaporization and inhalation of salvinorin A led to more rapid effects beginning at 30 seconds after exposure. These effects plateaued at 5 to 10 minutes and typically subsided after 20 to 30 minutes. In this study, ingestion of *S. divinorum* leaves did not produce the same effects as buccal or inhalational administration, leading to the theory that GI deactivation of salvinorin A occurs after ingestion.[137]

Kratom leaves are decocted into tea, chewed, or smoked.[79] Kratom leaves contain approximately 0.8% mitragynine by weight but can vary by geographic origin of trees, as well as season.[132] In addition, several commercially available kratom products have excessive quantities of 7-hydroxymitrogynine, suggesting that many of these products are likely being artificially adulterated with this alkaloid.[91] Neuropsychiatric effects are dose dependent and occur within 5 to 10 minutes of exposure, with effects lasting 4 to 6 hours.[144] Stimulant effects predominate at doses of 2 to 6 g, and sedation becomes more pronounced at doses above 7 g.

Nutmeg is usually ingested as a paste or mixed in a beverage; 15 to 20 g is required for clinical effects.[119] This dose is often unpalatable, and a case report of recreational use of encapsulated nutmeg is described.[126] Clinical effects begin 1 hour after nutmeg ingestion and persist for more than 24 hours after exposure.[119]

The belladonna alkaloids are most concentrated in the seeds of *Datura stramonium* (Jimson weed); each seed contains approximately 0.1 mg of atropine.[139] Ingestion of as few as 10 seeds produces hallucinations within 20- to minutes; these effects can last for 2 to 3 hours. Although the roots and seeds of *Brugmansia arborea* (Angel's trumpet) contain the highest alkaloid concentrations, users most often brew the blossom into a tea. Each blossom contains approximately 0.3 mg of atropine and 0.65 mg of scopolamine.[65] The elimination half-lives of atropine and hyoscyamine are 2.5 and 3.5 hours, respectively, and the elimination half-life of scopolamine is considerably longer, at 8 hours.[18]

PHARMACOLOGY

Although the lysergamide, indolealkylamine, and phenylethylamine hallucinogens are structurally distinct, the similarities in their effects on cognition support a common site of action on central serotonin receptors.[5,24,30,75,148] Serotonin modulates many psychological and physiologic processes, including mood, personality, affect, appetite, motor function, sexual activity, temperature regulation, pain perception, sleep induction and antidiuretic hormone (ADH) release. There are more than 14 known 5-HT receptor subtypes (Chap. 13); differing affinity for these subtypes occurs based on the structure of the hallucinogen and accounts for the subtle differences between their effects.

The lysergamide, indolealkylamine, and phenylethylamine hallucinogens all bind to the 5-HT$_2$ class of receptors. There is a good correlation between the affinity of both indolealkylamine and phenylethylamine hallucinogens for 5-HT$_2$ receptors in vitro and hallucinogenic potency in humans.[5,63,118,148] The 5-HT$_{2A}$ receptor subtype has the highest density in the cerebral cortex and represents the binding site for hallucinogens.[96] This is bolstered by an animal study that shows that a selective 5-HT$_{2A}$ antagonist inhibit the effects of LSD and a phenylethylamine, 2,5-dimethoxy-4-iodo-amphetamine (DOI).[97] The response to high doses of LSD and DOI suggest that both lysergamides and phenylethylamines are partial agonists at cortical 5-HT$_{2A}$ receptors.[62,96,125]

Although the majority of investigations have focused on the role of serotonin in drug-induced hallucinations, other neurotransmitters are also involved. Stimulation of 5-HT$_{2A}$ receptors enhances release of glutamate in the cortical layer V pyramidal cells.[5,11] Lysergic acid diethylamide and other lysergamides stimulate both D$_1$ and D$_2$ dopamine receptors.[10,60,161] In animal models, LSD and phenylethylamine hallucinogens modulate NMDA receptor-mediated effects and are suggested to have a protective effect against neurotoxicity secondary to PCP and ketamine.[11,52]

Another theory that incorporates these other neurotransmitters involves the concept of "thalamic filtering."[58] The thalamus receives input and output from the cortex and reticular activating system and functions to filter relevant sensory input. This theory has been explored as an explanation for organic psychosis and the effects of hallucinogenic xenobiotics. Multiple neurotransmitters, including dopamine, acetylcholine, γ-aminobutyric acid (GABA), and glutamate, exert their actions on the thalamus. Increased excitatory or decreased inhibitory neurotransmitters in this region of the brain leads to "sensory overload," which manifests itself clinically as symptoms of psychosis.[58] Experimental evidence also demonstrates electroencephalographic (EEG) abnormalities after administration of hallucinogens, confirming a cortical, rather the ophthalmologic, etiology for hallucinations.[51]

Salvinorin A, the psychoactive component of *S. divinorum*, is one of the most potent natural hallucinogens. The effect of Salvinorin A occurs via binding at the κ-opioid receptor, making it structurally and mechanistically unique (Fig. 79–4).[166] The κ-opioid receptor is distinct from the mu opioid receptor, stimulation of which generally causes euphoria and analgesia (Chap. 36). Salvinorin A does not have any serotonergic activity.[166]

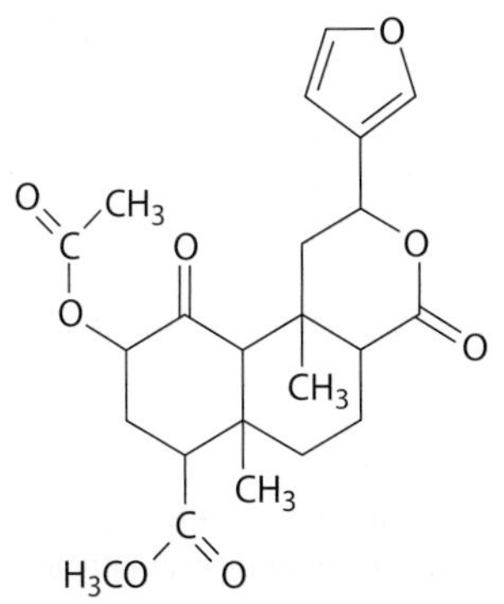

FIGURE 79-4. Structure of Salvinorin A.

The opioid effects of kratom are attributed to mitragynine.[132,165] The most prevalent of the kratom alkaloids, mitragynine, shares a structural similarity with yohimbine.[13] In vitro, mitragynine is active at both supraspinal opioid δ and μ receptors.[147] This μ-receptor activity results in analgesia and efficacy in treating opioid withdrawal symptoms. Additionally, mitragynine activates noradrenergic and serotonergic pathways.[100] Another kratom alkaloid, 7-hydroxymitragynine, has antinociceptive effects and high affinity for opioid receptors.[101] In animal studies, 7-hydroxymitragynine has more analgesic potency than morphine, even after oral administration.[99] This compound was found in commercial kratom products at concentrations that far exceed its natural occurrence in the plant, suggesting surreptitious adulteration of many these kratom products.[91]

Nutmeg contains a number of purportedly psychoactive compounds, including myristicin, elemicin, and safrole (Fig. 79–5). The psychoactive components of nutmeg include terpenes and alkyl benzyl derivatives (myristicin, elemicin, and safrole).[119]

It is theorized that the aromatics found in nutmeg are metabolized to amphetaminelike compounds that create hallucinogenic effects.[119] However, this mechanism is not supported in animal data.[126] Nutmeg contains myristicin and elemicin, both weak monoamine oxidase inhibitors that also demonstrate serotonergic activity, which likely accounts for the clinical effects of nutmeg.[126]

The pharmacology of atropine, a competitive central and peripheral antimuscarinic, and the most well-studied belladonna alkaloid, is discussed in detail in Antidotes in Depth: A35. Like atropine, scopolamine and hyoscyamine are tertiary amines that cross the blood–brain barrier. Scopolamine causes more sedation than atropine, and its transdermal availability led to its use in motion sickness patches. Hyoscyamine is more potent than atropine; it is used as an antispasmodic for GI conditions.

CLINICAL EFFECTS

Physiologic changes accompany and often precede the perceptual changes induced by lysergamides, tryptamines, and phenylethylamines. The physical effects are caused by direct drug effect or by a response to the disturbing or enjoyable hallucinogenic experience. Sympathetic effects mediated by the locus coeruleus include mydriasis, tachycardia, hypertension, tachypnea, hyperthermia, and diaphoresis. They occur shortly after ingestion and often precede the hallucinogenic effects. Other clinical findings that are reported include piloerection, dizziness, hyperactivity, muscle weakness,

ataxia, altered mental status, coma, and hippus (rhythmic pupillary dilation and constriction).[86] Nausea and vomiting often precede the psychedelic effects produced by psilocybin and mescaline. Potentially life-threatening complications, such as hyperthermia, hypertension, tachycardia, coma, respiratory arrest, and coagulopathy, were described in a report of 8 patients with a massive LSD overdose.[82] Sympathomimetic effects are generally less prominent in LSD toxicity than in phenylethylamine toxicity. Similar sympathetic symptoms are described after the use of 2C-B and 2C-T-7. Whereas low doses of 2C-B and 2C-T-7 produce hypertension, tachycardia, and visual hallucinations, larger doses are associated with shifts in color perception and enhanced auditory and visual stimulation. Three deaths are associated with 2C-T-7 use; in one case, death resulted from seizures or aspiration.[39,48] An analog of 2C-B, called 2C-B-FLY, or Bromo-dragonFLY, is implicated in finger necrosis requiring amputation secondary to potent peripheral vasospastic activity and sudden cardiac death.[114] Similar vasoconstrictive effects resulting in limb ischemia is induced by exposure to ergot containing alkaloids. Bromo-dragonFLY, like other 2-C compounds, is associated with agitated delirium and delayed onset of seizures.[163]

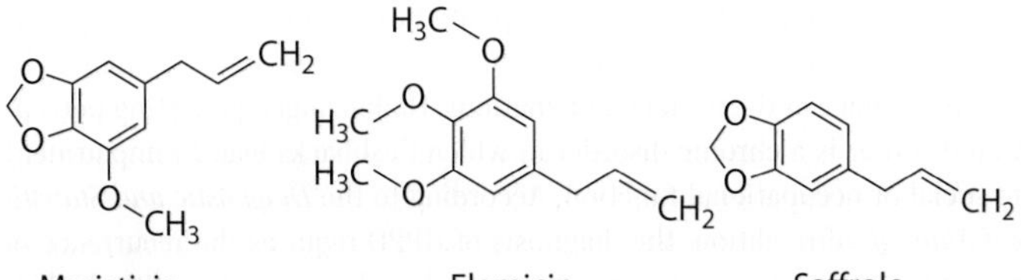

The psychological effects of hallucinogens seem to represent a complex and elusive interaction between different neurotransmitters, including the serotonergic and dopaminergic systems. Based on this serotonergic mechanism, serotonin toxicity could theoretically occur after the use of any of the lysergamide, indolealkylamine, or phenylethylamine hallucinogens. Animal studies documented LSD and tryptamine-induced serotonin toxicity.[138,158] Case reports link phenylethylamine use to fatal serotonin syndrome in recreational users.[20,110,160]

Tolerance to the psychological effects of LSD occurs within 2 or 3 days with daily dosing but rapidly dissipates if the drug is withheld for 2 days. Psychological cross-tolerance among mescaline, psilocybin, and LSD is reported in humans.[17] There is no evidence for physiologic tolerance, physiologic dependence, or a withdrawal syndrome after LSD use. Limited cross-tolerance is demonstrated between psilocybin and cannabinoids such as marijuana.[26]

Salvia divinorum use results in vivid hallucinations and synesthesia.[137] Additionally, its use causes diuresis, nausea and dysphoria. These aversive effects limit its long-term use.[13]

The dual stimulant and sedative properties of kratom contributed to its traditional use among manual laborers. However, its opioidlike activity led to a surge in contemporary use as an herbal treatment for opioid withdrawal among patients with chronic pain.[22,23] Anorexia, weight loss, and insomnia are reported among kratom-dependent individuals. Hyperpigmentation of the cheeks is also described among chronic users.[144]

Recreational nutmeg use results in the desired effects of euphoria and hallucinations, as well as the adverse effects of nausea, vomiting, dizziness, flushing, tachycardia, and hypotension. Two fatalities from nutmeg ingestion are reported.[33,140]

The belladonna alkaloids produce classic signs of anticholinergic toxicity, including hyperthermia, tachycardia, mydriasis, flushing, anhidrosis, urinary retention, and ileus. The central effects include restlessness, hallucinations, agitation, delirium, seizures, and coma.[35] The psychosis produced by belladonna alkaloids are profound; in one case, a young man autoamputated his tongue and penis after ingestion of tea made from *Brugmansia arborea*.[98]

The vast majority of morbidity from hallucinogen use stems from trauma. Hallucinogen users frequently report lacerations and bruises sustained during their "high." Additionally, dysphoria drives patients to react to stimuli with unpredictable and occasionally aggressive behavior. Many websites regarding hallucinogen use advise readers to take hallucinogens only while under the supervision of an observer."[49]

The psychological effects of hallucinogens are dose related and affect changes in arousal, emotion, perception, thought process, and self-image. The response is related to the person's mindset, emotions, or expectations at the time of exposure and are altered by the group or setting.[1] The person experiencing the effects of a hallucinogen is usually fully alert, oriented, and aware that he or she is under the influence of a drug. Euphoria, dysphoria, and emotional lability occur.

Myristicin   Elemicin   Saffrole

FIGURE 79-5. Structure of myristicin.

Illusions are common, typically involving distortion of body image and alteration in visual perceptions. Hallucinogen users display acute attention to details with excessive attachment of meaning to ordinary objects and events. Usual thoughts seem novel and profound. Many people report an intensification of their sensory perceptions such as sound magnification and distortion. Colors often seem brighter with halo-like lights around objects. Frequently, hallucinogen users relate a sense of depersonalization and separation from the environment, commonly called an "out-of-body" experience. Synesthesias, or sensory misperceptions, such as "hearing colors" or "seeing sounds" are commonly described. Hallucinations are visual, auditory, tactile, or olfactory.

Acute adverse psychiatric effects of hallucinogens include panic reactions, psychosis, and major depressive dysphoric reactions. Acute panic reactions, the most common adverse effect, present with frightening illusions, tremendous anxiety, apprehension, and a terrifying sense of loss of self-control.[46] These psychiatric effects cause patients to seek care in the emergency department (ED).

LABORATORY

Routine urine drug-of-abuse immunoassay screens do not detect LSD or other hallucinogens. Although LSD can be detected by radioimmunoassay of the urine, confirmation by high-performance liquid chromatography (HPLC) or gas chromatography is necessary for reliability. These tests are rarely used in the clinical setting but are commonly available for forensic purposes.[17,46] False-positive urine immunoassay test results for LSD are reported after exposure to several medications, including fentanyl, sertraline, haloperidol, and verapamil.[56,122]

Depending on their structure, phenylethylamines cause positive qualitative urine test results by immunoassay for amphetamines. However, amphetamine drug screening is associated with numerous false-positive results, particularly after the use of nonprescription medications that contain ephedrine, pseudoephedrine, or phenylpropanolamine.[142] Urine immunoassays do not detect 5-Meo-DiPT, DMT, AMT, 2C-T-7, and 2CB, but gas chromatography–mass spectrometry testing methods for detection of these compounds is available.[146] There are several websites that monitor the content of MDMA pills that are in distribution, such as pillreports.net and partyflock.nl, but these sites are inaccurate and fail to report contamination with other drugs.[159] Organizations such as DanceSafe promote safe drug use through user test kits, but it is unclear if this practice increases drug use or reduces harm.[45]

Routine urine drug immunoassay screens do not detect salvinorin A, mitragynine, or myristicin. High-performance liquid chromatography and liquid chromatography–mass spectrometry protocols are used for quantitative analysis of salvinorin A and B in plant matter and in ex vivo animal studies. Gas chromatography–mass spectrometry identified salvinorin A in urine and saliva obtained from 2 human volunteers who had smoked *S. divinorum.*[115] Myristicin testing is not widely available.[140]

TREATMENT

Most hallucinogen users rarely seek medical attention because either they experience only the desired effect of the drug or they minimize or cannot perceive the adverse effects. It is rare that hallucinogens produce life-threatening toxicity. Autonomic instability, seizures, hyperthermia, and excited delirium during severe hallucinations result in self harm and death. For any hallucinogen user presenting to the ED, initial treatment must begin with attention to airway, breathing, circulation, level of consciousness, and abnormal vital signs. Even in those in whom exposure to a hallucinogen is suspected, the basic approach for altered mental status should include dextrose, naloxone, and oxygen therapy as clinically indicated, as is the vigorous search for other etiologies. Because of their rapid absorption, GI decontamination with activated charcoal is of little value after clinical symptoms appear, and attempts may lead to further agitation. Sedation with benzodiazepines is usually sufficient to treat the hypertension, tachycardia, and hyperthermia which occur. The patient with a dysphoric reaction should be placed in a quiet location

with minimal stimuli. A nonjudgmental advocate should attempt to reduce the patient's anxiety, provide reality testing, and remind the individual that a drug was ingested and that the effect will dissipate in several hours. We recommend avoiding use of physical restraint when possible to prevent hyperthermia and rhabdomyolysis. Benzodiazepines remain the cornerstone of therapy for both autonomic instability and dysphoria because the sedating effect diminishes both endogenous and exogenous sympathetic effects.[105] Autonomic instability and hyperthermia are a feature of phenylethylamine use, as well as tryptamine use or massive LSD overdose.[55,82,105] Hyperthermia resulting from agitation or muscle rigidity requires urgent sedation with benzodiazepines and rapid ice bath cooling. Although CNS depression is unlikely to be severe enough to require endotracheal intubation in a patient with a pure hallucinogen exposure, intubation and paralysis are recommended in patients with life threatening hyperthermia.[19] Seizures that occur with tryptamine or phenylethylamine use should be initially treated with benzodiazepines. Seizures also result from hyponatremia in MDMA users and treatment with 3% (hypertonic) saline is recommended (Chap. 73).

The treatment of anticholinergic toxicity from the belladonna alkaloids involves several critical components: correction of abnormal vital signs, management of delirium, and rapid intervention for seizures or dysrhythmias. The mainstays of therapy are fluid resuscitation and benzodiazepines; however, physostigmine is recommended as antidotal therapy in cases of belladonna alkaloid poisoning. Physostigmine is efficacious in decreasing morbidity and length of hospital stay compared with benzodiazepines alone.[29,124] Based on the strength of this evidence, physostigmine is recommended for to patients with evidence of anticholinergic delirium or agitation if there are no contraindications. More information on physostigmine is found in Antidotes in Depth: A11.

Morbidity and mortality typically result from the complications of hyperthermia, including rhabdomyolysis and myoglobinuric acute kidney injury, hepatic necrosis, and disseminated intravascular coagulopathy. For the most part, however, hydration, sedation, a quiet environment, and meticulous supportive care prove adequate to prevent morbidity or mortality in recreational use or overdose.[32] Treatment of serotonin toxicity from phenylethylamine use is largely supportive and includes the avoidance of further administration of serotonergic medications. Specific therapy with cyproheptadine is recommended (Chap. 69).[21]

The role of antipsychotics in controlling hallucinogen-induced agitation is defined in detail in Chap. 26 and Special Considerations: SC4. Haloperidol, risperidone, and ziprasidone have utility in controlling the acutely agitated patient. However, haloperidol and risperidone worsen panic and visual symptoms and increase the incidence of HPPD (see later).[2] The safety of ziprasidone in hallucinogen users has not yet been reported yet. Although further study of these drugs is required, prolonged psychosis requires treatment with long-term antipsychotic therapy.

LONG-TERM EFFECTS

Long-term consequences of LSD use include prolonged psychotic reactions, severe depression, and exacerbation of preexisting psychiatric illness.[73,127] When LSD was initially popularized, some patients behaved in a manner similar to schizophrenia and required admission to psychiatric facilities. In volunteer studies, panic reactions, HPPD, and extended psychoses were noted. When the drug was used for alleviation of anxiety and personality abnormalities, flashbacks and extended psychosis were reported.[54] It is suggested that these individuals had preexisting compensated psychological disturbances.[5,95]

Flashbacks are reported in up to 15% to 80% of LSD users.[8] Anesthesia, alcohol intake, and medications precipitate flashbacks.[57] These perceptions are triggered during times of stress, illness, and exercise and are often a virtual recurrence of the initial hallucinations. Hallucinogen persisting perception disorder is a chronic disorder in which flashbacks lead to impairment in social or occupational function. According to the *Diagnostic and Statistical Manual,* fifth edition, the diagnosis of HPPD requires the recurrence of perceptual symptoms that were experienced while intoxicated with the hallucinogen that causes functional impairment and is not due to a medical condition.[9] The etiology of HPPD is still unknown, and the reported incidence varies widely. Symptoms are primarily visual, and reality testing is typically intact in HPPD. Common perceptual and visual disturbances in HPPD include geometric forms; false, fleeting perceptions in the peripheral fields; flashes of color; intensified color; and halos around objects.[95] One finding described after LSD use is palinopsia, or "trailing," which refers to the continued visual perception of an object after it has left the field of vision. These visual perceptions are associated with normal ophthalmologic examinations and abnormal EEG evaluations, suggesting a cortical cause for the visual symptoms. Lysergic acid diethylamide causes psychological but not physical dependence; therefore, it does not cause any physical withdrawal symptoms.

SUMMARY

- Hallucinogens are a diverse group of xenobiotics that alter and distort perception, thought, and mood without clouding the sensorium.
- The lysergamide, phenylethylamine, and tryptamine hallucinogens share a serotonergic mechanism of action; however, other neurotransmitters are responsible for the complex effects of these hallucinogens.
- Acute adverse psychiatric effects of hallucinogens include panic reactions, true hallucinations, psychosis, and major depressive dysphoric reactions.
- With severe poisoning, hallucinogens cause autonomic instability, seizures, and hyperthermia.
- Meticulous supportive care with attention to abnormal vital signs and sedation with a benzodiazepine are often the only therapies required.

Acknowledgement
Kavita Babu, MD, contributed to this chapter in a previous edition.

REFERENCES

1. Abraham HD, et al. The psychopharmacology of hallucinogens. *Neuropsychopharmacology.* 1996;14:285-298.
2. Abraham HD, Mamen A. LSD-like panic from risperidone in post-LSD visual disorder. *J Clin Psychopharmacol.* 1996;16:238-241.
3. US Drug Enforcement Administration. Pickard and Apperson convicted of LSD charges, largest LSD lab seizure in DEA history. https://www.dea.gov/pubs/states/newsrel/2003/sanfran033103.html.
4. US Drug Enforcement Administration. Pickard And Apperson sentenced on LSD charges, largest LSD lab seizure in DEA history. https://www.dea.gov/pubs/states/newsrel/2003/sanfran112403.html.
5. Aghajanian GK, Marek GJ. Serotonin and hallucinogens. *Neuropsychopharmacology.* 1999;21(2 suppl):16S-23S.
7. Al-Assmar SE. The seeds of the Hawaiian baby woodrose are a powerful hallucinogen. *Arch Intern Med.* 1999;159:2090.
8. Aldurra G, Crayton JW. Improvement of hallucinogen persisting perception disorder by treatment with a combination of fluoxetine and olanzapine: case report. *J Clin Psychopharmacol.* 2001;21:343-344.
9. American Psychiatric Association. *Diagnostic and Statistical Manual of Mental Disorders.* 5th ed. Washington, DC: American Psychiatric Association; 2013.
10. Antkiewicz-Michaluk L, et al. Ca2+ channel blockade prevents lysergic acid diethylamide-induced changes in dopamine and serotonin metabolism. *Eur J Pharmacol.* 1997;332:9-14.
11. Arvanov VL, et al. LSD and DOB: interaction with 5-HT2A receptors to inhibit NMDA receptor-mediated transmission in the rat prefrontal cortex. *Eur J Neurosci.* 1999;11:3064-3072.
12. Babu K, et al. Emerging drugs of abuse. *Clin Pediatr Emerg Med.* 2005;6:81-84.
13. Babu KM, et al. Opioid receptors and legal highs: Salvia divinorum and Kratom. *Clin Toxicol (Phila).* 2008;46:146-152.
14. Badham ER. Ethnobotany of psilocybin mushrooms, especially Psilocybe cubensis. *J Ethnopharmacol.* 1984;10:249-254.
15. Baselt RC, Cravey RH. *Disposition of Toxic Drugs and Chemicals in Man,* 4th ed. Foster City, CA, 1995, pp:44-47, 475-478.
16. Bellis MA, et al. The role of an international nightlife resort in the proliferation of recreational drugs. *Addiction.* 2003;98:1713-1721.
17. Blaho K, et al. Clinical pharmacology of lysergic acid diethylamide: case reports and review of the treatment of intoxication. *Am J Ther.* 1997;4:211-221.
18. Bliss M. Datura poisoning. *Clin Toxicol Rev.* 2001;23:1-2.
19. Borowiak KS, et al. Psilocybin mushroom (Psilocybe semilanceata) intoxication with myocardial infarction. *J Toxicol Clin Toxicol.* 1998;36:47-49.
20. Bosak A, et al. Recurrent seizures and serotonin syndrome following "2C-I" ingestion. *J Med Toxicol.* 2013;9:196-198.
21. Boyer E, Shannon M. Serotonin syndrome. *N Engl J Med.* 2005;352:1112-1120.
22. Boyer EW, et al. Self-treatment of opioid withdrawal using kratom (Mitragynia speciosa korth). *Addiction.* 2008;103:1048-1050.
23. Boyer EW, et al. Self-treatment of opioid withdrawal with a dietary supplement, Kratom. *Am J Addict.* 2007;16:352-356.
24. Brubacher JR, et al. Efficacy of digoxin specific Fab fragments (Digibind) in the treatment of toad venom poisoning. *Toxicon.* 1999;37:931-942.
25. Brush DE, et al. Monoamine oxidase inhibitor poisoning resulting from Internet misinformation on illicit substances. *J Toxicol Clin Toxicol.* 2004;42:191-195.
26. Buckholtz NS, et al. Serotonin2 agonist administration down-regulates rat brain serotonin2 receptors. *Life Sci.* 1988;42:2439-2445.
27. Buckman J. Brainwashing, LSD, and CIA: historical and ethical perspective. *Int J Soc Psychiatry.* 1977;23:8-19.
28. Bullis RK. Swallowing the scroll: legal implications of the recent Supreme Court peyote cases. *J Psychoactive Drugs.* 1990;22:325-332.
29. Burns MJ, et al. A comparison of physostigmine and benzodiazepines for the treatment of anticholinergic poisoning. *Ann Emerg Med.* 2000;35:374-381.
30. Burris KD, Sanders-Bush E. Unsurmountable antagonism of brain 5-hydroxytryptamine2 receptors by (+)-lysergic acid diethylamide and bromo-lysergic acid diethylamide. *Mol Pharmacol.* 1992;42:826-830.
31. Calabrese JD. Spiritual healing and human development in the Native American church: toward a cultural psychiatry of peyote. *Psychoanal Rev.* 1997;84:237-255.
32. Callaway CW, Clark RF. Hyperthermia in psychostimulant overdose. *Ann Emerg Med.* 1994;24:68-76.
33. Carstairs SD, Cantrell FL. The spice of life: an analysis of nutmeg exposures in California. *Clin Toxicol (Phila).* 2011;49:177-180.
34. Centers for Disease Control and Prevention. Deaths associated with a purported aphrodisiac—New York City, February 1993-May 1995. *MMWR Morb Mortal Wkly Rep.* 1995;44:853-855, 861.
35. Centers for Disease Control and Prevention. Suspected moonflower intoxication—Ohio, 2002. *MMWR Morb Mortal Wkly Rep.* 2003;52:788-791.
36. Cohen MM, et al. In vivo and in vitro chromosomal damage induced by LSD-25. *N Engl J Med.* 1967;277:1043-1049.
37. Congress.gov. H.R.3537—Dangerous Synthetic Drug Control Act of 2016. https://www.congress.gov/bill/114th-congress/house-bill/3537.
38. de la Torre R, et al. Human pharmacology of MDMA: pharmacokinetics, metabolism, and disposition. *Ther Drug Monit.* 2004;26:137-144.
39. DeBoer D, et al. Data about the new psychoactive drug 2C-B. *J Anal Toxicol.* 1999;23:227.
40. Demetriades AK, et al. Low cost, high risk: accidental nutmeg intoxication. *BMJ.* 2005;22:223-225.
41. Dennehy CE, et al. Evaluation of herbal dietary supplements marketed on the internet for recreational use. *Ann Pharmacother.* 2005;39:1634-1639.
42. Drug Abuse Prevention and Control, 893.03(2016). http://www.leg.state.fl.us/Statutes/index.cfm?App_mode=Display_Statute&URL=0800-0899/0893/Sections/0893.03.html.
43. Drug Regulations, 195.017.1(2016). http://www.moga.mo.gov/mostatutes/stathtml/19500000171.html.
44. Duffau B, et al. Analysis of 25 C NBOMe in Seized Blotters by HPTLC and GC-MS. *J Chromatogr Sci.* 2016;54:1153-1158.
45. Dundes L. DanceSafe and ecstasy: protection or promotion? *J Health Social Policy.* 2003;17:19-37.
46. Dupont R, Verebey K. The role of the laboratory in the diagnosis of LSD and ecstasy psychosis. *Psychiatr Ann.* 1994;24:142-144.
47. Eadie MJ. Convulsive ergotism: epidemics of the serotonin syndrome? *Lancet Neurol.* 2003;2:429-434.
48. Erowid. A Reported 2C-T-7 death. The Vaults of Erowid. http://www.erowid.org/chemicals/2ct7/2ct7_death1.shtml.
49. Erowid. Salvia divinorum basics. http://www.erowid.org/plants/salvia/salvia_basics.shtml.
50. Erowid. Terminology. The Vaults of Erowid. http://www.erowid.org/psychoactives/psychoactives_def.shtml.
51. Fairchild MD, et al. EEG effects of hallucinogens and cannabinoids using sleep-waking behavior as baseline. *Pharmacol Biochem Behav.* 1980;12:99-105.
52. Farber NB, et al. Serotonergic agents that activate 5HT2A receptors prevent NMDA antagonist neurotoxicity. *Neuropsychopharmacology.* 1998;18:57-62.
53. Fody EP, Walker EM. Effects of drugs on the male and female reproductive systems. *Ann Clin Lab Sci.* 1985;15:451-458.
54. Frankel FH. The concept of flashbacks in historical perspective. *Int J Clin Exp Hypn.* 1994;42:321-336.
55. Friedman SA, Hirsch SE. Extreme hyperthermia after LSD ingestion. *JAMA.* 1971;217:1549-1550.
56. Gagajewski A, et al. False-positive lysergic acid diethylamide immunoassay screen associated with fentanyl medication. *Clin Chem.* 2002;48:205-206.
57. Gaillard MC, Borruat FX. Persisting visual hallucinations and illusions in previously drug-addicted patients. *Klin Monatsbl Augenheilkd.* 2003;220:176-178.
58. Gaudreau JD, Gagnon P. Psychotogenic drugs and delirium pathogenesis: the central role of the thalamus. *Med Hypotheses.* 2005;64:471-475.
59. Gee P, et al. Case series: toxicity from 25B-NBOMe—a cluster of N-bomb cases. *Clin Toxicol.* 2016;54:141-146.

60. Giacomelli S, et al. Lysergic acid diethylamide (LSD) is a partial agonist of D2 dopaminergic receptors and it potentiates dopamine-mediated prolactin secretion in lactotrophs in vitro. *Life Sci.* 1998;63:215-222.

61. Glatstein M, et al. Belladonna alkaloid intoxication: the 10-year experience of a large tertiary care pediatric hospital. *Am J Ther.* 2016;23:e74-e77.

62. Glennon RA. Do classical hallucinogens act as 5-HT2 agonists or antagonists? *Neuropsychopharmacology.* 1990;3:509-517.

63. Glennon RA, et al. Evidence for 5-HT2 involvement in the mechanism of action of hallucinogenic agents. *Life Sci.* 1984;35:2505-2511.

64. Golub A, et al. Is the U.S. experiencing an incipient epidemic of hallucinogen use? *Subst Use Misuse.* 2001;36:1699-1729.

65. Gopel C, et al. Three cases of angel's trumpet tea-induced psychosis in adolescent substance abusers. *Nord J Psychiatry.* 2002;56:49-52.

66. GovTrack. S.3187 (112th): Food and Drug Administration Safety and Innovation Act. https://www.govtrack.us/congress/bills/112/s3187/text.

67. Gowda RM, et al. Toad venom poisoning: resemblance to digoxin toxicity and therapeutic implications. *Heart.* 2003;89:e14.

68. Grieshaber AF, et al. The detection of psilocin in human urine. *J Forensic Sci.* 2001;46:627-630.

69. Grob CS, et al. Pilot study of psilocybin treatment for anxiety in patients with advanced-stage cancer. *Arch Gen Psychiatry.* 2011;68:71-78.

70. Hallstrom H, Thuvander A. Toxicological evaluation of myristicin. *Nat Toxins.* 1997;5:186-192.

71. Halpern JH. Hallucinogens and dissociative agents naturally growing in the United States. *Pharmacol Ther.* 2004;102:131-138.

72. Halpern JH, et al. A review of hallucinogen persisting perception disorder (HPPD) and an exploratory study of subjects claiming symptoms of HPPD. *Curr Top Behav Neurosci.* 2018;36:333-360.

73. Halpern JH, Pope HG Jr. Do hallucinogens cause residual neuropsychological toxicity? *Drug Alcohol Depend.* 1999;53:247-256.

74. Hamilton RJ, et al. A descriptive study of an epidemic of poisoning caused by heroin adulterated with scopolamine. *J Toxicol Clin Toxicol.* 2000;38:597-608.

75. Harrington MA, et al. Molecular biology of serotonin receptors. *J Clin Psychiatry.* 1992;53 Suppl:8-27.

76. Hofmann A. *History of the Discovery of LSD.* New York, NY: Parthenon; 1994.

77. Isbell H, Gorodetzky CW. Effect of alkaloids of ololiuqui in man. *Psychopharmacologia.* 1966;8:331-339.

78. Jacobson CB, Berlin CM. Possible reproductive detriment in LSD users. *JAMA.* 1972;222:1367-1373.

79. Jansen KL, Prast CJ. Psychoactive properties of mitragynine (kratom). *J Psychoactive Drugs.* 1988;20:455-457.

80. Johnston L, et al. National Survey Results on Drug Abuse, the Monitoring the Future Study, 1975-1998. In: Abuse NIoD, ed. Volume I Secondary School Students. The University of Michigan Institute for Social Research National Institute on Drug Abuse 6001 Executive Boulevard Bethesda, Mary/and 20892 U.S. Department of Health and Human Services Public Health Service National Institutes of Health 1999. Vol NIH Publication No.98-43461999.

81. Kamour A, et al. Patterns of presentation and clinical toxicity after reported use of alpha methyltryptamine in the United Kingdom. A report from the UK National Poisons Information Service. *Clin Toxicol (Phila).* 2014;52:192-197.

82. Klock JC, et al. Coma, hyperthermia, and bleeding associated with massive LSD overdose, a report of eight cases. *Clin Toxicol.* 1975;8:191-203.

83. Kovar KA. Chemistry and pharmacology of hallucinogens, entactogens and stimulants. *Pharmacopsychiatry.* 1998;31(suppl 2):69-72.

84. Kulig K. LSD. *Emerg Med Clin North Am.* 1990;8:551-558.

85. Lake CR, Quirk RS. CNS stimulants and the look-alike drugs. *Psychiatr Clin North Am.* 1984;7:689-701.

86. Leikin JB, et al. Clinical features and management of intoxication due to hallucinogenic drugs. *Med Toxicol Adverse Drug Exp.* 1989;4:324-350.

87. Li JH, Lin LF. Genetic toxicology of abused drugs: a brief review. *Mutagenesis.* 1998;13:557-565.

88. Linden C, et al. Amphetamines. *Top Emerg Med.* 1985;7:18-32.

89. Long H, et al. Alpha-methyltryptamine revisited via easy Internet access. *Vet Hum Toxicol.* 2003;45:149.

90. Louria DB. Lysergic acid diethylamide. *N Engl J Med.* 1968;278:435-438.

91. Lydecker AG, et al. Suspected adulteration of commercial kratom products with 7-hydroxymitragynine. *J Med Toxicol.* 2016;12:341-349.

92. Lyttle T. Misuse and legend in the "toad licking" phenomenon. *Int J Addict.* 1993;28:521-538.

93. Lyttle T, et al. Bufo toads and bufotenine: fact and fiction surrounding an alleged psychedelic. *J Psychoactive Drugs.* 1996;28:267-290.

94. MacRae E. The ritual use of ayahuasca by three Brazilian religions. In: *Drug Use and Cultural Contexts—"Beyond the West": Tradition, Change and Post-Colonialism.* Coomber R. & South N., London, Free Association Books, 2004:27-45.

95. Madden JS. LSD and post-hallucinogen perceptual disorder. *Addiction.* 1994;89:762-763.

96. Marek GJ, Aghajanian GK. Indoleamine and the phenethylamine hallucinogens: mechanisms of psychotomimetic action. *Drug Alcohol Depend.* 1998;51:189-198.

97. Marek GJ, Aghajanian GK. LSD and the phenethylamine hallucinogen DOI are potent partial agonists at 5-HT2A receptors on interneurons in rat piriform cortex. *J Pharmacol Exp Ther.* 1996;278:1373-1382.

98. Marneros A, et al. Self-amputation of penis and tongue after use of Angel's Trumpet. *Eur Arch Psychiatry Clin Neurosci.* 2006;256:458-459.

99. Matsumoto K, et al. Antinociceptive effect of 7-hydroxymitragynine in mice: discovery of an orally active opioid analgesic from the Thai medicinal herb Mitragyna speciosa. *Life Sci.* 2004;74:2143-2155.

100. Matsumoto K, et al. Central antinociceptive effects of mitragynine in mice: contribution of descending noradrenergic and serotonergic systems. *Eur J Pharmacol.* 1996;317:75-81.

101. Matsumoto K, et al. Inhibitory effect of mitragynine, an analgesic alkaloid from Thai herbal medicine, on neurogenic contraction of the vas deferens. *Life Sci.* 2005;78:187-194.

102. McKenna DJ. Clinical investigations of the therapeutic potential of ayahuasca: rationale and regulatory challenges. *Pharmacol Ther.* 2004;102:111-129.

103. Meatherall R, Sharma P. Foxy, a designer tryptamine hallucinogen. *J Anal Toxicol.* 2003;27:313-317.

104. Mebs D, Schmidt K. Occurrence of tetrodotoxin in the frog Atelopus oxyrhynchus. *Toxicon.* 1989;27:819-822.

105. Miller PL, et al. Treatment of acute, adverse psychedelic reactions: "I've tripped and I can't get down." *J Psychoactive Drugs.* 1992;24:277-279.

106. Mithoefer MC, et al. The safety and efficacy of {+/-}3,4-methylenedioxymethamphetamine-assisted psychotherapy in subjects with chronic, treatment-resistant posttraumatic stress disorder: the first randomized controlled pilot study. *J Psychopharmacol.* 2011;25:439-452.

107. Moore K, et al. Do novel psychoactive substances displace established club drugs, supplement them or act as drugs of initiation? The relationship between mephedrone, ecstasy and cocaine. *Eur Addict Res.* 2013;19:276-282.

108. Moreno FA, et al. Safety, tolerability, and efficacy of psilocybin in 9 patients with obsessive-compulsive disorder. *J Clin Psychiatry.* 2006;67:1735-1740.

109. Most A. *Bufo Alvarius: The Psychedelic Toad of the Sonoran Desert.* Venom Press, Gila, Arizona: 1984.

110. Mueller PD, Korey WS. Death by "ecstasy": the serotonin syndrome? *Ann Emerg Med.* 1998;32(3 Pt 1):377-380.

111. National Drug Intelligence Center. Foxy Fast Facts. *Fast Facts,* September 2003. http://www.usdoj.gov/ndic/pubs6/6440/index.htm.

112. Neill JR. "More than medical significance": LSD and American psychiatry 1953 to 1966. *J Psychoactive Drugs.* 1987;19:39-45.

113. O'Malley P, et al. Adolescent substance use: epidemiology and implications for public policy. *Pediatr Clin North Am.* 1995;42:241-260.

114. Personne M, Hulten P. Bromo-dragonfly, a life threatening designer drug. *Clin Toxicol (Phila).* 2008;46:379.

115. Pichini S, et al. Quantification of the plant-derived hallucinogen Salvinorin A in conventional and non-conventional biological fluids by gas chromatography/mass spectrometry after Salvia divinorum smoking. *Rapid Commun Mass Spectrom.* 2005;19:1649-1656.

116. Prue B. Prevalence of reported peyote use 1985–2010 effects of the American Indian Religious Freedom Act of 1994. *Am J Addict.* 2014;23:156-161.

117. Results from the 2015 National Survey on Drug Use and Health ... Center for Behavioral Health Statistics and Quality. (2016). Key substance use and mental health indicators in the United States: Results from the 2015 National. Survey on Drug Use and Health (HHS Publication No. SMA 16-4984, NSDUH Series H-51).Substance Abuse and Mental Health Services Administration. Rockville, MD.

118. Rasmussen K, et al. Phenethylamine hallucinogens in the locus coeruleus: potency of action correlates with rank order of 5-HT2 binding affinity. *Eur J Pharmacol.* 1986;132:79-82.

119. Richardson WH, et al. Herbal drugs of abuse: an emerging problem. *Emerg Med Clinic North Am.* 2007;25:435-457.

120. Rickert VI, et al. Prevalence and risk factors for LSD use among young women. *J Pediatr Adolesc Gynecol.* 2003;16:67-75.

121. Riedlinger TJ. Wasson's alternative candidates for soma. *J Psychoactive Drugs.* 1993;25:149-156.

122. Ritter D, et al. Interference with testing for lysergic acid diethylamide. *Clin Chem.* 1997;43:635-637.

123. Ross S, et al. Rapid and sustained symptom reduction following psilocybin treatment for anxiety and depression in patients with life-threatening cancer: a randomized controlled trial. *JPsychopharmacol.* 2016;30:1165-1180.

124. Salen P, et al. Effect of physostigmine and gastric lavage in a Datura stramonium-induced anticholinergic poisoning epidemic. *Am J Emerg Med.* 2003;21:316-317.

125. Sanders-Bush E, et al. Lysergic acid diethylamide and 2,5-dimethoxy-4-methylamphetamine are partial agonists at serotonin receptors linked to phosphoinositide hydrolysis. *J Pharmacol Exp Ther.* 1988;246:924-928.

126. Sangalli B, Chiang W. Toxicology of nutmeg abuse. *J Toxicol Clin Toxicol.* 2000;38:671-678.

127. Schneier FR, Siris SG. A review of psychoactive substance use and abuse in schizophrenia. Patterns of drug choice. *J Nerv Ment Dis.* 1987;175:641-652.

128. Schultes R, Hofmann A. *Plants of the Gods.* Rochester, VT: Healing Arts Press; 1992.

129. Schultes RE. Hallucinogens of plant origin. *Science.* 1969;163:245-254.

130. Schwartz RH. LSD. Its rise, fall, and renewed popularity among high school students. *Pediatr Clin North Am.* 1995;42:403-413.
131. Shannon M. Methylenedioxymethamphetamine (MDMA, "Ecstasy"). *Pediatr Emerg Care.* 2000;16:377-380.
132. Shellard E. The alkaloids of Mitragyna with special reference. *Bull Narc.* 1974;26:41-55.
133. Shellard EJ. Ethnopharmacology of kratom and the Mitragyna alkaloids. *J Ethnopharmacol.* 1989;25:123-124.
134. Shulgin A. *Phenylethylamines I Have Known and Loved.* Berkley, CA: Transform Press; 1991.
135. Shulgin A, Shulgin A. *TiHKAL: A Continuation.* Berkley, CA: Transform Press; 1997.
136. Shulgin AT, Carter MF. N, N-diisopropyltryptamine (DIPT) and 5-methoxy-N, N-diisopropyltryptamine (5-MeO-DIPT). Two orally active tryptamine analogs with CNS activity. *Commun Psychopharmacol.* 1980;4:363-369.
137. Siebert DJ. Salvia divinorum and salvinorin A: new pharmacologic findings. *J Ethnopharmacol.* 1994;43:53-56.
138. Silbergeld EK, Hruska RE. Lisuride and LSD: dopaminergic and serotonergic interactions in the "serotonin syndrome." *Psychopharmacology (Berl).* 1979;65:233-237.
139. Spina SP, Taddei A. Teenagers with Jimson weed (Datura stramonium) poisoning. *CJEM.* 2007;9:467-468.
140. Stein U, et al. Nutmeg (myristicin) poisoning—report on a fatal case and a series of cases recorded by a poison information centre. *Forensic Sci Int.* 2001;118:87-90.
141. Stevens J. *Storming Heaven.* New York, NY: Harper and Row; 1987.
142. Stout PR, et al. Evaluation of ephedrine, pseudoephedrine and phenylpropanolamine concentrations in human urine samples and a comparison of the specificity of DRI amphetamines and Abuscreen online (KIMS) amphetamines screening immunoassays. *J Forensic Sci.* 2004;49:160-164.
143. Substance Abuse and Mental Health Services Administration. Office of Applied Studies. *The NSDUH Report: Use of Specific Hallucinogens.* Rockville, MD; 2006.
144. Suwanlert S. A study of kratom eaters in Thailand. *Bull Narc.* 1975;27:21-27.
145. Taber WA, Heacock RA. Location of ergot alkaloid and fungi in the seed of Rivea corymbosa (L.) Hall. f., "ololiuqui." *Can J Microbiol.* 1962;8:137-143.
146. Takahashi M, et al. Analysis of phenethylamines and tryptamines in designer drugs using gas chromatography mass spectrometry. *J Health Sci.* 2008;54:89-96.
147. Thongpradichote S, et al. Identification of opioid receptor subtypes in antinociceptive actions of supraspinally-administered mitragynine in mice. *Life Sci.* 1998;62:1371-1378.
148. Titeler M, et al. Radioligand binding evidence implicates the brain 5-HT2 receptor as a site of action for LSD and phenylisopropylamine hallucinogens. *Psychopharmacology (Berl).* 1988;94:213-216.
149. Ulrich RF, Patten BM. The rise, decline, and fall of LSD. *Perspect Biol Med.* 1991;34:561-578.
150. Uniform Controlled Substance Act, 16.4714. http://delcode.delaware.gov/title16/c047/sc02/index.shtml.
151. Unlawful production, manufacture, distribution, or possession of hallucinogenic plants, RS 40:989.1(2006). http://legis.la.gov/legis/Law.aspx?d=321523.
152. US Department of Health and Human Services. Results from the 2010 National Survey on Drug Use and Health: Summary of National Findings. http://www.samhsa.gov/data/NSDUH/2k10NSDUH/2k10Results.htm.
153. US Drug Enforcement Administration. Information Bulletin: Salvia Divinorum. *Microgram Bull.* 2003;36:122-125.
154. US Drug Enforcement Administration. Schedules of controlled substances: placement of alpha-methyltryptamine and 5-methoxy-N,N-diisopropyltryptamine into schedule I of the Controlled Substances Act. Final rule. *Fed Regist.* 2004;69:58950-58953.
155. Valdes LJ 3rd, et al. Ethnopharmacology of ska Maria Pastora (Salvia divinorum, Epling and Jativa-M.). *J Ethnopharmacol.* 1983;7:287-312.
156. Van Buskirk J, et al. Trends in new psychoactive substances from surface and "dark" net monitoring. *Lancet Psychiatry.* 4:16-18.
157. Van Hout MC, Hearne E. New psychoactive substances (NPS) on cryptomarket fora: an exploratory study of characteristics of forum activity between NPS buyers and vendors. *Int J Drug Policy.* 2017;40:102-110.
158. Van Oekelen D, et al. Role of 5-HT(2) receptors in the tryptamine-induced 5-HT syndrome in rats. *Behav Pharmacol.* 2002;13:313-318.
159. Vrolijk RQ, et al. Is online information on ecstasy tablet content safe? *Addiction.* 2017;112:94-100.
160. Vuori E, et al. Death following ingestion of MDMA (ecstasy) and moclobemide. *Addiction.* 2003;98:365-368.
161. Watts VJ, et al. LSD and structural analogs: pharmacological evaluation at D1 dopamine receptors. *Psychopharmacology (Berl).* 1995;118:401-409.
162. Weil AT, Davis W. Bufo alvarius: a potent hallucinogen of animal origin. *J Ethnopharmacol.* 1994;41:1-8.
163. Wood DM, et al. Delayed onset of seizures and toxicity associated with recreational use of Bromo-dragonFLY. *J Med Toxicol.* 2009;5:226-229.
164. Woolf A. Witchcraft or mycotoxin? The Salem witch trials. *J Toxicol Clin Toxicol.* 2000;38:457-460.
165. Yamamoto LT, et al. Opioid receptor agonistic characteristics of mitragynine pseudoindoxyl in comparison with mitragynine derived from Thai medicinal plant Mitragyna speciosa. *Gen Pharmacol.* 1999;33:73-81.
166. Yan F, Roth BL. Salvinorin A: a novel and highly selective kappa-opioid receptor agonist. *Life Sci.* 2004;75:2615-2619.
167. Yotsu-Yamashita M, et al. Tetrodotoxin and its analogues in extracts from the toad Atelopus oxyrhynchus (family: Bufonidae). *Toxicon.* 1992;30:1489-1492.

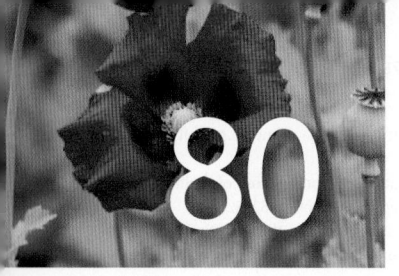

80

γ-HYDROXYBUTYRIC ACID (γ-HYDROXYBUTYRATE)

Rachel Haroz and Brenna M. Farmer

HISTORY AND EPIDEMIOLOGY

OH
|
$CH_2-CH_2-CH_2-C$ $\overset{O}{\underset{OH}{\|}}$

γ-Hydroxybutyric acid (GHB)

γ-Butyrolactone (GBL)

OH
|
$CH_2-CH_2-CH_2-CH_2$ OH

Butanediol

γ-Hydroxybutyric acid (GHB) was discovered in 1960 while searching for an analog for γ-aminobutyric acid (GABA).[38] Because of its central nervous system (CNS) depressive and amnestic properties, GHB was initially used as an anesthetic adjunct, especially in Europe, but never gained favor in the United States for this indication. Outside of the United States, GHB is still used for anesthesia or as an adjunct sedative for therapeutic hypothermia and wound care in children.[50,61] During the 1970s, a Food and Drug Administration (FDA) investigational new drug application (NDA) was submitted to test the use of GHB as a treatment for sleep disturbances. In the 1980s and 1990s, body builders popularized GHB as an anabolic dietary supplement because of its purported release of growth hormone. Its euphoric effects were recognized at this time, and it rapidly gained favor as a "club drug." Because it can cause coma and profound amnesia, GHB was reportedly used in drug-facilitated sexual assault, and in 1990, the FDA banned all use of non-prescription GHB because of this concern.[70]

Following the ban, the analogs γ-butyrolactone (GBL) and 1,4-butanediol (BD) were quickly substituted for GHB in dietary supplements. After the Samantha Reid and Hillory J. Farias Date-Rape Prevention Act of 1999 was passed in 2000, the Drug Enforcement Administration (DEA) classified GHB and its analogs as Schedule I substances, claiming that GHB was a hazard to public safety.[54,70] Also in 2000, an NDA was submitted to the FDA for GHB—under the generic name sodium oxybate and the trade name Xyrem—to reduce the incidence of cataplexy and improve the symptoms of daytime sleepiness in patients with narcolepsy.[35] This latter indication was approved in 2002 and given a Schedule III designation by the DEA,[83] which was expanded, in 2005, to include the treatment of excessive daytime sleepiness in patients with narcolepsy. In 2017, the generic sodium oxybate was approved for the same use. It is now also used "off label" for fibromyalgia, chronic fatigue syndrome, and depressive disorders, and shows promising results in treating spasmodic dysphonia.[6,63,65,74] However, in 2010 the FDA declined to approve GHB for fibromyalgia because of a lack of evidence of efficacy and concerns for safety, citing specifically concerns for respiratory depression, abuse or misuse, and potential unintentional exposure and overdose in children. In the case of narcolepsy, these medications are subject to a Risk Evaluation and Mitigation Strategy (REMS). This requires prescribers to be certified and that patients must be enrolled in certified pharmacies. These pharmacies ship the medications directly to the patients.[23,36] In Europe, specifically Austria and Italy, sodium oxybate is used both for alcohol withdrawal syndrome and for relapse prevention.[10]

In 2007, during an epidemic largely in England and Australia, 1,4-BD was identified in the sticky surface material of toy beads marketed under the names Bindeez or Aquadots. This led to inadvertent toxicity in children ingesting these beads.[30,64]

National statistics demonstrated a trend of escalating GHB abuse and poisoning throughout the 1990s. However, exposures reported to poison control centers has declined in recent years. In 2002, there were 1,386 exposures with GHB and its analogs and precursors reported to the American Association of Poison Control Centers (AAPCC)–Toxic Exposure Surveillance

System, representing more than a twofold increase from approximately 600 GHB cases reported in 1996. Among these, 1,181 exposures (85%) required treatment in a health care facility and resulted in 272 major outcomes and 3 deaths (Chap. 130).[82] From the 2015 the AAPCC, National Poison Data System (NPDS) reports 620 exposures involved GHB and its analogs and precursors. In 379 of these cases, GHB, its analogs and precursors were the single xenobiotic of exposure. Of the reported cases, 318 were treated in a health care facility, and 201 of the cases had moderate or major outcomes.[9] The Drug Abuse Warning Network's 2010 estimates revealed 1,787 emergency department (ED) visits for GHB exposures, similar to the number of visits from 2004 to 2009 with a range of 1,036 to 2,207 ED visits.[75] A retrospective review of deaths in 2011 related to GHB, GBL, and 1,4-BD showed that death from GHB toxicity was more likely to occur in men in their 20s. Thirty-four percent of these deaths were caused by GHB alone.[87]

The apparent trend of decreased GHB exposures in the United States after 2000 contrasts starkly with the increased use reported in some European countries and Australia.[14,17,37] γ-Hydroxybutyrate recently was found to be the fourth most common drug found in ED cases in a recent European publication.[21] More recent reports of large criminal seizures of GBL from Europe indicate the presence of large-scale manufacturing, shipment, and distribution concentrated in the Netherlands and associated with other synthetic drugs such as 3,4-methylenedioxy methamphetamine (MDMA).[20]

In Spain, a study of 505 consecutive GHB-poisoned patients presenting to one hospital from 2001 to 2007 revealed that these patients came to the hospital on the weekends in the early morning hours and require more treatment if ethanol, amphetamines or their derivatives, or cocaine was used concomitantly.[26]

A growing trend in South London coined "chemsex" refers to the recreational use of GHB, methamphetamine, and mephedrone to enhance sexual encounters. Described primarily among men who have sex with men, this practice is associated with an increase in GHB-related deaths. There were 61 deaths in London related to GHB between 2011 and 2015, which includes an increase of 119% between 2014 and 2015.[7,33]

PHARMACOLOGY

γ-Hydroxybutyrate is both a precursor and degradation product of GABA.[72] It has a dual pharmacologic profile, with the neuropharmacology of endogenous GHB being distinct and divergent from that of exogenously administered GHB. Whereas the principal difference is that the activity of endogenous GHB is mediated by the GHB receptor, the activity of exogenously administered GHB is most likely mediated by intrinsic activity at the $GABA_B$ receptor.[71,73]

ENDOGENOUS γ-HYDROXYBUTYRIC ACID

γ-Hydroxybutyrate is formed from GABA by the enzymes GABA transaminase and succinic semialdehyde reductase (Fig. 80–1).[46] γ-Hydroxybutyrate is also endogenously transformed from GBL by lactonases and from 1,4-BD by alcohol and aldehyde dehydrogenase. Endogenous GHB acts as a putative neurotransmitter and is found in highest concentrations in the hippocampus, basal ganglia, hypothalamus, striatum, and substantia nigra.[46,48,80] It has subcellular systems for synthesis, vesicular uptake, and storage in presynaptic terminals. It is released in a Ca^{2+}-dependent manner following depolarization of neurons.

After release, GHB binds to GHB-specific receptors that modulate other neurotransmitter systems. As noted, endogenous GHB acts predominantly on the GHB receptor, which is a G protein–linked receptor located presynaptically.[15,46,71] The GHB receptor is located in the synaptosomal membranes of neuronal cells, most highly concentrated in the pons and hippocampus followed by

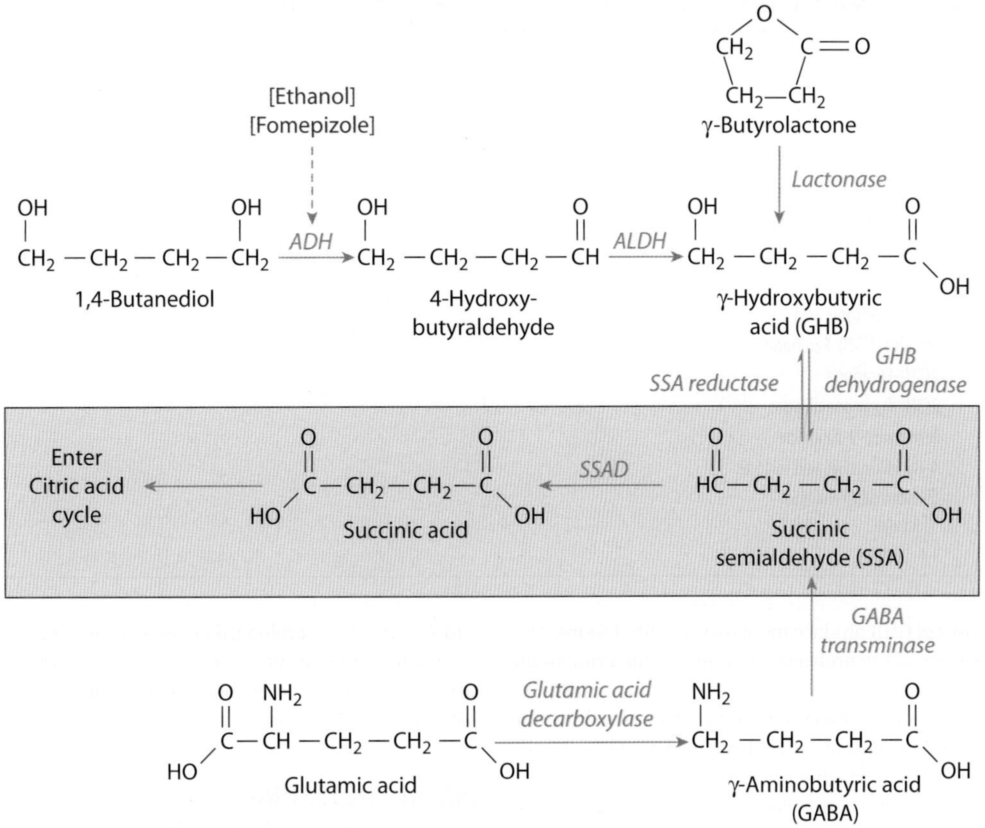

FIGURE 80–1. The synthesis and metabolism of γ-hydroxybutyric acid (GHB). ADH = alcohol dehydrogenase; ALDH = aldehyde dehydrogenase; SSAD = succinic semialdehyde dehydrogenase.

the cerebral cortex and caudate. The GHB receptor has no affinity for typical $GABA_A$ or $GABA_B$ agonists such as GABA and baclofen, respectively. Localized application of GHB produces a response that mimics the action of endogenous GHB.[4,51] γ-Hydroxybutyrate receptors are highly associated with dopaminergic neurons and increase the concentration of dopamine by stimulating tyrosine hydroxylase to synthesize dopamine.[46,73,77] γ-Hydroxybutyrate is also a neuromodulator of dopamine, acetylcholine, endogenous opioids, and glutamate.[46] It either increases (concentrations below 1 mM) or decreases (at higher concentrations) the release of dopamine throughout the mesolimbic system.[13] By contrast, GHB increases dopamine concentrations in the striatum and cortex in a dose-dependent manner by stimulating tyrosine hydroxylase to synthesize dopamine.[46,47,73] γ-Hydroxybutyrate also increases the turnover of serotonin in the brain by stimulating both serotonin synthesis and breakdown.[29,32] Furthermore, GHB decreases acetylcholine in the brain stem and corpus striatum, as well as in the hippocampus (via $GABA_B$ receptors).[52,73] γ-Butyrolactone, but not GHB itself, increases total-brain acetylcholine concentrations by decreasing firing of cholinergic neurons.[28,39,67]

Through an unclear mechanism, GHB increases the release of growth hormone by promoting slow-wave sleep without affecting total sleep time, and additional GHB release is enhanced.[79,81] Although GHB has no effect on total sleep time, it decreases latency to slow-wave sleep while also decreasing the time spent in stages 1 and 2 of the sleep cycle.[40] γ-Hydroxybutyric acid activity is terminated by active uptake from the synaptic cleft for metabolism by specific cytosolic and mitochondrial enzymes.

EXOGENEOUS γ-HYDROXYBUTYRIC ACID

Exogeneous GHB, which produces supraphysiologic GHB concentrations, acts predominantly on the $GABA_B$ receptor, which is found throughout the cerebral cortex, cerebellum, and thalamus.[27,62,84] Presynaptically and postsynaptically, these receptors signal the adenylate cyclase system to activate calcium channels and G protein–coupled inwardly rectifying K^+ channels.[5] Through $GABA_B$ receptor signaling pathways, both dopamine and

acetylcholine pathways are altered, leading to decreased dopamine release and decreased acetylcholine concentrations.[13,52] These effects of GHB are potentiated by baclofen, a $GABA_B$ receptor agonist. Further discussion of these receptors and pathways is found in Chap. 13.

γ-HYDROXYBUTYRIC ACID ANALOGS

γ-Butyrolactone, like GHB, exists in the mammalian brain.[16] Its pharmacologic properties are only evident after conversion to its active metabolite, GHB. Like GBL, 1,4-BD occurs naturally in the brain and exerts its pharmacologic and toxicologic properties only when converted to GHB by alcohol dehydrogenase (ADH).[59]

Table 80–1 lists other GHB analogs known to result in similar toxicity and lists synonyms for GHB, GBL, and 1,4-BD that are often found on the labels of commercial and illicit products.

PHARMACOKINETICS AND TOXICOKINETICS

The endogenous production and metabolism of GHB is shown in Figure 80–1. Exogeneous GHB is typically ingested in its sodium salt form. Oral bioavailability of exogeneous GHB is approximately 60% in rats.[41,42] It is rapidly absorbed from the gastrointestinal (GI) tract in 15 to 45 minutes and displays 2-compartment distribution in animals with an initial volume of distribution of 0.4 L/kg and final volume of distribution 0.6 L/kg.[18,41-43] It is lipid soluble and crosses the blood–brain barrier rapidly. It does not bind significantly to any plasma proteins.[55] γ-Hydroxybutyrate is metabolized mainly by succinic semialdehyde reductase (also known as GHB dehydrogenase) to succinic semialdehyde, which is subsequently metabolized to succinate and enters the citric acid cycle (Fig. 80–1). γ-Hydroxybutyrate is also metabolized directly to succinate via β oxidation in the liver.[57] γ-Hydroxybutyrate is subject to first-pass metabolism by the cytochrome P450 system. However, the specific enzyme is not known.[41] In adult volunteers, the elimination half-life is 20 to 53 minutes. Less than 5% of GHB is excreted unchanged in the urine.[55] In patients with HIV taking protease inhibitors, GHB first-pass metabolism is

TABLE 80-1	Common Synonyms for γ-Hydroxybutyric Acid and Analogs				
GHB (γ-Hydroxybutyrate)	**GBL (γ-Butyrolactone)**	**1,4-BD (1,4-Butanediol)**	**GHV (γ-Hydroxyvaleric Acid)**	**GVL (γ-Valerolactone)**	**THF Tetrahydrofuran**
4-Hydroxybutanoic acid	1,4-Butanolide	1,4-Butylene glycol	γ-Methyl-GHB	4,5-Dihydro-5-methyl-2(3H)-furanone	No other synonyms
4-Hydroxybutyric acid sodium salt	4-Butanolide	1,4-Dihydroxybutane		4-Hydroxypentanoicacid lactone	
γ-Hydroxybutyric acid	Butyric acid lactone	1,4-Tetramethylene glycol		γ-Methyl-GHB	
γ-Hydroxybutyric acid sodium salt	Butyrolactone				
Sodium 4-Hydroxybutyrate	Butyrolactone-γ				
Sodium oxybate	4-Butyrolactone				
	Butyryl lactone				
	4-Deoxytetronic acid				
	Dihydro-2(3H)-Furanone				
	2(3H)-Furanone				
	2(3H)-Furanone dihydro				
	Tetrahydro-2-furanone				
	4-Hydroxbutyric acid lactone				
	γ-Hydroxybutyric acid lactone				
	1,4-Lactone				

altered such that low doses of GHB produce more toxic manifestations. This results from the interactions of the protease inhibitors on the cytochrome P450 system.[1,31]

γ-Butyrolactone undergoes conversion to GHB by a lactonase.[59,60] Compared with GHB, GBL is more rapidly absorbed from the GI tract and has a longer duration of action, both of which result from higher lipid solubility. 1,4-Butanediol exerts its effects after conversion to GHB by ADH.[11,58] Coingestion with ethanol can therefore prolong the onset of clinical effects because of competitive inhibition of ADH.[53,66]

CLINICAL MANIFESTATIONS

The clinical manifestations of GHB are mainly caused by its effects on the CNS. Initial clinical effects of ingested GHB occur in 15 to 20 minutes and peak in 30 to 60 minutes.[8] The clinical manifestations of GHB follow a steep dose–response curve. Doses of 20 to 30 mg/kg create euphoria, memory loss, and drowsiness, and doses of 40 to 60 mg/kg result in coma.[24,48] Doses of 25 mg/kg given to naïve healthy participants result in mean serum GHB concentrations of 39.4 ± 25.2 mcg/mL (range, 4.7–76.3 mcg/mL).[8] Vital sign changes include bradycardia, hypotension, bradypnea, and hypothermia. Pupils are typically miotic and poorly responsive to light. Acute toxicity typically results in CNS depression or coma, respiratory depression, salivation, vomiting, and sometimes myoclonus.[18,45] Of these findings, the most concerning is respiratory depression because apnea is the primary cause of death.[12,44,86] Salivation and vomiting can complicate the respiratory and CNS depression and lead to pulmonary aspiration. Case series also report aggressive and combative behavior, which is characteristically exacerbated when assessing the airway and initiating endotracheal intubation in those patients with compromised consciousness.[18,85] Motor manifestations can be confusing. Although GHB induces seizures (electroencephalographic changes and convulsions) in animal models, this has never been demonstrated in humans. More commonly, in humans, GHB induces myoclonus, which is confused with seizures because of the altered consciousness.[22]

Other findings reported in patients taking prescribed therapeutic doses for narcolepsy include confusion, abnormal thought processes, and depression.[35] The most common adverse effects reported in these patients using prescribed GHB include nausea, dizziness, headache, vomiting, and urinary incontinence.[35]

Recovery from overdose occurs rapidly, typically in less than 6 to 8 hours, and patients often extubate themselves after rapid improvement of their level of consciousness. No sequelae should be expected if hypoxia or aspiration did not occur.

Frequent GHB users develop both tolerance and dependence to GHB.[25,70] In rats receiving doses of GHB every 3 hours for up to 6 days, tolerance was observed.[2] Dependent patients typically use GHB or one of its analogs every

2 to 4 hours over a prolonged period of time, with cumulative daily doses in the range of 10 g or more.[49] The majority of patients with dependence use GHB for its purported anabolic rather than for its psychoactive effects. In patients with dependence, withdrawal symptoms occur after discontinuation or a reduction in dose (see later).

DIAGNOSTIC TESTING

Routine "screens" for drugs of abuse do not typically include analysis for GHB. Specific testing for GHB and its related analogs usually is not requested unless there is suspicion of its use associated with drug-facilitated sexual assault. However, urine and serum testing can also be performed if needed for other forensic purposes. Gas chromatography–mass spectrometry is the test of choice for both urine and serum. γ-Hydroxybutyrate is typically detected in the urine up to 12 hours after use.[8] Interpretation of these tests must include cutoff concentrations because GHB and 1,4-BD also occur endogenously. γ-Butyrolactone does not occur endogenously. These cutoff concentrations must be able to distinguish endogenous production and therapeutic use (as in patients using prescribed GHB for narcolepsy) from abuse or misuse. Attempts to correlate concentrations with clinical effects in any individual are not valid when used chronically because of tolerance. Because of rapid metabolism and elimination, concentrations return to baseline shortly after drug-naïve patients become clinically normal. Normal urinary concentrations of endogenous GHB are less than 5 to 10 mcg/mL, and serum concentrations of endogenous GHB are less than 5 mcg/mL.[8] In patients receiving a 25-mg/kg dose of GHB, serum GHB concentrations ranged from 4.7 mcg/mL to 76.3 mcg/mL 20 to 45 minutes after administration, and urine concentrations ranged from below the detection limit to 840 mcg/mL. In general, loss of consciousness occurs when serum concentrations reach 50 mcg/mL, and deep coma occurs when concentrations rise above 260 mcg/mL.[68]

Screening for GHB is also routinely performed when specific genetic or metabolic disorders are of concern. In particular, elevated GHB concentrations on a urinary organic acid screen in a child is indicative a succinic semialdehyde dehydrogenase deficiency. These children have developmental delay, seizures, hypotonia, and elevated GHB concentrations in the blood, urine, and cerebrospinal fluid.[56] One case report describes a child with a serum GHB concentration of 775 mcg/mL, significantly higher than most patients with exogenous GHB poisoning.[34]

Other routine tests in patients with depressed levels of consciousness include a rapid evaluation of blood glucose, an ethanol concentration as clinically indicated, and an electrocardiogram (ECG). Electrocardiogram findings in reported GHB overdose include sinus bradycardia and prominent U waves, which may be related to the sinus bradycardia. Other standard laboratory test results are typically normal.[12] When intentional overdose or self-harm is suspected, a determination of serum acetaminophen concentration is also recommended. Other studies should be obtained based on the clinical condition of the patient.

MANAGEMENT

Supportive care is the mainstay of therapy for patients with GHB toxicity. All patients presenting to the hospital should have their airway, breathing, and circulation assessed immediately. Some patients with GHB toxicity require airway protection in the presence of profound coma and respiratory depression or apnea. However, many become combative during the intubation process. Supportive care with a nasal airway is often sufficient in a snoring patient who has an appropriate gag and respiratory function. The need for endotracheal intubation is a bedside clinical decision and should be based on the patient's ability to oxygenate and ventilate, especially when the diagnosis is known or highly suspected, as recovery is expected shortly. An intravenous (IV) catheter should be established and IV fluids infused as necessary for hypotension. It is reasonable to give atropine for severe bradycardia that results in hemodynamic compromise. However, in most instances, the bradycardia will not necessitate treatment in otherwise healthy patients. Patients should be warmed if they are hypothermic.

There is no role for gastric decontamination in patients with isolated GHB toxicity because GHB is rapidly absorbed from the GI tract. The increased risk of vomiting and aspiration also limits any beneficial role of gastric decontamination. If a coingestant is present, decontamination with activated charcoal is reasonable if there are no contraindications (Chap. 5).

Other therapies such as dextrose and thiamine should be administered as clinically indicated. Some proposed antidotes include physostigmine, naloxone, and flumazenil. All of these antidotes lack a pharmacologic basis for use and likely place the patient at increased risk because other drugs of abuse commonly used with GHB may interact with these xenobiotics. An animal model did not support the use of physostigmine in GHB toxicity,[3] nor did a systematic literature review.[78] Naloxone is recommended for patients with respiratory and CNS depression in the setting of unknown or presumed overdose. However, in patients with known GHB toxicity, naloxone administration is largely unsuccessful at improving clinical status and therefore is not recommended.[44]

Patients whose symptoms resolve are safe for discharge from the hospital after appropriate psychosocial evaluation for abuse and dependency. All patients who do not follow the expected course of resolution of their clinical manifestations (in ~6 hours) should be admitted to the hospital and investigated for other potential etiologies.

γ-HYDROXYBUTYRIC ACID WITHDRAWAL

Patients who use GHB or its analogs daily in large quantities develop tolerance and dependence.[25] Such patients are prone to withdrawal if they abruptly cease or decrease their daily dose. In patients prescribed GHB for narcolepsy, withdrawal rarely develops when the GHB is used as prescribed because the recommended doses are low and given only at night.[35,76]

γ-Hydroxybutyrate withdrawal is similar to ethanol and benzodiazepine withdrawal (Chap. 14). It can be severe and potentially life threatening. The onset of withdrawal typically occurs 1 to 6 hours after last use. In a descriptive analysis of patients with GHB withdrawal, 64% were male.[49] Manifestations of withdrawal include tachycardia, hypertension, tremors, agitation, dysphoria, nausea, vomiting, auditory and visual hallucinations, and seizures.[19,25,49,76]

For acute withdrawal symptoms, benzodiazepines and supportive care are the recommended mainstays of therapy[49,76] (Antidotes in Depth: A26). Rapid cooling, IV fluids, and evaluation for other medical or traumatic illnesses should be performed. Some patients require large doses of benzodiazepines to control symptoms. In patients with withdrawal symptoms refractory to benzodiazepines, barbiturates and propofol are reasonable.[49,69,76] Baclofen, a GABA$_B$ receptor agonist, is also a reasonable treatment choice in patients with severe GHB withdrawal, although research must be done to determine appropriate dosing and escalation of dosing.

SUMMARY

- γ-Hydroxybutyrate is a unique xenobiotic because it occurs naturally as an endogenous neurotransmitter and is both a licensed pharmaceutical (Schedule III) and a drug of abuse (Schedule I).
- γ-Hydroxybutyrate, GBL, and 1,4-BD result in GHB toxicity through complex neuropharmacological effects to rapidly produce CNS and respiratory depression that is characteristically of short duration.
- γ-Hydroxybutyrate toxicity rarely results in death when patients are treated with supportive care.
- In patients who are dependent on GHB or its analogs, a life-threatening withdrawal syndrome occurs with cessation or decreased use. This withdrawal syndrome should be treated in a manner similar to ethanol or sedative–hypnotic withdrawal.
- With appropriate care of both acute toxicity and withdrawal, patients recover without sequelae, but psychosocial care and referral for management of abuse or dependency are essential.

Acknowledgment

Lawrence S. Quang contributed to this chapter in a previous edition.

REFERENCES

1. Antoniou T, Tseng AL. Interactions between recreational drugs and antiretroviral agents. *Ann Pharmacother.* 2002;36:1598-1613.
2. Bania TC, et al. Gamma-hydroxybutyric acid tolerance and withdrawal in a rat model. *Acad Emerg Med.* 2003;10:697-704.
3. Bania TC, Chu J. Physostigmine does not effect arousal but produces toxicity in an animal model of severe gamma-hydroxybutyrate intoxication. *Acad Emerg Med.* 2005;12:185-189.
4. Benavides J, et al. A high-affinity, Na+-dependent uptake system for gamma-hydroxybutyrate in membrane vesicles prepared from rat brain. *J Neurochem.* 1982;38:1570-1575.
5. Bettler B, et al. Molecular structure and physiological functions of GABA(B) receptors. *Physiol Rev.* 2004;84:835-867.
6. Bosch OG, et al. Reconsidering GHB: orphan drug or new model antidepressant? *J Psychopharmacol.* 2012;26:618-628.
7. Bourne A, et al. "Chemsex" and harm reduction need among gay men in South London. *Int J Drug Policy.* 2015;26:1171-1176.
8. Brenneisen R, et al. Pharmacokinetics and excretion of gamma-hydroxybutyrate (GHB) in healthy subjects. *J Anal Toxicol.* 2004;28:625-630.
9. Bronstein AC, et al. 2011 Annual report of the American Association of Poison Control Centers' National Poison Data System (NPDS): 29th Annual Report. *Clin Toxicol (Phila).* 2012;50:911-1164.
10. Busardo FP, et al. Clinical applications of sodium oxybate (GHB): from narcolepsy to alcohol withdrawal syndrome. *Eur Rev Med Pharmacol Sci.* 2015;19:4654-4663.
11. Carai MA, et al. Central effects of 1,4-butanediol are mediated by GABA(B) receptors via its conversion into gamma-hydroxybutyric acid. *Eur J Pharmacol.* 2002;441:157-163.
12. Chin RL, et al. Clinical course of gamma-hydroxybutyrate overdose. *Ann Emerg Med.* 1998;31:716-722.
13. Cruz HG, et al. Bi-directional effects of GABA(B) receptor agonists on the mesolimbic dopamine system. *Nat Neurosci.* 2004;7:153-159.
14. Dietze PM, et al. Patterns and incidence of gamma-hydroxybutyrate (GHB)-related ambulance attendances in Melbourne, Victoria. *Med J Aust.* 2008;188:709-711.
15. Doherty JD, et al. Identification of endogenous gamma-hydroxybutyrate in human and bovine brain and its regional distribution in human, guinea pig and rhesus monkey brain. *J Pharmacol Exp Ther.* 1978;207:130-139.
16. Doherty JD, et al. A sensitive method for quantitation of gamma-hydroxybutyric acid and gamma-butyrolactone in brain by electron capture gas chromatography. *Anal Biochem.* 1975;69:268-277.
17. Drasbek KR, et al. Gamma-hydroxybutyrate--a drug of abuse. *Acta Neurol Scand.* 2006;114:145-156.
18. Dyer JE. Gamma-Hydroxybutyrate: a health-food product producing coma and seizurelike activity. *Am J Emerg Med.* 1991;9:321-324.
19. Dyer JE, et al. Gamma-hydroxybutyrate withdrawal syndrome. *Ann Emerg Med.* 2001;37:147-153.
20. European Monitoring Centre for Drugs and Drug Addiction. *Drug Markets Report: In-depth Analysis.* Lisbon, Portugal: European Monitoring Centre for Drugs and Drug Addiction; April 2016.
21. European Monitoring Centre for Drugs and Drug Addiction. *European Drug Report 2016: Trends and Developments.* Lisbon, Portugal: European Monitoring Centre for Drugs and Drug Addiction; 2013.
22. Entholzner E, et al. [EEG changes during sedation with gamma-hydroxybutyric acid]. *Anaesthesist.* 1995;44:345-350.
23. Food and Drug Administration. FDA approves a generic of Xyrem with a REMS program. https://www.fda.gov/Drugs/DrugSafety/ucm537281.htm.

24. Food and Drug Administration. Gamma-hydroxybutyric acid. *FDA News*. 1990:P90–P53.

25. Freese TE, et al. The effects and consequences of selected club drugs. *J Subst Abuse Treat*. 2002;23:151-156.

26. Galicia M, et al. Liquid ecstasy intoxication: clinical features of 505 consecutive emergency department patients. *Emerg Med J*. 2011;28:462-466.

27. Gervasi N, et al. Pathway-specific action of gamma-hydroxybutyric acid in sensory thalamus and its relevance to absence seizures. *J Neurosci*. 2003;23:11469-11478.

28. Giarman NJ, Schmidt KF. Some neurochemical aspects of the depressant action of gamma-butyrolactone on the central nervous system. *Br J Pharmacol Chemother*. 1963;20:563-568.

29. Gobaille S, et al. Gamma-hydroxybutyrate increases tryptophan availability and potentiates serotonin turnover in rat brain. *Life Sci*. 2002;70:2101-2112.

30. Gunja N, et al. Gamma-hydroxybutyrate poisoning from toy beads. *Med J Aust*. 2008;188:54-55.

31. Harrington RD, et al. Life-threatening interactions between HIV-1 protease inhibitors and the illicit drugs MDMA and gamma-hydroxybutyrate. *Arch Intern Med*. 1999;159:2221-2224.

32. Hedner T, Lundborg P. Effect of gammahydroxybutyric acid on serotonin synthesis, concentration and metabolism in the developing rat brain. *J Neural Transm*. 1983;57:39-48.

33. Hockenhull J, et al. An observed rise in gamma-hydroxybutyrate-associated deaths in London: Evidence to suggest a possible link with concomitant rise in chemsex. *Forensic Sci Int*. 2017;270:93-97.

34. Ishiguro Y, et al. The first case of 4-hydroxybutyric aciduria in Japan. *Brain Dev*. 2001;23:128-130.

35. Jazz Pharmaceuticals. XYREM (sodium oxybate) [prescribing information]. XYREM® (sodium oxybate) Oral Solution CIII. https://www.xyrem.com/hcp?gclid=Cj0KCQjwlMXMBRC1ARIsAKKGuwhAQTeGSu13oOrDok6yivoJPsxZl6z7qfz5_MADkB56NS78Yn63R5EaArxbEALw_wcB.

36. Kilgore E PO. Sodium Oxybate Fibromyalgia Indication Background Efficacy and Safety. 2014.

37. Knudsen K, et al. High mortality rates among GHB abusers in Western Sweden. *Clin Toxicol (Phila)*. 2008;46:187-192.

38. Laborit H. Sodium 4-Hydroxybutyrate. *Int J Neuropharmacol*. 1964;3:433-451.

39. Ladinsky H, et al. Mode of action of gamma-butyrolactone on the central cholinergic system. *Naunyn Schmiedebergs Arch Pharmacol*. 1983;322:42-48.

40. Lapierre O, et al. The effect of gamma-hydroxybutyrate on nocturnal and diurnal sleep of normal subjects: further considerations on REM sleep-triggering mechanisms. *Sleep*. 1990;13:24-30.

41. Lettieri J, Fung HL. Absorption and first-pass metabolism of 14C-gamma-hydroxybutyric acid. *Res Commun Chem Pathol Pharmacol*. 1976;13:425-437.

42. Lettieri J, Fung HL. Improved pharmacological activity via pro-drug modification: comparative pharmacokinetics of sodium gamma-hydroxybutyrate and gamma-butyrolactone. *Res Commun Chem Pathol Pharmacol*. 1978;22:107-118.

43. Lettieri JT, Fung HL. Dose-dependent pharmacokinetics and hypnotic effects of sodium gamma-hydroxybutyrate in the rat. *J Pharmacol Exp Ther*. 1979;208:7-11.

44. Li J, et al. A tale of novel intoxication: seven cases of gamma-hydroxybutyric acid overdose. *Ann Emerg Med*. 1998;31:723-728.

45. Liechti ME, et al. Clinical features of gamma-hydroxybutyrate and gamma-butyrolactone toxicity and concomitant drug and alcohol use. *Drug Alcohol Depend*. 2006;81:323-326.

46. Maitre M. The gamma-hydroxybutyrate signalling system in brain: organization and functional implications. *Prog Neurobiol*. 1997;51:337-361.

47. Mamelak M. Gammahydroxybutyrate: an endogenous regulator of energy metabolism. *Neurosci Biobehav Rev*. 1989;13:187-198.

48. Mamelak M, et al. Treatment of narcolepsy with gamma-hydroxybutyrate. A review of clinical and sleep laboratory findings. *Sleep*. 1986;9:285-289.

49. McDonough M, et al. Clinical features and management of gamma-hydroxybutyrate (GHB) withdrawal: a review. *Drug Alcohol Depend*. 2004;75:3-9.

50. Mourand I, et al. Feasibility of hypothermia beyond 3 weeks in severe ischemic stroke: an open pilot study using gamma-hydroxybutyrate. *J Neurol Sci*. 2012;316:104-107.

51. Muller C, et al. Evidence for a gamma-hydroxybutyrate (GHB) uptake by rat brain synaptic vesicles. *J Neurochem*. 2002;80:899-904.

52. Nava F, et al. gamma-Hydroxybutyric acid and baclofen decrease extracellular acetylcholine levels in the hippocampus via GABA(B) receptors. *Eur J Pharmacol*. 2001;430:261-263.

53. Nelson L. Butanediol and ethanol: a reverse Mickey Finn? *Int J Med Toxicol*. 2000;3:1-3.

54. Office of the Federal Register. Federal Register. Schedules of Controlled Substances: addition of gamma-hydroxybutyric acid to Schedule I. 21 CFR Part 1301. https://www.deadiversion.usdoj.gov/fed_regs/rules/2000/fr0313.htm.

55. Palatini P, et al. Dose-dependent absorption and elimination of gamma-hydroxybutyric acid in healthy volunteers. *Eur J Clin Pharmacol*. 1993;45:353-356.

56. Pearl PL, et al. Succinic semialdehyde dehydrogenase deficiency in children and adults. *Ann Neurol*. 2003;54(suppl 6):S73-S80.

57. Poldrugo F, Addolorato G. The role of gamma-hydroxybutyric acid in the treatment of alcoholism: from animal to clinical studies. *Alcohol Alcohol*. 1999;34:15-24.

58. Poldrugo F, Snead OC 3rd. 1,4-Butanediol and ethanol compete for degradation in rat brain and liver in vitro. *Alcohol*. 1986;3:367-370.

59. Roth RH, Giarman NJ. Evidence that central nervous system depression by 1,4-butanediol in mediated through a metabolite, gamma-hydroxybutyrate. *Biochem Pharmacol*. 1968;17:735-739.

60. Roth RH, et al. Dependence of rat serum lactonase upon calcium. *Biochem Pharmacol*. 1967;16:596-598.

61. Rousseau AF, et al. Clinical sedation and bispectral index in burn children receiving gamma-hydroxybutyrate. *Paediatr Anaesth*. 2012;22:799-804.

62. Rubin BA, Giarman NJ. The therapy of experimental influenza in mice with antibiotic lactones and related compounds. *Yale J Biol Med*. 1947;19:1017-1022.

63. Rumbach AF, et al. An open-label study of sodium oxybate in Spasmodic dysphonia. *Laryngoscope*. 2017;127:1402-1407.

64. Runnacles JL, Stroobant J. [gamma]-Hydroxybutyrate poisoning: Poisoning from toy beads. *BMJ*. 2008;336:110.

65. Russell IJ, et al. Sodium oxybate reduces pain, fatigue, and sleep disturbance and improves functionality in fibromyalgia: results from a 14-week, randomized, double-blind, placebo-controlled study. *Pain*. 2011;152:1007-1017.

66. Schneidereit T, et al. Butanediol toxicity delayed by preingestion of ethanol. *Int J Med Toxicol*. 2000;3:1-3.

67. Sethy VH, et al. Effect of anesthetic doses of gamma-hydroxybutyrate on the acetylcholine content of rat brain. *Naunyn Schmiedebergs Arch Pharmacol*. 1976;295:9-14.

68. Shannon M, Quang LS. Gamma-hydroxybutyrate, gamma-butyrolactone, and 1,4-butanediol: a case report and review of the literature. *Pediatr Emerg Care*. 2000;16:435-440.

69. Sivilotti ML, et al. Pentobarbital for severe gamma-butyrolactone withdrawal. *Ann Emerg Med*. 2001;38:660-665.

70. Smith KM, et al. Club drugs: methylenedioxymethamphetamine, flunitrazepam, ketamine hydrochloride, and gamma-hydroxybutyrate. *Am J Health Syst Pharm*. 2002;59:1067-1076.

71. Snead OC 3rd. Evidence for a G protein-coupled gamma-hydroxybutyric acid receptor. *J Neurochem*. 2000;75:1986-1996.

72. Snead OC 3rd, et al. In vivo conversion of gamma-aminobutyric acid and 1,4-butanediol to gamma-hydroxybutyric acid in rat brain. Studies using stable isotopes. *Biochem Pharmacol*. 1989;38:4375-4380.

73. Snead OC 3rd, Liu CC. Gamma-hydroxybutyric acid binding sites in rat and human brain synaptosomal membranes. *Biochem Pharmacol*. 1984;33:2587-2590.

74. Staud R. Sodium oxybate for the treatment of fibromyalgia. *Expert Opin Pharmacother*. 2011;12:1789-1798.

75. Substance Abuse and Mental Health Services Administration. Drug Abuse Warning Network, 2009: National Estimates of Drug-Related Emergency Department Visits. HHS Publication No. (SMA) 11-4659. Rockville, MD; 2011.

76. Tarabar AF, Nelson LS. The gamma-hydroxybutyrate withdrawal syndrome. *Toxicol Rev*. 2004;23:45-49.

77. Toide K, et al. Effects on 1,3-bis(tetrahydro-2-furanyl)-5-fluoro-2,4-pyrimidinedione(FD-1) on the central nervous system: 1. Effects on monoamines in the brain. *Arch Int Pharmacodyn Ther*. 1980;247:243-256.

78. Traub SJ, et al. Physostigmine as a treatment for gamma-hydroxybutyrate toxicity: a review. *J Toxicol Clin Toxicol*. 2002;40:781-787.

79. Van Cauter E, et al. Simultaneous stimulation of slow-wave sleep and growth hormone secretion by gamma-hydroxybutyrate in normal young men. *J Clin Invest*. 1997;100:745-753.

80. Vayer P, Maitre M. Regional differences in depolarization-induced release of gamma-hydroxybutyrate from rat brain slices. *Neurosci Lett*. 1988;87:99-103.

81. Vescovi PP, Coiro V. Different control of GH secretion by gamma-amino- and gamma-hydroxy-butyric acid in 4-year abstinent alcoholics. *Drug Alcohol Depend*. 2001;61:217-221.

82. Watson WA, et al. 2003 annual report of the American Association of Poison Control Centers Toxic Exposure Surveillance System. *Am J Emerg Med*. 2004;22:335-404.

83. Wears RL, Berg M. Computer technology and clinical work: still waiting for Godot. *JAMA*. 2005;293:1261-1263.

84. Wu Y, et al. Gamma-hydroxybutyric acid (GHB) and gamma-aminobutyric acidB receptor (GABABR) binding sites are distinctive from one another: molecular evidence. *Neuropharmacology*. 2004;47:1146-1156.

85. Zvosec DL, Smith SW. Agitation is common in gamma-hydroxybutyrate toxicity. *Am J Emerg Med*. 2005;23:316-320.

86. Zvosec DL, et al. Adverse events, including death, associated with the use of 1,4-butanediol. *N Engl J Med*. 2001;344:87-94.

87. Zvosec DL, et al. Case series of 226 gamma-hydroxybutyrate-associated deaths: lethal toxicity and trauma. *Am J Emerg Med*. 2011;29:319-332.

81 INHALANTS

Heather Long

HISTORY AND EPIDEMIOLOGY

Inhalant use is defined as the deliberate inhalation of vapors for the purpose of changing one's consciousness or becoming "high." It is also referred to as volatile substance use, which was first described in medical literature in 1951.[43] Inhalants are appealing to adolescents because they are inexpensive, readily available, and sold legally. Initially, inhalant use was viewed as physically harmless, but reports of "sudden sniffing death" began to appear in the 1960s.[13] Shortly thereafter, evidence surfaced of other significant morbidities, including organic brain syndromes, peripheral neuropathy, and withdrawal.

The demographics of inhalant use differ markedly from those of other traditional substances of use.[160] Age at initiation of illicit drug use is youngest for those choosing inhalants, and among students, the reported use of inhalants peaked among eighth graders.[117,159] For the first time since conducting its drug use survey, the Substance Abuse and Mental Health Services Administration (SAMSHA) reported a second peak in use among 18- to 25-year-old individuals; this may be because of inclusion of a new question specifically asking about inhalation of computer dusters (see later).

In the United States, the problem is greatest among children of lower socioeconomic groups. Non-Hispanic white adolescents are the most likely and black adolescents the least likely to use inhalants. Use among girls equals or surpasses boys.[160] Although inhalant use is a problem in both urban and rural communities, it is more prevalent in rural settings.[113,154] This may relate to the easier access that teens in urban areas have to other drugs of use. Disturbingly, a study of 279 youths who were lifetime inhalant users found 37% perceived experimental inhalant use of slight or no risk.[134]

Inhalant use includes the practices of sniffing, huffing, and bagging. *Sniffing* entails the inhalation of a volatile substance directly from a container, as occurs with modeling glue or rubber cement. *Huffing* involves pouring a volatile liquid onto fabric, such as a rag or sock, and placing it over the mouth, nose, or both while inhaling and is the method used by more than 60% of volatile-substance users.[113] *Bagging* refers to instilling a solvent into a plastic or paper bag and rebreathing from the bag several times; spray paint is among the inhalants commonly used with this method.

COMMON INHALANTS

There are myriad xenobiotics used as inhalants (Table 81–1). Hydrocarbons are organic compounds composed of carbon and hydrogen atoms and are divided into 2 basic categories: aliphatic (straight, branched, or cyclic chains) and aromatic. Most of the commercially available hydrocarbon products are mixtures of hydrocarbons; for example, gasoline is a mixture of aliphatic and aromatic hydrocarbons that consists of more than 1,500 compounds. Substituted hydrocarbons contain halogens or other functional groups such as hydroxyl or nitrite that are substituted for hydrogen atoms in the parent structure. Solvents are themselves a heterogeneous group of xenobiotics that are used to dissolve other chemical compounds or provide a vehicle for their delivery.

The most commonly inhaled hydrocarbons are fuels, such as gasoline, and solvents, such as toluene.[154] Other commonly inhaled hydrocarbon-containing products include spray paints, lighter fluid, air fresheners, and glue. In most reported cases of inhalant use, the inhalant is identified not by its chemical name (eg, butane, toluene) but rather by its intended use (eg, lighter fluid, paint thinner). Because exact components may vary among products, identification by the intended commercial use of the product is inaccurate and imprecise. The choice of xenobiotic used likely reflects its availability: cases from the 1970s frequently reported use of antiperspirants

and typewriter correction fluid; computer and electronics cleaners have largely replaced these products.

Dusting refers to the inhalation of compressed air cleaners containing halogenated hydrocarbons like 1,1-difluoroethane (eg, CRC Dust Off), marketed for cleaning computer keyboards and electronics equipment. Reports of such exposures, including deaths and ventricular dysrhythmias, have dramatically increased. From 2008 to 2012 at the San Diego County Medical Examiner's Office, 1,1-difluoroethane was detected in 17 postmortem tissues and cited as the cause of death in 13.[170] Of the 56 deaths attributed to recreational inhalant use in Washington State between 2003 and 2012, 54% involved difluoroethane from computer dusters, yet dusting is not perceived to be harmful by users, and surprisingly, many users do not consider it a form of inhalant use.[112,128]

Although intentional inhalation of the inert gas helium for its voice-altering effects is common, it has not traditionally been inhaled for potential euphoric effects. Among 723 adolescents, however, 11.5% reported inhaling helium with the intention of getting high, and of them, 34% reported they did get high from inhaling helium.[180]

Although volatile alkyl nitrites are technically substituted hydrocarbons, they have pharmacologic and behavioral effects, as well as patterns of use, that are distinct from the other volatile hydrocarbons. For this

TABLE 81–1	Common Inhalants and the Constituent Xenobiotics
Inhalant	**Chemical**
Carburetor cleaner	Methanol, methylene chloride, toluene, propane
Cigarette lighter fluid	Butane
Computer keyboard duster	Difluoroethane, tetrafluoroethane
Deodorizers (room)	Butyl nitrite, isobutyl nitrite, cyclohexyl nitrite
Dry cleaning agents, spot removers, degreasers	Tetrachloroethylene, trichloroethane, trichloroethylene
DVD and video cassette recorder head cleaner	Ethyl chloride
Freon (refrigerants)	Hydrofluorocarbons
Gasoline	Aliphatic and aromatic hydrocarbons
Glues and adhesives	Toluene, *n*-hexane, benzene, xylene, trichloroethane, trichloroethylene, tetrachloroethylene, ethyl acetate, methylethyl ketone, methyl chloride
Hair spray, deodorants, air fresheners	Butane, propane, fluorocarbons
Nail polish remover	Acetone
Paint thinner	Toluene, methylene chloride, methanol
"Poppers"	Amyl nitrite, isobutyl nitrite
Paints, lacquers, varnishes	Trichloroethylene, toluene, *n*-hexane
Spray paint	Toluene, butane, propane
Typewriter correction fluid	Trichloroethane, trichloroethylene
Whipped cream dispensers, "whippits"	Nitrous oxide

reason, researchers usually classify them as a separate category among used inhalants. Amyl nitrite is the prototypical volatile alkyl nitrite.[11] Amyl nitrite became popular in the 1960s with the appearance of "poppers," small glass capsules containing the chemical in a plastic sheath or gauze. When crushed, the ampules release the amyl nitrite. When nonprescription sales of amyl nitrite were restricted in 1968, sex and drug paraphernalia shops began selling small vials of butyl and isobutyl nitrites marketed as room deodorizers or liquid incense.[11,108] Because of further restrictions on sales of alkyl nitrites, most of these products now contain chemicals that are not technically alkyl nitrites, such as cyclohexyl nitrite.[11]

The most commonly used nonhydrocarbon inhalant is nitrous oxide (N_2O). Nitrous oxide, or "laughing gas," is used medicinally as an inhalational anesthetic. It is the propellant in supermarket-bought whipped cream canisters, and cartridges of the compressed gas are sold for home use in whipped cream dispensers. These battery-sized metal containers of compressed gas are known as "whippits." The container is punctured using a device known as a "cracker," and the escaping gas is either inhaled directly or collected in a balloon and then inhaled.

PHARMACOLOGY AND PHARMACOKINETICS

Although chemically heterogeneous, inhalants are generally highly lipophilic and gain rapid entrance into the central nervous system (CNS). Little is known about the cellular basis of the effects of inhalants. Evidence to date shows the most commonly used hydrocarbons have molecular mechanisms similar to those of other classic CNS depressants, frequently with common cellular sites of action. Their effects are probably best represented by the model for ethanol in which multiple different cellular mechanisms explain diverse pharmacologic and toxicologic effects.[11]

Volatile Hydrocarbons

The clinical effects of the volatile hydrocarbons are likely mediated through stimulation of inhibitory neurotransmission and antagonism of excitatory neurotransmission within the CNS. Like ethanol, toluene, trichloroethane (TCE), and trichloroethylene enhance γ-aminobutyric acid type A ($GABA_A$) receptor–mediated synaptic currents as well as glycine receptor–activated ion function. Stimulation of these receptors acts to increase chloride permeability, hyperpolarizing the neuronal cell membrane and inhibiting excitability.[17,80,148,156] Like inhaled anesthetics, these inhalants act presynaptically on the GABA nerve terminals. Toluene-induced increases in inhibitory synaptic current are blocked by dantrolene and ryanodine, suggesting toluene effects release of calcium from intracellular nerve terminal stores.[107] Despite very different molecular structures, ethanol, enflurane, chloroform, toluene, and TCE compete for binding sites at α_1 glycine receptors.[16] Like ethanol and subanesthetic concentrations of isoflurane, toluene, TCE, and benzene all interfere with glutamate-mediated excitatory neurotransmission by inhibiting N-methyl-D-aspartate (NMDA) receptor–mediated currents in a concentration dependent manner.[10,44,136,147] Furthermore, repeated toluene exposure increases NMDA receptors, suggesting that chronic exposure leads to upregulation of excitatory neurotransmission as occurs with ethanol.[10,184]

Toluene is the prototypical volatile hydrocarbon and the best studied. In animal models, differences in pharmacologic action are demonstrated between toluene and other alkylbenzenes, halogenated hydrocarbons such as TCE, and acetone (Chap. 105).[23,44,100,149,166] These differences represent evidence that specific cellular sites for their actions exist. Additionally, these differences may explain the variation in their use potential or their clinical effects.[11] Despite these distinctions, there are marked similarities in the behavioral and pharmacologic effects of the volatile hydrocarbons. Moreover, the clinical effect profile shared by the volatile hydrocarbons, subanesthetic concentrations of general anesthetics, ethanol, and benzodiazepines suggests that they share cellular mechanisms. Shared clinical effects include anxiolysis,[28] anticonvulsant effects,[187] impaired motor coordination,[120] and physical dependence upon withdrawal.[54,55]

Most research on inhalants has focused on the neural basis of their effects, yet it is the cardiotoxicity that is responsible for the majority of their lethal effects. In vivo, toluene reversibly inhibits myocardial voltage-activated sodium channels.[45] Similarly, it inhibits muscle sodium channels but with less potency.[63] Ethanol and toluene have opposite effects on potassium channels in vivo; whereas ethanol potentiates the large conductance, calcium-activated potassium channels, and certain G protein–coupled inwardly rectifying potassium channels, toluene inhibits them.[46] The combined inhibition of the sodium channels and the inwardly rectifying potassium channels is postulated to play a role in cardiac dysrhythmias and sudden sniffing death associated with the aromatic and halogenated hydrocarbons. Animal studies show toluene and 1,1,1-trichloroethane produce biphasic dose–response curves for motor activity: low concentrations yield motor excitation, and high concentrations produce sedation, motor impairment, and anesthesia.[24,178] Molecular mechanisms underlying motor excitation and cardiac dysrhythmias may maximize the risk and explain the observed clinical phenomenon described in sudden sniffing death (see below).

There are scant data on the pharmacokinetics of the inhalants. Most data are derived from studies on occupational and environmental exposures and have limited applicability to intentional inhalation. More relevant to the understanding of inhalants are the similarities with the inhalational anesthetics, many of which are also halogenated hydrocarbons. Factors determining pharmacokinetic and pharmacodynamic effects of a given inhalational anesthetic include its concentration in inspired air; partition coefficient; interaction with other inhaled substances, ethanol, and drugs; the patient's respiratory rate and blood flow; percent body fat; and individual variation in drug metabolism (Chap. 65).[67]

Partition coefficients measure the relative affinity of a gas for two different substances at equilibrium and are used to predict the rate and extent of uptake of an inhaled substance. The blood:gas partition coefficient is most commonly referenced. The higher the number, the more soluble the substance is in blood. Substances with a low blood:gas partition coefficient, like N_2O, are rapidly taken up by the brain and, conversely, are rapidly eliminated from the brain once exposure is ended (Table 81–2).

In a rodent model of inhalation use of toluene and acetone, the rapidity of onset and the extent of CNS depression were dependent on the concentration of the solvent inhaled.[32] There was a parallel relationship between brain concentration and pharmacologic effect during induction (inhalation) and postexposure. Brain and liver concentrations dropped rapidly after exposure; concentration in blood decreased at the slowest rate. Elimination was biphasic: rapid elimination during the first step was a result of tissue redistribution, alveolar ventilation, and metabolic clearance. During the second phase, there was a slow decrease in tissue concentrations as a result of the gradual mobilization from adipose tissue with subsequent exhalation or metabolism. Acetone, which is more water soluble than toluene, is less potent and slower acting than toluene but is eliminated much more slowly than toluene and has a much longer duration of action.[32] In a rat study designed to mimic use, initial distribution of 1,1-difluoroethane (DFE) was rapid with an average half-life during the uptake phase of 9 seconds, 18 seconds, and 27 seconds for blood, brain, and heart, respectively. Average elimination half-lives were 86 seconds, 110 seconds, and 168 seconds in the blood, brain, and heart, respectively. After a burst exposure mimicking inhalant use, all animals demonstrated CNS toxicity within 20 seconds with no detectable toxicity by 8 minutes and brain and serum concentrations nearing zero.[7] Positron emission tomography (PET) studies using (^{11}C) radiolabeled toluene, butane, and acetone in nonhuman primates showed rapid uptake of radioactivity in striatal and frontal regions of the cortex followed by rapid clearance from the brain.[64] Whole-body PET scans in mice showed excretion through the kidneys and liver.[65]

The inhalants are eliminated unchanged by the lungs, undergo hepatic metabolism, or both (Table 81–2). For some, the percentage that is metabolized versus eliminated unchanged varies with the exposure dose. Nitrous oxide and the aliphatic hydrocarbons are frequently eliminated unchanged in the expired air. The aromatic and halogenated hydrocarbons are metabolized

TABLE 81–2 Blood:Gas Partition Coefficients, Routes of Elimination, and Important Metabolites of Selected Inhalants

Xenobiotic	Blood:Gas Partition Coefficient (98.6°F {37°C})	Routes of Elimination	Important Metabolites
Acetone	243–300	Largely unchanged via exhalation 95% and urine 5%	None
n-Butane	0.019	Largely unchanged via exhalation	Metabolized to 2-butanol and 2-butanone
Carbon tetrachloride	1.6	50% unchanged via exhalation; 50% hepatic metabolism and urinary excretion	CYP2E1 to trichloromethyl radical, trichloromethyl peroxy radical, phosgene
n-Hexane	2	10%–20% exhaled unchanged; hepatic metabolism and urinary excretion	CYP2E1 to 2-hexanol, 2,5-hexanedione, γ-valerolactone
Methylene chloride	5–10	92% exhaled unchanged; hepatic metabolism and urinary excretion	1. CYP2E1 to CO and CO_2 2. Glutathione transferase to CO_2, formaldehyde, and formic acid
Nitrous oxide	0.47	>99% exhaled unchanged	None
Toluene	8–16	<20% exhaled unchanged; >80% hepatic metabolism and urinary excretion	CYP2E1 to benzoic acid, then 1. Glycine conjugation to form hippuric acid (68%) 2. Glucuronic acid conjugation to benzoyl glucuronide (insignificant pathway except after large exposure)
1,1,1-Trichloroethane	1–3	91% exhaled unchanged; hepatic metabolism and urinary excretion	CYP2E1 to trichloroethanol, then 1. Conjugated with glucuronic acid to formurochloralic acid or 2. Further oxidized to trichloroacetic acid
Trichloroethylene	9	16% exhaled unchanged; 84% hepatic metabolism and urinary excretion	CYP2E1 to epoxide intermediate (transient); chloral hydrate (transient); trichloroethanol (45%), trichloroacetic acid (32%). Urinary trichloroacetic acid peaks 2–3 days postexposure
1,2-Dichloro-1,1-difluoroethane	NA	NA	CYP2E1 to 2-chloro-2,2-difluoroethyl glucuronide, 2-2chloro-2,2-difluoroethyl sulfate, chlorodifluoroacetic acid, chlorodifluoroacetaldehyde hydrate, chlorodifluoroacetaldehyde-urea adduct, and inorganic fluoride; no covalently bound metabolites to liver proteins

NA = not applicable.

extensively via the cytochrome P450 (CYP) system, particularly CYP2E1, which has a substrate spectrum that includes a number of aliphatic, aromatic, and halogenated hydrocarbons.[21,75,76,189] Extrahepatic expression of CYP2E1 occurs to a lesser extent but is of toxicologic significance, particularly in the kidneys and the dopaminergic cells of the substantia nigra.[22,82,172] In humans, there appears to be no significant gender difference in CYP2E1 activity; however, it is polymorphic, and as such, allelic distributions vary among different human populations.[22,151] Moreover, this polymorphism explains the varying degrees of toxicity exhibited after inhalant use.

Reward and reinforcement effects of inhalants are readily demonstrated. Although the mechanisms underlying their reinforcement behavior remain poorly studied, activation of the dopaminergic neurons of the ventral tegmental area is thought to play an important role in solvent use, similar to more commonly studied drugs of use.[65,126,140,168,188] Interestingly, the reward and reinforcement effects of the toluene appear to vary with age of exposure, suggesting that physiologic as well as psychosocial factors play a role in the prevalence of inhalant use among adolescents compared with adults.[14,26,127] Furthermore, age at exposure differentially affects dendritic growth in the brain as well as subunit expression of both NMDA and GABA$_A$ receptors, suggesting that the adolescent brain is at greater risk for cognitive impairment after inhalant use.[61,127,130]

Volatile Alkyl Nitrites

Little still is known about the molecular basis of use of the volatile alkyl nitrites. Their effects are thought to be mediated through smooth muscle relaxation in the central and peripheral vasculature, and they share a common cellular pathway with other nitric oxide (NO) donors similar to nitroglycerin and sodium nitroprusside.[11,92] As occurs with other used substances, a rodent study found elevated dopamine release after exposure to isobutyl nitrite.[83] In rats, chronic exposure to alkyl nitrites impaired motor

coordination as well as memory acquisition and retention.[40] A rat model of inhalation of isobutyl nitrite found a half-life of 1.4 minutes with almost 100% biotransformation to isobutyl alcohol. Bioavailability after inhalation was estimated to be 43%.[91]

Nitrous Oxide

The pharmacokinetics and pharmacodynamics of N_2O use are derived from its use as an inhalational anesthetic (Chap. 65). In contrast to toluene and other used volatile solvents, N_2O mediate its stimulant effects through inhibition of excitatory NMDA-activated currents; in animal models, it does not have an effect on GABA-activated currents.[84,138,176] Nitrous oxide also stimulates dopaminergic neurons, but the significance of this in mediating its anesthetic effects remains unclear.[89,121]

Animal studies suggest the analgesic effects (or more accurately, the antinociceptive effects because it refers to animals) of N_2O appear to be mediated through κ-opioid receptors in the midbrain.[60] These antinociceptive effects can be reversed by the opioid antagonist naloxone.[19] However, in humans, the anesthetic effects are not attenuated by naloxone, nor are the subjective and psychomotor effects of N_2O extinguished.[152,191]

CLINICAL MANIFESTATIONS

Signs and symptoms of inhalant use may be subtle, tend to vary widely among individuals, and generally resolve within several hours of exposure. After acute exposure, there may be a distinct odor of the used inhalant on the patient's breath or clothing. Depending on the inhalant used and the method, there may be discoloration of skin around the nose and mouth. Mucous membrane irritation causes sneezing, coughing, and tearing. Patients may complain of dyspnea and palpitations. Gastrointestinal complaints include nausea, vomiting, and abdominal pain. After an initial period of euphoria, patients have residual headache and dizziness.

Volatile Hydrocarbons

The CNS is the intended target of the inhalants and is most susceptible to its adverse effects. Initial CNS effects include euphoria and hallucinations, that are both visual and auditory, as well as headache and dizziness. As toxicity progresses, CNS depression worsens, and patients develop slurred speech, confusion, tremor, and weakness. Transient cranial nerve palsies are reported.[162] Further CNS depression is marked by ataxia, lethargy, seizures, coma, and respiratory depression. These acute encephalopathic effects generally resolve spontaneously, and associated neuroimaging abnormalities are not reported.[57]

As can be expected, given the high lipophilicity of most inhalants, toxicity is manifested most strikingly in the CNS. Chronic users demonstrate impaired executive function compared with control participants.[163,164] Toluene leukoencephalopathy, characterized by dementia, ataxia, eye movement disorders, and anosmia, is the prototypical manifestation of chronic inhalant neurotoxicity. Patients with toluene leukoencephalopathy display characteristic neurobehavioral deficits reflecting white matter involvement, including inattention, apathy, and impaired memory and visuospatial skills with relative preservation of language.[57] Autopsy studies reveal white matter degeneration, including cerebral and cerebellar atrophy and thinning of the corpus callosum.[1,94,141] On microscopy, there is diffuse demyelination with relative sparing of the axons. Abundant perivascular macrophages containing coarse or laminar myelin debris found in areas of the greatest myelin loss is a characteristic pathologic feature.[1,57] This targeting of myelin, which is 70% lipid, is explained by the lipophilicity of toluene.[57] Because myelinization continues at least through the second decade of life, the typical toluene user who begins inhaling during adolescence will be particularly susceptible to its toxic CNS effects.[56] Advances in magnetic resonance imaging (MRI) with gadolinium, which allow enhanced visualization of the cerebral white matter, demonstrate that the extent of white matter injury in the brain directly corresponds to the clinical severity of toluene leukoencephalopathy.[57] Younger age at onset of use is associated with decreased frontal white-matter integrity on MRI.[190] Chronic inhalant use is associated with altered concentrations of antioxidant enzymes, including erythrocyte superoxide dismutase and plasma glutathione peroxidase, and it is postulated that reactive oxygen species generated either by toluene or its metabolite benzaldehyde induce lipid peroxidation in the brain.[51,110,139] Genetic polymorphisms and host susceptibility among chronic users are also hypothesized to play a role.[70]

Acute cardiotoxicity associated with hydrocarbon inhalation is manifested most dramatically in "sudden sniffing death." In witnessed cases, sudden death occurred when sniffing was followed by some physical activity. Examples include running or wrestling or a stressful situation such as being caught sniffing by parents or police.[13] It is thought that the inhalant "sensitizes the myocardium" by blocking the potassium current (I_{kr}), thereby prolonging repolarization.[124] This produces a substrate for dysrhythmia propagation; the activity or stress then causes a catecholamine surge that initiates the dysrhythmia (Chap. 15).[124] Cardiac dysrhythmias after the inhalation of hydrocarbons were documented with the halogenated inhalational anesthetics in the early 1900s, and this association was subsequently confirmed in both animal and human studies.[58,165]

More typically, the clinical presentation of a patient with hydrocarbon cardiotoxicity includes palpitations, shortness of breath, syncope, and electrocardiographic (ECG) abnormalities, including atrial fibrillation, premature ventricular contractions, QT interval prolongation, and U waves.

Multiple case reports of ventricular fibrillation and torsade de pointes follow intentional inhalation of other hydrocarbons such as butane fuel,[72,183] fluorinated hydrocarbons such as DFE,[8,38] and Glade Air Freshener (SC Johnson), which contains a mixture of short-chain aliphatic hydrocarbons.[103] Among 44 patients with a history of inhalant use, specifically toluene exposure, the QT interval and QT interval dispersion were significantly greater than in healthy control participants. Furthermore, the QT interval and QT interval dispersion were significantly greater in the 20 toluene users with a history of unexplained syncope than in asymptomatic users and control participants.[3] Although cardiotoxic effects

of inhalant use are generally acute, myocarditis and dilated cardiomyopathy are reported with use of toluene, trichloroethylene, and DFE.[31,38,48,114,186] Microscopy reveals evidence of chronic myocarditis with fibrosis.[186]

The most significant respiratory complication of inhalational use is hypoxia, which is either caused by displacement of inspired oxygen with the inhalant, reducing the fraction of inspired oxygen (FIO_2), or by rebreathing of exhaled air, as occurs with bagging. Direct pulmonary toxicity associated with inhalants is most often a result of inadvertent aspiration of a liquid hydrocarbon (Chap. 105). Aspiration injury is associated with the acute respiratory distress syndrome (ARDS), a continuum of lung injury characterized by increased permeability of the alveolar–capillary barrier and the resulting influx of edema into the alveoli, neutrophilic inflammation, and an imbalance of cytokines and other inflammatory mediators.[177] Chronic use of volatile solvents induces increased lung epithelial permeability, suggesting pulmonary alveolar–capillary membrane dysfunction independent of aspiration injury.[39] Reports of asphyxiation initially ascribed to inhalant use were later found caused by suffocation by a plastic bag, mask, or container pressed firmly to the face and not specifically by toxicity of the inhaled vapor.[13,35,175]

Irritant effects on the respiratory system are frequently transient, but some patients progress to chemical pneumonitis. This syndrome is characterized by tachypnea, fever, tachycardia, crackles, rhonchi, leukocytosis, and radiographic abnormalities, including perihilar densities, bronchovascular markings, increased interstitial markings, infiltrates, and consolidation. Acute eosinophilic pneumonia after use of a fabric protector containing 1,1,1-trichloroethane is also reported.[90] Barotrauma, from deep inhalation or breath-holding, presents as pneumothorax, pneumomediastinum, or subcutaneous emphysema.[143]

Hepatoxicity is associated with exposure to halogenated hydrocarbons, particularly carbon tetrachloride (CCl_4), but also chloroform, trichloroethane, trichloroethylene, and toluene.[109] Intentional inhalation of (CCl_4) is rarely reported, but its toxic metabolite, the trichloromethyl radical, created by the cytochrome CYP2E1, can covalently bind to hepatocyte macromolecules and cause lipid peroxidation[137] (Chap. 105). Two cases of centrilobular hepatic necrosis are reported after inhalation of trichloroethylene. In a case series of 34 serum-confirmed inhalant deaths, 2 of the 3 who died from trichloroethane and trichloroethylene inhalation had cirrhosis of the liver at autopsy. None of the victims of other inhalants had cirrhosis.[62] Inhalation of either toluene or one of the many halogenated hydrocarbons is associated with elevated liver enzymes and hepatomegaly that generally return to pre-exposure condition within 2 weeks of abstinence.[9,79,87,102]

Most reported kidney toxicity is associated with toluene inhalation. Prolonged toluene inhalation was said to cause a distal renal tubular acidosis (RTA), resulting in hypokalemia. However, whereas distal RTA is typically associated with a hyperchloremic metabolic acidosis and a normal anion gap, toluene use is associated with both normal and increased anion gap acidosis. Production of hippuric acid, a toluene metabolite, plays an important role in the genesis of the metabolic acidosis.[37] Hippurate excretion, usually expressed as a ratio to creatinine, rises dramatically with toluene inhalation.[115] The excretion of abundant hippurate in the urine unmatched by ammonium mandates an enhanced rate of excretion of sodium and potassium cations. Continued loss of potassium in the urine leads to hypokalemia. Toluene is rapidly metabolized to hippuric acid, and the hippurate anion is swiftly cleared by the kidneys, leaving the hydrogen ion behind. This prevents the rise in the anion gap that would normally occur with an acid anion other than chloride, resulting in a normal anion gap. In some cases, the loss of sodium causes extracellular fluid volume contraction and a fall in the glomerular filtration rate, which transforms the metabolic acidosis with a normal anion gap into one with a high anion gap caused by the accumulation of hippurate and other anions.[37] Other renal abnormalities of uncertain etiology are associated with toluene inhalation, including hematuria, albuminuria, and pyuria. Glomerulonephritis associated with hydrocarbon inhalation is also reported and is a result of antiglomerular basement membrane antibody-mediated immune complex deposition.[18,123,171,192]

Toluene using patients often present with profound hypokalemic muscle weakness. In a study of 25 patients admitted to the hospital after inhalant use, 9 presented with muscle weakness. The mean serum potassium concentration was 1.7 mEq/L, and 6 of these patients also had rhabdomyolysis. Four patients were quadriplegic on presentation, and initially, 2 of these were misdiagnosed with Guillain-Barré syndrome. The patients had inhaled toluene 6 to 7 hours per day for 4 to 14 days before presentation.[157] In a prospective study of 20 patients presenting to a single emergency department (ED) with acute toluene toxicity, 15 (75%) had had muscle weakness or paralysis. Three patients died from cardiac dysrhythmias, all of whom presented with altered mental status, hypokalemia, marked acidemia, and acute kidney injury.[36]

Acute dermatologic and upper airway toxicity is associated with the inhalation of fluorinated hydrocarbons. This is caused by the cooling of the gas as it rapidly expands on release from its pressurized container. First- and second-degree burns of the face, neck, shoulder and chest are reported in a 12-year-old-girl inhaling a computer duster containing difluoroethane.[118] Vesicular lesions of frostbite affect the tongue, lips, oral mucosa, airway, and hands as well as other areas that come in contact with dropped or discarded containers.[2,74,93,97] Massive, potentially life-threatening edema of the oropharyngeal, glottic, epiglottic, and paratracheal structures is also reported.[95,96,112,135,185] With chronic use of volatile hydrocarbons, some patients develop severe drying and cracking around the mouth and nose as a consequence of a defatting dermatitis known as "huffer's eczema" or "glue sniffer's rash." Other manifestations of chronic irritation include recurrent epistaxis, chronic rhinitis, conjunctivitis, halitosis, and ulceration of the nasal and oral mucosa.[115]

Bone mineral density was significantly lower in 25 adolescent chronic glue sniffers compared with that of healthy control participants.[50] In a mouse model, chronic exposure to toluene significantly reduced bone mineral density.[6] Skeletal fluorosis, manifested clinically by pain in affected bones and joints, hypertrophic nodules (Figs. 81–1 and 81–2), and decreased joint mobility, is reported following use of fluoride-containing inhalants (Fig. 8–13).[42,74,169]

Ophthalmologic toxicity, although more commonly associated with use of alkyl nitrites (see later), is reported in 2 men with chronic toluene use. Both had gradual vision loss, bilateral optic atrophy, and characteristic white matter changes on MRI.[73]

Methylene chloride (dichloromethane), most commonly found in paint removers and degreasers, is unique among the halogenated hydrocarbons in that it undergoes metabolism in the liver by CYP2E1 to carbon monoxide (CO).[12] In addition to acute CNS and cardiac manifestations, inhalation of methylene chloride is associated with delayed onset and prolonged duration of signs and symptoms of CO poisoning. The CO metabolite is generated 4 to 8 hours after exposure and its apparent half-life is 13 hours, significantly longer than that of CO following inhalation (Chap. 122).[12,158] Methanol toxicity is reported after intentional inhalation of methanol-containing carburetor cleaners and paint strippers.[59,101,104,111] Significant findings include hyperemic optic discs on funduscopic examination, metabolic acidosis, and CNS and respiratory depression (Chap. 106). Methanol-containing carburetor cleaners also contain significant amounts of toluene (43.8%), methylene chloride (20.5%), and propane (12.5%). These xenobiotics potentiate CNS depression and contribute to the toxicity associated with these products.

Chronic inhalation of the solvent n-hexane, a petroleum distillate found, for example, in rubber cement, causes a sensorimotor peripheral neuropathy. Toxicity is mediated via a metabolite, 2,5-hexanedione, which interferes with glyceraldehyde-3-phosphate dehydrogenase–dependent axonal transport, resulting in axonal death.[49] Numbness and tingling of the fingers and toes is the most common initial complaint; progressive, ascending loss of motor function with frank quadriparesis may ensue[41] (Chap. 105).

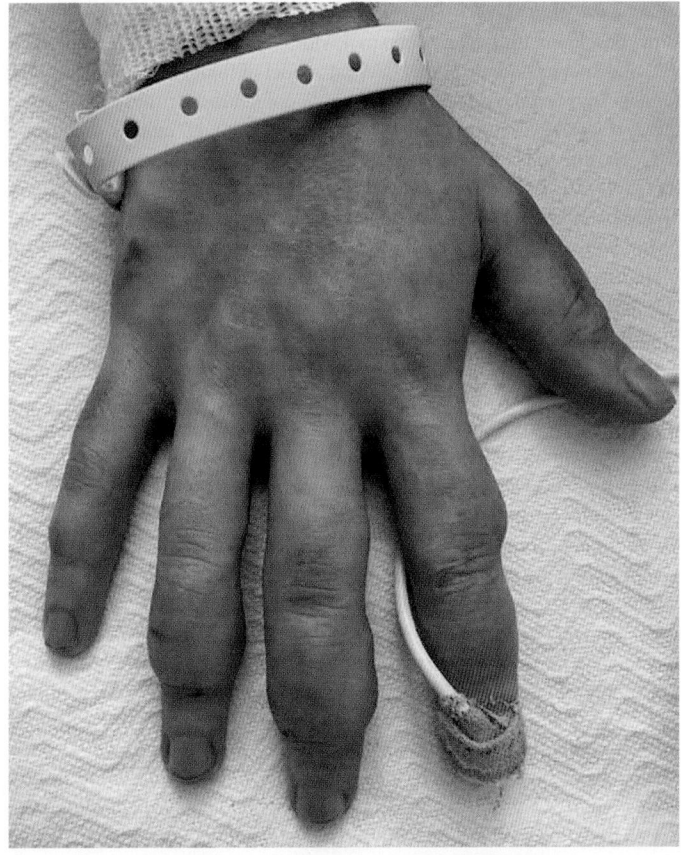

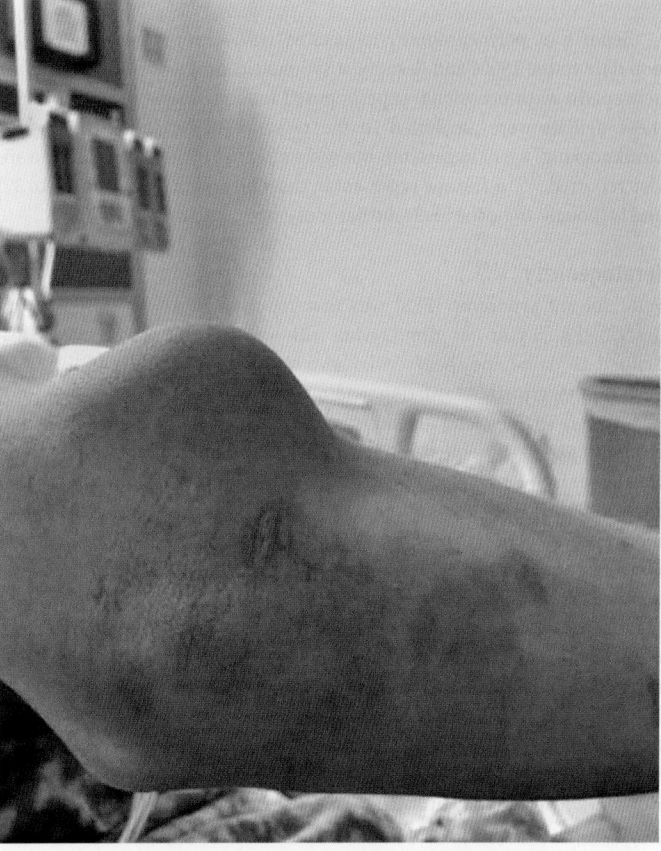

A   **B**

FIGURE 81–1. Hand (**A**) and knee (**B**) of a patient with skeletal fluorosis secondary to prolonged extensive inhalant use of fluorinated hydrocarbons. *(Used with permission from William Eggleston, PharmD, Department of Emergency Medicine, State University of New York, Upstate Medical University, Syracuse, NY.)*

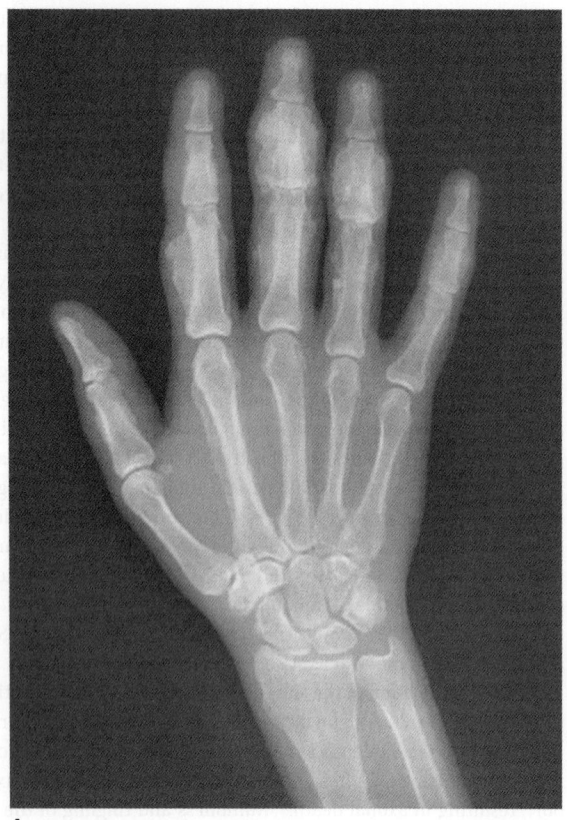

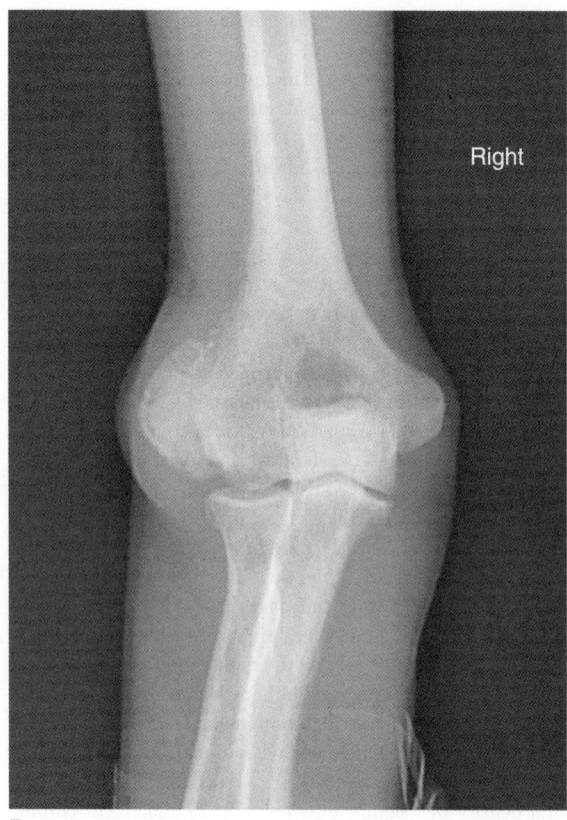

A   **B**

FIGURE 81–2. Radiograph of the hand (**A**) and elbow (**B**) with skeletal fluorosis. *(Used with permission from William Eggleston, PharmD, Department of Emergency Medicine, State University of New York, Upstate Medical University, Syracuse, NY.)*

Reports of polyneuropathy associated with chronic gasoline inhalation date to the 1960s and describe a symmetric, progressive, sensorimotor neuropathy with occasional superimposed mononeuropathies.[33,88] Initially, these deficits were attributed to the presence of tetraethyl lead as an "antiknocking" agent in gasoline, but cases after use of unleaded gasoline are also reported.[33,144] *n*-Hexane is present in gasoline in concentrations up to 3% and is thought to be the likely mediator of gasoline neuropathy.[179]

Teratogenicity

Fetal solvent syndrome (FSS) was first reported in 1979.[167] The authors described a 20-year-old primigravida with a 14-year history of solvent use defined as "daily" and "heavy" who gave birth to an infant exhibiting facial dysmorphia, growth retardation, and microcephaly, a constellation of findings that resembles fetal alcohol syndrome (FAS). A number of cases and case series were subsequently reported.[5,78,142,182] A general limitation of these case series is their reliance on self-reporting of substance use. In a number of cases included for analysis of teratogenic effects, mothers admit to use during pregnancy of other potential teratogens, including ethanol, cocaine, heroin, and phenobarbital.[5,182] Cases purported to represent inhalant use in the absence of other drug use, particularly ethanol, are not verified by laboratory testing. A small study of infants born to mothers with a self-reported history of chronic solvent use found 16% had major anomalies, 12.5% had facial features resembling FAS, and 3.6% had cleft palate.[142] Craniofacial abnormalities common to both FAS and FSS include small palpebral fissures, a thin upper lip, and midfacial hypoplasia. Features of FSS that distinguish it from FAS include micrognathia, low-set ears, abnormal scalp hair pattern, large anterior fontanelle, and downturned corners of the mouth.[167] Hypoplasia of the philtrum and nose are more characteristic of FAS.[131] Compared with matched control participants, infants born to mothers who report inhalant use are more likely to be premature, have low birth weight, have smaller birth length, and have small head circumference.[5,182] Follow-up studies of these infants

show developmental delay compared with children matched for age, race, sex, and socioeconomic status.[5,78] A rat model of toluene use embryopathy found a significant reduction in the number of neurons within each cortical layer, as well as abnormal neural migration.[69] In animal models of inhalant use, exposure to brief, repeated, high concentrations of toluene significantly increases rates of low birth weight, growth restriction, minor malformations, and impaired motor development as well as changes in regulation of metabolism, body composition, food intake, and weight gain.[25,81,85] In another rat model of maternal inhalant use, toluene concentrations in fetal brain tissue, the placenta, and amniotic fluid increased in a concentration-dependent manner.[27]

Withdrawal

Observed similarities in the acute effects of inhalants compared with other CNS depressants suggest similar patterns of tolerance and withdrawal. Rodent models of inhalant use with toluene and TCE show evidence of physical dependence that manifests as an increase in handling-induced seizures on cessation of inhalation.[55,181] Additionally, these studies demonstrate cross-tolerance of the benzodiazepine diazepam with the motor-stimulating effects of TCE and, to a lesser degree, with toluene. Inhalant users describe tolerance with weekly use in as little as 3 months.[71] Withdrawal symptoms, including irritability, both hypersomnia and insomnia, fatigue, craving, nausea, tremor, and dry mouth lasting 2 to 5 days after last use, are described.[133,146]

Volatile Alkyl Nitrites

Methemoglobinemia caused by inhalation of amyl, butyl, and isobutyl nitrites is well reported.[29,106] Nitrites are strong oxidants that induce hemoglobin oxidation from the ferrous (Fe^{2+}) to the ferric (Fe^{3+}) state. Patients with methemoglobinemia present with signs and symptoms that include shortness of breath, cyanosis, tachycardia, and tachypnea (Chap. 124). "Poppers retinopathy" characterized by eye pain; transient increased intraocular pressure; and central, bilateral visual loss is reported after use of alkyl nitrites. Optical coherence tomography, the preferred diagnostic modality, demonstrates disruption of the inner and outer segment layers of the fovea.[105,129,173]

Nitrous Oxide

Reported deaths associated with use of N_2O appear to be caused by secondary effects of N_2O, including asphyxiation and motor vehicle collisions while under the influence, and not a direct toxic effect.[161,175] Investigations after deaths associated with N_2O have found many of the dead were discovered with plastic bags over their heads in an apparent attempt to both prolong the duration of effect and increase the concentration of the inhalant.[175] Autopsy findings in these cases are consistent with asphyxiation, including ARDS, cardiac petechiae, and generalized visceral congestion.[161,175] Laboratory simulation of a reported death in which the victim was found with a plastic bag over his head with a belt fastened loosely around his neck and a spent whipped cream canister within the plastic bag showed that N_2O displaces oxygen in a closed space.[175] Additionally, N_2O concentrations in this simulation were greater than 60%; at concentrations of N_2O greater than 50%, the normal hypoxic response is diminished.[175] The combined effects of displaced oxygen and a blunted hypoxic drive likely increase the risk of asphyxia.

Chronic use of N_2O is associated with neurologic toxicity mediated via irreversible oxidation of the cobalt ion of cyanocobalamin (vitamin B_{12}). Oxidation blocks formation of methylcobalamin, a coenzyme in the production of methionine and S-adenosylmethionine, required for methylation of the phospholipids of the myelin sheaths. Additionally, cobalamin oxidation inhibits the conversion of methylmalonyl to succinyl coenzyme A. The resultant accumulation of methylmalonate and propionate results in synthesis of abnormal fatty acids and their subsequent incorporation into the myelin sheath (Chap. 65).[132] Case reports and small case series in humans after self-reported chronic, heavy use of N_2O found development of a myeloneuropathy resembling the subacute combined degeneration of the dorsal columns of the spinal cord of classic vitamin B_{12} deficiency.[20,99,174] Presenting signs and symptoms reflect varying involvement of the posterior columns, the corticospinal tracts, and the peripheral nerves. Numbness and tingling of the distal extremities is the most common presenting complaint. Physical examination reveals diminished sensation to pinprick and light touch, vibratory sensation and proprioception, gait disturbances, the Lhermitte sign (electric shock sensation from the back into the limbs with neck flexion), hyperreflexia, spasticity, urinary and fecal incontinence, and extensor plantar response.[34,132] Among reported patients with N_2O-associated neurotoxicity who had documented concentrations of vitamin B_{12}, approximately 50% were low.[4,20,52,99,145,155,174] Results were normal in the few patients who underwent a Schilling test, which evaluates the capacity to absorb vitamin B_{12} from the bowel using radiolabeled vitamin B_{12}.[99,174] Elevated concentrations of methylmalonic acid and homocysteine are often reported, even when vitamin B_{12} concentrations are normal.[4,52,145] Magnetic resonance imaging of the spinal cord may reveal symmetric enhancement and edema of the dorsal columns, referred to as the inverted V-sign (Fig. 65–3).[52,153] Nerve conduction studies and electromyography typically reveal a distal, axonal sensorimotor polyneuropathy.[34,99,174]

LABORATORY AND DIAGNOSTIC TESTING

Routine urine toxicology screens do not detect inhalants or their metabolites. Most volatile inhalants can be detected using gas chromatography as well as nuclear magnetic resonance spectroscopy (MRS). The likelihood of detection is limited by the dose, time to sampling, and method of specimen storage. Blood is the preferred specimen, but urinalysis for metabolites, including hippuric acid (the toluene metabolite) and methyl hippuric acid (the xylene metabolite), extend the time until the limit of detection is reached.[30,98] Furthermore, urinary hippuric acid is not specific for toluene exposure; the ratio of urine hippuric acid to urine creatinine must be considered. Specimens should be stored at a temperature between 23°F (−5°C) and 39.2°F (4°C).[30] Testing is not readily available at most institutions, and the need to send the specimen to a reference laboratory limits

TABLE 81–3	Inhalants With Unique Clinical Manifestations
Inhalant	**Clinical Manifestations**
Toluene	Hypokalemia Hepatotoxicity Leukoencephalopathy (chronic)
Difluoroethane, tetrafluoroethane	Frostbite Skeletal fluorosis (chronic)
1,1,1-Trichloroethane, trichloroethylene	Hepatotoxicity
Methylene chloride	Carbon monoxide poisoning
Carburetor cleaner	Methanol poisoning
n-Hexane	Peripheral neuropathy (chronic)
Alkyl nitrites (amyl, butyl, isobutyl)	Methemoglobinemia Vision loss
Nitrous oxide	Myeloneuropathy (chronic) Megaloblastic anemia (chronic) Skin hyperpigmentation (chronic)

the clinical utility in most situations. A thorough history and physical examination and careful questioning of the patient's friends and family are probably more helpful in cases of suspected inhalant use.

Depending on the patient's signs and symptoms, additional diagnostic testing is recommended, including an ECG, radiograph, electrolytes, liver enzymes, carboxyhemoglobin and blood pH. Inhalation of some xenobiotics presents unique diagnostic considerations (Table 81–3 and Fig. 81–2). Routine laboratory testing, including cerebrospinal fluid analysis, is unremarkable in patients with inhalant-induced leukoencephalopathy. A computed tomography (CT) scan of the head is generally normal until late in the disease, when diffuse hypodensity of white matter becomes evident. T2-weighted MRI with its superior resolution of white matter is the diagnostic study of choice. Standard MRI does not detect initial changes caused by toluene leukoencephalopathy; measurement of N-acetyl aspartate (NAA), a marker of CNS axons, with MRS assists with earlier detection. A decrease in NAA concentration, usually expressed as the ratio of NAA to creatinine (NAA:Cr), is suggested as a marker of axonal damage.[57] It is not currently routine or definitively valuable.

MANAGEMENT

Management begins with assessment and stabilization of the patient's airway, breathing, and circulation (the "ABCs"). The patient should be attached to a pulse oximeter and cardiac monitor. Oxygen should be administered if indicated. Early consultation with a regional poison control center or medical toxicologist is recommended to assist with identification of the xenobiotic and patient management.

Cardiac dysrhythmias associated with inhalant use carry a poor prognosis. Sudden death after use is not limited to novices, and there appears to be no premonitory signal.[13,68] Dysrhythmias, including ventricular fibrillation have been observed in the ED after witnessed exposures suggesting an ill-defined period of observation on cardiac monitor is warranted after initial exposure to inhalant. An evaluation for life-threatening electrolyte abnormalities is indicated and rapid correction is recommended in the patients presenting with dysrhythmias. Patients with nonperfusing rhythms should be managed after standard management with defibrillation. There are no evidence-based treatment guidelines for the management of inhalant-induced cardiac dysrhythmias, but β-adrenergic antagonists are thought to offer some cardioprotective effects to the sensitized myocardium.[124] Treatment with either propranolol or esmolol would be reasonable choices in managing ventricular dysrhythmias after inhalant use.[66,119]

Other complications, including methemoglobinemia, elevated carboxyhemoglobin, and methanol toxicity, should be managed with the appropriate antidotal therapy when present. Patients with respiratory symptoms that persist beyond the initial complaints of gagging and choking should be evaluated for hydrocarbon pneumonitis and treated supportively (Chap. 105).

With abstinence, cognitive and neuroimaging changes associated with toluene-induced leukoencephalopathy are initially partially reversible; beyond a poorly defined period, these changes are irreversible.[47,57] Cessation of use is the most important therapeutic intervention in patients with n-hexane–induced neuropathy and N_2O-induced myeloneuropathy; limited evidence supports the co-administration of vitamin B_{12} (1,000 mcg intramuscularly) and methionine (1 g orally) and 30 mg IV folinic acid in cases of N_2O induced myeloneuropathy and is a reasonable therapeutic intervention.[34,145,155]

Agitation, either from acute effects of the inhalant or from withdrawal, is safely managed with a benzodiazepine. In the vast majority of patients, symptoms resolve quickly, and hospitalization is not required. The potential toxicity of inhalants should be reinforced, and patients should be referred for counseling. Subsets of users, meeting the criteria for inhalant dependence and inhalant-induced psychosis, require inpatient psychiatric care. Pharmacotherapy with carbamazepine or the antipsychotics haloperidol, risperidone, and aripiprazole are reasonable for some patients with an inhalant-induced psychotic disorder.[53,77,116] Case reports suggest treating patients with inhalant dependence with lamotrigine, which inhibits excitatory glutamatergic tone, or with buspirone, an atypical anxiolytic.[125,150] There are limited data, suggesting that patients with inhalant withdrawal can be treated with baclofen in either single or divided doses of up to 50 mg/day.[86,122] Drug use treatment programs for inhalant use are scarce, and few providers have special training in this area.[15] Unfortunately there is limited evidence to support these therapeutic interventions and our standard approaches to psychosis will typically be the initial strategies.

SUMMARY

- Inhalants are a heterogeneous group of xenobiotics that include volatile hydrocarbons, the alkyl nitrites, and N_2O.
- The incidence of inhalant use is greatest among adolescents.
- The CNS is the intended target for the inhalant users; early effects include euphoria, hallucinations, headache, and dizziness.
- Chronic neurotoxicity, described best with toluene leukoencephalopathy, is characterized by dementia and ataxia.
- Muscle weakness, even paralysis, secondary to marked hypokalemia occurs with toluene use.
- Acute cardiotoxicity is manifested most dramatically in "sudden sniffing death."
- Diagnosis is largely clinical; further diagnostic testing should be guided by the patient's presenting complaint.
- Management begins with basic life support, and care is generally supportive.
- Cessation of use is the only known treatment for many manifestations of chronic toxicity.

REFERENCES

1. Al-Hajri Z, Del Bigio MR. Brain damage in a large cohort of solvent abusers. *Acta Neuropathol*. 2010;119:435-445.
2. Albright JT, et al. Upper aerodigestive tract frostbite complicating volatile substance abuse. *Int J Pediatr Otorhinolaryngol*. 1999;49:63-67.
3. Alper AT, et al. Glue (toluene) abuse: increased QT dispersion and relation with unexplained syncope. *Inhal Toxicol*. 2008;20:37-41.
4. Alt RS, et al. Severe myeloneuropathy from acute high-dose nitrous oxide (N2O) abuse. *J Emerg Med*. 2011;41:378-380.
5. Arnold GL, et al. Toluene embryopathy: clinical delineation and developmental follow-up. *Pediatrics*. 1994;93:216-220.
6. Atay AA, et al. Bone mass toxicity associated with inhalation exposure to toluene. *Biol Trace Elem Res*. 2005;105:197-203.
7. Avella J, et al. Uptake and distribution of the abused inhalant 1,1-difluoroethane in the rat. *J Anal Toxicol*. 2010;34:381-388.
8. Avella J, et al. Fatal cardiac arrhythmia after repeated exposure to 1,1-difluoroethane (DFE). *Am J Forensic Med Pathol*. 2006;27:58-60.
9. Baerg RD, Kimberg DV. Centrilobular hepatic necrosis and acute renal failure in "solvent sniffers." *Ann Intern Med*. 1970;73:713-720.
10. Bale AS, et al. Alterations in glutamatergic and gabaergic ion channel activity in hippocampal neurons following exposure to the abused inhalant toluene. *Neuroscience*. 2005;130:197-206.
11. Balster RL. Neural basis of inhalant abuse. *Drug Alcohol Depend*. 1998;51:207-214.
12. Baselt RC. *Biological Monitoring Methods for Industrial Chemicals*. Davis, CA: Biomedical Publications; 1982.
13. Bass M. Sudden sniffing death. *JAMA*. 1970;212:2075-2079.
14. Batis JC, et al. Differential effects of inhaled toluene on locomotor activity in adolescent and adult rats. *Pharmacol Biochem Behav*. 2010;96:438-448.
15. Beauvais F, et al. A survey of attitudes among drug user treatment providers toward the treatment of inhalant users. *Subst Use Misuse*. 2002;37:1391-1410.
16. Beckstead MJ, et al. Antagonism of inhalant and volatile anesthetic enhancement of glycine receptor function. *J Biol Chem*. 2001;276:24959-24964.
17. Beckstead MJ, et al. Glycine and gamma-aminobutyric acid(A) receptor function is enhanced by inhaled drugs of abuse. *Mol Pharmacol*. 2000;57:1199-1205.
18. Beirne GJ, Brennan JT. Glomerulonephritis associated with hydrocarbon solvents: mediated by antiglomerular basement membrane antibody. *Arch Environ Health*. 1972;25:365-369.
19. Berkowitz BA, et al. Nitrous oxide "analgesia": resemblance to opiate action. *Science*. 1976;194:967-968.
20. Blanco G, Peters HA. Myeloneuropathy and macrocytosis associated with nitrous oxide abuse. *Arch Neurol*. 1983;40:416-418.
21. Bolt HM, et al. The cytochrome P-450 isoenzyme CYP2E1 in the biological processing of industrial chemicals: consequences for occupational and environmental medicine. *Int Arch Occup Environ Health*. 2003;76:174-185.
22. Botto F, et al. Tissue-specific expression and methylation of the human CYP2E1 gene. *Biochem Pharmacol*. 1994;48:1095-1103.
23. Bowen SE, Balster RL. A comparison of the acute behavioral effects of inhaled amyl, ethyl, and butyl acetate in mice. *Fundam Appl Toxicol*. 1997;35:189-196.
24. Bowen SE, Balster RL. A direct comparison of inhalant effects on locomotor activity and schedule-controlled behavior in mice. *Exp Clin Psychopharmacol*. 1998;6:235-247.
25. Bowen SE, et al. Abuse pattern of gestational toluene exposure and early postnatal development in rats. *Neurotoxicol Teratol*. 2005;27:105-116.
26. Bowen SE, et al. Decreased sensitivity in adolescent vs. adult rats to the locomotor activating effects of toluene. *Neurotoxicol Teratol*. 2007;29:599-606.
27. Bowen SE, et al. Maternal and fetal blood and organ toluene levels in rats following acute and repeated binge inhalation exposure. *Reprod Toxicol*. 2007;24:343-352.
28. Bowen SE, et al. The effects of abused inhalants on mouse behavior in an elevated plus-maze. *Eur J Pharmacol*. 1996;312:131-136.
29. Bradberry SM, et al. Fatal methemoglobinemia due to inhalation of isobutyl nitrite. *J Toxicol Clin Toxicol*. 1994;32:179-184.
30. Broussard LA. The role of the laboratory in detecting inhalant abuse. *Clin Lab Sci*. 2000;13:205-209.
31. Brown C, Budhram G. Evaluation of left ventricular function by bedside ultrasound in acute toxic myocarditis. *J Emerg Med*. 2013;45:588-591.
32. Bruckner JV, Peterson RG. Evaluation of toluene and acetone inhalant abuse. I. Pharmacology and pharmacodynamics. *Toxicol Appl Pharmacol*. 1981;61:27-38.
33. Burns TM, et al. Gasoline sniffing multifocal neuropathy. *Pediatr Neurol*. 2001;25:419-421.
34. Butzkueven H, King JO. Nitrous oxide myelopathy in an abuser of whipped cream bulbs. *J Clin Neurosci*. 2000;7:73-75.
35. Byard RW, et al. Unusual facial markings and lethal mechanisms in a series of gasoline inhalation deaths. *Am J Forensic Med Pathol*. 2003;24:298-302.
36. Camara-Lemarroy CR, et al. Acute toluene intoxication—clinical presentation, management and prognosis: a prospective observational study. *BMC Emerg Med*. 2015;15:19.
37. Carlisle EJ, et al. Glue-sniffing and distal renal tubular acidosis: sticking to the facts. *J Am Soc Nephrol*. 1991;1:1019-1027.
38. Cates AL, Cook MD. Severe cardiomyopathy after huffing dust-off. *Case Rep Emerg Med*. 2016;2016:9204790.
39. Cayir D, et al. Evaluation of lung epithelial permeability in the volatile substance abuse using Tc-99m DTPA aerosol scintigraphy. *Ann Nucl Med*. 2011;25:554-559.
40. Cha HJ, et al. Neurotoxicity induced by alkyl nitrites: impairment in learning/memory and motor coordination. *Neurosci Lett*. 2016;619:79-85.
41. Chang AP, et al. Focal conduction block in n-hexane polyneuropathy. *Muscle Nerve*. 1998;21:964-969.
42. Chitkara M, et al. Multiple painless masses: periostitis deformans secondary to fluoride intoxication. *Skeletal Radiol*. 2014;43:529-530, 555-556.
43. Clinger OW, Johnson NA. Purposeful inhalation of gasoline vapors. *Psychiatr Q*. 1951;25:557-567.
44. Cruz SL, et al. Effects of the abused solvent toluene on recombinant N-methyl-D-aspartate and non-N-methyl-D-aspartate receptors expressed in Xenopus oocytes. *J Pharmacol. Exp. Ther*. 1998;286:334-340.
45. Cruz SL, et al. Inhibition of cardiac sodium currents by toluene exposure. *Br J Pharmacol*. 2003;140:653-660.

46. Del Re AM, et al. Effects of the abused inhalant toluene on ethanol-sensitive potassium channels expressed in oocytes. *Brain Res.* 2006;1087:75-82.

47. Dingwall KM, et al. Cognitive recovery during and after treatment for volatile solvent abuse. *Drug Alcohol Depend.* 2011;118:180-185.

48. Dinsfriend W, Rao K, Matulevicius S. Inhalant-abuse myocarditis diagnosed by cardiac magnetic resonance. *Tex Heart Ins. J.* 2016;43:246-248.

49. DiVincenzo GD, et al. Characterization of the metabolites of methyl n-butyl ketone, methyl iso-butyl ketone, and methyl ethyl ketone in guinea pig serum and their clearance. *Toxicol Appl Pharmacol.* 1976;36:511-522.

50. Dundaroz MR, et al. Evaluation of bone mineral density in chronic glue sniffers. *Turk J Pediatr.* 2002;44:326-329.

51. Dundarz MR, et al. Antioxidant enzymes and lipid peroxidation in adolescents with inhalant abuse. *Turk J Pediatr.* 2003;45:43-45.

52. Duque MA, et al. Nitrous oxide abuse and vitamin B12 Action in a 20-year-old woman: a case report. *Lab Med.* 2015;46:312-315.

53. Erdogan A, Yurteri N. Aripiprazole treatment in the adolescent patients with inhalant use disorders and conduct disorder: a retrospective case analysis. *Yeni Sympos.* 2010;48:229-233.

54. Evans EB, Balster RL. CNS depressant effects of volatile organic solvents. *Neurosci Biobehav Rev.* 1991;15:233-241.

55. Evans EB, Balster RL. Inhaled 1,1,1-trichloroethane-produced physical dependence in mice: effects of drugs and vapors on withdrawal. *J Pharmacol Exp Ther.* 1993;264:726-733.

56. Filley CM. Toluene abuse and white matter: a model of toxic leukoencephalopathy. *Psychiatr Clin North Am.* 2013;36:293-302.

57. Filley CM, et al. The effects of toluene on the central nervous system. *J Neuropathol Exp Neurol.* 2004;63:1-12.

58. Flowers NC, Horan LG. Nonanoxic aerosol arrhythmias. *JAMA.* 1972;219:33-37.

59. Frenia ML, Schauben JL. Methanol inhalation toxicity. *Ann Emerg Med.* 1993;22:1919-1923.

60. Fukagawa H, et al. kappa-Opioid receptor mediates the antinociceptive effect of nitrous oxide in mice. *Br J Anaesth.* 2014;113:1032-1038.

61. Furlong TM, et al. Toluene inhalation in adolescent rats reduces flexible behaviour in adulthood and alters glutamatergic and GABAergic signalling. *J Neurochem.* 2016.

62. Garriott J, Petty CS. Death from inhalant abuse: toxicological and pathological evaluation of 34 cases. *Clin Toxicol.* 1980;16:305-315.

63. Gauthereau MY, et al. A mutation in the local anaesthetic binding site abolishes toluene effects in sodium channels. *Eur J Pharmacol.* 2005;528:17-26.

64. Gerasimov MR, et al. Synthesis and evaluation of inhaled [11C]butane and intravenously injected [11C]acetone as potential radiotracers for studying inhalant abuse. *Nucl Med Biol.* 2005;32:201-208.

65. Gerasimov MR, et al. Toluene inhalation produces regionally specific changes in extracellular dopamine. *Drug Alcohol Depend.* 2002;65:243-251.

66. Gindre G, et al. [Late ventricular fibrillation after trichloroethylene poisoning]. *Ann Fr Anesth Reanim.* 1997;16:202-203.

67. Gompertz D. Solvents—the relationship between biological monitoring strategies and metabolic handling. A review. *Ann Occup Hyg.* 1980;23:405-410.

68. Goodheart RS, Dunne JW. Petrol sniffer's encephalopathy. A study of 25 patients. *Med J Aust.* 1994;160:178-181.

69. Gospe SM Jr, Zhou SS. Prenatal exposure to toluene results in abnormal neurogenesis and migration in rat somatosensory cortex. *Pediatr Res.* 2000;47:362-368.

70. Greenberg MM. The central nervous system and exposure to toluene: a risk characterization. *Environ Res.* 1997;72:1-7.

71. Grosse K, Grosse J. [Propane abuse. Extreme dose increase due to development of tolerance]. *Nervenarzt.* 2000;71:50-53.

72. Gunn J, et al. Butane sniffing causing ventricular fibrillation. *Lancet.* 1989;1:617.

73. Gupta SR, et al. Toluene optic neurotoxicity: magnetic resonance imaging and pathologic features. *Hum Pathol.* 2011;42:295-298.

74. Hanson H, et al. Acute systemic skeletal fluorosis confirmed with radiography and urine fluoride concentration in the setting of 1/1-difluoroethane abuse. *Clin Toxicol (Phila).* 2016;54.

75. Harris JW, Anders MW. Metabolism of the hydrochlorofluorocarbon 1,2-dichloro-1,1-difluoroethane. *Chem Res Toxicol.* 1991;4:180-186.

76. Herbst J, et al. Role of P4502E1 in the metabolism of 1,1,2,2-tetrafluoro-1-(2,2,2-trifluoroethoxy)-ethane. *Xenobiotica.* 1994;24:507-516.

77. Hernandez-Avila CA, et al. Treatment of inhalant-induced psychotic disorder with carbamazepine versus haloperidol. *Psychiatr Serv.* 1998;49:812-815.

78. Hersh JH, et al. Toluene embryopathy. *J Pediatr.* 1985;106:922-927.

79. Hutchens KS, Kung M. "Experimentation" with chloroform. *Am J Med.* 1985;78:715-718.

80. Ikeuchi Y, et al. Excitatory and inhibitory effects of toluene on neural activity in guinea pig hippocampal slices. *Neurosci Lett.* 1993;158:63-66.

81. Jarosz PA, et al. Effects of abuse pattern of gestational toluene exposure on metabolism, feeding and body composition. *Physiol Behav.* 2008;93:984-993.

82. Jenner P. Oxidative mechanisms in nigral cell death in Parkinson's disease. *Mov Disord.* 1998;13(suppl 1):24-34.

83. Jeon SY, et al. Abuse potential and dopaminergic effect of alkyl nitrites. *Neurosci Lett.* 2016;629:68-72.

84. Jevtovic-Todorovic V, et al. Nitrous oxide (laughing gas) is an NMDA antagonist, neuroprotectant and neurotoxin. *Nat Med.* 1998;4:460-463.

85. Jones HE, Balster RL. Neurobehavioral consequences of intermittent prenatal exposure to high concentrations of toluene. *Neurotoxicol Teratol.* 1997;19:305-313.

86. Kandasamy A, et al. Baclofen as an anti-craving agent for adolescent inhalant dependence syndrome. *Drug Alcohol Rev.* 2015;34:696-697.

87. Kaplan HG, et al. Hepatitis caused by halothane sniffing. *Ann Intern Med.* 1979;90:797-798.

88. Karani V. Peripheral neuritis after addiction to petrol. *Br Med J.* 1966;1:216.

89. Karuri AR, et al. Alterations in catecholamine turnover in specific regions of the rat brain following acute exposure to nitrous oxide. *Brain Res Bull.* 1998;45:557-561.

90. Kelly KJ, Ruffing R. Acute eosinophilic pneumonia following intentional inhalation of Scotchguard. *Ann Allergy.* 1993;71:358-361.

91. Kielbasa W, Fung HL. Pharmacokinetics of a model organic nitrite inhalant and its alcohol metabolite in rats. *Drug Metab Dispos.* 2000;28:386-391.

92. Kielbasa W, Fung HL. Relationship between pharmacokinetics and hemodynamic effects of inhaled isobutyl nitrite in conscious rats. *AAPS PharmSci.* 2000;2:E11.

93. Koehler MM, Henninger CA. Orofacial and digital frostbite caused by inhalant abuse. *Cutis.* 2014;93:256-260.

94. Kornfeld M, et al. Solvent vapor abuse leukoencephalopathy. Comparison to adrenoleukodystrophy. *J Neuropathol Exp Neurol.* 1994;53:389-398.

95. Kurbat RS, Pollack CV Jr. Facial injury and airway threat from inhalant abuse: a case report. *J Emerg Med.* 1998;16:167-169.

96. Kurniali PC, et al. Inhalant abuse of computer cleaner manifested as angioedema. *Am J Emerg Med.* 2012;30:265 e263-265.

97. Kuspis DA, Krenzelok EP. Oral frostbite injury from intentional abuse of a fluorinated hydrocarbon. *J Toxicol Clin Toxicol.* 1999;37:873-875.

98. Lavon O, Bentur Y. Acute inhaled xylene poisoning confirmed by methyl hippuric acid urine test. *J Toxicol Clin Toxicol.* 2012;50:354.

99. Layzer RB. Myeloneuropathy after prolonged exposure to nitrous oxide. *Lancet.* 1978;2:1227-1230.

100. Lee DE, et al. The effects of inhaled acetone on place conditioning in adolescent rats. *Pharmacol Biochem Behav.* 2008;89:101-105.

101. Lim CS, et al. Fatality after inhalation of methanol-containing paint stripper. *Clin Toxicol (Phila).* 2015;53:411.

102. Litt IF, Cohen MI. "Danger—vapor harmful": spot-remover sniffing. *N Engl J Med.* 1969;281:543-544.

103. LoVecchio F, Fulton SE. Ventricular fibrillation following inhalation of Glade Air Freshener. *Eur J Emerg Med.* 2001;8:153-154.

104. LoVecchio F, et al. Outcomes following abuse of methanol-containing carburetor cleaners. *Hum Exp Toxicol.* 2004;23:473-475.

105. Luis J, et al. Poppers retinopathy. *BMJ Case Rep.* 2016;2016.

106. Machabert R, et al. Methaemoglobinaemia due to amyl nitrite inhalation: a case report. *Hum Exp Toxicol.* 1994;13:313-314.

107. MacIver MB. Abused inhalants enhance GABA-mediated synaptic inhibition. *Neuropsychopharmacology.* 2009;34:2296-2304.

108. Maickel RP. The fate and toxicity of butyl nitrites. *NIDA Res Monogr.* 1988;83:15-27.

109. Marjot R, McLeod AA. Chronic non-neurological toxicity from volatile substance abuse. *Hum Toxicol.* 1989;8:301-306.

110. Mattia CJ, et al. Effects of toluene and its metabolites on cerebral reactive oxygen species generation. *Biochem Pharmacol.* 1991;42:879-882.

111. McCormick MJ, et al. Methanol poisoning as a result of inhalational solvent abuse. *Ann Emerg Med.* 1990;19:639-642.

112. McFee R, et al. "Dusting"—a new inhalant of abuse: office products containing difluoroethane. *J Toxicol Clin Toxicol.* 2007;45:632.

113. McGarvey EL, et al. Adolescent inhalant abuse: environments of use. *Am J Drug Alcohol Abuse.* 1999;25:731-741.

114. Mee AS, Wright PL. Congestive (dilated) cardiomyopathy in association with solvent abuse. *J R Soc Med.* 1980;73:671-672.

115. Meredith TJ, et al. Diagnosis and treatment of acute poisoning with volatile substances. *Hum Toxicol.* 1989;8:277-286.

116. Misra LK, et al. Treatment of inhalant abuse with risperidone. *J Clin Psychiatry.* 1999;60:620.

117. Monitoring the Future. https://www.drugabuse.gov/related-topics/trends-statistics/infographics/monitoring-future-2015-survey-results.

118. Moreno C, Beierle EA. Hydrofluoric acid burn in a child from a compressed air duster. *J Burn Care Res.* 2007;28:909-912.

119. Mortiz F, et al. Esmolol in the treatment of severe arrhythmia after acute trichloroethylene poisoning. *Intensive Care Med.* 2000;26:256.

120. Moser VC, Balster RL. Acute motor and lethal effects of inhaled toluene, 1,1,1-trichloroethane, halothane, and ethanol in mice: effects of exposure duration. *Toxicol Appl Pharmacol.* 1985;77:285-291.

121. Murakawa M, et al. Activation of the cortical and medullary dopaminergic systems by nitrous oxide in rats: a possible neurochemical basis for psychotropic effects and postanesthetic nausea and vomiting. *Anesth Analg.* 1994;78:376-381.

122. Muralidharan K, et al. Baclofen in the management of inhalant withdrawal: a case series. *Prim Care Companion J Clin Psychiatry.* 2008;10:48-51.

123. Nathan AW, Toseland PA. Goodpasture's syndrome and trichloroethane intoxication. *Br J Clin Pharmacol.* 1979;8:284-286.

124. Nelson LS. Toxicologic myocardial sensitization. *J Toxicol Clin Toxicol*. 2002;40: 867-879.

125. Niederhofer H. Treating inhalant abuse with buspirone. *Am J Addict*. 2007;16:69.

126. Nimitvilai S, et al. Differential effects of toluene and ethanol on dopaminergic neurons of the ventral tegmental area. *Front Neurosci*. 2016;10:434.

127. O'Leary-Moore SK, et al. Neurochemical changes after acute binge toluene inhalation in adolescent and adult rats: a high-resolution magnetic resonance spectroscopy study. *Neurotoxicol Teratol*. 2009;31:382-389.

128. Ossiander EM. Volatile substance misuse deaths in Washington State, 2003-2012. *Am J Drug Alcohol Abuse*. 2015;41:30-34.

129. Pahlitzsch M, et al. Poppers maculopathy: complete restitution of macular changes in OCT after drug abstinence. *Semin Ophthalmol*. 2016;31:479-484.

130. Pascual R, et al. Solvent inhalation (toluene and n-hexane) during the brain growth spurt impairs the maturation of frontal, parietal and occipital cerebrocortical neurons in rats. *J Dev Neurosci*. 2010;28:491-495.

131. Pearson MA, et al. Toluene embryopathy: delineation of the phenotype and comparison with fetal alcohol syndrome. *Pediatrics*. 1994;93:211-215.

132. Pema PJ, et al. Myelopathy caused by nitrous oxide toxicity. *AJNR Am J Neuroradiol*. 1998;19:894-896.

133. Perron BE, et al. The prevalence and clinical significance of inhalant withdrawal symptoms among a national sample. *Subst Abuse Rehabil*. 2011;2011:69-76.

134. Perron BE, Howard MO. Perceived risk of harm and intentions of future inhalant use among adolescent inhalant users. *Drug Alcohol Depend*. 2008;97:185-189.

135. Plumb J, Thomas RG. Sudden severe perioral swelling in an adolescent boy. *J Toxicol Clin Toxicol*. 2013;51:379-380.

136. Raines DE, et al. The N-methyl-D-aspartate receptor inhibitory potencies of aromatic inhaled drugs of abuse: evidence for modulation by cation-pi interactions. *J Pharmacol. Exp. Ther*. 2004;311:14-21.

137. Reynolds ES, et al. Metabolism of [14C]carbon tetrachloride to exhaled, excreted and bound metabolites. Dose-response, time-course and pharmacokinetics. *Biochem Pharmacol*. 1984;33:3363-3374.

138. Richardson KJ, Shelton KL. N-methyl-D-aspartate receptor channel blocker-like discriminative stimulus effects of nitrous oxide gas. *J Pharmacol Exp Ther*. 2015; 352:156-165.

139. Riegel AC, et al. Repeated exposure to the abused inhalant toluene alters levels of neurotransmitters and generates peroxynitrite in nigrostriatal and mesolimbic nuclei in rat. *Ann N Y Acad Sci*. 2004;1025:543-551.

140. Riegel AC, et al. The abused inhalant toluene increases dopamine release in the nucleus accumbens by directly stimulating ventral tegmental area neurons. *Neuropsychopharmacology*. 2007;32:1558-1569.

141. Rosenberg NL, et al. Toluene abuse causes diffuse central nervous system white matter changes. *Ann Neurol*. 1988;23:611-614.

142. Scheeres JJ, Chudley AE. Solvent abuse in pregnancy: a perinatal perspective. *J Obstet Gynaecol Can*. 2002;24:22-26.

143. Seaman ME. Barotrauma related to inhalational drug abuse. *J Emerg Med*. 1990;8:141-149.

144. Seshia SS, et al. The neurological manifestations of chronic inhalation of leaded gasoline. *Dev Med Child Neurol*. 1978;20:323-334.

145. Sethi NK, et al. Nitrous oxide "whippit" abuse presenting with cobalamin responsive psychosis. *J Med Toxicol*. 2006;2:71-74.

146. Shah R, et al. Phenomenology of gasoline intoxication and withdrawal symptoms among adolescents in India: a case series. *Am J Addict*. 1999;8:254-257.

147. Shelton KL. Discriminative stimulus effects of inhaled 1,1,1-trichloroethane in mice: comparison to other hydrocarbon vapors and volatile anesthetics. *Psychopharmacology (Berl)*. 2009;203:431-440.

148. Shelton KL, Nicholson KL. Benzodiazepine-like discriminative stimulus effects of toluene vapor. *Eur J Pharmacol*. 2013;720:131-137.

149. Shelton KL, Nicholson KL. GABA(A) positive modulator and NMDA antagonist-like discriminative stimulus effects of isoflurane vapor in mice. *Psychopharmacology (Berl)*. 2010;212:559-569.

150. Shen YC. Treatment of inhalant dependence with lamotrigine. *Prog. Neuropsychopharmacol Biol Psychiatry*. 2007;31:769-771.

151. Shimada T, et al. Interindividual variations in human liver cytochrome P-450 enzymes involved in the oxidation of drugs, carcinogens and toxic chemicals: studies with liver microsomes of 30 Japanese and 30 Caucasians. *J Pharmacol Exp Ther*. 1994;270:414-423.

152. Smith RA, et al. Naloxone has no effect on nitrous oxide anesthesia. *Anesthesiology*. 1978;49:6-8.

153. Sotirchos ES, et al. Neurological picture. Nitrous oxide-induced myelopathy with inverted V-sign on spinal MRI. *J Neurol Neurosurg Psychiatry*. 2012;83:915-916.

154. Spiller HA, Krenzelok EP. Epidemiology of inhalant abuse reported to two regional poison centers. *J Toxicol Clin Toxicol*. 1997;35:167-173.

155. Stacy CB, et al. Methionine in the treatment of nitrous-oxide-induced neuropathy and myeloneuropathy. *J Neurol*. 1992;239:401-403.

156. Stengard K, O'Connor WT. Acute toluene exposure decreases extracellular gamma-aminobutyric acid in the globus pallidus but not in striatum: a microdialysis study in awake, freely moving rats. *Eur J Pharmacol*. 1994;292:43-46.

157. Streicher HZ, et al. Syndromes of toluene sniffing in adults. *Ann Intern Med*. 1981;94:758-762.

158. Sturmann K, et al. Methylene chloride inhalation: an unusual form of drug abuse. *Ann Emerg Med*. 1985;14:903-905.

159. Substance Abuse and Mental Health Services Administration. http://www.samhsa.gov/data/sites/default/files/NSDUH-DetTabs-2015/NSDUH-DetTabs-2015/NSDUH-DetTabs-2015.pdf.

160. Substance Abuse and Mental Health Services Administration. http://www.samhsa.gov/data/sites/default/files/NSDUH-FRR1-2014/NSDUH-FRR1-2014.pdf.

161. Suruda AJ, McGlothlin JD. Fatal abuse of nitrous oxide in the workplace. *J Occup Med*. 1990;32:682-684.

162. Szlatenyi CS, Wang RY. Encephalopathy and cranial nerve palsies caused by intentional trichloroethylene inhalation. *Am J Emerg Med*. 1996;14:464-466.

163. Takagi M, et al. Verbal memory, learning, and executive functioning among adolescent inhalant and cannabis users. *J Stud Alcohol Drugs*. 2011;72:96-105.

164. Takagi MJ, et al. A signal detection analysis of executive control performance among adolescent inhalant and cannabis users. *Subst Use Misuse*. 2014;49:1920-1927.

165. Taylor GJ, Harris WS. Cardiac toxicity of aerosol propellants. *JAMA*. 1970;214:81-85.

166. Tegeris JS, Balster RL. A comparison of the acute behavioral effects of alkylbenzenes using a functional observational battery in mice. *Fundam Appl Toxicol*. 1994;22:240-250.

167. Toutant C, Lippmann S. Fetal solvents syndrome. *Lancet*. 1979;1:1356.

168. Tracy ME, et al. Negative allosteric modulation of GABAA receptors inhibits facilitation of brain stimulation reward by drugs of abuse in C57BL6/J mice. *Psychopharmacology (Berl)*. 2016;233:715-725.

169. Tucci JR, et al. Skeletal fluorosis due to inhalation abuse of a difluoroethane-containing computer cleaner. *J Bone Miner Res*. 2017;32:188-195.

170. Vance C, et al. Deaths involving 1,1-difluoroethane at the San Diego County Medical Examiner's Office. *J Anal Toxicol*. 2012;36:626-633.

171. Venkataraman G. Renal damage and glue sniffing. *Br Med J (Clin Res Ed)*. 1981;283:1467.

172. Viera I SM, Cresteil T. Developmental expression of CYP2E1 in the human liver. Hypermethylation control of gene expression during the neonatal period. *Eur J Biochem*. 1996;238:476-483.

173. Vignal-Clermont C, et al. Poppers-associated retinal toxicity. *N Engl J Med*. 2010; 363:1583-1585.

174. Vishnubhakat SM, Beresford HR. Reversible myeloneuropathy of nitrous oxide abuse: serial electrophysiological studies. *Muscle Nerve*. 1991;14:22-26.

175. Wagner SA, et al. Asphyxial deaths from the recreational use of nitrous oxide. *J Forensic Sci*. 1992;37:1008-1015.

176. Wakita M, et al. Nitrous oxide directly inhibits action potential-dependent neurotransmission from single presynaptic boutons adhering to rat hippocampal CA3 neurons. *Brain Res Bull*. 2015;118:34-45.

177. Ware LB, Matthay MA. The acute respiratory distress syndrome. *N Engl J Med*. 2000;342:1334-1349.

178. Warren DA, et al. Biphasic effects of 1,1,1-trichloroethane on the locomotor activity of mice: relationship to blood and brain solvent concentrations. *Toxicol Sci*. 2000;56:365-373.

179. Weaver NK. *Gasoline*. Philadelphia, PA: Williams & Wilkins; 1992.

180. Whitt A, Garland EL, Howard MO. Helium inhalation in adolescents: characteristics of users and prevalence of use. *J Psychoactive Drugs*. 2012;44:365-371.

181. Wiley JL, et al. Evaluation of toluene dependence and cross-sensitization to diazepam. *Life Sci*. 2003;72:3023-3033.

182. Wilkins-Haug L, Gabow PA. Toluene abuse during pregnancy: obstetric complications and perinatal outcomes. *Obstet Gynecol*. 1991;77:504-509.

183. Williams DR, Cole SJ. Ventricular fibrillation following butane gas inhalation. *Resuscitation*. 1998;37:43-45.

184. Williams JM, et al. Effects of repeated inhalation of toluene on ionotropic GABA A and glutamate receptor subunit levels in rat brain. *Neurochem Int*. 2005;46:1-10.

185. Winston A, et al. Air Duster abuse causing rapid airway compromise. *BMJ Case Rep*. 2015;2015.

186. Wiseman MN, Banim S. "Glue sniffer's" heart? *Br Med J (Clin Res Ed)*. 1987;294:739.

187. Wood RW, et al. Anticonvulsant and antipunishment effects of toluene. *J Pharmacol Exp Ther*. 1984;230:407-412.

188. Woodward JJ, Beckley J. Effects of the abused inhalant toluene on the mesolimbic dopamine system. *J Drug Alcohol Res*. 2014;3.

189. Yin H, et al. Metabolism of 1,2-dichloro-1-fluoroethane and 1-fluoro-1,2,2-trichloroethane: electronic factors govern the regioselectivity of cytochrome P450-dependent oxidation. *Chem Res Toxicol*. 1996;9:50-57.

190. Yucel M, et al. White-matter abnormalities in adolescents with long-term inhalant and cannabis use: a diffusion magnetic resonance imaging study. *J Psychiatry Neurosci*. 2010;35:409-412.

191. Zacny JP, et al. The subjective, behavioral and cognitive effects of subanesthetic concentrations of isoflurane and nitrous oxide in healthy volunteers. *Psychopharmacology (Berl)*. 1994;114:409-416.

192. Zimmerman SW, et al. Hydrocarbon exposure and chronic glomerulonephritis. *Lancet*. 1975;2:199-201.

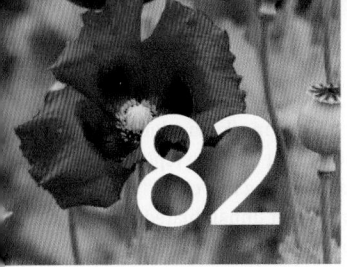

82 NICOTINE

Denise Fernández and Sari Soghoian

MW = 162 Da

Nicotine

HISTORY AND EPIDEMIOLOGY

Nicotine is the principal alkaloid derived from plants of the genus *Nicotiana*, collectively known as the tobacco plant, in the family *Solanaceae*. Other fruits and vegetables from the Solanaceae family, such as tomatoes, potatoes, eggplant, and cauliflower, also contain nicotine in amounts ranging from 3.8 to 100 ng/g.[29] The source of greatest toxicologic importance in human use is *Nicotiana tabacum*, and the primary method of exposure is cigarette smoking.

The tobacco plant is native to the Americas, and its use most likely predates the Mayan empire. In 1492, Christopher Columbus and his crew were given tobacco by the Arawaks but reportedly threw it away, not knowing any use for it. Ramon Pane, a monk who accompanied Columbus on his second voyage to America, is credited with introducing tobacco to Europe.[99]

Because of the highly addictive properties of nicotine, the global disease burden related to cigarette use today is staggering. Cigarette smoking increases rates of illnesses, such as chronic obstructive pulmonary disease (COPD), cardiovascular disease, pulmonary infections, macular degeneration, and cancers, and tobacco use causes more than 5 million deaths worldwide per year.[101] Chronic nicotine exposure causes cardiovascular damage related to catecholamine release and vasoconstriction and directly promotes angiogenesis, neuroteratogenicity, and possibly some cancers.[64] However, there are more than 3,000 components to tobacco smoke, and nicotine per se may not be the crucial determinant of the total health burden associated with its use.

Although the long-term effects of tobacco dependency are significant, this chapter is concerned with the sources, effects, and management of acute toxicity referable to nicotinic receptor stimulation and cholinergic activation. Compared with other xenobiotics, exposure to nicotine-containing products is a relatively rare cause of acute poisoning. For example, reviews of case data from the National Poison Data System (NPDS) suggest that cigarettes are by far the most common vehicle implicated in acute nicotine exposures and poisoning in the United States,[22] yet over a period of 27 years from 1983 to 2009, tobacco products accounted for 217,340 calls, or 0.37%, of all pediatric exposures reported to poison control centers in the United States[2] and accounted for only 0.7% of all unintentional poisoning cases in children treated in US hospital emergency departments.[36] More current data suggest that electronic cigarettes and liquid nicotine exposures are on the rise. In 2014, pediatric exposures to e-cigarettes and liquid nicotine accounted for approximately 59% of all calls reporting these exposures, a percentage that rose to 70% in 2015.[41] Consequential poisoning occurs, but most patients with nicotine exposure from tobacco products have a benign course, with only mild to moderate symptoms, and an infrequent need for hospitalization.

The frequency and severity of nicotine poisoning is changing with the rise of e-cigarette use, and associated increase in topical and oral exposures of more highly concentrated liquid nicotine preparations. According to NPDS data, pediatric nicotine exposure via e-cigarettes rose by more than 1,000% between 2012 and 2015.[52] During this time, cigarettes, other forms of tobacco, and e-cigarettes accounted for 60.1%, 16.4%, and 14.2% of pediatric nicotine exposure, respectively.[52] Other smoking cessation products containing nicotine or nicotinelike compounds are also increasingly available. Some of the more novel smokeless tobacco products have the appearance and flavor of candy, raising concern about the potential for unintentional poisoning of young children, in particular.[22]

Nicotine receptor partial agonists/antagonists are a relatively new class of drug mimicking the physiologic effects of nicotine. A 2-year review of poison control center data from the California Poison Control System found 36 calls regarding human exposures to varenicline which was approved in 2006 by the US Food and Drug Administration (FDA) as a smoking cessation aid.[58] Of these, 17 cases had no outcome data or involved coingestions. Nine of the remaining cases involved unintentional exposure in children younger than 6 years of age, one of whom was hospitalized; none experienced major adverse events. However, postmarketing safety reports of seizures[93] and neuropsychiatric effects, including anxiety, depression, and suicidal ideation,[100] drove the FDA to place a black box warning on varenicline in 2009.

Dermal exposure to tobacco plants during harvest remains an important source of occupational nicotine toxicity, known as green tobacco sickness (GTS). Green tobacco sickness was first reported in 1970 among tobacco workers in Florida.[105] In 1992, the US Centers for Disease Control and Prevention estimated the crude 2-month incidence rate of hospital treated GTS was 10 per 1,000 workers in a 5-county area in Kentucky.[77] Overall prevalence estimates among seasonal and migrant farmworkers are as high as 25% to 40% of workers.[3,5,88]

Insecticides containing nicotine and neonicotinoid compounds are also implicated in acute poisoning. These products and their role in human poisoning are discussed in Chap. 111 and are only briefly mentioned here. Tobacco extracts were first reported as effective for pest control in 1690, and in 1886, a mixture of tobacco and soapsuds was advocated for aphid control. The first commercial nicotine insecticides were developed in 1912. Crop dusting with nicotine sulfate began in 1917, although at the time, it was mostly accomplished by horse-drawn carriage.[84] The most widely known application of 40% nicotine sulfate, BlackLeaf 40, was discontinued in 1992. Nicotine-based insecticides are now restricted in the United States, although they are used in other countries, and a 14% preparation of nicotine is still marketed as a greenhouse smoke fumigator.[82] Because nicotine pesticides are highly concentrated, the ingestion of even small amounts produces serious toxicity, including catastrophic brain injury[90] and death.[60]

The neonicotinoids are a relatively new class of insecticide developed in the last quarter century, and epidemiologic data about their role in acute pesticide poisoning are still limited. A retrospective review of poison control center data from Thailand found no reports of neonicotinoid exposures before 1993.[86] Between 1993 and 2007 there were a total of 70 cases, including 2 deaths. The number of exposures reported annually increased dramatically after 2002, suggesting that neonicotinoid insecticides will likely continue to be an emerging cause of acute pesticide poisoning. However, in the year with the highest case incidence, these insecticides still represented fewer than 3% of all pesticide exposures reported. Neonicotinoid insecticides also carry environmental implications and are detrimental to pollinating insects such as bees.[42]

PHARMACOLOGY AND PHARMACOKINETICS

The pharmacologic characteristics of nicotine are listed in Table 82–1. Nicotine is well absorbed from the respiratory tract, mucosal surfaces, skin, and intestines. Nicotine is a weak base (pKa = 8.0) and is more readily absorbed in an alkaline environment. Many tobacco and nicotine replacement products are therefore buffered to alkaline pH to facilitate absorption.

TABLE 82–1	Pharmacology of Nicotine
Absorption	Lungs, oral mucosa, skin, intestinal tract; increased in more alkaline environments
Volume of distribution	2.6 L/kg
Protein binding	5%
Metabolism	80%–90% hepatic via CYP2A6 and CYP2D6, aldehyde oxidase, flavin monooxygenase, and by glycosylation; remainder in lung, kidney; principal (inactive) metabolite is cotinine
Half-life	Nicotine: 1–4 h, decreases with repeated exposure Cotinine: 20 h
Elimination	2%–35% excreted unchanged in urine

Nicotine from cigarette or cigar smoke is carried on inhaled tar particles into the lungs, where the pulmonary circulation rapidly absorbs the inhaled nicotine. After inhalation, studies show that peak nicotine concentration occurs within minutes. After 9 minutes of cigarette smoking, the nicotine concentration in the blood peaks within 10 minutes after cessation of use.[6] With e-cigarette use, nicotine concentrations peak within 5 minutes in naïve users; after more chronic use, peak nicotine concentrations rise along a similar timeline but surpass the concentration reached by naïve users.[45]

In the bloodstream, nicotine is about 69% ionized at a pH of 7.4, and less than 5% is bound to plasma proteins. Distribution to body tissues is rapid and extensive, with an average volume of distribution of about 2.6 L/kg.[12] Nicotine readily crosses the placental barrier and is secreted in breast milk. Metabolism occurs primarily in the liver via CYP2A6 and CYP2D6, aldehyde oxidase, flavin monooxygenase, and by glycosylation. About 70% of circulating nicotine is metabolized to cotinine, and much smaller amounts to nornicotine, nicotine-1-N-oxide, nicotine glucuronide, and 2′-hydroxynicotine.

Peak plasma concentrations of nicotine and cotinine are influenced most strongly by individual variations in clearance.[10,11] Hepatic nicotine metabolism is inducible and nicotine-dependent individuals metabolize the drug more rapidly than naïve ones.[48] Nicotine metabolism is also linked to race and sex. Asians and African Americans metabolize nicotine more slowly than whites, and they have prolonged cotinine clearance in the urine.[11,65,83] Women metabolize nicotine faster than men, which is further accelerated by oral contraceptive use and pregnancy, and is most likely mediated by an influence of estrogen on CYP2A6 activity.[48]

Renal excretion of unchanged nicotine accounts for 2% to 35% of total nicotine elimination,[14] and this is pH dependent. Nicotine is reabsorbed in the proximal tubule and acidification of the urine enhances elimination. The half-life of nicotine in the body is 1 to 4 hours, and it decreases with repeated nicotine exposure such as is associated with habitual cigarette smoking. Cotinine and trans-3′-hydroxycotinine are eliminated in the urine as glucuronide esters independent of urine pH. The elimination half-life of cotinine is approximately 20 hours, and therefore urinary cotinine is a more useful marker of nicotine exposure. The apparent elimination half-life of nicotine after transdermal patch removal is longer than that noted with nicotine exposure by other routes,[53] but this is most likely because a dermal reservoir of drug is established during patch use, from which absorption continues after removal.

Cigarette smoking modulates the bioavailability and effectiveness of numerous medications through effects on drug absorption, metabolism, or pharmacodynamics. Cigarette smoking induces CYP1A2 and accelerates the metabolism of caffeine, clozapine, olanzapine, tacrine, theophylline, and erlotinib.[46,51] This is not an effect of nicotine. For example, intravenous (IV) nicotine administration does not alter theophylline metabolism.[8] Smokers also have diminished effectiveness of opioids, benzodiazepines, β-adrenergic antagonists, and nifedipine[21] and are more likely to fail antacid and H$_2$-antagonist therapy for peptic ulcer disease.[8] However, an effect of nicotine is not clearly linked to these interactions.

The LD$_{50}$ of nicotine is usually estimated at 0.5 to 1 mg/kg in adults[38,40,65] but is much higher at about 6.5 to 13 mg/kg according to some reports.[70,71] Severe toxicity is reported with ingestion of less than 2 mg in a child,[74,94] and this dose is sufficient to produce mild symptoms in an unhabituated adult. However, the reported doses associated with toxicity varied widely. Children younger than 6 years of age who ingest one or more cigarettes, or 3 or more cigarette butts, generally develop symptoms of nicotine toxicity.[94] A retrospective review of 10 children who ingested cigarettes found that of the 4 patients with symptoms requiring medical evaluation and treatment, all ingested at least 2 entire cigarettes.[67] Two pediatric deaths associated with e-cigarettes (unknown nicotine doses) are also reported as well as a suicidal ingestion of up to 3 g of nicotine liquid by an adult.[17]

Acute tolerance to nicotine develops in smokers who take in small doses of nicotine regularly throughout the day. Sensitization to the effects of nicotine is restored with overnight abstinence.[6,48] Tolerance also develops in tobacco workers with regular exposure to tobacco plant leaves. However, the phenomenon of acute tolerance, along with considerable genetic variability in nicotine metabolism, implies a range of susceptibility to drug effect.

SOURCES AND USES OF NICOTINE

Cigarettes and Cigars

The amount of nicotine contained in a single cigarette is highly variable, ranging from less than 10 mg in a "low-nicotine" cigarette to 30 mg in some European cigarettes (Table 82–2). Because most nicotine is either lost in the sidestream (secondhand) smoke or left in the filter, the absorbed nicotine yield from a smoked cigarette is much less than this, on the order of 0.05 to 3 mg per cigarette.[35] The amount of nicotine absorbed by a particular individual from a single smoked cigarette is highly variable among smokers and depends on the puff rate, volume, the depth and duration of inhalation, and size of the residual.[68] Cigars have higher nicotine content than cigarettes (Table 82–2) and potentially greater absorption because cigar and pipe tobacco is typically air cured to achieve a high pH.

The potential for nicotine toxicity from smoking is limited because peak effects by this route occur within seconds and tend to limit further intake of drug. Most reports of acute nicotine toxicity referable to cigarette exposure are associated with cigarette and cigarette butt ingestion, usually by young children.[78,85,86] Although uncommon, severe toxicity from cigarette[13,94] ingestion is well reported and at least 3 deaths are associated with liquid nicotine.[17,54] Ingesting cigarette soakage water is recommended on the Internet as a "safe and effective" means of suicide, and several cases are reported.[24,91] Intravenous injection of cigarette soakage is also reported.[44]

TABLE 82–2	Commercial Sources of Nicotine	
Source	*Content (mg)*	*Delivered (mg)*
1 cigarette	10–30	0.05–3
1 cigarette butt	5–7	—
1 cigar	15–40	0.2–1
1 g snuff (wet)	12–16	2–3.5
1 g chewing tobacco	6–8	2–4
1 piece nicotine gum	2 or 4	1–2
1 nicotine patch	8.3–114	5–22 over 16–24 h
1 nicotine lozenge	2 or 4	2–4
1 nicotine nasal spray	0.5	0.2–0.4
30-mL bottle of 3.6% nicotine liquid refill for e-cigarette cartridges (30-, 50-, and 100-mL bottles also sold)	36 mg/mL	<43.2 mcg/100 mL "puff" of nicotine mist

Waterpipes, Hookah, and Shisha

Although the use of cigarettes has decreased in the United States, waterpipe use has become popular especially among college students with hookah bars opening all around the country. Waterpipes, also called hookah or shisha, refer to tobacco smoked through a pipe filled with water. A container holding 10 to 20 g of tobacco, often fruit flavored, is connected to the pipe and covered with aluminum foil paper.[50] Coal is used as a heat source and placed on top of the foil paper. The user then inhales the smoke produced from a mouthpiece at the end of a hose attached to the waterpipe. Waterpipes are perceived to be safer than smoking cigarettes, with 10% to 20% of US college students reporting its use.[32,87]

Toxins associated with waterpipe use include carbon monoxide, nicotine, and carcinogens. In a study including 16 participants who smoked a waterpipe with up to 32 mg of nicotine for a mean of 39 minutes, plasma nicotine concentrations peaked to 11.7 ng/mL and 28.4 ng/mL in waterpipe-only smokers and mixed tobacco users, respectively, 45 minutes after use.[50] These participants reached a systemic dose of 2.5 mg equal to that achieved after smoking 2 or 3 cigarettes, and the average carboxyhemoglobin in the waterpipe-only smokers was 6.2%. Several reports demonstrate overt carbon monoxide poisoning associated with waterpipes. In one case, a 24-year-old man who worked lighting hookahs at a hookah bar became unconscious with a carboxyhemoglobin level of 33.8% and an abnormal electrocardiogram.[75]

Given rising health concerns based on similar studies, in 2016, the FDA included waterpipes under the *Family Smoking Prevention and Tobacco Control Act of 2009*, which restricts tobacco sale to minors younger than 18 years of age, requires packaging to contain health warnings and product ingredients to be evaluated, and mandates FDA premarket review and authorization.[41,92]

Oral Tobacco

Snuff and chewing tobacco are still widely employed by users of smokeless tobacco products[22] despite clear associations with periodontal disease, dental cavities, and up to a 48 times greater risk of oropharyngeal cancers compared with people who do not use tobacco products.[23] Snuff, or dip, is a finely ground and sometimes flavored tobacco preparation often sold in small teabag-like pouches that users insert between their lower lips and gums. Chewing tobacco consists of shredded, twisted, or "bricked" dried tobacco leaves. Because nicotine is a weak base, smokeless tobacco is buffered to facilitate buccal absorption.

In one survey of major US brands, the pH of marketed oral tobacco products ranged from 5.24 to 8.35, and the nicotine content ranged from 3.37 to 11.04 mg/g.[76] Acute nicotine toxicity from smokeless tobacco is rarely reported in adults. A 14-month-old boy had muscle fasciculations and lethargy after ingesting material taken from his father's spittoon but recovered within 24 hours with supportive care.[40] Rectal administration of moist snuff as a treatment for migraine headache resulted in significant toxicity in one patient.[56] Presumably, the relatively alkaline environment of the rectum facilitated absorption of a high dose.

Oral tobacco has been popular on baseball fields for many decades. Despite a push to ban smokeless tobacco from baseball fields, the Major League Baseball organization has not prohibited its use. Recently, city and state governments have banned smokeless tobacco from baseball-related events and venues in 5 cities: San Francisco, Boston, Los Angeles, Chicago, and New York City.[55]

Gum

Nicotine gum has been available without a prescription as an aid to smoking cessation in the United States since 1996. It is sold in 2-mg and 4-mg strengths per piece. Approximately 53% to 72% of the nicotine in the gum is absorbed. It is buffered to an alkaline pH to facilitate buccal absorption. The gum is supposed to be chewed until mouth and throat tingling and a peppery taste develop, signaling the release of nicotine. The gum is then "parked" in the cheek until the sensation subsides, at which time it may be chewed again to release more drug.[81] If used correctly, serum nicotine concentrations rise gradually to a level slightly lower that normally achieved by cigarette smoking.[81] If the gum is swallowed whole, then serum concentrations rise even more slowly because the acidic environment of the stomach delays absorption.[8] Conversely, if the gum is chewed vigorously and saliva is swallowed, then nicotine concentrations rise rapidly, and adverse reactions occur.[94]

Lozenges

Nicotine lozenges containing 2 and 4 mg of nicotine are available for purchase without a prescription in the Unites States. The potential for rapid absorption of nicotine as a bolus dose from chewing the lozenge is a concern.

Transdermal Patches

Nicotine patches have been FDA approved for purchase without prescription in the United States since 1996. Most nicotine transdermal delivery systems are designed to deliver 7, 14, or 21 mg of nicotine over 24 hours.[43] Because many patch users have difficulty sleeping, experience vivid dreams, or have nightmares if they wear the patch overnight, systems designed to be applied for only 16 hours are now available. Several reports document consequential nicotine toxicity related to nicotine patch misuse. Toxicity occurs in people who continue to smoke cigarettes after beginning therapy with the nicotine patch. Children developed symptoms after exploratory self-application of one or more patches to the skin,[104,106] and concurrent use of multiple patches is used as a means of suicide.[59,95,105] Severe toxicity also occurs if patches are punctured—for example, by biting or tearing—thus allowing delivery of excessive quantities of nicotine.[106] The patch reservoirs contain an estimated 36 to 114 mg per patch.[80]

Spray or Inhaler

A nicotine spray has been available since 1996 to aid efforts at smoking cessation. The most commonly reported adverse effects during initiation of therapy are due to local irritation and include rhinorrhea, lacrimation, sneezing, and nasal and throat irritation.[49] One spray delivers 0.5 mg of nicotine and the recommended dose is 2 sprays every 30 to 60 minutes as needed. The absorption is about 50% of the delivered dose and is diminished or delayed by rhinitis or by α-adrenergic agonist decongestants.[63] No report of acute nicotine toxicity from nicotine inhalers has been published to date.

Electronic Cigarettes

Electronic cigarettes, or e-cigarettes, are a relatively new nicotine delivery product now widely available in various strengths and flavors.[20] The devices resemble cigarettes and contain a rechargeable battery pack along with a small heating element or atomizer attached to a reservoir of liquid nicotine. Currently, there are multiple generations of e-cigarettes with newer models combining the atomizer and the nicotine reservoir into one piece. An electronic airflow censor activates the heating element when the user inhales, allowing release of a "puff" of nicotine-containing vapor.

An FDA analysis of cartridges found that identically labeled products contained variable amounts of nicotine and a number of potentially harmful contaminants.[98] Personal vaporizers are newer models that allow nicotine delivery to be titrated based on the concentration of the liquid nicotine preparation being used.[96] Liquid nicotine is sold in different formulations with the highest strength preparations (3.6% nicotine) containing more than 1 g of nicotine per 30-mL bottle. This raises serious concerns about the risk of both unintentional and intentional toxic exposures. Additionally, large-volume liquid nicotine replacement fluid bottles (used to refill e-cigarette cartridges) are available, augmenting e-cigarettes' potential for harm.

Deaths from unintentional and intentional ingestion of e-cigarette liquid are reported.[17,92] Analysis of calls to US poison control centers about e-cigarette exposures shows a substantial increase between the years 2010 and 2014, with significantly greater adverse effects reported compared with calls about cigarette exposures.[16] Before 2016, the sale and use of e-cigarettes were not regulated in the United States. E-cigarette use increased in popularity among adolescents, both who had and those who had not smoked traditional cigarettes.[31] A study found that adolescents who use e-cigarettes are also more likely to try other tobacco products, including traditional cigarettes.[62]

In 2016, the rising concern for e-cigarettes' toxic potential lead the FDA to include e-cigarettes under the *Family Smoking Prevention and Tobacco Control Act of 2009*, thus regulating its sale to minors and requiring FDA approval for new e-cigarette products before entering the market.[92]

Partial Nicotine Receptor Agonists (Varenicline, Cytisine)

Partial nicotine receptor agonists are used to aid smoking cessation. Theoretically, they work by reducing smoking satisfaction (agonist/antagonism effect) while helping to maintain moderate concentrations of central dopamine release (partial agonist effect). Cytisine is a plant-derived xenobiotic with a chemical structure similar to nicotine that is used in East and Central Europe as a smoking cessation drug since the 1960s under the trade name Tabex (Sopharma Pharmaceuticals). Despite its widespread use, the safety, efficacy, pharmacokinetics, and pharmacodynamics of cytisine in humans are not well studied.[33] Varenicline was approved as a prescription-only aid to smoking cessation in 2006. Several randomized controlled trials demonstrated efficacy in controlling nicotine cravings and evidence suggests that varenicline increases the probability of successful abstinence from smoking.[15]

In 2009, the FDA mandated a black box warning due to an association with increased risk of depression or suicidal behavior. In 2011, the FDA updated the drug label for varenicline to include warning of its interaction with ethanol, including its association with decreased ethanol tolerance and increased aggressive behavior, as well as its potential to cause seizures.[34] There is now increasing experience with acute varenicline overdose, including effects such as nausea, vomiting, tachycardia, and hypertension, and one reported fatality after intentional overdose.[47,97]

Plants and Leaves

Green tobacco sickness (GTS) refers to nicotine-induced symptoms, including nausea, vomiting, headache, and dizziness, that occur when nicotine is topically absorbed during the handling of tobacco plants. Residual moisture or dew drops on tobacco leaves contains as much as 9 mg of nicotine per 100 mL.[39] Tobacco workers' hands tested for nicotine had concentrations between 4.1 and 27.1 mcg/cm^{-2} in one study.[25]

Tobacco workers are most at risk when their clothing comes in contact with moisture on the tobacco plants. Sweat wrung out of the shirts worn by workers during tobacco harvest in one study contained up to 98 mg/mL of nicotine.[39] Risk factors for GTS include decreased tolerance reflected by younger age and a relative lack of work experience as well as extent of exposure which increases with working with wet tobacco.[3,5,73,77] The use of impermeable garments or other barrier protection is the only protective factor consistently noted to be useful across multiple studies.[4,73,77]

Miscellaneous

In the pre-Columbian Americas, many tribes used tobacco extract and tobacco smoke enemas for both medicinal and spiritual purposes. They are still recommended by some naturopaths and folk healers as remedies for constipation, urinary retention, pinworm, and "hysterical convulsions." Nicotine was also recommended as a treatment for migraine on the basis of its vasoconstrictive properties.[103] "Therapeutic misadventures" resulted in nicotine poisoning in several documented cases.[38,56,57] For example, acute nicotine toxicity occurred in an 8 year-old boy after application of a homemade remedy for eczema made from a mixture of tobacco leaves, lime juice, and freeze-dried coffee.[27]

PATHOPHYSIOLOGY

Nicotine mimics the effects of acetylcholine by binding to nicotinic receptors (nAChRs) in the brain, spinal cord, autonomic ganglia, adrenal medulla, neuromuscular junctions, and chemoreceptors of the carotid and aortic bodies (Chap. 13). Activation of nAChRs in the CNS directly stimulates neurotransmitter release. When nicotine binds to this receptor, an ion channel opens, allowing an influx of cations, mostly sodium and calcium. Voltage-gated calcium channels are then activated, leading to further influx of calcium, and a variety of downstream effects, including depolarization.

At doses generally produced by cigarette smoking there is stimulation of the reticular activating system and an alerting pattern on the electroencephalogram.[107] Nicotine-stimulated release of dopamine occurs in the mesolimbic area, the corpus striatum, the prefrontal cortex, and in the nucleus accumbens; it is an important mediator of nicotine addiction.[69] Nicotine also stimulates glutaminergic activation and the GABA (γ-aminobutyric acid)-ergic inhibition of dopaminergic neurons in the hippocampus, basal forebrain, and ventral tegmental area of the midbrain.[7,30] These pathways, along with endogenous cannabinoid and opioid systems, are important neuromodulatory pathways for drug-induced reward, dependence, and withdrawal.[66,69,72] Norepinephrine, acetylcholine, GABA, serotonin, glutamate, and endorphins are all released by nicotine and are associated with cognitive and mood enhancement as well as appetite suppression, increased basal energy expenditures, and anxiety reduction.[7]

The clinical effects of nicotine are dose dependent. Low doses of nicotine and related compounds stimulate nicotinic receptors centrally and in autonomic and somatic motor nerve fibers, resulting in sympathetic agonism. At toxic concentrations, prolonged or excessive nicotinergic stimulation ultimately leads to receptor blockade (Chap. 66), with parasympathetic and neuromuscular-blocking effects.

At very high doses, nicotine induces seizures. In a mouse model, nicotine-induced seizures are blocked by the nicotine-receptor antagonists mecamylamine, methyllycaconitine citrate, and hexamethonium.[26] However, when given to mice at slightly higher doses, these nicotine receptor antagonists are epileptogenic. The specific mechanisms by which nicotine produces seizures are unknown. A disinhibition model is proposed in which desensitization or antagonism of central nicotinic cholinergic neurons blocks excitatory input to GABAergic neurons and reduces inhibitory GABAergic input to pyramidal cells, resulting in increased excitability and seizures.[1,18,28,37] An alternative hypothesis is that high doses of nicotine cause synchronous GABA-receptor mediated depolarization in hippocampal neurons to generate seizures.[28]

CLINICAL MANIFESTATIONS

Patients with nicotine exposure rarely display more than mild symptoms and typically have a benign course.

Exposure to nicotine in low doses comparable to cigarette smoking in nicotine-naïve patients produces fine tremor; cutaneous vasoconstriction; increased gastrointestinal motility; nausea; and increases in heart rate, respiratory rate, and blood pressure. Low-dose nicotine also increases mental alertness and produces euphoria. Because nicotine is poorly absorbed in the acid environment of the stomach, symptom onset occurs 30 to 90 minutes after ingestion of nicotine-containing products.

Early signs and symptoms of nicotine toxicity are referable to nicotinic cholinergic excess; increased salivation, nausea, vomiting, diaphoresis, and diarrhea all occur within minutes of systemic absorption. Vasoconstriction manifests with pallor and hypertension. Tachycardia also occurs, and nicotine gum chewing is implicated in the development of atrial fibrillation in several cases.[19,89] Neurologic signs and symptoms include headache, dizziness, ataxia, confusion, and perceptual distortions. Nicotine is an irritant, and ingestion of nicotine, including use of nicotine gum, causes a burning sensation and pain in the mouth, and constriction of the pharyngeal muscles. Similarly, application of nicotine patches generally results in dermal irritation.

Vomiting is the most common adverse effect reported, although agitation also commonly occurs. The relative rarity of life-threatening symptoms is caused by part to autodecontamination from vomiting. In addition, because most reported cases involve unintentional tobacco ingestion by young children, there is significant selection bias.

Data from poison control centers in the United States suggests that the increased availability of e-cigarettes and liquid nicotine is associated with an increased incidence of consequential poisoning. Most liquid nicotine exposures occur in children younger than 5 years of age,[102] and children exposed to liquid nicotine have 2.6 times higher odds of having severe outcomes than children exposed to traditional cigarettes including one reported death.[52] This is likely caused by larger nicotine concentrations available in

TABLE 82–3	Signs and Symptoms of Acute Nicotine Poisoning			
	Gastrointestinal	*Respiratory*	*Cardiovascular*	*Neurologic*
Early (0.25–1 h)	Nausea Vomiting Salivation Abdominal pain	Bronchorrhea Hyperpnea	Hypertension Tachycardia Pallor	Agitation Anxiety Dizziness Blurred vision Headache Hyperactivity Confusion Tremors Fasciculations Seizures
Late (0.5–4 h)	Diarrhea	Hypoventilation Apnea	Bradycardia Hypotension Dysrhythmias Shock	Lethargy Weakness Paralysis

liquid nicotine. Although less common, ingestion of novel smokeless tobacco preparations, such as gums and lozenges, is more likely to produce symptoms compared to cigarette ingestion because these are buffered to promote more rapid nicotine release.[94]

Because nicotine is rapidly metabolized, patients who develop only mild symptoms are expected to recover quickly. Most patients recover fully within 12 hours. An important exception to this rule is noted in patients with symptoms of nicotine toxicity after transdermal nicotine patch application because a reservoir of drug persists in the subcutaneous tissue after patch removal and can serve as a source of ongoing absorption. Removal of the patch and decontamination of these patients should remain paramount to limiting further absorption.

Clinical manifestations of severe poisoning are classically biphasic, reflecting early central stimulation followed by depression. Initial signs include cardiac dysrhythmias, seizures, and muscle fasciculations in addition to the cholinergic features described earlier. Bradycardia, hypotension, coma, and neuromuscular blockade with respiratory failure from muscular paralysis are a more delayed development (Table 82–3).

Exposure to fresh tobacco leaves produces GTS, which is likened to the experience of seasickness typically occurring within 3 to 17 hours after exposure. This syndrome, characterized by dizziness, headache, weakness, nausea, vomiting, diarrhea, abdominal cramps, chills, and in severe cases, signs of autonomic instability, often has a duration of several days.[72]

DIAGNOSTIC TESTING

Determination of serum or urinary concentrations of nicotine or its metabolites is unlikely to be helpful in the management of the acutely poisoned patient. Measurement can be made for confirmation purposes using various chromatographic techniques. Cigarette smokers typically maintain serum nicotine concentrations around 30 to 50 ng/mL during the day but can achieve concentrations as high as 100 ng/mL.[79] Postmortem analyses of nicotine concentrations in blood after fatal acute toxicity range from 5.5 to 800 mg/L.[24]

The presence of measurable concentrations of nicotine or cotinine in biologic samples often reflects coincidental or chronic exposure and does not necessarily imply acute toxicity. Urinary cotinine has a longer detection window than nicotine and is often used to document exposure to nicotine containing products, including exposure to secondhand smoke, or to guide dosage adjustments in nicotine replacement therapy.[7,61,79] Conversely, the absence of cotinine in the urine is used to document abstinence from tobacco products.

MANAGEMENT

Most patients with unintentional or low-dose nicotine exposures do not require medical treatment. Patients should be immediately referred for evaluation if they are symptomatic or have ingested any amount of nicotine- or neonicotinoid-containing liquid. Children who ingest one or more cigarettes or 3 or more cigarette butts should also be referred for evaluation without delay. Patients with mild or no symptoms can be observed for several hours and safely discharged home if there are no complicating circumstances such as significant comorbid cardiovascular illness or intent to self-harm.

Patients with dermal exposure to wet tobacco leaves or pesticides should be undressed completely and the skin washed thoroughly with soap and copious amounts of water. Medical staff charged with handling both clothing and patients before decontamination should wear personal protective gear and dispose of materials safely. Symptomatic patients should have any nicotine dermal patches removed immediately and the skin washed with soap and water.

Vomiting is the most commonly reported adverse effect in patients with acute nicotine toxicity and limits absorption in some cases. Induction of emesis because it is unlikely to be of added benefit and has the potential for harm. Orogastric lavage is reasonable in patients who present immediately after large intentional and potentially life-threatening ingestions of nicotine-containing products with the exception of liquid nicotine. Liquid nicotine formulations are more rapidly absorbed, making orogastric lavage less useful. Activated charcoal adsorbs nicotine and can reduce absorption, and therefore we recommend for consequential ingestions.

There is no specific antidote for nicotine toxicity. Treatment of acute nicotine toxicity is symptomatic and supportive. The first priority is to ensure airway protection and respiratory support. Atropine is used to treat symptoms associated with parasympathetic stimulation such as excess salivation, wheezing, or bradycardia. Endotracheal intubation is required for airway protection or to assist ventilation in severely poisoned patients. Seizures are treated with a benzodiazepine. Hypotension is treated with fluid boluses and infusion of 0.9% NaCl initially. Patients who fail to respond to volume infusion require treatment with a vasopressor such as norepinephrine. Dysrhythmias should be treated according to standard advanced cardiac life support protocols. Nicotine elimination is enhanced in acidic urine,[9] but the potential risks outweigh the benefits of this elimination strategy, so we recommend against this approach.

SUMMARY

- The primary source of nicotine is tobacco made from the leaves of *Nicotiana* species, but chemically related tobacco substitutes and pesticides are becoming increasingly available.
- Nicotine is well absorbed after inhalation, mucosal, or dermal exposure. It is rapidly distributed to the brain where it activates nicotinic acetylcholinergic receptors, stimulates the reticular activating system, and facilitates neurotransmitter release.
- Metabolism via the hepatic cytochrome oxidase system produces pharmacologically inactive metabolites slowly excreted in urine. The half-life of nicotine in the body is about 1 to 4 hours, with more rapid clearance in individuals who are chronically exposed.
- Clinical manifestations of nicotine toxicity are those of nicotinic cholinergic excess, most commonly including vomiting and agitation. Severe poisoning causes seizures, cardiac dysrhythmias, hypotension, and neuromuscular blockade with respiratory failure from muscular paralysis.
- There are no antidotes for nicotine, and acute toxicity should be managed with symptom directed, supportive care.

REFERENCES

1. Alkondon M, et al. Nicotine receptor activation in human cerebral cortical interneurons: a mechanism for inhibition and disinhibition of neuronal networks. *J Neurosci.* 2000;20:66-75.
2. Appleton S. Frequency and outcomes of accidental ingestion of tobacco products in young children. *Reg Tox Pharmacol.* 2011;61:210-214.

3. Arcury T, et al. A clinic-based, case-control comparison of green tobacco sickness among minority farmworkers: clues for prevention. *South Med J.* 2002;95:1008-1011.

4. Arcury T, et al. Predictors of incidence and prevalence of green tobacco sickness among Latino farmworkers in North Carolina, USA. *J Epidemiol Community Heal.* 2001;55:818-824.

5. Ballard T, et al. Green tobacco sickness: occupational poisoning in tobacco workers. *Arch Env Heal.* 1995;50:384-389.

6. Benowitz N. Clinical pharmacology of nicotine: implications for understanding, preventing, and treating tobacco addiction. *Clin Pharmacol Ther.* 2008;83:531-541.

7. Benowitz N. Neurobiology of nicotine addiction: implications for smoking cessation treatment. *Am J Med.* 2008;121:S3-S10.

8. Benowitz N. Pharmacologic aspects of cigarette smoking and nicotine addiction. *N Engl J Med.* 1988;319:1318-1330.

9. Benowitz N, Jacob P. Nicotine renal excretion rate influences nicotine intake during cigarette smoking. *J Pharmacol Exp Ther.* 1985;234:153-155.

10. Benowitz N, et al. CYP2D6 phenotype and the metabolism of nicotine and cotinine. *Pharmacogenetics.* 1996;6:239-242.

11. Benowitz N, et al. Female sex and oral contraceptive use accelerate nicotine metabolism. *Clin Pharmacol Ther.* 2006;79:480-488.

12. Benowitz NL, et al. Nicotine chemistry, metabolism, kinetics and biomarkers. *Handb Exp Pharmacol.* 2009;192:29-60.

13. Bonadio W, Anderson Y. Tobacco ingestions in children. *Clin Pediatr.* 1989;28:592-593.

14. Byrd G, et al. Evidence for urinary excretion of glucuronide conjugates of nicotine, cotinine, and trans-3′-hydroxycotinine in smokers. *Drug Metab Dispos.* 1992;20:192-197.

15. Cahill K, et al. Nicotine receptor partial agonists for smoking cessation (Review). *Cochrane Database Syst Rev.* 2007;1:CD006103.

16. Chatham-Stephens K, et al. Notes from the field: calls to poison centers for exposures to electronic cigarettes United States, September 2010-February 2014. *MMWR.* 2014;63:292-293.

17. Chen BC, et al. Death following intentional ingestion of e-liquid. *Clin Toxicol.* 2015;3650(March):1-3.

18. Chiodini F, et al. Modulation of synaptic transmission by nicotine and nicotinic antagonists in the hippocampus. *Brain Res Bull.* 1999;48:623-628.

19. Choragudi N, et al. Nicotine gum-induced atrial fibrillation. *Hear Dis.* 2003;5:100-101.

20. Yamin CK, et al. E-cigarettes: a rapidly growing internet phenomenon. *Ann Intern Med.* 2012;153:607.

21. Cone E, et al. Nicotine and tobacco. In: Mozayani A, Raymon L, eds. *Handbook of Drug Interactions: A Clinical and Forensic Guide.* Totwa, NJ: Humana Press; 2003:463-492.

22. Connolly G, et al. Unintentional child poisonings through ingestion of conventional and novel tobacco products. *Pediatrics.* 2010;125:896-899.

23. Consensus Conference: health applications of smokeless tobacco use. *JAMA.* 1986;255:1045-1048.

24. Corkery J, et al. Two UK suicides using nicotine extracted from tobacco employing instructions available on the Internet. *Forensic Sci Int.* 2010;199:e9-e13.

25. Curwin BD, et al. Nicotine exposure and decontamination on tobacco harvesters' hands. *Ann Occup Hyg.* 2005;49:407-413.

26. Damaj M, et al. Pharmacological characterization of nicotine-induced seizures in mice. *J Pharmacol Exp Ther.* 1999;291:1284–1291.

27. Davies P, et al. Acute nicotine poisoning associated with a traditional remedy for eczema. *Arch Dis Child.* 2001;85:500-502.

28. Dobelis P, et al. GABAergic systems modulate nicotinic receptor-mediated seizures in mice. *J Pharmacol Exp Ther.* 2003;206:1159-1166.

29. Domino E, et al. The nicotine content of common vegetables. *N Engl J Med.* 1993;329:437.

30. DuBois D, et al. Varenicline and nicotine enhance GABAergic synaptic transmission in rat CA1 hippocampal and medial septum/diagonal band neurons. *Life Sci.* 2013;92:337-344.

31. Durmowicz EL. The impact of electronic cigarettes on the paediatric population. *Tob Control.* 2014;23(suppl 2):ii41-ii46.

32. Eissenberg T, et al. Waterpipe tobacco smoking on a U.S. college campus: prevalence and correlates. *J Adolesc Heal.* 2008;42:526-529.

33. Etter J, et al. Cytisine for smoking cessation: a research agenda. *Drug Alcohol Depend.* 2008;92:3-8.

34. FDA updates label for stop smoking drug Chantix (varenicline) to include potential alcohol interaction, rare risk of seizures, and studies of side effects on mood, behavior, or thinking. http://www.fda.gov/Drugs/DrugSafety/ucm436494.htm.

35. Federal Trade Commission Report. Tar, nicotine, and carbon monoxide of the smoke of 1,294 varieties of domestic cigarettes for the year 1998. http://www.ftc.gov/opa/2000/07/t&n2000.shtm.

36. Franklin R, Rodgers G. Unintentional child poisonings treated in United States hospital emergency departments: national estimates of incident cases, population-based poisoning rates, and product involvement. *Pediatrics.* 2008;122:1244-1251.

37. Freund R, et al. Evidence for modulation of GABAergic neurotransmission by nicotine. *Brain Res.* 1988;453:215-220.

38. Garcia-Estrada H, Fischman C. An unusual case of nicotine poisoning. *Clin Toxicol.* 1977;10:391-393.

39. Gelbach S, et al. Nicotine absorption by workers harvesting tobacco. *Lancet.* 1975;1:478-480.

40. Goepferd S. Smokeless tobacco: a potential hazard to infants and children. *J Am Dent Assoc.* 1986;113:49-50.

41. Gonzales A. American Association of Poison Control Centers applauds the United States Food and Drug Administration's extension to regulate E-cigarette and additional nicotine products. American Association of Poison Control Centers news release; May 2016.

42. Goulson D. An overview of the environmental risks posed by neonicotinoid insecticides. *J Appl Ecol.* 2013;50:977-987.

43. Gupta S, et al. Bioavailability and absorption kinetics of nicotine following application of a transdermal system. *Br J Clin Pharmacol.* 1993;36:221-227.

44. Hagiya K, et al. Nicotine poisoning due to intravenous injection of cigarette soakage. *Hum Exp Toxicol.* 2010;29:427-429.

45. Hajek P, et al. Nicotine intake from electronic cigarettes on initial use and after 4 weeks of regular use. *Nicotine Tob Res.* 2015;17:175-179.

46. Hamilton M, et al. Effects of smoking on the pharmacokinetics of erlotinib. *Clin Cancer Res.* 2006;12:2166-2171.

47. Hedlund AJ, et al. Varenicline overdose in a teenager. *Clin Toxicol.* 2009;47:371.

48. Hukkanen J, et al. Metabolism and disposition kinetics of nicotine. *Pharmacol Rev.* 2005;57:79-115.

49. Hurt R, et al. Nicotine nasal spray for smoking cessation: pattern of use, side effects, relief of withdrawal symptoms, and cotinine levels. *Mayo Clin Proc.* 1988;73:118-125.

50. Jacob III P, Raddaha A, Dempsey D, et al. Nicotine, carbon monoxide, and carcinogen exposure after a single use of a waterpipe. *Cancer Epidemiol Biomarkers Prev.* 2011;20:2345-2353.

51. Jusko W. Influence of cigarette smoking on drug metabolism in man. *Drug Metab Rev.* 1979;9:221-236.

52. Kamboj A, et al. Pediatric exposure to E-cigarettes, nicotine, and tobacco products in the United States. *Pediatrics.* 2016;137.

53. Keller-Stanislawski B, et al. Transdermal nicotine substitution: pharmacokinetics of nicotine and cotinine. *Int J Clin Pharmacol Ther Toxicol.* 1993;31:417-421.

54. Kim JW, Baum CR. Liquid nicotine toxicity. *Pediatr Emerg Care.* 2015;31:517-521.

55. Baseball Deal Bans Smokeless Tobacco Use by New Players. Knock Tobacco Out of the Park website. https://tobaccofreebaseball.org/ Last accessed June 15, 2018.

56. Knudsen K, Strinholm M. A case of life-threatening rectal administration of moist snuff. *Clin Tox.* 2010;48:572-573.

57. Kravetz R. Tobacco enema. *Am J Gastroent.* 2002;43:1986-1991.

58. Kreshak A, et al. A retrospective poison center review of varenicline-exposed patients. *Ann Pharmacother.* 2009;43:1986-1991.

59. Labelle A, Boulay L. An attempted suicide using transdermal nicotine patches. *Can J Psychiatry.* 1999;44:190.

60. Lavioe F, Harris T. Fatal nicotine ingestion. *J Emerg Med.* 1991;9:133-136.

61. Lawson G, et al. Application of urine nicotine and cotinine excretion rates to assessment of nicotine replacement in light, moderate, and heavy smokers undergoing transdermal therapy. *J Clin Pharmacol.* 1998;38:510-516.

62. Leventhal A, et al. Association of electronic cigarette use with initiation of combustible tobacco product smoking in early adolescence. *JAMA.* 2015;314:700-707.

63. Lunell E, et al. Relative bioavailability of nicotine from a nasal spray in infectious rhinitis and after use of a topical decongestant. *Eur J Clin Pharmacol.* 1995;48:235-240.

64. Luo J, et al. Oral use of Swedish moist snuff (snus) and risk for cancer of the mouth, lung, and pancreas in male construction workers: a retrospective cohort study. *Lancet.* 2007;369:2015-2020.

65. Malaiyandi V, et al. Implications of CYP2A6 genetic variation for smoking behaviors and nicotine dependence. *Clin Pharmacol Ther.* 2006;77:480-488.

66. Maldonado R, Berrendero F. Endogenous cannabinoid and opioid systems and their role in nicotine addiction. *Curr Drug Targets.* 2010;11:440-449.

67. Malizia E, et al. Acute intoxication with nicotine alkaloids and cannabinoids in children from ingestion of cigarettes. *Hum Toxicol.* 1983;2:315-316.

68. Marion D, Fortmann S. Nicotine yield and measures of cigarette smoke exposure in a large population. *Am J Public Heal.* 1987;77:546-549.

69. Martin-Soelch C. Neuroadaptive changes associated with smoking: structural and functional neural changes in nicotine dependence. *Brain Sci.* 2013;3:159-176.

70. Matsushima D, et al. Absorption and adverse effect following topical and oral administration of three transdermal nicotine products to dogs. *J Pharm Sci.* 1995;84:365-369.

71. Mayer B. How much nicotine kills a human? Tracing back the generally accepted lethal dose to dubious self-experiments in the nineteenth century. *Arch Toxicol.* 2014;88:5-7.

72. McBride J, et al. Green tobacco sickness. *Tob Control.* 1998;7:294-298.

73. McKnight R, Spiller H. Green tobacco sickness in children and adolescents. *Public Heal Rep.* 2005;120:602-605.

74. Mensch A, Holden M. Nicotine overdose after a single piece of nicotine gum. *Chest.* 1984;86:801-802.

75. Misek R, Patte C. Carbon monoxide toxicity after lighting coals at a hookah bar. *J Med Toxicol.* 2014;10:295-298.

76. Centers for Disease Control and Prevention (CDC). Determination of nicotine, pH, and moisture content of six commercial moist snuff products—Florida, January-February 1999. *MMWR Morb Mortal Wkly Rep.* 1999;48:398-401.

77. Centers for Disease Control and Prevention (CDC). Green tobacco sickness in tobacco harvesters—Kentucky, 1992. *MMWR Morb Mortal Wkly Rep.* 1993;42:237-240.

78. Centers for Disease Control and Prevention (CDC). Ingestion of cigarettes and cigarette butts by children—Rhode Island, January 1994-July 1996. *MMWR Morb Mortal Wkly Rep.* 1997;46:125-128.

79. Moyer T, et al. Simultaneous analysis of nicotine, nicotine metabolites, and tobacco alkaloids in serum or urine by tandem mass spectrometry, with clinically relevant metabolic profiles. *Clin Chem.* 2002;48:1460-1471.

80. Nicoderm CQ [package insert]. 2006.

81. Nicorette [package insert]. 2002.

82. Ohio Vegetable Production Guide. Ohio State University Bulletin 672-08. http://ohioline.osu.edu/b672/index.html.

83. Perez-Stable E, et al. Nicotine metabolism and intake in black and white smokers. *JAMA.* 1998;280:152–156.

84. Pesticide Information Program, Clemson University. Fighting our insect enemies: achievements of professional entomology (1854–1954). http://www.clemson.edu/extension/pest_ed/histor.html.

85. Petridou E, et al. Childhood poisonings from ingestion of cigarettes (letter). *Lancet.* 1995;346:1296.

86. Phua D, et al. Neonicotinoid insecticides: an emerging cause of acute pesticide poisoning. *Clin Toxicol.* 2009;47:336-341.

87. Primack B, et al. Prevalence of and associations with waterpipe tobacco smoking among U.S. university students. *Ann Behav Med.* 2008;36:81-86.

88. Quandt S, et al. Migrant farmworkers and green tobacco sickness: new issues for an understudied disease. *Am J Ind Med.* 2000;37:307-315.

89. Rigotti N, Eagle K. Atrial fibrillation while chewing nicotine gum. *JAMA.* 1986;255:1018.

90. Rogers A, et al. Catastrophic brain injury after nicotine insecticide ingestion. *J Emerg Med.* 2004;26:169-172.

91. Schneider S, et al. Internet suicide guidelines: report of a life-threatening poisoning using tobacco extract. *J Emerg Med.* 2010;38:610-613.

92. US Food and Drug Administration. Family smoking prevention and tabacco control act. 2009. https://www.fda.gov/TobaccoProducts/Labeling/RulesRegulationsGuidance/ucm262084.htm Last accessed June 15, 2018.

93. Serafini A, et al. Varenicline-induced grand mal seizure. *Epileptic Disord.* 2010;12:338.

94. Smolinske S, et al. Cigarette and nicotine chewing gum toxicity in children. *Hum Toxicol.* 1988;7:27-31.

95. Solarino B, et al. Multidrug poisoning involving nicotine and tramadol. *Forensic Sci Int.* 2010;194:e17-e19.

96. St. Helen G, et al. Nicotine delivery, retention and pharmacokinetics from various electronic cigarettes. *Addiction.* 2016;111:535-544.

97. Stove CP, et al. Fatality following a suicidal overdose with varenicline. *Int J Legal Med.* 2013;127:85-91.

98. The Medical Letter. Electronic cigarettes for smoking cessation. *Med Lett Drugs Ther.* 2012;54:93-94.

99. The tobacco timeline. www.tobacco.org/History/TobaccoHistory.html.

100. Thomas K, et al. Smoking cessation treatment and risk of depression suicide, and self harm in the Clinical Practice Research Datalink: prospective chohort study. *BMJ.* 2013;347:15704.

101. Tobacco Fact Sheet. World Health Organization. http://www.who.int/mediacentre/factsheets/fs339/en/.

102. Vakkalanka JP, et al. Epidemiological trends in electronic cigarette exposures reported to U.S. Poison Centers. *Clin Toxicol (Phila).* 2014;52:542-548.

103. Gupta VK. Antimigraine action of nicotine: theoretical basis and potential clinical application. *Eur J Emerg Med.* 2007;14:243-244.

104. Wain A, Martin J. Can transdermal nicotine patch cause acute intoxication in a child? A case report and review of the literature. *Ulster Med J.* 2004;73:65-66.

105. Weizenecker R, Deal W. Tobacco cropper's sickness. *J Fla Med Assoc.* 1970;57:13-14.

106. Woolf A, et al. Childhood poisoning involving transdermal nicotine patches. *Pediatrics.* 1997;99:e4.

107. Zhang L, et al. Power spectral analysis of EEG activity during sleep in cigarette smokers. *Chest.* 2008;133:427-432.

PHENCYCLIDINE AND KETAMINE

Ruben E. Olmedo

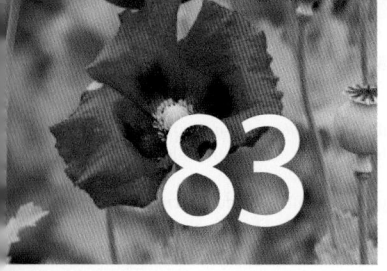

Phencyclidine (PCP)

Ketamine

Methoxetamine

Dextromethorphan

HISTORY AND EPIDEMIOLOGY

Phencyclidine (PCP) was discovered in 1926 but was not developed as a general anesthetic until the 1950s. At that time, the Parke Davis drug company was searching for an ideal intravenous (IV) anesthetic to rapidly achieve analgesia and anesthesia with minimal cardiovascular and respiratory depression.[39] Phencyclidine was marketed under the name Sernyl because it rendered an apparent state of serenity when administered to laboratory monkeys. Its human surgical use began in 1963, but it was rapidly discontinued when a 10% to 30% incidence of postoperative psychoses and dysphoria was documented over the subsequent 2-year period.[88] By 1967, the use of PCP was limited exclusively to veterinary medicine as a tranquilizer marketed under the name Sernylan.

Simultaneously, in the 1960s, PCP emerged as a street drug in San Francisco called "the PeaCe Pill."[74] Numerous street names have since been given to PCP: on the West Coast, it was called "angel dust," PCP, "crystal," "crystal joints" (CJs); Chicago called it "THC" or "TAC"; the East Coast opted for "the sheets," "Hog," or "elephant tranquilizer."[137] Ironically, PCP had limited popularity among drug users because of its dysphoric effects and unpredictable oral absorption.[177] However, with time, its use spread in a similar geographic pattern to that of marijuana and lysergic acid diethylamide (LSD), from the coastal United States to the Midwest region.[74]

Phencyclidine abuse became widespread during the 1970s.[28,207] The relatively easy and inexpensive synthesis coupled with the common marketing of PCP as LSD, mescaline, psilocybin, cocaine, amphetamine, or "synthetic THC" (tetrahydrocannabinol) added to its allure and consumption.[137] By the late 1970s, PCP abuse reached epidemic proportions.[10] The Drug Abuse Warning Network (DAWN) reported that the number of PCP-related emergencies and deaths had more than doubled from 1975 to 1977. In 1978, the National Institute of Drug Abuse reported that 13.9% of young adults (18–25 years old) had used PCP.[56] The manufacture of PCP was ultimately prohibited in 1978 when it was added to the list of federally controlled substances. Classifying PCP as a Schedule II drug led to its decrease in availability and, consequently, a decrease in its use. Although the 1980s brought about a cocaine epidemic that eclipsed PCP, PCP has remained consistently available, primarily regionalized to large cities in the northeastern United States and in the Los Angeles area,[112] where PCP use continues to rise and fall with societal trends. Because many of the PCP congeners made during the manufacturing process were being abused in place of PCP, the Controlled Substance Act of 1986 made these derivatives illegal and established that the use of the precursor of PCP, piperidine, necessitated mandatory reporting. With this new law in place, those possessing similar but not identical illegal substances could be prosecuted. This led to a further decline in the popularity of PCP. Beginning in 1984, the overall use of PCP declined sharply, reaching a nadir in 1994.[188,203] However, during the 8 years that followed, there was a small resurgence in reported PCP use but never reaching the epidemic proportions of the 1970s. Peak reported use reached an annual prevalence rate of 2.6% in 1996 among 12th graders. The Drug Abuse Warning Network reported that the highest number of PCP-related emergencies occurred in Washington, DC; Philadelphia; Los Angeles; Chicago; and Newark.[188,190,191] Since 2003, the use of PCP has declined, and its prevalence has remained low. During these years, the National Survey on Drug Use and Health (NSDUH) reported that the annual prevalence rate of PCP use for 12th graders fluctuated between 0.7% and 1.4% with the latest report of 1.4% in 2015. Lifetime prevalence of PCP use was highest among adults aged 29 to 30 years (3.9%).[113]

Laboratory investigation of PCP derivatives led to the discovery of ketamine, a chloroketone analog. Ketamine was introduced for general clinical practice in 1970 and was marketed for humans as Ketalar and Ketaject and for veterinary use as Ketavet. Because ketamine has approximately 10% of the potency of PCP and has a much shorter duration of action, it provides greater control in clinical use.[123,227] Forty-five years of clinical experience has established that ketamine provides adequate surgical anesthesia, a rapid recovery, and less prominent emergence reactions than PCP.[66,87,180,222] Because of the simplicity and efficacy of its use, it is regularly used in operating rooms, emergency departments (EDs), and throughout the developing world, where little clinical monitoring is available during surgical and emergency procedures.[60,86-89,181,221]

Abuse of ketamine was first noted in urban areas on the West Coast in 1971.[198] During the 1980s, there were reports of its abuse internationally, including among physicians.[6,76] The nonmedical use of dissociative anesthetics has continued to increase throughout the 1990s and into the 2000s despite the common complications associated with their use.[188,192] Unfortunately, these same pharmacologic qualities that make ketamine more popular than PCP clinically are responsible for its nonmedical popularity. Ketamine is regularly consumed at all-night "rave parties" and in nightclubs because of its "hallucinatory" and "out-of-body" effects, relatively inexpensive price, and short duration of effect: a single insufflation lasts between 15 and 20 minutes.[15,49,102,105,223]

The use of ketamine is not limited to the inner city. In the past 2 decades, the media reported police arrests for possession and sale of ketamine in affluent suburban communities, which is coupled to more in-depth and frequent reporting of its toxicity among users.[49,102,178,223] By contrast to PCP, ketamine is not manufactured illegally; rather, it is diverted from legitimate medical, dental, and veterinary sources. Additionally, with the advent of the Internet in the 1990s, its availability has dangerously grown nationwide from diverted legal or illicit international pharmaceutical companies; a sham "biotech" Internet company was seized by New York City police in 2000 for selling so-called date-rape drugs, including ketamine.[11]

TABLE 83–1	Common Phencyclidine (PCP) and Ketamine Analogs	
Name	*Chemical Name*	*Other Name*
PCP Analogs		
PCE	N-ethyl-1-phenylcyclohexylamine	Cyclohexamine
TCP	(1-(1-(Thiophen-2-yl)cyclohexyl) piperidine)	Tenocyclidine
PCPy	1-(1-Phenylcyclohexy)pyrrolidine	Rolicyclidine, PHP
Ketamine Analogs		
3-MeO-2-oxo-PCE	2-(3-Methoxyphenyl)-2-(ethylamino) cyclohexanone	Methoxetamine
3-MeO-PCE	2-(3-Methoxyphenyl)-2-(ethylamino) cyclohexane	Methoxieticyclidine
2-MK	2-(2-Methylphenyl)-2-(methylamino) cyclohexanone	2-MeO-ketamine
N-EK	2-(2-Chlorophenyl)-2-(ethylamino) cyclohexanone	N-ethylnorketamine

Adverse reactions do occur, although there are few reports of fatalities secondary to ketamine, even during this period (1990s and 2000s) of increased use.[80,125,131,156] Because of its abuse potential, ketamine was placed in Schedule III of the Controlled Substance Act in 1999.[180] The Drug Abuse Warning Network reported that there was a more than 2,000% increase in ketamine-related ED visits between 1994 and 2001. Despite any clear reason, after peaking in 2001, there was a decline in ketamine-related ED visits in the United States in 2002.[189,192] The use of ketamine has remained very low since 2006 with an annual prevalence rate at or below 1.4% for high school students and 0.7% for young adults in 2015.[113] The 2011 Central Registry of Drug Abuse by the government of Hong Kong reported that ketamine remained the most common psychotropic substance used among youth since 2001. The Hong Kong Poison Information Centre reported that ketamine drug-related ED visits rose from 16% in 2005 to 40% in 2008.[117]

In the past decade, several other PCP and ketamine analogs (eg, arylcyclohexylamines) were manufactured for their psychoactive effects (Table 83–1). These designer drugs have been synthesized as a means of evading law enforcement. There are several reports of toxicity and fatalities from the ketamine analog methoxetamine, (2-{3-methoxyphenyl}-2-{ethylamino} cyclohexanone or 3-MeO-2-oxo-PCE) since its production in 2010 by an underground pharmaceutical chemist. It is advertised as having less renal and hepatic adverse effects than ketamine. Toxicity and fatalities from methoxetamine are reported throughout Europe and Asia (Hong Kong, Taiwan, Korea, and Japan).[4] In the United States, its abuse was first reported in 2011; however, its prevalence is unknown.[55] The ban of arylcyclohexylamines in the United Kingdom in 2013 led to the use diarylethylamines as the next class of dissociatives to be abused.[163]

PHARMACOLOGY
Chemistry
The chemical name of PCP, 1-(1-phenylcyclohexyl)piperidine, provided the basis for its street acronym PCP. During its unlawful chemical synthesis, numerous analogs are made that have similar effects on the central nervous system (CNS) and are used as PCP substitutes. These "designer" arylcyclohexylamines are aliphatic- or aromatic-substituted amines, ketones, or halides and appear similar to the parent compound. More than 60 psychoactive analogs are known. These initial PCP analogs used piperidine as the synthetic precursor. They most likely resulted from a poor manufacturing process of legitimate research using piperidine as a synthetic precursor.[197] The most commonly available derivatives on the street as a white powder indistinguishable from PCP were TCP (1-(1-(Thiophen-2-yl)cyclohexyl)piperidine), PCE N-ethyl-1-phenylcyclohexylamine, and PCPy 1-(1-phenylcyclohexyl) pyrrolidine.[197] Phencyclidine, PCE, and PCPy are classified as Schedule I drugs, and the analog PCC is classified as a Schedule II drug.

Ketamine and tiletamine, two legal analogs of PCP, are used clinically for sedation and anesthesia. In larger quantities, both are also used in veterinary medicine for animal sedation. Tiletamine, in combination with zolazepam (Telazol), is commonly used for animal procedures in veterinary medicine. Ketamine is the only dissociative anesthetic product manufactured for human use for the purposes of anesthesia, conscious sedation, and the treatment of bronchospasm. The development of a mechanistic approach to pain therapy in the past 30 years has brought a renewed interest in the use of ketamine as an adjuvant to multimodal pain treatment. Ketamine is used therapeutically in children and adults in the management of postoperative pain. For the treatment of pain, ketamine is administered intravenously (median dose, 0.4 mg/kg; range, 0.1–1.6), orally, intramuscularly, rectally, subcutaneously, intraarticularly, caudally, epidurally, transdermally, or intranasally or added to a patient-controlled analgesia device.[69,90,98,119,184]

In the past 15 years, clinical studies support the rapid antidepressant effect of ketamine. Subanesthetic doses of 0.25 mg/kg to 0.5 mg/kg administered intravenously for 40 to 60 minutes to patients with refractory major depressive disorder provide a 25% to 85% antidepressant response lasting 3 to 7 days postinfusion. Positive results are also encountered in patients with bipolar depression, anxious depression, depression not responsive to electroconvulsive therapy, and posttraumatic stress disorder. The use of repeated infusions is also under investigation to measure the extended antidepressant effects of ketamine.[3] Although these studies report only transient neurocognitive and psychotomimetic effects with ketamine infusions, the dosing, maintenance of response, mode of delivery, and risk-to-benefit ratio of treatment sustainability are under investigation.[1]

The molecular structure of ketamine (2-{ortho-chlorophenyl}-2-methylaminocyclohexanone) contains a chiral center, producing a racemic mixture of 2 resolvable optical isomers or enantiomers, the S(+)-isomer and R(−)-isomer. Commercially available preparations of ketamine contain equal concentrations of the 2 enantiomers. These 2 molecules differ in their pharmacodynamic effects. In a randomized, double-blind evaluation of patients undergoing surgery, the S(+)-isomer of ketamine was a more effective anesthetic but manifested a higher incidence of psychotic emergence reactions than the R(−)-isomer. In other studies, the S(+)-isomer caused a greater increase in both blood pressure and pulse than the R(−)-isomer and had more bronchodilatory effects.[181,222] The R(-) ketamine enantiomers produce longer lasting antidepressant effects than the S(+) enantiomers.[234]

Ketamine analogs are "designer" dissociatives made by clandestine chemists. These new arylcyclohexylamides belong to the subclassification anisylcyclohexylamine and are more difficult to synthesize than the initial PCP analogs. Methoxetamine is a derivative of ketamine that is suggested to have a decreased anesthetic effect because of its 3-methoxy group. The addition of an ethyl group to its cyclic ring is thought to diminish urologic toxicity. However, because it is not a legally manufactured pharmaceutical, the only human experience is derived from its nonmedical reports. Less reported anilsylcyclohexylamines are 3-MeO-PCE (2-(3-methoxyphenyl)-2-{ethylamino}cyclohexane), 2-MK (2-MeO-deschloroketamine), and N-EK (N-ethylnorketamine). Diphenidine (1-{1,2-diphenethyl}piperidine) and 2-Me-O-diphenidine (1-{1-(2-methoxyphenyl)-2-phenylethyl}piperidine) are examples of diarylethylamines that have N-methyl-D-aspartate (NMDA) activity used in research.[163]

Pharmacokinetics and Toxicokinetics
Phencyclidine is a white, stable solid that is readily soluble in both water and ethanol. It is a weak base with a pK_a between 8.6 and 9.4 with a high lipid-to-water-partition coefficient (log D = 3.63). It is rapidly absorbed from the respiratory and the gastrointestinal (GI) tracts; as such, it is typically self-administered by the oral, nasal, inhalational, IV, or subcutaneous routes.

The effects of PCP are dependent on routes of delivery and dose. Its onset of action is most rapid from the IV and inhalational routes (2–5 minutes) and slowest (30–60 minutes) after GI absorption.[47,48] Sedation is commonly produced by doses of 0.25 mg intravenously; ingestion typically requires 1 to 5 mg to produce similar sedation. Signs and symptoms of toxicity usually last

4 to 6 hours, and large overdoses generally resolve within 24 to 48 hours, but effects persist in chronic users.[20,62,65,136,161,177] However, in PCP-toxic patients, the relationships between dose, clinical effects, and serum concentrations are neither reliable nor predictable.

There are several explanations for the protracted CNS effects of PCP. The large volume of distribution of 6.2 L/kg[47,230] and high lipid solubility account for its entry and storage in adipose and brain tissue. Also, on reaching the acidic cerebrospinal fluid (CSF), PCP becomes ionized, producing CSF concentrations approximately 6 to 9 times greater than those of serum.[153]

Phencyclidine undergoes first-order elimination over a wide range of doses. It has an apparent terminal elimination half-life of 21 ± 3 hours under both control and overdose settings.[47] Ninety percent of PCP is metabolized in the liver and 10% is excreted in the urine unchanged. Phencyclidine undergoes hepatic oxidative hydroxylation into 2 monohydroxylated and one dihydroxylated metabolites.[48] All 3 compounds are subsequently conjugated to form the more water-soluble glucuronide derivatives and then excreted in the urine. A variety of isoforms of CYP3A and CYP2B are involved in the metabolism of PCP. Hydroxylation at the piperidine ring is carried out by CYP1A and at the cyclohexyl ring by CYP3A.[130] Thiol adducts of PCP inactivate CYP2B6 in a mechanism-based manner.[115]

Urine pH is an important determinant of renal elimination of PCP. In acidic urine, PCP becomes ionized and then cannot be reabsorbed. Acidification of the urine increased renal clearance of PCP from 1.98 ± 0.48 L/h to 2.4 ± 0.78 L/h.[47] If the urine pH is decreased to less than 5.0, even higher renal clearance (8.04 ± 1.56 L/h) was noted.[14] Although this accounts for a 23% increase in the renal clearance, it only represents a 1.1% increase of the total clearance, and therefore we recommend against acidification. Additionally, in an agitated patient with rhabdomyolysis, acidification of the urine will worsen myoglobin clearance and therefore kidney function.

Ketamine is water soluble (log P 2.6) and has a high lipid solubility (log D = 2.01) that enables it to distribute to the CNS readily.[45] It has a pK_a of 7.5 and a volume of distribution of 1.8 ± 0.7 L/kg. Ketamine has approximately 10% of the potency of PCP.[87,106] Human trials demonstrate that similar to PCP, the clinical effects of ketamine are both route and dose dependent.[51,54,66,204] Peak blood concentrations occur within 1 minute of IV administration and within 5 minutes of a 5-mg/kg intramuscular (IM) injection.[222,235] Ketamine distributes rapidly into the CNS with the duration of its hypnotic and anesthetic effects extended by its slow redistribution from the brain to other tissues.[222] Recovery time averages 15 minutes for IV administration but is 30 and 120 minutes after IM administration. Oral and rectal doses are not well absorbed and undergo substantial first-pass metabolism.[181,222] In contrast to oral administration of ketamine in which clinical effects persist for 4 to 8 hours, after nasal administration, they last for 45 to 90 minutes.

Ketamine is extensively metabolized in the liver by CYP2B6 and to a lesser extent by CYP3A4 and CYP2C9.[232] Its biotransformation is complex with numerous metabolites described.[5,181,222] The major pathway involves its N-demethylation to norketamine, a metabolite with one-third the anesthetic potency of ketamine. Norketamine is hydroxylated at different sites within its hexanone ring, producing varying second chiral centers. The majority of these diastereoisomers are glucuronidated to more water-soluble derivatives that are then excreted in the urine.[87,181] Ketamine also undergoes ring hydroxylation before N-demethylation as a minor metabolic pathway. The elimination half-life, which reflects both metabolic and excretory phases, is 2.3 ± 0.5 hours and is prolonged when xenobiotics requiring hepatic metabolism are coadministered.[133] Because of the enzymatic metabolism, both tolerance and enzyme induction are reported after chronic administration.[87,181]

Methoxetamine is a white solid demonstrating aqueous and lipid solubility. Pharmacokinetic data for methoxetamine are obtained from in vivo animal studies and from in vitro studies with human hepatocytes and microsomes. The major metabolic pathway of methoxetamine is N-deethylation by cytochromes CYP2B6 and CYP3A4 into normethoxetamine. Minor pathways include O-demethylation (CYP2B6, and CYP2C19), hydroxylation (CYP2B6) and reduction reactions into the respective metabolites O-desmethylmethoxetamine, hydroxymethoxetamine, and dihydromethoxetamine. Urine analysis from patients with methoxetamine toxicity confirm these metabolites.[151]

Available Forms

Phencyclidine is available illicitly in a variety of forms, including powder, liquid, tablets, leaf mixtures, and rock crystal. Because of its uncontrolled illegal manufacture, the contents of products sold as PCP vary considerably, with powder often the purest form. A typical dose consumed contains approximately 5 mg.[175] Leaf mixtures are made by sprinkling approximately 1 to 10 mg of PCP onto parsley, oregano, mint, tobacco, or marijuana. A PCP joint (known as "crystal joint," "KJ," or "supergrass") is developed for smoking and contains about 1 mg of PCP/150 mg of plant product.[9] Mentholated cigarettes dipped into liquid PCP are known as "supercools."

Phencyclidine is included in the federal Controlled Substance Act of 1970, reducing its availability for incorporation into marijuana cigarettes. There are reports of marijuana cigarettes being adulterated with PCP and sold on the street under varying names such as "Illy" in Connecticut, "Hydro" in New York City, "Dip" in New Jersey, "Wet" in Philadelphia, and "Fry" in Texas.[100]

The cigarettes are purportedly treated with "embalming fluid," which allegedly enhances the euphoric effects of the drug. Rather, the embalming fluid or another organic solvent is used as a medium to allow a uniform distribution of PCP in these cigarettes.[100] Furthermore, the organic solvent is thought to be the remnant of the organic solvent used in the synthesis of PCP or one of its analogs. In either case, the ability to smoke the cigarette before drying after dipping in the solvent–PCP (nonaqueous) mixture accounts for some of its various names (eg, wet hydro). In most cases, this "enhanced" mixture appears to be purchased intentionally rather than having the PCP placed in these cigarettes surreptitiously.

On the street and on the Internet, ketamine is known as "vitamin K," "Special K," "Super K," "Ket," or simply "K." It is available in a liquid form that is dried into a pure-white crystalline powder and is typically self-administered by ingestion or insufflation in a fashion similar to PCP. It is rarely injected IV or IM in aqueous form.

When used by injection, there is an observed demographic and behavioral difference among those who initiate drug injection use with ketamine and those who initiate injection use with another xenobiotic and later transition into ketamine injection.[128] The majority of individuals whose initial injection drug use was ketamine administered it intramuscularly. These individuals almost solely used the liquid form. Those who initiated injection drug use with drugs other than ketamine did so intravenously.

Ketamine is primarily sold as tablets, capsules, or powder. These formulations are often adulterated with caffeine, methylenedioxymethamphetamine (MDMA), ephedrine, methamphetamine, heroin, and cocaine (a mixture known as CK or Calvin Klein).[63,185] In fact, in addition to ethanol, MDMA (39%), heroin (17%), and cocaine (14%) are the most frequently mentioned xenobiotics used with ketamine.[211] Exemplifying the commercial growth of ketamine, some of the tablets are even found to contain a "K" logo.[63] Common sedating doses are 75 to 300 mg orally (30–75 mg for insufflation). Higher doses, ranging between 300 and 450 mg orally (100–250 mg for insufflation), result in substantial CNS toxicity. These manifestations are similar to the clinical "emergence reactions" that patients experience after ketamine anesthesia.

New designer dissociatives (methoxetamine, 2-MK and N-EK) are currently sold through the Internet internationally as powders that are ingested, insufflated, or injected. Methoxetamine is used extensively in the United Kingdom and is referred to by various names, including MXE, M-ket, Kmax, Mexxy, Special-M, MEX, legal ketamine, and Minx. Case reports indicate that the clinical symptoms of patients with methoxetamine toxicity are similar to those reported from ketamine.[55,99,218,229] After the ban on arylcyclohexylamines in 2012 in the United Kingdom, the beige crystalline solid, 2-MK, and the white powder, N-EK, became available online in many countries where they are unscheduled.[163]

PATHOPHYSIOLOGY

The arylcyclohexylamines, are a group of anesthetics that functionally and electrophysiologically "dissociate" the somatosensory cortex from higher centers.[51,221] The precise mechanisms by which they achieve these effects are complex and not fully understood; however, investigation of the nature of PCP-induced psychosis has led to a substantial identification of the various sites of PCP activity.

Most studies demonstrate that arylcyclohexylamines bind with high affinity to sites located in the cortex and limbic structures of the brain.[140] They block the NMDA receptors at serum concentrations encountered clinically.[215,236] Analogs of PCP (TCP, PCE, PHP, ketamine) and the most potent, dizocilpine (MK-801), also interact with the NMDA receptors in a dose–response manner that corresponds with their neurobehavioral effect.[29,187,194,224] Binding to the NMDA receptor occurs at a site independent of glutamate.[106,111,140,187,226] This site is located within the ionotropic channel, partially overlapping the Mg^{2+} binding site, and it is often termed the PCP binding site. As such, they antagonize the action of glutamate on this channel and noncompetitively block Ca^{2+} influx (Fig. 13–14).

Arylcyclohexylamines also bind to the biogenic amine reuptake complex but with 10% to 20% of the affinity to which they bind to the NMDA receptor. Binding occurs at physiologic concentrations that normally take place after subanesthetic doses.[7,171] This weak inhibition of the catecholamine reuptake accounts for the respective sympathomimetic and psychomotor effects. An increase in blood pressure and heart rate is induced. Rapid IV infusion produces a more pronounced effect than by IM injection, with the S(+)-isomer having a greater effect than the R(−)-isomer.[222]

In large overdoses, arylcyclohexylamines also stimulate σ receptors at concentrations generally associated with coma, although with lower affinity than NMDA receptors.[205,225] Both D_2 and σ receptors have an inhibitory effect on the cholinergic receptor pathways.[225] At the higher concentrations, typically associated with death, arylcyclohexylamines bind to the nicotinic, opioid, and muscarinic cholinergic receptors.[214]

N-methyl-D-aspartate receptor antagonists produce effects on behavior, sensation, and cognition that resemble aspects of endogenous psychoses, particularly schizophrenia.[107,168] These behavioral abnormalities were first observed in studies in the late 1950s when PCP, administered to healthy volunteers, generated an organic psychosis that mimicked schizophrenia. When PCP was administered to patients with schizophrenia, it uniformly intensified their primary symptoms of profound disorganization, and some of these symptoms lasted for weeks.[136] Phencyclidine psychosis has such similarity clinically to schizophrenia that many psychiatrists cannot distinguish the entities without a prior indication of drug abuse history.[203] The multireceptor action of PCP and its link to schizophrenia are made more intriguing because various antipsychotics (eg, phenothiazines, thioxanthenes, and butyrophenones) are also σ agonists.[83]

Current interest in the role of excitatory neurotransmitter systems in the pathophysiology of schizophrenia produced similar observations in patients after ketamine administration. Subanesthetic doses of ketamine administered to both healthy and schizophrenic volunteers induced a mild, dose-related, short-lasting increase in psychotic symptoms. Although the normal and schizophrenic volunteers had different levels of baseline psychosis, the magnitude, time course, and dose–response changes in positive symptoms were similar between the 2 populations. Both groups experienced thought disorganization, such as concreteness and loose association, hallucinations, and delusions of varying intensity.[123,125-127]

There is a connection between PCP psychosis and sensory processing. Arylcyclohexylamines inhibit sensory perception in a dose-dependent manner. This processing in sensory information corresponds to their relative affinities to the NMDA receptor and not to the σ receptor.[9,171] Clinically, the impairment of sensory input produced by PCP resembles that of patients who are deprived of sensory stimulation.[147] When external stimulation was reduced by environmental sensory deprivation, the psychotomimetic effects of PCP were diminished,[44] giving credence to the theory that it is not anxiety that causes perceptual dysfunction in schizophrenia but the converse.

Many of the NMDA receptor antagonists have a negative effect on cognition and memory. Repeated administration of arylcyclohexylamines in many animal models results in cognitive and memory impairment.[95,109] They impair concentration, recall, learning, and retention of new information.[18,32,59,62,81,94-96,123,144,155,165] In human volunteers, ketamine selectively impairs explicit,[80] episodic,[58,158] and procedural memory[158] and disrupts frontal cortical function, as measured by the Wisconsin Card Sorting Task and verbal fluency,[123,144] in a dose-dependent manner. Learning and memory impairment in volunteers who were administered subanesthetic doses of ketamine (0.65 mg/kg) are independent of the subject's attention and related psychosis.[144] Testing performed on chronic ketamine users produces similar results that are long lasting and have more marked effects on semantic and episodic memory.[58,60,159,160] Accordingly, it is presumed that the acute and repeated NMDA receptor antagonism interferes with the functions that integrate interoceptive and exteroceptive input in which goal-directed action becomes possible, similar to the organic psychosis in schizophrenia. Because the rapid antidepressant effects have the potential for either continuous or repeated dosing, current research will of necessity address the long-term adverse effects.

Hypofunction of the NMDA receptor causes neuroanatomical and neurobehavioral effects. Animals exposed to NMDA antagonists such as PCP and dizocilpine transiently demonstrated neuronal vacuolar degeneration in the retrosplenial cortex and the posterior cingulate areas of the brain.[166,167] The major function of cingulate cortical neurons is to mediate affective responses to pain.[216] Single high doses (PCP, 18 mg/kg; ketamine, 40 mg/kg; tiletamine, 20 mg/kg) or repeated exposures to NMDA receptor antagonists are associated with a higher incidence of cellular death.[50,70,71,166] This injury seems to be related to the induction of selective expression of individual heat shock proteins in this anatomical area.[195] Such results raise concern over the use of ketamine for procedural sedation. However, several converging factors indicate its safety in humans. Doses used in animal studies are much higher than those used clinically. When higher doses are used clinically (ie, anesthesia), the sedating effects of ketamine occur as γ-aminobutyric acid (GABA) and σ receptors are activated, decreasing excitation. Also, human elimination kinetics of ketamine differ from those in animal studies. Excitatory amino acids are neurotransmitters responsible for mediating seizure activity in the brain. As NMDA inhibitors, the anticonvulsant properties of the arylcyclohexylamines are inconclusive. Animals administered PCP or PCP analogs progress through dose-related clonic activity followed by tonic–clonic convulsions, as is typical of classic convulsants.[171] Animal research also demonstrates wide interspecies variability of the electroencephalographic (EEG) effects of PCP.[65] In a murine seizure model, ketamine possessed selective anticonvulsant properties.[33] In addition, ketamine preserves learning proficiency in rats when administered shortly after onset of status epilepticus, an effect that is useful in the clinical setting when combined with conventional antiepileptics.[206]

In humans, although these dissociatives induce excitatory activity in the thalamus and limbic areas, they do not affect cortical regions.[53,54,66,77] Excitation, muscle twitching, posturing,[154] and tonic–clonic motor activity with or without EEG changes are reported with these subcortical EEG alterations.[36,52,77,154] In the clinical setting, many report ketamine to possess antiepileptic properties at clinically relevant doses that may be explained by an NMDA inhibitory effect.[36,52] This effect was used to treat patients with refractory status epilepticus in the critical care setting.[210]

The NMDA receptor is also responsible for the development of the neuronal organization of the CNS.[103,199,200] It is linked to hypoxic–ischemic brain injury by mediating calcium influx, a final pathway in cell death. The uninhibited firing of NMDA afferent neurons secondary to brain injury causes their death, as well as the death of efferent neurons downstream. In neonatal rats, ketamine increases the rate of neuronal apoptosis.[194] N-methyl D-aspartate receptor antagonists such as PCP block hypoxic brain injury from stroke and trauma.[21,135] In a rat model of ischemic stroke, PCP had a protective effect on the brain, demonstrated by a decreased rate of seizure activity.[21] This effect is transient and has not been studied in humans.

Neuronal development, plasticity, and connectivity are modulated by NMDA receptors. The phenotypic outcome of receptor malfunction is indicated by genetics, the extent and duration of malfunction (ie, from xenobiotic toxicity or illness), and neuroanatomical location (pre- and postsynaptic neuronal interactions or both). Polymorphisms of GRIN2B (encoding NMDA receptor's GluN2B subunit) are associated with schizophrenia. Animal studies using high doses of an NMDA receptor antagonist resulted in deleterious neuronal effects.[70,71,166] Postmortem and in vivo structural neuroimaging studies in patients with schizophrenia demonstrate a decreased number of dendritic spines, decreased axon dendrite arborization, reduced neuropil volume, and disarray of neuronal orientation in the cortex. It is thought that NMDA receptor hypofunction in mesolimbic areas of these patients leads to an excitatory feedback in the prefrontal cortex via GABAergic interneurons. This disrupted mesocorticolimbic connectivity underlies the cognitive and psychotomimetic impairment of this disease.[121] Stress and major depressive disorders also produce continuous glutaminergic states that cause neuronal atrophy, dendritic retraction, decreased spine density, reduced dendritic arborization, and synaptic strength in the prefrontal cortex. Treatment of depression with low dose ketamine is based on the premise that by blocking presynaptic disinhibition of glutamatergic neurons, a glutamine surge occurs that through a cascade of cellular events (involving postsynaptic α-amino-3-hydroxy-5-methyl-4isoxazoleproprionic acid {AMPA} receptors, extrasynaptic NMDA receptors and brain-derived neurotrophic factors {BDNF}, and mammalian target of rapamycin {mTORC1}) restore prefrontal connectivity.[3]

CLINICAL MANIFESTATIONS

The reported signs and symptoms of arylcyclohexylamine toxicity are variable. The variations are a result of differences in dosage, the multiple routes of administration, concomitant xenobiotic use, and other associated medical conditions. In accordance with their pharmacologic effect, arylcyclohexylamine toxicity is relatively similar producing signs and symptoms consistent with PCP but differing in potency and duration of action. Additionally, individual differences in xenobiotic susceptibility, the development of tolerance in chronic users, and contaminants in the drug manufacture account for erratic clinical findings.

Vital Signs

Body temperature is rarely affected directly by arylcyclohexylamines. In one large series of patients with PCP toxicity, only 2.6% demonstrated hyperthermia, defined as a temperature greater than 101.8°F (38.8°C).[148] In an experimental animal model, PCP failed to increase body temperature.[38,65] When hyperthermia does occur from agitation, all the known complications, including encephalopathy, rhabdomyolysis, myoglobinuria, acute kidney injury, electrolyte abnormalities, and liver failure, occur (Chap. 29).[12,22,43,173]

Most arylcyclohexylamine-toxic patients demonstrate mild sympathomimetic effects secondary to their monoamine reuptake inhibition.[138,139,181] Phencyclidine consistently increases both the systolic blood pressure (SBP) and diastolic blood pressure (DBP) in a dose-dependent fashion.[38,65] Doses of 0.06 mg/kg of IV PCP increased the SBP and DBP by 8 mm Hg, and 0.25 mg/kg produce a 26 and 19 mm Hg increase in SBP and DBP, respectively. Phencyclidine also inconsistently increases the heart rate.[92] Ketamine also produces mild increases in blood pressure, heart rate, and cardiac output via this same mechanism.[54,139,204,212,222] In fact, tachycardia was the most common finding on physical examination in a case series of ketamine users presenting to the ED.[220]

Cardiopulmonary

Cardiovascular catastrophes are rarely encountered in patients with PCP toxicity.[68,149] These complications result from direct vasospasm,[8,37] causing severe systemic hypertension, pulmonary edema, hypertensive encephalopathy,[69] and cerebral hemorrhage.[25] Hypertension, along with abnormal behavior, miosis, and nystagmus in children, strongly suggest toxicity caused by a dissociative anesthetic.[116]

The effect of PCP and ketamine on cardiac rhythm is controversial. Dysrhythmias are only observed in animals poisoned with very large doses of PCP. Ketamine both enhances and diminishes epinephrine-induced dysrhythmias in animals.[24,67,93,118] The considerable experience in the use of ketamine anesthesia on humans undergoing surgery or cardiac catheterization has not demonstrated prodysrhythmic effects.[73,162]

Because these dissociative anesthetics were designed to retain normal ventilation, hypoventilation is uncommon. In clinical studies, PCP increased the minute ventilation, tidal volume, and respiratory rate of volunteers.[92] Clinically, in PCP-toxic patients, irregular respiratory patterns occur with tachypnea much more often than with bradypnea.[12,148] Hypoventilation, when present, is usually secondary to the use of particularly high doses of PCP. Pulmonary edema secondary to respiratory depression is also a rare occurrence but was reported postmortem.[68] Large doses of PCP (20 mg/kg) administered to laboratory animals produced respiratory depression.[38] Although respiratory depression in humans is an uncommon event, it is reported with fast or high-dose infusions of ketamine.[85,222] A total of 8.3% of patients in whom ketamine was used for sedation in EDs needed to be intubated.[182] In fact, ketamine is successfully used to prevent intubation in patients with refractory asthma. Ketamine relaxes bronchial smooth muscles, decreases mean airway pressure and $PaCO_2$, and increases PaO_2.[79,183,209,222]

Neuropsychiatric

Most patients with arylcyclohexylamine toxicity who are brought to medical attention manifest diverse psychomotor abnormalities.[16,22,30,76,109,220] These xenobiotics impair responses to external stimuli by separating various elements of the mind. Consciousness, memory, perception, and motor activity appear dissociated from each other. This dissociation prevents the user from attaining cognition and properly assembling all information to construct "reality." Clinically, the person appears inebriated, either calm or agitated, and sometimes violent. In patients with large overdose, the anesthetic effect causes patients to develop stupor or coma. In recreational use, "dissociatives" are not taken for these effects but rather for out-of-body experiences. In addition, patients often have disordered thought processes (including disorientation as to time, place, and person) or amnesia, paranoia, and dysphoria.[75]

These manifestations of arylcyclohexylamine toxicity are better illustrated by the results of their effects in controlled human studies. Volunteers who took oral doses of up to 7.5 mg/d of PCP or 0.1 mg/kg of ketamine exhibited clinical toxicity, but higher doses (PCP >10 mg/d; ketamine 0.5 mg/kg) generally caused a more severe impairment of mental function.[65,123] Intravenous doses of 0.1 mg/kg of PCP[20,62,79,136,161,186] or 0.5 mg/kg of ketamine[123,171] diminish all sensory modalities (pain, touch, proprioception, hearing, taste, and visual acuity) in a dose-dependent fashion. Both xenobiotics also cause feelings of apathy, depersonalization, hostility, isolation, and alterations in body image.[20,62,78,110,143,160] The deficits in sensory modalities are evident before the development of the psychological effects of PCP, with pain perception disappearing first. This alteration in analgesic perception is caused by a blocking action on the thalamus and midbrain (Fig. 83–1).[161]

Abnormal stereognosis and proprioception occur in a dose-dependent manner. This disturbed perception results in body image distortions described as "numbness," "sheer nothingness," and "depersonalization." The decrease of proprioceptive sensation to gravity probably gives the sensation of "tripping" or "flying." Because all sensory modalities are affected, visual, auditory, and tactile illusions and delusions are common. This lack of stimuli from the surrounding environment is responsible for the "near-death experience" or the "near-birth experience" patients describe as their awareness wanes. Hallucinations are typically auditory rather than visual, which are more common with LSD use. The hallucinogenic effects of ketamine on healthy human volunteers are linearly related to steady-state concentrations between 50 and 200 ng/mL.[26] Ketamine users report experiencing a "k-hole" ("m-hole" in methoxetamine), a slang term for the intense psychological and somatic state experienced while under the influence of ketamine. This experience varies with the individual but can include buzzing, ringing,

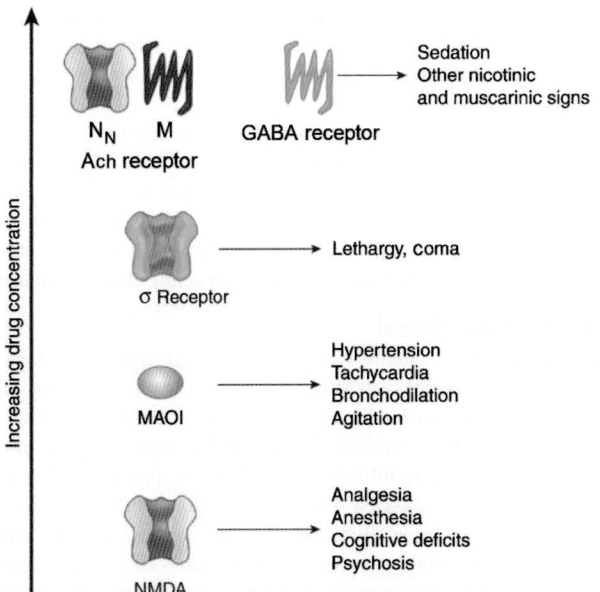

FIGURE 83–1. Clinical effects of the arylcyclohexylamines. The arylcyclohexylamines bind to different receptors in the central nervous system with varying degrees of affinity; that is, an increasing concentration is necessary to achieve the various clinical effects. ACh = acetylcholine; GABA = γ-aminobutyric acid; MAOI = monoamine oxidase inhibitor; N_N = nicotinic receptor; M = muscarinic receptor; NMDA = N-methyl-D-aspartate.

or whistling sounds; traveling through a dark tunnel; intense visions; and out-of-body or near-death sensations.[64,196]

The reaction to the misperceived or disconnected reality results in unintentional actions and violent behavior. The hallmark of PCP toxicity is the recurring delusion of superhuman strength and invulnerability resulting from both its anesthetic and dissociative properties. There are case reports of patients presenting with trauma from jumping from significant heights, fighting large crowds or the police, or self-mutilation. The true extent and incidence of violence is probably less than previously suggested.[27] These feelings of unreality and sedation are encountered in the clinical setting more commonly when low-dose ketamine is administered as an IV push as opposed to a low-dose infusion.[164]

Typical neurologic signs include horizontal, vertical, or rotatory nystagmus; ataxia; and altered gait. Initially, except for ataxia, movement is not impaired until the patient becomes unconscious. On physical examination, use of dissociative anesthetics typically produces relatively small pupils, nystagmus, and diplopia. In the largest case series reported to date, nystagmus and hypertension were noted in 57% of patients who had taken PCP.[148] Smaller and more limited studies found an incidence of nystagmus of 89% or higher.[22] In comparison, nystagmus was only found in 15% of patients with ketamine abuse.[220] Other cerebellar manifestations were also encountered, most notably dizziness, ataxia, dysarthria, and nausea. A pooled data compilation of 35 reports demonstrated that emesis occurred 8.5% of the time.[85] In fact, Internet chat groups devoted to substance abuse commonly direct users to "mix dissociatives with marijuana" for its antiemetic effect.

Larger doses of PCP produce loss of balance and confusion, the latter characterized by inability to repeat a set of objects, frequent loss of ideas, blocking, lack of concreteness, and disordered linguistic expression.[43,58,123,136,186] Similarly, ketamine users report a high incidence of incoordination, confusion, unusual thought content, and an inability to speak.[64] In general, dissociative anesthetics stimulate the CNS, but seizures rarely occur, except at high doses. The largest case series of PCP-toxic patients reported a 3.1% incidence of seizures.[148]

Although arylcyclohexylamine toxic patients also present with motor disturbances, it is unclear to what extent these dissociative drugs are actually responsible for these manifestations. The most common of the reported

disturbances are dystonic reactions: opisthotonos, torticollis, tortipelvis, and risus sardonicus (facial grimacing). Myoclonic movements, tremor, hyperactivity, athetosis, stereotypies, and catalepsy also occur.[16,31,76,148] A slight increase in muscle tone results from a dopaminergic effect.[136] Laryngospasm requiring intubation is reported after the use of ketamine anesthesia. The incidence of this complication is less than 0.017%.[87] In comparison, the incidence of laryngospasm after traditional general anesthesia is 2%.[169]

Cholinergic and Anticholinergic Effects

Both cholinergic and anticholinergic clinical manifestations occur in patients manifesting arylcyclohexylamine toxicity. Miosis or mydriasis, blurred vision, profuse diaphoresis, hypersalivation, bronchospasm, bronchorrhea, and urinary retention are reported.[16,22,132,147,148] Ketamine stimulates salivary and tracheobronchial secretions, both of which are equally and effectively inhibited by atropine and glycopyrolate.[157] Furthermore, in a randomized, double-blind trial, after infusion of 1.5 mg/kg of ketamine in healthy volunteers, physostigmine decreased nystagmus, blurred vision, and the time to recovery.[211]

Urologic and Hepatobiliary

Intense abdominal and pelvic pain is regularly reported in habitual ketamine users.[233] In the majority of cases, the cause is urologic. The first case series describing ketamine-associated urological dysfunction was reported in 2007. Symptoms consisted of a severe lower urinary tract syndrome (LUTS), including dysuria, frequency, urgency, urge incontinence, and painful hematuria (Fig. 83–2). When investigated by cystoscopy, patients with hematuria were frequently found to have ulcerative cystitis.[193]

Subsequent reports established LUTS as a complication in both recreational ketamine users as well as in a patient receiving ketamine therapeutically for chronic regional pain syndrome.[40,91,104] The incidence of ketamine-induced urologic dysfunction is not well established: whereas studies from the United Kingdom report an incidence of 20%, a study from Hong Kong reports the incidence of 32% and 92% in acute and chronic ketamine users, respectively.[146,228,233]

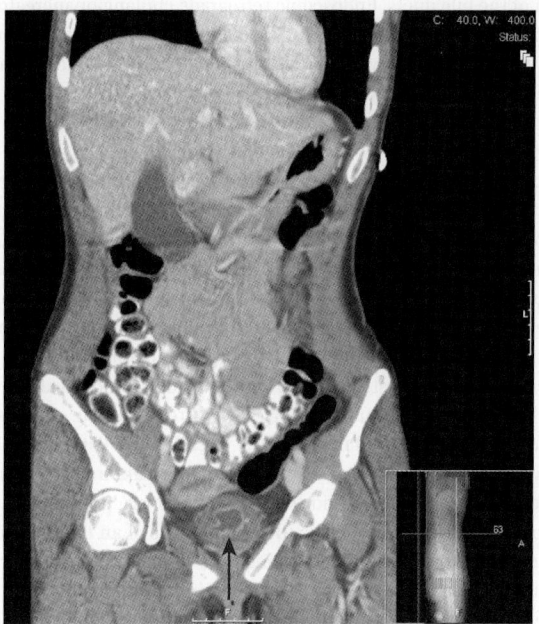

FIGURE 83–2. Ketamine-associated lower urinary tract syndrome. This abdominal-pelvic computed tomography (CT) scan was obtained in an 18-year-old girl who presented to the hospital with complaints of severe abdominal pain and hematuria. The image demonstrates a small bladder (↑) volume with an irregular thickened mucosal surface that enhances with contrast. (Used with permission from the Fellowship in Medical Toxicology, New York University School of Medicine, New York City Poison Center.)

The symptoms of ketamine-induced urologic dysfunction are secondary to an inflammatory process that reduces bladder size. Patients develop diminished voiding capacity of 20 to 200 mL, decreased bladder compliance, and detrusor overactivity as measured by urodynamic testing. A thickened bladder wall, a small bladder volume, and perivesicular stranding are usually detected by ultrasonography and computed tomography (CT) of the lower urological tract.[146] Cystoscopy demonstrates an erythematous bladder mucosa with various degrees of ulcerations. Bladder biopsies confer epithelium denudation and ulcerative cystitis. There is a marked lymphocytic infiltration with a variable number of eosinophils and fibrosis as well as squamous metaplasia and nephrogenic metaplasia. The loss of architectural reorganization encountered in fibrosis may be caused by a loss of expression of adhesion proteins in proximal tubule epithelial cells that is reported.[97] The exact mechanism by which ketamine or one its metabolites causes the destruction of the urinary tract remains unknown.[40,41,228,233]

There is a substantially lower incidence of LUTS reported in the United Kingdom (13%) compared with 51% in Hong Kong. The lower incidence is thought to be related to the early presentation of patients in the United Kingdom seeking medical attention as opposed to those living in Hong Kong. Intravenous urography and urography by CT reveal unilateral or bilateral ureteric narrowing. Bilateral hydronephrosis was reported in 44% to 50% of patients, and renal impairment is also described.[146,152] Biopsy of the ureter in a patient who underwent right nephrectomy with an ileal conduit anastomosis to the left renal pelvis demonstrated nephrogenic metaplasia throughout the ureter extending to the renal pelvis as well as ulceration with associated inflammatory changes as described by the bladder biopsies.[101] A murine model demonstrates the similarities between bladder and renal pathology induced by methoxetamine and ketamine.[61] The pathology of ketamine-induced urologic dysfunction is not confined to the lower urinary tract. Upper urinary tract involvement is variable.

Intense abdominal pain in frequent ketamine users is also suggestive of hepatobiliary dysfunction. Case series of patients who used ketamine illicitly or therapeutically report abnormal liver function test results and biliary tract abnormalities.[134] Computerized tomography revealed common bile duct dilation with a smooth, tapered end, a condition that mimics benign cystic dilation of the bile ducts. Endoscopic retrograde cholangiopancreatography and hepatobiliary iminodiacetic acid studies concur with these findings suggesting gallbladder wall dyskinesia. These biliary abnormalities are noted to subside with cessation of ketamine use.[134]

Emergence Reaction

The acute psychosis observed during the recovery phase of PCP anesthesia limited its clinical use. This bizarre behavior, characterized by confusion, vivid dreaming, and hallucinations, is termed an "emergence reaction." These reactions occur most frequently in middle-aged men, with a reported incidence of 17% and 30%.[92,114] The most violent emergence reactions follow an IV dose of approximately 0.25 mg/kg of PCP.[65] The mildest degrees of agitation produced by PCP resemble the effects of ethanol intoxication.

These same postanesthetic reactions also limit the clinical use of ketamine. The incidence of emergence reactions after ketamine administration is approximately 50% in adults and 10% in children.[87] Patients older than age 10 years; women; and persons who normally dream frequently or have a prior personality disorder, a prior history of psychosis, premorbid denial of presence of illness or anosognosia (denial presence of an illness), and paranoia incur the greatest risk.[87,150] Although the experience of vivid dreaming and visual illusions usually cease upon regaining consciousness, their recurrence weeks after ketamine administration in both children and adults is reported.[78] The origin of these altered visual experiences is thought to be ketamine's depressive action on auditory (inferior colliculus) and visual (medial geniculate) relay centers. Feelings of floating in space or body detachment and ataxia and dizziness occur because of a decreased perception to gravity. Added to this experience are feeling of ataxia and dizziness.[222] The incidence of the occurrence of emergence reactions appears to be exacerbated when dissociative anesthetics are rapidly administered IV, as well as in patients exposed to excessive stimuli during recovery. Although not demonstrated in a controlled study, reducing external stimuli during the recovery phase might reduce emergence reactions.

Ironically, the very characteristics that were thought to make PCP ideal for anesthesia—the preservation of muscle tone and cardiopulmonary function—exacerbate the difficulties in managing an individual who manifests dysphoria associated with an overdose. The course of delirium, stupor, and coma associated with PCP and ketamine is extremely variable, although the manifestations are much milder and shorter acting after ketamine use.

Tolerance and Withdrawal

Phencyclidine induces modest tolerance in rats and squirrel monkeys. The development of tolerance is mostly secondary to the pharmacologic effects of PCP rather than to biodispositional changes. Dependence was also observed in monkeys who self-administered PCP (10 mg/kg/d to serum concentrations of 100–300 ng/mL) over 1 month by the appearance of dramatic withdrawal signs when access was denied. Signs included vocalizations, bruxism, oculomotor hyperactivity, diarrhea, piloerection, difficulty remaining awake, tremors, and in one case convulsions.[19] These signs appeared within 8 hours of abstinence and were most severe at about 24 hours. When either PCP or ketamine (2.5 mg/kg/h) was readministered to the animals, PCP withdrawal symptoms were ameliorated, indicating cross-dependence between PCP and ketamine.[23,108,202]

Physiologic dependence in humans is not formally studied. It is implied to occur by the observation that chronic PCP users developed depression, anxiety, irritability, lack of energy, sleep disturbance, and disturbed thoughts after 1 day of abstinence from drug use.[179] Additionally, neonates whose mothers used PCP developed jitteriness, vomiting, and hypertonicity that lasted for at least 2 weeks.[208] These symptoms represent PCP withdrawal or intrinsic teratogenic effects on neurologic development.[84,103] Although there are no controlled studies observing the physiologic symptoms of withdrawal in humans who chronically use PCP or ketamine, there is a definite psychological dependence on the sensations experienced during recreational use.[198] There are a few cases of ketamine tolerance in which patients report a need to use an increased quantity of drug to achieve the same effects.[57,157,172] In a study of ketamine abstinence, patients characterized their withdrawal symptoms as anxiety, shaking, sweating, and palpitations.[159] In addition, ketamine impairs response inhibition, which is related to increases in subjective ratings of desire for the drug.[158]

DIAGNOSTIC TESTING

If it is necessary to confirm the suspicion of PCP usage, urine is most commonly used matrix for analysis, although serum, and possibly gastric contents, can also be used. Rarely is it essential to make this determination. Most hospital laboratories do not perform quantitative analysis of PCP, but many can perform a qualitative urine test for its presence. Qualitative testing is more important than a quantitative determination as serum concentrations do not correlate closely with the clinical effects. Phencyclidine is qualitatively detected by an enzyme immunoassay at a cutoff calibration of 25 ng/mL.[176] High-affinity antibodies were once studied as specific PCP antagonists to reverse PCP-induced toxicity.[170,213] The detection of PCP is thus dependent on the concentration of PCP in the body fluid tested and the affinity of the antibody for the PCP molecule. As such, the immunoassay antibody binding to a molecule similar to PCP can produce false-positive reactions. Metabolites of PCP, such as PCE, PHP, and TCP and its pyrrolizidine derivative TCPy, cross-react with the immunoassay at concentrations 30 times higher than those used to detect PCP. Because of its similar structure to PCP, dextromethorphan and its metabolite dextrorphan also cross-react with Syva enzyme-multiplied immunoassay and fluorescence polarization PCP assays (Chap. 7).[219]

Although nonspecific, laboratory findings associated with PCP use include leukocytosis, hypoglycemia, and elevated concentrations of muscle enzymes (CPK), myoglobin, blood urea nitrogen (BUN), and creatinine.[148] In patients administered ketamine, the EEG reveals diffuse slowing with θ and δ waves, which return to normal before the patient improves clinically.[36,53]

There is no commercially available quantitative immunoassay for ketamine or methoxetamine. When necessary, they are detected by gas chromatography and mass spectroscopy. The increase in popularity in ketamine use in certain parts of the world has led to the development of rapid-detection urine assays that are sensitive, specific, and accurate.[39,217] There is anecdotal evidence that ketamine also cross-reacts with the urine PCP immunoassay because of their structural similarity.[197] Other authors, including the manufacturer that tests the reactivity of the commercially available PCP immunoassay with ketamine, do not find such results.[34,220]

MANAGEMENT
Agitation

Conservative management is indicated for patients with arylcyclohexylamine toxicity and includes maintaining adequate respiration, circulation, and thermoregulation. The psychobehavioral symptoms observed during acute dissociative reactions and during the emergence reaction are similar. To treat the symptoms of agitation and alteration of mental status, it is helpful to recognize that both pharmacologic[2,42,46,72,87,89,141,145] and behavioral[44,46,87,124] modalities are used to diminish agitation and emergence phenomena during conscious sedation with ketamine. To prevent self-injury, a common form of PCP-induced morbidity and mortality, the patient must be safely restrained, initially physically, and then medically sedated. An IV catheter should be inserted and blood drawn for electrolytes, glucose, BUN, and creatinine concentrations. The use of 0.5 to 1.0 g/kg of body weight of dextrose and 100 mg of IV thiamine HCl should be administered as clinically indicated.

Hyperthermia occurs secondary to psychomotor agitation and should be rapidly identified. Treatment should be accomplished immediately with adequate sedation to control motor activity. At presentation, placing the patient in a quiet room with low sensory stimuli will help achieve this goal. Physical restraint should only be used temporarily, if necessary, until medical sedation is achieved. Rapid immersion in an ice water bath is recommended when body temperatures greater than 106°F (41.1°C) place the patient at great risk for end-organ injury.[129] These patients will need volume repletion and electrolyte supplementation because hyperthermia increases fluid loss from sweat.

In the pharmacologic treatment of emergence reactions, benzodiazepines are recommended as the first-line sedatives. A benzodiazepine such as diazepam, administered in titrated doses of up to 10 mg intravenously every 5 to 10 minutes until agitation is controlled, is usually safe and effective. Numerous studies demonstrate the benefits of benzodiazepines, but under certain conditions,[17,42] they prolong recovery time.[35,145] Additionally, in a double-blind, placebo-controlled study, lorazepam reduced the anxiety associated with ketamine without reducing the cognitive or psychotomimetic effects of ketamine (Antidotes in Depth: A26).[122] By contrast, phenothiazines lower the seizure threshold, and both phenothiazines and butyrophenones cause acute dystonic reactions. Phenothiazines also cause significant hypotension because of their α-adrenergic blocking effects on the vasculature, worsen hyperthermia, and exacerbate any anticholinergic effects and they should therefore be avoided.

Some behavioral modalities are implemented in the treatment. Early studies demonstrated that the psychotomimetic effects of PCP were diminished when external stimulation was reduced by environmental sensory deprivation.[44] When feasible, agitated patients should be placed in a single quiet room with minimal sensory stimulation to diminish potential harm to self, staff, or other patients. Conversely, it is observed in patients undergoing ketamine anesthesia that emergence reactions are less violent when patients are talked to or when music is played.[124,201]

Although it is always important to ask the patient the names, quantities, times, and route of all xenobiotics taken, the information obtained may be unreliable. Even when the patient is trying to cooperate and give an accurate history, many street psychoactive xenobiotics are mixtures, with the contents being unknown to the patient. Consequently, pharmacologic management is complex and often sign or symptom dependent. Although some authors have attempted to define the appropriate therapy for specific PCP congeners and for ketamine-induced psychosis, no single approach is consistently efficacious.[81,82,120,142]

Decontamination

Patients with a history of recent oral use of arylcyclohexylamines are candidates for GI decontamination. Although there is rarely, if ever, an indication for orogastric lavage, aggressive decontamination is indicated if potentially lethal coingestants are suspected. Activated charcoal (1 g/kg) is recommended as soon as possible and repeated in 4 hours for 2 doses as long as no contraindications exist. Activated charcoal effectively adsorbs PCP and increases its nonrenal clearance even without prior gastric evacuation. This approach is usually adequate.[174]

Theoretically, xenobiotics that are weak bases, such as PCP, can be eliminated more rapidly if the urine is acidified. Although urinary acidification with ammonium chloride was previously recommended,[13] we do not recommend this approach. The risks associated with acidifying the urine—simultaneously inducing an acidemia, thereby potentially increasing urinary myoglobin precipitation—outweigh any perceived benefits (Chap. 6).

As opposed to the problems in applying ion trapping to renal excretion, ion trapping results in the active mobilization of PCP into gastric secretions. Phencyclidine is in a substantially ionized (and therefore non–lipid-soluble) form in the acid of the stomach and is absorbed only when it reaches the more alkaline intestine. As a result, gastric suction can remove a significant amount of the xenobiotic and interrupt the gastroenteric circulation by which the xenobiotic is secreted into the acid environment of the stomach, only to be reabsorbed again in the small intestine.[13] However, continuous gastric suction is unnecessary and can be dangerous. Continuous suction results in trauma to the patient as well as in fluid and electrolyte loss, which further complicate management and possibly interfere with the efficacy of activated charcoal. For these reasons, the administration of single or multiple-dose activated charcoal rather than continuous nasogastric suction appears to be the safest and most effective way of removing ion trapped drug from the stomach in severely poisoned patients.

Most patients rapidly regain normal CNS function within 45 minutes to several hours after its use. However, those who have taken exceedingly high doses or who have an underlying psychiatric disorder may remain comatose or exhibit bizarre behavior for days or even weeks before returning to normal. Those who rapidly regain normal function should be monitored for several hours and then, after a psychiatric consultation, should receive drug counseling and additional social support as indicated. Patients whose recovery is delayed should be treated supportively and monitored carefully in an intensive care unit.

Many patients become depressed and anxious during the "post-high" period, and chronic users manifest a variety of psychiatric disturbances.[231] These individuals typically present with repeated drug use, hospitalizations, and poor psychosocial functioning in the long term.

The major toxicity of PCP appears to be behaviorally related: self-inflicted injuries, injuries resulting from exceptional physical exertion, and injuries sustained as a result of resisting the application of physical restraints are frequent. Patients appear to be unaware of their surroundings and sometimes even oblivious to pain because of the dissociative anesthetic effects. In addition to major trauma, rhabdomyolysis and resultant myoglobinuric acute kidney injury account in large measure for the high morbidity and mortality associated with PCP. If significant rhabdomyolysis[43,173] occurs, myoglobinuria will be present. Early fluid therapy should be used to avoid deposition of myoglobin to the kidneys. Urinary alkalinization as part of the treatment regimen for rhabdomyolysis would theoretically increase PCP reabsorption and deposition in fat stores and is not recommended.

Cystitis

The objectives of the management of ketamine-induced cystitis are establishing the diagnosis, decreasing symptoms, and maintaining kidney function. Urinalysis should be obtained on all symptomatic patients to exclude urinary tract infection, and a serum creatinine should be obtained to evaluate kidney function. However, initial urinalyses are typically sterile. For patients whose symptoms are mild, abstinence from ketamine use will be enough to reverse symptoms and pathology. Several therapeutic regimens have been tried with little success. They include antibiotics, nonsteroidal antiinflammatory drugs (NSAIDs), corticosteroids, and anticholinergics. Urologic evaluation and follow-up are necessary.[152]

Moderate and severe symptoms of LUTS are defined as daytime frequency greater than 6, nighttime frequency of one or more, regular urgency on voiding, and moderate bladder or pelvic pain. For patients with these symptoms, urologic consultation and repeated kidney function monitoring are essential. Ultrasonography and CT urography assist in detecting lower and upper tract abnormalities. In consultation with a urologist, urodynamic studies further quantify bladder voiding capacity and detrusor activity. Invasive procedures need to be undertaken in patients with impaired kidney function and deterioration. Cystoscopy aids in visualizing the bladder and exclude other causes of hematuria and LUTS. During this procedure, a bladder biopsy will further delineate mucosal pathology. Injury to the upper urologic tract imaged with CT urography. Nephrostomy insertions are necessary in patients who present with impaired kidney function secondary to ureteric narrowing. Refractory cases need to undergo surgical interventions such as augmentation enterocystoplasty, ureteroplasty, urinary diversion, cystectomy, or ileal neobladder formation.[41,101,146]

Toxic manifestations of ketamine and methoxetamine appear to be similar yet milder and shorter lived compared with PCP. In a study of 20 patients who presented with acute ketamine toxicity, all were treated conservatively and successfully with IV hydration, and sedation with benzodiazepines.[220]

SUMMARY

- Arylcyclohexylamines produce an "out-of-body experience" with seemingly hallucinatory effects.
- The action of these xenobiotics is largely mediated by the NMDA receptor.
- The neuropsychiatric toxicity is managed with supportive care and sedation.
- The popularity of ketamine is related to its lesser toxicity and milder distortion of the personality.
- A chronic effect of ketamine abuse toxicity not recognized after use of PCP is cystitis and bladder dysfunction.

REFERENCES

1. Aan Het Rot M, et al. Ketamine for depression: where do we go from here? *Biol Psychiatry.* 2012;72:537-547.
2. Abajian JC, et al. Effects of droperidol and nitrazepam on emergence reactions following ketamine anesthesia. *Anesth Analg.* 1973;52:385-389.
3. Abdallah CG, et al. Ketamine as a promising prototype for a new generation of rapid-acting antidepressants. *Ann NY Acad Sci.* 2015;1344:66-77.
4. Adamowicz P, Zuba D. Fatal intoxication with methoxetamine. *J Forensic Sci.* 2015;60(suppl 1):S264-S268.
5. Adams JD Jr, et al. Studies on the biotransformation of ketamine. 1-Identification of metabolites produced in vitro from rat liver microsomal preparations. *Biomed Mass Spectrom.* 1981;8:527-538.
6. Ahmed SN, Petchkovsky L. Abuse of ketamine. *Br J Psychiatry.* 1980;137:303.
7. Akunne HC, et al. [3H]1-[2-(2-thienyl)cyclohexyl]piperidine labels two high-affinity binding sites in human cortex: further evidence for phencyclidine binding sites associated with the biogenic amine reuptake complex. *Synapse.* 1991;8:289-300.
8. Altura BT, Altura BM. Phencyclidine, lysergic acid diethylamide, and mescaline: cerebral artery spasms and hallucinogenic activity. *Science.* 1981;212:1051-1052.
9. Anis NA, et al. The dissociative anaesthetics, ketamine and phencyclidine, selectively reduce excitation of central mammalian neurones by N-methyl-aspartate. *Br J Pharmacol.* 1983;79:565-575.
10. Anonymous. Phencyclidine: the new American street drug. *Br Med J.* 1980;281:1511-1512.
11. Anonymous. Police say web site was sham to sell drugs. *The New York Times.* Feb 25, 2000:6.
12. Armen R, et al. Phencyclidine-induced malignant hyperthermia causing submassive liver necrosis. *Am J Med.* 1984;77:167-172.
13. Aronow R, Done AK. Phencyclidine overdose: an emerging concept of management. *JACEP.* 1978;7:56-59.
14. Aronow R, et al. Clinical observations during phencyclidine intoxication and treatment based on ion-trapping. *NIDA Res Monogr.* 1978:218-228.
15. Awuonda M. Swedes alarmed at ketamine misuse. *Lancet.* 1996;348:122.
16. Bailey DN. Phencyclidine abuse. Clinical findings and concentrations in biological fluids after nonfatal intoxication. *Am J Clin Pathol.* 1979;72:795-799.
17. Bailey ME, et al. Pulmonary histopathology in cocaine abusers. *Hum Pathol.* 1994;25:203-207.
18. Bakker CB, Amini FB. Observations on the psychotomimetic effects of Sernyl. *Compr Psychiatry.* 1961;2:269-280.
19. Balster RL, Woolverton WL. Continuous-access phencyclidine self-administration by rhesus monkeys leading to physical dependence. *Psychopharmacology.* 1980;70:5-10.
20. Ban TA, et al. Observations on the action of Sernyl—a new psychotropic drug. *Can Psychiatr Assoc J.* 1961;6:150-157.
21. Barone FC, et al. Pharmacological profile of a novel neuronal calcium channel blocker includes reduced cerebral damage and neurological deficits in rat focal ischemia. *Pharmacol Biochem Behav.* 1994;48:77-85.
22. Barton CH, et al. Phencyclidine intoxication: clinical experience in 27 cases confirmed by urine assay. *Ann Emerg Med.* 1981;10:243-246.
23. Beardsley PM, Balster RL. Behavioral dependence upon phencyclidine and ketamine in the rat. *J Pharmacol Exp Ther.* 1987;242:203-211.
24. Bednarski RM, et al. Reduction of the ventricular arrhythmogenic dose of epinephrine by ketamine administration in halothane-anesthetized cats. *Am J Vet Res.* 1988;49:350-354.
25. Bessen HA. Intracranial hemorrhage associated with phencyclidine abuse. *JAMA.* 1982;248:585-586.
26. Bowdle TA, et al. Psychedelic effects of ketamine in healthy volunteers: relationship to steady-state plasma concentrations. *Anesthesiology.* 1998;88:82-88.
27. Brecher M, et al. Phencyclidine and violence: clinical and legal issues. *J Clin Psychopharmacol.* 1988;8:397-401.
28. Brown JK, Malone MH. Status of drug quality in the street-drug market—an update. *Clin Toxicol.* 1976;9:145-168.
29. Browne RG. Discriminative stimulus properties of PCP mimetics. *NIDA Res Monogr.* 1986;64:134-147.
30. Burns RS, Lerner SE. Perspectives: acute phencyclidine intoxication. *Clin Toxicol.* 1976;9:477-501.
31. Burrows FA, Seeman RG. Ketamine and myoclonic encephalopathy of infants (Kinsbourne syndrome). *Anesth Analg.* 1982;61:873-875.
32. Butelman ER. A novel NMDA antagonist, MK-801, impairs performance in a hippocampal-dependent spatial learning task. *Pharmacol Biochem Behav.* 1989;34:13-16.
33. Buterbaugh GG, Michelson HB. Anticonvulsant properties of phencyclidine and ketamine. *NIDA Res Monogr.* 1986;64:67-79.
34. Caplan YH, Levine B. Abbott phencyclidine and barbiturates abused drug assays: evaluation and comparison of ADx FPIA, TDx FPIA, EMIT, and GC/MS methods. *J Anal Toxicol.* 1989;13:289-292.
35. Cartwright PD, Pingel SM. Midazolam and diazepam in ketamine anaesthesia. *Anaesthesia.* 1984;39:439-442.
36. Celesia GG, et al. Effects of ketamine in epilepsy. *Neurology.* 1975;25:169-172.
37. Chen G, et al. Investigation on the sympathomimetic properties of phencyclidine by comparison with cocaine and desoxyephedrine. *J Pharmacol Exp Ther.* 1965;149:71-78.
38. Chen G, et al. The pharmacology of 1-(1-phenylcyclohexyl) piperidine-HCl. *J Pharmacol Exp Ther.* 1959;127:241-250.
39. Cheng JY, Mok VK. Rapid determination of ketamine in urine by liquid chromatography-tandem mass spectrometry for a high throughput laboratory. *Forensic Sci Int.* 2004;142:9-15.
40. Chu PS, et al. "Street ketamine"-associated bladder dysfunction: a report of ten cases. *Hong Kong Med J.* 2007;13:311-313.
41. Chu PS, et al. The destruction of the lower urinary tract by ketamine abuse: a new syndrome? *BJU Int.* 2008;102:1616-1622.
42. Chudnofsky CR, et al. A combination of midazolam and ketamine for procedural sedation and analgesia in adult emergency department patients. *Acad Emerg Med.* 2000;7:228-235.
43. Cogen FC, et al. Phencyclidine-associated acute rhabdomyolysis. *Ann Intern Med.* 1978;88:210-212.
44. Cohen BD, et al. Combined Sernyl and sensory deprivation. *Compr Psychiatry.* 1960;1:345-348.
45. Cohen ML, et al. Distribution in the brain and metabolism of ketamine in the rat after intravenous administration. *Anesthesiology.* 1973;39:370-376.
46. Cohen S. Angel dust. *JAMA.* 1977;238:515-516.
47. Cook CE, et al. Phencyclidine disposition after intravenous and oral doses. *Clin Pharmacol Ther.* 1982;31:625-634.
48. Cook CE, et al. Phencyclidine and phenylcyclohexene disposition after smoking phencyclidine. *Clin Pharmacol Ther.* 1982;31:635-641.
49. Cooper M. "Special K": rough catnip for clubgoers. *The New York Times.* January 28, 1996:6.
50. Corso TD, et al. Multifocal brain damage induced by phencyclidine is augmented by pilocarpine. *Brain Res.* 1997;752:1-14.
51. Corssen G, Domino EF. Dissociative anesthesia: further pharmacologic studies and first clinical experience with the phencyclidine derivative CI-581. *Anesth Analg.* 1966;45:29-40.

52. Corssen G, et al. Ketamine in the anesthetic management of asthmatic patients. *Anesth Analg.* 1972;51:588-596.
53. Corssen G, et al. Ketamine and epilepsy. *Anesth Analg.* 1974;53:319-335.
54. Corssen G, et al. Changing concepts in pain control during surgery: dissociative anesthesia with CI-581. A progress report. *Anesth Analg.* 1968;47:746-759.
55. Craig CL, Loeffler GH. The ketamine analog methoxetamine: a new designer drug to threaten military readiness. *Mil Med.* 2014;179:1149-1157.
56. Crider R. Phencyclidine: changing abuse patterns. *NIDA Res Monogr.* 1986;64:163-173.
57. Critchlow DG. A case of ketamine dependence with discontinuation symptoms. *Addiction.* 2006;101:1212-1213.
58. Curran HV, Monaghan L. In and out of the K-hole: a comparison of the acute and residual effects of ketamine in frequent and infrequent ketamine users. *Addiction.* 2001;96:749-760.
59. Curran HV, Morgan C. Cognitive, dissociative and psychotogenic effects of ketamine in recreational users on the night of drug use and 3 days later. *Addiction.* 2000;95:575-590.
60. Dachs RJ, Innes GM. Intravenous ketamine sedation of pediatric patients in the emergency department. *Ann Emerg Med.* 1997;29:146-150.
61. Dargan PI, et al. Three months of methoxetamine administration is associated with significant bladder and renal toxicity in mice. *Clin Toxicol (Phila).* 2014;52:176-180.
62. Davies BM, Beech HR. The effect of 1-arylcyclohexylamine (Sernyl) on twelve normal volunteers. *J Ment Sci.* 1960;106:912-924.
63. DEA. Unusual tablet combination (ephedrine, caffeine, ketamine, and phencyclidine). *Microgram Bull.* 2000;33:311.
64. Dillon P, et al. Patterns of use and harms associated with non-medical ketamine use. *Drug Alcohol Depend.* 2003;69:23-28.
65. Domino EF. Neurobiology of phencyclidine (Sernyl), a drug with an unusual spectrum of pharmacological activity. *Int Rev Neurobiol.* 1964;6:303-347.
66. Domino EF, et al. Pharmacologic effects of Ci-581, a new dissociative anesthetic, in man. *Clin Pharmacol Ther.* 1965;6:279-291.
67. Dowdy EG, Kaya K. Studies of the mechanism of cardiovascular responses to CI-581. *Anesthesiology.* 1968;29:931-943.
68. Eastman JW, Cohen SN. Hypertensive crisis and death associated with phencyclidine poisoning. *JAMA.* 1975;231:1270-1271.
69. Elia N, Tramer MR. Ketamine and postoperative pain—a quantitative systematic review of randomised trials. *Pain.* 2005;113:61-70.
70. Ellison G. Competitive and non-competitive NMDA antagonists induce similar limbic degeneration. *Neuroreport.* 1994;5:2688-2692.
71. Ellison G, Switzer RC 3rd. Dissimilar patterns of degeneration in brain following four different addictive stimulants. *Neuroreport.* 1993;5:17-20.
72. Erbguth PH, et al. The influence of chlorpromazine, diazepam, and droperidol on emergence from ketamine. *Anesth Analg.* 1972;51:693-700.
73. Faithfull NS, Haider R. Ketamine for cardiac catheterisation. An evaluation of its use in children. *Anaesthesia.* 1971;26:318-323.
74. Fauman B, et al. Psychiatric sequelae of phencyclidine abuse. *Clin Toxicol.* 1976;9:529-538.
75. Fauman B, et al. Psychosis induced by phencyclidine. *J Am Coll Emerg Physicians.* 1975;4:223-225.
76. Felser JM, Orban DJ. Dystonic reaction after ketamine abuse. *Ann Emerg Med.* 1982;11:673-675.
77. Ferrer-Allado T, et al. Ketamine-induced electroconvulsive phenomena in the human limbic and thalamic regions. *Anesthesiology.* 1973;38:333-344.
78. Fine J, Finestone SC. Sensory disturbances following ketamine anesthesia: recurrent hallucinations. *Anesth Analg.* 1973;52:428-430.
79. Fischer MM. Ketamine hydrochloride in severe bronchospasm. *Anaesthesia.* 1977;32:771-772.
80. Ghoneim MM, et al. Ketamine: behavioral effects of subanesthetic doses. *J Clin Psychopharmacol.* 1985;5:70-77.
81. Giannini AJ, et al. Treatment of phenylcyclohexylpyrrolidine (PHP) psychosis with haloperidol. *J Toxicol Clin Toxicol.* 1985;23:185-189.
82. Giannini AJ, et al. Acute ketamine intoxication treated by haloperidol: a preliminary study. *Am J Ther.* 2000;7:389-391.
83. Glennon RA. The enigmatic sigma receptors. *Cent Nerv Syst Agents Med Chem.* 2009;9:159-160.
84. Golden NL, et al. Angel dust: possible effects on the fetus. *Pediatrics.* 1980;65:18-20.
85. Green SM, et al. Inadvertent ketamine overdose in children: clinical manifestations and outcome. *Ann Emerg Med.* 1999;34(4 Pt 1):492-497.
86. Green SM, et al. Ketamine safety profile in the developing world: survey of practitioners. *Acad Emerg Med.* 1996;3:598-604.
87. Green SM, Johnson NE. Ketamine sedation for pediatric procedures: part 2, review and implications. *Ann Emerg Med.* 1990;19:1033-1046.
88. Green SM, et al. Predictors of adverse events with intramuscular ketamine sedation in children. *Ann Emerg Med.* 2000;35:35-42.
89. Green SM, et al. Ketamine sedation for pediatric procedures: part 1, a prospective series. *Ann Emerg Med.* 1990;19:1024-1032.
90. Green SM, et al. Intravenous ketamine for pediatric sedation in the emergency department: safety profile with 156 cases. *Acad Emerg Med.* 1998;5:971-976.
91. Gregoire MC, et al. A pediatric case of ketamine-associated cystitis (Letter-to-the-Editor RE: Shahani R, Streutker C, Dickson B, et al: Ketamine-associated ulcerative cystitis: a new clinical entity. Urology 69: 810-812, 2007). *Urology.* 2008;71:1232-1233.
92. Greifenstein FE, et al. A study of a 1-aryl cyclo hexyl amine for anesthesia. *Anesth Analg.* 1958;37:283-294.
93. Hamilton JT, Bryson JS. The effect of ketamine on transmembrane potentials of Purkinje fibres of the pig heart. *Br J Anaesth.* 1974;46:636-642.
94. Harborne GC, et al. The effects of sub-anaesthetic doses of ketamine on memory, cognitive performance and subjective experience in healthy volunteers. *J Psychopharmacol.* 1996;10:134-140.
95. Harris EW, et al. Long-term potentiation in the hippocampus involves activation of N-methyl-D-aspartate receptors. *Brain Res.* 1984;323:132-137.
96. Harris JA, et al. Attention, learning, and personality during ketamine emergence: a pilot study. *Anesth Analg.* 1975;54:169-172.
97. Hills CE, et al. "Special k" and a loss of cell-to-cell adhesion in proximal tubule-derived epithelial cells: modulation of the adherens junction complex by ketamine. *PloS One.* 2013;8:e71819.
98. Himmelseher S, Durieux ME. Ketamine for perioperative pain management. *Anesthesiology.* 2005;102:211-220.
99. Hofer KE, et al. Ketamine-like effects after recreational use of methoxetamine. *Ann Emerg Med.* 2012;60:97-99.
100. Holland JA, et al. Embalming fluid-soaked marijuana: new high or new guise for PCP? *J Psychoactive Drugs.* 1998;30:215-219.
101. Hopcroft SA, et al. Ureteric intestinal metaplasia in association with chronic recreational ketamine abuse. *J Clin Pathol.* 2011;64:551-552.
102. Hubel JA. Authorities cast a wary eye on raves. *The New York Times.* June 29, 1997:1.
103. Ikonomidou C, et al. Blockade of NMDA receptors and apoptotic neurodegeneration in the developing brain. *Science.* 1999;283:70-74.
104. Jalil R, Gupta S. Illicit ketamine and its bladder consequences: is it irreversible? *BMJ Case Rep.* 2012;2012.
105. Jansen KL. Non-medical use of ketamine. *BMJ.* 1993;306:601-602.
106. Javitt DC, Zukin SR. Recent advances in the phencyclidine model of schizophrenia. *Am J Psychiatry.* 1991;148:1301-1308.
107. Jentsch JD, Roth RH. The neuropsychopharmacology of phencyclidine: from NMDA receptor hypofunction to the dopamine hypothesis of schizophrenia. *Neuropsychopharmacology.* 1999;20:201-225.
108. Jentsch JD, et al. Altered frontal cortical dopaminergic transmission in monkeys after subchronic phencyclidine exposure: involvement in frontostriatal cognitive deficits. *Neuroscience.* 1999;90:823-832.
109. Jentsch JD, et al. Subchronic phencyclidine administration reduces mesoprefrontal dopamine utilization and impairs prefrontal cortical-dependent cognition in the rat. *Neuropsychopharmacology.* 1997;17:92-99.
110. Johnson BD. Psychosis and ketamine. *Br Med J.* 1971;4:428-429.
111. Johnson KM, et al. Pharmacologic regulation of the NMDA receptor-ionophore complex. *NIDA Res Monogr.* 1993;133:13-39.
112. Johnston L, et al. *National Survey Results on Drug Use from Monitoring the Future Survey, 1975-1993. NIH publication 93-3597.* Bethesda, MD: NIDA;1994.
113. Johnston L, et al. *Monitoring the Future National Results on Adolescent Drug Use: 1975-2015: Volume 2, College Students and Adults Ages 19-55. National Institute on Drug Abuse/National Institutes of Health.* Ann Arbor, MI: Institute for Social Research, University of Michigan; 2016.
114. Johnstone M, et al. Sernyl (CI-395) in clinical anaesthesia. *Br J Anaesth.* 1959;31:433-439.
115. Jushchyshyn MI, et al. Mechanism of inactivation of human cytochrome P450 2B6 by phencyclidine. *Drug Metab Dispos.* 2006;34:1523-1529.
116. Karp HN, et al. Phencyclidine poisoning in young children. *J Pediatr.* 1980;97:1006-1009.
117. KC Tsui T, et al. *Study of Patterns of Drugs of Abuse in New Territories East and West Clusters Drug of Abuse Clinic using Conventional and New Technologies.* Hong Kong: Central Registry of Drug Abuse, Narcotics Division, Security Bureau, HKSAR Government; July 29, 2011.
118. Koehntop DE, et al. Effects of pharmacologic alterations of adrenergic mechanisms by cocaine, tropolone, aminophylline, and ketamine on epinephrine-induced arrhythmias during halothane-nitrous oxide anesthesia. *Anesthesiology.* 1977;46:83-93.
119. Kronenberg RH. Ketamine as an analgesic: parenteral, oral, rectal, subcutaneous, transdermal and intranasal administration. *J Pain Palliat Car Pharmacother.* 2002;16:27-35.
120. Krystal JH, et al. Interactive effects of subanesthetic ketamine and haloperidol in healthy humans. *Psychopharmacology.* 1999;145:193-204.
121. Krystal JH, et al. NMDA receptor antagonist effects, cortical glutamatergic function, and schizophrenia: toward a paradigm shift in medication development. *Psychopharmacology.* 2003;169:215-233.
122. Krystal JH, et al. Interactive effects of subanesthetic ketamine and subhypnotic lorazepam in humans. *Psychopharmacology.* 1998;135:213-229.
123. Krystal JH, et al. Subanesthetic effects of the noncompetitive NMDA antagonist, ketamine, in humans. Psychotomimetic, perceptual, cognitive, and neuroendocrine responses. *Arch Gen Psychiatry.* 1994;51:199-214.
124. Kumar A, et al. The effect of music on ketamine induced emergence phenomena. *Anaesthesia.* 1992;47:438-439.
125. Lahti AC, et al. NMDA-sensitive glutamate antagonism: a human model for psychosis. *Neuropsychopharmacology.* 1999;21(S2):S158-S169.

126. Lahti AC, et al. Subanesthetic doses of ketamine stimulate psychosis in schizophrenia. *Neuropsychopharmacology*. 1995;13:9-19.

127. Lahti AC, et al. Effects of ketamine in normal and schizophrenic volunteers. *Neuropsychopharmacology*. 2001;25:455-467.

128. Lankenau SE, Clatts MC. Drug injection practices among high-risk youths: the first shot of ketamine. *J Urban Health*. 2004;81:232-248.

129. Laskowski LK, et al. Ice water submersion for rapid cooling in severe drug-induced hyperthermia. *Clin Toxicol (Phila)*. 2015;53:181-184.

130. Laurenzana EM, Owens SM. Metabolism of phencyclidine by human liver microsomes. *Drug Metab Dispos*. 1997;25:557-563.

131. Licata M, et al. A fatal ketamine poisoning. *J Forensic Sci*. 1994;39:1314-1320.

132. Liden CB, et al. Phencyclidine. Nine cases of poisoning. *JAMA*. 1975;234:513-516.

133. Lo JN, Cumming JF. Interaction between sedative premedicants and ketamine in man in isolated perfused rat livers. *Anesthesiology*. 1975;43:307-312.

134. Lo RS, et al. Cholestasis and biliary dilatation associated with chronic ketamine abuse: a case series. *Singapore Med J*. 2011;52:e52-55.

135. Lu YF, et al. Neuroprotective effects of phencyclidine on acute cerebral ischemia and reperfusion injury of rabbits. *Zhongguo Yao Li Xue Bao*. 1992;13:218-222.

136. Luby ED, et al. Study of a new schizophrenomimetic drug; Sernyl. *AMA Arch Neurol Psychiatry*. 1959;81:363-369.

137. Lundberg GD, et al. Phencyclidine: patterns seen in street drug analysis. *Clin Toxicol*. 1976;9:503-511.

138. Lundy PM, et al. The actions of ketamine on vascular smooth muscle. *Arch Int Pharmacodyn Ther*. 1976;220:213-230.

139. Lundy PM, et al. Differential effects of ketamine isomers on neuronal and extraneuronal catecholamine uptake mechanisms. *Anesthesiology*. 1986;64:359-363.

140. MacDonald JF, et al. The PCP site of the NMDA receptor complex. *Adv Exp Med Biol*. 1990;268:27-34.

141. Magbagbeola JA, Thomas NA. Effect of thiopentone on emergence reactions to ketamine anaesthesia. *Can Anaesth Soc J*. 1974;21:321-324.

142. Malhotra AK, et al. Clozapine blunts N-methyl-D-aspartate antagonist-induced psychosis: a study with ketamine. *Biol Psychiatry*. 1997;42:664-668.

143. Malhotra AK, et al. Ketamine-induced exacerbation of psychotic symptoms and cognitive impairment in neuroleptic-free schizophrenics. *Neuropsychopharmacology*. 1997;17:141-150.

144. Malhotra AK, et al. NMDA receptor function and human cognition: the effects of ketamine in healthy volunteers. *Neuropsychopharmacology*. 1996;14:301-307.

145. Martinez-Aguirre E, Sansano C. Comparison of midazolam (Ro 21-3981) and diazepam as complement of ketamine-air anesthesia in children. *Acta Anaesthesiol Belg*. 1986;37:15-22.

146. Mason K, et al. Ketamine-associated lower urinary tract destruction: a new radiological challenge. *Clin Radiol*. 2010;65:795-800.

147. McCarron MM, et al. Acute phencyclidine intoxication: clinical patterns, complications, and treatment. *Ann Emerg Med*. 1981;10:290-297.

148. McCarron MM, et al. Acute phencyclidine intoxication: incidence of clinical findings in 1,000 cases. *Ann Emerg Med*. 1981;10:237-242.

149. McMahon B, et al. Hypertension during recovery from phencyclidine intoxication. *Clin Toxicol*. 1978;12:37-40.

150. Melkonian DL, Meshcheriakov AV. [Possibility of predicting and preventing psychotic disorders during ketamine anesthesia]. *Anesteziol Reanimatol*. 1989:15-18.

151. Menzies EL, et al. Characterizing metabolites and potential metabolic pathways for the novel psychoactive substance methoxetamine. *Drug Test Anal*. 2014;6:506-515.

152. Middela S, Pearce I. Ketamine-induced vesicopathy: a literature review. *Int J Clin Pract*. 2011;65:27-30.

153. Misra AL, et al. Persistence of phencyclidine (PCP) and metabolites in brain and adipose tissue and implications for long-lasting behavioural effects. *Res Commun Chem Pathol Pharmacol*. 1979;24:431-445.

154. Modica PA, et al. Pro- and anticonvulsant effects of anesthetics (Part I). *Anesth Analg*. 1990;70:303-315.

155. Moerschbaecher JM, Thompson DM. Differential effects of prototype opioid agonists on the acquisition of conditional discriminations in monkeys. *J Pharmacol Exp Ther*. 1983;226:738-748.

156. Moore KA, et al. Tissue distribution of ketamine in a mixed drug fatality. *J Forensic Sci*. 1997;42:1183-1185.

157. Moore NN, Bostwick JM. Ketamine dependence in anesthesia providers. *Psychosomatics*. 1999;40:356-359.

158. Morgan CJ, et al. Ketamine impairs response inhibition and is positively reinforcing in healthy volunteers: a dose-response study. *Psychopharmacology*. 2004;172:298-308.

159. Morgan CJ, et al. Attentional bias to incentive stimuli in frequent ketamine users. *Psychol Med*. 2008;38:1331-1340.

160. Morgan CJ, et al. Long-term effects of ketamine: evidence for a persisting impairment of source memory in recreational users. *Drug Alcohol Depend*. 2004;75:301-308.

161. Morgenstern FS, et al. An investigation of drug induced sensory disturbances. *Psychopharmacologia*. 1962;3:193-201.

162. Morray JP, et al. Hemodynamic effects of ketamine in children with congenital heart disease. *Anesth Analg*. 1984;63:895-899.

163. Morris H, Wallach J. From PCP to MXE: a comprehensive review of the non-medical use of dissociative drugs. *Drug Test Anal*. 2014;6:614-632.

164. Motov S, et al. A prospective randomized, double-dummy trial comparing intravenous push dose of low dose ketamine to short infusion of low dose ketamine for treatment of moderate to severe pain in the emergency department. *Am J Emerg Med*. 2017.

165. Ng SH, et al. Emergency department presentation of ketamine abusers in Hong Kong: a review of 233 cases. *Hong Kong Med J*. 2010;16:6-11.

166. Olney JW, et al. Pathological changes induced in cerebrocortical neurons by phencyclidine and related drugs. *Science*. 1989;244:1360-1362.

167. Olney JW, et al. NMDA antagonist neurotoxicity: mechanism and prevention. *Science*. 1991;254:1515-1518.

168. Olney JW, et al. NMDA receptor hypofunction model of schizophrenia. *J Psychiatr Res*. 1999;33:523-533.

169. Olsson GL, Hallen B. Laryngospasm during anaesthesia. A computer-aided incidence study in 136,929 patients. *Acta Anaesthesiol Scand*. 1984;28:567-575.

170. Owens SM, Mayersohn M. Phencyclidine-specific Fab fragments alter phencyclidine disposition in dogs. *Drug Metab Dispos*. 1986;14:52-58.

171. Oye I, et al. Effects of ketamine on sensory perception: evidence for a role of N-methyl-D-aspartate receptors. *J Pharmacol Exp Ther*. 1992;260:1209-1213.

172. Pal HR, et al. Ketamine dependence. *Anaesth Intensive Care*. 2002;30:382-384.

173. Patel R, Connor G. A review of thirty cases of rhabdomyolysis-associated acute renal failure among phencyclidine users. *J Toxicol Clin Toxicol*. 1985;23:547-556.

174. Picchioni AL, Consroe PF. Activated charcoal—a phencyclidine antidote, or hog in dogs. *N Engl J Med*. 1979;300:202.

175. Pitts FN Jr, et al. Occupational intoxication and long-term persistence of phencyclidine (PCP) in law enforcement personnel. *Clin Toxicol*. 1981;18:1015-1020.

176. Poklis JL, et al. Evaluation of a new phencyclidine enzyme immunoassay for the detection of phencyclidine in urine with confirmation by high-performance liquid chromatography-tandem mass spectrometry. *J Anal Toxicol*. 2011;35:481-486.

177. Pradhan SN. Phencyclidine (PCP): some human studies. *Neurosci Biobehav Rev*. 1984;8:493-501.

178. Pristin T. Drug raids net 14 students. *The New York Times*. May 22, 1996:1.

179. Rawson RA, et al. Characteristics of 68 chronic phencyclidine abusers who sought treatment. *Drug Alcohol Depend*. 1981;8:223-227.

180. Rees D, Wasem S. The identification and quantitation of ketamine hydrochloride. *Microgram*. 2000;33:163.

181. Reich DL, Silvay G. Ketamine: an update on the first twenty-five years of clinical experience. *Can J Anaesth*. 1989;36:186-197.

182. Riddell J, et al. Ketamine as a first-line treatment for severely agitated emergency department patients. *Am J Emerg Med*. 2017;35:1000-1004.

183. Rock MJ, et al. Use of ketamine in asthmatic children to treat respiratory failure refractory to conventional therapy. *Crit Care Med*. 1986;14:514-516.

184. Roelofse JA, et al. Intranasal sufentanil/midazolam versus ketamine/midazolam for analgesia/sedation in the pediatric population prior to undergoing multiple dental extractions under general anesthesia: a prospective, double-blind, randomized comparison. *Anesth Prog*. 2004;51:114-121.

185. Rofael HZ, et al. Effect of ketamine on cocaine-induced immunotoxicity in rats. *Int J Toxicol*. 2003;22:343-358.

186. Rosenbaum G, et al. Comparison of Sernyl with other drugs: simulation of schizophrenic performance with Sernyl, LSD-25, and amobarbital (amytal) sodium; I. Attention, motor function, and proprioception. *AMA Arch Gen Psychiatry*. 1959;1:651-656.

187. Roth BL, et al. The ketamine analogue methoxetamine and 3- and 4-methoxy analogues of phencyclidine are high affinity and selective ligands for the glutamate NMDA receptor. *PloS One*. 2013;8:e59334.

188. Substance Abuse and Mental Health Services Administration. *Overview of Findings From the 2003 National Survey on Drug Use and Health. Office of Applied Studies, NSDUH Series H-24, Publication no. SMA 04-3963*. Rockville, MD: Substance Abuse and Mental Health Services Administration; 2004.

189. Substance Abuse and Mental Health Services Administration Office of the Assistant Secretary for Mental Health and Substance Use. *The DAWN Report, January. Trends in PCP-Related Emergency Department Visits*. Rockville, MD: Substance Abuse and Mental Health Services Administration; 2004.

190. Substance Abuse and Mental Health Services Administration Office of the Assistant Secretary for Mental Health and Substance Use. *Emergency Department Trends from the Drug Abuse Warning Network, Final Estimates 1994-2001, DAWN Series D-21. Publication no. SMA 02-3635*. Rockville, MD: Substance Abuse and Mental Health Services Administration; 2002.

191. Substance Abuse and Mental Health Services Administration Office of the Assistant Secretary for Mental Health and Substance Use. *The NSDUH Report. Substance Use and Dependence Following Initiation of Alcohol or Illicit Drug Use*. Rockville, MD: Substance Abuse and Mental Health Services Administration; 2008.

192. Substance Abuse and Mental Health Services Administration Office of the Assistant Secretary for Mental Health and Substance Use. *The NSDUH Report. Use of Specific Hallucinogens*. Rockville, MD: Substance Abuse and Mental Health Services Administration; 2008.

193. Shahani R, et al. Ketamine-associated ulcerative cystitis: a new clinical entity. *Urology*. 2007;69:810-812.

194. Shannon HE. Evaluation of phencyclidine analogs on the basis of their discriminative stimulus properties in the rat. *J Pharmacol Exp Ther*. 1981;216:543-551.

195. Sharp FR, et al. MK-801 and ketamine induce heat shock protein HSP72 in injured neurons in posterior cingulate and retrosplenial cortex. *Ann Neurol.* 1991;30:801-809.
196. Shields JE, et al. Methoxetamine associated reversible cerebellar toxicity: three cases with analytical confirmation. *Clin Toxicol (Phila).* 2012;50:438-440.
197. Shulgin AT, Mac Lean DE. Illicit synthesis of phencyclidine (PCP) and several of its analogs. *Clin Toxicol.* 1976;9:553-560.
198. Siegel RK. Phencyclidine and ketamine intoxication: a study of four populations of recreational users. *NIDA Res Monogr.* 1978:119-147.
199. Singer W. Development and plasticity of cortical processing architectures. *Science.* 1995;270:758-764.
200. Sircar R, Li CS. PCP/NMDA receptor-channel complex and brain development. *Neurotoxicol Teratol.* 1994;16:369-375.
201. Sklar GS, et al. Adverse reactions to ketamine anaesthesia. Abolition by a psychological technique. *Anaesthesia.* 1981;36:183-187.
202. Slifer BL, et al. Behavioral dependence produced by continuous phencyclidine infusion in rhesus monkeys. *J Pharmacol Exp Ther.* 1984;230:399-406.
203. Snyder SH. Phencyclidine. *Nature.* 1980;285:355-356.
204. Stanley V, et al. Cardiovascular and respiratory function with CI-581. *Anesth Analg.* 1968;47:760-768.
205. Steinpreis RE. The behavioral and neurochemical effects of phencyclidine in humans and animals: some implications for modeling psychosis. *Behav Brain Res.* 1996;74:45-55.
206. Stewart LS, Persinger MA. Ketamine prevents learning impairment when administered immediately after status epilepticus onset. *Epilepsy Behav.* 2001;2:585-591.
207. Stillman R, Petersen RC. The paradox of phencyclidine (PCP) abuse. *Ann Intern Med.* 1979;90:428-430.
208. Strauss AA, et al. Neonatal manifestations of maternal phencyclidine (PCP) abuse. *Pediatrics.* 1981;68:550-552.
209. Strube PJ, Hallam PL. Ketamine by continuous infusion in status asthmaticus. *Anaesthesia.* 1986;41:1017-1019.
210. Synowiec AS, et al. Ketamine use in the treatment of refractory status epilepticus. *Epilepsy Res.* 2013;105:183-188.
211. Toro-Matos A, et al. Physostigmine antagonizes ketamine. *Anesth Analg.* 1980;59:764-767.
212. Tweed WA, et al. Circulatory responses to ketamine anesthesia. *Anesthesiology.* 1972;37:613-619.
213. Valentine JL, et al. Antiphencyclidine monoclonal Fab fragments reverse phencyclidine-induced behavioral effects and ataxia in rats. *J Pharmacol Exp Ther.* 1996;278:709-716.
214. Vincent JP, et al. Interaction of phencyclidines with the muscarinic and opiate receptors in the central nervous system. *Brain Res.* 1978;152:176-182.
215. Vincent JP, et al. Interaction of phencyclidine ("angel dust") with a specific receptor in rat brain membranes. *Proc Nat Acad Sci U S A.* 1979;76:4678-4682.
216. Vogt BA. Cingulate cortex. *Association and Auditory Cortices.* Springer; 1985:89-149.
217. Wang KC, et al. Use of SPE and LC/TIS/MS/MS for rapid detection and quantitation of ketamine and its metabolite, norketamine, in urine. *Forensic Sci Int.* 2005;147:81-88.
218. Ward J, et al. Methoxetamine: a novel ketamine analog and growing health-care concern. *Clin Toxicol (Phila).* 2011;49:874-875.
219. Warner A. Dextromethorphan: analyte of the month. In: *Service Training and Continuing Education. Clinical Chemistry.* Vol 14. Washington, DC: 1993:27-28.
220. Weiner AL, et al. Ketamine abusers presenting to the emergency department: a case series. *J Emerg Med.* 2000;18:447-451.
221. Weingarten SM. Dissociation of limbic and neocortical EEG patterns in cats under ketamine anesthesia. *J Neurosurg.* 1972;37:429-433.
222. White PF, et al. Ketamine—its pharmacology and therapeutic uses. *Anesthesiology.* 1982;56:119-136.
223. Wilgoren J. Police arrest 14 in drug raid at a nightclub in Manhattan. *The New York Times.* Apr 18, 1999: 41.
224. Willetts J, Balster RL. Phencyclidine-like discriminative stimulus properties of MK-801 in rats. *Eur J Pharmacol.* 1988;146:167-169.
225. Wolfe SA Jr, De Souza EB. Sigma and phencyclidine receptors in the brain-endocrine-immune axis. *NIDA Res Monogr.* 1993;133:95-123.
226. Wong EH, Kemp JA. Sites for antagonism on the N-methyl-D-aspartate receptor channel complex. *Ann Rev Pharmacol Toxicol.* 1991;31:401-425.
227. Wong EH, et al. The anticonvulsant MK-801 is a potent N-methyl-D-aspartate antagonist. *Proc Nat Acad Sci U S A.* 1986;83:7104-7108.
228. Wood D, et al. Recreational ketamine: from pleasure to pain. *BJU Int.* 2011;107:1881-1884.
229. Wood DM, et al. Acute toxicity associated with the recreational use of the ketamine derivative methoxetamine. *Eur J Clin Pharmacol.* 2012;68:853-856.
230. Woodworth JR, et al. Phencyclidine (PCP) disposition kinetics in dogs as a function of dose and route of administration. *J Pharmacol Exp Ther.* 1985;234:654-661.
231. Wright HH, et al. Phencyclidine-induced psychosis: eight-year follow-up of ten cases. *Sout Med J.* 1988;81:565-567.
232. Yanagihara Y, et al. Involvement of CYP2B6 in n-demethylation of ketamine in human liver microsomes. *Drug Metab Dispos.* 2001;29:887-890.
233. Yiu-Cheung C. Acute and chronic toxicity pattern in ketamine abusers in Hong Kong. *J Med Toxicol.* 2012;8:267-270.
234. Zhang JC, et al. R (-)-ketamine shows greater potency and longer lasting antidepressant effects than S (+)-ketamine. *Pharmacol Biochem Behav.* 2014;116:137-141.
235. Zsigmond E, Domino E. Ketamine clinical pharmacology, pharmacokinetics and current clinical uses. *Anesth Rev.* 1980;7:13-33.
236. Zukin SR, Zukin RS. Specific [3H]phencyclidine binding in rat central nervous system. *Proc Nat Acad Sci U S A.* 1979;76:5372-5376.

CASE STUDY 9

History A 45-year-old man presented to the hospital complaining of hand and foot pain so severe that he was unable to drive his car. The man had been well until several weeks earlier, when he began having gastrointestinal distress that he thought was "heartburn" and mild weight loss, which he attributed to his dyspepsia. He denied fever, chills, nausea, vomiting, or diarrhea. He also related that on the day prior to admission he was unable to eat a meal because he thought it was spoiled after taking a few bites. The next morning, while driving, he pulled off the road and phoned emergency medical services. He was taking no medications and had no allergies.

Physical Examination In the emergency department, the patient appeared well developed and well nourished, but was complaining of severe pain in his hands and feet. Vital signs were: blood pressure, 124/68 mm Hg; pulse, 92 beats/min; respiratory rate, 14 breaths/min; oral temperature, 98.6°F (37.0°C); oxygen saturation, 99% on room air; and a rapid reagent glucose of 128 mg/dL. Physical examination was notable for pupils that were equal, round (4 mm), and reactive to light; normal extraocular movements; and the absence of nuchal rigidity. His chest was clear to auscultation, and his heart sounds were normal. His abdomen was soft and nontender, with normal bowel sounds and no organomegaly. He was awake, alert, and oriented with normal symmetrical strength and brisk reflexes. Although he complained of pain in his hands and feet, his two-point discrimination, proprioception, and vibration sensation appeared normal. His gait was slightly wide based and slow, but this was thought to be secondary to pain. Cranial nerves II through XII appeared intact, and cerebellar testing was normal.

Initial Management Although the patient appeared uncomfortable, there was no perception of an immediate life-threatening illness. An intravenous line was inserted, and blood was obtained for a complete blood count, electrolytes, and liver function testing. A urinalysis was requested as was an electrocardiogram and a chest radiograph. Acetaminophen was given for analgesia, without relief. The patient ultimately required parenteral opioids to diminish his pain, although he noted that the distribution had spread to include most of his legs and arms. He also became somnolent, and it was unclear if the ensuing somnolence was opioid related.

What Is the Differential Diagnosis? The major presenting symptom in this case is a painful sensory peripheral neuropathy (an uncommon clinical manifestation) associated with gastrointestinal symptoms (a common manifestation). Considerations include a variety of metabolic and endocrine disorders, infections, medications, and toxins. Severely painful symmetrical paresthesias are fairly uncommon and the differential diagnosis is limited. Considerations include freezing injury such as frostbite (Chap. 29), proximity to radioactive materials (Chap. 128), and dermal exposure to hydrofluoric acid (Chap. 104). A list of xenobiotics that can cause such findings following ingestion is found in Table CS9–1.

TABLE CS9–1	Differential Diagnosis of Sensory Peripheral Neuropathy With Gastrointestinal Complaints
Endocrine	Nitrous oxide
Diabetes mellitus	Organic phosphorus
Hypothyroidism	compounds
Nutritional	**Medications**
Alcoholism	Cisplatinum
B_{12} deficiency	Disulfiram
Thiamine deficiency	Isoniazid
Xenobiotics	Metronidazole
Alcohol	Phenytoin
Acrylamide	Pyridoxine
Hexane derivatives	Taxol
Metals (arsenic, gold, mercury, thallium)	Vinca alkaloids
	Connective tissue diseases

What Clinical and Laboratory Analyses Help Exclude Life-Threatening Causes of This Patient's Presentation? In addition to the above evaluation, a diagnosis of encephalitis was considered when the patient became somnolent, and a computed tomographic (CT) scan of the head was obtained without intravenous contrast. A lumbar puncture was performed after the CT scan was interpreted as normal. The lumbar puncture showed 2 red blood cells/mm³; 0 white blood cells/mm³; glucose, 85 mg/dL; and protein, 45 mg/dL, all within normal limits.

Unfortunately, over the next 48 hours, the patient's condition deteriorated and was characterized by encephalopathy with cranial nerve dysfunction and weakness with loss of deep tendon reflexes. A repeat lumbar puncture demonstrated elevated protein without abnormal cells and a CSF Gram stain was negative.

Further Diagnosis and Treatment A diagnosis of poisoning was considered, and a medical toxicology consult was obtained. The combination of gastrointestinal symptoms without significant diarrhea, severely painful ascending peripheral neuropathy and progression to encephalopathy with motor and cranial nerve findings strongly suggested metal poisoning, specifically thallium (Chap. 99). Treatment with Prussian Blue (Antidotes in Depth: A31) was recommended, and the original blood urine and cerebrospinal fluid were sent for thallium concentrations. Unfortunately, the patient's illness progressed rapidly, and he suffered a cardiac arrest shortly after the diagnosis was considered. Ultimately, a spot urine thallium concentration was reported as 50,000 mcg/L (normal < 5 mcg/L), and his serum was 8700 mcg/L (normal < 2 mcg/L).

Acknowledgment Postmortem findings and cerebrospinal fluid results of this case were reported in Sharma AN, Nelson LS, Hoffman RS: Cerebrospinal fluid analysis in fatal thallium poisoning: evidence for delayed distribution into the central nervous system. *Am J Forensic Med Pathol.* 2004;25:156-158.

ALUMINUM

Stephen A. Harding and Brenna M. Farmer

Aluminum (Al)

Atomic number	=	13
Atomic weight	=	26.98 Da
Normal concentrations		
Serum	<	2 mcg/L (0.074 µmol/L)
Whole blood concentration	<	12 mcg/L (0.445 µmol/L)
Urine (24-hour)	<	4–12 mcg/g creatinine
		(0.148–0.445 µmol/g creatinine)

CHEMISTRY

Aluminum (Al) is the most abundant metal in the crust of the earth, where it is found in many types of ores: bauxite, gibbite, boehmite, as alumina, and in gems such as ruby, sapphire, and turquoise. The most naturally occurring isotope is ^{33}Al. Aluminum is a nonessential element and a trace metal with a single oxidation state, Al^{3+}.

The aluminum industry is one of the largest industries in the world. Aluminum ores are converted to alumina and then reduced to aluminum metal. The first step usually involves refining bauxite at high temperature and pressure in a caustic soda to form alumina (aluminum oxide, Al_2O_3). The second step occurs by the Hall–Heroult process in potrooms and uses electrolytic reduction to form aluminum. Aluminum is then used alone or is processed into alloys to build a variety of products that are anticorrosive.[20] Aluminum is found in cookware, infant formula,[26] foil, vaccines as an adjuvant to boost immune response,[34] antiperspirants, antacids, and previously, in phosphate binders. It also contaminates hemodialysis (HD) fluids, intravenous (IV) fluids, total parenteral nutrition (TPN),[45] pharmaceutical albumin,[46] and is one component of alum solution (potassium aluminum sulfate or ammonium aluminum sulfate), which is used as an astringent for bladder irrigation.[112] In this chapter, aluminum metal is discussed as an occupational toxin with mainly lung manifestations. Aluminum salts, the more common form discussed in human toxicity, primarily act as neurotoxins, with both acute and chronic toxicity.

HISTORY AND EPIDEMIOLOGY

The first case of aluminum toxicity with neurologic findings was reported in 1921. This patient had memory loss, tremor, and impaired coordination.[100] Subsequently, a case series described occupational asthma in Norwegian aluminum (potroom) workers ("potroom asthma").[27] A pot is a large vessel in which aluminum is produced, and the building in which these pots are housed is known as a "potroom." In 1947, 26% of German potroom workers exposed to high concentrations of aluminum dust mixed with mineral oil–based lubricants developed pulmonary fibrosis or "aluminosis."[30] Some potroom workers also developed neurologic findings described as a progressive encephalopathy and termed "potroom palsy," with balance problems, intention tremors, decreased cognitive ability, and impaired memory, initially described in 1962.[53,60,83]

In the 1970s, encephalopathy in patients with chronic kidney disease (CKD) was attributed to using aluminum salt–containing phosphate binders or, more rarely, to aluminum-contaminated dialysis fluid. This clinical syndrome, known as "dialysis dementia," develop after years of HD.[90] By 1976, elevated serum aluminum concentrations were reported in encephalopathic HD patients.[77] Both the relation between aluminum and microcytic anemia

and the connection between aluminum and osteomalacia in dialysis patients were recognized in 1978.[21,103]

In 1982, alum (potassium aluminum sulfate or ammonium aluminum sulfate) was first used in the treatment of hemorrhagic cystitis.[75] Neurotoxicity develops if patients absorb alum systemically, especially if chronic kidney disease is present.

Subsequently, aluminum was linked to the spongiform leukoencephalopathy that in rare cases developed in heroin users who were "chasing the dragon." These patients inhaled the pyrolysate of heroin heated on aluminum or tin foil. A 2007 study showed elevated urinary aluminum concentrations in patients using heroin in this manner.[22] They developed bizarre behavior, slowed speech and movements, as well as cognitive abnormalities.[52]

There is also a concern over the relation between aluminum and Alzheimer disease. This linkage was studied because of the dialysis encephalopathy syndrome (dialysis dementia) and the association of aluminum with neuropsychiatric deficits and electroencephalographic (EEG) changes that occur in aluminum welders.[84] Although aluminum is a component of neurofibrillary tangles in senile plaques associated with Alzheimer disease, to date no studies have proven that aluminum is the cause of the disease.[67,77] Regardless, this association led several agencies in the United States and Canada, including the US Food and Drug Administration (FDA) and Health Canada, to decrease the amount of aluminum contamination allowable in food and water products.[108]

ALUMINUM-CONTAINING XENOBIOTICS

Antacids

Aluminum-containing products are rarely prescribed. However, patients take antacids containing aluminum hydroxide for symptomatic control of dyspepsia and gastroesophageal reflux disease. Aluminum hydroxide is usually packaged with magnesium hydroxide to counteract the induced delay of gastric emptying and constipation caused by aluminum hydroxide. These antacids are poorly absorbed and exit the stomach in about 30 minutes. The neutralizing effects of antacids last for 2 to 3 hours, especially in the presence of food.

Sucralfate

Sucralfate, an aluminum-containing salt with sucrose sulfate, is used for symptomatic control of ulcer disease, to accelerate healing of peptic ulcer disease, and as a protectant against stress ulcer formation. This sucrose aluminum complex is poorly absorbed from the gastrointestinal (GI) tract, and the little that is absorbed is excreted by the kidney without undergoing any metabolic changes. Although not approved by the FDA as a phosphate binder, it does have phosphate-binding properties.[12]

Alum

Alum is usually a 1% solution of potassium aluminum sulfate salt {KAl(SO$_4$)$_2$ * 12H$_2$O} or an ammonium aluminum sulfate salt {NH$_4$Al(SO$_4$)$_2$ * 12H$_2$O}, and is uncommonly used as an astringent for hemorrhagic cystitis and administered by bladder irrigation. It is poorly absorbed, although toxicity occurs.[94]

TOXICOKINETICS

Aluminum toxicokinetics are difficult to comprehend as many mechanisms remain to be elucidated. It is known that daily intake occurs, that absorption is limited, but that the concentrations of aluminum in urine and feces do not equal 100% of the exposure.[31] More research is necessary to expand current knowledge of toxicokinetics.

Absorption

Aluminum is ubiquitous in the food we eat and water we drink.[76] The daily intake of aluminum in the United States is estimated to be 2 to 25 mg from food and beverages, depending on the diet studied.[31] Gastrointestinal absorption mainly occurs in the proximal small bowel with uptake by the intestinal mucosal cells. Uptake occurs through both passive transport methods such as diffusion and active transport methods via transferrin as well as active methods shared by calcium.[31] Transferrin also mediates absorption into the blood from the mucosal cells.[31] The exact amount of aluminum absorption in humans is difficult to quantify because of the short half-lives of isotopes and lack of sensitive analysis techniques.[31] However, GI absorption and serum aluminum concentrations increase in the presence of citrate, other small organic acids, uremia, and iron deficiency anemia.[23,31,35,73,97] The GI absorption of aluminum is decreased in the presence of phosphorus and silicon.[35] There is negligible dermal absorption from the use of antiperspirants containing aluminum.[24,31] Pulmonary absorption of inhaled aluminum particulates is 1.5% to 2%, based on increased urinary aluminum excretion in workers exposed to aluminum-containing metal fumes.[31,68,95]

Distribution

The initial volume of distribution of aluminum is 0.06 L/kg with an equal distribution between plasma and red blood cells.[104] Aluminum then becomes 90% bound to transferrin, with approximately 10% bound to citrate.[101,107] From the blood, it distributes to many tissues, including 50% to the bone, where it is concentrated at the mineralization front,[111] and approximately 1% to the brain, primarily in the gray matter.[77] The remainder of the aluminum distributes variably to the heart, liver, kidney, and other organ systems. Citrate is the primary carrier in the cerebrospinal fluid (CSF).[107] Intracellularly, aluminum localizes in the lysosomes of brain neurons, liver (not the Kupffer cells), spleen, kidney epithelial tubules and glomerular mesangium cells, cardiac myocytes,[8,88] and in the mitochondria of osteoblasts.[19]

Metabolism/Excretion

Aluminum is not metabolized in the body and is considered to be greater than 95% excreted unchanged in the urine.[31,29] Citrate in the blood enhances the excretion of aluminum.[31,56] Less than 2% of aluminum is excreted by the bile.[47,80,109] Because aluminum is primarily excreted in the urine, patients with CKD have decreased aluminum excretion. The elimination half-life for aluminum is approximately 85 days in patients receiving dialysis.[89] Based on urinary excretion in workers (with preserved kidney function) with prolonged occupational exposure, the apparent half-life is extended to years.[51] This prolonged half-life may be related to deposits of aluminum metal dust in the lungs of workers with pulmonary fibrosis from exposure to aluminum dust. There is no normal reference point for elimination half-life.

PATHOPHYSIOLOGY

Little is known about the pathophysiology of aluminum toxicity. The information that follows is based on a summary of limited research. Some animal studies provide insight into the mechanisms that are responsible for the toxicity of aluminum, mainly citing oxidative stress on various tissues, but the studies are limited and do not offer a comprehensive understanding.[102] There remain many gaps in our knowledge of aluminum toxicity on specific organ systems.

Pulmonary System

In rats exposed to alumina and aluminum through intratracheal injection, fibrosis (aluminosis when secondary to aluminum) develops.[42,43] These animals develop epithelialization of alveoli, focal fibrosis occurring in the respiratory bronchioles and alveolar ducts, and alveolar proteinosis.[33,79]

Central Nervous System

Aluminum exposure is associated with acute encephalopathy, dialysis encephalopathy, seizures, and Alzheimer disease. The primary site of aluminum entry into the brain appears to be the cerebral microvasculature. Following IV administration in rats and rabbits, aluminum concentrations are higher in the frontal cortex than in the lateral ventricles. The cortex concentrations should result from blood supply, whereas the lateral ventricle concentration may be derived from the blood supply or the CSF, which bathes the lateral ventricles.[110,111] The mechanisms of entry are postulated to be transferrin mediated, endocytosis and other active processes.[27] Aluminum interacts with the acetylcholine pathways in the brain and decreases acetylcholine activity. High-affinity choline uptake in the brains of rats also decreases; the activity of choline acetyltransferase in rabbit brains is also decreased.[36,50] Rabbits treated with aluminum have significantly decreased acetylcholine outflow compared with controls, a finding that does not improve with potassium neuronal supplements. This finding suggests that aluminum attenuates the response of neurons to potassium-induced depolarization.[110] Adult rabbits exposed to aluminum also have a significant reduction in conditioned responses compared with rabbits exposed in utero or in the first or second month postpartum.[106]

Hematologic System

Early toxicity of aluminum affects hematopoiesis resulting in a microcytic hypochromic anemia before affecting the CNS. In rats, aluminum inhibits cell growth, while in humans hematopoietic cells are inhibited. In mice, aluminum decreases cell proliferation and hemoglobin synthesis.[5,64] Aluminum inhibits δ-aminolevulinic acid dehydrogenase in the heme synthesis pathway,[3,61] leading to the accumulation of erythrocyte protoporphyrins (Fig. 20–3). This effect is most noted in HD patients with aluminum overload.[14]

Musculoskeletal System

Vitamin D–resistant osteomalacia and osteopathy occur in patients with aluminum toxicity. It is characterized by hyperosteoidosis, minimal osteoblastic activity, and decreased mineralization. The metabolism and kinetics of calcium, magnesium, and phosphate do not appear to be affected in these patients.[17] Aluminum concentrates in the mitochondria of the osteoblasts at the mineralization front.[19] It is theorized that aluminum competes and replaces other cations in the bone, leading to osteopathy.[32] The osteomalacia is not caused solely by CKD but develops in the presence of aluminum exposure.[86] In rat studies, exogenous parathyroid hormone enhanced aluminum deposition into bone, leading to osteopathy.[57,58]

MANIFESTATIONS

Acute Toxicity

Regardless of pathophysiology, patients with acute aluminum toxicity typically develop encephalopathy, myoclonus, and seizures. The encephalopathy manifests as disorientation, confusion, and coma. All symptoms appear to develop within days to a few weeks of receiving massive systemic aluminum exposure (usually to an aluminum salt). Serum concentrations range from barely elevated to extremely elevated. Most patients who manifest toxicity have systemically absorbed aluminum, usually in the presence of CKD. In several case reports of acute aluminum toxicity, the initial exposure to aluminum was associated with alum bladder irrigations for hemorrhagic cystitis.[40,70,78] In 2 patients, these symptoms developed after only weeks of exposure to aluminum-containing phosphate binders in the presence of citrate.[44] Two neonates with uremia developed neurotoxicity after exposure over a 1- to 2-month period to infant formula with high aluminum content.[25] Although recovery occurs in patients promptly treated with deferoxamine and/or HD,[40,69,70] patients with unrecognized signs and/or a delay to treatment usually die (supportive care typically never able to restore a normal mental status).[44,90,94]

Chronic Toxicity

Two distinct types of chronic aluminum toxicity are reported: occupationally related lung disease, such as asthma and pulmonary fibrosis, and a multisystem syndrome most often noted in HD patients, which was initially described as dialysis encephalopathy syndrome or "dialysis dementia." These terms are not descriptive of the full effects of aluminum toxicity. Animal studies also report changes in cognitive development and memory following chronic exposure to aluminum salts.[6]

Pulmonary

Potroom asthma consists of dyspnea, cough, wheezing, bronchitis, and chest tightness.[62] These symptoms develop after only a few months of exposure to the metal fumes of aluminum and aluminum dust. The asthma often improves on cessation of exposure, although some workers never fully recover.[74] These manifestations cause for the high turnover among potroom workers, which, in turn, limits the quality of long-term follow-up.[38,99]

Pulmonary fibrosis from aluminum, termed aluminosis, is very similar to the other pneumoconiosis, like silicosis, and morbidity and mortality are consequential. This pathologic finding develops in workers exposed to aluminum dust. Patients experience cough, shortness of breath, and dyspnea on exertion, and they eventually develop restrictive lung disease.[48,63] Abnormal chest radiographic findings include increased pulmonary markings, distortion of pleura and diaphragms, and irregular opacities.[28,36,92] Recovery of lung function does not occur, and patients die from complications of pulmonary disease such as pneumonia.

Multisystem Toxicity

The other form of chronic aluminum toxicity has multisystem manifestations. It primarily affects 3 organ systems: hematopoietic, nervous, and musculoskeletal. In patients with CKD, the toxicity occurs after months to years of exposure to aluminum salt–contaminated dialysate and or aluminum salt–containing phosphate binders such as aluminum hydroxide and sucralfate. However, one review of 755 chronic dialysis patients in Australia found only 7 patients with significantly elevated aluminum concentrations, stating that modern techniques of reverse osmosis of water is substantially aluminum-free (nearly always <0.1 μmol/L).[91]

A similar clinical presentation developed over 3 months in a patient having used aluminum-coated cookware for 4 years to boil methadone for IV use.[26,112] Three industrial workers exposed to aluminum metal powder were reported to develop encephalopathy. One of these workers had a brain aluminum concentration 20 times normal.[53] Normal brain aluminum concentrations are reported as approximately 1.5 mcg/g dry weight, with a tendency to increase with age.[49,59] An infant with kidney insufficiency had 10 months of exposure to aluminum salt–containing phosphate binders and developed focal seizures, which eventually progressed to generalized seizures, hypotonia, poor head control, ataxia, and developmental delay in the presence of elevated serum aluminum concentration.[82]

The microcytic hypochromic anemia of aluminum poisoning is unresponsive to iron replacement therapy.[37] This clinical finding usually precedes encephalopathy and osteomalacia.[93] The encephalopathy is characterized by speech disturbances, EEG abnormalities, myoclonic jerks, and dementia.[98] The typical speech disturbances include dyspraxia, dysphasia, stuttering, and possibly mutism.[54,87,98] Electroencephalographic abnormalities include slowing of the normal rhythm and high-voltage biphasic or triphasic spikes.[55,98] The myoclonic activity includes uncontrolled twitching movements, myoclonus, or seizures.[98] The osteopathy and osteomalacia can lead to bone pain and fractures.[18,108] Death is common in these patients when aluminum toxicity is not recognized and treated.

DIAGNOSTIC TESTS

A normal serum aluminum concentration should be less than or equal to 2 mcg/L,[31] whereas a whole blood aluminum concentration should be less than 12 mcg/L.[96] Daily urinary excretion less than 4 to 12 mcg aluminum is considered normal.[31,72] Toxicity has occurred in patients with a wide range of serum and urine concentrations, with some dying of severe clinical manifestations with concentrations only slightly above normal.

Pulmonary function testing can be performed to evaluate for restrictive lung function, as occurs with aluminosis. A Finnish occupational study recommended spot urine aluminum measurements, proposing a maximum of 2.3 μmol/g creatinine after 2 exposure-free days as an actionable limit that prompts closer monitoring of aluminum exposure.[85]

MANAGEMENT

Patients with symptoms or with elevated aluminum concentrations should be removed from any aluminum exposure if identified. Exposure to aluminum in industry and exposure to antacids containing aluminum salts should also be limited. Patients with occupational asthma from aluminum exposure should be symptomatically treated with bronchodilators and steroids.

The only chelator with proven benefit is deferoxamine (DFO). Chelation therapy is recommended for both acute and chronic toxicity from aluminum salts. Chelation not only limits but also improves manifestations of neurotoxicity, anemia, and osteomalacia (Antidotes in Depth: A7). Other chelators such as D-penicillamine and 2,3-dimercapto-1-propanol (BAL) were tried in chronic HD patients without any improvement in their manifestations or aluminum concentrations and therefore we recommend that they not be used.[16] A review of numerous chelator studies revealed that no other chelator was an acceptable alternative to DFO.[105]

Acute Toxicity

A DFO dose of 15 mg/kg/d intravenously is recommended. Adults have received doses ranging from 1 to 2 g for aluminum toxicity. Deferoxamine chelates the aluminum to form aluminoxamine, which is excreted in the urine or removed by HD.[107] Chelation mobilizes aluminum from its storage sites in blood and increases its renal elimination. In dialysis-dependent patients, DFO is reported to precipitate aluminum encephalopathy and death, either from DFO redistribution of aluminum to brain tissue or aluminum oxide redistribution across the blood–brain barrier.

It is recommended that in patients with stage 5 chronic kidney disease that, 3 to 4 hours of HD is performed 6 to 8 hours after chelation in order to clear the aluminoxamine (the aluminum-DFO product) and prevent redistribution to vital tissues.[69] Patients with normal kidney function and urine output do not require HD, as the aluminoxamine is excreted in the urine (Antidotes in Depth: A7, "Deferoxamine,").

Chronic Toxicity

Chelation therapy with DFO reverses encephalopathy, osteomalacia, and anemia. Numerous case reports demonstrate the reversal of the neurotoxicity, vitamin D–resistant bone disease, and iron-resistant anemia.[7,11,15] The National Kidney Foundation provides guidelines for the treatment of dialysis encephalopathy. These guidelines of nephrologists recommend 4 months of once weekly DFO at 5 mg/kg over 1 hour given 5 hours before a regularly scheduled HD session in patients with serum aluminum concentrations greater than 300 mcg/L. In patients with serum aluminum concentrations between 50 and 300 mcg/L, DFO 5 mg/kg is given during the last hour of HD, once a week for 2 months. Serum aluminum concentrations are then monitored, and this therapy is repeated as needed based on renal function and neurologic symptoms.[71] A small study evaluated the effect of lower doses of DFO (2.5 mg/kg/week) for treatment of chronic toxicity in dialysis patients, and found similar therapeutic benefit compared to 5 mg/kg/week dosing, but stressed the need for further studies.[39]

Other Treatments

A myriad of other treatments were proposed and tested in animal models, though they were mainly small samples sizes and none have been tested in humans. Nearly all of the xenobiotics used reported benefit due to antioxidant properties and an overall decrease in oxidative stress. Substances with reported benefit have included, among others, zinc, copper, pomegranate peel, vitamin E, selenium, taurine, melatonin, coenzyme Q10, and fish oil, although there is not enough evidence to recommend the routine use of any of these substances at this time.[1,2,13,41,65,66,81]

SUMMARY

- Inhalational exposure to aluminum metal causes pulmonary toxicity, primarily manifested as bronchospasm, but progresses to restrictive lung disease.
- Acutely, aluminum salts are neurotoxins with manifestations of encephalopathy and seizures.

■ Chronically, aluminum salts affect at least 3 organ systems with manifestations of anemia, encephalopathy, dementia, and osteomalacia.

■ Treatment involves limiting or terminating exposure, chelation with DFO, and HD in patients with CKD.

REFERENCES

1. Abdel-Hamid GA. Effect of vitamin E and selenium against aluminum-induced nephrotoxicity in pregnant rats. *Folia Histochem Cytobiol.* 2013;51:312-319.

2. Abdel Moneim AE, et al. Pomegranate peel attenuates aluminum-induced hepatorenal toxicity. *Toxicol Mech Methods.* 2013;23:624-633.

3. Abdulla M, et al. Antagonistic effects of zinc and aluminum on lead inhibition of delta-aminolevulinic acid dehydratase. *Arch Environ Health.* 1979;34:464-469.

4. Abreo K, Glass J. Cellular, biochemical, and molecular mechanisms of aluminium toxicity. *Nephrol Dial Transplant.* 1993;8(suppl 1):5-11.

5. Abreo K, et al. Aluminum inhibits hemoglobin synthesis but enhances iron uptake in Friend erythroleukemia cells. *Kidney Int.* 1990;37:677-681.

6. Abu-Taweel GM, et al. Neurobehavioral toxic effects of perinatal oral exposure to aluminum on the developmental motor reflexes, learning, memory and brain neurotransmitters of mice offspring. *Pharmacol Biochem Behav.* 2012;101:49-56.

7. Ackrill P, et al. Successful removal of aluminium from patient with dialysis encephalopathy. *Lancet.* 1980;2:692-693.

8. Alfrey AC, et al. Metabolism and toxicity of aluminum in renal failure. *Am J Clin Nutr.* 1980;33:1509-1516.

9. Alfrey AC, et al. The dialysis encephalopathy syndrome. Possible aluminum intoxication. *N Engl J Med.* 1976;294:184-188.

10. Alfrey AC, et al. Syndrome of dyspraxia and multifocal seizures associated with chronic hemodialysis. *Trans Am Soc Artif Intern Organs.* 1972;18:257-261, 266-267.

11. Arze RS, et al. Reversal of aluminium dialysis encephalopathy after desferrioxamine treatment. *Lancet.* 1981;2:1116.

12. Axcan Scandipharm Inc. Carafate prescribing information [package insert]: Axcan Scandipharm Inc; 2005.

13. Bhasin P, et al. Protective role of zinc during aluminum-induced hepatotoxicity. *Environ Toxicol.* 2014;29:320-327.

14. Bia MJ, et al. Aluminum induced anemia: pathogenesis and treatment in patients on chronic hemodialysis. *Kidney Int.* 1989;36:852-858.

15. Brown DJ, et al. Treatment of dialysis osteomalacia with desferrioxamine. *Lancet.* 1982;2:343-345.

16. Burks JS, et al. A fatal encephalopathy in chronic haemodialysis patients. *Lancet.* 1976;1:764-768.

17. Burnatowska-Hledin MA, et al. Aluminum, parathyroid hormone, and osteomalacia. *Spec Top Endocrinol Metab.* 1983;5:201-226.

18. Cannata-Andia JB, Fernandez-Martin JL. The clinical impact of aluminium overload in renal failure. *Nephrol Dial Transplant.* 2002;17(suppl 2):9-12.

19. Clarkson E, et al. The effect of aluminium hydroxide on calcium, phosphorus, and aluminium balances, the serum parathyroid hormone concentration and the aluminium content of bone in patients with chronic renal failure. *Clin Sci.* 1972;43:519-531.

20. Dinman B. Aluminum, alloys, and compounds. *Encyclopedia of Occupational Health and Safety.* Vol. 11983:131-135.

21. Elliott HL, et al. Aluminium toxicity during regular haemodialysis. *Br Med J.* 1978;1:1101-1103.

22. Exley C, et al. Elevated urinary aluminium in current and past users of illicit heroin. *Addict Biol.* 2007;12:197-199.

23. Fernández Menéndez MJ, et al. Aluminium uptake by intestinal cells: effect of iron status and precomplexation. *Nephrol Dial Transplant.* 1991;6:672-674.

24. Flarend R, et al. A preliminary study of the dermal absorption of aluminium from antiperspirants using aluminium-26. *Food Chem Toxicol.* 2001;39:163-168.

25. Freundlich M, et al. Infant formula as a cause of aluminium toxicity in neonatal uraemia. *Lancet.* 1985;2:527-529.

26. Friesen MS, et al. Aluminum toxicity following IV use of oral methadone solution. *Clin Toxicol.* 2006;44:307-314.

27. Frostad E. Fluoride intoxication in Norwegian aluminum plant workers. *Tidsskr Nor Laegeforen.* 1936;56:179-182.

28. Gaffuri E, et al. Pulmonary changes and aluminium levels following inhalation of alumina dust: a study on four exposed workers. *Med Lav.* 1985;76:222-227.

29. Gitelman HJ. Aluminum exposure and excretion. *Sci Total Environ.* 1995;163:129-135.

30. Goralewski G. Die aluminumlunge: ein neue gewerbeerkrankung. *Z Gestamte Inn Med.* 1947;2:665-673.

31. Greger JL, Sutherland JE. Aluminum exposure and metabolism. *Crit Rev Clin Lab Sci.* 1997;34:439-474.

32. Griswold WR, et al. Accumulation of aluminum in a nondialyzed uremic child receiving aluminum hydroxide. *Pediatrics.* 1983;71:56-58.

33. Gross P, et al. Pulmonary reaction to metallic aluminum powders: an experimental study. *Arch Environ Health.* 1973;26:227-236.

34. Gupta RK, Relyveld EH. Adverse reactions after injection of adsorbed diphtheria-pertussis-tetanus (DPT) vaccine are not due only to pertussis organisms or pertussis components in the vaccine. *Vaccine.* 1991;9:699-702.

35. Health Canada. Guidelines for Canadian Drinking Water Quality. Supporting Documentation. Part II. Aluminum. Vol 22, Health Canada, Environmental Health Directorate; 1998.

36. Jederlinic PJ, et al. Pulmonary fibrosis in aluminum oxide workers. Investigation of nine workers, with pathologic examination and microanalysis in three of them. *Am Rev Respir Dis.* 1990;142:1179-1184.

37. Jeffery EH, et al. Systemic aluminum toxicity: effects on bone, hematopoietic tissue, and kidney. *J Toxicol Environ Health.* 1996;48:649-665.

38. Kaltreider NL, et al. Health survey of aluminum workers with special reference to fluoride exposure. *J Occup Med.* 1972;14:531-541.

39. Kan WC, et al. Comparison of low-dose deferoxamine versus-standard-dose deferoxamine for treatment of aluminium overload among haemodialysis patients. *Nephrol Dial Transplant.* 2010;25:1604-1608.

40. Kanwar VS, et al. Aluminum toxicity following intravesical alum irrigation for hemorrhagic cystitis. *Med Pediatr Oncol.* 1996;27:64-67.

41. AA Karabulut-Bulan O, et al. Role of exogenous melatonin on cell proliferation and oxidant/antioxidant system in aluminum-induced renal toxicity. *Biol Trace Elem Res.* 2015 Nov;168:141-149.

42. King EJ, et al. The effect of various forms of alumina on the lungs of rats. *J Pathol Bacteriol.* 1955;69:81-93.

43. King EJ, et al. The effect of aluminium and of aluminium containing 5 per cent of quartz in the lungs of rats. *J Pathol Bacteriol.* 1958;75:429-434.

44. Kirschbaum BB, Schoolwerth AC. Acute aluminum toxicity associated with oral citrate and aluminum-containing antacids. *Am J Med Sci.* 1989;297:9-11.

45. Klein GL, et al. Aluminum loading during total parenteral nutrition. *Am J Clin Nutr.* 1982;35:1425-1429.

46. Klein GL, et al. Elevated serum aluminum levels in severely burned patients who are receiving large quantities of albumin. *J Burn Care Rehabil.* 1990;11:526-530.

47. Kovalchik MT, et al. Aluminum kinetics during hemodialysis. *J Lab Clin Med.* 1978;92:712-720.

48. Kraus T, et al. Aluminium dust-induced lung disease in the pyro-powder-producing industry: detection by high-resolution computed tomography. *Int Arch Occup Environ Health.* 2000;73:61-64.

49. Krishnan SS, et al. Aluminum toxicity to the brain. *Sci Total Environ.* 1988;71:59-64.

50. Lai JC, et al. The effects of cadmium, manganese and aluminium on sodium-potassium-activated and magnesium-activated adenosine triphosphatase activity and choline uptake in rat brain synaptosomes. *Biochem Pharmacol.* 1980;29:141-146.

51. Ljunggren KG, et al. Blood and urine concentrations of aluminium among workers exposed to aluminium flake powders. *Br J Ind Med.* 1991;48:106-109.

52. Long H, et al. A fatal case of spongiform leukoencephalopathy linked to "chasing the dragon." *J Toxicol Clin Toxicol.* 2003;41:887-891.

53. Longstreth WT Jr, et al. Potroom palsy? Neurologic disorder in three aluminum smelter workers. *Arch Intern Med.* 1985;145:1972-1975.

54. Madison DP, et al. Communicative and cognitive deterioration in dialysis dementia: two case studies. *J Speech Hear Disord.* 1977;42:238-246.

55. Mahurkar SD, et al. Electroencephalographic and radionuclide studies in dialysis dementia. *Kidney Int.* 1978;13:306-315.

56. Maitani T, et al. Distribution and urinary excretion of aluminum injected with several organic acids into mice: relationship with chemical state in serum studied by HPLC-ICP method. *J Appl Toxicol.* 1994;14:257-261.

57. Mayor GH, et al. Parathyroid hormone-mediated aluminum deposition and egress in the rat. *Kidney Int.* 1980;17:40-44.

58. McDermott JR, et al. Aluminium and Alzheimer's disease. *Lancet.* 1977;2:710-711.

59. McDermott JR, et al. Brain aluminum in aging and Alzheimer disease: *Neurology.* 1979;29:809.

60. McLaughlin AI, et al. Pulmonary fibrosis and encephalopathy associated with the inhalation of aluminium dust. *Br J Ind Med.* 1962;19:253-263.

61. Meredith C, et al. The effect of Biostim (RU-41740) on the expression of cytokine mRNAs in murine peritoneal macrophages in vitro. *Toxicol Lett.* 1990;53:327-337.

62. Midttun O. Anaphylactic death caused by specific desensitization. *Acta Allergol.* 1954;7:186-192.

63. Mitchell J, et al. Pulmonary fibrosis in workers exposed to finely powdered aluminium. *Br J Ind Med.* 1961;18:10-23.

64. Mladenovic J. Aluminum inhibits erythropoiesis in vitro. *J Clin Invest.* 1988;81:1661-1665.

65. Mohammad NS, et al. Coenzyme Q10 and fish oil synergistically alleviate aluminum chloride-induced suppression of testicular steroidogenesis and antioxidant defense. *Free Radic Res.* 2015;49:1319-1334.

66. Moshtaghie AA, et al. Protective effects of copper against aluminum toxicity on acetylcholinesterase and catecholamine contents of different regions of rat's brain. *Neurol Sci.* 2013;34:1639-1650.

67. Murray JC, et al. Aluminum neurotoxicity: a reevaluation. *Clin Neuropharmacol.* 1991;14:179-185.

68. Mussi I, et al. Behaviour of plasma and urinary aluminium levels in occupationally exposed subjects. *Int Arch Occup Environ Health.* 1984;54:155-161.

69. Nakamura H, et al. Encephalopathy with seizures after use of aluminum-containing bone cement. *Lancet.* 1994;344:1647.

70. Nakamura H, et al. Acute encephalopathy due to aluminum toxicity successfully treated by combined intravenous deferoxamine and hemodialysis. *J Clin Pharmacol.* 2000;40:296-300.

71. National Kidney Foundation. K/DOQI clinical practice guidelines for bone metabolism and disease in chronic kidney disease. *Am J Kidney Dis.* 2003;42:S1-S201.

72. Nieboer E, et al. Health effects of aluminum: a critical review with emphasis on aluminum in drinking water. *Environ Rev.* 1995;3:29-81.

73. Nolan CR, et al. Aluminum and lead absorption from dietary sources in women ingesting calcium citrate. *South Med J.* 1994;87:894-898.

74. O'Connell T, et al. Potroom asthma: New Zealand experience and follow-up. *Am J Ind Med.* 1989;15:43-49.

75. Ostroff EB, Chenault OW Jr. Alum irrigation for the control of massive bladder hemorrhage. *J Urol.* 1982;128:929-930.

76. Pennington JA, Schoen SA. Estimates of dietary exposure to aluminium. *Food Addit Contam.* 1995;12:119-128.

77. Perl DP, Brody AR. Alzheimer's disease: X-ray spectrometric evidence of aluminum accumulation in neurofibrillary tangle-bearing neurons. *Science.* 1980;208:297-299.

78. Phelps KR, et al. Encephalopathy after bladder irrigation with alum: case report and literature review. *Am J Med Sci.* 1999;318:181-185.

79. Pigott GH, et al. Effects of long term inhalation of alumina fibres in rats. *Br J Exp Pathol.* 1981;62:323-331.

80. Priest ND, et al. Human metabolism of aluminium-26 and gallium-67 injected as citrates. *Hum Exp Toxicol.* 1995;14:287-293.

81. Qiao M, et al. Potential protection of taurine on antioxidant system and ATPase in brain and blood of rats exposed to aluminum. *Biotechnol Lett.* 2015;37:1579-1584.

82. Randall ME. Aluminium toxicity in an infant not on dialysis. *Lancet.* 1983;1:1327-1328.

83. Rifat SL, et al. Effect of exposure of miners to aluminium powder. *Lancet.* 1990;336:1162-1165.

84. Riihimaki V, et al. Behavior of aluminum in aluminum welders and manufacturers of aluminum sulfate—impact on biological monitoring. *Scand J Work Environ Health.* 2008;34:451-462.

85. Riihimäki V, Aitio A. Occupational exposure to aluminum and its biomonitoring in perspective. *Crit Rev Toxicol.* 2012 Nov;42:827-853.

86. Robertson JA, et al. Animal model of aluminum-induced osteomalacia: role of chronic renal failure. *Kidney Int.* 1983;23:327-335.

87. Rosenbek JC, et al. Speech and language findings in a chronic hemodialysis patient: a case report. *J Speech Hear Disord.* 1975;40:245-252.

88. Roth A, et al. Multiorgan aluminium deposits in a chronic haemodialysis patient. Electron microscope and microprobe studies. *Virchows Arch A Pathol Anat Histopathol.* 1984;405:131-140.

89. Schulz W, et al. On the differential diagnosis and therapy of dialysis osteomalacia under special consideration to a therapy with oral phosphate binders. *Trace Elem Med.* 1984;1:120-127.

90. Seear M. The Wilfred Fish Lecture. The professions: red light or green? *Br Dent J.* 1984;156:329-331.

91. Sharma AK, et al. Assessing the utility of testing aluminum levels in dialysis patients. *Hemodial Int.* 2015;19:256-262.

92. Shaver CG, Riddell AR. Lung changes associated with the manufacture of alumina abrasives. *J Ind Hyg Toxicol.* 1947;29:145-157.

93. Short AI, et al. Reversible microcytic hypochromic anaemia in dialysis patients due to aluminium intoxication. *Proc Eur Dial Transplant Assoc.* 1980;17:226-233.

94. Shoskes DA, et al. Aluminum toxicity and death following intravesical alum irrigation in a patient with renal impairment. *J Urol.* 1992;147:697-699.

95. Sjogren B, et al. Exposure and urinary excretion of aluminum during welding. *Scand J Work Environ Health.* 1985;11:39-43.

96. Sjogren B, et al. Aluminium in the blood and urine of industrially exposed workers. *Br J Ind Med.* 1983;40:301-304.

97. Slanina P, et al. Dietary citric acid enhances absorption of aluminum in antacids. *Clin Chem.* 1986;32:539-541.

98. Smith E, et al. Diagnosing dialysis dementia. *Dial Transplant.* 1978;7:1264-1274.

99. Smith M. The respiratory condition of potroom workers: the Australian experience. In: Hughes J, ed. *Health Protection in Primary Aluminum Production.* London: International Primary Aluminum Institute; 1977:79-86.

100. Spofforth J. Case of aluminum poisoning. *Lancet.* 1921;1:1301.

101. van Landeghem GF, et al. Al and Si: their speciation, distribution, and toxicity. *Clin Biochem.* 1998;31:385-397.

102. Vučetić-Arsić S, et al. Oxidative stress precedes mitochondrial dysfunction in gerbil brain after aluminum ingestion. *Environ Toxicol Pharmacol.* 2013;36:1242-1252.

103. Ward MK, et al. Osteomalacic dialysis osteodystrophy: evidence for a water-borne aetiological agent, probably aluminium. *Lancet.* 1978;1:841-845.

104. Wilhelm M, et al. Aluminium toxicokinetics. *Pharmacol Toxicol.* 1990;66:4-9.

105. Yokel RA. Aluminum chelation: chemistry, clinical, and experimental studies and the search for alternatives to desferrioxamine. *J Toxicol Environ Health.* 1994;41:131-174.

106. Yokel RA. Aluminum produces age related behavioral toxicity in the rabbit. *Neurotoxicol Teratol.* 1989;11:237-242.

107. Yokel RA. Brain uptake, retention, and efflux of aluminum and manganese. *Environ Health Perspect.* 2002;110(suppl 5):699-704.

108. Yokel RA. The toxicology of aluminum in the brain: a review. *Neurotoxicology.* 2000;21:813-828.

109. Yokel RA, et al. Prevention and treatment of aluminum toxicity including chelation therapy: status and research needs. *J Toxicol Environ Health.* 1996;48:667-683.

110. Yokel RA, et al. Studies of aluminum neurobehavioral toxicity in the intact mammal. *Cell Mol Neurobiol.* 1994;14:791-808.

111. Yokel RA, McNamara PJ. Aluminium toxicokinetics: an updated minireview. *Pharmacol Toxicol.* 2001;88:159-167.

112. Yong RL, et al. Aluminum toxicity due to intravenous injection of boiled methadone. *N Engl J Med.* 2006;354:1210-1211.

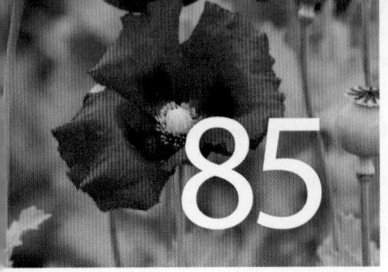

85 ANTIMONY

Asim F. Tarabar

Antimony (Sb)

Atomic number	=	51
Atomic weight	=	121.75 Da
Normal concentrations		
Serum	<	3 mcg/L (24.6 nmol/L)
Urine (24-hour)	<	6.2 mcg/L (50.1 nmol/L)
	<	3.5 mcg/g creatinine (28.7 nmol/g creatinine)

HISTORY AND EPIDEMIOLOGY

Antimony (Sb) and its compounds are among the oldest known remedies in the practice of medicine.[115,169] Because of a strong chemical similarity to arsenic, the features of antimony poisoning closely resemble arsenic poisoning (Chap. 86). Antimony poisoning also shares features common with other metal poisonings, described in the chapters that follow. Although relatively uncommon, antimony toxicity occurs, usually as a complication of the treatment of visceral leishmaniasis.[101] Acute overdose represents an even rarer, but potentially lethal event, most often recently as a result of a unconventional alcohol aversion treatment.[109,154]

Objects discovered during exploration of ancient Mesopotamian life (third and fourth millennium B.C.) suggest that both the Sumerians and the Chaldeans were able to produce pure antimony.[115,169] The reference to eye paint in the Old Testament suggested the use of antimony.[115] For several thousand years, Asian and Middle Eastern countries used antimony sulfide in the production of cosmetics, including rouge and black paint for eyebrows, also known as kohl or surma.[106,114] Because of the scarcity of antimony sulfide, lead replaced antimony as a main component in antiquated cosmetic preparations.

One of the first monographs on metals, written in the 16th century, included a description of antimony.[160] The medicinal use of antimony for the treatment of syphilis, whooping cough, and gout dates to the medieval period. Paracelsus was credited with establishing the therapeutic efficacy of antimony compounds and increasing their popularity. In spite of being aware of its toxic potential, many of the disciples of Paracelsus enthusiastically continued the use of antimony.[115] Various antimony compounds were also used as topical preparations for the treatment of herpes, leprosy, mania, and epilepsy.[169] Orally administered tartar emetic (antimony potassium tartrate) was used for treatment of fever, pneumonia, inflammatory conditions, and as a decongestant, emetic, and sedative, but it was abandoned because of its significant toxicity.[26,53,76,88] The use of antimony as a homicidal agent[155] continued well into the 20th century (Chap. 1).

The current medical use of antimony is limited to the treatments of leishmaniasis and schistosomiasis, and to sporadic use as aversive therapy for substance abuse.[109,154] Pentavalent compounds are used as antiparasitics because they are better tolerated. In the endemic regions of the world, generic pentavalent antimonials remain the mainstay of therapy because of their efficacy and low cost. The growing incidence of resistance is affecting their use,[119] forcing a shift toward the use of novel cost-effective delivery systems for antimonials and second-line agents as amphotericin B, miltefosine, and paromomycin (aminosidine).[75]

Some contemporary homeopathic[67] and anthroposophical[148] practices recommend the use of antimonial compounds as home remedies in rare cases.[115,169] In spite of its anticancer effects in vitro[53] and remarkable therapeutic efficacy in patients with acute promyelocytic leukemia,[143] there is no current accepted oncologic use of antimony. When compared with suramin, a well-known chemotherapeutic, sodium stibogluconate appears to be a better inhibitor, giving a foundation for future research of antimony-based chemotherapeutics.[143]

The elemental form of antimony has very few industrial uses because of its physical limitations, in particular the fact that it is not malleable. By contrast, its alloys with copper, lead, and tin have important applications. Various antimony compounds are used in the production of textiles, enamels, ceramics, fireworks, and pigments, and as catalysts in chemical reactions. Industrial and occupational exposure to antimony occurs mainly through the inhalation of dust or fumes during the processing or packaging of antimony compounds.[16,69] Workers involved in electronic waste recycling without adequate personal protective equipment develop elevated antimony concentrations in their hair, suggestive of significant exposure.[90] Smelters are at risk of occupational exposure to antimony as it is often present in arsenic-containing ore.[66] A time-weighted average over an 8-hour shift of the permissible exposure limit for antimony and its compounds is established by the Occupational Safety and Health Administration at 0.5 mg per cubic meter of air (mg/m³).[34] Antimony concentrations in cigarette smoke range from 10 to 60 mg/kg,[66,123] which is likely responsible for a substantial percentage of the antimony found in the lungs of smokers (Table 85–1).[66]

In developed countries, antimony poisoning rarely occurs following intentional ingestion of antimonials.[109,169] Most recent descriptions of antimony toxicity result from parenteral exposures during the treatment of schistosomiasis and leishmaniasis. Because of the infrequent use of therapeutic antimonials, health care providers in the United States are often not familiar with the standard dosing and administration procedures, placing their patients at risk for therapeutic misadventures.[95] An expected increase in the number of cases of domestically treated leishmaniasis resulted from the deployment of US troops to the Middle East.[170] Cutaneous leishmaniasis affected as many as 2% of troops deployed to Afghanistan and Iraq.[14]

Oral exposures usually occur following the use of antimonials containing potassium tartrate compounds.[109,154] Several cases were described after the use of old porcelain houseware or after the use of antimonials as home remedies.[4,99,118,154]

CHEMISTRY

Antimony is found in the same group on the periodic table as arsenic (As), and as such it has many similar chemical, physical, and toxicologic properties. Because it can react as both a metal and a nonmetal, antimony is classified as a metalloid (Chap. 10).[16,150] Pure antimony is a lustrous, silver-white, brittle, hard metal that is easily pulverized.[54,169] It is extremely rare to find elemental antimony in nature because of its ability to rapidly convert to either antimony oxide or antimony trioxide.[16] It is suggested that even its name originates from *anti monon* (enmity to solitude) because antimony is almost always found with some other metal.[115] Thus, for the purposes of this chapter, the term *antimony* refers to antimony ions.

In nature, antimony is found in more than 100 different minerals,[91,115] including stibnite, cervantite, valentine, and kermesite.[60] The sulfide ore (stibnite) is the most abundant form,[115] and Bolivia and South Africa are among the leading producers.[169] Like arsenic, antimony forms both organic and inorganic compounds with trivalent (3⁺) and pentavalent (5⁺) oxidation states. Common inorganic trivalent antimony compounds include antimony potassium tartrate ($C_8H_4K_2O_{12}Sb_2$), antimony trichloride ($SbCl_3$), antimony trioxide (Sb_2O_3), antimony trisulfide (Sb_2S_3), and stibine (SbH_3). Antimony pentasulfide (Sb_2S_5) and pentoxide (Sb_2O_5) are inorganic compounds that can act as oxidizing agents.[23] Antimony pentachloride ($SbCl_5$)

TABLE 85–1   Antimony Regulations and Advisories

Agency	Guidelines Description	Concentration
Air		
ACGIH (2004)	TLV (TWA) for antimony and inorganic antimony compounds	0.5 mg/m³
EPA IRIS (1999)	Inhalation Reference Concentration (RfC)	
	Antimony	Not established
	Antimony trioxide	2×10^{-4} mg/m³
NIOSH (1994)	REL (15-minute ceiling limit) for antimony and its compounds	0.5 mg/m³
	IDLH for antimony (as Sb)	50 mg/m³
OSHA (2012)	PEL (8-hour TWA) for antimony and compounds	0.5 mg/m³
29 CFR 1910.1000 Table Z-1	(General/Construction Industry/Shipyard Employment)	
Water		
EPA (2009)	National primary drinking water standards for antimony	
	MCL	0.006 mg/L (6 ppb)
	MCLG	0.006 mg/L (6 ppb)
FDA	Bottled drinking water	0.006 mg/L
WHO (2011)	Drinking water quality guidelines for antimony	0.02 mg/L (20 mcg/L)
ACGIH		
Human Carcinogenic Effect		
EPA/NTP	Not listed	
IARC (1999)	Group 2B (possibly carcinogenic to humans {antimony trioxide})	

ACGIH = American Conference of Governmental Industrial Hygienists; CFR = Code of Federal Regulations; DWEL = drinking water equivalent level; EPA = Environmental Protection Agency; FDA = Food and Drug Administration; IARC = International Agency for Research on Cancer; IDHL = immediately dangerous to life or health; IRIS = Integrated Risk Information System; MCL = maximum contaminant level; MCLG = maximum contaminant level goal; MW = molecular weight; NIOSH = National Institute for Occupational Safety and Health; NTP = National Toxicology Program; OSHA = Occupational Safety and Health Administration; PEL = permissible exposure limit; REL = recommended exposure limit; TLV = threshold limit value; TWA = time-weighted average; WHO = World Health Organization.

is used as a chemical reagent with acidic properties. It reacts with water, forming hydrochloric acid, which has a direct corrosive effect on the skin and mucous membranes.[43]

Besides amphotericin and paromomycin,[171] the standard treatment of cutaneous leishmaniasis, recommended by the World Health Organization (WHO) and the Centers for Disease Control and Prevention (CDC), is a 20-day course of 20 mg/kg/day of sodium stibogluconate.[170] The use of higher doses is associated with increased side effects.[170] One analytical approach measured a higher presence of trivalent antimony than previously reported with a pentavalent antimonial drug. It is postulated that trivalent antimony is released specifically in the acidic intracellular compartment targeting the *Leishmania* parasites. Released trivalent antimony could be responsible for the toxic effects of antiparasitic treatment.[141] The proposed mechanism of antimonial activity against the *Leishmania* parasites is the inhibition of try-panothione reductase that is essential for the parasite survival and virulence.[9]

From an industrial perspective, the most important application of antimony is the use of antimony oxychloride ($Sb_6O_6Cl_4$) as a flame retardant.[115] An investigation by the CDC of possible antimony toxicity in US firefighters who wear uniforms made from fabric containing antimony demonstrated no toxic link.[33]

Analysis of soil around firing ranges[104] and environmental examination around mines revealed elevated concentrations of antimony that can pose a significant health risk.[79,174] A public health concern was raised after reports of elevated antimony concentrations in water containers and commercial juices due to leaching from the packaging material or a flawed manufacturing process.[77,144]

Tartar emetic (antimony potassium tartrate) is an odorless trivalent antimony compound with a sweet metallic taste[78] and a potent emetic effect.[23] Antimony potassium tartrate is considered to be one of the most toxic antimony compounds, with minimal lethal doses reported between 200 mg[118] and 1,200 mg.[115] There are large species variations of the LD_{50} in experimental animals, with a reported range of 115 mg/kg in rabbits and rats to 600 mg/kg in mice. In comparison, because of low water solubility, antimony trioxide is considered to be nontoxic, with an LD_{50} greater than 20,000 mg/kg.[64]

PHARMACOLOGY

One proposed mechanism for the antiparasitic mechanisms of action of antimony is the inhibition of phosphofructokinase, which is the rate-limiting step in the glycolytic pathway of *Schistosoma* spp.[36] Trivalent antimony compounds inhibit phosphofructokinase, leading to energy failure from impaired adenosine triphosphate (ATP) synthesis.[31,169] It is also speculated that antimonial preparations exert their antiparasitic effect through selective targeting of guanosine diphosphate–mannose pyrophosphorylase, which interferes with nucleoside and mannose metabolism.[61] The result is that the parasites cannot synthesize purines and cannot survive without these mannose-containing glycoconjugates. A more recently proposed mechanism involves the inhibition of trypanothione reductase.[9] Even less is known about the effects of antimony on humans. It is proposed that, like other metals, antimony inactivates thiol-containing proteins and enzymes by binding to sulfhydryl groups.[48] Pentavalent antimony may act as a prodrug that is converted in acidic intracellular compartments into active and more toxic trivalent antimony.[141]

TOXICOKINETICS
Absorption

Antimony is absorbed by inhalation, ingestion, or transdermally. Absorption from the gastrointestinal tract begins immediately following ingestion, and the oral bioavailability of antimony ranges from 15% to 50%.[65,163] It is suggested that antimony absorption is a saturable process, given that several studies failed to demonstrate a dose–response relationship for absorption.[2,151] In fact, after a lethal ingestion of antimony tartrate, the total body antimony burden was only 5% of the ingested dose.[105] This poor gastrointestinal absorption in humans, in addition to the concomitant emesis, necessitates parenteral administration of many antimony-based pharmaceuticals.

Pulmonary absorption of many inorganic antimony compounds is very slow and limited by low water solubility.[115] By contrast, animal data suggest that inhaled trivalent antimony is well absorbed from the lungs, distributed to various organs, and subsequently excreted in the feces and urine.[52]

Transdermal absorption of antimony trioxide and pentoxide was documented in studies with rabbits;[122] however, dermal absorption in humans of antimony trioxide is considered negligible.[138] In an investigation of a possible outbreak of antimony exposure in firefighters, no significant transdermal absorption occurred from the antimony containing firefighter uniforms.[33]

Distribution

Distribution depends on the oxidation state of antimony. In animals, more than 95% of trivalent antimony is incorporated into the red blood cells within 2 hours of exposure, whereas 90% of pentavalent antimony remains in the serum in a similar time frame.[55]

When administered intravenously or orally, antimony is predominantly distributed among highly vascular organs, including the liver, kidneys, thyroid, and adrenals.[128,169] The antimony that is detected in the liver and spleen is predominantly in the pentavalent form, whereas the thyroid accumulates trivalent forms.[15] Uptake by the liver occurs through the mechanisms of diffusion and saturable binding.[147] In a hamster model, following a single injection of organic antimonials, the greatest concentration of antimony was found in the liver.[65] After inhalation, antimony accumulates predominantly in red blood cells and to a significantly lesser extent in the liver and spleen.[52,55] It is possible that inhaled antimony is retained in the lungs for a prolonged period of time without significant systemic absorption and distribution.[66] Animal data also demonstrated the accumulation of antimony in the skeletal system and in fur.[57,58]

After intramuscular (IM) administration of sodium stibogluconate, the antimony concentration versus time profile suggested a 2-compartment open model, with the rapid distribution phase and slower elimination half-life in the range of 10 hours.[175]

Metabolism

Although antimony and arsenic share many toxicokinetic properties, inorganic trivalent antimony, unlike arsenic, is not methylated in vivo.[8] Some microorganisms, however, are capable of biomethylation of antimony.[19] In humans, metabolic transformations of antimony are limited. Antimony is converted by binding to macromolecules, incorporation into lipids,[18] and covalent interactions with sulfhydryl groups and phosphates. Pentavalent antimony is either converted to trivalent compounds in the liver[169] or in the acidic intracellular environment of *Leishmania*-infected cells.[141]

Excretion

Trivalent antimony is excreted in the bile after conjugation with glutathione. A significant proportion of excreted antimony undergoes enterohepatic recirculation.[8] The remainder is excreted in urine. The overall elimination is very slow, with only 10% of a given dose cleared in the first 24 hours and 30% in the first week[12] although antimony is still detected in the urine 100 days after administration.[108,169] Pentavalent antimony is much more rapidly excreted by the kidneys than trivalent antimony (50%–60% vs 10% over the first 24 hours).[169] Renal excretion of sodium stibogluconate is as high as 90% within 6 hours of an IM administration.[135] However, urine and serum antimony concentrations remain elevated for several years following therapeutic use.[111] In workers, urine concentrations of pentavalent antimony correlate well with the extent of exposure.[8]

The clearance of tartar emetic has a biphasic pattern, with 90% being excreted within 24 hours after acute exposure, followed by a second slower phase with an estimated half-life of approximately 16 days.[57]

The renal elimination half-life of inhaled stibine was estimated at approximately 4 days following occupational exposure.[100]

PATHOPHYSIOLOGY

Antimony has no known biological functions and is considered to be toxic even at very low concentrations.[145] Like other toxic metals, antimony binds to sulfhydryl groups to inhibit a variety of metabolic functions.[37,48] Trivalent antimony compounds are more toxic than the pentavalent compounds because of their higher affinity for erythrocytes and sulfhydryl groups.[102] Tartar emetic and other antimony salts are gastrointestinal irritants. One proposed

mechanism for this local effect is the activation of enterochromaffin cells, which produce and secrete serotonin (5-HT). Released serotonin acts on the 5-HT$_3$ receptors, stimulating vagal sensory fibers and activating the vomiting center.[74,165] In addition, there is an apparent direct central medullary action, particularly after the administration of higher doses of antimony.[169]

CLINICAL MANIFESTATIONS

Data on human toxicity of antimony are very limited. They are largely extrapolated from occupationally exposed patients, adverse effects that have occurred during treatment of leishmaniasis and schistosomiasis, and very few case reports of intentional antimony exposures.[118] Serious adverse events and deaths resulting from treatment with sodium stibogluconate are very rare, and include cardiac dysrhythmias or pancreatitis.[170] Patients older than 50 years are at an increased risk for more serious reactions to meglumine antimonate used for the treatment of visceral leishmaniasis (Table 85–2).[51,125]

Workers with occupational exposures usually present with subtle delayed clinical manifestations as chronic toxicity develops. It is important to recognize that antimony ore contains a small concentration of arsenic, making it difficult to determine whether the effects on workers are caused by contaminants such as arsenic or by the antimony. Patients have side effects at therapeutic doses of prolonged treatment regimens with very large cumulative doses that result in acute and subacute clinical manifestations.[158] Therapeutic misadventures are possible, particularly in a setting in which antimony preparations are rarely used and health care providers are not familiar with the dosing regimen.[94]

Patients with acute ingestions usually present with signs and symptoms mimicking the toxicity of arsenic and other metal and metalloid salts.

Local Irritation

The most common manifestations of antimony toxicity involve local irritation. In sufficient concentration, antimony acts as an irritant to the eyes, skin, and mucosa. Ophthalmic exposure causes conjunctivitis.[21,60,136] Irritation of the upper respiratory tract leads to pharyngitis and frequent epistaxis.[168]

Antimony pentachloride is very irritating and causes local dermal and mucosal burns, as it reacts with water, releasing hydrochloric acid, heat, and antimony pentoxide (Sb_2O_5). Following ingestion, contact with the water in saliva produces sufficient hydrochloric acid to result in consequential gastrointestinal burns.

Ophthalmic exposure to Sb_2O_5 causes a typical caustic injury, resulting in blepharospasm, lacrimation, photophobia, and corneal burns. Exposure to antimony trichloride fumes causes similar ocular findings.[68]

Following systemic exposure, ophthalmic toxicity manifests in optic atrophy, uveitis, and retinal hemorrhage with exudates resulting in diminished visual acuity.[40,97] Some of these changes are permanent.[97] Interestingly, a metallic intraocular foreign body composed of antimony was removed 60 years after the initial injury with no evidence of metallosis. A postprocedural electroretinogram was normal.[146]

Thrombophlebitis is common after the intravenous (IV) use of antimony but it also occurs following oral exposure.[105]

Gastrointestinal

Following acute exposures, antimony rapidly produces anorexia, nausea, vomiting, abdominal pain, and diarrhea.[105,109,166] Some patients report a metallic taste in the mouth.[8,46] A garlic odor on the breath is often recognized but this may be due to concomitant arsenic exposure. In severe overdose, gastrointestinal irritation progresses to hemorrhagic gastritis.[105] Workers chronically exposed to antimony dusts have a much higher incidence of gastrointestinal ulcers in comparison to controls (63 per 1,000 vs 15 per 1,000).[27] Many patients develop pancreatitis following treatment with pentavalent antimonial salts.[47,63,116] Because most cases improved despite continuation of treatment, a mechanism other than direct pancreatic toxicity is presumed. In another series, several patients with human immunodeficiency virus (HIV) who were treated with high doses of meglumine antimonate developed severe pancreatitis and died.[49]

TABLE 85–2	Clinical Manifestations of Antimony Compounds Poisoning*					
Antimony Compound	Stibine	Antimony Potassium Tartrate	Antimony Trioxide	Antimony Pentachloride/Pentoxide	Meglumine Antimoniate	Sodium Stibogluconate
Formula	SbH_3	$C_8H_{10}K_2O_{15}Sb_2$	Sb_2O_3	$SbCl_5Sb_2O_5$	$C_7H_{18}NO_8Sb$	$C_{12}H_{38}Na_3O_{26}Sb_2$
Brand/common name		Tartar emetic			Glucantime	Pentostan
Common use			Flame retardant		Antileishmanial	Antileishmanial
Oxidation state	3+	3+	3+	5+	3+/5+	3+/5+
CLINICAL EFFECTS						
Local Irritation						
Conjunctival/mucosal irritant	++			++		
Corneal burns	+	+	+	+	+	+
Thrombophlebitis					+	+
Gastrointestinal						
Anorexia	+	+	+	+	+	+
N/V/D	+	+	+	+	+	+
Abdominal pain	+	+	+	+	+	+
Pancreatitis					+	+
Cardiovascular						
Prolonged QT interval					+	+
ST segment and T wave changes					+	+
Torsade de pointes					+	+
Ventricular dysrhythmias					+	+
Pericarditis					+	
Respiratory						
Laryngitis			+			
Tracheitis			+			
Pneumonitis						
ARDS				+		
Pneumoconiosis			+			
Metal fume fever			+	+ (Sb_2O_5)		
Renal						
Renal cell casts					+	+
Proteinuria					+	+
Increased BUN					+	+
Acute interstitial nephritis					+	+
Hematuria	+					
Hepatic						
Abnormal LFT's	+				+	+
Hepatic necrosis	+				+	+
Hematologic						
Anemia	+				+	+
Hemolysis	+					
Thrombocytopenia					+	+
Leukopenia/lymphopenia					+	+
Dermatologic						
Antimony spots	+		+			
Contact dermatitis	+		+		+	
Severe cutaneous reactions						

(Continued)

TABLE 85–2	Clinical Manifestations of Antimony Compounds Poisoning* (Continued)					
Antimony Compound	Stibine	Antimony Potassium Tartrate	Antimony Trioxide	Antimony Pentachloride/Pentoxide	Meglumine Antimoniate	Sodium Stibogluconate
Neurologic						
Vestibular-Cochlear toxicity					+	
Tinnitus					+	
Rotatory dizziness					+	
Peripheral sensory neuropathy						+
Cerebellar ataxia						+
Musculoskeletal						
Muscle and joint pain					+	+
Rhabdomyolysis						
Genotoxicity	+					
Carcinogenicity			+			

*The absence of a + indicates the absence of reported or recognized clinical manifestation.

Cardiovascular

In animals, antimony decreases myocardial contraction; lowers coronary vasomotor tone, producing decreased systolic pressure; and causes bradycardia.[45,169] The majority of reported human cardiac effects are related to the electrocardiographic (ECG) changes. Prolongation of the QT interval, inversion or flattening of T waves, and ST segment changes are frequently described during treatment of visceral leishmaniasis with pentavalent antimonial compounds (sodium stibogluconate and meglumine antimonate).[39,139,172] Torsade de pointes was described in patients treated with pentavalent antimonial preparations.[127,157] Prolongation of the cardiac action potential may be due to an increase in cardiac calcium currents.[103]

In some patients with underlying myocardial disease such as a cardiomyopathy, ECG changes occur even at subtherapeutic antimony doses.[73] These changes are not necessarily associated with deterioration in cardiac function.[80,82] However, it is important to recognize that pentavalent antimonial drugs used for the treatment of leishmaniasis are associated with sudden death, probably as a result of the development of ventricular dysrhythmias.[35,153] Cardiomyopathy followed by congestive heart failure and death is rare but is a reported adverse effect attributed to antimony.[125,152] Pericarditis, presenting with chest pain and typical ECG changes, is reported during the treatment with meglumine antimoniate.[56]

Chronic antimony exposure resulting in elevated concentrations of antimony in urine are associated with an increase in composite cardiovascular and cerebrovascular disease.[1]

Respiratory

Local irritation from antimony trioxide produces laryngitis, tracheitis, and pneumonitis.[66,136,156] Pneumonitis is usually reversible after exposure ceases and can be followed radiologically.[136] Acute respiratory distress syndrome was reported after acute inhalation of antimony pentachloride.[43,44]

Although antimony oxides are capable of causing metal fume fever,[6,59] this is much less common in comparison to exposure to zinc oxide (Chaps. 100 and 121).[6,59] Antimony metal fume fever is reported to occur even with air concentrations below 5 mg/m³.[42]

Workers chronically exposed to antimony compounds are at risk for developing "antimony pneumoconiosis."[41,114] Patients present with cough, wheezing, and exertional dyspnea, which can progress to obstructive lung disease. Radiologically, antimony pneumoconiosis appears as diffuse, dense, punctate nonconfluent opacities with a predominant distribution in the middle and lower lung lobes with or without pleural adhesions.[132] In the general population, increased urinary antimony concentrations are associated with higher odds of experiencing obstructive sleep apnea.[142]

Renal

Patients treated with sodium stibogluconate develop varied manifestations of nephrotoxicity ranging from renal cell casts, proteinuria, and increased blood urea nitrogen concentration[40] due to acute kidney injury (AKI).[10,133] Some patients also develop renal tubular acidosis[87] and acute tubular necrosis.[134] Older age and underlying chronic kidney disease are risk factors for the development of AKI that can progress to death.[112,125] Hemodialysis is reportedly helpful during the oliguric phase in acute overdose.[109]

Antimonials are also suggested as a possible cause of drug-induced acute interstitial nephritis responsive to treatment with steroids.[162]

Hepatic

Acute exposure to antimony results in severe acute liver injury.[109] Long-term therapeutic use of antimony compounds for the treatment of leishmaniasis causes hepatotoxicity that ranges from reversible elevations of aminotransferase concentrations to hepatic necrosis.[83,85,140,169] Elderly patients are at an increased risk for the development of significant hepatic failure.[125] Some pediatric patients treated for leishmaniasis develop fulminant hepatic failure after an initial positive response to antimony. The mechanism is unknown, but the condition may be due to a direct antimony effect in combination with immunologically mediated liver injury.[11,50]

Interestingly, in an animal study, concurrent administration of ascorbic acid (15 mg/kg/day) appeared to be hepatoprotective. Its activity reduced the extent of histologic changes, the apoptotic index, and the peroxidase activity.[98]

Hematologic

Severe anemia was reported in HIV-positive patients during treatment with sodium stibogluconate. Bone marrow biopsy documented transient severe marrow dyserythropoiesis, followed by complete recovery on discontinuation of the therapy.[84,110]

Patients treated with sodium stibogluconate for visceral leishmaniasis occasionally develop thrombocytopenia.[22,81,94] Rare cases of epistaxis are described during the treatment.[96] Visceral leishmaniasis is associated with pancytopenia, probably as a result of an increased destruction of peripheral blood cells.[131] It is difficult to determine whether this phenomenon is caused by the disease itself or is secondary to the treatment, although some authors suggested a drug-induced immune thrombocytopenia.[131]

Leukopenia is frequently observed in patients treated with antimonial compounds.[49,169,173] Some authors speculate that antimony-induced lymphopenia is associated with an increased frequency of herpes zoster in HIV-infected patients.[173] It is suggested that pentavalent antimony precipitates sickle cell crisis via a common glutathione pathway.[62] A homeopathic study suggested a procoagulant effect, leading some homeopathic practitioners to include antimony as a treatment for bleeding disorders.[86]

Dermatologic

Antimony spots[149] are papules and pustules that develop around sweat and sebaceous glands and resemble varicella. Chronically exposed patients typically develop eczema and lichenification of the arms, legs, and in the joint creases with sparing of the face, hands, and feet that typically occur in the summer.[114,136] A similar skin rash was described in the 18th century after the external application of antimony tartrate for medicinal use.[115] Curiously, these eruptions were usually interpreted as a sign of cure.[76] It is also suggested that antimony trioxide causes contact dermatitis.[120] A very high incidence of severe cutaneous reactions (37%) was reported in patients who were treated with meglumine antimonate at 20 mg/kg/day.[126] This high incidence was associated with high concentrations of other metals in the one particular drug lot. Herpes zoster was reported as a complication of antileishmaniasis treatment with associated leukopenia.[126,173] An isolated case of an infant who developed acute urticaria after her mother's parenteral use of meglumine antimoniate increases the possibility of antimony exposure via breast milk.[121]

Neurologic

Patients treated with sodium stibogluconate developed a reversible, peripheral sensory neuropathy,[29] and cerebellar ataxia in temporal association with exposure.[101] Reversible vestibular-cochlear toxicity was reported in a patient who presented with a significant increase in auditory threshold during the treatment with meglumine antimoniate. In addition, the patient experienced tinnitus and severe rotatory dizziness.[161]

Musculoskeletal

The therapeutic use of parenteral antimonials is associated with diffuse muscle and joint pain.[32,46,140,169] One of the most frequently reported clinical adverse effects of pentavalent antimonials was musculoskeletal pain.[126] The symptoms are sometimes so severe that they will require treatment interruption in about one third of patients. Patients who are not candidates for nonsteroidal antiinflammatory drug treatment are usually managed with glucocorticoids.[28]

Metabolic

Antimony is a recognized metalloestrogen,[38] and chronic exposure increases the risk of diabetes[117] through this hormonal disruption.

Immunologic

A case–control study of 100 patients and 300 controls showed a marked association between systemic sclerosis and antimony exposure in both male and female patients.[112] It is still unclear what the pathogenic mechanisms of antimony in development of systemic sclerosis are, although basic science research implied that antimony is capable of altering the epigenome, resulting in chromosomal aberration in cultured mammalian cells,[113] as well as in the excess production of reactive oxygen species and interference with the DNA repair system.[7] The use of meglumine antimoniate was reported to cause 2 different subsets of cutaneous hypersensitivity reactions: immunoglobulin E (IgE)–mediated allergic reactions (type-I) that presents immediately and can range from localized and generalized urticaria to anaphylaxis and delayed (type-IV) allergic reactions, including eczematous lesions and persistent subcutaneous nodules.[24]

Reproductive

In animal studies, antimony causes ovarian atrophy, uterine metaplasia, and impaired conception.[17] An association was found with spontaneous abortion and premature births reported in women who were occupationally exposed to antimony salts. Antimony was found in the blood, urine, placenta, amniotic fluid, and breast milk of these women.[17]

Carcinogenicity

Female rats developed lung tumors after the inhalation of antimony trioxide and antimony trisulfide.[20,72,164] A survey among antimony smelters suggested an excess of lung cancer, with a latency of 20 years, in comparison to a nonexposed population. However, concomitant exposure to arsenic and its effects could not be excluded, and the data were inadequately controlled for smoking habits.[93] In one group of workers who were exposed to antimony oxide over 9 to 31 years, there was no increased incidence of lung cancer.[132] Patients with schistosomiasis have an increased incidence of bladder tumors, and antimony compounds are considered to be one potential cause.[169] The International Agency for Research on Cancer classified antimony trioxide as possibly carcinogenic to humans (group 2B).[71]

Genotoxicity

Both stibine and trimethylstibine are capable of damaging DNA, presumably by the generation of reactive oxygen species. Other forms of antimony tested, including potassium antimony tartrate, potassium hexahydroxyantimonate, and trimethylantimony dichloride, were found to not be genotoxic.[5] Trivalent antimony interferes with proteins involved in nucleotide excision repair and partly impairs this pathway, pointing to an indirect mechanism in the genotoxicity of trivalent antimony.[71]

STIBINE

Antimony compounds react with nascent hydrogen, forming an extremely toxic gas, stibine (SbH_3), which resembles arsine (AsH_3) (Chap. 86). Stibine is probably the most toxic antimony compound. It is a colorless gas with a very unpleasant smell that rapidly decomposes at temperatures above 302°F (150°C).[70,169] Historically, stibine release was reported during the charging of lead storage batteries.[169] In addition to gastrointestinal effects that include nausea, vomiting, and abdominal pain, stibine has strong oxidative properties that results in massive hemolysis (Chap. 20). Similar to arsine,[137] severe stibine exposure results in hematuria, rhabdomyolysis, and death. Maintenance workers are advised to avoid use of drain cleaners containing sodium hydroxide, which is capable of releasing hydrogen in situations where antimony is present.[129]

DIAGNOSTIC TESTING

Standard laboratory testing to assess volume depletion and AKI is indicated for patients with acute antimony toxicity. A complete blood count, electrolytes, renal function studies, and a urinalysis should be obtained. When there is a known or suspected exposure to stibine, additional studies should include tests for hemolysis, such as determinations of bilirubin and haptoglobin. Blood should also be obtained for a blood type and cross-match, as transfusions are likely to be required.

An ECG should be obtained to evaluate for QT interval prolongation and dysrhythmias. Patients with known myocardial disease should have frequent evaluations of cardiac function,[73] and continuous ECG monitoring is recommended for all patients with significant toxicity or abnormal cardiovascular status. A chest radiograph should be performed in patients with respiratory symptoms and findings and evidence of hypoxia after significant inhalation exposure. In addition, an abdominal radiograph is reasonable in patients with ingestion to evaluate gastrointestinal antimony load and help guide decontamination.[30]

An antimony concentration in a 24-hour urine collection is used for the assessment of the intensity of exposure to either trivalent or pentavalent antimony.[8] A normal urinary antimony concentration in unexposed patients is reported as less than 6.2 mcg/L.[130,167] A serum antimony concentration cannot be determined in a timely fashion. The normal serum concentration of antimony is in the range of less than 3 mcg/L,[111] although some laboratories use higher values.[124]

TREATMENT

Decontamination

Following a significant acute ingestion, the majority of patients develop vomiting. Induction of emesis is unlikely to offer any additional benefit. By contrast, gastric lavage is reasonable, especially if performed before the onset of spontaneous emesis. Although it is unknown whether antimony is adsorbed to activated charcoal, based on experience with salts of arsenic, thallium, and mercury, administration of activated charcoal is recommended. Additionally, because antimony has a documented enterohepatic circulation, multiple-dose activated charcoal is reasonable if the patient can tolerate it.[8] Limited data on arsenic decontamination suggests the effectiveness of this method.[92] Based on experience with arsenic poisoning, whole-bowel irrigation (WBI) is also recommended with severe ingestions in patients who are able to tolerate it, especially if radiographs confirm radiopaque material.[3,30] It is suggested that WBI has no effectiveness after 48 hours from arsenic exposure,[92] but it is unclear whether this is applicable to antimony.

For patients exposed to stibine, removal from the exposure should be followed by the administration of high-flow oxygen. While theoretically patients with severe stibine exposures may benefit from exchange transfusion for the removal of the stibine–hemoglobin complex,[137] data are insufficient to routinely recommend this practice. Patients with dermal exposures, particularly to antimony tri- or pentachloride, should be decontaminated with soap and water. Prompt removal from the contaminated area is important for patients exposed to stibine. Rescuers need to take appropriate precautions to ensure their own safety (Chap. 132).

Supportive Care

The mainstay of treatment for antimony poisoning is good supportive care. Clinicians should anticipate massive volume depletion and begin rehydration with isotonic crystalloid solutions. Electrolytes, urine output, and renal and liver function[109] should be followed closely. A central venous pressure monitor is reasonable in patients with cardiovascular instability. Antiemetics are recommended both for patient comfort and to facilitate the administration of activated charcoal. Following stibine exposure, the hemoglobin concentration should be followed closely and blood should be transfused based on standard criteria.

Chelation

Human experience with regard to chelation of antimony is rather limited because of the scarcity of serious toxicity and the rarity of instances in which patients have received chelation. Most of the available data are based on animal experimentation. Dimercaprol, succimer, and dimercaptopropane-sulfonic acid (DMPS) all improve the survival of experimental animals.[13,25,89,159] A group from Shanghai demonstrated the ability of the sodium salt of succimer to increase the murine LD_{50} of tartar emetic 16-fold.[107] One animal study that compared survival after treatment with multiple chelators concluded that the most effective antidotes were DMPS and succimer.[13]

A single case series documented survival in 3 of 5 patients exposed to tartar emetic who were treated with intramuscular dimercaprol at a dose of 200 to 600 mg/day. All 5 patients had increased urinary excretion of antimony.[105] In another case report, a patient survived after chelation with dimercaprol but without evidence of enhanced urinary excretion of antimony.[8] Although specific recommendations are difficult to make, it is reasonable to begin therapy with IM dimercaprol until it is certain that antimony is removed from the gastrointestinal tract, at which time the patient can be switched to oral succimer. If the patient experiences cardiac or respiratory effects with associated ECG changes during administration of dimercaprol, treatment should be stopped.[109] Because chelation doses for antimony poisoning are not established, chelators should be administered in doses and regimens that are determined to be safe and effective for other metals such as arsenic given the similarities of these metals (Antidotes in Depth: A28 and A29).

SUMMARY

- Antimony toxicity should be suspected in patients with unexplained profuse nausea, vomiting, diarrhea, and abdominal pain, particularly in the setting of alcohol aversion treatment and acute kidney injury.
- Most patients will require only supportive therapy with decontamination.
- Multiple doses of activated charcoal are reasonable.

- Whole-bowel irrigation is recommended and likely most beneficial in the first 48 hours following oral exposure.
- Symptomatic patients should be admitted to telemetry for monitoring for cardiac dysrhythmias.
- Chelation with dimercaprol is reasonable in severe cases of acute overdose.
- Serious complications from treatment of leishmaniasis antimonial preparations are rare, related to the heart and pancreas, with age and underlying diseases constituting known risk factors.

REFERENCES

1. Agarwal S, et al. Heavy metals and cardiovascular disease: results from the National Health and Nutrition Examination Survey (NHANES) 1999-2006. *Angiology.* 2011;62: 422-429.
2. Ainsworth N, et al. Distribution and biological effects of antimony in contaminated grassland: 1—vegetation and soils. *Environ Pollution.* 1990;65:65-77.
3. American College of Medical Toxicology. Position paper: whole bowel irrigation. *J Toxicol.* 2004;42:843-854.
4. Andelman SL. Antimony poisoning—Illinois. *MMWR Morb Mortal Wkly Rep.* 1964;13:250.
5. Andrewes P, et al. Plasmid DNA damage caused by stibine and trimethylstibine. *Toxicol Appl Pharmacol.* 2004;194:41-48.
6. Anonymous. Metals and the lung. *Lancet.* 1984;2:903-904.
7. Asakura K, et al. Genotoxicity studies of heavy metals: lead, bismuth, indium, silver and antimony. *J Occup Health.* 2009;51:498-512.
8. Bailly R, et al. Experimental and human studies on antimony metabolism: their relevance for the biological monitoring of workers exposed to inorganic antimony. *Br J Ind Med.* 1991;48:93-97.
9. Baiocco P, et al. Molecular basis of antimony treatment in leishmaniasis. *J Med Chem.* 2009;52:2603-2612.
10. Balzan M, Fenech F. Acute renal failure in visceral leishmaniasis treated with sodium stibogluconate. *Trans R Soc Trop Med Hyg.* 1992;86:515-516.
11. Baranwal AK, et al. Post-treatment fulminant hepatic failure in an infant with visceral leishmaniasis: immune injury or stibogluconate toxicity? *Indian J Pediatr.* 2010;77: 107-108.
12. Bartter FC, et al. The fate of radioactive tartar emetic administered to human subjects. *Am J Trop Med Hyg.* 1947;27:403-416.
13. Basinger MA, Jones MM. Structural requirements for chelate antidotal efficacy in acute antimony(III) intoxication. *Res Commun Chem Pathol Pharmacol.* 1981;32:355-363.
14. Beaumier CM, et al. United States military tropical medicine: extraordinary legacy, uncertain future. *PLoS Negl Trop Dis.* 2013;7:e2448.
15. Beliles RP. The lesser metals. In: Oehme F, ed. *Toxicity of Heavy Metals in the Environment*, part II. New York, NY: Marcel Dekker; 1979:547-615.
16. Beliles RP. The metals: antimony. In: Clayton GD, et al., eds. *Patty's Industrial Hygiene and Toxicology.* Vol 2. New York, NY: John Wiley & Sons; 1994:1902-1913.
17. Belyaeva AP. The effect of antimony on the generative function [in Russian]. *Gig Tr Prof Zabol.* 1967;11:32-37.
18. Benson AA, Cooney RA. Antimony metabolites in marine algae. In: Craig PJ, Glockling F, eds. *Organometallic Compounds in the Environment. Principles and Reactions.* Harlow, UK: Longmans; 1988:135-137.
19. Bentley R, Chasteen TG. Microbial methylation of metalloids: arsenic, antimony, and bismuth. *Microbiol Mol Biol Rev.* 2002;66:250-271.
20. Beyersmann D, Hartwig A. Carcinogenic metal compounds: recent insight into molecular and cellular mechanisms. *Arch Toxicol.* 2008;82:493-512.
21. Bingham E, et al. *Patty's Toxicology.* Vol 2. 5th ed. New York, NY: John Wiley & Sons;1994.
22. Braconier JH, Miorner H. Recurrent episodes of thrombocytopenia during treatment with sodium stibogluconate. *J Antimicrob Chemother.* 1993;31:187-188.
23. Bradberry SM, et al. Antimony. http://www.inchem.org/documents/ukpids/ukpids/ ukpid40.htm. Published 1996. Accessed September 8, 2017.
24. Brasileiro A, et al. Allergic reactions to meglumine antimoniate while treating cutaneous leishmaniasis. *J Eur Acad Dermatol Venereol.* 2017;31:e59-e60.
25. Braun HA, et al. The efficacy of 2,3-dimercaptopropanol (BAL) in the therapy of poisoning by compounds of antimony, bismuth, chromium, mercury and nickel. *J Pharmacol Exp Ther.* 1946;87(4)(suppl):119-125.
26. Brieger GH. Therapeutic conflicts and the American medical profession in the 1860s. *Bull Hist Med.* 1967;41:215-222.
27. Brieger H, et al. Industrial antimony poisoning. *Ind Med Surg.* 1954;23:521-523.
28. Brostoff JM, Lockwood DN. Glucocorticoids as a novel approach to the treatment of disabling side effects of sodium stibogluconate. J Clin Pharm Ther. 2012;37:122-123.
29. Brummitt CF, et al. Reversible peripheral neuropathy associated with sodium stibogluconate therapy for American cutaneous leishmaniasis. *Clin Infect Dis.* 1996;22:878-879.
30. Buchanan JA, et al. Massive human ingestion of orpiment (arsenic trisulfide). J Emerg Med. 2013;44:367-372.
31. Bueding E, Fisher J. Factors affecting the inhibition of phosphofructokinase activity of *Schistosoma mansoni* by trivalent organic antimonials. *Biochem Pharmacol.* 1966;15: 1197-1211.

32. Castro C, et al. Severe arthralgia, not related to dose, associated with pentavalent antimonial therapy for mucosal leishmaniasis. *Trans R Soc Trop Med Hyg*. 1990;84:362.

33. Centers For Disease Control and Prevention. Pseudo-outbreak of antimony toxicity in firefighters—Florida. *MMWR Morb Mortal Wkly Rep*. 2009;58:1300-1302.

34. Centers for Disease Control and Prevention NIOSH. Occupational safety and health guideline for antimony and its compounds (as Sb). In: US Department of Health and Human Services, ed. http://www.cdc.gov/niosh/docs/81-123/pdfs/0036.pdf: CDC; 1988. Accessed September 11, 2017.

35. Cesur S, et al. Death from cumulative sodium stibogluconate toxicity on Kala-Azar. *Clin Microbiol Infect*. 2002;8:606.

36. Chai Y, et al. Complexation of antimony (Sb(V)) with guanosine 5'-monophosphate and guanosine 5'-diphospho-D-mannose: formation of both mono- and bis-adducts. *J Inorg Biochem*. 2005;99:2257-2263.

37. Chen G, et al. Trypanocidal activity and toxicity of antimonials. *J Infect Dis*. 1945;76:144-151.

38. Choe SY, et al. Evaluation of estrogenicity of major heavy metals. *Sci Total Environ*. 2003;312:15-21.

39. Chulay JD, et al. Electrocardiographic changes during treatment of leishmaniasis with pentavalent antimony (sodium stibogluconate). *Am J Trop Med Hyg*. 1985;34:702-709.

40. Chunge CN, et al. Complications of kala azar and its treatment in Kenya. *East Afr Med J*. 1984;61:120-127.

41. Cooper DA, et al. Pneumoconiosis among workers in an antimony industry. *Am J Roentgenol Radium Ther Nucl Med*. 1968;103:496-508.

42. Cooper Hand Tools/Cheraw Plant. Material safety data sheet for lead-free solder. http://core2062.com/wp-content/uploads/2012/12/Lead-Free-Solder.pdf. Published 1999. Accessed September 11, 2017.

43. Cordasco EM. Newer concepts in the management of environmental pulmonary edema. *Angiology*. 1974;25:590-601.

44. Cordasco EM, Stone FD. Pulmonary edema of environmental origin. *Chest*. 1973;64:182-185.

45. Cotton MD, Logan ME. Effects of antimony on the cardiovascular system and intestinal smooth muscle. *J Pharmacol Exp Ther*. 1966;151:7-22.

46. Davis A. Comparative trials of antimonial drugs in urinary schistosomiasis. *Bull World Health Organ*. 1968;38:197-227.

47. de Lalla F, et al. Acute pancreatitis associated with the administration of meglumine antimonate for the treatment of visceral leishmaniasis. *Clin Infect Dis*. 1993;16:730-731.

48. De Wolff FA. Antimony and health. *BMJ*. 1995;310:1216-1217.

49. Delgado J, et al. High frequency of serious side effects from meglumine antimoniate given without an upper limit dose for the treatment of visceral leishmaniasis in human immunodeficiency virus type-1-infected patients. *Am J Trop Med Hyg*. 1999;61:766-769.

50. di Martino L, et al. Fulminant hepatitis in an Italian infant with visceral leishmaniasis. *Trans R Soc Trop Med Hyg*. 1992;86:34.

51. Diniz DS, et al. The effect of age on the frequency of adverse reactions caused by antimony in the treatment of American tegumentary leishmaniasis in Governador Valadares, State of Minas Gerais, Brazil. *Rev Soc Bras Med Trop*. 2012;45:597-600.

52. Djuric D, et al. The distribution and excretion of trivalent antimony in the rat following inhalation. *Int Arch Gewerbepathol Gewerbehyg*. 1962;19:529-545.

53. Duffin J, Campling BG. Therapy and disease concepts: the history (and future?) of antimony in cancer. *J Hist Med Allied Sci*. 2002;57:61-78.

54. Duncan MW. *Antimony: Toxicology*. Chicago, IL: Industrial Medicine; 1937:285-290.

55. Edel J, et al. Metabolic behavior of inorganic forms of antimony in the rat. Paper presented at: Proceedings of Heavy Metal in the Environmental International Conference 1983; Heidelberg, Germany.

56. Eryilmaz A, et al. A case with two unusual findings: cutaneous leishmaniasis presenting as panniculitis and pericarditis after antimony therapy. *Int J Dermatol*. 2010;49:295-297.

57. Felicetti SA, et al. Metabolism of two valence states of inhaled antimony in hamsters. *Am Ind Hyg Assoc J*. 1974;35:292-300.

58. Felicetti SW, et al. Retention of inhaled antimony-124 in the beagle dog as a function of temperature of aerosol formation. *Health Phys*. 1974;26:515-531.

59. Finkel AJ. *Hamilton & Hardy's Industrial Toxicology*. Boston, MA: John Wright PSG; 1983.

60. Friberg L, et al. *Handbook on the Toxicology of Metals*. 2nd ed. Amsterdam, NY: Elsevier; 1986:27-42.

61. Garami A, Ilg T. Disruption of mannose activation in *Leishmania mexicana*: GDP-mannose pyrophosphorylase is required for virulence, but not for viability. *EMBO J*. 2001;20:3657-3666.

62. Garcerant D, et al. Possible links between sickle cell crisis and pentavalent antimony. *Am J Trop Med Hyg*. 2012;86:1057-1061.

63. Gasser RA Jr, et al. Pancreatitis induced by pentavalent antimonial agents during treatment of leishmaniasis. *Clin Infect Dis*. 1994;18:83-90.

64. Gebel T. Arsenic and antimony: comparative approach on mechanistic toxicology. *Chem Biol Interact*. 1997;107:131-144.

65. Gellhorn A, et al. The tissue-distribution and excretion of four organic antimonials after single or repeated administration to normal hamsters. *J Pharmacol Exp Ther*. 1946;87:169-180.

66. Gerhardsson L, et al. Antimony in lung, liver and kidney tissue from deceased smelter workers. *Scand J Work Environ Health*. 1982;8:201-208.

67. Gibson S, Gibson R. *Homoeopathy for Everyone*. Harmondsworth, UK: Penguin Books; 1987.

68. Grant WM, Schuman JS. *Toxicology of the Eye*. 4th ed. Chicago, IL: Charles C Thomas; 1993.

69. Great Britain Health and Safety Executive. *Antimony: Health and Safety Precautions*. London: HMSO; 1978.

70. Great Britain Health and Safety Executive. *Stibine: Health and Safety Precautions*. London: HMSO; 1978.

71. Grosskopf C, et al. Antimony impairs nucleotide excision repair: XPA and XPE as potential molecular targets. *Chem Res Toxicol*. 2010;23:1175-1183.

72. Groth DH, et al. Carcinogenic effects of antimony trioxide and antimony ore concentrate in rats. *J Toxicol Environ Health*. 1986;18:607-626.

73. Gupta P. Electrocardiographic changes occurring after brief antimony administration in the presence of dilated cardiomyopathy. *Postgrad Med J*. 1990;66:1089.

74. Hain TC. Emesis. http://www.tchain.com/otoneurology/treatment/emesis.html. Published 2001. Accessed Sept 8, 2017.

75. Haldar AK, et al. Use of antimony in the treatment of leishmaniasis: current status and future directions. *Mol Biol Int*. 2011;2011:571242.

76. Haller JS. The use and abuse of tartar emetic in the 19th century materia medica. *Bull Hist Med*. 1975;49:235-257.

77. Hansen C, et al. Elevated antimony concentrations in commercial juices. *J Environ Monit*. 2010;12:822-824.

78. Hawley GG. *The Condensed Chemical Dictionary*. New York, NY: Van Nostrand Reinhold; 1981.

79. He M, et al. Antimony pollution in China. *Sci Total Environ*. 2012;421-422:41-50.

80. Henderson A, Jolliffe D. Cardiac effects of sodium stibogluconate. *Br J Clin Pharmacol*. 1985;19:73-77.

81. Hepburn NC. Thrombocytopenia complicating sodium stibogluconate therapy for cutaneous leishmaniasis. *Trans R Soc Trop Med Hyg*. 1993;87:691.

82. Hepburn NC, et al. Cardiac effects of sodium stibogluconate: myocardial, electrophysiological and biochemical studies. *QJM*. 1994;87:465-472.

83. Hepburn NC, et al. Hepatotoxicity of sodium stibogluconate in leishmaniasis. *Lancet*. 1993;342:238-239.

84. Hernandez JA, et al. The irreplaceable image: acute toxicity in erythroid bone marrow progenitors after antimonial therapy. *Haematologica*. 2001;86:1319.

85. Herwaldt BL, et al. Sodium stibogluconate (Pentostam) overdose during treatment of American cutaneous leishmaniasis. *J Infect Dis*. 1992;165:968-971.

86. Heusser P, et al. Efficacy of homeopathically potentized antimony on blood coagulation. A randomized placebo controlled crossover trial. *Forsch Komplementmed*. 2009;16:14-18.

87. Horber FF, et al. Renal tubular acidosis, a side effect of treatment with pentavalent antimony. *Clin Nephrol*. 1991;36:213.

88. Hoyt DM. *Practical Therapeutics*. Mosby, 1914.

89. Hruby K, Donner A. 2,3-Dimercapto-1-propanesulphonate in heavy metal poisoning. *Med Toxicol Adverse Drug Exp*. 1987;2:317-323.

90. Huang Y, et al. Levels and risk factors of antimony contamination in human hair from an electronic waste recycling area, Guiyu, China. *Environ Sci Pollut Res Int*. 2015;22:7112-7119.

91. International Register of Potentially Toxic Chemicals. Antimony. Vol. Scientific Reviews of Soviet Literature on Toxicity and Hazards of Chemical. Moscow, Russia: United Nations Environmental Programme; 1984.

92. Isbister GK, et al. Arsenic trioxide poisoning: a description of two acute overdoses. *Hum Exp Toxicol*. 2004;23:359-364.

93. Jones RD. Survey of antimony workers: mortality 1961-1992. *Occup Environ Med*. 1994;51:772-776.

94. Just G, et al. Visceral leishmaniasis (kala-azar) in acquired immunodeficiency syndrome (AIDS) [in German]. *Dtsch Med Wochenschr*. 1988;113:1920-1922.

95. Just S, et al. Improving the safety of intravenous admixtures: lessons learned from a Pentostam® overdose. *Jt Comm J Qual Patient Saf*. 2006;32:366-372.

96. Kager PA, et al. Clinical, haematological and parasitological response to treatment of visceral leishmaniasis in Kenya. A study of 64 patients. *Trop Geogr Med*. 1984;36:21-35.

97. Kassem A, et al. Optic atrophy following repeated courses of tartar emetic for the treatment of bilharziasis. *Bull Ophthalmol Soc Egypt*. 1976;69:459-463.

98. Kato KC, et al. Hepatotoxicity of pentavalent antimonial drug: possible role of residual Sb(III) and protective effect of ascorbic acid. *Antimicrob Agents Chemother*. 2013;58:481-488.

99. Kenley JB, et al. Antimony poisoning—Virginia. *Mortal Morbid Wkly Rep*. 1965;14:27.

100. Kentner M, et al. External and internal antimony exposure in starter battery production. *Int Arch Occup Environ Health*. 1995;67:119-123.

101. Khalil EA, et al. Antimony-induced cerebellar ataxia. *Saudi Med J*. 2006;27:90-92.

102. Krachler M. Speciation of antimony for the 21st century: promises and pitfalls. *Trends Anal Chem*. 2001;20:79-90.

103. Kuryshev YA, et al. Antimony-based antileishmanial compounds prolong the cardiac action potential by an increase in cardiac calcium currents. *Mol Pharmacol*. 2006;69:1216-1225.

104. Laporte-Saumure M, et al. Characterization and metal availability of copper, lead, antimony and zinc contamination at four Canadian small arms firing ranges. *Environ Technol*. 2011;32:767-781.

105. Lauwers LF, et al. Oral antimony intoxications in man. *Crit Care Med*. 1990;18:324-326.

106. Leicester HM. *Discovery of the Elements*. Easton, PA: Mary Elvira Weeks; 1968.

107. Liang Y-I, et al. Studies on antibilharzial drugs. The antidotal effects of sodium dimeroaptosuccinate and BAL-gluooside against tartar emetic. *Acta Physiologica Sinica*. 1957;21:24-32.

108. Lippincott SW, et al. A study of the distribution and fate of antimony when used as tartar emetic and fouadin in the treatment of American soldiers with schistosomiasis japonica. *J Clin Invest*. 1947:370-378.

109. Macias Konstantopoulos W, et al. Case records of the Massachusetts General Hospital. Case 22-2012. A 34-year-old man with intractable vomiting after ingestion of an unknown substance. *N Engl J Med*. 2012;367:259-268.

110. Mallick BK. Hypoplasia of bone marrow secondary to sodium antimony gluconate. *J Assoc Physicians India*. 1990;38:310-311.

111. Mansour MM, et al. Anti-bilharzial antimony drugs. *Nature*. 1967;214:819-820.

112. Marie I, et al. Systemic sclerosis and exposure to heavy metals: a case control study of 100 patients and 300 controls. *Autoimmun Rev*. 2017;16:223-230.

113. Marie I, et al. Prospective study to evaluate the association between systemic sclerosis and occupational exposure and review of the literature. *Autoimmun Rev*. 2014;13: 151-156.

114. McCallum RI. The industrial toxicology of antimony. The Ernestine Henry lecture 1987. *J R Coll Physicians Lond*. 1989;23:28-32.

115. McCallum RI. *Antimony in Medical History*. Edinburgh, Scotland: Pentland Press; 1999.

116. McCarthy AE, et al. Pancreatitis occurring during therapy with stibogluconate: two case reports. *Clin Infect Dis*. 1993;17:952-953.

117. Menke A, et al. Metals in urine and diabetes in U.S. adults. *Diabetes*. 2016;65: 164-171.

118. Miller JM. Poisoning by antimony: a case report (Oliver Goldsmith). *South Med J*. 1982;75:592.

119. Mishra BB, et al. Alkaloids: future prospective to combat leishmaniasis. *Fitoterapia*. 2009;80:81-90.

120. Motolese A, et al. Contact dermatitis and contact sensitization among enamellers and decorators in the ceramics industry. *Contact Dermatitis*. 1993;28:59-62.

121. Mozafari O, et al. First report on infant acute urticaria after mother's parenteral use of meglumine antimoniate (glucantime): a case report. *Iran J Public Health*. 2016;45:1217-1219.

122. Myers R, et al. *Antimony Trioxide Range-Finding Toxicity Studies*. Pittsburgh, PA: Carnegie Mellon University; 1978.

123. Nadkarni RA, Ehmann WD. Transference studies of trace elements from cigarette tobacco into smoke condensate, and their determination by neutron activation analysis. Paper presented at: Proceedings of the Tobacco Health Conference 1970; University of Kentucky, Lexington.

124. National Medical Services. 24-Hour urine antimony reference value. In: Tietz NW, et al., ed: *Textbook of Clinical Chemistry*. Philadephia, PA: WB Saunders; 1986:1814.

125. Oliveira AL, et al. Severe adverse reactions to meglumine antimoniate in the treatment of visceral leishmaniasis: a report of 13 cases in the southwestern region of Brazil. *Trop Doct*. 2009;39:180-182.

126. Oliveira LF, et al. Systematic review of the adverse effects of cutaneous leishmaniasis treatment in the New World. *Acta Trop*. 2011;118:87-96.

127. Ortega-Carnicer J, et al. Pentavalent antimonial-induced torsade de pointes. *J Electrocardiol*. 1997;30:143-145.

128. Ozawa K. Studies on the therapy of schistosomiasis japonica. 1. On the fate and distribution of antimony in the body under the ordinary-treatment with sodium antimonyl tartrate. *Tohoku J Exp Med*. 1956;25:1-9.

129. Parish GG, et al. Acute arsine posioning in two workers cleaning a clogged drain. *Arch Environ Health*. 1979;34:224-227.

130. Paschal DC, Ting BG, Morrow JC, et al. Trace metals in urine of United States residents: reference range concentrations. *Environ Res*. 1998;76:53-59.

131. Pollack S, et al. Immunological studies of pancytopenia in visceral leishmaniasis. *Isr J Med Sci*. 1988;24:70-74.

132. Potkonjak V, Pavlovich M. Antimoniosis: a particular form of pneumoconiosis. I. Etiology, clinical and x-ray findings. *Int Arch Occup Environ Health*. 1983;51:199-207.

133. Rai US, et al. Renal dysfunction in patients of kala azar treated with sodium antimony gluconate. *J Assoc Physicians India*. 1994;42:383.

134. Rai US, et al. Acute renal failure and 9th, 10th nerve palsy in patient of kala-azar treated with stibanate. *J Assoc Physicians India*. 1994;42:338.

135. Rees PH, et al. Renal clearance of pentavalent antimony (sodium stibogluconate). *Lancet*. 1980;2:226-229.

136. Renes LE. Antimony poisoning in industry. *AMA Arch Ind Hyg Occup Med*. 1953;7: 99-108.

137. Romeo L, et al. Acute arsine intoxication as a consequence of metal burnishing operations. *Am J Ind Med*. 1997;32:211-216.

138. Roper CS, Stupart L. *The in vitro percutaneous absorption of diantimony trioxide through human skin*. Unpublished report on behalf of: International Antimony Oxide Industry Association; 2006.

139. Sadeghian G, et al. Electrocardiographic changes in patients with cutaneous leishmaniasis treated with systemic glucantime. *Ann Acad Med Singapore*. 2008;37: 916-918.

140. Saenz RE, et al. Efficacy and toxicity of pentostam against Panamanian mucosal leishmaniasis. *Am J Trop Med Hyg*. 1991;44:394-398.

141. Salaun P, Frezard F. Unexpectedly high levels of antimony(III) in the pentavalent antimonial drug Glucantime: insights from a new voltammetric approach. *Anal Bioanal Chem*. 2013;405:5201-5214.

142. Scinicariello F, et al. Antimony and sleep-related disorders: NHANES 2005-2008. *Environ Res*. 2017;156:247-252.

143. Sharma P, et al. Perspectives of antimony compounds in oncology. *Acta Pharmacol Sin*. 2008;29:881-890.

144. Shotyk W, Krachler M. Contamination of bottled waters with antimony leaching from polyethylene terephthalate (PET) increases upon storage. *Environ Sci Technol*. 2007;41:1560-1563.

145. Smichowski P. Antimony in the environment as a global pollutant: a review on analytical methodologies for its determination in atmospheric aerosols. *Talanta*. 2008;75: 2-14.

146. Smith JM, et al. Antimony intraocular foreign body with an intact electroretinogram. *Ophthalmology*. 2016;123:2224.

147. Smith SE. Uptake of antimony potassium tartrate by mouse liver slices. *Br J Pharmacol*. 1969;37:476-484.

148. Steiner R, Wegman I. *Fundamentals of Therapy: An Extension of the Art of Healing Through Spiritual Knowledge*. 4th ed. London: Rudolf Steiner Press; 1983.

149. Stevenson CJ. Antimony spots. *Trans St Johns Hosp Dermatol Soc*. 1965;51:40-48.

150. Sun H, et al. Interaction of antimony tartrate with the tripeptide glutathione implication for its mode of action. *Eur J Biochem*. 2000;267:5450-5457.

151. Sunagawa S. Experimental studies on antimony poisoning [in Japanese]. *Igaku Kenkyu*. 1981;51:129-142.

152. Sundar S, Chakravarty J. Antimony toxicity. *Int J Environ Res Public Health*. 2010;7: 4267-4277.

153. Sundar S, Sinha PR, Agrawal NK, et al. A cluster of cases of severe cardiotoxicity among kala-azar patients treated with a high-osmolarity lot of sodium antimony gluconate. *Am J Trop Med Hyg*. 1998;59:139-143.

154. Tarabar AF, et al. Antimony toxicity from the use of tartar emetic for the treatment of alcohol abuse. *Vet Hum Toxicol*. 2004;46:331-333.

155. Taylor AS. On poisoning by tartarized antimony; with medico-legal observations on the cases of Ann Palmer and others. In: Wilks S, ed. *Guy's Hospital Reports*. Vol III. London: Levy's Hospital; 1857.

156. Taylor PJ. Acute intoxication from antimony trichloride. *Br J Ind Med*. 1966;23:318-321.

157. Temprano Vazquez S, et al. Torsade de pointes secondary to treatment with pentavalent antimonial drugs [in Spanish]. *Med Clin (Barc)*. 1998;110:717.

158. Thakur CP, et al. Comparison of regimens of treatment with sodium stibogluconate in kala-azar. *Br Med J (Clin Res Ed)*. 1984;288:895-897.

159. Thompson RHS, Whittaker VP. Antidotal activity of British anti-Lewisite against compounds of antimony, gold and mercury. *Biochem J*. 1947;41:342-346.

160. Valentinus B. Triumph-Wagen des Antimonij (Triumphal Chariot of Antimony). A monograph on Antimony. 51. Stibium (Antimony) - Elementymology & Elements Multidict. 1604; Triumph-Wagen des Antimonij (Triumphal Chariot of Antimony). A monograph on Antimony: 1604 Basilius Valentinus (1565-1624).

161. Valete-Rosalino CM, et al. First report on ototoxicity of meglumine antimoniate. *Revista do Instituto de Medicina Tropical de São Paulo*. 2014;56:439-442.

162. Vikrant S, et al. Sodium stibogluconate-associated acute interstitial nephritis in a patient treated for visceral leishmaniasis. *Saudi J Kidney Dis Transpl*. 2015;26:757-760.

163. Waitz JA, et al. Physiological disposition of antimony after administration of 124Sb-labelled tartar emetic to rats, mice and monkeys, and the effects of tris (*p*-aminophenyl) carbonium pamoate on this distribution. *Bull World Health Organ*. 1965;33:537-546.

164. Watt WD. *Chronic Inhalation Toxicity of Antimony Trioxide: Validation of the Threshold Limit Value*. Detroit, MI: Wayne State University Press; 1983.

165. Weiss S, Hatcher RA. The mechanism of the vomiting induced by antimony and potassium tartrate (tartar emetic). *J Exp Med*. 1923;37:97-111.

166. Werrin M. Chemical food poisoning. *Bull Assoc Food Drug Office US*. 1963;27:38-45.

167. Wester PO. Trace elements in serum and urine from hypertensive patients before and during treatment with chlorthalidone. *Acta Med Scand*. 1973;194:505-512.

168. White GP Jr, et al. Dermatitis in workers exposed to antimony in a melting process. *J Occup Med*. 1993;35:392-395.

169. Winship KA. Toxicity of antimony and its compounds. *Adverse Drug React Acute Poisoning Rev*. 1987;6:67-90.

170. Wise ES, et al. Monitoring toxicity associated with parenteral sodium stibogluconate in the day-case management of returned travellers with New World cutaneous leishmaniasis [corrected]. *PLoS Negl Trop Dis*. 2012;6:e1688.

171. World Health Organization. Access to essential antileishmanial medicines and treatment. Leishmaniasis. Accessed August 1, 2017.

172. World Health Organization Expert Committee. *The Leishmaniasis. Report of a WHO Expert Committee*. Geneva: World Health Organization; 1984.

173. Wortmann GW, et al. Herpes zoster and lymphopenia associated with sodium stibogluconate therapy for cutaneous leishmaniasis. *Clin Infect Dis*. 1998;27:509-512.

174. Wu F, et al. Health risk associated with dietary co-exposure to high levels of antimony and arsenic in the world's largest antimony mine area. *Sci Total Environ*. 2011;409: 3344-3351.

175. Zaghloul IY, et al. Clinical efficacy and pharmacokinetics of antimony in cutaneous leishmaniasis patients treated with sodium stibogluconate. *J Clin Pharmacol*. 2010;50: 1230-1237.

86 ARSENIC

Stephen W. Munday

Arsenic (As)
Atomic number	=	33
Atomic weight	=	74.92 Da
Normal concentrations		
Whole blood	<	5 mcg/L (0.067 μmol/L)
Urine (24-hour)	<	50 mcg/L (0.67 μmol/L)
	<	100 mcg/g creatinine (1.33 μmol/g creatinine)

HISTORY AND EPIDEMIOLOGY

Arsenic poisoning can be unintentional, suicidal, homicidal, occupational, environmental, or iatrogenic.[114,115,150,177] Mass poisonings have occurred. Nearly 400 residents of Hong Kong fell ill after eating contaminated bread from the Esing Bakery in 1857, when 2 bakery foremen had tampered with the recipe.[94] In the 1900 Staffordshire beer epidemic in England, 6,000 beer drinkers fell ill and 70 died from beer brewed with sugar made with arsenic-contaminated sulfuric acid.[114] In Wakayama, Japan, 67 people were poisoned by eating intentionally contaminated curry at a festival in 1998.[235] In 2003, the largest recent outbreak of arsenic poisoning in the United States, occurred in New Sweden, Maine, when intentionally adulterated church coffee resulted in the death of one parishioner and the hospitalization of an additional 15 victims.[19] Arsenic trioxide (As_2O_3) reemerged as a treatment for acute promyelocytic leukemia (APML) in the 1990s after physicians in Harbin, China, found a high remission rate in patients given a crude As_2O_3 infusion.[135,251]

Contaminated soil, water, and food are the primary sources of arsenic for the general population. Pentavalent arsenic (As^{5+}) is the most common inorganic form in the environment.[61] Inorganic arsenic exposure from food is generally low and usually occurs from soil-derived foods such as rice and produce[32,211,265,273]; however, there is evidence that rice contamination is a significant source of arsenic exposure beyond drinking water.[113,125] Exposure to organic arsenic compounds of low toxicity occurs from consumption of algae, fish, and shellfish. In the past few decades, consumption of contaminated water has emerged as the primary cause of large-scale outbreaks of chronic arsenic toxicity. Arsenic leaches from certain minerals and ores, as well as from industrial waste.[157] In Bangladesh, millions of people have been poisoned by drinking water from wells contaminated with arsenic leached from ground minerals.[182] Ironically, the wells were dug to obtain safer groundwater. Hydroarsenicism is also reported in Chile, Taiwan, Brazil, India, Mexico, and Argentina.[35,54,61,107,157,182,251] In 2001, the US Environmental Protection Agency decreased the maximum contaminant concentration of arsenic in drinking water to 10 parts per billion (ppb), or 10 mcg/L, after statistical modeling indicated an increased risk of lung and bladder cancer from water contaminated with arsenic at the formerly acceptable concentration of 50 ppb.[70] The World Health Organization also recommends a maximum concentration of 10 ppb.

CHEMISTRY

Arsenic is a metalloid that exists in multiple forms: elemental, gaseous (arsine), organic, and inorganic (As^{3+} {trivalent, or arsenite} and As^{5+} {pentavalent, or arsenate}). Tables 86–1 and 86–2 list sources of arsenic and regulatory standards about arsenic, respectively. Arsenic metal is considered nonpoisonous because of its insolubility in water and, therefore, bodily fluids.[210] Arsine, which is highly toxic, is discussed in Chap. 121. Trivalent arsenicals include arsenic trioxide (As_2O_3), tetra-arsenic tetrasulfide (realgar; As_4S_4), and diarsenic trisulfide (orpiment; As_2S_3). Realgar and orpiment were used by the Chinese to treat malignancies, diarrhea, and infections of the chest and liver.[148] Organic arsenicals vary in toxicity. Arsenobetaine, which

is synthesized from inorganic arsenic by fish and crustaceans, and arsenosugars, which are synthesized by fish, crustaceans, and algae, have very low toxicity.[12,67,140] By contrast, the organoarsenical medication melarsoprol, used to treat the meningoencephalitic stage of African trypanosomiasis, is highly toxic and similar to inorganic arsenite.[27,199]

PHARMACOLOGY/PHYSIOLOGY

Arsenic trioxide is used to treat APML. The role of arsenic in our pharmacopeia is expanding. Its efficacy in treating various other leukemias, lymphomas, and multiple myeloma, as well as a variety of solid tumors such as breast cancer, colon cancer, lung cancer, hepatocellular carcinoma, colorectal cancer, renal cell carcinoma, and osteosarcoma is under study.[38,130,171]

Arsenic trioxide is administered therapeutically for treating APML in doses of 0.15 to 0.16 mg/kg/day by either the intravenous or oral route.[132,135,213,214,217] At this dose, its beneficial effects occur predominantly by initiating cellular apoptosis when arsenic concentrations reach 0.5 to 2.0 μmol/L. Apoptosis is triggered by several mechanisms. The trivalent arsenic (As^{3+}) ion binds to mitochondrial membrane sulfhydryl (SH) groups, damaging mitochondrial membranes and collapsing membrane potentials. Cytochrome C is released from the damaged mitochondria, with subsequent activation of

TABLE 86–1	Sources of Exposure to Arsenic

Inorganic
 Occupational/manufacturing
  Animal feed (additive)
  Brass/bronze
  Ceramics/glass
  Computer chips (same as semiconductors)
  Dyes/paints
  Electron microscopy
  Fireworks (Chinese)
  Fossil fuel combustion—coal
  Herbicides
  Insecticides/pesticides
  Metallurgy
  Mining
  Rodenticides
  Semiconductors (gallium arsenide)
  Smelting—copper, lead, zinc, sulfide minerals
  Soldering
  Wood preservatives
 Medications/contaminated xenobiotics
  Chemotherapeutics (acute promyelocytic leukemia)
  Depilatory
  Herbals/alternative medicines
  Homeopathic remedies
  Kelp
  "Moonshine" ethanol
  Opium
 Other
  Well water (contaminated)
  Candies/foods, eg, licorice (contaminated)

Organic
 Melarsoprol (trypanocidal)
 Thiacetarsamide (heartworm therapy in dogs)
 Seafood (arsenobetaine)

TABLE 86-2	Regulations and Guidelines Applicable to Arsenic and Arsenic Compounds		
Agency	**Guideline Description**	**Concentration**	**Source**
Air			
ACGIH	TLV (TWA) for arsenic and inorganic arsenic compounds	0.01 mg/m^3	ACGIH 2004
NIOSH	REL (15-min ceiling limit) for arsenic and inorganic compounds	0.002 mg/m^3	NIOSH 2005
	IDLH for arsenic and inorganic compounds	5 mg/m^3	NIOSH 2005
OSHA	PEL (8-hour TWA) for organic arsenic compounds (general industry, construction, and shipyard)	0.5 mg/m^3	OSHA 2005 29 CFR1910.1000; 1926.55; 1915.1000
	PEL (8-hour TWA) for general industry for inorganic arsenic compounds	10 mcg/m^3	OSHA 2005 29 CFR 1910.1018
Water			
EPA	National primary drinking water standards for arsenic		EPA 2002
	MCL	10 mcg/L (10 ppb)	EPA 2002
	MCLG	Zero	EPA 2002
FDA	Bottled drinking water	10 mcg/L	FDA 2005 21 CFR 165.110
WHO	Drinking water quality guidelines for arsenic	10 mcg/L	WHO 2004
Confirmed human carcinogen			
EPA/NTP			IRIS 2007/ NTP 2005
IARC			IARC 2007

ACGIH = American Conference of Governmental Industrial Hygienists; CFR = Code of Federal Regulations; DWEL = drinking water equivalent level; EPA = Environmental Protection Agency; FDA = Food and Drug Administration; IARC = International Agency for Research on Cancer; IDLH = immediately dangerous to life or health; IRIS = Integrated Risk Information System; MCL = maximum contaminant level; MCLG = maximum contaminant level goal; MW = molecular weight; NIOSH = National Institute for Occupational Safety and Health; NTP = National Toxicology Program; OSHA = Occupational Safety and Health Administration; PEL = permissible exposure limit; REL = recommended exposure limit; TLV = threshold limit value; TWA = time-weighted average; WHO = World Health Organization.

caspases 3, 8, and 9 and initiation of apoptosis. Cells are more susceptible if the intracellular concentrations of catalase and glutathione peroxidase (H_2O_2 scavenging enzymes) and glutathione-S-transferase (responsible for conjugating glutathione to xenobiotics) are reduced.[47,69,84,117,203] Arsenic trioxide also facilitates apoptosis by down-regulating gene expression of BCL2, a prosurvival protein that protects against apoptosis.[36] Finally, As_2O_3 arrests cells early in mitosis, subsequently leading to apoptosis.[97]

Low-dose As_2O_3 treatment (0.08 mg/kg/day) promotes cell differentiation of APL cells when arsenic concentrations reach 0.1 to 2.0 μmol/L. This differentiation is impaired by the promyelocytic leukemia–retinoic acid receptor α (PML-RARα) oncoprotein. This oncoprotein results from the APML-defining translocation of chromosomes 15 and 17. The PML portion of this oncoprotein plays a key role in leukemogenesis by interfering with RARα activity that is essential for normal myeloid cellular development. Trivalent arsenic degrades this PML portion, freeing RARα to facilitate cell differentiation.[47,164,173]

Melarsoprol is a trivalent organic arsenical compound used in Africa and parts of Europe to treat the meningoencephalitic stages of both species of African trypanosomes. It is ineffective against American trypanosomiasis and is available in the United States only directly from the Centers for Disease Control and Prevention (CDC), as it is not approved by the US Food and Drug Administration (FDA). The mechanism of action is still poorly understood but is related to inhibition of glycolysis and oxidation–reduction reactions. The pharmaceutical compound also contains dimercaprol (BAL), which seems to reduce toxicity without diminishing effectiveness. The therapeutic use of melarsoprol produces many of the toxic effects that occur with inorganic arsenic, including fever, encephalopathy, and acute cerebral edema with seizures and coma. Whether these effects are caused by drug toxicity or by an immune reaction elicited by trypanosomal antigens is unknown.[27,183,199] Other adverse effects include vomiting, abdominal pain, peripheral neuropathy with hypersensitivity reactions, hypertension, myocardial damage, and albuminuria. Hemolysis occurs in patients with glucose-6-phosphate dehydrogenase deficiency, and erythema nodosum occurs in patients with leprosy.[27,183] In a study of the usefulness of melarsoprol as a treatment for refractory or advanced leukemia, efficacy was very limited, and reported adverse effects included fatigue, vomiting, diarrhea, vertigo, fever, seizures, headache, back pain, and injection site pain.[218]

TOXICOLOGY/PATHOPHYSIOLOGY

Investigations of the pathophysiologic effects induced by toxic doses of arsenic are discussed below. The apoptotic mechanisms[30] thought to be responsible for some therapeutic effects of As_2O_3 are not well studied in toxicity models, but limited evidence suggests that cell necrosis may be more important.

Trivalent Arsenic

The primary biochemical effect of As^{3+} is inhibition of the pyruvate dehydrogenase (PDH) complex (Fig. 86–1). Normally, dihydrolipoamide is recycled to lipoamide, a necessary cofactor in the conversion of pyruvate to acetylcoenzyme A (acetyl-CoA). Trivalent arsenic (As^{3+}) binds the sulfhydryl groups of dihydrolipoamide, blocking lipoamide regeneration.[198] Acetyl-CoA is a central molecule in metabolism, and the resulting decrease leads to several deleterious effects:

- Decreased citric acid cycle activity and thus decreased adenosine triphosphate (ATP) production.
- Disruption of oxidative phosphorylation, which leads to production of hydrogen peroxide and oxygen radicals.
- Decreased gluconeogenesis that worsens hypoglycemia. Pyruvate carboxylase catalyzes the conversion of pyruvate to oxaloacetate (initial step in gluconeogenesis), and this reaction requires the carboxylation of biotin, a CO_2 carrier attached to pyruvate carboxylase. Biotin cannot be carboxylated unless acetyl-CoA is attached to the enzyme.[199,223]

In the citric acid cycle, oxidation of α-ketoglutarate to succinyl-CoA uses an α-ketoglutarate dehydrogenase complex that contains the same cofactors as the PDH complex, including lipoamide. Succinyl-CoA is necessary for production of porphyrins and amino acids, and deficiency contributes to the anemia and wasting that occurs with chronic arsenic poisoning. Arsenic inhibition of thiolase, the catalyst for the final step in fatty acid oxidation, also impairs ATP production. Diminished fatty acid oxidation results in decreased acetyl-CoA, in the loss of the reduced form of nicotinamide adenine dinucleotide (NADH) and the reduced form of flavin adenine dinucleotide ($FADH_2$) (electron carriers reduced during fatty acid breakdown whose subsequent oxidation yields ATP). Trivalent arsenic also inhibits glutathione synthetase, glucose-6-phosphate dehydrogenase (required to produce nicotinamide adenine dinucleotide phosphate {NADPH}), and glutathione reductase.[8] These inhibitions result in decreased concentrations of reduced

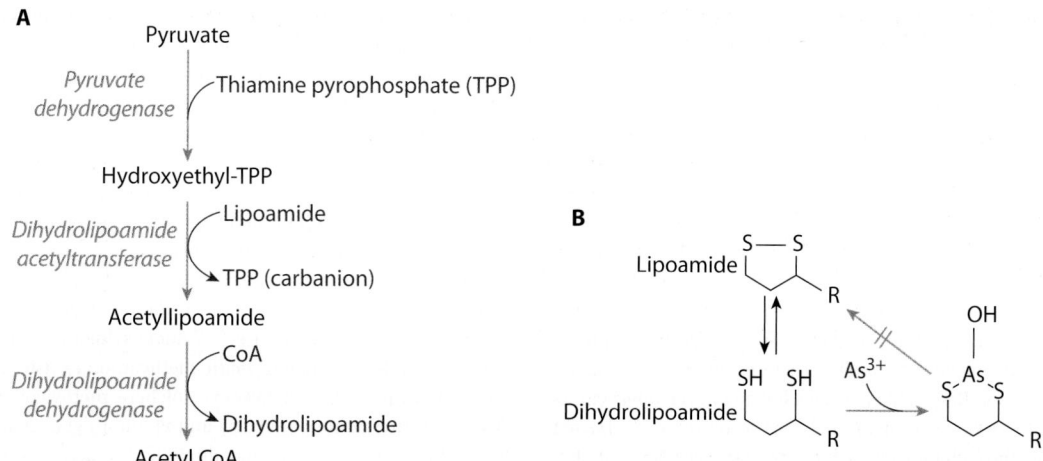

FIGURE 86–1. Effect of trivalent arsenicals (As³⁺) on pyruvate dehydrogenase (PDH) complex. (**A**) The PDH complex is composed of the 3 enzymes, which use thiamine pyrophosphate (TPP) and lipoamide as cofactors to decarboxylate pyruvate and form acetyl CoA. (**B**) Arsenic interferes with the regeneration of lipoamide from dihydrolipoamide, thereby altering the function of the PDH complex.

glutathione, which is required to facilitate arsenic metabolism, protect red blood cells (RBCs) from oxidative damage, maintain hemoglobin in the ferrous state, and scavenge hydrogen peroxide and other organic peroxides.

Arsenic affects cardiac repolarization currents. When toxicity occurs, the result is ventricular dysrhythmias, including torsade de pointes. An in vitro study of cells exposed to As³⁺ demonstrated blockade of the delayed rectifier channels I_{Ks} and I_{Kr}. Interestingly, activation of I_{K-ATP}, a weak inward rectifier channel, also occurred; this activation potentially counteracts some of the effects of As³⁺ on the I_{Ks} and I_{Kr} channels.[64] Recent epidemiologic evidence demonstrates a relationship between well water and urine arsenic concentrations and QT interval prolongation in women.[46]

Animal experiments with phenylarsine oxide, a trivalent arsenical, demonstrate inhibition of insulin-induced glucose transport involving vicinal (adjacent) sulfhydryl groups, as well as β cell damage in pancreatic islets attributed to inhibition of the α-ketoglutarate dehydrogenase complex.[25] The impaired glucose transport, plus the inhibited gluconeogenesis, leads to glycogen depletion and hypoglycemia.[200] Several animal experiments indicate improved central nervous system (CNS) glucose content[199] and increased survival time with glucose treatment.[199]

Effects on RBCs include decreased membrane fluidity and ATP depletion.[258] Chronic arsenic exposure is associated with vascular disease; in vitro studies demonstrate inhibition of endothelial cell proliferation and glycoprotein synthesis in addition to lipid peroxidation.[37] Evaluations of genetic polymorphisms showed an association between genetic variants and endothelial dysfunction.[261] A study on rodent and human platelets demonstrates increased platelet aggregation and arterial thrombosis.[142] Noncirrhotic hepatic portal fibrosis sometimes develops. In a controlled study where mice chronically ingested water containing equal parts As³⁺ and As⁵⁺ for up to 15 months, the development of portal fibrosis was preceded by decreased hepatic glutathione (GSH) concentration, increased lipid peroxidation, and diminished concentrations or activities of numerous enzymes involved in regenerating GSH or scavenging free radicals.[208] Proposed mechanisms by which arsenic induces cancer include DNA damage induced by a dimethyl sulfide (DMS)-derived peroxyl radical, gene amplification, replacing phosphate in DNA during replication, increased cell proliferation, and decreased DNA repair efficiency.[17,122,264] Experimental evidence and human studies support a number of etiologic or contributing factors for skin keratosis and cancer,[1] including chronic stimulation of keratinocyte-derived growth factors such as transforming growth factor-α (TGF-α), impaired methylation, mutation in the p53 tumor-suppressor gene, inhibition of poly(adenosine diphosphate {ADP}-ribose) polymerase vital for DNA repair, and interference with mitotic spindle and microtubular function.[7,86,111,146,260] Pigmentary changes also occur, and hyperpigmentation is attributed to increased melanin.

Pentavalent Arsenic

Several mechanisms contribute to the toxicity of As⁵⁺. Pentavalent arsenic is readily reduced to As³⁺.[112,243] Pentavalent arsenic also resembles phosphate chemically and structurally, may share a common transport system for cellular uptake with phosphate,[112] and inhibits oxidative phosphorylation by substituting for inorganic phosphate (P_i) in the glycolysis reaction catalyzed by glyceraldehyde 3-phosphate dehydrogenase (Fig. 86–2).[34,201] The resulting unstable product, 1-arseno-3-phosphoglycerate, spontaneously hydrolyzes to 3-phosphoglycerate, so glycolysis continues but the ATP normally produced during conversion of 1,3-bisphosphoglycerate to 3-phosphoglycerate is lost. Uncoupling also occurs if ADP forms ADP-arsenate, instead of ATP, in the presence of As⁵⁺. The ADP-arsenate rapidly hydrolyzes, thus uncoupling oxidative phosphorylation.

PHARMACOKINETICS AND TOXICOKINETICS
Absorption

Inorganic arsenic is tasteless and odorless and is absorbed by the gastrointestinal (GI), respiratory, intravenous, and mucosal routes. Gastrointestinal

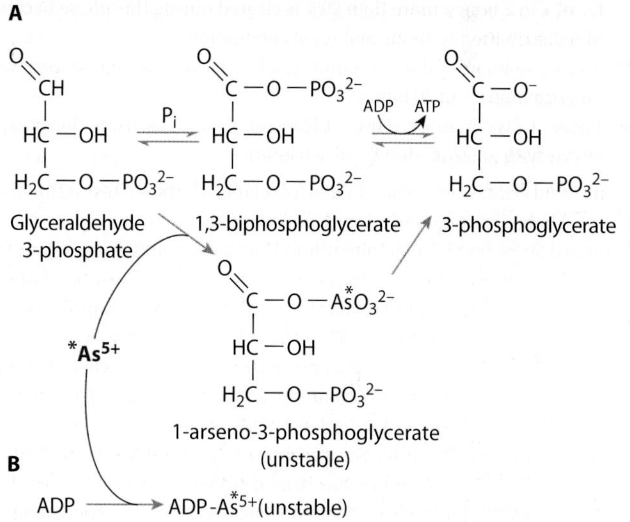

FIGURE 86–2. Pathophysiologic effects of As⁵⁺ (arsenate). (**A**) Arsenate (chemical formula AsO₄³⁻) substitutes for inorganic phosphate (Pi; the asterisk indicates substitutions), bypassing the formation of 1,3-bisphosphoglycerate (1,3-BPG), and thus losing the ATP formation that occurs when 1,3-BPG is metabolized to 3-phosphoglycerate. (**B**) Energy loss also occurs if arsenate substitutes for Pi and blocks the formation of ATP from ADP. ADP = adenosine diphosphate; ATP = adenosine triphosphate.

absorption is facilitated by increased solubility and smaller particle size, and it occurs predominantly in the small intestine, followed by the colon. Poorly soluble trivalent compounds such as As_2O_3 are less well absorbed than more soluble trivalent and pentavalent compounds that, in aqueous solution, have an oral bioavailability greater than 90%. Therefore, when placed in an aqueous solution, As_2O_3 is more toxic than an identical dose of undissolved As_2O_3 eaten in food because of its failure to dissolve, thereby limiting absorption.[240] Organic arsenicals tend to be well absorbed; for example, a rodent study demonstrated that approximately 70% GI absorption of the commonly used organic arsenical herbicide, dimethylarsinic acid (cacodylic acid).[220] Systemic absorption via the respiratory tract depends on the particulate size, as well as the arsenic compound and its solubility. Large, nonrespirable particles are cleared from the airways by ciliary action and swallowed, allowing GI absorption to occur. Respirable particles lodging in the lungs can be absorbed over days to weeks or remain unabsorbed for years.[28,255] Dermal penetration of arsenic through intact skin does not pose a risk for acute toxicity but potentially is problematic with chronic application. Arsenic acid (H_3AsO_4) applied to intact skin in rhesus monkeys resulted in absorption of a mean of 2.0% to 6.4% of the applied dose.[253] Skin irritation and damage increases systemic absorption.[83,202]

Pharmacokinetics of Arsenic Trioxide

Intravenous administration of a single 10-mg dose of As_2O_3 to 8 patients showed mean pharmacokinetic values as follows: maximum plasma concentration (Cp_{max}) of 6.85 μmol/L, α elimination half-life ($t_{1/2}$ α) of 0.89 ± 0.29 hours, and β elimination half-life ($t_{1/2}$ β) of 12.13 ± 3.31 hours.[214] In 6 patients, only 1% to 8% of the daily dose was eliminated in a 24-hour urine test. Repeat pharmacokinetic studies on day 30 of treatment were not statistically different.[214] Another study of patients receiving a single dose of 5 mg of As_2O_3 intravenously demonstrated mean pharmacokinetic values as follows: Cp_{max} of 2.6 μmol/L, $t_{1/2}$ α of 1.41 hours, $t_{1/2}$ β of 9.41 hours, serum clearance of 1.98 L/h, and area under the plasma drug concentration versus time curve (AUC) of 12.7 μmol/L/h. A single dose of 10 mg intravenously showed a Cp_{max} of 6.7 ± 0.3 μmol/L.[213] Arsenic trioxide 10 mg given orally for APML demonstrated total plasma and blood AUC values that were 99% and 87%, respectively, of the corresponding values reported for a 10-mg intravenous dose administered in the same 9 patients.[132]

A study in humans receiving intravenous radioarsenic isotope (^{74}As) showed arsenic clearing from the blood in 3 phases:

- Phase 1 (2–3 hours)—Arsenic is rapidly cleared from the plasma with a $t_{1/2}$ of 1 to 2 hours; more than 90% is cleared during this phase because of redistribution to tissue and renal elimination.
- Phase 2 (3 hours–7 days)—A more gradual plasma decline occurs, with an estimated $t_{1/2}$ of 30 hours.
- Phase 3 (10 or more days)—Clearance continues from the plasma slowly with an estimated $t_{1/2}$ of 300 hours.[159]

The rapid clearance in phases 1 and 2 explains why blood testing for arsenic is unreliable, except early in acute poisoning.

Initial distribution is predominantly to liver, kidney, muscle, and skin. The skin is rich in sulfhydryl groups; the elimination $t_{1/2}$ of arsenic by the skin was estimated to be one month in a rabbit study.[65] Distribution to brain also occurs quickly.[79] In the As (^{74}As) study, 0.3% of the administered dose was found in brain biopsy samples in the first hour postinfusion. This peak declined to 0.16% by day 7.[159] Ultimately, arsenic distributes to all tissues. In the single patient in this study who was followed for 18 days, 96.6% of the total injected arsenic dose was recovered in the urine. Fecal arsenic recovery was less than 1% of the total dose.[159] Other studies in humans demonstrate renal arsenic elimination of 46% to 68.9% within the first 5 days postingestion.[29,32,118,191] Approximately 30% is eliminated with a half-life of greater than one week, while the remainder is slowly excreted with a half-life of greater than one month.[29,158] Fecal elimination is considerably less, with reported amounts as much as 6.1% in humans.[225] Canine studies revealed that the mechanisms of urinary elimination of unchanged arsenic and its methylated metabolites are via glomerular filtration and tubular secretion; active reabsorption also occurs.[233]

Arsenic crosses the placenta and accumulates in the fetus,[149] but 3 studies of breast milk excretion from women exposed to drinking water with arsenic concentrations of approximately 200 mcg/L came to disparate conclusions. Breast milk arsenic concentrations were low in these studies, and only one of them demonstrated a correlation between maternal arsenic concentrations and concentrations in breast milk.[55,71,207] A single study suggests that breast feeding actually protects the infant from arsenic exposure.[71]

Metabolism, by adding methyl groups, occurs primarily in the liver, as well as in the kidneys, testes, and lungs (Fig. 86–3). If the arsenic is pentavalent, approximately 50% to 70% of As^{5+} will first be reduced to As^{3+}.[54,221,241] This bioactivation step requires the oxidation of glutathione[62] and can begin within 15 minutes of exposure.[241] S-Adenosylmethionine (SAM) is the primary methyl donor. Nonenzymatic methylation is also demonstrated in an in vitro study using human liver cytosol; here, methylcobalamin (methyl B_{12}) was the methyl donor.[270] Dietary and vitamin deficiencies, as well as high doses of inorganic arsenic, may diminish the ability to methylate arsenic, and folate supplementation lowers blood arsenic concentrations in a folate-deficient population.[15,80-82,98,102,103,188,190,242] However, a study in pregnant Bangladeshi women showed efficient arsenic methylation despite nutritional deficiencies.[145] Addition of one methyl group produces monomethylarsonic acid (MMA^{5+}); adding a second methyl group produces dimethylarsinic acid (DMA^{5+}). Production of a trivalent intermediate in this reaction, monomethylarsonous acid (MMA^{3+}), is catalyzed by MMA^{5+} reductase. In rabbits, this is the rate-limiting enzyme in the biotransformation pathway; however, no data exist to confirm a similar role in human metabolism.[239,271] Conversion of MMA^{5+} to DMA^{5+} is catalyzed by a methyltransferase. Genomic studies have begun to identify gene polymorphisms in these pathways that are associated with variations in arsenic metabolism and toxicity.[3,187]

These monomethylation and dimethylation steps were previously thought to detoxify arsenic, but is now questioned because of the generation of these trivalent intermediates, which are more toxic than the parent compounds.[237] Estimated human LD$_{50}$ (median lethal dose for 50% of test subjects) doses were reported to be As_2O_3, 1.43 mg/kg; MMA^{5+}, 50 mg/kg;

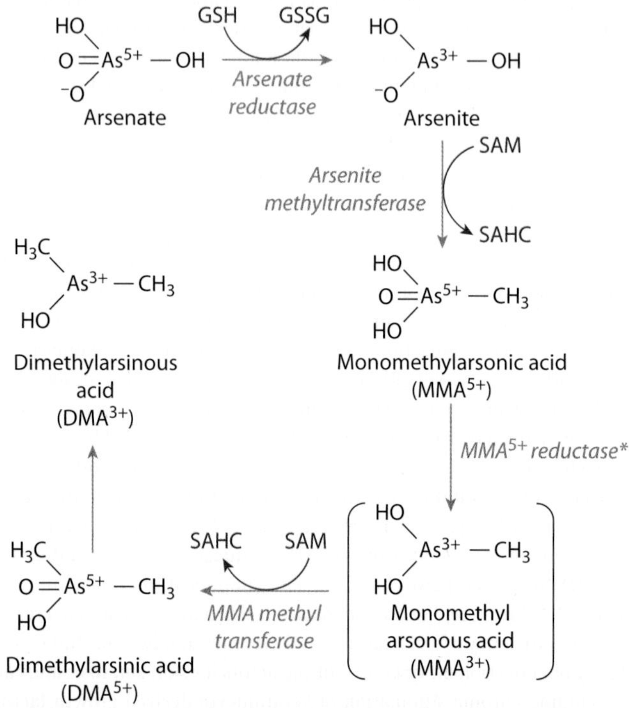

FIGURE 86-3. Metabolism of arsenate [As^{5+}] and arsenite [As^{3+}]. DMA = dimethylarsinic acid; GSH = glutathione; GSSG = oxidized glutathione MMA = monomethylarsonic acid; SAHC = S-adenosylhomocysteine; SAM = S-adenosylmethionine. The asterisk (*) denotes MMA^{5+} reductase, the rate-limiting enzyme in rabbit studies of arsenic metabolism; the analogy to humans is unknown.

and DMA^{5+}, 500 mg/kg. However, it is important to note that the doses cited for MMA and DMA apply to arsenic existing in the pentavalent form (As^{5+}). Studies in animals and cell cultures indicate that MMA^{3+} is more toxic than As^{3+}.[153,185,186] Cytotoxicity studies in human hepatocytes revealed descending toxicity of arsenic and its metabolites as follows: MMA^{3+} > arsenite > arsenate > MMA^{5+} = DMA^{5+}.[185] Thus, toxicity increases with the formation of MMA^{3+}.

There is some evidence that these findings have clinical relevance. In a study from a blackfoot disease hyperendemic area of Taiwan, lower capacity to methylate inorganic arsenic to DMA^{5+} is associated with increased risk of blackfoot disease. The capacity to methylate arsenic to DMA^{5+} was measured as the ratio of DMA^{5+} to MMA^{5+} and the ratio of MMA^{5+} to the sum of As^{3+} and As^{5+}.[231] Another study demonstrated an association between incomplete methylation capacity and carotid intima–media thickness.[44] Moreover a prospective study demonstrated an association between methylation capacity and heart disease risk.[45] In addition, a cohort study found that the odds of premalignant skin lesions increased with increasing urinary MMA^{5+} and decreasing urinary DMA^{5+}.[3] They also found that there was an increased risk of skin lesions associated with genetic polymorphisms of glutathione S-transferase and borderline increased risk with polymorphisms of methylenetetrahydrofolate reductase. The authors suggested that the conversion of MMA^{5+} to DMA^{5+} is saturable and that arsenic metabolism and toxicity are affected by genetics.[3] An additional nested case-controlled study of this cohort confirmed that folate deficiency and DNA hypomethylation were risk factors for skin lesions.[189]

Arsenobetaine (AsB) is also well absorbed orally and is excreted unchanged in the urine.[240] Elimination occurs more rapidly than with inorganic arsenic. In a study involving human volunteers, 25% was excreted within 2 to 4 hours, 50% by 20 hours, and 70% to 83.7% after 166 hours. A 2-compartment exponential model shows nearly 50% of the arsenobetaine eliminated, with a first compartment $t_{1/2}$ of 6.9 to 11.0 hours and a second compartment $t_{1/2}$ of 75.7 hours.[118]

CLINICAL MANIFESTATIONS

Inorganic Arsenicals

Toxic manifestations vary, depending on the amount and form, route, and chronicity of arsenic exposure. Other influencing factors include individual variations in methylation and excretion. Larger doses of a potent compound, such as As$_2$O$_3$, will rapidly produce manifestations of acute toxicity, whereas chronic ingestion of substantially lower amounts of As^{5+} in groundwater will result in different clinical findings over time. Manifestations of subacute toxicity can develop in patients who survive acute poisoning, as well as in patients who are slowly poisoned environmentally.

Acute Toxicity

Gastrointestinal signs and symptoms of nausea, vomiting, abdominal pain, and diarrhea, which occur 10 minutes to several hours following ingestion, are the earliest manifestations of acute poisoning by the oral route. The diarrhea is compared to cholera in that it resembles "rice water." Severe multisystem illness ensues with extensive exposure. Cardiovascular signs, ranging from sinus tachycardia and orthostatic hypotension to shock, can develop. Reported cases often mimic myocardial infarction or systemic inflammatory response syndrome, with intravascular volume depletion, capillary leak, myocardial dysfunction, and diminished systemic vascular resistance.[16,22,24,90,119,212] Acute encephalopathy develops and progress over several days, with delirium, coma, and seizures attributed to cerebral edema and microhemorrhages.[76,212] Seizures may be secondary to dysrhythmias, and the underlying cardiac rhythm should be assessed. Seizures apparently secondary to torsade de pointes associated with a prolonged QT interval developed 4 days to 5 weeks after acute arsenic ingestion.[22,88,219] Acute respiratory distress syndrome (ARDS) and respiratory failure, hepatitis, hemolytic anemia, acute kidney injury (AKI), rhabdomyolysis, ventricular dysrhythmias, and death are all reported.[24,74,93,167,234] Death occurs after suddenly developing bradycardia, followed by asystole.[24,119,150] Fever sometimes develops, misleading the practitioner to diagnose sepsis.[66,119] Hepatitis occurs and as a result of altered intrahepatic heme metabolism causing an increased synthesis of bilirubin or a result of altered protein transport between hepatocytes.[6] Acute kidney

injury occurs secondary to ischemia caused by hypotension, tubular deposition of myoglobin or hemoglobin, renal cortical necrosis, and direct renal tubular toxicity.[26,85,209,234] Glutathione depletion is contributory.[108] Unusual complications include phrenic nerve paralysis, unilateral facial nerve palsy, pancreatitis, pericarditis, and pleuritis.[18,271] Fetal demise is reported, with toxic arsenic concentrations found in the fetal organs.[24,149]

Acutely poisoned patients with less severe illness experience gastroenteritis and mild hypotension that persist despite antiemetic and intravenous crystalloid therapies. Hospitalization and continued intravenous fluids often are required for several days.[141] The prolonged character of the GI effects is atypical for most viral and bacterial enteric illnesses and should alert the physician to the possibility of arsenic poisoning, especially if there is a history of repetitive GI illnesses. A metallic taste or oropharyngeal irritation, mimicking pharyngitis, occurs.[24,105] Gastrointestinal ulcerative lesions and hemorrhage are reported.[76,90] Toxic erythroderma and exfoliative dermatitis result from a hypersensitivity reaction to arsenic.[226]

In the days and weeks following an acute exposure, prolonged or additional signs and symptoms in the nervous, GI, hematologic, dermatologic, pulmonary, and cardiovascular systems occur. Encephalopathic findings of headache, confusion, decreased memory, personality change, irritability, hallucinations, delirium, and seizures develop and persist.[66,79,204] Sixth cranial nerve palsy and bilateral sensorineural hearing loss are reported.[53,88] Peripheral neuropathy typically develops 1 to 3 weeks after acute poisoning, although in one series 9 patients developed maximal neuropathy within 24 hours of exposure.[53,105,141,253] Sensory symptoms develop first, with diminished to absent vibratory sense. Progressive signs and symptoms include numbness, tingling, and formication with physical findings of diminished to absent pain, touch, temperature, and deep-tendon reflexes in a stocking-glove distribution. Superficial touch of the extremities sometimes elicits severe or deep aching pains, a finding that also occurs with thallium poisoning (Chap. 99). Motor weakness often develops. The most severely affected patients manifest an ascending flaccid paralysis that mimics Guillain-Barré syndrome.[53,105,141] Respiratory findings include dry cough, crackles, hemoptysis, chest pain, and patchy interstitial infiltrates.[105,184] These findings are often misinterpreted as viral or bronchitic disease. Leukopenia, and less commonly anemia and thrombocytopenia, occur from days to 3 weeks after an acute exposure, but resolve as bone marrow function returns.[114,144]

Dermatologic lesions include patchy alopecia, oral herpetiform lesions, a diffuse pruritic macular rash, and a brawny nonpruritic desquamation (Chap. 17). Diaphoresis and edema of the face and extremities are reported.[1] Mees lines (transverse striate leuconychia of the nails) are 1- to 2-mm-wide horizontal nail bands that represent disturbed nail matrix keratinization (Fig. 86–4). They are uncommon in arsenic poisoning. A minimum of

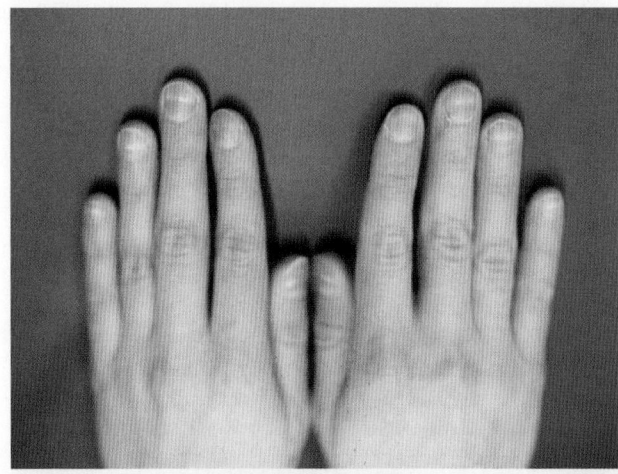

FIGURE 86–4. Mees lines, parallel white bands across the nails, result from exposures to metals, radiation, and chemotherapeutics, among others. *(Used with permission from the Fellowship in Medical Toxicology, New York University School of Medicine, New York City Poison Center.)*

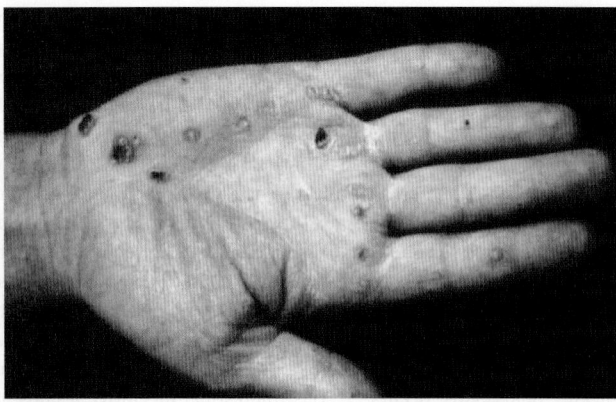

FIGURE 86–5. Characteristic hemorrhagic vesicles of arsenical dermatitis is shown. *(Used with permission from the New York University Department of Dermatology.)*

30 days after exposure is required for the lines to extend visibly beyond the nail lunulae.[105,260] Contact dermatitis is reported from topical exposure in an occupational setting. Other possible toxic manifestations of subacute inorganic arsenic toxicity include nephropathy, fatigue, anorexia with weight loss, torsade de pointes, and persistence of GI effects.[16,154]

Chronic Toxicity

Malignant and nonmalignant skin changes, hypertension, diabetes mellitus (DM), and peripheral cardiovascular and cerebral vascular disease, as well as lung, bladder, renal and hepatic malignancies are associated with drinking water containing arsenic that is consumed by study populations.[50,58,72,116,133,161,166,168,182,192,267] The skin is very susceptible to the toxic effects of arsenic; multiple dermatologic lesions are reported in populations suffering from hydroarsenicism.[157,267] Alterations in pigmentation occur first, with hyperpigmentation being the most common. Hypopigmentation ("raindrop" pattern) also occurs (Fig. 86–5). Hyperkeratoses typically develop on the palms and soles, but can be diffuse (Fig. 86–6). Squamous and basal cell carcinomas and Bowen's disease (intraepidermal squamous cell carcinoma) occur. Bowen's disease usually proliferates in multiple sites, especially on the trunk, and is noted for developing on sun-protected areas. Latency periods for developing keratoses, Bowen's disease, and squamous cell carcinoma were 28, 39, and 41 years, respectively, in 17 patients chronically exposed to environmental or medicinal arsenic.[60,259] Gastrointestinal signs and effects of nausea, vomiting, and diarrhea are less likely but do occur. Hepatomegaly was present in 120 of 156 patients with hydroarsenicism; liver biopsy in 45 cases revealed a noncirrhotic portal fibrosis in 91.1%.[157] Rodent

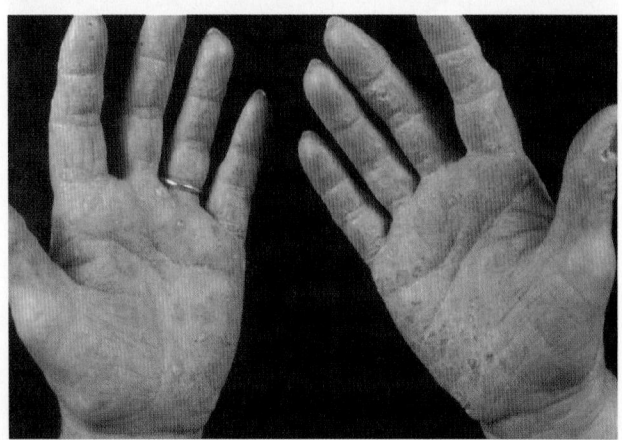

FIGURE 86–6. Characteristic vesicular xerotic arsenical dermatitis is shown. *(Used with permission from the New York University Department of Dermatology.)*

studies also demonstrate hepatic fibrosis from inorganic arsenic exposure.[208] Portal hypertension and hypersplenism occur.[157,208] Hepatic angiosarcomas are linked to arsenic exposure.[51,121,139]

Some, but not all, population studies in areas of Bangladesh, Taiwan, and the United States with arsenic-contaminated water show an increased prevalence of DM, pulmonary fibrosis, and other organ system effects.[39,124,194,195,232] A cross-sectional drinking water study from the United States revealed an odds ratio of 3.58 for prevalence of type 2 DM among those at the 80th percentile, as compared to those at the 20th percentile, despite a median total arsenic concentration of only 7.1 ppb.[138,172] However, a cross-sectional study in Bangladesh did not find a relationship between arsenic exposure and DM.[39] Animal studies demonstrate that arsenic decreases insulin-mediated uptake of glucose by cells and also disrupts insulin transcription factor signal transduction.[181,248] In a study from West Bengal, India, restrictive lung disease was reported in 9 of 17 patients, and a restrictive plus obstructive pattern occurred in another 7 cases.[157] Lung disease is also noted in other populations.[58,95] Proposed mechanisms include arsenic-induced inflammation and oxidative stress and endothelial dysfunction.[178,263] Aplastic anemia and agranulocytosis are documented in patients exposed to arsenic.[66] A dose–response relationship between arsenic exposure and vascular disease is reported in several populations.[250] After adjusting for age, sex, hypertension, DM, cigarette smoking, and ethanol consumption, a significant relationship was observed with cerebrovascular disease in a region of Taiwan.[50] Blackfoot disease, an obliterative arterial disease of the lower extremities, occurring in Taiwan, is linked to chronic arsenic exposure,[35,230] as is ischemic heart disease.[33,166] There is accumulating evidence that the vascular effects are related to endothelial dysfunction and that genetic polymorphisms moderate these effects.[261-263] The incidence of Raynaud phenomenon and vasospasm[35,230] was reported to be increased in smelter workers exposed to arsenic, compared with a control group.[137] Encephalopathy and peripheral neuropathy are the neurologic manifestations most commonly reported.[21,99] Electromyographic studies of 33 patients with chronic ingestion of arsenic-contaminated water[21] revealed 10 patients with findings consistent with sensory neuropathy. The minimum duration of exposure was 2 years. Interestingly, 3 of these patients consumed water with an arsenic concentration that only slightly exceeded the contaminant concentration of 50 ppb previously permissible in the United States.[107]

Arsenic is classified as a definite carcinogen by the International Agency for Research on Cancer (IARC, Group 1) and the National Toxicology Program (NTP). Cancers known to develop include lung, skin, and bladder.[12,52,113,207,216] Transitional cell bladder carcinoma was the most common type in one large epidemiologic study.[49] However, the exposure threshold of concern remains controversial.[160] A critical literature review of animal and human studies found that exposure to environmental arsenic was unlikely to cause reproductive or developmental toxicity.[63] However, a rodent study revealed fetal growth retardation and neurotoxicity at doses relevant to human exposure and in the absence of maternal toxicity.[249] More concerning, 2 drinking water cohort studies from Bangladesh showed small but statistically significant increases in birth defects and fetal loss.[134,194,238] In addition to possibly increasing the risk of birth defects, there is also cohort and cross-sectional evidence that in utero or early childhood exposure is associated with persistent neurocognitive effects in children.[31,39,57,99,100,124,229,246,251,252] Finally, there is evidence that in utero or early childhood exposure to arsenic in drinking water increases the risk of malignant and nonmalignant lung diseases in young adults.[216] In summary, there is accumulating evidence of persistent adverse effects from in utero or early childhood exposure, but additional prospective studies are needed to confirm these findings by decreasing the effects of confounding and bias that may explain the results.

Many of the questions regarding the chronic health effects of exposure to arsenic in drinking water are currently being investigated in the Health Effects of Arsenic Longitudinal Study (HEALS). This study is designed to evaluate the health effects of a full range of drinking water arsenic exposures, including mortality, premalignant and malignant skin tumors, pregnancy outcomes, and children's cognitive development.[5]

The HEALS study is a prospective cohort study in Araihazar, Bangladesh. Participants are between the ages of 18 and 75 years and married, although both members of a couple are not required to enroll. A total of 11,764 subjects enrolled, 6,704 women and 5,042 men. The participation rate in the initial enrollment was 97.5% of those approached.[5] Ninety-eight percent of those who agreed to participate completed an extensive questionnaire that included demographic and lifestyle components and a validated food-frequency questionnaire. They also participated in a clinical examination with an extensive skin evaluation. More than 90% of this group also provided blood and spot urine arsenic samples.[5]

Approximately one-third of the participants consumed water in each of 3 groups: greater than 100 mcg/L, 25 to 100 mcg/L, and less than 25 mcg/L. Average urinary concentrations of arsenic were approximately 140 mcg/L.

Many studies from this cohort are already published. Studies of persons with arsenic-induced skin lesions show increasing risk of disease as exposure increases.[4,13] Modification of risk was noted in relationship to nutritional status, sunlight exposure, smoking, and some occupational exposures such as fertilizers and pesticides.[41,42,162] A dose–response relationship was also found for other health effects, including total mortality,[14] cardiovascular disease,[40] respiratory symptoms,[179] proteinuria,[43] oral cavity lesions,[222] and neurologic effects.[96,180] Skin lesions are linked to lung cancer risk, and this risk is shown to be synergistic with cigarette smoking.[110] Biannual follow-up of this cohort continues.

Adverse Drug Effects: Arsenic Trioxide

The most common adverse effects are dermatologic (skin dryness, pigmentary changes, maculopapular eruptions with or without pruritus); GI (nausea, vomiting, anorexia, diarrhea, and dyspepsia); hematologic (leukemoid reactions); hepatic (elevation of aminotransferase concentrations typically less than or equal to 10 times the upper limit of normal values, with a reported incidence of 20% with low-dose and 31.9% with conventional-dose therapy[213]); cardiac (prolonged QT interval in 40%–63% of patients, first-degree atrioventricular block, ventricular ectopy, monomorphic nonsustained ventricular tachycardia, torsade de pointes, asystole, and death);[206,213,217,236,257] facial edema; and neurologic (paresthesias, peripheral neuropathy, and headache). All of these effects occurred more commonly in one case series with conventional-dose therapy (0.16 mg/kg/day) when compared to low-dose therapy. The majority of patients are treated symptomatically without discontinuing As_2O_3 treatment. Leukemoid reactions, defined as white blood cell counts greater than 50×10^9/L, develop in nearly 50% of patients between 14 and 42 days of beginning treatment. Such patients are at risk for intracerebral hemorrhage or infarction and for the APML syndrome. This syndrome is similar to the differentiation syndrome (DS), which was formerly known as the retinoic acid syndrome.[165] The remission-induction treatment phase is the period of greatest risk.[214] Common clinical findings in this syndrome include pulmonary interstitial infiltrates and/or pleural effusions, dyspnea, tachypnea, fluid retention, myalgias, arthralgias, fever, and weight gain; approximately 20% to 25% of patients treated with arsenic trioxide will develop one or more signs or symptoms of this syndrome.[155,171,206,213,214]

Although a theoretical concern, there is currently no evidence of increased risk of secondary malignancies in treated patients. Continued close follow-up will be necessary to evaluate whether secondary malignancy risk will increase over time.[69]

DIAGNOSTIC TESTING

Timing of testing for arsenic must be correlated with the clinical course of the patient and whether the poisoning is acute, subacute, chronic, or remote with residual clinical effects. To properly interpret laboratory measurements, confounding factors, such as food-derived organic arsenicals or accumulated arsenic (DMA and arsenobetaine) in patients with chronic kidney disease, must be evaluated.[59,275,276] Failure to understand potential confounders, as well as the time course of arsenic metabolism, clearance, and effect on laboratory parameters, can cause erroneous assessment of possible arsenic poisoning.

Urine and Blood

Diagnosis ultimately depends on finding an elevated urinary arsenic concentration. In an emergency, a spot urine sample for arsenic should be sent prior to beginning chelation therapy. A markedly elevated arsenic concentration verifies the diagnosis in a patient with characteristic history and clinical findings, but a low concentration does not exclude arsenic toxicity.[247] In 9 acutely symptomatic patients, initial spot urine arsenic concentrations ranged from 192 to 198,450 mcg/L.[123] Definitive diagnosis of arsenic exposure hinges on finding a 24-hour urinary concentration equal to or greater than 50 mcg/L, 100 mcg/g creatinine, or 100 mcg total arsenic. A study on arsenic exposure from drinking water showed excellent correlations between spot and 24-hour urine arsenic concentrations. There are not enough data to determine if this relationship holds true in acutely poisoned patients, so a 24-hour collection is still preferred.[32] Challenge testing with dimercaptopropane sulfonate (DMPS) has been performed in individuals exposed to arsenic in drinking water and clearly increases arsenic excretion; however, it also alters the percentages of the arsenic species recovered compared with controls and is not correlated with clinical effects.[11] All urine should be collected in metal-free polyethylene containers; acid-rinsed containers are not recommended since the acid alters the arsenic species.[73] If testing is performed by an outside reference laboratory, specimens from acutely ill patients should be sent via express transportation with a request for a rapid result.

When interpreting slightly elevated urinary arsenic concentrations, laboratory findings must also be correlated with the history and clinical findings, because seafood ingestion is reported to transiently elevate urinary total arsenic excretion up to 1700 mcg/L.[12] When seafood arsenic is a consideration, speciation of arsenic can be accomplished by high-performance liquid chromatography (HPLC) separation, followed by inductively coupled plasma–mass spectrometry (ICPMS), HPLC via ion-pair chromatography coupled with hydride-generation atomic fluorescence spectrometry (HGAFS), or by hydride generation coupled with cold-trap gas chromatography–atomic absorption spectrometry. These techniques separate arsenobetaine, As^{3+}, As^{5+}, MMA, and DMA.[73] Arsenobetaine can also be directly measured by silica-based cation-exchange separation, followed by atomic absorption spectrometry.[174] Two other methods, selective hydride-generation atomic absorption spectrometry (HGAAS) and resin-based ion exchange chromatography, do not directly measure arsenobetaine; instead, they indirectly derive this value by subtracting the sum of all measured arsenic species from the total arsenic concentration.[174] If arsenic speciation cannot be done, the patient should be retested after a one-week abstinence from fish, shellfish, and algae food products.

Conditions under which urine is stored affect total arsenic recovery, as well as proportionality of the species. The various arsenic species—arsenate (As^{5+}), arsenite (As^{3+}), MMA, DMA, and arsenobetaine—remain stable for 2 months in urine stored without preservatives at either −4°F (−20°C; freezer) or 39.2°F (4°C; refrigerator); AsB is stable for 8 months under these conditions. Storage for longer than 2 months can alter the recovery of various species. Addition of 0.1% hydrochloric acid (HCl) facilitates reduction of arsenate to arsenite and also decreases MMA and DMA concentrations. Acid-washed collection containers should not be used if measurement of the various arsenic species is planned. Total arsenic recovery is diminished by any of the following: specimen storage for greater than 2 months, acidification, or testing using HPLC-ICPMS and HPLC-HGAFS, because all these methods usually require that the samples be filtered prior to undergoing HPLC separation.[73]

Diagnostic evaluation of chronic toxicity should include laboratory parameters that typically become abnormal within days to weeks following an acute exposure. Tests should include a complete blood count, kidney and liver function tests, urinalysis, and 24-hour urinary arsenic determinations. Complete blood count findings can include a normocytic, normochromic, or megaloblastic anemia; an initial leukocytosis followed by development of leukopenia, with neutrophils depressed more than lymphocytes, and a relative eosinophilia; thrombocytopenia; and a rapidly declining hemoglobin, indicative of hemolysis or a GI hemorrhage.[136] Basophilic stippling of RBCs occurs, but this is reported in other toxic and clinical disorders. Karyorrhexis, a rupture of the RBC cell nucleus with chromatin disintegration into granules that are extruded from the cell, and dyserythropoiesis are reported in both lead- and arsenic-toxic patients. Both findings are caused by arsenic-induced inhibition of DNA synthesis and damage to the nuclear envelope.[68] The karyorrhexis occurs within 4 days and resolve by 2 weeks after poisoning, and is an early indication of arsenic toxicity.[136] Elevated serum creatinine, aminotransferases, and bilirubin, as well as depressed haptoglobin concentrations, develop. Urinalysis reveals proteinuria, hematuria, and pyuria. Cerebrospinal fluid examination in patients with CNS findings are often normal or exhibit mild protein concentration elevation, measured at 26.5 mg/dL in one case.[105] Urinary arsenic excretion in subacute and chronic cases varies inversely with the postexposure time period, but low concentration excretion for months after exposure is reported. In a study of 41 cases of arsenic-induced peripheral neuropathy, most patients with a neuropathy of 4 to 8 weeks' duration had total 24-hour urinary arsenic measurements of 100 to 400 mcg.[105]

Hair and Nail Testing

In cases of suspected arsenic toxicity, in which the urinary arsenic measurements fall to less than toxic concentrations, analysis of hair and nails may yield the diagnosis. Arsenic is detected in the proximal portions of hair within 30 hours of ingestion.[268] Inorganic arsenic is the form best absorbed by these tissues and the form most commonly found in human poisoning cases; small amounts of methylated metabolites are also be detected.[193] Arsenobetaine is not found in hair and tissues in human and animal studies.[265,266] Hair grows at rates varying from 0.7 to 3.6 cm per month, with a mean rate of 1 cm per month.[254] The Society of Hair Testing has made the following recommendations for collection of hair specimens: (1) collect approximately 200 mg of hair from the posterior vertex region of the scalp using scissors to cut as close to the scalp as possible, and (2) tie the hairs together, wrap in aluminum foil to protect from environmental contamination, and store at room temperature.[254] Although these recommendations are only validated for testing drugs of abuse, it is reasonable to follow them for hair testing of arsenic. Nails grow approximately 0.1 mm per day. Total replacement of a fingernail requires 3 to 4 months, whereas toenails require 6 to 9 months of growth. These facts, plus the frequency of hair cutting, should be evaluated when estimating the usefulness of measuring arsenic concentrations in these tissues. The normal concentration of the testing laboratory should be used to determine whether arsenic concentrations are elevated. In cases of remote toxicity, hair and nail arsenic concentrations are not always elevated, depending on the time elapsed since exposure. Sequential hair analysis to assess the time(s) of exposure can be performed by solid sampling graphite furnace atomic absorption spectrophotometry or by x-ray fluorescence spectrometry.[126,227,228]

Other Tests

Abdominal radiographs demonstrate radiopaque material in the GI tract soon after an ingestion.[2,45,90,91,106] However, even after an acute ingestion, the presence of radiopaque materials on abdominal radiographs may not be recognized.[56] Although it is reasonable to obtain radiographs, the incidence of positive radiographs after an ingestion is unknown, and a negative radiograph should not eliminate arsenic as a diagnostic consideration. Electrocardiographic changes reported include QRS complex widening, QT interval prolongation, ST segment depression, T-wave flattening, ventricular premature contractions, nonsustained monomorphic ventricular tachycardia, and torsade de pointes.[20,176,217,236] Nerve conduction studies (NCS) will confirm or diagnose clinical or subclinical axonopathy. Both the sensory nerve action potential (SNAP) and the motor compound muscle action potential (CMAP) measure the number of axons that are available to conduct impulses. Because the sensory studies are more sensitive than motor studies in detecting axonal degeneration and demyelination, decreased SNAP measurements better indicate subclinical neuropathy. In motor nerve studies, the amplitude (height

of the CMAP) is a more sensitive measure of the number of axons that are able to conduct impulses than is the conduction velocity; this is explained by the pattern of axonal destruction as opposed to myelin injury (which mainly affects conduction velocity). Nerve biopsies demonstrate disintegration of both axons and myelin in patients with arsenic-induced peripheral neuropathy; the axonal loss begins distally in the lower extremities and is initially scattered. Thus, conduction along the remaining functional axons can be sufficient to produce normal or only slightly decreased conduction measurements on NCS.[87,105,127,141,170,175]

MANAGEMENT

General

Acute arsenical toxicity is life threatening and mandates aggressive treatment. Advanced life support monitoring and therapies should be initiated when necessary, but with a few caveats. Careful attention to fluid balance is important because cerebral and pulmonary edema occur. Xenobiotics that prolong the QT interval, such as the class IA, class IC, and class III antidysrhythmics, should be avoided whenever possible (Chaps. 15 and 57). Potassium, magnesium, and calcium concentrations should be maintained within normal range to avoid exacerbating a prolonged QT interval. Glucose concentrations and glycogen stores should be maintained parenterally with dextrose and hyperalimentation solutions or with enteral feedings, in view of their beneficial effects in experimental models of arsenic poisoning.[147,199,200,223]

Gastrointestinal decontamination of patients acutely poisoned with arsenic is controversial. Arsenic is poorly adsorbed to activated charcoal, cholestyramine, and bentonite.[197] Moreover, significantly poisoned patients usually have nausea and vomiting and altered mental status, which make activated charcoal administration difficult. Despite these concerns, activated charcoal, in conjunction with airway protection if necessary, is recommended because of the relatively low likelihood of harming the patient and the hope that preventing even a small amount of absorption might prevent or lessen the potentially disastrous consequences of arsenic poisoning. If radiopaque material is visualized in the GI tract, whole-bowel irrigation is reasonable until the radiopaque material is no longer visualized on repeat abdominal radiograph. Continuing nasogastric suction removes arsenic resecreted in the gastric or biliary tract and is reasonable. Arsenite was still detectable in the gastric aspirate in 3 patients 5 to 7 days following an ingestion.[152] There is no clinical experience with the use of N-acetylcysteine to increase glutathione concentrations. Although an animal model suggested a protective effect, there are not enough data to recommend N-acetylcysteine for arsenic poisoning and treatment.[196]

In cases of chronic toxicity, patients should be removed from the arsenic source. It is reasonable to perform GI decontamination if there is evidence of arsenic in the GI tract. Arsenic can be readily removed from skin with soap, water, and vigorous scrubbing. In this situation, when homicidal intent is suspected, all hospital visitors should be closely monitored, and outside nutritional products should be forbidden.

Chelation Therapy

Chelators

Dimercaprol (BAL) and 2,3-dimercaptosuccinic acid (succimer) are the 2 chelators available to treat arsenic poisoning in the United States. A third drug, DMPS, is distributed by Heyl, a German pharmaceutical company, as Dimaval, but it is not approved or marketed in the United States (Antidotes in Depth: A28 and A29). All contain vicinal dithiol moieties that bind arsenic to form stable 1,2,5-arsadithiolanes (Fig. 86–7), and all are most effective when administered in doses equimolar to the arsenic burden.[169] Dosing regimens and adverse effects are listed in Table 86–3.

The decision to initiate chelation therapy should depend on the clinical condition of the patient as well as the laboratory results for arsenic in urine, hair, or nails. A severely ill patient with known or suspected acute arsenic poisoning should be chelated immediately, prior to laboratory confirmation. In the United States, dimercaprol remains the initial chelator for acute arsenical toxicity.[169] In a series of 33 patients who had coma, seizures, or both,

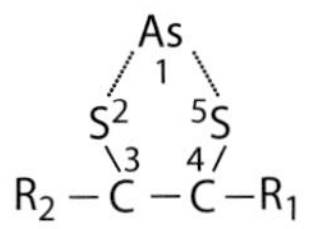

As
/1\
S² 5S
\3 4/
R₂ — C — C — R₁

Dimercaprol adduct
$R_1 = H, R_2 = CH_2OH$

DMPS adduct
$R_1 = H, R_2 = CH_2SO_2Na$

Succimer adduct
$R_1 = R_2 = COOH$

FIGURE 86–7. 1,2,5-Arsadithiolane adducts with dimercaprol (BAL), dimercaptopropane sulfonate (DMPS), and dimercaptosuccinic acid (DMSA).

24 patients were treated with dimercaprol within 6 hours (mean, 1 hour) and 75% survived, compared with a survival rate of 45% of 9 patients who were treated later (range, 9–72 hours; mean, 30 hours).[66] In cases of subacute and chronic toxicity, it is reasonable to await laboratory confirmation prior to beginning chelation, unless the clinical condition deteriorates.

In a cellular study of glucose uptake impaired by a lipophilic arsenical, dimercaprol was superior to succimer and DMPS in restoring cellular equilibrium.[169] A human case series found increased survival with early use of dimercaprol and improvement in encephalopathy within 24 hours of initiating therapy.[66] However, other acute cases treated promptly with dimercaprol developed peripheral neuropathy.[141] In a study of subacute cases with peripheral neuropathy, dimercaprol accelerated neurologic recovery but did not affect the overall recovery rate.[53] Despite starting dimercaprol therapy 8 hours postexposure, a man who had ingested 2.15 g of arsenic developed severe toxicity and neurologic deficits.[75] Most concerning are the animal experiments indicating that dimercaprol shifts arsenic into the brain and testes, 2 organs that have blood–organ barriers susceptible to this lipophilic drug.[10,109,129] It is clear that dimercaprol has limitations, and that a safer, more effective intracellular/extracellular parenteral chelator is needed.

Succimer is an oral hydrophilic analog of dimercaprol and is the chelator of choice for subacute and chronic toxicity. It has proven effective in animal studies and in reported human cases.[10,128,143,151,215] In mice exposed to sodium arsenite, succimer was more effective than either DMPS or dimercaprol in decreasing lethality and more potent than dimercaprol in restoring activity

in the pyruvate dehydrogenase complex.[10] It is equal or superior to dimercaprol in speeding arsenic elimination.[157] Liver function tests and essential metal concentrations should be monitored in patients requiring prolonged therapy.[78,92]

2,3-Dimercapto-1-propanesulfonic acid (DMPS) is also a water-soluble analog of dimercaprol. It is not approved for use in the United States. It is administered by the oral, intravenous, or intramuscular route. It is eliminated from the body more slowly than succimer and has the advantage of intracellular as well as extracellular distribution.[7] It predominantly binds MMA^{3+} and possibly removes the MMA^{3+} from endogenous ligands. The $DMPS–MMA^{3+}$ complex is eliminated in the urine.[9,11,84] It also works by synergistically increasing the nonenzymatic methylation of As^{3+}.[270] Two brothers ingested nearly pure arsenic trioxide (1 and 4 g each) and were treated with intravenous and oral DMPS. The brother who ingested 4 g developed hypotension, AKI, respiratory insufficiency, and asystolic cardiac arrest. 2,3-Dimercapto-1-propanesulfonic acid was started 32 hours postingestion, and the patient survived with normal kidney function and no neurologic dysfunction. His sibling had a milder course; DMPS was started 48 hours postingestion, and there were no neurologic sequelae on follow-up examination.[167] 2,3-Dimercapto-1-propanesulfonic acid significantly increased biliary excretion of arsenic in a guinea pig model but did not increase fecal excretion. The latter is most likely a result of enterohepatic recirculation of the DMPS–As complex.[197] However, in another guinea pig model, the addition of oral cholestyramine to either DMPS or DMSA but not to dimercaprol increased fecal arsenic excretion.[169]

D-Penicillamine has not demonstrated efficacy in chelating or reversing the biochemical lesions of arsenic and should not be used. Its previous advantage of oral administration is no longer relevant with the availability of succimer.

Because of the limitations of currently available chelators, research is ongoing to find better chelators to treat arsenic toxicity. For example, some analogs of succimer, especially its monoisoamyl ester, have increased intracellular penetration relative to the parent compound and increase survival in arsenic-poisoned rats.[77,120] In addition to improved chelators, other treatments for arsenic toxicity are being investigated. Some rodent studies suggest that certain micronutrients, such as zinc or selenium, decrease arsenic toxicity.[77] However, early findings from the HEALS cohort are mixed. A cross-sectional substudy from this group revealed an inverse relationship between the severity of skin lesions and dietary intake of folate, pyridoxine, riboflavin, and vitamins A, C, and E.[269] By contrast, another study from the same cohort did not find a statistically significant relationship between the severity of skin lesions and supplementation with vitamin E, selenium, or both.[245] Until more data are available, nutritional supplementation, in the absence of dietary deficiency, remains controversial.

Hemodialysis

Hemodialysis removes negligible amounts of arsenic, with or without concomitant dimercaprol therapy, and is not indicated in patients with normal kidney function.[23,101,156] In patients with AKI, hemodialysis clearance rates have ranged from 76 to 87.5 mL/min, with or without concomitant dimercaprol therapy.[244] In 2 acutely toxic patients with AKI, total arsenic removed during a 4-hour dialysis measured 4.68 mg in one and 3.36 mg in the other. Concomitant 24-hour urinary arsenic excretions were 3.12 mg and 2.03 mg, respectively. When kidney function returned, however, the 24-hour urinary excretion of arsenic far exceeded that recovered with dialysis, with reported amounts of 18.99 mg in the first patient and 75 mg in the second patient.[244] There are no published rigorous data regarding hemodialysis removal of a water-soluble complex such as DMPS–As.[131]

SUMMARY

- Environmental contamination of water sources is the major source of arsenic in many countries, including the United States.
- Arsenicals produce multisystem toxicity by a variety of pathophysiologic mechanisms.

TABLE 86–3	**Chelators for Arsenic Poisoning**
Dosage	**Adverse Effects**
Dimercaprol 3–5 mg/kg IM every 4–6 hours	Hypertension, febrile reaction, diaphoresis, nausea, vomiting, salivation, lacrimation, rhinorrhea, throat or chest pain, headache, painful injection, injection site sterile abscess, hemolysis in G6PD-deficient patients, chelation of essential metals (prolonged course)
Succimer 10 mg/kg/dose orally every 8 hours for 5 days, then 10 mg/kg/dose every 12 hours	Nausea, vomiting, diarrhea, abdominal gas and pain, transient elevations of hepatic aminotransferases and alkaline phosphatase concentrations, rash, pruritus, sore throat, rhinorrhea, drowsiness, paresthesias, thrombocytosis, eosinophilia
DMPS (not FDA approved) Dose: 5 mg/kg/dose IM, administered as a 5% solution Day 1: every 6–8 hours Day 2: every 8–12 hours Day 3 and thereafter: every 12–24 hours Regardless of the chelator used, the end point of chelation is a 24-hour urinary arsenic concentration of <50 mcg/L	Allergic reactions, increased copper and zinc excretion, nausea, pruritus, vertigo, weakness, toxic epidermal necrolysis

G6PD = glucose-6-phosphate dehydrogenase; IM = intramuscularly. DMPS = 2,3-dimercapto-1-propanesulfonic acid

- A thorough understanding of inorganic arsenic metabolism and excretion as well as the different clinical manifestations of acute, subacute, and chronic toxicity are necessary to avoid misdiagnosis.
- Chelation therapy with dimercaprol in the United States, or with DMPS elsewhere, if available, should be started immediately in the severely ill patient.
- For patients with subacute or chronic toxicity, it is reasonable to await laboratory results unless clinical deterioration occurs.

Acknowledgment

Marsha D. Ford, MD, contributed to this chapter in previous editions.

REFERENCES

1. Abernathy CO, Ohanian EV. Non-carcinogenic effects of inorganic arsenic. *Environ Geochem Health.* 1992;14:35-41.
2. Adelson L, et al. Acute arsenic intoxication shown by roentgenograms. *Arch Intern Med.* 1961;107:401-404.
3. Ahsan H, et al. Arsenic metabolism, genetic susceptibility and risk of premalignant skin lesions in Bangladesh. *Cancer Epidemiol Biomarkers Prev.* 2007;16:1270-1278.
4. Ahsan H, et al. Arsenic exposure from drinking water and risk of premalignant skin lesions in Bangladesh: baseline results from the Health Effects of Arsenic Longitudinal Study. *Am J Epidemiol.* 2006;163:1138-1148.
5. Ahsan H, et al. Health Effects of Arsenic Longitudinal Study (HEALS): description of a multidisciplinary epidemiologic investigation. *J Exp Sci Environ Epidemiol.* 2006;16:191-205.
6. Albores A, et al. Sodium arsenite induced alterations in bilirubin excretion and heme metabolism. *J Biochem Toxicol.* 1989;4:73-78.
7. Aposhian HV. Mobilization of mercury and arsenic in humans by sodium 2,3-dimercapto-1-propane sulfonate (DMPS). *Environ Health Perspect.* 1998;106(suppl 4):1017-1025.
8. Aposhian HV, Aposhian MM. Newer developments in arsenic toxicity. *J Am Coll Toxicol.* 1989;8:1297-1305.
9. Aposhian HV, et al. DMPS-arsenic challenge test. I: increased urinary excretion of monomethylarsonic acid in humans given dimercaptopropane sulfonate. *J Pharmacol Exp Ther.* 1997;282:192-200.
10. Aposhian HV, et al. DMSA, DMPS, and DMPA-As arsenic antidotes. *Fundam Appl Toxicol.* 1984;4:S58-S70.
11. Aposhian HV, et al. DMPS-arsenic challenge test. II. Modulation of arsenic species, including monomethylarsonous acid (MMA^{III}), excreted in human urine. *Toxicol Appl Pharmacol.* 2000;165:74-83.
12. Arbouine MW, Wilson HK. The effect of seafood consumption on the assessment of occupational exposure to arsenic by urinary arsenic speciation measurements. *J Trace Elem.* 1992;6:153-160.
13. Argos M, et al. A prospective study of arsenic exposure from drinking water and incidence of skin lesions in Bangladesh. *Am J Epidemiol.* 2011;174:85-194.
14. Argos M, et al. Arsenic exposure from drinking water, and all-cause and chronic-disease mortalities in Bangladesh (HEALS): a prospective cohort study. *Lancet.* 2010;376:252-258.
15. Argos M, et al. Dietary B vitamin intakes and urinary total arsenic concentration in the Health Effects of Arsenic Longitudinal Study (HEALS) cohort, Bangladesh. *Eur J Nutr.* 2010;49:473-481.
16. Armstrong CW, et al. Outbreak of fatal arsenic poisoning caused by contaminated drinking water. *Arch Environ Health.* 1984;39:276-279.
17. Banerjee M, et al. DNA repair deficiency leads to susceptibility to develop arsenic-induced premalignant skin lesions. *Int J Cancer.* 2008;123:283-287.
18. Bansal SK, et al. Phrenic neuropathy in arsenic poisoning. *Chest.* 1991;100:878-880.
19. Banville B, Kesseli D. State closes New Sweden arsenic case. *Bangor Daily News*, Bangor, ME; April 19, 2006.
20. Barbey JT, et al. Effect of arsenic trioxide on QT interval in patients with advanced malignancies. *J Clin Oncol.* 2003;21:3609-3615.
21. Beckett WS, et al. Acute encephalopathy due to occupational exposure to arsenic. *Br J Ind Med.* 1986;43:66-67.
22. Beckman KJ, et al. Arsenic-induced torsades de pointes. *Crit Care Med.* 1991;19:290-291.
23. Blythe D, Joyce DA. Clearance of arsenic by haemodialysis after acute poisoning with arsenic trioxide. *Intensive Care Med.* 2001;27:334.
24. Bolliger CT, et al. Multiple organ failure with the adult respiratory distress syndrome in homicidal arsenic poisoning. *Respiration.* 1992;59:57-61.
25. Boquist L, et al. Structural beta-cell changes and transient hyperglycemia in mice treated with compounds inducing inhibited citric acid cycle enzyme activity. *Diabetes.* 1988;37:89-98.
26. Bouletreau P, et al. Acute renal complications of acute intoxications. *Acta Pharmacol Toxicol.* 1977;41(suppl):49-63.
27. Bouteille B, et al. Treatment perspectives for human African trypanosomiasis. *Fundam Clin Pharmacol.* 2003;17:171-181.
28. Brune D, et al. Distribution of 23 elements in the kidney, liver and lungs of workers from a smeltery and refinery in North Sweden exposed to a number of elements and of a control group. *Sci Total Environ.* 1980;16:13-35.
29. Buchet JP, et al. Comparison of the urinary excretion of arsenic metabolites after a single oral dose of sodium arsenite, monomethylarsonate or dimethylarsinate in man. *Int Arch Occup Environ Health.* 1981;48:71-79.
30. Bustamante J, et al. The semiconductor elements arsenic and indium induce apoptosis in rat thymocytes. *Toxicology.* 1997;118:129-136.
31. Calderon J, et al. Exposure to arsenic and lead and neuropsychological development in Mexican children. *Environ Res.* 2001;85:69-76.
32. Calderon RL, et al. Excretion of arsenic in urine as a function of exposure to arsenic in drinking water. *Environ Health Perspect.* 1999;107:663-667.
33. Chang CC, et al. Ischemic heart disease mortality reduction in an arseniasis-endemic area in southwestern Taiwan after a switch in the tap-water supply system. *J Toxicol Environ Health A.* 2004;67:1353-1361.
34. Chen B, et al. In vivo ^{31}P nuclear magnetic resonance studies of arsenite induced changes in hepatic phosphate levels. *Biochem Biophys Res Commun.* 1986;139:228-234.
35. Chen C-J, et al. Malignant neoplasms among residents of a blackfoot disease-endemic area in Taiwan: high-arsenic artesian well water and cancers. *Cancer Res.* 1985;45:5895-5899.
36. Chen GQ, et al. In vitro studies on cellular and molecular mechanisms of arsenic trioxide (As_2O_3) in the treatment of acute promyelocytic leukemia: As_2O_3 induces NB4 cell apoptosis with downregulation of Bcl-2 expression and modulation of PMLRAR alpha/PML proteins. *Blood.* 1996;88:1052-1061.
37. Chen GS, et al. A possible pathogenesis for blackfoot disease: effects of trivalent arsenic (As_2O_3) on cultured human umbilical vein endothelial cells. *J Dermatol.* 1990;17:599-608.
38. Chen SJ, et al. From an old remedy to a magic bullet: molecular mechanisms underlying the therapeutic effects of arsenic in fighting leukemia. *Blood.* 2011;117:6425-6437.
39. Chen Y, et al. No association between arsenic exposure from drinking water and diabetes mellitus: a cross-sectional study in Bangladesh. *Environ Health Perspect.* 2010;118:1299-1305.
40. Chen Y, et al. Arsenic exposure from drinking water and mortality from cardiovascular disease in Bangladesh: prospective cohort study. *BMJ.* 2011;342:2431.
41. Chen Y, et al. Modification of risk of arsenic-induced skin lesions by sunlight exposure, smoking and occupational exposures in Bangladesh. *Epidemiology.* 2006;17:459-467.
42. Chen Y, et al. Arsenic exposure at low-to-moderate levels and skin lesions, arsenic metabolism neurological functions, and biomarkers for respiratory and cardiovascular diseases: review of recent findings from the Health Effects of Arsenic Longitudinal Study (HEALS) in Bangladesh. *Toxicol Appl Pharmacol.* 2009;239:184-192.
43. Chen Y, et al. Association between arsenic exposure from drinking water and proteinuria: results from Health Effects of Arsenic Longitudinal Study (HEALS) in Bangladesh. *Intl J Epidemiol.* 2011;40:828-835.
44. Chen Y, et al. Arsenic exposure from drinking water, arsenic methylation capacity and carotid intima-media thickness in Bangladesh. *Am J Epidemiol.* 2013;178:372-381.
45. Chen Y, et al. A prospective study of arsenic exposure, arsenic methylation capacity and risk of cardiovascular disease in Bangladesh. *Environ Health Perspect.* 2013;121:832-838.
46. Chen Y, et al. Arsenic exposure from drinking water and QT-interval prolongation: results from the health effects of arsenic longitudinal study. *Environ Health Perspect.* 2013;121:427-432.
47. Chen Z, et al. Treatment of acute promyelocytic leukemia with arsenic compounds: in vitro and in vivo studies. *Semin Hematol.* 2001;38:26-36.
48. Chernoff AI, Hartroft WS. Acute gastroenteritis. *Am J Med.* 1956;21:282-291.
49. Chiou HY, et al. Incidence of transitional cell carcinoma and arsenic in drinking water: a follow-up study of 8,102 residents in an arseniasis-endemic area in northeastern Taiwan. *Am J Epidemiol.* 2001;153:411-418.
50. Chiou HY, et al. Dose–response relationship between prevalence of cerebrovascular disease and ingested inorganic arsenic. *Stroke.* 1997;28:1717-1723.
51. Chiu HF, et al. Does arsenic exposure increase the risk for liver cancer? *J Toxicol Environ Health A.* 2004;67:1491-1500.
52. Chu HA, Crawford-Brown DJ. Inorganic arsenic in drinking water and bladder cancer: a meta-analysis for dose-response assessment. *Int J Environ Res Public Health.* 2006;3:316-322.
53. Chuttani PN, et al. Arsenical neuropathy. *Neurology.* 1967;17:269-274.
54. Concha G, et al. Metabolism of inorganic arsenic in children with chronic high arsenic exposure in northern Argentina. *Environ Health Perspect.* 1998;106:355-359.
55. Concha G, et al. Low-level arsenic excretion in breast milk of native Andean women exposed to high levels of arsenic in the drinking water. *Int Arch Occup Environ Health.* 1998;71:42-46.
56. Cullen NM, et al. Pediatric arsenic ingestion. *Am J Emerg Med.* 1995;13:432-435.
57. Dakeishi M, et al. Long-term consequences of arsenic poisoning during infancy due to contaminated milk powder. *Environ Health.* 2006;5:31.
58. Das D, et al. Chronic low-level arsenic exposure reduces lung function in male population without skin lesions. *Int J Public Health.* 2014;59:655-663.
59. De Kimpe J, et al. More than tenfold increase of arsenic in serum and packed cells of chronic hemodialysis patients. *Am J Nephrol.* 1993;13:429-434.
60. DeChaudhuri S, et al. Arsenic-induced health effects and genetic damage in keratotic individuals: involvement of p53 arginine variant and chromosomal aberrations in arsenic susceptibility. *Mutat Res.* 2008;659:118-125.
61. Del Razo LM, et al. The oxidation states of arsenic in well-water from a chronic arsenicism area of northern Mexico. *Environ Pollut.* 1990;64:143-153.
62. Delnomdedieu M, et al. Reduction and binding of arsenate and dimethylarsinate by glutathione: a magnetic resonance study. *Chem Biol Interact.* 1994;90:139-155.

63. DeSesso JM, et al. An assessment of the developmental toxicity of inorganic arsenic. *Reprod Toxicol.* 1998;12:385-433.

64. Drolet B, et al. Unusual effects of a QT-prolonging drug, arsenic trioxide, on cardiac potassium currents. *Circulation.* 2004;109:26-29.

65. Du Pont O, et al. The distribution of radioactive arsenic in the normal and tumor-bearing (Brown-Pearce) rabbit. *Am J Syph Gonorrhea Vener Dis.* 1941;26:96-118.

66. Eagle H, Magnuson HJ. The systemic treatment of 227 cases of arsenic poisoning (encephalitis, dermatitis, blood dyscrasias, jaundice, fever) with 2,3-dimercaptopropanol (BAL). *J Clin Invest.* 1946;25:420-441.

67. Edmonds JS, et al. Arsenic transformations in short marine food chains studied by HPLC-ICP MS. *Appl Organometal Chem.* 1997;11:281-287.

68. Eichner ER. Erythroid karyorrhexis in the peripheral blood smear in severe arsenic poisoning: a comparison with lead poisoning. *Am J Clin Pathol.* 1984;81:533-537.

69. Emadi A, Gore SD. Arsenic trioxide—an old drug rediscovered. *Blood Rev.* 2010;24:191-199.

70. Environmental Protection Agency. National primary drinking water regulations; arsenic and clarifications to compliance and new source contaminants monitoring. Proposed rules. 40 CFR Parts 141 and 142. *Fed Reg.* 2000;65:63027-63035.

71. Fangstrom B, et al. Breast-feeding protects against arsenic exposure in Bangladeshi infants. *Environ Health Perspect.* 2008;116:963-969.

72. Farzan S, et al. Gene-arsenic interaction in longitudinal changes of blood pressure: findings from the Health Effects of Arsenic Longitudinal Study (HEALS) in Bangladesh. *Toxicol Appl Pharmacol.* 2015;288:95-105.

73. Feldmann J, et al. Sample preparation and storage can change arsenic speciation in human urine. *Clin Chem.* 1999;45:1988-1997.

74. Fernandez-Sola J, et al. Acute arsenical myopathy: morphological description. *J Toxicol Clin Toxicol.* 1991;29:131-136.

75. Fesmire FM, et al. Survival following massive arsenic ingestion. *Am J Emerg Med.* 1988;6:602-606.

76. Fincher R-ME, Koerker RM. Long-term survival in acute arsenic encephalopathy: follow-up using newer measures of electrophysiologic parameters. *Am J Med.* 1987;82:549-552.

77. Flora SJS, et al. Arsenic and lead induced free radical generation and their reversibility following chelation. *Cell Mol Biol (Noisy-le-grand).* 2007;53:26-47.

78. Fournier L, et al. 2,3-Dimercaptosuccinic-acid treatment of heavy metal poisoning in humans. *Med Toxicol.* 1988;3:499-504.

79. Freeman JW, Crouch JR. Prolonged encephalopathy with arsenic poisoning. *Neurology.* 1978;28:853-855.

80. Gamble MV, et al. Folate and arsenic metabolism: a double-blind, placebo-controlled folic acid-supplementation trial in Bangladesh. *Am J Clin Nutr.* 2006;84:1093-1101.

81. Gamble MV, et al. Folate, homocysteine and arsenic metabolism in arsenic-exposed individuals in Bangladesh. *Environ Health Perspect.* 2005;113:1683-1688.

82. Gamble MV, et al. Folic acid supplementation lowers blood arsenic. *Am J Clin Nutr.* 2007;86:1202-1209.

83. Garb LG, Hine CH. Arsenical neuropathy: residual effects following acute industrial exposure. *J Occup Med.* 1977;19:567-568.

84. Gartenhaus RB, et al. Arsenic trioxide cytotoxicity in steroid and chemotherapy-resistant myeloma cell lines: enhancement of apoptosis by manipulation of cellular redox state. *Clin Cancer Res.* 2002;8:566-572.

85. Gerhardt RE, et al. Chronic renal insufficiency from cortical necrosis induced by arsenic poisoning. *Arch Intern Med.* 1978;138:1267-1269.

86. Germolec DR, et al. Arsenic enhancement of skin neoplasia by chronic stimulation of growth factors. *Am J Pathol.* 1998;153:1775-1785.

87. Goebel HH, et al. Polyneuropathy due to acute arsenic intoxication: biopsy studies. *J Neuropathol Exp Neurol.* 1990;49:137-149.

88. Goldsmith S, From AHL. Arsenic-induced atypical ventricular tachycardia. *N Engl J Med.* 1980;303:1096-1098.

89. Gong Z, et al. Determination of arsenic metabolic complex excreted in human urine after administration of sodium 2,3-dimercapto-1-propane sulfonate. *Chem Res Toxicol.* 2002;15:1318-1323.

90. Gousios AG, Adelson L. Electrocardiographic and radiographic findings in acute arsenic poisoning. *Am J Med.* 1959;27:659-663.

91. Gray JR, et al. Acute arsenic toxicity—an opaque poison. *Can Assoc Radiol J.* 1989;40:226-227.

92. Graziano JH, et al. The pharmacology of 2,3-dimercaptosuccinic acid and its potential use in arsenic poisoning. *J Pharmacol Exp Ther.* 1978;207:1051-1055.

93. Greenberg C, et al. Acute respiratory failure following severe arsenic poisoning. *Chest.* 1979;76:596-598.

94. Griffin JP. Famous names: the Esing Bakery, Hong Kong. *Adverse Drug React Toxicol Rev.* 1997;16:79-81.

95. Guha Mazumder DN. Arsenic and non-malignant lung disease. *J Environ Sci Health A Tox Hazard Subst Environ Eng.* 2007;42:1859-1867.

96. Hafeman DM, et al. Association between arsenic exposure and a measure of subclinical sensory neuropathy in Bangladesh. *J Occup Environ Med.* 2005;47:778-784.

97. Halicka HD, et al. Arsenic trioxide arrests cells early in mitosis leading to apoptosis. *Cell Cycle.* 2002;1:201-209.

98. Hall MN, et al. Influence on cobalamin on arsenic metabolism in Bangladesh. *Environ Health Perspect.* 2009;117:1724-1729.

99. Hamadani JD, et al. Pre- and postnatal arsenic exposure and child development at 18 months of age: a cohort study in rural Bangladesh. *Int J Epidemiol.* 2010;39:1206-1216.

100. Hamadani JD, et al. Critical windows of exposure for arsenic-associated impairment of cognitive function in pre-school girls and boys: a population-based cohort study. *Int J Epidemiol.* 2011;40:1593-1604.

101. Hantson P, et al. Acute arsenic poisoning treated by intravenous dimercaptosuccinic acid (DMSA) and combined extrarenal epuration techniques. *J Toxicol Clin Toxicol.* 2003;41:1-6.

102. Heck JE, et al. Consumption of folate-related nutrients and metabolism of arsenic in Bangladesh. *Am J Clin Nutr.* 2007;85:1367-1374.

103. Heck JE, et al. Dietary intake of methionine, cysteine and protein and urinary arsenic excretion in Bangladesh. *Environ Health Perspect.* 2009;117:99-104.

104. Hessl SM, Berman E. Severe peripheral neuropathy after exposure to monosodium methylarsonate. *J Toxicol Clin Toxicol.* 1982;19:281-287.

105. Heyman A, et al. Peripheral neuropathy caused by arsenical intoxication: a study of 41 cases with observations on the effects of BAL (2,3-dimercaptopropanol). *N Engl J Med.* 1956;254:401-409.

106. Hilfer RJ, Mandel A. Acute arsenic intoxication diagnosed by roentgenograms. *N Engl J Med.* 1962;266:663-664.

107. Hindmarsh JT, et al. Electromyographic abnormalities in chronic environmental arsenicalism. *J Anal Toxicol.* 1977;1:270-276.

108. Hirata M, et al. Effects of glutathione depletion on the acute nephrotoxic potential of arsenite and on arsenic metabolism in hamsters. *Toxicol Appl Pharmacol.* 1990;106:469-481.

109. Hoover TD, Aposhian HV. BAL increases the arsenic-74 content of rabbit brain. *Toxicol Appl Pharmacol.* 1983;70:160-162.

110. Hsu LI, et al. Use of arsenic-induced palmoplantar hyperkeratosis and skin cancers to predict risk of subsequent internal malignancy. *Am J Epidemiol.* 2013;177:202-212.

111. Hsueh YM, et al. Serum beta-carotene level, arsenic methylation capability, and incidence of skin cancer. *Cancer Epidemiol Biomarkers Prev.* 1997;6:589-596.

112. Huang R-N, Lee T-C. Cellular uptake of trivalent arsenite and pentavalent arsenate in KB cells cultured in phosphate-free medium. *Toxicol Appl Pharmacol.* 1996;136:243-249.

113. Huang Y, et al. Induction of cytoplasmic accumulation of p53: a mechanism for low levels of arsenic exposure to predispose cells for malignant transformation. *Cancer Res.* 2008;68:9131-9136.

114. Hunt E, et al. Arsenic poisoning seen at Duke Hospital, 1965–1998. *N C Med J.* 1999;60:70-74.

115. Hutton JT, et al. Arsenic poisoning. *N Engl J Med.* 1982;307:1080.

116. Jiang J, et al. Association between arsenic exposure from drinking water and longitudinal change in blood pressure among HEALS cohort participants. *Environ Health Perspect.* 2015;123:806-812.

117. Jing Y, et al. Arsenic trioxide selectively induces acute promyelocytic leukemia cell apoptosis via a hydrogen peroxide-dependent pathway. *Blood.* 1999;94:2102-2111.

118. Johnson LR, Farmer JG. Use of human metabolic studies and urinary arsenic speciation in assessing arsenic exposure. *Bull Environ Contam Toxicol.* 1991;46:53-61.

119. Jolliffe DM, et al. Massive acute arsenic poisoning. *Anaesthesia.* 1991;46:288-290.

120. Kalia K, Flora SJS. Strategies for safe and effective therapeutic measures for chronic arsenic and lead poisoning. *J Occup Health.* 2005;47:1-21.

121. Kasper ML, et al. Hepatic angiosarcoma and bronchioloalveolar carcinoma induced by Fowler's solution. *JAMA.* 1984;252:3407-3408.

122. Kenyon EM, Hughes MF. A concise review of the toxicity and carcinogenicity of dimethylarsinic acid. *Toxicology.* 2001;160:227-236.

123. Kersjes MP, et al. An analysis of arsenic exposures referred to the Blodgett regional poison center. *Vet Hum Toxicol.* 1987;29:75-78.

124. Khan K, et al. Manganese exposure from drinking water and children's academic achievement. *Neurotoxicology.* 2012;33:91-97.

125. Kippler M, et al. Elevated childhood exposure to arsenic despite reduced drinking water concentrations—a longitudinal cohort study in rural Bangladesh. *Environ Intl.* 2016;86:119-125.

126. Koons RD, Peters CA. Axial distribution of arsenic in individual human hairs by solid sampling graphite furnace AAS. *J Anal Toxicol.* 1994;18:36-40.

127. Kreiss K, et al. Neurologic evaluation of a population exposed to arsenic in Alaskan well water. *Arch Environ Health.* 1983;38:116-121.

128. Kreppel H, et al. Antidotal efficacy of newly synthesized dimercaptosuccinic acid (DMSA) monoesters in experimental arsenic poisoning in mice. *Fund Appl Toxicol.* 1995;26:239-245.

129. Kreppel H, et al. Efficacy of various dithiol compounds in acute As$_2$O$_3$ poisoning in mice. *Arch Toxicol.* 1990;64:387-392.

130. Kritharis A, et al. The evolving use of arsenic in pharmacotherapy of malignant disease. *Ann Hematol.* 2013;92:1-11.

131. Kruszewska S, et al. The use of haemodialysis and 2,3-propanesulphonate (DMPS) to manage acute oral poisoning by lethal dose of arsenic trioxide. *Int J Occup Med Environ Health.* 1996;9:111-115.

132. Kumana CR, et al. Systemic availability of arsenic from oral arsenic-trioxide used to treat patients with hematological malignancies. *Eur J Clin Pharmacol.* 2002;58:521-526.

133. Kuo CC, et al. Arsenic exposure, arsenic metabolism, and incident diabetes in the strong heart study. *Diabetes Care.* 2015;38:620-627.

134. Kwok RK, et al. Arsenic in drinking water and reproductive health outcomes: a study of participants in the Bangladesh Integrated Nutrition Programme. *J Health Popul Nutr.* 2006;24:190-205.

135. Kwong YL. Arsenic trioxide in the treatment of haematological malignancies. *Expert Opin Drug Saf.* 2004;3:589-597.

136. Kyle RA, Pease GL. Hematologic aspects of arsenic intoxication. *N Engl J Med.* 1965;271:18-23.

137. Lagerkvist BE, et al. Arsenic and Raynaud's phenomenon. Vasospastic tendency and excretion of arsenic in smelter workers before and after the summer vacation. *Int Arch Occup Environ Health.* 1988;60:361-364.

138. Lai MS, et al. Ingested inorganic arsenic and prevalence of diabetes mellitus. *Am J Epidemiol.* 1994;139:484-492.

139. Lander JJ, et al. Angiosarcoma of the liver associated with Fowler's solution (potassium arsenite). *Gastroenterology.* 1975;68:1582-1586.

140. Le XC, et al. Human urinary arsenic excretion after one-time ingestion of seaweed, crab, and shrimp. *Clin Chem.* 1994;40:617-624.

141. Le Quesne PM, McLeod J. Peripheral neuropathy following a single exposure to arsenic: clinical course in four patients with electrophysiological and histological studies. *J Neurol Sci.* 1977;32:437-451.

142. Lee MY, et al. Enhancement of platelet aggregation and thrombus formation by arsenic in drinking water: a contributing factor to cardiovascular disease. *Toxicol Appl Pharmacol.* 2002;179:83-88.

143. Lenz K, et al. 2,3-Dimercaptosuccinic acid in human arsenic poisoning. *Arch Toxicol.* 1981;47:241-243.

144. Lerman BB, et al. Megaloblastic, dyserythropoietic anemia following arsenic ingestion. *Ann Clin Lab Sci.* 1980;10:515-517.

145. Li L, et al. Nutritional status has marginal influence on the metabolism of inorganic arsenic in pregnant Bangladeshi women. *Environ Health Perspect.* 2008;116:315-321.

146. Li Y, et al. Serum levels of the extracellular domain of the epidermal growth factor receptor in individuals exposed to arsenic in drinking water in Bangladesh. *Biomarkers.* 2007;12:256-265.

147. Liebl B, et al. Influence of glucose on the toxicity of oxophenylarsine in MDCK cells. *Arch Toxicol.* 1995;69:421-424.

148. Lu DP, Wang Q. Current study of APL treatment in China. *Int J Hematol.* 2005;202(suppl 1): 316-318.

149. Lugo G, et al. Acute maternal arsenic intoxication with neonatal death. *Am J Dis Child.* 1969;117:328-330.

150. Mackell MA, et al. An unsuspected arsenic poisoning murder disclosed by forensic autopsy. *Am J Forensic Med Pathol.* 1985;6:358-361.

151. Maehashi H, Murata Y. Arsenic excretion after treatment of arsenic poisoning with DMSA or DMPS in mice. *Jpn J Pharmacol.* 1986;40:188-190.

152. Mahieu P, et al. The metabolism of arsenic in humans acutely intoxicated by As_2O_3: its significance for the duration of BAL therapy. *Clin Toxicol.* 1981;18:1067-1075.

153. Mass MJ, et al. Methylated trivalent arsenic species are genotoxic. *Chem Res Toxicol.* 2001;14:355-361.

154. Massey EW, et al. Arsenic: homicidal intoxication. *South Med J.* 1984;77:848-851.

155. Mathews V, et al. Arsenic trioxide in the treatment of newly diagnosed acute promyelocytic leukemia: a single center experience. *Am J Hematol.* 2002;70:292-299.

156. Mathieu D, et al. Massive arsenic poisoning—effect of hemodialysis and dimercaprol on arsenic kinetics. *Intensive Care Med.* 1992;18:47-50.

157. Mazumder DN, et al. Chronic arsenic toxicity in west Bengal—the worst calamity in the world. *J Indian Med Assoc.* 1998;96:4-7, 18.

158. McKinney JD. Metabolism and disposition of inorganic arsenic in laboratory animals and humans. *Environ Geochem Health.* 1992;14:43-48.

159. Mealey J, et al. Radioarsenic in plasma, urine, normal tissues, and intracranial neoplasms. *Arch Neurol Psychiatry.* 1959;8:310-320.

160. Meliker JR, et al. Lifetime exposure to arsenic in drinking water and bladder cancer: a population-based case-control study in Michigan, USA. *Cancer Causes Control.* 2010;21: 745-757.

161. Meliker JR, et al. Arsenic in drinking water and cerebrovascular disease, diabetes mellitus, and kidney disease in Michigan: a standardized mortality ratio analysis. *Environ Health.* 2007;6:4.

162. Melkonian S, et al. Intakes of several nutrients are associated with incidence of arsenic-related keratotic skin lesions in Bangladesh. *J Nutr.* 2012;142:2128-2134.

163. Melkonian S, et al. Urinary and dietary analysis of 18470 Bangladeshis reveal a correlation of rice consumption with arsenic exposure and toxicity. *PLoS One.* 2013;8:e80691.

164. Melnick A, Licht JD. Deconstructing a disease: RARα, its fusion partners, and their roles in the pathogenesis of acute promyelocytic leukemia. *Blood.* 1999;93:3167-3215.

165. Montesinos P, et al. Differentiation syndrome in patients with acute promyelocytic leukemia treated with all-trans retinoic acid and anthracycline chemotherapy: characteristics, outcome, and prognostic factors. *Blood.* 2009;113:775-783.

166. Moon KA, et al. Association between low to moderate arsenic exposure and incident cardiovascular disease. A prospective cohort study. *Ann Intern Med.* 2013;159: 649-659.

167. Moore DF, et al. Acute arsenic poisoning: absence of polyneuropathy after treatment with 2,3-dimercaptopropanesulphonate (DMPS). *J Neurol Neurosurg Psychiatry.* 1994;57: 1133-1135.

168. Mostafa MG, Cherry N. Arsenic in drinking water and renal cancers in rural Bangladesh. *Occup Environ Med.* 2013;70:768-773.

169. Muckter H, et al. Are we ready to replace dimercaprol (BAL) as an arsenic antidote? *Hum Exp Toxicol.* 1997;16:460-465.

170. Mukherjee SC, et al. Neuropathy in arsenic toxicity from groundwater arsenic contamination in West Bengal, India. *J Environ Sci Health A Tox Hazard Subst Environ Eng.* 2003;38:165-183.

171. Murgo AJ. Clinical trials of arsenic trioxide in hematologic and solid tumors: overview of the National Cancer Institute Cooperative Research and Development Studies. *Oncologist.* 2001;6(suppl 2):22-28.

172. Navas-Acien A, et al. Arsenic exposure and prevalence of type 2 diabetes in US adults. *JAMA.* 2008;300:814-822.

173. Niu C, et al. Studies on treatment of acute promyelocytic leukemia with arsenic trioxide: remission induction, follow-up, and molecular monitoring in 11 newly diagnosed and 47 relapsed acute promyelocytic leukemia patients. *Blood.* 1999;94:3315-3324.

174. Nixon DE, Moyer TP. Arsenic analysis II. Rapid separation and quantification of inorganic arsenic plus metabolites and arsenobetaine from urine. *Clin Chem.* 1992;38:2479-2483.

175. Oh SJ. Electrophysiological profile in arsenic neuropathy. *J Neurol Neurosurg Psychiatry.* 1991;54:1103-1105.

176. Ohnishi K, et al. Prolongation of the QT interval and ventricular tachycardia in patients treated with arsenic trioxide for acute promyelocytic leukemia. *Ann Intern Med.* 2000;133:881-885.

177. Park MJ, Currier M. Arsenic exposures in Mississippi: a review of cases. *South Med J.* 1991;84:461-464.

178. Parvez F, et al. Nonmalignant respiratory effects of chronic arsenic exposure from drinking water among never-smokers in Bangladesh. *Environ Health Perspect.* 2008;116:190-195.

179. Parvez F, et al. A prospective study of respiratory symptoms associated with chronic arsenic exposure in Bangladesh: findings from the Health Effects of Arsenic Longitudinal Study (HEALS). *Thorax.* 2010;65:528-533.

180. Parvez F, et al. Arsenic exposure and motor function among children in Bangladesh. *Environ Health Perspect.* 2011;119:1665-1670.

181. Paul DS, et al. Molecular mechanisms of the diabetogenic effects of arsenic: inhibition of insulin signaling by arsenite and methylarsonous acid. *Environ Health Perspect.* 2007;115:734-741.

182. Paul PC, et al. Histopathology of skin lesions in chronic arsenic toxicity—grading of changes and study of proliferative markers. *Indian J Pathol Microbiol.* 2000;43:257-264.

183. Pepin J, Milord F. African trypanosomiasis and drug-induced encephalopathy: risk factors and pathogenesis. *Trans R Soc Trop Med Hyg.* 1991;85:222-224.

184. Peters HA, et al. Seasonal arsenic exposure from burning chromium-copper-arsenate treated wood. *JAMA.* 1984;251:2393-2396.

185. Petrick JS, et al. Monomethylarsonous acid (MMA^III) is more toxic than arsenite in Chang human hepatocytes. *Toxicol Appl Pharmacol.* 2000;163:203-207.

186. Petrick JS, et al. Monomethylarsonous acid (MMA^III) and arsenite: LD_{50} in hamsters and in vitro inhibition of pyruvate dehydrogenase. *Chem Res Toxicol.* 2001;14:651-656.

187. Pierce BL, et al. Genome-wide association study identifies chromosome 10q24.32 variants associated with arsenic metabolism and toxicity phenotypes in Bangladesh. *PLoS Genet.* 2012;8:1-10.

188. Pilsner JR, et al. Associations of plasma selenium with arsenic and genomic methylation of leukocyte DNA in Bangladesh. *Environ Health Perspect.* 2011;119:113-118.

189. Pilsner JR, et al. Folate deficiency, hyperhomocysteinemia, low urinary creatinine and hypomethylation of leukocyte DNA are risk factors for arsenic-induced skin lesions. *Environ Health Perspect.* 2009;117:254-260.

190. Pilsner JR, et al. Genomic methylation of peripheral blood leukocyte DNA: influences of arsenic and folate in Bangladesh adults. *Am J Clin Nutr.* 2007;86:1179-1186.

191. Pomroy C, et al. Human retention studies with ⁷⁴As. *Toxicol Appl Pharmacol.* 1980;53:550-556.

192. Pu YS, et al. Urinary arsenic profile affects the risk of urothelial carcinoma even at low arsenic exposure. *Toxicol Appl Pharmacol.* 2007;218:99-106.

193. Raab A, Feldmann J. Arsenic speciation in hair extracts. *Anal Bioanal Chem.* 2005;381:332-338.

194. Rahman A, et al. Association of arsenic exposure during pregnancy with fetal loss and infant death: a cohort study in Bangladesh. *Am J Epidemiol.* 2007;165:1389-1396.

195. Rahman M, et al. Diabetes mellitus associated with arsenic exposure in Bangladesh. *Am J Epidemiol.* 1998;148:198-203.

196. Ramos O, et al. Arsenic increased lipid peroxidation in rat tissues by a mechanism independent of glutathione levels. *Environ Health Perspect.* 1995;103(suppl 1):85-88.

197. Reichl F-X, et al. Effect of DMPS and various adsorbents on the arsenic excretion in guinea-pigs after injection with As_2O_3. *Arch Toxicol.* 1995;69:712-717.

198. Reichl F-X, et al. Pyruvate and lactate metabolism in livers of guinea pigs perfused with chelation agents after repeated treatment with As_2O_3. *Arch Toxicol.* 1991;65:235-238.

199. Reichl F-X, et al. Effect of glucose treatment on carbohydrate content in various organs in mice after acute As_2O_3 poisoning. *Vet Hum Toxicol.* 1991;33:230-235.

200. Reichl F-X, et al. Effects of arsenic on carbohydrate metabolism after single or repeated injection in guinea pigs. *Arch Toxicol.* 1988;62:473-475.

201. Rein KA, et al. Arsenite inhibits β-oxidation in isolated rat liver mitochondria. *Biochim Biophys Acta.* 1979;574:487-494.

202. Robinson TJ. Arsenical polyneuropathy due to caustic arsenical paste. *Br Med J.* 1975;3:139.

203. Rojewski MT, et al. Depolarization of mitochondria and activation of caspases are common features of arsenic(III)-induced apoptosis in myelogenic and lymphatic cell lines. *Chem Res Toxicol.* 2004;17:119-128.

204. Rosado JL, et al. Arsenic exposure and cognitive performance in Mexican schoolchildren. *Environ Health Perspect.* 2007;115:1371-1375.

205. Roses OE, et al. Mass poisoning by sodium arsenite. *J Toxicol Clin Toxicol.* 1991;29:209-213.

206. Rust DM, Soignet SL. Risk/benefit profile of arsenic trioxide. *Oncologist.* 2001;6(suppl 2):29-32.

207. Samanta G, et al. Arsenic in the breast milk of lactating women in arsenic affected areas of West Bengal, India and its effect on infants. *J Environ Sci Health A Tox Hazard Subst Environ Enf.* 2007;42:1815-1825.

208. Santra A, et al. Hepatic damage caused by chronic arsenic toxicity in experimental animals. *J Toxicol Clin Toxicol.* 2000;38:395-405.

209. Sanz P, et al. Rhabdomyolysis in fatal arsenic trioxide poisoning. *JAMA.* 1989;262:3271.

210. Savory J, Sedor FA. Arsenic poisoning. In: Brown SS, ed. *Clinical Chemistry and Chemical Toxicology of Metals.* New York, NY: Elsevier/North Holland; 1977:271-286.

211. Schoof RA, et al. A market basket survey of inorganic arsenic in food. *Food Chem Toxicol.* 1999;37:839-846.

212. Schoolmeester WL, White DR. Arsenic poisoning. *South Med J.* 1980;73:198-208.

213. Shen Y, et al. Studies on the clinical efficacy and pharmacokinetics of low-dose arsenic trioxide in the treatment of relapsed acute promyelocytic leukemia: a comparison with conventional dosage. *Leukemia.* 2001;15:735-741.

214. Shen ZX, et al. Use of arsenic trioxide (As_2O_3) in the treatment of acute promyelocytic leukemia (APL): II. Clinical efficacy and pharmacokinetics in relapsed patients. *Blood.* 1997;89:3354-3360.

215. Shum S, et al. Chelation of organoarsenate with dimercaptosuccinic acid. *Vet Hum Toxicol.* 1995;37:239-242.

216. Smith AH, et al. Increased mortality from lung cancer and bronchiectasis in young adults after exposure to arsenic in utero and in early childhood. *Environ Health Perspect.* 2006;114:1293-1296.

217. Soignet SL, et al. United States multicenter study of arsenic trioxide in relapsed acute promyelocytic leukemia. *J Clin Oncol.* 2001;19:3852-3860.

218. Soignet SL, et al. Clinical study of an organic arsenical, melarsoprol, in patients with advanced leukemia. *Cancer Chemother Pharmacol.* 1999;44:417-421.

219. St. Petery J, et al. Ventricular fibrillation caused by arsenic poisoning. *Am J Dis Child.* 1970;120:367-371.

220. Stevens JT, et al. Disposition of ^{14}C and/or ^{74}As cacodylic acid in rats after intravenous, intratracheal, or peroral administration. *Environ Health Perspect.* 1977;19:151-157.

221. Styblo M, et al. Comparative in vitro methylation of trivalent and pentavalent arsenicals. *Toxicol Appl Pharmacol.* 1995;135:172-178.

222. Syed EH, et al. Arsenic exposure and oral cavity lesions in Bangladesh. *J Occup Environ Med.* 2013;55:59-66.

223. Szinicz L, Forth W. Effect of As_2O_3 on gluconeogenesis. *Arch Toxicol.* 1988;61:444-449.

224. Szuler IM, et al. Massive variceal hemorrhage secondary to presinusoidal portal hypertension due to arsenic poisoning. *CMAJ.* 1979;120:168-171.

225. Tam GK, et al. Metabolism of inorganic arsenic (^{74}As) in humans following oral ingestion. *Toxicol Appl Pharmacol.* 1979;50:319-322.

226. Tay CH, Seah CS. Arsenic poisoning from anti-asthmatic herbal preparations. *Med J Aust.* 1975;2:424-428.

227. Toribara TY. Analysis of single hair by XRF discloses mercury in-take. *Hum Exp Toxicol.* 2001;20:185-188.

228. Toribara TY, et al. Nondestructive x-ray fluorescence spectrometry for determination of trace elements along a single strand of hair. *Anal Chem.* 1982;54:1844-1849.

229. Tsai SY, et al. The effects of chronic arsenic exposure from drinking water on the neurobehavioral development in adolescence. *Neurotoxicology.* 2003;24:747-753.

230. Tseng CH, et al. Dose–response relationship between peripheral vascular disease and ingested inorganic arsenic among residents in blackfoot disease endemic villages in Taiwan. *Atherosclerosis.* 1996;120:125-133.

231. Tseng CH, et al. Arsenic exposure, urinary arsenic speciation, and peripheral vascular disease in blackfoot disease-hyperendemic villages in Taiwan. *Toxicol Appl Pharmacol.* 2005;206:299-308.

232. Tseng CH, et al. Long-term arsenic exposure and incidence of non-insulin-dependent diabetes mellitus: a cohort study in arseniasis-hyperendemic villages in Taiwan. *Environ Health Perspect.* 2000;108:847-851.

233. Tsukamoto H, et al. Metabolism and renal handling of sodium arsenate in dogs. *Am J Vet Res.* 1983;44:2331-2335.

234. Tsukamoto H, et al. Nephrotoxicity of sodium arsenate in dogs. *Am J Vet Res.* 1983;44:2324-2330.

235. Uede K, Furukawa F. Skin manifestations in acute arsenic poisoning from the Wakayama curry-poisoning incident. *Br J Dermatol.* 2003;149:757-762.

236. Unnikrishnan D, et al. Torsades de pointes in 3 patients with leukemia treated with arsenic trioxide. *Blood.* 2001;97:1514-1516.

237. Vahter M. Genetic polymorphism in the biotransformation of inorganic arsenic and its role in toxicity. *Toxicol Lett.* 2000;112-113:209-217.

238. Vahter M. Health effects of early life exposure to arsenic. *Basic Clin Pharmacol Toxicol.* 2008;102:204-211.

239. Vahter M. Mechanisms of arsenic biotransformation. *Toxicology.* 2002;181-182:2111-2117.

240. Vahter M. Metabolism of arsenic. In: Fowler BA, ed. *Biological and Environmental Effects of Arsenic.* New York, NY: Elsevier; 1983:171-198.

241. Vahter M. Methylation of inorganic arsenic in different mammalian species and population groups. *Sci Prog.* 1999;82(pt 1):69-88.

242. Vahter M, Marafante E. Effects of low dietary intake of methionine, choline or proteins on the biotransformation of arsenite in the rabbit. *Toxicol Lett.* 1987;37:41-46.

243. Vahter M, Marafante E. Intracellular interaction and metabolic fate of arsenite and arsenate in mice and rabbits. *Chem Biol Interact.* 1983;47:29-44.

244. Vaziri ND, et al. Hemodialysis clearance of arsenic. *Clin Toxicol.* 1980;17:451-456.

245. Verret WJ, et al. Effects of vitamin E and selenium on arsenic-induced skin lesions. *J Occup Environ Med.* 2005;47:1026-1035.

246. Von Ehrenstein OS, et al. Children's intellectual function in relation to arsenic exposure. *Epidemiology.* 2007;18:44-51.

247. Wagner SL, Weswig P. Arsenic in blood and urine of forest workers. *Arch Environ Health.* 1974;28:77-79.

248. Walton FS, et al. Inhibition of insulin-dependent glucose uptake by trivalent arsenicals: possible mechanism of arsenic-induced diabetes. *Toxicol Appl Pharmacol.* 2004;198:424-433.

249. Wang A, et al. Reproductive and developmental toxicity of arsenic in rodents: a review. *Int J Toxicol.* 2006;25:319-331.

250. Wang CH, et al. A review of the epidemiologic literature on the role of the environmental arsenic exposure and cardiovascular diseases. *Toxicol Appl Pharmacol.* 2007;222:315-326.

251. Wasserman GA, et al. Water arsenic exposure and children's intellectual function in Araihazar, Bangladesh. *Environ Health Perspect.* 2004;112:1329-1333.

252. Wasserman GA, et al. Water arsenic exposure and intellectual function in 6-year-old children in Araihazar, Bangladesh. *Environ Health Perspect.* 2007;115:285-289.

253. Wax PM, Thornton CA. Recovery from severe arsenic-induced peripheral neuropathy with 2,3-dimercapto-1-propanesulphonic acid. *J Toxicol Clin Toxicol.* 2000;38:777-780.

254. Wennig R. Potential problems with the interpretation of hair analysis results. *Forensic Sci Int.* 2000;107:5-12.

255. Wester PO, et al. Arsenic and selenium in lung, liver, and kidney tissue from dead smelter workers. *Br J Ind Med.* 1981;38:179-184.

256. Wester RC, et al. In vivo and in vitro percutaneous absorption and skin decontamination of arsenic from water and soil. *Fundam Appl Toxicol.* 1993;20:336-340.

257. Westervelt P, et al. Sudden death among patients with acute promyelocytic leukemia treated with arsenic trioxide. *Blood.* 2001;98:266-271.

258. Winski SL, Carter DE. Arsenate toxicity in human erythrocytes: characterization of morphologic changes and determination of the mechanism of damage. *J Toxicol Environ Health A.* 1998;53:345-355.

259. Wong SS, et al. Cutaneous manifestations of chronic arsenicism: review of seventeen cases. *J Am Acad Dermatol.* 1998;38(2, pt 1):179-185.

260. Woollons A, Russell-Jones R. Chronic endemic hydroarsenicism. *Br J Dermatol.* 1998;139:1092-1096.

261. Wu F, et al. Interaction between arsenic exposure from drinking water and genetic polymorphisms on cardiovascular disease in Bangladesh: a prospective case-cohort study. *Environ Health Perspect.* 2015;123:451-457.

262. Wu F, et al. Interaction between arsenic exposure from drinking water and genetic susceptibility in carotid intima-media thickness in Bangladesh. *Toxicol Appl Pharmacol.* 2014;276:195-203.

263. Wu F, et al. Association between arsenic exposure from drinking water and plasma levels of cardiovascular markers. *Am J Epidemiol.* 2012;175:1252-1261.

264. Yamanaka K, et al. Dimethylated arsenics induce DNA strand breaks in lung via the production of active oxygen in mice. *Biochem Biophys Res Commun.* 1989;165:43-50.

265. Yamato N. Concentrations and chemical species of arsenic in human urine and hair. *Bull Environ Contam Toxicol.* 1988;40:633-640.

266. Yamauchi H, Yamamura Y. Concentration and chemical species of arsenic in human tissue. *Bull Environ Contam Toxicol.* 1983;31:267-270.

267. Yoshida T, et al. Chronic health effects in people exposed to arsenic via the drinking water: dose–response relationships in review. *Toxicol Appl Pharmacol.* 2004;198:243-252.

268. Young EG, Smith RP. Arsenic content of hair and bone in acute and chronic arsenical poisoning: review of 2 cases examined posthumously from medico-legal aspect. *Br Med J.* 1942;1:251-253.

269. Zablotska LB, et al. Protective effects of B vitamins and antioxidants on the risk of arsenic-related skin lesions in Bangladesh. *Environ Health Perspect.* 2008;116:1056-1062.

270. Zakharyan RA, Aposhian HV. Arsenite methylation by methylvitamin B_{12} and glutathione does not require an enzyme. *Toxicol Appl Pharmacol.* 1999;154:287-291.

271. Zakharyan RA, Aposhian HV. Enzymatic reduction of arsenic compounds in mammalian systems: the rate-limiting enzyme of rabbit liver arsenic biotransformation is MMA^V reductase. *Chem Res Toxicol.* 1999;12:1278-1283.

272. Zaloga GP, et al. Case report: unusual manifestations of arsenic intoxication. *Am J Med Sci.* 1985;289:210-214.

273. Zavala YJ, et al. Arsenic in rice: II. Arsenic speciation in USA grain and implications for human health. *Environ Sci Technol.* 2008;42:3861-3866.

274. Zhang P, et al. Treatment of 72 cases of acute promyelocytic leukemia by intravenous arsenic trioxide. *Chin J Hematol.* 1996;17:58-62.

275. Zhang X, et al. Accumulation of arsenic species in serum of patients with chronic renal disease. *Clin Chem.* 1996;42(8, pt 1):1231-1237.

276. Zhang X, et al. Chemical speciation of arsenic in serum of uraemic patients. *Analyst.* 1998;123:13-17.

A28

DIMERCAPROL (BRITISH ANTI-LEWISITE OR BAL)

Mary Ann Howland

H—C—OH
|
H—C—SH
|
H—C—SH
|
H

(structural formula)

INTRODUCTION

British anti-Lewisite (BAL) (2,3-dimercaptopropanol; dimercaprol) is a metal chelator used clinically in conjunction with edetate calcium disodium (CaNa$_2$EDTA) for lead encephalopathy and severe lead poisoning as well as other metals and metalloids.[26,34] In severe lead poisoning, dimercaprol should precede the first dose of CaNa$_2$EDTA by 4 hours to prevent redistribution of lead to the central nervous system (CNS).[17,18] Dimercaprol has a narrow therapeutic index and is only administered intramuscularly (IM) because it is formulated in peanut oil. Oral succimer is used for patients with less severe lead toxicity. The roles for dimercaprol in arsenic and mercury poisoning have diminished since the development of succimer and the investigational chelator 2,3-dimercaptopropane sulfonate (DMPS). Dimercaprol remains indicated when the gastrointestinal tract is compromised.

HISTORY

Investigation into the use of sulfur donors as antidotes was precipitated by the World War II threat of chemical warfare with Lewisite (dichloro{2-chlorovinyl} arsine) and mustard gas (dichlorodiethyl sulfide {ClCH$_2$CH$_2$}$_2$S).[1,35,36] Both are vesicants that cause tissue damage when combined with protein sulfhydryl groups (Chap. 126).[39] The investigations of Stocken and Thompson at Oxford led to the discovery of the dithiol 2,3-dimercaptopropanol (or BAL) that combines with Lewisite to form a stable 5-membered ring.[44,47]

PHARMACOLOGY

Chemistry

Dimercaprol has a molecular weight of 124.2 Da and a specific gravity of 1.21.[37] It is an oily liquid with only 6% weight/volume water solubility, 5% weight/volume peanut oil solubility, and a disagreeable odor. Aqueous solutions are easily oxidized and therefore unstable. Peanut oil stabilizes dimercaprol and benzyl benzoate (in the ratio of one part dimercaprol to 2 parts of benzyl benzoate), which renders the dimercaprol miscible in peanut oil.[40]

Mechanism of Action

The sulfhydryl groups of dimercaprol form chelates with certain metals, which are then excreted in the urine. Lead, arsenic, and inorganic mercury salts are the metals most amenable to chelation with dimercaprol.

Pharmacokinetics

The limited information available about the pharmacokinetics of dimercaprol was determined in the 1940s.[1,28] Serum concentrations of dimercaprol peak about 30 minutes after IM administration, and distribution occurs rapidly.[40,43] Within 2 hours after IM administration to rabbits, serum concentrations rapidly fall. Urinary excretion of dimercaprol metabolites, perhaps partially as glucuronic acid conjugates, accounted for nearly 45% of the dose within 6 hours and 81% of the dose within 24 hours.[40,42] Very little is excreted unchanged in the urine.[40] Dimercaprol is concentrated in the kidney, liver,

and small intestine.[38] Dimercaprol is also found in the feces, suggesting that an enterohepatic circulation exists. Hemodialysis is useful in removing the dimercaprol–metal chelate in cases of kidney failure.[26,33,46]

ROLE OF DIMERCAPROL IN ARSENIC POISONING

Animal Studies

The fear of Lewisite attack causing skin lesions led researchers to investigate the potential for cutaneous application of dimercaprol.[44] This was based on the limited water solubility and high lipid solubility of dimercaprol. In a rodent model, low concentrations of topical dimercaprol were very effective both in preventing Lewisite-induced toxicity and in reversing toxicity when administered within one hour of skin exposure.[37,39] In rabbits, ophthalmic application of dimercaprol proved effective in preventing corneal destruction if applied within 20 minutes of exposure.[26] Additionally, urinary arsenic concentrations were significantly increased after the application of dimercaprol.[39]

The effectiveness of both parenteral single-dose and multiple-dose dimercaprol against lewisite and other arsenicals was studied in rabbits. When begun within 2 hours of lewisite exposure, dimercaprol injections of 4 mg/kg every 4 hours led to a 50% survival of exposed rabbits. This dosing regimen was demonstrated to be one-seventh of the maximum tolerated dose of dimercaprol.[20]

The most recent animal studies demonstrate that although dimercaprol increases the LD$_{50}$ (median lethal dose for 50% of test subjects) of sodium arsenite, the therapeutic index of dimercaprol is low and arsenic redistribution to the brain occurs.[4,6,7,23,41] In these same animal models, succimer and DMPS also increased the LD$_{50}$ but with better therapeutic indices and without causing redistribution to the brain.[3,4]

Ophthalmic damage caused by Lewisite is partly a result of the liberation of hydrochloric acid, which results in an acid injury causing localized superficial opacities of the cornea and deep penetration of lewisite into the cornea and aqueous humor with resultant rapid necrosis. In an experimental model, a 5% dimercaprol ointment or solution applied within 2 minutes of exposure prevented the development of a significant reaction; application at 30 minutes limited the reaction, but did not prevent permanent damage.[24]

Human Studies

Experiments in human volunteers who were given minute amounts of arsenic demonstrated that dimercaprol increased urinary arsenic concentration by approximately 40%, with maximum excretion occurring 2 to 4 hours after dimercaprol administration.[49] Dimercaprol was subsequently used in the treatment of arsenical dermatitis resulting from organic arsenicals used to treat syphilis. When applied to affected skin, topical dimercaprol produced erythema, pruritus, and dysesthesias, without adverse effects on unaffected skin. Dimercaprol (IM) produced both subjective and objective improvement, limited the duration of the arsenical dermatitis, and increased urinary arsenic elimination.[15,31,32]

In a study of 227 patients with inorganic arsenic poisoning, maximal efficacy and minimal toxicity were achieved when 3 mg/kg of dimercaprol was administered IM every 4 hours for 48 hours and then twice daily for 7 to 10 days. This regimen resulted in complete recovery in 6 of 7 patients with severe arsenical encephalopathy and demonstrated the importance of administering dimercaprol as soon as possible after an exposure. Of 33 patients with severe arsenical encephalopathy, 18 of 24 (75%) treated within 6 hours survived, whereas only 4 of 9 (44%) treated after a delay of greater than 72 hours survived.[19] Furthermore, the effectiveness of dimercaprol was demonstrated in 3 patients who were treated successfully after mistakenly receiving 10 to 20 times the therapeutic dose of oxophenarsine hydrochloride an arsenical primarily used for the treatment of syphilis. A fourth patient, treated with inadequate doses of dimercaprol, died.[19] These cases support the effectiveness of dimercaprol in treating arsenic-induced agranulocytosis, encephalopathy, dermatitis, and probably arsenical fever.[18]

When dimercaprol first became more widely available, 42 children were treated following arsenic ingestions, and their results were compared with a historical group of 111 untreated children who had also ingested arsenic.[50] The percentage of children exhibiting symptoms on presentation were similar between groups (46%), but in the group of children treated with dimercaprol there were fewer deaths (zero vs 3), a shorter average hospital stay (1.6 vs 4.2 days), and fewer cases of persistent symptoms at 12 hours (0% vs 29.3%).

ROLE OF DIMERCAPROL IN MERCURY POISONING

Because mercury also reacts with sulfhydryl groups, animal studies were performed to assess the affinity and ability of thiols to competitively chelate inorganic mercury and prevent toxicity. As in the case of arsenic, the dithiol dimercaprol was more effective than the monothiol 1-thiosorbitol in preventing mercury-induced death and uremia.[22] The clinical efficacy of dimercaprol in treating inorganic mercury poisoning was substantiated in patients who ingested mercuric chloride.[29,30] Thirty-eight patients ingesting more than 1 g of mercuric chloride who were treated with dimercaprol within 4 hours of exposure were compared with historical controls.[29] There were no deaths in the 38 patients treated with dimercaprol as compared to 27 deaths in the 86 untreated patients. Death typically resulted from hemorrhagic gastritis and kidney failure.[29] Dimercaprol is particularly useful for patients who ingested a mercuric salt, as the associated gastrointestinal toxicity of the mercuric salt limits the potential of an orally administered antidote such as succimer.[48]

Animal models demonstrate that when dimercaprol is administered following poisoning from elemental mercury vapor or short-chain organic mercury compounds, brain concentrations of mercury increase.[10,14] As a result, dimercaprol therapy is not recommended in these circumstances (Chap. 95).[2,5,26]

ROLE OF DIMERCAPROL IN LEAD POISONING

Dimercaprol is used in combination with $CaNa_2EDTA$ to treat patients with severe lead poisoning. In all other cases, succimer is the chelator of choice. When treating patients with lead encephalopathy, it is essential to administer the dimercaprol first, followed 4 hours later by $CaNa_2EDTA$ with a second dose of dimercaprol. This regimen prevents the $CaNa_2EDTA$ from redistributing lead into the brain.[17,18] Providing 2 different chelators also reduces the blood lead concentration significantly faster than either one alone, and maintains a better molar ratio of chelator to lead.[17] Once the mobilization of lead is initiated, it is essential to provide uninterrupted therapy to prevent redistribution of lead to the brain (Chap. 93).[17] In the event that $CaNa_2EDTA$ is not available, succimer has been used successfully with and without dimercaprol.[8,45]

ADVERSE EFFECTS AND SAFETY ISSUES

Dimercaprol has an LD_{50} in mice via intraperitoneal administration of 90 to 180 mg/kg, which is significantly lower than that of $CaNa_2EDTA$ at 4,000 to 6,000 mg/kg, succimer at 2,480 mg/kg, and DMPS at 1,100 to 1,400 mg/kg.[2]

Among 700 patients who received 2.5 mg/kg of BAL IM every 4 to 6 hours for 4 doses, less than 1% developed minor reactions, such as pain at the injection site.[15] When doses of 4 and 5 mg/kg were given, the incidence of adverse effects rose to 14% and 65%, respectively.[19] At these higher doses, the following symptoms were reported in decreasing order of frequency: nausea; vomiting; headache; burning sensation of lips, mouth, throat, and eyes; lacrimation; rhinorrhea; salivation; muscle aches; burning and tingling of extremities; tooth pain; diaphoresis; chest pain; anxiety; and agitation.[31] These effects were maximal within 10 to 30 minutes of dosing and usually

subsided within 30 to 50 minutes.[19] Elevations in systolic and diastolic blood pressure and tachycardia were common and correlated with increasing doses.[26,34] Thirty percent of children given dimercaprol developed a fever that persisted throughout the therapeutic period.[26] In addition, in children, a transient reduction in the percentage of polymorphonuclear leukocytes also occured.[26] We recommend not to administer doses above 5 mg/kg because of the high risk of adverse reactions. Doses above 25 mg/kg often resulted in a hypertensive encephalopathy with convulsions and coma.[50]

Dimercaprol is not very effective in the presence of arsenic-induced hepatotoxicity.[32] Moreover, in rats, preexistent hepatotoxicity was exacerbated when dimercaprol was used for treatment of arsenic poisoning. Therefore, unless the hepatotoxicity is considered to be arsenic induced, hepatic dysfunction is a contraindication to dimercaprol use.[39] Dimercaprol should not be used for patients poisoned by methylmercury because animal studies demonstrate a redistribution of mercury to the brain.[5,26] In a rabbit model of sodium arsenite poisoning, dimercaprol increased the concentration of arsenic in the brain whereas succimer did not alter the concentration and DMPS reduced the concentration.[4,27]

Because dissociation of the dimercaprol–metal chelate will occur in acidic urine, we recommend that the urine of patients receiving dimercaprol be alkalinized with hypertonic sodium bicarbonate to a pH of 7.5 to 8.0 to prevent liberation of the metal (Antidotes in Depth: A5).[9,26] Dimercaprol causes hemolysis in 2 children with glucose-6-phosphate dehydrogenase (G6PD) deficiency.[25] Because G6PD deficiency syndromes are variably expressed, patients at risk should be carefully monitored for hemolysis. In addition, chelators are relatively nonspecific and bind metals other than those desired, thus causing essential metal deficiencies. For example, dimercaprol given to mice increased copper elimination to 3 times normal.[13] Dimercaprol is formulated in peanut oil; therefore, the patient should be questioned regarding any known peanut allergy and a risk–benefit analysis undertaken. Limited evidence suggests that iron supplements should not be given to patients while receiving dimercaprol because the dimercaprol–iron complex causes severe vomiting and decreases metal chelation.[17,18,21]

Unintentional intravenous (IV) infusion of dimercaprol could theoretically produce fat embolism (peanut oil), lipoid pneumonia, chylothorax, and associated hypoxia.[42]

Pregnancy and Lactation

Dimercaprol is pregnancy category C.[9] There are no animal studies evaluating the effects of dimercaprol on reproduction. It is unknown whether dimercaprol is harmful to a fetus or is capable of affecting reproduction capability.[9] There are no data in human poisoning in pregnancy, and dimercaprol should only be administered to a pregnant woman after addressing a risk–benefit analysis with the patient.[9]

No data address whether dimercaprol or its chelates are excreted in human breast milk. It is not known whether succimer is excreted in human milk, but breast feeding is a contraindication[11] in some sources and is a caution in the package insert.[28] However in the 2010 CDC Guidelines for the identification and management of lead exposure in pregnant and breast-feeding women, the CDC suggests allowing breastfeeding for mothers with BLLs of less than or equal to 40 mcg/dL.[16] Mothers with BLLs of greater than 40 mcg/dL are encouraged to pump and discard their breast milk until their BLLs drop to less than 40 mcg/dL. Because dimercaprol is only indicated for BLLs greater than 40, we encourage the latter.

DOSING AND ADMINISTRATION

No clinical trial has been performed to identify the appropriate dose of dimercaprol. The dosing for dimercaprol is expressed in both milligrams per square meter body surface area (mg/m²) and milligrams per kilogram body weight (mg/kg) (Table A28–1). Dimercaprol should be administered only by deep IM injection. The dose of dimercaprol for lead encephalopathy is 75 mg/m² IM every 4 hours for 5 days in children (Table 93–8).[17,18] As noted earlier, we recommend that the first dose of dimercaprol precede the first dose of $CaNa_2EDTA$ by 4 hours. Thereafter, IV $CaNa_2EDTA$, in a dose of 1500 mg/m²/day (up to a

TABLE A28–1	Calculations for Average Deep Intramuscular (IM) Dimercaprol Use When Using Body Surface Area (m²)				
Child	Average Height (in.)	Average Weight (lb)	m²	75 mg/m² Every 4 hours IM[a]	50 mg/m² Every 4 hours IM[b]
2-year-old boy	36	30.5	0.593	44.5 mg	30 mg
2-year-old girl	35	29	0.57	43 mg	28.5 mg
4-year-old boy	42	39.75	0.73	55 mg	36.5 mg
4-year-old girl	41.75	38.75	0.72	54 mg	36 mg

[a]Approximately 4 mg/kg. [b]Approximately 3 mg/kg.

maximum of 2–3 g) as a continuous infusion, or divided into 2 to 4 doses, is recommended. A continuous infusion is reasonable because the half-life of CaNa$_2$EDTA is short. For adults, the dose of dimercaprol is 4 mg/kg every 4 hours (Table 93–8).[9] We recommend shortening the duration of dimercaprol to 3 days if there is prompt resolution of the encephalopathy and the blood lead concentration decreases to below 50 mcg/dL while the CaNa$_2$EDTA continues for the remainder of the 5 days.

The dose of dimercaprol for arsenic poisoning is not established. One regimen for severe arsenic poisoning suggests the use of 3 mg/kg IM every 4 hours for 48 hours and then every 12 hours for 10 days or until complete recovery for severe poisoning.[19] In this large case series in adults, arsenic poisoning was a result of the treatment of syphilis with arsenic (oxophenarsine) and *severe* was defined as encephalopathy, exfoliative dermatitis, blood dyscrasia, or massive injection of the arsenical. In this same series, 2.5 mg/kg IM for each of 4 daily doses spaced every 4 hours for the first 2 days and then reduced to one or 2 injections daily for 10 days or until complete recovery was suggested for mild arsenic toxicity defined as fever, rash, and mild arsenical dermatitis. Another regimen uses 3 to 5 mg/kg IM every 4 to 6 hours on the first day and then tapers the dose and frequency, depending on the patient's symptomatology. A third regimen reduces the number of injections by day 2 from 6 to 4 and then from 3 to 2 to 1 and terminates therapy within 5 to 7 days.[50] Based on this limited data, we recommend the first regimen cited in this paragraph.

The dose of dimercaprol for patients exposed to inorganic mercuric salts is 5 mg/kg IM initially, followed by 2.5 mg/kg every 12 to 24 hours until the patient appears clinically improved, up to a total of 10 days.[9] Dimercaprol is for deep IM use only.

As noted above, we recommend that the urine be alkalinized to avoid dissociation of the dimercaprol–metal chelate.[12,26]

FORMULATION AND ACQUISITION

Commercially available dimercaprol is a yellow, viscous liquid with a sulfur odor. It is available in 3-mL ampules containing 100 mg/mL of dimercaprol, 200 mg/mL of benzyl benzoate, and 700 mg/mL of peanut oil.[9]

SUMMARY

■ Dimercaprol is a metal chelator used clinically in conjunction with CaNa$_2$EDTA for lead encephalopathy and severe lead toxicity.[26,34]

■ In patients with severe lead poisoning, we recommend that dimercaprol precede the first dose of CaNa$_2$EDTA by 4 hours.

■ When dimercaprol is not available, succimer with CaNa$_2$EDTA or even succimer alone in resource-poor areas appears adequate.

■ The roles of dimercaprol in arsenic and mercury poisonings are being supplanted by oral succimer and the investigational chelator DMPS, which are reasonable unless the gastrointestinal tract is compromised.

REFERENCES

1. Aaseth J. Recent advances in the therapy of metal poisonings with chelating agents. *Hum Toxicol*. 1983;2:257-272.
2. Andersen O. Principles and recent developments in chelation treatment of metal intoxication. *Chem Rev*. 1999;99:2683-2710.
3. Aposhian HV, Aposhian MM. Arsenic toxicology: five questions. *Chem Res Toxicol*. 2006;19:1-15.
4. Aposhian HV, et al. DMSA, DMPS, and DMPA as arsenic antidotes. *Fundam Appl Toxicol*. 1984;4:S58-S70.
5. Aposhian HV, et al. Mobilization of heavy metals by newer, therapeutically useful chelating agents. *Toxicology*. 1995;97:23-38.
6. Aposhian HV, et al. Anti-Lewisite activity and stability of meso-dimercaptosuccinic acid and 2,3-dimercapto1-propanesulfonic acid. *Life Sci*. 1982;31:2149-2156.
7. Aposhian HV, et al. Protection of mice against the lethal effects of sodium arsenite—a quantitative comparison of a number of chelating agents. *Toxicol Appl Pharmacol*. 1981;61:385-392.
8. Arnold J, Morgan B. Management of lead encephalopathy with DMSA after exposure to lead-contaminated moonshine. *J Med Toxicol*. 2015;11:464-467.
9. BAL in oil ampules (dimercaprol injection USP) [package insert]. Decatur, IL: Taylor Pharmaceuticals; 2006.
10. Berlin M, Ullberg S. Increased uptake of mercury in mouse brain caused by 2,3-dimercaptopropanol. *Nature*. 1963;197:84-85.
11. Briggs GG, et al. *Drugs in Pregnancy and Lactation: A Reference Guide to Fetal and Neonatal Risk*. 11th ed. Philadelphia, PA: Lippincott Williams & Wilkins; 2017.
12. Byrns MC, Penning TM. Environmental toxicology: carcinogens and heavy metals. In: Brunton LL, Chabner BA, Knollmann BC, eds. *Goodman & Gilman's The Pharmacological Basis of Therapeutics*. chap. 7. 12th ed. New York, NY: McGraw-Hill; 2011. http://accesspharmacy.mhmedical.com/Book.aspx?bookid=1613. Accessed October 2, 2017.
13. Cantilena LR, Klaassen CD. The effect of chelating agents on the excretion of endogenous metals. *Toxicol Appl Pharmacol*. 1982;63:344-350.
14. Canty AJ, Kishimoto R. British anti-Lewisite and organ-mercury poisoning. *Nature*. 1972;253:123-125.
15. Carleton AB, et al. Clinical uses of 2,3-dimercaptopropanol (BAL): VI. The treatment of complications of arseno-therapy with BAL. *J Clin Invest*. 1946;25:497-527.
16. Centers for Disease Control and Prevention (CDC). Guidelines for the identification and management of lead exposure in pregnant and lactating women, 2010. http://www.cdc.gov/nceh/lead/publications/LeadandPregnancy2010.pdf. Accessed October 2, 2017.
17. Chisolm JJ Jr. The use of chelating agents in the treatment of acute and chronic lead intoxication in childhood. *J Pediatr*. 1968;73:1-38.
18. Committee on Drugs. Treatment guidelines for lead exposure in children. *Pediatrics*. 1995;96:155-160.
19. Eagle H, Magnuson HJ. The systemic treatment of 227 cases of arsenic poisoning (encephalitis, dermatitis, blood dyscrasias, jaundice, fever) with 2,3-dimercaptopropanol (BAL). *Am J Syph Gonorrhea Vener Dis*. 1946;30:420-441.
20. Eagle H, et al. Clinical uses of 2,3-dimercaptopropanol (BAL): I. The systemic treatment of experimental arsenic poisoning (Mapharsen, lewisite, phenyl arsenoxide) with BAL. *J Clin Invest*. 1946;25:451-466.
21. Edge WD, Somers GF. The effect of dimercaprol (BAL) in acute iron poisoning. *Q J Pharm Pharmacol*. 1948;21:364-369.
22. Gilman A, et al. Clinical uses of 2,3-dimercaptopropanol (BAL): X. The treatment of acute systemic mercury poisoning in experimental animals with BAL, thiosorbitol and BAL glucoside. *J Clin Invest*. 1946;25:549-556.
23. Hoover TD, Aposhian HV. BAL increases the arsenic-74 content of rabbit brain. *Toxicol Appl Pharmacol*. 1983;70:160-162.
24. Hughes WF. Clinical uses of 2,3-dimercaptopropanol (BAL): IX. The treatment of lewisite burns of the eye with BAL. *J Clin Invest*. 1946;25:541-548.
25. Janakiraman N, et al. Hemolysis during BAL chelation therapy for high blood lead levels in two G6PD-deficient children. *Clin Pediatr (Phila)*. 1978;17:485-487.
26. Klaassen CD. Heavy metals and heavy metal antagonists. In: Hardman JG, Limbird LE, eds. *The Pharmacological Basis of Therapeutics*. 10th ed. New York, NY: Macmillan; 2001:1851-1875.
27. Kosnett MJ. The role of chelation in the treatment of arsenic and mercury poisoning. *J Med Toxicol*. 2013;9:347-354.
28. Kosnett MJ. Unanswered questions in metal chelation. *J Toxicol Clin Toxicol*. 1992;30:529-547.
29. Longcope WT, Luetscher JA. The use of BAL (British anti-Lewisite) in the treatment of the injurious effects of arsenic, mercury and other metallic poisons. *Ann Intern Med*. 1949;31:545-554.
30. Longcope WT, et al. Clinical uses of 2,3-dimercaptopropanol (BAL): XI. The treatment of acute mercury poisoning by BAL. *J Clin Invest*. 1946;25:557-567.
31. Longcope WT, et al. Clinical uses of 2,3-dimercaptopropanol (BAL): VII. The treatment of arsenical dermatitis with preparations of BAL. *J Clin Invest*. 1946;25:528-533.
32. Luetscher JA, et al. Clinical uses of 2,3-dimercaptopropanol (BAL): VIII. The effect of BAL on the excretion of arsenic in arsenical intoxication. *J Clin Invest*. 1946;25:534-540.
33. Maher JF, Schreiner GE. The dialysis of mercury and mercury-BAL complex. *Clin Res*. 1959;7:298.
34. Mahieu P, et al. The metabolism of arsenic in humans acutely intoxicated by As$_2$O$_3$: its significance for the duration of BAL therapy. *J Toxicol Clin Toxicol*. 1981;18:1067-1075.
35. Oehme FW. British anti-Lewisite (BAL): the classic heavy metal antidote. *Clin Toxicol*. 1972;5:215-222.
36. Pearson RG. Hard and soft acids and bases; NSAB. Part II. Underlying theories. *J Chem Educ*. 1968;45:643-648.
37. Peters RA. Biochemistry of some toxic agents. *J Clin Invest*. 1955;34:1-20.

38. Peters RA, et al. The use of British anti-Lewisite containing radioactive sulfur for metabolism investigations. *Biochem J.* 1947;41:370-373.

39. Peters RA, et al. British anti-Lewisite (BAL). *Nature.* 1945;156:616-618.

40. Randall RV, Seeler AO. BAL. *N Engl J Med.* 1948;239:1004-1009; 1040-1048.

41. Schafer B, et al. Effect of oral treatment with BAL, DMPS or DMSA arsenic in organs of mice injected with arsenic trioxide. *Arch Toxicol.* 1991;14(suppl):228-230.

42. Seifert SA, et al. Accidental, intravenous infusion of a peanut oil-based medication. *J Toxicol Clin Toxicol.* 1998;36:733-736.

43. Spray GM, et al. Further investigations on the metabolism of 2,3-dimercaptopropanol. *Biochem J.* 1947;41:363-366.

44. Stocken LA, Thompson RM. Reactions of British anti-Lewisite with arsenic and other metals in living systems. *Physiol Rev.* 1949;29:168-194.

45. Thurtle N, et al. Description of 3,180 courses of chelation with dimercaptosuccinic acid in children ≤5 y with severe lead poisoning in Zamfara, Northern Nigeria: a retrospective analysis of programme data. *PLoS Med.* 2014;11:e1001739.

46. Vaziri ND, et al. Hemodialysis clearance of arsenic. *Clin Toxicol.* 1980;17:451-456.

47. Vilensky J, Redman K. British anti-Lewisite (dimercaprol): an amazing history. *Ann Emerg Med.* 2003;41:378-383.

48. Wang E, et al. Successful treatment of potentially fatal heavy metal poisoning. *J Emerg Med.* 2007;32:289-294.

49. Wexler J, et al. Clinical uses of 2,3-dimercaptopropanol (BAL): II. The effect of BAL on the excretion of arsenic in normal subjects after minimal exposure to arsenical smoke. *J Clin Invest.* 1946;25:467-473.

50. Woody NC, Kometani JT. BAL in the treatment of arsenic ingestion of children. *Pediatrics.* 1948;1:372-378.

51. Zimmer LJ, Carter DE. The effect of 2,3-dimercaptopropanol and D-penicillamine on methyl mercury-induced neurological signs and weight loss. *Life Sci.* 1978;23:1025-1034.

87 BISMUTH

Rama B. Rao

HISTORY AND EPIDEMIOLOGY

Elemental bismuth is nontoxic. Bismuth salts have therapeutic uses and are responsible for the toxicities described in this chapter. Thus, the term *bismuth* in this chapter refers to bismuth salts. Nearly 300 years ago, bismuth was recognized as medicinally valuable. It was included in topical salves and oral preparations for various gastrointestinal (GI) disorders. Nephrotoxicity was first described as early as 1802. In the early 20th century, acute kidney injury was reported in children administered intramuscular bismuth salts for the treatment of gingivostomatitis.[8,28,51,52] Administration of bismuth thioglycollate and its related water-soluble compounds, triglycollamate and trithioglycollamate, were responsible for the kidney failure, which occurred with as little as one or 2 doses.[9,13,32,37,41,59] Children with kidney failure would typically present with abdominal pain, oliguria, anuria, malaise, depressed mental status, and vomiting. Alterations in consciousness usually abated with chelation or resolution of the uremia. After the use of intramuscular injections was abandoned, this form of bismuth-induced kidney failure became rare. Syphilis was previously treated with intramuscular bismuth. A rash known as "erythema of the 9th day," consisting of a diffuse macular rash of the trunk and extremities, occasionally occurred and resolved without intervention.[17]

In patients administered "Analbis" antipyretic rectal suppositories, hepatic failure was described histopathologically as yellow atrophy with vacuolization.[4,25] An investigation of the suppositories suggested that diallylacetic acid, a xenobiotic that is no longer marketed in the United States, and not bismuth, was the hepatotoxin.

Today, bismuth is one of many xenobiotics commonly used in prescription and nonprescription oral preparations for treatment of traveler's diarrhea, nausea, and vomiting. In addition, bismuth-impregnated surgical packing paste is used for the treatment of the flatus and odor associated with ileostomies and colostomies,[10,61] and as an adjunct in the treatment of oral and gastrointestinal ulcers.[15,18] In the GI tract, bismuth binds to sulfhydryl groups and decreases fecal odor through formation of bismuth sulfide.[54] Sulfhydryl binding is also the proposed mechanism for the antimicrobial effect of bismuth, causing lysis of *Helicobacter pylori*, the causative bacteria in peptic ulcer formation. Bismuth also inhibits bacterial enzyme function, as well as prevent adhesion of *H. pylori* to the gastric mucosa.[60]

Epidemics of bismuth-induced encephalopathy, particularly among patients with ileostomies or colostomies, were reported from France, Britain, and Australia.[7,11,29,31,35] As a result, some countries banned or restricted bismuth preparations to prescription only. Bismuth subsalicylate, which is currently available in the United States as a nonprescription remedy, is still periodically responsible for cases of encephalopathy.[16,19,33] Other reported causes of bismuth-induced encephalopathy include systemic absorption from bismuth-impregnated surgical packing paste and transdermal absorption from long-term application of a bismuth-containing skin cream.[27]

In 2006, the United States Food and Drug Administration (FDA) issued a warning on an alternative health product known as "bismacine" or "chromacine." This alternative medicine product was not FDA approved, but was used by some practitioners as an injectable treatment for Lyme disease, for which efficacy data are lacking. The product contains bismuth citrate and was associated with at least one death and other adverse events.[2]

CHEMISTRY AND TOXICOLOGY

Bismuth is present in nature in both the trivalent and pentavalent forms. The trivalent form of bismuth is used for all medicinal purposes, usually as the bismuthyl (BiO) moiety generated by hydrolysis of trivalent bismuth compounds to yield a low-solubility alkaline salt. Bismuth salts are divided into 4 groups based on their water or lipid solubility; or whether they are organic or inorganic (Table 87-1). Most orally administered bismuth remains in the GI tract, and is subsequently excreted in the feces, and with only 0.2% is systemically absorbed.[22] Absorption of some bismuth preparations such as colloidal bismuth subcitrate increases as gastric pH increases.[39] The time to peak absorption ranges between 15 and 60 minutes with high intra- and interindividual variation.[26,28] The serum-to-blood ratio of bismuth is 1.55.[5] The distribution and elimination of orally administered bismuth follows a complex, multicompartmental model. The volume of distribution in humans is unknown.[6,46,47]

Novel research of bismuth uptake in human cells indicates that up to 90% of bismuth is passively absorbed and binds to glutathione and is transported by a multidrug-resistant protein into vesicles. In the same in vitro model, human cells depleted of glutathione and exposed to bismuth had reduced cell survival.[20]

Once in the circulation, bismuth binds to α_2-macroglobulin, IgM, β-lipoprotein, and haptoglobin. Bismuth rapidly enters liver, kidney, lungs, and bone.[55] It crosses the placenta and enters the amniotic fluid and fetal circulation.[57] It also readily crosses the blood–brain barrier.[38] Evidence in a rat model suggests that, when administered intramuscularly, bismuth enters the central nervous system (CNS) via retrograde axonal transport.[53] In both animal models and human reports, bismuth is identified in the fenestrated membranes of synaptosomes,[41,44] localizing in the thalamus and cerebellum with diffuse cortical uptake as well.[28,38] Ninety percent of absorbed bismuth is eliminated through the kidneys, where it induces the production of its own metal-binding protein.[55]

Three different half-lives describe the pharmacokinetics of orally administered therapeutic doses of bismuth.[6,46] The first, the distribution half-life, is approximately 1 to 4 hours. The second, the apparent plasma half-life, lasts 5 to 11 days. The third is the apparent half-life of urinary excretion lasting between 21 and 72 days[5] with urinary bismuth detected as late as 5 months after the last oral dose.[26]

PATHOPHYSIOLOGY

Like other metals, bismuth toxicity involves multiple organ systems. The effect of different bismuth salts can be categorized into 4 groups based on solubility and GI absorption (Table 87–1).[46,47] The highly lipid-soluble compounds such as bismuth subsalicylate or bismuth subgallate are most commonly associated with neurotoxicity.

Bismuth-induced encephalopathy likely results from neuronal sulfhydryl binding. In patients who die of bismuth encephalopathy, the gray-matter concentration of bismuth is nearly twice that of white-matter.[28] In a patient with bismuth encephalopathy dying from concomitant sepsis, the autopsy revealed loss of cerebellar Purkinje cells, which would be unexpected from sepsis.[29] The factors predisposing some individuals to encephalopathy from lipid soluble bismuth salts, however, are not well defined. Age, gender, and duration of

TABLE 87–1	The Physicochemical Characteristics of Bismuth Salts		
Group	Chemistry	Toxicity	Examples
I	Water insoluble Inorganic	Minimal Neurologic	Bismuth subnitrate Bismuth subcarbonate
II	Lipid soluble Organic	Neurologic Renal	Bismuth subsalicylate Bismuth subgallate
III	Water soluble Organic	Renal	Bismuth triglycollamate Dicitratobismuthate
IV	Hydrolyzable Water soluble Organic	Minimal	Bismuth bicitropeptide

TABLE 87–2	Differential Diagnosis of Bismuth Encephalopathy
Akinetic status epilepticus	
Creutzfeldt–Jacob disease	
Delirium tremens	
Hyperglycemic hyperosmolar syndrome	
Lithium toxicity (chronic)	
Malignant catatonia	
Myxedema coma	
Neurodegenerative leukoencephalopathies	
NMDA receptor antibody encephalitis	
Paradichlorobenzene encephalopathy	
Postanoxic and posthypoglycemic encephalopathies	
Progressive multifocal ataxia	
Tetanus/strychnine	
Viral encephalopathies	

NMDA = *N*-methyl-D-aspartate.

therapeutic use do not predict the likelihood of developing encephalopathy, but typically these patients were chronically treated (Table 87–1).

CLINICAL MANIFESTATIONS

Acute

Acute kidney injury is primarily due to exposure to the water-soluble bismuth salts (group III).[37,42] Massive overdoses of water-soluble bismuth salts result in abdominal pain and oliguria or anuria. In reported cases, overdoses of colloidal bismuth subsalicylate or tripotassium dicitratobismuthate (TDC) caused acute tubular necrosis.[1,21,23,51,52,56] Histopathologically, bismuth causes degeneration of the proximal tubule, similar to other metals. Although these xenobiotics are potentially neurotoxic, signs of encephalopathy are generally absent.[12,19] In one case, a patient with bismuth-induced kidney failure was described as having diminished deep tendon reflexes, muscle weakness, and myoclonus, without an alteration in consciousness.[21]

Neurotoxicity in the acute and subacute setting is less common, but also occurs. Bismuth subnitrate iodoform–impregnated surgical packs for oral surgery are implicated in neurotoxicity, occurring within as little as 9 days of exposure (Table 87–1).[3]

A young woman who reported ingesting 8 tablets of bismuth subsalicylate every 2 hours for up to 20 days developed hearing loss, tinnitus, and altered mental status within 5 days of her last dose. She subsequently developed chronic neurologic impairments.[48]

Chronic

The most common toxicologic finding associated with repeated therapeutic doses of oral bismuth compounds is a diffuse, progressive myoclonic encephalopathy.[12,19] Affected patients exhibit neurobehavioral changes, such as apathy and irritability. With continued exposure, these patients develop difficulty concentrating, diminished short-term memory, and occasionally, visual hallucinations.[30,31] A movement disorder characterized by muscle twitching, myoclonus, ataxia, and tremors ensues.[12] Weakness and, rarely, seizures ultimately advance to immobility.[33,35] With continued bismuth administration, these patients develop coma and die.

Rarely, patients recovering from severe encephalopathy complain of scapular, humeral, or vertebral pain because of fractures caused by severe neuromuscular manifestations such as myoclonus.[14]

Like several other metals, bismuth often causes a generalized pigmentation of skin. Deposition of bismuth sulfide into the mucosa causes a blue-black discoloration of gums.[62] This occurs in the absence of toxic effects. Formation of the same compound in the GI tract causes blackening of the stool. Liver failure is rarely reported, except in patients with multisystem organ failure from fatal neurotoxicity.

DIAGNOSIS

The clinician must have an index of suspicion based on the acute or chronic nature of the exposure. For oral exposures, the class of bismuth salt ingested will determine primary organ toxicity. Patients with acute massive overdoses should be evaluated for acute kidney injury. Formation of nuclear inclusion bodies can be identified on renal biopsy or on postmortem examination.[13,43]

The diagnosis of bismuth-induced encephalopathy is based on a history of exposure coupled with diffuse neuropsychiatric and motor findings.[31] Other causes of encephalopathy should be entertained and excluded (Table 87–2). An abdominal radiograph will likely demonstrate radiopacities of bismuth in the intestines. Stool likely will be black and test negative for occult blood.

The presence of bismuth in the blood is confirmatory of exposure, but absolute concentrations correlate poorly with morbidity.[6] In a review of 310 patients with bismuth-induced encephalopathy, 288 (93%) had a blood concentration greater than 10 mcg/dL, with the majority of these blood concentrations between 10 and 100 mcg/dL.[30] Twenty-two patients had encephalopathy at blood concentrations lower than 10 mcg/dL.[30] In another report, 2 patients with encephalopathy had blood concentrations of 90 and 250 mcg/dL, both of whom recovered when their concentrations fell below 50 mcg/dL.[7] Just as blood concentrations do not reflect severity of illness, tissue concentrations also correlate poorly with severity of illness. This is demonstrated by a patient who recovered from a severe bismuth encephalopathy. On discharge, he had a low blood bismuth concentration and died 3 months later of unrelated trauma. At autopsy, he had an elevated CNS bismuth concentration but no reported symptoms at the time of the trauma.[11]

The electroencephalographic (EEG) findings of patients with bismuth encephalopathy generally demonstrate nonspecific slow-wave changes.[16,21] In one study, the EEG findings were described in association with blood concentrations. At less than 5 mcg/dL, the EEG was normal or demonstrated diffuse slowing. In patients with blood concentrations up to 150 mcg/dL, the findings of sharp-wave abnormalities were noted. At higher concentrations (>200 mcg/dL), some patients with neurologic events, such as myoclonic jerks, did not have corresponding EEG changes. The authors proposed that an elevated body burden might have an inhibitory effect on the cerebral cortex paradoxically affecting EEG findings.[11]

In encephalopathic patients with blood concentrations greater than 200 mcg/dL, diagnostic imaging such as computed tomography demonstrates a diffuse cortical hyperdensity of the gray matter.[11] These findings tend to resolve with recovery. Magnetic resonance image was normal in another encephalopathic patient.[16]

TREATMENT

Typically, cessation of bismuth exposure and supportive care results in a complete recovery. For toxicity from bismuth-iodoform–impregnated surgical packing, removal is warranted.[3] For oral bismuth exposures, some authors suggest GI decontamination with activated charcoal and polyethylene glycol solution.[49] Administration of polyethylene glycol solution is recommended until the rectal effluent is clear. Although evidence for activated charcoal is lacking, one dose, especially in patients with severe encephalopathy from oral exposure, is reasonable once the airway it protected. In patients with kidney failure, resolution is generally observed with supportive care. The use of chelators in patients with acute overdose without neurotoxicity is probably not indicated.

It is uncertain whether different chelators affect the clinical course of patients with bismuth encephalopathy (see Chelation below). Withdrawal of the source of bismuth results in complete reversal of effects within days to weeks, even in those patients who are severely ill. Prevention is the most effective means of avoiding neurotoxicity. Blood concentrations of bismuth are not routinely performed nor readily available, but a bismuth concentration above 10 mcg/dL or symptoms at lower concentrations warrant withdrawal of bismuth therapy.

Although novel data on the role of glutathione in bismuth uptake are described,[20] the clinical significance of this finding is unknown. The role of intravenous N-acetylcysteine to replete glutathione is not known at this time. In life-threatening cases of severe bismuth poisoning, it is reasonable to administer N-acetylcysteine at doses typically used for the treatment of acetaminophen toxicity.

CHELATION

In general, the data regarding chelation are limited and in vitro, and animal models are not clearly predictive of human response. Chelation therapy with dimercaprol (BAL) is beneficial in experimental models,[49,52] reportedly beneficial in humans,[34] and often recommended by others, although clear evidence of efficacy is lacking. Dimercaprol undergoes biliary elimination, offering a major advantage over other chelators in patients who develop acute kidney injury. Based on the limited data available, it is reasonable to administer dimercaprol in encephalopathic patients with kidney failure in whom no neurologic improvement is noted within 48 hours of whole-bowel irrigation and bismuth withdrawal (Antidotes in Depth: A28).

One report of a patient with bismuth-induced kidney injury advocated the addition of dimercaptopropane sulfonate (DMPS), as BAL did not affect hemodialysis clearance, but the addition of DMPS to patients needing hemodialysis was effective in enhancing elimination.[52] It is uncertain whether the clinical course of the patients was improved. In human volunteers given colloidal bismuth subcitrate, succimer and DMPS, both at a dose of 30 mg/kg, increased urinary elimination of bismuth by 50-fold.[50] The availability of DMPS and indications for use are limited (Antidotes in Depth: A29). Although succimer can be added to severe cases, there is no current data that outcomes are changed once the offending source of bismuth is withheld or removed.

In an animal model, D-penicillamine was most efficacious in enhancing elimination of bismuth. In a human volunteer model using therapeutic doses of tripotassium-dicitrato-bismuthate, however, a single dose of D-penicillamine did not enhance urinary excretion.[36] Based on the above information, we recommend withdrawal of bismuth therapy and whole-bowel irrigation as a first intervention. Although data on chelation efficacy is lacking, BAL is reasonable in patients with life-threatening encephalopathy unresponsive to initial measures after 48 hours.

BISMUTH DRUG INTERACTIONS AND REACTIONS

The coadministration of proton pump inhibitors (PPIs) increases the absorption of some bismuth preparations. In a prospective evaluation of patients receiving different treatment regimens for H. pylori–induced dyspepsia or peptic ulcer disease, individuals taking PPIs had a statistically significant elevation in their blood bismuth concentrations, with 3 patients exceeding 5,000 mcg/dL, compared with a similar group administered bismuth without PPIs. The authors suggest that the bismuth preparation used, colloidal bismuth subcitrate, is more soluble and absorbable at the higher gastric pH of patients on PPIs.[22] All these patients received short courses of therapy (2 weeks). Although the investigators did not attempt to follow neurobehavioral or neuropsychiatric changes, none of the patients had clinically evident bismuth toxicity.[39]

Based on this investigation, coadministration of PPIs with longer courses of colloidal bismuth subcitrate should be avoided or only offered with extreme caution. Ranitidine, which is frequently prescribed with a bismuth compound for dyspepsia or ulcer disease, does not affect the pharmacokinetics of bismuth absorption.[26]

In the United States, where bismuth subsalicylate is the most common oral bismuth-containing compound, up to 90% of the salicylate is absorbed.[40,45] Salicylate toxicity is rare but reported, and salicylate concentrations should be determined in both acute and chronic exposures.[45,51] Methemoglobinemia from subnitrate salt of bismuth is uncommonly described.[24]

SUMMARY

- Bismuth toxicity manifests as nephrotoxicity following exposure to group III water soluble bismuth salts.
- Myoclonic encephalopathy, myoclonices, and coma occur following chronic exposure to Group II (lipophilic) bismuth salts.
- Supportive care, whole-bowel irrigation, and withdrawal of the bismuth-containing compound are the mainstays of treatment.
- Dimercaprol is reasonable in patients with life threatening encephalopathy unresponsive to initial measures after 48 hours.
- Salicylate concentrations are elevated in some cases of chronic bismuth subsalicylate poisoning.

REFERENCES

1. Akpolat I, et al. Acute renal failure due to overdose of colloidal bismuth. *Nephrol Dial Transplant.* 1996;11:1890-1898.
2. Anonymous. Warning on bismacine. *FDA Consum.* 2006;40:5.
3. Atwal A, Cousin GCS. Bismuth toxicity in patients treated with bismuth iodoform paraffin packs. *Br J Oral Maxillo Surg.* 2016;54:111-112.
4. Barnett RN. Reactions to a bismuth compound. Toxic manifestations following the use of the bismuth salt of heptadienecarboxylic acid in suppositories. *JAMA.* 1947;135:28-30.
5. Benet LZ. Safety and pharmacokinetics: colloidal bismuth subcitrate. *Scand J Gastroenterol.* 1991;25(suppl 185):29-35.
6. Bennet JE, et al. Modeling trough plasma bismuth concentrations. *J Pharmacokinet Biopharm.* 1997;25:79-106.
7. Bes A, et al. Encephalopathie toxique par les sels de bismuth. *Rev Med Toulouse.* 1976;12:810-813.
8. Bierer DW. Bismuth subsalicylate: history chemistry, and safety. *Rev Infect Dis.* 1990; 12:S3-S8.
9. Boyette DP, Ahiskie NC. Bismuth nephrosis with anuria in an infant. *J Pediatr.* 1946;28:493-497.
10. Bridgeman AM, Smith AC. Iatrogenic bismuth poisoning: case report. *Aust Dental J.* 1994;39:279-281.
11. Buge A, et al. Epileptic phenomena in bismuth toxic encephalopathy. *J Neurol Neurosurg Psychiatry.* 1981;44:62-67.
12. Burns R, et al. Reversible encephalopathy possibly associated with bismuth subgallate ingestion. *Br Med J.* 1974;1:220-223.
13. Czerwinski AW, Ginn HE. Bismuth nephrotoxicity. *Am J Med.* 1964;37:969-975.
14. Emile J, et al. Osteoarticular complications in bismuth encephalopathy. *Clin Toxicol.* 1981;18:1285-1290.
15. Goldenberg MM, et al. Antinauseant and antiemetic properties of bismuth subsalicylate in dogs and humans. *J Pharmacol Sci.* 1976;65:1398-1400.
16. Gordon MF, et al. Bismuth subsalicylate toxicity as a cause of prolonged encephalopathy with myoclonus. *Mov Disord.* 1995;10:220-222.
17. Gryboski JD, Gotoff SP. Bismuth nephrotoxicity. *N Engl J Med.* 1961;265:1289-1291.
18. Hansen PB, Penkowa M. Bismuth adjuvant ameliorates adverse effects of high dose chemotherapy in patients with multiple myeloma, and malignant lymphoma undergoing autologous stem cell transplantation: a randomized double-blind, prospective study. *Support Care Cancer.* 2017;25:1279-1289.
19. Hasking GJ, Duggan JM. Encephalopathy from bismuth subsalicylate. *Med J Aust.* 1982;2:167.
20. Hong Y, et al. Glutathione and MDR protein transporter mediate self-propelled disposal of bismuth in human cells. *Proc Natl Acad Sci U S A.* 2015;112:3211-3216.
21. Hudson M, Mowat NAG. Reversible toxicity in poisoning with colloidal bismuth subcitrate. *BMJ.* 1989;299:159.
22. Hundal O, et al. Absorption of bismuth from two bismuth compounds before and after healing of peptic ulcers. *Hepatogastroenterology.* 1999;46:2882-2886.
23. Huwez F, et al. Acute renal failure after overdose of colloidal bismuth subcitrate. *Lancet.* 1992;340:1298.
24. Jacobsen JB, Huttel MS. Methemoglobin after excessive intake of a subnitrate containing antacid. *Ugeskr Laeger.* 1982;144:2340-2350.
25. Karelitz S, Freedman AD. Hepatitis and nephrosis due to soluble bismuth. *Pediatrics.* 1951;8:772-776.

26. Koch KM, et al. Pharmacokinetics of bismuth and ranitidine following multiple doses of ranitidine bismuth citrate. *Br J Clin Pharmacol.* 1996;42:207-211.

27. Kruger G, et al. Disturbed oxidative metabolism in organic brain syndrome caused by bismuth in skin creams. *Lancet.* 1976;1:485-487.

28. Lambert JR. Pharmacology of bismuth-containing compounds. *Rev Infect Dis.* 1991;13:S691-S695.

29. Liessens JL, et al. Bismuth encephalopathy. *Act Neurol Belg.* 1978;78:301-309.

30. Martin-Bouyer G, et al. Epidemiological study of encephalopathies following bismuth administration per os. Characteristics of intoxicated subjects: comparison with a control group. *Clin Toxicol.* 1981;18:1277-1283.

31. Martin-Bouyer G, Weller M. Neuropsychiatric symptoms following bismuth intoxication. *Postgrad Med J.* 1988;64:308-310.

32. McClendon SJ. Toxic effects with anuria from a single injection of a bismuth preparation. *Am J Dis Child.* 1941;61:339-341.

33. Mendelowitz PC, et al. Bismuth absorption and myoclonic encephalopathy during bismuth subsalicylate therapy. *Ann Intern Med.* 1990;112:140-141.

34. Molina JA, et al. Myoclonic encephalopathy due to bismuth salts: treatment with dimercaprol and analysis of CSF transmitters. *Acta Neurol Scand.* 1989;79:200-203.

35. Monseu G, et al. Bismuth encephalopathy. *Acta Neurol Belg.* 1976;76:301-308.

36. Nwokolo CU, Pounder RE. D-penicillamine does not increase urinary bismuth excretion in patients treated with tripotassium dicitrato bismuthate. *Br J Clin Pharmacol.* 1990;30:648-650.

37. O'Brien D. Anuria due to bismuth thioglycollate. *Am J Dis Child.* 1959;97:384-386.

38. Pamphlett R, et al. Uptake of bismuth in motor neurons of mice after single oral doses of bismuth compounds. *Neurotoxicol Teratol.* 2000;22:559-563.

39. Phillips RH, et al. Is eradication of *Helicobacter pylori* with colloidal bismuth subcitrate quadruple therapy safe? *Helicobacter.* 2001;6:151-156.

40. Pickering LK, et al. Absorption of salicylate and bismuth from a bismuth subsalicylate containing compound (Pepto-Bismol). *J Pediatr.* 1981;99:654-656.

41. Pollet S, et al. Bismuth intoxication: bismuth level in pig brain lipids and in subcellular fractions. *Toxicol Eur Res.* 1979;2:123-125.

42. Randall RE, et al. Bismuth nephrotoxicity. *Ann Intern Med.* 1972;77:481-482.

43. Rodilla V, et al. Exposure of human cultured proximal tubule cells to cadmium, mercury, zinc, and bismuth: toxicity and metallothionein induction. *Chem Biol Interact.* 1998;115:71-83.

44. Ross JF, et al. Highest brain bismuth levels and neuropathology are adjacent to fenestrated blood vessels in mouse brain after intraperitoneal dosing of bismuth subnitrate. *Toxicol Appl Pharmacol.* 1994;124:191-200.

45. Sainsbury SJ. Fatal salicylate toxicity from bismuth subsalicylate. *West J Med.* 1991;155:637-639.

46. Serfontein WJ, Mekel R. Bismuth toxicity in man II. Review of bismuth blood and urine levels in patients after administration of therapeutic bismuth formulations in relation to the problem of bismuth toxicity in man. *Res Commun Chemical Pathol Pharmacol.* 1979;26:391-411.

47. Serfontein WJ, et al. Bismuth toxicity in man I: bismuth blood and urine levels in patients after administration of a bismuth protein complex (bictropeptide). *Res Commun Chem Pathol Pharmacol.* 1979;26:383-389.

48. Siram R, et al. Chronic encephalopathy with ataxia, myoclonus, and auditory neuropathy: a case of bismuth poisoning. *Neuro India.* 2017;65:186-187.

49. Slikkerveer A, et al. Development of a therapeutic procedure for bismuth intoxication with chelating agents. *J Lab Clin Med.* 1992;119:529-537.

50. Slikkerveer A, et al. Comparison of enhanced elimination of bismuth in humans after treatment with meso-2,3 dimercaptosuccinic acid and d,l-2,3-dimercaptopropane-1-sulfonic acid. *Analyst.* 1998;123:91-92.

51. Stevens PE, Bierer DW. Bismuth subsalicylate: history chemistry, and safety. *Rev Infect Dis.* 1990;12:S3-S8.

52. Stevens PE, et al. Significant elimination of bismuth by haemodialysis with a new heavy metal chelating agent. *Nephrol Dial Transplant.* 1995;10:696-698.

53. Stoltenberg M, et al. Retrograde axonal transport of bismuth: an autometallographic study. *Acta Neuropathol.* 2001;101:123-128.

54. Suarez FL, et al. Bismuth subsalicylate markedly decreases hydrogen sulfide release in the human colon. *Gastroenterology.* 1998;114:923-929.

55. Szymanska JA, et al. Some aspects of bismuth metabolism. *Clin Toxicol.* 1981;18:1291-1298.

56. Taylor EG, Klenerman P. Acute renal failure after bismuth subcitrate overdose. *Lancet.* 1990;335:670-671.

57. Thompson HE, et al. The transfer of bismuth into fetal circulation after maternal administration of sobisimol. *Am J Syp.* 1941;25:725-730.

58. Tremaine WJ, et al. Bismuth carbomer foam enemas for chronic pouchitis: a randomized, double-blind, placebo-controlled trial. *Aliment Pharmacol Ther.* 1997;11:1041-1046.

59. Urizar R, Vernier RL. Bismuth nephropathy. *JAMA.* 1966;198:207-209.

60. Walsh JH, Peterson WL. Drug therapy: the treatment of *Helicobacter pylori* infection in the management of peptic ulcer disease. *N Engl J Med.* 1995;333:984-991.

61. Wilson APR. The dangers of BIPP. *Lancet.* 1994;334:1313-1314.

62. Zala L, et al. Pigmentation following long-term bismuth therapy for pneumatosis cystoides intestinalis. *Dermatology.* 1993;187:288-289.

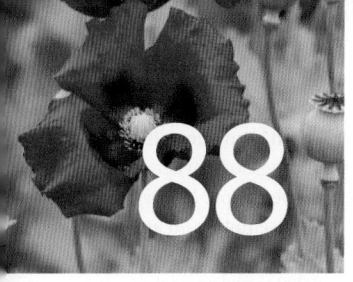

88 CADMIUM

Stephen J. Traub and Robert S. Hoffman

Cadmium (Cd)
Atomic number = 48
Atomic weight = 112.4 Da
Normal concentrations
   Whole blood   < 5 mcg/L (44.5 nmol/L)
   Urine   < 3 mcg/g creatinine
         < 26.7 nmol/g creatinine

HISTORY AND EPIDEMIOLOGY

Cadmium, atomic number 48, is a transition metal in IUPAC group 12 of the modern periodic table. In its pure atomic form, it is a bluish solid at room temperature. It is readily oxidized to a divalent ion, Cd^{2+}. Naturally occurring cadmium commonly exists as cadmium sulfide (CdS), a trace contaminant of zinc-containing ores.[39]

Cadmium sulfide, cadmium oxide, and other cadmium-containing compounds are refined to produce elemental cadmium, which is used for industrial purposes. When combined with other metals, cadmium forms alloys of relatively low melting points, which accounts for its extensive use in solders and brazing rods. Today, cadmium is primarily used as a reagent in electroplating and in the production of nickel-cadmium batteries. Other uses of cadmium include as a pigment in patient and as a neutron absorber in nuclear reactors. Cadmium salts were once also used as veterinary antihelminthics.[14]

As cadmium processing has increased, so has the incidence of cadmium toxicity. Cadmium toxicity usually occurs after environmental, occupational, or hobby work exposure.

Environmental Exposure

Environmental exposure to cadmium generally occurs through the consumption of foods grown in cadmium-contaminated areas. Because cadmium is fairly common as an impurity in ores, areas where mining or refining of ores takes place are the most likely to contain cadmium-contaminated soil.

In the 1950s, a mine near the Jinzu River basin in Japan discharged large amounts of cadmium into the environment, contaminating the rice that was a staple of the local food supply. An epidemic of painful osteomalacia followed, affecting hundreds of people, particularly postmenopausal multiparous women.[70] The afflicted were prone to develop pathologic fractures, and were reported to call out "itai-itai" ("ouch-ouch") as they walked because of the severity of their pain.[30] These symptoms were ultimately linked to cadmium, and the event came to be known as the Itai-Itai epidemic. Less consequential environmental cadmium exposures are also reported from Sweden,[49] Belgium,[12] and China.[51] Smokers have higher blood cadmium concentrations than nonsmokers,[96] probably as a result of contamination of soil where the tobacco is grown. This is noteworthy, in that cadmium and tobacco are reported to be synergistic causes of chronic pulmonary disease.[66]

Occupational and Hobby Exposure

Welders, solderers, and jewelry workers who use cadmium-containing alloys are at risk for developing acute cadmium toxicity due to inhalation of cadmium oxide fumes. Other workers who do not work with metals per se are at risk for chronic cadmium toxicity through exposure to cadmium-containing dust.

Hobbyists who work with cadmium solders have exposures similar to occupational metalworkers. Significant cadmium toxicity in this population is usually the result of metalworking in a closed space with inadequate ventilation and/or improper respiratory precautions.

TOXICOKINETICS

There is no known biologic role for cadmium. Ingested cadmium salts are poorly bioavailable (5%–20%), whereas inhaled cadmium fumes (cadmium oxide) are readily bioavailable (up to 90%).[104] As the only data on cadmium toxicokinetics are derived from work with cadmium salts and oxides, the term "cadmium" in the following discussions refers to these species unless otherwise noted.

After exposure, cadmium is absorbed into the bloodstream, where it is bound to α_2-macroglobulin and albumin.[105] It is then quickly and preferentially redistributed to the liver and kidney, and to a lesser extent to other organs such as the pancreas, spleen, heart, lung, and testes.[27] Cadmium enters target organs via 3 possible mechanisms: zinc and calcium transporters; uptake of cadmium–glutathione or cadmium–cysteine complexes by transport proteins; and/or endocytosis of cadmium–protein complexes.[111]

After incorporation into the liver and kidney, cadmium forms a complex with metallothionein, an endogenous thiol-rich protein that is produced in both organs. Metallothionein binds and sequesters cadmium. Over time, hepatic stores of the cadmium–metallothionein complex (Cd-MT) are slowly released. Circulating Cd-MT is filtered by the glomerulus but reabsorbed and concentrated in proximal tubular cells,[21,91,92] explaining why the kidney is a principal target organ in cadmium toxicity.

There is no evidence that cadmium ions are oxidized, reduced, methylated, or otherwise biotransformed in vivo. The volume of distribution (V_d) of cadmium is unknown, but is presumably quite large as a consequence of significant hepatic sequestration. Cadmium distribution and elimination are complex, and an 8-compartment kinetic model is proposed.[57] The slow release of cadmium from metallothionein-complexed hepatic stores accounts for its very long biologic half-life of 10 or more years.

PATHOPHYSIOLOGY
Cellular Pathophysiology

Cadmium toxicity results from interactions of the free cations with target cells.[27,38,64,69,92] Complexation with metallothionein is cytoprotective,[24,64] and metallothionein functions as a natural chelator with a strong affinity for cadmium.[20,58] Although metallothionein plays a role in proximal tubular concentration of cadmium, kidney damage is attenuated by metallothionein, as metallothionein-deficient mice are more susceptible to cadmium toxicity than controls.[64]

There are several mechanisms by which cadmium interferes with cellular function. Cadmium binds to sulfhydryl groups, denaturing proteins and/or inactivating enzymes. The mitochondria are severely affected by this process,[1] which results in an increased susceptibility to oxidative stress.[50] Generally, cadmium affects processes involved in DNA repair, generation of reactive oxygen species, and induction of apoptosis.[80] Specifically, cadmium interferes with mediators of cell adhesion such as E-cadherin, N-cadherin, and β-catenin,[76-78] and interacts with other proteins such as kinesin[10] and amyloid beta protein 1-42.[71] Finally, the demonstrated interference of cadmium with calcium transport mechanisms[101,102] leads to intracellular hypercalcemia and, ultimately, apoptosis

Specific Organ System Injury (Table 88–1)
Kidney

The kidney damage caused by cadmium develops over years. Proteinuria is the most common clinical finding and correlates with proximal tubular dysfunction, which manifests as urinary loss of low-molecular-weight proteins

TABLE 88–1	Major Acute and Chronic Organ System Effects of Cadmium	
Organ	*Acute*	*Chronic*
Kidney		Proteinuria
		Nephrolithiasis
Bone		Osteomalacia
Lung	Pneumonitis	Cancer
Gastrointestinal system	Caustic injury	

such as β_2-microglobulin and retinol-binding protein. Cadmium also produces hypercalciuria,[88] possibly also via damage to the proximal tubule.

Musculoskeletal

Cadmium-induced osteomalacia is a result of abnormalities in calcium and phosphate homeostasis, which, in turn, result from renal proximal tubular dysfunction. In one autopsy study, the severity of osteomalacia in cadmium exposed subjects correlated with a decline in the serum calcium-phosphate product.[95]

Pulmonary

Acute cadmium pneumonitis is characterized by infiltrates on chest radiograph and hypoxia. Human autopsy studies[35,75,89,106] generally show degeneration and/or loss of bronchial and bronchiolar epithelial cells.

Gastrointestinal Tract

Based on case reports,[13,107] ingested cadmium salts are caustic with the potential to induce significant nausea, vomiting, and abdominal pain, and result in GI hemorrhage, necrosis, and perforation. With respect to their effect on the GI mucosa, cadmium salts act similar to mercuric salts (Chap. 95).

CLINICAL MANIFESTATIONS

Acute Poisoning

Pulmonary/Cadmium Fumes

Cadmium pneumonitis results from inhalation of cadmium oxide fumes. The acute phase of cadmium pneumonitis mimics metal fume fever (Chap. 121), but the 2 entities are distinctly different. Whereas metal fume fever is benign and self-limited, acute cadmium pneumonitis progresses to hypoxia, respiratory insufficiency, and death.

Published case reports of patients who develop acute cadmium pneumonitis[4,5,34,75,89,98,106,110] are strikingly similar in their presentation. Within 6 to 12 hours of soldering or brazing with cadmium alloys in a closed space, patients typically develop constitutional symptoms, such as fever and chills, as well as a cough and respiratory distress.

On initial presentation, patients often have a normal physical examination, oxygenation, and chest radiograph. This relatively mild presentation potentially leads both to the misdiagnosis of metal fume fever and an underestimation of the severity of illness. As the pneumonitis progresses to acute respiratory distress syndrome (ARDS) (Chap. 121), crackles and rhonchi develop, oxygenation becomes impaired, and the chest radiograph develops a pattern consistent with alveolar filling. In fulminant cases, death usually occurs within 3 to 5 days.[35,75,89,106]

Patients who survive an episode of acute cadmium pneumonitis are at increased risk for developing chronic pulmonary disorders, including restrictive lung disease,[4,5] diffusion abnormalities,[4] and pulmonary fibrosis,[98] although recovery without sequelae is also reported.[110]

Oral/Cadmium Salts

Most acute cadmium exposures are inhalational, and acute ingestions are rare. Based on case report data, GI injury is likely to be the most significant clinical finding after acute ingestion, although other presentations are possible.

In one case,[13] a 17-year-old student ingested approximately 150 g of cadmium chloride that she obtained from her school science stockroom. She presented to the emergency department with hypotension and edema of the face,

pharynx, and neck. Her condition quickly deteriorated, and she suffered a respiratory arrest. She was intubated and underwent orogastric lavage, chelation with an unspecified chelator, and charcoal hemoperfusion. Multisystem organ failure ensued, and she died within 30 hours of presentation. At autopsy, the most significant finding was hemorrhagic necrosis of the upper GI tract. Her blood cadmium concentration was more than 2,000 times normal.

In a second reported case, a 23-year-old man ingested approximately 5 g of cadmium iodide in a suicide attempt and presented with acute hemorrhagic gastroenteritis.[107] His condition deteriorated, and despite treatment with calcium disodium ethylenediaminetetraacetic acid ($CaNa_2EDTA$) and supportive measures, he died on hospital day 7. Autopsy did not reveal a specific cause of death.

A 51-year-old man taking multiple nutritional supplements who had no history to suggest cadmium exposure presented with a one-month history of fatigue, with laboratory findings suggestive of autoimmune hemolytic anemia. He was treated aggressively for that condition, but developed progressive multisystem organ failure and expired one week after presentation. His blood cadmium concentrations were extraordinarily high, suggesting an acute ingestion, although the source of cadmium was never determined.[81]

Chronic Poisoning

Nephrotoxicity

The most common finding in chronic cadmium poisoning is proteinuria. Low-molecular-weight proteinuria is usually more significant than, and generally precedes, glomerular dysfunction, although some cadmium-exposed workers manifest predominantly glomerular proteinuria.[7] There is a dose–response relationship between total body cadmium burden and kidney dysfunction,[12,47,49,70,100] although this relationship weakens at low doses.[42] Patients with diabetes mellitus are reported to be particularly susceptible to the nephrotoxic effects of cadmium.[40] In most cases, proteinuria is considered to be irreversible even after removal from exposure,[41,55,84] but improvement is sometimes reported.[63,99] Less clear is the question of whether kidney dysfunction progresses after removal from exposure, with studies showing both stable[41] and deteriorating[45,83,84] function in cadmium-exposed workers who are removed from exposure. The routes and duration of exposure, as well as blood and urine cadmium concentrations, differ markedly among these studies, limiting wider applicability of any analysis. Occupational cadmium exposure is also associated with nephrolithiasis,[48,87] likely as a result of hypercalciuria.[88]

Pulmonary Toxicity

Large studies of workers chronically exposed to relatively low concentrations of cadmium fail to demonstrate consistent effects on the lung. In one study of 57 workers with sufficient exposure to cadmium oxide to produce kidney dysfunction, there was no evidence of pulmonary dysfunction, even in those with the greatest cumulative cadmium exposure.[29] By contrast, other studies report both restrictive[19] and obstructive[23,86] changes on pulmonary function tests. Interestingly, a follow-up study of the group with restrictive lung disease showed improvements after cadmium exposure was reduced.[18] The discrepancies in these results are due in part to markedly different doses and durations of exposure among the various groups. Cadmium is also associated with pulmonary neoplasia; the carcinogenicity of cadmium is discussed separately (see Cancer below).

Musculoskeletal Toxicity

Cadmium-induced osteomalacia usually occurs in the setting of environmental exposure;[46] although mentioned in case reports,[8,56] osteomalacia is generally not a prominent feature of occupational exposure to cadmium. Gender and age differences explain part of this apparent difference: victims of the original Itai-Itai epidemic were mostly older women, whereas occupational cadmium exposures typically occur in younger men. In addition, differences in cumulative dosing and in route of exposure (oral vs pulmonary) partly account for the unique prominence of osteomalacia in patients with environmental exposures. Cadmium exposure is associated with osteopenia and osteoporosis even in areas (such as the United States) where widespread environmental exposure is unlikely.[108]

Hepatotoxicity

Although the liver stores as much cadmium as any other organ, hepatotoxicity is not a prominent feature in humans with cadmium exposure, probably because hepatic cadmium is usually complexed to metallothionein.[40] The liver is a potential target organ, however, as hepatotoxicity is easily inducible in animals.[1,25,26,77]

Neurologic Toxicity

Cadmium exposure is linked to olfactory disturbances,[67,85,94] impaired higher cortical function,[103] and parkinsonism.[72,103]

Cardiovascular

Cadmium induces hypertension in rats,[62] but human studies have only yielded unconvincing and conflicting results.[33,61,73,97] Cadmium is associated with the development of atherosclerotic plaques[34] as well as heart failure.[11]

Other Organ Systems

Although there is evidence that cadmium causes immunosuppression affecting both humoral and cell-mediated immunity in animals,[26] a single human study showed no overt immunopathology in an occupationally exposed cohort.[54] The testes are clearly a target organ in animal exposures,[60] but they are not considered a major target organ in humans.

Cancer

Cadmium induces tumors in multiple animal organs, an effect that is exacerbated by zinc deficiency.[104] In humans, cadmium exposure is principally associated with lung cancer.[74] The strength of this association is questioned, as most studies have methodologic problems such as coexposure to arsenic, a known pulmonary carcinogen.[9,56] Despite these confounding coexposures, cadmium is designated as a human carcinogen by the International Agency for Research on Cancer.[44]

DIAGNOSTIC TESTING

Other than to confirm exposure, cadmium concentrations have limited usefulness in the management of the acutely exposed patient. Diagnosis and treatment are based on the history, physical examination, and symptoms, and in acute exposures ancillary tests (such as pulse oximetry and chest radiography) are more useful than actual cadmium concentrations.

In the patient chronically exposed to cadmium, both cadmium concentrations and ancillary testing are recommended. Urinary cadmium concentrations, which reflect the slow, steady-state turnover and release of metallothionein-bound cadmium from the liver, are a better reflection of the total body cadmium burden than are whole blood concentrations. In a 22-year follow-up study, mortality was higher in those with elevated urine cadmium concentrations, although it was impossible to determine if the cadmium was causative or served as a marker for another process.[79]

Cadmium is a significant workplace toxin. In the United States, the Permissible Exposure Limit (PEL), expressed as the concentration of cadmium in air as an 8-hour time-weighted average exposure (TWA), is 5 mcg/m³. Workers must also be provided with lunchroom facilities in which the concentration of cadmium in air must be below 2.5 mcg/m³.

Yearly biologic monitoring plays an important role in the surveillance of workplace cadmium toxicity, and involves testing not only for urinary and blood levels of cadmium but for indices of renal function as well. Abnormalities in monitoring data require 90-day follow-up testing; if subsequent testing meets action levels, the worker must be medically removed from exposure to cadmium. Workers with higher cadmium indices on initial evaluation have lower thresholds for removal based on 90-day follow-up testing. Testing and removal thresholds for workplace cadmium testing are noted in Table 88–2.

The values noted for industrial hygiene are reasonable in light of the fact that kidney dysfunction is reported to occur at cadmium concentrations as low as 5 mcg/g urinary creatinine,[22,47] a concentration significantly higher than that of the general US population (95% of whom have concentrations that are less than 3 mcg/g urinary creatinine).[17]

TABLE 88–2	Workplace Cadmium Exposure Risk Assessment Values		
Biologic Index	Initial Low Risk Level	Initial High Risk Level	90-Day Medical Removal Level
Urine Cadmium (mcg/g Cr)	3		15
		7	7
Beta₂-Microglobulin (mcg/g Cr)	300		1,500
		750	750
Whole Blood Cadmium (mcg/L)	5		15
		10	10

MANAGEMENT

Acute Exposure

Oral Exposure/Cadmium Salts

After the patient's airway, breathing, and circulation are secured, attention should be given to GI decontamination. Although large ingestions of soluble cadmium salts are rare, they are potentially fatal,[13,107] with the lowest reported human lethal dose being 5 g. In light of this, if a significant ingestion occurs but emesis has not occurred, gastric lavage is recommended. In this situation, a small nasogastric tube should suffice, as inorganic cadmium salts are powders, not pills.

Given the relative lack of experience with acute oral cadmium poisoning, all patients with known exposures and/or abnormal findings consistent with cadmium toxicity or exposure should be admitted to the hospital for supportive care, monitoring of renal and hepatic function, and possibly evaluation of the GI tract for injury.

Although it seems logical to use chelation therapy in any patient with an acute life-threatening ingestion of a metal compound, the benefit of chelation in acute cadmium exposure is unproven. Multiple chelators have been studied, all in animal models, with inconsistent results.

The ideal chelator for treatment of oral cadmium toxicity would be well tolerated, and would decrease GI absorption of cadmium and decrease the concentration of cadmium in organs such as the kidney and liver, while not increasing cadmium concentrations in other critical organs such as the brain. Of the chelators studied for cadmium toxicity, succimer comes closest to fulfilling these criteria. In models of acute oral cadmium toxicity, succimer decreases the GI absorption of cadmium,[3,6] without increasing cadmium burdens in target organs, and improves survival.[2,6,53]

In a patient thought to have acutely ingested potentially lethal amounts of cadmium, treatment with succimer is reasonable but unproven. Succimer should be given as soon as possible after the ingestion, as the effectiveness of chelators decreases dramatically over time in experimental models of cadmium poisoning.[16]

It must be stressed, however, that supporting data for chelation are solely derived from animal models. Succimer dosing in human cadmium poisoning is unstudied. Doses that are well tolerated (10 mg/kg/dose 3 times a day) are reasonable.

Other chelators with potential benefits include diethylenetriaminepentaacetic acid (DTPA)[6,15] and 2,3-dimercaptopropane sulfonate (DMPS),[13,53] both of which reduce tissue burdens and increase survival but for which further investigation is needed.

Most other chelators are either ineffective or detrimental, including dimercaprol (British anti-Lewisite {BAL}),[15,21,52] penicillamine,[15,65] cyclic tetramines (such as cyclam and tACPD),[93] detergent formula chelators (such as sodium tripolyphosphate {STPP} and nitrilotriacetic acid {NTA}),[31,32] CaNa₂EDTA,[68] and dithiocarbamates.[3,35]

Pulmonary/Cadmium Fumes

The patient who is ill after exposure to cadmium fumes (generally cadmium oxide) presents with predominantly respiratory complaints and constitutional symptoms. The patient's airway should be assessed and appropriate oxygenation ensured, although hypoxia is commonly delayed.

Corticosteroids are used in most reported cases (although there are no studies to support their efficacy), and a standard dose of methylprednisolone (1 mg/kg up to 60 mg) is reasonable. Because cadmium inhalation injuries are neither benign nor self-limited, all patients with acute inhalational exposures to cadmium should be admitted to the hospital for observation and supportive care until respiratory symptoms have resolved. All such patients should have long-term follow-up arranged with a pulmonologist to assess the possibility of chronic lung injury, even following a single exposure.

Chelation is not recommended as an option for patients with single acute exposures to cadmium fumes, as these patients do not appear to develop extrapulmonary injury.[4,5,98,110]

Chronic Exposure

Patients chronically exposed to cadmium frequently come to attention during routine screening, as those who work with cadmium are under close medical surveillance (Chap. 131). These patients may have developed proteinuria or, less commonly, chronic pulmonary complaints.

Management is challenging. Cessation of cadmium exposure is the first intervention. However, as mentioned earlier, chronic cadmium-induced kidney and lung changes are largely irreversible.

We recommend again chelation for chronic cadmium toxicity. There is no evidence that chelation of chronically poisoned animals improves long-term outcomes, and one study in humans found no improvement in cadmium-induced kidney dysfunction with periodic CaNa$_2$EDTA chelation.[109] Furthermore, in a chronically exposed patient, the majority of cadmium is bound to intracellular metallothionein, which greatly reduces its toxicity. Any attempt to remove cadmium from these deposits risks redistributing cadmium to other organs, possibly exacerbating toxicity, as is known to occur with BAL therapy.[25]

Of all the chelators tested thus far in animal models of chronic cadmium toxicity, the dithiocarbamates have shown the most success in reducing total body cadmium burdens. Unfortunately, these chelators tend to cause redistribution of cadmium to the brain; the lipophilicity that allows them to cross cell membranes into hepatocytes (to access stored cadmium) also promotes their uptake into the lipid-rich central nervous system (CNS).[37] Numerous dithiocarbamates have been synthesized and studied with regard to cadmium decorporation, however, and several species effectively reduce whole-body, kidney, and liver cadmium concentrations without an increase in CNS cadmium.[59,90] Thus, at present, there is insufficient evidence to justify the use of any chelator in the treatment of patients with chronic cadmium toxicity.

SUMMARY

- Cadmium toxicity is largely dependent on the route of and chronicity of exposure.
- After acute oral exposure, GI injury predominates.
- After acute inhalation, a severe chemical pneumonitis can ensue.
- With chronic environmental or occupational exposure, nephrotoxicity (usually manifested by proteinuria) is the most significant finding, although other organ systems, such as the lungs, can be affected.
- Treatment for all patients with suspected cadmium poisoning consists of removal from the source, decontamination if possible, and supportive care.
- In the rare instance of a potentially life-threatening acute cadmium salt ingestion, treatment with succimer is reasonable.
- At this time, we recommend against chelation in the patient with chronic cadmium poisoning.

REFERENCES

1. Al-Nasser IA. Cadmium hepatotoxicity and alterations of the mitochondrial function. *J Toxicol Clin Toxicol.* 2000;38:407-413.
2. Andersen O, Nielsen JB. Oral cadmium chloride intoxication in mice: effects of penicillamine, dimercaptosuccinic acid and related compounds. *Pharmacol Toxicol.* 1988;63:386-389.
3. Anderson O, et al. Oral cadmium chloride intoxication in mice: diethyldithiocarbamate enhances rather than alleviates acute toxicity. *Toxicology.* 1988;52:331-342.
4. Anthony JS, et al. Abnormalities in pulmonary function after brief exposure to toxic metal fumes. *CMAJ.* 1978;119:586-588.
5. Barnhart S, Rosenstock L. Cadmium chemical pneumonitis. *Chest.* 1984;86:791.
6. Basinger MA, et al. Antagonists for acute oral cadmium chloride intoxication. *J Toxicol Environ Health.* 1988;23:77-89.
7. Bernard A, et al. Characterization of the proteinuria of cadmium-exposed workers. *Int Arch Occup Environ Health.* 1976;38:19-30.
8. Blainey JD, et al. Cadmium-induced osteomalacia. *Br J Ind Med.* 1980;37:278-284.
9. Bofetta P. Methodological aspects of the epidemiological association between cadmium and cancer in humans. *IARC Sci Publ.* 1992;118:425-434.
10. Böhm KJ. Kinesin-dependent motility generation as target mechanism of cadmium intoxication. *Toxicol Lett.* 2014;224:356-361.
11. Borné Y, et al. Cadmium exposure and incidence of heart failure and atrial fibrillation: a population-based prospective cohort study. *BMJ Open.* 2015;5:e007366.
12. Buchet JP, et al. Renal effects of cadmium body burden of the general population. *Lancet.* 1990;336:699-702.
13. Buckler HM, et al. Self-poisoning with oral cadmium chloride. *Br Med J.* 1986;292:1559-1560.
14. Budavari S, et al., eds. *The Merck Index.* Whitehouse Station, NJ: Merck & Company; 1996:1665.
15. Cantilena LR, Klaassen CD. Comparison of the effectiveness of several chelators after single administration on the toxicity, excretion, and distribution of cadmium. *Toxicol Appl Pharmacol.* 1981;58:452-460.
16. Cantilena LR, Klaassen CD. Decreased effectiveness of chelation therapy with time after acute cadmium poisoning. *Toxicol Appl Pharmacol.* 1982;63:173-180.
17. Centers for Disease Control and Prevention. Second national report on human exposure to environmental chemicals. NCEH Pub. No. 02-0716. March 2003:13-16. Atlanta.
18. Chan OY, et al. Respiratory function in cadmium battery workers—a follow-up study. *Ann Acad Med Singapore.* 1988;17:283-287.
19. Chan OY, et al. Respiratory function in cadmium battery workers. *Singapore Med J.* 1986;27:108-119.
20. Cherian MG, et al. Cadmium-metallothionein-induced nephropathy. *Toxicol Appl Pharmacol.* 1976;38:399-408.
21. Cherian MG, Rodgers K. Chelation of cadmium from metallothionein in vivo and its excretion in rats repeatedly injected with cadmium chloride. *J Pharmacol Exp Ther.* 1982;222:699-704.
22. Chia KS, et al. Renal tubular function of cadmium exposed workers. *Ann Acad Med Singapore.* 1992;21:756-759.
23. Cortona G, et al. Occupational exposure to cadmium and lung function. *IARC Sci Publ.* 1992;118:205-210.
24. Coyle P, et al. Tolerance to cadmium toxicity by metallothionein and zinc: in vivo and in vitro studies with MT-null mice. *Toxicology.* 2000;150:53-67.
25. Dalhamn T, Friberg L. Dimercaprol (2,3-dimercaptopropanol) in chronic cadmium poisoning. *Acta Pharmacol Toxicol.* 1955;11:68-71.
26. Dan G, et al. Humoral and cell-mediated immune response to cadmium in mice. *Drug Chem Toxicol.* 2000;23:349-360.
27. Dudley RE, et al. Cadmium-induced hepatic and renal injury in chronically exposed rats: likely role of hepatic cadmium-metallothionein in nephrotoxicity. *Toxicol Appl Pharmacol.* 1985;77:414-426.
28. Dudley RE, et al. Acute exposure to cadmium causes severe liver injury in rats. *Toxicol Appl Pharmacol.* 1982;65:302-313.
29. Edling C, et al. Lung function in workers using cadmium containing solder. *Br J Ind Med.* 1986;43:657-662.
30. Emmerson BT. "Ouch-ouch" disease: the osteomalacia of cadmium nephropathy. *Ann Intern Med.* 1970;73:854-855.
31. Engstrom B. Influence of chelating agents on toxicity and distribution of cadmium among tissues of mouse liver and kidney following oral or subcutaneous exposure. *Acta Pharmacol Toxicol.* 1981;48:108-117.
32. Engstrom B, Nordberg GF. Effects of detergent formula chelating agents on the metabolism and toxicity of cadmium in mice. *Acta Pharmacol Toxicol.* 1978;43:387-397.
33. Engvall J, Perk J. Prevalence of hypertension among cadmium-exposed workers. *Arch Environ Health.* 1985;40:185-190.
34. Fagerberg B, et al. Cadmium exposure and atherosclerotic carotid plaques—results from the Malmö diet and Cancer study. *Environ Res.* 2015;136:67-74.
35. Fuortes L, et al. Acute respiratory fatality associated with exposure to sheet metal and cadmium fumes. *J Toxicol Clin Toxicol.* 1991;29:279-283.
36. Gale GR, et al. Comparative effects of diethyldithiocarbamate, dimercaptosuccinate, and diethylenetriaminepentaacetate on organ distribution and excretion of cadmium. *Ann Clin Lab Sci.* 1983;13:33-44.
37. Gale GR, et al. Mechanism of diethyldithiocarbamate, dihydroxyethyldithiocarbamate, and dicarboxymethyldithiocarbamate action on distribution and excretion of cadmium. *Ann Clin Lab Sci.* 1983;13:474-481.
38. Goyer RA, et al. Non-metallothioneinbound cadmium in the pathogenesis of cadmium nephrotoxicity in the rat. *Toxicol Appl Pharmacol.* 1989;101:232-244.
39. Hammond CR. Cadmium. In: Lide DR, ed. *CRC Handbook of Chemistry and Physics.* 80th ed. Boca Raton, FL: CRC Press; 1989:4-8.
40. Haswell-Elkins M, et al. Striking association between urinary cadmium level and albuminuria among Torres Strait Islander people with diabetes. *Environ Res.* 2008;106:379-383.
41. Hotz P, et al. Renal effects of low-level environmental cadmium exposure: 5-year follow-up of a subcohort from the Cadmibel study. *Lancet.* 1999;354:1508-1513.

42. Ikeda M, et al. Urinary alpha$_1$-microglobulin, beta$_2$-microglobulin, and retinol-binding protein levels in general populations in Japan with references to cadmium in urine, blood, and 24-hour food duplicates. *Environ Res.* 1995;70:35-46.

43. Ikeda M, et al. The integrity of the liver among people environmentally exposed to cadmium at various levels. *Int Arch Occup Environ Health.* 1997;69:379-385.

44. International Agency for Research on Cancer. Cadmium. http://www-cie.iarc.fr/htdocs/monographs/vol58/mono58-2.htm. Accessed January 5, 2005.

45. Iwata K, et al. Renal tubular function after reduction of environmental cadmium exposure: a ten-year follow-up. *Arch Environ Health.* 1993;48:157-163.

46. Järup L, Alfvén T. Low level cadmium exposure, renal and bone effects—the OSCAR study. *Biometals.* 2004;17:505-509.

47. Järup L, Elinder CG. Dose-response relations between urinary cadmium and tubular proteinuria in cadmium-exposed workers. *Am J Ind Med.* 1994;26:759-769.

48. Järup L, Elinder CG. Incidence of renal stones among cadmium exposed battery workers. *Br J Ind Med.* 1993;50:598-602.

49. Järup L, et al. Low-level exposure to cadmium and early kidney damage: the OSCAR study. *Occup Environ Med.* 2000;57:668-672.

50. Jimi S, et al. Mechanisms of cell death induced by cadmium and arsenic. *Ann N Y Acad Sci.* 2004;1011:325-331.

51. Jin T, et al. Osteoporosis and renal dysfunction in a general population exposed to cadmium in China. *Environ Res.* 2004;96:353-359.

52. Jones MM, et al. A comparative study on the influence of vicinal dithiols and a dithiocarbamate on the biliary excretion of cadmium in rat. *Toxicol Appl Pharmacol.* 1991;110:241-250.

53. Jones MM, et al. The relative effectiveness of some chelating agents as antidotes in acute cadmium poisoning. *Res Commun Chem Pathol Pharmacol.* 1978;22:581-588.

54. Karakaya A, et al. An immunological study on workers occupationally exposed to cadmium. *Hum Exp Toxicol.* 1994;13:73-75.

55. Kazantis G. Renal tubular dysfunction and abnormalities of calcium metabolism in cadmium workers. *Environ Health Perspect.* 1979;28:155-159.

56. Kazantis G, et al. Is cadmium a human carcinogen? *IARC Sci Publ.* 1992;118:435-446.

57. Kjellstrom T, Nordberg GF. A kinetic model of cadmium metabolism in the human being. *Environ Res.* 1978;16:248-269.

58. Klaassen CD, et al. Metallothionein: an intracellular protein to protect against cadmium toxicity. *Annu Rev Pharmacol Toxicol.* 1999;39:267-294.

59. Kojima S, et al. Effect of N-benzyl-D-glucamine dithiocarbamate on the renal toxicity produced by subacute exposure to cadmium in rats. *Toxicol Appl Pharmacol.* 1989;98:39-48.

60. Kojima S, et al. Effects of dithiocarbamates on testicular toxicity in rats caused by acute exposure to cadmium. *Toxicol Appl Pharmacol.* 1992;116:24-29.

61. Kurihara I, et al. Association between exposure to cadmium and blood pressure in Japanese peoples. *Arch Environ Health.* 2004;59:711-716.

62. Lall SB, et al. Cadmium-induced nephrotoxicity in rats. *Indian J Exp Biol.* 1997;35:151-154.

63. Liang Y, et al. Renal function after reduction in cadmium exposure: an 8-year follow-up on residents in cadmium-polluted areas. *Environ Health Perspect.* 2012;120:223-228.

64. Liu J, et al. Susceptibility of MT null mice to chronic CdCl$_2$-induced nephrotoxicity indicates that renal injury is not mediated by the CdMT complex. *Toxicol Sci.* 1998;46:197-203.

65. Lyle WH, et al. Enhancement of cadmium nephrotoxicity by penicillamine in the rat. *Postgrad Med J.* 1968;Suppl:18-21.

66. Mannino DM, et al. Urinary cadmium levels predict lower lung function in current and former smokers: data from the Third National Health and Nutrition Examination Survey. *Thorax.* 2004;59:194-198.

67. Mascagni P, et al. Olfactory function in workers exposed to moderate airborne cadmium levels. *Neurotoxicology.* 2003;24:717-724.

68. McGivern J, Mason J. The effect of chelation on the fate of intravenously administered cadmium in rats. *J Comp Pathol.* 1979;89:1-9.

69. Min K-S, et al. Renal accumulation of cadmium and nephropathy following long-term administration of cadmiummetallothionein. *Toxicol Appl Pharmacol.* 1996;141:102-109.

70. Nogawa K, et al. Dose-response relationship for renal dysfunction in a population environmentally exposed to cadmium. *IARC Sci Publ.* 1992;118:311-318.

71. Notarachille G, et al. Heavy metals toxicity: effect of cadmium ions on amyloid beta protein 1-42. Possible implications for Alzheimer's disease. *Biometals.* 2014;27:371-388.

72. Okuda B, et al. Parkinsonism after acute cadmium poisoning. *Clin Neurol Neurosurg.* 1997;99:263-265.

73. Ostergaard K. Cadmium and hypertension. *Lancet.* 1977;8013:677-678.

74. Park R, et al. Cadmium and lung cancer mortality accounting for simultaneous arsenic exposure. *Occup Environ Med.* 2012;69:303-309.

75. Patwardhan JR, Finckh ES. Fatal cadmium-fume pneumonitis. *Med J Aust.* 1976;1:962-966.

76. Pearson CA, et al. Effects of cadmium on E-cadherin and VE-cadherin in mouse lung. *Life Sci.* 2003;72:1303-1320.

77. Prozialeck WC. Evidence that E-cadherin may be a target for cadmium toxicity in epithelial cells. *Toxicol Appl Pharmacol.* 2000;164:231-249.

78. Prozialeck WC, et al. Cadmium alters the localization of N-cadherin, E-cadherin, and beta-catenin in the proximal tubule epithelium. *Toxicol Appl Pharmacol.* 2003;189:180-195.

79. Qian L, et al. Relationship between urinary cadmium and mortality in habitants of a cadmium-polluted area: a 22-year follow-up study in Japan. *Chin Med J.* 2011;124:3504-3509.

80. Rani A, et al. Cellular mechanisms of cadmium-induced toxicity: a review. *Int J Environ Health Res.* 2014;24:378-399.

81. Raval G, et al. Unexplained hemolytic anemia with multiorgan failure. *Clin Chem.* 2011;57:1485-1489.

82. Rikans LE, Yamano T. Mechanisms of cadmium-mediated acute hepatotoxicity. *J Biochem Mol Toxicol.* 2000;14:110-117.

83. Roels H, et al. Evolution of cadmium-induced renal dysfunction in workers removed from exposure. *Scand J Work Environ Health.* 1982;8:191-200.

84. Roels HA, et al. Health significance of cadmium-induced renal dysfunction: a five-year follow-up. *Br J Ind Med.* 1989;46:755-764.

85. Rose CS, et al. Olfactory impairment after chronic occupational cadmium exposure. *J Occup Med.* 1992;34:600-605.

86. Sakurai H, et al. Cross-sectional study of pulmonary function in cadmium alloy workers. *Scand J Work Environ Health.* 1982;8(suppl 1):122-130.

87. Scott R, et al. The importance of cadmium as a factor in calcified upper urinary tract stone disease—a prospective 7-year study. *Br J Urol.* 1982;54:584-589.

88. Scott R, et al. Hypercalciuria related to cadmium exposure. *Urology.* 1978;11:462-465.

89. Seidal K, et al. Fatal cadmium-induced pneumonitis. *Scand J Work Environ Health.* 1993;19:429-431.

90. Singh PK, et al. Selective removal of cadmium from aged hepatic and renal deposits: N-substituted talooctamine dithiocarbamates as cadmium mobilizing agent. *Chem Biol Interact.* 1990;74:79-91.

91. Squibb KS, et al. Cadmium-metallothionein nephropathy. Relationships between ultrastructural/biochemical alterations and intracellular cadmium binding. *J Pharmacol Exp Ther.* 1984;229:311-321.

92. Squibb KS, et al. Early cellular effects of circulating cadmium-thionein on kidney proximal tubules. *Environ Health Perspect.* 1979;28:287-296.

93. Srivasta RC, et al. Comparative evaluation of chelating agents on the mobilization of cadmium: a mechanistic approach. *J Toxicol Environ Health.* 1996;47:173-182.

94. Suruda AJ. Measuring olfactory dysfunction from cadmium in an occupational and environmental medicine office practice. *J Occup Environ Med.* 2000;42:337.

95. Takebayashi S, et al. Cadmium induces osteomalacia mediated by proximal tubular atrophy and disturbances of phosphate reabsorption. A study of 11 autopsies. *Pathol Res Pract.* 2000;196:653-663.

96. Telisman S, et al. Cadmium in the blood and seminal fluid of nonoccupationally exposed adult male subjects with regard to smoking habits. *Int Arch Occup Environ Health.* 1997;70:243-248.

97. Tellez-Plaza M, et al. Cadmium exposure and hypertension in the 1999-2004 National Health and Nutrition Examination Survey (NHANES). *Environ Health Perspect.* 2008;116:51-56.

98. Townshend RH. Acute cadmium pneumonitis: a 17-year follow up. *Br J Ind Med.* 1982;39:411-412.

99. Tsychya K. Proteinuria of cadmium workers. *J Occup Med.* 1976;18:463-466.

100. van Sittert NJ, et al. A nine-year follow-up study of renal effects in workers exposed to cadmium in a zinc ore refinery. *Br J Ind Med.* 1993;50:603-612.

101. Verbost PM, et al. Cadmium inhibition of the erythrocyte Ca^{2+} pump. *J Biol Chem.* 1989;264:5613-5615.

102. Verbost PM, et al. Nanomolar concentrations of Cd^{2+} inhibit Ca^{2+} transport systems in plasma membranes and intracellular Ca^{2+} stores in intestinal epithelium. *Biochim Biophys Acta.* 1987;902:247-252.

103. Viaene MK, et al. Neurobehavioural effects of occupational exposure to cadmium: a cross-sectional epidemiological study. *Occup Environ Med.* 2000;57:19-27.

104. Waalkes MP. Cadmium carcinogenesis in review. *J Inorg Biochem.* 2000;79:241-244.

105. Watkins SR, et al. Cadmium-binding serum protein. *Biochem Biophys Res Commun.* 1977;74:1403-1410.

106. Winston RM. Cadmium fume poisoning. *Br Med J.* 1971;758:401.

107. Wisniewska-Knypl JM, et al. Binding of cadmium on metallothionein in man: an analysis of a fatal poisoning by cadmium iodide. *Arch Toxicol.* 1971;28:46-55.

108. Wu Q, et al. Urinary cadmium, osteopenia, and osteoporosis in the US population. *Osteoporos Int.* 2010;21:1449-1454.

109. Wu X, et al. Lack of reversal effect of EDTA treatment on cadmium induced renal dysfunction. A fourteen-year follow-up. *Biometals.* 2004;17:435-441.

110. Yates DH, Goldman KP. Acute cadmium poisoning in a foreman plant welder. *Br J Ind Med.* 1990;47:429-431.

111. Zalups RK, Ahmad S. Molecular handling of cadmium in transporting epithelia. *Toxicol Appl Pharmacol.* 2003;186:163-188.

89 CESIUM

Zhanna Livshits

Cesium (Cs)

Atomic number	=	55
Atomic weight	=	132.91 Da
Normal concentrations		
Whole blood	=	<10 mcg/L (75.42 nmol/L)
Urine	=	<20 mcg/L (150.48 nmol/L)

HISTORY AND EPIDEMIOLOGY

The name "cesium" derives from the Latin word for "sky," *caelum*. Cesium (Cs) is among the most rare and reactive alkali metals. Elemental cesium (Cs^0) is silvery white, soft, and malleable. It has a relatively low melting point of 82.4°F (28°C) and thus exists as both solid and liquid at room temperature. Elemental cesium (Cs^0) ignites violently when exposed to moist air or water but forms stable salt complexes. The greatest concentration of naturally occurring cesium (32%), the compound cesium oxide (Cs_2O), is found in the ore pollucite.[1,81,83] Since Cs^0 is so highly reactive and short-lived, the name "cesium" will refer to cesium salts in the following discussion, unless specifically noted otherwise.

Radionuclides of cesium were identified in the 1940s by the American scientist and Nobel Prize winner Glenn Seaborg and his student Margaret Melhase.[63] Radioactive cesium isotopes are products of nuclear fission of uranium and plutonium.[85] Both [134]Cs and ^{137}Cs decay via β particle emission; however, ^{137}Cs also emits γ rays.[81] Because ^{137}Cs has a long half-life of 30 years, it serves not only as an "atomic clock" but also poses potential radiological hazard as it deposits and complexes in earth and water. Of the numerous cesium radioisotopes that are identified to date, only [133]Cs is stable.[9]

Several releases of radioactive cesium have occurred in the past century, resulting in large-scale contamination and human exposure. Examples include the nuclear weapons use in Hiroshima and Nagasaki; nuclear weapons testing in Bikini Atoll[11] and Republic of Georgia;[26] poor nuclear waste management in Goiânia,[36,60,68] Tammiku,[37] and Camp Lilo in the Republic of Georgia;[26] as well as critical nuclear power plant malfunctions in Chernobyl[71] and Fukushima Daiichi.[42]

Occupational exposure to radiocesium occurs routinely in nuclear power plant employees and people who live and work in close proximity to a nuclear facility. Both ^{137}Cs and [131]Cs are used as sources of external and internal radiation for treatment of numerous malignancies. Internal radiotherapy with [131]Cs seed implantation, called brachytherapy, is approved by the US Food and Drug Administration (FDA).[23] Physicians and staff working with these isotopes are at risk of occupational exposure.[24,61]

Cesium compounds are employed in scintillation counters, photoelectric cells, vacuum tubes, optical instruments, semiconductors and extensively in alternative medicine.[1] They serve as catalysts for organic synthesis and are utilized for laboratory experiments in animal models of ventricular dysrhythmias. Nonradioactive cesium chloride is promoted as a supplement or an alternative treatment for cancer, despite no scientific support for this claim. Its increasing popularity in cancer treatment stems from a theory that cesium chloride increases the intracellular pH of tumor cells, resulting in cell death.[7,73] This theory was first proposed in a paper describing the effects of cesium, rubidium, and potassium in cancer cells and its effects in mice.[7] Although the extent of its popularity is unknown, cesium chloride is promoted as a treatment for cancers on various websites and can be easily found for sale on the Internet. There is no scientific evidence that cesium chloride is effective for cancer treatment in humans, and it has the potential for grave toxicity. Cesium chloride is also suggested for treatment of depression on some internet websites, however dosing and mechanism of action are unclear. Cesium chloride was also proposed, but not implemented, as a preventive therapy for potential radiocesium exposure.[6]

PHARMACOLOGY

Like thallium (Chap. 99), cesium has a molecular structure that resembles potassium, and similarly, it either mimics or antagonizes potassium in cellular processes.[44] Because cesium blocks the delayed rectifier (I_{kr}) channel in the cardiac myocyte and prolongs repolarization (Chap. 15), it is used in animal models to induce QT interval prolongation and subsequent ventricular ectopy and ventricular dysrhythmias.[57,74]

Although radiocesium is indistinguishable from nonradioactive cesium in biological and chemical reactions, radiocesium damages tissues via emission of β particles and γ rays during its decay (Chap. 128). [134]Cesium decays to a stable isotope by emission of β particles. [137]Cesium initially emits β particles to form the unstable intermediate barium isotope [137m]Ba, which then further emits γ rays to form stable [137]Ba. Radiocesium is such a potent emitter that lethal doses of radiation are delivered following exposures that are too small to cause cardiac effects.

Oral and intravenous cesium chloride preparations are used as an alternative cancer therapy. There is a significant risk for cardiac toxicity and no proven therapeutic benefit. Dysrhythmias and death are reported following intravenous, oral, and subcutaneous administration.

PHARMACOKINETICS AND TOXICOKINETICS

Pharmacokinetic data following radiocesium injection and ingestion are limited and derived from radiotracer studies in animals and a few reports in human volunteers.

Exposure to cesium occurs through ingestion, inhalation,[55] injection, and dermal contact. Animal studies with a guinea pig model demonstrate rapid absorption via inhalation, intraperitoneal injection, and ingestion.[77] Human volunteer studies demonstrate 98% to 99% absorption of ingested cesium salts.[69,70] Absorption through intact skin is minimal. One case estimated 20% dermal absorption of radiocesium through burned skin.[85]

Once absorbed, cesium is rapidly distributed to the blood compartment, followed by subsequent distribution to various organs. Animal studies with rat, dog, and guinea pig models demonstrate that cesium is initially distributed to the myocardial, renal, pulmonary, and hepatic tissue followed by subsequent accumulation in the skeletal muscle.[43,51,77,80]

Data from human volunteers suggest that once ingested, cesium is absorbed from the small intestine,[32,44] distributes to the blood compartment and various organs. Initial accumulation occurs in the salivary glands following ingestion, and in the liver both following ingestion and injection of radiocesium; subsequent distribution to the myocardium, spleen, adrenals, gastrointestinal (GI) tract, bone, and lungs, with elevated concentration in the skeletal muscle approximately 10 days postexposure.[35,69]

Cesium undergoes enterohepatic circulation limiting fecal elimination. As such, urinary excretion accounts for 80% to 90% and fecal excretion for 2% to 10% of elimination of an ingested dose.[47,49,65] Some elimination occurs in the feces independent of whether cesium is injected or ingested, likely due to hepatic elimination.[69] Only a small amount of cesium is eliminated through sweat or respiratory secretions.[22,49,86]

The biological elimination half-life ranges from 50 to 150 days,[9,31,34,35,49,52,67,70,82] with a few cases up to 200 days[35] following ingestion. The biological half-life increases with age[4,8] and male sex[4] and decreases with pregnancy.[94] The half-life in children and infants is significantly shorter than that of adults.[52]

[137]Cesium elimination follows first-order kinetics.[45,47] Pharmacokinetic analysis in a woman who developed cardiac toxicity from nonradioactive cesium suggested first-order elimination using a 2-compartment model.[91]

Radiocesium transfers to placenta and maternal breast milk.[3,25,30,53,89] Modeling based on estimates and human studies demonstrates approximately 0.5%, 10%, and 24% transfer of ^{137}Cs through maternal milk during the stages of early pregnancy, late pregnancy, and lactation respectively.[30]

PATHOPHYSIOLOGY

[137]Cesium undergoes radioactive decay. Beta particles have very limited dermal penetration and effects from external exposure are limited to dermal irritation and burns (Chap. 128). Release of β particles within the body, as typically occurs after inhalation, ingestion, or dermal absorption, harms internal organs. Gamma rays penetrate the skin with external exposure and cause organ toxicity.

As noted above, cardiotoxicity is the principal and most life-threatening clinical effect of nonradioactive cesium. QT interval prolongation occurs rapidly and predisposes individuals to torsade de pointes (TdP) and other ventricular dysrhythmias. In animal models, especially in canines, cesium is one of the more reliable methods to induce and study nonischemic ventricular dysrhythmias. Prolongation of the QT interval in the cardiac myocyte results from antagonism at the delayed rectifier I_{kr} channel.[93] This delays the repolarization phase of the cardiac action potential, thus prolonging the action potential duration.[29] Additionally, it promotes early after-depolarizations (EADs), which are cellular depolarizations that occur during phases 2 and 3 of the cardiac action potential prior to completion of repolarization.[19,29,46] This generation of EADs leads to TdP,[13,19,20,27,78] as cesium chloride–induced EADs precede the development of dysrhythmias in a canine model.[46,62]

Cesium-induced ventricular dysrhythmias are potentiated by bradycardia.[5,38,62] This is explained by either potentiation of EAD formation[38] or increase in temporal variability of the refractory period throughout the cardiac muscle.[28] Overdrive pacing abolishes both EADs and ventricular dysrhythmias in an isolated canine cardiac tissue.[17,46,62] In addition to bradycardia, EADs are induced by hypokalemia[21] and metabolic acidosis[12] (Chaps. 15 and 16). These EADs are modulated by L-type calcium channel currents,[2,38] and calcium channel blockers, such as verapamil, suppress cesium-induced ventricular dysrhythmias in dogs.[16,57]

Sodium channel modulation also may be contributory in cesium-induced ventricular dysrhythmias. Low concentrations of tetrodotoxin, a sodium channel antagonist, terminate EADs induced by cesium chloride.[5,40] Lidocaine abolishes cesium-induced ventricular dysrhythmias in a canine model.[57]

CLINICAL MANIFESTATIONS

Radiation injuries are discussed in detail in Chap. 128. The following discussion focuses on nonradioactive cesium toxicity observed with oral and intravenous CsCl preparation used by patients as an alternative form of cancer therapy. The case reports for cesium chloride use and toxicity are limited to cancer therapy.

Cardiovascular Toxicity

Prolongation of the QT interval and subsequent ventricular dysrhythmias are the principal cardiac effects, described with cumulative oral ingested doses ranging from 3 g/day[33,48,72,90] to 10 g/day.[15,92] Time from daily oral cesium exposure to development of dysrhythmias ranged from 1 week to 3 months. Rapid onset of dysrhythmias is reported following injection of a 9 mL of oral preparation of cesium chloride into a breast mass.[75] The patient died within 1 week after failing to have a neurologic recovery.[75] Most patients with ventricular ectopy, TdP, or ventricular dysrhythmias developed syncope or "seizures." A prolonged QT interval was present and either resistant to potassium repletion or was challenging to correct. Serum and urine cesium concentrations were markedly elevated in all case reports ranging from 2,400 mcg/dL[59] to 28,000 mcg/dL,[33] and 130,000 mcg/L[33] to 360,000 mcg/L[59] respectively.

Whole blood cesium concentration were reported in 2 cases; 100,000 mcg/L[75] and 160,000 mcg/L.[15] The QT interval normalized and dysrhythmias ceased after termination of cesium chloride exposure.[10,14,15,48,59,64,72,90,91]

Intravenous injection of cesium chloride in 2 patients with metastatic kidney and lung cancer resulted in death. Forensic records indicate that the first patient had chills and seizures during the first session and went into cardiac arrest during the second session. The second patient collapsed during the infusion.[9] Postmortem whole blood concentration of cesium was 84,000 mcg/L for first patient and 28,100 mcg/L for second patient. Another case report described an 8-year-old boy who developed bradycardia, premature ventricular depolarizations, and TdP that terminated without intervention.[14] Cesium concentrations were not obtained.

Gastrointestinal Effects

Patients receiving alternative oral therapies of 3 to 10 g of cesium chloride per day for diverse neoplasms developed nausea, vomiting, diarrhea, and abdominal cramping.[10,15,48,59,72,92]

Electrolyte Abnormalities

Some patients taking cesium chloride alternative cancer therapy develop hypokalemia and hypomagnesemia. Serum potassium concentrations ranged from 2.7 mEq/L[75] to 3.4 mEq/L/L[92] and serum magnesium concentrations were reported as low as 1.4 mEq/L/dL.[90] Both corrected with electrolyte repletion. Electrolyte imbalance likely reflects GI loss through vomiting and/or diarrhea.[10,15,48,64,72,90]

Neurologic Effects

A heightened sense of perception as well as facial and acral tingling are described following self-administration of 6 g of cesium chloride daily for 36 consecutive days.[58] Reports of syncope[10,48,59,64,90,91] and "seizures"[9,15] should be interpreted with caution because a nonperfusing cardiac rhythm is the most likely etiology for both clinical presentations.

DIAGNOSTIC TESTING

Radioactive cesium is detected by whole-body counters using γ-ray spectrometry and β counting.[81] Shielding of the room where testing is performed is sometimes necessary to reduce background radiation. Urine and feces are analyzed for ^{137}Cs and/or [134]Cs in a similar manner.

Analysis of nonradioactive cesium in blood, urine, feces, or tissue samples is performed by spectrometric methods such as flame atomic emission spectrometry, inductively coupled plasma–mass spectrometry (ICP-MS), or instrumental neutron activation analysis.[1]

Computed tomography (CT) imaging of the brain was obtained in a patient with metastatic breast cancer to the brain who presented to the hospital following a seizure following the receipt of intravenous cesium chloride as an alternative chemotherapeutic.[41] The CT findings showed diffusely increased attenuation of brain parenchyma. She died within 48 hours of hospitalization. Patient also had elevated post-mortem brain cesium concentration of 780 mg/kg.

MANAGEMENT

Radiocesium and Cesium

Patient management following radiation exposure is outlined in detail in Chap. 128 and Antidotes in Depth: A31. Although most data are obtained following cesium exposures in animals and humans, the treatment of patients with radiocesium-induced toxicity is similar. Recognition of radiocesium exposure and decontamination is critical in all cases of exposure and toxicity due to the potential radiation injuries.

Gastrointestinal decontamination is likely of limited value and is not recommended following cesium ingestion. Cesium is not well adsorbed to activated charcoal,[88] and patients who present with significant cesium toxicity often have vomiting or altered mental status. Administration of antiemetics and repletion of volume loss with intravenous fluids is central to supportive management of patients who present with nausea and vomiting. Caution is warranted with use of 5HT$_3$ antagonists such as ondansetron given their potential for QT interval prolongation. Serum potassium and magnesium concentrations should be carefully monitored and supplemented as needed.

All patients with suspected cesium salt ingestion should have an electrocardiogram (ECG) and be attached to a continuous cardiac monitor. Their QT intervals should be monitored closely and documented often with serial ECGs. Intravenous magnesium and overdrive pacing should be used to prevent recurrent episodes torsade de pointes. It is recommended to use synchronous cardioversion in unstable rhythms. Lidocaine is also a reasonable choice. Amiodarone is not routinely recommended given its propensity to prolong the QT interval. Even though amiloride decreased the need for supplemental potassium supplementation in a case report,[33] it is not recommended at this time given paucity of data and potential for adverse effects.

Because isolated seizures are not reported, syncope and "seizurelike activity" should heighten concern for hypoperfusion or potential cardiac dysrhythmias.

The following therapies have been attempted after radiocesium exposure and have not been effective: activated charcoal, diuretics, enhanced sweating, and disodium ethylenediaminetetraacetate (EDTA).[22,87] The paucity of literature makes it impossible to conclusively recommend or reject hemodialysis as a modality for enhanced cesium elimination.[39,87]

Prussian Blue

Prussian blue, ferric hexacyanoferrate(II), is a blue crystal lattice composed of iron and cyanide molecules. In 2003, the insoluble form of Prussian blue was approved by the FDA for oral treatment of radioactive cesium and/or radioactive or nonradioactive thallium (Antidotes in Depth: A31).[66] The insoluble crystal lattice adsorbs cesium[18] in the intestinal lumen, and enhances both elimination and gut dialysis.[56] A systematic analysis of published literature on the use of Prussian blue in the treatment of radiocesium poisoning suggests that it reduces the half-life of radiocesium by as much as 43%.[79]

Although the majority of Prussian blue literature focuses on radiocesium elimination,[47,50,54,76,79] it was also used for a patient with cesium chloride toxicity. Prussian blue was started on hospital day 7 in a patient with cardiac toxicity following cesium ingestion. She received 3 g 3 times per day for 4 weeks. Cesium half-life was decreased by 47.7% (from 61.7 days to 29.4 days).[10]

Because laboratory confirmation of cesium will be substantially delayed, Prussian blue is recommended on suspicion of cesium toxicity. Although the optimal dose and interval are unknown, the package insert for Prussian blue, which recommends 3 g orally 3 times per day, for a total daily dose of 9 g in adults and adolescents is reasonable. A dose of 1 g orally 3 times per day is recommended in children for a total daily dose of 3 g. Cesium concentration and clinical effects should guide the duration of therapy.

SUMMARY

- Radioactive cesium is a strong β-particles and γ-ray emitter that is released following normal operation of power plants and/or nuclear incidents.
- Because of the availability of commercial and therapeutic sources of radioactive cesium, human exposure is also likely either through unintentional exposure to discarded equipment or through acts of terrorism.
- Exposure to nonradioactive cesium salts occurs through intentional use as an alternative therapy for cancer.
- The principal toxicity of nonradioactive cesium is ventricular dysrhythmias and TdP that result from blockade of cardiac potassium channels.
- In addition to supportive care, Prussian blue is used for both radioactive and nonradioactive cesium toxicity.

REFERENCES

1. Agency for Toxic Substances and Disease Registry. Toxicological profile for cesium. http://www.atsdr.cdc.gov/toxprofiles/tp157.pdf. Accessed April 20, 2013.
2. Bailie DS, et al. Magnesium suppression of early afterdepolarizations and ventricular tachyarrhythmias induced by cesium in dogs. *Circulation.* 1988;77:1395-1402.
3. Boni AL. Correlation of ^{137}Cs concentrations in milk, urine and the whole body. *Health Phys.* 1966;12:501-508.
4. Boni AL. Variations in the retention and excretion of ^{137}Cs with age and sex. *Nature.* 1969;222:1188-1189.
5. Brachmann J, et al. Bradycardia-dependent triggered activity: relevance to drug-induced multiform ventricular tachycardia. *Circulation.* 1983;68:846-856.
6. Braverman ER, et al. Cesium chloride: preventive medicine for radioactive cesium exposure? *Med Hypotheses.* 1988;26:93-95.
7. Brewer KA. The high pH therapy for cancer tests on mice and humans. *Pharmacol Biochem Behav.* 1984;21:1-5.
8. Cahill DF, Wheeler JK. The biological half-life of cesium-137 in children determined by urinary assay. *Health Phys.* 1968;14:293-297.
9. Centeno JA, et al. Blood and tissue concentration of cesium after exposure to cesium chloride. *Biol Trace Elem Res.* 2003;94:97-104.
10. Chan CK, et al. Life-threatening torsades de pointes resulting from "natural" cancer treatment. *Clin Toxicol.* 2009;47:592-594.
11. Conrad RA. Fallout: the experiences of a medical team in the care of a Marshallese population accidentally exposed to fallout radiation. Office of Health, Safety and Security. United States Department of Health. http://www.hss.energy.gov/HealthSafety/IHS/marshall/collection/data/ihp2/0379_.pdf. Accessed August 4, 2012.
12. Coraboeuf F, et al. Acidosis-induced abnormal repolarization and repetitive activity in isolated dog Purkinje fibers. *J Physiol.* 1980;76:97-106.
13. Cranefield PF, Aronson RS. Torsades de pointes and early afterdepolarizations. *Cardiovasc Drugs Ther.* 1991;5:531-537.
14. Curry TB, et al. Acquired long QT syndrome and elective anesthesia in children. *Paediatr Anaesth.* 2006;16:471-478.
15. Dalal AK, et al. Acquired long QT syndrome and monomorphic ventricular tachycardia after alternative treatment with cesium chloride for brain cancer. *Mayo Clin Proc.* 2004;79:1065-1069.
16. D'Alonzo AJ, et al. Effects of intracoronary cromakalin, pinacidil, or diltiazem on cesium chloride-induced arrhythmias in anesthetized dogs under conditions of controlled coronary blood flow. *J Cardiovasc Pharmacol.* 1993;21:677-683.
17. Damiano BP, Rosen MR. Effects of pacing on triggered activity induced by early afterdepolarizations. *Circulation.* 1984;69:1013-1025.
18. Dresow B, et al. In vivo binding of radiocesium by two forms of Prussian blue and by ammonium hexacyanoferrate (II). *Clin Toxicol.* 1993;31:563-569.
19. Eckardt L, et al. Experimental models of torsade de pointes. *Cardiovasc Res.* 1998;39:178-193.
20. El-sherif N. Early afterdepolarizations and arrhythmogenesis. Experimental and clinical aspects. *Arch Mal Coeur Vaiss.* 1991;84:227-234.
21. El-sherif N, Turitto G. Electrolyte disorders and arrhythmogenesis. *Cardiol J.* 2011;18:233-245.
22. Farina R, et al. Medical aspects of ^{137}Cs decorporation: the Goiânia radiological accident. *Health Phys.* 1991;60:63-66.
23. Food and Drug Administration. Cesium implant devices. http://www.accessdata.fda.gov/cdrh_docs/pdf6/K062384.pdf. Accessed August 5, 2012.
24. Forsberg B, et al. Radiation exposure to personnel in departments of gynaecologic oncology in Sweden. *Acta Oncol.* 1987;26:113-123.
25. Gori G, et al. Radioactivity in breast milk and placenta after Chernobyl accident. *Am J Obstet Gynecol.* 1988;158:1243-1244.
26. Gottlöber P, et al. The radiation accident in Georgia: clinical appearance and diagnosis of cutaneous radiation syndrome. *J Am Acad Dermatol.* 2000;42:453-458.
27. Habbab MA, El Sherif N. Drug-induced torsades de pointes: role of early afterdepolarizations and dispersion of repolarization. *Am J Med.* 1990;89:241-246.
28. Han J, et al. Temporal dispersion of recovery of excitability in atrium and ventricle as a function of heart rate. *Am Heart J.* 1966;71:481-487.
29. Hanich RF, et al. Autonomic modulation of ventricular arrhythmia in cesium chloride-induced long QT syndrome. *Circulation.* 1988;77:1149-1161.
30. Harrison JD, et al. Infant doses from the transfer of radionuclides in mother's milk. *Radiat Prot Dosimetry.* 2003;105:251-256.
31. Häsänen E, Rahola T. The biological half-life of ^{137}Cs and ^{24}Na in man. *Ann Clin Res.* 1971;3:236-240.
32. Henrichs K, et al. Measurements of Cs absorption and retention in man. *Health Phys.* 1989;4:571-578.
33. Horn S, et al. Cesium-associated hypokalemia successfully treated with amiloride. *Clin Kidney J.* 2015;8:335-338.
34. Iinuma T, et al. Cesium turnover in man following single administration of ^{132}Cs. I. Whole body retention and excretion pattern. *J Radiat Res.* 1965;6:73-81.
35. Iinuma T, et al. Comparative studies of ^{132}Cs and ^{86}Rb turn-over in man using a double-tracer method. *J Radiat Res.* 1967;8:100-115.
36. International Atomic Energy Agency. Dosimetric and medical aspects of the radiological accident in Goiânia in 1987. http://www-pub.iaea.org/MTCD/publications/PDF/te_1009_prn.pdf. Accessed August 4, 2012.
37. International Atomic Energy Agency. The radiological accident in Tammiku. Vienna, 1998. http://www-pub.iaea.org/MTCD/publications/PDF/Pub1053_web.pdf. Accessed August 4, 2012.
38. January CT, Moscucci A. Cellular mechanisms of early afterdepolarizations. *Ann N Y Acad Sci.* 1992;644:23-32.
39. Josefsson D, et al. The effect of dialysis on radiocesium in man. *Sci Total Environ.* 1995;173-174:407-411.
40. Kaseda S, et al. Depressant effect of magnesium on early afterdepolarizations and triggered activity induced by cesium, quinidine, and 4-aminopyridine in canine cardiac Purkinje fibers. *Am Heart J.* 1989;118:458-466.

41. Khangure SR, et al. CT brain findings in a patient with elevated brain cesium level. *Neuroradiol J*. 2013;26:607-609.

42. Koizumi A, et al. Preliminary assessment of ecological exposure of adult residents in Fukushima Prefecture to radioactive cesium through ingestion and inhalation. *Environ Health Prev Med*. 2012;17:292-298.

43. Krulík R, et al. Distribution of cesium in the organism and its effect on the nucleotide metabolism enzymes. *Int Pharmacopsychiatry*. 1980;15:157-165.

44. Leggett RW, Williams LR. A physiologically based biokinetic model for cesium in the human body. *Sci Total Environ*. 2003;317:235-255.

45. Legett RW. Biokinetic models for radiocesium and its progeny. *J Radiol Prot*. 2013;33:123-1.

46. Levine JH, et al. Cesium chloride-induced long QT syndrome: demonstration of afterdepolarizations and triggered activity in vivo. *Circulation*. 1985;72:1092-1103.

47. Lipsztein JL, et al. Studies of Cs retention in the human body related to body parameters and Prussian blue administration. *Health Phys*. 1991;60:57-61.

48. Lyon AW, Mayhew WJ. Cesium toxicity: a case of self-treatment by alternate therapy gone awry. *Ther Drug Monit*. 2003;25:114-116.

49. Madshus K, Strömme A. Cesium behavior and distribution in man following a single dose of ^{137}Cs. *Z Naturforsch B*. 1964;19:690-692.

50. Madshus K, Strömme A. Increased excretion of ^{137}Cs in humans by Prussian blue. *Z Naturforsch B*. 1968;23:391-392.

51. Matthews CM, et al. Distribution of caesium, rubidium and potassium isotopes in the dog and measurement of coronary flow. *J Nucl Biol Med*. 1969;13:49-63.

52. McCraw TF. The half-time of cesium 137 in man. *Radiol Health Data*. 1965;6:711-718.

53. Messiha FS. A toxicology evaluation of postnatal maternal exposure to cesium. *Physiol Behav*. 1989;46:85-88.

54. Melo DR, et al. ^{137}Cs internal contamination involving a Brazilian accident, and the efficacy of Prussian blue treatment. *Health Phys*. 1994;66:245-252.

55. Miller CE. Retention and distribution of ^{137}Cs after accidental inhalation. *Health Phys*. 1964;10:1065-1070.

56. Moore W Jr, Comar CL. Absorption of caesium 137 from the gastrointestinal tract of the rat. *Int J Radiat Biol*. 1962;5:247-254.

57. Nayebpour M, Nattel S. Pharmacologic response of cesium-induced ventricular tachyarrhythmias in anesthetized dogs. *J Cardiovasc Pharmacol*. 1990;15:552-561.

58. Neulieb R. Effect of oral intake of cesium chloride: a single case report. *Pharmacol Biochem Behav*. 1984;21:15-16.

59. O'Brien CE, et al. Cesium-induced QT-Interval prolongation in an adolescent. *Pharmacotherapy*. 2008;28:1059-1065.

60. Oliveira AR, et al. Medical and related aspects of the Goiânia accident: an overview. *Health Phys*. 1991;60:17-24.

61. Parashar B, et al. Cesium-131 permanent seed brachytherapy: dosimetric evaluation and radiation exposure to surgeons, radiation oncologists, and staff. *Brachytherapy*. 2011;10:508-513.

62. Patterson E, et al. Early and delayed afterdepolarizations associated with cesium chloride-induced arrhythmias in the dog. *J Cardiovasc Pharmacol*. 1990;15:323-331.

63. Patton DD. How Cesium-137 was discovered by an undergraduate student. *J Nucl Med*. 1999;40:18N, 31N.

64. Pinter A, et al. Cesium-induced torsades de pointes. *N Engl J Med*. 2002;346:383-384.

65. Rääf CL, et al. Human metabolism of radiocesium revisited. *Radiat Prot Dosimetry*. 2004;112:395-404.

66. Radiogardase package insert. Haupt Pharma, Berlin GmbH, March 2008.

67. Richmond CR, et al. Long-term retention of radiocesium by man. *Los Alamos Sci*. 1961;2627:163-167.

68. Roberts L. Radiation accident grips Goiânia. *Science*. 1987;238:1028-1031.

69. Rosoff B, et al. Cesium-137 metabolism in man. *Radiat Res*. 1963;19:643-654.

70. Rundo J. The metabolism of biologically important radionuclides. VI. A survey of the metabolism of caesium in man. *Br J Radiol*. 1964;37:108-114.

71. Saenko V, et al. The Chernobyl accident and its consequences. *Clin Oncol*. 2011;23:234-243.

72. Saliba W, et al. Polymorphic ventricular tachycardia in a woman taking cesium chloride. *Pacing Clin Electrophysiol*. 2001;24:515-517.

73. Sartori HE. Cesium therapy in cancer patients. *Pharmacol Biochem Behav*. 1984;21:11-13.

74. Senges JC, et al. Cesium chloride induced ventricular arrhythmias in dogs: three-dimensional activation patterns and their relation to the cesium dose applied. *Basic Res Cardiol*. 2000;95:152-162.

75. Sessions D, et al. Fatal cesium chloride toxicity after alternative cancer treatment. *J Altern Complement Med*. 2013;19:973-975.

76. Stather JW, Smith H. Treatment of accidental intakes of ^{137}Cs. *Health Phys*. 1982; 42:239-240.

77. Strara JF. Tissue distribution and excretion of Cesium-137 in the guinea pig after administration by three different routes. *Health Phys*. 1965;11:1195-1202.

78. Surawicz B. Electrophysiologic substrate of torsade de pointes: dispersion of repolarization or early afterdepolarizations? *J Am Coll Cardiol*. 1989;14:172-184.

79. Thompson DF, Church CO. Prussian blue treatment of radiocesium poisoning. *Pharmacotherapy*. 2001;21:1364-1367.

80. Tourlonias E, et al. Distribution of ^{137}Cs in rat tissues after various schedules of chronic ingestion. *Health Phys*. 2010;99:39-48.

81. Toxnet. Cesium compounds. http://toxnet.nlm.nih.gov/cgi-bin/sis/search/f?./temp/~NFCpS3:3. Accessed August 3, 2012.

82. Uchiyama M. Estimation of ^{137}Cs body burden in Japanese II. The biological half-life. *J Radiat Res*. 1978;19:246-261.

83. United States Department of Energy. Cesium. http://www.evs.anl.gov/pub/doc/esium.pdf. Accessed August 4, 2012.

84. United States Environmental Protection Agency. Cesium. http://www.epa.gov/rpdweb00/radionuclides/cesium.html. Accessed August 3, 2012.

85. Vasilenko IIa. Injury caused by radioactive cesium. *Voen Med Zh*. 1989;5:37-39.

86. Vellar OD, Madshus K. Excretion of radiocesium (^{137}Cs) in sweat from humans. *Z Naturforsch B*. 1970;25:213-216.

87. Verzijl JM, et al. Hemodialysis as a potential method for decontamination of persons exposed to radiocesium. *Health Phys*. 1995;69:543-548.

88. Verzijl JM, et al. In vitro binding characteristics for cesium of two qualities of Prussian blue, activated charcoal, and Resonium-A. *Clin Toxicol*. 1992;30:215-222.

89. von Zallinger C, Tempel K. Transplacental transfer of radionuclides. A review. *Zentralbl Veterinarmed A*. 1998;45:581-590.

90. Vyas H, et al. Acquired long QT syndrome secondary to cesium chloride supplement. *J Altern Complement Med*. 2006;12:1011-1014.

91. Wiens M, et al. Cesium chloride-induced torsades de pointes. *Can J Cardiol*. 2009; 25:e329-e331.

92. Young F, Bolt J. Torsades de pointes—a report of a case induced by caesium taken as a complementary medicine, and the literature review. *J Clin Pharm Ther*. 2013;38:254-257.

93. Zhang S, et al. Modulation of human ether-à-go-go-related K$^+$ (HERG) channel inactivation by Cs$^+$ and K$^+$. *J Physiol*. 2003;548:691-702.

94. Zundel WS, et al. Short half-times of caesium-137 in pregnant women. *Nature*. 1969;221:89-90.

CHROMIUM

Steven B. Bird

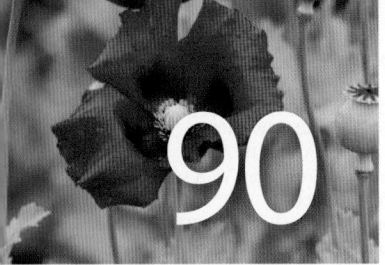

INTRODUCTION

Chromium toxicity results from occupational exposure, environmental exposure, or a combination of both routes. Like many metals, the clinical manifestations of chromium toxicity depend upon whether the exposure is acute or chronic and on the chemical form of chromium. Acute toxicity is more likely to involve multiple-organ failure, whereas chronic exposure is more likely to lead to cancer.

HISTORY AND EPIDEMIOLOGY

Chromium (from the Greek word for color, *chroma*) is a naturally occurring element that is found in oxidation states of –2 to +6, but it primarily exists in the trivalent (Cr^{3+}) and hexavalent (Cr^{6+}) forms. It was first discovered in 1797 in the form of Siberian red lead (crocoite: $PbCrO_4$), and occurs only in combination with other elements, primarily as halides, oxides, or sulfides (Table 90–1). Elemental chromium (Cr^0) does not occur naturally but is extracted commercially from ore. Chromium is found most abundantly in chromite ore ($FeCr_2O_4$).[7]

Elemental chromium is a blue-white metal that is hard and brittle. It is typically polished to a fine, shiny surface, affords significant protection against corrosion, and added to steel to form stainless steel (an alloy of chromium, nickel, and iron). One of the most important uses of chrome plating is to apply a hard, smooth, surface to machine parts such as crankshafts, printing rollers, ball bearings, and cutting tools. This is known as "hard" chrome plating. Elemental chromium is also used in armor plating safes, and is used

TABLE 90–1	Common Forms of Chromium		
Name	Chemical Formula	Oxidation State	Uses
Barium chromate	$BaCrO_4$	6^+	Safety matches, anticorrosive, paint pigment
Calcium chromate	$CaCrO_4$	6^+	Batteries, metallurgy
Chromic acid	H_2CrO_4	6^+	Electroplating, oxidizer
Chromic chloride	$CrCl_3$	3^+	Supplement in total parenteral nutrition
Chromic fluoride	CrF_3	3^+	Mordant in dye industry, mothproofing for wool
Chromic oxide	Cr_2O_3	3^+	Metal plating, wood treatment
Chromite ore	$FeCr_2O_4$	3^+	Water tower treatment
Chromium picolinate	$C_{18}H_{12}CrN_3O_6$	3^+	Nutritional supplement
Lead chromate	$PbCrO_4$	6^+	Yellow pigment for paints and dye
Potassium dichromate	$K_2Cr_2O_7$	6^+	Oxidizer of organic compounds, leather tanning, porcelain painting

in forming brick molds because of its high melting point and moderate thermal expansion.

The carcinogenic potential of hexavalent chromium was first recognized as a cause of nasal tumors in Scottish chrome pigment workers in the late 1800s. In the 1930s, the pulmonary carcinogenicity of hexavalent chromium was first described in German chromate workers.[10]

PHARMACOLOGY

Chromium is an essential element involved in glucose metabolism. The mechanism appears to be either facilitation of insulin binding to insulin receptors or by amplification of the effects of insulin on carbohydrate and lipid metabolism.[19]

The chemical properties and health risks of chromium depend mostly on its oxidative state, and on the solubility of the chromium compound. Chromium is found naturally in the hexavalent (Cr^{6+}) or in the trivalent (Cr^{3+}) valence states, the species most relevant to human exposures. However, chromium has very different properties in the Cr^{6+} and Cr^{3+} oxidation states. The relationship between these oxidative states is described by the following equation[12]:

$$Cr_2O_7^{2-} + 14\ H^+ + 6\ electrons \rightarrow 2Cr^{3+} + 7H_2O + 1.33\ eV$$

This difference of 1.33 eV in electric potential between the Cr^{6+} (in $Cr_2O_7^{2-}$) and Cr^{3+} states reflects both the significant oxidizing potential of Cr^{6+} and the high energy required for the oxidation of Cr^{3+} to Cr^{6+}. Reduction of Cr^{6+} to Cr^{3+} occurs in vivo by abstraction of electrons from cellular constituents such as proteins, lipids, DNA, RNA, and plasma transferrin and accounts for the toxicity of Cr^{6+}.[37]

The rapidity and completeness of the reduction of Cr^{6+} is the subject of considerable scientific debate. Hexavalent chromium is reduced to Cr^{3+} in saliva, the gastrointestinal tract, respiratory tract epithelium and pulmonary macrophages, and in blood.[2,32] During this reduction, several other oxidative states transiently occur (namely Cr^{4+} and Cr^{5+}) and contribute to the cytotoxicity, genotoxicity, and carcinogenicity of Cr^{6+} chromium compounds.[46]

Although most Cr^{6+} is rapidly reduced on entering the gastrointestinal tract, ingestion of Cr^{6+} in drinking water leads to measurable chromium concentrations in plasma, red blood cells, and urine. Hexavalent chromium accumulates in most body tissues, raising concerns that chromium-induced toxicity and carcinogenesis are more widespread than was previously appreciated.[10]

Environmental Exposure

The processing of chromium ores primarily releases Cr^{3+} into the environment. However, some hexavalent chromium is released from chromate manufacturing and coal-based power plants. The most significant environmental sources of Cr^{6+} are chromate production, ferrochrome pigment manufacturing, chrome plating, and certain types of welding.

The general population is exposed to chromium via drinking water, food and food supplements (eg, chromium picolinate), joint arthroplasty, coronary artery stents, and cigarettes. Chromium is used extensively to prevent equipment and piping corrosion in industrial cooling towers and air conditioning (trivalent chromium). Dermal exposure occurs from use of tanned leather products or wood treated with CCA (copper, chromate, and arsenate), which contains hexavalent chromium that is reduced to trivalent chromium by organic compounds once incorporated in wood. Lumber treated with CCA was voluntarily removed from the US consumer market in 2003, because of possible health concerns resulting from exposure to the arsenic and chromium. No specific adverse health effects related to

CCA-treated lumber were reported by the Environmental Protection Agency before the voluntary withdrawal. A reanalysis of cancer mortality and hexavalent chromium–contaminated drinking water from Liaoning Province, China, demonstrated an increase in stomach cancer rate in communities with chromium-contaminated drinking water.[5] Significant exposure from more than 160 chromate production waste sites within Hudson County, New Jersey, was discovered in the late 1980s.[17] A final report published by the Agency for Toxic Substances and Disease Registry in 2008 found an increased risk of lung cancer in populations living in proximity to historic chromium ore–processing residue sites, although the increases were not statistically significant.[33]

Occupational Exposure

Workers in industries that use chromium are exposed to 100 times greater concentrations of chromium than the general population. Chromium pigmentation production and leather tanning use significantly more Cr^{6+} compounds, whereas metal finishing, wood preservation, and cooling towers use Cr^{3+} compounds (Table 90–2).

Several studies focus on the risk of chromium exposure in welders.[41,42] Stainless steel welding liberates significantly more hexavalent chromium than do other types of welding. Although the lung cancer rate of stainless steel (containing chromium) welders was not found to be different from that in regular steel welders, in 2006 the Occupational Safety and Health Administration (OSHA) lowered the permissive exposure limit of hexavalent chromium by 10-fold for welders. More recently, a meta-analysis of occupational exposures demonstrated a statistically significant increase in both lung and stomach cancer in workers with exposure to hexavalent chromium.[50]

Medical Device Exposure

Recent concerns and media attention are directed to the use of metal on metal (MoM) implants for total hip arthroplasty and surface refinishing. Unlike non-MoM implants in which the articular surfaces are made of ceramic or polyethylene, these metal implants have metal rubbing on metal. For more than 20 years, it has been known that blood concentrations of metal ions increase in patients with MoM hip arthroplasty. One-year postoperative blood chromium concentrations increased by 21 times over the preoperative concentrations.[21] Metal release will cause some tiny metal particles to wear off of the device around the implant, which causes damage to bone and/or soft tissue surrounding the implant and joint. Although some patients with failed MoM hip implants report memory difficulties, chronic pain, and pain in the implanted hip, the true incidence and nature of adverse health outcomes due to release of chromium ions and particles from these implants is not yet established. Currently, there is insufficient evidence to conclusively demonstrate that with regard to chromium, MoM hip implants produce side effects beyond those that may occur at the site of implantation. There is no consensus on what might be the significance of elevated blood chromium concentrations,

TABLE 90–2	Occupations at Risk for Chromium Exposure
Cement workers	
Chromite ore workers	
Electroplaters	
Foundry workers	
Galvanized steel workers	
Glass polishers and glazers	
Lithographers	
Machinists	
Painters	
Photograph developers	
Tanners	
Textile dyers	
Welders	
Wood preservers	

nor are there data to specify the concentration of chromium necessary to produce adverse systemic effects. Further discussion of orthoprosthetic cobaltism is found in the chapter on cobalt effects in MoM Hip implants. (Chap. 91).[16]

PHARMACOKINETICS AND TOXICOKINETICS

Because they possess significantly different properties, Cr^{3+} and Cr^{6+} must be evaluated separately.

Absorption

Trivalent Chromium Compounds

Oral absorption of Cr^{3+} salts is limited. Approximately 98% is recovered in the feces, just 0.1% is excreted in the bile, and 0.5% to 2.0% is excreted in the urine.[14,16] Human case reports and animal studies also corroborate the generally poor absorption of Cr^{3+} salts by the oral, inhalational, and dermal routes, except through burns and other disrupted mucosal or epithelial surfaces.[27]

Hexavalent Chromium Compounds

Cr^{6+} is modestly absorbed after ingestion partly as a result of the structural similarity between hexavalent chromium compounds and phosphate and sulfate.[11] These 3 chemicals undergo facilitated diffusion through non-specific anion channels as well as active transport. In human volunteers, approximately 10% of an ingested dose of sodium chromate was absorbed; duodenal administration increased this to roughly 50%.[14] This difference likely relates to the reduction of the hexavalent chromium to trivalent chromium in the acidic environment of the stomach. Similarly, 3 hours after the ingestion of a lethal amount of potassium dichromate (hexavalent), greater than 80% of the chromium was reduced to the trivalent state in the blood.[20] Hexavalent chromium compounds are generally not well absorbed after dermal exposure. Whatever the route of exposure, Cr^{6+} is absorbed much more readily than Cr^{3+}, but the Cr^{6+} is then rapidly reduced to Cr^{3+} after absorption.

Epidemiologically, inhalation of Cr^{6+} is the most consequential route of exposure. Furthermore, the greatest health consequences from Cr^{6+} exposure are due to inhalation. The exact rate of absorption is unknown, but is dependent on the solubility of the specific Cr^{6+} compound, the size of the particles, the phagocytic activity of the pulmonary macrophages, and the general health of the lungs. In animal studies roughly 50% to 85% of small (<5 μm) inhaled Cr^{6+} potassium dichromate particles are absorbed.[34]

Distribution

Because most of the Cr^{6+} is rapidly reduced on absorption by the gastrointestinal tract and by red blood cells (RBCs), Cr^{3+} accounts for virtually the entire body burden of chromium. Trivalent chromium accumulates to the greatest extent in the kidneys, bone marrow, lungs, lymph nodes, liver, spleen, and testes. The kidneys and liver alone account for approximately 50% of the total body burden.[11]

Elimination

Urinary excretion of trivalent chromium occurs rapidly. Roughly 80% of parenterally administered Cr^{6+} is excreted as Cr^{3+} in the urine and 2% to 20% in the feces.[31] The urinary excretion half-life of Cr^{6+} ranges from 15 to 41 hours.[22] Because Cr^{6+} undergoes reduction to Cr^{3+} following uptake by RBCs, an apparent slow compartment is created, with the elimination half-life dependent on the life span of erythrocytes. Small amounts of chromium are detectable in sweat, breast milk, nails, and hair.

PATHOPHYSIOLOGY

Trivalent Chromium

Trivalent chromium is an essential trace metal required for the metabolism of glucose and fats. The complex nutritional interactions of trivalent chromium with numerous metabolic pathways are not understood, and remain the subject of much debate among researchers. However, it is clear that dietary chromium deficiency leads to insulin resistance with elevated insulin concentrations, hypercholesterolemia, hyperglycemia, increased body fat, and the attendant risks of these metabolic derangements. Trivalent chromium enhances insulin sensitivity and glucose disappearance concomitantly with lower insulin concentrations in an obese rat model, with no difference in lean controls.[9]

Chromium picolinate is a popular Cr^{3+} dietary supplement. There is a dearth of rigorous science concerning the efficacy or safety of chromium picolinate. However, organ deposition of Cr^{3+} occurs.[40] There is no strong evidence of any significant end-organ toxicity due to exposure to Cr^{3+}, perhaps because Cr^{3+} is so poorly absorbed. There is little or no rigorous evidence that exposure to Cr^{3+} compounds increases cancer risk. Animal work and epidemiologic studies of workers exposed to Cr^{3+} compounds fail to demonstrate a statistically significant increased incidence of cancer.[3]

Hexavalent Chromium

Hexavalent chromium is a powerful oxidizing agent that has corrosive and irritant effects. The greatest toxicity from Cr^{6+} lies in its ability to produce oxidative DNA damage. Strand breaks with DNA, DNA–DNA and DNA–protein crosslinks, and nucleotide modifications all occur.[12] Although the exact mechanisms of how Cr^{6+} is genotoxic are unknown, transient toxic chromium intermediates such as Cr^{4+} and Cr^{5+} are probably responsible.[39]

Inconsistent data suggest that either immunostimulation or immunosuppression result from chronic chromium exposure. At least one study suggests that chromium induced immunosuppression is responsible for implant associated infections in patients after hip or knee arthroplasty.[39] Although human data are incomplete, adverse developmental effects, including cleft palate, hydrocephalus, and neural tube defects, are demonstrated in animals.[13]

CLINICAL MANIFESTATIONS

The clinical manifestations of chromium poisoning depend on the valence of chromium, the source and route of exposure, and the duration of exposure. The clinical manifestations of chromium exposure are best divided into acute and chronic (low-level exposure) effects.

Acute

Manifestations of acute, massive Cr^{6+} ingestions are similar to other caustic metal ingestions. Gastrointestinal hemorrhage, with or without bowel perforation, occurs acutely.[51] Because of the strong oxidative properties of Cr^{6+}, intravascular hemolysis with disseminated intravascular coagulation is also observed. Renal effects include acute tubular necrosis leading to acute kidney injury.[49] Metabolic abnormalities after acute, massive, exposure include metabolic acidosis with elevated lactate concentration, hyperkalemia, and uremia. Acute respiratory distress syndrome (ARDS) develops up to 3 days after exposure. Although Cr^{6+} is generally not well absorbed after dermal exposure, it is a caustic that causes skin inflammation and ulceration, which ultimately increases dermal absorption. Dermal chromic acid (H_2CrO_4) burns lead to severe systemic toxicity with as little as 10% body surface area involvement.

Chronic

Because most chronic exposures are inhalational, the respiratory tract is the organ most affected after chronic chromium exposure. When inhaled, Cr^{6+} is a respiratory tract irritant that causes inflammation and, with continued exposure, ulceration including nasal septum perforation.[23] Furthermore, the sensitizing effects of Cr^{6+} leads to chronic cough, shortness of breath, occupational asthma, bronchospasm, and anaphylactoid reactions. Chronic deposition of chromium dust is also associated with pneumoconiosis.[38]

Epidemiologic studies of chromate workers in the 1980s indicated a significantly increased risk of lung cancer in those individuals exposed to Cr^{6+} compounds.[24,35] Small cell and poorly differentiated carcinomas are the most common types, although nearly all pathologic types of lung cancer are associated with inhalational Cr^{6+} exposure.[1] The latency between exposure and development of lung cancer ranges from 13 to 30 years, although cases are reported after as few as 2 years.[6]

Although conclusive evidence is lacking, it appears that chronic exposure to Cr^{6+} via all routes causes mild to moderate elevation in hepatic aminotransferases and abnormal liver architecture, visible on histologic

specimens.[51] Unlike acute exposures, low-dose chronic chromium exposure occasionally causes transiently elevated urinary β_2-microglobulin concentrations, with no obvious lasting effects.[49]

Type IV (delayed-type) hypersensitivity reactions occur after acute exposure to hexavalent chromium compounds. Chronic hexavalent chromium exposures also occur via dermal contact. Up to 24% of cement workers who have frequent contact with wet cement (which contains Cr^{6+}), automobile part handlers, and locksmiths develop skin sensitivity to chromium compounds.[26,28]

Occupational chromium exposure leads to contact dermatitis in as many as 10% to 20% of chromium workers.[44] There remains considerable debate over the relative sensitization abilities of Cr^{3+} and Cr^{6+}. Furthermore, what was initially thought to be sensitization to Cr^{3+} exposure was more likely exposure to Cr^{6+} with subsequent in vivo reduction to Cr^{3+}. It is likely, however, the Cr^{6+} is a more potent sensitizer than Cr^{3+}, and that there is limited cross-reactivity between the 2 forms of chromium.[15] Similarly, exposure to chromium-containing gaming table felt has led to hand dermatitis referred to as "blackjack disease," and virtually all occupations that involve exposure to inhaled chromium can lead to painless, scarring skin and nasal septum ulcerations, referred to as "chrome holes".[25]

DIAGNOSTIC TESTING

Chromium is detected in blood, urine, and hair of exposed individuals. Because of the great difficulty in speciation, differentiation between Cr^{3+} and Cr^{6+} is generally not performed; instead, the total chromium concentration is usually reported. Needles used for phlebotomy and plastic containers used for sample storage generally contain significant amounts of chromium. Unfortunately, there are no commercially available chromium-free needles. Modern, highly sensitive assay equipment, such as graphite furnace atomic absorption spectrometry, neutron activation analysis, and graphite spark atomic emission spectrometry, require diligence in sample handling to ensure that biological samples are not contaminated.

Because of the inherent difficulties in quantifying trace elements such as chromium, and the lack of standard chromium reference materials, the reported normal serum and urine chromium concentrations in unexposed people have varied by more than 5,000-fold over the last 50 years.[34] Consequently, older reference ranges should be interpreted with caution. Lastly, although cigarette smoke contains chromium, no studies have quantified the effect of smoking on serum, blood, or urinary chromium concentrations.

Blood or Serum

Chromium is distributed evenly between the serum and erythrocytes. Serum chromium concentrations are reflective of recent exposure to both Cr^{3+} and Cr^{6+}. Serum concentrations in people without occupational exposure to chromium are reported to be from 0.05 mcg/L (1 nmol/L)[8] up to more than 2.8 mcg/L (54 nmol/L).[34] It is not certain whether concentrations above these values should be considered potentially toxic, as no clear correlation has been found between serum or blood concentrations and physiologic effects.

Urine

Although urine chromium concentrations reflect the acute absorption of chromium over the previous 1 to 2 days, wide individual variation in metabolism and total body burden limit the value of urinary chromium monitoring. Urine should be collected over a 24-hour period because of diurnal variation in excretion. Data from the third National Health and Nutrition Examination Survey (NHANES III) demonstrated mean and median urinary chromium concentrations in approximately 500 individuals without known exposure to chromium of 0.22 mcg/L (4.2 nmol/L) and 0.13 mcg/L (2.5 nmol/L). When corrected for creatinine, the values were 0.21 and 0.12 mcg/g creatinine, respectively.[30]

Hair and Nails

Hair and nail samples are not reliable indicators of exposure to chromium because of the difficulty distinguishing between chromium contamination of the hair sample from chromium incorporated into the hair during normal hair protein synthesis. Chromium found in hair is not due to contamination or exposure to shampoo or tap water.[18] Chromium concentrations in hair are up to 1,000 times higher than those found in serum.

Ancillary Tests

After confirmed or suspected acute chromium exposure, complete blood count, serum electrolytes, blood urea nitrogen, creatinine, urinalysis, and liver enzymes testing should be performed. If signs of systemic toxicity are evident, serial determination of coagulation function and disseminated intravascular coagulation may be useful to guide therapy.

MANAGEMENT

Acute chromium ingestions are infrequent, but often severe, with significant morbidity and mortality. Consequently, after adequate airway, breathing, and circulatory support are addressed, attention should be given to decontamination.

Decontamination

Because of its serious but very limited toxicity, Cr^{3+} compounds require limited decontamination measures. Decontamination with soap and water is recommended after skin contact. No specific pulmonary decontamination is required.

Hexavalent chromium is caustic and profuse vomiting and hematemesis usually follow acute ingestions. Nasogastric lavage is reasonable after Cr^{6+} ingestions if the patient presents to the emergency department within several hours of exposure and no vomiting has occurred. There are no data regarding the use of activated charcoal in acute chromium ingestions and endoscopic visualization will be more difficult after administration of activated charcoal. Therefore, we recommend using activated charcoal in order to obtain adequate endoscopic visualization.

Oral N-acetylcysteine increases the renal excretion of chromium in rats,[4] but there are no human data to support this therapy. Years of clinical experience using N-acetylcysteine for other indications and the very low incidence of adverse effects, however, makes the administration of oral N-acetylcysteine in the setting of acute chromium toxicity reasonable.

Although ascorbic acid facilitates reduction of Cr^{6+} to Cr^{3+} in vitro, there are no data to substantiate decreased absorption.[44] There is some evidence that topical ascorbic acid reduces dermal Cr^{6+} exposure, but this was not demonstrated in controlled trials.[39] Therefore, the routine use of ascorbic acid cannot be recommended at this time.

Chelation Therapy

Currently available chelators do not appear efficacious at either lowering serum or blood chromium concentrations or ameliorating chromium toxicity in experimental models. Specifically, calcium ethylenediaminetetraacetic acid (CaEDTA) had no effect on urinary chromium excretion in experimental animals[48] and dimercaprol (British anti-Lewsite {BAL}) was not beneficial in an animal model of chromium poisoning.[29]

In a single study, dimercaptopropane sulfonate (DMPS) had no effect on urinary chromium excretion in humans.[45] D-Penicillamine also failed to increase urinary excretion of chromium.[29] There are no studies of chromium chelation with 2,3-dimercaptosuccinic acid (succimer). Therefore, at this time, there is no evidence to support the use of any chelation therapy after acute Cr^{6+} or Cr^{3+} poisoning.

Extracorporeal Elimination

Hemodialysis, hemofiltration, and peritoneal dialysis do not efficiently remove chromium. Studies in animals and human case reports indicate that as little as 1% of chromium is removed by hemodialysis or hemofiltration after acute dichromate (a hexavalent compound) exposure.[20,43] Limited data in dialysis patients demonstrate some ability of peritoneal dialysis and hemodialysis to remove intravenously administered chromium.[36] Therefore, in the setting of normal renal function, extracorporeal means of eliminated chromium are not likely to be of benefit. In the setting of acute

kidney injury or chronic kidney disease, peritoneal dialysis or hemodialysis is a reasonable therapeutic choice to attempt to reduce serum chromium concentrations, although there are no data that clinical outcomes are affected.

SUMMARY

- Hexavalent chromium remains an uncommon, but serious, cause of acute metal poisoning, whereas trivalent chromium is minimally toxic.
- Acute ingestion of Cr^{6+} chromium salts causes gastrointestinal hemorrhage, hepatic necrosis, and acute kidney injury.
- Toxicity after chronic Cr^{6+} chromium exposure includes ulcerations of the skin and nasopharynx ("chrome holes"), and more significantly, lung and stomach cancer. Definitive data regarding other types of cancer resulting from chronic Cr^{6+} exposure are unavailable.
- Regardless of the time course of the poisoning, treatment for chromium exposure includes removal of the patient from the source of exposure, gastrointestinal decontamination, and supportive care.
- There is insufficient evidence to support the use of chelators in either acute or chronic chromium poisoning.

REFERENCES

1. Abe S, et al. Chromate lung cancer with special reference to its cell type and relation to the manufacturing process. *Cancer.* 1982;49:783-787.
2. Aitio A, et al. Urinary excretion of chromium as an indicator of exposure to trivalent chromium sulphate in leather tanning. *Int Arch Occup Environ Health.* 1984;54:241-249.
3. Axelsson G, et al. Mortality and incidence of tumours among ferrochromium workers. *Br J Ind Med.* 1980;37:121-127.
4. Banner W Jr, et al. Experimental chelation therapy in chromium, lead, and boron intoxication with N-acetylcysteine and other compounds. *Toxicol Appl Pharmacol.* 1986;83:142-147.
5. Beaumont JJ, et al. Cancer mortality in a Chinese population exposed to hexavalent chromium in drinking water. *Epidemiology.* 2008;19:12-23.
6. Becker N. Cancer mortality among arc welders exposed to fumes containing chromium and nickel. Results of a third follow-up: 1989-1995. *J Occup Environ Med.* 1999;41:294-303.
7. Bencko V. Chromium: a review of environmental and occupational toxicology. *J Hyg Epidemiol Microbiol Immunol.* 1985;29:37-46.
8. Brune D, et al. Normal concentrations of chromium in serum and urine—a TRACY project. *Scand J Work Environ Health.* 1993;19(suppl 1):39-44.
9. Cefalu WT, et al. Oral chromium picolinate improves carbohydrate and lipid metabolism and enhances skeletal muscle glut-4 translocation in obese, hyperinsulinemic (JCR-LA corpulent) rats. *J Nutr.* 2002;132:1107-1114.
10. Cohen MD, et al. Mechanisms of chromium carcinogenicity and toxicity. *Crit Rev Toxicol.* 1993;23:255-281.
11. Costa M. Toxicity and carcinogenicity of Cr(VI) in animal models and humans. *Crit Rev Toxicol.* 1997;27:431-442.
12. Dayan AD, Paine AJ. Mechanisms of chromium toxicity, carcinogenicity and allergenicity: review of the literature from 1985 to 2000. *Hum Exp Toxicol.* 2001;20:439-451.
13. Domingo JL. Metal-induced developmental toxicity in mammals: a review. *J Toxicol Environ Health.* 1994;42:123-141.
14. Donaldson RM Jr, Barreras RF. Intestinal absorption of trace quantities of chromium. *J Lab Clin Med.* 1966;68:484-493.
15. Eisler R. *Handbook of Chemical Risk Assessment: Health Hazards to Humans, Plants, and Animals.* Boca Raton, FL: CRC Press; 2000.
16. FDA. FDA safety communication: metal-on-metal hip implants. http://www.fda.gov/MedicalDevices/Safety/AlertsandNotices/ucm335775.htm. Published 2013. Accessed July 24, 2017.
17. Freeman NC, et al. Exposure to chromium dust from homes in a Chromium Surveillance Project. *Arch Environ Health.* 1997;52:213-219.
18. Hambidge KM, et al. Hair chromium concentration: effects of sample washing and external environment. *Am J Clin Nutr.* 1972;25:384-389.
19. Hua Y, et al. Molecular mechanisms of chromium in alleviating insulin resistance. *J Nutr Biochem.* 2012;23:313-319.
20. Iserson KV, et al. Failure of dialysis therapy in potassium dichromate poisoning. *J Emerg Med.* 1983;1:143-149.
21. Jacobs JJ, et al. Metal degradation products: a cause for concern in metal-metal bearings? *Clin Orthop Relat Res.* 2003:139-147.
22. Kerger BD, et al. Ingestion of chromium(VI) in drinking water by human volunteers: absorption, distribution, and excretion of single and repeated doses. *J Toxicol Environ Health.* 1997;50:67-95.
23. Koutkia P, Wang RY. Electroplaters. In: Greenberg MI, et al., eds. *Occupational, Industrial, and Environmental Toxicology.* Boston, MA: Mosby; 2003:126-139.
24. Langard S, Vigander T. Occurrence of lung cancer in workers producing chromium pigments. *Br J Ind Med.* 1983;40:71-74.

25. Lee HS, Goh CL. Occupational dermatosis among chrome platers. *Contact Dermatitis.* 1988;18:89-93.

26. Liden C, et al. Deposition of nickel, chromium, and cobalt on the skin in some occupations—assessment by acid wipe sampling. *Contact Dermatitis.* 2008;58:347-354.

27. Matey P, et al. Chromic acid burns: early aggressive excision is the best method to prevent systemic toxicity. *J Burn Care Rehabil.* 2000;21:241-245.

28. Newhouse ML. A cause of chromate dermatitis among assemblers in an automobile factory. *Br J Ind Med.* 1963;20:199-203.

29. Nowak-Wiaderek W. Influence of various drugs on excretion and distribution of chromium-51 in acute poisoning in rats. *Mater Med Pol.* 1975;7:308-310.

30. Paschal DC, et al. Trace metals in urine of United States residents: reference range concentrations. *Environ Res.* 1998;76:53-59.

31. Paustenbach DJ, et al. Observation of steady state in blood and urine following human ingestion of hexavalent chromium in drinking water. *J Toxicol Environ Health.* 1996;49:453-461.

32. Proctor DM, et al. Is hexavalent chromium carcinogenic via ingestion? A weight-of-evidence review. *J Toxicol Environ Health A.* 2002;65:701-746.

33. Registry Agency for Toxic Substances and Disease. *Analysis of Lung Cancer Incidence Near Chromium-Contaminated Sites in New Jeresy (a/k/a Hudson County Chromium Sites) Jersey City, Hudson County, New Jersey.* September 30, 2008.

34. Registry. Agency for Toxic Substances and Disease. Toxicologic profile for chronmium compounds. Atlanta, GA: US Department of Health and Human Services, Public Health Service, ATSDR; 2000.

35. Satoh K, et al. Epidemiological study of workers engaged in the manufacture of chromium compounds. *J Occup Med.* 1981;23:835-838.

36. Schiffl H, et al. Dialysis treatment of acute chromium intoxication and comparative efficacy of peritoneal versus hemodialysis in chromium removal. *Miner Electrolyte Metab.* 1982;7:28-35.

37. Shrivastava R, et al. Effects of chromium on the immune system. *FEMS Immunol Med Microbiol.* 2002;34:1-7.

38. Sluis-Cremer GK, Du Toit RS. Pneumoconiosis in chromite miners in South Africa. *Br J Ind Med.* 1968;25:63-67.

39. Stearns DM, et al. Reduction of chromium(VI) by ascorbate leads to chromium-DNA binding and DNA strand breaks in vitro. *Biochemistry.* 1995;34:910-919.

40. Stearns DM, et al. Chromium(III) picolinate produces chromosome damage in Chinese hamster ovary cells. *FASEB J.* 1995;9:1643-1648.

41. Stern RM, et al. In vitro toxicity of welding fumes and their constituents. *Environ Res.* 1988;46:168-180.

42. Stern RM. In vitro assessment of equivalence of occupational health risk: welders. *Environ Health Perspect.* 1983;51:217-222.

43. Stift A, et al. Liver transplantation for potassium dichromate poisoning. *N Engl J Med.* 1998;338:766-767.

44. Suzuki Y. Reduction of hexavalent chromium by ascorbic acid in rat lung lavage fluid. *Arch Toxicol.* 1988;62:116-122.

45. Torres-Alanis O, et al. Urinary excretion of trace elements in humans after sodium 2,3-dimercaptopropane-1-sulfonate challenge test. *J Toxicol Clin Toxicol.* 2000;38:697-700.

46. Vasant C, et al. Apoptosis of lymphocytes in the presence of Cr(V) complexes: role in Cr(VI)-induced toxicity. *Biochem Biophys Res Commun.* 2001;285:1354-1360.

47. Wang JY, et al. Prosthetic metals impair murine immune response and cytokine release in vivo and in vitro. *J Orthop Res.* 1997;15:688-699.

48. Waters MD, et al. Metal toxicity for rabbit alveolar macrophages in vitro. *Environ Res.* 1975;9:32-47.

49. Wedeen RP, Qian LF. Chromium-induced kidney disease. *Environ Health Perspect.* 1991;92:71-74.

50. Welling R, et al. Chromium VI and stomach cancer: a meta-analysis of the current epidemiological evidence. *Occup Environ Med.* 2015;72:151-159.

51. Wood R, et al. Acute dichromate poisoning after use of traditional purgatives. A report of 7 cases. *S Afr Med J.* 1990;77:640-642.

91 COBALT

Gar Ming Chan

Cobalt (Co)

Atomic number	=	27
Atomic weight	=	58.9 Da
Normal concentrations		
Serum	=	0.1–1.2 mcg/L (1.7–20.4 nmol/L)
Urine	=	0.1–2.2 mcg/L (1.7–37.3 nmol/L)

HISTORY AND EPIDEMIOLOGY

The name cobalt (Co) originates from, "kobold" (German for "goblin"), and was given to the cobalt-containing ore cobaltite (CoAsS), because it made exposed miners ill. However, the miners' illness had more likely resulted from the arsenic exposure than that of the cobalt. Georg Brandt discovered cobalt in 1753 during an attempt to prove that an element other than bismuth gave glass a blue hue.

With an atomic number of 27 and a molecular weight of 58.93 Da, cobalt is a light metal that has a melting point of 1,768.2° K and a boiling point of 3,373° K. These attributes make elemental Co (Co^0) very useful in industry, in which it is primarily incorporated into hard, high-speed, high-temperature cutting tools. When aluminum and nickel are blended with cobalt, an alloy (Alnico) with magnetic properties is formed. Other uses for cobalt include electroplating because of its resistance to oxidation and as an artist's pigment owing to its bright blue color.

A Co^{3+} ion is at the center of cyanocobalamin (vitamin B_{12}), which is synthesized only by microorganisms and is not found in plants. Common dietary sources are fish, eggs, chicken, pork, and seafood. A diet deficient in cyanocobalamin results in pernicious anemia. Hydroxocobalamin, a Co^{3+}-containing precursor to cyanocobalamin, is used as an antidote for cyanide poisoning (Antidotes in Depth: A41).

Medicinally, cobalt chloride was combined with iron salts and marketed in the 1950s as Roncovite, for the treatment of anemia because of its ability to stimulate erythropoiesis. As recently as 1976, physicians still used cobalt salts to reduce transfusion requirements in anemic patients in spite of concomitant adverse effects.[47] The other common medical use of cobalt is as a radioactive isotope, cobalt-60 (^{60}Co). This gamma emitter was formerly used in the radiotherapy of cancers but was largely replaced by linear accelerators in the Western world. Radiotherapy devices are a source of radioactive material that could be used by terrorist groups.

Epidemics of cardiomyopathy and goiter termed "beer drinker's cardiomyopathy"[18] and "cobalt-induced goiter"[33,104] occurred between the 1950s and the 1970s. During that period, cobalt sulfate was added to beer as a foam stabilizer. In the 1970s, these epidemics were halted with the discontinued use of cobalt sulfate for this purely aesthetic purpose.[119]

Current sources of cobalt exposure include chemistry sets,[80] weather indicators,[80] antiquated anemia therapies,[80] cement,[88] fly ash,[88] dyes,[56] mineral wool,[88] asbestos,[88] molds for ceramic tiles,[52] the production of Widia-steel (utilized in the wood industry),[159] mining,[81] porcelain paint,[140] orthopedic implants,[79] dental hardware,[9] and as a nutritional supplement.[177] The most recent area of concern is "arthroprosthetic cobaltism,"[109,128,145,175,176] which results from cobalt-containing orthopedic implants.[2] The prevalence of arthroprosthetic cobaltism is largely unknown, and likely underreported. The usage of metal-on-metal implants began in the 1990s and since has been was voluntarily recalled as a result of the high rate of implant failure in 2010.[97] Determining the at-risk population is both difficult and dynamic due to the associated reporting practices and potential litigation activity. Metal-on-metal implants are considered the highest-risk prostheses; however, there are cases that include exposure to other types of metal-containing implants.[30] A proposed risk stratification algorithm uses patient factors, such as female sex and high levels of activity, and implant factors such as diameter of femoral heads (≥36 mm).[96]

The largest source, however, arises through the formation of cemented tungsten carbide, a "hard metal." In tungsten carbide factories, powdered cobalt and tungsten are combined through an intense sintering process that exposes these metals to hydrogen heated to 1,000°C. The first published investigation of these factories reported a 10-fold increase in workspace cobalt concentrations compared to atmospheric concentrations.[49] These respiratory exposures produced pulmonary toxicity, known as "hard-metal disease." As a result of this report, occupational studies and preventive measures have greatly reduced the acceptable cobalt exposure concentration in the workplace.

CHEMISTRY

Like other metals, cobalt occurs in elemental, inorganic, and organic forms. The clinical effects of each form are less well defined than the more common transition metals such as lead, mercury, or arsenic. Elemental cobalt (Co^0) toxicity is reported through both inhalational[173] and oral exposures.[74] Inorganic cobalt salts typically occur in one of 2 oxidation states: cobaltous (Co^{2+}) or cobaltic (Co^{3+}). Inorganic cobalt salts, such as cobaltous chloride ($CoCl_2$) and cobaltous sulfate ($CoSO_4$), were historically used for the treatment of anemias[19,62,70,139,186] and were implicated in the "beer drinker's cardiomyopathy" epidemics, respectively.[4,113,121]

Organic cobalt exposure results from cyanocobalamin (vitamin B_{12}) ingestion, but as a result of its limited oral absorption and its rapid renal elimination it is considered of low toxicity.[136] Comparing organic and inorganic forms of cobalt in animal models, inorganic cobalt salts are more toxic than the organic forms such as cobalt stearate.[25]

TOXICOKINETICS

Based on animal studies, oral absorption of cobalt oxides, salts, and metal is highly variable, with a reported bioavailability of 5% to 45%.[89,103] In human studies, both iron deficiency and iron overload (hemochromatosis) enhance radio-labeled $^{57}CoCl_2$ absorption in the small bowel.[127] Similarly, inhaled cobalt oxide is about 30% bioavailable,[103] but the volume of distribution and elimination half-life are not well defined.

The distribution of cobalt is influenced by plasma proteins, mainly albumin,[26,27] and is the basis of the U.S. Food and Drug Administration (FDA) approved the Albumin Cobalt Binding test (ACB test) for myocardial ischemia. Transferrin, another plasma protein, which normally binds iron, also binds cobalt, explaining its erythropoietic effect.[82] Following distribution, cellular uptake is mediated by the P2X7 transporter[179] and the active divalent metal transporter 1 (DMT1).[27]

Most (50%–88%) absorbed cobalt (organic and inorganic) is eliminated renally, and the remainder is eliminated in the feces.[157] Acutely, an increase in inorganic cobalt concentrations will result in an increased renal elimination.[86] However, this initial increased elimination decreases rapidly in spite of a large body burden.[5,127]

The elimination of cobalt correlates with the patterns of occupational exposure.[173] For example, a worker with a standard (Monday to Friday) work week will have much higher urine cobalt concentrations on Friday morning compared to Monday morning.[173] However, this finding that Monday afternoon urine cobalt concentrations are higher than Friday morning concentrations is due to the rapid elimination that occurs following an initial exposure.[5,173] Based on these findings, the exposure over time must be considered when interpreting urinary cobalt concentrations in occupationally exposed individuals.[14]

PATHOPHYSIOLOGY

Like other transition metals, cobalt is a multiorgan toxin. Divalent cobalt inhibits several key enzyme systems and interferes with the initiation of protein synthesis.[15] Polynucleotide phosphorylase, an essential enzyme in RNA synthesis, requires Mg^{2+} to function normally. In vitro, this enzyme only functions at 50% that of normal in the presence of Co^{2+}.[15] It is hypothesized that Co^{2+} is capable of displacing Mg^{2+} from the cofactor site of this enzyme.[15]

Cobalt salts interfere with the citric acid cycle mitochondrial enzyme, α-ketoglutarate dehydrogenase. Because of this inhibition, Co^{2+} increases the rate of anaerobic glycolysis and at the same time decreases oxygen consumption,[36] and thus inhibits aerobic metabolism. In vitro studies demonstrate that other divalent cations, Zn^{2+}, Cd^{2+}, Cu^{2+}, and Ni^{2+}, also inhibit α-ketoglutarate dehydrogenase (Chap. 11).[183] When compared with these divalent cations, Co^{2+} is not considered a potent inhibitor.[183] However, this in vitro model demonstrates that Co^{2+} is capable of almost entirely inhibiting the reaction when nicotinamide adenine dinucleotide (NADH) is added.[183] This study suggests that NADH abundance, such as occurs with chronic ethanol use, potentiates the inhibition of α-ketoglutarate dehydrogenase.[184]

Moreover, cobalt salts are capable of inhibiting α lipoic acid and dihydrolipoic acid by complexing with its sulfhydryl groups.[38,183] These reactions result in the inability to convert both pyruvate into acetyl-CoA and α-ketoglutarate into succinyl-CoA (Chap. 11 and Antidotes in Depth: A27). These combined interactions offer explanations as to why chronic ethanol use and cobalt exposure result in cardiomyopathy (Chap. 53).[183]

In addition to enzyme inhibition, $CoCl_2$ induces oxidant-mediated pulmonary toxicity (see below)[124] and neurotoxicity.[27] Xenobiotics implicated in free radical–mediated pulmonary injury are capable of accepting an electron from a reductant and subsequently transferring the electron to oxygen, forming a superoxide free radical (Chap. 10). Cobalt is then capable of accepting another electron, which starts the cycle over again—a process known as redox cycling. This leads to an accumulation of free radicals in the lung due to the abundance of oxygen ready to receive electrons and results in injury.

Within the endocrine system, $CoCl_2$ inhibits tyrosine iodinase.[92] This enzyme is responsible for combining iodine (I_2) with tyrosine to form monoiodotyrosine and serves as the first step in the synthesis of thyroid hormone (Chap. 53). This inhibition decreases circulating T_3 and T_4, which results in hypothyroidism (see below).

The hematopoietic system is also affected by Co salts. Multiple animal models demonstrate that $CoCl_2$ administration results in reticulocytosis, polycythemia, and erythropoiesis.[55,90,118,129,130,186] These events occur in both the bone marrow and extramedullary locations.[19,59] Although the pathogenesis remains largely unknown,[38] one theory is that cobalt ion binds to iron-binding sites such as transferrin,[82] resulting in impaired oxygen transport to renal cells, which in turn induces erythropoietin production. A second theory in which cobalt is thought to stimulate erythropoiesis is through improving iron availability. In an animal model of anemia, a greater degree of gastrointestinal iron uptake occurs in cobalt-treated rats compared to rats with either hypoxia or nephrectomy.[59] A similar study of injected cobalt chloride in mice suggested that the increase in iron uptake exceeded that following exogenous erythropoietin.[6] Moreover, human data demonstrate $CoCl_2$ in vivo induce hypoxia inducible factor-1 alpha (HIF-1α) protein expression, transcription factors responsible for hypoxia-linked effects.[152]

Finally, within the nervous system, $CoCl_2$ inhibits neuromuscular transmission by competing with Ca^{2+}, another divalent ion. Co^{2+} is 20 times more potent than magnesium with regard to its ability to compete with calcium for a site on the motor nerve terminal.[182] Additionally, the formation of free radicals is theorized as a cause of cobalt associated neurotoxicity.[27]

TOXICITY

The single acute minimal toxic dose of cobalt salts is not well defined, and comparable doses have variable effects in different patients. Patients with "beer drinker's cardiomyopathy" received an average daily dose of 6 to 8 mg of $CoSO_4$ (over weeks to months) and developed toxic effects of acidemia, cardiomyopathy, shock, and death,[87,121] whereas infants being treated for anemia who received much higher daily cobalt doses of an iron-cobalt preparation (40 mg of $CoCl_2$ and 75 mg of $FeSO_4$) for 3 months did not develop toxicity.[147] The inconsistency of these findings suggests that multiple factors are responsible for the development of the clinical manifestations; in this case the role of ethanol metabolism and/or nutritional status is an important variable.[26,80]

CLINICAL MANIFESTATIONS

Organ systems affected by acute cobalt poisoning include endocrine,[74] gastrointestinal,[47,62] central[62,156] and peripheral nervous system,[156] hematologic,[55,90,118,186] cardiovascular,[74] ophthalmic,[12,13,83,126] and metabolic.[74] Chronic inhalational exposures affect the pulmonary system[31,37,49,94,95,143,165] and dermatologic system.[53,150,185] In the past, the following section was divided into acute and chronic clinical manifestations; however, there is substantial temporal cross-over and these presentations have systemic diversity. These distinctions suggest a deterministic outcome whereas stochastic processes are just as probable. The clinical manifestations will be described by organ system and chronic occupational manifestations. The 2 major organ systems cardiovascular and soft tissue will be illustrated by "beer drinker's cardiomyopathy" and arthroprosthetic cobaltism respectively despite these special populations having a myriad of shared manifestations.

Cardiovascular

"Beer drinker's cardiomyopathy." In 1966, a Veterans Affairs (VA) Hospital in Nebraska cared for 28 white men with a history of beer drinking who presented with tachycardia, dyspnea, and metabolic acidosis with elevated lactate concentrations, and congestive heart failure.[113] The mortality rate for these cases was 38% and death occurred rapidly within 72 hours of presentation, because of severe metabolic acidosis and cardiac failure.[113] Of the survivors, most responded immediately to supportive care and thiamine supplementation, and a lack of response was found to be secondary to complications; most commonly, symptomatic pericardial effusions or embolic events.[113] Epidemiologic evaluation of this case series revealed that these men habitually drank large quantities of beer.

Ultimately, 64 cases and 30 fatalities were reported from Nebraska.[172] Twenty-six of the 30 deaths received autopsies. Common post-mortem findings were dilated cardiomyopathy and cellular degeneration with vacuolization and edema with a lack of inflammation or fibrosis.[113] When cobalt was implicated in the pathogenesis of these deaths, preserved cardiac tissue of 8 decedents revealed cobalt concentrations 10 times greater than that of controls.[172]

Within a year of the Nebraska cases, reports began to emerge from Quebec.[121] Forty-eight beer drinkers (only 2 of whom were women) developed unexplained cardiomyopathy, with a mortality rate of 46%.[121] The only association between these patients was the common consumption of Dow Beer, originally anonymized as "XXX" beer.[121] The producers of this beer had factories in Quebec City and Montreal. The only difference between the Nebraska brewery and the one in Quebec was that the latter added 10 times the amount of $CoSO_4$ to the beer as a foam stabilizer.[119] Clinical findings in these cases included tachycardia, tachypnea, polycythemia, and low-voltage electrocardiograms (ECGs).[120] Cases began to appear 1 month after beer with the higher amount $CoSO_4$ was released onto the market, and no new cases were reported in Quebec after this beer with more $CoSO_4$ was removed from the market.[119]

Between the years 1964 and 1967, 20 additional cases occurred in Minneapolis with similar findings of tachycardia, dyspnea, pericardial effusion, polycythemia, and metabolic acidosis with elevated lactate concentrations, and there was a mortality rate of 18% acutely and 43% over a 3-year period.[4]

Similar to the previous cases, all were associated with the addition of $CoSO_4$ as a foam stabilizer in beer.

Because the clinical findings resemble the cardiomyopathy associated with chronic alcoholism[51] and infantile malnutrition,[137] a debate persists as to whether cobalt is the sole cause of this syndrome. Cardiomyopathies due to poor protein intake, vitamin deficiency, and cobalt toxicity have similar histologic findings. For example, myocardial biopsy of dogs with cobalt-induced cardiac failure revealed diffuse cytosolic vacuolization, loss of cross-striations, and interstitial edema,[154] all of which are similar to findings of malnutrition.[51,137] However, some other findings are more specific to cobalt associated-cardiomyopathy. For example, a small retrospective analysis revealed myocyte atrophy and myofibril loss to be present in people with cobalt-associated cardiomyopathy significantly more often than in those with idiopathic dilated cardiomyopathy.[28]

Some animal models of cobalt cardiomyopathy were only able to reproduce pathologic and ECG findings if cobalt and ethanol[10] were coadministered whereas others required protein deficiency.[148] Contrary to these studies, several murine and canine models of cobalt poisoning demonstrated cardiac lesions,[68,153,154] cardiac failure,[71,153,154] and ECG abnormalities while receiving nutritional supplementation.[69,153]

Despite the implication that cobalt-induced cardiomyopathy requires malnutrition or alcoholism, a case of cardiac toxicity following acute cobalt poisoning is reported.[74] However, it is difficult to identify other cases reported outside of the aforementioned small epidemics in beer drinkers. In a controlled study of occupationally exposed subjects evaluated with echocardiograms, significantly more cobalt exposed workers had diastolic dysfunction when compared to controls.[101] However, none of these subjects under study developed congestive heart failure.[101] Of the few reported cases of cardiomyopathy associated with arthroprosthetic cobaltism, patients are typically older than those with the "beer drinker's cardiomyopathy" cohort, and their nutritional status and ethanol use are unreported.[128,135] There are rare reports of cardiomyopathy in chronically exposed workers,[17,35,85] which suggests that the cardiomyopathy reported in the "beer drinkers" cohort is multifactorial and not solely due to cobalt.

Another source of criticism of the role of cobalt in the development of cardiomyopathy is the relatively low dose of cobalt needed to induce heart failure in these patients.[87] In patients receiving 20 to 75 mg/day of $CoCl_2$ for various red cell dysplasias, there were no reports of heart failure[87] whereas the "beer drinker's cardiomyopathy" group reportedly consumed only 6 to 8 mg/day of $CoSO_4$ while drinking 24 pints of cobalt-containing beer.[87,119] All patients who developed cardiomyopathies were malnourished, which supports the theory that a multifactorial nutritional deficiency in the presence of excessive cobalt is necessary for the development of cardiomyopathy.[87]

Within the cases of arthroprosthetic cobaltism reported so far, few have detailed cardiac manifestations reported despite the presence of cardiomyopathy; this is most likely due to cardiomyopathy being common in the age group receiving hip arthroplasties. Of the 3 cases[7,65,122] within this cohort reporting histopathology, the common features are myocyte hypertrophy,[7,122] dilated atrial and ventricular chambers,[57] deposits of electron-dense material,[65] interstitial fibrosis,[7,122] cytoplasmic vacuoles,[7,122] and without evidence of infiltrative or infective cardiomyopathy.[7,65,122] Interestingly, heart failure was so profound that 2 of these cases went on to receive cardiac transplants.[7,122]

Endocrine

Both acute and chronic cobalt exposures are associated with thyroid hyperplasia and goiter. A series of patients with severe sickle cell anemia treated with cobalt salts developed goiters with varying degrees of thyroid dysfunction[70,91] including clinical hypothyroidism.[92] In 1 patient, the goiter was so severe that airway obstruction developed.[91]

Older occupational data suggest that inhalational exposure to cobalt metals, salts, and oxides results in abnormalities in thyroid function studies.[173] When 82 workers in a cobalt refinery were compared to age- and sex-matched controls, exposed workers had significantly lower T_3 concentrations.[173] Studies of cobalt-exposed workers in environments that limit exposure do not demonstrate any changes in serum thyroid markers,[99] supporting occupationally imposed limits.

Within the previously mentioned beer drinker's cardiomyopathy cohort, 11 of 14 decedents had abnormal thyroid histology.[149] Among them, the most common findings were follicular cell abnormalities and colloid depletion, which did not exist on thyroid analysis from 11 randomly selected autopsies that served as controls.[149] Of the patients with arthroprosthetic cobaltism, many had abnormal thyroid function studies with or without clinical symptoms of hypothyroidism[128,135,189]

Hematologic

Anemias of the newborn,[32,84,139] erythrocyte hypoplasia,[158] red cell aplasia,[180] and kidney failure–associated anemia[62] were all successfully treated with cobalt salts. Patients undergoing $CoCl_2$ therapy for these diseases had increased hemoglobin,[62,139] hematocrit,[62,139] and red cell counts.[62,139]

A published series of Peruvian cobalt miners working in an open pit at 4,300 m (2.7 miles) elevation developed clinical effects including headache, dizziness, weakness, mental fatigue, dyspnea, insomnia, tinnitus, anorexia, cyanosis, polycythemia, and conjunctival hyperemia consistent with acute mountain sickness.[81] When the study group was compared to age-, height-, and weight-matched high-altitude controls, the study group had higher chronic mountain sickness scores.[81] The only difference detected was elevated serum cobalt concentrations in the study group.[81]

In addition to effects on red cells, mice develop transient hemolysis, methemoglobinemia, and methemoglobinuria from subcutaneous $CoCl_2$ exposure.[75] These findings explain reports of dark urine following cobalt exposure in other animal models.[66,167] However, similar human cases are not reported.

Other

Gastrointestinal distress is reported following the ingestion of "therapeutic" doses of cobalt salts[156] and elemental cobalt.[80] Decreased proprioception, impaired cranial nerve VIII function, and nonspecific peripheral nerve findings are reported with acute oral $CoCl_2$ exposures.[156] Patients with arthroprosthetic cobaltism have seizures, cerebellar deficits, retinopathy,[12,126] hearing loss, cognitive deficits, and peripheral neuropathy, and some of whom had concomitant elevations of cerebrospinal fluid cobalt concentrations.[27,109,128,175,176] Retinal effects were noted in at least 2 case reports of patients with cobalt-containing arthroprostheses.[10,11] The pathophysiology of these cases is poorly understood and confounded by comorbidities typical in this cohort of patients. Radioactive ^{60}Co used for radiation therapy is associated with radiation burns (Chap. 128). Unlike acute toxicity, chronic cobalt exposure is not associated with an increased mortality; a cohort study evaluating more than 1,100 persons with pulmonary exposures to cobalt salts and oxides over a 30-year period was unable to demonstrate an increased mortality rate.[110]

Arthroprosthetic Cobaltism

Soft Tissue

It has been known for some time that metal-on-metal alloy orthopedic implants result in elevations of the associated metal concentration in blood, urine, and hair.[27] Serum cobalt concentrations become elevated 3 weeks after surgery and remain elevated through a 5-year study period, which contradicts earlier theories of elevated concentrations being related to the life of the implant.[20] Despite the elevation of both chromium and cobalt in measured samples, it appears that the constellation of clinical findings is more consistent with cobalt rather than chromium toxicity.[1] Additionally, the toxicity of chromium develops more slowly than that of cobalt.[1]

Reported cases of toxicity follow revisions, dislocations, or first-time arthroplasties of cobalt-containing prosthetics.[97,156,157] The association of having a cobalt-containing prosthetic, an elevated marker of cobalt burden, and findings of end-organ toxicity has been coined "arthroprosthetic cobaltism." Before these clinical manifestations occur, cobalt ions are deposited in the soft tissue. Gross deposition of metal in surrounding soft tissue is termed metallosis. Metallosis is accompanied by other clinical findings such as discoloration of synovial fluid[65] and pseudotumor[7,60,122] formation. Pseudotumor is also described as an aseptic lymphocyte-dominated vasculitis-associated lesion (ALVAL). The specific findings on histopathology show an invasion of lymphocytes and plasma cells forming a perivascular lymphocytic infiltrate.[181] It is hypothesized that these findings are a type IV mediated immune response to metal ions, which correlates highly for these patients having a positive patch clamp skin test.[174] A newer entity is trunnionosis,[117,164] the erosion of metal at the level of the trunnion—the location of where the neck of the arthroplasty inserts into the femoral head implant. Trunnionosis occurs at a higher rate of metal-on-metal implants, but is also reported with metal-on-polyethylene implants. Both metallosis and trunnionosis are findings suggestive of implant failure and thought to place the patient at risk for systemic toxicity if left to progress.

Some of the common presentations of local soft tissue reactions are pain, swelling, and painful gait not attributed to recent surgery. These symptoms are a common presentation leading the clinician to suspect a local reaction to the metal-containing prosthesis. The presence of the above findings leads the clinician to suspect implant failure and, more consequentially, risk of developing cobalt toxicity.

Cases of implant failure and local tissue reactions are common but arthroprosthetic cobaltism remains a rarely reported entity, considering the hundreds of thousands of implants performed annually. Because of the concern of implant failure and systemic absorption of metal ions, government agencies from the United States, Canada, United Kingdom, European Union, and Australia have made recommendations regarding investigation of problematic implants.[1-3,142] However, these guidelines are not uniform, vary regionally, and subject to dated information.

Of the reported cases, some arthroplasties had excessive wear[115] or were placed following a ceramic arthroplasty, resulting in metallosis.[100] Lumbar metal-on-metal total disk replacements are associated with smaller elevations in serum cobalt concentrations when compared with hip resurfacing or total hip arthroplasties,[19] there are no reported cases of clinical cobaltism with lumbar implants.

Renal

A single report associates reversible acute kidney injury with the chronic administration of $CoCl_2$ as treatment for anemia.[156] Some animal models of cobalt cardiomyopathy demonstrate cellular changes in renal tissue.[67] However, when 26 exposed hard-metal workers were evaluated for urinary albumin, retinol binding protein, beta$_2$-microglobulin, and tubular brush border antigens, no detectable differences could be found between the study group and controls.[58] Additionally, patients with cobalt-containing total hip arthroplasties were followed over 2 years with elevated serum cobalt concentrations without any significant effect on serum creatinine over this study period.[16] Based on these few reports, it appears that acute and chronic exposure to cobalt has little effect on the kidneys.

Reproduction

In pregnant rats, $CoCl_2$ exposure neither results in teratogenicity nor fetal toxicity.[132] In a case report of a pregnant woman with hard-metal disease, the woman was able to bring the pregnancy to term and deliver without complication.[141] In another case report, a woman with a cobalt-containing hip arthroplasty had repeated joint aspirations, dislocations, and revisions before and during her pregnancy.[60] Cobalt concentrations of this mother were 138 to 143 mcg/L throughout the pregnancy; cord blood concentration was 75 mcg/L; and infant blood concentration at 8 weeks was 13 mcg/L. Despite these elevated concentrations, there was no clinical evidence of toxicity.[60] It is hypothesized that only exposures that are toxic to the mother result in fetal toxicity.[46]

In mice, chronic exposure to cobalt results in impaired spermatogenesis and decreased fertility without affecting follicular stimulating hormone or luteinizing hormone, whereas acute exposures did not demonstrate similar reproductive effects.[134] Additional murine studies discuss the possible interactions between cobalt with iron and zinc, which are both essential elements

for spermatogenesis.[8] Despite these findings, there are no reported human cases that associate cobalt exposure with teratogenicity or impaired fertility.

Carcinogenesis

Animal experiments with injection of $CoCl_2$ into soft tissue resulted in soft tissue sarcomas, leading the International Agency for Research on Cancer (IARC) to consider cobalt metal without tungsten carbide, cobalt sulfate, and other soluble cobalt(II) salts possibly carcinogenic to humans (group 2B).[18,33,44,152,167] Cobalt metal associated with tungsten carbide is probably carcinogenic to humans (group 2A).[167] There are case reports and cohort studies that suggest that pulmonary exposure to Co^{2+} increases the risk of lung cancer. However, these studies were unable to control for other known carcinogens such as arsenic.[33] In the largest occupational cohort study to date, which followed more than 1,100 workers for more than 38 years, there was no increase in the prevalence of lung cancer.[109] Finally, in 2 of the largest population studies to date, researchers were unable to demonstrate a higher cancer rate for individuals with metal-on-metal implants when compared to the general population;[22,108] however, because of the relatively recent nature of the implants, these studies suffer from length-time bias and do not capture the needed time between exposure to carcinogenesis.

Chronic Occupational Exposure
Pulmonary

Both asthma and "hard-metal disease" are associated with cobalt exposure. Occupational asthma is reported in hard-metal workers with a prevalence of 2% to 5%[31,94,95] at exposure concentrations as low as 50 mcg/m^3.[95] As is the case with most causes of occupational asthma, cobalt hypersensitivity–induced asthma is most likely immune mediated rather than toxicologic.[34,94,165] Most hard-metal workers are exposed to other metals, such as tungsten (W) and nickel (Ni), in addition to cobalt, and these other metals account for some of the occupational asthma that is attributed to cobalt.[162,163] However, in a small but well-performed study in patients with cobalt-associated asthma, intradermal cobalt chloride resulted in a positive wheal response in all subjects and 50% of patients had a positive radioallergosorbent test (RAST) scores, which correlated to the wheal size[161] and suggests cobalt salts elicit an immune response independent of the other metals.

Cobalt-associated pulmonary toxicity was first noted in tungsten carbide workers,[49,72] and was subsequently referred to as "hard-metal disease." Exposures result from the process by which tungsten-carbide is sintered with cobalt. Signs and symptoms of hard-metal disease include upper respiratory tract irritation, exertional dyspnea, severe dry cough, wheezing, and interstitial lung disease ranging from alveolitis to progressive fibrosis. The prevalence of hard-metal disease is largely unknown. In one study, 11 of 290 (3.8%) exposed workers were diagnosed with interstitial infiltrates on chest radiographs but only 2 (0.7%) had a decrease in predicted total lung capacity.[168]

Certain individuals who are exposed to large doses of hard metal for prolonged periods never develop disease; which suggests that a susceptible population exists. A glutamate substitution for lysine in position 69 of the beta unit HLA-DP has a strong association with hard-metal disease, similar to chronic beryllium disease.[138] Clinically, hard-metal disease is difficult to distinguish from berylliosis, although an occupational history is helpful.

Histopathologic findings of hard-metal disease include multinucleated giant cells and interstitial pneumonitis with bronchiolitis.[11] Elevated concentrations of cobalt in lung tissue are detected,[144,166] even as long as 4 years after exposure.[144] In patients with interstitial lung disease, bronchoalveolar lavage commonly reveals multinucleated giant cells, type II alveolar cells, and alveolar macrophages.[37] The finding of multinucleated giant cells from bronchoalveolar lavage washing is characteristic of hard-metal disease.[34,39,40,114,178]

A cross-sectional study of more than a 1,000 tungsten carbide-exposed workers found an increased odds ratio of 2.1 for having a work-related wheeze, when exposed to greater than 50 mcg/m^3 of Co.[169] In the same study, workers with exposures recorded at greater than 100 mcg/m^3 had higher odds (OR 5.0) of having a chest radiograph perfusion score of greater than or equal to 1/0.[169] This perfusion score, established by the United Nations agency, the International Labor Organization (ILO), is a grading system for pneumoconioses. When used to grade radiographs of asbestosis, this score correlates strongly with mortality risk,[111] reduced diffusing capacity, and decreased ventilatory capacity.[73,123] Additional studies have similarly concluded that pulmonary disease occurs when individuals are exposed to concentrations of cobalt that approach 100 mcg/m³.[93] Thus, with a margin of safety, the current threshold limit value (TLV) is less than 50 mcg/m³.

Until 1984, all reported cases of hard-metal disease were associated with the combination of cobalt and other metals, such as nickel, cadmium, and tungsten.[11,72,95,169] When diamond polishers initiated the use of high-speed grinding disks coated with abrasive microdiamonds embedded in a matrix of cobalt powder,[98] case reports ensued demonstrating similar clinical[98] and pathologic findings to hard-metal disease, strengthening the association with cobalt.[34,39,125] Some authors still contend that the presence of other metals[11,72,95,169] and diamond dust[39,63,125] are confounding factors.[173] Like hard-metal disease, most reported cases show resolution of symptoms following removal from the exposure,[39] although this is not always sufficient.[125]

There are very few reports of isolated cobalt exposures. In an age-matched and sex-matched study of 82 workers with respiratory exposures to cobalt oxides, cobalt salts, cobalt metal, and no other metal, researchers were unable to detect a difference between exposed (mean of 8 years, time-weighted average 125 mcg/m³, 25% >500 mcg/m³) and unexposed workers with any objective measured pulmonary tests.[173] Neither group had any abnormality in chest radiography that would suggest pulmonary fibrosis.[173] The only significant pulmonary differences detected were a higher reported rate of dyspnea both on exertion and at rest and the presence of wheezing in the exposed group.[173] These authors concluded that cobalt contributes to the development of pulmonary disease but is not independently responsible for the development of pulmonary fibrosis.[173]

Despite the progressive and debilitating nature of hard-metal disease, most signs and symptoms improve with cessation of exposure.[110,115,188] Moreover, the length and dose of exposure do not appear to correlate with the presence or severity of illness, suggesting that individual susceptibility is the key determinant for developing illness.[110,151]

Dermatology

In a study of 1,782 construction workers, 23.6% developed dermatitis and 11.2% developed oil acne while using cobalt-containing cement, fly ash, or asbestos.[88] As in hard-metal disease, it is difficult to isolate cobalt as the sole contributor to the development of dermatitis. Nickel (Chap. 96) is the classic xenobiotic causing dermatitis. Commonly found in some of these construction occupations, nickel is implicated in the development of cutaneous manifestations.[53,150] However, consumer products such as piercings, tattoo ink, plastics, clothing dye, makeup, and dental treatments are implicated in cobalt-induced allergic contact dermatitis.[56] Additionally, within the arthroprosthetic cobaltism cohort, dermatitis is found to present both in proximity and remotely from the cobalt reservoir, and diffusely.[187] Furthermore, in vitro studies demonstrate that cobalt induces production of both Th1- and Th2-type cytokines in peripheral blood mononuclear cells—the same pathway implicated in nickel contact dermatitis.[116] Thus, it appears that cobalt induces a hypersensitivity reaction independent of the presence of nickel. Within the arthroprosthetic cobaltism group, cases of both local and remote dermatitis are reported, but because of poor reporting details of its nature, the pathophysiology of these particular cases is unclear.[170,176]

DIAGNOSTIC TESTING

Currently, body fluid cobalt concentrations are not readily available and therefore cannot be used to direct emergent clinical care. Some adjunctive testing that supports a clinical diagnosis of cobalt toxicity should include complete blood count (CBC), reticulocyte count, erythropoietin (EPO) concentration, and thyroid-stimulating hormone (TSH) concentration. The results of these tests reflect the level of exposure or potential toxic manifestations.

Cardiac Studies

Electrocardiogram, echocardiogram, and radionuclide angiocardiography with ^{99}Tc(RNA) are useful screening tests for detecting abnormalities associated with cobalt cardiomyopathy and/or pulmonary hypertension due to hard-metal disease.[35] Magnetic resonance imaging is used to exclude other causes of cardiomyopathy.[7,122] In a single case report, a cardiac MRI demonstrated extensive hyperenhancement, diffuse edema, and was instrumental in excluding other causes of heart failure.[122] The true sensitivity and specificity of these cardiac tests for cobalt-induced cardiomyopathy is unknown.

Pulmonary Testing

Patients with hard-metal lung disease demonstrate bilateral upper lobe interstitial lung disease on chest radiograph. However, patients have signs and symptoms of disease without specific radiographic findings.[141] Pulmonary function testing in occupationally exposed workers shows decreased vital capacity[141] and a decrease in transfer factor for carbon monoxide, both of which are useful in identifying patients at risk for developing pulmonary fibrosis.[171] An inversion of CD4/CD8 ratio in bronchoalveolar lavage washings is a useful tool for diagnosis and evaluation of progression of illness and that normalization is a marker for improvement.[143] Despite these available tests, a definitive diagnosis of hard-metal disease requires a tissue sample with findings of multinucleated giant cells in the setting of interstitial pulmonary fibrosis.

Soft Tissue Imaging

Specifically with regard to failed cobalt-containing implants, some groups recommend plain radiographs for the assessment of metallosis, osteolysis, and other subtle findings of implant failure.[96] However, ultrasonography combined with metal artifact reduction sequence MRI has come to the forefront as the more sensitive and specific radiologic study for cobalt-containing implants, revealing soft tissue reactions, metallosis, and pseudotumor, and assist in revision planning.[96] These tests, however, do not assist in the diagnosis of cobalt toxicity, but merely reveal the presence of local reactions that would place the patient at risk of systemic toxicity. Various governing bodies made recommendations/guidelines for physicians caring for patients with hip arthroplasties in which cobalt poisoning is a risk. The American Association of Hip and Knee Surgeons, the American Academy of Orthopaedic Surgeons, and the Hip Society endorse a stratifying schema placing patients into low-, medium-, and high-risk groups based on characteristics that are not prospectively validated.[96] In addition to these guidelines, government oversight bodies for medical devices all over the world have varying recommendations from biologic testing to treatment. It is advised that the reader refer to their regional medical device oversight body (eg, FDA, Medicines and Healthcare products Regulatory Agency)[1-3,24] for current recommendations.

Cobalt Testing

Cobalt, as stated above, is primarily eliminated in the urine and to a lesser extent in the feces, making urine cobalt evaluation most appropriate.[103] The difficulty lies in the interpretation of the result. Cobalt is detectable in the urine after inhalational exposure and reflects elimination kinetics that are rapid during an initial exposure but which slow after prolonged exposure.[103,155] Because of this variable elimination pattern, it is difficult to interpret both urine and blood concentrations unless the dose and length of exposure are precisely known. Furthermore, the defined patterns are applicable to shift workers exposed to soluble forms of cobalt.[103]

Further complicating the interpretation of urinary cobalt concentrations is the abundance of organic cobalt in the form of vitamin B_{12}. A detailed vitamin supplementation history is needed before the interpretation of a urine or blood cobalt concentration, as a diet regimen high in vitamin B_{12} increases urine cobalt concentrations. For this reason, speciation of cobalt should be investigated. The ratio of inorganic to organic cobalt is higher in occupationally exposed workers (2.3) when compared to controls (1.01) independent of the wide variations of urinary cobalt concentrations.[61] This is a promising area of study for the evaluation of cobalt-exposed workers.

Further complicating the meaning of a cobalt concentration is the availability of plasma, serum, and whole blood cobalt testing.[133] Evidence suggests whole blood cobalt reflects total body metal burden more accurately because it takes albumin into consideration.[26] Toxic concentrations of cobalt in serum and urine are poorly defined. Published literature on "normal values" is fraught with variability, which reflects differences in the population under study and the techniques and fluids used for measurement. Normal serum concentrations of cobalt are frequently reported as 0.1 to 1.2 mcg/L.[5,18,74,78,160] In a cohort of patients with asymptomatic cobalt-containing hip implants, the peak serum cobalt concentration did not exceed 11.5 mcg/L, baring 1 outlier of 35 mcg/L at 1 year postprocedure.[16,21,23] Based on this data, some recommend suspecting arthroprosthetic cobaltism when a blood concentration exceeds 10 mcg/L.[3,175] In comparison, a single acutely poisoned patient had a reported serum concentration of 41 mcg/L.[74] In the arthroprosthetic cobaltism group, serum cobalt concentrations ranged from 23 to 1,085 mcg/L.[7,60,65,77,109,122,128,135,146,170,176] Interestingly, a cobalt concentration of more than 7 mcg/L in whole blood "indicates potential for soft tissue reaction" according to the Medicines and Healthcare products Regulatory Agency in the United Kingdom,[3] whereas the FDA has no threshold concentration of concern, but allows the clinician to interpret these findings and take appropriate actions.[2] Despite the lack of uniformity in recommendations, most agencies currently recommend whole blood cobalt concentrations as the preferred form of testing.[2,3]

Normal reference urine cobalt concentrations are between 0.1 and 2.2 mcg/L.[5,18,74,78,131,160] In contrast, a patient with an acute elemental cobalt ingestion had a concentration of 1,700 mcg/L on a spot urinalysis several days after the exposure.[74] In the arthroprosthetic cobaltism group, 1 patient had a urine cobalt concentration of 16,500 mcg/L.[128]

Chronic exposures should be evaluated differently as discussed above (see Toxicokinetics). Exposed workers, without clinical disease, have reported spot urine concentrations that range from ten to several hundred micrograms per liter.[76]

TREATMENT

Acute Management

Patients with acute cobalt poisoning require aggressive therapy. It is reasonable to conclude that the same decontamination principles used for other metals apply to cobalt. There are no studies examining the benefit of gastric emptying, activated charcoal, or whole-bowel irrigation (WBI) following acute ingestion. It is reasonable to attempt WBI for radiopaque solid forms of cobalt prior to endoscopic or surgical removal.[74] Regardless of the decontamination procedure used, we recommend against chelation therapy until the gastrointestinal cobalt source is removed. If there is a large stomach burden of a solid, endoscopic or surgical removal is reasonable, keeping in mind that the administration of activated charcoal prior to surgical removal will obscure visualization of the surgical field (Chap. 5). After decontamination, reduction of tissue burden and prevention of end organ toxicity is the next crucial step.

The data on chelation therapy is unfortunately limited to animal models[41-46,105-107] and human case reports.[74,135] The basis of chelation therapy originates from the mid-1900s when oral protein intake was found to result in a reduction of cobalt toxicity in calves[48] and rats.[68] Certain sulfur-containing proteins serve as good chelators for some transition metals.

In a series of animal models of acute cobalt toxicity, several potential chelators, N-acetylcysteine (NAC), succimer, calcium disodium ethylenediaminetetraacetic acid CaNa$_2$(EDTA), glutathione, and diethylenetriaminepentaacetic acid (DTPA) were evaluated for their ability to enhance urinary and fecal elimination of cobalt.[105] Succimer and EDTA were able to enhance fecal elimination.[105] Glutathione and DTPA were able to enhance urinary elimination, and NAC was able to enhance elimination by both routes.[105]

In 2 separate animal studies, NAC reduced the tissue burden and injury due to cobalt in the liver and spleen.[45,105] Glutathione, another sulfur-containing protein, also reduced tissue concentrations of cobalt, but only in the spleen.[105]

The sulfur-containing proteins, NAC,[42,45] L-cysteine,[41,42] L-methionine,[42] and L-histidine,[46] were studied for their ability to reduce mortality in rats that were administered an LD$_{50}$ of CoCl$_2$ orally and intraperitoneally. N-acetylcysteine, L-cysteine and L-histidine[46] therapy were more effective than L-methionine in protecting against mortality, offering almost 100% protection. In a similar fashion, CaNa$_2$EDTA was effective in reducing mortality.[44] In all of these therapies, the successful reduction in mortality from these therapies is predicated on its early administration.[41,42,44-46]

In a murine model, L-cysteine, NAC, glutathione, L-histidine, sodium salicylate, D,L-penicillamine, succimer, N-acetylpenicillamine (NAPA), diethyldithiocarbamate (DDC), dimercaprol, 4,5-dihydroxy-1,3-benzene disulfonic acid, Na$_3$CaDTPA, CaNa$_2$EDTA, and deferoxamine were each evaluated for exposures to an LD$_{50}$ and an LD$_{99}$ of CoCl$_2$.[107] Potential chelators that were ineffective at improving survival following an LD$_{50}$ were sodium salicylate, NAPA, DOC, dimercaprol, 4,5-dihydroxy-1,3-benzene disulfonic acid and deferoxamine.[107] Chelators that were seemingly effective at LD$_{50}$ and not at LD$_{99}$ were L-histidine and D,L-penicillamine.[106] N-acetylcysteine, L-cysteine, and succimer were able to improve survival by 40% to 50%.[107] The most effective chelators at LD$_{99}$ were CaNa$_2$EDTA and DTPA.[106,107] An expanded analysis of these data revealed that CaNa$_2$EDTA and DTPA had better therapeutic indices when compared with succimer.[107] In another in vitro study, dimercaprol was unable to chelate Co^{2+} that was already bound to α-ketoglutarate.[183]

Data on chelation in humans is available from 6 case reports.[57,64,65,74,135,146] In 1 case, a child ingested multiple elemental cobalt-containing magnets, resulting in a serum cobalt concentration of 41 mcg/L.[74] Five days of 50 mg/kg/day of intravenous CaNa$_2$EDTA enhanced renal elimination of cobalt, and the patient's metabolic acidosis and the cardiac dysfunction resolved simultaneously.[74] All other cases studied are as a result of arthroprosthetic cobaltism.

Clinical symptoms and serum cobalt reduction respond well to arthroplasty revision[100,128,135,176] and potentially chelation therapy.[64,135] A 56-year-old man developed arthroprosthetic cobaltism with elevated serum (506 mcg/L), cerebrospinal fluid concentrations (8.5 mcg/L) of cobalt, hypothyroidism, cardiomyopathy with pericardial effusion, polycythemia, and both central and peripheral neuropathy.[135] Unlike the previous case report, this patient was treated with 2,3-dimercaptopropane-1-sulfonate (DMPS) at a dose of 14 mg/kg for 6 days and followed by 4 mg/kg for 5 days for a total of 10 gm of antidote. Serum cobalt concentrations were reduced 26% in 1 month following treatment.[135] However, despite removal of the prosthesis and chelation therapy, the patient had permanent hearing loss and a persistently elevated serum concentration,[135] most likely because of a delay of 7 months from onset of symptoms and metallosis of tissue.

Another human case receiving chelation therapy was a 58-year-old woman with a hip prosthesis, symptoms of cobaltism, and cobalt blood concentrations of 549 mcg/L, cerebrospinal fluid concentrations of 11.4 mcg/L, and urine concentrations of 11.4 mcg/L.[146] Initial chelation with CaNa$_2$EDTA resulted in a decrease in cobalt concentrations, but without a significant change in her symptoms.[146] After several months, she had resection of the arthroplasty and only then did she have gradual improvements in her symptoms.[146] Quantitative concentrations were not reported subsequent to chelation, and it is unclear whether she had continued chelation following the initial dosing before, during, or after revision surgery.[146]

Contrasting the previous cases, there is a single human case report describing the use of dimercaprol in a patient with evidence of arthroprosthetic cobaltism and elevated blood cobalt concentrations.[65] This is a curious choice of chelators because evidence demonstrates its ineffectiveness at reducing cobalt burden in animal models.[107] However, cobalt concentration reduced by 33% and the patient went on to have the arthroplasty resected, resulting in a further 40% reduction of cobalt.[65] Unfortunately, despite the resection and chelation, the patient was unable to be weaned from balloon pump and care was withdrawn.[65]

There is one case report of arthroprosthetic cobaltism with ventricular dysfunction and rapid clinical deterioration following relocation of a dislocated hip.[57] The patient had progressive elevations of her cobalt concentrations and worsening left ventricular function and a metabolic acidosis with elevated lactate concentration. Treatment was initiated with NAC and she was due to receive a revision, but subsequently died with worsening acidemia and heart failure prior to revision.[57] Because of insufficient data, it is unclear if the NAC had assisted in the reduction of cobalt concentrations.[57] In contrast to this aforementioned case, a 75-year-old patient with arthroprosthetic cobaltism had resolution of both ventricular dysfunction and a pericardial effusion, and reduction of blood cobalt concentrations with intravenous and oral NAC as the sole chelator without concomitant hip revision.[64] There is such variability in the human case reports and chelation approaches that it is difficult to draw any evidence-based recommendations at this point.

In conclusion, based on human case reports, several animal studies, and safety profiles: CaNa$_2$EDTA and NAC are reasonable chelating choices. Despite a paucity of data, reasonable indications for chelation include patients who demonstrate end organ manifestations of toxicity. This includes acidemia and cardiac failure. Other manifestations of severe cobalt toxicity such as pericardial effusion, clinically significant goiter, and hyperviscosity syndrome should be treated as aggressively as are patients from other etiologies—pericardiocentesis, airway protection, and phlebotomy, respectively. Based on years of experience with lead, we recommend the regimen for CaNa$_2$EDTA at doses of 1,000 mg/m^2/day by continuous infusion for 5 days. If the diagnosis is confirmed and signs of cardiac failure and acidemia persist after 5 days, an alternate chelator (succimer or DTPA) can be started. Similarly, we recommend NAC dosing based on the acetaminophen (APAP) experience. The 20-hour intravenous NAC protocol should be initiated, and continued as in the case of fulminant hepatic failure (Antidotes in Depth: A3) for as long as the patient can tolerate therapy, or continued if cardiac failure or acidemia persists. If there are contraindications to intravenous NAC, oral NAC should be administered using one of the APAP treatment regimens. Thiamine hydrochloride should be administered to all patients presenting independent of whether the patient is an alcoholic, had heart failure, or is malnourished. The dose of thiamine is not well defined but should be based on its safety and clinical experience with the treatment of Wernicke encephalopathy. We recommend the administration of 500 mg intravenously of thiamine 3 times daily for 2 to 3 days and 250 mg intravenously daily for the next 3 to 5 days for life-threatening manifestations (cardiac failure and acidemia) (Antidotes in Depth: A27).

Arthroprosthetic Cobaltism

The key to treatment of this entity is early clinical suspicion with the constellation of findings of cardiomyopathy, hypothyroidism, polycythemia, and peripheral and central nervous system impairment. Early arthroprosthetic revision supports the decontamination tenets within this text and published in case reports;[20,112,128,135,176] however emergent revisions may not be practical in a patient who is acutely ill. Therefore, the only modality of treatment other than a supportive one is chelation. However, based on the limited literature, it is unclear if chelation eliminates significant quantities of cobalt in the presence of a large reservoir of metal.

Occupational/Chronic Exposure

As is always the case of occupational poisonings, prevention is of paramount importance. The use of skin and respiratory protection and improvement of personal hygiene reduces exposure and subsequently the amount of urinary cobalt in occupationally exposed workers.[102] Barrier and emollient creams cannot prevent the dermatitis associated with cobalt metal exposures.[54]

Large statistically significant reductions in urinary cobalt concentrations were demonstrated after the implementation of aspirator systems over machines in the production of Widia-steel.[29] These aspirators were found to reduce ambient cobalt concentrations by as much as a factor of 6.[50]

SUMMARY

- Acute cobalt toxicity results in multiorgan toxicity, including the cardiac, endocrine, hematopoietic, gastrointestinal, and neurologic systems.
- The literature regarding metal-containing hip prostheses is focused on preventing, detecting, and treating implant failures and does not address toxicity.
- Arthroprosthetic cobaltism is unique in that there is a large reservoir of metal, and the clinical presentation is subacute and often mistaken for other disease processes.
- The evaluation and treatment of all patients will be determined by the cobalt source and type (elemental, inorganic, or organic), route of poisoning, and time and duration of exposure.
- Treatment of patients with chronic occupational exposures is mainly symptomatic and is often dependent on improving industrial hygiene and removal from the source.
- Acute poisoning with end-organ manifestations requires aggressive decontamination and chelation therapy utilizing CaNa$_2$EDTA and NAC and at times succimer is reasonable.

REFERENCES

1. Australian Government-Department of Health Therapeutic Goods Adminisration. Metal-on-metal hip replacement implants—information for general practitioners, orthopaedic surgeons and other health professionals, 2012.
2. US Food & Drug Administration. Concerns about metal-on-metal hip implants. https://www.fda.gov/MedicalDevices/ProductsandMedicalProcedures/ImplantsandProsthetics/MetalonMetalHipImplants/ucm241604.htm. Accessed March 18, 2017.
3. Medicines and Healthcare products Regulatory Agency. Management recommendations for patients with metal-on-metal hip replacement implants 2012.
4. Alexander CS. Cobalt-beer cardiomyopathy. A clinical and pathologic study of twenty-eight cases. *Am J Med.* 1972;53:395-417.
5. Alexandersson R. Blood and urinary concentrations as estimators of cobalt exposure. *Arch Environ Health.* 1988;43:299-303.
6. Alippi RM, et al. Higher erythropoietin secretion in response to cobaltous chloride in post-hypoxic than in hypertransfused polycythemic mice. *Haematologica.* 1992;77:446-449.
7. Allen LA, et al. Clinical problem-solving. Missing elements of the history. *N Engl J Med.* 2014;370:559-566.
8. Anderson MB, et al. Histopathology of testes from mice chronically treated with cobalt. *Reprod Toxicol.* 1992;6:41-50.
9. Andreasen GF, Barrett RD. An evaluation of cobalt-substituted nitinol wire in orthodontics. *Am J Orthod.* 1973;63:462-470.
10. Anonymous. Synergism of cobalt and ethanol. *Nutr Rev.* 1971;29:43-45.
11. Anttila S, et al. Hard metal lung disease: a clinical, histological, ultrastructural and X-ray microanalytical study. *Eur J Respir Dis.* 1986;69:83-94.
12. Apel W, et al. Cobalt-chromium toxic retinopathy case study. *Doc Ophthalmol.* 2013;126:69-78.
13. Apostoli P, et al. High doses of cobalt induce optic and auditory neuropathy. *Exp Toxicol Pathol.* 2013;65:719-727.
14. Apostoli P, et al. Urinary cobalt excretion in short time occupational exposure to cobalt powders. *Sci Total Environ.* 1994;150:129-132.
15. Babinet C, et al. Metal ions requirement of polynucleotide phosphorylase. *Biochem Biophys Res Commun.* 1965;19:95-101.
16. Back DL, et al. How do serum cobalt and chromium levels change after metal-on-metal hip resurfacing? *Clin Orthop Relat Res.* 2005;438:177-181.
17. Barborik M, Dusek J. Cardiomyopathy accompaning industrial cobalt exposure. *Br Heart J.* 1972;34:113-116.
18. Barceloux DG. Cobalt. *J Toxicol Clin Toxicol.* 1999;37:201-206.
19. Berk L, et al. Erythropoietic effect of cobalt in patients with or without anemia. *N Engl J Med.* 1949;240:754-761.
20. Bernstein DT, et al. Eighty-six percent failure rate of a modular-neck femoral stem design at 3 to 5 years: lessons learned. *J Bone Joint Surg Am.* 2016;98:e49.
21. Bisseling P, et al. Metal ion levels in patients with a lumbar metal-on-metal total disc replacement: should we be concerned? *J Bone Joint Surg Br.* 2011;93:949-954.
22. Brewster DH, et al. Risk of cancer following primary total hip replacement or primary resurfacing arthroplasty of the hip: a retrospective cohort study in Scotland. *Br J Cancer.* 2013;108:1883-1890.
23. Brodner W, et al. Serum cobalt levels after metal-on-metal total hip arthroplasty. *J Bone Joint Surg Am.* 2003;85-A:2168-2173.
24. Health Canada. Metal-on-metal hip implants—information for orthopaedic surgeons regarding patient management following surgery—for health professionals. 2012. http://www.healthycanadians.gc.ca/recall-alert-rappel-avis/hc-sc/2012/15835a-eng.php. Accessed March 17, 2017.
25. Carson B, et al. *Toxicology and Biological Monitoring of Metals in Humans.* Chelsea, MI: Lewis Publishers Inc; 1986.
26. Catalani S, et al. The role of albumin in human toxicology of cobalt: contribution from a clinical case. *ISRN Hematol.* 2011;2011:690620.
27. Catalani S, et al. Neurotoxicity of cobalt. *Hum Exp Toxicol.* 2012;31:421-437.
28. Centeno JA, et al. An analytical comparison of cobalt cardiomyopathy and idiopathic dilated cardiomyopathy. *Biol Trace Elem Res.* 1996;55:21-30.
29. Cereda C, et al. Widia tool grinding: the importance of primary prevention measures in reducing occupational exposure to cobalt. *Sci Total Environ.* 1994;150:249-251.

30. Cheung AC, et al. Systemic cobalt toxicity from total hip arthroplasties: review of a rare condition Part 1—history, mechanism, measurements, and pathophysiology. *Bone Joint J.* 2016;98:6-13.

31. Coates EO Jr, et al. Hypersensitivity bronchitis in tungsten carbide workers. *Chest.* 1973;64:390.

32. Coles BL, James U. The effect of cobalt and iron salts on the anaemia of prematurity. *Arch Dis Child.* 1954;29:85-96.

33. Crawford JD, et al. Cobalt-induced myxedema; report of a case. *N Engl J Med.* 1956;255:955-957.

34. Cugell DW, et al. The respiratory effects of cobalt. *Arch Intern Med.* 1990;150:177-183.

35. D'Adda F, et al. Cardiac function study in hard metal workers. *Sci Total Environ.* 1994;150:179-186.

36. Daniel M, et al. The biological action of cobalt and other metals. I. The effect of cobalt on the morphology and metabolism of rat fibroblasts in vitro. *Br J Exp Pathol.* 1963;44:163-176.

37. Davison AG, et al. Interstitial lung disease and asthma in hard-metal workers: bronchoalveolar lavage, ultrastructural, and analytical findings and results of bronchial provocation tests. *Thorax.* 1983;38:119-128.

38. de Moraes S, Mariano M. Biochemical aspects of cobalt intoxication. Cobalt ion action on oxygen uptake. *Med Pharmacol Exp Int J Exp Med.* 1967;16:441-447.

39. Demedts M, et al. Cobalt lung in diamond polishers. *Am Rev Respir Dis.* 1984;130:130-135.

40. Demedts M, Gyselen A. The cobalt lung in diamond cutters: a new disease [in Dutch]. *Verh K Acad Geneeskd Belg.* 1989;51:559-581.

41. Domingo JL, Llobet JM. The action of L-cysteine in acute cobalt chloride intoxication. *Rev Esp Fisiol.* 1984;40:231-236.

42. Domingo JL, Llobet JM. Treatment of acute cobalt intoxication in rats with L-methionine. *Rev Esp Fisiol.* 1984;40:443-448.

43. Domingo JL, et al. A study of the effects of cobalt administered orally to rats. *Arch Farmacol Toxicol.* 1984;10:13-20.

44. Domingo JL, et al. The effects of EDTA in acute cobalt intoxication in rats. *Toxicol Eur Res.* 1983;5:251-255.

45. Domingo JL, et al. *N*-acetyl-L-cysteine in acute cobalt poisoning. *Arch Farmacol Toxicol.* 1985;11:55-62.

46. Domingo JL, et al. Effects of cobalt on postnatal development and late gestation in rats upon oral administration. *Rev Esp Fisiol.* 1985;41:293-298.

47. Duckham JM, Lee HA. The treatment of refractory anaemia of chronic renal failure with cobalt chloride. *Q J Med.* 1976;45:277-294.

48. Ely R, et al. Cobalt toxicity in calves resulting from high oral administration. *J Anim Sci.* 1948;7:239-243.

49. Fairhall LT, et al. Cobalt and dust environment of the cemented tungsten carbide industry. *Public Health Rep.* 1949;64:485-490.

50. Ferdenzi P, et al. Cobalt powdersintering industry (stone cutting diamond wheels): a study of environmental-biological monitoring, workplace improvement and health surveillance. *Sci Total Environ.* 1994;150:245-248.

51. Ferrans VJ. Alcoholic cardiomyopathy. *Am J Med Sci.* 1966;252:89-104.

52. Ferri F, et al. Exposure to cobalt in the welding process with stellite. *Sci Total Environ.* 1994;150:145-147.

53. Fischer T, Rystedt I. Cobalt allergy in hard metal workers. *Contact Dermatitis.* 1983;9:115-121.

54. Fischer T, Rystedt I. Skin protection against ionized cobalt and sodium lauryl sulphate with barrier creams. *Contact Dermatitis.* 1983;9:125-130.

55. Fisher JW, Langston JW. Effects of testosterone, cobalt and hypoxia on erythropoietin production in the isolated perfused dog kidney. *Ann N Y Acad Sci.* 1968;149:75-87.

56. Forte G, et al. Metal allergens of growing significance: epidemiology, immunotoxicology, strategies for testing and prevention. *Inflamm Allergy Drug Targets.* 2008;7:145-162.

57. Fox KA, et al. Fatal cobalt toxicity after total hip arthroplasty revision for fractured ceramic components. *Clin Toxicol (Phila).* 2016;54:874-877.

58. Franchini I, et al. Does occupational cobalt exposure determine early renal changes? *Sci Total Environ.* 1994;150:149-152.

59. Fried W, Kilbridge T. Effect of testosterone and of cobalt on erythropoietin production by anephric rats. *J Lab Clin Med.* 1969;74:623-629.

60. Fritzsche J, et al. Case report: High chromium and cobalt levels in a pregnant patient with bilateral metal-on-metal hip arthroplasties. *Clin Orthop Relat Res.* 2012;470:2325-2331.

61. Gallorini M, et al. Cobalt speciation in urine of hard metal workers. A study carried out by nuclear and radioanalytical techniques. *Sci Total Environ.* 1994;150:153-160.

62. Gardner FH. The use of cobaltous chloride in the anemia associated with chronic renal disease. *J Lab Clin Med.* 1953;41:56-64.

63. Gennart JP, Lauwerys R. Ventilatory function of workers exposed to cobalt and diamond containing dust. *Int Arch Occup Environ Health.* 1990;62:333-336.

64. Giampreti A, et al. Chelation in suspected prosthetic hip-associated cobalt toxicity. *Can J Cardiol.* 2014;30:465.e13.

65. Gilbert CJ, et al. Hip pain and heart failure: the missing link. *Can J Cardiol.* 2013;29:639.e1-639.e2.

66. Giovannini E, et al. Early effects of cobalt chloride treatment on certain blood parameters and on urine composition. *J Pharmacol Exp Ther.* 1978;206:398-404.

67. Greenberg SR. The beer drinker's kidney. *Nephron.* 1981;27:155.

68. Grice HC, et al. Myocardial toxicity of cobalt in the rat. *Ann N Y Acad Sci.* 1969;156:189-194.

69. Grice HC, et al. Experimental cobalt cardiomyopathy: correlation between electrocardiography and pathology. *Cardiovasc Res.* 1970;4:452-456.

70. Gross RT, et al. The hematopoietic and goitrogenic effects of cobaltous chloride in patients with sickle cell anemia. *Pediatrics.* 1955;15:284-290.

71. Haga Y, et al. Impaired myocardial function following chronic cobalt exposure in an isolated rat heart model. *Trace Elements Electrolytes.* 1996;13:69-74.

72. Harding HE. Notes on the toxicology of cobalt metal. *Br J Ind Med.* 1950;7:76-78.

73. Harkin TJ, et al. Differentiation of the ILO boundary chest roentgenograph (0/1 to 1/0) in asbestosis by high-resolution computed tomography scan, alveolitis, and respiratory impairment. *J Occup Environ Med.* 1996;38:46-52.

74. Henretig F. Case presentation: an 11-year-old boy develops vomiting, weakness, weight loss and a neck mass. *Internet J Med Toxicol.* 1998;1:13.

75. Horiguchi H, et al. Acute exposure to cobalt induces transient methemoglobinuria in rats. *Toxicol Lett.* 2004;151:419-466.

76. Ichikawa Y, et al. Biological monitoring of cobalt exposure, based on cobalt concentrations in blood and urine. *Int Arch Occup Environ Health.* 1985;55:269-276.

77. Ikeda T, et al. Polyneuropathy caused by cobalt-chromium metallosis after total hip replacement. *Muscle Nerve.* 2010;42:140-143.

78. Iyengar V, Woittiez J. Trace elements in human clinical specimens: evaluation of literature data to identify reference values. *Clin Chem.* 1988;34:474-481.

79. Jacobs JJ, et al. Cobalt and chromium concentrations in patients with metal on metal total hip replacements. *Clin Orthop.* 1996:S256-263.

80. Jacobziner H, Raybin HW. Poison control...accidental cobalt poisoning. *Arch Pediatr.* 1961;78:200-205.

81. Jefferson JA, et al. Excessive erythrocytosis, chronic mountain sickness, and serum cobalt levels. *Lancet.* 2002;359:407-408.

82. Jones HD, Perkins DJ. Metal-ion binding of human transferrin. *Biochim Biophys Acta.* 1965;100:122-127.

83. Kang JY, et al. A case of acute retinal toxicity caused by an intraocular foreign body composed of cobalt alloy. *Cutan Ocul Toxicol.* 2014;33:91-93.

84. Kato K. Iron-cobalt treatment of physiologic and nutritional anemia in infants. *J Pediatr.* 1937;11:385-396.

85. Kennedy A, et al. Fatal myocardial disease associated with industrial exposure to cobalt. *Lancet.* 1981;1:412-414.

86. Kent NL, McCance RA. The absorption and excretion of "minor" elements by man. *Biochem J.* 1941;35:837-844.

87. Kesteloot H, et al. An enquiry into the role of cobalt in the heart disease of chronic beer drinkers. *Circulation.* 1968;37:854-864.

88. Kiec-Swierczynska M. Occupational dermatoses and allergy to metals in Polish construction workers manufacturing prefabricated building units. *Contact Dermatitis.* 1990;23:27-32.

89. Kirchgessner M, et al. Endogenous excretion and true absorption of cobalt as affected by the oral supply of cobalt. *Biol Trace Elem Res.* 1994;41:175-189.

90. Kleinberg W, et al. Effect of cobalt on erythropoiesis in anemic rabbits. *Proc Soc Exp Biol Med.* 1939;42:119-120.

91. Klinck GH. Thyroid hyperplasia in young children. *JAMA.* 1955;158:1347-1348.

92. Kriss JP, et al. Hypothyroidism and thyroid hyperplasia in patients treated with cobalt. *JAMA.* 1955;157:117-121.

93. Kusaka Y, et al. Effect of hard metal dust on ventilatory function. *Br J Ind Med.* 1986;43:486-489.

94. Kusaka Y, et al. Epidemiological study of hard metal asthma. *Occup Environ Med.* 1996;53:188-193.

95. Kusaka Y, et al. Respiratory diseases in hard metal workers: an occupational hygiene study in a factory. *Br J Ind Med.* 1986;43:474-485.

96. Kwon YM, et al. Risk stratification algorithm for management of patients with metal-on-metal hip arthroplasty: consensus statement of the American Association of Hip and Knee Surgeons, the American Academy of Orthopaedic Surgeons, and the Hip Society. *J Bone Joint Surg Am.* 2014;96:e4.

97. Laaksonen I, et al. Outcomes of the recalled articular surface replacement metal-on-metal hip implant system: a systematic review. *J Arthroplasty.* 2017;32:341-346.

98. Lahaye D, et al. Lung diseases among diamond polishers due to cobalt? *Lancet.* 1984;1:156-157.

99. Lantin AC, et al. Absence of adverse effect on thyroid function and red blood cells in a population of workers exposed to cobalt compounds. *Toxicol Lett.* 2011;201:42-46.

100. Leikin JB, et al. Outpatient toxicology clinic experience of patients with hip implants. *Clin Toxicol (Phila).* 2013;51:230-236.

101. Linna A, et al. Exposure to cobalt in the production of cobalt and cobalt compounds and its effect on the heart. *Occup Environ Med.* 2004;61:877-885.

102. Linnainmaa M, Kiilunen M. Urinary cobalt as a measure of exposure in the wet sharpening of hard metal and stellite blades. *Int Arch Occup Environ Health.* 1997;69:193-200.

103. Lison D, et al. Biological monitoring of workers exposed to cobalt metal, salt, oxides, and hard metal dust. *Occup Environ Med.* 1994;51:447-450.

104. Little JA, Sunico R. Cobalt-induced goiter with cardiomegaly and congestive failure. *J Pediatr.* 1958;52:284-288.

105. Llobet JM, et al. Comparative effects of repeated parenteral administration of several chelators on the distribution and excretion of cobalt. *Res Commun Chem Pathol Pharmacol.* 1988;60:225-233.

106. Llobet JM, et al. Comparison of antidotal efficacy of chelating agents upon acute toxicity of Co(II) in mice. *Res Commun Chem Pathol Pharmacol.* 1985;50:305-308.

107. Llobet JM, et al. Comparison of the effectiveness of several chelators after single administration on the toxicity, excretion and distribution of cobalt. *Arch Toxicol.* 1986; 58:278-281.

108. Makela KT, et al. Risk of cancer with metal-on-metal hip replacements: population based study. *BMJ.* 2012;345:e4646.

109. Mao X, et al. Cobalt toxicity—an emerging clinical problem in patients with metal-on-metal hip prostheses? *Med J Aust.* 2011;194:649-651.

110. Mariano A, et al. Evolution of hard metal pulmonary fibrosis in two artisan grinders of woodworking tools. *Sci Total Environ.* 1994;150:219-221.

111. Markowitz SB, et al. Clinical predictors of mortality from asbestosis in the North American Insulator Cohort, 1981 to 1991. *Am J Respir Crit Care Med.* 1997;156:101-108.

112. Matharu GS, et al. Failure of a novel ceramic-on-ceramic hip resurfacing prosthesis. *J Arthroplasty.* 2015;30:416-418.

113. McDermott PH, et al. Myocardosis and cardiac failure in men. *JAMA.* 1966;198:253-256.

114. Migliori M, et al. Hard metal disease: eight workers with interstitial lung fibrosis due to cobalt exposure. *Sci Total Environ.* 1994;150:187-196.

115. Miller CW, et al. Pneumoconiosis in the tungsten-carbide tool industry; report of three cases. *A M A Arch Ind Hyg Occup Med.* 1953;8:453-465.

116. Minang JT, et al. Nickel, cobalt, chromium, palladium and gold induce a mixed Th1- and Th2-type cytokine response in vitro in subjects with contact allergy to the respective metals. *Clin Exp Immunol.* 2006;146:417-426.

117. Mistry JB, et al. Trunnionosis in total hip arthroplasty: a review. *J Orthop Traumatol* 2016;17:1-6.

118. Morelli L, et al. Effect of acute and chronic cobalt administration on carotid body chemoreceptors responses. *Sci Total Environ.* 1994;150:215-216.

119. Morin Y, Daniel P. Quebec beer-drinkers' cardiomyopathy: etiological considerations. *Can Med Assoc J.* 1967;97:926-928.

120. Morin Y, et al. Cobalt cardiomyopathy: clinical aspects. *Br Heart J.* 1971;33(suppl):175-178.

121. Morin YL, et al. Quebec beer-drinkers' cardiomyopathy: forty-eight cases. *Can Med Assoc J.* 1967;97:881-883.

122. Mosier BA, et al. Progressive cardiomyopathy in a patient with elevated cobalt ion levels and bilateral metal-on-metal hip arthroplasties. *Am J Orthop (Belle Mead NJ).* 2016;45:E132-E135.

123. Murphy RL Jr, et al. Crackles in the early detection of asbestosis. *Am Rev Respir Dis.* 1984;129:375-379.

124. Nemery B, et al. Cobalt and possible oxidant-mediated toxicity. *Sci Total Environ.* 1994; 150:57-64.

125. Nemery B, et al. Rapidly fatal progression of cobalt lung in a diamond polisher. *Am Rev Respir Dis.* 1990;141:1373-1378.

126. Ng SK, et al. Hip-implant related chorio-retinal cobalt toxicity. *Indian J Ophthalmol.* 2013;61:35-37.

127. Olatunbosun D, et al. Alteration of cobalt absorption in portal cirrhosis and idiopathic hemochromatosis. *J Lab Clin Med.* 1970;75:754-762.

128. Oldenburg M, et al. Severe cobalt intoxication due to prosthesis wear in repeated total hip arthroplasty. *J Arthroplasty.* 2009;24:825.e15-825.e20.

129. Orten J. Blood volume studies in cobalt polycythemia. *J Am Biol Chem.* 1933;1936:457-463.

130. Orten J. On the mechanism of the hematopoietic action of cobalt. *Am J Physiol.* 1936;114:414-422.

131. Paschal DC, et al. Trace metals in urine of United States residents: reference range concentrations. *Environ Res.* 1998;76:53-59.

132. Paternain JL, et al. Developmental toxicity of cobalt in the rat. *J Toxicol Environ Health.* 1988;24:193-200.

133. Paustenbach DJ, et al. Interpreting cobalt blood concentrations in hip implant patients. *Clin Toxicol (Phila).* 2014;52:98-112.

134. Pedigo NG, et al. Effects of acute and chronic exposure to cobalt on male reproduction in mice. *Reprod Toxicol.* 1988;2:45-53.

135. Pelclova D, et al. Severe cobalt intoxication following hip replacement revision: clinical features and outcome. *Clin Toxicol (Phila).* 2012;50:262-265.

136. Pitkin RM. *Dietary Reference Intakes: For Thiamin, Riboflavin, Niacin, Vitamin B₆, Folate, Vitamin B₁₂, Pantothenic Acid, Biotin, and Choline.* Washington, DC: Institute of Medicine; 1998.

137. Piza J, et al. Myocardial lesions and heart failure in infantile malnutrition. *Am J Trop Med Hyg.* 1971;20:343-355.

138. Potolicchio I, et al. Susceptibility to hard metal lung disease is strongly associated with the presence of glutamate 69 in HLA-DP beta chain. *Eur J Immunol.* 1997;27:2741-2743.

139. Quilligan JJ Jr. Effect of a cobalt-iron mixture on the anemia of prematurity. *Tex State J Med.* 1954;50:294-296.

140. Raffn E, et al. Health effects due to occupational exposure to cobalt blue dye among plate painters in a porcelain factory in Denmark. *Scand J Work Environ Health.* 1988;14:378-384.

141. Ratto D, et al. Pregnancy in a woman with severe pulmonary fibrosis secondary to hard metal disease. *Chest.* 1988;93:663-665.

142. Scientific Committee on Emerging and Newly Identified Health Risks. The safety of Metal-on-Metal joint replacements with a particular focus on hip implants. European Union; 2014.

143. Rivolta G, et al. Hard metal lung disorders: analysis of a group of exposed workers. *Sci Total Environ.* 1994;150:161-165.

144. Rizzato G, et al. Trace of metal exposure in hard metal lung disease. *Chest.* 1986; 90:101-106.

145. Rizzetti MC, et al. Cobalt toxicity after total hip replacement: a neglected adverse effect? *Muscle Nerve.* 2011;43:146-147; author reply 147.

146. Rizzetti MC, et al. Loss of sight and sound. Could it be the hip? *Lancet.* 2009;373:1052.

147. Rohn RJ, Bond WH. Observations on some hematological effects of cobalt-iron mixtures. *J Lancet.* 1953;73:317-324.

148. Rona G. Experimental aspects of cobalt cardiomyopathy. *Br Heart J.* 1971;33(suppl): 171-174.

149. Roy PE, et al. Thyroid changes in cases of Quebec beer drinkers myocardosis. *Am J Clin Pathol.* 1968;50:234-239.

150. Rystedt I, Fischer T. Relationship between nickel and cobalt sensitization in hard metal workers. *Contact Dermatitis.* 1983;9:195-200.

151. Sabbioni E, et al. The European Congress on Cobalt and Hard Metal Disease. Conclusions, highlights and need of future studies. *Sci Total Environ.* 1994;150:263-270.

152. Samelko L, et al. Cobalt-alloy implant debris induce HIF-1alpha hypoxia associated responses: a mechanism for metal-specific orthopedic implant failure. *PLoS One.* 2013; 8:e67127.

153. Sandusky GE, et al. Experimental cobalt cardiomyopathy in the dog: a model for cardiomyopathy in dogs and man. *Toxicol Appl Pharmacol.* 1981;60:263-278.

154. Sandusky GE, et al. Histochemistry and ultrastructure of the heart in experimental cobalt cardiomyopathy in the dog. *Toxicol Appl Pharmacol.* 1981;61:89-98.

155. Scansetti G, et al. Urinary cobalt as a measure of exposure in the hard metal industry. *Int Arch Occup Environ Health.* 1985;57:19-26.

156. Schirrmacher UO. Case of cobalt poisoning. *Br Med J.* 1967;1:544-545.

157. Schroeder HA, Nason AP. Trace-element analysis in clinical chemistry. *Clin Chem.* 1971;17:461-474.

158. Seaman AJ. Acquired erythrrocyte hypoplasia: a recovery during cobalt therapy. *Acta Haematol.* 1953;9:153-171.

159. Sesana G, et al. Cobalt exposure in wet grinding of hard metal tools for wood manufacture. *Sci Total Environ.* 1994;150:117-119.

160. Shannon M. Differential diagnosis and evaluation: an 11-year-old boy develops vomiting, weakness, weight loss, and a neck mass. *Internet J Med Toxicol.* 1988;1:14.

161. Shirakawa T, et al. Occupational asthma from cobalt sensitivity in workers exposed to hard metal dust. *Chest.* 1989;95:29-37.

162. Shirakawa T, et al. Hard metal asthma: cross immunological and respiratory reactivity between cobalt and nickel? *Thorax.* 1990;45:267-271.

163. Shirakawa T, et al. Specific IgE antibodies to nickel in workers with known reactivity to cobalt. *Clin Exp Allergy.* 1992;22:213-218.

164. Shulman RM, et al. Trunnionosis: the latest culprit in adverse reactions to metal debris following hip arthroplasty. *Skeletal Radiol.* 2015;44:433-440.

165. Sjogren I, et al. Hard metal lung disease: importance of cobalt in coolants. *Thorax.* 1980;35:653-659.

166. Skluis-Cremer GK, et al. Hard-metal lung disease. A report of 4 cases. *S Afr Med J.* 1987;71:598-600.

167. Sobel H, et al. Effect of cobalt ion, nickel ion, an zinc ion on corticoid excretion by the guinea pig. *Proc Soc Exp Biol Med.* 1960;104:86-88.

168. Sprince NL, et al. Respiratory disease in tungsten carbide production workers. *Chest.* 1984;86:549-557.

169. Sprince NL, et al. Cobalt exposure and lung disease in tungsten carbide production. A cross-sectional study of current workers. *Am Rev Respir Dis.* 1988;138:1220-1226.

170. Steens W, et al. Severe cobalt poisoning with loss of sight after ceramic-metal pairing in a hip—a case report. *Acta Orthop.* 2006;77:830-832.

171. Suardi R, et al. Health survey of workers occupationally exposed to cobalt. *Sci Total Environ.* 1994;150:197-200.

172. Sullivan J, et al. Tissue cobalt content in "beer drinkers' myocardiopathy." *J Lab Clin Med.* 1968;71:893-911.

173. Swennen B, et al. Epidemiological survey of workers exposed to cobalt oxides, cobalt salts, and cobalt metal. *Br J Ind Med.* 1993;50:835-842.

174. Thomas P, et al. Increased metal allergy in patients with failed metal-on-metal hip arthroplasty and peri-implant T-lymphocytic inflammation. *Allergy.* 2009;64: 1157-1165.

175. Tower SS. Arthroprosthetic cobaltism associated with metal on metal hip implants. *BMJ.* 2012;344:e430.

176. Tower SS. Arthroprosthetic cobaltism: neurological and cardiac manifestations in two patients with metal-on-metal arthroplasty: a case report. *J Bone Joint Surg Am.* 2010;92:2847-2851.

177. Tvermoes BE, et al. Effects and blood concentrations of cobalt after ingestion of 1 mg/d by human volunteers for 90 d. *Am J Clin Nutr.* 2014;99:632-646.

178. van den Eeckhout AV, et al. Pulmonary pathology due to cobalt and hard metals [in French]. *Rev Mal Respir.* 1989;6:201-207.

179. Virginio C, et al. Effects of divalent cations, protons and calmidazolium at the rat P2X7 receptor. *Neuropharmacology.* 1997;36:1285-1294.

180. Voyce MA. A case of pure red-cell aplasia successfully treated with cobalt. *Br J Haematol.* 1963;9:412-18.

181. Watters TS, et al. Aseptic lymphocyte-dominated vasculitis-associated lesion: a clinicopathologic review of an underrecognized cause of prosthetic failure. *Am J Clin Pathol.* 2010;134:886-893.

182. Weakly JN. The action of cobalt ions on neuromuscular transmission in the frog. *J Physiol.* 1973;234:597-612.

183. Webb M. The biological action of cobalt and other metals. IV. Inhibition of alpha-oxoglutarate dehydrogenase. *Biochim Biophys Acta.* 1964;89:431-446.

184. Wiberg GS. The effect of cobalt ions on energy metabolism in the rat. *Can J Biochem.* 1968;46:549-554.

185. Wigren A. Cobalt allergy reaction after knee arthroplasty with a Walldius prosthesis [in German]. *Z Orthop Ihre Grenzgeb.* 1982;120:17.

186. Wintrobe M, et al. The anemia of infection. VI. The influence of cobalt on the anemia associated with inflammation. *Blood.* 1947;2:323-331.

187. Wong CC, Nixon RL. Systemic allergic dermatitis caused by cobalt and cobalt toxicity from a metal on a metal hip replacement. *Contact Dermatitis.* 2014;71:113-114.

188. Zanelli R, et al. Uncommon evolution of fibrosing alveolitis in a hard metal grinder exposed to cobalt dusts. *Sci Total Environ.* 1994;150:225-229.

189. Zywiel MG, et al. Systemic cobalt toxicity from total hip arthroplasties: review of a rare condition Part 2. measurement, risk factors, and step-wise approach to treatment. *Bone Joint J.* 2016;98-B:14-20.

92 COPPER

Lewis S. Nelson

Copper (Cu)

Atomic number	=	29
Atomic weight	=	63.5 Da
Normal concentrations		
Whole blood	=	70–140 mcg/dL (11–22 mmol/L)
Total serum	=	120–145 mcg/dL (18.8–22.8 mmol/L)
Free serum	=	0.1–7 mcg/dL (0.02–1.1 mmol/L)
Ceruloplasmin	=	20–50 mg/dL (1–4 mmol/L)
Urine	=	25–50 mcg/d (0.4–0.8 mmol/24 d)

HISTORY AND EPIDEMIOLOGY

Copper is available in available in nature as elemental copper or as one of its sulfide or oxide ores. Important ores include malachite ($CuCO_3 \cdot (OH)_2$), chalcocite (Cu_2S), cuprite (Cu_2O), and chalcopyrite ($CuFeS_2$ or $Cu_2S \cdot Fe_2S_3$). Chalcopyrite, a yellow sulfide ore, is the source of 80% of the world's copper production. The smelting, or separation, of copper ores began about 7,000 years ago; copper gradually assumed its current level of importance at the start of the Bronze Age, around 3000 B.C. Smelting begins with roasting to dry the ore concentrate, which, in more modern times, is further purified by electrolysis to a 99.5% level of purity. The sulfide ores have naturally high arsenic content, which is released during the extraction process, posing a risk to those who smelt copper.

Although acute copper poisoning is uncommon in the United States, the historical role of copper as a therapeutic remains noteworthy. Copper sulfate was used in burn wound debridement until cases of systemic copper poisoning including hemolysis were reported.[50] In one report, each wound debridement procedure was associated with an 8% to 10% fall in the hematocrit. In the 1960s, copper sulfate (250-mg dose, containing 100 mg copper ion) ironically was recommended as an emetic, typically for use in children following potentially toxic exposures.[59] It was recognized for its speed of onset and effectiveness, and it compared favorably with syrup of ipecac. However, copper-induced emesis was rapidly identified to be extremely dangerous, and this practice was generally discontinued,[67] although fatal cases still occur. Copper salts are administered in religious rituals as a blue-green-colored "spiritual water," containing 100–150 g/L of copper sulfate as an emetic to "expel one's sins."[109]

Copper sulfate is used as a fungicide and algicide, and to eradicate tree roots that invade septic, sewage, and drinking water systems. Copper oxide, in combination with salts of chromium and arsenic (chromated cupric arsenate {CCA}), was used as an outdoor wood preservative, despite concerns over environmental arsenic contamination and has since been removed from the market.[20] Copper sulfate is the most readily available compound and is the form involved in the majority of nonindustrial copper exposures. Copper sulfate was a favorite ingredient in many home chemistry sets because of its brilliant blue color when dissolved in water. Although serious poisoning, particularly in children, led regulatory agencies in the United States to restrict its use, it accounts for the most consequential chemistry set–related toxic exposures reported in other countries.[78] Similarly, homegrown copper sulfate crystals from kits are occasionally responsible for fatal poisonings.[42]

Acute or chronic copper poisoning occurs when the metal is leached from copper pipes or copper containers. This occurs when carbon dioxide gas, used for postmix soft drink carbonation, backflows into the tubing transporting water to the soda dispensers, creating an acidic solution of carbonic acid that leaches copper from the equipment pipes.[121] Similarly, storage of acidic potable substances, such as orange or lemon juice, in copper vessels causes copper poisoning. A particularly dangerous situation occurs when acidic water is inadvertently used for hemodialysis.[33,73] In this circumstance, the leached copper avoids the normal gastrointestinal barrier and is delivered parenterally to the patient's circulation. In one case series, the copper concentration in the dialysis water was 650 mcg/L, causing several poisonings and the death of a patient with a whole blood copper concentration of 2,095 mcg/L.[34] Similarly, stagnant water or hot water, even if not highly acidic, can accumulate copper ions from pipes and cause poisoning.[8,34]

Although most natural water contains a small quantity of copper (4–10 mcg/L), it is tightly bound to organic matter and therefore not orally bioavailable. Copper pipes typically add about 1 mg of copper to the daily intake of an adult. The Environmental Protection Agency guidelines permit up to 1.3 mg/L of copper in drinking water.[28,89]

Metallic copper is ideal for electrical wiring because it is highly malleable. Its electrical conductivity is only exceeded by silver. Similarly, copper's excellent heat conductivity accounts for its widespread use in cookware. Although the metal is reactive with air, it forms a resistant surface of insoluble copper carbonate on its surface. This water- and air-resistant compound accounts for the green coloration of ornamental roofing and statues. Because copper is a soft metal, it must be strengthened prior to use in structural applications or as a coinage metal. This is most commonly done by the creation of copper alloys. Brass is an alloy of copper that is compounded with as much as 35% zinc. Similarly, bronze contains copper combined with up to 14% tin. Gun metal is an alloy that contains 88% copper, 10% tin, and 2% zinc. Sterling silver and white gold also contain copper.

There is a growing body of knowledge linking copper to the promotion of both physiologic and malignant angiogenesis.[46] In this latter case, copper may enable tumor expansion, invasion, and metastasis. Additionally, copper binding to amyloid fibers in the brain of patients with Alzheimer disease may lead to local oxidative damage and cause the characteristic neurodegeneration.[21] Copper is similarly implicated in the pathogenesis of both Parkinson disease and autism.[23,125]

CHEMICAL PRINCIPLES

Elemental copper (Cu^0) is a metal although not in itself poisonous, reacts in acidic environments to release copper ions to form either cuprous (I) or cupric (II) compounds. The elemental copper contraceptive intrauterine device (IUD) derives its efficacy from the local release of copper ions.[14] Elemental copper bracelets worn by patients with rheumatoid arthritis and other ailments purportedly derive their far-reaching "antiinflammatory effect" through dermal copper ion absorption and distribution to affected tissues.[118] Empiric support for this effect is lacking.[97] Local copper ion release is responsible for the occasional case of dermatitis that occurs following skin exposure to copper metal.[51] Ingestion of large amounts of metallic copper, for example as coins, rarely produces acute copper poisoning.[96,124] Poisoning under these circumstances is a result of the release of large amounts of copper ion from copper alloy by acidic gastric contents. Also, inhalation of finely divided metallic copper dust or bronze powder, used in industry and for gilding, produces life-threatening bronchopulmonary irritation, presumably as a consequence of the local release of ions.[44]

The majority of patients suffering from acute copper poisoning are exposed to ionic copper. In copper sulfate, also known as cupric sulfate, the copper atom is in the +2 oxidation state. Cuprous salts, containing copper in the +1 oxidation state, are unstable in water and readily oxidize to the cupric

TABLE 92–1   Important Copper Compounds

Chemical Name	Chemical Structure	Common Name	Notes
Chalcopyrite	$CuFeS_2$	Copper iron sulfide	Copper ore; source of 80% of world's copper
Chromated cupric arsenate	35% CuO 20% CrO_3 45% As_2O_5	CCA	Wood preservative[a]
Copper octanoate	$Cu\{CH_3(CH_2)_6COO\}_2$	Copper soap	Fungicide in home garden products, paint, rot-proof rope, and roofing
Copper triethanolamine complex	$Cu\{(HOCH_2CH_2)_3N\}_2$	Chelated copper	Algicide
Cupric acetoarsenite	$Cu(C_2H_3O_2)_2 \cdot 3Cu(AsO_2)_2$	Paris or Vienna green	Insecticide, wood preservative, pigment[a]
Cupric arsenite	$CuHAsO_3$	Swedish or Scheele green	Wood preservative, insecticide[a]
Cupric chloride	$CuCl_2$		Catalyst in petrochemical industry
Cupric chloride, basic	$CuCl_2 \cdot 3Cu(OH)_2$	Basic copper chloride; copper oxychloride	Fungicide
Cupric hydroxide	$Cu(OH)_2$	Copper hydroxide	Fungicide
Cupric oxide	CuO	Black copper oxide; tenorite	Glass pigment, flux, polishing agent
Cupric sulfate	$CuSO_4$	Roman vitriol, blue vitriol, bluestone, hydrocyanite	Fungicide, plant growth regulator, white wash, homegrown crystals
Cupric sulfate, basic	$CuSO_4 \cdot 3Ca(OH)_2 \cdot 3CaSO_4$	Bordeaux solution	Fungicide
Cuprous cyanide	$CuCN$	Cupricin	Electroplating solutions
Cuprous oxide	Cu_2O	Red copper oxide, cuprite	Antifouling paint

[a]No longer used in the United States.

form. There are numerous copper salts with varying oxidation states used in industry and agriculture (Table 92–1), many of which are not poisonous. Because those salts that are water soluble are more likely to be toxic, it is important to determine the nature of the copper compound implicated in an exposure. Analogously, when interpreting the literature, it is critical to discern which form of copper is involved in the study or case report before applying the results to clinical practice.

PHARMACOLOGY AND PHYSIOLOGY

Copper is an essential metal with total body stores of 100-150 mg. Daily requirements for copper are approximately 50 mcg/kg in infants and 30 mcg/kg in adults. The average daily intake of copper in the United States noted in NHANES III is about 1.2 mg.[35]

The daily nutritional requirement is satisfied by eating nuts, fish, and green vegetables such as legumes, although our largest source is generally from drinking water. Copper deficiency is exceedingly rare even in the poorest communities, and most frequently results from excessive zinc intake.[82] A Genetic disorder, Menkes "kinky-hair" syndrome, results in impaired intestinal copper absorption. Menkes syndrome is characterized by mental retardation, thermoregulatory dysfunction, hypopigmentation, connective tissue abnormalities, and pili torti (kinky hair). Interestingly, with the increased focus on the role of copper in neurodegenerative disorders and cancer, some authors suggest intentionally depleting patients of their copper stores with tetrathiomolybdate, an experimental copper chelator.[39] There is currently inadequate evidence to support this approach.

Copper is absorbed by an active process involving a copper adenosine triphosphatase (CuATPase) in the small intestinal mucosal cell membrane, also known as the Menkes ATPase (see below). The gastrointestinal absorption varies with the copper intake and the food source and is as low as 12% in patients with high copper intake.[47] In the presence of damaged mucosa, such as following acute overdose, the fractional absorption is likely to be significantly higher.[68] Once absorbed, copper is rapidly bound to high-affinity

carriers such as ceruloplasmin, and low-affinity carriers such as albumin, for transport to the liver and other tissues.[119] The amount of unbound ionized copper in the blood under normal circumstances is well below 1%. After being released locally in the reduced form from its carrier, copper uptake by the hepatic cells occurs via a specific uptake pump.[99] This process, which is facilitated by the reducing agent ascorbic acid, provides a potential window, however brief, for elimination of the ion by chelators. In acute overdose, a high fraction of the plasma copper remains bound to low-affinity proteins, such as albumin, and thus is biologically active. The volume of distribution of copper is 2 L/kg.

In the hepatocyte, complex trafficking systems exist (involving ceruloplasmin, metallothionein, and other metallochaperones {carrier proteins} within the cytoplasm) to prevent copper toxicity and to aid delivery to the appropriate enzymes.[94] A distinct CuATPase, located on certain subcellular organelles such as the *trans*-Golgi network or pericanalicular lysosomes, assists in the appropriate localization and elimination, respectively, of the metal ion.[120] By this mechanism, copper is either incorporated into enzymes or released, as a metallothionein–copper complex, directly into the biliary system for fecal elimination.

Some copper released from the liver is bound primarily to ceruloplasmin, an α_2-sialoglycoprotein with a molecular weight of 132,000 Da. Ceruloplasmin-bound copper accounts for approximately 90% to 95% of serum copper. Ceruloplasmin is a multifunctional protein that binds 6 copper ions per molecule. Copper bound to this carrier has a plasma half-life of approximately 24 hours. Ceruloplasmin is also involved in the mobilization of iron from its storage sites, and it serves an analogous role as a ferroxidase during the ferrous–ferric conversion. Copper in the Cu$^+$ form is oxidized directly by ceruloplasmin, thereby bypassing the generation of reactive oxygen species.

There are several important copper-containing enzymes in humans (Table 92–2). The common link among these enzymes is their participation in redox (reduction–oxidation) reactions in which a molecule, typically

TABLE 92–2	Important Copper-Containing Enzymes and Proteins and Their Functions
Enzyme or Protein	**Function**
Alcohol dehydrogenase	Alcohol metabolism
Catalase	Peroxide detoxification
Ceruloplasmin enzymes	Copper transport, ferroxidase
Cytochrome C oxidase	Complex IV of electron transport chain
Dopamine β-hydroxylase	Dopamine conversion to norepinephrine
Factor V	Coagulation system cofactor
Lysyl oxidase	Cross-linkage of collagen and elastin precursors
Monoamine oxidase	Primary amine deamination
Superoxide dismutase	Free radical detoxification
Tyrosinase	Melanin production (rate-limiting step)

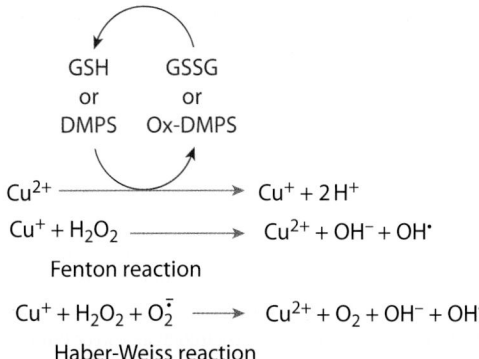

FIGURE 92–1. In the cupric or Cu^{2+} state, copper is reduced by sulfhydryl-containing compounds such as glutathione (GSH) or the chelator 2,3-dimercapto-1-propanesulfonic acid (DMPS) to its cuprous form (Cu^+), forming disulfide links in the process. Oxidized glutathione (GSSG) is subsequently enzymatically reduced by glutathione reductase to regenerate GSH. Superoxide anions O_2^-, formed when molecular oxygen (O_2) acquires an additional electron, are continually generated by mitochondria. Both the Fenton and the Haber–Weiss reactions use the cuprous form of copper as a catalyst to convert hydrogen peroxide or superoxide radical into the more biologically consequential hydroxyl radical (OH).

oxygen, donates or shares its electrons with another compound. In this respect, the physiology, chemistry, and toxicology of copper are most similar to that of iron. In fact, "blue-blooded" animals, such as octopi and spiders, use copper in hemocyanin, a blue pigment, in an analogous manner that "red-blooded" animals use iron in hemoglobin.

The elimination of copper occurs predominantly through biliary excretion following complexation with ceruloplasmin. Biliary excretion approximates gastrointestinal absorption, and averages 2 mg/24 h.[94] Renal elimination under normal conditions is trivial, accounting for approximately 5 to 25 mcg/24 h. The elimination $t_{1/2}$ of erythrocyte copper is 26 days.

Copper in water is tasted at concentrations of 1 to 5 mg/L, and a blue-green discoloration is imparted when the concentrations are greater than 5 mg/L.[32] Acute gastrointestinal symptoms occur when drinking water contains more than 25 mg/L,[52] although concentrations as low as 3 mg/L are associated with abdominal pain and vomiting in many, without a rise in the serum copper concentrations.[93] In one blinded, randomized study comparing copper-adulterated water to pure water, women appeared more sensitive than men to copper, but both groups were symptomatic when the copper concentration in the water was 6 mg/L.[7]

TOXICOLOGY AND PATHOPHYSIOLOGY
Redox Chemistry
Because copper is a transition metal, it is capable of assuming one of several different oxidation (or valence) states, and it is an active participant in redox reactions. In particular, participation in the Fenton reaction and the Haber–Weiss reaction explains the toxicologic effects of copper as a generator of oxidative stress and inhibitor of several key metabolic enzymes (Table 10–2).[56] In the presence of sulfhydryl-rich cell membranes, such as those on erythrocytes, cupric ions are reduced to cuprous ions, which are capable of generating superoxide radicals in the presence of oxygen.[63] This one-electron reduction of oxygen regenerates the cupric ion, allowing redox cycling and continuous generation of reactive oxygen species (Fig. 92–1). In particular, the mitochondrial electron transport chain and lipid membranes serve as ready sources of electrons for copper reduction, establishing a chain of events that ultimately leads to mitochondrial or membrane dysfunction, respectively.[81]

Erythrocytes
Cupric ion inhibits sulfhydryl groups on enzymes in important antioxidant systems, including glucose-6-phosphate dehydrogenase and glutathione reductase.[102] However, although support for these effects is only indirect, intraerythrocytic concentrations of reduced glutathione fall demonstrably following copper exposure. This effect is presumably part of the

protective role that glutathione, a nucleophile or reducing agent, normally has on oxidants, such as either cupric ions or the reactive oxygen species they generate.[75,76] Thus, in the setting of copper poisoning, in which excessive quantities of oxidants are produced, the depletion of glutathione presumably augments peroxidative membrane damage.

The importance of hemoglobin-derived reactive oxygen species is demonstrated by the lack of hemolysis in the presence of copper under anaerobic conditions or in an environment saturated with carbon monoxide.[11] The in vitro hemolytic activity of copper sulfate is reduced by albumin and several sulfhydryl containing compounds, including D-penicillamine and succimer.[1] Interestingly, 2,3-dimercapto-1-propanesulfonic acid (DMPS), another sulfhydryl containing compound often used as a chelator, exacerbates copper-induced hemolysis. This paradoxical effect is variably attributed to concomitant inhibition of superoxide dismutase, an important antioxidant enzyme, or to the ability of DMPS to efficiently reduce either membrane dithiols or cupric ions, in either case increasing the generation of superoxide.[2]

Hemolysis frequently occurs within 24 hours following acute copper salt poisoning.[109] This rapidity of hemolysis differs markedly from most other oxidant stressors, which usually take several days, and is likely a result of the differing nature of the erythrocyte insult. That is, the hemolysis following most oxidant exposures is caused by precipitation of hemoglobin as Heinz bodies and subsequent erythrocyte destruction by the reticuloendothelial system. Hemoglobin precipitation can also occur in the setting of acute copper poisoning, particularly following less substantial exposure. Additionally, and accounting for the early hemolysis, copper also directly oxidizes the erythrocyte membrane, thereby initiating red cell lysis independently of the reticuloendothelial system.[101] Oxidant-induced disulfide cross-links in the erythrocyte membrane reduce its stability and flexibility, thereby predisposing to early cell rupture.[3]

Copper-induced oxidation of the heme iron within the erythrocyte produces methemoglobinemia.[79] Given the high incidence of hemolysis, the methemoglobin is commonly released within the plasma. In this situation, methylene blue does not reliably reduce the ferric iron.[115,123]

Liver
Although most of the accumulated copper ions in hepatocytes are rapidly complexed with metallothionein, unsequestered copper ions participate in redox reactions. Hepatic cells are protected from copper toxicity in vitro after induction of metallothionein with zinc or cadmium salts or by the infusion of metallothionein prior to exposure. These interventions demonstrate the toxicologic significance of free intracellular ionic copper. These findings also

explain the therapeutic use of zinc acetate in patients suffering from Wilson disease. This benefit derives from the fact that reliably zinc induces the synthesis of hepatic metallothionein whereas ionic copper itself does not.

Copper ions also generate hydroxyl radicals, which are potent inducers of both lipid peroxidation and other reactive oxygen species. The peroxidative effect on biologic membranes is more significant in animals deficient in vitamin E and is prevented by vitamin E replacement, presumably because of the role of vitamin E as a free radical scavenger.[107] These effects are most pronounced in mitochondria, perhaps as a consequence of the reduction of cupric to cuprous ion in these organelles.[41,108] Ionic copper also accumulates in the cellular nuclei, where localized production of hydroxyl radicals forms DNA adducts and causes apoptosis.[100] Histologically, liver damage follows a centrilobular pattern of necrosis (Chap. 21).

The sequelae of the potent hepatotoxic effects of copper are not isolated to the liver. Once liver necrosis occurs, massive release of ionic copper into the blood occurs, which at times is of sufficient magnitude to cause hemolysis. This sequence of events is common during the crises of Wilson disease, and allows for an understanding of the delayed secondary episode of hemolysis that occurs in some ionic copper-poisoned patients.

Kidney

The kidneys bioaccumulate ionic copper although it is primarily bound to metallothionein. Reactive oxygen species are probably also responsible for the nephrotoxic effects of unbound copper. Pathologic analyses of the kidneys of oliguric or anuric copper poisoned patients typically reveal acute tubular necrosis and demonstrate hemoglobin casts. These findings suggest that kidney failure results indirectly from the hemoglobinuria induced by the massive release of free extracellular hemoglobin. The urinary hemoglobin, like myoglobin, will undergo conversion to ferriheme or release its iron, both of which result in oxidative stress on the renal tubular epithelial cells. Additionally, free extracellular hemoglobin causes renal vasoconstriction through the local scavenging of nitric oxide within the renal arterioles.

Central Nervous System

Charged entities such as copper ions do not readily cross the blood–brain barrier, whereas elevated cerebrospinal fluid ionic copper concentrations are characteristic of chronic copper overload conditions such as Wilson disease.[110] This accumulation is accomplished through carrier-mediated transport of albumin-bound, not ceruloplasmin-bound, ionized copper into the central nervous system. Once in the central nervous system, oxidative damage, as occurs in other tissues, results in cellular dysfunction and destruction.[95]

CLINICAL MANIFESTATIONS

Acute Copper Poisoning

The acute lethal dose following a single ingestion of copper sulfate is estimated to be 0.15 to 0.3 g/kg, but this is unverified.[6] Gastrointestinal irritation is the most common initial manifestation of copper salt poisoning. This syndrome includes the rapid onset of emesis and abdominal pain, possibly followed by gastroduodenal hemorrhage, ulceration, or perforation. Blue coloration of the vomitus does occur following the ingestion of certain copper salts, particularly copper sulfate.[80] Blue vomitus is not, however, pathognomonic for copper poisoning and also occurs in patients who ingest boric acid, methylene blue, paraquat (due to an additive), or food dyes. Other common symptoms include retrosternal chest pain and a metallic taste.

Given its location within the gastrointestinal tract, the liver receives the most substantial systemic exposure to ingested ionized copper. In patients with more severe acute copper sulfate poisoning, hepatotoxicity is a frequent, although rarely an isolated, manifestation. Jaundice, while among the most common clinical and biochemical findings following overdose, can be hepatocellular necrosis or hemolytic in origin.[9]

Hemolysis is more common than hepatotoxicity, and occurs invariably in those patients with liver damage.[106] As noted, copper-induced hemolysis often occurs rapidly following exposure (see Pathophysiology above

and Chap. 20). In most reported cases, significant methemoglobinemia occurs early in the patient's clinical course and is rapidly followed by hemolysis. Because free methemoglobin is filterable, methemoglobinuria occurs, although it cannot be differentiated from other heme forms in the urine without specialized testing.

Kidney and lung toxicities occur occasionally and represent extraerythrocytic manifestations of the oxidative effects of the copper ions. In spite of massive intravascular hemolysis, hemoglobinuric acute kidney injury is uncommon in patients who receive adequate volume-replacement therapy.[26]

Hypotension and cardiovascular collapse occur in patients with the most severe poisoning and is likely multifactorial in origin.[105] Undoubtedly, intravascular volume depletion from vomiting and diarrhea is involved. However, the severity and poor patient outcome despite appropriate volume repletion suggest that direct effects of ionized copper on vascular and myocardial cells are also involved. Sepsis, as a result of transmucosal bacterial invasion from the gastrointestinal tract, can also be partially responsible.[68]

Depressed mental status, which ranges from lethargy to coma, or seizures following acute poisoning, is likely an epiphenomenon related to damage to other organ systems. These findings are particularly common in patients with hepatic failure and are comparable to those of hepatic encephalopathy from other causes. In patients with chronic copper poisoning, such as Wilson disease, neurologic manifestations are prominent, and typically involve movement disorders (see Chronic Copper Poisoning below).

Intravenous injection of copper sulfate produces a clinical syndrome identical to that which occurs following ingestion, although the gastrointestinal findings are less pronounced.[13] Subcutaneous administration of a veterinary copper glycinate solution in a patient with a suicide attempt produced localized skin necrosis.[87]

Inhalation of copper oxide fumes, generated during welding or other industrial processes, can produce metal fume fever, a syndrome historically called "brass chills" or "foundry workers' ague." Patients with this syndrome present with cough, chills, chest pain, or fever that are most likely immunologic, and not toxicologic, in origin (Chap. 121). However, copper oxide formation, unlike zinc oxide, only occurs at extremely high temperatures, accounting for the relative infrequency of the copper-induced metal fume fever.

Chronic Copper Poisoning

Although hepatolenticular degeneration, known as Wilson disease, is a condition of chronic copper overload, there are qualitative similarities to acute copper salt poisoning. Wilson disease is an inherited, autosomal recessive disorder of copper metabolism affecting approximately 1 in 40,000 persons. The gene implicated in this disease (*ATP7B*, copper-transporting ATPase 2) codes for a hepatocyte membrane-bound copper-binding protein that is required for the maturation of ceruloplasmin and the biliary excretion of copper. Transgenic replacement models, in which human *ATP7B* is expressed in deficient animals, demonstrate normalization of copper excretion.[74] The absence of this gene and the resultant increase in hepatic copper concentrations produce continuing oxidative stress on the hepatocyte and cellular necrosis with the inevitable development of cirrhosis. Patients undergo periodic fluctuations in the extent of their copper-induced hepatotoxicity, and episodes of severe hepatotoxicity are frequently associated with hemolysis as stored copper is released from dying hepatocytes.

The adverse effects of ionized copper deposition in the lenticular nucleus in the basal ganglia cause movement disorders such as ataxia, tremor, parkinsonism, dysphagia, and dystonia.[69,85] No other forms of copper salt poisoning are associated with substantial or direct neurotoxicity. Psychiatric manifestations, such as behavioral changes or mood disorders, also occur. Accumulation of copper within the cornea accounts for the characteristic green-brown Kayser-Fleischer rings. Although the patient's serum copper concentrations are decreased, the individuals typically have a reduced ceruloplasmin concentration and an elevated urinary copper concentration. Treatment involves lifelong therapy with chelators such as D-penicillamine, trientine (triethylene tetramine), or molybdenum salts if the patient is

D-penicillamine sensitive. Zinc acetate, U.S. Food and Drug Administration (FDA) approved as a maintenance therapy, induces the formation of intestinal metallothionein and thereby blocks copper absorption by enhancing intestinal mucosal cell sequestration. Orthotopic liver transplantation results in improvement in nearly all aspects of the disease, including the central nervous system and ophthalmic manifestations.[98]

Chronic exogenous copper poisoning is uncommon in adults, but is reported following the use of copper-containing dietary supplements.[84] However, subacute or chronic exposure is common in children in some parts of the world. This condition, commonly called childhood cirrhosis in India or idiopathic copper toxicosis elsewhere, generally occurs in the setting of excessive dietary intake of copper because of copper-contaminated water from brass vessels used to store milk. These children have a genetic predisposition to copper accumulation, as signs of chronic liver disease develop by several months of age and progress rapidly.[55,83] Both serum copper and ceruloplasmin concentrations are markedly elevated, which differentiates this disease from Wilson disease. The incidence of the disease has fallen dramatically, probably as a result of improved nutrition and replacement of copper utensils and storage containers with those made of steel. One family of four developed abdominal pain, malaise, tachycardia, and anemia after approximately one month of eating home-grown vegetables treated with copper oxychloride pesticide.[43] Each patient had anemia and a slightly elevated (or upper limit of normal) serum copper concentration.

"Vineyard sprayer's lung," first described in 1969, refers to the occupational pulmonary disease that occurred among Portuguese vineyard workers applying Bordeaux solution, a 1% to 2% copper sulfate solution containing both hydrated lime {Ca(OH)$_2$} and calcium sulfate.[90] The patients developed interstitial pulmonary fibrosis and histiocytic granulomas containing copper. Many of these workers also developed pulmonary adenocarcinoma, hepatic angiosarcoma, and micro-nodular cirrhosis, raising the possibility of a carcinogenic effect of long-term copper exposure.[91] There is also a suggestion of an increased incidence of pulmonary adenocarcinoma among smelters, who are, however, exposed to many other xenobiotics, including arsenic, a known carcinogen.[70] No forms of copper are on the list of suspected carcinogens compiled by the International Agency of Research on Cancer.

Ophthalmic effects of copper salts, primarily following occupational exposure, include irritation of the corneal, conjunctival, or adnexal structures. Chronic ophthalmic exposure to particulate elemental copper or one of its alloys results in chalcosis lentis, from the Greek word *chalkos*, or copper. This chronic exposure manifests as a green-brown discoloration of the lens or cornea, similar to Kayser–Fleischer rings.

DIAGNOSTIC TESTING

Real-time testing for copper is impractical, and almost all management decisions must be based on clinical criteria. Copper concentrations are often obtained for confirmatory or investigative purposes. Although never adequately studied, whole-blood copper concentrations appear to correlate better with clinical findings than do serum copper concentrations.[4] The rapid movement of copper from serum into the erythrocyte presumably explains this finding. However, although there is a statistical relationship between the whole-blood copper concentrations and the severity of poisoning,[4,117] there is little correlation between clinical findings at any given copper concentration, regardless of which biologic tissue is measured. Similarly, other than at extremely high or low concentrations, there is no concentration at which the prognosis is definitively established. Reported serum copper concentrations in patients with hemolysis range from 96 to 747 mcg/dL, and those following severe poisoning have values of 6,600 mcg/dL[42] and 8,267 mcg/dL.[27] Serum copper concentrations in 11 patients with copper-induced acute kidney injury ranged from 115 to 390 mcg/dL.[25] The normal urinary copper excretion per 24 hours is up to approximately 25 mcg, and is reportedly as high as 628 mcg/24 h in patients with copper poisoning.

Occasionally serum copper concentrations reveal a secondary rise, which likely results from release during hepatocellular necrosis. This secondary rise typically occurs only in patients with life-threatening poisoning, and clinical evaluation is far more important and relevant than serial copper concentrations.[106]

Elevated copper concentrations are also noted in patients with inflammatory conditions, biliary cirrhosis, pregnancy, and estrogenic oral contraceptive use.[22] These conditions are associated with an elevated ceruloplasmin, and while the serum copper concentrations rise, the fraction of bound copper in the serum remains normal. Copper concentrations in the erythrocyte remain normal. Patients with Wilson disease have elevated hepatocyte copper content, but their serum copper concentrations are generally below normal unless hepatic necrosis is occurring.[71]

Although serum ceruloplasmin concentrations rise in patients with acute copper poisoning,[117] presumably reflecting increased hepatic synthesis, the ceruloplasmin concentration cannot be used to define the patient's prognosis. Tissue metallothionein concentrations also commonly rise after copper poisoning, but the implication of this finding, which is limited by the inability to rapidly obtain tissue samples, is unknown.[65] Ceruloplasmin concentrations are low in patients with Wilson disease, reflecting aberrant enzymatic activity.

Routine laboratory testing following acute copper salt poisoning should include an assessment for both hemolysis and hepatotoxicity. Differentiation of these etiologies as a cause for jaundice is made by standard methodology, such as comparison of the bilirubin fractions and an assessment of the hepatic enzymes and hemoglobin; that is, indirect bilirubin is proportionally elevated in patients with hemolysis, whereas the direct fraction rises in patients with hepatocellular necrosis. An assessment of the patient's electrolyte and hydration status is warranted. The prothrombin time can be prolonged in the absence of liver injury or disseminated intravascular coagulopathy and is likely the result of a direct effect of copper ions on the coagulation cascade.[79] In addition, many reports document an abnormal glucose 6-phosphate dehydrogenase (G6PD) activity, suggesting causation for hemolysis. However, interpretation of this test result is difficult, as copper poisoning interferes with the measurement of G6PD.[36]

Although copper metal embedded in the skin is clearly visible, topically applied copper salts are not visualized.[15] The clinical usefulness of radiographs to identify ingested copper salt solutions is unstudied. Obtaining an abdominal radiograph, while probably of limited benefit, is justified because it occasionally demonstrates the presence of radiopaque material in the gastrointestinal tract. Early efforts to use magnetic resonance imaging to identify Wilson disease are under way.[95]

MANAGEMENT

Supportive care is the cornerstone to the effective management of patients with acute copper salt poisoning, emphasizing antiemetic therapy, fluid and electrolyte correction, and normalization of vital signs prior to the evaluation for chelation therapy. Gastrointestinal decontamination is of limited concern because the onset of emesis generally occurs within minutes of ingestion and is often protracted. In patients who present for health care prior to vomiting following ingestion of a liquid copper solution, aspiration with a nasogastric tube to remove copper ion is a reasonable option. In one case, even after extensive vomiting, nasogastric aspiration still removed blue solution, but removing this remaining volume is unlikely to provide significant clinical benefit and should not be done.[17] Although oral activated charcoal is unlikely to be harmful, it is of unproved benefit, and it will hinder the ability to perform gastrointestinal endoscopy to evaluate the corrosive effects of a copper salt on the mucosal surface.[17] For this reason, even though activated charcoal may adsorb the remaining copper in the proximal gastrointestinal tract, we recommend against administering it to patients with isolated copper salt exposures. The potential benefit of *N*-acetylcysteine has not been studied, although its usefulness in many forms of fulminant hepatic failure support its empiric use. Advanced therapy for patients with acute kidney injury includes hemodialysis, using the usual criteria. For patients with life-threatening hepatic failure, liver transplantation is a reasonable option, but specific criteria for transfer to a specialized liver unit or for transplant, other than those that are applicable for Wilson disease or other more common, noncopper etiologies, are undefined.

Chelation Therapy

Chelation therapy is recommended when hepatic or hematologic compromise or other concerning or severe manifestations of poisoning are present. Studies on the efficacy of chelation therapy following acute copper salt poisoning are limited. Even when chelation is initiated early and appropriately, organ damage and death still occur. Application of the data from the existing literature is difficult because of the lack of controlled therapeutic studies of human copper salt poisoning. Although experimental animal models and uncontrolled human data exist, the results are frequently contradictory. Fortunately, exhaustive research into diseases of copper metabolism, particularly Wilson disease, which has periodic exacerbations similar to acute copper poisoning, has provided insight into managing patients with acute copper salt poisoning. However, direct applicability remains uncertain.

Three chelators are clinically available, and most data regarding dosing and efficacy are derived either from their use in the treatment of patients with Wilson disease or from their effects on copper elimination during chelation of patients manifesting toxicity from other metals.

D-Penicillamine, a structurally distinct metabolite of penicillin, is an orally bioavailable monothiol chelator. It is used in the treatment of lead, mercury, and copper poisoning, as well as in the management of rheumatoid arthritis and scleroderma. It has also been investigated for its antiangiogenesis effects in cancer therapy, which occur by chelation of copper that serves as a cofactor for certain growth factors, such as fibroblast growth factor.[113] D-Penicillamine is effective in preventing copper-induced hemolysis in patients with Wilson disease. Its protective mechanism is primarily mediated through chelation of unbound ionized copper, rendering them inaccessible to participate in redox reactions,[61] and dramatically increasing their urinary elimination.[116] The D-penicillamine–copper complex undergoes rapid renal clearance in patients with competent kidneys.

The use of D-penicillamine is not formally studied in the patients with acute copper salt poisoning, but case studies and animal models suggest that copper elimination is enhanced.[19,40,50] For this reason, D-penicillamine is the drug of choice for acute copper salt poisoning. The recommended dose is 1 to 1.5 g/d given orally in 4 divided doses. D-Penicillamine is also indicated for the treatment of chronic copper salt poisoning, such as Indian childhood cirrhosis. Initiation early in the course of disease and discontinuation of the exposure are associated with hepatic recovery and dramatically improved survival rates.[12]

Although D-penicillamine is effective, it is associated with several significant complications. In nearly 50% of patients treated with D-penicillamine for Wilson disease, there is worsening of the neurologic manifestations.[16] Subacute toxicities of D-penicillamine include aplastic anemia, agranulocytosis, renal and pulmonary disease, and loss of trace metals.[53] Long-term use of D-penicillamine is also associated with the development of cutaneous lesions and immunologic dysfunction. However, in the brief treatment necessary for acutely poisoned patients, the major risk is the potential for hypersensitivity reactions that occur in 25% of patients who are penicillin allergic. This hypersensitivity reaction is likely related to contamination of the pharmaceutical preparation with penicillin, rather than immunologic cross-reactivity.[49,58] The use of D-penicillamine during pregnancy is associated with congenital abnormalities, although all of the data are derived from women with Wilson disease who were receiving long-term therapy.[92]

Trientine (triethylenetetramine), another orally bioavailable chelator, is the second-line agent for patients with Wilson disease, but it is generally better tolerated.[54] However, unlike D-penicillamine, its use in patients with acute copper salt poisoning is unstudied. It was studied for its role as a copper chelator in patients with Alzheimer disease.[30] Trientine is generally safe, although colitis is reported.[18] One concern with trientine, as with penicillamine, is an initial neurologic worsening in about 25% of the patients who receive it for Wilson disease.[48]

Although intramuscular British anti-Lewisite (BAL) is likely to be less effective than other chelators described above, its use is appropriate in patients in whom vomiting or gastrointestinal injury prevents oral D-penicillamine administration.[111] Furthermore, because the dimercaprol–copper complex primarily undergoes biliary elimination, whereas D-penicillamine undergoes renal elimination, dimercaprol should be used in patients with acute kidney injury. When tolerated, D-penicillamine therapy should be started simultaneously or shortly after the initiation of therapy with dimercaprol (Antidotes in Depth: A28).

Calcium disodium ethylenediaminetetraacetate (CaNa$_2$EDTA) reduces the oxidative damage induced by ionized copper in experimental models.[122] However, it does not greatly enhance the elimination of copper ions when used for the chelation of other metals.[112] In addition, short-term use of CaNa$_2$EDTA inactivates dopamine β-hydroxylase in humans, presumably by chelating the copper moiety from its active site.[31] However, because the in vivo activity of this enzyme is restored on the addition of copper salt supplement, the potential for inhibition of the formation of neuronal norepinephrine during the treatment of acute poisoning is unknown. Successful clinical use of CaNa$_2$EDTA is reported making its use appropriate if other options are not available.[37,86] Interestingly, CuCaEDTA is used as a copper supplement in animals, and overdose of this formulation results in copper poisoning, suggesting that its chelating ability is limited (Antidotes in Depth: A30).[38]

Succimer is sometimes described as an ineffective copper chelator, although it is able to triple the baseline copper elimination in a murine model. Given its ease of use, ready availability, relative safety, and benefit in experimental models,[1] succimer can often be used in lieu of D-penicillamine or trientine in patients with less consequential poisoning, particularly when there is difficulty in obtaining penicillamine. Under these circumstances, it is reasonable to utilize standard lead poisoning succinic dosing regimens. (Chap. 93 and Antidotes in Depth: A29).

Dimercaptopropane sulfonate, an experimental chelator that is gaining popularity for the treatment of arsenic poisoning, prevents acute tubular necrosis in copper-poisoned mice.[77] 2,3-Dimercapto-1-propanesulfonic acid also proved to be the most effective of a panel of chelators in a murine model of copper sulfate poisoning,[57] and it substantially increased urinary copper elimination in nonpoisoned individuals.[114] However, DMPS, unlike D-penicillamine, forms intramolecular disulfide bridges, which, in so doing, liberates an electron. Although this accounts for its potency as a reducing agent, it also probably explains its propensity to worsen copper-induced hemolysis in vitro.[2] Because an adequate analysis of risk versus benefit is unavailable we recommend against using DMPS to chelate copper-poisoned patients.

Administration of zinc to induce metallothionine synthesis, which is also of proven, but limited, efficacy in Wilson disease, has an unknown role in the treatment of acute copper poisoning.[103] The need for several weeks of zinc therapy prior to realizing full efficacy makes its therapeutic use in acutely poisoned patients questionable. Although large oral doses of zinc salts can limit the absorption of copper ion, the concomitant gastrointestinal irritant effects of zinc ion make this therapy impractical.

Tetrathiomolybdate, an FDA-recognized chelator with orphan drug status although not marketed, can be available through compounding pharmacies, typically as ammonium tetrathiomolybdate. Tetrathiomolybdate is suggested to benefit copper-poisoned animals in uncontrolled studies,[88] but its use in acute copper poisoning in humans is unstudied and is unlikely to be beneficial. Tetrathiomolybdate depleted the copper stores in a patient with cancer who purchased the compound over the Internet as an "alternative" antiangiogenesis therapy.[66] We do not recommend the use of this inadequately studied antidote.

Clioquinol, a xenobiotic used 50 years ago as an antiparasitic, was discontinued because of an epidemic of optic neuropathy that may have been due to its ability to chelate copper ions.[104] Clioquinol has been more recently investigated as a therapy for Alzheimer disease.[10] It has not been studied for patients with acute or chronic copper poisoning and is not recommended.

Extracorporeal Elimination

There are limited data regarding the extent to which copper ion is eliminated by various extracorporeal means. Hemodialysis membranes undoubtedly allow the passage of copper ions, based on the epidemics in which hemodialysis using copper-rich water inadvertently resulted in copper poisoning.[33] Although copper should be cleared by hemodialysis, its relatively large volume of distribution limits the potential clinical usefulness of this technique. Furthermore, copper ions are highly protein bound, and the dialyzable concentration is typically less than 1 pmol/L, suggesting that hemodialysis would have little clinical usefulness. This fact is supported by case reports in which serum, tissue, or dialysate concentrations of copper were assessed.[5,86] Furthermore, given the propensity of hemodialysis to lyse erythrocytes, which will release stored copper and potentially worsen toxicity, hemodialysis is not recommended to enhance copper elimination, but it should be used for the standard nephrologic indications.

Molecular Adsorbents Recirculating System (MARS) and Single Pass Albumin Dialysis (SPAD), modified forms of hemodialysis in which albumin is included in the dialysate, are reported to rapidly and substantially lower the serum copper concentrations in patients with fulminant Wilson disease, allowing a bridge to hepatic transplantation.[24,29] One patient was treated with albumin dialysis using a 44 g/L albumin-containing dialysate and a slow dialysate flow rate (1–2 L/h) in a manner similar to routine continuous venovenous hemodiafiltration reportedly removed 105 mg of copper and normalized the serum copper concentration.[62] Caution should be used when extrapolating therapy from Wilson disease to exogenous copper poisoning, but it seems reasonable to utilize this technique if readily available. No evidence exists to support its use in patients with acute copper poisoning and the risk associated with hemolysis likely remains, preventing a recommendation for its use.

Exchange transfusion is of undefined, but probably limited, benefit in acute copper sulfate poisoning.[72,123] Plasma exchange enhanced the elimination of copper in patients with fulminant Wilson disease.[60,62] Copper removal ranged from 3 to 12 mg per treatment, but it is unclear if either of these removal techniques would be beneficial following an ingestion of gram quantities of copper sulfate. The same aforementioned risks of iatrogenic red cell lysis apply. However, in some settings exchange transfusion may be the only available practical therapy and it seem reasonable to attempt.

Peritoneal dialysis is not useful in patients with fulminant Wilson disease.[64] Peritoneal dialysis removed less than 700 mcg in a copper sulfate–poisoned child whose copper concentration was 207 mcg/dL.[45] However, in the same patient, the addition of albumin to the dialysate removed 9 mg of copper at a time when the child's serum copper concentration had already fallen substantially. Given the limited potential for removal of copper ion, this technique is not recommended.

There are no controlled data on the treatment of acute copper poisoning in pregnancy. The available data on pregnant women with Wilson disease document that D-penicillamine is teratogenic and that zinc is the preferred treatment.

SUMMARY

- The toxic effects of copper salts are primarily mediated by oxidative stress on the erythrocyte and hepatocyte, and this similarity to iron salt poisoning adds a framework for the conceptual understanding of the pathophysiology.

- Chelation is most commonly performed with D-penicillamine if the patient can tolerate oral medications and does not have renal failure, or dimercaprol if either of these findings are present. Both of these chelators have significant adverse effects.

- Succimer is more familiar to most clinicians and has fewer associated adverse effects; therefore, it is a reasonable alternative chelator.

- For patients with findings of impending hepatic failure, consultation or transfer to a liver transplantation center should be initiated.

REFERENCES

1. Aaseth J, et al. Hemolytic activity of copper sulfate as influenced by epinephrine and chelating thiols. *Acta Pharamacol Sinica.* 1998;19:203-206.
2. Aaseth J, et al. The interaction of copper (Cu++) with the erythrocyte membrane and 2,3-dimercaptopropanesulphonate in vitro: a source of activated oxygen species. *Pharmacol Toxicol.* 1987;61:250-253.
3. Adams KF, et al. The effect of copper on erythrocyte deformability: a possible mechanism of hemolysis in acute copper intoxication. *Biochim Biophys Acta.* 1979;550:279-287.
4. Adelstein SJ, Vallee BL. Copper metabolism in man. *N Engl J Med.* 1961;265:892897.
5. Agarwal BN, et al. Ineffectiveness of hemodialysis in copper sulphate poisoning. *Nephron.* 1975;15:74-77.
6. Akintonwa A, et al. Fatal poisonings by copper sulfate ingested from "spiritual water." *Vet Hum Toxicol.* 1989;31:453-454.
7. Araya M, et al. Community-based randomized double-blind study of gastrointestinal effect and copper exposure in drinking water. *Environ Health Perspect.* 2004; 112:1068-1073.
8. Arens P. Factors to be considered concerning the corrosion of copper tubes. *Eur J Med Res.* 1999;4:243-245.
9. Ashraf I. Hepatic derangements (biochemical) in acute copper sulphate poisoning. *J Indian Med Assoc.* 1970;55:341-342.
10. Bareggi SR, Cornelli U. Clioquinol: review of its mechanisms of action and clinical uses in neurodegenerative disorders. *CNS Neurosci Ther.* 2012;18:41-46.
11. Barnes G, Frieden E. Oxygen requirement for cupric ion induced hemolysis. *Biochem Biophys Res Commun.* 1983;115:680-684.
12. Bavdekar AR, et al. Long term survival in Indian childhood cirrhosis treated with D-penicillamine. *Arch Dis Child.* 1996;74:32-35.
13. Behera C, et al. An unusual suicide with parenteral copper sulphate poisoning: a case report. *Med Sci Law.* 2007;47:357-358.
14. Beltran-Garcia MJ, et al. Formation of copper oxychloride and reactive oxygen species as causes of uterine injury during copper oxidation of Cu-IUD. *Contraception.* 2000;61:99-9103.
15. Bentur Y, et al. An unusual skin exposure to copper; clinical and pharmacokinetic evaluation. *J Toxicol Clin Toxicol.* 1988;26:371-380.
16. Berger B, et al. Epileptic status immediately after initiation of D-penicillamine therapy in a patient with Wilson's disease. *Clin Neurol Neurosurg.* 2014;127:122-124.
17. Blundell S, et al. Blue lips, coma and haemolysis. *J Paediatr Child Health.* 2003;39:67-68.
18. Boga S, et al. Trientine induced colitis during therapy for Wilson disease: a case report and review of the literature. *BMC Pharmacol Toxicol.* 2015;16:30.
19. Botha CJ, et al. The cupruretic effect of two chelators following copper loading in sheep. *Vet Hum Toxicol.* 1993;35:409-413.
20. Breuer C, et al. Successful detoxification and liver transplantation in a severe poisoning with a chemical wood preservative containing chromium, copper, and arsenic. *Transplantation.* 2015;99:e29-e30.
21. Brewer GJ. Alzheimer's disease causation by copper toxicity and treatment with zinc. *Front Aging Neurosci.* 2014;6:92.
22. Buchwald A. Serum copper elevation from estrogen effect, masquerading as fungicide toxicity. *J Med Toxicol.* 2008;4:30-32.
23. Chauhan A, et al. Oxidative stress in autism: increased lipid peroxidation and reduced serum levels of ceruloplasmin and transferrin—the antioxidant proteins. *Life Sci.* 2004;75:2539-2549.
24. Chiu A, et al. Use of the molecular adsorbents recirculating system as a treatment for acute decompensated Wilson disease. *Liver Transpl.* 2008;14:1512-1516.
25. Chugh KS, et al. Acute renal failure following copper sulphate intoxication. *Postgrad Med J.* 1977;53:18-23.
26. Chugh KS, et al. Acute renal failure due to intravascular hemolysis in the North Indian patients. *Am J Med Sci.* 1977.
27. Chugh KS, et al. Letter: Methemoglobinemia in acute copper sulfate poisoning. *Ann Intern Med.* 1975;82:226-227.
28. Cockell KA, et al. Regulatory frameworks for copper considering chronic exposures of the population. *Am J Clin Nutr.* 2008;88(suppl):6.
29. Collins KL, et al. Single pass albumin dialysis (SPAD) in fulminant Wilsonian liver failure: a case report. *Pediatr Nephrol.* 2008;23:1013-1016.
30. Cooper GJS. Therapeutic potential of copper chelation with triethylenetetramine in managing diabetes mellitus and Alzheimer's disease. *Drugs.* 2011;71:1281-1320.
31. De Paris P, Caroldi S. In vivo inhibition of serum dopamine-beta-hydroxylase by CaNa$_2$ EDTA injection. *Hum Exp Toxicol.* 1994;13:253-256.
32. Dietrich AM, et al. Health and aesthetic impacts of copper corrosion on drinking water. *Water Sci Technol.* 2004;49:55-62.
33. Eastwood JB, et al. Heparin inactivation, acidosis and copper poisoning due to presumed acid contamination of water in a hemodialysis unit. *Clin Nephrol.* 1983;20:197-201.
34. Eife R, et al. Chronic poisoning by copper in tap water: II. Copper intoxications with predominantly systemic symptoms. *Eur J Med Res.* 1999;4:224-228.
35. Ervin RB, et al. Dietary intake of selected minerals for the United States population: 1999-2000. *Adv Data.* 2004:1-5.
36. Fairbanks VF. Copper sulfate-induced hemolytic anemia. Inhibition of glucose-6-phosphate dehydrogenase and other possible etiologic mechanisms. *Arch Intern Med.* 120:428-432.
37. Franchitto N, et al. Acute copper sulphate poisoning: a case report and literature review. *Resuscitation.* 2008;78:92-96.

38. Giuliodori MJ, et al. Acute copper intoxication after a Cu-Ca EDTA injection in rats. *Toxicology.* 1997;124:173-177.

39. Goodman VL, et al. Copper deficiency as an anti-cancer strategy. *Endocr Relat Cancer.* 2004;11:255-263.

40. Gooneratne SR, Christensen DA. Effect of chelating agents on the excretion of copper, zinc and iron in the bile and urine of sheep. *Vet J.* 1997;153:171-178.

41. Gu M, et al. Oxidative-phosphorylation defects in liver of patients with Wilson's disease. *Lancet.* 2000;356:469-474.

42. Gulliver JM. A fatal copper sulfate poisoning. *J Anal Toxicol.* 1991;15:341-342.

43. Gunay N, et al. A series of patients in the emergency department diagnosed with copper poisoning: recognition equals treatment. *Tohoku J Exp Med.* 2006;209:243-248.

44. Haggerty RJ, Harris GB. Toxic hazards; bronze-powder inhalation. *N Engl J Med.* 1957;256:40-41.

45. Hamlyn AN, et al. Fulminant Wilson's disease with haemolysis and renal failure: copper studies and assessment of dialysis regimens. *Br Med J.* 1977;2:660-663.

46. Harris ED. A requirement for copper in angiogenesis. *Nutr Rev.* 2004;62:60-64.

47. Harvey LJ, et al. Copper absorption from foods labelled intrinsically and extrinsically with Cu-65 stable isotope. *Eur J Clin Nutr.* 2005;59:363-368.

48. Hedera P. Update on the clinical management of Wilson's disease. *Appl Clin Genet.* 2017;10:9-19.

49. Herbst D. Detection of penicillin G and ampicillin as contaminants in tetracyclines and penicillamine. *J Pharm Sci.* 1977;66:1646-1648.

50. Holtzman NA, et al. Copper intoxication. Report of a case with observations on ceruloplasmin. *N Engl J Med.* 1966;275:347-352.

51. Hostynek JJ, Maibach HI. Copper hypersensitivity: dermatologic aspects*. *Dermatol Ther.* 2004;17:328-333.

52. Hoveyda N, et al. A cluster of cases of abdominal pain possibly associated with high copper levels in a private water supply. *J Environ Health.* 2003;66:29-32.

53. Huang L, et al. Metal element excretion in 24-h urine in patients with Wilson disease under treatment of D-penicillamine. *Biol Trace Elem Res.* 2012;146:154-159.

54. Hunt DP, et al. Case records of the Massachusetts General Hospital. Case 30-2014. A 29-year-old man with diarrhea, nausea, and weight loss. *N Engl J Med.* 2014;371:1238-1247.

55. Johncilla M, Mitchell KA. Pathology of the liver in copper overload. *Semin Liver Dis.* 2011;31:239-244.

56. Jomova K, Valko M. Advances in metal-induced oxidative stress and human disease. *Toxicology.* 2011;283:65-87.

57. Jones MM, et al. The relative effectiveness of some chelating agents in acute copper intoxication in the mouse. *Res Commun Chem Pathol Pharmacol.* 1980;27:571-577.

58. Juhlin L, et al. Antibody reactivity in penicillin-sensitive patients determined with different penicillin derivatives. *Int Arch Allergy Appl Immunol.* 1977;54:19-28.

59. Karlsson B, Noren L. Ipecacuanha and copper sulphate as emetics in intoxications in children. *Acta Paediatr Scand.* 1965;54:331-335.

60. Kiss JE, et al. Effective removal of copper by plasma exchange in fulminant Wilson's disease. *Transfusion.* 1998;38:327-331.

61. Klein D, et al. Dissolution of copper-rich granules in hepatic lysosomes by D-penicillamine prevents the development of fulminant hepatitis in Long-Evans cinnamon rats. *J Hepatol.* 2000;32:193-201.

62. Kreymann B, et al. Albumin dialysis: effective removal of copper in a patient with fulminant Wilson disease and successful bridging to liver transplantation: a new possibility for the elimination of protein-bound toxins. *J Hepatol.* 1999;31:1080-1085.

63. Kumar KS, et al. Copper-induced generation of superoxide in human red cell membrane. *Biochem Biophys Res Commun.* 1978;83:587-592.

64. Kuno T, et al. Severely decompensated abdominal Wilson disease treated with peritoneal dialysis: a case report. *Acta Paediatr Jpn.* 1998;40:85-87.

65. Kurisaki E, et al. Copper-binding protein in acute copper poisoning. *Forensic Sci Int.* 1988;38:3-11.

66. Lang TF, et al. Iatrogenic copper deficiency following information and drugs obtained over the Internet. *Ann Clin Biochem.* 2004;41(pt 5):417-420.

67. Liu J, et al. Death following cupric sulfate emesis. *Clin Toxicol.* 2001;39:161-163.

68. Liu Z, Chen B. Copper treatment alters the barrier functions of human intestinal Caco-2 cells: involving tight junctions and P-glycoprotein. *Hum Exp Toxicol.* 2004;23:369-377.

69. Lorincz MT. Neurologic Wilson's disease. *Ann N Y Acad Sci.* 2010;1184:173-187.

70. Lubin JH, et al. Respiratory cancer and inhaled inorganic arsenic in copper smelters workers: a linear relationship with cumulative exposure that increases with concentration. *Environ Health Perspect.* 2008;116:1661-1665.

71. Mak CM, Lam C-W. Diagnosis of Wilson's disease: a comprehensive review. *Crit Rev Clin Lab Sci.* 2008;45:263-290.

72. Malik M, Mansur A. Copper sulphate poisoning and exchange transfusion. *Saudi J Kidney Dis Transpl.* 2011;22:1240-1242.

73. Manzler AD, Schreiner AW. Copper-induced acute hemolytic anemia. A new complication of hemodialysis. *Ann Intern Med.* 1970;73:409-412.

74. Meng Y, et al. Restoration of copper metabolism and rescue of hepatic abnormalities in LEC rats, an animal model of Wilson disease, by expression of human ATP7B gene. *Biochim Biophys Acta.* 2004;1690:208-219.

75. Metz EN, Sagone AL. The effect of copper on the erythrocyte hexose monophosphate shunt pathway. *J Lab Clin Med.* 1972;80:405-413.

76. Milne L, et al. Effects of glutathione and chelating agents on copper-mediated DNA oxidation: pro-oxidant and antioxidant properties of glutathione. *Arch Biochem Biophys.* 1993;304:102-109.

77. Mitchell WM, et al. Antagonism of acute copper(II)-induced renal lesions by sodium 2,3-dimercaptopropanesulfonate. *Johns Hopkins Med J.* 1982;151:283-285.

78. Mucklow ES. Chemistry set poisoning. *Int J Clin Pract.* 1997;51:321-323.

79. Nagaraj MV, et al. Copper sulphate poisoning, hemolysis and methaemoglobinemia. *J Assoc Physicians India.* 1985;33:308-309.

80. Naha K, et al. Blue vitriol poisoning: a 10-year experience in a tertiary care hospital. *Clin Toxicol.* 2012;50:197-201.

81. Nakatani T, et al. Redox state in liver mitochondria in acute copper sulfate poisoning. *Life Sci.* 1994;54:967-974.

82. Nations SP, et al. Denture cream: an unusual source of excess zinc, leading to hypocupremia and neurologic disease. *Neurology.* 2008;71:639-643.

83. Nayak NC, Chitale AR. Indian childhood cirrhosis (ICC) & ICC-like diseases: The changing scenario of facts versus notions. *Indian J Med Res.* 2013.

84. O'Donohue J, et al. A case of adult chronic copper self-intoxication resulting in cirrhosis. *Eur J Med Res.* 1999;4:252-252.

85. Oder W, et al. Wilson's disease: evidence of subgroups derived from clinical findings and brain lesions. *Neurology.* 1993;43:120-124.

86. Oldenquist G, Salem M. Parenteral copper sulfate poisoning causing acute renal failure. *Nephrol Dial Transplant.* 1999;14:441-443.

87. Oon S, et al. Acute copper toxicity following copper glycinate injection. *Intern Med J.* 2006;36:741-743.

88. Ortolani EL, et al. Acute sheep poisoning from a copper sulfate footbath. *Vet Hum Toxicol.* 2004;46:315-318.

89. Pal A, et al. An urgent need to reassess the safe levels of copper in the drinking water: lessons from studies on healthy animals harboring no genetic deficits. *NeuroToxicology.* 2014;44:58-60.

90. Pimentel JC, Marques F. "Vineyard sprayer's lung": a new occupational disease. *Thorax.* 1969;24:678-688.

91. Pimentel JC, Menezes AP. Liver disease in vineyard sprayers. *Gastroenterology.* 1977;72:275-283.

92. Pinter R, et al. Infant with severe penicillamine embryopathy born to a woman with Wilson disease. *Am J Med Genet.* 2004;128A:294-298.

93. Pizarro F, et al. Acute gastrointestinal effects of graded levels of copper in drinking water. *Environ Health Perspect.* 1999;107:117-121.

94. Prohaska JR, Gybina AA. Intracellular copper transport in mammals. *J Nutr.* 2004;134:1003-1006.

95. Ranjan A, et al. MRI and oxidative stress markers in neurological worsening of Wilson disease following penicillamine. *NeuroToxicology.* 2015;49:45-49.

96. Rebhandl W, et al. In vitro study of ingested coins: leave them or retrieve them? *J Pediatr Surg.* 2007;42:1729-1734.

97. Richmond SJ, et al. Copper bracelets and magnetic wrist straps for rheumatoid arthritis – analgesic and anti-inflammatory effects: a randomised double-blind placebo controlled crossover trial. *PLoS One.* 2013;8:e71529-e71529.

98. Rosencrantz R, Schilsky M. Wilson disease: pathogenesis and clinical considerations in diagnosis and treatment. *Semin Liver Dis.* 2011;31:245-259.

99. Safaei R, et al. The role of copper transporters in the development of resistance to Pt drugs. *J Inorg Biochem.* 2004;98:1607-1613.

100. Sagripanti JL, et al. Interaction of copper with DNA and antagonism by other metals. *Toxicol Appl Pharmacol.* 1991;110:477-485.

101. Salhany JM, et al. Evidence suggesting direct oxidation of human erythrocyte membrane sulfhydryls by copper. *Biochem Biophys Res Commun.* 82:1294-1299.

102. Sansinanea AS, et al. Glucose-6-phosphate dehydrogenase activity in erythrocytes from chronically copper-poisoned sheep. *Comp Biochem Physiol C Pharmacol Toxicol Endocrinol.* 1996;114:197-200.

103. Santiago R, et al. Zinc therapy for Wilson disease in children in French pediatric centers. *J Pediatr Gastroenterol Nutr.* 2015;61:613-618.

104. Schaumburg H, Herskovitz S. Copper deficiency myeloneuropathy: a clue to clioquinol-induced subacute myelo-optic neuropathy? *Neurology.* 2008;71:622-623.

105. Schwartz E, Schmidt E. Refractory shock secondary to copper sulfate ingestion. *Ann Emerg Med.* 1986;15:952-954.

106. Singh MM, Singh G. Biochemical changes in blood in cases of acute copper sulphate poisoning. *J Indian Med Assoc.* 50:549-554.

107. Sokol RJ, et al. Oxidant injury to hepatic mitochondrial lipids in rats with dietary copper overload. Modification by vitamin E deficiency. *Gastroenterology.* 1990;99:1061-1071.

108. Sokol RJ, et al. Abnormal hepatic mitochondrial respiration and cytochrome C oxidase activity in rats with long-term copper overload. *Gastroenterology.* 1993;105:178-187.

109. Sontz E, Schwieger J. The "green water" syndrome: copper-induced hemolysis and subsequent acute renal failure as consequence of a religious ritual. *Am J Med.* 1995;98:311-315.

110. Stuerenburg HJ. CSF copper concentrations, blood-brain barrier function, and ceruloplasmin synthesis during the treatment of Wilson's disease. *J Neural Transm.* 2000;107:321-329.

111. Takeda T, et al. Cupric sulfate intoxication with rhabdomyolysis, treated with chelating agents and blood purification. *Intern Med.* 2000;39:253-255.

112. Thomas DJ, Chisolm J. Lead, zinc and copper decorporation during calcium disodium ethylenediamine tetraacetate treatment of lead-poisoned children. *J Pharmacol Exp Ther*. 1986;239:829-835.

113. Tisato F, et al. Copper in diseases and treatments, and copper-based anticancer strategies. *Med Res Rev*. 2010;30:708-749.

114. Torres-Alanís O, et al. Urinary excretion of trace elements in humans after sodium 2,3-dimercaptopropane-1-sulfonate challenge test. *J Toxicol Clin Toxicol*. 2000;38: 697-700.

115. Umbreit J. Methemoglobin—it's not just blue: a concise review. *Am J Hematol*. 2007; 82:134-144.

116. Vieira J, et al. Urinary copper excretion before and after oral intake of D-penicillamine in parents of patients with Wilson's disease. *Dig Liver Dis*. 2012;44:323-327.

117. Wahal PK, et al. Study of whole blood, red cell and plasma copper levels in acute copper sulphate poisoning and their relationship with complications and prognosis. *J Assoc Physicians India*. 1976;24:153-158.

118. Walker WR, Keats DM. An investigation of the therapeutic value of the "copper bracelet"—dermal assimilation of copper in arthritic/rheumatoid conditions. *Agents Actions*. 1976;6:454-459.

119. Walshe JM. Serum "free" copper in Wilson disease. *Q J Med*. 2012;105:419-423.

120. Wang Y, et al. Advances in the understanding of mammalian copper transporters. *Adv Nutr*. 2011;2:129-137.

121. Witherell LE, et al. Outbreak of acute copper poisoning due to soft drink dispenser. *Am J Public Health*. 1980;70:1115.

122. Yamamoto H, et al. Mechanism of enhanced lipid peroxidation in the liver of Long-Evans cinnamon (LEC) rats. *Arch Toxicol*. 1999;73:457-464.

123. Yang CC, et al. Prolonged hemolysis and methemoglobinemia following organic copper fungicide ingestion. *Vet Hum Toxicol*. 2004;46:321-323.

124. Yelin G, et al. Copper toxicity following massive ingestion of coins. *Am J Forensic Med Pathol*. 1987;8:78-85.

125. Zecca L, et al. The role of iron and copper molecules in the neuronal vulnerability of locus coeruleus and substantia nigra during aging. *Proc Natl Acad Sci U S A*. 2004; 101:9843-9848.

# 93 LEAD

Diane P. Calello and Fred M. Henretig

Lead (Pb)

Atomic number	=	82
Atomic weight	=	207.21 Da
Whole blood	<	5 mcg/dL (<0.24 mmol/L)

HISTORY AND EPIDEMIOLOGY

The low melting point and high malleability of lead made it one of the first metals smelted and used by humans. Ancient Egyptians and Hebrews used lead, and the Phoenicians established lead mines in Spain circa 2000 B.C. The Greeks and Romans released lead during the process of extracting silver from ore. Roman society found many uses for lead, including pipes, cooking utensils, and ceramic glazes, and a common practice was to use sapa, a grape syrup simmered down in lead vessels, as a sweetener and preservative.[139] Postindustrial lead use increased dramatically, and today lead is used widely for its waterproofing and electrical- and radiation-shielding properties.[96] Use of both lead-based paint for house paint and leaded gasoline has been essentially eliminated by regulation in the United States since the 1980s, but is still a concern in many nations, and persistence of lead paint in older US homes and water-supply systems still constitutes an enormous environmental challenge.[4,5,80]

Recognition of the clinical effects of excess lead exposure can be traced back to antiquity. Dioscorides, a Greek physician in the second century B.C., observed adverse cognitive effects, and Pliny cautioned the Romans of the danger of inhaled fumes from lead smelting.[134] Modern authors suggest that extensive use of sapa in Roman aristocratic society contributed to the downfall of Roman dominance.[139] Lead poisoning was also recognized in American colonial times. Benjamin Franklin observed in 1763 the "dry gripes" (abdominal colic) and "dangles" (wrist drop) that afflicted tinkers, painters, and typesetters, as well as the "gripes" caused by rum distillation in leaden condensing coils.[123] Lead salts, particularly lead acetate (sugar of lead), were used medicinally in the early 19th century to control bleeding and diarrhea. With the 19th-century Industrial Revolution, lead poisoning became a common occupational disease. The reproductive effects of lead poisoning were recognized by the turn of the 20th century, including the high rate of stillbirths, infertility, and abortions among women in the pottery industry or who were married to pottery workers.

The majority of health effects that occur today in the United States concern childhood lead poisoning due to residential house paint. In this chapter we will use the synonyms lead poisoning and plumbism interchangeably. The modern history of childhood plumbism can be traced to the recognition of lead-paint poisoning in Brisbane, Australia, in 1897.[134] Lead poisoning was reported in American children in 1917, and by 1943, it was established that children who recovered from clinical plumbism were frequently left with neurologic sequelae and intellectual impairment. Symptomatic childhood lead poisoning was a frequent occurrence in American pediatric medical centers throughout the 1950s and 1960s, a period during which research established effective chelation therapy protocols with British anti-Lewisite (dimercaprol) and edetate calcium disodium (CaNa$_2$EDTA).[36,207] From the 1970s to the present, the research thrust in childhood lead poisoning has centered on the recognition and quantification of more subtle neurocognitive impairment caused by subclinical lead poisoning.[19,135] Over this time period, the US Centers for Disease Control and Prevention (CDC) has steadily revised downward the definitions of an elevated blood lead concentration or thresholds of concern in children, from 60 mcg/dL in the early 1960s to 5 mcg/dL today.[28]

Numerous sources of lead exposure exist and are generally classified as perinatal, environmental, occupational, or additional (somewhat "exotic") sources. Perinatal lead exposures relate to placental transfer and subsequent breast feeding for infants whose mothers have elevated blood lead concentrations.[25] Environmental exposures affect the entire population, particularly young children. Elevated lead concentrations in drinking water are being detected with increasing frequency as plumbing infrastructure ages. However, the health impact of these elevations in drinking water is not yet clear.[14,80] Most environmental lead poisoning of consequence in the United States still results from exposure to residential lead paint (Table 93–1).

Lead pigments (typically lead carbonate) account for up to 40% by weight of many white house paints from the pre–World War II era.[134] Since 1978, paint intended for interior or exterior residential surfaces, toys, or furniture in the United States is allowed, by law, to contain no more than 0.06% lead. However, an estimated 3 million tons of lead remain in 57 million US homes built before 1980 and painted with lead-based paint. This aging housing stock has created an enormous environmental hazard of lead exposure to children and to adult homeowners, house painters, and construction workers who become involved in sanding, scraping, and restoration of painted surfaces in these homes. Furthermore, lead-based paint is still allowed for industrial, military, marine, and some outdoor uses, such as structural components of bridges and highways; occasionally, some of this paint is inadvertently used in homes. Attempts to abate lead-painted outdoor structures can pollute entire communities.[104]

Although paint-derived lead exposure results from overt pica of lead paint chips in some children, most lead paint exposure in childhood relates to the crumbling, peeling, flaking, or chalking of aging paint.[5] These fine paint particles are incorporated into household dust and yard soil, where ordinary childhood hand–mouth activity results in ingestion.[5] Seasonal variations in house dust contamination occur, with higher house dust lead concentrations and increased blood lead concentrations in exposed preschool children noted during the summer.

Adults with occupational exposures to lead constitute another large group of persons at risk. It is estimated that more than 3 million workers in

TABLE 93–1	Environmental Lead Sources
Source	**Comment**
Air	Leaded gasoline (pre-1976 United States; still prevalent worldwide), industrial emissions
Dust	House dust from deteriorated lead paint
Food	Lead solder in cans (pre-1991 United States; still prevalent in imported canned foods); "natural" dietary supplements; "moonshine" whiskey and lead foil–covered wines; contaminated flour, paprika, other imported foods and candy; lead leached from leaded crystal, ceramics, vinyl lunch boxes
Other	Complementary and alternative medicines, children's toys and jewelry (especially imported products), cosmetics, leaded ink, vinyl mini-blinds
Paint	Especially pre-1978 homes
Soil	From yards contaminated by deteriorated lead paint, lead industry emissions, roadways with high leaded gasoline usage
Water	Leached from leaded plumbing (pipes, solder), cooking utensils, water coolers

the United States, employed in more than 100 occupations, are exposed to lead.[98] The most important route of absorption in occupational settings is inhalation of lead dust and fumes. In addition, ingestion also results when workers eat, drink, or smoke in lead dust–contaminated areas. However, the presence of lead in the workplace, per se, does not imply a significant risk of poisoning. Some types of lead-related work are more hazardous than others (Table 93–2).[2] For example, lead smelting is categorized as primary (from raw ore) and secondary (reclamation, such as from used car batteries). Secondary lead production workers are at higher risk of poisoning because this job more typically involves small, sometimes "backyard," operations that are less likely to adhere to industry safety regulations than large, well-regulated primary smelters.[47] A significant hazard exists for workers at firearm shooting ranges, where workplace conditions frequently fail on several fronts to protect workers from lead dust hazards. This is particularly true with the use of unjacketed bullets, the handling of targets after practice that contain splintered fragments and lead dust, and shooting in a prone position.[10,68]

For convenience, environmental and occupational or recreational lead exposures are discussed separately, although there is considerable overlap. For example, workers who fail to change lead dust–covered work clothes or shoes inevitably bring this occupational lead hazard home and secondarily contaminate their children's environment.[161]

Finally, numerous additional sources of lead exposure are also reported, including contaminated folk medications or cosmetics,[95,207] imported food,[79] ingested lead foreign bodies,[124,193] and retained bullets.[58,110,169] Ayurveda and other folk medicine, specifically "rasa shastra," where heavy metals are incorporated into products for their medicinal value, is a frequent source of lead exposure in children and adults.[26,94,127,164] Since 2010, an outbreak of lead encephalopathy from artisanal gold mining in Nigeria has claimed hundreds of lives, with the toll still growing.[77,184]

Some potential exposures raised considerable community concern and media coverage in recent years—for example, the discovery of lead contamination of some artificial turfs,[31] imported toys coated with lead paint,[111] the disposition of electronic waste,[100] and elevated drinking water concentrations.[14,80] These, too, are highlighted separately in Table 93–2.

Several recent national and regional surveys evaluated current US population-based trends in blood lead concentrations and sociodemographic correlates. The CDC and individual experts estimate that 450,000 to 500,000 children aged 1 to 5 years have blood lead concentrations greater than 5 mcg/dL.[11,32] The 2012 revised reference value representing primarily excessive household exposure, and that in 2013 approximately 5,200 adults are reported each year with blood lead concentrations greater than 24 mcg/dL typically reflecting excessive occupational exposure.[2] Although such numbers are impressive, they represent a considerable decrease from prevalence rates reported in prior decades,[11] and it is certainly the observed clinical experience that symptomatic lead poisoning in children, in particular, is far less common than it was a generation ago. Nevertheless, for children who reside in the deteriorating cities of the United States, the battle is far from won. The CDC reported in 2000 that children enrolled in Medicaid had a prevalence of elevated blood lead concentrations 3 times greater than those not enrolled.[22] Refugee, immigrant, and foreign-born adopted children remain at particularly high risk,[24] and remarkable cases of extremely elevated blood lead concentrations (>100 mcg/dL) are still be detected on routine screening.[46]

CHEMICAL PRINCIPLES

Lead is a silvery-gray, soft metal ubiquitous element in the Earth's crust, with an atomic weight of 207.21 Da and an atomic number of 82. It has a low melting point, 621.3°F (327.4°C), and boils at 2,948°F (1,620°C) at atmospheric pressure.[192] It occurs principally as 2 isotopes: ^{206}Pb and ^{208}Pb. Metallic lead is relatively insoluble in water and dilute acids but dissolves in nitric, acetic, and hot, concentrated sulfuric acids. In compounds, lead assumes valence states of +2 and +4. Inorganic lead compounds are often brightly colored and vary widely in water solubility; several are used extensively as pigments in paints such as lead chromate (yellow) and lead oxide (red). Lead also forms organic compounds, of which 2, tetramethyl and tetraethyl lead (TEL), were used commercially as gasoline additives.[96] These are essentially insoluble in water but readily soluble in organic solvents.[165] Lead complexes with ligands containing sulfur, oxygen, or nitrogen as electron donors. It thus forms stable complexes with several ligands common to biologic molecules, including –OH, –SH, and –NH_2. Complexes with endogenous sulfhydryl (–SH) groups are the most toxicologically important. There is no known physiologic role for lead, and thus any lead presence in human tissue represents contamination.

TABLE 93–2 Occupational and Recreational Lead Sources

High-Risk Occupations
- Automobile radiator repairers
- Crystal glass makers
- Firing range instructors, bullet salvagers
- Lead smelters, refiners
- Metal welders, cutters (includes bridge and highway reconstruction workers)
- Painters, construction workers (sanding, scraping, or spraying of lead paint; demolition of lead-painted sites)
- Polyvinyl chloride plastic manufacturers
- Shipbreakers
- Storage battery manufacturers, repairers, recyclers

Moderate-Risk Occupations
- Automobile factory workers and mechanics
- Enamelers
- Glass blowers
- Lead miners
- Plumbers
- Pottery glazers
- Ship repairers
- Shot makers
- Solderers
- Type founders
- Varnish makers
- Wire and cable workers

Possible Increased-Risk Occupations
- Electronics manufacturers
- Jewelers
- Pipefitters
- Printers
- Rubber product manufacturers
- Traffic police officers, taxi drivers, garage workers, turnpike tollbooth operators, gas station attendants (exposed to leaded gasoline exhaust fumes; unlikely now in the United States but still a hazard in developing countries)

Recreational and Hobby Sources
- Ceramic crafts
- Furniture refinishing, restoring
- Home remodeling, refinishing
- Painting (fine artist's pigments)
- Repair of automobiles, boats
- Stained-glass making
- Target shooting, recasting lead for bullets

Additional Sources
- Ingested lead foreign bodies and retained lead bullets
- Illicit substance abuse (heroin, methamphetamine, leaded gasoline "huffing")
- Burning batteries, leaded paper, or wood for fuel
- Hand–mouth contact with pool cue chalk, glazes, leaded ink

PHARMACOLOGY
Inorganic and Metallic Lead
Absorption

Gastrointestinal (GI) absorption is less efficient than pulmonary absorption. Adults absorb an estimated 10% to 15% of ingested lead in food, and children have a higher GI absorption rate, averaging 40% to 50%.[1,72] In animal studies, this varies by type of lead compound studied.[8] However, it should be noted that fasting and diets deficient in iron, calcium, and zinc—factors that are frequent among groups of young children—enhance GI absorption of lead.[72,116,175] The role of essential trace elements in decreasing lead absorption is assumed to be a consequence of competitive absorption processes, particularly of the apical divalent metal transporter (DMT1) in the small intestine.[100] Metallic lead, such as potentially encountered in fishing weights swallowed by young children or retained bullets in gunshot victims, is also absorbed, albeit less readily than most lead compounds.[8] The rate of absorption of ingested metallic lead is related to particle size, total surface area, and GI tract location; whereas gastric acidity favors dissolution, the small bowel is likely the site of maximal absorption.[193]

The overall absorption of inhaled lead averages 30% to 40%. Of note, both minute ventilation and the concentration of lead in air determine airborne lead exposure, so a worker engaged in vigorous physical activity will absorb considerably more lead than a person in the same atmosphere at rest. Likewise, children, having relatively greater volume of inhaled air per unit of body size because of higher metabolic rates, are proportionally at greater risk in a given degree of atmospheric lead pollution. It is estimated that children have a 2.7-fold higher lung deposition rate of lead than do adults.[1]

Cutaneous absorption of inorganic lead has been traditionally considered low; one study found an average absorption of 0.06% through intact skin.[129] However, a few more recent studies have questioned this dogma and suggest that cutaneous exposure is a potential source of exposure in workers.[61,63,181] Anecdotal cases exist of pediatric lead toxicity ascribed to application of lead-contaminated ethnic cosmetics.[27,128,144] Some of these exposures likely also involve occult conjunctival absorption and ingestion,[144] but given especially the thinner skin of children, it seems plausible that some dermal absorption is occurring in such cases. Soft tissue absorption of metallic lead follows exposure to retained bullets, and similar to ingested lead foreign bodies, also depends on particle size, total surface area, and location; multiple small shot and location in which particles are bathed by synovial, serosal, or spinal fluid favor a more rapid increase in blood lead concentration.[58,110,169] This is most likely due to increased solvency of lead in organic acids, such as hyaluronic acid in synovial fluid, as well as mechanical forces from joint motion.

Transplacental lead transfer is critical in fetal and neonatal lead exposure. Lead readily crosses the placental barrier throughout gestation, and lead uptake is cumulative until birth.[25,154] Breast milk also contains lead in relatively low concentration, and it is a significant source of neonatal exposure at maternal blood lead concentrations of approximately 40 mcg/dL or greater.[9] One study demonstrated that the relationship between breast milk and maternal blood and plasma lead was not linear, although overall breast milk concentrations were still quite low (see also Management, Adults, Pregnancy and Lactation).[53]

Distribution

Absorbed lead enters the bloodstream, in which at least 99% is bound to erythrocytes.[113] From blood, lead is distributed into both a relatively labile soft tissue pool and into a more stable bone compartment. This classic 3-compartment model is somewhat of an oversimplification. At least 2 bone compartments are recognized: a more labile pool in trabecular bone and a more stable pool in cortical bone. In adults, approximately 95% of the body lead burden is stored in bone versus only 70% for children. The remainder is distributed to the major soft tissue lead-storage sites, including the liver, kidney, bone marrow, and brain. Lead uptake into soft tissues occurs in a complex fashion that depends on numerous factors, including blood lead concentrations, external exposure factors, and specific tissue kinetics. Most of the toxicity associated

with lead is a result of soft tissue uptake, so that the relative decrease in bone storage is another comparative disadvantage for children.

Lead in the central nervous system (CNS) is of particular toxicologic importance. Lead preferentially concentrates in gray matter and certain nuclei.[73] Fetal brain uptake is relatively higher than that which occurs with postnatal exposure in animal models. The highest brain concentrations are found in the hippocampus, cerebellum, cerebral cortex, and medulla.

Unlike soft tissue storage, bone lead accumulates throughout life. Bone storage begins in utero and occurs across all ranges of exposure, so that there is no threshold for bone lead uptake.[1] Bone lead was thought to be relatively metabolically inert, but it can be mobilized from the more labile compartments and contributes as much as 50% of the blood lead content. This is of particular importance during times of rapid bone turnover such as pregnancy and lactation, in elderly persons with osteoporosis,[174] and in children with immobilization.[121] Lead also accumulates in the teeth, particularly the dentine of children's teeth, a phenomenon that has been used to quantify cumulative lead exposure in young children.[135]

Excretion

Absorbed lead that is not retained is primarily excreted in urine (approximately 65%) and bile (approximately 35%).[1] A miniscule amount is lost via sweat, hair, and nails. Children excrete less of their daily uptake than adults, with an average retention of 33% versus 1% to 4%, respectively.[208] Biologic half-lives for lead are estimated as follows: blood 25 days (adults, short-term experiments) and 10 months (children, natural exposure); soft tissues (adults, short-term exposure), 40 days; bone (labile, trabecular pool), 90 days; and bone (cortical, stable pool), 10 to 20 years.[1,118,155] As mentioned, trace amounts of lead are also excreted in breast milk.[9,53]

Organic Lead

Alkyl lead compounds are lipid soluble and have unique pharmacokinetics that are less well characterized than those of inorganic lead.[12] Animal studies and human clinical experience with acute ingestions and leaded gasoline sniffing demonstrate TEL absorption through ingestion, inhalation, and intact skin, with subsequent distribution to lipophilic tissues, including the brain.[165,182,203] Tetraethyl lead is metabolized to triethyl lead, which is likely the major toxic compound. Alkyl lead also slowly releases lead as the inorganic form, with subsequent kinetics as noted above.[12]

PATHOPHYSIOLOGY
General Mechanisms

Similar to many metals, lead is a complex xenobiotic exerting numerous pathophysiologic effects in many organ systems.[113] Furthermore, genetic polymorphism impacts an individual's susceptibility to lead.[142] Several examples of such include the genes for apolipoprotein E, the vitamin D receptor, Na^+,K^+-ATPase (adenosine triphosphatase), δ-aminolevulinic acid, and protein kinase C.[168] At the biomolecular level, lead functions in 3 general ways. First, its affinity for biologic electron-donor ligands, especially sulfhydryl groups, allows it to bind and impact numerous enzymatic, receptor, and structural proteins. Second, lead is chemically similar to the divalent cations calcium, magnesium, and zinc, and it interferes with numerous calcium and perhaps magnesium and zinc mediated metabolic pathways, particularly in mitochondria and in second-messenger systems regulating cellular energy metabolism.[107,178] Lead-induced mitochondrial injury results in apoptosis, a phenomenon particularly well studied in animal models of retinal cells.[107] Lead also functions as an antagonist or agonist of calcium-dependent processes. For example, lead inhibits neuronal voltage-sensitive calcium channels[8] and membrane-bound Na^+,K^+-ATPase (adenosine triphosphatase)[176] but activates calcium-dependent protein kinase C.[119] These effects adversely impact neurotransmitter function.[198] Third, lead affects nucleic acids by mechanisms not fully understood, though some evidence exists for alteration of DNA methylation.[106,206] It exhibits mutagenic and mitogenic effects in mammalian cells in vitro and is carcinogenic in rats and mice.[51] There is mechanistic plausibility and some epidemiologic evidence for at least a facilitative role of lead in human carcinogenesis,[87] and the International

Agency for Research on Cancer (IARC) has assigned inorganic lead compounds to the group 2A category, which is the class probably carcinogenic to humans.[86]

Neurotoxicity

The neurotoxicity of lead involves multiple targets, including cerebrovascular endothelium, mitochondria, neural cell adhesion molecules, neurotransmitter and second-messenger function, regulation of apoptosis, and myelin formation.[107,156,198] Lead-induced dysfunction in several neurotransmitter systems is linked to its calcium-mimetic properties. Through blockade of calcium influx at voltage-sensitive calcium channels, lead inhibits depolarization-triggered release of acetylcholine, dopamine, and γ-aminobutyric acid (GABA) but augments the background rate of spontaneous release.[41,91,107,113,198] The dampening of the evoked neurotransmitter response in conjunction with enhanced background release results in a decreased "signal-to-noise" ratio.[69,91] In addition, lead decreases calcium currents at the N-methyl-D-aspartate (NMDA) glutamate receptor and directly activates the intracellular second-messenger protein kinase C.[91] These effects on neurotransmitter release, receptor activity, and intracellular signaling adversely affect "synaptic pruning" in the developing brain, a process by which the volume of excessive synaptic connections is selectively reduced. This disruption results in suboptimal cortical microarchitecture and function, and it particularly affects the hippocampus, an important locus of learning and memory.[69,91,198]

Lead also interferes with the 78-kDa chaperone glucose-regulated protein (GRP78) in astrocytes, which results in adverse protein conformational effects that are thought to be associated with conditions such as Alzheimer disease and parkinsonism.[198] In severe cases, pathologic changes in cerebral microvasculature result in cerebral edema and increased intracranial pressure (ICP), which are associated with the clinical syndrome of acute lead encephalopathy (Fig. 93–1). Peripheral neuropathy is a classic effect of lead poisoning in adults, and is reported rarely in lead-exposed children with associated sickle cell disease.[52] The neuropathology in humans is poorly characterized. In animal models, it is associated with Schwann cell destruction, segmental demyelination, and axonal degeneration.[113] Sensory nerves are rarely affected.

Hematologic Toxicity

Lead is hematotoxic in several ways, including via potent inhibition of several enzymes in the heme biosynthetic pathway (Chap. 20 and Fig. 20–3). It also induces a defect in erythropoietin function secondary to associated kidney damage.[76] A shortened erythrocyte life span is caused by increased membrane fragility with resultant hemolysis. Inhibition of Na^+,K^+-ATPase and pyrimidine-5′-nucleotidase impair erythrocyte membrane stability by altering energy metabolism. The inhibition of pyrimidine-5′-nucleotidase also underlies the appearance of basophilic stippling in erythrocytes, representing clumping of degraded RNA, which is normally eliminated by this enzyme[143] (Fig. 93–2).

Nephrotoxicity

Functional changes associated with acute lead nephropathy include decreased energy-dependent transport, resulting in a Fanconilike syndrome of aminoaciduria, glycosuria, and phosphaturia. These changes are related to disturbed mitochondrial respiration and phosphorylation and are reversible with discontinuation of exposure or treatment.[136] A pathologic finding is characteristic nuclear inclusion bodies in renal tubular cells composed of lead–protein complex. Chronic high-dose lead poisoning is associated with progressive interstitial fibrosis.[136] Lead is a renal carcinogen in rodent models, but its status in humans is uncertain.[51]

The association of plumbism with gout ("saturnine gout") was noted more than 100 years ago. Lead competitively decreases uric acid excretion in the distal tubule, resulting in elevated blood urate concentrations and urate crystal deposition in joints. Kidney function is virtually always impaired in patients with saturnine gout.[44]

Cardiotoxicity

The most important manifestation of lead toxicity on the cardiovascular system is hypertension. This is likely caused by altered calcium-activated changes in contractility of vascular smooth muscle cells secondary to decreased Na^+,K^+-ATPase activity and stimulation of the Na^+-Ca^{2+} exchange pump. Lead also affects blood vessels by altering neuroendocrine input or sensitivity to such stimuli or by increasing reactive oxygen species that enhance nitric oxide inactivation.[109] Elevated serum renin activity is found with moderate toxicity but is normal or decreased in chronic severe

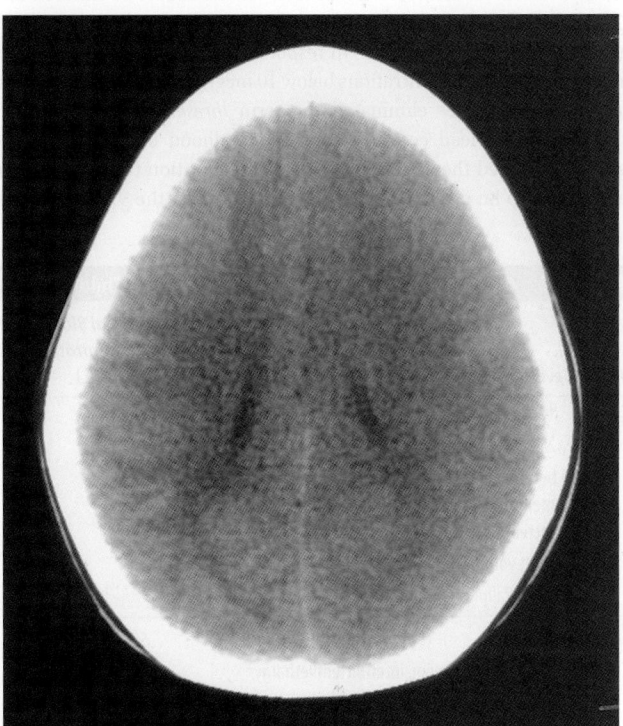

FIGURE 93–1. Computed tomography scan of the brain reveals diffuse cerebral edema and loss of gray–white matter differentiation on day 1 of hospitalization of a 3-year-old boy. He had presented with a brief prodrome of vomiting and altered mental status followed by status epilepticus, characteristic of acute lead encephalopathy. His blood lead concentration was 220 mcg/dL. *(Used with permission from Department of Radiology, St. Christopher's Hospital for Children, Philadelphia, PA.)*

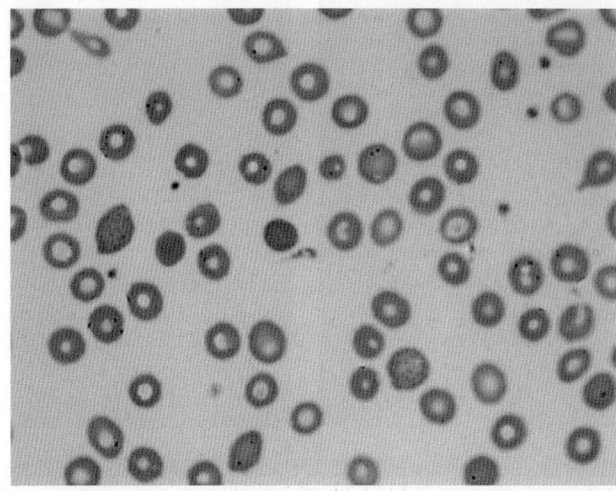

FIGURE 93–2. This peripheral smear of blood examined under high-power microscopy demonstrates the classic basophilic stippling associated with lead poisoning. The patient's blood lead concentration was >100 mcg/dL. *(Used with permission from the Fellowship in Medical Toxicology, New York University School of Medicine, New York City Poison Center.)*

plumbism.[194] Rarely, direct cardiotoxicity is reported.[134,157] Animal models demonstrate increased sensitivity to norepinephrine-induced dysrhythmias and decreased myocardial contractility, protein phosphorylation, and high-energy phosphate generation.[99] Lead-induced impairment of intracellular calcium metabolism impacts cardiac electrophysiology.[7]

Reproductive Toxicity

Impairment of both male and female reproductive function is associated with overt plumbism. Gametotoxic effects in animals of both sexes and chromosomal abnormalities in workers with blood lead concentrations above 60 mcg/dL are reported.[113] Male infertility arises from 3 mechanisms: hypothalamic–pituitary–testicular axis disruption, impairment of spermatogenesis, and inhibition of sperm function, at blood lead concentrations of 40 mcg/dL and above.[66,159]

Endocrine Toxicity

Reduced thyroid and adrenopituitary function are found in adult lead workers.[62,163] Children with elevated blood lead concentrations have a depressed secretion of human growth hormone and insulinlike growth factor.[85]

Skeletal Toxicity

In addition to the importance of the skeletal system as the largest repository of lead body burden, studies suggest that bone metabolism also is adversely affected by lead.[113] Hormonal response is altered by reduced 1,25-dihydroxyvitamin D_3 concentrations and by inhibition of osteocalcin. Both new bone formation and coupling of normal osteoblast and osteoclast function can thus be impaired.[113] Bands of increased metaphyseal density on radiographs of long bones ("lead lines") in young children with heavy lead exposure represent increased calcium deposition (not primarily lead) in the zones of provisional calcification (Fig. 93–3). Impaired bone growth and shortened stature are associated with childhood lead poisoning. Impaired calcium or cyclic adenosine monophosphate (cAMP) messenger systems underlie these cellular effects.[151]

Gastrointestinal Toxicity

Lead toxicity causes constipation, anorexia, and colicky abdominal pain. Although the mechanisms are not fully elucidated, theories include impaired intestinal motility, alterations in luminal ion transport, and spasmodic contraction of intestinal wall smooth muscle.[45,165]

CLINICAL MANIFESTATIONS

Inorganic Lead

The numerous observed lead-induced pathophysiologic effects accurately predict that the clinical manifestations of lead poisoning are diverse. These manifestations of lead toxicity are characterized into distinct acute and chronic syndromes (Tables 93–3 and 93–4). In most cases, these distinctions really describe a continuum of dose- and time-related severity, and the occurrence of overt clinical effects in lead poisoning is, in most cases, the culmination of a long-term lead exposure. As the total dose increases, these effects are usually preceded first by biochemical and physiologic impairment followed, in turn, by subtle prodromal clinical effects that only become apparent in hindsight. In general, children are considered to be more susceptible than adults to toxicity for a given measured blood lead concentration, a distinction that applies primarily to CNS effects.

Asymptomatic Children

Children with *elevated body lead burdens but without overt symptoms* represent the largest group of persons at risk for chronic lead toxicity. The subclinical toxicity of lead in this population centers around subtle effects on growth, hearing, and neurocognitive development. This last effect, in particular, is the subject of intense research interest and scrutiny. Numerous population-based studies report significant inverse associations with blood lead concentration and IQ, with an overall magnitude of 1 to 2 IQ points for chronic blood lead concentration increases from 10 to 20 mcg/dL.[149] A landmark study evaluating IQ in children from 6 months to 5 years of age found that blood lead concentrations were inversely correlated with IQ at 3 and 5 years of age and that the magnitude of effect for all subjects was an average 4.6-point decrement in IQ for each 10-mcg/dL increase in blood lead concentration.[19] Of particular concern, this effect was even greater, with an estimated 7.4-point loss, for the subset of children in the 1- to 10-mcg/dL blood lead concentration range, which other epidemiologic studies also reported.[19,92,105] In response to this steeper dose–response curve at blood lead concentrations below 10 mcg/dL, the CDC and American Academy of Pediatrics eliminated the term *threshold*, declared there to be no safe blood lead concentration for childhood intellectual development, and lowered the action blood lead concentration to 5 mcg/dL, a reference value to be evaluated every 4 years based on the 97.5 percentile in

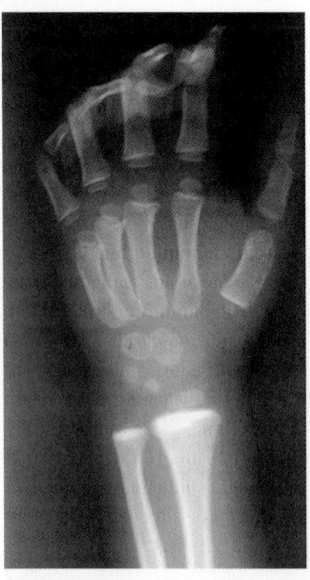
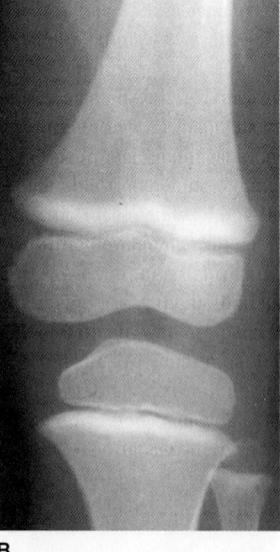

A   B

FIGURE 93–3. (A) Radiograph of the wrist reveals increased bands of calcification ("lead lines") in the same patient as in Fig. 93–1. **(B)** Similar radiographic findings in another patient at the knee. *(Part A used with permission from Department of Radiology, St. Christopher's Hospital for Children, Philadelphia, PA. Part B used with permission from Richard Markowitz, MD, Department of Radiology, Children's Hospital of Philadelphia, Philadelphia, PA.)*

TABLE 93–3	Clinical Manifestations of Lead Poisoning in Children
Clinical Severity	*Typical Blood Lead Concentrations (mcg/dL)*
Severe	>70–100
CNS: Encephalopathy (coma, altered sensorium, seizures, bizarre behavior, ataxia, apathy, incoordination, loss of developmental skills, papilledema, cranial nerve palsies, signs of increased ICP)	
GI: Persistent vomiting	
Hematologic: Pallor (anemia)	
Moderate	50–70
CNS: Hyperirritable behavior, intermittent lethargy, decreased interest in play, "difficult" child	
GI: Intermittent vomiting, abdominal pain, anorexia	
Mild	≤49
CNS: Impaired cognition, behavior, balance, fine-motor coordination	
Miscellaneous: Impaired hearing, impaired growth	

CNS = central nervous system; GI = gastrointestinal; ICP = intracranial pressure.

TABLE 93–4	Clinical Manifestations of Lead Poisoning in Adults
Clinical Severity	**Typical Blood Lead Concentrations (mcg/dL)**
Severe	>100
CNS: Encephalopathy (coma, seizures, obtundation, delirium, focal motor disturbances, headaches, papilledema, optic neuritis, signs of increased ICP)	
PNS: Foot drop, wrist drop	
GI: Abdominal colic	
Hematologic: Pallor (anemia)	
Renal: Nephropathy	
Moderate	70–100
CNS: Headache, memory loss, decreased libido, insomnia	
PNS: Peripheral neuropathy	
GI: Metallic taste, abdominal pain, anorexia, constipation	
Kidney: Arthritis due to saturnine gout (impaired urate excretion)	
Miscellaneous: Mild anemia, myalgias, muscle weakness, arthralgias	
Mild	20–69[a]
CNS: Fatigue, somnolence, moodiness, lessened interest in leisure activities	
Miscellaneous: Adverse effects on cognition, reproduction, kidney function, or bone density; hypertension and cardiovascular disease; possible increased risk of bladder, lung and stomach cancer	

[a]Chronic lead exposure at lower blood lead concentrations leads to cumulative body burdens of lead associated with these clinical findings.

CNS = central nervous system; GI = gastrointestinal; ICP = intracranial pressure; PNS = peripheral nervous system.

most recent NHANES data.[5,28] Nevertheless, it should be noted that some recent reviewers of this body of work, including the National Health and Medical Research Council of Australia, citing methodologic flaws such as uncontrolled confounding in many studies, questioned the evidence for a causal relationship between very low lead concentrations (<10 mcg/dL) and negative impact on IQ and academic achievement.[133,204] Additional consequences of low-level lead exposure include increased propensity for a variety of behavioral problems as well as dental caries.[114,200]

Symptomatic Children

Subencephalopathic symptomatic plumbism usually occurs in children 1 to 5 years of age and is associated with blood lead concentrations above 70 mcg/dL but may occur with concentrations as low as 50 mcg/dL. Unfortunately, common behavioral and abdominal manifestations in well children of this age, including the "terrible twos" temperamental outbursts, functional constipation, abdominal pain, and not eating as much as parents expect, often overlap with the milder range of reported symptoms of lead poisoning. Frequently, parents of children diagnosed by routine blood screening recognize milder symptoms only in hindsight after chelation treatment results in clinical improvement ("it seemed as if the child was going through a phase").[64] Other uncommon clinical presentations are described, including isolated seizures without encephalopathy (indistinguishable from idiopathic epilepsy), chronic hyperactive behavior disorder, isolated developmental delay, progressive loss of cortical function simulating degenerative cerebral disease, peripheral neuropathy (reported particularly in children with sickle cell hemoglobinopathy), and the occurrence of GI effects (colicky abdominal pain, vomiting, constipation) with myalgias of the trunk and proximal girdle muscles.[36,52]

Acute lead encephalopathy is the most severe presentation of pediatric plumbism (Table 93–3). It is associated with cerebral edema and increased intracranial pressure (ICP) in severe cases (Fig. 93–1). Encephalopathy is characterized by severe vomiting and apathy, bizarre behavior, loss of recently acquired developmental skills, ataxia, incoordination, seizures, altered sensorium, or coma. Physical examination often reveals papilledema, oculomotor or facial nerve palsy, diminished deep tendon reflexes, or other evidence of increased ICP.[20,201]

Milder but ominous findings that portend incipient encephalopathy include anorexia, constipation, intermittent abdominal pain, sporadic vomiting, hyperirritable or aggressive behavior, periods of lethargy interspersed with lucid intervals, and decreased interest in play activities. Patients frequently seek medical advice for vomiting and lethargy during the 2 to 7 days before onset of frank encephalopathy.[36,147] Physical examination of such children usually reveals no specific abnormalities beyond, possibly, pallor reflecting concomitant anemia.

Encephalopathy usually occurs in children ages 15 to 30 months; is associated with blood lead concentrations above 100 mcg/dL, although it is reported with blood lead concentrations as low as 70 mcg/dL; and tends to occur more commonly in summer months, when blood lead concentrations peak.[147] A cohort of 972 Nigerian children demonstrated overt neurologic features with blood lead concentrations above 80 mcg/dL, although the majority occurred over 100 mcg/dL. Additional risk factors in this study included age 1 to 2 years and concomitant malaria infection.[77] Mortality caused by encephalopathy was 65% in the prechelation era, decreasing to below 5% with the advent of effective chelation. The incidence of permanent neurologic sequelae, including mental retardation, seizure disorder, blindness, and hemiparesis, is 25% to 30% in patients who develop encephalopathic symptoms before the onset of chelation (Fig. 93–4).[36]

Adults

Adults with occupational lead exposure typically manifest numerous signs and symptoms representing disorders of several organ systems. Severity of

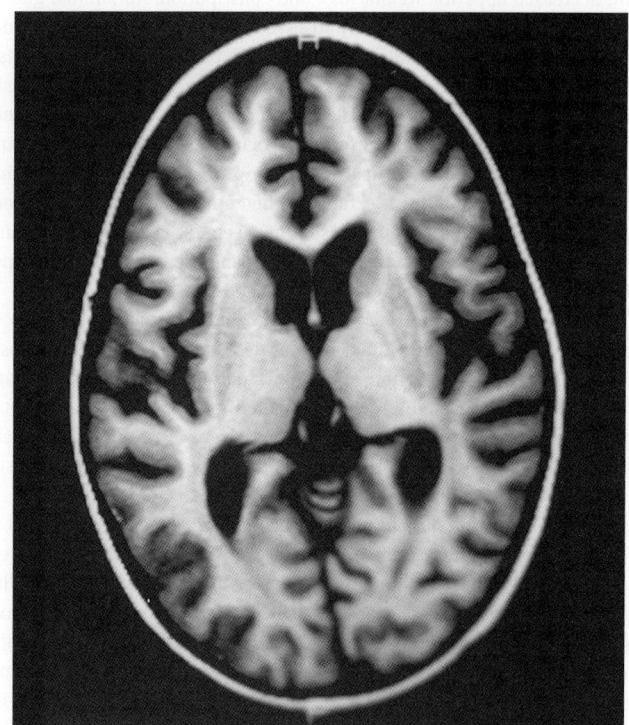

FIGURE 93–4. Magnetic resonance image of the brain reveals cortical atrophy and multiple areas of cerebral infarction in the same patient as in Fig. 93–1, done on hospital day 22. At this time, the child's clinical status was notable for choreoathetoid movements and generalized hypotonia, inability to localize visual or auditory stimuli, and nonpurposeful movements of the extremities. *(Used with permission from Eric Faerber, MD, Department of Radiology, St. Christopher's Hospital for Children, Philadelphia, PA.)*

symptoms correlates roughly with blood lead concentrations, although many conditions thought to be associated with low-dose chronic lead exposure are better correlated with markers of cumulative dose, such as bone lead or the cumulative blood lead index (area under the curve of blood lead concentrations versus time)[84,103] (Table 93–4). True acute poisoning occurs rarely, after very high inhalational,[96] large oral,[137] or intravenous (IV) exposures.[138] Clinical manifestations in such patients include colicky abdominal pain, hepatitis, pancreatitis, hemolytic anemia, and encephalopathy over days or weeks. Most adult plumbism is related to chronic respiratory exposure, although some authors have used the term "acute poisoning" to include patients with such exposure whose symptoms are severe and of relatively recent onset (within 6 weeks of presentation) and whose exposure is relatively brief (average, one year or less).[43]

In severe plumbism, the hallmark of toxicity is acute encephalopathy, which has been rarely reported in adults since the 1920s.[43] The majority of modern cases are actually not associated with occupational exposures but rather with more exotic exposures, such as ingestion of lead-contaminated illicit "moonshine" whiskey and ethnic alternative medications.[94,179] Encephalopathy in adults is usually associated with very high blood lead concentrations (typically >150 mcg/dL) and is manifested by seizures (75% of cases), obtundation, confusion, focal motor disturbances, papilledema, headaches, and optic neuritis.[122,199] In addition, adult patients with severe plumbism often manifest attacks of abdominal colic, are virtually always anemic, and are at significant risk for severe peripheral neuropathy that manifests as wrist drop and foot drop. Nephrotoxic effects include a Fanconilike syndrome, impaired kidney function, and progressive interstitial fibrosis. Rarely, ventricular dysrhythmias are reported, and long-standing lead toxicity is associated with prolonged QT intervals and widened QRS complexes.[56,157]

Moderate plumbism in adults typically involves CNS, peripheral nerves, hematologic, kidney, GI, rheumatologic, endocrine or reproductive, and cardiovascular findings.[65,96,165] At blood lead concentrations higher than 70 mcg/dL, such symptoms include headache, memory loss, decreased libido, and insomnia. Gastrointestinal symptoms include metallic taste, abdominal pain, decreased appetite, weight loss, and constipation. Abdominal guarding and tenderness are occasionally observed. Musculoskeletal and rheumatologic complaints at this stage include muscle pain and joint tenderness. Patients with saturnine gout have typical joint findings of acute arthritis. In contrast to gouty arthritis not associated with lead, there is a more equal gender ratio and increased tendency for polyarticular involvement, particularly in the knee.[44] Peripheral neuropathy occurs, primarily motor, manifesting initially in the wrist and finger extensors, then other muscular involvement including foot drop and tremor. Sensory involvement is generally minimal. Many patients at this stage have mild anemia, and those with chronic exposure are at risk for nephropathy as described above.

Mild plumbism manifests as minor CNS findings, such as changes in mood and cognition. Subtle abnormalities detectable by careful neuropsychiatric testing are found in both adults and children with modest elevations in blood concentrations and include impaired memory span, rapid motor tapping, visual motor coordination, and grip strength.[43] Studies document abnormal psychometrics and nerve conduction in workers recently exposed to lead as blood lead concentrations increased to above 30 mcg/dL.[117] Early psychiatric effects, manifesting at blood lead concentrations of 40 to 70 mcg/dL, include increased tiredness at the end of the day, disinterest in leisure-time pursuits, falling asleep easily, moodiness, and irritability. Chronic lead exposure is associated with higher depressive and phobic anxiety scores on surveys in premenopausal women.[57] The physical examination is usually normal,[47] or hypertension is present. A bluish-purple gingival lead line (Burton line), representing lead sulfide precipitation in patients with poor dentition, is rarely described. Ophthalmic lead toxicity results in myriad abnormalities including cataract formation, optic neuritis, optic atrophy, pigmented retinal deposits, and increased thickness of retinal, macular, and choroidal fibers, which lead to amblyopia, decreased visual acuity, ophthalmoplegia, decreased color vision, and scotoma.[50]

Effects on reproductive function are also apparent in this range of exposure. Historically, infertility and stillbirths were common among heavily exposed women lead workers. More recent studies found reduced sperm counts, impaired motility, and abnormal morphology in men who work in the battery industry with blood lead concentrations above 40 mcg/dL[6,66] and an increased incidence of menstrual irregularity and spontaneous abortion in lead-exposed women who worked in China[90] and Mexico.[13] Prematurity is more common in children of pregnancies associated with elevated maternal blood lead concentrations.[112]

Increased blood pressure is probably the most prevalent adverse health effect observed from lead toxicity in adults. Epidemiologic studies document significant associations between hypertension and body lead burdens. The association is particularly strong for adult men aged 40 to 59 years, with an approximate 1.5- to 3.0–mm Hg increase in systolic pressure for every doubling of blood lead concentration beginning at 7 mcg/dL.[148,187] Additional studies correlate body lead burden with several other disorders of aging, including a decline in cognitive ability,[173] essential tremor,[49] cardiac and cerebrovascular events,[88,103] electrocardiographic abnormalities,[34] chronic kidney disease,[103,109] osteoporosis,[18] cataract prevalence,[166] and all-cause and cardiovascular mortality.[197]

Organic Lead

Clinical symptoms of TEL toxicity are usually nonspecific initially and include nausea, vomiting, anorexia, insomnia, and emotional instability.[12,165] Patients exhibit tremor and increased deep tendon reflexes, as well as hepatic or renal injury. In more severe cases, these symptoms progress to encephalopathy with delusions, hallucinations, and hyperactivity, which resolve or deteriorate to coma and, occasionally, death. Because many reported patients were exposed via intentional abuse of leaded gasoline, much of the literature reporting this syndrome is confounded by accompanying volatile hydrocarbon toxicity.[182] Of note, in contrast to inorganic lead poisoning, patients with significant TEL toxicity do not consistently manifest hematologic abnormalities or elevations of heme synthesis pathway biomarkers. In addition, significant neurotoxicity occurs at blood lead concentrations considerably lower than those typically associated with inorganic lead poisoning.[81] A case report details the clinical course of a 13-year-old boy who unintentionally ingested a mouthful of fuel stabilizer containing 80% to 90% TEL. He developed progressive tremor, weakness, hallucinations, myoclonus, and hyperreflexia and required mechanical ventilation for 2 days and prolonged hospitalization for management of persistent hallucinations, weakness, dysphagia, and urinary and fecal incontinence. His blood lead concentration peaked on the third day after ingestion at only 62 mcg/dL.[203]

DIAGNOSTIC TESTING
Clinical Diagnosis in Symptomatic Patients

The medical evaluation should first include a comprehensive medical history. Further inquiry should elicit environmental, occupational, or recreational sources of exposure as detailed earlier (Tables 93–1 and 93–2). Plumbism is more likely in a child between the ages of 1 and 5 years with prior plumbism or noted elevated blood lead concentrations; history of pica or acute unintentional ingestions;[78] aural, nasal, or esophageal foreign bodies;[202] history of iron-deficiency anemia; residence in a pre-1960s–built home, especially with deteriorated paint, or one that has undergone recent remodeling; family history of lead poisoning; or foreign-born status.[5] Affected children manifest persistent vomiting, lethargy, irritability, clumsiness, or loss of recently acquired developmental skills; afebrile seizures; or evidence of child abuse or neglect.[60,170] In adults, the history should focus on occupational and recreational activities involving lead exposure (Table 93–2), a history of plumbism, and gunshot wounds with retained bullets.

The differential diagnosis of plumbism is broad. Adult patients are misdiagnosed as having carpal tunnel syndrome, Guillain-Barré syndrome, sickle cell crisis, acute appendicitis, renal colic, or infectious encephalitis. Children are often initially considered to have viral gastroenteritis or even to have insidious symptoms passed off as a difficult developmental phase.

A patient who presents to the emergency department with potential lead encephalopathy presents the physician with a dilemma: severe lead toxicity requires urgent diagnosis, but confirmatory blood lead assays are not usually rapidly available.[141] For adults, a history of occupational exposure is often available from medical records or family members, and lead encephalopathy can be strongly considered with positive supportive laboratory findings such as anemia, basophilic stippling, elevated erythrocyte protoporphyrin (especially >250 mcg/dL, sometimes available on an urgent basis), and abnormal urinalysis. In this context, it is reasonable to institute presumptive chelation therapy while awaiting a blood lead concentration. In children, a similar indication for presumptive treatment would be suggested by a constellation of clinical features and ancillary studies, such as age 1 to 5 years, a prodromal illness of several days' to weeks' duration (suggestive of milder lead-related symptoms), history of pica and source of lead exposure, the laboratory features noted above (which are equally helpful in young children), and suggestive radiologic findings (detailed below) such as dense metaphyseal "lead lines" or ingested foreign bodies. In both adults and children, the decision to institute empiric chelation treatment should not deter additional emergent diagnostic efforts to exclude or to confirm other important entities while blood lead concentrations are pending. An important consideration in this context is the suspicion of an acute, potentially treatable CNS infection (eg, bacterial meningitis or herpetic encephalitis). Lumbar puncture should be generally avoided in patients with suspected lead encephalopathy because of the risk of cerebral herniation.[40] If there is a significant suspicion of such CNS infection, we recommend empiric treatment be instituted while awaiting blood lead concentration results, and a delayed lumbar puncture be considered if the blood lead concentration is normal.[141]

Laboratory Evaluation

In patients suspected of having plumbism, laboratory testing is used to augment the evaluation of both lead exposure and lead toxicity. The whole blood lead concentration is the principal measure of lead exposure available in clinical practice, reflecting both recent and remote exposure. In any patient suspected of symptomatic plumbism, whole blood should be collected by venipuncture into special lead-free evacuated tubes. The most accurate method for measurement of blood lead concentration is inductively coupled plasma mass spectrometry (ICP-MS); however, many laboratories still utilize atomic absorption spectrophotometry, graphite furnace spectrophotometry, and anodic stripping voltammetry, with variable performance at very low blood lead concentrations near the CDC threshold.[16] A commonly used point-of-care testing device was recalled for inaccurate results on venous samples, prompting the CDC to recommend re-screening many children.[30,188]

For asymptomatic children, blood lead concentration screening is often performed by capillary blood testing for convenience; however, venous confirmation of elevated capillary lead concentrations, unless extremely high (eg, ≥70 mcg/dL) or unless the patient is clearly symptomatic, is still warranted before chelation or other significant interventions. Hair and urine

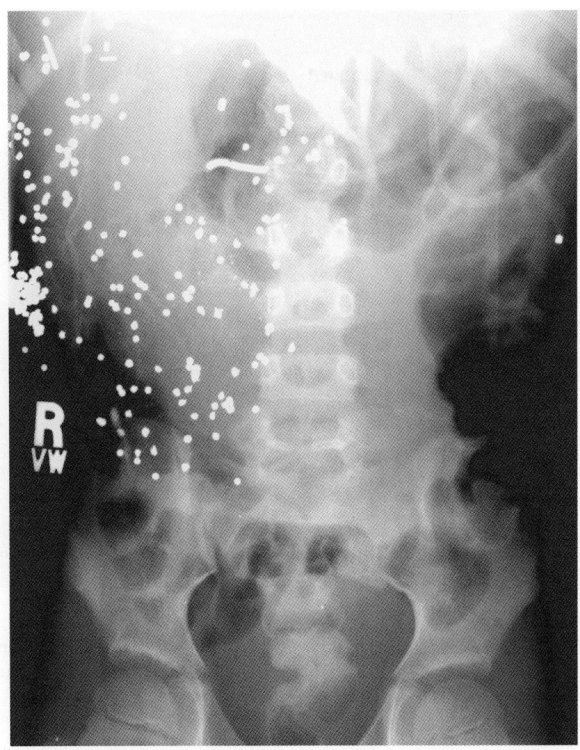

FIGURE 93–5. Abdominal radiograph of an 8-year-old child who sustained a shotgun wound to the right paraspinal area, with resultant paraplegia and multiple visceral injuries. The blood lead concentration was found to be 60 mcg/dL at 11 weeks after injury, and chelation therapy was commenced. *(Used with permission from Children's Hospital of Philadelphia, Department of Radiology, Philadelphia, PA.)*

lead concentrations have no clinical utility. The erythrocyte protoporphyrin concentration reflects inhibition of the heme synthesis pathway (Chap. 20) and was used as a screening tool in the past, but it is no longer considered sufficiently sensitive. The erythrocyte protoporphyrin concentration tests are useful for tracking response to therapy and in distinguishing acute from chronic lead poisoning; as an adjunct to the emergency diagnosis of symptomatic plumbism if emergent blood lead concentration determination is not available and, rarely, in the evaluation of suspected factitious plumbism. Routine serum chemistries, kidney function tests, liver function tests, urinalysis, and complete blood count are recommended in patients who are symptomatic or about to undergo chelation therapy. Radiographic studies should be

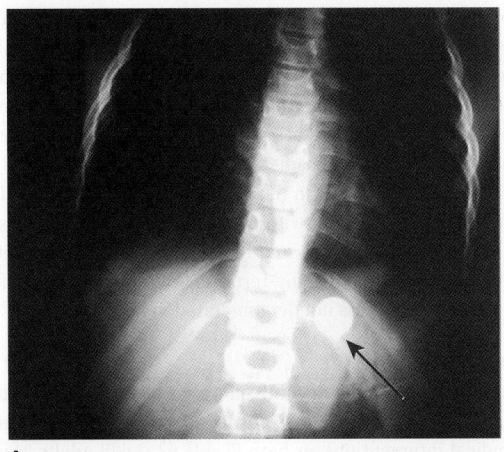

A

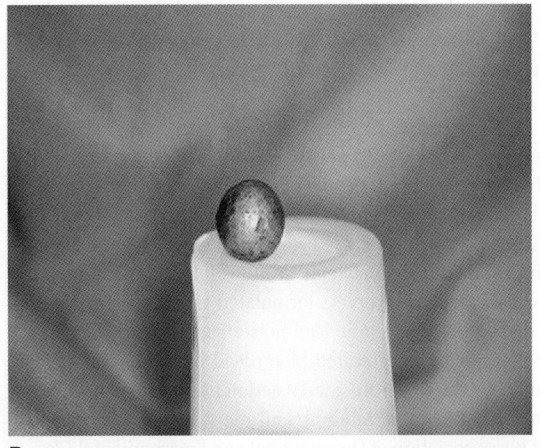

B

FIGURE 93–6. An unusual source of lead poisoning. (**A**) Radiograph of the abdomen reveals (↑) ingested metallic foreign body. (**B**) The ingested foreign body was a Civil War–era musketball from the collection of the patient's father. *(Used with permission from Evaline Alessandrini, MD, Division of Emergency Medicine, Children's Hospital of Philadelphia, Philadelphia, PA.)*

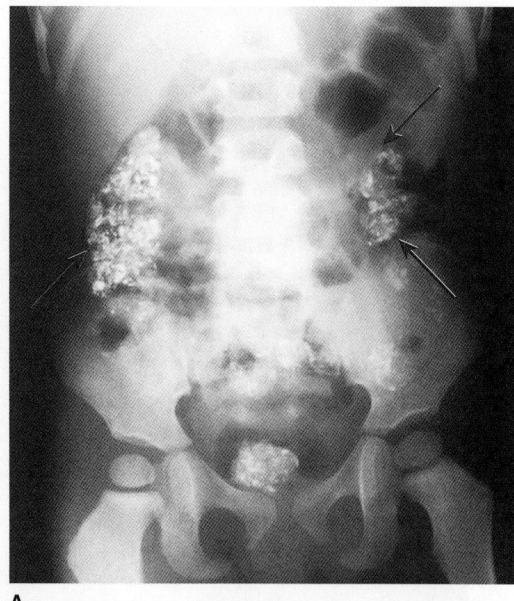 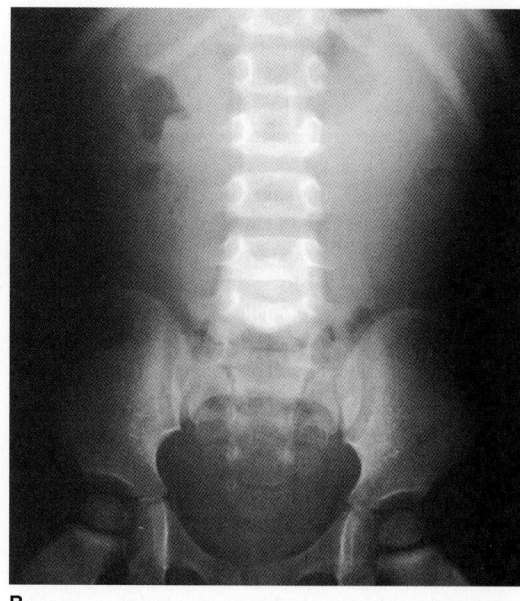

FIGURE 93–7. (A) Abdominal radiograph of a child who had massive paint chip ingestion. The dispersed radiodense (white) fragments are noted (↖) to follow the outline of the large intestine. **(B)** No remaining lead is seen on follow-up radiograph after whole-bowel irrigation. *(Used with permission from Department of Radiology, St. Christopher's Hospital for Children, Philadelphia, PA.)*

obtained according to relevant history, to determine the presence of ingested foreign bodies, retained bullets or shrapnel (Figs. 93–5, 93–6, 93–7).[58,110,169] In addition, the presence of "lead lines" can strengthen the clinical diagnosis of childhood plumbism before blood lead concentrations are available (Fig. 93–3), although dense metaphyseal bands are sometimes caused by other causes, including other metals (arsenic, bismuth, and mercury), healing rickets, and recovery from scurvy.[153,203] Cerebrospinal fluid examination in lead encephalopathy reveals characteristic findings such as increased protein concentration, lymphocytic pleocytosis, and increased intracranial pressure (ICP);[40,141] however, as discussed above, lumbar puncture is not recommended for routine diagnosis because of risk of herniation.

Two measures of cumulative lead exposure are available. X-ray fluorescence technology measures bone lead, and thus indirectly estimates total body lead burden. The cumulative blood lead index, derived from several blood lead concentrations measured over the presumed course of lifetime lead exposure, calculated as an area under the concentration curve, is also described.[84] Both techniques are used in research studies of issues concerning past chronic lead exposure and a variety of current health outcomes.[83,196] Another putative measure of body lead burden is the use of provoked challenge urine testing, in which urinary lead is measured after the administration of chelator. We recommended against its use as results are difficult to interpret and often misleading.[162]

SCREENING

Screening is an essential public health practice for the prevention of severe plumbism in children, pregnant women, and other adults from high-risk settings. Table 93–5 outlines the current CDC[28,32] pediatric guidelines, which also are endorsed by the American Academy of Pediatrics and we recommend as well.[5] Likewise, the Occupational Safety and Health Administration (OSHA) maintains a lead standard for US workers formulated to reduce workplace exposure to lead, decrease symptomatic lead poisoning, and provide quality medical care to workers with elevated blood lead concentrations.[189-192] Table 93–6A summarizes the OSHA-mandated action blood lead concentration values for worker notification, removal, and reinstatement. An expert panel convened by the Association of Occupational and Environmental Clinics (AOEC) published an alternative set of health-based management recommendations for lead-exposed workers, which we support. The AOEC authors propose that their recommendations are more reflective of recent research

linking adverse health outcomes to chronic, low-dose lead exposure.[103] These guidelines are summarized in Table 93–6B.

MANAGEMENT

There are several caveats about the management of patients with lead poisoning. First, the most important aspect of treatment is removal from further exposure to lead. Unfortunately, effective implementation of this therapy is often beyond the control of the clinician but rather depends on a complex interplay of public health, social, and political actions. Currently, the ability to control exposure is generally more applicable to adults with occupational exposures than to children exposed to residential hazards. Second, in children for whom some residual lead exposure potentially continues, optimization of nutritional status is vital in order to minimize absorption. Finally, pharmacologic therapy with chelators, although a mainstay of therapy for symptomatic patients, is an inexact science, with numerous unanswered questions despite more than 50 years of clinical use.[3,101] The rationale for chelation therapy of lead-poisoned patients is that chelators complex with lead, forming a chelate that is excreted in urine, feces, or both. Chelation therapy increases lead excretion, reduces blood concentrations, and reverses hematologic markers of toxicity during therapy. Reports from the 1950s found symptomatic improvement in adults chelated for lead colic.[195] The institution of effective combination chelation treatment of childhood lead encephalopathy in the 1960s contributed to the dramatic decline in mortality and morbidity of that devastating degree of plumbism.[36] However, the same era saw major advances in pediatric critical care in general and medical management of increased ICP in particular. The situation of chelation therapy for asymptomatic patients with mildly to moderately increased body burdens of lead is even less clear, and many questions regarding efficacy and safety remain.[37,101,146] To date, long-term reduction of target tissue lead content or reversal of toxicity is not demonstrated in human trials.[48,120,160]

Decreasing Exposure

All patients with significantly elevated blood lead concentrations warrant identification of the lead exposure source, and specific environmental and medical interventions, or both (Table 93–7). In adults, this usually involves worksite changes.[47,103,165] The risk of occupational lead exposure correlates with several factors that contribute to the occurrence of respirable lead fumes or dust particles in the worksite atmosphere.[165] First, there are hazards

TABLE 93–5 Pediatric Screening and Follow-up Guidelines[5,29,32]

Screening

1. Screening is recommended for all children who are Medicaid eligible at age 1 and 2 years (and those ages 3–6 years who have not been screened previously). Children who may not be Medicaid eligible but whose families participate in any poverty assistance program should also be screened.

2. Certain local health departments (eg, New York, Chicago, and Philadelphia) recommend screening at younger ages or more frequently. Such recommendations include starting at age 6–9 months, testing every 6 months for children younger than 2 years, and provision of additional education and more rapid follow-up testing for children younger than 12 months whose blood lead concentrations are 6–9 mcg/dL.

3. In addition, children who are not Medicaid eligible but are designated high-risk by their state or local health departments should be screened as per these local policies.[a]

4. For children who are neither Medicaid eligible nor live in areas with locale-specific health department guidelines, recommendations are less clear. The AAP supports universal screening of such children as well.[b]

5. Recent immigrants, refugees, or international adoptee children should be screened on arrival to the United States.

Follow-Up

Blood Lead Concentration (mcg/dL)	Recommended Action and Confirmatory Testing Schedule
≤5	Retest in one year, or more frequently if at high risk for lead exposure[c]; anticipatory guidance
5–14	Retest in 1–3 months; education, environmental history, nutritional counseling[5]
15–19	Retest in 1–4 weeks; education; if the blood lead concentration is 15–19 mcg/dL twice, refer for case management; consider abdominal radiograph if excessive mouthing behaviors[5]
20–44	Clinical evaluation; education; environmental investigation and lead hazard control; obtain abdominal film, iron studies, and hemoglobin/hematocrit[32]
45–69	Clinical evaluation and case management within 48 hours; education; environmental investigation and lead hazard control; abdominal film, iron studies and hemoglobin/hematocrit; chelation therapy[5,23]
≥70	Hospitalize child; obtain studies as above; immediate chelation therapy; education; environmental investigation and lead hazard control

[a]Many relevant state and city health department contacts may be located at: http://www.cdc.gov/nceh/lead/about/program.htm. [b]The 1997 CDC guidance[21] allowed for targeted screening of some children of low-risk geographic and demographic background based on a personal risk questionnaire. A listing of potential risk factors is instructive and is summarized here. [c]Screening was recommended if a child had any of the following high-risk factors:

Housing: Lives in or regularly visits a home built before 1960; lives in or regularly visits a home built before 1978 undergoing remodeling or renovation (or renovated within 6 months).

Medical history: Pica for paint chips or dirt; iron deficiency.

Personal, family, and social history: Personal, family, or playmate history of lead poisoning; parental occupational, industrial, hobby exposures; live in proximity to major roadway; use of hot tap water for consumption; use of complementary remedies, cosmetics, ceramic food containers; trips or residence outside United States; parents are migrant farm workers, receive poverty assistance.

Educational interventions as per Table 93–7.

Chelation therapy as per Table 93–8.

AAP = American Academy of Pediatrics; BPb = venous blood lead; CDC = Centers for Disease Control and Prevention.

TABLE 93–6A Occupational Safety and Health Administration General Industry[a] Standards for Various Blood Lead Concentrations

Number of Tests	Blood Lead Concentration (mcg/dL)	Action Required
1	≥40	Notification of worker in writing; medical examination of worker and consultation
3 (average)	≥50	Removal of worker from job with potential lead exposure
1	≥60	Removal of worker from job with potential lead exposure
2	<40	Reinstatement of worker in job with potential lead exposure

[a]The construction industry standard is similar for worker notification (at 40 mcg/dL) and reinstatement (<40 mcg/dL twice) but requires worker removal for a single value ≥50 mcg/dL.

Data from US Department of Labor, Occupational Safety and Health Administration: Medical Surveillance Guidelines—1910.1025 App C.

http://www.osha.gov/pls/oshaweb/owadisp.show_document?p_table=STANDARDS&p_id=10033 and US Department of Labor, Occupational Safety and Health Administration: Medical Surveillance Guidelines. Lead—1926.

protective clothes and equipment, and thorough housekeeping. Remedial actions include improvements in ventilation, modification of personal hygiene habits, and optimal use of respiratory apparatus. It is vital to prohibit smoking, eating, and drinking in a lead-exposed work area. Work clothes should be changed after each shift and should not be lockered together with street clothes.

In patients with plumbism or consequential elevated blood lead concentrations believed due to retained bullets, surgical removal of this lead source is recommended when anatomically feasible.[33,110,126] Table 93–7 also summarizes several specific educational guidelines that should be offered to parents of lead-exposed children.[5,17,23] Overarching principles include home lead paint abatement (done preferably by professionals, with the family out of the home), home dust reduction techniques, decreasing soil lead exposure, and nutritional evaluation and counseling. Patients manifesting iron deficiency

TABLE 93–6B Health-Based Occupational Surveillance Recommendations[a]

Blood Lead Concentration (mcg/dL)	Recommendation
<10	Check every month for 3 months and then every 6 months (unless exposure increases); if blood lead concentration increases >4 mcg/dL, exposure evaluation or reduction effort; exposure evaluation or reduction if blood lead concentration 5–9 mcg/dL for women who are or may become pregnant
10–19	As for blood lead concentration <10 mcg/dL and check every 3 months; exposure evaluation and reduction effort; consider removal if no improvement with exposure reduction or complicating medical condition;[b] resume check every 6 months if 3 blood level concentrations <10 mcg/dL
≥19	Remove from exposure if blood lead concentration >30 mcg/dL or repeat blood lead concentration in 4 weeks; check every month; consider return to work after blood lead concentration <15 mcg/dL twice

[a]All potentially lead-exposed workers warrant preemployment clinical evaluation, baseline blood lead concentration, and serum creatinine concentration. [b]Such conditions include chronic kidney disease, hypertension, neurologic disorders, and cognitive dysfunction.

Data from Kosnett MJ, Wedeen RP, Rothenberg SJ, et al. Recommendations for medical management of adult lead exposure. *Environ Health Perspect.* 2007 Mar;115(3):463-471.

inherent in the work process itself, including high temperatures; significant aerosol, dust, or fume production; and a less mechanized workplace (with resulting greater "hands-on" employee exposure). Second, the adequacy of dust elimination, such as local and general ventilation, is critical. The third category is that of worksite and personal hygiene, including proper use of

TABLE 93–7	Evaluation and Management of Patients with Lead Exposure

Adults

Implement careful lead exposure monitoring (Table 93–6A and 6B)

Improve ventilation

Use a respiratory protective apparatus

Wear protective clothing; change from work clothes before leaving worksite

Modify personal hygiene habits

Prohibit eating, drinking, and smoking at the worksite

Evaluate possible sources beyond occupational setting (Tables 93–1 and 93–2)

Children

Notify the local health department to initiate home inspection and abatement as needed

Home lead paint abatement (professional contractors if possible; use plastic sheeting, low dust-generating paint removal; replacement of lead-painted windows, floor treatment; final cleanup with high-efficiency particle air vacuum, wet mopping)

Avoid most hazardous areas of the home and yard

Dust control: Wet mopping, sponging with high-phosphate detergent; frequent hand, toy, and pacifier washing

Soil lead exposure reduction by planting grass and shrubs around the house

Use only cold, flushed tap water for consumption

Optimize nutrition to reduce lead absorption: avoid fasting; give an iron-, calcium-, vitamin C–sufficient diet; supplement iron and calcium as necessary

Avoid food storage in open cans

Avoid imported ceramic containers for food and beverage use

Evaluate parental occupations and hobbies and eliminate high-risk activity

Evaluate possible sources beyond lead paint exposure (Tables 93–1 and 93–2)

should be treated, and for others, ensuring a diet sufficient in trace nutrients, particularly iron, calcium and vitamin C, is reasonable.[5,175] Clinicians who have primary responsibility for children with elevated blood lead concentrations should refer to the exhaustive monograph developed by the CDC and recent American Academy of Pediatrics (AAP) guidance, both of which detail such pediatric case management.[5,23]

Occasionally, children require urgent GI decontamination to reduce ongoing acute lead exposure. We recommend the prompt institution of whole-bowel irrigation (WBI) for those patients with large burdens of lead paint chips (Fig. 93–6) (Antidotes in Depth: A2). Another unique situation arises when children ingest solid lead foreign bodies, such as fishing sinkers, bullets, or curtain weights. Several case reports document rapid absorption in this scenario, with significantly elevated blood lead concentrations measured within 24 hours of ingestion.[124,132,193] Such patients warrant a baseline blood lead concentration determination and frequent repeat evaluation. We recommend prompt endoscopic removal for gastric foreign bodies, particularly with increasing blood lead concentrations. Proton pump inhibitor and prokinetic therapy are also reasonable adjuncts for gastric foreign bodies to decrease gastric acidity, retention time, and resultant lead dissolution.[59] For foreign bodies in the small bowel, a trial of WBI is reasonable but has not been uniformly successful.[132,193] Endoscopic or surgical removal is also recommended for such foreign bodies, if there is delayed passage, failure of WBI, or rapid elevations in blood lead concentrations.[59,193] The issue of concomitant chelation therapy in patients with significant GI lead burdens is addressed in the following section.

Chelation Therapy

The indications for and specifics of chelation therapy are determined by the age of the patient, the blood lead concentration, and clinical symptomatology (Table 93–8). Three chelators are currently recommended for the treatment of lead poisoning: dimercaprol (Antidotes in Depth: A28) and edetate calcium disodium (CaNa$_2$EDTA) (Antidotes in Depth: A30) are used parenterally for more severe cases, and succimer (Antidotes in Depth: A29) is available for oral therapy. A fourth drug, D-penicillamine, was used orally for patients with

mild to moderate excess lead burdens. Unfortunately, D-penicillamine has a toxicity profile that includes life-threatening hematologic disorders and reversible, but serious, dermatologic and kidney effects; consequently, since 1991, its role in lead poisoning treatment at most centers has been largely replaced by succimer. Currently, D-penicillamine use is only recommended when unacceptable adverse reactions to both succimer and CaNa$_2$EDTA occur, and it remains important to continue chelation.[3]

Chelation is not a panacea for lead poisoning. It is a relatively inefficient process, with a typical course of therapy decreasing body content of metal by only 1% to 2%.[101,131] Furthermore, there is little evidence that chelators have significant access to critical sites in target organs, particularly in the brain.[42] Assumptions that reducing blood lead concentration will improve subtle neurocognitive dysfunction or other subclinical organ toxicity are appealing theoretically but unproven.[48,160]

Children

Lead encephalopathy is an acute life-threatening emergency and should be treated under the guidance of a multidisciplinary team in the intensive care unit of a hospital experienced in the management of critically ill children. The recommended treatment for encephalopathy is combination parenteral chelation therapy with maximum-dose dimercaprol and CaNa$_2$EDTA along with meticulous supportive care.[3,23,36] Such combination therapy has a dramatic effect on decreasing blood lead concentration—to 50% or less of baseline within 15 hours and to 75% to 80% of baseline by 48 to 72 hours. It is far superior to monotherapy with CaNa$_2$EDTA in this regard.[36]

Chelation is instituted with 450 mg/m^2/day (or 25 mg/kg/day) of intramuscular (IM) dimercaprol in 6 divided doses.[3,23] The second dose of dimercaprol is given 4 hours later followed immediately by IV CaNa$_2$EDTA, in maximum concentration of 0.5% solution, at 1,500 mg/m^2/day (or 50 mg/kg/day) as a continuous infusion or in divided-dose infusions over several hours.[3,23,147] The delay in initiating CaNa$_2$EDTA infusion is based on past observations of clinical deterioration in encephalopathic patients treated with CaNa$_2$EDTA alone.[3,36] Therapy is typically continued with both antidotes for 5 days, although in milder cases with prompt resolution of encephalopathy and decrease of blood lead concentration to below 50 mcg/dL, it is reasonable to discontinue dimercaprol after 3 days, with continuation of CaNa$_2$EDTA alone for 2 more days.

The presence of radiopaque material in the GI tract on radiography has raised concern that parenteral chelation might enhance absorption of residual gut lead. This issue is not settled fully,[37] but we recommend the initiation of parenteral chelation without delay in seriously symptomatic patients. It seems reasonable in such cases to simultaneously attempt WBI with a polyethylene glycol preparation.[3] One case report described the successful use of parenteral chelation therapy begun simultaneously with WBI, followed by enteral succimer on day 3 for a child with lead encephalopathy and an extraordinarily high blood lead concentration of 550 mcg/dL.[70] This issue applies as well to ingested lead foreign bodies, as noted above.[124,193] Generally, oral fluids, feedings, and medications are withheld for at least the first several days. Careful provision of adequate IV fluids optimizes kidney function while avoiding overhydration and the risk of exacerbating cerebral edema. The occurrence of the syndrome of inappropriate secretion of antidiuretic hormone (SIADH) is associated with lead encephalopathy,[36,180] so urine volume, urine osmolarity, specific gravity, and serum electrolytes should be closely monitored, especially as fluids are gradually liberalized with clinical improvement (Chap. 12). In the context of lead encephalopathy, this approach would need to be tempered by the requirement for maintaining good urine output to optimize chelation efficacy.

Intravenous benzodiazepines are recommended as initial therapy to achieve seizure control. Although, in general, phenytoin or fosphenytoin is the second-line therapy for pediatric status epilepticus, in the context of toxin-induced status, we recommend sequential use of benzodiazepines, phenobarbital, or propofol,[201] followed by valproate or levetiracetam and, if needed, inhalational anesthetics.[71,97] This should be

TABLE 93–8   Chelation Therapy Guidelines[3,5,23,96,147,150] for Initial Course of Treatment[a]

Condition, Blood Lead Concentration (mcg/dL)	Dose	Regimen/Comments
Adults		
Encephalopathy	Dimercaprol 450 mg/m²/d[a,b] and	75 mg/m² IM every 4 hours for 5 days
	CaNa₂EDTA 1,000–1,500 mg/m²/d[a]	Continuous infusion or 2–4 divided IV doses for 5 days (start 4 hours after dimercaprol)
Symptoms suggestive of encephalopathy or >100	Dimercaprol 300–450 mg/m²/d[a,b] and	50–75 mg/m² IM every 4 hours for 3–5 days (base dose, duration on blood lead concentration, severity of symptoms; see text)
	CaNa₂EDTA 1,500 mg/m²/d[a]	Continuous infusion or 2–4 divided IV doses for 5 days (start 4 hours after dimercaprol)
		Lab: Baseline CT scan; CBC, Ca²⁺, blood lead concentration, BUN, Cr, LFTs, U/A; repeat CBC, Ca²⁺, BUN, Cr, LFTs, U/A daily; blood lead concentration on days 3 and 5
Mild symptoms or 70–100	Succimer 700–1,050 mg/m²/d	350 mg/m² 3 times per day orally for 5 days, then twice per day for 14 days. Remove from exposure (Table 93–7)
		Lab: CBC, blood lead concentration, BUN, Cr, LFTs, U/A; repeat CBC, LFTs, blood lead concentration on days 7 and 21
Asymptomatic and <70	Usually not indicated	–
Children		
Encephalopathy	Dimercaprol 450 mg/m²/d[a] and	75 mg/m² IM every 4 hours for 5 days
	CaNa₂EDTA 1,500 mg/m²/d[a]	Continuous infusion or 2–4 divided IV doses for 5 days (start 4 hours after dimercaprol)
		Lab: Baseline AXR, CT scan, CBC, Ca²⁺, Na⁺, blood lead concentration, BUN, Cr, LFTs, U/A; repeat CBC, Ca²⁺, Na⁺, BUN, Cr, LFTs, U/A daily; blood lead concentration on days 3 and 5
Symptomatic (without encephalopathy) or >69	Dimercaprol 300–450 mg/m²/d[a] and	50–75 mg/m² IM every 4 hours for 3–5 days (base dose, duration on blood lead concentration, severity of symptoms; see text)
	CaNa₂EDTA 1,000–1,500 mg/m²/d[a]	Continuous infusion or 2–4 divided IV doses for 5 days (start 4 hours after dimercaprol)
		Lab: Baseline AXR, CBC, Ca²⁺, blood lead concentration, BUN, Cr, LFTs, U/A; repeat CBC, Ca²⁺, BUN, Cr, LFTs, U/A on days 3 and 5 and blood lead concentration day 5
Asymptomatic: 45–69	Succimer 700–1,050 mg/m²/d[a] or	350 mg/m² 3 times per day orally for 5 days and then twice per day for 14 days
		Lab: Baseline AXR, CBC, blood lead concentration, LFTs; repeat CBC, LFTs, blood lead concentration days 7 and 21
	CaNa₂EDTA, 1,000 mg/m²/d[a]	Continuous infusion or 2–4 divided IV doses for 5 days (see text)
		Lab: Baseline AXR, CBC, Ca²⁺, blood lead concentration, BUN, Cr, LFTs, U/A; repeat Ca²⁺, BUN, Cr, LFTs, U/A on days 3 and 5 and blood lead concentration on day 5
20–44	Routine chelation not indicated (see text)	If succimer used, same regimen as per above group (Table 93–7)
<20	Chelation not indicated	(Table 93–7)

[a]Subsequent treatment regimens should be based on post-chelation blood lead concentration and clinical symptoms (see text).

Approximate equivalent doses are expressed in milligrams per kilogram of body weight: dimercaprol 450 mg/m²/d (~24 mg/kg/d); 300 mg/m²/d (~18 mg/kg/d).

CaNa₂EDTA 1,000 mg/m²/d (~25–50 mg/kg/d); 1,500 mg/m²/d (~50–75 mg/kg/d); adult maximum dose 2–3 g/d; succimer 350 mg/m² (~10 mg/kg).

[b]Some clinicians recommend CaNa₂EDTA alone in these contexts (see text).

AXR = abdominal radiography; BPb = venous blood lead; BUN = blood urea nitrogen; Ca = calcium; CaNa₂EDTA = edetate calcium disodium; CBC = complete blood count; Cr = creatinine, CT scan = computed tomography scan of the brain; IM = intramuscular; IV = intravenous; Lab = suggested laboratory and radiologic evaluation; LFTs = hepatic aminotransferases; U/A = urinalysis with microscopy (frequent monitoring of urine dipstick analysis for hematuria and proteinuria also advised during CaNa₂EDTA therapy).

done in conjunction with pediatric neurology consultation and bedside EEG monitoring.[71,97] Modern approaches to the management of cerebral edema and increased ICP have not been critically evaluated in the context of lead encephalopathy. As noted previously, we recommend lumbar puncture be avoided in concern for cerebral herniation if lead encephalopathy is highly suspected. Of note, repeated lumbar puncture was used as an adjunct to the treatment of lead encephalopathy associated with increased ICP in the 1950s, but was complicated by proximate death when signs of impending herniation were present.[40] It seems reasonable to utilize noninvasive measures considered today in the context of intracranial hypertension associated with severe head trauma, in consultation with pediatric intensive care and neurosurgical teams, such as prevention of hypoxia and hypercarbia with tracheal intubation and controlled ventilation, maintenance of intravascular volume to provide effective cerebral perfusion pressure, seizure control, and neutral head positioning with elevation of the head of the bed to 30 degrees.[125] If such measures are not adequate, hyperosmolar therapy with mannitol or hypertonic saline is also reasonable, particularly mannitol if cerebral edema is complicated by SIADH or impaired kidney function.[40] Whether more aggressive measures, including acute hyperventilation for impending herniation, drainage of ventricular cerebrospinal fluid, or decompressive craniectomy, would

decrease mortality or morbidity further in advanced lead encephalopathy is unknown.[125]

For children with milder effects or who are asymptomatic with blood lead concentration greater than or equal to 70 mcg/dL, chelation with a 2-drug regimen similar to that used for encephalopathy is recommended. It is likely that this group of patients will require only 3 days of dimercaprol in addition to 5 days of CaNa₂EDTA.[3] For asymptomatic patients in this group, particularly those with blood lead concentrations lower than 100 mcg/dL, some authors have suggested CaNa₂EDTA alone,[205] succimer plus CaNa₂EDTA, or even succimer alone in resource-limited locales. However, if resources allow, we recommend chelation with both dimercaprol and CaNa₂EDTA. Most recently a large cohort of 3,130 Nigerian children with moderate to severe lead poisoning were managed with succimer alone. Although data concerning long-term efficacy is still emerging, this appears to be a safe alternative if circumstances preclude standard 2-drug chelation.[184] Intensive care monitoring is reasonable for such patients as well, particularly those with blood lead concentrations greater than or equal to 70 mcg/dL, at least during the initiation of chelation therapy.

Chelation therapy is recommended for asymptomatic children with blood lead concentrations between 45 and 69 mcg/dL.[3,23] For children without overt symptoms, we recommend treatment with succimer alone, which has documented efficacy in lowering blood lead concentrations and short-term safety since its approval by the US Food and Drug Administration in 1991.[75] Succimer is initiated at 30 mg/kg/day (or 1,050 mg/m^2/day) orally in 3 divided doses; this is continued for 5 days and then decreased to 20 mg/kg/day (or 700 mg/m^2/day) in 2 divided doses for 14 additional days.[3,74] The original data establishing this empiric dosing regimen were based on body surface area rather than weight.[74] For younger children, the alternative dosing by body weight results in suboptimal dosing.[158] Although the ability to chelate children orally with succimer makes it tempting to prescribe routinely for outpatient therapy and some animal evidence suggests succimer does not enhance enteral lead absorption,[93] clinical experience has shown that children must be protected from continued lead exposure during succimer chelation.[38,39] Home abatement and reinspection should be accomplished before initiation of ambulatory succimer therapy; if this is not feasible, hospitalization is still warranted. Alternative regimens (for rare patients with succimer intolerance or allergy or because of parental noncompliance) include parenteral chelation with CaNa$_2$EDTA at 25 mg/kg/day for 5 days.[3]

After initial chelation therapy, decisions to repeat treatment are based on clinical symptoms and follow-up blood lead concentrations. For patients with encephalopathy or any severe symptoms or with an initial blood lead concentration above 100 mcg/dL we recommend repeated courses of treatment. It is reasonable that at least 2 days elapse before restarting chelation.[147] The precise regimen and dosing of chelator are determined by ongoing symptomatology and the repeat blood lead concentrations (Table 93–8). A third course of chelation is rarely necessary sooner than 5 to 7 days after the second course ends.[147] For patients with milder degrees of plumbism (eg, asymptomatic, initial blood lead concentration <70 mcg/dL), it is reasonable to allow 10 to 14 days of reequilibration before restarting treatment according to the indications outlined in Table 93–8.[2]

The management of asymptomatic children with blood lead concentrations of 20 to 44 mcg/dL is controversial.[38,130,186] The National Institutes of Health–sponsored Treatment of Lead-exposed Children (TLC) trial found only modest efficacy of succimer in reducing blood lead concentrations. Furthermore, at 3 years post-enrollment, no benefit was noted in treated patients on measures of cognition, neuropsychiatric function, or behavior.[160] This large study enrolled 780 children in a multicenter, randomized, placebo-controlled, double-blind trial, but is still criticized, particularly for using a single chelator and having failed to lower blood lead concentrations significantly over time between treated and control groups.[171] Of note, small but statistically significant decrements in growth velocity were noted in the treatment group, which might reflect trace mineral depletion.[146] Since its initial publication, the primary findings of the TLC trial on lack of cognitive improvement were confirmed in a 7 year follow-up study.[48] In addition, a reanalysis of the original data found that decreasing blood concentrations did correlate with improved cognitive scores over the initial 36-month trial period (approximately 4 IQ points for each 10-mcg/dL decrease in blood lead concentration), but only in the placebo group.[115] Nevertheless, we believe it is reasonable to perform chelation for such children with blood lead concentrations at the higher end of the range (eg, 35–44 mcg/dL), especially if they remain the same or increase over several months after rigorous environmental controls, in younger children (eg, younger than 2 years), in children with evidence of biochemical toxicity (an elevated erythrocyte protoporphyrin concentration after iron supplementation, for example), or any hint of subtle symptoms. Currently, the CDC[19] and the American Academy of Pediatrics[3,5] recommend neurodevelopmental assessment, aggressive environmental assessment and lead hazard reduction, laboratory evaluation and abdominal radiograph, along with routine nutritional interventions with close monitoring of blood lead concentrations, without routine chelation therapy, for such children. While the efficacy of aggressive home environment control efforts in reducing lead exposure to young children remains unproven,[140] these measures should be instituted

as good practice to both minimize exposure and facilitate family engagement in lead hazard reduction.

For children with blood lead concentrations of 5 to 19 mcg/dL, we recommend general measures of anticipatory guidance and nutritional counseling, along with environmental assessments, with follow-up monitoring of blood lead concentrations, as endorsed by the AAP and CDC.[3,5,23] The educational approaches outlined earlier should be included in the case management of all children with even modestly elevated lead concentrations. These interventions are summarized in Table 93–7.

Adults
General Considerations
The first principle in the treatment of adults with lead poisoning is that chelation therapy is not a substitute for adherence to OSHA lead standards at the worksite and should never be given prophylactically.[47,96] In addition to the guidelines for decreasing lead exposure noted earlier, chelation therapy is recommended for adults with significant symptoms (encephalopathy, abdominal colic, severe arthralgias, or myalgias), evidence of target organ damage (neuropathy or nephropathy), and possibly in asymptomatic workers with markedly elevated blood lead concentrations or evidence of biochemical toxicity.[103,165] Table 93–8 outlines recommended chelation therapy regimens for adults. For encephalopathic adult patients, we recommend combined dimercaprol and CaNa$_2$EDTA therapy, just as for children, although some clinicians suggest that adults with severe lead poisoning may be successfully treated with CaNa$_2$EDTA alone in doses of 2 to 4 g/day by continuous IV infusion.[102] Recent reports support the use of succimer in adult patients with mild to moderate plumbism after environmental and occupational remedies are instituted.[108,150] Chelation therapy using similar clinical and blood lead concentration–based guidelines is recommended in the perioperative period for patients undergoing surgical removal of retained bullets or débridement of adjacent lead-contaminated tissue.[110,126,169] Treatment of patients with acute TEL toxicity is largely supportive, with sedation as necessary. For patients evaluated soon after a large-volume ingestion, nasogastric suction is recommended with airway protection performed as needed. In general, chelation therapy for TEL toxicity is associated with enhanced lead excretion[15] but has not been found to be clinically efficacious.[165,182,203] However, for symptomatic, especially encephalopathic, patients (in whom there may be a significant component of metabolically derived inorganic lead toxicity) or those with very elevated blood lead concentrations, we do recommend chelation therapy.

Pregnancy, Neonatal, and Lactation Issues
An area of particular concern in the management of adult plumbism involves decisions regarding therapy during pregnancy. As noted previously, lead freely passes the placental barrier and accumulates in the fetus throughout gestation. Screening of pregnant women for lead exposure, although not universal, is indicated in the presence of certain risk factors. Women of lower socioeconomic status and some ethnic groups (South American, Mexican, Asian, African American) are reported to engage in pica behavior, specifically geophagia (eating dirt or clay) at much higher rates than other groups, up to 30%.[183] Ayurvedic and other folk remedies are intended to improve fetal health, but reports of lead contamination are frequent.[26] Maternal bone stores are also a potential endogenous source of elevated blood lead concentrations in pregnancy, and contribute to modest increases in blood lead concentration during the third trimester, particularly in women with low calcium intake.[25,82] Screening should be conducted at prenatal visits and blood lead concentration obtained if any concern arises. Guidelines from the CDC and American College of Obstetrics and Gynecology outline appropriate screening and follow-up of elevated blood lead concentrations in pregnancy.[25] In general, any pregnant woman with a blood lead concentration of greater than 5 mcg/dL requires close follow-up testing, along with careful environmental and occupational exposure investigation and nutritional counseling. Appropriate calcium intake (2,000 mg/day) through adequate diet or supplementation should be ensured because its use is associated with decreased bone resorption during pregnancy, which likely lessens fetal lead

exposure.[89] Adequate maternal iron intake is also associated with lower neonatal blood lead concentration.[167] Iron-deficient patients should be treated; otherwise an iron-sufficient diet should be advised. Women with blood lead concentrations greater than 10 mcg/dL should be reported to the lead poisoning program of the local health department, and if an occupational source is suspected, a consult to an occupational medicine specialist obtained. Pregnant patients with blood lead concentrations greater than 45 mcg/dL should undergo medical toxicology and high-risk pregnancy consultation.

Chelation therapy during early pregnancy poses theoretical problems of teratogenicity, particularly that caused by enhanced excretion of potentially vital trace elements, or translocation of lead from mother to fetus (Antidotes in Depth: A28, A29, and A30). However, of some reassurance regarding fetal health, a case series and 25-year literature review of lead poisoning during pregnancy found no reports of chelation-associated birth defects in the handful of published cases.[172] It should be noted that despite decreases in maternal blood lead concentration in most treated women, the effect on cord or neonatal blood lead concentrations is more variable, and in some cases these approximate the pretreatment maternal blood lead concentration.[25] In general, there currently seems little support for routine chelation therapy in asymptomatic pregnant women with only moderate increases in blood lead concentration (eg, <45 mcg/dL), particularly during the first-trimester period of fetal organogenesis. Symptomatic women and those with blood lead concentrations greater than or equal to 70 mcg/dL should undergo chelation, regardless of trimester. For pregnant patients whose blood lead concentrations are 45 to 69 mcg/dL, medical toxicology and high-risk obstetric consultation is recommended[25] as well as for women with lower blood lead concentrations for whom substantial questions exist about source of lead exposure, or for whom blood lead concentrations are rising significantly during their pregnancy on follow-up testing.

Postnatally, infant blood lead concentrations usually decline over time without chelation, but this occurs very slowly, and the course is variable. For example, in 2 reported neonates exposed to prenatal maternal chelation who were then monitored for 2 weeks postpartum, the blood lead concentration remained stable or increased until chelation therapy was instituted.[145,185] In 2 additional cases of neonates whose mothers were not treated prepartum, blood lead concentrations also remained stable or increased for 17 days to 3 weeks.[67,177] Thus, postpartum chelation therapy should be conducted for neonates, according to blood lead concentrations, as per the guidelines described above for older children. For overtly symptomatic neonates or those with extremely elevated blood lead concentrations, both chelation therapy and exchange transfusion are reasonable treatment modalities.[35] However, many practitioners are unfamiliar with exchange transfusion, and there are several reports of safe and effective chelation therapy with edetate calcium disodium, dimercaprol, and/or succimer in the newborn.[152,172] Taking these considerations into account, for the majority of neonates with blood lead concentration at or above 45 mcg/dL, we recommend chelation.

Lastly, the issue of allowing mothers with elevated blood lead concentrations to breastfeed their infants will arise. Breast milk from heavily exposed mothers is a potential source of lead exposure.[9,53,54] One small case series found that breast milk from 2 women with blood lead concentrations of 34 and 29 mcg/dL, respectively, had clinically insignificant lead content (<0.01 mcg/mL).[9] Another study calculated the estimated rise in infant blood lead concentration at 1 month postpartum to be expected from breastfeeding, suggesting a rise of 0.12 mcg/dL for each mcg/dL of maternal blood lead concentration.[54] Given these considerations, the majority of lead-exposed mothers should still be encouraged to breastfeed with monitoring of the infant's blood lead concentration.[53] For mothers with blood lead concentrations of less than or equal to 40 mcg/dL, breastfeeding should be encouraged with close follow-up of maternal and infant blood lead concentrations (Table 93–9).[25,53] We also recommend maternal calcium supplementation (1,200 mg/day of elemental calcium as calcium carbonate), a simple intervention that reduces breast milk lead content by 5% to 10%.[55]

TABLE 93–9   Summary of Guidelines for Breastfeeding with Perinatal Lead Exposure[a]

Recommendations for Initiation of Breastfeeding[b]

- Measurement of concentrations of lead in breast milk is not recommended.
- Mothers with blood lead concentrations <40 mcg/dL should breastfeed if there are no other contraindications.
- Mothers with confirmed blood lead concentrations ≥40 mcg/dL should begin breastfeeding when their blood lead concentrations drop below 40 mcg/dL. Until then, they should pump and discard their breast milk (chelation therapy of mother with blood lead concentration ≥45 mcg/dL is reasonable[b])
- These recommendations are likely not appropriate in countries where infant mortality from infectious diseases is high.

Recommendations for Continuation of Breastfeeding[b]

- Breastfeeding should continue for infants with blood level concentrations below 5 mcg/dL.
- Infants born to mothers with blood lead concentration ≥5 mcg/dL, but <40 mcg/dL can continue to breastfeed unless there are indications that the breast milk is contributing to elevating blood lead concentrations. These infants should have blood lead concentration tests at birth and be followed, according to the following schedule:

Infant blood lead concentration 5–24 mcg/dL: Follow-up test, within 1 month (we recommend at 1 and 3 weeks until trend established)[b]

Infant blood lead concentration 25–44 mcg/dL: Follow-up blood lead concentration within 2 weeks (we recommend at 1 week, then weekly during first month)[b]

Infant blood lead concentration ≥45 mcg/dL: Follow-up test within 24 hours and then frequently (also see above if maternal blood lead concentrations >40 mcg/dL)[b]

For infants whose blood lead concentrations are rising or failing to decline by 5 mcg/dL or more, environmental and other sources of lead exposure should be evaluated. If no external source is identified, and maternal blood lead concentrations are >20 mcg/dL and infant blood lead concentration ≥5 mcg/dL, then breast milk should be suspected as the source, and breastfeeding should be temporarily interrupted until maternal blood lead concentrations decline.[b]

[a]Data from Centers for Disease Control and Prevention. Guidelines for the identification and management of lead exposure in pregnant and lactating women. http://www.cdc.gov/nceh/lead/publications/LeadandPregnancy2010.pdf. Published 2010.[25]

Comments in italics are the opinions of the authors. It should be noted that these guidelines were developed at a time when the CDC threshold of concern for infant blood lead concentration was 10 mcg/dL. In light of the new lowered threshold to 5 mcg/dL, more conservative guidelines may be developed in the foreseeable future.

[b]Owing to the complexity of these cases and varied data regarding the contribution of maternal blood lead concentration and breast milk to infant exposure and clinical effects, pediatric toxicology consultation is advised to assist with risk assessment, interpretation, and management.

SUMMARY

- Lead is a widely distributed element that has long been used by humans for a variety of purposes, including waterproofing; electrical and radiation shielding; and the production of ammunitions, paints, plastics, ceramics, glass, and explosives.

- Lead poisoning, or plumbism, has an equally long history, but today it is primarily manifest in young children exposed to deteriorated lead paint and as an occupational toxic exposure for adult workers.

- Lead causes multiorgan toxicity, affecting especially the hematologic and neurologic systems in patients of all ages and causing hypertension in adults. The broad spectrum of clinical effects range from subtle neurocognitive insults to vague constitutional symptoms to acute encephalopathy, intracranial hypertension, cerebral edema, and death.

- The mainstays of treatment are removal from exposure for all patients, and chelation therapy for patients with symptoms or significantly elevated blood lead concentrations. Defining a group of asymptomatic patients that will benefit from chelation therapy has been difficult and controversial.

- Parenteral chelation with $CaNa_2EDTA$ and dimercaprol is efficacious in lowering blood lead concentrations and reducing mortality and morbidity from severe lead poisoning. Succimer, an oral chelator, also has efficacy in reducing blood lead concentrations in asymptomatic children, although the neurocognitive benefit of doing so is unproven.

REFERENCES

1. Agency for Toxic Substances and Disease Registry. *The Nature and Extent of Lead Poisoning in Children in the United States: A Report to Congress.* Atlanta, GA: Agency for Toxic Substances and Disease Registry; 1988.
2. Alarcon WA. Elevated blood lead levels among employed adults—United States, 1994-2013. *MMWR Morb Mortal Wkly Rep.* 2016;63:59-65.
3. American Academy of Pediatrics Committee on Drugs. Treatment guidelines for lead exposure in children. *Pediatrics.* 1995;96:155-160.
4. American Academy of Pediatrics Committee on Environmental Health. Lead exposure in children: prevention, detection and management. *Pediatrics.* 2005;116:1036-1046.
5. American Academy of Pediatrics Council on Environmental Health. Prevention of childhood lead toxicity. *Pediatrics.* 2016;138.
6. Assennato G, et al. Sperm count suppression without endocrine dysfunction in lead-exposed men. *Annu Rev Pharmacol Toxicol.* 1986;41:387-390.
7. Audesirk G. Electrophysiology of lead intoxication: effects on voltage-sensitive ion channels. *Neurotoxicology.* 1993;14:137-147.
8. Barltrop D, Meek F. Absorption of different lead compounds. *Postgrad Med J.* 1975;51:805-809.
9. Baum CR, Shannon MW. Lead in breast milk. *Pediatrics.* 1996;97:932.
10. Beaucham C, et al. Indoor firing ranges and elevated blood lead levels—United States, 2002-2013. *MMWR Morb Mortal Wkly Rep.* 2014;63:347-351.
11. Bellinger DC, et al. Establishing and Achieving National Goals for Preventing Lead Toxicity and Exposure in Children. *JAMA Pediatr.* 2017;171:616-618.
12. Bolanowska W, et al. Triethyl lead in the biologic material in cases of acute tetraethyl lead poisoning. *Arch Toxicol.* 1967;22:278-282.
13. Borja-Aburto VH, et al. Blood lead levels measured prospectively and risk of spontaneous abortion. *Am J Epidemiol.* 1999;150:590-597.
14. Brown MJ, Margolis S. Lead in drinking water and human blood lead levels in the United States. *MMWR Morb Mortal Wkly Rep Suppl.* 2012;61:1-9.
15. Burns CB, Currie B. The efficacy of chelation therapy and factors influencing mortality in lead intoxicated petrol sniffers. *Aust N Z J Med.* 1995;25:197-203.
16. Caldwell KL, et al. Measurement challenges at low blood lead levels. *Pediatrics.* 2017;140.
17. Campbell C, Osterhoudt KC. Prevention of childhood lead poisoning. *Curr Opin Pediatr.* 2000;12:428-437.
18. Campbell JR, Auginer P. The association between blood lead levels and osteoporosis among adults—results from the Third National Health and Nutrition Examination Survey (NHANES III). *Environ Health Perspect.* 2007;115:1018-1022.
19. Canfield RL, et al. Intellectual impairment in children with blood lead concentrations below 10 μg per deciliter. *N Engl J Med.* 2003;348:1517-1526.
20. Centers for Disease Control and Prevention. Fatal pediatric poisoning from leaded paint-Wisconsin, 1990. *MMWR Morb Mortal Wkly Rep.* 1991;40:193-195.
21. Centers for Disease Control and Prevention. Screening young children for lead poisoning: guidance for state and local public health officials. Atlanta, GA: Centers for Disease Control and Prevention; 1997.
22. Centers for Disease Control and Prevention. Recommendations for blood lead screening of young children enrolled in Medicaid: targeting a group at high risk. *MMWR Morb Mortal Wkly Rep.* 2000;49:1-13.
23. Centers for Disease Control and Prevention. Managing elevated blood lead levels among young children: recommendations from the Advisory Committee on Childhood Lead Poisoning Prevention. Atlanta, GA: Centers for Disease Control and Prevention; 2002.
24. Centers for Disease Control and Prevention. Elevated blood lead levels in refugee children-New Hampshire, 2003-2004. *MMWR Morb Mortal Wkly Rep.* 2005;54:42-46.
25. Centers for Disease Control and Prevention. Guidelines for the identification and management of lead exposure in pregnant and lactating women. http://www.cdc.gov/nceh/lead/publications/LeadandPregnancy2010.pdf. Published 2010. Accessed August 7, 2017.
26. Centers for Disease Control and Prevention. Lead poisoning in pregnant women who used Ayurvedic medications from India—New York City, 2011–2012. *MMWR Morb Mortal Wkly Rep.* 2012;61:641-646.
27. Centers for Disease Control and Prevention. Childhood lead exposure associated with the use of kajal, an eye cosmetic from Afghanistan—Albuquerque, New Mexico, 2013. *MMWR Morb Mortal Wkly Rep.* 2013;62:917-919.
28. Centers for Disease Control and Prevention. Blood lead levels in children aged <5 years—United States, 2007-2013. *MMWR Morb Mortal Wkly Rep.* 2016;63:66-72.
29. Centers for Disease Control and Prevention. Childhood blood lead levels in children aged <5 years—United States, 2009–2014. *MMWR Morb Mortal Wkly Rep.* 2017;66:1-10.
30. Centers for Disease Control and Prevention. Potential for falsely low blood lead test results from LeadCare Analyzers. https://emergency.cdc.gov/han/han00403.asp. Published 2017. Accessed August 10, 2017.
31. Centers for Disease Control and Prevention. Potential exposure to lead in artificial turf. *CDC Health Alert Network (HAN) Advisory,* June 18, 2008.
32. Centers for Disease Control and Prevention Advisory Committee on Childhood Lead Poisoning Prevention. Low level lead exposure harms children: a renewed call for primary prevention. January 4, 2012.
33. Chan GM, et al. Get the lead out. *Ann Emerg Med.* 2004;44:551-552.
34. Cheng Y, et al. Electrocardiographic conduction disturbances in association with low-level lead exposure (The Normative Aging Study). *Am J Cardiol.* 1998;82:594-599.
35. Chinnakaruppan NR, Marcus SM. Asymptomatic congenital lead poisoning—case report. *Clin Toxicol (Phila).* 2010;48:563-565.
36. Chisholm JJ Jr. The use of chelating agents in the treatment of acute and chronic lead intoxication in childhood. *J Pediatr.* 1968;73:1-38.
37. Chisholm JJ Jr. Mobilization of lead by calcium disodium edetate: a reappraisal. *Am J Dis Child.* 1987;141:1256-1257.
38. Chisholm JJ Jr. BAL, EDTA, DMSA, and DMPS in the treatment of lead poisoning in children. *J Toxicol Clin Toxicol.* 1992;30:493-504.
39. Chisholm JJ Jr. Safety and efficacy of meso-2,3-dimercaptosuccinic acid (DMSA) in children with elevated blood lead concentrations. *J Toxicol Clin Toxicol.* 2000;38:365-375.
40. Chisholm JJ Jr, Harrison HE. The treatment of acute lead encephalopathy in children. *Pediatrics.* 1957;19:2-20.
41. Cory-Slechta DA. Relationships between lead-induced learning impairments and changes in dopaminergic, cholinergic, and glutamatergic neurotransmitter system functions. *Annu Rev Pharmacol Toxicol.* 1995;35:391-415.
42. Cremin JJ, et al. Efficacy of succimer chelation for reducing brain lead in a primate model of human lead exposure. *Toxicol Appl Pharmacol.* 1999;161:283-293.
43. Cullen MR, et al. Adult inorganic lead intoxication: presentation of 31 new cases and a review of the literature. *Medicine (Baltimore).* 1983;62:221-247.
44. Dalvi SR, Pillinger MH. Saturnine gout, redux: a review. *Am J Med.* 2013;126:450.e451-450.e458.
45. Dasani BM, Kawanishi H. The gastrointestinal manifestations of gunshot-induced lead poisoning. *J Clin Gastroenterol.* 1994;19:296-299.
46. Davoli CT, et al. Asymptomatic children with venous lead levels >100 μg/dL. *Pediatrics.* 1996;98:965-968.
47. DeRoos FJ. Smelters and metal reclaimers. In: Greenberg MI, et al, eds. *Occupational, Industrial and Environmental Toxicology.* 2nd ed. St. Louis, MO: Mosby-Year Book; 2003:388-397.
48. Dietrich KN, et al. Effect of chelation therapy on the neuropsychological and behavioral development of lead-exposed children after school entry. *Pediatrics.* 2004;114:19-26.
49. Dogu O, et al. Elevated blood lead concentrations in essential tremor: a case-control study in Mersin, Turkey. *Environ Health Perspect.* 2007;115:1564-1568.
50. Ekinci M, et al. Occupational exposure to lead decreases macular, choroidal, and retinal nerve fiber layer thickness in industrial battery workers. *Curr Eye Res.* 2014;39:853-858.
51. Environmental Protection Agency. *Evaluation of Potential Carcinogenicity of Lead and Lead Compounds.* EPA/600/8-89/0454A. Washington, DC: US Environmental Protection Agency, Office of Health and Environmental Assessment; 1989.
52. Erenberg G, et al. Lead neuropathy and sickle cell disease. *Pediatrics.* 1974;54:438-441.
53. Ettinger AS, et al. Maternal blood, plasma, and breast milk lead: lactational transfer and contribution to infant exposure. *Environ Health Perspect.* 2014;122:87-92.
54. Ettinger AS, et al. Levels of breast milk lead and their relation to maternal blood and bone lead levels at one-month postpartum. *Environ Health Perspect.* 2004;112:926-931.
55. Ettinger AS, et al. Influence of maternal bone lead burden and calcium intake on levels of lead in breast milk over the course of lactation. *Am J Epidemiol.* 2006;163:48-56.
56. Eum KD, et al. Prospective cohort study of lead exposure and electrocardiographic conduction disturbances in the department of veterans affairs normative aging study. *Environ Health Perspect.* 2011;119:940-944.
57. Eum KD, et al. Relation of cumulative low-level lead exposure to depressive and phobic anxiety symptom scores in middle-age and elderly women. *Environ Health Perspect.* 2012;120:817-823.
58. Farrell SE, et al. Blood lead levels in emergency department patients with retained bullets and shrapnel. *Acad Emerg Med.* 1999;6:208-212.
59. Fergusson L, et al. Lead foreign body ingestion in children. *J Paediatr Child Health.* 1997;33:542-544.
60. Flaherty EG. Risk of lead poisoning in abused and neglected children. *Clin Pediatr (Phila).* 1995;43:128-132.
61. Florence TM, et al. Skin absorption of lead. *Lancet.* 1988;2:157-158.
62. Fortin MC, et al. Increased lead biomarker levels are associated with changes in hormonal response to stress in occupationally exposed male participants. *Environ Health Perspect.* 2011;120:278-283.
63. Franken A, et al. In vitro permeation of metals through human skin: a review and recommendations. *Chem Res Toxicol.* 2015;28:2237-2249.
64. Friedman JA, Weinberger HL. Six children with lead poisoning. *Am J Dis Child.* 1990;144:1039-1044.
65. Friedman LS, et al. Case records of the Massachusetts General Hospital. Case 12-2014. A 59-year-old man with fatigue, abdominal pain, anemia, and abnormal liver function. *N Engl J Med.* 2014;370:1542-1550.
66. Gandhi J, et al. Impaired hypothalamic-pituitary-testicular axis activity, spermatogenesis, and sperm function promote infertility in males with lead poisoning. *Zygote.* 2017;25:103-110.
67. Ghafour SY, et al. Congenital lead intoxication with seizures due to prenatal exposure. *Clin Pediatr (Phila).* 1984;23:282-283.
68. Goldman RH, et al. Gun marksmanship and youth lead exposure: a practice-oriented approach to prevention. *Clin Pediatr (Phila).* 2017;56:1068-1071.
69. Goldstein GW. Neurologic concepts of lead poisoning in children. *Pediatr Ann.* 1992;21:384-388.

70. Gordon RA, et al. Aggressive approach in the treatment of acute lead encephalopathy with an extraordinarily high concentration of lead. *Arch Pediatr Adolesc Med.* 1998;152:1100-1104.

71. Gorelick MH, Gray MP. Neurologic emergencies. In: Shaw KN, Bachur RG, eds. *Fleisher and Ludwig's Textbook of Pediatric Emergency Medicine.* 7th ed. Philadelphia, PA: Wolters Kluwer; 2016:914-933.

72. Goyer RA. Lead toxicity: current concerns. *Environ Health Perspect.* 1993;100:177-187.

73. Goyer RA. Toxic effects of metals. In: Klaassen CD, ed. *Casarett and Doull's Toxicology: the Basic Science of Poisons.* 5th ed. New York, NY: McGraw-Hill; 1996:691-709.

74. Graziano JH, et al. Dose-response study of oral 2,3-dimercaptosuccinic acid in children with elevated blood lead concentrations. *J Pediatr.* 1988;113:751-757.

75. Graziano JH, et al. Controlled study of meso-2,3-dimercaptosuccinic acid for the management of childhood lead intoxication. *J Pediatr.* 1992;120:133-139.

76. Graziano JH, et al. Depressed serum erythropoietin in pregnant women with elevated blood lead. *Arch Environ Health.* 1991;46:347-350.

77. Greig J, et al. Association of blood lead level with neurological features in 972 children affected by an acute severe lead poisoning outbreak in Zamfara State, northern Nigeria. *PLoS One.* 2014;9:e93716.

78. Hammer LD, et al. Increased lead absorption in children with accidental ingestions. *Am J Emerg Med.* 1985;3:301-304.

79. Handley MA, et al. Globalization, binational communities, and imported food risks: Results of an outbreak investigation of lead poisoning in Monterey County, California. *Am J Public Health.* 2007;97:900-906.

80. Hanna-Attisha M, et al. Elevated blood lead levels in children associated with the flint drinking water crisis: a spatial analysis of risk and public health response. *Am J Public Health.* 2016;106:283-290.

81. Hansen KS, Sharp FR. Gasoline sniffing, lead poisoning and myoclonus. *JAMA.* 1978;240:1375-1376.

82. Hertz-Picciotto I, et al. Patterns and determinants of blood lead during pregnancy. *Am J Epidemiol.* 2000;152:829-837.

83. Hu H, et al. The use of K x-ray fluorescence for measuring lead burden in epidemiological studies: high and low lead burdens and measurement uncertainty. *Environ Health Perspect.* 1991;94:107-110.

84. Hu H, et al. The epidemiology of lead toxicity in adults: measuring dose and consideration of other methodologies. *Environ Health Perspect.* 2007;115:455-462.

85. Huseman CA, et al. Neuroendocrine effects of toxic and low blood lead levels in chidlren. *Pediatrics.* 1992;90:186-189.

86. IARC (International Agency for Research on Cancer). Monograph on inorganic and organic lead compounds. *IARC Monogr Eval Carcinog Risks Hum.* 2006;87:370-378.

87. Ilychova SA, Zaridze DG. Cancer mortality among female and male workers occupationally exposed to inorganic lead in the printing industry. *Occup Environ Med.* 2011;69:87-92.

88. Jain NB, et al. Lead levels and ischemic heart disease in a prospective study of middle-aged and elderly men: the VA normative aging study. *Environ Health Perspect.* 2007;115:871-875.

89. Jarakiraman V, et al. Calcium supplements and bone resorption in pregnancy: a randomized crossover trial. *Am J Prev Med.* 2003;24:260-264.

90. Jiang X, et al. Studies of lead exposure on reproductive system: a review of work in China. *Biomed Environ Sci.* 1992;5:266-275.

91. Johnston MV, Goldstein GW. Selective vulnerability of the developing brain to lead. *Curr Opin Neurol.* 1988;11:688-693.

92. Jusko TA, et al. Blood lead concentrations < 10 µg/dL and child intelligence at 6 years of age. *Environ Health Perspect.* 2007;116:243-248.

93. Kapoor SC, et al. Influence of 2,3-dimercaptosuccinic acid on gastrointestinal lead absorption and whole body lead retention. *Toxicol Appl Pharmacol.* 1989;97:525-529.

94. Kari SK, et al. Lead encephalopathy due to traditional medicines. *Curr Drug Saf.* 2008;3:54-59.

95. Karwowski MP, et al. Toxicants in folk remedies: implications of elevated blood lead in an American-born infant due to imported diaper powder. *Environ Geochem Health.* 2017;39:1133-1143.

96. Keogh JP. Lead. In: Sullivan JB, Krieger GR, eds. *Hazardous Materials Toxicology: Clinical Principles of Environmental Health.* Baltimore, MD: Williams & Wilkins; 1992:834-844.

97. Kimia AA, Chiang VW. Seizures. In: Shaw KN, Bachur RG, eds. *Fleisher and Ludwig's Textbook of Pediatric Emergency Medicine.* Philadelphia, PA: Wolters Kluwer; 2016:465-471.

98. Koh D-H, et al. Lead exposure in US Worksites: a literatuer review and development of an occupational lead exposure database from the published literature. *Am J Ind Med.* 2015;58:605-616.

99. Kopp SJ, et al. The influence of chronic low-level cadmium and/or lead feeding on myocardial contractility related to phosphorylation of cardiac myofibrillar proteins. *Toxicol Appl Pharmacol.* 1980;54:48-56.

100. Kordas K. Iron, lead, and children's behavior and cognition. *Annu Rev Nutr.* 2010; 30:123-148.

101. Kosnett MJ. Unanswered questions in metal chelation. *J Toxicol Clin Toxicol.* 1992; 30:529-547.

102. Kosnett MJ. Lead. In: Brent J, eds. *Critical Care Toxicology: Diagnosis and Management of the Critically Poisoned Patient.* 2nd ed. Switzerland: Springer International Publishing; 2016:1-30.

103. Kosnett MJ, et al. Recommendations for medical management of adult lead exposure. *Environ Health Perspect.* 2007;115:463-471.

104. Landrigan PJ, et al. Exposure to lead from the Mystic River bridge: the dilemma of deleading. *N Engl J Med.* 1982;306:673-676.

105. Lanphear BP, et al. Low-level environmental lead exposure and children's intellectual function: an international pooled analysis. *Environ Health Perspect.* 2005; 113:894-899.

106. Li C, et al. Epigenetic marker (LINE-1 promoter) methylation level was associated with occupational lead exposure. *Clin Toxicol (Phila).* 2013;51:225-229.

107. Lidsky TI, Schneider JS. Lead neurotoxicity in children: basic mechanisms and clinical correlates. *Brain.* 2003;126:5-19.

108. Lifshitz M, et al. The effect of 2,3-dimercaptosuccinic acid in the treatment of lead poisoning in adults. *Ann Med.* 1997;29:83-85.

109. Lin JL, et al. Environmental lead exposure and progression of chronic renal disesaes in patients without diabetes. *N Engl J Med.* 2003;348:277-286.

110. Linden MA, et al. Lead poisoning from retained bullets: pathogenesis, diagnosis and management. *Ann Surg.* 1982;195:305-313.

111. Lipton ES, Barboza D. As more toys are recalled, trail ends in China. *The New York Times.* June 19, 2007.

112. Liu J, et al. Lead exposure at each stage of pregnancy and neurobehavioral development of neonates. *Neurotoxicology.* 2014;44:1-7.

113. Liu J, et al. Toxic effects of metals. In: Klaassen CD, ed. *Casarett & Doull's Toxicology: The Basic Science of Poisons.* 7th ed. New York, NY: McGraw-Hill; 2008:931-981.

114. Liu J, et al. Blood lead concentrations and children's behavioral and emotional problems: a cohort study. *JAMA Pediatr.* 2014;168:737-745.

115. Liu X, et al. Do children with falling blood lead levels have improved cognition? *Pediatrics.* 2002;110:787-791.

116. Mahaffey KR. Nutrition and lead: strategies for public health. *Environ Health Perspect.* 1995;103:191-196.

117. Mantere P, et al. A prospective follow-up study on psychological effects in workers exposed to low levels of lead. *Scand J Work Environ Health.* 1984;10:43-50.

118. Marcus AH. Multicompartment kinetic modules for lead: linear kinetics and variable absorption in humans without excessive lead exposures. *Environ Res.* 1985; 36:459-472.

119. Markovac J, Goldstein GW. Picomolar concentrations of lead stimulate brain protein kinase C. *Nature.* 1988;334:71-73.

120. Markowitz ME, et al. Effects of calcium disodium versenate (CaNa$_2$EDTA) chelation in moderate childhood lead poisoning. *Pediatrics.* 1993;92:265-271.

121. Markowitz ME, Weinberger HL. Immobilization-related lead toxicity in previously lead-poisoned children. *Pediatrics.* 1990;86:455-457.

122. Maslinski PG, Loeb JA. Pica-associated cerebral edema in an adult. *J Neurol Sci.* 2004;225:149-151.

123. McCord CP. Lead and lead poisoning in early America. Benjamin Franklin and lead poisoning. *Indust Med Surg.* 1953;22:394-399.

124. McKinney PE. Acute elevation of blood lead levels within hours of ingestion of large quantities of lead shot. *J Toxicol Clin Toxicol.* 2000;38:435-440.

125. McManemy JK, Jea A. Neurotrauma. In: Shaw KN, Bachur RG, eds. *Fleisher and Ludwig's Textbook of Pediatric Emergency Medicine.* Philadelphia, PA: Wolters Kluwer; 2016:1280-1287.

126. Meggs WJ, et al. The treatment of lead poisoning from gunshot wounds with succimer (DMSA). *J Toxicol Clin Toxicol.* 1994;32:377-385.

127. Mehta V, et al. Lead intoxication due to ayurvedic medications as a cause of abdominal pain in adults. *Clin Toxicol (Phila).* 2017;55:97-101.

128. Mojdehi GM, Gurtner J. Childhood lead poisoning through kohl. *Am J Public Health.* 1996;86:587-588.

129. Moore MR, et al. The percutaneous absorption of lead-203 in humans from cosmetic preparations containing lead acetate, as assessed by whole-body counting and other techniques. *Food Cosmet Toxicol.* 1980;18:399-405.

130. Mortensen ME. Succimer chelation: what is known?. *J Pediatr.* 1994;125:233-234.

131. Mortensen ME, Walson PD. Chelation therapy for childhood lead poisoning—the changing scene in the 1990s. *Clin Pediatr (Phila).* 1993;32:284-291.

132. Mowad E, et al. Management of lead poisoning from ingested fishing sinkers. *Arch Pediatr Adolesc Med.* 1998;152:485-488.

133. National Health and Medical Research Council. 2015 NHMRC Information Paper: Evidence on the Effects of Lead on Human Health. http://www.nhmrc.gov.au/guidelines/publications/eh58. Published 2015. Accessed August 17, 2017.

134. Needleman HL. The persistent threat of lead: medical and sociological issues. *Curr Probl Pediatr.* 1988;18:702-744.

135. Needleman HL, et al. Deficits in psychological and classroom performance of children with elevated dentine lead levels. *N Engl J Med.* 1979;300:689-695.

136. Nolan CV, Shaikh ZA. Lead nephrotoxicity and associated disorders: biochemical mechanisms. *Toxicology.* 1992;73:127-146.

137. Nortier JWR, et al. Acute lead poisoning with hemolysis and liver toxicity after ingestion of red lead. *Vet Hum Toxicol.* 1980;22:145-147.

138. Norton RL, et al. Acute intravenous lead poisoning in a drug abuser: associated complications of hepatitis, pancreatitis, hemolysis and renal failure [abstract]. *Vet Hum Toxicol.* 1989;31:340.

139. Nriagu JO. Saturnine gout among Roman aristocrats. *N Engl J Med.* 1983;308:660-663.

140. Nussbaumer-Streit B, et al. Household interventions for preventing domestic lead exposure in children. *Cochrane Database Syst Rev.* 2016;10:CD006047.

141. O'Donnell KA, et al. Toxicologic Emergencies. In: Shaw KN, et al, eds. *Fleisher & Ludwig's Textbook of Pediatric Emergency Medicine.* 7th ed. Philadelphia, PA: Wolters Kluwer; 2016:1061-1114.

142. Onalaja AO, Claudio L. Genetic susceptibility to lead poisoning. *Environ Health Perspect.* 2000;108(suppl 1):23-28.

143. Paglia DE, et al. Effects of low level lead exposure on pyrimidine-5' nucleotidase and other erythrocyte enzymes. *J Clin Invest.* 1976;56:1164-1169.

144. Parry C, Eaton J. Kohl: a lead-hazardous eye makeup from the Third World to the First World. *Environ Health Perspect.* 1991;94:121-123.

145. Pearl M, Boxt LM. Radiographic findings in congenital lead poisoning. *Radiology.* 1980;136:83-84.

146. Peterson KE, et al. Effect of succimer on growth of preschool children with moderate blood lead levels. *Environ Health Perspect.* 2004;112:233-237.

147. Piomelli S, et al. Management of childhood lead poisoning. *J Pediatr.* 1984;105:523-532.

148. Pirkle JL, et al. The relationship between blood lead levels and blood pressure and its cardiovascular risk implications. *Am J Epidemiol.* 1985;121:246-258.

149. Pocock SJ, et al. Environmental lead and children's intelligence: a systematic review of the epidemiological evidence. *Br Med J.* 1994;309:1189-1197.

150. Porru S, Alessio L. The use of chelating agents in occupational lead poisoning. *Occup Med.* 1996;46:41-48.

151. Pounds JG, et al. Cellular and molecular toxicity of lead in bone. *Environ Health Perspect.* 1991;91:17-32.

152. Powell ST, et al. Succimer therapy for congenital lead poisoning from maternal petrol sniffing. *Med J Aust.* 2006;184:84-85.

153. Raber SA. The dense metaphyseal band sign. *Radiology.* 1999;211:773-774.

154. Rabinowitz MB, Needleman HL. Temporal trends in the lead concentrations of umbilical cord blood. *Science.* 1982;216:1429-1431.

155. Rabinowitz MB, et al. Kinetic analysis of lead metabolism in healthy humans. *J Clin Invest.* 1976;58:260-270.

156. Regan CM. Neural cell adhesion molecules, neuronal development and lead toxicity. *Neurotoxicology.* 1993;14:69-74.

157. Restek-Samarzija N, et al. Ventricular arrhythmia in acute lead poisoning: a case report [abstract]. EAPCCT XVI International Congress; 1994; Vienna, Austria.

158. Rhoads GG, Rogan WJ. Treatment of lead-exposed children. *Pediatrics.* 1996;98:162-163.

159. Rodamilans M, et al. Lead toxicity on endocrine testicular function in an occupationally exposed population. *Hum Toxicol.* 1988;7:125-128.

160. Rogan WJ, et al; For the Treatment of Lead-Exposed Chidlren (TLC) Trial Group. The effect of chelation therapy with succimer on neuropsychological development in children exposed to lead. *N Engl J Med.* 2001;344:1421-1426.

161. Royce SE, Needleman HL. Case studies in environmental medicine. Lead toxicity. In: Agency for Toxic Substances and Disease Registry, ed. Atlanta 1992.

162. Ruha AM. Recommendations for provoked challenge urine testing. *J Med Toxicol.* 2013;9:318-325.

163. Sandstead HH, et al. Lead intoxication and the thyroid. *Arch Intern Med.* 1969; 123:632-635.

164. Saper RB, et al. Lead, mercury, and arsenic in US- and Indian-manufactured ayurvedic medicines sold via the Internet. *JAMA.* 2008;300:915-923.

165. Saryan LA, Zenz C. Lead and its compounds. In: Zenz C, et al, eds. *Occupational Medicine.* 3rd ed. St. Louis, MO: Mosby; 1994:506-541.

166. Schaumberg DA, et al. Accumulated lead exposure and risk of age-related cataract in men. *JAMA.* 2004;292:2750-2754.

167. Schell LM, et al. Maternal blood lead concentration, diet during pregnancy, and anthropometry predict neonatal blood lead in a socioeconomically disadvantaged population. *Environ Health Perspect.* 2002;111:195-200.

168. Schwartz BS, Hu H. Adult lead exposure: time for change. *Environ Health Perspect.* 2007;115:451-454.

169. Selbst SM, et al. Lead poisoning in a child with a gunshot wound. *Pediatrics.* 1986;77:413-416.

170. Selbst SM, et al. Lead encephalopathy in a child with sickle cell disease. *Clin Pediatr (Phila).* 1985;24:280-285.

171. Shannon MW. Lead poisoning treatment—a continuing need. *J Toxicol Clin Toxicol.* 2001;39:661-663.

172. Shannon MW. Severe lead poisoning in pregnancy. *Ambul Pediatr.* 2003;3:37-39.

173. Shih RA, et al. Cumulative lead dose and cognitive function in adults: a review of studies that measured both blood lead and bone lead. *Environ Health Perspect.* 2007;115:483-492.

174. Silbergeld EK, et al. Lead and osteoporosis: mobilization of lead from bone in post-menopausal women. *Environ Res.* 1988;47:79-94.

175. Sim CS, et al. Iron deficiency increases blood lead levels in boys and pre-menarche girls surveyed in KNHANES 2010-2011. *Environ Res.* 2014;130:1-6.

176. Simons TJB. Cellular interactions between lead and calcium. *Br Med Bull.* 1986; 42:431-434.

177. Singh N, et al. Neonatal lead intoxication in a prenatally exposed infant. *J Pediatr.* 1978;93:1019-1021.

178. Srivastava D, et al. Lead- and calcium-mediated inhibition of bovine rod cGMP phosphodiesterase: interactions with magnesium. *Toxicol Appl Pharmacol.* 1995; 134:43-52.

179. Staes C, et al. Lead poisoning deaths in the United States, 1979-1988. *JAMA.* 1995; 273:847-848.

180. Suarez CR, et al. Elevated lead levels in a patient with sickle cell disease and inappropriate secretion of antidiuretic hormone. *Pediatr Emerg Care.* 1992;8:88-90.

181. Sun CC, et al. Percutaneous absorption of inorganic lead compounds. *AIHA J.* 2002;63:641-646.

182. Tenenbein M. Leaded gasoline abuse: the role of tetraethyl lead. *Hum Exp Toxicol.* 1997;16:217-222.

183. Thihalolipavan S, et al. Examining pica in NYC pregnant women with elevated blood lead levels. *Matern Child Health J.* 2013;17:49-55.

184. Thurtle N, et al. Description of 3,180 courses of chelation with dimercaptosuccinic acid in children </= 5 y with severe lead poisoning in Zamfara, Northern Nigeria: a retrospective analysis of programme data. *PLoS Med.* 2014;11:e1001739.

185. Tinapu AE, et al. Congenital lead intoxication. *J Pediatr.* 1979;94:765-767.

186. Treatment of Lead-Exposed Children (TLC) Trial Group. Safety and efficacy of succimer in toddlers with blood lead levels of 20-44 ug/dL. *Pediatr Res.* 2000;48:593-599.

187. Tyroler HA. Epidemiology of hypertension as a public health problem: an overview as background for evaluation of blood lead-blood pressure relationship. *Environ Health Perspect.* 1988;78:3-8.

188. US Food and Drug Administration. Magellan Diagnostics Inc. expands recall for LeadCare Testing Systems due to inaccurate test results. https://www.fda.gov/MedicalDevices/Safety/ListofRecalls/ucm561936.htm. Published 2017. Accessed August 10, 2017.

189. US Department of Labor Occupational Safety and Health Administration. Occupational health and safety standard: occupational exposure to lead (29 CFR 1910.1025). *Fed Regist.* 1978;42:52952-53014.

190. US Department of Labor Occupational Safety and Health Administration. *Lead Standard (20 CFR 1910.1025; revised July 1, 1990).* Washington, DC: US Government Printing Office; 1990.

191. US Department of Labor Occupational Safety and Health Administration. Lead exposure in construction—interim final rule (29 CFR part 1926.62). *Fed Regist.* May 4, 1993.

192. US Department of the Interior. *Minerals Yearbook for 1990.* vol 1. Washington, DC: US Government Printing Office; 1991.

193. VanArsdale JL, et al. Lead poisoning from a toy necklace. *Pediatrics.* 2004;114:1096-1099.

194. Vander AJ. Chronic effects of lead on renin-angiotensin system. *Environ Health Perspect.* 1988;78:77-83.

195. Wade JF Jr, Burnum JF. Treatment of acute and chronic lead poisoning with disodium calcium versenate. *Ann Intern Med.* 1955;42:251-259.

196. Wedeen RP, et al. Clinical application of in vivo tibial K-XRF for monitoring lead stores. *Arch Environ Health.* 1995;50:355-361.

197. Weisskopf MG, et al. A prospective study of bone lead concentration and death from all causes, cardiovascular diseases, and cancer in the Department of Veterans Affairs Normative Aging Study. *Circulation.* 2009;120:1056-1064.

198. White LD, et al. New and evolving concepts in the neurotoxicology of lead. *Toxicol Appl Pharmacol.* 2007;225:1-27.

199. Whitfield CL, et al. Lead encephalopathy in adults. *Am J Med.* 1972;52:289-297.

200. Wiener RC, et al. Blood levels of the heavy metal, lead, and caries in children aged 24-72 months: NHANES III. *Caries Res.* 2015;49:26-33.

201. Wiley J, et al. Status epilepticus and severe neurologic impairment from lead encephalopathy [abstract]. *J Toxicol Clin Toxicol.* 1995;33:529-530.

202. Wiley JF, et al. Blood lead levels in children with foreign bodies. *Pediatrics.* 1992;89:593-596.

203. Wills BK, et al. Tetraethyl lead intoxication. *J Med Toxicol.* 2010;6:31-34.

204. Wilson IH, Wilson SB. Confounding and causation in the epidemiology of lead. *Int J Environ Health Res.* 2016;26:467-482.

205. Woolf AD, et al. Update on the clinical management of childhood lead poisoning. *Pediatr Clin North Am.* 2007;54:271-294.

206. Wright RO, et al. Biomarkers of lead exposure and DNA methylation within retrotransposons. *Environ Health Perspect.* 2010;118:790-795.

207. Ying XL, et al. Pediatric lead poisoning from folk prescription for treating epilepsy. *Clin Chim Acta.* 2016;461:130-134.

208. Ziegler EE, et al. Absorption and retention of lead by infants. *Pediatr Res.* 1978; 12:29-34.

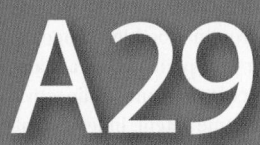

Antidotes in Depth

A29

SUCCIMER (2,3-DIMERCAPTOSUCCINIC ACID) AND DMPS (2,3-DIMERCAPTO-1-PROPANESULFONIC ACID)

Mary Ann Howland

Succimer
2,3-Dimercaptosuccinic acid

DMPS
2,3-Dimercapto-1-propanesulfonic acid

INTRODUCTION

Succimer (meso-2,3-dimercaptosuccinic acid, DMSA) is an orally active metal chelator that is approved by the US Food and Drug Administration (FDA) for the treatment of lead poisoning in children with blood lead concentrations greater than 45 mcg/dL. Succimer is also used to treat patients poisoned with arsenic and mercury. Succimer has a wider therapeutic index and exhibits many advantages over dimercaprol and ethylenediaminetetraacetic acid calcium disodium (CaNa$_2$EDTA), the 2 other chelators used for similar clinical problems. Animal studies demonstrate that succimer does not redistribute lead or arsenic to the central nervous system. The role of succimer alone and in conjunction with other chelators to treat lead encephalopathy continues to be defined.[64,78,107]

HISTORY

Succimer was initially synthesized in 1949 in England.[76] In 1954, antimony-a,a′-dimercaptopotassium succinate (TWSb) was developed to treat schistosomiasis.[45] Antimony-a,a′-dimercaptopotassium succinate is antimony bound to the potassium salt of succimer in a 2:3 ratio, forming a water-soluble xenobiotic with 50 times less toxicity than the previously employed antimony compound, tartar emetic. Chinese investigators subsequently demonstrated the ability of the sodium salt of succimer to increase the LD$_{50}$ of tartar emetic 16-fold in mice (Chap. 85).[119] An early review of the Chinese experience with intravenous (IV) succimer in the treatment of occupational lead and mercury poisoning suggested efficacy similar to IV CaNa$_2$EDTA in increasing urinary lead and to intramuscular (IM) DMPS (racemic-2,3-dimercapto-1-propanesulfonic acid) for mercury, with little observed toxicity.[105] This experience, the subsequent widespread use in Asia[80,83,95,115,116,122] and Europe,[18,37,43,46,67,105] and the realization that succimer could be used orally,[7,52] led to US-based animal experiments, human trials, and FDA approval in 1991 for the treatment of lead-poisoned children.

PHARMACOLOGY
Chemistry
Succimer is a white crystalline powder with a molecular weight of 182 Da and a characteristic sulfur odor and taste.[6] Succimer is the highly polar and water soluble form of 2,3-dimercaptosuccinic acid.

Related Chelators
Racemic-2,3-dimercapto-1-propanesulfonic acid (DMPS) is a chelator that, like succimer, is a water-soluble analog of dimercaprol (British anti-Lewisite

{BAL}).[7,9,25] A dose of 15 mg/kg of DMPS is equimolar to 12 mg/kg of succimer. 2,3-Dimercapto-1-propanesulfonic acid has been used in the Soviet Union since the late 1950s and continues to be used in Russia and Eastern Europe. 2,3-Dimercapto-1-propanesulfonic acid, which is an investigational drug in the United States, is marketed in both oral and parenteral forms in Germany as Dimaval. Dimercaptopropane sulfonate seems promising in mercury and arsenic poisoning.[3,5,7,9,11,14,25,48] Dimercaptopropane sulfonate is associated with an increase in the urinary excretion of copper and the development of Stevens-Johnson syndrome.[28,111] Like succimer, DMPS does not appear to redistribute mercury or lead to the brain. Additional research is needed to determine whether DMPS is more advantageous than succimer, given its lower LD$_{50}$ in mice (5.22 mmol/kg versus 13.58 mmol/kg for succimer) when administered intraperitonealy.[4]

Mechanisms of Action
Succimer contains 4 ionizable hydrogen ions, giving it 4 different pK$_a$s—2.31, 3.69, 9.68, and 11.14—with the dissociation of the 2 lower values representing the carboxyl groups and the 2 higher values the sulfur groups.[4] Lead and cadmium bind to the adjoining sulfur and oxygen atoms, whereas arsenic and mercury bind to the 2 sulfur moieties, forming pH-dependent water-soluble complexes (Fig. A29–1).[90]

Pharmacokinetics and Pharmacodynamics
Succimer is highly protein bound to albumin through a disulfide bond. Subhuman primate studies of IV and oral[24] succimer indicate that following an IV dose, radiolabeled succimer is eliminated almost exclusively via the kidney, with only trace amounts (<1%) excreted via feces or expired air.[24,76] Following the administration of a single oral dose of 10 mg/kg, succimer is rapidly and extensively metabolized.[73] Approximately 20% of the administered oral dose is recovered in the urine, presumably reflecting the low bioavailability of the drug.[10] Of the total drug eliminated in the urine (20%), 89% is altered and in the form of disulfides of L-cysteine. The majority of the altered succimer is in the form of a mixed disulfide with 2 molecules of L-cysteine to one molecule of succimer.[8] The remaining 11% is excreted as unaltered free succimer.[73] Maximal excretion of succimer occurs in urine specimens collected between 2 and 4 hours after administration. Surprisingly, the blood only contains albumin-bound succimer and no evidence of the altered disulfide moieties, which suggests that the kidney is involved in the biotransformation of succimer. It is likely that succimer gains entry to the kidney via an active organic anion transporter.[9,22,121]

The pharmacokinetics of a single oral dose of succimer were determined in 3 children and 3 adults with lead poisoning and in 5 healthy adult

FIGURE A29–1. The chelation of cadmium, lead, and mercury with succimer.

volunteers.[36] Children received 350 mg/m² of succimer, and adults received 10 mg/kg of succimer. The peak concentration and the time to peak blood concentration of total succimer (parent plus altered oxidized metabolites) were similar for all 3 groups. The half-life of total succimer was 1.5 times longer in the children than in either adult group. The renal clearance of total succimer was greater in healthy adults (Cl_{Cr} > 77 mL/min) than in lead-poisoned adults (Cl_{cr} = 25 mL/min) and children (Cl_{cr} = 17 mL/min) with reduced creatinine clearances. Distribution of succimer (parent and/or oxidized metabolites) into erythrocytes appeared greater in poisoned patients than in the healthy adults, whereas another study in human volunteers revealed no distribution into the red blood cells.[36,72]

The metabolism of succimer was studied in lead-poisoned children and in normal adults.[15] The results indicate that succimer undergoes an enterohepatic circulation facilitated by gastrointestinal (GI) microbiome. Similar to the previous pharmacokinetic study, moderate lead exposure impaired the renal elimination of succimer.

A simulation model of the plasma pharmacokinetics of succimer was developed in 2016. This model[113] was then expanded to predict the efficacy of succimer in reducing blood lead concentrations when prechelation concentrations were between 99 and 150 mcg/dL[112] and the duration of lead exposure is known. This model is likely to have utility when blood lead concentrations are not easily obtained.

ROLE IN LEAD POISONING

In addition to precise analysis of metal elimination kinetics, measures of clinical outcome are essential for an understanding of the utility of this chelator. The Treatment of Lead-Exposed Children (TLC) trial was a step in that direction.[109] The TLC trial was a randomized, multicenter, double-blind, placebo-controlled study of 780 children to examine the effects of succimer on cognitive development, behavior, stature, and blood pressure in children 1 to 3 years of age with blood lead concentrations between 20 and 44 mcg/dL.[91] The children received up to 3 courses of 26 days each of succimer compared to placebo. For the first 7 days, the children received 350 mg/m² 3 times a day and for the remaining 19 days they received 350 mg/m² twice a day. The largest drop in blood lead occurred within the first week of therapy with succimer and then rebounded somewhat. This pattern recurred with subsequent courses. However, at the end of one year, there was no difference in the blood lead concentrations between the succimer and the placebo groups. There was also no difference in test scores on cognition, behavior, or neuropsychological function.[91] A follow-up study conducted on those children at age 7 confirmed the lack of benefit in chelating children with succimer whose blood lead concentrations were 20 to 44 mcg/dL, at ages 1 to 3 years.[38] Similarly, succimer showed no benefit on growth in children aged 12 to 33 months with blood lead concentrations of 20 to 44 mcg/dL.[87]

Several groups are studying the efficacy of succimer in reducing blood, brain, and tissue lead by using rat and nonhuman primate models of childhood and adult lead poisoning.[96,98,100] Although monkeys most closely resemble humans in their lead-associated toxicity, using them in studies is costly;[82] the rat model is economical but limited because of species differences in lead and succimer metabolism and efficacy.

The validity of using blood lead concentrations as a marker of brain lead was studied in the adult rhesus monkey. Lead was administered orally for 5 weeks to achieve a target blood lead concentration of 35 to 40 mcg/dL.[35] Five days after the cessation of lead exposure, succimer chelation was initiated in the currently approved dosage regimen. Two IV doses of radioactive lead tracer were administered prior to succimer chelation to study the kinetics of recent versus chronic lead uptake and distribution. Four areas of the brain, as well as blood and bone, were assayed for lead. Merely stopping further lead exposure significantly reduced blood lead concentrations by 63% and brain lead concentrations by 34% compared with pretreatment concentrations, a finding that was not statistically different from succimer administration after halting exposure. However, when an integrated area under the serum lead concentration versus time curve (AUC) blood analysis was used over the 19-day succimer treatment course, instead of a single blood

lead concentration, the differences between succimer and control were statistically significant. The clinical significance of these differences is unclear. Succimer-treated animals showed the greatest drop in blood lead concentrations over the first 5 days, whereas a similar end point was gradually achieved in the control. The lead from both the recent exposure (radioactive tracer lead) and chronic exposure declined to the same extent, independent of treatment with succimer. A better correlation was found between brain prefrontal cortex lead concentrations and an integrated blood lead analysis than with a single blood lead measurement.

Similarly, a study in neonatal rats demonstrated that increasing the duration of succimer chelation from 7 to 21 days decreased brain lead concentrations without a corresponding decrease in blood lead concentrations.[96] The authors proposed that a slow rate of egress of brain lead to the blood was responsible for the demonstrable benefit of prolonging therapy to 21 days. In this study, succimer decreased blood lead concentration by approximately 50% when compared with the vehicle as the control, and this difference persisted for the 21 days of treatment. With succimer treatment, brain lead concentration decreased by 38% at 7 days and by 68% at 21 days. This same group also demonstrated that rats exposed to lead from postnatal days 1 to 30, then treated with succimer, demonstrated reductions in blood and brain lead concentrations and an improvement in cognitive deficits.[101] Previous animal studies demonstrated the ability of succimer to enhance urinary lead elimination[44,52,100] and to reduce blood,[17,32,41,42,57,85,98,100,102,104] brain,[17,32,85,103,104] liver,[100] and kidney lead concentrations,[17,32,41,57,85,104] while either reducing[17,57,85,104] or demonstrating no effect on bone lead concentrations.[32,100] These studies differ in the amounts and duration of lead administration prior to chelation, as well as in route, dose, and duration of chelation; however, several months after a course of succimer chelation, tissue lead concentrations had returned to concentrations found in the pretreatment stage.[32] Given the limited absolute amount of lead that is actually eliminated by chelation in comparison to the total body burden, particularly bone, these transient effects are not surprising.

Under a variety of experimental conditions in animals, succimer prevents the deleterious effect of lead on heme synthesis,[17,52,85] blood pressure,[61] and behavior.[102]

The use of succimer in both children and adults with chronic lead poisoning demonstrated consistent findings.[19,29,53–55,68,81] During the first 5 days of succimer chelation (1,050 mg/m²/day in children and 30 mg/kg/day in adults, both in 3 divided doses), the blood lead concentration dropped precipitously by approximately 60% to 70%. This blood lead concentration remained unchanged during the next 14 to 23 days of continued therapy. Increases in urinary lead excretion are concurrent with the reduction in blood lead concentration, with maximal excretion occurring on day 1.[29,54] Urinary lead excretion exceeds estimated blood content, which suggests that some lead is being removed from soft tissues as a concentration gradient is established from tissue to blood to urine.[29,55] Typically, 2 weeks after the completion of succimer, the blood lead concentration rebounds to values 20% to 40% lower than pretreatment values. In the one randomized, double-blind, placebo-controlled trial of succimer use in children with pretreatment blood lead concentrations of 30 to 45 mcg/dL, follow-up at one month and at 6 months showed no differences between succimer-treated children and controls.[81] Succimer restored red blood cell Delta-aminolevulinic acid dehydratase activity, decreased erythrocyte protoporphyrin, and decreased urinary excretion of Delta-aminolevulinic acid and coproporphyrin.[19,29,54,55,81]

There is a large body of evidence documenting on usage and safety profile of succimer in adults with chronic lead poisoning.[13,18,29,43,46,47,50,51,62,65,74,88,106,110] The published experience outside the United States with the use of oral succimer for metal poisoning includes nearly 100 adult cases and contributes considerably to the supporting evidence. At least 74 additional individuals were successfully treated parenterally (IM or IV) with the sodium salt of succimer.[13,18,43,46]

Role in Lead Encephalopathy

The experience with the use of succimer in severely lead-poisoned patients, including those with encephalopathy, is limited to case studies and a large retrospective analysis.[43,46,54,107] Three children with mean blood lead concentrations higher than 70 mcg/dL who were treated with 5 days of succimer achieved comparable declines in blood lead concentration to 2 similar children who had been treated previously with a combination of dimercaprol for 3 days and CaNa$_2$EDTA for 5 days.[54] Three adult patients with encephalopathy achieved significant improvement following succimer chelation.[43] An adult woman presented to the ED with seizures of unknown origin that resolved.[15] Two weeks later, she presented to another ED with worsening headache, weakness, and confusion and a CT scan of the brain that showed cerebral edema. She was intubated and ventilated for almost 2 weeks after extubation and with a persistent altered mental status a heavy metal screen revealed a lead concentration of 148 mcg/dL. One dose of dimercaprol was administered followed by succimer since CaNa$_2$EDTA was unavailable. Within 4 days her mental status returned to baseline and her weakness resolved. An analysis of her blood lead concentrations demonstrated an initial rise to 164 mcg/dL after succimer was administered followed by a steep decline to 102 mcg/dL in a day and 56 mcg/dL after 8 days. A 3-year-old child with a massive lead exposure superimposed on chronic lead poisoning and a blood lead concentration of 550 mcg/dL was given dimercaprol and CaNa$_2$EDTA for 5 days, with whole-bowel irrigation (WBI) was performed during the first 3 days and succimer following WBI beginning on day 3 and continuing for 19 days. When blood lead concentration was reduced from 550 to 70 mcg/dL on day 5, but rebounded to 99 mcg/dL 2 days after dimercaprol and CaNa$_2$EDTA were discontinued but not the succimer was discontinued.[49] Most recently, a retrospective analysis of more than 3,000 children with moderate to severe lead poisoning in resource-poor Nigeria were treated with succimer alone.[107] About one-third of the children had lead concentrations greater than 80 mcg/dL, 6% had concentrations >120 mcg/dL, and 24 had lead encephalopathy. The geometric mean of the postcourse blood lead concentration divided by the precourse blood lead concentration in patients treated with succimer and a precourse blood lead concentration greater than 120 mcg/dL was 68%. In the 3 months before the institution of succimer, there were 400 fatalities attributed to lead compared with 6 deaths during the 13 months when succimer was used.

ROLE IN ARSENIC POISONING

Succimer was used for arsenic toxicity in China and the Soviet Union since 1965.[7,13] Animal[63] studies with sodium arsenite and lewisite demonstrate the ability of succimer to improve the LD$_{50}$ with a good therapeutic index, lack of redistribution of arsenic to the brain as compared to dimercaprol or control, and reduced kidney and liver arsenic concentrations.[7,13,66,86,92] A few case reports of concentrations following ingestion of arsenic trioxide ant bait by toddlers attest to the ability of succimer to enhance the urinary excretion of arsenic,[34,93] and after 2 to 7 weeks of chelation, urinary arsenic returned to normal.[117] A randomized, placebo-controlled trial of succimer to treat 21 patients with chronic arsenic poisoning in India who had stopped ingesting arsenic contaminated water 5 months previously demonstrated improved clinical results and enhanced urinary excretion of arsenic in both the treatment and placebo groups, but no statistical differences could be demonstrated.[75] A comparison of dimercaprol, succimer, and DMPS as arsenic antidotes demonstrated higher therapeutic indices for succimer and DMPS over dimercaprol in chronic arsenic poisoning.[79]

ROLE IN MERCURY POISONING

Succimer enhances the elimination of mercury and has been used to treat patients poisoned with inorganic, elemental, and methylmercury. It improves survival, decreases kidney damage, and enhances the elimination of mercury in animals following exposure to inorganic mercury[4,24,57,60,69,89,120] and methylmercury.[1,2,9,70] However, one study in mice subjected to intraperitoneal mercuric chloride demonstrated an enhanced deposition of mercury in motor neurons following chelation with succimer or DMPS.[40] Of 53 construction workers who were exposed to mercury vapor, 11 received succimer and N-acetyl-D,L-penicillamine in a crossover study.[21] Mercury elimination was increased during the period of succimer administration compared with the period of N-acetyl-D,L-penicillamine administration. Because the chelators

were administered for only 2 weeks and late in the clinical course, therapeutic benefit could not be evaluated. When succimer was given to victims of an extensive Iraqi methylmercury exposure, blood methylmercury half-life decreased from 63 days to 10 days.[7] Animal studies suggest that succimer is not able to reduce brain mercury concentrations following inhalation of elemental mercury vapor although renal mercury concentrations did decrease.[63]

ADVERSE EVENTS AND SAFETY ISSUES

Succimer is generally well tolerated, with few serious adverse events reported.[29,30,91,108] Common adverse events are typically GI in nature, including nausea, vomiting, flatus, diarrhea, and a metallic taste in 10% to 20% of patients. Rashes are reported in about 4% of patients.[26] Fever and oropharyngeal ulcers with rash or rash alone are uncommon and are theorized to be fixed drug eruptions.[114] Some of these adverse events required discontinuation of the succimer. Mild elevations in aspartate aminotransferase and alanine aminotransferase considerations are reported.[22,28,30,55,68,84] In the Nigeria experience, ALT did not exceed 500 U/L and no hepatic failure was noted.[107,121] Rarely, chills, fever, urticaria, reversible neutropenia, and eosinophilia are reported.[19,29,30,50] Because neutropenia was observed in some patients taking succimer and because bone marrow effects are reported with other drugs in the same chemical class, we recommend a complete blood count with a differential and a platelet count before initiating treatment and weekly during treatment.[26] Therapy should be discontinued if the absolute neutrophil count drops to less than 1,200/μL.[26] During the latest open label prospective study in children, apparently unrelated adverse events included an elevation in bone-derived alkaline phosphatase, eosinophils, and elevated serum aminotransferases.[29] One patient developed severe hyperthermia and hypotension reportedly related to succimer administration.[84]

Chinese clinicians reported a high incidence of more serious adverse effects (including dizziness and weakness) in response to either IV or IM succimer.[116,122] This discrepancy is undoubtedly related to the substantially greater dose of succimer delivered from parenteral administration compared with the relatively low (20%)[76] oral bioavailability of succimer as a result of first-pass metabolism.

Incidental chelation of essential elements is always a concern with the use of chelators. A number of studies using succimer demonstrate no rise in urinary zinc, copper, iron, or calcium.[29,43,46,53–55] Urinary excretion of essential elements was the focus of a study in a primate model of childhood lead poisoning.[98] Infant rhesus monkeys were exposed to lead for the first year of life to achieve blood lead concentrations of 40 to 50 mcg/dL. Succimer was administered in the standard dosage regimen and complete urine collections over the first 5 days were analyzed for calcium, cobalt, copper, iron, magnesium, manganese, nickel, and zinc. Only when the data were analyzed collectively for all 8 elements on all 5 days was there a statistically significant increased urinary elimination. These results raise concern that children subjected to repeated succimer chelation are also be at risk for enhanced elimination of essential elements.[29,98,100] Therefore, children should be monitored and repleted with these essential elements as needed based on measured concentrations. There is still relatively limited clinical experience with succimer, particularly with regard to long-term administration.

A 3-week course of succimer administered to control rats produced a significant and long-lasting dysfunction in cognition and affect that was comparable to effects that occurred in rats exposed to high concentrations of lead.[97,101] The explanation for this finding is unknown but may be related to chelation of essential trace metals.

One concern with administering succimer orally is that outpatient management might permit continued unintentional lead exposure and the possibility for succimer-facilitated lead absorption. Studies with D-penicillamine, dimercaprol,[58] and CaNa$_2$EDTA demonstrate enhanced lead absorption and elevated blood lead concentrations.

Most blood lead concentrations are measured by graphite furnace atomic absorption spectrophotometry, in which case succimer does not interfere with the measurement. However, if blood lead concentrations were to be measured by anodic stripping voltammetry, succimer affects the results by chelating the mercury in the electrode.[26] Succimer is reported to cause a false-positive result for urinary ketones when tests using nitroprusside reagents are used, and falsely decreased serum uric acid and creatine phosphokinase concentrations.[26]

Animal studies suggest that succimer does not promote lead retention in the setting of continued exposure unless lead exposure is overwhelming.[52,59,85] A radiolabeled lead tracer administered to adult volunteers suggested that succimer increased the net absorption of lead from the GI tract and have distributed it to other tissues, as well as having enhanced urinary elimination.[99] Absorption is bimodal and consistent with an initial phase, followed by a delayed increase attributable to an enterohepatic effect. Succimer-enhanced urinary lead elimination often exceeds enhanced lead absorption.[86] However, this was not supported by a more recent study using a juvenile nonhuman primate model of moderate childhood lead poisoning. Oral succimer administered for multiple days after the oral administration of an oral lead tracer significantly reduced the gastrointestinal absorption of lead and enhanced the renal elimination of lead.[33] One study reported 2 children with environmental exposure and dramatic rises in blood lead concentrations while receiving succimer which is further supported by the epidemic lead poisoning in Zamfara, Nigeria ... although the compliance with succimer was unclear in one of these patients.[29] In the event of exposure to a new oral lead source, decontamination of the GI tract should complement oral succimer.[77]

Although iron supplementation cannot be given concomitantly with dimercaprol, because the dimercaprol–iron complex is a potent emetic, iron has been given concomitantly to patients receiving oral succimer without any adverse events.[56] The prevalence of both iron deficiency and elevated blood lead concentrations is highest among poor, inner-city children.[71] Because heme is a constituent of all cells, including those of the brain, it appears clinically indicated to provide iron supplementation during chelation therapy, when the heme pathway is freed of the inhibitory effects of lead. The timing of administration of the iron should be separate from administration of the succimer by a few hours.[29]

Overdoses of succimer are rarely reported. A case report describes a 3-year-old child who reportedly ingested 185 mg/kg of succimer and was asymptomatic.[94] Rodent models suggest doses of 2 gm/kg caused ataxia, seizures, labored breathing, and death.[26]

PREGNANCY AND LACTATION

Succimer is FDA pregnancy category C. There are no adequate studies in pregnant women. The use of succimer in pregnancy is restricted to women who warrant therapy based on their symptoms.[29] There was a dose-dependent effect of succimer on early and late fetal resorption and on fetal body weight and length when succimer was administered to pregnant mice during organogenesis. No observed teratogenic effects were noted when 410 mg/kg, or approximately 5% of the acute LD_{50}, of succimer was administered subcutaneously.[39] However, doses of 410 to 1,640 mg/kg/day of succimer administered subcutaneously to pregnant mice during organogenesis are teratogenic and fetotoxic, and doses of more than 510 mg/kg/day to pregnant rats also showed problems with reflexes in the offspring.[26] Succimer 30 to 60 mg/kg/day was administered by gavage to lead-poisoned rats from days 6 to 21 of gestation.[27] These doses of succimer decreased embryonic and fetal blood lead concentrations and normalized offspring body weight at 13 weeks. Although succimer was able to reverse some lead-induced immunotoxic effects, succimer itself caused problems with the immune system that persisted into adulthood.[27] Female mice exposed to lead in utero and then administered succimer from the fourth day of gestation to parturition demonstrated decreased blood lead concentrations; however, fetal liver and bone concentrations increased and worsened neural development in the offspring.[118] The exact mechanism for these effects is unknown, but disturbances in zinc and copper are hypothesized to be involved.[23] The use of succimer during pregnancy should only be undertaken if the potential benefit to the mother justifies the potential risk to the fetus.[26] It is not known whether succimer is excreted in human milk, but breast feeding is a contraindication in some sources and is discouraged in the package insert.[26] However, in the 2010 Centers for Disease Control and Prevention (CDC) Guidelines for the identification and management of lead exposure in pregnant and breastfeeding women the CDC suggests allowing breast feeding for mothers with blood lead concentrations of less than or equal to 40 mcg/dL. Mothers with BLLs of greater than 40 mcg/dL are encouraged to pump and discard their breast milk until their blood lead concentrations are reduced to less than 40 mcg/dL.

COMBINED CHELATION THERAPY

Succimer can be combined with $CaNa_2EDTA$ to take advantage of the ability of succimer to remove lead from soft tissues, including the brain, while capitalizing on the ability of $CaNa_2EDTA$ to mobilize lead from bone.[32] This combination is recommended in patients in whom dimercaprol would be indicated but is not available. A number of rodent models have examined this combination and found it to be superior to either drug alone in enhancing the elimination of lead, in reducing tissue concentrations of lead, and in remediating some lead-induced biochemical abnormalities.[41,42,103] Although the addition of succimer to $CaNa_2EDTA$ prevented the redistribution of lead to the brain caused by $CaNa_2EDTA$ alone, the combination also increased urinary excretion of zinc, calcium, and iron.[103,104] A retrospective review comparing dimercaprol plus $CaNa_2EDTA$ to succimer plus $CaNa_2EDTA$ in children with blood lead concentrations greater than 45 mcg/mL, demonstrated a similar reduction in blood lead concentrations at the end of treatment and at 14 and 33 days following the termination of treatment.[20] Blood lead concentration reductions were approximately 75%, 40%, and 37% at the end of therapy and at 14 and 33 days posttreatment, respectively. The succimer plus $CaNa_2EDTA$ combination was better tolerated.

DOSING AND ADMINISTRATION

The recommended dosage is 350 mg/m² in children, 3 times a day for 5 days, followed by 350 mg/m² twice a day for 14 days. In adults, the recommended dosage is 10 mg/kg 3 times a day for 5 days followed by 10 mg/kg twice a day for 14 days. At approximately 5 years of age, dosing based on body surface area approximates the 10-mg/kg dose, whereas for children younger than 5 years dosing by body surface area, as was done during the premarketing trials, resulted in higher doses and is recommended.[31,78] Repeated courses may be needed depending on the blood lead concentration (Chap. 93 and Table 93–8). However, a minimum of 2 weeks between courses is recommended unless blood lead concentrations are initially greater than 100 mcg/dL or the patient has lead encephalopathy.[26] For patients who cannot swallow the capsule whole, it can be separated immediately prior to use and the contents sprinkled into a small amount of juice or on apple sauce, ice cream, or any soft food, or placed on a spoon and followed by a fruit drink (Table A29–1).

FORMULATION AND ACQUISITION

Succimer is available as 100-mg bead-filled capsules. Povidone, sodium starch glycolate, starch, and sucrose are the inactive ingredients in the beads. The capsule contains gelatin, iron oxide, titanium dioxide, and other ingredients as inactive ingredients.

SUMMARY

- Succimer (meso-2,3-dimercaptosuccinic acid) is an orally active metal chelator that is FDA approved for the treatment of lead poisoning in children with blood lead concentrations greater than 45 mcg/dL.
- There is no evidence at this time that succimer improves cognitive performance in patients with blood lead concentrations less than 45 mcg/dL.
- Succimer is also used to treat patients poisoned with arsenic and mercury.
- The advantages of succimer use include oral administration, limited effects on trace metals such as zinc, enhanced patient tolerance, limited toxicity, and the ability to coadminister iron (if needed). It is acceptable to use in glucose-6-phosphate dehydrogenase–deficient patients.

TABLE A29–1A and B   Examples of Dosing Calculations

A. Succimer (available as 100-mg bead-filled capsules)

	Avg. Height (in.)	Avg. Weight (lb.)	m^2	350 mg/m^{2a}	10 mg/kg^a
Child					
2-year-old boy	36	30.5	0.593	189 mg	
2-year-old girl	35	29	0.57	200 mg	
4-year-old boy	42	39.75	0.73	255 mg	
4-year-old girl	41.75	38.75	0.72	250 mg	
Adult					
50-kg					500 mg
70-kg					700 mg
90-kg					900 mg

B. Chemet (Succimer) Pediatric Dosing Chart

Pounds	Kilograms	Dose (mg)^a	Number of Capsules^a
18–35	8–15	100	1
36–55	16–23	200	2
56–75	24–34	300	3
76–100	35–44	400	4
100	>45	500	5

^{a}To be administered every 8 hours for 5 days, followed by dosing every 12 hours for 14 days.

■ By contrast to CaNa$_2$EDTA, succimer does not redistribute lead to the brain of poisoned animals.[11,32]

■ Succimer was used in Nigeria, a resource-poor area without access to either dimercaprol or CaNa$_2$EDTA, for patients with moderate to severe lead poisoning including some patients with lead encephalopathy with apparent efficacy and safety.

REFERENCES

1. Aaseth J. Treatment of mercury and lead poisonings with dimercaptosuccinic acid and sodium dimercaptopropanesulfonate. *Analyst.* 1996;120:853-854.
2. Aaseth J, Friedheim EA. Treatment of methyl mercury poisoning in mice with 2,3-dimercaptosuccinic acid and other complexing thiols. *Acta Pharmacol Toxicol.* 1978;42:248-252.
3. Andersen O. Principles and recent developments in chelation treatment of metal intoxication. *Chem Rev.* 1999;99:2683-2710.
4. Aposhian HV. Succimer and DMPS—water-soluble antidotes for heavy metal poisoning. *Annu Rev Pharmacol Toxicol.* 1983;23:193-215.
5. Aposhian HV, Aposhian M. Aresenic toxicology: five questions. *Chem Res Toxicol.* 2006;19:1-15.
6. Aposhian HV, Aposhian MM. Meso-2,3-dimercaptosuccinic acid: chemical, pharmacological and toxicological properties of an orally effective metal chelating agent. *Annu Rev Pharmacol Toxicol.* 1990;30:279-306.
7. Aposhian HV, et al. Succimer, DMPS and DMPA—as arsenic antidotes. *Fundam Applied Toxicol.* 1984;4:S58-S70.
8. Aposhian HV, et al. Urinary excretion of meso-2,3 dimercaptosuccinic acid in human subjects. *Clin Pharmacol Ther.* 1989;45:520-526.
9. Aposhian HV, et al. Mobilization of heavy metals by newer, therapeutically useful chelating agents. *Toxicology.* 1995;97:23-38.
10. Aposhian HV, et al. Human studies with the chelating agents, DMPS and succimer. *J Toxicol Clin Toxicol.* 1992;30:505-528.
11. Aposhian M, et al. Sodium 2,3-dimercapto-1-propanesulfonate (DMPS) treatment does not redistribute lead or mercury to the brain of rats. *Toxicology.* 1996;109:49-55.
12. Aposhian HV, et al. Anti-lewisite activity and stability of meso-dimercaptosuccinic acid and 2,3-dimercapto-1-propanesulfonic acid. *Life Sci.* 1982;31:2149-2156.
13. Aposhian HV, et al. Protection of mice against the lethal effects of sodium arsenite: a quantitative comparison of a number of chelating agents. *Toxicol Appl Pharmacol.* 1981;61:385-392.
14. Aposhian HV, et al. DMPS-arsenic challenge test. *Toxicol Appl Pharmacol.* 2000;165:74-83.
15. Arnold J, Morgan B. Management of lead encephalopathy with DMSA after exposure to lead-contaminated moonshine. *J Med Toxicol.* 2015;11:464-467.
16. Asiedu P, et al. Metabolism of meso-2,3-dimercaptosuccinic acid in lead-poisoned children and normal adults. *Environ Health Perspect.* 1995;103:734-739.
17. Bankowska J, Hine C. Retention of lead in the rat. *Arch Environ Contam Toxicol.* 1985;14:621-629.
18. Bentur Y, et al. Meso-2,3-dimercaptosuccinic acid in the diagnosis and treatment of lead poisoning. *J Toxicol Clin Toxicol.* 1987;25:39-51.
19. Besunder JB, et al. Short-term efficacy of oral dimercaptosuccinic acid in children with low to moderate lead intoxication. *Pediatrics.* 1995;96:683-687.
20. Besunder JB, et al. Comparison of dimercaptosuccinic acid and calcium disodium ethylenediaminetetraacetic acid versus dimercaptopropanol and ethylenediaminetetraacetic acid in children with lead poisoning. *J Pediatr.* 1997;130:966-971.
21. Bluhm RE, et al. Elemental mercury vapour toxicity, treatment, and prognosis after acute, intensive exposure in chloralkali plant workers. I: history, neuropsychological findings and chelator effects. *Hum Exp Toxicol.* 1992;11:201-210.
22. Bradberry S, Vale A. Dimercaptosuccinic acid (succimer, DMSA) in inorganic lead poisoning. *Clin Tox (Phila).* 2009;47:617-631.
23. Briggs GG, et al. *Drugs in Pregnancy and Lactation: A Reference Guide to Fetal and Neonatal Risk.* 11th ed. Philadelphia, PA: Lippincott Williams & Wilkins; 2017.
24. Buchet JP, Lauwerys RR. Influence of 2,3 dimercaptopropane-1-sulfonate and dimercaptosuccinic acid on the mobilization of mercury from tissues of rats pretreated with mercuric chloride, phenylmercury acetate or mercury vapors. *Toxicology.* 1989;54:323-333.
25. Campbell JR, et al. The therapeutic use of 2,3-dimercaptopropane-1-sulfonate in two cases of inorganic mercury poisoning. *JAMA.* 1986;256:3127-3130.
26. Chemet (succimer) [package insert]. Deerfield, IL: Manufactured by Kremers Urban Pharmaceuticals Inc. Seymour, IN for Recordati Rare Diseases, Inc Lebanon, NJ, April 25, 2016.
27. Chen S, et al. Persistent effect of in utero meso-2,3-dimercaptosuccinic acid (DMSA) on immune function and lead-induced immunotoxicity. *Toxicology.* 1999;132:67-69.
28. Chisolm JJ. BAL, EDTA, DMSA and DMPS in the treatment of lead poisoning in children. *J Toxicol Clin Toxicol.* 1992;30:493-504.
29. Chisolm JJ. Safety and efficacy of meso-2,3-dimercaptosuccinic acid (DMSA) in children with elevated blood lead concentrations. *J Toxicol Clin Toxicol.* 2000;38:365-375.
30. Committee on Drugs. Treatment guidelines for lead exposure in children. *Pediatrics.* 1995;96:155-160.
31. Committee on Environmental Health. Lead exposure in children: prevention, detection and management. *Pediatrics.* 2005;116:1036-1046.
32. Cory-Slechta DA. Mobilization of lead over the course of DMSA chelation therapy and long-term efficacy. *J Pharmacol Exp Ther.* 1988;246:84-91.
33. Cremin JD, et al. Oral succimer decreases the gastro-intestinal absorption of lead in juvenile monkeys. *Environ Health Perspect* 2001;109:613-619.
34. Cullen NA, et al. Pediatric arsenic ingestion. *Am J Emerg Med.* 1995;13:432-435.
35. Cremin JD, et al. Efficacy of succimer chelation for reducing brain lead in a primate model of human exposure. *Toxicol Appl Pharmacol.* 1999;161:283-293.
36. Dart RC, et al. Pharmacokinetics of meso-2,3-dimercaptosuccinic acid in patients with lead poisoning and in healthy adults. *J Pediatr.* 1994;125:309-316.
37. Devars DuMayne JF, et al. Lead poisoning treated with 2,3-dimercaptosuccinic acid. *Presse Med.* 1984;13:2209.
38. Dietrich K, et al. Effect of chelation therapy on the neuropsychological and behavioral development of lead exposed children after school entry. *Pediatrics.* 2004;114:19-26.
39. Domingo JL, et al. Developmental toxicity of subcutaneously administered meso-2,3-dimercaptosuccinic acid in mice. *Fundam Appl Toxicol.* 1986;11:715-722.
40. Ewan KB, Pamphlett R. Increased inorganic mercury in spinal motor neurons following chelating agents. *Neurotoxicology.* 1996;17:343-349.
41. Flora GJS, et al. Therapeutic efficacy of combined meso-2,3-dimercaptosuccinic acid and calcium disodium edetate treatment during acute lead intoxication in rats. *Hum Exp Toxicol.* 1995;14:410-413.
42. Flora SJS, et al. Combined therapeutic potential of meso-2,3-dimercaptosuccinic acid and calcium disodium versenate on the mobilization and distribution of lead in experimental lead intoxication in rats. *Fundam Appl Toxicol.* 1995;25:233-240.
43. Fournier L, et al. 2,3-Dimercaptosuccinic acid treatment of heavy metal poisoning in humans. *Med Toxicol.* 1988;3:499-504.
44. Friedheim E, et al. Meso-dimercaptosuccinic acid, a chelating agent for the treatment of mercury and lead poisoning. *J Pharm Pharmacol.* 1976;28:711-712.
45. Friedheim E, DaSilva JR. Treatment of schistosomiasis mansonii with antimony a,a'-dimercapto-potassium succinate (TWSb). *Am J Trop Med Hyg.* 1954;3:714-727.
46. Friedheim E, et al. Treatment of lead poisoning by 2,3-dimercaptosuccinic acid. *Lancet.* 1978;2:1234-1235.
47. Glotzer DE. The current role of 2,3-dimercaptosuccinic acid (succimer) in the management of childhood lead poisoning. *Drug Saf.* 1993;9:85-92.
48. Gonzalez-Ramirez D, et al. DMPS (2,3-dimercaptopropane-1-sulfonate, Dimaval) decreases the body burden of mercury in humans exposed to mercurous chloride. *J Pharm Exp Ther.* 1998;287:8-12.
49. Gordon R, et al. Aggressive approach in the treatment of acute lead encephalopathy with an extraordinarily high concentration of lead. *Arch Pediatr Adolesc Med.* 1998;152:1100-1104.
50. Grandjean P, et al. Chronic lead poisoning treated with dimercaptosuccinic acid. *Pharmacol Toxicol.* 1991;68:266-269.

51. Graziano JH. Role of 2,3-dimercaptosuccinic acid in the treatment of heavy metal poisoning. *Med Toxicol.* 1986;1:155-162.

52. Graziano JH, et al. 2,3-Dimercaptosuccinic acid: a new agent for the treatment of lead poisoning. *J Pharm Exp Ther.* 1978;206:696-700.

53. Graziano JH, et al. A dose–response study of oral 2,3-dimercaptosuccinic acid (succimer) in children with elevated blood lead concentrations. *J Pediatr.* 1988;113:751-757.

54. Graziano JH, et al. Controlled study of meso-2,3-dimercaptosuccinic acid for the management of childhood lead intoxication. *J Pediatr.* 1992;120:133-139.

55. Graziano JH, et al. 2,3-Dimercaptosuccinic acid as an antidote for lead intoxication. *Clin Pharmacol Ther.* 1985;37:431-438.

56. Haust HL, et al. Intramuscular administration of iron during long-term chelation therapy with 3,2-dimercaptosuccinic acid in a man with severe lead poisoning. *Clin Biochem.* 1989;22:189-196.

57. Jones M, et al. Effect of chelate treatment on kidney, bone, and brain levels of lead-intoxicated mice. *Toxicology.* 1994;89:91-100.

58. Jugo S, et al. Influence of chelating agents on the gastrointestinal absorption of lead. *Toxicol Appl Pharmacol.* 1975;34:259-263.

59. Kapoor SC, et al. Influence of 2,3-dimercaptosuccinic acid on gastrointestinal lead absorption and whole body lead retention. *Toxicol Appl Pharmacol.* 1989;97:525-529.

60. Keith RL, et al. Utilization of renal slices to evaluate the efficacy of chelating agents for removing mercury from the kidney. *Toxicology.* 1997;116:67-75.

61. Khalil-Manesh F, et al. Effect of chelation treatment with dimercaptosuccinic acid (succimer) on lead-related blood pressure changes. *Environ Res.* 1994;65:86-99.

62. Klaassen CD. Heavy metals and heavy-metal antagonists. In: Gilman AG, et al, eds. *Goodman and Gilman's the Pharmacological Basis of Therapeutics.* 7th ed. New York, NY: Macmillan; 1985:1605-1627.

63. Kosnett MJ. The role of chelation in the treatment of arsenic and mercury poisoning. *J Med Toxicol.* 2013;9:347-354.

64. Kosnett MJ. Unanswered questions in metal chelation. *J Toxicol Clin Toxicol.* 1992;304:529-547.

65. Kosnett M, et al. Recommendations for medical management of adult lead exposure. *Environ Health Perspect.* 2007;115:463-471.

66. Kreppel H, et al. Therapeutic efficacy of new dimercaptosuccinic acid (succimer) analogues in acute arsenic trioxide poisoning in mice. *Arch Toxicol.* 1993;67:580-585.

67. Lenz K, et al. 2,3-Dimercaptosuccinic acid in human arsenic poisoning. *Arch Toxicol.* 1981;47:241-243.

68. Liebelt E, Shannon M. Oral chelators for childhood lead poisoning. *Pediatr Ann.* 1994;23:616-626.

69. Magos L. The effects of dimercaptosuccinic acid on the excretion and distribution of mercury in rats and mice treated with mercuric chloride and methylmercury chloride. *Br J Pharmacol.* 1976;56:479-484.

70. Magos L, et al. Postexposure preventive treatment of methylmercury intoxication in rats with dimercaptosuccinic acid. *Toxicol Appl Pharmacol.* 1978;45:463-475.

71. Mahaffey KR. Factors modifying susceptibility to lead. In: Mahaffey KR, ed. *Dietary and Environmental Lead: Human Health Effects.* New York, NY: Elsevier; 1985:373-419.

72. Maiorino RM, et al. Determination and metabolism of dithiol chelating agents: X. In humans, meso-2,3-dimercaptosuccinic acid is bound to plasma proteins via mixed disulfide formation. *J Pharmacol Exp Ther.* 1990;254:570-577.

73. Maiorino RM, et al. Determination and metabolism of dithiol chelating agents: VI. Isolation and identification of the mixed disulfides of meso-2,3-dimercaptosuccinic acid with L-cysteine in human urine. *Toxicol Appl Pharmacol.* 1989;97:338-349.

74. Mann KV, Travers JD. Succimer, an oral lead chelator. *Clin Pharm.* 1991;10:914-922.

75. Mazumder DN, et al. Chronic arsenic toxicity in West Bengal—the worst calamity in the world. *J Indian Med Assoc.* 1998;96:4-7, 18.

76. McGown EL, et al. Biological behavior and metabolic fate of the BAL analogues succimer and DMPS. *Proc West Pharmacol Soc.* 1984;27:169-176.

77. McKinney PE. Acute elevation of blood lead levels within hours of ingestion of large quantities of lead shot. *J Toxicol Clin Toxicol.* 2000;38:435-440.

78. Mortensen ME. Succimer chelation: what is known? *J Pediatr.* 1994;125:233-234.

79. Muckter H, et al. Are we ready to replace dimercaprol (BAL) as an arsenic antidote? *Hum Exp Toxicol.* 1997;16:460-465.

80. Ni W, et al. A study of oral succimer in the treatment of lead poisoning. Personal communication, 1989.

81. O'Connor ME, Rich D. Children with moderately elevated lead levels: is chelation with succimer helpful? *Clin Pediatr (Phila).* 1999;38:325-331.

82. O'Flaherty EJ, et al. Plasma and blood lead concentrations, lead absorption and lead excretion in sub-human primates. *Toxicol Appl Pharmacol.* 1996;138:121-130.

83. Okonishnokova IE, Rosenberg EE. Succimer as a means of chemoprophylaxis against occupational poisonings of workers handling mercury. *Gig Tr Prof Zabol.* 1971;15:29-32.

84. Okose P, et al. Untoward effects of oral dimercaptosuccinic acid in the treatment of lead poisoning [abstract]. *Vet Hum Toxicol.* 1991;33:376.

85. Pappas JB, et al. Oral dimercaptosuccinic acid and ongoing exposure to lead: effects on heme synthesis and lead distribution in a rat model. *Toxicol Appl Pharmacol.* 1995;133:121-129.

86. Pappas JB, et al. The effect of oral succimer on ongoing exposure to lead [abstract]. *Vet Hum Toxicol.* 1992;34:361.

87. Peterson K, et al. Effect of succimer on growth of preschool children with moderate blood lead levels. *Environ Health Perspect.* 2004;112:233-237.

88. Piomelli S, et al. Management of childhood lead poisoning. *J Pediatr.* 1984;105:523-532.

89. Planas-Bohne F. The influence of chelating agents on the distribution and biotransformation of methylmercuric chloride in rats. *J Pharmacol Exp Ther.* 1981;217:500-504.

90. Rivera M, et al. Determination and metabolism of dithiol-containing agents VIII. Metal complexes of mesodimercaptosuccinic acid. *Toxicol Appl Pharmacol.* 1989;100:96-106.

91. Rogan WJ, et al; Treatment of Lead-Exposed Children Trial Group. The effect of chelation therapy with succimer on neuropsychological development in children exposed to lead. *N Engl J Med.* 2001;344:1421-1426.

92. Schafer B, et al. Effect of oral treatment with BAL, DMPS or succimer in organs of mice injected with arsenic trioxide. *Arch Toxicol.* 1991;14(suppl):228-230.

93. Shum S, et al. Chelation of organoarsenate with dimercaptosuccinic acid. *Vet Hum Toxicol.* 1995;37:239-242.

94. Sigg T, et al. A report of pediatric succimer overdose. *Vet Hum Toxicol.* 1998;40:90-91.

95. Singh PK, et al. Mobilization of lead by esters of meso-2,3-dimercaptosuccinic acid. *J Toxicol Environ Health.* 1989;27:423-434.

96. Smith D, et al. Efficacy of succimer chelation for reducing brain Pb levels in a rodent model. *Environ Res.* 1998;78:168-176.

97. Smith D, Strupp BJ. The scientific basis for chelation: animal studies and lead chelation. *J Med Toxicol.* 2013;9:326-338.

98. Smith DR, et al. Succimer and the urinary excretion of essential elements in a primate model of childhood lead exposure. *Toxicol Sci.* 2000;54:473-480.

99. Smith DR, et al. Methodological considerations for the accurate determination of lead in human plasma and serum. *Am J Ind Med.* 1998;33:430-438.

100. Smith DR, et al. Succimer and the reduction of tissue lead in juvenile monkeys. *Toxicol Appl Pharmacol.* 2000;166:230-240.

101. Stangle D, et al. Succimer chelation improves learning, attention, and arousal recognition in lead exposed rats but produces lasting cognitive impairment in the absence of lead exposure. *Environ Health Perspect.* 2007;115:201-209.

102. Stewart PW, et al. Acute and longer term effects of meso-2,3 dimercaptosuccinic acid (succimer) on the behavior of lead-exposed and control mice. *Physiol Behav.* 1996;59:849-855.

103. Tandon SK, et al. Efficacy of combined chelation in lead intoxication. *Chem Res Toxicol.* 1994;7:585-589.

104. Tandon SK, et al. Mobilization of lead by calcium versenate and dimercaptosuccinate in the rat. *Clin Exp Pharmacol.* 1998;25:686-692.

105. Thomas G, et al. Nail dystrophy and dimercaptosuccinic acid. *J Toxicol Clin Exp.* 1987;7:285-287.

106. Thomas PS, Ashton C. An oral treatment for lead toxicity. *Postgrad Med J.* 1991;67:63-65.

107. Thurtle N, et al. Description of 3,180 courses of chelation with dimercaptosuccinic acid in children ≤5 y with severe lead poisoning in Zamfara, Northern Nigeria: a retrospective analysis of programme data. *PLoS Med.* 2014;11:e1001739.

108. Treatment of Lead-Exposed Children (TLC) Trial Group. Safety and efficacy of succimer in toddlers with blood lead levels 20-44 µg/dL. *Pediatr Res.* 2000;48:593-599.

109. Treatment of Lead-Exposed Children (TLC) Trial Group. The Treatment of Lead-Exposed Children (TLC) trial: design and recruitment for a study of the effect of oral chelation on growth and development in toddlers. *Pediatr Perinat Epidemiol.* 1998;12:313-333.

110. Tuntunji MF, al-Mahasneh QM. Disappearance of heme metabolites following chelation therapy with meso 2,3-dimercaptosuccinic acid (succimer). *J Toxicol Clin Toxicol.* 1994;32:267-276.

111. Van Der Linde A, et al. Stevens-Johnson syndrome in a child with chronic mercury exposure and 2,3-dimercaptopropane-1-sulfate (DMPS) therapy. *Clin Toxicol.* 2008;46:479-481.

112. van Eijkeren JC, et al. Modeling the effect of succimer (DMSA; dimercaptosuccinic acid) chelation therapy in patients poisoned by lead. *Clin Toxicol (Phila).* 2017;55:133-141.

113. van Eijkeren JC, et al. Modelling dimercaptosuccinic acid (DMSA) plasma kinetics in humans. *Clin Toxicol (Phila).* 2016;54:833-839.

114. Varma A, et al. Rash and pyrexia after succimer (dimercaptosuccinic acid; DMSA). *Clin Toxicol (Phila).* 2017;55:680.

115. Wang SC, et al. Chelating therapy with NaDMS in occupational lead and mercury intoxication. *Chin Med J.* 1965;84:437-439.

116. Xue H, et al. Comparison of lead excretion of patients after injection of five chelating agents. *Chung Kuo Yao Li Hsuch Pao.* 1982;3:41-44.

117. Yarris J, et al. Acute arsenic trioxide ant bait ingestion by toddlers. *Clin Toxicol.* 2008;46:785-789.

118. Yu F, et al. Effects of in utero meso-2,3-dimercaptosuccinic acid with calcium and ascorbic acid on lead induced fetal development. *Arch Toxicol.* 2008;82:453-459.

119. Yu-I L, et al. Studies on antibilharzial drugs VI: the antidotal effects of sodium dimercaptosuccinate and BAL-glucoside against tartar emetic. *Acta Physiol Sinica.* 1957;21:24-32.

120. Zalups RK. Influence of 2,3-dimercaptopropoane-1-sulfonate (DMPS) and meso-2,3-dimercaptosuccinic acid (succimer) on the renal disposition of mercury in normal and uninephrectomized rats exposed to inorganic mercury. *J Pharmacol Exp Ther.* 1993;267:791-799.

121. Zalups RK, Bridges CC. Relationships between the renal handling of DMPS and DMSA and the renal handling of mercury. *Chem Res Toxicol.* 2012;25:1825-1838.

122. Zhang J. Clinical observations in ethyl mercury chloride poisoning. *Am J Ind Med.* 1984;5:251-258.

A30 EDETATE CALCIUM DISODIUM (CaNa$_2$EDTA)

Mary Ann Howland

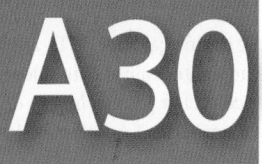

INTRODUCTION

Edetate calcium disodium (CaNa$_2$EDTA) is a chelator that is primarily used for the management of patients with severe lead poisoning (blood lead concentrations >70 mcg/dL) in conjunction with dimercaprol (British anti-Lewisite {BAL}). Edetate calcium disodium was replaced by succimer for the treatment of patients with lead concentrations between 45 and 70 mcg/dL. In a clinical trial with much criticism, disodium EDTA (Na$_2$EDTA) reduced adverse cardiovascular outcomes in patients with a history of myocardial infarction.[3,22,36,41] We recommend against using this preparation (Na$_2$EDTA) for lead chelation because of the potential for life-threatening hypocalcemia.

HISTORY

Ethylenediaminetetraacetic acid (EDTA) was discovered and synthesized in the 1930s and approved by the US Food and Drug Administration (FDA) as a food additive in the 1940s. Investigations on CaNa$_2$EDTA for lead toxicity and for Na$_2$EDTA for the reversal of cardiovascular disease began in the 1950s.

PHARMACOLOGY

Chemistry

Edetate calcium disodium is an ionic, water-soluble compound with an anhydrous molecular weight of 374.27 Da. It is also referred to as calcium disodium versenate, calcium disodium EDTA, or calcium disodium ethylenediaminetetraacetic acid.

Mechanism of Action

Edetate calcium disodium belongs to the family of polyaminocarboxylic acids. Although it is capable of chelating many metals, its current use is almost exclusively in the management of lead poisoning. The term *chelate* has its origin in the Greek word *chele*, which means "claw," implying an ability to tightly grasp the metal.[52] Implicit in chelation is the formation of a ring-structured complex. When CaNa$_2$EDTA chelates lead, the calcium is displaced and the lead takes its place, forming a stable ring compound.[34] Bone is the primary source of lead chelated by CaNa$_2$EDTA. The blood lead concentration drops due to urinary elimination; however, once chelation is stopped, redistribution to soft tissues, including the brain, and then bone occurs.[11] Although zinc, iron, manganese, copper, and mercury are also capable of displacing calcium and forming a stable chelate, for a number of reasons, only the effect on zinc is clinically significant.

PHARMACOKINETICS AND PHARMACODYNAMICS

Edetate calcium disodium is a highly polar drug with a small volume of distribution (V$_d$) due to its polar nature and approximates that of the extracellular fluid compartment regardless of renal function.[29,34,42] In one study of 14 patients the V$_d$ was 0.05 to 0.23 L/kg.[42] Edetate calcium disodium appears to penetrate erythrocytes poorly,[2,29] and less than 5% of CaNa$_2$EDTA gains access to the spinal fluid.[29,34] Oral administration of CaNa$_2$EDTA is not practical because the bioavailability is less than 5%. The half-life is about 20 to 60 minutes.[6,29,34] When CaNa$_2$EDTA combines with lead, it forms a stable, soluble, nonionized compound subsequently excreted in the urine. Following CaNa$_2$EDTA administration, urinary lead excretion is increased 20- to 50-fold.[14,43] Renal elimination approximates the glomerular filtration rate,[40] which correlates with creatinine clearance,[9] resulting in the excretion of 50% of CaNa$_2$EDTA in the urine within 1 hour, and more than 95% within 24 hours.[29,34] Elimination is entirely via the kidney with no appreciable metabolism.

ROLE IN LEAD EXPOSURE

Animals

A mouse study demonstrated a decrease in tissue lead stores, including brain concentrations, when measurements are performed following CaNa$_2$EDTA therapy.[32] A rat study examining the effect of a single dose of CaNa$_2$EDTA on brain lead concentrations demonstrated a significant increase in brain lead concentrations,[22] suggesting that CaNa$_2$EDTA initially mobilizes lead and facilitates adverse redistribution to the brain. Additional doses enhanced lead elimination, reduced blood lead concentrations, and subsequently reduced brain lead concentrations to prechelation concentrations but without any net loss from the brain.[22] The initial increase in brain lead offers an explanation to why some human case reports demonstrate worsening lead encephalopathy when CaNa$_2$EDTA is used without concomitant dimercaprol (BAL) chelation therapy.[19,43]

Humans

The CaNa$_2$EDTA mobilization test was once widely recommended as a diagnostic aid for assessing the potential benefits of chelation therapy, but has since been abandoned.[15,19,22,38,39] Criticisms of the mobilization test include difficulties with administration of the antidote, unreliability as a predictor of total-body lead burden, expense, and the risk of worsening toxicity through redistribution of lead to either the kidney or the brain.[19]

Edetate calcium disodium is capable of reducing blood lead concentrations, enhancing renal excretion of lead, and reversing the effects of lead on hemoglobin synthesis.[19] With chronic lead exposure, blood lead concentrations rebound considerably in the days to weeks following cessation of CaNa$_2$EDTA.[1,2,31] No rigorous clinical studies were ever performed to evaluate whether CaNa$_2$EDTA reverses the neurobehavioral effects of lead.[20,21] Chelators are incapable of dramatically decreasing the body burden of lead, because only several milligrams of lead are eliminated during chelation.[14,16,44] Children evaluated with blood lead concentrations of 25 to 50 mcg/dL who were given CaNa$_2$EDTA for 5 days revealed very little difference in blood lead, or bone lead, or erythrocyte protoporphyrin concentrations, when compared to pretreatment values in unchelated patients.[37] A study in children demonstrated no additional benefits of CaNa$_2$EDTA on cognitive performance beyond that which was achieved by limiting further lead exposure and correcting iron deficiency anemia.[43,45] A follow-up study in children with initial blood lead concentrations between 25 and 55 mcg/dL also suggested an interaction between initial iron stores, blood lead concentration, and an improvement in perceptual motor performance over a 6-month period. Both the correction of iron deficiency and a reduction in blood lead concentration (accomplished with limiting further exposure and or CaNa$_2$EDTA chelation) contributed to the improvement, emphasizing a critical need to correct iron deficiency anemia as well as limit lead exposure.[46]

ADVERSE EVENTS AND SAFETY ISSUES

The principal toxicity of $CaNa_2EDTA$ is related to the metal chelates it forms. In mice, the intraperitoneal (IP) LD_{50} values of various $CaNa_2EDTA$ metal chelates are $CaNa_2EDTA$, 14.3 mmol/kg; lead EDTA, 3.1 mmol/kg; and mercury EDTA, 0.01 mmol/kg.

When $CaNa_2EDTA$ is given to patients with lead poisoning, the resultant sites of major renal toxicity are the proximal convoluted tubule, the distal convoluted tubule, and the glomeruli, possibly caused by the release of lead in the kidneys during excretion.[7,11,19,34] We recommend monitoring urine output, proteinuria, serum creatinine, and BUN. Of the 130 children who received both dimercaprol and $CaNa_2EDTA$, 13% had biochemical evidence of nephrotoxicity, and 3% developed acute oliguric kidney injury, which resolved over time; none needed hemodialysis.[39] Because lead toxicity causes kidney damage independent of chelation, it is important to monitor kidney function closely during $CaNa_2EDTA$ administration and to adjust the dose and schedule appropriately.[11,40] Nephrotoxicity is minimized by limiting the total daily dose of $CaNa_2EDTA$ to 1 g in children or to 2 g in adults, although higher doses are recommended to treat lead encephalopathy.[43] Continuous infusion while maintaining good hydration increases efficacy and decreases toxicity.[40] Because the administration of disodium EDTA, a grave medical error can lead to life-threatening hypocalcemia and death,[23,27] $CaNa_2EDTA$ is the preparation of choice for lead toxicity and the risk of hypocalcemia is no longer a clinical concern.[4,9] Other adverse clinical effects of $CaNa_2EDTA$, most of which are uncommon, include malaise, fatigue, thirst, chills, fever, myalgias, headache, anorexia, urinary frequency and urgency, sneezing, nasal congestion, lacrimation, glycosuria, anemia, transient hypotension, increased prothrombin time, and inverted T waves on the ECG.[11,34] Various mucocutaneous lesions described in 2 patients included cheilosis and sore throat, magenta tongue, and extensive papular lesions attributed to zinc deficiency.[7] Typically reversible, mild increases in alanine aminotransferase and aspartate aminotransferase, and decreases in alkaline phosphatase are frequently reported. Extravasation resulted in the development of painful calcinosis at the injection site.[43,47] Depletion of endogenous metals, particularly zinc, results from chronic therapy.[12,50] An animal study suggests that gastrointestinal lead absorption is enhanced by either IP or oral administration of $CaNa_2EDTA$;[33] consequently, removal of lead from the environment should always remain the first strategy in the management of lead toxicity. In the event of exposure to a new lead source, decontamination of the gastrointestinal tract should complement chelation.[38]

PREGNANCY AND LACTATION

Although $CaNa_2EDTA$ is FDA pregnancy category B, there are no adequate and well-controlled studies in pregnant women and a risk-to-benefit analysis must be made prior to use. Lead encephalopathy is life threatening, and chelation should be commenced regardless of the trimester.[13] It is not known whether $CaNa_2EDTA$ is excreted in human milk, but breastfeeding is a contraindication[8] in some sources and is listed as a caution in the package insert.[11] However, in the 2010 Centers for Disease and Prevention (CDC) Guidelines for the identification and management of lead exposure in pregnant and breastfeeding women, the CDC suggests allowing breastfeeding for mothers with blood lead concentrations of less than or equal to 40 mcg/dL. Mothers with blood lead concentrations of greater than 40 mcg/dL are encouraged to pump and discard their breast milk until their BLLs drop to less than 40 mcg/dL.

In a model of lead poisoning in pregnant rats, fetal resorption decreased and the number of live fetuses increased when $CaNa_2EDTA$ was used, although the placental concentrations of lead were increased.[25] Zinc concentrations were not affected. However, another study found that when $CaNa_2EDTA$ was given to pregnant rats not poisoned with lead, increases in submucous clefts, cleft palate, adactyly/syndactyly, curly tail, and abnormal ribs and vertebrae resulted.[10] These teratogenic effects occurred with doses of $CaNa_2EDTA$ comparable to human doses and without causing noticeable

changes in the mother except for weight gain. Use of zinc calcium EDTA and zinc EDTA preparations in pregnant rats caused no teratogenic effects at low doses, but resulted in the development of submucous cleft palates in 30% of the offspring receiving the higher dose of zinc calcium EDTA.[10] Another study in rats with doses 25 to 40 times that used in humans revealed fetal malformations that were prevented by simultaneous zinc supplementation.[11]

Of 7 cases reported by the CDC of pregnant women who received chelation therapy, all but one was chelated in the seventh or eighth month. Six patients received $CaNa_2EDTA$, with one of those also receiving dimercaprol for a maternal BLL of 104 mcg/dL. One patient received succimer alone. The dosage regimens were variable as was the time from chelation to delivery. Four of 6 newborns had cord blood concentrations lower than the maternal prechelation concentration. Six of 7 newborns appeared healthy at delivery. One premature infant was born following an antepartum hemorrhage with subsequent developmental delay and hearing deficits after 36 hours of chelation to a mother with a pretreatment lead concentration of 104 mcg/dL.[13]

DOSING AND ADMINISTRATION

There has never been a clinical trial to identify the best dose of $CaNa_2EDTA$ or how best to administer the dose. The most commonly recommended dose is determined by the patient's by surface area or weight (up to a maximum dose), the severity of the poisoning, and kidney function (Chap. 93; Tables 93–8 and A30–1).[19,37,43] For patients with lead encephalopathy, the dose of $CaNa_2EDTA$ recommended is 1,500 mg/m²/day, approximately 50 to 75 mg/kg/day, by continuous IV infusion, starting 4 hours after the first dose of dimercaprol. The initiation of an adequate urine flow is recommended before administering $CaNa_2EDTA$.[14,18,19,43] The dose in obese patients has not been studied. A maximum dose of 3 g is reasonable. Simultaneous dimercaprol and $CaNa_2EDTA$ therapy is typically administered for 5 days, followed by a rest period of at least 2 to 4 days, which permits lead redistribution. For adults with lead nephropathy, the following dosage regimen is recommended: 500 mg/m² every 24 hours for 5 days for patients with a serum creatinine of 2 to 3 mg/dL; every 48 hours for 3 doses for a serum creatinine of 3 to 4 mg/dL; and one dose for a serum creatinine concentration greater than 4 mg/dL.[11] Previous recommendations were to limit the daily dose to 50 mg/kg when $CaNa_2EDTA$ is used in patients with kidney dysfunction.[29,40,42] The data supporting the use of folic acid, pyridoxine, and thiamine to increase the efficacy of $CaNa_2EDTA$[48] is inadequate to recommend routine administration. A blood lead concentration should be measured no sooner than one hour after the $CaNa_2EDTA$ infusion is discontinued in order to avoid falsely elevated blood lead concentrations.

In symptomatic children without manifestations of lead encephalopathy, the recommended dose of $CaNa_2EDTA$ is 1,000 mg/m²/day, approximately 25 to 50 mg/kg/day, in addition to dimercaprol at 50 mg/m² every 4 hours.[43] The demonstrated ability of succimer to reduce brain lead concentrations in animals led to the replacement of $CaNa_2EDTA$ by succimer as the chelator of choice in lead-poisoned children without encephalopathy and lead concentration less than 70 mcg/dL.[16,31] Adding to the evidence supporting succimer is a retrospective analysis of more than 3,000 children in a resource-poor area of Nigeria with moderate to severe lead poisoning. Treatment with succimer alone appeared safe and effective although long-term efficacy is still being determined.[51]

Because of the pain associated with intramuscular (IM) administration, it is recommended that $CaNa_2EDTA$ be administered at concentrations of approximately 0.5% by continuous IV infusion in 5% dextrose or 0.9% NaCl over 24 hours. Higher concentrations may lead to thrombophlebitis.[19] The package insert recommends infusing the dose over 8 to 12 hours.[11] In light of the short half-life of $CaNa_2EDTA$, we think it is reasonable to infuse the dose continuously over 24 hours. Edetate calcium disodium is incompatible with other solutions. Careful attention to total fluid requirements in children and patients who have, or who are at risk for lead encephalopathy is paramount.[34,43] Rapid IV infusions in patients with lead encephalopathy is likely to increase intracranial pressure and cerebral edema. In children with acute lead encephalopathy, starting dimercaprol 4 hours prior to $CaNa_2EDTA$ is

TABLE A30–1	Calculations for IV Edetate Calcium Disodium Infusion Over 24 hours						
	Avg. Height (in.)	Avg. Weight (lb)	m^2	1,000 mg/m^2 Over 24 hours IV	Dilute in D₅W or NS and Infuse Over 24 Hours[a]	1,500 mg/m^2 Over 24 Hours IV	Dilute in D₅W or NS and Infuse Over 24 Hours[a]
Child[b]							
2-year-old boy	36	30.5	0.593	593 mg	200 mL	890 mg	300 mL
2-year-old girl	35	29	0.57	570 mg	200 mL	855 mg	300 mL
4-year-old boy	42	39.75	0.73	730 mg	250 mL	1,095 mg	400 mL
4-year-old girl	41.75	38.75	0.72	720 mg	250 mL	1,080 mg	400 mL
Adult[c,d]							
50-kg			1.5	1,500 mg	500 mL	2,250 mg	750 mL
70-kg			1.8	1,800 mg	600 mL	2,700 mg	1,000 mL
90-kg			2.1	2,100 mg	700 mL	3,000 mg	1,000 mL

Edetate calcium disodium comes in 5-mL ampules of 200 mg/mL.

[a]Dilute in D₅W or 0.9% NaCl to concentrations of less than 0.5% to avoid thrombophlebitis with IV administration. Be mindful of total fluid requirements if encephalopathic to avoid cerebral edema. If fluid overload is possible intramuscular injection is reasonable, otherwise infuse IV over 24 hours. [b]Do not exceed the adult dose. [c]For adults with lead nephropathy, the following dosing regimen has been suggested: 500 mg/m^2 every 24 hours for 5 days for patients with serum creatinine concentrations of 2–3 mg/dL, every 48 hours for three doses for patients with creatinine concentrations of 3–4 mg/dL, and once weekly for patients with creatinine concentrations above 4 mg/dL. [d]The dose in obese patients has not been studied. A maximum dose of 3 g seems reasonable.

D₅W = 5% dextrose in water; IV = intravenous; NS = 0.9% sodium chloride solution.

more effective than starting CaNa₂EDTA prior to and simultaneously with dimercaprol.[14,15,19,43] In addition, treating with 2 chelators also reduces the blood lead concentration significantly faster than CaNa₂EDTA alone, while maintaining a better molar ratio of chelator to lead.[16]

If CaNa₂EDTA is to be administered IM to avoid the use of an IV and fluid overload, then either procaine or lidocaine is added to the CaNa₂EDTA in a dose sufficient to produce a final concentration of 0.5% (5 mg/mL). This can be accomplished by mixing 1 mL of a 1% procaine or 1% lidocaine solution with each milliliter of chelator.[11,34] The procaine or lidocaine minimizes pain at the injection site.

COMBINATION THERAPY WITH SUCCIMER OR DMPS

The possible benefit of combining CaNa₂EDTA with succimer or 2,3-dimercapto-1-propane-sulfonic acid (DMPS) is under investigation in animals.[24,26,49] The combination of CaNa₂EDTA with succimer is more potent than either individual chelator in promoting urine and fecal lead excretion, and decreasing blood and liver lead concentrations.[24,26] However, this approach increases zinc depletion.[24,26,49]

A retrospective analysis compared the combination of dimercaprol and CaNa₂EDTA with succimer and CaNa₂EDTA in children with blood lead concentrations of 35 to 70 mcg/dL (<90 mcg/dL for the dimercaprol group).[5] Equivalent reductions in blood lead concentrations were demonstrated with fewer adverse events in the succimer group. One case report of a child with lead encephalopathy and an extremely high blood concentration of 550 mcg/dL employed initially a combination of dimercaprol and CaNa₂EDTA followed by succimer alone, but a rebound increase in the lead concentration resulted in the addition of CaNa₂EDTA.[30] More data are needed to confirm this approach.

FORMULATION

Edetate calcium disodium is available as calcium disodium versenate in 5-mL ampules containing 200 mg of CaNa₂EDTA per milliliter (1 g per ampule).[34] Disodium edetate (sodium EDTA) should not be used as an alternative to CaNa₂EDTA because of the risk of life-threatening hypocalcemia and death associated with sodium EDTA use.

SUMMARY

- Edetate calcium disodium reduces blood lead concentrations, enhances urinary lead excretion, and reverses lead-induced hematologic effects.
- Edetate calcium disodium remains the standard of care for patients with lead encephalopathy when used in conjunction with dimercaprol.

- In patients with lead encephalopathy, the first dose of dimercaprol should precede the first dose of CaNa₂EDTA by 4 hours to prevent redistribution of lead to the brain.
- When dimercaprol is unavailable, it is reasonable to substitute succimer.
- Recommended doses and schedules should not be exceeded and should be reduced when the creatinine clearance is reduced.
- Patients should be well hydrated to achieve an adequate urine flow prior to and during CaNa₂EDTA therapy.

REFERENCES

1. Angle CR. Childhood lead poisoning and its treatment. *Annu Rev Pharmacol Toxicol.* 1993;32:409-434.
2. Aposhian HV, et al. Mobilization of heavy metals by newer, therapeutically useful chelating agents. *Toxicology.* 1995;97:23-38.
3. Bauchner H, et al. Evaluation of the Trial to Assess Chelation Therapy (TACT): the scientific process, peer review, and editorial scrutiny. *JAMA.* 2013;309:1291-1292.
4. Baxter AJ, Krensolek EP. Pediatric fatality secondary to EDTA chelation. *Clin Toxicol (Phila).* 2008;46:1083-1084.
5. Besunder J, et al. Comparison of dimercaptosuccinic acid and calcium disodium ethylenediaminetetraacetic acid versus dimercaptopropanol and ethylenediaminetetraacetic acid in children with lead poisoning. *J Pediatr.* 1997;130:966-971.
6. Bowzazi P, et al. Pharmacokinetic studies of EDTA in rats. *Eur J Drug Metab Pharmacokinet.* 1981;6:21-26.
7. Bradberry S, Vale A. A comparison of sodium calcium edentate (edentate calcium disodium) and succimer (DMSA) in the treatment of inorganic lead poisoning. *Clin Toxicol (Phila).* 2009;47:841-858.
8. Briggs GG, et al. *Drugs in Pregnancy and Lactation. A Reference Guide to Fetal and Neonatal Risk.* 11th ed. Philadelphia, PA: Lippincott Williams & Wilkins; 2017.
9. Brown MJ, et al. Deaths resulting from hypocalcemia after administration of edetate disodium: 2003-2005. *Pediatrics.* 2006;118:e534-e536.
10. Brownie CF, et al. Teratogenic effect of Ca EDTA in rats and the protective effect of zinc. *Toxicol Appl Pharmacol.* 1986;82:426-443.
11. Calcium disodium versenate edetate calcium disodium–injection [package insert]. Manufactured for Medicis, The Dermatology Company, Scottsdale, AZ, by CP Pharmaceuticals 10/12.
12. Cantilena LR, Klaassen CD. The effect of chelating agents on the excretion of endogenous metals. *Toxicol Appl Pharmacol.* 1982;63:344-350.
13. Centers for Disease Control and Prevention. Guidelines for the identification and management of lead exposure in pregnant and lactating women. https://www.cdc.gov/nceh/lead/publications/leadandpregnancy2010.pdf. Published 2010. Accessed October 2, 2017.
14. Chisolm JJ Jr. The use of chelating agents in the treatment of acute and chronic lead intoxication in childhood. *J Pediatr.* 1968;73:1-38.
15. Chisolm JJ Jr. Mobilization of lead by calcium disodium edetate. *Am J Dis Child.* 1987;141:1256-1257.
16. Chisolm JJ Jr. BAL, EDTA, DMSA and DMPS in the treatment of lead poisoning in children. *J Toxicol Clin Toxicol.* 1992;30:493-504.

17. Chisolm JJ Jr. Safety and efficacy of meso-2,3-dimercaptosuccinic acid (DMSA) in children and elevated blood lead concentrations. *J Toxicol Clin Toxicol.* 2000;38:365-375.

18. Coffin R, et al. Treatment of lead encephalopathy in children. *J Pediatr.* 1966;69:198-206.

19. Committee on Drugs. Treatment guidelines for lead exposure in children. *Pediatrics.* 1995;96:155-160.

20. Corey-Slechta DA. Relationships between lead-induced learning impairments and changes in dopaminergic, cholinergic, and glutamatergic neurotransmitter system functions. *Annu Rev Pharmacol Toxicol.* 1995;35:391-415.

21. Cory-Slechta DA, Weiss B. Efficacy of the chelating agent CaEDTA in reversing lead-induced changes in behavior. *Neurotoxicology.* 1989;10:685-698.

22. Cory-Slechta DA, et al. Mobilization and redistribution of lead over the course of calcium disodium ethylenediamine tetraacetate chelation therapy. *J Pharmacol Exp Ther.* 1987;243:804-813.

23. Ernst E. Fatalities after CAM: an overview. *Br J Gen Pract.* 2011;61:404-405.

24. Flora GJS, et al. Therapeutic efficiency of combined meso-2,3-dimercaptosuccinic acid and calcium disodium edetate treatment during acute lead intoxication in rats. *Hum Exp Toxicol.* 1995;14:410-413.

25. Flora SJ, Tandon SK. Influence of calcium disodium edetate on the toxic effects of lead administration in pregnant rats. *Indian J Physiol Pharmacol.* 1987;31:267-272.

26. Flora SJS, et al. Combined therapeutic potential of meso-2,3-dimercaptosuccinic acid and calcium disodium edetate on the mobilization and distribution of lead in experimental lead intoxication in rats. *Fundam Appl Toxicol.* 1995;25:233-240.

27. FDA, US Food and Drug Administration. Edetate Disodium (marketed as Endrate and generic products)—Full Version, Podcast. https://www.fda.gov/Drugs/DrugSafety/DrugSafetyPodcasts/ucm078387.htm. Accessed October 2, 2017.

28. FDA, US Food and Drug Administration. Public Health Advisory. Edetate Disodium (marketed as Endrate and generic products). https://www.fda.gov/Drugs/DrugSafety/PostmarketDrugSafetyInformationforPatientsandProviders/ucm051138.htm. Accessed October 2, 2017.

29. Foreman H, Trujillo T. The metabolism of ^{14}C labeled ethylenediaminetetraacetic acid in human beings. *J Lab Clin Med.* 1954;43:566-571.

30. Gordon RA, et al. Aggressive approach in the treatment of acute lead encephalopathy with an extraordinarily high concentration of lead. *Arch Pediatr Adolesc Med.* 1998;152:1100-1104.

31. Graziano JH, et al. 2,3-Dimercaptosuccinic acid: a new agent for the treatment of lead poisoning. *J Pharmacol Exp Ther.* 1978;206:696-700.

32. Jones MM, et al. Effect of chelate treatments on kidney, bone and brain lead levels of lead-intoxicated mice. *Toxicology.* 1994;89:91-100.

33. Jugo S, et al. Influence of chelating agents on the gastrointestinal absorption of lead. *Toxicol Appl Pharmacol.* 1975;34:259-263.

34. Klaassen CD. Heavy metals and heavy metal antagonists. In: Gilman AG, et al, eds. *Goodman and Gilman's the Pharmacological Basis of Therapeutics.* 11th ed. New York, NY: McGraw-Hill; 1996:1753-1775.

35. Lamas GA, et al. Design of the Trial to Assess Chelation Therapy (TACT). *Am Heart J.* 2012;163:7-12.

36. Lamas GA, et al. Effect of disodium EDTA chelation regimen on cardiovascular events in patients with previous myocardial infarction: the TACT randomized trial. *JAMA.* 2013;309:1241-1250.

37. Markowitz M, et al. Effects of calcium disodium versenate (CaNa$_2$-EDTA) chelation in moderate childhood lead poisoning. *Pediatrics.* 1993;92:265-271.

38. McKinney PE. Acute elevation of blood lead levels within hours of ingestion of large quantities of lead shot. *J Toxicol Clin Toxicol.* 2000;38:435-440.

39. Moel DI, Kumark N. Reversible nephrotoxic reactions to a combined 2,3-dimercapto-1-propanol and calcium disodium ethylene diaminetetraacetic acid regimen in asymptomatic children with elevated blood lead levels. *Pediatrics.* 1982;70:259-262.

40. Morgan JW. Chelation therapy in lead nephropathy. *South Med J.* 1975;68:1001-1006.

41. Nissen SE. Concerns about reliability in the Trial to Assess Chelation Therapy (TACT). *JAMA.* 2013;309:1293-1294.

42. Osterloh J, Becker CE. Pharmacokinetics of CaNa$_2$-EDTA and chelation of lead in renal failure. *Clin Pharmacol Ther.* 1986;40:686-693.

43. Piomelli S, et al. Management of childhood lead poisoning. *J Pediatr.* 1984;105:523-532.

44. Rosen JF, Markowitz ME. Trends in the management of childhood lead poisonings. *Neurotoxicology.* 1993;14:211-217.

45. Ruff HA, et al. Declining blood levels and cognitive changes in moderately lead-poisoned children. *JAMA.* 1993;269:1641-1646.

46. Ruff H, Markowitz M, Bijur P, Rosen J. Relationships among blood lead levels, iron deficiency, and cognitive development in two-year-old children. *Environ Health Perspect.* 1996;104:180-185.

47. Schumacher HR, et al. Calcinosis at the site of leakage from extravasation of calcium disodium edetate intravenous chelator therapy in a child with lead poisoning. *Clin Orthop.* 1987;219:221-225.

48. Tandon SK, et al. Chelation in metal intoxication: influence of various components of vitamin B complex on the therapeutic efficacy of CaEDTA in lead intoxication. *Pharmacol Toxicol.* 1987;60:62-65.

49. Tandon SK, et al. Efficiency at combined chelation in lead intoxication. *Chem Res Toxicol.* 1994;7:585-589.

50. Thomas DJ, Chisolm J. Lead, zinc, copper decorporation during Ca EDTA treatment of lead poisoned children. *J Pharmacol Exp Ther.* 1986;229:829-835.

51. Thurtle N, et al. Description of 3,180 courses of chelation with dimercaptosuccinic acid in children ≤ 5 y with severe lead poisoning in Zamfara, Northern Nigeria: a retrospective analysis of programme data. *PLoS Med.* 2014;11:e1001739.

52. Williams DR, Halstead BW. Chelating agents in medicine. *J Toxicol Clin Toxicol.* 1982;19:1081-1115.

94 MANGANESE

Elizabeth Q. Hines and Sari Soghoian

Manganese (Mn)		
Atomic number	=	25
Atomic weight	=	54.94 Da
Normal concentrations		
Whole blood	=	4–15 mcg/L (72.8–273 nmol/L)
Serum	=	0.4–0.85 mcg/L (7.3–15.5 nmol/L)
Urine	<	10 mcg/L (<182 nmol/L)

HISTORY AND EPIDEMIOLOGY

Manganese is the 12th most abundant element in the Earth's crust (0.106%). The name manganese derives from *Magnesia*, a prefecture of Thessaly in ancient Greece. Ores from this region are particularly abundant in manganese oxides and carbonates. Manganese salts are brightly pigmented, and the earliest known uses were artisanal. Manganese dioxide was found in prehistoric paints and was used as a decolorant in glassmaking during the Roman Empire.

Adding manganese to iron produces a stronger metal alloy, and manganese-iron alloys are found in weapons from ancient Sparta. By the early 19th century, manganese became an important component in the manufacture of steel, which remains the largest industrial use of manganese today. Currently, more than 85% of manganese is used in the production of ferromanganese alloys. Manganese chloride is used in dry-cell battery manufacture and the metal is a catalyst for chlorination of organic compounds. Manganese dioxide is used in batteries and glass production, and manganese sulfate is used to make ceramics, fungicides, and pesticides.

Most reported cases of manganese toxicity, or manganism, are associated with chronic occupational exposure. Manganism was first described in 1837, when the development of a characteristic neuropsychiatric syndrome in French pyrolusite mill workers was linked with exposure to high concentrations of manganese oxide dusts.[23] The release of manganese, primarily in the form of oxides, during mining, and inhalation exposure to dusts from grinding manganese ore has historically been the most important source of manganese toxicity. Inhalation of inorganic manganese compounds also occurs during smelting, welding, or burning of coal, oil, or fuel containing manganese compounds. A neuropsychiatric syndrome in welders is attributed to the inhalation of manganese oxide fumes.[16,18,42,54,79]

Manganism is also described in several nonoccupational settings. Manganese chloride and manganese sulfate are employed as nutritional supplements,[11] and manganese toxicity is well documented in patients receiving excessive doses in total parenteral nutrition.[28,61,67] Infants, young children, and patients with impaired clearance from chronic liver disease are particularly at risk. More recently, epidemic manganese toxicity was reported from the use of intravenous psychostimulant drugs such as methcathinone and a "Russian cocktail" prepared from pseudoephedrine-containing cough and cold products in the presence of potassium permanganate as a strong oxidizer.[49,86,91]

Environmental exposure to excessive manganese in drinking water is linked to neurodevelopmental deficiencies in children, including effects on cognition, behavior, memory, and motor function.[15,21,45] Concerns are also raised about the potential environmental health risks of methylcyclopentadienyl manganese tricarbonyl (MMT), an antiknock agent added to gasoline as an alternative to lead.[26,35] Methylcyclopentadienyl manganese tricarbonyl was allowed in Canada since 1976 and in the United States since 1995; however, more research is needed to understand its contribution to the environmental burden of manganese and to human health.[87]

Permanganates were first discovered to be strong oxidizers in the 18th century. Weak solutions of potassium permanganate (0.01%) are still used in medicine as topical drying and antiseptic skin preparations. Potassium, sodium, and barium permanganate also have uses in the pharmaceutical, chemical, and photographic industries. The toxicity of permanganates is mostly related to their oxidizing effects and is not discussed here.

CHEMISTRY

Manganese is a transition metal with atomic number 25, located between chromium and iron in the periodic table. It is dark-gray, brittle paramagnetic, and occurs in several mineral forms. Most manganese in the environment is found complexed to oxygen, carbon, or chloride. The most economically important ore is pyrolusite, or manganese dioxide (MnO_2), from which metallic manganese was first isolated in 1774.

Manganese can exist in oxidation states from –3 to +7. Divalent manganese (Mn^{2+}) is the most common, the most bioavailable, and the most physiologically important form. Trivalent manganese ion (Mn^{3+}) is also biologically important and is, for example, the form of manganese in superoxide dismutase. Elemental Mn^0 is benign and ionized manganese exists in diverse states.

PHARMACOLOGY AND PHYSIOLOGY

Manganese is an essential dietary element found in nuts, grains, legumes, fruits, and vegetables. Most people consume 2 to 9 mg of manganese compounds per day, but vegetarians often consume more. Manganese salts in well water also contribute to dietary intake.[83] Manganese is present in human breast milk in its trivalent form bound to lactoferrin, which is readily absorbed via receptors in the small intestine. Manganese salts—usually manganese sulfate or manganese chloride—are typically added to infant formulas, processed foods, and dietary supplements, although these are less well absorbed.

Manganese is considered an essential dietary element because it is a cofactor in many human enzyme systems, including superoxide dismutase, hexokinase, xanthine oxidase, arginase, 3-hydroxymethylglutaryl-CoA (HMG) CoA reductase, and glutamine synthase. It is also present in several metalloproteins involved in the metabolism of amino acids, carbohydrates, and lipids.[11] Although deficiency in humans is not reported, experimental manganese restriction produced a scaling, erythematous, pruritic rash; alterations in calcium homeostasis (eg, hypercalcemia, hyperphosphatemia); and increased alkaline phosphatase in healthy volunteers.[31]

Normally, less than 5% of dietary manganese is absorbed throughout the length of the small intestine. However, enteral manganese absorption is altered depending on the dietary needs of the host and the presence of similarly charged compounds in the diet. For example, divalent manganese ion (Mn^{2+}) forms complexes with a variety of ligands in the body and substitutes for Mg^{2+}, Ca^{2+}, and Fe^{2+} in complexes with proteins and enzymes.[63] Because manganese ions compete with iron for binding sites on transferrin, the absorption of manganese is dependent on iron status, increasing in the presence of iron deficiency and decreasing when iron stores are adequate. Radioisotope studies demonstrate that absorption of dietary manganese is doubled in individuals with anemia.[11,30] Manganese absorption from the gastrointestinal tract is also inversely proportional to the amount of calcium in the diet, most likely because of competition between divalent cations for transport.[11]

About 85% of manganese in whole blood is bound to hemoglobin in erythrocytes, and normal measured whole blood concentrations are as much as 5 times higher than those measured in serum.[74] The remaining manganese in plasma is mostly bound to transferrin, β_1-globulin, and albumin.[5]

Manganese is widely distributed to all tissues, and crosses both the placental[11] and the blood–brain barriers.[16] Transport in the body is facilitated by transport proteins and for Mn^{2+} by the divalent metal transporter.[11]

Manganese is primarily eliminated via the bile in feces, which requires normal hepatic function for healthy manganese homeostasis. It accumulates in bile against a concentration gradient, which suggests an active transport mechanism, possibly by hepatic metal ion ZIP transporter protein.[8,55] Renal excretion is negligible, whereas 67% of a radio-labeled manganese dose injected intravenously is recovered in feces within 48 hours, and less than 0.1% appears in the urine within 5 days of administration.[48]

The elimination half-life of manganese from the body is approximately 40 days,[60] with high variability among individuals. Elimination of manganese is prolonged in young women with high ferritin stores[30] or after the initiation of oral iron therapy for anemia.[60] This effect is most likely due to increased hepatic sequestration from increased production of iron transport and storage proteins. High concentrations of manganese are found in patients with hemochromatosis, supporting the idea that increased or abnormal iron storage proteins will also lead to increased hepatic manganese stores.[1]

PATHOPHYSIOLOGY

Manganese toxicity typically results from either overexposure or impaired elimination. Because of its low enteral absorption, excessive dietary ingestion of manganese is unlikely to cause toxicity in adults with normal elimination. However, parenteral administration of either nutritional supplements or xenobiotics containing manganese presents a greater toxicologic risk. The major occupational route of exposure is inhalation of manganese dusts or fumes. Inhalation acutely elevates blood concentrations, and possibly creates pulmonary manganese deposits that effectively prolong the exposure and absorption even following patient removal from the environmental source.[68] Whereas normal liver function protects against accumulation of manganese in soft tissue, patients with hepatic disease are at risk for manganese bioaccumulation and toxicity from normal dietary intake.[81,84]

Although manganese is widely distributed in the body, major clinical features of manganese toxicity are primarily related to its accumulation in brain, where it concentrates in the basal ganglia and, to a lesser extent, in the caudate and putamen. People with hereditary mutations in the cell membrane manganese exporter protein SLC30A10 develop manganism in the absence of elevated environmental or occupational exposure, as a result of a relative deficit in manganese efflux from cells.[73,95] The exact mechanisms of manganese uptake into and efflux from neurons, and its transport within the brain, are still being elucidated, but involve multiple transport mechanisms. Transferrin receptor–mediated endocytosis of transferrin-bound manganese is thought to be the major route of entry under normal conditions.[6] However, for unclear reasons, nonprotein-bound manganese crosses the blood–brain barrier more quickly than protein-bound manganese.[66,78] Therefore, exposure to manganese in excess of blood ligand-binding capacity promotes its distribution to the brain. Transferrin also plays an important part in manganese accumulation in the basal ganglia, specifically, because these are areas of high transferrin-receptor density.[5,27] The divalent-metal transporter is most likely also important, but more research is needed to understand its role.

The specific mechanisms of ionized manganese neurotoxicity are also not well established, although oxidative stress, mitochondrial dysfunction, neuroinflammation, and alterations in neurotransmitter metabolism are all likely implicated. Ionized manganese (Mn^{2+}) concentrates in mitochondria and inhibits both mitochondrial F1-ATPase and complex I in the electron transport chain, thereby disrupting oxidative phosphorylation and contributing to energy failure and cytotoxicity.[19,32,33,99,100] Like other transition metals, manganese causes local damage by generating reactive oxygen species during redox cycling between the divalent (Mn^{2+}) and trivalent (Mn^{3+}) forms. The participation of manganese in Fenton reactions also occurs and results in oxidative tissue damage (Chap. 10). Manganese also promotes sustained inflammatory neuronal injury by activating microglia and astrocytes, potentiating the release of nitric oxide, prostaglandin E1, tumor necrosis factor

alpha (TNF-α), nuclear factor κB (NF-κB), and other inflammatory mediators from activated glial cells.[29,47,56,65]

The clinical features of manganism share many similarities with idiopathic Parkinson disease. However, neuroimaging and neurochemical studies suggest that the neurodegenerative patterns are different. Degeneration of nigrostriatal dopaminergic neurons is clearly implicated in Parkinson disease, and single-photon emission computed tomography (SPECT) and positron emission tomography (PET) studies in patients with Parkinson disease show decreased presynaptic dopamine terminal markers in the striatum and reduced dopa decarboxylase activity. By contrast, newer evidence indicates a lack of degeneration among midbrain dopaminergic neurons, with normal dopamine synthesis and transporters, and a marked degeneration of basal ganglia structures, in particular the globus pallidus, in patients with manganese-related motor dysfunction.[34] Although neuroimaging and neurochemical studies in patients with manganism are limited, the hypothesis that manganese does not cause presynaptic nigrostriatal neurodegeneration but rather a more widespread pattern of subcortical damage bears further exploration.[44]

CLINICAL MANIFESTATIONS

Early reports of manganism in German manganese workers[11] and Chilean miners[85] described an acute phase characterized by psychiatric symptoms known as "manganese madness" and included visual hallucinations, behavioral changes, anxiety, impotence, and decreased libido.[11] Currently accumulated evidence indicates that psychiatric and/or cognitive abnormalities such as deficits in attention and memory are common. However, classic manganism is best typified by a late-presenting syndrome of extrapyramidal movement abnormalities, including marked bradykinesia, rigidity, postural instability, loss of facial expression, impaired speech, and pronounced gait disturbance.[10] Signs and symptoms vary with duration and level of exposure, are often insidious in onset, and do not become apparent for several years (Table 94–1). Neurodevelopmental deficits are reported in children with chronic manganese exposure, and numerous studies correlate elevated home water manganese concentrations with poor academic performance and lower IQ scores.[13,15,21,45,72] More work is needed to describe how these clinical features evolve, as well as to understand the relevance of subtle preclinical neuropsychological signs for predicting sequelae.

In a longitudinal study of 14 former chronic Ephedrone abusers, the first symptom developed 6 to 12 months after intravenous drug abuse. Dysarthria was the initial symptom in 31% of patients, with 1 patient presenting with manganese madness. Dystonia, tremor, and postural instability began later, but all symptoms demonstrated progression.[86]

TABLE 94–1	Typical Features of Chronic Manganism	
System	**Early Manifestations**	**Late Manifestations**
Constitutional	Asthenia, lethargy	—
Gastrointestinal	Anorexia	—
Neurologic	Fine intention tremor	Coarse intention tremor
	Headaches	Visual hallucinations
		Cognitive impairment
		Loss of facial expression
		Dysphagia
		Micrographia
		Gait instability[a]
		Low-volume speech
Psychiatric	Apathy	Decreased libido or impotence
	Irritability	Anxiety
	Emotional lability	Additional behavioral changes
Musculoskeletal	Arthralgias	Muscle rigidity

[a]Decreased arm swing, toe walking, and inability to turn or walk backward without falling.

Although the movement disorder that typically occurs in patients with manganism is similar to that which occurs in cases of idiopathic Parkinson disease, including a typical "cock walk" on the balls of the feet, there are several distinguishing clinical features, including the lack of a typical tremor, a particular tendency to fall backward, and an absence of severe progressive dementia.[34,43] Oculomotor abnormalities are also similar to those that occur in idiopathic Parkinson disease but have distinctive features.[14] Unlike Parkinson disease, the histologic hallmark Lewy bodies are absent in manganism.[17,57] In addition, an absent or transient clinical response to levodopa therapy is considered a criterion for establishing a diagnosis of probable manganism.[70] Although symptomatic improvement with levodopa therapy was reported is some patients,[22,62,79] most evidence indicates that dopamine supplementation does not improve signs and symptoms of parkinsonian in patients with manganese-associated neurotoxicity.[34,50,59,91]

Acute inhalational exposure to high concentrations of manganese oxides can cause metal fume fever (Chaps. 100 and 121), with characteristic fever, chills, nausea, headache, myalgias, and arthralgias.[11] Chronic occupational exposure to manganese oxide fumes is associated with chemical pneumonitis and increased rates of bronchitis and pneumonia, but it does not cause pulmonary fibrosis.[58,80] Manganese exposure is also associated with hypertension.[53]

DIAGNOSTIC TESTING

Manganism is often difficult to differentiate from other neurodegenerative disorders. Several tests help establish the diagnosis, but each has important limitations. Careful evaluation of plausible sources of exposure, findings on neurologic and neuropsychologic examinations, and determining hepatic function and iron reserve status are important. If movement abnormalities are present, then failure of sustained response to levodopa therapy is highly suggestive of manganism. Because genetic mutations in the manganese transporter SLC30A10 are linked to a neurodegenerative syndrome, a family history should also be explored.[77,95]

Normal reference values for manganese in blood and urine are published (see above) and measurements are helpful, but concentrations are poorly correlated with total body manganese burden. Whole blood manganese concentrations are the most reliable values for biomonitoring purposes, although they only correlate with group and not with individual exposures.[9,11] Additionally, manganese concentrations vary with age, gender, and during pregnancy. Neonates have concentrations up to 3 times the traditional upper limit of normal, probably because of concomitant iron status and erythropoiesis.[71,89] Manganese concentrations are most commonly determined by flame or furnace atomic absorption spectrophotometry. Manganese concentrations should be elevated after acute overexposure, but abnormal concentrations are neither sensitive nor specific for chronic manganese toxicity because manganese is rapidly cleared from the blood.[98] Signs and symptoms of manganism are insidious and typically occur long after concentrations in urine or blood have normalized.

Urine manganese concentrations are not well correlated with either symptoms or extent of exposure.[9] Increased urinary elimination of manganese after chelation challenge with calcium disodium ethylenediaminetetraacetic acid (CaNa$_2$EDTA) occurs but cannot be interpreted. In most situations, it is unclear whether the increased excretion signifies mobilization of physiologic manganese, an increased body burden of manganese, or toxicity. The utility of hair, nail clippings, and saliva as biomarkers of chronic manganese exposure is not clearly established.[9,52,90,96]

Patients with manganese-associated movement disorders often have a characteristic pattern of abnormalities on magnetic resonance imaging (MRI) that includes a bilateral, symmetric, hyperintense signal in the basal ganglia, particularly in the globus pallidus, on T1-weighted images.[4,42,43,69,91] The paramagnetic quality of manganese directly affects the MRI spin state in regions of deposition causing T1-hyperintensity.[46] This pattern is also reported in patients with iatrogenic manganism from long-term parenteral nutrition,[12,28,41,64,93] is sometimes seen in cirrhotic patients with impaired dietary manganese elimination,[36,76,88] and in chronic methcathinone abusers.[44,86] Magnetic resonance imaging studies in patients receiving

total parenteral nutrition (TPN) have shown a positive correlation between the concentration of manganese in TPN mixtures and the intensity of increased basal ganglia signal on T1-weighted MRI images.[12,93] An increased T1-weighted MRI signal throughout the basal ganglia was demonstrated in welders and correlates with the length of welding exposure.[24] These changes on MRI are reversible with TPN discontinuation in patients without neurologic symptoms.[64,93] Although highly suggestive of manganism in the correct clinical context, an increased T1-weighted signal in the basal ganglia is a nonspecific finding that may also reflect iron, copper, or lipid deposition; hemorrhage; or neurofibromatosis.[11]

By contrast to these radiographic abnormalities, MRI findings in Parkinson disease typically demonstrate a hypointense signal in the substantia nigra on T2-weighted images.[7,51] SPECT and PET facilitate differentiating Parkinson disease from chronic manganese exposure. For example, molecular imaging studies of patients with chronic manganese exposure and extrapyramidal symptoms have largely failed to demonstrate abnormal nigrostriatal dopaminergic activity and projections, although these are clearly abnormal in patients with Parkinson disease.[34,69,97]

TREATMENT

Treatment for manganese toxicity is primarily supportive. Discovery and removal from the source of exposure is paramount, although clinical manifestations often progress as manganese body stores fall.[40] Antiparkinsonian therapy is generally ineffective or has limited benefit in relieving motor symptoms. Antioxidant therapy is proposed by some authors, based on the hypothesis that oxidant stress and mitochondrial dysfunction contribute to manganese-induced cellular damage,[19,20,37] but because human data are lacking, these therapies are reasonable but not recommended at this time.

The clinical utility of chelation therapy in patients with manganese toxicity is not well studied and remains controversial. Treatment with CaNa$_2$EDTA was reportedly useful in some cases (Antidotes in Depth: A30).[38] More often, chelation improves urinary excretion of manganese and decreases concentrations in blood without affecting neurologic manifestations of toxicity.[17,25,91] It is a nonetheless reasonable therapy, particularly in acutely poisoned patients or those with elevated whole blood concentrations. Chelation with succimer had no effect on either manganese concentrations in blood and urine or on clinical signs of manganism in 2 patients.[2]

Iron supplementation is another therapy proposed to reduce manganese concentrations in blood and lower total body burden. Iron supplementation in addition to chelation therapy improved neurologic symptoms in one patient,[95] and is reasonable in patients with iron deficiency or acute exposures. Conversely, treatment with the iron chelator deferoxamine is theoretically counterproductive since iron and manganese tend to compete for ligands, and iron sequestration might leave more ion transporters available for manganese uptake. In vitro studies demonstrate increased rates of cellular apoptosis after co-incubation with manganese and deferoxamine compared to incubation with manganese alone.[82] Human data are lacking but treatment with deferoxamine is not recommended.

Additionally, hemodialysis did not prove beneficial in a case of massive intravenous manganese salt overdose. There was no evidence of enhancement of manganese elimination by analysis of extraction ratio or dialysate concentration, and the patient had a rapid fall in whole blood concentration, suggesting tissue distribution. This hypothesis was supported by positive basal ganglia MRI findings on day 2.[39] Hemodialysis is therefore also not recommended.

SUMMARY

- Accumulation of manganese in the brain produces a characteristic neurologic disorder, manganism, with cognitive, psychiatric, and movement abnormalities.
- The movement disorder has many features in common with Parkinson disease, including bradykinesia, rigidity, postural instability, gait abnormalities, and hypophonia, but neither tremor nor dementia are characteristically present, and patients with manganism do not typically respond to levodopa therapy.

■ An increased signal in the globus pallidus on T1-weighted MRI is typically but not invariably seen.

■ Elevated whole blood manganese concentrations help differentiate the cause, but rapid clearance of manganese from the blood makes this a less sensitive test in cases where exposure is remote from the onset of symptoms.

■ Treatment is primarily supportive because neither any chelation regimen nor hemodialysis is shown to alter the clinical course.

REFERENCES

1. Altstatt LB, et al. Liver manganese in hemochromatosis. *Exp Biol Med (Maywood)*. 1967;124:353-355.
2. Angle CR. Dimercaptosuccinic acid (DMSA): negligible effect on manganese in urine and blood. *Occup Environ Med*. 1995;52:846.
3. Aposhian HV, et al. Transport and control of manganese ions in the central nervous system. *Environ Res*. 1999;80:96-98.
4. Arjona A, et al. Diagnosis of chronic manganese intoxication by magnetic resonance imaging. *N Engl J Med*. 1997;336:964-965.
5. Aschner M. Manganese: brain transport and emerging research needs. *Environ Health Perspect*. 2000;108:429-432.
6. Aschner M. Manganese homeostasis in the CNS. *Environ Res*. 1999;80:105-109.
7. Atasoy HT, et al. T2-weighted MRI in Parkinson's disease; substantia nigra pars compacta hypointensity correlates with the clinical scores. *Neurol India*. 2004;52:332-337.
8. Aydemir TB, et al. Metal transporter deletion in mice increases manganese deposition and produces neurotoxic signatures and diminished motor activity. *J Neurosci*. 2017;37:5996-6006.
9. Bader M, et al. Biomonitoring of manganese in blood, urine and axillary hair following low-dose exposure during the manufacture of dry cell batteries. *Int Arch Occup Environ Health*. 1999;72:521-527.
10. Barbeau A. Manganese and extrapyramidal disorders (a critical review and tribute to Dr. George C. Cotzias). *Neurotoxicology*. 1984;5:13-36.
11. Barceloux DG, et al. American Academy of Clinical Toxicology Practice Guidelines on the Treatment of Ethylene Glycol Poisoning. Ad Hoc Committee. *J Toxicol Clin Toxicol (Phila)*. 1999;37:537-560.
12. Bertinet DB, et al. Brain manganese deposition and blood levels in patients undergoing home parenteral nutrition. *JPEN J Parenter Enteral Nutr*. 2000;24:223-227.
13. Björklund G, et al. Manganese exposure and neurotoxic effects in children. *Environ Res*. 2017;155:380-384.
14. Bonnet C, et al. Eye movements in ephedrine-induced parkinsonism. *PLoS One*. 2014;9:e104784.
15. Bouchard MF, et al. Intellectual impairment in school-age children exposed to manganese from drinking water. *Environ Health Perspect*. 2010;119:138-143.
16. Bowler RM, et al. Neuropsychological sequelae of exposure to welding fumes in a group of occupationally exposed men. *Int J Hyg Environ Health*. 2003;206:517-529.
17. Calne DB, et al. Manganism and idiopathic parkinsonism: Similarities and differences. *Neurology*. 1994;44:1583-1586.
18. Chandra SV, et al. An exploratory study of manganese exposure to welders. *Clin Toxicol (Phila)*. 2008;18:407-416.
19. Chen J-Y, et al. Differential cytotoxicity of Mn(II) and Mn(III): special reference to mitochondrial [Fe-S] containing enzymes. *Toxicol Appl Pharmacol*. 2001;175:160-168.
20. Chtourou Y, et al. Improvement of cerebellum redox states and cholinergic functions contribute to the beneficial effects of silymarin against manganese-induced neurotoxicity. *Neurochem Res*. 2011;37:469-479.
21. Claus Henn B, et al. Associations of early childhood manganese and lead coexposure with neurodevelopment. *Environ Health Perspect*. 2011;120:126-131.
22. Cotzias GC, et al. Metabolic modification of Parkinson's disease and of chronic manganese poisoning. *Annu Rev Med*. 1971;22:305-326.
23. Couper J. On the effects of black oxide of manganese when inhaled into the lungs. *Br Ann Med Pharmacol*. 1837;1:41-42.
24. Criswell SR, et al. Basal ganglia intensity indices and diffusion weighted imaging in manganese-exposed welders. *Occup Environ Med*. 2012;69:437-443.
25. Crossgrove JS, Zheng W. Manganese toxicity upon overexposure. *NMR Biomed*. 2004;17:544-553.
26. Crump KS. Manganese exposures in Toronto during use of the gasoline additive, methylcyclopentadienyl manganese tricarbonyl. *J Expo Anal Environ Epidemiol*. 2000;10:227-239.
27. Erikson KM, et al. Manganese neurotoxicity: a focus on the neonate. *Pharmacol Ther*. 2007;113:369-377.
28. Fell JME, et al. Manganese toxicity in children receiving long-term parenteral nutrition. *Lancet*. 1996;347:1218-1221.
29. Filipov NM, Dodd CA. Manganese absorption and retention by young women is associated with serum ferritin concentration. *J Appl Toxicol*. 2012;32:310-317.
30. Finley JW. Manganese absorption and retention by young women is associated with serum ferritin concentration. *Am J Clin Nutr*. 1999;70:37-43.
31. Friedman BJ, et al. Manganese balance and clinical observations in young men fed a manganese-deficient diet. *J Nutr*. 1987;117:133-143.
32. Galvani P, et al. Vulnerability of mitochondrial complex I in PC12 cells exposed to manganese. *Eur J Pharmacol*. 1995;293:377-383.
33. Gavin CE, et al. Mn^{2+} sequestration by mitochondria and inhibition of oxidative phosphorylation. *Toxicol Appl Pharmacol*. 1992;115:1-5.
34. Guilarte TR. Manganese and Parkinson's disease: a critical review and new findings. *Environ Health Perspect*. 2010;118:1071-1080.
35. Gulson B, et al. Changes in manganese and lead in the environment and young children associated with the introduction of methylcyclopentadienyl manganese tricarbonyl in gasoline—preliminary results. *Environ Res*. 2006;100:100-114.
36. Hauser RA, et al. Blood manganese correlates with brain magnetic resonance imaging changes in patients with liver disease. *Can J Neurol Sci*. 2015;23:95-98.
37. Hazell AS, et al. Alzheimer type II astrocytic changes following sub-acute exposure to manganese and its prevention by antioxidant treatment. *Neurosci Lett*. 2006;396:167-171.
38. Herrero Hernandez E, et al. Follow-up of patients affected by manganese-induced Parkinsonism after treatment with CaNa$_2$EDTA. *Neurotoxicology*. 2006;27:333-339.
39. Hines EQ, et al. Massive intravenous manganese overdose due to compounding error: minimal role for hemodialysis. *Clin Toxicol (Phila)*. 2016;54:523-525.
40. Huang CC, et al. Long-term progression in chronic manganism: ten years of follow-up. *Neurology*. 1998;50:698-700.
41. Iinuma Y, et al. Whole-blood manganese levels and brain manganese accumulation in children receiving long-term home parenteral nutrition. *Pediatr Surg Int*. 2003;19:268-272.
42. Jankovic J. Searching for a relationship between manganese and welding and Parkinson's disease. *Neurology*. 2005;64:2021-2028.
43. Josephs KA, et al. Neurologic manifestations in welders with pallidal MRI T1 hyperintensity. *Neurology*. 2005;64:2033-2039.
44. Juurmaa J, et al. Grey matter abnormalities in methcathinone abusers with a Parkinsonian syndrome. *Brain Behav*. 2016;6:e00539.
45. Khan K, et al. Manganese exposure from drinking water and children's academic achievement. *Neurotoxicology*. 2012;33:91-97.
46. Kim Y, et al. Increase in signal intensities on T1-weighted magnetic resonance images in asymptomatic manganese-exposed workers. *Neurotoxicology*. 1999;20:901-907.
47. Kirkley KS, et al. Microglia amplify inflammatory activation of astrocytes in manganese neurotoxicity. *J Neuroinflammation*. 2017;14:99.
48. Klaassen C. Biliary excretion of manganese in rats, rabbits, and dogs. *Toxicol Appl Pharmacol*. 1974;29:458-468.
49. Koksal A, et al. Chronic manganese toxicity due to substance abuse in Turkish patients. *Neurol India*. 2012;60:224.
50. Koller WC, et al. Effect of levodopa treatment for parkinsonism in welders: a double-blind study. *Neurology*. 2004;62:730-733.
51. Kosta P, et al. MRI evaluation of the basal ganglia size and iron content in patients with Parkinson's disease. *J Neurol*. 2005;253:26-32.
52. Laohaudomchok W, et al. Toenail, blood and urine as biomarkers of occupational exposure to manganese. *Epidemiology*. 2011;22:S93-S94.
53. Lee B-K, Kim Y. Relationship between blood manganese and blood pressure in the Korean general population according to KNHANES 2008. *Environ Res*. 2011;111:797-803.
54. Lees-Haley PR, et al. Methodological problems in the neuropsychological assessment of effects of exposure to welding fumes and manganese. *Clin Neuropsychol*. 2004;18:449-464.
55. Lin W, et al. Hepatic metal ion transporter ZIP8 regulates manganese homeostasis and manganese-dependent enzyme activity. *J Clin Invest*. 2017;127:2407-2417.
56. Liu X. Manganese-induced neurotoxicity: the role of astroglial-derived nitric oxide in striatal interneuron degeneration. *Toxicol Sci*. 2006;91:521-531.
57. Livingstone C. Manganese provision in parenteral nutrition: an update. *Nutr Clin Pract*. 2017 Apr 1:884533617702837. [Epub ahead of print]
58. Lloyd Davies TA, Harding HE. Manganese pneumonitis; further clinical and experimental observations. *Br J Ind Med* 1949;6:82-90.
59. Lu CS, et al. Levodopa failure in chronic manganism. *Neurology*. 1994;44:1600-1602.
60. Mahoney JP, Small WJ. The biological half-life of radiomanganese in man and factors which affect this half-life. *J Clin Invest*. 1968;47:643-653.
61. Masumoto K, et al. Manganese intoxication during intermittent parenteral nutrition: report of two cases. *JPEN J Parenter Enteral Nutr*. 2016;25:95-99.
62. Mena I, et al. Modification of chronic manganese poisoning. *N Engl J Med*. 1970;282:5-10.
63. Michalke B, et al. Speciation and toxicological relevance of manganese in humans. *J Environ Monit*. 2007;9:650.
64. Mirowitz SA, Westrich TJ. Basal ganglial signal intensity alterations: reversal after discontinuation of parenteral manganese administration. *Radiology*. 1992;185:535-536.
65. Moreno JA, et al. Manganese potentiates nuclear factor-κB-dependent expression of nitric oxide synthase 2 in astrocytes by activating soluble guanylate cyclase and extracellular responsive kinase signaling pathways. *J Neurosci Res*. 2008;86:2028-2038.
66. Murphy VA, et al. Saturable transport of manganese(II) across the rat blood-brain barrier. *J Neurochem*. 1991;57:948-954.
67. Nagatomo S, et al. Manganese intoxication during total parenteral nutrition: report of two cases and review of the literature. *J Neurol Sci*. 1999;162:102-105.

68. Newland MC. Animal models of manganese's neurotoxicity. *Neurotoxicology.* 1999;20:415-432.

69. Olanow CW. Manganese-induced parkinsonism and Parkinson's disease. *Ann N Y Acad Sci.* 2004;1012:209-223.

70. Ostiguy C, et al. The emergence of manganese-related health problems in Quebec: An integrated approach to evaluation, diagnosis, management and control. *Neurotoxicology.* 2006;27:350-356.

71. Oulhote Y, et al. Neurobehavioral function in school-age children exposed to manganese in drinking water. *Environ Health Perspect.* 2014;122:1343-1350.

72. Oulhote Y, et al. Sex- and age-differences in blood manganese levels in the U.S. general population: national health and nutrition examination survey 2011-2012. *Environ Health.* 2014;13:87.

73. Peres TV, et al. Manganese-induced neurotoxicity: a review of its behavioral consequences and neuroprotective strategies. *BMC Pharmacol Toxicol.* 2016;17:57.

74. Pleban PA, Pearson KH. Determination of lead in whole blood and urine using Zeeman effect flameless atomic absorption spectroscopy. *Anal Lett.* 1979;12:935-950.

75. Pomier-Layrargues G, et al. Increased manganese concentrations in pallidum of cirrhotic patients. *Lancet.* 1995;345:735.

76. Pujol A, et al. Hyperintense globus pallidus on T1-weighted MRI in cirrhotic patients is associated with severity of liver failure. *Neurology.* 1993;43:65-69.

77. Quadri M, et al. Mutations in SLC30A10 cause parkinsonism and dystonia with hypermanganesemia, polycythemia, and chronic liver disease. *Am J Hum Genet.* 2012;90:467-477.

78. Rabin O, et al. Rapid brain uptake of manganese(II) across the blood-brain barrier. *J Neurochem.* 2006;61:509-517.

79. Racette BA, et al. Welding-related parkinsonism: clinical features, treatment, and pathophysiology. *Neurology.* 2001;56:8-13.

80. Roels H, et al. Epidemiological survey among workers exposed to manganese: effects on lung, central nervous system, and some biological indices. *Am J Ind Med.* 1987;11:307-327.

81. Rose C, et al. Manganese deposition in basal ganglia structures results from both portal-systemic shunting and liver dysfunction. *Gastroenterology.* 1999;117:640-644.

82. Roth JA, et al. Effect of the iron chelator desferrioxamine on manganese-induced toxicity of rat pheochromocytoma (PC12) cells. *J Neurosci Res.* 2002;68:76-83.

83. Sahni V, et al. Case report: a metabolic disorder presenting as pediatric manganism. *Environ Health Perspect.* 2007;115:1776-1779.

84. Schaumburg HH, et al. Occupational manganese neurotoxicity provoked by hepatitis C. *Neurology.* 2006;67:322-323.

85. Schuler P, et al. Manganese poisoning; environmental and medical study at a Chilean mine. *Ind Med Surg.* 1957;26:167-173.

86. Selikhova M, et al. Analysis of a distinct speech disorder seen in chronic manganese toxicity following Ephedrone abuse. *Clin Neurol Neurosurg.* 2016;147:71-77.

87. Silbergeld EK. MMT: science and policy. *Environ Res.* 1999;80:93-95.

88. Spahr L. Increased blood manganese in cirrhotic patients: relationship to pallidal magnetic resonance signal hyperintensity and neurological symptoms. *Hepatology.* 1996;24:1116-1120.

89. Spencer A. Whole blood manganese levels in pregnancy and the neonate. *Nutrition.* 1999;15:731-734.

90. Sriram K, et al. Manganese accumulation in nail clippings as a biomarker of welding fume exposure and neurotoxicity. *Toxicology.* 2012;291:73-82.

91. Stepens A, et al. A Parkinsonian syndrome in methcathinone users and the role of manganese. *N Engl J Med.* 2008;358:1009-1017.

92. Takagi Y, et al. On-off study of manganese administration to adult patients undergoing home parenteral nutrition: new indices of in vivo manganese level. *JPEN J Parenter Enteral Nutr.* 2016;25:87-92.

93. Takagi Y, et al. Evaluation of indexes of in vivo manganese status and the optimal intravenous dose for adult patients undergoing home parenteral nutrition. *Am J Clin Nutr.* 2002;75:112-118.

94. Tuschl K, et al. Syndrome of hepatic cirrhosis, dystonia, polycythemia, and hypermanganesemia caused by mutations in SLC30A10, a manganese transporter in man. *Am J Hum Genet.* 2012;90:457-466.

95. Tuschl K, et al. Manganese and the brain. *Int Rev Neurobiol.* 2013;110:277-312.

96. Wang D, et al. Alteration of saliva and serum concentrations of manganese, copper, zinc, cadmium and lead among career welders. *Toxicol Lett.* 2008;176:40-47.

97. Wolters EC, et al. Positron emission tomography in manganese intoxication. *Ann Neurol.* 1989;26:647-651.

98. Young RJ, et al. Fatal acute hepatorenal failure following potassium permanganate ingestion. *Hum Exp Toxicol.* 2016;15:259-261.

99. Zwingmann C, et al. Brain energy metabolism in a sub-acute rat model of manganese neurotoxicity: an ex vivo nuclear magnetic resonance study using [1-13C]glucose. *Neurotoxicology.* 2004;25:573-587.

100. Zwingmann C, et al. Energy metabolism in astrocytes and neurons treated with manganese: relation among cell-specific energy failure, glucose metabolism, and intercellular trafficking using multinuclear NMR-spectroscopic analysis. *J Cereb Blood Flow Metab.* 2016;23:756-771.

95 MERCURY

Young-Jin Sue

Mercury (Hg)

Atomic number	=	80
Atomic weight	=	200.59 Da
Normal concentrations		
Whole blood	<	10 mcg/L (50 nmol/L)
Urine	<	20 mcg/L (100 nmol/L)

HISTORY AND EPIDEMIOLOGY

Mercury is a metal that is widely toxic to multiple organ systems. Its toxicologic manifestations are well known as a result of thousands of years of medicinal applications, industrial use, and environmental disasters.[69,112] Mercury occurs naturally in small amounts as the elemental (Hg^0) silver-colored liquid (quicksilver); as inorganic compounds such as mercuric (Hg^{2+}) sulfide (cinnabar), mercurous (Hg^+) chloride (calomel), mercuric chloride (corrosive sublimate), and mercuric oxide; and as organic compounds (methylmercury and dimethylmercury). Mercury's gastroenteric irritant effects led to its use as a therapy for constipation. In recent (16th–19th), centuries, mercury-containing preparations, advocated for their potent diuretic and sialogogic properties, were widely used to treat syphilis to "flush" the "virus" out.[81] The musician Paganini was one of several famous persons whose gingivitis, dental decay, ptyalism (excessive salivation), and erethism (pathologic irritability and emotional instability) were attributed to mercury therapy.[80] In the 1800s, the United States witnessed an epidemic of "hatters' shakes" or "Danbury shakes" and "mercurial salivation" in hat industry workers.[123] Danbury, Connecticut, was a US center of felt hat manufacturing in which mercuric nitrate was used to mat animal furs into felt.[112,123]

In the early 1900s, acrodynia, a painful dusky pink discoloration of the hands and feet, or "pink disease," was described in children who received calomel for ascariasis or teething discomfort.[16] Vividly described in a series of 41 children, the development of acrodynia was more common in younger children, did not seem to correlate with mercury dose, and was not necessarily related to urine concentrations of mercury.[122]

One of the most devastating epidemics of mercury poisoning occurred as the result of a decade of contamination of Minamata Bay in Japan by a nearby vinyl chloride plant during the 1940s. Methylmercury accumulated in the bay's marine life and poisoned the inhabitants of the local fishing community. Although officially only 121 victims were reported, thousands more are believed to have been affected by what has subsequently been named Minamata disease.[88,113] The largest outbreak of methylmercury poisoning to date occurred in Iraq in late 1971. Approximately 95,000 tons of seed grain intended for planting and treated with methylmercury as a fungicide were baked into bread for direct consumption, resulting in widespread neurologic symptoms, 6,530 hospital admissions, and more than 400 deaths.[5,23,96]

In 1990, the US Environmental Protection Agency (EPA) banned mercury-containing compounds from interior paints.[3] However, mercury-containing paints manufactured before that ruling may still be on interior walls, and mercury-containing paint can still be sold for outdoor use. In 1997, a scientist succumbed to delayed, progressive neurologic deterioration after a minute dermal exposure to dimethylmercury.[77] Contemporary exposures occur in the form of mercury-tainted seafood, mercury-based preservatives (thimerosal), and artisanal gold mining.[36]

However, a once widely feared source of potential poisoning, mercury-containing dental amalgam does not result in clinical poisoning.[14] Occasionally, exposure to mercury from broken thermometers leads to poisoning in the home, but such thermometers are becoming less common because of recent efforts to replace mercury with digital thermometers and other electronic devices.[78]

More recently, the ongoing movement to replace incandescent light bulbs with compact fluorescent bulbs has once again raised the concern of exposure to mercury in the home and environment. Promoted to reduce greenhouse gas emissions, each bulb contains about 4 mg of elemental mercury.[2]

Table 95–1 lists some potential sources of mercury exposure.

FORMS OF MERCURY AND TOXICOKINETICS

The 3 clinically important forms of mercury—elemental, inorganic, and organic—differ with respect to their toxicodynamics and toxicokinetics (Table 95–2). Each produces distinct clinical patterns of poisoning

TABLE 95–1	Exposures to Mercury		
	Elemental	**Inorganic**	**Organic**
Manufacturing/ Industrial	Barometers	Batteries	Agriculture
	Bronzing	Chemistry sets	Embalming
	Ceramics	Dyes	Fungicides
	Chlorine manufacture	Explosives	Laboratory reagents
	Electroplating	Fireworks	Pesticides
	Jewelry	Laboratory reagents	Wood preservatives
	Metal refineries	Tanneries	
	Paints	Taxidermy	
	Paper pulp	Vinyl chloride manufacture	
	Photography		
Medical/ Medicinal	Amalgam	Antiseptics	Bactericidals
	Sphygmomanometry	Calomel	Pharmaceuticals
	Tissue fixatives	Disinfectants	Preservatives
	Thermometers	Laxatives	
	Weighted nasogastric tubes	Nonprescription medications	
Food/Other	Ritualistic, complementary	Aesthetic, cosmetic Ayurvedic	Grains (contaminated) Seafood

TABLE 95–2	Classes of Mercury Compounds	
	Nomenclature	**Example**
Elemental	Hg^0	Quicksilver
Inorganic	Hg^+	Mercurous ion
	HgCl	Calomel, mercurous chloride
	Hg^{2+}	Mercuric ion
	$HgCl_2$	Mercuric chloride
Organic	Short-chain alkyl–mercury compounds	Methylmercury
	Long-chain mercury compounds	Ethylmercury
		Dimethylmercury
		Methoxyethylmercury
	Aryl mercury compounds	Phenylmercury

TABLE 95–3	Differential Characteristics of Mercury Exposure		
	Elemental	**Inorganic**	**Organic**
Primary route of exposure	Inhalation	Oral	Oral
Primary tissue distribution	CNS, kidney	Blood (transient, acute) Kidney CNS (delayed)	CNS, kidney, liver, blood, hair
Clearance	Kidney, GI	Kidney, GI	Methyl: GI Aryl: kidney, GI
Clinical effects			
CNS	Tremor	Tremor, erethism	Paresthesias, ataxia, tremor, tunnel vision, dysarthria
Pulmonary	+++	–	–
Gastrointestinal	+	+++ (caustic)	+
Renal	+	+++ (ATN)	+
Acrodynia	+	++	–
Therapy	BAL, succimer	BAL, succimer	Succimer (early)

ATN = acute tubular necrosis; BAL = British anti-Lewisite; CNS = central nervous system; GI = gastrointestinal; + to +++ = present with increasing importance; - = absent.

stemming in part from their unique kinetic features (Table 95–3). For each form, the specific manifestations are determined by the route of exposure, rate of exposure, distribution, biotransformation of mercury within the body, and relative accumulation or elimination of mercury by the target organ systems. Whereas elemental mercury produces pulmonary toxicity, inorganic mercury initially causes gastrointestinal (GI) symptoms followed by nephrotoxicity. A nearly pure neurologic toxicity results from organic (methylmercury) exposure.

ABSORPTION

Elemental Mercury

Elemental mercury (Hg^0) is absorbed primarily via inhalation of vapor, although slow absorption after aspiration, subcutaneous deposition, and direct intravenous (IV) embolization occurs.[60,74,121] Volatility, moderate at room temperature, increases significantly with heating or aerosolization, both of which occur with vacuuming.[44,102] When inhaled by human volunteers, 75% to 80% of mercury vapor is absorbed.[44] However, elemental mercury is negligibly absorbed from an anatomically and functionally normal GI tract, and it is usually considered nontoxic when ingested. Abnormal GI motility prolongs mucosal exposure to elemental mercury, and massive ingestion increases subsequent ionization to more readily absorbed forms. Similarly, anatomic GI abnormalities such as fistulae or perforation are associated with extravasation of mercury into the peritoneal in which where elemental mercury is oxidized to more readily absorbed inorganic forms.

Inorganic Mercury

The principal route of absorption for inorganic mercury is the GI tract. Approximately 10% of soluble divalent (Hg^{2+}) mercuric salts such as mercuric chloride ($HgCl_2$) are absorbed following ingestion and dissociation.[66] Absorption of a relatively insoluble monovalent (Hg^+) mercurous compound, such as mercurous chloride (calomel; HgCl), is dependent on its oxidation to the divalent form.[79] Inorganic mercury is also absorbed across the skin and mucous membranes, as evidenced by urinary excretion of mercury after dermal application of skin-lightening mercurial ointments and powders containing HgCl.[106,122]

The degree of dermal absorption varies by the concentration of mercury, skin integrity, and lipid solubility of the vehicle. With substantial dermal exposures to mercury salts, skin absorption may be difficult to distinguish from concomitant absorption via other routes, such as ingestion.

Organic Mercury

As in the case of inorganic mercury, organic mercury is primarily absorbed from the GI tract. Methylmercury, considered the prototype of the short-chain alkyl compounds, is approximately 90% absorbed from the gut. Aryl and long-chain alkyl compounds have more than 50% GI absorption.[79] Although both dermal and inhalational absorption of organic mercury is reported, precise quantitation and exclusion of concomitant absorption by ingestion are difficult to determine.

DISTRIBUTION AND BIOTRANSFORMATION

After absorption, mercury distributes widely to all tissues, predominantly the kidneys, liver, spleen, and central nervous system (CNS). The initial distributive pattern into nervous tissue of elemental and organic mercury differs from that of the inorganic compounds because of their greater lipid solubility.

Elemental Mercury

Although peak concentrations of elemental mercury are delayed in the CNS as compared with other organs (2–3 days versus 1 day),[44] significant accumulation in the CNS occurs after an acute, intense exposure to elemental mercury vapor. Conversion of elemental mercury to the charged mercuric (Hg^{2+}) cation within the CNS favors retention and local accumulation. Because elemental mercury does not covalently bind to other compounds, its toxicity depends on its oxidation initially to the mercurous ion (Hg^+) and then to the mercuric ion (Hg^{2+}) by the enzyme catalase.[66] Because this oxidation–reduction reaction favors the mercuric cation at steady state, the distribution and late manifestations of metallic mercury toxicity eventually resemble those of inorganic mercury poisoning. Conversely, and to a lesser extent, inorganic mercuric ions are reduced to the elemental state (Hg^0), although the site and mechanism of this reaction are not well understood.[79]

Inorganic Mercury

The greatest concentration of mercuric ions is found in the kidneys, particularly within the renal tubules. At least in animal studies, administration of mercury induces the renal synthesis of metallothionein, a compound that binds to and detoxifies mercuric ions.[12] Very little mercury is found as free mercuric ions. In blood, mercuric ions are found both within the red blood cells (RBCs) and bound to plasma proteins in approximately equal proportions. Blood concentrations are greatest immediately after inorganic mercury exposure, with rapid waning as distribution to other tissues occurs. Although penetration of the blood–brain barrier is poor because of low lipid solubility, slow elimination and prolonged exposure contribute to significant CNS accumulation of mercuric ions. Within the CNS, mercuric ions concentrate in the cerebellum and hippocampus, and to a lesser degree, the cerebral cortex.[35] Although inorganic mercurials undergo organification in marine life, as in the Minamata Bay disaster,[9,85] the importance of this conversion in humans is unknown. Animal studies demonstrate that the placenta functions as an effective barrier to mercuric ions.[79]

Organic Mercury

Once absorbed, aryl (phenyl mercury) and long-chain alkyl mercury compounds differ from the short-chain organic mercury compounds (methylmercury) in an important way—the former possess a labile carbon–mercury bond, which is subsequently cleaved, releasing the inorganic mercuric ion. Thus, the distribution pattern and toxicologic manifestations produced by the aryl and long-chain alkyl compounds that occur beyond the immediate postabsorptive phase are comparable to those of inorganic mercury, but organification has facilitated absorption and reduced the local caustic effects.[79] In contrast, short-chain alkyl mercury compounds possess relatively stable carbon–mercury bonds that survive the absorptive phase, although conversion to the inorganic mercuric cation at a rate of less than 1% per day occurs after absorption.[124] Because it is lipophilic, methylmercury readily distributes across all tissues, including the blood–brain barrier and placenta.[46] An important consequence of this property is the devastating neurologic degeneration that develops in prenatally exposed infants with Minamata disease. The rapid decline of blood mercury concentrations in both suckling rats and breastfeeding human infants is attributed to rapid growth of body volume combined with limited transport of mercury by milk.[76,97,98]

After methylmercury is distributed to brain tissue, its fate is uncertain. Animal evidence indicates that methylmercury is converted to inorganic mercury in brain tissue.[63] Primates fed oral methylmercury daily for periods exceeding 1 year and then killed within days of the last exposure demonstrated an average brain inorganic mercury fraction of only 19%. By contrast, when the postexposure period was extended to between 150 and 650 days, the inorganic mercury fraction increased to 88%. Similarly, long-term survivors of methylmercury poisoning had a higher ratio of inorganic mercury to total mercury in their brains.[29] In one patient who survived 22 years after methylmercury ingestion, autopsy revealed that the brain mercury was nearly completely in the inorganic form.

Methylmercury concentrates in RBCs to a much greater degree than do mercuric ions, with an RBC-to-plasma ratio of about 10:1 (in contrast to 1:1 RBC-to-plasma ratio for inorganic mercury).[124] However, despite this apparent affinity for nervous tissue and RBCs, the greatest methylmercury concentrations are found in the kidneys and liver. In addition, because of the extensive sulfhydryl bonds in hair, methylmercury deposits in hair at concentrations approximately 250 times that found in whole blood.[55]

ELIMINATION
Elemental Mercury and Inorganic Mercury
Mercuric ions are excreted through the kidney by both glomerular filtration and tubular secretion and in the GI tract by transfer across gut mesenteric vessels into feces. Small amounts are reduced to elemental mercury vapor and volatilized from skin and lungs. The total-body half-life of elemental mercury and inorganic mercury was previously estimated at approximately 30 to 60 days.[22,66] However, a recent review of case studies indicates that the half-life of inorganic mercury in human brains is on the order of several years to several decades.[92]

Organic Mercury
In contrast to elemental mercury and inorganic mercury, the elimination of short-chain alkyl mercury compounds (such as methylmercury) is predominantly fecal. Enterohepatic recirculation contributes to its somewhat longer total body half-life of about 70 days. Less than 10% of methylmercury is excreted in urine and feces as the mercuric cation.[124]

PATHOPHYSIOLOGY
The pervasive disruption of normal cell physiology by mercury arises from its avid covalent binding to sulfur, replacing the hydrogen ion in the body's ubiquitous sulfhydryl groups. Mercury also reacts with phosphoryl, carboxyl, and amide groups, resulting in widespread dysfunction of enzymes, transport mechanisms, membranes, and structural proteins.

Because mercury deposits in all tissues, the clinical manifestations of mercury toxicity involve multiple organ systems with variable features and intensity. Necrosis of the GI mucosa and proximal renal tubules, which occurs shortly after mercury salt poisoning, is thought to result from the direct oxidative effect of mercuric ions. An immune mechanism is attributed to membranous glomerulonephritis and acrodynia associated with the use of mercurial ointments.[13]

Neurologic manifestations of methylmercury poisoning correlate with pathologic findings in the brains of both adults and children who were prenatally exposed.[68,113] Grossly, atrophy of the brain is more severe in children who had prenatally or postnatally acquired methylmercury compared with the brains of those exposed as adults. In the adult brain, neuronal necrosis and glial proliferation are most prominent in the calcarine cortex of the cerebrum

and in the cerebellar cortex. In fetal Minamata disease, similar lesions are present but in a more diffuse and severe form. Atrophy of the cerebellar hemispheres, postcentral gyri, and calcarine area of the brain demonstrated on magnetic resonance images in organic mercury–poisoned patients correlates with clinical findings of ataxia, sensory neuropathy, and visual field constriction, respectively.[58] Neuropathologic examination of the brain of a scientist who died after unintentional dermal exposure to dimethylmercury revealed lesions in the cerebellum, temporal lobe, and visual cortex.[105]

In rats, neuronal cytotoxicity of methylmercury may result partly from muscarinic receptor–mediated calcium release from smooth endoplasmic reticulum of cerebellar granule cells.[62] There is animal evidence that methylmercury may trigger reactive oxygen species production. In addition, methylmercury inhibits astrocyte uptake of cysteine, the rate-limiting step in the production of glutathione, a major antioxidant in mammalian cell systems.[104] Cultured astrocytes accumulated methylmercury and exhibited increased mitochondrial permeability and oxidative injury.[125] Complexing of methylmercury with L-cysteine may enhance brain uptake by mimicry of methionine, a substrate of the endogenous L amino acid transport system. Uptake of the L-isomer significantly exceeds that of methylmercury–D-cysteine. Careful selection of stereospecific thiol complexing agents may lead to strategies to limit brain uptake of methylmercury.[56,70]

CLINICAL MANIFESTATIONS
Elemental Mercury
Symptoms of acute elemental mercury inhalation occur within hours of exposure and consist of cough, chills, fever, and shortness of breath. Gastrointestinal complaints include nausea, vomiting, and diarrhea accompanied by a metallic taste, dysphagia, salivation, weakness, headaches, and visual disturbances. Chest radiography during the acute phase reveals interstitial pneumonitis and both patchy atelectasis and emphysema. Symptoms either resolve with lesser exposures or progress to acute respiratory distress syndrome (ARDS) with respiratory failure and death. Some survivors of severe pulmonary toxicity develop interstitial fibrosis and residual restrictive pulmonary disease. The acute respiratory symptoms occur concomitantly with or precede the development of subacute inorganic mercury poisoning manifested by tremor, kidney dysfunction, and gingivostomatitis.[17,54,94] Thrombocytopenia is also reported to occur during the acute phase.[38]

Although acute exposure to elemental mercury vapor occurs most commonly in the occupational setting, poisonings caused by mishandling of the metal in the home are well reported.[19,29,50,72,108] In fact, attempts at home metallurgy using metallic mercury have resulted in fatalities with ambient air concentrations of mercury as high as 0.9 mg/m³. The current US Occupational Safety and Health Administration permissible exposure limit (PEL) for mercury vapor is 0.1 mg/m³ of air as a ceiling limit.[82]

As with other inhaled toxins, children are likely to be more sensitive to the pulmonary toxicity of mercury vapor because of their ratio of minute ventilation volume to body size.[72] Although pulmonary toxicity from elemental mercury usually results from inhalation of vapor, massive endobronchial hemorrhage followed by death has occurred secondary to direct *aspiration of metallic mercury* into the tracheobronchial tree.[127] Gradual volatilization of elemental mercury results in chronic toxicity from improper handling, such as vacuuming spilled mercury.[102]

The clinical importance of volatilized metallic mercury from dental amalgams for both the dentist and patient is controversial. The preponderance of evidence refutes the idea that dental amalgam causes mercury poisoning. Several comprehensive reviews of the subject conclude that (1) occupational exposure to mercury from dental amalgam is acceptably low, provided that recommended preventive measures such as adequate ventilation are adhered to; (2) the quantity of mercury vaporized from dental amalgam by mechanical forces, such as chewing, is clinically insignificant; and (3) only in exceedingly rare cases will immunologic hypersensitivity to mercury amalgam (manifested as cutaneous signs and symptoms and confirmed by patch testing) necessitate removal of the amalgam.[33,34,37,61,107]

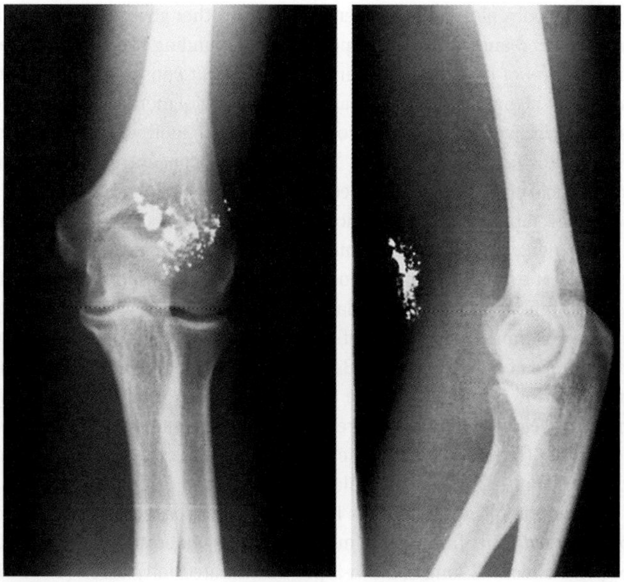

FIGURE 95–1. Anteroposterior (**A**) and lateral (**B**) views of the elbow after an unsuccessful suicidal gesture involving an attempted intravenous injection of elemental mercury in the antecubital fossa. Note the extensive subcutaneous mercury deposition, which was partially removed by surgical intervention. (*Used with permission from Diane Sauter, MD.*)

Unusual cases of chronic toxicity have resulted from intentional subcutaneous or IV injection of elemental mercury (Figs. 8–6 and 95–1).[49,74] Aside from management of systemic mercury toxicity, local wound care and excision of deposits of mercury are additional therapeutic challenges presented by these cases. Serial or repeat radiographs are useful in guiding the removal of the radiopaque deposits.

Inorganic Mercury

Acute ingestion of mercuric salts produces a characteristic spectrum from severe irritant to caustic gastroenteritis. Immediately after the ingestion, a grayish discoloration of mucous membranes and metallic taste typically accompany local oropharyngeal pain, nausea, vomiting, and diarrhea followed by abdominal pain, hematemesis, and hematochezia. The lethal dose of mercuric chloride is estimated to be 30 to 50 mg/kg.[116] The life-threatening manifestations of severe acute mercuric salt ingestion are hemorrhagic gastroenteritis, massive fluid loss resulting in shock, and acute kidney failure.[100]

Oropharyngeal injury, nausea, hematemesis, hematochezia, and abdominal pain were the most prominent symptoms in a series of 54 patients who presented after ingesting up to 4 g of mercuric chloride.[116] In this series, fatality was associated with the early development of oliguria (within 3 days) likely due in large part to lack of routinely available hemodialysis at that time. The development of anuria appeared to be related to the dose of mercuric chloride ingested. The histopathologic finding of proximal tubular necrosis after mercuric salt poisoning results both from direct toxicity to renal tubules and from renal hypoperfusion caused by shock. Consequently, aggressive fluid therapy to maintain perfusion is recommended.[101]

Acute ingestion of mercuric salts is usually intentional, but unintentional ingestion occurs sporadically in both children and adults.[51] Although ingestion of older button batteries containing mercuric oxide was associated with a greater incidence of fragmentation than with other batteries, clinically significant systemic mercury toxicity by this route was not reported.[64,67] Mercuric chloride–containing stool preservatives are another potential source of unintentional inorganic mercury poisoning. Ingestion of 10 to 20 mL of a polyvinyl alcohol preservative that contained 4.5% mercuric chloride resulted in bloody gastroenteritis and proteinuria.[103] Nonprescription[49] and Ayurvedic[99] medicines are also associated with unintentional inorganic mercury poisoning (Chap. 43).[53] These xenobiotics are not subject to US Food

and Drug Administration (FDA) regulation, available without prescription, of variable composition, and are often inadequately labeled (Chap. 43).

Subacute or chronic mercury poisoning occurs after inhalation, aspiration, or injection of elemental mercury; ingestion or application of mercury salts; or ingestion of aryl or long-chain alkyl mercury compounds. Slow in vivo oxidation of elemental mercury and dissociation of the carbon–mercury bond of aryl or long-chain alkyl mercury compounds result in the production of the inorganic mercurous and mercuric ions.

The predominant manifestations of subacute or chronic mercury toxicity include GI symptoms, neurologic abnormalities, and renal dysfunction. Gastrointestinal symptoms consist of a metallic taste and burning sensation in the mouth, loose teeth and gingivostomatitis, excessive salivation (ptyalism), and nausea.[122] The neurologic manifestations of chronic inorganic mercurialism include tremor, as well as the syndromes of neurasthenia and erethism. Neurasthenia is a symptom complex that includes fatigue, depression, headaches, hypersensitivity to stimuli, psychosomatic complaints, weakness, and loss of concentrating ability. Erethism, derived from the Greek word *red*, describes the easy blushing and extreme shyness of affected individuals. Other symptoms of erethism include anxiety, emotional lability, irritability, insomnia, anorexia, weight loss, and delirium. Mercury produces a characteristic central intention tremor (Chap. 22) that is abolished during sleep. In the most severe forms of mercury-associated tremor, choreoathetosis and spasmodic ballismus are also reported. Other neurologic manifestations of inorganic mercurialism include a mixed sensorimotor neuropathy, ataxia, concentric constriction of visual fields ("tunnel vision"), and anosmia.

Chronic poisoning with mercuric ions is associated with renal dysfunction, which ranges from asymptomatic, reversible proteinuria to nephrotic syndrome with edema and hypoproteinemia. An idiosyncratic hypersensitivity to mercury ions is thought to be responsible for acrodynia, or "pink disease," which is an erythematous, edematous, and hyperkeratotic induration of the palms, soles, and face, and a pink papular rash that was first described in a subset of children exposed to mercurous chloride powders.[122] The rash is described as morbilliform, urticarial, vesicular, and hemorrhagic. This symptom complex also includes excessive sweating, tachycardia, irritability, anorexia, photophobia, insomnia, tremors, paresthesias, decreased deep tendon reflexes, and weakness. The acral rash frequently progresses to desquamation and ulceration. The prognosis is favorable after withdrawal from mercury exposure. Childhood acrodynia has become uncommon since the abandonment of mercurial teething powders and diaper rinses. Occasional case reports still implicate improperly disposed fluorescent light bulbs and phenylmercuric acetate–containing paint.[3,117]

Thimerosal is an example of an aryl mercury compound that results in chronic inorganic mercury toxicity. It is a compound that was widely used as a preservative in the pharmaceutical industry (Chap. 46). Although initial kinetics suggested a stable ethyl–mercury bond, the later elimination phase more closely resembles that of the inorganic mercury compounds. Thimerosal is approximately 50% mercury by weight. Although generally considered safe, toxicity and death can occur after both intentional overdose and excessive therapeutic application of merthiolate (0.1% thimerosal or 600 mcg/mL mercury).[87,95]

Concern that the cumulative dose of thimerosal in childhood immunizations exceeded federally recommended maximum mercury doses (EPA, 0.1 mcg/kg/day; Agency for Toxic Substances and Disease Registry, 0.3 mcg/kg/day; FDA, 0.4 mcg/kg/day) led to a call by the American Academy of Pediatrics to reduce or eliminate thimerosal from vaccines.[4] Thimerosal continues to be used in medically underserved nations as a preservative in multidose vials in areas with inadequate refrigeration.[31] Nevertheless, since 2001, routinely administered childhood vaccines in the United States no longer contain thimerosal.[4,47]

Although sensitization after use in vaccinations has been reported in atopic children,[86] clinical mercury toxicity has not been reported in appropriately immunized children. The claim that thimerosal-containing vaccines causes autism has been refuted by numerous studies and meta-analyses.[8,65,84,109] No causal association with early thimerosal exposure and adverse neuropsychological outcomes was shown in children tested at 7 to 10 years of age.[115] Clearly, the risk to child health from the diseases targeted for prevention by vaccines far exceeds the risk from thimerosal preservative in vaccines.[39,114,119] In 2010, US courts rejected a causal relationship between thimerosal and autism.[32]

Organic Mercury Compounds

In contrast to the inorganic mercurials, methylmercury produces an almost purely neurologic disease that is usually permanent except in the mildest of cases. Although the predominant syndrome associated with methylmercury is that of a delayed neurotoxicity, acute GI symptoms, tremor, respiratory distress, and dermatitis are also reported.[124] In addition, ST segment changes on electrocardiography and renal tubular dysfunction are associated with this poisoning.[45] However, no increase in cardiovascular disease risk was reported with mercury exposure in a large cohort of US adults.[73]

The lipophilic property and slower elimination of methylmercury likely contribute to its profound neurologic effects. Characteristically, clinical manifestations occur after the initial poisoning by a latent period of weeks to months. Consequently, the lethal dose of methylmercury is difficult to determine. As noted previously, infants exposed prenatally to methylmercury were the most severely affected individuals in Minamata. Often born to mothers with little or no manifestation of methylmercury toxicity themselves, exposed infants exhibited decreased birth weight and muscle tone, profound developmental delay, seizure disorders, deafness, blindness, and severe spasticity.

Several weeks after methylmercury contaminated grain was ingested in Iraq, patients began to appear with paresthesias involving the lips, nose, and distal extremities. Symptomatic patients also noted headaches, fatigue, and tremor. More serious cases progressed to ataxia, dysarthria, visual field constriction, and blindness. Other neurologic deficits included hyperreflexia, hearing disturbances, movement disorders, salivation, and dementia. The most severely affected patients lay in a mute, rigid posture punctuated only by spontaneous crying, primitive reflexive movements, or feeding efforts.[96]

Although the outlook for methylmercury neurotoxicity is generally considered dismal, observations over the subsequent 2 years in 49 Iraqi children poisoned during the 1971 outbreak revealed complete resolution or partial improvement in all but the most severely affected.[5] Of the 40 symptomatic children, 33 mildly to severely affected children showed partial to complete resolution of symptoms, but the 7 children classified as "very severely poisoned" remained dysarthric, ataxic, blind, and bedridden.

An important route of organic mercury exposure is through seafood consumption. The safe amount of methylmercury in seafood remains controversial. The FDA action concentration of 1 ppm for methylmercury in fish was set to limit consumption of methylmercury to less than 1/10th of amounts found in cases of symptomatic poisoning. The EPA established a reference dose for methylmercury of 0.1 mcg/kg/day.[90,118] Although elevated blood concentrations (19–53 mcg/L) of mercury were found in one group of self-reported high consumers of seafood, increased incidence of cognitive and GI complaints were not.[52] Even so, concentrations at which fetuses experience adverse effects are unknown. Longitudinal studies of fish-eating populations are conflicting. No effect of a high prenatal fish diet was found on developmental markers in children followed to 19 years of age in the Seychelles Islands.[27,28,120]

However, in the studies done in the Faroe Islands and New Zealand, a subtle but significant effect on neuropsychological development was reported.[25,42,110] In the Faroe Islands, this effect persisted when children were retested at 22 years of age.[30,31]

One reason for the discrepancy that occurs between the 2 populations may be the different patterns of seafood consumption and concentrations of methylmercury in the seafood consumed by each. The Faroese consume low level mercury–containing fish 1 to 3 times a week with episodic feasts of highly contaminated pilot whale, whereas the Seychellois consume a more steady diet of low level–contaminated fish on average 12 times per week. The pilot whales consumed in the Faroe Islands are also contaminated with neurotoxic polychlorinated biphenyls (PCBs), although these compounds were measured and considered a potential confounding variable. The mean concentration of methylmercury in the whale meat consumed in the Faroe Islands was 1.6 mcg/g, and the mean concentration of mercury found in New Zealand shark was 2.2 mcg/g. By contrast, the mean methylmercury content of Seychellois fish was 0.3 mcg/g.[75] The threshold concentration for neuropsychological effects may lie between these concentrations.

The development of neurologic symptoms in infants exclusively breast-fed by women exposed to methylmercury after delivery and the detection of mercury in the milk of lactating women implies a risk for mercury poisoning via breast milk.[57] In one series of lactating women, mercury concentrations in milk were approximately 30% of the concentrations found in blood.[83] Perhaps because of high levels of PCBs in pilot whale meat, 7-year-old children from the Faroe Islands, who have a diet traditionally high in the mercury-containing sea mammals and were breast-fed as infants, exhibited a diminished benefit (but not deficit) on neuropsychological testing when compared with their counterparts fed formula.[48]

Further complicating findings in a cohort of Faroese children, the neurobehavioral deficits from methylmercury may be underestimated unless the protective effects of long-chain n-3 polyunsaturated fatty acids (n-3 PUFA, also found in fish) are included in the analysis.[21] Likewise, the Seychelles Child Development Study Nutrition Cohort 2 found no overall adverse association between prenatal methylmercury exposure and neurodevelopmental outcomes in children with high maternal n-3 PUFA concentrations.[111] The net neuropsychological effects of prenatal and dietary methylmercury result from dose and timing of fish in the diet as well as the concentrations of methylmercury, neurotoxic PCBs, and neuroprotective PUFA in the consumed fish.[111]

The FDA recommends that at-risk populations (pregnant women and women who may become pregnant, nursing mothers, and young children) avoid large predator fish (shark, swordfish, tilefish, and king mackerel) that contain concentrations of methylmercury approaching 1 ppm (1 mcg/g). The 2004 FDA/EPA consumer advisory emphasizes the health benefits of eating fish and allow for up to 12 ounces per week of fish and shellfish lower in mercury such as shrimp, canned light tuna, salmon, pollock and catfish and up to 6 ounces of albacore tuna per week. Given the beneficial effects of seafood, efforts should be aimed at decreasing anthropogenic release of mercury rather than elimination of dietary exposure.[91]

Although methylmercury has greater importance worldwide, the extreme toxicity of another organic mercurial, dimethylmercury, was tragically demonstrated by the delayed fatal neurotoxicity that developed in a chemist who inadvertently spilled dimethylmercury on a break in the gloves on her hands.[77] Over a period of several days, she developed progressive difficulty with speech, vision, and gait. Despite chelation and exchange transfusion, she died of mercury neurotoxicity within several months of the exposure.

DIAGNOSTIC TESTING

The dual findings of unexplained neuropsychiatric and kidney abnormalities in an individual should alert the clinician to the possibility of mercurialism, as should an at-risk occupation or access by the patient to a mercurial product (Table 95–1). Occupational or environmental exposure and a consistent clinical scenario are suggestive of mercury poisoning, but demonstration of mercury in blood, urine, or tissues is necessary for confirmation of exposure. Of the many methods available to measure mercury, cold atomic absorption spectrometry is rapid, sensitive, and accurate but cannot distinguish the various forms of mercury. Thin-layer and gas chromatographic techniques are recommended to distinguish organic from inorganic mercury. Whole blood should be collected into a trace element collection tube obtained from the laboratory performing the assay. Urine should be collected for 24 hours into an acid-washed container obtained from a laboratory. Spot collections must be adjusted for creatinine concentration. Attempts to measure or otherwise handle the specimen should be avoided to prevent external contamination (Table 95–4).

There is considerable overlap among concentrations of mercury found in the normal population, asymptomatic exposed individuals, and patients

TABLE 95–4	Diagnostic Testing for Mercury			
	Whole Blood	**24-hour Urine**	**Hair**	**Clinical**
Elemental/ Inorganic	(+)	(++)	(+)	(+)
	Acute, transient	Confirm exposure	Reflects past exposure and external adsorption	Poor correlation to TBB
		Monitor chelation		Early detection
		Poor correlation to TBB		
Organic	(++)	(−)	(+)	(+)
	Best reflects TBB	Fecal elimination	Reflects past exposure and external adsorption	Poor correlation to TBB
				Reflects irreversible CNS toxicity
				Early detection

CNS = central nervous system; TBB = total body burden; + to ++ = useful testing specimen; − = lack of utility.

with clinical evidence of poisoning. There is no definitive correlation between either whole blood or urine mercury concentration and mercury toxicity. However, mercury serves no useful role in human physiology, and concentrations of 1.0 mcg/L or less for whole blood and 0.5 mcg/L for urine are generally considered to reflect background exposure in nonpoisoned individuals. The inconsistencies of the values found in the literature for mercury exposure are a recurrent issue in metal testing. A credible and qualified laboratory should be employed and their reference ranges accepted when testing is desired.[20]

For inorganic mercury poisoning, urine mercury concentrations correlate roughly with exposure severity and neuropsychiatric symptoms,[93] but the relationship to total body burden is probably poor. Urine mercury determinations have their greatest usefulness in confirming exposure and monitoring the efficacy of chelation therapy. Whole blood mercury concentrations reflect intense, acute inorganic mercury exposure but become less reliable as redistribution to tissues takes place.

Because organic mercury is eliminated via the fecal route, urine mercury concentrations are not useful in methylmercury poisoning. Because methylmercury concentrates in RBCs, the total-body methylmercury burden is best reflected acutely by whole-blood concentrations. As methylmercury distributes to and accumulates in brain, the severity of clinical manifestations probably more closely reflects the degree of the irreversible neuronal destruction that has taken place rather than the current body burden of mercury. Correlation of increasing whole-blood mercury concentrations with prevalence of paresthesias was suggested in a population of Iraqis studied early in the course of methylmercury poisoning.[24] However, in another group of patients, whole-blood concentrations did not correlate with severity of methylmercury poisoning.[96] This apparent discrepancy may have resulted from the finding that paresthesias are among the earliest reported symptoms of methylmercury poisoning.

Because mercury accumulates in the hair, hair analysis has been used as a tool for measuring mercury burden. However, because metal incorporation reflects past exposure and hair avidly binds to noningested environmental mercury, the reliability of this method is questionable and is not recommended.[89] In addition to mercury assays, neuropsychiatric testing, nerve conduction studies, and urine assays for N-acetyl-β-D-glucosaminidase and β$_2$-microglobulin are advocated for early detection of subclinical inorganic and organic mercury toxicity.[34,45,93]

GENERAL MANAGEMENT

After the initial assessment and stabilization, the early toxicologic management of a patient with mercury poisoning includes termination of exposure by removal from vapors, washing exposed skin, GI decontamination, supportive measures (eg, hydration, humidified oxygen), baseline diagnostic studies (eg, complete blood count, serum chemistries, venous blood gas, radiography, ECG), specific analysis of whole blood and urine for mercury, evaluation of possible cointoxicants, and meticulous monitoring.

Elemental Mercury

Inhalation of mercury vapors or aspiration of metallic mercury may result in life-threatening respiratory failure; in this situation, stabilization of cardiorespiratory function is the initial priority. Postural drainage and endotracheal suction are a reasonable technique to attempt to remove aspirated metallic mercury. Parenteral deposition of subcutaneous or intramuscular (IM) mercury is amenable to surgical excision, if well localized (Fig. 95–1).

An adjunct to the initial management of patients with mercury poisoning is environmental decontamination. Elemental mercury that spills onto solid surfaces should be adsorbed to sand and the resulting mixture then swept into tightly sealed containers. Ideally, a mercury decontamination kit should be used. The kit consists of calcium polysulfide, which contains excess sulfur to convert mercury to water-insoluble mercuric sulfide. Absorbent surfaces, such as carpets, should be removed. Spilled mercury compounds should not be vacuumed because vacuuming could volatilize the mercury.[18] Broken compact fluorescent light bulbs should be handled and disposed of according to EPA guidelines and local requirements.[2]

Recommendations for decontamination after breakage include opening windows to release vapor, using adhesive tape to pick up visible fragments, and discarding contaminated material in double-wrapped bags. Guidance for decontamination of major spills and disposal of materials can be provided by local and federal hazardous materials agencies.

Inorganic Mercury

Because ingestion of inorganic mercuric may lead to cardiovascular collapse caused by severe gastroenteritis and third-space fluid loss, fluid resuscitation is a priority. Gastrointestinal decontamination of ingested inorganic mercury is particularly problematic because of its causticity and risk for perforating injury. Nevertheless, one series of patients with mercuric chloride ingestion of up to 4 g reported recovery without long-term GI sequelae in patients who did not succumb to kidney failure.[116] Therefore, unless there is high suspicion for penetrating GI mucosal injury, removal of mercury from absorptive surfaces should take priority over endoscopic evaluation. The prominence of vomiting makes gastric lavage unnecessary for most patients with inorganic mercury poisoning.

Metals are among the substances that are often considered to be poorly adsorbed to activated charcoal. Nevertheless, the serious nature of late sequelae after mercury absorption, the typically small quantities of mercury ingested, and evidence that inorganic mercuric salts actually have substantial adsorption to activated charcoal (800 mg mercuric chloride can be adsorbed to 1 g activated charcoal) justify the routine administration of activated charcoal.[6] Whole-bowel irrigation with polyethylene glycol solution is a reasonable adjunct to remove residual mercury, and its progress can be followed with serial radiographs.

Organic Mercury

Organic mercury exposures do not typically present as single acute ingestions but rather as chronic or subacute ingestion of contaminated food. Therefore, GI decontamination is generally moot with respect to organic mercury poisoning. Nevertheless, its irreversible toxicity coupled with unsatisfactory treatments calls for aggressive decontamination when acute ingestions or dermal exposures occur.

CHELATION

After initial stabilization and decontamination, early institution of chelators minimizes or prevents the widespread effects of poisoning. Dimercaprol was developed during World War II as an antidote against lewisite, an arsenical warfare agent. The water-soluble analogs DMPS and succimer were developed in the 1950s, and the 3 chelators have remained the mainstay of therapy for mercury poisoning.[59] A high degree of protein binding and distribution to the brain are responsible for the lack of efficacy of other measures to increase mercury clearance, such as peritoneal dialysis and hemodialysis.[100] In one report of the use of continuous venovenous hemodiafiltration in combination with a chelator in a patient with severe inorganic mercury poisoning, 12.7% of the ingested dose was recovered in the ultrafiltrate.[26] Hemodialysis may nevertheless ultimately be necessary because of the acute kidney failure that often occurs after mercuric chloride poisoning.

Chelators have thiol groups that compete with endogenous sulfhydryl groups for the binding of mercury, thereby preventing inactivation of sulfhydryl-containing enzymes and other essential proteins (Antidotes in Depth: A28 and A29). A history of significant mercury exposure combined with the presence of typical symptoms of mercury poisoning is an appropriate indication for the institution of chelation therapy. Elevated whole-blood and urine mercury concentrations help support the decision to begin chelation therapy in unclear cases and can also be used to guide the duration of therapy. Provocative chelation, in which urinary mercury excretion before and after a chelating dose is compared to determine the degree of mercury poisoning, is of no value.[52] Chelation tends to increase urinary elimination of mercury, regardless of exposure history and baseline excretion.

Elemental Mercury and Inorganic Mercury Salts

For patients with symptomatic acute inorganic mercury poisoning, dimercaprol should be administered for 10 days in dosages of 5 mg/kg/dose every 4 hours IM for 48 hours, then 2.5 mg/kg every 6 hours for 48 hours, followed by 2.5 mg/kg every 12 hours for 7 days. It is reasonable to adjust this dosing regimen, which was derived from lead poisoning, according to clinical response and the occurrence of adverse reactions.

When a patient can take oral medications, we recommend that dimercaprol be replaced with succimer at 10 mg/kg orally 3 times a day for 5 days, then twice a day for 14 days if the GI tract is clear. Because headache, nausea, vomiting, abdominal pain, and diaphoresis are common reactions during dimercaprol chelation therapy, oral succimer is recommended in patients who are not acutely ill or who have been chronically poisoned.

Either dimercaprol or succimer is considered the treatment of choice for inorganic mercury poisoning in the United States, but a few other chelators deserve mention. 2,3-Dimercapto-1-propanesulfonic acid (DMPS) is a water-soluble dimercaprol derivative that is used in Europe. It is administered both IV and orally. D-Penicillamine is an orally administered monothiol. Its adverse events—GI distress, rashes, leukopenia, thrombocytopenia, and proteinuria—although uncommon in therapeutic doses, seriously limit the usefulness of the drug. N-acetyl-D,L-penicillamine (NAP), an investigational analog of D-penicillamine, is thought to be a more effective chelator of mercury than is D-penicillamine, perhaps because of its greater stability.[11,40,43]

Organic Mercury Compounds

The neurotoxicity of methylmercury and other organic mercury compounds is resistant to treatment, and therapeutic options are less than satisfactory. In rats, both dimercaprol and D-penicillamine effectively reduced tissue mercury and prevented neurologic toxicity if administered within the first day of a methylmercury injection.[126] Neither treatment reversed neurologic toxicity when administered 12 days after methylmercury injection. 2,3-Dimercapto-1-propanesulphonate, D-penicillamine, NAP, and a thiolated resin all led to a marked reduction of blood half-life of mercury (ie, 10, 24, 23, and 19 days, respectively, versus 60 days) during the outbreak of methylmercury poisoning in Iraq in 1971.[24] Clinical improvement was not observed in any treatment group, but it is reasonable to postulate that reducing the total-body burden of methylmercury may prevent or limit the progression of disease.

When studied in mice poisoned with methylmercury,[1] succimer was superior to NAP, DMPS, and a thiolated resin in decreasing brain mercury and increasing urinary excretion. Brain mercury was decreased to 35% of control, and the total-body burden fell to 19%. Some animal evidence suggests that dimercaprol increases mercury mobilization into the brain.[7,10,15] For this reason, and the lack of serious GI symptoms necessitating parenteral chelation, We recommend against the use of dimercaprol the treatment of patients with organic mercury poisoning.

Because the neurologic impairment associated with methylmercury is both profound and essentially irreversible, early recognition of poisoning and prevention of neurotoxicity are essential to a successful outcome. At this time, succimer is the most reasonable treatment for methylmercury poisoning because of its apparently low toxicity and reported efficacy in animal trials.

SUMMARY

- Mercury poisoning by any of the 3 major forms—elemental, inorganic, and organic—presents a complex toxicologic problem associated with a large variety of clinical presentations.

- An ever present awareness of the signs and symptoms coupled with the knowledge of the differing clinical forms is essential for both early recognition and effective treatment.

- Although some chelators show promise in the treatment of mercury poisoning, neurologic sequelae, particularly those resulting from organic mercury exposures, remain largely irreversible.

- Dietary fish remains an important source of mercury exposure and mercurial neuropsychologic illness.

- There is no evidence for the role of mercury in the pathogenesis of autism.

- Promotion of public education regarding the dangers of mercury, its avoidance, and proper disposal may aid in the prevention of mercury poisoning.

REFERENCES

1. Aaseth J, Frieheim EA. Treatment of methyl mercury poisoning in mice with 2,3-dimercaptosuccinic acid and other complexing thiols. *Acta Pharmacol Toxicol (Copenh)*. 1978;42:248-252.
2. Agency USEP. Cleaning up a broken CFL. http://www2.epa.gov/cfl/cleaning-broken-cfl.
3. Agocs MM, et al. Mercury exposure from interior latex paint. *N Engl J Med*. 1990; 323:1096-1101.
4. American Academy of Pediatrics Committee on Infectious Diseases and Committee on Environmental Health. Thimerosal in vaccines—an interim report to clinicians. *Pediatrics*. 1999;104:570-574.
5. Amin-zaki L, et al. Methylmercury poisoning in Iraqi children: clinical observations over two years. *Br Med J*. 1978;1:613-616.
6. Andersen A. Experimental studies on the pharmacology of activated charcoal. III: adsorption from gastrointestinal contents. *Acta Pharmacol Toxicol*. 1948;4:275-284.
7. Andersen O, Aaseth J. Molecular mechanisms of in vivo metal chelation: implications for clinical treatment of metal intoxications. *Environ Health Perspect*. 2002; 110(suppl 5):887-890.
8. Andrews N, et al. Thimerosal exposure in infants and developmental disorders: a retrospective cohort study in the United Kingdom does not support a causal association. *Pediatrics*. 2004;114:584-591.
9. Poulain AJ, Barkay T. Cracking the mercury methylation code. *Science*. 2013;339:1280.
10. Aposhian HV, et al. Mobilization of heavy metals by newer therapeutically useful chelating agents. *Toxicology*. 1995;97:23-38.
11. Aronow R, Fleischmann LE. Mercury poisoning in children. The value of N-acetyl-D, L-penicillamine in a combined therapeutic approach. *Clin Pediatr (Phila)*. 1976;15:936-937, 943-945.
12. Asano S, et al. Review article: acute inorganic mercury vapor inhalation poisoning. *Pathol Int*. 2000;50:169-174.
13. Becker CG, et al. Nephrotic syndrome after contact with mercury. A report of five cases, three after the use of ammoniated mercury ointment. *Arch Intern Med*. 1962;110:178-186.
14. Bellinger DC, et al. Neuropsychological and renal effects of dental amalgam in children. A randomized clinical trial. *JAMA*. 2006;295:1775-1783.
15. Berlin M, Rylander R. Increased brain uptake of mercury induced by 2,3-dimercaptopropanol (BAL) in mice exposed to phenylmercuric acetate. *J Pharmacol Exp Ther*. 1964;146:236-240.
16. Black J. The puzzle of pink disease. *J R Soc Med*. 1999;92:478-481.

17. Bluhm RE, et al. Elemental mercury vapour toxicity, treatment, and prognosis after acute, intensive exposure in chloralkali plant workers. Part I: history, neuropsychological findings and chelator effects. *Hum Exp Toxicol.* 1992;11:201-210.

18. Caldwell KL, et al. Total blood mercury concentrations in the U.S. population: 1999–2006. *Int J Hyg Environ Health.* 2009;212:588-598.

19. Centers for Disease Control and Prevention. Epidemiologic notes and reports elemental mercury poisoning in a household—Ohio, 1989. *MMWR Morb Mortal Wkly Rep.* 1990;39:424-425.

20. Centers for Disease Control and Prevention. *Fourth National Report on Human Exposure to Environmental Chemicals.* July 26, 2012. 2009.

21. Choi AL, et al. Negative confounding by essential fatty acids in methylmercury neurotoxicity associations. *Neurotoxicol Teratol.* 2014;42:85-92.

22. Clarkson T. Mercury. *J Am Coll Toxicol.* 1989;8:1291-1296.

23. Clarkson TW, et al. An outbreak of methylmercury poisoning due to consumption of contaminated grain. *Fed Proc.* 1976;35:2395-2399.

24. Clarkson TW, et al. Tests of efficacy of antidotes for removal of methylmercury in human poisoning during the Iraq outbreak. *J Pharmacol Exp Ther.* 1981;218:74-83.

25. Crump KS, et al. Influence of prenatal mercury exposure upon scholastic and psychological test performance: benchmark analysis of a New Zealand cohort. *Risk Anal.* 1998;18:701-713.

26. Dargan PI, et al. Case report: severe mercuric sulphate poisoning treated with 2,3-dimercaptopropane-1-sulphonate and haemodiafiltration. *Crit Care.* 2003;7:R1-R6.

27. Davidson PW, et al. Fish consumption and prenatal methylmercury exposure: cognitive and behavioral outcomes in the main cohort at 17 years from the Seychelles child development study. *Neurotoxicology.* 2011;32:711-717.

28. Davidson PW, et al. Fish consumption, mercury exposure, and their associations with scholastic achievement in the Seychelles Child Development Study. *Neurotoxicology.* 2010;31:439-447.

29. Davis LE, et al. Methylmercury poisoning: long-term clinical, radiological, toxicological, and pathological studies of an affected family. *Ann Neurol.* 1994;35:680-688.

30. Debes F, et al. Impact of prenatal methylmercury exposure on neurobehavioral function at age 14 years. *Neurotoxicol Teratol.* 2006;28:536-547.

31. Debes F, et al. Cognitive deficits at age 22 years associated with prenatal exposure to methylmercury. *Cortex.* 2016;74:358-369.

32. Dyer C. Thiomersal does not cause autism, US court finds. *BMJ.* 2010;340:c1518.

33. Eley BM, Cox SW. Mercury from dental amalgam fillings in patients. *Br Dent J.* 1987;163:221-226.

34. Eti S, et al. Slight renal effect of mercury from amalgam fillings. *Pharmacol Toxicol.* 1995;76:47-49.

35. Feng W, et al. Mercury and trace element distribution in organic tissues and regional brain of fetal rat after in utero and weaning exposure to low dose of inorganic mercury. *Toxicol Lett.* 2004;152:223-234.

36. Fraser B. Peru's gold rush prompts public-health emergency. *Nature.* 2016;534:162.

37. Fung YK, Molvar MP. Toxicity of mercury from dental environment and from amalgam restorations. *J Toxicol Clin Toxicol.* 1992;30:49-61.

38. Fuortes LJ, et al. Immune thrombocytopenia and elemental mercury poisoning. *J Toxicol Clin Toxicol.* 1995;33:449-455.

39. Gadad BS, et al. Administration of thimerosal-containing vaccines to infant rhesus macaques does not result in autism-like behavior or neuropathology. *Proc Natl Acad Sci U S A.* 2015;112:12498-12503.

40. Gledhill RF, Hopkins AP. Chronic inorganic mercury poisoning treated with *N*-acetyl-D-penicillamine. *Br J Ind Med.* 1972;29:225-228.

41. Global Alliance for Vaccines and Immunisation. *Report to the GAVI Alliance Board Report of the Chief Executive Officer.* 2012.

42. Grandjean P, et al. Cognitive deficit in 7-year-old children with prenatal exposure to methylmercury. *Neurotoxicol Teratol.* 1997;19:417-428.

43. Hryhorczuk DO, et al. Treatment of mercury intoxication in a dentist with *N*-acetyl-D,L-penicillamine. *J Toxicol Clin Toxicol.* 1982;19:401-408.

44. Hursh JB, et al. Clearance of mercury (HG-197, HG-203) vapor inhaled by human subjects. *Arch Environ Health.* 1976;31:302-309.

45. Iesato K, et al. Renal tubular dysfunction in Minamata disease: detection of renal tubular antigen and beta-2-microglobulin in the urine. *Ann Intern Med.* 1977;86:731-737.

46. Inouye M, Kajiwara Y. Developmental disturbances of the fetal brain in guinea-pigs caused by methylmercury. *Arch Toxicol.* 1988;62:15-21.

47. Jacobson R. Vaccine safety. *Immunol Allergy Clin North Am.* 2003;23:589-603.

48. Jensen TK, et al. Effects of breast feeding on neuropsychological development in a community with methylmercury exposure from seafood. *J Expo Anal Environ Epidemiol.* 2005;15:423-430.

49. Johnson HR, Koumides O. Unusual case of mercury poisoning. *Br Med J.* 1967;1:340-341.

50. Jung RC, Aaronson J. Death following inhalation of mercury vapor at home. *West J Med.* 1980;132:539-543.

51. Kahn A, et al. Accidental ingestion of mercuric sulphate in a 4-year-old child. Management with BAL and peritoneal dialysis. *Clin Pediatr (Phila).* 1977;16:956-958.

52. Kales SN, Goldman RH. Mercury exposure: current concepts, controversies, and a clinic's experience. *J Occup Environ Med.* 2002;44:143-154.

53. Kang-Yum E, Oransky SH. Chinese patent medicine as a potential source of mercury poisoning. *Vet Hum Toxicol.* 1992;34:235-238.

54. Kanluen S, Gottlieb CA. A clinical pathologic study of four adult cases of acute mercury inhalation toxicity. *Arch Pathol Lab Med.* 1991;115:56-60.

55. Katz SA, Katz RB. Use of hair analysis for evaluating mercury intoxication of the human body: a review. *J Appl Toxicol.* 1992;12:79-84.

56. Kerper LE, et al. Methylmercury transport across the blood-brain barrier by an amino acid carrier. *Am J Physiol.* 1992;262(5, pt 2):R761-R765.

57. Koos BJ, Longo LD. Mercury toxicity in the pregnant woman, fetus, and newborn infant. A review. *Am J Obstet Gynecol.* 1976;126:390-409.

58. Korogi Y, et al. MR findings in seven patients with organic mercury poisoning (Minamata disease). *AJNR Am J Neuroradiol.* 1994;15:1575-1578.

59. Kosnett MJ. The role of chelation in the treatment of arsenic and mercury poisoning. *J Med Toxicol.* 2013;9:347-354.

60. Krohn IT, et al. Subcutaneous injection of metallic mercury. *JAMA.* 1980;243:548-549.

61. Langan DC, et al. The use of mercury in dentistry: critical review of the recent literature. *J Am Dent Assoc.* 1987;115:867-879.

62. Limke TL, et al. Acute exposure to methylmercury causes Ca^{2+} dysregulation and neuronal death in rat cerebellar granule cells through an M3 muscarinic receptor-linked pathway. *Toxicol Sci.* 2004;80:60-68.

63. Lind B FL, Nylander M. Preliminary studies on methylmercury biotransformation and clearance in the brain of primates: II. Demethylation of mercury in brain. *J Trace Elem Exp Med.* 1988;1:49-56.

64. Litovitz T, Schmitz BF. Ingestion of cylindrical and button batteries: an analysis of 2382 cases. *Pediatrics.* 1992;89:747-757.

65. Madsen KM, et al. Thimerosal and the occurrence of autism: negative ecological evidence from Danish population-based data. *Pediatrics.* 2003;112:604-606.

66. Magos L. Mercury. In: Seiler HG, ed. *Handbook on Toxicity of Inorganic Compounds.* New York, NY: Marcel Dekker; 1988:419-436.

67. Mant TGK, et al. Mercury poisoning after disc-battery ingestion. *Hum Toxicol.* 1987;6:179-181.

68. Matsumoto H, et al. Fetal Minamata disease: a neuropathological study of two cases of intrauterine intoxication by a methyl mercury compound. *J Neuropathol Exp Neurol.* 1964;24:563-574.

69. Maurissen J. History of mercury and mercurialism. *N Y State J Med.* 1981;81:1902-1909.

70. Mokrzan EM, et al. Methylmercury-thiol uptake into cultured brain capillary endothelial cells on amino acid system L. *J Pharmacol Exp Ther.* 1995;272:1277-1284.

71. Mostafazadeh B, et al. Mercury exposure of gold mining workers in the northwest of Iran. *Pak J Pharm Sci.* 2013;26:1267-1270.

72. Moutinho ME, et al. Acute mercury vapor poisoning. Fatality in an infant. *Am J Dis Child.* 1981;135:42-44.

73. Mozaffarian D, et al. Mercury exposure and risk of cardiovascular disease in two U.S. cohorts. *N Engl J Med.* 2011;364:1116-1125.

74. Murray KM, Hedgepeth JC. Intravenous self-administration of elemental mercury: efficacy of dimercaprol therapy. *Drug Intell Clin Pharm.* 1988;22:972-975.

75. Myers G. Prenatal methylmercury exposure from ocean fish consumption in the Seychelles child development study. *Lancet.* 2003;361:1686-1692.

76. Newland MC, Reile PA. Blood and brain mercury levels after chronic gestational exposure to methylmercury in rats. *Toxicol Sci.* 1999;50:106-116.

77. Nierenberg DW, et al. Delayed cerebellar disease and death after accidental exposure to dimethylmercury. *N Engl J Med.* 1998;338:1672-1676.

78. NIST. End of an era: NIST to cease calibrating mercury thermometers. February 02, 2011 https://www.nist.gov/news-events/news/2011/02/end-era-nist-cease-calibrating-mercury-thermometers. Created February 01, 2011. Updated September 21, 2016.

79. Nordberg GF, Skerfving S. Metabolism. In: Friberg L, Vostal J, eds. *Mercury in the Environment: An Epidemiological and Toxicological Appraisal.* Cleveland, OH: CRC Press; 1972:29-90.

80. O'Shea J. Was Paganini poisoned with mercury? *J R Soc Med.* 1988;81:594-597.

81. O'Shea JG. Two minutes with venus, two years with mercury—mercury as an antisyphilitic chemotherapeutic agent. *J R Soc Med.* 1990;83:392-395.

82. Occupational Safety and Health Administration. *Occupational Safety and Health Guideline for Mercury Vapor. Occupational Safety and Health Guidelines.* http://www.osha.gov/SLTC/healthguidelines/mercuryvapor/recognition.html.

83. Oskarsson A, et al. Exposure to toxic elements via breast milk. *Analyst.* 1995;120:765-770.

84. Parker SK, et al. Thimerosal-containing vaccines and autistic spectrum disorder: a critical review of published original data. *Pediatrics.* 2004;114:793-804.

85. Parks JM, et al. The genetic basis for bacterial mercury methylation. *Science.* 2013;339:1332-1335.

86. Patrizi A, et al. Sensitization to thimerosal in atopic children. *Contact Dermatitis.* 1999;40:94-97.

87. Pfab R, et al. Clinical course of severe poisoning with thimerosal. *J Toxicol Clin Toxicol.* 1996;34:453-460.

88. Powell P. Minamata disease: a story of mercury's malevolence. *South Med J.* 1991; 84:1352-1358.

89. Queipo Abad S, et al. Evidence of the direct adsorption of mercury in human hair during occupational exposure to mercury vapour. *J Trace Elem Med Biol.* 2016;36:16-21.

90. Rice D. Methods and rationale for derivation of a reference dose for methylmercury by the US EPA. *Risk Anal.* 2003;23:107-115.

91. Rice DC. The US EPA reference dose for methylmercury: sources of uncertainty Backgrounder for the 2004 FDA/EPA Consumer Advisory: what you need to know about mercury in fish and shellfish. *Environ Res*. 2004;406-413. http://water.epa.gov/scitech/swguidance/fishshellfish/outreach/factsheet.cfm.

92. Rooney JP. The retention time of inorganic mercury in the brain—a systematic review of the evidence. *Toxicol Appl Pharmacol*. 2014;274:425-435.

93. Rosenman KD, et al. Sensitive indicators of inorganic mercury toxicity. *Arch Environ Health*. 1986;41:208-215.

94. Rowens B, et al. Respiratory failure and death following acute inhalation of mercury vapor. A clinical and histologic perspective. *Chest*. 1991;99:185-190.

95. Royhans J, et al. Mercury toxicity following Merthiolate ear irrigations. *J Pediatr*. 1984;104:311-313.

96. Rustam H, Hamdi T. Methyl mercury poisoning in Iraq. A neurological study. *Brain*. 1974;97:500-510.

97. Sakamoto M, et al. Evaluation of changes in methylmercury accumulation in the developing rat brain and its effects: a study with consecutive and moderate dose exposure throughout gestation and lactation periods. *Brain Res*. 2002;949:51-59.

98. Sakamoto M, et al. Declining risk of methylmercury exposure to infants during lactation. *Environ Res*. 2002;90:185-189.

99. Saper RB, et al. Lead, mercury, and arsenic in US- and Indian-manufactured Ayurvedic medicines sold via the Internet. *JAMA*. 2008;300:915-923.

100. Sauder P, et al. Acute mercury chloride intoxication. Effects of hemodialysis and plasma exchange on mercury kinetic. *J Toxicol Clin Toxicol*. 1988;26:189-197.

101. Schnellmann R. Toxic responses of the kidney. In: Klaassen CD, Casarett LJ, eds. *Casarett and Doull's Toxicology: The Basic Science of Poisons*. 6th ed. New York, NY: McGraw-Hill; 2001:491-514.

102. Schwartz JG, et al. Toxicity of a family from vacuumed mercury. *Am J Emerg Med*. 1992;10:258-261.

103. Seidel J. Acute mercury poisoning after polyvinyl alcohol preservative ingestion. *Pediatrics*. 1980;66:132-134.

104. Shanker G, Aschner M. Identification and characterization of uptake systems for cystine and cysteine in cultured astrocytes and neurons: evidence for methylmercury-targeted disruption of astrocyte transport. *J Neurosci Res*. 2001;66:998-1002.

105. Siegler RW, et al. Fatal poisoning from liquid dimethylmercury: a neuropathologic study. *Hum Pathol*. 1999;30:720-723.

106. Sin KW, Tsang HS. Large-scale mercury exposure due to a cream cosmetic: community-wide case series. *Hong Kong Med J*. 2003;9:329-334.

107. Snapp KR, et al. The contribution of dental amalgam to mercury in blood. *J Dent Res*. 1989;68:780-785.

108. Snodgrass W, et al. Mercury poisoning from home gold ore processing. Use of penicillamine and dimercaprol. *JAMA*. 1981;246:1929-1931.

109. Stehr-Green P. Autism and thimerosal-containing vaccines: lack of consistent evidence for an association. *Am J Prev Med*. 2003;25:101-106.

110. Stern A, et al. Do recent data from the Seychelles Islands alter the conclusions of the NRC report on the toxicologic effects of methylmercury? *Environ Health*. 2004;3.

111. Strain JJ, et al. Prenatal exposure to methyl mercury from fish consumption and polyunsaturated fatty acids: associations with child development at 20 mo of age in an observational study in the Republic of Seychelles. *Am J Clin Nutr*. 2015;101:530-537.

112. Sunderman FW. Perils of mercury. *Ann Clin Lab Sci*. 1988;18:89-101.

113. Takeuchi T. Pathology of Minamata disease. With special reference to its pathogenesis. *Acta Pathol Jpn*. 1982;32(suppl 1):73-99.

114. Taylor LE, et al. Vaccines are not associated with autism: an evidence-based meta-analysis of case-control and cohort studies. *Vaccine*. 2014;32:3623-3629.

115. Thompson W, et al. Early Thimerosal exposure and neuropsychological outcomes at 7-10 years. *N Engl J Med*. 2007;357:1281-1292.

116. Troen P, et al. Mercuric bichloride poisoning. *N Engl J Med*. 1951;244:459-463.

117. Tunnessen WW Jr, et al. Acrodynia: exposure to mercury from fluorescent light bulbs. *Pediatrics*. 1987;79:786-789.

118. United States Environmental Protection Agency. *Characterization of Human Health and Wildlife Risks from Anthropogenic Mercury Emissions in the United States*. Washington, DC: US EPA; 1997.

119. Uno Y, et al. Early exposure to the combined measles-mumps-rubella vaccine and thimerosal-containing vaccines and risk of autism spectrum disorder. *Vaccine*. 2015;33:2511-2516.

120. van Wijngaarden E, et al. Prenatal methyl mercury exposure in relation to neurodevelopment and behavior at 19 years of age in the Seychelles Child Development Study. *Neurotoxicol Teratol*. 2013;39:19-25.

121. Wallach L. Aspiration of elemental mercury—evidence of absorption without toxicity. *N Engl J Med*. 1972;287:178-179.

122. Warkany J, Hubbard DM. Adverse mercurial reactions in the form of acrodynia and related conditions. *AMA Am J Dis Child*. 1951;81:335-373.

123. Wedeen R. Were the hatters of New Jersey "mad"? *Am J Ind Meds*. 1989;16:225-233.

124. Winship K. Organic mercury compounds and their toxicity. *Adverse Drug React Toxicol Rev*. 1986;3:141-180.

125. Yin Z, et al. Methylmercury induces oxidative injury, alterations in permeability and glutamine transport in cultured astrocytes. *Brain Res*. 2007;1131:1-10.

126. Zimmer L, Carter DE. The effect of 2,3-dimercaptopropanol and D-penicillamine on methyl mercury induced neurological signs and weight loss. *Life Sci*. 1978;23:1025-1034.

127. Zimmerman JE. Fatality following metallic mercury aspiration during removal of a long intestinal tube. *JAMA*. 1969;208:2158-2160.

96 NICKEL

John A. Curtis

Nickel (Ni)

Atomic number	=	28
Atomic weight	=	58.7 Da
Normal concentrations		
Serum	<	1.1 mcg/L (17 nmol/L)
Urine	<	6 mcg/L (102 nmol/L)

HISTORY AND EPIDEMIOLOGY

Nickel is a ubiquitous metal commonly found in both home and industry. It exists in a variety of chemical forms, from naturally occurring ores to synthetically produced nickel carbonyl. Elemental nickel is a white, lustrous metal, the name being derived from the German word "kupfernickel" or "devil's copper." Swedish chemist Baron Axel Fredrik Cronstedt first identified kupfernickel in 1751 in a mineral known as niccolite, and named it nickel in 1754. The fifth most abundant element on Earth, Nickel comprises 0.008% of the Earth's crust and is found in diverse locations, ranging from meteorites and soil to bodies of fresh- and saltwater.

First produced by the Chinese, nickel has been used as a component in a variety of metal alloys for more than 1,700 years. The first malleable nickel was produced by Joseph Wharton following the American Civil War. Wharton went on to sell bulk quantities of nickel to the United States government for the minting of 3-cent coins, and later donated the equivalent of 3.3 million of these coins to help fund what is known today as the Wharton School of Business.[44] The modern United States 5 cent piece, the "nickel," is actually only approximately 25% nickel by weight, and all currently United States coins except the penny are made of nickel-containing alloys.[7]

Nickel ores typically consist of accumulations of nickel sulfide minerals of relatively low nickel content. Although there are a variety of technical methods for extracting nickel from ore, one method of special note was developed in 1890 by Ludwig Mond, who is credited with the discovery of nickel carbonyl (also called nickel tetracarbonyl). The Mond process for the extraction of nickel involves passing carbon monoxide over smelted ore. This creates nickel carbonyl, which then decomposes at high temperatures to produce purified nickel and carbon monoxide.[44]

There have been 2 notable occupational disasters associated with exposure to nickel carbonyl. The Gulf Oil Company refinery incident in Port Austin, Texas, in 1953 resulted in more than 100 workers' being exposed, with 31 hospitalizations and 2 deaths. The Toa Gosei Chemical company incident in Nagoya, Japan, in 1969, resulted in 156 male workers' being exposed to nickel carbonyl, with 137 developing signs and symptoms but no fatalities reported.[44]

Currently, most nickel is imported into the United States from other nickel-rich countries, such as Canada, Russia, and Australia. After a more than 30-year period in which there was no domestic nickel mining in the United States, there is now one active US nickel mine: the Eagle Mine opened in Michigan in 2014, and produced 25,000 metric tons of nickel in 2016.[53]

Nickel is a siderophoric material that forms naturally occurring alloys with iron, a property that has made it useful for many centuries in the production of coins, tools, and weapons. Today, most nickel is used in the production of stainless steel, a highly corrosion-resistant alloy containing 8% to 15% nickel by weight.

Occupational exposure to nickel and nickel-containing compounds occurs in a variety of industries, including nickel mining, refining, reclaiming, and smelting. Chemists, magnet makers, jewelry makers, oil hydrogenator workers, battery manufacturers, petroleum refinery workers, electroplaters, stainless steel and alloy workers, and welders are at increased risk for exposure to nickel and nickel-containing compounds. Most nonindustrial human exposures to nickel are from dietary and environmental sources, although cigarette smoking is an important source of nickel exposure and elevates urinary nickel concentrations.[41] In the occupational setting, nickel carbonyl is responsible for the majority of acute nickel toxicity, whereas in clinical practice, the most common health issue related to nickel is the development of allergic dermatitis from jewelry and clothing, as well as cosmetics and complementary and alternative medicines. It is estimated that 10% to 15% of people have a metal allergy, with nickel being the most frequent, affecting about 10% to 15% of women and 2% to 3% of men. The incidence of metal allergy is increased in those with autoimmune diseases.[35]

TOXICOKINETICS

Exposure

Nickel occurs naturally in soil, volcanic dust, and fresh and saltwater, but it also enters the environment from the combustion of fuel oil, municipal incineration, nickel-refining processes, and the production of steel and other nickel alloys that allow aerosolized nickel to be disseminated into the environment.

The specific form of nickel emitted to the atmosphere depends on the source. Complex nickel oxides, nickel sulfate, and metallic nickel are associated with combustion incineration, smelting, and refining processes. Consequently, ambient air concentrations of these forms of nickel tend to be higher in urban areas, and concentrations of nickel in urban household dust is elevated under certain circumstances and thus poses variable exposure risk for young children who crawl or sit on floors.

Nickel carbonyl, $Ni(CO)_4$, deserves special mention. This colorless, highly volatile and potentially dangerous liquid nickel compound is a product of the reaction of nickel and carbon monoxide and is commonly used in nickel refining and petroleum processing, and as a chemical reagent. Its high vapor pressure and high lipid solubility lead to rapid systemic absorption through the lungs. In the air and in the body, it decomposes into metallic nickel and carbon monoxide and its toxicity is often compared with hydrogen cyanide.[35] Even at potentially harmful concentrations, nickel carbonyl has only a mild "sooty" or "musty" odor, and therefore environmental monitoring is necessary.[43] Previously mentioned disasters, such as the Gulf Oil Company refinery and the Toa Gosei Chemical company incidents, illustrate that clinical effects associated with serious toxicity were often delayed, again highlighting the need for monitoring.[44]

However, nonoccupational exposures to nickel are usually environmental and dietary. Ambient air nickel concentrations are typically around 2.2 ng/m³, whereas soil usually has nickel concentrations of 4 to 80 parts per million, with some regional variations based on both geography and man-made inputs, and local concentrations in some areas being as high as 5,000 ppm in soils derived from serpentine rock and up to 24,000 ppm near metal refineries.[17,18] Concentrations of metallic nickel in drinking water in the United States average 2 to 4 parts per billion, but higher concentrations of nickel in household and other potable and nonpotable water sources results from corrosion and leaching of nickel alloys present in various plumbing fixtures, including valves and faucets.[18] It is reported that the first water drawn from a hot-water tap plated with nickel may contain 1 to 1.3 mg/L of nickel.[3] Further, it is demonstrated that hot water contains more nickel than cold tap water, and the first 250 mL drawn from the tap contain more nickel than after pipes are flushed for 5 minutes.[1] Although many water suppliers in the United States monitor nickel concentrations in their water, there is currently no US Environmental Protection Agency (EPA) regulation regarding how much nickel is permissible in drinking water.

Dietary intake is a recognized source of nickel exposure for humans. Foods high in nickel include nuts, legumes, cereals, licorice, and chocolate. In addition, certain homeopathic medications, ginseng products, Indian herbal teas, Nigerian herbal remedies, and Chinese herbal plants are high in nickel content.[13] Nickel is not definitively an essential element for human health and dietary recommendations for nickel are not established. Normal consumption is between 0.3 and 0.6 mg/day. A Danish meta-analysis of 17 studies suggested that up to 1% of individuals develop allergic contact dermatitis at the low concentration of oral nickel exposure represented by dietary and drinking water sources.[22] Although estimates vary widely, the total body burden for a 70-kg reference human is about 10 mg of nickel, giving an average body concentration of 0.14 ppm.[18]

Absorption

Nickel enters the body through the skin, lungs, and gastrointestinal tract. The amount and rate of absorption are dependent on the water solubility of the nickel compound. Once in the body, nickel exists primarily as the divalent cation (Ni^{2+}). Independent of the particular nickel compound involved in the exposure, it is nickel ion (Ni^{2+}) that is typically measured in the serum or urine.

Following inhalational exposure, nickel accumulates in the lungs, but only 20% to 35% of nickel deposited in the human lung is systemically absorbed.[18] The remainder of the inhaled material is swallowed, expectorated, or deposited in the upper respiratory tract. Subsequent systemic absorption from the respiratory tract is dependent on the solubility of the specific nickel compound in question. Soluble nickel salts (nickel sulfate and nickel chloride) are more easily absorbed, whereas the less-soluble oxides and sulfides of nickel are absorbed to a lesser extent.

Because water-soluble nickel compounds tend to be more readily absorbed from the respiratory tract when compared with poorly soluble nickel compounds, exposure to the soluble nickel chloride or nickel sulfate results in higher urinary nickel concentrations than does exposure to less-soluble nickel oxide or nickel subsulfide, whereas the less soluble compounds have longer apparent half-lives. This likely at least partially represents a longer absorption phase.

The gastrointestinal absorption of nickel compounds varies with the particular nickel compound as well as coingestants. For example, approximately 27% of the total nickel in nickel sulfate given to humans in drinking water is absorbed, whereas only approximately 1% is absorbed when given in food. Serum nickel concentrations peak between 1.5 and 3 hours following ingestion.[46] As noted above, the presence of food in the gastrointestinal tract appears to reduce the absorption of nickel, and most ingested nickel remains in the gut and is excreted in the feces.

Although some systemic absorption of nickel occurs through skin contact, much of the applied nickel remains in the keratinized skin, with limited absorption by keratinocytes.[25]

Distribution

In human serum, the exchangeable pool of primarily divalent nickel is bound to albumin, L-histidine, and α_2-macroglobulin. A nonexchangeable pool of nickel that is tightly bound to a transport protein known as nickeloplasmin also exists in the serum. Nickel crosses the placenta and is present in breast milk.

Nickel is also concentrated in various solid organs. An autopsy study of individuals not occupationally exposed to nickel reported the highest concentrations of nickel in the lungs, followed by the thyroid, adrenals, kidneys, heart, liver, brain, spleen, and pancreas.[34] Nickel concentrations in the nasal mucosa are higher in workers exposed to less-soluble nickel compounds relative to soluble nickel compounds,[51] indicating that, following inhalation exposure, less-soluble nickel compounds remain deposited on the nasal mucosa.

Elimination

In humans, most ingested nickel is excreted in the feces; however, because more than 90% of ingested nickel does not leave the gut, most of the nickel found in feces represents the unabsorbed fraction rather than the elimination of body nickel.[46] Absorbed nickel is primarily excreted in the urine and, to a lesser degree, other bodily fluids.

Regardless of the route of exposure, workers occupationally exposed to nickel have increased urinary concentrations of nickel.[19] In nickel refinery workers, urinary excretion increased from the beginning to the end of the shift, indicating that a fraction of absorbed nickel is rapidly eliminated.[51] Similarly, urinary excretion increased as the work week progressed, indicating the presence of a fraction that is excreted more slowly. In fact, after a massive inhalational welding exposure, the apparent half-life of nickel in urine and blood followed a biphasic exponential decay pattern of excretion, and was 25 and 610 days in urine, and 30 and 240 days in blood, indicating potential saturation of elimination pathways and delayed absorption and redistribution of nickel.[36]

Studies of workers who unintentionally ingested water contaminated with nickel sulfate and nickel chloride reported a mean apparent serum half-life of 60 hours, but this decreased substantially (≤27 hours) when the workers were treated with intravenous fluids.[45]

The available literature supports the view that systemically absorbed nickel is excreted through the kidneys, with some excretion of insoluble compounds in the feces. Because of the previously mentioned factors affecting absorption, the apparent half-life following exposure likely reflects continuing absorption and will therefore depend on the route of exposure and the particular nickel species involved.

CLINICAL MANIFESTATIONS

Acute

The clinical manifestations associated with acute exposure to nickel depend on the particular compound and route of exposure. Inhalation of nickel-containing aerosolized particles tends to affect the lungs and upper airways directly, whereas ingestion and intravenous administration results in systemic toxicity, usually involving the nervous system (Table 96–1).

The most common disorder associated with exposure to nickel, by far, is an allergic dermatitis. Although acute toxicity is reported following various routes of exposure, the most important source of acute nickel toxicity is inhalational exposure to nickel carbonyl, which is associated with pulmonary, neurologic, and hepatic dysfunction.[44]

Nickel Allergy and Dermatitis

Nickel dermatitis was first reported in the late 1800s in nickel-plating workers and was recognized as an allergic reaction in 1925. Since then, nickel has been recognized as a common cause of allergic contact dermatitis. Divalent nickel is not itself antigenic but acts as a hapten, binding larger proteins and inducing conformational changes such that these become recognized as non–self antigens.[21]

TABLE 96–1	Symptoms and Signs of Nickel Carbonyl Poisoning[39]
Symptoms and Signs in 179 Cases	**Frequency, %**
Chest pain/tightness	67
Dizziness	66
Nausea	64
Weakness	54.8
Headache	54
Cough	43.6
Dyspnea	8.9
Vomiting	7.3
Fever	6.7
Somnolence	5.1
Abdominal pain	1.7

TABLE 96-2	Findings Suggestive of Nickel Dermatitis

Previous history of allergic response to jewelry

Multiple body piercings

Eruptions at the site of metal contact, or flexor areas if generalized

Eruptions following placement of orthodontic appliances containing high concentrations of nickel (unusual)

Seasonal dermatitis in warm months (increased metal–skin contact and increased sweating)

Facial dermatitis in mobile phone users

The allergic reaction caused by contact with nickel is a type IV delayed hypersensitivity immune response that typically occurs in 2 phases. In the first phase, sensitization occurs when nickel enters the body. The second phase occurs when the body is re-exposed to nickel, at which time allergy manifests. The diagnosis of nickel allergy is suggested by specific historical findings listed in Table 96–2 (Chap. 17).

The North American Contact Dermatitis Group reports that nickel has been the most frequently positive of the 65 tested allergens in patch-testing since 1992.[26] The 5-fold greater prevalence of nickel allergy in women is presumably a consequence of their higher rates of body piercing and more frequent wearing of jewelry, both of which are risk factors for nickel sensitization. Denmark in 2001 and later the European Union as a whole initiated nickel regulations. These laws forbade the use of nickel in piercings during the period of epithelialization, in accessories such as watches and jewelry to be in prolonged contact with skin, and even limited use of nickel when plated with another metal unless liberation of nickel was less than 0.5 mcg/cm^2/week.[14] It is unclear if these regulations succeeded in reducing rates of nickel sensitivity although this is suggested in several studies.[50]

Nickel dermatitis is classified into 2 types: primary and secondary. The more common primary dermatitis presents as a typical eczematous reaction in the area of skin that is in contact with nickel. It is characterized initially by erythematous papules that progress to lichenification because of pruritus and scratching. These eruptions reportedly mimic basal cell carcinoma.[25] Areas typically involved are the wrists, as a result of wearing watches and bracelets, the ears from earrings, and the periumbilical area at the site of contact with jewelry, nickel-containing buttons on jeans, or nickel-containing belt buckles (Fig. 96–1). Approximately 50% of all belt buckles and 10% of buttons on blue jeans contain nickel.[10] The most common cause for nickel dermatitis in women is direct contact from jewelry, garments, wristwatches, cosmetics, and occupational contact in the metal, hairdressing, tailoring, hotel, and restaurant industries. In men, nickel dermatitis is often occupational but in some individuals, is also related to jewelry, body piercing, garments, or even metal guitar strings.

The secondary form involves a more widespread dermatitis as a result of other exposures, such as ingestion or inhalation of nickel compounds, and implantation of metal medical devices, and is regarded as a systemic contact

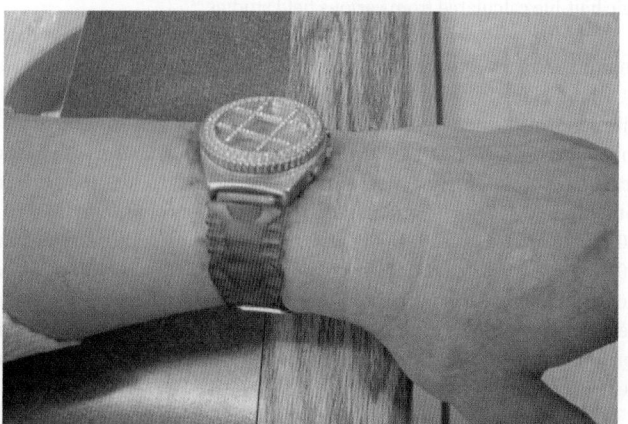

FIGURE 96-1. Nickel dermatitis from jewelry. (Used with permission from Brian Wexler.)

dermatitis elicited by nickel. Secondary eruptions are typically symmetrically distributed and localized in the elbow flexure, on the eyelids, on the sides of the neck, and face and can become widespread.

Nickel in foods, excessive skin contact, and certain orthodontic appliances with high nickel content are all linked to this eczematous eruption. Nonetheless, orthodontic exposure to nickel-containing alloys is unlikely to induce hypersensitivity reactions in patients without prior sensitization, and such reactions are still infrequent even in those sensitized.[33]

Other types of medical devices containing nickel have the potential to induce either primary or local nickel dermatitis. Occlusion of a biliary stent was reported as related to nickel allergy, and increased rates of restenosis of bare metal and cobalt-chromium cardiac stents are linked to nickel sensitization, although other studies have found no such correlation, and drug-eluting stents may mitigate any effect of metal allergy.[29]

One study showed that following skin application, nickel salts are retained in the skin for an extended period of time,[25] which could lead to prolonged antigen processing and consequent immune responses in dermal tissue. There may also be a genetic basis for nickel sensitization.[35,49] Development of an allergy, like most of toxicology, is probably dose and duration dependent, and this is the basis of the recent EU regulations to limit consumer exposure to nickel.

INHALATIONAL EXPOSURE
Nickel Carbonyl

Nickel carbonyl is the most harmful form of nickel and the majority of acute occupational nickel exposures involve nickel carbonyl. Nickel carbonyl is described as having a "musty" or "sooty" odor, although thresholds for detection vary considerably and potentially harmful exposures cannot be excluded simply by a reported lack of odor. Exposure to concentrations of 100 mg/m^3 is fatal in rats after 20 minutes.[23,47] Once dissociated, nickel carbonyl is oxidized in tissues to Ni^{2+}.

Nickel carbonyl exposure causes both immediate and delayed symptoms. In a series of 179 exposures, approximately 40% of patients reported symptoms within 1 hour of exposure; however, it is important to note that symptoms were delayed for approximately 1 week in 20% of patients, and even some patients with mild initial symptoms developed severe delayed symptoms, although usually within the next 2 days.[39] In patients who developed symptoms shortly following exposure, the initial manifestations involved nonspecific complaints, including respiratory tract irritation, chest pain, cough, dyspnea, frontal headache, dizziness, weakness, and nausea. Patients manifesting only these initial signs are categorized as mildly toxic.

Manifestations of severe acute nickel carbonyl poisoning generally develop over the course of several hours to days and are associated with acute respiratory distress syndrome and interstitial pneumonitis. Myocarditis, marked by persistent (time) changes on electrocardiography, including ST- and T-wave changes, as well as QT interval prolongation, are reported.[39] Neurologic symptoms associated with severe poisoning include altered mental status, seizures, and extreme weakness that sometimes necessitate mechanical ventilation. A moderate leukocytosis (10,000–15,000 white blood cells/mm^3), nonspecific opacities on chest radiography, and elevation of aminotransferase concentrations also occur, but these tend to resolve over the course of several weeks. Deaths from nickel carbonyl are typically caused by interstitial pneumonitis and cerebral edema occurring within 2 weeks of initial exposure.[47] Autopsy studies of those dying after nickel carbonyl exposure demonstrate diffuse pulmonary consolidation, organizing fibrosis, cerebral edema or hemorrhage, and cardiac dilation.[37] Survivors usually recover completely, although in some cases the development of a prolonged neurasthenic syndrome occurs which lasts for months.[39] Clinical features of nickel carbonyl poisoning are found in Table 96–1.

Noncarbonyl Nickel

There are few human cases of inhalational nickel poisoning. However, from the available data, the primary concerns appear to be pulmonary, neurologic, and, perhaps, renal.

A case report described seizure activity in 2 patients following occupational inhalational exposure to noncarbonyl nickel. Both patients exhibited elevated urinary nickel concentrations, with no recurrence of seizure activity upon removal from exposure.[15] Seizures were previously documented in animal studies, although the mechanisms are unclear and are hypothesized to involve inhibition of the glutamate transporter.[27] Interstitial pneumonia is also associated with inhalational exposure while spray painting high-temperature nickel-chromium alloys.[20] As previously mentioned, inhalational exposure to metallic nickel particles/nanoparticles can induce acute respiratory distress syndrome as well as acute tubular necrosis.[32]

Parenteral Administration

Acute parenteral toxicity from nickel-containing compounds occurred following the use of water for hemodialysis that was heated in a nickel-plated tank.[55] The concentration of nickel in the delivered water was 0.25 mg/L, and measured serum concentrations exceeded 3 mg/L. Through back-extrapolation, peak serum concentrations were estimated to be as high as 9 mg/L. These patients developed nonspecific effects, including headache, nausea, and vomiting, similar to nickel carbonyl poisoning, although no respiratory complaints were reported. The effects resolved after several hours, and the patients recovered without sequelae.

Ingestion

Acute ingestions of contaminated water containing 1.63 g Ni^{2+}/L caused nausea, vomiting, diarrhea, weakness, and headache, as well as pulmonary findings, including cough and dyspnea, lasting up to 48 hours.[45] Estimated ingested doses of nickel (as Ni^{2+}) were 0.5 to 2.5 g, and serum concentrations as high as 13.4 mcg/L were reported.

Dermal Absorption

Although transdermal absorption is typically of minor clinical significance, disruption of the normal integument likely allows for more efficient systemic absorption. A metal refinery worker suffered a 40% body surface area partial-thickness chemical injury resulting from exposure to a chemical mixture that included nickel carbonate and nickel sulfate.[30] Prior to the incident, this individual's measured serum nickel concentration was 0.023 μmol/L (1.35 mcg/L). On the sixth day following the injury, the serum concentration was 0.490 μmol/L (28.8 mcg/L). Two 5-day courses of chelation with edetate calcium disodium ($CaNa_2EDTA$) were begun for concomitant cobalt poisoning, and the patient's serum and urine nickel concentrations were within normal limits by 21 days postexposure. He subsequently recovered without manifesting signs of nickel toxicity.

Chronic Nickel Exposure

Chronic inhalational exposure to nickel is associated with injury characterized by specific histologic changes in the nasopharynx and upper respiratory tract, including atrophy of the olfactory epithelium, rhinitis, sinusitis, nasal polyps, and nasal septal damage.[8] Pulmonary effects include asthma[28] and pulmonary fibrosis.[6]

The International Agency for Research on Cancer classifies nickel compounds as a group 1 carcinogen (carcinogenic to humans). The potential for and mechanisms of carcinogenesis of nickel depend heavily on the specific compounds studied. Although nickel-induced carcinogenesis is fairly well established for nickel compounds, the role of metallic nickel is less clear.

In Taiwan, an increased incidence of oral cancer is associated with geographic areas containing higher concentrations of nickel in farming soil.[42] Although earlier studies of occupationally exposed workers, primarily electroplaters and refinery workers, also showed increased rates of nasal and pulmonary tumors, more recent studies of nickel-exposed workers in more modern environments with lower permissible limits of nickel exposure do not show a significantly increased risk of cancer or any cause of mortality.[40]

Although the exact mechanism of any possible carcinogenesis remains to be firmly elucidated, studies indicate several potential mechanisms. Animal studies show a threshold dose–response curve for inflammation with soluble

TABLE 96–3	United States Nickel Exposure Limits	
	Concentration (mg/m³)	Parts per million
ACGIH TLV-TWA		
Elemental	1.5	
Soluble inorganic	0.1	
Insoluble inorganic	0.2	
Nickel subsulfide	0.1	
Nickel carbonyl	0.35	0.05
OSHA PEL-TWA		
Noncarbonyl nickel	1	
Nickel carbonyl	0.007	0.001
NIOSH REL-TWA		
Noncarbonyl nickel	0.015	
Nickel carbonyl	0.007	0.001

ACGIH = American Conference of Governmental Industrial Hygienists; NIOSH = National Institute for Occupational Safety and Health; OSHA = Occupational Safety and Health Administration;

TLV = Threshold Limit Values; TWA = Time-Weighted Average; REL = Recommended Exposure Limit; PEL = Permissible Exposure Limit.

compounds (nickel sulfate), and similar curves describe the risks of pulmonary cancers with the less-soluble nickel oxides and nickel subsulfide.[38]

Depending on the particular nickel compounds studied, carcinogenesis is hypothesized to be due to genetic, epigenetic, or inflammatory mechanisms. The more potent carcinogenic effects of insoluble nickel compounds are suggested to be a consequence of their increased cellular uptake.[12]

Based on concerns about long-term health effects, exposure limits for various nickel compounds were proposed (Table 96–3).

DIAGNOSTIC TESTING

Although nickel is widely distributed to many body fluids and tissues, urine and blood are the most commonly analyzed samples. Urine collection should ideally use acid-washed, metal-free containers. Some authors recommend correcting urinary nickel concentration per gram of urine creatinine, but it is not clear that this offers any particular advantage in clinical decision making. The average nickel concentration in serum is less than 1.1 mcg/L (17 nmol/L), whereas the value in urine ranges from 1 to 3 mcg/L (102 nmol/L),[48] although substantially higher values are reported even in non–occupationally exposed populations. Concentrations in serum and urine of workers occupationally exposed to nickel are substantially higher, but do not directly correlate with adverse health effects.

Nickel concentrations rise in urine, serum, and whole blood following oral administration. In these studies, serum concentrations were slightly higher than whole blood. Urine and blood concentrations primarily reflect exposure occurring within the previous 48 hours,[11] which is roughly the biologic half-life calculated from various field studies.[52]

Urine nickel concentrations are used more commonly than blood for monitoring of workplace exposures and for prognostic and therapeutic decision making in nickel carbonyl exposures. An 8-hour collection is typically performed, and the average urinary excretion of nickel (in these nickel workers) is 2 mcg/L, with an upper limit of normal of 5 mcg/L. In cases of nickel carbonyl poisoning, concentrations of less than 100 mcg/L in the initial-8-hour specimen implies mild toxicity. Concentrations of 100 to 500 mcg/L are classified as moderate, whereas concentrations higher than 500 mcg/L are categorized as severe poisonings.[47] These classifications are used in guiding treatment decisions. Urine nickel concentrations rise prior to the onset of symptoms in nickel carbonyl poisoning, making this determination a potentially useful screening tool for both workforce surveillance and the management of acute exposures.

Testing for allergic contact dermatitis due to nickel is performed using patch testing, as for other types of contact dermatitis. "Strip" patch testing, in which the stratum corneum is thinned by repeated application and removal of adhesive tape prior to application of the test substance, is more sensitive than standard patch testing by 16%.[16] Testing metal surfaces for free nickel is possible and sometimes necessary in the evaluation and treatment of nickel dermatitis. Patients with clinically important sensitivity or suspect medical histories can order an inexpensive, commercially packaged dimethylglyoxime spot test, allowing them to test metal objects for the presence of free nickel.[10]

TREATMENT

The first step in treatment of nickel-related medical problems is eliminating the exposure, which includes detection and removal of the source. In the case of acute exposures to nickel carbonyl, removal of clothing to prevent continued exposure and thorough skin decontamination is recommended.

Symptomatic treatment for pulmonary symptoms associated with hypoxia includes the administration of supplemental oxygen. The use of bronchodilators and corticosteroids are reasonable interventions for the treatment of concomitant bronchospasm. Mechanical ventilation will be required in the most severe cases. Extracorporeal membrane oxygenation is not reported for nickel poisoning, but would be reasonable if needed for oxygenation or hemodynamic support.

The administration of intravenous fluids to promote diuresis reduces the half-life of orally ingested nickel chloride by approximately 50%.[45] Because of high levels of protein binding, hemodialysis does not effectively remove nickel from the serum.[55]

Chelation

Because there are no controlled human trials, specific recommendations for the use of chelation to treat nickel toxicity are not currently supported by the literature. As a result, extrapolation from animal studies and case reports form the basis for most treatment regimens. Most studies and reports involving treatment focused on workers exposed to nickel carbonyl.

Several drugs are proposed as potential treatments for nickel carbonyl exposures. Studies in rats with various chelators show some protection by administration of dimercaprol and D-penicillamine,[57] whereas $CaNa_2EDTA$ had no protective effect.[56] Although dimercaprol was being used in the past,[47] the most recent literature has focused on the use of diethyldithiocarbamate (DDC) (Chaps. 78 and 99).

Diethyldithiocarbamate is a chelator formerly used as the color reagent for urine nickel measurements. Rats exposed to several times the LD_{50} (median lethal dose for 50% of subjects) for nickel carbonyl had dramatically reduced mortality when pretreated with DDC; however, the antidotal efficacy decreased with increasing delay to treatment.[5] A proposed treatment regimen for exposed workers focuses on analysis both of the exposure and of the initial 8-hour urine collection.[47] Patients with suspected severe poisonings are typically given the first gram of DDC in divided oral doses. When less-severe exposures are suspected, treatment decisions are based on the urinary nickel concentration. At urinary concentrations lower than 100 mcg/L, no initial therapy is recommended as delayed symptoms are unlikely to develop. At urinary concentrations between 100 and 500 mcg/L, an oral regimen consisting of 1 g DDC initially, 0.8 g at 4 hours, 0.6 g at 8 hours, and 0.4 g at 16 hours is used. Diethyldithiocarbamate is continued at a dose of 0.4 g every 8 hours until there is symptomatic improvement and urine nickel concentration is normal. Severe exposures with urinary nickel concentrations more than 500 mcg/L are treated using the same regimen, although these patients frequently require closer monitoring. Critically ill patients should be given parenteral DDC starting at a dose of 12.5 mg/kg. However, given the animal data that the route and timing of administration are important to survival, if available, parenteral DDC should be given as soon as possible following nickel carbonyl poisoning.[9] Although typically well-tolerated, DDC induces a disulfiram reaction (Chap. 78) if taken with ethanol, and there are concerns about using DDC when there is concurrent cadmium exposure, at least by the oral route.[2] As in the case of many chelators, there is also debate about whether the redistribution of nickel by chelators is detrimental by increasing brain and organ concentrations.[31]

Disulfiram is metabolized into 2 molecules of DDC. Given that DDC is not pharmaceutically available in the United States, there is some interest in the use of disulfiram as an antidote for nickel carbonyl. Although case reports describe successful treatment of nickel carbonyl toxicity with disulfiram,[35] concern exists because animal studies show that disulfiram increased nickel concentration in brain tissue.[4] Disulfiram cannot be considered a standard of care, because of the lack of convincing evidence, but would be reasonable because of its theoretical efficacy. One suggested treatment regimen is 750 mg given orally every 8 hours for 24 hours, followed by 250 mg every 8 hours.[24]

Considering most of the literature and almost all human case reports of nickel carbonyl refer to the use of DDC, it is considered the treatment of choice for nickel toxicity. Although commonly available as a reagent, pharmaceutical-grade DDC is not produced commercially. Although based on less robust evidence, given the fact that disulfiram is essentially a prodrug for the unavailable DDC, treatment of nickel carbonyl poisonings with disulfiram would be reasonable.

Contact dermatitis from nickel is treated with avoidance, topical corticosteroids, and oral antihistamines. Some patients also benefit from dietary reduction of nickel intake, including running hot water faucets to flush pipes before using water for human consumption. Although sometimes advised, there does not appear to be a role for avoiding stainless steel cookware to reduce the nickel content of food.

SUMMARY

- Nickel is a ubiquitous metal, found in jewelry, electronics, stainless steel, and currencies, as well as in food and water.
- Allergic dermatitis due to hypersensitivity is the most common type of nickel-related disease.
- Acute nickel toxicity is rare and most often related to nickel carbonyl.
- Diethyldithiocarbamate (DDC) is the most studied chelator of nickel for nickel carbonyl exposures, but is currently not pharmaceutically available. It is reasonable to treat with disulfiram, a prodrug of DDC, in the setting of serious nickel carbonyl exposures.
- Chronic, excessive exposures to nickel compounds, particularly subsulfide nickel, increases the risk of sinonasal and lung cancers.

Acknowledgments

Michael I. Greenberg, MD, and David A. Haggerty, MD, contributed to this chapter in previous editions.

REFERENCES

1. Andersen KE, et al. Nickel in tap water. *Contact Dermatitis.* 1983;9:140-143.
2. Andersen O, et al. Oral cadmium chloride intoxication in mice: diethyldithiocarbamate enhances rather than alleviates acute toxicity. *Toxicology.* 1988;52:331-342.
3. Barceloux DG. Nickel. *J Toxicol Clin Toxicol.* 1999;37:239-258.
4. Baselt RC, Hanson VW. Efficacy of orally-administered chelating agents for nickel carbonyl toxicity in rats. *Res Commun Chem Pathol Pharmacol.* 1982;38:113-124.
5. Baselt RC, et al. Comparisons of antidotal efficacy of sodium diethyldithiocarbamate, D-penicillamine and triethylenetetramine upon acute toxicity of nickel carbonyl in rats. *Res Commun Chem Pathol Pharmacol.* 1977;18:677-688.
6. Berge SR, Skyberg K. Radiographic evidence of pulmonary fibrosis and possible etiologic factors at a nickel refinery in Norway. *J Environ Monit.* 2003;5:681-688.
7. Boland MA. *Nickel-makes Stainless Steel Strong: U.S. Geological Survey Fact Sheet 2012-3024.* Washington, DC: US Geological Survey; 2012.
8. Boysen M, et al. Nasal histology and nickel concentration in plasma and urine after improvements in the work environment at a nickel refinery in Norway. *Scand J Work Environ Health.* 1982;8:283-289.
9. Bradberry SM, Vale JA. Therapeutic review: do diethyldithiocarbamate and disulfiram have a role in acute nickel carbonyl poisoning? *J Toxicol Clin Toxicol.* 1999;37:259-264.
10. Byer TT, Morrell DS. Periumbilical allergic contact dermatitis: blue jeans or belt buckles? *Pediatr Dermatol.* 2004;21:223-226.
11. Christensen OB, Lagesson V. Nickel concentration of blood and urine after oral administration. *Ann Clin Lab Sci.* 1981;11:119-125.
12. Costa M, Mollenhauer HH. Carcinogenic activity of particulate nickel compounds is proportional to their cellular uptake. *Science.* 1980;209:515-517.
13. de Medeiros LM, et al. Complementary and alternative remedies: an additional source of potential systemic nickel exposure. *Contact Dermatitis.* 2008;58:97-100.
14. Delescluse J, Dinet Y. Nickel allergy in Europe: the new European legislation. *Dermatology.* 1994;189(suppl 2):56-57.
15. Denays R, et al. First epileptic seizure induced by occupational nickel poisoning. *Epilepsia.* 2005;46:961-962.

16. Dickel H, et al. Increased sensitivity of patch testing by standardized tape stripping beforehand: a multicentre diagnostic accuracy study. *Contact Dermatitis*. 2010;62:294-302.

17. Environmental Protection Agency: Office of Health and Environmental Assessment. Project summary health assessment document for nickel. Washington, DC: EPA; 1990.

18. Fay M. *Toxicological Profile for nickel*. Atlanta, GA: Agency for Toxic Substances and Disease Registry; 2005:1-351.

19. Hassler E, et al. Urinary and fecal elimination of nickel in relation to air-borne nickel in a battery factory. *Ann Clin Lab Sci*. 1983;13:217-224.

20. Hisatomi K, et al. Interstitial pneumonia caused by inhalation of fumes of nickel and chrome. *Respirology*. 2006;11:814-817.

21. Hostynek JJ. Sensitization to nickel: etiology, epidemiology, immune reactions, prevention, and therapy. *Rev Environ Health*. 2006;21:253-280.

22. Jensen CS, et al. Systemic contact dermatitis after oral exposure to nickel: a review with a modified meta-analysis. *Contact Dermatitis*. 2006;54:79-86.

23. Kincaid JF, et al. Nickel poisoning; 1. Experimental study of the effects of acute and subacute exposure to nickel carbonyl. *AMA Arch Ind Hyg Occup Med*. 1953;8:48-60.

24. Kurta DL, et al. Acute nickel carbonyl poisoning. *Am J Emerg Med*. 1993;11:64-66.

25. Lacy SA, et al. Distribution of nickel and cobalt following dermal and systemic administration with *in vitro* and *in vivo* studies. *J Biomed Mater Res*. 1996;32:279-283.

26. Lu LK, et al. Prevention of nickel allergy: the case for regulation? *Dermatol Clin*. 2009;27:155-161, vi-vii.

27. Mafra RA, et al. Glutamate transport in rat cerebellar granule cells is impaired by inorganic epileptogenic agents. *Neurosci Lett*. 2001;310:85-88.

28. Malo JL, et al. Occupational asthma caused by nickel sulfate. *J Allergy Clin Immunol*. 1982;69(1, pt 1):55-59.

29. Nakazawa G, et al. Sirolimus-eluting stents suppress neointimal formation irrespective of metallic allergy. *Circ J*. 2008;72:893-896.

30. Neligan PC. Transcutaneous metal absorption following chemical burn injury. *Burns*. 1996;22:232-233.

31. Nielsen GD, Andersen O. Effect of tetraethylthiuramdisulphide and diethyldithiocarbamate on nickel toxicokinetics in mice. *Pharmacol Toxicol*. 1994;75:285-293.

32. Phillips JI, et al. Pulmonary and systemic toxicity following exposure to nickel nanoparticles. *Am J Ind Med*. 2010;53:763-767.

33. Rahilly G, Price N. Nickel allergy and orthodontics. *J Orthod*. 2003;30:171-174.

34. Rezuke WN, et al. Reference values for nickel concentrations in human tissues and bile. *Am J Ind Med*. 1987;11:419-426.

35. Saito M, et al. Molecular mechanisms of nickel allergy. *Int J Mol Sci*. 2016;17.

36. Schaller KH, et al. Elimination kinetics of metals after an accidental exposure to welding fumes. *Int Arch Occup Environ Health*. 2007;80:635-641.

37. Seet RC, et al. Inhalational nickel carbonyl poisoning in waste processing workers. *Chest*. 2005;128:424-429.

38. Seilkop SK, Oller AR. Respiratory cancer risks associated with low-level nickel exposure: an integrated assessment based on animal, epidemiological, and mechanistic data. *Regul Toxicol Pharmacol*. 2003;37:173-190.

39. Shi ZC. Acute nickel carbonyl poisoning: a report of 179 cases. *Br J Ind Med*. 1986;43:422-424.

40. Sorahan T. Mortality of workers at a plant manufacturing nickel alloys, 1958-2000. *Occup Med (Lond)*. 2004;54:28-34.

41. Stojanovic D, et al. The level of nickel in smoker's blood and urine. *Cent Eur J Public Health*. 2004;12:187-189.

42. Su CC, et al. Incidence of oral cancer in relation to nickel and arsenic concentrations in farm soils of patients' residential areas in Taiwan. *BMC Public Health*. 2010;10:67.

43. Sunderman FW. Efficacy of sodium diethyldithiocarbamate (dithiocarb) in acute nickel carbonyl poisoning. *Ann Clin Lab Sci*. 1979;9:1-10.

44. Sunderman FW. A pilgrimage into the archives of nickel toxicology. *Ann Clin Lab Sci*. 1989;19:1-16.

45. Sunderman FW Jr, et al. Acute nickel toxicity in electroplating workers who accidently ingested a solution of nickel sulfate and nickel chloride. *Am J Ind Med*. 1988;14:257-266.

46. Sunderman FW Jr, et al. Nickel absorption and kinetics in human volunteers. *Proc Soc Exp Biol Med*. 1989;191:5-11.

47. Sunderman FW Sr. Use of sodium diethyldithiocarbamate in the treatment of nickel carbonyl poisoning. *Ann Clin Lab Sci*. 1990;20:12-21.

48. Templeton DM, et al. Tentative reference values for nickel concentrations in human serum, plasma, blood, and urine: evaluation according to the TRACY protocol. *Sci Total Environ*. 1994;148:243-251.

49. Thyssen JP, et al. Nickel sensitization, hand eczema, and loss-of-function mutations in the filaggrin gene. *Dermatitis*. 2008;19:303-307.

50. Thyssen JP, et al. Nickel allergy in Danish women before and after nickel regulation. *N Engl J Med*. 2009;360:2259-2260.

51. Torjussen W, Andersen I. Nickel concentrations in nasal mucosa, plasma, and urine in active and retired nickel workers. *Ann Clin Lab Sci*. 1979;9:289-298.

52. Tossavainen A, et al. Application of mathematical modelling for assessing the biological half-times of chromium and nickel in field studies. *Br J Ind Med*. 1980;37:285-291.

53. US Geological Survey. Mineral commodity summaries 2017. Washington, DC: US Geological Survey; 2017.

54. Verma R, et al. Molecular biology of nickel carcinogenesis: identification of differentially expressed genes in morphologically transformed C3H10T1/2 Cl 8 mouse embryo fibroblast cell lines induced by specific insoluble nickel compounds. *Mol Cell Biochem*. 2004;255:203-216.

55. Webster JD, et al. Acute nickel intoxication by dialysis. *Ann Intern Med*. 1980;92:631-633.

56. West B, Sunderman FW. Nickel poisoning. VI. A note concerning the ineffectiveness of edathamil calcium-disodium (calcium disodium ethylenediaminetetraacetic acid). *AMA Arch Ind Health*. 1958;18:480-482.

57. West B, Sunderman FW. Nickel poisoning. VII. The therapeutic effectiveness of alkyl dithiocarbamates in experimental animals exposed to nickel carbonyl. *Am J Med Sci*. 1958;236:15-25.

97 SELENIUM

Diane P. Calello

Selenium (Se)

Atomic number	=	34
Atomic weight	=	78.96 Da
Normal concentrations		
Whole blood	=	0.1–0.34 mg/L (1.27–4.32 µmol/L)
Serum	=	0.04–0.6 mg/L (0.51–7.6 µmol/L)
Urine		<0.03 mg/L (0.38 µmol/L)
Hair	=	5.1–17.7 nmol/g

INTRODUCTION

Selenium was discovered by Jöns Berzelius in 1817 as a contaminant in sulfuric acid vats that caused illness in Swedish factory workers. He originally believed it to be the element tellurium (from the Latin *tellus*, meaning "earth"); however, on finding it to be an entirely new, yet similar, element, he named it from the Greek *selene*, meaning "moon." Selenium has unusual light-sensitive electrical conductive properties, leading to its widespread use in industry. The long-term health benefits and risks of selenium are the subject of much recent investigation. It is both an essential component of the human diet and a poison.

In the 1970s, the role of selenium as an essential cofactor of the enzyme glutathione peroxidase was discovered. Keshan disease, an endemic cardiomyopathy, was described in 1979 in Chinese women and children who chronically consumed a selenium-poor diet.[15] Kashin-Beck disease, a disease causing shortened stature from chondrocyte necrosis, is described in young children in Russia, China, and Korea; although other etiologies are also likely responsible, selenium supplementation results in partial improvement.[4,23] Selenium was investigated for the prevention and treatment of a myriad of conditions, including autoimmune thyroiditis, cancer, Alzheimer disease, and tropical leishmaniasis.[43] However, it is now clear that selenium supplementation increases the risk of diabetes, amyotrophic lateral sclerosis, depression, and some forms of malignancy.[2,12,25,51]

The recommended daily allowance (RDA) in the United States of selenium for adults was established in 1980 and remains today at 55 mcg/day.[22] This was determined based on the degree of supplementation required to achieve optimal glutathione peroxidase activity in selenium-deficient study populations, and the amounts required to cause overt toxicity. Deficiency occurs when daily intake falls below 20 mcg/day.[15]

Chronic selenium toxicity, or selenosis, was first described in animals. It manifested as the acute syndrome of "blind staggers," and the more chronic "alkali disease" affected livestock eating plants grown in highly seleniferous soil. Findings included blindness, walking in circles, anorexia, weight loss, ataxia, and dystrophic hooves. Humans in seleniferous areas of China and Venezuela develop similar integumentary symptoms (dermatitis, hair loss, and nail changes) at an intake of approximately 6,000 mcg/day.[7,46] Several outbreaks of chronic selenium toxicity were related to improperly formulated dietary supplements.[3,10,52]

Selenium is widely distributed throughout the Earth's crust, usually substituting for sulfur in sulfide ores such as marcasite (FeS_2), arsenopyrite (FeAsS), and chalcopyrite ($CuFeS_2$). It is found in the soil, where it has leached from bedrock, in groundwater, and in volcanic gas. The highest soil concentrations of selenium in the United States are in the Midwest and the West, specifically areas of the Dakotas, Wyoming, Nebraska, Kansas, Utah, Colorado, Arizona, and New Mexico.[4] Dietary selenium is easily obtained through meats, grains, and cereals. Brazil nuts, grown in the foothills of the highly seleniferous Andes Mountains, contain the highest concentration measured in food, but chronic selenium toxicity from Brazil nuts is not reported.[4,27]

In industry, selenium is generated primarily as a by-product of electrolytic copper refining and in the combustion of rubber, paper, municipal waste, and fossil fuels. Selenium compounds are used in glass manufacture and coloring, photography, xerography, rubber vulcanization, and as insecticides and fungicides. Selenium sulfide is the active ingredient in many antidandruff shampoos. Gun bluing solution, used in the care of firearms to restore the natural color to the gun barrel, is composed of selenious acid in combination with cupric sulfate in hydrochloric acid, nitric acid, copper nitrate, or methanol. Tables 97–1 and 97–2 list features and regulatory standards of common selenium compounds.

CHEMICAL PRINCIPLES

Selenium is a nonmetal element of group 16/VIA of the periodic table along with oxygen, sulfur, tellurium, and polonium. Selenium exists in elemental, organic, and inorganic forms, with 4 important oxidation states: selenide (Se^{2-}), elemental (Se^0), selenite (Se^{4+}), and selenate (Se^{6+}). Water solubility generally increases with oxidation state. Selenium behaves similarly to sulfur in its tendency to form compounds and to participate extensively in biologic systems[4] and is both photovoltaic (able to convert light to electricity) and photoconductive (conducts electricity faster in bright light), which has led to its use in photography, xerography, and solar cells.

At least 3 solid allotropes of elemental selenium are described, including "gray selenium," which is predominant at room temperature, red crystalline selenium, and a red amorphous powder.[4] In general, toxicity from elemental selenium is rare and only occurs from long-term exposure. Hydrogen selenide (H_2Se) is formed from the reaction of water or acids with metal selenides or from the reaction of hydrogen with soluble selenium compounds; at room

TABLE 97–1	Selenium Compounds		
Name	**Chemical Formula**	**Oxidation State**	**Uses**
Selenium (elemental)	Se	0	Photography, catalyst, dietary supplement, xerography
Selenium sulfide	SeS_2	2⁻	Antidandruff shampoo, fungicide
Hydrogen selenide	H_2Se	2⁻	A by-product of metal selenides reaction with water; no commercial use
Dimethylselenide	CH_3SeCH_3	2⁻	Metabolite, garlic odor
Selenium dioxide	SeO_2	4⁺	Catalyst, photography, glass decolorizer, vulcanization of rubber, xerography
Selenium oxychloride	$SeOCl_2$	4⁺	Solvent, plasticizer
Selenious acid	H_2SeO_3	4⁺	Gun bluing solution
Sodium selenite	Na_2SeO_3	4⁺	Glass and porcelain manufacture
Selenium hexafluoride	SeF_6	6⁺	Gaseous electrical insulator
Sodium selenate	Na_2SeO_4	6⁺	Glass manufacture, insecticide

TABLE 97–2	Selenium Regulations and Advisories	
Oral—Recommended Intake and Exposure Limits		
RDA (2000)	55 mcg/day[a]	(0.8 mcg/kg/day)
NAS-TUL	400 mcg/day	(5.7 mcg/kg/day)
ATSDR-chronic oral	5 mcg/kg/day	
MRL[b]		
Water—Limits		
WHO	Drinking water	0.01 mg/L
FDA	Bottled water	0.05 mg/L
EPA	MCL, drinking	0.05 mg/L
Air—Limits[c]		
NIOSH		
REL (TWA)		0.2 mg/m³
IDLH		1.0 mg/m³
OSHA		
PEL (TWA)		0.2 mg/m³

[a] Values differ for pregnant and lactating women, children, and neonates. [b] No acute or intermediate MRL is established. Chronic ≥ 365 days. [c]Ambient background air concentrations are usually in the nanograms per cubic millimeter (ng/m³) range.

AHTSDR = American Toxic Surveillance and Disease Registry; EPA = Environmental Protection Agency; FDA = Food and Drug Administration; IDLH = immediately dangerous to life or health; MCL = maximum contaminant level; MRL = minimal risk level; NAS = National Academy of Sciences; NIOSH = National Institute for Occupational Safety and Health; OSHA = Occupational Safety and Health Administration; PEL = permissible exposure limit; RDA = recommended daily allowance; REL = recommended exposure limit; TUL = tolerable upper limit; TWA = time-weighted average; WHO = World Health Organization.

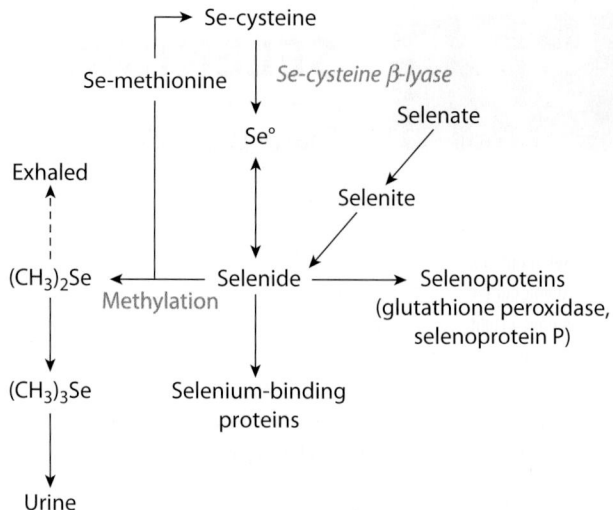

FIGURE 97–1. Metabolism of selenium. The selenide anion is central in selenium metabolism. Organic selenocysteine is converted via the β-lyase enzyme to elemental selenium and then to selenide. Selenomethionine either undergoes transsulfuration to selenocysteine or methylation to excretable metabolites. The selenate and selenite salts are reduced to selenide. Selenide then undergoes one of 3 processes: methylation, incorporation into selenoproteins, or binding by nonspecific plasma proteins.[1]

temperature, it exists in gaseous form, which results in industrial inhalation exposures. The organic alkyl selenides (dimethylselenide, trimethylselenide) are the least toxic and are by-products of endogenous selenium detoxification (methylation). Inorganic salts and acids are responsible for all cases of acute toxicity. Selenious acid (H_2SeO_3), generated from the reaction of selenium dioxide with water, is the most toxic form of selenium; ingestion of selenious acid is often fatal.[21,35,40,49]

PHARMACOLOGY

Selenium exists in one of 3 forms in the body. First, *selenoproteins* contain selenocysteine residues and have specific selenium-dependent roles primarily in oxidation–reduction reactions.[8] Second, nonspecific plasma proteins bind and aid in transport of selenium, either by directly binding selenium (albumin, globulins) or incorporating it as selenocysteine or selenomethionine in place of cysteine and methionine, respectively.[8] Third, there are several inorganic forms of selenium in transit throughout the body, such as selenate, alkyl selenides, and elemental selenium (Se^0).[8]

There are at least 25 selenoproteins—which include glutathione peroxidases, iodothyronine 5-deiodinases, and thioredoxin reductase—each of which contain a selenocysteine or selenomethionine residue at the active site.[43] The most studied of these is glutathione peroxidase I, which is responsible for detoxification of reactive oxygen species. Using reduced glutathione (GSH) as a substrate, glutathione peroxidase catalyzes the reduction of hydrogen peroxide to water and oxidized glutathione (GSSG, or glutathione disulfide); the reaction occurs by concomitant oxidation of the selenocysteine unit on the enzyme.[5] Other selenocysteine-containing proteins, such as thioredoxin reductase, have antioxidant properties. The selenocysteine-containing thyroid hormone deiodinases are responsible for the conversion of thyroxine (T_4) to the active triiodothyronine (T_3) form (Chap. 53).

PHARMACOKINETICS AND TOXICOKINETICS

Gastrointestinal (GI) absorption varies with the type of selenium, and human data are limited. Elemental selenium is the least bioavailable (≤50%), followed by inorganic selenite and selenate salts (75%).[33] Selenious acid is well absorbed from the lungs and GI tract (~85%) in animal studies.[13] Organic

selenium compounds are the best absorbed (~90%) as determined by isotope tracers in human studies.[4,29] A breastfed infant developed selenosis exclusively from maternal overexposure, suggesting transmission through breast milk.[53]

Inhalational absorption was reported in a group of workers exposed to selenium dioxide and hydrogen selenide gas,[4,19] but quantitative inhalation studies in humans are not available. Dermal absorption is limited. Selenium disulfide shampoos are not systemically absorbed as measured by urinary selenium concentrations[13] except in cases of repeated use on excoriated skin.[41]

The toxic dose of selenium varies widely among selenium compounds, as demonstrated by LD_{50} (median lethal dose for test subjects: 50%) animal studies,[46] making milligram per kilogram exposure estimates difficult to interpret. Elemental selenium has no reported adverse effects in acute overdose, although long-term overexposure is harmful. The selenium salts, particularly selenite, are more acutely toxic, as is selenium oxide (SeO_2) through its conversion to selenious acid in the presence of water. Selenious acid was lethal in children following ingestion of as little as a tablespoon of 4% solution.[35]

Metabolic conversion of all forms of selenium to the selenide anion occurs through various means (Fig. 97–1), after which the selenide ion undergoes one of 3 fates: (1) incorporation into selenoproteins such as glutathione peroxidase and triiodothyronine, (2) binding by nonspecific plasma proteins such as albumin or globulins, or (3) hepatic methylation into nontoxic, excretable metabolites. Trimethylselenide is the primary metabolite and is excreted by the kidneys, the major elimination pathway for selenium. Fecal elimination also occurs. Dimethylselenide production is usually minor but increases with exposure; this compound is volatilized through exhalation and sweat and is responsible for the garlic odor of patients exposed to excess selenium. The remaining selenium in the body is greater than 95% protein bound within 24 hours.[1,46] Toxicokinetic data are limited and vary by compound.

PATHOPHYSIOLOGY

In selenium deficiency, glutathione peroxidase activity is decreased, and GSH and glutathione S-transferases are increased.[9] Consequently, selenium-deficient rats are more resistant to substances detoxified by glutathione S-transferase, such as acetaminophen and aflatoxin B, and less resistant to other prooxidants, such as nitrofurantoin, diquat, and paraquat.[9] In animal studies of metal toxicity, selenium also appears to modify the effects of silver, cadmium, arsenic, copper, zinc, mercury, and fluoride; conversely, vanadium, tellurium, and arsenic modify the effects of selenium deficiency or excess.[6,20,24,46] Although it is proposed that this is accomplished through the formation of insoluble selenium–metal complexes, these relationships are not entirely understood.[18]

Less is known about the biochemical mechanism of selenium toxicity, and what is known is generally from in vitro data. Paradoxically, excess selenium causes oxidative stress, presumably as a result of prooxidant selenide (R-Se⁻) anions. In addition, the replacement of sulfur by selenium in enzymes of cellular respiration causes mitochondrial disruption, and the substitution of selenomethionine in place of methionine interferes with protein synthesis. Integumentary effects are also most likely a result of selenium interpolation into disulfide bridges of structural proteins such as keratin.[50]

CLINICAL MANIFESTATIONS
Acute
Dermal and Ophthalmic Exposure
Dermal exposure to selenious acid or to selenium dioxide (which is converted to selenious acid) and to selenium oxychloride (a vesicant hydrolyzed to hydrochloric acid) causes painful caustic burns.[16] Excruciating pain results from accumulation under fingernails. Corneal injury with severe pain, lacrimation, and conjunctival edema are reported after exposure to selenium dioxide sprayed unintentionally into the face.[34] In chronic exposures, "rose eye," a red discoloration of eyelids with palpebral conjunctivitis, is also described.

Inhalational Exposure
When inhaled, all selenium compounds have the potential to be respiratory irritants, although inhaled elemental selenium dusts are less injurious than those compounds that are converted to selenious acid.[1] Toxicity from hydrogen selenide inhalation is reported throughout the industrial literature.[11,17] Hydrogen selenide is oxidized to elemental selenium, so acute toxic exposures are limited to confined spaces where the hazardous gas accumulates; however, similar to hydrogen sulfide (H₂S), its ability to cause olfactory fatigue, rendering the exposed persons anosmic to the toxic fumes, poses a significant hazard (Chap. 25).[11] Acute exposure to high concentrations of hydrogen selenide gas produces respiratory and mucosal irritation, which in some cases persists for years as residual restrictive and obstructive disease.[44]

By contrast, selenium dioxide and selenium oxide fumes cause more injury through conversion to selenious acid in the presence of water in the respiratory tract. Upper respiratory irritation, bronchospasm, and transient hemodynamic instability developed in 28 workers in a selenium rectifier plant who were inadvertently exposed to smoke and high concentrations of selenium oxide in an enclosed area.[54] Some developed chemical pneumonitis, fever, chills, headache, vomiting, and diarrhea. Five patients required hospitalization for respiratory support, with fever, leukocytosis, and bilateral infiltrates. All patients recovered without sequelae.

Selenium hexafluoride is a caustic gas used in industrial settings as an electrical insulator. Its caustic properties are derived from its conversion to elemental selenium and hydrofluoric acid in the presence of water. Severe pain and burning of the eyes, skin, and respiratory tract similar to that seen with hydrofluoric acid exposure can occur after inhalation of selenium hexafluoride (Chap. 104).[36]

Oral Exposure
Acute fulminant selenium toxicity occurs after ingestion of inorganic selenium compounds, the most toxic of which is selenious acid in the form of gun bluing solution. Similar toxicity results from selenium oxide and dioxide, which are converted to selenious acid as well as sodium selenite and selenate. The underlying mechanism for this often fatal syndrome is not well understood, but may stem from a multifocal disruption of cellular oxidative processes and antioxidant defense mechanisms. Elemental selenium and organic selenium compounds do not cause acute toxicity.

Some authors have proposed a "triphasic" course of acute inorganic selenium toxicity, with GI, skeletal muscle, and circulatory symptoms as the toxic effects progress.[49] In reality, acute inorganic selenium poisoning is often rapid and fulminant, with onset of symptoms within minutes and, in some cases, death within one hour of ingestion. Gastrointestinal symptoms are the most commonly described and the first to occur and include abdominal pain, diarrhea, nausea, and vomiting. Caustic esophageal and gastric burns are sometimes the cause of these symptoms but not in all cases. Patients frequently have a garlic odor. Skeletal muscle involvement is characterized by weakness, hyporeflexia, myoclonus, fasciculations, and elevated creatine phosphokinase concentrations with normal myocardial band (MB) fraction. Acute kidney injury is also reported and presumably results from myoglobinuria and hemolysis. More severely poisoned patients exhibit lethargy, delirium, and coma.

Circulatory failure is the hallmark of serious inorganic selenium toxicity. Patients present with dyspnea, chest pain, tachycardia, and hypotension. Reported initial electrocardiographic (ECG) abnormalities include ST segment elevation, a prolonged QT interval, and T-wave inversions. Refractory hypotension occurs both as a result of decreased myocardial contractility from toxic cardiomyopathy and decreased peripheral vascular resistance. Pulmonary edema, ventricular dysrhythmias, myocardial and mesenteric infarction, and metabolic acidosis all contribute to poor outcome in these patients.[35,39,54] Death results from circulatory collapse in the setting of pump failure, hypotension, and ventricular dysrhythmias, often within 4 hours of ingestion.[21,26,40,48] Other less frequent abnormalities include hypokalemia, hyperkalemia, coagulopathy, leukocytosis, hemolysis, thrombocytopenia, and metabolic acidosis with an elevated lactate concentration.[45,49]

Chronic
Chronic elemental selenium toxicity, or selenosis, is most commonly reported in the present day as a result of improperly formulated selenium-containing dietary supplements. In 2008, at least 200 people developed painful skin lesions, diarrhea, alopecia, fever, fatigue, memory loss, and nail deformities after use of the supplement.[3,32,52] The manufacturer voluntarily recalled the product, and a US Food and Drug Administration investigation revealed that the liquid supplement contained approximately 200 times the concentration stated on the packaging.[14] The patients consumed approximately 40,000 mcg/d while taking the supplement, or 1,000 times the US RDA.[3] A similar outbreak occurred from a super-potent supplement in 1983, affecting at least 13 patients, all of whom recovered after discontinuation of the supplement.[10]

Selenosis is similar to arsenic toxicity, with the most consistent manifestations being nail and hair abnormalities. As in the case of arsenic toxicity, nail or hair findings alone are unlikely to be the sole evidence of selenosis, but their absence makes the diagnosis unlikely. The hair becomes very brittle, breaking off easily at the scalp, with regrowth of discolored hair and the development of an exfoliative pruritic scalp eruption with acneiform papules.[31] The nails also break easily, with white or red ridges that can be either transverse or longitudinal; the thumb is usually involved first, and paronychia and nail loss often develops.[31,38] The skin becomes erythematous, swollen, and blistered, as well as slow to heal and has a persistent red discoloration. Increased dental caries are described.[31] Neurologic manifestations include hyperreflexia, peripheral paresthesia, anesthesia, and hemiplegia. Although cardiotoxicity is described with both selenium deficiency and acute poisoning, no such cases are reported with human selenosis from chronic exposure. Aside from one case described in which there was insufficient postmortem data, there are no reported deaths from chronic exposure.[55]

Selenosis is implicated in a number of long-term environmental exposures. Many descriptions come from inhabitants of the Hubei province of China from 1961 to 1964, the majority of whom developed clinical signs after an estimated average consumption of 5,000 mcg/d of selenium (but as little as 910 mcg/d) derived from local crops and vegetation.[55] Inhabitants of a seleniferous area of Venezuela, consuming approximately 300 to 400 mcg/d of selenium, also developed symptoms of selenium excess; however, the low socioeconomic and poor dietary status of the subjects is a confounding factor.[7] In contrast, US residents in a seleniferous area with a high selenium intake (724 mcg/d) over 2 years who were compared with a control population and monitored for symptoms and laboratory abnormalities remained asymptomatic, with only a clinically insignificant elevation of hepatic aminotransferases in the high-selenium group.[30] Average selenium concentrations were serum, 0.215 mg/L; whole blood, 0.322 mg/L; and urine, 0.17 mg/L. A similar cohort with comparable blood concentrations was also reported in the Brazilian Amazon.[27]

Selenosis is also reported in the industrial setting. Copper refinery workers develop garlic odor and GI and respiratory symptoms coincident with exposure to selenium dust and fumes.[19] Long before workplace biologic monitoring took place, intense garlic odor of the breath and secretions was recognized as a reason to remove a worker from selenium exposure until the odor subsided. Neuropsychiatric findings such as fatigue, irritability, and depression are reported throughout the industrial literature and are difficult to quantify. Early reports describe the selenium factory worker who "could not stand his children about him" at the end of the day.[16]

Although carcinogenicity is suggested by a number of animal studies, the available human data suggest, if anything, an inverse correlation between selenium intake and cancer risk. The International Agency for Research on Cancer does not list selenium as a known or suspected carcinogen.[4] Animal studies also suggest that selenium has embryotoxic and teratogenic properties.[18] A recent large randomized controlled trial of selenium supplementation reported an increased risk of diabetes mellitus with the ingestion of 200 mcg/d of elemental selenium-fed baker's yeast compared with placebo.[2,25,51]

DIAGNOSTIC TESTING

Over time, selenium is incorporated into blood and erythrocyte proteins, making serum the best measure of acute toxicity and whole blood preferable for the assessment of patients with chronic exposure. Patients with acute poisoning generally have an initial serum concentration greater than 2 mg/L, which falls below 1 mg/L within 24 hours, reflecting redistribution.[38] Patients with long-term elemental exposures are reported to have serum concentrations of 0.5 to 1.0 mg/L. However, there is no predictable relationship between selenium concentrations and exposure, toxicity, or time course. Population-based studies suggest an average serum concentration of 0.126 mg/L in the United States.[37]

Urine concentrations reflect very recent exposure because urinary excretion of selenium is maximal within the first 4 hours. In addition, urine concentrations are an imperfect measure because they can be affected by the most recent meal and hydration status. However, in general, a normal urinary concentration is less than 0.03 mg/L.[42] Freezing of urine specimens after collection is recommended to retard the enzymatic formation of volatile metabolites.[38]

Hair concentrations of selenium were measured in the Hubei Chinese populations of interest and during the contaminated supplement outbreak in 2008 and may be a useful qualitative measure of chronic exposure.[31,47,55] However, the usefulness of hair selenium is limited in countries such as the United States where the use of selenium sulfide shampoos is widespread.

Other ancillary tests to assess selenium toxicity include ECG, thyroid function, platelet counts, aminotransferases, creatinine, and creatine phosphokinase concentrations. These are abnormal in some patients (eg, patients with selenious acid poisoning) and are not indicated in patients not expected to develop systemic toxicity.

MANAGEMENT

Pain

Aside from standard pain management strategies, a number of topical remedies for selenium burns are reported historically with little evidence supporting their use. For example, a 10% sodium thiosulfate solution or ointment to reduce selenium dioxide to elemental selenium is mentioned as a potential therapy for painful skin, nail bed, or ocular burns.[16] In one series, workers exposed to selenium dioxide fumes reported similar relief from inhalation of vapor from ammonium hydroxide–soaked sponges.[54] However, the mechanism and efficacy of these therapies are unproven, and we recommend they not be administered.

For workers exposed to selenium hexafluoride gas, it is reasonable to apply calcium gluconate gel to the affected areas. This is the same treatment as in hydrofluoric acid exposures, which is discussed in Chap. 104.

Decontamination

As in the case of any toxic exposure, prompt removal from the source is required if possible. Patients with dermal exposure should have their skin irrigated immediately. There are limited data to support the use of aggressive GI decontamination after the ingestion of most elemental selenium–containing xenobiotics because little expected acute toxicity is present. However, in xenobiotics with the potential for producing systemic toxicity, such as the selenite salts, decontamination with orogastric lavage and activated charcoal is reasonable.

Special mention should be made of the ingestion of selenious acid. Given its toxicity, the judicious use of small nasogastric lavage would be reasonable based on the time since ingestion, the amount and concentration ingested, the presence or absence of spontaneous emesis, the likelihood of caustic esophageal injury, and the clinical condition of the patient.

Chelation and Antidotal Therapy

There are no proven antidotes for selenium toxicity. Animal studies and scant human data suggest that chelation with dimercaprol (BAL), edetate calcium disodium ($CaNa_2EDTA$), or succimer is not advised because they form nephrotoxic complexes with selenium, do not speed clinical recovery, and in fact, worsen toxicity.[28,29] Arsenical compounds appear to ameliorate selenium toxicity through enhanced biliary excretion,[11,18,19,28] but in light of their inherent toxicity and unproven efficacy, they are not indicated.

Extracorporeal removal techniques such as hemodialysis or hemofiltration decrease selenium concentrations in patients undergoing the procedure regularly for chronic kidney disease, so theoretically, this could be effective in lowering toxic serum selenium concentrations. However, because of extensive protein binding, this benefit is likely minor and only relevant to patients undergoing frequent dialysis. Nonetheless, although there are only scant reports of hemodialysis in acute selenium poisoning, it would be reasonable in patients with severe toxicity.[24,26]

Supportive Care

This is the mainstay of therapy in selenium poisoning. In particular, patients with selenious acid toxicity require intensive monitoring and multisystem support to survive.

SUMMARY

- Selenium is an essential trace element and is required in the diet of both animals and humans.
- Ingestion of selenious acid is often fatal.
- Other selenium compounds cause variable toxicity, usually in the setting of occupational exposure. Topical and inhalational exposure causes burns and pulmonary irritation, respectively. Acute systemic exposure results in gastrointestinal, muscular, and circulatory toxicity.
- Long-term exposure to elemental selenium leads to selenosis, of which alopecia is the most consistent finding.
- Although it is possible to obtain blood, urine, and hair selenium concentrations to confirm exposure, no clear relationship exists between concentration and clinical outcome.
- Supportive therapy remains the standard of care.

REFERENCES

1. Agency for Toxic Substances and Disease Registry. *Toxicological Profile for Selenium.* Atlanta, GA: Agency for Toxic Substances and Disease Registry; 2003.
2. Albanes D, et al. Plasma tocopherols and risk of prostate cancer in the Selenium and Vitamin E Cancer Prevention Trial (SELECT). *Cancer Prev Res (Phila).* 2014;7:886-895.
3. Aldosary BM, et al. Case series of selenium toxicity from a nutritional supplement. *Clin Toxicol (Phila).* 2012;50:57-64.
4. Barceloux DG. Selenium. *J Toxicol Clin Toxicol.* 1999;37:146-172.
5. Berg JM, et al. *Biochemistry.* 5th ed. New York, NY: W. H. Freeman; 2002.
6. Bjorklund G. Selenium as an antidote in the treatment of mercury intoxication. *Biometals.* 2015;28:605-614.
7. Bratter P, et al. Selenium status of children living in seleniferous areas of Venezuela. *J Trace Elem Electrolytes Health Dis.* 1991;5:269-270.
8. Burk RF, Hill KE. Regulation of selenium metabolism and transport. *Annu Rev Nutr.* 2015;35:109-134.

9. Burk RF, Lane JM. Modification of chemical toxicity by selenium deficiency. *Fundam Appl Toxicol.* 1983;3:218-221.

10. Centers for Disease Control and Prevention. Selenium intoxication—New York. *MMWR Morb Mortal Wkly Rep.* 1984;33:157-158.

11. Cerwenka EA, Cooper WC. Toxicology of selenium and tellurium and their compounds. *Arch Environ Health.* 1961;3:189-200.

12. Colangelo LA, et al. Selenium exposure and depressive symptoms: the Coronary Artery Risk Development in Young Adults Trace Element Study. *Neurotoxicology.* 2014; 41:167-174.

13. Cummins LM, Kimura ET. Safety evaluation of selenium sulfide anti-dandruff shampoos. 1971;20:89-96.

14. F.D.A. completes final analysis of "Total Body Formula" and "Total Body Mega Formula" products. 2008; https://wayback.archive-it.org/7993/20170113085654/ http://www.fda.gov/NewsEvents/Newsroom/PressAnnouncements/ucm116892.htm. Accessed October 4, 2017.

15. Ge K, et al. Keshan disease—an endemic cardiomyopathy in China. *Virchows Arch.* 1983;401:1-15.

16. Glover JR. Selenium and its industrial toxicology. *Ind Med Surg.* 1970;39:50-54.

17. Goen T, et al. Biological monitoring of exposure and effects in workers employed in a selenium-processing plant. *Int Arch Occup Environ Health.* 2015;88:623-630.

18. Goyer RA, Clarkson TW. *Toxic Effects of Metals.* 6th ed. New York, NY: McGraw-Hill; 2000.

19. Holness DL, et al. Health status of copper refinery workers with specific reference to selenium exposure. *Arch Environ Health.* 1989;44:291-297.

20. Huang Z, et al. Low selenium status affects arsenic metabolites in an arsenic exposed population with skin lesions. *Clin Chim Acta.* 2008;387:139-144.

21. Hunsaker DM, et al. Acute selenium poisoning: suicide by ingestion. *J Forensic Sci.* 2005;50:942-946.

22. Institute of Medicine (US) Panel on Dietary Oxidants and Related Compounds. *Dietary reference intakes for vitamin C, vitamin E, selenium, and carotenoids.* Washington, DC: National Academy of Sciences; 2000.

23. Jirong Y, et al. Sodium selenite for treatment of Kashin-Beck disease in children: a systematic review of randomised controlled trials. *Osteoarthritis Cartilage.* 2012;20:605-613.

24. Kise Y, et al. Acute oral selenium intoxication with ten times the lethal dose resulting in deep gastric ulcer. *J Emerg Med.* 2004;26:183-187.

25. Klein EA, et al. Vitamin E and the risk of prostate cancer: the selenium and vitamin E cancer prevention trial (SELECT). *JAMA.* 2011;306:1549-1556.

26. Koppel C, et al. Fatal poisoning with selenium dioxide. *J Toxicol Clin Toxicol.* 1986; 24:21-35.

27. Lemire M, et al. No evidence of selenosis from a selenium-rich diet in the Brazilian Amazon. *Environ Int.* 2012;40:128-136.

28. Levander OA. Metabolic interrelationships and adaptations in selenium toxicity. *Ann N Y Acad Sci.* 1972;192:181-192.

29. Lombeck I, et al. Acute selenium poisoning of a 2-year-old child. *Eur J Pediatr.* 1987; 146:308-312.

30. Longnecker MP, et al. Selenium in diet, blood, and toenails in relation to human health in a seleniferous area. *Am J Clin Nutr.* 1992;53:1288-1294.

31. Lopez RE, et al. Ingestion of a dietary supplement resulting in selenium toxicity. *J Am Acad Dermatol.* 2009;63:168-169.

32. MacFarquhar JK, et al. Acute selenium toxicity associated with a dietary supplement. *Arch Intern Med.* 2010;170:256-261.

33. McAdam PA, et al. Absorption of selenite and L-selenomethionine in healthy young men using a 74selenium tracer [abstract]. *Fed Proc.* 1985;44:1670.

34. Middleton JM. Selenium burn of the eye. Review of a case with review of the literature. *Arch Ophthalmol.* 1947;38:806-811.

35. Nantel AJ, et al. Acute poisoning by selenious acid. *Vet Hum Toxicol.* 1985;27:531-533.

36. National Research Council (US) Committee on Toxicology. *Nineteenth Interim Report of the Committee on Acute Exposure Guideline Levels: Part A.* Washington, DC: National Academy of Sciences; 2011.

37. Niskar AS, et al. Serum selenium levels in the US population: Third National Health and Nutrition Examination Survey, 1988-1994. *Biol Trace Elem Res.* 2003;91:1-10.

38. Nuttall KL. Evaluating selenium poisoning. *Ann Clin Lab Sci.* 2006;36:406-420.

39. Pentel P, et al. Fatal acute selenium toxicity. *J Forensic Sci.* 1985;30:556-562.

40. Quadrani DA, et al. A fatal case of gun blue ingestion in a toddler. *Vet Hum Toxicol.* 2000;42:96-98.

41. Ransome JW. Selenium sulfide intoxication. *N Engl J Med.* 1961;264:384-385.

42. Robberecht HJ, Deelstra HA. Selenium in human urine: Concentration levels and medical implications. *Clin Chim Acta.* 1984;136:107-120.

43. Sanmartin C, et al. Selenium and clinical trials: new therapeutic evidence for multiple diseases. *Curr Med Chem.* 2011;18:4635-4650.

44. Schecter A, et al. Acute hydrogen selenide inhalation. *Chest.* 1980;77:554-555.

45. See KA, et al. Accidental death from acute selenium poisoning. *Med J Aust.* 2006; 185:388-389.

46. Shamberger RJ. *Biochemistry of Selenium.* New York, NY: Plenum Press; 1983.

47. Shamberger RJ. Validity of hair mineral testing. *Biol Trace Elem Res.* 2002;87:1-28.

48. Sioris LJ, Pentel PR. Acute selenium poisoning. *Vet Hum Toxicol.* 1980;22:364.

49. Spiller HA, Pfiefer E. Two fatal cases of selenium toxicity. *Forensic Sci Int.* 2007; 171:67-72.

50. Stadtman T. Selenium biochemistry. *Science.* 1974;183:915-922.

51. Stranges S, et al. Effects of long-term selenium supplementation on the incidence of type 2 diabetes. *Ann Intern Med.* 2007;147:217-223.

52. Sutter ME, et al. Selenium toxicity: a case of selenosis caused by a nutritional supplement. *Ann Intern Med.* 2008;148:970-971.

53. Webb A, Kerns W. What is the origin of these nail changes in an otherwise healthy young patient? *J Med Toxicol.* 2009;5:39-40.

54. Wilson HM. Selenium oxide poisoning. *N C Med J.* 1962;23:73-75.

55. Yang G, et al. Endemic selenium intoxication of humans in China. *Am J Clin Nutr.* 1983; 37:872-881.

98

SILVER

Melisa W. Lai-Becker and Michele M. Burns

Silver (Ag)

Atomic number	=	47
Atomic weight	=	107.9
Normal concentrations		
Serum	<	0.5 mcg/L (<10 nmol/L)
Urine (24-hour)	<	1 mcg/L (<20 nmol/L)

HISTORY

Although the symbol of silver, Ag, is derived from the Latin and Greek words for silver—*argentum* and *argyros*—the word we use in English is derived from Slavic and Germanic *Silubr* and *Sirebro*, as well as Old English *Seolfor*. The alchemy symbol of silver (a crescent moon) and dalton symbol (a coinlike circumscribed letter S) convey the impression of silver as a valued and precious element.

In Asia Minor and on islands in the Aegean Sea, dumps of slag (scum formed by molten metal surface oxidation) demonstrate that silver was likely separated from lead circa 4000 B.C. The use of silver as a precious metal with trade value appears to have begun around 600 B.C., when weighed pieces of silver were exchanged for goods. Silver coinage debuted circa 550 B.C. in the Mediterranean, and was adopted by various empires, dynasties, and nation-states thereafter. Today, only Mexico uses silver in circulating coinage.

The Phoenicians and early Greeks knew to store water, wine, and vinegar in silver-lined vessels during long sea voyages, just as later American pioneers added silver coins to water barrels and jugs of milk to keep them fresh.[56] The phrase "born with a silver spoon in his mouth" referred originally to health and not wealth, as silver pacifiers and baby spoons were used to help ward off childhood illnesses.

A traded commodity on the world's markets, silver was used as an abstract financial standard for various economies throughout modern banking history until the late 19th century. Although the United States incorporates silver purely in commemorative and proof coins, the state of Utah passed the "Legal Tender Act of 2011" to allow its residents to use silver and gold coins produced by the US Mint as cash with value based on weight rather than minted face value.[71,85]

Beyond the economic role of silver, the electrical and thermal conductive properties of the element make it an invaluable material for scientific instrument manufacture and engineering. Because silver contacts neither corrode nor overheat, silver is commonly used in electronic devices and appliances. Silver was a key component of early telecommunications—it was the choice for Morse's first telegraph contacts in 1844—and made the jet age possible, as only silver-plated bearings have the adequate dry lubricity necessary for safe engine shutdown without volatile oil lubricants. Today, washing machines, cars, smartphones, and many types of consumer electronics—from televisions to toaster ovens—use small amounts of silver throughout their mechanical and electronic parts. Silver also remains relevant in advancing technologies of the Information Age. Silver nanoparticles (AgNPs) decorated on graphene layers combined in a pencillike tool provide the ability to literally draw conducting lines on new portable, foldable, and disposable "paper" circuit boards.[52] Likewise, integrating silver nanowire (AgNW) with conducting films polymerized to cloth is allowing for development of wearable electronics that can maintain thermal, chemical, and mechanical stability.[65,86]

Silver is also used to "make rain": silver iodide crystals, whose lattice structure is similar to ice, are released into "supercooled" (7°F–25°F) clouds, causing water droplets in clouds to attach and form ice crystals that become large and heavy enough to drop from the clouds and melt into raindrops en route to earth.

The medicinal value of silver has been greatly exaggerated and is suggested by some to be a "cure-all." In the late 19th and early 20th century, claims were made that oral administration of colloidal silver proteins (CSPs) (gelatinous suspensions of finely divided elemental silver) would successfully treat diverse diseases, mostly without evidence.[21,81] However, in 1960, the United States Dispensary stated that "there is no justification for this internal use, either theoretically or practically," and silver was banned in all nonprescription drugs.[19] In 1999, the US Food and Drug Administration (FDA) issued a Final Rule declaring that all nonprescription (over-the-counter {OTC}) drugs containing colloidal silver or silver salts are "not recognized as safe and effective and are misbranded."[20] However, CSPs and other silver-containing "natural" products were reintroduced for use as health and dietary supplements and as such are not subject to FDA regulation under the Dietary Supplement Health and Education Act of 1994 (DSHEA) as long as they make no claim to treat or prevent any disease.[21] After the anthrax terrorist acts of 2001, the mayor of Tampa, Florida, called for CSPs to be mixed into the town's water supply as a protective "elixir" without scientific justification.[4] Throughout the late 20th century, companies even tried to market silver acetate—containing products such as lozenges, gums, and sprays for use as smoking-cessation aids due to production of an unpleasant taste when combined with tobacco.[36] Since the turn of the 21st century, there has been a small resurgence of case reports of argyria—a permanent bluish-gray discoloration of the skin from chronic silver overexposure—due to silver-containing products continuing to be marketed and sold online as "natural" health supplements, with few warnings about the possible development of argyria.[24]

EPIDEMIOLOGY

Humans are exposed to minute amounts of silver in various occupations. Silver is released into the environment during silver nitrate manufacture for use in photography (diminishing), mirrors, plating, inks and dyes, and porcelain; as well as for germicides, antiseptics, caustics, and analytical reagents. Silver-salt catalysts, used for oxidation–reduction and polymerization reactions, are another source of silver exposure, as are silver powder pigments and paints.[43] Workplace exposure is often via transdermal, transmucosal, or inhalational routes as silver particles are liberated during various mining, refining, and manufacturing processes.

Both the National Institute for Occupational Safety and Health (NIOSH) and the Occupational and Safety Health Administration (OSHA) established the safe occupational exposure limit to silver metal and soluble compounds as 10 mcg/m^3 air per 8-hour work shift. The estimated oral intake of silver from average environmental exposure for humans not working in silver-related industries ranges from 10 to 88 mcg/d.[18]

Additionally, industrial exposure of workers involved in silver mining and manufacturing increases the workplace risk of generalized argyria, although development of signs of argyria from uninterrupted occupational exposure reportedly takes up to 24 years.[14] Employees are susceptible to localized argyria and corneal argyrosis (permanent ashen-gray discoloration of the conjunctiva) following repeated topical exposure from working with smaller amounts of silver in specific applications. These localized forms of argyria occur in workers who coat metallic films on glass and china, manufacture electroplating and photographic processing solutions, prepare artificial pearls, and even those who simply primarily cut and polish silver.

PHARMACOLOGY

Following absorption, silver is transported by globulins in blood and stored mainly in skin and liver, with average daily excretion via bile and elimination in the feces (up to 30–80 mcg/day), with a smaller amount excreted in the urine (up to 10 mcg/day).[19] Silver elimination through the feces occurs in 2 phases: the initial phase has a relatively short $t_{1/2}$ ranging from 1 to 2.4 days, varying with route of administration (apparent $t_{1/2}$ is: oral, 1 day; inhalational, 1.7 days; and intravenous, 2.4 days),[19,22,54] and second has an elimination $t_{1/2}$ of 48 to 52 days, which is thought to represent liver deposition and clearance.[47,55]

Although study of a single human showed 18% of an orally administered silver acetate salt was retained after 30 weeks, animal studies show little silver absorption from gastrointestinal (GI) tract, with 90% of ingested silver excreted within 2 days of ingestion.[18] Humans retain only 0% to 10% of their daily silver exposure of 10 to 88 mcg/day.[83] Minute amounts of silver accumulate in humans throughout life, with a possible estimated lifetime accumulation of 230 to 480 mg by 50 years of age.[18] Silver has a $1^+(Ag^+)$ valence when bonding with other elements and compounds to form complex ions and salts. Because of the antimicrobial effects of silver cations at low concentrations,[70] silver is used for potential medicinal and bactericidal effects.

The antimicrobial activity of silver is related to both direct binding to biologic molecules and disruption of hydrogen ions and, thus, pH balance. Silver ions bind to electron donor groups of proteins (sulfhydryl, amine, carboxyl, phosphate, and imidazole) to inhibit enzymatic activities and provoke protein denaturation and precipitation.[21] Silver also intercalates with DNA without destroying the double helix, thereby inhibiting fungal DNAse.[19a] Silver ions induce proton leakage through a bacterial (*Vibrio cholerae*) membrane, leading to loss of the proton motor force in oxidative phosphorylation, with subsequent energy loss and cell death.[13] Bacterial resistance to silver was not reported until the mid-1970s, followed shortly thereafter by the identification of the genes for silver resistance in bacteria.[70]

Although banned from routine administration via intravenous, intramuscular, and oral routes in the United States, silver salts are approved for use in topical medications, either as a caustic styptic (hemostatic) or as an antimicrobial for burn care. Approved medicinal uses for silver in the United States apply only to silver salts and specifically preclude use of elemental silver (Table 98–1).

Today silver is used in water filtration cartridges and supermarket products for washing vegetables. It is also used as a low cost nonfiltration point-of-use-water-treatment (PoUWT) technology by embedding silver in ceramic tablets that can be placed in a water storage container to release low steady concentrations of disinfecting silver ions.[16] Incorporation of silver is also used as a means of preventing biofilm formation in dental unit water lines.[27] Silver was also used to sterilize recycled drinking water on the Russian MIR space station and NASA space shuttle.[70] Silver dressings used on burns speed healing and reduce scarring,[46] perhaps because of hormesis of epithelial cells;[72] and silver sulfadiazine added to burn dressings is bacteriocidal and increases the rate of reepithelialization across partial-thickness wounds.[12] However, more recent animal model research demonstrates that these findings may not be applicable to nonburn excisional wounds.[57]

Central venous catheters impregnated with silver sulfadiazine and silver-impregnated Foley catheters are used to lower rates of infection.[29,48] For example, extraventricular drains (EVDs) impregnated with silver have had half the CSF infection risk as plain catheters.[35] Also, silver-lined endotracheal tubes reduce the risk of ventilator-assisted pneumonia (VAP) by up to 51%, including specifically drug-resistant pathogens such as methicillin-resistant *Staphylococcus aureus*, *Pseudomonas aeruginosa*, and *Acinetobacter baumanii*.[66]

Multiple new antibacterial applications are under investigation, ranging from applying a silver-containing coating to prevent biofilm formation on titanium orthopedic implants, to the use of silver to treat osteomyelitis.[42,74] Additionally, in the realm of oral and dental health, silver nanoparticles eliminate *Enterococcus faecalis* following root canal surgery and are effective

TABLE 98–1 Medicinal Silver Containing Products

Product Name/Device	Route of Administration/ Exposure	Applications
Silver nitrate (1% AgNO$_3$)	Ophthalmic	Prevention of gonorrheal ophthalmia neonatorum.
Silver nitrate (10% AgNO$_3$)	Cutaneous	Chemical cautery of nasal mucosa and exuberant granulations (eg, in podiatry for corns, calluses, impetigo vulgaris, plantar warts, and papillomatous growths).
Silver sulfadiazine (0.2% or 1% micronized silver sulfadiazine)	Cutaneous	Antimicrobial adjunct for prevention and treatment of wound infection for patients with second- and third-degree burns.
Silver-impregnated catheters and tubes	Nanoparticle coating	Antimicrobial adjunct for use in catheters (Foley catheters, central venous catheters, extra ventricular drains, and endotracheal tubes).
Silver acetate	Mucocutaneous (oral)	Used in gum, sprays, and lozenges as smoking cessation adjunct. Silver combined with smoke creates an unpleasant metallic taste in the user's mouth.[36]

in preventing dental caries in children when infused as pit and fissure sealants.[2,61] However, in spite of the disinfectant characteristics of silver, concerns persist with regard to the long-term toxicity of silver.[10,78]

PATHOPHYSIOLOGY

In great enough quantities, silver manifests cardiovascular, hepatic, and hematopoietic toxicity. Acutely, administration of 50 mg or more of particulate metallic (colloidal) silver intravenously in humans is fatal, leading to pulmonary edema, acute respiratory distress syndrome (ARDS), hemorrhage, and necrosis of bone marrow, liver, and kidneys.[19] The mechanism for this acute toxicity was studied only in the water flea (*Daphnia magna*) where silver blocks Na$^+$,K$^+$-ATPase activity.[6] A summary of silver toxicity manifested in animals and humans is described in Table 98–2.

Silver is not classified with regard to human carcinogenicity. It has not been found to be mutagenic, and no current data link therapeutic use of silver to human cancer.[18] Although animal studies show that silver implanted subcutaneously leads to local sarcoma formation, the EPA has deemed this reaction questionable with regard to human carcinogenicity, as implantation of other insoluble solids—such as plastic and smooth ivory—in animals produces similar results.[18] Colloidal silver injected into rats induces growths at injection sites, but intramuscular injections of silver powder have not induced cancer.[23]

Local inflammatory responses notwithstanding, silver is considered an inert substance and not a human carcinogen. In fact, silver nanoparticles (AgNPs) (Chap. 125) are increasingly being shown to possess antitumor properties through inhibition of transcription factors that promote cancer cell growth and angiogenesis.[11] Continued research of the antimicrobial properties of silver has led to further inquiry into its apparent specific cytotoxicity against ovarian cancer cells[3] and ovarian cancer stem cells[84] as well as a chemotherapeutic adjunct by providing a delivery scaffold for chemotherapeutics.[38] As a result of these new insights into AgNP cytotoxicity, more research is being conducted to assess the effects of silver nanoparticles on reproductive toxicity[17,33,39] and the formation of neural tube defects.

TABLE 98–2	Silver Toxicity: Systemic Manifestations
Cardiovascular	Rats given 0.1% silver nitrate in drinking water for 218 days developed ventricular hypertrophy that was not attributable to silver deposition in the heart despite advanced pigmentation in other body organs.[51]
Dermatologic	Generalized argyria, localized argyria, and argyrosis (silver deposition in the eyes) developed after chronic administration of silver.
Hematologic	Topical application of silver (human) correlated with bone marrow depression with subsequent leukopenia or aplastic anemia.[9]
Hepatic	Vitamin E and selenium-deficient rats developed hepatic necrosis with ultrastructural changes after administration of silver salts.[9,13,77] Silver can induce selenium deficiency that consequently inhibits synthesis of the selenoenzyme glutathione peroxidase.
Neurologic	Silver deposits in peripheral nerves, basal membranes, macrophages, and elastic fibers were found in one reported case of a 55-year-old woman with progressive vertigo, cutaneous hypoesthesia, and weakness after self-administration of silver salts to treat oral mycosis for 9 years.[80] Seizures were reported in a schizophrenic patient who ingested >20 mg silver daily for 40 years. Serum silver concentrations were elevated (12 mcg/L). Seizures resolved concurrently with discontinuation of silver ingestion and a subsequent decrease in silver serum concentration.[50]
Renal	Tubular lesions are demonstrated in animals, and acute tubular necrosis is rarely reported in humans.[44]

In vitro, silver nanoparticles are effective in inhibiting islet amyloid polypeptide (IAPP) aggregation associated with type 2 diabetes, perhaps opening a promising new application for nanotechnologies aimed at mitigating such an amyloid-mediated pathology.[79] However, although this IAPP inhibition may be extrapolated to other amyloid-mediated diseases like Alzheimer dementia in vitro,[53] in vivo exposure in murine models has instead demonstrated potential neurodegenerative progression.[40]

Argyria

The most significant effect of silver overexposure in humans is argyria, a permanent bluish-gray discoloration of skin resulting from silver throughout the integument (Figs. 98–1 and 98–2).

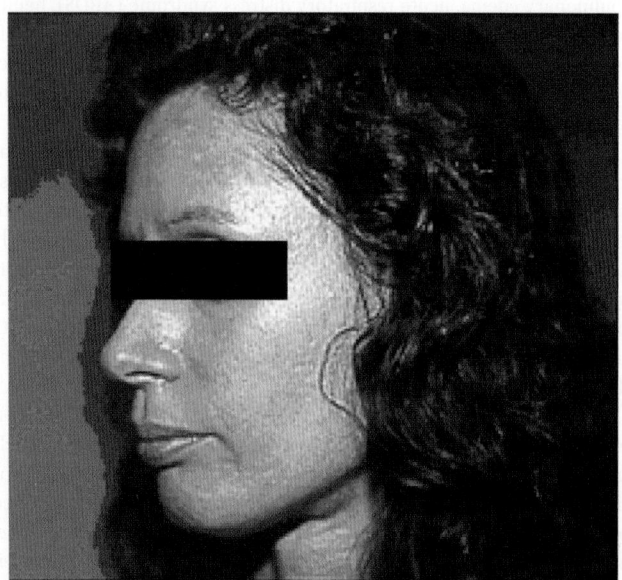

FIGURE 98–1. Argyria, the slate or silver discoloration of the skin that results from silver overexposure is demonstrated in this image of Rosemary Jacobs, who developed the condition after use of colloidal silver nasal drops for 3 years as a teenager. *(Used with permission from Rosemary Jacobs. We thank Ms. Rosemary Jacobs for her support and her permission to use the featured photographs.)*

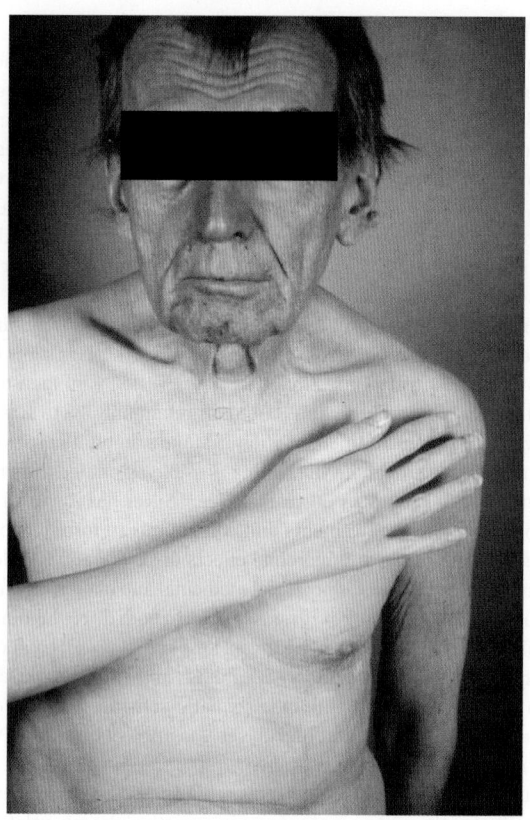

FIGURE 98–2. Long-term exposure to AgNO$_3$ in the workplace led to this patient's characteristic pigment changes of argyria. A normally pigmented arm is across the patient's chest. *(Used with permission from the New York University Department of Dermatology.)*

Generalized argyria develops in stages, beginning with an initial gray-brown staining of gingiva, progressing to hyperpigmentation and bluish-gray discoloration in sun-exposed areas. Later, nail beds, sclerae and mucous membranes become hyperpigmented; on autopsy, viscera are noted to be blue.

Cases of argyria have been reported in the medical literature since at least the early 19th century. One of the most famous cases of argyria is that of the Barnum and Bailey Circus' "Blue Man" who died at New York's Bellevue hospital in 1923 and was described on autopsy as follows: "The color of the skin was of an unusually deep blue and from a distance appeared almost black. This deep color was almost uniform throughout the entire body, although it was more intense over the exposed skin areas."[26] An American woman who developed argyria as a teenager during the 1950s from the use of a nasal CSP for allergies described her story on the Internet to warn others of the effects of prolonged contact with, or ingestion of, silver salts.[31] Her appearance was documented as an Image in Clinical Medicine in the *New England Journal of Medicine*.[8] In 2002, libertarian party Montana legislator Stan Jones became known as the "blue" lawmaker who promoted the use of colloidal silver health supplements and developed argyria after manufacturing his own colloidal silver at home out of fears that the Y2K (year 2000) problem might cause a shortage of antibiotics.[5,59]

Generalized argyria can result from either simple mechanical impregnation of skin by silver particles or inhalational and oral absorption of particulate silver. Local routes of silver absorption are through the conjunctiva or oral mucous membranes after long-term topical treatment with silver salts.

Argyria occurs at doses much lower than those associated with acutely toxic effects of silver; the degree of discoloration is directly proportional to the amount of silver absorbed or ingested.[25] The threshold dose for silver accumulation and retention resulting in generalized argyria varies considerably. Discoloration is reported from as little as a cumulative 1 g of metallic silver administered intravenously (from 4 g of silver arsphenamine used to treat syphilis over a 2-year period in the early 1900s), whereas others tolerated infusions containing up to 5 g of elemental silver over 9 months before clinical change was noted.[25]

In 2002, a 42-year-old European man developed argyria after just 4 years of weekly application of a topical nasal vasoconstrictor (Coldargan, manufactured by Siegfried, Sweden) available in Austria. The patient used this product to treat his rhinitis medicamentosa (rebound nasal congestion brought on by extended use of topical decongestants); each drop of medication contained 0.85 mg silver protein—considerably more than expected in chronic occupational exposure.[75] More directly, colloidal silver protein ingestion for "health supplementation" leads to body burdens of silver that can produce argyria. In 1933, argyria was reported in a 33-year-old woman who ingested 48 mg/day of elemental silver (from silver nitrate capsules) during alternating 2-week periods (2 weeks on—2 weeks off) over 1 year to treat chronic gastrointestinal symptoms.[7] Her serum silver concentrations remained at 500 mcg/L for 3 months after discontinuation of the capsules, indicating significant silver deposition in tissues.

Mechanical impregnation of silver produces localized argyria following repeated contact with metallic silver or silver salts.[34] Localized argyria is reported from both implanted acupuncture needles and short-contact acupuncture, when particle deposition occurs from silver needles used repeatedly during brief therapeutic sessions.[37] Silver sulfadiazine use produces localized argyria in and around wound scars.[22,78] Localized argyria of the tongue and gingiva is described in patients with silver dental amalgams.[32,60] Some of these patients also have elevated tissue concentrations of silver, but there are no known cases of significant absorption resulting in generalized argyria.[15] Even long-standing wearing of silver earrings has resulted in local contact argyria.[45,73,76] Corneal argyrosis was frequently reported from prolonged use of colloidal silver disinfectant eyedrops, but as these drops are no longer used, the condition has become an occupational disease caused by both inadequate eye personal protection and worker self-contamination of their eyes with hands contaminated by silver particles.[62,64,87]

Histopathology of Argyria

There are no inflammatory reactions noted because of silver deposition or impregnation. Rather, the skin discoloration of argyria comes from the silver itself and from the induction of increased melanin production. Silver granules are initially found within fibroblasts and macrophages, then extracellularly along the basement membrane of blood vessels, sweat glands, dermoepidermal junction, and beside erector pili muscles (Chap. 17). Patients with argyria commonly manifest increased pigmentation over sun-exposed skin. Although the mechanism for this process is not yet fully understood, it is proposed that silver-complexed proteins are reduced to their elemental form via photoactivation from sunlight, similar to photographic image development. Silver and light then further stimulate melanogenesis, increasing melanin in light-exposed areas and enhancing this cycle.

Evidence demonstrates how silver is deposited in the skin. Ingested silver nanoparticles dissolve in the acidic environment of the stomach, forming silver ions that are transported by glutathione and other biomolecules to the dermis. These ions are reduced by sunlight and sulfur. Subsequently, selenium ions align or colocate alongside silver atoms creating blue discoloration.[41] Skin biopsy can confirm the diagnosis of argyria, showing brown-black clusters of silver granules in the dermis.

Diagnostic Testing

Urine and serum concentrations of silver are measured as indices of silver exposure. Hair is also tested for silver, but airborne silver particles bind to hair and contaminate samples, potentially invalidating the results.

In individuals without a history of medicinal silver ingestion or occupational exposure, the normal serum silver concentration is less than or equal to 0.5 nmol/L, normal urinary silver concentration is less than or equal to 21 nmol/L and normal fecal silver concentration less than or equal to 1.5 mcg/g.[14] These values are in contrast to workers who smelt and refine silver and who prepare silver salts for use in the photographic industry, who have mean serum concentrations measured of 234 nmol/L, urine silver concentrations of less than 0.005 mcg/g, and fecal silver concentrations of 15 mcg/g.[14]

Treatment of Argyria

Chelators are ineffective in treating both silver toxicity and argyria.[19] Dermatologic conventional wisdom has suggested that topical hydroquinone 5% reduces the number of silver granules in the dermis and around sweat glands, as well as diminishes the number of melanocytes.[9] Sunscreens and opaque cosmetics prevent further pigmentation darkening from sun exposure. Successful treatment of argyria using laser technology is also reported and appears promising with one case report of a full cure.[28,58]

As oxidant deficiencies enhance silver toxicity, antioxidants, such as selenium and vitamin E, limit the effects of silver exposure. Selenium-dependent glutathione peroxidase synthesis is diminished when silver binds to selenium and thus reduces intracellular selenium.[9,77] Supplemental vitamin E and selenium increase tolerance for silver in rats and chickens.[10]

Selenium has been considered a potentially effective treatment for argyria. Although colocation of selenium with silver nanoparticles promotes argyria, paradoxically it to precipitates or chelates silver by forming silver selenide complexes. Furthermore, silver selenide is insoluble in vivo and should reduce the availability of monovalent silver to interfere with normal enzymatic activities.[1,49,63] Hence, increased selenium intake is theorized to bind silver for excretion rather than skin deposition. Similarly, sulfur has been investigated for effects comparable to those of selenium, although the silver—sulfur complex is not as stable.[63] At this time, there are no recommendations for dosages or duration of treatment with vitamin E, selenium or sulfur for reversing argyria.

EMERGENCY MANAGEMENT

Although systemic toxicity of silver is predominantly a result of chronic exposure, clinicians rarely encounter a patient who has ingested a colloidal silver product, a silver-containing medicinal product, or a silver salt. Emergency management should take into consideration the type of silver ingested.

Cutaneous burns from silver salt cautery should be managed as thermal burns; ingested cautery should be treated as a caustic. Patients who ingest elemental silver should be managed supportively, as elemental silver should pass through the GI tract unchanged. Silver salt ingestion (such as silver nitrate) should be treated as a caustic ingestion (Chap. 103). There is no evidence to support gastric lavage or administration of activated charcoal as a decontamination method, so neither of these decontamination methods is recommended.

SUMMARY

■ Silver toxicity—primarily argyria and burns—is still occasionally encountered.[30,74,81,82] The workplace environment and health and nutritional supplements are the main sources of exposure.

■ Despite frequent therapeutic use of elemental silver and silver salts, there is no evidence of silver mutagenicity or carcinogenicity in humans.

■ Significant toxicity is very rare, although when argyria results from chronic silver use, it is invariably permanent.

■ There are no proven effective means for removing accumulated silver and reversing argyria.

REFERENCES

1. Aaseth J, et al. Chelation of silver in argyria. *Acta Pharmacol Toxicol.* 1986;59(suppl 7): 471-474.
2. Afkhami F, et al. Entrococcus faecalis elimination in root canals using silver nanoparticles, photodynamic therapy, diode laser, or laser-activated nanoparticles: an in vitro study. *J Endod.* 2016;43:279-282.
3. AshaRani PV, et al. Cytotoxicity and genotoxicity of silver nanoparticles in human cells. *ACS Nano.* 2009;3:279-290.
4. Associated Press. Silver-tongued mayor's anthrax "cure" rebutted. *St. Petersburg Times.* November 24, 2001.

5. BBC News. True-blue bids for Senate. http://news.bbc.co.uk/2/hi/americas/2297471 .stm. Published online October 3, 2002. Accessed on May 5, 2017.

6. Bianchini A, Wood CM. Mechanism of acute silver toxicity in *Daphnia magna*. *Environ Toxicol Chem*. 2003;22:1361-1367.

7. Blumberg H, Carey TN. Argyremia: detection of unsuspected and obscure argyria by the spectrographic demonstration of high blood silver. *JAMA*. 1934;103:1521-1524.

8. Bouts BA. Images in clinical medicine. Argyria. *N Engl J Med*. 1999;340:1554.

9. Browning JC, Levy ML. Argyria attributed to silvadene application in a patient with dystrophic epidermolysis bullosa. *Dermatol Online J*. 2008;14:9.

10. Bunyan J, et al. Vitamin E and stress: 8. Nutritional effects of dietary stress with silver in vitamin E-deficient chicks and rats. *Br J Nutr*. 1968;22:165-182.

11. Choi YJ, et al. Differential cytotoxic potential of silver nanoparticles in human ovarian cancer cells and ovarian cancer stem cells. *Int J Mol Sci*. 2016;17:pii: E2077.

12. Demling RH, et al. The rate of re-epithelialization across meshed skin grafts is increased with exposure to silver. *Burns*. 2002;28:264-266.

13. Dibrov P, et al. Chemiosmotic mechanism of antimicrobial activity of Ag(+) in *Vibrio cholerae*. *Antimicrob Agents Chemother*. 2002;46:2668-2670.

14. DiVincenzo GD, et al. Biologic monitoring of workers exposed to silver. *Int Arch Occup Environ Health*. 1985;56:207-215.

15. Drasch G, et al. Silver concentrations in human tissues: their dependence on dental amalgam and other factors. *J Trace Elem Med Biol*. 1995;9:82-87.

16. Ehdaie B, et al. Evaluation of a silver-embedded ceramic tablet as a primary and secondary point-of-use water purification technology in Limpopo Province, S. Africa. *PLoS One*. 2017;12:e0169502.

17. Ema M, et al. A review of reproductive and developmental toxicity of silver nanoparticles in laboratory animals. *Reprod Toxicol*. 2017;67:149-164.

18. Environmental Protection Agency: Silver (CASRN 7440–22–4). US Environmental Protection Agency Integrated Risk Information System (IRIS). https://cfpub.epa.gov/ncea/iris2/chemicalLanding.cfm?substance_nmbr=99. Accessed May 5, 2017.

19. European Union European Commission Health & Consumer Protection Directorate General Scientific Committee on Medicinal Products and Medical Devices: Opinion on Toxicological data on colouring agents for medicinal products: E 174 Silver. 2000. 17.

19a. Fisher NM, Marsh E, Lazova R: Scar-localized argyria secondary to silver sulfadiazine cream. *J Am Acad Dermatol*. 2003;49:730-732.

20. Food and Drug Administration. *FDA Issues Final Rule on OTC Drug Products Containing Colloidal Silver*. Rockville, MD: US Department of Health and Human Services, Food and Drug Administration, August 17, 1999.

21. Fung MC, Bowen DL. Silver products for medical indications: risk-benefit assessment. *J Toxicol Clin Toxicol*. 1996;34:119-126.

22. Furchner JE, et al. Comparative metabolism of radionuclides in mammals—IV. Retention of silver-110m in the mouse, rat, monkey, and dog. *Health Phys*. 1968;15:505-514.

23. Furst A, Schlauder MC. Inactivity of two noble metals as carcinogens. *J Environ Pathol Toxicol*. 1978;1:51-57.

24. Gaslin MT, et al. Silver nasal sprays: misleading Internet marketing. *Ear Nose Throat J*. 2008;87:217-220.

25. Gaul LE, Staud AH. Seventy cases of generalized argyrosis following organic and colloidal silver medication including a biospectrometric analysis of ten cases. *JAMA*. 1935; 104:1387-1390.

26. Gettler AO, et al. A contribution to the pathology of generalized argyria with a discussion of the fate of silver in the human body. *Am J Pathol*. 1927;3:631-652.

27. Gitipour A, et al. Nanosilver as a disinfectant in dental unit waterlines: assessment of the physicochemical transformations of the AgNPs. *Chemosphere*. 2017;173:245-252.

28. Han TY, et al. Successful treatment of argyria using a low-fluence Q-switched 1064-nm Nd:YAG laser. *Int J Dermatol*. 2011;50:751-753.

29. Heidari Zare H, et al. Efficacy of silver/hydrophilic poly(*p*-xylylene) on preventing bacterial growth and biofilm formation in urinary catheters. *Biointerphases*. 2017;12:011001.

30. Hori K, et al. Believe it or not—Silver still poisons! *Vet Hum Toxicol*. 2002;44:291-292.

31. Jacobs R. Rosemary's story—if my doctor had read the medical literature instead of the ads I wouldn't look like this today. http://rosemaryjacobs.com. Published 1998. Accessed May 5, 2017.

32. Janner M, et al. Localized intramural silver impregnation of the tongue. Differential diagnosis from malignant melanoma [German]. *Hautarzt*. 1980;31:510-512.

33. Jiang X, et al. Interference of steroidogenesis by gold nanorod core/silver shell nanostructures: implications for reproductive toxicity of silver nanomaterials. *Small*. 2017;13: Epub 2016 Dec 23.

34. Kapur N, et al. Localized argyria in an antique restorer. *Br J Dermatol*. 2001;144: 191-192.

35. Keong NC, et al. The SILVER (Silver Impregnated Line Versus EVD Randomized trial): a double-blind, prospective, randomized, controlled trial of an intervention to reduce the rate of external ventricular drain infection. *Neurosurgery*. 2012;71:394-403.

36. Lancaster T, Stead LF. Silver acetate for smoking cessation. *Cochrane Database Syst Rev*. 2012;9:CD000191.

37. Legat FJ, et al. Argyria after short-contact acupuncture. *Lancet*. 1998;352:241.

38. Li Y, et al. Polyethylenimine-functionalized silver nanoparticle-based co-delivery of paclitaxel to induce HepG2 cell apoptosis. *Int J Nanomedicine*. 2016;11:6693-6702.

39. Li Z, et al. Association between titanium and silver concentrations in maternal hair and risk of neural tube defects in offspring: a case-control study in north China. *Reprod Toxicol*. 2016;66:115-121.

40. Lin HC, et al. Transcriptomic gene-network analysis of exposure to silver nanoparticle reveals potentially neurodegenerative progression in mouse brain neural cells. *Toxicol In Vitro*. 2016;34:289-299.

41. Liu J, et al. Chemical transformations of nanosilver in biological environments. *ACS Nano*. 2012;6:9887-9899. http://pubs.acs.org/doi/abs/10.1021/nn303449n?source=cen. Published online October 9, 2012. Accessed May 5, 2017.

42. Lu M, et al. An effective treatment of experimental osteomyelitis using the antimicrobial titanium/silver-containing nHP66 (nano-hydroxyapatite/polyamide-66) nanoscaffold biomaterials. *Sci Rep*. 2016;6:39174.

43. Mackison FW. *NIOSH/OSHA—Occupational Health Guidelines for Chemical Hazards*. Washington, DC: US Government Printing Office; 1981.

44. Maher JF. Toxic nephropathy. In: Brenner BM, Rector FC Jr, eds. *The Kidney*. Philadelphia, PA: WB Saunders; 1976:1355-1395.

45. Morton CA, et al. Localized argyria caused by silver earrings. *Br J Dermatol*. 1996; 135:484-485.

46. Munteanu A, et al. A modern method of treatment: the role of silver dressings in promoting healing and preventing pathological scarring in patients with burn wounds. *J Med Life*. 2016;9:306-315.

47. Newton D, Holmes A. A case of accidental inhalation of zinc-65 and silver-110m. *Radiat Res*. 1966;29:403-412.

48. Newton T, et al. A comparison of the effect of early insertion of standard latex and silver-impregnated latex Foley catheters on urinary tract infections in burn patients. *Infect Control Hosp Epidemiol*. 2002;23:217-218.

49. Nuttall KL. A model for metal selenide formation under biological conditions. *Med Hypotheses*. 1987;24:217-221.

50. Ohbo Y, et al. Argyria and convulsive seizures caused by ingestion of silver in a patient with schizophrenia. *Psychiatry Clin Neurosci*. 1996;50:89-90.

51. Olcott CT. Experimental argyrosis. V. Hypertrophy of the left ventricle of the heart in rats ingesting silver salts. *Arch Pathol*. 1950;49:138-149.

52. Park JH, et al. Dry writing of highly conductive electrodes on papers by using silver nanoparticle-graphene hybrid pencils. *Nanoscale*. 2017;9:555-561.

53. Parveen R, et al. Nanoparticles-protein interaction: role in protein aggregation and clinical implications. *Int J Biol Macromol*. 2017;94(pt A):386-395.

54. Phalen RF, Morrow PE. Experimental inhalation of metallic silver. *Health Phys*. 1973;24:509-518.

55. Polachek AA, et al. Metabolism of radioactive silver in a patient with carcinoid. *J Lab Clin Med*. 1960;56:499-505.

56. Powell J, Margarf H. Silver: emerging as our mightiest germ fighter. *Sci Dig*. 1978; March:57-60.

57. Qian LW, et al. Silver sulfadiazine retards wound healing and increases hypertrophic scarring in a rabbit ear excisional wound model. *J Burn Care Res*. 2017;38:e418-e422.

58. Rhee DY, et al. Treatment of argyria after colloidal silver protein ingestion using Q-switched 1,064-nm Nd:YAG laser. *Dermatol Surg*. 2008;34:1427-1430.

59. Ritter SK. Blue in the face, fiber fat fighter. *Chem Eng News*. 2013;91:40.

60. Rusch-Behrend GD, Gutmann JL. Management of diffuse tissue argyria subsequent to endodontic therapy: report of a case. *Quintessence Int*. 1995;26:553-557.

61. Salas-López EK, et al. Effect of silver nanoparticle-added pit and fissure sealant in the prevention of dental caries in children. *J Clin Pediatr Dent*. 2017;41:48-52.

62. Sanchez-Huerta V, et al. Occupational corneal argyrosis in art silver solderers. *Cornea*. 2003;22:604-611.

63. Sato S, et al. Two unusual cases of argyria: the application of an improved tissue processing method for X-ray microanalysis of selenium and sulphur in silver-laden granules. *Br J Dermatol*. 1999;140:158-163.

64. Scroggs MW, et al. Corneal argyrosis associated with silver soldering. *Cornea*. 1992; 11:264-269.

65. Seo JW, et al. Facilitated embedding of silver nanowires into conformally-coated iCVD polymer films deposited on cloth for robust wearable electronics. *Nanoscale*. 2017;9:3399-3407.

66. Shorr AF. Impact of a silver-coated endotracheal tube on ventilator-associated pneumonia due to resistant pathogens. *Am J Respir Crit Care Med*. 2008;177:A530. As reported by Smith M: American Thoracic Society (ATS): Silver Lining Prevents Ventilator Pneumonia. http://www.medpagetoday.com/MeetingCoverage/ATS/9556. Accessed May 5, 2017.

70. Silver S. Bacterial silver resistance: molecular biology and uses and misuses of silver compounds. *FEMS Microbiol Rev*. 2003;27:341-353.

71. State of Utah Legal Tender Act of 2011. Utah Code Section 59-1-1501. Part 15. Legal Tender Act. http://le.utah.gov/~2011/bills/hbillint/hb0317s01.htm. Accessed May 5, 2017.

72. Sthijns MM, et al. Silver nanoparticles induce hormesis in A549 human epithelial cells. *Toxicol In Vitro*. 2017;40:223-233.

73. Sugden P, et al. Argyria caused by an earring. *Br J Plast Surg*. 2001;54:252-253.

74. Tomi NS, et al. A silver man. *Lancet*. 2004;363:532.

75. Ueno M, et al. Silver-containing hydroxyapatite coating reduces biofilm formation by methicillin-resistant staphylococcus aureus in vitro and in vivo. *Biomed Res Int*. 2016; 2016:8070597.

76. van den Nieuwenhuijsen IJ, et al. Localized argyria caused by silver earrings. *Dermatologica*. 1988;177:189-191.

77. Wagner PA, et al. Alleviation of silver toxicity by selenite in the rat in relation to tissue glutathione peroxidase. *Proc Soc Exp Biol Med*. 1975;148:1106-1110.

78. Wan AT, et al. Determination of silver in blood, urine, and tissues of volunteers and burn patients. *Clin Chem*. 1991;37:1683-1687.

79. Wang M, et al. Differential effects of silver and iron oxide nanoparticles on IAPP amyloid aggregation. *Biomater Sci*. 2017;5:485-493.

80. Westhofen M, Schafer H. Generalized argyrosis in man: neurotological, ultrastructural and X-ray microanalytical findings. *Arch Otorhinolaryngol*. 1986;243:260-264.

81. White JM, et al. Severe generalized argyria secondary to ingestion of colloidal silver protein. *Clin Exp Dermatol*. 2003;28:254-256.

82. Wickless SC, et al. Medical mystery—the answer. *N Engl J Med*. 2004;351:2349-2350.

83. World Health Organization. 13. Inorganic constituents and physical parameters. In: WHO, ed. *Guidelines for Drinking-Water Quality, vol. 2: Health Criteria and Other Supporting Information*. 2nd ed. Geneva: World Health Organization: 1996:153-157.

84. Yang T, et al. Silver nanoparticles inhibit the function of hypoxia-inducible factor-1 and target genes: insight into the cytotoxicity and antiangiogenesis. *Int J Nanomedicine*. 2016;11:6679-6692.

85. Yardley W. Utah law makes coins worth their weight in gold (or silver). *The New York Times*. http://www.nytimes.com/2011/05/30/us/30gold.html?pagewanted=all&_r=0. Published May 29, 2011. Accessed May 5, 2017.

86. Yu X, et al. Growth of a large-area, free-standing, highly conductive and fully foldable silver film with inverted pyramids for wearable electronics applications. *ACS Appl Mater Interfaces*. 2017;9:5312-5318.

87. Zografos L, et al. Unilateral conjunctival–corneal argyrosis simulating conjunctival melanoma. *Arch Ophthalmol*. 2003;121:1483-1487.

99 THALLIUM

Maria Mercurio-Zappala and Robert S. Hoffman

HISTORY AND EPIDEMIOLOGY

Thallium (Tl^0), a metal with atomic number 81, is located between mercury and lead on the periodic table. Elemental thallium is a soft, pliable metal that melts at 572°F (300°C), boils at 26,99.6°F (1,482°C), and is essentially nontoxic. Thallium forms univalent thallous (Tl^{1+}) and trivalent thallic (Tl^{3+}) salts, which are highly toxic. Thallium is a commonly found constituent of granite, shale, volcanic rock, and pyrites used to make sulfuric acid and is also recovered as flue dust from iron, lead, cadmium, and copper smelters.[28]

In the early 1900s, thallium salts were used medicinally to treat syphilis, gonorrhea, tuberculosis, and as a depilatory for ringworm of the scalp.[7,73] Although the usual oral dose given for ringworm was 7 to 8 mg/kg, fatal doses ranged from 6 to 40 mg/kg.[16,62] Many cases of severe thallium poisoning (thallotoxicosis) resulted from this treatment, with one author summarizing nearly 700 cases and 46 deaths.[75]

Because thallium sulfate is odorless, tasteless, and highly toxic it became commercially available as a rodenticide and was sold as Thalgrain, Echol's Roach Powder, Mo-Go, Martin's Rat Stop liquid, and Senco Corn Mix. As a consequence of numerous case reports of unintentional poisonings,[75,87] the use of thallium salts as a household rodenticide was restricted in the United States in 1965. Ultimately, even the commercial use of thallium salts as a rodenticide was banned in the United States in 1972 because of continued reports of human toxicity.

Life-threatening unintentional poisoning continues to occur in other countries, especially where thallium salts are still commonly used as rodenticides.[2,15,58,85,89,94,104,113] Additional cases of thallium poisoning are reported in the United States and other countries as a result of the use of thallium for suicide,[101] homicide,[23,57,66,71,79,81,91,100] through contamination of herbal products,[18,97] and illicit drugs such as heroin, opium,[1,34,84] and cocaine.[48] Although occupational exposures to consequential amounts of thallium salts are uncommon, occupational toxicity is well described.[42] Additionally, although small amounts of thallium salts (<1 mcg) are used as radioactive contrast to image tumors and to permit the visualization of cardiac function, the doses used are insignificant and pose no risk for thallium toxicity.[73]

The following discussion of thallium toxicity is based on exposures to inorganic thallium salts, which represents virtually the entire literature on thallium poisoning. Although exceedingly rare, exposures to organic thallium compounds are reported[4] and should be assessed and managed in a fashion similar to that used for patients with inorganic exposures.

TOXICOKINETICS

Exposures usually occur via one of 3 routes: inhalation, ingestion, and absorption through intact skin. Thallium is rapidly absorbed following all routes of exposure. Bioavailability is greatest after ingestion and exceeds 90%.[44] Distribution follows 3-compartment toxicokinetics (Chap. 9),[86] achieving a final volume of distribution that is estimated to be about 3.6 L/kg.[21] Thallium toxicity is manifested in virtually all organs; however, it is distributed unevenly, with the highest concentrations found in the large and small intestine, liver, kidney, heart, brain, and muscle.[8,56] In animals, the highest concentrations of thallium are found in the kidney.[3,56]

The toxicokinetics of thallium is described in the following 3-phase model. The first phase occurs within 4 hours after oral exposure, during which time thallium is distributed to the central compartment and to well-perfused peripheral organs such as the kidney, liver, and muscle. In the second phase, which lasts between 4 and 48 hours, thallium is distributed into the central nervous system (CNS).[86] Whereas some literature suggests that this distribution phase is generally completed within 24 hours of ingestion,[86] one human case suggests slower distribution into the CNS as evidenced by increasing cerebrospinal fluid (CSF) concentrations in the days after exposure when blood concentrations were declining, which likely excludes ongoing absorption.[100] The third or elimination phase usually begins within 24 hours after ingestion. The primary mechanism of thallium elimination is secretion into the intestine, but enteral reabsorption of thallium that is present in the bile subsequently reduces the fecal elimination.[21,71] Thallium is excreted primarily via the feces (51.4%) and the urine (26.4%).[61] It is filtered by the glomerulus, with approximately 50% being reabsorbed in the tubules. Thallium is also secreted into the tubular lumen in a manner similar to potassium.[7] The duration of the elimination phase depends on the route of exposure, dose, and treatment. Unlike many other metals, thallium does not have a major anatomic reservoir. For this reason, reported elimination half-lives are as short as 1.7 days in humans with thallium poisoning.[46]

PATHOPHYSIOLOGY

The mechanism of thallium toxicity is not well established. Thallium behaves biologically in a manner similar to potassium because both have similar ionic radii (1.47 Å for thallium and 1.33 Å for potassium). Because cell membranes cannot differentiate between thallous (Tl^{+1}) and potassium (K^+) ions, thallous ions accumulate in areas with high potassium concentrations, such as the central and peripheral nervous system, liver, and muscle.[67,113] This accumulation is the fundamental principle that governs the use of radioactive thallium in cardiac imaging studies. Thallium replaces potassium in the activation of potassium-dependent enzymes.[67] In low concentrations, thallium stimulates these enzyme systems, but in high concentrations, inhibition occurs.[9,69] Pyruvate kinase, a magnesium-dependent glycolytic enzyme that requires potassium to achieve maximum activity, has 50 times greater affinity for thallous ions than potassium ions.[52] Succinate dehydrogenase, a citric acid cycle enzyme, is inhibited by small doses of thallium in rats.[41] Sodium-potassium adenosine triphosphatase (Na^+,K^+-ATPase), which is responsible for active transport of monovalent ions across cell membranes, can use thallous ions at extremely low concentrations because of an affinity that is 10-fold greater than that for potassium, ions,[10,33] but is inhibited by thallium at higher concentrations.[49]

Thallium also impairs depolarization of muscle fibers.[73] Mitochondrial energy is decreased as a result of the inhibition of pyruvate kinase and succinate dehydrogenase, resulting in a decrease of adenosine triphosphate (ATP) generation via oxidative phosphorylation. Oxidative stress results in opening of the mitochondrial permeability transition pore.[27] This results in swelling and vacuolization of the mitochondria.[57,102] At low concentrations, thallium activates other potassium-dependent enzymes such as phosphatase, homoserine dehydrogenase, vitamin B_{12}–dependent diol dehydrogenase, L-threonine dehydrogenase, and adenosine monophosphate (AMP) deaminase.[73] The net result of these processes is a failure of energy production. In the central nervous system, there is evidence that damage is also caused by activation of glutaminergic transmission by the *N*-methyl-D-aspartate (NMDA) receptor, because as an antagonist, dizocilpine (MK-801), limits injury in rats by preventing this transmission.[78]

Thallous ions are used to isolate riboflavin from milk in the form of a reversible precipitate. Thallous ions may also form insoluble complexes and cause intracellular sequestration of riboflavin in vivo.[14] Riboflavin is the vitamin precursor of the flavin coenzyme flavin adenine dinucleotide (FAD). Because of a decrease in riboflavin, metabolic reactions dependent on flavoproteins decrease, causing disruption of the electron transport chain and a subsequent further decrease or impairment in the generation of cellular energy.[14] This decrease in cellular energy may lead to a decrease in mitotic activity and cessation of hair follicle formation, resulting in the clinical sign of alopecia. Subsequent hair loss is the result of combined arrested formation and local destruction of hair shaft cells in the hair bulb and is known as anagen effluvium (Chap. 17).[12,14,18,87] Unfortunately, riboflavin supplementation was not beneficial in one animal model of thallium poisoning.[6] Data also demonstrate that the dermatologic, neurologic, and cardiovascular effects of thallium toxicity mirror the manifestations of thiamine deficiency (beriberi), highlighting the inhibitory effect of thallium on glycolytic enzymes.[14,73] It is unclear whether thiamine administration has any beneficial effect in patients with thallium poisoning.

Thallium has a high affinity for the sulfhydryl groups present in many other enzymes and proteins. Keratin, a structural protein, consists of many cysteine residues that crosslink and form disulfide bonds. These disulfide bonds add strength to keratin. Thallium interferes with the formation of disulfide bonds, which likely contributes to the development of alopecia and defects in nail growth, resulting in Mees lines (Fig. 86–4).[37,73,79,93,94] Additionally, the complexation of sulfhydryl groups with thallium results in a decrease in both the production of glutathione and the reduction of oxidized glutathione.[39,114] This results in oxidative damage[31] and the accumulation of lipid peroxides in the brain (which is most prominent in the cerebellum) and appears as dark, pigmented areas.[40] The complexity and presumable multifactorial nature of thallium poisoning are further demonstrated by the inability of *N*-acetylcysteine (NAC)—induced augmentation of glutathione stores to protect against toxicity in an animal model.[6]

Thallium also adversely affects protein synthesis in animals by damaging ribosomes, particularly the 60S subunit.[47] Although ribosomes are primarily dependent on potassium and magnesium, thallium is substituted if present. In an experimental model, low concentrations of thallium are protective against hypokalemia-induced ribosomal inactivation. As thallium concentrations increase, the protective effects diminish, resulting in progressive destabilization and destruction of the ribosomes.

Pathologic studies of the CNS in patients with thallium poisoning reveal localized areas of edema in the cerebrum and brain stem. Chromatolytic changes are prominent in neurons of the motor cortex, third nerve nuclei, substantia nigra, and pyramidal cells of the globus pallidus. In chronic exposures, there are signs of edema of the pial and arachnoidal membranes and chromatolysis, swelling, and fatty degeneration in the ganglion cells of the ventral and dorsal horns of the spinal cord.[8,87]

The peripheral nervous system, which is usually clinically affected before the CNS, develops a diffuse axonopathy in a classic dying back or Wallerian degeneration pattern (Chap. 22).[7,8,19,25,68] Fragmentation and degeneration of associated myelin sheaths are accompanied by activation of Schwann cells.[8,13,14] Because thallium affects the longer peripheral fibers—first sensory, then motor, and finally the shorter fibers—toxic effects occur initially in the lower extremities.[60,77,120]

CLINICAL MANIFESTATIONS

Many of the effects of thallium poisoning are nonspecific and occur throughout the acute and chronic phases of an exposure.[59] When combined, however, a clear toxic syndrome is defined (Table 99–1). Alopecia and a painful ascending peripheral neuropathy are the most characteristic findings.[7,30,71,77] Because of the delayed development of alopecia, the diagnosis of thallotoxicosis is often delayed. In fact, with acute exposures, a dose-dependent latent period of hours to days may precede initial symptoms.[59,73] When death

occurs, it is usually the result of coma with loss of airway protective reflexes, respiratory paralysis, and cardiac arrest.

Unlike most other metal salt poisonings, diarrhea is often modest or even absent following thallium exposure.[16] The most common symptom is abdominal pain, which is often accompanied by vomiting and either diarrhea or constipation.[23,54,59,69,93,115,116] Constipation is presumed to be a result of decreased intestinal motility and peristalsis caused by direct involvement of the vagus nerve[16,73] Rarely, severe manifestations occur, such as hematemesis, bloody diarrhea, or ulceration of the mucosal lining.

Pleuritic chest pain was described in a small series of poisoned patients.[66] Another patient was reported to have developed chest tightness shortly after drinking thallium-poisoned tea.[71] Although the etiology for this finding is uncertain, a more recent case report describing the development of pleural and pericardial effusions in an otherwise healthy young man with a suicidal ingestion of thallium monobromide may sheds light on one possible etiology of this symptom.[101]

Tachycardia and hypertension frequently occur in patients with thallotoxicosis and usually develop during the first or second week after acute ingestion. A persistent and pronounced tachycardia is associated with a poor prognosis. No exact mechanism has been determined for these cardiovascular effects of thallium toxicity. Some authors theorize that they result from autonomic neuropathic dysfunction directly related to involvement of the vagus nerve,[77] but others have noted early electrocardiographic (ECG) changes, such as prolongation of the QT interval, T wave flattening or inversion, and nonspecific ST segment abnormalities, which might suggest direct myocardial injury.[8,13,69,73,90] Another theory suggests that the direct stimulation of ATPase in the chromaffin cells by thallium leads to increased output of catecholamines, resulting in sinus tachycardia.[5,71]

Neurologic effects usually appear 2 to 5 days after exposure. Patients develop severely painful, rapidly progressive, ascending peripheral neuropathies.[7,8,25,66] Pain and paresthesias are present in the lower extremities (especially the soles of the feet), and although numbness is present in the fingers and toes, there is also decreased sensation to pinprick, touch, temperature, vibration, and proprioception.[7,97] The weight of bedsheets on the lower extremities is sometimes sufficient to cause excruciating pain.[66] Motor weakness is always distal in distribution, with the lower limbs more affected than the upper limbs.[13,73]

Confusion, delirium, psychosis, hallucinations, seizures, headache, insomnia, anxiety, tremor, ataxia, and choreoathetosis are common. The onset of these clinical findings is variable and most likely dependent on dose. Insomnia occurs in most patients and progresses to total reversal of sleep rhythms. Coma occurs following large exposures.[13,59,73,93] All cranial nerves can probably be affected by thallium, although abnormalities of cranial nerves I, V, and VIII have not been reported. Cranial nerve III involvement, as evidenced by ptosis, is common and may be asymmetric.[13] Nystagmus, another common finding, demonstrates involvement of cranial nerves IV and VI.[13] Cognitive abnormalities often persist for months after exposure.[64]

Thallium is toxic to both the retinal fibers and the neural retina.[98] In cases of a large, single ingestion of thallium, approximately 25% of patients develop severe lesions of the optic nerve.[73,93] Optic neuropathy can progress to optic atrophy and a permanent decrease in visual acuity. In the early stages, the optic disk shows signs of neuritis, which is red and poorly defined, and later develops pallor from resultant optic nerve atrophy. In patients exposed to multiple small doses, nearly 100% suffer optic nerve injury.[69] Visual complaints are often significantly delayed in comparison to other neurologic findings,[98] typically include decreased acuity and central scotomata, and sometimes are not noted until after recovery from coma. Other described ophthalmic effects are noninflammatory keratitis, cataracts, and the color vision defect of tritanomaly (blue color defect).[106,107]

Kidney function remains normal in mild cases of thallium poisoning, even though the kidney has greater bioaccumulation than any other organ. Proteinuria is often the earliest or only finding of kidney injury. Changes in kidney function in patients with severe thallotoxicosis include oliguria, diminished creatinine clearance, elevated blood urea nitrogen,

TABLE 99–1   Clinical Manifestations of Thallium Poisoning

Organ System	Onset of Effects			
	Immediate (<6 hours)	Intermediate (Rarely in the first few days; within 2 weeks)	Late (>2 weeks)	Residual Effects‡
Gastrointestinal				
Nausea	†			
Vomiting	†			
Diarrhea	†			
Constipation	†	†		
Cardiovascular				
Nonspecific ECG changes	†	†		
Hypertension		†		
Sinus tachycardia		†		
Pleural and pericardial effusions		†		
Respiratory				
Pleuritic chest pain	†	†		
Respiratory depression		†	†	
Renal				
Albuminuria		†		
Acute kidney injury			†	
Dermatologic				
Dry skin		†		
Alopecia		†		†
Mees lines			†	†
Neurologic				
Sensory neuropathy (painful ascending with paresthesias, and numbness)		†	†	†
Motor neuropathy (distal and ascending)		†	†	†
Cranial nerve abnormalities (ptosis, bulbar dysfunction)		†		
Delirium, psychosis, coma		†		†
Memory and cognitive deficits			†	†
Optic neuritis	†	†		†

† = Typical onset of clinical effects. The predicted time course if often accelerated with extremely large doses. When † appears in 2 adjacent columns, the time course is highly variable and likely dose dependent. With small ingestions, many of the effects listed above are evident. ‡ = Effects that persist long after exposure, possibly permanently.

and proteinuria.[5,66,69,73] These findings correlate with morphologic studies in thallium poisoned rats, demonstrating abnormalities in the renal medulla, mainly in the thick ascending limb of the loop of Henle, that occur by the second day after exposure and resolve by the 10th day.[5]

Alopecia is the most characteristic manifestation of thallium toxicity.[71,110] In patients with chronic exposure, hair loss is often the first recognizable symptom and typically is present at approximately 10 days and is maximal within 1 month.[30,71,75] With acute or massive exposure, hair loss can occur earlier. Facial and axillary hair, especially the inner third of the eyebrows, is often spared, but in some cases, full beards, as well as all scalp hair, are lost.[87] Microscopic inspection of the hair reveals a diagnostic pattern of black pigmentation of the hair roots of the scalp in approximately 95% of poisoned patients,[11,18,71,93,110] which can be found within 3 to 5 days of initial exposure[11,69] (Fig. 99–1). In patients with recurrent exposures, several bands are noted on the hair shaft, demonstrating multiple exposures. Initial hair regrowth is very fine and unpigmented but usually returns to normal after mild exposures.[69] In some patients with severe exposures, alopecia is permanent. Other dermatologic effects that are observed include acne, palmar erythema, and dry scaly skin that results from sebaceous gland damage.[110] Mees lines appear within 2 to 4 weeks after exposure[71,79,93] (Fig. 86–4).

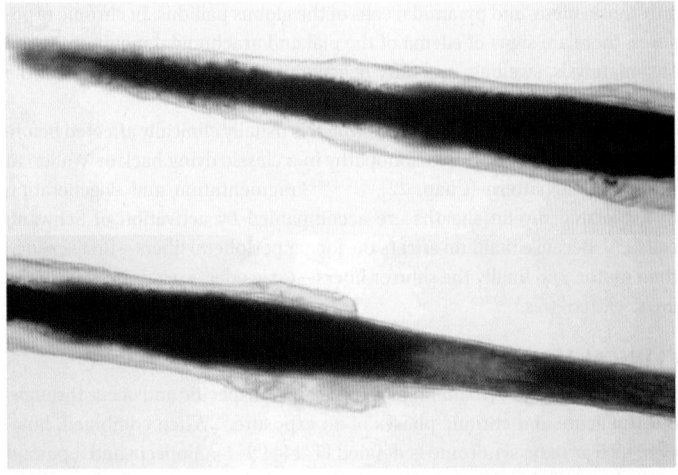

FIGURE 99–1. Hair from a patient with severe thallium poisoning (top) compared to a normal (bottom). Note the dark pigmented granules around the root of the poisoned patient. (*Used with permission from the Fellowship in Medical Toxicology, New York University School of Medicine, New York City Poison Center.*)

Other less common findings include hepatotoxicity,[48] hyperchloremic metabolic acidosis,[93] anemia, and thrombocytopenia.[60,93]

Teratogenicity

In animal models, thallium is teratogenic.[36,38] In humans, one study evaluated 297 children born in a region in which the population's urine thallium concentrations were higher than normal because of industrial contamination of their environment.[24] Urine thallium concentrations in the exposed children were as high as 76.5 mcg/L. Although these children had a slightly higher than expected incidence of congenital abnormalities, no causal relation could be established with regard to thallium exposure.[24] More recently, a case–control study evaluating more than 1,000 infants born in a region of China with high environmental concentrations of thallium demonstrated an association between thallium exposure and low birth weight.[119]

There are few human reports of acute thallium poisoning during pregnancy. A comprehensive literature review demonstrated 25 cases, which included acute and chronic exposures that occurred during all trimesters.[43] Thallium slowly traverses the placenta and is able to cause characteristic fetal toxicity,[26,76] which manifests initially as decreased fetal movement, possibly as a consequence of fetal paralysis. Findings consistent with thallium poisoning are described both in the fetus after abortion and in the neonate after viable delivery.[26,69,76,85] However, normal infants are also reported despite being born to mothers with significant maternal toxicity.[26,50] The only consistent finding is a trend toward prematurity and low birth weight, especially in children exposed during the first trimester.[43] One author recommends continuing the pregnancy as long as the mother is clinically improving.[26]

These few case reports and animal studies provide confusing and sometimes contradictory results. It seems that fetal outcome is determined by both the trimester of pregnancy and the extent of maternal toxicity. It is reasonable to conclude that a fetus exposed to thallium during organogenesis has the potential for permanent injury. Those exposed later in pregnancy may recover without deficit if their exposures are limited and the mother recovers. If the exposure occurs closer to term, some children will be born with overt toxicity such as alopecia, dermatitis, nail growth disturbances, and permanent CNS injury.[69] However, because there are insufficient data to predict the outcome of pregnancy complicated by maternal thallium poisoning, no specific course of action can be recommended other than extensive fetal monitoring and aggressive treatment for the mother. When a viable child is delivered, it is important to note that thallium is eliminated in breast milk, and that ongoing evaluation of maternal toxicity is essential because nursing will result in continued exposure for the child.[43]

ASSESSMENT

Most patients with acute thallium toxicity seek health care soon after exposure because of either alterations in their gastrointestinal (GI), cardiovascular, and neurologic function. Establishing the correct diagnosis at this early stage is essential to maximize the likelihood of for a satisfactory outcome. Unfortunately, many patients with either smaller acute exposures or chronic thallium poisoning first present days to weeks after their initial exposure and diagnosis is often further delayed. In these instances, many valuable epidemiologic aspects of the exposure history become difficult to obtain. Gastrointestinal findings may not have occurred or their consequence or etiology unrecognized because of their nonspecific, mild, and transient nature. Many patients with small acute or chronic exposures usually seek care because of alopecia or neuropathy.

The differential diagnosis of the neuropathy includes poisoning by arsenic, colchicine, vinca alkaloids, and disorders such as botulism, thiamine deficiency, and Guillain-Barré syndrome. Both the sensory neuropathy and the preservation of reflexes help differentiate thallium-induced neuropathy from Guillain-Barré syndrome and most other causes of acute neuropathy.[13] When GI manifestations are present in addition to a neuropathy and other end-organ manifestations, possible poisoning with metal salts such as arsenic and mercury should be evaluated (Chaps. 86 and 95). The differential diagnosis of rapid-onset alopecia is more restricted and includes arsenic,

selenium, colchicine, and vinca alkaloid poisoning as well as radiation injury (Chap. 17). When present, Mees lines indicate past exposure to metals, mitotic inhibitors, or antimetabolites and as such are nonspecific for thallium poisoning (Chaps. 17, 86, and 95).

Diagnostic Testing

Radiographs of tampered food products[66] or of the abdomen[37] can document the presence of a metal such as thallium, which is radiopaque. Although abdominal radiography has potential utility shortly after a suspected exposure, the sensitivity and specificity of this test is unknown. Similarly, the yield from other routine studies, such as the complete blood count, electrolytes, urinalysis, and ECG, is limited in that these other studies are often normal or at most, merely demonstrate nonspecific abnormalities. Although microscopic inspection of the hair is intriguing, this test is unlikely to be conclusive for inexperienced observers.

The definitive clinical diagnosis of thallium poisoning can only be established by demonstrating elevated thallium concentrations in various body fluids or organs. Thallium can be recovered in the hair, nails, feces, saliva, CSF, blood, and urine, and standard assays and normal concentrations for most of these sources are published.[73] Qualitative point of care urine spot tests notoriously give false negative results and require the use of dangerous chemicals that are not routinely available (20% nitric acid) and therefore should be avoided.[93] The standard toxicologic testing method is to assay a 24-hour urine sample for thallium by atomic absorption spectroscopy.[17,117] Normal urine concentrations are lower than 5 mcg/L. Some authors suggest a potassium mobilization test to enhance urinary elimination (similar to the edetate calcium disodium mobilization test), to assist in the diagnosis of thallium exposure.[11,48,93] We recommend against this practice because of its lack of proven usefulness and its potential to exacerbate neurologic toxicity (see Potassium below).

MANAGEMENT

The treatment goals for a patient with thallium poisoning are initial stabilization, prevention of absorption, and enhanced elimination. After the initial assessment and stabilization of the patient's airway, breathing, and circulatory status, GI decontamination is recommended in all patients with suspected thallium ingestions because of the morbidity and mortality associated with a significant exposure.

Decontamination

Orogastric or nasogastric lavage is recommended for patients who have not had spontaneous emesis and present within 1 to 2 hours after ingestion (Chap. 5). If the patient presents more than 2 hours after ingestion or has had considerable spontaneous emesis, gastric emptying is unnecessary unless the ingestion is known to be massive.

Thallium salts are substantially adsorbed to activated charcoal (AC) in vitro.[45,54] Additionally, because thallium undergoes enterohepatic recirculation, AC will be useful both to prevent absorption after a recent ingestion and also to enhance elimination of thallium in patients who present in the postabsorptive phase.[109] In fact, a rat model of thallium poisoning demonstrated that multiple-dose AC (given as 0.5 g/kg twice daily for 5 days) increased the fecal elimination of thallium by 82% and substantially improved survival.[61] Other data demonstrate that AC alone is superior to either forced diuresis or potassium chloride therapy.[55]

In some patients with severe thallium toxicity, constipation will be prominent, so the addition of oral mannitol[63,103,115] or another cathartic to the first dose of AC is reasonable. Although no studies address the efficacy of whole-bowel irrigation with polyethylene glycol electrolyte lavage solution, we recommend this technique when radiopaque material is demonstrated in the GI tract (Antidotes in Depth: A2).

Potassium

The similarities between the cellular handling of potassium ions and thallium ions led to the investigation of a possible role for potassium in the treatment of thallium poisoning. In humans, parenteral potassium administration is associated with an increase in urinary thallium elimination.[16,32,80] The magnitude of this increase is on the order of 2- to 3-fold.[80] This is supported by animal models that demonstrate some benefit in terms of either enhanced thallium elimination or animal survival.[33,55,61] Potassium administration is believed to both block tubular reabsorption of thallium and mobilize thallium from tissue stores, thereby increasing thallium concentrations available for glomerular filtration.[74,93] However, the mobilization of the thallium is of concern. Many authors report either the development of acute neurologic symptoms or the significant exacerbation of neurologic manifestations during potassium administration.[7,32,66,80,90,111] Others cite data demonstrating that the augmentation of thallium elimination by potassium administration in humans is quite limited.[53] Additionally, animal models demonstrate that potassium loading enhances lethality and permits thallium redistribution into the CNS.[40] For these reasons, we recommend against the use of potassium loading. Some authors recommend forced diuresis, especially in conjunction with potassium chloride.[22,108] However, no convincing experimental or clinical evidence can support the use of forced diuresis with or without potassium at this time.

Likewise, the similarities between thallium and potassium might suggest a role for administration of sodium polystyrene sulfonate (SPS) as a sodium—thallium exchange resin. Despite excellent in vitro binding of thallium by SPS, it is unlikely to be clinically useful because of preferential binding between potassium and SPS and a comparatively large reservoir of potassium in the body and SPS is therefore not recommended.[45]

Prussian Blue

Prussian blue is approved by the US Food and Drug Administration for thallium toxicity (Antidotes in Depth: A31).[109] When given orally, Prussian blue acts as an ion exchanger for univalent cations, with its affinity increasing as the ionic radius of the cation increases. As such, Prussian blue interferes with the enterohepatic recirculation of thallium by exchanging potassium ions from its lattice for thallium ions in the GI tract. This results in the formation of a concentration gradient, causing an increased movement of thallium into the GI tract.

Humans with thallium exposure are routinely given Prussian blue, with apparent clinical benefits, enhanced fecal elimination, and decreasing thallium concentrations.[17,20,66,83,103,111,112,115,116] One series of 11 thallium-poisoned patients demonstrated both tolerability of Prussian blue and substantially increased fecal thallium elimination.[103] Unfortunately, because there have been no controlled trials in humans that compare Prussian blue with other drugs and because many of the patients reported above received multiple therapies, the actual efficacy of Prussian blue is unknown.

The dose of Prussian blue is 250 mg/kg/day orally via a nasogastric tube in 2 to 4 divided doses.[103] For patients who are constipated, the Prussian blue may have greater benefit if dissolved in 50 mL of 15% mannitol.[108] Although any cathartic is theoretically useful, most authors have used mannitol, possibly because of concerns regarding repeated use of magnesium-containing cathartics in patients with neurologic findings and the use of sorbitol in patients with poor GI mobility (Antidotes in Depth: A31).

Extracorporeal Drug Removal

Extracorporeal drug removal has at most a limited beneficial role in patients with thallium exposure, especially if initiated shortly after the initial exposure while serum concentrations remain high before effective tissue distribution. Because a frequently quoted review attests to the benefits of hemodialysis,[69] many patients still receive this therapy.[68] The actual data, however, show that hemodialysis, at various stages of poisoning, is no better than forced diuresis.[20,82] Reported thallium removal rates by hemodialysis are trivial: 143 mg of thallium was removed by 120 hours,[83] 222.8 mg was removed by 121 hours,[20] and 128 mg was removed by 54 hours of hemodialysis.[20] These quantities are placed in perspective knowing that the minimum lethal adult dose of thallium is estimated to be on the order of 1 g,[73] and that many reported doses exceed that by a factor of 10. Data from one hemodialysis case suggests that by using high blood flow rates (300 mL/min), clearances as high as 90 to 150 mL/min could be obtained.[63] Although these clearances seem encouraging, they should be interpreted with an appreciation of the large volume of distribution that thallium achieves in the postabsorptive phase. With lower

blood flow rates, charcoal hemoperfusion is 2 to 3 times more efficient than hemodialysis, providing clearance rates as high as 139 mL/min.[20] Combined hemoperfusion and hemodialysis were used in several cases[4,20,22] and were reported to remove as much as 93 mg of thallium within 3 hours of therapy.[4] Although extracorporeal therapy alone is probably insufficient for patients with significant poisoning and unnecessary in those with small exposures, some benefit seems likely when used in combination with other therapies, especially in patients with either underlying chronic kidney disease or acute kidney injury from thallium poisoning, and those with early massive, and presumed lethal, exposures. As is the case with other xenobiotics, thallium is probably not effectively removed by peritoneal dialysis.[53] A multidisciplinary consensus work group recently supported extracorporeal (HD + HP) therapy in patients with acute exposure when blood thallium concentrations are greater than 400 mcg/L (if rapidly available) or, if in the absence of laboratory support, severe signs and symptoms are present and treatment can be initiated within 24 to 48 hours of ingestion.[35] Table 99–2 summarizes the suggested therapy for thallium-exposed patients.

Chelation

Patients with thallium toxicity do not respond to traditional chelation therapy. Studies demonstrate that the use of EDTA and diethylenetriamine pentaacetic acid are without benefit.[70,93] Dimercaprol (British anti-Lewisite {BAL}) and D-penicillamine also fail to enhance thallium excretion in experimental models.[70,93] In one model in which D-penicillamine was able to enhance thallium elimination, the resultant substantial thallium redistribution into vital organs was a significant disadvantage.[88] A rodent model of combined use of Prussian blue with DL-penicillamine not only suggested a survival advantage for combined therapy but demonstrated reduced thallium concentrations in vital organs, including the brain.[70] Sulfur-containing compounds such as cysteine and NAC are not beneficial.[61,65] Another chelator, diphenylthiocarbazone (dithizone), forms a minimally toxic complex with thallium, resulting in a 33% increase in fecal elimination of thallium in rats.[99] Unfortunately, dithizone is goitrogenic and diabetogenic in animal studies.[61,73,108] Dithiocarb (sodium diethyldithiocarbamate), an intermediate metabolite of tetraethylthiuram disulfide (disulfiram, or Antabuse) (Chap. 78), also increases the urinary excretion of thallium.[99,105] Before thallium is eliminated, however, the formation of a lipophilic thallium—diethyldithiocarbamate complex likely results in the redistribution

---

TABLE 99–2   Treatment for Thallium Exposure

Early (patients who present in the first 1–2 hours postexposure)
- Stabilize airway, breathing, and circulation if necessary.
- Perform orogastric or nasogastric lavage if the patient has not vomited.
- Perform whole-bowel irrigation with polyethylene glycol electrolyte lavage solution for large ingestions or the presence of radiopaque material on abdominal radiographs.
- Begin multiple-dose activated charcoal (MDAC) therapy; add a cathartic (preferably oral mannitol) to the first dose if no recent bowel movements. Discontinue MDAC when Prussian blue can be administered.
- Give 250 mg/kg/d of Prussian blue orally in 2 or 4 divided doses dissolved in water or 50 mL of 15% mannitol if no recent bowel movements.
- Add simultaneous charcoal hemoperfusion and hemodialysis or hemodialysis alone, especially if in the presence of chronic kidney disease or acute kidney injury.

Delayed (patients who present more than 2–4 hours after acute exposure or with chronic toxicity)
- Stabilize airway, breathing, and circulation if necessary.
- Begin MDAC therapy; add a cathartic (preferably oral mannitol) to the first dose if no recent bowel movement. Discontinue MDAC when Prussian blue can be administered.
- Give 250 mg/kg/day of Prussian blue orally in 2 or 4 divided doses dissolved in water or 50 mL of 15% mannitol if no recent bowel movements.
- Add simultaneous charcoal hemoperfusion and hemodialysis or hemodialysis alone if in the presence of chronic kidney disease or acute kidney injury or life-threatening clinical manifestations or a thallium concentration 400 mcg/L.

of thallium into the CNS.[51,105] After decomposition of the chelate complex, thallium remains in the CNS, potentially exacerbating neurologic manifestations.[51,92] Because of the significant adverse effects of dithizone and the redistribution of thallium after dithiocarb use, neither chelator is recommended in the treatment of patients with thallium poisoning.

There is some interest in the water-soluble analogs of dimercaprol (DMPS (2,3-dimercapto-1-propanesulfonic acid) and succimer) for the treatment of thallium toxicity. However, in an animal model, DMPS failed to decrease tissue concentrations of thallium.[72] Similarly, in another animal model, although succimer improved survival over control subjects, the benefit was less than that achieved for Prussian blue and was at the cost of an increase in brain thallium concentrations.[92] Preliminary animal investigations demonstrate reduction in serum thallium concentrations after administration of the iron chelators deferoxamine and deferasirox.[29,95,96] Although worthy of additional study, these results are too preliminary to recommend either drug antidotes in thallium-poisoned patients. Similarly, experimental evidence from combined use of Zn-DTPA and Prussian blue is insufficient to recommend use in humans.[118]

SUMMARY

- Thallium is a multiorgan system toxin whose effects result from cellular mimicry for potassium and avid binding to sulfhydryl groups.
- The removal of thallium salts from depilatories and rodenticides has substantially reduced the incidence of both intentional and unintentional thallium toxicity in the United States.
- Cases of significant poisoning still occur in countries where thallium-containing rodenticides remain in use, as well as in this country, from suicide, attempted homicide, and by personal injury from contamination of foods and illicit xenobiotics.
- Early recognition of the characteristic signs and symptoms of thallium poisoning, such as a painful ascending sensory neuropathy and alopecia, followed by prompt initiation of safe and appropriate therapy will substantially improve the prognosis.
- Orogastric or nasogastric lavage is recommended for patients with acute oral poisonings if they present early and have not had significant emesis and/or at least one dose of oral AC followed by either multiple-dose activated charcoal (MDAC) or Prussian blue, if available. Oral mannitol can be added to either MDAC or Prussian blue when constipation is present.
- In severe acute poisoning, the addition of hemodialysis or combined hemodialysis and hemoperfusion in series is reasonable and offers a limited additional benefit.

REFERENCES

1. Afshari R, et al. Thallium poisoning: one additional and unexpected risk of heroin abuse. *Clin Toxicol (Phila)*. 2012;50:791-792.
2. Al Hammouri F, et al. Acute thallium poisoning: series of ten cases. *J Med Toxicol*. 2011;7:306-311.
3. Aoyama H. Distribution and excretion of thallium after oral and intraperitoneal administration of thallous malonate and thallous sulfate in hamsters. *Bull Environ Contam Toxicol*. 1989;42:456-463.
4. Aoyama H, et al. Acute poisoning by intentional ingestion of thallous malonate. *Hum Toxicol*. 1986;5:389-392.
5. Appenroth D, et al. Functional and morphological aspects of thallium-induced nephrotoxicity in rats. *Toxicology*. 1995;96:203-215.
6. Appenroth D, Winnefeld K. Is thallium-induced nephrotoxicity in rats connected with riboflavin and/or GSH?—Reconsideration of hypotheses on the mechanism of thallium toxicity. *J Appl Toxicol*. 1999;19:61-66.
7. Bank WJ. Thallium. In: Spencer PS, Schaumburg HH, eds. *Experimental and Clinical Neurotoxicology*. Baltimore, MD: Williams & Wilkins; 1980:570-577.
8. Bank WJ, et al. Thallium poisoning. *Arch Neurol*. 1972;26:456-464.
9. Bostian K, et al. Thallium activation and inhibition of yeast aldehyde dehydrogenase. *FEBS Lett*. 1975;59:88-91.
10. Britten JS, Blank M. Thallium activation of the (Na⁺—K⁺)-activated ATPase of rabbit kidney. *Biochim Biophys Acta*. 1968;159:160-166.
11. Burnett JW. Thallium poisoning. *Cutis*. 1990;46:112-113.
12. Campbell C, et al. Anagen effluvium caused by thallium poisoning. *JAMA Dermatol*. 2016;152:724-726.
13. Cavanagh JB. What have we learnt from Graham Frederick Young? Reflections on the mechanism of thallium neurotoxicity. *Neuropathol Appl Neurobiol*. 1991;17:3-9.
14. Cavanagh JB, et al. The effects of thallium salts, with particular reference to the nervous system changes. A report of three cases. *Q J Med*. 1974;43:293-319.
15. Chakrabarti AK, et al. Thallium poisoning—a case report. *J Trop Med Hyg*. 1985;88:291-293.
16. Chamberlain PH, et al. Thallium poisoning. *Pediatrics*. 1958;22:1170-1182.
17. Chandler HA, et al. Excretion of a toxic dose of thallium. *Clin Chem*. 1990;36:1506-1509.
18. Curto-Barredo L, et al. Anagen effluvium due to thallium poisoning derived from the intake of Chinese herbal medicine and rodenticide containing thallium salts. *J Dermatol*. 2015;42:1027-1029.
19. Davis LE, et al. Acute thallium poisoning: toxicological and morphological studies of the nervous system. *Ann Neurol*. 1981;10:38-44.
20. De Backer W, et al. Thallium intoxication treated with combined hemoperfusion-hemodialysis. *J Toxicol Clin Toxicol*. 1982;19:259-264.
21. de Groot G, van Heijst AN. Toxicokinetic aspects of thallium poisoning. Methods of treatment by toxin elimination. *Sci Total Environ*. 1988;71:411-418.
22. de Groot G, et al. An evaluation of the efficacy of charcoal haemoperfusion in the treatment of three cases of acute thallium poisoning. *Arch Toxicol*. 1985;57:61-66.
23. Desenclos JC, et al. Thallium poisoning: an outbreak in Florida, 1988. *South Med J*. 1992;85:1203-1206.
24. Dolgner R, et al. Repeated surveillance of exposure to thallium in a population living in the vicinity of a cement plant emitting dust containing thallium. *Int Arch Occup Environ Health*. 1983;52:79-94.
25. Dumitru D, Kalantri A. Electrophysiologic investigation of thallium poisoning. *Muscle Nerve*. 1990;13:433-437.
26. English JC. A case of thallium poisoning complicating pregnancy. *Med J Aust*. 1954;41:780-782.
27. Eskandari MR, et al. Toxicity of thallium on isolated rat liver mitochondria: the role of oxidative stress and MPT pore opening. *Environ Toxicol*. 2015;30:232-241.
28. Ewers U. Environmental exposure to thallium. *Sci Total Environ*. 1988;71:285-292.
29. Fatemi SJ, et al. Clinical evaluation of desferrioxamine (DFO) for removal of thallium ions in rat. *Int J Artif Organs*. 2007;30:902-905.
30. Feldman J, Levisohn DR. Acute alopecia: clue to thallium toxicity. *Pediatr Dermatol*. 1993;10:29-31.
31. Galvan-Arzate S, et al. Delayed effects of thallium in the rat brain: regional changes in lipid peroxidation and behavioral markers, but moderate alterations in antioxidants, after a single administration. *Food Chem Toxicol*. 2005;43:1037-1045.
32. Gastel B. Clinical conferences at the Johns Hopkins Hospital. Thallium poisoning. *Johns Hopkins Med J*. 1978;142:27-31.
33. Gehring PJ, Hammond PB. The interrelationship between thallium and potassium in animals. *J Pharmacol Exp Ther*. 1967;155:187-201.
34. Ghaderi A, et al. Thallium exists in opioid poisoned patients. *Daru*. 2015;23:39.
35. Ghannoum M, et al. Extracorporeal treatment for thallium poisoning: recommendations from the EXTRIP Workgroup. *Clin J Am Soc Nephrol*. 2012;7:1682-1690.
36. Gibson JE, Becker BA. Placental transfer, embryotoxicity, and teratogenicity of thallium sulfate in normal and potassium-deficient rats. *Toxicol Appl Pharmacol*. 1970;16:120-132.
37. Grunfeld O, Hinostroza G. Thallium poisoning. *Arch Intern Med*. 1964;114:132-138.
38. Hall BK. Critical periods during development as assessed by thallium-induced inhibition of growth of embryonic chick tibiae in vitro. *Teratology*. 1985;31:353-361.
39. Hanzel CE, et al. Glutathione metabolism is impaired in vitro by thallium(III) hydroxide. *Toxicology*. 2005;207:501-510.
40. Hasan M, Ali SF. Effects of thallium, nickel, and cobalt administration of the lipid peroxidation in different regions of the rat brain. *Toxicol Appl Pharmacol*. 1981;57:8-13.
41. Hasan M, et al. Biochemical and electrophysiologic effects of thallium poisoning on the rat corpus striatum. *Toxicol Appl Pharmacol*. 1977;41:353-359.
42. Hirata M, et al. A probable case of chronic occupational thallium poisoning in a glass factory. *Ind Health*. 1998;36:300-303.
43. Hoffman RS. Thallium poisoning during pregnancy: a case report and comprehensive literature review. *J Toxicol Clin Toxicol*. 2000;38:767-775.
44. Hoffman RS. Thallium toxicity and the role of Prussian blue in therapy. *Toxicol Rev*. 2003;22:29-40.
45. Hoffman RS, et al. Comparative efficacy of thallium adsorption by activated charcoal, prussian blue, and sodium polystyrene sulfonate. *J Toxicol Clin Toxicol*. 1999;37:833-837.
46. Hologgitas J, et al. Thallium elimination kinetics in acute thallotoxicosis. *J Anal Toxicol*. 1980;4:68-75.
47. Hultin T, Naslund PH. Effects of thallium (I) on the structure and functions of mammalian ribosomes. *Chem Biol Interact*. 1974;8:315-328.
48. Insley BM, et al. Thallium poisoning in cocaine abusers. *Am J Emerg Med*. 1986;4:545-548.
49. Inturrisi CE. Thallium-induced dephosphorylation of a phosphorylated intermediate of the (sodium plus thallium-activated) ATPase. *Biochim Biophys Acta*. 1969;178:630-633.
50. Johnson W. A case of thallium poisoning during pregnancy. *Med J Aust*. 1960;47:540-542.
51. Kamerbeek HH, et al. Prussian blue in therapy of thallotoxicosis. An experimental and clinical investigation. *Acta Med Scand*. 1971;189:321-324.
52. Kayne FJ. Thallium (I) activation of pyruvate kinase. *Arch Biochem Biophys*. 1971;143:232-239.

53. Koshy KM, Lovejoy FH. Thallium ingestion with survival: ineffectiveness of peritoneal dialysis and potassium chloride diuresis. *Clin Toxicol (Phila).* 1981;18:521-525.

54. Lehmann PA, Favari L. Parameters for the adsorption of thallium ions by activated charcoal and Prussian blue. *J Toxicol Clin Toxicol.* 1984;22:331-339.

55. Leloux MS, et al. Experimental studies on thallium toxicity in rats. II—the influence of several antidotal treatments on the tissue distribution and elimination of thallium, after subacute intoxication. *J Toxicol Clin Exp.* 1990;10:147-156.

56. Leung KM, Ooi VE. Studies on thallium toxicity, its tissue distribution and histopathological effects in rats. *Chemosphere.* 2000;41:155-159.

57. Li S, et al. Human fatality due to thallium poisoning: autopsy, microscopy, and mass spectrometry assays. *J Forensic Sci.* 2015;60:247-251.

58. Lopez Segura N, et al. Thallium poisoning in an adolescent girl [in Spanish]. *Med Clin (Barc).* 2013;141:557-558.

59. Lovejoy FH. Thallium. *Clin Toxicol Rev.* 1982;4:1-2.

60. Lukacs M. Thallium poisoning induced polyneuropathy—clinical and electrophysiological data [in Hungarian]. *Ideggyogy Sz.* 2003;56:407-414.

61. Lund A. The effect of various substances on the excretion and the toxicity of thallium in the rat. *Acta Pharmacol Toxicol (Copenh).* 1956;12:260-268.

62. Lynche GR, et al. The toxicology of thallium. *Lancet.* 1930;12:1340-1344.

63. Malbrain ML, et al. Treatment of severe thallium intoxication. *J Toxicol Clin Toxicol.* 1997;35:97-9100.

64. McMillan TM, et al. Neuropsychology of thallium poisoning. *J Neurol Neurosurg Psychiatry.* 1997;63:247-250.

65. Meggs WJ, et al. Effects of potassium in a murine model of thallium poisoning [abstract]. *J Toxicol Clin Toxicol.* 1995;33:559.

66. Meggs WJ, et al. Thallium poisoning from maliciously contaminated food. *J Toxicol Clin Toxicol.* 1994;32:723-730.

67. Melnick RL, et al. Uncoupling of mitochondrial oxidative phosphorylation by thallium. *Biochem Biophys Res Commun.* 1976;69:68-73.

68. Misra UK, et al. Thallium poisoning: emphasis on early diagnosis and response to haemodialysis. *Postgrad Med J.* 2003;79:103-105.

69. Moeschlin S. Thallium poisoning. *Clin Toxicol (Phila).* 1980;17:133-146.

70. Montes S, et al. Additive effect of DL-penicillamine plus Prussian blue for the antidotal treatment of thallotoxicosis in rats. *Environ Toxicol Pharmacol.* 2011;32:349-355.

71. Moore D, et al. Thallium poisoning. Diagnosis may be elusive but alopecia is the clue. *BMJ.* 1993;306:1527-1529.

72. Mulkey JP, Oehme FW. Are 2,3-dimercapto-1-propanesulfonic acid or Prussian blue beneficial in acute thallotoxicosis in rats? *Vet Hum Toxicol.* 2000;42:325-329.

73. Mulkey JP, Oehme FW. A review of thallium toxicity. *Vet Hum Toxicol.* 1993;35:445-453.

74. Mullins LJ, Moore RD. The movement of thallium ions in muscle. *J Gen Physiol.* 1960;43:759-773.

75. Munch JC. Human thallotoxicosis. *JAMA.* 1934;102:1929-1933.

76. Neal JB, et al. An unusual occurrence of thallium poisoning. *N Y State J Med.* 1935;35:657-659.

77. Nordentoft T, et al. Initial sensorimotor and delayed autonomic neuropathy in acute thallium poisoning. *Neurotoxicology.* 1998;19:421-426.

78. Osorio-Rico L, et al. The *N*-methyl-D-aspartate receptor antagonist MK-801 prevents thallium-induced behavioral and biochemical alterations in the rat brain. *Int J Toxicol.* 2015;34:505-513.

79. Pai V. Acute thallium poisoning. Prussian blue therapy in 9 cases. *West Indian Med J.* 1987;36:256-258.

80. Papp JP, et al. Potassium chloride treatment in thallotoxicosis. *Ann Intern Med.* 1969;71:119-123.

81. Pau PW. Management of thallium poisoning. *Hong Kong Med J.* 2000;6:316-318.

82. Paulson G, et al. Thallium intoxication treated with dithizone and hemodialysis. *Arch Intern Med.* 1972;129:100-103.

83. Pedersen RS, et al. Thallium intoxication treated with long-term hemodialysis, forced diuresis and Prussian blue. *Acta Med Scand.* 1978;204:429-432.

84. Questel F, et al. Thallium-contaminated heroin. *Ann Intern Med.* 1996;124:616.

85. Rangel-Guerra R, et al. Thallium poisoning. Experience with 50 patients [in Spanish]. *Gac Med Mex.* 1990;126:487-494.

86. Rauws AG. Thallium pharmacokinetics and its modification by Prussian blue. *Naunyn Schmiedebergs Arch Pharmacol.* 1974;284:294-306.

87. Reed D, et al. Thallotoxicosis. Acute manifestations and sequelae. *JAMA.* 1963;183:516-522.

88. Rios C, Monroy-Noyola A. D-Penicillamine and prussian blue as antidotes against thallium intoxication in rats. *Toxicology.* 1992;74:69-76.

89. Riyaz R, et al. A fatal case of thallium toxicity: challenges in management. *J Med Toxicol.* 2013;9:75-78.

90. Roby DS, et al. Cardiopulmonary effects of acute thallium poisoning. *Chest.* 1984; 85:236-240.

91. Rusyniak DE, et al. Thallium and arsenic poisoning in a small midwestern town. *Ann Emerg Med.* 2002;39:307-311.

92. Rusyniak DE, et al. Dimercaptosuccinic acid and Prussian blue in the treatment of acute thallium poisoning in rats. *J Toxicol Clin Toxicol.* 2003;41:137-142.

93. Saddique A, Peterson CD. Thallium poisoning: a review. *Vet Hum Toxicol.* 1983;25:16-22.

94. Saha A, et al. Erosion of nails following thallium poisoning: a case report. *Occup Environ Med.* 2004;61:640-642.

95. Saljooghi A, Fatemi SJ. Removal of thallium by deferasirox in rats as biological model. *J Appl Toxicol.* 2011;31:139-143.

96. Saljooghi AS, et al. Chelation of thallium by combining deferasirox and desferrioxamine in rats. *Toxicol Ind Health.* 2016;32:83-88.

97. Schaumburg HH, Berger A. Alopecia and sensory polyneuropathy from thallium in a Chinese herbal medication. *JAMA.* 1992;268:3430-3431.

98. Schmidt D, et al. A case of localized retinal damage in thallium poisoning. *Int J Ophthalmol.* 1997;21:143-147.

99. Schwetz BA, et al. Effects of diphenylthiocarbazone and diethyldithiocarbamate on the excretion of thallium by rats. *Toxicol Appl Pharmacol.* 1967;10:79-88.

100. Sharma AN, et al. Cerebrospinal fluid analysis in fatal thallium poisoning: evidence for delayed distribution into the central nervous system. *Am J Forensic Med Pathol.* 2004;25:156-158.

101. Sojakova M, et al. Thallium intoxication. Case report. *Neuro Endocrinol Lett.* 2015; 36:311-315.

102. Spencer PS, et al. Effects of thallium salts on neuronal mitochondria in organotypic cord-ganglia-muscle combination cultures. *J Cell Biol.* 1973;58:79-95.

103. Stevens W, et al. Eleven cases of thallium intoxication treated with Prussian blue. *Int J Clin Pharmacol.* 1974;10:1-22.

104. Sun TW, et al. Management of thallium poisoning in patients with delayed hospital admission. *Clin Toxicol (Phila).* 2012;50:65-69.

105. Sunderman FW. Diethyldithiocarbamate therapy of thallotoxicosis. *Am J Ophthalmol.* 1967;2:107-118.

106. Tabandeh H, et al. Ophthalmologic features of thallium poisoning. *Am J Ophthalmol.* 1994;117:243-245.

107. Tabandeh H, Thompson GM. Visual function in thallium toxicity. *BMJ.* 1993;307:324.

108. Thompson DF. Management of thallium poisoning. *Clin Toxicol (Phila).* 1981;18: 979-990.

109. Thompson DF, Callen ED. Soluble or insoluble prussian blue for radiocesium and thallium poisoning? *Ann Pharmacother.* 2004;38:1509-1514.

110. Tromme I, et al. Skin signs in the diagnosis of thallium poisoning. *Br J Dermatol.* 1998;138:321-325.

111. van der Merwe CF. The treatment of thallium poisoning. A report of 2 cases. *S Afr Med J.* 1972;46:560-561.

112. Vergauwe PL, et al. Near fatal subacute thallium poisoning necessitating prolonged mechanical ventilation. *Am J Emerg Med.* 1990;8:548-550.

113. Villanueva E, et al. Poisoning by thallium. A study of five cases. *Drug Saf.* 1990;5:384-389.

114. Villaverde MS, et al. In vitro interactions of thallium with components of the glutathione-dependent antioxidant defence system. *Free Radic Res.* 2004;38:977-984.

115. Vrij AA, et al. Successful recovery of a patient with thallium poisoning. *Neth J Med.* 1995;47:121-126.

116. Wainwright AP, et al. Clinical features and therapy of acute thallium poisoning. *Q J Med.* 1988;69:939-944.

117. Wakid NW, Cortas NK. Chemical and atomic absorption methods for thallium in urine compared. *Clin Chem.* 1984;30:587-588.

118. Wang Y, et al. Detoxification effects of two drugs in thallium-poisoned mice [in Chinese]. *Zhongguo Wei Zhong Bing Ji Jiu Yi Xue.* 2012;24:338-341.

119. Xia W, et al. A case-control study of prenatal thallium exposure and low birth weight in China. *Environ Health Perspect.* 2016;124:164-169.

120. Yokoyama K, et al. Distribution of nerve conduction velocities in acute thallium poisoning. *Muscle Nerve.* 1990;13:117-120.

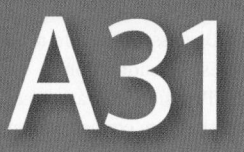

PRUSSIAN BLUE

Robert S. Hoffman

INTRODUCTION

Poisoning with salts of thallium or cesium are uncommon causes of life-threatening toxicity in which supportive care is often insufficient to alter outcome. Radioactive cesium is either released as part of a nuclear incident[13,22,68] or dispersed as a "dirty bomb,"[4,16] producing radiation exposure with subtoxic cesium doses. Prussian blue is an orally available cation exchange resin that enhances elimination of thallium and cesium in humans and animals and improves survivability in animals.

HISTORY

Prussian blue, the first artificially synthesized pigment, was discovered unintentionally by Diesbach in 1704 while attempting to make another pigment, cochineal red lake. Although immediately popular in art and later in printing, it took approximately 250 years to recognize that Prussian blue attracted monovalent alkali metals into its crystal lattice. Subsequently, in 1963, Nigrovic demonstrated that Prussian blue enhanced cesium elimination from the gastrointestinal tract of rats given either oral or intraperitoneal cesium.[44] In 2003, the US Food and Drug Administration (FDA) approved Prussian blue (as Radiogardase) for the treatment of thallium and radioactive cesium poisoning.

The Prussian blue literature is complicated by many confusing chemical and physical terms. The product synthesized by Diesbach, $Fe_4\{Fe(CN)_6\}_3$, iron(III) hexacyanoferrate(II), commonly known as insoluble Prussian blue, is assigned the Chemical Abstracts Service (CAS) number 14038-43-8 and is the FDA-approved product Radiogardase (Fig. A31–1). Synonyms for Prussian blue include Berlin blue, Hamburg blue, mineral blue, Paris blue, Turnbull's blue, and Pigment blue 27, among others.[66] These names are often used interchangeably to refer to both insoluble Prussian blue and a soluble (colloidal) Prussian blue that either has the molecular formula $KFe\{Fe(CN)_6\}_3$ or $K_3Fe\{Fe(CN)_6\}_3$. Thus "Prussian blue" also carries 2 additional CAS numbers: 25869-98-1 and 12240-15-2.[45] Compounds containing the same basic core structure, such as $NH_4Fe\{Fe(CN)_6\}_3$ (ammonium ferric ferrocyanide or Chinese blue) and sodium ferric ferrocyanide, may have similar efficacy in binding monovalent cations and are also sometimes incorrectly called Prussian blue. For the purpose of clarity, general statements that follow use the term "Prussian blue." In many instances, the terms "insoluble" and "soluble" are chosen to highlight differences between the compounds. Unfortunately,

because many studies do not specify which Prussian blue is used, some inherent ambiguity persists in the literature. Radiogardase, the currently available pharmaceutical preparation, is the insoluble form of Prussian blue, possibly selected preferentially for its efficacy in cesium poisoning.

PHARMACOLOGY

The crystal lattice of Prussian blue typically binds cationic potassium ions from the surrounding environment. However, because its affinity increases as the ionic radius of the monovalent cation increases, Prussian blue preferentially binds cesium (ionic radius: 1.69 Å) and thallium (ionic radius: 1.47 Å) over potassium (ionic radius: 1.33 Å).[10,23] Additionally, strong binding for rubidium (ionic radius: 1.48 Å) is demonstrated.[55] Thus, when given orally, Prussian blue binds unabsorbed thallium or cesium in the gastrointestinal tract, preventing absorption and reversing the concentration gradient to enhance elimination through enteroenteric circulation (gastrointestinal dialysis). Prussian blue also interferes with enterohepatic circulation, causing a further reduction in tissue stores.

Insoluble Prussian blue remains almost exclusively in the gastrointestinal tract and is eliminated nearly entirely in feces at a rate determined by gastrointestinal (GI) transit time. In a radiolabeled study of healthy pigs, 99% of a single ingested dose was recovered unchanged in the stool.[42] In contrast, soluble Prussian blue is slightly absorbed based on the clinical finding of a blue discoloration that develops in the sweat and tears of patients undergoing prolonged therapy.[18] This discoloration appears to be without clinical significance and resolves within days when therapy ceases. No significant food or drug interactions are known to exist.

THALLIUM

In Vitro Adsorption

The chemical formulation of Prussian blue influences the in vitro and, presumably, the in vivo adsorption of thallium ions. An early investigation demonstrated that the soluble form more effectively adsorbs thallium than the insoluble form.[12] In a more rigorous study, the in vitro adsorptions of both forms were similar when thallium concentrations remained low.[21] However, as thallium concentrations increased, the colloidal (soluble) form demonstrated far greater adsorptive capacity. Although not proven, this difference may occur because the soluble form contains more potassium and can therefore exchange proportionally more cation. Furthermore, the actual size of the crystal lattice alters its efficacy. When laboratory-synthesized Prussian blue (with a crystal size of 176.8 Å) was compared with a commercial preparation (with a crystal size of 311.9 Å), the laboratory-synthesized product adsorbed more thallium in vitro because its smaller size increased its surface area.[23] In vitro analysis of the FDA-approved antidote demonstrated that pH and hydration state greatly influenced adsorption, with the maximal adsorptive capacity (MAC) predicted to be as high as 1,400 mg of thallium/g at pH 7.5.[78]

In Vitro Comparison of Prussian Blue and Activated Charcoal

In one in vitro study, thallium was well adsorbed to Norit brand activated charcoal.[21] Although numerical data are not supplied in the body of the paper, the 10% to 20% adsorption to activated charcoal demonstrated in a figure was far less than the results achieved with several different forms of Prussian blue tested simultaneously.[21] Two other binding studies showed results different from the Norit activated charcoal study. One investigation determined

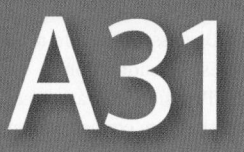

FIGURE A31–1. The chemical structure of insoluble Prussian blue. The Roman numerals II and III denote the valence state of iron. Although in most current nomenclature this would be expressed as Fe^{2+} and Fe^{3+}, the figure is drawn this way for consistency with most available references, which employ the older nomenclature.

that the MAC of activated charcoal was 124 mg of thallium/g, whereas the MAC for Prussian blue was only 72 mg of thallium/g.[24] In another study, a MAC of only 59.7 mg of thallium/g was calculated for CharcoAid activated charcoal, compared with a higher MAC for insoluble Prussian blue of 72.7 mg of thallium/g.[19] Although the MACs for Prussian blue in these 2 studies are nearly identical, they differ significantly from the MAC reported above for the FDA-approved formulation, possibly as a result of different experimental conditions.[78] Similarly, the variable results for activated charcoal may also be a function of the study pH or the different types of activated charcoal used.

Animal Data: Kinetics, Tissue Concentrations, and Survival
Thallium

Sublethal doses of thallium were used to evaluate the effects of various antidotes in rats over an 8-day period.[24] Although the control group only eliminated 53% of the administered dose of thallium, 93% of the dose was eliminated in the activated charcoal, and 82% was eliminated in the insoluble Prussian blue groups. In contrast, other investigators demonstrated only a modest increase in thallium elimination in rats treated with oral activated charcoal while demonstrating a consistent benefit of Prussian blue.[25]

Multiple studies demonstrate that Prussian blue not only decreases the half-life of thallium in animals but also lowers thallium content in critical organs such as the brain and the heart.[17,38,39,54,56] Half-lives are typically reduced by approximately 50% when Prussian blue is given with or without a cathartic. The rationale for the cathartic is that constipation is invariably present in humans and animals with severe thallium poisoning.

Only a few studies evaluated the effects of Prussian blue on survival. In these studies, a statistically significant survival advantage is shown in thallium-poisoned rats[23,56] and mice[29] treated with Prussian blue. The experimental benefit was a 31% increase in the LD_{50} (median lethal dose for 50% of poisoned animals).[57] Although most chelators have a limited or detrimental effect in thallium poisoning (Chap. 99) and DL-penicillamine has no demonstrable benefit as a single antidote, in an animal model the combined use of Prussian blue and DL-penicillamine not only decreased thallium concentration in critical tissues such as the brain but also enhanced survival.[2,36] Although interesting, these data are too preliminary to recommend the routine use of combined DL-penicillamine and Prussian blue in poisoned humans.

Radioactive Thallium

There is no published experience describing human poisoning with radioactive thallium. Prussian blue has demonstrable efficacy in an animal model of radioactive thallium poisoning, as would be expected because the ionic radii of isotopes are generally similar. In one small study, insoluble Prussian blue decreased the biologic half-life of radioactive thallium in rats by approximately 40%.[5] Many humans receive radioactive thallium (^{201}Tl) chloride as part of myocardial scintigraphy, with a typical adult dose of 110 megabecquerels (MBq). Concerns about excess radiation exposure following the termination of diagnostic testing have led to the evaluation of Prussian blue to enhance post-imaging elimination. In vitro evidence suggests a MAC of 5,000 MBq/g.[3] In a controlled trial, in which Prussian blue was given to a patient post myocardial scintigraphy, radioactivity was reduced 18% and 30% after 24 and 48 hours, respectively.[3]

Thallium Poisoning in Humans

A thorough analysis of the efficacy of Prussian blue in thallium poisoning is severely hampered by many factors. First, and most importantly, there are no controlled human trials. Second, although multiple patients have received Prussian blue in the setting of thallium poisoning, many were simultaneously treated with a variety of therapies, including forced potassium diuresis, single- or multiple-dose activated charcoal, and either hemodialysis or hemoperfusion. Thus, it is impossible to determine the specific effects of Prussian blue on morbidity or mortality, and even toxicokinetic data must be interpreted with caution. Third, many reports fail to specify the exact type of Prussian blue used. Those investigations that do specify the type of Prussian blue typically used the soluble form, which is presently unavailable as a

pharmaceutical preparation in the United States. Discussions of the available data in the following sections are limited by these considerations.

Three patients, in 1971, were the first to receive Prussian blue as a treatment for thallium poisoning.[21] Although daily fecal thallium concentrations were not determined in 2 of the 3 patients because of severe constipation, an approximately 7-fold increase in fecal thallium elimination over baseline was attributed to Prussian blue therapy in the third patient. Subsequently, many humans with thallium poisoning have received Prussian blue, with or without a cathartic, as part of their therapy.[1,7,9,10,15,21,48,51,52,58,61,63,70,71,75] Unfortunately, other components of therapy that may have confounded the effects of Prussian blue in these cases include single- or multiple-dose activated charcoal and the use of D-penicillamine, dimercaprol, ethylenediaminetetraacetic acid (EDTA), succimer, 2,3-dimercaptopropane-1-sulfate (DMPS), forced potassium diuresis, and either hemodialysis or hemoperfusion. There are no controlled human trials of any of these modalities alone or in combination, and most of the data presented are based on single case reports or small case series.

One of the largest series was composed of 11 thallium-poisoned patients who were treated with soluble Prussian blue.[63] This report not only demonstrated the tolerability of Prussian blue, but also was the first to systematically evaluate its fecal elimination. In all individuals studied, fecal elimination remained high, even when urinary elimination fell, suggesting selective redistribution of thallium into the gut.[63] Although the authors commented on clinical improvement in these patients, the lack of controlled data makes these subjective observations difficult to interpret. Similarly, a substantial reduction in thallium half-life was demonstrated when Prussian blue was compared with no therapy at all in patients with thallium poisoning.[10] Another series of 14 patients with delayed presentation (9–19 days) were reported. These patients were treated with DMPS, followed by Prussian blue and hemodialysis, and 13 survived. Data are insufficient to make inferences about the effects of Prussian blue alone or as part of this treatment regimen.[64]

Dosage and Administration

The dosage of Prussian blue has never been investigated systematically in either humans or animals. In most of the case reports and series mentioned above, a total dose of 150 to 250 mg/kg/day was administered orally or via a nasogastric tube in 2 to 4 divided doses.[63] Because constipation or obstipation is often present or expected, Prussian blue is generally administered dissolved in 50 mL of 15% mannitol.[65] Although any cathartic may be appropriate, mannitol is used most frequently, possibly because of concerns over the risks associated with repeated doses of magnesium or sorbitol (Antidotes in Depth: A2). The manufacturer of Radiogardase recommends that adults and adolescents with thallium poisoning receive a total dose of 9 g divided daily (3 g every 8 hours) and that children receive a total dose of 3 g divided daily (1 g every 8 hours). Although the manufacturer does not recommend using a cathartic, a high fiber diet is advocated when constipation is present. Because Prussian blue is well tolerated, the editors of this text continue to favor the 150- to 250-mg/kg/day dosing because it provides more antidote with limited adverse consequence and most of the published experience has used this dose with essentially no adverse effects. In addition, because many severely poisoned patients cannot tolerate swallowing large numbers of capsules, it is recommended to open the capsules and mix them with food or liquids when needed. This will often result in a benign blue discoloration of the mouth and teeth. The use of a cathartic is reasonable when constipation is consequential.

The end point of therapy is similarly poorly defined. By convention, Prussian blue is usually continued until total urinary thallium concentrations fall below 0.5 mg/day. Although this end point is not a perfect measurement of total body thallium burden, as small amounts of fecal elimination continue, even when urinary elimination has diminished,[63] most laboratories are not equipped to measure fecal thallium concentrations. In patients who remain significantly symptomatic, it is reasonable to continue Prussian blue therapy for a short period past the 0.5-mg/day endpoint on an individual basis.

CESIUM

The radioactive isotope of cesium (^{137}Cs), a common byproduct of nuclear fission reactions, is a strong β and γ emitter with a physical half-life of more than 30 years and a biologic half-life of about 110 days. Another isotope (^{134}Cs) is only produced by neutron activation of the stable isotope (^{133}Cs) and has a physical half-life of about 2 years and a biologic half-life comparable to ^{137}Cs. Cesium is absorbed in the small bowel, distributes like potassium, and undergoes enteric recirculation in a manner comparable to thallium.[37] Approximately 80% of a given dose of cesium is eliminated in the urine, with 20% cleared in the feces.

The isotope ^{137}Cs is used clinically as a radiotherapy source in nuclear medicine and to irradiate banked blood. Although uncommon, radiologic disasters such as Fukushima, Chernobyl, and Goiânia (see human data below) have resulted in lethal incorporation exposures. Additionally, concerns over the use of ^{137}Cs in "dirty bombs" have increased the potential need to treat patients with radioactive cesium poisoning. Toxicity from nonradioactive cesium is also reported. Cases of QT interval prolongation, torsade de pointes, and death are reported in patients taking cesium chloride either as a dietary supplement or for its alleged antineoplastic effects.[6,8,27,47,53,59,67]

In Vitro Adsorption

Standard binding studies compared the ability of activated charcoal, sodium polystyrene sulfonate (SPS), and both soluble and insoluble Prussian blue to adsorb ^{137}Cs over a range of gastrointestinal pHs.[73] Unlike thallium, the adsorption of cesium to activated charcoal was negligible. Comparable to thallium, SPS offered no benefit, likely because of preferential effects on potassium. Although both forms of Prussian blue adsorbed cesium, the insoluble form was consistently superior. A pH of 7.5 was selected to represent the pH of the small bowel lumen, the location where most adsorption would occur. At this pH, a MAC of 238 mg of ^{137}Cs/g of insoluble Prussian blue was determined. In an interesting extension, when the same authors bound insoluble Prussian blue to a hemoperfusion column, they demonstrated a clearance of approximately 100 mL/min of ^{137}Cs from plasma and projected that a 4-hour treatment would adsorb about 0.3 terabecquerel (TBq) of radioactive cesium.[74] When the FDA-approved antidote was analyzed, like thallium, pH and hydration introduced significant variations in binding, with a MAC of 715 mg of cesium/g noted at pH 7.5.[14]

Animal Data: Kinetics, Tissue Concentrations, and Survival

Small animal investigations with either ^{134}Cs or ^{137}Cs consistently demonstrate that Prussian blue therapy reverses the urine-to-stool elimination ratio from 8:1 to 0.3:1 and reduces the biologic half-life and the total body area under the curve by as much as 60%.[40,43,44,55,62] For example, rats given oral ^{134}Cs retained 84.7% of the ingested dose at 7 days. Treatment with insoluble or soluble Prussian blue, as well as Chinese blue, produced significant reductions in retained cesium (only 6.36%, 2.63%, and 2.43% of the dose was retained at 7 days, respectively).[11]

In addition to human toxicity, concern over radioactive cesium incorporation into cattle milk and meat resulted in a number of large animal model investigations. Daily Prussian blue therapy reduced radioactive cesium concentrations in sheep by as much as 42%.[20,50] Likewise, radioactive cesium transfer to milk was reduced by 85% in cows.[69] When dogs were contaminated with ^{137}Cs, Prussian blue reduced the total body burden by as much as 51%.[32] Similar efficacy in reducing the amount of cesium was demonstrated in meat from pigs fed ^{134}Cs-contaminated whey, with insoluble Prussian blue reducing activity from 359 to 11 Bq/kg over 27 days.[11]

Human Volunteer Studies

Two human volunteers ingested meals contaminated with ^{134}Cs to compare the efficacy of both the soluble and insoluble forms of Prussian blue with controls.[11] At 14 days after exposure and without therapy, the volunteers retained 94.7% of the ingested dose, compared with retention of only 5.1% following therapy with insoluble Prussian blue and 4.9% following soluble

Prussian blue. In another study, 2 volunteers demonstrated that Prussian blue decreased the biologic half-life of ingested radioactive cesium by approximately 33%.[28] Finally, in 2 volunteers, the effects of pretreatment were compared with simultaneous posttreatment Prussian blue. When a single dose of Prussian blue was administered 10 minutes before ^{134}Cs, absorption decreased from 100% (without therapy) to 3% to 10%. However, simultaneous administration of 0.5 or 1 g of Prussian blue with ^{134}Cs resulted in 38% to 63% absorption. Finally, when Prussian blue was given daily at a dose of 0.5 g every 8 hours in the postabsorptive phase, the biologic half-life of ^{134}Cs was reduced from 106 to 44 days.[42]

Radioactive Cesium Poisoning in Humans

There are no controlled trials of Prussian blue in radioactive cesium poisoning. Experience is derived exclusively from treating disaster victims. In 1987, a number of people in Goiânia, Brazil, were incorporated with radioactive cesium from a discarded radiotherapy unit.[46] Although the reported total number of individuals treated is uncertain because of multiple reports that probably include the same patient several times, one group describes 37 patients who were given insoluble Prussian blue in doses ranging from 3 g/d in children up to 10 g/d in adults. Untreated, elimination kinetics were first order, and half-lives varied extensively from 39 to 106 days in adults (mean: 65.5 days in women and 83 days in men). Half-lives were shorter in children. Therapy with insoluble Prussian blue reduced half-lives by a mean of 32%,[26] and reduced the retained cesium dose from between 51% and 84% of the total dose.[30]

The nuclear disaster at Chernobyl, Ukraine, resulted in many cases of acute radiation exposure as well as incorporation into the population of radioactive iodine, cesium, and strontium. In one trial, insoluble Prussian blue was given to 3 victims of radioactive cesium incorporation many weeks after their exposure. The reported reduction in biologic half-life ranged from 12% to 52%.[33] The authors of this paper include data from the Chinese literature describing another 6 patients who demonstrated a similar reduction in the biologic half-life of cesium following Prussian blue therapy. Kinetic modeling based on all available data suggest that although Prussian blue is most effective if given nearly immediately post exposure. However, administration as late as 30 days post exposure, and perhaps even one year post exposure will substantially reduce the biological half-life of ^{137}Cs.

Nonradioactive Cesium Poisoning in Humans

Three cases describe the use of Prussian blue for patients with nonradioactive cesium poisoning. A 58-year-old woman presented with syncope, polymorphic ventricular tachycardia, hypokalemia, and a QT interval of 590 ms after taking cesium chloride as an alternative therapy for cancer. The apparent half-life of cesium was reported as 7.9 days during Prussian blue therapy in comparison to 86.6 days after therapy. The authors state that there were no adverse effects of therapy.[67] Similarly, a 65-year-old woman presented with syncope and was found to have multiple episodes of torsade de pointes, hypokalemia, and a QT interval of 620 ms after taking cesium chloride for 6 weeks. Therapy with insoluble Prussian blue (3 g/d) was associated with a reduction in the apparent half-life for cesium from 61.7 to 29.4 days.[6] The final case describes a 61-year-old woman who injected cesium chloride subcutaneously around a mass and suffered a cardiac arrest. She was resuscitated, found to have a prolonged QT interval (>700 ms) and a very high blood cesium concentration. She received Prussian blue but the regimen and effect on cesium elimination are not clearly defined.[60]

Dosage and Administration

We agree with the manufacturer of Radiogardase recommendation that for radioactive cesium poisoning, adults and adolescents 13 years or older receive a total daily dose of 9 g divided into 3 g, 3 times per day. Children aged 2 through 12 years should receive a total daily dose of 3 g divided into 1 g, 3 times per day. Although the manufacturer offers no recommendation in children under the age of 2 years, administering 150 to 250 mg/kg/day in divided doses are appropriate. Although these are the same doses used for thallium poisoning, therapy for cesium poisoning should be continued for at least 30 days. Even though there are no recommendations of other criteria to determine the end point of therapy, quantitative and radiologic evaluations of cesium elimination should be performed. Capsules can be opened and mixed in liquids and given via nasogastric tube for patients unable to swallow. Since constipation does not commonly occur with either radioactive or nonradioactive cesium poisoning, neither routine cathartic administration nor the use of a high-fiber diet is recommended.

ADVERSE EFFECTS AND SAFETY ISSUES

Animal studies show no adverse effects of therapeutic doses.[49] Oral lethal doses are not known or projected for humans, but are likely to be astronomic given that there is no or minimal absorption of Prussian blue and the absence of local toxicity in the GI tract. The only significant adverse effects reported in humans receiving therapeutic doses are constipation and hypokalemia,[65] and the constipation is likely to be related more to the thallium toxicity than to Prussian blue.

Although there is some concern regarding the potential for cyanide liberation from Prussian blue, this release appears to be quantitatively minimal. Cyanide release from soluble Prussian blue was less than 3 mg/24 h in simulated gastric fluid.[72] When 3 human volunteers were given 500 mg of soluble Prussian blue (radiolabeled with ^{59}Fe, either in the ferric or ferrous position and with ^{14}C on the CN), only 2 mg of cyanide were absorbed.[41] Over the physiological range of potential gastrointestinal pH, the maximal cyanide release from insoluble Prussian blue is only 135 mcg/g at pH 1.[76,77] When extrapolated even for repeated therapeutic doses, only a trivial amount of cyanide would be liberated.

PREGNANCY AND LACTATION

Insoluble Prussian blue is listed as pregnancy category C. Because of the severe consequences of poisoning from radioactive cesium and thallium, both of which cross the placenta, and the lack of systemic absorption of insoluble Prussian blue, a risk-to-benefit analysis would favor the use of the antidote in all poisoned pregnant patients. Both cesium and thallium are excreted in breast milk. Prussian blue's confinement in the GI tract would make excretion in breast milk unlikely. In any event, women contaminated with cesium or thallium should not breastfeed.

FORMULATION AND ACQUISITION

Insoluble Prussian blue (Radiogardase) is available as a 0.5-g blue powder in gelatin capsules for oral administration manufactured from Haupt Pharma Berlin GmbH for distribution by HEYL Chemisch-pharmazeutische Fabrik GmbH & Co. KG, Berlin (281-395-7040; fax 281-395-2320; see information at www.heyltex.com). Prussian blue is part of the US Strategic National Stockpile, which can be accessed at CDC emergency response hotline: 770-488-7100; and is also stored at REAC/TS, Oak Ridge: emergency number 865-576-1005. Thirty capsules retail for about $100 and have a listed 5-year shelf-life. Although data suggest that Prussian blue is stable well beyond the 5-year label,[34,35] recommendations for use after longer storage periods cannot be made without formal evaluation by the shelf-life extension program.

SUMMARY

- Prussian blue is a crystalline lattice that adsorbs radioactive and nonradioactive isotopes of thallium and cesium.
- Animal data demonstrate the ability of Prussian blue to prevent absorption, enhance elimination, and improve survival following thallium or cesium administration.
- Although human data are limited, the use of Prussian blue appears beneficial in case reports and small case series.
- Because Prussian blue is essentially nontoxic, it should be used whenever severe thallium or cesium poisoning is suspected.
- If Prussian blue is unavailable, activated charcoal can be substituted for thallium poisoning, but not for cesium poisoning.

Acknowledgment

Part of this chapter was adapted, with permission from the publisher, from Hoffman RS: Thallium toxicity and the role of Prussian blue in therapy. *Toxicol Rev.* 2003;22:29–40.

REFERENCES

1. Atsmon J, et al. Thallium poisoning in Israel. *Am J Med Sci.* 2000;320:327-330.
2. Barroso-Moguel R, et al. Combined D-penicillamine and Prussian blue as antidotal treatment against thallotoxicosis in rats: evaluation of cerebellar lesions. *Toxicology.* 1994;89:15-24.
3. Bhardwaj N, et al. Dynamic, equilibrium and human studies of adsorption of 201Tl by Prussian blue. *Health Phys.* 2006;90:250-257.
4. Blair JD. Why the dirty bomb is still ticking. *J Healthc Prot Manage.* 2014;30:109-115.
5. Borisov VP, et al. Effectiveness of ferrocin in decreasing the resorption of radioactive thallium [in Russian]. *Med Radiol (Mosk).* 1984;29:15-18.
6. Chan CK, et al. Life-threatening torsades de pointes resulting from "natural" cancer treatment. *Clin Toxicol (Phila).* 2009;47:592-594.
7. Chandler HA, et al. Excretion of a toxic dose of thallium. *Clin Chem.* 1990;36(8, pt 1): 1506-1509.
8. Dalal AK, et al. Acquired long QT syndrome and monomorphic ventricular tachycardia after alternative treatment with cesium chloride for brain cancer. *Mayo Clin Proc.* 2004;79:1065-1069.
9. De Backer W, et al. Thallium intoxication treated with combined hemoperfusion-hemodialysis. *J Toxicol Clin Toxicol.* 1982;19:259-264.
10. de Groot G, van Heijst AN. Toxicokinetic aspects of thallium poisoning. Methods of treatment by toxin elimination. *Sci Total Environ.* 1988;71:411-418.
11. Dresow B, et al. In vivo binding of radiocesium by two forms of Prussian blue and by ammonium iron hexacyanoferrate (II). *J Toxicol Clin Toxicol.* 1993;31:563-569.
12. Dvorak P. Colloidal hexacyanoferrates (II) as antidotes in thallium poisoning [in German]. *Z Gesamte Exp Med.* 1969;151:89-92.
13. Evangeliou N, et al. Reconstructing the Chernobyl Nuclear Power Plant (CNPP) accident 30 years after. A unique database of air concentration and deposition measurements over Europe. *Environ Pollut.* 2016;216:408-418.
14. Faustino PJ, et al. Quantitative determination of cesium binding to ferric hexacyanoferrate: Prussian blue. *J Pharm Biomed Anal.* 2008;47:114-125.
15. Ghezzi R, Bozza Marrubini M. Prussian blue in the treatment of thallium intoxication. *Vet Hum Toxicol.* 1979;21(suppl):64-66.
16. Goffman T. Lack of strategic insight: the "dirty bomb" effort. *Am J Disaster Med.* 2009; 4:181-183.
17. Heydlauf H. Ferric-cyanoferrate (II): an effective antidote in thallium poisoning. *Eur J Pharmacol.* 1969;6:340-344.
18. Hoffman RS. Thallium toxicity and the role of Prussian blue in therapy. *Toxicol Rev.* 2003;22:29-40.
19. Hoffman RS, et al. Comparative efficacy of thallium adsorption by activated charcoal, Prussian blue, and sodium polystyrene sulfonate. *J Toxicol Clin Toxicol.* 1999;37: 833-837.
20. Ioannides KG, et al. Reduction of cesium concentration in ovine tissues following treatment with Prussian blue labeled with 59Fe. *Health Phys.* 1996;71:713-718.
21. Kamerbeek HH, et al. Prussian blue in therapy of thallotoxicosis. An experimental and clinical investigation. *Acta Med Scand.* 1971;189:321-324.
22. Kanapilly GM, et al. Characterization of an aerosol sample from the auxiliary building of the Three Mile Island reactor. *Health Phys.* 1983;45:981-989.
23. Kravzov J, et al. Relationship between physicochemical properties of Prussian blue and its efficacy as antidote against thallium poisoning. *J Appl Toxicol.* 1993;13:213-216.
24. Lehmann PA, Favari L. Parameters for the adsorption of thallium ions by activated charcoal and Prussian blue. *J Toxicol Clin Toxicol.* 1984;22:331-339.
25. Leloux MS, et al. Experimental studies on thallium toxicity in rats. II—The influence of several antidotal treatments on the tissue distribution and elimination of thallium, after subacute intoxication. *J Toxicol Clin Exp.* 1990;10:147-156.
26. Lipsztein JL, et al. Studies of Cs retention in the human body related to body parameters and Prussian blue administration. *Health Phys.* 1991;60:57-61.
27. Lyon AW, Mayhew WJ. Cesium toxicity: a case of self-treatment by alternate therapy gone awry. *Ther Drug Monit.* 2003;25:114-116.
28. Madshus K, Stromme A. Increased excretion of ^{137}Cs in humans by Prussian Blue. *Z Naturforsch B.* 1968;23:391-392.
29. Meggs WJ, et al. Effects of Prussian blue and N-acetylcysteine on thallium toxicity in mice. *J Toxicol Clin Toxicol.* 1997;35:163-166.
30. Melo DR, et al. ^{137}Cs internal contamination involving a Brazilian accident, and the efficacy of Prussian blue treatment. *Health Phys.* 1994;66:245-252.
31. Melo DR, et al. Efficacy of Prussian blue on ^{137}Cs decorporation therapy. *Health Phys.* 2014;106:592-597.
32. Melo DR, et al. Prussian blue decorporation of ^{137}Cs in beagles of different ages. *Health Phys.* 1996;71:190-197.
33. Ming-hua T, et al. Measurement of internal contamination with radioactive caesium released from the Chernobyl accident and enhanced elimination by Prussian blue. *J Radiol Protect.* 1988;8:25-28.

34. Mohammad A, et al. Long-term stability study of Prussian blue—a quality assessment of water content and thallium binding. *Int J Pharm.* 2014;477:122-127.

35. Mohammad A, et al. A long-term stability study of Prussian blue: a quality assessment of water content and cesium binding. *J Pharm Biomed Anal.* 2015;103:85-90.

36. Montes S, et al. Additive effect of DL-penicillamine plus Prussian blue for the antidotal treatment of thallotoxicosis in rats. *Environ Toxicol Pharmacol.* 2011;32:349-355.

37. Moore W Jr, Comar CL. Absorption of caesium 137 from the gastro-intestinal tract of the rat. *Int J Radiat Biol.* 1962;5:247-254.

38. Mulkey JP, Oehme FW. A review of thallium toxicity. *Vet Hum Toxicol.* 1993;35:445-453.

39. Mulkey JP, Oehme FW. Are 2,3-dimercapto-1-propanesulfonic acid or prussian blue beneficial in acute thallotoxicosis in rats? *Vet Hum Toxicol.* 2000;42:325-329.

40. Muller WH, et al. Long-term treatment of cesium 137 contamination with colloidal and a comparison with insoluble Prussian blue in rats. *Strahlentherapie.* 1974;147:319-322.

41. Nielsen P, et al. Bioavailability of iron and cyanide from oral potassium ferric hexacyanoferrate(II) in humans. *Arch Toxicol.* 1990;64:420-422.

42. Nielsen P, et al. Inhibition of intestinal absorption and decorporation of radiocaesium in humans by hexacyanoferrates(II). *Int J Radiat Appl Instrument B Nucl Med Biol.* 1991;18:821-826.

43. Nigrovic V. Enhancement of the excretion of radiocaesium in rats by ferric cyanoferrate. II. *Int J Radiat Biol Relat Stud Phys Chem Med.* 1963;7:307-309.

44. Nigrovic V. Retention of radiocaesium by the rat as influenced by Prussian blue and other compounds. *Phys Med Biol.* 1965;10:81-92.

45. O'Neil MJ, et al. *The Merck Index.* Whitehouse Station, NJ: Merck & Co & Inc; 2004 [http://themerckindex.cambridgesoft.com/TheMerckIndex/default.asp?formgroup=basenp_form_group&dataaction=db&dbname=TheMerckIndex. updated 2001.]

46. Oliveira AR, et al. Medical and related aspects of the Goiania accident: an overview. *Health Phys.* 1991;60:17-24.

47. Olshansky B, Shivkumar K. Patient—heal thyself? Electrophysiology meets alternative medicine. *Pacing Clin Electrophysiol.* 2001;24(4, pt 1):403-405.

48. Pai V. Acute thallium poisoning. Prussian blue therapy in 9 cases. *West Indian Med J.* 1987;36:256-258.

49. Pearce J. Studies of any toxicological effects of Prussian blue compounds in mammals—a review. *Food Chem Toxicol.* 1994;32:577-582.

50. Pearce J. The effects of prussian blue provided by indwelling rumen boli on the tissue retention of dietary radiocaesium by sheep. *Sci Total Environ.* 1989;85:349-355.

51. Pedersen RS, et al. Thallium intoxication treated with long-term hemodialysis, forced diuresis and Prussian blue. *Acta Med Scand.* 1978;204:429-432.

52. Pelclova D, et al. Two-year follow-up of two patients after severe thallium intoxication. *Hum Exp Toxicol.* 2009;28:263-272.

53. Pinter A, et al. Cesium-induced torsades de pointes. *N Engl J Med.* 2002;346:383-384.

54. Rauws AG. Thallium pharmacokinetics and its modification by Prussian blue. *Naunyn Schmiedebergs Arch Pharmacol.* 1974;284:294-306.

55. Richmond CR, Bunde DE. Enhancement of cesium-137 excretion by rats maintained chronically on ferric ferrocyanide. *Proc Soc Exp Biol Med.* 1966;121:664-670.

56. Rios C, et al. Efficacy of Prussian blue against thallium poisoning: effect of particle size. *Proc West Pharmacol Soc.* 1991;34:61-63.

57. Rios C, Monroy-Noyola A. D-Penicillamine and Prussian blue as antidotes against thallium intoxication in rats. *Toxicology.* 1992;74:69-76.

58. Riyaz R, et al. A fatal case of thallium toxicity: challenges in management. *J Med Toxicol.* 2013;9:75-78.

59. Saliba W, et al. Polymorphic ventricular tachycardia in a woman taking cesium chloride. *Pacing Clin Electrophysiol.* 2001;24(4, pt 1):515-517.

60. Sessions D, et al. Fatal cesium chloride toxicity after alternative cancer treatment. *J Altern Complement Med.* 2013;19:973-975.

61. Sojakova M, et al. Thallium intoxication. Case report. *Neuro Endocrinol Lett.* 2015;36:311-315.

62. Stather JW. Influence of prussian blue on metabolism of ^{137}Cs and ^{86}Rb in rats. *Health Phys.* 1972;22:1-8.

63. Stevens W, et al. Eleven cases of thallium intoxication treated with Prussian blue. *Int J Clin Pharmacol Ther Toxicol.* 1974;10:1-22.

64. Sun TW, et al. Management of thallium poisoning in patients with delayed hospital admission. *Clin Toxicol (Phila).* 2012;50:65-69.

65. Thompson DF. Management of thallium poisoning. *Clin Toxicol.* 1981;18:979-990.

66. Thompson DF, Callen ED. Soluble or insoluble Prussian blue for radiocesium and thallium poisoning? *Ann Pharmacother.* 2004;38:1509-1514.

67. Thurgur LD, et al. Non-radioactive cesium toxicity: a case of treatment using Prussian Blue.[abstract]. *Clin Toxicol (Phila).* 2006;44:730-731.

68. Tsubokura M, et al. Estimated association between dwelling soil contamination and internal radiation contamination levels after the 2011 Fukushima Daiichi nuclear accident in Japan. *BMJ Open.* 2016;6:e010970.

69. Unsworth EF, et al. Investigations of the use of clay minerals and Prussian blue in reducing the transfer of dietary radiocaesium to milk. *Sci Total Environ.* 1989;85:339-347.

70. van der Merwe CF. The treatment of thallium poisoning. A report of 2 cases. *S Afr Med J.* 1972;46:560-561.

71. van der Stock J, de Schepper J. The effect of Prussian blue and sodium-ethylenediaminetetraacetic acid on the faecal and urinary elimination of thallium by the dog. *Res Vet Sci.* 1978;25:337-342.

72. Verzijl JM, et al. In vitro cyanide release of four Prussian blue salts used for the treatment of cesium contaminated persons. *J Toxicol Clin Toxicol.* 1993;31:553-562.

73. Verzijl JM, et al. In vitro binding characteristics for cesium of two qualities of Prussian blue, activated charcoal and Resonium-A. *J Toxicol Clin Toxicol.* 1992;30:215-222.

74. Verzijl JM, et al. In vitro binding of radiocesium to Prussian blue coated strips and Prussian blue containing hemoperfusion columns as a potential tool for the treatment of persons internally contaminated with radiocesium. *Artif Organs.* 1995;19:86-93.

75. Wainwright AP, et al. Clinical features and therapy of acute thallium poisoning. *Q J Med.* 1988;69:939-944.

76. Yang Y, et al. Quantitative measurement of cyanide released from Prussian blue. *Clin Toxicol (Phila).* 2007;45:776-781.

77. Yang Y, et al. Validation of an in vitro method for the determination of cyanide release from ferric-hexacyanoferrate: Prussian blue. *J Pharm Biomed Anal.* 2007;43:1358-1363.

78. Yang Y, et al. Quantitative determination of thallium binding to ferric hexacyanoferrate: Prussian blue. *Int J Pharm.* 2008;353:187-194.

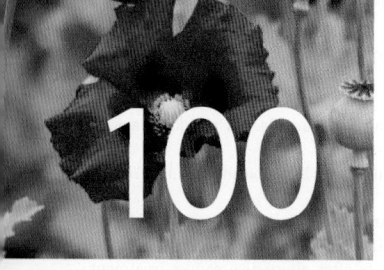

100

ZINC

Nima Majlesi

Zinc (Zn)

Atomic number	=	30
Atomic weight	=	65.37 Da
Normal concentrations		
Blood	=	600–1,000 mcg/dL (91.8–153 mmol/L)
Serum	=	109–130 mcg/dL (16.7–19.9 mmol/L)
Urine (24-hour)	=	<500 mcg/d (<7.65 mmol/d)

HISTORY AND EPIDEMIOLOGY

The Babylonians used zinc alloys more than 5,000 years ago,[2] and references to zinc oxide as a lotion to heal lesions around the eye can be found in the Ebers papyrus, written in 1500 BC.[18] Zinc oxide and zinc sulfate were used in Western Europe during the late 1700s and early 1800s for gleet (urethral discharge), vaginal exudates, and convulsions. In the late 1800s, brass workers who inhaled zinc oxide fumes were noted to develop "zinc fever," "brass founders' ague," and "smelter shakes," all of which are now identified as metal fume fever (Chap. 121).[70]

Throughout history, humans have contaminated the environment with zinc. For example, release of zinc from mines such as those in southern China and the former Soviet Union elevated concentrations in the water supply and vegetation, which lead to elevated tissue zinc concentrations and clinical effects in the population.[54,64]

The antiinflammatory effects of zinc sulfate were studied in the late 1970s for acne vulgaris with mixed results. However, a double-blinded controlled study found no difference between zinc and placebo.[75] The more recent use of zinc supplementation as an alternative preventive and treatment strategy for upper respiratory infections exposes large numbers of patients to undefined risks for unclear benefits.

An epidemic of hematologic and, more importantly, neurologic impairment resulting from large unintentional exposures to zinc denture creams occurred. This syndrome, sometimes referred to as "Zinc swayback," is described below.[3,11,42,58]

The nanotoxicology associated with zinc will not be discussed here (Chap. 125).

CHEMISTRY

Zinc, a transition metal, has 2 common oxidation states, Zn^0 (elemental or metallic) and Zn^{2+}. The pure element exists as a blue to white shiny metal. Zinc combines with other elements to form many compounds such as zinc chloride ($ZnCl_2$), zinc oxide (ZnO), zinc sulfate ($ZnSO_4$), and zinc sulfide (ZnS). Once metallic zinc is exposed to moisture, it becomes coated with zinc oxide or carbonate ($ZnCO_3$).[85]

Like the other transition metals iron (Chap. 45) and copper (Chap. 92), zinc ions participate in reactions that result in the generation of reactive oxygen species such as superoxide radicals or hydroxyl radicals that damage both local and remote tissues (Chap. 10).

PHARMACOLOGY AND PHYSIOLOGY

Zinc is an essential nutrient and found in more than 200 metalloenzymes, including acid phosphatase, alkaline phosphatase, alcohol dehydrogenase, carbonic anhydrase, superoxide dismutase, and DNA and RNA polymerases.[85] The average daily intake of zinc in the United States is 5.2 to 16.2 mg; foods that contain zinc include leafy vegetables (2 ppm), meats, fish, and poultry (29 ppm).[85] The recommended daily allowance is 11 mg/day for men and 8 mg/day for women. Pregnant and nursing women require 12 mg/day. Zinc accumulates in erythrocytes resulting in whole blood concentrations 6- to 7-fold higher than those in the serum.[72] Zinc and copper concentrations generally have an inverse relationship in the serum with elevated zinc concentrations resulting in decreased copper concentrations (Chap. 92).

Zinc contributes to gene expression and chelates with either cysteine or histidine in a tetrahedral configuration, forming looped structures known as "zinc fingers," which bind to specific DNA regions.[12,105] Other functions of zinc include membrane stabilization, vitamin A metabolism, and the development and maintenance of the nervous system. Zinc is important for fetal growth. When 29 pregnant mothers who were at risk for small for gestational age babies were given zinc citrate, zinc sulfate, or zinc aspartate, no intrauterine growth retardation was observed.[91] Subsequent studies demonstrated that zinc supplementation in women with low serum zinc concentrations in early pregnancy is associated with greater infant birth weights and head circumferences.[37]

Zinc is important in maintaining olfactory and gustatory function (Chap. 25). Serum, urine, and salivary zinc concentrations are lower in patients with dysfunctional senses of smell or taste. This is thought to be related to an abnormality in a salivary growth factor known as gustin/carbonic anhydrase VI.[43] Because this enzyme is zinc dependent, oral zinc produced subjective improvement in taste and smell in patients with a known decrease in parotid gustin/carbonic anhydrase VI complex.[44] Oral zinc sulfate also improved subjective findings in a group of 25 patients with post-traumatic olfactory disorders.[6]

Zinc gluconate supplementation, when added to corticosteroid therapy, was beneficial in patients with sudden sensorineural hearing loss when compared to corticosteroid treatment alone. The antioxidant and antiinflammatory effect on the cochlea is thought to be the mechanism for this benefit.[107]

The role of zinc in the immune system is undefined. Zinc therapy remains controversial for nonspecific infectious diarrhea.[80] However, it appears to be beneficial specifically in the management of *Shigella* spp by improving the shigellacidal antibody response and increasing circulating B lymphocytes and plasma cells.[82,83]

Zinc gluconate and zinc acetate containing lozenges are sold as dietary supplements with conflicting evidence that they shorten the duration of the "common cold."[50,66] One placebo-controlled study found that zinc nasal gel shortened the duration of viral syndromes when applied within 24 hours of the onset of symptoms.[45] A subsequent systematic review concluded that zinc administration within 24 hours of onset of symptoms reduces the duration and severity of the common cold in healthy people. In addition, when supplemented for at least 5 months, it reduces cold incidence, school absenteeism, and prescription of antibiotics in children.[92]

Zinc deficiency, or hypozincemia, is a well described clinical entity. It is either inherited as an autosomal recessive pattern known as acrodermatitis enteropathica, or develops due to a defect in zinc absorption in the gastrointestinal (GI) tract.[77] Additional patients at risk for acquiring the disorder include patients who receive total parenteral nutrition without adequate zinc supplementation, patients who have undergone intestinal bypass procedures, those with Crohn's disease, and premature infants with low zinc stores. A nationwide shortage of injectable zinc resulted in the development of dermatitis in the diaper region, perioral erosions, and bullae on the dorsal surfaces of the hands and feet in premature infants requiring parenteral nutrition due to severe cholestasis.[1] Excessive ingestion of phytates the primary storage of phosphates) in whole grains, legumes, nuts, and seeds also decreases zinc absorption.[40] Physical findings that suggest the diagnosis of zinc deficiency, regardless of etiology, include the triad of dermatitis (acral and perioral), diarrhea, and alopecia. Zinc salts, in initial doses of 5 to 10 mg/kg/day of elemental zinc followed by maintenance doses of 1 to 2 mg/kg/day, are highly effective as a treatment regimen. In fact, skin lesions typically heal within 2 to 4 weeks, and hair growth is also reestablished during this time frame.

The US Food and Drug Administration (FDA) approved zinc acetate in 1997 for maintenance therapy of Wilson disease, a disorder associated with copper overload.[13,63] Its use in this disorder is related to the ability of zinc to induce the formation of metallothionein, which assists in the elimination of copper from the blood and body tissues (Chap. 92).[7]

TOXICOKINETICS AND PATHOPHYSIOLOGY

Following ingestion, the main site of zinc absorption is the jejunum, although absorption occurs throughout the intestine. Binding to metallothionein, which is a zinc protein complex found in the luminal cells, facilitates this absorption.[104] Metallothioneins are family of specific metal binding proteins with diverse and complex functions considered essential to metal homeostasis. Metallothioneins are relatively low molecular weight (3,500–14,000 Da) and are rich in thiol ligands; it is these ligands that allow high affinity binding to metals such as zinc, copper, cadmium, mercury, and silver. Metallothioneins regulate the peripheral utilization of zinc and copper once they are bound.[33] Excess zinc absorption leads to upregulation of metallothioneins as a counterregulatory mechanism to prevent excess plasma absorption. However, the affinity of other metals, especially copper, is higher for metallothioneins, resulting in excessive copper elimination and hence decreased absorption. The primary route of excretion of the copper and zinc metallothioneins complexes is fecal. In addition, sequestration of copper in the absorptive cells of the enterocytes also plays a role in the decreased peripheral utilization of copper.[24] Very little metallothionein is bound to zinc or copper in the blood as it is primarily an intracellular cytosolic molecule.[8] Albumin binds about two-thirds of zinc in the plasma, and the remainder is bound to α_2-globulins.[85] Zinc concentrations in the body show a great variability by organ, with the prostate having the highest concentration because of the presence of the zinc-containing enzyme acid phosphatase.[9]

Zinc salts are used to enhance the solubility of pharmaceuticals such as insulin. Certain salts, such as zinc oxide, are used in baby powder, sun blocks, and topical burn preparations, and are also used on both latex and latex-free gloves. In contrast, the use of oral zinc salts within 3 hours of cephalexin administration decreased peak serum concentrations, which is suggested to result from its inhibitory effects on intestinal transport peptides. This finding may imply that the absorption of all orally administered β-lactam antibiotics are altered as they are all dependent on these intestinal transport peptides.[26]

CLINICAL MANIFESTATIONS

The toxicity of zinc is dependent on the route of exposure. Each zinc compound has similar toxic manifestations following oral and dermal exposure. However, they have unique inhalational toxicities. The metallic form of zinc is not toxic per se, and only the salt forms are considered here unless otherwise specifically mentioned. The acute and chronic toxic doses of each compound and route of exposure are difficult to define because of a lack of human studies.

Acute

The hallmark of acute oral zinc salt (Zn^{2+}) toxicity is GI distress, including nausea, vomiting, abdominal pain, and gastrointestinal hemorrhage.[9] In initial studies that evaluated the oral use of zinc sulfate ($ZnSO_4$) as an acne therapy, epigastric distress occurred in 33% of patients.[28,36] Zinc chloride solutions in concentrations greater than 20% are particularly corrosive when ingested. Partial- and full-thickness burns to the oral mucosa, pharynx, esophagus, and stomach, as well as to the laryngo-tracheal tree, occur even following small unintentional ingestions of zinc chloride by children.[22,56,71] Delayed gastric stricture is reported after acute[71] or chronic zinc chloride consumption.[20,98] Pancreatitis was noted in a piglet model[34] and also in a 24-year-old man who inadvertently ingested liquid zinc chloride.[22]

Hyperamylasemia, acute respiratory distress syndrome (ARDS), hypotension, vomiting, diarrhea, jaundice, anemia, thrombocytopenia, and subsequent death occurred following an unintentional 60-hour intravenous infusion of 7.4 g of zinc sulfate in a total parenteral nutrition formula. The patient's serum zinc concentration was 4,184 mcg/dL.[13] A 14-week premature neonate received a 1,000-fold error increase in the concentration of zinc in her total parenteral nutrition. Rather than 330 mcg/dL, she received 330 mg/dL, which resulted in hypotension, respiratory failure, and death despite the administration of edetate calcium disodium ($CaNa_2EDTA$).[38]

The degree of inhalational toxicity is dependent on the type of zinc salt involved in an exposure. The water solubility of the various zinc salts plays an important role in the extent and time to onset of pulmonary toxicity. The solubility of zinc chloride in water at 77°F (25°C) is 432 g/100 mL, whereas that of zinc oxide at 84°F (29°C) is 0.00016 g/100 mL.[85] Acute inhalation of zinc chloride from smoke bombs produces lacrimation, rhinitis, dyspnea, stridor, and retrosternal chest pain. Upper respiratory tract inflammation and ARDS occur, generally without renal or hepatic manifestations of systemic absorption.[35,47,48,68] Morbidity and mortality increase when the exposure to a zinc chloride smoke bomb occurs in an enclosed space.[88] Of 70 individuals exposed to a zinc chloride smoke bomb in a tunnel during World War II, 10 died within 4 days. Ambient zinc concentrations in the tunnel were measured at 33,000 mg/m³.[30] Inhalation of zinc oxide, a far less water-soluble zinc salt, is associated with metal fume fever and not pneumonitis or ARDS despite similar ambient zinc concentrations (Chap. 121).[9]

Despite the importance of zinc in gustatory function, there is an association of intranasal zinc use and anosmia.[93] Animal research suggests that intranasal zinc sulfate use causes transient or persistent anosmia as a consequence of anatomic disruption of functional connections between the olfactory bulb and the olfactory epithelium.[69] Topical zinc sulfate is used experimentally in murine models to induce anosmia.[102] Multiple patients, ages 31 to 55 years, who developed a burning sensation after intranasal zinc gluconate application to the olfactory epithelium for therapeutic purposes later developed either a long-lasting or permanent anosmia and olfactory dysfunction.[53] The mechanism of zinc-induced hyposmia and anosmia is thought to be a direct result of proteolytic destruction of the olfactory receptor cells.[25]

United States pennies (97.5% Zn and 2.5% Cu) lodged in the distal esophagus release zinc ions following exposure to gastric acids and can damage the local esophageal tissue.[17] The phenomenon of acid dissolution is demonstrated in animal[4] and in vitro models.[74]

Rare reports of renal complications exist. Hematuria was observed in a 24-year-old man who ingested liquid zinc chloride, but kidney function remained otherwise normal.[22] Intravenous zinc sulfate administration can result in acute tubular necrosis and acute kidney injury.[13]

Certain zinc salts, such as zinc oxide, found in baby powders and calamine lotion, are usually nonirritating for intact skin.[5] Although older studies suggested the possibility of pruritic, pustular rashes in workers who are exposed to zinc oxide, other causative factors, including personal hygiene, were not considered.[100] One case report describes urticaria and angioedema in a 34-year-old welder following contact with zinc oxide fumes at a smelting plant.[31] The patient was asymptomatic once he was removed from the environment and had no further difficulty during the welding process when appropriate personal protective equipment was employed.

Chronic

Several individual case reports demonstrate the significant implications of chronic zinc exposure. Chronic zinc toxicity following nutritional supplements and the ingestion of coins produces a reversible sideroblastic anemia manifested by anemia and granulocytopenia associated with bone marrow demonstrating vacuolated myeloid and erythroid precursors and ringed sideroblasts.[14] The mechanism for this reversible sideroblastic anemia appears to be a zinc-induced copper deficiency.[32]

A 55-year-old schizophrenic patient with a 15-year history of pica typically of metal objects and frequently zinc-containing pennies, presented with pancytopenia, including a hemoglobin of 3 g/dL and a white blood cell count of 1,300/mm³. He had a serum zinc concentration of 280 mcg/mL and low serum copper concentration of less than 0.05 mcg/mL.[57] The patient refused surgery to remove the coins, which formed a massive bezoar in his GI tract. The patient continued to ingest coins and ultimately died of sepsis and multiorgan failure. An autopsy revealed a coin mass, almost all of which were pennies, weighing 1,870 g in his stomach and another bezoar at the site of a sigmoid volvulus.

Over a 6- to 7-month period, a 17-year-old boy used significant doses of oral vitamins and mineral supplements containing zinc to treat acne and developed copper deficiency and anemia, leukopenia, and neutropenia.[87] A 28-month-old boy developed anemia, neutropenia, and developmental delay after 11 months of parental administration of 314 mg/day of oral zinc gluconate (3.6 mg/kg/day of elemental zinc).[96] Hyperzincemia and hypocupremia were present and improved after discontinuation of zinc without copper supplementation.

It is suggested that zinc and other transition metals are important in the pathogenesis of demyelinating diseases.[59,81] Clusters of cases of multiple sclerosis (MS) were described in northern New York in a factory where zinc was the primary occupational exposure. One hypothesis is that the allele frequency for transferrin (an iron- and zinc-binding protein) differs in these MS subjects.[89,95] Another cluster was found in Canada where excess metals, including zinc, were found in the soil and water.[39,51,52] A conclusive link to MS, however, has not been established.

Because the prostate contains the highest concentration of zinc in the human body, the role of zinc in the development of prostate cancer has been investigated. Specifically, American men participating in the Health Professionals Follow-Up Study were followed for 14 years, from 1986 to 2000. Of the 46,974 in the cohort, 2,901 new cases of prostatic cancer were diagnosed, with 434 of them considered to be in an advanced stage.[63] Men who used zinc supplementation at a dose greater than 100 mg/day had a relative risk of 2.29 for advanced prostate cancer, and those using zinc for longer than 10 years had a relative risk of 2.37. Neither the International Agency for Research on Cancer (IARC) nor the Environmental Protection Agency (EPA) currently classify zinc as a carcinogen.

The Third National Health and Nutrition Examination Survey examined the association of higher dietary zinc intake on the risk of kidney stone disease. Dietary zinc intake of greater than 15 mg/day was associated with a significantly increased risk of kidney stones compared to those with a dietary zinc intake less than 7 mg/day. More rigorous studies are required to determine causality and a potential underlying mechanism for this association.[97]

A neurologic syndrome of progressive myeloneuropathy called "swayback" is defined by a spastic gait, usually a prominent sensory ataxia, and hematologic manifestations.[58,59,61,62] These cases involve patients with copper deficiency and typically elevated serum zinc concentrations. A history of excess zinc exposure is obtained in some but not all patients. The potential of an inherited zinc overload syndrome was considered.[41] A 46-year-old man presented with evidence of bone marrow suppression followed by sensory ataxia and a progressive myelopathy. His neuroimaging evaluation was normal. His only remarkable laboratory studies included an elevated serum zinc concentration of 184 mcg/dL (28.1 μmol/L) and a low copper concentration of less than 10 mcg/dL (<1.57 μmol/L). There was no known occupational exposure or supplementation of zinc by history. Although his copper deficit improved with copper therapy, hyperzincemia persisted for more than the 3 years that he was followed. More recently, an unusual source of high zinc concentrations was related to denture creams, which contained as much as 34 g of zinc per gram of cream. Four patients with chronic exposure to excess denture cream developed neurologic abnormalities in the setting of hyperzincemia with associated hypocupremia.[73] Multiple other reports have confirmed the relationship between denture cream, hyperzincemia, hypocupremia, and the development of this progressive myeloneuropathy. The history in these patients often reveals poor fitting dentures as well as use of dentures during sleep.[3,11,42,94]

Patients with underlying Wilson disease are also at risk for chronic zinc overload syndromes due to treatment. Reports express concern

over increased use of zinc in the treatment of Wilson disease, with recommendations for more frequent monitoring of zinc and copper blood concentrations.[49,84,106]

Chronic inhalation of zinc oxide lowers blood copper and serum calcium concentrations. However, no long-term effect on ventilatory function or chest radiography is reported.[29]

Occupational Exposures

Since 1983, the US penny is composed of 97.5% zinc and 2.5% copper.[101] Zinc is widely used in industry because it enhances the durability of iron and steel alloys; it also is commonly used in construction. Galvanization involves coating an iron product with metallic zinc to prevent it from oxidizing (rusting). Electroplaters, smelters, jewelers, artists working on stained glass or sculpting metal, as well as aircraft manufacturing workers, are routinely exposed to zinc. Zinc chloride is an essential component of flux, which can be used for soldering of galvanized iron.

Zinc is present in drinking water and beverages stored in metal containers or that flow through pipes coated with zinc. Zinc concentrations in air are typically low; average zinc concentrations in the United States are less than 1 mcg/m³. Air concentrations near industrial zones can be higher, and are typically substantially greater in certain occupational settings such as mining and smelting. The currently accepted occupational threshold limit value (TLV)-time-weighted average (TWA) is 1 mg/m³.[85]

Metal Fume Fever

Metal fume fever typically occurs within 12 hours after an exposure to metal oxide fumes. Patients develop fever, chills, cough, myalgias, muscle cramping, chest pain, dyspnea, dry throat, and a metallic taste in the mouth. Although exposure to zinc oxide fumes is the commonest zinc etiology, other zinc salts are implicated. Although the chest radiograph is often normal, infiltrates are common finding. Hypoxia and tachycardia are rare, but reported. Overall, however, the syndrome is relatively benign, with tolerance developing within days.[29] An immune mechanism is suggested, and chronic exposure leads to sensitization (Chap. 121).[23]

DIAGNOSTIC TESTING

Because zinc is ubiquitous in the environment and laboratory, great care must be taken to avoid contamination of any samples intended for investigation.[85] Because elevated zinc concentrations cause copper deficiency, a serum copper and ceruloplasmin concentration should be obtained in patients with suspected zinc poisoning.

Urine zinc concentrations are not well defined. In a cohort of non–occupationally exposed patients, the mean urine concentrations were 450 mcg/L, with a maximum concentration up to 1,300 mcg/L.[72] In the United States, normal urine concentrations are generally accepted as less than 500 mcg/d. The National Institute for Occupational Safety and Health established detection limits in urine and blood or tissue as low as 0.1 mcg per sample and 1 mcg/100 g, respectively. Testing requires extraction of the metals from urine with polydithiocarbamate resin prior to digestion with concentrated acids and analysis.[85]

Errors are caused by incorrect sample collection, equipment malfunction or miscalibration, inadequate reagent purity, and atmospheric deposition. Zinc oxide powder in some gloves can contaminate specimens, as can the rubber stoppers in certain blood collection tubes. Specific tubes are recommended with exceptionally low concentrations of trace elements.[19] During sample analysis, laminar flow is recommended to prevent airborne particles from interfering.

Abdominal radiographs have limited utility in determining the gastrointestinal burden of zinc, except following ingestions of pennies. Findings should be used to guide the decision to continue gastrointestinal decontamination in certain circumstances.[16] (See Management below.)

Neuroimaging in patients with chronic zinc exposure and secondary copper deficiency reveals characteristic findings. The MRI typically reveals increased T2 signal in the dorsal columns of the cervical spinal cord similar to that found in B₁₂ deficiency.[60] These lesions are thought to represent

Wallerian degeneration and demyelination of white matter. One case showed evidence of bilateral subcortical hyperintense T2 abnormalities on an MRI of the brain.[73] These findings are the result of copper deficiency and not necessarily zinc toxicity.

MANAGEMENT

Treatment for acute oral zinc salt toxicity is primarily supportive. Efforts should focus on hydration and antiemetic therapy. Histamine$_2$ receptor antagonists or proton pump inhibitors can relieve abdominal discomfort when given for several days following the zinc salt ingestion and are recommended.[9]

We recommend whole-bowel irrigation (WBI) for gastrointestinal decontamination after zinc salt ingestion. A radiograph in a 16-year-old boy who ingested 50 (500 mg) zinc sulfate tablets noted no change in tablet position 4 hours after gastric emptying with induced emesis followed by orogastric lavage. Within one hour of institution of WBI therapy, zinc tablets were present in the rectal effluent.[16] Zinc-containing penny ingestion can provide a unique challenge. A schizophrenic patient required laparotomy and gastrotomy to remove a total of 275 coins.[76]

The data regarding the efficacy of chelation therapy for zinc is limited in humans. Edetate calcium disodium (CaNa$_2$EDTA) was used successfully in several cases, including a child[79] and a 24-year-old man who were exposed to zinc chloride as a component of soldering flux.[22] The combination of CaNa$_2$EDTA and dimercaprol (British anti-Lewisite {BAL}) was used successfully in a 16 month-old 74 hours after ingestion.[71] However, the potential of BAL to increase copper elimination should limit its clinical use.

Both DTPA (diethylenetriaminepentaacetic acid) and CaNa$_2$ EDTA (ethylenediaminetetraacetic acid) were effective in enhancing the urinary excretion of zinc in a rodent model of zinc acetate poisoning.[27] Diethylenetriaminepentaacetic acid had its greatest antidotal efficacy when given within 30 minutes of the intraperitoneal injection of zinc acetate.[65] The urinary excretion of zinc increased 1.6- to 44-fold following a 3-mg/kg intravenous dose of DMPS (2,3-dimercaptopropane-1-sulfonate) in one human study where metal toxicity in patients with dental amalgams was the focus.[99] Two potential zinc-selective chelators, DPESA (4-{[2-(bis-pyridin-2-ylmethylamino) ethylamino]-methyl}phenyl) methanesulfonic acid) sodium salt, as well as TPESA(4-{[2-bis-pyridin-2-ylmethylamino) ethyl]pyridin-2-ymethylamino}-methyl)phenyl]methanesulfonic acid) sodium salt, rapidly chelate zinc in vitro, but further detailed in vivo studies are needed before their clinical use can be considered.[55] Finally, an iron chelator, deferiprone, was incidentally noted to decrease serum zinc concentrations when it was used to lower iron concentrations in patients with transfusion overload (Antidotes in Depth: A7).[103] A subsequent prospective trial showed enhanced urinary excretion of zinc in children with thalassemia major who had received multiple blood transfusions.[10]

Many of the clinical manifestations and metabolic effects of zinc toxicity are due to its ability to cause copper deficiency. In patients with zinc overload–related copper deficiency, the supplementation of oral copper alone improved the hematopoietic effects and prevented further neurologic deterioration without chelation therapy.[86] The route of copper supplementation may be dependent on tolerability and reliability of gastrointestinal absorption. Initial recommended starting doses are 2 mg intravenously or 6 mg orally of elemental copper once per day. A decrease in dose by 2 mg each week is recommnded with the goal of eventually giving 2 mg orally once per day until complete resolution of toxicity and normalization of blood concentrations occur.

Though treatment with copper sulfate alone can be adequate for patients with neurologic sequelae and mild hematopoietic effects, chelation will be required for patients with hemodynamic compromise or other consequential systemic manifestations. Limited experience exists with regard to treatment of these patients; however, 1,000 mg/m^2/day IV CaNa$_2$EDTA divided every 6 hours seems to be the most reasonable choice based on case reports of successful use.

Intravenous N-acetylcysteine (NAC) increased the urinary zinc excretion in a patient who had inhaled zinc chloride fumes.[78] Two individuals

with inhalational zinc chloride–induced ARDS had simultaneous transient decreases in serum zinc concentrations and increases in urinary zinc excretion when treated with intravenous and nebulized NAC.[47] However, these individuals succumbed at days 25 and 32 after inhalation. Although an increase in urinary zinc excretion was noted in one rat model, 10 healthy volunteers who were treated with oral NAC for 2 weeks had no significant change in either their serum or urine zinc concentrations.[46] As a result of these findings, NAC therapy cannot be recommended at this time.

Supportive care is used for patients with inhalational zinc exposures, including oxygen therapy and bronchodilators as clinically indicated; however, the seriously ill will necessitate ventilatory support. Exposure to zinc oxide fumes by rescuers is usually minimal, although respiratory protective equipment should be worn.[90] In a case series of 5 soldiers exposed to zinc chloride smoke bombs during military training, the 2 individuals not wearing gas masks developed ARDS;[47] the others remained clinically well. A 23-year-old man developed severe ARDS after inhalation of zinc chloride from a smoke bomb during a military drill. After extensive ventilatory supportive efforts, tube thoracostomy, intravenous antibiotics, and intravenous corticosteroids, the patient continued to deteriorate. The patient was placed on extracorporeal life support (ECLS), weaned off the ventilator by day 30, and survived. If ECLS is available, its use is reasonable based on clinical grounds. More prospective studies are required to determine the extent of the benefit of ECMO.[21]

Metal fume fever is typically self-limited. Nonsteroidal antiinflammatory drugs are usually sufficient to relieve the transient discomfort. Personal protective equipment and or adequate engineering design and strategies may allow the individual to continue to work in the particular occupational site. Personal protective equipment (PPE) is essential in preventing inhalational exposure to zinc chloride. The National Institute of Safety and Health (NIOSH) has recommended the following PPE based upon ambient air concentrations. Up to 10 mg/m^3, the recommendation is use of N95, R95, or P95 filter particulate respirators. Up to 25 mg/m^3, a continuous-flow respirator is required. Up to 50 mg/m^3, an air-purifying full facepiece respirator with N100, R100, or P100 filter is required.

Dermal decontamination is paramount to prevent direct epidermal effects or systemic absorption of zinc salts.[15] However, water should not be used to perform dermal decontamination of patients exposed to metallic zinc because zinc metal ignites when wet. Treatment in these situations includes mechanical removal of any metallic particles with forceps and the application of mineral oil to the affected skin to protect the metal from ambient moisture.

SUMMARY

- Zinc exposures in humans occur due to diet, medicinal uses, nutritional supplements, and the occupational settings.
- The clinical manifestations of zinc toxicity include acute, life-threatening gastrointestinal and pulmonary effects, which are generally effectively treated with supportive care.
- Chronic zinc toxicity manifests primarily as copper deficiency.
- Copper supplementation alone often corrects systemic manifestations.
- Chelation therapy is reasonable for patients with severe zinc toxicity.

REFERENCES

1. Abdel-Mageed AB, Oehme FW. A review of the biochemical roles, toxicity and interactions of zinc, copper and iron: I. Zinc. *Vet Hum Toxicol*. 1990;32:34-39.
2. Afrin LB. Fatal copper deficiency from excessive use of zinc-based denture adhesive. *Am J Med Sci*. 2010;340:164-168.
3. Agnew DW, et al. Zinc toxicosis in a captive striped hyena (*Hyaena hyaena*). *J Zoo Wildl Med*. 1999;30:431-434.
4. Agren MS. Percutaneous absorption of zinc from zinc oxide applied topically to intact skin in man. *Dermatologica*. 1990;180:36-39.
5. Aiba T, et al. Effect of zinc sulfate on sensorineural olfactory disorder. *Acta Otolaryngol Suppl*. 1998;538:202-204.
6. Askari FK, et al. Treatment of Wilson's disease with zinc. XVIII. Initial treatment of the hepatic decompensation presentation with trientine and zinc. *J Lab Clin Med*. 2003;142:385-390.
7. Babula P, et al. Mammalian metallothioneins: properties and functions. *Metallomics*. 2012;4:739-750.

8. Barceloux D. Zinc. *J Toxicol Clin Toxicol*. 1999;37:279-292.

9. Bartakke S, et al. Effect of deferiprone on urinary zinc excretion in multiply transfused children with thalassemia major. *Indian Pediatr*. 2005;42:150-154.

10. Barton AL, et al. Zinc poisoning from excessive denture fixative use masquerading as myelopolyneuropathy and hypocupraemia. *Ann Clin Biochem*. 2011;48:383-385.

11. Berg JM, Shi Y. The galvanization of biology: a growing appreciation for the roles of zinc. *Science*. 1996;271:1081-1085.

12. Brocks A, et al. Acute intravenous zinc poisoning. *Br Med J*. 1977;1:1390-1391.

13. Broun ER, et al. Excessive zinc ingestion. A reversible cause of sideroblastic anemia and bone marrow depression. *JAMA*. 1990;264:1441-1443.

14. Burgess JL, et al. Emergency department hazardous material protocol for contaminated patients. *Ann Emerg Med*. 1999;34:205-212.

15. Burkhart KK, et al. Whole bowel irrigation as treatment for zinc sulfate overdose. *Ann Emerg Med*. 1990;19:1167-1170.

16. Cantu S Jr, Conners GP. The esophageal coin: is it a penny? *Am Surg*. 2002;68:417-420.

17. Cassel GH. Zinc: a review of current trends in therapy and our knowledge of its toxicity. *Del Med J*. 1978;50:323-328.

18. Centers for Disease Control and Prevention. Notes from the field: zinc deficiency dermatitis in cholestatic extremely premature infants after a nationwide shortage of injectable zinc—Washington, DC, December 2012. *MMWR Morb Mortal Wkly Rep*. 2013;62:136-137.

19. Chan S, et al. The role of copper, molybdenum, selenium, and zinc in nutrition and health. *Clin Lab Med*. 1998;18:673-685.

20. Chew LS, et al. Gastric stricture following zinc chloride ingestion. *Singapore Med J*. 1986;27:163-166.

21. Chian CF, et al. Acute respiratory distress syndrome after zinc chloride inhalation: survival after extracorporeal life support and corticosteroid treatment. *Am J Crit Care*. 2010;19:86-90.

22. Chobanian S. Accidental ingestion of liquid zinc chloride: local and systemic effects. *Ann Emerg Med*. 1981;10:91-93.

23. Cohen MD. Pulmonary immunotoxicology of select metals: aluminum, arsenic, cadmium, chromium, copper, manganese, nickel, vanadium, and zinc. *J Immunotoxicol*. 2004;1:39-69.

24. Cousins RJ. Absorption, transport, and hepatic metabolism of copper and zinc: special reference to metallothionein and ceruloplasmin. *Physiol Rev*. 1985;65:238-309.

25. Davidson TM, Smith WM. The Bradford Hill criteria and zinc-induced anosmia: a causality analysis. *Arch Otolaryngol Head Neck Surg*. 2010;136:673-676.

26. Ding Y, et al. The effect of staggered administration of zinc sulfate on the pharmacokinetics of oral cephalexin. *Br J Clin Pharmacol*. 2012;73:422-427.

27. Domingo JL, et al. Acute zinc intoxication: comparison of the antidotal efficacy of several chelating agents. *Vet Hum Toxicol*. 1988;30:224-228.

28. Dreno B, et al. Multicenter randomized comparative double-blind controlled clinical trial of the safety and efficacy of zinc gluconate versus minocycline hydrochloride in the treatment of inflammatory acne vulgaris. *Dermatology*. 2001;203:135-140.

29. El Safty A, et al. Zinc toxicity among galvanization workers in the iron and steel industry. *Ann N Y Acad Sci*. 2008;1140:256-262.

30. Evans. Casualties following exposure to zinc chloride smoke. *Lancet*. 1945;2:368-370.

31. Farrell FJ. Angioedema and urticaria as acute and late phase reactions to zinc fume exposure, with associated metal fume fever-like symptoms. *Am J Ind Med*. 1987;12:331-337.

32. Fiske DN, et al. Zinc-induced sideroblastic anemia: a report of a case, review of the literature, and description of the hematologic syndrome. *Am J Hematol*. 1994;46:147-150.

33. Fosmire GJ. Zinc toxicity. *Am J Clin Nutr*. 1990;51:225-227.

34. Gabrielson KL, et al. Zinc toxicity with pancreatic acinar necrosis in piglets receiving total parental nutrition. *Vet Pathol*. 1996;33:692-696.

35. Gil F, et al. A fatal case following exposure to zinc chloride and hexachloroethane from a smoke bomb in a fire simulation at a school. *Clin Toxicol*. 2008;46:563-565.

36. Glover SC, White MI. Zinc again. *Br Med J*. 1977;2:640-641.

37. Goldenberg RL, et al. The effect of zinc supplementation on pregnancy outcome. *JAMA*. 1995;274:463-468.

38. Grissinger M. A fatal zinc overdose in a neonate: confusion of micrograms with milligrams. *P T*. 2011;36:393-409.

39. Hader WJ, et al. A cluster-focus of multiple sclerosis at Henribourg, Saskatchewan. *Can J Neurol Sci*. 1990;17:391-394.

40. Hambidge KM, et al. Zinc bioavailability and homeostasis. *Am J Clin Nutr*. 2010;91:1478S-1483S.

41. Hedera P, et al. Myelopolyneuropathy and pancytopenia due to copper deficiency and high zinc levels of unknown origin: further support for existence of a new zinc overload syndrome. *Arch Neurol*. 2003;60:1301-1306.

42. Hedera P, et al. Myelopolyneuropathy and pancytopenia due to copper deficiency and high zinc levels of unknown origin II. The denture cream is a primary source of excessive zinc. *Neurotoxicology*. 2009;30:996-999.

43. Henkin RI, et al. Decreased parotid saliva gustin/carbonic anhydrase VI secretion: an enzyme disorder manifested by gustatory and olfactory dysfunction. *Am J Med Sci*. 1999;18:380-391.

44. Henkin RI, et al. Efficacy of exogenous oral zinc in treatment of patients with carbonic anhydrase VI deficiency. *Am J Med Sci*. 1999;18:392-405.

45. Hirt M, et al. Zinc nasal gel for the treatment of common cold symptoms: A double-blind, placebo-controlled trial. *Ear Nose Throat J*. 2000;79:778-780.

46. Hjortso E, et al. Does *N*-acetylcysteine increase the excretion of trace metals (calcium, magnesium, iron, zinc and copper) when given orally? *Eur J Clin Pharmacol*. 1990;39:29-31.

47. Hjortso E, et al. ARDS after accidental inhalation of zinc chloride smoke. *Intensive Care Med*. 1988;14:17-24.

48. Homma S, et al. Pulmonary vascular lesions in the adult respiratory distress syndrome caused by inhalation of zinc chloride smoke: a morphometric study. *Hum Pathol*. 1992;23:45-50.

49. Horvath J, et al. Zinc-induced copper deficiency in Wilson disease. *J Neurol Neurosurg Psychiatry*. 2010;81:1410-1411.

50. Hulisz D. Efficacy of zinc against common cold viruses: an overview. *J Am Pharm Assoc*. 2004;44:594-603.

51. Irvine DG, et al. Geotoxicology of multiple sclerosis: the Henribourg, Saskatchewan, cluster focus II: the soil. *Sci Total Environ*. 1988;77:175-188.

52. Irvine DG, et al. Geotoxicology of multiple sclerosis: the Henribourg, Saskatchewan, cluster focus I: the water. *Sci Total Environ*. 1989;84:45-59.

53. Jafek BW, et al. Anosmia after intranasal zinc gluconate use. *Am J Rhinol*. 2004;18:137-141.

54. Kachur AN, et al. Environmental conditions in the Rudnaya River watershed—a compilation of Soviet and post-Soviet era sampling around a lead smelter in the Russian Far East. *Sci Total Environ*. 2003;303:171-185.

55. Kawabata E, et al. Design and synthesis of zinc-selective chelators for extracellular applications. *J Am Chem Soc*. 2005;127:818-819.

56. Knapp JF, et al. A toddler with caustic ingestion. *Pediatr Emerg Care*. 1994;10:54-58.

57. Kumar A, Jazieh AR. Case report of sideroblastic anemia caused by ingestion of coins. *Am J Hematol*. 2001;66:126-129.

58. Kumar N. Copper deficiency myelopathy (human swayback). *Mayo Clin Proc*. 2006;81:1371-1384.

59. Kumar N, Ahlskog JE. Myelopolyneuropathy due to copper deficiency or zinc excess? *Arch Neurol*. 2004;61:604-605.

60. Kumar N, et al. Imaging features of copper deficiency myelopathy: a study of 25 cases. *Neuroradiology*. 2006;48:78-83.

61. Kumar N, et al. Copper deficiency myelopathy. *Arch Neurol*. 2004;61:762-766.

62. Kumar N, et al. Myelopathy due to copper deficiency. *Neurology*. 2003;61:273-274.

63. Leitzmann MF, et al. Zinc supplement use and risk of prostate cancer. *J Natl Cancer Inst*. 2003;95:1004-1007.

64. Liu H, et al. Metal contamination of soils and crops affected by the Chenzhou lead/zinc mine spill (Hunan, China). *Sci Total Environ*. 2005;339:153-166.

65. Llobet JM, et al. Comparison of the antidotal efficacy of polyamincarboxylic acids (CDTA and DTPA) with time after acute zinc poisoning. *Vet Hum Toxicol*. 1989;31:25-28.

66. Macknin ML, et al. Zinc gluconate lozenges for treating the common cold in children: a randomized controlled trial. *JAMA*. 1998;279:1962-1967.

67. Marrs TC, et al. The repeated dose toxicity of a zinc oxide/hexachloroethane smoke. *Arch Toxicol*. 1988;1988:123-132.

68. Matarese SL, Matthews JI. Zinc chloride (smoke bomb) inhalational lung injury. *Chest*. 1986;89:308-309.

69. McBride K, et al. Does intranasal application of zinc sulfate produce anosmia in the mouse? An olfactometric and anatomical study. *Chem Senses*. 2003;28:659-670.

70. McCord CP, Friedlander A. An occupational syndrome among workers in zinc. *Am J Public Health (N Y)*. 1926;16:274-280.

71. McKinney PE, et al. Acute zinc chloride ingestion in a child: local and systemic effects. *Ann Emerg Med*. 1994;23:1383-1387.

72. Minoia C, et al. Trace element reference values in tissues from inhabitants of the European Community I. A study of 46 elements in urine, blood, and serum of Italian subjects. *Sci Total Environ*. 1990;95:89-105.

73. Nations SP, et al. Denture cream: an unusual source of excess zinc, leading to hypocupremia and neurologic disease. *Neurology*. 2008;71:639-643.

74. O'Hara SM, et al. Gastric retention of zinc-based pennies: radiographic appearance and hazards. *Radiology*. 1999;213:113-117.

75. Orris L, et al. Oral zinc therapy of acne. Absorption and clinical effect. *Arch Dermatol*. 1978;114:1018-1020.

76. Pawa S, et al. Zinc toxicity from massive and prolonged coin ingestion in an adult. *Am J Med Sci*. 2008;336:430-433.

77. Perafán-Riveros C, et al. Acrodermatitis enteropathica: case report and review of the literature. *Pediatr Dermatol*. 2002;19:426-431.

78. Pettilä V, et al. Zinc chloride smoke inhalation: a rare cause of severe acute respiratory distress syndrome. *Intensive Care Med*. 2000;26:215-217.

79. Potter J. Acute zinc chloride ingestion in a young child. *Ann Emerg Med*. 1981;10:267-269.

80. Prasad AS. Zinc: role in immunity, oxidative stress and chronic inflammation. *Curr Opin Clin Nutr Metab Care*. 2009;12:646-652.

81. Prodan CI, Holland NR. CNS demyelination from zinc toxicity? *Neurology*. 2000;54:1705-1706.

82. Rahman MJ, et al. Effects of zinc supplementation as adjunct therapy on the systemic immune responses in shigellosis. *Am J Clin Nutr*. 2005;81:495-502.

83. Raqib R, et al. Effect of zinc supplementation on immune and inflammatory responses in pediatric patients with shigellosis. *Am J Clin Nutr*. 2004;79:444-450.

84. Roberts EA. Zinc toxicity: from "no, never" to "hardly ever." *Gastroenterology*. 2011;140:1132-1135.

85. Roney N, et al. ATSDR evaluation of potential for human exposure to zinc. *Toxicol Ind Health*. 2007;23:247-308.

86. Rowin J, Lewis SL. Copper deficiency myeloneuropathy and pancytopenia secondary to overuse of zinc supplementation. *J Neurol Neurosurg Psychiatry*. 2005;76:750-751.

87. Salzman MB, et al. Excessive oral zinc supplementation. *J Pediatr Hematol Oncol*. 2002;24:582-584.

88. Schenker MB, et al. Acute upper respiratory symptoms resulting from exposure to zinc chloride aerosol. *Environ Res*. 1981;25:317-324.

89. Schiffer RB. Zinc and multiple sclerosis. *Neurology*. 1994;44:1987-1988.

90. Schultz M, et al. Simulated exposure of hospital emergency personnel to solvent vapors and respirable dust during decontamination of chemically exposed patents. *Ann Emerg Med*. 1995;26:324-329.

91. Simmer K, et al. A double-blind trial of zinc supplementation in pregnancy. *Eur J Clin Nutr*. 1991;45:139-144.

92. Singh M, Das RR. Zinc for the common cold. *Cochrane Database Syst Rev*. 2013;6:CD001364.

93. Smith WM, et al. Toxin-induced chemosensory dysfunction: a case series and review. *Am J Rhinol Allergy*. 2009;23:578-581.

94. Sommerville RB, Baloh RH. Anemia, paresthesias, and gait ataxia in a 57-year-old denture wearer. *Clin Chem*. 2011;57:1103-1106.

95. Stein EC, et al. Multiple sclerosis and the workplace: report of an industry-based cluster. *Neurology*. 1987;37:1672-1677.

96. Sugiura T, et al. Chronic zinc toxicity in an infant who received zinc therapy for atopic dermatitis. *Acta Paediatr*. 2005;94:1333-1335.

97. Tang J, et al. Dietary zinc intake and kidney stone formation: evaluation of NHANES III. *Am J Nephrol*. 36:549-553.

98. Tayyem R, et al. Gastric stricture following zinc chloride ingestion. *Clin Toxicol*. 2009;47:689-690.

99. Torres-Alanis O, et al. Urinary excretion of trace elements after sodium 2,3-dimercaptoproprane-1-sulfonate challenge test. *J Toxicol Clin Toxicol*. 2000;38:697-700.

100. Turner JA. An occupational dermatoconiosis among zinc oxide workers. *Public Health Rep*. 1921;36:2727-2732.

101. United States Department of the Treasury USM. The Composition of the Cent. http://usmint.gov/about_the_mint/fun_facts/index.cfm?flash=no&action=fun_facts2. 2004.

102. van Denderen JC, et al. Zinc sulphate-induced anosmia decreases the nerve fibre density in the anterior cerebral artery of the rat. *Auton Neurosci*. 2001;10:102-108.

103. Victor Hoffbrand A. Deferiprone therapy for transfusional iron overload. *Best Pract Res Clin Haematol*. 2005;18:299-317.

104. Walsh CT, et al. Zinc. Health effects and research priorities for the 1990s. *Environ Health Perspect*. 1994;102:5-46.

105. Wang R, et al. Identification of genes encoding zinc finger motifs in the cardiovascular system. *J Mol Cell Cardiol*. 1997;86:281-287.

106. Weiss KH, et al. Zinc monotherapy is not as effective as chelating agents in treatment of Wilson disease. *Gastroenterology*. 2011;140:1189-1198, e1181.

107. Yang CH, et al. Zinc in the treatment of idiopathic sudden sensorineural hearing loss. *Laryngoscope*. 2011;121:617-621.

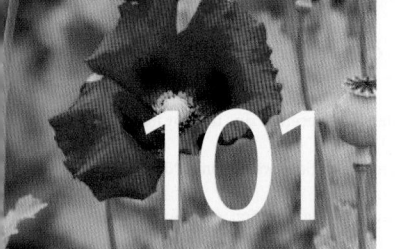

J. Household Products

101

ANTISEPTICS, DISINFECTANTS, AND STERILANTS

Ashley Haynes and Paul M. Wax

HISTORY AND EPIDEMIOLOGY

Joseph Lister, often considered the father of modern surgery, revolutionized surgical treatment and dramatically reduced surgical mortality by introducing the concept of antisepsis to the surgical theatre.[50] It was Lister's understanding that microorganisms contributed to infection and sepsis from even the most trivial wounds that led to his search for chemicals that would prevent such infection. Lister demonstrated that phenol, a chemical that was used to treat foul-smelling sewage, could be used to clean dirty wounds of patients with compound fractures and dramatically increase survival rates. Soon thereafter, the use of phenol was expanded to surgical instrument cleaning and as a surgical hand scrub wash, ushering in the modern surgical era.

Antiseptics, disinfectants, and sterilants are a diverse group of germicides used to prevent the transmission of microorganisms to patients (Table 101–1). Although these terms are sometimes used interchangeably and some of these xenobiotics are used for both antisepsis and disinfection, the distinguishing characteristics between the groups are important to emphasize. An *antiseptic* is a chemical that is applied to living tissue to kill or inhibit microorganisms. Iodophors, chlorhexidine, and the alcohols (ethanol and isopropanol) are commonly used antiseptics. A *disinfectant* is a chemical that is applied to inanimate objects to kill microorganisms. Bleach (sodium hypochlorite), phenolic compounds, formaldehyde, hydrogen peroxide liquid, *ortho*-phthalaldehyde, and quaternary ammonium compounds are examples of currently used disinfectants. Neither antiseptics nor disinfectants have complete sporicidal activity. A *sterilant* is a chemical that is applied to inanimate objects to kill all microorganisms as well as spores. Ethylene oxide, glutaraldehyde, hydrogen peroxide gas, and peracetic acid are examples of sterilants. Many of the xenobiotics used to kill microorganisms also demonstrate considerable human toxicity.[18,69,180]

The choice of disinfectant or sterilant depends on the degree of risk for infection involved in use of medical and surgical instruments and patient care items. Surgical instruments and cardiac and urinary catheters that enter the vascular system or other sterile tissues (so-called critical items) must be cleaned with a sterilant while instruments that contact mucous membranes or nonintact skin such as gastrointestinal (GI) endoscopes and laryngoscope blades (semicritical items) are cleaned with a high-level disinfectant such as *ortho*-phthalaldehyde or 7.5% hydrogen peroxide. Noncritical items such as bedpans, blood pressure cuffs, crutches, and computers are those that come in contact with intact skin but not mucous membranes and are cleaned with intermediate-level and low-level disinfectants such as bleach or phenol. Whether a chemical is classified as a sterilant or disinfectant depends on how it is used. Device sterilization with glutaraldehyde 3% requires a 10-hour cleaning cycle whereas high-level disinfection using the same chemical requires a 25-minute cleaning cycle.

The use of these xenobiotics evolved during the 20th century as their toxicity and the principles of microbiology became better understood. Two of the more toxic antiseptics—iodine and phenol—were gradually replaced by the less toxic iodophors and substituted phenols. The use of mercuric chloride was superseded by the organic mercurials such as merbromin and thimerosal, which also proved toxic. In recent years, newer xenobiotics, such as quaternary ammonium compounds, ethylene oxide, glutaraldehyde, and a peracetic acid–hydrogen peroxide mixture, are more extensively used.

ANTISEPTICS

Chlorhexidine

This cationic biguanide has had extensive use as an antiseptic since the early 1950s. It is found in a variety of skin cleansers, usually as a 4% emulsion, and is also found in some mouthwash.

Clinical Effects

Few cases of deliberate ingestion of chlorhexidine are reported. Symptoms are usually mild, and GI irritation is the most likely effect after ingestion.[25] Chlorhexidine has poor enteral absorption. In one case, ingestion of 150 mL of a 20% chlorhexidine gluconate solution resulted in oral cavity edema and significant irritant injury of the esophagus.[130] In the same case, liver enzyme concentrations rose to 30 times normal on the fifth day after ingestion. Liver biopsy showed lobular necrosis and fatty degeneration. In another case, the ingestion of 30 mL of a 4% solution by an 89-year-old woman did not result in any GI injury.[52] An 80-year-old woman with dementia ingested 200 mL of a 5% chlorhexidine solution and subsequently aspirated.[79] She rapidly developed hypotension, respiratory distress, coma, and died 12 hours following ingestion.

Intravenous administration of chlorhexidine is associated with acute respiratory distress syndrome (ARDS)[90] and hemolysis.[28] Inhalation of vaporized chlorhexidine causes methemoglobinemia, likely as a consequence of the conversion of chlorhexidine to *p*-chloraniline.[211] Methemoglobinemia due to this degradation product was also reported after the ingestion of a 0.5% chlorhexidine in 70% ethanol solution.[107] This patient was successfully treated with methylene blue. In one patient, the rectal administration of 4% chlorhexidine resulted in acute colitis with ulcerations.[68]

Topical absorption of chlorhexidine is negligible. Contact dermatitis is reported in up to 8% of patients who received repetitive topical applications of chlorhexidine.[69] More ominously, anaphylactic reactions, including shock, are associated with dermal application.[7,148] Some of these cases of chlorhexidine-related anaphylaxis occurred during surgery, appearing 15 to 45 minutes after application of the antiseptic.[13] Eye exposure results in corneal damage.[205]

Management

Treatment guidelines for chlorhexidine exposure are similar to those for other potential caustics (Chap. 103). Patients with significant symptoms should undergo endoscopy, but the need for such extensive evaluation is uncommon.

Hydrogen Peroxide

Hydrogen peroxide, an oxidizer with weak antiseptic properties, has a long history of use as an antiseptic and a disinfectant.[215] This oxidizer is generally available in 2 strengths: dilute, with a concentration of 3% to 9% by weight (usually 3%), sold for home use; and concentrated, with a concentration greater than 10%, used primarily for industrial purposes. Commercial-strength hydrogen peroxide is commonly found in solutions varying from 27.5% to 70%. Home uses for dilute hydrogen peroxide include cerumen removal, mouth gargle, vaginal douche, enema, and hair bleaching. Dilute hydrogen peroxide is also used as a veterinary emetic. Commercial uses of the more concentrated solutions include bleaching and cleansing textiles and wool, and producing foam rubber and rocket fuel.

TABLE 101–1	Antiseptics, Disinfectants, Sterilants, and Related Xenobiotics				
Xenobiotic	*Commercial Product*	*Use*	*Toxic Effects*	*Therapeutics and Evaluation*
Acids				
Boric acid	Borax	Antiseptic	Blue-green emesis and diarrhea	Orogastric lavage
	Sodium perborate	Mouthwash	Boiled lobster appearance of skin	Hemodialysis (rare)
	Dobell solution	Eyewash	Central nervous system (CNS) depression;	
		Roach powder	kidney failure	
Alcohols				
(Chaps. 76 and 106)				
Ethanol	Rubbing alcohol (70% ethanol)	Antiseptic	CNS depression	Supportive
		Disinfectant	Respiratory depression	
			Dermal irritant	
Isopropanol	Rubbing alcohol (70% isopropanol)	Antiseptic	CNS depression	Supportive
		Disinfectant	Respiratory depression	Hemodialysis (rare)
			Ketonemia, ketonuria	
			Gastritis/hemorrhage	
			Hemorrhagic tracheobronchitis	
Aldehydes				
Formaldehyde	Formalin	Disinfectant	Caustic	Orogastric lavage
	(37% formaldehyde,	Fixative	CNS depression	Hemodialysis
	12%–15% methanol)	Urea-formaldehyde	Carcinogen	Sodium bicarbonate
		insulation		Endoscopy
				Folinic acid
Glutaraldehyde	Cidex (2% glutaraldehyde)	Sterilant	Mucosal and dermal irritant	Supportive
ortho-Phthalaldehyde (OPA)	Cidex OPA (<1% OPA)	Sterilant	Mucosal and dermal irritant	Supportive
Chlorinated Compounds				
Chlorhexidine	Hibiclens	Antiseptic	GI irritation	Supportive
Chlorates	Sodium chlorate	Antiseptic (obsolete)	Hemolysis	Exchange transfusion
	Potassium chlorate	Matches	Methemoglobinemia	Hemodialysis
		Herbicide	Kidney failure	
Chlorine		Disinfectant	Irritant	Supportive
Chlorophors (sodium hypochlorite)	Household bleach (5% NaOCl)	Disinfectant	Mild GI irritation	Endoscopy (rare)
	Dakin solution (1 part 5% NaOCl,	Decontaminating		
	10 parts H$_2$O)	solution		
Ethylene Oxide		Sterilant	Irritant	Supportive
		Plasticizer	CNS depression	
			Peripheral neuropathy	
			Carcinogen, mutagen	
Mercurials	Merbromin 2% (Mercurochrome)	Antiseptic (obsolete)	CNS	Orogastric lavage, activated charcoal dimercaprol, succimer
(Chaps. 46 and 95)	Thimerosal (Merthiolate)		Kidney	
Iodinated Compounds				
Iodine	Tincture of iodine (2% iodine, 2%	Antiseptic	Caustic	Orogastric lavage Milk, starch,
	sodium iodide, and 50% ethanol)			sodium thiosulfate
	Lugol solution (5% iodine)			Endoscopy
Iodophors	Povidone-iodine (Betadine)	Antiseptic	Limited	Same as iodine
	(0.01% iodine)			
Oxidants				
Hydrogen peroxide	H$_2$O$_2$ 3%—household	Disinfectant	Oxygen emboli	Orogastric lavage
	H$_2$O$_2$ 30%—industrial		Caustic	Radiographic evaluation
				Endoscopy
Potassium permanganate	Crystals, solution	Antiseptic	Oxidizer, caustic, increased serum manganese	Decontamination
				Endoscopy
Phenols				
Nonsubstituted	Phenol	Disinfectant	Caustic	Decontamination: polyethylene glycol or water
			Dermal burns	
			Cutaneous absorption	Endoscopy
			CNS effects	
Substituted	Hexachlorophene	Disinfectant	CNS effects	Supportive
Quaternary Ammonium Compounds				
Benzalkonium chloride	Zephiran	Disinfectant	Caustic	Endoscopy as needed

A 35% hydrogen peroxide solution is also available to the general public in health food stores and is sold as "hyperoxygenation therapy" and as an additive to oxygenate health food drinks.[86] This potentially dangerous therapy is suggested as a treatment for a variety of conditions, including AIDS and cancer.

Toxicity from hydrogen peroxide occurs after ingestion, inhalation, injection, wound irrigation, rectal administration, dermal exposure, and ophthalmic exposure.[215] Hydrogen peroxide has 2 main mechanisms of toxicity: local tissue injury and gas formation. The extent of local tissue injury and amount of gas formation are determined by the concentration of the hydrogen peroxide. Dilute hydrogen peroxide is an irritant, and concentrated hydrogen peroxide is a caustic. Gas formation results when hydrogen peroxide interacts with tissue catalase, liberating molecular oxygen, and water. At standard temperature and pressure, 1 mL of 3% hydrogen peroxide liberates 10 mL of oxygen, whereas 1 mL of the more concentrated 35% hydrogen peroxide liberates more than 100 mL of oxygen. Gas formation results in life-threatening embolization. The ingestion of "2 sips" of 33% hydrogen peroxide resulted in cerebral gas embolization and hemiplegia.[173] Gas embolization is a result of dissection of gas under pressure into the tissues or of liberation of gas in the tissue or blood following absorption. The use of hydrogen peroxide in partially closed spaces, such as operative wounds, or its use under pressure during wound irrigation increases the likelihood of embolization.

Clinical Effects

Airway compromise manifested by stridor, drooling, apnea, and radiographic evidence of subepiglottic narrowing occurs.[44] The combination of local tissue injury and gas formation from the ingestion of concentrated hydrogen peroxide causes abdominal bloating, abdominal pain, vomiting, and hematemesis.[55,123] Endoscopy shows esophageal edema and erythema and significant gastric mucosal erosions.[162,182]

Symptoms consistent with sudden oxygen embolization include rapid deterioration in mental status, cyanosis, respiratory failure, seizures, ischemic ECG changes, and acute paraplegia.[57,119] A 2-year-old boy died after ingesting 120 to 180 mL of 35% hydrogen peroxide.[30] Antemortem chest radiography showed gas in the right ventricle, mediastinum, and portal venous system. Portal vein gas is also a prominent feature in other cases.[55,85,155] Arterialization of oxygen gas embolization results in cerebral infarction.[189] Encephalopathy with cortical visual impairment[23] and bilateral hemispheric infarctions detected by MRI imaging occurred after ingestion of concentrated hydrogen peroxide.[89] In a case of acute paraplegia after the ingestion of 50% hydrogen peroxide, MRI revealed discrete segmental embolic infarctions of the cervical and thoracic spinal cord as well as both cerebral hemispheres and left cerebellar hemisphere.[119]

Death from intravenous injection of 35% hydrogen peroxide is also reported.[112] The application of a concentrated hydrogen peroxide solution to the scalp and hair as part of a hair highlighting procedure resulted in a severe scalp injury, including necrosis of the galea aponeurotica.[183]

Clinical sequelae from the ingestion of dilute hydrogen peroxide are usually much more benign.[44,76] Nausea and vomiting are the most common symptoms.[44] A whitish discoloration is noted in the oral cavity. Gastrointestinal injury is usually limited to superficial mucosal irritation, but multiple gastric and duodenal ulcers, accompanied by hematemesis, and diffuse hemorrhagic gastritis are reported.[76,136] Portal venous gas embolization occurs as a result of the ingestion of 3% hydrogen peroxide.[31,136,166]

The use of 3% hydrogen peroxide for wound irrigation results in significant complications. Extensive subcutaneous emphysema occurred after a dog bite to a human's face was irrigated under pressure with 60 mL of 3% hydrogen peroxide.[192] Systemic oxygen embolism, causing hypotension, cardiac ischemia, and coma, resulted from the intraoperative irrigation of an infected herniorrhaphy wound.[12] Gas embolism, resulting in intestinal gangrene, was reported to occur following colonic lavage with 1% hydrogen peroxide during surgical treatment of meconium ileus.[187] Multiple cases of acute colitis are reported as a complication of administering 3% hydrogen peroxide

enemas.[132] The use of 3% hydrogen peroxide as a mouth rinse is associated with the development of oral ulcerations.[170] Ophthalmic exposures result in conjunctival injection, burning pain, and blurry vision.[44,131] Optic neuropathy including transient blindness (ability to visualize shadows only) and subsequent optic atrophy from possible inhalational of hydrogen peroxide is described.[45] Cough, wheezing, and shortness of breath is associated with occupational exposure to peracetic acid–hydrogen peroxide mixtures used to clean endoscopic equipment.[36]

Diagnosis

A careful examination should be performed to detect any evidence of gas formation. A chest radiograph is recommended to assess for gas in the cardiac chambers, mediastinum, or pleural space. Likewise, an abdominal radiograph is also recommended to assess for gas in the GI tract or portal system and define the extent of bowel distension. Magnetic resonance imaging and CT imaging are reasonable to detect brain and spinal cord lesions secondary to gas embolism and should be obtained if patient experiences neurologic effects.[5,89,119] For those with clinical presentations consistent with esophageal, gastric or intestinal injury, endoscopic evaluation is recommended.[162]

Management

The treatment of patients with hydrogen peroxide ingestions depends, to a large degree, on whether the patient has ingested a diluted or concentrated solution. Those with ingestions of concentrated solutions require expeditious evaluation. There is not enough evidence to support the dilution with milk or water. Nasogastric or orogastric aspiration of hydrogen peroxide is reasonable to consider if the patient presents immediately after ingestion. Induced emesis and activated charcoal are contraindicated. Gastric suctioning for patients with abdominal distension from gas formation is recommended. Place patients with clinical or radiographic evidence of gas in the heart in the Trendelenburg position to prevent gas from blocking the right ventricular outflow tract. Careful aspiration of intracardiac air through a central venous line is recommended in patients in extremis.[30] Hyperbaric therapy is recommended in cases of life-threatening gas embolization after hydrogen peroxide ingestion.[55,85,119,138,155,211] We recommend home observation for asymptomatic patients who unintentionally ingest small amounts of 3% hydrogen peroxide.

Iodine and Iodophors

Iodine is one of the oldest topical antiseptics.[184] Iodine usually refers to molecular iodine, also known as I_2, free iodine, and elemental iodine, which is the active ingredient of iodine-based antiseptics. The use of ethanol as the solvent, such as in tincture of iodine, allows substantially more concentrated forms of I_2 to be available. Iodine (I_2) and tincture of iodine ingestions are much less common than in the past as a result of the change in antiseptic use from iodine to iodophor antiseptics.[46]

Iodophors have molecular iodine compounded to a high-molecular-weight carrier or to a solubilizing xenobiotic. Povidone-iodine, a commonly used iodophor, consists of iodine linked to polyvinylpyrrolidone (povidone). Iodophors, which limit the release of molecular iodine and are generally less toxic, are the current standard iodine-based antiseptic preparations. Iodophor preparations are formulated as solutions, ointments, foams, surgical scrubs, wound-packing gauze, and vaginal preparations. The most common preparation is a 10% povidone-iodine solution that contains 1% "available" iodine (referring to all oxidizing iodine species), but only 0.001% free iodine (referring only to molecular iodine).[18,69]

Iodine is used to disinfect medical equipment and drinking water. Iodine is effective against bacteria, viruses, protozoa, and fungi, and is used both prophylactically and therapeutically.[42] Iodine is cytotoxic and also an oxidant. It is thought to work by binding amino and heterocyclic nitrogen groups, oxidizing sulfhydryl groups, and saturating double bonds. Iodine also iodinates tyrosine groups.[69] It appears to induce apoptosis through oxidative stress.[95]

Significant systemic absorption of iodine from topical iodine or iodophor preparations is rare.[157] Markedly elevated iodine concentrations occur in patients who receive topical iodophor treatments to areas of dermal break-down, such as burn injuries.[109] Significant absorption occurs when iodophors are applied to the vagina, perianal fistulas, umbilical cords, and the skin of low-birth-weight neonates.[212] The mucosal application of povidone-iodine during a hysteroscopy procedure resulted in acute kidney injury (AKI) that transiently required hemodialysis.[14] A fatality following intraoperative irriga-tion of a hip wound with povidone-iodine was also reported.[37] In this latter case, the postmortem serum iodine concentration was 7,000 mcg/dL (nor-mal: 5–8 mcg/dL).

Clinical Effects

Problems associated with the use of iodine include unpleasant odor, skin irritation, allergic reactions, and clothes staining. Ingestion of iodine causes abdominal pain, vomiting, diarrhea, GI bleeding, delirium, hypovolemia, anuria, and circulatory collapse. Severe caustic injury of the GI tract occurs. The ingestion of approximately 45 mL of a 10% iodine solution resulted in death from multisystem failure 67 hours after ingestion.[48] In another case, the ingestion of 200 mL of tincture of iodine containing 60 mg/mL iodine and 40 mg/mL potassium iodide in 70% v/v ethanol resulted in AKI and severe hemolysis.[126]

Reports of adverse consequences from iodophor ingestions are rare. In one case report, a 9-week-old infant died within 3 hours of receiving povidone-iodine by mouth.[106] In this unusual case, the child was adminis-tered 15 mL of povidone-iodine mixed with 135 mL of polyethylene glycol by nasogastric tube over a 3-hour period for the treatment of infantile colic. Postmortem examination showed an ulcerated and necrotic intestinal tract. A blood iodine concentration of 14,600 mcg/dL was recorded. Significant toxicity from intentional ingestions of iodophors in adults is not documented.

Acid–base disturbances are among the most significant abnormalities associated with iodine and iodophors. Metabolic acidosis occurred in sev-eral burn patients after receiving multiple applications of povidone-iodine ointment.[109,158] These patients had elevated serum iodine concentrations and normal lactate concentrations. The exact etiology of the acidosis remains unclear. Postulated mechanisms for the acidosis include the povidone-iodine itself (pH 2.43), bicarbonate consumption from the conversions of I_2 to NaI, and decreased renal elimination of H^+ as a consequence of iodine toxicity.[158] Metabolic acidosis associated with an elevated lactate concentration after iodine ingestion likely reflects tissue destruction.[42]

Electrolyte abnormalities also occur following the absorption of iodine. A patient with decubitus ulcers who received prolonged wound care with povidone-iodine–soaked gauze developed hypernatremia, hyperchloremia, metabolic acidosis, and AKI.[37] The hyperchloremia was thought to be caused by a spurious elevation of measured chloride ions as a consequence of the interference of iodine with the chloride assay. This interference occurs on the Technicon STAT/ION autoanalyzer, but does not occur when the silver halide precipitation assay is used.[42] Spurious hyperchloremia from iodine (or iodide) results in the calculation of a low or negative anion gap (Chaps. 7 and 12).[24,54] The spurious effect of iodide on chloride and anion gap occurs even with very low serum iodide concentrations (<1 mEq/L) and the degree of anion gap deviation does not reliably predict the amount of iodide present.[105]

Other problems associated with topical absorption of iodine-containing preparations are hypothyroidism (particularly in neonates),[24,193] hyperthyroidism,[169,174] elevated liver enzyme concentrations, neutropenia, anaphylaxis,[1] and hypoxemia.[42] Because of the lack of consistency between iodine concentrations and clinical manifestations, and because many of these patients had significant secondary medical problems that contributed to their symptoms, the exact relationship between iodine absorption and the development of a specific clinical syndrome remains speculative. However, a clinical controlled trial that compared preterm infants exposed to either top-ical iodinated antiseptics or to chlorhexidine-containing antiseptics showed that the infants exposed to topical iodine-containing antiseptics were more likely to have higher TSH concentrations and elevated urine iodine concen-trations than were those in the chlorhexidine group.[116]

Contact dermatitis can result from repetitive applications of iodophors.[127] A dermal burn results from the trapping of an iodophor solution under the body of a patient in a pooled dependent position or under a tourniquet.[118,142] Aspiration pneumonitis is rarely described following the intraoperative application of povidone-iodine prior to craniofacial surgeries.[27] These patients generally recover with supportive care.

Management

The patient who ingests iodine requires expeditious evaluation, stabi-lization, and decontamination. If signs of perforation are absent, it is reasonable to proceed with careful nasogastric or orogastric aspiration and lavage to limit the caustic effect of the iodine. In symptomatic patients, irrigation with a starch solution is recommended to convert iodine to the much less toxic iodide and, in the process, turn the gastric effluent dark blue-purple. This change in color is a useful guide in determining when lavage can be terminated. If starch is not available, milk or 100 mL of a solution of 1% to 3% sodium thiosulfate is a reasonable alternative to convert any remaining iodine to iodide. We recommend early endoscopy in patients with significant symptoms to help assess the extent of the GI injury. Hemodialysis and continuous venovenous hemodiafiltration were used successfully to enhance elimination of iodine in a patient with CKD with iodine toxicity who developed renal deterioration after undergoing continuous mediastinal irrigation with povidone-iodine.[99] The benefit of hemodialysis or continuous venovenous hemodiafiltration is unknown in patients with normal kidney function and therefore not routinely recom-mended at this time.

Most patients with iodophor ingestion require only supportive manage-ment. The use of starch or sodium thiosulfate is reasonable in symptomatic patients.

Potassium Permanganate

Potassium permanganate ($KMnO_4$) is a violet water-soluble xenobiotic that is usually sold as crystals or tablets or as a 0.01% dilute solution.[96] Histori-cally, it was used as an abortifacient, urethral irrigant, lavage fluid for alka-loid poisoning, and snakebite remedy. Currently, potassium permanganate is most often used in baths and wet bandages as a dermal antiseptic, particu-larly for patients with eczema.

Potassium permanganate is a strong oxidizer, and poisoning results in local and systemic toxicity.[195] Upon contact with mucous membranes, potas-sium permanganate reacts with water to form manganese dioxide, potas-sium hydroxide, and molecular oxygen. Local tissue injury is the result of contact with the nascent oxygen, as well as the caustic effect of potassium hydroxide. A brown-black staining of the tissues occurs from the manganese dioxide. Systemic toxicity occurs from free radicals generated by absorbed permanganate ions.[221]

Clinical Effects

Dermal contact leads to cutaneous staining. Following ingestion, initial symptoms include nausea and vomiting. Laryngeal edema and ulceration of the mouth, esophagus, and, to a lesser extent, the stomach, result from the caustic effects. Airway obstruction and fatal GI perforation and hemorrhage are reported.[43,133,150] Esophageal strictures and pyloric stenosis are potential late complications.[103]

Although potassium permanganate is not well absorbed from the GI tract, systemic absorption occurs, resulting in life-threatening toxicity. Systemic effects include hepatotoxicity, AKI, methemoglobinemia, hemo-lysis, hemorrhagic pancreatitis, airway obstruction, ARDS, disseminated intravascular coagulation, and cardiovascular collapse.[114,125,133,150] Elevation in blood and serum manganese concentrations also occurs, confirming sys-temic absorption.

Chronic ingestion of potassium permanganate results in classic manga-nese poisoning (manganism) characterized by behavioral changes, halluci-nations, and delayed onset of parkinsonian-like symptoms. A 66-year-old man who ingested 10 g of potassium permanganate instead of potassium iodate over a 4-week period (because of medication mislabeling) developed impaired concentration and autonomic and visual symptoms. He also developed abdominal pain, gastric ulceration, and alopecia. Serum manganese concentration was elevated. Nine months later, the patient had extrapyramidal signs consistent with parkinsonism (Chap. 94).[83]

Management
Because the consequential effects of potassium permanganate ingestion are a result of the liberation of strong alkalis, immediate assessment for evidence of airway compromise should be performed in such a patient. Dilution with milk or water is reasonable. Patients with symptoms consistent with caustic injury should undergo early upper–GI tract endoscopy.[96] Corticosteroids are recommended if laryngeal edema is present. When systemic toxicity is suspected, of liver enzymes, blood urea nitrogen, creatinine, lipase, serum manganese, and methemoglobin concentrations all will help in the evaluation. We recommend methylene blue for clinically significant methemoglobinemia (Antidotes in Depth: A43). Dermal irrigation with dilute oxalic acid removes cutaneous staining.[195] The administration of N-acetylcysteine (Antidotes in Depth: A3) to increase reduced glutathione production, thereby limiting free radical–mediated oxidative injury in cases of systemic potassium permanganate poisoning, is suggested, but there is inadequate evidence to support routine use at this time.[221]

OTHER ANTISEPTICS
Alcohols
Ethanol and isopropanol (Chaps. 76 and 106) are commonly used as skin antiseptics. When sold as rubbing alcohol, the standard concentration for these solutions is usually 70%. In recent years, alcohol-based hand sanitizers containing 60% to 95% ethyl or isopropyl alcohol have become ubiquitous throughout patient care units, jails, and some public buildings as a primary infection control measure. Their antiseptic action is a result of their ability to coagulate proteins. Isopropanol is slightly more germicidal than ethanol.[69] The alcohols have limited efficacy against viruses or spores. Isopropanol tends to be more irritating than ethanol and causes more pronounced central nervous system depression.[213] Unfortunately, readily available alcohol-based sanitizers are a tempting source for patients admitted with alcohol abuse disorders.[51,217] In one report, a patient was admitted to the hospital with chest pain. While in the hospital the patient became hypotensive and delirious. He was later found in the bathroom drinking an alcohol-based hand wash that contained 63% isopropanol.[51] The clinical effects and treatment for alcohol poisoning are discussed in Chaps. 76 and 106.

Chlorine and Chlorophors
Chlorine, one of the first antiseptics, is still used in the treatment of the community water supply and in swimming pools. Chlorine is a potent pulmonary irritant that can cause severe bronchospasm and ARDS. Chapter 121 contains a further discussion of chlorine.

Sodium hypochlorite (NaClO), found in household bleaches and in Dakin solution, remains a commonly used disinfectant. First used in the late 1700s to bleach clothes, its usefulness arises from its oxidizing capability, measured as "available chlorine," and its ability to release hypochlorous acid (HClO) slowly. It is used to clean blood spills and to sterilize certain medical instruments. A 0.5% hypochlorite solution is sometimes recommended for dermal and soft-tissue wound decontamination after exposure to biologic and chemical warfare agents (Chaps. 126 and 127).[86] Toxicity from hypochlorite is mainly a result of its irritant effects. The ingestion of large amounts of household liquid bleach (5% sodium hypochlorite) on rare occasions can result in esophageal burns with subsequent stricture formation.[56] In a cat model of bleach ingestion, a high incidence of mucosal injury and stricture formation was noted.[216] However, the vast majority of household bleach ingestions in humans do not cause significant GI injuries.[159] Accordingly, we recommend not performing routine endoscopic evaluation when assessing asymptomatic patients with household liquid bleach ingestions. Endoscopy is reasonable in symptomatic patients. Endoscopy is recommended in symptomatic

patients who ingest a more concentrated "industrial strength" bleach preparation such as 35% sodium hypochlorite, because of the increased likelihood of local tissue injury (Chap. 103).

Mercurials
Both inorganic mercurials, such as mercuric bichloride ($HgCl_2$), and organic mercurials, such as merbromin ($C_{20}H_8Br_2HgNa_2O_6$) (mercurochrome) and thimerosal ($C_9H_9HgNaO_2S$) (merthiolate), which both contain 49% mercury, were previously used as topical antiseptics. The usefulness of mercurials is significantly limited because of their relatively weak bacteriostatic properties and the many concerns associated with mercury toxicity (Chap. 95). Repeated application of topical mercurial causes significant absorption and systemic toxicity.[139,176] The use of high-dose hepatitis B immunoglobulin (HBIG) causes mercury toxicity because of the use of thimerosal as a preservative in the HBIG preparation.[121] In one case, a 44-year-old man received 250 mL of HBIG (containing about 30 mg of thimerosal) over 9 days following liver transplantation.[121] He developed speech difficulties, tremor, and chorea. His whole blood mercury concentration was 104 mcg/L (normal <10 mcg/L).

DISINFECTANTS
Formaldehyde
Formaldehyde is a water-soluble, highly reactive gas at room temperature. Formalin consists of an aqueous solution of formaldehyde, usually containing approximately 37% formaldehyde and 12% to 15% methanol. Formaldehyde is irritating to the upper airways, and its odor is readily detectable at low concentrations. Lethality in adults follows ingestion of as little as 30 to 60 mL of formalin.[49]

Formerly used as a disinfectant and fumigant, its role as a disinfectant is now largely confined to the maintenance of hemodialysis machines. Nonetheless, formaldehyde has many other applications. Formaldehyde is widely used in construction including wood processing and the manufacturing of furniture, textiles, and carpeting.[101] Health care workers are probably most familiar with the use of formaldehyde as a tissue fixative and embalming agent. Medical students are routinely exposed to formalin in the anatomy laboratory.[167]

Exposure to formaldehyde, a potent tissue fixative results in both local and systemic symptoms, causing coagulation necrosis, protein precipitation, and tissue fixation. Ingestions of formalin results in significant gastric injury, including hemorrhage, diffuse necrosis, perforation, and stricture.[3,11] The most extensive damage appears in the stomach, with only occasional involvement of the small intestine and colon.[220] Chemical fixation of the stomach occurs. Esophageal involvement is not very prominent and, if present, is usually limited to its distal segment.

The most striking and rapid systemic manifestation of formaldehyde poisoning is anion gap metabolic acidosis, resulting both from tissue injury and from the conversion of formaldehyde to formic acid. Although the methanol component of the formalin solution is readily absorbed and produces methanol concentrations reportedly as high as 40 mg/dL,[22,49] the rapid metabolism of formaldehyde to formic acid is responsible for much of the metabolic acidosis (Chap. 106).

Clinical Effects
Patients presenting after formalin ingestions complain of the rapid onset of severe abdominal pain, vomiting, and diarrhea. Altered mental status and coma usually follow rapidly. Physical examination demonstrates epigastric tenderness, hematemesis, cyanosis, hypotension, and tachypnea. Profound hypotension is due to decreased myocardial contractility, as well as hypovolemic shock.[78,203] Early endoscopic findings include ulceration, necrosis, perforation, and hemorrhage of the stomach, with infrequent esophageal involvement. Chemical pneumonitis occurs after significant inhalational exposure.[161] Intravascular hemolysis is described in hemodialysis patients whose dialysis equipment contained residual formaldehyde after undergoing routine cleaning.[152,165]

Occupational and environmental exposure to formaldehyde receives considerable attention. In particular, there is concern over the potential off-gassing of formaldehyde from the widely used urea formaldehyde building insulation and particle board.[149] Headache, nausea, skin rash, sore throat, nasal congestion, and eye irritation are associated with the use of these polymers.[39] Formaldehyde, at concentrations as low as 1 ppm, causes significant irritation to mucous membranes of the upper respiratory tract and conjunctivae.[82,120] Formaldehyde is also a potential sensitizer for immune-mediated reversible bronchospasm.[75] The exact immunologic mechanism is not yet elucidated, although it is likely that formaldehyde acts as a hapten. In addition, formaldehyde is a dermal sensitizer.[194]

Concerns about the health effects from the off-gassing of formaldehyde in trailers used by the Federal Emergency Management Agency (FEMA) after Hurricane Katrina illustrates the potential public health issues related to low-level formaldehyde exposure.[124] A Centers for Disease Control and Prevention (CDC) investigation revealed that air formaldehyde concentrations in closed, unventilated trailers are, in fact, high enough to cause acute symptoms in some people.[4] Long-term effects after these exposures remain undefined.

Formaldehyde exposure is associated with an increased incidence of nasopharyngeal carcinoma.[2,71,156,177] Although its role in the pathogenesis of cancer in humans is the subject of much debate,[33,128] formaldehyde is classified as a Group 1, *known*, carcinogen by the International Agency for Research on Cancer (IARC).

Management

Dilution with water is reasonable for the immediate management of a patient who has ingested formalin. Gastric aspiration with a small-bore nasogastric or orogastric tube is also reasonable to limit systemic absorption. Activated charcoal should not be used. Significant acidemia is treated with sodium bicarbonate and folinic acid (Chap. 106). Immediate hemodialysis removes the accumulating formic acid as well as the parent molecules formaldehyde and methanol and is reasonable in refractory acidemia (Antidotes in Depth: A33 and A34).[6,49] Early endoscopy is recommended for all patients with significant GI manifestations to assess the degree of burn injury. Surgical intervention is required for those with suspected severe burns, tissue necrosis and/or perforation.[220] Emergent gastrectomy, as well as late surgical intervention to relieve formaldehyde-induced gastric outlet obstruction, is rarely required.[72,104]

Phenol

Phenol is one of the oldest antiseptics. It is rarely used as an antiseptic today, because of its toxicity, and is replaced by the many phenolic derivatives. Currently, phenol is used as a disinfectant and chemical intermediary. The concentration of phenol in consumer products can vary significantly, from 0.1% to 4.7% in various lotions, ointments, gels, gargles, lozenges, and throat sprays and up to 89% in nail cauterizer solution.[69] Although many cases of phenol poisoning were reported in the past, acute oral overdoses of phenol-containing solutions are uncommon today.[62]

Phenol acts as a caustic causing cell wall disruption, protein denaturation, and coagulation necrosis. It also acts as a central nervous system (CNS) stimulant. Intentional ingestion of concentrated phenol, ingestion of phenol-containing water, occupational exposure to aerosolized phenol, dermal contact, and parenteral administration result in symptomatic phenol poisoning. Phenol demonstrates excellent skin penetration and causes severe dermal burns, resulting in potentially fatal systemic toxicity within minutes to hours.[16,113] Deaths from parenteral administration of phenol are reported. The lethal oral dose is as little as 1 g.[84]

Clinical Effects

Clinical manifestations can be divided into local and systemic symptoms. Systemic symptoms from GI or dermal absorption of phenol are usually more dangerous than the local effects. Manifestations of systemic toxicity include CNS and cardiac manifestations. Central nervous system effects include central stimulation, seizures, lethargy, and coma.[65] In a study of patients who

had ingested Creolin (26% phenol), CNS toxicity predominated.[196] Of the 52 patients who were evaluated at the hospital, 9 developed lethargy and 2 developed coma. Seizures were not reported. Cardiac signs and symptoms from phenol include tachycardia, bradycardia, and hypotension.[65] Parenteral absorption of 10 mL concentrated 89% phenol resulted in hypoxemia, ARDS, pulmonary nodular opacities, and AKI requiring intubation and hemodialysis.[64] This last case was associated with a phenol concentration of 87 mg/dL (normal <2 mg/dL).

Other systemic effects include hypothermia, metabolic acidosis, methemoglobinemia, and rabbit syndrome.[84,97] Rabbit syndrome is most commonly observed as a distinctive extrapyramidal effect from antipsychotics and is characterized by fine rapid repetitive movements of the perioral musculature resembling a rabbit's chewing movements. Increased acetylcholine release and a relative dopaminergic hypofunction explain the development of rabbit syndrome after phenol exposure.[97]

Local toxicity to the GI tract from the ingestion of phenol results in nausea, painful oral lesions, vomiting, severe abdominal pain, bloody diarrhea, and dark urine.[8,94] Serious GI burns are uncommon, and strictures are rare. White patches in the oral cavity occur. In the Creolin study cited above, only 1 of 17 patients who underwent endoscopy had a significant esophageal burn.[196] Dermal exposures to phenol usually result in a light-brown staining of the skin. Excessive dermal absorption of phenol during chemical peeling procedures is associated with dysrhythmias and many of the other toxic manifestations.[208,214]

Markedly elevated blood and urine concentrations of phenol are detected after ingestion, or dermal absorption, of phenol and phenol-containing compounds.[16,84]

Management

When phenol is mixed with water, a bilayer with unique properties is created that makes it difficult to remove from tissues. A variety of treatments are suggested for dermal and gastric decontamination of phenol. A study using a rat model showed that cutaneous decontamination with a low-molecular-weight polyethylene glycol solution decreased mortality, systemic effects, and dermal burns.[21] Although this study suggested that polyethylene glycol (PEG) was superior to water as a decontamination, a subsequent study using a swine model could not demonstrate a difference between these 2 therapies.[164] In another swine model, PEG 400 and 70% isopropanol were both superior to water washes and equally effective in decreasing dermal burn.[135] Given the lack of definitive efficacy data, either low-molecular-weight PEG, for example, PEG 300 or 400 (not to be confused with high-molecular-weight PEG that is used for whole-bowel irrigation), or high-flow water are reasonable for dermal irrigation and careful gastric decontamination. Endoscopic evaluation, for symptomatic patients to determine the extent of GI injury is recommended.

Substituted Phenols and Other Related Compounds

Hexachlorophene, a trichlorinated *bis*-phenol, is considered generally less tissue-toxic than phenol. During the 1970s, an association was observed between repetitive whole-body washing of premature infants with 3% hexachlorophene and the development of vacuolar encephalopathy and cerebral edema.[129] There are also multiple reports of significant neurologic toxicity and death in children who became toxic after ingesting hexachlorophene.[77] In addition, fatalities also occurred after patients absorbed substantial amounts of hexachlorophene during the treatment of burns.[29] The use of hexachlorophene has declined significantly. Currently used substituted phenols include a sodium solution of octylphenoxyethoxyethyl ether sulfonate, chloroxylenol and cresol.

Clinical Effects

A sodium solution of octylphenoxyethoxyethyl ether sulfonate and lanolin is a safe antiseptic. Irritative effects such as nausea, vomiting, and diarrhea are the main adverse effects following ingestion.

In a study of poisoning admissions to Hong Kong hospitals, the ingestion of a household disinfectant that contained 4.8% chloroxylenol, 9% pine oil, and 12% isopropanol accounted for 10% of admissions.[26] Aspiration (perhaps, in part, because of the pine oil) occurred in 8% of these patients, resulting in upper airway obstruction, pneumonia, and ARDS. More common symptoms included nausea, vomiting, sore mouth, sore throat, drowsiness, abdominal pain, and fever. Dermal contact with Dettol results in full-thickness chemical burns.[40]

Cresol, a mixture of 3 isomers of methylphenol, has better antiseptic activity than phenol and is a commonly used disinfectant. Exposure to concentrated cresol results in significant local tissue injury, hemolysis, AKI, hepatic injury, and CNS and respiratory depression.[40,70,98,219] Phenol concentrations, as well as cresol concentrations, serve as markers of exposure.[219]

Management
Treatment is supportive care emphasizing decontamination.

Quaternary Ammonium Compounds
Quaternary ammonium compounds, positively charged compounds where 4 organic groups are linked to a nitrogen atom (NR_4^+), are cationic surfactants (surface-active agent) that are used as disinfectants, detergents, and sanitizers. Chemically, the quaternary ammonium compounds are synthetic derivatives of ammonium chloride, and structurally similar to other quaternary ammonium derivatives, such as carbamate cholinesterase inhibitors and neuromuscular blockers. Other cationic surfactants include the pyridinium compounds and the quinolinium compounds. Benzalkonium chloride was one of the most commonly employed quaternary ammonium compounds in the past. Many newer quaternary ammonium compounds have supplanted its use. However, nebulized solutions used for the treatment of asthma, including albuterol and ipratropium bromide, contain small amounts of benzalkonium chloride.

Clinical
Quaternary ammonium compounds are usually less toxic than phenol or formaldehyde. Most of the infrequent complications that are described result from ingestions of benzalkonium chloride. Complications of these ingestions include burns to the mouth and esophagus, CNS depression, elevated liver enzyme concentrations, metabolic acidosis, and hypotension.[80,147,210] Paralysis is also occasionally described as a complication of these ingestions and is presumably a result of cholinesterase inhibition at the neuromuscular junction.[62] Chronic inhalational exposure is associated with occupational asthma.[17] Topical use of the quaternary ammonium compounds causes contact dermatitis.[190] Ingestion of a 2.25% ammonium chloride solution, marketed as a bacteriostatic for algae and odor humidifier treatment, results in serious GI and pulmonary injury.[67]

Ingestions of other cationic surfactants, such as the pyridinium-derived cetrimonium bromide are associated with corrosive burns to the mouth, lips, and tongue.[137] Peritoneal irrigation with cetrimonium bromide produces metabolic abnormalities, hypotension, and methemoglobinemia.[9,134] Intravenous administration of cetrimonium bromide leads to hemolysis, muscle paralysis, and cardiac arrest.[58]

Management
Treatment recommendations following the ingestion of the quaternary ammonium compounds and other cationic surfactants are similar to those for other potentially caustic ingestions. Emergency department evaluation is recommended for all patients who ingest more than a taste of a dilute (<1%) solution. Therapy is mainly supportive care. Endoscopy is indicated if signs and symptoms suggest the possibility of a burn.

STERILANTS
Ethylene Oxide
Ethylene oxide (C_2H_4O) is a gas that is commonly used to sterilize heat-sensitive material in health care facilities. Unlike antiseptics and disinfectants, which generally do not exhibit full sporicidal activity, sterilants, such as ethylene oxide, inactivate all organisms. Ethylene oxide is also used in the synthesis of many chemicals, including ethylene glycol, surfactants, rocket propellants, and petroleum demulsifiers, and is used as a fumigant. Ethylene oxide has a cyclic ester structure that acts as an alkylating agent, reacting with most cellular components, including DNA and RNA.

Medical attention regarding ethylene oxide toxicity has centered on its mutagenic and possible carcinogenic effects.[108] Approximately 270,000 workers (including 96,000 hospital workers) in the United States are at risk for occupational exposure to ethylene oxide.[199] Retrospective studies suggest a possible excess incidence of leukemia and gastric cancer in ethylene oxide exposed workers.[81,199] The 2008 IARC updated monographs concluded that there was limited evidence for carcinogenicity in humans, with an association with lymphatic, hematopoietic, and breast cancers. However, sufficient evidence for the carcinogenicity of ethylene oxide was found in experimental animals. Evidence suggests direct-acting alkylating effects leading to genotoxicity. Ethylene oxide was subsequently placed in IARC group I—carcinogenic to humans.[87] An increased incidence of spontaneous abortions is associated with occupational exposure to ethylene oxide.[74]

Clinical Effects
The acute toxicity of ethylene oxide is mainly the result of its irritant effects, including conjunctival, upper respiratory tract, GI, and dermal irritation. Dermal burns from acute exposure to ethylene oxide are reported. Acute exposure to a broken ethylene oxide ampule (17 g) by a 43-year-old recovery room nurse resulted in nausea, lightheadedness, malaise, syncope, and recurrent seizures.[181] There were no long-term complications. In another case of acute exposure, coma was followed by an irreversible parkinsonism.[10]

Chronic exposure to high concentrations of ethylene oxide causes mild cognitive impairment and motor and sensory neuropathies.[20,63,146] Hazard studies of occupational exposure have demonstrated no increased incidence of cancer in exposed populations over the expected occurrence rate.[32,198,204]

Management
Treatment for patients with ethylene oxide exposure is supportive.

Glutaraldehyde
Glutaraldehyde is a liquid solution used in the cold sterilization of nonautoclavable endoscopic, surgical, and dental equipment. It is also employed as a tissue fixative, embalming fluid, preservative, and tanning agent, in radiographic solutions, and in the treatment of warts.[60] Glutaraldehyde ($C_5H_8O_2$) is a dialdehyde with 2 active carbonyl groups that is less volatile than formaldehyde. It kills all microorganisms, including viruses and spores. The sterilant ability of glutaraldehyde results from the alkylation of sulfhydryl, hydroxyl, carboxyl, and amino groups, within microbes interfering with RNA, DNA, and protein synthesis.[179] It is prepared as a 2% alkaline solution in 70% isopropanol. Health care workers are exposed to glutaraldehyde vapors when equipment is processed in poorly ventilated areas, or in open immersion baths or after spills. Under these circumstances, the evaporation of glutaraldehyde results in the increase in ambient air concentrations that exceeds recommended limits. Approximately 35,000 workers are occupationally exposed to glutaraldehyde annually.[160] To prevent exposure, OSHA recommends the use of personal protective equipment with elbow-length gloves of butyl rubber or nitrile, gowns and eye protection. Local exhaust ventilation at the point of release should include either a local exhaust hood or ductless hood. Enclosed processing is also recommended when available. Respirators should be available in the event that ventilation fails for any reason.[153] Patients are exposed when diagnostic instruments are inadequately rinsed following cold sterilization with glutaraldehyde.

Clinical
Clinical signs and symptoms are comparable to those of formaldehyde exposure, although human toxicity data are limited. Animal studies show that the inhalational and dermal toxicity of glutaraldehyde are similar to those of formaldehyde at equivalent doses.[202]

Glutaraldehyde is a mucosal irritant. Coryza, epistaxis, headache, asthma, chest tightness, palpitations, tachycardia, and nausea are all associated with glutaraldehyde vapor exposure.[15,34,143,154] Occupational asthma, contact dermatitis, and ocular inflammation also occur.[38,151,186] Colitis is reported following the use of endoscopes contaminated with residual glutaraldehyde solution.[188] Patients with glutaraldehyde-induced colitis typically present with fever, chills, severe abdominal pain, bloody diarrhea, and an elevated white blood cell count within 48 hours after colonoscopy or sigmoidoscopy.

The IARC has not ranked the carcinogenic potential of glutaraldehyde.

Management

Treatment recommendations are similar to those for patients with formaldehyde exposure. Prompt removal from the exposure is essential. Copious irrigation with water is recommended for dermal decontamination. Severe inhalational exposures require hospital admission for observation, supportive care, and treatment of bronchospasm.

In recent years, some hospitals have started using *ortho*-phthalaldehyde (OPA) or a mixture of hydrogen peroxide and peracetic acid as alternatives to glutaraldehyde for high-level disinfection.[172] These alternative disinfectants do not appear to have the pulmonary or dermal sensitizing properties associated with glutaraldehyde, although they do cause some irritation to skin and mucous membranes.[172] A single case of occupational asthma related to OPA exposure was reported in 2014, proven with a specific inhalation challenge, and represents the only reported case in the literature.[175] Oropharyngeal and laryngeal burns are also reported in a patient exposed to residual OPA during transesophageal echocardiography.[185]

OTHER PRODUCTS
Boric Acid

Boric acid is an odorless, transparent crystal, although it is most commonly available as a finely ground white powder. It is also available as a 2.5% to 5% aqueous solution. Boric acid (H_3BO_3), prepared from borax (sodium borate; $Na_2B_4O_7 \cdot 10 H_2O$), was first used as an antiseptic by Lister in the late 19th century. Although used extensively over the years for antisepsis and irrigation, boric acid is only weakly bacteriostatic. As a result of its germicidal limitations and its inherent toxicity, boric acid is nearly obsolete in modern antiseptic therapy. Nonetheless, it continues to be used as an antimicrobial to treat such conditions as vulvovaginal candidiasis.[88,100,163] Boric acid is also employed in the treatment of cockroach infestation and as a soap, contact lens solution, toothpaste, and food preservative.[66] Recently, do-it-yourself recipes for children's slime, a squishy colorful play material, include boric acid as a major ingredient.[47]

Boric acid is readily absorbed through the GI tract, wounds, abraded skin, and serous cavities. Absorption does not occur through intact skin. Boric acid is predominantly eliminated unchanged by the kidney. Small amounts are also excreted into sweat, saliva, and feces.[59] Boric acid is concentrated in the brain and liver.

The exact mechanism of action of toxicity remains unclear. Although it is an inorganic acid, it is not a caustic. Local effects are limited to tissue irritation.

Over the years, boric acid developed a reputation as an exceptionally potent toxin. This reputation derived in great part from a series of reports involving neonatal exposures to boric acid resulting in high morbidity and mortality. Life-threatening toxicity resulted from the repetitive topical application of boric acid for the treatment of diaper rash or the use of infant formulas unintentionally contaminated with boric acid.[59,218] Fatality rates greater than 50% were reported in some series.[218] Although infants appear to be the most sensitive to the toxic effects of boric acid, many cases of significant toxicity are also reported in adults. These cases date predominantly from the first half of the 20th century when boric acid was widely used as an irrigant. Routes of exposure to boric acid, resulting in fatalities, include wound irrigation, pleural irrigation, rectal washing, bladder irrigation, and vaginal packing.[209]

Clinical Effects

Boric acid poisoning usually involves multiple exposures over a period of days. Gastrointestinal, dermal, CNS, and renal manifestations predominate.

The initial effects—nausea, vomiting, diarrhea, and occasionally crampy abdominal pain—are frequently confused with an acute gastroenteritis. At times, the emesis and diarrhea are greenish blue.[218] Following the onset of GI signs and symptoms, the majority of patients develop a characteristic intense generalized erythroderma.[218] This rash, described as producing a "boiled lobster" appearance, appears indistinguishable from toxic epidermal necrolysis or staphylococcal scalded skin syndrome in the neonate.[122,178] The rash is especially noticeable on the palms, soles, and buttocks.[59] Typically, extensive desquamation takes place within 1 to 2 days. On occasion, prominent mucous membrane involvement of the oral cavity and conjunctivae is also apparent.[218] At the time of development of the erythroderma, patients, particularly young infants, develop prominent signs of CNS irritability, resembling meningeal irritation. Seizures, delirium, and coma occur.[59] Acute kidney injury is common, both as a result of the renal elimination of this compound and prerenal azotemia from GI losses.[59] Other complications of boric acid poisoning include hepatic injury, hyperthermia, and cardiovascular collapse. A marked decrease in the incidence of significant boric acid poisoning is attributed to the abandonment of boric acid as an irrigant and particularly its removal from the nursery setting.

Two retrospective studies on boric acid ingestions suggest that a single acute ingestion of boric acid is generally quite benign.[115,117] In these studies, 79% to 88% of patients remained asymptomatic. Symptoms, when present, primarily consist of nausea and vomiting. None of the 1,184 patients in these 2 studies manifested the generalized erythroderma so commonly described in previous reports. Central nervous system manifestations of acute overdose were infrequent and limited to occasional lethargy and headache. Kidney injury did not occur following single acute ingestions.

Fatalities from massive acute ingestion of boric acid are reported in both unintentional ingestions in children and intentional ingestions in adults.[66,171] Fatality resulted from a single ingestion of 2 cups (280 g) of boric acid crystals dissolved in water by a 45-year-old man. Signs and symptoms on presentation (2 days after ingestion) included nausea, vomiting, green diarrhea, lethargy, hypotension, AKI, and a prominent "boiled lobster" rash on his trunk and extremities. In another case, the ingestion of 30 g of boric acid by a 77-year-old man resulted in similar symptoms and death 63 hours postingestion, despite hemodialysis.[91]

Long-term chronic exposure to boric acid results in alopecia in adults and seizures in children.[145] A 32-year-old woman who over a 7-month period ingested commercial mouthwash products containing boric acid developed progressive hair loss.[201] The chronic application of a commercial preparation of borax and honey mixture to pacifiers resulted in the development of recurrent seizures in 9 infants, which resolved after the mixture was withheld.[61,145]

Management

Treatment of boric acid toxicity is supportive care. Activated charcoal is not recommended because of its relatively poor adsorptive capacity for boric acid.[41] Because boric acid has a low molecular weight and relatively small volume of distribution, in cases of massive oral overdose or AKI, hemodialysis, or perhaps exchange transfusion in infants, is reasonable in shortening the half-life of boric acid.[35,117,141,206] Although forced diuresis is suggested by others to enhance renal elimination, this is highly unlikely to be successful and is not recommended.[207]

Chlorates

Sodium chlorate is a strong oxidizer. At one time, the chlorate salts sodium chlorate and potassium chlorate were used as medicinals to treat inflammatory and ulcerative lesions of the oral cavity and could be found in various mouthwash, toothpaste, and gargle preparations.[197] Although their use as local antiseptics is obsolete, chlorates are used as herbicides and in the manufacture of matches, explosives, and dyestuffs.[92] Historically, cases have included dispensing errors that confused sodium chlorate with sodium sulfate or sodium chloride.[92] Sodium chlorate in the form of white crystals was mistaken for table sugar in one case.[73] A case of significant toxicity from the inhalation of atomized chlorates is also reported.[92] More recent cases of chlorate poisoning continue to result from the ingestion of sodium chlorate–containing weed killers[168,197] and industrial chemicals.[111]

Sodium chlorate is rapidly absorbed from the GI tract and eliminated predominantly unchanged from the kidneys.[93] Its systemic effects are chiefly hematologic and renal. The major mechanism of toxicity of chlorate is its ability to oxidize hemoglobin and increase red blood cell membrane rigidity.[191] Consequently, significant methemoglobinemia and hemolysis result. Methemoglobinemia occurs prior to or after the development of hemolysis.[144,200] The hemolysis and the resultant hemoglobinuria secondarily causes disseminated intravascular coagulation and potential renal toxicity. Chlorates are also directly toxic to the proximal renal tubule.[110] The worsening kidney function is especially problematic because of its adverse effect on chlorate elimination. Chlorates also act locally as a GI irritant and cause mild CNS depression after absorption (Chap. 124).[62]

Clinical

Clinical signs and symptoms of chlorate poisoning usually begin 1 to 4 hours after ingestion.[102] The earliest manifestations are nausea, vomiting, diarrhea, and crampy abdominal pain. Subsequently, the patient exhibits cyanosis from the methemoglobinemia and black-brown urine from the hemoglobinuria. Obtundation and anuria ensue. Laboratory studies demonstrate methemoglobinemia, anemia, Heinz bodies, ghost cells, fragmented spherocytes, metabolic acidosis, thrombocytopenia, and abnormal coagulation.[53] Hyperkalemia is particularly problematic if the patient ingests potassium chlorate preparations.[140] In a case of chlorate poisoning from the ingestion of 120 potassium chlorate–containing matchsticks, an MRI revealed symmetric abnormal signal intensity within the deep gray matter and medial temporal lobes.[140] This finding can be explained by the increased vulnerability to oxygen deprivation of the basal ganglia. Follow-up MRI 2 months later was normal.

Management

In symptomatic patients with chlorate ingestions, it is reasonable to pursue GI decontamination.[73] The utility of methylene blue in the treatment of symptomatic chlorate-induced methemoglobinemia has been questioned as a consequence of the inactivation by chlorates of glucose-6-phosphate dehydrogenase, an enzyme that is required for methylene blue to effectively reduce methemoglobin.[191,200] Nevertheless, more recent experience suggests that early use of methylene blue prior to the onset of hemolysis is beneficial due to the necessity of the intact erythrocyte for methylene blue to be efficacious and thus a reasonable treatment.[19,111] Exchange transfusion and hemodialysis are reasonable in the treatment of patients with severe chlorate poisoning.[144,200] Because the chlorate ion is easily dialyzable, hemodialysis will be effective in removal of chlorate as well as in treating concomitant AKI.[92,102,110]

SUMMARY

- Many of the more toxic xenobiotics, such as iodine, phenol, and chlorates, are no longer commonly used as cleansers but are still available in some health care and occupational settings.
- Formaldehyde exposures, though also uncommon, cause significant respiratory toxicity and is potentially carcinogenic.
- Frequently employed antiseptics, are chlorhexidine, octylphenoxyethoxyethyl ether sulfonate, and many of the currently used quaternary ammonium compounds. Iodine, phenol, and quaternary ammonium compounds are caustic when ingested.
- Ingestions of the iodophors do not usually cause significant toxicity, but absorption through other routes produces significant adverse effects.
- Ingestion of concentrated hydrogen peroxide results in life-threatening injuries. Boric acid causes a dermatitis.

REFERENCES

1. Adachi A, et al. Anaphylaxis to polyvinylpyrrolidone after vaginal application of povidone-iodine. *Contact Dermatitis.* 2003;48:133-136.
2. Albert RE, et al. Gaseous formaldehyde and hydrogen chloride induction of nasal cancer in the rat. *J Natl Cancer Inst.* 1982;68:597-603.
3. Allen RE, et al. Corrosive injuries of the stomach. *Arch Surg.* 1970;100:409-413.
4. Anonymous. An update and revision of ATSDR's February 2007 health consultation: formaldehyde sampling of FEMA temporary-housing trailers, Baton Rouge, Louisiana, September-October, 2006. https://www.atsdr.cdc.gov/substances/formaldehyde/pdfs/revised_formaldehyde_report_1007.pdf. Published 2007. Accessed April 1, 2017.
5. Ashdown BC, et al. Hydrogen peroxide poisoning causing brain infarction: neuroimaging findings. *AJR Am J Roentgenol.* 1998;170:1653-1655.
6. ATSDR. Medical management guidelines for formaldehyde. https://www.atsdr.cdc.gov/mmg/mmg.asp?id=216&tid=39. Published 2014. Accessed June 25, 2017.
7. Autegarden JE, et al. Anaphylactic shock after application of chlorhexidine to unbroken skin. *Contact Dermatitis.* 1999;40:215.
8. Baker EL, et al. Phenol poisoning due to contaminated drinking water. *Arch Environ Health.* 1978;33:89-94.
9. Baraka A, et al. Cetrimide-induced methaemoglobinaemia after surgical excision of hydatid cyst. *Lancet.* 1980;2:88-89.
10. Barbosa ER, et al. Parkinsonism secondary to ethylene oxide exposure: case report [in Portuguese]. *Arq Neuropsiquiatr.* 1992;50:531-533.
11. Bartone NF, et al. Corrosive gastritis due to ingestion of formaldehyde: without esophageal impairment. *JAMA.* 1968;203:50-51.
12. Bassan MM, et al. Near-fatal systemic oxygen embolism due to wound irrigation with hydrogen peroxide. *Postgrad Med J.* 1982;58:448-450.
13. Beaudouin E, et al. Immediate hypersensitivity to chlorhexidine: literature review. *Eur Ann Allergy Clin Immunol.* 2004;36:123-126.
14. Beji S, et al. Acute renal failure following mucosal administration of povidone iodine [in French]. *Presse Med.* 2006;35(1, pt 1):61-63.
15. Benson WG. Exposure to glutaraldehyde. *J Soc Occup Med.* 1984;34:63-64.
16. Bentur Y, et al. Prolonged elimination half-life of phenol after dermal exposure. *J Toxicol Clin Toxicol.* 1998;36:707-711.
17. Bernstein JA, et al. A combined respiratory and cutaneous hypersensitivity syndrome induced by work exposure to quaternary amines. *J Allergy Clin Immunol.* 1994;94(2, pt 1):257-259.
18. Block S. *Definition of Terms.* 5th ed. Philadelphia, PA: Lippincott Williams & Wilkins; 2001.
19. Bradberry SM. Occupational methaemoglobinaemia. Mechanisms of production, features, diagnosis and management including the use of methylene blue. *Toxicol Rev.* 2003;22:13-27.
20. Brashear A, et al. Ethylene oxide neurotoxicity: a cluster of 12 nurses with peripheral and central nervous system toxicity. *Neurology.* 1996;46:992-998.
21. Brown VK, et al. Decontamination procedures for skin exposed to phenolic substances. *Arch Environ Health.* 1975;30:1-6.
22. Burkhart KK, et al. Formate levels following a formalin ingestion. *Vet Hum Toxicol.* 1990;32:135-137.
23. Cannon G, et al. Hydrogen peroxide neurotoxicity in childhood: case report with unique magnetic resonance imaging features. *J Child Neurol.* 2003;18:805-808.
24. Chabrolle JP, Rossier A. Goitre and hypothyroidism in the newborn after cutaneous absorption of iodine. *Arch Dis Child.* 1978;53:495-498.
25. Chan TY. Poisoning due to Savlon (cetrimide) liquid. *Hum Exp Toxicol.* 1994;13:681-682.
26. Chan TY, et al. Serious complications associated with Dettol poisoning. *Q J Med.* 1993;86:735-738.
27. Chepla KG, Gosain AK. Interstitial pneumonitis after betadine aspiration. *J Craniofac Surg.* 2012;23:1787-1789.
28. Cheung J, O'Leary JJ. Allergic reaction to chlorhexidine in an anaesthetised patient. *Anaesth Intensive Care.* 1985;13:429-430.
29. Chilcote R, et al. Hexachlorophene storage in a burn patient associated with encephalopathy. *Pediatrics.* 1977;59:457-459.
30. Christensen DW, et al. Fatal oxygen embolization after hydrogen peroxide ingestion. *Crit Care Med.* 1992;20:543-544.
31. Cina SJ, et al. Hydrogen peroxide: a source of lethal oxygen embolism. Case report and review of the literature. *Am J Forensic Med Pathol.* 1994;15:44-50.
32. Coggon D, et al. Mortality of workers exposed to ethylene oxide: extended follow up of a British cohort. *Occup Environ Med.* 2004;61:358-362.
33. Collins JJ, et al. An updated meta-analysis of formaldehyde exposure and upper respiratory tract cancers. *J Occup Environ Med.* 1997;39:639-651.
34. Connaughton P. Occupational exposure to glutaraldehyde associated with tachycardia and palpitations. *Med J Aust.* 1993;159:567.
35. Corradi F, et al. A case report of massive acute boric acid poisoning. *Eur J Emerg Med.* 2010;17:48-51.
36. Cristofari-Marquand E, et al. Asthma caused by peracetic acid-hydrogen peroxide mixture. *J Occup Health.* 2007;49:155-158.
37. D'Auria J, et al. Fatal iodine toxicity following surgical debridement of a hip wound: case report. *J Trauma.* 1990;30:353-355.
38. Dailey JR, et al. Glutaraldehyde keratopathy. *Am J Ophthalmol.* 1993;115:256-258.
39. Dally KA, et al. Formaldehyde exposure in nonoccupational environments. *Arch Environ Health.* 1981;36:277-284.
40. DeBono R, Laitung G. Phenolic household disinfectants—further precautions required. *Burns.* 1997;23:182-185.

41. Decker WJ, et al. Adsorption of drugs and poisons by activated charcoal. *Toxicol Appl Pharmacol.* 1968;13:454-460.

42. Dela Cruz F, et al. Iodine absorption after topical administration. *West J Med.* 1987;146:43-45.

43. Dhamrait RS. Airway obstruction following potassium permanganate ingestion. *Anaesthesia.* 2003;58:606-607.

44. Dickson KF, Caravati EM. Hydrogen peroxide exposure—325 exposures reported to a regional poison control center. *J Toxicol Clin Toxicol.* 1994;32:705-714.

45. Domac FM, et al. Optic neuropathy related to hydrogen peroxide inhalation. *Clin Neuropharmacol.* 2007;30:55-57.

46. Dyck RF, et al. Iodine/iodide toxic reaction: case report with emphasis on the nature of the metabolic acidosis. *CMAJ.* 1979;120:704-706.

47. Earl J. 11-year-old girl's hands covered in third-degree burns after making "slime." http://www.cbsnews.com/news/girls-hands-third-degree-burns-making-slime/. Published 2017. Accessed May 21, 2017.

48. Edwards NA, et al. Death by oral ingestion of iodine. *Emerg Med Australas.* 2005;17:173-177.

49. Eells JT, et al. Formaldehyde poisoning. Rapid metabolism to formic acid. *JAMA.* 1981;246:1237-1238.

50. Ellis H. Joseph Lister: father of modern surgery. *Br J Hosp Med (Lond).* 2012;73:52.

51. Emadi A, Coberly L. Intoxication of a hospitalized patient with an isopropanol-based hand sanitizer. *N Engl J Med.* 2007;356:530-531.

52. Emerson D, Pierce C. A case of a single ingestion of 4% Hibiclens. *Vet Hum Toxicol.* 1988;30:583.

53. Eysseric H, et al. A fatal case of chlorate poisoning: confirmation by ion chromatography of body fluids. *J Forensic Sci.* 2000;45:474-477.

54. Fischman RA, et al. Iodide and negative anion gap. *N Engl J Med.* 1978;298:1035-1036.

55. French LK, et al. Hydrogen peroxide ingestion associated with portal venous gas and treatment with hyperbaric oxygen: a case series and review of the literature. *Clin Toxicol (Phila).* 2010;48:533-538.

56. French RJ, et al. Esophageal stenosis produced by ingestion of bleach: report of two cases. *South Med J.* 1970;63:1140-1144.

57. Giberson TP, et al. Near-fatal hydrogen peroxide ingestion. *Ann Emerg Med.* 1989;18:778-779.

58. Gode GR, et al. Accidental intravenous injection of cetrimide. A case report. *Anaesthesia.* 1975;30:508-510.

59. Goldbloom RB, Goldbloom A. Boric acid poisoning; report of four cases and a review of 109 cases from the world literature. *J Pediatr.* 1953;43:631-643.

60. Goncalo S, et al. Occupational contact dermatitis to glutaraldehyde. *Contact Dermatitis.* 1984;10:183-184.

61. Gordon AS, et al. Seizure disorders and anemia associated with chronic borax intoxication. *CMAJ.* 1973;108:719-721 passim.

62. Gosselin RE, et al. *Clinical Toxicology of Commercial Products.* 5th ed. Baltimore, MD: Williams & Wilkins; 1984.

63. Gross JA, et al. Ethylene oxide neurotoxicity: report of four cases and review of the literature. *Neurology.* 1979;29:978-983.

64. Gupta S, et al. Acute phenol poisoning: a life-threatening hazard of chronic pain relief. *Clin Toxicol (Phila).* 2008;46:250-253.

65. Haddad LM, et al. Phenol poisoning. *JACEP.* 1979;8:267-269.

66. Hamilton RA, Wolf BC. Accidental boric acid poisoning following the ingestion of household pesticide. *J Forensic Sci.* 2007;52:706-708.

67. Hammond K, et al. A complicated hospitalization following dilute ammonium chloride ingestion. *J Med Toxicol.* 2009;5:218-222.

68. Hardin RD, Tedesco FJ. Colitis after Hibiclens enema. *J Clin Gastroenterol.* 1986;8:572-575.

69. Harvey S. Antiseptics and disinfectants; fungicides; ectoparasiticides. In: Gilman AG, et al, eds. *Goodman and Gilman's The Pharmacological Basis of Therapeutics.* 7th ed. New York, NY: Pergamon Press; 1985.

70. Hashimoto T, et al. Marked increases of aminotransferase levels after cresol ingestion. *Am J Emerg Med.* 1998;16:667-668.

71. Hauptmann M, et al. Mortality from solid cancers among workers in formaldehyde industries. *Am J Epidemiol.* 2004;159:1117-1130.

72. Hawley CK, Harsch HH. Gastric outlet obstruction as a late complication of formaldehyde ingestion: a case report. *Am J Gastroenterol.* 1999;94:2289-2291.

73. Helliwell M, Nunn J. Mortality in sodium chlorate poisoning. *Br Med J.* 1979;1:1119.

74. Hemminki K, et al. Spontaneous abortions in hospital staff engaged in sterilising instruments with chemical agents. *Br Med J (Clin Res Ed).* 1982;285:1461-1463.

75. Hendrick DJ, Lane DJ. Occupational formalin asthma. *Br J Ind Med.* 1977;34:11-18.

76. Henry MC, et al. Hydrogen peroxide 3% exposures. *J Toxicol Clin Toxicol.* 1996;34:323-327.

77. Herskowitz J, Rosman NP. Acute hexachlorophene poisoning by mouth in a neonate. *J Pediatr.* 1979;94:495-496.

78. Hilbert G, et al. Circulatory shock in the course of fatal poisoning by ingestion of formalin. *Intensive Care Med.* 1997;23:708.

79. Hirata K, Kurokawa A. Chlorhexidine gluconate ingestion resulting in fatal respiratory distress syndrome. *Vet Hum Toxicol.* 2002;44:89-91.

80. Hitosugi M, et al. A case of fatal benzalkonium chloride poisoning. *Int J Legal Med.* 1998;111:265-266.

81. Hogstedt C, et al. Epidemiologic support for ethylene oxide as a cancer-causing agent. *JAMA.* 1986;255:1575-1578.

82. Holness DL, Nethercott JR. Health status of funeral service workers exposed to formaldehyde. *Arch Environ Health.* 1989;44:222-228.

83. Holzgraefe M, et al. Chronic enteral poisoning caused by potassium permanganate: a case report. *J Toxicol Clin Toxicol.* 1986;24:235-244.

84. Horch R, et al. Phenol burns and intoxications. *Burns.* 1994;20:45-50.

85. Horowitz BZ. Massive hepatic gas embolism from a health food additive. *J Emerg Med.* 2004;26:229-230.

86. Hurst C. Decontamination. In: Sidell FR, et al, eds. *Medical Aspects of Chemical and Biological Warfare, Part I.* Washington, DC: Office of the Surgeon General; 1997.

87. IARC Working Group on the Evaluation of Carcinogenic Risks to Humans. 1,3-Butadiene, ethylene oxide and vinyl halides (vinyl fluoride, vinyl chloride and vinyl bromide). *IARC Monogr Eval Carcinog Risks Hum.* 2008;97:3-471.

88. Iavazzo C, et al. Boric acid for recurrent vulvovaginal candidiasis: the clinical evidence. *J Womens Health (Larchmt).* 2011;20:1245-1255.

89. Ijichi T, et al. Multiple brain gas embolism after ingestion of concentrated hydrogen peroxide. *Neurology.* 1997;48:277-279.

90. Ishigami S, et al. Intravenous chlorhexidine gluconate causing acute respiratory distress syndrome. *J Toxicol Clin Toxicol.* 2001;39:77-80.

91. Ishii Y, et al. A fatal case of acute boric acid poisoning. *J Toxicol Clin Toxicol.* 1993;31:345-352.

92. Jackson RC, et al. Sodium-chlorate poisoning complicated by acute renal failure. *Lancet.* 1961;2:1381-1383.

93. Jansen H, Zeldenrust J. Homicidal chronic sodium chlorate poisoning. *Forensic Sci.* 1972;1:103-105.

94. Jarvis SN, et al. Illness associated with contamination of drinking water supplies with phenol. *Br Med J (Clin Res Ed).* 1985;290:1800-1802.

95. Joanta AE, et al. Iodide excess exerts oxidative stress in some target tissues of the thyroid hormones. *Acta Physiol Hung.* 2006;93:347-359.

96. Johnson TB, Cassidy DD. Unintentional ingestion of potassium permanganate. *Pediatr Emerg Care.* 2004;20:185-187.

97. Kamijo Y, et al. Rabbit syndrome following phenol ingestion. *J Toxicol Clin Toxicol.* 1999;37:509-511.

98. Kamijo Y, et al. Hepatocellular injury with hyperaminotransferasemia after cresol ingestion. *Arch Pathol Lab Med.* 2003;127:364-366.

99. Kanakiriya S, et al. Iodine toxicity treated with hemodialysis and continuous venovenous hemodiafiltration. *Am J Kidney Dis.* 2003;41:702-708.

100. Khameneie KM, et al. Fluconazole and boric acid for treatment of vaginal candidiasis—new words about old issue. *East Afr Med J.* 2013;90:117-123.

101. Kim KH, et al. Exposure to formaldehyde and its potential human health hazards. *J Environ Sci Health C Environ Carcinog Ecotoxicol Rev.* 2011;29:277-299.

102. Knight RK, et al. Suicidal chlorate poisoning treated with peritoneal dialysis. *Br Med J.* 1967;3:601-602.

103. Kochar R, et al. Potassium permanganate induced esophageal stricture. *Human Toxicol.* 1986;5:393-394.

104. Koppel C, et al. Suicidal ingestion of formalin with fatal complications. *Intensive Care Med.* 1990;16:212-214.

105. Kraut JA, Madias NE. Serum anion gap: its uses and limitations in clinical medicine. *Clin J Am Soc Nephrol.* 2007;2:162-174.

106. Kurt TL, et al. Fatal iatrogenic iodine toxicity in a nine-week old infant. *J Toxicol Clin Toxicol.* 1996;34:231-234.

107. Kuypers MI, et al. A case of methemoglobinemia after ingestion of a chlorhexidine in alcohol solution in an alcohol-dependent patient. *Clin Toxicol (Phila).* 2016;54:604.

108. Landrigan PJ, et al. Ethylene oxide: an overview of toxicologic and epidemiologic research. *Am J Ind Med.* 1984;6:103-115.

109. Lavelle KJ, et al. Iodine absorption in burn patients treated topically with povidone-iodine. *Clin Pharmacol Ther.* 1975;17:355-362.

110. Lee DB, et al. Haematological complications of chlorate poisoning. *Br Med J.* 1970;2:31-32.

111. Lee E, et al. Severe chlorate poisoning successfully treated with methylene blue. *J Emerg Med.* 2013;44:381-384.

112. Leiken J, et al. Fatality from intravenous use of hydrogen peroxide for home "superoxygenation therapy" [abstract]. *Vet Hum Toxicol.* 1993;35:342.

113. Lewin JF, Cleary WT. An accidental death caused by the absorption of phenol through skin. A case report. *Forensic Sci Int.* 1982;19:177-179.

114. Lifshitz M, et al. Fatal potassium permanganate intoxication in an infant. *J Toxicol Clin Toxicol.* 1999;37:801-802.

115. Linden CH, et al. Acute ingestions of boric acid. *J Toxicol Clin Toxicol.* 1986;24:269-279.

116. Linder N, et al. Topical iodine-containing antiseptics and subclinical hypothyroidism in preterm infants. *J Pediatr.* 1997;131:434-439.

117. Litovitz TL, et al. Clinical manifestations of toxicity in a series of 784 boric acid ingestions. *Am J Emerg Med.* 1988;6:209-213.

118. Liu FC, et al. Chemical burn caused by povidone-iodine alcohol solution—a case report. *Acta Anaesthesiol Sin.* 2003;41:93-96.

119. Liu TM, et al. Acute paraplegia caused by an accidental ingestion of hydrogen peroxide. *Am J Emerg Med.* 2007;25:90-92.

120. Loomis TA. Formaldehyde toxicity. *Arch Pathol Lab Med.* 1979;103:321-324.

121. Lowell JA, et al. Mercury poisoning associated with high-dose hepatitis-B immune globulin administration after liver transplantation for chronic hepatitis B. *Liver Transpl Surg.* 1996;2:475-478.

122. Lung D, Clancy C. "Boiled lobster" rash of acute boric acid toxicity. *Clin Toxicol (Phila)*. 2009;47:432.

123. Luu TA, et al. Portal vein gas embolism from hydrogen peroxide ingestion. *Ann Emerg Med*. 1992;21:1391-1393.

124. Madrid PA, et al. Building integrated mental health and medical programs for vulnerable populations post-disaster: connecting children and families to a medical home. *Prehosp Disaster Med*. 2008;23:314-321.

125. Mahomedy MC, et al. Methaemoglobinaemia following treatment dispensed by witch doctors. Two cases of potassium permanganate poisoning. *Anaesthesia*. 1975;30:190-193.

126. Mao YC, et al. Acute hemolysis following iodine tincture ingestion. *Hum Exp Toxicol*. 2011;30:1716-1719.

127. Marks JG Jr. Allergic contact dermatitis to povidone-iodine. *J Am Acad Dermatol*. 1982;6(4, pt 1):473-475.

128. Marsh GM, et al. Pharyngeal cancer mortality among chemical plant workers exposed to formaldehyde. *Toxicol Ind Health*. 2002;18:257-268.

129. Martinez AJ, et al. Acute hexachlorophene encephalopathy: clinico-neuropathological correlation. *Acta Neuropathol*. 1974;28:93-103.

130. Massano G, et al. Striking aminotransferase rise after chlorhexidine self-poisoning. *Lancet*. 1982;1:289.

131. Memarzadeh F, et al. Corneal and conjunctival toxicity from hydrogen peroxide: a patient with chronic self-induced injury. *Ophthalmology*. 2004;111:1546-1549.

132. Meyer CT, et al. Hydrogen peroxide colitis: a report of three patients. *J Clin Gastroenterol*. 1981;3:31-35.

133. Middleton SJ, et al. Haemorrhagic pancreatitis—a cause of death in severe potassium permanganate poisoning. *Postgrad Med J*. 1990;66:657-658.

134. Momblano P, et al. Metabolic acidosis induced by cetrimonium bromide. *Lancet*. 1984;2:1045.

135. Monteiro-Riviere NA, et al. Efficacy of topical phenol decontamination strategies on severity of acute phenol chemical burns and dermal absorption: in vitro and in vivo studies in pig skin. *Toxicol Ind Health*. 2001;17:95-104.

136. Moon JM, et al. Hemorrhagic gastritis and gas emboli after ingesting 3% hydrogen peroxide. *J Emerg Med*. 2006;30:403-406.

137. Mucklow ES. Accidental feeding of a dilute antiseptic solution (chlorhexidine 0.05% with cetrimide 1%) to five babies. *Hum Toxicol*. 1988;7:567-569.

138. Mullins ME, Beltran JT. Acute cerebral gas embolism from hydrogen peroxide ingestion successfully treated with hyperbaric oxygen. *J Toxicol Clin Toxicol*. 1998;36:253-256.

139. Mullins ME, Horowitz BZ. Iatrogenic neonatal mercury poisoning from Mercurochrome treatment of a large omphalocele. *Clin Pediatr (Phila)*. 1999;38:111-112.

140. Mutlu H, et al. Cranial MR imaging findings of potassium chlorate intoxication. *AJNR Am J Neuroradiol*. 2003;24:1396-1398.

141. Naderi AS, Palmer BF. Successful treatment of a rare case of boric acid overdose with hemodialysis. *Am J Kidney Dis*. 2006;48:e95-e97.

142. Nahlieli O, et al. Povidone-iodine related burns. *Burns*. 2001;27:185-188.

143. Norback D. Skin and respiratory symptoms from exposure to alkaline glutaraldehyde in medical services. *Scand J Work Environ Health*. 1988;14:366-371.

144. O'Grady J, Jarecsni E. Sodium chlorate poisoning. *Br J Clin Pract*. 1971;25:38-39.

145. O'Sullivan K, Taylor M. Chronic boric acid poisoning in infants. *Arch Dis Child*. 1983;58:737-739.

146. Ohnishi A, Murai Y. Polyneuropathy due to ethylene oxide, propylene oxide, and butylene oxide. *Environ Res*. 1993;60:242-247.

147. Okan F, et al. A rare and preventable cause of respiratory insufficiency: ingestion of benzalkonium chloride. *Pediatr Emerg Care*. 2007;23:404-406.

148. Okano M, et al. Anaphylactic symptoms due to chlorhexidine gluconate. *Arch Dermatol*. 1989;125:50-52.

149. Olsen JH, Dossing M. Formaldehyde induced symptoms in day care centers. *Am Ind Hyg Assoc J*. 1982;43:366-370.

150. Ong KL, et al. Potassium permanganate poisoning—a rare cause of fatal self poisoning. *J Accid Emerg Med*. 1997;14:43-45.

151. Ong TH, et al. A case report of occupational asthma due to glutaraldehyde exposure. *Ann Acad Med Singapore*. 2004;33:275-278.

152. Orringer EP, Mattern WD. Formaldehyde-induced hemolysis during chronic hemodialysis. *N Engl J Med*. 1976;294:1416-1420.

153. OSHA. Best practices for the safe use of glutaraldehyde in health care. https://www.osha.gov/Publications/glutaraldehyde.pdf. Published 2006. Accessed June 1, 2017.

154. Palczynski C, et al. Occupational asthma and rhinitis due to glutaraldehyde: changes in nasal lavage fluid after specific inhalatory challenge test. *Allergy*. 2001;56:1186-1191.

155. Papafragkou S, et al. Treatment of portal venous gas embolism with hyperbaric oxygen after accidental ingestion of hydrogen peroxide: a case report and review of the literature. *J Emerg Med*. 2012;43:e21-e23.

156. Partanen T. Formaldehyde exposure and respiratory cancer—a meta-analysis of the epidemiologic evidence. *Scand J Work Environ Health*. 1993;19:8-15.

157. Pennington JA. A review of iodine toxicity reports. *J Am Diet Assoc*. 1990;90:1571-1581.

158. Pietsch J, Meakins JL. Complications of povidone-iodine absorption in topically treated burn patients. *Lancet*. 1976;1:280-282.

159. Pike DG, et al. A re-evaluation of the dangers of Clorox ingestion. *J Pediatr*. 1963;63:303-305.

160. Pinnas JL, Meinke GC. Other aldehydes. In: Sullivan JB, Krieger GR, eds. *Hazardous Material Toxicology*. Baltimore, MD: Williams & Wilkins; 1992.

161. Porter JA. Letter: acute respiratory distress following formalin inhalation. *Lancet*. 1975;2:603-604.

162. Pritchett S, et al. Accidental ingestion of 35% hydrogen peroxide. *Can J Gastroenterol*. 2007;21:665-667.

163. Prutting SM, Cerveny JD. Boric acid vaginal suppositories: a brief review. *Infect Dis Obstet Gynecol*. 1998;6:191-194.

164. Pullin TG, et al. Decontamination of the skin of swine following phenol exposure: a comparison of the relative efficacy of water versus polyethylene glycol/industrial methylated spirits. *Toxicol Appl Pharmacol*. 1978;43:199-206.

165. Pun KK, et al. Acute intravascular hemolysis due to accidental formalin intoxication during hemodialysis. *Clin Nephrol*. 1984;21:188-190.

166. Rackoff WR, Merton DF. Gas embolism after ingestion of hydrogen peroxide. *Pediatrics*. 1990;85:593-594.

167. Raja DS, Sultana B. Potential health hazards for students exposed to formaldehyde in the gross anatomy laboratory. *J Environ Health*. 2012;74:36-40.

168. Ranghino A, et al. A case of acute sodium chlorate self-poisoning successfully treated without conventional therapy. *Nephrol Dial Transplant*. 2006;21:2971-2974.

169. Rath T, Meissl G. Induction of hyperthyroidism in burn patients treated topically with povidone-iodine. *Burns Incl Therm Inj*. 1988;14:320-322.

170. Rees TD, Orth CF. Oral ulcerations with use of hydrogen peroxide. *J Periodontol*. 1986;57:689-692.

171. Restuccio A, et al. Fatal ingestion of boric acid in an adult. *Am J Emerg Med*. 1992;10:545-547.

172. Rideout K, et al. Considering risks to healthcare workers from glutaraldehyde alternatives in high-level disinfection. *J Hosp Infect*. 2005;59:4-11.

173. Rider SP, et al. Cerebral air gas embolism from concentrated hydrogen peroxide ingestion. *Clin Toxicol (Phila)*. 2008;46:815-818.

174. Robertson P, et al. Thyrotoxicosis related to iodine toxicity in a paediatric burn patient. *Intensive Care Med*. 2002;28:1369.

175. Robitaille C, Boulet LP. Occupational asthma after exposure to ortho-phthalaldehyde (OPA). *Occup Environ Med*. 2015;72:381.

176. Rohyans J, et al. Mercury toxicity following merthiolate ear irrigations. *J Pediatr*. 1984;104:311-313.

177. Roush GC, et al. Nasopharyngeal cancer, sinonasal cancer, and occupations related to formaldehyde: a case-control study. *J Natl Cancer Inst*. 1987;79:1221-1224.

178. Rubenstein AD, Musher DM. Epidemic boric acid poisoning simulating staphylococcal toxic epidermal necrolysis of the newborn infant: Ritter's disease. *J Pediatr*. 1970;77:884-887.

179. Russell AD. Glutaraldehyde: current status and uses. *Infect Control Hosp Epidemiol*. 1994;15:724-733.

180. Rutala WA, Weber DJ; Centers for Disease Control (US). *Guideline for Disinfection and Sterilization in Healthcare Facilities, 2008*. Washington, DC: Centers for Disease Control (US); 2008.

181. Salinas E, et al. Acute ethylene oxide intoxication. *Drug Intell Clin Pharm*. 1981;15:384-386.

182. Sansone J, et al. Unintentional ingestion of 60% hydrogen peroxide by a six-year-old child. *J Toxicol Clin Toxicol*. 2004;42:197-199.

183. Schroder CM, et al. Necrotizing toxic contact dermatitis of the scalp from hydrogen peroxide [in German]. *Hautarzt*. 2008;59:148-150.

184. Selvaggi G, et al. The role of iodine in antisepsis and wound management: a reappraisal. *Acta Chir Belg*. 2003;103:241-247.

185. Senchak AJ, et al. Oropharyngeal and laryngeal burn resulting from exposure to endoscope disinfectant: a case report. *Ear Nose Throat J*. 2008;87:580-581.

186. Shaffer MP, Belsito DV. Allergic contact dermatitis from glutaraldehyde in health-care workers. *Contact Dermatitis*. 2000;43:150-156.

187. Shaw A, et al. Gas embolism produced by hydrogen peroxide. *N Engl J Med*. 1967;277:238-241.

188. Sheibani S, Gerson LB. Chemical colitis. *J Clin Gastroenterol*. 2008;42:115-121.

189. Sherman SJ, et al. Cerebral infarction immediately after ingestion of hydrogen peroxide solution. *Stroke*. 1994;25:1065-1067.

190. Shmunes E, Levy EJ. Quaternary ammonium compound contact dermatitis from a deodorant. *Arch Dermatol*. 1972;105:91-93.

191. Singelmann E, Steffen C. Increased erythrocyte rigidity in chlorate poisoning. *J Clin Pathol*. 1983;36:719.

192. Sleigh JW, Linter SP. Hazards of hydrogen peroxide. *Br Med J (Clin Res Ed)*. 1985;291:1706.

193. Smerdely P, et al. Topical iodine-containing antiseptics and neonatal hypothyroidism in very-low-birthweight infants. *Lancet*. 1989;2:661-664.

194. Sneddon I. Dermatitis in an intermittent haemodialysis unit. *Br Med J*. 1968;1:183-184.

195. Southwood T, et al. Ingestion of potassium permanganate crystals by a three-year-old boy. *Med J Aust*. 1987;146:639-640.

196. Spiller HA, et al. A five year evaluation of acute exposures to phenol disinfectant (26%). *J Toxicol Clin Toxicol*. 1993;31:307-313.

197. Stavrou A, et al. Accidental self-poisoning by sodium chlorate weed-killer. *Practitioner*. 1978;221:397-399.

198. Steenland K, et al. Mortality analyses in a cohort of 18 235 ethylene oxide exposed workers: follow up extended from 1987 to 1998. *Occup Environ Med*. 2004;61:2-7.

199. Steenland K, et al. Mortality among workers exposed to ethylene oxide. *N Engl J Med.* 1991;324:1402-1407.

200. Steffen C, Wetzel E. Chlorate poisoning: mechanism of toxicity. *Toxicology.* 1993;84:217-231.

201. Stein KM, et al. Toxic alopecia from ingestion of boric acid. *Arch Dermatol.* 1973;108:95-97.

202. Stonehill AA, et al. Buffered glutaraldehyde—a new chemical sterilization solution. *Am J Hosp Pharm.* 1963;20:458-465.

203. Strubelt O, et al. Experimental studies on the acute cardiovascular toxicity of formalin and its antidotal treatment. *J Toxicol Clin Toxicol.* 1990;28:221-233.

204. Swaen GM, et al. Mortality study update of ethylene oxide workers in chemical manufacturing: a 15 year update. *J Occup Environ Med.* 2009;51:714-723.

205. Tabor E, et al. Corneal damage due to eye contact with chlorhexidine gluconate. *JAMA.* 1989;261:557-558.

206. Teshima D, et al. Clinical management of boric acid ingestion: pharmacokinetic assessment of efficacy of hemodialysis for treatment of acute boric acid poisoning. *J Pharmacobiodyn.* 1992;15:287-294.

207. Teshima D, et al. Usefulness of forced diuresis for acute boric acid poisoning in an adult. *J Clin Pharm Ther.* 2001;26:387-390.

208. Unlu RE, et al. Phenol intoxication in a child. *J Craniofac Surg.* 2004;15:1010-1013.

209. Valdes-Dapena MA, Arey JB. Boric acid poisoning: three fatal cases with pancreatic inclusions and a review of the literature. *J Pediatr.* 1962;61:531-546.

210. van Berkel M, de Wolff FA. Survival after acute benzalkonium chloride poisoning. *Hum Toxicol.* 1988;7:191-193.

211. Vander Heide SJ, Seamon JP. Resolution of delayed altered mental status associated with hydrogen peroxide ingestion following hyperbaric oxygen therapy. *Acad Emerg Med.* 2003;10:998-1000.

212. Vorherr H, et al. Vaginal absorption of povidone-iodine. *JAMA.* 1980;244:2628-2629.

213. Wallgren H. Relative intoxicating effects on rats of ethyl, propyl and butyl alcohols. *Acta Pharmacol Toxicol (Copenh).* 1960;16:217-222.

214. Warner MA, Harper JV. Cardiac dysrhythmias associated with chemical peeling with phenol. *Anesthesiology.* 1985;62:366-367.

215. Watt BE, et al. Hydrogen peroxide poisoning. *Toxicol Rev.* 2004;23:51-57.

216. Weeks RS, Ravitch MM. Esophageal injury by liquid chlorine bleach: experimental study. *J Pediatr.* 1969;74:911-916.

217. Weiner SG. Changing dispensers may prevent intoxication from isopropanol and ethyl alcohol-based hand sanitizers. *Ann Emerg Med.* 2007;50:486.

218. Wong LC, et al. Boric acid poisoning: report of 11 cases. *CMAJ.* 1964;90:1018-1023.

219. Wu ML, et al. Concentrated cresol intoxication. *Vet Hum Toxicol.* 1998;40:341-343.

220. Yanagawa Y, et al. A case of attempted suicide from the ingestion of formalin. *Clin Toxicol (Phila).* 2007;45:72-76.

221. Young RJ, et al. Fatal acute hepatorenal failure following potassium permanganate ingestion. *Hum Exp Toxicol.* 1996;15:259-261.

Camphor   Naphthalene   Paradichlorobenzene

Many different products have been used as moth repellents. In the United States, paradichlorobenzene has largely replaced both camphor and naphthalene as the most common active component of moth repellent and moth flakes because of its lower toxicity. However, life-threatening camphor and naphthalene toxicity still occurs, especially in immigrant communities, from exposures to imported camphor or naphthalene-containing products.[3,48,65,80] Therefore, toxicity of camphor, naphthalene, and paradichlorobenzene all remain possible following exposure to moth repellents.

CAMPHOR

History and Epidemiology

Camphor (2-bormanone, 2-camphonone), a cyclic ketone of the terpene group, is an essential oil originally distilled from the bark of the camphor tree, *Cinnamomum camphora*. Today, camphor is synthesized from the hydrocarbon pinene, a derivative of turpentine oil. Camphor has been used for centuries as an aphrodisiac, fumigant, contraceptive, abortifacient, suppressor of lactation, analeptic, cardiac stimulant and antiseptic.[1,56,72,96,108] Camphor is a commonly used ingredient found in many nonprescription remedies for cold symptoms, cold sores, and in muscle liniments.[2,75,77,93] Camphor is also rarely abused as a stimulant (Chap. 42).[70]

Camphorated oil and camphorated spirits contain varying concentrations of camphor. Historically, most camphorated oil was prepared as a 20% weight (of solute) per weight (of solvent) (w/w) solution of camphor with cottonseed oil, and most camphorated spirits contained 10% w/w camphor with isopropyl alcohol. Toxicity and death following ingestion of camphorated oil, which was confused with castor oil and cod liver oil, prompted the FDA to ban the nonprescription sale of camphorated oil in the United States in 1980.[76,123,126] The FDA ban of camphorated oil was followed in 1983 by a restriction on camphor concentration to less than 11% in nonprescription camphor-containing products.[126] However, camphorated oil is still used as a herbal remedy and muscle liniment, and products containing greater than 11% camphor can be purchased in local stores of various ethnic communities in the United States and in other countries.[48,65,118]

Common camphor-containing products include ointments used for herpes simplex on the lips (usually <1% camphor), muscle liniments, rubefacients (usually 4%–7% camphor), and camphor spirits (usually 10% camphor). Paregoric, camphorated tincture of opium, contains a combination of anhydrous morphine (0.4 mg/mL), ethanol (46%), benzoic acid (4 mg/mL), and a small amount of camphor.[69] For industrial uses, strengths up to 100% camphor are sold legally in the United States. Occupational exposures to camphor occur during the manufacture of plastic, celluloid, lacquer, varnish, explosives, embalming fluids, numerous pharmaceuticals and cosmetics.[69]

Although products containing lower concentrations of camphor are implicitly safer, life-threatening toxicity and death still result from misuse or intentional overdose. Most reported cases of acute camphor poisoning are unintentional ingestions of camphor-containing products mistaken for other medications or therapeutic misadventures from nonprescription products, including home remedies.[3,50,65,99,119] According to data obtained by the American Association of Poison Control Centers (AAPCC), there are approximately 13,000 exposures to camphor-containing products each year, with a majority of the exposure, approximately 80%, occurring in children under the age of 5 years (Chap. 130).

Prior to the FDA ban of camphorated oil and restriction on camphor content in nonprescription products, there was a high incidence of systemic manifestations such as vertigo, confusion, delirium, seizures and coma reported in children younger than 5 years.[131] In a group of 530 patients with camphor exposures, 15% presented with systemic effects and 4% had seizures.[41,93] Unfortunately, limited data are available with regard to the true incidence of symptoms associated with camphor toxicity since the FDA ruling in 1983. According to AAPCC data, 8 reported deaths (1 child and 7 adults) were attributable to camphor over the past 25 years. Although a majority of the patients with unintentional exposures remain asymptomatic and do not present to a health care facility, significant morbidity from unintentional camphor exposures continue to occur in children.[3,48,65,118] The public health implication of camphor exposure in children is of great concern because of the simultaneous lack of therapeutic value of their products and their potential life-threatening toxicity.

Pharmacology

Camphor is a colorless glassy solid. Its pharmacologic activity is not well studied, and its mechanism of action remains unclear. Therapeutic use of camphor as an expectorant is limited, and its anti-infective property is being explored. Camphor, a major component in the essential oil of many plant species, demonstrates bacteriostatic and fungistatic activities against select microorganisms (eg, *Enterococcus hirae*, *Staphylococcus aureus*, and *Candida albicans*) in several in vitro studies.[64,105,120,132] Imine derivatives of camphor under investigation have antiviral effects against influenza virus (A and H1N1 subtypes) through inhibition of viral hemagglutinin.[113-115] No therapeutic benefit of camphor is proven in any well-controlled clinical trials although camphor provides limited local analgesic and antipruritic effects, much safer alternatives are available for these indications.

Pharmacokinetics and Toxicokinetics

There are limited pharmacokinetic and toxicokinetic data for camphor. Ingestion is the most common route of exposure that results in significant camphor toxicity.[3,65,70,80] However, toxicity also occurs following inhalation, intranasal instillation, intraperitoneal administration, dermal, and from transplacental transfer, resulting in fetal death.[48,65,97,110] Camphor is a highly lipophilic compound that is rapidly absorbed from the gastrointestinal tract and is detected in the blood within 15 to 20 minutes following ingestion.[93,101] Because of the lack of experimental data, the bioavailability from each route of exposure is unknown. A peak blood camphor concentration was achieved in 90 minutes when rats were administered an oral dose of 1 g/kg.[35] A significant amount of camphor is absorbed through normal skin. Dermal absorption of camphor is slow, but can produce systemic toxicity up to 72 hours following exposure.[48,65] The volume of distribution is estimated at 2 to 4 L/kg with protein binding of approximately 61%.[69,70]

Camphor is predominantly metabolized in the liver and eliminated by the kidneys. Up to 59% of the camphor is eliminated in urine as glucuronides, but unchanged camphor (<1%) and other oxidative metabolites are also found in the urine.[70,103,108] Five inactive metabolites are produced by hydroxylation of a methylene group (the predominant pathway) and reduction of the oxo group.[103] Inactive metabolites, 3-hydroxycamphor, 5-hydroxycamphor (major metabolite), 8-hydroxycamphor, 9-hydroxycamphor, and borneol, are either conjugated with glucuronic acid or further oxidized and eliminated by the kidneys.[70,103] The exact site of camphor metabolism is unknown, but CYP 2A6 and NADPH-P450 reductase are known to be involved.[49,84] A volunteer study in which 200 mg of camphor with Tween 80 as a solvent (10 mL) or without the solvent was ingested demonstrated, in humans, plasma elimination half-lives of 93 minutes and 167 minutes, respectively following oral administration.[69] A comparable elimination half-life of 144 minutes was found in an animal model.[35] Small amounts of camphor are eliminated by exhalation, as noted by characteristic breath odor but no studies have assessed the significance of this route of elimination.[70,75]

The reported toxic dose of camphor is highly variable.[50,112] A potential lethal dose of 50 to 500 mg/kg of camphor is often cited for humans.[41,80,93] Yet, as little as 1 g of camphor resulted in death in a 19-month-old infant, whereas up to 42 g of camphor was ingested by an adult who recovered.[2,112] There are insufficient data to suggest a clear toxic dose range of camphor. However, there is evidence to suggest that camphor causes life-threatening toxicity at low doses (estimated exposure of 700–1,500 mg) based on a series of case reports in both adults and children.[75,93,112,118]

Workplace standards determined by the Occupational Safety and Health Administration (OSHA) has set the permissible exposure limit (PEL) at 2 mg/m³.[125] The American Conference of Governmental Industrial Hygienists (ACGIH) threshold limit value (TLV) is 12 mg/m³ (2 ppm), whereas the short-term exposure limit (STEL) is 19 mg/m³ (3 ppm). The National Institute for Occupational Safety and Health (NIOSH) Immediately Dangerous To Life or Health Concentration (IDLH) is 200 mg/m³.[124]

Pathophysiology

The mechanism of toxicity of camphor is unknown. Camphor is an irritant. Pathologic changes following ingestion include cerebral edema, neuronal degeneration, fatty changes in the liver, centrilobular congestion of the liver, and hemorrhagic lesions in the skin, gastrointestinal tract, and kidneys.[62,112,139]

Clinical Manifestations

Exposure to camphor can often be detected by its characteristic aromatic odor (Chap. 25). Ingestion of camphor typically produces oropharyngeal irritation, nausea, vomiting, and abdominal pain. Generalized tonic–clonic seizures usually occur within 1 to 2 hours of ingestion.[13,17] The onset of systemic toxicity, particularly CNS toxicity, occurs as early as 5 minutes after ingestion.[30,33,75,112] Most seizures are brief and self-limited, although some patients experience multiple seizures, including status epilepticus.[43,48,68,111] Delayed seizures are reported occurring up to 9 hours following ingestion and up to 72 hours following dermal exposure.[49,105] Central nervous system (CNS) depression is common, but camphor rarely compromises respiratory function.[29,68] Other neurologic manifestations include headache, lightheadedness, transient visual changes, confusion, myoclonus, and hyperreflexia.[65,102] Psychiatric manifestations include agitation, anxiety, and hallucinations.[51,65,68] Dermal effects include flushing and petechiae.[29,55] Camphor does not typically cause life-threatening cardiovascular effects, although a case of myocarditis is reported.[19] Deaths are reported secondary to status epilepticus.[16,29,77,110] Transient elevation of hepatic aminotransferases concentrations were observed in acute ingestion of camphor.[62,101,110] Chronic administration of camphor to a child caused altered mental status and elevated hepatic aminotransferase concentrations suggestive of Reye syndrome.[62] When hepatotoxicity occurs, however, camphor does not typically produce morphologic changes in the liver characteristic of Reye syndrome. Albuminuria was also reported.[112]

Camphor crosses the placenta. Both fetal demise and delivery of healthy neonates are reported in mothers following intentional and unintentional ingestion.[19,101,139] Specific dose-related toxicity cannot be determined from these case reports.

Inhalational and dermal exposures to camphor typically result in mucous membrane and dermal irritation, respectively.[47]

Diagnostic Testing

No specific diagnostic test is available or indicated when managing patients with camphor toxicity. Camphor and its metabolites can be identified in blood and urine,[70,103] but these tests are not clinically useful.[53,70,103]

Management

Gastric decontamination is not well studied in patients with acute camphor ingestion. Camphor is rapidly absorbed from the gastrointestinal tract because of its high lipophilicity and vomiting is common. The benefit of gastrointestinal decontamination rapidly diminishes with time following acute ingestion. Gastric lavage was commonly performed in patients with acute camphor ingestions, but it is no longer routinely performed or recommended.[41,93] The utility of activated charcoal in acute camphor ingestion is unknown. One animal study showed the administration of activated charcoal (2 g/kg; 2:1 activated charcoal to toxin ratio) immediately following camphor ingestion did not alter the gastrointestinal absorption of camphor.[35] There are no human data in support of the use of activated charcoal in camphor ingestions. It remains reasonable to administer activated charcoal following a large recent ingestion if no contraindications exist.

Patients who should be evaluated in a health care facility after an acute ingestion include those who have signs or symptoms consistent with camphor toxicity, those who ingest more than 30 mg/kg of camphor, suicidal patients, and any patient with a significant occupational exposure.[77]

There is no antidote for camphor. Most patients survive with supportive care. Although the management of camphor-induced seizures is not well studied, the first-line therapy recommended for camphor-induced seizures are a benzodiazepines. Repeat doses of benzodiazepines are often needed to control seizures. If benzodiazepines fail to control seizures, other sedative-hypnotics, including propofol or pentobarbital, should be administered. Case reports suggest that most patients who develop life-threatening camphor toxicity develop symptoms within a few hours postexposure. Based on this, an observation period of at least 4 hours is reasonable following a potentially toxic ingestion. In case reports, hemodialysis with a lipid dialysate and either hemoperfusion using an Amberlite resin or charcoal hemoperfusion successfully removed camphor.[42,68,69,78] However, isolated lipid hemodialysis or lipid dialysis in combination with hemoperfusion is neither routinely recommended nor widely available.

NAPHTHALENE

History and Epidemiology

Naphthalene, an aromatic bicyclic hydrocarbon, is commonly found in products such as moth repellents, toilet-bowl and diaper-pail deodorizers, and soil fumigants.[116] It is the single most abundant component of coal tar, approximately 11% by weight, and is used in the manufacture of numerous commercial and industrial products.[25,116] Both crude oil and refined products such as gasoline and diesel fuels contain naphthalene.

Historically, naphthalene toxicity resulted from its use as an antihelminthic and an antiseptic.[111] In more recent years, unintentional and intentional ingestions of mothballs containing naphthalene became the major etiology of naphthalene toxicity.[73,108,117,138] A single naphthalene mothball can contain between 0.5 and 5 g of naphthalene depending on its size.[4] Toilet-bowl and diaper-pail deodorizers containing naphthalene also cause toxicity.[29,148] Chronic exposure to naphthalene occurs in occupational setting with variable amounts of exposure depending on the industry. The most common use of naphthalene is in the production of phthalic anhydride, a compound used in chemical feedstock.[46] Other industrial uses of naphthalene include carbamate insecticides, dye intermediates, synthetic resins, bathroom (urinal) air fresheners, fuel additives, plasticizers, and the manufacture of other chemicals.[46,116] Naphthalene is also generated as a by-product of combustion and is present in ambient air at low concentrations.[46]

Most unintentional exposures to naphthalene-containing moth repellents occur in children and do not cause life-threatening toxicity. According to data from the AAPCC, there are 1,200 to 1,900 naphthalene exposures annually. During the past 25 years, one death occurred from suicide whereas reports of "major toxicity" occurred rarely (Chap. 130). Mothball vapors are also intentionally inhaled as a form of "recreational" inhalant abuse.[71,138]

Pharmacology, Pharmacokinetics, and Toxicokinetics

Naphthalene is a white, flakey crystalline solid with a noxious odor. Synonyms include white tar and tar camphor. Naphthalene toxicity is reported following ingestion, dermal application, and inhalation.[34,106,129] The absorption of naphthalene is not well studied. Naphthalene metabolism is complex and varies considerably among species and different anatomical regions.[21] For instance, an in vitro study using human liver microsomes showed that multiple CYP450 enzymes are involved in naphthalene metabolism: 1A1, 1A2, 1B1, 2A6, 2B6, 2C19, 2D6, 2E1, and 3A4.[27] Metabolic pathways involve several intermediates and generate multiple reactive metabolites: 1,2-naphthalene oxide, 1,4-naphthoquinone, 1,2-naphthoquinone, and 1,2-dihydroxy-3,4-epoxy-1,2,3,4-tetrahydronaphthalene[4,21,22] (Fig. 102–1).

Naphthalene is initially metabolized to an unstable epoxide intermediate, naphthalene 1,2-oxide, in both human and animals.[4,22,116] 1,2-Naphthalene oxide reacts with cellular components such as DNA and protein to form covalent adducts or can be spontaneously converted to 1-naphthol and 2-naphthol, which undergo glucuronidation or sulfation to form conjugates that are subsequently eliminated in urine.[4,21,22] Glutathione-*S*-transferase and glutathione play an important role in detoxification of 1,2-naphthalene oxide by converting the reactive epoxide to nonreactive mercapturic acid metabolites.[21,22,76] The depletion of glutathione prior to naphthalene exposure increases acute injury in lung Clara cells, one of the target organs of naphthalene toxicity in mice.[94,95]

Reactive hepatic metabolites, 1-naphthol (α-naphthol), 1,2-naphthoquinone, and 1.4-naphthoquinone, are cytotoxins that deplete intracellular glutathione stores and generate reactive oxygen species.[4,116,147] They are responsible for the oxidative stress leading to naphthalene-induced hemolysis and methemoglobinemia.

The toxic amount of naphthalene reported is highly variable. As little as one naphthalene mothball resulted in hemolysis in an infant.[40,148] Workplace standards include the OSHA PEL, which is 50 mg/m³ (10 ppm), ACGIH TLV, which is 52 mg/m³ (10 ppm), and the ACGIH STEL, which is 79 mg/m³ (15 ppm); NIOSH IDLH is 250 ppm (US Department of Labor OSHA).[125]

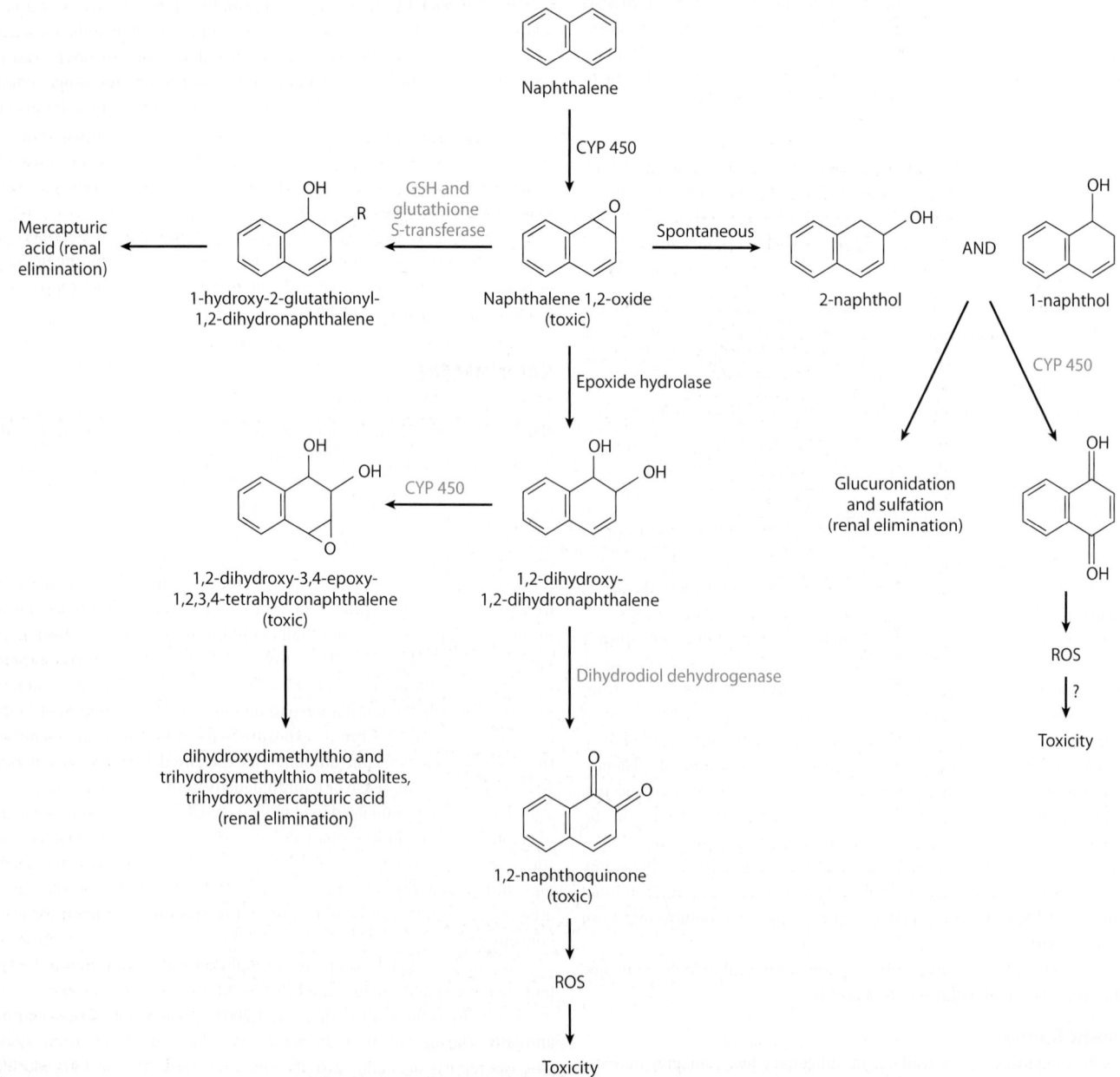

FIGURE 102–1. Hepatic metabolism of naphthalene and its respective metabolites. GSH = reduced glutathione; ROS = reactive oxygen species; R=2-glutathionyl. *(Data from Buckpitt, et al 2002; Bogen, et al 2008; Agency for Toxic Substances and Disease Registry 2005.)*

Pathophysiology

Naphthalene-induced (via oxidative metabolites: 1-naphthol, 1,2-naphtho-quinone, and 1,4-naphthoquinone) hemolysis and methemoglobinemia result when physiologic compensatory mechanisms to oxidative stress are overwhelmed. It is important to understand how oxidant stress affects erythrocytes and the normal mechanisms that erythrocytes use to prevent and reverse the effects of oxidant stress.

Oxidant stressors cause methemoglobinemia and/or hemolysis. When oxidant stress causes an iron atom from any of the 4 globin chains of hemo-globin to be oxidized from the ferrous state (Fe^{2+}) to the ferric state (Fe^{3+}), methemoglobin is formed (Chap. 124). When oxidant stress causes hemo-globin denaturation, the heme groups and the globin chains dissociate and precipitate in the erythrocyte, forming Heinz bodies. An erythrocyte with denatured hemoglobin is more susceptible to hemolysis (Chap. 20).

Hemolysis and methemoglobinemia can occur independently or simul-taneously in patients with either normal or deficient glucose-6-phosphate dehydrogenase (G6PD) activity.[58,129,148] Patients with G6PD deficiency are at much greater risk of hemolysis rather than methemoglobinemia because of their decreased glutathione stores.[79,129,147] Glucose-6-phosphate dehydro-genase affects all races, but is most prevalent in patients of African, Medi-terranean, and Asian descent. The gene that codes for G6PD is X-linked; consequently, men are affected more often than women.

Infants are also at increased risk of methemoglobinemia because fetal hemoglobin is more susceptible to the formation of methemoglobin. Moreover, cytochrome-b_5 reductase (a nicotinamide adenine dinucleotide {NADH}-dependent enzyme) activity in infants is approximately 50% lower than adults, impairing the reduction of methemoglobin to hemoglobin.[45,54,63]

Injuries to other organs, that is, eyes, lungs, and liver, occurred in ani-mals after exposure to naphthalene.[39,89,98,116,130] However, there is a significant interspecies variation in the degree of toxicity. Human data on organ toxicity beyond hematologic effects of naphthalene are limited. A few case reports link the development of cataracts to occupational exposure; however, the causal relationship remains questionable.[89] Oxidative destruction of lens proteins is theorized to result in cataract formation.[116] Animal studies show that oxidative stress from naphthalene results in pulmonary epithelial necro-sis and hepatic injury by lipid peroxidation.[39,98,116] However, there is no report of hepatotoxicity or pulmonary toxicity in humans following naphthalene exposure.

Clinical Manifestations

Clinically significant toxicity from naphthalene exposure occurs rarely. How-ever, if present, both acute and chronic exposures to naphthalene result in similar toxicity.[29,86,147] Ingestion and inhalational exposures to naphthalene commonly cause headache, nausea, vomiting, diarrhea, abdominal pain, fever, and altered mental status.[29,74,91] Dermal exposure results in dermatitis.[44]

Hemolysis and methemoglobinemia, caused by naphthalene metabolite 1-naphthol, occurs infrequently as a result of naphthalene exposure. They become clinically evident as early as 24 to 48 hours postexposure, but more typically on the third day postexposure because of the time necessary for the hepatic metabolism of naphthalene.[34,73] Anemia secondary to hemolysis often does not reach its nadir until 3 to 5 days postexposure.[9,121]

Signs and symptoms of hemolysis and methemoglobinemia include tachycardia, tachypnea, shortness of breath, cyanosis, jaundice, dark urine, generalized weakness, decreased exercise tolerance, and altered mental status (Chap. 124). Acute kidney injury is reported as a complication of naphthalene-induced hemolysis and hemoglobinuria. Naphthalene and its metabolites cross the placenta.[11] Naphthalene pica during pregnancy causes both maternal and fetal toxicity. Hemolytic anemia in children born to moth-ers who had naphthalene toxicity at the time of delivery is believed to be related to the maternal naphthalene exposure.[147] Data on the development cataracts following naphthalene exposure in human are inconclusive.[82]

Based on animal data on carcinogenicity, naphthalene is classified by the International Agency for Research on Cancer (IARC) as a Group 2B carcino-gen (possibly carcinogenic to humans) and by the EPA as a Group C possible

human carcinogen.[46,60] The data supporting human carcinogenicity of naph-thalene are limited. There are several case reports that associate exposure with laryngeal cancer in East Germany and colorectal cancer in Nigeria, but causal relationship cannot be determined.[7,46]

Diagnostic Testing

No specific diagnostic testing is indicated, although both naphthalene and its metabolites are identifiable in blood and urine. Identification of 1-naphthol and 2-naphthol in the urine confirms exposure to naphthalene. Qualitative or quantitative testing for naphthalene or its metabolites is not clinically indicated when managing a patient with an acute overdose.[92]

The presentation of naphthalene-induced hemolysis is similar to that of hemolysis from other causes. Hyperbilirubinemia from hemolysis is charac-terized by an elevation of the unconjugated (indirect) bilirubin and a rela-tively normal conjugated (direct) fraction. Serum haptoglobin is usually low because the haptoglobin–hemoglobin complex is cleared by the kidneys. Both the direct and indirect Coombs tests are negative in naphthalene-induced hemolytic anemia. Lactate dehydrogenase is elevated due to its release from hemolyzed red blood cells. Hemoglobinuria is suggested by a urine dipstick that reacts strongly positive for hemoglobin with a paucity or absence of red blood cells on microscopic examination of the urine sediment. Hemoglobinemia is differentiated from myoglobinuria, which has a compa-rable urine sediment, by measuring the serum creatine phosphokinase and myoglobin which will be elevated in patients with rhabdomyolysis and myo-globinuria but not in those with hemolysis and hemoglobinuria.

Examination of a peripheral blood smear is useful in identifying hemo-lysis before a patient develops clinical or laboratory evidence of anemia. Hemolysis is present when red blood cell (RBC) abnormalities are present including schistocytes, anisocytosis, microspherocytosis, reticulocytosis, nucleated RBCs, Blister cells, and Heinz body (Chap. 20). Peripheral smear abnormalities and anemia often occurs within the first 24 hours following ingestion.[29,107,147,148] Testing for G6PD activity is not recommended during an acute episode of hemolysis. Reticulocytes have higher G6PD activity than do older RBCs. If G6PD activity is measured during an episode of hemolysis when many of the older RBCs have already been destroyed, false elevation or normal G6PD activity is observed. It is best to delay testing for G6PD activ-ity for a few months following an episode of hemolysis. Family members of patients with life-threatening G6PD deficiency should also be tested.

Naphthalene-induced methemoglobinemia is similar in presentation to methemoglobinemia from other xenobiotics. The percentage of methemo-globin is rapidly determined using a cooximeter (Chap. 124).

Management

Most patients with an unintentional exposure to no more than one naphthalene-containing mothball do not require medical evaluation. Patients who should be evaluated in a health care facility following an acute ingestion include those who recently ingested more than one naphthalene-containing mothball equivalent, those with signs or symptoms of toxicity, especially hemolysis and/or methemoglobinemia, those with known or sus-pected G6PD deficiency, all intentional ingestions, and those patients with substantial inhalational exposures, particularly those occurring in an occu-pational setting.

Gastrointestinal decontamination is not well studied in patients who have ingested naphthalene. Most patients with unintentional exposures do not require gastrointestinal decontamination. Administration of activated charcoal, 1 g/kg, although not of proven efficacy, is reasonable because it is considered safe. Repeat doses of activated charcoal 0.5 g/kg and/or whole-bowel irrigation with polyethylene glycol electrolyte lavage solution would only reasonable for patients with large ingestions of naphthalene who are expected to have significant ongoing gastrointestinal absorption.

Diagnostic testing within the first 24 to 48 hours postexposure will detect the onset of methemoglobinemia and/or hemolysis before a patient becomes symptomatic. Most low-risk patients who are asymptomatic within the first 24 to 48 hours postexposure and who have no laboratory evidence of hemolysis or methemoglobinemia should be managed as outpatients if reevaluation within 24 to 48 hours can be arranged. Patients who are discharged should be instructed to return if they become symptomatic. Admission recommended for high-risk patients, those with laboratory evidence of hemolysis and/or methemoglobinemia, and those who cannot be reliably managed as outpatients.

Patients with life-threatening hemolysis and anemia should be transfused with packed red blood cells. However, most healthy patients will be able to compensate for the hemolysis and will not require a transfusion. For patients with symptomatic methemoglobinemia methylene blue 1 to 2 mg/kg (0.1–0.2 mL/kg of a 1% solution) is recommended intravenously. Repeat doses may be necessary (Antidotes in Depth: A43).

PARADICHLOROBENZENE

History and Epidemiology

Paradichlorobenzene (1,4-dichlorobenzene) is widely used as a deodorizer, disinfectant, repellent, fumigant, insecticide, fungicide, and industrial solvent. Today, paradichlorobenzene is the most common component of moth repellents and deodorants for restrooms in the United States. Low-level exposure to paradichlorobenzene in the United States is extremely common as a result of environmental contamination from release of paradichlorobenzene to air by industrial facilities.[90] The primary route of human exposure is inhalation in either an occupational setting or from indoor air where paradichlorobenzene is used as a deodorizer or moth repellent.[90] Paradichlorobenzene is also found in both water and numerous food items, including pork and fresh vegetables, from environmental contamination.[90,102,133] Consequently, approximately 96% to 98.3% of the US population, including children as young as 2 years old, have detectable 2,5-dichlorophenol, a metabolite of paradichlorobenzene, in the urine.[57,58,144] Analysis of urine samples from the participants of National Health and Nutrition Examination Survey (NHANES) showed that urinary 2,5-dichlorobenzene concentrations decreased between the 2003–2004 and 2009–2010 survey periods. However, highest urinary concentrations were noted among 6- to 11-year-old children and adults older than 60 years.[144] The health effects of the low-level paradichlorobenzene exposure from environmental contamination are unclear. Recent population-based (NHANES) studies suggest a dose-dependent increase in the prevalence of diabetes, thyroid dysfunction, metabolic syndrome, obesity, earlier age of menarche, and food allergies.[22,23,61,123,134-137] These findings do not establish a clear causal relationship, but further research is warranted to investigate the relationship between environmental paradichlorobenzene exposure and its potential adverse health effects.

Approximately 150 paradichlorobenzene exposures are reported annually. The majority of the cases are unintentional exposures to paradichlorobenzene-containing moth repellents, predominantly occurring in children (<5 years old), which do not cause toxicity. According to the AAPCC data, no deaths or major toxicity were reported between 1995 and 2015, and only 15 cases of paradichlorobenzene exposures experienced moderate toxicity during the same period (Chap. 130).

Pharmacology, Pharmacokinetics, Toxicokinetics, and Pathophysiology

Paradichlorobenzene is a colorless solid with a noxious odor. It is available as pure white crystals, as a solid in combination with other chemicals, or as a liquid dissolved in volatile solvents or oil.[10] Paradichlorobenzene is well absorbed via ingestion, inhalation, and dermal exposure. Inhalation toxicokinetics show that there is rapid distribution and accumulation in tissues, specifically in adipose tissue.[14,27,55,146] This contributes to sustained serum paradichlorobenzene concentrations and clinical toxicity after cessation of chronic exposure, a phenomenon known as "coasting."[56,36] Starvation increases paradichlorobenzene release owing to utilization of adipose tissues.[13,52] Paradichlorobenzene undergoes hepatic metabolism by several CYP450 enzymes including 1A1, 1A2, 2B1, 2E1 (primary isoenzyme), and 3A1 and 3A4 to its primary metabolite, 2,5-dichlorophenol.[20,36,52,56] With several other minor metabolites (2,5-dichlorohydroquinone, 2,5-dichlorophenylmethyl sulfide, 2,5-dichlorophenylmethyl sulfone), 2,5-dichlorophenol is eliminated primarily via urinary excretion as either sulfated or glucuronidated conjugates.[14,36,52,146]

The mechanism of the toxicologic effect of paradichlorobenzene has not been studied to date. Although rare, paradichlorobenzene toxicity is reported following ingestion and inhalation.[59,81]

Workplace standards include the OSHA PEL, which is 450 mg/m³ (75 ppm) time-weighted average (TWA), ACGIH TLV, which is 60 mg/m³ (10 ppm) TWA, and the ACGIH STEL, which is 675 mg/m³ (110 ppm); NIOSH IDLH is 150 ppm.[126]

Clinical Manifestations

Paradichlorobenzene is considered to have less toxicity than camphor and naphthalene. However, cases of clinical toxicity from paradichlorobenzene are reported ranging from hemolytic anemia to toxic leukoencephalopathy following acute and/or chronic exposure.[13,27,37,38,56] Although paradichlorobenzene is absorbed following inhalation, ingestion and cutaneous exposures, ingestion, and inhalation are the routes of exposure that lead to toxicity.[37,38,56,83] Acute unintentional exposure to paradichlorobenzene typically causes limited transient clinical effects such as nausea and vomiting, headache, and mucous membrane irritation.[32,59] However, significant neuropsychiatric dysfunction, specifically cerebellar dysfunction, motor weakness, behavioral changes, and cognitive decline, is reported following chronic intentional and occupational exposure.[37,38,56] In most cases, neurologic and cognitive deficits associated with paradichlorobenzene developed after several months of exposure and seldom had complete resolution after cessation of paradichlorobenzene exposure.[13,36,56,83] Other clinical signs and symptoms from chronic exposure include pulmonary granulomatosis, hepatotoxicity, acute kidney injury, an ichthyosislike dermatosis, aplastic anemia, and dyspnea.[37,38,85,140]

Hemolytic and aplastic anemias are reported, as well as methemoglobinemia, following acute paradichlorobenzene ingestion.[53,109]

Paradichlorobenzene is classified by IARC as a Group 2B, possibly carcinogenic to humans, based on evidence of carcinogenicity from experimental animal studies. In mice and rats, chronic exposure was associated with the development of both hepatocellular carcinomas and adenomas in male and female mice, and renal tubular cell adenocarcinoma and mononuclear cell leukemia developed in male mice.[5,6,16,87,88,143] Evidence for carcinogenicity in humans from paradichlorobenzene exposure is limited. One case series reported 5 cases of leukemia that were associated with paradichlorobenzene exposure.[88,142] No additional epidemiologic data on human carcinogenesis from paradichlorobenzene exposure is available.

Diagnostic Testing

Both paradichlorobenzene and its primary metabolite, 2,5-dichlorophenol, can be identified in blood and urine following exposure.[14,59] However, detectable serum or urine concentrations of paradichlorobenzene or 2,5-dichlorobenzene are difficult to interpret as they are universally present in healthy adults and children as a common environmental contaminant.[56,57,146] In one study, a sample of 1,000 adults in the United States had detectable concentrations of 2,5-dichlorophenol and paradichlorobenzene in their urine and blood, 98% and 96%, respectively, without evidence of clinical toxicity. The mean 2,5-dichlorophenol and paradichlorobenzene concentrations in urine and blood were 200 and 2.1 mcg/L, respectively. A similar frequency of detectable 2,5-dichlorophenol concentrations in urine was also detected in healthy children.[57] Quantifying the amount of paradichlorobenzene in the urine of workers is useful for monitoring occupational exposures.[40] Overall, qualitative or quantitative testing for paradichlorobenzene or its metabolites is not generally indicated when managing a patient with an acute overdose. Structural CNS abnormalities, including toxic leukoencephalopathy, are occasionally noted on imaging studies such as MRI.[13] Hyperintense signals are seen in specific anatomic locations including periventricular white matter, corpus callosum, deep cerebellar nuclei, the parieto-occipital region and internal capsule.[13,27,56]

Management

Most unintentional exposures to paradichlorobenzene do not cause severe or life-threatening toxicity. It is reasonable to manage asymptomatic patients with unintentional exposures as outpatients. Patients who should be evaluated in a health care facility include those with clinical signs or symptoms, suicidal patients, and patients who have had a large exposure.

Gastrointestinal decontamination has not been studied in patients who ingest paradichlorobenzene. Most patients with unintentional exposures do not require gastrointestinal decontamination. However, administration of activated charcoal, 1 g/kg, is reasonable for patients with large, intentional ingestions. If present, gastrointestinal effects such as nausea and vomiting should be managed with supportive care, including fluid resuscitation and antiemetics. Laboratory testing is generally not helpful in the acute setting unless there is clinical evidence for hemolysis or methemoglobinemia. Transfusion of packed RBCs is recommended for symptomatic anemia resulting from acute hemolysis. Methylene blue is recommended for symptomatic methemoglobinemia.

It is reasonable for asymptomatic patients to follow up as outpatients for reevaluation in 24 to 48 hours postexposure as delayed development of hemolysis or methemoglobinemia is possible, but rare. Careful discharge instructions should be provided to patients should they become symptomatic.

Management of paradichlorobenzene-induced neurotoxicity such as encephalopathy, cerebellar dysfunction, psychomotor retardation and cognitive decline from chronic exposure is mainly supportive. Improvement of neuropsychiatric symptoms is variable; complete recovery is possible, although infrequent, after cessation of exposure, but residual neurotoxic effects are frequently present.[36,56,83]

MOTH REPELLENT RECOGNITION

Health care providers occasionally must determine whether a mothball is made of naphthalene, paradichlorobenzene, or camphor because management and prognosis for each is different. When the container is unavailable, as is often the case, mothballs are difficult to distinguish based on appearance, odor, texture, or size. Most mothballs are white, crystalline, and have a noxious odor.[141] Camphor moth repellents are more oily than both naphthalene and paradichlorobenzene mothballs. If controls are available, moth repellents are frequently differentiated based on their odor and texture.[8] Although most new paradichlorobenzene moth repellents are slightly larger than most new naphthalene moth repellents, all moth repellents shrink over time when exposed to air, making size an unreliable differentiating characteristic. Identifying a moth repellent as paradichlorobenzene often permits outpatient management, saving both hospital resources and unnecessary concern. The tests described in Table 102–1 and shown in Fig. 102–2 might

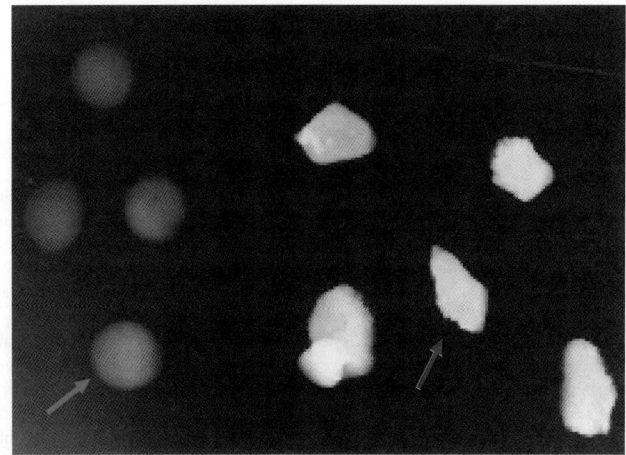

FIGURE 102–2. Radiograph of mothballs. Paradichlorobenzene (⟶) is densely radiopaque, whereas naphthalene (⟶) is faintly radiopaque.

allow rapid identification of the component of an unknown moth repellent. When performing these tests, it is most helpful to have camphor, naphthalene, and paradichlorobenzene controls available for comparison.

SUMMARY

- Paradichlorobenzene has largely replaced both camphor and naphthalene as a moth repellent in the United States, but exposures to all 3 compounds occur, especially in immigrant communities.
- It is reasonable to administer activated charcoal in patients with large ingestions if no contraindications are present, such as CNS depression, active vomiting, or seizures.
- Seizures commonly occur after camphor ingestion, and deaths due to status epilepticus are reported. Camphor-induced seizures are responsive to benzodiazepines, propofol, and barbiturates.
- Hemolytic anemia and methemoglobinemia occur after naphthalene and, less frequently, following paradichlorobenzene ingestions. Appropriate supportive care, packed red blood cell transfusions, and methylene blue administration are recommended for symptomatic patients.
- Simple radiography and buoyance tests are helpful in identifying the unknown moth repellent.

Acknowledgment

Edward K. Kuffner, MD, contributed to this chapter in previous editions.

TABLE 102–1	Moth Repellents: Laboratory Differentiation[8,72,141]		
Characteristic	*Camphor*	*Naphthalene*	*Paradichlorobenzene*
Water solubility (g/L)	1.2	0.03	0.08
Buoyancy in water	Floats	Sinks	Sinks
Buoyancy in water saturated with table salt	Floats	Floats	Sinks
Radiopacity	Radiolucent	Faintly radiopaque	Densely radiopaque
Melting point	350.6°F (177°C)	176°F (80°C)	127.4°F (53°C)
Boiling point	399.2°F (204°C)	424.4°F (218°C)	345.2°F (174°C)
In chloroform	Untested	Blue color	No reaction
Place on copper wire in a flame	Untested	Flame is yellow-orange	Initially flame is yellow-orange then bright green
Solubility in turpentine	Untested	Fast	Slow

REFERENCES

1. American Academic of Pediatrics Committee on Drugs. Camphor: who needs it? *Pediatrics.* 1978;62:404-406.
2. American Academy of Pediatrics Committee on Drugs. Camphor revisited: focus on toxicity. *Pediatrics.* 1994;94:127-128.
3. Agarwal A, Malhotra HS. Camphor ingestion: an unusual cause of seizure. *J Assoc Physicians India.* 2008;56:123-124.
4. Agency for Toxic Substances and Disease Registry. United States Department of Health and Human Services: toxicological profile for naphthalene, 1-methylnaphthalene, and 2-methylnaphthalene. http://www.atsdr.cdc.gov/toxprofiles/tp.asp?id=240&tid=43. Published 2005. Accessed November 15, 2012.
5. Aiso S, et al. Thirteen-week inhalation toxicity of *p*-dichlorobenzene in mice and rats. *J Occup Health.* 2005;47:249-260.
6. Aiso S, et al. Carcinogenicity and chronic toxicity in mice and rats exposed by inhalation to *para*-dichlorobenzene for two years. *J Vet Med Sci.* 2005;67:1019-1029.
7. Ajao OG, et al. Colorectal carcinoma in patients under the age of 30 years: a review of 11 cases. *J R Coll Surg Edinb.* 1988;33:277-279.
8. Ambre J, et al. Mothball composition: three simple tests for distinguishing paradichlorobenzene from naphthalene. *Ann Emerg Med.* 1986;15:724-726.
9. Annamali KC, et al. Acute naphthalene toxicity presenting with metabolic acidosis: a rare complication. *J Acute Dis.* 2012;1:75-76.
10. Anonymous. *Ortho-, meta-,* and *para*-dichlorobenzene. *Rev Environ Contam Toxicol.* 1988;106:51-68.
11. Anziulewicz JA, et al. Transplacental naphthalene poisoning. *Am J Obstet Gynecol.* 1959;78:519-521.
12. Aronow R, Spigiel RW. Implications of camphor poisoning: therapeutic and administrative. *Drug Intell Clin Pharm.* 1976;10:631-634.
13. Avila E, et al. Pica with paradichlorobenzene mothball ingestion associated with toxic leukoencephalopathy. *J Neuroimaging.* 2006;16:78-81.
14. Azouz WM, et al. Studies in detoxication. 62. The metabolism of halogenobenzenes; *ortho-* and *para*-dichlorobenzenes. *Biochem J.* 1955;59:410-415.
15. Barker F. A case of poisoning by camphorated oil. *BMJ.* 1910;1:921.
16. Barter JA, Sherman JH. An evaluation of the carcinogenic hazard of 1,4-dichlorobenzene based on internationally recognized criteria. *Regul Toxicol Pharmacol.* 1999;29:64-79.
17. Benz RW. Camphorated oil poisoning with no mortality: report of twenty cases. *JAMA.* 1919;72:1217-1218.
18. Bhaya M, Beniwal R. Camphor induced myocarditis: a case report. *Cardiovasc Toxicol.* 2007;7:212-214.
19. Blackmon WP, Curry HB. Camphor poisoning; report of case occurring during pregnancy. *J Fla Med Assoc.* 1957;43:999-1000.
20. Bogaards JJ, et al. Human cytochrome P450 enzyme selectivities in the oxidation of chlorinated benzenes. *Toxicol Appl Pharmacol.* 1995;132:44-52.
21. Bogen KT, et al. Naphthalene metabolism in relation to target tissue anatomy, physiology, cytotoxicity and tumorigenic mechanism of action. *Regul Toxicol Pharmacol.* 2008;51:S27-S36.
22. Buckpitt A, et al. Naphthalene-induced respiratory tract toxicity: metabolic mechanisms of toxicity. *Drug Metab Rev.* 2002;34:791-820.
23. Buser MC, et al. Association of urinary phenols with increased body weight measures and obesity in children and adolescents. *J Pediatr.* 2014;165:744-749.
24. Buttke DE, et al. Exposures to endocrine-disrupting chemicals and age of menarche in adolescent girls in NHANES (2003-2008). *Environ Health Perspect.* 2012;120:1613-1618.
25. California Office of Environmental Health Hazard Assessment. Chronic toxicity summary: naphthalene. http://oehha.ca.gov/air/chronic_rels/pdf/91203.pdf. Accessed November 12, 2012.
26. Chen W, et al. Camphor—a fumigant during the Black Death and a coveted fragrant wood in ancient Egypt and Babylon—a review. *Molecules.* 2013;18:5434-5454.
27. Cheong R, et al. Mothball withdrawal encephalopathy: case report and review of paradichlorobenzene neurotoxicity. *Subst Abus.* 2006;27:63-67.
28. Cho TM, et al. In vitro metabolism of naphthalene by human liver microsomal cytochrome P450 enzymes. *Drug Metab Dispos.* 2006;34:176-183.
29. Chusid E, Fried CT. Acute hemolytic anemia due to naphthalene ingestion. *AMA Am J Dis Child.* 1955;89:612-614.
30. Clark TL. Fatal case of camphor poisoning. *Br Med J.* 1924:467.
31. Cock TC. Acute hemolytic anemia in the neonatal period. *AMA J Dis Child.* 1957;94:77-79.
32. Cotter LH. Paradichlorobenzene poisoning from insecticides. *N Y State J Med.* 1953;53:1690-1692.
33. Craig JO. Poisoning by the volatile oils in childhood. *Arch Dis Child.* 1953;28:475-483.
34. Dawson JP, et al. Acute hemolytic anemia in the newborn infant due to naphthalene poisoning: report of two cases, with investigations into the mechanism of the disease. *Blood.* 1958;13:1113-1125.
35. Dean BS, et al. In vivo evaluation of the adsorptive capacity of activated charcoal for camphor. *Vet Hum Toxicol.* 1992;34:297-300.
36. Dubey D, et al. *Para*-Dichlorobenzene toxicity—a review of potential neurotoxic manifestations. *Ther Adv Neurol Disord.* 2014;7:177-187.
37. Feuillet L, et al. Twin girls with neurocutaneous symptoms caused by mothball intoxication. *N Engl J Med.* 2006;355:423-424.
38. Friedman BJ, et al. A fatal case of mothball intoxication presenting with refractory pruritus and ichthyosis. *Arch Dermatol.* 2012;148:404-405.
39. Germansky M, Jamall IS. Organ-specific effects of naphthalene on tissue peroxidation, glutathione peroxidases and superoxide dismutase in the rat. *Arch Toxicol.* 1988;61:480-483.
40. Ghittori S, et al. Urinary elimination of *p*-dichlorobenzene (*p*-DCB) and weighted exposure concentration. *G Ital Med Lav.* 1985;7:59-63.
41. Gibson DE, et al. Camphor ingestion. *Am J Emerg Med.* 1989;7:41-43.
42. Ginn HE, et al. Camphor intoxication treated by lipid dialysis. *JAMA.* 1968;203:230-231.
43. Gouin S, Patel H. Unusual cause of seizure. *Pediatr Emerg Care.* 1996;12:298-300.
44. Greene RR, Ivy AC. The effect of camphor in oil on lactation. *JAMA.* 1938;110:641-642.
45. Greer FR, Shannon M. Infant methemoglobinemia: the role of dietary nitrate in food and water. *Pediatrics.* 2005;116:784-786.
46. Griego FY, et al. Exposure, epidemiology and human cancer incidence of naphthalene. *Regul Toxicol Pharmacol.* 2008;51:S22-S26.
47. Gronka PA, et al. Camphor exposures in a packaging plant. *Am Ind Hyg Assoc J.* 1969;30:276-279.
48. Guilbert J, et al. Anti-flatulence treatment and status epilepticus: a case of camphor intoxication. *Emerg Med J.* 2007;24:859-860.
49. Gyoubu K, Miyazawa M. In vitro metabolism of (−)-camphor using human liver microsomes and CYP2A6. *Biol Pharm Bull.* 2007;30:230-233.
50. Haft HH. Camphor liniment poisoning. *JAMA.* 1925;84:1571.
51. Harden RA, Baetjer AM. Aplastic anemia following exposure to paradichlorobenzene and naphthalene. *J Occup Med.* 1978;20:820-822.
52. Hawkins DR, et al. The distribution excretion and biotransformation of *p*-dichloro[¹⁴C]benzene in rats after repeated inhalation, oral and subcutaneous doses. *Xenobiotica.* 1980;10:81-95.
53. Heard JD, Brooks RC. A clinical and experimental investigation of the therapeutic value of camphor. *Am J Med Sci.* 1913;145:238-253.
54. Hegesh E, et al. Congenital methemoglobinemia with a deficiency of cytochrome b₅. *N Engl J Med.* 1986;314:757-761.
55. Hernandez SH, et al. Case files of the New York City poison control center: paradichlorobenzene-induced leukoencephalopathy. *J Med Toxicol.* 2010;6:217-229.
56. Herrmann AP. Camphorated oil: health, history and hazard. *Am Pharm.* 1978;18:15.
57. Hill RH Jr, et al. *p*-Dichlorobenzene exposure among 1,000 adults in the United States. *Arch Environ Health.* 1995;50:277-280.
58. Hill RH, et al. Residues of chlorinated phenols and phenoxy acid herbicides in the urine of Arkansas children. *Arch Envrion Contam Toxicol.* 1989;18:469-474.
59. Hollingsworth RL, et al. Toxicity of paradichlorobenzene; determinations on experimental animals and human subjects. *AMA Arch Ind Health.* 1956;14:138-147.
60. International Agency for Research on Cancer. Some traditional herbal medicines, some mycotoxins, naphthalene and styrene. *IARC Monographs on the Evaluation of Carcinogenic Risks to Humans.* Vol 82. Lyon, France: IARC Press; 2002:590.
61. Jerschow E, et al. Dichlorophenol-containing pesticides and allergies: results from the US National Health and Nutrition Examination Survey 2005-2006. *Ann Allergy Asthma Immunol.* 2012;109:420-425.
62. Jimenez JF, et al. Chronic camphor ingestion mimicking Reye's syndrome. *Gastroenterology.* 1983;84:394-398.
63. Johnson CJ, et al. Fatal outcome of methemoglobinemia in an infant. *JAMA.* 1987;257:2796-2797.
64. Juteau F, et al. Antibacterial and antioxidant activities of *Artemisai annua* essential oil. *Fitoterapia.* 2002;73:532-535.
65. Khine H, et al. A cluster of children with seizures caused by camphor poisoning. *Pediatrics.* 2009;123:1269-1272.
66. Klingensmith WR. Poisoning by camphor. *JAMA.* 1934;102:2182-2183.
67. Kong JT, Schmiesing C. Concealed mothball abuse prior to anesthesia: mothballs, inhalants, and their management. *Acta Anaesthesiol Scand.* 2005;49:113-116.
68. Kopelman R, et al. Camphor intoxication treated by resin hemoperfusion. *JAMA.* 1979;241:727-728.
69. Koppel C, et al. Hemoperfusion in acute camphor poisoning. *Intensive Care Med.* 1988;14:431-433.
70. Koppel C, et al. Camphor poisoning—abuse of camphor as a stimulant. *Arch Toxicol.* 1982;51:101-106.
71. Kuczkowski KM. Mothballs and obstetric anesthesia. *Ann Fr Anesth Reanim.* 2006;25:464-465.
72. Lahoud CA, et al. Campho-Phenique ingestion: an intentional overdose. *South Med J.* 1997;90:647-648.
73. Lim HC, Poulose V, Tan HH. Acute naphthalene poisoning following the non-accidental ingestion of mothballs. *Singapore Med J.* 2009;50:e298-e301.
74. Linick M. Illness associated with exposure to naphthalene in mothballs—Indiana. *MMWR Morb Mortal Wkly Rep.* 1983;32:34-35.
75. Love JN, et al. Are one or two dangerous? Camphor exposure in toddlers. *J Emerg Med.* 2004;27:49-54.
76. Mackell JV, et al. Acute hemolytic anemia due to ingestion of naphthalene moth balls. I. Clinical aspects. *Pediatrics.* 1951;7:722-728.
77. Manoguerra AS, et al. Camphor poisoning: an evidence-based practice guideline for out-of-hospital management. *Clin Toxicol (Phila).* 2006;44:357-370.

78. Mascie-Taylor BH, et al. Camphor intoxication treated by charcoal haemoperfusion. *Postgrad Med J.* 1981;57:725-726.

79. Melzer-Lange M, Walsh-Kelly C. Naphthalene-induced hemolysis in a black female toddler deficient in glucose-6-phosphate dehydrogenase. *Pediatr Emerg Care.* 1989;5:24-26.

80. Michiels EA, Mazor SS. Toddler with seizures due to ingesting camphor at an Indian celebration. *Pediatr Emerg Care.* 2010;26:574-575.

81. Miyai I, et al. Reversible ataxia following chronic exposure to paradichlorobenzene. *J Neurol Neurosurg Psychiatry.* 1988;51:453-454.

82. Molloy EJ, et al. Perinatal toxicity of domestic naphthalene exposure. *J Perinatol.* 2004;24:792-793.

83. Murray SB, et al. Mothball induced encephalopathy presenting as depression: it's all in the history. *Gen Hosp Psychiatry.* 2010;32:341.e7-341.e9.

84. Nakahashi H, Miyazawa M. Biotransformation of (–)-camphor by *Salmonella typhimurium* OY1002/2A6 Expressing Human CYP2A6 and NADPH-P450 Reductase. *J Oleo Sci.* 2011;60:545-548.

85. Nalbandian RM, Pearce JF. Allergic purpura induced by exposure to *p*-dichlorobenzene. Confirmation by indirect basophil degranulation test. *JAMA.* 1965;194:828-829.

86. Nash FL. Naphthalene poisoning. *BMJ.* 1903;1:251-259.

87. National Toxicology Program. NTP toxicology and carcinogenesis studies of 1,4-dichlorobenzene (CAS No. 106-46-7) in F344/N rats and B6C3F1 mice (gavage studies). *Natl Toxicol Program Tech Rep Ser.* 1987;319:1-198.

88. National Toxicology Program. 1,4-Dichlorobenzene. *Rep Carcinog.* 2011;12:139-141.

89. National Toxicology Program. Naphthalene. *Rep Carcinog.* 2011;12:276-278.

90. National Toxicology Program. United States Department of Health and Human Services. 12th Report on carcinogens. http://ntp.niehs.nih.gov/?objectid=03C9AF75-E1BF-FF40-DBA9EC0928DF8B15. Published 2011. Accessed November 13, 2012.

91. Ostlere L, et al. Haemolytic anaemia associated with ingestion of naphthalene-containing anointing oil. *Postgrad Med J.* 1988;64:444-446.

92. Owa JA, et al. Quantitative analysis of 1-naphthol in urine of neonates exposed to mothballs: the value in infants with unexplained anaemia. *Afr J Med Med Sci.* 1993;22:71-76.

93. Phelan WJ 3rd. Camphor poisoning: over-the-counter dangers. *Pediatrics.* 1976;57:428-431.

94. Phimister AJ, et al. Consequences of abrupt glutathione depletion in murine Clara cells: ultrastructural and biochemical investigations into the role of glutathione loss in naphthalene cytotoxicity. *J Pharmacol Exp Ther.* 2005;314:506-513.

95. Plopper CG, et al. Early events in naphthalene-induced acute Clara cell toxicity. II. Comparison of glutathione depletion and histopathology by airway location. *Am J Respir Cell Mol Biol.* 2001;24:272-281.

96. Rabl W, et al. Camphor ingestion for abortion (case report). *Forensic Sci Int.* 1997;89:137-140.

97. Rampini SK, et al. Camphor intoxication after cao gio (coin rubbing). *JAMA.* 2002;288:45-45.

98. Rao GS, Pandya KP. Biochemical changes induced by naphthalene after oral administration in albino rats. *Toxicol Lett.* 1981;8:311-315.

99. Reid FM. Accidental camphor ingestion. *JACEP.* 1979;8:339-340.

100. Reygagne A, et al. Encephalopathy due to repeated voluntary inhalation of paradichlorobenzene. *J Toxicol Clin Exp.* 1992;12:247-250.

101. Riggs J, et al. Camphorated oil intoxication in pregnancy: report of a case. *Obstet Gynecol.* 1965;25:255-258.

102. Rius MA, et al. Influence of volatile compounds on the development of off-flavours in pig back fat samples classified with boar taint by a test panel. *Meat Sci.* 2005;71:595-602.

103. Robertson JS, Hussain M. Metabolism of camphors and related compounds. *Biochem J.* 1969;113:57-65.

104. Ruha A-M, et al. Late seizure following ingestion of Vicks VapoRub. *Acad Emerg Med.* 2003;10:691.

105. Santoyo S, et al. Chemical composition and antimicrobial activity of *Rosmarinus officinalis* L. essential oil obtained via supercritical fluid extraction. J Food Prot. 2005;68:790-795.

106. Schafer WB. Acute hemolytic anemia related to naphthalene; report of a case in a newborn infant. *Pediatrics.* 1951;7:172-174.

107. Shannon K, Buchanan GR. Severe hemolytic anemia in black children with glucose-6-phosphate dehydrogenase deficiency. *Pediatrics.* 1982;70:364-369.

108. Siegel E, Wason S. Camphor toxicity. *Pediatr Clin North Am.* 1986;33:375-379.

109. Sillery JJ, et al. Hemolytic anemia induced by ingestion of paradichlorobenzene mothballs. *Pediatr Emerg Care.* 2009;25:252-254.

110. Skoglund RR, et al. Prolonged seizures due to contact and inhalation exposure to camphor. A case report. *Clin Pediatr (Phila).* 1977;16:901-902.

111. Smillie WG. Betanaphthol poisoning in the treatment of hookworm disease. *JAMA.* 1920;74:1503-1506.

112. Smith AG, Margolis G. Camphor poisoning; anatomical and pharmacologic study; report of a fatal case; experimental investigation of protective action of barbiturate. *Am J Pathol.* 1954;30:857-869.

113. Sokolova AS, et al. Antiphatic and alicyclic camphor imines as effective inhibitors of influenza virus H1N1. *Eur J Med Chem.* 2017;127:661-670.

114. Sokolova AS, et al. Camphor-based symmetric diimines as inhibitors of influenza virus reproduction. *2014 Bioorg Med Chem.* 2014;22:2141-2148.

115. Sokolova AS, et al. Discovery of a new class of antiviral compounds: camphor imine derivatives. *Eur J Med Chem.* 2015;105:263-273.

116. Stohs SJ, et al. Naphthalene toxicity and antioxidant nutrients. *Toxicology.* 2002;180:97-105.

117. Tarnow-Mordi WO, et al. Risk of brain damage in babies from naphthalene in mothballs: call to consider a national ban. *Med J Aust.* 2011;194:150.

118. Theis JG, Koren G. Camphorated oil: still endangering the lives of Canadian children. *CMAJ.* 1995;152:1821-1824.

119. Tidcombe F. Sever symptoms following the administration of a small teaspoonful of camphorated oil. *Lancet.* 1897;150:660.

120. Tirillini B, et al. Chemical composition and antimicrobial activity of essential oil of *Piper angustifolium.* Planta Med. 1996;62:372-373.

121. Todisco V, et al. Hemolysis from exposure to naphthalene mothballs. *N Engl J Med.* 1991;325:1660-1661.

122. Trestrail JH, Spartz ME. Camphorated and castor oil confusion and its toxic results. *Clin Toxicol.* 1977;11:151-158.

123. Twum C, Wei Y. the association between urinary concentrations of dichlorophenol pesticides and obesity in children. *Rev Environ Health.* 2011;26:215-219.

124. United States Department of Labor Occupational Safety and Health Administration. Camphor. Safety and health topics. http://www.osha.gov/dts/chemicalsampling/data/CH_224600.html. Accessed March 3, 2009.

125. United States Department of Labor Occupational Safety and Health Administration. Naphthalene. Chemical sampling Information. http://www.osha.gov/dts/chemical-sampling/data/CH_255800.html. Accessed March 21, 2009.

126. United States Department of Labor Occupational Safety and Health Administration. p-Dichlorobenzene. Chemical sampling information. http://www.osha.gov/dts/chemicalsampling/data/CH_232900.html. Accessed March 21, 2009.

127. United States Food and Drug Administration. External analgesic drug products for over-the-counter human use: reopening of the administrative record. *Fed Regist.* 1980;45:63878-63879.

128. United States Food and Drug Administration. Proposed rules: external analgesic drug products for over-the-counter human use; tentative final monograph. *Fed Regist.* 1983;48:5852-5869.

129. Valaes T, et al. Acute hemolysis due to naphthalene inhalation. *J Pediatr.* 1963;63:904-915.

130. van Heyningen R. Naphthalene cataract in rats and rabbits: a resume. *Exp Eye Res.* 1979;28:435-439.

131. Verhulst HL, et al. Camphor. *Am J Dis Child.* 1961;101:536-537.

132. Viljoen A, et al. *Osmitopsis asteriscoides* (Asteraceae)—the antimicrobial activity and essential oil composition of a Cape-Dutch remedy. *J Ethnopharmacol.* 2003;88:137-143.

133. Wang MJ, Jones KC. Occurrence of chlorobenzenes in nine United Kingdom retail vegetables. *J Agric Food Chem.* 1994;42:2322-2328.

134. Wei Y, Zhu J. Urinary concentrations of 2,5-dichlorophenol and diabetes in US adults. *J Expo Sci Envrion Epidemiol.* 2016;26:92-100.

135. Wei Y, Zhu J. *para*-Dichlorobenzene exposure is associated with thyroid dysfunction in US adolescents. *J Pediatr* 2016;177:238-243.

136. Wei Y, Zhu J. Associations between urinary concentrations of 2,5-dichlorophenol and metabolic syndrome among non-diabetic adults. *Environ Sci Pollut Res Int.* 2016;23:581-588.

137. Wei Y, et al. Urinary concentrations of dichlorophenol pesticides and obesity among adult participants in the U.S. National Health and Nutrition Examination Survey (NHANES) 2005-2008. *Int J Hyg Environ Health.* 2014;217:294-299.

138. Weintraub E, et al. Medical complications due to mothball abuse. *South Med J.* 2000;93:427-429.

139. Weiss J, Catalano P. Camphorated oil intoxication during pregnancy. *Pediatrics.* 1973;52:713-714.

140. Weller RW, Crellin AJ. Pulmonary granulomatosis following extensive use of paradichlorobenzene. *AMA Arch Intern Med.* 1953;91:408-413.

141. Winkler JV, et al. Mothball differentiation: naphthalene from paradichlorobenzene. *Ann Emerg Med.* 1985;14:30-32.

142. World Health Organization. Some industrial chemicals and dyestuffs: summary of data reported and evaluation. *IARC Monogr Eval Carcinog Risk Chem Hum.* 1982;29:213-238.

143. World Health Organization. Dichlorobenzenes. *IARC Monogr Eval Carcinog Risk Chem Hum.* 1999;73:223-276.

144. Ye X, et al. Urinary concentrations of 2,4-dichlorophenol and 2,5-dichlorophenol in the U.S. population (National Health Nutrition Examination Survey, 2003-2010): trends and predictors. *Environ Health Perspect.* 2014;122:351-355.

145. Yoshida T, et al. Urinary 2,5-dichlorophenol as biological index for *p*-dichlorobenzene exposure in the general population. *Arch Environ Contam Toxicol.* 2002;43:481-485.

146. Yoshida T, et al. Inhalation toxicokinetics of *p*-dichlorobenzene and daily absorption and internal accumulation in chronic low-level exposure to humans. *Arch Toxicol.* 2002;76:306-315.

147. Zinkham WH, Childs B. A defect of glutathione metabolism in erythrocytes from patients with a naphthalene-induced hemolytic anemia. *Pediatrics.* 1958;22:461-471.

148. Zuelzer WW, Apt L. Acute hemolytic anemia due to naphthalene poisoning; a clinical and experimental study. *JAMA.* 1949;141:185-190.

103 CAUSTICS

Rachel S. Wightman and Jessica A. Fulton

HISTORY AND EPIDEMIOLOGY

A caustic is a xenobiotic that causes both functional and histologic damage on contact with tissue surfaces. As early as 1927, legislation in the United States governing the packaging of alkali- and acid-containing products mandated that warning labels be placed on these products. In response to the recognition that caustic exposures were more frequent in children, the Federal Hazardous Substances Act and Poison Prevention Packaging Act were passed in 1970. These acts mandated that all caustics with a concentration greater than 10% be sold in child-resistant containers. By 1973, the household concentration triggering mandatory child-resistant packaging was lowered to 2%. In addition, the subsequent development of poison prevention education dramatically decreased the incidence of unintentional caustic injuries in children in the United States. The positive impact of both regulatory legislation and public health intervention is evident when observing the decreasing number of significant exposures in the United States compared to the number of exposures in developing nations that lack these policies.

In the United States, even though legislation limiting the concentration of caustics has existed since the early 20th century, exposures to both acids and alkalis continue to be significant. Data collected from the 5 most recent years of the American Association of Poison Control Centers Annual Reports of the National Poison Data System revealed 37,272 acid exposures and 18,801 alkali exposures. Of these, 4,405 (12%) of acid and 3,153 (17%) of alkali exposures resulted in moderate to major outcomes and a total of 26 deaths occurred (Chap. 130).

Caustic exposures follow a bimodal age distribution pattern with peak occurrences in the pediatric population age 1 to 5 years and again in adulthood. In children, exposures usually consist of household products and occur most often in an unsupervised setting. In adults, exposures to household or industrial products result from occupational exposure, suicide attempts, and assaults. Although less frequent, intentional exposures by adults are invariably more significant. One study noted that although children comprised 39% of admissions for caustic ingestions, adults comprised 81% of patients requiring treatment.[38]

Exposure to caustics occurs via the dermal, ocular, respiratory, and gastrointestinal route. Caustics cause diverse histologic and functional damage on contact with tissues depending on the tissue and caustic involved. Table 103–1 lists common caustics and the products that contain them. Many are available for home use, in both solid and liquid forms, with variations in viscosity, concentration, and pH.

The severity of a caustic injury is often not immediately evident in patients who present shortly after exposure. Predicting which patients will require rapid interventions to prevent morbidity and mortality requires the determination and evaluation of multiple clinical and laboratory parameters. This chapter reviews the pathophysiology and approach to patients with potentially serious exposures.

PATHOPHYSIOLOGY

Although there are many ways to categorize caustics, they are most typically classified as acids or alkalis. An acid is a proton donor and causes significant injury, generally at a pH below 3. An alkali is a proton acceptor and causes significant injury, generally when the pH is above 11. Chapter 10 contains a more detailed discussion of the chemistry of acids and bases. The extent of injury is modulated by duration of contact; ability of the caustic to penetrate tissues; volume, pH, and concentration; the presence or absence of food in the stomach; and a property known as titratable

acid/alkaline reserve (TAR). Titratable acid/alkaline reserve quantifies the amount of neutralization needed to bring the pH of a caustic to that of physiologic tissues. Neutralization of caustics takes place at the expense of the tissues, resulting in the release of thermal energy, producing burns. Generally, as the TAR of a caustic increases, so does the ability to produce tissue damage.[5,42] Some caustics, such as zinc chloride and phenol, have a high TAR and are capable of producing severe burns even though their pH is near physiologic. Beyond tissue damage, some caustics have the potential to cause systemic toxicity.

TABLE 103–1	Sources of Common Caustics
Caustic	**Common Applications**
Acetic acid	Permanent wave neutralizers, photographic stop bath, concentrated solution for food purposes
Ammonia (ammonium hydroxide)	Toilet bowl cleaners, metal cleaners and polishes, hair dyes and tints, antirust products, jewelry cleaners, floor strippers, glass cleaners, wax removers
Benzalkonium chloride	Detergents
Boric acid	Roach powders, water softeners, germicides
Formaldehyde, formic acid	Deodorizing tablets, plastic menders, fumigants, embalmers
Hydrochloric acid (muriatic acid)	Metal and toilet bowl cleaners
Hydrofluoric acid	Antirust products, glass etching, microchip etching
Iodine	Antiseptics
Mercuric chloride ($HgCl_2$)	Preservatives
Methylethyl ketone peroxide	Industrial synthetic
Oxalic acid	Disinfectants, household bleaches, metal polishes, antirust products, furniture refinishers
Phenol (creosol, creosote)	Antiseptics, preservatives
Phosphoric acid	Toilet bowl cleaners
Phosphorus	Matches, fireworks, rodenticides, methamphetamine synthesis
Potassium permanganate	Illicit abortifacients, antiseptic solutions
Potassium hydroxide	Oven cleaners, hair products, manufacture of biodiesel, soaps
Selenious acid	Gun bluing agents
Sodium hydroxide (lye)	Detergents, paint removers, drain cleaners and openers, oven cleaners
Sodium borates, carbonates, phosphates, and silicates	Detergents, electric dishwasher preparations, water softeners
Sodium hypochlorite	Bleaches, cleansers
Sulfuric acid	Automobile batteries, drain cleaners
Zinc chloride	Soldering flux

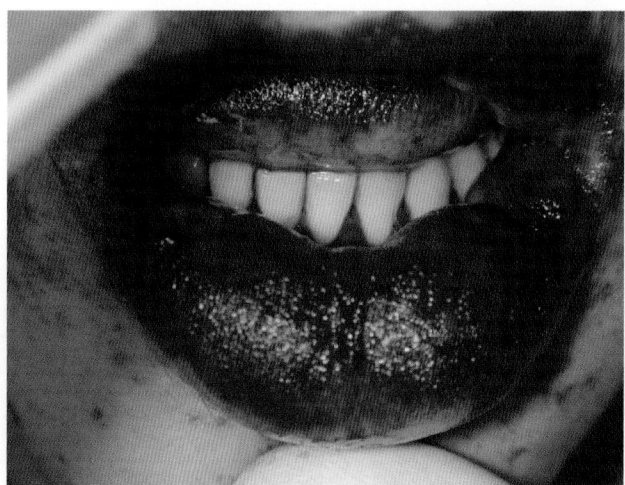

FIGURE 103-1. Photograph demonstrating burns to the lips and tongue of a 20-year-old man following ingestion of sodium hydroxide. *(Used with permission from the Fellowship in Medical Toxicology, New York University School of Medicine, New York City Poison Center.)*

Alkalis

Following exposure to an alkaline xenobiotic, dissociated hydroxide (OH⁻) ions penetrate tissue surfaces, producing a histologic pattern of liquefactive necrosis (Figs. 103-1 and 103-2). This process includes protein dissolution, collagen destruction, fat saponification, cell membrane emulsification, transmural thrombosis, and cell death.[5] Animal studies of alkali exposure to the eye[41] demonstrate rapid formation of corneal epithelial defects with eventual deep penetration that may lead to perforation. Similarly, animal studies of the esophagus demonstrate that erythema and edema of the mucosa occur within seconds followed by an inflammatory reaction extending to the submucosa and muscular layers. The alkali, such as sodium hydroxide ("lye"), continues to penetrate until the OH⁻ concentration is sufficiently neutralized by the tissues.[5,55]

Although federal regulations have lowered the maximal available household concentration of many caustics, 2 industrial-strength products seem to be readily available and therefore warrant special mention: ammonium hydroxide and sodium hypochlorite. Ammonia (ammonium hydroxide) products are weak bases—partially dissociated in water—that cause significant esophageal burns, depending on the concentration and volume ingested.[38] Household ammonium hydroxide ranges in concentration from 3% to 10%. Strictures are reported in patients who ingested 28% solutions.[71] Sodium hypochlorite is the major component in most industrial and household bleaches. Severe injuries typically only occur in patients with large-volume ingestions of concentrated products and most other patients do well with supportive care.[15,38] A series of 393 patients with household bleach ingestions demonstrated no stricture

formation.[5] Likewise, a canine model found that although vomiting was commonly associated with bleach ingestion, no esophageal lesions were noted, and perforation occurred only following prolonged contact.[54]

Ingestion of button batteries were once considered a unique caustic exposure. Composed of metal salts and a variety of alkaline xenobiotics, such as sodium and potassium hydroxide, leakage of battery contents was a legitimate concern. In recent years, however, new techniques used in the production of button batteries that effectively prevent leakage have shifted the concern following their ingestion from that of a caustic to a foreign body exposure with the significant potential for electrical injury.

Household detergents, such as laundry powders, laundry detergent pods (LDPs),[83] and dishwasher detergents, contain silicates, carbonates, and phosphates and have the potential to induce caustic burns and strictures, even when ingested unintentionally.[16] Although airway compromise rarely occurs after ingestion of traditional detergents,[16,23,59] the majority of exposures to traditional products result in only minor toxicity and usually do not require hospitalization. Compared to children with traditional non-LDP exposures, LDP exposures are associated with a higher incidence of adverse health effects, including mental status depression and respiratory compromise.[10,26,49] At this time it is unclear if the adverse health effects observed with LDP versus non-LDP exposures are due to unique contents or differences in pH, concentration, tensile strength, or the delivery vehicle.

Cationic detergents include quinolinium compounds, pyridinium compounds, and quaternary ammonium salts. These are frequently found in products developed for industrial use, as well as household fabric softeners. A concentration greater than 7.5% can cause severe burns.[58]

Acids

In contrast to alkaline exposures, following exposure to an acid, hydrogen (H⁺) ions desiccate epithelial cells, producing an eschar and resulting in a histologic pattern of coagulation necrosis. This process leads to edema, erythema, mucosal sloughing, ulceration, and necrosis of tissues. Dissociated anions of the acid (Cl⁻, SO₄²⁻, PO₄³⁻) also act as reducing agents, further injuring tissue. Ophthalmic exposure to acid results in coagulative necrosis that tends to prevent further penetration into deeper layers of the eye.

In most series, following an acid ingestion, both the gastric and esophageal mucosa are equally affected.[21,103] On occasion, the esophagus is spared damage while severe injury is noted in the stomach[29,38] (Fig. 103-3). This result tends to be a rarer finding than concomitant injury to both stomach and esophagus and is probably related to the rapid transit time of liquid acids through the upper gastrointestinal tract. Skip lesions from acid ingestions are reported and presumed to be a function of viscosity and contact

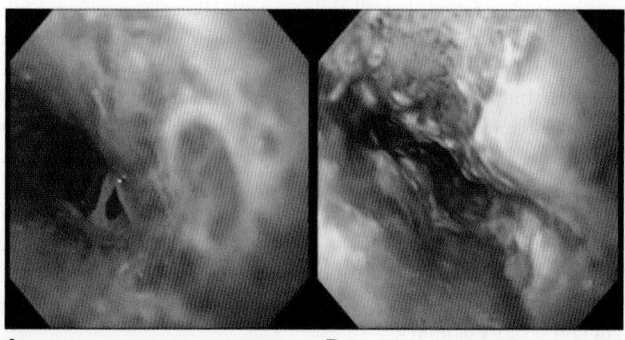

A   B

FIGURE 103-2. Endoscopic images of a 20-year-old man following ingestion of sodium hydroxide. (**A**) Grade IIa noncircumferential burn of the midesophagus. (**B**) Grade IIb circumferential burn of the distal esophagus. *(Used with permission from the Fellowship in Medical Toxicology, New York University School of Medicine, New York City Poison Center.)*

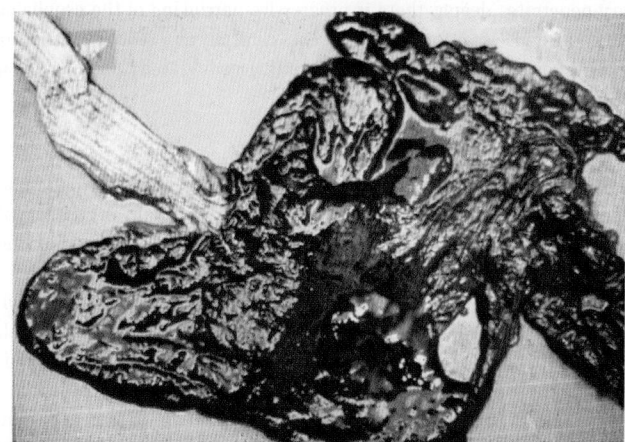

FIGURE 103-3. Postmortem specimen from a man with an intentional ingestion of a mixture of phosphoric and hydrochloric acid that was used as a brick cleaner. Note the relative sparing of the esophagus in contrast to full-thickness injury with perforation of the stomach. *(Used with permission from the Fellowship in Medical Toxicology, New York University School of Medicine, New York City Poison Center.)*

TABLE 103–2   Evaluation of Caustic Injuries and Their Management[3,19,38,93,103]

Grading of Injury by Endoscopic Visualization	Tissue Findings	Likelihood of Stricture Formation	Suggested Nutritional Support	Indication for Corticosteroids	Indications for Antibiotics	Indication for Stenting
I	Hyperemia or edema of mucosa without ulcer formation	None	Resume diet as tolerated	None (unless airway edema mandates short course)	None	None No stricture risk
IIa	Submucosal lesions, ulcers, exudates that are not circumferential	Low	Soft diet as tolerated or tube feeds (following nasogastric tube placement under direct visualization)	None (unless airway edema mandates short course)	Identified infection	None No stricture risk
IIb	Submucosal lesions, ulcers, exudates that are near-circumferential	High, 75%	Because of risk of perforation, feeding via gastrostomy, jejunostomy, or total parenteral nutrition are recommended as rapidly as possible	Short course	Identified infection	Intraluminal stents, nasogastric tubes are reasonable interventions to prevent strictures
III	Deep ulcers and necrosis into periesophageal tissues	High, near 100%	Because of risk of perforation, feeding via gastrostomy, jejunostomy, or total parenteral nutrition are recommended as rapidly as possible	Contraindicated (unless airway edema mandates short course)	Identified infection	Intraluminal stents, nasogastric tubes are reasonable interventions to prevent inevitable strictures

time.[38] Additionally, acid-induced pylorospasm is reported to lead to gastric outlet obstruction, antral pooling, and perforation.[21,102] A cat model of the effects of sulfuric acid on the esophagus revealed a coagulative necrosis of the mucosa with whitish discoloration of the tissues and underlying smooth muscle spasm.[5] Other animal models demonstrate chronic generalized esophageal motility dysfunction and shortening.[86,88]

Chapters 95, 101, and 104 contain a more detailed discussion of mercury, phenol, and hydrofluoric acid, respectively, each a unique caustic.

Classification and Progression of Caustic Injury

Esophageal burns, secondary to both alkali and acid exposures, are classified based on endoscopic visualization that employs a grading system similar to that used with dermal burns (Table 103–2).[19,28,33,102] Human case reports, postmortem studies, histologic inspection of surgical specimens, and experimental animal models reveal a consistent pattern of injury and repair following caustic injury.[80] As wound healing of gastrointestinal tract tissue occurs, neovascularization and fibroblast proliferation take place, laying down new collagen and replacing the damaged tissue with granulation tissue. A similar pattern of repair occurs following caustic injuries of the eye.

Burns of the esophagus typically persist for up to 8 weeks as remodeling takes place and is often followed by esophageal shortening. If the initial injury penetrates deeply, there is progressive narrowing of the esophageal lumen. The dense scar formation presents clinically as a stricture. Strictures can evolve over a period of weeks to months, leading to dysphagia and significant nutritional deficits.

CLINICAL MANIFESTATIONS

The gastrointestinal tract, respiratory tract, eyes, and skin of the patient are potential sites of caustic injury. Caustics produce severe pain on contact with any of these tissues. By far, the majority of long-term morbidity and mortality from caustic exposure results from ingestion.

In general, despite variation in the mechanism of injury, patients who have ingested either alkalis or acids present and are managed in a similar manner. Depending on the type, amount, and formulation (solid vs liquid) as well as the percentage of tissue exposed, ingestion has the potential to produce severe pain of the lips, mouth, throat, chest, or abdomen. Oropharyngeal edema and burns lead to drooling and rapid airway compromise. Symptoms and findings of esophageal involvement include dysphagia and odynophagia, whereas epigastric pain and hematemesis are typical of gastric involvement.

Respiratory tract damage occurs through direct inhalation or aspiration of vomitus, leading to the clinical manifestations of hoarseness, stridor, and respiratory distress. Injury results in epiglottitis, laryngeal edema and ulceration, pneumonitis, and impaired gas exchange. Tachypnea or hyperpnea results from either direct injury or as a compensatory response to a metabolic acidosis, which often is associated with elevated lactate concentrations from necrotic tissue or hemodynamic compromise.

Visual changes, eye pain, redness, burns, or ulceration of the eyes suggest ophthalmic exposure. Skin contact with caustics can result in pain, burns, and/or ulceration.

Predictors of Injury

The severity of injury following a caustic ingestion varies from mild with complete recovery to severe with associated morbidity and mortality. Many attempts have been made to define a method for clinical identification of patients with severe esophageal injuries based on signs and symptoms at presentation in an effort to avoid unnecessary procedures and admission for patients with less severe injury, while identifying patients at risk for severe complications. Various studies, mostly involving alkaline xenobiotics, examine the predictive value of stridor, oropharyngeal burns, drooling, vomiting, and abdominal pain.

One prospective study of 79 children evaluated for vomiting, drooling, and stridor found that a combination of 2 or more of these signs was predictive of significant esophageal injury as visualized on endoscopy.[19] Another study found that drooling, buccal mucosal burns, and an elevated white blood cell count elevation were significant independent predictors of severe gastrointestinal tract injury following acid ingestions.[37] Two additional retrospective studies found that all children with clinically significant injury had symptoms on presentation, but that no single symptom or combination of symptoms could identify all patients with esophageal injury.[15,35] A prospective study of alkali ingestions in both adults and children found that stridor was 100% specific for significant esophageal injury, but this was based on only 3 patients with this finding.[33] However, other authors have found signs or symptoms at presentation to lack prognostic utility in caustic ingestions. A retrospective study of 378 children admitted for a caustic injury found that signs or symptoms could not be used to predict significant esophageal injury.[28] A prospective evaluation of 41 patients after caustic ingestion found that signs and symptoms were unreliable in predicting the extent and severity of injury.[103]

Variation in findings between studies may be due to the population studied (pediatric vs adult), differences in the type of caustic ingested (acid vs alkali), and/or the circumstances associated with the ingestion (intentional vs unintentional). Additionally, studies evaluating the presence or absence of oropharyngeal burns as a predictor of distal esophagogastric injury repeatedly found this finding to be poorly predictive.[1,19,28,33,76,90] In one study, esophageal injury was present 51.5% of the time in the absence of oropharyngeal lesions, and 22.2% of these were second- and third-degree burns.[76]

Based on these findings, endoscopy, a standard diagnostic tool used in the management of caustic ingestions, is recommended in all patients with intentional ingestions. Endoscopy is also recommended in any patient with an unintentional ingestion in the presence of stridor and in any patient with 2 or more of the following findings: pain, vomiting, and drooling.[19,77] Children with unintentional caustic ingestions who remain completely asymptomatic and tolerate liquids after a few hours of observation probably require no further medical care.

The abdominal examination is likewise an unreliable indicator of the severity of injury. The presence of abdominal pain suggests tissue injury, but the absence of pain or findings on abdominal examination does not preclude life-threatening gastrointestinal damage.[24,99,103] Esophageal perforations result in mediastinitis and are commonly associated with fever, dyspnea, chest pain, and subcutaneous emphysema of the neck and chest. Although indicative of viscus perforation, abdominal peritoneal signs are late findings.

In addition to the direct effects that occur with tissue contact, systemic absorption and/or direct contact after perforation of acids results in damage to the spleen, liver, biliary tract, pancreas, and kidneys. This also produces a metabolic acidosis, hemolysis, and, ultimately, death.[44] Significant complications occur at various stages of wound recovery. Most importantly, these include airway compromise, hemodynamic instability secondary to hemorrhage from vascular erosion or septic shock, perforations of the gastrointestinal tract with the development of mediastinitis or peritonitis, and other overwhelming infections from bacteria residing in the oropharynx. A patient who survives acute injury with an acid or an alkali is at risk to subsequently develop stricture formation, gastric atony, decreased acid secretion, pseudodiverticula, and gastric outlet obstruction.[31,103]

Other complications include dysmotility of the pharynx and esophagus,[20] formation of aorto- and tracheo-esophageal fistulas resulting in delayed massive hemorrhage from erosion into a great vessel, and pulmonary thrombosis.[9,38,68,85] Those patients surviving a few weeks after a grade IIb or III injury who subsequently form strictures present with dysphagia and vomiting. Some strictures result in esophageal motility disorders caused by impaired smooth muscle reactivity. Manometric studies of the esophagus help with the early assessment and long-term prognosis by providing precise information about the severity of the initial injury.[30]

Long-term survivors of moderate and severe caustic injury of the esophagus have a risk of esophageal carcinoma that is estimated to be 1,000 times higher than that of the general population and appears to present with a latency of up to 40 years.[4]

DIAGNOSTIC TESTING
Laboratory
Laboratory assessment in patients with caustic ingestion has limited clinical utility, but can aid in management planning and evaluation of systemic toxicity and hemorrhage. Thus, all patients with presumed serious caustic ingestion should have an evaluation of serum pH, blood type and cross-match, complete blood count, coagulation parameters, and electrolytes. Elevated coagulation markers,[44] as well as a venous or arterial pH lower than 7.22,[13] are associated with severe caustic injury, but these findings are neither sensitive nor specific. One study evaluating 32 children with caustic ingestion found no difference in the mean leukocyte count or CRP between children with mild versus severe esophageal injury.[12]

Absorption of nonionized acid from the stomach mucosa results in acidemia. Following ingestion of hydrochloric acid, hydrogen and chloride ions (both of which are accounted for in the measurement of the anion gap) dissociate in the serum, resulting in a hyperchloremic (normal anion gap) metabolic acidosis. Other acids, such as sulfuric acid, result in an elevated anion gap metabolic acidosis because the sulfate anion (SO_4^{2-}) is not measured in the calculation of the anion gap. Although alkalis are not absorbed

systemically, significant necrosis of tissue results in a metabolic acidosis with an elevated lactate concentration.

A gastric pH greater than 7.30 correlated retrospectively with severe alkaline injury. The prospective usefulness of this information is limited, as obtaining gastric secretions without direct visualization is dangerous. One prospective study in children also found an increase in uric acid and decreases in phosphate and alkaline phosphatase concentrations to be useful in predicting the presence of esophageal injuries.[73]

Radiology
Chest and abdominal radiographs are useful in the initial stages of assessment to detect gross signs of esophageal or gastric perforation. Signs of alimentary tract perforation visualized on plain radiographs include pneumomediastinum, pneumoperitoneum, and pleural effusion. However, these studies have a limited sensitivity, and an absence of findings does not preclude perforation.[99] Free intraperitoneal air is best visualized on an upright chest radiograph. Occasionally, free air is only visible on the lateral view. In patients too ill to obtain an upright chest radiograph, an abdominal radiograph obtained with the patient in a left-side-down position is useful to evaluate free intraperitoneal air adjacent to the liver. Additionally, bedside ultrasound has potential utility in the diagnosis of free air and is based entirely on the lack of visualization of the usual intraperitoneal structures.[11,70] Computed tomography (CT) scanning is considerably more sensitive than both radiography and ultrasound for detecting viscus perforation and is recommended for patients if endoscopy is unavailable or if the patient is critically ill.[25,97] In settings in which CT scan is not readily available, a contrast esophagram can be performed if endoscopy is unavailable.

The role for CT scans in caustic ingestions has not been prospectively investigated. In the acute stage, CT has great sensitivity at detecting extraluminal air in the mediastinum or peritoneal cavity as a sign of perforation. In addition, CT visualizes the esophagus and stomach distal to severe caustic burns that cannot be safely visualized using endoscopy, one retrospective study suggests that CT grading of esophageal injuries is superior to endoscopy for prediction of the degree of esophageal damage and the development of stricture formation.[82] These results suggest a promising future role for this noninvasive study following caustic ingestions. Other imaging modalities are proposed for assessing esophageal injury after ingestion of a caustic, including technetium 99m-labeled sucralfate swallow for the presence of injury[65] and esophageal ultrasonography for determining the depth of injury.[67]

Another use of radiographic imaging is to noninvasively follow the patient after initial evaluation and stabilization. For example, contrast radiography is routinely used in the weeks or months following a caustic ingestion to detect esophageal narrowing representing stricture formation (Fig. 103–4).[87,91]

Endoscopy
Endoscopy is recommended for all patients with intentional ingestions, regardless of symptoms, as well as in patients with unintentional ingestions who demonstrate stridor, or 2 or more of the findings of pain, vomiting, and drooling.[19,33] Early endoscopy serves multiple purposes. It offers a rapid means of obtaining diagnostic and prognostic information while shortening the period of time that patients forego nutritional support, permitting more precise treatment regimens. Patients found to have minimal or no evidence of gastroesophageal injury can be discharged. A nasogastric tube may be passed under direct visualization in appropriate patients to facilitate caloric intake. Endoscopy is ideally performed within 12 hours and generally not later than 24 hours postingestion. Numerous case series demonstrate that the procedure is safe during this period.[15,24,28,57,64,77,84,95,102] We recommend against the use of endoscopic assessment after 24 hours and it should be avoided between 48 hours and 2 weeks postingestion; at this time, tissue strength is most compromised and the risk of perforation is greatest.

The choice of rigid versus flexible endoscopy is dependent on the comfort and experience of the endoscopist. The flexible endoscope has a smaller diameter but requires gentle insufflation of air to achieve or enhance visualization. We agree with a prospective evaluation of the role of fiberoptic endoscopy in the management of caustic ingestions that recommended

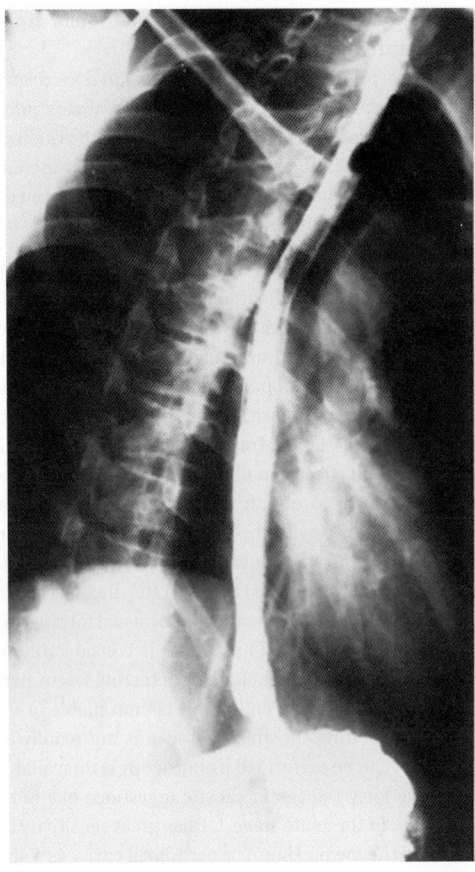

A

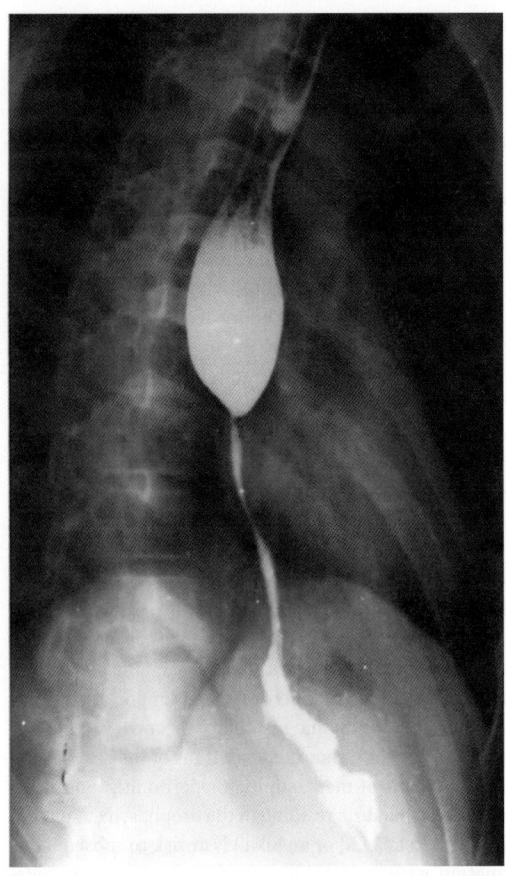

B

FIGURE 103–4. (**A**) Barium swallow several days after ingestion of liquid lye shows the esophagus to be atonic. There is poor coating of the esophagus, suggesting edema and intramural penetration. Note that the initial evaluation immediately following a caustic ingestion to assess the extent of injury is esophagoscopy, rather than a contrast esophagram. (**B**) Four months later, a repeat barium esophagram shows a severe stricture below the middle third of the esophagus. The barium barely passes the stricture, and the remainder of the esophagus is pencil thin. *(Used with permission from Emil J. Balthazar, MD, Professor of Radiology, New York University.)*

the following guidelines: (a) direct visualization of the esophagus prior to advancing the instrument, (b) minimal insufflation of air, (c) passage into the stomach unless there is a severe (particularly circumferential) esophageal burn, and (d) avoidance of retroversion or retroflexion of the instrument within the esophagus. Provided that the patient is hemodynamically stable and endoscopy is indicated, every attempt should be made to visualize the esophagus, stomach, and proximal duodenum as soon as possible after a caustic ingestion.[103] The absence of burns in the esophagus does not imply that severe necrosis and ulcerations do not exist in the stomach[65,96,102] and duodenum. In the case of termination of endoscopy because of grade IIb or grade III esophageal burns, we recommend water-soluble contrast studies,[77] CT scan, or surgical exploration to visualize remaining structures.

Endoscopy permits limited evaluation of gastrointestinal injury. For example, the endoscopist is able to appreciate only the mucosal surface of tissues, not the serosal side. This is especially evident in stomach ulcerations, which often appear black and necrotic from a true burn through the layers of the stomach or from the effect of stomach acid on the blood exposed from a shallow lesion. As mentioned above, in these cases, endoscopic ultrasonography or CT scan improves assessment of injury depth.[8,52] Often, however, only direct visualization of serosal and mucosal tissues with laparoscopy or laparotomy allows for definitive evaluation.

Most cases of perforation clearly linked to endoscopy have occurred when the endoscope was advanced through an esophagus with severe grade IIb or III lesions—a violation of current endoscopic standards.[97] In addition, perforations are also more likely to occur when rigid instruments are used in children or in uncooperative patients. Thus, the use of the flexible endoscope and adequate procedural sedation has decreased the complications

from endoscopic evaluation.[77] Some authors advocate the presence of a surgeon during endoscopy to assist in the assessment for potential surgical intervention.

MANAGEMENT
Acute Management
As in the case of any patient presenting with a toxicologic emergency, the health care provider must first adhere to universal precautions using early decontamination. Decontamination should include removal of clothing isolating it in a plastic bag for appropriate disposal and careful, copious irrigation of the patient's skin and eyes when indicated to remove any residual caustic and to prevent contamination of other patients, staff, and equipment. Concurrently, initial stabilization should include airway inspection and protection if indicated as well as basic resuscitation principles. Examination of the oropharynx should look for signs of injury, drooling, and vomitus, as well as careful auscultation of the neck and chest for stridor. Careful and constant attention to signs and symptoms of respiratory distress and airway edema, such as a change in voice, are essential and should prompt early intubation as airway edema characteristically rapidly progress over minutes to hours. Although not studied, dexamethasone 10 mg (intravenous) in adults and 0.6 mg/kg up to a total dose of 10 mg in children is reasonable for patients with these or other signs of caustic-induced airway compromise.

If airway involvement is significant enough to warrant intubation, it is best to mobilize a team of the most skilled physicians early in case of unforeseen complications. A delay in prophylactic airway protection often makes subsequent attempts at intubation or bag–valve–mask ventilation difficult or impossible. Direct visual inspection of the vocal cords with a fiberoptic laryngoscope, nasopharyngoscope, or intubating scope can be used to evaluate impending airway compromise when clinical signs and symptoms are unclear. Patients necessitating intubation are best served by direct visualization of the airway either via direct laryngoscopy or fiberoptic endoscopy, as perforation of edematous tissues of the pharynx and larynx is a grave complication that may occur during blind nasotracheal intubation attempts.

Nonsurgical airway placement is recommended whenever possible as both cricothyrotomy and tracheostomy interfere with the surgical field if esophageal repair is required.[58] Some patients with significant ingestions, however, require emergent surgical airway intervention. The decision to perform a surgical airway is dependent on the status of the patient, the ability to orotracheally or nasotracheally intubate via a fiberoptic endoscope, and operator skill.

Following definitive airway management, large-bore intravenous access should be secured and volume resuscitation initiated. Both acid and alkali ingestions cause "third spacing" of intravascular fluid to the interstitial space, which can result in hypotension. Empiric volume resuscitation with clinical assessment should be used to guide individual fluid requirements. In addition to third spacing hypotension can also result from gastrointestinal tract perforation leading to peritonitis, or mediastinitis, infection, or hemorrhagic shock from vascular erosion. In patients with caustic ingestions, significant complications can occur acutely on presentation or in a delayed fashion on admission. Serial physical examinations and constant monitoring of the vital signs, acid–base status, and urine output to assess the severity of the exposure and the progression in clinical status throughout the ED and/or hospital admission are imperative in patients with suspected serious caustic ingestion.

Gastrointestinal Decontamination, Dilution, and Neutralization

Gastrointestinal decontamination is usually limited in patients with a caustic ingestion with rare exceptions discussed below. Induced emesis is contraindicated, as it may cause reintroduction of the caustic to the upper gastrointestinal tract and airway. Activated charcoal is also not recommended, as it will interfere with tissue evaluation by endoscopy and preclude a subsequent management plan. Most caustics are not adsorbed to activated charcoal. Exceptions, such as cationic detergents, that do bind well to activated charcoal[58] have not been evaluated with a large series. For this reason, therapy with activated charcoal following any caustic ingestion cannot be recommended, with rare exceptions discussed below. Gastric emptying via cautious placement of a narrow nasogastric tube with gentle suction is reasonable to remove the remaining acid in the stomach only in patients with large, life-threatening, intentional ingestions of acid who present within 30 minutes. Although this technique has never been studied and carries the risk of perforation, the outcome for this particular group of patients with massive exposure is often grave, and options for treatment are limited. Therefore, preventing absorption of some portion of the ingested acid has the potential benefit in reducing systemic toxicity. Although the procedure also has the potential to induce injury, a risk-to-benefit analysis favors gastric emptying following a presumed lethal ingestion. In contrast, gastric emptying is contraindicated with alkaline and unknown caustic ingestions as blind passage of a nasogastric tube carries the risk of perforation of damaged tissues, a risk that outweighs the benefit.

Exceptions to the general rules of gastrointestinal decontamination of caustics exist in the management of zinc chloride ($ZnCl_2$) and mercuric chloride ($HgCl_2$). Both are caustics with severe systemic toxicity in the form of cationic metal injury.[14,32,53,62,63,69,89,101] The local caustic effects, though of great concern, are less consequential than the manifestations of systemic absorption. Therefore, prevention of systemic absorption should be addressed primarily, followed by the direct assessment and management of the local effects of these xenobiotics. Initial management to prevent systemic absorption includes aggressive decontamination with gentle nasogastric tube aspiration and administration of activated charcoal. In vitro data exist to suggest adequate activated charcoal adsorption of ionic mercury.[2]

The use of dilutional therapy was examined using in vitro, ex vivo, and in vivo models in an attempt to assess its efficacy in caustic ingestions. An early in vitro model demonstrated a dramatic increase in temperature when either water or milk was added to a lye-containing crystal drain opener (NaOH).[81] Another in vitro model found less consequential increases in temperature despite large volumes of diluent. Results of both studies suggested that dilutional therapy was of limited benefit.[61] Dilutional therapy was also associated with an increase in temperature in an ex vivo study of harvested rat esophagi that examined the histopathologic effects of saline dilution after an alkali injury. Additionally, the usefulness of dilution appeared to be inversely related to the length of time from exposure, with minimal efficacy when delay to initiation was as short as 30 minutes.[44,46] In contrast, an in vivo canine model of alkaline injury demonstrated that water dilution did not cause an increase in either temperature or intraluminal pressures.[47]

The extrapolation of these variable results to humans with caustic ingestions is limited and suggests that histologic damage can only be attenuated by milk or water when administered within the first seconds to minutes following ingestion.[5,43,44,46,47,55] For solid, as opposed to liquid, substances (eg, crystal lye), there is a theoretical value for delayed dilutional therapy, as tissue contact time is increased with solids and their concentration is distributed over a small surface area. However, dilutional therapy is limited in its ability to change pH, risks the spread of the caustic, and adds concerns of producing an exothermic reaction. Experimentally, milk is the best diluent with regard to an ability to attenuate the heat generated by a caustic. Caution should be used in advising patients or family members about the use of diluents. A child who refuses to swallow or take oral liquids should never be forced to do so. In general, dilutional therapy should be limited to the first few minutes after ingestion in patients without airway signs or compromise; are not complaining of significant pharyngeal, chest, or abdominal pain; are not vomiting; and are alert. Dilutional therapy should be avoided in patients with nausea, drooling, stridor, or abdominal distention as it stimulates vomiting and results in reintroduction of the caustic into the upper gastrointestinal tract.[81]

Attempts at neutralization of ingested caustics are contraindicated. This technique has the potential to worsen tissue damage by forming gas and generating an exothermic reaction. In vitro and ex vivo models demonstrate that neutralization of caustics generates heat, requires a large volume to attain physiologic pH, and had limited usefulness in preventing histologic damage if delayed beyond the first several minutes following caustic exposure.[45,81] In one in vivo canine model, orange juice was used to neutralize sodium hydroxide–induced gastric injury and demonstrated no change in temperature or intraluminal pressure.[47] Despite this study, neutralization is contraindicated; there are no other data demonstrating that clinical outcome is improved.

Surgical Management

The decision to perform surgery in patients with caustic ingestions is generally clear in the presence of either endoscopic or diagnostic imaging evidence of perforation,[99] severe abdominal rigidity, or persistent hypotension. Hypotension is a grave finding and often indicates perforation or significant blood loss. Additionally, elevated PT and PTT,[99] as well as acidemia,[13,50,100] are correlated with severe caustic injury.

Many patients will not have an obvious indication for surgical intervention despite impending perforation, necrosis, sepsis, or delayed hemorrhage. Although more challenging to diagnose, all these sequelae are potentially avoidable if surgery is performed early[58] as morbidity and mortality increase in patients whose surgery is delayed.[20,40,63] Multiple studies have attempted to codify the signs and symptoms necessary or sufficient to rapidly identify patients who would benefit from surgery but who lack clear clinical indications. Several retrospective and prospective series of caustic ingestions found that patients with large ingestions (>150 mL), shock, acidemia, or coagulation disorders tended to have severe findings on surgical exploration. These studies also reinforce that the abdominal examination was frequently unreliable in predicting the need for surgery.[21,99,103] It should be noted, again, that patients with severe acid injuries often lack abdominal pain, but generally have positive findings on diagnostic imaging.[21,103]

It is recommended to consult with a surgeon who is familiar with caustic ingestions for patients with grade IIb and III esophageal burns identified on endoscopy in case of progression of injury and surgery is required.[24,64]

Adjunctive Therapies

Steroids

The recommendations for steroid use in patients with caustic injury vary according to the grade of caustic injury. Although corticosteroid therapy is theorized to arrest the process of inflammatory repair and potentially prevent stricture formation, there is evidence that patients with grade III burns, in particular, will progress to stricture formation regardless of therapy.[3,38,96] Additionally, the use of corticosteroids in the management of patients with grade III burns has the potential to mask infection and make the friable, necrotic esophageal tissue more prone to perforation.[75] No study has found benefit for routine use of steroid therapy in grade I or IIa caustic injury. For these reasons, corticosteroid therapy is contraindicated for grade I, IIa, and III esophageal burns. When required in these patients for other indications such as caustic-induced airway inflammation, short-term corticosteroids are recommended.

Currently, some controversy exists regarding the use of corticosteroid therapy in the management of grade IIb circumferential esophageal burns. A recent prospective study of 83 children with grade IIb esophageal burns compared a short (3 day) course of high-dose methylprednisolone to placebo and found a statistically significant decrease in stricture formation in the group that received a short course of high-dose steroids.[93] Prior to this study, the medical literature suggested no benefit of steroids and occasionally harm for patients with grade IIb caustic injury. Two prospective studies to evaluate the efficacy of corticosteroid therapy for caustic injuries to the esophagus failed to show a benefit of corticosteroid therapy, and one even suggested harm.[3,51] A meta-analysis of studies completed from 1956 to 1991, with a total of 361 patients, evaluated the efficacy of corticosteroid therapy and found that in patients with grade II and III esophageal burns, strictures formed in 19% of the corticosteroid-treated group and in 41% of the untreated group.[48] Another meta-analysis of studies from 1991 to 2003, with a total of 211 patients, was unable to find a benefit in treating patients with corticosteroids with grade II and III esophageal burns.[75] A systematic pooled analysis of studies from 1956 to 2006, with a total of 328 patients, attempted to reevaluate the usefulness of corticosteroid therapy in grade II esophageal burns. Although methodologically limited, this study found no benefit in treating patients with steroids with grade II esophageal burns.[75] In addition, a multitude of case series failed to clearly differentiate between grade IIa, IIb, and III lesions, making clinical application of their results difficult.[3,17,96] However, prior to the more recent study noted above, all preceding studies were either retrospective or failed to differentiate between grades of lesions, making interpretation of the data difficult. Despite the imbalance of the quantity of studies demonstrating no benefit (or even harm) versus benefit for the use of steroids in the treatment of grade IIb lesions, the quality of the single prospective study supports our recommendation of a short course of methylprednisolone ($1g/1.73\ m^2$/day for 3 days) and ranitidine, ceftriaxone, and total parenteral nutrition in these patients.[93]

Antibiotics

No major outcome studies have investigated the use of antibiotics alone as prophylactic treatment for stricture prevention, but it is reasonable to reserve antibiotics for patients with an identified source of infection.

H₂ Antagonists/Proton Pump Inhibitors

Histamine₂ antagonists or proton pumps inhibitors theoretically help reduce acid production and injury after caustic ingestion and are thus reasonable as adjunctive therapy in discussion with a gastroenterologist despite a lack of studies to demonstrate their efficacy.

Stents and Feeding Tubes

A variety of other management strategies have been used in an attempt to prevent strictures and esophageal obstruction. In both animal models[79] and in human case series,[24,66,78] intraluminal stents and nasogastric tubes[66] made

of silicone rubber tubing successfully maintain the patency of the esophageal lumen. For nutritional support, the stents are usually attached to a feeding tube secured in the nasopharynx through which the patient can receive feedings without interfering with esophageal repair. These tubes are left in place for 3 weeks[78,79] and are often used with concomitant corticosteroid and antibiotic therapy. In animal models, the use of a stent for 3 weeks is superior in maintaining esophageal patency when compared to corticosteroids and antibiotics alone.[79] Potential disadvantages of esophageal stents include mechanical trauma at the site and increased reflux, both of which may inhibit healing.[87] A feline model of esophageal exposure to sodium hydroxide used stents but reported deaths from aspiration and mediastinitis.[79] One series of 251 humans exposed to caustics who were managed with silicone rubber stents found that the procedure was successful in preventing stricture formation.[7] Stents and feeding tubes provide the benefit of enteral nutrition and potential to prevent stricture formation and are reasonable on a case-by-case basis in discussion with surgery and gastroenterology consultants.

Additional Considerations

Additionally, a plethora of animal models have attempted to identify therapies that attenuate oxidative damage, inhibit synthesis, or stimulate breakdown of collagen and thereby prevent stricture formation. β-Amino propionitrile,[60] penicillamine,[29] *N*-acetylcysteine,[56] halofuginone,[34,74] vitamin E, sphingosylphosphorylcholine, colchicine, erythropoietin,[6] mitomycin C,[92] ozone,[36] fibroblast growth factor,[72] 5-fluorouracil,[22] ibuprofen,[39] and retinoic acid[18] are some of these xenobiotics. These treatments are inadequately studied in humans and cannot be routinely recommended at this time.

Disposition

The extent of tissue injury dictates the subsequent management and disposition of patients with caustic ingestions.

Grade I Esophageal Injuries

Patients with isolated grade I injuries of the esophagus do not develop strictures and are not at increased risk of carcinoma. Their diet can be resumed as tolerated. No further therapy is required. These patients can be discharged from the emergency department as long as they are able to eat and drink and their psychiatric status is stable.

Grade IIa Esophageal Injuries

If endoscopy reveals grade IIa lesions of the esophagus and sparing of the stomach, a soft diet can be resumed as tolerated or a nasogastric tube can be passed under direct visualization. If oral intake or feeding via a nasogastric tube is not feasible, feeding via gastrostomy, jejunostomy, or total parenteral nutrition is recommended as rapidly as possible. Providing interim enteral support is imperative as metabolic demands are increased in any patient with a significant caustic injury.

Grades IIb and III Esophageal Injuries

Patients with grades IIb and III lesions must be followed for the complications of perforation, infection, and stricture development. Strictures are a debilitating complication of both acid and alkali ingestions that evolve over a period of weeks or months. Strictures form as a result of the natural process by which the body repairs injured tissue through the production of collagen with resultant scar formation. In addition to stricture formation, patients with grade III burns are also at high risk for other complications, including fistula formation, infection, and perforation with associated mediastinitis and peritonitis.

Chronic Treatment of Strictures

Commonly, the management of patients with esophageal strictures includes endoscopic dilation, for which a variety of types of dilators are available. Contrast CT can be used to determine maximal esophageal wall thickness, which can then be used to predict response, as well as the number of sessions required to achieve adequate dilation. Multiple dilations are often necessary. In one study, patients with a maximal esophageal wall thickness of 9 mm or greater required more than 7 sessions to achieve adequate dilation.

This was significantly higher than in patients with a lesser maximal wall thickness. Measurement of maximal wall thickness is useful in determining long-term follow-up, type of nutritional support, and the potential need for surgical repair as an alternative to dilation. It also provides an indication for those who should undergo dilation under fluoroscopy to limit the risk of perforation.

The risk of perforation from esophageal dilation is decreased if the initial procedure is delayed beyond 4 weeks postingestion, when healing, remodeling, and potential stricture formation in the esophagus have already taken place. Several series report perforation secondary to esophageal dilation.[38,97] Following perforation, patients develop dyspnea or chest pain in the setting of associated subcutaneous emphysema or pneumomediastinum. Diagnostic imaging is recommended to identify the perforation and provide information for emergent surgical repair if the diagnosis is unclear. Patients with stricture formation require long-term endoscopic follow-up for the presence of neoplastic changes of the esophagus that may occur with a delay of several decades.[4,94]

Management of Ophthalmic Exposures

Ophthalmic exposures occur from splash injuries and malicious events as well as from the alkaline by-products of sodium azide released in automobile air bag deployment and rupture.[98] The mainstay of therapy for these patients is immediate irrigation of the eye for a minimum of 15 minutes with 0.9% sodium chloride, lactated Ringer solution, or tap water, if it is the only therapy immediately available. Several liters of irrigation fluid are recommended. The normal pH of ophthalmic secretions is approximately 6.5 to 7.6. This can be tested colorimetrically by using a urine dipstick, which can test a range of pH from 5 to 9.6; litmus paper can be used in the same fashion. Another useful option in acid exposures is Nitrazine (phenaphthazine) paper, which changes color from yellow to dark blue at a pH above 6.5.[25] These different test strips should be applied to the ophthalmic secretions to test the baseline pH and followed with intermittent evaluations after 15 minutes of lavage to determine the adequacy of irrigation. If these testing materials are not readily available, irrigation should not be delayed, as the depth of penetration of the caustic will determine outcome. If anterior chamber irrigation is required it should be performed emergently by an ophthalmologist. A thorough eye examination should be completed, and follow-up should be arranged. Chapter 24 and Special Considerations: SC2 contain a more detailed description of the evaluation and management of caustic injuries of the eye.

SUMMARY

- Initial management of all patients with caustic exposures begins with universal precautions in an effort to prevent further contamination of staff, other patients, and equipment.
- In patients with caustic ingestions, airway assessment and stabilization are of primary importance.
- It is recommended to not perform induced emesis, lavage, activated charcoal, neutralization, or dilutional therapy in patients with caustic ingestions with rare exceptions.
- Significant caustic injury should be suspected in all patients with intentional ingestions and in patients with unintentional ingestions presenting with stridor or 2 or more of the following: vomiting, drooling, and pain in the oropharynx, chest, or abdomen.
- All patients with suspected significant ingestions should undergo endoscopy or CT emergently so that effective treatment strategies are initiated expeditiously.
- Surgeons should be involved in the initial assessment of all patients with suspected significant ingestions and those who have an acute abdomen or hypotension so that any surgical intervention deemed necessary is performed promptly.

Acknowledgments

Robert S. Hoffman, MD, and Rama B. Rao, MD, contributed to this chapter in previous editions.

REFERENCES

1. Alford BR, Harris HH. Chemical burns of the mouth, pharynx and esophagus. *Ann Otol Rhinol Laryngol.* 1959;68:122-128.
2. Andersen AH. Experimental studies on the pharmacology of activated charcoal. III. Adsorption from gastro-intestinal contents. *Acta Pharmacol Toxicol (Copenh).* 2009;4:275-284.
3. Anderson KD, et al. A controlled trial of corticosteroids in children with corrosive injury of the esophagus. *N Engl J Med.* 1990;323:637-640.
4. Appelqvist P, Salmo M. Lye corrosion carcinoma of the esophagus: a review of 63 cases. *Cancer.* 1980;45:2655-2658.
5. Ashcraft KW, Padula RT. The effect of dilute corrosives on the esophagus. *Pediatrics.* 1974;53:226-232.
6. Bakan V, et al. The protective effect of erythropoietin on the acute phase of corrosive esophageal burns in a rat model. *Pediatr Surg Int.* 2010;26:195-201.
7. Berkovits RN, et al. Caustic injury of the oesophagus. Sixteen years experience, and introduction of a new model oesophageal stent. *J Laryngol Otol.* 1996;110:1041-1045.
8. Bernhardt J, et al. Caustic acid burn of the upper gastrointestinal tract: first use of endosonography to evaluate the severity of the injury. *Surg Endosc.* 2002;16:1004.
9. Borja AR, et al. Lye injuries of the esophagus. Analysis of ninety cases of lye ingestion. *J Thorac Cardiovasc Surg.* 1969;57:533-538.
10. Centers for Disease Control and Prevention (CDC). Health hazards associated with laundry detergent pods—United States, May-June 2012. *MMWR Morb Mortal Wkly Rep.* 2012;61:825-829.
11. Chen S-C, et al. Selective use of ultrasonography for the detection of pneumoperitoneum. *Acad Emerg Med Off J Soc Acad Emerg Med.* 2002;9:643-645.
12. Chen T-Y, et al. Predictors of esophageal stricture in children with unintentional ingestion of caustic agents. *Chang Gung Med J.* 2003;26:233-239.
13. Cheng Y-J, Kao E-L. Arterial blood gas analysis in acute caustic ingestion injuries. *Surg Today.* 2003;33:483-485.
14. Chobanian SJ. Accidental ingestion of liquid zinc chloride: local and systemic effects. *Ann Emerg Med.* 1981;10:91-93.
15. Christesen HB. Prediction of complications following unintentional caustic ingestion in children. Is endoscopy always necessary? *Acta Paediatr Oslo Nor 1992.* 1995; 84:1177-1182.
16. Clausen JO, et al. Admission to Danish hospitals after suspected ingestion of corrosives. A nationwide survey (1984-1988) comprising children aged 0-14 years. *Dan Med Bull.* 1994;41:234-237.
17. Cleveland WW, et al. The effect of prednisone in the prevention of esophageal stricture following the ingestion of lye. *South Med J.* 1958;51:861-864.
18. Corduk N, et al. Effects of retinoic acid and zinc on the treatment of caustic esophageal burns. *Pediatr Surg Int.* 2010;26:619-624.
19. Crain EF, et al. Caustic ingestions. Symptoms as predictors of esophageal injury. *Am J Dis Child. 1960.* 1984;138:863-865.
20. Dantas RO, Mamede RC. Esophageal motility in patients with esophageal caustic injury. *Am J Gastroenterol.* 1996;91:1157-1161.
21. Dilawari JB, et al. Corrosive acid ingestion in man—a clinical and endoscopic study. *Gut.* 1984;25:183-187.
22. Duman L, et al. The efficacy of single-dose 5-fluorouracil therapy in experimental caustic esophageal burn. *J Pediatr Surg.* 2011;46:1893-1897.
23. Einhorn A, et al. Serious respiratory consequences of detergent ingestions in children. *Pediatrics.* 1989;84:472-474.
24. Estrera A, et al. Corrosive burns of the esophagus and stomach: a recommendation for an aggressive surgical approach. *Ann Thorac Surg.* 1986;41:276-283.
25. Fadoo F, et al. Helical CT esophagography for the evaluation of suspected esophageal perforation or rupture. *AJR Am J Roentgenol.* 2004;182:1177-1179.
26. Forrester MB. Comparison of pediatric exposures to concentrated "pack" and traditional laundry detergents. *Pediatr Emerg Care.* 2013;29:482-486.
27. Fulton JA, Hoffman RS. Steroids in second degree caustic burns of the esophagus: a systematic pooled analysis of fifty years of human data: 1956-2006. *Clin Toxicol Phila Pa.* 2007;45:402-408.
28. Gaudreault P, et al. Predictability of esophageal injury from signs and symptoms: a study of caustic ingestion in 378 children. *Pediatrics.* 1983;71:767-770.
29. Gehanno P, Guedon C. Inhibition of experimental esophageal lye strictures by penicillamine. *Arch Otolaryngol Chic Ill 1960.* 1981;107:145-147.
30. Genç A, Mutaf O. Esophageal motility changes in acute and late periods of caustic esophageal burns and their relation to prognosis in children. *J Pediatr Surg.* 2002;37:1526-1528.
31. Gillis DA, et al. Gastric damage from ingested acid in children. *J Pediatr Surg.* 1985;20:494-496.
32. Giunta F, et al. Severe acute poisoning from the ingestion of a permanent wave solution of mercuric chloride. *Hum Toxicol.* 1983;2:243-246.
33. Gorman RL, et al. Initial symptoms as predictors of esophageal injury in alkaline corrosive ingestions. *Am J Emerg Med.* 1992;10:189-194.
34. Günel E, et al. Effect of antioxidant therapy on collagen synthesis in corrosive esophageal burns. *Pediatr Surg Int.* 2002;18:24-27.
35. Gupta SK, et al. Is esophagogastroduodenoscopy necessary in all caustic ingestions? *J Pediatr Gastroenterol Nutr.* 2001;32:50-53.

36. Guven A, et al. The efficacy of ozone therapy in experimental caustic esophageal burn. *J Pediatr Surg*. 2008;43:1679-1684.

37. Havanond C, Havanond P. Initial signs and symptoms as prognostic indicators of severe gastrointestinal tract injury due to corrosive ingestion. *J Emerg Med*. 2007;33:349-353.

38. Hawkins DB, et al. Caustic ingestion: controversies in management. A review of 214 cases. *Laryngoscope*. 1980;90:98-109.

39. Herek O, et al. Protective effects of ibuprofen against caustic esophageal burn injury in rats. *Pediatr Surg Int*. 2010;26:721-727.

40. Hill JL, et al. Clinical technique and success of the esophageal stent to prevent corrosive strictures. *J Pediatr Surg*. 1976;11:443-450.

41. Hirst LW, et al. Controlled trial of hyperbaric oxygen treatment for alkali corneal burn in the rabbit. *Clin Experiment Ophthalmol*. 2004;32:67-70.

42. Hoffman RS, et al. Comparison of titratable acid/alkaline reserve and pH in potentially caustic household products. *J Toxicol Clin Toxicol*. 1989;27:241-246.

43. Homan CS, et al. Effective treatment of acute alkali injury of the rat esophagus with early saline dilution therapy. *Ann Emerg Med*. 1993;22:178-182.

44. Homan CS, et al. Histopathologic evaluation of the therapeutic efficacy of water and milk dilution for esophageal acid injury. *Acad Emerg Med Off J Soc Acad Emerg Med*. 1995;2:587-591.

45. Homan CS, et al. Effective treatment for acute alkali injury to the esophagus using weak-acid neutralization therapy: an ex-vivo study. *Acad Emerg Med Off J Soc Acad Emerg Med*. 1995;2:952-958.

46. Homan CS, et al. Therapeutic effects of water and milk for acute alkali injury of the esophagus. *Ann Emerg Med*. 1994;24:14-20.

47. Homan CS, et al. Thermal effects of neutralization therapy and water dilution for acute alkali exposure in canines. *Acad Emerg Med Off J Soc Acad Emerg Med*. 1997;4:27-32.

48. Howell JM, et al. Steroids for the treatment of corrosive esophageal injury: a statistical analysis of past studies. *Am J Emerg Med*. 1992;10:421-425.

49. Huntington S, et al. Serious adverse effects from single-use detergent sacs: report from a U.S. statewide poison control system. *Clin Toxicol Phila Pa*. 2014;52:220-225.

50. Javed A, et al. Surgical management and outcomes of severe gastrointestinal injuries due to corrosive ingestion. *World J Gastrointest Surg*. 2012;4:121-125.

51. Jovic-Stosic J, et al. Steroid treatment of corrosive injury. *J Toxicol Clin Toxicol*. 42:417-418.

52. Kamijo Y, et al. Alkaline esophagitis evaluated by endoscopic ultrasound. *J Toxicol Clin Toxicol*. 2001;39:623-625.

53. Kondo T, et al. An autopsy case of zinc chloride poisoning. *Leg Med Tokyo Jpn*. 2016;21:11-14.

54. Landau GD, Saunders WH. The effect of chlorine bleach on the esophagus. *Arch Otolaryngol Chic Ill 1960*. 1964;80:174-176.

55. Leape LL, et al. Hazard to health—liquid lye. *N Engl J Med*. 1971;284:578-581.

56. Liu AJ, Richardson MA. Effects of *N*-acetylcysteine on experimentally induced esophageal lye injury. *Ann Otol Rhinol Laryngol*. 1985;94(5, pt 1):477-482.

57. Lowe JE, et al. Corrosive injury to the stomach: the natural history and role of fiberoptic endoscopy. *Am J Surg*. 1979;137:803-806.

58. Mack RB. Decant the wine, prune back your long-term hopes. Cationic detergent poisoning. *N C Med J*. 1987;48:593-595.

59. Madarikan BA, Lari J. Ingestion of dishwasher detergent by children. *Br J Clin Pract*. 1990;44:35-36.

60. Madden JW, et al. Experimental esophageal lye burns. II. Correcting established strictures with beta-aminopropionitrile and bougienage. *Ann Surg*. 1973;178:277-284.

61. Maull KI, et al. Liquid caustic ingestions: an in vitro study of the effects of buffer, neutralization, and dilution. *Ann Emerg Med*. 1985;14:1160-1162.

62. McKinney PE, et al. Acute zinc chloride ingestion in a child: local and systemic effects. *Ann Emerg Med*. 1994;23:1383-1387.

63. McKinney PE, et al. Zinc chloride ingestion in a child: exocrine pancreatic insufficiency. *Ann Emerg Med*. 1995;25:562.

64. Meredith JW, et al. Management of injuries from liquid lye ingestion. *J Trauma*. 1988;28:1173-1180.

65. Millar AJ, et al. Detection of caustic oesophageal injury with technetium 99m-labelled sucralfate. *J Pediatr Surg*. 2001;36:262-265.

66. Mills LJ, et al. Avoidance of esophageal stricture following severe caustic burns by the use of an intraluminal stent. *Ann Thorac Surg*. 1979;28:60-65.

67. Mitani M, et al. Endoscopic ultrasonography in corrosive injury of the upper gastrointestinal tract by hydrochloric acid. *J Clin Ultrasound JCU*. 1996;24:40-42.

68. Mutaf O, et al. Management of tracheoesophageal fistula as a complication of esophageal dilatations in caustic esophageal burns. *J Pediatr Surg*. 1995;30:823-826.

69. Newton JA, et al. Plasma mercury during prolonged acute renal failure after mercuric chloride ingestion. *Hum Toxicol*. 1983;2:535-537.

70. Nirapathpongporn S, et al. Pneumoperitoneum detected by ultrasound. *Radiology*. 1984;150:831-832.

71. Norton RA. Esophageal and antral strictures due to ingestion of household ammonia: report of two cases. *N Engl J Med*. 1960;262:10-12.

72. Okata Y, et al. Topical application of basic fibroblast growth factor reduces esophageal stricture and esophageal neural damage after sodium hydroxide-induced esophagitis in rats. *Pediatr Surg Int*. 2012;28:43-49.

73. Otçu S, et al. Biochemical indicators of caustic ingestion and/or accompanying esophageal injury in children. *Turk J Pediatr*. 2003;45:21-25.

74. Ozçelik MF, et al. The effect of halofuginone, a specific inhibitor of collagen type 1 synthesis, in the prevention of esophageal strictures related to caustic injury. *Am J Surg*. 2004;187:257-260.

75. Pelclová D, Navrátil T. Do corticosteroids prevent oesophageal stricture after corrosive ingestion? *Toxicol Rev*. 2005;24:125-129.

76. Previtera C, et al. Predictive value of visible lesions (cheeks, lips, oropharynx) in suspected caustic ingestion: may endoscopy reasonably be omitted in completely negative pediatric patients? *Pediatr Emerg Care*. 1990;6:176-178.

77. Ramasamy K, Gumaste VV. Corrosive ingestion in adults. *J Clin Gastroenterol*. 2003;37:119-124.

78. Reyes HM, Hill JL. Modification of the experimental stent technique for esophageal burns. *J Surg Res*. 1976;20:65-70.

79. Reyes HM, et al. Experimental treatment of corrosive esophageal burns. *J Pediatr Surg*. 1974;9:317-327.

80. Ritter FN, et al. A clinical and experimental study of corrosive burns of the stomach. *Ann Otol Rhinol Laryngol*. 1968;77:830-842.

81. Rumack BH, Burrington JD. Caustic ingestions: a rational look at diluents. *Clin Toxicol*. 1977;11:27-34.

82. Ryu HH, et al. Caustic injury: can CT grading system enable prediction of esophageal stricture? *Clin Toxicol Phila Pa*. 2010;48:137-142.

83. Scharman EJ. Liquid "laundry pods": a missed global toxicosurveillance opportunity. *Clin Toxicol Phila Pa*. 2012;50:725-726.

84. Schild JA. Caustic ingestion in adult patients. *Laryngoscope*. 1985;95:1199-1201.

85. Scott JC, et al. Caustic ingestion injuries of the upper aerodigestive tract. *Laryngoscope*. 1992;102:1-8.

86. Shirazi S, et al. Motility changes in opossum esophagus from experimental esophagitis. *Dig Dis Sci*. 1989;34:1668-1676.

87. Sinar D, et al. Acute acid-induced esophagitis impairs esophageal peristalsis in baboons. *Gastroenterology*. 80:1286.

88. Sinar DR, et al. Prostaglandin E1 effects on resting and cholinergically stimulated lower esophageal sphincter pressure in cats. *Prostaglandins*. 1981;21:581-590.

89. Singer AJ, et al. Mercuric chloride poisoning due to ingestion of a stool fixative. *J Toxicol Clin Toxicol*. 1994;32:577-582.

90. Tewfik TL, Schloss MD. Ingestion of lye and other corrosive agents—a study of 86 infant and child cases. *J Otolaryngol*. 1980;9:72-77.

91. Thompson JN. Corrosive esophageal injuries. I. A study of nine cases of concurrent accidental caustic ingestion. *Laryngoscope*. 1987;97:1060-1068.

92. Türkyilmaz Z, et al. Mitomycin C decreases the rate of stricture formation in caustic esophageal burns in rats. *Surgery*. 2009;145:219-225.

93. Usta M, et al. High doses of methylprednisolone in the management of caustic esophageal burns. *Pediatrics*. 2014;133:E1518-1524.

94. Uygun I. Caustic oesophagitis in children: prevalence, the corrosive agents involved, and management from primary care through to surgery. *Curr Opin Otolaryngol Head Neck Surg*. 2015;23:423-432.

95. Viscomi GJ, et al. An evaluation of early esophagoscopy and corticosteroid therapy in the management of corrosive injury of the esophagus. *J Pediatr*. 1961;59:356-360.

96. Webb WR, et al. An evaluation of steroids and antibiotics in caustic burns of the esophagus. *Ann Thorac Surg*. 1970;9:95-102.

97. White CS, et al. Esophageal perforation: CT findings. *AJR Am J Roentgenol*. 1993;160:767-770.

98. White JE, et al. Ocular alkali burn associated with automobile air-bag activation. *CMAJ Can Med Assoc J J Assoc Medicale Can*. 1995;153:933-934.

99. Wu MH, Lai WW. Surgical management of extensive corrosive injuries of the alimentary tract. *Surg Gynecol Obstet*. 1993;177:12-16.

100. Wu MH, Wu HY. Perioperative evaluation of patient outcomes after severe acid corrosive injury. *Surg Res Pract*. 2015;2015:545262.

101. Yoshida M, et al. Acute mercury poisoning by intentional ingestion of mercuric chloride. *Tohoku J Exp Med*. 1997;182:347-352.

102. Zargar SA, et al. The role of fiberoptic endoscopy in the management of corrosive ingestion and modified endoscopic classification of burns. *Gastrointest Endosc*. 1991;37:165-169.

103. Zargar SA, et al. Ingestion of corrosive acids. Spectrum of injury to upper gastrointestinal tract and natural history. *Gastroenterology*. 1989;97:702-707.

104

HYDROFLUORIC ACID AND FLUORIDES

Mark K. Su

HISTORY AND EPIDEMIOLOGY

Hydrofluoric acid has been known for centuries for its ability to dissolve silica. The Nuremberg artist Schwanhard is given credit for the first attempt in 1670 to use HF vapors to etch glass.[47] Today, hydrofluoric acid (HF) is widely used throughout industry. In addition to glass etching, HF is used in brick cleaning, etching microchips in the semiconductor industry, electroplating, leather tanning, rust removal, and the cleaning of porcelain.[47] From 2011 to 2015, the American Association of Poison Control Centers (AAPCC) reported 2,761 single-substance exposures to HF and 6 deaths (Chap. 130). The hands are the commonest part of the body injured. Exposures to HF often occur as unintentional occupational hazards. The actual number of work-related poisonings from HF appears difficult to quantitate because of limitations in International Classification of Diseases (ICD) medical coding and the lack of notification of regional poison control centers by worksites.[10]

Hydrofluoric acid is also the commonest cause of fluoride poisoning, although other forms of fluoride, including sodium fluoride (NaF), ammonium bifluoride (NH_4HF_2), and sodium or zinc fluorosilicate, also produce significant toxicity. Historically, NaF was used as an insecticide, rodenticide, an antihelminthic for swine, and a delousing powder for poultry and cattle. Ammonium bifluoride is mainly used in industrial inorganic chemistry, especially in the processing of alloys and in glass etching. Other fluoride salts are widely used in, for example, the steel industry, drinking water, toothpaste additives, electroplating, lumber treatment, and the glass and enamel industries.

The widespread use of HF and fluoride-containing compounds results in significant toxicity. In 1988, an oil refinery in Texas released a cloud of hydrogen fluoride gas that resulted in 939 people seeking hospital treatment and 94 of these patients requiring admission.[100] The petroleum industry has since been plagued by similar HF incidents.[100] In 2015, Washington State reported one death and 48 occupational HF burns associated with car and truck washing between 2001 and 2013.[78] Sodium fluoride was responsible for the poisoning of 263 people and 47 fatalities when it was mistaken for powdered milk and unintentionally combined with scrambled eggs.[55] Following ingestion, this and other fluoride salts are converted to HF in vivo, resulting in significant fluoride toxicity.

CHEMISTRY

Hydrofluoric acid is synthesized as the product of gaseous sulfuric acid and calcium fluoride, which is subsequently cooled to a liquid.[56] Aqueous HF is a weak acid, with a pK_a of 3.17; as such, it is approximately 1,000 times less dissociated than equimolar hydrochloric acid, a strong acid. Hydrofluoric acid generally ranges in concentrations from 3% to 40%, for use in both industry and the home. Anhydrous HF is highly concentrated (>70%) and used almost exclusively for industrial purposes. Hydrofluoric acid has unique properties that can cause life-threatening complications following seemingly trivial exposure.

Sodium fluoride is commonly synthesized by the reaction of sodium hydroxide (NaOH) with HF, with subsequent purification by recrystallization. Sodium fluoride is highly water soluble and readily dissociates.[4]

To synthesize ammonium bifluoride (NH_4HF_2), ammonium fluoride (NH_4F) is first formed by the reaction of ammonium hydroxide (NH_4OH) with HF. Ammonium fluoride is then converted to bifluoride by dehydrating the aqueous solution.

Fluorine is the most electronegative element in the Periodic Table of the Elements owing to its relatively large number of protons in the nucleus compared to its molecular size, and the minimal amount of screening or shielding by inner electrons. Other halides possess lesser electronegative properties. Consequently, the corresponding anion of fluorine, the fluoride ion (F^-), is a weak base because it possesses only a limited ability to donate its electrons. Liberation of the fluoride ion from the previously mentioned compounds is believed to be the major determinant of toxicity.

PATHOPHYSIOLOGY

Exposures to HF occur via dermal, ophthalmic, inhalation, oral, and rectal routes.[18] A permeability coefficient of 1.4×10^{-4} cm/sec allows HF to penetrate deeply into tissues prior to dissociating into hydrogen ions and highly electronegative fluoride ions.[34] These fluoride ions avidly bind to extracellular and intracellular stores of calcium (Ca^{2+}) and magnesium (Mg^{2+}), depleting them, and ultimately leading to cellular dysfunction and cell death.[11,54,64] The alteration in local calcium homeostasis causes neuroexcitation and accounts for the development of neuropathic pain. Furthermore, ischemia related to calcium dysregulation–mediated localized vasospasm is likely an additional contributory factor to the development of pain.[42,91]

Formation of insoluble calcium fluoride (CaF_2) is proposed as the etiology for both the precipitous fall in serum calcium concentration and the severe pain associated with tissue toxicity. There are several theories regarding the actual fate of calcium and fluoride ions in tissues. In vitro evidence suggests that fluorapatite is formed in the presence of phosphate and hydroxyapatite, which is a more likely pathway for disposition of the fluoride ion.[11] Fluorapatite, like calcium fluoride, is insoluble and its formation contributes to the clinical findings recognized following HF toxicity.

Fluoride also binds magnesium and manganese ions and there is in vitro evidence that this interferes with many enzyme systems. In the anhydrous form, the high concentration of hydrogen ions in HF also produces a caustic burn similar to that caused by strong acids (Chap. 103). The minimal lethal oral dose in humans is approximately 5 to 10 g of NaF.[5]

CLINICAL EFFECTS
Local Effects
Dermal

The extent of tissue injury following dermal exposure is determined by the volume, concentration, and contact time with the tissues. Following dermal exposure, the concentration of HF is directly related to the onset of pain at the contact site.[31,56,90] High concentrations (>20%) cause immediate pain with visible tissue damage.[84] Exposure to household rust-removal products (6% and 12% HF) is often associated with a typical latency of several hours, before pain develops.[31,85,95,96] The initial site of injury typically appears relatively benign despite significant subjective complaints of pain. Over time, the tissue becomes hyperemic, with subsequent blanching and coagulative necrosis. As calcium complexes precipitate, a white discoloration of the affected area appears[74] (Fig. 104–1). Ulceration is dependent on the concentration and duration of contact.[27,48,57] If more than 2.5% of the body surface area (BSA) is burned with highly concentrated HF, life-threatening systemic toxicity should be expected.[20,71,73,84,90] Small body surface area exposures to low concentrations (<20%) typically do not result in life-threatening systemic toxicity, although fatalities have resulted with dermal exposures to concentrated HF covering less than 5% body surface area.[89]

Gastrointestinal

Intentional ingestion of concentrated HF (or other fluoride salts) causes significant gastritis yet often spares the remainder of the gastrointestinal tract. Patients promptly develop vomiting and abdominal pain. Although systemic

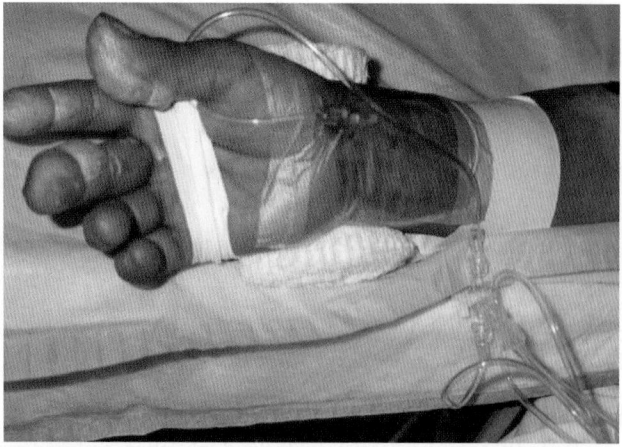

FIGURE 104–1. Severe injury to the fingers resulted from exposure to hydrofluoric acid. Note the arterial line in place for administration of calcium. *(Used with permission from the Fellowship in Medical Toxicology, New York University School of Medicine, New York City Poison Center.)*

absorption is rapid and almost invariably fatal, there is at least one report of a patient who ingested a low concentration (8%) of HF and suffered multiple episodes of ventricular fibrillation but was successfully resuscitated.[87] Following HF ingestion, patients often present with altered mental status, airway compromise, and dysrhythmias.[13,55,59,87]

Ophthalmic

Hydrofluoric acid results in more extensive injury to the eye than most other acids.[65] Ophthalmic exposures from liquid splashes or hydrogen fluoride gas rapidly denudes the corneal and conjunctival epithelium, and lead to stromal corneal edema, conjunctival ischemia, sloughing, and chemosis.[47] Fluoride ions penetrate deeply to affect anterior chamber structures.[47] The effects are usually noted within one day.[47] Other possible findings include corneal revascularization, recurrent epithelial erosions, and, sometimes, keratoconjunctivitis sicca (dry eye) develops as a long-term complication with subsequent corneal ulcers.[7,65,80]

Pulmonary

Patients with inhalational exposures present with a variety of signs and symptoms depending on the concentration and exposure time. Thirteen oil refinery workers exposed to a low-concentration HF mist experienced minor upper respiratory tract irritation.[52] By contrast, in a mass inhalational exposure to HF, throat burning and shortness of breath were among the more common chief complaints.[100] Some of these patients developed hypoxemia and hypocalcemia and had altered pulmonary function tests. Stridor, wheezing, rhonchi, and erythema and ulcers of the upper respiratory tract were described. Eye pain was also noted, reinforcing the fact that ophthalmic injury often accompanies inhalational and/or dermal exposures.[52,62,79,100]

ASSESSING SEVERITY OF SYSTEMIC EFFECTS

Significant systemic toxicity occurs via any route of exposure because of the ability of HF to penetrate tissues. The potential for systemic toxicity is an important consideration in management necessitating rapid decontamination and treatment.[12,16,33,83,84,92,93] Fatal exposures to HF by any route share the similar features of hypocalcemia, hypomagnesemia, and, in many cases, hyperkalemia as preterminal events.[4,13,19,23,33,56,59,66,67,90] In some circumstances, the hypocalcemia severely disrupts the coagulation cascade, resulting in significant anticoagulation, even on postmortem examination.[59,69,70]

Fatalities from HF occur as a result of either sudden-onset myocardial conduction failure or ventricular fibrillation. Although the evidence regarding the mechanism of myocardial irritability is inconclusive, electrolyte disturbances that lead to ventricular dysrhythmias including ventricular fibrillation are the most likely primary cause of death in patients with severe

systemic fluoride poisoning.[20,72,84,90,104] Although one postmortem human case reveals significant structural myocardial injury,[63] interestingly, histologic abnormalities of the myocardium do not occur in canine models of HF poisoning.[25,69]

Systemic fluoride toxicity results in hypocalcemia, by mechanisms not fully elucidated. Fluoride causes calcium ions to accumulate intracellularly, leading to an efflux of potassium ions into the extracellular space.[25,54,69] One in vitro study performed with human erythrocytes demonstrated that fluoride inhibition of Na^+,K^+-ATPase and Na^+,Ca^{2+} exchange leads to an increase in intracellular calcium.[68] The subsequent hyperkalemia alters the automaticity and resting potential of the heart, leading to fatal dysrhythmias (Chap. 15).[66] Dogs treated with quinidine, a potassium efflux blocker, are protected from lethal doses of intravenous NaF.[25] Likewise, amiodarone, which also blocks potassium efflux has demonstrable efficacy in both in vitro and in vivo models of fluoride toxicity.[88] However, efficacy in humans has not been studied. Furthermore, the mechanism of toxicity is likely much more complicated.[106] A child with systemic fluoride toxicity, who was appropriately replenished with calcium, and had normal electrolytes still experienced nonfatal ventricular fibrillation.[12,106] Perhaps this is because serum potassium, calcium, and magnesium concentrations only partly represent tissue concentrations.[11,12,25,66,67] Furthermore, HF directly impairs myocardial function. Rabbits exposed to topical HF over 2% of their total body surface area developed focal necrosis of myocardial fibers, as well as significant elevations in cardiac enzymes that persisted for almost 5 days after injury.[105]

Assessing Severity of Clinical Exposures. Historical and clinical features of an exposure usually determine which HF exposures are life-threatening. All oral and inhalational exposures are potentially fatal, as should burns of the face and neck, regardless of HF concentration. Inhalational exposure should be assumed for all patients with skin burns of greater than 5% body surface area, any exposure to HF concentrations greater than 20%, and head and neck burns.[46] Patients presenting with altered mental status directly related to HF are critically ill and necessitate rapid therapy.

Hydrofluoric acid concentrations greater than 20% have potential for significant toxicity in any patient, even if only a small surface area is exposed.[61] As a general rule, patients who experience severe pain within minutes of contact are most likely exposed to a very high concentration of HF and their condition should be expected to rapidly deteriorate. Some otherwise well-appearing patients have a precipitous demise without any clinical manifestations of hypocalcemia. Furthermore, it is possible that systemic toxicity will occur following seemingly minimal exposure. A 36-year-old man was exposed to 20% HF over a 3% BSA and subsequently developed hypocalcemia, hypomagnesemia, and cardiac arrest 16 hours later.[102] A 2-year-old girl ingested some "fingers full" of an ammonium bifluoride glass etching cream and had prolonged hypocalcemia refractory to calcium gluconate up to 24 hours after ingestion.[58] Consequently, patients will require prolonged electrolyte and cardiac monitoring following significant fluoride exposures.

DIAGNOSTIC TESTING

No monitoring or testing is required for uncomplicated small BSA exposures to low concentrations of HF. Diagnostic testing for systemic fluoride poisoning is currently based on monitoring of serum electrolytes. Calcium, magnesium and potassium concentrations should be serially monitored.[33] As systemic toxicity progresses, a metabolic acidosis will likely develop necessitating a venous or arterial blood gas analysis.[11] Serum fluoride concentrations are not readily available in a clinically relevant time frame. Although a serum fluoride concentration of 0.3 mg/dL was reported as fatal, one patient survived with a serum fluoride concentration of 1.4 mg/dL.[90,106]

Electrocardiographic findings of both hypocalcemia (prolonged QT interval) and hyperkalemia (peaked T waves, etc) are often reliable indicators of toxicity (Chap. 15).[4,16,33,36,41,70,90] In fact, ECG findings of peaked T waves from hyperkalemia preceded the onset of ventricular dysrhythmias in reported cases, thus potentially serving as a marker of severe fluoride toxicity.[12,67] It should be noted that in some cases of HF poisoning, hypokalemia is reported[26,32,102] and for unclear reasons, are specifically related to sodium fluoride toxicity.[97]

MANAGEMENT

General

For patients with more than localized exposure to low concentration (<20%) HF or any exposures to high concentration (>50%) HF, the mainstay of management is to prevent or limit systemic absorption, assess for systemic toxicity, and rapidly correct any electrolyte imbalances. Intravenous access should be obtained. An ECG should be obtained and examined for dysrhythmias and signs of hypocalcemia, hypomagnesemia, and hyperkalemia. The patient should be attached to continuous cardiac monitoring and have a rapid assessment of serum electrolyte concentrations.

Rapid airway assessment and protection should occur early in patients with inhalation or ingestion, respiratory distress, ingestion with vomiting, or burns significant enough to cause a change in mental status or phonation. If an unstable patient requires intubation, the depolarizing neuromuscular blocking agent, succinylcholine, should not be used because of potential hyperkalemia.

For patients with less significant dermal exposures, studies have focused on alternatives to irrigation with water or saline as decontamination techniques. The compound "hexafluorine" is promoted for dermal and ophthalmic decontamination of HF splashes.[60,86] Hexafluorine is a proprietary name whose chemical formula is not disclosed and papers that report success have strong ties to the manufacturer. In a controlled and blinded experimental study, Hexafluorine treatment was less effective than irrigation with water followed by the application of topical calcium.[40] In a follow-up animal study, water irrigation was as effective as Hexafluorine in preventing systemic toxicity from HF.[43] At this time, until further objective data are available, we do not recommend the use Hexafluorine for initial decontamination of patients with HF exposures.

An iodine-containing preparation was evaluated in a guinea pig model of HF-induced burns and found to be associated with significant reductions in ulceration area.[101] Iodine is hypothesized to inhibit apoptosis and has protective effects against burns from various alkylating agents, including mustard gas.[101] Because experience with iodine treatment of human HF burns is lacking, it cannot be recommended at this time.

The most important therapy for skin exposures is the rapid removal of clothing and irrigation of the affected area with copious amounts of water or saline, whichever is more readily available.[2,51,53,57]

One report describes a woman who was dying from severe HF toxicity who was treated by amputation of the affected limb, and survived. Although this may be an alternative measure for patients who are critically ill and demonstrate an inadequate response to all other therapeutic modalities, we do not recommend such aggressive measures.[15,49]

Dermal Toxicity

Several therapeutic options have been studied in animal models for treatment of topical HF burns. Unfortunately, many study designs use histologic or subjective wound inspection as outcome parameters,[17,75] some with unblinded inspection.[14,29,49,51,72] These animal models do not address the clinically important parameters of pain reduction, cosmesis, and functionality (Antidotes in Depth: A32).

We recommend that a topical calcium gel be applied to the affected area. A commercial gel is available in the United States but an acceptable substitute is reasonable and easily prepared. This is accomplished by mixing 3.5 g of calcium gluconate powder in 150 mL of sterile water-soluble lubricant, or 25 mL of 10% calcium gluconate in 75 mL of sterile water-soluble lubricant.[2,17,46] If calcium gluconate is unavailable, it is reasonable to use calcium chloride or calcium carbonate in a similar formulation.[21] This topical therapy for severe and non–life-threatening toxicity scavenges fluoride ions. After irrigation, we recommend a gel solution of calcium carbonate or gluconate be applied directly to the affected area or mixed directly into a sterile surgical glove and then placed on the patient's burned hand for 30 minutes.

Two case series report limited success with this therapy.[2,21] Some patients describe prompt and dramatic relief of pain. Alternatively or simultaneously, analgesics are recommended orally or parenterally as needed, but preferably not to the point of sedation, because local pain response is used to guide therapy. Digital nerve blocks with subcutaneous lidocaine or bupivacaine is also reasonable for patients with significant pain presenting 12 to 24 hours after the injury from a low concentration of HF and with no systemic signs of toxicity since that time topical calcium salts are unlikely to be effective.[28] An animal study examining the efficacy and mechanism of topical calcium gel therapy found that the fluoride ion concentration in the calcium gel was significantly higher than non–calcium-containing gel controls. Although this was a limited study, these animals also had a decrease in urinary fluoride ion concentration as compared to controls, suggesting less overall tissue absorption of the HF.[51] Delivery of calcium transcutaneously is enhanced by various means. In a rodent study of HF burns, iontophoretic (facilitated transport using an electromotive force) delivery of calcium ions appeared to increase calcium concentrations in vitro and improve pathologic changes in vivo.[103] Significant limitations to this study are time to administration of therapy and feasibility in patients with complex burns.[81] Human data are lacking. Dimethyl sulfoxide (DMSO) mixed with topical calcium salts facilitates the transport of calcium ions through the skin to penetrate deeply into the tissues. Dimethyl sulfoxide also is able to act as a scavenger of free radicals, thus limiting inflammation and ongoing injury.[36] Although one group of authors advocates for the combined use of DMSO and calcium,[36] concerns remain over reported adverse effects of DMSO.[47] There are currently inadequate data to support the routine use of DMSO in the treatment of HF burns.

Three other therapies have had variable success in human exposures: the application of calcium via intradermal, intravenous, and intraarterial routes. If topical gel therapy fails within the first few minutes of application, intradermal therapy with dilute calcium gluconate is a reasonable next step. Unfortunately, this treatment has limited usefulness and is not recommend in nondistensible spaces such as fingertips. Histologic studies in animal models demonstrate that 10% calcium chloride solution is damaging to the tissues and is not recommended.[28,35] The preferred method is to approach the wound from a distal point of injury and inject intradermally no more than 0.5 mL/cm^2 of 5% calcium gluconate. Although one author recommends a palmar fasciotomy whenever this method of treatment is used in the hand,[2] this practice is not recommended unless a compartment syndrome is present. The potential for iatrogenic injury exceeds the potential benefit of injections in the hand. The limits of intradermal injection include the potential to increase soft-tissue damage without adequate relief, infection, and inadequate space to safely inject without causing a compartment syndrome.

Effective pain relief is especially problematic for nailbed involvement, leading some authors to suggest removal of the nail. This approach has some advantages in accessing the affected area; however, it is a painful procedure that is often cosmetically undesirable and the outcome is not always significantly improved. We therefore do not routinely recommend this procedure.

If the wound is large or on a section of the fingerpad or an area that is not amenable to intradermal injections, intraarterial calcium gluconate is the next most reasonable step.[95] This procedure delivers calcium directly to the affected tissue from a proximal artery. Placement should be ipsilateral and proximal to the affected area, usually in the radial or brachial artery. The method of obtaining access is debated. Because of the potential to damage the endothelial lining of the artery, and because extravasation can have potentially devastating consequences, angiographic confirmation or direct visualization of the vessel was formerly recommended. This practice is still prudent if cannulation of the artery is expected to be difficult because of prior surgery or if an anatomic deformity is suspected. If the arterial line is carefully placed in a single attempt, and a good confirmatory arterial tracing is obtained, the infusion can be started. We recommend adding 10 mL of 10% calcium gluconate to either 40 mL of D$_5$W (dextrose 5% in water) or 0.9% sodium chloride solution infused continuously over 4 hours.[1,2,76,85,94,95] This results in a 2% calcium gluconate solution. An animal model examined the effect of undiluted 10% calcium gluconate intraaortically. Although the model did not involve exposure to HF, there was significant tissue injury in the vessel wall as compared to a 2% calcium gluconate solution.[28] Calcium chloride has also been used successfully, although the potential for vessel injury and extravasation are significant and there is no defined benefit over calcium gluconate.[94,107] The complications associated with the use of intraarterial calcium infusion in several case series were relatively benign, and include transient radial artery spasm, hematoma, inflammation at the puncture site, and a fall in serum magnesium concentration.[82,95] After the infusion is initiated, patients typically experience significant pain relief. Patients requiring an arterial line for treatment should be admitted to the hospital, as the majority will require more than one treatment, and some patients require as many as 5 separate infusions of calcium gluconate. Although wounds may require débridement,[2] some authors suggest that following intraarterial calcium infusion, tissue can be salvaged that initially would not have been considered viable.[96] There are no reported cases of clinically significant hypercalcemia following infusion as the total dose infused is quite low, although serum calcium concentrations were not routinely recorded in some cases.

Magnesium salts are an alternative or adjunctive therapy to the administration of calcium salts for patients with dermal HF burns. Application of magnesium hydroxide and magnesium gluconate gel show histologic evidence of efficacy in rabbit models of dermal HF burns.[17] Two other animal models of intravenous magnesium for dermal HF burns also suggest efficacy in terms of wound healing.[24,99] Magnesium was suggested as an antidote for fluoride poisoning because magnesium fluoride is more water soluble than calcium fluoride and magnesium is readily excreted by the kidneys.[100] However, these magnesium models inadequately address the disadvantage of magnesium salt solubility, and both topical and intravenous magnesium therapy remain incompletely evaluated in humans and therefore is not routinely recommended.

Another reported therapy for localized HF poisoning is an intravenous Bier block technique that uses 25 mL of 2.5% calcium gluconate. In one case, the effects lasted 5 hours and there were no adverse events.[39] In 2 other cases of patients exposed to HF, a 6% calcium gluconate solution administered using this procedure resulted in rapid and complete analgesia with minimal tissue necrosis.[82] Although the intravenous Bier block technique is not reported as being used in a substantial number of patients, it is reasonable, particularly when intraarterial infusion is problematic.[82] Further data are required before this therapy is routinely recommended.

We routinely observe all patients with digital exposures to HF over 4 to 6 hours, as the pain often recurs and reapplication of the gel or an alternative therapy will be necessary. Even if successful pain control is achieved, the patient will require specialized follow-up and wound care.

Inhalational Toxicity

Patients exposed to a low concentration of HF and treated with 4 mL of a 2.5% nebulized calcium gluconate solution demonstrated a subjective decrease in irritation with no adverse effects.[52] Another report demonstrated a good outcome following nebulization of a 5% calcium gluconate solution in a patient with an inhalational exposure.[50] Because nebulized calcium gluconate is a relatively benign therapy, we recommend that all patients with symptomatic inhalational exposures to any concentration of HF be administered a dilute solution of calcium gluconate.[30]

Ingestions

In patients with intentional ingestions of HF, gastrointestinal decontamination poses a dilemma. Induction of emesis is potentially harmful and therefore contraindicated. Because aqueous HF is a weak acid, the risk of perforation by passage of a small nasogastric tube may be lower than the risk of death from systemic absorption.[4,59] In the acidic environment of the stomach, more of the weak acid solution remains nonionized, thus penetrating the gastric mucosa and causing rapid systemic poisoning. Moreover, activated charcoal is unlikely to adsorb the relatively small fluoride ions. Although placement of a nasogastric tube to perform gastric lavage is

clearly associated with risks to the patient, insertion of a nasogastric tube is beneficial under specific circumstances if done safely and in a timely manner. Consequently, gastric emptying via a nasogastric tube is reasonable in the absence of significant spontaneous emesis because these exposures are almost universally fatal.[4,13,59,70] Health care providers should exercise extreme caution during this procedure because secondary dermal or inhalational exposures to the provider is possible in the absence of appropriate personal protective equipment. If there is a possibility of inhalation by the provider, the area should be well ventilated. Acceptable forms of hand protection include gloves made of nitrile, butyl rubber, polyvinyl chloride, or Neoprene. Latex gloves should not be used.

Following ingestion, we recommend a solution of a calcium or magnesium salt be administered orally as soon as possible to prevent HF penetration into the stomach and to provide an alternative source of cations for the damaging electronegative fluoride ions.

When comparing the efficacy of calcium to magnesium salts, calcium is better than magnesium in reducing the bioavailability of fluoride as described in a murine model.[38] Magnesium citrate in a standard cathartic dose, magnesium sulfate, or any of the calcium solutions can be administered orally to prevent absorption (Antidotes in Depth: A16). Although intuitive, evidence for the benefit of oral calcium or magnesium salts is limited. In a mouse model of oral HF toxicity, administration of calcium- or magnesium-containing solutions did not change average survival time.[37] The study results, however, were limited because the calcium and magnesium salts were premixed together with the HF during administration, thus being an inadequate model for the study of HF ingestion. In another study, the survival rate of mice poisoned with NaF was significantly greater when treated with either high doses of oral $CaCl_2$ or $MgSO_4$.[45] Given the current information, we recommend oral calcium salts for oral ingestion; however, if calcium salts are unavailable, magnesium salts are reasonable should be given.

Ophthalmic Toxicity

Patients with ophthalmic exposures should have each eye irrigated with 1 L of 0.9% sodium chloride solution, lactated Ringer solution, or water.[65] Although there are limited data, repetitive or prolonged irrigation appears to worsen outcome.[65] A complete ophthalmic examination should be performed after the patient is deemed stable, and an ophthalmology consultation should be obtained (Chap. 24). One case report demonstrated a good outcome following ocular HF exposure with the use of 1% calcium gluconate eye drops.[7] Although 2 reviews also recommend the use of 1% calcium gluconate for this purpose,[30,36] calcium salts tend to be irritating to the eye and this therapy is not adequately studied; consequently, use is not recommended at this time. There is no role for gel therapy or ophthalmic injection for these patients, because most calcium and magnesium salts are potentially toxic to ophthalmic tissues and may actually worsen outcome.[6,65]

Systemic Toxicity

If there is a clinical suspicion of severe toxicity, the immediate intravenous administration of both calcium and magnesium salts is recommended. Calcium gluconate is preferred over calcium chloride because of the risks associated with extravasation (Antidotes in Depth: A32). Patients often require several grams of calcium to treat severe HF toxicity.[33] We recommend that intravenous magnesium be administered to adults as 20 mL of a 20% magnesium sulfate solution (4 g) over 20 to 30 minutes. An approach that uses intravenous calcium or magnesium, and local calcium or magnesium gels to limit absorption protects against life-threatening hypocalcemia and hyperkalemia. Because of the numerous adverse effects of systemic fluoride poisoning, administration of calcium and magnesium salts alone is often insufficient in improving survival from systemic fluoride poisoning.[22] Furthermore, an animal model of hydrogen fluoride toxicity found that maintaining a normal acid–base balance was protective against HF toxicity.[98] Moreover, in a study of patients receiving enflurane, an inhalational anesthetic metabolized by the liver to fluoride ions, urine alkalinization improved the excretion of fluoride.[77] Thus, it is beneficial to correct any significant acidemia with hydration and IV sodium bicarbonate (calcium salts and sodium bicarbonate cannot be mixed). Because standard treatment for systemic fluoride toxicity includes administration of calcium salts and sodium bicarbonate, hyperkalemia is simultaneously addressed.

Treatment with large quantities of calcium and magnesium do not generally result in significant hypercalcemia or hypermagnesemia.[30] Several explanations are proposed. First, in systemically HF-poisoned patients, total body calcium and magnesium stores are severely decreased so that large doses are required for adequate repletion. In addition, most patients who are exposed to HF are young and healthy, with intact kidney function.[30] Administration of calcium also results in antidiuretic hormone antagonism on renal tubular reabsorption resulting in polyuria which facilitates the urinary excretion of calcium and magnesium.[30]

Because most of the fluoride ions are eliminated renally,[8,44,51,83] hemodialysis is reasonable in patients with severe HF poisoning and acute kidney injury. There are several reported cases of successful clearance of fluoride ions via hemodialysis, with one case also using continuous venovenous hemodialysis.[3,8,9] Because the reported clearance rate did not differ significantly from normally functioning kidneys, it is unclear whether hemodialysis alters outcome in patients with normal kidney function. Furthermore, prolonged hemodialysis, beyond the standard 4-hour course, is unnecessary for most patients unless they have kidney failure.[3]

Although the use of quinidine, a potassium channel blocker, is protective in dogs,[69] it has not been studied or used in humans, and at this time cannot be recommended, but in the presence of life-threatening ventricular dysrhythmias, quinidine (or any other class III antidysrhythmic) is reasonable.

SUMMARY

■ Although HF has a pKa of 3.17 and is considered a weak acid, it causes local and systemic toxicity because of fluoride binding to cations.

■ Dermal exposure to HF causes severe pain, often before any physical manifestations are evident.

■ In patients with greater than 2.5% BSA HF burns we recommend periodic assessment of serum calcium, magnesium, and potassium concentrations. Admission is required for prolonged electrolyte and cardiac monitoring.

■ Therapy for local toxicity includes topical calcium and magnesium salts and systemic analgesia. In some cases, intradermal or intraarterial administration of calcium is required.

■ Therapy for systemic toxicity includes all treatments for local toxicity plus intravenous calcium and magnesium salts, sodium bicarbonate, and potentially hemodialysis.

REFERENCES

1. Achinger R, et al. A new treatment method of hydrofluoric acid burns of the extremities [in German]. *Chir Forum Exp Klin Forsch*. 1979:229-231.
2. Anderson WJ, Anderson JR. Hydrofluoric acid burns of the hand: mechanism of injury and treatment. *J Hand Surg Am*. 1988;13:52-57.
3. Antar-Shultz M, et al. Use of hemodialysis after ingestion of a mixture of acids containing hydrofluoric acid. *Int J Clin Pharmacol Ther*. 2011;49:695-699.
4. Baltazar RF, et al. Acute fluoride poisoning leading to fatal hyperkalemia. *Chest*. 1980;78:660-663.
5. Baselt RC. *Disposition of Toxic Drugs and Chemicals in Man*. 9th ed. Seal Beach, CA; Biomedical Publications; 2011.
6. Beiran I, et al. The efficacy of calcium gluconate in ocular hydrofluoric acid burns. *Hum Exp Toxicol*. 1997;16:223-228.
7. Bentur Y, et al. The role of calcium gluconate in the treatment of hydrofluoric acid eye burn. *Ann Emerg Med*. 1993;22:1488-1490.
8. Berman L, et al. Inorganic fluoride poisoning: treatment by hemodialysis. *N Engl J Med*. 1973;289:922.
9. Bjornhagen V, et al. Hydrofluoric acid-induced burns and life-threatening systemic poisoning—favorable outcome after hemodialysis. *J Toxicol Clin Toxicol*. 2003;41:855-860.
10. Blodgett DW, et al. Fatal unintentional occupational poisonings by hydrofluoric acid in the U.S. *Am J Ind Med*. 2001;40:215-220.
11. Boink AB, et al. The mechanism of fluoride-induced hypocalcaemia. *Hum Exp Toxicol*. 1994;13:149-155.
12. Bordelon BM, et al. Systemic fluoride toxicity in a child with hydrofluoric acid burns: case report. *J Trauma*. 1993;34:437-439.
13. Bost RO, Springfield A. Fatal hydrofluoric acid ingestion: a suicide case report. *J Anal Toxicol*. 1995;19:535-536.
14. Bracken WM, et al. Comparative effectiveness of topical treatments for hydrofluoric acid burns. *J Occup Med*. 1985;27:733-739.
15. Buckingham FM. Surgery: a radical approach to severe hydrofluoric acid burns. A case report. *J Occup Med*. 1988;30:873-874.
16. Burke WJ, et al. Systemic fluoride poisoning resulting from a fluoride skin burn. *J Occup Med*. 1973;15:39-41.
17. Burkhart KK, et al. Comparison of topical magnesium and calcium treatment for dermal hydrofluoric acid burns. *Ann Emerg Med*. 1994;24:9-13.
18. Cappell MS, Simon T. Fulminant acute colitis following a self-administered hydrofluoric acid enema. *Am J Gastroenterol*. 1993;88:122-126.
19. Chan KM, et al. Fatality due to acute hydrofluoric acid exposure. *J Toxicol Clin Toxicol*. 1987;25:333-339.
20. Chela A, et al. Death due to hydrofluoric acid. *Am J Forensic Med Pathol*. 1989;10:47-48.
21. Chick LR, Borah G. Calcium carbonate gel therapy for hydrofluoric acid burns of the hand. *Plast Reconstr Surg*. 1990;86:935-940.
22. Coffey JA, et al. Limited efficacy of calcium and magnesium in a porcine model of hydrofluoric acid ingestion. *J Med Toxicol*. 2007;3:45-51.
23. Cordero SC, et al. A fatality due to ingestion of hydrofluoric acid. *J Anal Toxicol*. 2004;28:211-213.
24. Cox RD, Osgood KA. Evaluation of intravenous magnesium sulfate for the treatment of hydrofluoric acid burns. *J Toxicol Clin Toxicol*. 1994;32:123-136.
25. Cummings CC, McIvor ME. Fluoride-induced hyperkalemia: the role of Ca²⁺-dependent K+ channels. *Am J Emerg Med*. 1988;6:1-3.
26. Dalamaga M, et al. Hypocalcemia, hypomagnesemia, and hypokalemia following hydrofluoric acid chemical injury. *J Burn Care Res*. 2008;29:541-543.
27. Dibbell DG, et al. Hydrofluoric acid burns of the hand. *J Bone Joint Surg Am*. 1970;52:931-936.
28. Dowbak G, et al. A biochemical and histologic rationale for the treatment of hydrofluoric acid burns with calcium gluconate. *J Burn Care Rehabil*. 1994;15:323-327.
29. Dunn BJ, et al. Hydrofluoric acid dermal burns. An assessment of treatment efficacy using an experimental pig model. *J Occup Med*. 1992;34:902-909.
30. Dunser MW, et al. Critical care management of major hydrofluoric acid burns: a case report, review of the literature, and recommendations for therapy. *Burns*. 2004;30:391-398.
31. el Saadi MS, et al. Hydrofluoric acid dermal exposure. *Vet Hum Toxicol*. 1989;31:243-247.
32. Gallerani M, et al. Systemic and topical effects of intradermal hydrofluoric acid. *Am J Emerg Med*. 1998;16:521-522.
33. Greco RJ, et al. Hydrofluoric acid-induced hypocalcemia. *J Trauma*. 1988;28:1593-1596.
34. Gutknecht J, Walter A. Hydrofluoric and nitric acid transport through lipid bilayer membranes. *Biochim Biophys Acta*. 1981;644:153-156.
35. Harris JC, et al. Comparative efficacy of injectable calcium and magnesium salts in the therapy of hydrofluoric acid burns. *Clin Toxicol (Phila)*. 1981;18:1027-1032.
36. Hatzifotis M, et al. Hydrofluoric acid burns. *Burns*. 2004;30:156-159.
37. Heard K, Delgado J. Oral decontamination with calcium or magnesium salts does not improve survival following hydrofluoric acid ingestion. *J Toxicol Clin Toxicol*. 2003;41:789-792.
38. Heard K, et al. Calcium neutralizes fluoride bioavailability in a lethal model of fluoride poisoning. *J Toxicol Clin Toxicol*. 2001;39:349-353.
39. Henry JA, Hla KK. Intravenous regional calcium gluconate perfusion for hydrofluoric acid burns. *J Toxicol Clin Toxicol*. 1992;30:203-207.
40. Hojer J, et al. Topical treatments for hydrofluoric acid burns: a blind controlled experimental study. *J Toxicol Clin Toxicol*. 2002;40:861-866.
41. Holstege C, et al. The electrocardiographic toxidrome: the ECG presentation of hydrofluoric acid ingestion. *Am J Emerg Med*. 2005;23:171-176.
42. Huisman LC, et al. An atypical chemical burn. *Lancet*. 2001;358:1510.
43. Hulten P, et al. Hexafluorine vs. standard decontamination to reduce systemic toxicity after dermal exposure to hydrofluoric acid. *J Toxicol Clin Toxicol*. 2004;42:355-361.
44. Juncos LI, Donadio JV Jr. Renal failure and fluorosis. *JAMA*. 1972;222:783-785.
45. Kao WF, et al. Ingestion of low-concentration hydrofluoric acid: an insidious and potentially fatal poisoning. *Ann Emerg Med*. 1999;34:35-41.
46. Kirkpatrick JJ, Burd DA. An algorithmic approach to the treatment of hydrofluoric acid burns. *Burns*. 1995;21:495-499.
47. Kirkpatrick JJ, et al. Hydrofluoric acid burns: a review. *Burns*. 1995;21:483-493.
48. Klauder JV, et al. Industrial uses of compounds of fluorine and oxalic acid; cutaneous reaction and calcium therapy. *AMA Arch Ind Health*. 1955;12:412-419.
49. Kohnlein HE, et al. Hydrogen fluoride burns: experiments and treatment. *Surg Forum*. 1973;24:50.
50. Kono K, et al. Successful treatments of lung injury and skin burn due to hydrofluoric acid exposure. *Int Arch Occup Environ Health*. 2000;73(suppl):S93-S97.
51. Kono K, et al. An experimental study on the treatment of hydrofluoric acid burns. *Arch Environ Contam Toxicol*. 1992;22:414-418.
52. Lee DC, et al. Treatment of inhalational exposure to hydrofluoric acid with nebulized calcium gluconate. *J Occup Med*. 1993;35:470.
53. Leonard LG, et al. Chemical burns: effect of prompt first aid. *J Trauma*. 1982;22:420-423.

54. Lepke S, Passow H. Effects of fluoride on potassium and sodium permeability of the erythrocyte membrane. *J Gen Physiol.* 1968;51:365-372.

55. Lidbeck WL, et al. Acute sodium fluoride poisoning. *JAMA.* 1943;121:826-827.

56. MacKinnon MA. Hydrofluoric acid burns. *Dermatol Clin.* 1988;6:67-74.

57. MacKinnon MA. Treatment of hydrofluoric acid burns. *J Occup Med.* 1986;28:804.

58. Maddry JK, et al. Prolonged hypocalcemia refractory to calcium gluconate after ammonium bifluoride ingestion in a pediatric patient. *Am J Emerg Med.* 2017;35:378.e371-378.e372.

59. Manoguerra AS, Neuman TS. Fatal poisoning from acute hydrofluoric acid ingestion. *Am J Emerg Med.* 1986;4:362-363.

60. Mathieu L, et al. Efficacy of hexafluorine for emergent decontamination of hydrofluoric acid eye and skin splashes. *Vet Hum Toxicol.* 2001;43:263-265.

61. Matsuno K. The treatment of hydrofluoric acid burns. *Occup Med (Lond).* 1996;46:313-317.

62. Mayer L, Guelich J. Hydrogen fluoride (Hf) inhalation and burns. *Arch Environ Health.* 1963;7:445-447.

63. Mayer TG, Gross PL. Fatal systemic fluorosis due to hydrofluoric acid burns. *Ann Emerg Med.* 1985;14:149-153.

64. McClure F. A review of fluorine and its physiologic effects. *Physiol Rev.* 1933;13:277-300.

65. McCulley JP, et al. Hydrofluoric acid burns of the eye. *J Occup Med.* 1983;25:447-450.

66. McIvor M, et al. Hyperkalemia and cardiac arrest from fluoride exposure during hemodialysis. *Am J Cardiol.* 1983;51:901-902.

67. McIvor ME. Delayed fatal hyperkalemia in a patient with acute fluoride intoxication. *Ann Emerg Med.* 1987;16:1165-1167.

68. McIvor ME, Cummings CC. Sodium fluoride produces a K^+ efflux by increasing intracellular Ca^{2+} through Na^+-Ca^{2+} exchange. *Toxicol Lett.* 1987;38:169-176.

69. McIvor ME, et al. Sudden cardiac death from acute fluoride intoxication: the role of potassium. *Ann Emerg Med.* 1987;16:777-781.

70. Menchel SM, Dunn WA. Hydrofluoric acid poisoning. *Am J Forensic Med Pathol.* 1984;5:245-248.

71. Mullett T, et al. Fatal hydrofluoric acid cutaneous exposure with refractory ventricular fibrillation. *J Burn Care Rehabil.* 1987;8:216-219.

72. Murao M. Studies on the treatment of hydrofluoric acid burn. *Bull Osaka Med Coll.* 1989;35:39-48.

73. Muriale L, et al. Fatality due to acute fluoride poisoning following dermal contact with hydrofluoric acid in a palynology laboratory. *Ann Occup Hyg.* 1996;40:705-710.

74. Noonan T, et al. Epidermal lipids and the natural history of hydrofluoric acid (HF) injury. *Burns.* 1994;20:202-206.

75. Paley A, Seifter J. Treatment of experimental hydrofluoric acid corrosion. *Exp Biol Med.* 1941;46:190-192.

76. Pegg SP, et al. Intra-arterial infusions in the treatment of hydrofluoric acid burns. *Burns Incl Therm Inj.* 1985;11:440-443.

77. Proudfoot AT, et al. Position paper on urine alkalinization. *J Toxicol Clin Toxicol.* 2004;42:1-26.

78. Reeb-Whitaker CK, et al. Occupational hydrofluoric acid injury from car and truck washing—Washington State, 2001-2013. *MMWR Morb Mortal Wkly Rep.* 2015;64:874-877.

79. Rose L. Further evaluation of hydrofluoric acid burns of the eye. *J Occup Med.* 1984;26:483, 486.

80. Rubinfeld RS, et al. Ocular hydrofluoric acid burns. *Am J Ophthalmol.* 1992;114:420-423.

81. Rutan R, et al. Electricity and the treatment of hydrofluoric acid burns—the wave of the future or a jolt from the past? *Crit Care Med.* 2001;29:1646.

82. Ryan JM, et al. Regional intravenous calcium—an effective method of treating hydrofluoric acid burns to limb peripheries. *J Accid Emerg Med.* 1997;14:401-402.

83. Sadove R, et al. Total body immersion in hydrofluoric acid. *South Med J.* 1990;83:698-700.

84. Sheridan RL, et al. Emergency management of major hydrofluoric acid exposures. *Burns.* 1995;21:62-64.

85. Siegel DC, Heard JM. Intra-arterial calcium infusion for hydrofluoric acid burns. *Aviat Space Environ Med.* 1992;63:206-211.

86. Soderberg K, et al. An improved method for emergent decontamination of ocular and dermal hydrofluoric acid splashes. *Vet Hum Toxicol.* 2004;46:216-218.

87. Stremski ES, et al. Survival following hydrofluoric acid ingestion. *Ann Emerg Med.* 1992;21:1396-1399.

88. Su M, et al. Amiodarone attenuates fluoride-induced hyperkalemia in vitro. *Acad Emerg Med.* 2003;10:105-109.

89. Takase I, et al. Fatality due to acute fluoride poisoning in the workplace. *Leg Med (Tokyo).* 2004;6:197-200.

90. Tepperman PB. Fatality due to acute systemic fluoride poisoning following a hydrofluoric acid skin burn. *J Occup Med.* 1980;22:691-692.

91. Thomas D, et al. Intra-arterial calcium gluconate treatment after hydrofluoric acid burn of the hand. *Cardiovasc Intervent Radiol.* 2009;32:155-158.

92. Trevino MA, et al. Treatment of severe hydrofluoric acid exposures. *J Occup Med.* 1983;25:861-863.

93. Upfal M, Doyle C. Medical management of hydrofluoric acid exposure. *J Occup Med.* 1990;32:726-731.

94. Upton J, et al. Major intravenous extravasation injuries. *Am J Surg.* 1979;137:497-506.

95. Vance MV, et al. Digital hydrofluoric acid burns: treatment with intraarterial calcium infusion. *Ann Emerg Med.* 1986;15:890-896.

96. Velvart J. Arterial perfusion for hydrofluoric acid burns. *Hum Toxicol.* 1983;2:233-238.

97. Vohra R, et al. Recurrent life-threatening ventricular dysrhythmias associated with acute hydrofluoric acid ingestion: observations in one case and implications for mechanism of toxicity. *Clin Toxicol (Phila).* 2008;46:79-84.

98. Whitford GM, et al. Acute fluoride toxicity: influence of metabolic alkalosis. *Toxicol Appl Pharmacol.* 1979;50:31-39.

99. Williams JM, et al. Intravenous magnesium in the treatment of hydrofluoric acid burns in rats. *Ann Emerg Med.* 1994;23:464-469.

100. Wing JS, et al. Acute health effects in a community after a release of hydrofluoric acid. *Arch Environ Health.* 1991;46:155-160.

101. Wormser U, et al. Protective effect of topical iodine preparations upon heat-induced and hydrofluoric acid-induced skin lesions. *Toxicol Pathol.* 2002;30:552-558.

102. Wu ML, et al. Survival after hypocalcemia, hypomagnesemia, hypokalemia and cardiac arrest following mild hydrofluoric acid burn. *Clin Toxicol (Phila).* 2010;48:953-955.

103. Yamashita M, et al. Iontophoretic delivery of calcium for experimental hydrofluoric acid burns. *Crit Care Med.* 2001;29:1575-1578.

104. Yamaura K, et al. Recurrent ventricular tachyarrhythmias associated with QT prolongation following hydrofluoric acid burns. *J Toxicol Clin Toxicol.* 1997;35:311-313.

105. Yan F, et al. An experimental study of myocardial injury by hydrofluoric acid in burned rabbits [in Chinese]. *Zhonghua Shao Shang Za Zhi* 2000;16:237-240.

106. Yolken R, et al. Acute fluoride poisoning. *Pediatrics.* 1976;58:90-93.

107. Yosowitz P, et al. Peripheral intravenous infiltration necrosis. *Ann Surg.* 1975;182:553-556.

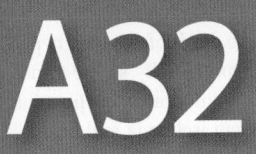
CALCIUM

Silas W. Smith and Mary Ann Howland

INTRODUCTION

Calcium is a divalent cation that is essential to maintain the normal function of the heart, vascular smooth muscle, the skeletal system, the nervous system, and intracellular signaling. It is vital in enzymatic reactions, neurohormonal transmission, blood coagulation, and the maintenance of cellular integrity.[12] The endocrine system maintains calcium homeostasis. Hypercalcemia raises the threshold for nerve and muscle excitation, resulting in muscle weakness, lethargy, cardiac conduction disturbances, and coma. Hypocalcemia can result in hyperreflexia, muscle spasms, tetany, seizures, and QT interval prolongation (Chaps. 12 and 15).[12]

HISTORY

Sir Humphry Davy used his pioneering work in electrolysis to isolate potassium and sodium from their hydroxides in 1807. In 1808, using slightly moistened lime, $Ca(OH)_2$, Davy succeeded again, in a series of experiments using electrolysis, to isolate calcium.[25] Ringer performed controlled animal experiments in the 1880s demonstrating the importance of calcium in sustaining and resuscitating cardiac ventricular contraction.[96,97] As the clinical use of calcium chloride antedated 1938, it was "grandfathered" under the Food, Drug, and Cosmetic Act; calcium gluconate was approved in 1941.[37,115]

PHARMACOLOGY
Chemistry/Preparation

Calcium has an atomic number of 20, a molecular weight of 40.08 Da, and a valence of 2. For clinical use, calcium is prepared typically in combination with gluconate or chloride. Calcium as calcium chloride ($CaCl_2$) is used in its dihydrate form $CaCl_2 \cdot 2H_2O$, with a molecular weight of 147.02 Da when accounting for water. It is a white odorless fragments or granules that are freely soluble in water.[1] Calcium as calcium gluconate is provided as calcium D-gluconate (1:2) monohydrate, $C_{12}H_{22}CaO_{14} \cdot H_2O$, with a molecular weight of 448.39 Da.[37] It is a clear and colorless to slightly yellow solution.

Related Agents

Calcium as calcium chloride or gluconate is a component of electrolyte, parenteral nutrition, dialysis, and cardioplegic solutions.[115] Calcium acetate is used orally to treat hyperphosphatemia, particularly in patients with end-stage kidney disease.[10] Other oral calcium salts such as calcium carbonate, citrate, lactate, glubionate, glycerophosphate, and polycarbophil are variously used as cariostatics, food additives, mineral supplements, and stool stabilizers.

Pharmacokinetics

Calcium is the fifth most abundant element and the most abundant mineral in the body, and the third most common plasma cation after sodium and potassium.[1,31] More than 99% of the 1 to 2 kg of calcium in the adult human is located in bone.[12] Calcium is variously reported in units of mg/dL, mmol/L (mM), and mEq/L, as well as both in total and ionized values. To convert mg/dL to mM, multiply by 0.25; to convert mg/dL to mEq/L, multiply by 0.5. Antidotal calcium is also variously reported as grams of the salt or mEq (mM) of calcium. One gram of calcium chloride contains 13.6 mEq (6.8 mM, 272.5 mg) of elemental calcium; one gram of calcium gluconate contains 4.64 mEq (2.32 mM, 93 mg) of calcium. In blood, the total calcium concentration is normally 8.5 to 10.6 mg/dL (2.13–2.65 mM, 4.25–5.3 mEq/L), of which approximately half is ionized and active, that is, 4.65 to 5.30 mg/dL (1.16–1.33 mM, 2.33–2.65 mEq/L).[39] The remaining calcium is bound to negatively charged proteins (such as albumin and immunoglobulins) or loosely associated with anions such as phosphate, citrate, sulfate, lactate, and bicarbonate.[12] Because of this calcium binding to albumin, the total calcium is typically corrected or adjusted as follows:

$$Calcium_{corrected}\,(mg/dL) = Serum\ calcium_{measured}\,(mg/dL) + [\kappa \times (normal\ albumin - measured\ albumin)],$$

where κ is typically ascribed a value of 0.8 and a "normal" albumin is arbitrarily 4 g/dL.[88] However, this formula underestimates calcium for albumin values greater than 4 g/dL, limiting its utility in cases of hyperalbuminemia.[86] Calcium concentrations are also affected by pH, with increases in pH causing a decrease in ionized calcium and vice versa.[103] Intracellular cytosolic free calcium concentrations are many orders of magnitude (~10,000-fold) lower than ionized calcium concentrations in the blood and extracellular fluid, creating a significant gradient.[12] Calcium is excreted fecally as insoluble salts (80%) and renally (20%).[1] Non–albumin-bound calcium is filterable at the glomerulus and is reabsorbed in the proximal tubule (60%–70%), in the thick ascending limb of Henle (20%–30%), and in the distal convoluted tubule (10%).[35]

Following establishment of the principle that ionized calcium was critical for myocardial inotropy and conduction, calcium preparations were evaluated for their kinetics and effects. In a placebo-controlled trial of 30 consecutive adults receiving cardiopulmonary bypass and citrated blood products, calcium chloride via intermittent IV bolus (5 mg/kg) or as a constant infusion (0.5 mg/kg/min) raised ionized calcium concentrations from 1.48±0.30 to 1.79±0.28 mEq/L (0.74±0.15 to 0.89±0.14 mM), but did not produce a detectible hemodynamic effect.[4] In a prospective, randomized, double-blind trial of calcium chloride in 36 cardiac surgery patients emerging from cardiopulmonary bypass, calcium chloride (200 mg/dose) increased serum ionized calcium by 6% to 8%.[57] In a prospective, randomized, blinded, crossover designed study of 12 postoperative aortocoronary bypass surgery patients, calcium chloride (10 mg/kg bolus followed by 2 mg/kg/h infusion) raised ionized calcium concentrations from 2.12±0.06 to 2.88±0.1 mEq/L (1.06±0.03 to 1.44±0.05 mM), and raised arterial pressure without elevating cardiac index.[126] In a single-arm, placebo-controlled study of 43 preterm infants, calcium gluconate (100 mg/kg over 30–60 minutes) raised total and ionized serum calcium concentrations 3 to 6 hours after infusion from 3.16±0.06 to 3.4±0.1 mEq/L (1.58±0.03 to 1.70±0.05 mM) and 1.34±0.06 to 1.6±0.04 mEq/L (0.67±0.03 to 0.80±0.02 mM), respectively.[93]

The issue of interchangeability arose because calcium gluconate was thought to both have a lower bioavailability and to require gluconate metabolism for ionized calcium release.[123] In 49 hypocalcemic critically ill children, calcium chloride produced slightly larger increases in ionic calcium than infusions of calcium gluconate in central venous infusions (not controlled for rate of administration), with no survival difference.[13] Other studies challenged the notion of calcium gluconate metabolism. In 15 adults undergoing extracorporeal perfusion with a citrated priming solution, there were no significant differences in ionized calcium between calcium chloride or calcium gluconate.[123] In animals instrumented with a calcium-selective catheter electrode in the aorta, there was no significant difference in plasma calcium ion concentrations between calcium gluconate and calcium chloride administered intravenously.[48] Similar results were found in human in vitro experiments, in which calcium gluconate and calcium chloride added to blood samples produced identical rises in plasma calcium ion concentrations.[48] In 10 children undergoing burn excision and grafting, calcium chloride and calcium gluconate produced identical ionized calcium changes at 0, 0.5, 1, 3, 5, and 10 minutes when injected over the same period of time.[23] Animal studies with calcium chloride (4, 8, 12 mg/kg) and calcium gluconate (14, 28, 42 mg/kg) produced similar ionized calcium concentrations when measured as early as 30 seconds to 45 minutes.[23] In a pivotal human trial during the intraoperative period in liver transplant patients in which no liver was present, administration of equivalent molar doses of calcium found in calcium chloride (1 g CaCl$_2$ 10%) and calcium gluconate (3 g Ca gluconate 10%) produced similar serum ionized calcium concentrations, with both peaks occurring within 30 seconds.[77] These results support the concept that simple dissociation of calcium from gluconate is responsible for releasing calcium, rather than hepatic metabolism.[37]

Pharmacodynamics and Mechanisms of Action

The roles and functions of calcium are more completely reviewed in Chaps. 12, 13, 15, 16, and 20. Calcium is fundamental to neurotransmission, cardiovascular physiology, muscle performance, bone maintenance, coagulation, cellular exocytosis, and signaling. Cardiac excitation-contraction coupling is accomplished via sodium-triggered calcium influx through voltage-activated L-type calcium channels (Ca$_v$1.2), which triggers ryanodine receptor type-2 (RyR2) calcium release, calcium binding to and activation of cardiac troponin C, and initiation of myofilament contraction.[66] Calcium is labeled for use in children and adults for the treatment of acute symptomatic hypocalcemia and conditions requiring a prompt increase in plasma calcium.[1,37]

ROLE IN CALCIUM CHANNEL BLOCKER TOXICITY

Calcium enters cells in numerous ways. In cardiac and smooth muscles the voltage-dependent L-type channels are inhibited by the calcium channel blockers (CCBs) available in the United States.[7,106] Patients with CCB overdose (Chap. 60) typically develop nausea, vomiting, hypotension, bradycardia, myocardial depression, sinus arrest, atrioventricular (AV) block, cardiovascular collapse, and metabolic acidosis, hyperglycemia, shock, pulmonary edema, altered mental status, and seizures.[59,89] Because CCBs do not alter either receptor-operated channels or the release of calcium from intracellular stores,[113] the serum calcium concentration remains normal in overdose.

Intravenous administration of calcium to dogs poisoned with verapamil or diltiazem improved cardiac output secondary to increased inotropy.[44] The heart rate and cardiac conduction were affected minimally, if at all.[38,44] Case reports and reviews of the literature suggest similar minimal or variable findings in human calcium channel blocker overdose, although some cases report benefit in severe bradycardia or asystole.[2,3,14,21,27,34,36,45,59,74,94,95,108] Pretreatment with 10 mL of 10% calcium chloride prevented hypotension associated with intravenous verapamil (average verapamil dose 6.25 ± 1.52 mg) administered for supraventricular tachycardia.[43] Calcium gluconate provided prior to or following intravenous verapamil demonstrated similar efficacy.[122] Several other clinical trials validated the efficacy of calcium salts to preclude verapamil-induced hypotension.[6,63,80,101] A statistically significant benefit in preventing hypotension was not observed with calcium pretreatment in diltiazem administration.[61]

As a relatively simple intervention, calcium is recommended for symptomatic patients with CCB overdoses.[53,65,73] Unfortunately, the most seriously ill patients respond inadequately, and other measures are often required. The dose of calcium needed to treat patients with CCB overdose is unknown. In animal experiments, there appears to be a dose-related improvement.[14] Several authors have successfully treated patients with a total of 18-30 g of calcium gluconate or 13 g of calcium chloride over 0.5-12 hours, either by intermittent bolus dose or infusion, without apparent adverse

effects.[14,53,65,73,74] However, following the use of large doses of calcium, hypercalcemia is expected, which is associated with potentially severe consequences including altered mental status, gut atony, myocardial depression, and intense vasoconstriction leading to multiorgan ischemia and death.[105] Introduction of high-dose insulin (Antidotes in Depth: A21) in the treatment of CCB overdose has diminished the need for extensive calcium administration. The provision of massive calcium doses should therefore be limited, and if used, meticulous monitoring of ionized calcium is advised to avoid hypercalcemia (Table A32–1).

Because calcium chloride is extremely irritating to small vessels, subcutaneous tissue, and muscle, and causes necrosis following extravasation, it is usually only administered through a central venous line. The customary approach is to administer an initial IV dose of 3 g of calcium gluconate (30 mL of 10% calcium gluconate) or 1 g of calcium chloride (10 mL of 10% calcium chloride) to adults.[89] Based on case reports, it is reasonable to repeat this dose every 10–20 minutes for up to 3–4 doses as necessary. The hypothesis is that sufficient calcium must be present to compete with the CCB for binding to the L-type calcium channel. This approach is reportedly beneficial even in moribund cases. One author used a total of 10 g of calcium gluconate as 1 g boluses over 12 minutes after diltiazem induced asystole and another 2.5 g of calcium gluconate minutes later for a second asystolic event, with a resultant serum calcium concentration of 3.36 mM (6.72 mEq/L) approximately 1 hour after administration of the calcium gluconate.[55] Other authors reported smaller dose requirements (eg, 2 g calcium gluconate) in diltiazem-induced asystole.[21] Table A32–1 provides recommended dosing.

The administration of calcium to a patient with toxicity from cardioactive steroids such as digoxin is potentially harmful.[42,120] In the event of concurrent overdose with both a cardioactive steroid and a CCB, the early use of digoxin-specific antibody fragments (Antidotes in Depth: A22) will permit the subsequent safe use of calcium (Chap. 62).

Therapy in children poisoned by CCBs is based on more limited data. The American Heart Association pediatric guidelines did not review calcium administration in calcium channel blocker exposure in the 2015 update to the 2010 guidelines.[26] The 2010 guidelines preferentially suggested calcium chloride based on a single study mentioned above that compared the chloride to the gluconate salt in critically ill children with hypocalcemia.[13] The 2015 guidelines comment that calcium administration is of variable efficacy.[26] It is reasonable to administer calcium gluconate in pediatric CCB toxicity, particularly if only peripheral venous access is available.[60]

TABLE A32–1	Calcium Salts for Intravenous Use	
	Calcium Gluconate[a]	**Calcium Chloride (CaCl$_2$)**[a,b]
10% solution	10 mL = 1 g of Ca^{2+} gluconate 10 mL = 4.64 mEq = 93 mg = 2.32 mmol of elemental Ca^{2+} *or* 1 mL = 0.465 mEq = 9.3 mg = 0.23 mmol of elemental Ca^{2+}	10 mL = 1 g of CaCl$_2$ 10 mL = 13.6 mEq = 273 mg = 6.8 mmol of elemental Ca^{2+} *or* 1 mL = 1.36 mEq = 27.3 mg = 0.68 mmol of elemental Ca^{2+}
Adult dose	3 g (30 mL of 10% solution) over 10 minutes (unless in extremis—deliver over 60 seconds) Repeat every 10–20 minutes up to 3–4 doses as necessary	1 g (10 mL of 10% solution) over 10 minutes (unless in extremis—deliver over 60 seconds) Repeat every 10–20 minutes up to 3–4 doses as necessary
Pediatric dose (not to exceed the adult dose)	60 mg/kg (0.6 mL/kg) of 10% solution infused over 5–10 minutes (unless in extremis—deliver over 60 seconds) Repeat every 10–20 minutes up to 3–4 doses as necessary	20 mg/kg (0.2 mL/kg) infused over 5–10 minutes (unless in extremis—deliver over 60 seconds) Repeat every 10–20 minutes up to 3–4 doses as necessary

[a]Monitor calcium concentration after several doses. [b]Use of a central venous line is recommended to avoid extravasation.

ROLE IN β-ADRENERGIC ANTAGONIST TOXICITY

In vitro studies suggest that the negative inotropic action of β-adrenergic antagonists are related to interference with both the forward and reverse transport of calcium in the sarcoplasmic reticulum and the inhibition of microsomal and mitochondrial calcium uptake (Chap. 59).[28,67,84] In isolated rat hearts, higher calcium concentrations blunted the adverse effects of β-adrenergic antagonists.[29,67] In a canine model of propranolol poisoning, the administration of calcium chloride improved mean arterial pressure, the change in maximal left ventricular pressure over time, and peripheral vascular resistance, but it had no significant effect on bradycardia or QRS complex prolongation.[72] With a dose of both propranolol and verapamil that produced death in all controls, calcium chloride pretreatment in mice and posttreatment in rabbits and swine led to survival of all animals.[118] Several case reports attest to the beneficial effects of intravenous calcium in β-adrenergic antagonist overdose alone or in combination with CCBs.[11,50,58,92,102] Because distinguishing an overdose of a CCB from that of a β-adrenergic antagonist is often clinically difficult and the 2 classes are sometimes ingested simultaneously, a trial of IV calcium is reasonable for a presumed β-adrenergic antagonist overdose if cardioactive steroid toxicity is excluded.

ROLE IN HYPOCALCEMIA SECONDARY TO ETHYLENE GLYCOL

Following ethylene glycol poisoning (Chap. 106), metabolism of the parent molecule generates oxalic acid, which complexes with calcium and subsequently precipitates in the kidneys, brain, and elsewhere, resulting in hypocalcemia.[54,87,106,110] Although one more recent study found hypocalcemia to be uncommon and to correlate poorly with changes in serum pH, it may yet be severe enough to warrant treatment.[51] After exposure to ethylene glycol, it is reasonable to monitor the ionized calcium concentration in addition to repeated examinations for signs of hypocalcemia such as QT interval prolongation, hyperreflexia, muscle spasms, tetany, and seizures (Chap. 12). Intravenous calcium is recommended in the customary doses (as above) to patients with these findings.

ROLE IN HYPOCALCEMIA SECONDARY TO HYDROFLUORIC ACID AND FLUORIDE-RELEASING XENOBIOTICS

Deaths from dermal, gastrointestinal, and inhalational hydrofluoric acid (HF) exposures are well documented in the literature.[17,41,119] In these cases, hypocalcemia is invariably present. Any body contact with HF (Chap. 104) can result in severe burns and death, depending on concentration, area exposed, and duration of exposure. The toxicity results from (a) release of free hydrogen ions; (b) complexation of fluoride with calcium and magnesium to interfere with many enzyme systems and to form insoluble salts, which cause cellular necrosis; (c) liberation of potassium ions and permeability of cell membranes for potassium ions, and other mechanism.[16,33,75,78,121] Soluble salts of fluoride and bifluoride (eg, sodium, potassium, and ammonium) have all the toxicity associated with HF and should be managed accordingly.

Following HF exposure, calcium gluconate is recommended topically and subcutaneously to manage minor to moderate cutaneous burns, intravenously to treat systemic hypocalcemia, and intraarterially to manage significant burns.[2,16,17,18,22,33,41,75,78,83,90,98,104,117,119,125] Experimental studies demonstrate that when concentrated HF burns are immediately flushed with water and then treated with topical calcium, burn size, severity, and depth are significantly reduced.[9,15] A 2.5% topical calcium gluconate topical gel is marketed. In the event that the commercial preparation is inaccessible, a topical calcium gel can be prepared from calcium carbonate tablets, calcium gluconate powder or solution, and a water-soluble jelly or surgical lubricant (mix 3.5 g calcium gluconate powder or 35 mL of a 10% calcium gluconate solution or 10 g of calcium carbonate tablets or seven 500-mg crushed calcium gluconate tablets with 5 oz of water-soluble jelly). The chloride salt is also acceptable for topical therapy. However, calcium chloride should never be injected into tissues (subcutaneously, intramuscularly), because severe tissue necrosis can result. While an experimental study in rats demonstrated that iontophoretic delivery of calcium chloride enhanced the delivery of calcium and

significantly reduced the burn area if applied within 30 minutes,[100,124] practical considerations have limited use.

Repeated intrabrachial arterial perfusion of calcium gluconate was described in 1979.[56] Use of intravenous regional analgesia (the "Bier's method" or "Bier block") for hydrofluoric acid poisoning was reported in 1992.[49] In patients with severe topical HF exposures, aggressive administration of regional IV calcium using a Bier block technique (10 mL of 10% calcium gluconate in a total volume of 40 mL) or intraarterial calcium (10 mL of 10% calcium gluconate in 50 mL in a total volume of 5% dextrose solution over 4 hours) is reasonable (Chap. 104).[46,71,111] One patient who was massively exposed to HF required 211 mEq (4.2 g) of calcium (equivalent to 15.5 g of calcium chloride) infused within the first 5 hours, with an additional 55.8 mEq (1.1 g) of calcium gluconate injected below the burn eschar.[41] For moderate to severe burns (generally from HF concentrations >20%) of the fingers and hands or other areas such as the face, an intraarterial calcium infusion is reasonable and more effective than local or IV therapy, although it is more invasive and more hazardous.[83,90,104,111,117,119] In a series of 7 cases who failed topical therapy, 4 patients had complete pain relief with Bier's technique and one patient had partial relief, with 3 patients requiring intraarterial therapy.[40] A calcium gluconate solution (10 mL of 10%) mixed in 40 to 50 mL of 5% dextrose solution creates a reasonable concentration to be infused intraarterially over 4 hours, followed by subsequent 40 to 50 mL intraarterial infusions after 4 hours when pain persists.[116]

In patients with life-threatening poisoning and particularly HF inhalation, it is reasonable to simultaneously administer IV, oral, and nebulized 2.5% calcium gluconate[68] to facilitate the availability of the maximum amount of calcium. To prepare nebulized calcium gluconate, mix 1.5 mL of 10% calcium gluconate solution with 4.5 mL of sterile water or 0.9% sodium chloride to make a 2.5% solution. Serum calcium, potassium, and magnesium concentrations should be carefully monitored in all severely poisoned patients, as well as coagulation parameters, which are disrupted by calcium depletion.[121]

Hypocalcemia from the ingestion of household fluoride-containing dental products such as dental fluoride rinses and sodium fluoride tablets rarely occurs and is dose dependent. Hypocalcemia and significant morbidity and mortality occur with ingestion of industrial-strength fluoride cleaners or fluoride releasers such as ammonium bifluoride used for cleaning white wall tires. Patients with these exposures should be treated with calcium in a manner similar to the hypocalcemia from other causes.

ROLE IN HYPOCALCEMIA SECONDARY TO PHOSPHATE EXPOSURES

Inappropriate use of oral and rectal phosphates as a laxative can result in hypocalcemia, hyperphosphatemia, and hyperkalemia with resultant morbidity and mortality.[5,30] Furthermore, even routine high phosphorus supplementation (1 g/day) in healthy adults adversely affects calcium metabolism.[112] Intravenous calcium is recommended for life-threatening hypocalcemia. However, because administration of calcium in the presence of hyperphosphatemia risks precipitation of calcium phosphate throughout the body (most commonly in cases of chronic phosphate exposure),[30] in non–life-threatening cases, the risks and benefits of calcium administration versus hemodialysis and other therapies should be weighed in consultation with a nephrologist.

ROLE IN HYPERMAGNESEMIA

Hypermagnesemia causes both direct and indirect depression of skeletal muscle, resulting in neuromuscular blockade, loss of reflexes, and profound muscular paralysis, with attendant ventilatory failure (Chap. 12 and Antidotes in Depth: A16).[31,64,81] Excess magnesium also causes prolongation of the PR interval and QRS complex on electrocardiography (ECG) and depression of the sinoatrial node, leading to a bradycardic arrest. Intravenous calcium serves as a physiologic competitive antagonist to these adverse effects of magnesium and is recommended as indicated in Table A32–1.

ROLE IN HYPERKALEMIA

Hyperkalemia causes significant myocardial depression. The resultant ECG changes are well defined. The height of the T wave increases, and lengthening of the PR interval and QRS complex develop; ultimately, a sine wave pattern precipitating cardiac arrest occurs (Chaps. 12 and 15).[79,99] Calcium makes the membrane threshold potential less negative, restoring the resting and threshold potential difference so that a larger stimulus is required to depolarize the cell from the resting potential. This stabilization antagonizes the hyperexcitability caused by modest hyperkalemia.[79] However, when severe hyperkalemia exists, voltage-gated sodium channels are inactivated and cannot be depolarized, regardless of the strength of the impulse. Calcium transforms the voltage sensor of the sodium channel from inactive to closed, thus allowing the sodium channel to be opened with depolarization.[52] The typical initial dose is 1 g (10 mL) of IV calcium gluconate. The onset of action is within minutes, but the duration of action is only 30-60 minutes. Data do not support any definitive recommendations for repeat calcium administration; experts recommend up to 2 additional doses.[99] If hyperkalemia is secondary to the toxic effects of cardioactive steroids on the Na+,K+-adenosine triphosphatase (ATPase) pump, IV calcium can potentially exacerbate an already excessive intracellular calcium concentration, making IV calcium potentially harmful (Chap. 62). Although the consequences of inadvertent administration have been somewhat mitigated by animal and clinical experience, digoxin-specific antibody fragments (Antidotes in Depth: A22) should be given for cardioactive steroid-induced hyperkalemia.[42,69,120]

ROLE IN CITRATE TOXICITY

Citrate binds divalent cations. This property is useful therapeutically (eg, to mitigate renal calcium stone disease) and analytically (eg, to facilitate laboratory anticoagulation studies). Citrate is hepatically metabolized via the citric acid cycle and participates in many other pathways, including conversion to glucose via gluconeogenesis.[32,82] In a process dating back to 1914–1915, blood products contain citrate to prevent coagulation, and thus citrate is transfused into the patient.[32] In massive transfusions, with citrate use in extracorporeal circuits, and in patients with liver disease (who metabolize citrate more slowly), excess citrate causes toxicity (hypocalcemia and more rarely, hypomagnesemia).[4,32,82,91] Signs and symptoms range from mild perioral paresthesias and digital numbness to tetany, myocardial depression, and cardiac dysrhythmias.[24,47] Calcium correction should be guided by clinical signs and ionized calcium determinations. Calcium should not be directly added to blood products, as this can cause clotting, but rather provided via a separate infusion line.

ADVERSE EFFECTS AND SAFETY ISSUES

Severe hypercalcemia is defined by a serum calcium concentration greater than 14.0 mg/dL (3.5 mmol/L) in a patient with a normal albumin concentration.[19] The adverse effects of hypercalcemia (independent of the rate of administration) include nausea, vomiting, constipation, ileus, polyuria, polydipsia, nephrolithiasis, cognitive alterations, hyporeflexia, coma, vascular alterations, and dysrhythmias.[114] Excessively aggressive calcium infusions in a patient with channel blocker overdose have led to death.[105] Neither calcium chloride nor calcium gluconate should be combined and administered intravenously with sodium bicarbonate because calcium carbonate, a precipitate, is formed. Calcium gluconate is not physically compatible with fluids containing phosphate and will result in precipitation if mixed with solutions of these compounds.[37] Calcium gluconate should not be mixed with ceftriaxone, because of formation of ceftriaxone-calcium precipitates that may act as emboli.[37] Calcium should not be given concurrently with minocycline, as it complexes with minocycline, rendering it inactive.[37] Calcium chloride is an acidifying salt, and it is extremely irritating to tissue. It should never be given intramuscularly, subcutaneously, or perivascularly, and is typically administered via central venous access. In a series of 96 patients receiving IV calcium chloride solution peripherally for symptomatic hypocalcemia after parathyroidectomy, 3 suffered skin necrosis.[70] Calcium gluconate is less irritating, but care should also be taken to avoid

extravasation. Calcinosis cutis—dermal deposits of calcium salts—which can lead to tissue necrosis, ulceration, and secondary infection is reported with calcium gluconate.[37] The best reason for choosing calcium gluconate in almost all clinical situations is that the risk of tissue injury is far less. If extravasation occurs, subcutaneous injection of aliquots of hyaluronidase is reasonable to inject around the site to diminish tissue injury (Special Considerations: SC8). In pediatric patients intraosseous calcium chloride administration along with other vasopressors is rarely associated with acute limb ischemia, presumably due to calcium extravasation, which resulted in amputation.[85,109]

PREGNANCY AND LACTATION

Calcium injection is U.S. Food and Drug Administration pregnancy category C. Animal reproductive studies have not been conducted. Benefit is expected to outweigh risk when indicated as life-saving therapy for the mother. The World Health Organization guidelines recommend calcium supplementation as part of antenatal care to reduce maternal mortality.[76] Calcium is excreted as a natural component in human breast milk, but no definitive evaluations have been performed on potential adverse effects in the breastfed child following maternal intravenous calcium administration.

DOSING AND ADMINISTRATION

Intravenous calcium must be administered slowly, at a rate not exceeding 0.7 to 1.8 mEq (14–36.1 mg) per minute, which equates to approximately one-half to one 10-mL vial of calcium chloride or one-and-one-half to three 10-mL vials of calcium gluconate over 10 minutes in adults, unless the patient is in extremis. The package label recommends not to exceed 200 mg/min calcium gluconate in adult patients or 100 mg/min in pediatric patients.[37] More rapid administration can lead to vasodilation, hypotension, bradycardia, dysrhythmias, syncope, and cardiac arrest.[8,20,62,107] In cases of life-threatening hypocalcemia or for a patient in extremis, a slow IV push is reasonable. Repeat doses are administered every 10 to 20 minutes up to 3 to 4 doses as clinically indicated. Total and ionized calcium should be frequently monitored, particularly in light of the acid–base disturbances that occur in poisoned patients. Topical, nebulized, and intraarterial administration is specifically addressed in the section on the role of calcium in the management of HF. If time permits, calcium solutions should be warmed to body temperature to minimize pain. Although intraosseous administration of calcium was used for vascular collapse, ensuring correct needle placement and the gluconate formulation are recommended, given the previous reports of limb ischemia.[85,109] Pediatric dosing is provided in Table A32–1.

FORMULATION AND ACQUISITION

A variety of calcium salts are available for parenteral administration. The 2 most commonly used are calcium chloride (10%) and calcium gluconate (10%) (Table A32–1). Calcium chloride 10% injection contains 100 mg of calcium chloride per mL, which contains 27.3 mg (1.36 mEq) of elemental calcium per mL.[115] Calcium gluconate 10% injection contains 100 mg of calcium gluconate per mL, which contains 9.3 mg (0.464 mEq) of elemental calcium per mL.[37] Calcium chloride 10% injection has a pH of 6.3 (5.5–7.5); calcium gluconate 10% injection has a pH of 6.0 to 8.2.

A topical calcium gluconate gel (2.5%) 25 g is available. Topical preparations can be made extemporaneously as described in the section above on hydrofluoric acid. A commercially prepared emergency eyewash calcium gluconate 1% solution is available in 120-mL squirt bottles.

SUMMARY

- Calcium serves as a physiologic antagonist to the cardiac and/or neurologic effects of hypermagnesemia and hyperkalemia and counteracts some of the effects of CCB overdoses.
- Calcium is beneficial in the treatment of some β-adrenergic antagonist overdoses, and since coingestion with CCBs occurs, is reasonable to administer.
- Intravenous calcium infusion is an effective antidote for the hypocalcemia induced by ethylene glycol, phosphate, HF, and fluoride-releasing xenobiotics.

- Equivalent molar calcium doses found in appropriate volumes of calcium gluconate and calcium chloride deliver equal amounts of ionized calcium.
- Calcium gluconate is preferred for peripheral administration because extravasation of calcium chloride causes tissue necrosis.
- Electrocardiographic monitoring and frequent ionized calcium concentration measurements are required to prevent iatrogenic toxicity.

REFERENCES

1. Abbot Laboratories. 10% Calcium chloride, USP [label]. Chicago, IL; 2000.
2. Anderson WJ, Anderson JR. Hydrofluoric acid burns of the hand: mechanism of injury and treatment. *J Hand Surg Am.* 1988;13:52-57.
3. Ashraf M, et al. Massive overdose of sustained-release verapamil: a case report and review of literature. *Am J Med Sci.* 1995;310:258-263.
4. Auffant RA, et al. Ionized calcium concentration and cardiovascular function after cardiopulmonary bypass. *Arch Surg.* 1981;116:1072-1076.
5. Azzam I, et al. Life threatening hyperphosphataemia after administration of sodium phosphate in preparation for colonoscopy. *Postgrad Med J.* 2004;80:487-488.
6. Barnett JC, Touchon RC. Short-term control of supraventricular tachycardia with verapamil infusion and calcium pretreatment. *Chest.* 1990;97:1106-1109.
7. Bean BP. Classes of calcium channels in vertebrate cells. *Annu Rev Physiol.* 1989; 51:367-384.
8. Berliner K. The effect of calcium injections on the human heart. *Am J Med Sci.* 1936;191:117-121.
9. Bracken WM, et al. Comparative effectiveness of topical treatments for hydrofluoric acid burns. *J Occup Med.* 1985;27:733-739.
10. Braintree Laboratories I. PhosLo® Capsules (Calcium Acetate) [prescribing information]. Braintree, MA: Braintree Laboratories, Inc; 2001.
11. Brimacombe JR, et al. Propranolol overdose—a dramatic response to calcium chloride. *Med J Aust.* 1991;155:267-268.
12. Bringhurst F, et al. Bone and mineral metabolism in health and disease. In: Kasper D, et al, eds. *Harrison's Principles of Internal Medicine.* 19th ed. New York, NY: McGraw-Hill; 2014.
13. Broner CW, et al. A prospective, randomized, double-blind comparison of calcium chloride and calcium gluconate therapies for hypocalcemia in critically ill children. *J Pediatr.* 1990;117:986-989.
14. Buckley N, et al. Slow-release verapamil poisoning. Use of polyethylene glycol whole-bowel lavage and high-dose calcium. *Med J Aust.* 1993;158:202-204.
15. Burkhart KK, et al. Comparison of topical magnesium and calcium treatment for dermal hydrofluoric acid burns. *Ann Emerg Med.* 1994;24:9-13.
16. Caravati EM. Acute hydrofluoric acid exposure. *Am J Emerg Med.* 1988;6:143-150.
17. Chan KM, et al. Fatality due to acute hydrofluoric acid exposure. *J Toxicol Clin Toxicol.* 1987;25:333-339.
18. Chick LR, Borah G. Calcium carbonate gel therapy for hydrofluoric acid burns of the hand. *Plast Reconstr Surg.* 1990;86:935-940.
19. Cho KC. Electrolyte & acid-base disorders. In: Papadakis MA et al, eds. *Current Medical Diagnosis & Treatment.* New York, NY: McGraw-Hill; 2018.
20. Clarke NE. The action of calcium on the human electrocardiogram. *Am Heart J.* 1941;22:367-373.
21. Connolly DL, et al. Massive diltiazem overdose. *Am J Cardiol.* 1993;72:742-743.
22. Conway EE Jr, Sockolow R. Hydrofluoric acid burn in a child. *Pediatr Emerg Care.* 1991;7:345-347.
23. Cote CJ, et al. Calcium chloride versus calcium gluconate: comparison of ionization and cardiovascular effects in children and dogs. *Anesthesiology.* 1987;66:465-470.
24. Cote CJ, et al. Ionized hypocalcemia after fresh frozen plasma administration to thermally injured children: effects of infusion rate, duration, and treatment with calcium chloride. *Anesth Analg.* 1988;67:152-160.
25. Davy H. Electro-chemical researches, on the decomposition of the earths; with observations on the metals obtained from the alkaline earths, and on the amalgam procured from ammonia. *Phil Trans R Soc Lond.* 1808;98:333-370.
26. de Caen AR, et al. Part 12: pediatric advanced life support: 2015 American Heart Association Guidelines Update for Cardiopulmonary Resuscitation and Emergency Cardiovascular Care. *Circulation.* 2015;132:S526-S542.
27. DeWitt CR, Waksman JC. Pharmacology, pathophysiology and management of calcium channel blocker and beta-blocker toxicity. *Toxicol Rev.* 2004;23:223-238.
28. Dhalla NS, Lee SL. Comparison of the actions of acebutolol, practolol and propranolol on calcium transport by heart microsomes and mitochondria. *Br J Pharmacol.* 1976;57:215-221.
29. Dhalla NS, et al. Effects of acebutolol, practolol and propranolol on the rat heart sarcolemma. *Biochem Pharmacol.* 1977;26:2055-2060.
30. Domico MB, et al. Severe hyperphosphatemia and hypocalcemic tetany after oral laxative administration in a 3-month-old infant. *Pediatrics.* 2006;118:e1580-e1583.
31. Dube L, Granry JC. The therapeutic use of magnesium in anesthesiology, intensive care and emergency medicine: a review. *Can J Anaesth.* 2003;50:732-746.
32. Dzik WH, Kirkley SA. Citrate toxicity during massive blood transfusion. *Transfus Med Rev.* 1988;2:76-94.
33. Edinburg M, Swift R. Hydrofluoric acid burns of the hands: a case report and suggested management. *Aust N Z J Surg.* 1989;59:88-91.
34. Erickson FC, et al. Diltiazem overdose: case report and review. *J Emerg Med.* 1991;9:357-366.
35. Felsenfeld AJ, et al. Pathophysiology of calcium, phosphorus, and magnesium dysregulation in chronic kidney disease. *Semin Dial.* 2015;28:564-577.
36. Ferner RE, et al. Pharmacokinetics and toxic effects of diltiazem in massive overdose. *Hum Toxicol.* 1989;8:497-499.
37. Fresenius Kabi. Calcium gluconate injection, for intravenous use [prescribing information]. Lake Zurich, IL: Fresenius Kabi; 2017.
38. Gay R, et al. Treatment of verapamil toxicity in intact dogs. *J Clin Invest.* 1986;77:1805-1811.
39. Goltzman D. Approach to hypercalcemia. In: De Groot LJ, et al, eds. *Endotext.* South Dartmouth, MA: MDText.com, Inc; 2016.
40. Graudins A, et al. Regional intravenous infusion of calcium gluconate for hydrofluoric acid burns of the upper extremity. *Ann Emerg Med.* 1997;30:604-607.
41. Greco RJ, et al. Hydrofluoric acid-induced hypocalcemia. *J Trauma.* 1988;28:1593-1596.
42. Hack JB, et al. The effect of calcium chloride in treating hyperkalemia due to acute digoxin toxicity in a porcine model. *J Toxicol Clin Toxicol.* 2004;42:337-342.
43. Haft JI, Habbab MA. Treatment of atrial arrhythmias. Effectiveness of verapamil when preceded by calcium infusion. *Arch Intern Med.* 1986;146:1085-1089.
44. Hariman RJ, et al. Reversal of the cardiovascular effects of verapamil by calcium and sodium: differences between electrophysiologic and hemodynamic responses. *Circulation.* 1979;59:797-804.
45. Harris NS. Case records of the Massachusetts General Hospital. Case 24-2006. A 40-year-old woman with hypotension after an overdose of amlodipine. *N Engl J Med.* 2006;355:602-611.
46. Hatzifotis M, et al. Hydrofluoric acid burns. *Burns.* 2004;30:156-159.
47. Hegde V, et al. Prophylactic low dose continuous calcium infusion during peripheral blood stem cell (PBSC) collections to reduce citrate related toxicity. *Transfus Apher Sci.* 2016;54:373-376.
48. Heining MP, et al. Choice of calcium salt. A comparison of the effects of calcium chloride and gluconate on plasma ionized calcium. *Anaesthesia.* 1984;39:1079-1082.
49. Henry JA, Hla KK. Intravenous regional calcium gluconate perfusion for hydrofluoric acid burns. *J Toxicol Clin Toxicol.* 1992;30:203-207.
50. Henry M, et al. Cardiogenic shock associated with calcium-channel and beta blockers: reversal with intravenous calcium chloride. *Am J Emerg Med.* 1985;3:334-336.
51. Hodgman M, et al. Serum calcium concentration in ethylene glycol poisoning. *J Med Toxicol.* 2017;13:153-157.
52. Hofer CA, et al. Verapamil intoxication: a literature review of overdoses and discussion of therapeutic options. *Am J Med.* 1993;95:431-438.
53. Hung YM, Olson KR. Acute amlodipine overdose treated by high dose intravenous calcium in a patient with severe renal insufficiency. *Clin Toxicol (Phila).* 2007;45:301-303.
54. Introna F Jr, Smialek JE. Antifreeze (ethylene glycol) intoxications in Baltimore. Report of six cases. *Acta Morphol Hung.* 1989;37:245-263.
55. Isbister GK. Delayed asystolic cardiac arrest after diltiazem overdose; resuscitation with high dose intravenous calcium. *Emerg Med J.* 2002;19:355-357.
56. Jacobitz K, et al. A new treatment method for hydrochloric acid burns of the hand [in German]. *Handchirurgie.* 1979;11:81-85.
57. Johnston WE, et al. Is calcium or ephedrine superior to placebo for emergence from cardiopulmonary bypass? *J Cardiothorac Vasc Anesth.* 1992;6:528-534.
58. Jones JL. Metoprolol overdose. *Ann Emerg Med.* 1982;11:114-115.
59. Kerns W 2nd. Management of beta-adrenergic blocker and calcium channel antagonist toxicity. *Emerg Med Clin North Am.* 2007;25:309-331.
60. Kleinman ME, et al. Part 14: pediatric advanced life support: 2010 American Heart Association Guidelines for Cardiopulmonary Resuscitation and Emergency Cardiovascular Care. *Circulation.* 2010;122:S876-S908.
61. Kolkebeck T, et al. Calcium chloride before i.v. diltiazem in the management of atrial fibrillation. *J Emerg Med.* 2004;26:395-400.
62. Kuhn M. Severe bradyarrhythmias following calcium pretreatment. *Am Heart J.* 1991;121:1812-1813.
63. Kuhn M, Schriger DL. Low-dose calcium pretreatment to prevent verapamil-induced hypotension. *Am Heart J.* 1992;124:231-232.
64. Kutsal E, et al. Severe hypermagnesemia as a result of excessive cathartic ingestion in a child without renal failure. *Pediatr Emerg Care.* 2007;23:570-572.
65. Lam YM, et al. Continuous calcium chloride infusion for massive nifedipine overdose. *Chest.* 2001;119:1280-1282.
66. Landstrom AP, et al. Calcium signaling and cardiac arrhythmias. *Circ Res.* 2017;120:1969-1993.
67. Langemeijer J, et al. Calcium interferes with the cardiodepressive effects of beta-blocker overdose in isolated rat hearts. *J Toxicol Clin Toxicol.* 1986;24:111-133.
68. Lee DC, et al. Treatment of inhalational exposure to hydrofluoric acid with nebulized calcium gluconate. *J Occup Med.* 1993;35:470.
69. Levine M, et al. The effects of intravenous calcium in patients with digoxin toxicity. *J Emerg Med.* 2011;40:41-46.
70. Lin CY, et al. Skin necrosis after intravenous calcium chloride administration as a complication of parathyroidectomy for secondary hyperparathyroidism: report of four cases. *Surg Today.* 2007;37:778-781.

71. Lin TM, et al. Continuous intra-arterial infusion therapy in hydrofluoric acid burns. *J Occup Environ Med.* 2000;42:892-897.

72. Love JN, et al. Hemodynamic effects of calcium chloride in a canine model of acute propranolol intoxication. *Ann Emerg Med.* 1996;28:1-6.

73. Luscher TF, et al. Calcium gluconate in severe verapamil intoxication. *N Engl J Med.* 1994;330:718-720.

74. MacDonald D, Alguire PC. Case report: fatal overdose with sustained-release verapamil. *Am J Med Sci.* 1992;303:115-117.

75. MacKinnon MA. Hydrofluoric acid burns. *Dermatol Clin.* 1988;6:67-74.

76. Martin SL, et al. Adherence-specific social support enhances adherence to calcium supplementation regimens among pregnant women. *J Nutr.* 2017;147:688-696.

77. Martin TJ, et al. Ionization and hemodynamic effects of calcium chloride and calcium gluconate in the absence of hepatic function. *Anesthesiology.* 1990;73:62-65.

78. McCulley JP. Ocular hydrofluoric acid burns: animal model, mechanism of injury and therapy. *Trans Am Ophthalmol Soc.* 1990;88:649-684.

79. Meroney WH, Herndon RF. The management of acute renal insufficiency. *J Am Med Assoc.* 1954;155:877-883.

80. Miyagawa K, et al. Administration of intravenous calcium before verapamil to prevent hypotension in elderly patients with paroxysmal supraventricular tachycardia. *J Cardiovasc Pharmacol.* 1993;22:273-279.

81. Moe SM. Disorders involving calcium, phosphorus, and magnesium. *Prim Care.* 2008;35:215-237, v-vi.

82. Monchi M. Citrate pathophysiology and metabolism. *Transfus Apher Sci.* 2017;56:28-30.

83. Nguyen LT, et al. Treatment of hydrofluoric acid burn to the face by carotid artery infusion of calcium gluconate. *J Burn Care Rehabil.* 2004;25:421-424.

84. Noack E, et al. The effect of propranolol and its analogs on Ca^{++} transport by sarcoplasmic reticulum vesicles. *J Pharmacol Exp Ther.* 1978;206:281-288.

85. Oesterlie GE, et al. Crural amputation of a newborn as a consequence of intraosseous needle insertion and calcium infusion. *Pediatr Emerg Care.* 2014;30:413-414.

86. Parent X, et al. "Corrected" calcium: calcium status underestimation in non-hypoalbuminemic patients and in hypercalcemic patients [in French]. *Ann Biol Clin (Paris).* 2009;67:411-418.

87. Parry MF, Wallach R. Ethylene glycol poisoning. *Am J Med.* 1974;57:143-150.

88. Payne RB, et al. Interpretation of serum calcium in patients with abnormal serum proteins. *Br Med J.* 1973;4:643-646.

89. Pearigen PD, Benowitz NL. Poisoning due to calcium antagonists. Experience with verapamil, diltiazem and nifedipine. *Drug Saf.* 1991;6:408-430.

90. Pegg SP, et al. Intra-arterial infusions in the treatment of hydrofluoric acid burns. *Burns Incl Therm Inj.* 1985;11:440-443.

91. Perkins HA, et al. Calcium ion activity during rapid exchange transfusion with citrated blood. *Transfusion.* 1971;11:204-212.

92. Pertoldi F, et al. Electromechanical dissociation 48 hours after atenolol overdose: usefulness of calcium chloride. *Ann Emerg Med.* 1998;31:777-781.

93. Porcelli PJ Jr, Oh W. Effects of single dose calcium gluconate infusion in hypocalcemic preterm infants. *Am J Perinatol.* 1995;12:18-21.

94. Proano L, et al. Calcium channel blocker overdose. *Am J Emerg Med.* 1995;13:444-450.

95. Ramoska EA, et al. A one-year evaluation of calcium channel blocker overdoses: toxicity and treatment. *Ann Emerg Med.* 1993;22:196-200.

96. Ringer S. Regarding the action of hydrate of soda, hydrate of ammonia, and hydrate of potash on the ventricle of the frog's heart. *J Physiol.* 1882;3:195-202.

97. Ringer S, Buxton DW. Concerning the action of calcium, potassium, and sodium salts upon the eel's heart and upon the skeletal muscles of the frog. *J Physiol.* 1887;8:15-19.

98. Roberts JR, Merigian KS. Acute hydrofluoric acid exposure. *Am J Emerg Med.* 1989;7:125-126.

99. Rossignol P, et al. Emergency management of severe hyperkalemia: guideline for best practice and opportunities for the future. *Pharmacol Res.* 2016;113:585-591.

100. Rutan R, et al. Electricity and the treatment of hydrofluoric acid burns—the wave of the future or a jolt from the past? *Crit Care Med.* 2001;29:1646.

101. Salerno DM, et al. Intravenous verapamil for treatment of multifocal atrial tachycardia with and without calcium pretreatment. *Ann Intern Med.* 1987;107:623-628.

102. Sangster B, et al. A case of acebutolol intoxication. *J Toxicol Clin Toxicol.* 1983;20:69-77.

103. Seamonds B, et al. Determination of ionized calcium in serum by use of an ion-selective electrode. I. Determination of normal values under physiologic conditions, with comments on the effects of food ingestion and hyperventilation. *Clin Chem.* 1972;18:155-160.

104. Siegel DC, Heard JM. Intra-arterial calcium infusion for hydrofluoric acid burns. *Aviat Space Environ Med.* 1992;63:206-211.

105. Sim MT, Stevenson FT. A fatal case of iatrogenic hypercalcemia after calcium channel blocker overdose. *J Med Toxicol.* 2008;4:25-29.

106. Simpson E. Some aspects of calcium metabolism in a fatal case of ethylene glycol poisoning. *Ann Clin Biochem.* 1985;22(pt 1):90-93.

107. Smallwood RA. Some effects of the intravenous administration of calcium in man. *Australas Ann Med.* 1967;16:126-131.

108. Spiller HA, et al. Delayed onset of cardiac arrhythmias from sustained-release verapamil. *Ann Emerg Med.* 1991;20:201-203.

109. Tareq AA. Gangrene of the leg following intraosseous infusion. *Ann Saudi Med.* 2008;28:456-457.

110. Tarr BD, et al. Low-dose ethanol in the treatment of ethylene glycol poisoning. *J Vet Pharmacol Ther.* 1985;8:254-262.

111. Thomas D, et al. Intra-arterial calcium gluconate treatment after hydrofluoric acid burn of the hand. *Cardiovasc Intervent Radiol.* 2009;32:155-158.

112. Trautvetter U, et al. Consequences of a high phosphorus intake on mineral metabolism and bone remodeling in dependence of calcium intake in healthy subjects—a randomized placebo-controlled human intervention study. *Nutr J.* 2016;15:7.

113. Triggle DJ. Calcium-channel antagonists: mechanisms of action, vascular selectivities, and clinical relevance. *Cleve Clin J Med.* 1992;59:617-627.

114. Turner JJO. Hypercalcaemia—presentation and management. *Clin Med (Lond).* 2017;17:270-273.

115. US Food and Drug Administration. *Medical Officer's Review of NDA 21-117.* Silver Spring, MD: US Food and Drug Administration; 2000. https://www.accessdata.fda.gov/drugsatfda_docs/nda/2000/021117_10%calciumchlorideinjectionuspin10mlsyringe_medr_p1.pdf. Accessed August 16, 2017.

116. Vance MV, et al. Digital hydrofluoric acid burns: treatment with intraarterial calcium infusion. *Ann Emerg Med.* 1986;15:890-896.

117. Velvart J. Arterial perfusion for hydrofluoric acid burns. *Hum Toxicol.* 1983;2:233-238.

118. Vick JA, et al. Reversal of propranolol and verapamil toxicity by calcium. *Vet Hum Toxicol.* 1983;25:8-10.

119. Vohra R, et al. Recurrent life-threatening ventricular dysrhythmias associated with acute hydrofluoric acid ingestion: observations in one case and implications for mechanism of toxicity. *Clin Toxicol (Phila).* 2008;46:79-84.

120. Wagner J, Salzer WW. Calcium-dependent toxic effects of digoxin in isolated myocardial preparations. *Arch Int Pharmacodyn Ther.* 1976;223:4-14.

121. Wang X, et al. A review of treatment strategies for hydrofluoric acid burns: current status and future prospects. *Burns.* 2014;40:1447-1457.

122. Weiss AT, et al. The use of calcium with verapamil in the management of supraventricular tachyarrhythmias. *Int J Cardiol.* 1983;4:275-284.

123. White RD, et al. Plasma ionic calcium levels following injection of chloride, gluconate, and gluceptate salts of calcium. *J Thorac Cardiovasc Surg.* 1976;71:609-613.

124. Yamashita M, et al. Iontophoretic delivery of calcium for experimental hydrofluoric acid burns. *Crit Care Med.* 2001;29:1575-1578.

125. Zachary LS, et al. Treatment of experimental hydrofluoric acid burns. *J Burn Care Rehabil.* 1986;7:35-39.

126. Zaloga GP, et al. Calcium attenuates epinephrine's beta-adrenergic effects in postoperative heart surgery patients. *Circulation.* 1990;81:196-200.

105

HYDROCARBONS

Morgan A. A. Riggan and David D. Gummin

HISTORY AND EPIDEMIOLOGY

The modern world could not exist without hydrocarbons. Virtually everything we touch is either coated with or made up primarily of hydrocarbon products. Organic chemistry originated during the Industrial Revolution, largely as a result of advances in coal tar technology. In the coking process, bituminous (soft) coal is heated to liberate coal gas. This gas contains volatile hydrocarbons that are captured and separated into a variety of natural gases. The viscous residue left over from the coking process forms coal tar, which is distilled into kerosene and other hydrocarbon mixtures. Over the years, petroleum replaced coal tar as the principal source of commercial organic compounds.

Crude oil processing involves heating to a set temperature within processors that separate (distill) hydrocarbon fractions by vapor (or boiling) point. Because of the relationship between boiling point and molecular weight, distillation roughly divides hydrocarbons into like-sized molecules. The most volatile fractions come off early as gases, and these are used primarily as heating fuels. The least volatile fractions (larger than about 10 or 12 carbons) are used chiefly for lubricants or as paraffins, petroleum jelly, or asphalt. The remaining midsized fractions (5 to 10 carbons) are those most commonly used in combustion fuels and as solvents. Petroleum distillates are also used as raw materials in the production of finished products.

For decades in the United States, kerosene ingestion in children was a major public health concern.[108] Only through public education, consumer product safety initiatives, and modernization of the use and distribution of cooking and heating fuels has this problem been largely eliminated. However, in the developing world, these same challenges have yet to be resolved, with large numbers of children ingesting kerosene from poorly labeled and poorly secured containers.[1,14,15,40,57,82,97,111,124]

Public attention and debate surround the hydrocarbon exposures following environmental spills. One of the most notable events in recent years was the April 20, 2010, explosion of the BP Deepwater Horizon oil platform in the Gulf of Mexico. This resulted in the release of millions of barrels of oil into the Gulf. The human health consequences of disasters of this nature are categorized as related to worker safety; toxicologic effects in workers, visitors, and community members; mental health effects due to social and economic disruption; and ecosystem effects that have health effects on humans.[52] Even more controversial is the practice of "induced hydraulic fracturing" of rock or shale, commonly called "fracking." Fracking is performed on up to 60% of oil and gas wells drilled today, to liberate pockets of trapped gas or oil from within the fractured rock.[92,145] The intent is to capture and collect trapped hydrocarbons, but some escape into nearby aquifers, thereby entering water supplies or otherwise contaminating human environments. Critics are concerned about the composition of the hydraulic fluids used, as these often contain methanol, ethylene glycol, benzene, or other hydrocarbons. Components of these fluids are found in area groundwater, with resultant risk of human exposure[56,153] and untoward health effects.[87] In addition to the toxicity associated with direct hydrocarbon exposure, the combustion of hydrocarbons leads to other long-term health effects such as chronic lung disease, coronary artery disease, and malignancy.[33] This is a major concern when massive quantities of oil are burned such as in Kuwait, Nigeria, and Venezuela, and areas of the Middle East plagued by terrorism.[117]

The true epidemiology of hydrocarbon exposure and illness is difficult to ascertain from available data sources. Three populations appear to be at particular risk for hydrocarbon-related illness: children with unsupervised ingestions that result in pulmonary aspiration; workers with inhalational and dermal occupational exposures; and adolescents or young adults who intentionally abuse solvents by inhalation. High-risk occupations include petrochemical workers, plastics and rubber workers, printers, laboratory workers, painters, and hazardous waste workers. Most hydrocarbon exposures do not involve ingestion, and most do not result in illness. Exposures range from self-pumping gasoline, painting a spare bedroom, or applying or removing fingernail polish. Hydrocarbon solvents are often volatile, making inhalation common in these exposures. Lipid solubility results in dermal absorption when skin is exposed.[59] Data from US poison control centers suggest that about 30% of reported exposures to hydrocarbons are in children younger than 6 years (Chap. 130). Largely not captured in these data is an alarming rate of intentional misuse of volatile solvents by adolescents, which is discussed in more depth in Chap. 81.

Most commonly encountered hydrocarbons are mixtures of compounds, often obtained from a common petroleum distillation fraction. The many applications for these in consumer and household products include paints and thinners, furniture polish, lamp oils, and lubricants. Table 105–1 lists frequently encountered hydrocarbon compounds and their common uses. This chapter focuses principally on toxicity of hydrocarbons present in these commercially available mixtures. Individual hydrocarbons are discussed only when they are commonly available in purified form, or when specific xenobiotics result in unique toxicologic concerns.

TABLE 105–1	Classification and Viscosity of Common Hydrocarbons	
Compound	*Common Uses*	*Viscosity (SUS)*[a]
Aliphatics		
Gasoline	Motor vehicle fuel	30
Naphtha	Charcoal lighter fluid	29
Kerosene	Heating fuel	35
Turpentine	Paint thinner	33
Mineral spirits	Paint and varnish thinner	30–35
Mineral seal oil	Furniture polish	30–35
Heavy fuel oil	Heating oil	>450
Aromatics		
Benzene	Solvent, reagent, gasoline additive	31
Toluene	Solvent, spray paint solvent	28
Xylene	Solvent, paint thinner, reagent	28
Halogenated		
Methylene chloride	Solvent, paint stripper, propellant	27
Carbon tetrachloride	Solvent, propellant refrigerant	30
Trichloroethylene	Degreaser, spot remover	27
Tetrachloroethylene	Dry cleaning solvent, chemical intermediate	28

[a]Direct values for kinematic viscosity in Saybolt Universal seconds (SUS) were not available for the following compounds: naphtha, xylene, methylene chloride, carbon tetrachloride, trichloroethylene, perchloroethylene, and toluene. Saybolt universal seconds was calculated for these hydrocarbons by converting from available measurements in centipoise viscosity and/or centistokes viscosity using the following conversions: the value in centistokes is estimated by dividing centipoise by density at 68°F (20°C); SUS (Y) is approximated from centistokes (X) using $y = 3.2533x + 26.08$ ($R^2 = 0.9998$). Centipoise viscosity for naphtha was estimated from the value for butylbenzene. Centipoise viscosity for xylene is the average of *o-*, *m-*, and *p-*xylene.

CHEMISTRY

A *hydrocarbon* is an organic compound made up primarily of carbon and hydrogen atoms, typically ranging from 1 to 60 carbon atoms in length. This definition includes products derived from plants (terpenes such as pine oil and triglyceresin vegetable oil), animal fats (cod liver oil), natural gas, petroleum, or coal tar. There are 2 basic types of hydrocarbon molecules, *aliphatic* (straight or branched chains) and *cyclic* (closed ring), each with its own subclasses. The aliphatic compounds include the *paraffins* (*alkanes*, with a generic formula C_nH_{2n+2}); the *olefins* (*alkenes* have one double bond and *alkadienes* have 2 double bonds); *acetylenes* (alkynes) with at least one triple bond; and the *acyclic terpenes* (polymers of isoprene, C_5H_8). Some aliphatic compounds have branches with carbon atoms in the subchain; both the chain and branches are essentially straight.

The cyclic hydrocarbons include *alicyclic* (3 or more carbon atoms in a ring structure, with properties similar to the aliphatics), and *aromatic* compounds, as well as the *cyclic terpenes.* The alicyclics are further divided into *cycloparaffins* (*naphthenes*) such as cyclohexane, and the *cycloolefins* (2 or more double bonds) such as cyclopentadiene. Aromatic hydrocarbons are divided into the *benzene* group (one ring), *naphthalene* group (2 rings), and the *anthracene* group (3 rings). *Polycyclic aromatic hydrocarbons* (polynuclear aromatic hydrocarbons) have multiple, fused benzenelike rings. Aromatic organic compounds may also be *heterocyclic* (in which oxygen or nitrogen substitutes for carbon in the ring). The *cyclic terpenes* are the principal components of the variety of plant-derived essential oils (Chap. 43), often providing color, odor, and flavor. *Limonene* in lemon oil, *menthol* in mint oil, *pinene* in turpentine, and *camphor* are terpenes.

Saturated hydrocarbons contain carbon atoms that exist only in their most reduced state. This means that each carbon is bound to either hydrogen or to another carbon, with no double or triple bonds. Conversely, *unsaturated* compounds are those with hydrogens removed, in which double or triple bonds exist.

Solvents are a heterogenous class of xenobiotics used to dissolve and provide a vehicle for delivery of other xenobiotics. The most common industrial solvent is water. The solvents most familiar to toxicologists are *organic solvents* (containing one or more carbon atoms), and most of these are composed of hydrocarbons. Most are liquids in the conditions under which they are used. Specifically named solvents (Stoddard solvent, white naphtha, ligroin) represent mixtures of hydrocarbons emanating from a common petroleum distillation fraction.

Physical properties of hydrocarbons vary by the number of carbon atoms and by molecular structure. Unsubstituted, aliphatic hydrocarbons that contain up to 4 carbons are gaseous at room temperature, 5 to 19 carbon molecules are liquids, and longer-chain molecules tend to be tars or solids. Branching of chains tends to destabilize intermolecular forces, so that less energy is required to separate the molecules. The result is that for a given molecular size, highly branched molecules have lower melting and boiling points and tend to be more volatile.

The various definitions of paraffin warrant discussion. In chemistry, *paraffin* is a general term for any alkane. In North American common use, paraffin describes either medicinal paraffin or paraffin wax. *Medicinal paraffin* is the same as mineral oil, a viscous mixture of longer-chained alkanes (typically 15–50 carbon atoms per molecule) derived from a petroleum source. The molecules in *medicinal paraffin* are considerably branched, making it a viscous liquid at room temperature and pressure. *Paraffin wax* molecules are nearly identical in size to *medicinal paraffin*, but due to less branching it forms a waxy solid at room temperature. Outside North America, the term *paraffin* often refers to kerosene—a mixture of medium-chain alkanes typically used for lighting and heating.

Gasoline is a mixture of alkanes, alkenes, naphthenes, and aromatic hydrocarbons, predominantly 5 to 10 carbon atoms in size. Gasoline is separated from crude oil in particular distillation fractions and then blended with several other fractions in refinery processors. More than 1,500 individual molecular species are present in commercial gasoline grades, but most analytical methods isolate only 150 to 180 constituent compounds. Notably, *n*-hexane is present at up to 6%, and benzene is present between 1% and 6%, depending on the origin and processing technique. A number of additives may go into the final formulation: alkyl leads, ethylene dichloride, and ethylene dibromide in leaded gasoline, and oxygenates such as methyl *t*-butyl ether (MTBE), as well as methanol, ethanol, and detergents.

Organic halides contain one or more halogen atoms (fluorine, chlorine, bromine, iodine) substituted for a hydrogen atom in the parent structure. Examples include chloroform, trichloroethylene, and the freons.

Oxygenated hydrocarbons demonstrate toxicity specific to the oxidation state of the carbon, as well as to the atoms adjacent to it (the "R" groups). The *alcohols* are widely used as solvents in industry and in household products. Their toxicity is discussed in Chaps. 76 and 106. *Ethers* contain an oxygen atom bound on either side by a carbon atom. Acute toxicity from ethers tends to mirror that of the corresponding alcohols. *Aldehydes* and *ketones* contain one carbon–oxygen double bond (C=O), the former at a terminal carbon, the latter on a nonterminal carbon. Organic *acids, esters, amides*, and *acyl halides* represent more oxidized states of carbon; human toxicity is xenobiotic specific.

Phenols consist of benzene rings with an attached hydroxyl (alcohol) group. The parent compound, phenol, has only one hydroxyl group attached to benzene. The toxicity of phenol is dramatically altered by addition of other functional groups to the benzene ring (Chap. 101). Cresols, catechols, and salicylate are examples of substituted phenols.

A variety of amines, amides, nitroso and nitro compounds, as well as phosphates, sulfites, and sulfates are used commercially and industrially. The addition of these functional groups to hydrocarbons dramatically alters the characteristics, including the toxicity of the compound.

PHARMACOLOGY

The effects of hydrocarbons on humans are chiefly related to interactions with lipid bilayers in cellular membranes. Acute central nervous system (CNS) toxicity from inhalational occupational overexposure or recreational abuse parallels the effect of administering an inhaled general anesthetic. Inhaled solvent vapor produces unconsciousness in 50% of subjects, when the partial pressure in the lung reaches its median effective dose (ED_{50}). The ED_{50} in occupational terms is effectively the same as the MAC in anesthesiology terms (Chap. 65).

The physical property of an inhaled anesthetic that correlates most closely with its ability to extinguish nociception is its lipid solubility. The Meyer-Overton lipid solubility theory implies that the potency of an anesthetic correlates directly with its lipid solubility (Chap. 65).

Unfortunately, this theory is too simplistic. Numerous protein receptor interactions also occur. Halothane, isoflurane, sevoflurane, enflurane, and desflurane inhibit fast sodium channels.[104] Toluene, trichloroethylene, perchloroethylene, and others inhibit neuronal calcium currents.[101,122] The halogenated hydrocarbons increase the outward potassium rectifying current[123] and decrease exocytosis of neuronal synaptic vesicles.[62] Specific ligand-receptor interactions also occur,[36] such as the inhibition of receptor function at nicotinic,[146] and at glutamate receptors,[35] as well as enhancement of type-A γ-aminobutyric acid ($GABA_A$) and glycine receptor currents.[13]

Pharmacodynamic properties of inhaled hydrocarbons and other volatile xenobiotics (Chap. 65) suggest some receptor–ligand interaction, and a growing body of evidence suggests that the Meyer–Overton lipid solubility theory cannot explain the many neurochemical activities demonstrated by this broad class of xenobiotics.[64] Perhaps a more elegant approach to the lipid bilayer interaction is termed the "modern lipid hypothesis." The hypothesis is thermodynamically derived, purporting an increase in lateral pressure on protein receptors within the neuronal bilayer. Lateral pressure leads to conformational changes in membrane ion channels, modulating the capacity for activation.[27] Although this hypothesis is mechanistically plausible, no in vitro or in vivo work has yet substantiated it. Thus, no single mechanism fully explains the pharmacologic and toxicologic activity of volatile hydrocarbons on neuronal tissues.

TOXICOKINETICS

Hydrocarbons are variably absorbed by ingestion, inhalation, or by dermal routes. Human toxicokinetic data are lacking for most of these xenobiotics, so much of our understanding derives from in vitro studies and animal research. Partition coefficients are useful predictors of the rate and extent of the absorption and distribution of hydrocarbons into tissues. A partition coefficient for a given chemical species is the ratio of concentrations achieved between 2 different media at equilibrium. The blood-to-air, tissue-to-air, and tissue-to-blood coefficients directly relate to the pulmonary uptake and distribution of hydrocarbons. The tissue-to-blood partition coefficient is commonly derived by dividing the tissue-to-air coefficient by the blood-to-air coefficient.[107] The higher the value, the greater the potential for distribution into tissue. Table 105–2 lists partition coefficients for commonly encountered hydrocarbons. Where human data are limited, rat data are presented in the table, because human and rat data often correlate.[107]

Inhalation is a major route of exposure for volatile hydrocarbons. Most cross the alveolar membrane by passive diffusion. The driving force is the difference in vapor concentration between the alveolus and the blood. The absorbed dose is determined by the air concentration, duration of exposure, minute ventilation, and the blood-to-air partition coefficient. Hydrocarbons that are highly soluble in blood and tissues are readily absorbed, and blood concentrations rise rapidly following inhalation exposure. Although aromatic species are generally well absorbed, absorption of aliphatic hydrocarbons varies by molecular weight: aliphatic hydrocarbons with between 5 and 16 carbons are readily absorbed through inhalation, whereas those with more than 16 carbons are less extensively absorbed.

Absorption of aliphatic hydrocarbons through the digestive tract is inversely related to molecular weight, ranging from complete absorption at lower molecular weights, to approximately 60% for C-14 hydrocarbons, 5% for C-28 hydrocarbons, and essentially no absorption for aliphatic hydrocarbons with more than 32 carbons. Oral absorption of aromatic hydrocarbons with between 5 and 9 carbons ranges from 80% to 97%. Oral absorption of aromatics with more than 9 carbons is poorly characterized.

Although the skin is a common area of contact with solvents, the dose of dermally absorbed hydrocarbons is small compared to other routes such as inhalation. The skin is composed of both hydrophilic (proteinaceous portion of cells) and lipophilic (cell membranes) regions (Chap. 17). Although many hydrocarbons can remove lipids from the stratum corneum, permeability is not simply the result of lipid removal; permeability also increases with hydration of the skin. The rate of skin absorption is highest when xenobiotics have a water-to-lipid partition coefficient near one. Solvents that contain both hydrophobic and hydrophilic moieties (eg, glycol ethers, dimethylformamide, dimethylsulfoxide) are particularly well absorbed through skin. Other factors that determine penetration across the skin include the thickness of the skin layer, the difference in concentration of the solvent on either side of the epithelium, the diffusion constant, and skin integrity (ie, normal versus cut or abraded).

The dose absorbed through skin is proportional to the exposed surface area and the duration of contact. Although highly volatile compounds typically have a short duration of skin contact because of evaporation, skin absorption also occurs from contact with hydrocarbon vapor. In studies with human volunteers exposed to varying concentrations of hydrocarbon vapors, the dermal dose accounted for 0.1% to 2% of the inhalation dose. With massive exposure (eg, whole-body immersion), dermal absorption contributes significantly to toxicity. Significant dermal absorption with resultant toxicity is described with carbon tetrachloride,[68] tetrachloroethylene,[59] and phenol.[80]

Once absorbed into the central compartment, hydrocarbons are distributed to target and storage organs based on their tissue-to-blood partition coefficients and on the rate of perfusion of the tissue with blood. During the onset of systemic exposure, hydrocarbons accumulate in tissues that have tissue-to-blood coefficients greater than 1 (eg, for toluene, the fat-to-blood partition coefficient is 60). Table 105–2 lists the distribution half-lives of selected hydrocarbons.

Hydrocarbons can be eliminated from the body unchanged, for example, through expired air, or can be metabolized to more polar compounds, which are then excreted in urine or bile. Table 105–2 lists the blood elimination half-lives (for first-order elimination processes) and metabolites of selected hydrocarbons. Some hydrocarbons are metabolized to toxic compounds (eg, methylene chloride, carbon tetrachloride, n-hexane, methyl-n-butyl ketone). The specific toxicities of these metabolites are discussed later in this chapter.

TABLE 105–2	Kinetic Parameters of Selected Hydrocarbons					
	Partition Coefficients[a]		**t₁/₂**			
	Blood-to-Air	**Fat-to-Air**	**α**	**β**	**Elimination**	**Relevant Metabolites**
Aliphatics						
n-Hexane	2	159	0.17 hours	1.7 hours	10%–20% exhaled; liver metabolism by CYP2E1	2-Hexanol, 2,5-hexanedione, 'Y-valerolactone
Paraffin/tar	Not absorbed or metabolized	—	—	—		
Aromatics						
Benzene	8.19	499	8 hours	90 hours	12% exhaled; liver metabolism to phenol	Phenol, catechol, hydroquinone, and conjugates
Toluene	8-16	1021	4–5 hours	15–72 hours	Extensive liver extraction and metabolism	80% metabolized to benzyl alcohol; 70% renally excreted as hippuric acid
o-Xylene	34.9	1877	0.5–1 hour	20–30 hours	Liver CYP2E1 oxidation	Toluic acid, methyl hippuric acid
Halogenated						
Methylene chloride	5-10	120	Apparent t₁/₂ of COHb 13 hours	0.7 hours	92% exhaled unchanged Low doses metabolized; high doses exhaled Two liver metabolic pathways	(a) CYP2E1 to CO and CO₂ (b) Glutathione transferase to CO₂, formaldehyde, formic acid
Carbon tetrachloride	1.6	359	~1.5 hours	1.5–8 hours	Liver CYP2E1, some lung exhalation (dose-dependent)	Trichloromethyl radical, trichloromethyl peroxy radical, phosgene
Trichloroethylene	9	554	3 hours	30 hours	Liver CYP2E1—epoxide intermediate; trichloroethanol is glucuronidated and excreted	Chloral hydrate, trichloroethanol, trichloroacetic acid
1,1,1-Trichloroethane	1-3	263	0.7 hours	53 hours	91% exhaled; liver CYP2E1	Trichloroacetic acid, trichloroethanol
Tetrachloroethylene	10.3	1638	2.7 hours	33 hours	80% exhaled; liver CYP2E1	Trichloroacetic acid, trichloroethanol

[a]Fat-to-blood partition coefficient is obtained by dividing the fat-to-air coefficient by the blood-to-air coefficient, as determined in rat models. All coefficients are determined at 98.6°F (37°C).

PATHOPHYSIOLOGY AND CLINICAL FINDINGS

Respiratory

Several factors are associated with pulmonary toxicity after hydrocarbon ingestion. These include specific physical properties of the xenobiotics ingested, the volume ingested, and the occurrence of vomiting. Physical properties of viscosity, surface tension, and volatility are primary determinants of aspiration potential.

Dynamic (or absolute) viscosity is the measurement of the ability of a fluid to resist flow. This property is measured with a rheometer and is typically given in units of pascal-seconds. More frequently, engineers work with *kinematic viscosity*, measured in square millimeters per second, or centistokes. Dynamic viscosity is converted to kinematic viscosity by dividing the dynamic viscosity by the density of the fluid. An older system for measuring viscosity was initially popularized by the petroleum industry and expresses kinematic viscosity in units of Saybolt Universal seconds (SUS). Unfortunately, many policy statements were developed in an era when SUS units were popular, and many still describe viscosity in SUS units. Various tables and calculators are available to convert kinematic viscosity to SUS units. Table 105–1 shows kinematic viscosity of common hydrocarbons, measured in SUS. An approximate unit conversion is given in the footnote of tables.

Hydrocarbons with low viscosities (<60 SUS; eg, turpentine, gasoline, naphtha) have a higher tendency for aspiration in animal models. The US Consumer Products Safety Commission issued a rule in 2001, requiring child-resistant packaging for products that contain 10% or more hydrocarbon by weight and have a viscosity less than 100 SUS.

Surface tension is a cohesive force generated by attraction due to the Van der Waals forces between molecules. This influences adherence of a liquid along a surface ("its ability to creep"). The lower the surface tension, the more effectively the liquid will creep, leading to a higher aspiration risk.[49]

Volatility is the tendency for a liquid to become a gas. Hydrocarbons with high volatility tend to vaporize, displace oxygen, and potentially lead to transient hypoxia.

Early reports conflicted in their attempts to relate risk of pulmonary toxicity[1] to the amount of hydrocarbon ingested[12] or to the presence or absence of vomiting. One prospective study addressed both these variables. The cooperative kerosene poisoning (COKP) study was a multicenter study that enrolled 760 patients with hydrocarbon ingestion. Of these, 409 individuals could provide an estimate of the amount ingested. Patients who reportedly ingested more than 30 mL had a 52% chance of developing pulmonary complications, compared with 39% of those who ingested less than 10 mL. The risk of central nervous complications was 41%, compared with 24% using the same criterion. There was a 53% incidence of pulmonary toxicity when vomiting occurred, compared with 37% when there was no history of vomiting.[108] Although this knowledge may help modify the index of suspicion regarding possible pulmonary toxicity, none of these parameters is completely predictive. Severe hydrocarbon pneumonitis sometimes occurs after ingestion of "low-risk" hydrocarbons.[118] Some patients develop severe lung injury after low-volume (<5 mL) ingestions, as well as after ingestions with no history of coughing, gagging, or vomiting.[5]

It is widely held that aspiration is the main route of injury from ingested simple hydrocarbons. The mechanism of pulmonary injury, however, is not fully understood. Intratracheal instillation of 0.2 mL/kg of kerosene causes physiologic abnormalities in lung mechanics (decreased compliance and total lung capacity) and pathologic changes such as interstitial inflammation, polymorphonuclear exudates, intraalveolar edema and hemorrhage, hyperemia, bronchial and bronchiolar necrosis, and vascular thrombosis.[56] These changes most likely reflect both direct toxicity to pulmonary tissue and disruption of the lipid surfactant layer.[149]

Most patients who develop pulmonary toxicity following hydrocarbon ingestion will have an initial episode of coughing, gagging, or choking. This usually occurs within 30 minutes after ingestion and is presumptive evidence of aspiration. The majority of patients who have respiratory signs and symptoms in addition to the initial history of gagging, choking, and coughing

develop radiographic evidence of pneumonitis. Pulmonary toxicity manifests as crackles, rhonchi, bronchospasm, tachypnea, hypoxemia, hemoptysis, acute respiratory distress syndrome (hemorrhagic or nonhemorrhagic), or respiratory distress. Cyanosis develops in approximately 2% to 3% of patients. The etiology of cyanosis is multifactorial and includes the simple asphyxiant effects of volatilized hydrocarbons, ventilation–perfusion mismatch, or, rarely, from methemoglobinemia (aniline, nitrobenzene, or nitrite-containing hydrocarbons). Clinical findings often worsen over the first several days but typically resolve within a week. Death is distinctly uncommon and typically occurs after a severe, progressive respiratory insult marked by hypoxia, ventilation–perfusion mismatch, and barotrauma.[69,81,157]

Intravenous (IV), subcutaneous, and even intrapleural injection of hydrocarbons are reported.[39,115,144] Severe hydrocarbon pneumonitis occurs following IV exposure. Animal experiments show that intravascular hydrocarbons injure the first capillary bed encountered.[113,151] The clinical course after IV hydrocarbon injection is comparable to that of aspiration injury.

Radiographic evidence of pneumonitis develops in 40% to 88% of patients admitted following aspiration.[12,38,102] Findings develop as early as 15 minutes or as late as 24 hours after exposure (Fig. 105–1).[18,47,108] Chest radiographs performed immediately on initial presentation are not useful in predicting infiltrates in either symptomatic or asymptomatic patients.[5] Ninety percent of patients who develop radiographic abnormalities do so by 4 hours postingestion.[18] Clinical signs of pneumonia (eg, crackles, rhonchi) are evident in 40% to 50% of patients.[38] A small percentage (<5%) are completely asymptomatic after a period of observation, yet go on to have radiographic findings.[5,102]

Specific radiologic findings include perihilar densities, bronchovascular markings, bibasilar infiltrates, and pneumonic consolidation.[50] Right-sided involvement occurs in 75% of cases and bilateral involvement in approximately 50%. Upper-lobe involvement is uncommon. Pleural effusions develop in 3% of cases, with one-third appearing within 24 hours.[88] Pneumothorax, pneumomediastinum, and pneumatoceles occur uncommonly.[6,16,72] Initial upright chest radiographs after ingestion rarely reveal 2 liquid densities in the stomach, known as the "double-bubble" sign. This represents an air–fluid (hydrocarbon or water) and a hydrocarbon–water interface, as the hydrocarbon is not miscible with gastric (aqueous) fluid and may have a specific gravity less than that of water.[32]

Radiographic resolution does not correlate with clinical improvement but rather lags behind by several days to weeks. There are few reports of long-term follow-up on patients with hydrocarbon pneumonitis.[58,138] Frequent respiratory tract infections are described after hydrocarbon pneumonitis, but these studies are not well controlled.[47,141] Delayed formation of pneumatoceles occurs in isolated reports.[16,72] Bronchiectasis and pulmonary fibrosis are reported but appear to be uncommon.[54,111] In one study, 82% of patients examined 8 to 14 years after hydrocarbon-induced pneumonitis had asymptomatic minor pulmonary function abnormalities. The abnormalities were consistent with small-airway obstruction and loss of elastic recoil.[58]

Cardiac

The most concerning cardiac effect from hydrocarbon exposure is precipitation of dysrhythmias through myocardial sensitization.[98] Malignant dysrhythmias occur after exposure to high concentrations of volatile inhalants or inhaled anesthetics. Such events are described with all classes of hydrocarbons, but halogenated compounds are most frequently implicated, followed by aromatic compounds.[9,112] Atrial fibrillation, ventricular tachycardias, junctional rhythms, ventricular fibrillation, and cardiac arrest are reported.[93,99,112] When this occurs in the context of inhalant abuse, it is termed the "sudden sniffing death syndrome."[10] Prolongation of the QT interval in some cases raises additional concern for the development of torsade de pointes.[10,120]

Cardiac sensitization is incompletely understood.[98] Halothane and isoflurane inactivate sodium channels,[129] whereas chloroform and others attenuate potassium efflux through voltage-gated channels.[120] Sensitization is mediated by slowed conduction velocity through membrane gap junctions.[69]

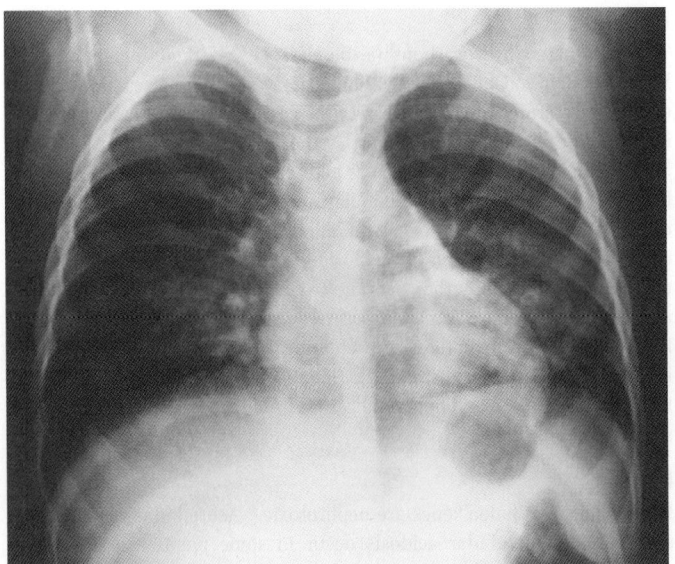

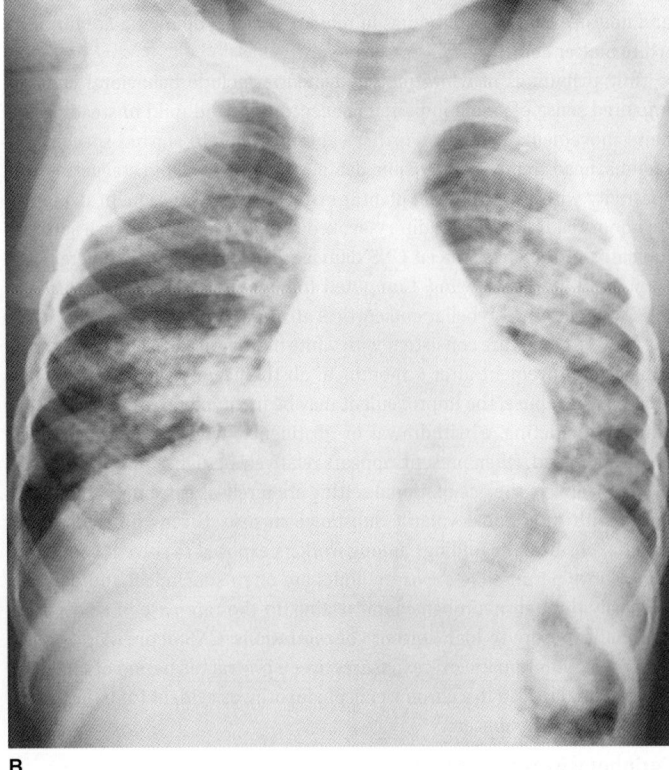

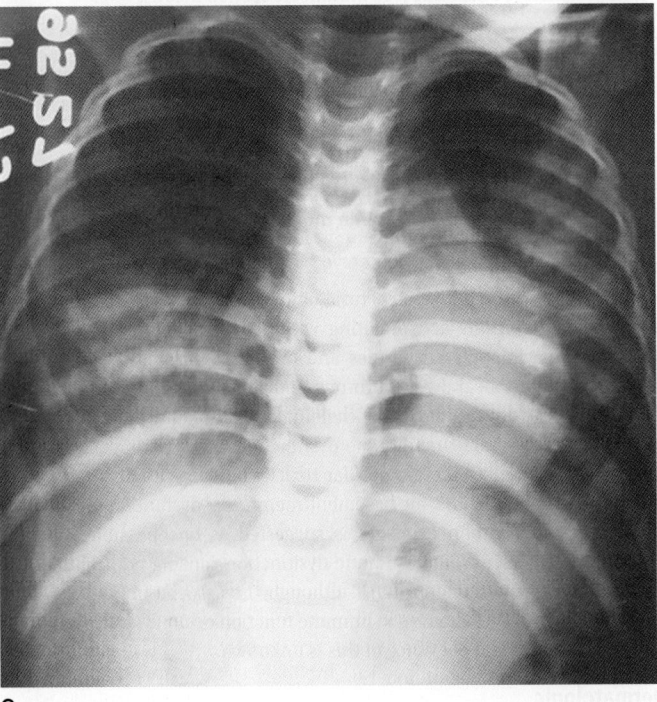

FIGURE 105–1. Three sequential radiographs of a young girl with severe hydrocarbon aspiration. (A) Initial: Patchy densities appear in the basilar areas of both lung fields with increased interstitial markings and peribronchial thickening. (B) Day 2: More extensive diffuse alveolar infiltrates are apparent. (C) Day 6: Dense consolidation and atelectasis are evident in the right lower lobe. (Used with permission from Nancy Genieser, MD, Professor of Radiology, New York University.)

Gap junction channels are composed of 2 hemichannels (connexons), each composed of 6 subunits (connexins). Halothane modulates gap-junction channels to the closed state in a dose-specific and connexin-specific manner, thus altering conductance.[61] Halocarbons, in the presence of epinephrine, cause dephosphorylation of the gap junction protein connexin-43, thereby increasing resistance and slowing conduction velocity in myocardial tissue.[70,90]

All routes of exposure to hydrocarbons are potentially cardiotoxic. Classically, sudden death follows an episode of sudden exertion, presumably associated with an endogenous catecholamine surge.[10] Tachydysrhythmias, cardiomegaly, and myocardial infarction are rarely reported after ingestion of hydrocarbons.[66] A retrospective follow-up cohort of exposed methylene chloride workers did not find evidence of excess long-term cardiac disease.[103]

Central Nervous System

Transient CNS excitation occurs after acute hydrocarbon inhalation or ingestion, but more commonly, CNS depression or general anesthesia

occurs.[38] In cases of aspiration, hypoxemia from pulmonary damage may contribute to CNS depression.[81,152] Coma and seizures are reported in 1% to 3% of cases.[102,110,156] Chronic occupational exposure or volatile substance use leads to a chronic neurobehavioral syndrome, the painter syndrome, most notably described after toluene overexposure as toluene leukoencephalopathy which also occurs after inhalational abuse. Clinical features include ataxia, spasticity, dysarthria, and dementia, consistent with leukoencephalopathy.[44,46] Autopsy studies of the brains of chronic toluene abusers show atrophy and mottling of the white matter, as though the lipid-based myelin were dissolved away. Microscopic examination shows a consistent pattern of myelin and oligodendrocyte loss with relative preservation of axons.[75] Animal models of toluene poisoning reveal norepinephrine and dopamine depletion. The severity and reversibility of this syndrome depends on the intensity and duration of toluene exposure.[119] Infrequent exposure rarely produces clinical neurologic signs, whereas severe (daily) use can lead to significant neurologic impairment after as little as 1 year, but more commonly after 2 to 4 years of continuous exposure. The specific cognitive and neuropsychological findings in toluene-induced dementia are termed a white matter dementia.[44,46]

Initial findings of white matter dementia include behavioral changes, impaired sense of smell, impaired concentration, and mild unsteadiness of hand movements and gait. Further exposure leads to slurred speech, nystagmus, head tremor, poor vision, deafness, stiff-legged and staggering gait, spasticity with hyperreflexia, plantar extension, and subsequent dementia. An abnormal brain stem auditory-evoked response appears to be a sensitive indicator of toluene-induced CNS damage. The electroencephalogram can show mild, diffuse slowing. Computed tomography in severe cases shows mild to moderate cerebellar and cortical atrophy. Magnetic resonance imaging (MRI) findings are consistent with white matter disease. Most cases show clinical improvement after 6 months of abstinence; however, with moderate to severe abuse, the improvement may be incomplete. Although toluene abuse is addicting, a withdrawal or abstinence syndrome is surprisingly uncommon and, when present, appears relatively benign.[44,46]

Exposures in the occupational setting are rarely as extreme as those that occur with intentional volatile substance misuse. Given the significantly lesser exposures, the findings among workers exposed to solvent concentrations above permissible exposure limits are often subclinical and detected primarily through neurobehavioral testing. In the rare case of acute occupational exposure to high solvent concentrations, CNS depression is likely. Repeated, symptomatic overexposures over a protracted period of time have the potential to lead to a chronic encephalopathy, as evident from the experience with solvent abusers.[45]

Peripheral Nervous System

Peripheral neuropathy is well described following occupational exposure to n-hexane or methyl-n-butyl ketone (MBK).[20] This axonopathy results from a common metabolic intermediate, 2,5-hexanedione. The mechanism by which this intermediate causes peripheral neuropathy probably relates to decreased phosphorylation of neurofilament proteins, with disruption of the axonal cytoskeleton. Methyl ethyl ketone may exacerbate this neurotoxicity, probably by interfering with metabolic pathways of n-hexane and MBK.[4,116] Axonopathy from MBK or n-hexane exposure typically begins in the distal extremities and progresses proximally (a classic, "dying-back" neuropathy) (Chap. 22).[53] Exposure to one of these hydrocarbons should be included in the differential diagnosis of the patient with Guillain-Barré syndrome (GBS), although sensory findings are present with MBK and absent in GBS.[127] The longest axons appear to be affected initially, so that the patient manifests a "length-dependent polyneuropathy." With discontinuation of exposure many of the effects reverse over weeks to months.[65] Alternatively, the phenomenon of "coasting" occurs, in which neuropathy progresses for a time (weeks to months) after discontinuation of the toxic insult.[127] A reversible peripheral neuropathy occurred in 40% of chronic toluene abusers and was characterized by severe motor weakness without sensory deficits or areflexia.[134] However, it is possible that the toluene in this series was contaminated by n-hexane or MBK.[4]

Other organic solvents, such as carbon disulfide, acrylamide, and ethylene oxide, are reported to cause a similar peripheral axonopathy.[53] Cranial and peripheral neuropathies occur after acute and chronic exposure to trichloroethylene (TCE).[42,71,79,135] Pathologically, TCE appears to induce a myelinopathy.[42,53] Trichloroethylene exposure is also associated with trigeminal neuralgia.[42,79] Symptoms can develop within 12 hours of a single intense exposure and persist for many years.[42] Trigeminal nerve damage was documented by evoked potentials following 15 minutes of TCE inhalation.[79] Some evidence suggests that decomposition products or impurities in TCE are responsible for cranial neuropathy.[29,41]

Gastrointestinal

Hydrocarbons irritate gastrointestinal mucous membranes. Nausea and vomiting are common after ingestion. As discussed earlier, vomiting increases the risk of pulmonary toxicity.[100,102] Hematemesis was reported in 5% of cases in one study.[100]

Hepatic

The chlorinated hydrocarbons (Table 105–1) and their metabolites are hepatotoxic. In most cases, activation occurs via a phase I reaction to form a reactive intermediate (Chap. 11). In the case of carbon tetrachloride, this intermediate is the trichloromethyl radical. This radical forms covalent bonds with hepatic macromolecules and initiates lipid peroxidation.[22] Carbon tetrachloride causes centrilobular necrosis after inhalational, oral, or dermal exposure.[22] Hepatotoxicity in animals is ranked for common hydrocarbons as follows: carbon tetrachloride is greater than benzene, and trichloroethylene is greater than pentane.[150] Vinyl chloride is a liver carcinogen, and trichloroethylene, tetrachloroethylene, and 1,1,1-trichloroethane are less acutely hepatotoxic than vinyl chloride.[89] Hepatotoxicity rarely follows ingestion of petroleum distillates.[67] Hepatic injury, manifested as aminotransferase elevation and hepatomegaly, is usually reversible except in massive exposures.[71]

Renal

Haloalkanes and haloalkenes are nephrotoxic.[31] Acute kidney injury (AKI) and distal renal tubular acidosis occur in some painters and volatile-substance abusers.[11] Toluene causes a renal tubular acidosislike syndrome (see Toluene later in the chapter). Hydrocarbon exposure is also associated with Goodpasture syndrome (see Immulogic section below).

Hematologic

Hemolysis is sporadically reported to occur following hydrocarbon ingestion.[3] One retrospective study of 12 patients showed hemolysis in 3 individuals and disseminated intravascular coagulation in another.[3] Although one patient required transfusion, hemolysis is usually mild and typically does not require red blood cell transfusion (also see discussion of the effects of benzene on bone marrow, under Benzene later in the chapter).

Immunologic

Hydrocarbons disturb the structural and functional integrity of membrane lipid bilayers by accumulating within the membrane and disrupting membrane lipopolysaccharides and proteins. This results in swelling and increased permeability to protons and other ions.[125] Resultant toxicity directly destroys capillary endothelium.[21] Additionally, there appears to be significant basement membrane dysfunction, and this is postulated to underlie both alveolar and glomerular toxicity of hydrocarbons.[131] Immune mechanisms may account for basement membrane dysfunction in chronic exposures. Hydrocarbon exposure is suggested as one possible cause of the Goodpasture syndrome (immune dysfunction causing both pulmonary damage and glomerulonephritis),[19] although the association is not widely accepted. Measurable changes in immune function occur after hydrocarbon exposure;[8] the clinical relevance of this is unknown.

Dermatologic

Most hydrocarbon solvents cause nonspecific irritation of skin and mucous membranes. Repeated, prolonged contact can dry and crack the skin. The mechanism of dermal injury appears to be defatting of the lipid layer of the stratum corneum. Up to 9% of workers develop contact dermatitis.[154] Solvent abusers demonstrate a classic "glue sniffer's rash" or "huffer's eczema." Limonene and turpentine contain sensitizers that can rarely result in contact allergy (Chap. 17).

Hydrocarbons are irritating to skin. Acute, prolonged exposure causes dermatitis and even full-thickness dermal damage.[60] Severity is proportional to duration of exposure. Chronic dermal exposure to kerosene or diesel fuel causes oil folliculitis.[143] A specific cutaneous lesion called chloracne is associated with exposure to chlorinated aromatic hydrocarbons with highly specific stereochemistry such as dioxins and polychlorobiphenyls.[37]

Soft tissue injection of hydrocarbon is locally toxic, leading to necrosis.[39] Secondary cellulitis, abscess formation, and fasciitis can occur. Infectious complications are treated by meticulous wound care, with surgical débridement as necessary. Particularly destructive lesions result from high-pressure injection gun injury. These injuries typically involve the extremities, with high-pressure

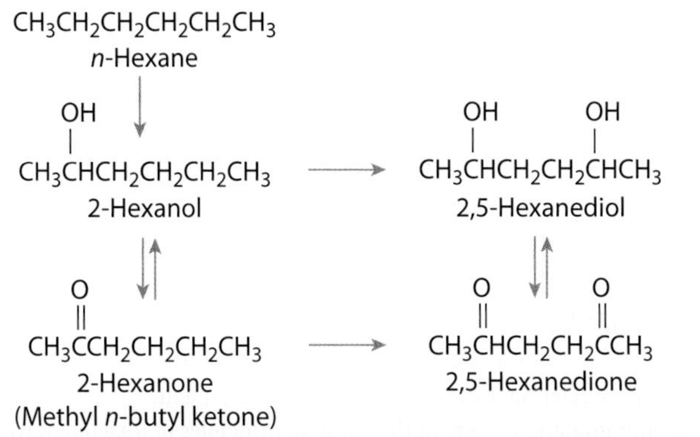

CH₃CH₂CH₂CH₂CH₂CH₃
n-Hexane

$$CH_3CH_2CH_2CH_2CH_2CH_3$$
n-Hexane

FIGURE 105–2. The metabolism of both organic solvents *n*-hexane and methyl *n*-butyl ketone produces the same common metabolite, 2,5-hexanedione.

injection of grease or paint into the fascial planes and tendon sheaths. Emergent surgical débridement is necessary in most of these cases.[43,95]

HYDROCARBONS WITH SPECIFIC AND UNIQUE TOXICITY

n-Hexane

Hexane is a 6-carbon simple aliphatic hydrocarbon. It is a constituent of some brake-cleaning fluids, rubber cement, glues, spray paints, coatings, and silicones. Outbreaks of *n*-hexane–related neurotoxicity have occurred in printing plants, sandal shops, furniture factories, and automotive repair shops.[30] Human exposure occurs primarily by inhalation. As discussed above, both *n*-hexane and MBK are well-known peripheral neurotoxins because of their common metabolic intermediate: 2,5-hexanedione. Similar 5- and 7-carbon species do not induce a comparable neurotoxicity, except those that are direct precursor intermediates in the metabolic pathway producing 2,5-hexanedione[137] (Fig. 105–2).

Methylene Chloride

Methylene chloride is commonly found in paint removers, cleansers, degreasers, and aerosol propellants. Like other halogenated hydrocarbons, it can rapidly induce general anesthesia by inhalation or ingestion. Unlike other hydrocarbons, methylene chloride and similar one-carbon halomethanes such as methylene dibromide are metabolized by CYP2E1 mixed-function oxidase to carbon monoxide.[2] Significant delayed and prolonged carboxyhemoglobinemia can occur[109] (Table 105–2 and Chap. 122).

Carbon Tetrachloride

Carbon tetrachloride (CCl₄), although not actually a hydrocarbon, has been used as an industrial solvent and reagent. Its use in the United States declined dramatically since recognition of its toxicity caused the Environmental Protection Agency to restrict its commercial use. Absorption occurs by all routes, including dermal. Carbon tetrachloride is an irritant to skin and mucous membranes and gastric mucosa when ingested. As in the case of other halogenated hydrocarbons, aspiration can result in pneumonitis, and systemic absorption may result in ventricular dysrhythmias.

Carbon tetrachloride exposures are hepatotoxic and nephrotoxic. Both occur more commonly with repetitive occupational exposure.[68,139] Toxicity follows phase-I dehalogenation of the parent compound, which produces free radicals and causes lipid peroxidation and the production of protein adducts.[22] Localization of specific phase I hepatic enzymes in the centrilobular area of the liver results in regionalized (zone 3) centrilobular injury after CCl₄ exposure (Chap. 21). Hepatotoxicity is typically manifested as reversible aminotransferase concentration elevations with or without hepatomegaly. Cirrhosis is reported in both animal models and in humans with prolonged excessive exposures. Nephrotoxicity is less studied but may result from a similar mechanism. Carbon tetrachloride is a suspected human carcinogen.[96]

Trichloroethylene

Trichloroethylene is a commonly used industrial solvent, cleanser, and degreaser. Systemically absorbed TCE, as might occur in the occupational setting, competitively inhibits aldehyde dehydrogenase. Concomitant ethanol consumption results in a disulfiramlike reaction that is termed "degreaser's flush"[132] (Chap. 78).

Trichloroethylene was used for years as a general anesthetic, and hundreds of disposal sites in the United States remain sources of ongoing human exposure. The use of TCE as a general anesthetic was abandoned because of associated acute cardiotoxicity.[51] Trichloroethylene is also hepatotoxic, neurotoxic, and nephrotoxic in humans and animals.[51] Trichloroethylene exposure is linked to the development of neurodegenerative diseases, such as parkinsonism.[48] Evidence suggests that TCE is a human carcinogen.[105]

Benzene

Benzene is hematotoxic and associated with acute hemolysis or with the delayed development of aplastic anemia and acute myelogenous leukemia.[76,106,114] Other aromatic hydrocarbons that are reported to cause similar hematologic effects most likely are contaminated with benzene. Benzene is an IARC group I carcinogen linked to chronic myelocytic leukemia, acute myeloid leukemia, acute nonlymphocytic leukemia, multiple myeloma, myelodysplastic syndromes, and lymphoma.[140] Chromosomal changes are believed to provide a marker for carcinogenicity.[142] Because of the carcinogenic risk, most benzene-based solvents were removed from the US market, and the Occupational Safety and Health Administration has limited the permissible worker exposure concentration to 1 ppm.

Toluene

Toluene has essentially replaced benzene as the primary organic solvent in many commercial products. Many oil paints and stains primarily contain toluene as solvent. As such, it is readily available and abused as an inhalant. The CNS sequelae of chronic solvent inhalation are most frequently related to chronic toluene exposure.

Chronic toluene abuse can also cause a syndrome that resembles transient distal renal tubular acidosis (RTA).[136] Although the mechanism is incompletely understood, the acidosis results in great part from the urinary excretion of hippuric acid (Table 105–2).[28] Renal potassium loss results in symptomatic hypokalemia.[73] Clinical findings are a hyperchloremic metabolic acidosis, hypokalemia, and aciduria. Transient azotemia, proteinuria, and an active urine sediment are reported.[147] Some also report a proximal RTA, or the Fanconi syndrome.[94] A metabolic acidosis resulting from the metabolism of toluene to benzyl alcohol through alcohol dehydrogenase to benzoic acid may be an adequate explanation for the serum and urine acid–base disturbances.

Pine Oil and Terpenes

Pine oil is an active ingredient in many household cleaning products. It is a mixture of unsaturated hydrocarbons composed of terpenes, camphenes, and pinenes. The major components are terpenes, which are found in plants and flowers. Wood distillates including pine oil and turpentine are derived from pine trees. Patients who ingest pine oil often emit a strong pine odor. Wood distillates are readily absorbed from the gastrointestinal tract, and ingestion causes CNS and pulmonary toxicity without aspiration.

The clinical features of pine oil ingestion include CNS depression, respiratory failure, and gastrointestinal dysfunction, which are rarely fatal.[74] Aspiration pneumonitis remains the primary clinical concern. Rare reported complications of wood distillate ingestion include turpentine-associated thrombocytopenic purpura, AKI, and hemorrhagic cystitis.[148]

Lipoid Pneumonia

Ingestion of low-viscosity hydrocarbons poses risk of pulmonary aspiration with subsequent acute pneumonitis. Conversely, viscous hydrocarbons rarely lead to pulmonary aspiration. However, inhalation of aerosolized oil droplets occurs in various occupational settings, resulting in lipoid pneumonia. The most common xenobiotics involved are mineral or vegetable oils.[17]

Initially, inhaled oil droplets are emulsified in the alveoli by surfactant, and then engulfed by alveolar macrophages. Unfortunately, macrophages are unable to readily process the internalized, exogenous oil. Microscopically, persistent cytoplasmic droplets give a "foamy" appearance to these "lipophages" that may persist for weeks to years. Symptoms of lipoid pneumonia are limited or even subclinical, but once they arise, illness may be prolonged from months to years. Ultimately, irreversible proliferative fibrosis may develop.[128]

Silicone-based polymers share structural similarities and some physical properties with long-chain hydrocarbons. Silicone polymers such as dimethicone exist as oily, viscous liquids at room temperature and are widely used as lubricants, antifoaming agents, and even as medicine and food additives. Pulmonary aspiration or inhalation of aerosolized silicone droplets causes clinical pneumonitis that is indistinguishable from that caused by their viscous hydrocarbon counterparts. The time course of lung injury is similarly protracted, and complications result.[126]

Tar and Asphalt Injury

Tar and asphalt injuries are common occupational hazards among construction workers. Asphalt workers are at risk for toxic gas exposure to hydrogen sulfide, carbon monoxide, propane, methane, and volatilized hydrocarbons.[64] In addition, cutaneous exposure to these hot hydrocarbon mixtures causes severe burns. The material quickly hardens and is very difficult to remove. However, immediate cooling with cold water is important to limit further thermal injury. Complete removal is essential to ensure proper burn management and to limit infectious complications. Attempts to remove hardened tar or asphalt mechanically cause further damage. Dissolving the material with mineral oil, petroleum jelly, or antibacterial ointments are met with variable success. Surface-active compounds combined with an ointment (De-Solv-it, Tween-80, Polysorbate 80) are more effective.[34,133]

DIAGNOSTIC TESTING

Laboratory and ancillary testing for hydrocarbon toxicity should be guided by available information regarding the specific xenobiotic, the route of exposure, and the best attempt at quantifying the exposure. Inhalation or ingestion of hydrocarbons associated with pulmonary aspiration is most likely to result in pulmonary toxicity. The use of pulse oximetry and arterial blood gas testing in this group of patients is warranted in symptomatic patients. Early radiography is indicated in patients who are severely symptomatic; however, radiographs performed immediately after hydrocarbon ingestion have a poor predictive value for the occurrence of aspiration pneumonitis.[5] In the asymptomatic patient, early radiography is not cost effective. Patients observed for 6 hours after an ingestion, who demonstrate adequate oxygenation, are not tachypneic, demonstrate no abnormal pulmonary findings, and have a normal chest radiograph obtained after the 6-hour observation period have a good medical prognosis with very low risk of subsequent deterioration.[5]

The choice of specific diagnostic laboratory tests to assess organ system toxicity or function following exposure to a hydrocarbon depends on the patient's clinical condition, as well as the dose, route, and intent (intentional self-harm versus unintentional). Always exercise caution and assume potentially severe toxicity with any intentional self-harm exposure. Useful clinical tests include pulse oximetry, ECG, arterial blood gas, serum or urine electrolytes, complete blood counts, and creatinine phosphokinase. If a hydrocarbon has specific target organ toxicities (eg, benzene/bone marrow, CCl_4/liver, or n-hexane/peripheral nervous system), evaluating and monitoring target organ system function is indicated.

Specific diagnostic testing for hydrocarbon poisoning can be performed with bioassays for the specific hydrocarbon or its metabolites in blood, breath, or urine. These bioassays are not available in a clinically relevant time frame and should not be used to guide initial management of suspected hydrocarbon poisoning in the emergency setting. Bioassays can be useful to assist with a differential diagnosis (eg, testing for CCl_4 in a comatose patient with unexplained hepatic and renal toxicity or a carboxyhemoglobin determination in a paint stripper with chest pain), in workers compensation situations (eg, testing for urinary trichloroethanol and trichloroacetic acid in a worker exposed to TCE with unexplained bouts of dizziness), or for forensic purposes (eg, sudden death in a huffer).

Chronic overexposures to hydrocarbons, as occurs with volatile substance use, results in persistent damage to the CNS. Damage can be detected and quantified using neuroimaging methods such as MRI or positron emission tomography. Major MRI findings in patients with chronic toluene abuse include atrophy, white matter T2 hyperintensity, and T2 hypointensity involving the basal ganglia and thalamus.[26,155] Neurobehavioral testing can be used to detect subtle central nervous system effects following chronic occupational overexposures.

MANAGEMENT

Identification of the specific type, route, and amount of hydrocarbon exposure is rarely essential to achieve effective management.

Decontamination is one of the cardinal principles of toxicology, with priority that is second only to stabilization of the cardiopulmonary status. Safe decontamination prevents further absorption and also avoids secondary casualties among those providing care. Protection of rescuers with appropriate personal protective equipment and rescue protocols is paramount, especially in situations in which the victim has lost consciousness. The principle of removing the patient from the exposure (eg, vapor or gaseous hydrocarbon) or the exposure from the patient (eg, hydrocarbon liquid on skin or clothing), while protecting the rescuer, implies that appropriate personal protective equipment be applied at each level of the health care delivery system.

Exposed clothing should be removed and safely discarded as further absorption or inhalation of hydrocarbons from grossly contaminated clothing can worsen systemic toxicity. Decontamination of the skin is a high priority in patients with massive hydrocarbon exposures, particularly those exposures involving highly toxic hydrocarbons. Soap and water should be the initial method of skin decontamination for the majority of hydrocarbons. The exception to this is phenol, for which water is often inadequate and polyethylene glycol 400 (PEG 400) solution is recommended.[91] Note that PEG 400 is not interchangeable with polyethylene glycol with electrolytes (PEG-ELS) used for bowel irrigation. The caregiver should remain aware that certain hydrocarbons are highly flammable posing a fire risk to hospital staff (Chap. 131 and Special Considerations: SC2).

Several studies have attempted to evaluate the role of gastric emptying with gastric lavage or syrup of ipecac after hydrocarbon ingestion. Results were largely inconclusive and in some instances showed a trend toward harm.[12,25,69,108] Because of the high incidence of spontaneous emesis and the risk of aspiration in hydrocarbon ingestion, we recommend against routine attempts at gastric emptying.

Activated charcoal (AC) has limited ability to decrease gastrointestinal absorption of hydrocarbons and may distend the stomach and predispose patients to vomiting and aspiration.[77] Given the risk of spontaneous emesis and aspiration, we likewise recommend against the routine use of activated charcoal.

Antibiotics were once frequently administered in the setting of hydrocarbon pneumonitis to treat possible bacterial superinfection,[25] and they are still occasionally used today as fever and infiltrates are common. Although animal models rapidly demonstrate superinfection, prophylactic antibiotics only appear to alter pulmonary flora.[23] Prophylactic antibiotics did not affect length of stay or otherwise impact the outcome of 48 pediatric patients admitted for respiratory distress from hydrocarbon poisoning.[69] A randomized controlled study of pediatric patients with mild respiratory symptoms (history of cough or dyspnea, age-specific tachypnea, chest indrawing, stridor, or wheeze) due to kerosene-induced pneumonitis did not show any benefit of prophylactic amoxicillin in reducing the rate of clinical deterioration (treatment failure), duration of hospitalizations or signs and symptoms at follow-up.[7] However, this study excluded all patients judged to be too ill to withhold antibiotics, as determined by requiring more than 2 L/min of oxygen by nasal prongs, intermittent or continuous positive-pressure ventilation, or those with a fever greater than 40°C. Given the available evidence, we recommend against routine antibiotic use in the management of patients with mild hydrocarbon pneumonitis.

Corticosteroids, like antibiotics, have been prophylactically administered in the setting of hydrocarbon pulmonary toxicity.[54,138] The rationale for their use is prevention and limitation of the pulmonary inflammatory response after hydrocarbon injury. Animal models do not show any benefit of corticosteroid administration,[130] and corticosteroids may increase the risk of bacterial superinfection. Furthermore, a controlled human trial failed to show a benefit from corticosteroid administration.[84] It is clear that corticosteroid use does not improve the acute course of hydrocarbon pulmonary toxicity, although some authors suggest improved outcome with delayed corticosteroid therapy despite little supporting evidence.[72] Coupled with the possible increased risk of bacterial superinfection, we recommend against the routine use of corticosteroids for hydrocarbon pulmonary toxicity.

Patients with severe hydrocarbon toxicity pose unique problems for management. Respiratory distress requiring mechanical ventilation in this setting may be associated with a large ventilation–perfusion mismatch. The use of positive end-expiratory pressure (PEEP) in this setting is often beneficial. However, when very high levels of PEEP are required there is an increased risk of barotrauma.[119] High-frequency jet ventilation (HFJV), using very high respiratory rates (220–260) with small tidal volumes, has helped to decrease the need for PEEP.[24] Patients who continue to have severe ventilation–perfusion mismatch despite PEEP and HFJV have benefited from extracorporeal membrane oxygenation (ECMO).[118] Extracorporeal membrane oxygenation appears to be a useful option in severe pulmonary toxicity after other treatments have failed. Although there are case reports of clinical improvement of hydrocarbon pneumonitis with early administration of surfactant therapy, the evidence is poor and we do not recommend routine use of surfactant.[86]

Cyanosis is uncommon after hydrocarbon toxicity. Although this is most often caused by severe hypoxia, methemoglobinemia associated with hydrocarbon exposure is reported.[78] The potential for methemoglobinemia should be investigated in patients who remain cyanotic following normalization of arterial oxygen tension (Chap. 124).

Hypotension in severe hydrocarbon toxicity raises additional concerns. The etiology of hypotension in this setting is often due to compromise of cardiac output because of high levels of PEEP. Hydrocarbons do not have significant direct cardiovascular effects, and decreasing the PEEP may improve hemodynamics. The use of β-adrenergic agonists such as dopamine, epinephrine, isoproterenol, and norepinephrine should be avoided if possible, as certain hydrocarbons predispose to dysrhythmias.[98,112] The recommended first-line treatments for hypotension is fluid resuscitation and minimizing PEEP, with phenylephrine used for refractory hypotension.

Management of dysrhythmias associated with hydrocarbon toxicity includes evaluation and correction of electrolyte and acid–base abnormalities such as hypokalemia and acidosis resulting from toluene, hypoxemia, hypotension, and hypothermia. Ventricular fibrillation poses a specific concern, as common resuscitation algorithms recommend epinephrine administration to treat this rhythm. If it is ascertained that the dysrhythmia emanates from myocardial sensitization by a hydrocarbon solvent, catecholamines should be avoided. In this setting, we recommend short-acting β-adrenergic antagonists such as esmolol as the treatment of choice for hydrocarbon induced dysrhythmias.[93]

Hyperbaric oxygen (HBO) was studied in a rat model of severe kerosene-induced pneumonitis.[121] Hyperbaric oxygen at 4 ATA showed some benefit in 24-hour survival rates; however, no follow-up studies were performed. Hyperbaric oxygen also decreased CCl_4-induced hepatic necrosis in a rat model when given within 6 hours, after which HBO augmented necrosis.[85] Given the lack of human studies and the risks associated with hyperoxia, we do not routinely recommend HBO for the treatment of CCl_4 poisoning.

In the past, hospital admission was routinely recommended for patients who ingested hydrocarbons, because of concern over possible delayed symptom onset and progression of toxicity. Several reports documented patients with relatively asymptomatic presentations who rapidly decompensated with respiratory compromise. However, progressive symptoms after hydrocarbon ingestion are rare,[5,83] and these recommendations predate noninvasive assessments of gas exchange. In a retrospective study of 950 patients,[5] 800 patients were asymptomatic on initial evaluation with normal chest radiographs, remained asymptomatic after 6 to 8 hours of observation, and had a normal repeat radiograph. No patient in this group of 800 had progressive symptoms,

and all were discharged from the emergency department (ED) without clinical deterioration. A total of 150 patients were diagnosed with hydrocarbon pneumonitis based on a history of hydrocarbon ingestion and either abnormalities on physical examination or an abnormal chest radiograph, and these patients were admitted to hospital for observation. Seventy-nine of the 150 hospitalized patients (53%) were symptomatic on presentation to the ED, and 71 patients (47%) were asymptomatic at the time of their ED evaluation. All were reported to have had symptoms prior to ED arrival. Furthermore, 36 of the 71 had an abnormal chest radiograph, and 35 were admitted because of the history of prehospital respiratory symptoms. Of the 36 patients with abnormal chest radiographs, 2 (6%) developed progression of pulmonary symptoms during the 6-hour observation period. Of the 35 who had a normal radiograph, 2 (6%) developed pulmonary symptoms and radiographic pneumonitis during the 6-hour observation period. The 4 patients who were hospitalized for progression of symptoms became asymptomatic over the next 24 hours and had no complications. Overall, 136 patients (91%) had no progression of their pulmonary disease and uneventful hospitalizations. Only 14 of the 150 hospitalized patients (9.3%) had progression of pulmonary toxicity.[5] Of these 14 patients, 7 had persistence of symptoms for less than 24 hours. Overall, 1.5% of all patients presenting with a history of hydrocarbon exposure had progression of their pulmonary symptoms.

A separate poison control center–based study evaluated 120 asymptomatic patients over an 18-hour telephone follow-up period.[83] Sixty-two patients had initial pulmonary symptoms that quickly resolved. One of the 62 patients (1.6%) developed progressive pulmonary toxicity. This patient was hospitalized and had resolution of symptoms within 24 hours without complications.

A number of investigators offer protocols for determining which patients can be safely discharged.[5,83] None of these protocols are prospectively validated. However, rational guidelines for hospitalization can be recommended. We recommend hospitalization for those patients who have clinical evidence of toxicity, and most individuals with intentional ingestions. Patients who do not have any initial symptoms, have normal chest radiographs obtained at least 6 hours after ingestion, and who do not develop symptoms during the 6-hour observation period can be safely discharged. Patients who are asymptomatic on initial assessment but who have radiographic evidence of hydrocarbon pneumonitis can be safely discharged if they remain asympomatic after a 6-hour observation period and able to be reassessed in 24 hours. Patients who have initial respiratory symptoms but quickly become asymptomatic during medical evaluation and remain so after a 6-hour observation period who have a normal 6-hour chest radiograph can be discharged home.

SUMMARY

- Hydrocarbons are a diverse group of xenobiotics that cause toxicity by inhalation, ingestion, or dermal absorption.
- Populations at particular risk for toxicity include unsupervised children who ingest hydrocarbon compounds, workers who are occupationally exposed by inhalation or dermal absorption, and youths who intentionally inhale volatile hydrocarbons.
- Aspiration pneumonitis is the primary concern after hydrocarbon ingestion, with the risk of aspiration dependent on many factors, including viscosity, volatility, surface tension, amount ingested, and the history or presence of emesis.
- Many hydrocarbons are poorly absorbed from the gastrointestinal tract and unlikely to produce systemic poisoning. Acute systemic toxicity is unlikely to occur in the absence of CNS effects such as excitation or sedation.
- An exposed child who is asymptomatic after 6 hours of observation and who has a normal chest radiograph taken after 6 hours of observation is most likely safe for discharge.

REFERENCES

1. Abu-Ekteish F. Kerosene poisoning in children: a report from northern Jordan. *Trop Doct.* 2002;32:27-29.
2. Ahmed AE, et al. Halogenated methanes: metabolism and toxicity. *Fed Proc.* 1980;39:3150-3155.

3. Algren JT, Rodgers GC. Intravascular hemolysis associated with hydrocarbon poisoning. *Pediatr Emerg Care.* 1992;8:34-35.

4. Altenkirch H, et al. Experimental studies on hydrocarbon neuropathies induced by methyl-ethyl-ketone (MEK). *J Neurol.* 1978;219:159-170.

5. Anas N, et al. Criteria for hospitalizing children who have ingested products containing hydrocarbons. *JAMA.* 1981;246:840-843.

6. Baldachin BJ, Melmed RN. Clinical and therapeutic aspects of kerosene poisoning: a series of 200 cases. *Br Med J.* 1964;2:28-30.

7. Balme KH, et al. The efficacy of prophylactic antibiotics in the management of children with kerosene-associated pneumonitis: a double-blind randomised controlled trial. *Clin Toxicol (Phila).* 2015;53:789-796.

8. Ban M, et al. Effect of inhaled industrial chemicals on systemic and local immune response. *Toxicology.* 2003;184:41-50.

9. Bass M. Death from sniffing gasoline. *N Engl J Med.* 1978;299:203-203.

10. Bass M. Sudden sniffing death. *JAMA.* 1970;212:2075-2079.

11. Batlle DC, et al. On the mechanism of toluene-induced renal tubular acidosis. *Nephron.* 1988;49:210-218.

12. Beamon RF, et al. Hydrocarbon ingestion in children: a six-year retrospective study. *JACEP.* 1976;5:771-775.

13. Beckstead MJ, et al. Glycine and gamma-aminobutyric acid(A) receptor function is enhanced by inhaled drugs of abuse. *Mol Pharmacol.* 2000;57:1199-1205.

14. Belonwu RO, Adeleke SI. A seven-year review of accidental kerosene poisoning in children at Aminu Kano Teaching Hospital, Kano. *Niger J Med.* 2008;17:380-382.

15. Benois A, et al. Clinical and therapeutic aspects of childhood kerosene poisoning in Djibouti. *Trop Doct.* 2009;39:236-238.

16. Bergeson PS, et al. Pneumatoceles following hydrocarbon ingestion. Report of three cases and review of the literature. *Am J Dis Child.* 1975;129:49-54.

17. Betancourt SL, et al. Lipoid pneumonia: spectrum of clinical and radiologic manifestations. *AJR Am J Roentgenol.* 2010;194:103-109.

18. Blattner RJ, et al. Hydrocarbon pneumonitis. *Pediatr Clin North Am.* 1957:243-253.

19. Bombassei GJ, Kaplan AA. The association between hydrocarbon exposure and anti-glomerular basement membrane antibody-mediated disease (Goodpasture's syndrome). *Am J Ind Med.* 1992;21:141-153.

20. Bos PM, et al. Critical review of the toxicity of methyl n-butyl ketone: risk from occupational exposure. *Am J Ind Med.* 1991;20:175-194.

21. Bratton L, Haddow JE. Ingestion of charcoal lighter fluid. *J Pediatr.* 1975;87:633-636.

22. Brent JA, Rumack BH. Role of free radicals in toxic hepatic injury. II. Are free radicals the cause of toxin-induced liver injury? *J Toxicol Clin Toxicol.* 1993;31:173-196.

23. Brown J, et al. Experimental kerosene pneumonia: evaluation of some therapeutic regimens. *J Pediatr.* 1974;84:396-341.

24. Bysani GK, et al. Treatment of hydrocarbon pneumonitis. High frequency jet ventilation as an alternative to extracorporeal membrane oxygenation. *Chest.* 1994;106:300-303.

25. Cachia EA, Fenech FF. Kerosene poisoning in children. *Arch Dis Child.* 1964;39:502-504.

26. Caldemeyer KS, et al. The spectrum of neuroimaging abnormalities in solvent abuse and their clinical correlation. *J Neuroimaging.* 1996;6:167-173.

27. Cantor RS. The lateral pressure profile in membranes: a physical mechanism of general anesthesia. *Biochemistry.* 1997;36:2339-2344.

28. Carlisle EJ, et al. Glue-sniffing and distal renal tubular acidosis: sticking to the facts. *J Am Soc Nephrol.* 1991;1:1019-1027.

29. Cavanagh JB, Buxton PH. Trichloroethylene cranial neuropathy: is it really a toxic neuropathy or does it activate latent herpes virus? *J Neurol Neurosurg Psychiatry.* 1989;52:297-303.

30. Centers for Disease Control and Prevention. *n*-Hexane-related peripheral neuropathy among automotive technicians—California, 1999-2000. *MMWR Morb Mortal Wkly Rep.* 2001;50:1011-1013.

31. Cristofori P, et al. Three common pathways of nephrotoxicity induced by halogenated alkenes. *Cell Biol Toxicol.* 2015;31:1-13.

32. Daffner RH, Jimenez JP. The double gastric fluid level in kerosene poisoning. *Radiology.* 1973;106:383-384.

33. Dellinger B, et al. Report: combustion byproducts and their health effects: summary of the 10th International Congress. *Environ Eng Sci.* 2008;25:1107-1114.

34. Demling RH, et al. Management of hot tar burns. *J Trauma.* 1980;20:242.

35. Dildy-Mayfield JE, et al. Anesthetics produce subunit-selective actions on glutamate receptors. *J Pharmacol Exp Ther.* 1996;276:1058-1065.

36. Dilger JP. The effects of general anaesthetics on ligand-gated ion channels. *Br J Anaesth.* 2002;89:41-51.

37. Dunagin WG. Cutaneous signs of systemic toxicity due to dioxins and related chemicals. *J Am Acad Dermatol.* 1984;10:688-700.

38. Eade NR, et al. Hydrocarbon pneumonitis. *Pediatrics.* 1974;54:351-357.

39. Eskandarlou M, Moaddab AH. Chest wall necrosis and empyema resulting from attempting suicide by injection of petroleum into the pleural cavity. *Emerg Med J.* 2010;27:616-618.

40. Fagbule DO, Joiner KT. Kerosene poisoning in childhood: a 6-year prospective study at the University of Ilorin Teaching Hospital. *West Afr J Med.* 1992;11:116-121.

41. Feldman RG, et al. Blink reflex latency after exposure to trichloroethylene in well water. *Arch Environ Health.* 1988;43:143-148.

42. Feldman RG, et al. Long-term follow-up after single toxic exposure to trichloroethylene. *Am J Ind Med.* 1985;8:119-126.

43. Fialkov JA, Freiberg A. High pressure injection injuries: an overview. *J Emerg Med.* 1991;9:367-371.

44. Filley CM. Toluene abuse and white matter: a model of toxic leukoencephalopathy. *Psychiatr Clin North Am.* 2013;36:293-302.

45. Filley CM. Toxic leukoencephalopathy. In: *The Behavioral Neurology of White Matter.* 2nd ed. New York, NY: Oxford University Press; 2013:163-185.

46. Filley CM, et al. The effects of toluene on the central nervous system. *J Neuropathol Exp Neurol.* 2004;63:1-12.

47. Foley JC, et al. Kerosene poisoning in young children. *Radiology.* 1954;62:817-829.

48. Gash DM, et al. Trichloroethylene: Parkinsonism and complex 1 mitochondrial neurotoxicity. *Ann Neurol.* 2008;63:184-192.

49. Gerarde HW. Toxicological studies on hydrocarbons. IX. The aspiration hazard and toxicity of hydrocarbons and hydrocarbon mixtures. *Arch Environ Health.* 1963;6:329-341.

50. Gershon-Cohen J, et al. Roentgenography of kerosene poisoning, chemical pneumonitis. *Am J Roentgenol Radium Ther Nucl Med.* 1953;69:557-562.

51. Gist GL, Burg JR. Trichloroethylene—A review of the literature from a health effects perspective. *Toxicol Ind Health.* 1995;11:253-307.

52. Goldstein BD, et al. The Gulf oil spill. *N Engl J Med.* 2011;364:1334-1348.

53. Graham DG. Neurotoxicants and the cytoskeleton. *Curr Opin Neurol.* 1999;12:733-737.

54. Graham JR. Pneumonitis following aspiration of crude oil and its treatment by steroid hormones. *Trans Am Clin Climatol Assoc.* 1955;67:104-112.

55. Gross P, et al. Kerosene pneumonitis: an experimental study with small doses. *Am Rev Respir Dis.* 1963;88:656-663.

56. Gross SA, et al. Analysis of BTEX groundwater concentrations from surface spills associated with hydraulic fracturing operations. *J Air Waste Manag Assoc.* 2013;63:424-432.

57. Gupta P, et al. Kerosene oil poisoning—a childhood menace. *Indian Pediatr.* 1992;29:979-984.

58. Gurwitz D, et al. Pulmonary function abnormalities in asymptomatic children after hydrocarbon pneumonitis. *Pediatrics.* 1978;62:789-794.

59. Hake CL, Stewart RD. Human exposure to tetrachloroethylene: inhalation and skin contact. *Environ Health Perspect.* 1977;21:231-238.

60. Hansbrough JF, et al. Hydrocarbon contact injuries. *J Trauma.* 1985;25:250-252.

61. He DS, Burt JM. Mechanism and selectivity of the effects of halothane on gap junction channel function. *Circ Res.* 2000;86:E104-E109.

62. Hemmings HC, et al. The general anesthetic isoflurane depresses synaptic vesicle exocytosis. *Mol Pharmacol.* 2005;67:1591-1599.

63. Himmel HM. Mechanisms involved in cardiac sensitization by volatile anesthetics: general applicability to halogenated hydrocarbons? *Crit Rev Toxicol.* 2008;38:773-803.

64. Hoidal CR, et al. Hydrogen sulfide poisoning from toxic inhalations of roofing asphalt fumes. *Ann Emerg Med.* 1986;15:826-830.

65. Huang CC, et al. Biphasic recovery in *n*-hexane polyneuropathy. A clinical and electrophysiological study. *Acta Neurol Scand.* 1989;80:610-615.

66. James FW, et al. Cardiac complications following hydrocarbon ingestion. *Am J Dis Child.* 1971;121:431-433.

67. Janssen S, et al. Impairment of organ function after oral ingestion of refined petrol. *Intensive Care Med.* 1988;14:238-240.

68. Javier Perez A, et al. Acute renal failure after topical application of carbon tetrachloride. *Lancet.* 1987;1:515-516.

69. Jayashree M, et al. Predictors of outcome in children with hydrocarbon poisoning receiving intensive care. *Indian Pediatr.* 2006;43:715-719.

70. Jiao Z, et al. A possible mechanism of halocarbon-induced cardiac sensitization arrhythmias. *J Mol Cell Cardiol.* 2006;41:698-705.

71. Joron GE, et al. Massive necrosis of the liver due to trichlorethylene. *Can Med Assoc J.* 1955;73:890-891.

72. Kamijo Y, et al. Pulse steroid therapy in adult respiratory distress syndrome following petroleum naphtha ingestion. *J Toxicol Clin Toxicol.* 2000;38:59-62.

73. Kao KC, et al. Hypokalemic muscular paralysis causing acute respiratory failure due to rhabdomyolysis with renal tubular acidosis in a chronic glue sniffer. *J Toxicol Clin Toxicol.* 2000;38:679-681.

74. Koppel C, et al. Acute poisoning with pine oil—metabolism of monoterpenes. *Arch Toxicol.* 1981;49:73-78.

75. Kornfeld M, et al. Solvent vapor abuse leukoencephalopathy. Comparison to adrenoleukodystrophy. *J Neuropathol Exp Neurol.* 1994;53:389-398.

76. Kwong YL, Chan TK. Toxic occupational exposures and paroxysmal nocturnal haemoglobinuria. *Lancet.* 1993;341:443-443.

77. Laass W. Therapy of acute oral poisoning by organic solvents: treatment by activated charcoal in combination with laxatives. *Arch Toxicol Suppl.* 1980;4:406-409.

78. Lareng L, et al. Acute, toxic methemoglobinemia from accidental ingestion of nitrobenzene [in French]. *Eur J Toxicol Environ Hyg.* 1974;7:12-16.

79. Leandri M, et al. Electrophysiological evidence of trigeminal root damage after trichloroethylene exposure. *Muscle Nerve.* 1995;18:467-468.

80. Liao JT, Oehme FW. Literature reviews of phenolic compounds, IV, *o*-Phenylphenol. *Vet Hum Toxicol.* 1980;22:406-408.

81. Lifshitz M, et al. Hydrocarbon poisoning in children: a 5-year retrospective study. *Wilderness Environ Med.* 2003;14:78-82.

82. Lucas GN. Kerosene oil poisoning in children: a hospital-based prospective study in Sri Lanka. *Indian J Pediatr.* 1994;61:683-687.

83. Machado B, et al. Accidental hydrocarbon ingestion cases telephoned to a regional poison center. *Ann Emerg Med.* 1988;17:804-807.

84. Marks MI, et al. Adrenocorticosteroid treatment of hydrocarbon pneumonia in children—A cooperative study. *J Pediatr.* 1972;81:366-369.

85. Marzella L, et al. Effect of hyperoxia on liver necrosis induced by hepatotoxins. *Virchows Arch B Cell Pathol Incl Mol Pathol.* 1986;51:497-507.

86. Mastropietro CW, Valentine K. Early administration of intratracheal surfactant (calfactant) after hydrocarbon aspiration. *Pediatrics.* 2011;127:1600-1604.

87. McKenzie LM, et al. Human health risk assessment of air emissions from development of unconventional natural gas resources. *Sci Total Environ.* 2012;424:79-87.

88. McNally WD. Kerosene poisoning in children; a study of 48 cases. *J Med Assoc State Ala.* 1957;27:53-55.

89. Meredith TJ, et al. Diagnosis and treatment of acute poisoning with volatile substances. *Hum Toxicol.* 1989;8:277-286.

90. Miyata Y, et al. Prophylactic antiarrhythmic effect of anesthetics at subanesthetic concentration on epinephrine-induced arrhythmias in rats after brain death. *Biomed Res Int.* 2015;2015:575474.

91. Monteiro-Riviere NA, et al. Efficacy of topical phenol decontamination strategies on severity of acute phenol chemical burns and dermal absorption: in vitro and in vivo studies in pig skin. *Toxicol Ind Health.* 2001;17:95-104.

92. Montgomery CT, Smith MB. Hydraulic fracturing. History of an enduring technology. *JPT Online* (Society of Petroleum Engineers). http://www.spe.org/jpt/print/archives/2010/12/10Hydraulic.pdf. Accessed June 12, 2013.

93. Mortiz F, et al. Esmolol in the treatment of severe arrhythmia after acute trichloroethylene poisoning. *Intensive Care Med.* 2000;26:256.

94. Moss AH, et al. Fanconi's syndrome and distal renal tubular acidosis after glue sniffing. *Ann Intern Med.* 1980;92:69-70.

95. Mrvos R, et al. High pressure injection injuries: a serious occupational hazard. *J Toxicol Clin Toxicol.* 1987;25:297-304.

96. Nagano K, et al. Inhalation carcinogenicity and chronic toxicity of carbon tetrachloride in rats and mice. *Inhal Toxicol.* 2007;19:1089-1103.

97. Nagi NA, Abdullah ZA. Kerosene poisoning in children in Iraq. *Postgrad Med J.* 1995;71:419-422.

98. Nelson LS. Toxicologic myocardial sensitization. *J Toxicol Clin Toxicol.* 2002;40:867-879.

99. Nierenberg DW, et al. Mineral spirits inhalation associated with hemolysis, pulmonary edema, and ventricular fibrillation. *Arch Intern Med.* 1991;151:1437-1440.

100. Nouri L, al-Rahim K. Kerosene poisoning in children. *Postgrad Med J.* 1970;46:71-75.

101. Okuda M, et al. Inhibitory effect of 1,1,1-trichloroethane on calcium channels of neurons. *J Toxicol Sci.* 2001;26:169-176.

102. Olstad RB, Lord RM Jr. Kerosene intoxication. *AMA Am J Dis Child.* 1952;83:446-453.

103. Ott MG, et al. Health evaluation of employees occupationally exposed to methylene chloride. *Scand J Work Environ Health.* 1983;9(suppl 1):1-38.

104. Ouyang W, et al. Comparative effects of halogenated inhaled anesthetics on voltage-gated Na+ channel function. *Anesthesiology.* 2009;110:582-590.

105. Page NN. Assessment of trichloroethylene as an occupational carcinogen. *IARC Sci Publ.* 1979:75-79.

106. Paustenbach DJ, et al. Benzene toxicity and risk assessment, 1972-1992: implications for future regulation. *Environ Health Perspect.* 1993;101(suppl 6):177-200.

107. Pierce CH, et al. Partition coefficients between human blood or adipose tissue and air for aromatic solvents. *Scand J Work Environ Health.* 1996;22:112-118.

108. Press E, et al. Cooperative kerosene poisoning study: evaluation of gastric lavage and other factors in the treatment of accidental ingestion of petroleum distillate products. *Pediatrics.* 1962;29:648-674.

109. Raphael M, et al. Acute methylene chloride intoxication—A case report on domestic poisoning. *Eur J Emerg Med.* 2002;9:57-59.

110. Reed E, et al. Kerosene intoxication. *Am J Dis Child.* 1950;15:623-632.

111. Reed RP, Conradie FM. The epidemiology and clinical features of paraffin (kerosene) poisoning in rural African children. *Ann Trop Paediatr.* 1997;17:49-55.

112. Reinhardt CF, et al. Epinephrine-induced cardiac arrhythmia potential of some common industrial solvents. *J Occup Med.* 1973;15:953-955.

113. Richardson JA, Pratt-Thomas HR. Toxic effects of varying doses of kerosene administered by different routes. *Am J Med Sci.* 1951;221:531-536.

114. Rinsky RA, et al. Benzene and leukemia. An epidemiologic risk assessment. *N Engl J Med.* 1987;316:1044-1050.

115. Rush MD, et al. Skin necrosis and venous thrombosis from subcutaneous injection of charcoal lighter fluid (naphtha). *Am J Emerg Med.* 1998;16:508-511.

116. Saida K, et al. Peripheral nerve changes induced by methyl *n*-butyl ketone and potentiation by methyl ethyl ketone. *J Neuropathol Exp Neurol.* 1976;35:207-225.

117. Salgado S. When the oil fields burned. *New York Times*, 2016.

118. Scalzo AJ, et al. Extracorporeal membrane oxygenation for hydrocarbon aspiration. *Am J Dis Child.* 1990;144:867-871.

119. Schaumburg HH. Toluene. In: Spencer PS, et al, eds. *Experimental and Clinical Neurotoxicology.* 2nd ed. New York: Oxford University Press; 2000:1183-1189.

120. Scholz C, et al. In vitro modulation of HERG channels by organochlorine solvent trichloromethane as potential explanation for proarrhythmic effects of chloroform. *Toxicol Lett.* 2006;165:156-166.

121. Schwartz SI, et al. Effects of drugs and hyperbaric oxygen environment on experimental kerosene pneumonitis. *Dis Chest.* 1965;47:353-359.

122. Shafer TJ, et al. Perturbation of voltage-sensitive Ca^{2+} channel function by volatile organic solvents. *J Pharmacol Exp Ther.* 2005;315:1109-1118.

123. Shin WJ, Winegar BD. Modulation of noninactivating K^+ channels in rat cerebellar granule neurons by halothane, isoflurane, and sevoflurane. *Anesth Analg.* 2003;96:1340-1344.

124. Shotar AM. Kerosene poisoning in childhood: a 6-year prospective study at the Princess Rahmat Teaching Hospital. *Neuro Endocrinol Lett.* 2005;26:835-838.

125. Sikkema J, et al. Mechanisms of membrane toxicity of hydrocarbons. *Microbiol Rev.* 1995;59:201-222.

126. Silicone Environmental Health and Safety Council of North America. Guidance for aerosol applications of silicone-based materials (2001). http://www.sehsc.com/PDFs/Guidance for Aerosol Applications-Sep 01.pdf. Accessed June 12, 2013.

127. Smith AG, Albers JW. *n*-Hexane neuropathy due to rubber cement sniffing. *Muscle Nerve.* 1997;20:1445-1450.

128. Spickard A, Hirschmann JV. Exogenous lipoid pneumonia. *Arch Intern Med.* 1994;154:686-692.

129. Stadnicka A, et al. Effects of halothane and isoflurane on fast and slow inactivation of human heart hH1a sodium channels. *Anesthesiology.* 1999;90:1671-1683.

130. Steele RW, et al. Corticosteroids and antibiotics for the treatment of fulminant hydrocarbon aspiration. *JAMA.* 1972;219:1434-1437.

131. Stevenson A, et al. Biochemical markers of basement membrane disturbances and occupational exposure to hydrocarbons and mixed solvents. *QJM.* 1995;88:23-28.

132. Stewart RD, et al. Degreaser's flush. *Arch Environ Health.* 1974;29:1-5.

133. Stratta RJ, et al. Management of tar and asphalt injuries. *Am J Surg.* 1983;146:766-769.

134. Streicher HZ, et al. Syndromes of toluene sniffing in adults. *Ann Intern Med.* 1981;94:758-762.

135. Szlatenyi CS, Wang RY. Encephalopathy and cranial nerve palsies caused by intentional trichloroethylene inhalation. *Am J Emerg Med.* 1996;14:464-466.

136. Taher SM, et al. Renal tubular acidosis associated with toluene "sniffing." *N Engl J Med.* 1974;290:765-768.

137. Takeuchi Y, et al. A comparative study on the neurotoxicity of *n*-pentane, *n*-hexane, and *n*-heptane in the rat. *Br J Ind Med.* 1980;37:241-247.

138. Taussig LM, et al. Pulmonary function 8 to 10 years after hydrocarbon pneumonitis. Normal findings in three children carefully studied. *Clin Pediatr (Phila).* 1977;16:57-59.

139. Tomenson JA, et al. Hepatic function in workers occupationally exposed to carbon tetrachloride. *Occup Environ Med.* 1995;52:508-514.

140. Travis LB, et al. Hematopoietic malignancies and related disorders among benzene-exposed workers in China. *Leuk Lymphoma.* 1994;14:91-9102.

141. Truemper E, et al. Clinical characteristics, pathophysiology, and management of hydrocarbon ingestion: case report and review of the literature. *Pediatr Emerg Care.* 1987;3:187-193.

142. Turkel B, Egeli U. Analysis of chromosomal aberrations in shoe workers exposed long term to benzene. *Occup Environ Med.* 1994;51:50-53.

143. Upreti RK, et al. Dermal exposure to kerosene. *Vet Hum Toxicol.* 1989;31:16-20.

144. Vaziri ND, et al. Toxicity with intravenous injection of naphtha in man. *Clin Toxicol (Phila).* 1980;16:335-343.

145. Vidic RD, et al. Impact of shale gas development on regional water quality. *Science.* 2013;340:1235009-1235009.

146. Violet JM, et al. Differential sensitivities of mammalian neuronal and muscle nicotinic acetylcholine receptors to general anesthetics. *Anesthesiology.* 1997;86:866-874.

147. Voigts A, Kaufman CE Jr. Acidosis and other metabolic abnormalities associated with paint sniffing. *South Med J.* 1983;76:443-447, 452.

148. Wahlberg P, Nyman D. Turpentine and thrombocytopenic purpura. *Lancet.* 1969;2:215-216.

149. Widner LR, et al. Artificial surfactant for therapy in hydrocarbon-induced lung injury in sheep. *Crit Care Med.* 1996;24:1524-1529.

150. Wirtschafter ZT, Cronyn MW. Free radical mechanism for solvent toxicity. *Arch Environ Health.* 1964;9:186-191.

151. Wolfsdorf J. Experimental kerosene pneumonitis in primates: relevance to the therapeutic management of childhood poisoning. *Clin Exp Pharmacol Physiol.* 1976;3:539-544.

152. Wolfsdorf J, Paed D. Kerosene intoxication: an experimental approach to the etiology of the CNS manifestations in primates. *J Pediatr.* 1976;88:1037-1040.

153. Wright PR, et al. Groundwater-quality and quality-control data for two monitoring wells near Pavillion, Wyoming, April and May 2012. http://pubs.usgs.gov/ds/718/DS718_508.pdf.

154. Yakes B, et al. Occupational skin disease in newspaper pressroom workers. *J Occup Med.* 1991;33:711-717.

155. Yucel M, et al. Toluene misuse and long-term harms: a systematic review of the neuropsychological and neuroimaging literature. *Neurosci Biobehav Rev.* 2008;32:910-926.

156. Zieserl E. Hydrocarbon ingestion and poisoning. *Compr Ther.* 1979;5:35-42.

157. Zucker AR, et al. Management of kerosene-induced pulmonary injury. *Crit Care Med.* 1986;14:303-304.

CASE STUDY 10

History A 38-year-old woman was transported to the hospital by EMS directly from the airport because she complained of shortness of breath immediately after exiting the airplane. She had a history of depression and took amitriptyline and zolpidem and admitted to daily alcohol use. She also had a history of hypertension but did not recall the name of her medication. She reported that she was well prior to getting on the flight and only drank 2 beers about 6 hours apart. During the flight, she noted some abdominal and back pain, followed by difficulty breathing. She denied other ingestions or suicidal ideations.

Physical Examination On arrival to the hospital, she was noted to be severely short of breath with the following vital signs: blood pressure, 156/92 mm Hg; pulse, 140 beats/min; respiratory rate, 42 breaths/min; temperature, 98.2°F (36.8°C); oxygen saturation, 100% on a 100% non-rebreather mask. Her head was without signs of trauma, and her pupils were equal, round, and sluggishly reactive to light. Her neck was supple, and her chest was clear. She had a regular tachycardia, no murmurs, rubs, thrills, or gallops. Her abdomen was soft with normal bowel sounds and no organomegaly. She was slightly tender in all 4 quadrants, but without guarding or rebound. Her extremities were without clubbing, cyanosis, or edema, and a neurologic examination was without deficit or focality.

Initial Management The patient was immediately intubated, sedated with midazolam, and attached to a mechanical ventilator. A rapid bedside glucose was reported as 50 mg/dL, and she was given 25 g of $D_{50}W$ and 100 mg of thiamine intravenously. An arterial blood gas revealed a pH of 6.80, a PCO_2 of 24 mm Hg, and a PO_2 of 106 mm Hg on 21% oxygen. A CT scan of the chest was negative for pulmonary embolus. Standard laboratories are shown in Table CS10–1.

What Is the Differential Diagnosis? The laboratory analysis shows a severe metabolic acidosis with elevated anion gap (40 mEq/L). Of the many mnemonics used to help recall the differential diagnosis, one of the most popular is MUDPILES: (Methanol, Uremia, Diabetic and other ketoacidoses, Phenformin and metformin, Iron and isoniazid, Lactate, Ethylene glycol, Salicylates) (Chap. 12). It should be remembered that this is an imperfect mnemonic in that it is easy to forget cyanide, theophylline, and a number of other xenobiotics that are not directly noted. Instead, a mnemonic that is more comprehensive and helps to guide laboratory analysis is KULTS: (Ketones, Uremia, Lactate, Toxic Alcohols, and Salicylate).

What Clinical and Laboratory Analyses Can Help Identify the Etiology? A rapid clinical assessment will help to narrow the differential diagnosis. For example, iron poisoning is almost always associated with vomiting (Chap. 45), and isoniazid rapidly produces seizures (Chap. 56). Uremia is excluded based on the BUN and creatinine. Likewise, the presentation glucose concentration helps diminish the probability of diabetic ketoacidosis.

At this point, additional rapid tests are useful. A urinalysis showing ketones would be helpful in cases of alcoholic ketoacidosis (Chap. 76) or salicylates (Chap. 37) and might show oxalate crystals or fluorescence following ethylene glycol poisoning (Chap. 106). A lactate concentration would be elevated in patients with metformin toxicity (Chap. 47) and might be falsely elevated from glycolate accumulation following ethylene glycol poisoning (Chap. 106). Additionally, most laboratories can determine salicylate concentrations rapidly. An ethanol concentration is exceedingly helpful in that it might be low in those with alcoholic ketoacidosis and if elevated essentially excludes methanol or ethylene glycol poisoning because it would be protective. Finally, if ethanol and methanol concentrations are not available, an osmol gap can be calculated, although caution is advised when interpreting the results especially in this case (Chap. 12).

Further Diagnosis and Treatment Additional studies revealed the following: urine was negative for ketones and crystals; a serum lactate was 6 mmol/L; ethanol and salicylate concentrations were negative. Despite receiving fluids, thiamine, and glucose (empiric treatment for alcoholic ketoacidosis), the patient's metabolic acidosis persisted. Because of the severity of the anion gap acidosis and the lack of alternative diagnoses, a loading dose of fomepizole was administered (Antidotes in Depth: A33) for presumed toxic alcohol (methanol or ethylene glycol) ingestion. Intravenous hypertonic sodium bicarbonate was infused for presumed methanol poisoning (Antidotes in Depth: A5), as a repeat creatinine concentration was slightly improved prior to fomepizole administration, making ethylene glycol poisoning less likely (Chap. 106).

Nephrology was consulted for hemodialysis, and two 4-hour hemodialysis treatments were performed 8 hours apart. A second dose of fomepizole was given in between the hemodialysis treatments. After the second treatment, her anion gap was 8 mEq/L, and sedation was weaned. The patient was extubated easily a few hours later, and her mental status and neurologic examination were normal. The next day her presentation methanol concentration was reported from the reference laboratory as 45 mg/dL. A formal ophthalmology evaluation was unremarkable, and the patient was transferred to psychiatry for what was ultimately decided was her suicidal behavior.

TABLE CS10–1	Laboratory Analyses						
Sodium, mEq/L	Potassium, mEq/L	Chloride, mEq/L	Bicarbonate, mEq/L	BUN, mg/dL	Creatinine, mg/dL	Glucose,* mg/dL	Calcium, mg/dL
149	3.4	104	5	14	1.4	124	8.9

*The glucose was obtained after $D_{50}W$ was given.

106 TOXIC ALCOHOLS

Sage W. Wiener

Ethylene glycol Isopropanol Methanol

Ethylene Glycol
MW = 62 Da
Isopropanol
MW = 60 Da
Methanol
MW = 32 Da

HISTORY AND EPIDEMIOLOGY

Methanol was a component of the embalming fluid used in ancient Egypt. Robert Boyle first isolated the molecule in 1661 by distilling boxwood, calling it *spirit of box*.[29] The molecular composition was determined in 1834 by Dumas and Peligot, who coined the term "methylene" from the Greek roots for "wood wine."[215] Industrial production began in 1923, and today most methanol is used for the synthesis of other chemicals. Methanol-containing consumer products that are commonly encountered include model airplane and model car fuel, windshield washer fluid, solid cooking fuel for camping and chafing dishes, photocopying fluid, colognes and perfumes, and gas line antifreeze ("dry gas"). Methanol is also used as a solvent by itself or as an adulterant in "denatured" alcohol.[141] Most reported cases of methanol poisoning in the United States involve ingestions of one of the above products, with more than 60% involving windshield washer fluid,[58] although most inhalational exposures involve carburetor cleaner.[86] In a Tunisian series, ingested cologne was the most common etiology.[30] In a Turkish series, cologne was also most common, accounting for almost 75% of ingestions.[132] Perfume was one of several exposures in a patient with methanol poisoning in a report from Spain,[183] and methanol poisoning from cologne was also reported in India.[12] There are sporadic epidemics of mass methanol poisoning, most commonly involving tainted fermented beverages.[23,133] These epidemics are a continuing problem in many parts of the world (Table 106–1).[102,216] Abuse of hydraulic fracturing ("fracking") fluid is another more recent source of methanol poisoning.[50] Methyl acetate in non-acetone nail polish removers is hydrolyzed to methanol in acidic environments, but it is unclear to what extent this occurs in vivo.[184]

Ethylene glycol was first synthesized in 1859 by Charles-Adolphe Wurtz and first widely produced as an engine coolant during World War II, when its precursor ethylene oxide became readily available.[69] Today its primary use remains as an engine coolant (antifreeze) in car radiators. Because of its sweet taste, it is often unintentionally consumed by animals and children. Aversive bittering agents are often added to ethylene glycol-containing antifreeze to try to prevent ingestions by making the antifreeze unpalatable, an approach that manufacturers now voluntarily employ throughout the United States, and that is required by law in many states.[128] However, there is no evidence that this strategy is effective, and comparisons in poison control center data between ethylene glycol ingestions in which bittering agents were required and or not revealed no significant differences in frequency or volume of ingestion, or any other outcome variable (Chap. 129).[128,272,273]

Isopropanol is primarily available as rubbing alcohol. Typical household preparations contain 70% isopropanol. It is also a solvent used in many

		Affected people	Reported deaths
TABLE 106–1	**International Methanol Poisoning Epidemics Since 1998**[102]		
Year	Location	Affected people	Reported deaths
1998	Phnom Penh, Cambodia	>400	60
1998	Nis, Serbia	>90	43
1998	Shanxi Province, China	>200	27
2000	Nairobi, Kenya	661	140
2000	San Salvador, El Salvador	>200	117
2000	Feni, Bangladesh	>100	56
2001	Pärnu, Estonia	154	68
2001	Bombay, India	>120	27
2002	Antananarivo, Madagascar	40	11
2002-2004	Norway	59	17
2003	Botswana	>45	9
2004	Shiraz, Iran	62	17
2005	Kenya	174	49
2006	Nicaragua	801	48
2006	Urals, Russia	60	3
2008	Karnataka/Tamil Nadu, India	285	150
2009	Central Uganda	77	27
2009	Ahmedabad, Gujarat, India	>275	136
2009	Bali/Lombok, Indonesia	45	25
2009	Kampala, Uganda	189	89
2011	Khartoum, Sudan	>137	71
2011	Los Rios, Ecuador	>770	51
2011	West Bengal, India	>370	170
2011	Haiti	40	18
2011	Kolkata, India	>167	143
2012	Orissa, India	100	31
2012	Cambodia	367	49
2012	Tegucigalpa, Honduras	48	24
2012	Czech Republic and Slovakia	>105	33
2013	Rafsanjan, Iran	694	8
2013	Tripoli, Libya	1066	101
2014	Kenya	467	126
2016	Irkutsk, Russia	107	74

Adapted with permission from Hassanian-Moghaddam H, Nikfarjam A, Mirafzal A, et al. Methanol mass poisoning in Iran: role of case finding in outbreak management. *J Public Health (Oxf)*. 2015 Jun;37(2):354-359.

household, cosmetic, and topical pharmaceutical products. Perhaps because it is so ubiquitous, inexpensive, and with a common name that contains the word "alcohol," isopropanol ingestions are by far the most common toxic alcohol exposure reported to poison control centers in the United States every year, typically in cases in which it was used as an ethanol substitute (Chap. 130).

CHEMISTRY

Alcohols are hydrocarbons that contain a hydroxyl (–OH) group. The term "toxic alcohol" refers to alcohols other than ethanol that are not intended for ingestion. In a sense, this is arbitrary, since all alcohols are toxic, causing inebriation and end-organ effects if taken in excess. The most common clinically relevant toxic alcohols are methanol and ethylene glycol (1,2-ethanediol). Primary alcohols, such as methanol and ethanol, contain a hydroxyl group on the end of the molecule (the terminal carbon), whereas secondary alcohols, such as isopropanol, contain hydroxyl groups bound to middle carbons. Ethylene glycol contains 2 hydroxyl groups; molecules with this characteristic are termed diols or glycols because of their sweet taste. Other common toxic alcohols include isopropanol (isopropyl alcohol or 2-propanol), benzyl alcohol (phenylmethanol), and propylene glycol (1,2-propanediol). Glycol ethers are glycols with a hydrocarbon chain bound to one or more of the hydroxyl groups (forming the basic structure $R_1O\text{-}CH_2\text{-}CH_2\text{-}OR_2$ or $R_1O\text{-}CH_2\text{-}CH_2\text{-}OR_2$). Glycol ethers commonly encountered include ethylene glycol butyl ether (also known as 2-butoxyethanol, ethylene glycol monobutyl ether, or butyl Cellosolve), ethylene glycol methyl ether (2-methoxyethanol), and diethylene glycol (2,2'-dihydroxydiethyl ether). Poisoning with these xenobiotics has some clinical similarities with toxic alcohol poisoning, and diethylene glycol is discussed in detail in Special Considerations: SC9.

TOXICOKINETICS/TOXICODYNAMICS

Absorption

Ingestion

Alcohols are rapidly absorbed after ingestion,[73,87] but are not completely bioavailable because of metabolism by gastric alcohol dehydrogenase (ADH), as well as by first-pass hepatic metabolism. Occasionally, delayed or prolonged absorption occurs.[66] Ethylene glycol has an oral bioavailability 92% to 100%.[73] The bioavailabilities of methanol and isopropanol are not described, but are likely to be similar.

Inhalation

Although methanol is absorbed in significant amounts by inhalation, poisoning by this route is uncommon. In workers exposed to methanol fumes from industrial processes for up to 6 hours at concentrations of 200 ppm (Occupational Health and Safety Administration {OSHA} permissible exposure limit {PEL}), there was no significant accumulation of methanol or its metabolite formate.[152] Another study showed that with methanol use in the semiconductor industry, ambient methanol concentrations generally do not approach this OSHA limit even in a room with poor ventilation and with no local exhaust ventilation.[77] However, a total of 5 patients in 2 case series of smartphone manufacturing workers had chronic exposures and developed permanent visual and neurologic sequelae.[46,219] Surprisingly, concentrations far in excess of the OSHA PEL are present within the passenger compartment of a car when using the windshield wipers with methanol-containing windshield washing fluid.[21] No cases of human poisoning are reported from this type of exposure, probably because these concentrations are not sustained over a long time. Two patients with occupational inhalational exposure aboard a tanker carrying methanol developed toxicity, including the death of one; both patients reportedly used appropriate personal protective equipment.[142] Additionally, cases of inhalational poisoning are reported with intentional inhalation of methanol as a drug of abuse, typically in the form of carburetor-cleaning fluid ("huffing") (Chap. 81), and with massive exposures of rescue workers responding to the scene of an overturned rail car filled with methanol.[14,74,86,166,262,269] Two case series suggest that patients who present after chronic inhalation of methanol generally do not have severe

poisoning,[20,166] but in another series, patients with inhalational exposure were as likely to require extensive therapy as patients with methanol ingestion,[86] and permanent visual sequelae and death are reported.[142,162,219]

Ethylene glycol has low volatility and is not reported to cause poisoning by inhalation. In one study, human volunteers inhaled vaporized ethylene glycol at a concentration of 1,340 to 1,610 ppm for 4 hours to simulate an industrial exposure. Afterward, the volunteers had detectable but not clinically significant concentrations of ethylene glycol and its metabolites.[261]

Transdermal

Most alcohols have some dermal absorption, although isopropanol and methanol penetrate the skin much more effectively than ethylene glycol.[62,158,266] Most reported cases of toxic alcohol poisoning by this route involve infants[57] because of their greater body surface area–volume ratio and differences in permeability of infant skin compared to adults, and likely this also involved simultaneous inhalation. When transdermal methanol exposure is prolonged, severe toxicity is reported.[134] One reported case of transdermal methanol poisoning involved a 51-year-old woman, but details of the exposure were not reported.[245] Another case involved a 52-year-old woman who reportedly frequently massaged with methanol-containing cologne and spirit over the course of 3 days. That patient had significant visual and neurologic sequelae despite aggressive treatment with ethanol and hemodialysis.[2] One methanol fatality was deemed to be caused by transdermal absorption (in addition to blunt trauma) when high tissue methanol concentrations were measured in the absence of detectable methanol in the gastrointestinal tract,[15] but inhalational exposure could have also conceivably contributed. Transdermal methanol absorption is responsible for multiple cases of consequential poisoning in Turkey, where methanol-soaked bandages or clothing are used as a traditional or alternative remedy for musculoskeletal pain.[105,260] When human volunteers were exposed to 100% ethylene glycol applied to a 66 cm² area of skin under an occlusive dressing for 6 hours, detectable but not clinically significant amounts were absorbed.[261]

Distribution

Once absorbed, alcohols are rapidly distributed to total body water. In human volunteers given an oral dose of methanol on an empty stomach, the measured volume of distribution was 0.77 L/kg, with a distribution half-life of about 8 minutes.[87] This is only slightly longer than the absorption half-life, so serum concentrations often peak soon after ingestion and then begin to fall. However, this is not necessarily the case in patients with large ingestions or with food in their stomachs prior to ingestion. The volume of distribution of ethylene glycol with IV administration in a rat model was 0.60 L/kg.[73] The reported volume of distribution of isopropanol is 0.45 to 0.55 L/kg.[242]

Metabolism and Elimination

Without intervention, toxic alcohols are metabolized through successive oxidation by ADH and aldehyde dehydrogenase (ALDH), each of which is coupled to the reduction of NAD^+ to NADH. Methanol is metabolized to formaldehyde, then to formic acid (Fig. 106–1). The formate metabolite is then bound by tetrahydrofolate and undergoes metabolism by 10-formyltetrahydrofolate dehydrogenase to carbon dioxide and water. Ethylene glycol has 2 hydroxyl groups that are serially oxidized by ADH and ALDH, producing, in turn, glycoaldehyde, glycolic acid, glyoxylic acid, and finally oxalic acid (Fig. 106–2). Like ethanol, metabolism follows zero-order kinetics, with a rate of approximately 10 mg/dL/h.[49,120,179] Additionally, this rate is apparently unchanged in chronic ethanol users.[97,98] Alternate minor metabolic pathways such as catalase exist for methanol and ethylene glycol.

Ethylene glycol is also metabolized to ketoadipate and glycine using thiamine and pyridoxine as cofactors.[189] Because of the low toxicity of these ethylene glycol metabolites, enhancing these normally minor metabolic pathways is theoretically beneficial in poisoned patients.

Methanol and ethylene glycol are also eliminated from the body as unchanged parent compounds. When kidney function is normal, ethylene glycol is cleared with a half-life of approximately 17 hours.[28,45,240] In patients with renal impairment, the half-life is prolonged (34 ± 13 hours) in the absence

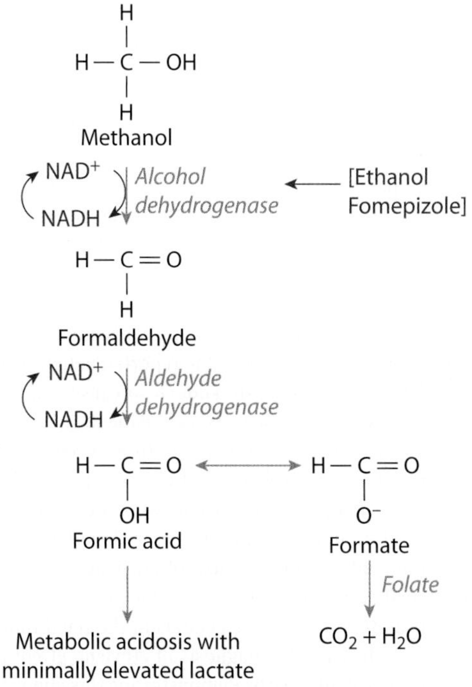

H
|
H — C — OH
|
H
Methanol

NAD⁺ → NADH, Alcohol dehydrogenase ← [Ethanol Fomepizole]

H — C = O
|
H
Formaldehyde

NAD⁺ → NADH, Aldehyde dehydrogenase

H — C = O
|
OH
Formic acid

↔

H — C = O
|
O⁻
Formate

Folate

Metabolic acidosis with minimally elevated lactate ← | → CO₂ + H₂O

FIGURE 106–1. Major pathway of methanol metabolism.

OH
|
H₃C — CH — CH₃   Isopropanol

NAD⁺ → NADH, Alcohol dehydrogenase

O
||
H₃C — C — CH₃   Acetone

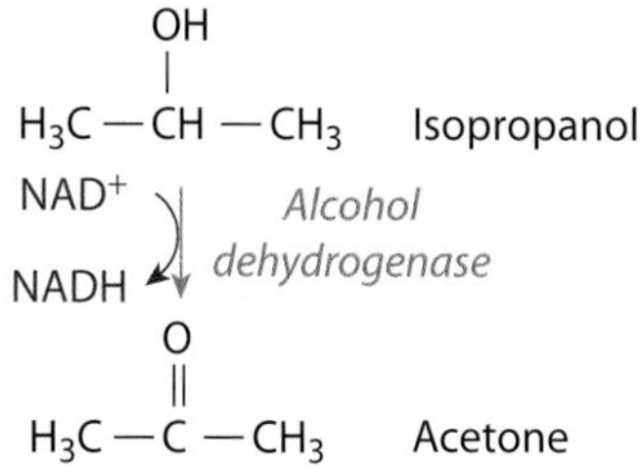

FIGURE 106–3. Isopropanol metabolism.

of renal function) and about 49 h in those with impaired kidney function (Cr>1.2).[240] Methanol does not have significant renal elimination (about 1% of the ingested dose in patients with intact hepatic metabolism) and is cleared much more slowly than is ethylene glycol, presumably as a vapor in expired air (half-life 52 hours, with a longer half-life at very high concentrations).[32,111,147,198]

Isopropanol is metabolized by alcohol dehydrogenase to acetone. Because acetone is a ketone, not an aldehyde, it cannot be further metabolized by ALDH and is eliminated in the urine and in expired air (Fig. 106–3).

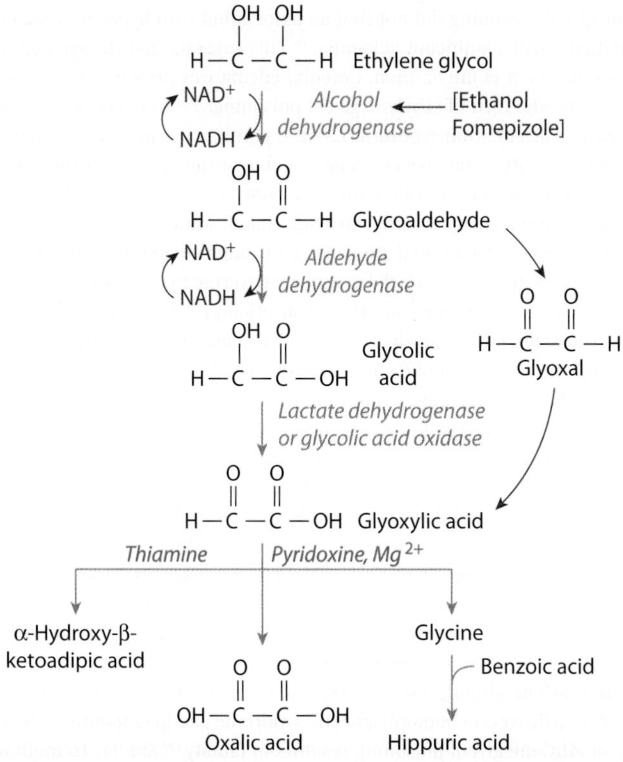

OH OH
| |
H — C — C — H   Ethylene glycol

NAD⁺ → NADH, Alcohol dehydrogenase ← [Ethanol Fomepizole]

OH O
| ||
H — C — C — H   Glycoaldehyde

NAD⁺ → NADH, Aldehyde dehydrogenase

OH O
| ||
H — C — C — OH   Glycolic acid

O O
|| ||
H — C — C — H   Glyoxal

Lactate dehydrogenase or glycolic acid oxidase

O O
|| ||
H — C — C — OH   Glyoxylic acid

Thiamine | Pyridoxine, Mg²⁺

α-Hydroxy-β-ketoadipic acid

O O
|| ||
OH — C — C — OH   Oxalic acid

Glycine

Benzoic acid

Hippuric acid

FIGURE 106–2. Pathways of ethylene glycol metabolism. Thiamine and pyridoxine enhance formation of nontoxic metabolites.

PATHOPHYSIOLOGY AND CLINICAL MANIFESTATIONS

Acute Central Nervous System Effects

All alcohols cause inebriation, depending on the dose. Based on limited animal data, the higher-molecular-weight alcohols are more intoxicating than lower-molecular-weight alcohols on a molar basis (therefore, isopropanol approximates ethylene glycol < which is greater than ethanol < which is greater than methanol).[270] However, the absence of apparent inebriation does not exclude ingestion, particularly if the patient chronically drinks ethanol and is thereby tolerant to its central nervous system (CNS) effects.[250] Additionally, serum methanol concentrations of 25 to 50 mg/dL are associated with toxicity, whereas one may legally drive a car in the US with a blood ethanol concentration of up to 80 mg/dL.

The CNS manifestations of toxic alcohol poisoning are incompletely understood. It is assumed by analogy that inebriation is similar to that of ethanol, in which effects are mediated through increased γ-aminobutyric acid (GABA)–ergic tone both directly and through inhibition of presynaptic GABA, $GABA_A$ receptors as well as inhibition of the N-methyl-D-aspartic acid glutamate receptors.[9,40,89,107,182] Although the CNS effects of other alcohols are clinically similar, there is no direct evidence that they are mechanistically the same.

Metabolic Acidosis

Metabolic acidosis with an elevated anion gap is a hallmark of toxic alcohol poisoning. This is a consequence of the metabolism of the alcohols to toxic organic acids. The acids have no rapid natural metabolic pathway of elimination, and therefore they accumulate. In methanol poisoning, formic acid is responsible for the acidosis, whereas in ethylene glycol poisoning, glycolic acid is the primary acid responsible for the acidosis, with other metabolites making a minor contribution.[123] An exception to the formation of an acid metabolite is isopropanol, which is metabolized to acetone. Because acetone cannot be metabolized by ALDH, isopropanol has no organic acid metabolite and does not cause metabolic acidosis. In fact, ketosis without acidosis is essentially diagnostic of isopropanol poisoning. Occasionally, a non–anion gap (hyperchloremic) metabolic acidosis is present with ethylene glycol poisoning (almost 18% in one series), often concurrently with anion gap acidosis.[244] The mechanism for this is unclear, but a similar pattern is observed in diabetic ketoacidosis, alcoholic ketoacidosis, and toluene poisoning. Different volumes of distribution of bicarbonate and the anion are a potential explanation for the phenomenon.

End-Organ Manifestations

Additional end-organ effects depend on which alcohol is involved. Methanol causes visual impairment, ranging from blurry or hazy vision or defects in color vision, to "snowfield vision" or total blindness in severe poisoning. Although it is counterintuitive, vision loss is often asymmetric.[47,169] On physical examination, central scotoma are sometimes present on visual field testing, and both hyperemia and pallor of the optic disc, papilledema, and an afferent papillary defect are described as characteristic findings.[23,194,290] In a retrospective study, optic disk cupping developed in at least one eye in 22 of 50 consecutive patients with vision loss due to methanol poisoning, and 43 of 100 eyes.[79] Scotopic (monochromatic vision in low-light conditions) and photopic (color vision under well-lit conditions) function are both impaired after methanol poisoning in a rat model.[163] Electroretinography demonstrates a diminished b-wave,[258] a marker of bipolar cell dysfunction, and optical coherence tomography (OCT), similar in principle to ultrasound, but using reflected light waves to image translucent tissues, demonstrates peripapillary nerve fiber swelling and intraretinal fluid accumulation.[76] These OCT changes are best assessed at 2 months after discharge, when retinal edema resolves, to prevent false negative results. Formate is a mitochondrial toxin, inhibiting cytochrome oxidase and it thereby interferes with oxidative phosphorylation.[67,190,191] Although it is unclear why this results in ocular toxicity whereas other tissues are relatively spared, retinal pigmented epithelial cells and optic nerve cells appear to be uniquely susceptible.[64,175,257,258] Proteomic analysis of retinas in rats poisoned by methanol showed that concentrations of 24 proteins were different from baseline (14 increased, 10 decreased),[44] so the underlying pathophysiology of retinal toxicity from methanol is likely more complex than is currently understood. Years after exposure, optic nerve atrophy, disc pallor, and severe cupping often persist, even with normal intraocular pressure.[79,236] In fact, optic nerve axonal degeneration continues to progress over at least 2 years after exposure to methanol.[283]

Interestingly, neurons in the basal ganglia appear to be similarly susceptible to this toxicity. Bilateral basal ganglia lesions, bilateral necrosis of the putamen (with or without hemorrhage), and less commonly, caudate nucleus are characteristically abnormal visualized on cerebral computed tomography (CT) or magnetic resonance imaging (MRI) after methanol poisoning.[134,232,253] Although lesions of this type are nonspecific, and also occur in hypoxia, hypotension, and carbon monoxide poisoning, in methanol poisoning they occur in the absence of hypotension and hypoxia,[177] suggesting a direct toxic mechanism. Some patients develop parkinsonism after poisoning by methanol, a finding consistent with lesions in the basal ganglia.[91,176,209] In one series, typical radiological lesions were present in 6 of 9 cases.[232] Other CNS lesions reported include necrosis of the corpus callosum,[137] infarcts of other areas of the brain,[95] and intracranial hemorrhage.[13,231] Pathologic examination of the brain reveals lesions similar to those found radiologically.[135] Increased glial fibrillary acidic protein and decreased CD34 expression are pathologic markers in affected tissues, although how these relate to the underlying pathophysiology is not yet clear.[259] Serum leukotrienes are also elevated in patients with methanol poisoning, and patients with the worst neurologic outcomes have the least elevated leukotrienes.[279] The role of leukotrienes is incompletely understood, but this could be explained by leukotriene-related inflammation as part of the pathophysiology of neurodegeneration.

Both retinal and neurologic toxicity in patients with methanol poisoning are often permanent. Among 86 survivors of a methanol poisoning outbreak in Estonia in 2001, 26 had died 6 years later (many from ethanol intoxication) and 33 could not be located. Of the 5 patients who could be located of the 20 patients who were discharged with retinal or neurologic sequelae, all had persistent effects. Interestingly, 8 of the 22 patients located who were discharged without sequelae had newly identified neurologic and visual sequelae 6 years later (among 66 initially discharged without sequelae), possibly because they were present initially but missed because of lack of ophthalmologic evaluation, but more likely because they had progressive findings or reexposure to methanol. New neurologic abnormalities were probably due to ongoing ethanol consumption.[197] In another series from Iran, 37 of 50 survivors of methanol poisoning with retinal toxicity were followed 1 year later; 16 patients improved before discharge from the hospital. Seven patients had their visual disturbance resolve within 2 weeks; 5 were blind at discharge but partially recovered within 3 to 4 weeks; 5 were blind at discharge and had no improvement 1 year later; and 4 were blind at discharge, had partial recovery within 1 month, but then had worsening vision within the subsequent 9 months.[225] In a series of patients from a 2012 methanol poisoning outbreak in the Czech Republic, 42 of 101 hospitalized patients presented with visual disturbances. Only 16 of these 42 (38%) survived without sequelae.[289] In a subsequent study of these patients, 8 of 37 who were discharged with no visual complaints after methanol poisoning subsequently had visual damage after additional testing at follow-up.[285] Further testing showed progressive axonal injury over 2 years.[283] In another study of 50 patients from the same outbreak, major neurologic sequelae were uncommon, but cognitive deficits in executive function and verbal memory compared

to controls persisted 2 years later.[25] Clearly, long-term outcomes of retinal and neurologic toxicity are difficult to predict from the initial presentation, especially when complicated by persistent alcoholism and thiamine deficiency.

Injury to other tissues also occurs. Both acute kidney injury (AKI) and pancreatitis are reported after methanol poisoning.[101,143] One case series showed a much higher incidence of pancreatitis (50%)[101] and in another, 11 of 15 patients had pancreatitis,[265] but this is not typical. Of note, all of the patients in the first series and 13 of 15 patients in the second series had been treated with ethanol. Some of the AKI that results from methanol poisoning likely results from myoglobinuria.[90] In one series of methanol-poisoned patients with AKI, about half had associated myoglobinuria, presumably because of atraumatic rhabdomyolysis and prolonged immobilization associated with inebriation, or to seizures. One reported patient with methanol poisoning had rhabdomyolysis severe enough to cause compartment syndrome in both legs, requiring fasciotomies.[70] Patients with AKI were also more likely than a control group of patients to have severe poisoning, as manifested by low initial serum pH, high initial osmolality, and high peak formate concentration.[265] Pathologic abnormalities of the liver, esophagus, and gastric mucosa are also found in some fatal cases of methanol poisoning.[4,42]

The most prominent end-organ effect of ethylene glycol is nephrotoxicity. The oxalic acid metabolite forms a complex with calcium to precipitate as calcium oxalate monohydrate crystals in the renal tubules, leading to AKI.[72,92,93,178,205,249,254] In fact, the diagnosis of ethylene glycol poisoning is sometimes established at autopsy by demonstrating this abnormality;[10,156] in another case, the diagnosis was established by kidney biopsy.[137] Although the intermediate products of ethylene glycol metabolism, and possibly ethylene glycol itself, are directly toxic to the renal tubules in some studies,[48,72,204,207] this appears not to occur at clinically relevant concentrations.[92] Currently no explanation exists for the presence of necrotic lesions to the glomerular basement membrane on some pathology specimens[72] as oxalic acid generally does not cause glomerular injury.[127]

Ethylene glycol can occasionally affect other organ systems. In severe poisoning, the oxalic acid metabolite causes hypocalcemia by precipitation as calcium oxalate. Hypocalcemia results in prolongation of the QT interval on the electrocardiogram and ventricular dysrhythmias.[230] However, a retrospective review of serum calcium concentrations in patients with ethylene glycol poisoning did not find an association with hypocalcemia, even in patients with significant acidemia.[106] This suggests that though hypocalcemia occurs, it is uncommon. Cerebral edema was present on CT scan in 2 patients who died of ethylene glycol poisoning.[75,254] In contrast, reversible osmotic demyelination syndrome (central pontine myelinolysis) occurred in one patient with a massive ethylene glycol ingestion despite normal serum sodium; the patient had full neurologic recovery several weeks later.[3] Two reported patients had delayed neurologic manifestations. One patient developed increased intracranial pressure, with papilledema and an abducens (CN VI) palsy approximately 9 days after recovering from acute ethylene glycol poisoning and without another clear etiology.[59] Another patient developed the same cluster of delayed effects (increased intracranial pressure, papilledema, and an abducens palsy) on day 13 of hospitalization, after fomepizole, thiamine, pyridoxine, and hemodialysis. He subsequently developed a facial (CN VII) palsy, sensory neuropathy, and autonomic neuropathy, including postural hypotension and gastroparesis.[208] Precipitation of calcium oxalate crystals in the brain was found on autopsy after severe ethylene glycol poisoning[7,72,75] and likely accounts for the multiple cranial nerve abnormalities that occasionally develop,[59,68,246] although there is as yet no direct evidence of causation. Peripheral polyradiculoneuropathy was diagnosed by electromyography and nerve conduction studies in cases of ethylene glycol poisoning,[6,16] and intracranial hemorrhage involving the globus pallidus also occurs.[37] A leukemoid reaction is reported in some patients with severe ethylene glycol poisoning, but the mechanism remains unclear.[168,187] One pediatric case of hemophagocytic syndrome and liver failure in the setting of ethylene glycol poisoning resulted in fatality.[150] Similar to methanol poisoning, parkinsonism also occurs.[209] Two severe cases of unintentional ethylene glycol ingestion in the United Kingdom resulted in blindness and deafness; one with associated cranial neuropathies and one with multiple peripheral neuropathies.[39,61] One patient had a myocardial infarction with ST segment elevation while poisoned with ethylene glycol, but survived after cardiac catheterization and placement of 5 stents, as well as treatment with ethanol and hemodialysis.[252] However, this was most likely due to the stress of poisoning in a patient with underlying cardiovascular disease rather than a direct toxic effect. Finally, death is reported from massive ethylene glycol ingestion with no elevation of its metabolites, suggesting direct toxicity of the alcohol, probably through respiratory depression.[80]

Hemorrhagic gastritis is associated with isopropyl alcohol toxicity. Although this is often assumed to be caused by a local irritant effect, one reported case of hemorrhagic gastritis after percutaneous isopropanol exposure suggests that this is not the only mechanism, and could in fact be a specific end-organ effect.[63] Hemorrhagic tracheobronchitis is reported in fatal cases of isopropanol aspiration.[5] The acetone metabolite of isopropyl alcohol also interferes with some creatinine assays, causing a falsely elevated result,[139] but it does not actually cause AKI.

DIAGNOSTIC TESTING

Toxic Alcohol and Metabolite Concentrations

Serum methanol, formate, ethylene glycol, oxalate, and isopropanol concentrations (as appropriate) would be the ideal tests to perform shortly after suspected toxic alcohol poisoning. However, these concentrations are most commonly measured by gas chromatography with or without mass spectrometry confirmation, methodologies that are not available in most hospital laboratories on a 24-hour basis, if at all. In fact, in many hospitals these are only available as "send out" tests, so results arrive too late for meaningful clinical decision making.[136] Enzymatic assays for methanol, formic acid, ethylene glycol, and glycolic acid use newer methology,[26,99,212,228,247,268] and these may lead to more readily available clinical tests in the future. One commercial assay currently only approved for veterinary use is effective for confirming the qualitative presence of ethylene glycol in human poisoning, although false positives may occur with propylene glycol.[165] At least one medical center has adopted the veterinary product for clinical use. Over 4 years, no false negatives occurred (most negative tests did not have GC performed for confirmation, but chart review did not identify any missed cases).[140,213] There were only 25 false positives out of 222 samples, most due to propylene glycol in lorazepam or in activated charcoal.[214] In a murine model, a commercially available ethanol in saliva point of care test detected the presence of a low concentration of methanol but not ethylene glycol.[96] Unfortunately, it would not distinguish between methanol and ethanol, limiting the clinical utility of this test. A group in Finland described a point of care breath test for methanol, using a portable Fourier transform infrared (FT-IR) analyzer similar to the "breathalyzers" used by law enforcement agents.[151] Although analyzers like this are used to detect methanol as a combustion product in industry, they are not yet approved for medical use in the United States. Once approved, they would be useful for early clinical decision making because they are easy to use and provide a rapid result. They also can provide continuous monitoring of concentrations, a feature that would be very helpful during hemodialysis. Unfortunately, this methodology could not be used to detect ethylene glycol because of its low volatility. A newer dry chemistry "dipstick" technology for formate detection shows promise for rapid detection of cases of methanol poisoning with minimal equipment or skilled laboratory personnel.[112] Patients with significant serum concentrations of ethanol generally do not have measurable formate concentrations even when there are significant serum concentrations of methanol,[170] so serial testing of these patients would be necessary if methanol poisoning is suspected.

Patients presenting late after ingestion have already metabolized all parent compound to toxic metabolites and thus have low or no measurable toxic alcohol concentrations. The enzymatic assay for ethylene glycol is also capable of detecting glycolic acid, although as mentioned, this assay is approved only for veterinary use. Some authors actually advocate for routine testing for glycolic acid in addition to testing for the parent compound when ethylene glycol poisoning is suspected.[207] Serum and urine oxalate concentrations

can also be determined,[248] but they are unlikely to be clinically useful. In a postmortem study, patients who died of ethylene glycol poisoning had similar oxalate concentrations to some negative controls who died of causes unrelated to ethylene glycol, and 2 of 6 patients who died of ethylene glycol poisoning had very low urine oxalate concentrations.[267] By contrast, a formate concentration would be valuable when a patient presents late after methanol ingestion.[117,195] Formate was detected in blood samples from 97% of patients who died of methanol poisoning in one series; all of these patients also had detectable blood or vitreous methanol concentrations.[129] Based on a series of 38 patients from the Czech methanol epidemic, serum formate concentrations greater than 4.0 mmol/L (18 mg/dL) were associated with clinical signs of visual toxicity, and concentrations greater than 11 mmol/L (49.5 mg/dL) were associated with permanent visual and neurologic sequelae. Concentrations greater than 17.5 mmol/L (78.8 mg/dL) were potentially lethal.[280] Newer capillary electrophoresis methodology has the potential to rapidly determine serum formate concentrations with a small sample size and lower cost.[148,149] Clearly, a low or undetectable toxic alcohol concentration must be interpreted within the context of the history and other clinical data, such as the presence of acidosis and end-organ toxicity, with glycolate and formate concentrations as potentially valuable additions.

Samples must be handled correctly for accurate toxic alcohol results. Particularly with the more volatile alcohols methanol and isopropanol, evaporation from sample tubes that are not airtight lowers serum concentrations in those tubes so that they do not accurately reflect the serum concentration in the patient. This results in falsely low results if alcohol concentrations are done as "add on" tests to samples already opened for electrolyte or osmol determinations.

Other alcohols such as benzyl alcohol and propylene glycol are not routinely assayed for by gas chromatography. Thus, these xenobiotics present a much greater diagnostic challenge than methanol and ethylene glycol. Enzymatic assays for methanol or ethylene glycol would also fail to detect these, although false positive ethylene glycol tests may occur if propylene glycol is present. Thus, a high index of suspicion is critical to establishing the diagnosis in these cases. If suspected on the basis of history, specific toxic alcohol testing should be performed.

Once alcohol concentrations are obtained, their interpretation represents a further point of controversy. Traditionally, a methanol or ethylene glycol concentration greater than 25 mg/dL was considered toxic, but the evidence supporting this as a threshold is often questioned. In a case series of methanol-poisoned patients from the 1950s, a methanol concentration of 52 mg/dL was the lowest associated with vision loss.[23] This is the origin of the 25-mg/dL threshold, incorporating a 50% reduction as a margin of safety. However, the patient with the 52-mg/dL concentration presented 24 hours after his initial ingestion, and therefore was much more severely poisoned than suggested by his serum concentration at that point. In fact, almost all reported cases of methanol poisoning involve patients with delayed presentations who already have a metabolic acidosis.[144] A 6-week-old infant, the only reported patient who went untreated after presenting early with an elevated methanol concentration (45.6 mg/dL), never developed acidosis or end-organ toxicity.[31,144] A systematic review found that 126 mg/dL was the lowest methanol concentration resulting in metabolic acidosis in a patient who arrived early after ingestion and met the inclusion criteria. The authors concluded that the available data are currently insufficient to apply a 25-mg/dL treatment threshold in a patient presenting early after ingestion without metabolic acidosis.[144] However, until better data are available demonstrating the safe application of a higher concentration, it seems prudent to use a conservative concentration such as 25 mg/dL as a threshold for treatment.

Because of the problems with obtaining and interpreting actual serum concentrations, many surrogate markers are used to assess the patient with suspected toxic alcohol poisoning. The initial laboratory evaluation should include serum electrolytes, including calcium, blood urea nitrogen, serum creatinine concentrations, urinalysis, measured serum osmolality, and a serum ethanol concentration. Blood gas analysis with a lactate concentration is also helpful in the initial evaluation of ill-appearing patients.

Anion Gap and Osmol Gap

For a full discussion of the anion gap concept, refer to Chap. 12. As previously discussed, anion gap elevation is a hallmark of toxic alcohol poisoning. In fact, the possibility of methanol or ethylene glycol poisoning is often first considered when patients present with an anion gap metabolic acidosis of unknown etiology, frequently with no history of ingestion. Unless clinical information suggests otherwise, it is important to exclude metabolic acidosis with elevated lactate concentration and ketoacidosis, which are the most common causes of anion gap metabolic acidosis, before pursuing toxic alcohols in these patients. This is because of the extensive evaluation required and expensive, potentially invasive course of therapy to which they are otherwise committed. However, elevated lactate concentrations are often present in the setting of both methanol and ethylene glycol poisoning.[173,180,234]

The unmeasured anions in toxic alcohol poisoning are the dissociated organic acid metabolites discussed above. The metabolic acidosis takes time to develop, sometimes up to 16 to 24 hours for methanol. Thus, the absence of an anion gap elevation early after reported toxic alcohol ingestion does not exclude the diagnosis. If ethanol is present in the body, the development of metabolic acidosis will not begin to occur until enough ethanol has been metabolized that it can no longer effectively inhibit ADH (see Ethanol Concentration, below).

A potential early surrogate marker of toxic alcohol poisoning is an elevated osmol gap (the principles and the calculations are discussed in detail in Chap. 12). However, it is important to recognize that osmol gap elevation is neither sensitive nor specific for toxic alcohol poisoning. Because a baseline osmol gap is generally not available when evaluating a patient (with rare exceptions),[115] and a normal osmol gap ranges from –14 to +10 mOsm/L, so-called "normal" osmol gaps cannot exclude toxic alcohol poisoning.[109] For example, in a patient with a baseline osmol gap of –10, a current gap of +5 mOsm/L potentially represents a methanol concentration of 47 mg/dL or an ethylene glycol concentration of 93 mg/dL, values that might require hemodialysis. Inversely, a moderately elevated osmol gap (+10 to +20 mOsm/L) is not necessarily diagnostic of toxic alcohol poisoning because other disorders such as alcoholic ketoacidosis and metabolic acidosis with elevated lactate concentration will raise the osmol gap.[229] Furthermore, mean osmol gaps vary within populations over time, further limiting their utility.[145] However, a markedly elevated osmol gap (>50 mOsm/L) is difficult to explain by anything other than a toxic alcohol.

Further complicating matters, the anion gap and osmol gap have a reciprocal relationship over time. This is because soon after ingestion, the alcohols present in the serum raise the osmol gap but do not affect the anion gap because metabolism to the organic acid anion has not yet occurred. As the alcohols are metabolized to organic acid anions, the anion gap rises while the osmol gap falls, because the metabolites are negatively charged particles that have already been accounted for in the calculated osmolarity by doubling of the sodium. Thus patients who present early after ingestion have a high osmol gap and normal anion gap, whereas those who present later have the reverse.[113,119] Figure 106–4 depicts a more intuitive visual representation of this process.

One retrospective and one prospective study attempted to evaluate the performance characteristic of the osmol gap as a diagnostic test. Although in both cases, the osmol gap performed fairly well, the studies were small, 20 patients with toxic alcohol poisoning in the retrospective study and 28 patients with methanol poisoning in the prospective study, and the prospective study identified 3 patients with significant poisoning and metabolic acidosis but "normal" osmol gaps, defined in the study as less than 25 mOsm/L.[113,172] Therefore, these data do not eliminate the concern that a patient with significant poisoning could be missed by relying on the osmol gap alone to exclude poisoning. One reported patient had his diagnosis delayed by 2 days because of false reassurance from a "normal" osmol gap.[11]

Ethanol Concentration

A serum ethanol concentration is an important part of the assessment of the patient with suspected toxic alcohol poisoning. As discussed in Chap. 12, the ethanol concentration is necessary to calculate osmolarity. In addition,

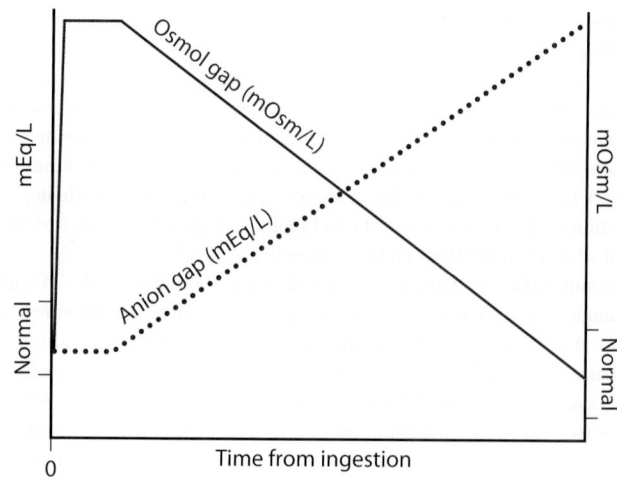

FIGURE 106–4. The reciprocal relationship of anion gap and osmol gap over time (hours). Note that patients presenting early may have a normal anion gap while patients who present late may have a normal osmol gap.

because ethanol is the preferred substrate of ADH (4:1 over methanol and 8:1 over ethylene glycol on a molar basis), a significant concentration would be protective if coingested with a toxic alcohol. In fact, ethanol concentrations near 100 mg/dL virtually preclude toxic alcohols as the cause of an unknown anion gap metabolic acidosis because the presence of such a concentration should have prevented metabolism to the organic acid. A possible exception would be ingestion of ethanol several hours after ingestion of a toxic alcohol.[108] If a breath alcohol analyzer is used to determine ethanol concentration, significant methanol concentrations can cause a false positive ethanol, without an indication from the machine that an interfering substance is present (as there is with acetone).[38] Therefore, even if a prehospital breath alcohol analyzer indicates a significant ethanol concentration, this should be confirmed by determining the serum ethanol concentration.

Lactate Concentration

Both methanol and ethylene glycol poisoning can result in elevated lactate concentrations, for different reasons. Formate, as an inhibitor of oxidative phosphorylation, leads to anaerobic metabolism and resultant lactate elevation. Additionally, metabolism of all alcohols results in an increased $NADH/NAD^+$ ratio, which favors the conversion of pyruvate to lactate. Furthermore, hypotension and organ failure in severely poisoned patients also produces an elevated lactate concentration. Finally, the fact that these patients are often alcoholics who are nutritionally deprived and thiamine depleted also contributes to the elevated lactate concentration. However, lactate production by these mechanisms is rarely greater than 5 mmol/L.

In ethylene glycol poisoning, the glycolate metabolite also causes a false positive lactate elevation when measured by some analyzers, particularly with whole blood arterial blood gas analyzers. The Radiometer ABL series (625, 700, 725, 825, 835) is most widely reported to result in a false positive lactate. Other specific models implicated to varying degrees of false positive lactate results include Beckman LX 20, Siemens Rapidlab series (860, 865), all Roche models, Architect c8000, Vitros Fusion 5.1, IL GEM 4000 Premium, Abbott iSTAT and Hitachi 911 analyzers. The Vitros 950, Vitros 250, Siemens Dimension Vista, Siemens Dimension RxL, Abbott Aeroset, or Abbott Architecht C8000 do not produce false positive results. Reports are conflicting on the Beckman Coulter DxC-800 chemistry analyzer.[34,43,52,71,173,180,186,206,200,227,256,276] In such cases, the degree of lactate elevation directly correlates with the concentration of glycolate present,[173,180] and the artifact results from the lack of specificity of the lactate oxidase enzyme used in these machines,[180,186,206,276] although direct oxidation of glycolate at the analyzer anode is also a possible mechanism.[237] In general, assays that use a lactate dehydrogenase enzyme instead of lactate oxidase, or assays that use lactate oxidase with colorimetry instead of amperometry, are less prone to give a false positive lactate result.[256] This artifact can be exploited, using the presence of a "lactate gap" to diagnose ethylene glycol poisoning in hospitals where lactate assays are available with and without sensitivity to glycolate (eg, the lactate assay using lactate oxidase on the blood gas machine and the plasma lactate assay using lactate dehydrogenase), or 2 lactate assays with different sensitivities to glycolate.[237,264] Ingestion of propylene glycol also results in elevated lactate concentrations, but in this case, it is not a false positive lactate but rather an accurate measurement of lactate, the principal metabolite of propylene glycol.[130,131]

Other Diagnostics

Serum glucose concentration is generally obtained as part of routine laboratory analysis. Hyperglycemia, defined as serum glucose greater than 140 mg/dL (7.77 mmol/L) in nondiabetic patients, portended a greater risk of death after methanol poisoning, with an odds ratio of 6.5 in one retrospective study.[224] This has not yet been prospectively validated.

The urine provides some information in the assessment of the patient with suspected ethylene glycol poisoning. Calcium oxalate monohydrate (spindle-shaped) and dihydrate (envelope-shaped) crystals are often seen when the urine sediment is examined by microscopy, although this finding is neither sensitive nor specific.[78,120,185] In fact, calcium oxalate crystals were present in the urine of 63% (12 of 19) of patients with proven ethylene glycol ingestion in one series.[33]

Some brands of antifreeze contain fluorescein to facilitate the detection of radiator leaks. If one of these products is ingested and the urine is examined with a Woods lamp within the first 6 hours, there will often be urinary fluorescence.[275] False positive fluorescence also results from examining the urine in glass or plastic containers because of the inherent fluorescence of these materials, so if this test is performed, an aliquot of the urine should be poured onto a piece of white gauze or paper. Unfortunately, the utility of this test is quite limited. In one study, almost all children had urinary fluorescence, and there was poor interrater agreement in determining fluorescence of specimens.[41,199] Gastric aspirate also sometimes demonstrates fluorescence.[55]

The evaluation of patients with known or suspected ethylene glycol poisoning should also include serum calcium and creatinine concentrations. Patients with methanol poisoning and abdominal pain also warrant an assessment of liver function tests and serum lipase because of the possibility of associated hepatitis and pancreatitis. In one study, 4 of 13 patients had an elevation of serum troponin, but no further cardiac testing of these patients was reported.[220] Until more data are available, there is likely little role for serum troponin screening in patients without ischemic symptoms or suggestive ECG findings.

Although characteristic brain CT and MRI abnormalities are frequently reported in the setting of methanol poisoning, it is unclear what role they have in the routine evaluation of these patients. The presence of putaminal hemorrhage or insular subcortex white matter necrosis was associated with a greater odds ratio of death (8 and 10, respectively) in one study of patients with methanol poisoning.[253] However, in the absence of neurologic abnormalities on physical examination, routine CT or MRI is not routinely recommended.

Various electrocardiographic abnormalities are reported in the setting of methanol poisoning (more than 80% had some kind of abnormality in one series), including sinus tachycardia, prolonged QT interval, right bundle branch block, prolonged PR interval, and nonspecific T-wave changes. However, none correlates well with clinical outcomes, and changes generally normalize as patients recover.[99,126]

Diagnostic Testing and Risk Assessment

Many pediatric patients with toxic alcohol exposures have not actually ingested the product with which they are found. Because of this, pediatric patients tend to do better than adults with similar exposures.[161] However, children who actually do ingest toxic alcohols can be just as sick as adults and smaller-volume ingestions are required to reach consequential serum concentrations, so risk assessment is particularly important for these patients. It can also be important for managing adults, particularly in allocating resources during poisoning epidemics.

If the ingested dose of a toxic alcohol is known, an estimate of the projected maximum serum concentration can be determined using the formula:

$$C = D/V_D$$

where C is the estimated concentration projected, D is the dose in grams, and V_D is the volume of distribution (typically estimated at 0.6 L/kg, though this may lead to an underestimate of the projected concentration for isopropanol and an overestimate for methanol) multiplied by the patient's weight in kilograms. Care must be taken with units to avoid 10-, 100-, or 1000-fold errors. Once the projected serum concentration is calculated and converted to mg/dL, it can be compared to typical thresholds for treatment (see Management below) to decide whether the ingestion could potentially lead to a concerning serum concentration.

Increases in both anion gap and osmolar gap are useful for risk stratification in methanol poisoning, and a venous or arterial blood gas with lactate is recommended. Formate concentrations should also be obtained, if available. A review of reported toxic alcohol cases attempted to identify risk factors for mortality in adults with methanol or ethylene glycol poisoning. For methanol poisoning, no patient with an anion gap less than 30 mEq/L or an osmolar gap less than 49 mOsm/L died. A pH less than 7.22 was an even better predictor of mortality, as no patient with a pH greater than 7.22 died. For ethylene glycol, the tests were less useful. One patient with an osmolar gap of only 25 mOsm/L died, no patient with an anion gap less than 20 mEq/L died, and pH did not predict mortality with statistical significance.[53] This study was criticized for missing a substantial number of patients,[222] and for selection bias,[171] and it still needs to be validated in another population. A more recent retrospective study of 121 patients with ethylene glycol poisoning suggests pH has more promise. A pH higher than 7.37 predicted survival without prolonged kidney injury with a sensitivity of 95% and a specificity of 76%, whereas a pH less than 7 had a sensitivity of 36% and specificity of 95% for death or prolonged kidney injury. Other markers of poor outcomes in this study were initial creatinine higher than 1.65 mg/dL (sensitivity 41%, specificity 97%), seizure, and coma.[171] Another retrospective study of risk factors for poor outcomes in methanol poisoning only found that pH less than 7 (as well as coma or a greater than 24-hour delay to presentation) was associated with death.[103] In a large series from several epidemics of methanol poisoning, a pH less than 7 and coma were again identified as risk factors associated with death. In patients with a pH less than 7, PCO_2 greater than or equal to 23.3 mm Hg was also a risk factor.[196] In another series, 50% of those who were comatose at presentation died, and no patients who were not comatose died.[281] Another study of 32 methanol-poisoned patients found no statistically significant relationship between pH and mortality, but did find an association between low GCS, hypothermia and elevated serum creatinine with mortality.[153] In methanol-poisoned patients unlikely to die, the pH is of some use in predicting retinal toxicity. A retrospective study examined markers for poor visual outcome after methanol poisoning and again found pH to be the best predictor, with a pH greater than 7.2 associated with a high likelihood of only transient visual sequelae.[60] Formate, as discussed above, was a good predictor of outcome in one series, with concentrations less than 18 mg/dL associated with good outcomes and concentrations higher than 78.8 mg/dL associated with a 90% risk of mortality. The same study showed that lactate greater than 7 mmol/L and/or pH less than 6.87 carried the same 90% risk of mortality.[280] All of these studies, while interesting, are of limited utility in decision making about an individual patient because of wide variability of the studied markers, often with overlapping ranges and wide confidence intervals.[210] Markers are a guide to inform clinical judgment, but decisions about management should be based on the entirety of clinical and laboratory data.

MANAGEMENT

As always, immediate resuscitation of critically ill patients starts with management of the airway, breathing, and circulation. Because alcohols cause respiratory depression and coma, intubation and mechanical ventilation are commonly necessary for patients with severe poisoning. Alcohol-induced vasodilation combined with vomiting often leads to hypotension, and many patients will require fluid resuscitation with intravenous crystalloid. Gastrointestinal decontamination is rarely, if ever, indicated for toxic alcohols because of their rapid absorption and limited binding to activated charcoal. However, placement of a nasogastric tube and aspiration of any gastric contents is reasonable in intubated patients, as absorption is sometimes delayed after a large dose.[66]

Alcohol Dehydrogenase Inhibition

The most important part of the initial management of patients with known or suspected toxic alcohol poisoning (after initial resuscitation) is blockade of ADH. This allows time for the establishment of a definitive diagnosis and arrangement for hemodialysis while preventing the formation of toxic metabolites. Additionally, in some cases ADH blockade will itself serve as definitive therapy.

Teleologically, ADH exists for the purpose of metabolizing ethanol, so it is not surprising that the enzyme has a higher affinity for ethanol than for other alcohols. Alcohol dehydrogenase metabolizes ethanol with a K_M that is 15 to 20 times lower in vitro than its K_M for methanol metabolism and 67 times lower than its K_M for ethylene glycol metabolism.[54,201,202] Thus, significant concentrations of ethanol prevent metabolism of other alcohols to their toxic products. Ethanol is the traditional method of ADH inhibition and is still the only option in most of the world, although it is rarely used in the United States. Orally administered ethanol is effective and may be reasonable when intensive monitoring is unavailable, particularly in rural areas where there is likely a significant delay in getting the patient to a hospital.[84] A 10% solution is administered through a central venous catheter or peripheral vein if a central vein canulation is not easily accomplished and titrated to maintain a serum concentration of 100 mg/dL (Antidotes in Depth: A34). Complications of the infusion include hypotension, respiratory depression (with supratherapeutic concentrations), CNS depression and inebriation, flushing, hypoglycemia, hyponatremia, pancreatitis, and gastritis, so patients receiving intravenous ethanol require admission to an intensive care unit. The true incidence of these adverse events is unclear. In one study, complications of ethanol infusion in children were uncommon.[217] However, in another review of 49 adults treated with ethanol infusions for toxic alcohol poisoning, 92% of patients had at least one adverse event.[271] In a prospective study from the United Kingdom, 12% of 131 patients treated with ethanol had an adverse event.[255] Both orally and parenterally administered ethanol are effective and generally safe, but it is challenging to maintain the serum concentration in the therapeutic range, and the risk of medication errors is also a concern.[255,282]

Fomepizole is a competitive antagonist of ADH that has many advantages over ethanol. It reliably inhibits ADH when administered as an intravenous bolus diluted and administered over 30 mins every 12 hours, and concentrations do not need to be monitored as with an ethanol infusion.[32,33] It does not cause inebriation and is associated with fewer adverse effects and fewer medication errors, so it does not require intensive care unit monitoring.[18,19,32,33,155,255] For these reasons, it has become the preferred method of ADH blockade in the United States, despite being significantly more expensive than ethanol.[239] In theory, the savings in intensive care unit (ICU) monitoring and laboratory costs probably compensate for the higher drug cost of fomepizole, unless the patient requires intensive monitoring regardless based on the severity of illness.[28] However, one study showed that even after fomepizole was introduced to their hospital, 95% of patients received ICU admission and hemodialysis,[88] so this may not be a large area of savings. Additionally, the cost difference will vary depending on the setting of poisoning and the health care delivery system of the country involved. A series in Belgium found that treating with ethanol and dialysis was much less expensive than fomepizole without dialysis within their system.[8] In the 2012 Czech outbreak of methanol poisoning, the sickest patients were treated with fomepizole, whereas others were treated with ethanol because of limited availability of fomepizole, yet the outcomes in both groups were similar.[281,286]

The dose of fomepizole is 15 mg/kg intravenously as an initial loading dose followed by 10 mg/kg every 12 hours. Fomepizole infusion rarely causes bradycardia and hypotension, so vital signs should be monitored closely during and after each dose.[154] After 48 hours of therapy, fomepizole induces its own metabolism, so the dose must be increased to 15 mg/kg every 12 hours. Although one review advocates giving doses as high as 20 mg/kg every 12 hours with no adjustment for induced metabolism,[24] this dosing regimen is not supported by the manufacturer or any current clinical guideline. A review of reported cases in which fomepizole was used in children suggests that it is safe and effective with the same weight-based dosing as in adults.[31] When treating chronic alcoholics with fomepizole, it is important to be vigilant of signs of alcohol withdrawal, because unlike ethanol, fomepizole does not prevent withdrawal.[281] Pharmacokinetic data from a human volunteer study show that there is no significant difference in serum concentrations between oral and intravenous fomepizole.[174] However, there is currently no oral preparation of fomepizole on the market in the United States (Antidotes in Depth: A33).

Indications for fomepizole or ethanol therapy are based on the history or on laboratory data. It is reasonable to treat a patient with a history of methanol or ethylene glycol ingestion until concentrations are available because, as previously discussed, early signs and symptoms, and laboratory markers other than serum concentrations are frequently absent. In addition, we recommend treating any patient with an anion gap metabolic acidosis without another explanation or a markedly elevated osmol gap. Once concentrations are available, we recommend continuing therapy until the serum toxic alcohol concentration is predicted or measured to be below 25 mg/dL, although as discussed previously, this value is based more on consensus opinion than on data.

The antiretroviral medication abacavir is a substrate for ADH and seemed to delay metabolism of methanol in one case.[83] It was suggested that abacavir could have potential as an alternative to fomepizole in places where fomepizole is unavailable.[226] Similarly, ranitidine is an inhibitor of gastric and hepatic ADH, and in a rat model, ranitidine improved pH, formate concentrations, and retinal histopathology.[65] Although both of these are intriguing possibilities, there are currently no data to support the use of either abacavir or ranitidine in human poisoning.

Hemodialysis

The definitive therapy for symptomatic patients poisoned by toxic alcohols is hemodialysis. Hemodialysis clears both the alcohols and their toxic metabolites from the blood and corrects the acid–base disorder. The indications for hemodialysis have become more restricted with the advent of fomepizole because of its effectiveness combined with its low incidence of adverse effects. Particularly for ethylene glycol, which can generally be expected to be cleared within a few days once ADH is blocked, as long as the glomerular filtration rate is normal.[35,157,263] Some have argued that the risks of an invasive and costly procedure such as hemodialysis are not warranted in minimally symptomatic patients with normal kidney function and without metabolic acidosis.[36,81] However, a single treatment of hemodialysis is less expensive than a day in the hospital, and the complication rate is exceedingly low.[27] While fomepizole alone is reasonable for ethylene glycol poisoning in a setting in which a patient might need to be transferred for hemodialysis or in a patient who cannot tolerate vascular access or hemodialysis, hemodialysis remains a reasonable option when available. Even a patient with a moderately elevated serum methanol concentration, 80 mg/dL (2.5 mmol/L), was successfully treated with fomepizole alone,[218] though the 4 days in the hospital and 8 doses of fomepizole would be prohibitively expensive in many settings. Based on toxicokinetic data, some patients with methanol poisoning might be treated without dialysis or with delayed dialysis, particularly in epidemic scenarios, in which the need for hemodialysis exceeds the availability.[114] However, patients with end-organ toxicity or severe acidemia have significant amounts of toxic metabolites (a problem not addressed by ADH blockade) and acidemia is associated with poor prognosis.[164] Additionally, although formate is normally cleared rapidly once ADH is blocked, the apparent half-life increases with higher serum methanol concentrations and varies from 2.5 to 12.5 hours.[100,111] In one very atypical patient with severe poisoning, formate was eliminated at an extremely slow rate with an apparent half-life of 77 hours until hemodialysis was initiated,[116] underscoring the importance of hemodialysis in patients with significant metabolic acidosis. In addition, patients with AKI will not eliminate the parent compound once ADH is blocked, except very slowly in expired air in the case of methanol. Therefore, the consensus is that metabolic acidosis, signs of end-organ toxicity, including coma and seizures, and AKI are indications for hemodialysis. A "toxic concentration" and possibly a very high osmol gap[203] are more relative indications for hemodialysis, and decisions must be based on the judgment of the clinician for the specific clinical scenario, considering the available resources. Some authors advocate using toxic metabolite concentrations if available as additional criteria for hemodialysis. In data from one case series, an elevated formate concentration appears to be a better predictor of clinically important toxicity than methanol concentrations.[195] Similarly, glycolate concentrations are a better predictor of death and AKI than ethylene glycol concentrations.[207] However, although clearance of formate by hemodialysis is substantial,[124,125,138] the overall clearance in one case series did not appear to increase significantly above endogenous clearance in patients also treated with folate and bicarbonate.[138] Some question the data quality in this series, pointing out that (a) the predialysis clearance in 2 patients was calculated using only 2 data points and in the 3 others was calculated using 3 points, generally considered the minimum; (b) several patients actually had decreased clearance during dialysis, contradicting all previous data; and (c) 2 of the patients had variable blood flow during dialysis.[114,277]

The Extracorporeal Treatments in Poisoning (EXTRIP) group has published interdisciplinary consensus guidelines for dialysis in methanol poisoning (Table 106–2).[211] The AACT guidelines for ethylene glycol actually advise against hemodialysis for a concentration alone without clinical indications such as metabolic acidosis, AKI, end-organ effects, or worsening clinical status,[19] and rates of hemodialysis for early ethylene glycol poisoning have declined in recent years.[84] Still, ethylene glycol remains the second most common xenobiotic to be removed by hemodialysis in the United States,[110] and hemodialysis for ethylene glycol remains a reasonable choice for the treatment of ethylene glycol poisoning depending on local resources. In addition, decisions about treatment should also be informed by the availability of ethanol and fomepizole, the cost of each, the cost of hemodialysis and intensive care, and the turnaround time for serum toxic alcohol concentrations in any given clinical setting, as well as consensus recommendations.[8,56,274]

TABLE 106–2	EXTRIP Guidelines for Extracorporeal Treatment in Methanol Poisoning[211]

Hemodialysis Recommended:

1. Severe methanol poisoning
   a) coma
   b) seizures
   c) new vision deficit
   d) metabolic acidosis
      i) blood pH ≤ 7.15
      ii) persistent metabolic acidosis despite adequate support measures and antidotes
   e) serum anion gap ≥ 24 calculated by serum [Na⁺] − ([Cl⁻] + [HCO₃⁻])
2. Serum methanol concentration
   a) >70 mg/dL in the context of fomepizole therapy
   b) >60 mg/dL in the context of ethanol treatment
   c) >50 mg/dL in the absence of an ADH antagonist
   d) in the absence of a serum methanol concentration, the osmol gap may be informative
3. In the context of impaired renal function

To optimize the outcomes of extracorporeal treatment:

4. Intermittent hemodialysis is the modality of choice in methanol poisoning. Continuous modalities are acceptable alternatives if intermittent hemodialysis is unavailable.
5. Alcohol dehydrogenase inhibitors and folic acid are to be continued during hemodialysis.
6. Extracorporeal treatment can be terminated when the methanol concentration is <20 mg/dL and a clinical improvement is observed.

Modified with permission from Roberts DM, Yates C, Megarbane B, et al. Recommendations for the role of extracorporeal treatments in the management of acute methanol poisoning: a systematic review and consensus statement. *Crit Care Med.* 2015 Feb;43(2):461-472.

Although hemodialysis effectively clears isopropanol and acetone from the blood, it is rarely if ever indicated for this purpose. Because isopropanol does not cause a metabolic acidosis and very rarely results in significant end-organ effects, the risks of hemodialysis likely outweigh the benefits.

Many patients will require multiple courses of hemodialysis to clear the toxic alcohol estimated. The dialysis time required can be calculated using the formula:

$$t = [-V \ln(5/A)]/0.06k$$

where t is the dialysis time required to reach a 5 mmol/L toxic alcohol concentration, V is the estimate of total body water (liters), A is the initial toxic alcohol concentration (mmol/L), and k is 80% of the manufacturer-specified dialyzer urea clearance (mL/min) at the observed initial blood flow rate.[104,278] The main problem with this formula is that it relies on an initial toxic alcohol concentration, which is often not available when hemodialysis needs to be initiated. If practicing in a setting where rapid determination of toxic alcohol concentrations is available, the need for further hemodialysis should be guided by the posthemodialysis concentration. Normalization of the osmol gap is another strategy to guide the required duration of hemodialysis, and though not validated, seems reasonable.[118] The important point with all of these strategies is that the duration of hemodialysis required is often much longer than a standard 4-hour course that would be used routinely in a patient with kidney failure, necessitating multiple or very long courses of hemodialysis. Regardless of how the duration of dialysis is determined, we recommend continuing ADH blockade during and after hemodialysis until a subsequent concentration of the offending toxic alcohol is below 20 mg/dL. Ethanol infusion rates must be increased during hemodialysis to maintain a therapeutic serum concentration as the ethanol is cleared (Antidotes in Depth: A34). Fomepizole should be redosed every 4 hours during hemodialysis to maintain therapeutic serum concentrations.[18,19]

Continuous renal replacement therapy (CRRT) such as venovenous hemodiafiltration is used in some patients with toxic alcohol poisoning. Hemodialysis is much more efficient at clearing xenobiotics than CRRT and is the modality of choice if available.[211,287,288] However, if there is a contraindication to hemodialysis, such as hemodynamic instability or severe cerebral edema,[85,251] or if hemodialysis is unavailable, continuous modalities are acceptable alternatives.[211] In a pharmacokinetic model, the addition of CRRT to hemodialysis can decrease the treatment time by 40%.[54]

Because methanol poisoning is sometimes complicated by coagulopathy, anticoagulations during hemodialysis is at least a theoretical concern because of the potential risk of bleeding. In patients with laboratory evidence of coagulopathy, it is reasonable to perform hemodialysis or CRRT without systemic anticoagulation.

Adjunctive Therapy

There are several therapeutic adjuncts to ADH blockade with or (especially) without hemodialysis that we recommend for these patients. One of the differences invoked to explain the absence of retinal toxicity from methanol in some species is the relative abundance of hepatic folate stores in these species such as the rat. Folate and leucovorin enhance the clearance of formate in animal models.[192,193] Thiamine enhances the metabolism of ethylene glycol to ketoadipate, and pyridoxine enhances its metabolism to glycine and ultimately hippuric acid (Fig. 106–2).[189] Although all of these modalities offer theoretical advantages, they have yet to be proven to change outcome in humans. However, there is one human case report showing enhanced formate elimination with folinic acid therapy.[122] Additionally, the apparent lack of an increase in formate clearance by hemodialysis in one study could be because it was dwarfed by the effectiveness of folate supplementation in both the study group and the control group.[138] In a study of 79 patients who survived methanol poisoning, patients treated with folate or folinic acid had better visual outcomes that those untreated, despite sicker patients in the treated group, but these differences were not statistically significant.[284] For unclear reasons, folate treatment for methanol poisoned patients has declined in recent years.[160] However, because of the safety of vitamin supplementation and the fact that many of these patients are chronic alcoholics who require folate and thiamine anyway, we recommend the use of folate, thiamine and pyridoxine in toxic alcohol poisoning (Antidotes in Depth: A12, A15, and A27).

Formate is much less toxic than undissociated formic acid, likely because formic acid has a much higher affinity for cytochrome oxidase in the mitochondria, the ultimate target site for toxicity.[159] In addition, the undissociated form is better able to diffuse into target tissues.[125] Alkalinization with a bicarbonate infusion shifts the equilibrium to favor the less toxic, dissociated form, in accordance with the Henderson-Hasselbalch equation. This also enhances formate clearance in the urine by ion trapping.[125] Data from uncontrolled case series demonstrate that patients treated with bicarbonate alone had better than expected outcomes after severe methanol poisoning,[188] but the results are equivocal in patients also treated with ADH blockade and hemodialysis.[32,121,181] Additionally, the severity of the metabolic acidosis after methanol poisoning is a good predictor of severe neurologic effects such as coma and seizures,[164] although it is not proven that alkalinization prevents these effects. However, in the absence of contraindications to a bicarbonate infusion (eg, hypokalemia, volume overload), alkalinization is reasonable in the patient with suspected methanol poisoning and a significant acidemia. A blood pH greater than 7.20 is a reasonable endpoint. Alkalinization is also reasonable for patients with ethylene glycol poisoning and life-threatening metabolic acidosis.

Aluminum citrate has potential promise as an adjunctive therapy for ethylene glycol poisoning. It interacts with the surface of calcium oxalate monohydrate crystals and prevents their aggregation. This decreases tissue damage from calcium oxalate monohydrate crystals in an in vitro model of human proximal tubule cells.[94] However, there are not yet any in vivo human studies or even case reports, so it cannot be recommended for clinical use.

Some have suggested a possible benefit of corticosteroids for retinal injury following methanol poisoning. In an uncontrolled case series, 13 of 15 patients showed improvement in their vision after treatment with 1 g of methylprednisolone daily for 3 days, with one having worsening vision and one unchanged.[238] A patient in another case report had permanent vision loss despite corticosteroid therapy using the same regimen.[76] Another uncontrolled case series used a slightly different dosing regimen, with 250 mg of intravenous methylprednisolone administered every 6 hours followed by oral prednisolone 1 mg/kg daily for 10 days. After treatment, the mean best corrected visual acuity improved, but methanol concentrations were not reported so exposure was not confirmed, and acuity data were not reported for individual patients, so it is unclear whether any worsened.[1,223] Another series of 4 patients with mild methanol poisoning given the same treatment regimen showed some improvement in vision.[243] An uncontrolled case series with delayed presentations, incomplete follow-up, and an inconsistent corticosteroid regimen showed improvement in some patients.[221,235] In a series of 63 patients with methanol poisoning from a 2009 epidemic in India, all patients with evidence of optic neuritis (at least 60% of 46 survivors), were treated with retrobulbar injections of triamcinolone (dose not reported); 75% had some improvement.[233] Currently, although limited data support the routine use of corticosteroids in methanol poisoning,[241] it is reasonable to give 1 gm of methylprednisone for 3 days given the low risk and possible benefit for a devastating clinical outcome.

Stem cell transplantation is an emerging therapy that shows promise for treating vision loss from methanol poisoning. One case series of 5 patients with complete blindness from methanol poisoning between were treated with stem cells ranging from 1 week to 12 weeks after exposure. All showed significant recovery of their vision.[17]

SPECIAL CONSIDERATIONS
Poisoning Epidemics
As discussed earlier, toxic alcohol poisoning epidemics can at times overwhelm local capacity to provide antidotal therapy and hemodialysis, necessitating triage decisions in allocating resources. Equally important is early recognition of an epidemic and effective communication with the population to try to identify affected people. Reaching patients before they become severely ill can potentially prevent bad outcomes. During an outbreak in Iran in 2013, multiple strategies were used, including text messaging, radio broadcasting, encouraging patients to find their drinking partners, and loudspeaker announcements near health care facilities, to encourage people to spread the word about contaminated alcoholic beverages, while emergency operation centers coordinated the medical response and distribution of patients to local dialysis centers. Mortality during the epidemic was much lower than other recent outbreaks, although the lack of methanol concentrations in affected patients makes the actual denominator unclear.[102] Where available, syndromic surveillance is another strategy for early identification of an epidemic. In places where it is politically possible, shutting down local bars and liquor shops is effective at limiting the extent of an outbreak of methanol poisoning,[216] though data on admissions for ethanol withdrawal after instituting this approach were not reported. Another strategy to mitigate harm from methanol epidemics is empiric prehospital oral ethanol administration in patients with suspected methanol poisoning.[282,289]

Pregnant Women and Perinatal Exposure
There are very few reported cases of pregnant women with toxic alcohol poisoning, but some conclusions can be drawn from the available data. Toxic alcohols readily cross the placenta, and perinatal maternal methanol ingestion has resulted in death of a newborn.[22] One woman was initially misdiagnosed with eclampsia after ingesting ethylene glycol and presenting with seizures and metabolic acidosis in her 26th week of pregnancy. An emergency cesarean section was performed, and she was later treated with hemodialysis and ethanol once the correct diagnosis was recognized. The child was severely ill, with an initial pH of 6.63 and an initial serum ethylene glycol concentration of 220 mg/dL. The baby was treated with exchange transfusion and ultimately survived without sequelae after a long hospital course.[146] In rat but not rabbit models of chronic high-dose ethylene glycol exposure, fetal axial skeletal malformations occur and are thought to be caused by glycolate.[51] No human case of chronic exposure has yet been reported.

OTHER ALCOHOLS
Propylene Glycol
Propylene glycol is commonly used as an alternative to ethylene glycol in "environmentally safe" antifreeze. It is also used as a diluent for many pharmaceuticals (such as phenytoin and lorazepam). This alcohol is successively metabolized by ADH and ALDH to lactate, so a metabolic acidosis results. This can result in extremely high lactate concentrations typically that would be incompatible with life if generated by any disease process. In other diseases associated with lactate accumulation and metabolic acidosis, the lactate is a reflection of underlying anaerobic metabolism, a marker of severe illness rather than part of the underlying pathophysiology. Lactic acidosis from propylene glycol is surprisingly well tolerated because it represents nothing more sinister than its own metabolism, and it is rapidly cleared by oxidation to pyruvate, which then undergoes normal carbohydrate metabolism (Chap. 46).

Benzyl Alcohol
Benzyl alcohol is used as a preservative for intravenous solutions. Although it is no longer used in neonatal medicine, it was responsible for "neonatal gasping syndrome," involving multiorgan system dysfunction, metabolic acidosis, and death because of its metabolism to benzoic acid and hippuric acid (Chap. 46).[82,167]

SUMMARY
- Early manifestations of toxic alcohol poisoning includes inebriation, and subsequent toxicity results from metabolism to organic acid anions that cause metabolic acidosis and end-organ effects. Only very high concentrations of methanol cause inebriation.

- The time required for metabolism results in a delay before toxicity is clinically manifest.
- Until serum concentrations are available, the serum anion gap and osmol gap help with decision making, but do not exclude toxicity if the history is concerning.
- Therapy consists of ADH antagonism with fomepizole or ethanol, as well as adjunctive therapy with bicarbonate, folate or folinic acid, pyridoxine, and thiamine.
- Hemodialysis is the definitive therapy for clinically ill patients as it removes the alcohol as well as toxic metabolites while correcting the metabolic acidosis and electrolyte abnormalities.

Acknowledgments

Neal E. Flomenbaum, MD, Mary Ann Howland, PharmD, Neal A. Lewin, MD, and Adhi N. Sharma, MD, contributed to this chapter in previous editions.

REFERENCES

1. Abrishami M, et al. Therapeutic effects of high-dose intravenous prednisolone in methanol-induced toxic optic neuropathy. *J Ocul Pharmacol Ther.* 2011;27:261-263.
2. Adanir T, et al. Percutaneous methanol intoxication: case report. *Eur J Anaesthesiol.* 2005;22:560-561.
3. Ahmed A, et al. Massive ethylene glycol poisoning triggers osmotic demyelination syndrome. *J Emerg Med.* 2014;46:e69-e74.
4. Akhgari M, et al. Fatal methanol poisoning: features of liver histopathology. *Toxicol Ind Health.* 2013;29:136-141.
5. Alexander CB, et al. Isopropanol and isopropanol deaths—ten years' experience. *J Forensic Sci.* 1982;27:541-548.
6. Alzouebi M, et al. Acute polyradiculoneuropathy with renal failure: mind the anion gap. *J Neurol Neurosurg Psychiatry.* 2008;79:842-844.
7. Anderson TJ, et al. Neurologic sequelae of methanol poisoning. *CMAJ.* 1987;136:1177-1179.
8. Anseeuw K, et al. Methanol poisoning: the duality between "fast and cheap" and "slow and expensive." *Eur J Emerg Med.* 2008;15:107-109.
9. Ariwodola OJ, Weiner JL. Ethanol potentiation of GABAergic synaptic transmission may be self-limiting: role of presynaptic GABA(B) receptors. *J Neurosci.* 2004;24:10679-10686.
10. Armstrong EJ, et al. Homicidal ethylene glycol intoxication: a report of a case. *Am J Forensic Med Pathol.* 2006;27:151-155.
11. Arora A. The "gap" in the "plasma osmolar gap." *BMJ Case Rep.* 2013;2013.
12. Arora V, et al. MRI findings in methanol intoxication: a report of two cases. *Br J Radiol.* 2007;80:e243-e246.
13. Askar A, Al-Suwaida A. Methanol intoxication with brain hemorrhage: catastrophic outcome of late presentation. *Saudi J Kidney Dis Transpl.* 2007;18:117-122.
14. Aufderheide TP, et al. Inhalational and percutaneous methanol toxicity in two firefighters. *Ann Emerg Med.* 1993;22:1916-1918.
15. Avella J, et al. Percutaneous absorption and distribution of methanol in a homicide. *J Anal Toxicol.* 2005;29:734-737.
16. Baldwin F, Sran H. Delayed ethylene glycol poisoning presenting with abdominal pain and multiple cranial and peripheral neuropathies: a case report. *J Med Case Rep.* 2010;4:220.
17. Bansal H, et al. Reversal of methanol-induced blindness in adults by autologous bone marrow-derived stem cells: a case series. *J Stem Cells.* 2015;10:127-139.
18. Barceloux DG, et al. American Academy of Clinical Toxicology practice guidelines on the treatment of methanol poisoning. *J Toxicol Clin Toxicol.* 2002;40:415-446.
19. Barceloux DG, et al. American Academy of Clinical Toxicology Practice Guidelines on the treatment of ethylene glycol poisoning. Ad Hoc Committee. *J Toxicol Clin Toxicol.* 1999;37:537-560.
20. Bebarta VS, et al. Inhalational abuse of methanol products: elevated methanol and formate levels without vision loss. *Am J Emerg Med.* 2006;24:725-728.
21. Becalski A, Bartlett KH. Methanol exposure to car occupants from windshield washing fluid: a pilot study. *Indoor Air.* 2006;16:153-157.
22. Belson M, Morgan BW. Methanol toxicity in a newborn. *J Toxicol Clin Toxicol.* 2004;42:673-677.
23. Bennett IL Jr, et al. Acute methyl alcohol poisoning: a review based on experiences in an outbreak of 323 cases. *Medicine (Baltimore).* 1953;32:431-463.
24. Bestic M, et al. Fomepizole: a critical assessment of current dosing recommendations. *J Clin Pharmacol.* 2009;49:130-137.
25. Bezdicek O, et al. Cognitive sequelae of methanol poisoning involve executive dysfunction and memory impairment in cross-sectional and long-term perspective. *Alcohol (Fayetteville, NY).* 2017;59:27-35.
26. Blomme B, et al. Cobas Mira S endpoint enzymatic assay for plasma formate. *J Anal Toxicol.* 2001;25:77-80.
27. Bouchard J, et al. Availability and cost of extracorporeal treatments for poisonings and other emergency indications: a worldwide survey. *Nephrol Dial Transplant.* 2017;32:699-706.
28. Boyer EW, et al. Severe ethylene glycol ingestion treated without hemodialysis. *Pediatrics.* 2001;107:172-173.
29. Boyle R. *The Sceptical Chymist.* London: J.M. Dent & Sons; 1911.
30. Brahmi N, et al. Methanol poisoning in Tunisia: report of 16 cases. *Clin Toxicol (Phila).* 2007;45:717-720.
31. Brent J, et al. Methanol poisoning in a 6-week-old infant. *J Pediatr.* 1991;118(4, pt 1):644-646.
32. Brent J, et al. Fomepizole for the treatment of methanol poisoning. *N Engl J Med.* 2001;344:424-429.
33. Brent J, et al. Fomepizole for the treatment of ethylene glycol poisoning. Methylpyrazole for Toxic Alcohols Study Group. *N Engl J Med.* 1999;340:832-838.
34. Brindley PG, et al. Falsely elevated point-of-care lactate measurement after ingestion of ethylene glycol. *CMAJ.* 2007;176:1097-1099.
35. Buchanan JA, et al. Massive ethylene glycol ingestion treated with fomepizole alone—a viable therapeutic option. *J Med Toxicol.* 2010;6:131-134.
36. Buller GK, Moskowitz CB. When is it appropriate to treat ethylene glycol intoxication with fomepizole alone without hemodialysis? *Semin Dial.* 2011;24:441-442.
37. Caparros-Lefebvre D, et al. Bipallidal haemorrhage after ethylene glycol intoxication. *Neuroradiology.* 2005;47:105-107.
38. Caravati EM, Anderson KT. Breath alcohol analyzer mistakes methanol poisoning for alcohol intoxication. *Ann Emerg Med.* 2010;55:198-200.
39. Carr S, et al. Outcomes with bilateral cochlear implantation following sudden dual sensory loss after ethylene glycol poisoning. *Cochlear Implants Int.* 2011;12:173-176.
40. Carta M, et al. Alcohol enhances GABAergic transmission to cerebellar granule cells via an increase in Golgi cell excitability. *J Neurosci.* 2004;24:3746-3751.
41. Casavant MJ, et al. Does fluorescent urine indicate antifreeze ingestion by children? *Pediatrics.* 2001;107:113-114.
42. Cascallana JL, et al. Severe necrosis of oesophageal and gastric mucosa in fatal methanol poisoning. *Forensic Sci Int.* 2012;220:e9-e12.
43. Chaudhry SD, et al. Lactate gap and ethylene glycol poisoning. *Eur J Anaesthesiol.* 2008;25:511-513.
44. Chen JM, et al. Proteomic analysis of rat retina after methanol intoxication. *Toxicology.* 2012;293:89-96.
45. Cheng JT, et al. Clearance of ethylene glycol by kidneys and hemodialysis. *J Toxicol Clin Toxicol.* 1987;25:95-108.
46. Choi JH, et al. Neurological complications resulting from non-oral occupational methanol poisoning. *J Korean Med Sci.* 2017;32:371-376.
47. Chung TN, et al. Unilateral blindness with third cranial nerve palsy and abnormal enhancement of extraocular muscles on magnetic resonance imaging of orbit after the ingestion of methanol. *Emerg Med J.Emerg Med J.* 2010;27:409-410.
48. Clay KL, Murphy RC. On the metabolic acidosis of ethylene glycol intoxication. *Toxicol Appl Pharmacol.* 1977;39:39-49.
49. Clay KL, et al. Experimental methanol toxicity in the primate: analysis of metabolic acidosis. *Toxicol Appl Pharmacol.* 1975;34:49-61.
50. Collister D, et al. A methanol intoxication outbreak from recreational ingestion of fracking fluid. *Am J Kidney Dis.* 2017;69:696-700.
51. Corley RA, et al. Mode of action: oxalate crystal-induced renal tubule degeneration and glycolic acid-induced dysmorphogenesis—renal and developmental effects of ethylene glycol. *Crit Rev Toxicol.* 2005;35:691-702.
52. Cornes MP, et al. The lactate gap revisited: variable interference with lactate analyses in ethylene glycol poisoning. *Br J Biomed Sci.* 2010;67:148-150.
53. Coulter CV, et al. Methanol and ethylene glycol acute poisonings—predictors of mortality. *Clin Toxicol (Phila).* 2011;49:900-906.
54. Coulter CV, et al. The pharmacokinetics of methanol in the presence of ethanol: a case study. *Clin Pharmacokinet.* 2011;50:245-251.
55. Darracq MA, Ly BT. Gastric aspirate fluorescence in ethylene glycol poisoning. *J Emerg Med.* 2012;43:e457-e458.
56. Darracq MA, et al. Cost of hemodialysis versus fomepizole-only for treatment of ethylene glycol intoxication. *Clin Toxicol (Phila).* 2013;51:188.
57. Darwish A, et al. Investigation into a cluster of infant deaths following immunization: evidence for methanol intoxication. *Vaccine.* 2002;20:3585-3589.
58. Davis LE, et al. Methanol poisoning exposures in the United States: 1993-1998. *J Toxicol Clin Toxicol.* 2002;40:499-505.
59. Delany C, Jay WM. Papilledema and abducens nerve palsy following ethylene glycol ingestion. *Semin Ophthalmol.* 2004;19:72-74.
60. Desai T, et al. Methanol poisoning: predictors of visual outcomes. *JAMA Ophthalmol.* 2013;131:358-364.
61. Dezso A, et al. Bilateral cochlear implantation after ethylene glycol intoxication: a case report. *Cochlear Implants Int.* 2011;12:170-172.
62. Driver J, et al. In vitro percutaneous absorption of [14C] ethylene glycol. *J Expo Anal Environ Epidemiol.* 1993;3:277-284.
63. Dyer S, et al. Hemorrhagic gastritis from topical isopropanol exposure. *Ann Pharmacother.* 2002;36:1733-1735.
64. Eells JT, et al. Development and characterization of a rodent model of methanol-induced retinal and optic nerve toxicity. *Neurotoxicology.* 2000;21:321-330.
65. El-Bakary AA, et al. Ranitidine as an alcohol dehydrogenase inhibitor in acute methanol toxicity in rats. *Hum Exp Toxicol.* 2010;29:93-101.
66. Elwell RJ, et al. Delayed absorption and postdialysis rebound in a case of acute methanol poisoning. *Am J Emerg Med.* 2004;22:126-127.

67. Erecińska M, Wilson DF. Inhibitors of cytochrome c oxidase. *Pharmacol Ther.* 1980;8:1-20.

68. Eroglu E, et al. Unusual clinical presentation of ethylene glycol poisoning: unilateral facial nerve paralysis. *Case Rep Med.* 2013;2013:460250.

69. Ethylene glycol: chemeurope.com information service. http://www.chemie.de/lexikon/e/Ethylene_glycol. Accessed August 8, 2008.

70. Figueras Coll G, et al. Bilateral compartment syndrome in thighs and legs by methanol intoxication: a case report. *Emerg Med J.Emerg Med J.* 2008;25:540-541.

71. Fijen JW, et al. False hyperlactatemia in ethylene glycol poisoning. *Intensive Care Med.* 2006;32:626-627.

72. Frang D, et al. Kidney damage caused by ethylene glycol poisoning [in German]. *Z Urol Nephrol.* 1967;60:465-471.

73. Frantz SW, et al. Pharmacokinetics of ethylene glycol. I. Plasma disposition after single intravenous, peroral, or percutaneous doses in female Sprague-Dawley rats and CD-1 mice. *Drug Metab Dispos.* 1996;24:911-921.

74. Frenia ML, Schauben JL. Methanol inhalation toxicity. *Ann Emerg Med.* 1993;22:1919-1923.

75. Froberg K, et al. The role of calcium oxalate crystal deposition in cerebral vessels during ethylene glycol poisoning. *Clin Toxicol (Phila).* 2006;44:315-318.

76. Fujihara M, et al. Methanol-induced retinal toxicity patient examined by optical coherence tomography. *Jpn J Ophthalmol.* 2006;50:239-241.

77. Gaffney S, et al. Worker exposure to methanol vapors during cleaning of semiconductor wafers in a manufacturing setting. *J Occup Environ Hyg.* 2008;5:313-324.

78. Gaines L, Waibel KH. Calcium oxalate crystalluria. *Emerg Med J.Emerg Med J.* 2007;24:310.

79. Galvez-Ruiz A, et al. Cupping of the optic disk after methanol poisoning. *Br J Ophthalmol.* 2015;99:1220-1223.

80. Garg U, et al. A fatal case involving extremely high levels of ethylene glycol without elevation of its metabolites or crystalluria. *Am J Forensic Med Pathol.* 2009;30:273-275.

81. George M, et al. Re: ethylene glycol ingestion treated only with fomepizole (*Journal of Medical Toxicology*: volume 3, number 3, September 2007; 125-128). *J Med Toxicol.* 2008;4:67.

82. Gershanik J, et al. The gasping syndrome and benzyl alcohol poisoning. *N Engl J Med.* 1982;307:1384-1388.

83. Ghannoum M, et al. Lack of toxic effects of methanol in a patient with HIV. *Am J Kidney Dis.* 2010;55:957-961.

84. Ghannoum M, et al. Trends in toxic alcohol exposures in the United States from 2000 to 2013: a focus on the use of antidotes and extracorporeal treatments. *Semin Dial.* 2014;27:395-401.

85. Gilbert C, et al. Continuous venovenous hemodiafiltration in severe metabolic acidosis secondary to ethylene glycol ingestion. *South Med J.* 2010;103:846-847.

86. Givens M, et al. Comparison of methanol exposure routes reported to Texas poison control centers. *West J Emerg Med.* 2008;9:150-153.

87. Graw M, et al. Invasion and distribution of methanol. *Arch Toxicol.* 2000;74:313-321.

88. Green R. The management of severe toxic alcohol ingestions at a tertiary care center after the introduction of fomepizole. *Am J Emerg Med.* 2007;25:799-803.

89. Grobin AC, et al. The role of GABA(A) receptors in the acute and chronic effects of ethanol. *Psychopharmacology (Berl).* 1998;139:2-19.

90. Grufferman S, et al. Methanol poisoning complicated by myoglobinuric renal failure. *Am J Emerg Med.* 1985;3:24-26.

91. Guggenheim MA, et al. Motor dysfunction as a permanent complication of methanol ingestion. Presentation of a case with a beneficial response to levodopa treatment. *Arch Neurol.* 1971;24:550-554.

92. Guo C, et al. Calcium oxalate, and not other metabolites, is responsible for the renal toxicity of ethylene glycol. *Toxicol Lett.* 2007;173:8-16.

93. Guo C, McMartin KE. The cytotoxicity of oxalate, metabolite of ethylene glycol, is due to calcium oxalate monohydrate formation. *Toxicology.* 2005;208:347-355.

94. Guo C, McMartin KE. Aluminum citrate inhibits cytotoxicity and aggregation of oxalate crystals. *Toxicology.* 2007;230:117-125.

95. Gupta N, et al. A rare presentation of methanol toxicity. *Ann Indian Acad Neurol.* 2013;16:249-251.

96. Hack JB, et al. An alcohol oxidase dipstick rapidly detects methanol in the serum of mice. *Acad Emerg Med.* 2007;14:1130-1134.

97. Haffner HT, et al. The kinetics of methanol elimination in alcoholics and the influence of ethanol. *Forensic Sci Int.* 1997;89:129-136.

98. Haffner HT, et al. The elimination kinetics of methanol and the influence of ethanol. *Int J Legal Med.* 1992;105:111-114.

99. Hanton SL, Watson ID. An enzymatic assay for the detection of glycolic acid in serum as a marker of ethylene glycol poisoning. *Ther Drug Monit.* 2013;35:836-843.

100. Hantson P, et al. Formate kinetics in methanol poisoning. *Hum Exp Toxicol.* 2005;24:55-59.

101. Hantson P, Mahieu P. Pancreatic injury following acute methanol poisoning. *J Toxicol Clin Toxicol.* 2000;38:297-303.

102. Hassanian-Moghaddam H, et al. Methanol mass poisoning in Iran: role of case finding in outbreak management. *J Public Health (Oxf).* 2015;37:354-359.

103. Hassanian-Moghaddam H, et al. Prognostic factors in methanol poisoning. *Hum Exp Toxicol.* 2007;26:583-586.

104. Hirsch DJ, et al. A simple method to estimate the required dialysis time for cases of alcohol poisoning. *Kidney Int.* 2001;60:2021-2024.

105. Hizarci B, et al. Transdermal methyl alcohol intoxication: a case report. *Acta Derm Venereol.* 2015;95:740-741.

106. Hodgman M, et al. Serum calcium concentration in ethylene glycol poisoning. *J Med Toxicol.* 2017;13:153-157.

107. Hoffman PL. NMDA receptors in alcoholism. *Int Rev Neurobiol.* 2003;56:35-82.

108. Hoffman RJ, et al. Ethylene glycol toxicity despite therapeutic ethanol level [abstract]. *J Toxicol Clin Toxicol.* 2001;39:302.

109. Hoffman RS, et al. Osmol gaps revisited: normal values and limitations. *J Toxicol Clin Toxicol.* 1993;31:81-93.

110. Holubek WJ, et al. Use of hemodialysis and hemoperfusion in poisoned patients. *Kidney Int.* 2008;74:1327-1334.

111. Hovda KE, et al. Methanol and formate kinetics during treatment with fomepizole. *Clin Toxicol (Phila).* 2005;43:221-227.

112. Hovda KE, et al. A novel bedside diagnostic test for methanol poisoning using dry chemistry for formate. *Scand J Clin Lab Invest.* 2015;75:610-614.

113. Hovda KE, et al. Anion and osmolal gaps in the diagnosis of methanol poisoning: clinical study in 28 patients. *Intensive Care Med.* 2004;30:1842-1846.

114. Hovda KE, Jacobsen D. Expert opinion: fomepizole may ameliorate the need for hemodialysis in methanol poisoning. *Hum Exp Toxicol.* 2008;27:539-546.

115. Hovda KE, et al. Studies on ethylene glycol poisoning: one patient—154 admissions. *Clin Toxicol (Phila).* 2011;49:478-484.

116. Hovda KE, et al. Extremely slow formate elimination in severe methanol poisoning: a fatal case report. *Clin Toxicol (Phila).* 2007;45:516-521.

117. Hovda KE, et al. Increased serum formate in the diagnosis of methanol poisoning. *J Anal Toxicol.* 2005;29:586-588.

118. Hunderi OH, et al. Use of the osmolal gap to guide the start and duration of dialysis in methanol poisoning. *Scand J Urol Nephrol.* 2006;40:70-74.

119. Jacobsen D, et al. Anion and osmolal gaps in the diagnosis of methanol and ethylene glycol poisoning. *Acta Med Scand.* 1982;212:17-20.

120. Jacobsen D, et al. Ethylene glycol intoxication: evaluation of kinetics and crystalluria. *Am J Med.* 1988;84:145-152.

121. Jacobsen D, et al. Studies on methanol poisoning. *Acta Med Scand.* 1982;212:5-10.

122. Jacobsen D, McMartin KE. Methanol and ethylene glycol poisonings. Mechanism of toxicity, clinical course, diagnosis and treatment. *Med Toxicol.* 1986;1:309-334.

123. Jacobsen D, et al. Glycolate causes the acidosis in ethylene glycol poisoning and is effectively removed by hemodialysis. *Acta Med Scand.* 1984;216:409-416.

124. Jacobsen D, et al. Toxicokinetics of formate during hemodialysis. *Acta Med Scand.* 1983;214:409-412.

125. Jacobsen D, et al. Methanol and formate kinetics in late diagnosed methanol intoxication. *Med Toxicol Adverse Drug Exp.* 1988;3:418-423.

126. Jaff Z, et al. Impact of methanol intoxication on the human electrocardiogram. *Cardiol J.* 2014;21:170-175.

127. Jeghers H, Murphy R. Practical aspects of oxalate metabolism. *N Engl J Med.* 1945;233:208-215.

128. Jobson MA, et al. Clinical features of reported ethylene glycol exposures in the United States. *PLoS One.* 2015;10:e0143044.

129. Jones GR, et al. The relationship of methanol and formate concentrations in fatalities where methanol is detected. *J Forensic Sci.* 2007;52:1376-1382.

130. Jorens PG. Ethylene glycol poisoning and lactate concentrations. *J Anal Toxicol.* 2009;33:395; author reply 396.

131. Jorens PG. Falsely elevated lactate and ethylene glycol. *Clin Toxicol (Phila).* 2009;47:691.

132. Kalkan S, et al. Acute methanol poisonings reported to the Drug and Poison Information Center in Izmir, Turkey. *Vet Hum Toxicol.* 2003;45:334-337.

133. Kane RL, et al. A methanol poisoning outbreak in Kentucky. A clinical epidemiologic study. *Arch Environ Health.* 1968;17:119-129.

134. Karaduman F, et al. Bilateral basal ganglionic lesions due to transdermal methanol intoxication. *J Clin Neurosci.* 2009;16:1504-1506.

135. Karayel F, et al. Methanol intoxication: pathological changes of central nervous system (17 cases). *Am J Forensic Med Pathol.* 2010;31:34-36.

136. Kearney J RS, Chiang WK. Availability of serum methanol and ethylene glycol levels: a national survey [abstract]. *J Toxicol Clin Toxicol (Phila).* 1997;35:509.

137. Keiran S, et al. Ethylene glycol toxicity. *Am J Kidney Dis.* 2005;46:e31-33.

138. Kerns W 2nd, et al. Formate kinetics in methanol poisoning. *J Toxicol Clin Toxicol.* 2002;40:137-143.

139. Killeen C, et al. Pseudorenal insufficiency with isopropyl alcohol ingestion. *Am J Ther.* 2011;18:e113-e116.

140. Kim JL, et al. Letter in response to: "Use of a Rapid Ethylene Glycol Assay: a 4-Year Retrospective Study at an Academic Medical Center." *J Med Toxicol.* 2016;12:324-325.

141. Kinoshita H, et al. Methanol: toxicity of the solvent in a commercial product should also be considered. *Hum Exp Toxicol.* 2005;24:663-664.

142. Kleiman R, et al. Medical toxicology and public health—update on research and activities at the Centers for Disease Control and Prevention, and the Agency for Toxic Substances and Disease Registry inhalational methanol toxicity. *J Med Toxicol.* 2009;5:158-164.

143. Korchanov LS, et al. Treatment of patients with acute kidney insufficiency caused by methyl alcohol poisoning [in Russian]. *Urol Nefrol (Mosk).* 1970;35:66-67.

144. Kostic MA, Dart RC. Rethinking the toxic methanol level. *J Toxicol Clin Toxicol.* 2003;41:793-800.

145. Krahn J, Khajuria A. Osmolality gaps: diagnostic accuracy and long-term variability. *Clin Chem.* 2006;52:737-739.

146. Kralova I, et al. Ethylene glycol intoxication misdiagnosed as eclampsia. *Acta Anaesthesiol Scand.* 2006;50:385-387.

147. Kraut JA, Kurtz I. Toxic alcohol ingestions: clinical features, diagnosis, and management. *Clin J Am Soc Nephrol.* 2008;3:208-225.

148. Kuban P, Bocek P. Direct analysis of formate in human plasma, serum and whole blood by in-line coupling of microdialysis to capillary electrophoresis for rapid diagnosis of methanol poisoning. *Anal Chim Acta.* 2013;768:82-89.

149. Kuban P, et al. Capillary electrophoresis with contactless conductometric detection for rapid screening of formate in blood serum after methanol intoxication. *J Chromatogr A.* 2013;1281:142-147.

150. Kuskonmaz B, et al. Hemophagocytic syndrome and acute liver failure associated with ethylene glycol ingestion: a case report. *Pediatr Hematol Oncol.* 2006;23:427-432.

151. Laakso O, et al. FT-IR breath test in the diagnosis and control of treatment of methanol intoxications. *J Anal Toxicol.* 2001;25:26-30.

152. Leaf G, Zatman LJ. A study of the conditions under which methanol may exert a toxic hazard in industry. *Br J Ind Med.* 1952;9:19-31.

153. Lee CY, et al. Risk factors for mortality in Asian Taiwanese patients with methanol poisoning. *Ther Clin Risk Manag.* 2014;10:61-67.

154. Lepik KJ, et al. Bradycardia and hypotension associated with fomepizole infusion during hemodialysis. *Clin Toxicol (Phila).* 2008;46:570-573.

155. Lepik KJ, et al. Adverse drug events associated with the antidotes for methanol and ethylene glycol poisoning: a comparison of ethanol and fomepizole. *Ann Emerg Med.* 2009;53:439.e410-450.e410.

156. Leth PM, Gregersen M. Ethylene glycol poisoning. *Forensic Sci Int.* 2005;155:179-184.

157. Levine M, et al. Ethylene glycol elimination kinetics and outcomes in patients managed without hemodialysis. *Ann Emerg Med.* 2012;59:527-531.

158. Lewin GA, et al. Coma from alcohol sponging. *J Am Coll Emerg Phys.* 1977;6:165-167.

159. Liesivuori J, Savolainen H. Methanol and formic acid toxicity: biochemical mechanisms. *Pharmacol Toxicol.* 1991;69:157-163.

160. Lim CS, Bryant SM. Forgoing the folate? Contemporary recommendations for methanol poisoning and evidence review. *Am J Ther.* 2016;23:e850-e854.

161. Lim CS, et al. Management of unintentional methanol ingestions—kids aren't little adults? *Clin Toxicol (Phila).* 2013;51:455.

162. Lim CS, et al. Fatality after inhalation of methanol-containing paint stripper. *Clin Toxicol (Phila).* 2015;53:411.

163. Liu DM, et al. The intoxication effects of methanol and formic acid on rat retina function. *J Ophthalmol.* 2016;2016:4087096.

164. Liu JJ, et al. Prognostic factors in patients with methanol poisoning. *J Toxicol Clin Toxicol.* 1998;36:175-181.

165. Long H, et al. A rapid qualitative test for suspected ethylene glycol poisoning. *Acad Emerg Med.* 2008;15:688-690.

166. LoVecchio F, et al. Outcomes following abuse of methanol-containing carburetor cleaners. *Hum Exp Toxicol.* 2004;23:473-475.

167. Lovejoy FH Jr. Fatal benzyl alcohol poisoning in neonatal intensive care units. A new concern for pediatricians. *Am J Dis Child.* 1982;136:974-975.

168. Lovric M, et al. Ethylene glycol poisoning. *Forensic Sci Int.* 2007;170:213-215.

169. Lu JJ, et al. Unilateral blindness following acute methanol poisoning. *J Med Toxicol.* 2010;6:459-460.

170. Lukasik-Glebocka M, et al. Usefulness of blood formic acid detection in the methanol poisoning in the practice of clinical toxicology department-preliminary assessment [in Polish]. *Przegl Lek.* 2014;71:475-478.

171. Lung DD, et al. Predictors of death and prolonged renal insufficiency in ethylene glycol poisoning. *J Intensive Care Med.* 2015;30:270-277.

172. Lynd LD, et al. An evaluation of the osmole gap as a screening test for toxic alcohol poisoning. *BMC Emerg Med.* 2008;8:5.

173. Manini AF, et al. Relationship between serum glycolate and falsely elevated lactate in severe ethylene glycol poisoning. *J Anal Toxicol.* 2009;33:174-176.

174. Marraffa J, et al. Oral administration of fomepizole produces similar blood levels as identical intravenous dose. *Clin Toxicol (Phila).* 2008;46:181-186.

175. Martin-Amat G, et al. Methyl alcohol poisoning. II. Development of a model for ocular toxicity in methyl alcohol poisoning using the rhesus monkey. *Arch Ophthalmol.* 1977;95:1847-1850.

176. Massoumi G, et al. Methanol poisoning in Iran, from 2000 to 2009. *Drug Chem Toxicol.* 2012;35:330-333.

177. McLean DR, et al. Methanol poisoning: a clinical and pathological study. *Ann Neurol.* 1980;8:161-167.

178. McMartin KE, Cenac TA. Toxicity of ethylene glycol metabolites in normal human kidney cells. *Ann N Y Acad Sci.* 2000;919:315-317.

179. McMartin KE, et al. Methanol poisoning. I. The role of formic acid in the development of metabolic acidosis in the monkey and the reversal by 4-methylpyrazole. *Biochem Med.* 1975;13:319-333.

180. Meng QH, et al. Elevated lactate in ethylene glycol poisoning: true or false? *Clin Chim Acta.* 2010;411:601-604.

181. Meyer RJ, et al. Methanol poisoning. *N Z Med J.* 2000;113:11-13.

182. Mihic SJ. Acute effects of ethanol on GABAA and glycine receptor function. *Neurochem Int.* 1999;35:115-123.

183. Minguela JI, et al. Methanol poisoning. Evolution of blood levels with high-flux haemodialysis. *Nefrologia.* 2011;31:120-121.

184. Minns AB, et al. Examining the risk of methanol poisoning from methyl acetate-containing products. *Am J Emerg Med.* 2013;31:964-966.

185. Morfin J, Chin A. Images in clinical medicine. Urinary calcium oxalate crystals in ethylene glycol intoxication. *N Engl J Med.* 2005;353:e21.

186. Morgan TJ, et al. Artifactual elevation of measured plasma L-lactate concentration in the presence of glycolate. *Crit Care Med.* 1999;27:2177-2179.

187. Mycyk MB, et al. Leukemoid response in ethylene glycol intoxication. *Vet Hum Toxicol.* 2002;44:304-306.

188. Naraqi S, et al. An outbreak of acute methyl alcohol intoxication. *Aust N Z J Med.* 1979;9:65-68.

189. Nath R, et al. Role of pyridoxine in oxalate metabolism. *Ann N Y Acad Sci.* 1990;585:274-284.

190. Nicholls P. Formate as an inhibitor of cytochrome c oxidase. *Biochem Biophys Res Commun.* 1975;67:610-616.

191. Nicholls P. The effect of formate on cytochrome aa3 and on electron transport in the intact respiratory chain. *Biochim Biophys Acta.* 1976;430:13-29.

192. Noker PE, et al. Methanol toxicity: treatment with folic acid and 5-formyl tetrahydrofolic acid. *Alcohol Clin Exp Res.* 1980;4:378-383.

193. Noker PE, Tephly TR. The role of folates in methanol toxicity. *Adv Exp Med Biol.* 1980;132:305-315.

194. Onder F, et al. Acute blindness and putaminal necrosis in methanol intoxication. *Int Ophthalmol.* 1998;22:81-84.

195. Osterloh JD, et al. Serum formate concentrations in methanol intoxication as a criterion for hemodialysis. *Ann Intern Med.* 1986;104:200-203.

196. Paasma R, et al. Risk factors related to poor outcome after methanol poisoning and the relation between outcome and antidotes—a multicenter study. *Clin Toxicol (Phila).* 2012;50:823-831.

197. Paasma R, et al. Methanol poisoning and long term sequelae—a six years follow-up after a large methanol outbreak. *BMC Clin Pharmacol.* 2009;9:5.

198. Palatnick W, et al. Methanol half-life during ethanol administration: implications for management of methanol poisoning. *Ann Emerg Med.* 1995;26:202-207.

199. Parsa T, et al. The usefulness of urine fluorescence for suspected antifreeze ingestion in children. *Am J Emerg Med.* 2005;23:787-792.

200. Pernet P, et al. False elevation of blood lactate reveals ethylene glycol poisoning. *Am J Emerg Med.* 2009;27:132.e131-132.e132.

201. Pietruszko R. Human liver alcohol dehydrogenase—inhibition of methanol activity by pyrazole, 4-methylpyrazole, 4-hydroxymethylpyrazole and 4-carboxypyrazole. *Biochem Pharmacol.* 1975;24:1603-1607.

202. Pietruszko R, et al. Alcohol dehydrogenase from human and horse liver—substrate specificity with diols. *Biochem Pharmacol.* 1978;27:1296-1297.

203. Pizon AF, Brooks DE. Hyperosmolality: another indication for hemodialysis following acute ethylene glycol poisoning. *Clin Toxicol (Phila).* 2006;44:181-183.

204. Poldelski V, et al. Ethylene glycol-mediated tubular injury: identification of critical metabolites and injury pathways. *Am J Kidney Dis.* 2001;38:339-348.

205. Pomara C, et al. Calcium oxalate crystals in acute ethylene glycol poisoning: a confocal laser scanning microscope study in a fatal case. *Clin Toxicol (Phila).* 2008;46:322-324.

206. Porter WH, et al. Interference by glycolic acid in the Beckman Synchron method for lactate: a useful clue for unsuspected ethylene glycol intoxication. *Clin Chem.* 2000;46(6, pt 1):874-875.

207. Porter WH, et al. Ethylene glycol toxicity: the role of serum glycolic acid in hemodialysis. *J Toxicol Clin Toxicol.* 2001;39:607-615.

208. Rahman SS, et al. Autonomic dysfunction as a delayed sequelae of acute ethylene glycol ingestion: a case report and review of the literature. *J Med Toxicol.* 2012;8:124-129.

209. Reddy NJ, et al. Two cases of rapid onset Parkinson's syndrome following toxic ingestion of ethylene glycol and methanol. *Clin Pharmacol Ther.* 2007;81:114-121.

210. Roberts DM, et al. The authors reply. *Crit Care Med.* 2015;43:e211-e212.

211. Roberts DM, et al. Recommendations for the role of extracorporeal treatments in the management of acute methanol poisoning: a systematic review and consensus statement. *Crit Care Med.* 2015;43:461-472.

212. Robson AF, et al. Validation of a rapid, automated method for the measurement of ethylene glycol in human plasma. *Ann Clin Biochem.* 2017;54:481-489.

213. Rooney SL, et al. Reply to Dr. Kim and colleagues regarding use of a rapid ethylene glycol assay. *J Med Toxicol.* 2016;12:326-327.

214. Rooney SL, et al. Use of a rapid ethylene glycol assay: a 4-year retrospective study at an academic medical center. *J Med Toxicol.* 2016;12:172-179.

215. Roscoe HE, Schorlemmer C. *A Treatise on Chemistry.* London: Macmillan and Co; 1884.

216. Rostrup M, et al. The methanol poisoning outbreaks in Libya 2013 and Kenya 2014. *PLoS One.* 2016;11:e0152676.

217. Roy M, et al. What are the adverse effects of ethanol used as an antidote in the treatment of suspected methanol poisoning in children? *J Toxicol Clin Toxicol.* 2003;41:155-161.

218. Rozenfeld RA, Leikin JB. Severe methanol ingestion treated successfully without hemodialysis. *Am J Ther.* 2007;14:502-503.

219. Ryu J, et al. Two cases of methyl alcohol intoxication by sub-chronic inhalation and dermal exposure during aluminum CNC cutting in a small-sized subcontracted factory. *Ann Occup Environ Med.* 2016;28:65.

220. Salek T, et al. Metabolic disorders due to methanol poisoning. *Biomed Pap the Med Fac Univ Palacky Olomouc Czech Repub.* 2014;158:635-639.

221. Sanaei-Zadeh H. Is high-dose intravenous steroid effective on preserving vision in acute methanol poisoning? *Optom Vis Sci.* 2012;89:244.

222. Sanaei-Zadeh H. Response to "Methanol and ethylene glycol acute poisonings—predictors of mortality." *Clin Toxicol (Phila).* 2012;50:225; author reply 226.

223. Sanaei-Zadeh H. What are the therapeutic effects of high-dose intravenous prednisolone in methanol-induced toxic optic neuropathy? *J Ocul Pharmacol Ther.* 2012;28:327-328.

224. Sanaei-Zadeh H, et al. Hyperglycemia is a strong prognostic factor of lethality in methanol poisoning. *J Med Toxicol.* 2011;7:189-194.

225. Sanaei-Zadeh H, et al. Outcomes of visual disturbances after methanol poisoning. *Clin Toxicol (Phila).* 2011;49:102-107.

226. Sanaei-Zadeh H, et al. Can fomepizole be substituted by abacavir in the treatment of methanol poisoning? *J Med Toxicol.* 2011;7:179-180.

227. Sandberg Y, et al. Falsely elevated lactate in severe ethylene glycol intoxication. *Neth J Med.* 2010;68:320-323.

228. Sankaralingam A, et al. Assessment of a semi-quantitative screening method for diagnosis of ethylene glycol poisoning. *Ann Clin Biochem.* 2017;54:501-503.

229. Schelling JR, et al. Increased osmolal gap in alcoholic ketoacidosis and lactic acidosis. *Ann Intern Med.* 1990;113:580-582.

230. Scully R, et al. Case records of the Massachusetts General Hospital. Weekly clinicopathological exercises. Case 38-1979. *N Engl J Med.* 1979;301:650-657.

231. Sebe A, et al. Intracranial hemorrhage associated with methanol intoxication. *Mt Sinai J Med.* 2006;73:1120-1122.

232. Sefidbakht S, et al. Methanol poisoning: acute MR and CT findings in nine patients. *Neuroradiology.* 2007;49:427-435.

233. Shah S, et al. Study of 63 cases of methyl alcohol poisoning (hooch tragedy in Ahmedabad). *J Assoc Physicians India.* 2012;60:34-36.

234. Shahangian S, Ash KO. Formic and lactic acidosis in a fatal case of methanol intoxication. *Clin Chem.* 1986;32:395-397.

235. Sharma R, et al. Methanol poisoning: ocular and neurological manifestations. *Optom Vis Sci.* 2012;89:178-182.

236. Shin YW, Uhm KB. A case of optic nerve atrophy with severe disc cupping after methanol poisoning. *Korean J Ophthalmol.* 2011;25:146-150.

237. Shirey T, Sivilotti M. Reaction of lactate electrodes to glycolate. *Crit Care Med.* 1999;27:2305-2307.

238. Shukla M, et al. Intravenous methylprednisolone could salvage vision in methyl alcohol poisoning. *Indian J Ophthalmol.* 2006;54:68-69.

239. Sivilotti ML. Ethanol: tastes great! Fomepizole: less filling! *Ann Emerg Med.* 2009;53:451-453.

240. Sivilotti ML, et al. Toxicokinetics of ethylene glycol during fomepizole therapy: implications for management. For the Methylpyrazole for Toxic Alcohols Study Group. *Ann Emerg Med.* 2000;36:114-125.

241. Skolnik AB, et al. Recommendations regarding management of methanol toxicity. *Ann Emerg Med.* 2012;60:816-817, author reply 817.

242. Slaughter RJ, et al. Isopropanol poisoning. *Clin Toxicol (Phila).* 2014;52:470-478.

243. Sodhi PK, et al. Methanol-induced optic neuropathy: treatment with intravenous high dose steroids. *Int J Clin Pract.* 2001;55:599-602.

244. Soghoian S, et al. Ethylene glycol toxicity presenting with non-anion gap metabolic acidosis. *Basic Clin Pharmacol Toxicol.* 2009;104:22-26.

245. Soysal D, et al. Transdermal methanol intoxication: a case report. *Acta Anaesthesiol Scand.* 2007;51:779-780.

246. Spillane L, et al. Multiple cranial nerve deficits after ethylene glycol poisoning. *Ann Emerg Med.* 1991;20:208-210.

247. Standefer J, Blackwell W. Enzymatic method for measuring ethylene glycol with a centrifugal analyzer. *Clin Chem.* 1991;37(10, pt 1):1734-1736.

248. Stapenhorst L, et al. Hyperoxaluria after ethylene glycol poisoning. *Pediatr Nephrol.* 2008;23:2277-2279.

249. Stokes MB. Acute oxalate nephropathy due to ethylene glycol ingestion. *Kidney Int.* 2006;69:203.

250. Symington L, et al. Toxic alcohol but not intoxicated—a case report. *Scott Med J.* 2005;50:129-130.

251. Szmigielska A, et al. Hemodiafiltration efficacy in treatment of methanol and ethylene glycol poisoning in a 2-year-old girl. *Dev Period Med.* 2015;19:174-177.

252. Szponar J, et al. Myocardial infarction in the course of ethylene glycol poisoning—a case report [in Polish]. *Przegl Lek.* 2012;69:603-605.

253. Taheri MS, et al. The value of brain CT findings in acute methanol toxicity. *Eur J Radiol.* 2010;73:211-214.

254. Takahashi S, et al. Brain death with calcium oxalate deposition in the kidney: clue to the diagnosis of ethylene glycol poisoning. *Legal Med (Tokyo).* 2008;10:43-45.

255. Thanacoody RH, et al. Management of poisoning with ethylene glycol and methanol in the UK: a prospective study conducted by the National Poisons Information Service (NPIS). *Clin Toxicol (Phila).* 2016;54:134-140.

256. Tintu A, et al. Interference of ethylene glycol with (L)-lactate measurement is assay-dependent. *Ann Clin Biochem.* 2013;50(pt 1):70-72.

257. Treichel JL, et al. Formate, the toxic metabolite of methanol, in cultured ocular cells. *Neurotoxicology.* 2003;24:825-834.

258. Treichel JL, et al. Retinal toxicity in methanol poisoning. *Retina.* 2004;24:309-312.

259. Turkmen N, et al. Glial fibrillary acidic protein (GFAP) and CD34 expression in the human optic nerve and brain in methanol toxicity. *Adv Ther.* 2008;25:123-132.

260. Uca AU, et al. An undercovered health threat in Turkey: transdermal methanol intoxication. *Clin Neuropharmacol.* 2015;38:52-54.

261. Upadhyay S, et al. Inhalation and epidermal exposure of volunteers to ethylene glycol: kinetics of absorption, urinary excretion, and metabolism to glycolate and oxalate. *Toxicol Lett.* 2008;178:131-141.

262. Velez LI, et al. Inhalational methanol toxicity in pregnancy treated twice with fomepizole. *Vet Hum Toxicol.* 2003;45:28-30.

263. Velez LI, et al. Ethylene glycol ingestion treated only with fomepizole. *J Med Toxicol.* 2007;3:125-128.

264. Verelst S, et al. Ethylene glycol poisoning presenting with a falsely elevated lactate level. *Clin Toxicol (Phila).* 2009;47:236-238.

265. Verhelst D, et al. Acute renal injury following methanol poisoning: analysis of a case series. *Int J Toxicol.* 2004;23:267-273.

266. Vicas IM, Beck R. Fatal inhalational isopropyl alcohol poisoning in a neonate. *J Toxicol Clin Toxicol.* 1993;31:473-481.

267. Viinamaki J, et al. Ethylene glycol and metabolite concentrations in fatal ethylene glycol poisonings. *J Anal Toxicol.* 2015;39:481-485.

268. Vinet B. An enzymic assay for the specific determination of methanol in serum. *Clin Chem.* 1987;33:2204-2208.

269. Wallace EA, Green AS. Methanol toxicity secondary to inhalant abuse in adult men. *Clin Toxicol (Phila).* 2009;47:239-242.

270. Wallgren H. Relative intoxicating effects on rats of ethyl, propyl and butyl alcohols. *Acta Pharmacol Toxicol.* 1960;16:217-222.

271. Wedge MK, et al. The safety of ethanol infusions for the treatment of methanol or ethylene glycol intoxication: an observational study. *CJEM.* 2012;14:283-289.

272. White NC, et al. The impact of bittering agents on pediatric ingestions of antifreeze. *Clin Pediatr (Phila).* 2009;48:913-921.

273. White NC, et al. The impact of bittering agents on suicidal ingestions of antifreeze. *Clin Toxicol (Phila).* 2008;46:507-514.

274. Wiles D, et al. Comment on treatment methods for ethylene glycol intoxication. *Neth J Med.* 2014;72:383-384.

275. Winter ML, et al. Urine fluorescence using a Wood's lamp to detect the antifreeze additive sodium fluorescein: a qualitative adjunctive test in suspected ethylene glycol ingestions. *Ann Emerg Med.* 1990;19:663-667.

276. Woo MY, et al. Artifactual elevation of lactate in ethylene glycol poisoning. *J Emerg Med.* 2003;25:289-293.

277. Yip L, Jacobsen D. Endogenous formate elimination and total body clearance during hemodialysis. *J Toxicol Clin Toxicol.* 2003;41:257-258; author reply 259-260.

278. Youssef GM, Hirsch DJ. Validation of a method to predict required dialysis time for cases of methanol and ethylene glycol poisoning. *Am J Kidney Dis.* 2005;46:509-511.

279. Zakharov S, et al. Leukotriene-mediated neuroinflammation, toxic brain damage, and neurodegeneration in acute methanol poisoning. *Clin Toxicol (Phila).* 2017;55:249-259.

280. Zakharov S, et al. Is the measurement of serum formate concentration useful in the diagnostics of acute methanol poisoning? A prospective study of 38 patients. *Basic Clin Pharmacol Toxicol.* 2015;116:445-451.

281. Zakharov S, et al. Fomepizole in the treatment of acute methanol poisonings: experience from the Czech mass methanol outbreak 2012-2013. *Biomed Pap the Med Fac Univ Palacky Olomouc Czech Repub.* 2014;158:641-649.

282. Zakharov S, et al. Fluctuations in serum ethanol concentration in the treatment of acute methanol poisoning: a prospective study of 21 patients. *Biomed Pap the Med Fac Univ Palacky Olomouc Czech Repub.* 2015;159:666-676.

283. Zakharov S, et al. Factors predicting optic nerve axonal degeneration after methanol-induced acute optic neuropathy: a 2-year prospective study in 54 patients. *Monatsh Chem.* 2016;147:251-261.

284. Zakharov S, et al. Acute methanol poisonings: folates administration and visual sequelae. *J Appl Biomed.* 2014;12:309-316.

285. Zakharov S, et al. Long-term visual damage after acute methanol poisonings: longitudinal cross-sectional study in 50 patients. *Clin Toxicol (Phila).* 2015;53:884-892.

286. Zakharov S, et al. Fomepizole versus ethanol in the treatment of acute methanol poisoning: comparison of clinical effectiveness in a mass poisoning outbreak. *Clin Toxicol (Phila).* 2015;53:797-806.

287. Zakharov S, et al. Intermittent hemodialysis is superior to continuous veno-venous hemodialysis/hemodiafiltration to eliminate methanol and formate during treatment for methanol poisoning. *Kidney Int.* 2014;86:199-207.

288. Zakharov S, et al. Efficiency of acidemia correction on intermittent versus continuous hemodialysis in acute methanol poisoning. *Clin Toxicol (Phila).* 2017;55:123-132.

289. Zakharov S, et al. Czech mass methanol outbreak 2012: epidemiology, challenges and clinical features. *Clin Toxicol (Phila).* 2014;52:1013-1024.

290. Ziegler S. The ocular menace of wood alcohol poisoning. *JAMA.* 1921;77:1160-1166.

FOMEPIZOLE

Mary Ann Howland

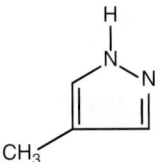

INTRODUCTION

Fomepizole, a competitive inhibitor of alcohol dehydrogenase (ADH), prevents the formation of toxic metabolites from ethylene glycol and methanol. It also has a role in halting the disulfiram–ethanol reaction and in limiting the toxicity from a variety of xenobiotics that rely on ADH for metabolism to toxic metabolites. In addition, as both an inducer and an inhibitor of certain cytochrome P450 CYP enzymes, the presence of fomepizole leads to drug interactions.

HISTORY

In 1963, Theorell described the inhibiting effect of pyrazole on the horse ADH nicotinamide adenine dinucleotide (NAD⁺) enzyme–coenzyme system.[83,106] Pyrazole blocked ADH by complexation, and the administration of pyrazole to animals poisoned with methanol and ethylene glycol improved survival.[107] However, pyrazole also inhibited other liver enzymes, including catalase and the microsomal ethanol-oxidizing system.[75] Additional adverse effects of pyrazole administration resulted in bone marrow, liver, and kidney toxicity, and these effects increased in the presence of ethanol and methanol.[87] These factors led to the search for less toxic compounds with comparable mechanisms of action.

In 1969, Li and Theorell found that both pyrazole and 4-methylpyrazole (fomepizole) inhibited ADH in human liver preparations,[74] and studies in rodents found that fomepizole, unlike pyrazole, was relatively nontoxic regardless of the presence or absence of ethanol.[14] Subsequent studies of fomepizole in monkeys and humans poisoned with methanol and ethylene glycol confirmed both the inhibitory effect and relative safety of fomepizole.[21,22,87]

PHARMACOLOGY

Chemistry

Fomepizole has a molecular weight of 82 Da, and a pK_a of 2.91 at low concentrations and a pK_a of 3.0 at high concentrations. The free base is used in the United States, whereas the salts are used in Europe. The free base is chemically equivalent to the chloride and sulfate salts at physiologic pH.[28]

Mechanism of Action

Fomepizole is a potent competitive inhibitor of ADH with a very high affinity for ADH, thereby blocking the metabolism of methanol and ethylene glycol to their respective toxic metabolites.[88]

Values for K_m are estimated for the toxic alcohols and the K_i with fomepizole. The smaller the K_m, the higher the affinity of the substrate (alcohol) for the enzyme, and the lower the concentration of the substrate to achieve V_{max} (maximum velocity of the reaction of 50%) of the enzyme. The K_i is the inhibition constant for the inhibitor. Studies in monkey and human liver tissue demonstrate that fomepizole is a competitive inhibitor of alcohol dehydrogenase.[78,96] In monkey liver, fomepizole demonstrated very similar K_i's for both

ethanol and methanol at 7.5 and 9.1 μmol/L, respectively.[78] The affinity was 10 times higher when human liver was used.[95] Studies in monkeys demonstrate that a fomepizole concentration of 9 to 10 μmol/L (0.74–0.8 mcg/mL) is needed to inhibit the metabolism of methanol to formate.[14,87] In human liver, the concentration needed to achieve inhibition is about 0.9 to 1 μmol/L.[74,95] The most recent trial using intravenous (IV) fomepizole attempted to maintain a serum fomepizole concentration above 10 μmol/L. Current dosing calls for a serum fomepizole concentration of 100 to 300 μmol/L to ensure a margin of safety.[1]

Cytochrome P450 (CYP) 2E1 oxidizes ethanol and a number of other xenobiotics, including acetaminophen, carbon tetrachloride, nitrosamines, and benzene to toxic metabolites. Fomepizole, like ethanol and isoniazid, induces CYP2E1 in rat liver and kidney, but not in the lung, through a posttranscriptional mechanism via stabilization and not involving increase in messenger RNA.[90] However, when fomepizole is present, CYP2E1 is inhibited. It is not until after fomepizole is eliminated that the consequences of induction are manifest.[18,112,113] In hepatocyte culture, fomepizole stabilizes and maintains the induced metabolic activity of the isoenzyme for about one week.[114]

Pharmacokinetics

The volume of distribution of fomepizole is about 0.6 to 1 L/kg; it is metabolized to 4-carboxypyrazole, an inactive metabolite that accounts for 80% to 85% of the administered dose.[84,90] In healthy human volunteers, oral doses of fomepizole are rapidly absorbed and demonstrate saturation and nonlinear kinetics.[55,80,90] The K_m was estimated to be 75 μmol/L in 2 studies, and 0.94 μmol/L at a dose of 15 mg/kg to 2.49 μmol/L at a dose of 7 mg/kg in 2 analyses, although the reason for the discrepancy is not known.[55,80,81,90] First-order kinetics were exhibited at concentrations below the K_m, whereas zero-order elimination occurred at concentrations 100% to 200% of the K_m.[55] Thus, elimination of fomepizole at doses of 10, 20, 50, and 100 mg/kg was 3.66, 5.05, 10.3, and 14.9 μmol/L/h, respectively.[55] Classical Michaelis-Menten kinetics would predict that the elimination rate should be comparable at the 2 higher doses. The authors speculate that the differences are attributable to the existence of other metabolic pathways with different affinities that predominate at different fomepizole concentrations. Following multiple doses, the elimination of fomepizole increases at 36 to 48 hours, most likely because of autoinduction.[90] After 96 hours fomepizole elimination apparently changed to first order elimination with a half-life of 1.5 to 2 hours, from zero order elimination. At a single dose of 20 mg/kg, the apparent half-life of fomepizole calculated from the linear portion of the curve was 5.2 hours and occurred when serum concentrations were less than 100 μmol/L. Peak concentrations after oral administration were achieved within 2 hours and were 132, 326, 759, and 1,425 μmol/L following 10, 20, 50, and 100 mg/kg doses, respectively. Every increase of 10 mg/kg in the oral dose of fomepizole raised the serum concentration 130 to 160 μmol/L.[55] The renal clearance was low (0.016 mL/min/kg), and only 3% of the administered dose was excreted unchanged in the urine.[55]

In the 2 pharmacokinetic studies in healthy volunteers, oral administration produced similar serum concentrations to IV fomepizole.[80,90] The pharmacokinetics of IV fomepizole were studied in 14 patients being treated for ethylene glycol toxicity.[84] A mean peak concentration of 342 μmol/L (200–400 μmol/L) was achieved following a loading dose of 15 mg/kg (183 μmol/kg).[84,102] A significant weakness of this toxicokinetic study is that the effect of simultaneous serum ethanol concentrations was not analyzed. The lowest serum fomepizole concentration of 105 μmol/L was present at 8 hours after the loading dose. The rate of elimination was determined to be zero order at 16 μmol/L/h compared with a first-order elimination half-life of 3 hours during hemodialysis (HD). Other authors have reported similar fomepizole clearances (13 μmol/L/h).[25] A pharmacokinetic analysis in patients poisoned with methanol or ethylene glycol demonstrated a mean peak fomepizole concentration of 226 μmol/L (19 mcg/mL), an apparent half-life of 14.5 hours (in the presence of methanol or ethylene glycol), and an apparent half-life of 40 hours in the presence of ethanol, in addition to methanol or ethylene glycol.[110] In the sole death, hepatic tissue contained 12 mcg/g of fomepizole, even when the serum concentration was less than 1 mcg/mL (12 μmol/L).[110]

The hemodialysis clearance of fomepizole ranges from 50 to 137 mL/min.[37,62] An analysis of the concentration of fomepizole in dialysis fluid revealed an extraction ratio of approximately 75% and a dialysance of 117 mL/min, which was very similar to a simultaneous ethylene glycol determination.[37] The dialysance was similar to urea in a pig model and suggests no significant protein binding of fomepizole.[56]

The pharmacokinetic interactions between fomepizole and ethanol were studied in a double-blind crossover design in healthy human volunteers.[60] Fomepizole was given orally in doses of 10, 15, and 20 mg/kg 1 hour prior to oral ethanol at 0.5 to 0.7 g/kg as a 20% solution in orange juice. Fomepizole decreased the elimination rate of ethanol by approximately 40%, from 12 to 16 mg/dL/h to about 7 to 9.5 mg/dL/h. When fomepizole was administered IV at 5 mg/kg over 30 minutes and ethanol was administered orally at doses to achieve a concentration of 50 to 150 mg/dL for 6 hours beginning at the end of the fomepizole infusion, the elimination of fomepizole was decreased by approximately 50%.[60] This decrease occurred without a change in the amount or fraction of unchanged fomepizole appearing in the urine. The authors suggested that the ethanol probably inhibited the metabolism of fomepizole to 4-carboxypyrazole. A single low dose of fomepizole given to humans had a maximal effect on ethanol metabolism at 1.5 to 2 hours.[13] Thus, ethanol and fomepizole mutually inhibit the elimination of the other, thereby maintaining higher serum concentrations than otherwise expected.[79,85] Methanol also decreases the elimination of fomepizole by approximately 25% in the monkey.[87]

ROLE IN METHANOL TOXICITY

In Vitro and Animal Studies
Studies using human livers demonstrate the inhibitory effect of fomepizole on alcohol dehydrogenase.[95] Studies in monkeys, the animal species that most closely resembles humans in metabolizing methanol, also demonstrate the inhibitory effect of fomepizole in preventing the accumulation of formate.[12,30,87,89]

Human Experience
The 2 largest fomepizole case series to date involved 11 and 8 patients, respectively, who were given IV fomepizole in the approved US dosing regimen.[20,22] Following administration, formate concentrations in all patients fell, and the arterial pH increased.[22] Case reports demonstrate similar findings.[25,42,45]

Effect on Methanol and Formate Concentrations
Methanol exhibits dose-dependent kinetics.[59] At low doses (0.08 g/kg), which achieve serum concentrations of about 10 mg/dL, methanol elimination is first order, with a half-life of about 2.5 to 3 hours.[63,68] In concentrations of approximately 100 to 200 mg/dL, methanol exhibits zero-order kinetics and is eliminated at about 8.5 to 9 mg/dL/h in untreated humans[61] and 4.4 to 7 mg/dL/h in untreated monkeys.[35,92] When monkeys were given 3 g/kg of methanol with resultant serum concentrations of about 500 mg/dL, the elimination of methanol exhibited apparent first-order kinetics. This alteration is likely caused by the greater contribution of other first-order pathways, such as pulmonary and urinary elimination, which account for a greater fraction of the total body clearance under these circumstances.[59] Once fomepizole was administered, the elimination of methanol became first order in

humans, and the half-life of methanol was about 54 hours but the range was from 22 to 87 hours.[22,49] When the metabolism of methanol to formate is blocked, formate is eliminated with a half-life dependent on formate concentration, folate stores, kidney function, urinary pH, and exogenous folate and bicarbonate therapies. When formate was administered to monkeys in the absence of methanol, formate half-life was 30 to 50 minutes.[30] In monkeys given methanol followed by fomepizole, the formate concentrations decreased by more than 80% in 2 hours.[12] An analysis of formate concentrations in 6 patients with methanol poisoning treated with fomepizole, folate, and sodium bicarbonate revealed a formate half-life of 235 ± 83 minutes.[64] A more recent analysis involving 8 patients with methanol poisoning treated with fomepizole and sodium bicarbonate revealed a formate half-life of 156 minutes.[49]

ROLE IN ETHYLENE GLYCOL TOXICITY

In Vitro and Animal Studies
Monkeys given 3 g/kg of ethylene glycol intraperitoneally recovered without treatment, whereas those given 4 g/kg died without therapy. All those given 4 g/kg of ethylene glycol with fomepizole 50 mg/kg intraperitoneally survived.[29]

Human Experience
The first 3 patients treated with oral fomepizole improved clinically and tolerated the therapy.[4] Subsequent case reports and case series using fomepizole orally or IV, with or without hemodialysis, also demonstrated the effectiveness of fomepizole in preventing glycolate accumulation.[5,16,21,24,43,46,48,62,91,94,102]

Effect on Ethylene Glycol and Glycolate Concentrations in Humans
Kidney function is essential for the elimination of ethylene glycol. With normal kidney function, the half-life of ethylene glycol is about 8.6 hours.[102] Based on pooled human data, the half-life of ethylene glycol after alcohol dehydrogenase is blocked by fomepizole is about 14 to 17 hours in patients with normal kidney function, and about 49 hours in patients with impaired kidney function defined as a serum creatinine greater than 1.2 mg/dL.[4,46,73,102] Based on a limited number of determinations, the renal clearance of ethylene glycol averaged 31.5 mL/min during the first 2 days; the corresponding creatinine clearance was 112 mL/min, and estimated total body clearance during fomepizole therapy was 57 mL/min.[5] These calculations suggest that the renal clearance of ethylene glycol accounted for only 55% of estimated total body clearance. In a study where neither kidney function was defined nor the amount of glycolate excreted unchanged by the kidneys described, glycolate had a mean half-life of 10 ± 8 hours in patients treated with fomepizole before hemodialysis, and a mean half-life of less than 3 hours during hemodialysis.[57,65,91]

ROLE IN TOXICITY FROM DIETHYLENE GLYCOL, DISULFIRAM, AND OTHER XENOBIOTICS
Fomepizole successfully terminated the adverse reactions resulting from the use of disulfiram administered to volunteers pretreated with a small dose of ethanol, in a chronic alcoholic surreptitiously given disulfiram by his wife, and in 2 patients who intentionally ingested ethanol in addition to an overdose of disulfiram.[76,99] Pretreatment with oral fomepizole was also successful in preventing the facial flushing and tachycardia typically associated with ethanol administration in ethanol-sensitive Japanese volunteers.[53,54]

Several animal studies and a few case reports suggest that fomepizole is effective in limiting the toxicity secondary to diethylene glycol (DEG), triethylene glycol, and 1,3-difluoro-2-propanol.[10,16,38,100,101,108] In particular an analysis of DEG concentrations and its metabolites in stored serum, urine and CSF from the Panama epidemic in 2006 revealed the presence of elevated 2-hydroxyethoxyacetic acid (HEAA) in serum and CSF and of diglycolic acid in serum, urine, and CSF in patients compared to controls.[101] It is hypothesized that these metabolites are most likely responsible for the nephrotoxicity and neurotoxicity associated with DEG.[31,66,67,97,101] Fomepizole blocks the metabolism of DEG to these toxic metabolites and is recommended as early as possible after ingestion before metabolism of DEG occurs[10,88] along with urgent HD.

The role of fomepizole in overdoses secondary to 2-butoxyethanol (ethylene glycol monobutyl ether, butyl Cellosolve) is unclear,[52] but fomepizole is reasonable for administration within several hours of ingestion and before rapid metabolism of butoxyethanol to butoxyacetic acid occurs.[82,93] Isopropanol is metabolized in part by alcohol dehydrogenase, but fomepizole therapy is not indicated, as this intervention would prolong the metabolism of isopropanol to acetone without any clinical benefit.[1,69]

COMPARISON TO ETHANOL

Ethanol effectively inhibits the metabolism of methanol and ethylene glycol to their respective toxic metabolites and has been used for many years.[44,109,116] Although very inexpensive, ethanol has many disadvantages, compared to fomepizole.[7,71,105,111] The affinity of ethanol for ADH is much lower than fomepizole, and rather than compete with the active site on ADH, it acts as a competitive substrate.[88] Ethanol causes central nervous system depression that is at least additive to that of the methanol or ethylene glycol, and dosing difficulties occur as a result of the rapid and often unpredictable rate of ethanol metabolism (Antidotes in Depth: A34).[7,9,111,115] Fomepizole has the advantage of being a very potent competitive inhibitor of alcohol dehydrogenase without producing CNS depression. Fomepizole dosing is much easier and does not require therapeutic monitoring of its serum concentration; administration and monitoring errors occur more frequently with ethanol.[72,105] Limited adverse effects of fomepizole include local reactions at the site of infusion when concentrations exceeding 25 mg/mL are used, nausea, dizziness, anxiety, headache, rash, transiently elevated aminotransferases, and eosinophilia. Fomepizole is preferred to ethanol for all of the above reasons. Ethanol is recommended for use when fomepizole is not readily available with the exception that ethanol is most likely preferred in a mass casualty situation until sufficient supplies of fomepizole could be procured.[72,103]

ADVERSE EFFECTS AND SAFETY ISSUES

Retinol dehydrogenase, an isoenzyme of ADH is responsible for converting retinol to retinal in the retina. For this reason, it was essential to study whether fomepizole would inhibit this enzyme and produce retinal damage.[87,89] Studies in several animal species demonstrated that fomepizole has limited toxicity, with no ophthalmic toxicity.[12] Two of the largest case series and 2 case reports confirm the lack of retinal toxicity with fomepizole and demonstrate the reversibility of methanol-induced visual toxicity when patients are treated with fomepizole and hemodialysis before permanent ophthalmic damage developed.[21,22,36,104]

The LD_{50} (median lethal dose for 50% of test subjects) of fomepizole in mice and rats is 3.8 mmol/kg after IV administration and 7.9 mmol/kg following oral administration.[77] An oral placebo-controlled, double-blind, single-dose, randomized, sequential, ascending-dose study was performed in healthy volunteers to determine fomepizole tolerance at 10 to 100 mg/kg.[59] There were no adverse effects in the 10- and 20-mg/kg groups, whereas at 50 mg/kg, 3 of 4 subjects experienced slight to moderate nausea and dizziness within 2.5 hours of fomepizole administration. All subjects reported these same symptoms at 100 mg/kg, which lasted for 30 hours in one individual without vital sign or laboratory abnormalities. The most common adverse effects of the use of fomepizole reported by the manufacturer (in a total of 78 patients and 63 volunteers) were headache (14%), nausea (11%), and dizziness, increased drowsiness, and dysgeusia or metallic taste (6%).[1,39] Other less commonly observed adverse effects include phlebitis, rash, fever, and eosinophilia. A case report of a patient severely poisoned with ethylene glycol suggested a temporal association between IV fomepizole administration during hemodialysis and the development of bradycardia and hypotension. However, this patient was severely acidemic, and when the patient received the fomepizole postdialysis no such adverse effects were noted.[70] Divided daily doses of fomepizole up to 20 mg/kg for 5 days were administered without any demonstrable toxicity.[86] The most common laboratory abnormality after fomepizole administration is a transient elevation of aminotransferase concentrations, which was reported in 6 of 15 healthy volunteers.[58] In the 2 largest case series of patients treated with fomepizole for toxic alcohol poisoning, there were no adverse events classified as "definitely" or "probably" related to fomepizole.[21,22] One patient received fomepizole 99 times for repetitive ethylene glycol self-poisoning without adverse effects.[51] Fomepizole safety and effectiveness in pediatric patients is not established, but children who have ingested ethylene glycol and methanol were treated successfully.[6,17,19,26,32,33,40,47,110]

PREGNANCY AND LACTATION

Fomepizole is pregnancy category C. Animal studies have not been conducted. One case report of a pregnant woman treated twice with fomepizole for inhalation of a carburetor cleaner containing methanol is reported in the literature but follow-up information on the fetus was never obtained. The risks of methanol and ethylene glycol poisoning are so consequential (including neonatal death) that it is recommended that fomepizole be administered when toxicity is present or anticipated with these toxic alcohols.[8,15,23,34,88] If fomepizole is not available, then ethanol is recommended. There are no studies that have examined the amount of fomepizole in breast milk although the low molecular weight suggests that it will be excreted into breast milk. It is likely that the toxic alcohol for which the fomepizole is being used would also be excreted into breast milk.[23] Therefore it is recommended that breast feeding be temporarily discontinued until fomepizole is predicted to be eliminated from the body (about 24 hours after the last dose) and the toxic alcohol has been eliminated.

DOSING AND ADMINISTRATION

The loading dose of fomepizole is 15 mg/kg IV, followed in 12 hours by 10 mg/kg every 12 hours for 4 doses. If therapy is necessary beyond 48 hours, the dose is then increased to 15 mg/kg every 12 hours, for as long as necessary. This increase is recommended because fomepizole stimulates its own metabolism.[76] Patients undergoing hemodialysis require additional doses of fomepizole to replace the amount removed during hemodialysis.

The manufacturer recommends dosing fomepizole every 4 hours during hemodialysis.[1,39] We recommend the administration of fomepizole at the beginning of hemodialysis if the last dose was given more than 6 hours earlier. At the completion of hemodialysis, we recommend the administration of the next scheduled dose if more than 3 hours have transpired, or one-half of the dose if 1 to 3 hours have passed. Following hemodialysis dosing of fomepizole every 12 hours is reinstituted.

It is expected that patients undergoing continuous renal replacement therapy (CRRT) such as continuous venovenous hemodialysis (CVVHD) or continuous venovenous hemodiafiltration (CVVHDF) would also require an increase in the dose of fomepizole. Theoretically since the amount of removal with these CRRT modalities is not as extensive as with HD, a reasonable recommendation would be to administer the fomepizole every 8 hours during the CVVHD or CVVHDF.

Fomepizole must be diluted in 100 mL of 0.9% sodium chloride solution or 5% dextrose in water (D_5W) before IV administration, and then infused over 30 minutes to avoid venous irritation and thrombophlebitis. Once diluted, fomepizole remains stable for 24 hours when stored in a refrigerator or at room temperature.[1]

Fomepizole therapy should be continued until the methanol or ethylene glycol is no longer present in sufficient concentrations to produce toxicity. We recommend continuing therapy until the serum toxic alcohol concentration is predicted or measured to be below 25 mg/dL in the absence of any acid–base disturbances.[1-3]

The threshold concentrations for hemodialysis for methanol or ethylene glycol can be based on measurements when analyses can be done in a timely fashion. The duration of fomepizole therapy in the absence of hemodialysis can be estimated based on the assumption of half-life of the toxic alcohol when blocked with fomepizole. The half-life of methanol is approximately 54 hours in the presence of fomepizole with a range of 22 to 87 hours.[20,49]

The half-life of ethylene glycol in the presence of fomepizole is approximately 14 to 17 hours in patients with normal kidney function, and 49 hours in patients with impaired kidney function.[4,48,102]

The need for hemodialysis is based on the presence of toxic metabolites inferred by the presence of metabolic acidosis and end-organ damage; the ability of the kidney to eliminate ethylene glycol, glycolic acid and formate, the risk benefit of hemodialysis, and the length of time to remain hospitalized for elimination of the remaining methanol and ethylene glycol.[50,98]

FORMULATION AND ACQUISITION

Fomepizole is marketed in branded and generic formulations in 1.5-mL vials of 1 g/mL. Temperatures of less than 77°F (25°C) cause the contents of the fomepizole vials to solidify. Warming reliquifies the product without adversely affecting its potency.

SUMMARY

- Fomepizole is a potent competitive inhibitor of ADH that inhibits the metabolism of methanol, ethylene glycol, diethylene glycol and other xenobiotics that use ADH in the formation of toxic metabolites.

- Once ADH is blocked and sustained, the decision to use hemodialysis depends on how much damage has occurred to the organs of elimination, the acid-base status of the patient, and how well the body can eliminate both the parent compound and the toxic metabolites formed prior to fomepizole administration.

- Fomepizole is safe and, although it has been used successfully orally, only an IV dosing regimen is approved and available.

- Fomepizole is more costly than ethanol, but its many advantages over ethanol, including the ability to deliver care outside an intensive care unit, which makes fomepizole the preferred antidote in most circumstances.

- Ethanol is likely to be preferred in a mass casualty situation until sufficient supplies of fomepizole are procured.

REFERENCES

1. Antizol (Fomepizole) injection [package insert]. Dover, DE: Paladin Labs; 2009.
2. Barceloux DG, et al. American Academy of Clinical Toxicology practice guidelines on the treatment of methanol poisoning. *J Toxicol Clin Toxicol.* 2002;40:415-446.
3. Barceloux DG, et al. American Academy of Clinical Toxicology practice guidelines on the treatment of ethylene glycol poisoning. Ad Hoc Committee. *J Toxicol Clin Toxicol.* 1999;37:537-560.
4. Baud F, et al. 4-Methylpyrazole may be an alternative to ethanol therapy for ethylene glycol intoxication in man. *J Toxicol Clin Toxicol.* 1986;24:463-483.
5. Baud F, et al. Treatment of ethylene glycol poisoning with intravenous 4-methylpyrazole. *N Engl J Med.* 1988;319:97-110.
6. Baum CR, et al. Fomepizole treatment of ethylene glycol poisoning in an infant. *Pediatrics.* 2000;106:1489-1491.
7. Beatty L, et al. A systematic review of ethanol and fomepizole use in toxic alcohol ingestions. *Emerg Med Int.* 2013;2013:1-14.
8. Belson M, Morgan BW. Methanol toxicity in a newborn. *J Toxicol Clin Toxicol.* 2004; 42:673-677.
9. Berberet B, et al. Discontinuation of 5% alcohol in 5% dextrose injection: implications for antidote stocking. *Am J Health Syst Pharm.* 2008;65:2200, 2203.
10. Besenhofer LM, et al. Inhibition of metabolism of diethylene glycol prevents target organ toxicity in rats. *Toxicol Sci.* 2010;117:25-35.
11. Blair AH, Vallee BL. Some catalytic properties of human liver alcohol dehydrogenase. *Biochemistry.* 1966;5:2026-2034.
12. Blomstrand R, Ingelmansson S. Studies on the effect of 4-methylpyrazole on methanol poisoning using the monkey as an animal model: with particular reference to the ocular toxicity. *Drug Alcohol Depend.* 1984;13:343-355.
13. Blomstrand R, Theorell H. Inhibitory effect on ethanol oxidation in man after administration of 4-methylpyrazole. *Life Sci.* 1970;9:631-640.
14. Blomstrand R, et al. Pyrazoles as inhibitors of alcohol oxidation and as important tools in alcohol research: an approach to therapy against methanol poisoning. *Proc Natl Acad Sci U S A.* 1979;76:3499-3503.
15. Bolon B, et al. Phase-specific developmental toxicity in mice following maternal methanol inhalation. *Fundam Appl Toxicol.* 1993;21:508-516.
16. Borron SW, Mégarbane B, Baud FJ. Fomepizole in treatment of uncomplicated ethylene glycol poisoning. *Lancet.* 1999;354:831.
17. Boyer EW, et al. Severe ethylene glycol ingestion treated without hemodialysis. *Pediatrics.* 2001;107:172-173.
18. Brennan RJ, et al. 4-Methylpyrazole blocks acetaminophen hepatotoxicity in the rat. *Ann Emerg Med.* 1994,23:487-494.
19. Brent J. Fomepizole for the treatment of pediatric ethylene glycol and diethylene glycol, butoxyethanol, and methanol poisonings. *Clin Toxicol.* 2010;48:401-406.
20. Brent J, et al. 4-Methylpyrazole (fomepizole) therapy of methanol poisoning: preliminary results of the META trial. *J Toxicol Clin Toxicol.* 1997;35:507.
21. Brent J, et al. Fomepizole for the treatment of ethylene glycol poisoning. *N Engl J Med.* 1999;340:832-838.
22. Brent J, et al. Fomepizole for the treatment of methanol poisoning. *N Engl J Med.* 2001;344:424-429.
23. Briggs GG, Freeman RK. Drugs in pregnancy and lactation: a reference guide to fetal and neonatal risk. Fomepizole monograph, 2015. Last accessed August 7, 2017.
24. Buchanan JA, et al. Massive ethylene glycol ingestion treated with fomepizole alone-a viable therapeutic option. *J Med Toxicol.* 2010;6:131-134.
25. Burns MJ, et al. Treatment of methanol poisoning with intravenous 4-methylpyrazole. *Ann Emerg Med.* 1997;30:829-832.
26. Caravati EM, et al. Treatment of severe pediatric ethylene glycol intoxication without hemodialysis. *J Toxicol Clin Toxicol.* 2004;42:255-259.
27. Cheng JT, et al. Clearance of ethylene glycol by kidneys and hemodialysis. *J Toxicol Clin Toxicol.* 1987;25:95-108.
28. Chilukuri DM, Shah JC. pKa of 4MP and chemical equivalence in formulations of free base and salts of 4MP. *PDA J Pharm Sci Technol.* 1999;53:44-47.
29. Clay KL, Murphy RC. On the metabolic acidosis of ethylene glycol intoxication. *Toxicol Appl Pharmacol.* 1977;39:39-49.
30. Clay KL, et al. Experimental methanol toxicity in the primate: analysis of metabolic acidosis. *Toxicol Appl Pharmacol.* 1975;13:319-333.
31. Conrad T, et al. Diglycolic acid, the toxic metabolite of diethylene glycol, chelates calcium and produces renal mitochondrial dysfunction in vitro. *Clin Toxicol (Phila).* 2016;54:501-511.
32. De Brabander N, et al. Fomepizole as a therapeutic strategy in paediatric methanol poisoning. A case report and review of the literature. *Eur J Pediatr.* 2005;164:158-161.
33. Detaille T, et al. Fomepizole alone for severe infant ethylene glycol poisoning. *Pediatr Crit Care Med.* 2004;5:490-491.
34. Dorman DC, et al. Role of formate in methanol-induced exencephaly in CD-1 mice. *Teratology.* 1995;52:30-40.
35. Eells JT, et al. Methanol poisoning and formate oxidation in nitrous oxide-treated rats. *J Pharmacol Exp Ther.* 1981;217:57-61.
36. Essama Mbia JJ, et al. Fomepizole therapy for reversal of visual impairment after methanol poisoning: a case documented by visual evoked potentials investigation. *Am J Ophthalmol.* 2002;134:914-916.
37. Faessel H, et al. 4-Methylpyrazole monitoring during haemodialysis of ethylene glycol intoxicated patients. *Eur J Clin Pharmacol.* 1995;49:211-213.
38. Feldwick MS, et al. The biochemical toxicology of 1,3-difluoro-2-propanol, the major ingredient of the pesticide Gliftor: the potential of 4-methylpyrazole as an antidote. *J Biochem Mol Toxicol.* 1998;12:41-52.
39. Fomepizole package insert manufactured for X-Gen Big Flats, NY Dec 2016.
40. Frémont D, et al. Loading dose of fomepizole is safe in children with presumed toxic alcohol exposure—a case series. *Basic Clin Pharmacol Toxicol.* 2014;115:229-230.
41. Gilfillan C, et al. Management of poisoning with ethylene glycol and methanol in the UK: a prospective study conducted by the National Poisons Information Service (NPIS). *Clin Toxicol (Phila).* 2016;54:134-140.
42. Girault C, et al. Fomepizole (4-methylpyrazole) in fatal methanol poisoning with early CT scan cerebral lesions. *J Toxicol Clin Toxicol.* 1999;35:777-780.
43. Goldfarb DS. Fomepizole for ethylene-glycol poisoning. *Lancet.* 1999;354:1646.
44. Grauer GF, et al. Comparison of the effects of ethanol and 4-methylpyrazole on the pharmacokinetics and toxicity of ethylene glycol in the dog. *Toxicol Lett.* 1987;35:307-314.
45. Hantson P, et al. Two cases of acute methanol poisoning partially treated by oral 4-methylpyrazole. *Intensive Care Med.* 1999;25:528-531.
46. Hantson PH, et al. Ethylene glycol poisoning treated by intravenous 4-methylpyrazole. *Intensive Care Med.* 1998;24:736-739.
47. Harry P, et al. Ethylene glycol poisoning in a child treated with 4-methylpyrazole. *Pediatrics.* 1998;102:E31.
48. Harry P, et al. Efficacy of 4-methylpyrazole in ethylene glycol poisoning. Clinical and toxicokinetic aspects. *Hum Exp Toxicol.* 1994;13:61-64.
49. Hoda KE, et al. Methanol and formate kinetics during treatment with fomepizole. *Clin Toxicol.* 2005;43:221-227.
50. Hovda KE, Jacobsen D. Expert opinion: fomepizole may ameliorate the need for hemodialysis in methanol poisoning. *Hum Exp Ther.* 2008;27:539-546.
51. Hovda KE, et al. Studies on ethylene glycol poisoning: one patient—154 admissions. *Clin Toxicol (Phila).* 2011;49:478-484.
52. Hung T, et al. Fomepizole fails to prevent progression of acidosis in 2-butoxyethanol and ethanol coingestion. *Clin Toxicol.* 2010;48:569-571.
53. Inoue K, et al. Accumulation of acetaldehyde in alcohol-sensitive Japanese: relation to ethanol and acetaldehyde oxidizing capacity. *Alcohol Clin Exp Res.* 1984;8:319-322.
54. Inoue K, et al. Suppression of acetaldehyde accumulation by 4-methylpyrazole in alcohol-hypersensitive Japanese. *Jpn J Pharmacol.* 1985;38:43-48.
55. Jacobsen D, et al. Nonlinear kinetics of 4-methylpyrazole in healthy human subjects. *Eur J Clin Pharmacol.* 1989;37:599-604.
56. Jacobsen D, et al. 4-Methylpyrazole (4-MP) is effectively removed by hemodialysis in the pig model. *Vet Hum Toxicol.* 1992;34:362.

57. Jacobsen D, et al. Glycolate causes the acidosis in ethylene glycol poisoning and is effectively removed by hemodialysis. *Acta Med Scand.* 1984;216:409-416.

58. Jacobsen D, et al. Effects of 4-methylpyrazole, methanol/-ethylene glycol antidote, in healthy humans. *J Emerg Med.* 1990;8:455-461.

59. Jacobsen D, et al. 4-methylpyrazole: a controlled study of safety in healthy human subjects after single ascending doses. *Alcohol Clin Exp Res.* 1988;12:516-522.

60. Jacobsen D, et al. Kinetic interactions between 4-methylpyrazole and ethanol in healthy humans. *Alcohol Clin Exp Res.* 1996;20:804-809.

61. Jacobsen D, et al. Methanol and formate kinetics in late diagnosed methanol intoxication. *Med Toxicol.* 1988;3:418-423.

62. Jobard E, et al. 4-Methylpyrazole and hemodialysis in ethylene glycol poisoning. *J Toxicol Clin Toxicol.* 1996;34:373-377.

63. Jones AW. Elimination half-life of methanol during hangover. *Pharmacol Toxicol.* 1987;60:217-220.

64. Kerns W 2nd, et al; META Study Group. Methylpyrazole for toxic alcohols. Formate kinetics in methanol poisoning. *J Toxicol Clin Toxicol.* 2002;40:137-143.

65. Knepshield JH, et al. Dialysis of poisons and drugs—annual review. *Trans Am Soc Artif Intern Organs.* 1973;19:590-633.

66. Landry GM, et al. Diglycolic acid inhibits succinate dehydrogenase activity in human proximal tubule cells leading to mitochondrial dysfunction and cell death. *Toxicol Lett.* 2013;221:176-184.

67. Landry GM, et al. Diglycolic acid is the nephrotoxic metabolite in diethylene glycol poisoning inducing necrosis in human proximal tubule cells in vitro. *Toxicol Sci.* 2011;124:35-44.

68. Leaf G, Zatman LJ. A study of the conditions under which methanol may exert a toxic hazard in industry. *Br J Ind Med.* 1952;9:19-31.

69. Lee SL, et al. Oxidation of methanol, ethylene glycol, and isopropanol with human alcohol dehydrogenases and the inhibition by ethanol and 4-methylpyrazole. *Chem Biol Interact.* 2011;30;191:26-31.

70. Lepik KJ, et al. Bradycardia and hypotension associated with fomepizole infusion during hemodialysis. *Clin Toxicol.* 2008;46:570-573.

71. Lepik KJ, et al. Adverse drug events associated with the antidotes for methanol and ethylene glycol poisoning: a comparison of ethanol and fomepizole. *Ann Emerg Med.* 2009;53:439-450.

72. Lepik KJ, et al. Medication errors associated with the use of ethanol and fomepizole as antidotes for methanol and ethylene glycol poisoning. *Clin Toxicol (Phila).* 2011;49:391-401.

73. Levine M, et al. Ethylene glycol elimination kinetics and outcomes in patients managed without hemodialysis. *Ann Emerg Med.* 2012;59:527-531.

74. Li TK, Theorell H. Human liver alcohol dehydrogenase: inhibition by pyrazole and pyrazole analogs. *Acta Chem Scand.* 1969;23:892-902.

75. Lieber C, et al. Effects of pyrazole on hepatic function and structure. *Lab Invest.* 1970;22:615-621.

76. Lindros KO, et al. The disulfiram (Antabuse)-alcohol reaction in male alcoholics: its efficient management by 4-methylpyrazole. *Alcohol Clin Exp Res.* 1981;5:528-530.

77. Magnusson G, et al. Toxicity of pyrazole and 4-methylpyrazole in mice and rats. *Experientia.* 1972;28:1198-1200.

78. Makar AB, Tephly TR. Inhibition of monkey liver alcohol dehydrogenase by 4-methylpyrazole. *Biochem Med.* 1975;13:334-342.

79. Makar AB, et al. Methanol metabolism in the monkey. *Mol Pharmacol.* 1968;4:471-483.

80. Marraffa J, et al. Oral administration of fomepizole produces similar blood levels as identical intravenous dose. *Clin Toxicol.* 2008;46:181-186.

81. Mayersohn M, et al. 4-Methylpyrazole disposition in the dog: evidence for saturable elimination. *J Pharm Sci.* 1985;74:895-896.

82. McKinney PE, et al. Butoxyethanol ingestion with prolonged hyperchloremic metabolic acidosis treated with ethanol therapy. *J Toxicol Clin Toxicol.* 2000;38:787-793.

83. McMartin KE. Antidotes for alcohol and glycol toxicity: translating mechanisms into treatment. *Clin Pharmacol Ther.* 2010;88:400-404.

84. McMartin KE, Brent J; META Study Group. Pharmacokinetics of fomepizole (4MP) in patients [abstract]. *J Toxicol Clin Toxicol.* 1998;36:450-451.

85. McMartin KE, Collins TD. Distribution of oral 4-methylpyrazole in the rat: inhibition of elimination by ethanol. *J Toxicol Clin Toxicol.* 1988;26:451-466.

86. McMartin KE, Heath A. The treatment of ethylene glycol poisoning with intravenous 4-methylpyrazole. *N Engl J Med.* 1989;320:125.

87. McMartin KE, et al. Studies on the metabolic interactions between 4-methylpyrazole and methanol using the monkey as an animal model. *Arch Biochem Biophys.* 1980;199:606-614.

88. McMartin K, et al. Antidotes for poisoning by alcohols that form toxic metabolites. *Br J Clin Pharmacol.* 2016;81:505-515.

89. McMartin KE, et al. Methanol poisoning I. The role of formic acid in the development of metabolic acidosis in the monkey and the reversal by 4-methylpyrazole. *Biochem Med.* 1975;13:319-333.

90. McMartin KE, et al. Kinetics and metabolism of fomepizole in healthy humans. *Clin Toxicol.* 2012;50:375-383.

91. Moreau CL, et al. Glycolate kinetics and hemodialysis clearance in ethylene glycol poisoning. *J Toxicol Clin Toxicol.* 1998;36:659-666.

92. Noker PE, et al. Methanol toxicity: treatment with folic acid and 5-formyl-tetrahydrofolic acid. *Alcohol Clin Exp Res.* 1980;4:378-383.

93. Osterhoudt KC. Fomepizole therapy for pediatric butoxyethanol intoxication. *J Toxicol Clin Toxicol.* 2002;40:929-930.

94. Parry MF, Wallach R. Ethylene glycol poisoning. *Am J Med.* 1974;57:143-150.

95. Pietruszko R. Human liver alcohol dehydrogenase inhibition of methanol activity by pyrazole, 4-methylpyrazole, 4-hydroxymethylpyrazole and 4-carboxypyrazole. *Biochem Pharmacol.* 1975;24:1603-1607.

96. Pietruszko R, et al. Alcohol dehydrogenase from human and horse liver–substrate specificity with diols. *Biochem Pharmacol.* 1978;27:1296-1297.

97. Robinson CN, et al. In-vivo evidence of nephrotoxicity and altered hepatic function in rats following administration of diglycolic acid, a metabolite of diethylene glycol. *Clin Toxicol (Phila).* 2017;55:196-205.

98. Rozenfeld RA, Leikin JB. Severe methanol ingestion treated successfully without hemodialysis. *Am J Ther.* 2007;14:502-503.

99. Sande M, et al. Fomepizole for severe disulfiram-ethanol reactions. *Am J Emerg Med.* 2012;262.e3–262.e5.

100. Schep LJ, et al. Diethylene glycol poisoning. *Clin Toxicol.* 2009;47:525-535.

101. Schier JG, et al. Characterizing concentrations of diethylene glycol and suspected metabolites in human serum, urine, and cerebrospinal fluid samples from the Panama DEG mass poisoning. *Clin Toxicol (Phila).* 2013;51:923-929.

102. Sivilotti M, et al. Toxicokinetics of ethylene glycol during fomepizole therapy: implications for management. *Ann Emerg Med.* 2000;36:114-125.

103. Sivilotti ML. Ethanol: tastes great! Fomepizole: less filling! *Ann Emerg Med.* 2009;53:451-453.

104. Sivilotti ML, et al. Reversal of severe methanol-induced visual impairment: no evidence of retinal toxicity due to fomepizole. *J Toxicol Clin Toxicol.* 2001;39:627-631.

105. Thanacoody RH, et al. Management of poisoning with ethylene glycol and methanol in the UK: a prospective study conducted by the National Poisons Information Service (NPIS). *Clin Toxicol (Phila).* 2016;54:134-140.

106. Theorell H, et al. On the effects of some heterocyclic compounds on the enzymatic activity of liver alcohol dehydrogenase. *Acta Chem Scand.* 1969;23:255-260.

107. Van Stee E, et al. The treatment of ethylene glycol toxicosis with pyrazole. *J Pharmacol Exp Ther.* 1975;192:251-259.

108. Vassiliadis J, et al. Triethylene glycol poisoning treated with intravenous ethanol infusion. *J Toxicol Clin Toxicol.* 1999;37:773-776.

109. Wacker WEC, et al. Treatment of ethylene glycol poisoning with ethyl alcohol. *JAMA.* 1965;194:1231-1233.

110. Wallemacq PE, et al. Plasma and tissue determination of 4-methylpyrazole for pharmacokinetic analysis in acute adult and pediatric methanol/ethylene glycol poisoning. *Ther Drug Monit.* 2004;26:258-262.

111. Wedge MK, et al. The safety of ethanol infusions for the treatment of methanol or ethylene glycol intoxication: an observational study. *CJEM.* 2012;14:283-289.

112. Wu D, Cederbaum AI. Characterization of pyrazole and 4-methylpyrazole induction of cytochrome P4502E1 in rat kidney. *J Pharmacol Exp Ther.* 1994;270:407-413.

113. Wu D, Cederbaum AI. Induction of liver cytochrome P4502E1 by pyrazole and 4-methylpyrazole in neonatal rats. *J Pharmacol Exp Ther.* 1993;263:1468-1473.

114. Wu DF, et al. Rapid decrease of cytochrome P45011E1 in primary hepatocyte culture and its maintenance by added 4-methylpyrazole. *Hepatology.* 1990;12:1379-1389.

115. Zakharov S, et al. Fluctuations in serum ethanol concentration in the treatment of acute methanol poisoning: a prospective study of 21 patients. *Biomed Pap Med Fac Univ Palacky Olomouc Czech Repub.* 2015;159:666-676.

116. Zakharov S, et al. Fomepizole versus ethanol in the treatment of acute methanol poisoning: comparison of clinical effectiveness in a mass poisoning outbreak. *Clin Toxicol (Phila).* 2015;53:797-806.

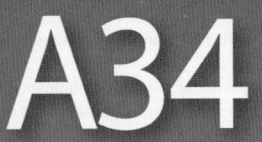
ETHANOL

Mary Ann Howland

H—C—C—OH (with H atoms shown around the two carbons)

INTRODUCTION

Ethanol is used therapeutically as a competitive substrate for xenobiotics metabolized by alcohol dehydrogenase, thus limiting the bioactivation of those xenobiotics to toxic metabolites. Methanol and ethylene glycol are potentially lethal xenobiotics metabolized by this pathway.[16,17] Ethanol also inhibits the metabolism of short-chain polyethylene glycols, such as di- and triethylene glycol,[70] and competes with monofluoroacetate and fluoroacetamide for binding to the citric acid cycle. Ethanol also affects the cytochrome (CYP) enzyme system, especially CYP2E1, for which it has biphasic properties as an inducer and an inhibitor similar to fomepizole and isoniazid. The competitive relationship of ethanol with toxic xenobiotics is used to therapeutic advantage, but the effect of ethanol on the CYP system often leads to unwanted drug interactions and pharmacokinetic tolerance after several days of administration.

HISTORY

Ethanol has been used as an antidote for methanol poisoning since the 1940s and for ethylene glycol since the 1960s.[2]

PHARMACOLOGY

Mechanism of Action

Ethanol works as a competitive substrate for alcohol dehydrogenase, inhibiting the metabolism of xenobiotics such as methanol and ethylene glycol that employ this enzyme.

Affinity for Alcohol Dehydrogenase

The dose of ethanol necessary to achieve competitive inhibition depends on the relative concentrations of the toxic alcohols and their affinity for the enzyme. An affinity constant, K_m, is used to express the degree of affinity: the lower the K_m value, the stronger the affinity. The following equates millimoles or milligrams for alcohols: 1 mmol ethanol equals 46 mg, 1 mmol methanol equals 32 mg, and 1 mmol ethylene glycol equals 64 mg. A millimolar concentration means millimoles per liter (mM). A summary of in vitro experiments using human liver cells demonstrated a K_m for alcohol dehydrogenase of 30 mM for ethylene glycol, 7 mM for methanol, and 0.45 mM for ethanol.[40,55,56] This means that the molar affinity of ethanol for alcohol dehydrogenase is 67 times that of ethylene glycol and 15.5 times that of methanol. Using human alcohol dehydrogenase and a simulation model the oxidation of 50 mM of methanol and ethylene glycol were inhibited by 20 mM (92 mg/dL) of ethanol and 50 mM (4 mg/dL) of fomepizole.[38] Studies in methanol-poisoned monkeys revealed that when ethanol was administered at a molar ethanol-to-methanol ratio (E/M) of 1:4, the metabolism of methanol was reduced by 70%; at a 1:1 E/M ratio, metabolism was reduced by greater than 90%.[43] In these experiments, the dose of methanol was kept constant at about 1 g/kg (32 mmol/kg), whereas the dose of ethanol was varied. Although the serum methanol concentration was not measured, a calculation using this

dose and a volume of distribution (V_d) of 0.6 L/kg would predict a serum concentration of about 166 mg/dL. Even in molar ratios as high as 1:8, methanol did not inhibit ethanol metabolism. When ethylene glycol and methanol are administered together in a 0.5:1 molar ratio, ethylene glycol did not inhibit methanol metabolism.[43] When compared with methanol, smaller amounts of ethanol are required to block the metabolism of ethylene glycol, as the affinity of ethylene glycol for alcohol dehydrogenase is less than that of methanol.[30,40,55,56,59,68] We agree with most authors[1,30,68] who recommend either a serum ethanol concentration of 100 mg/dL, or at least a 1:4 molar ratio of ethanol to methanol or ethylene glycol, whichever is greater. Using this ratio, 100 mg/dL (approximately 22 mmol/L) of ethanol protects against 88 mmol/L (286 mg/dL) of methanol or 88 mmol/L (546 mg/dL) of ethylene glycol. Inhibiting the metabolism of methanol and ethylene glycol impedes the formation of toxic metabolites and prevents the development of metabolic acidosis.[18,21,29,68] After this toxic metabolic pathway is blocked with ethanol, renal, pulmonary, and extracorporeal routes of toxic alcohol removal become the sole mechanisms for elimination.

PHARMACOKINETICS

Ethanol administered orally is rapidly absorbed and achieves peak concentrations in about 1 to 1.5 hours.[13,20,41,69] The amount of ethanol absorbed after oral administration is highly variable and dependent on a number of factors, such as ethanol dose, fasting, nutritional status, accelerated gastric emptying, gender, genetics, chronic alcohol use, lean body mass, and increasing age, as well as the presence of certain H_2-receptor antagonists.[10,14,20,33,37,66,72,75] Sufficient concentrations are generally achieved when 0.8 g/kg of ethanol is given orally over 20 minutes.[10,13,14,20,37,69]

Given that the V_d for ethanol is approximately 0.6 L/kg,[15,77] the loading dose of ethanol is obtained by the following formula:

$$
\begin{aligned}
\text{Loading dose} &= C_p \times V_d \\
&= 1 \text{ g/L (100 mg/dL)} \times 0.6 \text{ L/kg} \\
&= 0.6 \text{ g/kg} \\
C_p &= \text{plasma concentration, which is comparable to the} \\
&\quad \text{serum concentration}
\end{aligned}
$$

For a 70-kg person, the loading dose would be 42 g (70 kg × 0.6 g/kg) of ethanol, or 420 mL of 10% V/V (volume-to-volume) ethanol. This calculation assumes that the specific gravity of ethanol is 1 g/mL. However, a 0.8 g/kg or 8 mL/kg loading dose of a 10% ethanol solution is recommended in order to provide a margin of safety because of the variabilities in V_d and the ongoing metabolism that occurs during administration.[34,57] The intravenous (IV) loading dose should be administered over 20 to 60 minutes, as tolerated by the patient. The 10% ethanol concentration is preferable to the 5% concentration to limit the volume of fluid administered. It is also recommended not to use more concentrated solutions to limit local venous irritation and avoid postinfusion phlebitis. Because of the free water content and significant hypertonicity of the 10% solution, the patient should be closely observed for the development of hyponatremia.

To maintain an ethanol concentration of 100 mg/dL, ethanol replacement must equal ongoing elimination (66–130 mg/kg/h). The average hourly dose for a 70 kg person is 4.6 g, but higher doses are required in ethanol-tolerant patients (100–150 mg/kg/h) or others who may have induced enzymes, and in those undergoing hemodialysis (250–350 mg/kg/h) (Chap. 6).[17,30,44,53,54]

ROLE IN METHANOL AND ETHYLENE GLYCOL TOXICITY

When administered in a timely fashion after methanol and ethylene glycol ingestion and before the accumulation of the toxic metabolites, case reports and utilization in mass poisonings confirm the efficacy of ethanol in preventing sequelae.[12,14,32,36,50,67,73,81,82] A half-life of 46.5 hours for methanol was reported in a patient who had received a sufficient blocking quantity of ethanol,[53] which is quite similar to the 54 hours reported in a case series of methanol poisoned patients treated only with fomepizole.[8,32] In another case series of 3 methanol poisoned patients treated with ethanol, the median methanol half-life was 43.1 hours (range 30.3–52.0 hours).[51] In the presence of sufficient inhibitory concentrations of ethanol, the half-life of ethylene glycol in 2 patients with normal kidney function was 17.5 hours, which was comparable with 17 hours in a case series of ethylene glycol poisoned patients receiving only fomepizole with normal kidney function.[12,66] An ethylene glycol half-life of 15.4 hours was reported in one woman with repetitive poisoning who was treated 60 separate times with ethanol.[27,80]

ADVERSE EFFECTS AND SAFETY ISSUES

Problems encountered with the administration of ethanol include further risk of central nervous system (CNS) depression, behavioral disturbances, or ethanol-related toxicity, such as nausea, emesis, hepatitis, pancreatitis, hypoglycemia, dehydration, various administration and monitoring errors resulting in fluctuating serum concentrations (subtherapeutic and supratherapeutic ethanol concentrations and premature discontinuation), and potential drug interactions resulting in disulfiramlike reactions.[3,19,24,39,45,47,50,52,74,78]

PREGNANCY AND LACTATION

Ethanol (injection) is US Food and Drug Administration pregnancy category C. Ethanol crosses the placenta and reaches the fetus. Ethanol is teratogenic, and the American Academy of Pediatrics (AAP) recommends that pregnant women abstain from all alcohol consumption. It is likely that the short duration of ethanol therapy, when used to compete with alcohol dehydrogenase, during the second or third trimester, has a minimal risk of inducing fetal alcohol syndrome. Ethanol should only be used following a risk-benefit analysis, particularly in the first trimester.[9] Ethanol has been used to manage methanol poisoning in pregnancy when fomepizole was unavailable.[6,22] Because of the potentially devastating maternal and fetal effects of methanol or ethylene glycol,[4,6,35] if an antidote is required in a pregnant woman to treat an overdose and fomepizole is not available, then ethanol is recommended,[47] until fomepizole and/or hemodialysis can be effected.[71] Ethanol crosses into breast milk and, depending on the dose of ethanol and the time since ingestion, causes CNS depression and ethanol toxicity in the breast-fed infant. We recommend that breast-feeding should be temporarily discontinued until the ethanol is eliminated as well as the toxic alcohol for which it is being used.

DOSING AND ADMINISTRATION

Ethanol is given either orally or IV (Tables A34–1 and A34–2). Concentrations of 20% to 30% orally and 5% to 10% IV are well tolerated. Intravenous administration has the advantages of complete absorption[34] and avoidance of most gastrointestinal symptoms, and is recommended in an unconscious or uncooperative patient. The disadvantages of IV ethanol include difficulty in obtaining and preparing an IV ethanol solution, which results in significant delays in administration, the hyperosmolarity of a 10% ethanol solution approximately 1,900 mOsm/L, and the possibilities of osmotic dehydration, hyponatremia, and venous irritation.

Regardless of route, the objective is to rapidly achieve and maintain a serum ethanol concentration of at least 100 mg/dL, which is adequate for enzyme inhibition in most cases. Inhibition is best achieved by administering a loading dose of ethanol, followed by a maintenance dose.

Because ethanol elimination varies in each individual, frequent serum ethanol determinations should be obtained to ensure adequate dosing while also monitoring blood glucose and fluid and electrolyte status. In addition, any increase in the anion gap or decrease in bicarbonate concentration implies that the ethanol concentration is inadequate to achieve blockade of alcohol dehydrogenase and the ethanol dosing should be increased.

TABLE A34–1	Intravenous Administration of 10% Ethanol					
	Volume (mL)[b] (given over 1 hour as tolerated)					
Loading Dose[a]	10 kg	15 kg	30 kg	50 kg	70 kg	100 kg
0.8 g/kg of 10% ethanol	80	120	240	400	560	800
	mL/h for various weights[d]					
Maintenance Dose[c]	10 kg	15 kg	30 kg	50 kg	70 kg	100 kg
Ethanol naïve						
80 mg/kg/h	8	12	24	40	56	80
110 mg/kg/h	11	16	33	55	77	110
130 mg/kg/h	13	19	39	65	91	130
Ethanol tolerant						
150 mg/kg/h	—	—	—	75	105	150
During hemodialysis						
250 mg/kg/h	25	38	75	125	175	250
300 mg/kg/h	30	45	90	150	210	300
350 mg/kg/h	35	53	105	175	245	350

[a]A 10% V/V concentration yields approximately 100 mg/mL. [b]For a 5% concentration, multiply the amount by 2. [c]Infusion to be started immediately following the loading dose. Concentrations above 10% are recommended not to be used for intravenous administration. The dose schedule is based on the premise that the patient initially has a zero ethanol concentration. The aim of therapy is to maintain a serum ethanol concentration of 100-150 mg/dL, but constant monitoring of the ethanol concentration is required because of wide variations in endogenous metabolic capacity. Ethanol will be removed by hemodialysis, and the infusion rate of ethanol must be increased during hemodialysis. Prolonged ethanol administration may lead to hypoglycemia. [d]Rounded to the nearest milliliter.

Adapted with permission from Roberts JR, Hedges J. *Clinical Procedures in Emergency Medicine*. Philadelphia, PA: WB Saunders; 1985.

TABLE A34–2	Oral Administration of 20% Ethanol					
	Volume (mL)					
Loading Dose[a]	**10 kg**	**15 kg**	**30 kg**	**50 kg**	**70 kg**	**100 kg**
0.8 g/kg of 20% ethanol, diluted in juice (administered orally or via nasogastric tube)	40	60	120	200	280	400
	mL/h for various weights[c,d]					
Maintenance Dose[b]	**10 kg**	**15 kg**	**30 kg**	**50 kg**	**70 kg**	**100 kg**
Ethanol naïve						
80 mg/kg/h	4	6	12	20	28	40
110 mg/kg/h	6	8	17	27	39	55
130 mg/kg/h	7	10	20	33	46	66
Ethanol tolerant						
150 mg/kg/h	—	—	—	38	53	75
During hemodialysis						
250 mg/kg/h	13	19	38	63	88	125
300 mg/kg/h	15	23	46	75	105	150
350 mg/kg/h	18	26	53	88	123	175

[a]A 20% V/V concentration yields approximately 200 mg/mL. [b]Concentrations above 30% (60 proof) are not recommended for oral administration. The dose schedule is based on the premise that the patient initially has a zero ethanol concentration. The aim of therapy is to maintain a serum ethanol concentration of 100–150 mg/dL, but constant monitoring of the ethanol concentration is required because of wide variations in endogenous metabolic capacity. Ethanol will be removed by hemodialysis, and the dose of ethanol must be increased during hemodialysis. Prolonged ethanol administration may lead to hypoglycemia. [c]Rounded to the nearest milliliter. [d]For a 30% concentration, multiply the amount by 0.66.

Adapted with permission from Roberts JR, Hedges J. *Clinical Procedures in Emergency Medicine*. Philadelphia, PA: WB Saunders; 1985.

FORMULATION AND ACQUISITION

A practical problem often involves preparing the ethanol to be given since commercial preparations of 5% ethanol in 5% dextrose are no longer available in the US for IV administration.[5] Not having a commercially available preparation increases the delay to administration of IV ethanol and the potential for a medication error in preparation. Sterile ethanol USP (absolute ethanol, dehydrated, preservative free) 98% can be added to 5% dextrose to make a solution of approximately 10% ethanol concentration; 55 mL of absolute ethanol is added to 500 mL of 5% dextrose to produce a total volume of 555 mL (10% = 10 mL in 100 mL; in this case, 55 mL in 555 mL or 55/555). In almost all circumstances (eg, except in which the gastrointestinal tract cannot be used or mental status changes preclude oral administration), oral ethanol is recommended over the extemporaneous preparation of IV ethanol. Ethanol in a 20% concentration is administered either orally or via a nasogastric tube. If oral administration is chosen, then it is important to remember that in the United States the "proof" number on the label is double the concentration; that is, "100-proof" ethanol is 50% ethanol by volume (50 mL/100 mL). Vodka is usually 40% (80 proof) and can be diluted one to one to make a 20% concentration. If fomepizole is unavailable recommend that the pharmacy have vodka on the premises to use as an alternative. Stocking vodka should not excuse the failure to obtain fomepizole once the shortage of fomepizole is over.

COMPARISON TO FOMEPIZOLE

Although ethanol was the standard antidote for toxic alcohols for many years in both adults and children,[61,79] and has the advantages of easy accessibility to oral ethanol and low acquisition cost, fomepizole is a very potent inhibitor of alcohol dehydrogenase with many important advantages.[23,25,31,42,46-48,58,62] Although the acquisition cost of fomepizole is greater than for ethanol, the many advantages of fomepizole over ethanol make fomepizole the preferable antidote in most circumstances, and overall hospital costs including critical care resources, hemodialysis, and laboratory analyses are equivalent or less, depending on the health care and reimbursement system[7,11,64,66,76] (Antidotes in Depth: A33 and Chap. 106).[39,65,74] Ethanol is easier to deploy, particularly in the prehospital setting, in mass poisonings,[36,50,60,63,81,82] or resource-poor settings.

SUMMARY

- The disadvantages of ethanol compared with fomepizole (when available) make ethanol an outmoded antidote under most circumstances.
- When administered appropriately, ethanol prevents further metabolism of methanol and ethylene glycol to their respective toxic metabolites.
- Neither fomepizole nor ethanol affects the toxic metabolites already present in the body.
- Once alcohol dehydrogenase is blocked, the decision whether to use hemodialysis depends on the degree of end-organ damage that has occurred, how well the body can eliminate the parent compound without the benefit of hemodialysis, and the extent to which toxic metabolites are already present.
- With the use of either ethanol or fomepizole without subsequent hemodialysis, the increase in hospital length of stay in an intensive care unit or on a medical floor is substantial for methanol poisoned patients or those poisoned with ethylene glycol who have poor kidney function.[26,28,62]
- Ethanol is recommended in a mass casualty situation until sufficient supplies of fomepizole are procured.[36,50,81,82]

REFERENCES

1. Agner K, et al. The treatment of methanol poisoning with ethanol. *J Stud Alcohol*. 1949;9:515-522.
2. Barceloux DG, et al. American Academy of Clinical Toxicology Practice Guidelines on the treatment of ethylene glycol poisoning. Ad Hoc Committee. *J Toxicol Clin Toxicol*. 1999;37:537-560.
3. Beatty L, et al. A systematic review of ethanol and fomepizole use in toxic alcohol ingestions. *Emerg Med Int*. 2013;2013:1-14.
4. Belson M, Morgan BW. Methanol toxicity in a newborn. *J Toxicol Clin Toxicol*. 2004;42:673-677.
5. Berberet B, et al. Discontinuation of 5% alcohol in 5% dextrose injection: implications for antidote stocking. *Am J Health Syst Pharm*. 2008;65:2200-2203.
6. Bharti D. Intrauterine cerebral infarcts and bilateral frontal cortical leukomalacia following chronic maternal inhalation of carburetor cleaning fluid during pregnancy. *J Perinatol*. 2003;23:693-696.
7. Boyer EW, et al. Severe ethylene glycol ingestion treated without hemodialysis. *Pediatrics*. 2001;107:172-173.

8. Brent J, et al. Fomepizole for the treatment of methanol poisoning. *N Engl J Med.* 2001;344:424-429.

9. Briggs GG, Freeman RK. *Ethanol in Drugs in Pregnancy and Lactation: A Reference Guide to Fetal and Neonatal Risk.* 10th ed. Philadelphia, PA: Lippincott Williams & Wilkins; 2015.

10. Caballeria L. First-pass metabolism of ethanol: its role as a determinant of blood alcohol levels after drinking. *Hepatogastroenterology.* 1992;39:62-66.

11. Cannarozzi AA, Mullins ME. A cost analysis of treating patients with ethylene glycol poisoning with fomepizole alone versus hemodialysis and fomepizole [abstract]. *Clin Toxicol.* 2010;48:299-300.

12. Cheng JT, et al. Clearance of ethylene glycol by kidneys and hemodialysis. *J Toxicol Clin Toxicol.* 1987;25:95-108.

13. Cobaugh DJ, et al. A comparison of the bioavailabilities of oral and intravenous ethanol in healthy male volunteers. *Acad Emerg Med.* 1999;6:984-988.

14. Cole-Harding S, Wilson JR. Ethanol metabolism in men and women. *J Stud Alcohol.* 1987;48:380-387.

15. Cowan JM Jr, et al. Determination of volume of distribution for ethanol in male and female subjects. *J Anal Toxicol.* 1996;20:287-290.

16. Davis DP, et al. Ethylene glycol poisoning: case report of a record-high level and a review. *J Emerg Med.* 1997;15:653-667.

17. Ekins BR, et al. Standardized treatment of severe methanol poisoning with ethanol and hemodialysis. *West J Med.* 1985;142:337-340.

18. Faci A, et al. Chloral hydrate enhances ethanol-induced inhibition of methanol oxidation in mice. *Toxicology.* 1998;131:1-7.

19. Fillmore MT, Vogel-Sprott M. Behavioral impairment under alcohol: cognitive and pharmacokinetic factors. *Alcohol Clin Exp Res.* 1998;22:1476-1482.

20. Fraser AG, et al. Ranitidine, cimetidine, famotidine have no effect on post-prandial absorption of ethanol (0.8 g/kg) taken after an evening meal. *Aliment Pharmacol Ther.* 1992;6:693-700.

21. Grauer G, et al. Comparison of the effects of ethanol on 4-methylpyrazole on the pharmacokinetics and toxicity of ethylene glycol in the dog. *Toxicol Lett.* 1987;35:307-314.

22. Hantson P, et al. Methanol poisoning during late pregnancy. *J Toxicol Clin Toxicol.* 1997;35:187-191.

23. Hantson P, et al. Two cases of acute methanol poisoning partially treated by oral 4-methylpyrazole. *Intensive Care Med.* 1999;25:528-531.

24. Hantson P, et al. Ethanol therapy for methanol poisoning: duration and problems. *Eur J Emerg Med.* 2002;9:278-279.

25. Hauser J, Szabo S. Extremely long protection by pyrazole derivatives against chemically induced gastric mucosal injury. *J Pharmacol Exper Ther.* 1991;256:592-598.

26. Hovda K, Jacobsen D. Expert opinion: fomepizole may ameliorate the need for hemodialysis in methanol poisoning. *Hum Exp Ther.* 2008;27:539-546.

27. Hovda KE, et al. Studies on ethylene glycol poisoning: one patient—154 admissions. *Clin Toxicol (Phila).* 2011;49:478-484.

28. Jacobsen D, et al. Ethylene glycol intoxication: evaluation of kinetics and crystalluria. *Am J Med.* 1988;84:145-152.

29. Jacobsen D, et al. Studies on methanol poisoning. *Acta Med Scand.* 1982;212:5-10.

30. Jacobsen D, McMartin KE. Methanol and ethylene glycol poisonings: mechanism of toxicity, clinical course, diagnosis and treatment. *Med Toxicol.* 1986;1:309-334.

31. Jacobsen D, et al. Effects of 4-methylpyrazole, methanol/-ethylene glycol antidote, in healthy humans. *J Emerg Med.* 1990;8:455-461.

32. Jacobsen D, et al. Methanol and formate kinetics in late diagnosed methanol intoxication. *Med Toxicol.* 1988;3:418-423.

33. Jones AW, et al. Effect of high-fat, high-protein, and high-carbohydrate meals on the pharmacokinetics of a small dose of ethanol. *Br J Clin Pharmacol.* 1997;44:521-526.

34. Julkunen RJ, et al. First pass metabolism of ethanol: an important determinant of blood levels after alcohol consumption. *Alcohol.* 1985;2:437-441.

35. Jung H, et al. A rare case of fatal materno-fetal methanol poisoning. Volatile congeners analysis as forensic evidence. *Rom J Leg Med.* 2014;22:63-68.

36. Karlson-Stiber C, Persson H. Ethylene glycol poisoning: experiences from an epidemic in Sweden. *J Toxicol Clin Toxicol.* 1992;30:565-574.

37. Korman MG, Bolin TD. Alcohol and H$_2$-receptor antagonists. *Med J Aust.* 1992;157:730-731.

38. Lee SL, et al. Oxidation of methanol, ethylene glycol, and isopropanol with human alcohol dehydrogenases and the inhibition by ethanol and 4-methylpyrazole. *Chem Biol Interact.* 2011;191:26-31.

39. Lepik KJ, et al. Adverse drug events associated with the antidotes for methanol and ethylene glycol poisoning: a comparison of ethanol and fomepizole. *Ann Emerg Med.* 2009;53:439-450.

40. Li TK, Theorell H. Human liver alcohol dehydrogenase: inhibition by pyrazole and pyrazole analogs. *Acta Chem Scand.* 1969;23:892-902.

41. Lieber CS. Gastric ethanol metabolism and gastritis: interactions with other drugs, *Helicobacter pylori*, and antibiotic therapy (1957-1997)—a review. *Alcohol Clin Exp Res.* 1997;21:1360-1366.

42. Makar AB, Tephly TR. Inhibition of monkey liver alcohol dehydrogenase by 4-methylpyrazole. *Biochem Med.* 1975;13:334-342.

43. Makar AB, et al. Methanol metabolism in the monkey. *Mol Pharmacol.* 1968;4:471-483.

44. McCoy HG, et al. Severe methanol poisoning: application of a pharmacokinetic model for ethanol therapy and hemodialysis. *Am J Med.* 1979;67:804-807.

45. McKnight AJ, et al. Estimating blood alcohol level from observable signs. *Accid Anal Prev.* 1997;29:247-255.

46. McMartin KE, et al. Studies on the metabolic interactions between 4-methylpyrazole and methanol using the monkey as an animal model. *Arch Biochem Biophys.* 1980;199:606-614.

47. McMartin K, et al. Antidotes for poisoning by alcohols that form toxic metabolites. *Br J Clin Pharmacol.* 2016;81:505-515.

48. McMartin KE, et al. Methanol poisoning I. The role of formic acid in the development of metabolic acidosis in the monkey and the reversal by 4-methylpyrazole. *Biochem Med.* 1975;13:319-333.

49. Norberg A, et al. Role of variability in explaining ethanol pharmacokinetics research and forensic applications. *Clin Pharmacokinet.* 2003;42:1-31.

50. Paasma R, et al. Methanol mass poisoning in Estonia: outbreak in 154 patients. *Clin Toxicol.* 2007;45:152-157.

51. Palatnick W, et al. Methanol half-life during ethanol administration: implications for management of methanol poisoning. *Ann Emerg Med.* 1995;26:202-207.

52. Papineau KL, et al. Electrophysiological assessment (the multiple sleep latency test) of the biphasic effects of ethanol in humans. *Alcohol Clin Exp Res.* 1998;22:231-235.

53. Peterson C. Oral ethanol doses in patients with methanol poisoning. *Am J Hosp Pharm.* 1981;38:1024-1027.

54. Peterson CD, et al. Ethylene glycol poisoning: pharmacokinetics during therapy with ethanol and hemodialysis. *N Engl J Med.* 1981;304:21-23.

55. Pietruszko R. Human liver alcohol dehydrogenase inhibition of methanol activity by pyrazole, 4-methylpyrazole, 4-hydroxymethylpyrazole and 4-carboxypyrazole. *Biochem Pharmacol.* 1975;24:1603-1607.

56. Pietruszko R, et al. Alcohol dehydrogenase from human and horse liver—substance specificity with diols. *Biochem Pharmacol.* 1978;27:1296-1297.

57. Rainey PM. Relation between serum and whole-blood ethanol concentrations. *Clin Chem.* 1993;39:2288-2292.

58. Rietjens SJ, et al. Ethylene glycol or methanol intoxication: which antidote should be used, fomepizole or ethanol? *Neth J Med.* 2014;72:73-79.

59. Roe O. Methanol poisoning: its clinical course, pathogenesis and treatment. *Acta Med Scand.* 1946;126(suppl 182):1-253.

60. Rostrup M, et al. The methanol poisoning outbreaks in Libya 2013 and Kenya 2014. *PLoS One.* 2016;11:e0152676.

61. Roy M, et al. What are the adverse effects of ethanol used as an antidote in the treatment of suspected methanol poisoning in children? *J Toxicol Clin Toxicol.* 2003;44:155-161.

62. Rozenfeld R, Leikin J. Severe methanol ingestion treated successfully without hemodialysis. *Am J Ther.* 2007;14:502-503.

63. Rulisek J, et al. Cost-effectiveness of hospital treatment and outcomes of acute methanol poisoning during the Czech Republic mass poisoning out-break. *J Crit Care.* 2017; 39:190-198.

64. Shiew CM, et al. An economic analysis: Is fomepizole really more expensive than ethanol for the treatment of ethylene glycol poisoning? *Clin Toxicol.* 2005;43:690.

65. Sivilotti M. Ethanol: tastes great! Fomepizole: less filling! *Ann Emerg Med.* 2009;53: 451-453.

66. Sivilotti ML. Toxicokinetics of ethylene glycol during fomepizole therapy: implications for management. For the Methylpyrazole for Toxic Alcohols Study Group. *Ann Emerg Med.* 2000;36:114-125.

67. Sullivan M, et al. Absence of metabolic acidosis in toxic methanol ingestion: a case report and review. *Del Med J.* 1999;71:421-426.

68. Tarr B, et al. Low-dose ethanol in the treatment of ethylene glycol poisoning. *J Vet Pharmacol Ther.* 1985;8:254-262.

69. Tomaszewski C, et al. Effect of acute ethanol ingestion on orthostatic vital signs. *Ann Emerg Med.* 1995;25:636-641.

70. Vassiliadis J, et al. Triethylene glycol poisoning treated with intravenous ethanol infusion. *J Toxicol Clin Toxicol.* 1999;37:773-776.

71. Velez LI, et al. Inhalational methanol toxicity in pregnancy treated twice with fomepizole. *Vet Hum Toxicol.* 2003;45:28-30.

72. Vestal RE, et al. Aging and ethanol metabolism. *Clin Pharmacol Ther.* 1975;21:343-353.

73. Wacker WE, et al. Treatment of ethylene glycol poisoning with ethyl alcohol. *JAMA.* 1965;194:173-175.

74. Wedge MK, et al. The safety of ethanol infusions for the treatment of methanol or ethylene glycol intoxication: an observational study. *CJEM.* 2012;14:283-289.

75. Whitfield JB. ADH and ALDH genotypes in relation to alcohol metabolic rate and sensitivity. *Alcohol Alcohol Suppl.* 1994;2:59-65.

76. Wiles D, et al. Comment on treatment methods for ethylene glycol intoxication. *Neth J Med.* 2014;72:383-384.

77. Wilkinson P. Pharmacokinetics of ethanol: a review. *Alcohol Clin Exp Res.* 1980;4:6-21.

78. Williams CS, Woodcock KR. Do ethanol and metronidazole interact to produce a disulfiram-like reaction? *Ann Pharmacother.* 2000;34:255-257.

79. Wu AH, et al. Definitive identification of an exceptionally high methanol concentration in an intoxication of a surviving infant: methanol metabolism by first-order elimination kinetics. *J Forensic Sci.* 1995;40:315-320.

80. Zakharov S, et al. Fluctuations in serum ethanol concentration in the treatment of acute methanol poisoning: a prospective study of 21 patients. *Biomed Pap Med Fac Univ Palacky Olomouc Czech Repub.* 2015;159:666-676.

81. Zakharov S, et al. Positive serum ethanol concentration on admission to hospital as the factor predictive of treatment outcome in acute methanol poisoning. *Monatsh Chem.* 2017;148:409-419.

82. Zakharov S, et al. Use of out-of-hospital ethanol administration to improve outcome in mass methanol outbreaks. *Ann Emerg Med.* 2016;68:52-61.

DIETHYLENE GLYCOL

Capt. Joshua G. Schier

$$HO-CH_2-CH_2-O-CH_2-CH_2-OH$$

HISTORY AND EPIDEMIOLOGY

Diethylene glycol (DEG) is a solvent with physical and chemical properties similar to propylene glycol, a xenobiotic that is used throughout the chemical industry. Pharmaceutical-grade propylene glycol is a safe and commonly used solvent for water-insoluble pharmaceuticals (Chap. 46). However, unlike propylene glycol, DEG is a potent nephrotoxic and neurotoxic chemical. Substitution of DEG for propylene glycol and other diluents such as glycerin in oral pharmaceutical elixirs has repeatedly caused epidemics of mass poisoning (Chap. 2). This substitution usually occurred early in the pharmaceutical manufacturing process because of a variety of reasons, including the intentional mislabeling of DEG as an inexpensive replacement diluent for pharmaceutical-grade glycerin, for financial gain and various other reasons.[37,45] As medication-associated DEG mass poisonings recurred over time, numerous quality assurance and control guidelines were developed to identify DEG-contaminated materials. Failure to adhere to these guidelines throughout the pharmaceutical manufacturing and distribution process contributes to this persistent public health problem.[45] In DEG poisoning, patients develop acute kidney injury (AKI) that often rapidly progresses to kidney failure. Patients who developed AKI and do not die quickly after exposure, often become dialysis dependent. A subset who survive the initial poisoning also develop neurological signs and symptoms. These patients either deteriorate further after the onset of neurologic signs and symptoms and die, or they recover from their initial poisoning event, but suffer neurologic sequelae that tends to improve with time.[42,47]

The metabolism of DEG and the pathophysiology of DEG-associated disease are incompletely understood and most of what is known comes from animal studies. Indeed, very little data regarding DEG and its metabolites are available from biological samples of humans poisoned by DEG. It was once thought that DEG was metabolized to 2 ethylene glycol molecules, which, when metabolized to glycolic acid and oxalic acid, caused AKI; this theory has been disproven.[20] Current evidence supports that the terminal DEG metabolite diglycolic acid (DGA) is the nephrotoxin.[10,28,38] Diglycolic acid is neurotoxic as well based on a single published case report of DGA ingestion.[40] This Special Consideration will provide a brief history and epidemiology of DEG poisoning, describe existing pharmacokinetic and toxicokinetic data collected primarily from animal studies, and then discuss available information on the toxic dose, pathophysiology, clinical manifestations, testing and treatment for DEG poisoning. When specific doses of DEG in the literature were reported in milliliters per kilogram, they were converted to grams per kilogram by taking into account the density of DEG (1.118 g/mL) and the concentration. If information on concentration was not provided, then a 100% concentration was assumed. For the reader's convenience, the original dose (if it was in milliliters per kilogram) and commensurate DEG concentration are provided following the converted dose in grams per kilogram or milligrams per kilogram.

Diethylene glycol is produced by the condensation of 2 ethylene glycol molecules forming an ether bond,[1] which yields a compound with a molecular weight of 106 g/mol.[1,42] It was first identified in 1869 and is used in industry and manufacturing.[1] Currently, DEG is used as an antifreeze, as a finishing agent for wool, cotton, silk, and other fabrics, as well as in dye manufacturing. It is also often used as an intermediate in the production of polymers, higher glycols, morpholine, and dioxane.[31] Diethylene glycol is chemically inert and has a higher boiling point than ethylene glycol. Its other physical properties are quite similar to ethylene glycol, including a sweet taste.[19,50] Its physical properties enable it to serve as an excellent solvent for delivery of water-insoluble substances. Unfortunately, its use as a diluent for various pharmaceuticals intended for human consumption resulted in the vast majority of reported cases of poisoning.[5,7,8,12,15-17,25,33-35,37,46,47] In these recurring events, DEG was substituted for a safe and appropriate diluent such as glycerin or propylene glycol. Diethylene glycol poisoning is also reported from the intentional addition of DEG to wine as a sweetener,[48,49] consumption as a substitute for ethanol,[52] and following topical application of DEG-containing medicinal products.[8,11] Finally, there are numerous isolated case reports of DEG poisoning resulting from the consumption of DEG-containing products such as radiator fluid or antifreeze,[52] brake fluid,[6] Sterno,[39] "fog solution,"[18] cleaning solutions,[1] and wallpaper stripper.[30]

PHARMACOKINETICS/TOXICOKINETICS

Absorption and Distribution

In rodents, DEG is highly greater than or equal to 75% and almost immediately absorbed after ingestion. It is distributed primarily based on blood flow, with the kidneys receiving the most DEG, followed by the brain, the spleen, liver, and muscles. The degree of protein binding and the volume of distribution (V_d) in humans is unknown but the V_d in the rat is approximately 1 L/kg.[19] Maximal DEG plasma concentrations occur within 4 hours of ingestion: the ratio of DEG in plasma to red blood cells is 3:2 (approximately 60% of a dose is found in the plasma).[3,19,50] In animal studies, diethylene glycol readily crosses the blood–brain barrier, and concentrations peak in brain tissue (CSF concentration not reported) within 3 to 4 hours of exposure.[19]

Metabolism

Existing animal data demonstrate that as much as 40% of an ingested dose undergoes hepatic metabolism, with most of that eliminated in the urine.[19,29,32] Diethylene glycol is metabolized by alcohol dehydrogenase (ADH) to 2-hydroxyethoxyacetaldehyde, which is then further metabolized by aldehyde dehydrogenase (ALDH) to 2-hydroxyethoxyacetic acid (HEAA).[3,20] This is either renally excreted, oxidized to DGA (also known as 2,2-oxybisacetic acid) or converted to 1,4-dioxan-2-one under extremely acidic conditions.[20] The predominant pathway depends on numerous factors such as dose, degree of kidney function, and acid–base status of the patient.[2,20,28,29] The DEG ether bond linking the 2 ethylene glycol molecules is stable and is not hydrolyzed. Ingestion of DEG and subsequent metabolism does not therefore result in ethylene glycol release.[2,20,31] However, a small amount of ethylene glycol is formed as an intermediate after formation of 2-hydroxyethoxyacetaldehyde. This likely originates from either the aldehyde or HEAA metabolites (Fig. SC9–1).[2] Serum HEAA concentrations peak approximately 4 hours following small DEG ingestions (2 g/kg), but a delayed peak at 8 to 24 hours occurs with larger exposures (10 g/kg) in rodents. Rats that ingest relatively small doses of DEG (2 g/kg) and rats given larger amounts of DEG with coadministration of an ADH blocker (10 g/kg + fomepizole) do not accumulate DGA in their serum over time. Blood DGA concentrations in rats dosed with 10 g/kg of DEG and fomepizole are not significantly different from control rat blood DGA concentrations. Furthermore, DEG elimination half-lives in

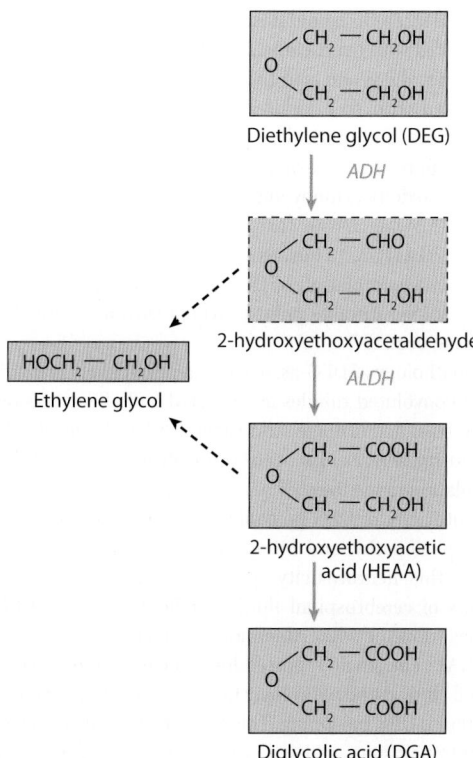

FIGURE SC9–1. Metabolic pathway for DEG based on animal studies and on the results presented in this report. Metabolites in solid boxes are observed following administration of DEG to animals; those in dashed boxes are theoretical intermediates. Because fomepizole reduced the amount of EG in the urine, its origin is shown as coming from the aldehyde or acid intermediate, rather than from DEG itself. ALDH = aldehyde dehydrogenase. Diglycolic acid is also known as oxybisacetic acid. *(Reproduced with permission from Besenhofer LM, Adegboyega PA, Bartels M, et al. Inhibition of metabolism of diethylene glycol prevents target organ toxicity in rats. Toxicol Sci. 2010 Sep;117(1):25-35.)*

the 2 groups dosed with 10 g/kg (one with fomepizole and without) were not significantly different, and almost the entire DEG dose given to the DEG plus fomepizole group was recovered in the urine. This suggests that elimination from the body is mainly controlled by urinary elimination of DEG, rather than by metabolism. Larger doses (10 g/kg) in rat studies, without simultaneous coadministration of an ADH inhibitor, are associated with clinically significant serum DGA concentrations that peak at 24 hours postingestion. If kidney function is impaired, concentrations of both HEAA and DGA continue to climb in a dose-dependent manner.[3]

Elimination

Animal studies utilizing DEG with radiolabeled carbon report that (>60%) of a dose is eliminated within 24 hours of ingestion and all (>90%) within 72 hours.[29,31] The majority of a DEG dose is eliminated unchanged in the urine (>60%).[19,29] The proportion of DEG excreted in the urine increases when compared to metabolites as the dose increases, probably because of saturation of hepatic metabolism.[29,31] This effect persists for approximately 24 hours following exposure. This effect was not demonstrable beyond 24 hours either because the dose was small enough such that it was rapidly eliminated or because the dose was large enough to induce AKI.[29] As the dose increases, the probability of developing AKI increases, which results in decreased elimination of both DEG and its metabolites. Up to 30% of a DEG dose is eliminated via the kidneys as HEAA.[2,13,20,29] Many initial investigations did not either look for or detect DGA, probably because of small exposures in the range of 1.1 g/kg, which did not result in substantial DGA generation.[20] For those reasons, DGA metabolic data was not available until more recently.[2,3] Both HEAA and DGA are transported into the liver and

the kidneys in a dose-dependent manner. Kidney tissue concentrations of HEAA are correlated directly with peak blood concentrations, but DGA concentrations are not. In fact, kidney tissue DGA concentrations are approximately 100 times greater than peak blood DGA concentrations, suggesting much greater accumulation in the kidney.[3] This accumulation explains the low concentrations of urinary DGA noted experimentally.[3] In rodent studies of DGA ingestion limited to 48 hours, DGA is detected in the urine, but at concentrations 50 times lower than HEAA.[2] However, biologic samples in DEG-poisoned humans many days after exposure and in the presence of AKI demonstrated a predominance of urinary DGA concentrations and a relative absence of urinary HEAA.[44] These findings are likely due to a number of different reasons such as the delayed blood peak of DGA when compared with HEAA, the greater time interval from exposure to sampling, which affords a greater likelihood of HEAA metabolism to DGA (compared with experimental animal data), and saturation of kidney tubule cell uptake of DGA. Finally, small amounts of a given DEG dose are eliminated in a dose-dependent fashion via fecal excretion (<3%) and exhalation (<7%).[19,29,31,42] Animal studies also demonstrate that small amounts of DEG with radiolabeled carbon are not eliminated, but rather are distributed to and collected in certain tissues such as muscle, fat, and skin (<4% each) and the intestines, liver, and kidneys (<2% each).[29,31]

Two studies reported data on apparent half-lives calculated from serial DEG concentrations. The first reported that oral doses of 6.7 and 13.4 g/kg (6 and 12 mL/kg of assumed 100% DEG) result ED in half-lives of 8 and 12 hours, respectively.[50] The second report suggests ED that when animals were given DEG doses of 1.1, 5.5, and 10.9 g/kg (1, 5, and 10 mL/kg of 97.5% DEG), most (64%, 87%, and 91%, respectively) of the dose is eliminated in the first 16 hours after exposure with calculated apparent half-lives of 3 to 4 hours. The remainder is then eliminated much more slowly with apparent half-lives ranging from 39 to 49 hours.[19]

Several rodent studies reported data on apparent elimination half-lives collected from serial urinary DEG measurements in pharmacokinetic investigations. These same studies demonstrated that a DEG dose-dependent osmotic diuresis occurs. As the ingested dose increases from 1.1 to 19.6 g/kg (1–17.5 mL/kg of >99% DEG), it induces a fourfold increase in urine production. This effect plateaus at approximately 19.6 g/kg (17.5 mL/kg of >99% DEG).[19] Diethylene glycol elimination undergoes zero order kinetics for the first 9 to 18 hours following ingestion. This correlates temporally with the osmotic diuresis that contributes to this phenomenon.[19,29] During this time, apparent elimination half-lives range from 6 hours at doses of 1.1 to 5.5 g/kg (1–5 mL/kg of 97.5% DEG) to 10 hours for doses of 10.9 g/kg (10 mL/kg of 97.5% DEG).[19] First-order kinetics ensue thereafter with apparent elimination half-lives that are dose-dependent and range from 3 to 13 hours[2,3,19,29] Based on limited animal data, 12 hours seems to be sufficient to eliminate 94% of a dose assuming an elimination half-life of 3 hours at doses of 1.1 to 5.5 g/kg (1–5 mL/kg of 97.5% DEG).[29,32] However, several other studies with similar exposures (2 g/kg) suggest apparent urinary elimination half-lives as high as 5 to 6 hours. This suggests that more than 12 hours is needed to eliminate the majority of a similar dose.[2,19] Apparent half-lives are prolonged to at least 13 hours in more substantial poisonings (10 g/kg)[3] and as kidney function becomes impaired, DEG and its metabolites are unable to be excreted effectively, thereby prolonging apparent elimination half-lives further. This information is of importance in determining the appropriate observation period for a patient with a suspected or known DEG exposure.

TOXIC DOSE

Rodent studies report that doses of up to 2 g/kg are minimally toxic and that doses of approximately 10 g/kg result in significant toxicity.[2] However, rodents are relatively resistant to the clinical effects of DEG poisoning compared to humans. Human data are limited, established primarily from the history of affected patients from mass poisonings, and usually represent an estimated cumulative exposure that occurred over a certain time period, rather than a single point of time. The median estimated toxic dose from the 1995 Haitian mass poisoning was approximately 1.5 g/kg (range, 0.25–4.94 g/kg) (1.34 mL/kg; range, 0.22–4.42 mL/kg of 100% DEG).[33] This estimation is similar to the doses reported for the elixir of sulfanilamide mass poisoning in the United States in the 1930s.[7] The estimated toxic dose (0.36 g/kg) based on patient recall in the 2006 DEG mass poisoning in was lower than previous mass poisonings for which data was available.[47] The reason for this lower toxic dose in this mass poisoning is unclear. One proposed explanation is that it involved an older population with more chronic diseases when compared with other mass poisonings that affected younger, presumably healthier persons. Postmortem DEG concentrations from an Argentinean mass poisoning reported a lethal dose ranging from 0.014 to 0.170 mg/kg,[12,14] although these data are most likely inaccurate, possibly by a factor of at least 1,000.[41] In addition, the analytical testing techniques used in this report may have been subject to error due to cross-reactivity with other metabolites formed as the result of normal postmortem processes.[41] These data also are inconsistent with the fact that polyethylene glycol solutions with trace DEG concentrations yielding average total DEG exposures of 11 mg (range, 2–22 mg) administered for whole-bowel irrigation in adults do not cause adverse effects. Thus, total cumulative DEG exposures of up to 22 mg in adults appear to be safe.[51] The trace DEG concentrations found in these polyethylene glycol solutions likely reflect a minor contamination or byproduct produced during the manufacturing process, however this issue is unstudied. Quantities far in excess of the Argentinean analysis are estimated to occur in adults from nonprescription health products containing trace amounts of DEG (maximum value, 6.3 mg) currently sold in the United States.[43] There were no reports of DEG poisoning associated with the products tested in this report.

In summary, the minimum toxic DEG dose in an acute, single-dose exposure is unclear but limited data suggest that single, small total exposures of less than or equal to 22 mg in an adult are not associated with adverse health effects. Analysis of past DEG mass poisoning incidents suggests that cumulative exposures of as little as 0.25 g/kg are associated with illness,[33] but this number cannot be used as a reliable cutoff to exclude poisoning.

The minimum toxic dose of DGA is unknown, but ingestion of 100 g in an adult was fatal. The actual absorbed dose is probably much less since the patient in this case report vomited immediately after ingestion but still died.[40]

PATHOPHYSIOLOGY

Accumulation of HEAA and DGA in the blood causes a metabolic acidosis that was prevented by early administration of an ADH inhibitor such as fomepizole.[2,3] Although there are no published reports examining the efficacy of ethanol to block DEG metabolism, it would also be expected to be efficacious. Inhibition of DEG metabolism with an ADH inhibitor prevents kidney and liver toxicity[2] and decreases lethality in rodents.[20] The parent compound (DEG) does not appear to be toxic based on these same studies.[2,20,27,28] Diglycolic acid is likely to be the major if not sole cause of nephrotoxicity in DEG poisoning. Animal studies consistently demonstrate an association between the presence of DGA with toxicity, and the absence of toxicity when DGA is not present.[26,38] Studies with human proximal tubule cells demonstrate that DGA-induced cell death is due to necrosis via uptake by a sodium-dicarboxylate-1 transporter, which probably occurs because of its structural similarities to citric acid cycle intermediates.[28] Additional studies demonstrate that DGA preferentially inhibits succinate dehydrogenase, but has no effect on the other citric acid cycle enzyme activities.[27] In vitro data suggest that the mechanism is likely related to the ability of DGA to chelate calcium and subsequently preventing substrate and reducing equivalent availability for oxidative phosphorylation.[10] These activities ultimately result in interruption of mitochondrial respiration, leading to decreased energy production (and subsequent availability) and proximal tubule cell necrosis.[10] These studies also suggest that neither DEG nor HEAA causes cellular toxicity in kidney tissue (in vitro proximal tubule cell testing) and that acidemia enhances DGA toxicity.[26-28] Elevations in blood urea nitrogen and plasma creatinine concentrations correlate moderately well with elevations in tissue DGA concentrations.[2] Diethylene glycol exhibits a steep threshold dose response. Doses of 2 and 5 g/kg were neither associated with overt clinical illness, nor were they associated with detectable kidney diglycolic acid tissue concentrations. This is in contrast to rodents dosed with 10 g/kg of DEG, which developed nephrotoxicity, metabolic acidosis, and markedly elevated kidney DGA tissue concentrations.[26] Furthermore, direct dosing of rodents with DGA exhibited a similar pattern. Severe toxicity (kidney and liver) was noted in animals receiving 300 mg/kg DGA, whereas no toxicity was noted in those animals that received 100 mg/kg DGA.[38] Thus, DEG doses capable of producing substantial target organ accumulation of DGA are needed for nephrotoxicity and there is likely some saturable point at which DGA accumulation in target organs begins to occur.[26,38]

The histopathology of DEG-associated nephrotoxicity primarily involves the proximal convoluted tubules as expected and affects the renal cortex, in which necrosis, hemorrhage, and vacuolization develop.[42] Elevations in hepatic aminotransferases also occur probably because of DEG, HEAA, and DGA accumulation in the liver.[3,30,31]

The neurotoxicity of DEG poisoning includes a severe peripheral neuropathy, encephalopathy, and other signs and symptoms.[42,47] The pathophysiology of this neurotoxicity spectrum is unclear; however, limited testing results of cerebrospinal fluid samples taken from DEG-poisoned patients cases from the 2006 Panama mass poisoning suggest an association with DGA.[44] The single reported human case of a pure DGA ingestion demonstrated clinical and pathologic findings, including severe neurotoxicity, very similar to DEG poisoning. This further supports the hypothesis that the aforementioned signs and symptoms of DEG-associated neurotoxicity are likely due to DGA.[40]

CLINICAL MANIFESTATIONS

The signs, symptoms, and severity of DEG poisoning are dependent on various factors such as duration of exposure, dose, and other intrinsic host factors such as the presence of comorbidities. Following ingestion, symptoms typical of ethanol intoxication such as lethargy, confusion, "drunkenness," and altered mental status begin rapidly and last for several hours.[4,42] Clinical signs and symptoms of a metabolic acidosis including tachypnea and hypernea are reported.[3,42] Although nausea, vomiting, abdominal pain, diarrhea, headache, and confusion are reported with DEG poisoning,[6,42] nephrotoxicity (acute kidney injury) remains the single consistent feature of all cases. This finding manifests over 1 to 3 days following ingestion as a progressive course of oliguria, anuria, or both.[37,42,47]

In some of the reported DEG mass poisonings, patients presented in AKI with profound metabolic acidosis and acidemia.[34] Many of these mass poisonings were in children who received relatively high DEG doses in the form of a pediatric pharmaceutical such as liquid acetaminophen.[33] In the 2006 Panama mass poisoning, the overwhelming majority of patients were adults who probably ingested smaller doses per unit body weight when compared to pediatric victims of past mass poisonings (although they were probably consumed for a longer period of time). Most of these patients presented to health care facilities with vague gastrointestinal or respiratory symptoms and were found to have AKI.[37,47] Many subsequently developed bilateral cranial nerve VII (facial nerve) paralysis and peripheral extremity weakness, often within several days. Finally, many also rapidly developed encephalopathy, coma, and death in the subsequent 24 to 48 hours.[47] This pattern of AKI, followed days later by the appearance of neurologic signs and symptoms such as unilateral or bilateral cranial nerve VII paresis or paralysis, peripheral neuropathy, encephalopathy, autonomic nervous system instability, and coma is frequently reported.[1,17,18,24,39,42,47]

Two case reports document primarily demyelinating peripheral neuropathies,[30,39] but data from the large numbers of patients who received nerve conduction testing from the Panama mass poisonings, as well as other case reports[18,24,47] demonstrate that axonal sensorimotor neuropathy with secondary demyelination is the typical clinical course. Only those DEG-poisoned patients who develop some degree of AKI are at risk for developing neurotoxicity.[24,36,42,47]

Long-term outcomes among DEG poisoning survivors are not well characterized. In one study, patients who remained hemodialysis-dependent after acute illness resolution generally remained hemodialysis dependent. Those who rapidly recovered from their initial AKI event appear to retain normal or at least adequate long-term kidney function for at least the 2 years following exposure. Patients with DEG-associated neurologic findings tended to improve over time. Delayed-onset (beyond the typical initial course of acute DEG poisoning) renal and neurological toxicity is unlikely to occur based on the single longitudinal study of DEG-poisoned survivors.[9]

DIAGNOSTIC TESTING

The clinician will have to rely on a high index of suspicion, a good exposure history and more commonly encountered "routine" testing methodologies including serum electrolytes, blood gas measurements, and kidney function studies upon initial presentation. Use of the osmol gap calculation for evaluating the potential of a toxic alcohol (including DEG) has limitations.[21,22] Generally, the osmol gap should never be used to exclude the possibility of a toxic alcohol ingestion. However, in the authors' experience, very large gaps (>30 mOsm/L), especially in the setting of a suspected or possible poisoning, are likely to be due to some exogenous, osmotically active, xenobiotic that was ingested or otherwise absorbed. The reader is referred to Chaps. 12 and 106 for a complete discussion on this topic. Nerve conduction studies are helpful in establishing the pattern of neuropathy if present. Otherwise, routine laboratory and diagnostic tests are used as needed to help evaluate end organ damage.

Although laboratory assays for DEG in whole blood, serum, plasma, and urine are commercially available at specialized toxicology testing laboratories, they are not available in most hospital laboratories. A study conducted during the 2006 Panama DEG mass poisoning demonstrated statistically significant differences in urinary DEG concentrations among cases (range, 50–4,000 ng/mL) and controls (undetectable). Biologic samples collected from the 2006 Panama investigation demonstrated that serum and urine DGA concentrations were significantly associated with patient status (OR > 999; $P < 0.0001$). Diglycolic acid holds promise as a potential biomarker for DEG poisoning, but further work validating the methodology is needed.[44] One study found that among 14 DEG-poisoned patients who presented without neurologic signs and symptoms, but who had initially elevated CSF protein concentrations (without pleocytosis), almost all (n=13; 93%) developed progressive neurologic sequelae within a few days following CSF collection.[47]

TREATMENT

Treatment options include observation, gastrointestinal decontamination, supportive care, administration of an ADH inhibitor therapy, and hemodialysis. There is no evidence of clinical benefit or even reduced bioavailability of DEG following orogastric or nasogastric lavage or the administration of oral activated charcoal.[23] Nevertheless, given the limited data regarding the role of gastrointestinal decontamination techniques in DEG poisoning, the profound dose-related clinical effects, and the liquid state of the xenobiotic, it is reasonable to perform nasogastric lavage for an individual who presents recently (within 1–2 hours) after ingestion for a large amount of a liquid product containing DEG in order to try to remove unabsorbed DEG in the stomach. It is also reasonable to administer a dose of activated charcoal if presentation is within 1 to 2 hours of ingestion.

Animal evidence suggests that the osmotic diuretic effect of DEG causes large urinary volume losses in the immediate postexposure period. Adequate volume repletion and resuscitation should be performed as soon as possible. The patient should be closely monitored for decreases in urine output and fluid input and output recorded. Fluids need to be adjusted if AKI develops. There is no evidence for using forced diuresis; however, we recommend that all patients are well hydrated (after appropriate resuscitation if needed) to ensure maintenance of euvolemia and a steady urine output. This is appropriate for several reasons, including (1) DEG is primarily eliminated unchanged in the urine via the kidneys; (2) inadequate resuscitation and/or suboptimal hydration beyond the initial fluid resuscitation period contributes

to prerenal azotemia, thereby decreasing elimination of unchanged DEG; (3) any impairment in kidney function will result in decreased elimination of unchanged DEG with a resultant increase in available DEG for metabolism to toxic metabolites such as DGA; and (4) animal studies suggest that when doses associated with adverse health effects (10 g/kg) are given in addition to fomepizole, almost the entire dose is eliminated unchanged in the urine.[2] Careful attention to acid–base status is essential because limited in vitro work with DGA and human proximal tubule cells suggest that acidemia enhances the toxicity of DGA.[27,28] The use of intravenous sodium bicarbonate therapy for controlling metabolic acidosis is unstudied and therefore not routinely recommended at this time.

An ADH inhibitor such as fomepizole is recommended in suspected or known DEG poisoning to prevent nephrotoxicity, although most of the supporting evidence is from animal studies (Antidotes in Depth: A33). This same evidence suggests that the parent compound is not nephrotoxic.[2,20,28] Neurotoxicity seems to only appear following DEG metabolite-associated AKI.[42] Therefore, based on current evidence, administration of a metabolism blocker such as fomepizole seems unlikely to contribute to neurotoxicity (a possible health risk if the parent compound were toxic). In the absence of human dosing data for fomepizole in DEG poisoning, the dosing regimen used for other toxic alcohols is reasonable. Hemodialysis is recommended if clinical evidence of acidemia or end organ toxicity is present. Although the minimal toxic dose of DEG is unknown, cumulative exposures at or above 250 mg/kg (the lower limit of the range reported in the Haiti mass poisoning) are potentially life threatening. A single report documented higher prehemodialysis and lower posthemodialysis concentrations of DEG suggesting that it is cleared by hemodialysis, although the gradient was relatively small (0 and 1.6 mg/dL).[6] Nevertheless, the volume of distribution and molecular weight of DEG suggest that hemodialysis would be effective.[19,42] The endpoint of fomepizole therapy or need for additional rounds of dialysis is unclear, but the relatively new commercial availability of techniques for the determination of whole blood, plasma, serum and urine DEG concentrations with careful attention to acid–base status will be helpful in guiding therapy. At this time, there is insufficient human data to conclude that fomepizole monotherapy (without hemodialysis) in human DEG poisoning is completely protective as the currently available, albeit limited, evidence shows it prevents nephrotoxicity and that the DGA metabolite is the most likely cause of the neurotoxicity that follows onset of AKI. Therefore it is a reasonable management approach to take for suspected or known DEG poisoning as discussed above. However, early nephrology consultation for hemodialysis in cases of suspected severe DEG poisoning is also recommended. Consultation with a medical toxicologist or poison control center will be helpful.

Exposures to amounts of DEG less than those known to be definitely associated with poisoning present management dilemmas. The following sections consist of reasonable treatment protocols, which will need to be modified depending on the individual situation. In all exposures, a medical toxicologist should be consulted as the circumstances surrounding the exposure are invariably different and may affect management.

Mass poisonings–derived toxic doses of DEG are not reliable measures for excluding poisoning. Patients with a reliable history of a minimal ingestion, such as an unintentional sip of a low-concentration DEG-containing product, are unlikely to be at risk for toxicity. For those individuals careful observation coupled with serial chemistries, blood gas measurements, and an osmol gap to rapidly identify onset of renal function and acid–base abnormalities is reasonable. Decisions are more complicated for those adult patients with slightly larger DEG ingestions of relatively low concentrations (5%) such as exposures consisting of more than a sip but less than a "mouthful." Although the true minimum toxic dose of DEG is unknown, an example of the aforementioned situation might involve an unintentional ingestion of 30 mL (approximately a mouthful) of a 5% DEG product by volume in an adult. This is approximately 1.5 mL of pure DEG, which is equivalent to about 1.7 g, which in an 80-kg adult is about 21 mg/kg. The lower end of the estimated toxic dose range in Haiti was 250 mg/kg, which is more than 10 times higher. Therefore careful observation is reasonable if the dose and product concentrations are reliable and there were no other potential risk factors for DEG-associated illness, such as preexisting kidney disease. Such an exposure in a 3-year-old child weighing 16 kg would yield a dose of 110 mg/kg, an exposure of greater concern that would warrant more aggressive treatment. Unfortunately, ascertainment of the true volume ingested and product concentration is usually difficult, which contributes to the problem of estimating risk based on patient history. If in doubt as to the extent or severity of dose and/or potential for toxicity, proceed with at least fomepizole therapy and follow-up DEG-specific testing.

Patients with signs or symptoms of alcohol intoxication, but who did not consume ethanol should be suspected of having a potentially life threatening DEG ingestion and treated as discussed in the previous section. Asymptomatic patients with ingestions beyond the "unintentional sip or taste" should be observed for at least 24 hours regardless of therapy protocol choice. Serial laboratory determinations to monitor acid–base status should be obtained and evaluated for at least 24 hours based on DEG toxicokinetics.

Unless laboratory testing documents a minimal or absent exposure, the patient's clinical, acid–base, and kidney function status should be followed for at least 24 hours for evidence of DEG poisoning. For patients receiving fomepizole, this 24-hour period should begin 12 hours following the last dose of fomepizole. If clinical evidence of nephrotoxicity or acidemia appears, then fomepizole is recommended in addition to hemodialysis.

For those patients presenting to health care facilities with an acidemia, oliguria or anuria within 24 to 36 hours of a DEG ingestion, fomepizole is recommended in addition to emergent hemodialysis. Regardless of the patient's acid–base and electrolyte status. This recommendation is based in part on animal studies showing that serum DGA concentrations peak at 24 hours following ingestion, DGA is nephrotoxic, sequesters in kidney tissue,[3,27,28] and its half-life increases with larger doses.[3] Early presentation to health care facilities (<10 hours from ingestion) and aggressive treatment (gastrointestinal decontamination, fomepizole, and hemodialysis) appeared to be associated with better outcomes in patients treated with fomepizole or ethanol for DEG exposure.[1,4,6,18,39] In one of these cases, a 15-year-old girl who was witnessed to ingest approximately 22.4 g of DEG (patient weight unknown) was managed with orogastric lavage and early (<3 hours) fomepizole therapy alone; the patient had a good outcome with no renal or neurologic dysfunction (other than inebriation).[4] For those patients presenting later than 36 to 48 hours after a DEG ingestion with the aforementioned signs and symptoms, fomepizole and hemodialysis are recommended. Although the ability of these therapies to limit the damage of DEG and its toxic metabolites will be less (vs earlier implementation), it will be of value with regard to correcting electrolyte imbalances and managing AKI.

Although there are no published reports examining the efficacy of ethanol in blocking DEG metabolism, it is expected to act similarly to fomepizole. Hence, it is a reasonable alternative therapy if fomepizole and hemodialysis are unavailable and a rapid transfer to another hospital is not possible.

SUMMARY

- Patients with suspected or known exposures to DEG present a diagnostic and therapeutic challenge.
- Emerging work demonstrates that the DEG metabolite DGA, and not the parent compound, is nephrotoxic and most likely neurotoxic.
- Alcohol dehydrogenase inhibitor therapies such as fomepizole have a role in treating DEG poisoning, and urgent hemodialysis is recommended for substantial ingestions and/or when evidence of acidemia and/or end-organ toxicity is present.
- Diethylene glycol poisoned patients who develop AKI are at risk for severe neurotoxicity.
- Diethylene glycol ingestion should be suspected in patients presenting with AKI and neurologic signs and symptoms such as cranial nerve VII paresis or paralysis, or extremity weakness consistent with a peripheral neuropathy.

Disclaimer

The findings and conclusions in this article are those of the author and do not necessarily represent the views of the Centers for Disease Control and Prevention or the Agency for Toxic Substances and Disease Registry.

REFERENCES

1. Alfred S, et al. Delayed neurologic sequelae resulting from epidemic diethylene glycol poisoning. *Clin Toxicol (Phila).* 2005;43:155-159.
2. Besenhofer LM, et al. Inhibition of metabolism of diethylene glycol prevents target organ toxicity in rats. *Toxicol Sci.* 2010;117:25-35.
3. Besenhofer LM, et al. Role of tissue metabolite accumulation in the renal toxicity of diethylene glycol. *Toxicol Sci.* 2011;123:374-383.
4. Borron SW, et al. Intravenous 4-methylpyrazole as an antidote for diethylene glycol and triethylene glycol poisoning: a case report. *Vet Hum Toxicol.* 1997;39:26-28.
5. Bowie MD, McKenzie D. Diethylene glycol poisoning in children. *S Afr Med J.* 1972; 46:931-934.
6. Brophy PD, et al. Childhood diethylene glycol poisoning treated with alcohol dehydrogenase inhibitor fomepizole and hemodialysis. *Am J Kidney Dis.* 2000;35:958-962.
7. Calvery HO, Klumpp TG. The toxicity for human beings of diethylene glycol with sulfanilamide. *South Med J.* 1939;32:1105-1109.
8. Cantarell MC, et al. Acute intoxication due to topical application of diethylene glycol. *Ann Intern Med.* 1987;106:478-479.
9. Conklin L, et al. Long-term renal and neurologic outcomes among survivors of diethylene glycol poisoning. *JAMA Intern Med.* 2014;174:912-917.
10. Conrad T, et al. Diglycolic acid, the toxic metabolite of diethylene glycol, chelates calcium and produces renal mitochondrial dysfunction in vitro. *Clin Toxicol (Phila).* 2016;54:501-511.
11. Devoti E, et al. Diethylene glycol poisoning from transcutaneous absorption. *Am J Kidney Dis.* 2015;65:603-606.
12. Drut R, et al. Pathologic findings in diethylene glycol poisoning [in Spanish]. *Medicina (B Aires).* 1994;54:1-5.
13. Durand A, et al. A study of mortality and urinary excretion of oxalate in male rats following acute experimental intoxication with diethylene-glycol. Preliminary report. *Eur J Intensive Care Med.* 1976;2:143-146.
14. Ferrari LA, Giannuzzi L. Clinical parameters, postmortem analysis and estimation of lethal dose in victims of a massive intoxication with diethylene glycol. *Forensic Sci Int.* 2005;153:45-51.
15. Geiling EMK, Cannon PR. Pathologic effects of elixir of sulfanilamide (diethylene glycol) poisoning. *JAMA.* 1938;111:919-926.
16. Hanif M, et al. Fatal renal failure caused by diethylene glycol in paracetamol elixir: the Bangladesh epidemic. *BMJ.* 1995;311:88-91.
17. Hari P, et al. Fatal encephalopathy and renal failure caused by diethylene glycol poisoning. *J Trop Pediatr.* 2006;52:442-444.
18. Hasbani MJ, et al. Encephalopathy and peripheral neuropathy following diethylene glycol ingestion. *Neurology.* 2005;64:1273-1275.
19. Heilmair R, et al. Toxicokinetics of diethylene glycol (DEG) in the rat. *Arch Toxicol.* 1993;67:655-666.
20. Wiener HL. Ethylene and diethylene glycol metabolism, toxicity and treatment. Dissertation, Ohio State University. 1986.
21. Hoffman RS, et al. Osmol gaps revisited: normal values and limitations. *J Toxicol Clin Toxicol.* 1993;31:81-93.
22. Holland MG, et al. Osmol gap method for the detection of diethylene glycol in human serum. *World J Emerg Med.* 2010;1:104-107.
23. Hulten BA, et al. Does alcohol absorb to activated charcoal? *Hum Toxicol.* 1986;5:211-212.
24. Imam YZ, et al. Neurological manifestation of recreational fatal and near-fatal diethylene glycol poisonings: case series and review of literature. *Medicine (Baltimore).* 2014;93:e62.
25. Junod SW. Diethylene glycol deaths in Haiti. *Public Health Rep.* 2000;115:78-86.
26. Landry GM, et al. Diethylene glycol-induced toxicities show marked threshold dose response in rats. *Toxicol Appl Pharmacol.* 2015;282:244-251.
27. Landry GM, et al. Diglycolic acid inhibits succinate dehydrogenase activity in human proximal tubule cells leading to mitochondrial dysfunction and cell death. *Toxicol Lett.* 2013;221:176-184.
28. Landry GM, et al. Diglycolic acid is the nephrotoxic metabolite in diethylene glycol poisoning inducing necrosis in human proximal tubule cells in vitro. *Toxicol Sci.* 2011;124:35-44.
29. Lenk W, et al. Pharmacokinetics and biotransformation of diethylene glycol and ethylene glycol in the rat. *Xenobiotica.* 1989;19:961-979.
30. Marraffa JM, et al. Diethylene glycol: widely used solvent presents serious poisoning potential. *J Emerg Med.* 2008;35:401-406.
31. Mathews JM, et al. Metabolism and disposition of diethylene glycol in rat and dog. *Drug Metab Dispos.* 1991;19:1066-1070.
32. Ming Xing H, et al. Pre-existing liver cirrhosis reduced the toxic effect of diethylene glycol in a rat model due to the impaired hepatic alcohol dehydrogenase. *Toxicol Ind Health.* 2011;27:742-753.
33. O'Brien KL, et al. Epidemic of pediatric deaths from acute renal failure caused by diethylene glycol poisoning. Acute Renal Failure Investigation Team. *JAMA.* 1998;279:1175-1180.

34. Okuonghae HO, et al. Diethylene glycol poisoning in Nigerian children. *Ann Trop Paediatr.* 1992;12:235-238.

35. Leech PN. Special article from the American Medical Association Chemical Laboratory. Elixir of sulfanilamide-massengill: chemical, pharmacologic, pathologic, and necropsy reports; preliminary toxicity reports on diethylene glycol and sulfanilamide. *JAMA.* 1937;109:1531-1539.

36. Reddy NJ, et al. Delayed neurological sequelae from ethylene glycol, diethylene glycol and methanol poisonings. *Clin Toxicol (Phila).* 2010;48:967-973.

37. Rentz ED, et al. Outbreak of acute renal failure in Panama in 2006: a case-control study. *Bull World Health Organ.* 2008;86:749-756.

38. Robinson CN, et al. In-vivo evidence of nephrotoxicity and altered hepatic function in rats following administration of diglycolic acid, a metabolite of diethylene glycol. *Clin Toxicol (Phila).* 2017;55:196-205.

39. Rollins YD, et al. Fulminant ascending paralysis as a delayed sequela of diethylene glycol (Sterno) ingestion. *Neurology.* 2002;59:1460-1463.

40. Roscher AA, et al. Fatal accidental diglycolic acid intoxication. *Toxicol Pathol.* 1975;3:3-13.

41. Schep LJ, Slaughter RJ. Comments on diethylene glycol concentrations. *Forensic Sci Int.* 2005;155:233.

42. Schep LJ, et al. Diethylene glycol poisoning. *Clin Toxicol (Phila).* 2009;47:525-535.

43. Schier JG, et al. Diethylene glycol in health products sold over-the-counter and imported from Asian countries. *J Med Toxicol.* 2011;7:33-38.

44. Schier JG, et al. Characterizing concentrations of diethylene glycol and suspected metabolites in human serum, urine, and cerebrospinal fluid samples from the Panama DEG mass poisoning. *Clin Toxicol (Phila).* 2013;51:923-929.

45. Schier JG, et al. Medication-associated diethylene glycol mass poisoning: a review and discussion on the origin of contamination. *J Public Health Policy.* 2009; 30:127-143.

46. Singh J, et al. Diethylene glycol poisoning in Gurgaon, India, 1998. *Bull World Health Organ.* 2001;79:88-95.

47. Sosa NR, et al. Clinical, laboratory, diagnostic, and histopathologic features of diethylene glycol poisoning—Panama, 2006. *Ann Emerg Med.* 2014;64:38-47.

48. van der Linden-Cremers PM, Sangster B. Medical sequelae of the contamination of wine with diethylene glycol [in Dutch]. *Ned Tijdschr Geneeskd.* 1985;129:1890-1891.

49. van Leusen R, Uges DR. A patient with acute tubular necrosis as a consequence of drinking diethylene glycol-treated wine [in Dutch]. *Ned Tijdschr Geneeskd.* 1987; 131:768-771.

50. Winek CL, et al. Ethylene and diethylene glycol toxicity. *Clin Toxicol.* 1978;13:297-324.

51. Woolf A, Pearson K. Presence of dietylene glycol in commerical polyethylene (PEG) solutions. *J Toxicol Clin Toxicol.* 1995;1995:490.

52. Wordley E. Diethylene glycol poisoning: report on two cases. *J Clin Pathol.* 1947; 1:44-46.

History A 2-year-old (12 kg) girl was transported to the hospital by ambulance after having a witnessed seizure at home. The child was healthy, born at term, and without any significant past medical history. Although her family had recently immigrated to the United States, she was followed in a primary care clinic and was fully vaccinated. She had one screening test for lead, which was "normal." Her mother relates that their house had problems with roaches, mice, and rats and she thinks her husband applied a chemical to deal with the problem.

About 20 minutes before the girl became ill, her mother saw the child pick up something from the corner of the room and immediately thereafter removed some material that looked like food from the child's mouth. The girl subsequently lost consciousness and began to shake. The mother called 9-1-1 and when EMS arrived the child was intermittently seizing. Lorazepam (1 mg IM) was administered and EMS gave the child supplemental oxygen for transport. The paramedics reported that the child stopped seizing during transport but started again upon arrival to the emergency department.

Physical Examination On arrival, the child was seizing with the following vital signs: blood pressure, 90/40 mm Hg; pulse, 160 beats/min, respiratory rate, 36 breaths/min; temperature, 100°F (37.7°C); oxygen saturation, 100% on a 100% nonrebreather mask and rapid reagent glucose of 160 mg/dL. There were no signs of trauma. The skin was moist, pupils were 4 to 5 mm and fixed, the chest was clear, heart sounds were regular, and her abdomen was soft. Neurologic examination revealed repetitive symmetrical movements of the limbs, slight eye deviation to the left, and a lack of responsiveness to stimulation.

Initial Management Another 1 mg dose of lorazepam was given IM, while an IV line was being inserted. Additional blood samples were obtained for complete blood count, electrolytes, liver function tests, and creatine phosphokinase. The child continued to seize and a 2-mg IV dose of lorazepam was administered that terminated the seizure. Repeat vital signs were notable for a pulse of 165 beats/min and a rectal temperature of 100.6°F (38.1°C). Blood cultures were sent and the child was given an empiric dose of ceftriaxone. An ECG was obtained and showed sinus tachycardia with normal axis and intervals.

What Is the Differential Diagnosis? In addition to infectious, structural, and traumatic causes for repeated seizures, the history is suggestive of pesticide poisoning. Pesticides are defined by the US Federal Insecticide, Fungicide, and Rodenticide Act (FIFRA) as "any substance or mixture of substances intended for preventing, destroying, repelling, or mitigating any pest, and any substance or mixture of substances intended for use as a plant regulator, defoliant, or desiccant." Since 1947, the production, use, and distribution of pesticides in the United States have been regulated under FIFRA and its subsequent amendments in 1972, 1975, and 1978. In 1970, the US Environmental Protection Agency (EPA) was given the authority to administer and enforce FIFRA regulations. Under FIFRA, all pesticides and their manufacturers must be registered with the EPA, and the pesticide must be classified for either general use or restricted use by licensed or certified applicators. Additionally, according to FIFRA, rodenticides are classified by their toxicities and must be labeled by signal words as designated in Table CS11–1. The WHO applies a similar classification scheme for all pesticides based on either oral or dermal LD_{50}.

Unfortunately, as is so commonly the case, not only was the mother unaware of the name or type of pesticide used, but also both the original container and label were missing. Furthermore, there was a possibility that the product used was brought from the parent's home country and was either illegal or unlicensed in the United States. As a result, clinicians are often forced to provide empirical treatment based largely on clinical diagnosis. An understanding of the likely possibilities in Tables CS11–2 improves both diagnostic utility and treatment decisions.

What Clinical and Laboratory Analyses Help in the Evaluation of This Patient's Presentation? The possible pesticides when ingested that are most likely to result in seizurelike activity or status epilepticus include organic phosphorus compounds and carbamates (Chap. 110), organic chlorines (Chap. 111), monofluoroacetate and fluoroacetamide (Chap. 113), strychnine (Chap. 114), thallium (Chap. 99), zinc and aluminum phosphide, and tetramine (Chap. 112). The absence of associated clinical manifestations helps eliminate some of the choices: organic phosphorus compounds and carbamates (eg, salivation, lacrimation, urination, defecation, bradycardia, bronchorrhea, miosis), thallium (the onset was rapid and there was an absence of painful peripheral neuropathy), strychnine (not true seizures, consciousness should be preserved until hyperthermia, hypoxia, or hypercarbia becomes severe), and aluminum phosphide (absence of vomiting with characteristic odor of rotten fish). Although routine laboratory testing has little utility here, the absence of a profound metabolic acidosis might suggest that monofluoroacetate and fluoroacetamide are not responsible for this clinical presentation. Certain dangerous rodenticides imported for illicit use include tetramine (status epilepticus) and aldicarb (a carbamate found in tres pasitos). Unfortunately, because there are no rapidly available tests to help establish this diagnosis, treatment will have to be based entirely on the clinical assessment.

Further Diagnosis and Treatment Shortly after the third dose of lorazepam, the child began to seize again and endotracheal intubation was performed. Following intubation, the child was placed

TABLE CS11–1	US Environmental Protection Agency Toxicity Classification of Pesticides				
Category and Signal Word	Oral LD_{50} (mg/kg)	Dermal LD_{50} (mg/kg)	Inhalation LC_{50} (mg/L)	Eye Irritation	Skin Irritation
I Danger	0–50	0–200	0–0.05	Corrosive: corneal opacity not reversible within 21 days	Corrosive
II Warning	50–500	200–2,000	0.05–0.5	Corneal opacity reversible within 8–21 days; irritation persisting for 7 days	Severe irritation at 72 hours
III Caution	500–5,000	2,000–20,000	0.5–5.0	Corneal opacity; irritation reversible within 7 days	Moderate irritation at 72 hours
IV None	>5,000	>20,000	>5.0	Irritation cleared within 24 hours	Mild or slight irritation at 72 hours

CASE STUDY 11 (CONTINUED)

on a continuous infusion of propofol. A nasogastric tube was inserted and 10 g of activated charcoal was instilled into the stomach. The child was transferred to the PICU and attached to a video EEG monitor, where intermittent seizure activity was noted over the next 12 to 16 hours. A non-contrast CT scan of the head was normal and a lumbar puncture was performed to exclude meningitis. The following day, the father brought in the original package and the product was identified as tetramine.

Over the subsequent 24 hours, the propofol infusion was titrated to a lower dose and then discontinued. The child was able to be extubated and appeared clinically normal. Because the package was brought from their home country and not imported, authorities were not notified. The parents were educated about safe use of pesticides, and a social worker was able to help coordinate legal exterminating efforts by the landlord.

Acknowledgments Authors from previous editions, including Neal E. Flomenbaum, Mary Ann Howland, Richard Weisman, Rebecca Tominack, and Susan Pond, contributed to the development of Tables CS11–2 as well as the discussion of FIFRA.

TABLE CS11–2   Management of Specific Rodenticide Ingestions

Rodenticide Name	Physical Characteristics	Toxic Mechanism	Estimated Fatal Dose	Signs and Symptoms	Onset	Antidotes and Other Treatments[a]
Highly Toxic Signal Word: DANGER[b] (LD$_{50}$ < 50 mg/kg)						
Thallium	White, crystalline, odorless, tasteless.	Combines with mitochondrial sulfhydryl groups; interferes with oxidative phosphorylation.	14 mg/kg	Anorexia, abdominal pain, diarrhea, painful neuropathy, delirium, coma, seizures, alopecia (late), Mees lines.	GI symptoms acutely; other symptoms 12–14 hours delay.	Activated charcoal, Prussian blue (Chap. 99).
Sodium monofluoroacetate (SMFA, compound 1080)	White, crystalline, odorless, tasteless, water soluble.	Fluoroacetate to fluorocitrate; interferes with tricarboxylic acid cycle.	3–7 mg/kg	Seizures, coma, tachycardia, PVCs, VT, VF, ST-T wave changes, rhabdomyolysis (hypocalcemia).	30 minutes–20 hours	Experimental regimens (Chap. 113).
Sodium fluoroacetamide (compound 1081)	Same as SMFA.	Same as SMFA; fluoride toxicity.	13–14 mg/kg	Same as SMFA.	Same as SMFA.	Same as SMFA.
Strychnine	Bitter taste.	Glycine receptor antagonist on spinal cord motor neurons.	Children: 15 mg Adults: 1–2 mg/kg	Restlessness, anxiety, twitching, hyperextension alternating with relaxation, intense pain, trismus or facial grimacing ("risus sardonicus"), inability to swallow, opisthotonos.	10–20 minutes	Quiet room, IV midazolam, diazepam, neuromuscular blockade (Chap. 114).
Zinc phosphide	Heavy, gray, crystalline powder, water insoluble, "rotten fish" or "phosphorus" odor; normally used as 1% concentration.	Inhibition of oxidative phosphorylation.	40 mg/kg in rats	Releases phosphine on contact with water or acid or in GI tract. "Rotten fish" breath odor, black vomitus, GI and cardiovascular toxicity, acute respiratory distress syndrome, agitation, coma, seizures, hepatic and renal toxicity.	Within hours; inhalation may have delayed onset.	Dilution with sodium bicarbonate water or milk (Chap. 108).
Elemental phosphorus (yellow or white phosphorus)	Yellow, waxy paste, fat soluble, water insoluble.	Local irritation and burns on contact followed by GI, liver, and kidney damage, and interferes with clotting.	1 mg/kg (more toxic if dissolved in alcohol, fats, oils).	Skin and GI burns, "smoking" luminescent vomitus and stools with garlic odor, jaundice, dysrhythmias, coma, delirium, seizures, cardiac arrest.	1–2 hours	Supportive care (Chap. 112).
Arsenic trioxide	White, crystalline powder.	Combines with sulfhydryl groups and interferes with a variety of enzymatic reactions.	1–4 mg/kg	Dysphagia, nausea and vomiting, bloody diarrhea, cardiovascular collapse (VT, torsade de pointes), garlic odor, altered mental status, late sensory/motor neuropathy.	Symptoms: 1 hour Death: 1–24 hours.	Succimer, dimercaprol until urine arsenic concentration <50 mcg/L Hemodialysis to remove chelation compound if acute kidney injury develops (Chap. 86).
Barium (soluble forms: carbonate, chloride, hydroxide)	Yellow, white, slightly lustrous.	Inhibits calcium activated potassium rectifier channels.	20–30 mg/kg	Headache, paresthesias, muscle weakness, paralysis, nausea, vomiting, diarrhea, abdominal pain, prolonged QT interval, dysrhythmias, cardiac and pulmonary failure. Hypokalemia, neuromuscular blockade.	1–8 hours	Orogastric lavage followed by oral magnesium sulfate at 250 mg/kg for children and 30 gm for adults, potassium replacement (Chap. 107).
PNU (N3-pyridylmethyl-N′-p-nitrophenyl urea; Vacor)	Yellow, resembling cornmeal or yellow green powder in bait; odor: peanuts.	Interferes with nicotinamide metabolism in pancreas (destroying pancreatic β cells), central and peripheral nervous system, and heart.	5 mg/kg	Nausea and vomiting, abdominal pain, severe orthostatic hypotension, hyperglycemia with or without ketoacidosis, gastrointestinal perforation, pneumonia, neuropathy.	4–48 hours	Nicotinamide (niacinamide) 500 mg IV or IM (historically used, but likely unavailable), manage diabetic ketoacidosis.
Tetramine (tetramethylene disulfotetramine, TETS, TEM)	White powder.	Noncompetitive, GABA antagonism by direct blockade of chloride ionophore.	5–10 mg/kg	Refractory status epilepticus, fainting, coma, coronary ischemia.	0.5–13 hours	Benzodiazepines, barbiturates, propofol, neuromuscular blockers.

Moderately Toxic Signal Word: WARNING[a] (LD$_{50}$, 50–500 mg/kg)

Compound	Formulation	Toxic Dose	Mechanism	Clinical Manifestations	Onset	Treatment
α-Naphthylthiourea (ANTU)	Odorless, slightly bitter, fine, blue-gray powder, water-insoluble.	>4 g/kg	Unknown	Hypothermia, dyspnea, crackles, clear pulmonary froth, cyanosis. Acute respiratory distress syndrome.	?	Supportive care.
Cholecalciferol (vitamin D$_3$)	0.075% pellets, 364 pellets/oz (1 pellet = 2308 U vitamin D).	?	Hypercalcemia.	Headache, lethargy, weakness, fatigue, polyuria, acute kidney injury and failure, hypertension, hypercalcemia.	Hours to days	Fluids; if severe: furosemide, prednisone, calcitonin, bisphosphonates hemodialysis (Chap. 44).

Low Toxicity Signal Word: CAUTION[a] (LD$_{50}$, 500–5,000 mg/kg)

Compound	Formulation	Toxic Dose	Mechanism	Clinical Manifestations	Onset	Treatment
Red squill	Bitter taste.	?	Cardioactive steroid poisoning. Inhibition of Na$^+$ K$^+$ ATPase	Myocardial irritability, blurred vision, hyperkalemia.	30 minutes–6 hours	Digoxin-specific Fab, atropine (Chap. 62).
Norbormide (dicarboximide)	Yellow cornmeal bait, peanut butter, 1% concentration.	Unknown, toxicity at < 300 mg.	Vasoconstriction and ischemia in rats only via specific norbormide receptor in rat smooth muscle.	Transient hypothermia and hypotension.	?	Supportive care.
Bromethalin	7.5% concentrate, green pellets, with Bitrex (denatonium benzoate).	?	Uncouples oxidative phosphorylation; interrupts nerve impulse conduction.	Muscle tremors, myoclonic jerks, flexion of major muscles, coma?, ataxia, focal motor seizures.	Immediate	Supportive care.

Anticoagulants: Short-Acting

Compound	Formulation	Toxic Dose	Mechanism	Clinical Manifestations	Onset	Treatment
Warfarin	Yellow cornmeal, rolled oats (0.025%).	>5–20 mg/day for > 5 days	Anticoagulation via interference with clotting factors II, VII, IX, X.	Elevated INR; bleeding death from hemorrhage.		Vitamin K, fresh-frozen plasma as indicated, prothrombin complex concentrate (Chap. 58 and Antidotes in Depth: A18).

Anticoagulants: Long-Acting
Hydroxycoumarins

Compound	Formulation	Toxic Dose	Mechanism	Clinical Manifestations	Onset	Treatment
4-Hydroxycoumarin (brodifacoum, difenacoum)	0.005% grain-based bait.		Anticoagulation via interference with clotting factors II, VII, IX, X.	Elevated INR; bleeding, death from uncertain hemorrhage.	Delayed several days.	Vitamin K, fresh-frozen plasma as indicated. Prothrombin complex concentrate.
Coumafuryl (warfacide)	0.5% for dilution to 0.025% white powder, tasteless, odorless.					

Indandiones

Compound	Formulation	Toxic Dose	Mechanism	Clinical Manifestations	Onset	Treatment
Pindone	Moldy, acrid odor, fluffy yellow powder, concentrations 0.005–2.5%.		Anticoagulation via interference with clotting factors II, VII, IX, X.	Chronic ingestion possibly produces cardiac and neurologic signs and symptoms, elevated INR; bleeding, death from uncertain hemorrhage.	Delayed several days.	Vitamin K, fresh-frozen plasma as indicated. Prothrombin complex concentrate.
Diphacinone	0.005%–2.0%					
Chlorophacinone	0.005%–2.5%					
Valone	0.005%–2.5%					

[a] Gastrointestinal decontamination should be provided as appropriate (Chap. 5); only unique or controversial aspects are discussed in this table. [b] The LD$_{50}$ values used in this table are derived from data on acute oral ingestions of the commercial product based on rats. In some cases, the commercial product contains a very small percentage of the active ingredient. The signal words that appear on labels of registered products may differ from the signal word assigned to the acute oral LD$_{50}$ test because the label may also reflect another study (acute dermal or inhalational LD$_{50}$) requiring a more severe signal word. See Table 110–1 for the Consumer Product Safety Commission definitions and use of signal words as indicators of potential hazard of toxicity. Peacock D, Biologist, Registrations Division Office of Pesticide Programs, EPA, Washington, DC.

107

BARIUM

Andrew H. Dawson

Barium (Ba)
Atomic number   =   56
Atomic weight   =   137.3 Da
Normal concentration
    Serum   <   0.2 mg/L (1.46 µmol/L)

HISTORY AND EPIDEMIOLOGY

Although barium is utilized in various forms in developed nations, exposure to barium salts is uncommon and clinically significant poisoning is rare. Acute, clinically relevant exposures occur most commonly following the intentional ingestion of the soluble salts found in rodenticides, insecticides, or depilatories.[10,11] Barium carbonate has an appearance similar to flour, which is reported to be responsible for most unintentional barium poisonings.[9,13]

Barium salts and barium hydroxide are extensively employed in industry particularly in thermoplastics and the manufacture of synthetic fibers, soap manufacture, and in lubricants (Table 107–1). Toxicity occurs following occupational exposure to barium salts through ingestion, inhalation,[34] or explosion of the propellant barium styphnate.[15] Despite the fact that barium sulfate is insoluble, rare cases of unintentional toxicity are reported during radiographic procedures and include complications associated with oral[24] and rectal administration.[14,19,22,27] Toxicity and death occurred when solutions were unintentionally contaminated with soluble contrast barium salts.[29]

CHEMISTRY

Barium is a soft metallic element that was first isolated by Sir Humphry Davy in 1808. With an atomic weight of 137.3 Da, barium is located at number 56 in the periodic table (between cesium and lanthanum). The metal oxidizes easily when exposed to water or alcohol, has a melting point of 1,341°F (727°C) and a boiling point of 3,398°F (1,870°C). Elemental barium is not found in nature; it normally occurs as an oxide, dioxide, sulfate (barite), or carbonate (witherite). Chemically, barium resembles calcium more than it resembles any other element. Although some barium salts are naturally occurring, most used commercially are produced from the more commonly found carbonates or oxides. Barium salts are typically classified as either water soluble or insoluble, but the solubility of all barium salts increases as pH falls. The soluble salts acetate, chloride, hydroxide, oxide, nitrate, and (poly) sulfide are the most commonly associated with toxicity (Table 107–1). Barium (poly) sulfide also produces toxicity through the formation of hydrogen sulfide when ingested and exposed to gastric hydrochloric acid. Poorly soluble barium carbonate is converted by gastric acid to highly soluble barium chloride. The other insoluble barium salts such as arsenate, chromate, fluoride, oxalate, and sulfate are rarely associated with toxicity.

TOXICOKINETICS

Toxicity can result from ingestion of as little as 200 mg of a barium salt. Oral lethal doses are reported to range from 1 to 30 g of a barium salt. Occupational exposure to barium fumes of greater than 0.02 mg/m³ are associated with health effects.[38] Exposure to inhaled particulate insoluble barium causes pulmonary baritosis, which consists of very fine punctate and annular lesions and some slightly larger nodular lesions.[38]

Following ingestion, 5% to 10% of soluble barium salts are absorbed,[16] with the rate of absorption dependent on the degree of water solubility of the salt. The time to peak serum concentration is 2 hours.[16]

The toxicokinetics are characterized by a rapid redistribution phase, followed by a slow decrease of serum barium concentrations, with a reported half-life ranging between 18 and 85 hours.[16,28] Renal elimination of the absorbed dose accounts for 10% to 28% of total barium excretion, with the predominant route of fecal elimination through the gastrointestinal tract.

In published case reports of symptomatic patients, serum barium concentrations range from 3.7 to 41.1 mg/L.[2,9,23,25,28,31,33] Death is uncommon following ingestion, but occurs most commonly in clinical settings with limited health care resources.[13] Death from an ingestion of barium chloride was associated with the following barium concentrations at autopsy: blood, 9.9 mg/L; bile, 8.8 mg/L; urine, 6.3 mg/L; and gastric contents, 10 g/L.[17]

Intravasation is a rare but serious complication of radiologic studies in which barium sulfate is administered under pressure, such as a barium enema. Following a small perforation, barium sulfate leaks into the peritoneal cavity or portal venous system.[22] Although sudden cardiovascular collapse occurs, it is unclear whether this is the result of venous occlusion

TABLE 107–1	Barium Salts: Solubility and Common Usages	
Barium Salt	*Solubility (mg/L at 20°C)*	*Common Uses*
Acetate	58.8	Textile dyes
Carbonate	0.02 increases in an acid pH; also, can be converted to barium chloride by gastric acid (HCl)	Rodenticide, welding fluxes, pigments, glass, ceramics, pyrotechnics, electronic devices, welding rods, ferrite magnet materials, optical glass, manufacture of caustic soda and other barium salts
Chloride	375	Textile dyes, pigments, boiler detergents, in purifying sugar, as mordant in dyeing and printing textiles, as water softener, in manufacture of caustic soda and chlorine, polymers, stabilizers
Fluoride	1.2	Welding fluxes
Nitrate	87	Optical glass, ceramic glazes, fireworks (green), explosives, antiseptic preparation
Oxide	34.8	In glass, ceramics, refining oils and sugar, as an additive in petroleum products and also as materials of plastics, pharmaceuticals, polymers, glass, and enamel industries
Styphnate	—	Propellant used in manufacture of explosive detonators
Sulfate	0.002	Radiopaque contrast solutions, manufacture of white pigments, paper making
Sulfide	Slightly soluble in H_2O	Depilatories, manufacture of fluorescent tubes

(pulmonary embolism), overwhelming sepsis, or barium toxicity.[7,32,37] In at least one case report of intravasation, signs and symptoms were consistent with barium toxicity and elevated barium concentrations were confirmed.[24] Under these circumstances if hypokalemia is present, then barium toxicity can be assumed.

Additionally, intravenous administration of barium sulfate has occurred as the result of unintentional administration. Recognition followed by aspiration through a central venous catheter was associated with a good outcome.[30]

PATHOPHYSIOLOGY

Hypokalemia is due to redistribution of potassium from the extracellular to intracellular compartment. This is thought to be due to 2 synergistic mechanisms. Barium inhibits calcium-activated potassium rectifier channels, reducing outward flow of potassium; this occurs in the context of persistent Na^+,K^+-ATPase pump electrogenesis leading to a shift of extracellular potassium into the cell.[3]

Intracellular trapping of potassium leads to depolarization and paralysis.[18] Additionally, the inhibition of potassium channels increases vascular resistance and reduces blood flow[4,6] and is the likely mechanism for hypertension and metabolic acidosis with an elevated lactate concentration.

Although severe hypokalemia contributes significantly to paralysis, some authors report that muscle weakness correlates better with barium concentrations than with potassium concentrations.[25,33] This suggests a possible direct effect of barium on either skeletal muscle or neuromuscular transmission.

CLINICAL MANIFESTATIONS

Abdominal pain, nausea, vomiting, and diarrhea commonly occur within 2 hours of ingestion.[13] Esophageal injury and hemorrhagic gastritis are also reported.[1,18]

Severe hypokalemia is the cardinal feature of barium toxicity and typically occurs within 2 hours following oral or parenteral exposure. Hypokalemia is exacerbated by blood transfusions, suggesting that fresh red blood cells provide a new reservoir for K^+ sequestration.[15] Progressive hypokalemia is associated with ventricular dysrhythmias, hypotension, profound flaccid muscle weakness, and respiratory failure (Chaps. 12, 15, and 22).[3]

Other effects less commonly reported include hypertension, metabolic acidosis with an elevated lactate concentration, hypophosphatemia, and rhabdomyolysis.[16] Altered level of consciousness, seizures,[8] and parkinsonism with findings on magnetic resonance imaging of bilateral hyperintensity of the basal ganglia are reported.[12] It is unclear whether these latter findings are due to direct toxicity, deposition of barium, or secondary to tissue ischemia.

DIAGNOSTIC TESTING

Barium can be measured by a variety of techniques. Mass spectrometry and graphite furnace atomic absorption spectrometry can quantitate barium in blood and urine.[18,20] Serum barium concentrations are not readily available, but values greater than 0.2 mg/L are considered abnormal.[5]

Following acute exposures, patients should have serum electrolytes (particularly potassium and phosphate) measured hourly while performing continuous electrocardiographic monitoring. Creatine phosphokinase (CK), acid–base status, and kidney function should also be measured. In one case, abdominal radiography showed barium, but the sensitivity and specificity of radiography for barium poisoning is unknown.[18]

MANAGEMENT

Toxicologic etiologies for flaccid paralysis such as hypermagnesemia, botulism, and the administration of neuromuscular blockers should be evaluated while the serum potassium concentration is being determined. Once the hypokalemia is diagnosed, other causes of acute hypokalemia (Chap. 12) associated with paralysis such as periodic hypokalemic paralysis, toluene toxicity, and diuretic use are included in the differential diagnosis if there is no history or laboratory confirmation of barium exposure.

Patients who are asymptomatic at 6 hours following ingestion with normal potassium concentrations can be discharged. Patients with signs or symptoms of toxicity should be admitted to an intensive care unit with expectant management of respiratory compromise and cardiovascular instability.

DECONTAMINATION

Activated charcoal is unlikely to be effective. Orogastric lavage is reasonable in patients who present early after ingestion, but lavage is unlikely to provide substantial benefit in patients who are already symptomatic or who have had spontaneous emesis. Oral sodium sulfate administration theoretically prevents absorption by precipitating unabsorbed barium ions as insoluble, nontoxic barium sulfate. Oral magnesium sulfate has had similar efficacy.[21] Early administration of oral magnesium sulfate is a reasonable intervention; the dose is 250 mg/kg for children and 30 g for adults.[23] Intravenous magnesium sulfate or sodium sulfate is not recommended because of its potential to produce acute kidney injury due to precipitation of barium in the renal tubules.[25,36]

Patients in respiratory failure should receive assisted ventilation. Expeditious correction of hypokalemia is important to minimize the risk or to treat cardiac dysrhythmias. It should be anticipated that large doses of potassium replacement (400 mEq in 24 hours) will be required to correct serum potassium although as noted above repletion of potassium alone may be inadequate to improve the resting membrane potential or muscle strength[18] (Chap. 12). As hypokalemia is due to intracellular sequestration of potassium, potassium supplementation increases the total body potassium load. In this situation, rebound hyperkalemia should be expected when barium is eliminated, especially in patients with acute or chronic kidney disease. Observation and serial evaluation for this clinical complication is essential.

Elimination Enhancement

If hypokalemia is unable to be corrected or if the correction of hypokalemia does not restore normal motor function and muscle strength, hemodialysis is recommended. Case reports suggest that hemodialysis for the management of severe barium toxicity is associated with rapid clinical improvement.[2,28,31,35] Additionally, in a case report, continuous veno-venous hemodiafiltration provided a clinically significant increase in measured barium elimination, stabilized serum potassium concentrations, and was associated with rapidly improved motor strength.[18]

Management of Intravasation

Following intravasation of oral barium sulfate patients should be admitted to an intensive care unit. Expectant management should include evaluation of intraabdominal sepsis, hemorrhage and trauma, pulmonary embolus, and barium toxicity.[22] Prophylactic antibiotics use appears reasonable and serial determinations of serum potassium concentrations are warranted. Computed tomography scanning of the chest and abdomen can demonstrate both the location and extent of the barium sulfate administered.[32]

SUMMARY

- Although poisoning by barium salts is rare, these salts are widely used in industry and therefore represent a substantial risk for human exposure.
- The hallmark of barium salt toxicity is rapidly developing and severe hypokalemia with attendant weakness progressing to paralysis.
- In addition to supportive care, the mainstay of treatment is rapid correction of hypokalemia.
- Hypokalemia results from an intracellular shift of potassium. As toxicity resolves and potassium redistributes into the extracellular space, cautious evaluation for the development of hyperkalemia is essential.
- Extracorporeal therapies are reasonable in cases of refractory hypokalemia.

REFERENCES

1. Aks SE, et al. Barium sulfide ingestions in an urban correctional facility population. *J Prison Jail Health* 1993;12:3-12.
2. Bahlmann H, et al. Acute barium nitrate intoxication treated by hemodialysis. *Acta Anaesthesiol Scand.* 2005;49:110-112.

3. Bhoelan BS, et al. Barium toxicity and the role of the potassium inward rectifier current. *Clin Toxicol (Phila)* 2014;52:584-593.

4. Chilton L, Loutzenhiser R. Functional evidence for an inward rectifier potassium current in rat renal afferent arterioles. *Circ Res.* 2001;88:152-158.

5. Crafoord B, Ekwall B. Time-related lethal blood concentrations from acute human poisoning of chemicals. Part 2: The Monographs. No. 37 Barium.

6. Dawes M, et al. Barium reduces resting blood flow and inhibits potassium-induced vasodilation in the human forearm. *Circulation.* 2002;105:1323-1328.

7. de Feiter PW, et al. Rectal perforations after barium enema: a review. *Dis Colon Rectum.* 2006;49:261-271.

8. Deixonne B, et al. A case of barium-peritoneum with neurological involvement. Importance of barium determination in biological fluids. *J Chir (Paris).* 1983;120:611-613.

9. Deng JF, et al. The essential role of a poison center in handling an outbreak of barium carbonate poisoning. *Vet Human Toxicol.* 1991;33:173-175.

10. Dhamija RM, et al. Acute paralysis due to barium carbonate. *J Assoc Physicians India.* 1990;38:948-949.

11. Downs JC, et al. Suicidal ingestion of barium-sulfide-containing shaving powder. *Am J Forensic Med Pathol.* 1995;16:56-61.

12. Fogliani J, et al. Voluntary barium poisoning. *Ann Fr Anesth Reanim.* 1993;12:508-511.

13. Ghose A, et al. Mass barium carbonate poisoning with fatal outcome, lessons learned: a case series. *Cases J.* 2009;2:9069.

14. Gross GF, Howard MA. Perforations of the colon from barium enema. *Am Surg.* 1972;38:583-585.

15. Jacobs IA, et al. Poisoning as a result of barium styphnate explosion. *Am J Ind Med.* 2002;41:285-288.

16. Johnson CH, VanTassell VJ. Acute barium poisoning with respiratory failure and rhabdomyolysis. *Ann Emerg Med.* 1991;20:1138-1142.

17. Jourdan S, et al. Suicidal poisoning with barium chloride. *Forensic Sci Int.* 2001;119:263-265.

18. Koch M, et al. Acute barium intoxication and hemodiafiltration. *J Toxicol Clin Toxicol.* 2003;41:363-367.

19. Lewis JW Jr, et al. Barium granuloma of the rectum: an uncommon complication of barium enema. *Ann.Surg.* 1975;181:418-423.

20. Lukasik-Głębocka, et al. Barium determination in gastric contents, blood and urine by inductively coupled plasma mass spectrometry in the case of oral barium chloride poisoning. *J Anal Toxicol.* 2014;38:380-382.

21. Mills K, Kunkel D. Prevention of severe barium carbonate toxicity with oral magnesium sulfate. *Vet Human Toxicol.* 1993;35:342.

22. O'Hara DE, et al. Barium intravasation during an upper gastro-intestinal examination: a case report and literature review. *Am Surg.* 1995;61:330-333.

23. Payen C, et al. Intoxication by large amounts of barium nitrate overcome by early massive K supplementation and oral administration of magnesium sulphate. *Hum Exp Toxicol.* 2011;30:34-37.

24. Pelissier-Alicot AL, et al. Fatal poisoning due to intravasation after oral administration of barium sulfate for contrast radiography. *Forensic Sci Int.* 1999;106:109-113.

25. Phelan DM, et al. Is hypokalaemia the cause of paralysis in barium poisoning? *BMJ (Clin Res Ed).* 1984;289:882.

26. Rhyee SH, Heard K. Acute barium toxicity from ingestion of "snake" fireworks. *J Med Toxicol.* 2009;5:209-213.

27. Salvo AF, et al. Barium intravasation into portal venous system during barium enema examination. *JAMA.* 1976;235:749-751.

28. Schorn TF, et al. Barium carbonate intoxication. *Intensive Care Med.* 1991;17:60-62.

29. Silva RF. Barium toxicity after exposure to contaminated contrast solution—Goias State, Brazil, 2003. *MMWR Morb Mortal Wkly Rep.* 2003;52:1047-1048.

30. Soghoian S, et al. Unintentional intravenous injection of barium sulfate in a child. *Clin Toxicol.* 2008;46:387.

31. Szajewski J. High-potassium haemodialysis in barium poisoning. *J Toxicol Clin Toxicol.* 2004;42:117.

32. Takahashi M, et al. Nonfatal barium intravasation into the portal venous system during barium enema examination. *Intern Med.* 2004;43:1145-1150.

33. Thomas M, et al. Acute barium intoxication following ingestion of ceramic glaze. *Postgrad Med J.* 1998;74:545-546.

34. Tsai CY, et al. Acute barium intoxication following accidental inhalation of barium chloride. *Intern Med J.* 2011;41:293-295.

35. Wells JA, Wood KE. Acute barium poisoning treated with hemodialysis. *Am J Emerg Med.* 2001;19:175-177.

36. Wetherill SF, et al. Acute renal failure associated with barium chloride poisoning. *Ann Intern Med.* 1981;95:187-188.

37. White JS, et al. Intravasation of barium sulphate at barium enema examination. *Br J Radiol.* 2006;79:e32-e35.

38. World Health Organization: *Environmental Health Criteria 107: Barium.* IPCS INCHEM. 1-1-1990. 7-2-2005.

108 FUMIGANTS

Shahin Shadnia and Kambiz Soltaninejad

HISTORY AND EPIDEMIOLOGY

The proper use of pesticides has a beneficial role in human health by increasing the quality and quantity of crops. Alternatively, acute and chronic pesticide poisoning are significant causes of morbidity and mortality worldwide, especially in developing countries, making pesticide poisoning a global public health problem.[78,191]

Fumigants are nonspecific pesticides applied to kill and control rodents, nematodes, insects, weed seeds, and fungi anywhere in soil, in structures, crops, grains, and commodities.[37] They represent a diverse group of pesticides that are dissimilar in their chemical structures, physical properties, and mechanisms of toxicity (Tables 108–1 and 108–2). Many fumigants, particularly the halogenated solvents, have been largely abandoned because of their toxicity. In the 1987 Montreal Protocol, an international agreement was adopted to phase out ozone-depleting chemicals, such as methyl bromide, which was scheduled to be discontinued in 2005. Unfortunately, many agricultural companies received exemptions, as satisfactory substitutes for some of methyl bromide uses have not emerged.

Because fumigants exist as solids that release toxic gases on reacting with water (zinc phosphide, aluminum phosphide) or with acids (sodium or calcium cyanide), as liquids (ethylene dibromide, dibromochloropropane, formaldehyde) that can vaporize at ambient temperature, or as gases (methyl bromide, hydrogen cyanide, ethylene oxide), inhalation is the most common route of exposure (Table 108–1). In their gaseous forms, fumigants are generally heavier than air and will be found concentrated just above the ground surface and lower floors of buildings.

Their exposure risk is enhanced by their general lack of warning properties, non–species-selective effects, and high potency. Although xenobiotics from many different chemical classes were used in the past as fumigants, only a few remain in use today in the United States. This chapter summarizes the remaining US fumigants and also highlights important fumigants that are in use in developing countries.

METAL PHOSPHIDES AND PHOSPHINE

Introduction

In addition to the organic phosphorus and organic chlorine compounds, metal phosphides (aluminum, zinc, magnesium, and calcium) have been used as rodenticides and fumigants around the world for many years. The metal phosphides are advantageous because of their low cost, high effectiveness in destroying harmful insects and rodents, freedom from toxic residue, and lack of adverse effects on seed viability. Metal phosphides are used to protect grain held in silos, in the holds of ships, and during transportation by rail. They are generally admixed with the grain at a predetermined

rate at the initiation of storage.[163] Following exposure to ambient moisture, the metal phosphides release phosphine gas (PH_3). Exposure to water results in rapid release, highlighting the concern for their use as chemical weapons.[25] Phosphine gas itself is also used in the synthesis of flame retardants, organic phosphorus compounds, pharmaceuticals, and in the production of semiconductors.[170]

History and Epidemiology

Over the last decades, cases of PH_3 and metal phosphide poisonings have escalated, carrying a high mortality rate, likely related to the use of these chemicals for suicides.[42,64,93,98,131,179,190,197] Unintentional poisoning as a result of negligence or ignorance are also reported.[54,120,160,172] Aluminum phosphide (AlP) poisoning is one of the commonest causes of poisoning both in adults and children in agricultural societies and developing countries, such as India, Sri Lanka, and Iran.[68,72,110,148,173,177] The incidence of AlP poisoning is low in developed countries;[155,160] however, PH_3 poisoning has increased in frequency as it is a by-product of the use of red phosphorus in the synthesis of methamphetamines.[33,215]

Physicochemical Properties

Commercially, AlP (molecular weight of 57.95 Da) is most widely available as a greenish-gray tablet or pellet bag and granular form that has a garlic odor. The 3-g tablet usually contains AlP (56%), ammonium carbamate, and urea, which liberates PH_3 (up to 1 g), ammonia, and carbon dioxide. Each pellet (0.6 g) releases 0.2 g PH_3.

Zinc phosphide (Zn_3P_2; molecular weight of 258.1 Da) is available as a dark-gray powder or as quadrilateral crystals that have an odor of acetylene or rotten fish. Calcium phosphide (Ca_3P_2; molecular weight of 182.2 Da) is available as a reddish-brown crystal powder. Magnesium phosphide (Mg_3P_2; molecular weight of 134.8 Da) is a white crystalline solid.[15,143]

In the presence of moisture or acid, metal phosphides are converted to PH_3 (hydrogen phosphide, phosphorus trihydride, molecular weight of 34 Da):

$$AlP + 3H_2O = Al(OH)_3 + PH_3$$
$$Zn_3P_2 + 6H_2O = 3Zn(OH)_2 + 2PH_3$$
$$Mg_3P_2 + 6H_2O = 3Mg(OH)_2 + 2PH_3$$

or

$$AlP + 3H^+ = Al^{3+} + PH_3$$
$$Zn_3P_2 + 6H^+ = 3Zn^{2+} + 2PH_3$$
$$Mg_3P_2 + 6H^+ = 3Mg^{2+} + 2PH_3$$

The release of PH_3 is even more vigorous after contact with an aqueous acid, such as hydrochloric acid. The residue, $Al(OH)_3$, is nontoxic.[15,170] Phosphine gas is flammable, and other by-products of commercial tablets (diphosphine gas) are spontaneously flammable in air concentrations above the lower explosive limit (LEL) of 1.8% v/v.[100,130,175,201,214,216] In aqueous solutions, PH_3 produces phosphinic, phosphonic and phosphoric acids, which are all corrosive and produce exothermic reactions.[130,170]

Although PH_3 is colorless and odorless in pure form up to toxic concentrations (200 parts per million {ppm}), the presence of substituted phosphines and diphosphines imparts a decaying fish or garlic odor that is detectable at concentrations of as little as 2 ppm.[159,163,170]

Toxicokinetics

Following ingestion—the most common route of exposure—metal phosphides react with acidic fluid in the gastrointestinal (GI) tract to release PH_3,

TABLE 108–1	Physical Properties and Industrial Uses of Fumigants				
Fumigant	Color	State	Flammability	Odor	Use
Phosphine	Colorless	Gas	High	Rotten fish Garlic	Rodenticide
Methyl bromide	Colorless	Gas	No	None at low concentrations. Sweet chloroformlike at high concentrations	Soil Structural Crop
Dichloropropene	Yellow	Liquid	No	Garlic	Soil
Sulfuryl fluoride	Colorless	Gas	No	None	Structural

TABLE 108–2	Comparison of Clinical Effects of Fumigants

Fumigant	Mucous Membrane Irritation	Dermatitis	Burns (Frostbite)	Gastrointestinal: Nausea, Vomiting, Abdominal Pain	Hepatic Dysfunction	Chest Pain	Adult Respiratory Distress Syndrome	Nephrotoxicity	Hypotension	Dysrhythmias	Mental Status Changes
Phosphine	++	−		+	+	+	+	+	++	+	+
Methyl bromide	± High concentration	+	+	+	+	+	+	+	+	+	+
Dichloropropene	+	+	−	+	+	+	+		+	+	+
Sulfuryl fluoride	± High concentration	+	+	+	−	−	+	+	++	−	+

− = Absent; + = Present; ++ = Very substantial; ± = Variable.

which is rapidly absorbed. Metal phosphides may be absorbed as microscopic particles of unhydrolyzed salt and subsequently converted to PH_3. Phosphine gas is also absorbed from respiratory tract mucosa if inhaled. Dermal absorption is insignificant.[15]

There are no data about distribution of PH_3 in humans, but it would be expected that as a small soluble molecule PH_3 is widely distributed.[15,163] Its half-life ranges from 5 to 24 hours based on various factors.[209] Phosphine gas is detectable in the blood of severely poisoned patients and is also found in the kidney, brain, and liver of decedents following ingestion.[11,49] In vitro studies demonstrated that PH_3 interacts irreversibly with free hemoglobin and hemoglobin in intact erythrocytes (rat and human) that results in the production of Heinz bodies and hemichromes, which are methemoglobin derivatives.[40,161] Rare clinical presentations such as intravascular hemolysis and methemoglobinemia support the involvement of erythrocytes in the biotransformation of PH_3 in humans.[163]

Phosphate, hypophosphite, and phosphite are identified in the urine, whereas PH_3 itself is exhaled.[81,163]

Toxicodynamics

The toxicity of metal phosphides is due to PH_3 release. Phosphine gas is a protoplasmic toxin. The mechanisms of toxicity include blocking the electron transport chain and oxidative phosphorylation through noncompetitive inhibition of cytochrome-c oxidase.[9,182] Phosphine gas decreases the activities of mitochondrial complexes I, II, IV, V. This inhibits cellular respiration and ATP production and leads to the formation of highly reactive hydroxyl radicals that cause additional damage.[10,26,59,60,102,170,182,185] Phosphine gas also inhibits catalase, induces superoxide dismutase, and reduces the glutathione (GSH) concentration. All of these effects combine to result in lipid peroxidation, protein denaturation of cell membranes, and DNA damage, leading to widespread cellular damage and ion channel dysfunction.[10,47,48,50,60,82,94,102,109,170,185,200,203]

Because PH_3 is corrosive, it directly injures the alveolar capillary membrane in addition to producing oxidative injury, leading to an acute respiratory distress syndrome (ARDS).[81,179] Although both AlP and PH_3 inhibit cholinesterase activity, this effect is unlikely to have substantial clinical relevance.[6,127,128,142,162]

Toxic Dose

Ingestion of 1 g of zinc phosphide can causes toxicity in humans, and death is reported after ingestion of 4 g. Ingestion of 500 mg of AlP can be fatal.[16] The recommended exposure limit (REL) of PH_3 in the workplace is less than 0.3 ppm as a time-weighted average (TWA) for up to 10 hours per day during a 40-hour work week, and 1 ppm as a 15-minute short-term exposure limit (STEL) that should not be exceeded at any time during a workday. The National Institute of Occupational Safety and Health established 50 ppm as the concentration that is immediately dangerous to life or health (IDLH) for PH_3.[153,196] Workplace standards are not available for AlP specifically.[196]

Clinical Manifestations

The smell of garlic or decaying fish on the breath is a common finding and results from oral or inhalational poisoning with metal phosphides and PH_3.[160] The clinical manifestations are dependent on the dose, route of entry, and time since exposure.[81] After ingestion, the onset of toxicity usually is slightly more rapid for AlP (10–15 minutes) than for zinc phosphide (20–40 minutes).[80,108] In patients with mild poisoning, nausea, repeated vomiting, thirst, diarrhea, abdominal discomfort or pain, especially epigastric pain, and tachycardia are common clinical manifestations. In those with moderate to severe effects, palpitations, tachypnea, GI manifestations, dysrhythmias, ARDS, hypotension, shock, and cardiovascular collapse, occur rapidly.[72,93,98,106,109,110,131,146,163,177,197]

Restlessness, anxiety, dizziness, ataxia, numbness, paresthesias, and tremor are universally observed, but central nervous system (CNS) manifestations are not prominent until a secondary event, such as hypoxia occurs.[93,110,197] Late and severe neurologic findings include delirium, convulsions, ischemic/hemorrhagic stroke and coma.[1,27,55]

Following limited PH_3 inhalational exposure, patients commonly have airway irritation and breathlessness.[170] Other features include chest tightness, tachycardia, headache, nausea, vomiting, diarrhea, numbness, muscle weakness, and diplopia.[72,80,196]

Uncommon complications of metal phosphides and PH_3 poisoning include gastroduodenitis, hepatitis,[51] ascites,[22] pancreatitis,[211] myocardial infarction,[104,111] acute pericarditis,[44] pleural effusion,[67,198] rhabdomyolysis,[163] acute tubular necrosis, adrenocortical congestion, hemorrhage and/or necrosis,[12] and delayed esophageal stricture or tracheoesophageal fistulas.[23,105,113,123,152,210] Liver and kidney failure, as well as disseminated intravascular coagulation (DIC), are also rarely reported following acute poisoning.[22,54,72,163,196]

Diagnostic Testing

Initial investigations should include electrocardiography (ECG) and continuous cardiac monitoring, chest radiograph, blood glucose, blood gases, serum electrolytes, complete blood count (CBC), liver, and kidney function studies.

Hypokalemia is common after oral poisoning.[98,131,163] Magnesium concentrations are reported as normal, increased, or decreased.[10,41,43,45,46,180,181,183,197] Hypoglycemia as a result of impaired gluconeogenesis, glycogenolysis, and possibly due to adrenal insufficiency is common and at times severe and persistent.[52,66,107,137] Hyperglycemia and metabolic acidosis are also reported.[93,134,135,177,197] Hemolysis, methemoglobinemia, leukopenia, and hyperbilirubinemia are unusual complications of metal phosphides poisonings.[112,116,146,156,170,176,188,193]

Electrocardiographic abnormalities are very common, but highly variable, and include rhythm disturbances, ST segment and T wave changes, QRS complex widening, and conduction defects that revert to a normal pattern within several days.[43,103,170,179,189] During the first 3 to 6 hours after poisoning, sinus tachycardia is predominant, followed over the next 6 to 12 hours by ST segment and T wave changes, conduction disturbances, and dysrhythmias.[187] Ventricular tachycardia, ventricular fibrillation, supraventricular tachycardia, and atrial flutter/fibrillation are the most common consequential dysrhythmias.[184] Echocardiography typically reveals cardiac dysfunction, dilation, and hypokinesia or akinesia of the left ventricle that typically resolves over several days.[5,24,25,79]

Chest radiography shows diffuse infiltration, pulmonary edema, ARDS, and atelectasis.[143,170] As aluminum and PH$_3$ both inhibit cholinesterase,[6,127,128,162] measurement of cholinesterase activity in the presence of cholinergic findings is recommended.[110]

Toxicological Analyses

Chemical analysis for PH$_3$ in blood or urine is not recommended and is not typically helpful as PH$_3$ is rapidly oxidized to phosphite and hypophosphite.[15,81,163] The presence of PH$_3$ is suggested by a positive silver nitrate test on gastric contents or exhaled breath. In this test, which is a simple and sensitive method to detect PH$_3$, paper impregnated with silver nitrate will turn black (silver phosphide) in the presence of PH$_3$.[141] The detection limit of the test is 0.05 ppm for PH$_3$.

The ammonium molybdate test is another chemical method that is used for the qualitative or quantitative analysis of phosphorus, PH$_3$, and phosphides in the stomach contents and postmortem samples. Formation of canary yellow precipitates confirms the presence of PH$_3$ or phosphides.[65,114]

Headspace gas chromatographic with a nitrogen-phosphorous detector (HS-GC/NPD) is a specific and sensitive test for PH$_3$ or phosphides.[149] Headspace gas chromatography coupled with mass spectrometry (HS-GC-MS) was described for the analysis of the PH$_3$ metabolites in biological samples. The detection limit of this method for PH$_3$ is 0.2 mcg/mL.[217] Unfortunately, none of these tests are available in a time frame to permit their clinical utility.

Prognosis

The mortality rate following ingestion of metal phosphides is reportedly 31% to 77%.[41-43,63,98,109,121,131,174,177,197] Most of the deaths occur within 12 to 24 hours and are due to cardiovascular collapse.[8,189] After 24 hours, most of the deaths are due to refractory shock, severe acidemia, and ARDS.[213] Fulminant hepatic failure develops within 72 hours after poisoning and is another cause of delayed death.[12]

In some studies of acute AlP poisoning, vomiting after ingestion was significantly more common in survivors. Nonsurvivors ingested significantly higher doses of AlP and had greater delays from exposure to treatment initiation. In nonsurvivors blood pressure and level of consciousness were significantly altered on admission.[93,173,177,197] The Acute Physiology and Chronic Health Evaluation (APACHE) Score and Simplified Acute Physiology Score (SAPS) are significantly higher in nonsurvivors than survivors.[98,131,174]

Metabolic acidosis with an elevated lactate concentration is an index of severity of AlP poisoning. It was demonstrated that there is significant correlation between blood lactate concentration and time of death in the nonsurvivors. Also, derived from this study, the line of best fit connecting the blood lactate concentration of 5.4 mmol/L at 4 hours and 2.8 mmol/L at 24 hours post ingestion was used to predict the likelihood of death.[63]

Treatment

The victim should immediately be removed from the area of exposure to fresh air, and supplemental oxygen should be provided as needed.[81,163] Clinical staff and other health care professionals should use universal precautions, including gloves, goggles, N95 respirators and other PPE as indicated (Special Considerations: SC2),[141] with the understanding that a particulate mask will not protect against PH$_3$. Staff should also be aware of the risk for spontaneous ignition.[175,214] As PH$_3$ is absorbed cutaneously, the patient's clothes should be removed and the skin and eyes decontaminated with water as early as possible.[72]

In oral exposure, gastric emptying is reasonable if it is done within a few hours of ingestion and significant emesis has not already occurred (Chap. 5). The acidic content of stomach facilitates the conversion of metal phosphides

to PH$_3$. As a result, some authors suggest the oral administration of sodium bicarbonate (88 mEq), but this is not supported by clinical trials, and therefore not recommended at this time.[4,81,82,84,93,110,124,200] Potassium permanganate (KMnO$_4$) (1:10,000) was used as an adjunct to gastric lavage to oxidize PH$_3$ to nontoxic phosphate.[4,82,84,93,124,158,197,200] Neither this approach nor the use of boric acid[186] is recommended because of multiple associated risks and no proven benefit.[140]

There is limited evidence that activated charcoal (AC) (Chap. 5 and Antidotes in Depth: A1) fails to reduces GI absorption even if administered rapidly following ingestion.[84,93,110] Its use is therefore not routinely recommended.[124]

In vitro studies suggest that lipid, mainly vegetable oils and liquid paraffin, inhibit PH$_3$ release from the ingested AlP.[4,76,93,165,171,187] Unfortunately, aspiration is a significant risk with oil ingestion and these data are too premature to recommend the routine use of oils at this time.

Management should be rapidly initiated based on a history and clinical examination that support metal phosphides or PH$_3$ poisoning, and should not be delayed for a confirmatory diagnosis.[81] Standard supportive care to address ventilatory and vital sign abnormalities should be administered. If necessary, norepinephrine or phenylephrine are recommended.[81,84]

As there is no known specific antidote, management remains primarily intensive monitoring and supportive treatment, to allow sufficient time for the poison to be eliminated. Hypoglycemia, hypokalemia, and ARDS, should be managed conventionally.[81,84,163] Aggressive correction of severe acidemia in acute AlP poisoning with IV sodium bicarbonate theoretically improves the outcome,[84,106,125] and is reasonable as long as the sodium load can be tolerated.

In view of the role of oxidative stress in toxicity from metal phosphides or PH$_3$, antioxidants such as N-acetylcysteine (NAC), vitamin C, vitamin E, magnesium, melatonin, and methylene blue were investigated both in experimental and clinical studies.[38,50]

The beneficial effects of NAC in animal studies are variable.[13,71] In a human study, NAC administration at a dose of 140 mg/kg IV infusion as a loading dose and 70 mg/kg IV infusion every 4 hours up to 17 doses significantly decreased the plasma malondialdehyde (MDA) concentration as a biomarker of lipid peroxidation, the duration of hospitalization, and rate of intubation. In that study, the mortality rate in NAC treatment and control groups were 36% and 60%, respectively.[200] In another clinical study, NAC administration significantly decreased the mortality rate and increased the duration of survival in fatal cases in the treatment group.[3] For these reasons, we recommend the utilization of NAC at these doses (Antidotes in Depth: A3).

Administration of vitamin E (alpha tocopherol) at a dose of 400 mg IM, every 12 hours for 72 hours in a human study, significantly decreased the plasma MDA concentration and the necessity for, and duration of, intubation and mechanical ventilation. This treatment also significantly decreased the mortality rate from 50% in control group to 15% in treatment group.[82] Given these encouraging results and limited safety concerns, it is reasonable to administer vitamin E in cases of life-threating toxicity, if it is available.

In a limited study, the use of oral liothyronine with a dose of 50 mcg in the first 6 hours of poisoning as an adjuvant therapy in acute AlP poisoning was suggested to decrease lipid peroxidation and improve systolic blood pressure and arterial blood pH.[73] There is inadequate evidence to recommend routine utilization at this time.

The use of magnesium sulfate (MgSO$_4$) in metal phosphides or PH$_3$ poisoning remains controversial and unsubstantiated.[81,163,183] Because of the low risk of the use of MgSO$_4$ in metal phosphides or PH$_3$ poisoning and the recent study showing its usefulness,[177] it is reasonable to utilize MgSO$_4$ utilization at standard intravenous doses.[84] Dysrhythmias should be treated with standard antidysrhythmics.[84,102,136,166]

The benefit of highdose insulin (HDI) treatment (Antidotes in Depth: A21) is suggested by preliminary investigations in that insulin promotes energy production from carbohydrates, restores calcium flux, and improves myocardial contractility.[85] There is inadequate evidence to routinely recommend this intervention; however, in cases of refractory shock, a trial of HDI is reasonable.

The use of an intraaortic balloon pump in circulatory failure due to acute AlP poisoning is reported.[21,61,138,178] It is only recommended following failure of all other procedures.

Clinical studies showed the beneficial effects of venoarterial extracorporeal membrane oxygenation (VA-ECMO) with regard to improvement of short-term survival patients with acute AlP poisoning. If available, VA-ECMO is recommended in the management of a subset of acute AlP-poisoned patients with severe left ventricular dysfunction (LV ejection fraction ≤35%), refractory cardiogenic shock, and severe acidemia (pH ≤7) who do not respond to conventional treatment.[61,86,139,144,145]

One study reported the beneficial effect of IV administration of lipid emulsion (20%) at a dose of 10 mL/hour in 2 cases with AlP poisoning.[19] Given the lack of beneficial evidence for intravenous lipid emulsion (ILE) in oral overdoses, its complication rate, and its ability to interfere with ECMO, we recommend not to use ILE in this setting unless there are no other options in cardiac resuscitation available (Antidotes in Depth: A23). High-dose L-carnitine (1 g 3 times a day for 10 days) was given as an essential cofactor in fatty acid metabolism.[61]

Because the experimental and clinical evidence shows that both PH$_3$ and aluminum inhibit acetylcholinesterase,[6,127,128,162] atropine and pralidoxime have theoretical roles in management.[110] Further studies are recommended to confirm usefulness of oximes.[142] Neither atropine nor oximes are routinely recommended at this time.

In another experimental study, the protective role of iron sucrose as an electron receiver was shown potentially be a competitor with mitochondrial respiratory chain complexes.[185] Once again these data are too preliminary to recommend the use of this approach.

Experimental data suggest that hyperbaric oxygenation (HBO) improves the survival time of poisoned rats, with no change in the mortality rate.[164] There is inadequate evidence to recommend the use of HBO for this toxin.

Hemodialysis is not very effective in removing PH$_3$,[83,151] but is recommended in patients with acute kidney failure, severe metabolic acidemia, or fluid overload.[61,81]

The sole recognized approach remains intensive care monitoring and supportive treatment.

METHYL BROMIDE

History and Epidemiology

Methyl bromide was used as an anesthetic in the early 1900s, but fatalities halted this practice. Today, methyl bromide is used widely as a fumigant for all types of dry food stuffs, in grain elevators, mills, ships, warehouses, greenhouses, and food-processing facilities for the control of nematodes, fungi, and weeds. It is also used as an insecticide, fire extinguisher, and refrigerant, although its domestic use was banned in 1987. Methyl bromide is also used as a methylating chemical in manufacturing and as a low-boiling solvent for extracting oils from nuts, seeds, and flowers. It is termed a structural or commodity fumigant, which is a class term from the Environmental Protection Agency.

Historically, poisonings involving the general public were mainly associated with the methyl bromide used in fire extinguishers. Other poisoning involved unauthorized entry into buildings being fumigated with methyl bromide.[20,87,117]

Occupational and environmental exposures to methyl bromide as a fumigant are most common. Hazardous materials incidents are reported for methyl bromide, during manufacture or as a result of use and transport,[28,32,69] but they are relatively uncommon in plant employees or residents living adjacent to agricultural fields where methyl bromide is applied.[32,36] Before 1955, the majority of methyl bromide poisonings resulted from chemical manufacture and filling operations. Since then, fumigation has become the major source of fatalities and fumigators, and greenhouse workers are the highest-risk group. In many countries, the use of methyl bromide is restricted to trained and licensed personnel.[62]

Methyl bromide has a threshold limit value–time weighted average (TLV-TWA) of 5 ppm and the IDLH concentration is 2,000 ppm. The Occupational Safety and Health Administration (OSHA) permissible exposure limit is 20 ppm.

Methyl bromide (CH$_3$Br) is a halogenated aliphatic hydrocarbon. It is a colorless gas at room temperature and standard pressure.[34] It is 3 times heavier than air. It is odorless except at high concentrations, when it has a burning taste and sweet, chloroformlike smell. Commercially, it is available as a liquefied gas. Some formulations also contain chloropicrin or amyl acetate as a warning agent.

Toxicokinetics

Inhalation is the primary route of exposure, although methyl bromide is rapidly absorbed through the dermal and oral routes. After absorption, methyl bromide or metabolites are rapidly distributed to many tissues, including the lungs, adrenals, kidneys, liver, brain, testis, and fat. The major organs of distribution observed immediately after exposure includes fat, lungs, liver, adrenals, and kidneys.

The metabolism of methyl bromide is not completely elucidated. Methyl bromide is partially converted to inorganic bromide in man and bromide concentrations in blood and target organs increase after exposure to methyl bromide.[20,36] It is metabolized to methyl glutathione by the enzyme glutathione S-transferase (GST) and is then converted into the neurotoxic metabolites of methanethiol and formaldehyde.[119]

Depending on the route of exposure, 16% to 40% is eliminated as metabolized methyl bromide in the urine and only 4% to 20% is eliminated in the expired air as parent compound. Biliary excretion accounts for about 46% of the elimination, generally within 24 hours following oral exposure.[7,132,133] Methyl bromide is hydrolyzed and produces methanol and hydrobromic acid in animal models.

Toxicodynamics

The mode of action of methyl bromide is still not understood. Several mechanisms of toxicity are postulated, including the direct cytotoxic effect of the intact methyl bromide molecule or toxicity due to one of its metabolites.

Methyl bromide is a potent alkylating agent with high affinity for sulfhydryl and amino groups. It reacts in vitro with a number of sulfhydryl-containing enzymes and causes irreversible inhibition of microsomal metabolism.[20,75,192] It binds to amine groups in amino acids, interfering with protein synthesis and function. Also it may methylate many other cellular components such as GSH, proteins, DNA, and RNA.[31,194] The methanethiol and formaldehyde metabolites may have a role in neurologic and visual changes. The bromide ion concentrations are insufficient to explain methyl bromide toxicity.

Clinical Manifestations

Inhalation of more than 10,000 ppm for more than a few minutes is sufficient to cause death.[87] Severe poisoning produces tremor, convulsion, rapid loss of consciousness, dysrhythmias, and death. Convulsions generally occur in fatal cases, but ARDS leading to respiratory failure or cardiovascular collapse is the leading cause of death. Pulmonary symptoms begin with cough or shortness of breath that rapidly progresses to bronchitis, pneumonitis, and ARDS.[91] In contrast, following low concentration exposure, a characteristic delay of up to 48 hours in the onset of manifestations is expected. Headache, dizziness, abdominal pain, nausea, vomiting, chest pain, and difficulty breathing are the manifestations of mild to moderate exposure. Some individuals initially manifest irritant symptoms of the eye, nasopharynx, and oropharynx, which are misdiagnosed as influenza or another viral illness. Visual disturbances such as blurred or double vision are also reported.[39,74]

The neurologic effects of methyl bromide poisoning are the most consequential and often occur without antecedent irritant effects. Initial CNS signs and symptoms that manifest in the first few hours after exposure include headache, dizziness, numbness, drowsiness, euphoria, confusion, diplopia, dysmetria, dysarthria, agitation and mood disorders, or inappropriate affect. Those findings progress rapidly in the first day or manifest over the next few days include ataxia, intention tremor, fasciculation, myoclonus, delirium, seizures, and coma.[14,34,56-58]

Methyl bromide also causes severe irritation, erythema, corrosive skin injury, blisters, and vesicles predominantly in moist areas or pressure points such as groin, axilla and wrist.[92,218] Liver and kidney damage are also described.[20,87]

Most patients who develop seizures or coma will not survive, and in those who survive, recovery typically takes months. Permanent sequelae such as neuropsychiatric impairment, ataxia, muscular weakness, irritability, blurred vision, myoclonus, and electroencephalographic (EEG) disturbances are frequent.[30,204]

Diagnostic Testing

The standard laboratory evaluations such as CBC, serum electrolytes, blood urea nitrogen (BUN), creatinine, ammonia concentration, blood gases, urinalysis, hepatic enzymes, chest radiography, and ECG, should be obtained after an acute exposure.

Although a serum bromide concentration will help to confirm the diagnosis, it is not readily available in most laboratories. Furthermore, it does not always correlate with the severity of the exposure and does not facilitate clinical management. Serum bromide concentrations are reported to remain elevated for a week or more following an acute exposure.[95] Hemoglobin adducts are used as a biologic index for exposure to methyl bromide.[101] Hemoglobin adducts have a life span of about 2 months, so workers who even have only intermittent exposure to methyl bromide benefit from testing.

The findings on magnetic resonance imaging following methyl bromide toxicity are symmetric T2 signal abnormalities in posterior putamen, subthalamic nuclei, restiform bodies, vestibular nuclei, inferior colliculi, and periaqueductal gray matter and also symmetric involvement of inferior colliculi and periaqueductal gray, as well as dentate nuclei, dorsal pons, and inferior olives.[70]

Treatment

The poisoned or exposed individual should be immediately removed from the area of exposure to fresh air. Rescue and decontamination should be performed only by personnel wearing personal protective equipment. In patients with respiratory and cardiac arrest, cardiopulmonary resuscitation should be initiated immediately when it is safe to perform. The clothing should be removed carefully, as methyl bromide adheres to clothing, including rubber and leather, and placed in plastic bags and disposed appropriately. The affected skin should be washed with soap and water. Decontamination includes irrigation of the eyes with copious amounts of 0.9% sodium chloride solution or water. It is also reasonable to administer at least one dose of oral AC following ingestion, although there is no supporting documentation for any benefit. Medical management should proceed as it would for any hazardous materials event (Chap. 132).

Management is primarily general and supportive care, and often requires intensive care unit management of coma, seizures, ARDS, and hepatic and kidney failure. Administer supplemental oxygen and treat bronchospasm, ARDS, and seizures. Seizures are common and difficult to control with traditional anticonvulsants such as benzodiazepines. Pentobarbital, high-dose thiopental, and propofol are required in many cases.[95] All exposed patients should be monitored for a minimum of 24 to 48 hours to detect delayed effects, especially ARDS.

Although dimercaprol was used for the treatment of methyl bromide poisoning, its effectiveness is only reported in less severely affected patients[87] and there is inadequate evidence to support the use of dimercaprol. The use of NAC is not studied in controlled prospective trials, but its effectiveness is reported in mild to moderate poisonings.[95] For this reason and the benignity of NAC, we recommend the utilization of NAC at standard doses.

There are no data indicating the benefit of alkalinization or hemoperfusion. Hemodialysis can rapidly clear serum bromide, but tissue injury following exposure occurs as the bromide is released into the serum, suggesting that the methylation of neuronal proteins and neurologic injury has already occurred. Post hemodialysis, neurologic improvement is reported, but severe disabilities typically remain. Thus, there is inadequate evidence to support the use of hemodialysis.

DICHLOROPROPENE

History and Epidemiology

1,3-Dichloropropene is a volatile chlorinated aliphatic hydrocarbon that was introduced in 1945 and is primarily used as a soil fumigant for nematodes. Its use escalated after the restriction of ethylene dibromide, methyl bromide, and dibromochloropropane in 1956. The current formulation contains dichloropropene solubilized in soybean oil.[205]

Exposures are reported during production, application, and ingestion, most commonly in occupational settings where formulations are manufactured or applied. Unintentional releases during transport resulted in several poisonings.[126] The OSHA standard TLV-TWA for dermal exposure is 1 ppm.[118]

Toxicokinetics

Dichloropropene is rapidly absorbed by the oral, inhalational, and dermal routes. Oral exposure is theoretically possible through contaminated groundwater, but this is not reported in humans. Inhalation is the primary route of human exposure and dichloropropene is rapidly absorbed from the lungs.[29,207]

No human data describe systemic distribution, but animal studies show that tissue concentrations after dichloropropene ingestion were highest in the stomach, followed by the blood, bone, brain, heart, kidneys, liver, bladder, skin, skeletal muscle, spleen, ovaries, testes, and fat.[18]

The metabolism of dichloropropene is similar to that of other chlorinated hydrocarbon solvents such as carbon tetrachloride and chloroform (Chap. 105). In humans, dichloropropene is metabolized in liver via oxidation in a phase I biotransformation,[17,129,195] which is catalyzed by CYP2E1[77] and then glutathione-dependent biotransformation.[29,207,212] Toxicity is proposed to result from metabolism via an electrophilic epoxide intermediate.[208] Most of the glutathione-conjugated form of dichloropropene is eliminated by the kidneys, and smaller amounts are eliminated in the feces.[53,96,205]

Toxicodynamics

Human and animal health effects include damage to the liver, kidney, lung, CNS, myocardium, GI tract, skin, and mucous membranes. The exact mechanisms of toxicity are not clear, but data suggest that there is more than one mechanistic pathway in humans.

Glutathione depletion is documented in the rat model. The dose and route of dichloropene correlated with toxicity and outcome in rodent models. At 100 mg/kg in mice, hepatotoxicity occurred by the intraperitoneal route, but not after oral gavage. At 700 mg/kg administered by the intraperitoneal route, hepatic failure and death resulted.[17] The higher dose correlated with a 130-fold increase in dichloropropene epoxide formation. Interestingly, in a rat hepatocyte model, pretreatment with the antioxidant, α-tocopherol, prevented cell death.[199]

Clinical Manifestations

Signs and symptoms of acute oral or inhalational exposure include nausea, vomiting, bloody diarrhea, pancreatitis, hepatotoxicity, tachycardia and hypotension,[90] dyspnea,[97] ARDS,[90] CNS depression,[126] acute kidney injury (acute tubular necrosis),[90] and muscle pain and weakness.[126] Coagulopathy and thrombocytopenia, hyperglycemia, severe metabolic acidosis,[90] and intravascular fluid depletion secondary to hemorrhage are reported. Dermal manifestations include contact hypersensitivity,[87,205,206] erythema,[126] and profuse sweating.[90] Mucous membrane irritation including erythema, edema, and irritation of the eyes, ears, nose, and throat occurs.[126,205] Concentrations above 1,000 ppm cause lacrimation.[2] Hematologic malignancies including lymphoma and histiocytic lymphoma were reported after prolonged (6 years) dichloropropene exposure.[126]

Radiographic abnormalities typically lag behind clinical signs. It may take up to 8 hours before abnormalities appear on chest radiography, even in symptomatic patients.[90]

Weight loss, hyperemia and superficial ulcerations of the nasal mucosa, inflammation of the pharynx, bleeding from swollen gums,[126] hepatic aminotransferase elevations, and kidney function abnormalities[29] are reported after chronic exposure to dichloropropene.

Diagnostic Testing

Liver and kidney function should be monitored following acute poisoning.[90] No additional or specific tests are recommended beyond those needed for supportive care. Biomonitoring for exposure to dichloropropene is under development.[29] Hepatic gamma-glutamyl transpeptidase (GGT) concentrations are increased in fumigators, but the increase is not statistically significant. However, this finding suggests hepatic enzyme induction. In fumigators, erythrocyte GST and GSH concentrations decreased with increased serum creatinine concentrations and increased urine concentrations of albumin and retinol-binding protein when compared with controls.[29]

Treatment

Because of the volatility of dichloropropene, caution should be used to avoid continued inhalational and dermal exposure for both the patient and the health care professionals. Symptomatic and supportive care should be provided as for methyl bromide. Following ingestion, oral AC is reasonable, but there is no proven value. Orogastric lavage is also reasonable in a patient presenting shortly following ingestion. Exposed eyes should be irrigated with copious amounts of water or 0.9% sodium chloride solution for at least 15 minutes, and exposed skin should be similarly washed with soap.[115]

There are no data to support specific therapies beyond supportive care, although the use of antioxidant therapy and NAC warrants further study. The patients should be monitored for at least 24 hours after exposure.

SULFURYL FLUORIDE

History and Epidemiology

Sulfuryl fluoride has been used since 1957 as a structural fumigant insecticide to control wood-boring insects such as termites in homes. Structure or tent fumigation is performed by completely enclosing a house or other structure in plastic or a tarpaulin, and then sulfuryl fluoride is pumped in as a compressed gas. Chloropicrin is typically added as a warning agent. Although sulfuryl fluoride is commonly used in Florida, California,[147,157] and Washington, a 5-year review of fumigant illness did not contain any reports of sulfuryl fluoride toxicity.[32]

Toxicokinetics and Toxicodynamics

Sulfuryl fluoride gas is colorless, odorless, and heavier than air. The TLV-TWA for sulfuryl fluoride is 5 ppm; TLV-STEL is 10 ppm; IDLH is 200 ppm.[154]

Little is known about the toxicokinetics of sulfuryl fluoride in humans, and the exact mechanism of toxicity is not understood. The respiratory, central nervous, and cardiovascular systems are the primary target organ systems.[168] The measurable fluoride concentrations in patients with sulfuryl fluoride poisoning and the development of fluorosis in models of chronic, low-concentration exposures suggest that the release of fluoride is of major pathophysiologic consequence.[157] Fluoride complexes with calcium and magnesium, resulting in hypocalcemia and hypomagnesemia (Chap. 104).[88]

Clinical Manifestations

Case reports of sulfuryl fluoride exposure describe acute and subacute clinical courses that share many similarities to methyl bromide poisoning. Initial manifestations, especially in limited exposures, include nausea, vomiting, diarrhea, abdominal pain, cough, and dyspnea. Irritation of mucosal surfaces produces salivation and nasopharyngitis, lacrimation, and conjunctival injection. Central nervous system manifestations include paresthesias, irritability, agitation, tetany, refractory seizures, and coma. Finally, fluoride toxicity results in profound shock, cardiac dysrhythmias, wide QRS complexes, prolongation of the QT interval, torsade de pointes, hyperkalemia, and ARDS (Chap. 104).[157,167]

Memory and dexterity testing were abnormal in structural fumigation workers exposed to both methyl bromide and sulfuryl fluoride.[35]

Diagnostic Testing

Patients with sulfuryl fluoride exposure require monitoring of serum calcium, magnesium, and potassium concentrations. Patients should have an ECG performed and be attached to continuous cardiac monitoring to observe for QRS complex widening, QT interval prolongation, and dysrhythmias. Serum fluoride concentrations, although not helpful for acute management, may help as a confirmatory diagnostic test.

Treatment

In patients with inhalational exposure, after removal from the scene to fresh air, the patients should be partially disrobed to avoid further exposure to any liberated sulfuryl fluoride gas.

In treating sulfuryl fluoride poisoning, aggressive treatment of hypocalcemia with calcium gluconate or calcium chloride should be expected (Antidotes in Depth: A32). Similar to the management of methyl bromide, intensive care is often required for seizures, dysrhythmias, bronchospasm, and ARDS. As the fluoride ion is excreted in the urine, fluid resuscitation is recommended to maintain a steady urine output.[202]

METHYL IODIDE

Iodomethane or methyl iodide is a monohalomethane and mainly used as a chemical reagent in the manufacturing of different pharmaceuticals and pesticides.[89,169] It is proposed as a fumigant to replace methyl bromide.

Human poisoning with methyl iodide is rare. Recently there are reports of dermal exposure with severe burns, respiratory insufficiency, and delayed neuropsychiatric sequel. Cerebellar and Parkinson findings followed by the development of cognitive impairment and the late appearance of psychiatric disturbances (personality change) are reported.[89,99,122,150,169]

There is no antidote for the treatment of methyl iodide poisoning. Successful treatment requires early diagnosis and cessation of exposure. It is difficult to distinguish the neurotoxic syndromes due to methyl iodide poisoning from other neurodegenerative conditions, infectious processes, and psychiatric disorders, especially when there is a lag time between exposure and onset of clinical manifestations.[122]

SUMMARY

- Exposure to fumigants follow inhalation, dermal exposure, or ingestion depending on the specific fumigant and the physical state.
- The fumigants are associated with multiorgan failure and, following acute exposure, adversely affect the cardiovascular, respiratory, and central nervous systems.
- Treatment involves removal from exposure and removal of outer clothing. Dermal decontamination is not generally needed given the volatile nature of most fumigants.
- First-responder protection from inhalation is important to prevent poisoning for these health care workers.

Acknowledgment

Keith K. Burkhart, MD, contributed to this chapter in previous editions.

REFERENCES

1. Abedini M, et al. Ischemic stroke as a rare manifestation of aluminum phosphide poisoning: a case report. *Acta Medica Iranica.* 2014;52:947-949.
2. ACGIH. *Threshold Limit Values and Biological Exposure Indices for 1989-1990.* Cincinnati, OH: American Conference of Government Industrial Hygienists; 1989.
3. Agarwal A, et al. Oxidative stress determined through the levels of antioxidant enzymes and the effect of *N*-acetylcysteine in aluminum phosphide poisoning. *Indian J Crit Care Med.* 2014;18:666-671.
4. Agrawal VK, et al. Aluminum phosphide poisoning: possible role of supportive measures in the absence of specific antidote. *Indian J Crit Care Med.* 2015;19:109-112.
5. Akkaoui M, et al. Reversible myocardial injury associated with aluminium phosphide poisoning. *Clin Toxicol.* 2007;45:728-731.
6. Al-Azzawi MJ, et al. In vitro inhibitory effects of phosphine on human and mouse serum cholinesterase. *Toxicol Environ Chem.* 1990;29:53-56.
7. Alonzo MC. International Program on Chemical Safety (IPCS): methyl bromide. http://www.inchem.org/documents/pims/chemical/methbrom.htm. Accessed May 15, 2017.
8. Alter P, et al. Lethal heart failure caused by aluminum phosphide poisoning. *Intensive Care Med.* 2001;27:327.
9. Amores E, et al. Letter to the editor: Comment on "Cytochrome-c oxidase inhibition in 26 aluminum phosphide poisoned patients." *Clin Toxicol.* 2007;45:461.
10. Anand R, et al. Effect of acute aluminum phosphide exposure on rats: a biochemical and histological correlation. *Toxicol Lett.* 2012;215:62-69.

11. Anger F, et al. Fatal aluminum phosphide poisoning. *J Anal Toxicol.* 2000;24:90-92.

12. Arora B, et al. Histopathological changes in aluminium phosphide poisoning. *J Indian Med Assoc.* 1995;93:380-381.

13. Azad A, et al. Effect of *N*-acetylcysteine and L-NAME on aluminium phosphide induced cardiovascular toxicity in rats. *Acta Pharmacol Sin.* 2001;22:298-304.

14. Balagopal K, et al. Methyl bromide poisoning presenting as acute ataxia. *Neurol India.* 2011;59:768-769.

15. Balali M; International Program on Chemical Safety (IPCS). *Phosphine.* http://www .inchem.org/documents/pims/chemical/pim865.htm. Accessed May 15, 2017.

16. Banjaj R, Wasir HS. Epidemic aluminium phosphide poisoning in northern India. *Lancet.* 1988;1:820-821.

17. Bartels MJ, et al. Mechanistic aspects of the metabolism of 1,3-dichloropropene in rats and mice. *Chem Res Toxicol.* 2000;13:1096-1102.

18. Bartels MJ, et al. Pharmacokinetics and metabolism of ^{14}C-1,3-dichloropropene in the Fischer 344 rat and the B6C3F1 mouse. *Xenobiotica.* 2004;34:193-213.

19. Baruah U, et al. Successful management of aluminium phosphide poisoning using intravenous lipid emulsion: report of two cases. *Indian J Crit Care Med.* 2015;19: 735-738.

20. Baselt R. *Disposition of Toxic Drugs and Chemicals in Man.* 2nd ed. Davis, CA: Biochemical Publications; 1982:516-517.

21. Baud FJ, et al. Clinical review: aggressive management and extracorporeal support for drug-induced cardiotoxicity. *Crit Care.* 2007;11:207.

22. Bayazit AK, et al. A child with hepatic and renal failure caused by aluminum phosphide. *Nephron.* 2000;86:517.

23. Bhargava S, et al. Esophagobronchial fistula—a rare complication of aluminum phosphide poisoning. *Ann Thorac Med.* 2011;6:41-42.

24. Bhasin P, et al. An echocardiographic study in aluminium phosphide poisoning [abstract]. *J Assoc Physicians India.* 1991;39:851.

25. Bogle RG, et al. Aluminium phosphide poisoning. *Emerg Med J.* 2006;23:e3.

26. Bolter CJ, Chefurka W. Extramitochondrial release of hydrogen peroxide from insect and mouse liver mitochondria using the respiratory inhibitors phosphine, myxothiazol, and antimycin and spectral analysis of inhibited cytochromes. *Arch Biochem Biophys.* 1990;278:65-72.

27. Brautbar N, Howard J. Phosphine toxicity: report of two cases and review of the literature. *Toxicol Ind Health.* 2002;18:71-75.

28. Breeman W. Methylbromide intoxication: a clinical case study. *Adv Emerg Nurs J.* 2009; 31:153-160.

29. Brouwer EJ, et al. Biological effect monitoring of occupational exposure to 1,3-dichloropropene: effects on liver and renal function and on glutathione conjugation. *Br J Ind Med.* 1991;48:167-172.

30. Buchwald AL, Muller M. Late confirmation of acute methyl bromide poisoning using *S*-methylcysteine adduct testing. *Vet Hum Toxicol.* 2001;43:208-211.

31. Bulathsinghala AT, Shaw IC. The toxic chemistry of methyl bromide. *Hum Exp Toxicol.* 2014;33:81-91.

32. Burgess JL, et al. Fumigant-related illness: Washington State's five-year experience. *J Toxicol Clin Toxicol.* 2000;38:7-14.

33. Burgess JL. Phosphine exposure from a methamphetamine laboratory investigation. *J Toxicol Clin Toxicol.* 2001;39:165-168.

34. Büyükçoban S, et al. A case report of toxic brain syndrome cause by methyl bromide. *Turk J Anaesthesiol Reanim.* 2015;43:134-137.

35. Calvert GM, et al. Health effects associated with sulfuryl fluoride and methyl bromide exposure among structural fumigation workers. *Am J Public Health Nations Health.* 1998;88:1774-1780.

36. Centers for Disease Control and Prevention (CDC). Illness associated with exposure to methyl bromide-fumigated produce—California, 2010. *MMWR Morb Mortal Wkly Rep.* 2011;60:923-926.

37. Centers for Disease Control and Prevention (CDC). Pesticide exposures. https:// ephtracking.cdc.gov/showpesticideFumigants. Accessed May 15, 2017.

38. Chaudhry D, Rai AS. *N*-Acetyl cysteine in aluminum phosphide poisoning: myth or hope. *Indian J Crit Care Med.* 2014;18:646-647.

39. Chavez CT, et al. Methyl bromide optic atrophy. *Am J Ophthalmol.* 1985;99:715-719.

40. Chin KL, et al. The interaction of phosphine with haemoglobin and erythrocytes. *Xenobiotica.* 1992;22:599-607.

41. Chugh SN, et al. Electrocardiographic abnormalities in aluminium phosphide poisoning with special reference to its incidence, pathogenesis, mortality and histopathology. *J Indian Med Assoc.* 1991;89:32-35.

42. Chugh SN, et al. Incidence & outcome of aluminium phosphide poisoning in a hospital study. *Indian J Med Res.* 1991;94:232-235.

43. Chugh SN, et al. Magnesium levels in acute cardiotoxicity due to aluminium phosphide poisoning. *Indian J Med Res.* 1991;94:437-439.

44. Chugh SN, Malhotra KC. Acute pericarditis in aluminium phosphide poisoning. *J Assoc Physicians India.* 1992;40:564.

45. Chugh SN, et al. Magnesium status and parenteral magnesium sulphate therapy in acute aluminum phosphide intoxication. *Magnes Res.* 1994;7:289-294.

46. Chugh SN, et al. Efficacy of magnesium sulphate in aluminium phosphide poisoning—comparison of two different dose schedules. *J Assoc Physicians India.* 1994;42:373-75.

47. Chugh SN, et al. Lipid peroxidation in acute aluminium phosphide poisoning. *J Assoc Physicians India.* 1995;43:265-266.

48. Chugh SN, et al. Free radical scavengers and lipid peroxidation in acute aluminium phosphide poisoning. *Indian J Med Res.* 1996;104:190-193.

49. Chugh SN, et al. Serial blood phosphine levels in acute aluminium phosphide poisoning. *J Assoc Physicians India.* 1996;44:184-185.

50. Chugh SN, et al. A critical evaluation of anti-peroxidant effect of intravenous magnesium in acute aluminium phosphide poisoning. *Magnes Res.* 1997;10:225-230.

51. Chugh SN, et al. Multiorgan failure in acute aluminium phosphide poisoning. *J Assoc Physicians India.* 1998;46:983.

52. Chugh SN, et al. Hypoglycemia in acute aluminium phosphide poisoning. *J Assoc Physicians India.* 2000;48:855-856.

53. Climie I, et al. Glutathione conjugation in the detoxification of (*Z*)-1,3-dichloropropene (a component of the nematocide D-D) in the rat. *Xenobiotica.* 1979;9:149-156.

54. Dadpour B, et al. An outbreak of aluminium phosphide poisoning in Mashhad, Iran. *Arh Hig Rada Toksikol.* 2016;67:65-66.

55. Dave HH, et al. Delayed haemorrhagic stroke following accidental aluminium phosphide ingestion. *J Assoc Physicians India.* 1994;42:78-79.

56. De Haro L, et al. Central and peripheral neurotoxic effects of chronic methyl bromide intoxication. *J Toxicol Clin Toxicol.* 1997;35:29-34.

57. Deschamps FJ, Turpin JC. Methyl bromide intoxication during grain store fumigation. *Occup Med.* 1996;46:89-90.

58. De Souza A, et al. The neurological effects of methyl bromide intoxication. *J Neurol Sci.* 2013;335:36-41.

59. Dua R, Gill KD. Effect of aluminium phosphide exposure on kinetic properties of cytochrome oxidase and mitochondrial energy metabolism in rat brain. *Biochim Biophys Acta.* 2004;1674:4-11.

60. Dua R, et al. Impaired mitochondrial energy metabolism and kinetic properties of cytochrome oxidase following acute aluminium phosphide exposure in rat liver. *Food Chem Toxicol.* 2010;48:53-60.

61. Elabbassi W, et al. Severe reversible myocardial injury associated with aluminium phosphide toxicity: a case report and review of literature. *J Saudi Heart Assoc.* 2014;26:216-221.

62. Environmental Health Criteria (EHC). Methyl bromide. IPCS/UNEP/ILO/WHO; 1994.

63. Erfantalab P, et al. Trend of blood lactate level in acute aluminum phosphide poisoning. *World J Emerg Med.* 2017;8:116-120.

64. Etemadi-Aleagha A, et al. Aluminum phosphide poisoning-related deaths in Tehran, Iran, 2006 to 2013. *Medicine (Baltimore).* 2015;94:1-7.

65. Flanagan RJ, et al. *Basic Analytical Toxicology.* Geneva: WHO; 1995.

66. Frangides CY, Pneumatikos IA. Persistent severe hypoglycemia in acute zinc phosphide poisoning. *Intensive Care Med.* 2002;28:223.

67. Garg K, et al. Pleural effusion in aluminum phosphide poisoning. *Lung India.* 2012;29:370-372.

68. Gargi J, et al. Current trend of poisoning—a hospital profile. *J Indian Med Assoc.* 2006;104:72-73.

69. Gaskin S, et al. Dermal absorption of fumigant gases during HAZMAT incident exposure scenarios—methyl bromide, sulfuryl fluoride, and chloropicrin. *Toxicol Ind Health.* 2017;33:547-554.

70. Geyer HL, et al. Methyl bromide intoxication causes reversible symmetric brainstem and cerebellar MRI lesions. *Neurology.* 2005;64:1279-1281.

71. Gheshlaghi F, et al. *N*-Acetylcysteine, ascorbic acid, and methylene blue for the treatment of aluminium phosphide poisoning: still beneficial? *Toxicol Int.* 2015;22:40-44.

72. Goel A, Aggarwal P. Pesticide poisoning. *Natl Med J India.* 2007;20:182-191.

73. Goharbari MH, et al. Therapeutic effects of oral liothyronine on aluminum phosphide poisoning as an adjuvant therapy: a clinical trial. *Hum Exp Toxicol.* 2018;37:107-117.

74. Goldman LR, et al. Acute symptoms in persons residing near a field treated with soil fumigants methyl bromide and chloropicrin. *West J Med.* 1987;147:95-98.

75. Gosselin RE, et al. *Clinical Toxicology of Commercial Products.* 5th ed. Baltimore, MD: William & Wilkins; 1984:III–280, III–284, II–158.

76. Goswami M, et al. Fat and oil inhibit phosphine release from aluminium phosphide—its clinical implication. *Indian J Exp Biol.* 1994;32:647-649.

77. Guengerich FP, et al. Role of human cytochrome P-450 IIE1 in the oxidation of many low molecular weight cancer suspects. *Chem Res Toxicol.* 1991;4:168-179.

78. Gunnell D, et al. The global distribution of fatal pesticide self-poisoning: systemic review. *BMC Public Health.* 2007;7:357-371.

79. Gupta MS, et al. Cardiovascular manifestations in aluminium phosphide poisoning with special reference to echocardiographic changes. *J Assoc Physicians India.* 1995;43:773-774.

80. Gupta S, Alhawat SK. Aluminum phosphide poisoning: a review. *J Toxicol Clin Toxicol.* 1995;33:19-24.

81. Gurjar M, et al. Managing aluminum phosphide poisonings. *J Emerg Trauma Shock.* 2011;4:378-384.

82. Halvaei Z, et al. Vitamin E as a novel therapy in the treatment of acute aluminum phosphide poisoning. *Turkish J Med Sci.* 2017;47:795-800.

83. Hakimoğlu S, et al. Successful management of aluminium phosphide poisoning resulting in cardiac arrest. *Turk J Anaesth Reanim.* 2015;43:288-290.

84. Hashemi-Domeneh B, et al. A review of aluminium phosphide poisoning and a flowchart to treat it. *Arh Hig Rada Toksikol.* 2016;67:183-193.

85. Hassanian-Moghaddam H, Zamani N. Therapeutic role of hyperinsulinemia/euglycemia in aluminum phosphide poisoning. *Medicine (Baltimore).* 2016;95:e4349.

86. Hassanian-Moghaddam H, et al. Successful treatment of aluminium phosphide poisoning by extracorporeal membrane oxygenation. *Basic Clin Pharmacol Toxicol.* 2016;118:243-246.

87. Hayes W Jr, Laws E Jr. *Handbook of Pesticide Toxicology.* Vol. 2. San Diego, CA: Academic Press Inc; 1991;668-671.

88. Heard K, et al. Calcium neutralizes fluoride bioavailability in a lethal model of fluoride poisoning. *J Toxicol Clin Toxicol.* 2001;39:349-353.

89. Held M, et al. Methyl iodide exposure presenting as severe chemical burn injury with neurological complications and prolonged respiratory insufficiency. *J Burn Care Res.* 2016;37:e592-e594.

90. Hernandez AF, et al. Clinical and pathological findings in fatal 1,3-dichloropropene intoxication. *Human Exp Toxicol.* 1994;13:303-306.

91. Herzstein J, Cullen MR. Methyl bromide intoxication in four field-workers during removal of soil fumigation sheets. *Am J Ind Med.* 1990;17:321-326.

92. Hezemans-Boer M, et al. Skin lesions due to exposure to methyl bromide. *Arch Dermatol.* 1988;124:917-921.

93. Hosseinian A, et al. Aluminum phosphide poisoning known as rice tablet: a common toxicity in North Iran. *Indian J Med Sci.* 2011;65:143-150.

94. Hsu CH, et al. Phosphine-induced oxidative damage in rats: role of glutathione. *Toxicology.* 2002;179:1-8.

95. Hustinx WNM, et al. Systemic effects of inhalational methyl bromide poisoning: a study of nine cases occupationally exposed due to inadvertent spread during fumigation. *Br J Ind Med.* 1993;50:155-159.

96. Hutson DH, et al. The excretion and retention of components of the soil fumigant D-D, and their metabolites in the rat. *Food Cosmet Toxicol.* 1971;9:677-680.

97. IARC. *Monographs on the Evaluation of the Carcinogenic Risk of Chemicals to Humans: Some Halogenated Hydrocarbons and Pesticide Exposure.* Lyon, France: International Agency for Research on Cancer; 1986:113-147.

98. Inbanathan J, Karimungi RN. A study of simplified acute physiological score (SAPSII) in the prediction of acute aluminium phosphide poisoning outcome on MICU: a hospital based study. *Int J Chem and LifeSci.* 2014;3:1317-1321.

99. Iniesta I, et al. Methyl iodide rhombencephalopathy: clinico-radiological features of a preventable, potentially fatal industrial accident. *Pract Neurol.* 2013;13:393-395.

100. International Program on Chemical Safety for Phosphine and Selected Metal Phosphides. *Environmental Health Criteria 73.* Geneva: WHO; 1988. http://www.inchem.org/documents/ehc/ehc/ehc73.htm. Accessed May 15, 2017.

101. Iwasaki K, et al. Biological exposure monitoring of methyl bromide workers by determination of hemoglobin adducts. *Indust Health.* 1989;27:181-183.

102. Jafari A, et al. An electrocardiographic, molecular and biochemical approach to explore the cardioprotective effect of vasopressin and milrinone against phosphide toxicity in rats. *Food Chem Toxicol.* 2015;80:182-192.

103. Jain SM, et al. Electrocardiography changes in aluminum phosphide poisoning. *J Assoc Physicians India.* 1985;33:406-409.

104. Jain MK, et al. Electrocardiographic diagnosis of atrial infarction in aluminium phosphide poisoning. *J Assoc Physicians India.* 1992;40:692-693.

105. Jain RK, et al. Esophageal complications following aluminium phosphide ingestion: an emerging issue among survivors of poisoning. *Dysphagia.* 2010;25:271-276.

106. Jaiswal S, et al. Aluminum phosphide poisoning: effect of correction of severe metabolic acidosis on patient outcome. *Indian J Crit Care Med.* 2009;13:21-24.

107. Jamshed N, et al. Severe hypoglycemia as a presenting feature of aluminum phosphide poisoning. *Ann Saudi Med.* 2014;34:189.

108. Jayaraman KS. Death pills from pesticide. *Nature.* 1991;353:377.

109. Kariman H, et al. Aluminium phosphide poisoning and oxidative stress. *J Med Toxicol.* 2012;8:281-284.

110. Kariyappa M, et al. Phosphide poisoning in children in tertiary care hospital of south India: a retrospective study. *Int J Sci Stud.* 2015;3:5-9.

111. Kaushik RM, et al. Subendocardial infarction in a young survivor of aluminium phosphide poisoning. *Hum Exp Toxicol.* 2007;26:457-460.

112. Khurana V, et al. Microangiopathic hemolytic anemia following disseminated intravascular coagulation in aluminium phosphide poisoning. *Indian J Med Sci.* 2009;63:257-259.

113. Kochhar R, et al. Clinical profile and outcome of aluminum phosphide-induced esophageal strictures. *J Med Toxicol.* 2010;6:301-306.

114. Koreti S, et al. Aluminium phosphide poisoning in children—challenges in diagnosis and management. *Sch Acad J Biosci.* 2014;2:505-509.

115. Kowalczyk M. International Program on Chemical Safety (IPCS): 1,3-Dichloropropene, http://www.inchem.org/documents/pims/chemical/pim025.htm. Accessed May 15, 2017.

116. Lakshmi B. Methemoglobinemia with aluminum phosphide poisoning. *Am J Emerg Med.* 2002;20:130-132.

117. Lecailtel S, et al. How unclogging a sink can be lethal: case report of an accidental methyl bromide poisoning leading to a multiple organ failure. *J Intensive Care.* 2015;3:12.

118. Lewis RJ Sr. *Hazardous Chemicals Desk Reference.* 5th ed. New York: John Wiley & Sons; 2002:401.

119. Lifshitz M, Gavrilov V. Central nervous system toxicity and early peripheral neuropathy following dermal exposure to methyl bromide. *Clin Toxicol.* 2000;38:799-801.

120. Loddé B, et al. Acute phosphine poisoning on board a bulk carrier: analysis of factors leading to a fatal case. *J Occup Med Toxicol.* 2015;10:10.

121. Louriz M, et al. Prognostic factors of acute aluminium phosphide poisoning. *Indian J Med Sci.* 2009;63:227-234.

122. Mackenzie Ross S. Delayed cognitive and psychiatric symptoms following methyl iodide and manganese poisoning: potential for misdiagnosis. *Cortex.* 2016;74:427-439.

123. Madan K, et al. Corrosive-like strictures caused by ingestion of aluminium phosphide. *Natl Med J India.* 2006;19:313-314.

124. Maitai CK, et al. Investigation of possible antidotal effects of activated charcoal, sodium bicarbonate, hydrogen peroxide and potassium permanganate in zinc phosphide poisoning. *East Central Afr J Pharm Sci.* 2002;5:38-41.

125. Marashi SM, Nasri-Nasrabadi Z. Can sodium bicarbonate really help in treating metabolic acidosis caused by aluminium phosphide poisoning? *Arh Hig Rada Toksikol.* 2015;66:83-84.

126. Markovitz A, Crosby WH. Chemical carcinogenesis: a soil fumigant, 1,3-dichloropropene, as possible cause of hematologic malignancies. *Arch Intern Med.* 1984;144:1409-1411.

127. Marquis JK, Lerrick AJ. Noncompetitive inhibition by aluminum, scandium and yttrium of acetylcholinesterase from electrophorus electricus. *Biochem Pharmacol.* 1982;31:1437-1440.

128. Marquis JK. Aluminum inhibition of human serum cholinesterase. *Bull Environ Contam Toxicol.* 1983;31:164-169.

129. Martelli A, et al. Cytotoxic and genotoxic activity of 1,3-dichloropropene in cultured mammalian cells. *Tox Appl Pharm.* 1993;120:144-149.

130. Material Safety Data Sheet. United Phosphorus, Inc. http://www.sfm.state.or.us/CR2K_SubDB/MSDS/WEEVIL_CIDE_PELLETS.PDF. Accessed May 15, 2017.

131. Mathai A, Bhanu MS. Acute aluminium phosphide poisoning: can we predict mortality? *Indian J Anaesth.* 2010;54:302-307.

132. Medinsky M, et al. Disposition of ¹⁴C-methyl bromide in rats after inhalation. *Toxicology.* 1984;32:187-196.

133. Medinsky M, et al. Uptake and excretion of ¹⁴C-methyl bromide as influenced by exposure concentration. *Toxicol Appl Pharmacol.* 1985;78:215-225.

134. Mehrpour O, et al. Hyperglycemia in acute aluminum phosphide poisoning as a potential prognostic factor. *Hum Exp Toxicol.* 2008;27:591-595.

135. Mehrpour O, et al. Evaluation of histopathological changes in fatal aluminum phosphide poisoning. *Indian J Forensic Med Toxicol.* 2008;2:34-36.

136. Mehrpour O, et al. Successful treatment of aluminum phosphide poisoning with digoxin: a case report and review of literature. *Int J Pharmacol.* 2011;7:761-764.

137. Mehrpour O, et al. Severe hypoglycemia following acute aluminum phosphide (rice tablet) poisoning; a case report and review of the literature. *Acta Medica Iranica.* 2012;50:568-571.

138. Mehrpour O, et al. Successful treatment of cardiogenic shock with an intraaortic balloon pump following aluminium phosphide. *Arh Hig Rada Toksikol.* 2014;65:121-127.

139. Merin O, et al. Salvage ECMO deployment for fatal aluminum phosphide poisoning. *Am J Emerg Med.* 2015;33:1718.e1-1718.e3.

140. Mirakbari SM. Hot charcoal vomitus in aluminum phosphide poisoning—a case report of internal thermal reaction in aluminum phosphide poisoning and review of literature. *Indian J Anaesth.* 2015;59:433-436.

141. Mital HS, et al. A study of aluminium phosphide poisoning with special reference to its spot diagnosis by silver nitrate test. *J Assoc Physicians India.* 1992;40:473-474.

142. Mittra S, et al. Cholinesterase inhibition by aluminium phosphide poisoning in rats and effects of atropine and pralidoxime chloride. *Acta Pharmacol Sin.* 2001;22:37-39.

143. Moghadamnia AA. An update on toxicology of aluminum phosphide. *DARU.* 2012;20:25.

144. Mohan B, et al. Role of extracorporeal membrane oxygenation in aluminum phosphide poisoning-induced reversible myocardial dysfunction: a novel therapeutic modality. *J Emerg Med.* 2015;49:651-656.

145. Mohan B, et al. Outcome of patients supported by extracorporeal membrane oxygenation for aluminum phosphide poisoning: an observational study. *Indian Heart J.* 2016;68:295-301.

146. Mostafazadeh B, et al. Blood levels of methemoglobin in patients with aluminum phosphide poisoning and its correlation with patient's outcome. *J Med Toxicol.* 2011;7:40-43.

147. Mulay PR, et al. Notes from the field: acute sulfuryl fluoride poisoning in a family—Florida, august 2015. *MMWR Morb Mortal Wkly Rep.* 2016;65:698-699.

148. Murali R, et al. Acute pesticide poisoning: 15 years experience of a large North-West Indian hospital. *Clin Toxicol.* 2009;47:35-38.

149. Musshoff F. A gas chromatographic analysis of phosphine in biological material in a case of suicide. *Forensic Sci Int.* 2008;177:e35-38.

150. Nair JR, Chatterjee K. Methyl iodide poisoning presenting as a mimic of acute stroke: a case report. *J Med Case Rep.* 2010;4:177.

151. Nasa P, et al. Use of continuous renal replacement therapy in acute aluminum phosphide poisoning: a novel therapy. *Ren Fail.* 2013;35:1170-1172.

152. Nijhawan S, et al. Aluminum phosphide-induced esophageal stricture: an unusual complication. *Endoscopy.* 2006;38:E23.

153. NIOSH. Preventing phosphine poisoning and explosions during fumigation. Publication No. 99-126. http://www.cdc.gov/niosh/docs/99-126/pdfs/99-126.pdf. Accessed May 15, 2017.

154. NIOSH. *Pocket Guide to Chemical Hazards.* National Institute of Occupational Safety and Health. Publication No. 2002-140. Washington, DC: US Government Printing Office; 2002.

155. Nocera A, et al. Dangerous bodies: a case of fatal aluminium phosphide poisoning. *Med J Aust.* 2000;173:133-135.

156. Ntelios D, et al. Aluminium phosphide-induced leukopenia. *BMJ Case Rep.* 2013;2013.

157. Nuckolls JG, et al. Fatalities resulting from sulfuryl fluoride exposure after home fumigation—Virginia. *JAMA.* 1987;258:2041-2042.

158. Pajoumand A, et al. Survival following severe aluminium phosphide poisoning. *J Pharm Pract Res.* 2002;32:297-299.

159. Pepelko B, et al. Worker exposure standard for phosphine gas. *Risk Anal.* 2004;24:1201-1213.

160. Popp W, et al. Phosphine gas poisoning in a German office. *Lancet.* 2002;359:1574.

161. Potter WT, et al. Phosphine-mediated Heinz body formation and hemoglobin oxidation in human erythrocytes. *Toxicol Lett.* 1991;57:37-45.

162. Potter WT, et al. Radiometric assay of red cell and plasma cholinesterase in pesticide appliers from Minnesota. *Toxicol Appl Pharmacol.* 1993;119:150-155.

163. Proudfoot AT. Aluminium and zinc phosphide poisoning. *Clin Toxicol.* 2009;47:89-100.

164. Saidi H, et al. Effects of hyperbaric oxygenation on survival time of aluminum phosphide intoxicated rats. *J Res Med Sci.* 2011;16:1306-1312.

165. Saidi H, Shojaie S. Effect of sweet almond oil on survival rate and plasma cholinesterase activity of aluminum phosphide-intoxicated rats. *Hum Exp Toxicol.* 2012;31:51822.

166. Sanaei-Zadeh H, Farajidana H. Is there a role for digoxin in the management of acute aluminum phosphide poisoning? *Med Hypotheses.* 2011;76:765-766.

167. Scheuerman EH. Case report: suicide by exposure to sulfuryl fluoride. *J Forensic Sci.* 1986;31:1154-1158.

168. Schneir A, et al. Systemic fluoride poisoning and death from inhalational exposure to sulfuryl fluoride. *Clin Toxicol (Phila).* 2008;46:850-854.

169. Schwartz MD, et al. Acute methyl iodide exposure with delayed neuropsychiatric sequelae: report of a case. *Am J Ind Med.* 2005;47:550-556.

170. Sciuto AM, et al. Phosphine toxicity: a story of disrupted mitochondrial metabolism. *Ann N Y Acad Sci.* 2016;1374:41-51.

171. Shadnia S, et al. Successful treatment of acute aluminium phosphide poisoning: possible benefit of coconut oil. *Hum Exp Toxicol.* 2005;24:215-218.

172. Shadnia S, et al. Unintentional poisoning by phosphine released from aluminum phosphide. *Hum Exp Toxicol.* 2008;27:87-89.

173. Shadnia S, et al. A retrospective 7-years study of aluminum phosphide poisoning in Tehran: opportunities for prevention. *Hum Exp Toxicol.* 2009;28:209-213.

174. Shadnia S, et al. Simplified acute physiology score in the prediction of acute aluminum phosphide poisoning outcome. *Indian J Med Sci.* 2010;64:532-539.

175. Shadnia S, Soltaninejad K. Spontaneous ignition due to intentional acute aluminum Phosphide poisoning. *J Emerg Med.* 2011;40:179-181.

176. Shadnia S, et al. Methemoglobinemia in aluminum phosphide poisoning. *Hum Exp Toxicol.* 2011;30:250-253.

177. Sharma AD, et al. Aluminum phosphide (Celphos) poisoning in children: a 5-year experience in a tertiary care hospital from northern India. *Indian J Crit Care Med.* 2014;18:33-36.

178. Siddaiah L, et al. Intra-aortic balloon pump in toxic myocarditis due to aluminium phosphide poisoning. *J Med Toxicol.* 2009;5:80-83.

179. Singh S, et al. Aluminium phosphide ingestion. *Br Med J (Clin Res Ed).* 1985;290:1110-1111.

180. Singh RB, et al. Can aluminium phosphide poisoning cause hypermagnesaemia? A study of 121 patients. *Magnes Trace Elem.* 1990;9:212-218.

181. Singh RB, et al. Hypermagnesemia following aluminum phosphide poisoning. *Int J Clin Pharmacol Ther Toxicol.* 1991;29:82-85.

182. Singh S, et al. Cytochrome-c oxidase inhibition in 26 aluminum phosphide poisoned patients. *Clin Toxicol.* 2006;44:155-158.

183. Siwach SB, et al. Serum and tissue magnesium content in patients of aluminium phosphide poisoning and critical evaluation of high dose magnesium sulphate therapy in reducing mortality. *J Assoc Physicians India.* 1994;42:107-110.

184. Siwach SB, et al. Cardiac arrhythmias in aluminium phosphide poisoning studied by on continuous holter and cardioscopic monitoring. *J Assoc Physicians India.* 1998;46:598-601.

185. Solgi R, et al. Electrophysiological and molecular mechanisms of protection by iron sucrose against phosphine-induced cardiotoxicity: a time course study. *Toxicol Mech Methods.* 2015;25:249-257.

186. Soltani M, et al. Proposing boric acid as an antidote for aluminium phosphide poisoning by investigation of the chemical reaction between boric acid and phosphine. *J Med Hypotheses Ideas.* 2013;7:21-24.

187. Soltaninejad K, et al. Aluminum phosphide intoxication mimicking ischemic heart disease led to unjustified treatment with streptokinase. *Clin Toxicol.* 2009;47:908-909.

188. Soltaninejad K, et al. Unusual complication of aluminum phosphide poisoning: development of hemolysis and methemoglobinemia and its successful treatment. *Indian J Crit Care Med.* 2011;15:117-119.

189. Soltaninejad K, et al. Electrocardiographic findings and cardiac manifestations in acute aluminum phosphide poisoning. *J Forensic Legal Med.* 2012;19:291-293.

190. Soltaninejad K, et al. Fatal aluminum phosphide poisoning in Tehran-Iran from 2007 to 2010. *Indian J Med Sci.* 2012;66:66-70.

191. Soltaninejad K, Shadnia S. History of the use and epidemiology of organophosphorus poisoning. In: Balali-Mood M, Abdollahi M, eds., *Basic and Clinical Toxicology of Organophosphorus Compounds.* London: Springer-Verlag; 2014:25-45.

192. Squier MV, et al. Case report: neuropathology of methyl bromide intoxication. *Neuropathol Appl Neurobiol.* 1992;18:579-584.

193. Srinivas R, et al. Intravascular haemolysis due to glucose-6-phosphate dehydrogenase deficiency in a patient with aluminium phosphide poisoning. *Emerg Med J.* 2007;24:67-69.

194. Starratt AN, Bond EJ. In vitro methylation of DNA by the fumigant methyl bromide. *J Environ Sci Health B.* 1988;23:513-525.

195. Stott WT, Kastl PE. Inhalation pharmacokinetics of technical grade 1,3-dichloropropene in rats. *Toxicol Appl Pharmacol.* 1986;85:332-341.

196. Sudakin DL. Occupational exposure to aluminium phosphide and phosphine gas? a suspected case report and review of the literature. *Hum Exp Toxicol.* 2005;24: 27-33.

197. Sulaj Z, et al. Fatal aluminum phosphide poisoning in Tirana (Albania), 2009-2013. *DARU.* 2015;23:8.

198. Suman RL, Savani M. Pleural effusion—a rare complication of aluminium phosphide poisoning. *Indian Pediatr.* 1999;36:1161-1163.

199. Suzuki T, et al. Cytotoxicity of 1,3-dichloropropene and cellular phospholipids peroxidation in isolated rat hepatocytes, and its prevention by alpha-tocopherol. *Biol Pharm Bull.* 1994;17:1351-1354.

200. Tehrani H, et al. Protective effects of *N*-acetylcysteine on aluminum phosphide-induced oxidative stress in acute human poisoning. *Clin Toxicol.* 2013;51:23-28.

201. The National Institute for Occupational Safety and Health. PHOSPHINE: lung damaging agent. The Emergency Response Safety and Health Database, Centers for Disease Control and Prevention. http://www.cdc.gov/niosh/ershdb/emergencyresponsecard_29750035.html. Accessed May 15, 2017.

202. TOXNET. Sulfuryl fluoride. https://toxnet.nlm.nih.gov/cgi-bin/sis/search/a?dbs+hsdb:@term+@DOCNO+828. Accessed May 15, 2017.

203. Türkez H, Toğar B. Aluminium phosphide-induced genetic and oxidative damages in vitro: attenuation by *Laurus nobilis* L. leaf extract. *Indian J Pharmacol.* 2013;45: 71-75.

204. Uncini A, et al. Methyl bromide myoclonus: an electrophysiological study. *Acta Neurol Scand.* 1990;81:159-164.

205. US EPA. *Environmental Fate Data Requirements Used to Evaluate Groundwater Contamination Potential for Reregistration.* Washington, DC: US Environmental Protection Agency; 1992.

206. Van Joost T, de Jong G. Sensitization to DD soil fumigant during manufacture. *Contact Dermatitis.* 1988;18:307-308.

207. Van Welie RTH, et al. Thioether excretion in urine of applicators exposed to 1,3-dichloropropene: a comparison with urinary mercapturic acid excretion. *Br J Ind Med.* 1991;48:492-498.

208. Van Welie RTH, et al. Mercapturic acids, protein adducts, and DNA adducts as biomarkers of electrophilic chemicals. *Crit Rev Tox.* 1992;22:271-306.

209. Verma VK, et al. Aluminium phosphide poisoning: a challenge for the physician. *JK Science.* 2001;3:13-20.

210. Verma RK, et al. Aluminium phosphide poisoning: late presentation as oesophageal stricture. *JK Sci.* 2006;8:235-236.

211. Verma SK, et al. Acute pancreatitis: a lesser-known complication of aluminum phosphide poisoning. *Hum Exp Toxicol.* 2007;26:979-981.

212. Vos M, et al. Genetic deficiency of human class mu glutathione *S*-transferase enzymes in relation to urinary excretion of the mercapturic acids of *Z*- and *E*-1,3-dichloropropene. *Arch Toxicol.* 1991;65:95-99.

213. Wahab A, et al. Acute aluminium phosphide poisoning: an update. *Hong Kong J Emerg Med.* 2008;15:152-155.

214. Wahab A, et al. Spontaneous self-ignition in a case of acute aluminium phosphide poisoning. *Am J Emerg Med.* 2009;27:752.e5-752.e6.

215. Willers-Russo LJ. Three fatalities involving phosphine gas, produced as a result of methamphetamine manufacturing. *J Forensic Sci.* 1999;44:647-652.

216. Yadav J, et al. Spontaneous ignition in case of Celphos poisoning. *Am J Forensic Med Pathol.* 2007;28:353-355.

217. Yan H, et al. Diagnosis of aluminum phosphide poisoning using a new analytical approach: forensic application to a lethal intoxication. *Int J Legal Med.* 2017; 131:1001-1007.

218. Zwaveling JH, et al. Exposure of the skin to methyl bromide: a study of six cases occupationally exposed to high concentrations during fumigation. *Hum Toxicol.* 1987;6:491-495.

109 HERBICIDES

Darren M. Roberts

HISTORY, CLASSIFICATION, AND EPIDEMIOLOGY

Herbicides, defined as any chemical that regulates the growth of a plant, encompass a large number of xenobiotics of varying characteristics. Herbicides are used around the world for the destruction of plants in the home environment and also in agriculture in which weeds are particularly targeted. Poisoning follows acute (intentional or unintentional poisoning) or chronic (such as occupational) exposures. Depending on the herbicide and the characteristics of the exposure, this may lead to clinically significant poisoning, including death. This chapter focuses on the most widely used herbicides and also those associated with significant clinical toxicity. In particular, risk assessment and the management of patients with a history of acute herbicide poisoning are emphasized.

Prior to the 1940s, the main method of weed control and field clearance was manual labor, which was time consuming and expensive. A range of xenobiotics were tested, including metals and inorganic compounds; however, their efficacy was limited. The first herbicide marketed was 2,4-dichlorphenoxyacetic acid (2,4-D) during the 1940s, followed by other phenoxy acid compounds. Paraquat was marketed in the early 1960s, followed by dicamba later that decade. The development of new herbicides is an active area of research and new herbicides and formulations are frequently released into the market. This includes a number of novel structural compounds for which clinical toxicology data are unavailable. Hundreds of xenobiotics are classified as herbicides and a much larger number of commercial preparations are marketed. Some commercial preparations contain more than one herbicide to potentiate plant destruction. From another perspective, crops are being developed that are resistant to particular herbicides to maximize the selective destruction of weeds without reducing crop production.

Herbicides are the most widely sold pesticides in the world; in 2007 they accounted for approximately 40% of the total world pesticide market and 48% of the pesticide market in the United States. Home and garden domestic use accounts for 7% of the overall herbicide use in the United States, whereas the remainder is used in agriculture, government (eg, vegetation control on highways and railways), and industry. In each of the US market sectors, herbicides were 4 of the top 5 used pesticides in 2012, including glyphosate, atrazine, metolachlor-S, and 2,4-D.[33]

Not all herbicide exposures are clinically significant. In developed countries, most acute herbicide exposures are unintentional and the majority of patients do not require admission to a hospital. The National Poisoning Database System (NPDS) of the American Association of Poison Control Centers (AAPCC) describes approximately 10,000 herbicide exposures each year. Over the last 12 years, there were approximately 5 deaths per year and 20 patients per year with clinical outcomes categorized as "major" that were attributed to herbicide poisoning (Chap. 130). Most deaths were due to paraquat and diquat, although recently glyphosate and phenoxy acid compounds are more commonly implicated. Cases of severe poisoning that required hospitalization usually followed intentional self-poisoning. Significant toxicity including death also occurs with unintentional (eg, storage of an herbicide in food or drink containers) or criminal exposures.

Classification

Hundreds of xenobiotics have herbicidal activity and they are subclassified by a number of methods. Most commonly they are categorized in terms of their spectrum of activity (selective or nonselective), chemical structure, mechanism of action (contact herbicides or hormone dysregulators), use (preemergence or postemergence), or their toxicity to rats such as the amount of that xenobiotic killing 50% of exposed animals (LD$_{50}$). Certain

xenobiotics are classified as plant growth regulators rather than herbicides, but in this chapter all are considered to be herbicides.

Table 109–1 lists the extensive range of herbicides in current use.[49] By convention, they are subclassified according to their chemical class and their World Health Organization (WHO) hazard classification. Unfortunately, the utility of these (or any other) methods of classification to predict the hazard to humans with self-poisoning is not proven.

The WHO categorizes pesticides by their LD$_{50}$. This system does not consider morbidity or the effect of treatments. Further, the calculated LD$_{50}$ varies among studies in the same type of animal, and between different species. For example, in the case of paraquat, the LD$_{50}$ in rats, monkeys, and guinea pigs is reported as 125, 50, and 25 mg/kg, respectively.[83] It should be emphasized that the intended application of the WHO hazard classification was for the risk assessment following occupational exposures to operators using the product as intended. Furthermore, the LD$_{50}$ is determined by using the pure herbicide compound, whereas human poisoning follows exposure to proprietary formulations that also contain coformulants, and these often contribute to the overall toxicity. Preparations that decrease human toxicity without compromising herbicidal activity are also being developed, for example, paraquat containing lysine salicylate.

Herbicides within a single chemical class can manifest different clinical toxicity; for example, glyphosate is an organic phosphorus compound that does not inhibit acetylcholinesterase, which contrasts with insecticides of a similar structure. The mechanism of action of herbicides in plants usually differs from the mechanism of toxicity in humans; indeed, for some herbicides the mechanism of human toxicity is poorly described.

Contribution of Coformulations

Commercial herbicide formulations are identified by their active ingredients but they almost always contain coformulants that often contribute to clinical toxicity. Hydrocarbon-based solvents and surfactants improve the contact of the herbicide with the plant and enhance penetration. Coformulants are generally considered "inactive" or "inert" because they lack herbicidal activity; however, increasingly their contribution to the human toxicity of a formulation is being appreciated.

The most widely discussed example of a coformulant dominating the toxicity of an herbicide product is that of glyphosate-containing products, which is discussed below. Another example is imazapyr, which has an LD$_{50}$ in rats of 1,500 mg/kg intraperitoneally (IP) compared with 262 mg/kg IP when administered as the product Arsenal. This difference is attributed to the surfactant nonylphenol ethoxylate used in this product, which has an LD$_{50}$ of 75 mg/kg IP. In vitro studies with a number of formulations demonstrate increased cardiovascular toxicity compared with the technical herbicides.[13] Similarly, coformulants increase the in vitro toxicity from phenoxyacetic acid derivatives and glufosinate.

Impurities generated during manufacture or storage of the herbicide formulation also contribute to toxicity. For example, phenolic by-products from the manufacture of phenoxyacetic acid herbicides are reported in commercial formulations. Some proprietary products contain a combination of herbicidal compounds that probably have additive effects, further complicating the risk assessment of an acute exposure.

Epidemiology

The incidence of poisoning with individual herbicides depends on their availability. Availability is associated with local marketing practices and is reflected in sales in the domestic sector. For example, paraquat poisonings

TABLE 109–1 Characteristics of the Major Herbicides Categorized by Chemical Class and WHO Hazard Classification

Chemical Class[a]	Applications, Usage Data, and Mechanism of Action in Plants, If Known[b]	Compounds Included	WHO Hazard Class[c]	Clinical Effects, Treatments, and Supportive Care
Alcohol and aldehyde	Broad-spectrum contact herbicide	Allyl alcohol (prop-2-en-1-ol) and acrolein (the metabolite of allyl alcohol)	Ib	Local irritation, cardiotoxicity, pulmonary edema, and death. Administer N-acetylcysteine or mesna.
Amide, Fig. 109–1	Selective for grasses pre- or postemergence. In 2012, acetochlor, propanil, metolachlor, and metolachlor-S were among the top herbicides used in the United States. Multiple mechanisms of action, including inhibition of photosynthesis at photosystem II and/or inhibition of dihydropteroate synthase and/or inhibition of cell division through inhibition of the synthesis of very-long-chain fatty acids and/or inhibition of acetolactate synthase (interferes with branched amino acid synthesis) and/or inhibition of microtubule assembly. Some compounds are also included in other chemical classes, including asulam (carbamate); oryzalin (dinitroaniline); clomeprop (phenoxy); diclosulam, flumetsulam, and metosulam (triazolopyrimidines).	*Anilide derivatives:* Acetochlor, alachlor, dimethachlor, flufenacet, mefluidide, metolachlor, propachlor, propanil (DCPA) *Nonanilide derivatives:* Chlorthiamid, diphenamid *Anilide derivatives:* Butachlor, clomeprop, diclosulam, flamprop, flumetsulam, metosulam, mefenacet, metazachlor, pentanochlor, pretilachlor *Nonanilide derivatives:* Asulam, bromobutide, dimethenamid, isoxaben, napropamide, oryzalin, propyzamide, tebutam	III U	See text for anilide derivatives. There are limited human data about the non-anilide derivatives. Lethargy or sedation preceded death in animals exposed to chlorthiamid. Behavioral changes, ataxia, and prostration were noted in animals exposed to diphenamid. Drowsiness and tachypnea were noted in goats following acute poisoning with napropamide. Oryzalin inhibits human carbonic anhydrase. Methemoglobinemia results, the treatment of which is methylene blue (Antidotes in Depth: A43).
Aromatic acid	In 2012, dicamba was the eighth most used herbicide in the domestic sector in the United States. Dicamba is commonly coformulated with phenoxyacetic acid compounds. Inhibits acetolactate synthase and/or inhibition of microtubule assembly and/or indole acetic acid–like (synthetic auxins).	Dicamba, 2,3,6-trichlorobenzoic acid (2,3,6-TBA) Bispyribac, chloramben (amiben), chlorthal, clopyralid, pyriminobac, pyrithiobac, quinclorac, quinmerac	III U	Bispyribac causes gastrointestinal irritation, sedation and death (case fatality 1.8%; asystolic arrest reported).[30] Minimal toxicity from dicamba, but some products are corrosive to the gut, and rhabdomyolysis and acute pancreatitis are reported.[87] Human data are limited for the other compounds, particularly single-agent exposures. In animals, myotonia, dyspnea, and death are reported with dicamba and 2,3,6-TBA poisoning.
Arsenical	Unknown	Dimethylarsinic acid (cacodylic acid), methylarsonic acid (MAA or MSMA)	III	Chap. 86
Benzothiazole	Indole acetic acid–like (synthetic auxins) and/or inhibits photosynthesis at photosystem II.	Benazolin, methabenzthiazuron	U	Limited human data.
Bipyridyl	Nonselective, postemergence, contact herbicide Photosystem I electron diversion These compounds are part of a larger group of quaternary ammonium herbicides, including difenzoquat, which is also a pyrazole compound (see below).	Paraquat, diquat	II	See text for paraquat and diquat.
Carbanilate	Inhibits photosynthesis at photosystem II and/or inhibits mitosis or microtubule organization	Carbetamide, desmedipham, phenmedipham, propham	U	Limited human data.
Cyclohexane oxime	Postemergence, selective for grasses Inhibits acetyl-CoA carboxylase (lipid biosynthesis inhibitors)	Butroxydim, sethoxydim, tralkoxydim Alloxydim, cycloxydim, cyhalofop	III U	Limited human data.

(Continued)

TABLE 109–1 Characteristics of the Major Herbicides Categorized by Chemical Class and WHO Hazard Classification *(Continued)*

Chemical Class[a]	Applications, Usage Data, and Mechanism of Action in Plants, If Known[b]	Compounds Included	WHO Hazard Class[c]	Clinical Effects, Treatments, and Supportive Care
Dinitroaniline	Preemergence, selective for grasses In 2012, trifluralin and pendimethalin were among the top 20 herbicides used in the United States overall, while trifluralin and pendimethalin were among the top 10 used in the domestic sector Inhibits microtubule assembly.	Fluchloralin, pendimethalin Benfluralin (benefin), butralin, dinitramine, ethalfluralin, oryzalin, prodiamine, trifluralin	III U	Pendimethalin induces mild clinical toxicity in most cases, but gastroduodenal injury, sedation, seizures, hypotension and death due to respiratory failure are reported, usually within 24 hours. Limited human data for the others Aniline metabolites are reported from trifluralin and oryzalin, which induce methemoglobinemia and hemolysis with prolonged exposures. For which methylene blue, blood transfusions and supportive care are recommended (Antidotes in Depth: A43). In rats, fluchloralin induces hyperexcitability, tremors, and convulsions prior to death. Agitation, trembling, and fatigue occur in rats following lethal doses of trifluralin. Many of these compounds are poorly absorbed and some are subject to enterohepatic recycling.
Dinitrophenol	Uncoupling (membrane disruption)	Dinoterb, DNOC (4,6-dinitro-*o*-cresol)	Ib	Limited human data; methemoglobinemia is reported in animals. Dinitrophenol uncouples oxidative phosphorylation.
Diphenylether	Postemergence (particularly broad leaves) Contact herbicide, inhibits protoporphyrinogen oxidase, and/or inhibits carotenoid biosynthesis Aclonifen is also an amine compound.	Acifluorfen, fluoroglycofen Aclonifen, bifenox, chlomethoxyfen, oxyfluorfen	III U	Limited human data.
Halogenated aliphatic	Inhibit lipid synthesis	Dalapon, fluopropanate	U	Limited human data.
Imidazolinone	Inhibit acetolactate synthase, interfering with branched amino acid synthesis	Imazamethabenz, imazapyr, imazaquin, imazethapyr	U	Limited human data. In a small case series, imazapyr induced sedation, respiratory distress, metabolic acidosis, hypotension, and hepatorenal dysfunction.
Inorganic	Nonselective	Sodium chlorate Ammonium sulfamate	III U	Nausea, vomiting, diarrhea, metabolic acidosis, kidney failure, hemolysis, methemoglobinemia, rhabdomyolysis, and disseminated intravascular coagulation. Treatment includes hemodialysis and erythrocyte and plasma transfusion. Methemoglobinemia is usually unresponsive to methylene blue (a single report suggested benefit when used within 6 hours of exposure[63]) Limited human data.
Nitrile	Preemergence, selective for grasses Inhibits photosynthesis at photosystem II and/or inhibition of cell wall (cellulose) synthesis Commonly coformulated with phenoxyacetic acid compounds	Bromoxynil, ioxynil Dichlobenil	II U	Limited human data of single-substance exposures. In animals, it uncouples oxidative phosphorylation and induces CNS toxicity. Similar clinical effects noted in humans.
Organic phosphorus	Bensulide: preemergence selective for grasses. Glyphosate and glufosinate are nonselective postemergence herbicides. In 2012, glyphosate was the most used pesticide in the United States and the second most used in the domestic sector. Bialaphos and glufosinate inhibit glutamine synthetase, bensulide inhibits lipid synthesis, and glyphosate inhibits EPSP synthase, which interferes with aromatic amino acid synthesis.	Butamifos, bialaphos (bilanafos), anilofos, bensulide, piperophos Glufosinate Fosamine, glyphosate	II III U	Limited human data. Bialaphos is metabolized to glufosinate in plants, but in humans only the metabolite L-amino-4-hydroxymethyl-phosphonoyl-butyric acid has been found. Clinical effects of poisoning include apnea, amnesia, and metabolic acidosis. Anilofos and bensulide are shown to inhibit acetyl cholinesterase. See text for glufosinate and Fig. 109–5 See text for glyphosate and Fig. 109–7; Limited human data for fosamine.

Class	Description	Toxicity class	Compounds	Comments
Phenoxy (Fig. 109–8)	Postemergence, selective for grasses. In 2012, 2,4-D was the fifth most used herbicide in the United States but the most used in the domestic sector (mecoprop was third and MCPA ninth).	II	Phenoxyacetic derivatives: 2,4-D	See text for phenoxyacetic derivatives; similar clinical features of toxicity are noted for the chlorinated nonphenoxyacetic acid compounds. Mild clinical toxicity from fenoxaprop-ethyl in acute overdose.[132]
	Inhibits acetyl-CoA carboxylase (lipid biosynthesis; fops) or indole acetic acid–like (auxin growth regulators; chlorinated compounds)	III	Nonphenoxyacetic derivatives: haloxyfop, quizalofop-P	Limited human data on poisoning for others.
			Phenoxyacetic derivatives: MCPA, 2,4,5-T	Fluazifop 0.07 mg/kg was safely administered to humans in a volunteer study.
			Nonphenoxyacetic derivatives: Bromofenoxim, 2,4-DB, dichlorprop, diclofop, fluazifop, MCPB, mecoprop (MCPP), quizalofop, propaquizafop	
	Clomeprop is also an amide compound.	U	Nonphenoxyacetic derivatives: Clomeprop, fenoxaprop-ethyl	
Pyrazole	Inhibition of 4-hydroxyphenyl-pyruvate dioxygenase or photosystem I electron diversion (difenzoquat is also a quaternary ammonium compound)	II	Difenzoquat	Limited human data.
		III	Pyrazoxyfen, pyrazolynate	
		U	Azimsulfuron	
Pyridazine	Preemergence application. Inhibits photosynthesis at photosystem II	III	Pyridate	Limited human data.
Pyridazinone	Inhibits photosynthesis at photosystem II or inhibits carotenoid biosynthesis at the phytoene desaturase step.	U	Chloridazon, norflurazon	Limited human data. In animals, chloridazon interferes with mitochondrial function. Respiratory distress, seizures, and paralysis precede death.
Pyridine	Inhibits carotenoid biosynthesis at the phytoene desaturase step and/or inhibits microtubule assembly and/or indole acetic acid–like (synthetic auxins).	III	Triclopyr	Limited human data on poisoning, but triclopyr appears to be low toxicity,[87] except for one case of acute poisoning with metabolic acidosis, coma and cardiotoxicity; yet, recovery was complete. Triclopyr 0.5 mg/kg was safely administered to humans in a volunteer study. Picloram 5 mg/kg was safely administered to humans in a volunteer study.
		U	Diflufenican, dithiopyr, fluroxypyr, fluthiacet, picloram	
Thiocarbamate	Preemergence, selective for grasses. Inhibits lipid synthesis	II	EPTC, molinate, pebulate, prosulfocarb, thiobencarb, vermolate	Molinate 5 mg was orally administered to volunteers. Limited human data, including effects on cholinesterase. Some compounds display variable inhibition of nicotinic receptors, esterases, and aldehyde dehydrogenase in animals. Cycloate induces neurotoxicity in rats.
		III	Cycloate, esprocarb, triallate	
		U	Tiocarbazil	
Triazine (Fig. 109–9)	Mostly preemergence and nonselective. In 2007 atrazine was the second most used herbicide in the United States. Inhibits photosynthesis at photosystem II	II	Cyanazine, terbumeton	See text.
		III	Ametryn, desmetryn, dimethametryn, simetryn	
		U	Atrazine, prometon, prometryn, propazine, simazine, terbuthylazine, terbutryn, trietazine	
Triazinone	Inhibits photosynthesis at photosystem II	II	Metribuzin, hexazinone	Limited human data. With hexazinone, rats and guinea pigs experience lethargy and ataxia, progressing to clonic seizures prior to death, while dogs were not particularly sensitive. Goats experience sedation, lethargy, and impaired respiration with metamitron poisoning.
		III	Metamitron	
Triazole	Postemergent, nonselective. Commonly coformulated with ammonium thiocyanate. Inhibits lycopene cyclase; chlorophyll or carotenoid pigment inhibitor	U	Amitrole (aminotriazole)	Limited human data on single-agent exposures. Ingestion of 20 mg/kg in a human and > 4,000 mg/kg in rats did not induce symptoms.
Triazolone	Inhibits acetolactate synthase	U	Flucarbazone	Limited human data.
Triazolopyrimidine	Inhibits acetolactate synthase. These herbicides are also amide compounds.	U	Diclosulam, flumetsulam, metosulam	Limited human data. Asthma is reported from occupational exposures to flumetsulam.

(Continued)

TABLE 109–1 Characteristics of the Major Herbicides Categorized by Chemical Class and WHO Hazard Classification *(Continued)*

Chemical Class[a]	Applications, Usage Data, and Mechanism of Action in Plants, If Known[b]	Compounds Included	WHO Hazard Class[c]	Clinical Effects, Treatments, and Supportive Care
Uracil	Mostly preemergence. Inhibit photosynthesis at photosystem II	Bromacil, lenacil, terbacil	U	Limited human data.
Urea	Both pre- and postemergence	Isoproturon, isouron, tebuthiuron	III	Limited human data. Some urea herbicides are metabolized to aniline compounds, which induce methemoglobinemia and hemolysis (similar to propanil, see text). Given the limited experience in treating poisonings with urea herbicides, it is reasonable to apply treatments described for amide herbicide poisoning (see text); success with methylene blue is reported. Wheezing is reported from occupational exposures to chlorimuron.
	Inhibits acetolactate synthase (interferes with branched amino acid synthesis) and/or inhibits photosynthesis at photosystem II and/or inhibition of carotenoid biosynthesis	Bensulfuron, chlorbromuron, chlorimuron, chlorotoluron, cinosulfuron, cyclosulfamuron, daimuron, dimefuron, diuron, fenuron, fluometuron, linuron, methyldymron, metobromuron, metoxuron, metsulfuron, monolinuron, neburon, nicosulfuron, metsulfuron, monolinuron, neburon, nicosulfuron, primisulfuron, pyrazosulfuron, rimsulfuron, siduron, sulfometuron, thifensulfuron, triasulfuron, tribenuron, triflusulfuron	U	Animal studies suggest that isoproturon causes CNS depression and tebuthiuron causes lethargy, ataxia, and anorexia.
Miscellaneous	Clomazone: may be coformulated with propanil	Clomazone, endothal	II	Limited human data; in one case vomiting and gastric and pulmonary hemorrhage preceded death. Animal studies suggest that clomazone inhibits acetylcholinesterase and endothal induces lethargy, respiratory, and hepatic dysfunction. In vitro, clomazone induces oxidative stress and inhibits acetylcholinesterase.
	Clomazone and fluridone: chlorophyll or carotenoid pigment inhibitor	Bentazone, quinoclamine	III	
	Bentazone: pre- and postemergence for control of broadleaf plants. Inhibits photosynthesis	Benfuresate, cinmethylin, ethofumesate, fluridone, flurochloridone, oxadiazon	U	Bentazone: gastrointestinal irritation, hepatic failure, acute kidney injury, dyspnea, muscle rigidity, confusion, death
	Fluridone: chlorophyll or carotenoid pigment inhibitor			Limited human data.

[a]Many of these classes can be further subclassified on the basis of chemical structure; however, the relationship between structure and clinical effects is not adequately described. The classification listed here is adapted from http://www.alanwood.net/pesticides/class_herbicides.html. Accessed December 9, 2012. [b]The mechanism by which a number of herbicides regulate plant growth is not fully described. The mechanisms listed here are adapted from http://www.plantprotection.org/HRAC/MOA.html (Accessed December 9, 2012) and http://www.ces.purdue.edu/extmedia/WS/WS-23-W.html (Accessed December 9, 2012). [c]WHO Hazard Classification scale for oral liquid exposures of the technical grade ingredient based on rat LD$_{50}$ (mg/kg body weight): Ia = "extremely hazardous," <20 mg/kg; Ib = "highly hazardous," 20–200 mg/kg; II = "moderately hazardous," 200–2,000 mg/kg; III = "slightly hazardous," > 2,000 mg/kg; and U = "technical grade active ingredients of pesticides unlikely to present acute hazard in normal use."

CNS = central nervous system; WHO = World Health Organization.

are now comparatively rare in the United States (it remains the 23rd most commonly used pesticide in the United States[33]), whereas the incidence of glyphosate poisoning has increased. Similarly, after paraquat was banned in Japan (late 1980s) and Korea (2012), there was an increase in the number of glufosinate poisonings.

Herbicide poisoning is a major issue in developing countries of the Asia-Pacific region where subsistence farming is common and herbicide use is relatively high. By contrast, the incidence of severe herbicide poisoning is less in developed countries because the population is concentrated in urban areas where access is limited to lower-toxicity herbicides that are sold in smaller volumes as diluted formulations intended for household use (Chaps. 110 and 136).

Regulatory Considerations

When properly used, most herbicide formulations have a low toxic potential for applicators because they are poorly absorbed across the skin and respiratory membranes. When inappropriately used, in particular when there is enteral (or rarely parenteral) exposure, toxicity is more pronounced.

The toxicity on herbicides varies among individual xenobiotics and many are intrinsically more toxic than medications when ingested with suicidal intent. Restrictions of the availability and formulation of toxic herbicides by regulatory authorities improve outcomes from herbicide poisoning. For example, in the context of self-poisoning, in Sri Lanka the replacement of highly toxic pesticides with less toxic compounds decreased the overall mortality[97] without altering agricultural outputs.[72] Prospective cohort studies are useful for estimating the case fatality of individual herbicides in the context of intentional self-poisoning, particularly when encountered in the same clinical environment. For example, in Sri Lanka the following herbicide case fatalities are reported: fenoxaprop-P-ethyl, 0%;[132] bispyribac, 1.8%;[30] glyphosate, 3.2%;[100] 4-chloro-2-methylphenoxyacetic acid (MCPA), 4.4%;[98] propanil, 3.1% to 10.7%;[99] and paraquat, 50% to 70%.[128] This information is of interest to regulatory authorities in their control of the marketing, sales, and formulation of herbicides.

Regulatory bodies must also evaluate other factors, including the cost and efficacy of herbicides and their fate in the environment. An ideal herbicide is one that is selective for the target plant and does not migrate far from the site of application. Selective targeting occurs when the herbicide is rapidly inactivated or binds strongly to soil components. For example, paraquat and glyphosate are inactivated when they contact soil, which is favorable because they remain in the region of application. By contrast, atrazine is more mobile, allowing it to leach into groundwater and migrate great distances. While the concentration of atrazine at distant sites is low, there is concern that it has the potential to alter the growth and development of nontarget plants and animals.[104]

GENERAL COMMENTS FOR THE MANAGEMENT OF ACUTE HERBICIDE POISONING

Diagnosis

Herbicide poisoning is diagnosed following a specific history or other evidence of exposure (such as an empty or partially used bottle) and associated clinical symptoms. A detailed history, including the type of herbicide, amount, time since poisoning, and symptoms, is essential. It is necessary to determine the actual brand in many cases because of variability in salts, concentrations, and coformulants. Furthermore, in some cases it is also necessary to determine the specific type of a brand; for example, the product called Roundup contains glyphosate but it is sold in different formulations worldwide within market sectors.

Depending on local laboratory resources, the diagnosis is confirmed using a specific assay, such as paraquat and glufosinate, but these are not usually available in a clinically meaningful time frame.

The low incidence of herbicide poisoning in some regions often means that it is not considered in the differential diagnosis when a history is not available. Therefore, a high index of suspicion is necessary and clinicians should be familiar with the features of herbicide poisoning.

The pathophysiology of acute herbicide poisoning, and therefore the clinical manifestations, vary between individual compounds. Some herbicides induce multisystem toxicity due to interactions with a number of physiologic systems. The mechanism of toxicity and pathophysiological changes in humans are discussed below for each herbicide individually.

Initial Management

An accurate risk assessment is necessary for the proper triage and subsequent management of patients with acute herbicide poisoning. Risk assessment involves an understanding of the dose ingested, time since ingestion, clinical features, patient factors, and availability of medical facilities. All intentional exposures should be assumed significant. If a patient presents to a facility that is unable to provide sufficient medical and nursing care or does not have ready access to necessary antidotes, then arrangements should be made to rapidly and safely transport the patient to an appropriate health care facility.

For many herbicides, the initial management of an acute poisoning follows standard guidelines. All patients should receive prompt resuscitation emphasizing the airway, breathing, and circulation. Gastrointestinal toxicity, such as nausea, vomiting, and diarrhea, is common, leading to salt and water depletion that requires the administration of antiemetics and intravenous fluids.

Gastrointestinal decontamination decreases absorption of the herbicide from the gut, reducing systemic exposure. We generally recommend not to perform gastric lavage in acute poisoning because patients usually present too late or have self-decontaminated from vomiting and diarrhea. However, gastric lavage is reasonable for patients presenting shortly after an ingestion of a liquid formulation for which treatment options are limited. Ingestion of a corrosive product is a relative contraindication. Depending on the procedure used, this treatment is potentially harmful and should only be conducted by an experienced clinician when the airway is protected. Oral activated charcoal is recommended if the patient presents within 1 to 2 hours of ingestion of an herbicide known to cause significant poisoning. In the case of herbicides with prolonged absorption (eg, propanil, MCPA), later administration of activated charcoal is reasonable. Specific antidotes are available for only a few herbicides, which reflect their ill-defined mechanisms of toxicity. Extracorporeal techniques, including hemoperfusion and hemodialysis, decrease the systemic exposure by increasing the rate of elimination. The role of these treatments is discussed below for each pesticide.

Dermal decontamination is recommended if the patient has incurred cutaneous exposure. The patient should be washed with soap and water, and contaminated clothes, shoes, and leather materials should be removed and safely discarded.

Laboratory investigations are useful for determining the evolution of organ toxicity, including serial measurement of liver and kidney function, electrolytes, and acid–base status. Abnormalities should be corrected when possible. Respiratory distress and hypoxia with focal respiratory crackles soon after presentation are likely to result from aspiration pneumonitis, which should be confirmed on chest radiography.

We recommend a minimum of 6 hours of observation for patients with a history of acute ingestion, unless otherwise stated below. For patients with a history of intentional ingestion and gastrointestinal symptoms, we recommend at least 24 hours of observation depending on the herbicide, given that clinical toxicity will progress or be delayed in some cases.

Occupational and Secondary Exposures (Including Nosocomial Poisoning)

Concern has been expressed regarding the risk of nosocomial poisoning to staff and family members who are exposed to patients with acute herbicide poisoning. However, the risk to health care staff providing clinical care is low compared with other occupations, such as agricultural workers in whom acute toxicity is rarely observed. Universal precautions using nitrile gloves are recommended to provide sufficient protection for staff members.

Few cases of secondary poisoning, if any, are confirmed, and effects in these potentially exposed individuals were generally mild, such as nausea, dizziness, weakness, and headaches, probably relating to inhalation of the hydrocarbon solvent. These symptoms usually resolve after exposure to fresh air. Biomarkers for monitoring occupational exposures, as in the case of pesticide applicators, are outside the scope of this chapter.

Amide Compounds, Particularly Anilide Derivatives

Anilide compounds are the most widely used amide herbicides, of which propanil (3′4′-dichloropropionanilide {DCPA}), alachlor (2-chloro-2′,6′-diethyl-*N*-methoxymethylacetanilide), and butachlor (*N*-butoxymethyl-2-chloro-2′,6′-diethylacetanilide) are particularly common. Other amide herbicides and available toxicity data are listed in Table 109–1. In 2012, acetochlor, propanil, metolachlor, and metolachlor-S were among the most commonly used herbicides in the United States.[33] Anilide compounds are selective herbicides used mostly in rice cultivation in many parts of the world. Acute self-poisoning is reported particularly in Asia where subsistence farming is common. Toxicity data are limited for most compounds, except for propanil, butachlor, metachlor, and alachlor. The case fatality of propanil exceeds 10%, compared with a combined mortality of less than 3% for butachlor, metachlor, and alachlor in case series from Asia.

Pharmacology

Most of the clinical manifestations of propanil poisoning are mediated by its metabolites. 3,4-Dichlorophenylhydroxylamine is the most toxic metabolite and it directly induces methemoglobinemia and hemolysis in a dose-related manner. 3,4-Dichlorophenylhydroxylamine is cooxidized with oxyhemoglobin (Fe^{2+}) in erythrocytes to produce methemoglobin (Fe^{3+}).

However, toxicity is not solely due to methemoglobinemia. Isolated methemoglobin levels exceeding 50% are usually required for fatal outcomes, but fatal propanil poisoning is reported with methemoglobin levels as low as 40%.[17,86,129,130] Therefore, other toxic mechanisms must contribute to clinical outcomes. Rats show signs of toxicity despite inhibition of the hydrolytic enzymes that metabolize propanil (Fig. 109–1) and in the absence of methemoglobinemia, supporting direct toxicity from propanil itself.[115] Dose-dependent kidney and liver cytotoxicity are noted in mice with chronic dosing. Coformulants may also contribute.

The hydroxylamine metabolite depletes glutathione, although this is not consistently reported. Other possible toxicities from the metabolism of propanil include nephrotoxicity, lipid peroxidation, myelotoxicity, and immune dysfunction; the significance of these toxicities is poorly defined.

Para-hydroxylated aniline and other compounds are products of alachlor, butachlor, and acetochlor (2-chloro-*N*-ethoxymethyl-6′-ethylacet-*o*-toluidide)

A. Common Anilide Xenobiotics

Amide   Butachlor   Alachlor

B. Bioconversion of Propanil

Propanil   3,4-dichloroaniline   3,4-dichlorophenyl-hydroxylamine

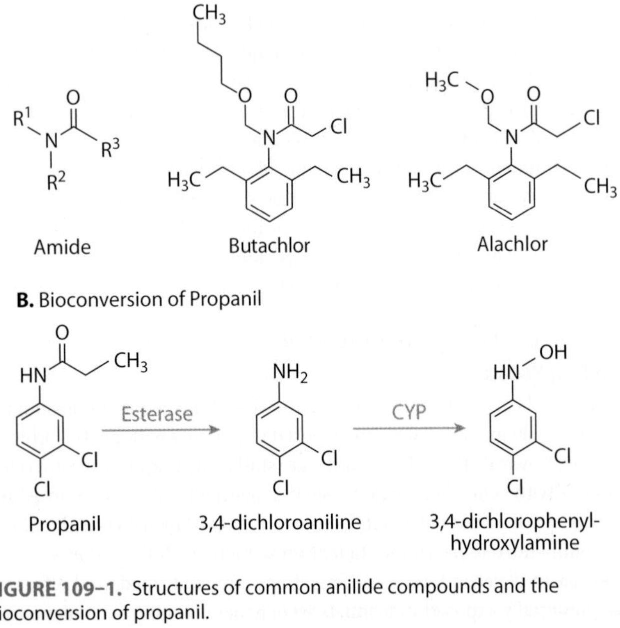

FIGURE 109–1. Structures of common anilide compounds and the bioconversion of propanil.

metabolism and reduces glutathione and induce hepatotoxicity or cancer, particularly in rats.

Pharmacokinetics and Toxicokinetics

Absorption is rapid in animals, with a peak serum concentration expected one hour postingestion. The volume of distribution (V_d) of propanil is not defined, but is expected to be large given that both propanil and 3,4-dichloroaniline are highly lipid soluble. This V_d is consistent with data in the channel catfish in which uptake and distribution of propanil were noted to be extensive.

Anilide compounds undergo sequential metabolic reactions that produce toxic xenobiotics (Fig. 109–1). The first reaction is hydrolysis of the anilide to an aniline compound. This reaction is catalyzed by an esterase known as arylamidase, which has a high capacity in humans compared to rats ($K_m = 473$ μM and 271 μM, respectively) and sometimes by the cytochrome P450 system. Examples include the bioconversion of propanil to 3,4-dichloroaniline and also conversion of alachlor and butachlor to 2,6-diethylaniline. These aniline intermediates are then oxidized by cytochrome P450, although the responsible enzyme is not defined. *N*-Hydroxylation of 3,4-dichloroaniline produces the hydroxylamine compound that induces hemolysis and methemoglobinemia, which are the most obvious manifestations of propanil poisoning.[76,77,115]

These bioactivation reactions appear to be fairly rapid, whereas 3,4-dichloroaniline and methemoglobin are formed within 2 to 3 hours of parenteral administration of propanil to animals. The hydroxylation of 3,4-dichloroaniline is saturable ($K_m = 120$ μM in rats) and slower than arylamidase, leading to a prolonged elimination of 3,4-dichloroaniline following large exposures. In the case of alachlor, butachlor, and acetochlor, parahydroxylated aniline compounds are produced, which appear to be carcinogens in rats.

These metabolic reactions are similar to those of dapsone, which are well characterized: the severity of methemoglobinemia relates to the amount of the dapsone hydroxylamine, metabolite, which varies with dose, and cytochrome P450 activity (Chap. 124).

Propanil displays nonlinear toxicokinetics in humans with prolonged absorption continuing for approximately 10 hours following ingestion. Bioconversion to 3,4-dichloroaniline occurs largely within 6 hours, although it is particularly variable, which reflects interindividual differences in esterase activity, dose, or coexposure to cholinesterase inhibitors.[99] The median apparent elimination half-life of propanil is 3.2 hours compared with 3,4-dichloroaniline, which has a highly variable elimination profile. In general, the concentration of 3,4-dichloroaniline exceeds that of propanil and remains elevated for a longer period.[99] In a case of coingestion of carbaryl, the peak 3,4-dichloroaniline concentration was observed at 24 hours,[42] whereas in a fatal case the concentration of 3,4-dichloroaniline continued to increase until at least 30 hours postingestion.[99] By 36 hours postingestion, the concentration of 3,4-dichloroaniline is low in survivors, so clinical toxicity is unlikely to increase beyond this time.[99]

Pathophysiology

The predominant clinical manifestation in acute poisoning is methemoglobinemia. Methemoglobin is unable to bind and transport oxygen, inducing a relative hypoxia at the cellular level despite adequate dissolved arterial oxygen content. This leads to end-organ dysfunction, including central nervous system depression, hypotension, and acidemia. Because the plasma concentration of 3,4-dichloroaniline remains elevated, the potential production of methemoglobin persists for a protracted period of time.[42,86,129] Sedation due to the direct effect of propanil or a hydrocarbon coformulant solvent causes hypoventilation, which contributes to cellular hypoxia. Failure to correct these abnormalities may lead to irreversible injury and death.

Clinical Manifestations

Methemoglobinemia, hemolysis and anemia, coma, and death are reported following acute propanil poisoning. These occur in the clinical context of cyanosis, acidemia, and progressive end-organ dysfunction. A case fatality as high as 10.7% is reported and the median time to death was 36 hours. Patients who die tend to be older with a depressed Glasgow Coma Scale score and elevated concentration of propanil. Nausea, vomiting, diarrhea, tachycardia, dizziness, and confusion are also reported in patients who do not develop severe poisoning.[99] However, with earlier recognition and improved use of methylene blue and a color chart for categorizing severity of methemoglobinemia, mortality decreased to 3.1%.

Alachlor, metachlor, and butachlor are less toxic than propanil, with a case fatality less than 3% with self-poisoning.[71,112] The manifestations of acute poisoning are usually mild, including gastrointestinal symptoms, agitation, dyspnea, and abnormal liver enzymes.[71,112] Major symptoms include seizures, rhabdomyolysis, acidemia, kidney failure, and cardiac dysrhythmias; hypotension and coma preceded death.[71,112] Methemoglobinemia was not reported in these studies. Hepatic dysfunction was reported following dermal occupational exposure to butachlor.

Cyanosis was reported following acute ingestion of mefenacet (2-benzothiazol-2-yloxy-N-methylacetanilide) and imazosulfuron (1-{2-chloroimidazo-(1,2-a) pyridin-3-ylsulfonyl}-3-{4,6-dimethoxypyrimidin-2-yl}urea) in the context of normal cooximetry. This was attributed to formation of a green pigment (green-colored urine was also reported), and no other symptoms of toxicity were observed.[114]

Acute metolachlor (2-chloro-N-{6-ethyl-o-tolyl}-N-{(1RS)-2-methoxy-1-methylethyl}acetamide) poisoning in goats induced predominantly neuromuscular symptoms, including tremors, ataxia, and myoclonus, which progressed rapidly to death. Kidney and hepatocellular toxicity were also noted. Acute acetochlor exposures in rats induced methemoglobinemia and hepatocellular toxicity.

Diagnostic Testing

Patients with a history of propanil poisoning should be investigated for the presence of methemoglobinemia (Chap. 124). In the absence of co-oximetry, simple color charts can be used to support the diagnosis and severity of methemoglobinemia and to direct the use of antidotes at the bedside.

While the concentrations of propanil and 3,4-dichloroaniline reflect clinical outcomes, this relationship is less marked for 3,4-dichloroaniline during the first 6 hours, which probably relates to the time for bioconversion from propanil.[99] However, propanil and 3,4-dichloroaniline assays are not commercially available and this observation was not validated. Further, the relationship between concentration and outcomes may depend on patient comorbidities.

Management

The minimum toxic dose has not been determined and the potential for severe poisoning and death is high, so all patients with amide herbicide ingestions should be treated as significant and monitored for a minimum of 12 hours. Patients with symptomatic ingestions should be treated cautiously, including continuous monitoring for 24 to 48 hours, preferably in an intensive care unit.

Routine clinical observations are sufficient to detect signs of poisoning, in particular sedation and cyanosis, which are noted early postingestion. The time to death is usually greater than 24 hours so there is an opportunity to initiate treatment. There are no controlled clinical or laboratory data available on the effect of any specific treatment in acute symptomatic propanil poisoning, so management is largely focused on reversal of methemoglobinemia and supportive care.

Resuscitation and Supportive Care

Prompt resuscitation and close observation are required in all patients. Patients should be monitored clinically including pulse oximetry, and receive supportive care including supplemental oxygen, intravenous fluids, and ventilatory and hemodynamic support as required. In the absence of cooximetry analysis, significant methemoglobinemia should be suspected when cyanosis does not correct with high-flow oxygen and ventilatory support. Bedside visual assessment, using blood added to absorbent paper, is an accurate method to quantify the degree of methemoglobinemia.[113] Euglycemia should be ensured since adequate glucose concentrations are required for reversal of methemoglobin. Hemoglobin concentrations should be monitored to detect hemolysis, and folate supplementation is recommended during the recovery phase if anemia is significant.

Gastrointestinal Decontamination

Toxicokinetic studies of propanil demonstrate a prolonged absorption phase, so it is reasonable to administer activated charcoal to the patient a number of hours postingestion.

Extracorporeal Removal

Data are extremely limited and based on a single report it does not have a role in routine care. A report of combined hemodialysis and hemoperfusion noted a propanil elimination half-life of one hour,[86] but similar half-lives are reported in patients who have not received this treatment.[99] Exchange transfusion has the potential to decrease the concentration of propanil and free hemoglobin, while replacing reduced hemoglobin and hemolyzed erythrocytes. Exchange transfusion may be particularly useful in the treatment of patients who also have glucose-6-phosphate dehydrogenase (G6PD) deficiency. However, the function of transfused erythrocytes is temporarily impaired posttransfusion because of depletion of 2,3-bisphosphoglycerate and G6PD during storage. Further, transfusion reactions such as acute respiratory distress syndrome (ARDS) are a concern, particularly when oxygenation is already impaired. In the absence of controlled studies, the role of such treatments in the routine management of acute propanil poisoning is poorly defined and cannot be recommended at this time (Chap. 6).

Antidotes

Methylene blue (Antidotes in Depth: A43) is the first-line treatment for methemoglobinemia. Methylene blue has a half-life of 5 hours, which is commonly shorter than that of 3,4-dichloroaniline, so rebound poisoning (ie, an increase in methemoglobin following an initial recovery postadministration of methylene blue) is anticipated and has been observed with a bolus regimen. This is prevented by administration of methylene blue as a constant infusion.

Other potential treatments for methemoglobinemia from propanil include toluidine blue, N-acetylcysteine, ascorbic acid, and cimetidine, but no clinical studies have assessed the role of these potential antidotes in the management of propanil poisoning.

BIPYRIDYL COMPOUNDS, PARAQUAT AND DIQUAT

Bipyridyl compounds are nonselective contact herbicides. The most widely used is paraquat (1,1'-dimethyl-4,4'-bipyridinium), but diquat (1,1'-ethylene-2,2'-bipyridyldiylium) is also commonly used (Fig. 109–2). Paraquat is one of the most toxic pesticides available. Ingestion of as little as 10 to 20 mL of the 20% wt/vol solution is sufficient to cause death. Overall, the mortality rate varies between 50% and 90%; however, in cases of intentional self-poisoning with concentrated formulations, mortality approaches 100%. An increasing number of countries are banning the sale of paraquat in view of its high toxicity. Diquat is less toxic than paraquat, so it is frequently coformulated with paraquat (allowing a lower concentration of paraquat) or used as an alternative in countries where paraquat is severely restricted. Nevertheless, deaths are still reported from intentional and unintentional diquat poisoning in the United States. Because more data are available on paraquat than diquat, much of the following discussion and information relates particularly to paraquat.

Pharmacology

Paraquat and diquat formulations are highly irritating and often corrosive, causing direct injury. They induce intracellular toxicity by the generation of

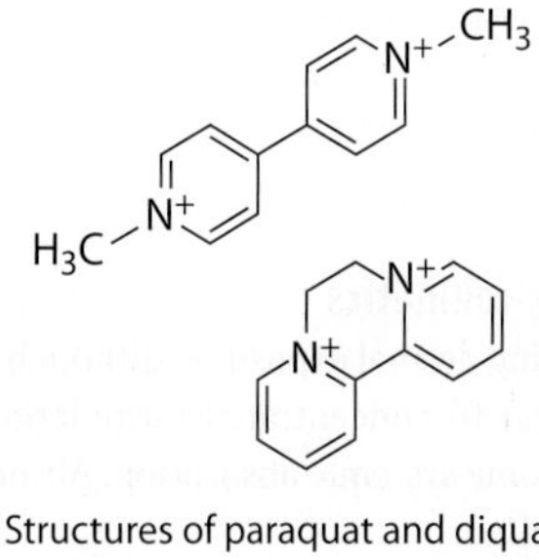

FIGURE 109–2. Structures of paraquat and diquat.

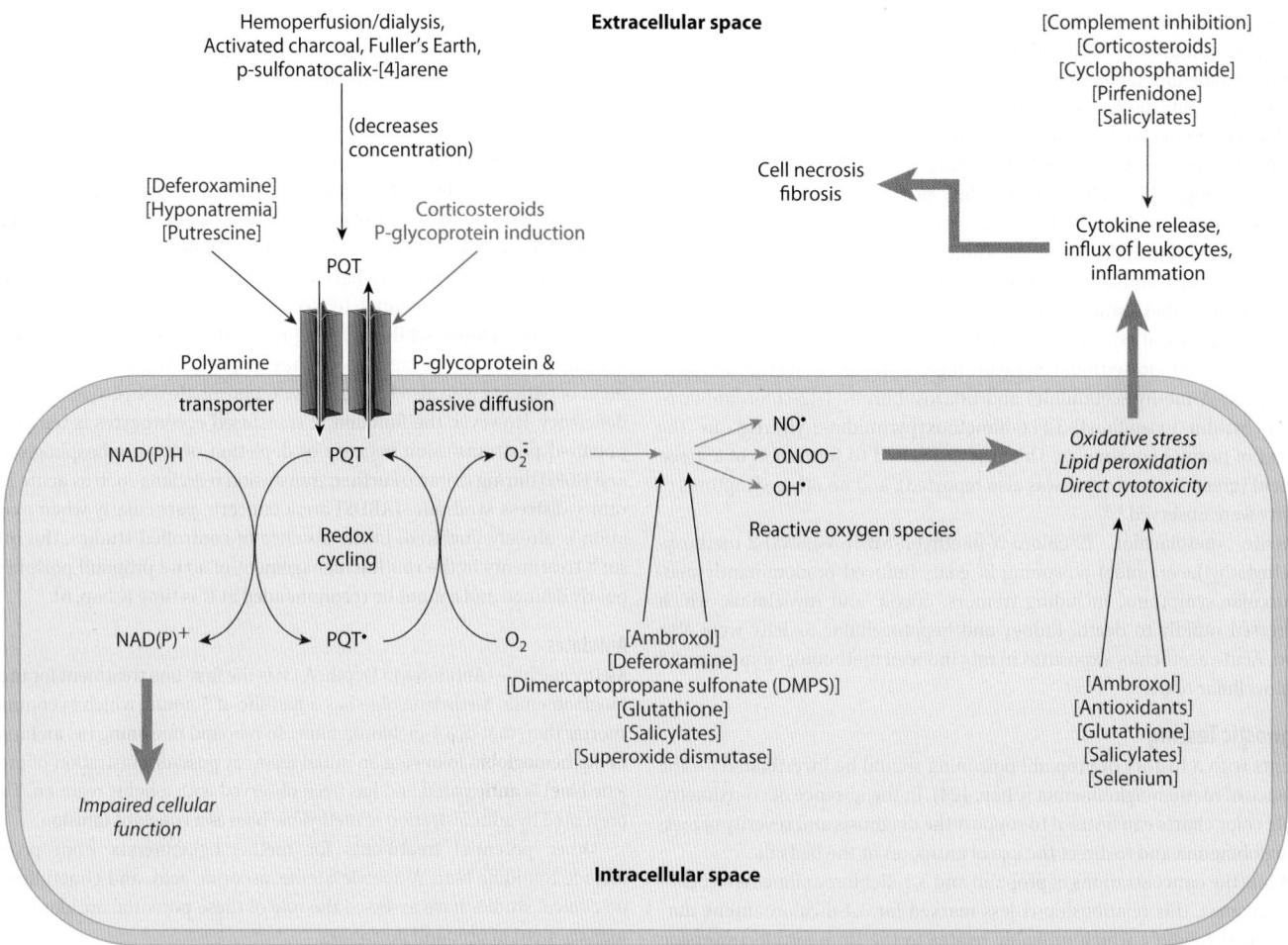

FIGURE 109–3. Toxicology of paraquat (PQT) and proposed mechanisms of action of potential treatments. Antioxidants include vitamins C and E and glutathione donors (particularly *N*-acetylcysteine, *S*-carboxymethylcysteine). PQT· = paraquat radical; NO· = nitric oxide; ONOO⁻ = peroxynitrite; OH· = hydroxyl radical.

reactive oxygen species that nonspecifically damage the lipid membrane of cells, inducing cellular injury and death. Once paraquat enters the intracellular space it is oxidized to the paraquat radical. This radical is subsequently reduced by diaphorase in the presence of nicotinamide adenine dinucleotide phosphate (NADPH) to re-form the parent paraquat compound and superoxide radical, a reactive oxygen species. This process is known as redox cycling (Fig. 109–3). The superoxide radical is susceptible to further reactions by other intracellular processes, leading to formation of other reactive oxygen species, including hydroxyl radicals and peroxynitrite. Reactive oxygen species are potent cytotoxics. Paraquat redox cycling continues if NADPH and oxygen are available. Depletion of NADPH prevents recycling of glutathione and interferes with other intracellular processes, including energy production and active transporters, exacerbating toxicity. Intracellular protective mechanisms, such as glutathione, superoxide dismutase, and catalase, are overwhelmed or depleted following large exposures. Taken together, these cytotoxic reactions induce cellular necrosis, which is followed by an influx of neutrophils and macrophages. The reactions contribute to the inflammatory response and promote fibrosis and destruction of normal tissue architecture over a number of days.[2,18]

Supplemental oxygen probably increases the generation of reactive oxygen species.

Pharmacokinetics and Toxicokinetics

Absorption is limited following dermal exposures, although prolonged exposures (at least several hours) to concentrated formulations degrades the epithelial barrier, allowing some systemic absorption. Absorption across the respiratory epithelium is limited.

The oral bioavailability of paraquat in humans is estimated to be less than 5%,[16] yet an oral exposure of as little as 10 mL of the 20% wt/vol formulation is sufficient for significant poisoning to occur. Absorption is rapid and the peak concentration occurs within one hour. The peak parquat plasma concentration correlates with the amount ingested. Paraquat was reformulated with an emetic along with an alginate (Gramoxone Inteon) that formed a gelatinous mixture on contact with gastric acid, limiting release of the paraquat into the stomach. This formulation reduced paraquat absorption in animals[37] and initially appeared to improve outcomes from self-poisoning in humans (mortality of 64% compared with 74% with the standard preparation),[126] but this observation was not sustained.[128]

Paraquat binds minimally to plasma proteins. Paraquat and diquat rapidly distribute to all tissues and then redistribute back to the central circulation.[84] In humans, the distribution half-life is approximately 5 hours. Paraquat is taken up by alveolar cells through an active energy-dependent polyamine transporter. Paraquat accumulates in alveolar cells, peaking at around 6 hours postingestion in patients with normal kidney function, but later in the context of kidney impairment.[5] Paraquat slowly redistributes from the lungs into the systemic circulation as the plasma concentration falls. By contrast, diquat uptake occurs to a limited extent.

Paraquat and diquat are not metabolized. Elimination is primarily renal with more than 90% of a dose being excreted within the first 24 hours of poisoning if kidney function is maintained.[45] Systemic clearance initially exceeds that of GFR because of active secretion.[12] Impaired kidney function commonly occurs with paraquat and diquat poisoning, particularly beyond 24 to 48 hours postingestion, which decreases excretion and potentiates poisoning. Elimination is prolonged in this setting with a terminal half-life of around 80 hours in humans.[45] Paraquat is detected in the urine of surviving patients beyond 30 days despite plasma concentrations being quite low 48 hours postingestion.[3]

Pathophysiology

Paraquat and diquat induce nonspecific cellular necrosis. Lung and kidney injuries are prominent in acute paraquat poisoning because of the high concentrations found in these cells.

Acute pneumonitis and hemorrhage, followed by ongoing inflammation and progressive pulmonary fibrosis, reduces oxygen diffusion and induces dyspnea and hypoxia, which interferes with normal cellular function.[22]

Paraquat induces acute tubular necrosis due to direct toxicity to the proximal tubule in particular, and to a lesser degree distal structures. Other factors contributing to the development of acute kidney injury include hypoperfusion from hypovolemia and/or hypotension and direct glomerular injury. Varying degrees of oliguria, proteinuria, hematuria, and glycosuria are reported.[12] Acute kidney injury interferes with normal fluid and electrolyte homeostasis, as well as interfering with paraquat elimination, which promotes systemic toxicity.

Necrosis of the gastrointestinal tract limits absorption and causes fluid shifts that contribute to hypotension induced by direct vascular toxicity. Hypotension impairs tissue perfusion and if uncorrected progresses to irreversible shock. Failure to correct these abnormalities leads to irreversible organ injury and death.

Clinical Manifestations

Topical exposures induce painful irritation to the eyes (including formation of a conjunctival pseudomembrane) and skin, progressing to ulceration or desquamation depending on the concentration of the solution, duration of exposure, and adequacy of decontamination. Intravenous administration induces severe poisoning from small exposures.

Most ingestions of bipyridyl compounds induce poisoning, in which ingestion of as little as 5 mL of paraquat 20% wt/vol causes death in more than 50% of cases. Outcomes are more favorable in pediatric patients because of the higher proportion with unintentional poisoning. Gastrointestinal toxicity occurs early, including nausea, vomiting, and abdominal and oral pain. Diarrhea, ileus, and pancreatitis are also reported. Necrosis of mucous membranes, occasionally referred to as pseudodiphtheria,[117] and ulceration are prominent findings that occur within 12 hours. Oromucosal injury without systemic features is observed following brief oral exposures without swallowing. Dysphagia and odynophagia follow larger exposures and progress to esophageal rupture, pneumomediastinum and mediastinitis, subcutaneous emphysema, and pneumothorax, which are usually preterminal events. Death is more likely in those patients who experience a peripheral burning sensation.[29]

Respiratory symptoms are prominent in patients with paraquat poisoning, including acute respiratory distress syndrome manifesting as dyspnea, hypoxia, and increased work of breathing. Ingestions of greater than 50 mL of 20% wt/vol formulation causes multiorgan dysfunction with rapid onset of death within days of ingestion in most patients. Features include hypotension, acute kidney and liver injury, severe diarrhea, and hemolytic anemia.

By contrast, ARDS is less marked with diquat ingestion or following smaller exposures of paraquat (<15–20 mL of 20% wt/vol formulations). In the case of paraquat, the acute respiratory impairment is often followed by progressive pulmonary fibrosis and death weeks or months postingestion. Varying degrees of acute kidney injury and hepatic dysfunction occur.[6,48] Acute kidney injury peaks around 5 days postingestion and resolves within 3 weeks in survivors.[54] Paraquat-induced pulmonary injury is reported to resolve to near-normal function over months to years in survivors.[66]

Diquat does not concentrate in the pneumocytes as readily as paraquat. Therefore, if the patient survives the multiorgan dysfunction, pulmonary fibrosis is less likely to occur.[131] Seizures are reported with diquat poisoning and uncommonly with paraquat.

Ingestion of the adjuvant for Gramoxone Inteon (20% methanol, 20% sodium lignosulfonate, 10% alkylaryl polyoxyethylene ether) induces minor gastrointestinal adverse effects, an elevated serum osmolar gap, and metabolic acidosis with hyperlactatemia, but outcomes are favorable.[80]

Diagnostic Testing

Paraquat poisoning is diagnosed when there is a history of exposure and the recognized clinical features, so a high index of clinical suspicion is required. Differential diagnoses include other caustic exposures, sepsis, or other cellular poisons such as phosphine, colchicine, or iron.

The presence of a bipyridyl compound in blood confirms exposure but availability of these assays is increasingly limited. The urinary dithionite test is a simple and quick method for confirming (or excluding) paraquat and diquat poisoning. Various methods are reported, including the addition of 1 g of sodium bicarbonate and 1 g of sodium dithionite, or 1 to 2 mL of 1% sodium dithionite in 1 to 2 M sodium hydroxide, to 10 mL of urine. A color change (blue for paraquat and green for diquat) confirms ingestion—the darker the color, the higher the concentration.[3,58,103] If the test is negative on urine beyond 6 hours after ingestion, a large exposure is unlikely, but repeat testing should be conducted over 24 hours. When the dithionite test is conducted on plasma (eg, add 200 μL of 1% sodium dithionite in 2 M sodium hydroxide to 2 mL plasma from the patient), a positive result is specific for death, but a negative test does not exclude severe poisoning or death.[58]

Given that outcomes from paraquat poisoning are generally poor, diagnostic tests help differentiate patients who are likely to survive compared to those in whom death is almost certain. The dose of paraquat is a well-established predictor of death, although this information often is not accurately known at the time of admission. Investigations in patients with acute paraquat poisoning have attempted to determine the severity of poisoning and better define prognosis. Unfortunately, few are validated so their predictive ability is unconfirmed. A range of prognostic tests has been reviewed[24] and a selection of these are discussed below.

Quantitative analysis of the concentration of paraquat in plasma is useful for prognostication, and a number of similar nomograms have been developed to assist with this process (eg, Fig. 109–4). The paraquat concentration must be interpreted relative to the time since ingestion, and each method performs similarly.[110] The Severity Index of Paraquat Poisoning (SIPP) is also calculated with this information, by multiplying the plasma concentration (mg/L) by the time since ingestion (hours). Here, SIPP less than 10 predicts survival, SIPP 10 to 50 predicts death from lung fibrosis, and SIPP more than 50 predicts death from circulatory failure.[107] Determination of the concentration of paraquat in the urine of exposed patients also predicts outcomes. Barriers to the use of these methods include the limited availability of quantitative paraquat assays (leading to a long turnaround time) and the accuracy of the time of ingestion.

Other methods for predicting outcomes from paraquat poisoning have used combinations of simple laboratory tests, including blood gas analysis, complete blood count, electrolytes, uric acid, pancreatitis, kidney function, and liver function tests.[24] Various specific changes are proposed to predict death (eg, metabolic acidosis with an elevated lactate concentration) and increasingly complicated algorithms are being developed, but few are validated. In general, any abnormal result raises the suspicion of a significant poisoning and serial testing is warranted.

An elevated admission creatinine concentration or albuminuria predicts death but is neither sensitive nor specific, although the higher the creatinine concentration, the higher the risk of death.[31,54,58,102]

The rate of increase in creatinine concentration is a simple and practical test to predict prognosis. An increase less than 0.03 mg/dL/h (3 μmol/L/h) over 5 hours predicts survival,[95] or greater than 0.05 mg/dL/h (4.3 μmol/L/h) over 12 hours (sensitivity 100%, specificity 85%, likelihood ratio 7) predicts death.[102] A similar relationship was noted for cystatin C, in which a rate of increase in cystatin C greater than 0.009 mg/L/h over 6 hours (sensitivity 100%, specificity 91%, likelihood ratio 11) predicted death.[102] This method of prognostication is advantageous because it is determined irrespective of the time of poisoning. Paraquat and diquat interfere with creatinine assays using the Jaffe method, but this is mostly an issue with concentrations exceeding

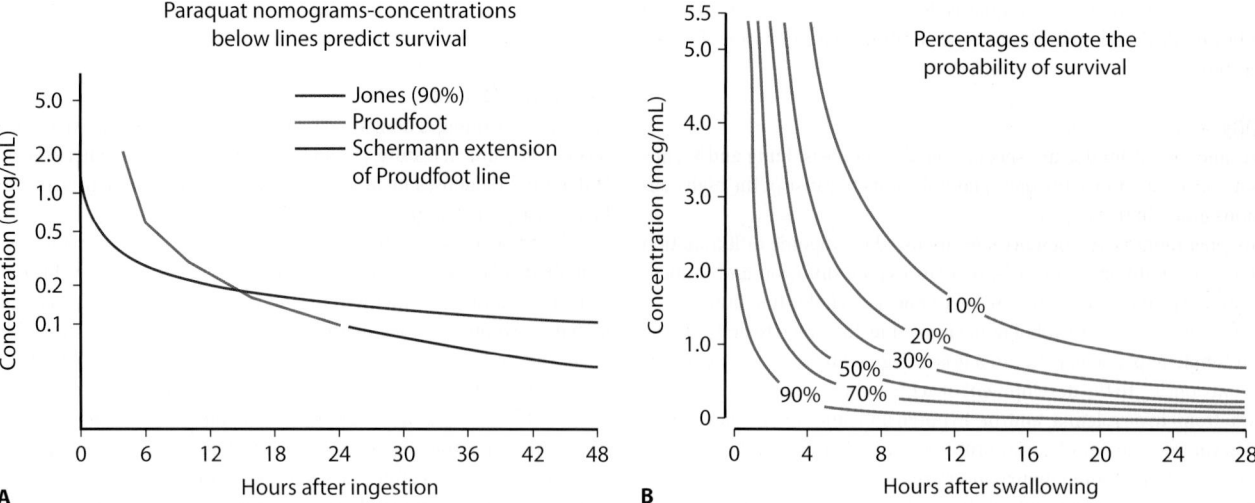

FIGURE 109–4. Nomograms for plasma paraquat concentrations. (**A**) Compilation of 3 nomograms proposed by Proudfoot et al,[94] Scherrmann et al,[108] and Jones et al.[52] (**B**) Hart paraquat nomogram.[36] In *A*, concentrations below lines predict survival. In *B*, lines link concentrations of equal probability of survival. *(Reproduced with permission from Eddleston M, Wilks MF, Buckley NA. Prospects for treatment of paraquat-induced lung fibrosis with immunosuppressive drugs and the need for better prediction of outcome: a systematic review. QJM. 2003 Nov;96(11):809-824.)*

100 mg/L, which are rarely observed and would be associated with severe clinical toxicity.[92] Other biomarkers of kidney function have been explored but their role in clinical management is not confirmed, nor did they improve on existing methods.

Computed tomography provides prognostic information based on the proportion of lung with ground-glass opacification. For example, ground-glass opacities in 11% to 12% of lung within 4 to 6 days postingestion predicted death in two studies, but in another less than 20% predicted survival and greater than 40% predicted death. Progression of consolidation, fibrosis, and pleural effusion over 2 to 3 days are also strong indicators of poor prognosis.

Management

Because death follows ingestion of as little as 5 mL of the 20% wt/vol paraquat, all exposures should be treated as potentially life threatening. Patients suspected of ingesting paraquat should be observed in hospital for at least 6 hours postingestion or until a urinary dithionite test is conducted.

Many medical interventions are proposed for the treatment of patients with acute paraquat poisoning but data supporting their efficacy are lacking. Dose–response studies for most of these interventions are also unavailable, and although cell-based and animal studies provide insights into the dose–response, this does not readily translate to human therapeutics.

Given the high likelihood of death from acute paraquat poisoning, many publications report concurrent administration of a number of therapies in the hope of a benefit, including activated charcoal, acetylcysteine, vitamins C and E, immunosuppressants, and hemodialysis and/or hemoperfusion. Xuebijing (a preparation made from 5 traditional Chinese medicines reported to have antiinflammatory properties) and ulinastatin are used in some hospitals in China and supported by animal studies. The literature is complicated by case reports describing survival in patients who were administered one or a combination of these and other therapies, despite apparently poor prognosis. Various other treatments have been studied in animals including pirfenidone, complement inhibition, sivelestat, bosentan, *p*-sulfonatocalix-[4]arene, dimercaptopropane sulfonate, ambroxol, sucralfate, bone marrow mesenchymal stem cell transplantation and selenium, but human data are lacking. We have no evidence to recommend treatment with any of these regimens.

The choice of which interventions should be administered to a patient is made on a case-by-case basis by the treating physician in consultation with relevant resources. In the context of the anticipated prognosis (see above), detailed discussion with the patient and relatives early in the presentation is recommended to determine their preference for treatment. In general, a comprehensive treatment regimen is reasonable in patients who present

very early (within 2 hours of poisoning) or those with a faintly positive dithionite urinary test. Here, treatments that reduce the exposure to paraquat by either reducing absorption or increasing clearance must be initiated promptly. In contrast, active treatment is not recommended in patients in whom this test is strongly positive, or those with hemodynamic compromise or evolving lung injury. Instead, palliation should be the priority, including supplemental oxygen for hypoxia and morphine for dyspnea and oropharyngeal and abdominal pain.

Serial pulse oximetry measurements and chest radiographs will demonstrate onset and progression of lung injury. Lung transplantation has been tried in patients with delayed respiratory failure, but it was largely unsuccessful because of the prolonged elimination half-life of paraquat.[6] However, successful lung transplantation was reported when performed 56 days postpoisoning after 12 days of extracorporeal membrane oxygenation therapy. Patients developing acute kidney injury should receive hemodialysis or hemofiltration per usual guidelines if active treatment is to be pursued, and these treatments also enhance elimination of herbicide if commenced promptly (see below).

Resuscitation and Supportive Care

All patients should receive prompt routine resuscitation and close observation. Supplemental oxygen should only be administered to patients for palliation when there is confirmed hypoxia and/or prognosis is extremely poor. Although controlled hypoxia does not prevent the development of pulmonary injury, unnecessary supplemental oxygen theoretically hastens the progression of injury. In patients with established lung injury, ventilatory support is reasonable to improve oxygenation and reduce dyspnea.

Intravenous fluids should be administered to patients who are volume depleted from reduced intake, diarrhea, or third-space shifts, as this reduces the severity of acute kidney injury and promotes renal clearance of paraquat. Care is required with volume resuscitation in the context of acute kidney injury to prevent fluid overload. Electrolyte abnormalities should be corrected as required.

Ongoing management includes regular clinical observations including urine output quantification, daily routine laboratory tests (or more frequently if clinically indicated) in patients receiving active treatment and supportive care. Analgesia for oral and abdominal pain should be administered as required, including intravenous opioids, such as morphine, and possibly topical anesthetics, such as lidocaine. Plain radiographs or a CT of the chest provide information on lung and esophageal injury, which may be prognostic as noted above.

Gastrointestinal Decontamination

Activated charcoal is recommended for all patients presumed to have ingested paraquat as soon as possible, within 2 hours of exposure. Paraquat is coformulated with an emetic so a degree of self-decontamination frequently occurs by the time of presentation to hospital. Fuller's Earth and activated charcoal decrease absorption of paraquat to a similar extent but Fuller's Earth is in limited supply.[4] Because paraquat is rapidly absorbed, decontamination must be commenced within a few hours of ingestion to be useful. Gastric lavage is not shown to improve outcomes overall.[127]

Extracorporeal Removal

Extracorporeal techniques, in particular hemoperfusion and hemodialysis, increase the elimination of paraquat, which decreases the systemic exposure, and potentially toxicity. Although published data regarding the efficacy of these treatments are contradictory or limited, extracorporeal treatments are recommended in cases of large exposures if the treatment can be initiated within a few hours of ingestion.

Paraquat clearance by hemoperfusion is similar to endogenous clearance but exceeds it when there is impaired kidney function.[53,67] Hemoperfusion is more efficient than hemodialysis, and elimination is maximized when treatment is initiated within the first couple of hours because the plasma concentration is high.[39] Further, given that paraquat rapidly distributes from the circulation, prompt treatment is necessary to limit the uptake into pulmonary and other tissues.[89]

Experimentally, hemoperfusion reduces mortality in dogs only when it is commenced within a few hours of poisoning, and repeated treatments did not significantly increase clearance.[89] Other animal studies have suggested benefits from hemoperfusion when performed within one hour, including a decrease in paraquat exposure, less end-organ damage and a reduction in inflammatory cytokines, but no mortality benefit.

Past experience suggested that extracorporeal treatments do not sufficiently improve mortality in humans, particularly when the concentration is greater than 3 mg/L.[35] Hemoperfusion followed by continuous venovenous hemofiltration prolonged the time to death compared with hemoperfusion alone without changing the overall mortality in nonrandomized studies and a meta-analysis that included three randomized controlled trials (n = 290 patients). However, increasing publications from eastern Asia suggest a clinical benefit from these therapies if commenced early, within 4 to 6 hours of ingestion and possibly with repeat treatment or with concurrent hemodialysis.

The risk of harm from extracorporeal techniques reflects the requirement for central venous access, metabolic disequilibrium, or increased clearance of antidotes, although such risks are low.

Antidotes

A large number of potential antidotes are under study in the treatment of acute paraquat poisoning. The combination of antidotes (if any) that will improve outcomes is not known, so it is not possible to recommend specific antidotes or dosages in routine clinical care.

Antidotes attempt to counteract the effects of paraquat by targeting various steps in the pathogenesis of organ dysfunction or to alter cellular uptake (Fig. 109–3). Unfortunately, despite their potential promise in animal studies, none of these antidotes are proven to reduce mortality in humans. Some of the interventions that decrease paraquat exposure by decreasing absorption[126] or increasing elimination[57] were shown to prolong the time to death. Therefore, clinicians commonly combine these treatments as part of a multimodal approach in the hope that it will reduce mortality. There are insufficient published data to support this approach, but in view of the high mortality from paraquat this approach is not generally considered to add to patient's risk. Therefore, such a multimodal approach to treatment may be reasonable in certain cases, such as early presentations of less than 50 mL of 20% wt/vol formulations when extracorporeal treatments are also available. Examples of specific potential antidotes are detailed here.

Immunosuppression with corticosteroids (dexamethasone or methylprednisolone) and cyclophosphamide are the most extensively studied antidotes in humans. Early randomized controlled trial data (3 trials, n = 164 patients) suggested a benefit from these treatments but because of limitations in study design these results were not considered conclusive.[68] This was followed by a larger randomized controlled trial (n = 298) that reported no mortality benefit from high-dose immunosuppression (cyclophosphamide, methylprednisolone, dexamethasone) in patients with acute paraquat poisoning.[28] Therefore, although nonrandomized studies support a potential benefit, this immunosuppressive regimen is not recommended.

Generation of reactive oxygen species is an important step in the pathogenesis of paraquat poisoning (Fig. 109–3). This leads to cytotoxicity, the extent of which depends on the concentration of paraquat and the efficiency of endogenous protective mechanisms such as vitamin C (ascorbic acid), vitamin E (α-tocopherol), and glutathione. Administration of these vitamins and/or a glutathione donor (eg, N-acetylcysteine, S-carboxymethylcysteine, captopril) or other scavenging agents such as superoxide dismutase and amifostine and deferoxamine is not routinely recommended because they are not proven to be beneficial, and potentially vitamin C might increase oxidative toxicity.[22]

Some treatments influence the toxicokinetics of paraquat at the cellular level. Xenobiotics that decrease the uptake of paraquat into pneumocytes were studied such as putrescine, spermidine, and deferoxamine, but their effect is limited and they do not alter efflux. Corticosteroids, particularly dexamethasone and methylprednisolone, were shown in animal models to induce P-glycoprotein, which increases the cellular efflux and excretion of paraquat although data regarding the extent to which paraquat is a substrate for P-glycoprotein are conflicting. Therefore, these treatments are not routinely recommended.

Salicylates are proposed to inhibit multiple steps in the pathogenesis of paraquat poisoning, including decreasing production of reactive oxygen species, inhibition of NF-κB, antithrombotic effects, and chelation of paraquat.[20,21] Sodium salicylate 200 mg/kg decreased reactive oxygen species production and inflammation and improved survival in rats.[20] Similarly, lysine acetylsalicylate 200 mg/kg improved survival in rats in a dose-finding study.[23,46] A small pilot study noted a delayed time to death in patients receiving intravenous acetylsalicylic acid. Other antidotes and treatments have also been proposed, but less information regarding their effects is available. Therefore, these treatments are not routinely recommended.

Treatment Recommendations

Most clinical studies have not demonstrated favorable outcomes, in contrast to animal studies. This reflects larger poisonings, increased sensitivity or delayed institution of therapy in human reports. Because some studies report a delayed time to death in patients who receive an intervention, this has suggested a possible effect and prompted further research into dose–response and the effect of combination therapy. In patients with a poor prognosis, active treatment, particularly with invasive modalities such as hemoperfusion/dialysis, will interfere with end-of-life care. Based on these principles, our recommendations favor intervention when there is a hope of recovery, while avoiding unfounded experimental technologies.

The prognosis in patients presenting more than 12 hours after ingesting 50 mL or more of paraquat 20% wt/vol, those with a positive plasma dithionite test, or those with a SIPP greater than 50 is so poor that treatment should focus on symptom control and end-of-life support and palliation.

The prognosis in patients presenting within 6 hours of ingesting less than 50 mL of paraquat, those with a faint-positive dithionite test, or those with a SIPP less than 50 is also poor, but prompt multimodal treatment with volume resuscitation, oral activated charcoal (or Fuller's Earth), hemoperfusion or hemodialysis, intravenous corticosteroids, acetylsalicylate, N-acetylcysteine, deferoxamine, and vitamin E can be considered on a case-by-case basis. It cannot be overemphasized that potential benefits of these treatments (if any) is time-critical so they must be commenced immediately. If any of these treatments are not available at the initial treatment center it is reasonable to transfer the patient to a center that can provide them within the stated time frame. Excluding dermal exposures, other exposures not yet mentioned are associated with poor prognosis and unlikely to respond to treatment. However, if resources are available and psychosocial or cultural factors support aggressive treatment then the previous-mentioned treatment regimen can be attempted (but a benefit is not anticipated). In particular, it is not recommended that such patients be transferred to another center to receive active treatment.

It is unfortunate that paraquat is so inexpensive and effective as an herbicide when outcomes from unintentional and intentional poisoning are so devastating despite maximal medical treatment. Ultimately, the key focus to reducing deaths from paraquat poisoning is to ban its sale (or at least highly restrict its availability to commercial operators), which is supported by outcome data from a number of countries.

GLUFOSINATE

Glufosinate (Fig. 109–5) is a nonselective herbicide used predominantly in Japan and Korea, but it is the 25th most commonly used pesticide in the United States.[33] Commercial preparations contain 14% to 30% glufosinate as the ammonium or sodium salt, with anionic surfactants. Case fatalities between 6.1% and 17.7% are reported from glufosinate poisoning, and increasing age is a risk factor.[74]

Pharmacology

Glufosinate is neurotoxic, although the specific mechanism is incompletely described. Because it is structurally similar to glutamate, studies have explored whether it interferes with glutamate networks in the central nervous system. Studies in rats demonstrate both agonism and antagonism to glutamate receptors and no effect on other receptors in the brain.[34] Glufosinate also interferes with glutamine synthetase activity, which induces hyperammonemia. Ammonia concentrations were not markedly altered in rats,[34] but hyperammonemia is observed following self-poisoning.[34,60,73,124]

Cellular toxicity appears to be persistent; for example, mouse studies note that effects persists beyond 2 weeks after an acute exposure.

Glufosinate was not found to inhibit cholinesterase enzymes in rat studies,[34] although this is reported in humans on occasion, including one case in which it decreased to 40% of the lower limit of normal with subsequent recovery.[124]

The extent to which the surfactant contributes to clinical toxicity is not confirmed. Rat studies suggest that hemodynamic changes due to glufosinate ammonium formulations are entirely caused by the surfactant component rather than glufosinate itself.[59] Surfactants may also cause uncoupling of oxidative phosphorylation, although this was not demonstrated in the study of a single case of glufosinate ammonium poisoning.[70]

Pharmacokinetics and Toxicokinetics

Kinetic analysis of glufosinate is limited to animal studies and a few human case reports. Minor differences in kinetics of the D- and L-glufosinate enantiomers are observed between patients, the clinical implications of which are not known.

The peak concentration is observed 1 hour postingestion in mice administered the formulated product, and less than 15% of a dose is absorbed by rats.

Glufosinate does not appear to bind to plasma proteins to a significant extent. The V_d was calculated to be 1.44 L/kg in a case of acute poisoning by assuming that the renal excretion of glufosinate is similar to animals.[38] Glufosinate distributes into the central nervous system, but the rate of distribution to the cerebrospinal fluid has not been characterized. It is theorized that glufosinate distributes into the central nervous system, slowly, perhaps due to active transporters, where it accumulates, which is why the onset of respiratory depression is delayed.[44] Indeed, seizures have occurred in some patients after glufosinate was no longer detectable in the blood.[124] However, this theory was not supported in a case in which glufosinate was not detected in the cerebrospinal fluid 6 hours after a seizure that occurred 30 hours postingestion.[121] Yet in another case of acute poisoning, the cerebrospinal fluid concentration was one-third the serum concentration 27 hours postingestion. Seizures occur 3 hours after the administration of intracerebral glufosinate in rats, which further challenges the theory that distribution kinetics influence the delayed onset of seizures in humans.[34]

Glufosinate is subject to minimal metabolism and the majority of the bioavailable dose of glufosinate is excreted unchanged in urine.

The elimination half-life is 4 hours in rats, whereas in rabbits elimination is biphasic with a terminal elimination half-life of 1.9 hours, which is not dose dependent. Kinetic data in humans are limited to a small number of cases of acute intentional poisoning in which the elimination profile appeared biphasic with a distribution half-life of 2 to 4 hours and a terminal elimination of 10 to 18 hours.[38,41,118]

Pathophysiology

It is not known whether the manifestations of glufosinate poisoning represent a primary (toxic) or secondary (downstream) effect. The most important manifestations are neurologic, with respiratory impairment that reduces oxygen delivery and subsequently compromises cellular function. Hypotension also impairs tissue perfusion and if uncorrected progresses to shock. Failure to correct these abnormalities leads to irreversible cellular injury and death.

Clinical Manifestations

Nausea and vomiting are early features of acute poisoning. An altered level of consciousness precedes severe neurotoxicity, which occurs between 4 and 50 hours postingestion, but usually within 24 hours, and includes seizures and central respiratory failure requiring ventilatory support.[60,73,74] These toxicities often persist for a number of days. In rats, following the intraperitoneal administration of glufosinate, the onset of seizures is also delayed by a number of hours and the time to onset decreases in a dose-dependent manner.[75]

Other manifestations of acute poisoning include cardiac dysrhythmias, fever, amnesia (both antegrade and retrograde), diabetes insipidus, and rhabdomyolysis. Refractory hypotension is often preterminal.[60,73,74]

Diagnostic Testing

Glufosinate poisoning is diagnosed clinically in the context of a history of exposure. Glufosinate assays are available for clinical use in Japan and a nomogram was developed for predicting clinical outcomes (Fig. 109–6).[40] Clinical chemistry assays including kidney function, blood gases, electrolytes, creatine kinase, and ammonia concentrations support clinical management.

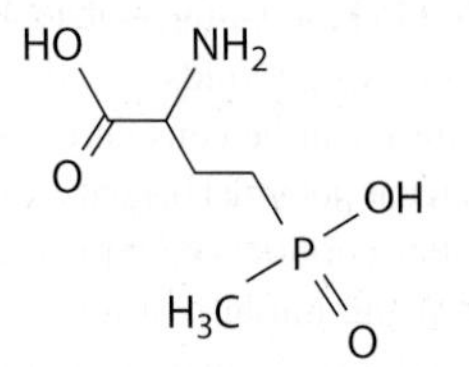

FIGURE 109–5. Structure of glufosinate.

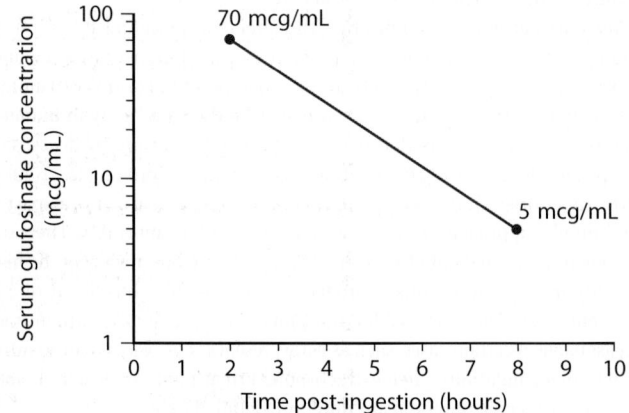

FIGURE 109–6. Glufosinate nomogram as described by Hori et al.[40] Concentrations above the line are associated with more severe poisoning.

Metabolic acidosis is more common with severe poisoning.[74] The ammonia concentration peaks 24 to 48 hours postingestion and increasing concentrations suggest an increased risk of neurotoxicity.[34,60,73] An increase in serum S100B protein precedes the onset of neurotoxicity.

Management

Toxicity is not consistently dose-dependent and severe symptoms are reported following unintentional ingestion, so all patients with oral exposures should be carefully monitored. Patients with confirmed exposures should be monitored for a minimum of 48 hours because the onset of clinical toxicity is often delayed. Prior to discharge, each patient should be carefully screened to identify those with cognitive impairment.

Resuscitation and Supportive Care

Routine resuscitation, close observation, and supportive care are required. Careful monitoring for the onset of respiratory failure is necessary and early intubation and ventilation is recommended in symptomatic patients. Given that glufosinate and metabolites are primarily renally cleared, intravenous fluids to maintain a consistent urine output is reasonable. Seizures should be treated in a standard manner initially with benzodiazepines as first-line therapy, which was effective in animal studies. Biochemical and acid–base abnormalities should be corrected as per usual care.

Gastrointestinal Decontamination

In most reports of glufosinate poisoning, gastric lavage and activated charcoal were administered, but it is not possible to determine whether these interventions improved clinical outcomes. The high incidence of both seizures and respiratory failure from glufosinate poisoning are relative contraindications to the administration of activated charcoal to patients with an unprotected airway.

Extracorporeal Removal

Hemodialysis and hemoperfusion were both used and hemodialysis was superior in terms of extraction of glufosinate from whole blood in vitro, with an extraction ratio of 80%. The clearance by hemodialysis is less than 60% of renal clearance in patients with normal kidney function. Although prompt hemodialysis in patients promotes a decrease in the concentration of glufosinate and probably ammonia, it is not known if this prevents the occurrence of neurotoxicity such as seizures, so its role in routine management is poorly defined. It is reasonable to administer these treatments in patients with severe poisoning and also in those with impaired kidney function.

Antidotes

Specific antidotes are not available. Benzodiazepines should be first-line therapy for seizures.

GLYPHOSATE

Glyphosate (Fig. 109–7) is a nonselective postemergence herbicide. It is used extensively worldwide, most commonly as the isopropylamine salt but also a potassium salt. Glyphosate-containing herbicides are available in various formulations: 1% to 5% glyphosate (ready to use) or 30% to 50% (concentrate requiring dilution before use). In 2012, glyphosate was the most frequently used herbicide in the United States and the second most commonly used herbicide in the domestic sector.[33] Products containing glyphosate trimesium are less widely used and differ with respect to their toxicity profile. Glyphosate is banned in some countries because of data suggesting that it is a

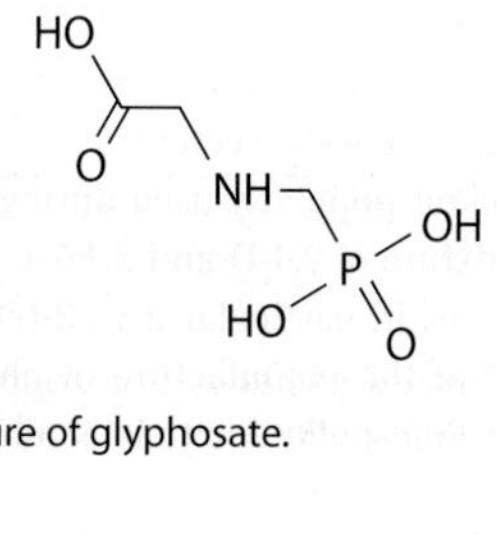

FIGURE 109–7. Structure of glyphosate.

carcinogen. However, this topic is extensively debated, and in March 2017 the EPA concluded that glyphosate is not likely to be carcinogenic to humans.

Pharmacology

Glyphosate inhibits 5-enolpyruvylshikimate-3-phosphate synthase in plants, which interferes with their aromatic amino acid synthesis; this enzyme is not present in humans.

The mechanism of toxicity of glyphosate-containing herbicides to humans is not adequately described. The formulation is irritating and high concentrations are corrosive, causing direct injury to the gastrointestinal tract. Despite being an organic phosphorus compound, glyphosate does not inhibit acetylcholinesterase. Patients with severe poisoning manifest multisystem effects, suggesting that the formulation is either nonspecific in its action or that it interferes with a physiologic process common to a number of systems. Proposed mechanisms include disruption of cellular membranes and uncoupling of oxidative phosphorylation, which are interrelated. Indeed, the mechanism of toxicity varies between different glyphosate salts. In 2 cases of glyphosate trimesium poisoning, cardiopulmonary arrest occurred within minutes of ingestion.[81,116] Because this is not reported from glyphosate isopropylamine, it is possible that these products differ in the mechanism of toxicity.

Experimentally, there is minimal (if any) mammalian toxicity from glyphosate itself. Glyphosate is categorized as WHO class "U" (unlikely to present acute hazard in normal use; the dose of a xenobiotic predicted to kill 50% of exposed animals $LD_{50} > 4,000$ mg/kg).[49] Surfactant coformulants are likely the more toxic component in glyphosate-containing herbicides. Polyoxyethyleneamine (tallow amine; LD_{50} equal to 1,200 mg/kg) is the most common surfactant formulated in these products, but others are also used. Systemic exposure to surfactants induces hypotension, which is primarily due to direct effects on the heart and blood vessels.[13] Surfactants directly disrupt cellular and subcellular membranes, including those of mitochondria, which has the potential to lead to systemic symptoms.[32] Coformulated potassium and isopropylamine contribute to toxicity. Isopropylamine has a rat LD_{50} of 111 to 820 mg/kg, decreases vascular resistance, and either increases or decreases cardiac contractility and rate.[50,93]

Pharmacokinetics and Toxicokinetics

The kinetics of the surfactant are not described. The relevance of the kinetics of glyphosate is questioned because its contribution to clinical toxicology is minimal; however, it is summarized here for completeness. Glyphosate does not penetrate the skin to a significant extent. Up to 40% of an oral dose is absorbed in rats, although this could increase when ingested as a concentrated solution with injury to the gastrointestinal epithelium. The peak glyphosate plasma concentration occurs within 2 hours of ingestion and distribution appears to be limited. Glyphosate does not readily cross the placenta according to an ex vivo model.[82] Glyphosate has an elimination half-life of less than 4 hours and is excreted unchanged in the urine.[7,9,43,100,125]

Pathophysiology

It is not known whether the manifestations of glyphosate poisoning represent a primary (toxic) or secondary (downstream) effect. Disruptions of oxidative phosphorylation globally impair normal cellular function as a result of limited energy supply (discussed further with the pathophysiology of phenoxy herbicides). Similarly, direct toxicity to cell membranes (including those of the mitochondria) interferes with normal cellular processes such as ion channels. Both disruptions induce multiorgan toxicity. Hypotension and dysrhythmias impair tissue perfusion, and liver and kidney injuries induce metabolic disequilibria and acidemia, which impair normal physiologic processes. Pulmonary toxicity induces hypoxia, which further compromises normal cellular functioning. Failure to correct these abnormalities leads to irreversible cellular toxicity and death.

Clinical Manifestations

Abdominal pain with nausea, vomiting, and/or diarrhea are the most common manifestations of acute poisoning. These are mild and self-resolving except in patients with severe poisoning due to inflammation, ulceration, or infarction of the gut wall. Severe diarrhea and recurrent vomiting result in dehydration. Gastrointestinal burns and necrosis occur with high doses of concentrated formulations and are associated with hemorrhage. Extensive erosion of the upper gastrointestinal tract is associated with more severe systemic poisoning and prolonged hospitalizations.[14,15,47,79,100]

Severe poisoning manifests as multiorgan failure, including hypotension, cardiac dysrhythmias, kidney and liver dysfunction, hyperkalemia, pancreatitis, pulmonary edema or pneumonitis, altered level of consciousness including encephalopathy, seizures, and metabolic acidosis. These effects range from transient to severe, progressing over 12 to 72 hours to resistant shock, respiratory failure, and death. Hypotension relates to both hypovolemia (fluids shifts and increased losses) and/or direct cardiovascular toxicity.[7,15,65,69,79,100,111,120]

Intravenous self-administration of glyphosate-containing herbicide caused hemolysis in one patient, and intramuscular self-administration caused rhabdomyolysis in another.

A large prospective study reported a case fatality of 3.2% in patients presenting to rural hospitals in Asia in which resources are limited,[100] but mortality reported in other studies varied from 2% to 30%.[15] These differences in outcomes likely reflect differences in timely access to health care services, available medical facilities, variability in glyphosate formulations, or selection bias related to case-referral. Proposed risk factors for death include a large exposure, delayed presentation to hospital, elevated glyphosate concentration, and increasing age.[15,79,100,111]

Respiratory, ocular, and dermal effects occur following occupational use of these preparations but are usually of minor severity.

Diagnostic Testing

Acute poisoning with a glyphosate-containing herbicide is diagnosed on the basis of a history of exposure and clinical findings. The differential diagnoses are wide, including any xenobiotic or medical condition associated with gastrointestinal effects and progressive multisystem toxicity.

A number of clinical criteria for the classification of severity are suggested, but none are validated.[7,100,120,122] There are no readily available specific clinical investigations to guide management or estimate prognosis in acute poisoning. Higher plasma glyphosate concentrations are associated with more severe poisoning, for example concentrations greater than 734 mg/L predicted death in one study.[100] A review noted that severe poisoning is associated with concentrations greater than 1,000 mg/L.[7] These concentrations probably reflect the amount of exposure, because glyphosate is minimally toxic. Quantitative glyphosate assays are not routinely available for clinical use.

Targeted laboratory and radiologic investigations should be conducted in patients demonstrating anything more than mild gastrointestinal symptoms. Pulse oximetry and blood gas measurements detect metabolic disequilibria and respiratory impairment. Electrolytes should be measured early because some formulations contain glyphosate as a potassium salt and severe hyperkalemia and electrocardiographic changes are reported.

Patients who develop marked nonspecific organ toxicity (eg, acute kidney injury, pulmonary edema, metabolic acidosis (including an elevated lactate concentration, sedation, dysrhythmias, hypotension) are more likely to die.[15,62,64,79,100]

Endoscopy identifies erosions or ulceration following exposures to the concentrated formulation, although this will not prompt a change in management. Further, endoscopy of an inflamed viscus presents a risk of perforation.

Management

Retrospective studies suggest a correlation between ingestion, severity of poisoning, and death.[64,100,106,122] All patients except for those with trivial exposures should be observed for a minimum of 6 hours. In particular, patients presenting with intentional self-poisoning or ingestion of a concentrated formulation must be carefully monitored. If gastrointestinal symptoms are noted then the patient should be observed for a minimum of 24 hours given

that clinical toxicity may progress. Because the toxicity of individual surfactants was not determined, treatment does not vary depending on specific coformulants.

Resuscitation and Supportive Care

All patients should receive prompt resuscitation, close observation, and routine supportive care; other treatments are largely empiric. The airway is usually maintained but respiratory distress and failure occur, which require supplemental oxygen and possibly mechanical ventilation. The optimal management of hypotension is complicated because its etiology is potentially related to hypovolemia, negative inotropy, and/or reduced vascular resistance. A detailed clinical review is required, followed by cautious administration of intravenous fluids to the patient. If the response to prompt administration of 20 to 30 mL/kg intravenous fluid to the patient is insufficient or there is increasing pulmonary congestion, then vasopressors are recommended. Other investigations such as echocardiography and central venous pressure will guide management, if available.

Biochemical and acid–base abnormalities, such as hyperkalemia, should be corrected where possible. The contribution of uncoupling of oxidative phosphorylation to clinical toxicity and death is proposed, but no specific treatment is available. In the context of acute poisoning with glyphosate-containing herbicides, signs suggestive of uncoupling of oxidative phosphorylation, such as hyperthermia, metabolic acidosis with elevated lactate concentration, and hypoglycemia, often represent a preterminal event. Hemodialysis or hemofiltration should be administered to patients developing acute kidney injury per usual guidelines if active treatment is to be pursued. Survival is reported with severe glyphosate poisoning (respiratory failure, persistent ventricular tachycardia and shock refractory to inotropes, and acidemia) using extracorporeal membrane oxygenation therapy.

Gastrointestinal Decontamination

No data exist to support the role of gastrointestinal decontamination in acute poisoning with glyphosate-containing herbicides beyond the usual recommendations discussed above.

Extracorporeal Removal

The role of extracorporeal removal in routine care is not known, but we recommend using it in patients with severe poisoning. Patients who received hemodialysis have survived severe poisoning; however, other patients have died despite this treatment. There are limited quantitative data reporting direct clearances, and uncertainty regarding which compound to measure.

Antidotes

No specific antidotes are proposed or tested for the treatment of acute poisoning with glyphosate-containing herbicides, which relates in part to the unknown mechanism of toxicity.

PHENOXY HERBICIDES (PHENOXYACETIC DERIVATIVES), INCLUDING 2,4-D AND MCPA

Phenoxy compounds are selective herbicides that are widely used in both developing and developed countries. A large number of compounds are included in this category; however, the most widely used are the phenoxyacetic derivatives. This includes 2,4-dichlorophenoxyacetic acid (2,4-D), 4-chloro-2-methylphenoxyacetic acid (MCPA), 2,4,5-trichlorophenoxyacetic acid (2,4,5-T; no longer available), and mecoprop (MCPP; 2-{4-chloro-2-methylphenoxy}propionic acid; Fig. 109–8). Other phenoxy herbicides and available toxicity data are listed in Table 109–1. In 2012, 2,4-D was the fifth most commonly used herbicide in the United States but the most commonly used herbicide in the domestic sector (MCPP was third and MCPA the ninth most commonly used in the domestic sector).[33]

Agent Orange, a defoliant popularly used during the Vietnam War, was composed of an equal mixture of 2,4-D and 2,4,5-T. This product also contained contaminant dioxins, in particular 2,3,7,8-tetrachlorodibenzodioxin which was a by-product of the manufacture of phenoxy herbicides. This dioxin is a persistent organic pollutant that is alleged to induce chronic

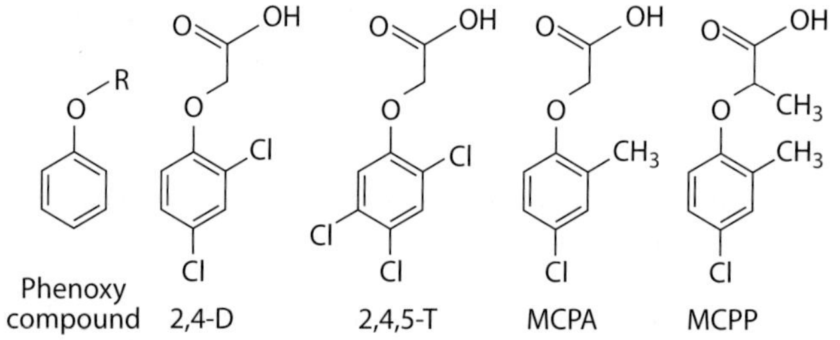

FIGURE 109–8. Structures of common phenoxy herbicides.

health conditions and cancer, although this is debated. This chapter discusses only the outcomes of acute exposures to phenoxy herbicides.

Pharmacology

The mechanism of toxicity of phenoxy compounds is not well described. The formulation is irritating or caustic, causing direct injury to the gastrointestinal tract. Patients with severe poisoning manifest multisystem effects, suggesting that the formulation is either nonspecific in its action or that it interferes with a physiological process common to a number of systems. As with other herbicide preparations, this reflects the uncertain contributions of coformulants such as bromoxynil, ioxynil or surfactants.

In rats, high plasma concentrations of MCPA damage cell membranes and induce toxicity, but the correlation between plasma concentrations, membrane damage, and toxicity is poor. Dose-dependent acute kidney injury from 2,4-D is observed in rats.

Uncoupling of oxidative phosphorylation also contributes to the development of severe clinical toxicity. Phenoxyacetic derivatives demonstrate concentration-dependent uncoupling of rat mitochondria in vitro, although the specific process that is disrupted is not sufficiently described.[10,133] Features of uncoupling of oxidative phosphorylation were observed antemortem in clinical studies of patients with large phenoxy herbicide exposures.[98]

Phenoxy acid compounds inhibit the voltage-gated chloride channel (CLC-1) in skeletal muscles, which is thought to contribute to the neuromuscular toxicity of these compounds. Dysfunction of CLC-1 induces myotonia due to hyperpolarization of the cell membrane. Other CLC channels are important for normal renal physiology. There are differences in the degree of inhibition between individual phenoxy acid compounds, which likely contributes to the variability in animal LD_{50} and possibly clinical features.

Other possible mechanisms of toxicity relate to their similarity to acetic acid, interfering with the utilization of acetylcoenzyme A (acetyl-CoA), or action as a false messenger at cholinergic receptors.[8]

Pharmacokinetics and Toxicokinetics

Animal studies and human case reports demonstrate nonlinear kinetics for the phenoxy herbicide compounds. Dose-dependent changes in absorption, protein binding, and clearance all occur, and each will influence the concentration-time profile.

Absorption is usually first order;[1] however, the time to peak concentration is delayed with increasing doses, which suggests saturable absorption and is supported by cell culture studies that demonstrate active absorption of these herbicides by a hydrogen ion-linked monocarboxylic acid transporter.[55,61,101,123]

As the dose of MCPA increases, there is a change in the semilogarithmic plasma concentration–time profile from linear to a biphasic convex profile. The inflection of this elimination curve in rats is approximately 200 mg/L,[25,26,101,123] which appears to reflect saturation of albumin binding. As the plasma concentration exceeds this point, the proportion of herbicide that is free (unbound) increases.[101] This increases the V_d and prolongs the apparent plasma elimination half-life.

Another contributing mechanism to the observed biphasic convex concentration-time profile is saturation of renal clearance for which there is some interspecies variability. Dose-dependent renal clearance is attributed

to saturation of an active transport process or direct nephrotoxicity. Renal clearance also varies with urine production because of reabsorption from the distal tubule.

Similar to data from animal studies, the semilogarithmic plasma concentration–time curve of phenoxy herbicides in humans with acute poisoning is generally convex, with an apparent inflection from a longer (but highly variable) to shorter elimination half-life between 200 and 300 mg/L. The elimination half-lives are prolonged, contributing to the persistence of clinical toxicity and occurrence of death a number of days postingestion of a phenoxyacetic herbicide.[98,101]

Alterations in blood pH theoretically change tissue distribution because phenoxyacetic herbicides are weak acids (pK_a approximately 3). Here, acidemia increases the proportion that is nonionized, and therefore lipophilic, which increases tissue binding and distribution. This is observed in vitro and is similar to that observed for salicylates (Chap. 37). Similarly, an alkaline plasma pH is expected to decrease tissue (and probably receptor) binding and increase plasma concentrations.

Experience with acute human poisonings noted a poor correlation between plasma concentrations and peak toxicity.[98] This probably reflects a discordance between plasma (measured) and intracellular (eg, mitochondrial) concentrations.

Pathophysiology

Direct injury to the gastrointestinal tract causes vomiting and diarrhea, which induces hypovolemia and electrolyte abnormalities.[8] Nonspecific cellular toxicity and uncoupling of oxidative phosphorylation interfere with normal function of ion channels and other cellular functions, preventing normal physiological processes.

Uncoupling of oxidative phosphorylation disrupts mitochondrial function, and causes inefficiency in energy production. Here, there is an increase in heat production out of proportion to the generation of ATP. Varying degrees of uncoupling of oxidative phosphorylation occur. The initial physiological response to uncoupling is to increase mitochondrial respiration to maintain the supply of ATP, which increases heat production and respiratory rate. As ATP falls there is an increase in glycolysis, causing hypoglycemia and metabolic acidosis with an elevated lactate concentration. If the mitochondrial defect persists then there will be hyperthermia and insufficient ATP for essential cellular functions, including active transport pumps such as Na^+,K^+-ATPase. This is followed by a loss of cellular ionic and volume regulation, which if persistent, is irreversible and cell death occurs. Because mitochondria are the primary supplier of ATP for most physiologic systems, uncoupling of oxidative phosphorylation is expected to induce multisystem toxicity.

Clinical Manifestations

Severe toxicity is more commonly reported in patients ingesting herbicide preparations containing both a phenoxy acid derivative with bromoxynil or ioxynil.

Vomiting, myotonia, confirmed on electromyography, and miosis are prominent features of 2,4-D poisoning in dogs. Severity varies in a dose-dependent manner, peaking 12 to 24 hours postingestion and persisting for a number of days.

Gastrointestinal toxicity including nausea, vomiting, abdominal or throat pain, and diarrhea are common. Other clinical features include neuromuscular findings (myalgia, rhabdomyolysis, weakness, myopathy, myotonia, and fasciculations), central nervous system effects (agitation, sedation, confusion, miosis), tachycardia, hypotension, acute kidney injury, and hypocalcemia. In some patients, these effects persist for a number of days.[98]

Tachypnea with respiratory alkalosis occurs in patients with phenoxy herbicide poisoning, some of whom died, which is consistent with increased mitochondrial respiration from mild uncoupling. More severe poisoning is characterized by metabolic acidosis, hyperventilation, hyperthermia, elevated creatine kinase, generalized muscle rigidity, progressive hypotension, pulseless electrical activity, or asystole.[8,19,85,98]

The mortality from acute phenoxy herbicide poisoning is high. A systematic review of all acute phenoxy herbicide poisoning described severe clinical toxicity in most patients, including death in one-third of the cases.[8] Subsequently, a prospective study of MCPA exposures demonstrated minor toxicity in greater than 80% of patients and a mortality of 4.4% (8 of 181 patients).[98] When death occurs, it is usually delayed by 24 to 48 hours postingestion and results from cardiorespiratory arrest. The exact mechanism of death is inadequately described, but appears to relate to uncoupling of oxidative phosphorylation or other metabolic dysfunction including acute kidney injury, as discussed above.

Diagnostic Testing

Commercial assays for the specific measurement of phenoxy herbicides are not available to assist in the diagnosis of acute poisoning. Further, their role in the management of acute poisoning is not confirmed because the relationship between plasma phenoxy herbicide concentration and clinical toxicity appears to be poor.[98] Sedation is reported with a plasma phenoxy concentration above 80 mg/L,[96] whereas concentrations more than 500 mg/L are associated with severe toxicity.[27] A patient survived severe MCPA poisoning (hypotension and limb myotonia) with a plasma concentration of 546 mg/L. The myotonia persisted for days and resolved when the MCPA plasma concentration was less than 100 mg/L.[109] By contrast, death following MCPA poisoning is reported at plasma concentrations as low as 107 mg/L to 230 mg/L.[51,90,98]

Monitoring of electrolytes, kidney function, pulse oximetry, and blood gases is recommended to detect progression of organ toxicity. Hypoalbuminemia predisposes to severe poisoning.[101] Creatine kinase should be determined because rhabdomyolysis is reported following acute poisoning. Urinalysis will identify myoglobinuria. There are insufficient data describing the role of these measurements for prognostication.

Management

All patients with significant poisonings, particularly those with symptomatic oral ingestions, should be treated cautiously, including continuous monitoring for 24 to 48 hours preferably in an intensive care unit. Initial mild toxicity such as gastrointestinal symptoms with normal vital signs and level of consciousness does not preclude subsequent severe toxicity and death.[98]

Animal studies suggest that phenoxy herbicide toxicity increases when elimination is impaired. Empirically, this supports the use of treatments that reduce exposure by either decreasing absorption or increasing elimination. Unfortunately, there is insufficient evidence to recommend specific interventions in patients with acute phenoxy herbicide poisoning. However, an adequate urine output (>1 mL/kg/h) optimizes the renal excretion of phenoxy herbicides as well as decreasing renal toxicity from rhabdomyolysis. Because signs consistent with uncoupling of oxidative phosphorylation are associated with a poor outcome, when present more advanced treatments such as hemodialysis should be used.[8,98]

Resuscitation and Supportive Care

All patients should receive routine resuscitation, close observation, and supportive care. It is reasonable to correct electrolyte abnormalities, and acidemia as acidemia promotes the distribution of weak acids and increases the intracellular concentration.

Gastrointestinal Decontamination

Gastrointestinal decontamination is recommended to patients per the guidelines listed in Chap. 5. However, administration of activated charcoal beyond the usual time frame is reasonable given that absorption appears to be saturable.

Extracorporeal Removal

Urgent hemodialysis is recommended in patients with severe poisoning. Because phenoxy compounds are small and water soluble, and subject to saturable protein binding with large exposures (increasing the free concentration), they are likely to be cleared by extracorporeal techniques.

Extracorporeal elimination using resin hemoperfusion, hemodialysis, or plasmapheresis was studied in a few cases, with clearances approaching 75 mL/min.

Antidotes

There are no specific antidotes for phenoxy herbicides, but sodium bicarbonate or other alkalinizing agents favorably alter the kinetics of phenoxy herbicides.

Data from animal studies and case reports suggest that urinary alkalinization increases the elimination of phenoxy herbicides due to "ion trapping." For example, renal 2,4-D clearance was increased from 5.1 to 63 mL/min when urine pH increased from 5.0 to 8.0.[91] Compared with a total clearance of approximately 30 mL/minute or less in volunteer studies,[56,105] this increase in renal clearance is potentially significant. Prospective, randomized studies are required to confirm the efficacy of urinary alkalinization in humans. Plasma alkalinization theoretically limits the distribution of phenoxy compounds from the central circulation by "ion trapping."

It is reasonable to alkalinize the urine to a pH greater than 7.5 in patients who are symptomatic, particularly if there are features of uncoupling of oxidative phosphorylation or metabolic acidosis. Alkalinization is rarely associated with adverse effects when administered to patients with care and close observation (Antidotes in Depth: A5).

TRIAZINE COMPOUNDS, INCLUDING ATRAZINE

The 1,3,5-triazine or s-triazine compound (Fig. 109–9) is central to a large number of compounds, including herbicides, other pesticides (eg, cyromazine), resins (eg, melamine), explosives (RDX or C-4), and antiinfectives. Triazine herbicides are widely used, and in 2012 atrazine was the second most used pesticide in the United States.[33] However, cases of acute poisoning are infrequent. Other herbicides included in this group are listed in Table 109–1. These selective herbicides are used pre- or post-emergence for weed control.

The safety of atrazine from an environmental health perspective is debated because of its persistence and propensity to spread across water systems and potential toxicity from chronic exposure. This led to restrictions on the use of triazine compounds in the European Union.

Pharmacology

The mechanism of toxicity is not fully determined, although it might relate to uncoupling of oxidative phosphorylation. Atrazine is a direct arteriolar vasodilator. Some metabolites of atrazine, particularly those remaining chlorinated, are thought to retain biologic activity.[2] Similarly, clinical features of prometryn poisoning resolved posthemodialysis despite persistence of the parent herbicide, suggesting that toxic metabolites or coformulants were eliminated.[11]

Pharmacokinetics and Toxicokinetics

Approximately 60% of an oral atrazine dose is absorbed in rats and the concentration peaks beyond 3 hours.[78] The absorption phase of triazine compounds appears to be prolonged in humans in which the serum or plasma concentration continues to increase during treatment with hemodialysis.[11,88] Atrazine is rapidly dealkylated to a metabolite that binds strongly to hemoglobin and plasma proteins, allowing it to be detected in the blood for months. Metabolites are excreted in the urine, and around 25% of them are conjugated to glutathione.[78]

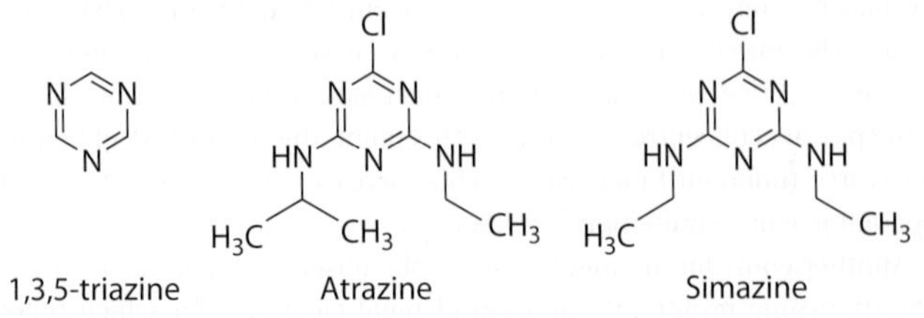

FIGURE 109–9. Structures of common triazine herbicides.

The metabolism of atrazine has been studied in humans following occupational exposures, and animals, and a range of metabolites are described, in particular glutathione conjugates. Other metabolic products from dealkylation and oxidation are also present.

Dermal absorption of atrazine is incomplete but increases with exposure to the proprietary formulation. Atrazine metabolites are readily measured in the urine of atrazine applicators.

Clinical Manifestations

There are limited cases of triazine herbicide poisoning. Vomiting, depressed levels of consciousness, tachycardia, hypertension, acute kidney injury, and metabolic acidosis with an elevated lactate concentration were described in a patient with acute prometryn and ethanol poisoning.[11] Similar clinical signs, in addition to hypotension with a low peripheral vascular resistance, were noted in a case of poisoning with atrazine, amitrole (Table 109–1), ethylene glycol, and formaldehyde. This was followed by progressive multiorgan dysfunction and death due to refractory shock 3 days later.[88] Death following acute ametryn poisoning (coformulated with xylene and cyclohexanone) is reported, but the mechanism of death was not apparent.[119]

Diagnostic Testing

In a single case report, clinical toxicity did not directly relate to the concentration of prometryn, but the relationship to the concentration of metabolites was not determined.[11] Routine biochemistry and blood gases are useful for monitoring for the development of systemic toxicity.

Management

The limited number of publications of triazine herbicide poisoning are inadequate to guide specific management of patients with acute triazine poisoning.

Resuscitation and Supportive Care

Routine resuscitation, close observation, and supportive care should be provided to all patients. Ventilatory support and correction of hypotension and metabolic disequilibria are appropriate.

Gastrointestinal Decontamination.

It is reasonable to administer activated charcoal to patients beyond one hour because of the slow absorption of these compounds.

Extracorporeal Removal

Hemodialysis corrected metabolic acidosis in a case of prometryn poisoning without decreasing the serum concentration of prometryn. In the absence of direct measurements of clearance, the efficacy of hemodialysis in removing prometryn cannot be determined, but is probably limited.[11] Hemodialysis clearance of atrazine was 250 mL/minute (extraction ratio 76%), but only 0.1% of the dose was removed after 4 hours of treatment. Further, similar to the previous case, atrazine concentrations continued to increase during the treatment.[88]

Antidotes

No antidotes are available for the treatment of triazine herbicide poisoning.

SUMMARY

- A large number of heterogeneous xenobiotics are classified as herbicides; the toxicity in humans is not completely described for many of these xenobiotics.
- Coformulants, such as surfactants and solvents, probably contribute to clinical toxicity in commercial preparations.
- Many herbicides induce multisystem toxicity for which treatments are often unsatisfactory, although some compounds induce organ-specific toxicity.
- All patients with acute intentional poisoning should be carefully observed for the development of poisoning.
- The priorities of treatment include prompt resuscitation, consideration of antidotes, a detailed history, ongoing monitoring, and supportive care.

- More research is required to better define the clinical syndromes associated with herbicide poisoning, the toxicokinetics of relevant compounds, and the efficacy of treatments including antidotes.
- Prospective case series are useful for describing the toxicity of herbicides in humans. These guide clinicians in the management of poisoning, and also inform regulatory agencies regarding the relative toxicity of different herbicides, which prompt actions that reduce risk to human health.
- Regulatory agencies should monitor data research describing outcomes from unintentional and intentional self-poisoning, and actively ban or severely restrict the availability of highly toxic herbicides, in particular those for which an antidote is not available.

Acknowledgment

Rebecca L. Tominack, MD, and Susan M. Pond, MD, contributed to this chapter in previous editions.

REFERENCES

1. Arnold EK, Beasley VR. The pharmacokinetics of chlorinated phenoxy acid herbicides: a literature review. *Vet Hum Toxicol*. 1989;31:121-125.
2. Barr DB, et al. Assessing exposure to atrazine and its metabolites using biomonitoring. *Environ Health Perspect*. 2007;115:1474-1478.
3. Berry DJ, Grove J. The determination of paraquat (I,I'-dimethyl-4,4'-bipyridylium cation) in urine. *Clin Chim Acta*. 1971;34:5-11.
4. Berry DJ, et al. Adsorptive properties of activated charcoal and Fuller's Earth used for treatment of paraquat ingestion. Proceedings of the 6th Annual Congress of the Asia Pacific Association of Medical Toxicology, Thailand. 2007:130.
5. Bismuth C, et al Elimination of paraquat. *Hum Toxicol*. 1987;6:63-67.
6. Bismuth C, et al. Paraquat poisoning. An overview of the current status. *Drug Saf*. 1990;5:243-251.
7. Bradberry SM, et al. Glyphosate poisoning. *Toxicol Rev*. 2004;23:159-167.
8. Bradberry SM, et al. Poisoning due to chlorophenoxy herbicides. *Toxicol Rev*. 2004;23:65-73.
9. Brewster DW, et al. Metabolism of glyphosate in Sprague-Dawley rats: tissue distribution, identification, and quantitation of glyphosate-derived materials following a single oral dose. *Fundam Appl Toxicol*. 1991;17:43-51.
10. Brody TM. Effect of certain plant growth substances on oxidative phosphorylation in rat liver mitochondria. *Proc Soc Exp Biol Med*. 1952;80:533-536.
11. Brvar M, et al. Metabolic acidosis in prometryn (triazine herbicide) self-poisoning. *Clin Toxicol*. 2008;46:270-273.
12. Chan BS, et al. The renal excretory mechanisms and the role of organic cations in modulating the renal handling of paraquat. *Pharmacol Ther*. 1998;79:193-203.
13. Chan YC, et al. Cardiovascular effects of herbicides and formulated adjuvants on isolated rat aorta and heart. *Toxicol In Vitro*. 2007;21:595-603.
14. Chang CY, et al. Clinical impact of upper gastrointestinal tract injuries in glyphosate-surfactant oral intoxication. *Hum Exp Toxicol*. 1999;18:475-478.
15. Chen YJ, et al. The epidemiology of glyphosate-surfactant herbicide poisoning in Taiwan, 1986-2007: a poison center study. *Clin Toxicol*. 2009;47:670-677.
16. Conning DM, et al. Paraquat and related bipyridyls. *Br Med Bull*. 1969;25:245-249.
17. De Silva WA, Bodinayake CK. Propanil poisoning. *Ceylon Med J*. 1997;42:81-84.
18. Denicola A, Radi R. Peroxynitrite and drug-dependent toxicity. *Toxicology*. 2005;208:273-288.
19. Dickey W, et al. Delayed sudden death after ingestion of MCPP and ioxynil: an unusual presentation of hormonal weedkiller intoxication. *Postgrad Med J*. 1988;64:681-682.
20. Dinis-Oliveira RJ, et al. Full survival of paraquat-exposed rats after treatment with sodium salicylate. *Free Rad Biol Med*. 2007;42:1017-1028.
21. Dinis-Oliveira RJ, et al. Reactivity of paraquat with sodium salicylate: formation of stable complexes. *Toxicology*. 2008;249:130-139.
22. Dinis-Oliveira RJ, et al. Paraquat poisonings: mechanisms of lung toxicity, clinical features, and treatment. *CRC Crit Rev Toxicol*. 2008;38:13-71.
23. Dinis-Oliveira RJ, et al. An effective antidote for paraquat poisonings: the treatment with lysine acetylsalicylate. *Toxicology*. 2009;255:187-193.
24. Eddleston M, et al. Prospects for treatment of paraquat-induced lung fibrosis with immunosuppressive drugs and the need for better prediction of outcome: a systematic review. *Q J Med*. 2003;96:809-824.
25. Elo H. Distribution and elimination of 2-methyl-4-chlorophenoxyacetic acid (MCPA) in male rats. *Acta Pharmacol Toxicol (Copenh)*. 1976;39:58-64.
26. Elo HA, Ylitalo P. Distribution of 2-methyl-4-chlorophenoxyacetic acid and 2,4-dichlorophenoxyacetic acid in male rats: evidence for the involvement of the central nervous system in their toxicity. *Toxicol Appl Pharmacol*. 1979;51:439-446.
27. Flanagan RJ, et al. Alkaline diuresis for acute poisoning with chlorophenoxy herbicides and ioxynil. *Lancet*. 1990;335:454-458.
28. Gawarammana I, et al. A randomised controlled trial of high-dose immunosuppression in paraquat poisoning [abstract 15]. *Clin Toxicol*. 2012;50:278.

29. Gawarammana IB, Dawson AH. Peripheral burning sensation: a novel clinical marker of poor prognosis and higher plasma-paraquat concentrations in paraquat poisoning. *Clin Toxicol (Phila)*. 2010;48:347-349.

30. Gawarammana IB, et al. Acute human self-poisoning with bispyribac-containing herbicide Nominee: a prospective observational study. *Clin Toxicol*. 2010;48:198-202.

31. Gil HW, et al. Clinical implication of urinary neutrophil gelatinase-associated lipocalin and kidney injury molecule-1 in patients with acute paraquat intoxication. *Clin Toxicol*. 2009;47:870-875.

32. Goldstein DA, et al. Mechanism of toxicity of commercial glyphosate formulations: how important is the surfactant? *Clin Toxicol*. 2005;43:423-424.

33. Atwood D, Paisley-Jones C. *Pesticides Industry Sales and Usage—2008-2012 Market Estimates*. Washington, DC: US Environmental Protection Agency; 2017.

34. Hack R, et al. Glufosinate ammonium—some aspects of its mode of action in mammals. *Food Chem Toxicol*. 1994;32:461-470.

35. Hampson EC, Pond SM. Failure of haemoperfusion and haemodialysis to prevent death in paraquat poisoning. A retrospective review of 42 patients. *Med Toxicol Adverse Drug Exp*. 1988;3:64-71.

36. Hart TB, et al. A new statistical approach to the prognostic significance of plasma paraquat concentrations. *Lancet*. 1984;2:1222-1223.

37. Heylings JR, et al. Identification of an alginate-based formulation of paraquat to reduce the exposure of the herbicide following oral ingestion. *Toxicology*. 2007;241:1-10.

38. Hirose Y, et al. A toxicokinetic analysis in a patient with acute glufosinate poisoning. *Hum Exp Toxicol*. 1999;18:305-308.

39. Hong SY, et al. Effect of haemoperfusion on plasma paraquat concentration in vitro and in vivo. *Toxicol Indust Health*. 2003;19:17-23.

40. Hori Y, et al. Determination of glufosinate ammonium and its metabolite, 3-methylphosphinicopropionic acid, in human serum by gas chromatography-mass spectrometry following mixed-mode solid-phase extraction and t-BDMS derivatization. *J Anal Toxicol*. 2001;25:680-684.

41. Hori Y, et al. Enantioselective analysis of glufosinate using precolumn derivatization with (+)-1-(9-fluorenyl)ethyl chloroformate and reversed-phase liquid chromatography. *J Chromatogr B Analyt Technol Biomed Life Sci*. 2002;776:191-198.

42. Hori Y, et al. Simultaneous determination of propanil, carbaryl and 3,4-dichloroaniline in human serum by HPLC with UV detector following solid phase extraction [in Japanese]. *Yakugaku Zasshi*. 2002;122:247-251.

43. Hori Y, et al. Determination of the herbicide glyphosate and its metabolite in biological specimens by gas chromatography-mass spectrometry. A case of poisoning by Roundup(r) herbicide. *J Analytical Toxicol*. 2003;27:162-166.

44. Hori Y, et al. Toxicokinetics of DL-glufosinate enantiomer in human BASTA poisoning. *Biol Pharma Bull*. 2003;26:540-543.

45. Houze P, et al. Toxicokinetics of paraquat in humans. *Hum Exp Toxicol*. 1990;9:5-12.

46. Huang WD, et al. Lysine acetylsalicylate ameliorates lung injury in rats acutely exposed to paraquat. *Chin Med J (Engl)*. 2011;124:2496-2501.

47. Hung DZ, et al. Laryngeal survey in glyphosate intoxication: a pathophysiological investigation. *Hum Exp Toxicol*. 1997;16:596-599.

48. Hunt K, Thomas SHL. Renal impairment following low dose intravenous and oral diquat administration. *Clin Toxicol*. 2006;44:572-573.

49. IPCS. *The WHO Recommended Classification of Pesticides by Hazard and Guidelines to Classification 2000–2002*. Geneva: World Health Organisation; 2002.

50. Ishizaki T, et al. Cardiovascular actions of a new metabolite of propranolol: isopropylamine. *J Pharmacol Exp Ther*. 1974;189:626-632.

51. Johnson HR, Koumides O. A further case of MCPA poisoning. *BMJ*. 1965:629-630.

52. Jones AL, et al. Multiple logistic regression analysis of plasma paraquat concentrations as a predictor of outcome in 375 cases of paraquat poisoning. *Q J Med*. 1999;92:573-578.

53. Kang MS, et al. Comparison between kidney and hemoperfusion for paraquat elimination. *J Korean Med Sci*. 2009;24:S156-S160.

54. Kim SJ, et al. The clinical features of acute kidney injury in patients with acute paraquat intoxication. *Nephrol Dial Transplant*. 2009;24:1226-1232.

55. Kimura O, et al. Transepithelial transport of 4-chloro-2-methylphenoxyacetic acid (MCPA) across human intestinal Caco-2 cell monolayers. *Basic Clin Pharmacol Toxicol*. 2012;110:530-536.

56. Kohli JD, et al. Absorption and excretion of 2,4-dichlorophenoxyacetic acid in man. *Xenobiotica*. 1974;4:97-100.

57. Koo JR, et al. Failure of continuous venovenous hemofiltration to prevent death in paraquat poisoning. *Am J Kidney Dis*. 2002;39:55-59.

58. Koo JR, et al. Rapid analysis of plasma paraquat using sodium dithionite as a predictor of outcome in acute paraquat poisoning. *Am J the Med Sci*. 2009;338:373-377.

59. Koyama K, Goto K. Cardiovascular effects of a herbicide containing glufosinate and a surfactant: in vitro and in vivo analyses in rats. *Toxicol Appl Pharmacol*. 1997;145:409-414.

60. Kyong YY, et al. "Hyperammonemia following glufosinate-containing herbicide poisoning: a potential marker of severe neurotoxicity" by Yan-Chido Mao et al., *Clin Toxicol (Phila)*. 2011;49:48-52. *Clin Toxicol (Phila)*. 2011;49:510-513.

61. Lappin GJ, et al. Absorption, metabolism and excretion of 4-chloro-2-methylphenoxyacetic acid (MCPA) in rat and dog. *Xenobiotica*. 2002;32:153-163.

62. Lee CH, et al. The early prognostic factors of glyphosate-surfactant intoxication. *Am J Emerg Med*. 2008;26:275-281.

63. Lee E, et al. Severe chlorate poisoning successfully treated with methylene blue. *J Emerg Med*. 2013;44:381-384.

64. Lee HL, et al. Clinical presentations and prognostic factors of a glyphosate-surfactant herbicide intoxication: a review of 131 cases. *Acad Emerg Med*. 2000;7:906-910.

65. Lee HL, et al. Comparative effects of the formulation of glyphosate-surfactant herbicides on hemodynamics in swine. *Clin Toxicol*. 2009;47:651-658.

66. Lee KH, et al. Marked recovery from paraquat-induced lung injury during long-term follow-up. *Korean J Internal Med*. 2009;24:95-100.

67. Li GQ, et al. Paraquat (PQ) clearance through continuous plasma perfusion in PQ poisoning patients: a clinical study [in Chinese]. *Zhongguo Wei Zhong Bing Ji Jiu Yi Xue*. 2011;23:588-592.

68. Li LR, et al. Glucocorticoid with cyclophosphamide for paraquat-induced lung fibrosis. *Cochrane Database Syst Rev*. 2014;8:CD008084.

69. Lin CM, et al. Cardiogenic shock in a patient with glyphosate-surfactant poisoning. *J Formos Med Assoc*. 1999;98:698-700.

70. Lluis M, et al. Severe acute poisoning due to a glufosinate containing preparation without mitochondrial involvement. *Hum Exp Toxicol*. 2008;27:519-524.

71. Lo YC, et al. Acute alachlor and butachlor herbicide poisoning. *Clin Toxicol*. 2008;46:716-721.

72. Manuweera G, et al. Do targeted bans of insecticides to prevent deaths from self-poisoning result in reduced agricultural output? *Environ Health Perspect*. 2008;116:492-495.

73. Mao YC, et al. Hyperammonemia following glufosinate-containing herbicide poisoning: a potential marker of severe neurotoxicity. *Clin Toxicol (Phila)*. 2011;49:48-52.

74. Mao YC, et al. Acute human glufosinate-containing herbicide poisoning. *Clin Toxicol (Phila)*. 2012;50:396-402.

75. Matsumura N, et al. Glufosinate ammonium induces convulsion through N-methyl-D-aspartate receptors in mice. *Neurosci Lett*. 2001;304:123-125.

76. McMillan DC, et al. Propanil-induced methemoglobinemia and hemoglobin binding in the rat. *Toxicol Appl Pharmacol*. 1990;105:503-507.

77. McMillan DC, et al. Role of metabolites in propanil-induced hemolytic anemia. *Toxicol Appl Pharmacol*. 1991;110:70-78.

78. McMullin TS, et al. Pharmacokinetic modeling of disposition and time-course studies with [14 C]atrazine. *J Toxicol Environ Health Part A*. 2003;66:941-964.

79. Moon JM, Chun BJ. Predicting acute complicated glyphosate intoxication in the emergency department. *Clin Toxicol (Phila)*. 2010;48:718-724.

80. Moon JM, Chun BJ. Acute intoxication with the adjuvant itself for Gramoxone INTEON. *Hum Exp Toxicol*. 2012;31:18-23.

81. Mortensen OS, et al. Forgiftninger med ukrudtsbek'mpelsesmidlerne glyphosat og glyphosat-trimesium. *Ugeskr Laeger*. 2000;162:4656-4659.

82. Mose T, et al. Placental passage of benzoic acid, caffeine, and glyphosate in an ex vivo human perfusion system. *J Toxicol Environ Health A*. 2008;71:984-991.

83. Murray RE, Gibson JE. A comparative study of paraquat intoxication in rats, guinea pigs and monkeys. *Exp Mol Pathol*. 1972;17:317-325.

84. Murray RE, Gibson JE. Paraquat disposition in rats, guinea pigs and monkeys. *Toxicol Appl Pharmacol*. 1974;27:283-291.

85. O'Reilly JF. Prolonged coma and delayed peripheral neuropathy after ingestion of phenoxyacetic acid weedkillers. *Postgrad Med J*. 1984;60:76-77.

86. Ohashi N, et al. DCPA (propanil) and NAC (carbaryl) herbicide poisoning. *Japanese J Toxicol*. 1996;9:437-440.

87. Park JS, et al. Clinical outcome of acute intoxication due to ingestion of auxin-like herbicides. *Clin Toxicol (Phila)*. 2011;49:815-819.

88. Pommery J, et al. Atrazine in plasma and tissue following atrazine-aminotriazole-ethylene glycol-formaldehyde poisoning. *J Toxicol Clin Toxicol*. 1993;31:323-331.

89. Pond SM, et al. Kinetics of toxic doses of paraquat and the effects of hemoperfusion in the dog. *J Toxicol Clin Toxicol*. 1993;31:229-246.

90. Popham RD, Davies DM. A case of M.C.P.A poisoning. *Br Med J*. 1964;1:677-678.

91. Prescott LF, et al. Treatment of severe 2,4-D and mecoprop intoxication with alkaline diuresis. *Br J Clin Pharmacol*. 1979;7:111-116.

92. Price LA, et al. Paraquat and diquat interference in the analysis of creatinine by the Jaffe reaction. *Pathology*. 1995;27:154-156.

93. Privitera PJ, et al. Nicotinic-like effects and tissue disposition of isopropylamine. *J Pharmacol Exp Ther*. 1982;222:116-121.

94. Proudfoot AT, et al. Paraquat poisoning: significance of plasma-paraquat concentrations. *Lancet*. 1979;2:330-332.

95. Ragoucy-Sengler C, Pileire B. A biological index to predict patient outcome in paraquat poisoning. *Hum Exp Toxicol*. 1996;15:265-268.

96. Reingart JR, Roberts JR. Chlorophenoxy herbicides. *Recognition and Management of Pesticide Poisonings*. 5th ed. Washington: US Environmental Protection Agency; 1999:94-98.

97. Roberts DM, et al. Influence of pesticide regulation on acute poisoning deaths in Sri Lanka. *Bull World Health Organization*. 2003;81:789-798.

98. Roberts DM, et al. Intentional self-poisoning with the chlorophenoxy herbicide 4-chloro-2-methylphenoxyacetic acid (MCPA). *Ann Emerg Med*. 2005;46:275-284.

99. Roberts DM, et al. Clinical outcomes and kinetics of propanil following acute self-poisoning: a prospective case series. *BMC Clin Pharmacol*. 2009;9:3.

100. Roberts DM, et al. A prospective observational study of the clinical toxicology of glyphosate-containing herbicides in adults with acute self-poisoning. *Clin Toxicol*. 2010;48:129-136.

101. Roberts DM, et al. Toxicokinetics, including saturable protein binding, of 4-chloro-2-methyl phenoxyacetic acid (MCPA) in patients with acute poisoning. *Toxicol Lett.* 2011;201:270-276.
102. Roberts DM, et al. Changes in the concentrations of creatinine, cystatin C and NGAL in patients with acute paraquat self-poisoning. *Toxicol Lett.* 2011;202:69-74.
103. Salazar A, et al. Colorimetric detection of urinary diquat: in vitro demonstration. *Clin Toxicol.* 2007;45:381-382.
104. Sass JB, Colangelo A. European Union bans atrazine, while the United States negotiates continued use. *Int J Occup Environ Health.* 2006;12:260-267.
105. Sauerhoff MW, et al. The dose-dependent pharmacokinetic profile of 2,4,5-trichlorophenoxy acetic acid following intravenous administration to rats. *Toxicol Appl Pharmacol.* 1976;36:491-501.
106. Sawada Y, et al. Probable toxicity of surface-active agent in commercial herbicide containing glyphosate. *Lancet.* 1988;1:299.
107. Sawada Y, et al. Severity index of paraquat poisoning. *Lancet.* 1988;1:1333.
108. Scherrmann JM, et al. Prognostic value of plasma and urine paraquat concentration. *Hum Toxicol.* 1987;6:91-93.
109. Schmoldt A, et al. Massive ingestion of the herbicide 2-methyl-4-chlorophenoxyacetic acid (MCPA). *Clin Toxicol.* 1997;35:405-408.
110. Senarathna L, et al. Prediction of outcome after paraquat poisoning by measurement of the plasma paraquat concentration. *Q J Med.* 2009;102:251-259.
111. Seok SJ, et al. Surfactant volume is an essential element in human toxicity in acute glyphosate herbicide intoxication. *Clin Toxicol (Phila).* 2011;49:892-899.
112. Seok SJ, et al. Acute oral poisoning due to chloracetanilide herbicides. *J Korean Med Sci.* 2012;27:111-114.
113. Shihana F, et al. A simple quantitative bedside test to determine methemoglobin. *Ann Emerg Med.* 2010;55:184-189.
114. Shim YS, et al. A case of green urine after ingestion of herbicides. *Korean J Intern Med.* 2008;23:42-44.
115. Singleton SD, Murphy SD. Propanil (3,4-dichloropropionanilide)-induced methemoglobin formation in mice in relation to acylamidase activity. *Toxicol Appl Pharmacol.* 1973;25:20-29.
116. Sorensen FW, Gregersen M. Rapid lethal intoxication caused by the herbicide glyphosate-trimesium (Touchdown). *Hum Exp Toxicol.* 1999;18:735-737.
117. Stephens DS, et al. Pseudodiphtheria: prominent pharyngeal membrane associated with fatal paraquat ingestion. *Ann Intern Med.* 1981;94:202-204.
118. Takahashi H, et al. A case of transient diabetes insipidus associated with poisoning by a herbicide containing glufosinate. *Clin Toxicol.* 2000;38:153-156.
119. Takayasu T, et al. Postmortem distribution of ametryn in the blood and organ tissues of an herbicide-poisoning victim. *J Anal Toxicol.* 2010;34:287-291.
120. Talbot AR, et al. Acute poisoning with a glyphosate-surfactant herbicide ("roundup"): a review of 93 cases. *Hum Exp Toxicol.* 1991;10:1-8.
121. Tanaka J, et al. Two cases of glufosinate poisoning with late onset convulsions. *Vet Hum Toxicol.* 1998;40:219-222.
122. Tominack RL, et al. Taiwan National Poison Center survey of glyphosate—surfactant herbicide ingestions. *J Toxicol Clin Toxicol.* 1991;29:91-109.
123. van Ravenzwaay B, et al. Absorption, distribution, metabolism and excretion of 4-chloro-2-methylphenoxyacetic acid (MCPA) in rats. *Food Chem Toxicol.* 2004;42:115-125.
124. Watanabe T, Sano T. Neurological effects of glufosinate poisoning with a brief review. *Hum Exp Toxicol.* 1998;17:35-39.
125. Wester RC, et al. Glyphosate skin binding, absorption, residual tissue distribution, and skin decontamination. *Fundam Appl Toxicol.* 1991;16:725-732.
126. Wilks MF, et al. Improvement in survival after paraquat ingestion following introduction of a new formulation in Sri Lanka. *PLoS Med.* 2008;5:250-259.
127. Wilks MF, et al. Influence of gastric decontamination on patient outcome after paraquat ingestion. *J Med Toxicol.* 2008;4:212-213.
128. Wilks MF, et al. Formulation changes and time trends in outcome following paraquat ingestion in Sri Lanka. *Clin Toxicol.* 2011;49:21-28.
129. Yamashita M, Hukuda T. The pitfall of the general treatment in acute poisoning [in Japanese]. *Kyukyu Igaku.* 1985;9:65-71.
130. Yamazaki M, et al. Pesticide poisoning initially suspected as a natural death. *J Forensic Sci.* 2001;46:165-170.
131. Yoshioka T, et al. Effects of concentration reduction and partial replacement of paraquat by diquat on human toxicity: a clinical survey. *Hum Exp Toxicol.* 1992;11:241-245.
132. Zawahir S, et al. Acute intentional self-poisoning with a herbicide product containing fenoxaprop-P-ethyl, ethoxysulfuron, and isoxadifen ethyl: a prospective observational study. *Clin Toxicol.* 2009;47:792-797.
133. Zychlinski L, Zolnierowicz S. Comparison of uncoupling activities of chlorophenoxy herbicides in rat liver mitochondria. *Toxicol Lett.* 1990;52:25-34.

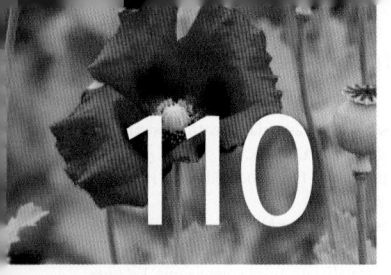

110

INSECTICIDES: ORGANIC PHOSPHORUS COMPOUNDS AND CARBAMATES

Michael Eddleston

INTRODUCTION

Globally and historically, pesticide poisoning has killed approximately 150,000 people each year, with anticholinesterase compounds responsible for about two-thirds of these deaths. Most deaths occur in rural Asia where intentional self-harm is common and where highly toxic organic phosphorus (OP) insecticides are still widely used in agriculture and available in households at times of stress.[67,104] Severe occupational or unintentional poisoning also happens where these highly toxic insecticides are used,[241] but deaths are generally less common.

Anticholinesterase poisoning is uncommon in industrialized countries where access to toxic pesticides is more controlled and a far smaller proportion of the population works in agriculture. However, when anticholinesterase poisoning does occur, patients often require intensive care with long hospital stays.[85,117,199] A further threat is the terrorist use of OP insecticides such as parathion to poison a water supply or flour used in bread baking. Food-borne poisoning occurs regularly in rural Asia;[57,180] such poisoning occurring in industrialized countries would result in hundreds of casualties being treated by clinicians with little experience of this frequently lethal toxic syndrome.

HISTORY AND EPIDEMIOLOGY

The first potent synthetic organic phosphorus (OP) anticholinesterase, tetraethylpyrophosphate (TEPP), was synthesized by Clermont in 1854. In 1932, Lange and Krueger wrote of choking and blurred vision following inhalation of dimethyl and diethyl phosphorofluoridates. Their account inspired Schrader in Germany to begin investigating these compounds, initially as pesticides, and later as warfare agents (Chap. 126). During this research, Schrader's group synthesized hundreds of compounds, including the pesticide parathion and the chemical weapons sarin, soman, and tabun.[115] Since that time, it is estimated that more than 50,000 OP compounds have been synthesized and screened for pesticidal activity, with dozens being produced commercially.[39]

Carbamates were first identified by Western scientists in the 19th century when the use of the Calabar bean (*Physostigma venenosum*) was recognized in tribal cultural practice in West Africa.[114] In 1864, Jobst and Hesse isolated an active alkaloid component they named physostigmine, which was used medicinally to treat glaucoma in 1877.[114] The synthesis of aliphatic esters of carbamic acid in the 1930s led to the development of carbamate pesticides, marketed initially as fungicides. In 1953 the Union Carbide Corporation first marketed carbaryl, the insecticide being prepared at the plant in Bhopal during the catastrophic release of methyl isocyanate in 1984 (Chap. 2).[7]

Although the term *organophosphate* is often used in both clinical practice and literature to refer to all phosphorus-containing pesticides that inhibit cholinesterase, phosphates are compounds in which the phosphorus atom is surrounded by 4 oxygen atoms, which is not the case for most OP compounds. Some chemicals, such as parathion, contain thioesters, whereas others are vinyl esters. Those cholinesterase-inhibiting (anticholinesterase) insecticides that contain phosphorus are collectively termed *organic phosphorus* compounds in this chapter. Those that contain the OC=ON linkage are termed carbamates.

Anticholinesterase pesticides are broadly grouped according to their toxicity by the World Health Organization's Classification of Pesticides into 5 groups,[248] from Class Ia "Extremely hazardous" through to "Active ingredients unlikely to present acute hazard in normal use" (Table 110–1). This classification is based upon comparative rat oral lethal dose for 50% of those exposed (LD_{50}) data of the active ingredient and is useful in its ability to distinguish very toxic OPs (such as parathion, rat oral LD_{50} 13 mg/kg) that have killed many thousands of people from relatively safe OPs (such as temephos, rat oral LD_{50} 8,600 mg/kg) that have not been reported to cause harm in humans. However, the rat LD_{50} is less useful in distinguishing between pesticides within the same class. Here, differential toxicity is likely to be due to differences in response to treatment, speed of onset, or co-formulants.[52,74]

The case fatality for OP and carbamate poisoning varies according to the insecticides used in local agriculture (and therefore taken for self-harm) and the health care services available. Where fast-acting, highly toxic pesticides are used for self-harm, deaths will occur before patients present to hospital. Hospital-based data therefore will have a falsely low case fatality, although often still high at 10% to 30%.[67] However, during the 1980 to 1990s, the case fatality for parathion poisoning in Munich's toxicology intensive care units (ICUs) was approximately 40%.[85,253] This was likely because ambulances were able to reach the patients early, before death, but after the patients had become symptomatic with this fast-acting OP. Some had already aspirated or suffered hypoxic brain injury prior to arrival of medical care. Despite resuscitation at the scene, many patients died from these complications of the prehospital events (in particular, loss of consciousness leading to aspiration and hypoxic brain injury) rather than from direct cholinergic effects of the OP insecticide. Few of these patients would have survived to hospital admission in lower-income countries. More recently, because parathion has become less common in Germany after its ban, the case fatality of OP-poisoned patients admitted to the Munich intensive unit has fallen to 5/33 (15%).[117] However, the case fatality for parathion poisoning remained high (3/7, 43%).

Although a major clinical problem in the developing world, the current annual estimate of at least 100,000 deaths is substantially less than previous estimate from the 1990 to 2000s of 200,000 per year due to a major migration from rural to urban areas in China and Taiwan,[40,178] reducing access to highly hazardous pesticides, and the implementation of highly effective pesticide regulation in countries such as Sri Lanka, Bangladesh, and South Korea.[37,41a,105,137]

As the most toxic WHO Toxicity Class 1a and 1b insecticides (such as parathion, methyl-parathion, monocrotophos) are gradually being withdrawn from agriculture across the world, the case fatality for OP and carbamate pesticide poisoning is declining. The 100,000 deaths annually probably represent around 1 to 2 million admissions for anticholinesterase poisoning. It is not yet clear that the reduction in mortality is reflected in reduced health care costs—an increasing number of survivors who required intensive care will increase costs as this is the most important health care cost for managing poisoned patients.[242] Much of this intensive care is required for respiratory failure and pulmonary injury.[119] Modeling in 2007 suggested that the

TABLE 110–1	WHO Classification of Pesticide Toxicity[248]				
		LD_{50} for the rat (mg/kg body weight)			
		Oral		Dermal	
	Class	Solids	Liquids	Solids	Liquids
Ia	Extremely hazardous	≤5	≤20	≤10	≤40
Ib	Highly hazardous	5–50	20–200	10–100	40–400
II	Moderately hazardous	50–500	200–2,000	100–1,000	400–4,000
III	Slightly hazardous	>500	>2,000	>1,000	>4,000

20% to 30% of patients who develop respiratory failure cumulatively received 1.1 to 2.3 million days of ventilation every year, requiring the constant use of 3,000 to 6,000 ventilators worldwide.[104] These figures for acute poisoning undoubtedly omit numerous unreported and possibly unrecognized illnesses resulting from lower level occupational and environmental exposure to these chemicals.

Typically, patients present following unintentional or suicidal ingestion of anticholinesterase insecticides or after working in areas recently treated with these compounds. Children and adults develop toxicity while playing in or inhabiting a residence recently sprayed or fogged with OP compounds by a pesticide applicator. Direct dermal contact with highly hazardous insecticides is dangerous.[10,108] Outbreaks of mass poisoning regularly occur in the developing world,[57,180] and less commonly in the United States,[28] from contamination of crops or food. Epidemics of toxicity are also reported among groups illegally importing and using the potent carbamate aldicarb.[27] Unfortunately, OPs and carbamates are also used for homicide.

PHARMACOLOGY
Organic Phosphorus Compounds

Organic phosphorus compound poisoning results in a rise in the concentration of acetylcholine (ACh) at muscarinic and nicotinic cholinergic synapses, which, in turn, leads to the syndrome of cholinergic excess. Figure 110–1 shows the basic formula for cholinesterase-inhibiting OP compounds. The "X" or "leaving group" determines many of the characteristics of the compound and provides a means of classifying OP insecticides into 4 main groups (Table 110–2). Group 1 compounds contain a quaternary nitrogen at the X position, and are collectively termed phosphorylcholines. These chemicals were originally developed as warfare agents, are powerful cholinesterase inhibitors, and can directly stimulate cholinergic receptors, presumably because of their structural resemblance to ACh. Group 2 compounds are called fluorophosphates because they possess a fluorine molecule as the leaving group. Like group 1 compounds, these compounds are volatile and highly toxic, making them well suited as warfare agents. The leaving group of group 3 compounds is a cyanide molecule or a halogen other than fluorine. The best-known compounds in this group are cyanophosphates such as the warfare agent tabun.

The fourth group is the broadest and comprises various subgroups based on the configuration of the R_1 and R_2 groups (Fig. 110–1), with the majority falling into the category of either a dimethoxy or diethoxy compound. Most of the insecticides in use today are in Group 4.

Direct-acting OP compounds (oxons) inhibit acetylcholinesterase (AChE) without needing to be metabolized in the body. However, many pesticides, such as parathion and malathion, are indirect inhibitors (prodrugs or thions) requiring partial metabolism (to paraoxon and malaoxon, respectively) within the body to become active. Desulfuration to the oxon occurs in the intestinal mucosa and liver following absorption.[216]

The OPs bind to a hydroxyl group at the active site deep inside a cleft in the AChE enzyme. As the leaving group of the OP insecticide is split off by AChE, a stable but reversible bond results between the remaining substituted phosphorus of the OP and AChE, effectively inactivating the enzyme (Figs. 110–2 and 110–3).

Although splitting of the choline-enzyme bond in normal ACh metabolism is completed within microseconds, the severing of the OP compound–enzyme bond is prolonged. The half-life of this reaction depends on the chemistry of the substituted phosphate. The in vitro half-life for spontaneous reactivation of human AChE inhibited by dimethoxy OPs is 0.7 to 0.86 hours,

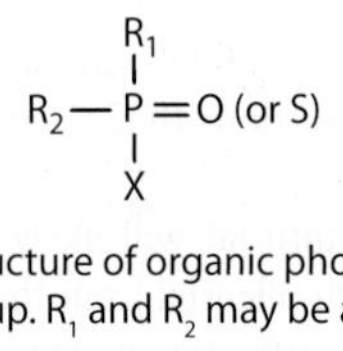

that of diethoxy inhibition 31 to 57 hours.[87] Spontaneous reactivation is therefore far quicker with dimethoxy OPs; however, this is only clinically relevant in patients with more moderate OP toxicity because, in patients with high OP concentrations, the reactivated AChE is simply reinhibited again.

Oximes, such as pralidoxime or obidoxime, markedly speed up the rate of reactivation.[87] However, if the phosphorus is allowed to remain bound to the AChE, because of late or inadequate administration of oximes, an alkyl group is nonenzymatically lost (Fig. 110–3), a process called "aging." Once aging occurs, the AChE can no longer be reactivated by oximes. Again, the half-life of this reaction is determined by the substituted phosphorus. The in vitro half-life of human AChE after poisoning with dimethoxy OPs is 3.7 hours, compared to 31 hours after diethoxy poisoning.[87] Clinically, this means that patients who present to a hospital 4 hours after poisoning with a dimethoxy OP will already have 50% of their AChE irreversibly inhibited; after 14 hours, the patients will be refractive to oxime therapy.[80,87] In contrast, patients poisoned by diethoxy OPs presenting within 14 hours will have little aged AChE and should be responsive to oximes.[80,87] De novo synthesis of AChE is required to replenish its supply once aging has occurred (see Diagnostic Testing section below).[221]

Organic phosphorus compounds also vary by lipid solubility,[19] rate of activation (conversion from thion to oxon) and rate of AChE inhibition,[87] and relative potency of inhibition of AChE and of the plasma enzyme butyrylcholinesterase (BuChE).

A few OP compounds do not fulfill the usual dimethoxy or diethoxy classification and have one of the alkyl groups linked to the phosphate by a sulfur molecule, rather than oxygen (eg, profenofos, prothiofos, methamidophos). Aging seems to be particularly rapid for these OPs, so that oximes have poor efficacy.[81]

Carbamates

Carbamate insecticides are *N*-methyl carbamates derived from carbamic acid (Fig. 110–4). Medicinal carbamate compounds that inhibit cholinesterases include physostigmine, pyridostigmine, and neostigmine. By contrast, thiocarbamate fungicides and herbicides (eg, maneb, mancozeb) do not inhibit AChE and so do not produce the cholinergic toxic syndrome.

When exposed to carbamates, AChE undergoes carbamylation in a manner similar to phosphorylation by OP compounds,[244] allowing ACh to accumulate in synapses. However, aging does not occur and the carbamate-AChE bond hydrolyzes spontaneously, reactivating the enzyme. As such, the duration of cholinergic symptoms in carbamate poisoning is generally less than 24 hours. However, complications that result from the cholinergic syndrome, in particular, pulmonary complications of the acute poisoning, can last much longer.

PHARMACOKINETICS AND TOXICOKINETICS
Organic Phosphorus Compounds

Organic phosphorus compounds are well absorbed from the lungs, gastrointestinal tract, mucous membranes, and conjunctiva following inhalation, ingestion, or topical contact.[93] Although absorption through intact skin appears to be relatively low,[99] percutaneous exposure to highly toxic compounds can cause severe toxicity.[42,240] The presence of broken skin, dermatitis, and higher environmental temperatures further enhances cutaneous absorption.[93]

Acute and chronic poisonings occur. The difficulty in removing these compounds from the skin and clothing explains some chronic poisonings; inadequate skin and respiratory protection during pesticide application is responsible for many cases of occupational poisonings.

The time to peak plasma concentration after self-poisoning is unknown. Human volunteer studies, using very low doses of chlorpyrifos, found Cmax to be around 6 hours after oral ingestion.[176] However, patients ingesting large amounts of oxon or fast-acting thion OPs often become symptomatic within minutes,[85,151] suggesting that absorption is rapid. In addition, the chlorpyrifos study[176] was performed with pure chlorpyrifos, not the formulated agricultural pesticide with solvents and surfactants that would be ingested

$$R_2 - \underset{\underset{X}{|}}{\overset{\overset{R_1}{|}}{P}} = O \text{ (or S)}$$

FIGURE 110–1. General structure of organic phosphorus compounds. X represents the leaving group. R_1 and R_2 may be aromatic or aliphatic groups that can be identical.

TABLE 110–2   The Classification of Organic Phosphorus Compounds by Groups, Showing Leaving Groups and Examples of Each Group

Group 1–phosphorylcholines
    Leaving group: substituted quaternary nitrogen
    Echothiophate iodide

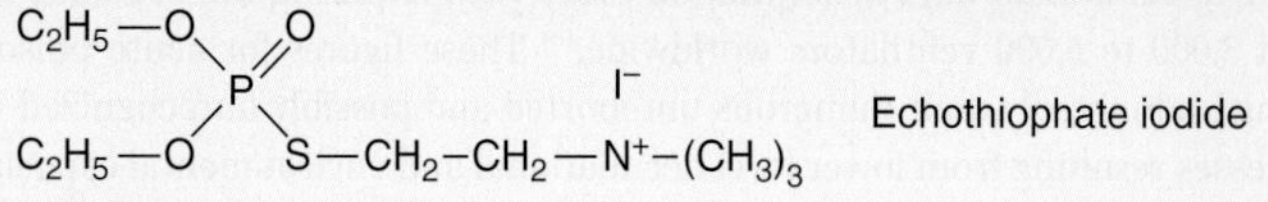

Group 2–fluorophosphates
    Leaving group: fluoride
    Dimefox, sarin, mipafox

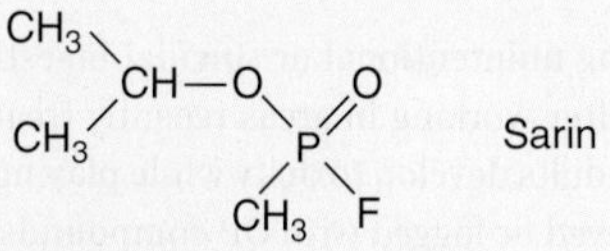

Group 3–cyanophosphates, other halophosphates
    Leaving group: CN-, SCN-, OCN-, halogen other than fluoride
    Tabun

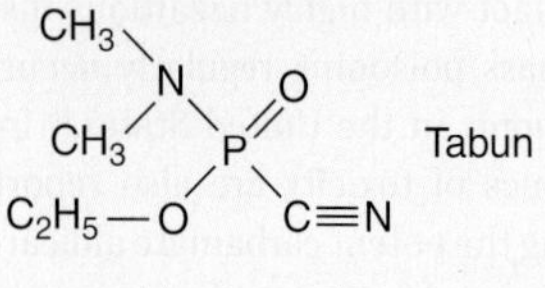

Group 4–multiple constituents
    Leaving group:
    Dimethoxy
        Azinphos-menthyl, bromophos, chlorothion, crotoxyphos, dicapthon, dichlorvos,
        dicrotophos, dimethoate, fenthion, malathion, mevinphos, parathion-methyl,
        phosphamidon, temephos, trichlorfon
    Diethoxy
        Carbophenothion, chlorfenvinphos, chlorpyriphos, coumaphos, demeton, diazinon,
        dioxathion, disulfoton, ethion, methosfolan, parathion, phorate, phosfolan, TEPP
    Other dialkoxy
        Isopropyl paraoxon, isopropyl parathion
    Diamino
        Schradan
    Chlorinated and other substituted dialkoxy
        Haloxon
    Trithioalkyl
        Merphos
    Triphenyl and substituted triphenyl
        Triorthocresyl phosphate (TOCP)
Mixed substituent
    Crufomate, cyanofenphos

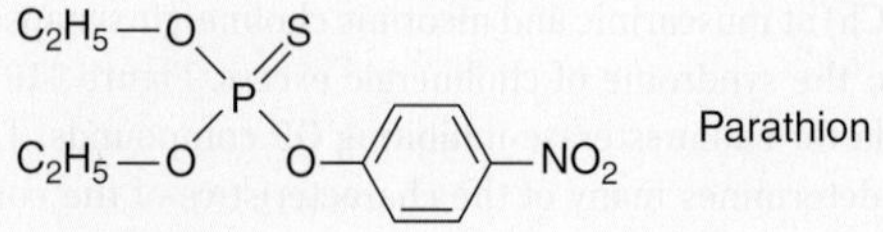

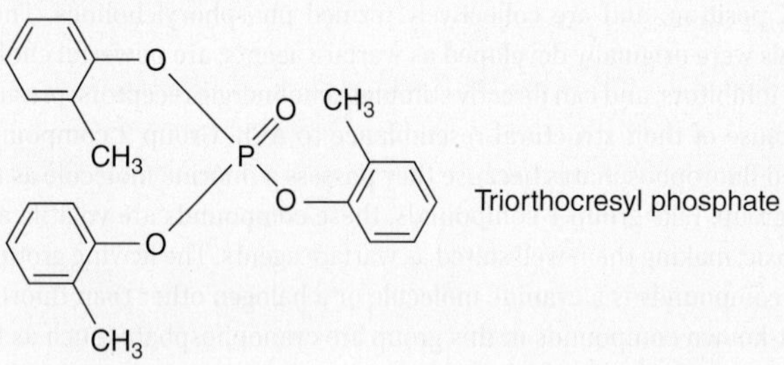

Echothiophate iodide

Sarin

Tabun

Parathion

Triorthocresyl phosphate

for self-harm. These solvents potentially change the toxicokinetics of the OP compound.

Most OP compounds are lipophilic,[19] with a large volume of distribution, and therefore rapidly distribute into tissue and fat, where they are protected

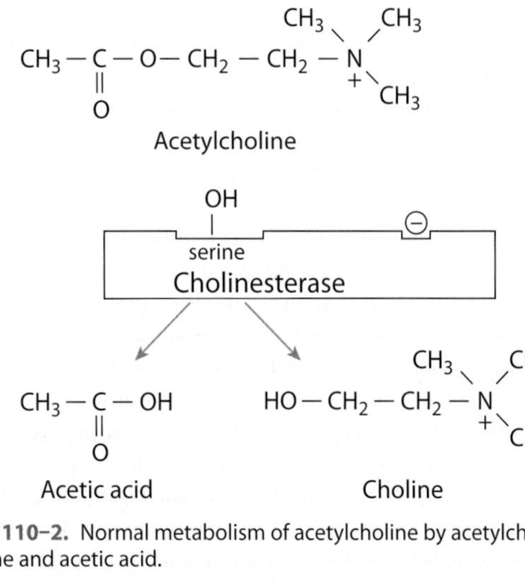

FIGURE 110–2. Normal metabolism of acetylcholine by acetylcholinesterase to choline and acetic acid.

from metabolism. Radiolabeled parathion injected into mice distributes most rapidly into the cervical brown fat and salivary glands, with high concentrations also measured in the liver, kidneys, and ordinary adipose tissue.[91] Adipose tissue gradually accumulates the highest concentrations. Redistribution from these stores allows measurement of circulating OP compound concentrations for up to 48 days post ingestion.[50,94]

The quantity of patient fat, as well as the lipophilicity of the OP compound, affects the outcome of poisoning. A Korean study of overweight patients (BMI >25) showed a longer duration of ventilation, intensive care, and hospital admission after poisoning with highly lipophilic OP insecticides compared to nonlipophilic OP insecticides.[145] This difference between highly lipophilic and nonlipophilic OP compounds did not occur in patients with a BMI of 25 or less.

The cholinergic crisis sometimes recurs in patients if unmetabolized OPs are mobilized from fat stores.[93] Highly lipophilic compounds such as fenthion and dichlofenthion (both with a Log Kow octanol/water coefficient >4) are particularly likely to cause this phenomenon.[50,74,161] Dimethoate, methamidophos and oxydemeton methyl are 3 common OPs that are not lipophilic (Log Kow <1), with small volumes of distribution and high plasma OP concentrations that do not appear to cause recurrent cholinergic crises.

The distribution of OPs into fat will likely include both activated and inactivated compound. When released from the fat hours to days later, the inactivated thion will require activation to cause clinical features.

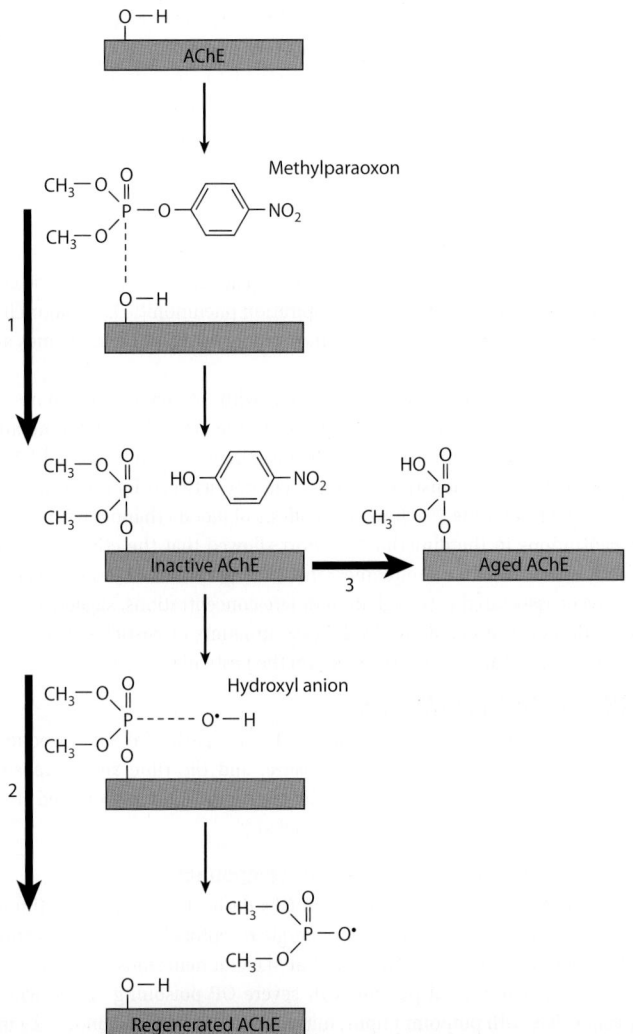

FIGURE 110–3. Mechanism of inhibition of acetylcholinesterase by an organic phosphorus compound. A dimethylated organic phosphorus pesticide (eg, methylparaoxon) inhibits AChE function by phosphorylating the serine hydroxyl group at the enzyme's active site (reaction 1). This reaction occurs very quickly. Active AChE is subsequently regenerated by a hydroxyl ion attacking the acetylated serine residue, removing the phosphate moiety, and releasing active enzyme (reaction 2). This regenerative process, however, is much slower than inhibition, requiring hours to days to occur (spontaneous reactivation $t_{1/2} \sim 0.7$ hours for dimethyl and 30 hours for diethyl compounds). While in the inactive state, the enzyme is prone to "aging" (reaction 3) in which one alkyl side-chain of the phosphoryl moiety is removed nonenzymatically, leaving a hydroxyl group in its place. Aged AChE can no longer react with water and regeneration no longer occurs. This reaction occurs considerably faster with enzymes that are inhibited by dimethylated pesticides ($t_{1/2} \sim$ 3.3 hours) than those inhibited by diethylated pesticides ($t_{1/2} \sim 30$ hours). The slower the regenerative process, the greater the quantity of inactive AChE available for aging. Pralidoxime catalyzes the regeneration of active acetylcholinesterase by exerting a nucleophilic attack on the phosphoryl group, transferring it from the enzyme to itself. By speeding up reaction 2, it reduces the quantity of inactive AChE available for ageing. However, because ageing occurs more rapidly with dimethylated OP compounds, pralidoxime is only useful before about 12 hours with dimethylated enzyme. *(Data from Eddleston M, Szinicz L, Eyer P, et al. Oximes in acute organophosphorus pesticide poisoning: a systematic review of clinical trials. QJM. 2002 May;95(5):275-283.)[88]*

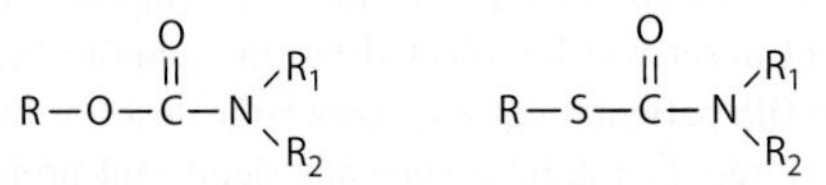

$$ R-O-\overset{\overset{\displaystyle O}{\|}}{C}-N\overset{\displaystyle R_1}{\underset{\displaystyle R_2}{<}} \qquad R-S-\overset{\overset{\displaystyle O}{\|}}{C}-N\overset{\displaystyle R_1}{\underset{\displaystyle R_2}{<}} $$

FIGURE 110–4. General structure of carbamate insecticides.

Thion OPs are activated by cytochrome P450 enzymes in the liver and intestinal mucosa. The precise CYP450s responsible vary according to the concentration of OP. For example, at low concentrations, chlorpyrifos, diazinon, parathion, and malathion are all metabolized and activated in vitro by CYP1A2 and 2B6.[30,31] However, at the higher concentrations more likely to occur after self-poisoning, CYP3A4 becomes dominant. The CYP450 enzymes involved in metabolism of active oxons to inactive metabolites are less clear.

Studies indicate that the activity of the human plasma enzyme paraoxonase (PON) is related to susceptibility to some acute and chronic effects of OP poisoning.[43,210,212] Paraoxonase is an A-esterase that can hydrolyze the active (oxon) metabolites of some but not all OP insecticides. Activity differs significantly among animal species. Animal models of OP poisoning demonstrate protection from toxicity when exogenous PON is administered, and greater susceptibility to poisoning when enzyme-deficient animals (such as genetically engineered knockout mice) are exposed.[210] Some authors propose that genetic polymorphisms in human PON activity lead to variations in interindividual susceptibility to some OP compounds.[43] However, the clinical relevance of these polymorphisms after poisoning are unclear.

Carbamates

Carbamate insecticides are absorbed across skin and mucous membranes, and by inhalation and ingestion. Peak cholinesterase inhibition occurred within 30 minutes of oral administration in rats.[177] Most carbamates undergo hydrolysis, hydroxylation, and conjugation in the liver and intestinal wall, with 90% excreted in the urine within 3 to 4 days.[16]

There is a view that carbamates, unlike OPs, do not easily enter the brain.[12] However, carbamates cause CNS depression in humans,[193] have lipophilic Log Kow values,[19] and rat studies show inhibition of brain cholinesterases with multiple carbamates.[177] Furthermore, post mortem studies demonstrate high concentrations of carbamates in cerebrospinal fluid and brain.[112,167] The evidence at present therefore suggests that they do not differ markedly from OPs in this aspect.

One important distinction between carbamates and OPs is that the carbamate-cholinesterase bond does not "age." Acetylcholinesterase inhibition is reversible, with spontaneous hydrolysis occurring usually within several hours. In addition, there appears to be less variation between carbamates than occurs between OP compounds. In a prospective case series of 1,288 patients who ingested carbosulfan, fenobucarb, or carbofuran, toxicity did not appear to vary markedly according to the carbamate ingested; the case fatality did however vary according to the concentration and formulation of the insecticide.[143]

PATHOPHYSIOLOGY
Cholinesterase Inhibition

Acetylcholine is a neurotransmitter found at both parasympathetic and sympathetic ganglia, skeletal neuromuscular junctions, terminal junctions of all postganglionic parasympathetic nerves, postganglionic sympathetic fibers to most sweat glands, and at some nerve endings within the central nervous system (Fig. 110–5). As the axon terminal is depolarized, vesicles containing ACh fuse with the nerve terminal, releasing ACh into the synapse or neuromuscular junction (NMJ). Acetylcholine then binds postsynaptic receptors, leading to activation (G proteins for muscarinic receptors and ligand-linked ion channels for the nicotinic receptors). Activation alters the flow of K^+, Na^+, and Ca^{2+} ionic currents on nerve cells, and alters the membrane potential of the postsynaptic membrane, resulting in propagation of the action potential.

Organic phosphorus and carbamate compounds are inhibitors of carboxylic ester hydrolases within the body, including acetylcholinesterase (AChE, EC 3.1.1.7), butyrylcholinesterase (plasma or pseudocholinesterase, BuChE, EC 3.1.1.8), plasma and hepatic carboxylesterases (aliesterases), paraoxonases (A-esterases), chymotrypsin, and other nonspecific proteases.[33]

Acetylcholinesterase hydrolyzes ACh into 2 inert fragments: acetic acid and choline (Fig. 110–2). Under normal circumstances, virtually all ACh released by the axon is hydrolyzed rapidly, with choline undergoing reuptake into the presynaptic terminal where it is reused to synthesize ACh.

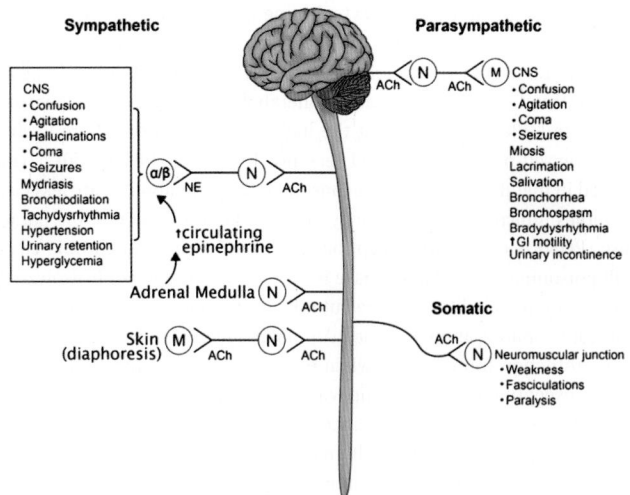

FIGURE 110–5. Pathophysiology of cholinergic syndrome as it affects the autonomic and somatic nervous systems.

Acetylcholinesterase is found in human nervous tissue and skeletal muscle, and on erythrocyte (ie, red blood cell {RBC}) cell membranes.[157]

Butyrylcholinesterase is a liver-derived protein found in human plasma, liver, heart, pancreas, and brain. Although the function of this enzyme is not well understood, its activity can be easily measured and has important clinical implications in anesthesia (Chap. 66).

Inhibition of AChE at synapses is generally thought to account for all, or the majority, of clinical features of both OP and carbamate compound poisoning. However, these compounds also inhibit many other enzymes;[33] the clinical effects of these interactions are not yet understood.

Markers of oxidative stress are raised after OP poisoning [47,194,232] leading some to suggest a pathogenic role for mitochondrial dysfunction and oxidative stress in OP poisoning[134] and trials of antioxidants such as acetylcysteine.[83,208] However, whether oxidative stress is simply an association or pathogenic in OP-poisoned patients is not yet clear.

Effect of Coformulants and Alcohol

Patients who drink agricultural pesticides in self-harm actually ingest formulated pesticides rather than the pure anticholinesterase compound or "active ingredient" (AI). Organic phosphorus compounds sold for agricultural use are typically emulsifiable concentrates (EC) in which the AI (eg, dimethoate) is mixed with an organic solvent such as xylene or cyclohexanone and a surfactant/emulsifier. Unfortunately, the compounds used for coformulation are highly variable, being optimized by each pesticide manufacturer for each OP. As a result, coformulants often differ between the same OP produced by 2 companies, and for different OPs produced by one company. Coformulants are much less likely to be a problem when people are exposed to agricultural insecticides that have been diluted for use, as occurs in sprayers exposed to their spray.

The clinical effect of self-poisoning with these coformulants, in addition to the carbamate or OP AI, is not yet clear. Complications of surfactant poisoning are well described in glyphosate poisoning[25] (Chap. 109) but not with OP or carbamate insecticides. The acute toxicity of the solvents appears to be low—for example, the rat oral LD_{50}s for xylene and cyclohexanone are 4,000 to 5,000 and 1,620 mg/kg, respectively. However, in a minipig model of acute oral dimethoate 40% emulsifiable concentrate (EC40) poisoning, early respiratory arrest occurred at a point when red blood cell AChE was little inhibited, suggesting a non-AChE mechanism.[79] Early work showed that dimethoate toxicity could be increased markedly by changing solvent;[34] more recent work with chlorpyrifos demonstrates a modest change in toxicity after changing the solvent.[227] The minipig model indicates that the toxicity of dimethoate EC40 requires both the dimethoate AI and the cyclohexanone solvent, with changes in the solvent reducing toxicity.[79] Although potentially

important, the major differences in the clinical syndrome noted in patients between dimethoate EC40, chlorpyrifos EC40, and fenthion EC50 cannot be attributed to the solvent because most pesticides in that study were generic, using 40% xylene as the solvent.[74] Further clinical studies with accurate measurement of all elements of the formulation in the plasma are required to address the importance of coformulants in human self-poisoning.

A further effect of the solvent/surfactant occurs after aspiration. Ingestion of large quantities of OPs or carbamates causes rapid loss of consciousness and respiratory arrest, increasing the risk of aspiration with pesticide AI, solvent, surfactant, and gastric contents. The relative role of gastric contents and pesticide is not yet clear. Aspiration pneumonitis is a major clinical problem in OP poisoning and cannot simply be treated with oximes and atropine.[66]

Pesticides are frequently coingested with ethanol, particularly by men,[229] raising questions about the effect of the alcohol on outcome after OP poisoning.[70] Two cohorts, of people ingesting either dimethoate EC40 or profenofos EC50, demonstrated an association between ingestion of ethanol and poor outcome.[59,76] However, analysis of blood ethanol and pesticide concentrations in the dimethoate cohort showed that the ethanol did not directly affect the clinical outcome;[76] instead, high ethanol blood concentrations were associated with high dimethoate concentrations, suggesting that inebriation caused people to drink larger amounts of pesticide, worsening outcome due to the direct toxic effects of the pesticide.

CLINICAL MANIFESTATIONS

Clinical manifestations vary according to the particular OP insecticide involved, the dose and route of exposure, and the time since exposure. Features are classified as acute (usually less than 24 hours), delayed (from 24 hours to 2 weeks), and late (after 2 weeks).[191]

Acute Toxicity—Organic Phosphorus Compounds

Clinical findings of acute toxicity from OPs derive from excessive stimulation of muscarinic and nicotinic cholinergic receptors by ACh in the central and autonomic nervous systems, and at skeletal neuromuscular junctions (Fig. 110–5). The typical patient with severe OP poisoning is one who is unresponsive, with pinpoint pupils, muscle fasciculations, diaphoresis, emesis, diarrhea, salivation, lacrimation, urinary incontinence, and (after self-poisoning) an odor of garlic or solvents.

Timing of Clinical Features

The timing of onset of symptoms varies according to the route, the degree of exposure, and the particular OP involved. This is important because more rapid onset of poisoning will reduce the likelihood of the patient reaching health care safely, before onset of respiratory failure or of complications such as aspiration. Out-of-hospital cardiorespiratory arrest in most parts of the world will result in the patient's death; in a Korean study, with an effective emergency ambulance system, only 22% and 10% of insecticide-poisoned patients with an out-of-hospital cardiac arrest survived to admission and discharge, respectively.[182] In other parts of the rural developing world, with longer distances and weaker emergency care systems, survival will be even lower.

Some patients ingesting large quantities of concentrated agricultural formulations become symptomatic as soon as 5 minutes following ingestion. Most patients with acute poisoning become symptomatic within a few hours of exposure, and practically all who will become ill show some features within 24 hours.

Oxon OP compounds (such as mevinphos and monocrotophos) are already active on exposure and patients become symptomatic quickly. Since some thion OPs are very rapidly converted to oxons, these OPs also rapidly produce symptoms—patients ingesting parathion can be unconscious within minutes.[85] In contrast, patients ingesting thions that are slowly converted to active oxons (such as fenthion) often do not show symptoms for hours.[74]

The speed of onset will be affected by the quantity ingested and the toxicity[87] of the OP: patients ingesting very large doses or highly toxic pesticides will more rapidly inhibit a clinically significant proportion of their AChE and exhibit features earlier.

Lipid solubility also likely affects time to onset. Fat-soluble OPs (with log Kow of >3-4) will rapidly distribute to fat stores, in the process reducing their concentration in extracellular fluid, where they impart their clinical effect (eg, fenthion[74]). Significant poisoning with such OPs is commonly delayed—respiratory failure with fenthion for example typically occurs after 24 hours in contrast to less fat soluble OPs.[78]

Symptoms following OP exposure last for variable lengths of time, again based on the compound and the circumstances of the poisoning. For example, highly lipophilic compounds, such as dichlofenthion or fenthion, cause recurrent cholinergic effects for many days in some patients following oral ingestion as they are released from fat stores.[50,161,190]

Clinical Features

Patients usually present awake and alert, complaining of anxiety, restlessness, insomnia, headache, dizziness, blurred vision, depression, tremors, and/or other nonspecific symptoms.[15,174] In moderate-severe poisoning, the level of consciousness then deteriorates rapidly to confusion, lethargy, and coma. Where careful observational studies have been done, convulsions appear to be uncommon in adult OP pesticide poisoning compared to OP nerve agent poisoning.[74,235] The convulsions that do occur are likely due to hypoxia as a complication of acute cholinergic poisoning.

The effects of excessive ACh on the autonomic nervous system is variable because cholinergic receptors are found in both the sympathetic and parasympathetic nervous systems (Fig. 110–5). Excessive muscarinic activity is characterized by several mnemonics, including "SLUD" (salivation, lacrimation, urination, defecation) and "DUMBBELS" (defecation, urination, miosis, bronchospasm or bronchorrhea, emesis, lacrimation, salivation). Of these, miosis is the most consistently encountered sign. Profuse bronchorrhea mimics pulmonary edema.[174] Excessive fluid loss results in salt and water depletion. Body temperature is often low acutely, rising to normal or higher with treatment and time.[163]

Although muscarinic findings are emphasized in these mnemonics, muscarinic signs are not always clinically dramatic or initially predominant. Parasympathetic effects can be offset by excessive autonomic activity from stimulation of nicotinic adrenal receptors (resulting in catecholamine release) and postganglionic sympathetic fibers.[221] Mydriasis, bronchodilation, and urinary retention can occur as a result of sympathetic activity. Increased sympathetic activity usually precipitates white blood cell demargination, resulting in leukocytosis.[172,174]

Excessive adrenergic influences on metabolism cause glycogenolysis[222] with hyperglycemia and ketosis that have been mistaken for diabetic ketoacidosis.[159,251] Transient glycosuria was reported in 16 of 23 (69%) of OP or carbamate poisoned patients in one series.[211] Hyperglycemia at presentation is associated with worse outcome;[165] however, in a small study, a medical history of diabetes mellitus was not associated with worse outcome.[150]

Hyperamylasemia appears to be relatively common in OP poisoning, occurring in 4/47 (9%) adults in one series[204] and 5/17 (29%) children in a second.[239] However, both included various anticholinesterase pesticides; a series of only malathion-poisoned patients reported hyperamylasemia in 47/75 (63%).[46] The amylase is likely pancreatic because animal studies show OP-induced damage[120] and human poisoning cases show associated pancreatic edema and/or rarely necrotizing pancreatitis.[181] The incidence of subclinical and clinical pancreatitis varies according to the OP ingested and perhaps the coformulants. Acute poisoning is associated with multiple temporary effects on thyroid and pituitary hormones.[65,106]

Cardiovascular manifestations reflect mixed effects on the autonomic nervous system (including increased sympathetic tone), together with the consequences of OP-induced hypoxia and hypovolemia. Troponin rises are reported, as well as ST segment elevation.[38,129] Admission heart rate is usually normal, with relatively few patients showing a tachycardia greater than 100 beats/min or bradycardia less than 60 beats/min. Patients who receive atropine before admission are infrequently tachycardic.

The literature is filled with reports of QT interval prolongation and ventricular dysrhythmias.[13,100,136,202,203] However, these reports are complicated by the fact that many patients had their ECG done before they received any atropine or were so ill that atropine was ineffective. The first is illustrated by a description of 46 patients with OP or carbamate poisoning in which "ECG recordings [were] taken on arrival ... before the start of atropine treatment."[203] The reported cardiac rhythms are confounded by the hypoxia and hypovolemia that characterize the cholinergic syndrome. In another study, 29 of the 35 patients with such dysrhythmias died.[154]

In contrast, when 1950 Sri Lanka patients poisoned with WHO Class II OP or carbamate compounds were evaluated, serious dysrhythmias were very rare in patients adequately resuscitated with atropine, intravenous fluids and when available oxygen.[139] In a case series of oxygenated and atropinized OP-poisoned patients in intensive care (27/33 due to aspiration pneumonia it is mixed group of OP compounds QT interval prolongation was noted in 9/33 (27.3%) of patients, but in only 5 was the corrected QT (QTc) interval greater than 500 ms.[117] The median QTc interval in fatal cases was only 497 ms versus 428 ms in survivors. However, bradycardia and torsade de pointes occurred after stopping atropine in 5 patients, suggesting that atropine had been treating a potential complication of OP compound poisoning.

Hypotension occurs because of stimulation of vascular receptors by excessive circulating ACh, severe volume loss, or myocardial dysfunction.[8,131] Severe hypotension is a particularly significant problem in poisoning with the unusually fat-insoluble OP dimethoate.[51,74] In these cases, fatal poisoning is characterized by early respiratory failure followed by hypotension that only transiently responds to vasopressors. Such a syndrome is not reported after poisoning with fat-soluble OPs such as chlorpyrifos and fenthion.[74] The exact role of direct cardiotoxicity and peripheral vasodilation is unclear, and whether this syndrome occurs with other fat-insoluble OPs, such as methamidophos and oxydemeton methyl.[51] There is evidence to suggest that the solvent in dimethoate EC40, cyclohexanone, is partially responsible for this severe hypotension.[79]

Acute respiratory complications of OP poisoning (Figs. 110–6 and 110–7) include the direct pulmonary effects of bronchorrhea and bronchoconstriction, NMJ failure in the diaphragm and intercostal muscles, and loss of central respiratory drive.[54,119] If severe and occurring before patients reach medical care, these effects will lead to hypoxemia and respiratory arrest, the most common cause of death after OP poisoning. Both bronchorrhea and bronchoconstriction respond to adequate atropine therapy. Unfortunately, neither NMJ failure nor loss of central respiratory drive responds to atropine, and patients must be ventilated until respiratory function recovers.

An additional early respiratory complication is hydrocarbon aspiration that may occur after ingestion of commercially formulated pesticides (Fig. 110–6). The incidence of aspiration and the consequences of aspiration—whether chemical pneumonitis, pneumonia, or acute respiratory distress syndrome—are not yet known and likely differ according to the OP, dose, and coformulants. In one German case series of patients requiring intensive care, 27/33 (81.8%) had aspiration pneumonia.[117]

Acetylcholine stimulation of nicotinic receptors also governs skeletal muscle activity. The effects of excessive cholinergic stimulation at the NMJ are similar to that of a depolarizing neuromuscular blocker (succinylcholine) and initially result in fasciculations or weakness. Severe poisoning results in paralysis.[236] Rarely, patients present with paralysis from nicotinic effects without any other initial signs and symptoms suggestive of OP toxicity.[90,97]

Extrapyramidal parkinsonian effects such as rigidity and choreoathetosis are reported after severe anticholinesterase poisoning,[22] persisting for several days after cholinergic features have resolved. They occur in severely ill patients requiring intensive care for more than a week.[195] However, the appearance of frank parkinsonism during acute poisoning is uncommon.[130]

Liver and kidney injury are not considered common features of OP or carbamate poisoning.[174] Liver injury occurred in poisoned patients receiving obidoxime.[11] Although severe acute kidney injury (AKI) requiring hemodialysis occurs,[36] a prospective Indian case series of 400 patients found no cases of acute kidney injury.[219] Substantial muscle injury also seems rare, although modest rises in creatine kinase are recognized in OP-poisoned patients in ICUs, possibly due to muscle injury from sustained paralysis and

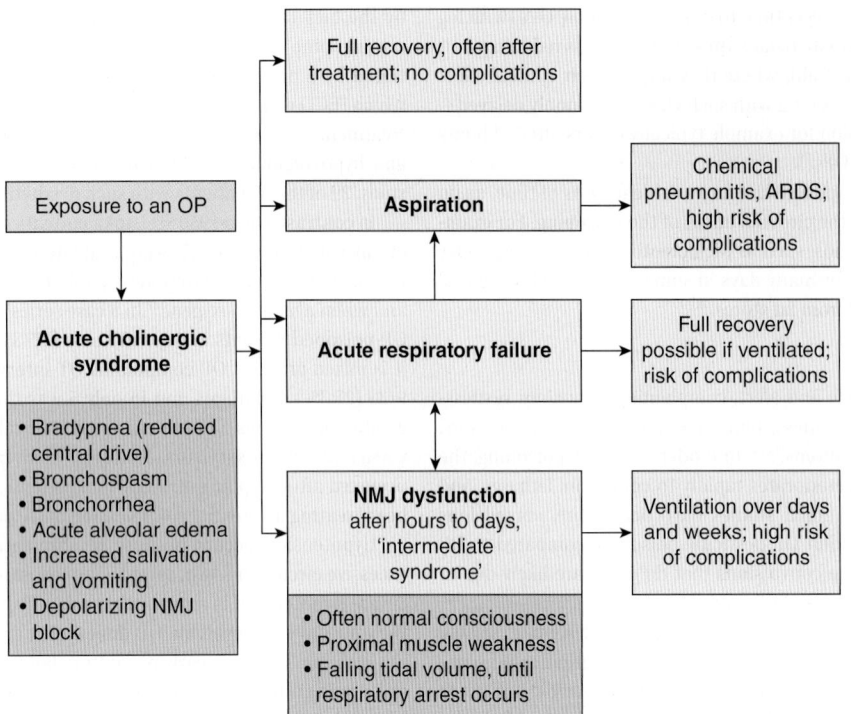

FIGURE 110–6. Respiratory system toxicity secondary to organic phosphorus compound poisoning. ARDS = acute respiratory distress syndrome; NMJ = neuromuscular junction of OP = organic phosphorus compound. *(Reproduced with permission from Hulse EJ, Davies JO, Simpson AJ, et al. Respiratory complications of organophosphorus nerve agent and insecticide poisoning. Implications for respiratory and critical care. Am J Respir Crit Care Med. 2014 Dec 15;190(12):1342-1354.)*

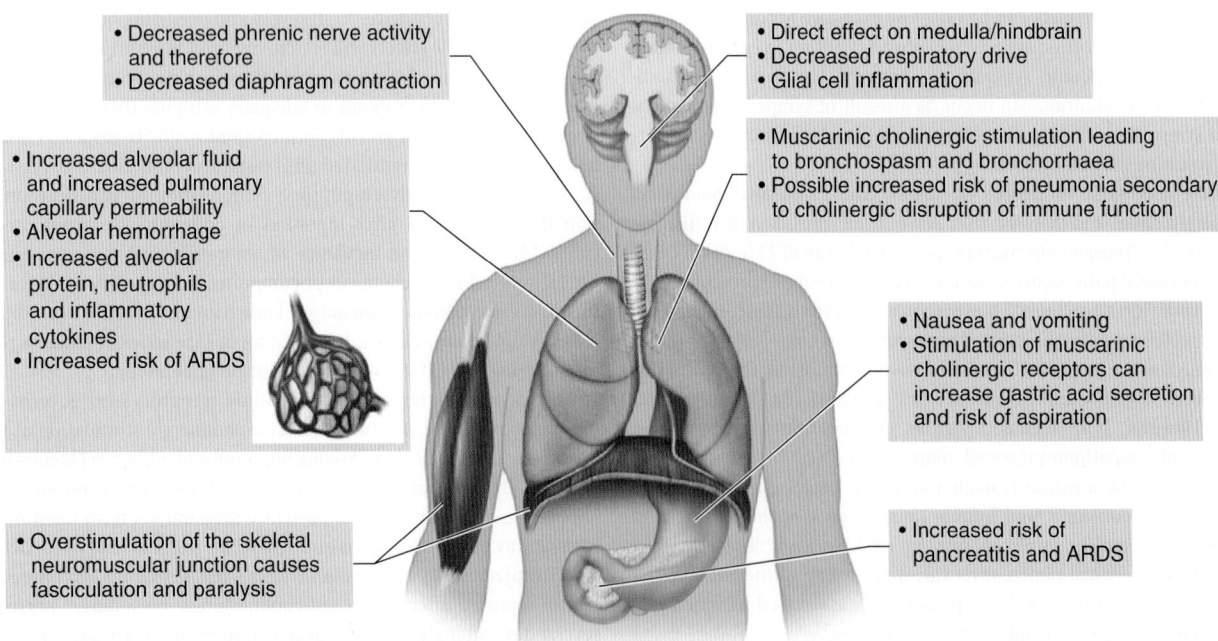

FIGURE 110–7. Pulmonary complications of organic phosphorus (OP) poisoning. Exposure to OP compounds causes the acute cholinergic syndrome characterized by reduction in central respiratory drive, bronchospasm, and hypoxia due to bronchorrhea and alveolar edema, and depolarizing neuromuscular junction (NMJ) block. This either resolves or progresses to acute respiratory failure that would be fatal without medical input. Reduced consciousness and loss of airway control in the cholinergic syndrome increases the risk of aspiration, resulting in chemical pneumonitis that will worsen oxygenation and progress to ARDS. Overstimulation of the NMJ causes chronic peripheral dysfunction that occurs simultaneously with the acute cholinergic syndrome or after it has resolved with normal cerebral function (then termed the "intermediate syndrome"). This NMJ dysfunction often requires days and weeks of mechanical ventilation with associated risk of ventilator-associated pneumonia and barotrauma. *(Reproduced with permission from Hulse EJ, Davies JO, Simpson AJ, et al. Respiratory complications of organophosphorus nerve agent and insecticide poisoning. Implications for respiratory and critical care. Am J Respir Crit Care Med. 2014 Dec 15;190(12):1342-1354.)*

little movement.[123] Two cases of rhabdomyolysis and AKI followed severe monocrotophos poisoning.[96] It is also possible that renal or muscle injury is due to solvents in the insecticides, such as cyclohexanone.[184]

Acute Toxicity—Carbamates

The acute effects of poisoning from carbamate insecticides are similar to those of OP insecticides, with coma and acute respiratory failure occurring after substantial exposure. Cholinergic features tend to last for shorter durations after poisoning, often for a matter of hours, rather than days. Persistent cholinergic features over many days are not reported for carbamate poisoning; however, complications of toxicity such as aspiration pneumonia can last for many days.[143]

Delayed Syndromes

Neuromuscular Junction Dysfunction (Intermediate Syndrome)

A syndrome of delayed muscle weakness without cholinergic features or fasciculations resulting in respiratory failure was first reported by Wadia in 1974 as type II paralysis[236] and further refined by Senanayake and Karalliedde in 1987 as the intermediate syndrome.[206] The syndrome is defined as occurring 24 to 96 hours after acute OP poisoning, and after resolution of the cholinergic crisis.[1,132,206,236] Patients develop proximal muscle weakness, especially of the neck flexors, and cranial nerve palsies, and progress to respiratory failure that lasts for up to several weeks.[132] Consciousness is preserved unless complicated by hypoxia or pneumonitis. The syndrome is important since apparently well patients suddenly develop respiratory failure; patients must be carefully observed for proximal muscle weakness if deaths are to be prevented.[18,183] The first sign is often weakness of neck flexion such that patients cannot lift their head off the bed. It is also recognized as occurring rarely with carbamate poisoning.[121]

Although the exact pathophysiology of the syndrome is unknown, it is clearly due to NMJ dysfunction, with respiratory failure resulting from weakness affecting the diaphragm and intercostal muscles. Preservation of consciousness suggests that the central respiratory drive is not involved. One theory is that overwhelming NMJ stimulation causes downregulation of the NMJ synaptic machinery.[53,206] This would require time to be repaired, even after the pesticide is removed from the body, explaining the long duration of ventilation needed by many patients.[78]

Cases and small case series of NMJ dysfunction suggest that it is more common with certain OPs, such as parathion, methyl parathion, malathion, and fenthion. Unfortunately, large cohorts of poisoning with specific OPs receiving standardized treatments are rarely reported, making comparisons of incidence between OPs difficult. However, 2 cohorts indicate that the intermediate syndrome causing respiratory failure is more common in fenthion poisoning than chlorpyrifos, malathion, or fenitrothion poisoning.[78,235]

Clinical examination for proximal muscle weakness remains the most reliable means of identifying the occurrence of intermediate syndrome.[132] Electromyograms often show tetanic fade, and suggest both pre- and postsynaptic involvement.[132] Characteristic electrophysiological features appear before onset of neurologic features and respiratory paralysis.[122] The majority of patients developing weakness do not progress to respiratory failure, indicating that intermediate syndrome is a spectrum disorder.

Another study of severely poisoned patients suggested that the occurrence of intermediate syndrome strongly correlated with the initial degree of cholinergic crisis, and seemed to be a continuum with the neuromuscular paralysis resulting from the early stages of poisoning.[123] This view is supported by early work[53] and a more recent study of dimethoate poisoning, which showed that peripheral NMJ dysfunction can occur simultaneously with the cholinergic syndrome.[78] Patients with moderate to severe dimethoate poisoning typically require intubation for respiratory failure soon after ingestion, during the acute cholinergic syndrome. However, this is relatively short-lived and patients recover consciousness after a few days. As the cholinergic syndrome settles and the patients regain consciousness, with presumed recovery of the central respiratory drive, they are still unable to ventilate. Similar to patients with classical intermediate syndrome, they require ventilatory support for

several weeks until their NMJ recovers function. In contrast, this case series showed that the classic intermediate syndrome—respiratory failure after resolution of the cholinergic syndrome—sometimes occurs before 24 hours and after 96 hours.[78]

These studies suggest that the original intermediate syndrome is just one important aspect of OP-induced peripheral NMJ dysfunction. It seems likely that the relative incidence and timing of the intermediate syndrome or delayed NMJ dysfunction for different OPs is determined by the rapidity and quantity of AChE inhibition. Where inhibition is intense, with fat-insoluble OPs like dimethoate that have very high plasma concentrations, NMJ dysfunction comes on early, before recovery from the cholinergic crisis. Fat-soluble OPs, such as fenthion, cause a more protracted AChE inhibition, likely explaining why fenthion induced NMJ dysfunction and respiratory failure occur later.[78]

Some authors suggest that insufficient oxime therapy explains the intermediate syndrome.[20] The occurrence of NMJ dysfunction in chlorpyrifos poisoning may well be due to inadequate oxime therapy. However, adequate oxime therapy after, for example, malathion poisoning[215] is probably irrelevant because AChE inhibited by this dimethyl OP shows poor biochemical reactivation after oxime therapy. Regardless, delayed NMJ dysfunction is possibly due to ineffective AChE reactivation, whether due to inadequate oxime doses or to poisoning with OP insecticides that do not respond to oxime therapy.

Animal studies of dimethoate poisoning have shed some light on this condition. These studies produced NMJ dysfunction and showed that it did not occur after poisoning with dimethoate active ingredient alone. Instead, it occurred after poisoning with the agricultural EC40 formulation that included both the dimethoate active ingredient and the solvent, cyclohexanone.[79] This raises the possibility that NMJ dysfunction is due to an interaction of solvent and active ingredient. All reported cases have occurred after self-poisoning by drinking agricultural formulations of OP insecticides; further human studies are required to clarify the role of solvents and the possible mechanisms of effect.

Organic Phosphorus Compound-Induced Delayed Neuropathy

Peripheral neuropathies occur with chronic OP compound exposures days to weeks following acute exposures, due to phosphorylation and inhibition of the enzyme neuropathy target esterase (NTE, now identified as a lysophospholipase) within nervous tissue.[95,124] This enzyme catalyzes breakdown of endoplasmic reticulum-membrane phosphatidylcholine, the major phospholipid of eukaryotic cell membranes. Neuropathic OPs (such as chlorpyrifos, dichlorvos, isofenphos, methamidophos[153]) cause a transient loss of NTE activity, putatively disrupting membrane phospholipid homeostasis, axonal transport, and glial–axonal interactions.[95]

Such neuropathies sometimes result from exposure to OPs that do not inhibit RBC cholinesterase or produce clinical cholinergic toxicity.[35] The more commonly implicated chemicals include triaryl phosphates, such as triorthocresyl phosphate (TOCP), and dialkyl phosphates, such as mephosfolan, mipafox, and chlorpyrifos.[125] Pathologic findings demonstrate effects primarily on large distal neurons, with axonal degeneration preceding demyelination.

Contaminated foods and beverages were responsible for epidemics of OP compound–induced delayed polyneuropathies and encephalopathy. In the 1930s, thousands of individuals in the United States became weak or paralyzed after drinking a supplement containing TOCP—an outbreak nicknamed "Ginger Jake paralysis" (Chap. 22).[166] Contaminated cooking and mineral oils were responsible for outbreaks of delayed polyneuropathies in Vietnam and Sri Lanka.[56,205] Vague distal muscle weakness and pain are often the presenting symptoms and progress to paralysis.[102] The administration of atropine or pralidoxime does not alter the onset and clinical course of these symptoms.[231] Pyramidal tract signs appear weeks to months after acute exposures. Electromyograms and nerve conduction studies are helpful in diagnosis by identifying the type of neuropathy (such as axonopathy, myelinopathy, or transmission neuropathy) and differentiating it from similar presentations such as Guillain-Barré syndrome.[3] Recovery of these patients is variable and occurs over months to years, with residual deficits common.[166,205]

Delayed neuropathies are not usually associated with carbamate insecticides. One reason for this difference is presumed to be that aging of the neuropathy target esterase pesticide complex is a requirement for neuronal degeneration. Paradoxically, one study suggested that subgroups of carbamates actually bind neuropathy target esterase and exert a protective effect against more toxic OP compounds.[4] However, delayed neuropathy does occur rarely after poisoning with carbamates.[61,228,249] These cases involved ingestions of carbaryl, *m*-tolyl methyl carbamate, and carbofuran, included both sensory and motor tracts, and tended to resolve over 3 to 9 months. Electromyogram findings were variable.

Behavioral Toxicity

Behavioral changes also occur after acute or chronic exposure to OP compounds.[86,213] Signs and symptoms include confusion, psychosis, anxiety, drowsiness, depression, fatigue, and irritability. Electroencephalographic changes last for weeks in some cases.[101] Single-photon emission computed tomography (SPECT) scanning revealed morphologic changes in the basal ganglia of one child following poisoning.[24] A deficit in cognitive processing was noted after acute OP self-poisoning that lasts for at least 6 months and is not found in matched patients who poisoned themselves with paracetamol.[48,49] Although multiple small studies have shown some effect,[86,169,201] thus far there is no clear evidence for neuropsychiatric deficits resulting from subclinical exposure to OPs.

Chronic Toxicity

Illness results from chronic exposure to excessive amounts of OP compounds. Chronic exposure most commonly occurs in workers who have regular contact with OPs, but also occurs in individuals who have repeated contact with insecticides in their living environment. Cholinergic ophthalmic preparations have led to toxicity.[155] Although tolerance to acute cholinergic systemic effects of OP insecticides (including death in rats) is observed with long-term exposures,[93] persons who have repeated contact have developed symptoms after many months. These effects range from vague neurologic complaints, such as weakness and blurred vision, to miosis, nausea, vomiting, diarrhea, diaphoresis, and other cholinergic effects (eg. DUMBELS, SLUD).[5,6,155,214] Butyrylcholinesterase activity is usually the most sensitive measure of exposure, and workers in contact with these chemicals should have baseline BuChE testing for comparison and monitoring.[113]

Studies have linked the onset of Parkinson's disease with chronic exposure to pesticides including OP compounds.[60] Although statistics derived from some epidemiologic studies suggest a connection with pesticide exposure,[84] others studies have failed to a find an association between OP compounds and Parkinson's disease (for example ref [220]). Overall, the studies have been retrospective in nature and confounded by recall bias. However, a recent case–control study using a geographic information system–based exposure assessment tool to estimate ambient exposure to OPs in central California found an adjusted odds ratio of 2.24 (95% confidence intervals 1.58–3.19).[237]

DIAGNOSTIC TESTING
Organic Phosphorus Compounds

When faced with a patient in cholinergic crisis who presents with a history of acute exposure to an OP cholinesterase inhibitor insecticide, the diagnosis is straightforward. Although textbooks list a variety of clinical signs for the cholinergic crisis (eg, DUMBELS, SLUD), most patients with significant poisoning are simply identified by the presence of pinpoint pupils, excessive sweat, and breathing difficulty.[72] However, when the history is unreliable or does not suggest poisoning, the physician must turn to other means to confirm the diagnosis of OP or carbamate poisoning. However, treatment of an ill patient with a cholinergic syndrome should not await confirmation of the diagnosis.

The most appropriate laboratory tests for confirming cholinesterase inhibition by insecticides are tests that measure (1) specific insecticides and active metabolites in biologic tissues and (2) cholinesterase activity in plasma or blood. Unfortunately, although urine and serum assays for OP compounds and their metabolites are available,[109,141] such testing is rarely obtainable within hours. Moreover, toxic concentrations are not established for most compounds. Currently, therefore, verifying cholinesterase inhibitor poisoning relies on measurement of cholinesterase activity.[69,93]

Cholinesterase Activity

The 2 cholinesterases commonly measured are butyrylcholinesterase (BuChE, plasma cholinesterase, EC 3.1.1.8) and red blood cell (RBC) acetylcholinesterase (AChE, EC 3.1.1.7). The former is produced by the liver and then secreted into the blood, where it metabolizes xenobiotics, including succinylcholine, pyrethroid insecticides, and cocaine. Red blood cell AChE is expressed from the same gene as the enzyme found in neuronal synapses. The main difference is in their mechanism of membrane attachment, which is due to posttranslational modification (RBC AChE is glycophosphatidylinositol linked to the RBC whereas neuronal AChE forms dimers and tetramers that are attached to the postsynaptic membrane by other proteins).[157] Inhibition of either RBC AChE or BuChE only serves as a marker for cholinesterase inhibitor poisoning, because inhibition of these enzymes specifically does not contribute to signs and symptoms of poisoning.

There is tremendous variability between OP compounds in the degree and duration with which they affect particular cholinesterases.[75,140,164] After a significant exposure, BuChE activity usually falls first, followed by a decrease in RBC AChE activity. The sequence is highly variable, but by the time patients present with acute symptoms, activities of both cholinesterase have usually fallen well below baseline values.[174] Of note, the presence of BuChE, AChE, and other esterases varies markedly between species,[146] complicating the interpretation of animal studies. Furthermore, AChE occurs at very low concentrations in human plasma;[146] therefore, papers citing human serum AChE activity are likely measuring serum BuChE.

Butyrylcholinesterase

Butyrylcholinesterase activity usually recovers before RBC AChE activity, returning to normal within a few days after a mild exposure in the absence of a repeat exposure.[44] However, BuChE activity is less specific for exposure than is RBC AChE activity. Low BuChE activity is also found in patients with a number of disorders, including hereditary deficiency of the enzyme, malnutrition, hepatic parenchymal disease, chronic debilitating illnesses, and iron deficiency anemia.[133]

The wide normal range of BuChE activity allows for patients with high normal values to suffer significant falls in activity, yet still register near normal BuChE activity on assay.[44] Additionally, day-to-day variation in the activity of this enzyme in healthy individuals may be as high as 20%.[110]

Furthermore, because BuChE inhibition varies between OPs and does not cause clinical effects, an admission value by itself is of little value in predicting outcome. An admission value will only predict outcome if the ingested OP is known and its clinical usefulness has been studied specifically for this OP.[75] For example, most patients who die with chlorpyrifos poisoning have a BuChE activity of around zero on admission; however, because chlorpyrifos is a very potent BuChE inhibitor, many other chlorpyrifos-poisoned patients who do not die also present with zero BuChE activities. In contrast, because dimethoate is a poor inhibitor of BuChE, the majority of patients who die from dimethoate poisoning have a BuChE activity on admission that is higher than many chlorpyrifos-poisoned patients who remain clinically well.[75]

Red Blood Cell Acetylcholinesterase

Red blood cell AChE activity is thought to more accurately reflect nervous tissue AChE activity than plasma BuChE, with Namba proposing that inhibition of greater than 50% is required for clinical features.[174] Acutely, for some OPs, RBC AChE activity correlates closely with nervous system AChE activity, with NMJ dysfunction associated with greater than 70% inhibition.[226] However, this is not always be the case. Patients with acute profenofos poisoning have complete inhibition of their RBC AChE activity without any apparent cholinergic or neuromuscular signs.[81] Similarly, in an animal model, RBC AChE activity did not reflect clinical severity, perhaps due to the role of co-formulated solvents.[79] It is therefore unclear at present how useful RBC AChE activity is in grading poisoning severity and measurement of AChE activity should not be used to predict outcome or guide management.[89]

One advantage of RBC AChE over BuChE is that its activity should be related to blood hemoglobin (Hb) concentration, reducing variation due to varying hematocrits.[245] Most Caucasians have a normal value of 600–700 mUnit/micromol Hb; a small study of Caucasians reported a mean of 651 with a SD of +/-18 mUnit/micromol Hb.[245]

After poisoning, and in the absence of oximes, RBC AChE takes many weeks to recover because erythrocytes in circulation at the time of OP exposure must be replaced. An average of 66 days is necessary for RBC AChE activity to recover following severe inhibition (assuming no treatment with oxime), and activity may take up to 100 days to return to normal. Rat studies suggest that neuronal AChE activity returns to normal more rapidly than RBC AChE.[103]

Depressed RBC AChE activity also results from exposures or conditions other than OP or carbamate poisoning, for example, pernicious anemia and during therapy with antimalarial or antidepressant medicines (Table 110–3).[135,168]

Blood samples for cholinesterase activity must be obtained in the appropriate blood tubes. Tubes containing fluoride will permanently inactivate the enzymes, yielding falsely low activities, and should never be used. Specimens for RBC AChE are usually drawn into tubes containing a chelating anticoagulant such as EDTA to prevent clot formation. Butyrylcholinesterase does not require an anticoagulant and can be drawn into a tube without chelators or anticoagulants.

Organic phosphorus compounds and oximes in collected blood samples will continue to interact with RBC AChE; small differences in time between sampling and assay results in marked artificial variation in results. The most accurate way to take blood for AChE activity measurement is to immediately dilute it 1:20 or 1:100 at the bedside into saline or water cooled to 4°C, before rapidly freezing the sample. This process slows down both inhibitory and reactivating reactions in the tube, allowing more uniform results.[69,245] Such rapid reactions do not occur with BuChE and bedside dilution and cooling are not therefore required.

Protein Adducts

Current research is attempting to find ways of detecting OP exposure many weeks after the event. New techniques using mass spectrometry aim to identify phosphorylated proteins, such as albumin or BuChE, in blood samples.[146a,186,217]

Carbamates

Carbamates inhibit neuronal AChE, RBC AChE, and BuChE. The relative ease with which spontaneous decarbamylation of AChE takes place results in the measurement of relatively normal RBC AChE activity despite severe cholinergic symptoms if the assay is not performed within several hours of sampling.[175] This emphasizes the importance of cooling and then freezing the blood sample within minutes of collection (see above). As with OP pesticide poisoning, the wide "normal" range of BuChE activity makes interpretation of BuChE activity difficult at times when the patient's baseline values are unknown. Red blood cell AChE inhibition is short-lived after carbamate poisoning, returning to normal within hours compared to days after OP insecticide poisoning.[230]

Atropine Challenge

An atropine challenge (administration of a 0.6–1 mg of atropine to test for cholinergic features responsive to atropine) has long been recommended. However, there are no studies of the sensitivity and specificity of the test, or of its predictive values. Patients with substantial poisoning will show no response to the small dose of atropine; in contrast, patients with either mild poisoning or no poisoning will develop antimuscarinic features. In the light of this lack of clarity on usefulness, we recommend against this approach to diagnosis.

Electromyogram Studies

Although measuring cholinesterase activity is the test most often used to estimate tissue and neuronal AChE activity, small studies support the use of repetitive nerve stimulation testing as an accurate method of quantifying AChE inhibition at the neuromuscular junction.[9,21,122] Further studies are required to determine the role of EMG studies in the diagnosis of anticholinesterase poisoning.

Differential Diagnosis

The differential diagnosis for cholinergic poisoning includes 3 main categories (Table 110–4). The first comprises insecticides and other noninsecticidal cholinesterase inhibitors including the medicinal anticholinesterases such as neostigmine and pyridostigmine. This entire group of xenobiotics often produce low BuChE and low RBC AChE activity. Newer pharmaceuticals used to treat Alzheimer disease, such as donepezil and rivastigmine, inhibit AChE but symptomatic overdose of these xenobiotics appears rare.[144,209]

TABLE 110–3	Interpreting Cholinesterase Activity Values	
	Red Blood Cell Acetylcholinesterase	**Butyrylcholinesterase**
Advantage	Better reflection of synaptic inhibition	Easier to assay, declines faster
Site	RBC	CNS white matter, plasma, liver, pancreas, heart
Regeneration (untreated)	1% per day	25%–30% in the first 7–10 days
Normalization (untreated with oxime)	35–100 days	28–42 days
Use	Unsuspected prior exposure with normal butyrylcholinesterase	Acute exposure
False depression	Pernicious anemia, hemoglobinopathies, antimalarial treatment, oxalate blood tubes	Liver dysfunction, malnutrition, hypersensitivity reactions, drugs (succinylcholine, codeine, morphine), pregnancy or deficiency

TABLE 110–4	Categories of Cholinergic Poisoning
Cholinesterase inhibitors	
Organic phosphorus insecticides	
Organic phosphorus ophthalmic medications	
Carbamate insecticides	
Carbamate medications	
Cholinomimetics	
Pilocarpine	
Carbachol	
Aceclidine	
Methacholine	
Bethanechol	
Muscarine-containing mushrooms	
Nicotine alkaloids	
Coniine	
Lobeline	
Nicotine	

The second category includes xenobiotics with cholinomimetic activity. These cholinomimetics directly stimulate muscarinic or nicotinic cholinergic receptors, but do not inhibit AChE. In exposed individuals, BuChE and RBC AChE activity should be normal. Cholinomimetics include preparations of carbachol, methacholine, pilocarpine, and bethanechol. Nonpharmaceuticals such as muscarine-containing mushrooms are also cholinomimetic (Chap. 117).

Finally, a third category of xenobiotics, the nicotine alkaloids (eg, nicotine, lobeline, and coniine), acts on nicotinic ACh receptors and causes CNS, autonomic, and skeletal muscle symptoms similar to those occurring in OP and carbamate toxicity, but without causing cholinesterase inhibition (Chap. 82). Poisoning with noncholinergic pesticides such as neonicotinoids sometimes causes increased secretions that may be mistaken for anticholinesterase poisoning.[58]

MANAGEMENT
Organic Phosphorus Compounds
The primary cause of death after anticholinesterase poisoning is respiratory failure and hypoxemia. This results from muscarinic effects on the cardiovascular and pulmonary systems (bronchospasm, bronchorrhea, aspiration, bradydysrhythmias, or hypotension), nicotinic effects on skeletal muscles (weakness and paralysis), loss of central respiratory drive, and rarely seizures (Figs. 110-6 and 110-7). Therefore, initial treatment for a patient exposed to OP compounds should be directed at ensuring an adequate airway and ventilation, and at stabilizing cardiorespiratory function by reversing excessive muscarinic effects.[69,72] Seizures not secondary to hypoxemia should be treated with standard benzodiazepine anticonvulsant.

Maintenance of the patient's airway should be ensured by early endotracheal intubation and positive-pressure ventilation in patients who are comatose, have significant weakness, or who are unable to handle copious secretions. Only a neuromuscular blocker that is not primarily metabolized by cholinesterases should be used to induce pharmacologic paralysis if needed. The duration of action of the depolarizing agent succinylcholine and the nondepolarizing agent mivacurium, for example, will be extended in the presence of low BuChE activity, causing paralysis lasting for several hours.[207]

Antimuscarinic Therapy
Excessive muscarinic activity should be controlled at the same time as resuscitation to aid respiration and oxygenation. The muscarinic antagonist atropine competitively blocks ACh at muscarinic receptors to reverse excessive secretions, miosis, bronchospasm, vomiting, diarrhea, diaphoresis, and urinary incontinence.[92,111]

For adolescents and adults, an intravenous loading bolus of between 1 and 3 mg (depending on the severity of symptoms) is recommended; doses for children should start at 0.05 mg/kg up to adult doses. Doses should be titrated against effect, individualizing therapy for the patient. Although previously guidelines had recommended repeating doses of 1 to 5 mg every 2 to 20 minutes until "atropinization" had occurred,[68] the most rapid method of controlling excessive cholinergic activity is to give doubling doses every 5 minutes if the response to the previous dose is inadequate.[68,72]

This approach, of doubling or incremental doses, was tested against a standard bolus dose approach in a randomized controlled trial.[2] Patients were randomized to receive either 2 to 5 mg of atropine (depending on severity), repeated every 10 to 15 minutes as required, or 1.8 to 3 mg of atropine (depending on severity) followed by doubling doses every 5 minutes as required. Atropine doses were continued until all clinical signs of "atropinization" (see below) were clearly evident; atropine was then given as further bolus doses at increasing intervals or as a constant infusion, respectively. All patients received pralidoxime (1–2 g every 8–12 hours). The incremental approach was associated with reaching atropinization at a median of 24 minutes versus 152 minutes with standard bolus dosing, despite administration of similar total doses of atropine (136 vs 109 mg, respectively). This faster administration of atropine was associated with more rapid

resuscitation and stabilization as shown by the improved outcome: mortality with bolus atropine was 22.5% (18/80) and with incremental atropine was 8% (6/75) ($P < .05$). Incremental dosing was also associated with less atropine toxicity, less NMJ failure, and less requirement for ventilation.[2]

"Atropinization" is classically said to occur when patients exhibit dry skin and mucous membranes, decreased or absent bowel sounds, tachycardia, reduced secretions, no bronchospasm (in absence of other causes such as aspiration), and usually, mydriasis.[68] However, patients die from cardiorespiratory compromise, not wet skin or miosis. As a result, cardiorespiratory parameters, not pupil size or the presence of sweating, should guide administration of atropine. Atropine dosing should aim to reverse bronchorrhea and bronchospasm, and to provide adequate blood pressure and heart rate for tissue oxygenation (eg, systolic blood pressure >90 mm Hg and heart rate >80 beats/min). All variables are easily and rapidly assessed.

Once atropinization occurs, an infusion of atropine, is recommended initially giving 10% to 20% of the total loading dose per hour (usually maximum 2 mg/h). Regular checks for signs of under- or overatropinization should guide the use of further boluses followed by changes in the infusion rate, or discontinuation of the infusion.[72] Infusions have been used for as long as 32 days in patients poisoned by fat-soluble OPs that continue to redistribute from the fat and freshly inhibit AChE.[94]

Some texts recommend not giving atropine until oxygen is administered because of the risk of inducing ventricular tachydysrhythmias. If true, this would have serious implications for patients in low-income countries or remote regions where oxygen is frequently unavailable and where the advice would delay administration of potentially life-saving atropine. Administration of atropine during resuscitation without oxygen to a cohort of 1900 OP or carbamate insecticide self-poisoned patients in Sri Lanka was not associated with tachydysrhythmias.[139] A review of the evidence base for this statement revealed that it originated from just 2 human case reports and from dog studies of limited relevance.[139] We therefore disagree with this recommendation. All patients showing signs of cholinergic toxicity should receive titrated atropine dosing whether oxygen is available or not.

The presence of marked tachycardia (>120–140 beats/min in a well-hydrated patient not withdrawing from alcohol), mydriasis, absent bowel sounds, and urinary retention after atropine administration indicates over-atropinization or atropine toxicity. This is unnecessary and possibly dangerous because of associated hyperthermia, confusion, and agitation.[72] Tachycardia is not however an absolute contraindication to atropine therapy because it can result from hypoxia, hypovolemia, aspiration pneumonitis, or agitation.

Large doses of atropine may be needed to reverse the bronchospasm, bronchorrhea, and bradycardia associated with severe OP compound toxicity.[174] Some patients with mild symptoms need only 1 or 2 mg of atropine to reverse cholinergic toxicity, but moderately poisoned adults often require total doses as large as 40 mg.[63,68] Some adults received more than 1,000 mg of atropine in 24 hours (with adequate pralidoxime dosing) without demonstrating antimuscarinic effects, and total doses as high as 11,000 mg during the course of treatment are reported.[116] However, the additional benefit of such extreme doses over more modest doses is unclear. A study from German ICUs, in which supportive care was likely optimized, reported that much smaller doses of around 1 mg/h were associated with adequate control of muscarinic features after initial atropinization.[224]

Atropine does not reverse nicotinic effects. Therefore, patients who improve after receiving atropine should be closely monitored in a critical care setting for impending respiratory failure from delayed NMJ dysfunction. Patients should be clinically examined regularly for proximal muscle weakness (particularly neck flexor weakness); once recognized, tidal volume or negative inspiratory force measurements should be made at least every 4 to 6 hours to detect impending respiratory failure and allow early initiation of ventilatory support.

When antimuscarinic CNS toxicity becomes evident yet peripheral cholinergic findings necessitate the administration of more atropine (eg, bradycardia, bronchorrhea), some authors recommend substituting glycopyrrolate for atropine because its quaternary ammonium structure limits CNS penetration.[196] One randomized clinical trial (RCT) compared atropine with glycopyrrolate in ICU management of OP poisoning, but was too small to detect any difference between regimens.[14] The initial intravenous dose of glycopyrrolate for adults and adolescents is 1–2 mg, repeated as needed, or in children 0.025 mg/kg up to adult doses. As with atropine, some patients with severe poisoning require higher doses of glycopyrrolate. Although scopolamine (hyoscine) has been used in place of atropine,[142,196] it may cause more pronounced CNS effects. The use of penehyclidine, a relatively M_1-, M_3-, and M_4-specific muscarinic antagonist with reduced cardiac effects, is recommended instead of atropine in China;[45,250] if it becomes widely available, larger studies are required to compare its effectiveness to atropine.

However, it is not clear that such approaches are required. In a large case series of patients treated by necessity outside of a critical care unit, atropinization without CNS toxicity could be safely accomplished by titrating the dose to clinical features and slowing atropine infusions whenever absent bowel sounds, confusion, or hyperthermia were detected.[72] We do not recommend the routine use of glycopyrrolate, scopolamine, or penehyclidine for anticholinesterase-poisoned patients.

The anticholinergic and α_1 adrenergic receptor antagonist anisodamine (7β-hydroxyhyoscyamine) is used in China for OP poisoning.[82] Its use has been recommended when high-dose atropine is considered insufficient;[238] however, in this study atropinization took a mean of 29.2 and 24.3 hours in the patients receiving atropine, or atropine plus anisodamine, respectively, suggesting an inadequate atropine dosing regimen. It is again not clear whether additional drugs are required if atropine administration is done appropriately.

Oximes

Phosphorylated AChE undergoes hydrolytic regeneration at a very slow rate. However, this process can be enhanced by using an oxime such as pralidoxime chloride (2-PAM) or obidoxime (Fig. 110–3).[87] Regeneration of AChE lowers ACh concentrations, improving both muscarinic and nicotinic effects. An immediate rise in RBC AChE activity, hopefully paralleling a rise in neuronal AChE activity, occurs after effective administration of oximes.[74,225]

As discussed above, phosphorylated AChE becomes aged, and therefore unresponsive to oximes, at different rates according to the chemistry of the OP.[87] Oximes therefore are recommended early, within 3 to 4 hours of exposure, after dimethoxy OP poisoning. In contrast, they can still be highly efficacious 48 hours after diethoxy OP poisoning, with some effect even when given several days after exposure. In cases of poisoning with highly fat-soluble OP insecticides, in which OP leaking out of fat stores can freshly inhibit AChE, oximes might be efficacious for weeks.[243] Case reports support this reasoning by noting dramatic effects in reversing paralysis, weakness, and cholinergic symptoms after late administration of pralidoxime.[161,173]

However, the clinical effectiveness of oximes in large-dose OP insecticide self-poisoning is still unclear.[80,247] The first clinical experience with pralidoxime was reported in the late 1950s by Namba, who treated 5 patients with occupational parathion poisoning.[173] All patients responded well to pralidoxime 1 g IV. As expected from occupational inhalational exposure, none of the patients were severely ill. Namba subsequently reported the use of much higher doses of pralidoxime, of 1- to 2-g bolus loading doses followed by 0.5 g/h, in patients with severe parathion poisoning.[171] He also noted that some OPs, including malathion, did not respond well to pralidoxime.[172] These caveats were subsequently lost, with the use of pralidoxime 1 g, followed by a second 1-g bolus after a few hours as necessary, being recommended for all cases.

Extensive clinical experience of bolus pralidoxime regimens in Asia led to widespread doubt about their efficacy for self-poisoning.[80] Asian clinicians have traditionally used 1 g of pralidoxime every 4 to 6 hours for 1 to 3 days, producing high peaks and deep troughs in blood pralidoxime concentration. In a 1992 ecological study, Sri Lankan doctors reported finding no difference in OP insecticide case fatality during a 6-month period when pralidoxime was not available in their hospital, compared to periods when it was available.[55] They argued that pralidoxime was of little clinical benefit

and, because it was expensive, should not be routinely used for treating OP-poisoned patients. European clinician researchers responded that the doses being used were too low and that higher doses, more akin to Namba's second regimen, were required.[127] Two further trials from south India reported no effect[128] or even harm[41] from pralidoxime therapy.

All these clinical trials aimed for a plasma oxime concentration of around 4 mcg/mL, a target based on a single study with a single nerve agent in cats[218] that should not have been extrapolated to human OP pesticide poisoning in general.[87] In vitro studies with human RBCs suggest that a higher concentration of around 100 micromolar (approximately 20 mcg/mL) is required for sustained reactivation,[87,225] resulting in the recommendation from a WHO group that all patients receive a loading dose of at least 30 mg/kg pralidoxime chloride, followed by at least 8 mg/kg/h.[126] A subsequent RCT from India showed that very high doses of pralidoxime iodide, a 2-g loading dose followed by 1 g/h, reduced death and length of ventilation in moderately poisoned patients who presented early and were treated in an ICU.[185] However, similar doses of pralidoxime chloride do not reactivate AChE in severe poisoning with dimethoate and other dimethoxy pesticides.[74]

A second RCT from Sri Lanka was unable to demonstrate a benefit from similarly high doses of pralidoxime in symptomatic patients of all severity treated in a resource-poor hospital.[73] This trial compared no pralidoxime chloride with a 2-g bolus over 20 minutes followed by 0.5 g/h for up to 7 days or when atropine was no longer required, in addition to standard therapy. Although the study was stopped earlier than planned, pralidoxime was associated with an adjusted hazard ratio {HR} of 1.69 (95% confidence interval 0.88–3.26, P = .12) for death.

Although a subsequent Cochrane review concluded that current evidence was insufficient to indicate whether oximes are harmful or beneficial,[29] it is possible that some of the difference between the outcomes in the 2 major trials is due to the very high level of supportive care available in India. Despite being less severely poisoned, 66% of Indian patients were intubated at baseline compared to 17% of Sri Lankan patients. This high level of supportive care is not available in rural resource-poor district hospitals that see most OP-poisoned patients globally.

Another reason for the apparent lack of efficacy of oximes may be the very large doses of OP insecticide ingested during self-harm. For example, a typical ingested dose of 100 mL of a 40% parathion formulation contains 40 g of active ingredient. This equals 666 mg/kg parathion for a 60-kg adult, a dose 51-fold greater than the rat oral LD_{50} for parathion of 13 mg/kg.[248] It is perhaps not surprising that standard doses of oximes are unable to counter such huge doses, with any reactivated oxime simply being reactivated by the high concentration of OP in the blood.[80]

All the clinical trials included in the Cochrane review assessed pralidoxime salts. Obidoxime[87] is used in some countries, including Germany[85,225] and Iran,[11] with reportedly beneficial effects. Although use of high-dose obidoxime is associated with liver injury,[11] this does not seem to be the case when doses of 250 mg as a loading dose followed by 750 mg per 24 hours are used.[87] The use of newer oximes such as HI-6 and HLo-7 has not yet been reported in pesticide-poisoned patients. However, in vitro studies suggest that they will not be highly effective for human AChE inhibited by a range of OP pesticides.[246]

The exact role of oximes is currently unclear. However, we recommend that oximes be given as soon as possible after exposure to increase the chance of benefit. The difference between Indian and Sri Lankan studies suggests that they should be administered in a critical care environment to reduce the risk of serious complications. The duration of use is unclear. It is reasonable to stop oxime administration when atropine is no longer clinically required. Electrophysiological and clinical observation may allow the benefit of oxime administration to be assessed before atropine is stopped. Transiently stopping the infusion after 2 to 3 days and carefully observing for clinical or electrophysiological deterioration is a reasonable approach to deciding whether to continue oxime therapy.

Titrated-dose pralidoxime regimens have been recommended, due to reduced case fatality in a study with historical controls[64] and in a small

RCT.[147] However, titration was performed against BuChE activity after prali-doxime doses, which is problematic because BuChE is rarely reactivated by oximes and its inhibition is not pathologic.[140] It is possible that titrated regi-mens may offer benefit, but more data are required and this approach is not currently recommended.

Some aspects of oximes are not well understood. Their quaternary ammonium compound structure is thought to reduce their passage across the blood–brain barrier and prevent CNS effects.[221] However, obidoxime has been detected in cerebrospinal fluid,[87] and at least one case report describes pralidoxime-induced improvements in mental status and electroencephalo-grams not attributable to improved ventilation or perfusion.[152]

Benzodiazepines
Animal studies demonstrate that administering benzodiazepines along with oximes in the treatment of poisoning with OP nerve agents or the insecti-cide dichlorvos increases survival and decreases the incidence of seizures and neuropathy.[62] Diazepam also decreases cerebral morphologic damage resulting from OP compound–related seizures.[158] One study suggests that diazepam attenuates OP-induced respiratory depression,[62] postulating that the benzodiazepines attenuate the overstimulation of central respiratory centers caused by OP compounds. However, seizures are uncommon in large case series of patients poisoned by OP insecticides,[74,235] and no clini-cal studies have been performed yet to determine whether benzodiazepines offer benefit to humans.[156] In the absence of this evidence, benzodiazepines should be used to treat OP-related seizures and agitation and to aid intuba-tion, but should not be given routinely to all cases.[156]

The treatment of intermediate syndrome is supportive with airway protection and mechanical ventilation. There are no data demonstrating that pralidoxime or atropine is effective in treating this disorder, although patients require these medications to control concurrent cholinergic symp-toms. The weakness and paralysis commonly resolve in 5 to 18 days.[78,122,123]

Other Drug Treatments
The therapies discussed above affect only limited mechanisms involved in OP poisoning. Multiple additional therapies have been tested in animals but none have been shown to be beneficial in large clinical trials and none are used widely in clinical practice.[71,189] Future clinical trials may identify patients for whom they would be beneficial. Treatments that have been pro-posed include magnesium[17,179,233] or clonidine[188] to reduce presynaptic acetyl-choline release, fresh-frozen plasma as a source of BuChE for scavenging OP pesticides,[107,192] and sodium bicarbonate.[197] A systematic review found eight clinical studies or trials of magnesium sulfate that suggested benefit but all were too small to provide definitive evidence.[26a] Lipid emulsions has also been suggested because of the high lipid solubility of most OP insecticides and their solvents;[162,252] however, an in vitro study suggested that the lipid actually stabilizes the OP from degradation.[234] More definitive studies are required; none of these therapies are currently recommended for anticho-linesterase poisoning.

Decontamination
Cutaneous absorption of OP pesticides and carbamates requires removal of all clothing as soon as possible after resuscitation and administration of atropine and oxygen. Medical personnel should avoid self-contamination by wearing neoprene or nitrile gloves. Skin should be triple-washed with water, soap, and water, and rinsed again with water. Although alcohol-based soaps are sometimes recommended to dissolve hydrocarbons, these products can be difficult to find, and rapid skin cleansing is the primary goal. Cutaneous absorption also results from contact with OP and carbamate compounds in vomitus and diarrhea if the initial exposure was by ingestion. Oily insecti-cides may be difficult to remove from thick or long hair, even with repeated shampooing, and shaving scalp hair may be necessary. Exposed leather clothing or products should be discarded because decontamination is very difficult once impregnation has occurred.

Military institutions are now experimenting with cholinesterase sponges for cutaneous OP decontamination.[98] The sponge consists of a cholinesterase enzyme covalently linked and immobilized in a polyurethane matrix. The sponge is reportedly effective in removing OP compounds from skin and surfaces.[98]

In potentially life-threatening acute ingestions, if emesis has not occurred, the patient presents within 2 hours, and the airway can be protected, the stomach contents should be evacuated by lavage using a nasogastric tube. Although there are data suggesting that activated charcoal adsorbs some OP insecticides, a study of 1,310 Sri Lankan patients with OP or carbamate poison-ing found no clear benefit from the use of multiple-dose activated charcoal.[77] For patients with anticholinesterase poisoning in whom the airway can be protected we recommend a single dose of 1 g/kg activated charcoal.

Health care providers must always maintain caution when coming into contact with stomach contents or other body fluids when managing these cases.[148] Bystanders were poisoned by providing mouth-to-mouth resusci-tation to a victim of an intentional ingestion of diazinon.[138] There are also reports of nosocomial poisoning in ED staff. However, in only one paper were BuChE activities tested[32] to support the hypothesis of nosocomial poison-ing, and none showed any evidence of inhibition. Clinical experience from South Asia suggests that nosocomial poisoning with OP pesticides is unlikely as long as standard universal precautions are followed.[198] It is possible that any nonspecific illnesses and anxiety are due to the solvents coformulated with the pesticides.[148]

Overall, the current view is best summarized by an Australian consensus statement on nosocomial poisoning that found little evidence that health care workers were at risk of such poisoning. In particular, it noted that timely resuscitation and medical assessment should take precedence over decontamination.[148]

Extracorporeal Elimination
Hemodialysis and/or hemoperfusion are sometimes recommended for OP and carbamate insecticide–poisoned patients, particularly in East Asia.[23,118,149] The EXTRIP group has not yet published an opinion on this subject. Such approaches might offer some benefit if provided early for poisoning with OP insecticides such as dimethoate[170] and dichlorvos[187] that have small volumes of distribution[200] or where solvents are a substantial component of the overall toxicity. However, at present, there is insufficient data to recommend extra-corporeal purification for anticholinesterase insecticide poisoning.

Disposition
After atropinization, patients with cholinesterase inhibitor poisoning should be carefully and frequently observed for evidence of (1) deteriorating neuro-logic function and potential paralysis and (2) need for an increase or reduc-tion in atropine dosing.

Cholinesterase activities can be measured to monitor their recovery.[85,223] However, clinical assessment is a more reliable marker of recovery because cholinesterase activities are often substantially reduced for many days after poisoning. We do not recommend using cholinesterase activities to make decisions on discharge. It is reasonable to discharge a patient who becomes asymptomatic and has not required atropine for 1 to 2 days. Although recur-rent cholinergic crises and/or respiratory failure can occur after several days, such patients have usually previously shown clinical signs of toxicity. Patients should not be allowed to go home wearing clothing that was worn when the poisoning occurred.

Carbamates
The treatment of patients with carbamate insecticide poisoning is similar to treatment of patients with OP poisoning. Urgent resuscitation and titrated dosing of atropine should be performed for all patients.

The efficacy of oximes for carbamate poisoning is unclear. Murine studies with pralidoxime and carbaryl indicate that the oxime dose used is important for outcome.[160] However, guinea pig studies of atropine and pralidoxime for aldicarb and methomyl poisoning showed no in vitro reactivation of AChE and no additional effect of oxime above that of atropine.[26] Human experi-ence is limited; a case series of aldicarb-poisoned patients reported the use of low-dose pralidoxime (mean dose of 400 mg over the first 10 hours) but pro-vided no evidence for efficacy.[193] Fortunately, because of the rapid hydrolysis of the carbamate-AChE complex (see above), symptoms, including weakness and paralysis, usually resolve within 24 to 48 hours without oxime therapy. We do not recommend the routine administration of oximes to patients poisoned by carbamate insecticides.

However, administering pralidoxime to a poisoned patient in a cholinergic crisis is appropriate when it is not known whether the patient is suffering from OP or carbamate pesticide poisoning.

Significant inhibition of RBC AChE and BuChE by carbamates generally does not last for more than 1 to 2 days, assuming absorption is complete. Patients exposed to carbamates usually have normal cholinesterase activities by the time of discharge. There are no reported cases of recurrent or delayed poisonings following carbamate insecticide poisoning. However, of note, complications of poisoning with carbamates, such as aspiration and hypoxic brain injury, can last many days.[143]

SUMMARY

- Organic phosphorus and carbamate compounds kill approximately 100,000 people each year.
- Poisoning with these pesticides is not uniform: they differ markedly in their human toxicity, pharmacokinetics, associated clinical syndromes, and response to therapy.
- Symptoms result from inhibition of AChE and overstimulation of muscarinic and nicotinic receptors in synapses of the autonomic and central nervous systems and at the NMJ.
- Patients with substantial poisoning present with the cholinergic crisis and have pinpoint pupils, excessive sweating and salivation, and respiratory failure due to bronchospasm, bronchorrhea, loss of central respiratory drive, and dysfunction of neuromuscular junction.
- Atropine is recommended in doubling doses to attain atropinization before being continued as an infusion at a dose individualized for the patient.
- Patients may develop NMJ dysfunction that progresses to respiratory failure; such patients often require ventilatory support for weeks.
- The effectiveness of oximes is unclear for pesticide self poisoning; it is dependent on the dose and type of OP ingested and the time to oxime administration. Where available, oximes are recommended as soon as possible after ingestion and in concert with atropine.
- Cholinergic features can recur many days after ingestion of highly fat-soluble compounds such as fenthion due to redistribution from fat stores.
- Patients should be carefully observed to ensure that the dose of atropine is not inadequate or excessive, any recurrence of cholinergic toxicity is identified and treated quickly, and NMJ dysfunction is recognized early, before the onset of respiratory failure.

REFERENCES

1. Abdollahi M, Karami-Mohajeri S. A comprehensive review on experimental and clinical findings in intermediate syndrome caused by organophosphate poisoning. *Toxicol Appl Pharmacol.* 2012;258:309-314.
2. Abedin MJ, et al. Open-label randomized clinical trial of atropine bolus injection versus incremental boluses plus infusion for organophosphate poisoning in Bangladesh. *J Med Toxicol.* 2012;8:108-117.
3. Abou-Donia MB, Lapadula DM. Mechanisms of organophosphorus ester-induced delayed neurotoxicity: type I and type II. *Annu Rev Pharmacol Toxicol.* 1990;30:405-440.
4. Ahmed MM, Glees P. Neurotoxicity of tricresylphosphate (TCP) in slow loris (*Nycticebus coucang coucang*). *Acta Neuropathol.* 1971;19:94-98.
5. Anon. Neurological findings among workers exposed to fenthion in a veterinary hospital: Georgia. *MMWR Morb Mortal Wkly Rep.* 1985;34:402-403.
6. Anon. Organophosphate toxicity associated with flea-dip products: California. *MMWR Morb Mortal Wkly Rep.* 1988;37:329-336.
7. Anonymous. Calamity at Bhopal. *Lancet.* 1984;2:1378-1379.
8. Asari Y, et al. Changes in the hemodynamic state of patients with acute lethal organophosphate poisoning. *Vet Hum Toxicol.* 2004;46:5-9.
9. Avasthi G, Singh G. Serial neuro-electrophysiological studies in acute organophosphate poisoning—correlation with clinical findings, serum cholinesterase levels and atropine dosages. *J Assoc Physicians India.* 2000;48:794-799.
10. Baker EL, et al. Epidemic malathion poisoning in Pakistan malaria workers. *Lancet.* 1978;i:31-34.
11. Balali-Mood M, Shariat M. Treatment of organophosphate poisoning. Experience of nerve agents and acute pesticide poisoning on the effects of oximes. *J Physiol (Paris).* 1998;92:375-378.
12. Ballantyne B, Marrs TC. Overview of the biological and clinical aspects of organophosphates and carbamates. In: Ballantyne B, Marrs TC, eds. *Clinical And Experimental Toxicology of Organophosphates and Carbamates.* Oxford, UK: Butterworth Heinemann; 1992:3-14.
13. Bar-Meir E, et al. Guidelines for treating cardiac manifestations of organophosphate poisoning with special emphasis on long QT and Torsades de Pointes. *Crit Rev Toxicol.* 2007;37:279-285.
14. Bardin PG, van Eeden SF. Organophosphate poisoning: grading the severity and comparing treatment between atropine and glycopyrrolate. *Crit Care Med.* 1990;18:956-960.
15. Bardin PG, et al. Organophosphate and carbamate poisoning. *Arch Intern Med.* 1994;154:1433-1441.
16. Baron RL. Carbamate insecticides. In: Hayes WJ, Laws ER, eds. *Handbook of Pesticide Toxicology.* San Diego, CA: Academic Press; 1991:1125-1189.
17. Basher A, et al. Phase II study of magnesium sulfate in acute organophosphate pesticide poisoning. *Clin Toxicol (Phila).* 2013;51:35-40.
18. Basnyat B. Organophosphate poisoning: the importance of the intermediate syndrome. *J Inst Med.* 2000;22:248-250.
19. Benfenati E, et al. Predicting log P of pesticides using different software. *Chemosphere.* 2003;53:1155-1164.
20. Benson B, et al. Is the intermediate syndrome in organophosphate poisoning the result of insufficient oxime therapy? *J Toxicol Clin Toxicol.* 1992;30:347.
21. Besser R, et al. End-plate dysfunction in acute organophosphate intoxication. *Neurology.* 1989;39:561-567.
22. Bhatt MH, et al. Acute and reversible parkinsonism due to organophosphate pesticide intoxication. Five cases. *Neurology.* 1999;52:1467-1471.
23. Bo L. Therapeutic efficacies of different hemoperfusion frequencies in patients with organophosphate poisoning. *Eur Rev Med Pharmacol Sci.* 2014;18:3521-3523.
24. Borowitz SM. Prolonged organophosphate toxicity in a twenty-six-month-old child. *J Pediatr.* 1988;112:302-304.
25. Bradberry SM, et al. Glyphosate poisoning. *Toxicol Rev.* 2004;23:159-167.
26. Brittain MK, et al. Efficacy of recommended prehospital human equivalent doses of atropine and pralidoxime against the toxic effects of carbamate poisoning in the Hartley guinea pig. *Int J Toxicol.* 2016;35:344-357.
26a. Brvar M, Chan MY, Dawson AH, Ribchester RR, Eddleston M. Magnesium sulfate and calcium channel blocking drugs as antidotes for acute organophosphorus insecticide poisoning - a systematic review and meta-analysis. *Clin Toxicol (Phila)* 2018; Mar 20: 1-12. [Epub ahead of print]
27. Bucaretchi F, et al. Poisoning by illegal rodenticides containing acetylcholinesterase inhibitors (Chumbinho): a prospective case series. *Clin Toxicol (Phila).* 2012;50:44-51.
28. Buchholz U, et al. An outbreak of food-borne illness associated with methomyl-contaminated salt. *JAMA.* 2002;288:604-610.
29. Buckley NA, et al. Oximes for acute organophosphate pesticide poisoning. *Cochrane Database Syst Rev.* 2011;2:CD005085.
30. Buratti FM, et al. Malathion bioactivation in the human liver: the contribution of different cytochrome P450 isoforms. *Drug Metab Dispos.* 2005;33:295-302.
31. Buratti FM, et al. CYP-specific bioactivation of four organophosphorothioate pesticides by human liver microsomes. *Toxicol Appl Pharmacol.* 2003;186:143-154.
32. Calvert GM, et al. Acute pesticide-related illness among emergency responders, 1993–2002. *Am J Ind Med.* 2006;49:383-393.
33. Casida JE, Quistad GB. Organophosphate toxicology: safety aspects of nonacetylcholinesterase secondary targets. *Chem Res Toxicol.* 2004;17:983-998.
34. Casida JE, Sanderson DM. Toxic hazard from formulating the insecticide dimethoate in methyl "Cellosolve." *Nature.* 1961;189:507-508.
35. Cavanagh JB, et al. Comparison of the functional effects of dyflos, tri-o-cresyl phosphate and tri-pethylphenyl phosphate in chickens. *Br J Pharmacol.* 1961;17:21-27.
36. Cavari Y, et al. Organophosphate poisoning-induced acute renal failure. *Pediatr Emerg Care.* 2013;29:646-647.
37. Cha ES, et al. Impact of paraquat regulation on suicide in South Korea. *Int J Epidemiol.* 2016;45:470-479.
38. Cha YS, et al. Features of myocardial injury in severe organophosphate poisoning. *Clin Toxicol (Phila).* 2014;52:873-879.
39. Chadwick JA, Oosterbaan RA. Actions on insects and other invertebrates. In: Koelle GB, ed. *Cholinesterases and Anticholinesterase Agents. Handbook Experimental Pharmak.* Vol. 15. Berlin: Springer-Verlag; 1963:299-373.
40. Chang SS, et al. Factors associated with the decline in suicide by pesticide poisoning in Taiwan: a time trend analysis, 1987-2010. *Clin Toxicol (Phila).* 2012;50:471-480.
41. Cherian AM, et al. Effectiveness of P2AM (PAM-pralidoxime) in the treatment of organophosphorus poisoning. A randomised, double blind placebo controlled trial. *J Assoc Physicians India.* 1997;45:22-24.
41a. Chowdhury FR, et al. Bans of WHO Class I pesticides in Bangladesh - suicide prevention without hampering agricultural output. *Int J Epidemiol.* 2018;47:175-184.
42. Clifford NJ, Bies AS. Organophosphate poisoning from wearing a laundered uniform previously contaminated with parathion. *JAMA.* 1989;262:3035-3036.

43. Costa LG, et al. Measurement of paraoxonase (PON1) status as a potential biomarker of susceptibility to organophosphate toxicity. *Clin Chim Acta*. 2005;352:37-47.

44. Coye MJ, et al. Clinical confirmation of organophosphate poisoning by serial cholinesterase analyses. *Arch Intern Med*. 1987;147:438-442.

45. Cui J, et al. Protective effects of penehyclidine hydrochloride on acute lung injury caused by severe dichlorvos poisoning in swine. *Chin Med J (Engl)*. 2013;126:4764-4770.

46. Dagli AJ, Shaikh WA. Pancreatic involvement in malathion anticholinesterase insecticide intoxication—a study of 75 cases. *Br J Clin Pract*. 1983;37:270-272.

47. Dandapani M, et al. Oxidative damage in intermediate syndrome of acute organophosphorous poisoning. *Indian J Med Res*. 2003;117:253-259.

48. Dassanayake T, et al. Cognitive processing of visual stimuli in patients with organophosphate insecticide poisoning. *Neurology*. 2007;68:2027-2030.

49. Dassanayake T, et al. Long-term event-related potential changes following organophosphorus insecticide poisoning. *Clin Neurophysiol*. 2008;119:144-150.

50. Davies JE, et al. Human pesticide poisonings by a fat soluble organophosphate pesticide. *Arch Environ Health*. 1975;30:608-613.

51. Davies JOJ, et al. Hypotension in severe dimethoate self-poisoning. *Clin Toxicol*. 2008;46:880-884.

52. Dawson AH, et al. Acute human lethal toxicity of agricultural pesticides: a prospective cohort study. *PLoS Med*. 2010;7:e1000357.

53. de Bleecker JL. The intermediate syndrome in organophosphate poisoning: an overview of experimental and clinical observations. *J Toxicol Clin Toxicol*. 1995;33:683.

54. de Candole CA, et al. The failure of respiration in death by anticholinesterase poisoning. *Br J Pharmacol*. 1953;8:466-475.

55. de Silva HJ, et al. Does pralidoxime affect outcome of management in acute organophosphate poisoning? *Lancet*. 1992;339:1136-1138.

56. Dennis DT. Jake walk in Vietnam. *Ann Intern Med*. 1977;86:665-666.

57. Dewan A, et al. Mass ethion poisoning with high mortality. *Clin Toxicol*. 2008;46:85-88.

58. Dewan G. Analysis of recent situation of pesticide poisoning in Bangladesh: is there a proper estimate? *Asia Pac J Med Toxicol*. 2014;3:76-83.

59. Dhanarisi HKJ, et al. Relationship between alcohol co-ingestion and outcome in profenofos self-poisoning—a retrospective case series. 2B-02. Paper presented at: 15th Asia Pacific Association of Medical Toxicology International Scientific Conference2016; Singapore.

60. Dick FD. Parkinson's disease and pesticide exposures. *Br Med Bull*. 2006;79-80:219-231.

61. Dickoff DJ, et al. Delayed neurotoxicity after ingestion of carbamate pesticide. *Neurology*. 1987;37:1229-1231.

62. Dickson EW, et al. Diazepam inhibits organophosphate-induced central respiratory depression. *Acad Emerg Med*. 2003;10:1303-1306.

63. du Toit PW, et al. Experience with the intensive care management of organophosphate insecticide poisoning. *S Afr Med J*. 1981;60:227-229.

64. Due P. Effectiveness of high dose pralidoxime for treatment of organophosphate poisoning. *Asia Pac J Med Toxicol*. 2014;3:97-103.

65. Dutta P, et al. Effects of acute organophosphate poisoning on pituitary target gland hormones at admission, discharge and three months after poisoning: a hospital based pilot study. *Indian J Endocrinol Metab*. 2015;19:116-123.

66. Eddleston M. The pathophysiology of organophosphorus pesticide self-poisoning is not so simple. *Neth J Med*. 2008;66:146-148.

67. Eddleston M. Patterns and problems of deliberate self-poisoning in the developing world. *Q J Med*. 2000;93:715-731.

68. Eddleston M, et al. Speed of initial atropinisation in significant organophosphorus pesticide poisoning—a systematic comparison of recommended regimens. *J Toxicol Clin Toxicol*. 2004;42:865-875.

69. Eddleston M, et al. Medical management of acute organophosphorus pesticide poisoning. *Lancet*. 2008;371:597-607.

70. Eddleston M, et al. Identification of strategies to prevent death after pesticide self-poisoning using a Haddon matrix. *Inj Prev*. 2006;12:333-337.

71. Eddleston M, Chowdhury FR. Pharmacological treatment of organophosphorus insecticide poisoning: the old and the (possible) new. *Br J Clin Pharmacol*. 2016;81:462-470.

72. Eddleston M, et al. Early management after self-poisoning with an organophosphorus or carbamate pesticide—a treatment protocol for junior doctors. *Crit Care*. 2004;8:R391-R397.

73. Eddleston M, et al. Pralidoxime in acute organophosphorus insecticide poisoning—a randomised controlled trial. *PLoS Med*. 2009;6:e1000104.

74. Eddleston M, et al. Differences between organophosphorus insecticides in human self-poisoning: a prospective cohort study. *Lancet*. 2005;366:1452-1459.

75. Eddleston M, et al. Predicting outcome using butyrylcholinesterase activity in organophosphorus pesticide self-poisoning. *Q J Med*. 2008;101:467-474.

76. Eddleston M, et al. Relationship between blood alcohol concentration on admission and outcome in dimethoate organophosphorus self-poisoning. *Br J Clin Pharmacol*. 2009;68:916-919.

77. Eddleston M, et al. Multiple-dose activated charcoal in acute self-poisoning: a randomised controlled trial. *Lancet*. 2008;371:579-586.

78. Eddleston M, et al. Respiratory failure in acute organophosphorus pesticide self-poisoning. *Q J Med*. 2006;99:513-522.

79. Eddleston M, et al. A role for solvents in the toxicity of agricultural organophosphorus pesticides. *Toxicology*. 2012;294:94-103.

80. Eddleston M, et al. Oximes in acute organophosphorus pesticide poisoning: a systematic review of clinical trials. *Q J Med*. 2002;95:275-283.

81. Eddleston M, et al. Poisoning with the S-Alkyl organophosphorus insecticides profenofos and prothiofos. *QJM*. 2009;102:785-792.

82. Eisenkraft A, Falk A. Possible role for anisodamine in organophosphate poisoning. *Br J Pharmacol*. 2016;173:1719-1727.

83. El-Ebiary AA, et al. *N*-Acetylcysteine in acute organophosphorus pesticide poisoning: a randomized, clinical trial. *Basic Clin Pharmacol Toxicol*. 2016;119:222-227.

84. Engel LS, et al. Parkinsonism and occupational exposure to pesticides. *Occup Environ Med*. 2001;58:582-589.

85. Eyer F, et al. Human parathion poisoning. A toxicokinetic analysis. *Toxicol Rev*. 2003;22:143-163.

86. Eyer P. Neuropsychopathological changes by organophosphorus compounds—a review. *Hum Exp Toxicol*. 1995;14:857-864.

87. Eyer P. The role of oximes in the management of organophosphorus pesticide poisoning. *Toxicol Rev*. 2003;22:165-190.

88. Eyer P, et al. The current status of oximes in the treatment of OP poisoning—comparing two regimes. *J Toxicol Clin Toxicol*. 2003;41:441-443.

89. Eyer P, et al. Paradox findings may challenge orthodox reasoning in acute organophosphate poisoning. *Chem Biol Interact*. 2010;187:270-278.

90. Fisher JR. Guillain-Barre syndrome following organophosphate poisoning. *JAMA*. 1977;238:1950-1951.

91. Fredriksson T, Bigelow JK. Tissue distribution of P32-labeled parathion. Autoradiographic technique. *Arch Environ Health*. 1961;2:663-667.

92. Freeman G, Epstein MA. Therapeutic factors in survival after lethal cholinesterase inhibition by phosphorus pesticides. *N Engl J Med*. 1955;253:266-271.

93. Gallo MA, Lawryk NJ. Organic phosphorus pesticides. In: Hayes WJ, Laws ER, eds. *Handbook of Pesticide Toxicology*. San Diego, CA: Academic Press; 1991:917-1123.

94. Gerkin R, Curry SC. Persistently elevated plasma insecticide levels in severe methyl-parathion poisoning [abstract]. *Vet Hum Toxicol*. 1987;29:483-484.

95. Glynn P. A mechanism for organophosphate-induced delayed neuropathy. *Toxicol Lett*. 2006;162:94-97.

96. Gokel Y. Subarachnoid hemorrhage and rhabdomyolysis induced acute renal failure complicating organophosphate intoxication. *Ren Fail*. 2002;24:867-871.

97. Goldman H, Teitel M. Malathion poisoning in a 34-month-old child following accidental ingestion. *J Pediatr*. 1958;52:76-81.

98. Gordon RK, et al. Organophosphate skin decontamination using immobilized enzymes. *Chem Biol Interact*. 1999;119-120:463-470.

99. Griffin P, et al. Oral and dermal absorption of chlorpyrifos: a human volunteer study. *Occup Environ Med*. 1999;56:10-13.

100. Grmec S, et al. Glasgow Coma Scale score and QTc interval in the prognosis of organophosphate poisoning. *Acad Emerg Med*. 2004;11:925-930.

101. Grob D, et al. The administration of diisopropyl fluorophosphate (DFP) to man. Effect on the central nervous system with special reference to the electrical activity of the brain. *Bull Johns Hopkins Hosp*. 1947;81:257.

102. Gross D. Clinical aspects: diagnosis and symptomatology. In: Albertini AV, et al, eds. *Triaryl-Phosphate Poisoning in Morocco 1959*. Stuttgart: George Thieme; 1968:53-81.

103. Grubic Z, et al. Recovery of acetylcholinesterase in the diaphragm, brain, and plasma of the rat after irreversible inhibition by soman: a study of cytochemical localization and molecular forms of the enzyme in the motor end plate. *J Neurochem*. 1981;37:909-916.

104. Gunnell D, et al. The global distribution of fatal pesticide self-poisoning: systematic review. *BMC Public Health*. 2007;7:357.

105. Gunnell D, et al. The impact of pesticide regulations on suicide in Sri Lanka. *Int J Epidemiol*. 2007;36:1235-1242.

106. Guven M, et al. Endocrine changes in patients with acute organophosphate poisoning. *Hum Exp Toxicol*. 1999;18:598-601.

107. Guven M, et al. The effects of fresh frozen plasma on cholinesterase levels and outcomes in patients with organophosphate poisoning. *J Toxicol Clin Toxicol*. 2004;42:617-623.

108. Halle A, Sloas DD. Percutaneous organophosphate poisoning. *South Med J*. 1987;80:1179-1181.

109. Hardt J, Angerer J. Determination of dialkyl phosphates in human urine using gas chromatography-mass spectrometry. *J Anal Toxicol*. 2000;24:678-684.

110. Hayes WJ. *Organic Phosphorus Insecticides: Pesticides Studied in Man*. Baltimore, MD: Williams & Wilkins; 1982.

111. Heath AJW, Meredith T. Atropine in the management of anticholinesterase poisoning. In: Ballantyne B, Marrs T, eds. *Clinical and Experimental Toxicology of Organophosphates and Carbamates*. Oxford: Butterworth Heinemann: 1992:543-554.

112. Hoizey G, et al. Thiodicarb and methomyl tissue distribution in a fatal multiple compounds poisoning. *J Forensic Sci*. 2008;53:499-502.

113. Holmes JH. Organophosphorus insecticides in Colorado. *Arch Environ Health*. 1964;9:445-453.

114. Holmstedt B. The ordeal bean of Old Calabar: the pageant of *Physostigma venenosum* in medicine. In: Swain T, ed. *Plants in the Development of Modern Medicine*. Cambridge, MA: Harvard University Press; 1972:303-360.

115. Holmstedt B. Pharmacology of organophosphorus cholinesterase inhibitors. *Pharmacol Rev*. 1959;11:567-688.

116. Hopmann G, Wanke H. Maximum dose atropine treatment in severe organophosphate poisoning [in German]. *Dtsch Med Wochenschr*. 1974;99:2106-2108.

117. Hrabetz H, et al. Organophosphate poisoning in the developed world—a single centre experience from here to the millennium. *Chem Biol Interact*. 2013;206:561-568.

118. Hu SL, et al. Therapeutic effectiveness of sustained low-efficiency hemodialysis plus hemoperfusion and continuous hemofiltration plus hemoperfusion for acute severe organophosphate poisoning. *Artif Organs.* 2014;38:121-124.

119. Hulse EJ, et al. Respiratory complications of organophosphorus nerve agent and insecticide poisoning. Implications for respiratory and critical care. *Am J Respir Crit Care Med.* 2014;190:1342-1354.

120. Ikizceli I, et al. Effect of interleukin-10 on pancreatic damage caused by organophosphate poisoning. *Regul Toxicol Pharmacol.* 2005;42:260-264.

121. Indira M, et al. Incidence, predictors, and outcome of intermediate syndrome in cholinergic insecticide poisoning: a prospective observational cohort study. *Clin Toxicol.* 2013;51:838-845.

122. Jayawardane P, et al. The spectrum of intermediate syndrome following acute organophosphate poisoning: a prospective cohort study from Sri Lanka. *PLoS Med.* 2008;5:e147.

123. John M, et al. Muscle injury in organophosphorous poisoning and its role in the development of intermediate syndrome. *Neurotoxicology.* 2003;24:43-53.

124. Johnson MK. The delayed neurotoxic effect of some organophosphorus compounds. Identification of the phosphorylation site as an esterase. *Biochem J.* 1969;114:711-717.

125. Johnson MK. Organophosphates and delayed neuropathy—is NTE alive and well? *Toxicol Appl Pharmacol.* 1990;102:385-399.

126. Johnson MK, et al. Evaluation of antidotes for poisoning by organophosphorus pesticides. *Emerg Med.* 2000;12:22-37.

127. Johnson MK, et al. Pralidoxime for organophosphorus poisoning [letter]. *Lancet.* 1992;340:64.

128. Johnson S, et al. Evaluation of two treatment regimens of pralidoxime (1gm single bolus dose vs 12gm infusion) in the management of organophosphorus poisoning. *J Assoc Physicians India.* 1996;44:529-531.

129. Joshi P, et al. Acute myocardial infarction: can it be a complication of acute organophosphorus compound poisoning? *J Postgrad Med.* 2013;59:142-144.

130. Kalyanam B, et al. A rare neurological complication of acute organophosphorous poisoning. *Toxicol Int.* 2013;20:189-191.

131. Kamijo Y, et al. A case of serious organophosphate poisoning treated by percutaneous cardiopulmonary support. *Vet Hum Toxicol.* 1999;41:326-328.

132. Karalliedde L, et al. Organophosphate-induced intermediate syndrome: aetiology and relationships with myopathy. *Toxicol Rev.* 2006;25:1-14.

133. Karalliedde L, et al. Variables influencing the toxic response to organophosphates in humans. *Food Chem Toxicol.* 2003;41:1-13.

134. Karami-Mohajeri S, Abdollahi M. Mitochondrial dysfunction and organophosphorus compounds. *Toxicol Appl Pharmacol.* 2013;270:39-44.

135. Katewa SD, Katyare SS. Antimalarials inhibit human erythrocyte membrane acetylcholinesterase. *Drug Chem Toxicol.* 2005;28:467-482.

136. Kiss Z, Fazekas T. Arrhythmias in organophosphate poisoning. *Acta Cardiol.* 1979;34:323-330.

137. Knipe DW, et al. Suicide in Sri Lanka 1975-2012: age, period and cohort analysis of police and hospital data. *BMC Public Health.* 2014;14:839.

138. Koksal N, et al. Organophosphate intoxication as a consequence of mouth-to-mouth breathing from an affected case. *Chest.* 2002;122:740-741.

139. Konickx LA, et al. Is oxygen required before atropine administration in organophosphorus or carbamate pesticide poisoning?—a cohort study. *Clin Toxicol (Phila).* 2014;52:531-537.

140. Konickx LA, et al. Reactivation of plasma butyrylcholinesterase by pralidoxime chloride in patients poisoned by WHO Class II toxicity organophosphorus insecticides. *Toxicol Sci.* 2013;136:274-283.

141. Kupfermann N, et al. Rapid and sensitive quantitative analysis of alkyl phosphates in urine after organophosphate poisoning. *J Anal Toxicol.* 2004;28:242-248.

142. Kventsel I, et al. Scopolamine treatment for severe extra-pyramidal signs following organophosphate (chlorpyrifos) ingestion. *Clin Toxicol.* 2005;43:877-879.

143. Lamb T, et al. High lethality and minimal variation after acute self-poisoning with carbamate insecticides in Sri Lanka—implications for global suicide prevention. *Clin Toxicol (Phila).* 2016;54:624-631.

144. Lee DH, et al. A case of rivastigmine toxicity caused by transdermal patch. *Am J Emerg Med.* 2011;29:695.e691-695.e692.

145. Lee DH, et al. Body mass index as a prognostic factor in organophosphate-poisoned patients. *Am J Emerg Med.* 2014;32:693-696.

146. Li B, et al. Butyrylcholinesterase, paraoxonase, and albumin esterase, but not carboxylesterase, are present in human plasma. *Biochem Pharmacol.* 2005;70:1673-1684.

146a. Li B, et al. Protein tyrosine adduct in humans self-poisoned by chlorpyrifos. *Toxicol Appl Pharmacol.* 2013;269:215-225.

147. Lin CC, et al. The effectiveness of patient-tailored treatment for acute organophosphate poisoning. *Biomed J.* 2016;39:391-399.

148. Little M, Murray L. Consensus statement: risk of nosocomial organophosphate poisoning in emergency departments. *Emerg Med Australas.* 2004;16:456-458.

149. Liu L, Ding G. Effects of different blood purification methods on serum cytokine levels and prognosis in patients with acute severe organophosphorus pesticide poisoning. *Ther Apher Dial.* 2015;19:185-190.

150. Liu SH, et al. Acute large-dose exposure to organophosphates in patients with and without diabetes mellitus: analysis of mortality rate and new-onset diabetes mellitus. *Environ Health.* 2014;13:11.

151. Lokan R, James R. Rapid death by mevinphos poisoning while under observation. *Forensic Sci Int.* 1983;22:179-182.

152. Lotti M, Becker CE. Treatment of acute organophosphate poisoning: evidence of a direct effect on central nervous system by 2-PAM (pyridine-2-aldoxime methyl chloride). *J Toxicol Clin Toxicol.* 1982;19:121-127.

153. Lotti M, Moretto A. Organophosphate-induced delayed polyneuropathy. *Toxicol Rev.* 2005;24:37-49.

154. Lyzhnikov EA, et al. Pathogenesis of disorders of cardiac rhythm and conductivity in acute organophosphate insecticide poisoning [in Russian]. *Kardiologiia.* 1975;15:126-129.

155. Manoguerra A, et al. Cholinergic toxicity resulting from ocular instillation of echothiophate iodide eye drops. *J Toxicol Clin Toxicol.* 1995;33:463-465.

156. Marrs TC. Diazepam in the treatment of organophosphorus ester pesticide poisoning. *Toxicol Rev.* 2003;22:75-81.

157. Massoulie J, et al. Acetylcholinesterase: C-terminal domains, molecular forms and functional localization. *J Physiol (Paris).* 1998;92:183-190.

158. McDonough JH Jr, et al. Atropine and/or diazepam therapy protects against soman-induced neural and cardiac pathology. *Fundam Appl Toxicol.* 1989;13:256-276.

159. Meller D, et al. Hyperglycemia in anticholinesterase poisoning. *Can Med Assoc J.* 1981;124:745-748.

160. Mercurio-Zappala M, et al. Pralidoxime in carbaryl poisoning: an animal model. *Hum Exp Toxicol.* 2007;26:125-129.

161. Merrill DG, Mihm FG. Prolonged toxicity of organophosphate poisoning. *Crit Care Med.* 1982;10:550-551.

162. Mir SA, Rasool R. Reversal of cardiovascular toxicity in severe organophosphate poisoning with 20% intralipid emulsion therapy: case report and review of literature. *Asia Pac J Med Toxicol.* 2014;3:169-172.

163. Moffatt A, et al. Hypothermia and fever after organophosphorus poisoning in humans—a prospective case series. *J Med Toxicol.* 2010;6:379-385.

164. Moon J, et al. Variable response of cholinesterase activities following human exposure to different types of organophosphates. *Hum Exp Toxicol.* 2015;34:698-706.

165. Moon JM, et al. Hyperglycemia at presentation is associated with in hospital mortality in non-diabetic patient with organophosphate poisoning. *Clin Toxicol (Phila).* 2016; 54:252-258.

166. Morgan JP, Penovich P. Jamaica ginger paralysis: forty-seven-year follow-up. *Arch Neurol.* 1978;35:530-532.

167. Moriya F, Hashimoto Y. Comparative studies on tissue distributions of organophosphorus, carbamate and organochlorine pesticides in decedents intoxicated with these chemicals. *J Forensic Sci.* 1999;44:1131-1135.

168. Muller TC, et al. Antidepressants inhibit human acetylcholinesterase and butyrylcholinesterase activity. *Biochim Biophys Acta.* 2002;1587:92-98.

169. Munoz-Quezada MT, et al. Chronic exposure to organophosphate (OP) pesticides and neuropsychological functioning in farm workers: a review. *Int J Occup Environ Health.* 2016;22:68-79.

170. Nagler J, et al. Combined hemoperfusion-hemodialysis in organophosphate poisoning. *J Appl Toxicol.* 1981;1:199-201.

171. Namba T, et al. Treatment of severe organophosphorus poisoning by large doses of PAM. *Naika no Ryoiki* [Domain of Internal Medicine] 1959;7:709-713.

172. Namba T, et al. Malathion poisoning. A fatal case with cardiac manifestations. *Arch Environ Health.* 1970;21:533-541.

173. Namba T, Hiraki K. PAM (pyridine-2-aldoxime methiodide) therapy of alkylphosphate poisoning. *JAMA.* 1958;166:1834-1839.

174. Namba T, et al. Poisoning due to organophosphate insecticides. *Am J Med.* 1971; 50:475-492.

175. Nelson LS, et al. Aldicarb poisoning by an illicit rodenticide imported into the United States: Tres Pasitos. *J Toxicol Clin Toxicol.* 2001;39:447-452.

176. Nolan RJ, et al. Chlorpyrifos: pharmacokinetics in human volunteers. *Toxicol Appl Pharmacol.* 1984;73:8-15.

177. Padilla S, et al. Time course of cholinesterase inhibition in adult rats treated acutely with carbaryl, carbofuran, formetanate, methomyl, methiocarb, oxamyl or propoxur. *Toxicol Appl Pharmacol.* 2007;219:202-209.

178. Page A, et al. Suicide by pesticide poisoning remains a priority for suicide prevention in China: analysis of national mortality trends 2006-2013. *J Affect Disord.* 2016;208:418-423.

179. Pajoumand A, et al. Benefits of magnesium sulfate in the management of acute human poisoning by organophosphorus insecticides. *Hum Exp Toxicol.* 2004;23:565-569.

180. Panda M, et al. A fatal waterborne outbreak of pesticide poisoning caused by damaged pipelines, Sindhikela, Bolangir, Orissa, India, 2008. *J Toxicol.* 2009;2009:692496.

181. Panieri E, et al. Severe necrotizing pancreatitis caused by organophosphate poisoning. *J Clin Gastroenterol.* 1997;25:463-465.

182. Park JH, et al. Epidemiology and outcomes of poisoning-induced out-of-hospital cardiac arrest. *Resuscitation.* 2012;83:51-57.

183. Parker PE, Brown FW. Organophosphate intoxication: hidden hazards. *South Med J.* 1989;82:1408-1410.

184. Passeron D, et al. Acute liver and kidney failure after the ingestion of cyclohexanone [in French]. *J Toxicol Clin Exp.* 1992;12:207-211.

185. Pawar KS, et al. Continuous pralidoxime infusion versus repeated bolus injection to treat organophosphorus pesticide poisoning: a randomised controlled trial. *Lancet.* 2006;368:2136-2141.

186. Peeples ES, et al. Albumin, a new biomarker of organophosphorus toxicant exposure, identified by mass spectrometry. *Toxicol Sci.* 2005;83:303-312.

187. Peng A, et al. Therapeutic efficacy of charcoal hemoperfusion in patients with acute severe dichlorvos poisoning. *Acta Pharmacol Sin.* 2004;25:15-21.

188. Perera PM, et al. A phase II clinical trial to assess the safety of clonidine in acute organophosphorus pesticide poisoning. *Trials.* 2009;10:73.

189. Peter JV, et al. Adjuncts and alternatives to oxime therapy in organophosphate poisoning—is there evidence of benefit in human poisoning? A review. *Anaesth Intensive Care.* 2008;36:339-350.

190. Peter JV, et al. In-laws, insecticide—and a mimic of brain death. *Lancet.* 2008;371:622.

191. Peter JV, et al. Clinical features of organophosphate poisoning: a review of different classification systems and approaches. *Indian J Crit Care Med.* 2014;18:735-745.

192. Pichamuthu K, et al. Bioscavenger therapy for organophosphate poisoning—an open-labeled pilot randomized trial comparing fresh frozen plasma or albumin with saline in acute organophosphate poisoning in humans. *Clin Toxicol (Phila).* 2010;48:813-819.

193. Ragoucy-Sengler C, et al. Aldicarb poisoning. *Hum Exp Toxicol.* 2000;19:657-662.

194. Ranjbar A, et al. Oxidative stress in acute human poisoning with organophosphorus insecticides; a case control study. *Environ Toxicol Pharmacol.* 2005;20:88-91.

195. Reji KK, et al. Extrapyramidal effects of acute organophosphate poisoning. *Clin Toxicol (Phila).* 2016;54:259-265.

196. Robenshtok E, et al. Adverse reaction to atropine and the treatment of organophosphate intoxication. *Isr Med Assoc J.* 2002;4:535-539.

197. Roberts D, Buckley NA. Alkalinisation for organophosphorus pesticide poisoning. *Cochrane Database Syst Rev.* 2005;CD004897.

198. Roberts D, Senarathna L. Secondary contamination in organophosphate poisoning. *Q J Med.* 2004;97:697-698.

199. Roberts DM, et al. Experiences of anticholinesterase pesticide poisonings in an Australian tertiary hospital. *Anaesth Intensive Care.* 2005;33:469-476.

200. Roberts DM, et al. Extracorporeal blood purification for acute organophosphorus pesticide poisoning. *J Intensive Care Med.* 2006.

201. Ross SM, et al. Neurobehavioral problems following low-level exposure to organophosphate pesticides: a systematic and meta-analytic review. *Crit Rev Toxicol.* 2013;43:21-44.

202. Roth A, et al. Organophosphates and the heart. *Chest.* 1993;103:576-582.

203. Saadeh AM, et al. Cardiac manifestations of acute carbamate and organophosphate poisoning. *Heart.* 1997;77:461-464.

204. Sahin I, et al. The prevalence of pancreatitis in organophosphate poisonings. *Hum Exp Toxicol.* 2002;21:175-177.

205. Senanayake N, Jeyaratnam J. Toxic polyneuropathy due to ginger oil contaminated with tri-cresyl phosphate affecting adolescent girls in Sri Lanka. *Lancet.* 1981;i:88-89.

206. Senanayake N, Karalliedde L. Neurotoxic effects of organophosphate insecticides: an intermediate syndrome. *N Engl J Med.* 1987;316:761-763.

207. Sener EB, et al. Prolonged apnea following succinylcholine administration in undiagnosed acute organophosphate poisoning. *Acta Anaesthesiol Scand.* 2002;46:1046-1048.

208. Shadnia S, et al. *N*-Acetylcysteine. A novel treatment for acute human organophosphate poisoning. *Int J Pharmacol.* 2011;7:732-735.

209. Shepherd G, et al. Donepezil overdose: a tenfold dosing error. *Ann Pharmacother.* 1999;33:812-815.

210. Shih DM, et al. Mice lacking serum paraoxanase are susceptible to organophosphate toxicity and atherosclerosis. *Nature.* 1998;394:284-287.

211. Shobha TR, Prakash O. Glycosuria in organophosphate and carbamate poisoning. *J Assoc Physicians India.* 2000;48:1197-1199.

212. Sozmen EY, et al. Effect of organophosphate intoxication on human serum paraoxonase. *Hum Exp Toxicol.* 2002;21:247-252.

213. Stallones L, Beseler CL. Assessing the connection between organophosphate pesticide poisoning and mental health: a comparison of neuropsychological symptoms from clinical observations, animal models and epidemiological studies. *Cortex.* 2016;74:405-416.

214. Steenland K, et al. Neurologic function among termiticide applicators exposed to chlorpyrifos. *Environ Health Perspect.* 2000;108:293-300.

215. Sudakin DL, et al. Intermediate syndrome after malathion ingestion despite continuous infusion of pralidoxime. *J Toxicol Clin Toxicol.* 2000;38:47-50.

216. Sultatos LG. Mammalian toxicology of organophosphorus pesticides. *J Toxicol Environ Health.* 1994;43:271-289.

217. Sun J, Lynn BC. Development of a MALDI-TOF-MS method to identify and quantify butyrylcholinesterase inhibition resulting from exposure to organophosphate and carbamate pesticides. *J Am Soc Mass Spectrom.* 2007;18:698-706.

218. Sundwall A. Minimum concentrations of *N*-methylpyridinium-2-aldoxime methane sulphonate (P2S) which reverse neuromuscular block. *Biochem Pharmacol.* 1961;8:413-417.

219. Sweni S, et al. Acute renal failure in acute poisoning: prospective study from a tertiary care centre of South India. *J Ren Care.* 2012;38:22-28.

220. Taylor CA, et al. Environmental, medical, and family history risk factors for Parkinson's disease: a New England-based case control study. *Am J Med Genet.* 1999;88:742-749.

221. Taylor P. Anticholinesterase agents. In: Brunton LL, et al, eds. *Goodman & Gilman's The Pharmacological Basis of Therapeutics.* 11th ed. New York, NY: McGraw-Hill; 2006:201-216.

222. Teimouri F, et al. Alteration of hepatic cells glucose metabolism as a non-cholinergic detoxication mechanism in counteracting diazinon-induced oxidative stress. *Hum Exp Toxicol.* 2006;25:696-703.

223. Thiermann H, et al. Red blood cell acetylcholinesterase and plasma butyrylcholinesterase status: important indicators for the treatment of patients poisoned by organophosphorus compounds. *Arh Hig Rada Toksikol.* 2007;58:359-366.

224. Thiermann H, et al. Atropine maintenance dosage in patients with severe organophosphate pesticide poisoning. *Toxicol Lett.* 2011;206:77-83.

225. Thiermann H, et al. Modern strategies in therapy of organophosphate poisoning. *Toxicol Lett.* 1999;107:233-239.

226. Thiermann H, et al. Correlation between red blood cell acetylcholinesterase activity and neuromuscular transmission in organophosphate poisoning. *Chem Biol Interact.* 2005;157-158:345-347.

227. Tsai MC, et al. Safety evaluation in rats of alternative solvents for pesticides formulated with emulsifiable concentrate. *Plant Prot Bull.* 2004;46:267-280.

228. Umehara F, et al. Polyneuropathy induced by *m*-tolyl methyl carbamate intoxication. *J Neurol.* 1991;238:47-48.

229. van der Hoek W, Konradsen F. Risk factors for acute pesticide poisoning in Sri Lanka. *Trop Med Int Health.* 2005;10:589-596.

230. Vandekar M, et al. Toxicity of carbamates for mammals. *Bull World Health Organ.* 1971;44:241-249.

231. Vasilescu C, et al. Delayed neuropathy after organophosphorus insecticide (Dipterex) poisoning: a clinical, electrophysiological, and nerve biopsy study. *J Neurol Neurosurg Psychiatry.* 1984;47:543-548.

232. Venkatesh S, et al. Progression of type I to type II paralysis in acute organophosphorous poisoning: is oxidative stress significant? *Arch Toxicol.* 2006;80:354-361.

233. Vijayakumar HN, et al. Study of effect of magnesium sulphate in management of acute organophosphorous pesticide poisoning. *Anesth Essays Res.* 2017;11:192-196.

234. Von Der Wellen J, et al. Investigations of kinetic interactions between lipid emulsions, hydroxyethyl starch or dextran and organophosphorus compounds. *Clin Toxicol (Phila).* 2013;51:918-922.

235. Wadia RS, et al. Neurological manifestations of three organophosphate poisons. *Indian J Med Res.* 1977;66:460-468.

236. Wadia RS, et al. Neurological manifestations of organophosphate insecticide poisoning. *J Neurol Neurosurg Psychiatry.* 1974;37:841-847.

237. Wang A, et al. The association between ambient exposure to organophosphates and Parkinson's disease risk. *Occup Environ Med.* 2014;71:275-281.

238. Wang W, et al. Efficiency of anisodamine for organophosphorus-poisoned patients when atropinization cannot be achieved with high doses of atropine. *Environ Toxicol Pharmacol.* 2014;37:477-481.

239. Weizman Z, Sofer S. Acute pancreatitis in children with anticholinesterase insecticide intoxication. *Pediatrics.* 1992;90:204-206.

240. Wesseling C, et al. Pesticide poisonings in Costa Rica. *Scand J Work Environ Health.* 1993;19:227-235.

241. Wesseling C, et al. Agricultural pesticide use in developing countries: health effects and research needs. *Int J Health Serv.* 1997;27:273-308.

242. Wickramasinghe K, et al. Cost to government health-care services of treating acute self-poisonings in a rural district in Sri Lanka. *Bull World Health Organ.* 2009;87:180-185.

243. Willems JL, et al. Cholinesterase reactivation in organophosphorus poisoned patients depends on the plasma concentrations of the oxime pralidoxime methylsulphate and of the organophosphate. *Arch Toxicol.* 1993;67:79-84.

244. Wilson IB, et al. Carbamylation of acetylcholinesterase. *J Biol Chem.* 1960;235:2312-2315.

245. Worek F, et al. Improved determination of acetylcholinesterase activity in human whole blood. *Clin Chim Acta.* 1999;288:73-90.

246. Worek F, et al. Kinetic analysis of interactions between human acetylcholinesterase, structurally different organophosphorus compounds, and oximes. *Biochem Pharmacol.* 2004;68:2237-2248.

247. Worek F, et al. Oximes in organophosphate poisoning: 60 years of hope and despair. *Chem Biol Interact.* 2016;259(pt B):93-98.

248. World Health Organization. *The WHO Recommended Classification of Pesticides by Hazard and Guidelines to Classification: 2009.* Geneva: WHO; 2010.

249. Yang PY, et al. Carbofuran-induced delayed neuropathy. *J Toxicol Clin Toxicol.* 2000;38:43-46.

250. Yu LQ, Zheng XQ. Clinical study of effect of penehyclidine hydrochloride and atropine sequential therapy in the treatment of severe acute organophosphorus pesticide poisoning [in Chinese]. *Zhongguo Wei Zhong Bing Ji Jiu Yi Xue.* 2012;24:349-351.

251. Zadik Z, et al. Organophosphate poisoning presenting as diabetic ketoacidosis. *J Toxicol Clin Toxicol.* 1983;20:381-385.

252. Zhou Y, et al. Intravenous lipid emulsions combine extracorporeal blood purification: a novel therapeutic strategy for severe organophosphate poisoning. *Med Hypotheses.* 2010;74:309-311.

253. Zilker T, Hibler A. Treatment of severe parathion poisoning. In: Szinicz L, et al, eds. *Role of Oximes in the Treatment of Anticholinesterase Agent Poisoning.* Heidelberg: Spektrum, Akademischer Verlag; 1996:9-17.

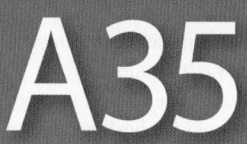

A35

ATROPINE

Mary Ann Howland

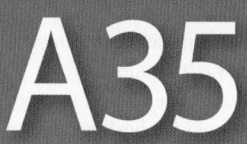

Atropine

INTRODUCTION

Atropine is the prototypical antimuscarinic xenobiotic. It is a competitive antagonist at both central and peripheral muscarinic receptors that is used to treat patients with symptoms following exposures to muscarinic agonists such as pilocarpine, *Clitocybe* and *Inocybe* mushroom species, and acetylcholinesterase inhibitors. The latter group includes pesticides, such as carbamate and organic phosphorus compounds, chemical weapons nerve agents, and some xenobiotics used to treat patients with Alzheimer disease, such as donepezil and rivastigmine.

HISTORY

Many plants contain the tropane alkaloids atropine and/or scopolamine. One notable example is *Atropa belladonna*, named by Linnaeus after Atropos, the goddess of fate in Greek mythology who could cut short a person's life. Belladonna means beautiful woman in Italian and comes from the practice by Italian women of placing belladonna extract in their eyes to produce aesthetically pleasing mydriasis.[14] In the early 1800s, atropine was isolated and purified from plants. In the 1860s, Fraser experimented with the dose–response relationship between atropine and physostigmine in various organs such as the heart and the eye.[28] Experiments in the 1940s with cholinesterase inhibitors demonstrated that atropine reversed many of the effects of these xenobiotics and protected animals against doses 2 to 3 times the dose necessary to kill 50% of the animals (LD_{50}).[62]

PHARMACOLOGY

Chemistry

Tropane alkaloids are bicyclic nitrogen-containing compounds that are naturally found in the plants of the families Solanaceae (eg, *Datura stramonium*) and Erythroxylaceae (eg, *Erythroxycom coca*) and have a long history of use as poisons and medicinals. Atropine (D,L-hyoscyamine), like scopolamine (L-hyoscine), is a tropane alkaloid with a tertiary amine structure that allows central nervous system (CNS) penetration. Only L-hyoscyamine is active and found in nature. Quaternary amine antimuscarinics such as glycopyrrolate, ipratropium, tiotropium, methylhomatropine, and methylatropine bromide are charged and do not cross the blood–brain barrier into the CNS (Fig. A35–1). The process of isolation results in racemization and forms D,L-hyoscyamine.

Mechanism of Action

Centrally acting muscarinic antagonists include atropine, scopolamine, and homatropine. Glycopyrrolate, ipratropium, and tiotropium act peripherally.

Scopolamine is approximately 10 times more potent than atropine.[40] Homatropine is approximately one-tenth as potent as atropine, depending on the measured outcome and route of administration.[38] Cholinergic receptors consist of muscarinic and nicotinic subtypes. Muscarinic receptors are coupled to G proteins and either inhibit adenylate cyclase (M_2, M_4) or increase phospholipase C (M_1, M_3, M_5). Muscarinic receptors are widely distributed throughout the peripheral and central nervous systems.[31]

The competitive blockade of muscarinic receptors in normal individuals results in dose-dependent clinical effects that vary by organ system based on the degree of endogenous parasympathetic tone.[14,31] In adults, low doses (0.5 mg) of atropine sometimes cause a paradoxical bradycardia of about 4 to 8 beats/min, not evident with rapid intravenous (IV) administration. The paradoxical bradycardia produced at low doses of atropine is attributed to the inhibition of peripheral M_1 presynaptic postganglionic parasympathetic neurons. Stimulation of these receptors by acetylcholine inhibits the further release of acetylcholine, and atropine interferes with this negative feedback.[14,60] Not all studies demonstrate this paradoxical decrease in heart rate.[9]

Higher doses of atropine in adults (2 mg) produce noticeable dryness of the mouth and sweat glands, feelings of warmth, flushing, tachycardia, reactive dilated pupils, blurred near vision, drowsiness, postural hypotension, and urinary hesitation. At even higher doses of atropine (3–5 mg) in adults all symptoms are exaggerated, with escalating degrees of hyperthermia, tachycardia, drowsiness, difficulty voiding, prolonged gastrointestinal transit time, and decreased peristalsis. Doses of greater than or equal to 10 mg of atropine produce incapacitation with hot, dry, flushed skin, dilated pupils, blurred vision, very dry mouth, tachycardia, urinary retention, constipation, increased drowsiness or disorientation, hallucinations, stereotypical movements, bursts of laughter, delirium, and finally, coma, and rarely death.[14,30]

Cholinesterase inhibitors prevent the breakdown of acetylcholine by acetylcholinesterase, thereby increasing the amount of acetylcholine available to stimulate cholinergic receptors at both muscarinic and nicotinic subtypes, although the degree of effect varies widely among the class. Atropine is a competitive antagonist of acetylcholine only at muscarinic receptors and not nicotinic receptors.[17]

Miosis from the topical ophthalmic administration of a cholinesterase inhibitor is not typically reversed by the systemic administration of atropine.[22,30] The systemic administration of 354 mg of atropine made one patient floridly

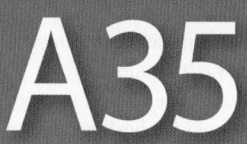

Atropine   Glycopyrrolate

FIGURE A35–1. The comparison of atropine, a tertiary amine structure which permits central nervous penetration, and glycopyrrolate, which is a quaternary amine structure and thus does not cross the blood–brain barrier.

anticholinergic, but did not counteract the ophthalmic effects following topical ophthalmic administration of a cholinesterase inhibitor.[30]

Pharmacokinetics and Pharmacodynamics

Atropine is absorbed rapidly from most routes of administration including inhalation, oral, and intramuscular (IM).[4] Ingestion of 1 mg of atropine produces maximal effects on heart rate and on salivary secretions in one and 3 hours, respectively. The duration of action lasts from 12 to 24 hours, depending on the dose.

The distribution half-life of atropine following IV administration is approximately one minute. The apparent volume of distribution (V_d) is about 2 to 2.6 L/kg.[38] As a result of the rapid distribution, within 10 minutes after IV administration less than 5% of the dose remains in the serum. The serum concentrations of atropine are similar at one hour following either 1 mg IV or IM in adults.[4,11] The elimination half-life is 6.5 hours.[50]

Following IM administration of 0.02 mg/kg in adults, the absorption rate and elimination rates are comparable for the racemic D,L-hyoscyamine and the active L-hyoscyamine at 8 minutes and 2.5 hours, respectively. The mean peak serum concentration and the area under the curve (AUC) are higher for the racemic mixture, indicating a stereochemical difference in pharmacokinetics.[38] Renal elimination accounts for 34% to 57% of the excretion of the dose, and the majority of renal elimination occurs within 6 hours.[4] Serum concentrations of L-hyoscyamine correlate with effects on heart rate and the antisialagogue effects. Serum concentrations of L-hyoscyamine below 0.5 mcg/L in an adult volunteer study were correlated with bradycardia, whereas higher concentrations caused tachycardia.[38]

A radioreceptor assay was developed to analyze the pharmacokinetics of the active enantiomer of atropine, referred to as (S)-L-hyoscyamine.[58] The sample for retrospective analysis of plasma concentrations was 6 organic phosphorus compound–poisoned patients from a previous clinical trial that included frequent blood samples and a detailed patient chart, and the atropine dose was linearly correlated with steady-state plasma concentrations. Elimination kinetics after an atropine bolus found a half-life of 1.5 hours, a V_d of 1.2 L/kg, a clearance of 13 mL/min/kg with a k_e of 0.536/h.

Intraosseous (IO) administration in minipigs demonstrated a pharmacokinetic profile similar to IV atropine.[45] The time to maximum concentration following a dose of 0.25 mg/kg was 2 minutes with both IV and IO injection, compared to 3.5 minutes for IM injection. Intraosseous administration in normal and hypovolemic swine demonstrated similar findings with very rapid absorption and distribution, although the hypovolemic swine had a comparatively longer half-life.[18] Atropine autoinjectors are now given to first responders for use during chemical weapons nerve agent attacks. The administration of 2 mg of atropine by autoinjector was compared with 2 mg administered by conventional needle and syringe into the deltoid of 6 adult subjects.[55] The onset of tachycardia and the time to maximal increase in heart rate occurred sooner with the autoinjector (16 minutes vs 23 minutes, and 34 minutes vs 41 minutes, respectively). An analysis of radiographs of contrast material injected by autoinjector or conventional IM administration into the leg of a dog demonstrated that the autoinjector appeared to "spray" the material into a larger tissue area, resulting in a faster rate of absorption.[55]

Ophthalmic administration of atropine causes cycloplegia and mydriasis by blocking the M_3 muscarinic receptor on the iris sphincter muscle.[44] The peak mydriatic effect occurs within 30 to 40 minutes and persists for 7 to 10 days. By contrast, the effects of topical homatropine on the eye occur sooner than topical atropine (10–30 minutes for mydriasis and 30–90 minutes for cycloplegia) and are shorter in duration (6–48 hours).

The effects on pupillary dilation after systemic atropine administration depend on the dose and route of administration. An IM dose of 0.01 mg/kg into the thigh of healthy adults produced no change in pupil size,[19] whereas subcutaneous administration into the upper arm of doses of 0.5, 1, and 2 mg per a 70-kg person produced a dose-dependent increase in pupil size. An oral dose of 0.02 mg/kg also produced pupillary dilation.[16,35]

An investigation of the bioavailability of atropine ophthalmic drops in healthy adults revealed approximately a 65% systemic absorption, but with a wide individual variability.[37] The time to maximum serum concentration was 30 minutes, and the apparent elimination half-life was 2.5 hours.

The pharmacokinetics of 3 inhaled doses of atropine from a metered dose nebulizer was compared with 2 mg of IM atropine in healthy adults.[32] Peak concentrations were comparable for the 2-mg inhaled and 2-mg IM atropine doses. The time to peak concentration following inhalation averaged 1.3 hours. Other dosage forms are being investigated as alternate ways to administer atropine in patients with organic phosphorus compound poisoning. Both a novel nanoatropine dry powder inhaler and a submicronic atropine in ethanol saline solution for nebulization are being evaluated to rapidly achieve blood concentrations of atropine in the hopes of circumventing IM administration.[43] Submicronic atropine sulfate nebulized solution, achieved therapeutic atropine concentrations in 5 minutes in healthy volunteers.[43] Another example is the development of a fast-disintegrating sublingual atropine sulfate tablet.[7]

ROLE IN ORGANIC PHOSPHORUS AND CARBAMATE TOXICITY

Atropine is recommended as the first line in therapy for the muscarinic effects of organic phosphorus and carbamate toxicity, which prevents patients from drowning in their own secretions.

One of the earliest descriptions of the effectiveness of atropine in parathion and tetraethylpyrophosphate insecticide poisoning was published in 1955.[29] Atropine improved survival when administered early and continued with adequate maintenance doses, intubation, and ventilation. Parathion and tetraethylpyrophosphate insecticide exposure led to heart block and bronchoconstriction in dogs, whereas humans were more likely to develop a relative bradycardia. Humans were more likely to die from respiratory causes resulting from central apnea, diaphragmatic weakness, and bronchorrhea.

In 1971, a landmark case series and review of organic phosphorus compound (OP) insecticide poisonings was published. Included was a table classifying the severity of poisoning along with treatment protocols for each level of severity.[46] This regimen served as the foundation of treatment regimens (atropine and pralidoxime) for many years.

In the 1930s and 1940s, the Germans synthesized OP insecticides (acetylcholinesterase inhibitors) that were further developed as chemical weapons nerve agents (Chap. 126).[54] Although these xenobiotics inhibit acetylcholinesterase in a manner similar to traditional OP insecticides, these so-called nerve agents also affect other cholinesterases, and at high doses directly affect nicotinic and muscarinic receptors. Atropine was chosen in the late 1940s as the standard antidote for these nerve agents. The dose of atropine needed to antagonize these nerve agents is much less than that needed to effectively antagonize traditional OP insecticides, largely because of differences in pharmacokinetics. The benefits of adding pralidoxime to atropine were noted in the 1950s, and in the 1960s, pralidoxime was established as a standard antidote in addition to atropine for these xenobiotics (Antidotes in Depth: A36).

ADVERSE EFFECTS AND SAFETY ISSUES

When atropine is used in the absence of a cholinergic agonist, adverse effects begin at 0.5 mg IV in the adult and include dry mouth and decreased sweat. However, in the presence of muscarinics or anticholinesterases, these effects do not typically occur until many milligrams of atropine are administered.

An unintentional atropine dose of 1,000 mg orally in one patient resulted in typical manifestations of anticholinergic poisoning that began within a short time and lasted 4 days.[2] In 2 hours, the patient went from feeling hot and flushed with blurred vision to stupor. Over the ensuing 24 hours he became tachycardic, hyperthermic, and comatose with mydriatic nonreactive pupils and shallow respirations. By 40 hours, he started to respond to his name and his temperature had normalized, but he had dry mucous membranes with mydriatic nonreactive pupils. He went from coma to restlessness, hallucinations, and paranoia. At 4 days, he regained a normal mental status with amnesia for the previous 4 days.

A survey of pediatric emergency departments in Israel reported on 240 children who unintentionally received atropine by autoinjections or autoinjector system administration, self-administration, needle injury, or delivery to an unintended site during the Persian Gulf crisis.[6] Half of the children developed systemic effects that correlated with the doses of atropine administered. Eight percent of effects were serious, but there were no seizures or deaths.

Systemic atropine toxicity also occurs when too large a dose of atropine, scopolamine, or homatropine is instilled in the eye, especially in children.[48] A medication error by a home hospice team led to the administration of atropine ophthalmic drops in the eye rather than a desired sublingual administration resulting in significant ophthalmic toxicity. A literature review dating from 1890 to 2004 identified 16 cases of seizures attributed to cycloplegic ophthalmic instillation with 9 of the cases secondary to atropine.[57] Excessive absorption from other routes of administration such as rectal or inhalation would also be expected to result in toxicity.[53] In the event of an atropine overdose, physostigmine, a reversible, CNS active, cholinesterase inhibitor, is the antidote of choice (Antidotes in Depth: A11).[47] Schizophrenic patients in the 1950s were often given atropine as a treatment. Within 15 to 20 minutes of getting 32 to 212 mg of IM atropine, patients became restless and often confused. This progressed to muscular incoordination, ataxia, weakness, and garbled speech.[27] These patients then progressed to disorientation with illusions, visual hallucinations, delirium, and coma. The coma often lasted for 4 to 6 hours, and then patients recovered in a manner that in some respects is similar to the reverse of the poisoning. Regardless of the dose of atropine required to induce the coma, physostigmine 4 mg IM completely reversed the toxicity within 20 minutes, although the reversal only lasted for 30 to 45 minutes.[27,47] One additional case describes a patient who ingested 10 mL of 1.5% atropine ophthalmic drops (for a total of 150 mg). He was treated in an ED with 1 mg physostigmine administered IV over 3 to 5 minutes to a total dose of 11 mg over 75 minutes. He then required 3 additional 1 mg doses of physostigmine in the ICU until complete recovery.[56]

In adults, low doses (0.5 mg) of atropine sometimes causes a paradoxical bradycardia of about 4 to 8 beats/min, not evident with rapid IV administration.[14,35] Other precautions or contraindications to consider when administering atropine include those associated with all antimuscarinics and include narrow angle closure glaucoma, obstructive uropathy, gastroparesis, pylorospasm, relaxation of the lower esophageal sphincter, and myasthenia gravis. Of course these complications must be weighed against the possible life-threatening nature of OP, carbamate, and chemical weapons nerve agent poisoning.

PREGNANCY AND LACTATION

Atropine is classified by the Food and Drug Administration (FDA) as pregnancy category C. Based on human data, atropine crosses the placenta and is recommended for use when indicated.[13,59] The American Academy of Pediatrics classifies atropine as compatible with breast-feeding.[13]

DOSING AND ADMINISTRATION

Although the dosage regimen of atropine for organic phosphorus compound poisoning in adults was evaluated in a randomized, controlled trial, and there is considerable variation in recommendations in the literature.[23,24] A prospective, observational study suggested that a dose doubling, titrated protocol provided equal efficacy and less atropine toxicity compared with an ad hoc dosing protocol.[49] Experience suggests that atropine should be initiated in adults in doses of 1 to 2 mg IV for mild to moderate poisoning and 3 to 5 mg IV for severe poisoning with unconsciousness.[46] We recommend that this dose be doubled every 3 to 5 minutes until improvement is observed, at which time dose doubling can stop and similar or smaller doses should be used as needed.[24,51] A recent open-label randomized trial conducted in Bangladesh compared conventional bolus-dose atropine (2–5 mg IV every 10–15 minutes) to a doubling-dose IV atropine protocol (1.8–3 mg IV initially and then doubled every 5 minutes until atropinization occurred, followed by an infusion of 10% to 20% of the total atropinization dose IV every hour). For inclusion in the study, patients had to have more than mild organic phosphorus compound toxicity. The time to atropinization decreased by more

than 90% from 152 to 24 minutes, atropine toxicity decreased from 28% to 12%, incidence of intermediate syndrome decreased, and survival increased. We believe that the most important end point for adequate atropinization is the resolution of bronchorrhea and secondarily the reversal of muscarinic toxicity. However, it is important not to confuse abnormal focal auscultatory sounds associated with pulmonary aspiration with those of extensive bronchorrhea.[24,51] We recommend achieving clear lungs, heart rate greater than or equal to 80 beats/min, and systolic blood pressure exceeding 90 mm Hg as the important goals of therapy. Dry axillae and the absence of pinpoint pupils are additional goals.[25] Once these end points are achieved, it is reasonable to establish a maintenance dose of atropine. Several groups suggest and we agree with administering 10% to 20% of the loading dose as an IV infusion every hour as a starting point with meticulous, frequent reevaluation and titration.[1,23,24] Atropine can be diluted in 0.9% sodium chloride, with rates of 0.5 to 1.5 mg/h of atropine commonly used.[49] For example, if a patient received atropine 2 mg IV, then 4 mg in 5 minutes, and 8 mg in 5 minutes, when improvement in bronchorrhea is noticeable, the total loading dose to initial control would be 14 mg in 10 minutes. The initial IV infusion dose of atropine would be 1.4 mg/h. This could be achieved by mixing 10 mg of atropine in 100 mL of 0.9% sodium chloride to make a concentration of 0.1 mg/mL and infusing it at 14 mL (1.4 mg)/h. If too much atropine is administered, the patient will demonstrate signs of peripheral and central anticholinergic toxicity as described above.

The IV/IO starting dose of atropine in children is 0.02 mg/kg up to the adult dose.[5,51,61] A continuous infusion of 0.025 mg/kg/h was successfully used in a 2-year-old child following a fenthion poisoning.[12] Although a minimum dose of 0.1 mg has been advocated, this dose would be toxic to infants less than 5 kg and is not recommended.[10]

Dosing for Chemical Weapons Nerve Agents

In the event that a person is exposed to a chemical weapons nerve agent, atropine is recommended in a dosage suitable for both the severity of the poisoning and the age of the patient. In a conscious adult with cholinergic effects, 2 mg of atropine IV or IM should be administered every 5 to 10 minutes until shortness of breath improves and drying of secretions occurs.[54] One adult autoinjector of atropine for IM administration, Mark 1 Nerve Agent Antidote Kit (NAAK), contains 2 mg of atropine, and therefore multiple injectors are often required. Similarly the autoinjector of atropine, AtroPen, comes in a variety of doses that are color coded with the green pen containing 2 mg and labeled for adults and children weighing more than 90 lb (usually corresponding to 10 years and older).[8]

Based on a limited amount of information, total doses of 2 to 4 mg of atropine are usually sufficient, which is much lower than the dose for most organic phosphorus compound exposures.[24,26,36,54] Patients who are unconscious or apneic require higher total doses, with 5 to 15 mg usually sufficing.[54] The appropriate total Mark 1 autoinjector doses of atropine for children depend on age and weight.[33,41] For ages 3 to 7 (13–25 kg), one autoinjector (2 mg) of atropine and one autoinjector of pralidoxime (600 mg) are recommended, resulting in a projected atropine dose of 0.08 to 0.15 mg/kg. For ages 8 to 14 years, 2 autoinjectors of atropine and 2 autoinjectors of pralidoxime are recommended, resulting in a projected atropine dose of 0.08 to 0.15 mg/kg. For patients older than 14 years, 3 autoinjectors of atropine and pralidoxime are recommended, resulting in a projected dose of atropine of less than 0.11 mg/kg. In an emergency for children younger than 3 years of age, a risk-to-benefit analysis would suggest injecting one autoinjector of atropine and one of pralidoxime. If time permits and only one autoinjector is available for use, it is recommended to transfer its contents to a small sterile vial for traditional IM administration with a needle and syringe.[34] We recommend that children younger than one year be administered one pediatric atropine autoinjector (0.5 mg), such as AtroPen (Meridian Medical Technologies, Inc), if available, and children older than one year be administered the Mark 1 autoinjector as described above.

When IV administration of atropine is not feasible, it is reasonable to administer IO at the standard IV dose. However, the dose for endotracheal administration in adults should be 2 to 2½ times the IV dose, diluted in 5 to 10 mL of 0.9% sodium chloride solution or sterile water. For children, we recommend following the 2015 American Heart Association guidelines for pediatric advanced life support, which recommend 0.04 to 0.06 mg/kg in a child endotracheally, followed by a flush of 5 mL of 0.9% sodium chloride solution and then 5 manual ventilations to enhance absorption.[5]

FORMULATION AND ACQUISITION

Atropine injection is available in many different strengths, with the following amounts in each 1 mL vial or ampule: 50 mcg, 300 mcg, 400 mcg, 500 mcg, 800 mcg, and 1 mg. Atropine is also available in prefilled 5- or 10-mL syringes with a concentration of 0.1 mg/mL for adults and in 5-mL syringes with a concentration of 0.05 mg/mL for children.[9]

The AtroPen Auto-Injector is a prefilled syringe designed for IM injection by an autoinjector into the outer thigh.[8] It is available in 4 strengths: 0.25 mg (yellow label), 0.5 mg (blue label), 1 mg (dark red label), and 2 mg (green label).

Atropine is also packaged in a kit designed for IM injection with a second autoinjector containing 600 mg of pralidoxime in 2 mL of sterile water for injection with 40 mg benzyl alcohol and 22.5 mg glycine. The pralidoxime injector is accompanied by an atropine autoinjector containing 2.1 mg of atropine in 0.7 mL of a sterile solution containing 12.47 mg glycerin and not more than 2.8 mg phenol. This particular combination kit is called a "Mark I Nerve Agent Antidote Kit" and is designed for IM use in case of a nerve agent attack. The needles are 0.8 inches in length.[42] The Mark I NAAK was replaced in great part by the DuoDote Autoinjector System and the analogous, military-designated Antidote Treatment Nerve Agent Autoinjector (ATNAA), which uses technology that sequentially administers 2.1 mg in 0.7 mL atropine followed by 600 mg in 2 mL pralidoxime chloride IM through the same syringe. The 23-gauge needle is 0.8 inches in length.[21]

Atropine is available orally in 300-, 400-, and 600-mcg tablets.

The expiration date for certain MARK I autoinjectors was extended because of drug shortages. In case of a shortage during an emergency, large numbers of atropine syringes can be compounded by a pharmacist from atropine powder using a standard syringe batching system.[39] In vitro evidence suggests that outdated atropine retains its potency and that an atropine solution prepared from powder is stable for at least 3 days.[20,52] Other sources of atropine to consider in an emergency during a shortage would be atropine eye drops, which come as a 1% concentration (10 mg/mL). Homatropine, available as eye drops in a 2% or 5% concentration, compared favorably with atropine in preventing lethality when administered IM in a pretreatment rodent model using dichlorvos. In this experimental model, homatropine appeared to be half as potent as atropine.[15] Glycopyrrolate and scopolamine are other atropine alternatives. Atropine is maintained as part of the Strategic National Stockpile (SNS) for formulary in repositories in numerous locations throughout the United States.

SUMMARY

- Atropine has many clinical uses as a competitive antagonist at both central and peripheral muscarinic receptor sites.
- The use of atropine is extensive for patients with bradycardias, in advanced cardiac life support, and in those exposed to acetylcholinesterase inhibitors in the workplace, in the home, and potentially on the battlefield.
- Atropine should be dosed to the resolution of bronchorrhea caused by the muscarinic toxidrome using a dose-titrated doubling protocol.

REFERENCES

1. Abedin M, et al. Open-label randomized clinical trial of atropine bolus injection versus incremental boluses plus infusion for organophosphate poisoning in Bangladesh. *J Med Toxicol.* 2012;8:108-117.
2. Alexander E, et al. Atropine poisoning: report of a case with recovery after ingestion of one gram. *N Engl J Med.* 1946;234:258-259.
3. Ali R, et al. Development and clinical trial of nano-atropine sulfate dry powder inhaler as a novel organophosphorous poisoning antidote. *Nanomedicine (Lond).* 2009;5:55-63.
4. Ali-Melkkila T, et al. Pharmacokinetics and related pharmacodynamics of anticholinergic drugs. *Acta Anaesthesiol Scand.* 1993;37:633-642.
5. American Heart Association. 2015 Guidelines for cardiopulmonary resuscitation and emergency cardiovascular care. Part 14: pediatric advanced life support. *Circulation.* 2010;122:S876-S908.
6. Amitai Y, et al. Atropine poisoning in children during the Persian Gulf crisis: a national survey in Israel. *JAMA.* 1992;268:630-632.
7. Aodah A, et al. Formulation and evaluation of fast-dissolving sublingual tablets of atropine sulfate: the effect of tablet dimensions and drug load on tablet characteristics. *AAPS PharmSciTech.* 2017;18:1624-1633.
8. AtroPen autoinjector-atropine sulfate injection [package insert]. Columbia, MD: Meridian Medical Technologies, Inc; 2016.
9. Atropine sulfate injection package insert by Hospira, Inc, Lake Forest, IL 60045.
10. Barrington KJ. The myth of a minimum dose for atropine. *Pediatrics.* 20121;127:783-784.
11. Berghem L, et al. Plasma atropine concentrations determined by radioimmunoassay after single-dose I.V. and I.M. administration. *Br J Anaesth.* 1980;52:597-601.
12. Borowitz SM. Prolonged organophosphate toxicity in a twenty-six-month-old child. *J Pediatr.* 1988;112:302-304.
13. Briggs G, et al. Atropine. In: Briggs GG, ed. *Drugs in Pregnancy and Lactation: A Reference Guide to Fetal and Neonatal Risk.* St. Louis, MO: Wolters Kluwer Health, Inc; 2011.
14. Brown JH, Laiken N. Muscarinic receptor agonists and antagonists. In: Brunton LL, et al., eds. *Goodman & Gilman's The Pharmacological Basis of Therapeutics.* 12th ed. New York, NY: McGraw-Hill; 2011:11.
15. Bryant S, et al. Intramuscular ophthalmic homatropine versus atropine to prevent lethality in rats with dichlorvos poisoning. *J Med Toxicol.* 2006;2:156-159.
16. Bye C, et al. Effects of systemically administered drugs with anticholinergic actions on the pupil and other organs. *Br J Clin Pharmacol.* 1978;5:366P-367P.
17. Caulfield MP, Birdsall NJ. International Union of Pharmacology: XVII. Classification of muscarinic acetylcholine receptors. *Pharmacol Rev.* 1998;50:279-290.
18. Cornell M, et al. Pharmacokinetics of sternal intraosseous atropine administration in normovolemic and hypovolemic swine. *Am J Disaster Med.* 2016;11:233-236.
19. Cozanitis D, et al. Atropine versus glycopyrrolate. A study of intraocular pressure and pupil size in man. *Anaesthesia.* 1979;34:236-238.
20. Dix J, et al. Stability of atropine sulfate prepared for mass chemical terrorism. *J Toxicol Clin Toxicol.* 2003;41:771-775.
21. DuoDote (atropine and pralidoxime chloride injection) Auto Injector [package insert]. Columbia, MD: Meridian Medical Technologies, Inc; 2017.
22. Durham WF, Hayes WJ Jr. Organic phosphorus poisoning and its therapy. With special reference to modes of action and compounds that reactivate inhibited cholinesterase. *Arch Environ Health.* 1962;5:21-47.
23. Eddleston M, et al. Speed of initial atropinisation in significant organophosphorus pesticide poisoning—a systematic comparison of recommended regimens. *J Toxicol Clin Toxicol.* 2004;42:865-875.
24. Eddleston M, et al. Management of acute organophosphorous pesticide poisoning. *Lancet.* 2008;371:597-607.
25. Eddleston M, et al. Early management after self-poisoning with an organophosphorus or carbamate pesticide—a treatment protocol for junior doctors. *Crit Care.* 2004;8:R391-R397.
26. Foltin G, et al. Pediatric nerve agent poisoning: medical and operational considerations for emergency medical services in a large American city. *Pediatr Emerg Care.* 2006;22:239-244.
27. Forrer GR, Miller JJ. Atropine coma: a somatic therapy in psychiatry. *Am J Psychiatry.* 1958;115:455-458.
28. Fraser TR. On the characters, action and therapeutic uses of the bean of Calabar. *Edinb Med J.* 1863;9:235-245.
29. Freeman G, Epstein MA. Therapeutic factors in survival after lethal cholinesterase inhibition by phosphorus insecticides. *N Engl J Med.* 1955;18;253:266-271.
30. Grob D. Anticholinesterase intoxication in man and its treatment. In: Koelle GB, ed. *Handbuch der Experimentellen Pharmakologie 15,* Suppl., Ch 22. New York, NY: Springer-Verlag; 1963:989-1027.
31. Gyermek L. *Pharmacology of Antimuscarinic Agents.* Boca Raton, FL: CRC Press; 1997.
32. Harrison LI, et al. Comparative absorption of inhaled and intramuscularly administered atropine. *Am Rev Respir Dis.* 1986;134:254-257.
33. Henretig FM, et al. Biological and chemical terrorism. *J Pediatr.* 2002;141:311-326.
34. Henretig FM, et al. Potential use of autoinjector-packaged antidotes for treatment of pediatric nerve agent toxicity. *Ann Emerg Med.* 2002;40:405-408.
35. Herxheimer A. A comparison of some atropine-like drugs in man, with a particular reference to their end organ specificity. *Brit J Pharmacol.* 1958;13:184-192.
36. Holstege CP, et al. Chemical warfare. Nerve agent poisoning. *Crit Care Clin.* 1997;13:923-942.
37. Kaila T, et al. Systemic bioavailability of ocularly applied 1% atropine eyedrops. *Acta Ophthalmol Scand.* 1999;77:193-196.
38. Kentala E, et al. Intramuscular atropine in healthy volunteers: a pharmacokinetic and pharmacodynamic study. *Int J Clin Pharmacol Ther Toxicol.* 1990;28:399-404.
39. Kozak R, et al. Rapid atropine synthesis for the treatment of massive nerve agent exposure. *Ann Emerg Med.* 2003;41:685-688.
40. Longo VG. Behavioral and electroencephalographic effects of atropine and related compounds. *Pharmacol Rev.* 1966;18:965-996.

41. Mark I. Nerve Agent Antidote Kit (NAAK) [package insert]. Columbia, MD: Meridian Medical Technologies, Inc; 2002.

42. Markenson D, Redlener I. Pediatric terrorism preparedness national guidelines and recommendations: findings of an evidenced-based consensus process. *Biosecur Bioterror.* 2004;2:301-319.

43. Mittal G, et al. Development and clinical study of submicronic-atropine sulphate respiratory fluid as a novel organophosphorous poisoning antidote. *Drug Deliv.* 2016;23:2255-2261.

44. Moroi SE, Lichter PR. Ocular pharmacology. In: Hardman JG, et al., eds. *Goodman and Gilman's the Pharmacologic Basis of Therapeutics.* 10th ed. New York, NY: McGraw-Hill; 2001:1821-1848.

45. Murray D, et al. Rapid and complete bioavailability of antidotes for organophosphorous nerve agent and cyanide poisoning in minipigs after intraosseous administration. *Ann Emerg Med.* 2012;60:424-430.

46. Namba T, et al. Poisoning due to organophosphate insecticides. Acute and chronic manifestations. *Am J Med.* 1971;50:475-492.

47. Nickalls RWD, Nickalls EA. The first use of physostigmine in the treatment of atropine poisoning. *Anaesthesia.* 1988;43:776-779.

48. Palmer EA. How safe are ocular drugs in pediatrics? *Ophthalmology.* 1986;93:1038-1040.

49. Perera P, et al. Comparison of two commonly practiced atropinization regimens in acute organophosphorous and carbamate poisoning, doubling doses versus ad hoc: a prospective observational study. *Hum Exp Toxicol.* 2008;27:513-518.

50. Pihlajamaki K, et al. Pharmacokinetics of atropine in children. *Int J Clin Pharmacol Ther Toxicol.* 1986;24:236-239.

51. Roberts D, Aaron C. Management of acute organophosphorous pesticide poisoning. *BMJ.* 2007;334:629-634.

52. Schier JG, et al. Preparing for chemical terrorism: stability of injectable atropine sulfate. *Acad Emerg Med.* 2004;11:329-334.

53. Sharony R, et al. Atropinism following rectal administration of a therapeutic atropine dose. *J Toxicol Clin Toxicol.* 1998;36:41-42.

54. Sidell FR. Nerve agents. In: Zajtchuk R, ed. *Textbook of Military Medicine: Medical Aspects of Chemical and Biological Warfare. Part I.* Office of the Surgeon General Department of the Army, United States of America; 1997:129-177.

55. Sidell FR, et al. Enhancement of drug absorption after administration by an automatic injector. *J Pharmacokinet Biopharm.* 1974;2:197-210.

56. Stellpflug S, et al. Massive atropine eye drop ingestion treated with high-dose physostigmine to avoid intubation. *West J Emerg Med.* 2012;13:77-79.

57. Tamara Wygnanski-Jaffe, et al. Epileptic seizures induced by cycloplegic eye drops. *Cutan Ocul Toxicol.* 2014;33:103-108.

58. Thiermann H, et al. Atropine maintenance dosage in patients with severe organophosphate pesticide poisoning. *Toxicol Lett.* 2011;206:77-83.

59. *USP DI Volume I. Drug Information for the Health Care Professional. 23rd ed.* Thomson Healthcare, Inc; 2004:3.

60. Wellstein A, Pitschner HF. Complex dose–response curves of atropine in man explained by different functions of M_1- and M_2-cholinoceptors. *Naunyn Schmiedebergs Arch Pharmacol.* 1988;338:19-27.

61. WHO Model Formulary for Children 2010. Based on the Second Model List of Essential Medicines for Children 2009. Geneva, Switzerland: WHO Press; 2010. http://apps.who.int/medicinedocs/documents/s17151e/s17151e.pdf. Accessed June 15, 2014.

62. Wills JH. Pharmacological antagonists of the anticholinesterase agents. In: Koelle GB, ed. *Handbuch der Experimenteller Pharmakologie.* New York, NY: Springer-Verlag; 1963:883-920.

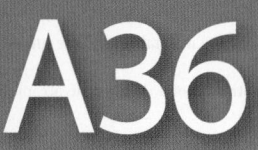

PRALIDOXIME

Mary Ann Howland

Pralidoxime

Obidoxime

Asoxime (HI-6)

INTRODUCTION

Pralidoxime chloride (2-PAM) is the only cholinesterase-reactivating xenobiotic currently available in the United States. It is used concomitantly with atropine in the management of patients poisoned by organic phosphorus (OP) compounds. Administration should be initiated as soon as possible after exposure, but can be effective even days later and therefore is recommended for all symptomatic patients independent of delay. Continuous infusion is preferable to intermittent administration for patients with serious toxicity, and a prolonged therapeutic course is required.

HISTORY

It was recognized that certain phosphate esters were potent and irreversible inhibitors of acetylcholinesterase (AChE).[94,95] Identification of an anionic site on AChE led to the theory that a compound could be developed that would bind to this site and remove the phosphate ester, thereby reactivating AChE. In 1951, Wilson demonstrated the key concept that cholinesterases inhibited by organic phosphorus compounds could be reactivated using hydroxylamine. Several hydroxylamine derivatives were studied and led to the design of pralidoxime (2-PAM), which American and British scientists independently synthesized as 2-PAM in 1955.[65,95]

PHARMACOLOGY
Chemistry

Pralidoxime chloride is a quaternary pyridinium oxime with a molecular weight of 173 Da. The chloride salt exhibits excellent water solubility and physiologic compatibility. Pralidoxime iodide has a molecular weight of 264 Da, is less water soluble, and can potentially induce iodism.[3]

Related Xenobiotics

Organic phosphorus pesticides and nerve agents both penetrate the central nervous system (CNS). A disadvantage of pralidoxime is that in vivo rat studies demonstrate only a 10% CNS penetration.[39,73] Strategies to enhance the penetration of oximes across the blood–brain barrier (BBB) include enhancing lipophilicity by adding a fluorine atom into the ring structure, designing a glucose-oxime drug that could use facilitated glucose transporters to cross the BBB, designing a prodrug of pralidoxime that could be oxidized to the active drug once it had crossed the BBB, conjugating the oxime with amidine, and by using a targeted nanoparticle drug delivery system.[56]

Obidoxime (Toxogonin, LuH-6) is an oxime used outside the United States that contains 2 active sites per molecule and is considered by some to be more effective than pralidoxime.[24,25,99] An in vitro study using human erythrocyte AChE supported the superiority of obidoxime to pralidoxime in reactivating AChE inhibited by the dimethyl phosphoryl (malaoxon, mevinphos) and diethyl phosphoryl OP compounds (paraoxon). On a molar basis, obidoxime is approximately 10 to 20 times more effective in reactivating AChE than pralidoxime.[99] A potential disadvantage is the concern that the phosphorylobidoxime generated from the reactivation of AChE by obidoxime could reinhibit AChE if not metabolized by a plasma enzyme similar or identical to human paraoxonase 1 (PON1). Paraoxonase exhibits polymorphism,[22] and one in 20 patients may not be able to metabolize this phosphorylobidoxime compound. Phosphorylpralidoxime is unstable and does not accumulate. A molecular docking simulation study demonstrated that pralidoxime had better positioning at the oxyanion hole compared to obidoxime, allowing better reactivation of methamidophos-inhibited AChE.[49] The H series of oximes (named after Hagedorn; HI-6, HIo-7) were developed to act against the chemical warfare nerve agents (Chap. 126).[6] These oximes have superior effectiveness against sarin, VX, and certain types of newer pesticides (eg, methyl-fluorophosphonylcholines).[3,11,41,46,50,72,99,100] Unfortunately, they are less efficacious for traditional OP insecticide poisoning, and their toxicity profile is inadequately defined.[11,41,46,50,72,99,100] In addition to reactivating AChEs, the Hagedorn oximes demonstrate direct central and peripheral anticholinergic effects at supratherapeutic concentrations.[72]

Mechanism of Action

Organic phosphorus compounds are powerful inhibitors of carboxylic esterase enzymes, including acetylcholinesterase (AChE; true cholinesterase, found in red blood cells, nervous tissue, and skeletal muscle) and plasma cholinesterase or butyrylcholinesterase (BuChE) (found in plasma, liver, heart, pancreas, and brain).[61] The OP binds firmly to the serine-containing esteratic site on the enzyme, inactivating it by phosphorylation (Fig. 110–3).[40,62,84] This reaction results in the accumulation of acetylcholine at muscarinic and nicotinic synapses in the peripheral and central nervous systems, leading to the clinical manifestations of OP poisoning. Following phosphorylation, the enzyme is inactivated and can undergo one of 3 processes; endogenous hydrolysis of the phosphorylated enzyme, reactivation by a strong nucleophile, such as pralidoxime, and aging, which involves biochemical changes that stabilize the inactivated phosphorylated molecule and render it incapable of reactivation by oximes.

Endogenous hydrolysis of the bond between the enzyme and the OP is generally extremely slow and is considered insignificant. This is in contrast to the rapid hydrolysis of the related bond between the enzyme and many carbamates. The positively charged quaternary nitrogen of pralidoxime is attracted to the negatively charged anionic site on the phosphorylated enzyme, bringing it close to the phosphorus moiety (Fig. 110–3). Pralidoxime then exerts a nucleophilic attack on the phosphate moiety, successfully releasing it from the AChE enzyme.[93] This action liberates the enzyme to a variable extent depending on the OP in question and restores enzymatic function.[51] The diethoxy organic phosphorus compounds (eg, chlorpyriphos, diazinon, ethyl parathion) take days to age ($t_{1/2}$, 33 hours to age) in comparison to hours ($t_{1/2}$, 3 hours to age) for the dimethoxy organic phosphorus compounds (eg, dimethoate, dichlorvos, fenthion, fenitrothion, malathion, monocrotophos) (Table 110–2).[18,26]

Pralidoxime is important at nicotinic sites where atropine is ineffective, most often typically improving muscle strength within 10 to 40 minutes after administration.[62,84] This effect is vital to maintaining the muscles of respiration. Pralidoxime is also synergistic with atropine; it liberates cholinesterase enzyme so that additional acetylcholine can be metabolized while atropine inhibits the effects of acetylcholine at cholinergic receptors. This suggests that pralidoxime has a synergistic effect with atropine in compromised patients.[25,62] Some OP compounds respond much better to pralidoxime than others, depending on the affinity of pralidoxime for the particular type of phosphorylated enzyme, its reactivating ability, concentrations of both the oxime and the OP, aging, and OP redistribution from a depot site such as fat.[24,99]

The CNS benefits of pralidoxime are controversial, as the molecule is a quaternary nitrogen compound and not expected to cross the BBB.[39,53,62] A rat experiment using a microdialysis technique demonstrated only 10% CNS penetration of pralidoxime.[73] Following exposure to IV fenitrothion, IV administration of pralidoxime in rats failed to improve survival or to reactivate brain cholinesterase, whereas with direct brain instillation pralidoxime partially restored brain cholinesterase and eliminated fatalities.[87] Intranasal oxime (obidoxime) delivery can circumvent the BBB and decreased mortality from 41% to zero in a murine paraoxon model.[45] Clinical observations have certainly suggested a CNS action of pralidoxime with a prompt return of consciousness reported in some cases.[61,62,70,93] A 3-year-old child who was comatose from parathion was given 500 mg of 2-PAM IV over 15 minutes with continuous electroencephalographic (EEG) monitoring. Within 2 minutes, there was a dramatic response on the EEG, followed rapidly by normalization of consciousness.[38]

Early work with feline models led to a proposal that a serum concentration of greater than or equal to 4 mcg/mL was a desired therapeutic concentration for pralidoxime.[82] However, more recent in vitro work with human erythrocytes and a mouse hemidiaphragm model suggests that higher serum concentrations are actually needed.[96,99] Twenty percent reactivation was achieved in 5 minutes with serum concentrations of 10 mcg/mL.[99] A simulation and analysis suggests that serum concentrations between 10 and 15 mcg/mL (50–100 μmol/L) are necessary for optimal treatment of severely poisoned patients.[22,101] These recommendations await validation in poisoned patients. Serum concentrations are not available in a timely manner, but may help in the design of future pralidoxime dosing protocols.

Organic phosphorus compounds inhibit BuChE (plasma cholinesterase) and AChE to different extents and are affected by oximes differently.[19] Butyrylcholinesterase is made in the liver and transported to the blood, where it metabolizes certain xenobiotics like cocaine and succinylcholine. Additionally, BuChE can be affected by disease states, and normal values show wide variation, making interpretation in any individual difficult without a preexposure concentration. Butyrylcholinesterase has no relationship to the manifestations of toxicity following an OP exposure. If performed correctly, and the OP does indeed inhibit BuChE, then the normalization can be utilized as a surrogate marker for OP or carbamate elimination from the body.[42] The benefit of this surrogate marker in contrast to monitoring manifestations of toxicity is a potential research tool. Likewise, the reactivation of BuChE by pralidoxime is dependent on the concentration of pralidoxime, often has a flat dose response, is quite variable, and is susceptible to aging.[44] For example, in an in vitro model of human blood taken from healthy volunteers and treated with paraoxon, pralidoxime was able to reactivate 1.3% and

18.1% of erythrocyte AChE at pralidoxime concentrations of 10 and 100 μmol, respectively, compared with only 1% and 5.5% of BuChE with 10 and 100 μmol concentrations of pralidoxime.[38]

By contrast to the usefulness of pralidoxime in the management of the cholinergic syndrome, current understanding of the pathophysiology of the intermediate syndrome is inadequate to determine whether pralidoxime can prevent its development (Chap. 110).[81] If cholinergic receptor desensitization due to ineffective AChE reactivation is responsible for the cause of the muscle weakness, then pralidoxime would only be likely to prevent the syndrome if the OP compound in question was responsive to pralidoxime (eg, chlorpyrifos) in the dose ingested, pralidoxime was administered before aging occurred and the solvent formulation of the compound was not contributory.[12,19]

In addition to the intermediate syndrome, certain OP compounds may lead to the development of delayed-onset neurotoxicity, which involves inhibition of neuropathy target esterases (now known as lysophospholipases). This delayed neurotoxicity cannot be prevented or treated by pralidoxime.[20,54]

Pharmacokinetics and Pharmacodynamics

Pralidoxime chloride pharmacokinetics are characterized by a 2-compartment model. Pharmacokinetics values vary depending on whether calculations are determined in healthy volunteers or poisoned patients. The volume of distribution (V_d) is larger in poisoned patients and most likely accounts for the prolonged elimination phase.[22]

In volunteers, the V_d is about 0.8 L/kg and the $t_{1/2}$ is 75 minutes.[35,68,79] Pralidoxime is renally excreted, and within 12 hours, 80% of the dose is recovered unchanged in the urine.[37,78]

A dose of 10 mg/kg of pralidoxime administered intramuscularly (IM) to volunteers results in peak serum concentrations of 6 mcg/mL (reached 5–15 minutes after IM injection) and a half-life of approximately 75 minutes.[78] Following a standard 30-minute IV infusion dose of 1 g of pralidoxime in a 70 kg man, the serum concentration fell to less than 4 mcg/mL (no longer thought to be considered a serum concentration goal) at 1.5 hours. In a simulated model, a continuous infusion of 500 mg/h of pralidoxime led to a concentration greater than 4 mcg/mL after 15 minutes, which could be maintained throughout the infusion.[85] In a human volunteer study, an IV loading dose of 4 mg/kg over 15 minutes followed by 3.2 mg/kg/h for a total of 4 hours maintained serum pralidoxime concentrations greater than 4 mcg/mL for 4 hours. The approximately same total dose, 16 mg/kg, administered over 30 minutes only maintained those concentrations for 2 hours.[55] In poisoned patients receiving continuous infusions of pralidoxime as opposed to intermittent infusions, both the V_d and the $t_{1/2}$ are increased.[78] A V_d of 2.77 L/kg, an elimination $t_{1/2}$ of 3.44 hours, and a clearance of 0.57 L/kg/h were reported in poisoned adults given a mean loading dose of 4.4 mg/kg followed by an infusion of 2.14 mg/kg/h.[93] In poisoned children and adolescents, the V_d varied with severity of poisoning from 8.8 L/kg in the severely poisoned patients to 2.8 L/kg in moderately poisoned patients.[75] After a mean loading dose of 29 mg/kg followed by a continuous infusion of about 14 mg/kg/h, a steady-state serum concentration of 22 mcg/mL, a $t_{1/2}$ of 3.6 hours, and a clearance of 0.88 L/kg/h were calculated.[75]

Oral administration of salts of pralidoxime (not used clinically because of OP poisoning–induced vomiting) demonstrated a peak concentration at 2 to 3 hours, a $t_{1/2}$ of 1.7 hours, and an average urine recovery of 27% of unchanged pralidoxime in humans.[43] Oral administration demonstrated clinical efficacy in a mice murine model.[8]

Autoinjector administration of 600 mg of pralidoxime chloride in an adult man (9 mg/kg) produced a concentration above 4 mcg/mL at 7 to 16 minutes, a maximum serum concentration of 6.5 mcg/mL at about 28 minutes, and a $t_{1/2}$ of 2 hours.[68,77] In 24 healthy volunteers, following 600 mg pralidoxime via the DuoDote autoinjector delivery system, a C_{max} of 7±3 mcg/mL, a $t_{1/2}$ of 2±1 hours and t_{max} of 28±15 minutes were achieved. When stratified by gender, the C_{max} was 36% higher in women, the $t_{1/2}$ was longer (153 minutes vs 107 minutes) and the t_{max} was achieved sooner (23 minutes vs 32 minutes).[16]

Using traditional needle and syringe IM administration requires a longer time to achieve comparable serum concentrations. The autoinjectors more widely disperse the medication in the tissues, resulting in faster absorption.[71,79]

ROLE IN ORGANIC PHOSPHORUS COMPOUND TOXICITY: EFFICACY RELATED TO TIME OF ADMINISTRATION AFTER POISONING

The sooner after exposure to an OP, the more likely pralidoxime is to be effective. Timely administration reduces the likelihood that aging of the OP–AChE complex has occurred and is completed. However, there is no absolute time limitation on reactivation function, as long as the patient remains symptomatic.

Early in vitro evidence suggested that the successful use of cholinesterase reactivators depended on administration within 24 to 48 hours of exposure to the OPs; afterward, the acetylcholinesterases would be irreversibly inactivated.[4,14,32,33,74] The 48-hour limit was derived from in vitro experiments using a small number of tightly bound compounds and reactivators and data from plasma cholinesterase enzyme activity, which is now recognized to be relatively resistant to oxime-nucleophilic attack. These early data were accepted without consideration of their relevance to human systems, the use of newer and less tightly bound OP compounds, temperature and pH variation, blood flow, fat solubility, active metabolites, and species specificity. Fat-soluble OP compounds redistribute from fat stores over time and can continue to newly inhibit AChE for days.

An in vitro experiment assessed the effect of aging on the ability of pralidoxime to regenerate rat erythrocyte and brain cholinesterases using 3 different OP compounds.[88] The rate of reactivation of erythrocyte and brain cholinesterases was significantly decreased over time for fenitrothion and methyl parathion, with no reactivation occurring at 48 hours. This is partly because dimethylated (dimethoxy) OP pesticides age more quickly than diethoxy phosphorylated compounds.[20] By contrast, a very high reactivation rate for ethyl parathion was still apparent at 48 hours. Thus, the structure of the OP compound is important in the rates of aging and reactivation with pralidoxime. Fenitrothion and methyl parathion are both o,o'-dimethoxy OP compounds as are dichlorvos, dimethoate, fenthion, and malathion whereas ethyl parathion is an o,o'-diethoxy OP compound, as are chlorpyriphos and diazinon.[88] Other studies also suggest that pralidoxime remains effective for more than 48 hours following exposure to diethyl OPs and to some fat-soluble OPs.[2,5,8,13,17,20,22,59,69,92]

ROLE IN ORGANIC PHOSPHORUS COMPOUND TOXICITY: HUMAN TRIALS

There are 4 randomized clinical trials examining the efficacy of pralidoxime for the management of OP poisoning. Two of these trials were done in the 1990s in India using doses of pralidoxime now considered to be inadequate.[20] Neither study demonstrated a benefit for pralidoxime and, in fact, suggested an increase in mortality in patients receiving the higher but still inadequate dose of pralidoxime. Criticisms include a delay in administration and an inadequate duration of treatment. The third clinical trial included 200 patients in India who were moderately to severely poisoned with an OP compound.[64] All patients received a 2-g loading dose of pralidoxime iodide over 30 minutes before being randomized to receive 1 g over 1 hour every 4 hours for 48 hours or a continuous infusion of 1 g/h for 48 hours. Beyond 48 hours, all patients received 1 g every 4 hours until no longer ventilator dependent. In the continuous pralidoxime infusion arm, there was a significant reduction in atropine requirements, a smaller number of patients require intubation, fewer days of intubation, and a reduction in mortality from 8% to 1%. It should be noted that the iodide salt of pralidoxime was used and would equate to about 650 mg/h of the chloride salt.[23] Even though the majority of the patients by history ingested dimethoate, a dimethoxy compound with high lethality and rapid aging, the time to admission and administration of pralidoxime was very short, with a median time of 2 hours. Criticisms of the study include a lack of blinding, no measurement of AChE or pesticide concentrations, and no objective monitoring of neuromuscular function.[23] By contrast, the most recent trial performed in Sri Lanka was unable to demonstrate a beneficial effect of pralidoxime in 121 patients compared to 114 patients treated with placebo.[21] There was no difference in mortality between groups, although

pralidoxime effectively reactivated red cell AChE inhibited by diethoxy OP insecticides. It also reactivated red cell AChE inhibited by dimethoxy OP insecticides, but less so, as expected. In comparison to the third study,[64] these patients arrived later (4.4 vs 2 hours), and the extent of supportive care was inferior. The exact reasons for these disparate results are unclear.

ROLE IN CARBAMATE TOXICITY

Acetylcholinesterases inactivated by most carbamates spontaneously reactivate with half-lives of 1 to 2 hours, and typical clinical recovery occurs in several hours. However, in severe cases, cholinergic findings may persist for 24 hours.[10,29] Pralidoxime is rarely indicated for carbamate poisoning, but it is not contraindicated as previously suggested. This erroneous conclusion was based solely on data regarding a single carbamate, carbaryl, and inappropriately applied to all carbamates. Pralidoxime decreased the rate of carbamylation of 16 insecticidal carbamates, though it modestly increased the rates for 3, one of which was carbaryl.[15] In another experiment, pralidoxime had no effect on the reactivation of human erythrocyte AChE carbamylated by aldicarb, methomyl, and carbaryl.[47] Furthermore, animal studies demonstrated the beneficial effects of pralidoxime in decreasing the lethality of several carbamate insecticides,[63,80] though it worsened the toxicity of carbaryl. An in vitro kinetic study demonstrated a 60% increased rate of inhibition with carbaryl and pralidoxime.[91] It was suggested that this is possibly because the carbamate–oxime complex may actually be a more potent cholinesterase inhibitor than carbaryl alone.[29,63,80] However, even in the presence of carbaryl, the combination of atropine plus an oxime, a more clinically relevant situation, resulted in survival data comparable to that of atropine alone.[29] Previous animal data may also be confounded by the use of excessive doses of pralidoxime.[57] The evidence in total suggests that pralidoxime is rarely a necessary adjunct to atropine for a patient with a pure carbamate overdose. However, there are cases reports, particularly with aldicarb, where pralidoxime appears to improve outcome.[10] Thus, pralidoxime should never be withheld in a seriously poisoned patient out of concern that a cholinergic xenobiotic is a carbamate.[47] Pralidoxime should be used in conjunction with atropine and rarely as the sole therapy in OP or carbamate poisoning.[34]

ADVERSE EFFECTS AND SAFETY ISSUES

At therapeutic doses of pralidoxime in humans, adverse effects are minimal.[27,28,60-62,70,85] Transient dizziness, blurred vision, and elevations in diastolic blood pressure appear to be related to the rate of administration.[35,55] Doses of 45 mg/kg produce blood pressure elevations that persist for several hours, but are reversed with IV phentolamine.[77] The most recent randomized clinical trial revealed a higher percentage of patients with tachycardia and hypertension associated with pralidoxime compared to placebo after both the loading dose and the continuous infusion (75% vs 49% and 30% vs 14%). Rapid IV administration has produced sudden cardiac and respiratory arrest as a result of laryngospasm and muscle rigidity,[36,66,76,97] whereas IM administration in volunteers produced diplopia, dizziness, headache, drowsiness, nausea, tachycardia, increased systolic blood pressure, hyperventilation, decreased kidney function, muscular weakness, and pain at the injection site.[68] Elevations in hepatic aminotransferase concentrations were observed in volunteers administered autoinjector doses of 1,200 to 1,800 mg; these enzyme concentrations returned to normal in 2 weeks.[68] An important safety issue is inadvertent provider or patient contact with the "active" needle end of autoinjectors or autoinjector systems, triggering unintended administration, self-administration, needle injury, or delivery to an unintended site.

PREGNANCY AND LACTATION

Pralidoxime is FDA pregnancy risk category C. Reproduction studies have not been done, and human case reports are limited. However, considering the maternal benefit of pralidoxime, it should be used as clinically indicated to protect the maternal fetal dyad. The use of pralidoxime should not be withheld because of pregnancy.[9] It is unknown whether pralidoxime is excreted into breast milk.

DOSING AND ADMINISTRATION

The optimal dosage regimen for pralidoxime is unknown. A loading dose of 2 g over 30 minutes followed by a maintenance dose in adults of 1 g/h of pralidoxime iodide was used in the study from India.[64] One gram of pralidoxime iodide is approximately equal to 650 mg of pralidoxime chloride.[64] The package insert, last updated in 2012, recommends a pediatric loading dose of 20 to 50 mg/kg (not to exceed 2,000 mg/dose) over 15 to 30 minutes followed by a continuous infusion of 10 to 20 mg/kg/h.[69] The package insert also recommends an adult dose of 1 to 2 g in 100 mL of 0.9% sodium chloride given intravenously over 15 to 30 minutes, with an additional dose in one hour if muscle weakness persists and then given every 10 to 12 hours if muscle weakness persists.[69] This dose is most likely insufficient in severely poisoned adult patients. The package insert then goes on to state that pharmacokinetic evidence suggests that a loading dose followed by a continuous infusion is more likely to maintain therapeutic serum concentrations as compared to intermittent dosing.[69] Difficulties arise because a target serum concentration in humans has not been established, although in vitro studies suggest a target concentration closer to 17 mcg/mL compared with the 4 mcg/mL previously suggested.[22,24,38] This is complicated by the possibility that there is a ceiling dose and that some OP compounds are more easily reactivated than others. In addition, pharmacokinetic studies in volunteers suggest that a continuous infusion maintains a target concentration with less variation compared with intermittent boluses.[55]

Based on all of the above, we recommend a loading dose of pralidoxime chloride of 30 mg/kg (up to 2 g) over 15 to 30 minutes followed by a maintenance infusion of 8 to 10 mg/kg/h for adults (up to 650 mg/h) and 10 to 20 mg/kg/h for children (up to 650 mg/h).[83]

The addition of 20 mL of sterile water for injection to the 1-g vial of pralidoxime chloride results in a 5% solution (50 mg/mL). Following reconstitution, the pralidoxime should be used within several hours. This solution can be further diluted to a volume of 100 mL of 0.9% sodium chloride solution for IV infusion, or a concentration of 10 to 20 mg/mL. The loading dose can be infused over 15 to 30 minutes. If pulmonary edema is present, the 1 g of pralidoxime in 20 mL can be infused slowly over not less than 5 minutes.[69]

Although IV administration is preferred, IM administration is acceptable using a 1-g vial of pralidoxime reconstituted with 3 mL of sterile water or 0.9% sodium chloride for injection to provide a solution containing 300 mg/mL (concentrations above 35% weight/volume produce muscle necrosis in animals).[78] This could be used until an IV site is established. Intraosseous administration is likely to be as effective or superior to IM delivery and was demonstrated to achieve excellent serum concentrations in a swine model.[89] Patients with reduced kidney function may require dosage adjustment, but there are no specific recommendations on how to accomplish this. In patients with ARDS, the dose can be given as a 5% solution by a slow IV injection over at least 15 to 30 minutes.[78]

Depending on the severity of a nerve agent exposure, one to 3 injections with a pair of autoinjectors containing atropine and pralidoxime or one to 3 injections of a DuoDote autoinjector that contains both atropine and pralidoxime in one device and injects both automatically should be administered into the outer thigh and held in place for 10 seconds (administration is similar to that of an EpiPen autoinjector). The number of autoinjector doses administered to a child depends on the age and weight of the child.[30,52] For children aged 3 to 7 years (13–25 kg), one autoinjector of atropine and one autoinjector of pralidoxime is recommended for administration, which should result in a projected pralidoxime dose of 24 to 46 mg/kg. For children aged 8 to 14 years, 2 autoinjectors of atropine and 2 autoinjectors of pralidoxime is recommended for administration. These injections should result in a projected pralidoxime dose of 24 to 46 mg/kg. For anyone older than 14 years of age, 3 autoinjectors of atropine and pralidoxime is recommended for administration. This results in a projected dose of pralidoxime of less than 35 mg/kg. For children younger than 3 years, during an emergency, one autoinjector of atropine and one of pralidoxime may be administered in accordance with a risk-to-benefit analysis. If time permits and only autoinjector doses are available, its contents may be transferred to a small sterile vial for traditional IM administration with a needle and syringe.[31]

Duration of Treatment

The signs and symptoms of OP poisoning usually manifest within minutes but infrequently are delayed up to 24 hours.[62] Delayed manifestations occur with the fat-soluble compounds, such as fenthion or chlorfenthion. The route of exposure also influences the onset of systemic symptoms. For example, there are delays following dermal contact, which does not occur following ingestion or inhalation. When symptoms are either delayed or prolonged, or when treatment is delayed, extended therapy with pralidoxime will usually be indicated.[1,7,59] In one case of poisoning with the fat soluble compound fenthion, 5 days elapsed before cholinergic symptoms appeared, and some symptoms then persisted for 30 days.[59] Pralidoxime and atropine were administered continuously in varying doses for the time that the patient was symptomatic. Therefore, the most practical recommendation is to continue the pralidoxime until symptoms have resolved and atropine has not been needed for 12 to 24 hours.[19] Other recommendations for estimating the duration of pralidoxime therapy include (1) measuring the serum or urinary concentration of the OP compound, (2) measuring serial determinations of plasma cholinesterase (increasing concentrations suggests the elimination of the OP compound), (3) incubating the patient's serum with an exogenous source of AChE or butyrylcholinesterase to assess inhibition, and (4) incubating the patient's inhibited red blood cell cholinesterase with a high concentration of oxime in vitro, to assess reactivation.[21] However, none of these measures are practical. Measurements of urinary concentrations of OP or AChE or BuChE are not likely to happen in real time. Furthermore, BuChE is not a good surrogate for OP inhibition.

In summary, duration of pralidoxime therapy is variable, dependent on the particular OP and dose ingested, and different for each patient. A reasonable approach would be to discontinue the pralidoxime when the patient has improved and no longer requires atropine. The patient must be observed carefully for recrudescence of toxicity potentially from a fat-soluble long-acting OP. If symptoms return, therapy with pralidoxime and atropine should be continued for at least an additional 24 hours.

FORMULATION AND ACQUISITION

Pralidoxime chloride (Protopam) is supplied in 20-mL vials containing 1 g of powder, ready for reconstitution with sterile water or 0.9% sodium chloride for injection.[67,69]

As noted above, pralidoxime chloride is also available for IM administration by an autoinjector containing 600 mg of pralidoxime in 2 mL of sterile water for injection with 20 mg of benzyl alcohol and 11.26 mg of glycine. The 2-PAM autoinjector is also packaged in a kit containing 600 mg of pralidoxime in 2 mL of sterile water for injection with 40 mg of benzyl alcohol and 22.5 mg of glycine, accompanied by an autoinjector containing 2.1 mg of atropine in 0.7 mL of a sterile solution containing 12.47 mg of glycerin and not more than 2.8 mg of phenol. This kit is called a "Mark I Nerve Agent Antidote Kit (NAAK)" and is designed to be used IM by first responders in case of a nerve agent attack. The needles extend 0.8 inches in length. The Mark I NAAK was replaced by the DuoDote Autoinjector System and the analogous, military-designated Antidote Treatment Nerve Agent Autoinjector (ATNAA), which use technology that sequentially administers 2.1 mg of atropine in 0.7 mL followed by 600 mg of pralidoxime chloride in 2 mL IM through the same syringe.[16] The 23-gauge needle is 0.8 inches in length. Pralidoxime is maintained as part of the Strategic National Stockpile (SNS) formulary in repositories in numerous locations throughout the United States.

SUMMARY

- Pralidoxime is an effective reactivator of AChE in many OP compound poisonings primarily reversing neuromuscular manifestations.
- The sooner pralidoxime is administered after the onset of OP toxicity, the more effective it is likely to be, although there is no absolute time limitation on reactivation function.
- Pralidoxime and atropine are synergistic and should be used together in the management of patients with OP poisonings.

- If a patient requires multiple doses of atropine for muscarinic symptoms or has neuromuscular weakness, then the use of 2-PAM is recommended.
- Because newer, highly fat-soluble OP compounds are currently available, it is necessary to administer atropine and 2-PAM for more prolonged periods of time than previously suggested.
- It is reasonable to stop 2-PAM when the patient is clinically well, atropine is no longer needed and neuromuscular weakness, if initially present, has recovered.

Acknowledgment

Cynthia K. Aaron, MD, contributed to this chapter in previous editions.

REFERENCES

1. Aaron CK, Smilkstein M. Intermediate syndrome or inadequate therapy [abstract]. *Vet Human Toxicol.* 1988;30:370.
2. Amos WC Jr, Hall A. Malathion poisoning treated with Protopam. *Ann Intern Med.* 1965;62:1013-1016.
3. Antonijevic B, Stojiljkovic M. Unequal efficacy of pyridinium oximes in acute organophosphate poisoning. *Clin Med Res.* 2006;5:71-82.
4. Blaber LC, Creasey NH. The mode of recovery of cholinesterase activity in vivo after organophosphorus poisoning: I. Erythrocyte cholinesterase. *Biochem J.* 1960;77:591-596.
5. Blaber LC, Creasey NH. The mode of recovery of cholinesterase activity in vivo after organophosphorus poisoning: II. Brain cholinesterase. *Biochem J.* 1960;77:597-604.
6. Bokowjic D, et al. Protective effects of oximes HI-6, and PAM 2, applied by osmotic minipumps in quinalphos poisoned rats. *Arch Int Pharmacodyn Ther.* 1987;288:309-318.
7. Borowitz SM. Prolonged organophosphate toxicity in a twenty-six-month-old child. *J Pediatr.* 1988;112:303-304.
8. Bowls BJ, et al. Oral treatment of organophosphate poisoning in mice. *Acad Emerg Med.* 2003;10:286-288.
9. Briggs GG, et al. *Drugs in Pregnancy and Lactation.* Philadelphia, PA: Lippincott Williams & Wilkins; 2011.
10. Burgess JL, et al. Aldicarb poisoning—a case report with prolonged cholinesterase inhibition and improvement after pralidoxime therapy. *Arch Intern Med.* 1994;154:221-224.
11. Clement JG, et al. The acetylcholinesterase oxime reactivator HI-6, in man: pharmacokinetics and tolerability in combination with atropine. *Biopharm Drug Dispos.* 1995;16:415-425.
12. Costa L. Current issues in organophosphate toxicology. *Clin Chim Acta.* 2006;366:1-13.
13. Davies DR, Green AL. The kinetics of reactivation, by oximes, of cholinesterase inhibited by organophosphorus compounds. *Biochemistry.* 1956;63:529-535.
14. Davison AN. Return of cholinesterase activity in the rat after inhibition by organophosphorus compounds: I. Diethyl *p*-nitrophenyl phosphate (E600 Paraoxon). *Biochem J.* 1953;54:583-590.
15. Dawson RM. Oximes in treatment of carbamate poisoning. *Vet Rec.* 1994;134:687.
16. DuoDote (atropine and pralidoxime chloride injection) Auto Injector [package insert]. Columbia, MD: Meridian Medical Technologies, Inc; 2017.
17. Durham WF, Hayes WJ Jr. Organic phosphorus poisoning and its therapy. *Arch Environ Health.* 1962;5:21-47.
18. Eddleston M. The pathophysiology of organophosphorus pesticide self-poisoning is not so simple. *Neth J Med.* 2008;66:146-148.
19. Eddelston M, et al. Management of acute organophosphorous pesticide poisoning. *Lancet.* 2008;371:597-607.
20. Eddleston M, et al. Oximes in acute organophosphorous pesticide poisoning: a systematic review of clinical trials. *Q J Med.* 2002;95:275-283.
21. Eddleston M, et al. Pralidoxime in acute organophosphorus insecticide poisoning—a randomized controlled trial. *PLoS Med.* 2009;6:1-12.
22. Eyer P. The role of oximes in the management of organophosphorus pesticide poisoning. *Toxicol Rev.* 2003;22:166-190.
23. Eyer P, Buckley N. Pralidoxime for organophosphate poisoning. *Lancet.* 2006; 368: 2110-2111.
24. Eyer P, et al. Testing of antidotes for organophosphorous compounds: experimental procedures and clinical reality. *Toxicology.* 2007;233:108-119.
25. Finkelstein Y, et al. CNS involvement in acute organophosphate poisoning: specific pattern of toxicity, clinical correlates and antidotal treatment. *Ital J Neurol Sci.* 1988;9:437-446.
26. Goel P, et al. Regeneration of red cell cholinesterase activity following pralidoxime (2-PAM) infusion in first 24 h in organophosphate poisoned patients. *Indian J Clin Biochem.* 2012;27:34-39.
27. Grob D, Jones RJ. Use of oximes in the treatment of intoxication by anticholinesterase compounds in normal subjects. *Am J Med.* 1958;24:497-511.
28. Hagerstrom-Portnoy G, et al. Effects of atropine and 2-PAM chloride on vision and performance in humans. *Aviat Space Environ Med.* 1987;10:47-53.
29. Harris LW, et al. The relationship between oxime-induced reactivation of carbamylated acetylcholinesterase and antidotal efficacy against carbamate intoxication. *Toxicol Appl Pharmacol.* 1989;98:128-133.
30. Henretig FM, et al. Biological and chemical terrorism. *J Pediatr.* 2002;141:311-326.
31. Henretig FM, et al. Potential use of autoinjector-packaged antidotes for treatment of pediatric nerve agent toxicity. *Ann Emerg Med.* 2002;40:405-408.
32. Hobbiger F. Chemical reactivation of phosphorylated human and bovine true cholinesterase. *Br J Pharmacol.* 1956;11:295-303.
33. Hobbiger F. Effect of nicotinehydroxamic acid methiodide on human plasma cholinesterase inhibited by organophosphates containing dialkylphosphate groups. *Br J Pharmacol.* 1955;10:356-362.
34. Hoffman RS, et al. Use of pralidoxime without atropine in rivastigmine (carbamate) toxicity. *Hum Exp Toxicol.* 2009;28:599-602.
35. Jager BV, Staff GN. Toxicity of diacetyl monoxime and of pyridine-2-aldoxime methiodide in man. *Bull Johns Hopkins Hosp.* 1958;102:203-211.
36. Jeong TO, et al. Respiratory arrest caused by accidental rapid pralidoxime infusion. *Clin Toxicol.* 2015;53:412.
37. John H, et al. Quantification of pralidoxime (2-PAM) in urine by ion pair chromatography-diode array detection: application to in vivo samples from minipig. *Drug Test Anal.* 2012;4:169-178.
38. Jun D, et al. Potency of several oximes to reactivate human acetylcholinesterase and butyrylcholinesterase inhibited by paraoxon in vitro. *Chem Biol Interact.* 2008;175:421-424.
39. Kalasz H, et al. Mini review on blood-brain barrier penetration of pyridinium aldoximes. *J Appl Toxicol.* 2015;35:116-123.
40. Karczmar A. Invited review. Anticholinesterases: dramatic aspects of their use and misuse. *Neurochem Int.* 1998;32:401-411.
41. Kassa J, Cabal J. A comparison of the efficacy of a new asymmetric bispyridinium oxime BI-6, with currently available oximes and H oximes against soman in in vitro and in vivo methods. *Toxicology.* 1999;132:111-118.
42. Khan S, et al. Neuroparalysis and oxime efficacy in organophosphate poisoning: a study of butyrylcholinesterase. *Hum Exp Toxicol.* 2001;20:169-174.
43. Kondritzer A, et al. Blood plasma levels and elimination of salts of 2-PAM in man after oral administration. *J Pharm Sci.* 1968;57:1142-1145.
44. Konickx L, et al. Reactivation of plasma butyrylcholinesterase by pralidoxime chloride in patients poisoned by WHO Class II Toxicity organophosphorus insecticides. *Toxicol Sci.* 2013;136:274-283.
45. Krishnan JK, et al. Intranasal delivery of obidoxime to the brain prevents mortality and CNS damage from organophosphate poisoning. *Neurotoxicology.* 2016;53:64-73.
46. Kusic R, et al. HI-6, in man: efficacy of the oxime in poisoning by organophosphorus insecticides. *Hum Exp Toxicol.* 1991;10:113-118.
47. Lifshitz M, et al. Carbamate poisoning and oxime treatment in children: a clinical and laboratory study. *Pediatrics.* 1994;93:652-655.
48. Lotti M, Becker C. Treatment of acute organophosphate-poisoning: evidence of a direct effect on central nervous system by 2-PAM (pyridine-2-aldoxime methyl chloride). *J Toxicol Clin Toxicol.* 1982;19:121-127.
49. Lugokenski TH, et al. Effect of different oximes on rat and human cholinesterases inhibited by methamidophos: a comparative in vitro and in silico study. *Basic Clin Pharmacol Toxicol.* 2012;111:362-370.
50. Lundy PM, et al. Comparison of several oximes against poisoning by soman, tabun and GF. *Toxicology.* 1992;72:99-105.
51. Luo C, et al. Phosphoryl oxime inhibition of acetylcholinesterase during oxime reactivation is prevented by edrophonium. *Biochemistry.* 1999;38:9937-9947.
52. Markenson D, Redlener I. Pediatric terrorism preparedness national guidelines and recommendations: findings of an evidenced-based consensus process. *Biosecur Bioterror.* 2004;2:301-319.
53. Matin M, Siddiqui R. Modification of the level of acetylcholinesterase activity by two oximes in certain brain regions and peripheral tissues of paraoxon treated rats. *Pharmacol Res Commun.* 1982;4:241-246.
54. Mattingly JE, et al. Intermediate syndrome after exposure to chlorpyrifos in a 16-month-old girl. *J Emerg Med.* 2003;25:379-381.
55. Medicis JJ, et al. Pharmacokinetics following a loading plus a continuous infusion of pralidoxime compared with the traditional short infusion regimen in human volunteers. *J Toxicol Clin Toxicol.* 1996;34:289-295.
56. Mercey G, et al. Reactivators of acetylcholinesterase inhibited by organophosphorus nerve agents. *Acc Chem Res.* 2012;45:756-766.
57. Mercurio-Zappala M, et al. Pralidoxime in carbaryl poisoning: an animal model. *Hum Exp Toxicol.* 2007;26:125-129.
58. Milosevic MP, Andjelkovic D. Reactivation of paraoxon-inactivated cholinesterase in the rat cerebral cortex by pralidoxime chloride. *Nature.* 1966;210:206.
59. Merrill D, Mihm F. Prolonged toxicity of organophosphate poisoning. *Crit Care Med.* 1982;10:550-551.
60. Namba T. Diagnosis and treatment of organophosphate insecticide poisoning. *Med Times.* 1972;100:100-126.
61. Namba T, Hiraki K. PAM (pyridine-2-aldoxime methiodide) therapy for alkyl-phosphate poisoning. *JAMA.* 1958;166:1834-1839.
62. Namba T, et al. Poisoning due to organophosphate insecticides: acute and chronic manifestations. *Am J Med.* 1971;50:475-492.
63. Natoff IL, Reiff B. Effect of oximes on the acute toxicology of acetylcholinesterase carbamates. *Toxicol Appl Pharmacol.* 1973;25:569-575.
64. Pawar K, et al. Continuous pralidoxime infusion versus repeated bolus injection to treat organophosphorous pesticide poisoning. A randomized trial. *Lancet.* 2006;368:2136-2141.

65. Petroianu GA. The history of pyridinium oximes as nerve gas antidotes: the British contribution. *Pharmazie*. 2013;68:916-918.

66. Pickering EN. Organic phosphate insecticide poisoning. *Can J Med Technol*. 1966;28:174-179.

67. Pralidoxime. In: Kastrup E, ed. *Facts and Comparisons*. Philadelphia, PA: JB Lippincott; 1983.

68. Pralidoxime Chloride injection (Auto-Injector) [package insert]. The antidote treatment–nerve agent, auto-injector (ATNAA) package insert. Columbia, MD: Meridian Medical Technologies, Inc; March 2017.

69. Protopam Chloride (pralidoxime chloride) for injection [package insert]. Deerfield, IL: Baxter Healthcare Corporation; 2012.

70. Quimby G. Further therapeutic experience with pralidoximes in organic phosphorus poisoning. *JAMA*. 1963;187:202-206.

71. Rotenberg J, Newmark J. Nerve agent attacks on children: diagnosis and management. *Pediatrics*. 2003;112:648-658.

72. Rousseaux CG, Du AK. Pharmacology of HI-6, an H-series oxime. *Can J Physiol Pharmacol*. 1989;67:1183-1189.

73. Sakurada K, et al. Pralidoxime iodide (2-PAM) penetrates across the blood–brain barrier. *Neurochem Res*. 2003;28:1401-1407.

74. Sanderson DM. Treatment of poisoning by anticholinesterase insecticides in the rat. *J Pharm Pharmacol*. 1961;13:435-442.

75. Schexnayder S, et al. The pharmacokinetics of continuous infusion pralidoxime in children with organophosphate poisoning. *J Toxicol Clin Toxicol*. 1998;36:549-555.

76. Scott RJ. Repeated asystole following PAM in organophosphate self-poisoning. *Anaesth Intensive Care*. 1986;4:458-460.

77. Sidell FR. Nerve agents. In: Zajtchuk R, ed. *Textbook of Military Medicine: Medical Aspects of Chemical and Biological Warfare, Part I*. Office of the Surgeon General Department of the Army, United States of America; 1997:129-179.

78. Sidell FR, Groff WA. Intramuscular and intravenous administration of small doses of 2-pyridinium aldoxime methylchloride to man. *J Pharm Sci*. 1971;60:1224-1228.

79. Sidell FR, et al. Enhancement of drug absorption after administration by an automatic injector. *J Pharm Sci*. 1974;2:197-210.

80. Sterri S, et al. Effect of toxogenin and P2S on the toxicity of carbamates and organophosphorus compounds. *Acta Pharmacol Toxicol*. 1979;45:9-15.

81. Sudakin D, et al. Intermediate syndrome after malathion ingestion despite continuous infusion of pralidoxime. *J Toxicol Clin Toxicol*. 2000;38:47-50.

82. Sundwall A. Minimum concentrations of *N*-methyl pyridinium-2-aldoxime methane sulphonate (PS2) which reverse neuromuscular block. *Biochem Pharmacol*. 1961;8:413-417.

83. Tang X, et al. Repeated pulse intramuscular injection of pralidoxime chloride in severe acute organophosphorus pesticide poisoning. *Am J Emerg Med*. 2013;31:946-949.

84. Taylor P. Anticholinesterase agents. In: Hardman JG, et al., eds. *Goodman and Gilman's The Pharmacological Basis of Therapeutics*. 9th ed. New York, NY: Macmillan; 1996:100-119.

85. Thompson DF, et al. Therapeutic dosing of pralidoxime chloride. *Drug Intell Clin Pharm*. 1987;21:1590-1593.

86. Tush G, Anstead M. Pralidoxime continuous infusion ion the treatment of organophosphate poisoning. *Ann Pharmacother*. 1997;31:441-444.

87. Uehara S, et al. Studies on the therapeutic effect of 2-pyridine aldoxime methiodide (2-PAM) in mammals following organophosphorous compound (OP)-poisoning (report III): distribution and antidotal effect of 2-PAM in rats. *J Toxicol*. 1993;18:265-275.

88. Uehara S, et al. Studies on the therapeutic effect of 2-pyridine aldoxime methiodide (2-PAM) in mammals following organophosphorous compound (OP)-poisoning (report II): aging of OP-inhibited mammalian cholinesterase. *J Toxicol*. 1993;18:179-183.

89. Uwaydah N, et al. Intramuscular versus intraosseous delivery of nerve agent antidote pralidoxime chloride in swine. *Prehosp Emerg Care*. 2016;20:485-492.

90. Wiener SW, Hoffman RS. Nerve agents: a comprehensive review. *J Intensive Care Med*. 2004;19:22-37.

91. Wille T, et al. Investigation of kinetic interactions between approved oximes and human acetylcholinesterase inhibited by pesticide carbamates. *Chem Biol Interact*. 2013;206:569-572.

92. Willems JL, et al. Cholinesterase reactivation in organophosphorus poisoned patients depends on the plasma concentrations of the oxime pralidoxime methylsulfate and of the organophosphate. *Arch Toxicol*. 1993;97:79-84.

93. Willems JL, et al. Plasma concentrations of pralidoxime methyl sulfate in organophosphorus poisoned patients. *Arch Toxicol*. 1992;66:260-266.

94. Wilson IB. Molecular complementarity and antidotes for alkylphosphate poisoning. *Fed Proc*. 1959;18(2, pt 1):752-758.

95. Wilson IB, Ginsburg B. A powerful reactivator of alkylphosphate-inhibited acetylcholinesterase. *Biochim Biophys Acta*. 1955;18:168-170.

96. Winter M, et al. Investigation of the reactivation kinetics of a large series of bispyridium oximes with organophosphate-inhibited human acetylcholinesterase. *Toxicol Lett*. 2016;244:136-142.

97. Wislicki L. Differences in the effect of oximes on striated muscle and respiratory centre. *Arch Int Pharmacodyn Ther*. 1960;120:1-19.

98. Wong L, et al. Mechanism of oxime reactivation of acetylcholinesterase analyzed by chirality and mutagenesis. *Biochemistry*. 2000;39:5750-5757.

99. Worek F, et al. Reappraisal of indications and limitations of oxime therapy in organophosphate poisoning. *Hum Exp Toxicol*. 1997;16:466-472.

100. Worek F, et al. Reactivation and aging kinetics of human acetylcholinesterase inhibited by organophosphonylcholines. *Arch Toxicol*. 2004;78:212-217.

101. Worek F, et al. Kinetic analysis of interactions between human acetylcholinesterase, structurally different organophosphorous compounds and oximes. *Biochem Pharmacol*. 2004;68:2237-2248.

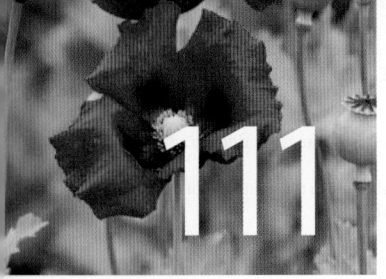

INSECTICIDES: ORGANIC CHLORINES, PYRETHRINS/PYRETHROIDS, AND INSECT REPELLENTS

Michael G. Holland

ORGANIC CHLORINE PESTICIDES

History and Epidemiology

Until the 1940s, commonly available pesticides included highly toxic arsenicals, mercurials, lead, sulfur, and nicotine. When Nobel Prize–winning chemist Paul Müller demonstrated the insecticidal properties of dichlorodiphenyltrichloroethane (DDT) in the early 1940s, a whole new class of pesticides was introduced. The organic chlorine insecticides (DDT, lindane, cyclodienes, and others) were inexpensive to produce, nonvolatile, environmentally stable, and had relatively low acute toxicity when compared to previous insecticides. Most organic chlorines have a negative temperature coefficient, making them more insecticidal at lower temperatures, and less toxic to warm-blooded organisms (Table 111–1).[168] Widespread use of these insecticides occurred from the 1940s until the mid-1970s. They were highly effective and revolutionized modern agriculture, allowing unprecedented crop output from each acre of arable land. Because of their stability, organic chlorines were used extensively in structural protection (termites, carpenter ants) and soil treatments. Medical and public health applications of DDT and its analogues were also found in the control of typhus body louse, and eradication of malaria in many countries by eliminating the mosquito vector.[36] By 1953, DDT alone was credited for saving an estimated 50 million lives, and with averting one billion cases of human disease, and is credited with eliminating malaria from the United States and Europe. It is suggested that because of this consequential impact on human health, DDT is the single most important factor in the world population explosion that occurred between 1950 and 1970.[48]

However, the properties that made these chemicals such effective insecticides were suspected as posing environmental hazards: they are slowly metabolized, lipid soluble, chemically stable, and environmentally persistent. In her 1962 book, *Silent Spring*,[17] Rachel Carson, a biologist with the US Fish and Wildlife Service, claimed that since organic chlorines are bioconcentrated and biomagnified up the food chain, this persistence could eventually lead to increases in cancer in the future, as well as having adverse effects on wildlife. The controversy arose when scientific opinions suggested that organic chlorine residues caused eggshell thinning and decreased reproductive success in predatory birds.[47] Although testing on domesticated birds,[18,26,126,166] when fed large amounts of DDT, showed little or no eggshell thinning, testing in mallard ducks did.[42,43] Hearings before the Environmental Protection Agency (EPA) regarding DDT registration focused also on the unproven fear of placing future generations at risk of cancer. This, and the demonstration of persistent DDT residues in all humans, even those living in areas where DDT was never utilized (eg, Native Alaskans) led to the severe restriction or total ban of DDT and most other organic chlorines in North America and Europe.[36] There is considerable evidence that since DDT was banned, less-effective replacements have placed many more millions at risk for malaria, and is at least in part responsible for millions of preventable deaths from this disease.[100,123,124] Dichlorodiphenyltrichloroethane is still considered a highly effective mosquito control agent with a low order of acute toxicity and is very inexpensive compared to newer replacement insecticides. For these reasons, the World Health Organization (WHO) exempted DDT from its list of banned pesticides, and it is still widely used for malaria control programs in many countries, because alternatives are more expensive and must be applied more frequently. Current use of DDT for indoor residual spraying is ongoing in endemic areas in Africa, and is considered safe and effective as a public health initiative to control malaria, even in areas with drug resistant strains.[131]

Organic chlorine pesticides are complex, cyclic polychlorinated hydrocarbons having molecular weights generally in the range of 300–550 Da. They are nonvolatile solids at room temperature. Most act as central nervous system stimulants.

The organic chlorine pesticides are grouped into 4 categories based on their chemical structures and similar toxicities: (a) DDT and related analogues; (b) cyclodienes (the related isomers aldrin, dieldrin, and endrin; and heptachlor, endosulfan) and related compounds (toxaphene, dienochlor) (c) hexachlorocyclohexane (still in clinical use as the pediculicide lindane) or "gamma-benzene hexachloride" (Table 111–1 and Fig. 111–1); and (d) mirex and chlordecone. These organic chlorine insecticide compounds differ substantially, both between and within groups, with respect to toxic doses, mechanism of action, skin absorption, fat storage, metabolism, and elimination.[36] The signs and symptoms of toxicity in humans, however, are remarkably similar within each group.

Toxicokinetics

Absorption

All of the organic chlorine pesticides are well absorbed orally and by inhalation; transdermal absorption is variable. Absorption by any route is affected by the vehicle and the physical state (solid or liquid) of the pesticide. None of the organic chlorines are water-soluble, and are usually either dissolved in organic solvents or manufactured as powders for dusting.

DDT and its analogues methoxychlor, dicofol, and chlorobenzilate are very poorly absorbed transdermally, unless the pesticide is dissolved in a suitable hydrocarbon solvent.[121] Dichlorodiphenyltrichloroethane has limited volatility, so that air concentrations are usually low, and toxicity by the respiratory route is unlikely.

All of the cyclodienes have significant transdermal absorption rates and extent. Cutaneous absorption of dieldrin is approximately 50% that of the oral route. Oral absorption of the cyclodienes is also high, and significant poisonings have occurred when foodstuffs were contaminated with these pesticides.[15,21] Toxaphene is poorly absorbed through the skin in both acute and chronic exposures.[136]

Lindane is well absorbed after skin application, and in adults has a documented forearm skin absorption rate of 9.3% of a topically applied dose over 24 hours.[57] Anatomic sites vary in their absorptive capacities: axillary rates are 3.6 times faster, and scrotal skin absorption is 42 times faster than that of forearm skin.[13,61,78,146] Animal studies and case reports suggest that the young, the malnourished, and those who receive repeated topical doses are at risk for increased accumulation and toxicity.[113] Hot baths, occlusive clothing or bandages, the vehicle for the lindane, and a disturbed cutaneous integrity, such as eczema, fissures, and other violations of the skin, all enhance dermal penetration.[145,146] The state of hydration of the skin also affects the amounts absorbed, so that bathing just prior to application enhances absorption and increases the likelihood of toxicity.[98,146] Lindane is a stable compound, and volatilizes easily when heated. It was previously used extensively in home vaporizers, and toxicity was common via inhalation, and when vaporizer tablets were unintentionally ingested by children. Review of data when lindane was ingested therapeutically as an anthelmintic demonstrates that 40 mg/day for 3–14 days generally produced no adverse effects.[36]

Mirex and chlordecone are efficiently absorbed via skin, by inhalation, and orally.[56]

TABLE 111–1   Classification of Organic Chlorine Pesticides

Classes of Organic Chlorines	Specific Organic Chlorine	Current EPA Registration (US)	Acute Oral* Toxicity (Man)	Dermal Absorption	Lipid Solubility	Specific Characteristics
Hexachlorocyclohexanes	Lindane (γ isomer)	Topical scabicide; agricultural use canceled 2006	Moderate	High	Low	Seizures, CNS excitation; musty odor
DDT and analogues	DDT— Dichlorodiphenyltrichloroethane	Banned 1972	Slightly to moderately	Low	Highest	Tremors, CNS excitation; odorless
	Methoxychlor	Banned 2003	Slightly	Low	Moderate	Less toxic DDT substitute
	Dicofol	Residential use banned 1998; cotton, citrus, apple	Slightly	Low	Low	
	Chlorobenzilate	Banned 1983	Slightly	Low	Low	Much less environmental persistence than DDT
Cyclodienes and related compounds	Aldrin	Banned 1974	Highly	High	High	Rapidly metabolized to dieldrin; mild "chemical" odor
	Dieldrin	Banned 1974	Highly	High	High	Stereoisomer of endrin; early and late seizures; odorless
	Endrin	Banned 1974	Very Highly	High	None	Most toxic organic chlorine; rapid onset seizures, status epilepticus
	Chlordane	Banned 1988	Moderately	High	High	Early and late seizures occur
	Endosulfan	RED^a 2002	Highly	High	Low	Strong sulfur odor
	Heptachlor	Restricted: fire ant control, soil treatment	Moderately	High	High	Toxic metabolite heptachlor epoxide; odor of camphor
	Isobenzan	Never Registered	Highly	Moderate	High	Also inhibits Mg^{2+}-ATPase; mild "chemical" odor
	Dienochlor	Banned	NA	Low	Low	Toxic metabolite binds to glutathione
	Toxaphene (polychlorinated camphene)	Banned 1982	Moderately to highly	Low	Low	Seizures; turpentinelike odor, often mixed with parathion
Chlordecone and Mirex	Chlordecone	Banned 1977	Moderately	High	High	"Kepone shakes"; seizures not seen, structurally similar to mirex
	Mirex	Banned 1976	Slightly	High	High	(?) Converted to chlordecone, toxicity identical

^{a}RED = Re-registration eligibility decision.

*ACUTE ORAL TOXICITY: (from EPA- https://www.epa.gov/pesticide-registration/label-review-manual July 2014, accessed January 26, 2017) (see SC-9-1)

Category I LD_{50} < 50 mg/kg Label Language: DANGER Skull and Crossbones Fatal if swallowed = very highly or highly toxic

Category II LD_{50} > 50 mg/kg < 500 mg/kg WARNING No symbol May be fatal if swallowed = moderately toxic

Category III LD_{50} > 500 mg/kg < 5,000 mg/kg CAUTION No symbol Harmful if swallowed = slightly toxic

Category IV LD_{50} > 5,000 mg/kg CAUTION or no signal word No symbol No hazard statement required; registrant may choose to use Category III statement

{947 US Environmental Protection Agency Office of Pesticide Programs 2016}

Distribution

All organic chlorines are lipophilics, a property that allows penetration to their sites of action in insects and mammals.[31] The fat-to-serum ratios at equilibrium are high, in the range of 660:1 for chlordane;[65] 220:1 for lindane;[137] and 150:1 for dieldrin.[37] Central nervous system redistribution of the organic chlorines to the blood and then to fat most likely accounts for the apparent rapid CNS recovery despite the persistent substantial total body burden. Not surprisingly, there is a direct correlation between the concentration of DDT or dieldrin in the brain of rats and the clinical signs produced after a single dose of the insecticide.[36,39]

Metabolism

The high lipid solubility and very slow metabolic disposition of DDT, DDE (dichlorodiphenyl dichloroethylene, the primary metabolite of DDT), dieldrin, heptachlor, chlordane, mirex, and chlordecone causes significant adipose tissue storage and increasing body burdens in chronically exposed populations.[56] Organic chlorines that are rapidly metabolized and eliminated, such as endrin (an isomer of dieldrin), endosulfan, lindane, methoxychlor, dienochlor, chlorobenzilate, dicofol, and toxaphene tend to have less persistence in body tissues, despite being highly lipid soluble.[121]

Most organic chlorines are metabolized by the hepatic microsomal enzyme systems by dechlorination and oxidation, with subsequent conjugation. However, for some insecticides metabolism results in the production of a metabolite with more toxicity than the parent compound, such as heptachlor to heptachlor epoxide, chlordane to oxychlordane, and aldrin to dieldrin.

In animals, most organic chlorine pesticides are capable of inducing the hepatic microsomal enzyme systems.[34,171] Enzyme induction changes the biodegradation of the pesticide in rodents.[151] In certain animal models the acute toxicity of organic phosphorus compounds and carbamates is to be reduced by the administration of organic chlorines, presumably by induction of the hepatic microsomal metabolism of the organic phosphorus compound. This effect is ameliorated by administering the liver microsomal enzyme system inhibitor piperonyl butoxide.[36,171] However, induction of hepatic enzymes is not described in man, except in rare cases of massive exposure with concomitant neurologic findings.[56,65]

Elimination

The half-lives of fat-stored compounds and poorly metabolized organic chlorines such as DDT and chlordecone are measured in months or years, compared to the elimination half-life of lindane, which is 21 hours in

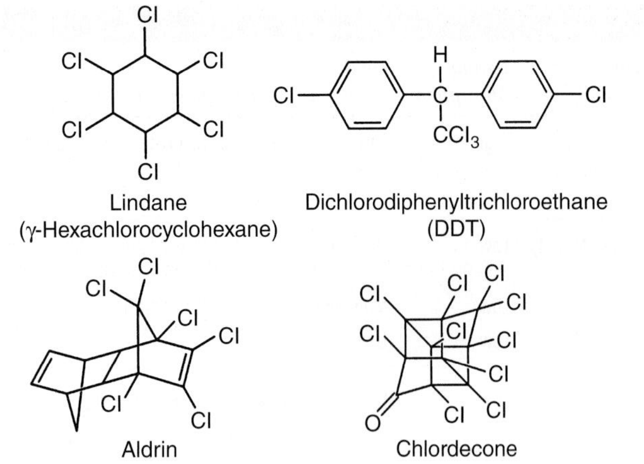

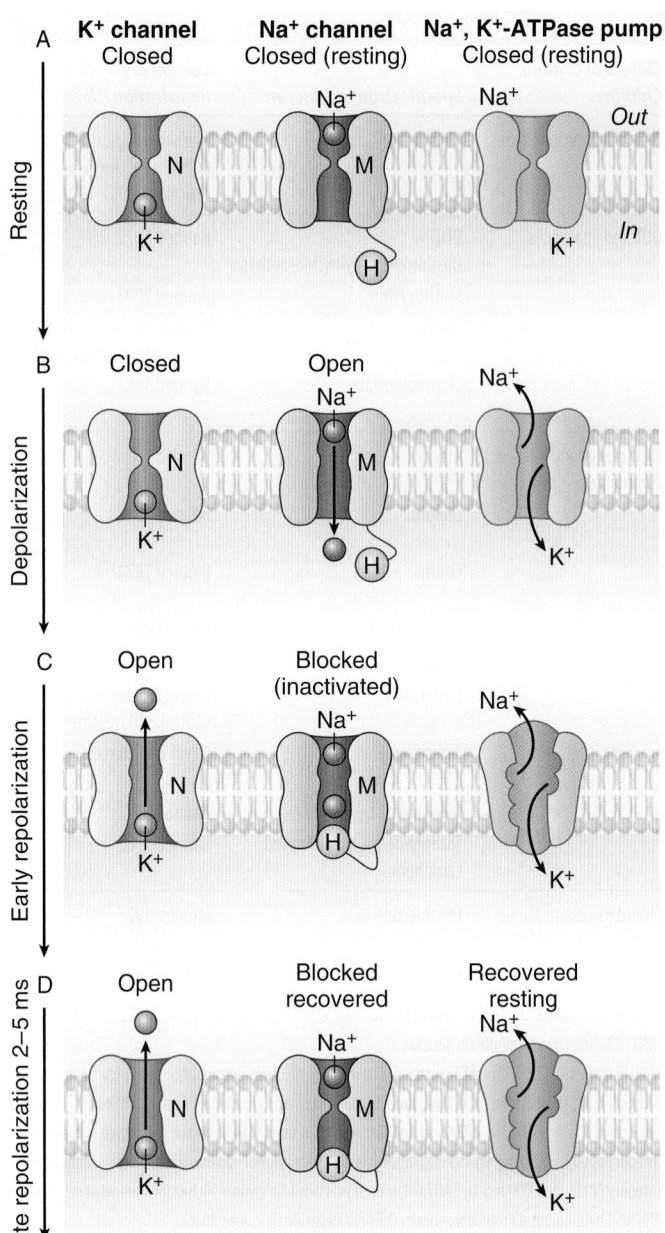

FIGURE 111–1. Structures of various organic chlorine pesticides.

adults.[99] The primary route of excretion of the organic chlorines is in the bile, but most also produce detectable urinary metabolites. However, as with other compounds excreted in bile, most of the organic chlorines, such as mirex and chlordecone, have significant enterohepatic or enteroenteric recirculation.[11,33,56] All of the lipophilic compounds are excreted in maternal milk.[128]

Mechanisms of Toxicity

The same neurotoxic properties that make the organic chlorines lethal to the target insects make them potentially toxic to higher forms of life. The organic chlorines exert their most important effects in both the central and peripheral nervous systems. Electrophysiologic studies demonstrate that the organic chlorine insecticides affect the membranes of excitable cells by either interfering with repolarization, by prolonging depolarization (both are Na^+ channel effects), or by impairing the maintenance of the polarized state of the neuron (gamma-aminobutyric acid ($GABA_A$) chloride ionophore effects). The end result is hyperexcitability of the nervous system and repetitive neuronal discharges with subsequent inhibition of further depolarization.[48]

The voltage-gated Na^+ channel is a common site of action for neurotoxins, both natural and synthetic. There are at least 10 separate binding sites on the Na^+ channel, including those for local anesthetics and anticonvulsants. Dichlorodiphenyltrichloroethane, as well as the pyrethroids (see below), bind at the same site on these channels (Fig. 111–2).

There are 2 primary gates in the Na^+ channel: the M gate and H gate. The extracellular entrance (the M gate) is voltage dependent, whereas the intracellular entrance (H gate) operates due to conformational changes in protein structure. Depolarization opens the voltage-dependent M gate, rapid influx of Na^+ then causes conformational change and closes the H gate, inactivating Na^+ influx. When repolarization restores polarity, the M gate closes and the H gate then re-opens, and the Na^+ channel returns to its resting state, ready to be activated again.

Dichlorodiphenyltrichloroethane and its analogues preferentially bind to the Na^+ channel when the M gate is open, allowing prolonged inward sodium conductance, repetitive action potentials, and extended tail currents. This occurs primarily in the peripheral nervous system with DDT and analogues, and prolonged axonal firing and repetitive stimulus eventually leads to nerve paralysis and death in target insects, whose Na^+ channels have much greater affinity for these insecticides than those in mammals.[35,41,104,105,107,147] In test animals, these Na^+ channel effects are manifested as exaggerated responses such as abnormal startle reflexes and tremors after low-level stimuli.[73,158] Further evidence of binding to the Na^+ channel and prolonging its open state as being the primary mechanism of action is the amelioration of DDT-induced tremor by pretreatment with phenytoin, a sodium channel blocker that acts by reducing the ability of voltage-dependent Na^+ channels to recover from inactivation.[73,159] Dichlorodiphenyltrichloroethane also inhibits Ca^{2+}-ATPase,

FIGURE 111–2. Sodium channel. Schematic drawing of voltage-gated neuronal Na^+ channel: demonstrating 4 phases of activation: (1) Closed, resting state: M gate closed, H gate open, cell is at normal polarized state, ready for activation. (2) Stimulus resulting in depolarization causes voltage-dependent M gate to open, allowing rapid Na^+ flow intracellularly, depolarizing the cell (H gate is open). (3) Inactivated (blocked) state: M gate still open, but depolarization causes a conformational change in the channel, and causes H gate to rapidly close (voltage independent), inactivating intracellular Na^+ flow. K^+ channels open to assist in repolarization (4) As repolarization is accomplished by Na^+,K^+-ATPase and K^+ channels, the voltage-dependent M gate closes again, conformational change reverts back to a recovered/resting position, and the H gate reopens. When the K^+ channel and Na^+, K^+-ATPase have completed repolarization the resting state (1) will be restored.

located on the external cell membrane. Inhibition of this pump likely contributes to membrane instability and repetitive discharges due to a reduction in external calcium concentrations.[35]

The cyclodienes and lindane act as GABA antagonists. They inhibit GABA binding at the $GABA_A$-receptor-chloride ionophore complex in the CNS, by interacting at the picrotoxin binding site.[102] In fact, the degree of binding at this site correlates well with the amount of Cl^- influx inhibited and the

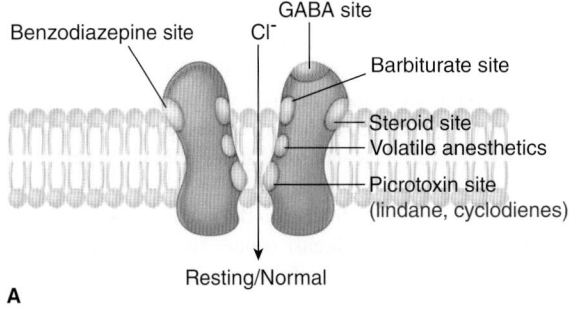

A Resting/Normal

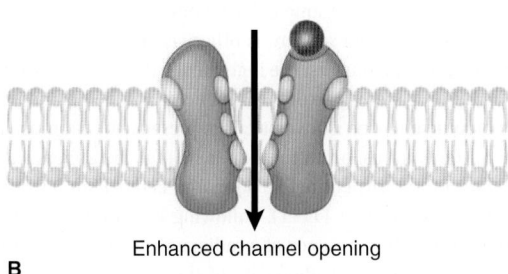

B Enhanced channel opening

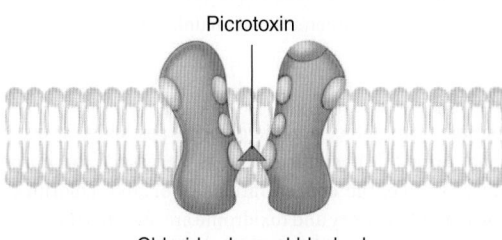

C Chloride channel blocked

FIGURE 111–3. Chloride channel. (A) Under resting conditions, a tonic influx of chloride maintains the nerve cell in a polarized state. (B) Binding of GABA or an indirect-acting GABA agonist (benzodiazepine, barbiturate, volatile anesthetic) opens the chloride channel. The subsequent chloride influx hyperpolarizes the cell membrane, making the neuron less likely to propagate an action potential in response to a stimulus. (C) GABA antagonists, such as picrotoxin, block the chloride channel, reducing chloride influx. The resulting decreased membrane polarity causes the neuron to become hyperexcitable to even those stimuli that are normally subthreshold in nature (Chap. 13).

relative neurotoxicity of each insecticide (Figs. 13–9, 13–10, and 111–3).[8,64] Indeed, development of cyclodiene resistance seems to be related to alterations of the GABA$_A$-receptor-chloride ionophore complex in these affected insects.[9,105] This also explains the efficacy of GABA agonists, such as benzodiazepines and phenobarbital, in treating the seizures and neurotoxicity of the cyclodienes[70] and lindane.[175] Toxaphene also inhibits GABA binding at the GABA$_A$ receptor-chloride ionophore complex.[136]

The mechanisms of action of mirex and chlordecone are not as well understood. They inhibit Na$^+$,K$^+$-ATPase, and Ca^{+2}-ATPase. However, lindane, DDT, and the cyclodienes also inhibit these enzymes yet produce very different symptoms of toxic effects, suggesting that these mechanisms aren't responsible for the clinical manifestations that occur in mirex and chlordecone poisoning. Phenytoin and serotonin agonists exacerbate the prominent tremor that occurs with chlordecone intoxication, but conversely attenuate the tremors in DDT poisoning, which further supports a different mechanism than the Na$^+$ channel effects of DDT.[48] Mirex and chlordecone are poor inhibitors of GABA binding at the GABA$_A$-receptor-chloride ionophore complex; therefore, their mechanism of action is likely not at this site,[56] and seizures are not described with mirex or chlordecone. Organic chlorines predispose test animals to cardiac dysrhythmias,[121] presumably via myocardial sensitization, similar to the chlorinated hydrocarbon solvents (Chaps. 15 and 105).

Drug Interactions

There are theoretical consequences of hepatic enzyme induction, such as enhanced metabolism of therapeutic drugs and/or reduced efficacy. Dysfunctional uterine bleeding was attributed to enhanced oral contraceptive metabolism induced by chlordane, but this report involved a single patient with weeks of excessive exposure to chlordane.[65] A large group of workers poisoned by chlordecone over many months had some increased hepatic microsomal activity, but no evidence of drug interactions or adverse clinical effects.[56] Thus, induction of the hepatic microsomal enzyme system by organic chlorines probably occurs only with extended, substantial exposure.[121] There are no definitive reports of enhanced metabolism of therapeutic drugs or adverse reactions because of microsomal enzyme induction in man.

Clinical Manifestations

Acute Exposure

In sufficient doses, organic chlorines lower the seizure threshold (DDT and related Na$^+$-channel agents) or remove inhibitory influences (antagonism to GABA effects) and produce peripheral and central nervous system stimulation, with resultant tremors, seizures, respiratory failure, and death.[35,70] After DDT exposure, tremor is often the only initial manifestation, except following extensive exposure. Nausea, vomiting, hyperesthesia of the mouth and face, paresthesias of face, tongue, and extremities, headache, dizziness, myoclonus, leg weakness, agitation, and confusion can follow after large exposures. Seizures only occur after very high exposures, usually following large intentional ingestions.[48,70] Dichlorodiphenyltrichloroethane has a relatively low order of acute toxicity, and high doses of DDT (>10 mg/kg) are usually necessary to produce effects.[70] However, with lindane, the cyclodienes, and toxaphene, there typically are no prodromal signs or symptoms, and more often than not, the first manifestation of toxicity is a generalized seizure.[35,70] If seizures develop, they often occur within 1 to 2 hours of ingestion when the stomach is empty, but delays of up to 5 to 6 hours are reported when the ingestion follows a substantial meal.[70]

Seizures related to dermal application of 1% lindane for treatment of ectoparasitic diseases are reported following a single inappropriate application[92,113,155] or, more commonly, after repetitive prolonged exposures.[89,118] The time from application to seizure onset varies from hours to days. The seizures are often self-limited, but recurrent seizures and even status epilepticus are reported. Analysis of an epidemic of lindane poisoning related to the unintentional substitution of lindane powder for sugar used in coffee demonstrated a delay of 20 minutes to 3 hours before the onset of nausea, vomiting, dizziness, facial pallor, severe cyanosis of the face and extremities, collapse, convulsions, and hyperthermia. Affected patients ingested an average of 86 mg/kg of lindane in a single dose.[36]

The cyclodienes are also notable for their propensity to cause seizures that often recur for several days following an acute exposure. If the seizures are brief and hypoxia has not occurred, recovery is usually complete. Electroencephalographic (EEG) abnormalities were recorded before, during, and following seizures showing that the cyclodienes affected seizure threshold/activity.[87] Hyperthermia secondary to central mechanisms, increased muscle activity, and/or aspiration pneumonia is common.[48]

Status epilepticus is a common occurrence in patients with intentional endosulfan ingestions. In 25 cases of endosulfan self-poisonings in Nepal, more than half of the patients developed refractory status epilepticus, and 8 died.[94]

The ingestion of combinations of xenobiotics has resulted in significantly increased toxicity, as demonstrated with DDT and lindane, and is probably the result of synergy.[70]

Lindane: Specific Risks

Patients are at risk for developing central nervous system toxicity from improper topical therapeutic use, such as excessive amounts used or applications, or after baths or under occlusive dressings; young children (<2 years) and the elderly appear to be at greatest risk. Toxicity also occurs after unintentional oral ingestion of topical preparations.[106]

Despite the availability of safer and equally or more effective treatments such as permethrin, lindane is still used because of its lower cost than permethrin and generally good safety profile, when used according to directions. However, less is being used[58] now that permethrin products are available in less-expensive generic forms and the cost advantage of lindane is gone.

An evaluation of published English-language case reports and those submitted to the US Food and Drug Administration (FDA) divided toxicity into those associated with concentrations of lindane greater than or less than 1%.[89] Only 6 of 26 cases could be considered probably related to 1% lindane;[3] 6 of these cases were the result of ingestion or inappropriate skin application.[3] However, a comprehensive review of all published adverse events associated with topical lindane (67 cases) showed that although most of the serious adverse reactions (16 deaths, 11 seizures) occurred following ingestions or excessive use, labeled use accounted for 11 seizures and 4 deaths.[106] In 1995, the FDA added a black-box warning to lindane emphasizing its potential for neurotoxicity, and it was relegated to second-line therapy for ectoparasitic skin infections.[162] In 2013, the FDA published a Postmarket Drug Safety Information for Patients and Providers, which restricted the sale of lindane and required extensive warning labels about adverse events even with labeled use.[58] The sale of lindane-containing products for use in humans was banned in California in 2004 because of its toxicity and environmental concerns,[15] and other states are considering it. In 2009, the American Academy of Pediatrics (AAP) recommended stopping the use of lindane for the treatment of lice or scabies, even as second-line therapy.

Chronic Exposure

Chlordecone (Kepone), unlike the other organic chlorines, produces an insidious picture of chronic toxicity related to its extremely long persistence in the body. Because of poor industrial hygiene practices in a makeshift chlordecone factory in Hopewell, Virginia, 133 workers were heavily exposed for 17 months in 1974–1975. They developed a clinical syndrome that became known as the "Hopewell epidemic," which consisted of a prominent tremor of the hands, a fine tremor of the head, and trembling of the entire body, known as the "Kepone Shakes." Other findings included weakness, opsoclonus (rapid, irregular, dysrhythmic ocular movements), ataxia, altered mental status, rash, weight loss, and elevated liver enzymes. Idiopathic intracranial hypertension, oligospermia, and decreased sperm motility were also found in some of these workers. Severely affected workers even exhibited an exaggerated startle response, remarkably similar to that seen in animal studies. The exposures were so intense that some workers went home covered with chlordecone, and several workers' wives developed neurologic symptoms, presumably from exposures while laundering their husbands' work clothes.[33,56]

There is much concern in environmental health centers on persistent organic chemicals, the organic chlorine residues and PCBs being prime examples. However, because many of these persistent pollutants have been outlawed in many processes and countries, human burden appears to be decreasing.[96]

DDT and Breast Cancer

Dichlorodiphenyltrichloroethane and other organic chlorine insecticides have estrogenic effects.[38,148] Because breast cancer incidence rates in the United States have steadily climbed 1% per year since the 1940s, coinciding with the worldwide use of DDT, it is postulated that women who have higher concentrations of estrogenic organic chlorine compounds (eg, DDT, polychlorinated biphenyls {PCBs}) are at risk for developing breast cancer.[132-134,174]

Several small case–control studies of women with breast cancer showed that women with the disease had higher average body burdens of DDT, DDE, and PCBs than their age-matched controls. These studies implicated the organic chlorines as a possible cause of human breast cancer. However, subsequent larger studies have shown no increased risk of breast cancer because of exposure to organic chlorines,[16] and that currently accepted hereditary and lifestyle risk factors were present in the patients with cancer.[76,90,132-134] In fact, other natural dietary estrogens such

as flavonoids, lignans, sterols, and fungal metabolites are present in the human diet, and these xenobiotics have much higher estrogenic potency; the organic chlorine contribution is probably minimal by comparison.[63] One interesting reported suggests age at first exposure, that is, age less than 14 years (prior to menarche), as having an association with later breast cancer.[32] However, most case–control studies do not supported an association between DDT and breast cancer.[14,66,77,80,142,143] A meta-analysis of 22 studies found strong evidence to discard the putative relationship between p,p'-DDE concentrations and breast cancer risk;[95] 2 more recent meta-analyses also confirmed the lack of any increased risk for breast cancer associated with DDT or DDE.[79,111]

Diagnostic Information

The history of exposure to an organic chlorine pesticide is the most critical piece of information, because exposure is otherwise rare. By law, the package label of these products must list the ingredients, the concentrations, and the vehicle. The EPA-registered use of the insecticide will be helpful in determining which organic chlorine is involved. The presence of an unusual odor in the mouth, in the vomitus, or on the skin is helpful. Toxaphene, a chlorinated pinene, has a mild turpentinelike odor, and endosulfan has a unique "rotten egg" sulfur odor (Table 111–1). Following ingestion, an abdominal radiographs often reveal the presence of a radiopaque chlorinated pesticide, because chlorine increases the radiopacity of the xenobiotics (Chap. 8). A large number of other xenobiotics lead to seizures as the first manifestation of toxicity, and must be in the differential of an unknown exposure (Chaps. 13 and 22).

Laboratory Testing

Gas chromatography can detect organic chlorine pesticides in serum, adipose tissue, and urine.[37,76] If confirmation is necessary for purposes of documentation of source, the concentrations of organic chlorines can be measured. If the patient's history and toxidrome are obvious, then laboratory evaluation is unnecessary, as this determination will not alter the course of management, and these blood tests are not available on an emergent basis. At present, there are no data correlating health effects and serum or tissue concentrations. Routine surveillance of serum concentrations in the occupationally exposed is not currently performed.[37]

Most humans studied have measurable concentrations of DDT in adipose tissue. In a study of a community with a very large exposure to DDT, serum DDT concentrations increased proportionally with age. These increasing concentrations were not associated with any apparent adverse health effects, but there was an association with increasing concentrations of the liver enzyme gamma-glutamyltransferase (GGT), although significant hepatotoxicity did not occur. The CDC's *Fourth National Report on Human Exposure to Environmental Chemicals* demonstrated the presence of numerous organic chlorine pesticide residues in the lipid fraction of serum of US residents. These concentrations tend to increase with patient age, consistent with the bio-accumulation and fat-storing properties of the chemicals.[19,24] More recently, studies of occupationally exposed pesticide applicators and persons living in targeted regions confirmed higher serum concentrations over those not exposed, but no ill health effects are documented.[131]

Serum lindane concentrations can be used to document exposure, and clinical signs and symptoms of toxicity correlated with average blood concentrations.[33] Lindane-exposed workers with chronic neurologic symptoms showed an average blood lindane concentration of 0.02 mg/L.[3,70] A limited series of patients with acute lindane ingestion suggests that a serum concentration of 0.12 mg/L correlates with sedation, and that 0.20 mg/L is associated with seizures and coma.[3] After cutaneous application, lindane concentrations in the CNS are 3 to 12 times higher than serum concentrations.[40,146] None of these tests are available in the acute care setting, and cannot aid in diagnosis or management.

Management

As with any patient who presents with an altered mental status, dextrose and thiamine in an adult should be administered as clinically indicated. Skin decontamination is essential, and clothing should be removed and placed in a plastic bag and disposed of appropriately as a biohazardous waste, and the skin washed with soap and water. Health care providers should be protected with rubber gloves and aprons. Because these pesticides are almost invariably liquids, a nasogastric tube is reasonable for suction and lavage gastric contents, if the ingestion was recent (Chap. 5). Because many mixtures contain petroleum distillates as their solvent vehicles, the benefit of AC is limited. Standard seizure management and control with benzodiazepines and barbiturates is recommended as needed, and additional medications such as propofol may also be necessary, due to the risk of recurrent seizures and status epilepticus. The use of cholestyramine, a nonabsorbable bile acid–binding anion exchange resin that was successfully used in chlordecone poisonings in humans (see below), showed a statistically significant benefit on decreasing seizure incidence and mortality in a murine experimental model.[85] Oil-based cathartics should never be used, as they may facilitate absorption. There is some evidence that sucrose polyester (ie, olestra, a nonabsorbed synthetic dietary oil substitute) increases excretion of a wide variety of fat-soluble organic chlorine chemicals, especially those undergoing enterohepatic recirculation, by fecal elimination.[81,101] This effect was demonstrated in dioxin-poisoned patients who were administered olestra in fat-free potato chips,[67] and was employed in treating Ukrainian president Viktor Yushchenko, among other therapeutic regimens.[149] Sucrose polyester is a reasonable inexpensive and more palatable alternative to cholestyramine to increase excretion in patients with chronic organic chlorine toxicity.

Cholestyramine or sucrose polyester resin is recommended for to all patients symptomatic from chlordecone, and possibly other organic chlorines. Chlordecone undergoes both enterohepatic and enteroenteric recirculation, which can be interrupted by cholestyramine at a dosage of 16 g/day. Cholestyramine increased the fecal elimination of chlordecone 3- to 18-fold in industrial workers exposed during the Hopewell epidemic, resulting in clinical improvement.[33] Sucrose polyester is a reasonable adjunct for enhancing excretion.

Chlorfenapyr

Chlorfenapyr is a member of a newer class of pesticides known as pyrroles.[75] It is not typically grouped with the organochlorines, even though it is an organic compound containing chlorine, but is structurally unrelated to the other OCs. The mechanism of action of chlorfenapyr is different from the typical Na^+-channel or $GABA_A$ antagonism mechanisms of the OC pesticides covered in this chapter. Chlorfenapyr itself is a pro-insecticide, and requires CYP enzyme metabolic activation by removal of the N-ethoxymethyl group, producing the free pyrrole (designated CL 303268) which is a lipophilic weak acid with very strong insecticidal activity. This pyrrole interferes with ATP production by uncoupling mitochondrial oxidative phosphorylation.[75] Acute ingestions have a high case-fatality ratio (8 of 24 in a 2004 case series in Japan).[49] A unique, consistent, yet disturbing feature of these poisonings is a long latency between ingestion and onset of toxic effects. Several case reports describe long relatively asymptomatic intervals after intentional suicidal ingestions lasting several days to a week or two before the onset of nausea, fever, and diaphoresis, which is usually followed by CNS manifestations (often with leukoencephalopathy on magnetic resonance imaging) and complete cardiovascular collapse and

death.[6,82,157] Some cases had relatively mild clinical effects of intermittent fever, thirst, and diaphoresis for a few days as the only abnormality prior to rapid collapse and death.[30] An agricultural worker died 7 days after spraying chlorfenapyr without wearing a respirator or personal protective garments; his presentation with fever, diaphoresis, and thirst for a week after exposure prior to collapse was remarkably similar to the suicidal ingestion cases.[74]

In insects, the microsomal enzyme inhibitor piperonyl butoxide antagonizes the insecticidal activity of chlorfenapyr by inhibiting the conversion into its active pyrrole metabolite. It is unknown whether CYP inhibitors would be useful in preventing conversion in human exposures, but to date GI decontamination and hemodialysis were not effective.

PYRETHRINS AND PYRETHROIDS

The natural pyrethrins are the active extracts from the flower *Chrysanthemum cinerariaefolium*. These insecticides are important historically, having been used in China since the first century A.D.,[36] and developed for commercial application by the 1800s. They are produced by organic solvent extraction from ground Chrysanthemum flowers. The resulting concentrates have greater than 90% purity. Pyrethrum, the first pyrethrin identified, consists of 6 esters derived from chrysanthemic acid and pyrethric acid. These insecticides are highly effective contact poisons, and their lipophilic nature allows them to readily penetrate insect chitin (exoskeleton) and paralyze the nervous system through interactions at the voltage-dependent Na^+ channel.[31,41,103,121,147] When applied properly, they have essentially no systemic mammalian toxicity because of their rapid hydrolysis. Pyrethrins break down rapidly in light and in water, and therefore have no environmental persistence or bioaccumulation. This fact makes the pyrethrins extremely safe after human exposures, but unsuitable for commercial agriculture, because the constant reapplication would be cost prohibitive.

The pyrethroids are the synthetic derivatives of the natural pyrethrins[144] (Table 111–2 and Fig. 111–4). They were developed in an effort to produce more environmentally stable products for use in agriculture. Originally, the pyrethroids were divided into 2 groups based on the toxic syndromes they elicited in test animals. The T syndrome (for tremor seen in rats) was produced by intravenous administration of pyrethrin and most (15 of 18) of the pyrethroids that did not contain a cyano group at the central ester linkage (see below). The CS syndrome (for choreoathetosis and salivation) was produced by 12 of the 17 pyrethroids that had an α-cyano group at the ester linkage. The original studies delineating the T or CS method of classification did not test several new currently registered pyrethroid pesticides, and the testing methods involved intravenous or intracerebral administration, which are not relevant to human exposures.[144]

The predominant classification scheme used today is based on the structure of the pyrethroid, their clinical manifestations in mammalian poisoning, its actions on insect nerve preparations, and its insecticidal activity. Type I pyrethroids have a simple ester bond at the central linkage without a cyano group. Commonly used type I pyrethroids include permethrin, allethrin, tetramethrin, and phenothrin. The type II pyrethroids have a cyano group at the carbon of this ester linkage. Type II pyrethroids in common use include cypermethrin, deltamethrin, fenpropathrin, fluvalinate, and fenvalerate. The cyano group greatly enhances neurotoxicity of the type II pyrethroids in both mammals and insects, and type II pyrethroids tend to produce the CS syndrome in test animals and are generally considered more potent and toxic than the type I pyrethroids (Fig. 111–4).[47,97,120,121,144]

The development of the pyrethroids can also be divided into "generations," based on efficacy and dates of introduction.[168] The first generation began in 1949, with the development of allethrin. The second generation began in 1965, with the introduction of tetramethrin. The major advance of the second generation was a dramatic increase in potency compared with the pyrethrins. The third generation, introduced in the 1970s, including fenvalerate and permethrin, were the first pyrethroids with practical agricultural use. They were more potent, and more environmentally stable, with efficacious crop residues lasting 4 to 7 days. The current fourth generation

TABLE 111–2   Synthetic Pyrethroids in Common Use

Pyrethroid Class	Generic Name	Generation of Pyrethroid, Dates Introduced (If Available)
Type I	Allethrin	1st generation; first synthetic pyrethroid, 1949
	Bioallethrin	2nd generation, 1969; trans isomer of allethrin
	Dimethrin	Not available
	Phenothrin	2nd generation, 1973
	Resmethrin	2nd generation, 1967; 20× strength of pyrethrum
	Bioresmethrin	2nd generation, 1967; 50× strength of pyrethrum, isomer of resmethrin
	Tetramethrin	2nd generation, 1965
	Permethrin	3rd generation, 1972; effective topical scabicide and miticide, low toxicity
	Bifenthrin	4th generation
	Prallethrin	4th generation
	Imiprothrin	3rd generation, 1998
Type II	Fenvalerate	3rd generation, 1973
	Acrinathrin	4th generation
	Cyfluthrin	4th generation
	Cyhalothrin	4th generation
	Cypermethrin	4th generation
	Deltamethrin	4th generation
	Esfenvalerate	4th generation
	Fenpropathrin	4th generation, 1989
	Flucythrinate 70124-77-5	4th generation
	Fluvalinate 102851-06-9	4th generation
	Imiprothrin 72963-72-5	4th generation, 1998
	Tefluthrin 79538-32-2	4th generation
	Tralomethrin 66841-25-6	4th generation

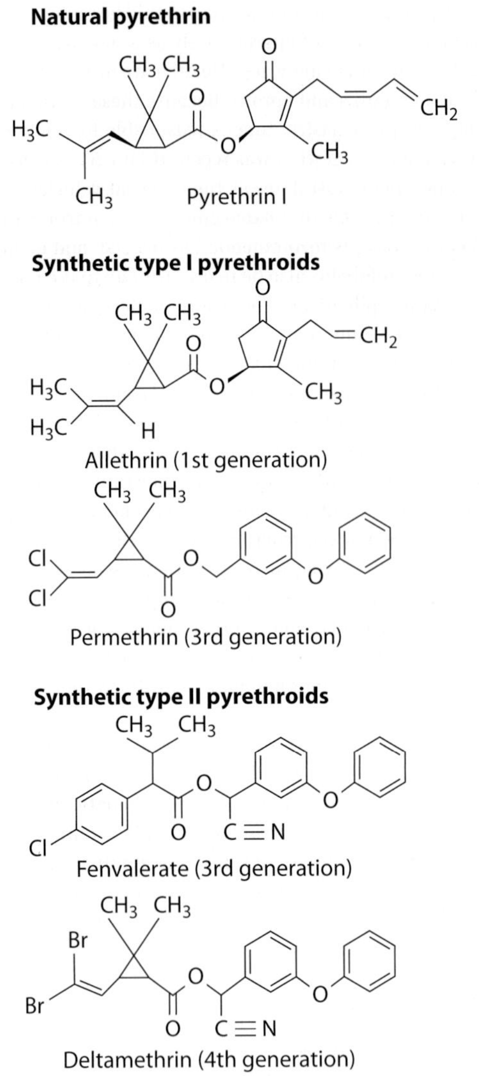

FIGURE 111–4. Representative structures of pyrethrin and pyrethroids.

includes mostly type II pyrethroids, which have greater insecticidal activity, are photostable, do not undergo photolysis "splitting" in sunlight, possess minimal volatility, and provide extended residual effectiveness for up to 10 days under optimum conditions.[97,168]

More than 1,000 pyrethroids have been synthesized, of which 16 to 20 are in widespread use today.[12,36] Pyrethrins and pyrethroids are found in more than 2,000 commercially available products. These insecticides have a rapid paralytic effect ("knock down") on insects.

Most mammalian species are relatively resistant, because the pyrethrins can be rapidly detoxified by ester cleavage and oxidation.[112] Toxicity of the pyrethrins and pyrethroids is enhanced in insects by combination with microsomal enzyme inhibitors such as piperonyl butoxide (a synthetic analogue of sesamin, the methylenedioxyphenyl component of sesame oil) or N-octyl bicycloheptene dicarboximide.[7,115]

Permethrin, a type I pyrethroid, is used medicinally for topical treatment of ectoparasitic conditions in humans, and impregnated in clothing and mosquito netting for its insect repellant properties. It has an excellent safety profile, with approximately 2% or less absorbed systemically through the skin.[98] Comprehensive reviews have confirmed that 5% permethrin is the drug of choice for scabies treatment, with the best efficacy versus safety profile of topical treatments for scabies and lice.[129,167]

West Nile virus was first identified in the United States in 1999 and rapidly spread to most US states by 2006. Outbreaks of encephalitis caused by West Nile virus (WNV) have occurred in the late summer and early autumn

months in the United States since 1999. Although birds are the reservoirs for WNV, transmission to humans occurs via mosquito bites, and hence many states and municipalities have increased their aerial spraying in an effort to control mosquito vectors of this disease. Most spraying programs use pyrethroid insecticides because of their favorable safety profile, and their efficacy against the adult mosquito. More recently, the CDC and Prevention has recommended several pyrethroids specifically for aerial spraying and indoor residual spraying for mosquito control in endemic Zika areas of the United States.[160] These widespread spraying programs have increased the potential for human exposures to these xenobiotics. A Centers for Disease Control and Prevention study of pyrethroid spraying for WNV did not reveal an increase in detectable pyrethroid metabolites in the general public living in the sprayed areas.[5] Another study of asthma surveillance showed no increases in emergency department visits because of asthma-related conditions for the periods after pyrethroid spraying.[83]

Toxicokinetics
Absorption
Pyrethrins are well absorbed orally and via inhalation, but skin absorption is poor. Piperonyl butoxide is also well absorbed orally, but likewise has poor dermal penetration.[115] The oral toxicity of pyrethrins in mammals is extremely low, because they are so readily hydrolyzed into inactive compounds. Their dermal toxicity is even lower, owing to their slow penetration and rapid metabolism.[48,112]

The pyrethroids are more stable than the natural pyrethrins, and significant systemic toxicity occurs following large ingestions.[71] An average of 35% (range 27%–57%) of orally administered cypermethrin is absorbed in human volunteers.[174] Most exposures are from dermal absorption, the rate of which varies depending on the solvent vehicle. In the same volunteer study noted above, a mean of 1.2% (range 0.85%–1.8%) of dermally applied cypermethrin in soybean oil vehicle was absorbed systemically.[174] Intradermal metabolism of pyrethroids is documented in test animals, and likely further limits systemic absorption.[12] Direct absorption of pyrethroids through the skin to the peripheral sensory nerves probably accounts for the facial paresthesias that occur in these cases, as symptoms are prominent in pesticide sprayers in areas of direct contact.[28,91] Absorption probably also occurs through the oral mucosa, as noted by a large study of Chinese insecticide sprayers who frequently used their mouths to clear clogged spray nozzles. The pyrethroids are also absorbed via inhalation; however, in these same sprayers, inhalation was not found to be a clinically significant route of exposure as analyzed by breathing zone assays.[28] The pyrethroids are not volatile compounds, so inhalation is always due to powders or sprayed mists, and mucosal and pulmonary toxicity can also be due to hydrocarbon solvent vehicles. Systemic absorption and resultant effects can follow massive exposures, such as occurs in enclosed spraying or other extreme conditions.

Distribution

The pyrethroids and pyrethrins are lipophilic and as such are rapidly distributed to the central nervous system. Because they are rapidly metabolized, there is no storage or bioaccumulation, which limits chronic toxicity.[47,48]

Metabolism

Natural pyrethrins are readily metabolized by mammalian microsomal enzymes, and hence are essentially nontoxic to humans. They can induce CYP3A and CYP2B enzymes in vitro in human cultured hepatocytes, but clinical significance is doubtful.[114]

The synthetic pyrethroids are readily metabolized in animals and man by hydrolases and the CYP microsomal system. The metabolites are of lower toxicity than the parent compounds.[144] Piperonyl butoxide, a CYP enzyme inhibitor in insects, enhances the potency of pyrethrins and pyrethroids 10- to 300-fold to target insects. It is often added to insecticide preparations to ensure lethality, as the initial "knock down" effect of a pyrethroid alone is not always lethal to the insect.[47] Testing of piperonyl butoxide on antipyrine metabolism (measure of CYP enzyme function) in humans at a dose exceeding 50 times that received in all-day confined space pesticide spraying revealed no effect on this enzyme system.[115]

Elimination

There is no evidence that the pyrethroids undergo enterohepatic recirculation. Deltamethrin disappeared from the urine of exposed workers within 12 hours, and fenvalerate disappeared within 24 hours.[28] Parent compounds, and metabolites of the pyrethroids, are found in the urine.[121] The pyrethroids have several common metabolites, some of which are also environmental breakdown products, that can be assayed.[93,152] Detection of these metabolites in the urine may be from a subject's exposure to the parent compound or from its metabolite in the environment.

Pathophysiology

Like DDT, pyrethrins and pyrethroids prolong the activation of the voltage-dependent Na$^+$ channel by binding to it in the open state, causing a prolonged depolarization, as evidenced by an extended tail current seen with squid axon voltage clamp experiments.[104,105] Although DDT affects primarily the insect peripheral nervous system (PNS), the pyrethroids affect the insect CNS as well as the PNS.[41] Because DDT and pyrethrin/pyrethroids bind to the same site on insect Na$^+$ channels, resistance to one class can often cause cross-resistance to the other class.[107] The voltage-sensitive Na$^+$-channel binding is responsible for the insecticidal activity and the toxicity of the pyrethroids to nontarget species. Natural pyrethrins and type I synthetic pyrethroids induce repetitive or "burst discharges" following a single stimulus, because they hold

the Na$^+$ channel in its open state. The actual amplitude of the tail current is determined by the concentration of the pyrethroids, regardless of type. Type II pyrethroids cause the Na$^+$ channel to remain open longer and allow a more prolonged period of depolarization of the resting membrane potential, causing a longer duration of the tail current, and eventual paralysis due to neurotransmitter depletion.[147,165] Type II pyrethroids are thus more potent, and lead to significant after-potentials and eventual nerve conduction block. The mammalian voltage-dependent Na$^+$ channel, unlike the insect, has many isoforms, which helps explain the relative resistance in mammalian species (>1,000-fold less susceptible). Different pyrethroids have varied effects on these mammalian Na$^+$ channels, and the effects are not additive, and in fact may be antagonistic.

Pyrethroids also have activity at certain isoforms of the voltage-sensitive Ca^{2+} channel, which would explain the neurotransmitter release that occurs in pyrethroid intoxication. Additionally, pyrethroids block voltage-sensitive Cl$^-$ channels in test animals, producing the salivation as part of the CS syndrome. These effects contribute to enhanced CNS toxicity,[144] and is likely responsible for the choreoathetosis that occurs in animal models of severe type II poisonings.[119] Some studies show some interference of the type II pyrethroids with the GABA$_A$-mediated inhibitory Cl$^-$ channels in high concentrations.[31,103] Antagonism of the GABA$_A$ Cl$^-$ channels likely has a significant role in human pyrethroid exposures, and probably contributes to the seizures following severe poisoning by type II pyrethyroids.[103,119] The pyrethroids also have activity at the peripheral benzodiazepine receptor, as evidenced by decreased salivation in test animals when this receptor was blocked.[117] The clinical significance of this in humans is currently unknown.

Natural pyrethrins and type I pyrethroids have a negative temperature coefficient, similar to DDT, and are more selectively toxic to non–warm-blooded target species, but also less effective at warmer environmental temperatures. Type II pyrethroids have a positive temperature coefficient, which makes them more insecticidal at higher ambient temperatures and thus more useful in agricultural applications.[103,168] However, this at least partly explains the greater toxicity of type II pyrethroids to warm-blooded species as compared to type I.[103]

Clinical Manifestations

Pyrethrum probably has an LD$_{50}$ of well over 1 g/kg in man, as extrapolated from animal data. Most cases of toxicity associated with the pyrethrins are the result of allergic reactions.[112,169] Theoretically, those at highest risk for allergic reactions would be patients who are sensitive to ragweed pollen, 50% of whom may cross-react with chrysanthemums (ragweed and chrysanthemum are in the same botanical family). These allergic reactions are postulated to be due to residual natural components present in the extracts.[121] However, recent reviews have cast some doubt on this explanation. First, there have been only 4 cases of life-threatening respiratory reactions reported in the literature, 3 of which were in known asthmatics.[115] Second, the presence of residual natural proteins is unlikely, as the purification procedures would allow little, if any, residuals.[62] Third, most reported cases of contact urticaria have been erroneously classified as type I hypersensitivity reactions.[62] The synthetic pyrethroids can cause histamine release in vitro,[44] but generally do not induce IgE-mediated allergic reactions.[15]

In animals, type I pyrethroid poisoning most closely resembles that of DDT, with extensive tremors, twitching, increased metabolic rate, and hyperthermia. Excluding the rare possibility of skin irritation or allergy, the type I pyrethroids are unlikely to cause systemic toxicity in humans. It has been shown experimentally that pyrethroids have greater than 1,000-fold more affinity for insect Na$^+$ channels than for those of mammals, explaining their low toxicity in higher life forms. This selectivity, along with the negative temperature coefficient and slower insect metabolism, combines to make the type I pyrethroids approximately 15,000 times more toxic in insects than humans.[105] The type II pyrethroids are generally more potent, and cause profuse salivation, ataxia, coarse tremor, choreoathetosis, and seizures in animals. In humans, poisoning with type II pyrethroids causes paresthesias (secondary to Na$^+$ channel's effects in cutaneous sensory nerves after topical exposure),[91] salivation, nausea, vomiting, dizziness, fasciculations, altered mental status, coma, seizures, and acute respiratory distress syndrome.[71] A review of more than 500 cases of acute pyrethroid poisoning from China highlights some similar manifestations between a massive acute type II pyrethroid overdose and an organic phosphorus compound overdose (salivation, vomiting, seizures). However, serious atropine toxicity and death has resulted when poisoning from a type II pyrethroid was mistaken for an organic phosphorus compound, and treatment was directed at these seemingly muscarinic signs.[71] Features such as acute respiratory distress syndrome can be caused by solvents and surfactants present in the agricultural products.[7] Although the type II pyrethroids contain a cyanide moiety, cyanide poisoning does not occur, and cyanide antidotal therapy is not indicated.

Most significant unintentional exposures are dermal, especially in occupational settings, and local symptoms predominate in the majority of these cases. Systemic effects from insecticidal sprayings are reported from wind drift or inappropriate handling, and the more potent type II pyrethroids predominate in case reports. An exposure of workers possibly affected by wind drift from a mixture of 32 ounces of the type II pyrethroid cyfluthrin mixed with 18.5 gallons of petroleum oil and 1,800 gallons of water was reported in California in 2006. Spraying occurred in a citrus grove, and 23 female workers in an adjacent vineyard were possibly exposed. These workers complained of a "chemical" odor, and felt ill with headaches, nausea, eye irritation, weakness, anxiety, and shortness of breath. They were all evaluated in hospitals and discharged home. Despite the fact that no cyfluthrin was detected on these workers' clothing or on foliage in the field where they were alleged to have been exposed, the report concluded that cyfluthrin was the cause; no estimate of the contribution of the petroleum vehicle to the symptoms was posited.[25] The predominant feature after significant cutaneous exposures is local paresthesias in the areas of skin contact, due to Na^+-channel effects on cutaneous sensory nerves. Local skin irritation occurred in up to 10% of workers spraying pyrethroid insecticides, but rarely occurs after medicinal use of the pyrethroid creams and shampoos. Some pyrethroid compounds can be very corrosive to the eyes.[121]

Intentional ingestions represent the most serious exposures, because of the higher doses involved, and the greater exposures to vehicles and solvents. However, a study of 48 cases of permethrin/xylene/surfactant mixtures (38 were suicidal ingestions) revealed that mild GI signs and symptoms predominated (73%: sore throat, mouth ulcerations, dysphagia, epigastric pain, vomiting). Pulmonary signs and symptoms were documented in 29%, and 8 patients (including 1 death) had aspiration pneumonitis. Thirty-three percent had CNS symptoms: confusion (13%), coma (21%), and seizures (8%). The involvement of the central nervous system and lungs was less common, but clinically more significant.[177] The relative contributions of the 70% xylene and 10% surfactant was likely responsible for much of the GI and pulmonary effects, though it was not discussed in the report.

Chronic Exposures

Because the pyrethroids are rapidly metabolized and are not biopersistent compounds, they are shown not to cause cumulative toxicity. A single case of motor neuron disease resulted from heavy daily inhalation exposure to pyrethroid mixtures in a combined space for 3 years, which resolved after exposure ceased.[45] Some investigators express concerns regarding possible neurotoxicity of the pyrethroids. However, a review noted that regulatory studies in multiple species showed no evidence supporting gross neurodevelopmental toxicity or adult neuronal loss in man.[119] In Germany, a unique situation exists where numerous civil lawsuits allege that multiple chemical sensitivity (MCS) is caused by pyrethroid exposures. Study of this phenomenon yields no scientific data to support this contention,[10] and the controversy is fueled by civil litigation, popular media sensationalizing, and subsequent public fear.[4]

Treatment

Initial treatment should be directed toward skin decontamination, as most poisonings occur from exposures by this route. For patients with intentional oral ingestions of a type II pyrethroid we recommend a single standard dose of AC, provided the diluent of the pyrethroid does not contain a petroleum solvent. Contact dermatitis and acute systemic allergic reactions should be treated in the usual manner, utilizing histamine blockers, corticosteroids, and inhalational beta-adrenergic agonists as clinically indicated.

Treatment of systemic toxicity is entirely supportive and symptomatic, because no specific antidote exists. Benzodiazepines should be used for tremor and seizures. Topical vitamin E oil (D,L-α-tocopherol) is especially effective in preventing and treating the cutaneous paresthesias due to topical pyrethroid exposures.[12,121]

ARTHROPOD REPELLENTS

Mosquitoes transmit more diseases to humans than any other biting insect. Worldwide, more than 700 million people are infected yearly by mosquito bites that transmit such diseases as malaria, viral encephalitis, yellow fever, dengue fever, bancroftian filariasis, and epidemic polyarthritis. Most recently, *Aedes aegypti* mosquitoes were found to transmit Zika virus and chikungunya. Novel approaches to mosquito control also includes impregnation of indoor house paints with various insecticides (organic phosphorus compounds) and insect growth regulators. WHO estimated 214 million cases of malaria worldwide in 2015, and an estimated 438,000 deaths, of which 306,000 deaths were of children younger than 5 years.[170]

Although malaria is not a significant risk in the United States, numerous mosquito-borne diseases are present, and the exposures are growing. Nearly 44,000 cases of West Nile virus (WNV) disease is reported in the United States since 1999 in 48 states, and more than 1,900 people have died. In 2015 alone, 2175 cases of WNV were reported to the CDC. Many more cases of illness go unreported.[23] More recently, the CDC has confirmed Zika virus infections in the continental United States from January 2015 through January 2017 as 246 local cases (not travel associated), but 34,249 locally acquired cases were registered in Puerto Rico.[22] Because of the severe birth defects associated with Zika and the severe illnesses associated with other arthropod-borne illnesses (chikungunya, dengue, etc.), mosquito repellents have become important public health tools. The *A aegypti* mosquito, vector of Zika, chikungunya, dengue fever, and yellow fever, is more difficult to avoid because they feed both day and night, and humans are their primary blood meal source, so they primarily breed in cities and crowded population areas. *N,N*-Diethyl-3-methylbenzamide (DEET) is the time-tested primary weapon for the past 5 decades. However, much controversy continues to surround DEET despite a remarkable safety profile with over a half-century of global use by billions of people. A growing trend in the United States and many Western cultures is a chemophobia against synthetic products like DEET. Many people favor plant-based "natural" or "organic" repellents, paralleling the increasing consumer preference for natural or organic foods. Several xenobiotics are proposed, but thus far few are shown by objective blinded studies to even approach the efficacy of DEET, much less surpass it. Numerous comprehensive reviews of the subject demonstrated the superiority of DEET in most cases, and it remains the insect repellent standard by which all others are measured (Table 111–3).

DEET

The topical insect repellent *N,N*-diethyl-3-methylbenzamide (DEET, former nomenclature *N,N*-diethyl-*meta*-toluamide) was patented by the US Army in 1946, and commercially marketed in the United States since 1956. Currently, it is used worldwide by more than 200 million persons annually. The EPA estimates that 38% of the US population uses DEET each year. Despite the current search for alternatives, DEET is still the most effective repellent available, and that with the most clinical toxicity information.[59,60]

Formulations of DEET can be purchased without prescription in concentrations ranging from 5% to 100%, and in multiple formulations of solutions, creams, lotions, gels, and aerosol sprays. Mosquitoes are attracted to their hosts by temperature and chemical attractants, principally CO_2 and lactate. The mechanism by which DEET repels insects was thought to be due to some interference with the chemoreceptors that detect lactic acid and CO_2.[59,116]

TABLE 111–3 Comparative Efficacy and Toxicity of Commonly Available Insect Repellents

Insect Repellent	EPA Approval	EPA Toxicity Rating[a]	Efficacy in Lab and Field Studies[b]	Notes
DEET	1957 (1980)	III	Most efficacious in lab and field studies; proven protection against ticks and mosquitoes	>50 years of experience, billions of users 10%–30% solution: safe, effective when used as directed
Picaridin (Bayrepel)	2001	IV	20% solution: Lab: Equivalent to DEET Field: Essentially equivalent to DEET	All studies done on 20% picaridin; no studies done with 7% US formula Recommended by CDC as a DEET alternative
IR3535 (substituted β amino acid)	1999	IV	Lab: Inferior to DEET Field: None available	Recommended by CDC as a DEET alternative
Oil of lemon eucalyptus (p-menthane diol)	2000	IV (I, ocular)	Equivalent to DEET for mosquitoes; not tested for tick bite prevention	Recommended by CDC as a DEET alternative
BioUD (2-undecanone)	2007	IV	Lab: Equivalent to 7% DEET Field: Equal to 25% and 30% DEET	Studies performed by patent holders and developers of IR, no impartial evidence
Citronella oil	1948	IV	Lab study: Ineffective	Candles only provide some repellency when within 1 meter

[a]EPA Acute Toxicity Ratings: Category I = very highly or highly toxic; Category II = moderately toxic; Category III = slightly toxic; Category IV = practically nontoxic. [b]Lab tests: arm-in-cage studies for mosquito repellency; Field studies: actual biting or tick attachment assays in natural conditions.

ACUTE ORAL TOXICITY: (from EPA- https://www.epa.gov/pesticide-registration/label-review-manual July 2014, accessed January 26, 2017)

Category I LD_{50} < 50 mg/kg Label Language: DANGER Skull and Crossbones Fatal if swallowed—very highly or highly toxic

Category II LD_{50} > 50 mg/kg < 500 mg/kg WARNING No symbol May be fatal if swallowed—moderately toxic

Category III LD_{50} > 500 mg/kg < 5,000 mg/kg CAUTION No symbol Harmful if swallowed—slightly toxic

Category IV LD_{50} > 5,000 mg/kg CAUTION or no signal word No symbol No hazard statement required; practically nontoxic -registrant may choose to use Category III statement

{947 US Environmental Protection Agency Office of Pesticide Programs 2016}

However, novel work demonstrated that DEET itself is actually detected by the mosquito's olfactory receptors and repels them independently of whether the normal physical or chemical attractants are present.[154] Formulations of DEET can feel greasy or sticky, and can dissolve or damage some plastics (eyeglass frames, watches) and synthetic fabrics.

Toxicokinetics

N,N-Diethyl-3-methylbenzamide is extensively absorbed via the GI tract.[163] Skin absorption is significant, depending on the vehicle and the concentration. Transdermal absorption of 30% to 45% DEET in ethanol is significantly higher than 100% DEET solution in an in vitro human skin model.[150] This has led to development of microencapsulated liposphere formulas and polyethylene glycol–based solutions that reduce absorption and increase repellent time and efficacy in animal models.[46]

N,N-diethyl-3-methylbenzamide does not bind to stratum corneum, and only 0.08% or less of a dose remains in the skin 8 hours after application.[116] DEET is lipophilic, and skin absorption usually occurs within 2 hours, although it is eliminated from plasma within 4 hours. The volume of distribution is large, in the range of 2.7 to 6.2 L/kg in animal studies. DEET is extensively metabolized by oxidation and hydroxylation by the hepatic microsomal enzymes, primarily by the isozymes CYP2B6, 3A4, 2C19, and 2A6.[163] DEET is excreted in the urine within 12 hours, mainly as metabolites, with 15% or less appearing as the parent compound.[60,116]

N,N-diethyl-3-methylbenzamide toxicity reports and studies are extensively reviewed in terms of acute and chronic toxicity. It is safe for use in pregnant and lactating women;[88] it has no specific target organ toxicity or oncogenicity in any observed rat, mouse, or dog studies;[140] and chronic DEET exposure together with other insecticides showed no increased cancer risks.[110]

Pathophysiology

The exact mechanism of DEET toxicity is unknown. Reviews of adverse reactions to DEET reported 26 cases with major morbidity, including encephalopathy, ataxia, convulsions, respiratory failure, hypotension, anaphylaxis, or death, particularly after ingestion or dermal exposure to large amounts.[20,60,108,109,156,164] These primarily neurologic adverse reactions occurred mainly in children, and most involved prolonged use and excessive dosing beyond what is currently recommended. One fatal case involved a child who was known to be heterozygous for ornithine carbamoyl transferase (OCT) deficiency, and death was because of a Reyelike syndrome with hyperammonemia. This child experienced prior episodes of hyperammonemia unrelated to DEET use, and DEET does not appear to affect, or be affected by, OCT activity in humans.[108] There is currently no evidence that enzyme polymorphism affects DEET metabolism or influences individual susceptibility to toxicity.

Although single, large, acute oral doses (1–3 g/kg) in rats produced seizures and CNS damage,[138,139] smaller acute doses (500 mg/kg and less) and chronic multigenerational dosing in another rat study produced no obvious toxicity.[139] Teratogenicity studies in rats and rabbits failed to demonstrate toxicity except at the highest doses,[140,176] and DEET was not found to be carcinogenic.[116,140] In view of the billions of applications, the number of reports of toxicity appears exceedingly small, and suggests a remarkably wide margin of safety.[60,68,108,109,125,153,164]

Clinical Manifestations

Most calls to poison control centers regarding DEET exposures involve minor or no symptoms, and symptomatic exposures occur primarily when DEET is sprayed in the eyes or inhaled.[164] Except for suicidal ingestions, most serious reactions consist of seizures in children overexposed via the dermal route; in fact, some of these cannot be definitely attributed to DEET.[68,108] Most symptoms resolve without treatment and the majority of patients with serious toxicity recover fully with supportive care. A single case report of severe poisoning developed in a man with extreme exposure. He used 30% DEET on his entire body several times daily for a prolonged time period, with an entire bottle used the day prior to admission. He developed weakness, and nausea that progressed to confusion and shortness of breath. Metabolic acidosis, elevated lactate concentration, acute kidney injury requiring hemodialysis, and worsening weakness requiring mechanical ventilation developed. His blood DEET concentration was 130 ppb (mcg/L). No seizures developed, and he experienced a full neurologic recovery after a prolonged hospitalization.[122] When toxicity data and the few cases of encephalopathy and death allegedly related to DEET use are closely analyzed, the actual role of DEET remains purely speculative.[29]

Treatment

Patients with DEET exposures are treated with supportive care aimed at the primarily neurologic symptoms. In cases of dermal exposures, skin decontamination should be a priority to prevent further absorption. For patients with intentional oral ingestions it is reasonable to give a single dose of AC if it has been less than 2 hours after ingestion and there are no contraindications such as seizures, decreased mental status, or vomiting.

An extensive review of the safety risk of DEET repellent use confirms its safe use for all populations when used according to labeling guidelines.[153] Despite its good safety profile, avoiding the overuse of DEET seems prudent. The American Academy of Pediatrics (AAP) revised its recommendations for insect repellent use due to the emergence of WNV infections and Zika and chikungunya (prior recommendations were for use of products with DEET <10%).[141] They found that DEET-containing products are the most effective mosquito repellents available, and are also effective against a variety of other insects, including ticks. Insect repellents with a DEET concentration from 10% to 30% (the maximum recommended for children) appear to be equally safe when used according to the directions on the product labels. The safety of DEET does not appear to relate to differences in these concentrations, and higher concentrations have longer durations of effects.[1] As indicated in the AAP handbook, repellents are not recommended for children younger than 2 months of age.[2]

The higher concentrations prolong the repellency period, but there is a plateau at about 50% DEET concentration, and about 6 hours is likely the maximum protection time from any single application of conventional formulations. Newer longer-acting DEET formulations in lipids or polymers cause the DEET to evaporate more slowly, which affords protection for greater than 6 hours and also less systemic absorption.[86,135] Because the lower concentrations recommended for children last approximately 2 hours, frequent reapplication is usually unnecessary. Most mosquitoes are most active for a few hours preceding and following dusk, and prior recommendations were to apply only during high-risk times. However, because *A aegypti* mosquito feeds both day and night, bite avoidance is important in areas where this vector and its diseases are a risk, so insect repellents are needed around the clock. DEET should be promptly washed off the child's skin when protection is no longer needed. Soaking the skin is not more effective and can contribute to toxicity. DEET should be applied only to exposed skin. Application on abraded skin or skin with rashes should be avoided. Care should be taken to avoid exposure to eyes and sensitive skin areas. Avoid use on children's hands, so that the child does not wipe on eyes, mouth, genitalia, and so on. Adults should apply DEET to their own hands and then wipe onto the child's face, rather than spraying onto a child's face.

Previous recommendations for conventional mosquito control were that DEET combination products that include sunscreen should not be used, because these combination products were found to mutually enhance the percutaneous absorption of each component in both a porcine in vivo study[84] and in an in vitro mouse skin model.[130] Because *A. aegypti* is most active during the day, combination products may be useful in this setting, but should be used judiciously. Other options for protection include mechanical means, such as mosquito netting, as well as permethrin-impregnated clothing for tick prevention.

NEWER INSECT REPELLENTS

The efficacy of any drug, treatment, or repellent is directly related to compliance with the treatment. Despite its demonstrated efficacy and safety, many people view chemical insect repellents such as DEET as potentially

harmful, and avoid their use. Several survey results in the United States and Canada revealed that 56% of people believe repellents are likely to be harmful to children, and 45% believed insect repellents are likely to sicken adults.[172] This has led to an intense search for effective alternatives to DEET-based repellents. Although their efficacy is not superior to DEET, their safety is likely at least equivalent to that of DEET. A review of the National Poison Data System from 2000 to 2015 of more than 68,000 exposures reveals that DEET, picaridin, and other non-DEET-containing insect repellents appear to have a low order of toxicity; the vast majority resulted in minimal effects after unintentional ingestions.[27]

Picaridin (Bayrepel, KBR3023)

Picaridin is also known as Bayrepel and KBR 3023 in Europe. It is a piperidine derivative, and has low acute oral, dermal, and inhalation toxicity. The EPA classifies it as toxicity category IV for acute inhalation toxicity and primary dermal irritation, the lowest rating available (class III for oral ingestion). It is not a dermal sensitizer, and no developmental toxicity was observed in chronic animal feeding studies. It was also not shown to be mutagenic in a battery of tests, and is not considered carcinogenic.[50] Picaridin is nearly as efficacious as DEET in comparison studies of the 20% solution used in Australia and Europe, and the 20% solution is now also available in the United States. Picaridin has significantly less percutaneous systemic absorption than DEET, even when mixed with sunscreens.[127]

Oil of Lemon Eucalyptus (PMD; *p*-Menthane-3,8-Diol)

Oil of lemon eucalyptus occurs naturally in the lemon eucalyptus plant (*Eucalyptus citriodora* also known as *Corymbia citriodora*). It is marketed in the United States under the brand name "OFF! Botanicals Insect Repellent." The natural oil can be extracted from the eucalyptus leaves and twigs; commercially the active ingredient, *p*-menthane-3,8-diol (PMD), is chemically synthesized, and is structurally similar to menthol. In its pure form, it is a solid at room temperature, and has a faint mintlike odor. *p*-Menthane-3,8-diol is placed into toxicity category IV for acute oral toxicity, dermal toxicity, and skin irritation, and toxicity category I for eye irritation (toxicity category II for the end-use product). It is not a skin sensitizer. The EPA has determined that there is reasonable certainty of no harm to the US population or subpopulations, including infants and children, as the result of the uses of *p*-menthane-3,8-diol to formulate insect repellents.[51] This compound, oil of lemon eucalyptus, is not to be confused with eucalyptus oil, a toxic essential oil containing 1,8-cineole, which has no insect repellent properties.

IR3535

IR3535 is a substituted beta-amino acid structurally similar to naturally occurring beta-alanine. The US EPA has classified IR3535 as a biochemical, based on the fact that it is functionally identical to naturally occurring beta alanine: both repel insects, the basic molecular structure is identical, the end groups are not likely to contribute to toxicity, and it acts to control the target pest via a nontoxic mode of action. It is a liquid that contains 98% active ingredient and 2% inert ingredients. It has been used as an insect repellent in Europe for more than 20 years with no substantial adverse effects. It is not as effective as DEET for mosquito control and is therefore not recommended for malaria-endemic areas,[69] and presumably also inadequate for protection against *A aegypti*. Toxicity tests show that IR3535 is not harmful when ingested, inhaled, or used on skin.[52,53] It is currently marketed in the United States by Avon Corporation as Skin-So-Soft Bug Guard Plus IR3535, at concentrations of 7.5% to 15%.

2-Undecanone (BioUD; Methyl Nonyl Ketone)

A newly formulated natural repellent, 2-undecanone, was approved for use as an insect repellent by the EPA in 2007, and is known by the brand name of BioUD. Its active ingredient is derived from the wild tomato plant, *Lycopersicon hirsutum* Dunal f. *glabratum* C. H. Mull.[172] 2-Undecanone (also known as methyl nonyl ketone) was originally registered in 1966 as a dog and cat repellent/training aid and an iris borer deterrent. It received EPA approval as a topical insect repellent in 2007. The EPA RED documents that in studies using laboratory animals, methyl nonyl ketone exhibited no toxicity via the oral and inhalation routes and was placed in toxicity category IV. Methyl nonyl ketone was slightly toxic (toxicity category III) for dermal toxicity, eye irritation, and dermal irritation and was a weak dermal sensitizer. Because it has a long history of safe use, is from a natural source, and is an approved food additive, it is considered essentially nontoxic. Methyl nonyl ketone is currently found in only one insect repellent in the form of both a lotion and a spray known as HOMS BiteBlocker Insect Repellent.[54] The manufacturer lists a nonpublished study on its Web site of a field test showing protection from mosquito bites surpassed that of a DEET 30% at 6 hours, and equivalent at 4 hours.[72] A 2008 study done by the inventors and patent holders showed it was only as efficacious as lower-DEET-concentration products in laboratory arm-in-cage trials, but field trials revealed efficacy equivalent to 25% to 30% DEET formulations.[172]

Oil of Citronella

Plant-derived essential oil products are considered minimum-risk pesticides and are exempt from EPA registration under section 25 (b) of the Federal Insecticide Fungicide and Rodenticide Act. Oil of Citronella has been used for more than 50 years as an insect repellent and as an animal repellent in candles and topical skin products. These products, which have little efficacy, are not expected to cause harm to humans, pets, or the environment when used according to the label.[55]

LEGAL STANDARDS FOR AN INSECTICIDE LABEL

The Federal Insecticide, Fungicide and Rodenticide Act of 1962 established criteria for a "signal word" on an insecticide label, which implies the degree of toxicity based on an oral LD_{50}. Also, the label on the original container of these products is usually instructive and should always be brought to the medical facility (Table CS11–1).

SUMMARY

- Organic chlorine insecticide agricultural use has largely been eliminated in the United States and Europe, but remains a problem in the developing world. DDT, with a low order of acute toxicity, remains an important tool for control of malaria vector mosquitoes and is approved for indoor spraying in Africa. Organic chlorines classically cause neurologic toxicity (tremors, seizures) when ingested.

- While pharmaceutical use of lindane for topical ectoparasitic infestations is still available in most US states, use has decreased greatly in favor of less-toxic permethrin preparations, and now accounts for only 2% of the prescriptions written for these conditions.

- Synthetic pyrethroid insecticides are the most commonly used insecticides for home use, and have a lower order of toxicity than organic chlorine or organic phosphorus insecticides. Their primary mechanism of action is similar to the DDT-type organic chlorines, acting on the insect voltage-gated sodium channel. The type II pyrethroids are more potent, and can cause systemic toxicity (CNS, pulmonary) when ingested, and $GABA_A$ antagonism may play a role in their toxicity, as well as the solvents and surfactants in the formulations.

- Athropod repellents containing DEET are still the most efficacious formulas and have many years of safe use in billions of people worldwide, when used as directed. Neurologic toxicity is described only after extreme exposure situations.

- Some newer insect repellents have efficacy approaching that of DEET, and few reported toxicities. As these newer repellents become more commonly used, significant toxicities are not expected.

REFERENCES

1. AAP Committee on Environmental Health. Follow safety precautions when using DEET on children. *AAP News.* 2003.
2. AAP Committee on Environmental Health. Pesticides. In: Etzel RA, ed. *Pediatric Environmental Health.* 2nd ed. Elk Grove Village, IL: American Academy of Pediatrics; 2003.
3. Aks SE, et al. Acute accidental lindane ingestion in toddlers. *Ann Emerg Med.* 1995; 26:647-651.
4. Altenkirch H. Multiple chemical sensitivity (MCS)—differential diagnosis in clinical neurotoxicology: a German perspective. *Neurotoxicology.* 2000;21:589-597.
5. Azziz-Baumgartner E. Mosquito control and exposure to pesticides, Virginia and North Carolina 2003. CDC Lecture Series 2003; http://www.cdc.gov/ncidod/dvbid/westnile/conf/pdf/Azziz_Baumgartner_6_04.pdf.
6. Baek BH, et al. Chlorfenapyr-induced toxic leukoencephalopathy with radiologic reversibility: a case report and literature review. *Korean J Radiol.* 2016;17:277-280.
7. Bateman DN. Management of pyrethroid exposure. *J Toxicol Clin Toxicol.* 2000; 38:107-109.
8. Bloomquist JR. Intrinsic lethality of chloride-channel-directed insecticides and convulsants in mammals. *Toxicol Lett.* 1992;60:289-298.
9. Bloomquist JR, et al. Reduced neuronal sensitivity to dieldrin and picrotoxinin in a cyclodiene-resistant strain of Drosophila melanogaster (Meigen). *Arch Insect Biochem Physiol.* 1992;19:17-25.
10. Bornschein S, et al. Pest controllers: a high-risk group for Multiple Chemical Sensitivity (MCS)? *Clin Toxicol (Phila).* 2008;46:193-200.
11. Boylan JJ, et al. Excretion of chlordecone by the gastrointestinal tract: evidence for a nonbiliary mechanism. *Clin Pharmacol Ther.* 1979;25:579-585.
12. Bradberry SM, et al. Poisoning due to pyrethroids. *Toxicol Rev.* 2005;24:93-106.
13. Brisson P. Percutaneous absorption. *Can Med Assoc J.* 1974;110:1182-1185.
14. Brody JG, et al. Breast cancer risk and historical exposure to pesticides from wide-area applications assessed with GIS. *Environ Health Perspect.* 2004;112:889-897.
15. Burkhart CG. Relationship of treatment-resistant head lice to the safety and efficacy of pediculicides. *Mayo Clin Proc.* 2004;79:661-666.
16. Calle EE, et al. Organochlorines and breast cancer risk. *CA Cancer J Clin.* 2002;52:301-309.
17. Carson R. Silent Spring. Houghton Mifflin; 1962.
18. Cecil HC, et al. Dietary p,p'-DDT, o,p'-DDT or p,p'-DDE and changes in egg shell characteristics and pesticide accumulation in egg contents and body fat of caged White Leghorns. *Poult Sci.* 1972;51:130-139.
19. Center for Disease Control and Prevention (CDC). Fourth National Report on Human Exposure to Environmental Chemicals—updated tables. 2015;2017.
20. Centers for Disease Control (CDC). Seizures temporally associated with use of DEET insect repellent—New York and Connecticut. *MMWR Morb Mortal Wkly Rep.* 1989;38:678-680.
21. Centers for Disease Control and Prevention (CDC). Acute convulsions associated with endrin poisoning—Pakistan. *MMWR Morb Mortal Wkly Rep.* 1984;33:687-688, 693.
22. Centers for Disease Control and Prevention (CDC). Zika Virus—case counts in the USA. 2017;2017.
23. Centers for Disease Control and Prevention (CDC). West Nile Virus. 2015;2017.
24. Centers for Disease Control and Prevention (CDC). *Fourth National Report on Human Exposure to Environmental Chemicals.* Atlanta, GA: Department of Health and Human Services (DHHS), Centers for Disease Control and Prevention (CDC), 2009.
25. Centers for Disease Control and Prevention (CDC). Worker illness related to ground application of pesticide—Kern County, California, 2005. *MMWR Morb Mortal Wkly Rep.* 2006;55:486-488.
26. Chang ES, Stokstad EL. Effect of chlorinated hydrocarbons on shell gland carbonic anhydrase and egg shell thickness in Japanese quail. *Poult Sci.* 1975;54:3-10.
27. Charlton NP, et al. The toxicity of picaridin containing insect repellent reported to the National Poison Data System. *Clin Toxicol (Phila).* 2016;54:655-658.
28. Chen SY, et al. An epidemiological study on occupational acute pyrethroid poisoning in cotton farmers. *Br J Ind Med.* 1991;48:77-81.
29. Chen-Hussey V, et al. Assessment of methods used to determine the safety of the topical insect repellent N,N-diethyl-m-toluamide (DEET). *Parasit Vectors.* 2014;7:173.
30. Choi JT, et al. Sensorimotor function and sensorimotor tracts after hemispherectomy. *Neuropsychologia.* 2010;48:1192-1199.
31. Coats JR. Mechanisms of toxic action and structure-activity relationships for organochlorine and synthetic pyrethroid insecticides. *Environ Health Perspect.* 1990; 87:255-262.
32. Cohn BA, et al. DDT and breast cancer in young women: new data on the significance of age at exposure. *Environ Health Perspect.* 2007;115:1406-1414.
33. Cohn WJ, et al. Treatment of chlordecone (Kepone) toxicity with cholestyramine. Results of a controlled clinical trial. *N Engl J Med.* 1978;298:243-248.
34. Conney AH, et al. Effects of pesticides on drug and steroid metabolism. *Clin Pharmacol Ther.* 1967;8:2-10.
35. Costa LG. The neurotoxicity of organochlorine and pyrethroid pesticides. *Handb Clin Neurol.* 2015;131:135-148.
36. Costa LG. Basic toxicology of pesticides. *Occup Med (Lond).* 1997;12:251-268.
37. Coye MJ, et al. Biological monitoring of agricultural workers exposed to pesticides: II. Monitoring of intact pesticides and their metabolites. *J Occup Med.* 1986;28:628-636.
38. Cummings AM. Methoxychlor as a model for environmental estrogens. *Crit Rev Toxicol.* 1997;27:367.
39. Dale WE, et al. Poisoning by DDT: relation between clinical signs and concentration in rat brain. *Science.* 1963;142:1474-1476.
40. Davies JE, et al. Lindane poisonings. *Arch Dermatol.* 1983;119:142-144.
41. Davies TG, et al. DDT, pyrethrins, pyrethroids and insect sodium channels. *IUBMB Life.* 2007;59:151-162.
42. Davison KL. Calcium-45 uptake by shell gland, oviduct, plasma and eggshell of DDT-dosed ducks and chickens. *Arch Environ Contam Toxicol.* 1978;7:359-367.

43. Davison KL, Sell JL. DDT thins shells of eggs from mallard ducks maintained on ad libitum or controlled-feeding regimens. *Arch Environ Contam Toxicol.* 1974;2:222-232.

44. Diel F, et al. In vitro effects of the pyrethroid *S*-bioallethrin on lymphocytes and basophils from atopic and nonatopic subjects. *Allergy.* 1998;53:1052-1059.

45. Doi H, et al. Motor neuron disorder simulating ALS induced by chronic inhalation of pyrethroid insecticides. *Neurology.* 2006;67:1894-1895.

46. Domb AJ, et al. Insect repellent formulations of *N,N*-diethyl-*m*-toluamide (DEET) in a liposphere system: efficacy and skin uptake. *J Am Mosq Control Assoc.* 1995;11:29-34.

47. Echobichon DJ. Toxic effects of pesticides. In: Klaassen CD, ed. *Casarett and Doull's Toxicology: The Basic Science of Poisons.* 5th ed. New York, NY: Macmillan; 1996:643-669.

48. Echobichon DJ, Joy RM. *Pesticides and Neurological Diseases.* Boca Raton, FL: CRC Press; 1994.

49. Endo Y, et al. Acute chlorfenapyr poisoning. *Chudoku Kenkyu.* 2004;17:89-93.

50. Environmental Protection Agency. Picaridin new pesticide fact sheet. US EPA, 2005.

51. Environmental Protection Agency. Registration eligibility document for *p*-menthane-3,8-diol (Oil of lemon eucalyptus). US EPA, 2000.

52. Environmental Protection Agency. 3-[*N*-Butyl-*N*-acetyl]-aminopropionic acid, ethylester (IR3535) fact sheet. US EPA, 2000.

53. Environmental Protection Agency. 3-[*N*-Butyl-*N*-acetyl]-aminopropionic acid, ethyl ester (IR3535) technical document. US EPA, 1997.

54. Environmental Protection Agency. Pesticide re-registration eligibility decision: methyl nonyl ketone (2-Undecanone). US EPA, 1995.

55. EPA. Citronella (Oil of Citronella) (021901) Fact Sheet. http://www.epa.gov/pesticides/biopesticides/ingredients/factsheets/factsheet_021901.htm.

56. Faroon O, et al. ATSDR evaluation of health effects of chemicals. II. Mirex and chlordecone: health effects, toxicokinetics, human exposure, and environmental fate. *Toxicol Ind Health.* 1995;11:1-203.

57. Feldmann RJ, Maibach HI. Percutaneous penetration of some pesticides and herbicides in man. *Toxicol Appl Pharmacol.* 1974;28:126-132.

58. Food and Drug Administration. Postmarket drug safety information for patients and providers—Lindane Shampoo and Lindane Lotion—Questions and Answers. 2013;2017.

59. Fradin MS, Day JF. Comparative efficacy of insect repellents against mosquito bites. *N Engl J Med.* 2002;347:13-18.

60. Fradin MS. Mosquitoes and mosquito repellents: a clinician's guide. *Ann Intern Med.* 1998;128:931-940.

61. Franz TJ. Kinetics of cutaneous drug penetration. *Int J Dermatol.* 1983;22:499-505.

62. Franzosa JA, et al. Cutaneous contact urticaria to pyrethrum-real?, common?, or not documented?: an evidence-based approach. *Cutan Ocul Toxicol.* 2007;26:57-72.

63. Gaido K, et al. Comparative estrogenic activity of wine extracts and organochlorine pesticide residues in food. *Environ Health Perspect.* 1998;106(suppl 6):1347-1351.

64. Gant DB, et al. Cyclodiene insecticides inhibit GABA$_A$ receptor-regulated chloride transport. *Toxicol Appl Pharmacol.* 1987;88:313-321.

65. Garrettson LK, et al. Subacute chlordane poisoning. *J Toxicol Clin Toxicol.* 1984; 22:565-571.

66. Gatto NM, et al. Serum organochlorines and breast cancer: a case-control study among African-American women. *Cancer Causes Control.* 2007;18:29-39.

67. Geusau A, et al. Severe 2,3,7,8-tetrachlorodibenzo-*p*-dioxin (TCDD) intoxication: kinetics and trials to enhance elimination in two patients. *Arch Toxicol.* 2002;76:316-325.

68. Goodyer L, Behrens RH. Short report: the safety and toxicity of insect repellents. *Am J Trop Med Hyg.* 1998;59:323-324.

69. Goodyer LI, et al. Expert review of the evidence base for arthropod bite avoidance. *J Travel Med.* 2010;17:182-192.

70. Hayes WJ. Chlorinated hydrocarbon insecticides. In: Hayes WJ, Lawes ER, eds. *Pesticides Studied in Man.* San Diego, CA: Academic Press; 1991:731-868.

71. He F, et al. Clinical manifestations and diagnosis of acute pyrethroid poisoning. *Arch Toxicol.* 1989;63:54-58.

72. Heal JD, Jones A. Field evaluation of two HOMS mosquito repellents to repel mosquitoes in Southern Ontario, 2006. http://www.bioud.com/Documents/HOMSfinalreport2006.pdf.

73. Herr DW, et al. Pharmacological modification of tremor and enhanced acoustic startle by chlordecone and *p,p'*-DDT. *Psychopharmacology (Berl).* 1987;91:320-325.

74. Hoshiko M, et al. Case report of acute death on the 7th day due to exposure to the vapor of the insecticide chlorfenapyr. *Chudoku Kenkyu.* 2007;20:131-136.

75. HSDB-TOXNET. HSDB: Chlorfenapyr. 2007;2017.

76. Hunter DJ, et al. Plasma organochlorine levels and the risk of breast cancer. *N Engl J Med.* 1997;337:1253-1258.

77. Ibarluzea J, et al. Breast cancer risk and the combined effect of environmental estrogens. *Cancer Causes Control.* 2004;15:591-600.

78. Idson B. Vehicle effects in percutaneous absorption. *Drug Metab Rev.* 1983;14:207-222.

79. Ingber SZ, et al. DDT/DDE and breast cancer: a meta-analysis. *Regul Toxicol Pharmacol.* 2013;67:421-433.

80. Iwasaki M, et al. Plasma organochlorine levels and subsequent risk of breast cancer among Japanese women: a nested case-control study. *Sci Total Environ.* 2008; 402:176-183.

81. Jandacek RJ, et al. Effects of yo-yo diet, caloric restriction, and olestra on tissue distribution of hexachlorobenzene. *Am J Physiol Gastrointest Liver Physiol.* 2005; 288:G292-G299.

82. Kang C, et al. A patient fatality following the ingestion of a small amount of chlorfenapyr. *J Emerg Trauma Shock.* 2014;7:239-241.

83. Karpati AM, et al. Pesticide spraying for West Nile virus control and emergency department asthma visits in New York City, 2000. *Environ Health Perspect.* 2004;112:1183-1187.

84. Kasichayanula S, et al. Percutaneous characterization of the insect repellent DEET and the sunscreen oxybenzone from topical skin application. *Toxicol Appl Pharmacol.* 2007;223:187-194.

85. Kassner JT, et al. Cholestyramine as an adsorbent in acute lindane poisoning: a murine model. *Ann Emerg Med.* 1993;22:1392-1397.

86. Katz TM, et al. Insect repellents: historical perspectives and new developments. *J Am Acad Dermatol.* 2008;58:865-871.

87. Klaassen CD. Nonmetallic environmental toxicants. In: Hardman JG, et al., eds. *Goodman and Gilman's The Pharmacologic Basis of Therapeutics.* 9th ed. New York, NY: McGraw-Hill; 1996:1684-1699.

88. Koren G, et al. DEET-based insect repellents: safety implications for children and pregnant and lactating women. *CMAJ.* 2003;169:209-212.

89. Kramer MS, et al. Operational criteria for adverse drug reactions in evaluating suspected toxicity of a popular scabicide. *Clin Pharmacol Ther.* 1980;27:149-155.

90. Krieger N, et al. Breast cancer and serum organochlorines: a prospective study among white, black, and Asian women. *J Natl Cancer Inst.* 1994;86:589-599.

91. Le Quesne PM, et al. Transient facial sensory symptoms following exposure to synthetic pyrethroids: a clinical and electrophysiological assessment. *Neurotoxicology.* 1981;2:1-11.

92. Lee B, Groth P. Scabies: transcutaneous poisoning during treatment. *Pediatrics.* 1977; 59:643.

93. Leng G, et al. Biomarker of pyrethrum exposure. *Toxicol Lett.* 2006;162:195-201.

94. Lohani S, et al. Abstract 146: Status epilepticus after acute endosulfan poisoning: a study of 25 cases. *Clin Toxicol (Phila).* 2012;50:574-720.

95. Lopez-Cervantes M, et al. Dichlorodiphenyldichloroethane burden and breast cancer risk: a meta-analysis of the epidemiologic evidence. *Environ Health Perspect.* 2004; 112:207-214.

96. Lucena RA, et al. A review of environmental exposure to persistent organochlorine residuals during the last fifty years. *Curr Drug Saf.* 2007;2:163-172.

97. Mestres R, Mestres G. Deltamethrin: uses and environmental safety. *Rev Environ Contam Toxicol.* 1992;124:1-18.

98. Morgan-Glenn PD. Scabies. *Pediatr Rev.* 2001;22:322-323.

99. Mortensen ML. Management of acute childhood poisonings caused by selected insecticides and herbicides. *Pediatr Clin North Am.* 1986;33:421-445.

100. Mouchet J, et al. Evolution of malaria in Africa for the past 40 years: impact of climatic and human factors. *J Am Mosq Control Assoc.* 1998;14:121-130.

101. Mutter LC, et al. Reduction in the body content of DDE in the Mongolian gerbil treated with sucrose polyester and caloric restriction. *Toxicol Appl Pharmacol.* 1988;92:428-435.

102. Narahashi T. Neuronal ion channels as the target sites of insecticides. *Pharmacol Toxicol.* 1996;79:1-14.

103. Narahashi T. Nerve membrane Na$^+$ channels as targets of insecticides. *Trends Pharmacol Sci.* 1992;13:236-241.

104. Narahashi T, et al. Sodium and GABA-activated channels as the targets of pyrethroids and cyclodienes. *Toxicol Lett.* 1992;64-65:429-436.

105. Narahashi T, et al. Differential actions of insecticides on target sites: basis for selective toxicity. *Hum Exp Toxicol.* 2007;26:361-366.

106. Nolan K, et al. Lindane toxicity: a comprehensive review of the medical literature. Pediatr Dermatol. 2012;29:141-146.

107. O'Reilly AO, et al. Modelling insecticide-binding sites in the voltage-gated sodium channel. *Biochem J.* 2006;396:255-263.

108. Osimitz TG, Murphy JV. Neurological effects associated with use of the insect repellent *N,N*-diethyl-*m*-toluamide (DEET). *J Toxicol Clin Toxicol.* 1997;35:435-441.

109. Osimitz TG, Grothaus RH. The present safety assessment of DEET. *J Am Mosq Control Assoc.* 1995;11:274-278.

110. Pahwa P, et al. Hodgkin lymphoma, multiple myeloma, soft tissue sarcomas, insect repellents, and phenoxyherbicides. *J Occup Environ Med.* 2006;48:264-274.

111. Park JH, et al. Exposure to dichlorodiphenyltrichloroethane and the risk of breast cancer: a systematic review and meta-analysis. *Osong Public Health Res Perspect.* 2014;5:77-84.

112. Paton DL, Walker JS. Pyrethrin poisoning from commercial-strength flea and tick spray. *Am J Emerg Med.* 1988;6:232-235.

113. Pramanik AK, Hansen RC. Transcutaneous gamma benzene hexachloride absorption and toxicity in infants and children. *Arch Dermatol.* 1979;115:1224-1225.

114. Price RJ, et al. Effect of pyrethrins on cytochrome P450 forms in cultured rat and human hepatocytes. *Toxicology.* 2008;243:84-95.

115. Proudfoot AT. Poisoning due to pyrethrins. *Toxicol Rev.* 2005;24:107-113.

116. Qiu H, et al. Pharmacokinetics, formulation, and safety of insect repellent *N,N*-diethyl-3-methylbenzamide (DEET): a review. *J Am Mosq Control Assoc.* 1998;14:12-27.

117. Ramadan AA, et al. Actions of pyrethroids on the peripheral benzodiazepine receptor. *Pestic Biochem Physiol.* 1988;32:106-113.

118. Rasmussen JE. The problem of lindane. *J Am Acad Dermatol.* 1981;5:507-516.

119. Ray DE, Fry JR. A reassessment of the neurotoxicity of pyrethroid insecticides. *Pharmacol Ther.* 2006;111:174-193.

120. Ray DE, Forshaw PJ. Pyrethroid insecticides: poisoning syndromes, synergies, and therapy. *J Toxicol Clin Toxicol.* 2000;38:95-101.

121. Reigart JR, Roberts JR. *Recognition and Management of Pesticide Poisonings.* EPA Document No. EPA 735-R-98-003. Washington, DC: Environmental Protection Agency; 1999.

122. Riley B, Bringhurst J. Abstract 200. DEET toxicity in a nudist. Abstracts of the 2011 North American Congress of Clinical Toxicology Annual Meeting, September 21-26, Washington, DC, USA. *Clin Toxicol.* 2011;49:515-627.

123. Roberts DR, et al. DDT house spraying and re-emerging malaria. *Lancet.* 2000; 356:330-332.

124. Roberts DR, et al. DDT, global strategies, and a malaria control crisis in South America. *Emerg Infect Dis.* 1997;3:295-302.

125. Roberts JR, Reigart JR. Does anything beat DEET? *Pediatr Ann.* 2004;33:443-453.

126. Robson WA, et al. Effect of DDE, DDT and calcium on the performance of adult Japanese quail (*Coturnix coturnix japonica*). *Poult Sci.* 1976;55:2222-2227.

127. Rodriguez J, Maibach HI. Percutaneous penetration and pharmacodynamics: wash-in and wash-off of sunscreen and insect repellent. *J Dermatolog Treat.* 2016;27:11-18.

128. Rogan WJ. Pollutants in breast milk. *Arch Pediatr Adolesc Med.* 1996;150:981-990.

129. Roos TC, et al. Pharmacotherapy of ectoparasitic infections. *Drugs.* 2001;61:1067-1088.

130. Ross EA, et al. Insect repellent [correction of repellant] interactions: sunscreens enhance DEET (*N,N*-diethyl-*m*-toluamide) absorption. *Drug Metab Dispos.* 2004;32:783-785.

131. Sadasivaiah S, et al. Dichlorodiphenyltrichloroethane (DDT) for indoor residual spraying in Africa: how can it be used for malaria control? *Am J Trop Med Hyg.* 2007;77:249-263.

132. Safe SH. Xenoestrogens and breast cancer. *N Engl J Med.* 1997;337:1303-1304.

133. Safe SH. Is there an association between exposure to environmental estrogens and breast cancer? *Environ Health Perspect.* 1997;105:675-678.

134. Safe SH. Environmental and dietary estrogens and human health: is there a problem? [see comment]. *Environ Health Perspect.* 1995;103:346-351.

135. Salafsky B, et al. Short report: study on the efficacy of a new long-acting formulation of *N,N*-diethyl-*m*-toluamide (DEET) for the prevention of tick attachment. *Am J Trop Med Hyg.* 2000;62:169-172.

136. Saleh MA. Toxaphene: chemistry, biochemistry, toxicity and environmental fate. *Rev Environ Contam Toxicol.* 1991;118:1-85.

137. Schenker MB, et al. Pesticides. In: Rom WN, ed. *Environmental and Occupational Medicine.* 3rd ed. Philadelphia, PA: Lippincott-Raven; 1998:1157-1172.

138. Schoenig GP, et al. Teratologic evaluations of *N,N*-diethyl-*m*-toluamide (DEET) in rats and rabbits. *Fundam Appl Toxicol.* 1994;23:63-69.

139. Schoenig GP, et al. Neurotoxicity evaluation of *N,N*-diethyl-*m*-toluamide (DEET) in rats. *Fundam Appl Toxicol.* 1993;21:355-365.

140. Schoenig GP, et al. Evaluation of the chronic toxicity and oncogenicity of *N,N*-diethyl-*m*-toluamide (DEET). *Toxicol Sci.* 1999;47:99-109.

141. Shelov SP. *Caring for Your Baby and Young Child: Birth to Age 5.* New York, NY: Bantam Books; 1994.

142. Siddiqui MK, et al. Biomonitoring of organochlorines in women with benign and malignant breast disease. *Environ Res.* 2005;98:250-257.

143. Snedeker SM. Pesticides and breast cancer risk: a review of DDT, DDE, and dieldrin. *Environ Health Perspect.* 2001;109:35-47.

144. Soderlund DM, et al. Mechanisms of pyrethroid neurotoxicity: implications for cumulative risk assessment. *Toxicology.* 2002;171:3-59.

145. Solomon BA, et al. Neurotoxic reaction to lindane in an HIV-seropositive patient. An old medication's new problem. *J Fam Pract.* 1995;40:291-296.

146. Solomon LM, et al. Gamma benzene hexachloride toxicity: a review. *Arch Dermatol.* 1977;113:353-357.

147. Song JH, et al. Interactions of tetramethrin, fenvalerate and DDT at the sodium channel in rat dorsal root ganglion neurons. *Brain Res.* 1996;708:29-37.

148. Soto AM, et al. The pesticides endosulfan, toxaphene, and dieldrin have estrogenic effects on human estrogen-sensitive cells. *Environ Health Perspect.* 1994;102:380-383.

149. Sterling JB, Hanke CW. Dioxin toxicity and chloracne in the Ukraine. *J Drugs Dermatol.* 2005;4:148-150.

150. Stinecipher J, Shah J. Percutaneous permeation of *N,N*-diethyl-*m*-toluamide (DEET) from commercial mosquito repellents and the effect of solvent. *J Toxicol Environ Health.* 1997;52:119-135.

151. Street JC, Chadwick RW. Ascorbic acid requirements and metabolism in relation to organochlorine pesticides. *Ann N Y Acad Sci.* 1975;258:132-143.

152. Sudakin DL. Pyrethroid insecticides: advances and challenges in biomonitoring. *Clin Toxicol (Phila).* 2006;44:31-37.

153. Sudakin DL, Trevathan WR. DEET: a review and update of safety and risk in the general population. *J Toxicol Clin Toxicol.* 2003;41:831-839.

154. Syed Z, Leal WS. Mosquitoes smell and avoid the insect repellent DEET. *Proc Natl Acad Sci U S A.* 2008;105:13598-13603.

155. Tenenbein M. Seizures after lindane therapy. *J Am Geriatr Soc.* 1991;39:394-395.

156. Tenenbein M. Severe toxic reactions and death following the ingestion of diethyltoluamide-containing insect repellents. *JAMA.* 1987;258:1509-1511.

157. Tharaknath VR, et al. Clinical and radiological findings in chlorfenapyr poisoning. *Ann Indian Acad Neurol.* 2013;16:252-254.

158. Tilson HA, et al. The effects of lindane, DDT, and chlordecone on avoidance responding and seizure activity. *Toxicol Appl Pharmacol.* 1987;88:57-65.

159. Tilson HA, et al. Effects of 5,5-diphenylhydantoin (phenytoin) on neurobehavioral toxicity of organochlorine insecticides and permethrin. *J Pharmacol Exp Ther.* 1985;233:285-289.

160. US CDC. Interim CDC recommendations for Zika vector control in the continental United States. 2016;2017.

161. US Environmental Protection Agency Office of Pesticide Programs. Label review manual. US Environmental Protection Agency Office of Pesticide Programs, 2016:71.

162. US FDA. FDA labeling changes for lindane. http://www.fda.gov/cder/drug/infopage/lindane/default.htm.

163. Usmani KA, et al. In vitro human metabolism and interactions of repellent *N,N*-diethyl-*m*-toluamide. *Drug Metab Dispos.* 2002;30:289-294.

164. Veltri JC, et al. Retrospective analysis of calls to poison control centers resulting from exposure to the insect repellent *N,N*-diethyl-*m*-toluamide (DEET) from 1985-1989. *J Toxicol Clin Toxicol.* 1994;32:1-16.

165. Vijverberg HP, van den Bercken J. Neurotoxicological effects and the mode of action of pyrethroid insecticides. *Crit Rev Toxicol.* 1990;21:105-126.

166. Waibel GP, et al. Effects of DDT and charcoal on performance of White Leghorn hens. *Poult Sci.* 1972;51:1963-1967.

167. Walker GJ, Johnstone PW. Interventions for treating scabies. *Cochrane Database Syst Rev.* 2007:CD000320.

168. Ware GW, Whitacre DM. *An Introduction to Insecticides.* 4th ed. (Extracted from *The Pesticide Book*, 6th ed*. (2004) Meister Media Worldwide. http://ipmworld.umn.edu/chapters/ware.htm.

169. Wax PM, Hoffman RS. Fatality associated with inhalation of a pyrethrin shampoo. *J Toxicol Clin Toxicol.* 1994;32:457-460.

170. WHO. Fact Sheet: World Malaria Day 2016. 2016;2017.

171. Williams CH, Casterline JL Jr. Effects of toxicity and on enzyme activity of the interactions between aldrin, chlordane, piperonyl butoxide, and banol in rats. *Proc Soc Exp Biol Med.* 1970;135:46-50.

172. Witting-Bissinger BE, et al. Novel arthropod repellent, BioUD, is an efficacious alternative to DEET. *J Med Entomol.* 2008;45:891-898.

173. Wolff MS, et al. Blood levels of organochlorine residues and risk of breast cancer. *J Natl Cancer Inst.* 1993;85:648-652.

174. Woollen BH, et al. The metabolism of cypermethrin in man: differences in urinary metabolite profiles following oral and dermal administration. *Xenobiotica.* 1992; 22:983-991.

175. Woolley DE. Differential effects of benzodiazepines, including diazepam, clonazepam, Ro 5-4864 and devazepide, on lindane-induced toxicity. *Proc West Pharmacol Soc.* 1994;37:131-134.

176. Wright DM, et al. Reproductive and developmental toxicity of *N,N*-diethyl-*m*-toluamide in rats. *Fundam Appl Toxicol.* 1992;19:33-42.

177. Yang PY, et al. Acute ingestion poisoning with insecticide formulations containing the pyrethroid permethrin, xylene, and surfactant: a review of 48 cases. *J Toxicol Clin Toxicol.* 2002;40:107-113.

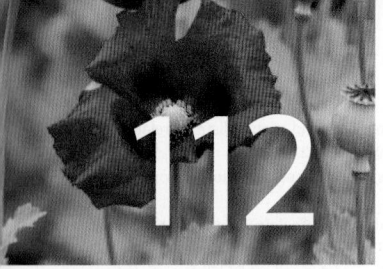

112 PHOSPHORUS

Michael C. Beuhler

Phosphorus (P)
Atomic number = 15
Atomic weight = 30.97 Da
Normal concentration
    Serum = 3–4.5 mg/dL (1–1.4 mmol/L) as phosphate

HISTORY AND EPIDEMIOLOGY

Phosphorus is a nonmetallic essential element discovered hundreds of years ago that exists in 3 forms, with white phosphorus being the most important from a toxicological standpoint. The word "phosphorus" means light-bearer, which originates from its property of glowing when exposed to air. Its luminescent and pyrotechnic qualities resulted in widespread use in matches and fireworks, and its toxic properties was historically used as a rodenticide. It is still encountered occasionally and remains in use for munitions and in chemical syntheses. Biologically, it is present in living organisms as the phosphate ion that is an entirely different entity than the elemental phosphorus and not considered in this chapter.

Phosphorus is a nonmetallic element not naturally found in its elemental form; the white allotropic form was isolated from urine by Hennig Brandt in 1669. White phosphorus has been used in munitions since World War I for its antipersonnel effect as well as its warning, incendiary, and smoke producing properties. It is also used in fireworks in countries other than the United States (where consumer-grade fireworks containing white phosphorus are illegal) and for some chemical synthetic processes. White phosphorus was used extensively in the past as a rodenticide but is no longer permitted for this purpose in the United States. Because of the potential use of phosphorus for illicit drug manufacturing of methamphetamines, its sale is monitored by the US Drug Enforcement Administration. Before modern regulation, it was used in scientifically unsubstantiated remedies primarily because its phosphorescent and reactive qualities suggested potency. Its occasional use for homicides was limited by its characteristic luminescent, smoking qualities; however, it remains a method of suicide in some countries.

At the beginning of the 20th century, phosphorus was used in millions of "strike anywhere" matches (lucifers). However, safety concerns with the matches and illnesses in the workers producing the matches prompted a shift from using the more dangerous white phosphorus in the match heads to substituting the safer red phosphorus in the strikers. Workers chronically exposed to white phosphorus developed "phossy jaw," an illness characterized by disfiguring osteonecrosis of the mandible along with multiple draining abscesses and bony loss. Although the disease was actually of low prevalence among phosphorus workers, the painful, visible deformities in otherwise healthy young people drew widespread attention.

CHEMISTRY AND PHARMACOLOGY

Phosphorus, atomic number 15, is in group 15 (CAS group VA) which is made up of nonmetals, metalloids, and metal elements; shares chemical properties with nitrogen (above) and arsenic (below) in the periodic table. Elemental phosphorus exists in several different allotropes (polymorphs); the 2 common forms considered in this chapter are red phosphorus and the highly reactive white phosphorus. The black allotrope is reasonably stable at standard conditions and has potential novel application in electronics because of its semiconductive planar crystalline structure and multiple anisotropic physical properties. However, the black allotrope is rarely encountered, relatively nontoxic, and will not be considered further.

White phosphorus is a waxy whitish to yellow solid with a melting point of 111.4°F (44.1°C); after ignition, it will have a gummy to liquid form. Often there is a small amount of red phosphorus in samples of white phosphorus, resulting in discoloration and explaining the term "yellow" phosphorus. The glow when exposed to air is due to the formation of reactive luminescent phosphorus oxides on its surface. White phosphorus is insoluble in water and often stored under it. It is soluble in carbon disulfide, which is the most common solvent used for dissolution as it is much less soluble in other organic solvents. White phosphorus is very reactive, igniting spontaneously in air at approximately 93°F (34°C), oxidizing to form phosphorus pentoxide (P_4O_{10}), phosphorus trioxide (P_4O_6), and potentially trace amounts of unreacted white phosphorus that usually appears as a white fume (smoke) having a garliclike smell. These anhydrous oxides of phosphorus are hydroscopic, reacting with water to form phosphorus-containing acids as well as with organic molecules in dehydrating reactions.

Red phosphorus is a red powdery compound of limited toxicologic significance. It is not luminescent, it does not combust in air, and its toxicity is orders of magnitude less than that of white phosphorus.

PHARMACOKINETICS AND TOXICOKINETICS

White phosphorus is well absorbed from the intestinal tract, and coingestion with fats, alcohol, and liquids increases toxicity, probably from increased absorption.[7,8] However, GI absorption is not always complete, which is quite evident when patients pass luminescent, smoking stools. White phosphorus is also well absorbed through the skin, with burns contributing to the absorption; however, fragments can remain unabsorbed in the skin for days.[22] Significant morbidity and mortality occur from large surface area burns. White phosphorus is also absorbed by inhalation, although this exposure route is rare with current industrial hygiene practices.

After ingestion, phosphorus is found in high concentrations within 3 hours in the liver (greatest concentration), blood, and kidneys.[4,13] The final amount of internalized phosphorus likely depends on the dose and its exact form, such as the particle size and the presence of a nonpolar solvent. The conversion of absorbed phosphorus to its oxidized forms is believed to be rapid, on the order of hours.[15] Absorbed phosphorus is eliminated after undergoing (likely nonenzymatic) oxidation to phosphate and probably other minor phosphorus acids; phosphorus may also form biological adducts, but this has not been determined.[15,21]

Internally absorbed white phosphorus has significant toxicity. A dose of only about 1 mg/kg in adults is likely to cause significant morbidity, but a lethal dose of 3 mg is reported in a child; part of the outcome variability may be due to differences between the exposure and the absorbed amount.[3] The mortality from white phosphorus ingestion is difficult to estimate, because the majority of reported cases occurred prior to the development of critical care. Historically, significant ingestions carried a 25% mortality rate.[11]

PATHOPHYSIOLOGY

The mechanism of dermal injury from white phosphorus differs significantly from that of ingested white phosphorus. Externally, white phosphorus reacts with oxygen (ie, burns) to form phosphorus pentoxide and other phosphorus oxides. Phosphorus pentoxide readily reacts with water in an exothermic reaction, producing corrosive phosphoric acid.[14] Additionally, phosphorus pentoxide reacts with (dehydrates) some organic molecules. These 3 mechanisms of exothermic, acid-producing, and dehydrating reactions all contribute to the tissue injury observed, although the most damaging mechanism is the thermal injury from the heat of the reaction, as evidenced by the relatively short distance of tissue penetration by the acid and the relatively large amount of available water.[6,26] The evidence for describing white phosphorus as a cytoplasmic poison is mostly derived from electron microscopy, which demonstrates an initial cytoplasmic injury of the rough endoplasmic reticulum rather than initial nuclear or mitochondrial changes, but white phosphorus has an effect on mitochondrial energetics and oxidant effects.[12,20]

A resurgence of toxicity and human injury indirectly related to red phosphorus resulted from the increase in North American domestic methamphetamine production. Red phosphorus is used in conjunction with elemental iodine to produce hydroiodic acid, the ultimate reducing agent required to convert ephedrine to methamphetamine. In this situation, red phosphorus contributes to human injury by causing fire because of its unintentional conversion to highly flammable white phosphorus. Toxicity occurs because during heating, the reaction products of iodine and red phosphorus often generate phosphine (PH_3), a pulmonary irritant and metabolic inhibitor gas (Chap. 108). Phosphine is only produced in significant amounts during an active methamphetamine "cook" using the red phosphorus method. This gas most likely contributes to some of the pulmonary effects occurring with chronic exposures in methamphetamine laboratories, as well as several of the deaths resulting from performing the synthesis in an area with limited ventilation in order to hide the characteristic odors.[27]

Red phosphorus has limited direct toxicologic significance. It can cause gastrointestinal (GI) irritation when ingested in significant amounts, but it is orders of magnitude less toxic than white phosphorus. All further references to phosphorus in this chapter refer to white phosphorus.

CLINICAL MANIFESTATIONS

General

The clinical manifestations of oral phosphorus poisoning are classically described in 3 stages. The initial effects are delayed for a few hours, and the degree of delay partially depends on the dose. During the first phase, patients experience vomiting, hematemesis, and abdominal pain, with hypotension and death occurring within 24 hours after large ingestions.[8] During the second stage, there is transient resolution of the toxic effects. During the third stage, the patient develops hepatic injury with coagulopathy, jaundice, and acute kidney injury with oliguria and uremia. Altered mental status and seizures, independent of electrolyte abnormalities, are also reported. However, clinical experience demonstrates that 3 distinct phases are the exception rather than the rule, with significant overlap or absence of the "quiescent" second stage and death potentially occurring within hours of ingestion.[7,17] In the first 6 hours postexposure, poor prognostic signs include altered sensorium, cyanosis, hypotension, metabolic acidosis, elevated prothrombin time, and hypoglycemia.[7] Survival to 3 days serves as a good prognostic sign. However, deaths also occur weeks later in the clinical course.[8] Recovery usually occurs over 1 to 2 weeks.

Gastrointestinal

Initial symptoms after ingestion of phosphorus include nausea, vomiting, and abdominal pain. Both diarrhea and constipation are reported but are much less common. The breath and vomitus are sometimes described as having a garlic or musty sweet odor. The vomitus and diarrhea are sometimes luminescent and smoking, but this specific finding occurs infrequently. The smoking effect is caused by the combustion of phosphorus upon its exposure to air after being eliminated unabsorbed from the GI tract. Phosphorus causes an inflammatory injury to the GI tract characterized by local hemorrhage and hematemesis, but generally perforation does not occur. Massive GI bleeding occurs later in the clinical course, particularly when hepatic failure and coagulopathy are present.[11]

Renal/Electrolytes

In a rat model of dermal burns from phosphorus, an initial diuresis occurs followed by acute kidney injury manifested by hyperkalemia, hyponatremia, and hyperphosphatemia.[1] Renal cell swelling and necrosis with vacuolar degeneration of proximal convoluted tubules was also observed.[1] Poisoned patients demonstrated an increase in urinary white and red blood cells with casts and proteinuria.[3] In humans, acute kidney injury from phosphorus is most likely acute tubular necrosis resulting from hypotension, salt and water depletion, and a direct toxic effect.[8]

Significant electrolyte disturbances result from both ingestion and dermal absorption of phosphorus. Hypocalcemia is common, but hypercalcemia is also occasionally reported.[14] Hyperphosphatemia reportedly accompanies the hypocalcemia but is not universal and can occur at any time in the clinical course.[3] The hyperphosphatemia is partially due to the conversion of absorbed phosphorus to phosphate. In an animal model, those that died had increased concentrations of phosphate, decreased concentrations of calcium, and hyperkalemia as early as one hour postexposure.[2] Hyperkalemia is occasionally reported in humans and may be secondary to tissue injury and acute kidney injury.[1] The electrolyte disturbances are likely a leading cause of early mortality from phosphorus.

Cardiovascular

When death occurs within 24 hours of the ingestion, it is likely the result of cardiovascular collapse. One series of 41 patients who attempted suicide demonstrated a variety of initial electrocardiographic (ECG) abnormalities. Abnormal T waves predominated in 24 patients, and there were also 2 cases of ventricular fibrillation. An increasing number of ECG abnormalities occurred in patients with larger ingestions, although electrolyte abnormalities were not described in many patients.[8] An animal model of phosphorus exposure demonstrated prolonged QT interval and ST segment changes along with electrolyte abnormalities, suggesting that many of the ECG changes might be due to electrolyte abnormalities.[2] A small study of phosphorus exposure in rats observed a decrease in amino acid uptake in myocytes suggesting a direct toxic effect. Human autopsies of several poisoned patients demonstrated fatty degeneration of the myocardium and vacuolated cytoplasm many hours postingestion.[25]

Hepatic

Phosphorus is a potent hepatotoxin. Increased prothrombin time, hyperbilirubinemia, and hypoglycemia usually occur within 3 days, with earlier signs of hepatic failure such as jaundice and coagulopathy indicative of a poor prognosis.[8,16] The increase in hepatic aminotransferases occurs over several days, usually peaking at or below 1,000 IU/L and almost invariably less than 3,000 IU/L.[11] Other biochemical effects demonstrated by experimental phosphorus toxicity include an increase in glucose-6-phosphate activity and impairment of triglyceride metabolism and protein synthesis. When death occurs after several days (as opposed to within 24 hours), hepatic injury is usually implicated. If survival occurs, the hepatic damage usually resolves over several months, although persistent periportal fibrosis is reported.[16]

With absorption of sufficient quantities, phosphorus causes a dose-related zone 1 or periportal hepatic injury, in contrast to the centrilobular pattern (zone 3) that occurs with many other hepatotoxins, such as acetaminophen and carbon tetrachloride (Chap. 21). Fatty degenerative changes and fatty infiltrates are also observed within 6 hours of ingestion.[7] Other histological changes include acute necrosis with large vacuoles and inflammatory changes. Some authors report microvesicular fatty degeneration of hepatocytes in patients who died early.[29] Electron microscopy in a rat model demonstrated an increase in the rough endoplasmic reticulum and an increase in the cytoplasmic fat without initial mitochondrial or nuclear injury.[12] Although the early pathologic effects appear to be predominantly cytoplasmic, the formation of nuclear vacuoles also occur.[16]

Nervous System

Central nervous system effects include headache, altered mental status, coma, and rarely seizures. The altered mental status is probably due partially to the presence of other organ dysfunction and shock; one example of the former is the encephalopathy secondary to hepatic injury. Patients with initial alterations in mental status or coma have an increased mortality rate independent of the presence of any electrolyte abnormalities.[17]

Dermal/Mucous Membranes

Dermal phosphorus exposure causes extensive burns, and this occurs most frequently in the military setting. The burns are described as emitting a garlic odor and displaying a yellow color that fluoresces under ultraviolet light.[5] Necrosis of the wounds is common when wound decontamination is incomplete. Depending on the release conditions, white phosphorus can be a solid or liquid but will be mostly liquid upon ignition. Liquid white phosphorus splatters and can penetrate clothing; burning clothing commonly exacerbates the burn area.[14,18] Dermal penetration is likely as a result of its lipophilicity and a compromised dermal barrier caused by the burn injury. The smoke produced by burning white phosphorus contains phosphorus pentoxide and is irritating to the conjunctiva and mucosa of the oropharynx and lungs.

Following a large burn, systemic illness manifested by electrolyte, cardiovascular, and hepatic abnormalities results from absorbed phosphorus.[1,2] A 12% to 15% body surface area burn in a rat was lethal 50% of the time; human morbidity from large skin burns is similarly high. Rats with dermal burns from phosphorus subsequently developed kidney and liver injury. Healing time from phosphorus burns is prolonged when compared with thermal burns.[8]

DIAGNOSTIC TESTING

Serum elemental phosphorus concentrations are not clinically available, and a serum phosphate concentration while potentially elevated does not reflect the serum elemental phosphorus concentration nor any body burden of elemental phosphorus. The diagnosis of phosphorus poisoning must rely on the history and physical examination. However, for optimal supportive care of the patient, many laboratory factors must be monitored, such as ECG, electrolytes, serum pH, hepatic function, glucose, kidney function, and coagulation parameters.

MANAGEMENT

Protection of Health Care Workers

At the absolute minimum, gloves and ocular protection (ie, face shield) should be used when managing a white phosphorus–poisoned patient until all elemental contamination is removed. Caution should be exercised with decontamination and subsequent storage of contaminated clothing. Following ingestion, vomitus and diarrhea must be considered potentially hazardous due to fire risk and should be carefully handled. Any phosphorus fragments removed from the patient as well as all potentially contaminated clothing items should be kept under water. Fires and explosions are reported during GI decontamination efforts, and the smoke from burning white phosphorus is irritating to the eyes and lungs and should be avoided.[19]

General

General supportive care is the mainstay of treatment. Cardiac monitoring; serial monitoring of calcium, phosphate, and potassium concentrations; and ECGs are essential for patients with a history of significant ingestion or overt toxicity as dysrhythmias can occur rapidly.[8] Electrolyte disturbances such as hyperkalemia, hypocalcemia, and hypercalcemia should be corrected. With a systemically absorbed toxic dose of phosphorus, hepatic injury will occur, and thus directed supportive care should be provided such as fresh-frozen plasma and vitamin K, when indicated. Adequate serum glucose concentrations are required to provide reducing equivalents through glycolysis and the glucose-6-phosphate dehydrogenase (G6PD) pathways, especially when there is evolving hepatic injury. Corticosteroids have not been shown to improve outcome following ingestions of white phosphorus and are not routinely recommended.[16] Direct contact of phosphorus with the eye can result in serious ophthalmic injury. Immediate copious ophthalmic decontamination with water rather than with copper sulfate is recommended (see Dermal Exposure).[24] A careful examination should be conducted by an ophthalmologist whenever possible.

Dermal Exposure

Initial treatment is to halt continuing injury by extinguishing combustion of the phosphorus. This should be performed by covering and lightly pressing down on any areas with a clean cloth (gauze) soaked in cool water or a 0.9% sodium chloride solution to limit the white phosphorus contact with atmospheric oxygen. Significant amounts of the white phosphorus will stick to the gauze or the cloth when removed 3 to 5 minutes later.[28] Clothing should be removed and fresh-soaked gauze immediately applied to skin areas beneath to prevent the remaining phosphorus that passed through the fabric from igniting. Subsequently, large amounts of cool water can be used to remove any phosphorus fragments. However, pouring water on burning phosphorus is very dangerous as burning phosphorus splashes unpredictably. Even with small amounts of dermal contamination caution should be exerted as spalling pieces of burning phosphorus originating from patient's wounds have injured health care workers; personal protective equipment including eye protection should be used. In the past, sodium bicarbonate decontamination solution was recommended, but because the tissue injury is not due to the production of acid and because no clinical benefit was demonstrated, specific neutralization fluids should not be used.[6,26] Water dilutes any phosphoric acid present and reacts with the phosphorus pentoxide to limit the damaging dehydrating reactions. All removed bandages and clothing should be kept wet or under water to prevent reignition.

Careful debridement is the next critical step as wounds that have not undergone adequate decontamination heal poorly, requiring additional debridement. Smoking pieces of phosphorus (ie, those emanating a white vapor) are not "burning" and not hot enough to cause thermal burns, but the oxidation process should be arrested. Fragments of phosphorus from the wound should be placed under water to prevent a fire hazard. Particles of phosphorus can be visualized by using a Woods lamp as the chemical burns have a yellowish fluorescence. One author recommends turning off the lights to look for the glow of the phosphorescent particles; presumably this will work only if copper or silver metal wash solution are not used, but due to lack of experience with this method along with problems of working in a completely dark area, this method is not routinely recommended.[9] Because of the increased solubility of phosphorus in hydrophobic solvents, it is important not to use ointments until the wound is completely decontaminated.

A copper(II) sulfate solution was previously recommended for "decontamination" (a misnomer in this case). Copper sulfate reacts with phosphorus to produce copper phosphide, a dark compound that is more easily visualized in the tissues. This dark material coats the particle, but the entire particle is not converted to copper phosphide. Additionally, this coating decreases the reaction of phosphorus with oxygen for a limited time and the particles should cease to smoke and will not phosphoresce. The application of high concentrations of copper sulfate solutions on damaged human tissue should not be done because of potential systemic toxicity such as hemolysis caused by the copper (Chap. 92).[24] This is especially concerning in patients at increased risk for oxidant injury, such as those with G6PD deficiency. The injurious solutions of copper sulfate historically used ranged from 2% to 5% and were applied for several hours to the wounds, resulting in substantial amounts of copper absorption and morbidity.

However, it is reasonable to utilize dilute copper sulfate solutions for the complete approach to the treatment of phosphorus wounds, acknowledging that this therapy is controversial, potentially harmful, especially in patients at risk for oxidant injury (G6PD deficiency) and not routinely available. It is possible that a dilute copper sulfate solution (0.5%–1.0%) applied once to the wound and then rinsed off with water will not result in the morbidity that occurred with the more concentrated rinses and will provide temporary neutralization of the outer surface of the phosphorus. This approach would be reasonable to assist in identification of the small pieces of phosphorus (after gross decontamination) that are difficult or impossible to visualize by darkening the fragments, especially in those with less experience débriding these wounds. Animal models suggest improved healing from the initial treatment with a copper solution, but a human case series did not find a difference in hospitalization days for those who were treated with copper sulfate compared with those who were not.[6] The copper phosphide–coated particles must be removed as they still react slowly, will release copper ions and will cause toxicity. It is important to restate that a single dilute copper sulfate solution wash is not a decontamination therapy but a temporizing treatment that allows for better visualization for physical debridement, and this solution must be rinsed away immediately after application.[9] Pads soaked in copper sulfate should not be used; this is because of the high concentration of copper, and the prolonged contact time that would promote a dangerous amount of systemic copper absorption.

Silver nitrate is suggested as a potential solution to replace the use of copper sulfate. It forms an insoluble, minimally reactive silver phosphide. Its use and preparation is similar to that described above and as such silver nitrate (1%–2% solution) is a temporary neutralization tool and not a decontamination therapy. It does not have the detrimental physiologic effects that internalized copper ions cause. However, there is very limited experience with this approach and no detailed human data, and although there may be some qualities that could make it more attractive than dilute copper solutions, it is not recommended at this time for lack of data. Silver forms an insoluble precipitate with chloride and cannot be combined with 0.9% sodium chloride solutions; therefore, the amount of soluble silver ion that reaches the imbedded phosphorus may be more limited than with copper because of the presence of relatively large amounts of chloride ion in living tissues.[23]

A reasonable approach is to begin by decontaminating the wound using a Woods lamp and/or a darkened room looking for phosphorescence. It would be reasonable to then apply a single transient dilute copper sulfate solution as described above with subsequent rinse to improve visualization and temporarily neutralize very small phosphorus particles. After decontamination, good wound care and burn management is required, because these burns (like other chemical burns) can be deep and require an extended period of time to heal. As discussed, incomplete decontamination is a common cause for delayed wound healing and there are cases of reactive fragments removed from the wound days after injury.[22] Patients with significant burns should be admitted to a burn intensive care unit for close monitoring of cardiovascular, kidney, and electrolyte status for several days at the minimum. Because of the potential instability of these patients, it is important to weigh the risk-to-benefit ratio of transfer to a specialized center. The experience of the receiving center with phosphorus burns in addition to the acuity and severity of the injury are important factors in making this decision.

Gastrointestinal Exposure

There is no good evidence that GI decontamination or antidotal therapy is efficacious following phosphorus ingestion. In the past, several different lavage fluids were recommended, ranging from the mostly benign (sodium bicarbonate) to the potentially dangerous (potassium permanganate). Milk might also be potentially harmful because of its lipophilic components due to the potential for increased phosphorus absorption. Some authors postulate better outcome with earlier GI decontamination by lavage, but no reliable studies are available.[16] There is the possibility that activated charcoal will bind to white phosphorus, although there are no human data to support its use and so it cannot be routinely recommend. However, despite the lack of data of efficacy, given the poor outcome of patients with large ingestions of phosphorus, gastric decontamination is recommended, even if there has already been vomiting. The tissue injury caused by phosphorus is not expected to cause early esophageal perforation, and so lavage is not contraindicated. Either an orogastric (OG) or nasogastric (NG) tube should be used, with the OG tube being preferred because of the variability in particle size in many products, although recognizing that an OG tube has greater risk associated with use than an NG tube (Chap. 5). Caution (gloves, eye protection at the minimum) should be exercised with any lavaged material to protect caregivers as spontaneous ignition can occur. Because of the risk of fire and explosion, it would be reasonable to keep the free end of the OG tube under water while inserting and instilling small amounts of water (not air) to check for proper placement, although this is only supported by one case report.[19]

It appears that the hepatic injury is much more likely with ingested phosphorus exposure than following dermal exposure. N-Acetylcysteine (NAC) would be reasonable as a potential adjunct in the treatment of phosphorus toxicity because of its antioxidant effects. Although NAC was used in a limited

human series, the numbers were small (n = 9 of 15) and there was no difference seen.[11] The use of superoxide dismutase in an animal model suggested benefit but did not limit morbidity, and a separate animal model suggested benefit from glutathione; therefore, limiting oxidant injury may play a role in treatment.[10] There is no theoretical harm in using NAC for phosphorus toxicity, and so it would be reasonable as part of the treatment regimen. Methionine was used many years ago in the treatment of a few patients, but the number of treated patients was too few to draw any conclusions and is not recommended.[7] When liver transplantation was performed for phosphorus-induced hepatic failure, outcomes have been suboptimal, probably because of concomitant toxicity occurring in the central nervous and cardiovascular systems.

SUMMARY

- White phosphorus was and is commonly used in warfare, causing morbidity through dermal burns.
- These burns require immediate quenching with wet cloths and adequate debridement while protecting health care workers.
- Following ingestion, typically in suicide attempts, morbidity remains quite high, and treatment options are limited to unproven decontamination therapies.
- Signs and symptoms of white phosphorus toxicity include vomiting, abdominal pain, confusion, dysrhythmias, hepatic injury, and acute kidney injury.
- As early mortality is believed to be due to electrolyte abnormalities and cardiac dysrhythmias, vigilant critical care is the mainstay of therapy.
- It would be reasonable to administer NAC, but it has not been shown to alter human outcomes.

Acknowledgments

Heikki E. Nikkanen, MD, and Michele M. Burns, MD, contributed to this chapter in previous editions.

REFERENCES

1. BenHur N, et al. Phosphorus burns—a pathophysiological study. *Br J Plast Surg*. 1972; 25:238-244.
2. Bowen TE, et al. Sudden death after phosphorus burns: experimental observations of hypocalcemia, hyperphosphatemia and electrocardiographic abnormalities following production of a standard white phosphorus burn. *Ann Surg*. 1971;174:779.
3. Brewer E, Haggerty R. Toxic hazards rat poisons II—phosphorus. *N Engl J Med*. 1958; 258:147-148.
4. Cameron J, Patrick RS. Acute phosphorus poisoning—the distribution of toxic doses of yellow phosphorus in the tissues of experimental animals. *Med Sci Law*. 1966;6:209-214.
5. Conner JC, Bebarta VS. White phosphorus dermal burns. *N Engl J Med*. 2007;357: 1530-1530.
6. Curreri PW, et al. The treatment of chemical burns: specialized diagnostic, therapeutic, and prognostic considerations. *J Trauma Acute Care Surg*. 1970;10:634-642.
7. Diaz-Rivera R, et al. Acute phosphorus poisoning in man: a study of 56 cases. *Medicine (Baltimore)*. 1950;29:269-298.
8. Diaz-Rivera R, et al. The electrocardiographs changes in acute phosphorus poisoning in man. *Am J Med Sci*. 1961;241:758-765.
9. Eldad A, Simon G. The phosphorous burn—a preliminary comparative experimental study of various forms of treatment. *Burns*. 1991;17:198-200.
10. Eldad A, et al. Phosphorous burns: evaluation of various modalities for primary treatment. *J Burn Care Res*. 1995;16:49-55.
11. Fernandez OUB, Canizares LL. Acute hepatotoxicity from ingestion of yellow phosphorus-containing fireworks. *J Clin Gastroenterol*. 1995;21:139-142.
12. Ganote CE, Otis J. Characteristic lesions of yellow phosphorus-induced liver damage. *Lab Invest*. 1969;21:207-213.
13. Ghoshal AK, et al. Isotopic studies on the absorption and tissue distribution of white phosphorus in rats. *Exp Mol Pathol*. 1971;14:212-219.
14. Konjoyan T. White phosphorus burns: case report and literature review. *Mil Med*. 1983;148:881-884.
15. Lee C-C, et al. *Mammalian Toxicity of Munition Compounds. Phase 1. Acute Oral Toxicity Primary Skin and Eye Irritation, Dermal Sensitization, and Disposition and Metabolism*. DTIC Document; 1975.
16. Marin GA, et al. Evaluation of corticosteroid and exchange-transfusion treatment of acute yellow-phosphorus intoxication. *N Engl J Med*. 1971;284:125-128.
17. McCarron MM, et al. Acute yellow phosphorus poisoning from pesticide pastes. *Clin Toxicol*. 1981;18:693-711.
18. Mozingo DW, et al. Chemical burns. *J Trauma Acute Care Surg*. 1988;28:642-647.

19. Pande T, Pandey S. White phosphorus poisoning-Explosive encounter. *J Assoc Physicians India.* 2004;52:249-250.

20. Pani P, et al. On the mechanism of fatty liver in white phosphorus-poisoned rats. *Exp Mol Pathol.* 1972;16:201-209.

21. Rubitsky HJ, Myerson RM. Acute phosphorus poisoning. *Arch Intern Med.* 1949; 83:164-178.

22. Saracoglu KT, et al. Delayed diagnosis of white phosphorus burn. *Burns.* 2013;39:825-826.

23. Song Z, et al. Treatment of yellow phosphorus skin burns with silver nitrate instead of copper sulfate. *Scand J Work Environ Health.* 1985;11:33.

24. Summerlin WT, et al. White phosphorus burns and massive hemolysis. *J Trauma Acute Care Surg.* 1967;7:476-484.

25. Talley RC, et al. Acute elemental phosphorus poisoning in man: cardiovascular toxicity. *Am Heart J.* 1972;84:139-140.

26. Walker J Jr, et al. *Quantitative Analysis of Phosphorus-Containing Compounds Formed in WP Burns.* DTIC Document; 1969.

27. Willers-Russo LJ. Three fatalities involving phosphine gas, produced as a result of meth-amphetamine manufacturing. *J Forensic Sci.* 1999;44:647-652.

28. Witkowski W, et al. Experimental comparison of efficiency of first aid dressings in burn-ing white phosphorus on bacon model. *Med Sci Monit.* 2015;21:2361-2366.

29. Yilmaz R, et al. An evaluation of childhood deaths in Turkey due to yellow phosphorus in firecrackers. *J Forensic Sci.* 2015;60:648-652.

113 SODIUM MONOFLUOROACETATE AND FLUOROACETAMIDE

Fermin Barrueto Jr.

HISTORY AND EPIDEMIOLOGY

Sodium monofluoroacetate (SMFA) occurs naturally in plants native to Brazil, Australia, and South and West Africa (eg, gifblaar {*Dichapetalum cymosum*}).[11] The highest concentration (8.0 mg/g) is found in the seeds of a South African plant, *Dichapetalum braunii*.[11] In the 1940s, SMFA was marketed as a rodenticide (CAS No. 62-74-8) and assigned the compound number 1080, which was registered as its trade name. Fluoroacetamide, a similar pesticide, is known as Compound 1081 (CAS No. 640-19-7). These compounds are widely effective as poisons against most mammals and some amphibians.[26] Both products were banned in the United States in 1972, except to protect sheep and cattle from coyotes. Collars embedded with SMFA are placed around the neck of livestock, the typical point of attack for coyotes.

Sodium monofluoroacetate is used extensively in New Zealand and Australia to control the possum population and other animal species considered pests that have no natural predators. In 1986, Compound 1080 was used to control the feral and free-ranging dogs in the Galapagos Islands due to their lack of a predator and their disruption of the sea turtle nests.[33] Its continued use is extremely controversial, but following a recent review of the ramifications of the use of 1080, the government of New Zealand retained both the aerosolized and collar applications. Reported cases of human poisoning with SMFA are uncommon, and the epidemiology is poorly understood. There have been only 68 reported cases from 1999 to 2017 with no deaths in the National Poisoning Database System of the American Association of Poison Control Centers (Chap. 130).

TOXICOKINETICS AND TOXICODYNAMICS

Sodium monofluoroacetate is an odorless and tasteless white powder with the consistency of flour. When dissolved in water, it is said to have a vinegarlike taste. Sodium monofluoroacetate and fluoroacetamide are well absorbed by the oral and inhalational routes.[10,11,12,27] Detailed toxicokinetic data are lacking in humans, but in sheep, up to 33% of an ingested dose is excreted unchanged in the urine over 48 hours. Glucuronide and glutathione conjugates were isolated.[11] Substantial defluorination is not thought to occur in vivo. The serum half-life is estimated to be 6.6 to 13.3 hours in sheep.[10] Sodium monofluoroacetate has a lethal dose of 50% of those exposed (LD_{50}) of 0.07 mg/kg in dogs.[19] The oral dose thought to be lethal to humans is 2 to 10 mg/kg.[3]

PATHOPHYSIOLOGY

Sodium monofluoroacetate, a structural analog of acetic acid (Fig. 113–1), is an irreversible inhibitor of the citric acid cycle (Fig. 11–3). Monofluoroacetic acid enters the mitochondria, where it is converted to

$$F-\overset{\overset{\displaystyle H}{|}}{\underset{\underset{\displaystyle H}{|}}{C}}-\overset{\overset{\displaystyle O}{\|}}{C}-O^- \ Na^+ \qquad \text{Sodium monofluoroacetate}$$

$$F-\overset{\overset{\displaystyle H}{|}}{\underset{\underset{\displaystyle H}{|}}{C}}-\overset{\overset{\displaystyle O}{\|}}{C}-NH_2 \qquad \text{Fluoroacetamide}$$

$$H-\overset{\overset{\displaystyle H}{|}}{\underset{\underset{\displaystyle H}{|}}{C}}-\overset{\overset{\displaystyle O}{\|}}{C}-CoA \qquad \text{Acetyl CoA}$$

FIGURE 113–1. Structural similarities among acetyl-CoA, sodium monofluoroacetate, and fluoroacetamide.

monofluoroacetyl-coenzyme A (CoA) by acetate thiokinase. Mitochondrial citrate synthase is then joined with the monofluoroacetyl-CoA complex with oxaloacetate to form fluorocitrate. Fluorocitrate then covalently binds aconitase, preventing the enzyme from any further metabolic activity in the citric acid cycle.[17] Thus, fluorocitrate acts as a "suicide inhibitor" of aconitase, producing a biochemical dead end. The net toxicity caused by fluorocitrate results from the increase in citric acid cycle substrates proximal to inhibition of aconitase and the depletion of substrates distal to the step catalyzed by aconitase. This inhibition of aconitase impairs energy production, leading to anaerobic metabolism and metabolic acidosis with an elevated lactate concentration. Additionally, other citric acid cycle intermediates increase in concentration, contributing to the toxicity. α-Ketoglutarate depletion, caused by the lack of isocitrate, leads to glutamate depletion since α-ketoglutarate is a precursor of glutamate synthesis. Glutamate depletion leads to urea cycle disruption and ammonia accumulation. Impaired fatty acid oxidation leads to ketosis. Excess citrate binds to divalent cations such as calcium causing hypocalcemia.

Disruption of the citric acid and urea cycles affects every system in the human body, but the most consequential effects occur in the central nervous system and the cardiovascular system. Fluoride toxicity from enzymatic defluorination of sodium monofluoroacetate and fluoroacetamide does not occur substantially in vivo and is of minor significance.

CLINICAL MANIFESTATIONS

The majority of the clinical experience with SMFA is associated with intentional self-poisoning; fluoroacetamide poisoning is presumed to have a similar presentation.[9,16,18,29] Most patients develop symptoms within 6 hours after exposure. In the largest case series of 38 Taiwanese patients who ingested SMFA, 7 died.[6] The most common clinical findings recorded at the time of emergency department (ED) presentation were nausea and vomiting (74%), diarrhea (29%), agitation (29%), and abdominal pain (26%).[6] The mean time to presentation to the hospital was 10.9 ± 5.7 hours for those who died and 3.4 ± 0.6 hours for the survivors. All deaths occurred within 72 hours of admission to the hospital. The presence of respiratory distress or seizures was a prognostic indicator of death. All 7 patients who died had systolic blood pressures less than 90 mm Hg on presentation to the ED, a finding noted in only 16% of the survivors.[6]

In a case series involving 2 patients, invasive hemodynamic monitoring revealed persistent low systemic vascular resistance and increased cardiac output despite adequate fluid resuscitation.[7] The authors theorized that the cardiovascular response was triggered by ATP depletion and inhibition of gluconeogenesis.[7] Anaerobic metabolism, mitochondrial inhibition, and sensitivity of the vasculature to SMFA are also confounding factors.

The initial neurologic manifestations consist of agitation and confusion with progression to seizures. Neurologic sequelae such as cerebellar dysfunction are likely permanent though there is a case report of reversible leukencephalopathy.[15,30,31,34,35] Another report describes a 15-year-old girl who survived an initial exposure to SMFA but later developed cerebellar dysfunction and cerebral atrophy, demonstrated by brain computed tomography (CT).[30] Prolongation of the QT interval, premature ventricular contractions, ventricular fibrillation, ventricular tachycardia, and other dysrhythmias are documented.[6] Sodium monofluoroacetate has negative inotropic effects, except in one case report that described episodic hypertension.[25] Signs and symptoms associated with severe poisoning include seizures, respiratory distress, and hypotension.

DIAGNOSTIC TESTING

The presence of SMFA and fluoroacetamide is confirmed in the blood and urine with gas chromatography–mass spectrometry and thin-layer chromatography.[1,5,20] Simultaneous analysis for other rodenticides that can induce seizures, for example, "tetramine," is reportedly performed by gas chromatography in China, where exposure to these xenobiotics is more probable.[2,4,32] Like tetramine, SMFA is classified as a potential chemical weapon.[13] An elevated serum citrate concentration was proposed as a useful marker for exposure to SMFA.[4] However, none of these analyses can be performed in a clinically relevant period. A combination of history, clinical signs and symptoms, and common laboratory tests can assist with the diagnosis.

Hypokalemia, anion gap metabolic acidosis, and an elevated creatinine concentration[8] are associated with severe poisoning but are very nonspecific.[6] The predominant electrolyte abnormality is hypocalcemia. Creatinine, aminotransferase and bilirubin concentrations are also elevated in some cases and likely result from multisystem organ toxicity. Ketones are present in urine and serum. A complete blood cell count will reveal leukocytosis. An electrocardiogram is valuable in the diagnosis of SMFA exposure; a prolonged QT interval, atrial fibrillation with a rapid ventricular response, ventricular tachycardia, and other dysrhythmias are reported.[6,28] An initial CT scan of the brain can be normal, but subsequent scans will reveal cerebral atrophy.[30] When compared to presentation a weighted magnetic resonance imaging (MRI) on day 7 post ingestion showed reversible symmetric high signal intensity in the cerebellar peduncles, corpus callosum, internal capsules, and corona radiata in an SMFA-poisoned patient with a sublethal ingestion.[15] Brain single photon emission computed tomogram (SPECT) was also normal 14 days later.

TREATMENT

Initial decontamination should include removal of clothes and cleansing of skin with soap and water. Because there is no proven antidote for SMFA or fluoroacetamide poisoning, orogastric lavage is reasonable for exposed patients who present to the ED prior to significant emesis. For patients who present within one to 2 hours of ingestion should receive we recommend 1 g/kg of activated charcoal (AC) orally. A rat study showed that colestipol is more effective than AC in binding SMFA.[21] Activated charcoal is more accessible, and the speed of administration would outweigh a theoretical benefit of increased binding of colestipol.

In a cat model, glycerol monoacetate (monacetin) at a dose of 0.5 mL/kg every 30 minutes prolonged survival. In this context, monacetin functions as an acetate donor for ultimate incorporation into citrate in place of fluoroacetate.[29] Both ethanol and glycerol monoacetate are converted to acetyl-CoA and compete with monofluoroacetyl-CoA for binding of citrate synthase. This prevents the "suicide-inhibition" of aconitase, subsequent increase in citrate, and the formation of the toxic metabolite fluorocitrate.[29] Availability of monacetin for human use is limited, and appropriate human dosing is unknown.

Ethanol was used in some human cases, although the appropriate dose is unknown.[6,7,24] A reasonable therapeutic dose is the amount of ethanol required to obtain and sustain an ethanol serum concentration of 100 mg/dL (Antidotes in Depth: A34). One intriguing case report involved a patient who ingested 240 mg of SMFA (typically a lethal dose) mixed with a Taiwanese wine (30% ethanol) and survived.[6] It is possible that the ethanol decreased or delayed the toxicity of SMFA.

In a mouse model, use of a combination of calcium salts, sodium succinate, and α-ketoglutarate improved survival.[22] The rationale of using these antidotes is to provide citric acid cycle intermediates distal to the inhibited aconitase in an attempt to improve energy production. These antidotes were not effective unless calcium was coadministered, emphasizing the importance of replenishing electrolytes, particularly the divalent cations chelated by citrate.[14,23,28] Access to α-ketoglutarate or sodium succinate for a human case would be limited and its use is reasonable; however, aggressive electrolyte replacement, especially the divalent

cations, is recommended and the importance is highlighted by this animal model.

If a patient develops hypotension and shock, rapid administration of intravenous 0.9% NaCl followed by a vasopressor, such as norepinephrine is recommended. Supportive care, correction of electrolyte abnormalities (especially calcium and potassium), ethanol infusion, and monitoring for dysrhythmias (prolonged QT interval) and seizures are the mainstays of treatment.

SUMMARY

- Sodium monofluoroacetate and fluoroacetamide are potent pesticides that inhibit the citric acid cycle, disrupting cellular energy production.
- Patients exposed to SMFA typically present with nausea, vomiting, agitation, and abdominal pain, which is followed by hypotension, respiratory distress, shock, seizures, and death.
- Hypokalemia, hypocalcemia, metabolic acidosis with an elevated lactate, and elevation of serum creatinine also occur.
- Treatment of SMFA and fluoroacetamide poisoning largely involves replenishing electrolytes, correcting hypotension with intravenous fluids and vasopressors if necessary, monitoring for dysrhythmias, and treating seizures.
- Ethanol is a therapy with a biological mechanism and theoretical benefit. It is relatively familiar, readily available, and can be administered safely.

REFERENCES

1. Allender WJ. Determination of sodium fluoroacetate (compound 1080) in biological tissues. *J Anal Toxicol.* 1990;14:45-49.
2. Barrueto F Jr, et al. Status epilepticus from an illegally imported Chinese rodenticide: "tetramine." *J Toxicol Clin Toxicol.* 2003;41:991-994.
3. Beasley M. Guidelines for the safe use of sodium fluoroacetate (1080). New Zealand Occupational Safety & Health Service, August 2002.
4. Bosakowski T, Levin AA. Serum citrate as a peripheral indicator of fluoroacetate and fluorocitrate toxicity in rats and dogs. *Toxicol Appl Pharmacol.* 1986;85:428-436.
5. Cai X, et al. Fast detection of fluoroacetamide in body fluid using gas chromatography-mass spectrometry after solid-phase microextraction. *J Chromatogr B Analyt Technol Biomed Life Sci.* 2004;802:239-245.
6. Chi CH, et al. Clinical presentation and prognostic factors in sodium monofluoroacetate intoxication. *J Toxicol Clin Toxicol.* 1996;34:707-712.
7. Chi CH, et al. Hemodynamic abnormalities in sodium monofluoroacetate intoxication. *Hum Exp Toxicol.* 1999;18:351-353.
8. Chung HM. Acute renal failure caused by acute monofluoroacetate poisoning. *Vet Hum Toxicol.* 1984;26(suppl 2):29-32.
9. Deng HY, et al. Management of severe fluoroacetamide poisoning with hemoperfusion in children. *Zhongguo Dang Dai Er Ke Za Zhi.* 2007;9:253-254.
10. Eason CT, et al. Persistence of sodium monofluoroacetate in livestock animals and risk to humans. *Hum Exp Toxicol.* 1994;13:119-122.
11. Eason CT. Sodium monofluoroacetate (1080) risk assessment and risk communication. *Toxicology.* 2002;181-182:523-530.
12. Eason CT, Turck P. A 90-day toxicological evaluation of Compound 1080 (sodium monofluoroacetate) in Sprague-Dawley rats. *Toxicol Sci.* 2002;69:439-447.
13. Holstege CP, et al. Unusual but potential agents of terrorists. *Emerg Med Clin North Am.* 2007;25:549-566.
14. Hornfeldt CS, Larson AA. Seizures induced by fluoroacetic acid and fluorocitric acid may involve chelation of divalent cations in the spinal cord. *Eur J Pharmacol.* 1990; 179:307-313.
15. Im TH, Yi HJ. The utility of early brain imaging (diffusion magnetic resonance and single photon emission computed tomography scan) in assessing the course of acute sodium monofluoroacetate intoxication. *J Trauma.* 2009;66:E72-E74.
16. Jones K. Two outbreaks of fluoroacetate and fluoroacetamide poisoning. *J Forensic Sci Soc.* 1965;12:76-79.
17. Liébecq C, Peters RA. The toxicity of fluoroacetate and the tricarboxylic acid cycle. 1949. *Biochim Biophys Acta.* 1989;1000:254-269.
18. Lin J, et al. Acute fluoroacetamide poisoning with main damage to the heart. *Zhonghua Lao Dong Wei Sheng Zhi Ye Bing Za Zhi.* 2002;20:344-346.
19. Meenken D, Booth LH. The risk to dogs of poisoning from sodium monofluoroacetate (1080) residues in possum (*Trichosurus vulpecula*). *N Z J Agric Res.* 1997;40:573-576.
20. Minnaar PP, et al. A high-performance liquid chromatographic method for the determination of monofluoroacetate. *J Chromatogr Sci.* 2000;38:16-20.
21. Norris WR, et al. Sorption of fluoroacetate (compound 1080) by colestipol, activated charcoal, and anion-exchange in resins in vitro and gastrointestinal decontamination in rats. *Vet Hum Toxicol.* 2000;42:269-275.

22. Omara F, Sisodia CS. Evaluation of potential antidotes for sodium fluoroacetate in mice. *Vet Hum Toxicol*. 1990;32:427-431.

23. Proudfoot AT, et al. Sodium fluoroacetate poisoning. *Toxicol Rev*. 2006;25:213-219.

24. Ramirez M. Inebriation with pyridoxine and fluoroacetate: a case report. *Vet Hum Toxicol*. 1986;28:154.

25. Robinson RF, et al. Intoxication with sodium monofluoroacetate (compound 1080). *Vet Hum Toxicol*. 2002;44:93-95.

26. Sherley M. The traditional categories of fluoroacetate poisoning signs and symptoms belie substantial underlying similarities. *Toxicol Lett*. 2004;151:399-406.

27. Singh M, et al. Acute inhalation toxicity study of 2-fluoroacetamide in rats. *Biomed Environ Sci*. 2000;13:90-96.

28. Taitelman U, et al. Fluoroacetamide poisoning in man: the role of ionized calcium. *Arch Toxicol Suppl*. 1983;6:228-231.

29. Taitelman U, et al. The effect of monoacetin and calcium chloride on acid-base balance and survival in experimental sodium fluoroacetate poisoning. *Arch Toxicol Suppl*. 1983;6:222-227.

30. Trabes J, et al. Computed tomography demonstration of brain damage due to acute sodium monofluoroacetate poisoning. *J Toxicol Clin Toxicol*. 1983;20:85-92.

31. Kim JB, et al. Reversible leukoencephalopathy in sodium monofluoroacetate intoxication. *Neurology*. 2014;82:1190-1191.

32. Wu Q, et al. Simultaneous determination of fluoroacetamide and tetramine by gas chromatography [in Chinese]. *Se Pu*. 2002;20:381-382.

33. Barnett BD. Eradication and control of feral and free-ranging dogs in the Galapagos Island. Proceedings of the 12th Vertebrate Pest conference. 1986.

34. Fukushima H. Case of sodium monofluoroacetic acid intoxication [in Japanese]. *Chudoku Kenkyu*. 2008;21:391-392.

35. Im TH, Yi HJ. The utility of early brain imaging (diffusion magnetic resonance and single photon emission computed tomography scan) in assessing the course of acute sodium monofluoroacetate intoxication. *J Trauma*. 2009;66:E72-E74.

114

STRYCHNINE

Yiu-Cheung Chan

HISTORY AND EPIDEMIOLOGY

Strychnine alkaloid occurs naturally in *Strychnos nux-vomica*, a tree native to tropical Asia and North Australia, and in *Strychnos ignatii* and *Strychnos tiente*, trees native to South Asia. The alkaloid was first isolated in 1818 by Pelletier and Caventou.[5,15] It is an odorless and colorless crystalline powder that has a bitter taste when dissolved in water. In addition to strychnine, the dried seeds of *S. nux-vomica* contain brucine, a structurally similar, although less potent, alkaloid.[87] Strychnine is available from commercial sources in its salt form, usually as nitrate, sulfate, or phosphate.

Strychnine was first introduced as a rodenticide in 1540, and in subsequent centuries was used medically as a cardiac, respiratory, and digestive stimulant,[44] as an analeptic,[90] and as an antidote to barbiturate[89] and opioid overdoses.[59] Nonketotic hyperglycemia,[9,80] sleep apnea,[76] and snake bites[15] were also once considered indications for strychnine use. In 1982, at least 172 commercial products were found to contain strychnine, including 77 rodenticides, 25 veterinary products, and 41 products made for human use.[83] In subsequent years, the use of strychnine significantly decreased; some countries such as the European Union banned its use as a rodenticide in 2006, and most of its prior medicinal indications are no longer utilized. Currently, strychnine is only widely used for moles, gophers, and pigeons and as a research tool for the study of glycine receptors. Most commercially available strychnine-containing products contain about 0.25% to 0.5% strychnine by weight.[83]

Between 1926 and 1928, strychnine killed more than 3 Americans every week.[5,27] In 1932, it was the most common cause of lethal poisoning in children,[5,83] and one-third of the unintentional poison-related deaths in children younger than 5 years were attributed to strychnine.[60] Currently, strychnine poisoning is rare and continues to decrease in the United States, although deaths are still reported. The Toxic Exposure Surveillance System (TESS) and National Poison Data System (NPDS) data of the American Association of Poison Control Centers (AAPCC) reported 1163 strychnine exposures including 5 deaths during the 10 years from 2006 to 2015 (Chap. 130).

In the modern era, strychnine poisoning typically results from deliberate exposure with suicidal and homicidal intent,[27,48] as well as from unintentional poisoning by a Chinese herbal medicine (Maqianzi)[16] and a Cambodian traditional remedy (slang nut).[46,48,51] Maqianzi is used to treat limb paralysis, severe rheumatism, inflammatory disease, and skeletal fluorosis[50] whereas slang nut is used to treat gastrointestinal diseases. The bitter taste of strychnine has led to its use as an adulterant in heroin[42] and cocaine.[13,22,64] There are also reports of strychnine poisoning from adulterated amphetamines,[22] 3,4-methylenedioxymethamphetamine (MDMA),[25] Spanish fly,[12] and from the ingestion of gopher bait.[52]

TOXICOKINETICS

Standard references list the lethal dose of strychnine as approximately 50 to 100 mg.[18,33,34,70,92] However, mortality resulting from doses as low as 5 to 10 mg and, conversely, survival following exposures of 1 to 15 g of strychnine are

reported.[6,18,82,95] Some of this variation likely results from differing routes of administration, with parenteral administration being more toxic than oral, the limitations of self-reported exposure quantities, and advances in supportive care.

Strychnine is rapidly absorbed from the gastrointestinal tract and mucous membranes. Poisoning is reported from dermal absorption of strychnine stored in an alkaline solution, in which strychnine exists in the nonionized, alkaloid form.[35] Protein binding is minimal, and strychnine is rapidly distributed to peripheral tissues[91] with a large volume of distribution (13 L/kg).[39] Based on postmortem findings, the highest concentrations of strychnine are found in the liver,[57,70,78] bile,[70] blood,[70] and gastric contents.[70,78] Relatively less strychnine is identified in kidney, urine, and brain.[78]

Strychnine is metabolized by hepatic cytochrome P450 enzymes, mainly CYP3A4[1,53,61] producing strychnine-*N*-oxide as the major metabolite,[1] the toxicity of which is about 1/10th of the original alkaloid.[55] This metabolism is increased by P450 induction.[43,47] Several urinary metabolites are identified,[65] and 1% to 30% of strychnine is excreted unchanged in urine,[10,38,69] in decreasing proportions when larger amounts are ingested.[81,91] Strychnine elimination follows first-order kinetics with an elimination half-life of 10 to 16 hours.[26,69,94]

PATHOPHYSIOLOGY

Glycine, one of the major inhibitory neurotransmitters in the spinal cord, opens a ligand-gated chloride (Cl⁻) channel, thus allowing the inward flow of Cl⁻ (Fig. 13–12).[20] As Cl⁻ moves inward, the cell becomes hyperpolarized, reducing neuronal excitability. Strychnine competitively inhibits the binding of glycine to the α-subunit of the glycinergic chloride channel.[13,19,94] Although strychnine affects all parts of the central nervous system in which glycine receptors are found, the most significant effect is in the spinal cord. With loss of the glycine inhibition at the motor neurons in the ventral horn, there is a loss of inhibitory influence on the normally suppressed reflex arc. The result is increased impulse transmission to the muscles, producing generalized muscular contraction. Rabbits pretreated with glycine had a 40% increase in the strychnine "seizure" threshold, illustrating the competitive nature of strychnine and glycine activity on the glycinergic chloride channel.[17,77] Tetanus toxin (tetanospasmin) causes an identical clinical syndrome of muscular contractions, but does so by preventing the release of presynaptic glycine and does not function as a competitive antagonist. In dogs, strychnine has positive chronotropic and inotropic effects on the heart,[84] but this effect is unlikely to exert a major effect in human poisoning.

CLINICAL MANIFESTATIONS

Oral strychnine poisoning is characterized by a rapid onset of signs and symptoms of toxicity beginning within 15 to 60 minutes of ingestion[32] and, although less well documented, effects occur sooner following parenteral or nasal administration. Delayed onset of clinical effects are rarely reported.[23,34] The typical findings of poisoning are involuntary, generalized muscular contractions resulting in neck, back, and limb pain. The contractions are easily triggered by trivial stimuli such as turning on a light, and each episode usually lasts for 30 to 120 seconds.[83] These episodes recur for as long as 12 to 24 hours. Differences in the strength of various opposing muscle groups result in the classic signs of opisthotonus, facial trismus, and risus sardonicus, with flexion of the upper limbs and extension of lower limbs predominating. Hyperreflexia, clonus, and nystagmus[11,62] are also evident on examination. Because strychnine affects glycine inhibition mainly in the spinal cord, the patient typically remains fully alert until metabolic complications occur. The combination of convulsive motor activity involving both sides of the body in the conscious patient often results in imprecise descriptions such as "conscious seizure" or "spinal seizure." Hemodynamically, both hypotension[24,26,64] and hypertension[13,29,63] in the presence of bradycardia[14,24,26,64] or tachycardia[13,14] are reported. Hyperthermia, presumably from increased muscular activity, is typical, and temperatures as high as 109.4°F (43°C) are reported.[13] Other nonspecific signs and symptoms include dizziness, vomiting, and chest and abdominal pain.[62]

Early in the course of strychnine poisoning, mortality is mainly due to hypoventilation and hypoxia secondary to muscular contractions.[29] Life-threatening complications include rhabdomyolysis, with subsequent myoglobinuria and acute kidney injury,[14] hypoxia or hyperthermia-induced multiorgan failure, aspiration pneumonitis,[85] anoxic brain injury, and pancreatitis.[41] Rarely, local neuromuscular sequelae such as weakness, myalgia, and anterior tibial compartment syndrome are reported.[13] As expected, the prognosis is directly correlated with the delay to care and the subsequent duration and magnitude of the episodes of muscle contractions.[31]

DIFFERENTIAL DIAGNOSIS

The diagnosis of strychnine poisoning is mainly established on clinical grounds, based on exposure history and compatible clinical manifestations, but can be confirmed by detection of strychnine in biological specimens. Several diagnoses are included, the most important of which is tetanus because it produces similar muscular hyperactivity. In a patient with tetanus, however, the onset of symptoms is more gradual and the duration of the complications much more protracted than in the case of strychnine poisoning. Frequently, the diagnosis of tetanus is suggested by a history of recent injury, injection drug use, or the presence of a wound. Additionally, patients with tetanus will often be unimmunized or have undocumented or incomplete tetanus immunization.

The motor activity associated with strychnine poisoning is best differentiated from generalized seizures by the presence of a normal sensorium during the period of diffuse convulsions. That is, most patients with bilateral convulsions are having generalized seizures, which by definition involves the reticular activating system, producing unconsciousness. It is conceivable, although extraordinarily rare, to have bilateral focal seizures producing apparent "generalized" convulsions. In the case of strychnine, because the reticular activating system is not be involved, the mental status of the patient is classically preserved. The presence of consciousness in a patient with a generalized convulsion is highly suggestive of a diagnosis of either strychnine poisoning or tetanus, at least in the early phase of the clinical course. As time progresses and management is delayed this finding will be obscured by metabolically induced alterations in sensorium.[17] When there is an alteration in the level of consciousness, an electroencephalogram (EEG) is recommended, to document the presence or absence of a seizure focus. A computed tomography (CT) scan of the head will help to exclude structural brain lesions, and a lumbar puncture is helpful to exclude meningitis or encephalitis. Hypocalcemia, hyperventilation, and myoclonus secondary to kidney or liver failure are evaluated by appropriate routine laboratory testing. Although a drug induced dystonic reaction is reasonable to include in the differential diagnosis when there is a relevant history, dystonic reactions are usually static, whereas strychnine poisoning results in dynamic muscular activity. Serotonin toxicity, malignant hyperthermia, neuroleptic malignant syndrome, and stimulant-associated toxicity all resemble late phases of strychnine poisoning, but other features of the history or physical examination usually help distinguish them from either strychnine or tetanus.

DIAGNOSTIC TESTING

Respiratory and metabolic acidosis both occur commonly in patients with strychnine poisoning. Metabolic acidosis is associated with elevated serum lactate concentrations,[13] whereas respiratory acidosis secondary to hypoventilation results from diaphragmatic and respiratory muscle failure. Survival of patients with serum pHs in the range of 6.5 to 6.6 is well

documented.[13,29,30,32,54,94] The lowest pH and highest lactate concentration reported in a patient with subsequent full recovery was 6.5 and 32 mmol/L,[13,94] respectively. Thus, profound acidemia in strychnine poisoning is not necessarily associated with a poor prognosis.[7,8,13,73] By contrast to the metabolic acidosis with elevated lactate concentration that occurs in shock, the elevated lactate concentration of strychnine poisoning results from overactivity of the muscle instead of undersupply or underutilization of oxygen and nutrients.

Besides acidemia, other laboratory abnormalities expected from prolonged muscular activity include hyperkalemia and those associated with rhabdomyolysis and acute kidney injury.[13] Other reported findings included stress-induced leukocytosis,[13,41] elevated aminotransferase concentrations,[41,62,88] hypocalcemia,[13,39] hypernatremia,[32] and hypokalemia.[28,62,84] The electrocardiogram is expected to remain normal or reflect changes consistent with the above electrolyte disturbances.[39] Chest radiography is appropriate to evaluate for aspiration pneumonitis or acute respiratory distress syndrome.

Strychnine can be detected by a variety of methods such as thin-layer chromatography,[66] high-performance liquid chromatography,[2] ultraviolet spectrometry,[66] a simple colorimetric reaction,[66] gas chromatography–mass spectrometry,[14,57,69,78] gas chromatography flame ionization detector,[92] and capillary electrophoresis.[96] With the exception of the bedside colorimetric reaction, none of these tests are routinely available in a time frame useful to assist in clinical decisions. Strychnine is also detectable in concentrations as low as 0.01 mg/L in tissue, and strychnine resists postmortem putrefaction.[2,21,58,72] Even when available, quantitative concentrations do not correlate with clinical toxicity. Reported blood strychnine concentrations in fatal poisoning ranged from 0.5 to 61 mg/L.[92] Conversely, the highest initial blood concentration associated with survival was 4.73 mg/L from blood drawn 1.5 hours postingestion;[93] a concentration as low as 0.06 mg/L was found in a patient who solely had muscular irritability.[26]

MANAGEMENT

In patients with strychnine poisoning, inducing vomiting is absolutely contraindicated because of the risk of aspiration and loss of airway control following rapid onset of muscle contractions. Orogastric lavage is reasonable in patients with early presentations and or life-threating ingestion histories (Chap. 5).[3] When orogastric lavage is reasonable, the airway should be protected and secured with an endotracheal tube before attempting lavage. Activated charcoal (AC) binds strychnine effectively at a ratio of approximately 1:1; 1 g of AC will bind 950 mg of strychnine.[4,87] In animal models, pretreatment[67] and posttreatment[71] with AC increase the median lethal dose in 50% of test subjects (LD$_{50}$) for strychnine. Clinical evidence of the effectiveness of AC for strychnine ingestion was first demonstrated in 1831, when Professor Touery survived the ingestion of a lethal dose of strychnine by using AC in a demonstration before the French Academy of Medicine, thus a single dose of 1 g/kg of oral AC is recommended.

Currently, there is no evidence to recommend the use of multiple-dose AC or whole-bowel irrigation for strychnine poisoning. Forced diuresis was previously suggested as an effective means of enhancing the elimination of strychnine,[87] subsequent data failed to demonstrate an increase in clearance,[81] and it is not recommended. Peritoneal dialysis, hemodialysis, and hemoperfusion are been extensively studied. However, because strychnine is rapidly distributed to the tissues[91] with a large volume of distribution (13 L/kg), extracorporeal drug elimination procedures are unlikely to be useful and therefore not justified.

Supportive treatment remains the most important aspect of management in the majority of cases. The focus of care is to stop the muscular hyperactivity as soon as possible to prevent the metabolic and respiratory complications. At all times, unnecessary stimuli and manipulation of the patient should be avoided, as these activities trigger muscle contractions. Benzodiazepines remain the first-line treatment for strychnine-induced muscular hyperactivity.[83,93] Although much of the evidence concerning the efficacy of benzodiazepines is based on clinical experience with diazepam,[37,45,64] any of the other commonly used benzodiazepines (midazolam or lorazepam) would likely have similar effects. The initial dose of the benzodiazepine chosen should be the standard dose used for other indications, although the use of doses greater than 1 mg/kg diazepam or its equivalent are reported to achieve control of convulsions.[40,56] Prior to establishing intravenous access, lorazepam or midazolam can be given intramuscularly or intraosseously. Dosing should be repeated at pharmacologically appropriate intervals until the patient demonstrates muscle relaxation and the contractions cease. In addition to benzodiazepines, propofol and barbiturates are also effective, although we recommend them as secondary therapies, in treating the strychnine-induced hyperactivity.[36,51,74,86] Benzodiazepines and barbiturates both work through agonism of γ-aminobutyric acid (GABA) receptor chloride complexes to increase the inhibitory neurotransmission to the spinal cord from the brain, and thus raise the reflex arc threshold.[79] If these measures fail to control the muscular hyperactivity, a nondepolarizing neuromuscular blocker (NMB) is recommended. Only nondepolarizing NMBs should be used, because succinylcholine itself, a depolarizing NMB, induces muscle contractions.[13,26,51,64,81] It is important to remember that strychnine has no direct effects on consciousness, so that sedation must always accompany neuromuscular blockade. Generally, therapy is continued for approximately 24 hours, at which time the benzodiazepines and/or NMBs can be tapered as tolerated.

The most important therapy for the metabolic complications of strychnine poisoning is to expeditiously stop the production of metabolic by-products by terminating the muscular hyperactivity. Hyperthermia should be treated rapidly by active cooling with ice water immersion, cooling blanket, or mist and fan, depending on the magnitude of temperature elevation (Chap. 29). Means to prevent rhabdomyolysis induced acute kidney injury include adequate fluid administration to ensure good urine output (>1 mL/kg/h), the use of urinary alkalinization with sodium bicarbonate (Antidotes in Depth: A5),[75] and temporary renal replacement therapy, if acute kidney failure occurs. Metabolic acidemia rapidly resolves when muscular activity is controlled.[13,68]

Effective management in the first few hours of strychnine poisoning is crucial for survival. If the patient is supported adequately for the first 6 hours, this is generally a good prognostic sign.[13,34] All significantly poisoned patients should be managed in an intensive care unit with the help of a regional poison control center or a medical toxicologist. For asymptomatic patients unintentionally exposed to strychnine, an observation period of 12 hours is sufficient to exclude significant risk.

SUMMARY

- Strychnine is a lethal poison that is no longer frequently encountered, except in areas where it is used as a rodenticide.
- A "conscious seizure" is the characteristic presentation of strychnine toxicity, and is rapidly followed by life threatening metabolic and respiratory consequences.
- The mainstay of treatment is supportive care with the goal of rapidly aborting muscular contractions, providing adequate airway management, and rapidly treating hyperthermia and or metabolic abnormalities.
- Although benzodiazepines are generally sufficient, neuromuscular paralysis with a nondepolarizing NMB are required in refractory cases.
- Generally, the prognosis of strychnine poisoning is good, if the patient is adequately supported and survives the first 6 hours of toxicity.

REFERENCES

1. Adamson RH, Fouts JR. Enzymatic metabolism of strychnine. *J Pharmacol Exp Ther*. 1959;127:87-91.
2. Alliot A, et al. Measurement of strychnine by high performance liquid chromatography. *J Chromatogr*. 1982;232:440-442.
3. American Academy of Clinical Toxicology, European Association of Poisons Centres and Clinical Toxicologists. Position statement: gastric lavage. *J Toxicol Clin Toxicol*. 2004; 42:933-943.
4. Anderson AH. Experimental studies on the pharmacology of activated charcoal. *Acta Pharmacol*. 1946;2:69-78.
5. Anonymous. The treatment of strychnine poisoning. *JAMA*. 1932;98:1992-1994.
6. Arena JM. Report from the Duke University Poison Control Center. *N C Med J*. 1962; 10:480-481.
7. Arieff AI, et al. Intracellular pH of brain: alterations in acute respiratory acidosis and alkalosis. *Am J Physiol*. 1976:230:804-812.
8. Arieff AI, et al. Pathophysiology of experimental lactic acidosis in dogs. *Am J Physiol Renal Physiol*. 1980;239:135-142.
9. Arneson D, et al. Strychnine therapy in nonketotic hyperglycemia. *Pediatrics*. 1979; 3:369-373.
10. Baselt RC. *Disposition of Toxic Drugs and Chemicals in Man*. 5th ed. Foster City, CA: Chemical Toxicology Institute; 2000.
11. Blain PG, et al. Strychnine poisoning: abnormal eye movements. *J Toxicol Clin Toxicol*. 1982;19:215-217.
12. *Boston Globe*. Warning is issued on Spanish fly. Anita Manning. August 26, 1991.
13. Boyd RE, et al. Strychnine poisoning. Recovery from profound lactic acidosis, hyperthermia, and rhabdomyolysis. *Am J Med*. 1983;74:507-512.
14. Burn DJ, et al. Strychnine poisoning as an unusual cause of convulsions. *Postgrad Med J*. 1989;65:563-564.
15. Campbell CH. Dr Mueller's strychnine cure of snakebite. *Med J Aust*. 1968;2:1-8.
16. Chan TY. Herbal medicine causing likely strychnine poisoning. *Hum Exp Toxicol*. 2002;21:467-468.
17. Ch'ien LT, et al. Glycine encephalopathy. *N Engl J Med*. 1978;298:687.
18. Cotton MS, Lane DH. Massive strychnine poisoning: a successful treatment. *J Miss State Med Assoc*. 1966;7:466-468.
19. Curtis DR, et al. The specificity of strychnine as a glycine antagonist in the mammalian spinal cord. *Exp Brain Res*. 1971;12:547-565.
20. Curtis DR, et al. A pharmacological study of the depression of spinal neurons by glycine and related amino acids. *Exp Brain Res*. 1968;6:1-18.
21. Decker W, Treuting J. Spot tests for rapid diagnosis of poisoning. *Clin Toxicol*. 1971;4:89-97.
22. Decker WJ, et al. Two deaths resulting from apparent parenteral injection of strychnine. *Vet Hum Toxicol*. 1982;24:161-162.
23. Dickson E, et al. Strychnine poisoning: an uncommon cause of convulsions. *Aust N Z J Med*. 1992;22:500-501.
24. Dittrich K, et al. A case of fatal strychnine poisoning. *J Emerg Med*. 1984;1:327-330.
25. Drugscope. Contaminated ecstasy. www.drugscope.org.uk/news_item.asp?a=1&intID=234. Published May 1, 2001. Accessed November 10, 2004.
26. Edmunds M, et al. Strychnine poisoning: clinical and toxicological observations on a non-fatal case. *J Toxicol Clin Toxicol*. 1986;24:245-255.
27. Ferguson MB, Vance MA. Payment deferred: strychnine poisoning in Nicaragua 65 years ago. *J Toxicol Clin Toxicol*. 2000;38:71-77.
28. Fernandez X, et al. Hypokalemia related to strychnine ingestion. *J Toxicol Clin Toxicol*. 2000;38:524.
29. Flood RG. Strychnine poisoning. *Pediatr Emerg Care*. 1999;15:286-287.
30. Goldstein MR. Recovery from severe metabolic acidosis. *JAMA*. 1975;234:1119.
31. Goodman LS, Gilman A. *The Pharmacological Basis of Therapeutics*. 3rd ed. New York, NY: Macmillan; 1965:345-348.
32. Gordon AM, Richards DW. Strychnine intoxication. *JACEP*. 1979;8:520-522.
33. Gosselin RE, et al. *Clinical Toxicology of Commercial Products*. 4th ed. Baltimore, MD: Williams & Wilkins; 1974:2.
34. Gosselin RE, et al. *Clinical Toxicology of Commercial Products*. 5th ed. Baltimore, MD: Williams & Wilkins; 1984:375-379.
35. Greene R, Meatherall R. Dermal exposure to strychnine. *J Anal Toxicol*. 2001;25: 344-347.
36. Haggard H, Greenberg L. Antidotes for strychnine poisoning. *JAMA*. 1983;98:1133-1136.
37. Hardin JA, Griggs RC. Diazepam treatment in a case of strychnine poisoning. *Lancet*. 1971;2:372-373.
38. Hatcher RA, Smith MI. The elimination of strychnine by the kidneys. *J Pharmacol Exp Ther*. 1916-1917;9:27-41.
39. Heiser JM, et al. Massive strychnine intoxication: serial blood levels in a fatal case. *J Toxicol Clin Toxicol*. 1992;30:269-283.
40. Herishanu Y Landau H. Diazepam in the treatment of strychnine poisoning. *Br J Anaesth*. 1972;44:747-748.
41. Hernandez AF, et al. Acute chemical pancreatitis associated with nonfatal strychnine poisoning. *J Toxicol Clin Toxicol*. 1998;36:67-71.
42. Hoffman RS. The toxic emergency—strychnine. *Emerg Med*. 1994;Feb:111-113.
43. Howes JF, Hunter WH. The stimulation of strychnine metabolism in rats by some anticonvulsant compounds. *J Pharm Pharmacol*. 1966;18:52S-57S.
44. Jackson G, Diggle G. Strychnine-containing tonics. *BMJ*. 1973;2:176-177.
45. Jackson G, et al. Strychnine poisoning treated successfully with diazepam. *BMJ*. 1971; 3:519-520.
46. Jacob J. Tarabar AF. A rare case of combined strychnine and propoxur toxicity from a single preparation. *Clin Toxicol*. 2012;50:224.
47. Kato R, et al. Increased activity of microsomal strychnine-metabolizing enzyme induced by phenobarbital and other drugs. *Biochem Pharmacol*. 1962;11:913-922.
48. Katz J, et al. Strychnine poisoning from a Cambodian traditional remedy. *Am J Emerg Med*. 1996;14:475-477.
49. Kodikara S. Strychnine in amoxicillin capsules: a means of homicide. *J Forensic Leg Med*. 2012;19:40-41.
50. Kong HY, et al. Safety of individual medication of Ma Qian Zi (semen strychni) based upon assessment of therapeutic effects of Guo's therapy against moderate fluorosis of bone. *J Tradit Chin Med*. 2011;31:297-302.

51. Libenson MH, Yang JM. Case 12-2001: a 16-year-old boy with altered mental status and muscle rigidity. *N Engl J Med.* 2001;344:1232-1239.

52. Lindsey T, et al. Strychnine overdose following ingestion of gopher bait. *J Anal Toxicol.* 2004;28:135.

53. Liu L, et al. In vitro metabolism of strychnine by human cytochrome P450 and its interaction with glycyrrhetic acid. *Chinese Herb Med.* 2012;4:118-125.

54. Loughhead M, et al. Life at pH 6.6. *Lancet.* 1978;2:952.

55. Ma C, et al. Strychnine and brucine compared with strychnine *N*-oxide and brucine *N*-oxide in toxicity [in Chinese]. *J Nanjing Univ Traditional Chinese Med.* 1994;10:37-38.

56. Maron BJ, et al. Strychnine poisoning successfully treated with diazepam. *J Pediatr.* 1971;78:697-699.

57. Marques EP, et al. Analytical method for the determination of strychnine in tissues by gas chromatography/mass spectrometry: two case reports. *Forensic Sci Int.* 2000; 110:145-152.

58. McConnell E, et al. A rapid test for the diagnosis of strychnine poisoning. *J S Afr Vet Med Assoc.* 1971;42:81-84.

59. McGarry RC, McGarry P. Please pass the strychnine: the art of Victorian pharmacy. *CMAJ.* 1999;161:1556-1558.

60. Metropolitan Life Insurance Company. *Stat Bull.* 1930;11:11.

61. Mishima M, et al. Metabolism of strychnine in vitro. *Drug Metab Dispos.* 1985;13:716-721.

62. Nishiyama T, Nagase M. Strychnine poisoning: natural course of a nonfatal case. *Am J Emerg Med.* 1995;13:172-173.

63. Oberpaur B, et al. Strychnine poisoning: an uncommon intoxication in children. *Pediatr Emerg Care.* 1999;1:264-265.

64. O'Callaghan WG, et al. Unusual strychnine poisoning and its treatment: report of eight cases. *BMJ (Clin Res Ed).* 1982;285:478.

65. Oguri K, et al. Metabolic fate of strychnine in rats. *Xenobiotica.* 1989;19:171-178.

66. Oliver JS, et al. Poisoning by strychnine. *Med Sci Law.* 1979;19:134-137.

67. Olkkola KT. Does ethanol modify antidotal efficacy of oral activated charcoal: studies in vitro and in experimental animals. *J Toxicol Clin Toxicol.* 1984;22:425-432.

68. Orringer C, et al. Natural history of lactic acidosis after grand mal seizures. *N Engl J Med.* 1977;297:697-699.

69. Palatnick W, et al. Toxicokinetics of acute strychnine poisoning. *J Toxicol Clin Toxicol.* 1997;35:617-620.

70. Perper JA. Fatal strychnine poisoning—a case report and review of the literature. *J Forensic Sci.* 1985;30:1248-1255.

71. Picchioni AL, et al. Activated charcoal vs "Universal Antidote" as an antidote for poisons. *Toxicol Appl Pharmacol.* 1966;8:447-454.

72. Platonow N, et al. Determination of strychnine in biological materials by gas chromatography. *J Forensic Sci.* 1970;15:433-446.

73. Posner JB, Plum F. Spinal fluid pH and neurologic symptoms in systemic acidosis. *N Engl J Med.* 1967;277:605-613.

74. Priest RE, Minn W. Strychnine poisoning successfully treated with sodium amytal. *JAMA.* 1938;110:1440.

75. Ralph D. Rhabdomyolysis and acute renal failure. *JACEP.* 1978;7:103-106.

76. Remmers JE, et al. Oropharyngeal muscle tone in obstructive sleep apnea before and after strychnine. *Sleep.* 1980;3:447-453.

77. Roches JC, et al. Effects of taurine, glycine and GABA on convulsions produced by strychnine in the rabbit. *Eur Neurol.* 1979;18:26-32.

78. Rosano TG, et al. Fatal strychnine poisoning: application of gas chromatography and tandem mass spectrometry. *J Anal Toxicol.* 2000;24:642-647.

79. Sangiah S. Effects of glycine and other inhibitory amino acid neurotransmitters on strychnine convulsive threshold in mice. *Vet Hum Toxicol.* 1985;27:97-99.

80. Sankaran K, et al. Glycine encephalopathy in a neonate: treatment with intravenous strychnine and sodium benzoate. *Clin Pediatr (Phila).* 1982;21:636-637.

81. Sgaragli GP, Mannaioni PF. Pharmacokinetic observations on a case of massive strychnine poisoning. *Clin Toxicol.* 1973;6:533-540.

82. Shadnia S, et al. A case of acute strychnine poisoning. *Vet Hum Toxicol.* 2004;46:76-79.

83. Smith BA. Strychnine poisoning. *J Emerg Med.* 1990;8:321-325.

84. Sofola OA, Odusote KA. Sympathetic cardiovascular effects of experimental strychnine poisoning in dogs. *J Pharmacol Exp Ther.* 1976;1:29-34.

85. Starretz-Hacham O, et al. Strychnine intoxication in a child. *Isr Med Assoc J.* 2003;5:531-532.

86. Swanson E. The antidotal effect of sodium amytal in strychnine poisoning. *J Lab Clin Med.* 1933;18:933-934.

87. Teitelbaum DT, Ott JE. Acute strychnine intoxication. *Clin Toxicol.* 1970;3:267-273.

88. Van Heerden PV, et al. Strychnine poisoning—alive and well in Australia! *Anaesth Intensive Care.* 1993;21:876-877.

89. Volynskaia EL. Use of large doses of strychnine and bemegride in barbiturate coma. *Klin Med (Mosk).* 1970;48:139-140.

90. Wax PM. Analeptic use in clinical toxicology: a historical appraisal. *J Toxicol Clin Toxicol.* 1997;35:203-209.

91. Weiss S, Hatcher RA. Studies on strychnine. *J Pharmacol Exp Ther.* 1922;14:419-482.

92. Winek CL, et al. Fatal strychnine ingestion. *J Anal Toxicol.* 1986;10:120-121.

93. Wood D, et al. Case report: survival after deliberate strychnine self-poisoning, with toxicokinetic data. *Crit Care.* 2002;6:456-459.

94. Woodbury DM. Convulsant drugs: mechanism of action. *Adv Neurol.* 1980;27:249-303.

95. Yamarick W, et al. Strychnine poisoning in an adolescent. *J Toxicol Clin Toxicol.* 1992; 30:141-148.

96. Zhang J, et al. Capillary electrophoresis with field-enhanced stacking for rapid and sensitive determination of strychnine and brucine. *Anal Bioanal Chem.* 2003;376:210-213.

115

L. Natural Toxins and Envenomations

ARTHROPODS

Daniel J. Repplinger and In-Hei Hahn

TAXONOMY

Arthropoda means "joint-footed" in Latin and describes the jointed bodies and legs connected to a chitinous exoskeleton of arthropods.[5] The majority of arthropods are benign to humans and environmentally beneficial. Some clinicians regard bites and stings as inconsequential and more of a nuisance than a threat to life. However, some spiders have toxic venoms that produce dangerous, painful lesions or significant systemic effects. Important clinical syndromes are produced by bites or stings from animals in the phylum Arthropoda, specifically the classes Arachnida (spiders, scorpions, and ticks) and Insecta (bees, wasps, hornets, and ants) (Table 115–1). Infectious diseases transmitted by arthropods, such as the various encephalitides, Rocky Mountain spotted fever, human anaplasmosis, babesiosis, ehrlichiosis, and Lyme disease, are not discussed in this chapter.

Arthropoda comprises the largest phylum in the animal kingdom. It includes more species than all other phyla combined (Fig. 115–1).[5] At least 1.5 million species are identified, and half a million or more are yet to be classified. Araneism (pertaining to spiders) or arachnidism (spiders including other arachnids) results from the envenomation caused by a spider bite. "Bites" are different from "stings." Bites are defined as creating a wound using the oral pole with the intention for either catching or envenomating prey or blood feeding,[93,194] or for the purpose of feeding such as in arthropods that have mouthparts for chewing or sucking. "Stings" occur from a modified ovipositor at the aboral pole that is also able to function in egg laying as in bees and wasps. In scorpions the sting is not a modified ovipositor and the "tail" is not a tail but the metasoma section of the abdomen. Stinging behavior typically is used for defense. Most spiders are venomous, and the venom weakens the prey, enabling the spider to secure and digest their prey. However, there is one family of spiders, Uloboridae, which does not have a venom gland, a venom duct, or duct opening in the fangs. Spiders in general are not aggressive toward humans unless they are provoked. The chelicerae (mouthparts composed of basal section and hinged fang) of many species have fangs that are too short to penetrate human skin.

Spiders are divided into categories based on whether they pursue their prey as hunters or trappers. Trappers snare their prey by spinning webs, then feed on their prey and enshrine excess victims in a cocoon silk to be eaten later. The order of spiders (Araneae) differs from other members of the class (Arachnida) because of various anatomic differences best assessed by an entomologist/arachnologist. Simplistically, the arachnids have 4 pairs of joined legs whereas insects have 3 pairs. The arachnid's body is divided into 2 parts (cephalothorax and unsegmented abdomen, except for some spiders in Mesothelae and also some Mygalomorph {tarantula-type} relatives that have abdominal plates) connected by a small pedicel and 2, 3, or 4 pairs (Mesothelae contain up to 6 pairs) of spinnerets from which silk is spun. Two pedipalps are attached anteriorly on the cephalothorax on either side of their chelicerae and are used for sensation, manipulation of food and objects, and in males are modified for sperm transfer. Spiders have 8 eyes and are quite myopic, although there are instances when they have 2, 4, 6, or even no eyes. Prey is localized by touch as they land in the spider's web, though not all spiders produce webs or use silk to capture prey. Most spiders use venom to kill or immobilize their prey. The spiders of medical importance in the United States include the widow spiders (*Latrodectus* spp), the violin spiders (*Loxosceles* spp), and the hobo spider (*Eratigena agrestis*). Although there is some disagreement as to the extent of the danger of hobo spiders in the United States, they are not considered dangerous in Europe. In Australia, the funnel web spider (*Atrax robustus*) and *Hadronyche* species cause serious illness and even death. In South America, the Brazilian Huntsmen (*Phoneutria fera*) and Brazilian armed spider, Aranha Armadeira (*Phoneutria nigriventer*) are threats to humans.

HISTORY AND EPIDEMIOLOGY

Since the time of Aristotle, spiders and their webs were used for medicinal purposes. Special preparations were concocted to cure a fantastic array of ailments, including earache, running of the eyes, "wounds in the joints," warts, gout, asthma, "spasmodic complaints of females," chronic hysteria, cough, rheumatic afflictions for the head, and stopping blood flow.[228]

One *Latrodectus* species has an infamous history of medical concern, hence the name *mactans*, which means "murderer" in Latin.[182] Hysteria regarding spider bites peaked during the 17th century in the Taranto region of Italy. The syndrome tarantism, which is characterized by lethargy, stupor, and a restless compulsion to walk or dance, was blamed on *Lycosa tarantula*, a spider that pounces on its prey like a wolf. Deaths were associated with these outbreaks. Dancing the rapid tarantella to music was the presumed remedy. The real culprit in this epidemic was *Latrodectus tredecimguttatus*.[182]

TABLE 115–1	North American Insects and Other Arthropods That Bite, Sting, or Nettle Humans
Arthropod	**Description**
Honeybee (*Apis mellifera*)	Hairy, yellowish brown with black markings
Bumblebee and carpenter bee (*Bombus* spp and *Xylocopa* spp)	Hairy, larger than honeybees and colored black and yellow
Vespids (yellow jackets, hornets, paper wasps)	Short-waisted, robust, black and yellow or white combination
Schecoids (thread-waisted wasps)	Threadlike waist
Nettling caterpillars (browntail, Io, hag, and buck moths, saddleback and puss caterpillars)	Caterpillar shaped
Southern fire ant (*Solenopsis* spp)	Ant shaped
Spiders (*Arachnida*) black widow, brown recluse	Body with 2 regions: cephalothorax and abdomen; 8 legs
Scorpions (*Centruroides*)	Eight-legged, crablike, stinger at the tip of the abdomen; pedipalps (pincers) highly developed (not a true insect)
Centipedes (*Chilopoda*)	Elongated, wormlike, with many jointed segments and legs; one pair of poison fangs behind head

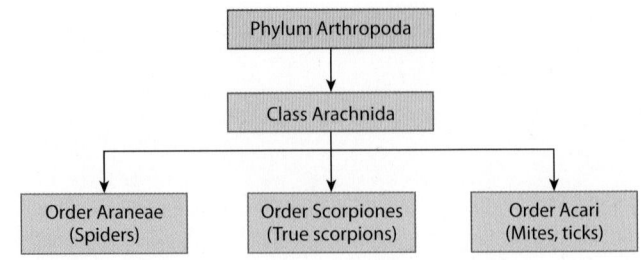

FIGURE 115–1. Taxonomy of the phylum Arthropoda.

TABLE 115–2	North American Spiders of Medical Importance
Genus	**Common Name**
Araneus spp	Orb weaver
Argiope spp	Orange argiope
Bothriocyrtum spp	Trap door spider
Chiracanthium spp	Running spider
Drassodes spp	Gnaphosid spider
Heteropoda spp	Huntsman spider
Latrodectus spp	Widow spider
Liocranoides spp	Running spider
Loxosceles spp	Brown, violin, or recluse spider
Lycosa spp	Wolf spider
Misumenoides spp	Crab spider
Neoscona spp	Orb weaver
Peucetia spp	Green lynx spider
Phiddipus spp	Jumping spider
Rheostica (Aphonopelma) spp	Tarantula
Steatoda grossa	False black widow spider
Eratigena spp	Hobo spider
Ummidia spp	Trap door spider

Other epidemics of arachnidism occurred in Spain in 1833 and 1841.[153] In North America, there was an increase in spider bites during the late 1920s; Rome reported large numbers in 1953; Yugoslavia reported a large number of cases between 1948 and 1953.[33,153] These epidemics may be related to actual reporting biases as well as climatic variations.[182] Spider bites are more numerous in warmer months, presumably because both spiders and humans are more active during that season.

Approximately 200 species of spiders are associated with envenomations.[191,195] Eighteen genera of North American spiders produce poisonings that require clinical intervention (Table 115–2). In one series of 600 suspected spider bites, 80% were determined to result from arthropods other than spiders, such as ticks, bugs, mites, fleas, moths, butterflies, caterpillars, flies, beetles, water bugs, and some members (ants, bees, wasps) of order Hymenoptera. Ten percent of the presumed bites actually were manifestations of other nonarthropod disorders.[193,195]

From 2011 through 2015, an annual average of approximately 8500 spider exposures and 34,000 insect exposures were reported to US poison control centers (Chap. 130). Over this time, only 5 fatalities were reported, 3 of which were from the Hymenoptera category. Overall, this represents a marked decline in reported cases over the last decade. From 2006 to 2007, an annual average of 14,000 spider exposures and 44,000 insect exposures were reported to US poison control centers. No more than 2 fatalities were reported per year. One was from the Hymenoptera category, and the other was an unknown spider exposure. Although the total number of reported cases has declined dramatically, the average number of fatal exposures remains stable (Chap. 130).

Most information on the clinical presentation of spider bites continues to be unreliable because it is based on case reports and case series. Frequently, the cases do not have any expert confirmation of the actual spider involved, which propagates misinformation about different spiders, particularly with necrotic arachnidism. For example, cutaneous anthrax was mistaken for a cutaneous necrotic spider bite.[190] Additionally, the white tail spider (*Lampona* spp) was suspected for more than 20 years to cause necrotic lesions. Ultimately a prospective study of confirmed spider bites refuted this myth by reporting more than 700 confirmed spider bites in Australia.[124-126] Because most arthropod-focused research involves characterizing the structure of spider toxins rather than verifying clinical presentations, it is important to produce clinical studies that have bites confirmed by the presence of the spider that is identified by an expert. Definite spider bites or stings are established by (1) evidence of a bite or sting soon after the incident or the creature is seen to bite or sting and (2) collection of the particular creature, either alive or dead, with positive identification of the creature by an expert biologist/taxonomist in the field relating to the creature.[125,127]

BLACK WIDOW SPIDER (*LATRODECTUS MACTANS;* HOURGLASS SPIDER)

Five species of widow spiders are found in the United States: *Latrodectus mactans* (black widow; Fig. 115–2A), *Latrodectus hesperus* (Western black widow), *Latrodectus variolus* (found in New England, Canada, south to Florida, and west to eastern Texas, Oklahoma, and Kansas), *Latrodectus bishopi* (red widow of the South), and *Latrodectus geometricus* (brown widow or brown button spider; Fig. 115–2B). They are present in every state except for Alaska. Dangerous widow spiders in other parts of the world include *L. geometricus* and *Latrodectus tredecimguttatus* (European widow spider found in southern Europe), *Latrodectus hasselti* (red back widow spider found in Australia, Japan, and India; Fig. 115–2C), and *Latrodectus cinctus* (found in South Africa). These spiders live in temperate and tropical latitudes in places such as stone walls, crevices, wood piles, outhouses, barns, stables, and rubbish piles. They molt multiple times and as a result can change colors. The ventral markings on the abdomen are species specific, and the classic red hourglass-shaped marking is noted in only *L. mactans*. Other species have variations on their ventral surface, such as triangles and spots.

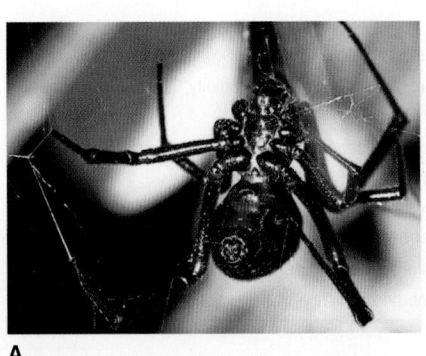
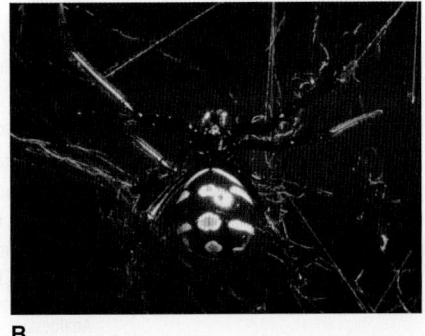
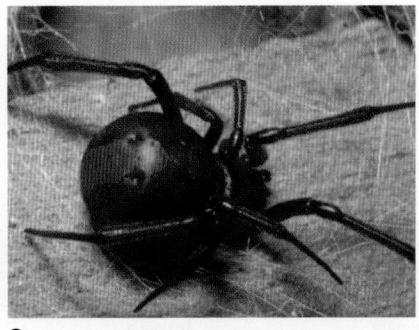

A   B   C

FIGURE 115–2. Widow spiders. (**A**) The North American black widow spider, *Latrodectus mactans*. Note the hourglass on the abdomen. (**B**) The brown widow spider, *Latrodectus geometricus*. (**C**) The Australian red back spider, *Latrodectus hasselti*. (*Used with permission from the American Museum of Natural History.*)

Typically, the female *L. mactans* is shiny, jet-black, and large (8–10 mm), with a rounded abdomen and a red hourglass mark on its ventral surface. Her larger size and ability of her fangs to penetrate human skin make her more venomous and toxic than the male spider, which resembles the immature spider in earlier stages of development and is smaller, lighter in color, and has a more elongated abdomen and fangs that usually are too short to envenomate humans (Table 115–3). Black widow females are trappers and inhabit large, untidy, irregularly shaped webs. Webs are placed in or close to the ground and in secluded, dimly lit areas that can trap flying insects, such as outdoor privies, barns, sheds, and garages.[5]

Pathophysiology

The venom is more potent on a volume-per-volume basis than the venom of a pit viper and contains 7 active components with molecular weights of 5,000 to 130,000 Da.[5] The 7 components are 5 latroinsectotoxins (α-, β-, γ-, δ-, ϵ-LITs) (insect-specific neurotoxins), α-latrocrustatoxin (α-LCT)

(crustacean-specific neurotoxin), and α-latrotoxin (vertebrate-specific neurotoxin).[102] α-Latrotoxin binds, with nanomolar affinity, to the specific presynaptic receptors neurexin I-α and Ca^{2+}-independent receptor for α-latrotoxin (CIRL), otherwise known as *latrophilin*.[30,111,123] The binding triggers a cascade of events: conformational change allowing pore formation by tethering the toxin to the plasma membrane; Ca^{2+} ionophore formation; translocation of the *N*-terminal domain of α-LTX into the presynaptic intracellular space, and intracellular activation of exocytosis of norepinephrine, dopamine, neuropeptides, acetylcholine, glutamate, and γ-aminobutyric acid (GABA), respectively. This massive release of neurotransmitters is what causes the clinical envenomation syndrome known as latrodectism.[5,169,193]

Clinical Manifestations

Widow spiders are shy and nocturnal. They usually bite when their web is disturbed or upon inadvertent exposure in shoes and clothing. A sharp pain typically described as a pinprick occurs as the victim is bitten. A pair of red

TABLE 115–3	Brown Recluse and Black Widow Spiders: Comparative Characteristics	
	Brown Recluse (Loxosceles spp)	**Black Widow (Latrodectus spp)**
Description of the spider	Female brown, 6–20 mm, violin-shaped mark on dorsum of cephalothorax; female greater toxicity than male	Female: jet black, 8–10 mm, red hourglass mark on ventral surface, female greater toxicity than male. Male: smaller and lighter in color, often with red or white markings on dorsal surface
Major venom component	Sphingomyelinase D	α-Latrotoxin
Pathophysiology of envenomation	Vascular injury, dermatonecrosis, hemolysis	Massive presynaptic discharge of neurotransmitters; lymphatic and hematogenous spread, neurotoxicity
Epidemiology	Bites more common in warmer months	Bites more common in warmer months in subtropical and temperate areas; perennial in tropics
	North America (southern and Midwestern states): *L. reclusa*	North America: *L. mactans*, *L. hesperus*, *L. geometricus*
	South America: *L. laeta*, *L. gaucho*	Europe: *L. tredecimguttatus*
	Europe: *L. rufescens*	Africa (southern): *L. indistinctus*
	Africa (southern): *L. parrami*, *L. spiniceps*, *L. pilosa*, *L. bergeri*	Australia: *L. hasselti*
	Asia/Australia: Rare	Asia/South America: Rare
Clinical effects	Cutaneous	Cutaneous
	Initial (0–2 hours after bite): Painless, erythema, edema	Initial (5 minutes–1 hour after bite): Local pain
	2–8 hours: Hemorrhagic, ulcerates, painful	1–2 hours: Puncture marks
	1 week: Eschar	Hours: Regional lymph nodes swollen, central blanching at bite site with surrounding erythema
	Months: Healing	
		CVS: Initial tachycardia followed by bradycardia, dysrhythmias, initial hypotension followed by hypertension
		GI: Nausea, vomiting, mimic acute abdomen
	Hematologic	Hematologic: Leukocytosis
	Methemoglobinemia, hemolysis, thrombocytopenia, disseminated intravascular coagulopathy	
		Resolution over several days
		Metabolic
		Hyperglycemia (transient)
		Musculoskeletal: Hypertonia, abdominal rigidity, "facies latrodectismica"
		Neurologic
		CNS: Psychosis, hallucinations, visual disturbance, seizures
		Peripheral nervous system: Pain at the site
		Autonomic nervous system: Increased secretions; sweating, salivation, lacrimation, diarrhea, bronchorrhea, mydriasis, miosis, priapism, ejaculation
	Renal: Kidney failure, acute tubular necrosis	Renal: Glomerulonephritis, oliguria, anuria
		Respiratory: Bronchoconstriction, acute respiratory distress syndrome
Treatment	Analgesia	Analgesia
	Wound care	Muscle relaxants
		Antivenom

spots often evolve at the site, although the bite is commonly unnoticed.[49,152] The bite mark itself tends to be limited to a small puncture wound or wheal and flare reaction that often is associated with a halo (Table 115–3). However, the bite from *L. mactans* produces *latrodectism*, a constellation of signs and symptoms resulting from systemic toxicity. Some cases do not progress; others show severe neuromuscular effects within 30 to 60 minutes. The effects from the bite spread contiguously. For example, if a person is bitten on the hand, the pain progresses up the arm to the elbow, shoulder, and then toward the trunk during systemic poisoning. Typically, a brief time to symptom onset denotes severe envenomation. One patient developed latrodectism following the intentional intravenous injection of a crushed whole black widow spider.[41]

One grading system divides the severity of the envenomation into 3 categories.[56] Grade 1 envenomations range from no symptoms to local pain at the envenomation site with normal vital signs. Grade 2 envenomations involve muscular pain at the site with migration of the pain to the trunk, diaphoresis at the bite site, and normal vital signs. Grade 3 envenomations include the grade 2 findings with abnormal vital signs; diaphoresis distant from the bite site; generalized myalgias to back, chest, and abdomen; and nausea, vomiting, and headache.

The myopathic syndrome of latrodectism involves muscle cramps that usually begin 15 to 60 minutes after the bite. The muscle cramps initially occur at the site of the bite, but later involves rigidity of other skeletal muscles, particularly muscles of the chest, abdomen, and face. The pain increases over time and occurs in waves that cause the patient to writhe. Large muscle groups are affected first. Classically, severe abdominal wall spasm occurs and is confused with a surgical abdomen, especially in children who cannot relate the history to the initial bite.[38] Muscle pain often subsides within a few hours but can recur for several days. Transient muscle weakness and spasms is reported to persist for weeks to months.

Additional clinical findings include "facies latrodectismica," which consists of sweating, contorted, grimaced face associated with blepharitis, conjunctivitis, rhinitis, cheilitis, and trismus of the masseters.[152] A fear of death, *pavor mortis*, is described.[152] Nausea, vomiting, sweating, tachycardia, hypertension, muscle cramping, restlessness, compartment syndrome at the site of the bite, and, rarely, priapism are also reported.[5,57,116,215] The mechanism of compartment syndrome developing after a black widow spider envenomation is unclear, but 2 postulated theories include rhabdomyolysis and the venom affecting the blood vessels leading to engorgement and obstruction of the venous outflow. In one case, the compartment syndrome was treated with antivenom, and the patient recovered without the need for a fasciotomy.[57] Recovery usually ensues within 24 to 48 hours, but clinical findings are reported to last several days with more severe envenomations. Life-threatening complications include severe hypertension, respiratory distress, myocardial infarction, cardiovascular failure, and gangrene.[41,56-78,163,178,182] In the past 20 years, more than 40,000 presumed black widow spider bites were reported to the American Association of Poison Control Centers (Chap. 130). Death is rarely reported. There were 2 reported fatalities in Madagascar from envenomation by *L. geometricus*, one from cardiovascular failure and the other from gangrene of the foot.[182] The most recent fatality reported from Greece resulted from myocarditis secondary to envenomation by *L. tredecimguttatus*,[181] confirmed by a local veterinarian. The patient developed severe dyspnea, hypoxemia, cyanosis, cardiomyopathy, and global hypokinesis of the left ventricle confirmed by echocardiography, followed by death 36 hours later; antivenom was not available. On autopsy, diffuse interstitial and alveolar edema, with mononuclear infiltrate of the myocardium and degenerative changes, were noted, and toxicologic analysis for xenobiotics, as well as all blood, urine, bronchial, serologic, and viral cultures, were negative. The paucity of death is presumed to result from the improvement in medical care, the availability of antivenom, or the limited toxicity of the spider.

Diagnostic Testing

Laboratory data generally are not helpful in management or predicting outcome. According to one study, the most common findings include

leukocytosis and increased creatine phosphokinase and lactate dehydrogenase concentrations.[56] Currently, no specific laboratory assay is capable of confirming latrodectism. However, the clinical situation, such as suspected compartment syndrome, would warrant the need to check laboratory tests and other studies to evaluate the sequelae of the black widow spider envenomation.

Management

Treatment involves establishing an airway and supporting respiration and circulation, if indicated. Wound evaluation and local wound care, including tetanus prophylaxis, are essential.[237] The routine use of antibiotics is not recommended.

Pain management is a substantial component of patient care and depends on the clinical findings. Using the grading system, grade 1 envenomations require only cold packs and orally administered nonsteroidal antiinflammatory drugs. For grade 2 and 3 envenomations, intravenous (IV) opioids and benzodiazepines are often reasonable for pain control and muscle spasm.

In the past, 10 mL 10% calcium gluconate solution was given IV to decrease cramping. However, a retrospective chart review of 163 patients envenomated by the black widow concluded that calcium gluconate was ineffective for pain relief compared with a combination of IV opioids and benzodiazepines.[56,138] Another study found greater neurotransmitter release when extracellular calcium concentrations were increased, suggesting that administration of calcium is irrational in patients suffering from latrodectism.[191] The mechanism of action of calcium remains unknown, and its efficacy is anecdotal; therefore, we do not recommend calcium administration for pain management.

Although often recommended, methocarbamol (a centrally acting muscle relaxant) and dantrolene also are ineffective for treatment of latrodectism.[138,196] A benzodiazepine, such as diazepam, is more effective for controlling muscle spasms and achieves sedation, anxiolysis, and amnesia. Management should primarily emphasize supportive care, with opioids and benzodiazepines for controlling pain and muscle spasms, because the use of antivenom risks anaphylaxis and serum sickness.

Latrodectus antivenom (Merck) is rapidly effective and curative. In the United States the antivenom formulation is effective for all species, but is available as a crude hyperimmune horse serum that is reported to cause anaphylaxis and serum sickness. The morbidity of latrodectism is high, with pain, cramping, and autonomic disturbances, but mortality is low. Hence controversy exists over when to administer the black widow antivenom (BW-AV). We recommend BW-AV for severe reactions (eg, hypertensive crisis or intractable pain), to high-risk patients (eg, pregnant women suffering from a threatened abortion), or for treatment of priapism.[138,182] The usual dose is one to two vials diluted in 50 to 100 mL 5% dextrose or 0.9% sodium chloride solution, with the combination infused over 1 hour (Antidotes in Depth: A37). Skin testing may elicit a hypersensitivity reaction to horse serum but the absence of a reaction does not exclude the occurrence of hypersensitivity reactions; therefore, we recommend against skin testing. An observational case series of 96 patients who received BW-AV found no cases of shortness of breath, angioedema, bronchospasm, hypotension, or death. In this series, adverse events occurred in 4% and were deemed mild to moderate and treated supportively.[172] However, an anaphylactic reaction to the BW-AV was reported after a negative skin test in both a boy and a man[121,166] who subsequently died from the anaphylactic reaction. Both were being treated for intractable pain after failing intravenous opioid management. Pretreatment with histamine H_1- or H_2-antagonists, or both, and epinephrine is beneficial in preventing histamine release and anaphylaxis. Patients with allergies to horse serum products and those who have received antivenom or horse serum products are at risk for immunoglobulin E (IgE)–mediated hypersensitivity reactions and, though efficacy is largely unproven, it is reasonable to pretreat with antihistamines and corticosteroids and have epinephrine available.

A purified F(ab′)$_2$ fragment *Latrodectus mactans* antivenom, Analatro, recently underwent a phase 2 clinical trial and is currently being investigated in a phase 3 trial (Antidotes in Depth: A37). Antivenin *Latrodectus* Equine Immune F(ab')₂ is currently available in Mexico but not yet FDA approved in the United States. This randomized trial included 24 patients and found no statistically significant difference in overall pain reduction compared to placebo, but the patients receiving antivenom had more rapid reduction of pain. No significant adverse events occurred in either group, specifically no incidence of anaphylaxis or anaphylactoid reactions.[67] However, as a phase 2 trial, this study was intended to examine efficacy and cannot be interpreted to establish safety.

In Australia, a purified equine-derived IgG-F(ab')₂ antivenom for the red back spider *L. hasselti* (RBS-AV) is available. The RBS-AV (CSL, Melbourne, Australia) is administered intramuscularly and given as first-line therapy to patients presenting with systemic signs or symptoms in Australia. Since its introduction in 1956, no deaths were reported, and the incidence of mild allergic reactions to RBS-AV was only 0.54% in 2,144 uses.[224]

However, an underpowered prospective cohort study of confirmed red back spider bites failed to show that intramuscular antivenom was better than no treatment when all patients were followed over a one-week period.[126] This study did note that only 17% of patients were pain-free at 24 hours with antivenom treatment. Therefore, intramuscular antivenom appears to be less effective than previously thought, and the route of administration requires review. A monoclonal Fab specific for the α-latroxin was demonstrated to be highly effective in neutralizing the toxin in vivo in mice and shows promise for study in humans for severe black widow spider envenomation.[12,39] Inadvertent use of RBS-AV successfully treated envenomations from the comb-footed spider (*Steatoda* spp),[127] and the *Steatoda* venom and clinical effects are similar to the *Latrodectus* venom but milder in clinical presentation.[100]

BROWN RECLUSE SPIDER (*LOXOSCELES RECLUSA*; VIOLIN OR FIDDLEBACK SPIDER)

Loxosceles reclusa was confirmed to cause necrotic arachnidism in 1957, although reports of systemic effects following brown spider bites have appeared since 1872.[10] This spider has a brown violin-shaped mark on the dorsum of the cephalothorax, 3 dyads of eyes arranged in a semicircle on top of the head, and legs that are 5 times as long as the body. It is small (6–20 mm long) and gray to orange or reddish brown (Fig. 115–3A). *Loxosceles* spiders weave irregular white, flocculent adhesive webs that line their retreats.[89] Spiders in the genus *Loxosceles* have a worldwide distribution. In the United States, other species of this genus, which include *L. rufescens*, *L. deserta*, *L. devia*, and *L. arizonica*, are prominent in the Southeast and Southwest.[9] *L. rufescens* was inadvertently introduced in several buildings in New York City. Though it is unclear how they initially arrived there, they were most likely transported on personal belongings and cartons of materials.[212] They are hunter spiders that live in dark areas (wood piles, rocks, basements), and their foraging is nocturnal. They are not aggressive but will bite if antagonized (Table 115–3). These spiders live up to 2 or more years. They are resilient and can survive up to 6 months without water or food and can tolerate temperatures from 46.4°F to 109.4°F (8°–43°C).[98] Like the black widow spider, the female is more dangerous than the male. *Loxosceles* venom has variable toxicity, depending on the species, with *Loxosceles intermedia* venom causing more severe clinical effects in humans.[15,16] The peak time for envenomation is from spring to autumn, and most victims are bitten in the morning. One study examined 182 patients enrolled over 23 months who presented to the emergency department (ED) for a chief complaint of spider bite. The study found that only 3% (7/182) were ultimately confirmed by their treating physician to have the diagnosis of a spider bite, whereas 84% (152/182) had a skin and soft tissue infection (SSTI), 9 patients were bitten by other animals; 6 patients were given other non-bite diagnoses, such as erythema multiforme, subcutaneous nodules, and folliculitis; and 8 patients had no diagnostic category recorded. Of the 7 patients who had a confirmed spider bite, only one brought the spider in for identification, whereas the others saw a spider or witnessed a bite, and one patient did not witness or feel a bite.[218] Community-acquired methicillin-resistant *Staphylococcus aureus*

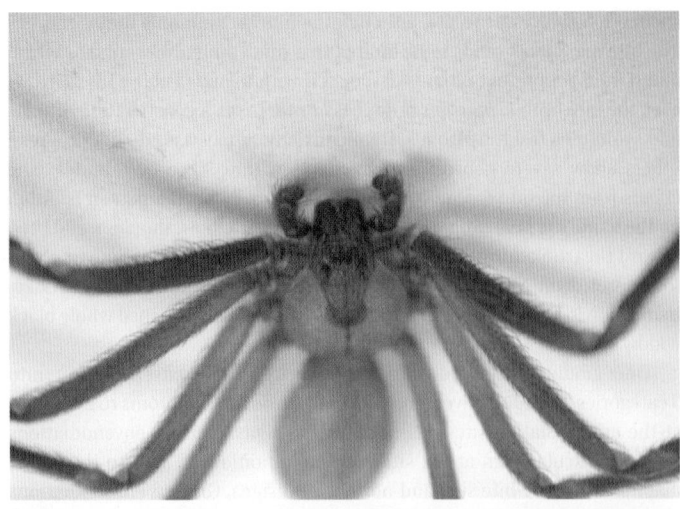

A

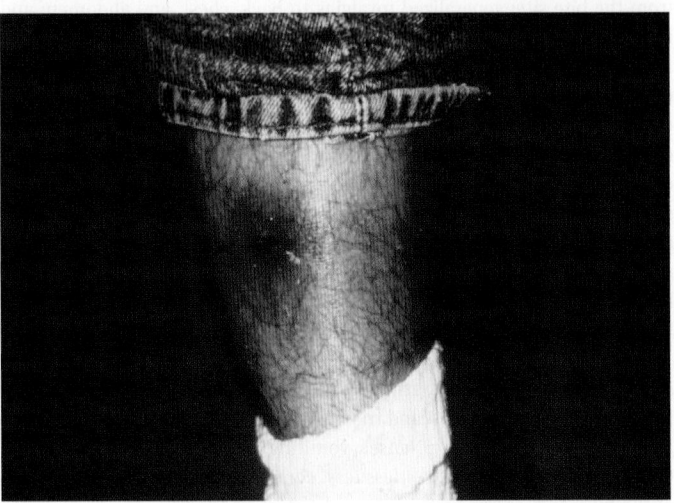

B

FIGURE 115–3. Brown recluse spider. (**A**) *Loxosceles reclusa*. Note the image of the violin, which gives the spider its common name, "the fiddleback spider." *(Image contributed by Progeny Products, www.brown-recluse.com.)* (**B**) A typical envenomation from the brown recluse spider. *(Used with permission from the Fellowship in Medical Toxicology, New York University School of Medicine, New York City Poison Center.)*

(MRSA) was the most common cause of skin and soft tissue injuries (SSTIs), accounting for 70% of positive wound cultures performed. Hence the spider bite diagnosis is frequently misused, and a diagnosis of dermatonecrotic wound of uncertain etiology would be more accurate.[218]

Pathophysiology

The venom is cytotoxic. The 2 main constituent enzymes of the venom are sphingomyelinase D and hyaluronidase, though other subcomponents include deoxyribonuclease, ribonuclease, collagenase, esterase, proteases, alkaline phosphatase, and lipase.[66,143,233] Hyaluronidase is a spreading factor that facilitates the penetration of the venom into tissue but does not induce lesion development.[143] Sphingomyelinase D is the primary constituent of the venom that causes necrosis and red blood cell hemolysis and also causes platelets to release serotonin.[143] Sphingomyelinase also reacts with sphingomyelin in the red blood cell membrane to release choline and *N*-acylsphingosine phosphate, which triggers a chain reaction, releasing inflammatory mediators, such as thromboxanes, leukotrienes, prostaglandins, and neutrophils, leading to vessel thrombosis, tissue ischemia, and skin loss.[143] Early perivascular collections of polymorphonuclear leukocytes with hemorrhage and edema progress to intravascular clotting. Coagulation and vascular occlusion of the microcirculation occurs, ultimately leading to necrosis.[208]

Clinical Manifestations

The clinical spectrum of loxoscelism is divided into 3 major categories. The first category includes bites in which very little, if any, venom is injected. A small erythematous papule appears, which then becomes firm before healing and is associated with a localized urticarial response. In the second category, the bite undergoes a cytotoxic reaction. The bite initially is reported to be painless or have a stinging sensation, followed by blistering, bleeding, and ulceration 2 to 8 hours later (Table 115–3). The lesion then increases in diameter, with demarcation of central hemorrhagic vesiculation, then ulceration, the development of violaceous necrosis surrounded by ischemic blanching of skin and outer erythema and, finally induration over 1 to 3 days. This is also known as the "red, white, and blue" reaction (Fig. 115–3B).[139,243] Necrosis of the central blister occurs in 3 to 4 days, with eschar formation between 5 and 7 days. After 7 to 14 days, the wound becomes indurated and the eschar falls off, leaving an ulceration that heals by secondary intention. Local necrosis is more extensive over fatty areas (thighs, buttocks, and abdomen).[143] The size of the ulcer determines the time for healing. Large lesions up to 30 cm require months or more to heal.

Upper airway obstruction was reported in a child who was bitten on his neck and subsequently developed progressive cervical soft tissue edema with airway obstruction and dermatonecrosis 40 hours later.[97] Another case reported stridor and respiratory distress following a brown recluse envenomation of the ear. Although the presentation is rare, respiratory status should be evaluated when an envenomation occurs on the head and neck.[92]

The third category consists of systemic loxoscelism, which is not predicted by the extent of cutaneous reaction, and occurs 24 to 72 hours after the bite. The young are particularly susceptible.[96,197] The clinical manifestations of systemic loxoscelism include fever, chills, weakness, edema, nausea, vomiting, arthralgias, petechial eruptions, rhabdomyolysis, disseminated intravascular coagulation, hemolysis that is reported to progress to hemoglobinuria, acute kidney injury, and death.[27,44,85,96,150,203,240] However, in North America, the incidence of systemic illness and mortality is rare.[7]

Diagnostic Testing

Bites from other spiders, such as *Cheiracanthium* (sac spider), *Phidippus* (jumping spider), and *Argiope* (orb weaver), also produce necrotic wounds. These spiders are often the actual culprits when the brown recluse is mistakenly blamed. Definitive diagnosis is achieved only when the biting spider is positively identified. No routine laboratory test for loxoscelism is available for clinical application, but several techniques are presently used for research purposes. The lymphocyte transformation test measures lymphocytes that have undergone blast transformation up to one month after exposure to *Loxosceles* venom. The lymphocytes incorporate thymidine into the nucleoprotein, providing a quantitative assay.[8] A passive hemagglutination inhibition test (PHAI) was developed in guinea pigs. The PHAI assay is based on the property of certain brown recluse spider venom components to spontaneously adsorb to formalin-treated erythrocyte membranes and the ability of the brown recluse spider venom to inhibit antiserum-induced agglutination of venom-coated red blood cells.[18] The test is 90% sensitive and 100% specific for 3 days postenvenomation and is useful for early diagnosis of brown recluse spider envenomation.[18] An enzyme-linked immunoassay (ELISA) test specific for *Loxosceles* venom in biopsied tissue can confirm the presence of venom for 4 days postenvenomation,[18] and in an experimental model using rabbits, the antigen was recoverable using the ELISA assay from 14 to 21 days.[155] The drawbacks of using a skin biopsy are the invasive nature of the procedure, which can result in further scarring with an increased potential for infection, and the lack of proof that skin biopsy is able to diagnose early envenomations prior to the development of dermatonecrosis. Another ELISA test utilizing serum for detection of venom antigens was developed that correctly discriminates the mice inoculated with antigens from *L. intermedia* venom. The ELISA immunoassay test and antivenom would become useful diagnostic tools if envenomation is proved or disproved early.[53] A venom-specific enzyme immunoassay that uses hair, skin biopsies, or aspirated

tissue near a suspected lesion to detect the presence of venom up to 7 days after injury is under investigation.[142,159] In Brazil, ELISA testing is used to detect the venom of *Loxosceles gaucho* in wounds and patient sera, but the technique is not in widespread clinical use.[49]

Clinical laboratory data include the findings of hemolysis, hemoglobinuria, and hematuria. Coagulopathy is often present, with laboratory data significant for elevated fibrin split products, decreased fibrinogen concentrations, and a positive D-dimer assay. Other tests include increased prothrombin time (PT) and partial thromboplastin time (PTT), leukocytosis (up to 20,000–30,000 cells/mm³), spherocytosis, Coombs-positive hemolytic anemia, thrombocytopenia, or abnormal kidney and liver function tests.[5,12,89,193,195,197,238]

Treatment

Optimal local treatment of the lesion is controversial. The most prudent management of the dermatonecrotic lesion is wound care, immobilization, tetanus prophylaxis, analgesics, and antipruritics as warranted (Table 115–4).[5,89,235,238] Early excision or intralesional injection of corticosteroids appears unwarranted.[188] Corrective surgery can be performed several weeks after adequate tissue demarcation has occurred. In one case series, the use of curettage of the lesion to remove necrotic and indurated tissue from the lesion, thus eliminating any continuing action of the lytic enzymes on the surrounding tissue.[114] These patients had wound healing without further necrosis and minimal scarring. Vacuum-assisted closure, otherwise known as negative-pressure wound therapy, is also described in a series of clinical cases in the surgical literature as a means to treat necrotic wounds caused by presumed brown recluse spider bites more quickly than the traditional methods, due to increased bacterial clearance and dermal perfusion, modulating the inflammatory response, extracting toxic substances, and accelerated rate of granulation tissue formation.[241] Electric shock delivered via stun guns was not found to be useful in a guinea pig envenomation model.[18] Cyproheptadine, a serotonin antagonist, was not beneficial in a rabbit model.[175] A randomized, controlled study evaluating the efficacy of topical nitroglycerin for envenomated rabbits showed no difference in preventing dermatonecrosis and suggested the possibility of increased systemic toxicity.[147] Additionally, intradermal injection of trypsin failed to show any benefit in a guinea pig model.[42] Antibiotics are recommended to treat cutaneous or systemic infections when present, but they are not recommended prophylactically.

Early use of dapsone (in patients who develop a central purplish bleb or vesicle within the first 6–8 hours) is reported to inhibit local infiltration of the wound by polymorphonuclear leukocytes.[139] The dosage previously recommended was 100 mg twice daily for 2 weeks.[186] However, prospective trials with large numbers of patients are lacking. One study compared the efficacy of erythromycin and dapsone therapy, erythromycin and antivenom therapy, and erythromycin, dapsone, and antivenom therapy (developed in rabbits based on a previous study).[185] Although the treatment groups were very small, all groups showed wound healing at approximately 20 days despite the different therapies used. The major limitation of the study includes the definition of a spider bite diagnosis (the study used the following criteria: a patient feeling the spider bite, seeing the spider, or having a clinically plausible necrotic

TABLE 115–4	Management of Brown Recluse Spider Bite	
General Wound Care	**Local Wound Care**	**Systemic**
Clean	Serial observations	Antipruritic/antianxiety and/or analgesics
Tetanus prophylaxis as indicated	Natural healing by granulation	
Immobilize and elevate bitten extremity	Delayed primary closure	Antibiotics for secondary bacterial infection
Apply cool compresses; avoid local heat	Delayed secondary closure with skin graft	Antivenom (experimental)
	Gauze packing, if applicable	

lesion). The study suggests that the use of dapsone may eliminate the need for surgery following bites and that antivenom therapy was most effective clinically if the patient never developed the necrotic lesion. However, there is not enough information to recommend the use of dapsone in the management of *Loxosceles* envenomation at this time. Hepatitis, methemoglobinemia (Chap. 124), and hemolysis are associated with dapsone use.[189]

An underpowered animal study evaluated the effects on the size of skin lesions induced by *Loxosceles* envenomation by treatment with hyperbaric oxygen therapy, dapsone, and combined hyperbaric oxygen therapy and dapsone.[112] The study concluded that there was no clinically significant change in necrosis or induration by these treatment modalities. Further evaluation of these interventions remains appropriate. Another study using hyperbaric oxygen for treatment of *Loxosceles*-induced necrotic lesions in rabbits revealed no clinical improvement in the size of the lesion; however, the histology of the lesions improved. Whether this finding is of consequence is unknown.[112,217] There is currently not enough evidence to recommend hyperbaric oxygen therapy for *Loxosceles* envenomation. Although the use of colchicine, a leukocyte inhibitor, was previously recommended, we do not advocate this treatment because of potential colchicine toxicity.[193] Rabbit-derived intradermal α-anti-*Loxosceles* Fab (α-Loxd) fragments attenuated the dermatonecrotic inflammation of rabbits injected with *L. deserta* venom in a time-dependent fashion.[94] At time 0 after envenomation, no lesion developed was blocked. At time 1 and 4 hours after envenomation, the α-anti-Loxd Fab antivenom continued to suppress lesion development, although the longer the delay in treatment, the smaller the difference in treatment and control lesion areas. At time 8 and 12 hours post-envenomation, there was no difference in lesion size. The typical 24-hour delay in lesion development makes the diagnosis difficult, and the antivenom would likely be useless if administered late in the clinical course. The antivenom is not available for commercial use.

One preclinical study investigating treatment of *Loxosceles* envenomations used an antiloxoscelic serum that was produced from recombinant sphingomyelinase D that was derived from the sphingomyelinase of the *L. intermedia* and *L. laeta* spiders. The isolated sphingomyelinase from the respective *Loxosceles* species carried the full biological effects of the entire venom. This antiloxoscelic serum, when administered IV into rabbits that were given intradermal injections of the loxoscelic venom from *L. laeta* and *L. intermedia*, had greater neutralizing activity than when compared to the existing antiarachnid serum, which is made by hyperimmunizing horses against the venom of *L. gaucho*, *P. nigriventer*, and the scorpion *Tityus serrulatus*. In Brazil and South America, most of the envenomations occur with the *L. laeta* and *L. intermedia*, not *L. gaucho*. Knowing which species envenomated the patient could help determine which antiserum is indicated.[70]

Patients manifesting systemic loxoscelism or those with expanding necrotic lesions should be admitted to the hospital. All patients should be monitored for evidence of hemolysis, acute kidney injury, or coagulopathy. If hemoglobinuria ensues, increased IV fluids and urinary alkalinization can be used in an attempt to prevent acute kidney injury. Hemolysis, if significant, can be treated with transfusions. Patients with coagulopathy should be monitored with serial complete blood cell count, platelet count, PT, PTT, fibrin split products, and fibrinogen. Disseminated intravascular coagulopathy requires treatment, based on severity.

HOBO SPIDER (*ERATIGENA AGRESTIS*, NORTHWESTERN BROWN SPIDER, WALCKENAER SPIDER)

Formerly known as *Tegenaria agrestis*, the hobo spider is native to Europe and was introduced to the northwestern United States (Washington, Oregon, Idaho) in the 1920s or 1930s.[234] These spiders build funnel-shaped webs within wood piles, crawl spaces, basements, and moist areas close to the ground. They are brown with gray markings and 7 to 14 mm long. They are most abundant in the midsummer through the fall. They bite if provoked or threatened but otherwise retreat quickly when disturbed.[23] The literature is sparse in reported hobo spider bites that are verified by a specialist. There is only one confirmed hobo spider bite resulting in a necrotic lesion.[59]

A 42-year-old woman with a history of phlebitis who felt a burning sensation on her ankle rolled her pants and found a crushed brown spider, which was later confirmed to be *E. agrestis*.[52] She complained of persistent pain, nausea, and dizziness, and a vesicular lesion developed within several hours. The vesicle ruptured and ulcerated the next day. The lesion initially was 2 mm, but over the next 10 weeks enlarged to 30 mm in diameter and was circumscribed with a black lesion, at which time she sought medical advice. She was given a course of antibiotics, which did not limit the progression of this ulcer. Subsequently, the patient was unable to walk, and she was found to have a deep venous thrombosis. The other cases implicating Hobo spiders as a cause for dermatonecrotic injuries are based on proximity of the Hobo spider or other large brown spiders that are unidentified. *Eratigena agrestis* venom implanted into rabbit skin produces hemorrhagic dermatonecrotic lesions dermally and systemically.[234,235]

The venom from European Hobo spiders and US Hobo spiders was analyzed using liquid chromatography to address the question of variability between the 2 spiders. *Eratigena agrestis* originating from Europe is considered medically harmless. Liquid chromatography (European Hobo *E. agrestis* from the United Kingdom and American Hobo *E. agrestis* from Washington State, United States) found little variability between the 2 venoms to account for their differential necrotic effects.[28] The authors suggest 4 possibilities for the discrepancy between the European Hobo and American Hobo spiders: (1) an evolutionary change accounted for the novel necrotic effects; (2) venom chemistry is similar but the habitat might account for the difference in behavior; (3) venom chemistry and habitat are similar but an extrinsic factor such as a bacterium found in the US Hobo spider might be the cause for the necrotic effects; (4) *E. agrestis* do not directly or indirectly cause necrotic arachnidism and are incorrectly analyzed.[28] The authors suggest that either a bacterium such as *Mycobacterium ulcerans*, known to cause slow-developing ulcers on human skin, might coexist on the chelicerae of the *E. agrestis*, which is highly unlikely because of the presence of antibacterial peptides in the venom,[110,242] or the more likely circumstance that *E. agrestis* is incorrectly suggested as being a cause for necrotic arachnidism. Further evidence to suggest that the *E. agrestis* is not likely to be a culprit for necrotic arachnidism is based on a study that evaluates the possibility of the ability of the spider to carry and transfer pathogenic bacteria including the MRSA and analyzes the hemolytic properties of the venom.[88] More than 100 *E. agrestis* adult spiders were collected, and a bacterial diversity assay was conducted to find a total of 6 gram-positive and 4 gram-negative bacteria genera identified, which was consistent with the bacteria found in the fauna of the natural environment of the Pacific Northwest and several occurring on human and animal skin. Spiders were then exposed to MRSA on polyethylene disks because the tissue lesions caused by this bacterium is often confounded with a necrotic arachnidism. No MRSA was found on either the spiders or the surfaces to which the MRSA-exposed spiders were subjected, although the MRSA was found to persist on the polyethylene disks. Finally, the hobo spider venom was analyzed to determine its hemolytic activity in vertebrate blood. Compared to the known *Loxosceles reclusa* hemolytic activity of 37%, the potential of *E. agrestis* venom hemolytic activity was negligible at 0.62% and 0.93% for male (n = 5) and female (n = 7) spiders, respectively. Misdiagnosis of spider bites is common. Wounds can be misleading and can occur from the reaction of other organisms such as ticks and other arthropods, superinfection with anthrax or another organism or underlying medical conditions like diabetes and leukemia or bacterial infections. The need to revisit the hobo spider toxicity syndrome with further studies that show direct evidence of *E. agrestis* causing necrotic arachnidism in humans is warranted before it is concluded that any necrotic arachnidism in the Pacific Northwest is caused by *E. agrestis*.

Pathophysiology

The toxin was fractionated, with 3 peptides identified as having potent insecticidal activity and no discernible effects in mammalian in vivo assays.[131] The peptide toxins TaITX-1, TaITX-2, and TaITX-3 exhibit potent insecticidal properties by acting directly in the insect central nervous system and not at the neuromuscular junction.[131] Insects envenomated with *E. agrestis* venom and the insecticidal toxins purified from the venom developed a slowly evolving spastic paralysis. Currently, little is known about the toxin and its mechanism of action in humans.

Clinical Manifestations

The toxicity of hobo spider venom is questionable; however, it occasionally causes dermatonecrosis secondary to infection. Other causes of dermatonecrotic lesions should be excluded. The most common symptom associated with the spider bite is a headache that persists for up to one week.[59] Other manifestations including nausea, vomiting, fatigue, memory loss, visual impairment, weakness, and lethargy, are reported.[59,235]

Diagnostic Testing

No specific laboratory assay confirms envenomation with *E. agrestis* spider.

Treatment

Treatment emphasizes local wound care and tetanus prophylaxis, although systemic corticosteroids are reasonable for hematologic complications. Surgical graft repair for severe ulcerative lesions is warranted when there is no additional progression of necrosis.[59]

TARANTULAS

Tarantulas are primitive mygalomorph spiders that belong to the family Theraphosidae, a subgroup of Mygalomorphae (Greek word *mygale* for field mouse).[54,201] There are more than 1,500 species, with 54 species found in the deserts of the western United States.[177] Because of their great size and reputation, tarantulas are often feared. They are the largest and hairiest spiders, popular as pets, and are found throughout the United States as well as in tropical and subtropical areas (Fig. 115–4). The life span of the female can exceed 15 to 20 years. They have poor eyesight and usually detect their victims by touch and vibrations. Their defense lies in either their painful bite with erect fangs or by barraging their victim with urticating hairs that are released on provocation.[54] Only the New World tarantulas (tarantulas indigenous to the Americas) have and use the urticating hairs to defend themselves.[54]

Tarantulas bite when provoked or roughly handled. Based on the few case reports, their venom has relatively minor effects in humans but can be deadly for canines and other small animals, such as rats, mice, cats, and birds.[38,128] Small prey might actually be killed by the physical nature of having fangs impaled many times through their bodies. A study from Australia covering

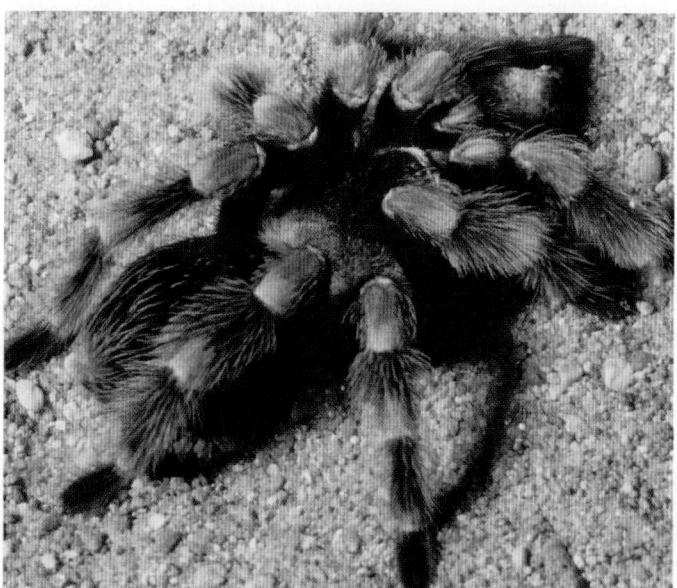

FIGURE 115–4. The Mexican redknee tarantula, *Brachypelma smithi. (Used with permission from the American Museum of Natural History.)*

a 25-year span reported only 9 confirmed bites by Theraphosid spiders in humans and 7 confirmed bites in canines—in 2 cases, the owner was bitten after the dog.[19,128] At least 4 genera of tarantulas (*Lasiodora*, *Grammostola*, *Acanthoscurria*, and *Brachypelma*) possess urticating hairs that are released in self-defense when the tarantulas rub their hind legs against their abdomen rapidly to create a small cloud.[93] There are 6 different types of urticating hairs. Type 1 hairs are found on tarantulas in the United States and are the only hairs that do not penetrate human skin. Type 2 hairs are incorporated into the silk web retreat but are not thrown off by the spider. Type 3 hairs can penetrate up to 2 mm into human skin. Type 4 hairs belong to the South American *Grammostola* spider and can cause severe respiratory inflammation. Urticarial hairs or setae are composed of chitin, lipoproteins, and mucopolysaccharides, which are recognized as foreign bodies triggering a humoral response in the mammalian immune system. Chitin is proinflammatory and activates T helper cells to stimulate activated macrophages to produce chitanases, which will break down the chitin but also trigger inflammation. Besides cell-mediated inflammation, spider setae also trigger IgE-mediated hypersensitivity.[19,51]

Pathophysiology

Tarantula venom, specifically the venoms of *Aphonopelma hentzi* (synonym of *Dugesiella hentzi* {Arkansas tarantula}) and other members of the genus *Aphonopelma* (Arizona or Texas brown tarantula), contains hyaluronidase, nucleotides (adenosine triphosphate {ATP}, adenosine diphosphate {ADP}, and adenosine monophosphate {AMP}), and polyamines (spermine, spermidine, putrescine, and cadaverine) that are essential to prey.[43,136,201] The role of spermine is unclear, but hyaluronidase is a spreading factor that allows more rapid entrance of venom toxin by destruction of connective tissue and intercellular matrix. Adenosine triphosphate potentiates death in mice exposed to the *A. hentzi* venom and lowers the LD_{50} in comparison to venom without ATP.[52,152] Both venoms cause skeletal muscle necrosis when injected intraperitoneally in mice.[87] The primary injury results in rupture of the plasma membrane, followed by the inability of mitochondria and sarcoplasmic reticulum to maintain normal concentrations of calcium in the cytoplasm leading to cell death. *Aphonopelma* venom is similar to scorpion venom in composition and clinical effects. Novel xenobiotics were discovered in the venom that can act on potassium channels, calcium channels, and the acid-sensing ion channels that elucidate the molecular mechanism of voltage-dependent channel gating and their respective physiologic roles.[79,80]

Clinical Manifestations

Although relatively infrequent in occurrence, bites present with puncture or fang marks. They range from being painless to a deep throbbing pain that are reported to last several hours without any inflammatory component.[128] Fever occurs in the absence of infection, suggesting a direct pyrexic action of the venom. Rarely, bites create a local histamine response with resultant itching, and hypersensitive individuals can have more severe reactions and, less commonly, mild systemic effects such as nausea and vomiting.[93,128] Contact reactions from the urticating hairs are more likely to be the health hazard than the spider bite. The urticating hairs provoke local histamine reactions in humans and are especially irritating to the eyes, skin, and respiratory tract. Tarantula urticating hairs cause intense inflammation that often remain pruritic for weeks. An allergic rhinitis is known to develop if the hairs are inhaled.[136] Tarantula hairs resemble sensory setae of caterpillars: both are type 3 hairs that can migrate relentlessly and cause multiple foci of ophthalmic inflammation.[118] *Ophthalmia nodosa*, a granulomatous nodular reaction to vegetable or insect hairs, is reported with casual handling of tarantulas.[22,26] Other ophthalmic findings include setae in the corneal stroma, anterior chamber inflammation, migration into the retina, and secondary glaucoma and cataracts.[31]

Treatment

Treatment is largely supportive. Cool compresses and analgesics should be given as needed. All bites should receive local wound care, including tetanus prophylaxis if necessary. If the hairs are barbed, as in some species, they can be removed by using adhesive such as duct tape or cellophane tape followed by compresses or irrigation with 0.9% sodium chloride solution. If the hairs are located in the eye, then surgical removal will be required, followed by medical management of inflammation. If the hairs are difficult to remove and the patient has persistent ophthalmic pain and discomfort, then a therapeutic pars plana vitrectomy is necessary to reduce the antigenic load and to improve clinical symptomatology.[115] Urticarial reactions should be treated with oral antihistamines and topical or systemic corticosteroids.

FUNNEL WEB SPIDERS

Australian funnel web spiders are a group of large Hexathelidae mygalomorphs that cause a severe neurotoxic envenomation syndrome in humans. The fang positions of funnel web spiders (as well as the tarantulas) are vertical relative to their body, which requires the spider to rear back and lift the body to attack. The length of fangs reach up to 5 mm. This spider bites tenaciously and occasionally requires extraction from the victim.[161] *Atrax* and *Hadronyche* species are found along the eastern seaboard of Australia. *Atrax robustus*, also called the Sydney funnel web spider, is the best known and is located around the center of Sydney, Australia.[161] Funnel web spiders tend to prefer moist, temperate environments.[161] They are primarily ground dwellers and live in burrows, crevices in rocks, and around foundations of houses. They build tubular or funnel-shaped webs.[93] At night, the spiders ascend the tubular web and wait for their prey. The Sydney funnel web spider is considered one of the most poisonous spiders. It was responsible for 14 deaths between 1927 and 1980, at which time an antivenom was introduced.[221,222]

Pathophysiology

Originally called robustoxin from *A. robustus* spider and versutoxin from the *Hadronyche versuta* spider, the toxin which is now referred to as atracotoxin or atraxin (δ-ACTX-Arl and δ-ACTX-Hvla, respectively) is the lethal protein component of *A. robustus* venom and is unique in its toxicity affecting primates and newborn mice, although other mammals are susceptible in higher doses.[161,220,222,239] Atracotoxin is a 42–amino acid peptide that targets mammals by increasing the ion conductance at voltage-gated sodium channels via trapping the voltage sensor domain IV S4 segment of the channel in an inward conformational change, preventing the closure of the ion channel, thereby evoking a fulminant neurotransmitter release at the autonomic and/or somatic synapses.[148,170] Hence δ-ACTX produces an autonomic storm, releasing acetylcholine, noradrenaline, and adrenaline. In monkeys, a 5 mcg/kg intravenous infusion dose of robustotoxin from male *A. robustus* spiders causes dyspnea, blood pressure fluctuations leading to severe hypotension, lacrimation, salivation, skeletal muscle fasciculation, and death within 3 to 4 hours.[167] Versutoxin, a toxin from the Blue Mountain funnel web spider, is closely related to robustotoxin and has demonstrated voltage-dependent slowing of sodium channel inactivation.[171]

Clinical Manifestations

A biphasic envenomation syndrome is described in humans and monkeys.[221,222] Phase 1 consists of localized pain at the bite site, perioral tingling, piloerection, and regional fasciculations (most prominent in the face, tongue, and intercostal muscles). Fasciculations progress to more overt muscle spasm; masseter and laryngeal involvement may threaten the airway.[220] Other features include tachycardia, hypertension, cardiac dysrhythmias, nausea, vomiting, abdominal pain, diaphoresis, lacrimation, salivation, and acute respiratory distress syndrome (ARDS), which often is the cause of death in phase 1.[239] Phase 2 consists of resolution of the overt cholinergic and adrenergic crisis; secretions dry up, and fasciculations, spasms, and hypertension resolve. This apparent improvement is occasionally followed by the gradual onset of refractory hypotension, apnea, and cardiac arrest.[222]

Treatment

Pressure immobilization using crepe bandage to limit lymphatic flow and immobilization of the bitten extremity is reported to inactivate the venom and is recommended to be applied if symptoms of envenomation are present. Funnel web venom is one of the few animal toxins known to undergo local inactivation. Monkey studies and a human case report support the utility of

pressure immobilization.[98,223] After injecting *A. robustus* venom subcutaneously in monkeys, pressure-immobilization technique increased survival by retarding the venom movement and also by allowing the local peripheral enzymes inactivating the venom.[221,223]

The patient should be transferred to the nearest hospital with the bandage in place and then stabilized and placed in a resuscitation facility with adequate ampules of antivenom readily available before the bandage is removed; otherwise, a precipitous envenomation will potentially occur during the removal of the pressure bandage. A purified IgG antivenom protective against *Atrax* envenomations was developed in rabbits.[221] One ampule of the antivenom contains 100 mg purified rabbit IgG or 125 units of neutralizing capacity per ampule.[239] It is shown to be effective for more than 40 humans bitten by the *Atrax* species.[223] The starting dose is 2 ampules if systemic signs of envenomations are present, and 4 ampules if the patient develops ARDS or decreased mental status. Doses are repeated every 15 minutes until clinical improvement occurs.[239] Up to 8 ampules is common in a severe envenomation. However, a recent study of 9 funnel web spider envenomations utilized a venom-specific enzyme immunoassay to measure venom concentrations in the serum before and after administration of antivenom. The results indicated that the starting dose of 2 ampules is sufficient to bind all free venom, but the envenomation may have irreversible effects such as myocarditis and ARDS.[158] Since anaphylaxis is not reported,[223] the manufacturer no longer recommends premedication. Serum sickness is rare after funnel web antivenom administration, with only one reported case in a patient who received 5 ampules of antivenom.[160]

SCORPIONS

Scorpions are invertebrate arthropods that have existed for more than 400 million years.[58] Of the 650 known living species, most of the lethal species are in the family Buthidae (Table 115–5). The genera of the family Buthidae include *Centruroides*, *Tityus*, *Leiurus*, *Androctonus*, *Buthus*, and *Parabuthus*.[58] Scorpions envenomate humans by stinging rather than biting. Their 5-segmented metasoma ("tail") contains a terminal bulbous segment called the *telson* that contains the venom apparatus (Fig. 115–5). More than 100,000 medically significant stings likely occur annually worldwide, predominantly in the tropics and North Africa.[1,25,70,103,129,141] According to American Association of Poison Control Centers data from 1995 to 2015, approximately 11,000 to 19,000 scorpion annual exposures occurred in the United States, mostly in the southwestern region. Only one death was reported during this period, involving a 3-year-old boy who expired despite receiving antivenom (Chap. 130). These members of the class Arachnida rarely cause mortality in victims older than 6 years.[188] The venomous scorpions in the United States are *Centruroides exilicauda* and *Centruroides vittatus*. The most important is *C. exilicauda*, previously called *Centruroides sculpturatus* Ewing and *Centruroides gertschii* (bark scorpion; Table 115–6).[83]

Pathophysiology

Components of scorpion venom are complex and species specific.[106,180,188,189] Buthidae venom is thermostable and consists of phospholipase, acetylcholinesterase, hyaluronidase, serotonin, and neurotoxins. Four neurotoxins,

TABLE 115–5	Scorpions of Toxicologic Importance[75,88]
Australia: *Lychas marmoreus, Lychas* spp, *Isometrus* spp, *Cercophonius squama, Urodacus* spp	
India: *Buthus tamulus*	
Mexico: *Centruroides* spp	
Middle East: *Androctonus crassicauda, Androctonus Australis, Buthus minax, Androctonus Australis, Buthus occitanus, Leiurus quinquestriatus*	
Spain: *Buthus occitanus*	
South Africa: *Androctonus crassicauda*	
South America: *Tityus serrulatus*	
United States: *Centruroides exilicauda*	

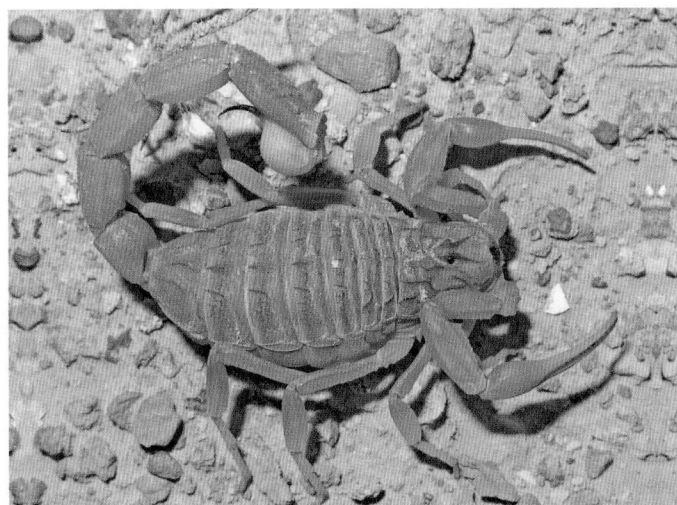

FIGURE 115–5. The Brazilian scorpion, *Tityus serrulatus*, shown here to demonstrate the typical features of scorpions. Note the telson (stinger) located on the tail. *(Used with permission from Dr. Michael Seiter, University of Vienna, Austria.)*

designated toxins I to IV, were isolated from *C. exilicauda*. Some of the toxins target excitable membranes,[67,82,104,156,198] especially at the neuromuscular junction, by opening sodium channels. The results are repetitive depolarization of nerves in both sympathetic and parasympathetic nervous systems causing catecholamine and acetylcholine release, respectively, and associated cardiac ischemia, and action at the juxtaglomerular apparatus, causing increased renin secretion.[64,188] The clinical effects of *Tityus* scorpion sting are related to elevated concentrations of interleukin (IL)-1β, IL-6, IL-8, IL-10, kinins,[86] and tumor necrosis factor (TNF)-α, which correlate with the severity of envenomation and hyperamylasemia.[63,87]

Clinical Manifestations

Scorpion stings produce a local reaction consisting of intense pain, erythema, tingling or burning, and occasionally discoloration and necrosis without tissue sloughing (Table 115–6). Envenomation from some scorpion species produces systemic effects that include autonomic storm consisting of cholinergic and adrenergic effects. Cardiotoxic effects include myocarditis, dysrhythmias, and myocardial infarction.[67,82,104,156,198] Electrocardiographic

(ECG) abnormalities are reported to persist for several days and include sinus tachycardia, sinus bradycardia, bizarre broad-notched biphasic T-wave changes with additional ST segment elevation or depression in the limb and precordial leads, appearance of tiny Q waves in the limb leads consistent with an acute myocardial infarction pattern, occasional electrical alternans, and prolonged QT interval.[104,106] Other reported effects include pancreatitis, coagulation disorders, ARDS, massive hemoptysis, cerebral infarctions in children, seizures, and a shock syndrome that occasionally precedes but usually follows the hypertensive phase.[24,73,82,104,105,198,210]

A 3-category classification system for scorpion envenomations worldwide was proposed. Category 1 is "mild" and involves local manifestations such as erythema, edema, sweating, numbness, and fasciculations. Category 2 is "moderate" and involves abdominal pain, vomiting, generalized diaphoresis, tachypnea, tachycardia or bradycardia, hypertension, agitation, hypersalivation, dysphagia, fever, and/or hyperglycemia. Category 3 is "severe" and indicates patients who present with cardiovascular complications such as congestive heart failure, dilated cardiomyopathy, cardiogenic shock, dysrhythmias, or severe hypertension. Severe envenomation also includes pulmonary manifestations such as pulmonary edema and ARDS; gastrointestinal findings such as acute pancreatitis or peptic ulceration; as well as neurologic manifestations such as hypertensive encephalopathy, coma, or seizures. The presence of diarrhea is associated with increased incidence of respiratory failure, neurologic failure, liver failure, and death.[200]

In the United States, *C. exilicauda* stings produce local paresthesias and pain that is accentuated by tapping over the envenomated area (tap test) without local skin evidence of envenomation.[58,188] Symptoms begin immediately after envenomation, progress to maximum severity in 5 hours, and may persist for up to 30 hours.[58,188] Autonomic findings include hypertension, tachycardia, diaphoresis, emesis, and bronchoconstriction. The somatic motor effects reported include ataxia, muscular fasciculations, restlessness, thrashing, and opsoclonus.[64,180]

Treatment

Because most envenomations do not produce severe effects, local wound care, including tetanus prophylaxis and pain management, usually is all that is warranted. In young children or patients who manifest severe toxicity, hospitalization is recommended. Treatment emphasizes support of the airway, breathing, and circulation. However, children rarely require respiratory support.[180] Corticosteroids, antihistamines, and calcium have been administered without any known benefit.[63] Continuous intravenous midazolam infusion is often used for *C. exilicauda* scorpion envenomation until resolution of the abnormal motor activity and agitation occurs.[91]

The clinical severity dictates the need to use antivenom for grade III and grade IV envenomations (Table 115–6).[63] When an equine-derived F(ab')$_2$ product called Alacramyn, developed in Mexico against the *Centruroides limpidus* venom, was administered to critically ill US children with neurotoxicity from scorpion stings, there was a rapid resolution of toxicity, decreased need for sedation, and reduced concentrations of circulating unbound venom.[34] This antivenom was subsequently approved in the United States in 2011 and called Anascorp (Bioclon, Mexico)[70] (Antidotes in Depth: A38). Because the neurotoxic syndrome occurs almost exclusively in children younger than 10 years, antivenom use is most likely to be considered in children. However, intractable pain in adults not responding to reasonable doses of opioids or other systemic effects that pose a danger to the patient or a fetus are reasonable indications for antivenom therapy.

Atropine has been used to reverse the excessive oral secretions in *C. exilicauda* scorpion envenomation, with some success in healthy children.[219] Routine use is not recommended and should be limited to species such as *Parabuthus transvaalicus* in southern Africa,[219] whose envenomations cause a prominent cholinergic crisis. Potentiation of the adrenergic effects causing cardiopulmonary toxicity is reported.[21] Atropine use to reverse the effects of stings from scorpions from India, South America, the Middle East, and Asia is contraindicated because these scorpions cause an "autonomic storm" with transient cholinergic stimulation followed by sustained adrenergic hyperactivity.[20,219]

TABLE 115–6	Envenomation Gradation for *Centruroides exilicauda* (Bark Scorpion)[63]
Grade	**Signs and Symptoms**
I	Site of envenomation
	Pain and/or paresthesias
	Positive tap test (severe pain increases with touch or percussion)
II	Grade I in addition to
	Pain and paresthesias remote from sting site (eg, paresthesias moving up an extremity, perioral "numbness")
III	One of the following:
	Somatic skeletal neuromuscular dysfunction: jerking of extremity(ies), restlessness, severe involuntary shaking and jerking, which may be mistaken for seizures
	Cranial nerve dysfunction: blurred vision, roving eye movements (opsoclonus) hypersalivation, dysphagia, tongue fasciculation, upper airway dysfunction, slurred speech
IV	Both cranial nerve dysfunction and somatic skeletal neuromuscular dysfunction

TICKS

In 1912, Todd described a progressive ascending flaccid paralysis after bites from ticks.[230] Three families of ticks are recognized: (1) Ixodidae (hard ticks), (2) Argasidae (soft ticks), and (3) Nuttalliellidae (a group that has characteristics of both hard and soft ticks and not thought to be parasitic compared to ixodids and argasids). The terms *hard* and *soft* refer to a dorsal scutum or "plate" that is present in the Ixodidae but absent in the Argasidae. Both types are characteristically soft and leathery, and both have clinical importance. Ixodidae females are capable of enormous expansion up to 50 times their weight in fluid and blood.[90] The paralytic syndrome is induced following envenomation during the larva, nymph, and adult stages and is related to the tick obtaining a blood meal. The following discussion focuses only on tick paralysis (TP) or tick toxicosis and not on any of the infectious diseases associated with tick bites. Most of the major tick-borne diseases in North America are transmitted by Ixodid ticks except for relapsing fever, which is spread by the soft tick of the genus *Ornithodorus* or *Pediculus humanus* (human louse).

In North America, *Dermacentor andersoni* (Rocky Mountain wood tick), *Dermacentor variabilis* (American dog tick), and *Amblyomma americanum* (Lone Star tick) are the most commonly implicated causes of TP.[96,230] Typically, tick toxicosis occurs in the Southeast, Rocky Mountain, and Pacific Northwest regions of the United States, but cases are also reported in the Northeast.[69] In Australia, the *Ixodes holocyclus* or Australian marsupial tick is the most common offender.[96,230] *Ixodes holocyclus* is the most potent of the paralyzing ticks in the world and is known to paralyze dogs, cats, sheep, mice, foals, pigs, chickens, and humans.[151]

Pathophysiology

Venom secreted from the salivary glands during the blood meal is absorbed by the host and systemically distributed. To allow successful feeding over several days, ticks need to overcome the host's hemostatic, inflammatory, and immune mechanisms by producing anticoagulants, fibrinolytic enzymes, antiplatelet, and vasodilator substances.[137,187] The saliva also contains some cement to anchor the tick to the host; however, the hypostome of the *I. holocyclus* reaches up to 980 microns into the host's skin and does not need cement support.[6] Paralysis results from the neurotoxin "ixobotoxin,"[165] which inhibits the release of acetylcholine at the neuromuscular junction and autonomic ganglia, very similar to botulinum toxin.[99,165] Both botulinum toxin and ixobotoxin demonstrate temperature dependence in rat models and show increased muscular twitching activity as the temperature is reduced.[60,151] The salivary toxin of *I. holocyclus* directly affects vascular and cardiac potassium channels by blockade, and this action differed from the respiratory distress caused by progressive muscle paralysis.[11] Cardiovascular function is decreased in dogs with TP. The dogs developed acute left-sided congestive heart failure and prolonged QT intervals.[47]

Clinical Manifestations

Usually the tick must remain on the person for 5 to 6 days in order to result in systemic effects. Several days must pass before tick salivary glands begin to secrete significant quantities of toxin. Once secreted, the toxin does not act immediately and undergoes binding and internalization, in a similar sequence to botulinum toxin.[18,60,133] Ticks typically attach to the scalp but are found on any part of the body, including the ear canals and anus. Children, particularly girls, and adult men in tick-infested areas are predominantly affected. One large series of 305 cases in Canada reported that 21% were adults older than 16 years.[205] Among the children, 67% were girls; in adults, 83% were male. The distribution was attributed to the difficulty of detecting ticks in long hair and the possible greater exposure of adult men to tick-infested environments. Children are reported to appear listless, weak, ataxic, and irritable for several days before they develop an ascending paralysis that begins in the lower limbs. Fever usually is absent. Other manifestations include sensory symptoms such as paresthesias, numbness, and mild diarrhea. These symptoms are followed by absent or decreased deep-tendon reflexes and an ascending generalized weakness that can progress to bulbar structures involving speech, swallowing, and facial expression within 24 to 48 hours, as well as fixed, dilated pupils and disturbances of extraocular movements.[99,205] Other atypical presentations are reported and include the following: a child presenting with double vision and being unable to see before the neuromuscular changes occurred, and a healthy elderly man presenting with unilateral weakness and numbness in the left arm for 2 days. Both patients fully recovered after the removal of the tick.[69] If the tick is not removed, respiratory weakness is reported to lead to hypoventilation, lethargy, coma, and death. Unlike the *Dermacentor* spp of North America, removal of the *I. holocyclus* tick does not result in dramatic improvement for several days to weeks. The maximal weakness is often not reached until 48 hours after the tick has been removed or drops off.[99] It is imperative to closely observe patients for possible deterioration. A recent 60-year meta-analysis of TP in the United States reviewed 50 well-documented cases from 1946 to 2006 supporting the above findings.[75] The demographics were analyzed and the following remained the same: (1) TP is a highly predictable regional disease found in the US Pacific Northwest (WA), the West (CA, CO), and the Southeast (GA, MS, NC, SC, VA), and very few cases occurred outside those areas; (2) TP remains a highly predictable seasonal disease occurring during the spring to summer seasons; (3) TP remains more common in females of all ages (80% female/male 4.9:1); (4) Tick attachment sites on the head and scalp continued to predominate over all other attachment sites, representing 48% of the reported attachment sites, 20% occur behind the ear; (5) The Rocky Mountain wood tick (*D. andersoni*) was the only TP vector in the western United States (CA, WA, CO) when reported, and *D. variabilis*, the American dog tick, was the only TP vector from the southeastern United States (GA, NC) when reported.

The differential diagnosis is extensive and includes Guillain-Barré syndrome (GBS), the Miller-Fisher variant of Guillain-Barré, poliomyelitis, botulism, transverse myelitis, myasthenia gravis, periodic paralysis, elapid snakebites, marine neurotoxin poisoning, acute cerebellar ataxia, and spinal cord lesions (Chap. 38). The cerebrospinal fluid remains normal, and the rate of progression is rapid, unlike GBS and poliomyelitis.[75,81,202] The edrophonium test to assess for myasthenia gravis is negative. Nerve conduction studies in patients with TP frequently resemble those of patients with early stages of GBS: findings in both conditions include prolonged latency of the distal motor nerves, diminished nerve conduction velocity, and reduction in the amplitudes of muscle and sensory-nerve action potentials.[81] With GBS, there is a prolongation of the F wave, however, that does not occur with TP, reflecting the more proximal demyelination of the nerve root.[101] The other causes for acute ascending flaccid paralysis should be eliminated by a complete history, including environmental exposure, hobbies, workplace, travel, ingestions, obtaining appropriate laboratory testing, psychiatric evaluations if needed, and of course a thorough physical examination.

Treatment

Other than removal of the entire tick, which is curative, treatment is entirely supportive. Proper removal of the tick is very important, otherwise infection or incomplete tick removal are able to occur. The tick should be grasped as close to the skin surface as possible with blunt curved forceps, tweezers, or gloved hands. Steady pressure without crushing the body should be used; otherwise, expressed fluid is reported to infect the patient and lead to inoculating the patient with a higher dose of toxin or infectious agent. After tick removal, the site should be disinfected. Traditional methods of tick removal using petroleum jelly, topical lidocaine, fingernail polish, isopropyl alcohol, or a hot match head are ineffective and often induces the tick to salivate or regurgitate into the wound.[168] It should be remembered that the very same vectors responsible for tick toxicosis also cause infectious illnesses such as babesiosis, Rocky Mountain spotted fever, anaplasmosis, ehrlichiosis, tularemia, Colorado tick fever, tick-borne relapsing fever, and Lyme disease. Since *I. holocyclus* of Australia is considerably more toxic and patients are more likely to deteriorate before they improve, close observation is required for several days until improvement is certain.[81]

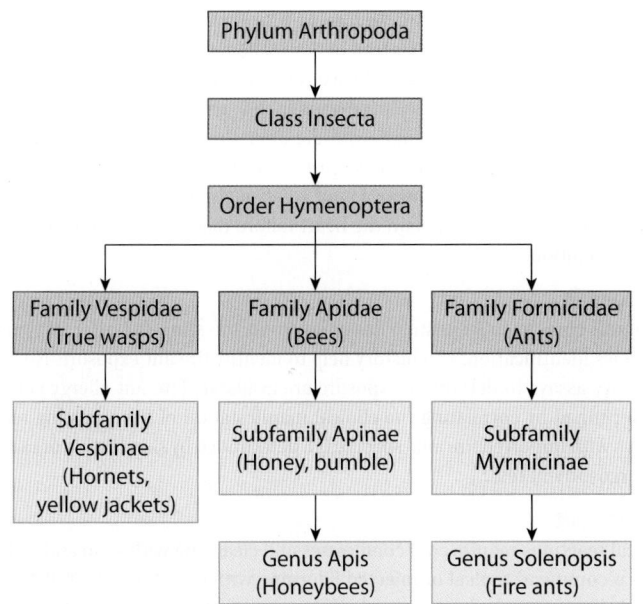

FIGURE 115–6. Taxonomy of the order Hymenoptera.

TABLE 115–7	Composition of Hymenoptera Venom	
Vespid (Wasps, Hornets, Yellow Jackets)	**Apids (Honeybees)**	**Formicids (Fire Ants)**
Biogenic amines (diverse)	Biogenic amines (diverse)	Biogenic amines (diverse)
Phospholipase A phospholipase B	Phospholipase A phospholipase B (?)	Phospholipase A_2
Hyaluronidase	Hyaluronidase	Hyaluronidase
Acid phosphatase	Acid phosphatase	Piperidines
Mast cell–degranulating peptide	Minimine	
Kinin	Mellitin	
	Apamin	
	Mast cell–degranulating peptide	

HYMENOPTERA: BEES, WASPS, HORNETS, YELLOW JACKETS, AND ANTS

Within the order Hymenoptera are 3 families of clinical significance: Apidae (honeybees and bumblebees), Vespidae (yellow jackets, hornets, and wasps), and Formicidae (ants, specifically fire ants). These insects (Fig. 115–6) are of great medical importance because their stings are the most commonly reported and can cause acute toxic and fatal allergic reactions. In the 1960s and 1970s, an estimated 40 deaths per year were attributed to anaphylaxis secondary to Hymenoptera stings in the United States.[17,209] However, from 2008 to 2015 there have been only 6 deaths related to envenomations from bees, wasps, and hornets reported to the National Poison Data System, probably due to increased public awareness of allergic reactions and easier access to medical care (Chap. 130).

Apis and *Bombus* species (honeybees and bumblebees) generally build nests away from humans and are passive unless disturbed, but nests of both the honeybees and bumblebees are also found in walls and rodent burrows near homes. Honeybee workers only sting once because their stinger is a modified ovipositor that resides in the abdomen and its shaft is barbed and has a venom sac attached. Once the stinger embeds into the skin, the stinger disembowels the bee. Bumblebees, however, can sting multiple times. Vespids, on the other hand, are more aggressive and build nests in human living areas, such as in trees and under awnings; yellow jackets inhabit shrubs, trees, and the ground. They, too, are able to sting multiple times.[93] The introduction of the Africanized honeybee in Brazil (because originally they were thought to be a more efficient honey producer) has caused significant economic and health issues. The bees have migrated toward the southern border of the United States and pose a greater threat to humans. Africanized honeybees are characterized by large populations, can make nonstop flights of at least 20 km, and have a tendency toward mass attack with little provocation.[162]

Pathophysiology

Several allergens (Table 115–7) and pharmacologically active compounds are found in honeybee venom. The 3 major venom proteins are found in the honeybee: melittin, phospholipase A_2, and hyaluronidase.[146] Other proteins include apamin, acid phosphatase, and other unidentified proteins. Phospholipase A_2 is the major antigen/allergen in bee venom.[32]

Melittin is the principal component of honeybee venom. It acts as a detergent to disrupt the cell membrane and liberate potassium and biogenic amines.[14] Histamine release by bee venom is largely mediated by mast cell

degranulation peptide. Apamin is a neurotoxin that acts on the spinal cord. Apamin binds to the Ca^{+2}-triggered K^+ channel and depresses delayed hyperpolarization to cause its toxicity, which is seen in the mouse model as uncoordinated movements leading to spasms, jerks, and convulsions of a spinal origin.[109] Adolapin inhibits prostaglandin synthase and has antiinflammatory properties that account for its use in arthritic therapy.[207] Phospholipase A_2 and hyaluronidase are the chief enzymes in bee venom.

The 3 major proteins in vespid venoms serve as allergens and are accompanied by a wide array of vasoactive peptides and amines.[146] The intense pain following vespid stings is largely caused by serotonin, acetylcholine, and wasp kinins. Antigen 5 is the major allergen in vespid venom.[163] Its biologic function is unknown. Mastoparans have action similar to mast cell degranulation peptide, but weaker.[14] Phospholipase A_2 is thought to be responsible for inducing coagulation abnormalities.[174]

Clinical Manifestations

Normally, the honeybee sting results in immediate pain, a wheal-and-flare reaction, and localized edema without a systemic reaction. Vomiting, diarrhea, and syncope occur with a higher dose of venom resulting from multiple stings.[35] Rarely, a sting in the oropharynx produces airway compromise.[209]

Toxic reactions occur with multiple stings (more than 500 stings are described as possibly fatal and occur with Africanized honeybees)[93] and include gastrointestinal (GI) effects, headache, fever, syncope and, rarely, rhabdomyolysis, acute kidney injury, and seizures.[35] Other rare complications include idiopathic intracranial hypertension,[227] cerebral infarction, and ischemic optic neuropathy[204] and parkinsonism[145] and are thought to occur because of the proximity of the sting near the head and neck. Bronchospasm and urticaria are typically absent.

This type of toxic reaction differs from the hypersensitivity reactions or anaphylactic reactions because it is not an IgE-mediated response, but rather a direct effect from the venom itself. Hypersensitivity reactions, including anaphylaxis, occur from Hymenoptera stings. These reactions are IgE mediated. The IgE antibodies attach to tissue mast cells and basophils in individuals who were previously sensitized to the venom. These cells are activated, allowing for progression of the cascade reaction of increased vasoactive substances, such as leukotrienes, eosinophil chemotactic factor-A, and histamine. An anaphylactic reaction is not dependent on the number of stings. Patients who are allergic to Hymenoptera venom develop a wheal-and-flare reaction at the site of the inoculum. The shorter the interval between the sting and symptom onset, the more likely the reaction will be severe. Fatalities can occur within several minutes; even initially mild symptoms are reported to be followed by a fulminant course. Generalized urticaria, throat and chest tightness, stridor, fever, chills, and cardiovascular collapse ensue.

Treatment

Application of ice at the site usually is sufficient to halt discomfort. Stingers from honeybees should be removed by scraping with a credit card or scalpel, as opposed to pulling, which potentially releases additional retained venom. Since the stinger in other bee species typically stays within the insect, this removal technique will not be necessary if other bee species are involved. Therapy is aimed at supportive care that includes standard therapy for anaphylaxis with epinephrine, diphenhydramine, and corticosteroids.

FIRE ANTS

There are native fire ants in the United States, but the imported fire ants *Solenopsis invicta* and *Solenopsis richteri* are significant pests that have no natural enemies. They are native to Brazil, Paraguay, Uruguay, and Argentina but were introduced into Alabama in the 1930s. They have spread rapidly throughout the southern United States, damaging crops, reducing biologic diversity, and inflicting severe stings to humans.[225] *Solenopsis invicta*, the most aggressive species, now infests 13 southern states and was introduced into Australia.[211,214] Allergic reactions to ant stings were limited to the jumper ant (*Myrmecia pilosula*, other *Myrmecia* spp) and the greenhead ant (*Rhytidoponera metallica*; *Odontomachus*, *Cerapachys*, and *Brachyponera* spp) in Australia until February 2001, when the imported red fire ant was identified at 2 sites in Brisbane.[211] The mode of introduction is unknown but are postulated to have originated from the transport of infested cargo. Fire ants range from 2 to 6 mm in size. They live in grassy areas, garden sites, and near sources of water. The nests are largely subterranean and have large, conspicuous, dome-shaped above-ground mounds (up to 45 cm above the ground), with many openings for traffic. The mounds can contain 80,000 to 250,000 workers and one or more queens that live for 2 to 6 years and produce 1,500 eggs daily.[236] Fire ants are named for the burning pain inflicted after exposure, and necrosis can result at the site. The imported fire ant attacks with little warning. By firmly grasping the skin with their mandibles, both the fire ant and the jumper ant can repeatedly inject venom from a retractile stinger at the end of the abdomen. Pivoting at the head, the fire ant injects an average of 7 or 8 stings in a circular pattern.[214]

Pathophysiology

The venom inhibits Na^+, K^+-ATPases, reduces mitochondrial respiration, uncouples oxidative phosphorylation, adversely affects neutrophil and platelet function, inhibits nitric oxide synthetase, and perhaps activates coagulation.[130,132] Unlike the venoms of wasps, bees, and hornets that contain mostly aqueous-containing proteins, the imported fire ant venom is 95% alkaloid, with a small aqueous fraction that contains soluble proteins.[149] Of the alkaloids, 99% is a 2,6-disubstituted piperidine that has hemolytic, antibacterial, insecticidal, and cytoxic properties.[71] There is also some *in vivo* evidence that the Solenopsin alkaloids inhibit nitric oxide synthetase activity and have direct cardiotoxic, convulsant, and respiratory depressant activities.[120,244] These alkaloids do not cause allergic reactions, but they produce a pustule and pain. The aqueous portion of the venom contains the allergenic activity of fire ant venom, Sol i I to IV.[113,214] The proteins identified in the venom include a phospholipase, a hyaluronidase, and the enzyme N-acetyl-β-glucosaminidase.[72,214]

Clinical Manifestations

In the United States, residents of health care facilities who are immobile or cognitively impaired are at risk for fire ant attacks, especially when the facility lacks pest control techniques for fire ants.[72] Three categories are suggested based on the reactions to the imported fire ant: local, large local, and systemic.[214] *Local reactions* occur in nonallergic individuals. *Large local reactions* are defined as painful, pruritic swelling at least 5 cm in diameter and contiguous with the sting site. *Systemic reactions* involve signs and symptoms remote from the sting site. The sting initially forms a wheal that is described as a burning itch at the site, followed by the development of sterile pustules. In 24 hours, the pustules umbilicate on an erythematous base. Pustules are reported to last 1 to 2 weeks.[93] Late cutaneous allergic reactions occur in some persons who experience indurated pruritic lumps at the site of subsequent stings.[71] Large reactions lead to tissue edema sufficient to compromise blood flow to an extremity. Anaphylaxis occurs in 0.6% to 6% of persons who have been stung.[214] Often, healing occurs with scarring in 10 to 14 days.

The majority of individuals who die after fire ant attacks succumb to heart failure.[72] These individuals primarily came from nursing homes; however, the solenopsins were found to strongly inhibit myocardial contractility, which might explain the heart failure that occurred after massive envenomations.[72,120]

Diagnosis

Clinical clues such as pustule development at the sting site after 24 hours, species identification, and history help to identify fire ant exposure. No laboratory assays to determine exposure are available. Fire ant allergy can be determined by correlating the clinical manifestation of fire ant sting reactions with imported fire ant–specific IgE determined by skin testing or radioallergosorbent test.

Treatment

Local reactions require cold compresses and cleansing with soap and water. We recommend topical or injected lidocaine with or without 1:100,000 epinephrine, and topical vinegar and salt mixtures to decrease pain at the site of the bite and sting.[37,117,154,192]

Large local reactions should be treated with oral corticosteroids, antihistamines, and analgesics. Secondary infections should be treated with antibiotics. It is reasonable for systemic reactions to be treated with subcutaneous or intravenous epinephrine.

BUTTERFLIES, MOTHS, AND CATERPILLARS

Butterflies and moths are insects of the order Lepidoptera. Several moth and butterfly families have species whose caterpillars are clinically important, that is, they contain spines or urticating hairs that secrete a poison that is irritating to humans on contact. *Lepidopterism* is a general term that describes the systemic adverse effects such as generalized urticaria, headache, pharyngitis, conjunctivitis, nausea, vomiting, bronchospasm, wheezing, and dyspnea that occur when humans are exposed to moths and butterflies.[164] Erucism is the term used when a cutaneous dermatitis results from contact with urticating caterpillars, the larval forms of the insect order Lepidoptera (moths and butterflies).[76] Caterpillar species from about 12 families of moths and rarely butterflies worldwide can inflict serious human injuries, including urticarial dermatitis, allergic reactions, consumptive coagulopathy, acute kidney injury, intracerebral hemorrhage, arthritis, joint deformity, and even altered mental status, ataxia, and dysarthria.[76,119]

Caterpillar, which means *hairy cat* in Latin, is the larval stage for moths and butterflies. In the United States, several significant stinging caterpillars are of note. Often the puss caterpillar (*Megalopyge opercularis*) is considered one of the most important toxic caterpillars in the United States because of the frequency with which reactions are reported, especially in Texas.[216] Other names for the puss caterpillar are woolly/hairy worm, wooly slug, opossum bug, tree asp, Italian asp, and "el perrito" in Spanish.[216] The caterpillars look furry and are covered in silky tan to brownish hairs that hide short spines containing an urticarial toxin. The spines are yellowish with black tips, and the hairs vary in color, ranging from pale yellow and gray to brown.[29] Other significant stinging caterpillars in the United States are the flannel moth caterpillar (*Megalopyge crispata*), the Io moth (*Automeris io*), the saddleback caterpillar (*Sibine stimulata*), and the hickory tussock caterpillar (*Lophocampa caryae*).[144] In South America, especially Brazil, *Lonomia obliqua* caterpillars are notorious for causing severe pain and a hemorrhagic syndrome.[48,65] In Australia, several caterpillars are of medical importance: mistletoe brown tail moth (*Euproctis edwardsi*), processionary caterpillars (*Ochrogaster lunifer*), cup moths (*Doratifera* spp), and the white-stemmed gum moth (*Chelepteryx collesi*).[13] Pine processionary caterpillars (*Thaumetopoea pityocampa*) are the most important defoliator of pine forests in the Mediterranean and central European countries, with significant consequential economic and occupational repercussions for workers who frequent these pine forests.[231] In Nigeria, the *Anaphe venata* caterpillar is an important resource for protein that can cause thiamine deficiency syndrome similar to dry beriberi.[3,4]

Finally, the dendrolimus caterpillars of China and the *Preolis semirufa* caterpillars in Brazil cause significant joint disease.

Pathophysiology

The pathophysiology of dendrolimiasis is not understood, but the tegument-produced venom contains formaldehyde and several uncharacterized histamine analogs with a tropism for receptors in bone, joints, and cartilage and during the acute phase results from IgE-mediated allergy to foreign proteins, and the chronic bone and joint disease is thought to be autoimmune mediated.[122] The composition of the venom varies according to the different caterpillar species. Some toxins contain proteins that cause histamine release, such as thaumetopoein isolated from *T. pityocampa* or pine processionary caterpillar.[231,232] Another protein isolated from the *Lonomia achelous* caterpillar causes coagulopathy. It is called lonomin V and is a proteolytic enzyme, which is isolated in the hairs, spines, and hemolymph of the *L. achelous*.[108] Its mechanism of action is not fully known, but it activates coagulation factors X and II, and there is some evidence that collagen degradation is responsible for platelet inhibition.[77,107,135] The venom and hair structure of *Lagoa crispata*, which has often been confused with the southern Texas puss caterpillar, is characterized. *Lagoa crispata* larvae have verrucal ridges containing poisonous spines along its filiform hairs.[144] The venom is stored at the base of the hollow setae (spines) where the poison sac and nervous tissue are located. Upon contact with these spines, the toxin, which is a protein or a substance that conjugates with proteins, is released.[84] The varying differences of caterpillar venom and their clinical effects emphasize the importance of positive identification of caterpillars.

Clinical Manifestations

The pathophysiologic effects of venomous caterpillar exposures are classified into 7 distinct clinical syndromes to guide clinicians in making earlier, more species-specific diagnoses to direct therapies, including (1) erucism, (2) lepidopterism, (3) dendrolimiasis, (4) ophthalmia nodosa, (5) consumptive coagulopathy with secondary fibrinolysis,[76] (6) seasonal ataxia, and (7) pararamose.[119] Erucism is the preferred term for caterpillar dermatitis caused by contact with caterpillar urticating hairs, spines, or toxic hemolymph. Lepidopterism is a systemic illness caused by a constellation of adverse effects resulting from direct or aerosol contact with caterpillar, cocoon, or moth urticating hairs, spines or body fluids and is characterized by generalized urticaria, headache, conjunctivitis, pharyngitis, nausea, vomiting, bronchospasm, wheezing, and, rarely, dyspnea. Dendrolimiasis is a chronic form of lepidopterism caused by direct contact with urticating hairs, spines, or hemolymph of living or dead central Asian pine-tree lappet moth caterpillars or their cocoons and is characterized by urticating maculopapular dermatitis, migratory inflammatory polyarthritis, migratory inflammatory polychondritis, chronic osteoarthritis, and, rarely, acute scleritis.[122] Ophthalmia nodosa is a chronic ocular condition characterized by initial conjunctivitis with subsequent panuveitis caused by corneal penetration and subsequent intraocular migration of urticating hairs from lymantriid caterpillars and moths and therapsid spiders (tarantulas).

The South American *Lonomia saturniid* moth caterpillars range from Venezuela to northern Argentina and pose a threat in Brazil because of the high fatality rates from venom-induced consumptive coagulopathy, intracerebral hemorrhage, and acute kidney injury, possibly due to a combination of venom nephrotoxicity and microcirculatory fibrin deposition.[40] A case reported from Brazil involved a patient who presented with persistent gingival bleeding, epistaxis, and ecchymoses to the upper extremities and abdomen 4 days after exposure. These manifestations persisted until day 8 postexposure, when the patient was treated with antivenom.[199] The hemorrhagic syndrome presents as a disseminating intravascular coagulopathy and as a secondary fibrinolysis with skin, mucosal, and visceral bleeding, acute kidney injury, and intracerebral hemorrhage.[48,135]

Seasonal ataxia is a syndrome of unsteady gait and dysarthria, which occurs after the ingestion of the caterpillar of *Anaphe venata*. This occurs in areas of Nigeria where the caterpillars are a source of protein.[3,4] Ingestion of the roasted larvae causes nausea and vomiting and progresses to dizziness, ataxia, and unsteady gait in more than 90% of victims. These findings may take weeks to months for resolution. Dysarthria and impaired consciousness are also reported. The pathogenesis is related to thiamine deficiency induced by thiaminases contained in the larvae.

Pararamose is similar to dendrolimiasis with pruritic or painful dermatitis associated with arthritis and joint deformity, arising from contact with the caterpillar of *Premolis semirufa*, which are found in the Brazilian Amazon rain forests. Rubber tree plantation workers are particularly at risk even when wearing protective gloves.[62,74]

The clinical effects of caterpillar exposure are generally separated into 2 types—stinging reaction and pruritic reaction—although overlap occurs. Stinging caterpillars, such as *M. opercularis*, envenomate by contact with their hollow spines containing venom. The reaction is characterized as a painful, burning sensation with local effects and, less commonly, systemic effects. The area becomes erythematous and swollen, and papules and vesicles may appear. A rash with a typical gridlike pattern develops within 2 to 3 hours of contact. Reported symptoms include nausea, vomiting, fever, headache, restlessness, tachycardia, hypotension, urticaria, seizures, and even radiating lymphadenitis and regional adenopathy.[176] Pruritic reactions occur upon exposure to the itchy caterpillars that have nonvenomous urticating hairs, which produce a mechanical irritation, allergic reaction, or a granulomatous reaction from the chronic presence of the hairs. Several species that cause allergic reactions are the white-stemmed moth (*C. collesi*), Douglas fir tussock moth (*Orgyria pseudotsugata*), and gypsy moth caterpillar (*Lymantria dispar*).[164] Caterpillar hairs can cause ophthalmic trauma, otherwise known as ophthalmia nodosa.[213] The range of ophthalmic pathology depends on the penetration factor and the effect of the released urticating toxins.[46] The ophthalmic spectrum is classified into 5 types.[46]

Type 1: Brief exposure time of 15 minutes. Symptoms of chemosis, inflammation, epiphora, and foreign body sensation are reported to last for weeks.
Type 2: Chronic mechanical keratoconjunctivitis (hairs in bulbar/palpebral conjunctivitis). Foreign body sensation is relieved by removal of hairs. Corneal abrasions are often present.
Type 3: Gray-yellow nodules or asymptomatic granulomas.
Type 4: Severe iritis with or without iritis nodules; hairs are in the anterior chamber and possible intralenticular foreign body.
Type 5: Vitreoretinal involvement. Hairs enter through the anterior chamber or iris lens or by transscleral migration. Causes vitreitis, cystoid macular edema, papillitis, or endophthalmitis.

Treatment

Management for most dermal caterpillar envenomations is entirely supportive and includes washing the area with soap and water; "no touch" drying of the sting site with a hair dryer; gentle stripping of the bite site with cellophane or adhesive duct tape; and application of ice packs with cooling enhanced by initial topical swabbing with isopropyl alcohol. Rings should be removed in anticipation for potential swelling of the extremity, and tetanus prophylaxis should be updated accordingly.[76]

Treatment of ophthalmic lesions depends upon the exposure classification and should be managed by an ophthalmologist. Most patients are classified as type 1 or 2. Irrigation with 0.9% sodium chloride solution should be followed by meticulous removal of setae, followed by topical steroids and antibiotics. Type 3 requires surgical excision of the nodules. Type 4 requires topical steroids with or without iridectomy for nodules or operative removal of setae. Type 5 requires local treatment with or without systemic steroids. Resistant cases require vitrectomy with removal of setae.

Opioids are recommended if minor analgesics do not provide relief. If muscle cramps develop, benzodiazepines are reasonable. One study recommended the use of 10 mL 10% calcium gluconate administered IV, which provided pain relief and is therefore reasonable to use in this circumstance.[157] Topical corticosteroids are reasonable to decrease local inflammation. Antihistamines such as diphenhydramine (25–50 mg for adults and 1 mg/kg, maximum 50 mg, in children) are recommended to relieve pruritus and urticaria.[157,176] Nebulized β-agonists and epinephrine administered subcutaneously should be used for more severe respiratory symptoms and anaphylactoid/anaphylactic-type reactions. Dendrolimiasis treatment consists of mostly supportive care with early surgical intervention recommended to excise draining sinus tracts and infected cartilage and to prevent permanent bone and joint deformities.[122] For hemorrhagic syndrome resulting from exposure to *L. obliqua* caterpillar, besides restoration of clotting factors, platelet, and cryoprecipitate infusions, an antidote called the antilonomic serum (SALon) is available and is used for treatment of the hemorrhagic syndrome in Brazil.[65] It is important to involve an experienced hematologist for suspected *Lonomia* envenomation and very important to distinguish *Lonomia obliqua* from *Lonomia achelous* because the cryoprecipitate, purified fibrinogen, and antifibrinolytic drugs, such as aprotinin and ε-aminocaproic acid, were used successfully in *Lonomia achelous* but exacerbated the hemorrhagic effects in *Lonomia obliqua* with fatal consequences.[55,95] Patients exposed to either species should neither receive whole blood nor fresh plasma, which aggravates the clinical effects. Treatment for the seasonal ataxia includes supportive care with the administration of thiamine 100 mg orally every 8 hours, which reversed symptoms within 48 hours without long-term sequelae in a double-blinded placebo-controlled trial.[2]

BLISTER BEETLES

Blister beetles are plant-eating insects that exude the blistering irritant cantharidin as a presumed defense mechanism. They are found in the eastern United States, southern Europe, Africa, and Asia. Most are from the order Coleoptera, family Meloidae. *Epicauta vittata* is the most common of more than 200 blister beetles identified in the United States.[134] When the beetles sense danger, they exude cantharidin by filling their breathing tubes with air, closing their breathing pores, and building up body fluid pressure until fluid is pushed out through one or more leg joints.[93] Cantharidin is found throughout all 10 stages of life of the blister beetle.[50] Cantharidin is produced only by the male blister beetle and is stored until mating. In the wild, the female repeatedly acquires cantharidin as copulatory gifts from her mates. However, the female blister beetle loses most of her reserves as she matures.[50] Cantharidin, also known popularly as *Spanish fly*, takes its name from the Mediterranean beetle *Cantharis vesicatoria*. It has been ingested as a sexual stimulant for millennia. The aphrodisiac properties are related to the ability of cantharidin to cause vascular engorgement and inflammation of the genitourinary tract upon elimination, hence the reports of priapism and pelvic organ engorgement.[229] Cantharidin was once used for treatment of bladder and kidney infections, stones, stranguria (bladder spasm), and various venereal diseases.[134] In the last century, cantharidin was commonly used for treatment of pleurisy, pneumonia, arthritis, neuralgias, and various dermatitides. A topical 1% commercial preparation is used for removal of warts and molluscum contagiosum.[61,206] Cantharidin poisoning is reported by cutaneous exposure,[36] unintentional inoculation,[179] and inadvertent ingestion of the beetle itself.[226] A case was reported of a child being treated for molluscum contagiosum with cantharidin preparation that included podophyllin and salicylic acid, also called Canthacur PS or Canthacur Plus.[206] The child developed varicelliform vesicular dermatitis in the distribution of the application of petrolatum. It is thought that the petrolatum used by the parents to moisturize her skin spread the lipophilic cantharidin preparation to the nearby areas, causing the blistering reaction. Canthacur PS should not be used for molluscum contagiosum but is reserved for verrucae vulgaris on acral areas. Canthacur or Cantharone contains plain cantharidin and can be used for the treatment of molluscum contagiosum. Fewer than 30 cases of Spanish fly poisoning are reported since 1900.[134]

Pathophysiology

Cantharidin is a natural, defensive, highly toxic terpenoid (lethal dose for humans 0.5 mg/kg) produced by blister beetles and shares a structural similarity with the herbicide Endothall.[146] Endothall causes corrosive effects to the GI tract; cardiomyopathy and vascular permeability, which has resulted in shock. A single case report of lethal poisoning with 7 to 8 g of Endothall led to the death of healthy young boy from hemorrhage of the GI tract and lung, which is clinically similar to the cantharidin exposures. Although the mechanism of action has not been elucidated, one mechanism based on an in vitro study suggests that cantharidin inhibits the activity of protein phosphatases type 1 and 2A. This inhibition alters endothelial permeability by enhancing the phosphorylation state of endothelial regulatory proteins and results in elevated albumin flux and dysfunction of the barrier.[140] Enhanced permeability of albumin is thought to be responsible for the systemic effects of cantharidin that lead to diffuse injury of the vascular endothelium and resultant blistering, hemorrhage, and inflammation.

Clinical Manifestations

The clinical effects are mostly attributed to the irritative effects on the exposed organ systems. The secretions of cantharidin from the beetle's leg joints cause an urticarial dermatitis that is manifested several hours later by burns, blisters, or vesiculobullae.[36] Symptoms are often immediate or sometimes delayed over several hours. In addition to the local effects, cantharidin can be absorbed through the lipid bilayer of the epidermis and cause systemic toxicity, with diaphoresis, tachycardia, hematuria, and oliguria from extensive dermal exposure.[229] If the periorbital region is contaminated, edema and blistering can evolve. Ophthalmic findings from direct contact with the beetle or hand contamination include decreased vision, pain, lacrimation, corneal ulcerations, filamentary keratitis, and anterior uveitis.[179] Most human exposures involve inadvertent contact with the beetle or its secretions, resulting in dermatitis, keratoconjunctivitis, and periorbital edema secondary to hand–eye involvement, also called the *Nairobi eye*.[179]

When cantharidin is ingested, severe GI disturbances and hematuria occur. Initial patient complaints typically include burning of the oropharynx, dysphagia, abdominal cramping, vomiting, hematemesis followed by lower GI tract hematochezia, and tenesmus. An inadvertent blister beetle ingestion by a child who thought it was the edible *Eulepida mashona* or white grub resulted in hematuria and abdominal cramping.[226] Genitourinary effects include dysuria, urinary frequency, hematuria, proteinuria, and acute kidney injury impairment. Most symptoms resolved over several weeks. However, death from acute kidney injury with acute tubular necrosis is reported.[229]

Diagnostic Testing

Cantharidin toxicosis is identified for equine and ruminant exposures by screening urine and gastric contents with high-performance liquid chromatography and gas chromatography–mass spectrometry.[183,184] This method is not used in clinical practice.

Treatment

Treatment is largely supportive. Wound care and tetanus status should be assessed. For keratoconjunctivitis, an ophthalmologist should be consulted early in the clinical course and the patient should be treated with topical corticosteroids (prednisolone 0.125%), mydriatics (cyclopentolate 1%), and antibiotics (ciprofloxacin 0.3%).

SUMMARY

- Health care providers should have an extensive knowledge regarding the identification of arthropods and their bites and stings to provide optimal care.
- Black widow: Latrodectism is a painful neurotoxic condition best known for causing intense muscle spasms associated with short-term autonomic and central nervous system dysfunction.
- Brown recluse: Loxoscelism is manifested by dermatonecrotic tissue loss, which is less often accompanied by systemic reactions such as hemolysis, coagulopathy, acute kidney injury, and death.
- Scorpions: Envenomation releases a neurotoxin that opens the sodium channels and causes local as well as systemic effects that activate the sympathetic and parasympathetic branches of the nervous system,

leading to intense pain, edema, erythema, as well as severe hypertension and tachy- or brady-dysrhythmias.

- Ticks: Ticks are vectors that are commonly known to transmit infectious diseases but in the setting of envenomations, one must remember tick toxicosis in the differential as a cause of progressive ascending flaccid paralysis that can be fatal if the tick is not removed.
- Caterpillars: Lepidopterism is another cause of common human envenomations including dermal and ophthalmic toxicity.

Acknowledgment

Neal A. Lewin, MD, contributed to this chapter in previous editions.

REFERENCES

1. Abroug F. Scorpion envenomation [in French]. *Tunis Med.* 2001;79:329-334.
2. Adamolekun B, et al. A double-blind, placebo-controlled study of the efficacy of thiamine hydrochloride in a seasonal ataxia in Nigerians. *Neurology.* 1994;44:549-551.
3. Adamolekun B, Ibikunle FR. Investigation of an epidemic of seasonal ataxia in Ikare, western Nigeria. *Acta Neurol Scand.* 1994;90:309-311.
4. Adamolekun B, Ndububa DA. Epidemiology and clinical presentation of a seasonal ataxia in western Nigeria. *J Neurol Sci.* 1994;124:95-98.
5. Allen C. Arachnid envenomations. *Emerg Med Clin North Am.* 1992;10:269-298.
6. Allen JR, et al. Histology of bovine skin reactions to *Ixodes holocyclus* Neumann. *Can J Comp Med.* 1977;41:26-35.
7. Anderson PC. Missouri brown recluse spider: a review and update. *Mo Med.* 1998;95:318-322.
8. Anderson PC. What's new in loxoscelism? *Mo Med.* 1973;70:711-712 passim.
9. Anderson PC. Spider bites in the United States. *Dermatol Clin.* 1997;15:307-311.
10. Atkins JA, et al. Probable cause of necrotic spider bite in the Midwest. *Science.* 1957;126:73.
11. Atwell RB, et al. Prospective survey of tick paralysis in dogs. *Aust Vet J.* 2001;79:412-418.
12. Babcock JL, et al. Immunotoxicology of brown recluse spider (*Loxosceles reclusa*) venom. *Toxicon.* 1986;24:783-790.
13. Balit CR, et al. Prospective study of definite caterpillar exposures. *Toxicon.* 2003;42:657-662.
14. Balit CR, et al. Randomized controlled trial of topical aspirin in the treatment of bee and wasp stings. *J Toxicol Clin Toxicol.* 2003;41:801-808.
15. Banks B. Immunotoxicology of the brown recluse spider venom. In: Koiznalik F, Mebs D, eds. *Proceedings of the 7th European Symposium on Animal, Plant, and Microbial Toxins.* Washington, DC: Pergamon Press; 1986:41.
16. Barbaro KC, et al. Identification and neutralization of biological activities in the venoms of Loxosceles spiders. *Braz J Med Biol Res.* 1996;29:1491-1497.
17. Barnard JH. Studies of 400 Hymenoptera sting deaths in the United States. *J Allergy Clin Immunol.* 1973;52:259-264.
18. Barrett SM, et al. Passive hemagglutination inhibition test for diagnosis of brown recluse spider bite envenomation. *Clin Chem.* 1993;39:2104-2107.
19. Battisti A, et al. Urticating hairs in arthropods: their nature and medical significance. *Annu Rev Entomol.* 2011;56:203-220.
20. Bawaskar HS, Bawaskar PH. Management of scorpion sting. *Heart.* 1999;82:253-254.
21. Bawaskar HS, Bawaskar PH. Role of atropine in management of cardiovascular manifestations of scorpion envenoming in humans. *J Trop Med Hyg.* 1992;95:30-35.
22. Belyea DA, et al. The red eye revisited: ophthalmia nodosa due to tarantula hairs. *South Med J.* 1998;91:565-567.
23. Bennett RG, Vetter RS. An approach to spider bites. Erroneous attribution of dermonecrotic lesions to brown recluse or hobo spider bites in Canada. *Can Fam Physician.* 2004;50:1098-1101.
24. Berg RA, Tarantino MD. Envenomation by the scorpion *Centruroides exilicauda* (*C sculpturatus*): severe and unusual manifestations. *Pediatrics.* 1991;87:930-933.
25. Bergman NJ. Clinical description of Parabuthus transvaalicus scorpionism in Zimbabwe. *Toxicon.* 1997;35:759-771.
26. Bernardino CR, Rapuano C. Ophthalmia nodosa caused by casual handling of a tarantula. *CLAO J.* 2000;26:111-112.
27. Bernstein B, Ehrlich F. Brown recluse spider bites. *J Emerg Med.* 1986;4:457-462.
28. Binford GJ. An analysis of geographic and intersexual chemical variation in venoms of the spider *Tegenaria agrestis* (Agelenidae). *Toxicon.* 2001;39:955-968.
29. Bishopp FC. The puss caterpillar and the effects of its sting on man. Washington, DC: US Department of Agriculture, Department Circular 288; 1923:1-14.
30. Bittner MA. Alpha-latrotoxin and its receptors CIRL (latrophilin) and neurexin 1 alpha mediate effects on secretion through multiple mechanisms. *Biochimie.* 2000;82:447-452.
31. Blaikie AJ, et al. Eye disease associated with handling pet tarantulas: three case reports. *BMJ.* 1997;314:1524-1525.
32. Blaser K, et al. Determinants and mechanisms of human immune responses to bee venom phospholipase A2. *Int Arch Allergy Immunol.* 1998;117:1-10.
33. Bogen E. Arachnidism, a study in spider poisoning. *JAMA.* 1926;86:1894-1896.
34. Bond GR. Antivenin administration for Centruroides scorpion sting: risks and benefits. *Ann Emerg Med.* 1992;21:788-791.
35. Bresolin NL, et al. Acute renal failure following massive attack by Africanized bee stings. *Pediatr Nephrol.* 2002;17:625-627.
36. Browne S. Cantharidin poisoning due to a blister beetle. *Br Med J.* 1960;2:1260-1291.
37. Bruce S, et al. Topical aluminum sulfate for fire ant stings. *Int J Dermatol.* 1984;23:211.
38. Bucherl W. *Spiders.* London: Academic Press; 1971.
39. Bugli F, et al. Monoclonal antibody fragment from combinatorial phage display library neutralizes alpha-latrotoxin activity and abolishes black widow spider venom lethality, in mice. *Toxicon.* 2008;51:547-554.
40. Burdmann EA, et al. Severe acute renal failure induced by the venom of Lonomia caterpillars. *Clin Nephrol.* 1996;46:337-339.
41. Bush SP, Naftel J. Injection of a whole black widow spider. *Ann Emerg Med.* 1996;27:532-533.
42. Cabaniss WW, et al. A randomized controlled trial of trypsin to treat brown recluse spider bites in guinea pigs. *J Med Toxicol.* 2014:10:266-268.
43. Cabbiness SG, et al. Polyamines in some tarantula venoms. *Toxicon.* 1980;18:681-683.
44. Cacy J, Mold JW. The clinical characteristics of brown recluse spider bites treated by family physicians: an OKPRN Study. Oklahoma Physicians Research Network. *J Fam Pract.* 1999;48:536-542.
45. Cadera W, et al. Ocular lesions caused by caterpillar hairs (ophthalmia nodosa). *Can J Ophthalmol.* 1984;19:40-44.
46. Campbell FE, Atwell RB. Long QT syndrome in dogs with tick toxicity (*Ixodes holocyclus*). *Aust Vet J.* 2002;80:611-616.
47. Caovilla JJ, Barros EJ. Efficacy of two different doses of antilonomic serum in the resolution of hemorrhagic syndrome resulting from envenoming by *Lonomia obliqua* caterpillars: a randomized controlled trial. *Toxicon.* 2004;43:811-818.
48. Cardoso JL, et al. Detection by enzyme immunoassay of *Loxosceles gaucho* venom in necrotic skin lesions caused by spider bites in Brazil. *Trans R Soc Trop Med Hyg.* 1990;84:608-609.
49. Carrel JE, et al. Cantharidin production in a blister beetle. *Experientia.* 1993;49:171-174.
50. Castro FF, et al. Occupational allergy caused by urticating hair of Brazilian spider. *J Allergy Clin Immunol.* 1995;95:1282-1285.
51. Centers for Disease Control and Prevention (CDC). Necrotic arachnidism—pacific northwest, 1988-1996. *MMWR Morb Mortal Wkly Rep.* 1996;45:433-436.
52. Chan TK, et al. Adenosine triphosphate in tarantula spider venoms and its synergistic effect with the venom toxin. *Toxicon.* 1975;13:61-66.
53. Chavez-Olortegui C, et al. ELISA for the detection of venom antigens in experimental and clinical envenoming by *Loxosceles intermedia* spiders. *Toxicon.* 1998;36:563-569.
54. Choi JT, Rauf A. Ophthalmia nodosa secondary to tarantula hairs. *Eye (Lond).* 2003;17:433-434.
55. Chudzinki-Tavassi A, Carrijo-Carvalho LC. Biochemical and biological properties of *Lonomia obliqua* bristle extract. *J Venom Anim Toxins Incl Trop Dis.* 2008;12:156-171.
56. Clark RF, et al. Clinical presentation and treatment of black widow spider envenomation: a review of 163 cases. *Ann Emerg Med.* 1992;21:782-787.
57. Cohen J, Bush S. Case report: compartment syndrome after a suspected black widow spider bite. *Ann Emerg Med.* 2005;45:414-416.
58. Connor D, Seldon BS. Scorpion envenomation. In: Auerbach P, ed. *Wilderness Medicine: Management of Wilderness and Environmental Emergencies.* St. Louis, MO: Mosby; 1995:831-842.
59. Centers for Disease Control and Prevention. Necrotic arachnidism—Pacific Northwest, 1988-1996. *MMWR Morb Mortal Wkly Rep.* 1996;45:433-436.
60. Cooper BJ, Spence I. Temperature-dependent inhibition of evoked acetylcholine release in tick paralysis. *Nature.* 1976;263:693-695.
61. Coskey RJ. Treatment of plantar warts in children with a salicylic acid-podophyllin-cantharidin product. *Pediatr Dermatol.* 1984;2:71-73.
62. Costa RM, et al. "Pararamose": an occupational arthritis caused by lepidoptera (Premolis semirufa). An epidemiological study. *Rev Paul Med.* 1993;111:462-465.
63. Curry SC, et al. Envenomation by the scorpion *Centruroides sculpturatus.* *J Toxicol Clin Toxicol.* 1983;21:417-449.
64. D'Suze G, et al. Relationship between plasmatic levels of various cytokines, tumour necrosis factor, enzymes, glucose and venom concentration following Tityus scorpion sting. *Toxicon.* 2003;41:367-375.
65. Da Silva WD, et al. Development of an antivenom against toxins of *Lonomia obliqua* caterpillars. *Toxicon.* 1996;34:1045-1049.
66. da Silveira RB, et al. Identification of proteases in the extract of venom glands from brown spiders. *Toxicon.* 2002;40:815-822.
67. Dart RC, et al. A randomized, double-blind, placebo-controlled trial of a highly purified equine F(ab)2 antibody black widow spider antivenom. *Ann Emerg Med.* 2013;61:458-467.
68. Das S, et al. Cardiac involvement and scorpion envenomation in children. *J Trop Pediatr.* 1995;41:338-340.
69. Daugherty RJ, et al. Tick paralysis: atypical presentation, unusual location. *Pediatr Emerg Care.* 2005;21:677-680.
70. Dehesa-Davila M, Possani LD. Scorpionism and serotherapy in Mexico. *Toxicon.* 1994;32:1015-1018.
71. deShazo RD, et al. Reactions to the stings of the imported fire ant. *N Engl J Med.* 1990;323:462-466.
72. deShazo RD, et al. Fire ant attacks on patients in nursing homes: an increasing problem. *Am J Med.* 2004;116:843-846.

73. Devi CS, et al. Defibrination syndrome due to scorpion venom poisoning. *Br Med J.* 1970;1:345-347.

74. Dias LB, de Azevedo MC. Pararama, a disease caused by moth larvae: experimental findings. *Bull Pan Am Health.* 1973;7:9.

75. Diaz JH. A 60-year meta-analysis of tick paralysis in the United States: a predictable, preventable, and often misdiagnosed poisoning. *J Med Toxicol.* 2010;6:15-21.

76. Diaz JH. The evolving global epidemiology, syndromic classification, management, and prevention of caterpillar envenoming. *Am J Trop Med Hyg.* 2005;72:347-357.

77. Donato JL, et al. *Lonomia obliqua* caterpillar spicules trigger human blood coagulation via activation of factor X and prothrombin. *Thromb Haemost.* 1998;79:539-542.

78. Erdur B, et al. Uncommon cardiovascular manifestations after a Latrodectus bite. *Am J Emerg Med.* 2007;25:232-235.

79. Escoubas P, et al. Novel tarantula toxins for subtypes of voltage-dependent potassium channels in the Kv2 and Kv4 subfamilies. *Mol Pharmacol.* 2002;62:48-57.

80. Escoubas P, et al. Structure and pharmacology of spider venom neurotoxins. *Biochimie.* 2000;82:893-907.

81. Felz MW, et al. A six-year-old girl with tick paralysis. *N Engl J Med.* 2000;342:90-94.

82. Fernandez-Bouzas A, et al. Brain infarcts due to scorpion stings in children: MRI. *Neuroradiology.* 2000;42:118-120.

83. Fet V, et al. *Catalog of the Scorpions of the World (1758-1998).* New York, NY: New York Entomological Society; 2000.

84. Foot N. Pathology of the dermatitis caused by the *Megalopyge opercularis*, a Texas caterpillar. *J Exp Med.* 1922;35:737-753.

85. Franca FO, et al. Rhabdomyolysis in presumed viscero-cutaneous loxoscelism: report of two cases. *Trans R Soc Trop Med Hyg.* 2002;96:287-290.

86. Fukuhara YD, et al. The kinin system in the envenomation caused by the *Tityus serrulatus* scorpion sting. *Toxicol Appl Pharmacol.* 2004;196:390-395.

87. Fukuhara YD, et al. Increased plasma levels of IL-1beta, IL-6, IL-8, IL-10 and TNF-alpha in patients moderately or severely envenomed by *Tityus serrulatus* scorpion sting. *Toxicon.* 2003;41:49-55.

88. Gaver-Wainwright MM, et al. Misdiagnosis of spider bites: bacterial associates, mechanical pathogen transfer, and hemolytic potential of venom from the hobo spider, *Tegenaria agrestis* (Araneae: Agelenidae). *J Med Entomol.* 2011;48:382-388.

89. Gendron BP. *Loxosceles reclusa* envenomation. *Am J Emerg Med.* 1990;8:51-54.

90. Gentile D. Tick-borne diseases. In: Auerbach P, ed. *Wilderness Medicine: Management of Wilderness and Environmental Emergencies.* St Louis, MO: Mosby; 1995:787-812.

91. Gibly R, et al. Continuous intravenous midazolam infusion for *Centruroides exilicauda* scorpion envenomation. *Ann Emerg Med.* 1999;34:620-625.

92. Ginsburg CM, Weinberg AG. Hemolytic anemia and multiorgan failure associated with localized cutaneous lesion. *J Pediatr.* 1988;112:496-499.

93. Goddard J. *Physician's Guide to Arthropods of Medical Importance.* 3rd ed. Boca Raton, FL: CRC Press; 2000.

94. Gomez HF, et al. Intradermal anti-Loxosceles Fab fragments attenuate dermonecrotic arachnidism. *Acad Emerg Med.* 1999;6:1195-1202.

95. Goncalves LR, et al. Efficacy of serum therapy on the treatment of rats experimentally envenomed by bristle extract of the caterpillar *Lonomia obliqua*: comparison with epsilon-aminocaproic acid therapy. *Toxicon.* 2007;50:349-356.

96. Gordon BM, Giza CC. Tick paralysis presenting in an urban environment. *Pediatr Neurol.* 2004;30:122-124.

97. Goto CS, et al. Upper airway obstruction caused by brown recluse spider envenomization of the neck. *Am J Emerg Med.* 1996;14:660-662.

98. Grant SJ, Loxton EH. Effectiveness of a compression bandage and antivene for Sydney funnel-web spider envenomation. *Med J Aust.* 1992;156:510-511.

99. Grattan-Smith PJ, et al. Clinical and neurophysiological features of tick paralysis. *Brain.* 1997;120(pt 11):1975-1987.

100. Graudins A, et al. Cross-reactivity of Sydney funnel-web spider antivenom: neutralization of the in vitro toxicity of other Australian funnel-web (Atrax and Hadronyche) spider venoms. *Toxicon.* 2002;40:259-266.

101. Greenstein P. Tick paralysis. *Med Clin North Am.* 2002;86:441-446.

102. Grishin EV. Black widow spider toxins: the present and the future. *Toxicon.* 1998;36:1693-1701.

103. Groshong TD. Scorpion envenomation in eastern Saudi Arabia. *Ann Emerg Med.* 1993;22:1431-1437.

104. Gueron M, et al. The cardiovascular system after scorpion envenomation. A review. *J Toxicol Clin Toxicol.* 1992;30:245-258.

105. Gueron M, Sofer S. Vasodilators and calcium blocking agents as treatment of cardiovascular manifestations of human scorpion envenomation. *Toxicon.* 1990;28:127-128.

106. Gueron M, Yaron R. Cardiovascular manifestations of severe scorpion sting. Clinico-pathologic correlations. *Chest.* 1970;57:156-162.

107. Guerrero B, et al. The effects of Lonomin V, a toxin from the caterpillar (*Lonomia achelous*), on hemostasis parameters as measured by platelet function. *Toxicon.* 2011;58:293-303.

108. Guerrero B, et al. Effect on platelet FXIII and partial characterization of Lonomin V, a proteolytic enzyme from *Lonomia achelous* caterpillars. *Thromb Res.* 1999;93:243-252.

109. Habermann E. Apamin. *Pharmacol Ther.* 1984;25:255-270.

110. Haeberli S, et al. Characterisation of antibacterial activity of peptides isolated from the venom of the spider *Cupiennius salei* (Araneae: Ctenidae). *Toxicon.* 2000;38:373-380.

111. Henkel AW, Sankaranarayanan S. Mechanisms of alpha-latrotoxin action. *Cell Tissue Res.* 1999;296:229-233.

112. Hobbs GD, et al. Comparison of hyperbaric oxygen and dapsone therapy for Loxosceles envenomation. *Acad Emerg Med.* 1996;3:758-761.

113. Hoffman DR. Allergens in Hymenoptera venom. XVII. Allergenic components of *Solenopsis invicta* (imported fire ant) venom. *J Allergy Clin Immunol.* 1987;80:300-306.

114. Hollabaugh RS, Fernandes ET. Management of the brown recluse spider bite. *J Pediatr Surg.* 1989;24:126-127.

115. Hom-Choudhury A, et al. A hairy affair: tarantula setae-induced panuveitis requiring pars plana vitrectomy. *Int Ophthalmol.* 2012;32:161-163.

116. Hoover NG, Fortenberry JD. Use of antivenin to treat priapism after a black widow spider bite. *Pediatrics.* 2004;114:e128-e129.

117. Horen WP. Insect and scorpion sting. *JAMA.* 1972;221:894-898.

118. Horng CT, et al. Caterpillar setae in the deep cornea and anterior chamber. *Am J Ophthalmol.* 2000;129:384-385.

119. Hossler EW. Caterpillars and moths: *Dermatol Ther.* 2009;22:353-366.

120. Howell G, et al. Cardiodepressant and neurologic actions of *Solenopsis invicta* (imported fire ant) venom alkaloids. *Ann Allergy Asthma Immunol.* 2005;94:380-386.

121. Hoyte CO, et al. Anaphylaxis to black widow spider antivenom. *Am J Emerg Med.* 2012;30:836.e1-836.e2.

122. Huang DZ. Dendrolimiasis: an analysis of 58 cases. *J Trop Med Hyg.* 1991;94:79-87.

123. Ichtchenko K, et al. A novel ubiquitously expressed alpha-latrotoxin receptor is a member of the CIRL family of G-protein-coupled receptors. *J Biol Chem.* 1999;274:5491-5498.

124. Isbister GK. Data collection in clinical toxinology: debunking myths and developing diagnostic algorithms. *J Toxicol Clin Toxicol.* 2002;40:231-237.

125. Isbister GK, Gray MR. A prospective study of 750 definite spider bites, with expert spider identification. *Q J Med.* 2002;95:723-731.

126. Isbister GK, Gray MR. Latrodectism: a prospective cohort study of bites by formally identified redback spiders. *Med J Aust.* 2003;179:88-91.

127. Isbister GK, Gray MR. Effects of envenoming by comb-footed spiders of the genera Steatoda and Achaearanea (family Theridiidae: Araneae) in Australia. *J Toxicol Clin Toxicol.* 2003;41:809-819.

128. Isbister GK, et al. Bites by spiders of the family Theraphosidae in humans and canines. *Toxicon.* 2003;41:519-524.

129. Ismail M. Treatment of the scorpion envenoming syndrome: 12-years experience with serotherapy. *Int J Antimicrob Agents.* 2003;21:170-174.

130. Javors MA, et al. Effects of fire ant venom alkaloids on platelet and neutrophil function. *Life Sci.* 1993;53:1105-1112.

131. Johnson JH, et al. Novel insecticidal peptides from *Tegenaria agrestis* spider venom may have a direct effect on the insect central nervous system. *Arch Insect Biochem Physiol.* 1998;38:19-31.

132. Jones T, et al. Ant venom alkaloids from *Solenopsis and Monomovian species venom.* *Tetrahedron.* 1982;38:1949-1958.

133. Kaire GH. Isolation of tick paralysis toxin from *Ixodes holocyclus. Toxicon.* 1966;4:91-97.

134. Karras DJ, et al. Poisoning from "Spanish fly" (cantharidin). *Am J Emerg Med.* 1996;14:478-483.

135. Kelen E, et al. Hemorrhagic syndrome induced by contact with caterpillars of the genus *Lonomia obliqua. J Toxicol Toxin Review.* 1995;14:283-308.

136. Kelley TD 3rd, Wasserman G. The dangers of pet tarantulas: experience of the Marseilles Poison Centre. *J Toxicol Clin Toxicol.* 1998;36:55-56.

137. Kemp DH, et al. Tick attachment and feeding: role of the mouthparts, feeding apparatus, salivary gland secretions and host response. In: Obenchain FD, Galun R, eds. *Physiology of Ticks.* Oxford: Pergamon Press; 1983:119-168.

138. Key GF. A comparison of calcium gluconate and methocarbamol (Robaxin) in the treatment of Latrodectism (black widow spider envenomation). *Am J Trop Med Hyg.* 1981;30:273-277.

139. King LE Jr, Rees RS. Dapsone treatment of a brown recluse bite. *JAMA.* 1983;250:648.

140. Knapp J, et al. The protein phosphatase inhibitor cantharidin alters vascular endothelial cell permeability. *J Pharmacol Exp Ther.* 1999;289:1480-1486.

141. Krifi MN, et al. Development of an ELISA for the detection of scorpion venoms in sera of humans envenomed by *Androctonus australis garzonii* (Aag) and *Buthus occitanus tunetanus* (Bot): correlation with clinical severity of envenoming in Tunisia. *Toxicon.* 1998;36:887-900.

142. Krywko DM, Gomez HF. Detection of *Loxosceles* species venom in dermal lesions: a comparison of 4 venom recovery methods. *Ann Emerg Med.* 2002;39:475-480.

143. Kurpiewski G, et al. Platelet aggregation and sphingomyelinase D activity of a purified toxin from the venom of *Loxosceles reclusa. Biochim Biophys Acta.* 1981;678:467-476.

144. Lamdin JM, et al. The venomous hair structure, venom and life cycle of *Lagoa crispata*, a puss caterpillar of Oklahoma. *Toxicon.* 2000;38:1163-1189.

145. Leopold NA, et al. Parkinsonism after a wasp sting. *Mov Disord.* 1999;14:122-127.

146. Lichtenstein LM, et al. Insect allergy: the state of the art. *J Allergy Clin Immunol.* 1979;64:5-12.

147. Lowry BP, et al. A controlled trial of topical nitroglycerin in a New Zealand white rabbit model of brown recluse spider envenomation. *Ann Emerg Med.* 2001;37:161-165.

148. Luch A. Mechanistic insights on spider neurotoxins. *EXS.* 2010;100:293-315.

149. MacConnell JG, et al. Fire ant venoms: chemotaxonomic correlations with alkaloidal compositions. *Toxicon.* 1976;14:69-78.

150. Malaque CM, et al. Clinical and epidemiological features of definitive and presumed loxoscelism in São Paulo, Brazil. *Rev Inst Med Trop Sao Paulo*. 2002;44:139-143.

151. Malik R, Farrow BR. Tick paralysis in North America and Australia. *Vet Clin North Am Small Anim Pract*. 1991;21:157-171.

152. Maretic Z. Latrodectism: variations in clinical manifestations provoked by *Latrodectus* species of spiders. *Toxicon*. 1983;21:457-466.

153. Maretic Z, Stanic M. The health problem of arachnidism. *Bull World Health Organ*. 1954;11:1007-1022.

154. Marshall TK. Wasp and bee stings. *Practitioner*. 1957;178:712-722.

155. McGlasson DL, et al. Duration of *Loxosceles reclusa* venom detection by ELISA from swabs. *Clin Lab Sci*. 2009;22:216-222.

156. Meki AR, et al. Significance of assessment of serum cardiac troponin I and interleukin-8 in scorpion envenomed children. *Toxicon*. 2003;41:129-137.

157. Micks DW. Clinical effects of the sting of the "puss caterpillar" (*Megalopyge opercularis* S & A) on man. *Tex Rep Biol Med*. 1952;10:399-405.

158. Miller M, et al. Towards rationalization of antivenom use in funnel-web spider envenoming: enzyme immunoassays for venom concentrations. *Clin Toxicol (Phila)*. 2016;54:245-251.

159. Miller MJ, et al. Detection of Loxosceles venom in lesional hair shafts and skin: application of a specific immunoassay to identify dermonecrotic arachnidism. *Am J Emerg Med*. 2000;18:626-628.

160. Miller MK, et al. Serum sickness from funnelweb spider antivenom. *Med J Aust*. 1999;171:54.

161. Miller MK, et al. Clinical features and management of Hadronyche envenomation in man. *Toxicon*. 2000;38:409-427.

162. Monsalve RI, et al. Expression of yellow jacket and wasp venom Ag5 allergens in bacteria and in yeast. *Arb Paul Ehrlich Inst Bundesamt Sera Impfstoffe Frankf A M*. 1999:181-188.

163. Moss HS, Binder LS. A retrospective review of black widow spider envenomation. *Ann Emerg Med*. 1987;16:188-192.

164. Mulvaney JK, et al. Lepidopterism: two cases of systemic reactions to the cocoon of a common moth, *Chelepteryx collesi*. *Med J Aust*. 1998;168:610-611.

165. Murnaghan MF. Site and mechanism of tick paralysis. *Science*. 1960;131:418-419.

166. Murphy CM, et al. Anaphylaxis with Latrodectus antivenin resulting in cardiac arrest. *J Med Toxicol*. 2011;7:317-321.

167. Mylecharane EJ, et al. Actions of robustoxin, a neurotoxic polypeptide from the venom of the male funnel-web spider (*Atrax robustus*), in anaesthetized monkeys. *Toxicon*. 1989;27:481-492.

168. Needham GR. Evaluation of five popular methods for tick removal. *Pediatrics*. 1985;75:997-1002.

169. Nicholson GM, Graudins A. Spiders of medical importance in the Asia-Pacific: atracotoxin, latrotoxin and related spider neurotoxins. *Clin Exp Pharmacol Physiol*. 2002;29:785-794.

170. Nicholson GM, et al. Structure and function of delta-atracotoxins: lethal neurotoxins targeting the voltage-gated sodium channel. *Toxicon*. 2004;43:587-599.

171. Nicholson GM, et al. Modification of sodium channel gating and kinetics by versutoxin from the Australian funnel-web spider *Hadronyche versuta*. *Pflugers Arch*. 1994;428:400-409.

172. Nordt SP, et al. Examination of adverse events following black widow antivenom use in California. *Clin Toxicol (Phila)*. 2012;50:70-73.

173. Petrenko AG, et al. Isolation and properties of the alpha-latrotoxin receptor. *EMBO J*. 1990;9:2023-2027.

174. Petroianu G, et al. Phospholipase A2-induced coagulation abnormalities after bee sting. *Am J Emerg Med*. 2000;18:22-27.

175. Phillips S, et al. Therapy of brown spider envenomation: a controlled trial of hyperbaric oxygen, dapsone, and cyproheptadine. *Ann Emerg Med*. 1995;25:363-368.

176. Pinson RT, Morgan JA. Envenomation by the puss caterpillar (*Megalopyge opercularis*). *Ann Emerg Med*. 1991;20:562-564.

177. Platnick N. The world spider catalog, version 9.5. In: *American Museum of Natural History*; 2009.

178. Pneumatikos IA, et al. Acute fatal toxic myocarditis after black widow spider envenomation. *Ann Emerg Med*. 2003;41:158.

179. Poole TR. Blister beetle periorbital dermatitis and keratoconjunctivitis in Tanzania. *Eye (Lond)*. 1998;12(pt 5):883-885.

180. Rachesky IJ, et al. Treatments for *Centruroides exilicauda* envenomation. *Am J Dis Child*. 1984;138:1136-1139.

181. Ramialiharisoa A, et al. Latrodectism in Madagascar [in French]. *Med Trop (Mars)*. 1994;54:127-130.

182. Rauber A. Black widow spider bites. *J Toxicol Clin Toxicol*. 1983;21:473-485.

183. Ray AC, et al. Etiologic agents, incidence, and improved diagnostic methods of cantharidin toxicosis in horses. *Am J Vet Res*. 1989;50:187-191.

184. Ray AC, et al. Evaluation of an analytical method for the diagnosis of cantharidin toxicosis due to ingestion of blister beetles (*Epicauta lemniscata*) by horses and sheep. *Am J Vet Res*. 1980;41:932-933.

185. Rees R, et al. The diagnosis and treatment of brown recluse spider bites. *Ann Emerg Med*. 1987;16:945-949.

186. Rees RS, et al. Brown recluse spider bites. A comparison of early surgical excision versus dapsone and delayed surgical excision. *Ann Surg*. 1985;202:659-663.

187. Ribeiro JM, Francischetti IM. Role of arthropod saliva in blood feeding: sialome and post-sialome perspectives. *Annu Rev Entomol*. 2003;48:73-88.

188. Rimsza ME, et al. Scorpion envenomation. *Pediatrics*. 1980;66:298-302.

189. Robertson FM, et al. Dapsone hepatitis following treatment of a brown recluse spider. *Comp Surg*. 1992;38:33-35.

190. Roche KJ, et al. Images in clinical medicine. Cutaneous anthrax infection. *N Engl J Med*. 2001;345:1611.

191. Rosenthal L, et al. Mode of action of alpha-latrotoxin: role of divalent cations in Ca2(+)-dependent and Ca2(+)-independent effects mediated by the toxin. *Mol Pharmacol*. 1990;38:917-923.

192. Ross EV Jr, et al. Meat tenderizer in the acute treatment of imported fire ant stings. *J Am Acad Dermatol*. 1987;16:1189-1192.

193. Russell FE. Arachnid envenomations. *Emerg Med Serv*. 1991;20:16-47.

194. Russell FE. Venomous animal injuries. *Curr Probl Pediatr*. 1973;3:1-47.

195. Russell FE, Gertsch WJ. For those who treat spider or suspected spider bites. *Toxicon*. 1983;21:337-339.

196. Ryan PJ. Preliminary report: experience with the use of dantrolene sodium in the treatment of bites by the black widow spider *Latrodectus hesperus*. *J Toxicol Clin Toxicol*. 1983;21:487-489.

197. Sams HH, et al. Necrotic arachnidism. *J Am Acad Dermatol*. 2001;44:561-573; quiz 573-576.

198. Santhanakrishnan BR. Scorpion sting. *Indian Pediatr*. 2000;37:1154-1157.

199. Santos JHA, et al. Severe hemorrhagic syndrome after Lonomia caterpillar envenomation in the western Brazilian Amazon: how many more cases are there? *Wilderness Environ Med*. 2017;28:46-50.

200. Santos MSV, et al. Clinical and epidemiological aspects of scorpionism in the world: a systematic review. *Wilderness Environ Med*. 2016;27:504-518.

201. Schanbacher FL, et al. Purification and characterization of tarantula, *Dugesiella hentzi* (Girard) venom hyaluronidase. *Comp Biochem Physiol B Biochem Mol Biol*. 1973;44:389-396.

202. Schaumburg HH, Herskovitz S. The weak child—a cautionary tale. *N Engl J Med*. 2000;342:127-129.

203. Schenone H, et al. Loxoscelism in Chile. Epidemiologic, clinical and experimental studies [in Spanish]. *Rev Inst Med Trop Sao Paulo*. 1989;31:403-415.

204. Schiffman JS, et al. Bilateral ischaemic optic neuropathy and stroke after multiple bee stings. *Br J Ophthalmol*. 2004;88:1596-1598.

205. Schmitt N, et al. Tick paralysis in British Columbia. *CMAJ*. 1969;100:417-421.

206. Shah A, et al. Spread of cantharidin after petrolatum use resulting in a varicelliform vesicular dermatitis. *J Am Acad Dermatol*. 2008;59:S54-S55.

207. Shkenderov S, Koburova K. Adolapin—a newly isolated analgetic and anti-inflammatory polypeptide from bee venom. *Toxicon*. 1982;20:317-321.

208. Smith CW, Micks DW. The role of polymorphonuclear leukocytes in the lesion caused by the venom of the brown spider, *Loxosceles reclusa*. *Lab Invest*. 1970;22:90-93.

209. Smoley BA. Oropharyngeal hymenoptera stings: a special concern for airway obstruction. *Mil Med*. 2002;167:161-163.

210. Sofer S, et al. Acute pancreatitis in children following envenomation by the yellow scorpion *Leiurus quinquestriatus*. *Toxicon*. 1991;29:125-128.

211. Solley GO, et al. Anaphylaxis due to red imported fire ant sting. *Med J Aust*. 2002;176:521-523.

212. Sorkin LN. *Loxosceles rufescens*' presence in New York City. Hahn I, private communication with LN Sorkin.

213. Sridhar MS, Ramakrishnan M. Ocular lesions caused by caterpillar hairs. *Eye (Lond)*. 2004;18:540-543.

214. Stafford CT. Hypersensitivity to fire ant venom. *Ann Allergy Asthma Immunol*. 1996;77:87-95; quiz 96-99.

215. Stiles AD. Priapism following a black widow spider bite. *Clin Pediatr (Phila)*. 1982;21:174-175.

216. Stipetic ME, et al. A retrospective analysis of 96 "asp" (*Megalopyge opercularis*) envenomations in Central Texas during 1996. *J Toxicol Clin Toxicol*. 1999;37:457-462.

217. Strain GM, et al. Hyperbaric oxygen effects on brown recluse spider (*Loxosceles reclusa*) envenomation in rabbits. *Toxicon*. 1991;29:989-996.

218. Suchard JR. "Spider bite" lesions are usually diagnosed as skin and soft-tissue infections. *J Emerg Med*. 2011;41:473-481.

219. Suchard JR, Hilder R. Atropine use in Centruroides scorpion envenomation. *J Toxicol Clin Toxicol*. 2001;39:595-598; discussion 599.

220. Sutherland SK. Genus Atrax Cambridge, the funnel web spiders. In: Sutherland S, ed. *Australian Animal Toxins*. Melbourne: Oxford University Press; 1983:255-298.

221. Sutherland SK. The management of bites by the Sydney funnel-web spider, *Atrax robustus*. *Med J Aust*. 1978;1:148-150.

222. Sutherland SK. Antivenom to the venom of the male Sydney funnel-web spider *Atrax robustus*: preliminary report. *Med J Aust*. 1980;2:437-441.

223. Sutherland SK, et al. Funnel-web spider (*Atrax robustus*) antivenom. 1. Preparation and laboratory testing. *Med J Aust*. 1981;2:522-525.

224. Sutherland SK, Trinca JC. Survey of 2,144 cases of red-back spider bites: Australia and New Zealand, 1963-1976. *Med J Aust*. 1978;2:620-623.

225. Taber S. *Fire Ants*. College Station, TX: Texas A&M University Press; 2000.

226. Tagwireyi D, et al. Cantharidin poisoning due to "blister beetle" ingestion. *Toxicon*. 2000;38:1865-1869.

227. Thapa R, et al. Hymenoptera sting complicated by pseudotumor cerebri in a 9-year-old boy. *Clin Toxicol (Phila).* 2008;46:1100-1101.

228. Thorp R, Woodson W. *Black Widow, America's Most Poisonous Spider.* Chapel Hill: North Carolina Press; 1945.

229. Till JS, Majmudar BN. Cantharidin poisoning. *South Med J.* 1981;74:444-447.

230. Vedanarayanan V, et al. Tick paralysis. *Semin Neurol.* 2004;24:181-184.

231. Vega J, et al. Occupational immunologic contact urticaria from pine processionary caterpillar (*Thaumetopoea pityocampa*): experience in 30 cases. *Contact Dermatitis.* 2004;50:60-64.

232. Vega JM, et al. Pine processionary caterpillar as a new cause of immunologic contact urticaria. *Contact Dermatitis.* 2000;43:129-132.

233. Veiga SS, et al. Identification of high molecular weight serine-proteases in *Loxosceles intermedia* (brown spider) venom. *Toxicon.* 2000;38:825-839.

234. Vest DK. Envenomation by *Tegenaria agrestis* (Walckenaer) spiders in rabbits. *Toxicon.* 1987;25:221-224.

235. Vest DK. Necrotic arachnidism in the northwest United States and its probable relationship to *Tegenaria agrestis* (Walckenaer) spiders. *Toxicon.* 1987;25:175-184.

236. Vinson S. Invasion of the red imported fire ant (Hymenoptera: Formicidae): spread, biology, and impact. *Ann Entomol.* 1997;43:23-39.

237. Wasserman GS. Wound care of spider and snake envenomations. *Ann Emerg Med.* 1988;17:1331-1335.

238. White J, et al. Clinical toxicology of spider bites. In: Meier J, White J, eds. *Handbook of Clinical Toxicology of Animal Venoms and Poisons.* Boca Raton, FL: CRC Press; 1995:259-329.

239. Wiener S. The Sydney funnel-web spider. *Med J Aust.* 1957;2:377-382.

240. Williams ST, et al. Severe intravascular hemolysis associated with brown recluse spider envenomation. A report of two cases and review of the literature. *Am J Clin Pathol.* 1995;104:463-467.

241. Wong SL, et al. Loxoscelism and negative pressure wound therapy (vacuum-assisted closure): a clinical case series. *Am Surg.* 2009;75:1128-1131.

242. Yan L, Adams ME. Lycotoxins, antimicrobial peptides from venom of the wolf spider *Lycosa carolinensis. J Biol Chem.* 1998;273:2059-2066.

243. Yarbrough B. Current treatment of brown recluse spiders. *Curr Concepts Wound Care.* 1987;10:4-6.

244. Yi GB, et al. Fire ant venom alkaloid, isosolenopsin A, a potent and selective inhibitor of neuronal nitric oxide synthase. *Int J Toxicol.* 2003;22:81-86.

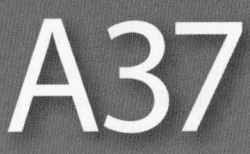

A37

ANTIVENOM: SPIDER

Michael A. Darracq and Richard F. Clark

INTRODUCTION

The terms "antivenom" and "antivenin" often are used interchangeably. Although the origin of the term "antivenom" is obvious, "venin" is French for venom and "antivenin" is traditionally used in certain parts of the world. Wyeth Pharmaceuticals, the maker of Crotaline and *Micrurus* antivenom, and Merck & Co, Inc, the maker of *Latrodectus* antivenom, adopted "antivenin" in the brand names for their products. Brand name recognition was largely responsible for the use of the term "antivenin" in place of "antivenom." In 1981, the World Health Organization determined the preferred terms for the English language to be "venom" and "antivenom."

HISTORY

Two of the most notable genera of spiders of medical importance in the United States are *Latrodectus* (*L. mactans*, *L. geometricus*, *L. variolus*, *L. hesperus*, and *L. bishopi* are native, whereas *L. geometricus* was introduced) and *Loxosceles*. Commercially available antivenom does not exist in the United States for treatment of *Loxosceles* envenomation. Currently, there is one commercially available *Latrodectus* antivenom in the United States. Black Widow Spider Antivenin (Merck & Co, Inc) (Merck BW-AV) has been available in the United States since its US Food and Drug Administration (FDA) approval in 1936.[3] The use of this antivenom in the treatment of *Latrodectus* envenomations remains controversial, as mortality from these bites is low in the United States,[8,9,31,33] and complications including death following antivenom administration are rarely reported.[8,22,32] Ongoing research and development of an F(ab')$_2$ antivenom may ameliorate concerns and limitations related to potential adverse events resulting from administration of the Merck antivenom and production shortages limiting availability.[12] As of June 2018, however, F(ab')$_2$ black widow antivenom has not been approved for use by the US Food and Drug Administration (FDA) but is in clinical trials under the trade name Analatro.

PHARMACOLOGY

Chemistry, Preparation, and Mechanism of Action

Antivenom for spiders is prepared in a similar manner as other antivenom products by first immunizing animals with nontoxic amounts of venom.[5,26] Monkeys, horses, goats, sheep, chicken, camels, and rabbits have been used historically to source antivenom.[29] The animals are placed on an inoculation schedule to allow gradual production of immunoglobulins, most importantly IgG. Sufficient antibody production usually occurs within 6 weeks. The species availability, financial considerations, and tradition rather than scientific modeling is typically responsible for animal choice for immune serum production. The majority of antivenom producers use horses, since they are relatively easy to maintain, and large volumes of serum can be obtained at one time without harming the animal. During antivenom production varying efforts are made to remove animal proteins such as albumin. Antivenoms target, bind, neutralize, and promote elimination or redistribution of toxins from body tissues. To date, no studies have compared immune sera of different animals for human compatibility or tolerance.

The antidotal fraction of an antivenom exists as either whole IgG, Fab, or F(ab')$_2$. The IgG molecule is composed of 2 antigen-binding fragments (Fab fragments) that are fused together and attached to the larger complement binding fragment (Fc fragment). It is the larger Fc portion that is generally considered to be the most responsible for immune-mediated reactions. Digestion of the disulfide bonds of an IgG molecule by pepsin will cleave the

Fc fragment, allowing isolation of pure F(ab')$_2$ fragments (2 fused Fab fragments with some intact hinge region). By contrast, digestion with papain cleaves the molecule more distally such that a larger Fc portion is removed from 2 separate Fab fragments. Both Fab and F(ab')$_2$ molecules are isolated with affinity chromatography, and the highly antigenic Fc portion discarded. Although Fab and F(ab')$_2$ are more expensive to produce than their whole immunoglobin counterparts, they are much less allergenic and therefore safer products.

Whole IgG antivenom is the easiest and least expensive to produce. It has a molecular weight of approximately 150 kDa, and is the largest of the 3 antivenom types. Because of its size, it is the least filterable at the glomerulus and has the smallest volume of distribution. Whole IgG has a longer elimination half-life than either Fab or F(ab')$_2$.[18]

F(ab')$_2$ antivenom has an intermediate size (~100 kDa) and elimination half-life. Although it lowers the risk of anaphylaxis compared to whole IgG, the F(ab')$_2$ portion retains much of the allosteric configuration of the original IgG molecule that is lost when Fab are formed. This configuration theoretically allows for tighter binding to venom. The Fab antivenom is the smallest (~50 kDa) molecule in size and is eliminated by the kidneys. It has the largest volume of distribution and a greater ability to reach extravascular compartments. Arachnid venoms that affect the central nervous system have low molecular weights and large volumes of distribution. Thus Fab and F(ab')$_2$ based antivenoms are theoretically best suited for this function.[18]

Immunoglobulin-based antivenoms can be given by the intramuscular, intravenous, or subcutaneous route. Intravenous administration achieves rapid peak plasma concentrations, and the infusion can be stopped in the event of an allergic reaction.[19] Intramuscular and intraosseous injection has been used when intravenous access is unobtainable.[20]

Pharmacokinetics and Pharmacodynamics

Currently, there is no published pharmacokinetic or pharmacodynamic information available on Merck BW-AV in humans or animals. One study colleagues demonstrated Western blot binding of *L. hasselti* (redback spider) Antivenom (RBS-AV) to purified α-latrotoxin and similar protein bands derived from multiple widow spiders (*L. mactans*, *L. hesperus*, *L. lugubris*, *L. tredecimguttatus*, and *L. hasselti*). When co-mixed with the venoms from these species prior to administration, RBS-AV prevented the development of a reproducible and rapid muscle contracture of an in vitro chicken nerve-muscle preparation. A dose–response relationship was observed with varying doses of RBS-AV administration.[17] This confirms a direct in vitro binding effect of RBS-AV against widow spider venoms.

Previous animal studies demonstrated that intramuscular administration of antivenom produced very low serum venom concentrations.[36,37] In these rabbit studies of intramuscular administration, F(ab')$_2$ and IgG had poor bioavailability (36%–42%) and delayed time to peak concentrations of 48 to 96 hours.

Pharmacokinetic and pharmacodynamic characteristics of equine-derived antivenoms differ between species studied. Equine-derived antivenom maximum concentrations were greater in cows than in horses, and steady-state distribution volumes were higher in cows than in horses in one study. Similar results were observed in rabbit models.[38] Pharmacokinetic and pharmacodynamic parameters observed in animal models should therefore be interpreted with caution with regard to behavior of antivenoms in humans.

Redback spider antivenom, available in Australia, has been administered intramuscularly to treat human envenomations, and clinical effectiveness equivalent to intravenous administration was reported.[22] Subsequent studies, however, demonstrated the absence of RBS-AV in circulating serum up to 5 hours following intramuscular administration. Serum concentrations of RBS-AV were detected within 30 minutes of administration following intravenous administration.[25] These results are consistent with animal studies demonstrating little if any effect on circulating venom when antivenoms are given intramuscularly. Additional studies on the pharmacokinetic and pharmacodynamic properties of RBS-AV, Merck Black Widow Antivenom, and F(ab')$_2$ based black widow antivenoms are needed.

ROLE IN *LATRODECTUS* SPECIES (*L. BISHOPI, L. GEOMETRICUS, L. HESPERUS, L. INDISTINCTUS, L. MACTANS, L. VARIOLUS*)

Although black widow bites are associated with severe muscle pain, cramping, and autonomic disturbances, mortality remains low.[7,8,31,34] Symptomatic treatment with muscle relaxants and opioid analgesics is generally effective, although the duration of symptoms following severe envenomation may necessitate hospitalization for 1 to 2 days or more.

The use of Merck BW-AV appears to shorten the length of symptoms dramatically, allowing outpatient care in some cases.[7,31,33,34,40] Studies of reported *Latrodectus*-envenomated patients in Australia, however, demonstrated little clinical difference between *Latrodectus* antivenom and placebo.[20,21] In addition, anaphylaxis and other adverse events following the administration of *Latrodectus* antivenom are reported.[7,20,21,31,32]

Because of low mortality and the potential for adverse events following administration, some authors question the use of BW-AV.[37] We still believe *Latrodectus* antivenom is safe and effective when used appropriately, and recommended it in cases of severe envenomation where muscle cramping, hypertension, diaphoresis, nausea, vomiting, myocardial infarction, or respiratory difficulty are present and appropriate use of opioid analgesia and muscle relaxants are ineffective.[7,9]

Latrodectus antivenom is also reported to successfully treat priapism complicating severe envenomation.[21] Although the safety of antivenom is not clearly established in the developing fetus, pregnancy is a reasonable indication for *Latrodectus* antivenom administration, as the stress of severe pain and muscle cramps may have adverse fetal effects.[4,39]

Antivenoms for a number of *Latrodectus* spiders are available worldwide (Table A37–1). A shortage of Merck BW-AV prompted the finding that antivenom against *L. hasseltii* (RBS-AV) also neutralizes the venom of *L. mactans* in a mouse model.[10] Analatro, a polyvalent F(ab')$_2$, is an equine-derived antivenom created for *L. mactans* in both Argentina and Mexico.

A randomized placebo-controlled multicenter trial of Analatro in the United States demonstrated similar overall reduction of pain between antivenom- and placebo-treated patients. Clinically significant reduction in pain, however, was more rapid with Analatro (30 minutes vs 90 minutes).[12]

In a review of 163 cases of presumed *L. hesperus* and *L. mactans* envenomations, Merck *Latrodectus* antivenom reduced the mean duration of symptoms from 22 to 9 hours. Symptoms usually subsided within 1 to 3 hours of antivenom administration. The hospital admission rate fell from 52% in those who were managed with opioids and muscle relaxants to 12% in those patients receiving antivenom.[8] A more recent review demonstrated immediate resolution of pain following BW-AV administration in suspected *L. mactans* envenomation.[35] Following administration of RBS-AV in redback spider envenomation, however, only 34% of recipients reported significant pain relief at 2 hours.[23]

ROLE IN FUNNEL-WEB SPECIES (*ATRAX* AND *HADRONYCHE*)

A rabbit IgG–based funnel-web spider (*Atrax robustus* and others) antivenom is available in Australia. Since the introduction of the antivenom, no deaths have been reported.[26] Complete response following administration of antivenom was reported in 97% of envenomations in one series.[25]

ROLE IN *LOXOSCELES* SPECIES (*L. RECLUSA, L. LAETA, L. RUFESCENS, L. ARIZONICA, L. UNICOLOR*)

Envenomation by the brown recluse spider *Loxosceles reclusa* is associated with low but significant morbidity, particularly in the midwest and southeast United States. Experimental anti-Loxosceles Fab blocked dermatonecrosis in a rabbit model, but only if provided within 24 to 48 hours of envenomation.[16,37] Although no commercially available antivenom exists in North America for treatment of *Loxosceles* envenomation, antivenom produced against South American *Loxosceles* spiders has cross-reactivity with North American species like *L. reclusa*.[13] The usual late presentation of patients with necrotic lesions from spider bites makes antivenom use for *Loxosceles* difficult to study. National laboratories in Brazil and Argentina produce antivenoms for *L. reclusa, L. boneti,* and *L. rufescens*.[5,13]

ADVERSE EFFECTS AND SAFETY ISSUES

Despite the apparent efficacy of antivenom, the decision to give horse serum for a disease with limited mortality is serious. Death from bronchospasm and anaphylaxis is a rarely reported complication of whole IgG BW-AV (Merck) administration,[8,23,34] as is serum sickness.[9] Serum sickness is dose-dependent and is less likely when the typical dose of one to 2 vials are administered. A detailed review of one case of death following antivenom administration[7] demonstrates that the antivenom was inappropriately prepared (not diluted) and inappropriately administered (intravenous push rather than slow infusion) to a patient with multiple drug allergies, atopy, and asthma. Resuscitation was further complicated by the development of a pneumothorax. A second death[34] was reported in a 37-year-old man with history of asthma who received antivenom as an infusion and developed cardiac arrest as a complication of severe anaphylaxis. He died 40 hours after presentation.[34]

In Australia, antivenom to the redback spider (*L. hasseltii*, CSL Ltd) is made by immunizing horses for production of F(ab')$_2$. Horse-derived F(ab')$_2$ has a lower reported incidence of allergic reactions, with early allergic reactions as infrequent as 0.5% to 0.8%. The incidence of serum sickness is reported at less than 5%.[23,43,44] Analatro, a similar F(ab')$_2$ product, is anticipated to be a safer antivenom than the currently available Merck whole IgG product. No serious adverse effects or deaths were observed in the previously described randomized controlled Analatro trial.[12]

A review of the US National Poison Data System (NPDS) demonstrated a 3.4% rate of adverse drug reactions (ADRs) following administration of the BW-AV.[33] This is consistent with previously reported rates of ADRs following BW-AV administration.[9] Directly attributing complications to administration of antivenom is difficult as these patients received multiple therapies, including opioids, benzodiazepines, and calcium salts preceding

TABLE A37–1	Worldwide Availability of Spider Antivenom
Atrax Species, Hadronyche Species	**Loxosceles Species**
(Funnel Web Spider)	(Brown spiders)
Argentina: Anti Latrodectus Antivenom, Instituto Nacional de Produccion de Biologicos, Equine IgG	Brazil: Antiloxosceles Serum, Centro de Producao e Pesquisas de Immun-biologicos. Equine IgG
Australia: Funnel Web Spider Antivenom, CSL Ltd. Rabbit IgG	Brazil: Soro Antiarachnidico, Instituto Butantan (contains *Loxosceles* spp, *Tityus* spp and *Phoneutria* spp Antivenom), Equine IgG
Latrodectus species	
(Black Widow Spider, Redback Spider)	
Australia: Red-backed spider Antivenom, CSL Ltd. Equine F(ab')$_2$	
Croatia: Antilatrodectus Mactans Tredecimguttatus Serum, Institute of Immunology, Equine IgG	Peru: Antiloxosceles Serum, Instituto Nacional de Salud, Centro Nacional de Production de Biologicos, Equine IgG
Mexico: Aracmyn, Instituto Bioclon, Equine F(ab')$_2$	
South Africa: SAIMR Spider Antivenom, SAIMR, Equine IgG	
USA: Antivenin *Latrodectus mactans*, Merck & Company, Equine IgG	

antivenom administration, and NPDS does not attribute an ADE to a specific therapy. Similarly, the nature of these ADEs is not described in NPDS. However, it is noteworthy that no deaths occurred in 374 instances of use and only 5 patients received antihistamines, suggesting acute hypersensitivity reactions to the Merck BW-AV to be uncommon and that this antivenom is generally safe. Similarly, a review of 96 assessable instances of BW-AV administration over a 10-year period in a single state similarly demonstrated a low rate of adverse reactions. Four patients in the series had adverse effects ascribed to antivenom administration. These reactions were generally mild and included myalgias, fatigue, generalized paresthesias, flushing, and urticarial rash. There were no cases of dyspnea, angioedema, bronchospasm, hypotension, or death.[35] This low rate of severe adverse reactions and lack of death suggests that Merck BW-AV is a safe product when prepared and administered correctly to patients without underlying atopy, asthma, or drug allergies.

PREGNANCY AND LACTATION

Black widow envenomations during pregnancy are relatively rare. In one study of 12,640 patients envenomated by a black widow spider, 97 (3%) were pregnant. When compared with nonpregnant women, no significant differences were observed in recommended or administered treatments including the use of antivenom.[6] There are 6 reported cases of *Loxosceles* envenomations in pregnant women. All were managed with supportive therapy including analgesics, antihistamines, and a short course of low-dose steroids. Pregnancy outcomes were favorable in all reported cases.[2,15] Merck BW-AV is Pregnancy Category C. It is not known whether antivenom is excreted in human milk.

DOSING AND ADMINISTRATION

The starting recommended dose of the Merck antivenom is one vial reconstituted with 2.5 mL sterile water for injection and then diluted in 50 mL of saline for intravenous administration over 15 min. Although BW-AV can also be given intramuscularly, this route carries the disadvantage of slower, more erratic absorption, less control over the rate of administration, and the inability to stop the administration should an allergic reaction occur. In addition, recent studies suggest intramuscular injection of antivenom may not yield significant serum concentrations.[27] For these reasons, the intramuscular route is not routinely recommended.

The initial dose of antivenom in funnel-web spider envenomation is 2 vials in patients with any signs or symptoms of envenomation. Patients with acute respiratory distress syndrome or decreased consciousness should receive 4 vials.[32] The following protocol is recommended for severe cases[32]: 2 vials (each containing 100 mg of rabbit IgG) of antivenom are administered very slowly intravenously. The dose can be repeated in 15 minutes if no improvement occurs. The dose recommended for more severe cases. A rapid response is expected. Repeated administration of antivenom is recommended until symptoms are completely reversed.[14] *Atrax robustus* envenomations are reported to require multiple infusions of antivenom.[14] The recommended dosage for children is the same as for adults.

FORMULATION AND ACQUISITION

Each vial of the Merck BW-AV contains 6,000 antivenom units standardized by biologic mouse assay. Because *Latrodectus* venoms are virtually identical by immunologic and electrophoretic mechanisms, antivenom created for *L. mactans* is presumed to be effective in other species of *Latrodectus* as well.[30]

Latrodectus antivenin is supplied as a white to gray crystalline powder in vials containing not less than 6,000 antivenin units with thimerosal 1:10,000 added as a preservative, along with a 2.5-mL vial of sterile diluent for reconstitution. The antivenin must be stored and shipped at 2°C to 8°C (36°F–46°F), but never frozen. The reconstituted antivenin color ranges from light straw to very dark iced tea, although color has no effect on potency.[2] A 1-mL vial of horse serum (1:10 dilution) for sensitivity testing is also included. We do not recommend utilization.

The Antivenom Index, maintained by the Association of Zoos and Aquariums (https://www.aza.org/antivenom-index/) and accessible by the nation's Poison Control Centers, might also serve as a resource.

SUMMARY

- The decision to use spider antivenom must be individualized to the patient's clinical manifestations.
- Because mortality following black widow envenomation is low, antivenom is reserved for cases in which symptoms are severe or do not respond to other therapies, and after a frank discussion with the patient of possible adverse effects.
- Although a large body of literature suggests that Merck BW-AV is safe when properly prepared and administered to patients without asthma, adverse effects including severe anaphylaxis and death are reported.
- A new, purified $F(ab')_2$ BW-AV is in clinical development, but is currently unavailable.

REFERENCES

1. Anderson PC. Loxoscelism threatening pregnancy; five cases. *Am J Obstet Gynecol.* 1991;165:1454-1456.
2. Antivenin (*Latrodectus mactans*) (Black Widow Spider Antivenin) Equine Origin [package insert]. Whitehouse Station, NJ: Merck & Co, Inc; 2018.
3. Armstrong C. Biologic products. *Public Health Rep.* 1936;51:248.
4. Bailey B. Are there teratogenic risks associated with antidotes used in the acute management of poisoned pregnant women? *Birth Defects Res A Clin Mol Teratol.* 2003;67:133-140.
5. Barbaro KC, et al. Enzymatic characterization, antigenic cross-reactivity and neutralization of dermonecrotic activity of five *Loxosceles* spider venoms of medical importance in the Americas. *Toxicon.* 2005;45:489-499.
6. Brown SA, et al. Management of envenomations during pregnancy. *Clin Toxicol.* 2013;51:3-15.
7. Bush SP, Davy JV. Troponin elevation after black widow spider envenomation. *CJEM.* 2015;17:571-575.
8. Clark RF, et al. Clinical presentation and treatment of black widow spider envenomation: a review of 163 cases. *Ann Emerg Med.* 1992;21:782-787.
9. Clark RF. The safety and efficacy of antivenin *Latrodectus mactans.* *J Toxicol Clin Toxicol.* 2001;39:125-127.
10. Clinical Toxicology Resources. http://www.toxinology.com/. Accessed March 20, 2013.
11. Daly FF, et al. Neutralization of *Latrodectus mactans* and *L. hesperus* venom by redback spider (*L. hasseltii*) antivenom. *J Toxicol Clin Toxicol.* 2001;39:119-123.
12. Dart RC, et al. A randomized, double-blind, placebo-controlled trial of a highly purified equine F(ab)2 antibody black widow spider antivenom. *Ann Emerg Med.* 2013;61:458-467.
13. de Roodt AR, et al. Toxicity of two North American *Loxosceles* (brown recluse spiders) venoms and their neutralization by antivenoms. *Clin Toxicol.* 2007;45:678-687.
14. Dieckmann J, et al. Efficacy of funnel-web spider antivenom in human envenomation by *Hadronyche* species. *Med J Aust.* 1989;151:706-707.
15. Elghblawi E. Loxoscelism in a pregnant woman. *Eur J Dermatol.* 2009;19:289.
16. Gomez HF, et al. Intradermal anti-loxosceles Fab fragments attenuate dermonecrotic arachnidism. *Acad Emerg Med.* 1999;6:1195-1202.
17. Graudins A, et al. Red-back spider (*Latrodectus hasselti*) antivenom prevents the toxicity of widow spider venoms. *Ann Emerg Med.* 2001;37:154-160.
18. Gutierrez JM, et al. Pharmacokinetic-pharmacodynamic relationships of immunoglobulin therapy for envenomation. *Clin Pharmacokinet.* 2003;42:721-741.
19. Heard K, et al. Antivenom therapy in the Americas. *Drugs.* 1999;5-15.
20. Hiller K, et al. Scorpion antivenom administered by alternative infusions. *Ann Emerg Med.* 2010;56:309-310.
21. Hoover NG, Fortenberry JD. Use of antivenin to treat priapism after black widow spider bite. *Pediatrics.* 2004;114:e128-e129.
22. Hoyte CO, et al. Anaphylaxis to black widow spider antivenom. *Am J Emerg Med.* 2012;30:836.e1-836.e2.
23. Isbister GK, et al. Randomized controlled trial of intravenous antivenom versus placebo for latrodectism: the second Redback Antivenom Evaluation (RAVE-II) study. *Ann Emerg Med.* 2014;64:620.e2-628.e2.
24. Isbister GK, et al. A randomized controlled trial of intramuscular vs. intravenous antivenom for latrodectism—the RAVE study. *Q J Med.* 2008;188:473-476.
25. Isbister GK, et al. Funnel-web spider bite: a systematic review of recorded clinical cases. *Med J Aust.* 2005;182:407-411.
26. Isbister GK, et al. Antivenom treatment in Arachnidism. *J Toxicol Clin Toxicol.* 2003;41:291-300.
27. Isbister GK, et al. A comparison of serum antivenom concentrations after intravenous and intramuscular administration of redback (widow) spider antivenom. *Br J Pharmacol.* 2008;65:139-143.
28. Krifi MN, et al. The improvement and standardization of antivenom production in developing countries: comparing antivenom quality therapeutical efficiency and cost. *J Venom Anim Toxins.* 1999;5:128-141.

29. Krifi MN, et al. Pharmacokinetic studies of scorpion venom before and after antivenom immunotherapy. *Toxicon.* 2005;45:187-198.

30. McCrone JD, Netzcoff ML. An immunological and electrophoretical comparison of the venoms of the North American *Latrodectus* spiders. *Toxicon.* 1965;3:107-110.

31. Meddeb-Mouelhi F, et al. Immunized camel sera and derived immunoglobulin subclasses neutralizing *Androctonus australis hector* scorpion toxins. *Toxicon.* 2003;42:785-791.

32. Miller MK, et al. Clinical features and management of *Hadronyche* envenomation in man. *Toxicon.* 2000:38:409-427.

33. Monte AA, et al. A US perspective of symptomatic *Latrodectus* spp. envenomation and treatment: a National Poison Data System review. *Ann Pharmacother.* 2011;45:1491-1498.

34. Murphy CM, et al. Anaphylaxis with *Latrodectus* antivenin resulting in cardiac arrest. *J Med Toxicol.* 2011;7:317-321.

35. Nordt SP, et al. Examination of adverse events following black widow antivenom use in California. *Clin Toxicol.* 2012;50:70-73.

36. O'Malley GF, et al. Successful treatment of latrodectism with antivenin after 90 hours. *N Engl J Med.* 1999;340:657.

37. Rees R, et al. The diagnosis and treatment of brown recluse spider bites. *Ann Emerg Med.* 1987;16:945-949.

38. Rivière G, et al. Effect of antivenom on venom pharmacokinetics in experimentally envenomed rabbits: toward an optimization of antivenom therapy. *J Pharmacol Exp Ther.* 1997;281:1-8.

39. Robertson WO. Black widow spider case. *Am J Emerg Med.* 1997;15:211.

40. Rojas A, et al. Role of the animal model on the pharmacokinetics of equine-derived antivenoms. *Toxicon.* 2013;70C:9-14.

41. Russell FE, et al. Black widow spider envenomation during pregnancy. *Toxicon.* 1979; 17:188-189.

42. Suntorntham S, et al. Dramatic clinical response to the delayed administration of black widow spider antivenom. *Ann Emerg Med.* 1994;24:1198-1199.

43. Sutherland SK, Trinca JC. Survey of 2144 cases of red back spider bites: Australia and New Zealand, 1963–1976. *Med J Aust.* 1978;2:620-623.

44. Sutherland SK. Antivenom use in Australia. Premedication, adverse reactions and the use of venom detection kits. *Med J Aust.* 1992;157:734-739.

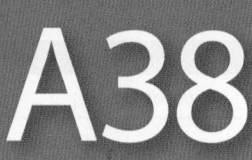

ANTIVENOM: SCORPION

Michael A. Darracq and Richard F. Clark

INTRODUCTION

Centruroides exilicauda (formerly known as *Centruroides sculpturatus*) is the only scorpion of medical importance in the United States. It is indigenous to the deserts of Arizona, but also can be found in Texas, New Mexico, California, and Nevada.[10] Occasionally, envenomations occur in nonindigenous areas of the country from "stowaway" scorpions in travelers' luggage.[34]

HISTORY

Poison control centers in Arizona receive several thousand calls annually for scorpion stings. Although the incidence of morbidity with these envenomations is significant, no deaths associated with the toxic effects of scorpion venom have been reported in the United States for almost 50 years. Antivenom for the *Centruroides* spp was first produced in horses in Mexico in the 1930s.[12] In 1947, antivenom was produced from rabbits and cats immunized with *C. sculpturatus* and *C. gertschi*.[31] The Antivenom Production Laboratory at Arizona State University (APL-ASU) began producing antivenom to *C. sculpturatus* in goats in 1965. This antivenom was used for treatment of scorpion stings in Arizona until 2004, when production ceased and stockpiles expired. In June 2000, Silanes Laboratory received orphan drug status for a *C.* scorpion antivenom, an equine F(ab')$_2$ derived from *C. limpidus*, *C. noxius*, *C. suffusus*, and *C. meisei* (formerly known as *C. elegans*) manufactured by Instituto Bioclon of Mexico, and sold as Anascorp. In August 2011, Anascorp was approved by the US Food and Drug Administration (FDA) for the treatment of *C. exilicauda* envenomations.[16]

PHARMACOLOGY

Antivenom for scorpions is prepared in the same manner as other antivenom products (Antidotes in Depth: A37 and A39).

Pharmacokinetics and Pharmacodynamics

In a study of 8 healthy patients (6 males and 2 females, age 17–26 years) without prior scorpion envenomation, an intravenous bolus dose of 47.5 mg of Anascorp was administered. Serial blood samples were collected over 21 days. Measured pharmacokinetic parameters (mean ± standard deviation) included area under the curve (AUC), 706 ± 352 mcg/mL; clearance, 83.5 ± 38.4 mL/h; half-life, 159 ± 57 hours; and steady-state volume of distribution (V$_{dss}$), 13.6 ± 5.4 L.[35]

ROLE IN CENTRUROIDES SPECIES

One vial of Anascorp antivenom contains sufficient F(ab')$_2$ to neutralize 150 mouse LD$_{50}$ of *Centruroides* venom.[26] Safety and efficacy are documented in both animals and humans.[1,8-10] In the FDA review and subsequent approval of Anascorp, 6 trials were submitted for evaluation. Only one study was prospective, randomized, double-blinded, and controlled. It demonstrated a clear benefit in reduction of signs and symptoms of scorpion envenomation by 4 hours post-administration (8/8 vs 1/7), reduction in quantity of sedative administered (mean midazolam dose of 0.1 mg/kg (0.0–0.2 mg/kg) in treated patients versus 4.6 mg/kg (0.1–16.7 mg/kg) in controls. It absence of free serum venom concentrations at one hour after administration (mean 0.0 in treated vs 2.65 ng/mL in controls).[8]

One retrospective trial using historical controls was included as representative of clinical outcomes in the absence of antivenom administration.

This trial demonstrated the need for exceedingly large dose of sedatives to treat the inability to walk and respiratory distress due to envenomation with a mean time to discharge of 12.6 hours without administration of scorpion antivenom.[12]

One large (n = 1,534), unpublished and open-label study was also included for review. The majority (1,204/1,534) of patients were children (0.7 months–18 years) and male (52.3%). In 1,396/1,425 patients, the mean time to resolution of clinically important signs of envenomation following Anascorp administration was 1.42 hours (0.2–20.5 hours). Children reportedly improved slightly faster than adults (1.28 ± 0.8 hours vs 1.91 ± 1.4 hours). Of the 1,534 patients included in the study, 95% had relief of systemic signs associated with *Centruroides* envenomation within 4 hours of Anascorp administration.[9,15]

Three additional open-label trials (AL-02/04-adult patients, AL-02/05-pediatric patients, and AL-02/06-pediatric patients) with the use of the Instituto Bioclon of Mexico product Alacramyn (Alacramyn is the Mexican equivalent of Anascorp) were reported by the study sponsors to demonstrate 100% resolution of symptoms by 4 hours following administration of antivenom.[15]

Because of the high cost of Anascorp ($3,750), some hospitals have adopted guidelines advocating for single-vial initial dose rather than the FDA-approved 3-vial initial dose. A more recent retrospective cohort of grade III or IV pediatric *Centruroides* envenomations comparing treatment with supportive care including benzodiazepines and opioids for agitation and pain, FDA approved dosing, and one- to 2-vial initial dose demonstrated no significant difference in emergency department lengths of stay or outcomes between groups. Clinical presentation however appeared to influence treatment as patients receiving antivenom had a higher envenomation grade than those receiving supportive care alone, and the 3-vial initial dose group was younger and had more respiratory distress than those receiving one- to 2-vial initial dose.[11]

ROLE IN *LEIURUS* SPECIES

The *Leiurus quinquestriatus* scorpion is indigenous to Africa, Asia, and the Middle East, including Egypt, Israel, Jordan, Kuwait, Lebanon, Oman, Qatar, Saudi Arabia, Syria, and Turkey. Antivenom to *L. quinquestriatus* is currently made in France, Germany, Israel, Saudi Arabia, Egypt, Tunisia, and Turkey (Table A38–1).

In observational studies, an intravenous infusion of 5 to 20 mL of *Leiurus* antivenom was needed to control venom effects, and only patients given antivenom within the first several hours demonstrated significant benefit.[2,21] The rate of allergic reactions for the Turkish antiscorpion antivenom is reported to be 1.6% to 6.6%.[21] The recommended dose of the Israeli *L. quinquestriatus* antivenom is 5 to 15 mL for intravenous use, although several authors report lack of clinical efficacy of this particular antivenom.[6,17,32]

Leiurus quinquestriatus antivenom was successfully used to treat a 2-year-old boy with envenomation by *Androctonus crassicauda*. Symptoms resolved 2 hours after antivenom administration.[30]

ROLE IN *TITYUS* SPECIES

Tityus species of scorpions are endemic to South America, particularly Brazil. An F(ab')$_2$ antivenom for *Tityus serrulatus* is available from Fundação Ezequiel Dias (FUNED), in Belo Horizonte, Brazil. The usual dose of the antivenom is 20 mL as an intravenous infusion.[14]

TABLE A38–1	**Worldwide Scorpion Antivenoms**			
Species	*Country*	*Name*	*Manufacturer*	*Antibody Type*
***Centruroides* species**				
(elegans, exilicauda, gertschi, limpidus, noxius, suffusus)	Mexico	Suero Antialacran Alacramyn	Instituto Bioclon	Equine F(ab′)$_2$
	United States	Anascorp Centruroides (Scorpion) Immune F(ab′)$_2$	Instituto Bioclon	Equine F(ab′)$_2$
***Androctonus* species**				
	Algeria	Antiscorpion Serum	Institut Pasteur d'Algerie	Equine F(ab′)$_2$
	Egypt	Purified Polyvalent Antiscorpion Serum	Egyptian Organization for Biological Products and Vaccines (VACSERA)	Equine F(ab′)$_2$
	France	ScorpiFAV	Aventis Pasteur	Equine F(ab′)$_2$
	Germany	Scorpion Antivenom	Twyford	Equine F(ab′)$_2$
	Iran	Polyvalent Scorpion Antivenom	Razi Vaccine and Serum Research Institute	Equine F(ab′)$_2$
	Tunisia	Scorpion Antivenom	Institut Pasteur de Tunis	Equine F(ab′)$_2$
	Turkey	Scorpion Antivenom	Refik Saydam Hygiene Center	Equine F(ab′)$_2$
***Buthus* species**				
	Algeria	Antiscorpion Serum	Institut Pasteur d'Algerie	Equine F(ab′)$_2$
	Egypt	Purified Polyvalent Antiscorpion Serum	VACSERA	Equine F(ab′)$_2$
	France	ScorpiFAV	Aventis Pasteur	Equine F(ab′)$_2$
	Germany	Scorpion Antivenom	Twyford	Equine F(ab′)$_2$
	India	Scorpion Venom	Haffkine Biopharmaceutical	Equine F(ab′)$_2$
	Saudi Arabia	Polyvalent Scorpion Antivenom	National Antivenom and Vaccine Production Center (NAVPC)	Equine F(ab′)$_2$
	Tunisia	Scorpion Antivenom	Institut Pasteur de Tunis	Equine F(ab′)$_2$
***Leiurus* species**				
	Egypt	Purified Polyvalent Antiscorpion Serum	VACSERA	Equine F(ab′)$_2$
	France	ScorpiFAV	Aventis Pasteur	Equine F(ab′)$_2$
	Saudi Arabia	Polyvalent Scorpion	NAVPC	Equine F(ab′)$_2$
	Tunisia	Scorpion Antivenom	Institut Pasteur de Tunis	Equine F(ab′)$_2$
	Turkey	Scorpion Antivenom	Refik Saydam Hygiene Center	Equine F(ab′)$_2$
***Mesobuthus* species**				
	India	Monovalent Scorpion Antivenom	Central Research Institute	Equine F(ab′)$_2$
	Iran	Polyvalent Scorpion Antivenom	Razi Vaccine and Serum Research Institute	Equine F(ab′)$_2$
Odontobuthus doriae				
	Iran	Polyvalent Scorpion Antivenom	Razi Vaccine and Serum Research Institute	Equine F(ab′)$_2$
***Palamnaeus* species**				
	India	Monovalent Scorpion Antivenom	Central Research Institute	Equine F(ab′)$_2$
***Parabuthus* species**				
	South Africa	SAIMR Scorpion Antivenom	South African Vaccine Producers	Equine F(ab′)$_2$
Scorpio maurus				
	Egypt	Purified Polyvalent Antiscorpion Serum	VACSERA	Equine F(ab′)$_2$
	France	ScorpiFAV	Aventis Pasteur	Equine F(ab′)$_2$
	Iran	Polyvalent Scorpion Antivenom	Razi Vaccine and Serum Research Institute	Equine F(ab′)$_2$
	Turkey	Scorpion Antivenom	Refik Saydam Hygiene Center	Equine F(ab′)$_2$

(Continued)

TABLE A38–1	Worldwide Scorpion Antivenoms (*Continued*)			
Species	Country	Name	Manufacturer	Antibody Type
Tityus species				
	Argentina	Scorpion Antivenom	Instituto Nacional	Equine Fab
	Brazil	Soro Antiscorpionico	Instituto Butantan	Equine Sera
	Brazil	Soro Antiarachnidico	Instituto Butantan,	Equine IgG (*antivenom, Loxosceles sp, Phoneutria sp, and Tityus sp*)
	Brazil	Antiscorpion Serum IVB	Instituto Vital Brazil S.A.	Equine IgG
	Brazil	Antiescopionico	Fundacao Ezequiel Dias	Equine F(ab')$_2$

In a series of 18 patients with *T. serrulatus* envenomation treated with antivenom, vomiting and local pain decreased within one hour, and cardiorespiratory manifestations disappeared within 6 to 24 hours in all patients except the 2 presenting with acute respiratory distress syndrome.[14] Sixteen patients recovered completely by 24 hours. The Instituto Buntantan in Brazil also produces Soro antiarachnidico and Soro antiscorpionico for treatment of *Tityus* spp.

Role in *Androctonus* Species

Scorpion antivenom in South Africa is an equine-derived antivenom available from the South African Vaccine Producers, formerly South African Institute for Medical Research (SAIMR), Johannesburg, South Africa. Scorpi-FAV, produced by Aventis Pasteur, is produced for treatment of *Androctonus* spp, *Buthus occitanus*, and *L. quinquestriatus*.

Buthus tamulus monovalent red scorpion antivenom serum produced by Central Research Institute of India is an equine-derived lyophilized antivenom for the venom of *Mesobuthus tamulus*. The manufacturer recommends a dosage of one vial, although a dose of 5 vials significantly decreased mortality in one study.[23,33]

Prazosin has also been used in the treatment of children with *Buthus tamulus* envenomation in Southern India. The addition of monovalent scorpion antivenom reduced the duration of clinical symptoms (sweating, salivation, cool extremities, priapism, hypertension or hypotension, tachycardia), percentage of children deteriorating into more severe symptoms, and the mean dose of prazosin received when compared with prazosin treatment alone.[4,28]

In Pakistan, the treatment of scorpion stings was modified in 1991 to include the administration of 5 vials of antivenom. A retrospective case series of 950 patients treated with and without antivenom was compared to 968 cases treated after the 5 vial protocol was initiated. A statistically significant decrease in mortality was demonstrated. The last recorded death in Pakistan resulting from a scorpion sting occurred in 1991 in a patient who did not receive antivenom.[33]

Parabuthus spp antivenom from South African Vaccine Producers is an equine-derived antivenom to *Parabuthus* spp. In one study, antivenom was unavailable for a period of time allowing for a unique design of matched pair of patients. Patients who received antivenom had a significant decrease in hospital stay after receiving one (5-mL) vial. Pain, hypersalivation, fasciculations, tremor, and bladder distension responded best to antivenom, whereas dysphagia, ptosis, and local swelling were more resistant.[7]

The unavailability of specific antivenoms often necessitates symptomatic treatment or use of a comparable foreign antivenom. In a study of 72 moderate scorpion stings in Para, Brazil, 33% of patients did not receive treatment because of unavailability of the antivenom.[29]

ADVERSE EFFECTS AND SAFETY ISSUES

Hypersensitivity reactions to Anascorp and other equine-derived antivenoms occasionally occur following administration. Adverse effects reported from cumulative clinical trial data revealed that 2.2% of patients experienced severe adverse reactions (respiratory distress, aspiration, hypoxia, ataxia, pneumonia, and eye swelling) following Anascorp administration. However, these symptoms occurred in the setting of acute *Centruroides* envenomation, limiting the direct attribution of symptoms to antivenom administration alone. The most common adverse effects reported included vomiting (4.7%), pyrexia (4.1%), rash (2.7%), nausea (2.1%), and pruritus (2%).[13] No deaths were reported in clinical trials of Anascorp. The presence of cresol as an injectable excipient may increase localized reactions and generalized myalgias following administration. Patients with known equine protein allergies or previous exposure to Anascorp or other equine-derived antivenoms or antitoxins may also be at increased risk because of previous sensitization. No drug interaction studies have been conducted with Anascorp.

PREGNANCY AND LACTATION

Anascorp is Pregnancy Category C. Animal reproduction studies have not been conducted, and it is unknown whether Anascorp causes fetal harm when administered to pregnant women. Reproductive capability postadministration similarly has not been assessed. Anascorp should only be administered in pregnant women if clearly needed for alleviation of symptoms and after other therapies have been utilized. It is unknown whether Anascorp is excreted in human breast milk.[13]

DOSING AND ADMINISTRATION

Anascorp is the only FDA–approved treatment for the clinical signs and symptoms of *Centruroides* scorpion envenomation. These include, but are not limited to, loss of motor control, roving or abnormal eye movements, slurred speech, respiratory depression, and excessive oral secretions. Package insert dosing recommendations (FDA) are 3 vials administered intravenously over 10 minutes after reconstitution (5 mL sterile 0.9% sodium chloride solution/vial) and dilution to a total volume of 50 mL; thereafter administer one additional vial at a time at 30- to 60-minute intervals as needed for symptom control. Do not use if the solution is turbid.

A cost-effectiveness study of Anascorp demonstrated a mean cost $10,708 (95% CI $10,556–$11,010) when antivenom was used as compared to a mean cost without scorpion antivenom of $3,178 (95% CI $1,627–$5,184). The mean success rate was 99.87% (95% CI 99.64%–99.98%) with scorpion antivenom and 94.31% (95% CI 91.10%–96.61%) without scorpion antivenom. These data suggest a very high rate of success with antivenom but at a very high cost. The authors of this study conclude that at current cost, scorpion antivenom in the United States cannot be justified for use in most clinical situations and is not cost-effective.[3]

FORMULATION AND ACQUISITION

Anascorp is supplied as a sterile lyophilized preparation in a single-use vial. When reconstituted, each vial contains not more than 24 mg per milliliter of protein, and not less than 150 mouse LD$_{50}$ neutralizing units. Anascorp should not be frozen, but stored at room temperature up to 25°C (77°F).[15]

The Antivenom Index, maintained by the Association of Zoos and Aquariums (https://www.aza.org/antivenom-index/) and accessible by the nation's Poison Control Centers, may serve as a resource in the event of difficulty obtaining antivenom. The World Health Organization's World Directory of Poison Control Centres (http://www.who.int/gho/phe/chemical_safety/poisons_centres/en/) might assist those outside of the United States to source more exotic antivenoms.

SUMMARY

- The indications for antivenom administration following scorpion stings remain controversial, in large part because of the current cost of the product.
- The decision to use antivenom should be individualized to the patient, weighing the risk of giving an immune serum, the level of available supportive care, the risks and costs of supportive care alone, and the cost of obtaining or importing antivenom.
- Scorpion antivenom administration for some species may not improve outcome.
- The preferred route of administration of these products is intravenous. The current FDA approved dosing for Anascorp is 3 vials to initiate therapy, followed by additional doses to alleviate symptoms.

REFERENCES

1. Alagon CA, Gonzalez JC. De la seroterapia a la faboterapia. *Foro Silanes.* 1998;2:8-9.
2. Amitai Y, et al. Scorpion sting in children: a review of 51 cases. *Clin Pediatr (Phila).* 1985;24:136-140.
3. Armstrong EP, et al. Is scorpion antivenom cost-effective as marketed in the United States? *Toxicon.* 2013;76:394-398.
4. Bawaskar HS, Bawaskar PH. Efficacy and safety of scorpion antivenom plus prazosin compared with prazosin alone for venomous scorpion (*Mesobuthus tamulus*) sting: randomised open label clinical trial. *BMJ.* 2011;342:c7136.
5. Bawaskar HS, Bawaskar PH. Utility of scorpion antivenin vs. prazosin in the management of severe *Mesobuthus tamulus* (Indian red scorpion) envenoming at rural setting. *J Assoc Physicians India.* 2007;55:14-21.
6. Belghith M, et al. Efficacy of serotherapy in scorpion sting: a matched-pair study. *J Toxicol Clin Toxicol.* 1999;37:51-57.
7. Bergman NJ. Clinical description of *Parabuthus transvaalicus* scorpionism in Zimbabwe. *Toxicon.* 1997;35:759-771.
8. Boyer LV, et al. Antivenom for critically ill children with neurotoxicity from scorpion stings. *N Engl J Med.* 2009;360:2090-2098.
9. Boyer LV, et al. Effectiveness of Centruroides scorpion antivenom compared to historical controls. *Toxicon.* 2013;76:377-385.
10. Calderon-Aranda ES, et al. Pharmacokinetics of the toxic fraction of *Centruroides limpidus limpidus* venom in experimentally envenomed rabbits and effects of immunotherapy with specific F(ab')₂. *Toxicon.* 1999;37:771-782.
11. Coorg V, et al. Clinical presentation and outcomes associated with different treatment modalities for pediatric bark scorpion envenomation. *J Med Toxicol.* 2017;13:66-70.
12. Curry SC, et al. Envenomation by the scorpion *Centruroides sculpturatus. J Toxicol Clin Toxicol.* 1984;21:417-449.
13. Daly FF, et al. Neutralization of *Latrodectus mactans* and *L. hesperus* venom by redback spider (*L. hasseltii*) antivenom. *J Toxicol Clin Toxicol.* 2001;39:119-123.
14. De Rezende NA, et al. Efficacy of antivenom therapy for neutralizing circulating venom antigens in patients stung by *Tityus serrulatus* scorpions. *Am J Trop Med Hyg.* 1995;52:277-280.
15. Food and Drug Administration (FDA): Anascorp® (Centruroides immune F(ab')₂ equine) Prescribing information. (2011). http://www.fda.gov/downloads/BiologicsBloodVaccines/BloodBloodProducts/ApprovedProducts/LicensedProductsBLAs/FractionatedPlasmaProducts/UCM266725.pdf. Accessed March 20, 2013.
16. Food and Drug Administration (FDA): FDA approves the first specific treatment for scorpion stings. http://www.fda.gov/NewsEvents/Newsroom/PressAnnouncements/ucm26611.htm. Accessed March 20, 2013.
17. Gueron M, Yaron R. Cardiovascular manifestations of severe scorpion sting. Clinicopathologic correlation. *Chest.* 1970;57:156-162.
18. Gutierrez JM, et al. Pharmacokinetic-pharmacodynamic relationships of immunoglobulin therapy for envenomation. *Clin Pharmacokinet.* 2003;42:721-741.
19. Heard K, et al. Antivenom therapy in the Americas. *Drugs.* 1999;585-595.
20. Ismail M, et al. Pharmacokinetics of ¹²⁵I-labelled *Walterinnesia aegyptia* venom and its distribution of the venom and its toxin versus slow absorption and distribution of IGG, F(AB')2 and F(AB) of the antivenin. *Toxicon.* 1998;36:93-114.
21. Ismail M. The treatment of the scorpion envenoming syndrome: the Saudi experience with serotherapy. *Toxicon.* 19994;32:1019-1026.
22. Krifi MN, et al. Effects of antivenom on *Buthus occitanus tunetanus* (Bot) scorpion venom pharmacokinetics: towards an optimization of antivenom immunotherapy in a rabbit model. *Toxicon.* 2001;39:1317-1326.
23. Krifi MN, et al. Evaluation of antivenom therapy in children severely envenomed by *Androctonus australis garzonii* (Aag) and *Buthus occitanus tunetanus* (Bot) scorpions. *Toxicon.* 1999;37:1627-1634.
24. Krifi MN, et al. The improvement and standardization of antivenom production in developing countries: comparing antivenom quality therapeutical efficiency and cost. *J Venom Anim Toxins.* 1999;5:128-141.
25. Meddeb-Mouelhi F, et al. Immunized camel sera and derived immunoglobulin subclasses neutralizing *Androctonus australis hector* scorpion toxins. *Toxicon.* 2003;42:785-791.
26. *Mexican Pharmacopeia*, 6th ed. 1994;163-164.
27. Natu VS, et al. Efficacy of species specific anti-scorpion venom serum (AScVS) against severe, serious scorpion stings (*Mesobuthus tamulus concanesis* Pocock)—an experience from rural hospital in western Maharashtra. *J Assoc Physicians India.* 2006;54:283-287.
28. Pandi K, et al. Efficacy of scorpion antivenom plus prazosin versus prazosin alone for *Mesobuthus tamulus* scorpion sting envenomation in children: a randomised controlled trial. *Arch Dis Child.* 2014;99:575-580.
29. Pardal PP, et al. Epidemiological and clinical aspects of scorpion envenomation in the region of Santarem, Para, Brazil. *Rev Soc Bras Med Trop.* 2003;36:349-353.
30. Pomeranz A, et al. Scorpion sting: successful treatment with nonhomologous antivenin. *Isr J Med Sci.* 1984;20:451-452.
31. Schnur L, Schnur P. A case of allergy to scorpion antivenin. *Ariz Med.* 1968;25:413-414.
32. Sofer S, Gueron M. Respiratory failure in children following envenomation by the scorpion *Leiurus quinquestriatus*: hemodynamic and neurological aspects. *Toxicon.* 1988;26:931-939.
33. Soomro RM, et al. A clinical evaluation of the effectiveness of anti-venom in scorpion envenomation. *J Coll Physicians Surg Pak.* 2001;11:297-299.
34. Trestrail JH. Scorpion envenomation in Michigan: Three cases of toxic encounters with poisonous stowaways. *Vet Hum Toxicol.* 1981;23:8-11.
35. Vazquez H, et al. Pharmacokinetics of a F(ab')₂ scorpion antivenom in healthy human volunteers. *Toxicon.* 2005;46:797-805.

116 MARINE ENVENOMATIONS

Eike Blohm and D. Eric Brush

Human contact with venomous marine creatures is common, with serious harm resulting from biological toxins or mechanical injury inflicted by the stinging apparatus. Envenomation occurs from both vertebrate and invertebrate animals. Venomous invertebrates include the phylum Cnidaria (jellyfish, anemones), Mollusca (snails, octopods), and Echinodermata (sea stars, sea urchins). Sea snakes and spiny fish are the common venomous vertebrates.

Our knowledge of the pathophysiology related to clinical syndromes in humans and the optimal therapies for human envenomation remain limited. Evidence for effective treatment is primarily derived from in vitro and in vivo animal research with few randomized controlled human trials. However, current research in toxinology coupled with clinical observations allows the development of cogent treatment guidelines for victims of marine envenomation.

INVERTEBRATES

Cnidaria

The phylum Cnidaria (formerly Coelenterata) originated in the Ediacaran period more than 750 million years ago and includes more than 9,000 species, of which approximately 100 are known to injure humans. Commonly referred to as jellyfish, they are the oldest lineage of venomous animals; however, their phylogenetic designations separate "true jellyfish" and other organisms into distinct classes (Table 116–1; Fig. 116–1A, B).

All species possess microscopic cnidae (the Greek *knide* means nettle), which are highly specialized organelles consisting of an encapsulated hollow barbed thread bathed in venom. Thousands of these stinging organelles, called nematocysts (or cnidocysts), are distributed along tentacles. A trigger mechanism called a cnidocil regulates nematocyst discharge. Pressure from contact with a victim's skin, or chemical triggers such as osmotic change, stimulates discharge of the thread and toxin from its casing.[140] Although all Cnidaria feature cnidae, only those whose barbed thread can penetrate the human epidermis for intradermal venom delivery to inflict injury. Among these are members of the subphylum Cubozoa (sea wasp, Irukandji jellyfish), Hydrozoa (Portuguese man-of-war, bluebottle), Scyphozoa (sea nettle, mauve stinger), and a class of Anthozoa (anemones) (Fig. 116–2).

Cubozoa

Members of Cubozoa are not true jellyfish. Animals of this subphylum have a cube-shaped bell with 4 corners, each supporting between 1 and 15 tentacles. Cubozoa species produce the greatest morbidity and mortality of all Cnidaria. The subphylum comprises 2 main families of toxicologic importance: Chirodropidae and Carybdeidae.

The Chirodropidae family is well known for the sea wasp (*Chironex fleckeri*, Greek *cheiro* means hand, Latin *nex* means death; therefore, "assassin's hand"). When full grown, the bell of the sea wasp, a type of box jellyfish, measures 25 to 30 cm in diameter and 15 tentacles are attached at each "corner" of the bell. These tentacles extend up to 3 m in length.

The Carybdeidae family is most notable for the Irukandji jellyfish (*Carukia barnesi*).[59] Its small size, with a bell diameter of only 2.5 cm, limits detection in open waters. Along with the common kingslayer (*Malo kingi*), the Irukandji jellyfish is known to cause Irukandji syndrome in its victims.

Hydrozoa

Members of the Hydrozoa class are also not true jellyfish. The order Siphonophorae (Physaliidae family) includes 2 unusual creatures of toxicologic concern: *Physalia physalis*, the Portuguese man-of-war, and its smaller counterpart, *Physalia utriculus*, the bluebottle. They are pelagic (floating) colonial Hydrozoa, meaning one "jellyfish" is actually a colony of multiple specialized animals (zooids) in a formed mass. The easily recognizable pneumatophore (blue sail) that floats above the surface of the water is filled with up to 13% carbon monoxide, 15% to 20% oxygen, and nitrogen for the remaining partial pressure.[164] Tentacles of *P. physalis* reach lengths exceeding 30 m and contain more than 750,000 nematocysts in each of its numerous tentacles (up to 40). *Physalia utriculus* has only one tentacle that measures up to 15 m.

The Anthomedusae order includes the sessile *Millepora alcicornis* (fire coral) that exists as a fixed colony of hydroids. It appears much like true coral and has a white to yellow-green lime carbonate exoskeleton. Small nematocyst-containing tentacles protrude through minute surface gastropores. The overall structure ranges from 10 cm to 2 m.

TABLE 116–1	Characteristics of Common Cnidaria	
Latin Name	*Common Name*	*Common Habitat (Coastal Waters)*
Cubozoa class		
Chironex fleckeri[a]	Sea wasp	Tropical Pacific Ocean, Indian Ocean, Gulf of Oman
Carukia barnesi[a]	Irukandji jellyfish	North Australian
Chiropsalmus spp[a]	Sea wasp or fire medusa	North Australian, Philippines, Japan, Indian Ocean, Gulf of Mexico, Caribbean
Chiropsalmus quadrigatus	Box jellyfish	
Chiropsalmus quadrumanus	Box jellyfish	
Carybdea alata	Hawaiian box jellyfish	Hawaii
Carybdea rastoni	Jimble	Australia
Hydrozoa class		
Physalia physalis[a]	Portuguese man-of-war	Eastern US from Florida to North Carolina, Gulf of Mexico, Australia (rare reports)
Physalia utriculus	Bluebottle	Tropical Pacific Ocean, particularly Australia
Millepora alcicornis	Fire coral	Widespread in tropical waters, including Caribbean
Scyphozoa class		
Chrysaora quinquecirrha	Sea nettle	Chesapeake Bay, widely distributed in temperate and tropical waters
Stomolophus meleagris	Cabbage head or cannonball jellyfish	Gulf of Mexico, Caribbean
Stomolophus nomurai[a]	Lion's mane	Yellow Sea between China and South Korea
Cyanea capillata	Lion's mane or hair jellyfish	Northwest US to Arctic Sea, Norway and Great Britain, Australia
Pelagia noctiluca	Mauve stinger or purple-striped jellyfish	Wide distribution in tropical zones
Linuche unguiculata	Thimble jellyfish	Florida, Mexico, and Caribbean
Anthozoa[b] class		
Anemonia sulcata	European stinging anemone	Eastern Atlantic, Mediterranean, Adriatic Sea
Actinodendron plumosum	Hell's fire anemone	South Pacific
Actinia equina	Beadlet anemone	Great Britain, Ireland

[a]Well-documented human fatalities.

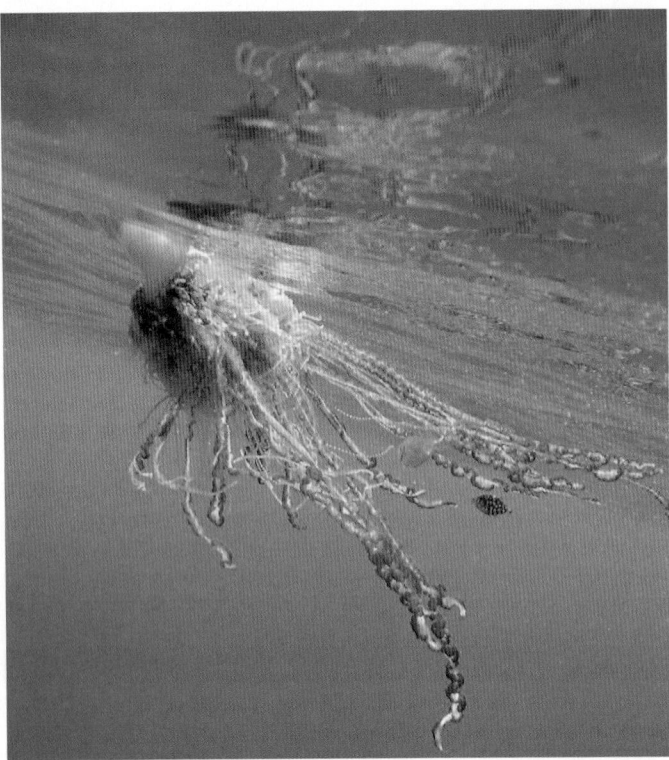

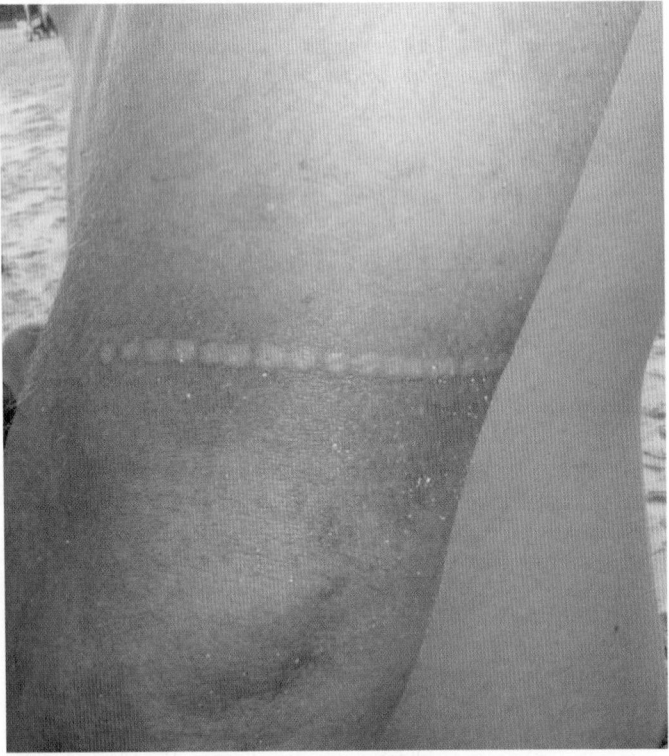

FIGURE 116–1. (**A**) North Atlantic Portuguese man-of-war *Physalia physalis* with multiple tentacles dangling in the water. The tentacles filled with venomous nematocysts extend several meters in length. *(Reproduced with permission from Knoop KJ, Stack LB, Storrow AB, et al. The Atlas of Emergency Medicine, 3rd ed. New York, NY: McGraw-Hill Inc; 2010. Photo contributor: Adam Laverty.)* (**B**) Linear eruption from contact with an unidentified jellyfish in the South Atlantic Ocean. *(Used with permission from David Goldfarb.)*

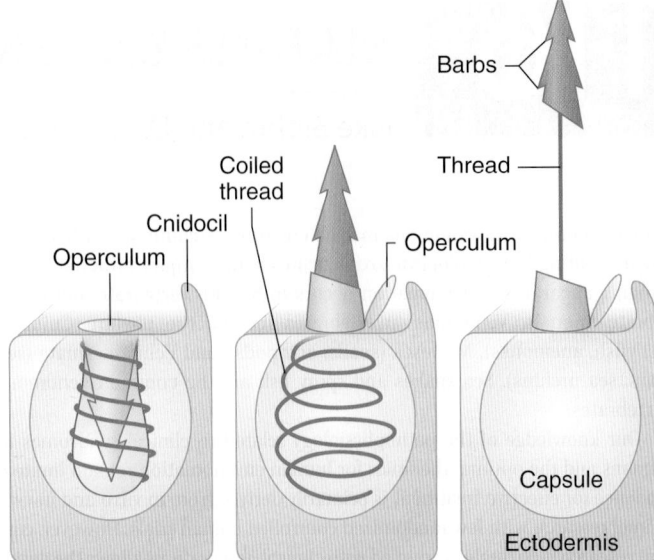

FIGURE 116–2. The structure and function of the nematocyst of the jellyfish (Cnidaria). The barbed thread rests inverted and spring-loaded in the nematocyst, which measures approximately 10–20 μm. Upon mechanical or osmotic stimulation of the trigger mechanism (called the cnidocil), the hinged operculum places the barb in its upright position and the thread uncoils, propelling itself outward. Venom stored in the capsule flows through the thread into the victim's tissue.

Scyphozoa

True jellyfish belong to the class Scyphozoa and are extremely diverse in size, shape, and color. Common varieties known to envenomate humans are *Cyanea capillata* (lion's mane or hair jelly), *Chrysaora quinquecirrha* (sea nettle), and *Pelagia noctiluca* (mauve stinger). The mauve stinger is easily recognized; it appears pink in daylight and phosphorescent at night. Larvae of *Linuche unguiculata* cause seabather's eruption (SBE).

Anthozoa

The Anthozoa class of Cnidaria does not feature a medusa ("jellyfish") stage in its life cycle and is thus marked by sessility. Its diverse membership includes true corals, soft corals, and anemones. Only the anemones are of toxicologic importance. They are common inhabitants of reefs and tide pools and attach themselves to rock or coral. Armed with modified nematocysts known as *sporocysts* and *basitrichous isorhiza* located on their tentacles, they produce stings similar to those of organisms from other Cnidaria classes.

Cnidaria common to the United States include the Portuguese man-of-war and sea nettle. Other species are widely distributed throughout the tropical and temperate waters of the globe (Table 116–1). Locations with documented Cnidaria-related deaths include the United States (Florida, North Carolina, Texas), Australia, the Indo-Pacific region (Malaysia, Langkawi Islands, Philippines, Solomon Islands, Papua New Guinea), and the coast of China. Since 1884, approximately 70 deaths in Australia are attributed to *C. fleckeri*. An estimated 2 to 3 deaths per year occur in Malaysia from contact with unknown species. Approximately 20 to 40 deaths are reported yearly in the Philippines from unidentified species of the Chirodropidae family. Three deaths are well documented from *P. physalis* in the United States (Florida, North Carolina). One death from *Chiropsalmus quadrumanus* occurred along the coast of Texas. Eight fatalities in the Bohai waters of China (Yellow Sea) are reported from *Stomolophus nomurai*. Although Chirodropidae are found off the western coast of Africa, no fatalities in that region are documented.

Cnidaria Dermatitis

Epidemiology

Stings from Cnidaria and subsequent dermal eruptions represent the overwhelming majority of marine envenomations. In Australia, approximately

10,000 stings per year are recorded from *Physalia* spp alone.[55] Most *Cnidaria* stings occur during the warmer months of the year. Stings occur with greatest frequency on hotter than average days with low winds, particularly during times of low precipitation. "Stinger nets" are used in high-risk areas of the Australian coastline. These nets often feature openings of 2 to 3 cm which prevent larger jellyfish from entering the protected area. Smaller jellyfish and severed tentacles continue to pose a threat. One study reported that 63% of stings requiring medical attention occurred within netted waters.[91] Along Australia's northern coastline, 70% of stings resulted from the box jellyfish envenomation; the remaining 30% involved other *Cubozoa* such as *C. barnesi*.[111] Although this finding indicates a predominance of box jellyfish as the cause of stings, it also suggests that stings from box jellyfish are more severe and require medical attention with greater frequency than stings from other species of Cnidaria.

Related to changes in ocean pH and temperature as a result of climate change, the size of jellyfish blooms and the subsequent incidence of Cnidaria envenomation has increased. In addition, the geographical distribution of venomous jellyfish is expanding.[76,78]

Pathophysiology

Dermal eruptions after *Cnidaria* envenomation occur due to both toxin and immune system mediated mechanisms. Toxins are subdivided into 4 types: Enzymes (Phospholipase A_2, metalloproteases), pore-forming toxins, neurotoxins, and nonprotein bioactive components (serotonin, histamine). The exact composition varies by class; *Cubozoa* only produce enzymes and pore-forming toxins, whereas Anthozoa produce all toxin types and are the only class that produces neurotoxins. Enzymes and nonprotein bioactive compounds produce significant dermal pathology: phospholipase A_2 enzymatically cleaves glycerophospholipids into arachidonic acid and thus induces inflammation. Metalloproteases are proteolytic enzymes that break down extracellular matrix and prevent hemostasis. Tissue edema with necrosis and blister formation ensues. Intradermal injection of both serotonin and histamine causes vasodilation and pain.[75] *Chironex fleckeri* venom also possesses dermatonecrotic and hemolytic fractions, although hemolysis is not documented in humans.[9] Two myotoxins from *C. fleckeri* cause powerful sustained muscle contractions in isolated muscle fibers.[42]

An immune-mediated response to venom explains some sting-related symptoms. Elevated serum anti–sea nettle immunoglobulins IgM, IgG, and IgE persist for years in patients with exaggerated reactions to stings compared with controls.[18] A direct correlation between titers against *Chrysaora* and *Physalia* and severity of a visible skin reaction to envenomation strongly suggests an allergic component.[129] Elevated IgG titers were demonstrated in one death from *P. physalis*.[139] Postenvenomation syndromes results from an exaggerated, prolonged, or aberrant T-cell response.[20,21] Erythema nodosum following a sting from *P. physalis* lends further support to an immunologic component.[3]

Clinical Manifestations

Most patients with stings are treated beachside and never require hospitalization. The vast majority of patients who seek medical care do so because of severe pain without evidence of systemic poisoning.[38] Envenomation by *C. fleckeri* inflicts the most severe pain and is frequently associated with systemic toxicity. Common symptoms include immediate severe pain, followed by an erythematous whiplike linear rash with a "frosted ladder" appearance. The pain often is excruciating and requires parenteral analgesia. Pain generally abates over several hours, although the rash typically persists for days. In a prospective series of *C. fleckeri* stings, 58% manifested delayed hypersensitivity reactions in the form of an itchy maculopapular rash at 7 to 14 days.[111] Most resolved spontaneously; some were treated with antihistamines and topical corticosteroids. Some patients experience flare-ups of an allergic dermatitis months to years after envenomation.[96]

Millepora alcicornis (fire coral) is a common cause of stings in southern United States and Caribbean waters. Although a member of the same phylogenetic class as *P. physalis*, it produces far less significant injuries. It is a nuisance to divers who touch the coral and suffer moderate burning pain for hours. Untreated pain generally lessens within 90 minutes, with skin wheals flattening at 24 hours and resolving within one week. Hyperpigmentation persists for up to 8 weeks.[14] The feather hydroid is the most numerous of the *Hydrozoa* and produces only mild stings.[100]

Following stings from sea anemones, victims develop either immediate or delayed pain. Skin findings range from mild erythema and itching to ulceration. A review of 55 stings from *Anemonia sulcata* presenting to a hospital in Yugoslavia (Adriatic Sea) revealed that, in addition to the local skin findings, many patients suffered nausea, vomiting, muscle aches, and dizziness.[97]

Diagnosis

Laboratory evaluation is warranted in patients suffering systemic toxicity following *Cnidaria* envenomation. Following severe stings from a variety of *Cnidaria*, urinalysis, hematocrit, and serum creatinine measurements serve to detect the presence of hemolysis and subsequent risk of kidney injury. Nonfatal elevation of hepatic enzyme concentrations following anemone sting also is reported.[23] Ocular exposure should be evaluated with slit lamp examination and fluorescein staining as corneal ulceration is a known complication.

Venom assays and serum antibody titers are not clinically useful.

Management

Initial interventions after *Cnidaria* envenomation are directed toward stabilization of cardiopulmonary abnormalities in cases of severe envenomation. Secondary measures are directed toward the prevention of further nematocyst discharge, which could intensify pain and enhance toxicity. Many topical therapies are used for this purpose, including sea water, vinegar, a commercial solution known as Stingose, methylated spirits, ethanol, isopropyl alcohol, dilute ammonium hydroxide, urine, sodium bicarbonate, papain, shaving cream, and sand.

Vinegar is a common first-line treatment for topical application following *Cnidaria* stings. In vitro trials with *C. fleckeri* tentacles demonstrate complete irreversible inhibition of nematocyst discharge following a 30-second application.[69] Additional study findings include massive nematocyst discharge with application of urine or ethanol, and no effect on discharge with use of sodium bicarbonate. Follow-up in vivo experiments demonstrate that vinegar is effective for other *Cubozoa*, including Morbakka (large Cubozoan in Australia),[46] *Carybdea rastoni*,[51] and *C. barnesi*.[50] Although massive nematocyst discharge occurs when vinegar is applied to *C. capillata* tentacles in vitro, clinical exacerbation following this treatment is not reported in humans.[47] Massive discharge also occurs with *C. quinquecirrha*.[53] A smaller degree of discharge (30%) occurs with *P. physalis*,[53] whereas nematocysts of *P. utriculus* are unaffected by application of vinegar.[69] Identification of the offending Cnidaria is often only possible by microscopic evaluation of skin scrapings. Hence, therapy must be guided by geographic location. In the United States, where *P. physalis* and *C. quinquecirrha* are of greatest consequence, sea water is recommended to aid in tentacle removal given that vinegar enhances nematocyst discharge in those species. In the Indo-Pacific region, where *C. fleckeri* and *C. barnesi* are of greatest concern, vinegar application confers greater advantage. If local species prevalence is unknown, it is reasonable to attempt vinegar application to a small area of affected skin and assess its effects before large surface area application.

Stingose is an aqueous solution of 20% aluminum sulfate and 1.1% surfactant. Its purported mechanism of action is denaturing of proteins and long-chain polysaccharides via interactions with the Al^{3+} ion, as well as osmotic removal of venom. A human volunteer trial involving stings from live tentacles of *C. fleckeri* demonstrated pain relief within 5 seconds of Stingose application.[72] Similar results were achieved following treatment of stings from *C. quinquecirrha*. A small randomized controlled trial found Stingose superior to salt water irrigation after Physalia envenomation.[154] A small volunteer study utilizing topical lidocaine reported successful treatment of stings via topical analgesia and reduced nematocyst discharge.[12]

Ice packs provided rapid, effective relief for patients with mild to moderate pain from *Cnidaria* stings in Australia. Patients with severe pain are less likely to benefit from ice packs. Many *Cnidaria* venoms are heat labile and are neutralized at supraphysiologic temperatures.

Hot water immersion (HWI) at 45°C for 20 minutes provided pain relief to 87% of victims of bluebottle (*P. utriculus*) stings in a randomized controlled trial.[94] In-vitro data support thermal denaturing of *C. fleckeri* cardiotoxin. We continue to recommend HWI despite theoretical concern that it leads to local vasodilation and subsequent enhanced systemic distribution of venom.[28] No human randomized controlled trials exist to assess the efficacy of HWI in *C. fleckeri* envenomation.

Pressure immobilization bandaging is a technique that applies sufficient pressure to a wound to impede lymphatic drainage and prevent the entrance of venom into systemic circulation. Given the rapid onset of symptoms, the utility of a technique that impedes lymphatic drainage is unlikely to provide benefit. Although the technique would be used only after tentacle removal, some microscopic nematocysts remain adherent to the skin after visible tentacles are removed. In vitro data investigating the effect of pressure on discharged nematocysts demonstrate not only that discharged nematocysts still contain venom, but that applying pressure forces more venom down the hollow tube.[114] This finding is correlated clinically as patients can deteriorate following pressure immobilization bandaging.[52] Given the lack of evidence suggesting benefit, coupled with clear in vitro evidence of increased venom delivery with this technique, we recommend against the use of pressure immobilization bandaging for treatment of Cnidaria stings. Because studies have not assessed the risks and benefits of proximal tourniquet application, it cannot be recommended at this time.

Cnidaria Cardiotoxicity
Epidemiology
The majority of victims do not present to health care facilities following *Cnidaria* envenomation. Old reports suggesting a 15% to 20% fatality rate[126] following *C. fleckeri* envenomation likely represent a gross overestimation given the low number of documented fatalities in the context of the extraordinary number of yearly stings. A prospective study of stings from *Cubozoa* over one year in Australia revealed no dysrhythmias, pulmonary edema, or death.[111] No patient received antivenom, and analgesia was the only pharmacotherapy implemented. Hospital admission was not required for any victim. Although most victims suffer only local severe pain, serious systemic toxicity occurs occasionally, and may include vertigo, ataxia, paralysis, delirium, syncope, respiratory distress, cardiogenic pulmonary edema, hypotension, and dysrhythmias. In a series of 10 reported deaths from *C. fleckeri*, all occurred in children, suggesting vulnerability due to lower body mass and thinner dermis.[38]

Pathophysiology
Cnidaria venoms contain a variety of components that induce cardiotoxicity. The cardiotoxin of *C. fleckeri* has not yet been fully identified, but is believed to be a pore-forming toxin of about 65 kDa.[130] This is supported by the nonspecific enhancement of cation conductance of isolated heart models exposed to *C. fleckeri* venom.[108] Other in vitro work confirms increased Na⁺ permeability in cardiac tissue.[61] Cardiovascular collapse results from osmotic dysregulation of endothelial and cardiac tissues following pore formation. A rat model demonstrated hemolysis, but this is not observed in envenomated patients.[75] Anthozoa and Hydrozoa feature actinoporins: proteins that insert themselves into the victim's cell membrane and then oligomerize to form an ungated, non-selective ion channel. Cardiac effects in animals include negative inotropy, conduction delays, ventricular tachycardia, and coronary artery vasoconstriction.[38,60] However, experiments using the purest venom extracts without contamination from tentacle material demonstrate cardiovascular collapse without electrocardiographic changes.[115]

Cardiotoxicity also results from blockade of voltage-gated sodium and potassium channels. Venom from *Physalia* spp blocks neural impulses in isolated frog sciatic nerve[82] and produces ventricular ectopy, cardiovascular collapse, hyperkalemia, and hemolysis in dogs.[70] *Physalia* spp venom inhibits Ca²⁺ entry into the sarcoplasmic reticulum.[82] Similar mechanisms

are proposed for *Chrysaora*, *Chiropsalmus*, and *Stomolophus*. *Chrysaora quinquecirrha* venom contains a 150-kDa polypeptide that induces atrioventricular block[17] and produces myocardial ischemia, hypertension, dysrhythmias, and nerve conduction block,[19] as well as hepatic and renal necrosis.[107]

Clinical Manifestations
Fatality is documented to occur with only 4 m of tentacle markings.[140] Death is rapid, preventing many victims from reaching medical care, or even the shore.[89] Cardiac arrest and cardiogenic pulmonary edema develops in young, healthy patients without prior cardiopulmonary disease.[95,161] Survival is possible with immediate cardiopulmonary resuscitation (CPR).[160] *Chiropsalmus quadrumanus*, a close relative of the box jellyfish, induces symptoms that are similar to *C. fleckeri* stings, including cardiogenic pulmonary edema and death.[11]

Diagnosis
Cnidaria cardiotoxicity should be suspected in all drowning victims with linear skin lesions. Onset of cardiovascular collapse occurs rapidly and is thus often confounded by saltwater aspiration and envenomation. Patients not in cardiac arrest present with hypotension and cardiac conduction abnormalities. An electrocardiogram is prudent to identify treatable dysrhythmias. Envenomation impairs coronary perfusion, and serial troponin assays are recommended.

Management
Rescuer efforts should focus on immediate nematocyst inactivation, tentacle removal, and basic life support. Box jellyfish antivenom is available as an ovine whole IgG raised against the "milked" venom of *C. fleckeri*. Combining *C. fleckeri* venom with box jellyfish antivenom prior to injection into pigs prevents all toxicity.[149] An isolated chick muscle experiment demonstrates that box jellyfish antivenom prevents the neurotoxicity and myotoxicity from *C. fleckeri* following pretreatment.[116] In vitro data demonstrate that box jellyfish antivenom neutralizes the dermatonecrotic, hemolytic, and lethal fractions of venom from *Chiropsalmus* spp; however, the venom of *Physalia physalis* and *Chrysaora quinquecirrha* were not neutralized.[10] Other in vitro and in vivo data demonstrate incomplete neutralization of *Chiropsalmus* spp venom.[10,116] A murine experiment with "rescue" administration of antivenom failed to show increased rates of survival, but prolonged time until death. This raises the possibility antivenom is underdosed under current guidelines.[41]

Distance from medical care limits the ability to obtain antivenom in a timely fashion.[38] Although box jellyfish antivenom can be administered by paramedics via intramuscular (IM) injection,[52] poor IM absorption and incomplete venom neutralization with antivenoms, as well as delayed peak serum concentrations, limit the utility of this approach.[123] The amount of antivenom required to neutralize twice the lethal dose in humans is estimated at 12 vials.[38] The manufacturer recommends treating initially with one vial intravenously (IV) diluted 1:10 with saline or 3 undiluted vials (1.5–4 mL each) IM at 3 separate sites, if IV access is unavailable. Some authors who have treated multiple patients with antivenom suggest treating coma, dysrhythmia, or respiratory depression with one vial IV, titrating up to 3 vials with continuation of CPR in patients with refractory dysrhythmias until a total of 6 vials are administered.[111] Serious adverse events or delayed sequelae following the use of IV antivenom are uncommon, although allergic reactions are a consideration.[142] Although available in Australia since 1970, to this date no survival is attributable to the administration of antivenom, and there are multiple fatalities despite its use.[38] If available, antivenom administration is recommended but does not replace supportive care.

Verapamil was evaluated as a treatment for *C. fleckeri* stings based on evidence that Ca²⁺ entry into cells represents an important mechanism of toxicity. One animal model demonstrated synergy with use of verapamil in combination with box jellyfish antivenom,[22] whereas another showed verapamil pretreatment as well as rescue prolonged survival.[16] This is in contrast to other models demonstrating that verapamil negates the benefits of antivenom[117] and increases mortality.[149] Verapamil administration to animals with *Chrysaora quinquecirrha* envenomation demonstrated no benefit.[107] Interestingly, addition of magnesium to antivenom for treatment of *C. fleckeri* envenomation in rats prevented cardiovascular collapse in 100%, suggesting that magnesium has a role in the treatment of stings from this species.[117] Given that animal data are inconsistent with regard to verapamil and that hypotension often develops with severe envenomation, use of calcium channel blockers is not currently recommended for treatment of *C. fleckeri* stings.

Although successfully utilized for the treatment of pain associated with *C. fleckeri* stings, HWI is unlikely to demonstrate benefit in the treatment of cardiotoxicity. Immersion in hot water is impractical for the critically ill patient, and penetrance of heat is limited to superficial tissues and will not denature circulating cardiotoxins.

Irukandji Syndrome
Epidemiology
Stings from the Portuguese man-of-war (*Physalia physalis*) and the Irukandji jellyfish (*Carukia barnesi*) are associated with the development of Irukandji syndrome. However, an unidentified species produced 3 cases of an Irukandjilike syndrome in the Florida Keys, and 6 cases were reported off the coast of Hawaii.[66,168] This suggests a more diverse geographical distribution and possibly multiple responsible organisms.

Pathophysiology
Carukia barnesi, the Irukandji jellyfish, likely induces its dramatic vasopressor effects via catecholamine release. In rats, the venom produces a pressor response that is blocked by α_1-adrenergic antagonism.[118] The pressor response is not dose dependent; therefore, catecholamines in the venom are an unlikely cause. In vitro experiments suggest a Na^+ channel modulator effect leading to massive catecholamine release.[163] Porcine studies with intravenous *C. barnesi* venom administration show a 4,000- and 1,000-fold increase in norepinephrine and epinephrine, respectively.[163] No electrocardiographic abnormalities occurred in envenomated rats.

Clinical Manifestations
Irukandji syndrome is a severe form of envenomation following Cubozoa stings from *Carukia barnesi*.[73] Individuals afflicted often notice a mild sting while they are in the water; however, skin findings typically are absent. Severe systemic symptoms develop after a latent period of 5 to 40 minutes and mimic a catecholamine surge including tachycardia, hypertension, piloerection, hyperpnea, headache, pallor, restlessness, apprehension, sweating, and a sense of impending doom. A prominent feature is severe diffuse muscle spasms that come in waves and preferentially affect the back. Spasms are described as unbearable and frequently require parenteral analgesia. Symptoms generally abate over several hours but can last up to 2 days. Admission rates in patients presenting to medical care exceed 50%.[91] Hypertension is universal and is severe, with systolic blood pressures well over 200 mm Hg. Two fatalities are described involving severe hypertension (280/150 mm Hg and 230/90 mm Hg) resulting in intracranial hemorrhage.[48,73] Hypotension frequently follows, requiring vasopressor support. Cardiogenic pulmonary edema can develop within hours. Echocardiograms consistently reveal global ventricular dysfunction.[92,98] Restored cardiac function typically returns after several days.[90] A retrospective review of 116 cases of Irukandji presenting to Cairns Base Hospital identified elevated troponin I measurements in 22% of patients.[73] Electrocardiographic changes are described as nonspecific.

Diagnosis
Irukandji syndrome is a clinical diagnosis based on the history of swimming in waters known to have Irukandji jellyfish and presentation compatible with hyperadrenergic state as described above. Complaint of headache or altered mental status should prompt cerebral imaging to assess for intracranial hemorrhage resulting from hypertensive crisis. Electrocardiogram, serial cardiac biomarkers, and echocardiography are recommended to screen for myocardial damage and Takotsubo (stress) cardiomyopathy.[150] Laboratory evaluation is recommended for rhabdomyolysis from severe muscle spasms and subsequent acute kidney injury (AKI).[28]

Management
Vinegar irrigation, or HWI, prevents further envenomation as discussed above and is recommended early in the course of treatment. Further treatment for Irukandji syndrome should focus on analgesia and blood pressure control. Several modalities for control of severe hypertension are reasonable and include phentolamine, IV magnesium sulfate, and nitroglycerin.[37,49] Dosing guidelines and efficacy following magnesium infusion for this indication are not established, and a small randomized controlled trial failed to demonstrate benefit, although external factors forced early termination of the study.[99] Because hypotension occurs in late stages of toxicity, clinicians should only administer short-acting titratable antihypertensives such as esmolol, nitroprusside, or nicardipine for control of initial hypertension. Case reports of box jellyfish antivenom use for *Carukia barnesi* stings demonstrate no apparent benefit.[44] A single case report details near-complete resolution of symptoms after a single dose of clonidine.[93] Although central α_2-agonism theoretically addresses the underlying pathophysiology, there is insufficient data to routinely recommend this therapy.

Seabather's Eruption
Epidemiology
Cases of Seabather's Eruption (SBE), a stinging rash evoked by contact with Cnidaria larvae, occur in clusters. Variation in intensity and frequency occurs from year to year as exemplified by a 25-year hiatus during which no cases were reported in Florida.[151] In 1992, more than 10,000 cases of SBE occurred in south Florida, with similar peaks in the 1940s and 1960s. Cases of SBE also are reported in Cuba, Mexico, Brazil, the Caribbean, and the coast of New York.

Pathophysiology
Seabather's Eruption is the result of envenomation by the larvae of *Linuche unguiculata* and *Edwardsiella lineata*. The larvae appear as pin-sized (0.5 mm) brown to green-brown spheres in the upper 2 inches of the water and are typically unnoticed. Discharge of the immature nematocyst of the larvae requires significant mechanical stimulation (friction between bathing suit and skin) or osmotic changes (taking a fresh-water shower after exiting the water). The eruption displays a characteristic delay in onset of symptoms and is effectively treated with steroids, suggesting a primary immune-mediated process. This is further supported by histopathology revealing the presence of perivascular and interstitial infiltrates with lymphocytes, neutrophils, and eosinophils.[165]

Clinical Manifestation
The pruritic papular eruption occurs mostly in areas covered by a bathing suit as a result of larvae trapped under the garments. Only 50% of people reported a stinging sensation while they were in the water, and 25% reported itching upon exiting the water.[165] The remainder of patients developed symptoms within 11 hours. Skin lesions develop within hours of itching and appear as discrete, closely spaced papules, with pustules, vesicles, and urticaria. Itching often is severe and prevents sleep. New lesions typically continue to develop over 72 hours. The average duration of symptoms is just under 2 weeks, and a small percentage of patients experience a recurrence of lesions several days later. Systemic symptoms such as chills, headache, nausea, vomiting, and malaise occur occasionally. Patients develop symptoms again when donning the same bathing suit unless it was decontaminated and washed with detergent.

Diagnosis
The diagnosis of SBE is based on history and physical examination. A pruritic, papular, erythematous rash in high-friction areas (skin folds, swim suit) that occurred after recent immersion in ocean waters suggests SBE. Although embedded nematocyst threads are at times be appreciated on skin biopsy, this is usually not required for diagnosis.

Management
Although not rigorously evaluated for the treatment of SBE, topical application of vinegar is known to deactivate nematocysts of *Linuche unguiculata*.

Topical application of vinegar is thus reasonable. A case series of 14 patients used antihistamines and topical corticosteroids as treatment, with resolution of symptoms within 7 days.[124] This approach to symptomatic control is recommended. Bacterial superinfection due to excoriation occurs rarely and should be treated with antibiotic therapy.

MOLLUSCA

The phylum Mollusca comprises Cephalopoda (octopus, squid, and cuttlefish) and Gastropoda (cone snails). Cephalopod species of toxicologic concern are limited to the blue-ringed octopus *Hapalochlaena maculosa* and the greater blue-ringed octopus *Hapalochlaena lunulata*. The blue-ringed and greater blue-ringed octopods are found in the Indo-Pacific region, primarily in Australian waters (Fig. 116–3). Of the 400 species of cone snails that belong to the genus Conus, 18 are implicated in human envenomations.

Cephalopoda

Epidemiology

The blue-ringed octopus is a relatively small (12–20 cm) animal that lives camouflaged in crevices and rock piles around Australia, the Indo-Pacific region, and Japan. It normally displays a yellow-brown color, but flashes iridescent blue rings aposematically to warn and repel predators. The species is not aggressive and only bites humans when handled. A 1983 review of reported octopus envenomations uncovered a total of 14 cases, all of which occurred in Australia.[156] There were 2 deaths and 4 serious envenomations. Other reviews suggest that up to 7 deaths occurred prior to 1969, some outside Australia.[40]

Pathophysiology

Symbiotic bacteria in the posterior salivary glands of the blue-ringed octopus produce a toxin originally designated maculotoxin and later identified as tetrodotoxin (TTX).[135] The parrotlike beak of the octopus creates small punctures in human skin through which venom is introduced. Tetrodotoxin blocks Na^+ conductance in neurons, leading to flaccid paralysis. Subsequent respiratory insufficiency results in hypoxic cardiac arrest without evidence of primary cardiotoxicity. Hypotension ensues due to reduction of vascular smooth muscle tone rather than poor cardiac output. This is likely due to lack of sympathetic nerve impulses to arteriolar vasoconstrictor muscles.[57] The venom does not affect mentation. If the murine LD_{50} of 9 mcg/kg translates to humans, an adult blue-ringed octopus carries enough TTX to kill 10 adults.[162] Venom also contains serotonin (5-HT), hyaluronidase, tyramine, histamine, tryptamine, octopine, taurine, acetylcholine, and dopamine.[142] Death occurs despite artificial respiration as a result of

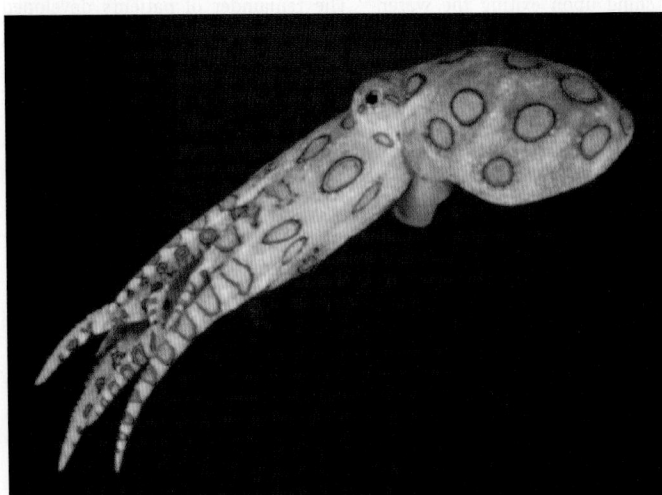

FIGURE 116–3. The blue-ringed octopus, *Hapalochlaena maculosa. (Used with permission from Dr. Roy Caldwell, Professor of Integrative Biology, University of California, Berkeley.)*

profound hypotension and subsequent global ischemia. Poisoning also occurs when the blue-ringed octopus is consumed as TTX is also highly concentrated in its integument.

Clinical Manifestations

The blue-ringed octopus creates one or 2 puncture wounds with its chitinous jaws, inflicting only minor discomfort. A wheal typically develops with erythema, tenderness, and pruritus as a result of the histamine content of the venom. Tetrodotoxin exerts a curarelike effect characterized by paralysis without depressing mental status. Symptoms include perioral and intraoral paresthesias, diplopia, aphonia, dysphagia, ataxia, weakness, nausea, vomiting, flaccid muscle paralysis, respiratory failure, and death. Detailed case reports describe rapid onset of symptoms within minutes.[27,156]

Complete paralysis requiring intubation with findings of fixed and dilated pupils is followed within 24 to 48 hours by near-complete recovery of neuromuscular function. In one reported death, a young man placed the octopus on his shoulder. He subsequently noted a small puncture wound, developed dry mouth, dyspnea, inability to swallow, and became apneic. Asystole occurred 30 minutes after arrival at the hospital despite mechanical ventilation.[58] Another similar bite resulted in symptom onset at 10 minutes, followed by death at 90 minutes, despite bystander CPR.[138] With less severe envenomations, cerebellar signs arise without paralysis. Near-total paralysis with intact mentation resolving over 24 hours occurred in humans.[141]

Diagnostic Testing

Although not a widely available assay, TTX can be detected in the urine or serum using high-performance liquid chromatography with subsequent fluorescence detection.[110] This is unlikely to yield results prior to death or resolution of symptoms. In vitro exposure of human red blood cells to blue-ringed octopus venom shows the development of sphero-echinocytosis mirroring observations in victims of snake envenomation.[56] No case reports exist to corroborate this finding in vivo. Unless the diagnosis of TTX exposure is clear from patient or bystander reports, other conditions such as botulism and Guillain–Barré syndrome should be investigated.

Management

Tetrodotoxin from blue-ringed octopus envenomations produces two potentially lethal conditions: respiratory arrest and peripheral vasodilation with profound hypotension. Patients with compromised respiratory effort require basic airway management and ventilator support, with expectation of weaning within 24 to 48 hours of envenomation based on cases reported in the literature. Although no randomized controlled human trials exist regarding the best approach to hypotension, animal studies indicate that phenylephrine and norepinephrine successfully raises blood pressure to physiologic levels. Interestingly, epinephrine and dopamine lacked efficacy.[57] Based on extrapolation of animal data, norepinephrine or phenylephrine are the recommended therapy to treat vasoplegia. Intravascular volume expansion with crystalloids is reasonable although effectiveness as monotherapy is unlikely based on underlying pathophysiology. Additional measures include local wound care and tetanus prophylaxis. Antivenom is not commercially available.

Gastropoda

Epidemiology

Cone snails predominantly inhabit the Indo-Pacific, including all parts of Australia, New Guinea, Solomon Islands, and the Philippines. Estimates of reported cone snail envenomations suggest only 16 human deaths have occurred worldwide. *Conus geographicus* (fish hunting cone) is the most common species implicated, and fatality is estimated in up to 25% of *C. geographicus* envenomations.[43] Mortality is difficult to assess because some patients do not present to health care facilities or die before eliciting a history of cone snail envenomation, or death is erroneously attributed to drowning. *Conus textile* also causes death in humans. Two deaths from *C. geographicus* occurred in Guam.[88]

Pathophysiology

Cone snails have a hollow proboscis that contains a disposable radular tooth bathed in venom. Similar to a harpoon, the barbed tooth is fired from the proboscis to hunt or in defense. Human envenomations occur when the shells are handled. Firing of the eyelash-sized tooth is powerful enough to penetrate a 5-mm neoprene wetsuit.[68] The proboscis extends the length of its shell, thereby envenomation is possible regardless how the shell is held. Any *Conus* species contains approximately 100 peptides or *conotoxins* in its venom along with hyaluronidases, proteases, and lipases that aid in local tissue breakdown and diffusion of venom.[155] There is significant interspecies variation of venom composition depending on prey preference. Conotoxins are divided into 3 superfamilies (A, M, and O). The A-superfamily of conotoxins acts as competitive nicotinic acetylcholine receptor antagonists and voltage-gated potassium channel blockers. The M-superfamily contains noncompetitive nicotinic acetylcholine receptor antagonists as well as voltage-gated sodium channel blockers. The O-superfamily blocks voltage-gated calcium, sodium, and potassium channels (Table 116–2).[85,104,112,148] Weakness and paralysis occur as a result of presynaptic voltage-gated calcium channel blockade with subsequent impaired acetylcholine release, as well as postsynaptic acetylcholine receptor blockade and inhibition of sodium-ion channels.[43]

Many of these peptides are used extensively in laboratory research for their ability to selectively target a variety of specific Ca^{2+}-channel subtypes. Venom from *Conus imperialis* (worm hunter) contains a substantial amount of 5-HT, a component not found in any other *Conus* venom tested thus far.[103] This species also contains a vasopressinlike peptide.[109] The neuropeptide omega-conotoxin, isolated from *Conus magnus*, is valued for its antinociceptive properties that arise from blockade of the N-type voltage-sensitive Ca^{2+} channel in spinal cord afferents.[102] The Food and Drug Administration approved ziconotide (Prialt, Elan Pharmaceuticals) in 2004 for intrathecal infusion in patients with severe chronic pain that require intrathecal therapy, and in whom other treatment modalities such as intrathecal morphine are not tolerated or ineffective. Frequent side effects such as dizziness, nausea, confusion, and memory impairment limit the broad application of this therapy.

Clinical Manifestations

Cone snail envenomation results from careless handling of the animal or rummaging through sand. Cone snails are nocturnal feeders, so they present more of a hazard to night divers. Localized symptoms range from a slight sting to excruciating pain, tissue ischemia, cyanosis, and numbness. Systemic symptoms include weakness, diaphoresis, diplopia, blurred vision, aphonia, dysphagia, generalized muscle paralysis, respiratory failure, cardiovascular collapse, and coma. Systemic symptoms occur within 30 minutes of envenomation; respiratory arrest occurs shortly thereafter.[68] Death is rapid and occurs within an hour.[43] Based on military medical records of more than 30 cases predating 1970, the mortality rate approaches 25%, with *Conus geographicus* causing the most deaths.[88] Other estimates suggest that, without medical care, mortality reaches 70%.[167] Given the rarity of severe human envenomations from cone snails, the manner of death, whether purely from respiratory insufficiency or direct cardiovascular toxicity, remains unknown.

Diagnostic Testing

Diagnosis of conotoxin envenomation is challenging. Whereas most venomous marine animals leave a visible injury, hypodermal injection by the radula toothlike structure produces minimal tissue injury easily missed on physical examination. Surrounding discoloration and local edema provide clues of envenomation. Typical points of entry are the hands (during shell handling) or the waist area (if held in pocket).[68] Laboratory assays for conotoxin are not routinely available. Based on the ion-channel blocking properties of some venom components, patients are at risk of dysrhythmias, which are reported with administration of ziconotide.[71] Hence, an electrocardiogram should be obtained in combination monitoring by telemetry until the patient is asymptomatic.

Management

Primary interventions include maintenance of airway, breathing, and circulation. The envenomation site should be irrigated and the patient's tetanus vaccination updated as appropriate. Some authors suggest HWI (113°–122°F, 45°–50°C) following cone snail stings for pain relief, but no data exist whether HWI enhances systemic distribution of conotoxins.[88] Antivenom is not available. Global flaccid paralysis requires short-term mechanical ventilation, but usually resolves within 24 hours.[43] Cardiac dysrhythmias require electrical cardioversion. Administration of antidysrhythmics that rely on sodium channel blockade for clinical effect could theoretically worsen the patient's dysrhythmia. Hypotension should be treated with intravenous fluids and norepinephrine as appropriate.

Echinodermata, Annelida, and Porifera

The Echinodermata phylum includes sea stars, brittle stars, sea urchins, sand dollars, and sea cucumbers. Annelida are segmented worms that include the Polychaetae family of bristle worms. Sponges are classified in the Porifera phylum. One feature that all 3 phyla share is the passive envenomation of people who mistakenly handle or step on the animals. Most stings from these creatures are mild.

Epidemiology

Echinoderms, annelids, and sponges are ubiquitous ocean inhabitants. The crown-of-thorns sea star (*Acanthaster planci*) is found in the warmest waters of Polynesia to the Red Sea and is a particularly venomous species because of its sharp spines that easily puncture human skin. Sea urchins inhabit all oceans of the world. They are nonaggressive, slow moving, bottom dwellers and human envenomation typically results from stepping on or handling the animal. The most venomous are species of *Diadema*, *Echinothrix*, and *Asthenosoma*. Bristle worms such as *Hermodice carunculata* typically inhabit tropical waters such as those of Florida and the Caribbean. However, some species thrive in the frigid waters of Antarctica. The fire sponge *Tedania ignis* is a brilliant yellow-orange sponge identified in large numbers off the coast of Hawaii and in the Florida Keys. Other common American sponges are *Neofibularia nolitangere* (poison-bun sponge or touch-me-not sponge) and *Microciona prolifera* (red sponge). *Neofibularia mordens* (Australian stinging sponge) is a common Southern Australian variety. In the Mediterranean, sponges are often colonized with sea anemones that inflict severe stings.[14]

Pathophysiology

Sea urchins are covered in spines and pedicellariae. The pedicellariae are pincerlike appendages used for feeding, cleaning, and defense. They generally contain more venom than the spines and are more difficult to remove from wounds. Urchins laden with pedicellariae can evoke more severe

TABLE 116–2 Conus Peptide Targets

Peptide	Receptor Type	Mechanism
Ligand-gated ion channels		
Conantokins	NMDA	Inhibits conductance
α-Conotoxin	Nicotinic	Competitive antagonism
σ-Conotoxin	5-HT$_3$	Noncompetitive antagonism
M1		Neuromuscular junction
M2		Neuronal receptors
Voltage-gated ion channels		
δ-Conotoxin		Delayed channel activation
κ-Conotoxin	K$^+$	Channel blockade
μ-Conotoxin	Na$^+$	Channel blockade
ω-Conotoxin	Ca^{2+}	Channel blockade
G-protein linked		
Conopressin-G	Vasopressin receptor	Receptor agonism
Contulakin-G	Neurotensin receptor	Receptor agonism

stings than urchins with less pedicellariae. Venom contained within the spines consists of steroid glycosides, 5-HT, hemolysin, protease, acetylcholinelike substances, and bradykininlike substances. Some species harbor neurotoxins.

Sea stars are less noxious because they generally have short, blunt spiny projections. The crown-of-thorns is the exception with its longer, sharp spines containing toxic saponins (plancitoxin I and II) with hemolytic and anticoagulant effects as well as histaminelike substances. The venom is hepatotoxic by an elusive mechanism. Animal studies reveal inhibition of glutathione S-transferase by crown-of-thorns venom; theoretically this leads to organ damage from failure to detoxify reactive molecules.[1]

Sea cucumbers excrete holothurin, a sulfated triterpenoid oligoglycoside, from the anus (organs of Cuvier) as a defense. The toxin inhibits neural conduction in fish, leading to paralysis. Some sea cucumbers eat Cnidaria and subsequently secrete their venom.

Bristle worms have many parapodia that have the appearance, but not the function, of legs. Several bristles extend from each parapodium giving the family (Polychaeta) its name (*poly* means many, *chaetae* means bristles). The bristles penetrate human skin, leading to envenomation with an unknown substance.

Sponges have an elastic skeleton with spicules of silicon dioxide or calcium carbonate. They attach to the sea floor or coral beds. Toxins include halitoxin, odadaic acid, and subcritine, the nature of which is uncertain.[15] Dried sponges are nontoxic; however, on rewetting they produce toxicity even after several years.[134,138]

Clinical Manifestations

Sea urchin envenomation presents as intense burning with local tissue reaction, including edema and erythema. Rarely, with multiple punctures, lightheadedness, numbness, paralysis, bronchospasm, and hypotension occur, although this is not documented in the peer-reviewed medical literature.[4] Reports of death are not well substantiated. The Pacific urchin *Tripneustes* produces a neurotoxin with a predilection for cranial nerves.[14] Mild elevations of hepatic enzymes are reported in one patient with foot cellulitis from an urchin sting.[166] Retention of sea urchin spine fragments predisposes the patient to development of painful granulomata.[67] Spine penetration of a joint induced synovitis.[125]

Small cuts on the skin from handling sea stars allow venom to penetrate, leading to contact dermatitis. The crown-of-thorns sea star causes severe pain, nausea, vomiting, and muscular paralysis.[100] Massive hemolysis and hepatic necrosis were reported after a single-stinger envenomation.[74] Its spines are brittle with a tendency to splinter off once embedded in the victim's tissues.

Cutaneous, scleral, or corneal exposure to sea cucumbers triggers contact dermatitis, intense corneal inflammation, and even blindness. Bristle worms are shrouded with bristles that produce a reddened urticarial rash. Symptoms typically are mild and resolve over several hours to days.

Contact with the fire sponge, poison-bun sponge, or red-moss sponge causes erythema, papules, vesicles, and bullae that generally subside within 3 to 7 days. Some victims develop fever, chills, and muscle cramps. Skin desquamation occurs at 10 days to 2 months,[4] with chronic skin changes lasting several months.[15] Erythema multiforme and anaphylaxis are uncommon complications associated with *Neofibularia* spp exposure.[14] Contact with sponges that are colonized with Cnidaria leads to dermatitis with skin necrosis, referred to as *sponge diver's disease*.

Diagnosis

Radiographic or ultrasonographic imaging of the affected body part is recommended to assess for the presence of remnant foreign bodies.[131] Elevated aminotransferase concentrations and hepatic necrosis are potential complications of crown-of-thorns envenomation, and plancitoxin I and II provoke hepatotoxicity in animal studies.[74,87] Phospholipase A_2 in the sea star's venom induces significant hemolysis in vitro.[83] Laboratory evaluation for these conditions is therefore reasonable.

Management

The primary objective following envenomation from sea urchins and crown-of-thorns starfish is analgesia. Submersion of the affected extremity in hot water (105°–115°F; 40.6°–46.1°C) and administration of oral analgesics often is sufficient as several components of the venom are thermolabile.[100] The hemolytic component of crown-of-thorns venom retains 50% of its hemolytic activity despite incubation to 100°C for 30 minutes in laboratory testing.[83] Hence, HWI alleviates local symptoms yet fails to prevent systemic toxicity.

Spines frequently crumble with attempted extraction and often require surgical exploration of the tract for complete removal. Intraarticular spines necessitate surgical removal. Patients' pain and systemic symptoms persist for months if spines are not removed.[131] Tetanus immune status must be addressed. Antibiotic prophylaxis is recommended for patients with immunosuppressive risk factors such as diabetes or other comorbidities. Although most infections likely are secondary to human skin flora, marine flora such as *Mycobacterium marinum* and *Vibrio parahaemolyticus* are potential wound contaminants, and *M. marinum* is associated with the formation for granulomata after sea urchin envenomation.[125]

Treatment of sponge exposures usually requires only removal of spicules using adhesive tape or the edge of a credit card. Antihistamines and topical corticosteroids often provide no relief from stinging sponges.[15]

VERTEBRATES

Snakes

Sea snakes are elapids and are divided into 2 subfamilies: Hydrophiinae and Laticaudinae. They are close relatives of the cobra and krait. Length typically does not exceed 1 m. Their tails are flattened, and their bodies often are brightly colored. Distinction from eels is made by the presence of scales and the absence of fins and gills. All 52 species of sea snakes are venomous and at least 6 species are implicated in human fatalities. The most common species cited in human envenomation are *Enhydrina schistosa*, the beaked sea snake, and *Pelamis platurus*, the yellow-bellied sea snake.

Epidemiology

Sea snakes are common to the tropical and temperate Indian and Pacific Oceans, but they are also found along the eastern Pacific Coast of Central and South America and the Gulf of California. In the eastern Pacific region, the yellow-bellied sea snake is the only species known. There are no venomous sea snakes in the Atlantic Ocean or Mediterranean. Sea snakes come ashore to replenish somatic water stores with fresh water.[86] The majority of envenomations occur along the coasts of Southeast Asia, the Persian Gulf, and the Malay Archipelago (Malaysia). Snakes tend to inhabit the turbid coastlines and deeper reefs of these regions. Workers of the fishing industry are at greatest risk as snakes frequently get trapped in fishing nets. Sea snakes generally are docile, except when provoked, or during the mating season. Two species, the Stokes' sea snake (*Astoria stokesii*) and Beaked sea snake (*Enhydrina schistosa*), are known for aggression.

The true incidence of sea snake envenomation is unknown because many bites are not recorded. Worldwide, the number of deaths per year approaches 150, with an overall mortality rate estimated between 3.2% and 30%.[144] In a review of 120 documented bites, 51.7% of victims were fishermen handling nets.[121] The remainder of victims were wading or swimming along the coastline. In a review of 101 bites occurring from 1957 to 1964 in Northwest Malaysia, more than 50% of bites were from the beaked sea snake, including 7 of the 8 fatal bites in that series, bringing the mortality to 8% prior to the availability of antivenom.[122] However, 31 "dry bites" were excluded, suggesting that the overall mortality is somewhat lower. Among the 20% of patients in that series suffering "serious envenomation," half died despite supportive care. A follow-up series of patients after the introduction of antivenom described 2 deaths out of 11 "serious envenomations," suggesting a decreased mortality resulting from this intervention. These were all retrospective reviews of published or personally communicated cases.

Pathophysiology

All sea snakes have small front fangs. Their venom is neurotoxic, myotoxic, nephrotoxic, and hemolytic. Known components of the venom include acetylcholinesterase, hyaluronidase, leucine aminopeptidase, 5′-nucleotidase, phosphodiesterase, and phospholipase A. The neurotoxin is a highly stable 6,000- to 8,000-Da protein similar to that of cobra and krait venom. The low molecular weight of sea snake toxins allows for high penetrance of membrane barriers.[145] In mice, beaked sea snake venom is 4 to 5 times more potent than cobra venom based on a microgram-per-kilogram ratio; however, cobra venom yield is greater.[26] Venom homology exists across many species. The neurotoxin targets postsynaptic acetylcholine (ACh) receptors, creating a blockade at the neuromuscular junction.[143] Presynaptic effects include initial enhanced ACh release and subsequent inhibition of ACh release.[157] In vitro research confirms direct nephrotoxicity of crude venom and partially explains the nephrotoxicity described clinically.[134] Rhabdomyolysis likely contributes to this clinical finding.

Clinical Manifestations

Bites typically are painless or inflict minimal discomfort initially despite significant envenomation as venom contains few inflammatory or necrotic factors.[81] Between one and 4 fang marks are common; however, up to 20 fang marks are possible as a result of multiple bites. The diagnosis often is obscured because victims do not associate the slight prick following the bite with later onset of ascending paralysis. Symptoms progress within minutes, although a delay of up to 6 hours is possible. Painful muscular rigidity and myoglobinuria are hallmarks of sea snake myotoxicity. Myoglobinuria develops between 30 minutes and 8 hours after the bite. This is followed by ascending paralysis from acetylcholine receptor blockade by the neurotoxic venom fraction and muscle destruction from myotoxic fraction. Massive potassium release from damaged muscle tissue coupled with impaired kidney function from myoglobin nephropathy predisposes to fatal dysrhythmias. Other classic symptoms include dysphagia, trismus, ptosis, aphonia, nausea, vomiting, fasciculations, and ultimately respiratory insufficiency, seizures, and coma.

Diagnostic Testing

Laboratory diagnostics are directed toward identifying hemolysis, myonecrosis, hyperkalemia, and acute kidney injury. Serum electrolytes, creatinine, and creatine phosphokinase, as well as hematocrit and urinalysis, should be obtained. Elevated concentrations of hepatic enzymes indicate severe envenomation. Serial measurement of these parameters is recommended. Testing for serum concentrations of venom is not routinely available. Electromyography (EMG) often shows myopathic features for several weeks after envenomation.[81] Muscle biopsy, although not typically needed for diagnosis, shows myonecrosis in up to 60% of muscle mass.[81]

Management

Prehospital management of sea snakebites mirrors treatment of terrestrial snakebites (Chap. 119) and includes immobilization of the extremity and consideration of a pressure immobilization bandage to impede lymphatic drainage. Currently no data regarding the efficacy of this technique for sea snake envenomations are available. Tourniquets that impede venous or arterial flow are not recommended. Airway and respiratory effort require close monitoring because paralysis develops rapidly.

Currently, only one antivenom specific to sea snake bites is available, produced by Commonwealth Serum Laboratories (CSL). The equine IgG Fab fragments are produced using the venom of beaked sea snake (*E. schistosa*) or terrestrial tiger snake (*Notechis scutatus*) (Table 116–3). In vitro experiments demonstrate that CSL sea snake antivenom is effective for neutralizing all species of sea snakes tested (*Praescutata viperina* in Thailand, *Pelamis platurus* in Central America, *Laticauda semifasciata* in the Philippines, *Laticauda laticaudata* in Japan, *Hydrophis cyanocinctus*, *Lapemis hardwickii*).[153] Optimal neutralization occurs within the subfamily Hydrophiinae, which contains *E. schistosa*; however, effective neutralization is demonstrated within the subfamily Laticaudinae. Commonwealth Serum Laboratories sea snake antivenom is relatively costly and requires continuous refrigeration during transport and storage. No controlled human trials have evaluated the efficacy of CSL sea snake antivenom, although case reports suggest improved outcomes and more rapid recovery with its use.[105,122] Anecdotal experience in Malaysia using CSL sea snake antivenom suggests slow recovery from myalgias and weakness over 48 hours, compared with resolution over 2 weeks without antivenom (2 cases, one control).[120]

In the event that sea snake antivenom is not available, several other treatment options exist because of the potential cross-reactivity of certain terrestrial antivenoms with sea snake venom. A murine rescue trial found Thai neuro polyvalent antivenom (NPAV) to be equipotent compared with Australian CSL sea snake antivenom after envenomation by the beaked sea snake or the spine-bellied sea snake (*Hydrophis curtus*).[145] Terrestrial tiger snake antivenom also neutralizes sea snake venom in vitro. Based on the volume of antivenom required, tiger snake antivenom was superior for neutralization of all sea snake venoms tested except that of the beaked sea snake, for which CSL sea snake antivenom was more effective.[7] In contrast to volume comparisons, measurements of unit dosing demonstrate CSL sea snake antivenom is more effective for all venoms tested. Another in vitro study comparing tiger snake and CSL sea snake antivenom against venom *E. schistosa* demonstrated tiger snake antivenom was 10 times more effective in terms of milligram of venom neutralized per milliliter of antivenom.[106] In the same study, the use of 17 different types of elapid antivenom resulted in poor neutralization of beaked sea snake venom.

In rescue experiments with mice using 11 sea snake venoms and 4 different antivenoms (*E. schistosa*, *E. schistosa-N. scutatus*, *N. scutatus*, and polyvalent sea snake *L. hardwickii*, *L. semifasciata*, *H. cyanocinctus*), tiger snake antivenom was superior to all others with respect to volume amount required to prevent death.[2,8,62] Another finding of the study was improved efficacy with early administration of antivenom.

Based on in vitro and in vivo research, selection of the optimal antivenom for treatment of sea snakebites is unclear. CSL sea snake antivenom, tiger snake antivenom, and NPAV are effective in neutralizing a wide variety of sea snake venoms. Therefore, the most readily available antivenom should be used when needed. The manufacturer's guidelines for use of monovalent CSL sea snake antivenom recommend administration of one vial (1,000 units) for systemic symptoms. However, because symptoms are often delayed and early administration is more likely to result in venom neutralization, antivenom is recommended if there is any evidence of envenomation. The antivenom requires a 1:10 dilution with 0.9% sodium chloride solution followed by intravenous administration over 30 minutes. A 1:5 dilution can be used for small children. Skin testing is not recommended. Epinephrine and antihistamines should be readily available. No upper limit is suggested for the number of vials to administer, although larger amounts are more likely to result in serum sickness. Patients have received up to 7 vials without adverse effect directly attributable to the antivenom.[105] Administration of one vial

TABLE 116–3	Antivenom, Initial Dosing by Route	
Organism	**Intravenous Dosing**	**Intramuscular Dosing**
Box jellyfish		
C. fleckeri	1 vial as 1:10 dilution[a]	3 vials (undiluted)
Sea snake		
E. schistose (beaked sea snake)	1-3 vials as 1:10 dilution,[a] up to 10 vials in severe cases	Not recommended
N. scutatus (terrestrial tiger snake)	1 vial as 1:10 dilution[a]	Not recommended
Stonefish		
S. trachynis	1 vial as 1:10 dilution,[a] high risk of anaphylactoid reaction	1 vial (undiluted) for every 2 punctures

[a]Dilution in pediatric patients 1:5 to avoid volume overload.

(3,000 units) of tiger snake antivenom is an alternative if CSL sea snake antivenom is unavailable. Other treatments should focus on wound care, tetanus prophylaxis, analgesia, and fluid administration to minimize nephrotoxicity from myoglobinuria.

Fish

Several fish utilize defensive venoms. Stingrays and spiny fish are known to pose a threat to fishermen, surfers, swimmers, waders, and divers. Although rare, death is typically the result of mechanical trauma rather than toxicological effects of venom, as was the case in the death of animal activist Steve Irwin. Stingrays are members of the class Chondrichthyes (order Rajiformes: skates and rays). Families include Dasyatidae (whip ray or sting ray), Urolophidae (round ray), Myliobatidae (batfish or eagle ray), Gymnuridae (butterfly ray), and Potamotrygonidae (river ray, freshwater).

Spiny fish of the family Scorpaenidae include a variety of venomous creatures (Table 116–4). Fish of the genus *Pterois* are commonly called *lionfish* (*P. volitans* and *P. lunulata*). Stonefish are grouped under the genus *Synanceja* and include *S. trachynis* (Australian estuarine stonefish), *S. horrida* (Indian stonefish), and *S. verrucosa* (reef stonefish). Stonefish display a mottled color and are covered in mucus that allows for growth of algae, making them well camouflaged among rocks and reefs (Fig. 116–4). Scorpionfish have a similar appearance and belong to the genus *Scorpaena* (eg, *S. guttata*: California sculpin). Other Scorpaenidae include *Notesthes robusta* (bullrout) and *Gymnapistes marmoratus* (cobbler). The European weeverfish produce toxicity similar to members of Scorpaenidae and are classified under the family Trachinidae. This includes *Trachinus vipera* (lesser weever) and *Trachinus draco* (greater weever, aka adderpike, stingfish, seacat). These bottom dwellers are smaller and have fewer spines than Scorpaenidae and are much less ghoulish in appearance. Catfish also envenomate humans. Although most live in freshwater, marine catfish such as *Plotosus lineatus* can inflict injury. Other venomous spiny fish include rabbitfish, stargazers, toadfish, ratfish, and even some sharks that have spines on their dorsal fins (Port Jackson shark, dogfish shark).

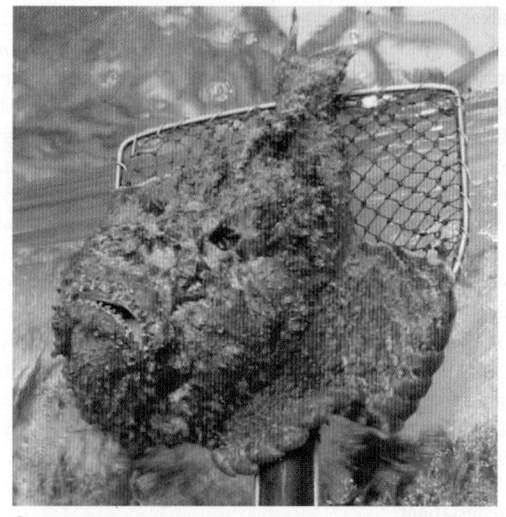

A

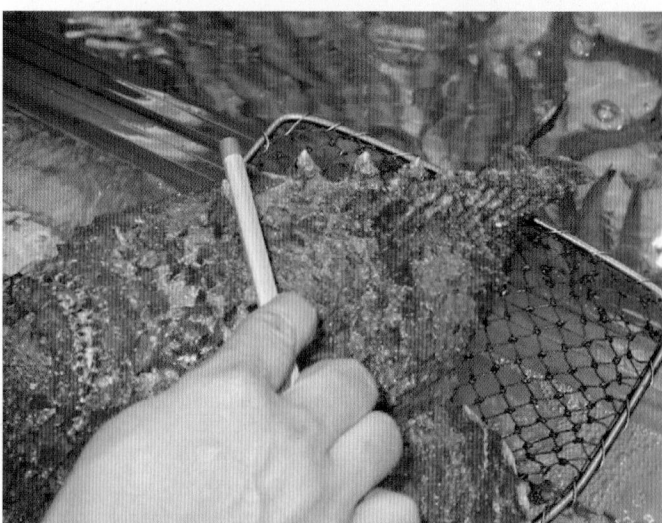

B

FIGURE 116–4. The stonefish, *Synanceja* spp. Note the stinging spines on the close-up. *(Used with permission from the Fellowship in Medical Toxicology, New York University School of Medicine, New York City Poison Center.)*

Epidemiology

There are 11 different species of stingrays in US coastal waters (7 in the Atlantic, 4 in the Pacific). In the southeastern United States, *Dasyatis americana* is a common inhabitant. *Urolophus halleri* is the most common species on the western coast of the United States. Some estimates suggest 1,500 to 2,000 stingray injuries occur yearly in the United States. Most envenomations occur when the animal is inadvertently stepped on. In one review, a total of 17 fatalities resulting from trunk wounds, hemorrhage, or tetanus were identified worldwide.[45] Another review of 603 cases of stingray injuries identified 2 deaths resulting from intraabdominal trauma.[127]

Three populations are at highest risk for spiny fish envenomation: fishermen sorting the catch from nets, waders, and aquarium enthusiasts. Only 5 deaths from Scorpaenidae are reported; all resulted from stonefish and are poorly documented.[36] No deaths from stonefish are reported in Australia, a country where they are commonly found in coastal waters.[38] The incidence of weeverfish stings is unknown, but they are a common occurrence in the summertime among Italian coastal towns.[25,137] Scorpaenidae inhabit waters throughout the tropical and temperate oceans. They exist as far north as the Gulf of Oman and Southern Japan and extend south beyond New Zealand. In the United States, Scorpaenidae stings occur in the Florida Keys, in the Gulf of Mexico, off the coast of California, and in Hawaii.

TABLE 116–4	Spiny Fish	
Latin Name	*Common Name*	*Habitat (Coastal Waters)*
Scorpaenidae family		
Pterois		
P. volitans	Lionfish (also zebrafish, turkeyfish, or red firefish)	Indo-Pacific region, Florida to North Carolina (nonnative to US coast)
P. lunulata	Lionfish or butterfly cod	
Synanceja		
S. trachynis	Australian estuarine stonefish	Indo-Pacific region (Pacific and Indian Oceans)
S. horrida	Indian stonefish	
S. verrucosa	Reef stonefish	
Scorpaena		
S. cardinalis	Red rock cod, scorpionfish	Australia
S. guttata	California sculpin, scorpionfish	California
Notesthes robusta	Bullrout	Australia
Gymnapistes marmoratus	Cobbler	Australia
Trachinidae family		
Trachinus		
T. vipera	Lesser weeverfish	Great Britain to Northwest Africa, throughout
T. draco	Greater weeverfish (also adderpike, stingfish, or seacat)	Mediterranean and Black Seas

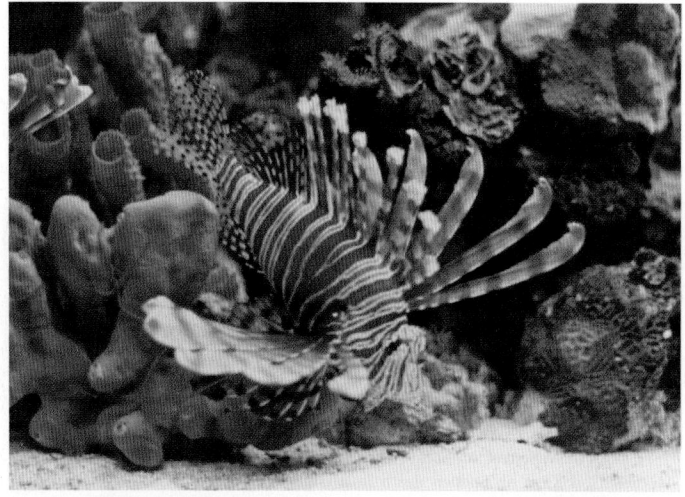

A

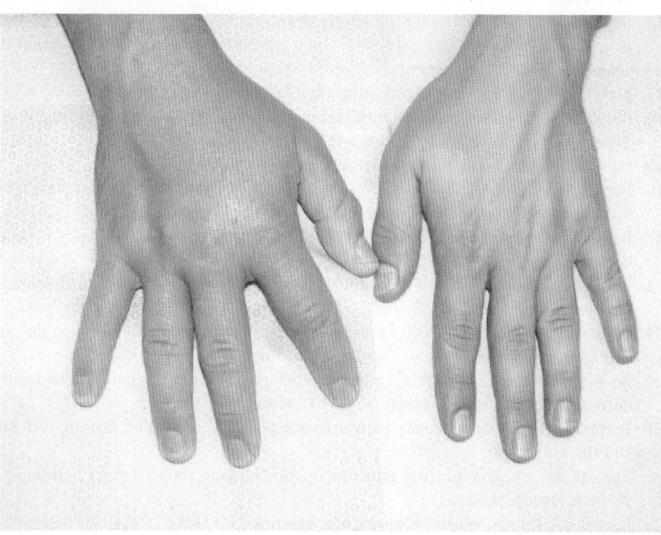

B

FIGURE 116–5. (**A**) The lionfish, *Pterois volitans*. (**B**) This patient's hand was envenomated by his pet lionfish while cleaning his aquarium. *(Used with permission from the Fellowship in Medical Toxicology, New York University School of Medicine, New York City Poison Center.)*

Lionfish (genus *Pterois*) (Fig. 116–5) are common to home aquariums and account for most poison control center calls involving spiny fish envenomation in the United States. The bullrout inhabits the eastern coast of Australia, along with the cobbler, which is found only in Australia. Weeverfish inhabit shallow temperate waters with sandy or muddy bottoms in the eastern Atlantic and Mediterranean, including the European Coast extending to the southern tip of Norway.[24] The marine catfish lives in the tropical Indo-Pacific waters.

Pathophysiology

Tapered, bilaterally retroserrated spines covered by an integumentary sheath emanate from the stingray tail. The ventrolateral groove contains venom glands that saturate the spine with venom and mucus. Puncture of the victim disrupts the integrity of the integument overlying the stinger. This releases the venom which contains several amino acids, serotonin, 5′-nucleotidase, and phosphodiesterase.[5] In animal models, venom induces local vasoconstriction, bradydysrhythmias, atrioventricular nodal block, subendocardial ischemia, seizures, coma, cardiovascular collapse, and death.[4,127] A rabbit model demonstrates initial vasodilation followed by vasoconstriction and cardiac standstill, suggesting a direct cardiac effect.[128] Wound specimens reveal necrotic muscle and neutrophilic infiltrates.[6] Other reports show central hemorrhagic necrosis with surrounding lymphoid and eosinophilic infiltrates indicating an immune-mediated cause of delayed wound healing.[64]

Scorpaenidae have 12 to 13 dorsal, 2 pelvic, and 3 anal spines that are covered with an integumentary sheath. Glands at the base contain 5 to 10 mg of venom each; the amount of venom released is proportional to the pressure applied to the spine. Ornate pectoral fins are not venomous. Venom can remain stable for 24 to 48 hours after the fish dies.[101] Three main toxins are isolated from various species of stonefish: stonustoxin (SNTX), verrucotoxin (VTX), and trachynilysin (TLY). SNTX, from *S. horrida*,[65] has 2 subunits, α and β (71,000 and 79,000 Da, respectively). It induces formation of hydrophilic pores in cell membranes.[29] Toxicity in animals includes hemolysis, local edema, vascular permeability, platelet aggregation, endothelium-dependent vasodilation, and hypotension. Decreased myocardial contractility occurs in rabbits.[132] Heating stonefish venom to 122°F (50°C) for 5 minutes prevents wound necrosis and hypotension in animal models.[159] Verrucotoxin, isolated from *S. verrucosa*, shares homology with SNTX in that both block cardiac Ca^{2+} channels.[63] trachynilysin, isolated from *S. trachynis*, is a 159-kDa protein that forms pores in cell membranes. It allows Ca^{2+} entry and causes Ca^{2+}-dependent release of ACh from nerve endings at motor end plates and increased catecholamine release.[79,113,133] *Synanceja trachynis* venom causes endothelium-dependent vasodilation and cardiovascular collapse in rats, which appears to be mediated by muscarinic and adrenergic receptors.[30] Hemolysis is demonstrated in animals but does not occur in humans.[80] Stonefish venom also contains a powerful hyaluronidase inducing local tissue destruction and systemic absorption of venom. Other venoms of Scorpaenidae include proteinase, phosphodiesterase, alkaline phosphomonoesterase, arginine esterase, arginine amidinase, 5′-nucleotidase, acetylcholinesterase, and biogenic amines. Crude venom from *G. marmoratus*, *P. volitans*, and *S. trachynis* leads to increased intracellular Ca^{2+} and muscle contracture in vivo.[33] Toxins from other spiny fish include dracotoxin (*T. draco*), trachinine (*T. vipera*), and nocitoxin (*N. robusta*).[32] Effects mirror those of Scorpaenidae toxins.[137]

Clinical Manifestations

Stepping on the body of a stingray causes a reflexive whip of the tail leading to wounds in the lower extremity. Intense pain out of proportion to the appearance of the wound is characteristic. Symptoms peak 30 to 90 minutes after injury and may persist for 48 hours. In a retrospective review of cases reported to the California Poison Control System, 9% of victims had retained stingers in their wound, and 9% of wounds became infected.[34] Local edema, cyanosis and ischemia due to vasospasm, erythema, and petechiae follow rapidly. Tissue hypoperfusion results in necrosis and ulceration. Symptoms include weakness, nausea, vomiting, diarrhea, vertigo, headache, syncope, seizures, muscle cramps, fasciculations, hypotension, and dysrhythmias. Chest and abdominal wounds, as well as tetanus, have caused death.[119]

Stings from stonefish produce immediate, severe pain with rapid wound cyanosis and edema that progresses up the injured extremity. Pain reaches a maximum after 30 to 90 minutes and usually resolves over 6 to 12 hours, although some patients experience pain for days. Headache, vomiting, abdominal pain, delirium, seizures, limb paralysis, hypertension, respiratory distress, dysrhythmias, congestive heart failure, and hypotension characterize systemic toxicity.[84] Wound healing requires months.

A poison control center case series from 1979 to 1988 identified 23 cases of *P. volitans* envenomation.[152] Reported symptoms included pain, swelling, nausea, numbness, joint pain, anxiety, headache, dizziness, and cellulitis. Another Poison Control Center series identified 51 Scorpaenidae stings (45 *P. pterois*, 6 *S. guttata*).[77] Intense pain was reported in 98%, extension of pain to the limb in 22%, swelling in 58%, and systemic signs (nausea, diaphoresis, dyspnea, chest pain, abdominal pain, weakness, hypotension, and syncope) in 13%. Thirteen percent of patients in the series developed wound infection; one patient's wound healing was delayed several weeks. Stings from weeverfish are similar to Scorpaenidae envenomation and rarely result in death.[13] Injury from catfish stings is comparable to that of other stinging fish.[39]

Diagnosis

The most commonly affected area is the lower extremities. Imaging of the affected body part is indicated because of the potential of retained foreign bodies. Stingray spines are denser than human tissue and easily identified on radiographs. However, if only the sheath of the spine remains in the wound, radiography is unlikely to reveal this foreign body. Ultrasonography is recommended for patients with a negative radiography. Stings from stone fish are associated with compartment syndrome. Compartment pressures should be evaluated for a patient with significant pain, pallor, poikilothermia, paresthesias, or loss of distal pulses. Disparate pulse oximetry measurements between an affected and unaffected extremity herald a developing compartment syndrome.[147]

Management

Wounds inflicted by stingrays and spiny fish should be carefully examined for imbedded foreign material. Stingray wounds have the potential to be extensive and require surgical attention for vascular or tendinous disruption. Tetanus immune status should be addressed. Prophylactic antibiotics decrease rates of wound infection; a quinolone and cefazolin are the recommended therapy.[35] In a series of 576 stings from *stingrays off the Californian coast*, 69% of patients reported significant relief of local pain with HWI.[34] In patients undergoing HWI due to stonefish envenomation, antibiotics should be administered early due to the theoretical increased rate of growth of *Vibrio vulnificus* and subsequent necrotizing fasciitis.[146] Although patients occasionally required a single dose of oral or parenteral analgesia, clinicians rarely prescribed analgesics on discharge. In a human volunteer study in which subjects received a subcutaneous injection of stingray venom, severe pain developed immediately, and was alleviated with water heated to 122°F (50°C).[127] Pain increased with application of cold water. Local lidocaine infiltration provides a reasonable alternate modality for pain control.[54] Severe vasospasm can generate limb-threatening ischemia. Infusion of prostaglandin E₁ has resulted in successful salvage of an ischemic leg,[136] but insufficient data exist to recommend this as routine therapy.

Stonefish antivenom, an equine-derived IgG Fab, is raised against the venom of *S. trachynis*. Each vial contains 2,000 units and neutralizes 20 mg venom. Between 1965 and 1981, antivenom was used in at least 267 cases.[38] Anecdotal reports suggest it provides effective relief from pain.[38,158] In a review of 26 documented cases in Australia where antivenom was administered IM, no acute adverse effects were identified.[142] Two of 15 patients who had follow-up visits suffered serum sickness. Rash develops several days postinjection.[158] In vitro and in vivo research with the antivenom demonstrates neutralization of venom from *G. marmoratus*[31] and *P. volitans*[32]; however, the application for human therapy remains untested.

The manufacturer recommends IM administration of stonefish antivenom, and advises against IV administration because of increased risk of anaphylactoid reaction. Administration is indicated for systemic toxicity or refractory pain. The number of puncture wounds guides therapy: one vial for one to 2 punctures, 2 vials for 3 to 4 punctures, and 3 vials for 5 or more punctures. Epinephrine and diphenhydramine should be readily available for treatment of anaphylactic reactions.

SUMMARY

- Fatalities from marine envenomations are rare. However, significant morbidity results from bites and stings, including severe pain, retained foreign bodies, infection, respiratory compromise, hemodynamic instability, and a variety of other end organ toxicities.

- Special attention is required when treating envenomations inflicted by box jellyfish or sea snakes. These injuries are common and result in serious harm or even death. Knowledge of the clinical manifestations and available antidotes will reduce morbidity.

- A thorough understanding of the mechanisms of toxicity and expected clinical course following envenomations from marine creatures will provide clinicians with the ability to manage these injuries effectively.

- Interventions should focus on patient comfort and recognition of potential complications.

- Hot water immersion provides adequate analgesia for a number of different species of *Cnidaria*, as well as stings from a variety of spiny fish.

REFERENCES

1. Aniya Y, et al. Effect of the spine venom from the crown-of-thorns starfish, *Acanthaster planci*, on drug-metabolizing enzyme in rat liver. *J Toxicol Sci*. 1998;23:419-423.
2. Audley I. A case of sea-snake envenomation. *Med J Aust*. 1985;143:532.
3. Auerbach PS, Hays JT. Erythema nodosum following a jellyfish sting. *J Emerg Med*. 1987;5:487-491.
4. Auerbach PS. Hazardous marine animals. *Emerg Med Clin North Am*. 1984;2:531-544.
5. Auerbach PS. Marine envenomations. *N Engl J Med*. 1991;325:486-493.
6. Barss P. Wound necrosis caused by the venom of stingrays. Pathological findings and surgical management. *Med J Aust*. 1984;141:854-855.
7. Baxter EH, Gallichio HA. Cross-neutralization by tiger snake (*Notechis scutatus*) antivenene and sea snake (*Enhydrina schistosa*) antivenene against several sea snake venoms. *Toxicon*. 1974;12:273-278.
8. Baxter EH, Gallichio HA. Protection against sea snake envenomation: comparative potency of four antivenenes. *Toxicon*. 1976;14:347-355.
9. Baxter EH, Marr AG. Sea wasp (*Chironex fleckeri*) venom: lethal, haemolytic and dermonecrotic properties. *Toxicon*. 1969;7:195-210.
10. Baxter EH, Marr GM. Sea wasp (*Chironex fleckeri*) antivenene: neutralizing potency against the venom of three other jellyfish species. *Toxicon*. 1974;12:223-229.
11. Bengtson K, et al. Sudden death in a child following jellyfish envenomation by *Chiropsalmus quadrumanus*. Case report and autopsy findings. *JAMA*. 1991;266:1404-1406.
12. Birsa LM, et al. Evaluation of the effects of various chemicals on discharge of and pain caused by jellyfish nematocysts. *Comp Biochem Physiol C Toxicol Pharmacol*. 2010;151:426-430.
13. Borondo JC, et al. Fatal weeverfish sting. *Hum Exp Toxicol*. 2001;20:118-119.
14. Brown CK, Shepherd SM. Marine trauma, envenomations, and intoxications. *Emerg Med Clin North Am*. 1992;10:385-408.
15. Burnett JW. Dermatitis due to stinging sponges. *Cutis*. 1987;39:476.
16. Burnett JW, Calton GJ. Response of the box-jellyfish (*Chironex fleckeri*) cardiotoxin to intravenous administration of verapamil. *Med J Aust*. 1983;2:192-194.
17. Burnett JW, Calton GJ. The chemistry and toxicology of some venomous pelagic coelenterates. *Toxicon*. 1977;15:177-196.
18. Burnett JW, Calton GJ. Use of IgE antibody determinations in cutaneous Coelenterate envenomations. *Cutis*. 1981;27:50-52.
19. Burnett JW, Goldner R. Effects of *Chrysaora quinquecirrha* (sea nettle) toxin on the rat cardiovascular system. *Proc Soc Exp Biol Med*. 1969;132:353-356.
20. Burnett JW, et al. Recurrent eruptions following unusual solitary coelenterate envenomations. *J Am Acad Dermatol*. 1987;17:86-92.
21. Burnett JW, et al. Lymphokine activity in coelenterate envenomation. *Toxicon*. 1986;24:104-107.
22. Burnett JW, et al. Verapamil potentiation of Chironex (box-jellyfish) antivenom. *Toxicon*. 1990;28:242-244.
23. Burnett JW. Human injuries following jellyfish stings. *Md Med J*. 1992;41:509-513.
24. Cain D. Weever fish sting: an unusual problem. *Br Med J (Clin Res Ed)*. 1983;287:406-407.
25. Carducci M, et al. Raynaud's phenomenon secondary to weever fish stings. *Arch Dermatol*. 1996;132:838-839.
26. Carey JE, Wright EA. The toxicity and immunological properties of some sea-snake venoms with particular reference to that of *Enhydrina schistosa*. *Trans R Soc Trop Med Hyg*. 1960;54:50-67.
27. Cavazzoni E, et al. Blue-ringed octopus (*Hapalochlaena* sp.) envenomation of a 4-year-old boy: a case report. *Clin Toxicol (Phila)*. 2008;46:760-761.
28. Cegolon L, et al. Jellyfish stings and their management: a review. *Mar Drugs*. 2013;11:523-550.
29. Chen D, et al. Haemolytic activity of stonustoxin from stonefish (*Synanceja horrida*) venom: pore formation and the role of cationic amino acid residues. *Biochem J*. 1997;325(pt 3):685-691.
30. Church JE, Hodgson WC. Dose-dependent cardiovascular and neuromuscular effects of stonefish (*Synanceja trachynis*) venom. *Toxicon*. 2000;38:391-407.
31. Church JE, Hodgson WC. Stonefish (*Synanceia* spp.) antivenom neutralises the in vitro and in vivo cardiovascular activity of soldierfish (*Gymnapistes marmoratus*) venom. *Toxicon*. 2001;39:319-324.
32. Church JE, Hodgson WC. The pharmacological activity of fish venoms. *Toxicon*. 2002;40:1083-1093.
33. Church JE, et al. Modulation of intracellular Ca²⁺ levels by Scorpaenidae venoms. *Toxicon*. 2003;41:679-689.
34. Clark AT, et al. A retrospective review of the presentation and treatment of stingray stings reported to a poison control system. *Am J Ther*. 2017;24:e177-e180.
35. Clark RF, et al. Stingray envenomation: a retrospective review of clinical presentation and treatment in 119 cases. *J Emerg Med*. 2007;33:33-37.
36. Cooper NK. Historical vignette—the death of an Australian army doctor on Thursday Island in 1915 after envenomation by a stonefish. *J R Army Med Corps*. 1991;137:104-105.
37. Corkeron MA. Magnesium infusion to treat Irukandji syndrome. *Med J Aust*. 2003;178:411.
38. Currie BJ. Marine antivenoms. *J Toxicol Clin Toxicol*. 2003;41:301-308.
39. de Haro L, Pommier P. Envenomation: a real risk of keeping exotic house pets. *Vet Hum Toxicol*. 2003;45:214-216.

40. Edmonds C. A non-fatal case of blue-ringed octopus bite. *Med J Aust.* 1969;2:601.

41. Endean R, Sizemore DJ. The effectiveness of antivenom in countering the actions of box-jellyfish (*Chironex fleckeri*) nematocyst toxins in mice. *Toxicon.* 1988;26:425-431.

42. Endean R. Separation of two myotoxins from nematocysts of the box jellyfish (*Chironex fleckeri*). *Toxicon.* 1987;25:483-492.

43. Fegan D, Andresen D. *Conus geographus* envenomation. *Lancet.* 1997;349:1672.

44. Fenner P, et al. Box jellyfish antivenom and "Irukandji" stings. *Med J Aust.* 1986; 144:665-666.

45. Fenner P. Marine envenomation: an update—a presentation on the current status of marine envenomation first aid and medical treatments. *Emerg Med.* 2008;12:295-302.

46. Fenner PJ, et al. "Morbakka," another cubomedusan. *Med J Aust.* 1985;143:550-1–554-5.

47. Fenner PJ, Fitzpatrick PF. Experiments with the nematocysts of *Cyanea capillata*. *Med J Aust.* 1986;145:174.

48. Fenner PJ, Hadok JC. Fatal envenomation by jellyfish causing Irukandji syndrome. *Med J Aust.* 2002;177:362-363.

49. Fenner PJ, Lewin M. Sublingual glyceryl trinitrate as prehospital treatment for hypertension in Irukandji syndrome. *Med J Aust.* 2003;179:655.

50. Fenner PJ, et al. Further understanding of, and a new treatment for, "Irukandji" (*Carukia barnesi*) stings. *Med J Aust.* 1986;145:569–572-4.

51. Fenner PJ, Williamson J. Experiments with the nematocysts of *Carybdea rastoni* ("Jimble"). *Med J Aust.* 1987;147:258-259.

52. Fenner PJ, et al. Successful use of Chironex antivenom by members of the Queensland Ambulance Transport Brigade. *Med J Aust.* 1989;151:708-710.

53. Fenner PJ, et al. First aid treatment of jellyfish stings in Australia. Response to a newly differentiated species. *Med J Aust.* 1993;158:498-501.

54. Fenner PJ, et al. Fatal and non-fatal stingray envenomation. *Med J Aust.* 1989;151:621-625.

55. Fenner PJ, Williamson JA. Worldwide deaths and severe envenomation from jellyfish stings. *Med J Aust.* 1996;165:658-661.

56. Flachsenberger W, et al. Sphero-echinocytosis of human red blood cells caused by snake, red-back spider, bee and blue-ringed octopus venoms and its inhibition by snake sera. *Toxicon.* 1995;33:791-797.

57. Flachsenberger WA. Respiratory failure and lethal hypotension due to blue-ringed octopus and tetrodotoxin envenomation observed and counteracted in animal models. *J Toxicol Clin Toxicol.* 1986;24:485-502.

58. Flecker H, Cotton BC. Fatal bite from octopus. *Med J Aust.* 1955;42:329-331.

59. Flecker H. Irukandji sting to North Queensland bathers without production of weals but with severe general symptoms. *Med J Aust.* 1952;2:89-91.

60. Freeman SE, Turner RJ. Cardiovascular effects of toxins isolated from the cnidarian *Chironex fleckeri* Southcott. *Br J Pharmacol.* 1971;41:154-166.

61. Freeman SE. Actions of *Chironex fleckeri* toxins on cardiac transmembrane potentials. *Toxicon.* 1974;12:395-404.

62. Fulde GW, Smith F. Sea snake envenomation at Bondi. *Med J Aust.* 1984;141:44-45.

63. Garnier P, et al. Cardiotoxicity of verrucotoxin, a protein isolated from the venom of *Synanceia verrucosa*. *Toxicon.* 1997;35:47-55.

64. Germain M, et al. The cutaneous cellular infiltrate to stingray envenomization contains increased TIA+ cells. *Br J Dermatol.* 2000;143:1074-1077.

65. Ghadessy FJ, et al. Stonustoxin is a novel lethal factor from stonefish (*Synanceja horrida*) venom. cDNA cloning and characterization. *J Biol Chem.* 1996;271:25575-25581.

66. Grady JD, Burnett JW. Irukandji-like syndrome in South Florida divers. *Ann Emerg Med.* 2003;42:763-766.

67. Haddad VJ, et al. Tropical dermatology: marine and aquatic dermatology. *J Am Acad Dermatol.* 2009;61:733-750; quiz 751-752.

68. Halford ZA, et al. Cone shell envenomation: epidemiology, pharmacology and medical care. *Diving Hyperb Med.* 2015;45:200-207.

69. Hartwick R, et al. Disarming the box-jellyfish: nematocyst inhibition in *Chironex fleckeri*. *Med J Aust.* 1980;1:15-20.

70. Hastings SG, et al. Effects of nematocyst toxin of *Physalia physalis* (Portuguese man-of-war) on the canine cardiovascular system. *Proc Soc Exp Biol Med.* 1967;125:41-45.

71. Heifets BD, et al. Acute cardiovascular toxicity of low-dose intrathecal ziconotide. *Pain Med.* 2013;14:1807-1809.

72. Henderson D, Easton RG. Stingose. A new and effective treatment for bites and stings. *Med J Aust.* 1980;2:146-150.

73. Huynh TT, et al. Severity of Irukandji syndrome and nematocyst identification from skin scrapings. *Med J Aust.* 2003;178:38-41.

74. Ihama Y, et al. Anaphylactic shock caused by sting of crown-of-thorns starfish (*Acanthaster planci*). *Forensic Sci Int.* 2014;236:e5-e8.

75. Jouiaei M, et al. Ancient venom systems: a review on cnidaria toxins. *Toxins (Basel).* 2015;7:2251-2271.

76. Kaffenberger BH, et al. The effect of climate change on skin disease in North America. *J Am Acad Dermatol.* 2017;76:140-147.

77. Kizer KW, et al. Scorpaenidae envenomation. A five-year poison center experience. *JAMA.* 1985;253:807-810.

78. Klein SG, et al. Irukandji jellyfish polyps exhibit tolerance to interacting climate change stressors. *Glob Chang Biol.* 2014;20:28-37.

79. Kreger AS, et al. Effects of stonefish (*Synanceia trachynis*) venom on murine and frog neuromuscular junctions. *Toxicon.* 1993;31:307-317.

80. Kreger AS. Detection of a cytolytic toxin in the venom of the stonefish (*Synanceia trachynis*). *Toxicon.* 1991;29:733-743.

81. Kularatne SAM, et al. *Enhydrina schistosa* (Elapidae: Hydrophiinae) the most dangerous sea snake in Sri Lanka: three case studies of severe envenoming. *Toxicon.* 2014;77:78-86.

82. Larsen JB, Lane CE. Direct action of Physalia toxin on frog nerve and muscle. *Toxicon.* 1970;8:21-23.

83. Lee C-C, et al. Hemolytic activity of venom from crown-of-thorns starfish *Acanthaster planci* spines. *J Venom Anim Toxins Incl Trop Dis.* 2013;19:22.

84. Lehmann DF, Hardy JC. Stonefish envenomation. *N Engl J Med.* 1993;329:510-511.

85. Lewis RJ, et al. Conus venom peptide pharmacology. *Pharmacol Rev.* 2012;64:259-298.

86. Lillywhite HB, et al. Sea snakes (*Laticauda* spp.) require fresh drinking water: implication for the distribution and persistence of populations. *Physiol Biochem Zool.* 2008;81:785-796.

87. Lin B, et al. A case of elevated liver function tests after crown-of-thorns (*Acanthaster planci*) envenomation. *Wilderness Environ Med.* 2008;19:275-279.

88. Linaweaver PG. Toxic marine life. *Mil Med.* 1967;132:437-442.

89. Lippmann JM, et al. Fatal and severe box jellyfish stings, including Irukandji stings, in Malaysia, 2000-2010. *J Travel Med.* 2011;18:275-281.

90. Little M, et al. Life-threatening cardiac failure in a healthy young female with Irukandji syndrome. *Anaesth Intensive Care.* 2001;29:178-180.

91. Little M, Mulcahy RF. A year's experience of Irukandji envenomation in far north Queensland. *Med J Aust.* 1998;169:638-641.

92. Little M, et al. Severe cardiac failure associated with presumed jellyfish sting. Irukandji syndrome? *Anaesth Intensive Care.* 2003;31:642-647.

93. Little M, Somerville A. Clonidine to treat Irukandji syndrome. *Emerg Med Australas.* 2016;28:756-757.

94. Loten C, et al. A randomised controlled trial of hot water (45 degrees C) immersion versus ice packs for pain relief in bluebottle stings. *Med J Aust.* 2006;184:329-333.

95. Lumley J, et al. Fatal envenomation by *Chironex fleckeri*, the north Australian box jellyfish: the continuing search for lethal mechanisms. *Med J Aust.* 1988;148:527-534.

96. Manabe Y, et al. A case of delayed flare-up allergic dermatitis caused by jellyfish sting. *Tokai J Exp Clin Med.* 2014;39:90-94.

97. Maretic Z, Russell FE. Stings by the sea anemone *Anemonia sulcata* in the Adriatic Sea. *Am J Trop Med Hyg.* 1983;32:891-896.

98. Martin JC, Audley I. Cardiac failure following Irukandji envenomation. *Med J Aust.* 1990;153:164-166.

99. McCullagh N, et al. Randomised trial of magnesium in the treatment of Irukandji syndrome. *Emerg Med Australas.* 2012;24:560-565.

100. McGoldrick J, Marx JA. Marine envenomations. Part 2: invertebrates. *J Emerg Med.* 1992;10:71-77.

101. McGoldrick J, Marx JA. Marine envenomations; Part 1: vertebrates. *J Emerg Med.* 1991; 9:497-502.

102. McIntosh JM, et al. Isolation and characterization of a novel conus peptide with apparent antinociceptive activity. *J Biol Chem.* 2000;275:32391-32397.

103. McIntosh JM, et al. Presence of serotonin in the venom of *Conus imperialis*. *Toxicon.* 1993;31:1561-1566.

104. McIntosh JM, Jones RM. Cone venom—from accidental stings to deliberate injection. *Toxicon.* 2001;39:1447-1451.

105. Mercer HP, et al. Envenomation by sea snake in Queensland. *Med J Aust.* 1981;1:130-132.

106. Minton SAJ. Paraspecific protection by elapid and sea snake antivenins. *Toxicon.* 1967;5:47-55.

107. Muhvich KH, et al. Pathophysiology of sea nettle (*Chrysaora quinquecirrha*), envenomation in a rat model and the effects of hyperbaric oxygen and verapamil treatment. *Toxicon.* 1991;29:857-866.

108. Mustafa MR, et al. The mechanism underlying the cardiotoxic effect of the toxin from the jellyfish *Chironex fleckeri*. *Toxicol Appl Pharmacol.* 1995;133:196-206.

109. Nielsen DB, et al. Isolation of Lys-conopressin-G from the venom of the worm-hunting snail, *Conus imperialis*. *Toxicon.* 1994;32:845-848.

110. O'Leary MA, et al. Use of high performance liquid chromatography to measure tetrodotoxin in serum and urine of poisoned patients. *Toxicon.* 2004;44:549-553.

111. O'Reilly GM, et al. Prospective study of jellyfish stings from tropical Australia, including the major box jellyfish *Chironex fleckeri*. *Med J Aust.* 2001;175:652-655.

112. Olivera BM, et al. Effects of Conus peptides on the behavior of mice. *Curr Opin Neurobiol.* 1999;9:772-777.

113. Ouanounou G, et al. Trachynilysin, a neurosecretory protein isolated from stonefish (*Synanceia trachynis*) venom, forms nonselective pores in the membrane of NG108-15 cells. *J Biol Chem.* 2002;277:39119-39127.

114. Pereira PL, et al. Pressure immobilisation bandages in first-aid treatment of jellyfish envenomation: current recommendations reconsidered. *Med J Aust.* 2000;173:650-652.

115. Ramasamy S, et al. Pharmacologically distinct cardiovascular effects of box jellyfish (*Chironex fleckeri*) venom and a tentacle-only extract in rats. *Toxicol Lett.* 2005;155:219-226.

116. Ramasamy S, et al. The in vitro effects of two chirodropid (*Chironex fleckeri* and *Chiropsalmus* sp.) venoms: efficacy of box jellyfish antivenom. *Toxicon.* 2003;41:703-711.

117. Ramasamy S, et al. The in vivo cardiovascular effects of box jellyfish *Chironex fleckeri* venom in rats: efficacy of pre-treatment with antivenom, verapamil and magnesium sulphate. *Toxicon.* 2004;43:685-690.

118. Ramasamy S, et al. The in vivo cardiovascular effects of the Irukandji jellyfish (*Carukia barnesi*) nematocyst venom and a tentacle extract in rats. *Toxicol Lett.* 2005;155: 135-141.

119. Rathjen WF, Halstead BW. Report on two fatalities due to stingrays. *Toxicon.* 1969; 6:301-302.

120. Reid HA. Sea-snake antivenene: successful trial. *Br Med J.* 1962;2:576-579.

121. Reid HA. Sea-snake bite research. *Trans R Soc Trop Med Hyg.* 1956;50:517–38; discussion 539-42.

122. Reid HA. Antivenom in sea-snake bit poisoning. *Lancet.* 1975;1:622-623.

123. Riviere G, et al. Effect of antivenom on venom pharmacokinetics in experimentally envenomed rabbits: toward an optimization of antivenom therapy. *J Pharmacol Exp Ther.* 1997;281:1-8.

124. Rossetto AL, et al. Seabather's eruption: report of fourteen cases. *An Acad Bras Cienc.* 2015;87:431-436.

125. Rossetto AL, et al. Sea urchin granuloma. *Rev Inst Med Trop Sao Paulo.* 2006;48:303-306.

126. Rosson CL, Tolle SW. Management of marine stings and scrapes. *West J Med.* 1989;150:97-100.

127. Russell FE, et al. Studies on the mechanism of death from stingray venom; a report of two fatal cases. *Am J Med Sci.* 1958;235:566-584.

128. Russell FE, van Harreveld A. Cardiovascular effects of the venom of the round stingray, *Urobatis halleri. Arch Int Physiol Biochim.* 1954;62:322-333.

129. Russo AJ, et al. The relationship of the possible allergic response to jellyfish envenomation and serum antibody titers. *Toxicon.* 1983;21:475-480.

130. Saggiomo SLA, Seymour JE. Cardiotoxic effects of venom fractions from the Australian box jellyfish *Chironex fleckeri* on human myocardiocytes. *Toxicon.* 2012;60:391-395.

131. Sato H, et al. Case of skin injuries due to stings by crown-of-thorns starfish (*Acanthaster planci*). *J Dermatol.* 2008;35:162-167.

132. Saunders PR, et al. Cardiovascular actions of venom of the stonefish *Synanceja horrida. Am J Physiol.* 1962;203:429-432.

133. Sauviat MP, et al. Effects of trachynilysin, a protein isolated from stonefish (*Synanceia trachynis*) venom, on frog atrial heart muscle. *Toxicon.* 2000;38:945-959.

134. Schmidt ME, et al. Nephrotoxic action of rattlesnake and sea snake venoms: an electron-microscopic study. *J Pathol.* 1976;118:75-81.

135. Sheumack DD, et al. Maculotoxin: a neurotoxin from the venom glands of the octopus *Hapalochlaena maculosa* identified as tetrodotoxin. *Science.* 1978;199:188-189.

136. Shiraev TP, et al. Threatened limb from stingray injury. *Vascular.* January 2016: 1708538116670315.

137. Skeie E. Toxin of the weeverfish (*Trachinus draco*). Experimental studies on animals. *Acta Pharmacol Toxicol (Copenh).* 1962;19:107-120.

138. Southcott RV, Coulter JR. The effects of the southern Australian marine stinging sponges, *Neofibularia mordens* and *Lissodendoryx* sp. *Med J Aust.* 1971;2:895-901.

139. Stein MR, et al. Fatal Portuguese man-o'-war (*Physalia physalis*) envenomation. *Ann Emerg Med.* 1989;18:312-315.

140. Strutton G, Lumley J. Cutaneous light microscopic and ultrastructural changes in a fatal case of jellyfish envenomation. *J Cutan Pathol.* 1988;15:249-255.

141. Sutherland SK, Lane WR. Toxins and mode of envenomation of the common ringed or blue-banded octopus. *Med J Aust.* 1969;1:893-898.

142. Sutherland SK. Antivenom use in Australia. Premedication, adverse reactions and the use of venom detection kits. *Med J Aust.* 1992;157:734-739.

143. Tamiya N, Yagi T. Studies on sea snake venom. *Proc Jpn Acad Ser B Phys Biol Sci.* 2011; 87:41-52.

144. Tan CH, et al. Venomics of the beaked sea snake, *Hydrophis schistosus*: a minimalist toxin arsenal and its cross-neutralization by heterologous antivenoms. *J Proteomics.* 2015;126:121-130.

145. Tan CH, et al. Antivenom cross-neutralization of the venoms of *Hydrophis schistosus* and *Hydrophis curtus*, two common sea snakes in Malaysian waters. *Toxins (Basel).* 2015;7:572-581.

146. Tang WM, et al. Rapidly progressive necrotising fasciitis following a stonefish sting: a report of two cases. *J Orthop Surg (Hong Kong).* 2006;14:67-70.

147. Tay TKW, et al. Stonefish envenomation of hand with impending compartment syndrome. *J Occup Med Toxicol.* 2016;11:23.

148. Terlau H, Olivera BM. Conus venoms: a rich source of novel ion channel-targeted peptides. *Physiol Rev.* 2004;84:41-68.

149. Tibballs J, et al. The effects of antivenom and verapamil on the haemodynamic actions of *Chironex fleckeri* (box jellyfish) venom. *Anaesth Intensive Care.* 1998;26:40-45.

150. Tiong K. Irukandji syndrome, catecholamines, and mid-ventricular stress cardiomyopathy. *Eur J Echocardiogr.* 2009;10:334-336.

151. Tomchik RS, et al. Clinical perspectives on seabather's eruption, also known as "sea lice." *JAMA.* 1993;269:1669-1672.

152. Trestrail JH, al-Mahasneh QM. Lionfish string experiences of an inland poison center: a retrospective study of 23 cases. *Vet Hum Toxicol.* 1989;31:173-175.

153. Tu AT, Salafranca ES. Immunological properties and neutralization of sea snake venoms. II. *Am J Trop Med Hyg.* 1974;23:135-138.

154. Turner B, Sullivan P. Disarming the bluebottle: treatment of Physalia envenomation. *Med J Aust.* 1980;2:394-395.

155. Violette A, et al. Recruitment of glycosyl hydrolase proteins in a cone snail venomous arsenal: further insights into biomolecular features of Conus venoms. *Mar Drugs.* 2012;10:258-280.

156. Walker DG. Survival after severe envenomation by the blue-ringed octopus (*Hapalochlaena maculosa*). *Med J Aust.* 1983;2:663-665.

157. Walker MJ, Peng-Nam-Yeoh. The in vitro neuromuscular blocking properties of sea snake (*Enhydrina schistosa*) venom. *Eur J Pharmacol.* 1974;28:199-208.

158. Wiener S. A case of stone-fish sting treated with antivenene. *Med J Aust.* 1965;1:191.

159. Wiener S. Observations on the venom of the stone fish (*Synanceja trachynis*). *Med J Aust.* 1959;46:620-627.

160. Williamson JA, et al. Serious envenomation by the Northern Australian box-jellyfish (*Chironex fleckeri*). *Med J Aust.* 1980;1:13-16.

161. Williamson JA, et al. Acute management of serious envenomation by box-jellyfish (*Chironex fleckeri*). *Med J Aust.* 1984;141:851-853.

162. Williamson JA. The blue-ringed octopus bite and envenomation syndrome. *Clin Dermatol.* 1987;5:127-133.

163. Winkel KD, et al. Cardiovascular actions of the venom from the Irukandji (*Carukia barnesi*) jellyfish: effects in human, rat and guinea-pig tissues in vitro and in pigs in vitro. *Clin Exp Pharmacol Physiol.* 2005;32:777-788.

164. Wittenberg JB. The source of carbon monoxide in the float of the Portuguese man-of-war, *Physalia physalis* L. *J Exp Biol.* 1960;37:698.

165. Wong DE, et al. Seabather's eruption. Clinical, histologic, and immunologic features. *J Am Acad Dermatol.* 1994;30:399-406.

166. Wu M-L, et al. Sea-urchin envenomation. *Vet Hum Toxicol.* 2003;45:307-309.

167. Yoshiba S. An estimation of the most dangerous species of cone shell, *Conus* (*Gastridium*) *geographus* Linne, 1758, venom's lethal dose in humans [in Japanese]. *Nihon Eiseigaku Zasshi.* 1984;39:565-572.

168. Yoshimoto CM, Yanagihara AA. Cnidarian (coelenterate) envenomations in Hawai'i improve following heat application. *Trans R Soc Trop Med Hyg.* 2002;96:300-303.

117 MUSHROOMS

Lewis R. Goldfrank

The diversity of mushroom species is evident in our grocery stores, our restaurant menus, and our environment. The enhanced culinary interest in mushrooms has led to experimentation by young and old—old citizens and our newest immigrants and our young children reaching for what might become an innocuous (common) or a serious (rare) ingestion. Rigor in analyzing the possible ingestion is indispensable for those treating a patient who has ingested a mushroom of concern. This chapter offers general information on the most consequential toxicologic groups of mushrooms and emphasizes clinical diagnosis over mushroom identification.

EPIDEMIOLOGY

Unintentional ingestions of mushrooms particularly in children represent a small but relatively constant percentage of consultations requested from poison control centers (Chap. 130). A summary of a quarter century of American Association of Poison Control Centers (AAPCC) data reveals that mushrooms represent less than 0.25% of the reported human exposures. Combined data accumulated by the AAPCC and the Mushroom Poisoning Registry of the North American Mycological Association indicates that approximately 5 patient exposures to toxic mushrooms are called into Poison Control Centers or reported to the Registry per 100,000 persons per year. Some variations result from geographic and climatic conditions and mycologic habitats.[141] Although the methods of codification of patients with mushroom exposure have changed over the past 35 years, cumulative AAPCC data consistently demonstrate the relative benignity of the vast majority of exposures. The inability of most health care providers to correctly identify the ingested mushroom and the rarity of lethal outcomes are also demonstrated by the accumulated data. In 75% to 95% of exposures, the exact species was unidentified[141] (Chap. 130). More than 50% of exposed individuals had no symptoms. Most patients were treated at home and rarely had major toxicity. During the 35 years covered by the AAPCC data, fewer than 100 patients died of their mushroom ingestion. Of the mushrooms associated with death, most were *Amanita* spp and several were hallucinogens, *Boletus* spp, or gyromitrin-containing mushrooms, while others remained unidentified. All reported deaths occurred in adults. Those containing either hallucinogens or gastrointestinal (GI) toxins were the most common reported exposures, yet they accounted for less than 10% of all mushroom exposures. All other presumed exposures represented less than 2% of those actually identified. A distinctly different analysis is presented by a retrospective study from the Krakow Department of Medical Toxicology suggesting that following mycological analysis 87% of their 457 adult poisoning cases over an 8-year period were related to edible species. They suggested that extended storage in plastic prior to preparation, long storage following cooking, or simply delay to use led to mild gastrointestinal manifestations.[60] Because more than 75% of mushrooms involved in exposures are never identified—more than 100,000 mushroom species exist, less than 0.1% of these are known to be toxic, and many species are poorly studied—a strategy for making significant decisions with incomplete data is essential.

CLASSIFICATION AND MANAGEMENT

This chapter does not address molds, mildews, and yeasts, which in addition to mushrooms are all categorized as fungi. The unifying principle for fungi is the lack of the photosynthetic capacity to produce nutrition. Survival is achieved by the enzymatic capacity of these organisms to integrate into living materials and digest them. Molds are ubiquitous and often associated with varied adverse health effects such as rhinitis, rashes, headaches, and asthma.[22] Trichothecenes are mold-related mycotoxins that are discussed in Chap. 127 as potential biological weapons. All other molds are not associated with toxicologic emergencies and are not addressed in this chapter.

Because mushroom species vary widely with regard to the xenobiotics they contain, and because identifying them with certainty is difficult, a system of classification based on clinical effects is more useful than one based on taxonomy (Table 117–1). The text and tables that follow associate the most common species with a particular syndrome or xenobiotic and are not meant to be inclusive of all the exceptionally diverse mushrooms associated with many xenobiotics. In many instances the taxonomy has changed, confusing readers and investigators. For example, the text will use the current nomenclature, whereas the citations will obviously use prior nomenclature. In many cases, management and prognosis can be determined with a high degree of confidence from the history and the geographic origin of the mushroom, the initial signs and symptoms, the organ system or systems involved, and coexistent factors or conditions.[32,65,84,121] Most unintentional ingestions in small children involve at the most tasting common backyard mushrooms, which almost invariably result in no symptoms and no risks. Identification of the mushroom by photography will permit enhancement of the toxicologists' efforts at reassurance.

GROUP I: CYCLOPEPTIDE-CONTAINING MUSHROOMS

α-Amanitin

Worldwide most mushroom fatalities are associated with cyclopeptide-containing species.[5,33,138] Approximately 50 to 100 cases are reported annually in Western Europe with fewer in Asia, Australia, Africa, and North and South America.[34] There are many fewer cases in the United States with far less certainty of amatoxin poisoning and with limited precise data of those patients ill enough to be transferred to transplant centers for acute liver injury or acute liver failure.[75] In North America, there are 2 distinct ranges of the *Amanita* species along the West Coast (California to British Columbia) and along the East Coast (Maryland to Maine).[157] These mushrooms include a number of *Amanita* species, including *A. verna*, *A. virosa*, and *A. phalloides*; *Galerina* spp, including *G. autumnalis*, *G. marginata*, and *G. venenata*; and *Lepiota* species, including *L. helveola*, *L. josserandi*, and *L. brunneoincarnata* (Fig. 117–1). Early differentiation of cyclopeptide poisonings from other types of mushroom poisoning is difficult (Fig. 117–2). Patients poisoned with cyclopeptides may be ill enough to seek health care for nausea, vomiting, abdominal pain, and diarrhea, which in the absence of a carefully focused history often is attributed to other causes as the patient improves with supportive care. Such patients are occasionally sent home, only to return moribund in 1 to 2 days. The delayed onset of more serious symptoms is typical of cyclopeptide toxicity and is a critical consideration in assessing the toxicologic potential of any exposure.

A. phalloides contains 15 to 20 cyclopeptides, each with an approximate weight of 900 Da. The amatoxins (cyclic octapeptides), phallotoxins (cyclic

TABLE 117–1   Mushroom Toxicity Overview

Representative Genus/ Species	Xenobiotic	Time of Onset of Symptoms	Primary Site of Toxicity	Clinical Findings	Mortality	Specific Therapy[a]

I
Amanita phalloides, A. tenuifolia, A. virosa Galerina autumnalis, G. marginata, G. venenata Lepiota josserandi, L. helveola
	Cyclopeptides Amatoxins Phallotoxins	5–24 h	Liver	Phase I: GI toxicity— N/V/D
				Phase II: Quiescent
				Phase III: N/V/D, jaundice, ↑ AST, ↑ ALT ↑ Bilirubin
					30%	Potential benefit early
						  Activated charcoal
						Hemoperfusion/hemodialysis
						  Silibinin
						  Polymyxin B
						Potential benefit late
						  N-acetylcysteine

II Gyromitra ambigua, G. esculenta, G. infula	Gyromitrin (metabolite: monomethylhydrazine)	5–10 h	CNS	Seizures, abdominal pain, N/V, weakness, hepatorenal failure	Rare	Benzodiazepines, pyridoxine 70 mg/kg IV (max 5 g)
III Clitocybe dealbata, Omphalotus olearius, most Inocybe spp Boletus eastwoodiae	Muscarine	0.5–2 h	Autonomic nervous system	Peripheral muscarinic effects— salivation, bradycardia, lacrimation, urination, defecation, diaphoresis	Rare	Atropine—Adults: 1–2 mg Children: 0.02 mg/kg with a minimum of 0.1 mg
IV Coprinopsis atramentaria C. insignis	Coprine (metabolite: 1- aminocyclopropanol)	0.5–2 h	Aldehyde dehydrogenase	Disulfiramlike effect with ethanol, tachycardia, N/V, flushing	Rare	Antiemetics Fluid resuscitation Fomepizole for refractory toxicity
V Amanita gemmata, A. muscaria, A. pantherina, Tricholoma muscarium	Ibotenic acid, muscimol	0.5–2 h	CNS	GABAergic effects, rare delirium, hallucinations, dizziness, ataxia	Rare	Benzodiazepines during excitatory phase
VI Psilocybe cyanescens, P. cubensis Gymnopilus spectabilis Psathyrella foenisecii	Psilocybin, psilocin	0.5–1 h	CNS	Ataxia, N/V, hyperkinesis, hallucinations, illusions	Rare	Benzodiazepines for agitation
VII Clitocybe nebularis Chlorophyllum molybdites, C. esculentum, Lactarius spp, Paxillus involutus	Various GI irritants	0.3–3 h	GI	Malaise, N/V/D	Rare	Symptomatic care
VIII Cortinarius orellanus, C. rubellus C. gentilis	Orellanine, orellinine	>1 d– weeks	Kidney	Phase I: N/V Phase II: Oliguria, Acute kidney injury	Rare	Hemodialysis for acute kidney injury
IX Amanita smithiana A. proxima, A. pseudoporphyria	Allenic norleucine	0.5–12 h	Kidney	Phase I: N/V Phase II: Oliguria, Acute kidney injury	None	Hemodialysis for acute kidney injury
X Tricholoma equestre (Europe) Russula subnigricans (Japan, China)	Cycloprop-2- enecarboxylic acid	24–72 h 0.5–2 h	Muscle (skeletal and cardiac)	Fatigue, nausea, vomiting, muscle weakness, myalgias, ↑ CK, facial erythema, diaphoresis, myocarditis	10%	Sodium bicarbonate, hemodialysis for acute kidney injury
XI Trogia venenata	2R-amino-4,5-hydroxy- 5-hexynoic acid	1–5 d	Cardiac and skeletal muscle	Tachycardia, GI symptoms, myalgias, tremor, seizures, dizziness, weakness, syncope, palpitations, ventricular fibrillation	High?	Intensive care monitoring
Amanita franchetti Ramaria rufescens		2–15 h 2–15 h				

(Continued)

TABLE 117–1 Mushroom Toxicity Overview *(Continued)*

Representative Genus/ Species	Xenobiotic	Time of Onset of Symptoms	Primary Site of Toxicity	Clinical Findings	Mortality	Specific Therapy[a]
XII						
Clitocybe acromelalga, C. amoenolens	Acromelic acids	24 h	Peripheral nervous system	Erythromelalgia paresthesias— hands and feet, dysesthesias, erythema, edema	None	Symptomatic care
XIII						
Pleurocybella porrigens	Unknown	1–31 d	CNS	Encephalopathy, convulsions, myoclonus in patients with chronic kidney failure	High (30%)	Hemodialysis
Hapalopilus rutilans	Polyporic acid	>12 h	GI, CNS	N/V, abdominal pain, vertigo, ataxia, drowsiness, encephalopathy	None	Symptomatic care
XIV						
Paxillus involutus, Clitocybe claviceps? Boletus luridus?	Involutin	Following repeated exposure 0.5–3 h	Red blood cell, kidney	Hemolytic anemia, acute kidney injury	Rare	Hemodialysis
XV						
Lycoperdon perlatum, L. pyriforme L. gemmatum	Spores	Hours	Pulmonary, GI	Cough, shortness of breath, fever, nausea, vomiting	None	Corticosteroids

[a]Supportive care (fluids, electrolytes, and antiemetics) as indicated.

AST/ALT = hepatic aminotransferases; CK = creatine phosphokinase; D = diarrhea; N = nausea; V = vomiting.

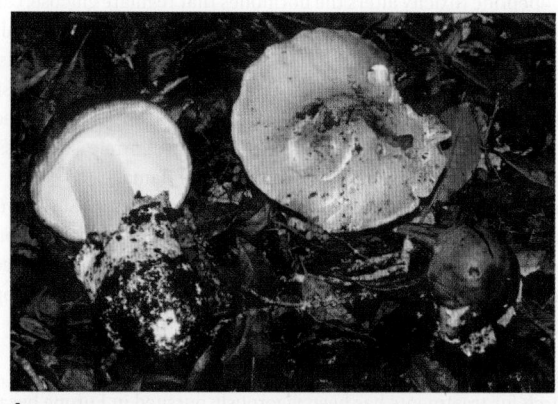

A

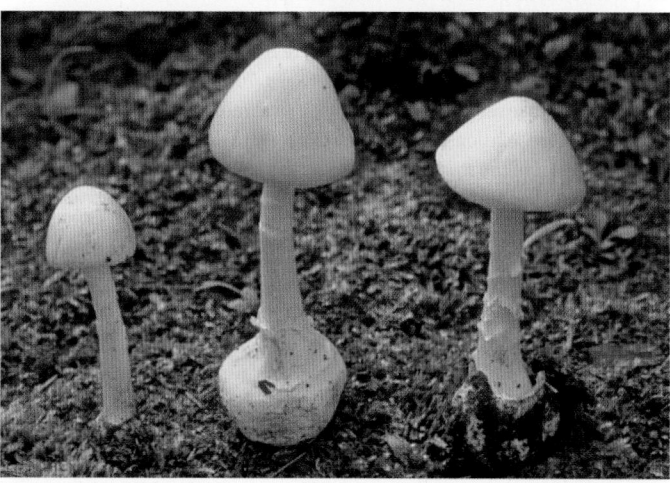

B

FIGURE 117–1. Group I: Cyclopeptide-containing mushrooms. **(A)** *Amanita phalloides* and **(B)** *Amanita virosa. (Used with permission from John Plischke III.)*

heptapeptides), and virotoxins (cyclic heptapeptides) are the best studied.[38,58,80,152] There is no evidence for the toxicity of virotoxins in humans. Of these 3 chemically similar cyclopeptide molecules, phalloidin (the principal phallotoxin) appears to be rapid-acting, whereas amanitin tends to cause more delayed manifestations.[125] Phalloidin crosses the sinusoidal plasma membranes of hepatocytes by a carrier-mediated process. This process is shared by bile salts and can be prevented in the presence of extracellular bile salts, suggesting competitive inhibition. A sodium-independent bile salt transporting system may be responsible for phalloidin hepatic uptake, elimination, and detoxification.[97] Phalloidin interrupts actin polymerization and impairs cell membrane function, but because of its very limited oral absorption it has minimal systemic toxicity, but results in the initial GI dysfunction noted following *Amanita* spp ingestion.

The amatoxins are the most toxic of the cyclopeptides, leading to liver, kidney, and central nervous system (CNS) damage. These polypeptides are heat stable.[36] α-Amanitin is the principal amatoxin responsible for human toxicity following ingestion. Approximately 1.5 to 2.5 mg of amanitin can be obtained from 1 g of dry *A. phalloides*, and as much as 3.5 mg/g can be obtained from some *Lepiota* spp.[107,111,152] A 20-g mushroom contains well in excess of the 0.1 mg/kg amanitin considered lethal for humans.[35] α-Amanitin and β-amanitin have comparable toxicity in animal models.[39]

The amanitins are highly bioavailable and rapidly absorbed from the GI tract.[70] Amatoxins show limited protein binding and are present in the plasma at low concentrations for 24 to 48 hours.[70] Hepatocellular entry of α-amanitin is facilitated by a sodium-dependent bile acid transporter. Several studies demonstrate that the sodium taurocholate cotransporter polypeptide, a member of the organic anion–transporter (OAT) polypeptide family localized in the sinusoidal membranes of human hepatocytes, facilitates hepatocellular α-amanitin uptake.[64,86] Once inside the cells, the cytotoxicity of amanitin results from its interference with RNA polymerase II, preventing the transcription of DNA thereby suppressing protein synthesis resulting in cell death.[89,133] α-Amanitin is enterohepatically recirculated. Target organs are those with the highest rate of cell turnover, including the GI tract epithelium, hepatocytes, and kidneys. Amatoxins do not cross the placenta, as demonstrated by the absence of fetal toxicity in severely poisoned pregnant women.[7,13,138]

In an intravenous radiolabeled amatoxin study in dogs, 85% of the amatoxin was recovered in the urine within the first 6 hours, whereas less than 1% was

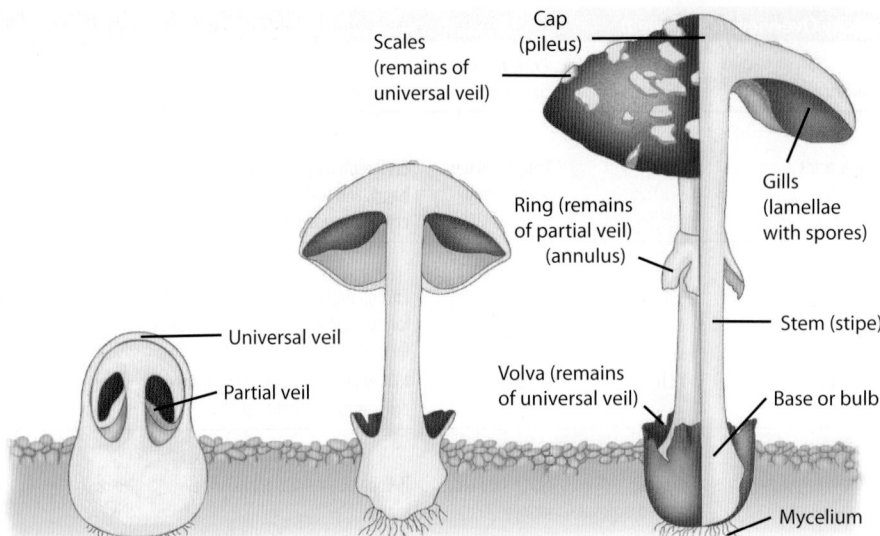

FIGURE 117–2. In the more highly specialized and evolved mushrooms, various protective tissues cover the fruit body and its constituent parts during its development. In the mushroom shown, an *Amanita* species, 2 veils of tissue are involved—one an outer enclosing bag, the universal veil, which ruptures as the fruit body expands to leave a volva at the base and fragments on the cap; the other an inner partial veil covering the developing gills that is pulled away as the cap opens to leave a ring on the stem. *(Adapted with permission from Kibby G. Mushrooms and Toadstools, A Field Guide: Oxford: Oxford University Press; 1979.)*

found in the blood at that time.[40] Some of the toxicokinetic analyses following unquantified ingestions demonstrate 12 to 23 mcg amanitin excretion in the urine over 24 to 66 hours, of which 60% to 80% occurred during the first 2 hours of collection. The extreme variabilities of the type and quantity of amanitin ingested, the host, the delay from the time of ingestion to collection, and the management make interpretations exceedingly difficult.[145] In another series, total maximal urinary α- and β-amanitin excreted over 6 to 72 hours were 3.19 and 5.21 mg, respectively. Two-thirds of the patients had total amanitin excretion greater than 1.5 mg.[70] Urinary amanitin excretion concentrations differ by several orders of magnitude. Whether the variation results from exposure dose, time following ingestion, or laboratory technique is unclear.

Several variable techniques for quantitative and qualitative evaluation of amatoxins are utilized. Amatoxins can be detected by high-performance liquid chromatography,[70] thin-layer chromatography, ion trap mass spectrometry,[44] and radioimmunoassay in gastroduodenal fluid, serum,[111] urine,[17,18] stool, and liver and kidney biopsies for several days following an ingestion.[38,39,79]

Clinical

Phase I of cyclopeptide poisoning resembles severe gastroenteritis, with profuse watery diarrhea that is delayed until 5 to 24 hours after ingestion. Some consider the early onset (< 8 hours) of diarrhea as a predictive factor for hepatic failure and the need for liver transplantation,[36] whereas this is not supported by most other case series reviewed. Early onset of gastrointestinal distress before 5 hours is strong support for another non-*Amanita* species or an etiology other than mushroom ingestion.

Transient improvement occurs during phase II from 12 and 36 hours after ingestion although hepatic injury begins during this phase.[111,159] Acute liver injury is defined by (a) a moderately severe coagulopathy (international normalized ratio {INR} ≥2.0), (b) presumed onset of acute illness less than 26 weeks, and (c) the absence of cirrhosis.[75,104] Acute liver failure can be defined as (a) the presence of hepatic encephalopathy of any degree, (b) evidence of moderately severe coagulopathy (INR ≥1.5), (c) presumed onset of illness of less than 26 weeks, and (d) the absence of cirrhosis.[104] Pathologic manifestations include steatosis, central zonal necrosis, and centrilobular hemorrhage, with viable hepatocytes remaining at the rims of the larger triads. Lobular architecture remains intact (Fig. 21–3).[5] Gastrointestinal manifestations including nausea, vomiting, abdominal pain and diarrhea may persist during the entirety of the clinical course.[66]

However, despite supportive care, phase III, manifested by hepatic and renal toxicity and death, may ensue 2 to 6 days after ingestion.[5] Although

hepatotoxicity begins within the second phase of toxicity, clinical hepatotoxicity (Chap. 21) with elevated concentrations of bilirubin, aspartate aminotransferase (AST), and alanine aminotransferase (ALT), hypoglycemia, jaundice, and hepatic coma are not manifest until 2 to 3 days after ingestion. Pancreatic toxicity rarely occurs.[51]

Cyclopeptide toxicity alters the hormones that regulate glucose, calcium, and thyroid homeostasis, resulting in widespread endocrine abnormalities.[76] Insulin and C-peptide concentrations are elevated at a stage of poisoning prior to hepatic and renal compromise.[30,76] These findings are suggestive of direct toxicity to pancreatic β cells, resulting in release of preformed hormone or induction of hormone synthesis. This insulin release necessitates vigilance for hypoglycemia prior to hepatocellular damage.

In a series of 10 patients exposed to diverse *Lepiota* spp, 50% developed a mixed sensory and motor polyneuropathy. Most of the patients spontaneously recovered within one year, although a single patient developed progressive clinical and electromyographic deterioration.[114] These neuropathic findings are not noted in other case reports.

Treatment

The search for treatments has been vigorously pursued in Europe because of the persistently large number of amatoxin exposures each year.[52] Survival rates in case series of variable numbers of patients poisoned by *A. phalloides* who received supportive care, fluid and electrolyte repletion, high-dose penicillin G, dexamethasone, or thioctic acid are between 70% and 100%.[52,62,69,100,105,116,159] Many of these case series have excellent survival rates with extremely variable therapeutic interventions, limiting the capacity to determine the need for or efficacy of most of the standard conservative therapeutic regimens.

Fluid and electrolyte repletion and treatment of hepatic compromise are essential. Intravenous 0.9% sodium chloride solution and electrolytes usually are necessary because of substantial fluid losses due to vomiting and diarrhea. Dextrose repletion titrating to serum glucose concentration (>100 mg/dL) is reasonable because of nutritional compromise, hepatic failure, or glycogen depletion. Activated charcoal both adsorbs the amatoxins and improves survival in laboratory animals.[39] Emesis, lavage, and catharsis are not necessary unless the patient presents within several hours after the ingestion because any substantial quantity of ingested toxin almost invariably induces emesis and catharsis. In an analysis[10] of the AAPCC Toxic Exposure Surveillance System (TESS) database of unintentional mushroom exposures in children from 1992 to 2005, it is suggested that a syrup of ipecac–treated subgroup compared to an activated charcoal or no intervention group showed the smallest percentage of moderate or major outcomes. Activated charcoal is safe, logical, and a valuable therapeutic strategy at least during the first 12 to 24 hours following mushroom ingestion. Although the clinical presentation often is delayed, 1 g/kg body weight of activated charcoal is reasonable for oral administration every 2 to 4 hours (if the patient is vomiting, an antiemetic is indicated) or by continuous nasogastric infusion. Continuous nasogastric duodenal aspiration is used by multiple groups (mainly European) to remove amatoxins secreted in the bile; others use an even more difficult biliary drainage approach to disrupt the enterohepatobiliary recirculation of the amatoxin.[95] Although there is theoretical support for early quantitative toxin removal due to substantial biliary concentration, the total quantity and actual gastroduodenal concentration remains low, offering inadequate clinical data to support high-risk invasive procedures such as gastroduodenal or biliary drainage.[71]

Thioctic (α-lipoic) acid previously was reported to be beneficial in treating the amatoxin-induced liver toxicity in several different animal models, and a number of uncontrolled clinical trials in humans followed.[5,82] Despite the initial success, thioctic acid was not effective in various other studies and is no longer recommended.[47,49]

A randomized murine model of intraperitoneal α-amanitin poisoning comparing treatment with rescue postexposure N-acetylcysteine, benzylpenicillin, cimetidine, thioctic acid, or silybin was unable to show benefit of any therapy with regard to hepatotoxic manifestations such as aminotransferase concentrations or histologic evidence of hepatonecrosis.[139]

Several laboratory investigations in mice and rats suggest that 1 g/kg penicillin G (1 g = 1,600,000 units) may have a time- and dose-dependent protective effect.[46,50] These results are limited because the amatoxins were administered intraperitoneally, resulting in the death of untreated animals 12 to 24 hours later. Additional investigations demonstrated that 1 g/kg penicillin G administered 5 hours after sublethal doses of α-amanitin decreased clinical and laboratory toxicity.[50] The mechanisms suggested include displacing α-amanitin from albumin, blocking its uptake from hepatocytes, binding circulating amatoxins, and preventing α-amanitin binding to RNA polymerase. None of these mechanisms is substantiated.[34] We no longer recommend penicillin G as a first-line regimen and it only recommend it if none of the following regimens are available.

The active complex of milk thistle (*Silybum marianum*) is silymarin, which is a lipophilic extract composed of 3 isomeric flavonolignans: silibinin, silychristin, and silydianin. Silibinin represents approximately 50% of the extract, but represents about 70% to 80% of the marketed products.[68] Silibinin, a mixture of Silibinin A and B, competitively inhibits the organic anion transporter (OATP1B3) that is responsible for the uptake and enterohepatic recycling of α-amanitin.

One of the earliest animal studies was conducted in mice using sublethal doses of *Amanita phalloides* extract administered intraperitoneally (IP) every 24 hours for 3 doses.[2] Silymarin was administered intravenously (IV) at 16 and 24 hours, with the highest dose resulting in a 58% survival compared to 11% in the control group. When the experiment was repeated using a purified α-amatoxin, time was the most important factor in predicting survival. All of the mice treated with silymarin one hour before exposure survived, whereas none survived when treatment was started 8 hours after exposure.[48] A similar study in mice treated with IP α-amatoxin followed 4 hours later with IP silibinin dosed every 4 to 6 hours for 48 hours was not able to show a benefit in reducing the increase in aminotransferases or a difference in the liver histopathology.[139]

Although in an experimental model of cultured canine hepatocytes silibinin was not able to reduce cytotoxicity, 2 experiments using cultured human hepatocytes demonstrated that the addition of silibinin was able to protect against lipid peroxidation and cytotoxicity, and also stimulate cell proliferation and attachment.[91-93]

Another study conducted in canines utilized an oral sublethal dose of *Amanita phalloides* extract and IV silymarin administered at 5 and 24 hours postingestion. Silymarin prevented or reduced the elevation in liver enzymes and the fall in clotting factors and reduced the severity of liver failure.[50] A similar protocol, but this time using silibinin instead of silymarin, demonstrated similar biochemical findings and a 100% survival.[147] These studies

suggest that silibinin diminishes α-amanitin enterohepatic circulation and may competitively inhibit the organic anion transporter.

A 20-year retrospective review of European and American case reports of more than 2,000 hospitalized patients with amatoxin-induced mushroom poisoning concluded that silibinin alone or in combination with N-acetylcysteine showed the most promise as hepatoprotective therapies.[34] The authors acknowledged the difficulty in determining efficacy of various therapies given the lack of randomized controlled trials. A more recent review included the data from the previous authors and any subsequent hospitalized patients. A multidimensional multivariate statistical analysis of the data reached a similar conclusion.[112]

Although silibinin is routinely available as a nonprescription supplement in most pharmacies and appears to be safe and well tolerated in patients with chronic liver disease, no reduction in mortality, improvement in histology at liver biopsy, or biochemical marker was identified in a systematic review and meta-analysis of diverse patients with chronic liver disease.[68] A dose of silibinin 20 to 50 mg/kg/d is suggested in humans, even though it is not approved as a therapeutic for hepatic disease by the Food and Drug Administration (FDA) in the United States.[79,150] Currently there is an amatoxin poisoning clinical trial utilizing Legalon SIL (silibinin) through an FDA-approved open treatment investigational new drug administration.[25] Legalon SIL, silibinin-C-2',3-dihydrogen succinate disodium salt, is a microcrystalline water-soluble powder for injection manufactured by Rottapharm/Madaus, a German pharmaceutical company.[63] Silibinin is a mixture of cis and trans diastereomers of silibinin A and B extracted from milk thistle fruit and then esterified with succinic anhydride to form the water-soluble salt. There are currently inadequate data to support recommending silibinin for *Amanita* poisoning.

Because of its hepatoprotective effects, N-acetylcysteine is recommended, but no evidence for any specific benefit as an antidote is demonstrated. When fulminant hepatic failure is present, it is reasonable to administer N-acetylcysteine in standardized dosing regimens for non–acetaminophen-poisoned patients until the patient recovers from the encephalopathy because of its presumptive benefits under these circumstances (Antidotes in Depth: A3).

In animals, cimetidine (a potent CYP2C9/2D6 inhibitor) may have a hepatoprotective effect against α-amanitin,[124] but it shows no protective effect against phalloidin toxicity.[125] Cimetidine is proposed as a therapeutic intervention,[123] but no available human data support its use, and it is not currently recommended.

In a response to the continuing quest for a successful antidote for α-amanitin poisoning, a group of investigators with computer modeling and simulation screened clinical drugs sharing bioisosterism with α-amanitin.[59] They subsequently found in an *in silico* study that polymyxin B had significant chemical similarities and molecular dynamics that successfully competed at the same interface and displaced α-amanitin from binding sites with RNA polymerase II. Polymyxin B was then used in vivo to demonstrate that all mice given a specified dose of α-amanitin died, whereas when polymyxin B was given simultaneously all mice survived. When polymyxin followed α-amanitin by 4, 8, and 12 hours, 50% of the mice survived up to 30 days.[59] Polymyxin B has potential to protect RNA polymerase II from inactivation, thereby preventing hepatic injury leading to survival. The investigators plan to utilize clinically approved polymyxin B dosing in suspected α-amanitin poisoning. This novel analysis and subsequent interesting success in mice appears to suggest a more rational strategy than most current antidotal interventions, and the authors' approach should stimulate extensive investigations. In the absence of any proven antidote, polymyxin B at a dose of at least 0.75 mg/kg body weight is reasonable to administer as a life-saving gesture when there is assuredness that *Amanita* species were ingested. Polymyxin is a highly nephrotoxic antibiotic when used parenterally for prolonged clinical treatments, which necessitates that fluid resuscitation is achieved and maintained during a course of therapy, which should be briefly occurring during the 12 to 24 hours following amanitin ingestions potentially limiting hepatotoxicity and nephrotoxicity. Roger L. Nation, PhD, Professor of Drug Disposition and Dynamics, Monash Institute of Pharmaceutical Sciences (written communication, July 21, 2016) stated that short-term therapy at the cited dose would not be expected to cause polymyxin B–associated nephrotoxicity. Although polymyxin B accumulates extensively in renal tubular cells, the concentration is lower in the liver. However, this novel research provides excellent evidence that polymyxin B reaches hepatocytes.[59]

Forced diuresis, hemodialysis, plasmapheresis,[71,72] hemofiltration, and hemoperfusion[42] are often considered shortly after ingestion, but most studies offer neither clinical evidence of benefit nor supportive pharmacokinetic data for any of these therapies.[79,110,111,128,145,149] "Shortly after" is not defined, although hemodialysis and hemoperfusion are reasonable for toxin removal within 24 hours of a documented ingestion.[43] Plasmapheresis, which is dependent on effective clearance, high plasma protein binding, and a low volume of distribution, does not remove more than 10 mcg of amatoxin. Because of the absence of prospective, controlled studies of exposure to amatoxins, in addition to the extreme variability of success with many regimens, multiple-dose activated charcoal, and supportive care remain the standard therapy. Early recognition (<24 hours) of exposure to amanitin is an indication for hemodialysis or hemoperfusion, but most patients at the time they develop clinical manifestations of toxicity likely will no longer have the potential for benefit.[72]

Future therapeutic interventions, such as the use of silibinin, may be dependent on improved understanding of the hepatocellular bile acid transporter, which is a member of the OAT polypeptide family.[64,83,86] The interesting theoretical benefit of the FDA-approved drug polymyxin B, which in in silico and in vivo animal models competed with and displaced α-amanitin from RNA polymerase II–binding sites makes this a mechanistically sound antidote.

Extracorporeal albumin dialysis,[41] molecular adsorbent recirculating system (MARS),[27,95,132,156] and fractionated plasma separation and adsorption system (FPSA; Prometheus system),[37,144,146] are variant detoxification techniques used in patients with fulminant hepatic failure to remove water-soluble and albumin-bound xenobiotics while providing renal support. The typical delayed time to onset of use of MARS and other extracorporeal liver assist devices in amanitin poisoning invariably limits the potential effects of these systems on correction or stabilization of hepatic dysfunction not to toxin removal. None of the available studies of these bridging systems are randomized or controlled. The clinical experience is solely in the care of patients with grave hepatotoxicity at a delayed stage limiting any potential for significant conclusions. These 2 techniques permit time for hepatic regeneration or sufficient bridging time to orthotopic liver transplantation.

The criteria and timing for liver transplantation following amatoxin poisoning are far less established than for fulminant viral hepatitis, where grade III or IV hepatic encephalopathy, marked hyperbilirubinemia, increased INR and azotemia are the well-established criteria for transplantation (Chap. 21).[109] From 1998 to 2014 the United States Acute Liver Failure Study group of 2,224 patients had only 18 patients (acute liver injury {5} and acute liver failure {13}) who were suggested to have had severe hepatotoxicity secondary to an amatoxin.[75] These data do not address those patients who died in the primary hospital of hepatic failure, those who had acute liver injury and survived without transfer. The authors recognize that this observational study represents an exceptionally small sample over many years, but many survived acute liver failure without transplant, and all those with liver transplant survived. Successful transplantations were performed in individuals whose resected livers showed 0% to 30% hepatocyte viability. In these cases, the authors did not wait for progression to exceed grade II encephalopathy or for development of azotemia or marked hyperbilirubinemia.[109] Criteria for patient selection are essential to avoid unnecessary risk while offering the potential for survival to appropriate candidates who have no functional liver. The grim prognosis associated with hepatic coma secondary to *Amanita* spp poisoning has led several transplant groups to consider hepatic transplantation for encephalopathic patients with prolonged INRs (>6), persistent hypoglycemia, metabolic acidosis, increased concentrations of serum ammonia and AST, and hypofibrinogenemia.[36,55-57,75,78,109,120] Each of these major studies has critical flaws including selection bias, retrospective observational series,

absence of controls, survival of those who did not receive transplantation, and lack of definitive evidence of amatoxin exposure. Most studies suggest that no circulating amatoxins are present by the time the need for transplantation is evident.[31] Therefore, there are no definitive transplant criteria for amatoxin-associated acute liver injury and acute liver failure, and the surgeon's judgment in a transplant center is essential. There are now case reports of successful liver transplantation for fulminant[70,74,109] hepatic failure from presumed *A. ocreata*,[78,158] *A. phalloides*, *A. virosa*,[16] *Lepiota helveola*,[98] and *L. brunneoincarnata* poisoning.[114]

To enhance the likelihood of success, individuals who manifest symptoms suggestive of hepatotoxic *Amanita*, *Galerina*, or *Lepiota* spp exposure should be told of the severity of their toxic exposure, the advantage of care in a center for those with liver failure, and the potential need for transplantation, and it is our belief that rapid transfer to a regional liver transplantation center offers the safest site for high-quality care and for decision making with regard to timing for liver transplantation in the face of advancing liver failure.[16,36,109]

GROUP II: GYROMITRIN-CONTAINING MUSHROOMS

$$H_3C \diagdown N - N = C \diagup H$$

Gyromitrin

Members of the gyromitrin group include *Gyromitra esculenta*, *G. ambigua*, and *G. infula*. *G. esculenta* enjoys a reputation of being edible in the Western United States but of being toxic in other areas. The most common error occurs in the spring, when an individual seeking the nongilled, brain-like *Morchella esculenta* (morel) finds the similar *G. esculenta* (false morel) (Fig. 117–3).

These mushrooms are found commonly in the spring under conifers and are easily recognized by their brainlike appearance. Poisonings with these mushrooms are exceptionally uncommon in the United States, representing less than 1% of all recognized events, whereas these poisonings are considered more common in Europe. Certain cooking methods may destroy the toxin, but because of the potential for toxicity, all members of this mushroom family should be avoided.

Gyromitra mushrooms contain the nonvolatile insoluble gyromitrin. Gyromitrin on hydrolysis yields a family of *N*-methyl-*N*-formyl hydrazones, which on subsequent hydrolysis split into aldehydes and

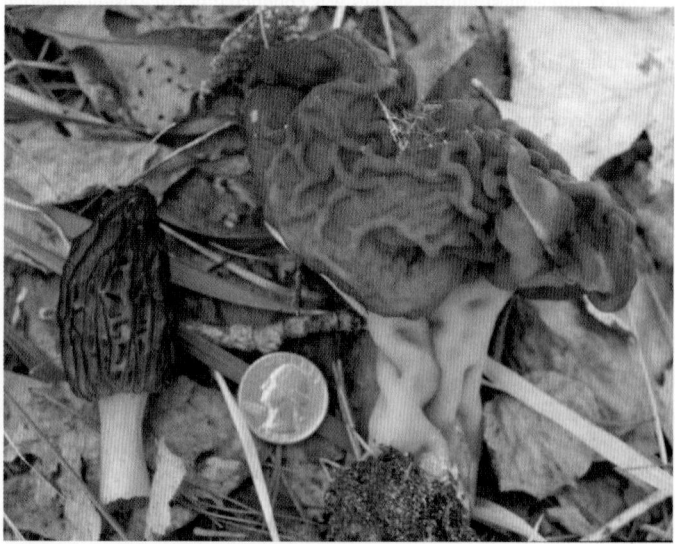

FIGURE 117–3. Group II: Gyromitrin-containing mushrooms. A true morel (*Morchella* spp) on the left is compared to a false morel (*Gyromitra esculenta*) on the right. (*Used with permission from John Trestrail.*)

$$H_3C \backslash N-N=C \diagdown CH_3 \quad \longrightarrow \quad H_3C \backslash N-NH_2 \quad \longrightarrow \quad H_3C \backslash N-NH_2$$

Gyromitrin   N-methyl-   Monomethylhydrazine
                          N-formylhydrazine

FIGURE 117–4. *Gyromitra* mushrooms contain gyromitrin, which undergoes hydrolysis to yield a family of *N*-methyl-formylhydrazines. These molecules on subsequent hydrolysis yield *N*-methyl-*N*-formylhydrazine and monomethylhydrazine.

N-methyl-*N*-formylhydrazine.[3] Subsequent hydrolysis of *N*-methyl-*N*-formylhydrazine yields monomethylhydrazine (Fig. 117–4). The hydrazine moiety reacts with pyridoxine, resulting in inhibition of pyridoxal phosphate–related enzymatic reactions (Figs. 56–2 and 56–3). This interference with pyridoxal phosphate synthesis impairs the production of the inhibitory neurotransmitter γ-aminobutyric acid (GABA).[84] This decrease in GABA is thought to contribute to the diverse neurologic manifestations typically associated with the ingestion of *Gyromitra* spp.

The initial signs and symptoms of toxicity from these mushrooms occur 5 to 10 hours after ingestion and include nausea, vomiting, diarrhea, and abdominal pain. Patients manifest headaches, weakness, and diffuse muscle cramping. Rarely in the first 12 to 48 hours, patients develop nystagmus, ataxia, delirium, stupor, convulsions, and coma. Most patients improve dramatically and return to normal function within several days.

Activated charcoal 1 g/kg body weight is recommended for administration. Benzodiazepines are appropriate for initial management of seizures. Under most circumstances, supportive care is adequate treatment. Pyridoxine (vitamin B_6) in doses of 70 mg/kg IV up to 5 g is recommended, as in the management of isoniazid poisoning, to limit seizures and other neurologic symptoms (Antidotes in Depth: A15).

There are no rapid diagnostic strategies in the laboratory, although thin layer chromatography, gas-liquid chromatography, and mass spectrometry can be used for subsequent identification of hydrazine and hydrazine metabolites.

GROUP III: MUSCARINE-CONTAINING MUSHROOMS

$$H_3C \diagup \underset{HO}{\diagdown} O \diagup CH_2-N^+(CH_3)_3 \quad \text{Muscarine}$$

$$H_3C-\underset{\underset{O}{\|}}{C} \diagup O-CH_2-CH_2-N^+(CH_3)_3 \quad \text{Acetylcholine}$$

Mushrooms that contain muscarine include numerous members of the *Clitocybe* species, such as *C. dealbata* (the sweater) and *C. illudens* (*Omphalotus olearius*) (Fig. 117–5A and 5B), and the *Inocybe* species, which include *I. iacera*, *I. lanuginosa*, and *I. geophylla*. *A. muscaria* and *A. pantherina* contain limited quantities of muscarine, although *A. muscaria* contains substantial amounts of muscimol.

Clinical manifestations, which typically are mild, usually develop within 0.25 to 2 hours, typically last several additional hours with complete resolution within 24 hours. Muscarine and acetylcholine are similar structurally and have comparable clinical effects at the muscarinic receptors. Peripheral manifestations typically include bradycardia, miosis, salivation, lacrimation, vomiting, diarrhea, bronchospasm, bronchorrhea, and micturition. Central muscarinic manifestations do not occur because muscarine, a quaternary ammonium compound, does not cross the blood–brain barrier. No nicotinic manifestations such as diaphoresis or tremor occur. The effects of muscarine often last longer than those of acetylcholine. Because muscarine lacks an ester bond, it is not hydrolyzed by acetylcholinesterase.

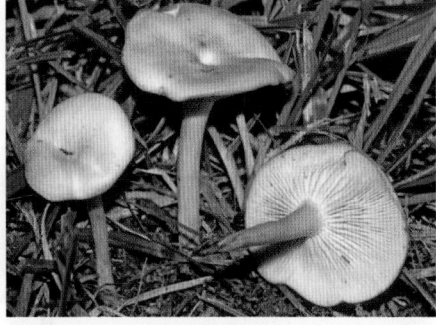

A

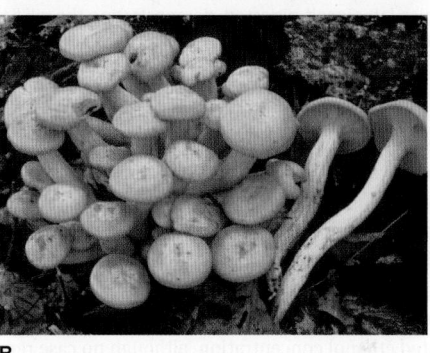

B

FIGURE 117–5. Group III: Muscarine-containing mushrooms. (**A**) *Clitocybe dealbata*. (**B**) *Omphalotus olearius*. (*Used with permission from John Plischke III.*)

Significant toxicity is uncommon, limiting the need for more than supportive care. Rarely, atropine (1–2 mg given IV slowly for adults or 0.02 mg/kg IV for children) is reasonable when titrated and repeated as frequently as indicated to reverse symptomatology. No current, clinically available, analytic techniques can identify muscarine, although high-performance liquid chromatography would be appropriate for investigative purposes.

GROUP IV: COPRINE-CONTAINING MUSHROOMS

$$\underset{H_2C}{\overset{H_2C}{\diagdown}} \underset{N}{\overset{OH}{\underset{|}{C}}} \underset{H}{-} \underset{\overset{\|}{O}}{C} - \underset{H_2}{C} - \underset{H_2}{C} - \underset{\overset{|}{H}}{\overset{NH_2}{C}} - \underset{\overset{\|}{O}}{C} - OH$$

Coprine

Coprinus mushrooms, particularly *C. atramentarius* (*Coprinopsis atramentaria*), contain the toxin coprine (Fig. 117–6A). These mushrooms grow abundantly in temperate climates in grassy or woodland fields. They are known as "inky caps" because the gills that contain a peptidase autodigest into an inky liquid shortly after picking. The edible member of this group, *Coprinus comatus* (shaggy mane) (Figs. 117–6B and 6C) is nontoxic, and probably its misidentification results in collectors' errors. Coprine, an amino acid, its primary metabolite, 1-aminocyclopropanol,[20,94,140] or, more likely, a secondary in vivo hydrolytic metabolite, cyclopropanone hydrate, has a disulfiramlike effect (Fig. 117–7 and Chap. 78).[155] Although both of these metabolites appear to inhibit aldehyde dehydrogenase, the most stable in vivo inhibitory effect is manifested by cyclopropanone hydrate.[155] Inhibition of acetaldehyde dehydrogenase results in accumulation of acetaldehyde and its associated adverse effects, which takes at least 0.5 to 2 hours if the patient ingests alcohol concomitantly or subsequent to eating a coprine-containing mushroom. For the subsequent 48 to 72 hours following coprine-containing mushroom ingestion, if ethanol ingestion occurs, toxicity ensues. Within 0.5 to 2 hours of ethanol ingestion, an acute disulfiram effect is noted, with tachycardia, flushing, nausea, and vomiting. The simultaneous ingestion of the mushroom and alcohol does not result

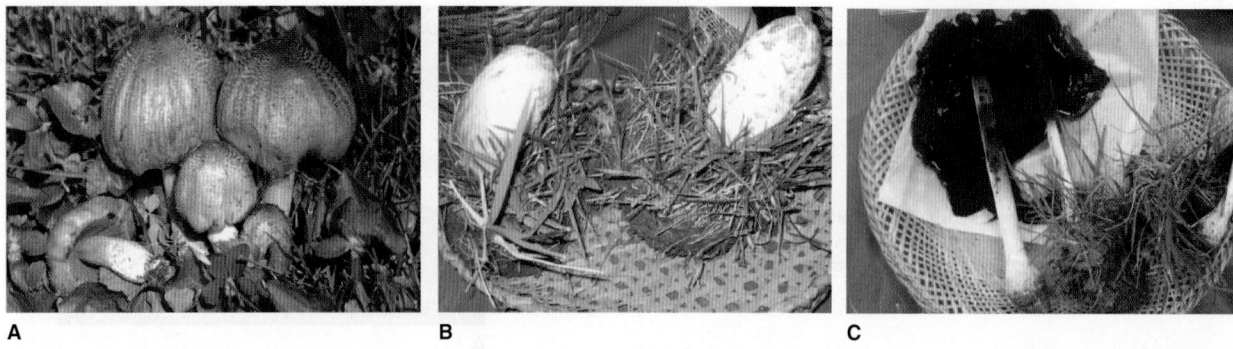

FIGURE 117–6. Group IV: Coprine-containing mushrooms. (**A**) *Coprinopsis atramentaria*; (**B**) and (**C**) show *Coprinus comatus* (shaggy mane). Image B shows an early form, which later is self-digested, demonstrating the gill liquefaction in image C. *(Image A Used with permission from John Plischke III, and images B and C used with permission from Lewis Nelson.)*

in immediate clinical manifestations because inhibition of aldehyde dehydrogenase occurs following coprine metabolism and the in vivo production of cyclopropane hydrate. Treatment is symptomatic with fluid repletion and antiemetics such as metoclopramide or ondansetron, although clinical manifestations usually are mild and resolve within several hours. Prophylactic use of fomepizole (Antidotes in Depth: A3) immediately following ingestion of ethanol and coprine-containing mushrooms would be reasonable, and therapeutic use would be appropriate if persistent toxicity occurs associated with an elevated ethanol concentration, although no case reports or studies are published. This group of mushrooms rarely causes fatalities.

GROUP V: IBOTENIC ACID– AND MUSCIMOL-CONTAINING MUSHROOMS

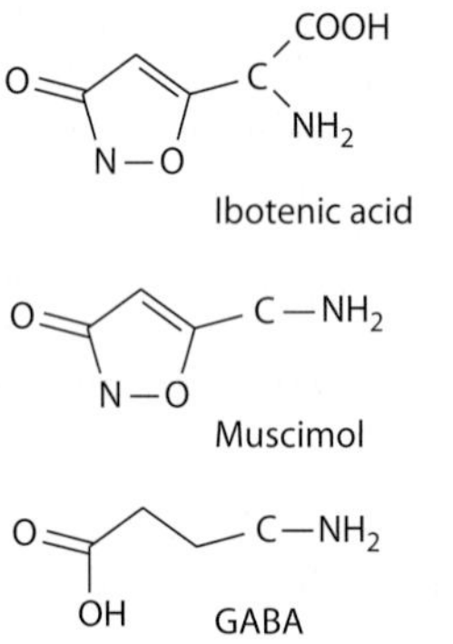

Ibotenic acid

Muscimol

GABA

Most of the mushrooms in this class are primarily in the *Amanita* species, which includes *A. muscaria* (fly agaric), *A. pantherina*, and *A. gemmata* (Fig. 117–8). They exist singly scattered throughout the US woodlands. The brilliant red or tan cap (pileus) is that of the mushroom commonly depicted in children's books and is easily recognized in the fields during summer and fall. These mushrooms have been used in religious ceremonies throughout history. Small variable quantities of the isoxazole derivative ibotenic acid and its decarboxylated metabolite muscimol are found in these mushrooms. Ibotenic acid is an amino acid that acts as a glutamate antagonist at *N*-methyl-D-aspartate (NMDA) receptors. Muscimol acts as a γ-aminobutyric acid type A (GABA$_A$) agonist.

Most patients who develop symptoms have intentionally ingested large quantities of these mushrooms while seeking a hallucinatory experience. Within 0.5 to 2 hours of ingestion, these mushrooms produce the GABAergic manifestations of somnolence, dizziness, auditory and visual hallucinations, dysphoria seizures and agitated delirium in adults, and the excitatory glutamatergic manifestations of myoclonic movements. Seizures and other neurologic findings predominate in children.[8]

Treatment is invariably supportive. Most symptoms respond solely to supportive care, although a benzodiazepine is recommended for excitatory CNS manifestations.

GROUP VI: PSILOCYBIN-CONTAINING MUSHROOMS

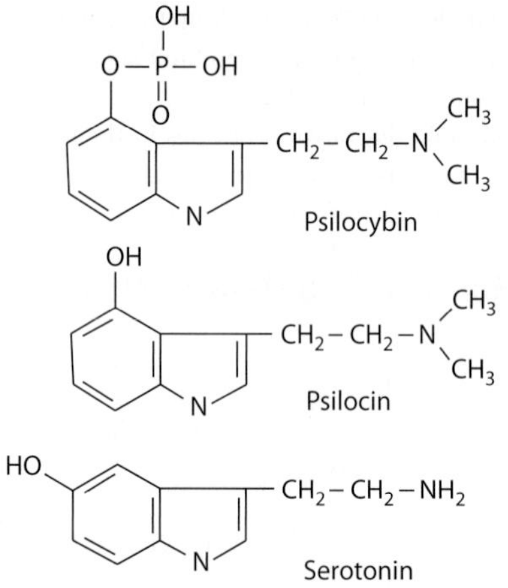

Psilocybin

Psilocin

Serotonin

Psilocybin-containing mushrooms include *Psilocybe cyanescens, Psilocybe cubensis, Conocybe cyanopus, Panaeolus cyanescens, Gymnopilus spectabilis,* and *Psathyrella foenisecii* (Fig. 117–9). These mushrooms have been used for native North and South American religious ceremonies for thousands of years. They grow abundantly in warm, moist areas of the United States. They are readily available through drug culture magazines and the Internet.

Toxicity from this group is probably directly correlated with the popularity of hallucinogens in the community.[11] Psilocybin is rapidly and completely

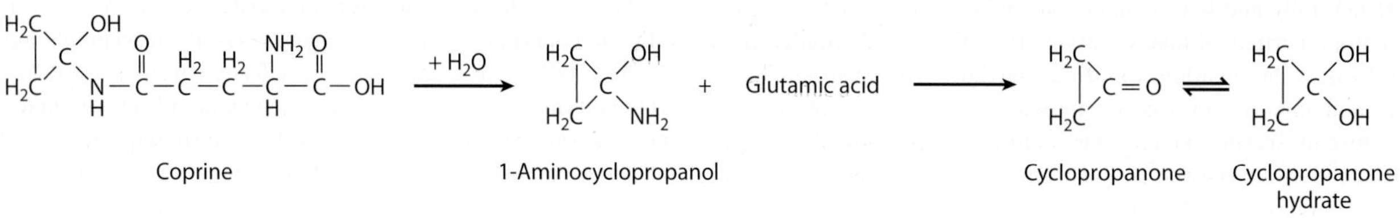

Coprine   1-Aminocyclopropanol   + Glutamic acid   Cyclopropanone   Cyclopropanone hydrate

FIGURE 117–7. The *Coprinus* mushrooms contain coprine, an amino acid, which is rapidly hydrolyzed to 1-aminocyclopropanol and subsequently cyclopropanone hydrate. It is this last metabolite that most likely has the disulfiramlike effect.

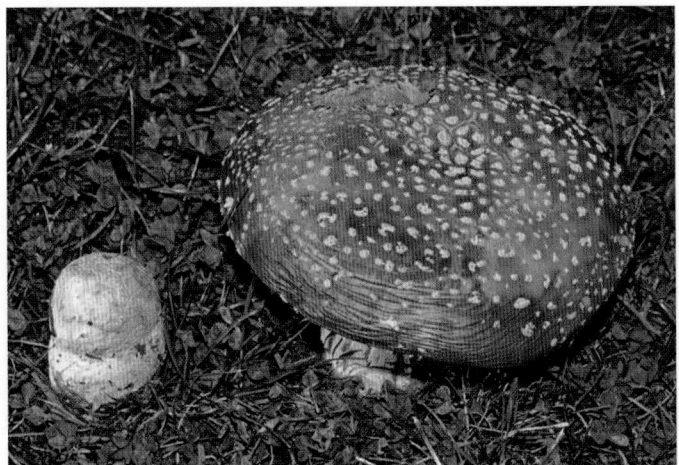

FIGURE 117–8. Group V: Muscimol-containing mushrooms. This image of *Amanita muscaria* highlights different development forms and colors. *(Used with permission from John Plischke III.)*

TABLE 117–2 Mushroom Toxicity: Correlation Between Organ System Affected, Time of Onset of Toxic Manifestations, and Mushroom Xenobiotic Responsible

Organ System	Time of Onset		
	Early: <5 h	*Middle: 5–24 h*	*Late: >24 h*
Cardiac muscle			2*R*-amino-4,5-hexynoic acid
Gastrointestinal	Allenic norleucine	Allenic norleucine	Orellanine and orellinine
	2*R*-amino-4, 5-hexynoic acid		
	Coprine	Amatoxin	
	Group VII	Gyromitrin	
	Psilocybin		
	Muscarine		
Liver			Amatoxin
Immunologic	Involutin		
	Spores		
Nervous	Ibotenic acid and muscimol	Gyromitrin	Acromelic acid
	Psilocybin		Gyromitrin
			Polyporic acid
Kidney			Allenic norleucine
			Orellanine and orellinine
Skeletal muscle	Cycloprop-2-enecarboxylic acid		

hydrolyzed to psilocin in vivo. Serotonin, psilocin, psilocybin, bufotenine, dimethyltryptamine, and lysergic acid diethylamide (LSD) are very similar structurally and presumably act at a similar 5-HT$_2$ receptor site. The effects of psilocybin as a serotonin agonist and antagonist are discussed in Chaps. 13 and 79.

The psilocybin and psilocin indoles, like those of LSD, rapidly (within one hour of ingestion) produce CNS effects, including ataxia, hyperkinesis, visual illusions, and hallucinations. Some patients manifest gastrointestinal distress, tachycardia, mydriasis, anxiety, lightheadedness, tremor, and agitation. Most manifestations are recognized within 4 hours of ingestion with a return to normalcy within 6 to 12 hours.[14] Rare cases of acute kidney failure,[53,113] seizures, and cardiopulmonary arrest[11] are associated with psilocybin-containing species. However, such associations should always be questioned when reported in a substance-using individual potentially simultaneously exposed to other xenobiotics.

A single patient who intravenously administered an extract of *Psilocybe* mushrooms experienced chills, weakness, dyspnea, headache, severe myalgia and vomiting associated with hyperthermia, hypoxemia, and mild methemoglobinemia.[28]

Treatment for hallucinations usually is supportive, although administering a benzodiazepine is reasonable when reassurance proves inadequate.

GROUP VII: GASTROINTESTINAL TOXIN–CONTAINING MUSHROOMS

By far the largest group of mushrooms is a diverse group that contains a variety of ill-defined GI toxins. Many of the hundreds of mushrooms in this group fall into the "little brown mushroom" category. Some *Boletus* spp, *Lactarius* spp, *O. olearius*, *Rhodophyllus* spp, *Tricholoma* spp, *Chlorophyllum molybdites*, and *Chlorophyllum esculentum* are mistaken for edible or

hallucinogenic species. A frequently reported error[4,54,143] is the confusion of the jack-o'-lantern (*Omphalotus olearius*) with the edible species of chanterelle (*Cantharellus cibarius*).

The toxins associated with this group are not identified. The malabsorption of proteins and sugars, such as trehalose, and the ingestion of a mushroom infected or partially digested by microorganisms or allergy may be responsible for symptoms. Gastrointestinal toxicity occurs 0.3 to 3 hours after ingestion when epigastric distress, malaise, nausea, vomiting, and diarrhea are evident. Treatment includes fluid resuscitation with control of vomiting and diarrhea. The clinical course is brief and the prognosis excellent. Those mushroom ingestions resulting in gastrointestinal toxicity more than 5 hours after ingestion are considered in Table 117–2. When symptoms seem to persist, the clinician must consider a mixed ingestion of another potentially toxic mushroom group.

Rarely, clinical presentations are life threatening, with hypovolemic shock necessitating fluids and vasopressors.[134] Resolution of symptoms usually occurs within 6 to 24 hours. The clinical courses associated with specific mushroom ingestions are variable.[8] Death is rare.

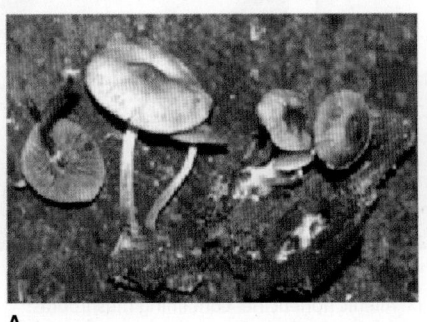
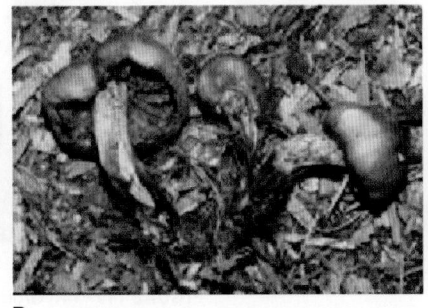
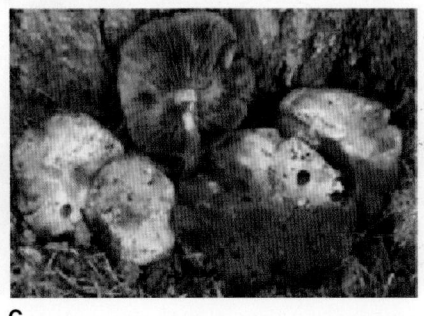

A   **B**   **C**

FIGURE 117–9. Group VI: Psilocybin-containing mushrooms. Three examples of hallucinogenic mushrooms: (**A**) *Psilocybe cyanescens*, (**B**) *Psilocybe caerulipes*, and (**C**) *Gymnopilus spectabilis*. *(Used with permission from John Plischke III.)*

GROUP VIII: ORELLANINE- AND ORELLININE-CONTAINING MUSHROOMS

Orellanine

Cortinarius mushrooms, such as *C. rubellus* (Fig. 117–10) and *C. orellanus*, are commonly found throughout North America and Europe.[19,73,126] The *C. orellanus* toxin orellanine is reduced by photochemical degradation to orellinine, a bipyridyl molecule that is further reduced to the nontoxic orelline.[2,33,106,117] The toxic compound orellanine is a hydroxylated bipyridine compound activated by its metabolism through the cytochrome P450 system. Toxicologically, these molecules are similar to paraquat and diquat and may have comparable mechanisms of action, although precise knowledge is limited (Chap. 109). Other nephrotoxins, such as cortinarines, are isolated from certain *Cortinarius* spp[123] and result in tubular damage, interstitial nephritis, and tubulointerstitial fibrosis.

Orellanine is rapidly removed from the plasma within 48 to 72 hours and concentrated in the urine in a soluble form. It can be detected in the plasma at the time of clinical symptoms by some[115] but not other investigators.[118] Thin-layer chromatography on renal biopsy material can detect orellanine long after clinical exposure.[115,118]

Initial manifestations occur 24 to 72 hours after ingestion and initially include headache, nausea, vomiting, and diarrhea followed by chills, polydipsia, anorexia, oliguria, and flank and abdominal pain. The largest case review demonstrated that numerous patients repetitively ingested the *Cortinarius* spp prior to diagnosis.[29] Oliguric kidney failure develops several days to weeks after initial symptoms.[12] The only initial laboratory abnormalities include hematuria, pyuria, and proteinuria. Nephrotoxicity is characterized by interstitial nephritis with tubular damage and early fibrosis of injured tubules with relative glomerular sparing.[19,126]

Hepatotoxicity is rarely reported.[12] Hemoperfusion, hemodialysis, and renal transplantation are used for the treatment of acute kidney failure.[12,29] No evidence suggests that secondary detoxification by plasmapheresis or hemoperfusion is of any benefit in preventing chronic kidney failure even when initiated in the first 48 hours.[29,79,115] The data are inadequate to define management or prognosis precisely, as many patients improve rapidly,

whereas some require temporary intermittent hemodialysis and others require chronic therapy for persistent kidney failure.[12] No laboratory or clinical parameters predicting the individual reactions to the toxins are available. Although case reports in the literature commonly lack definitive proof of ingestion or confirmation of toxin presence, the more rapid the onset of GI and kidney manifestations, the greater the risk of both acute and chronic kidney failure.[29]

GROUP IX: ALLENIC NORLEUCINE–CONTAINING MUSHROOMS

$$CH_2{=}C{=}CH{-}CH_2{-}CH{-}COOH$$
$$|$$
$$NH_2$$

Allenic norleucine

Amanita smithiana poisoning is reported in the Pacific Northwest and the Mediterranean area (Fig. 117–11).[77,85,142,148,151] Because the mature specimen often lacks any evidence of a partial or universal veil, these mushrooms are not recognized as *Amanita* species. It appears that all of the poisoned individuals were seeking the edible pine mushroom matsutake (*Tricholoma magnivelare*), a highly desirable lookalike. The *A. smithiana*, *A. proxima*, *A. abrupta*, and *A. pseudoporphyria* possess 2 amino acid toxins: allenic norleucine (2-amino-4,5-hexadienoic acid) and possibly 1,2-amino-4-pentynoic acid.[23,108,160] A case report following ingestion of *A. proxima* in Southern France also showed gastrointestinal and renal manifestations.[26] In vitro renal epithelial tissue cultured with allenic norleucine developed necrotic morphologic changes similar to those that occur following *A. smithiana* ingestion.[108] In mice, the extract of *A. abrupta* is hepatotoxic, which suggests that hepatotoxins and nephrotoxins are present in this species.[160]

Initial effects were noted from 0.5 to 12 hours following ingestion of either raw or cooked specimens. Gastrointestinal manifestations, including anorexia, nausea, vomiting, abdominal pain, and diarrhea, occurred frequently, accompanied by malaise, sweating, and dizziness. In some cases, vomiting and diarrhea persist for several days. The patients typically presented for care 3 to 6 days after ingestion, at which time they were oliguric or anuric. Acute kidney injury manifested 4 to 6 days following ingestion, with marked elevation of BUN and creatinine. Lactate dehydrogenase and ALT concentrations frequently were elevated, whereas amylase, AST, alkaline phosphatase, and bilirubin were only infrequently abnormal.

There is no known antidote for these nephrotoxins. Activated charcoal, although of no proven benefit, is recommended in standard doses when a patient in the northwest United States presents with early GI manifestations after mushroom ingestions. The clinician will be forced to consider the circumstances of ingestion to assess the probability of *A. smithiana* ingestion as opposed to ingestion of mushrooms containing a GI toxin.

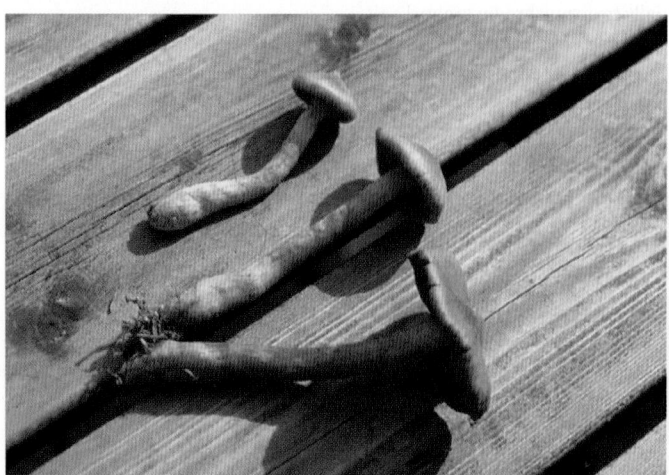

FIGURE 117–10. Group VIII: Orellanine- and orellinine-containing mushrooms: *Cortinarius rubellus. (Used with permission from Astrid Holmgren, Swedish Poisons Information Centre.)*

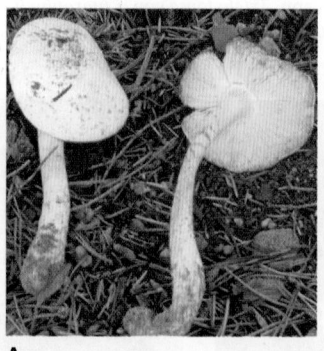 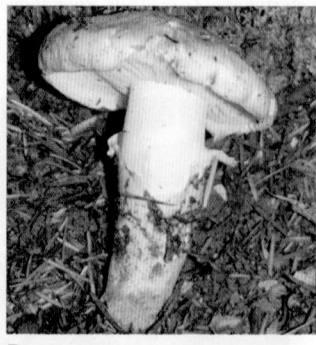

A   **B**

FIGURE 117–11. Group IX: Allenic norleucine–containing mushrooms: (**A**) *Amanita smithiana* compared to (**B**) *Tricholoma magnivelare* (matsutake, the mushroom with which it has been mistaken). *(Used with permission from John Plischke III.)*

In view of the substantial morbidity associated with *A. smithiana* ingestions, historic, clinical, and/or temporal evidence of this ingestion would be a reasonable indication for charcoal hemoperfusion or hemodialysis when the patient presents in the early phase (12–24 hours) of exposure. When a patient presents with renal compromise several days, as opposed to weeks, following mushroom ingestion and with a history of early, as opposed to delayed, GI manifestations, the clinician may be able to suggest *A. smithiana* as the etiology compared to *Cortinarius* spp exposure. Risk of toxicity was greatest in older patients and in patients with chronic kidney disease. Patients who required hemodialysis underwent the procedure 2 to 3 times per week for approximately one month until recovery. None of the patients in the 3 series died.

GROUP X: CYCLOPROP-2-ENECARBOXYLIC ACID–CONTAINING MUSHROOMS

There are several reports of *Tricholoma equestre* (*Tricholoma flavovirens*) ingestions in Poland and France, where although this mushroom is considered edible it has resulted in significant skeletal muscle myotoxicity.[24,103] In the first report, 12 patients who ingested *T. equestre* mushrooms for 3 consecutive days developed severe rhabdomyolysis that was lethal in 3 cases.[6] All patients developed fatigue, muscle weakness, and myalgias 24 to 72 hours following the last mushroom meal. The individuals also developed facial erythema, nausea without vomiting, and profuse sweating. The mean maximal creatine phosphokinase (CK) was 226,067 U/L in women and 34,786 U/L in men, with some values greater than 500,000 U/L. Electromyography and biopsies showed myofibrillar injury and edema consistent with an acute myopathy.

Dyspnea, muscle weakness, acute myocarditis, dysrhythmias, congestive heart failure, and death ensued in 3 patients. Autopsy demonstrated myocardial lesions identical to those found in the peripheral muscles. Although muscle toxicity was reproduced using *T. equestre* extracts in a mouse model, the etiology of the toxicity is not defined.[6] All the triterpenoids, sterols, indoles, and acetylenic compounds extracted from these mushrooms previously were assumed to be without toxicity. Currently all the clinical experience originates from Europe where these mushrooms are considered choice and eaten extensively; no cases are reported in the United States.

Similar clinical presentations are reported in China, Taiwan, and Japan associated with the ingestion of *Russula subnigricans*. Patients also manifest nausea, vomiting, diarrhea, malaise, fatigue, muscle weakness, dark urine, and oliguria. In these reports, rhabdomyolysis (CK in 100s–10,000s) and oliguric kidney failure necessitating hemodialysis occurred in several patients with rare deaths.[86] A toxin—cycloprop-2-enecarboxylic acid extracted from *R. subnigricans*—caused severe myotoxicity in mice,[96] but a mechanism is not defined and there are other proposed myotoxins also recognized in this species.

GROUP XI: 2R-AMINO-4,5-HYDROXY-5-HEXYNOIC ACID AND 2R-AMINO-5-HEXYNOIC ACID–CONTAINING MUSHROOMS

Two clinical syndromes both associated with diffuse myotoxicity with cardiac preference are described in China. They are associated with myocarditis and sudden cardiovascular collapse. The myocardial toxin and presumably skeletal muscle toxins found in *T. venenata* are 2R-amino-4,5-hydroxy-5-hexynoic acid and 2R-amino-5-hexynoic acid which are unsaturated amino acids. The first syndrome has been called Yunnan Sudden Unexplained Death (SUD) and has been recognized for 4 decades. Hundreds of individuals may have succumbed following the ingestion of an abundant flowerlike mushroom *Trogia venenata* that is typically eaten by many during the summer rainy season.[130] The few closely studied cases have minor gastrointestinal manifestations, including nausea and vomiting, followed by dizziness, dyspnea, myalgias, abdominal pain, dysesthesias, and tremor (myoclonic movements). Hypotension and syncope occur within several days of exposure. A number of these patients have presumably had ventricular fibrillation and sudden death. Most patients had significant leukocytosis, CK elevation (1,000–18,000), CKMB elevation (50–1,700), and a troponin I positivity on qualitative testing. Electrocardiographs were done infrequently and showed no conduction abnormalities. Although there is a high degree of suspicion and clinical correlation, others have had Yunnan SUD without ingestions, leading some investigators to suggest that viral etiologies, barium toxicity, and other foods as well as the previously unspeciated mushroom *T. venenata* were causative.[135,136,161]

The pathologic studies are limited; no skeletal muscle pathology was performed whereas mild myocardial necrosis with lymphocyte infiltration and focal myocardial interstitial hemorrhage was observed in several cases. The first of these amino acids was found at autopsy in an individual, and both hexynoic amino acids when administered to mice resulted in death.[129] The investigators suggest that these amino acids have a molecular similarity to hypoglycin A of the ackee fruit and that hypoglycemia occurred in the mice that succumbed. Hypoglycemia has not occurred in any of the patients with sudden deaths studied in China.[130] Since 2010, public health education has focused on the communities and their health care providers where these mushrooms are abundant.[129] There have been extensive public health interventions warning patients not to eat these mushrooms, and there have been no additional cases since this public health effort began.

A second epidemic with a similar clinical constellation of signs and symptoms occurred in Jiangxi Province with *Amanita franchetti* and *Ramaria rufescens* presumed to be etiologic.[67] In these cases, patients developed nausea, vomiting, malaise, dizziness, abdominal distress, myalgia, and tremors within 2 to 15 hours after ingestion. Within several days, they also developed tachycardia, hypotension, and experienced sudden death. There is less laboratory data in these cases, with little ECG evidence compared to SUD. There is little evidence to suggest a management approach other than observation, cardiac monitoring, and extensive cardiac evaluation, which has been limited in the Yunnan SUD heretofore.

GROUP XII: ACROMELIC ACID–CONTAINING MUSHROOMS

Acromelic acids D and E
D: R₁ = COOH; R₂ = H
E: R₁ = H; R₂ = COOH

Erythromelalgia is a poorly defined syndrome originally recognized in Japan,[99,102] recently in France[9] following the ingestion of various *Clitocybe* species (*C. acromelalga* and *C. amoenolens*), and not recognized currently in the United States. The toxic substances acromelic acids A to E have been isolated. These molecules are similar to kainic acid and are of the pyrrolidine dicarboxylic acid family, which act as ionotropic glutamate receptors. Erythromelalgia typically occurs more than 24 hours following ingestion. Patients develop paraesthesias of distal extremities followed by paroxysms of severe burning dysesthesias lasting several hours. The extremities show edema and erythema.

These manifestations respond variably to symptomatic and supportive care and resolve completely within several months. A single patient given nicotinic acid (niacin) at intermittent high IV doses initially demonstrated resolution of erythema and edema. The patient continued oral nicotinic acid as treatment for 3 months.[102] Varied hypotheses[101,127] for the improvement are suggested as related to nicotinic acid such as improved peripheral blood flow and resolution of neurovascular dysfunction associated with acromelic acid. The description of the evidence of resolution over a 3-month period is limited.

GROUP XIII: POLYPORIC ACID–CONTAINING MUSHROOMS

Two groupings of toxic mushroom ingestion syndromes result in encephalopathy. The first group of mushrooms associated with encephalopathy is the *Hapalopilus rutilans* reported in a German case series. More than 12 hours after ingestion, an adult and 2 children developed nausea, vomiting, and abdominal pain. Central nervous system abnormalities including vertigo, ataxia, visual disturbances, and somnolence were reported.[81,121] Aminotransferase and creatinine concentrations were elevated. In each case, the urine was a violet color, the color being noted when polyporic acid is placed in an alkaline solution. Polyporic acid, a dihydroquinone derivative (2,5-dihydroxy-3,6-diphenyl-1,4 benzoquinone), a constituent of these mushrooms, is a dihydroorotate dehydrogenase (an enzyme in the biosynthesis of pyrimidine) inhibitor that resulted in comparable clinical and biochemical manifestation when administered to rats.[81] Symptomatic treatment is indicated with more specific therapy should hepatic or renal compromise be significant.

In the second group, *Pleurocybella porrigens*, a mushroom species commonly eaten in Japanese miso soup, without any adverse effects, is suggested to be etiologic. However, their ingestion by patients with chronic kidney injury resulted in delayed manifestations of encephalopathy.[61] Three-quarters (24 of 32) of the affected patients were undergoing hemodialysis at the time of the presumed poisoning. The delay from time of ingestion to the development of an altered consciousness, convulsions, myoclonus, dysarthria, dysesthesias, ataxia, respiratory failure, or death was between 1 and 31 days. No prior toxic link or known xenobiotic in these commonly ingested mushrooms is recognized.

GROUP XIV: INVOLUTIN-CONTAINING MUSHROOMS

A small number of patients with ingestions of *Paxillus involutus*, and possibly *Clitocybe claviceps* and *Boletus luridus*, develop early-onset mild GI symptoms followed by an immune-mediated hemolytic anemia, hemoglobinuria, oliguria, and acute kidney injury. Immunoglobulin G antibodies to a *Paxillus* extract containing involutin[71] were detected by a hemagglutination test in these patients.[153,154] This syndrome occurs in Europe, typically among those who have eaten *P. involutus* on numerous occasions.

GROUP XV: LYCOPERDONOSIS

Puffball mushrooms (*Lycoperdon perlatum*, *Lycoperdon pyriforme*, or *Lycoperdon gemmatum*) are edible in the fall and can (upon decay or drying) release large numbers of spores following compression, fracture, or

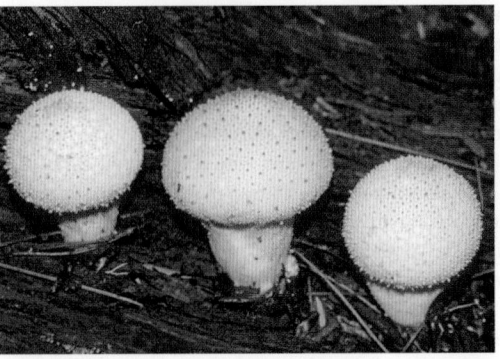

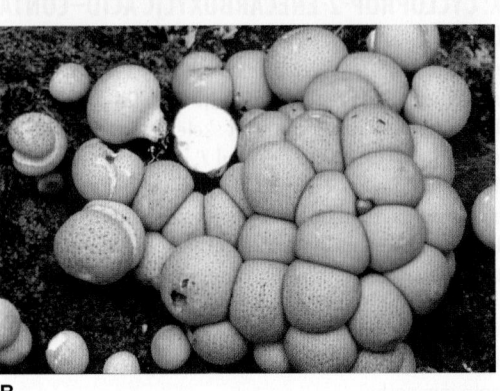

FIGURE 117–12. Puffballs: (**A**) *Lycoperdon pyriforme* and (**B**) *Lycoperdon perlatum*. *(Used with permission from John Plischke III.)*

shaking (Fig. 117–12). Lycoperdonosis is directly related to massive exposure to spores, although many consider the syndrome an allergic bronchoalveolitis. This syndrome occurs in patients following acute inhalation of spores as an alternative or complementary therapy for epistaxis[137] and in adolescents for various experimental reasons.[21] Massive inhalation, insufflation, and chewing of spores can lead to the development of nasopharyngitis, nausea, vomiting, and pneumonitis within hours. Over a period of several days, cough, shortness of breath, myalgias, fatigue, and fever develop. Rarely, patients require intubation because of pulmonary compromise associated with diffuse reticulonodular infiltrates.[21] Lung biopsy demonstrates an inflammatory process with the presence of *Lycoperdon* spores.[137] Patients treated with corticosteroids such as prednisone and antifungals such as amphotericin B recovered within several weeks without sequelae although there are no controlled studies of the merits of this approach.

GENERAL MANAGEMENT ISSUES

Because ingestion of certain mushrooms may lead to toxicity with substantial morbidity or mortality, patients with suspected mushroom ingestions require rigorous management. A serious effort at precise identification of the genus and species involved will make assessment, management, and follow-up easier and more logical. Unintentional ingestions in children "in their yards" are usually limited exposures to nontoxic mushrooms resulting in no symptoms necessitating solely reassurance by the certified specialist in Poison Information. Beuhler and coworkers utilizing the AAPCC Toxic Exposure Surveillance System suggest that the treatment of exposures to mushrooms in children with syrup of ipecac decreases morbidity.[10] It is unlikely that the syrup of the ipecac will be useful and it is not recommended. It is recommended that charcoal be administered if potentially toxic mushrooms are ingested. If nausea and vomiting persist, an antiemetic is recommended to ensure that the patient can retain activated charcoal. Appropriate life support measures recommended as necessary. Fluids, electrolytes, and dextrose repletion, as needed, are essential.

There is a wide variability in quantity and type of xenobiotic present in mushrooms according to geography, climate, and local conditions. The clinical course for *A. smithiana* poisoning has led us to suggest an alteration in the initial approach to patients in the northwest United States who have early onset (0.5–5 hours) of GI distress following mushroom ingestion as *A. smithiana* has a significant risk of kidney failure. Prior to the recognition of this mushroom poisoning, all patients who had early onset of nausea, vomiting, diarrhea, and abdominal cramps were presumed to be poisoned by a member of the groups containing either the GI toxins or muscarine. The more we learn and study, the more it is obvious that these clinical time courses as described in Table 117–2 are rough estimates of most likely estimates and the clinician should recognize that the quality of our understanding of mushroom toxicology is improving, but speciation, time course, actual mycologic chemistry, and management are based on limited evidence.

DISPOSITION

It is important to remember that many patients with mushroom ingestions present with mixed and incomplete signs and symptoms. Whereas some ingestions produce "purer" symptom complexes than others, some ingestions, such as those of *A. muscaria*, produce GI and CNS effects, and still other ingestions, such as those of *Cortinarius* spp, have acute GI and delayed kidney manifestations. Treatment or partial treatment may further confound the assessment. In addition, it is essential to remember that any acute GI disorder actually may be the manifestation of mushroom toxicity. In the spring and fall, in areas with temperate weather and humidity, it is particularly important to consider intentional or unrecognized exposure to mushroom toxins, although a logical approach to management is impossible in the absence of a precise history.

Because the clinical course of mushroom poisoning can be deceptive, all patients who manifest early gastrointestinal symptoms (<5 hours) and remain symptomatic for several hours despite supportive care (Tables 117–1 and 117–2) should be admitted to the hospital. In this group of patients inhabiting the Pacific northwest, *A. smithiana* is particular concern. Although acute kidney injuries will likely not occur for several days necessitating careful follow-up. Patients whose delayed initial presentation (≥5 hours) is suggestive of amatoxin exposure should be hospitalized, as should any patient postingestion who cannot be followed safely or reliably as an outpatient. Tables 117–1 and 117–2 list the characteristic times of appearance and evolution of symptoms caused by mushroom xenobiotics. Confusion may result from atypical clinical manifestations or, commonly, ingestion of several different mushrooms species, some of which may produce early symptoms and others delayed toxicity. Patients with certain types of ingestions may appear to improve initially with only supportive care. This latency period, which is characteristic of *Amanita* spp, may not be appreciated when several different species are eaten simultaneously. However, because hepatotoxicity leading to death may not appear until 2 to 3 days after ingestion (amatoxins) and nephrotoxicity may not appear for 3 to 21 days (orellanine and allenic norleucine), all patients with symptoms following unknown ingestions require subsequent follow-up.

IDENTIFICATION
General

Visualizing and analyzing the gross, microscopic, or chemical characteristics of the ingested mushroom remain vital strategies that are infrequently used. When the whole mushroom or parts are unavailable, the diagnosis must be based on the clinical presentation. No rapidly available studies in emergency departments or clinical chemistry laboratories are available to assist with identification. The development of a rapid clinical test for amatoxins,[17,18,79] gyromitrin, orellanine, and allenic norleucine would be useful and permit early use of hemodialysis or hemoperfusion and greater vigilance with regard

to use of hemodialysis. We have not yet achieved the ability to use thin-layer chromatography, high-performance liquid chromatography, gas chromatography, or gas chromatography–mass spectrometry in a clinically relevant manner. In Italy and Japan, real-time polymerase chain reaction (PCR) technology has been developed for multiple species for experimental evaluations of cooked mushrooms and gastric aspirates. Future development of this technique may prove clinically useful.[34,90]

Although mushroom identification is a difficult task, this section may be helpful to the clinician dealing with a suspected case of mushroom toxicity. However, it is generally best to rely on symptomatology, not mushroom appearances, to confirm a diagnosis. As a general rule, positive identification of the mushroom should be left to the mycologist or toxicologist.[45] The most important anatomic features of both edible and poisonous mushrooms are their pileus, stipe, lamellae or gills, and volva (Fig. 117–2).

- Pileus: Broad, caplike structure from which hang the gills (lamellae), tubes, or teeth.
- Stipe: Long stalk or stem that supports the cap; the stipe is not present in some species.
- Lamellae: Platelike or gilllike structures on the undersurface of the pileus that radiate out like the spokes of a wheel. The spores are found on the lamellae. Some mushrooms have pores or toothlike structures on their pili, which contain the spores. The mode of attachment of the lamellae to the stipe is noteworthy in making an identification.
- Volva: Partial remnant of the veil found around the base of the stipe in some species.
- Veil: Membrane that may completely or partially cover the lamellae, depending on the stage of development. The "universal" veil covers the underside, the spore-bearing surface of the pileus.
- Annulus: Ringlike structure that may surround the stipe at some point below the junction, with the cap that is a remnant of the partial veil.
- Spores: Microscopic reproductive structures that are resistant to extremes in temperature and dryness, produced in the millions on the spore-bearing surface (see Lamellae). Of all the characteristics of a particular mushroom species, spores are the least variable, although many mushrooms have similar-appearing spores. A spore print is helpful in establishing an identification. A spore print viewed microscopically is comparable to a bacterial Gram stain. Spore colors range from white to black and include shades of pink, salmon, buff, brown, and purple. Spore color in general is constant for a species.

THE UNKNOWN MUSHROOM

1. The most important determinant is whether the ingested mushroom is one of the high-morbidity varieties, especially *Amanita*.
2. An attempt should be made to obtain either the collected mushrooms, a photograph, or a detailed description of their features. Arrange for transport of the mushroom in a dry paper bag (not plastic). Ensure that the mushroom is neither moistened nor refrigerated, either of which will alter its structure. Remember that gastric contents may contain spores that are very difficult to find, but can be crucial for analysis.
3. If the mushroom cap is available, make a spore print by placing the pileus spore-bearing surface side down on a piece of paper for at least 4 to 6 hours in a windless area. The spores that collect on the paper can be analyzed for color. White spore prints can be visualized more easily on white paper by tilting the paper and looking at it from an angle.
4. Concomitant with step 3, contact a mycologist and use the best resources available for identification. A botanical garden usually has expert mycologists on staff, or a local mycology club can locate a mycologist. A regional poison control center almost always can provide this expertise or locate an expert.

POISONING PRINCIPLES: MYTHS AND SCIENCE

Differentiating myths from science is a difficult task in any field of medicine. This effort is even more complex when discussing mushrooms. The following principles are of great value in developing a logical approach to a potential ingestion.

1. Wild mushrooms should never be eaten unless an experienced mycologist can absolutely identify the mushroom. Even experts have trouble identifying some mushrooms, yet some foragers boldly indicate that distinguishing edible from toxic mushrooms is "as easy as telling brussels sprouts from broccoli." Remember the saying, "There are old mushroom hunters, and bold mushroom hunters; but there are no old, bold mushroom hunters."

2. The toxicology of any species can vary, depending on geographic location. This species confusion is obvious among American immigrants stating unequivocally that "this particular mushroom" was absolutely safe and routinely eaten in the individual's Asian or European country of origin.

3. If toxicity is suspected, attempt to obtain samples of the mushrooms eaten, and identify them. Every emergency department can have a readily available resource on mushrooms found on many Internet Web sites. The older, more comprehensive mycology field guides can be most useful as well.[1,15,87,88,119,131] In any case, identification is best made with the aid of the poison control center's consultant mycologist.

4. Mushrooms often are implicated as the cause of an illness when, in fact, infections or other diseases are responsible. Other etiologies include the mode of preparation (the sauce or wine) or the cooking utensil.

5. There are no absolute generic approaches for evaluating the potential toxicity of a mushroom. Myths suggesting the safety or lack of safety by staining of silver, presence of insects or slugs, peeling off the mushroom cap, or the area of mushroom growth are unreliable or false. Neither odor nor taste is a good predictor of toxicity. Pure white mushrooms, little brown mushrooms, large brown mushrooms, and red- or pink-spored boletus (a mushroom without lamellae) should be considered potentially toxic.

6. Cooking may inactivate some toxins contained in mushrooms but not others. In general, no wild mushroom should be eaten raw or in large quantities. Examples of toxicity associated with lack of cooking include *Armillariella mellea* (honey mushroom), which usually is well tolerated when cooked but not raw, and *Verpa bohemica* (a morellike mushroom), which is edible but causes illness if eaten in excess. Even the *Morchella esculenta*, the edible-choice morel, is well recognized to cause dizziness, tremor, and ataxia when eaten raw in large quantities.[122]

7. Associated phenomena may be responsible for or contribute to toxicity. Could insecticides have been sprayed on the mushrooms? Is it an alcohol-related response? Besides the well-known disulfiram-like reaction involving *C. atramentarius*, other good edibles, including the black morel (*Morchella angusticeps*) and the sulfur polypore (*Laetiporus sulfureus*), can cause adverse reactions if consumed with alcohol. The etiology of these adverse reactions is not understood.

8. "Edible" mushrooms that are allowed to deteriorate during collection, transport, and storage prior to or subsequent to preparation become toxic. Therefore, only young, recently matured specimens should be eaten when adequate mycologic support is available.

9. The finding that only some people who ate a mushroom species manifested characteristic toxicity should not exclude the diagnosis of mushroom poisoning. The degree of toxicity may be dose related or genetically determined, or a person may have a preexistent pathologic disposition to toxicity.

10. Mushroom allergy can manifest as an anaphylactic reaction.

11. Most poisonous mushrooms resemble edible mushrooms at some phase of their growth. For this reason, even careful examination of the ring, cap, consistency, form, and color may not reliably identify the edible species. Also, characteristic features of specific toxic mushrooms may not be present under certain conditions. Although the deadly *A. phalloides* and *A. virosa* usually have remnant patches of tissue from the universal veil that envelops the mushroom in its "button" stage, rain may wash these remnants away. Similarly, a subterranean basal cup may not be noticed if the mushroom is cut at the ground level by a novice forager (Fig. 117–1).

12. Even the new in-vogue "wild mushrooms" in the specialty markets may not be entirely safe (personal observations).

SUMMARY

- It is essential to determine whether the ingested mushroom is one of the high morbidity/mortality varieties such as the *Amanita* spp.
- The onset of GI symptoms within 5 hours of ingestion makes exposure to a hepatotoxic *Amanita* species less likely.
- Several mushroom species including *Amanita smithiana* containing allenic norleucine and *Cortinarius orellanus* containing orellinine and orellanine result in acute kidney injury more than 24 hours after ingestion.
- Silibinin, the active component of the milk thistle, is suggested to competitively inhibit the organic anion transporter polypeptide that is responsible for the uptake and enterohepatic recycling of α-amanitin thereby inhibiting α-amanitin hepatocellular penetration. The evidence is limited and we withhold recommendation.
- The potential morbidity and mortality associated with amanitin hepatotoxicity necessitates rapid assessment by a hepatic transplantation service, even though the clinical evolution is unpredictable and criteria for transplantation under these circumstances are not established.
- The novel research of Polymyxin B a US FDA approved antibiotic is a reasonable therapeutic intervention for presumed *Amanita* species ingestion. A brief course of 12-24 hours of Polymyxin B given as a single dose 0.75 mg/kg body weight has the potential to limit hepatotoxicity without significant risk of nephrotoxicity.

REFERENCES

1. Ammirati JF. *Poisonous Mushrooms of the Northern United States and Canada.* Minneapolis: University of Minnesota Press; 1985.
2. Antkowiak WZ, Gessner WP. Photodecomposition of orellanine and orellinine, the fungal toxins of *Cortinarius orellanus* fries and *Cortinarius speciossimus*. *Experientia.* 1985;41:769-771.
3. Arshadi M, et al. Gas chromatography-mass spectrometry determination of the penta-fluorobenzoyl derivative of methylhydrazine in false morel (*Gyromitra esculenta*) as a monitor for the content of the toxin gyromitrin. *J Chromatogr A.* 2006;1125:229-233.
4. Ayer WA, Browne LM. Terpenoid metabolites of mushrooms and related basidiomycetes. *Tetrahedron.* 1981;37:2197-2248.
5. Becker CE, et al. Diagnosis and treatment of *Amanita phalloides*-type mushroom poisoning: use of thioctic acid. *West J Med.* 1976;125:100-109.
6. Bedry R, et al. Wild-mushroom intoxication as a cause of rhabdomyolysis. *N Engl J Med.* 2001;345:798-802.
7. Belliardo F, et al. Amatoxins do not cross the placental barrier. *Lancet.* 1983;1:1381.
8. Benjamin DR. Mushroom poisoning in infants and children: the *Amanita pantherina/muscaria* group. *J Toxicol Clin Toxicol.* 1992;30:13-22.
9. Bessard J, et al. Mass spectrometric determination of acromelic acid a from a new poisonous mushroom: *Clitocybe amoenolens. J Chromatogr A.* 2004;1055:99-107.
10. Beuhler MC, et al. The outcome of north american pediatric unintentional mushroom ingestions with various decontamination treatments: an analysis of 14 years of TESS data. *Toxicon.* 2009;53:437-443.
11. Borowiak KS, et al. *Psilocybin* mushroom (*Psilocybe semilanceata*) intoxication with myocardial infarction. *J Toxicol Clin Toxicol.* 1998;36:47-49.
12. Bouget J, et al. Acute renal failure following collective intoxication by *Cortinarius orellanus. Intensive Care Med.* 1990;16:506-510.
13. Boyer JC, et al. Management of maternal *Amanita phalloides* poisoning during the first trimester of pregnancy: a case report and review of the literature. *Clin Chem.* 2001;47:971-974.
14. Brady LR. Toxins of higher fungi. *Lloydia.* 1975;38:36-56.
15. Bresinsky A, Besl H. *A Colour Atlas of Poisonous Fungi: A Handbook for Pharmacists, Doctors, and Biologists.* London: Wolfe Publishing; 1990.
16. Broussard CN, et al. Mushroom poisoning—from diarrhea to liver transplantation. *Am J Gastroenterol.* 2001;96:3195-3198.
17. Butera R, et al. Validation of the elisa test for urinary alpha-amanitin analysis in human *Amanita phalloides* poisoning. *J Toxicol Clin Toxicol (Phila).* 2004;42:535.
18. Butera R, et al. Diagnostic accuracy of urinary amanitin in suspected mushroom poisoning: a pilot study. *J Toxicol Clin Toxicol.* 2004;42:901-912.

19. Carder C, et al. Management of mushroom poisoning. *Clin Toxicol Consult.* 1983; 5:103-118.

20. Carlsson A, et al. On the disulfiram-like effect of coprine, the pharmacologically active principle of coprinus atramentarius. *Acta Pharmacol Toxicol (Copenh).* 1978;42:292-297.

21. Centers for Disease Control and Prevention. Respiratory illness associated with inhalation of mushroom spores—Wisconsin, 1994. *MMWR Morb Mortal Wkly Rep.* 1994;43:525.

22. Centers for Disease Control and Prevention. *Mold Prevention Strategies and Possible Health Effects in the Aftermath of Hurricanes and Major Floods.* Vol 55. US Department of Health and Human Services, Centers for Disease Control and Prevention; 2006.

23. Chilton W, et al. A naturally-occurring allenic amino acid. *Tetrahedron Lett.* 1968; 9:6283-6284.

24. Chodorowski Z, et al. Acute poisoning with *Tricholoma equestre. Przegl Lek.* 2002; 59:386-387.

25. ClinicalTrials.gov, Health UNIo. Intravenous milk thistle (silibinin-legalon) for hepatic failure induced by Amatoxin/Amanita mushroom poisoning. 2016; https://clinicaltrials.gov/ct2/show/NCT00915681.

26. Courtin P, et al. Renal failure after ingestion of *Amanita proxima. Clin Toxicol (Phila).* 2009;47:906-908.

27. Covic A, et al. Successful use of molecular absorbent regenerating system (mars) dialysis for the treatment of fulminant hepatic failure in children accidentally poisoned by toxic mushroom ingestion. *Liver Int.* 2003;23(suppl 3):21-27.

28. Curry SC, Rose MC. Intravenous mushroom poisoning. *Ann Emerg Med.* 1985;14:900-902.

29. Danel VC, et al. Main features of *Cortinarius* spp. poisoning: a literature review. *Toxicon.* 2001;39:1053-1060.

30. De Carlo E, et al. Effects of *Amanita phalloides* toxins on insulin release: in vivo and in vitro studies. *Arch Toxicol.* 2003;77:441-445.

31. Detry O, et al. Clinical use of a bioartificial liver in the treatment of acetaminophen-induced fulminant hepatic failure. *Am Surg.* 1999;65:934-938.

32. Diaz JH. Syndromic diagnosis and management of confirmed mushroom poisonings. *Crit Care Med.* 2005;33:427-436.

33. Dinis-Oliveira RJ, et al. Human and experimental toxicology of orellanine. *Hum Exp Toxicol.* 2016.;35:1016-1029.

34. Enjalbert F, et al. Treatment of amatoxin poisoning: 20-year retrospective analysis. *J Toxicol Clin Toxicol.* 2002;40:715-757.

35. Epis S, et al. Molecular detection of poisonous mushrooms in different matrices. *Mycologia.* 2010;102:747-754.

36. Escudie L, et al. *Amanita phalloides* poisoning: reassessment of prognostic factors and indications for emergency liver transplantation. *J Hepatol.* 2007;46:466-473.

37. Evenepoel P, et al. Prometheus versus molecular adsorbents recirculating system: comparison of efficiency in two different liver detoxification devices. *Artif Organs.* 2006;30:276-284.

38. Faulstich H. Structure of poisonous components of *Amanita phalloides. Curr Probl Clin Biochem.* 1977;7:1-10.

39. Faulstich H. New aspects of amanita poisoning. *Klin Wochenschr.* 1979;57:1143-1152.

40. Faulstich H, et al. Toxicokinetics of labeled amatoxins in the dog. *Arch Toxicol.* 1985;56:190-194.

41. Faybik P, et al. Extracorporeal albumin dialysis in patients with *Amanita phalloides* poisoning. *Liver Int.* 2003;23(suppl 3):28-33.

42. Feinfeld DA, et al. Poisoning by amatoxin-containing mushrooms in suburban New York—report of four cases. *J Toxicol Clin Toxicol.* 1994;32:715-721.

43. Feinfeld DA, et al. Three controversial issues in extracorporeal toxin removal. *Semin Dial.* 2006;19:358-362.

44. Filigenzi MS, et al. Determination of alpha-amanitin in serum and liver by multistage linear ion trap mass spectrometry. *J Agric Food Chem.* 2007;55:2784-2790.

45. Fischbein CB, et al. Digital imaging: a promising tool for mushroom identification. *Acad Emerg Med.* 2003;10:808-811.

46. Floersheim GL, et al. Curative potencies of penicillin in experimental *Amanita phalloides* poisoning. *Agents Actions.* 1971;2:138-141.

47. Floersheim GL. Rifampicin and cysteamine protect against the mushroom toxin phalloidin. *Experientia.* 1974;30:1310-1312.

48. Floersheim GL. Treatment of experimental poisoning produced by extracts of *Amanita phalloides. Toxicol Appl Pharmacol.* 1975;34:499-508.

49. Floersheim GL. Antagonistic effects against single lethal doses of *Amanita phalloides. Naunyn Schmiedebergs Arch Pharmacol.* 1976;293:171-174.

50. Floersheim GL, et al. Effects of penicillin and silymarin on liver enzymes and blood clotting factors in dogs given a boiled preparation of *Amanita phalloides. Toxicol Appl Pharmacol.* 1978;46:455-462.

51. Floersheim GL. Treatment of mushroom poisoning. *JAMA.* 1985;253:3252-3252.

52. Floersheim GL. Treatment of human *Amatoxin* mushroom poisoning. Myths and advances in therapy. *Med Toxicol.* 1987;2:1-9.

53. Franz M, et al. Magic mushrooms: hope for a "cheap high" resulting in end-stage renal failure. *Nephrol Dial Transplant.* 1996;11:2324-2327.

54. French AL, Garrettson LK. Poisoning with the North American Jack o'lantern mushroom, omphalotus illudens. *J Toxicol Clin Toxicol.* 1988;26:81-88.

55. Galler GW, et al. Mushroom poisoning: the role of orthotopic liver transplantation. *J Clin Gastroenterol.* 1992;15:229-232.

56. Ganzert M, et al. Indication of liver transplantation following amatoxin intoxication. *J Hepatol.* 2005;42:202-209.

57. Garcia de la Fuente I, et al. Amanita poisoning and liver transplantation: do we have the right decision criteria? *J Pediatr Gastroenterol Nutr.* 2011;53:459-462.

58. Garcia J, et al. *Amanita phalloides* poisoning: mechanisms of toxicity and treatment. *Food Chem Toxicol.* 2015;86:41-55.

59. Garcia J, et al. A breakthrough on *Amanita phalloides* poisoning: an effective antidotal effect by polymyxin B. *Arch Toxicol.* 2015;89:2305-2323.

60. Gawlikowski T, et al. Edible mushroom-related poisoning: a study on circumstances of mushroom collection, transport, and storage. *Hum Exp Toxicol.* 2015;34:718-724.

61. Gejyo F, et al. A novel type of encephalopathy associated with mushroom sugihiratake ingestion in patients with chronic kidney diseases. *Kidney Int.* 2005;68:188-192.

62. Giannini L, et al. Amatoxin poisoning: a 15-year retrospective analysis and follow-up evaluation of 105 patients. *Clin Toxicol (Phila).* 2007;45:539-542.

63. GmbH M. Legalon® sil [package insert]. Koln, Germany 2008.

64. Gundala S, et al. The hepatocellular bile acid transporter ntcp facilitates uptake of the lethal mushroom toxin alpha-amanitin. *Arch Toxicol.* 2004;78:68-73.

65. Hanrahan JP, Gordon MA. Mushroom poisoning. Case reports and a review of therapy. *JAMA.* 1984;251:1057-1061.

66. Hilty MP, et al. Ulcerating ileocolitis in severe amatoxin poisoning. *Case Rep Gastrointest Med.* 2015;2015:632085.

67. Huang L, et al. Outbreak of fatal mushroom poisoning with *Amanita franchetii* and ramaria rufescens. *BMJ Case Rep.* 2009;2009.

68. Jacobs BP, et al. Milk thistle for the treatment of liver disease: a systematic review and meta-analysis. *Am J Med.* 2002;113:506-515.

69. Jacobs J, et al. Serious mushroom poisonings in California requiring hospital admission, 1990 through 1994. *West J Med.* 1996;165:283-288.

70. Jaeger A, et al. Kinetics of amatoxins in human poisoning: therapeutic implications. *J Toxicol Clin Toxicol.* 1993;31:63-80.

71. Jander S, Bischoff J. Treatment of *Amanita phalloides* poisoning: I. Retrospective evaluation of plasmapheresis in 21 patients. *Ther Apher.* 2000;4:303-307.

72. Jander S, et al. Plasmapheresis in the treatment of *Amanita phalloides* poisoning: II. A review and recommendations. *Ther Apher.* 2000;4:308-312.

73. Judge BS, et al. Ingestion of a newly described North American mushroom species from Michigan resulting in chronic renal failure: *Cortinarius orellanosus. Clin Toxicol (Phila).* 2010;48:545-549.

74. Karakayali H, et al. Pediatric liver transplantation for acute liver failure. *Transplant Proc.* 2007;39:1157-1160.

75. Karvellas CJ, Tillman H, Leung AA, et al. Acute liver injury and acute liver failure from mushroom poisoning in North America. *Liver Int.* 2016;36:1043-1050.

76. Kelner MJ, Alexander NM. Endocrine hormone abnormalities in *Amanita* poisoning. *J Toxicol Clin Toxicol.* 1987;25:21-37.

77. Kirchmair M, et al. Amanita poisonings resulting in acute, reversible renal failure: new cases, new toxic amanita mushrooms. *Nephrol Dial Transplant.* 2012;27:1380-1386.

78. Klein AS, et al. Amanita poisoning: treatment and the role of liver transplantation. *Am J Med.* 1989;86:187-193.

79. Koppel C. Clinical symptomatology and management of mushroom poisoning. *Toxicon.* 1993;31:1513-1540.

80. Kostansek EC, et al. The crystal structure of the mushroom toxin beta-amanitin. *J Am Chem Soc.* 1977;99:1273-1274.

81. Kraft J, et al. Biological effects of the dihydroorotate dehydrogenase inhibitor polyporic acid, a toxic constituent of the mushroom *Hapalopilus rutilans*, in rats and humans. *Arch Toxicol.* 1998;72:711-721.

82. Kubicka J. Neue moglichkeiten in der behandlung von vergiftung mit dem grumen knollenblatterpilz—*Amanita phalloides. Mykol Mitteil.* 1963;7:92-94.

83. Kullak-Ublick GA, et al. Enterohepatic bile salt transporters in normal physiology and liver disease. *Gastroenterology.* 2004;126:322-342.

84. Lampe KF. Toxic fungi. *Annu Rev Pharmacol Toxicol.* 1979;19:85-104.

85. Leathem AM, et al. Renal failure caused by mushroom poisoning. *J Toxicol Clin Toxicol.* 1997;35:67-75.

86. Letschert K, et al. Molecular characterization and inhibition of amanitin uptake into human hepatocytes. *Toxicol Sci.* 2006;91:140-149.

87. Lincoff G, Mitchel DH. *Toxic and Hallucinogenic Mushroom Poisoning. A Handbook for Physicians and Mushroom Hunters.* New York, NY: Van Nostrand Reinhold Company; 1977.

88. Lincoff G. *The Audubon Society Field Guide to North American Mushrooms.* New York, NY: Knopf; 1981.

89. Lindell TJ, et al. Specific inhibition of nuclear RNA polymerase II by alpha-amanitin. *Science.* 1970;170:447-449.

90. Maeta K, et al. Rapid species identification of cooked poisonous mushrooms by using real-time PCR. *Appl Environ Microbiol.* 2008;74:3306-3309.

91. Magdalan J, et al. Failure of benzylpenicillin, N-acetylcysteine and silibinin to reduce alpha-amanitin hepatotoxicity. *In Vivo.* 2009;23:393-399.

92. Magdalan J, et al. Benzylpenicillin, acetylcysteine and silibinin as antidotes in human hepatocytes intoxicated with alpha-amanitin. *Exp Toxicol Pathol.* 2010;62:367-373.

93. Magdalan J, et al. Influence of commonly used clinical antidotes on antioxidant systems in human hepatocyte culture intoxicated with alpha-amanitin. *Hum Exp Toxicol.* 2011;30:38-43.

94. Marchner H, Tottmar O. A comparative study on the effects of disulfiram, cyanamide and 1-aminocyclopropanol on the acetaldehyde metabolism in rats. *Acta Pharmacol Toxicol (Copenh).* 1978;43:219-232.

95. Mas A. Mushrooms, amatoxins and the liver. *J Hepatol.* 2005;42:166-169.
96. Matsuura M, et al. Identification of the toxic trigger in mushroom poisoning. *Nat Chem Biol.* 2009;5:465-467.
97. Meier-Abt F, et al. Identification of phalloidin uptake systems of rat and human liver. *Biochim Biophys Acta.* 2004;1664:64-69.
98. Meunier BC, et al. Liver transplantation after severe poisoning due to amatoxin-containing lepiota—report of three cases. *J Toxicol Clin Toxicol.* 1995;33:165-171.
99. Minami T, et al. Acute and late effects on induction of allodynia by acromelic acid, a mushroom poison related structurally to kainic acid. *Br J Pharmacol.* 2004;142:679-688.
100. Moroni F, et al. A trend in the therapy of *Amanita phalloides* poisoning. *Arch Toxicol.* 1976;36:111-115.
101. Nakajima N, et al. Therapeutic potential of nicotinic acid in erythromelalgia associated with *Clitocybe acromelalga* intoxication. *Clin Toxicol (Phila).* 2013;51:815.
102. Nakajima N, et al. Erythromelalgia associated with *Clitocybe acromelalga* intoxication. *Clin Toxicol (Phila).* 2013;51:451-454.
103. Nieminen P, et al. Increased plasma creatine kinase activities triggered by edible wild mushrooms. *Food Chem Toxicol.* 2005;43:133-138.
104. O'Grady JG, et al. Acute liver failure: redefining the syndromes. *Lancet.* 1993;342:273-275.
105. Olson KR, et al. *Amanita phalloides*-type mushroom poisoning. *West J Med.* 1982; 137:282-289.
106. Oubrahim H, et al. Peroxidase-mediated oxidation, a possible pathway for activation of the fungal nephrotoxin orellanine and related compounds. ESR and spin-trapping studies. *Free Radic Res.* 1998;28:497-505.
107. Paydas S, et al. Poisoning due to amatoxin-containing *Lepiota* species. *Br J Clin Pract.* 1990;44:450-453.
108. Pelizzari V, et al. Partial purification and characterization of a toxic component of *Amanita smithiana*. *Mycologia.* 1994;86:555-560.
109. Pinson CW, et al. Liver transplantation for severe *Amanita phalloides* mushroom poisoning. *Am J Surg.* 1990;159:493-499.
110. Piqueras J, et al. Mushroom poisoning: therapeutic apheresis or forced diuresis. *Transfusion.* 1987;27:116-117.
111. Pond SM, et al. Amatoxin poisoning in northern california, 1982-1983. *West J Med.* 1986;145:204-209.
112. Poucheret P, et al. Amatoxin poisoning treatment decision-making: pharmaco-therapeutic clinical strategy assessment using multidimensional multivariate statistic analysis. *Toxicon.* 2010;55:1338-1345.
113. Raff E, et al. Renal failure after eating "magic" mushrooms. *CMAJ.* 1992;147:1339-1341.
114. Ramirez P, et al. Fulminant hepatic failure after lepiota mushroom poisoning. *J Hepatol.* 1993;19:51-54.
115. Rapior S, et al. Intoxication by *Cortinarius orellanus*: detection and assay of orellanine in biological fluids and renal biopsies. *Mycopathologia.* 1989;108:155-161.
116. Rengstorff DS, et al. Recovery from severe hepatitis caused by mushroom poisoning without liver transplantation. *Clin Gastroenterol Hepatol.* 2003;1:392-396.
117. Richard JM, et al. Nephrotoxicity of orellanine, a toxin from the mushroom *Cortinarius orellanus*. *Arch Toxicol.* 1988;62:242-245.
118. Rohrmoser M, et al. Orellanine poisoning: rapid detection of the fungal toxin in renal biopsy material. *J Toxicol Clin Toxicol.* 1997;35:63-66.
119. Rumack BH, Salzman E. *Mushroom poisoning: Diagnosis and treatment.* Boca Raton, FL: CRC Press; 1978.
120. Santi L, et al. Acute liver failure caused by *Amanita phalloides* poisoning. *Int J Hepatol.* 2012;2012:487480.
121. Saviuc P, Danel V. New syndromes in mushroom poisoning. *Toxicol Rev.* 2006;25:199-209.
122. Saviuc P, et al. Can morels (*Morchella* sp.) induce a toxic neurological syndrome? *Clin Toxicol (Phila).* 2010;48:365-372.
123. Schneider S, et al. Mushroom poisoning: recognition and emergency management. *Emerg Med Rep.* 1991;12:81-88.
124. Schneider SM, et al. Cimetidine protection against alpha-amanitin hepatotoxicity in mice: a potential model for the treatment of *Amanita phalloides* poisoning. *Ann Emerg Med.* 1987;16:1136-1140.
125. Schneider SM, et al. Failure of cimetidine to affect phalloidin toxicity. *Vet Hum Toxicol.* 1991;33:17-18.
126. Schumacher T, Hoiland K. Mushroom poisoning caused by species of the genus *Cortinarius* fries. *Arch Toxicol.* 1983;53:87-106.
127. Senthilkumaran S, et al. Nicotinic acid in erythromelalgia associated with *Clitocybe acromelalga* intoxication: theories and therapy. *Clin Toxicol (Phila).* 2013;51:814.
128. Serne EH, et al. *Amanita phalloides*, a potentially lethal mushroom: its clinical presentation and therapeutic options. *Neth J Med.* 1996;49:19-23.
129. Shi G, et al. Hypoglycemia and death in mice following experimental exposure to an extract of *Trogia venenata* mushrooms. *PLoS One.* 2012;7:e38712.
130. Shi GQ, et al. Clusters of sudden unexplained death associated with the mushroom, *Trogia venenata*, in rural Yunnan Province, China. *PLoS One.* 2012;7:e35894.

131. Smith A, Weber N. *The Mushroom Hunter's Field Guide.* Ann Arbor: University of Michigan Press Thunder Bay Press; 1980.
132. Sorodoc L, et al. Is MARS system enough for *A. phalloides*-induced liver failure treatment? *Hum Exp Toxicol.* 2010;29:823-832.
133. Sperti S, et al. Dissociation constants of the complexes between RNA-polymerase II and amanitins. *Experientia.* 1973;29:33-34.
134. Stenklyft PH, Augenstein WL. Chlorophyllum molybdites—severe mushroom poisoning in a child. *J Toxicol Clin Toxicol.* 1990;28:159-168.
135. Stone R. Epidemiology. Will a midsummer's nightmare return? *Science.* 2010;329: 132-134.
136. Stone R. Toxicology. Heart-stopping revelation about how Chinese mushroom kills. *Science.* 2012;335:1293.
137. Strand RD, et al. Lycoperdonosis. *N Engl J Med.* 1967;277:89-91.
138. Timar L, Czeizel AE. Birth weight and congenital anomalies following poisonous mushroom intoxication during pregnancy. *Reprod Toxicol.* 1997;11:861-866.
139. Tong TC, et al. Comparative treatment of alpha-amanitin poisoning with *N*-acetylcysteine, benzylpenicillin, cimetidine, thioctic acid, and silybin in a murine model. *Ann Emerg Med.* 2007;50:282-288.
140. Tottmar O, Lindberg P. Effects on rat liver acetaldehyde dehydrogenases in vitro and in vivo by coprine, the disulfiram-like constituent of coprinus atramentarius. *Acta Pharmacol Toxicol (Copenh).* 1977;40:476-481.
141. Trestrail JH 3rd. Mushroom poisoning in the united states—an analysis of 1989 united states poison center data. *J Toxicol Clin Toxicol.* 1991;29:459-465.
142. Tulloss R, Lindgren J. *Amanita smithiana*: taxonomy, distribution, and poisonings. *Mycotaxon (USA).* 1992;45:373-387.
143. Vanden Hoek TL, et al. Jack o'lantern mushroom poisoning. *Ann Emerg Med.* 1991; 20:559-561.
144. Vardar R, et al. Efficacy of fractionated plasma separation and adsorption system (prometheus) for treatment of liver failure due to mushroom poisoning. *Hepatogastroenterology.* 2010;57:573-577.
145. Vesconi S, et al. Therapy of cytotoxic mushroom intoxication. *Crit Care Med.* 1985; 13:402-406.
146. Vienken J, Christmann H. How can liver toxins be removed? Filtration and adsorption with the prometheus system. *Ther Apher Dial.* 2006;10:125-131.
147. Vogel G, et al. Protection by silibinin against *Amanita phalloides* intoxication in beagles. *Toxicol Appl Pharmacol.* 1984;73:355-362.
148. Warden CR, Benjamin DR. Acute renal failure associated with suspected *Amanita smithiana* mushroom ingestions: a case series. *Acad Emerg Med.* 1998;5:808-812.
149. Wauters JP, Rossel C, Farquet JJ. *Amanita phalloides* poisoning treated by early charcoal haemoperfusion. *Br Med J.* 1978;2:1465.
150. Wellington K, Jarvis B. Silymarin: a review of its clinical properties in the management of hepatic disorders. *BioDrugs.* 2001;15:465-489.
151. West PL, et al. *Amanita smithiana* mushroom ingestion: a case of delayed renal failure and literature review. *J Med Toxicol.* 2009;5:32-38.
152. Wieland T, et al. Amatoxins, phallotoxins, phallolysin, and antamanide: the biologically active components of poisonous amanita mushroom. *CRC Crit Rev Biochem.* 1978;5:185-260.
153. Winkelmann M, et al. Fatal immunohaemolytic anaemia after eating the mushroom paxillus involutus [author's translation, in German]. *Dtsch Med Wochenschr.* 1982;107:1190-1194.
154. Winkelmann M, et al. Severe hemolysis caused by antibodies against the mushroom paxillus involutus and its therapy by plasma exchange. *Klin Wochenschr.* 1986;64:935-938.
155. Wiseman JS, Abeles RH. Mechanism of inhibition of aldehyde dehydrogenase by cyclopropranone hydrate and the mushroom toxin coprine. *Biochemistry.* 1979; 18:427-435.
156. Wittebole X, Hantson P. Use of the molecular adsorbent recirculating system (MARS) for the management of acute poisoning with or without liver failure. *Clin Toxicol (Phila).* 2011;49:782-793.
157. Wolfe BE, et al. Distribution and abundance of the introduced ectomycorrhizal fungus *Amanita phalloides* in North America. *New Phytol.* 2010;185:803-816.
158. Woodle ES, et al. Orthotopic liver transplantation in a patient with amanita poisoning. *JAMA.* 1985;253:69-70.
159. Yamada EG, et al. Mushroom poisoning due to amatoxin. Northern california, winter 1996-1997. *West J Med.* 1998;169:380-384.
160. Yamaura Y, et al. Hepatotoxic action of a poisonous mushroom, *Amanita abrupta* in mice and its toxic component. *Toxicology.* 1986;38:161-173.
161. Zhang Y, et al. Evidence against barium in the mushroom *Trogia venenata* as a cause of sudden unexpected deaths in Yunnan, China. *Appl Environ Microbiol.* 2012;78:8834-8835.

118 PLANTS

Lewis S. Nelson and Lewis R. Goldfrank

Approximately 5% of all human exposures reported to poison control centers involve plants. The large number of exposures probably occur because plants are so accessible and attractive to youngsters. Approximately 80% of these cases involve individuals younger than 6 years. As indoor plants have become ever more popular, the incidence of plant exposures has increased. Data compiled by the American Association of Poison Control Centers (AAPCC) give some indication of which plants are more commonly involved (Chap. 130), but these plants typically have relatively limited toxicity. More than 80% of patients reported to the AAPCC as being exposed were asymptomatic, less than 20% had minor to moderate symptomatology, and less than 7% necessitated a health care visit. The benignity of these exposures in the United States, largely due to the unintentional nature of the event, is represented by a fatality rate of less than 0.001%. However, in other parts of the world, plant exposures, particularly those taken for self-harm and where health care is less accessible, carry a significant risk and public health burden.[12] This chapter addresses the toxicologic principles associated with the most potentially dangerous plants.

HISTORY AND CLASSIFICATION OF PLANT XENOBIOTICS

Aconitine, from monkshood, exemplifies the rich history of plant toxicology. It was believed by the Greeks to be the first poison—"lycotonum"—created by the goddess Hecate from the foam of the river Cerebrus. Alkaloid constituents are responsible for its toxic (and therapeutic) effects. Alkaloids represent one of several classes of organic molecules found in plants as defined by the science of pharmacognosy, which is the science of medicines derived from natural sources. The pharmacognosy approach is consistent with the literature of plant efficacy and is applied here to their toxicity (Table 118–1). Unfortunately, the science of pharmacognosy is not always straightforward, and systems of classification may vary depending on the pharmacognosist. Hence, our approach borrows primarily from 2 groups of authors to keep the classification as consistent as possible.[51,128] The major groups are as follows:

1. Alkaloids: Molecules that react as bases and contain nitrogen, usually in a heterocyclic structure. Alkaloids typically have strong pharmacologic activity that defines many major toxidromes.
2. Glycosides: Organic compounds that yield a sugar or sugar derivative (the glycone) and a nonsugar moiety (the aglycone) upon hydrolysis. The aglycone is the basis of subclassification into saponin or steroidal glycosides (including steroidal cardiac glycosides, cyanogenic glycosides, anthraquinone glycosides), and others such as atractyloside and salicin.
3. Terpenes and resins: Assemblages of 5-carbon units (isoprene unit) with many types of functional groups (eg, alcohols, phenols, ketones, and esters) attached. This is the largest group of secondary metabolites; approximately 20,000 are identified. Most essential oils are mixtures of monoterpenes, and the terpene name depends on the number of isoprene assemblages. Monoterpenes have 2 units ($C_{10}H_{16}$), sesquiterpenes have 3 isoprene units (C_{15}), diterpenes have 4 isoprene units (C_{20}), and triterpenes have 6 (C_{30}). These molecules often play an active role in plant defense mechanisms.
4. Proteins, peptides, and lectins: Proteins consist of amino acid units with various side chains, and peptides consist of linkages among amino acids. Lectins are glycoproteins classified according to the number of protein chains linked by disulfide bonds and by binding affinity for specific carbohydrate ligands, particularly galactosamines. The toxalbumins (eg, ricin) are lectins. These components tend to be neurotoxins, hemagglutinins, or cathartics.
5. Phenols and phenylpropanoids: Phenols contain phenyl rings and have one or more hydroxyl groups attached to the ring. Phenylpropanoids consist of a phenyl ring attached to a propane side chain. These compounds are devoid of nitrogen, even though some are derived from phenylalanine and tyrosine. They constitute a major group of secondary metabolites and among plant toxins include coumarins (lactone side chains), flavonoids (built upon a flavan 2,3-dihydro-2-phenylbenzopyran nucleus, such as naringenin and rutin), lignans (2 linked phenylpropanoids, such as podophyllin), lignins (complex polymers of lignans that bind cellulose for woody bark and stem), and tannins (polymers that bind to protein and can be further hydrolyzed or condensed).

Plant chemistry is complex. The simplified presentation of one xenobiotic per plant per symptom group used in Table 118–1 demphasizes the fact that plants contain multiple xenobiotics that work independently or in concert. Additionally, different plant families may contain similar, if not identical, xenobiotics (either from conservation of biochemical pathways inherited from a common ancestor or through convergent evolution). In some cases, xenobiotics remain unidentified and are grouped in the section Unidentified Toxins.

Our focus is on exposures to flowering plants (angiosperms) related to foraging, dietary, or occupational contact, except for some gymnosperms or algae and, rarely, medicinal contact (Chap. 43).[92] Because our understanding of plant xenobiotics is poor relative to that of pharmaceuticals, animal research is included to provide a more comprehensive foundation for comparison with human experiences that may otherwise go unrecognized without such precedent, or may likewise prove ultimately incorrect. The science of plant toxicology formally began in the United States as a response to significant poisonings of livestock. The overall quality of literature for human exposures is poor and primarily available as case reports. Many of these cases lack clear links between toxin exposure and illness, and qualitative or quantitative analyses are generally unavailable. Uncertainty is compounded by the fact that plants themselves are inherently variable, and potency and type of xenobiotic depend on the season, geography, growing environment, plant part, and methods of processing.

IDENTIFICATION OF PLANTS

Positive identification of the plant species should be attempted whenever possible, especially when the patient becomes symptomatic. Communication with an expert botanist, medical toxicologist, or poison control center is highly recommended and can be facilitated by transmission of digital images. Provisionally, simple comparison of the species in question with pictures or descriptions from a field guide of flora may help exclude the identity of the plant from among the most life-threatening in Table 118–1. A plant identification can also be compared with those searched in the PLANTOX database (http://www.accessdata.fda.gov/scripts/plantox/index.cfm) managed by the Food and Drug Administration (FDA). However, with some exceptions, laboratory analysis is generally not timely enough to be useful except as a tool in an investigatory or forensic analysis. As the state of analytical science advances, however, it is often possible to confirm a diagnosis based on DNA analysis of unidentifiable or degraded plant material.[106]

In cases where expert identification cannot be immediately achieved, preliminary recognition of taxonomic families of poisonous plants is the simplest first step to identify or exclude poisonous plants, but is most easily achieved when the plant is in flower or fruit. For instance, if the flower is described or looks like a flower from a tomato or potato, it probably is in the Solanaceae family. Plants of this family typically contain solanaceous

TABLE 118–1   Primary Toxicity of Common Important Plant Species

Plant Species (Family)	Typical Common Names	Primary Toxicity	Xenobiotic(s)	Class of Xenobiotic
Abrus precatorius (Euphorbiaceae)[a]	Prayer beans, rosary pea, Indian bean, crab's eye, Buddhist's rosary bead, jequirity pea	Gastrointestinal	Abrin	Protein, lectin, peptide, amino acid
Aconitum napellus and other Aconitum spp (Ranunculaceae)[a]	Monkshood Friar's cap Wolfsbane	Cardiac, neurologic	Aconitine and related xenobiotic	Alkaloid
Acorus calamus (Araliaceae)	Sweet flag, rat root, flag root, calamus	Gastrointestinal	Asarin	Phenol or phenylpropanoid
Aesculus hippocastanum (Hippocastanaceae)	Horse chestnut	Hematologic	Esculoside (6-β-D-glucopyranosyloxy-7-hydroxycoumarin)	Phenol or phenylpropanoid
Agave lecheguilla (Amaryllidaceae)	Agave	Dermatitis	Aglycones, smilagenin, sarsasapogenin	Saponin glycoside
Aloe barbadensis, Aloe vera, others (Liliaceae/Amaryllidaceae)	Aloagave	Gastrointestinal	Barbaloin, iso-barbaloin, aloinosides	Anthraquinone glycoside
Anabaena and Aphanizomenon[a]	Blue-green algae	Neurologic	Saxitoxinlike	Guanidinium
Anacardium occidentale, many others (Anacardiaceae)	Cashew, many others	Contact dermatitis	Urushiol oleoresins	Terpenoid
Anthoxanthum odoratum (Poaceae)	Sweet vernal grass	Hematologic	Coumarin	Phenol or phenylpropanoid
Areca catechu (Arecaceae)	Betel nut	Cholinergic	Arecoline	Alkaloid
Argemone mexicana (Papaveraceae)	Mexican pricklepoppy	Gastrointestinal	Sanguinarine	Alkaloid
Argyreia nervosa	Hawaiian baby woodrose seeds	Neurologic	Lysergic acid amide	Alkaloid
Argyreia spp (Convolvulaceae)	Morning glory	Neurologic	Lysergic acid derivatives	Alkaloid
Aristolochia reticulata, Aristolochia spp (Aristolochiaceae)[a]	Texan or Red River snake root	Renal, carcinogenic	Aristolochic acid	Alkaloid relative as derivative of isothebaine
Artemisia absinthium (Compositae/Asteraceae)[a]	Absinthe	Neurologic	Thujone	Terpenoid
Asclepias spp (Asclepiadaceae)[a]	Milk weed	Cardiac	Asclepin and related cardenolides	Cardioactive steroid
Astragalus spp (Fabaceae)[a]	Locoweed	Metabolic, neurologic	Swainsonine	Alkaloid
Atractylis gummifera (Compositae)[a]	Thistle	Hepatic	Atractyloside, gummiferine	Glycoside
Atropa belladonna (Solanaceae)[a]	Belladonna	Anticholinergic	Belladonna alkaloids	Alkaloid
Azalea spp (Ericaceae)[a,b]	Azalea	Cardiac, neurologic	Grayanotoxin	Terpenoid
Berberis spp (Ranunculaceae)	Barberry	Oxytocic, cardiovascular	Berberine	Alkaloid
Blighia sapida (Sapindaceae)[a]	Ackee fruit	Metabolic, gastrointestinal, neurotoxic	Hypoglycin	Protein, lectin, peptide, amino acid
Borago officinalis (Boraginaceae)[a]	Borage	Hepatic (venoocclusive disease)	Pyrrolizidine alkaloids	Alkaloid
Brassaia spp[b]	Umbrella tree	Dermatitis, mechanical and cytotoxic	Oxalate raphides	Carboxylic acid
Brassica nigra (Brassicaceae)	Black mustard	Dermatitis, irritant	Sinigrin	Glucosinolate (isothiocyanate glycoside)
Brassica oleracea var. capitata	Cabbage	Metabolic (precursor to goitrin, antithyroid compound)	Progoitrin	Isothiocyanate glycoside
Cactus spp[b]	Cactus	Dermatitis, mechanical	Nontoxic	None
Caladium spp (Araceae)[b]	Caladium	Dermatitis, mechanical and cytotoxic	Oxalate raphides	Carboxylic acid
Calotropis spp (Asclepiadaceae)[a]	Crown flower	Cardiac	Asclepin and related cardenolides	Cardioactive steroid

(Continued)

| | TABLE 118–1 | Primary Toxicity of Common Important Plant Species *(Continued)* | | | |

Plant Species (Family)	Typical Common Names	Primary Toxicity	Xenobiotic(s)	Class of Xenobiotic
Camellia sinensis (Theaceae)	Tea, green tea	Cardiac, neurologic	Theophylline, caffeine	Alkaloid
Cannabis sativa	Cannabis, marijuana, Indian hemp, hashish, pot	Neurologic	Tetrahydrocannabinol	Terpenoid, resin, oleoresin
Capsicum frutescens, Capsicum annuum, Capsicum spp (Solanaceae)[b]	Capsicum, cayenne pepper	Dermatitis, irritant	Capsaicin	Phenol or phenylpropanoid
Cascara sagrada, Rhamnus purshiana, Rhamnus cathartica (Rhamnaceae)	Cascara, sacred bark, Chittern bark, common buckthorn	Gastrointestinal	Cascarosides, *O*-glycosides, emodin	Anthraquinone glycoside
Cassia senna, Cassia angustifolia (Fabaceae)	Senna	Gastrointestinal	Sennosides	Anthraquinone glycoside
Catha edulis (Celastraceae)	Khat	Cardiac, neurologic	Cathinone	Alkaloid
Catharanthus roseus (formerly *Vinca rosea*) (Apocynaceae)	Catharanthus, vinca, madagascar periwinkle	Gastrointestinal	Vincristine	Alkaloid
Caulophyllum thalictroides (Berberidaceae)	Blue cohosh	Nicotinic	*N*-methylcytisine and related compounds	Alkaloid
Cephaelis ipecacuanha, Cephaelis acuminata (Rubiaceae)[a]	Syrup of ipecac	Gastrointestinal, cardiac	Emetine/cephaline	Alkaloid
Chlorophytum comosum[b]	Spider plant	Dermatitis, contact, and allergic	Urushiol oleoresins	Terpenoid
Chondrodendron spp, *Curarea* spp, *Strychnos* spp[a]	Tubocurare, curare	Neurologic	Tubocurarine	Alkaloid
Chrysanthemum spp, *Taraxacum officinale*, other Compositae (Asteraceae)[b]	Chrysanthemum, dandelion, other Compositaceae	Contact dermatitis	Sesquiterpene lactones	Terpenoid
Cicuta maculata (Apiaceae/ Umbelliferae)[a]	Water hemlock	Neurologic	Cicutoxin	Alcohol
Cinchona spp (Rubiaceae)[a]	Cinchona	Cardiac, cinchonism	Quinidine	Alkaloid
Citrus aurantium (Rutaceae)[a]	Bitter orange	Cardiac, neurologic	Synephrine	Alkaloid
Citrus paradisi (Rutaceae)	Grapefruit	Drug interactions	Bergamottin, naringenin, or naringen	Phenol or phenylpropanoid
Claviceps purpurea, Claviceps paspali (Claviceptacea = fungus)[a]	Ergot	Cardiac, neurologic, oxytocic	Ergotamine and related compounds	Alkaloid
Coffea arabica (Rubiaceae)	Coffee	Cardiac, neurologic	Caffeine	Alkaloid
Cola nitida, Cola spp (Sterculiaceae)	Kola nut	Cardiac, neurologic	Caffeine	Alkaloid
Colchicum autumnale (Liliaceae)[a]	Autumn crocus	Multisystem	Colchicine	Alkaloid
Conium maculatum (Apiaceae/ Umbelliferae)[a]	Poison hemlock	Nicotinic, neurologic, respiratory, renal	Coniine	Alkaloid
Convallaria majalis[a]	Lily of the valley	Cardiac	Convallatoxin, strophanthin (~40 others)	Cardioactive steroid
Coptis spp (Ranunculaceae)	Goldenthread	Oxytocic, cardiovascular	Berberine	Alkaloid
Crassula spp[b]	Jade plant	Gastrointestinal	Nontoxic	None
Crotalaria spp (Fabaceae)[a]	Rattlebox	Hepatic (venoocclusive disease)	Pyrrolizidine alkaloids	Alkaloid
Croton tiglium and *Croton* spp (Euphorbiaceae)	Croton	Carcinogen, gastrointestinal	Croton oil	Lipid and fixed oil, also contains tropane alkaloid and diterpene
Cycas circinalis[a]	Queen sago, indu, cycad	Neurologic	Cycasin	Glycosides
Cytisus scoparius (Fabaceae)[a]	Broom, Scotch broom	Nicotinic, oxytocic	Sparteine	Alkaloid

(Continued)

TABLE 118-1 Primary Toxicity of Common Important Plant Species (*Continued*)

Plant Species (Family)	Typical Common Names	Primary Toxicity	Xenobiotic(s)	Class of Xenobiotic
Datura stramonium (Solanaceae)[a]	Jimson weed, stramonium, locoweed	Anticholinergic	Belladonna alkaloids	Alkaloid
Delphinium spp (Ranunculaceae)[a]	Larkspur	Cardiac, neurologic	Methyllycaconitine	Alkaloid-related xenobiotic
Dieffenbachia spp (Araceae)[b]	Dieffenbachia	Dermatitis, mechanical and cytotoxic	Oxalate raphides	Carboxylic acid
Digitalis lanata[a]	Grecian foxglove	Cardiac	Digoxin, lanatosides A–E (contains ~70 cardiac glycosides)	Cardioactive steroid
Digitalis purpurea[a]	Purple foxglove	Cardiac	Digitoxin	Cardioactive steroid
Dipteryx odorata, Dipteryx oppositifolia (Fabaceae)	Tonka beans	Hematologic	Coumarin	Phenol or phenylpropanoid
Ephedra spp, especially *sinensis* (Ephedraceae/Gnetaceae = Gymnosperm)[a]	Ephedra, Ma-huang	Cardiac, neurologic	Ephedrine and related xenobiotics	Alkaloid
Epipremnum aureum (Araceae)[b]	Pothos	Dermatitis, mechanical, and cytotoxic	Oxalate raphides	Carboxylic acid
Erythroxylum coca	Coca	Neurologic, cardiac	Cocaine	Alkaloid
Eucalyptus globus or spp[b]	Eucalyptus	Dermatitis, contact, and allergic	Eucalyptol	Terpenoid
Euphorbia pulcherrima, Euphorbia spp (Eurphorbiaceae)[b]	Poinsettia	Dermatitis, contact, and allergic	Phorbol esters	Terpenoid
Galium triflorum (Rubiaceae)	Sweet-scented bedstraw	Hematologic	Coumarin	Phenol or phenylpropanoid
Ginkgo biloba (Ginkgoaceae)	Ginkgo	Dermatitis, contact, and allergic	Urushiol oleoresins	Terpenoid
		Hematologic	Ginkgolides A–C, M	Terpenoid
		Neurologic	4-Methoxypyridoxine in seeds only	Alkaloid, pyridine
Gloriosa superba (Liliaceae)[a]	Meadow saffron	Multisystem	Colchicine	Alkaloid
Glycyrrhiza glabra[a]	Licorice	Metabolic, renal	Glycyrrhizin	Saponin glycoside
Gossypium spp	Cotton, cottonseed oil	Metabolic	Gossypol	Terpenoid
Hedeoma pulegioides (Lamiaceae)[a]	Pennyroyal	Hepatic, neurologic, oxytoxic	Pulegone	Terpenoid
Hedera helix (Araliaceae)[b]	Common ivy	Not absorbed	Hederacoside C, α-hederin, hederagenin	Cardioactive steroid
Hedysarium alpinum (Fabaceae)	Wild potato	Metabolic, neurologic	Swainsonine	Alkaloid
Heliotropium spp (Compositae/Asteraceae)[a]	Ragwort	Hepatic (venoocclusive disease)	Pyrrolizidine alkaloids	Alkaloid
Helleborus niger[a]	Black hellebore, Christmas rose	Cardiac	Hellebrin	Cardioactive steroid
Hydrastis canadensis (Ranunculaceae)[a]	Goldenseal	Neurologic, oxytocic, cardiovascular, respiratory	Hydrastine, berberine	Alkaloid
Hyoscyamus niger (Solanaceae)[a]	Henbane, hyoscyamus	Anticholinergic	Belladonna alkaloids	Alkaloid
Hypericum perforatum (Clusiaceae)	St John's wort	Dermatitis, photosensitivity, neurologic, xenobiotic interactions	Hyperforin, hypericin	Terpenoid
Ilex paraguariensis (Aquifoliaceae)	Maté, Yerba Maté, Paraguay tea	Cardiac, neurologic	Caffeine	Alkaloid
Ilex spp berries (Aquifoliaceae)[b]	Holly	Gastrointestinal	Mixture. Alkaloids, polyphenols, saponins, steroids, triterpenoids	Unidentified
Illicium anisatum (Illiciaceae)[a]	Japanese Star anise	Neurologic	Anasatin	Terpenoid

(Continued)

TABLE 118–1	Primary Toxicity of Common Important Plant Species *(Continued)*			
Plant Species (Family)	*Typical Common Names*	*Primary Toxicity*	*Xenobiotic(s)*	*Class of Xenobiotic*
Ipomoea tricolor and other *Ipomoea* spp (Convolvulaceae)	Morning glory	Neurologic	Lysergic acid derivatives	Alkaloid
Jatropha curcas (Euphorbiaceae)	Black vomit nut, physic nut, purging nut	Gastrointestinal	Curcin	Protein, lectin, peptide, amino acid
Karwinskia humboldtiana[a]	Buckthorn, wild cherry, tullidora, coyotillo, capulincillo, others	Neurologic, respiratory	Toxin T-514	Phenol or phenylpropanoid
Laburnum anagyroides (syn. *Cytisus laburnum*; Fabaceae)[a]	Golden chain, laburnum	Nicotinic	Cytisine	Alkaloid
Lantana camara (Verbenaceae)	Lantana	Dermatitis, photosensitivity	Lantadene A and B, phylloerythrin	Terpenoid
Lathyrus sativus[a]	Grass pea	Neurologic, skeletal	β-N-oxalylamino-L-alanine (BOAA); β-aminopropionitrile (BAPN)	Protein, lectin, peptide, amino acid
Lobelia inflata (Campanulaceae)	Indian tobacco	Nicotinic	Lobeline	Alkaloid
Lophophora williamsii	Peyote or mescal buttons	Neurologic	Mescaline	Alkaloid
Lupinus latifolius and other *Lupinus* spp (Fabaceae)	Lupine	Nicotinic	Anagyrine	Alkaloid
Lycopersicon spp (Solanaceae)[a]	Tomato (green)	Gastrointestinal, neurologic, anticholinergic	Tomatine, tomatidine	Glycoalkaloid
Mahonia spp (Ranunculaceae)	Oregon grape	Oxytocic, cardiovascular	Berberine	Alkaloid
Mandragora officinarum (Solanaceae)[a]	European or true mandrake	Anticholinergic	Belladonna alkaloids	Alkaloid
Manihot esculentus (Euphorbiaceae)[a]	Cassava, manihot, tapioca	Metabolic, neurotoxic, motor spastic paresis and visual disturbances	Linamarin	Cyanogenic glycoside
Melilotus spp (Fabaceae/Legumaceae)	Sweet clover (spoiled moldy)	Hematologic	Dicumarol	Phenol or phenylpropanoid
Mentha pulegium (Lamiaceae)[a]	Pennyroyal	Hepatic, neurologic, oxytocic	Pulegone	Terpenoid
Microcystis and *Anabaena* spp	Blue-green algae (cyanobacteria)	Hepatotoxic, dermatitis, photosensitivity	Microcystin	Protein, lectin, peptide, amino acid
Myristica fragrans	Nutmeg, pericarp = mace	Neurologic (hallucinations)	Myristicin, elemicin	Terpenoid
Narcissus spp and other (Amaryllidaceae, Liliaceae)	Narcissus	Dermatitis, mechanical, and cytotoxic	Lycorine, homolycorin	Alkaloid
Nerium oleander[a]	Oleander	Cardiac	Oleandrin	Cardioactive steroid
Nicotiana tabacum, Nicotiana spp (Solanaceae)[a]	Tobacco	Nicotinic	Nicotine	Alkaloid
Oxytropis spp (Fabaceae)	Locoweed	Metabolic, neurologic	Swainsonine	Alkaloid
Papaver somniferum	Poppy	Neurologic	Morphine/other opium derivatives	Alkaloid
Paullinia cupana (Sapindaceae)	Guarana	Cardiac, neurologic	Caffeine	Alkaloid
Pausinystalia yohimbe (Rubiaceae)[a]	Yohimbe	Cardiac, cholinergic	Yohimbine	Alkaloid
Philodendron spp (Araceae)[b]	Philodendron	Dermatitis, mechanical, and cytotoxic	Oxalate raphides	Carboxylic acid
Phoradendron spp (Loranthaceae or Viscaceae)	American mistletoe	Gastrointestinal	Phoratoxin, ligatoxin	Protein, lectin, peptide, amino acid
Physostigma venenosum (Fabaceae)[a]	Calabar bean, ordeal bean	Cholinergic	Physostigmine	Alkaloid
Phytolacca americana (Phytolaccaceae)[a]	American cancer Pokeweed, poke	Gastrointestinal	Phytolaccotoxin	Protein, lectin, peptide, amino acid
Pilocarpus jaborandi, Pilocarpus pinnatifolius (Rutaceae)[a]	Pilocarpus, jaborandi	Cholinergic effects	Pilocarpine	Alkaloid

(Continued)

TABLE 118–1 Primary Toxicity of Common Important Plant Species *(Continued)*

Plant Species (Family)	Typical Common Names	Primary Toxicity	Xenobiotic(s)	Class of Xenobiotic
Piper methysticum[a]	Kava kava	Hepatic, neurologic	Kawain, methysticine yangonin, other kava lactones	Terpenoid, resin, oleoresin
Plantago spp	Plantago (seed husks)	Gastrointestinal	Psyllium	Carbohydrate
Podophyllum emodi (Berberidaceae)[a]	Wild mandrake	Gastrointestinal and neurologic effects	Podophyllin (lignan)	Phenol or phenylpropanoid
Podophyllum peltatum (Berberidaceae)[a]	Mayapple	Gastrointestinal and neurologic effects	Podophyllin (lignan)	Phenol or phenylpropanoid
Populus spp (Salicaceae)	Poplar species	Salicylism	Salicin	Glycoside
Primula obconica (Primulaceae)	Primrose	Dermatitis, contact, and allergic	Primin	Phenol or phenylpropanoid
Prunus armeniaca, Prunus spp, Malus spp (Rosaceae)[a]	Apricot seed pits, wild cherry, peach, plum, pear, almond, apple, and other seed kernels	Metabolic acidosis, respiratory failure, coma, death	Amygdalin, emulsin	Cyanogenic glycoside
Pteridium spp (Polypodiaceae)	Bracken Fern	Carcinogen, thiaminase	Ptaquiloside	Terpenoid
Pulsatilla spp (Ranunculaceae)	Pulsatilla	Dermatitis, contact	Ranunculin, protoanemonin	Glycoside
Quercus spp	Oak	Metabolic, livestock toxicity	Tannic acid	Phenol or phenylpropanoid
Ranunculus spp (Ranunculaceae)	Buttercups	Dermatitis, contact	Ranunculin, protoanemonin	Glycoside
Rauwolfia serpentine (Apocynaceae)	Indian snakeroot	Cardiac, neurologic	Reserpine	Alkaloid
Remijia pedunculata (Rubiaceae)[a]	Cuprea bark	Cardiac, cinchonism	Quinidine	Alkaloid
Rhamnus frangula (Rhamnaceae)	Frangula bark, alder buckthorn	Gastrointestinal	Frangulins	Anthraquinone glycoside
Rheum officinale, Rheum spp (Polygonaceae)	Rhubarb	Gastrointestinal / Metabolic	Rhein anthrones / Oxalic/Acid (soluble)	Anthraquinone glycoside / Carboxylic acid
Rheum spp (Polygonaceae)	Rhubarb species	Urologic	Oxalates	Carboxylic acid
Rhododendron spp (Ericaceae)[a]	Rhododendron	Cardiac, neurologic	Grayanotoxins	Terpenoid including resin and oleoresin
Ricinus communis (Euphorbiaceae)[a]	Castor or rosary seeds, purging nuts, physic nut, tick seeds	Gastrointestinal	Ricin, curcin	Protein, lectin, peptide, amino acid
Robinia pseudoacacia (Fabaceae)[a]	Black locust	Gastrointestinal	Robin (robinia lectin)	Protein, lectin, peptide, amino acid
Rumex spp (Polygonaceae)	Dock species	Urologic	Oxalates	Carboxylic acid
Salix spp (Salicaceae)	Willow species	Salicylism	Salicin	Glycosides, other
Sambucus spp (Caprifoliaceae)	Elderberry	Metabolic	Anthracyanins	Cyanogenic glycoside
Sanguinaria canadensis (Papaveraceae)	Sanguinaria, bloodroot	Gastrointestinal	Sanguinarine	Alkaloid
Schefflera spp (Araceae)[b]	Umbrella tree	Dermatitis, mechanical and cytotoxic	Oxalate raphides	Carboxylic acid
Schlumbergera bridgesii[b]	Christmas cactus	Dermatitis, mechanical	Nontoxic	None
Senecio spp (Compositae/Asteraceae)[a]	Groundsel	Hepatic (venoocclusive disease)	Pyrrolizidine alkaloids	Alkaloid
Sida carpinifolia (Malvaceae)	Locoweed	Metabolic, neurologic	Swainsonine	Alkaloid
Sida cordifolia (Malvaceae)[a]	Bala	Cardiac, neurologic	Ephedrine and related compounds	Alkaloid
Solanum americanum (Solanaceae)[a]	American nightshade	Gastrointestinal, neurologic, anticholinergic	Solasodine, soladulcidine, solanine, chaconine	Glycoalkaloid
Solanum dulcamara (Solanaceae)[a,b]	Bittersweet woody nightshade	Gastrointestinal, neurologic, anticholinergic	Solanine, chaconine, belladonna alkaloids	Alkaloid
Solanum nigrum (Solanaceae)[a]	Black nightshade, common nightshade	Gastrointestinal, neurologic, anticholinergic	Solanine, chaconine, belladonna alkaloids	Alkaloid

(Continued)

TABLE 118–1 Primary Toxicity of Common Important Plant Species *(Continued)*

Plant Species (Family)	Typical Common Names	Primary Toxicity	Xenobiotic(s)	Class of Xenobiotic
Solanum tuberosum (Solanaceae)[a]	Potato (green), leaves	Gastrointestinal, neurologic, anticholinergic	Solanine, chaconine	Alkaloid
Spathiphyllum spp (Araceae)[b]	Peace lily	Dermatitis, mechanical and cytotoxic	Oxalate raphides	Carboxylic acid
Spinacia oleracea (Chenopodiaceae)	Spinach, others	Urologic	Oxalates	Carboxylic acid
Strychnos nux-vomica, Strychnos ignatia (Loganiaceae)[a]	Nux vomica, Ignatia, St Ignatius bean, vomit button	Neurologic	Strychnine, brucine	Alkaloid
Swainsonia spp (Fabaceae)	Locoweed	Metabolic, neurologic	Swainsonine	Alkaloid
Symphytum spp (Boraginaceae)[a]	Comfrey	Hepatic (venoocclusive disease)	Pyrrolizidine alkaloids	Alkaloid
Tanacetum vulgare (= Chrysanthemum vulgare; Compositae/Asteraceae)[a]	Tansy	Neurologic	Thujone	Terpenoid
Taxus baccata, Taxus brevifolia, other *Taxus* spp (Taxaceae)[a]	English yew, Pacific yew	Cardiac	Taxine	Alkaloid
Theobroma cacao (Sterculiaceae)	Cocoa	Cardiac, neurologic	Theobromine	Alkaloid
Thevetia peruviana[a]	Yellow oleander	Cardiac	Thevetin	Cardioactive steroid
Toxicodendron radicans, Toxicodendron toxicarium, Toxicodendron diversilobum, Toxicodendron vernix, Toxicodendron spp, many others (Anacardaceae)[b]	Poison ivy, poison oak, poison sumac	Dermatitis, contact and allergic	Urushiol oleoresins	Terpenoid
Tribulus terrestris (Fabaceae)	Caltrop, puncture vine	Dermatitis, photosensitivity in animals	Steroidal saponins (aglycones, diosgenin, yamogenin)	Saponin glycoside
Trifolium pratense and other (Fabaceae/Legumaceae)	Red clover	Phytoestrogen, hematologic	Formononetin, Biochanin A, coumarin	Phenol (isoflavone)
Tussilago farfara (Compositae/Asteraceae)[a]	Coltsfoot	Hepatic (venoocclusive disease)	Pyrrolizidine alkaloids	Alkaloid
Urginea maritima, Urginea indica[a]	Red, or Mediterranean squill, Indian squill, sea onion	Cardiac	Scillaren A, B	Cardioactive steroid
Veratrum viride, Veratrum album, Veratrum californicum (Liliaceae)[a]	False hellebore, Indian poke, California hellebore	Cardiac	Veratridine	Alkaloid
Vicia fava, Vicia sativa (Fabaceae)	Fava bean, vetch	Hematologic	Vicine, convicine	Glycoside
Viscum album (Loranthaceae or Viscaceae)	European mistletoe	Gastrointestinal	Viscumin	Protein, lectin, peptide, amino acid, lignan, polypeptide
Wisteria floribunda (Fabaceae)	Wisteria	Gastrointestinal	Cystatin	Protein, lectin, peptide, amino acid

[a]Reports of life-threatening effects from plant use. [b]Plants reported commonly among calls to poison control centers.

alkaloids that produce gastrointestinal signs and symptoms following ingestion. This approach will be less useful for xenobiotics such as pyrrolizidine alkaloids that occur in numerous different families.

APPROACH TO THE EXPOSED PATIENT AND UNDERSTANDING RISK

Identified plant species most frequently reported to poison control centers are indicated in Table 118–1. In most cases, these species provide reassurance because most exposures result in benign outcomes, and only a few among these are regularly life threatening depending on the circumstances of the exposure. Given the relatively poor understanding of toxins and in the absence of complete information about an exposure, expectant management and supportive care are the rule. Even if a plant is not marked as life threatening or commonly reported, the patient should undergo a period of observation and follow-up, given the relatively immature science of plant toxicology relative to that of pharmaceuticals.

The difficult task in human plant toxicology is the lack of adequate data to determine risk (Chap. 133). Typically, evaluations of risk are based on poison control center data and usually cite the numerous calls without clinical consequence as a part of the risk equation (Chap. 130). However, poison control center data are predominantly unconfirmed exposures and cases with unsubstantiated clinical manifestations (Chap. 130). These cases often represent small or nonexistent exposures, and their inclusion in the database may mask actual risks by diluting hazardous exposures with trivial or nonexistent exposures.[69] Furthermore, misidentification of the plant can occur because of either similar appearance or similar nomenclature.

Basic decontamination and supportive care should be instituted as appropriate for the clinical situation, with poison control center consultation. The most consequential and dangerous plant xenobiotics for humans are discussed here, and those that can produce life-threatening signs acutely are denoted in Table 118–1.

Potential clinical effects listed in Table 118–1 are organized by plant name and the associated major organ system effects for quick reference as to the type of symptoms and their potential for morbidity or mortality. For instance, life-threatening effects such as dysrhythmias or seizures can be searched by "cardiac-" or "neurologic-" in the third column and compared with the plant(s) in question. The plants and xenobiotics that present life-threatening symptoms are so noted. Exposures associated with one of these plants or xenobiotics or major organ system symptoms dictate the need for possible prompt gastric emptying, decontamination, individualized therapy, and hospitalization. Nonspecific symptoms such as nausea and vomiting are listed only when they are a major cause of morbidity or mortality (toxalbumins such as ricin), but nausea and vomiting are exceptionally common in those individuals with consequential acute poisonings.

TOXIC CONSTITUENTS IN PLANTS, TAXONOMIC ASSOCIATIONS, AND SELECTED SYMPTOMS

Alkaloids

Alkaloids figure prominently in the history of human–plant interaction, ranging from epidemics of poisoning caused by ergot-infected rye bread in the Middle Ages to dependency on cocaine, heroin, and nicotine in contemporary time. Numerous examples of toxic constituents of these families are given in the following discussion, which begins with a description of the major toxidromes that involves alkaloids

Anticholinergic: Belladonna Alkaloids

The belladonna alkaloids are from the family Solanaceae and the plants are identified as members of this family by their characteristic flowers (most familiar from nightshade, potato, or tomato flowers). The belladonna alkaloids have potent antimuscarinic effects, manifested by tachycardia, hyperthermia, dry skin and mucous membranes, skin flushing, diminished bowel sounds, urinary retention, agitation, disorientation, and hallucinations (Chap. 3). Since the 1970s, the quest for recreational "highs" has surpassed unintentional ingestions as the main source of toxicity.[153] Hallucinatory effects are sought in seeds and teas, especially in late summer, when jimsonweed (*Datura stramonium*) seeds (Fig. 118–1) become available.

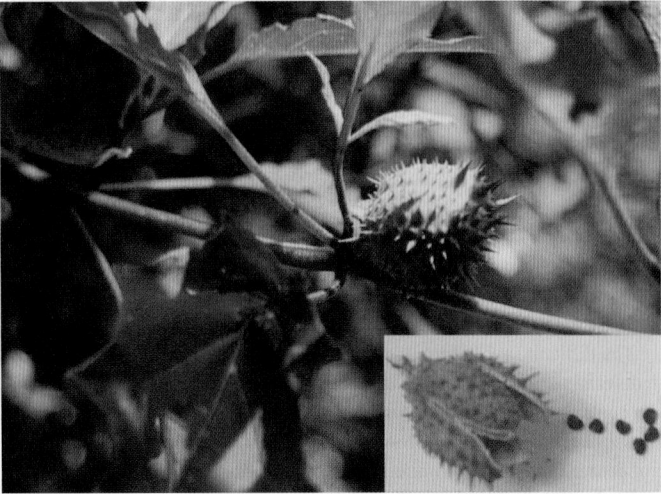

FIGURE 118–1. Jimsonweed (*Datura stramonium*) initially has a showy white tubular flower that becomes a prickly fruit (pod) following maturation. Inset: The pod (inset) of jimsonweed holds multiple small seeds containing atropine and scopolamine. *(Used with permission from the Fellowship in Medical Toxicology, New York University School of Medicine, New York City Poison Center.)*

One hundred of these seeds contain up to 6 mg atropine and related alkaloids, and an ingestion of this amount can be fatal.[21]

Although several anticholinergic alkaloid-containing species and even individual plants within species contain differing concentrations of several different phytochemicals, the clinical manifestations usually are similar. The onset of symptoms typically occurs one to 4 hours postingestion, and more rapidly if the plants are smoked or consumed as a brewed tea. The duration of effect is partly dose dependent and may last from a few hours to days.[25] The course of anticholinergic poisoning is not substantially altered by use of physostigmine, though this may be lifesaving in patients with seizures or an agitated delirium (Antidotes in Depth: A11).[43,135] Although methods for detection of atropine and scopolamine in clinical specimens are improving, anticholinergic toxicity is observed without detectable atropine, scopolamine, or hyoscyamine concentrations in biological fluids.

Solanine and chaconine are glycoalkaloids contained in many members of the Solanaceae family, but they are structurally and pharmacologically dissimilar to the belladonna alkaloids. The aglycone solanidine, which lacks the sugar moiety, is a steroidal alkaloid. Solanine inhibits cholinesterase in vitro, although cholinergic symptoms are not noted clinically. Nonetheless, reports of solanine-induced central nervous system (CNS) toxicity include hallucinations, delirium, and coma.[148] However, most symptomatic patients typically develop nausea, vomiting, diarrhea, and abdominal pain that begins 2 to 24 hours after ingestion, which, like CNS toxicity, infrequently persist for several days. Although solanine is present in most of the 1,700 species in the genus *Solanum*, solanine toxicity in humans is rarely encountered. The content of glycoalkaloids in tubers is usually 10 to 100 mg/kg and the maximum concentrations do not exceed 200 mg/kg. Green potatoes and the green potato plant itself are most commonly associated with toxicity, which is not surprising because the alkaloids are most concentrated in those items. The ingestion of 1 to 3 mg of glycoalkaloid per kilogram of body weight is likely to produce clinical symptoms.[133] Most reports of death come from the older literature,[2] and consumption of 2 to 5 g of green components of potatoes per kilogram of body weight per day is not predicted to cause acute toxicity.[120]

Nicotine and Nicotinelike Alkaloids: Nicotine, Anabasine, Lobeline, Sparteine, *N*-Methylcytisine, Cytisine, and Coniine

Nicotine toxicity (other than from inhaled sources) occurs via ingestion of leaves of *Nicotiana tabacum*, cigarettes and their remains, e-cigarette refill, organic insecticidal products, and transdermally among farm workers harvesting tobacco (green tobacco sickness) (Chap. 82).[17] A topical folk remedy made from the leaf of *Nicotiana glauca* (tree tobacco) caused anabasine toxicity in an infant.[113] The alkaloids of nicotine and anabasine are pale yellow oils at room temperature and readily penetrate the intact dermis. A dose of nicotine as small as 1 mg/kg of body weight can be lethal although it is more likely with doses >4 mg/kg.[101] Overstimulation of the nicotinic receptors by high doses of the alkaloid produces nicotinism, a toxidrome that progresses from gastrointestinal (GI) symptoms to diaphoresis, mydriasis, fasciculations, tachycardia, hypertension, hyperthermia, seizures, respiratory depression, and death (Chap. 82). Wearing of protective clothing is essential for tobacco farm workers to prevent green tobacco sickness.[7]

These manifestations are also produced by alkaloids other than nicotine. There are no recent reports of nicotinic toxicity from lobeline (found in all parts of *Lobelia inflata*), although its use in the 18th century resulted in morbidity and mortality.

Sparteine from broom (*Cytisus scoparius*) and *N*-methylcytisine from blue cohosh (*Caulophyllum thalictroides*)[124] are examples of alkaloids that produce nicotinelike effects. Laburnum or golden chain (*Cytisus laburnum*) contains cytisine, which reportedly is responsible for mass poisonings and fatalities in children and adults who eat the plants or parts thereof (even as little as 0.5 mg/kg, or a few peas).[111] Unfortunately, such reports have resulted in thousands of unnecessary hospital admissions for patients without morbidity and mortality after ingestion of this plant, demonstrating the difficulty in separating hazard from risk and in obtaining accurate dose–response information in the setting of plant exposures and human variability.

The most famous description of the end stages of nicotinic toxicity dates from approximately 2,400 years ago by an observer of Socrates' fatal ingestion of a decoction of poison hemlock (*Conium maculatum*).[125]

> *the person who had administered the poison went up to him and examined for some little time his feet and legs, and then squeezing his foot strongly asked whether he felt him. Socrates replied that he did not and said to us when the effect of the poison reached his heart, Socrates would depart.*

Birds do not experience coniine toxicity but provide a vector for poisoning. According to the book of Exodus, quail that fed on seeds (presumably from poison hemlock) became toxic and passed the toxicity on to the Israelites who ate the fowl.[19] In the 20th century, this is especially well documented in Italy, where the toxic alkaloid coniine was detected in bird meat, as well as in the blood, urine, and tissue of some individuals.[139]

The age of the plant seems to be directly correlated with increasing concentrations of coniine, whereas the toxin γ-coniceine occurs in greater amounts in new growth; hence, the plant remains toxic over the entire growing season. Fatal poisonings are reported on multiple continents frequently resulting from respiratory arrest. Of 17 poisoned Italian patients, all had elevated liver aminotransferases and myoglobin concentrations, and 5 had acute tubular necrosis.[127] Death developed 1 to 16 days following ingestion.

Cholinergic Alkaloids: Arecoline, Physostigmine, and Pilocarpine

Betel chewing has been a habitual practice in the tropical Pacific, Asia and East Africa. The "quid" consists of betel nut (*Areca catechu*) and other ingredients. The effects of acute exposure to arecoline, the major alkaloid, include sweating, salivation, hyperthermia, and rarely death.[40] Prolonged use is linked to dental decay and oral cancer. Physostigmine is an alkaloid derived from the Calabar bean (*Physostigma venenosum*), where it is present in concentrations of 0.15% (Antidotes in Depth: A11). Pilocarpine is derived from *Pilocarpus jaborandi* from South America. Its stimulatory effects on muscarinic receptors have proven valuable in the treatment of glaucoma. Reversal of toxicity can be achieved by atropine.

Psychotropic Alkaloids: Lysergic Acid and Mescaline

Hallucinations from the direct serotonin effects of lysergic acid diethylamide (LSD) and its derivatives, and from the amphetaminelike serotonin effects of the mescaline alkaloids are reported following ingestion of morning glory seeds (*Ipomoea* spp) and peyote cactus (*Lophophora williamsii*), respectively (Chap. 79). Despite their chemical relatedness to LSD, molecules such as lysergic acid amide and lysergic acid ethylamide, found in Hawaiian babywoodrose seeds (*Argyreia nervosa*) produce findings that may appear anticholinergic.[20]

Alkaloidal Central Nervous System Stimulants and Depressants: Ephedrine, Synephrine, Cathinone, and Opioids

The use of ephedrine-containing *Ephedra* spp in herbal dietary supplement products was banned by the FDA in 2004 because of the associated cardiovascular toxicity and deaths. Varieties of *Sida cordifolia* also contain ephedrine. Synephrine, a xenobiotic structurally related to ephedrine, occurs in bitter orange (*Citrus aurantium*), which is ingested as a plant, in foods such as marmalades, as a dietary supplement, or as a traditional medicine. Deaths and drug interactions can ensue from their use. Although illegal in the United States, another plant ingested for its CNS-stimulant activity is khat (*Catha edulis*). The plant contains cathinone (α-aminopropiophenone) and cathine ((+)-norpseudoephedrine). In addition, opioids derived from the poppy plant (*Papaver* spp) are prototypic CNS depressants and analgesics (Chap. 36).

Pyrrolizidine Alkaloids

Pyrrolizidine alkaloids are widely distributed both botanically and geographically. Approximately half of the 350 different pyrrolizidine alkaloids characterized to date are toxic when ingested. Pyrrolizidine alkaloids are found in 6,000 plants and in 13 plant families, but are most heavily represented within the Boraginaceae, Compositae, and Fabaceae families. Within these families,

the genera *Heliotropium*, *Senecio*, and *Crotalaria*, respectively, are particularly notable for their content of toxic pyrrolizidine alkaloids, including the unsaturated 1-hydroxymethyl pyrrolizidine.[59] The hepatic cytochrome P450 (CYP) system converts these compounds to highly reactive pyrroles in vivo. Chronic exposures stimulate the proliferation of the intima of hepatic vasculature and result in hepatic venoocclusive disease (HVOD). Poisonings occur as a result of the use of pyrrolizidine-rich plants for medicinal purposes and by contamination of food grain with seeds of pyrrolizidine-alkaloid-containing plants.[47] Acute hepatocellular toxicity can occur following ingestion of 10 to 20 mg of pyrrolizidine alkaloid and is probably caused by an oxidant effect producing hepatic necrosis. An estimated 20% of patients with acute pyrrolizidine alkaloid poisoning die, 50% recover completely, and the rest develop subacute or chronic manifestations of HVOD. Pyrrolizidine alkaloids are teratogenic and are also transmitted through breast milk. Pyrrolizidine alkaloids may be present in bee pollen and have been reported in honey. Other types of plant-associated hepatic disorders are discussed in Effects Shared Among Different Classes of Xenobiotics.

Isoquinoline Alkaloids: Sanguinarine, Berberine, and Hydrastine

Adverse effects on human health due to consumption of edible mustard oil adulterated with argemone oil are reported. Sanguinarine was detected in 26 family members who consumed a mustard oil contaminated with seeds of Mexican pricklypoppy (*Argemone mexicana*).[146] All patients suffered GI distress followed by peripheral edema (dropsy), skin darkening, erythema, skin lesions, perianal itching, anemia, and hepatomegaly. Ascites developed in 12%, and myocarditis and congestive heart failure occurred in approximately a third of affected individuals. Alterations in redox potentials and antioxidants in plasma are responsible for the histopathologic changes, including swollen hepatocytes and fluid accumulation in the spaces of Disse, and Kupffer cell hyperplasia.[11] Medicinally, sanguinarine is used for dental hygiene.[73] In North America, sanguinarine is found in bloodroot (*Sanguinaria canadensis*), which like *Argemone*, is in the Ranuculaceae family.

Berberine is structurally similar to sanguinarine and also has cardiac depressant effects.[89] A number of medicinal plants contain berberine, including goldenseal (*Hydrastis canadensis*), Oregon grape (*Mahonia* spp), and barberry (*Berberis* spp). It causes myocardial and respiratory depression and contraction of smooth muscle vasculature and the uterus. Strychninelike movement disorders are described following ingestion of hydrastine, which makes up 4% of goldenseal.

Other Alkaloids: Emetine/Cephaline, Strychnine/Curare, and Swainsonine

Emetine and cephaline are derived from *Cephaelis ipecacuanha*, a tropical plant native to the forests of Bolivia and Brazil. They are the principal active constituents in syrup of ipecac, which produces emesis. Chronic use of syrup of ipecac, typically by patients with eating disorders or Munchausen syndrome by proxy, has caused cardiomyopathy, smooth muscle dysfunction, myopathies, electrolyte, and acid–base disturbances related to excessive vomiting, and death. Poisoning in patients ingesting plant material is not reported.

Curare was used as an arrow poison derived from plants of the genus *Strychnos* as well as *Chondrodendron*, but the plants and their phytochemicals produce very different clinical effects. The convulsant alkaloids strychnine and brucine are found in various members of the genus *Strychnos*. Although used to produce arrow poison, the more widespread use of *Strychnos* spp in Africa was for trial by ordeal.[119] The seeds of *Strychnos nux-vomica* are especially rich in strychnine, which causes muscular spasms and rigidity by antagonizing glycine receptors in the spinal cord and brain stem. The plant is used as an herbal remedy for arthritis pain called "maqianzi," which if improperly processed produces muscle spasm and weakness, including respiratory muscles (Chap. 114).

Curare is an extract of the bark of *Chondrodendron tomentosum* and certain members of the genus *Strychnos*. The physiologically active xenobiotic of curare from *Chondrodendron* is D-tubocurarine chloride, a competitive antagonist of acetylcholine at nicotinic receptors in the neuromuscular junction. Curare is the molecule from which most nondepolarizing neuro-muscular blockers are derived (Chap. 66). Plant poisoning is recorded solely with its traditional use as a hunting poison.

Swainsonine is isolated from *Swainsonia canescens, Astragalus lentiginosis* (spotted locoweed), *Sida carpinifolia*, other species of *Swainsonia* and *Astragalus*, as well as several species in the genera *Oxytropis* and *Ipomoea*, and several fungi. After subsisting on seeds containing swainsonine for nearly 4 months, a naturalist forager manifested profound muscular weakness and died in the wilderness.[84] The compound is teratogenic and causes chronic neurologic disease called "locoism," with weakness and failure to thrive in livestock. Swainsonine inhibits the glycosylation of glycoproteins by α-mannosidase II of the Golgi apparatus, resulting in a lysosomal storage disease. Adverse effects included hepatic, pancreatic, and respiratory manifestations, as well as lethargy and nausea.

Glycosides

Glycosides yield a sugar or sugar derivative (the glycone) and a nonsugar moiety (the aglycone) upon hydrolysis. The nonsugar or aglycone group determines the subtype of glycoside. For instance, the cardiac glycosides have saponin (steroid) aglycone groups and are placed among the saponin glycosides.

Saponin Glycosides: Cardiac Glycosides, Glycyrrhizin, Ilex Saponins

Poisoning by virtually all cardioactive steroidal glycosides is clinically indistinguishable from poisoning by digoxin (Chap. 62), which itself is a cardioactive steroid derived from *Digitalis lanata*. However, compared with toxicity from *pharmaceutical* digoxin, toxicity resulting from the cardioactive steroidal glycosides found in plants has markedly different pharmacokinetic characteristics. For example, digitoxin in *Digitalis* species has a plasma half-life as long as 192 hours (average 168 hours).

The pharmacologic properties are true across taxonomic boundaries. Poisonings by *Digitalis* spp,[123,147] squill (*Urginea* spp),[161] lily of the valley,[3] oleander (*Nerium* spp),[168] yellow oleander (*Thevetia* spp),[44] and *Cerbera manghas*[45] are clinically similar (Fig. 118–2). The potency of these effects depends on the specific cardioactive glycoside constituents and their dose. For instance, lily of the valley is rarely associated with morbidity or mortality (except those mistaking lily of the valley for ramps {*Allium tricoccum*}) whereas ingestion of only 2 seeds of yellow oleander by adults can produce severe symptoms, and expected outcome is grave with several more.[44] Poisonings by oleander and yellow oleander occur predominantly in the Mediterranean and in the Near and Far East. These 2 plants are popular attractive ornamentals and commonly result in poisoning in the United States and Europe.

Patients experience vomiting within several hours, followed by hyperkalemia, cardiac conduction delays, and increased automaticity (bradycardia and tachydysrhythmias). Interestingly, the cardiac manifestations may be difficult to distinguish from those produced by plants containing sodium channel blockers (see section Sodium Channel Effects). Activated charcoal was beneficial in preventing death after suicide attempts with yellow oleander in Sri Lanka and its use should not be delayed in the face of uncertain plant identity.[38] Antibody therapy reduces mortality threefold from yellow oleander poisoning but is too expensive for developing countries, where oleander-induced mortality is highest.[46] In addition, various cardioactive steroids respond differently to therapeutic use of digoxin-specific antibody fragments. Use of very large doses of digoxin-specific antibody (up to 37 vials reported in one case[126]) may be necessary to capitalize on the therapeutic cross-reactivity between digoxin-specific antibody and the nondigoxin cardioactive steroids, such as oleander.[134] The potential for success should lead to use of antibody therapy without delay when available. Similarly, there is variable cross-reactivity among the individual plant cardioactive steroids with regard to the degree to which each elevates diagnostic polyclonal digoxin assay measurements in clinical laboratories.[35] These measurements can be used only as qualitative proof of exposure but not as quantitative indicators of the exposure, because the elevations can result in marked

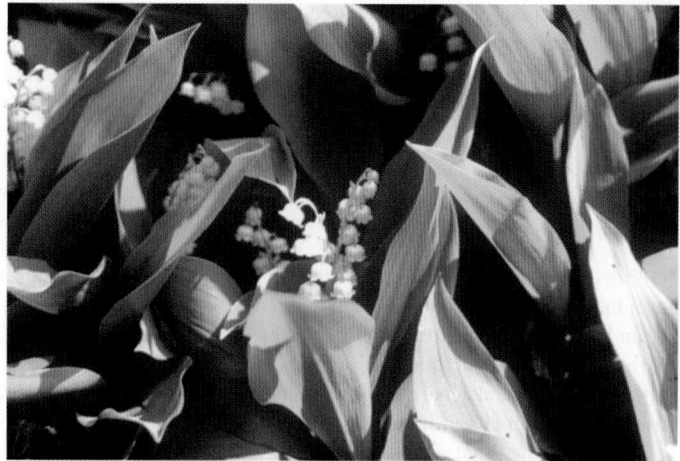

A

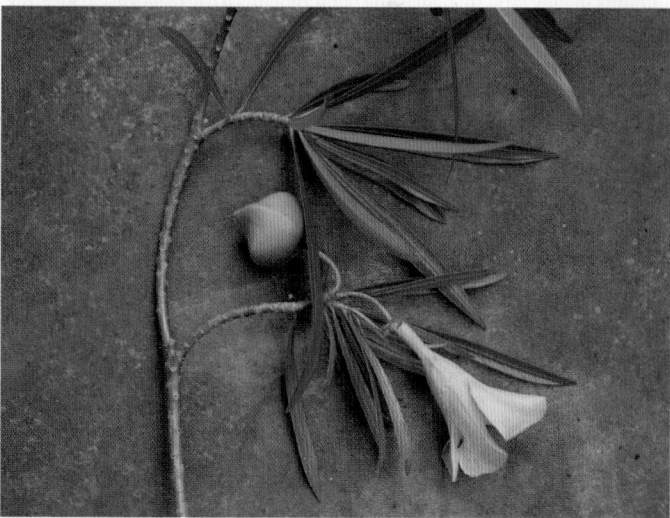

B

FIGURE 118–2. Saponin-glycoside containing plants: (**A**) Lily of the valley (*Convallaria majalis*) contains the cardioactive steroid convallatoxin. (**B**) Yellow oleander (*Thevetia peruviana*) contains a cardioactive steroid, thevetin. *(Used with permission from Darren Roberts, MD.)*

underestimation of the "functional digoxin concentrations." Until additional technologic advances occur, any positive digoxin concentration following exposure to a plant should be assumed to be significant.

Glycyrrhizin

Glycyrrhizin is a saponin glycoside derived from *Glycyrrhiza glabra* (licorice) and other *Glycyrrhiza* spp. Glycyrrhizin inhibits 11-β-hydroxysteroid dehydrogenase, an enzyme that converts cortisol to cortisone. When large amounts of licorice root are consumed chronically, cortisol concentrations rise, resulting in pseudo-hyperaldosteronism because of its affinity for renal mineralocorticoid receptors.[53] Chronic use eventually leads to hypokalemia with muscle weakness, sodium and water retention, hypertension, and dysrhythmias.[177] Assessment involves evaluation of the patient's fluid and electrolytes, and electrocardiogram. Potassium replacement is the most common necessary intervention.

Ilex Species

Holly berries from more than 300 *Ilex* spp are commonly ingested by children, especially during winter holidays. They contain a mixture of alkaloids, polyphenols, saponin glycosides, steroids, and triterpenes. Saponin glycosides appear to be responsible for GI symptoms such as nausea, vomiting, diarrhea, and abdominal cramping that result from ingestion of the berries. Central nervous system depression was reported in a case in which a child consumed a "handful" of berries; however, this child was also treated with syrup of ipecac.[130] The toxic quantity is undefined, but it is typically suggested that no untoward effects are to be expected for ingestions of fewer than 6 berries. Symptoms may be expected to be restricted to GI effects, and treatment is supportive.

Cyanogenic Glycosides: (S)-Sambunigrin, Amygdalin, Linamarin, and Cycasin
Cyanogenic glycosides yield hydrogen cyanide on complete hydrolysis. These glycosides are represented in a broad range of plant species.[164] The species that are most important to humans are cassava (*Manihot esculenta*), which contains linamarin, and *Prunus* spp, which contain amygdalin.[14] Cycad toxins are neurotoxic or pseudocyanogenic. Rare reports of cyanide poisoning associated with (S)-sambunigrin in European elderberry (*Sambucus nigra*; sambunigrin) are more severe when these ingestions include leaves as well as berries.[22]

Many North American species of plants contain cyanogenic compounds, including ornamental *Pyracantha*, *Passiflora*, and *Hydrangea* spp, which either do not release cyanide or are rarely consumed in quantities sufficient to result in toxicity. On the other hand, although the fleshy fruit of *Prunus* spp in the Rosaceae are nontoxic (apricots, peaches, pears, apples, and plums), the leaves, bark, and seed kernels contain amygdalin, which is metabolized to cyanide. Sufficient cyanide can be absorbed to cause acute poisoning.[156] Amygdalin was the active ingredient of Laetrile, an apricot pit extract promoted in the 1970s for its supposed selective toxicity to tumor cells. Its sale was restricted in the United States because it lacked efficacy and safety.[107,109] However, patients went to other countries for Laetrile therapy, which was marketed as "vitamin B-17," and available through alternative medicine providers. The manifestations of cyanide poisoning and treatment involving use of the cyanide antidote kit are detailed elsewhere (Chap. 123 and Antidotes in Depth: A41, A42).

Acute and chronic cyanide toxicity (including deaths) associated with consumption of inadequately prepared cassava (*M. esculenta*) are reported worldwide (Chap. 123).[1] Chronic manifestations include visual disturbances (amblyopia), upper motor neuron disease with spastic paraparesis, and hypothyroidism. These findings are associated with protein deficiency and the use of tobacco and alcohol. The ataxic neuropathy resembles that produced by lathyrism (see section Proteins, Peptides, and Lectins). A unifying hypothesis about the etiology of these 2 similar diseases from seemingly very different sources is that thiocyanate accumulation may lead to degeneration of the α-amino-3-hydroxy-5-methyl-isoxazole-4-propionic acid (AMPA)–containing neurons that are first stimulated and then destroyed in neurolathyrism.[151]

Similarly, seeds of cycads contain cycasin and neocycasin, which belong to the family of cyanogenic glycosides, as well as neurotoxins. The cyanogenic glycosides of cycads are pseudocyanogenic, with little potential to liberate hydrogen cyanide, but most typically produce violent vomiting 30 minutes to 7 hours after ingestion of one to 30 seeds.[28] On the island of Guam, indigenous peoples develop a devastating amyotrophic lateral sclerosis–parkinsonism dementia complex (ALS-PDC) that appears associated with ingestion of *Cycas circinalis* seeds or the flying foxes that feed extensively upon the cycads.[32] The implicated xenobiotic originally was believed to be an excitatory amino acid, but more recently is identified as a sterol glycoside. Research on the mechanism of this cycad-induced disease is ongoing, with the goal of understanding potential mechanisms of this disease and its links to ALS and Parkinson disease.[22,30]

Anthraquinone Glycosides: Sennoside and Others
Anthraquinone laxatives are regulated both as nonprescription pharmaceuticals and as dietary supplements. These glycosides, such as sennoside, are metabolized in the bowel to produce derivatives that stimulate colonic motility, probably by inhibiting Na^+,K^+-adenosine triphosphatase (ATPase) in the intestine, which also promote accumulation of water and electrolytes in the gut lumen, producing fluid and electrolyte shifts that can be life threatening.[155]

Other Glycosides: Salicin, Atractyloside, Carboxyatractyloside, Vicine, and Convicine
Salicin is an inactive glycoside until it is hydrolyzed to produce salicylic acid (Chap. 37). The glycosidic bond is relatively resistant to stomach acid, and the hydrolysis must be accomplished by gut flora. The ability of individual human flora to produce the necessary enzymes varies significantly, resulting in variable clinical effects for salicin or plant material that contains salicin. However, sufficient hydrolytic capacity for some transformation of the glycoside into salicylic acid occurs in all individuals.

Atractylis gummifera was a favorite agent for homicide during the reign of the Borgias. Atractyloside, the toxic xenobiotic, primarily inhibits oxidative phosphorylation in the liver by inhibiting the ADP/ATP antiporter blocking influx of adenosine diphosphate (ADP) into hepatic mitochondria and outflow of ATP to the rest of the cell (Chap. 11). Death or severe illness as a result of liver failure or hepatorenal disease following ingestion is reported.[34] *Callilepis laureola* is a South African medicinal plant that contains atractyloside and carboxyatractyloside and is reported to cause human poisonings. Cocklebur (*Xanthium strumarium*) is a herbaceous plant with worldwide distribution. The seeds contain the glycoside carboxyatractyloside. The toxic mechanism is similar to that for atractyloside, and seed ingestion has resulted in human fatalities. Nine patients presented with acute-onset abdominal pain, nausea and vomiting, drowsiness, palpitations, sweating, and dyspnea. Several patients developed hepatocellular damage, acute kidney injury, and myocardial injury and 3 developed convulsions followed by loss of consciousness and death.[162]

Favism is a potentially fatal disorder brought about by eating fava beans or vetch seeds (*Vicia faba*, *Vicia sativa*, respectively). These seeds contain the pyrimidine glycosides vicine and convicine (divicine is the aglycone of vicine). Consumption of these compounds by individuals with an inborn error of metabolism (glucose-6-phosphate dehydrogenase deficiency) can cause acute hemolytic crisis (Chap. 20).[143]

The effects of the glycosides sinigrin (from *Brassica nigra* seed and *Alliaria officinalis* {horseradish} root) and naringen (a polyphenolic glycoside from the grapefruit *Citrus paradisi*) are discussed in the sections on Plant-Induced Dermatitis and Plant–Xenobiotic Interactions, respectively.

Terpenoids and Resins: Ginkgolides, Kava Lactones, Thujone, Anisatin, Ptaquiloside/Thiaminase, and Gossypol
Ginkgolides in *Ginkgo biloba* result in antiplatelet aggregation effects. Reports of spontaneous bleeding associated with ingestion of Ginkgo leaf products as a herbal medicine are perhaps explained by this property.[131] Another xenobiotic found only in the seed, 4-methoxypyridoxine (pyridine alkaloid), is associated with seizures.[81] A mechanism similar to isoniazid-induced seizures is plausible, suggesting treatment with pyridoxine phosphate (Chap. 56 and Antidotes in Depth: A15). The dermal effects of *Ginkgo* are discussed in the section Plant-Induced Dermatitis.

Kava lactones are a family of terpene lactones found in kava (*Piper methysticum*) that cause central and peripheral nervous system effects. Kava has enjoyed a long, ceremonial history among islanders of the South Pacific, and observers visiting Oceania have recorded its acute and chronic effects (both pleasant and unpleasant) over the centuries. Importation of kava to Australia in 1983 was a measure to assist Aborigines with alcohol abuse problems. However, the kava itself became abused, and its subsequent ban has resulted in the growth of a black market for kava. Proposed mechanisms to explain the effects of kava lactones include effects at γ-aminobutyric acid type A ($GABA_A$) and $GABA_B$ receptors or local anesthetic effects.[137] Acute effects following ingestion include peripheral numbness, weakness, and sedation. Chronic use leads to kava dermopathy and weight loss. More than 70 cases of hepatotoxicity, several requiring liver transplantation, are associated with both acute and chronic effects of kava extracts on cytochrome oxygenases or other yet-to-be-defined etiologies and prompted regulatory health measures in Europe and North America.[159]

Thujone is one of many terpenes associated with seizures. It is found in the wormwood plant (*Artemisia absinthium*), in absinthe (the liquor flavored with *A. absinthium*), and in some strains of tansy (*Tanacetum vulgare*). The α- and β-isomers of thujone likely work similarly to camphor to produce CNS depression and seizures. Invoking the structural similarity of thujone to tetrahydrocannabinol (THC), one of the terpenoids of marijuana, to explain the psychoactive effects is controversial (Chap. 74).[105]

Absinthism is characterized by seizures and hallucinations, permanent cognitive impairment, and personality changes. Acute and chronic absinthism led to a worldwide ban of the alcoholic beverage absinthe, which contained thujone, in the early 1900s.[117] Over the past several years, there was a reexamination of the role of absinthe in the seizure disorders previously attributed to this liquor. Modern analytical procedures analyzed the thujone content of vintage absinthe and modern products made using vintage recipes. Results largely conclude that thujone content in the liquor was likely to be too low to have produced the claimed effects.[86] However, because the essential oil of wormwood is composed almost exclusively of thujone, it, but not absinthe, is a potent cause of seizures.[117] Wormwood oil for making homemade absinthe is currently available and is responsible for at least 2 reports of adverse reactions in people seeking its hallucinatory or euphoriant effects.[170]

Anisatin is found in *Illicium* spp. This terpenoid produces seizures as a noncompetitive GABA antagonist. The Chinese star anise (*Illicium verum*) is sometimes used in teas and occasionally is confused or contaminated with other species of *Illicium*, particularly Japanese star anise *Illicium anisatum*.[77] These contaminations caused small epidemics of tonic–clonic seizures, particularly, but not exclusively, in infants after use of the tea to treat their infantile colic. Recently, in the United States, a case series of at least 40 individuals who consumed teas brewed from "Star anise" experienced seizures, motor disturbances, other neurologic effects, and vomiting.[77] These cases include at least 15 infants treated for infantile colic with this home remedy. This trend prompted the FDA to issue an advisory regarding the health risk from remedies sharing the common name "star anise."

Ptaquilosides are found in the bracken fern (*Pteridium aquilinum*), a plant that is extending its range and density worldwide. In foraging animals, consumption of ptaquilosides results in acute hemorrhage secondary to profound thrombocytopenia, whereas thiaminases that are also found in the bracken fern result in cerebral disease.[50] Although no acute human poisonings are reported, these xenobiotics are transmitted through cow's milk and are associated with increased prevalence of gastric and esophageal cancer in areas where fern is endemic and consumed by cows whose milk is not diluted.[175] Chronic toxicity through spore inhalation also produces pulmonary adenomas in animals. More recently, research defined links between alimentary cancer in humans who previously consumed bracken fern fiddleheads.

Gossypol is a sesquiterpene that is derived from cottonseed oil. It was used experimentally as a reversible male contraceptive. The mechanism for its spermicidal effect is unclear, but the effects were attributed to inhibition of plasminogen activation and plasmin activity in acrosomal tissue. These effects are not currently reported to produce systemic bleeding. Gossypol also inhibits 11β-hydroxysteroid dehydrogenase, as does glycyrrhizin, and may result in hypokalemia.[176]

Proteins, Peptides, and Lectins: Ricin and Ricinlike, Pokeweed, Mistletoe, Hypoglycin, Lathyrins, and Microcystins

Lectins are glycoproteins that are classified according to their binding affinity for specific carbohydrate ligands, particularly galactosamines, and by the number of protein chains linked by disulfide bonds. Toxalbumins such as ricin and abrin are lectins that are such potent cytotoxins that they are used as biologic weapons (Chap. 133). Ricin, extracted from the castor bean (*Ricinus communis*; Fig. 118–3A), exerts its cytotoxicity by 2 separate mechanisms.[10] The compound is a large molecule that consists of 2 polypeptide chains bound by disulfide bonds. It must enter the cell to exert its toxic effect. The B chain binds to the terminal galactose of cell surface glycolipids and glycoproteins. The bound toxin then undergoes endocytosis and

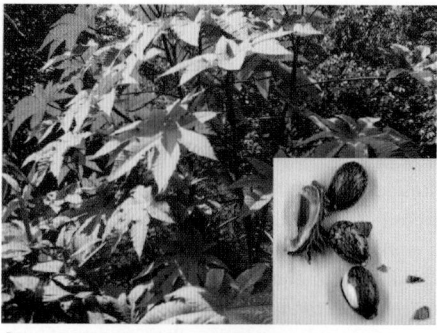

A

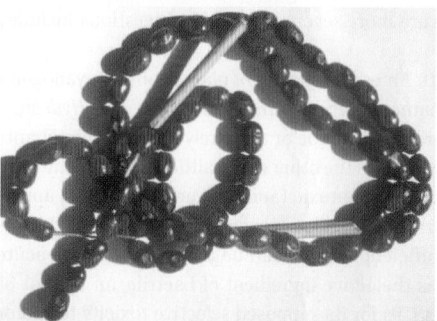

B

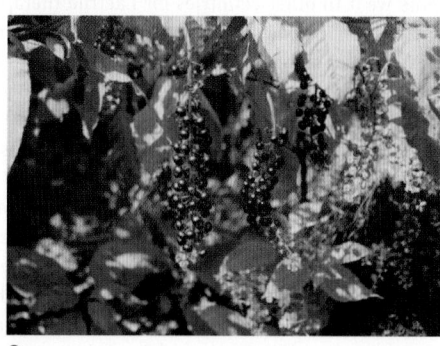

C

FIGURE 118–3. Protein-, peptide-, and lectin-containing plants: (**A**) The castor bean plant. The seedpods come in bunches, 2 of which appear near the center of the image. Each seedpod typically contains 3 seeds. Inset: Castor beans (*Ricinus communis*) which contain the toxalbumin ricin. By interfering with protein synthesis, ricin may cause multiorgan system failure when administered parenterally. However, its oral absorption is poor, and most oral poisonings cause gastroenteritis. (**B**) Rosary pea (*Abrus precatorius*) containing abrin, a toxalbumin that inhibits protein synthesis. The peas are shown strung together as a rosary. (**C**) Pokeweed (*Phytolacca americana*) has a large rootstock. The unripe berries contain phytolaccatoxin that produces gastroenteritis, but the mature, purple berries are often consumed. *(Used with permission from the Fellowship in Medical Toxicology, New York University School of Medicine, New York City Poison Center.)*

is transported via endosomes to the Golgi apparatus and the endoplasmic reticulum. There the A chain is translocated to the cytosol, where it stops protein synthesis by inhibiting the 28S subunit of the 60S ribosome. In addition to the GI manifestations of vomiting, diarrhea, and dehydration, ricin can cause cardiac, hematologic, hepatic, and renal toxicity. All contribute to death in humans and animals.[10] Despite the obvious toxicity of this compound, death probably can be prevented by early and aggressive fluid and electrolyte replacement after oral ingestion (but not injection or inhalation; Chap. 127). Allergic reactions to some of these lectin-bearing plants and their toxic constituents are noted. Given the potential for use in bioterrorism events, a vaccine is being developed primarily for military use.[121]

The highest concentration of xenobiotic in ornamental seeds is in the hard, brown-mottled seeds. These seeds are both tempting and available, even to children in the United States, because they are attractive enough to be used to make jewelry, and their parent plants are showy enough to be exported to many countries outside of their native India, including the United States, for horticultural purposes. Although mastication of one seed by a child liberates enough ricin to produce death, this outcome (or even serious toxicity) is uncommon, even if the seeds are chewed, probably because GI absorption of the ricin is poor and supportive care is effective.[6] Activated charcoal should be administered promptly following ingestion. Plasma exchange was utilized to remove ricin in 7 poisoned children with good effect.[166] However, the case data are uncontrolled and there are no analytical data on the presence of ricin, or its clearance, preventing a recommendation for its use.

Other ricinlike lectins are found in *Abrus precatorius* (jequirity pea, rosary pea (Fig. 118–3B),[41] *Jatropha* spp,[91] *Trichosanthes* spp (eg, *T. kirilowii* or Chinese cucumber), *Robinia pseudoacacia* (black locust),[76] *Phoradendron* spp (American mistletoe), *Viscum album* (European mistletoe), and *Wisteria* spp (wisteria). These all produce at least one double-chain lectin that binds to galactose-containing structures in the gut or inhibits protein synthesis in a manner similar to ricin.

The most commonly ingested toxic plant lectins in the United States are from pokeweed (*Phytolacca americana*) (Fig. 118–3C), which is eaten as a vegetable but rarely causes toxicity or death. The mature, deep purple berries are less toxic. Pokeweed leaves are consumed after boiling without toxic effect if the water is changed between the first and second boiling (parboiling). When this detoxification technique is not followed, as in preparation of poke salad or pokeroot tea, violent GI effects can ensue 0.5–6 hours after ingestion. Nausea, vomiting, abdominal cramping, diarrhea, hemorrhagic gastritis, and death may occur. In addition, bradycardia and hypotension, perhaps induced by an increase in vagal tone, may be associated with nausea and vomiting.[70,129] Phytolaccatoxin and pokeweed mitogen are found in all plant parts, but the highest concentrations are found in the plant root. Pokeweed mitogen is a single-chain protein that inhibits ribosomal RNA by removing purine groups.[16] It produces a lymphocytosis 2 to 4 days after ingestion that may last for 10 days, but this is without clinical consequence.

Mistletoe berries, both American and European, produce severe gastroenteritis, especially when delivered as teas or extracts, or particularly as parenteral antineoplastic medicinal agents in Europe. As festive holiday plants they become seasonally available for children. Poison control center data suggest that ingestion of 3 to 5 berries or one to 5 leaves of the American species may not cause toxicity, but these suggestions are based on limited evidence (Chap. 130). Despite single reports of seizure, ataxia, hepatotoxicity, and death, most authors performing such retrospective examinations conclude that mistletoe exposures are not a highly consequential risk.[152]

Hypoglycin A (β-methylene cyclopropyl-l-α-aminopropionic acid) and hypoglycin B (dipeptide of hypoglycin A and glutamic acid) are found in the unripe fruit and seeds of *Blighia sapida* (Euphorbiaceae), or ackee. The tree is native to Africa but was imported to Jamaica in 1778, and subsequently naturalized in Central America, southern California, and Florida. The scientific name of the plant derives from Captain William Bligh, the British explorer. Epidemics of illness (Jamaican vomiting sickness) associated with consumption of the unripe ackee fruit (raw and cooked) occur in Africa but are more common in Jamaica, where ackee is the national dish.[80] The most toxic part is the yellow oily aril of the fruit,[29] which contains 3 large, shiny black seeds. Cases of hypoglycin A poisoning are also associated with canned ackee fruit,[104] and recently to epidemic poisonings from litchi fruit in India.[144] Hypoglycin A is metabolized to methylene cyclopropyl acetic acid, which competitively inhibits the carnitine–acyl coenzyme (CoA) transferase system.[13] This prevents importation of long-chain fatty acids into the mitochondria, preventing their β-oxidation to precursors of gluconeogenesis. β-Oxidation and gluconeogenesis are further arrested by inhibition of various enzymes, such as glutaryl CoA dehydrogenase, which blocks the malate shunt (Chap. 11). In addition, increased concentrations of glutaric acid may inhibit glutamic acid decarboxylase, which produces GABA from glutamic acid. This not only depletes GABA but also increases concentrations of excitatory glutamate to produce seizures. Insulin concentrations remain unaffected by hypoglycin

and metabolites. Carboxylic and other organic acid substrates build up in the urine and serum as a result of these metabolic disturbances. Detection of these acids helps corroborate the diagnosis.[13] Jamaican vomiting sickness is characterized by epigastric discomfort and the onset of vomiting starting 2 to 6 hours after ingestion. Convulsions, coma, and death can ensue, with death occurring approximately 12 hours following consumption. Laboratory findings are notable for profound hepatic aminotransferase and bilirubin abnormalities, and aciduria and acidemia without ketonemia. Cholestatic hepatitis is reported with chronic use.[88] Autopsy reveals fatty degeneration of liver, particularly microvesicular steatosis, and other organs with depletion of glycogen stores. Left untreated, patient mortality reaches 80%, with 85% of the fatal cases suffering seizures. Treatment with dextrose and fluid replacement is essential. Benzodiazepines control seizures, but may fail if the seizures are related to depletion of GABA. In this situation, an alternative anticonvulsant, such as a barbiturate or propofol, should be utilized. L-Carnitine therapy may exert a theoretical therapeutic role similar to that noted with valproic acid toxicity (Chap. 48 and Antidotes in Depth: A10).[94] Its use, however, in this situation is not studied.

The lathyrins β-N-oxalylamino-L-alanine (BOAA) and β-aminopropionitrile (BAPN) are peptides from the grass pea (*Lathyrus sativus*) found in the seeds and leaves, respectively. β-N-Oxalylamino-L-alanine produces neurolathyrism and BAPN produces osteolathyrism in individuals with a dietary dependence on this plant. Neurolathyrism is nearly indistinguishable from spastic paresis associated with consumption of improperly prepared cassava (see section Cyanogenic Glycosides).[15,33] Thiol oxidation with depletion of nicotinamide adenine dinucleotide (NADH) dehydrogenase in neuronal mitochondria (ie, excitatory AMPA receptors) may be the common etiology.[151] Epidemics have occurred in Bangladesh, Ethiopia, Israel, and India. Exposure to BOAA results in degeneration of corresponding corticospinal pathways that becomes irreversible if consumption of undetoxified grass peas is not stopped early. β-N-Oxalylamino-L-alanine stimulates the AMPA class of glutamate receptors to provide constant neuronal stimulation, eventual degeneration, and hence spasticity.[174] β-Aminopropionitrile affects bone matrix and leads to bone pain and skeletal deformities that develop in adulthood. These diseases occur in areas where the plants are endemic, the food is consumed for 2 months or more, and when diets are otherwise poor in protein and possibly in zinc.[18,61]

Microcystins are found in several cyanobacteria (blue-green algae) belonging to various species of the genera *Microcystis*, *Anabaena*, *Nodularia*, *Nostoc*, and *Oscillatoria*. They elaborate a series of peptides called microcystins and nodularins (*Nodularia spumigena*).[42] These compounds produce hepatotoxicity by inhibiting phosphatases and causing deterioration of the microfilament function in hepatocytes, leading to cell shrinkage and bleeding into the hepatic sinusoids. Evidence indicates that these peptides are carcinogenic to humans. Although most cases of untoward effects from blue-green algae occur in animals, the potential for harm was demonstrated by use of microcystin-contaminated water in a dialysis unit in Brazil.[79] Unfiltered water was identified as the risk factor for liver disease in 100 patients who attended the dialysis center (Chap. 6). Fifty of these patients died of acute liver failure following early signs of nausea, vomiting, and visual disturbances. Of concern, certain species of *cyanobacteria* are harvested and consumed as health foods or may be consumed secondarily in fish.[62]

Phenols and Phenylpropanoids: Coumarins, Capsaicin, Karwinskia Toxins, Naringenin and Bergamottin, Asarin, Nordihydroguaiaretic Acid, Podophyllin, Psoralen, and Esculoside

Phenols and phenylpropanoids represent one of the largest groups of plant secondary metabolites. Coumarins and their isomers are phenylpropanoids that are discussed in Chap. 58. Some coumarins are warfarinlike in their activity and are capable of producing a bleeding diathesis when plants containing them are consumed in sufficiently large quantities.[74] Lignans are formed when phenylpropanoid side chains react to form bisphenylpropanoid derivatives. Lignins are high-molecular-weight polymers of phenylpropanoids that bind to cellulose and provide strength to cell walls of stem and bark. Tannins are polymers that bind to proteins and divide into 2 groups: hydrolyzable and condensed forms.

Capsaicin is derived from *Capsicum annuum* or other species of chili or cayenne peppers. Capsaicin is a simple phenylpropanoid that causes release of the neuropeptide substance P from sensory C-type nerve fibers that act upon transient receptor potential (TRP) channels in diverse human tissues.[165] The immediate response to capsaicin is intense local pain and is the rationale for its use as "pepper spray." Eventual depletion of substance P prevents local transmission of pain impulses from these receptors to the spinal cord, blocking perception of pain by the brain, explaining its use in postherpetic neuralgia.

Painful exposures to capsaicin-containing peppers are among the most common plant-related exposures presented to poison control centers. They cause burning or stinging pain to the skin. If ingested in large amounts by adults or small amounts by children, they can produce nausea, vomiting, abdominal pain, and burning diarrhea. Eye exposures produce intense tearing, pain, conjunctivitis, and blepharospasm. Fatality is rare, but is reported following inhalation and infusion.[150]

Skin irrigation, dermal aloe gel, analgesics, and oral antacids are therapeutic agents that may be helpful as appropriate, but patients can be reassured that the effects are transitory and produce no long-term damage. Irritated eyes should be treated with irrigation and, if severe, topical analgesia, but the pain generally resolve without sequelae within 24 hours.

Karwinskia toxins are found in plants commonly named Buckthorn, coyotillo, tullidora, wild cherry, or capulincillo (*Karwinskia humboldtiana*). These xenobiotics are identified by their molecular weights (T-514, T-496, T-516, T-544). Toxicity has been known for more than 200 years. In 1920, an epidemic of deaths was reported after 20% of 106 Mexican soldiers died following ingestion of foraged *Karwinskia* fruits.[100] The fruits are attractive to children. Epidemic poisonings have been reported in Central America and are possible wherever the shrub is found, typically in semidesert areas throughout the southwestern United States and in the Caribbean, Mexico, and Central America.[9] Uncoupling of oxidative phosphorylation or dysfunction of peroxisome assembly and integrity is described as the mechanism of action of T-514 on Schwann cells. Each xenobiotic exhibits similar cytotoxic effects at the cellular level, but with tropism for different organs in animal models.[100]

Within a few days of ingestion, a symmetric motor neuropathy ascends from the lower extremities to produce a bulbar paralysis that may lead to death. Deep-tendon reflexes are abolished in affected areas, but cranial nerve findings are absent. Distinction of this demyelinating motor neuropathy from Guillain-Barré syndrome, poliomyelitis, solvent, and other polyneuropathies is difficult without a history of the fruit ingestion,[115] but can be assisted by detection of T-514 in the blood of affected patients. The other recognized toxins are not detected in blood. Occasionally, axonal damage is observed, but demyelination is the predominant finding on biopsy. Nerve conduction studies generally demonstrate loss or abolition of function in fast-conducting axons. Cerebrospinal fluid demonstrates normal protein, glucose, and cytology. Treatment is supportive, with mechanical ventilation as needed, and recovery typically is slow.

Naringin and naringenin are flavonoid, whereas bergamottin and 6′,7′-dihydroxybergamottin are furanocoumarin, phenylpropanoids derived from grapefruit that inhibit CYP3A4 in gut and liver. Grapefruit juice consumption can increase circulating concentrations of drugs reliant on CYP3A4 for metabolic elimination, including carbamazepine, felodipine, and the statins. The most plausible mechanism is inhibition of enteric CYP3A4 and P-glycoprotein.[118] These effects are maximally achieved by a single glass of grapefruit juice.[98]

Comedication with St John's wort (*Hypericum perforatum*) resulted in decreased plasma concentrations of a number of xenobiotics.[99] Hyperforin is a phenylpropanoid found in St John's wort and is associated with plant–xenobiotic interactions through strong induction of CYP3A4 mediated drug metabolism as well as induction of P-glycoprotein. These combined mechanisms can cause subtherapeutic concentrations of xenobiotics metabolized via these pathways.

Asarin is a term sometimes used for the naturally occurring mixture of α- and β-asarones found in the root of *Asarum europaeum*, *Asarum arifolium*, and *Acorus calamus* (sweet flag). Essential oils of the plants have anthelminthic and nematocidal activity, but putative euphoric and hallucinogenic effects that motivate recreational ingestion are in contrast to confirmed reports of unpleasant GI effects.[163]

Nordihydroguaiaretic acid (NDGA) is associated with hepatotoxicity after ingestion of chaparral (*Larrea tridentata*).[64] Podophyllin and psoralens are phenylpropanoids discussed in the sections Antimitotic Alkaloids and Resins, and Plant-Induced Dermatitis, respectively.

Esculoside (also called esculin or aesculin) has triterpene saponin side chains and is believed to be the toxic component in horse chestnut (*Aesculus hippocastanum*). Horse chestnut extracts are used medicinally in patients with venous insufficiency. The therapeutic use of these extracts at high doses (>340 mcg/kg) is associated with acute kidney injury or a lupuslike syndrome.[65] Leaves, twigs, or horse chestnuts ingested by children or infused as teas result in a syndrome that resembles nicotine toxicity. The syndrome consists of vomiting, diarrhea, muscle twitching, weakness, lack of coordination, dilated pupils, paralysis, and stupor. The mechanism of toxicity is not defined.

Carboxylic Acids: Aristolochic Acids, Oxalic Acid, and Oxalate Raphides

Nitrophenanthrene carboxylic acids, collectively called aristolochic acids, are present in most members of the genus *Aristolochia*, including those used ornamentally and as traditional medicines. Consumption of these compounds can cause aristolochic acid nephropathy (AAN), a progressive renal interstitial fibrosis frequently associated with urothelial malignancies (Chap. 43).[39] Sources of exposure are via consumption of flour made from wheat contaminated with the seeds of *Aristolochia* clematis or other *Aristolochia* species (so called Balkan endemic nephropathy),[67] or through use of certain traditional Asian medicines made from *Aristolochia* spp (Chinese herb nephropathy).[36]

Oxalic acid is the strongest acid among the carboxylic acids found in living organisms. It forms poorly soluble chelates with calcium and other divalent cations. Higher plants have varying ability to accumulate these, include both soluble and insoluble oxalates, and many contain crystals of calcium oxalate called raphides. Certain plant families, such as the Araceae, Chenopodiaceae, Polygonaceae, and Amaranthaceae, and several of the grass families, are rich in oxalates. Human dietary sources include rhubarb, spinach, strawberries, chocolate, tea, and nuts. Human consumption of soluble oxalate-rich foods correlates with kidney stone formation.[93]

The insoluble calcium oxalate raphides that are present in certain plants, usually in the Araceae family, are found in conjunction with a protein toxin that increases the painful irritation to skin or mucous membranes. This special manifestation is discussed in greater detail in the section Plant-Induced Dermatitis.

Alcohols: Cicutoxin

Cicutoxin, a diacetylenic diol, is found in *Cicuta maculata* (water hemlock), *Cicuta douglasii* (western water hemlock), and *Oenanthe crocata* (hemlock water dropwort). *Oenanthe crocata* is native to Europe, where intoxications have been reported, and is now naturalized in the United States. Ingestion of any part of these plants constitutes the most common form of lethal plant ingestion in the United States. Hemlock is among the most prominent causes of plant-related fatalities among the most recent 10-year reviews of the AAPCC data and Centers for Disease Control and Prevention (CDC) plant poisoning records (Chap. 130).[85] In contrast to most plant exposures in humans, which tend to involve children, these ingestions usually involve adults who incorrectly identify the plant as wild parsnip, turnip, parsley, or ginseng.[142] All plant parts are poisonous at all times, but the tuber is especially toxic, and more so during the winter and early spring. Absorption of cicutoxin is rapid and occurs through the skin as well as through the gut. Although the mechanism is not fully understood, cicutoxin may noncompetitively inhibit GABA receptors or block potassium channels.[142]

Clinical findings of mild or early poisonings consist of GI symptoms (nausea, vomiting, epigastric discomfort) and begin as early as 15 minutes after ingestion. Diaphoresis, flushing, dizziness, excessive salivation, bradycardia, hypotension, bronchial secretions with respiratory distress, and cyanosis occur and rapidly progress to violent seizures. Ingestion of as little as a 2-cm section of the sweet-tasting root of *Cicuta* can produce status epilepticus.[142] Other complications include rhabdomyolysis with acute kidney injury and severe acidemia. Immediate gastric lavage should be performed if practical, and benzodiazepines should be administered for seizures. No specific antidote exists; supportive and symptomatic care should be provided.

Unidentified Toxins

Consistent with the inherent complexity of plants and the relatively early stage of the science, identification of the active ingredient(s) involved in poisoning is not always possible. An epidemic of the irreversible lung disease bronchiolitis obliterans developed in Taiwan in 1994 that involved more than 200 dieters who had been eating *Sauropus androgynus* as a weight-loss vegetable. The effects were dose related (usually approximately 100 g/d) and manifested by month 7 after approximately 10 weeks of use.[75] The cases were associated with at least 4 deaths and, in addition to pulmonary disease, resulting in lung transplantation.[97] Torsade de pointes occurred in 3 patients, consistent with the plant's high concentration of papaverine, which produces dysrhythmias in animals. Corticosteroid and bronchodilator therapy consistently failed to improve pulmonary symptoms. A report of a later outbreak in Japan followed consumption of uncooked plant.[116]

Milk sickness is a historic poisoning described by pioneer farmers. It was caused by transmission of the nontoxic ketone tremetone to humans via milk of animals grazing on white snake-root plants (*Ageratina altissima*, formerly *Eupatorium rugosum*). Tremetone is transformed into an unknown, unstable toxin by hepatic microsomal enzymes.[90] Toxicity is cumulative. Milk sickness can be fatal in one to 21 days or is associated with a slow recovery marked by weakness for months or years, relapsing sometimes to death. A delay in the development of the lactating animal's symptoms provided a lag time when xenobiotic-laden milk was taken from asymptomatic animals and thereby transmitted to humans before the problem was detected.

Ingestion of the air potato (*Breynia officinalis*) or bitter yam (*Dioscorea bulbifera*) is associated with hepatotoxicity.[96] Black cohosh (*Actaea racemosa*) hepatotoxicity is suggested in case reports, but causality is not established.[158]

Consumption of the star fruit (*Averrhoa carambola*) as a food in patients with chronic kidney disease is associated with development of intractable hiccups, vomiting, motor disabilities, paresthesias, confusion, seizures, and death unless patients receive supportive care and hemodialysis.[160] The unidentified toxin appears to be neuroexcitatory and may be oxalate.[24,52] Charcoal hemoperfusion is reported to be successful but clearance was not determined and causality not confirmed.[26] Given its limited availability and the poor potential outcomes, hemodialysis should be performed in affected patients.

EFFECTS SHARED AMONG DIFFERENT CLASSES OF XENOBIOTICS

Plant–Xenobiotic Interactions

By increasing the expression and function of CYP 3A4 enzymes and P-glycoprotein, hyperforin in St John's wort (*H. perforatum*) decreases concentrations of several drugs including amitriptyline, cyclosporine, digoxin, indinavir, irinotecan, warfarin, phenprocoumon, alprazolam, dextromethorphan, simvastatin, theophylline, and oral contraceptives.[122] Bergamottins and naringenin from grapefruit reduce activity of CYP 3A4 enzymes and increase drug concentrations. Other *Citrus* species also appear to increase drug concentrations.[72]

Pharmacodynamic interactions may be responsible for serotonin excess or mild serotonin syndrome when St John's wort is used concurrently with tryptophan or serotonin reuptake inhibitors.[140] Additive effects also appear

to be responsible for increased prothrombin time in patients taking *G. biloba* and various drugs that affect coagulation (eg, warfarin or aspirin) because the ginkgolides have antiplatelet activity.[37] Hawthorn (*Crataegus* spp), used medicinally for cardiac disorders, may produce an additive effect when taken concomitantly with digoxin, producing bradycardia. Excessive intake of broccoli provides enough vitamin K to competitively inhibit the effects of warfarin on vitamin K activation.

Sodium Channel Effects: Aconitine, Veratridine, Zygacine, Taxine, and Grayanotoxins

Several unrelated plants produce xenobiotics that affect the flow of sodium at the sodium channel. The mechanism of action depends on the individual alkaloid. For instance, aconitine and veratrum alkaloids tend to open the channels to influx of sodium, whereas others (eg, taxine) tend to block the flow, and grayanotoxins both increase and block sodium flow.[167] The sodium channel opener aconitine from *Aconitum* spp or *Delphinium* spp has the most persistent toxicity and the lowest therapeutic index among the many active alkaloid ingredients of these toxic plants called aconite. Some of the related alkaloids are controlled medicinal substances in the People's Republic of China and Taiwan.[27] Aconite has been abused for its psychoactive "out of body" effects and for suicide and homicide. These alkaloids should be suspected in potentially poisoned patients who manifest cardiac toxicity, paresthesias, and seizures.

Aconitine itself opens the voltage-dependent sodium channel at binding site 2 of the α-subunit, initially increasing cellular excitability.[58] By prolonging sodium current influx, neuronal and cardiac repolarization eventually slows. It also has calcium channel–opening effects. Those alkaloids are used in Asian prescription medicines to treat dysrhythmias and pain by reducing the excitability of the cardiac conducting system and sensory neurons, respectively.[27]

Approximately one teaspoon (2–5 g) of the root may cause death. The aconitine alkaloids are rapidly absorbed from the GI tract, and the calculated half-life of aconitine is 3 hours.[110] Central nervous system effects typically progress from paresthesias to CNS depression, respiratory muscle depression, paralysis, and seizures. Nausea, vomiting, diarrhea, and abdominal cramping occur.[95] Cardiotoxicity resembles that caused by cardioactive steroidal glycosides, and typically progresses from bradycardia with atrioventricular conduction blockade to increased ventricular automaticity resulting in diverse tachydysrhythmias. Multifocal premature ventricular contractions, bidirectional ventricular tachycardia,[149] torsade de pointes, and ventricular fibrillation may occur.[95]

A history of paresthesias or muscle weakness may be useful in differentiating aconitine toxicity from that caused by a cardioactive steroids. Aconite poisoning is confirmed by detection of the alkaloids in urine by liquid chromatography–mass spectrometry.

Antidysrhythmic success with lidocaine is limited, and amiodarone or flecainide are currently the antidysrhythmics of choice, with both drugs demonstrating more frequent return to sinus rhythms.[31,95] Orogastric lavage and/or administration of activated charcoal should be performed for any patient displaying signs or symptoms consistent with poisoning, or in those who are believed to have a potentially toxic exposures. Given the potential for rapid cardiovascular deterioration, equipment and staff for cardiac pacing, bypass, or balloon pump assist should be prepared and used for conventional indications.

Ingestion of veratridine and other veratrum alkaloids (from *Veratrum viride* and other *Veratrum* spp) generally results from foraging errors where the root appears similar to leeks (*Allium porrum*) and above-ground parts appear similar to gentian (*Gentiana lutea*) used for teas and wines in Europe.[141] Typical symptoms develop within an hour of ingestion and include headache followed by nausea, vomiting, and less frequently bradycardia and diarrhea. The mechanism of action is similar to that of aconitine (sodium channel opening) but the duration of effects is shorter.[167] Although severe toxicity is reported, management is supportive with fluids, atropine, and vasopressors. Deaths are rare.

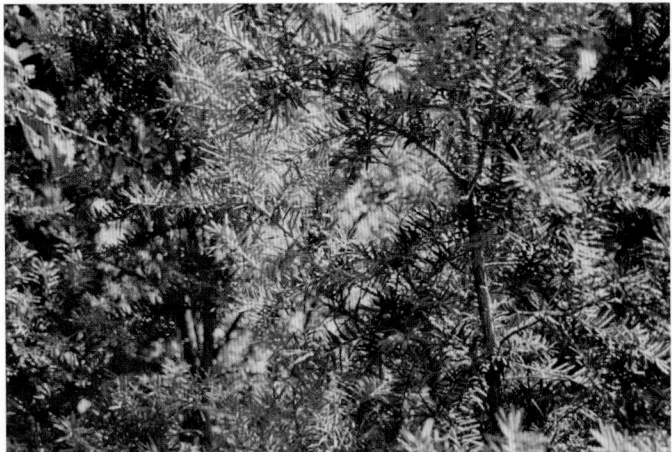

FIGURE 118–4. The Yew (*Taxus* sp.) is a common garden shrub that produces taxine, a cardiotoxin. Though the fleshy red aril is nontoxic, the hard seed it contains is toxic. *(Used with permission from the Fellowship in Medical Toxicology, New York University School of Medicine, New York City Poison Center.)*

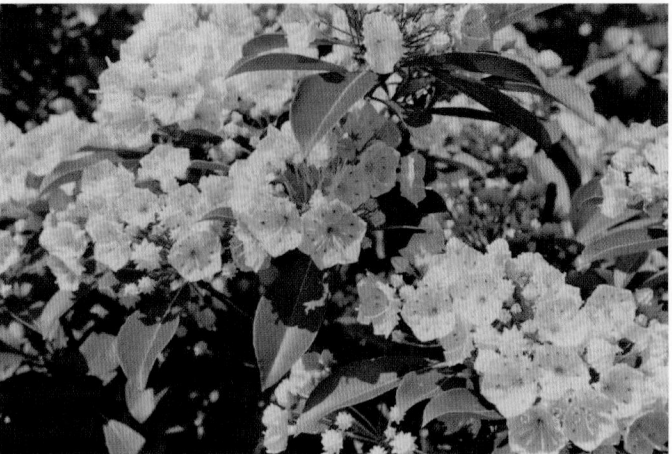

FIGURE 118–5. Mountain laurel (*Kalmia latifolia*), an evergreen shrub, contains the sodium channel opener grayanotoxin, which produces dysrhythmias. *(Used with permission from the Fellowship in Medical Toxicology, New York University School of Medicine, New York City Poison Center.)*

Zygacine from *Zigadenus* spp (death camas) and other members of the lily family produces the same toxic effects as veratridine alkaloids (vomiting, hypotension, and bradycardia).[171] Symptoms begin one to 2 hours after ingestion and usually result from errors while foraging for onions because of the plant's lookalike bulb.[154] Treatment options are the same as above with *Veratrum* alkaloids.

Taxine, derived from the yew, is another alkaloid mixture of sodium channel effectors that tend to close the channel (*Taxus baccata*) (Fig. 118–4). The toxicity of *Taxus* has been known since antiquity. Toxic alkaloids are contained within the bark, leaves, and hard central seed but not in the surrounding fleshy red aril, which partly explains the low rate of toxicity in reported cases of unintentional exposure.[173] Taxine-derived alkaloids (eg, taxine A and B, isotaxine B, paclitaxel), taxane-derived substances (eg, taxol A and B), and glycosides (eg, taxicatine) are responsible for the toxicity of *Taxus* spp. Lethal oral doses (LDmin) of yew leaves in humans are estimated to be 0.6 to 1.3 g/kg of body weight, or 3.0 to 6.5 mg taxines/kg of body weight.[172,173] Suicide using leaves is reported despite the large number of leaves required.[169] Clinical manifestations of yew poisoning include dizziness, nausea, vomiting, diffuse abdominal pain, tachycardia (initially), and convulsions followed by bradycardia, respiratory paralysis, and death. Several small European series report fatal and nonfatal cases with precise documentation of the yew alkaloids and metabolites in various tissues and their elimination half-lives.[83]

Paclitaxel (Taxol) is an alkaloid component of the relatively rare Pacific yew (*Taxus brevifolia*) that is used as an antitumor chemotherapeutic xenobiotic because of its ability to promote the assembly of microtubules and to inhibit the tubulin disassembly process in mitotic cells. Within one hour after ingestion, toxicity progresses from nausea, abdominal pain, bradycardia, and cardiac conduction delays to wide-complex ventricular dysrhythmias, paresthesias, ataxia, and depressed mental status.[66] Four prisoners who drank an extract of yew experienced profound hypokalemia, and 2 died of cardiac arrest.[54] Animal models indicate that bradycardia is responsive to atropine, but wide-complex tachydysrhythmias are unresponsive to sodium bicarbonate.[132]

Grayanotoxins (formerly termed andromedotoxins) are a series of 18 toxic diterpenoids present in leaves of various species of *Rhododendron*, *Azalea*, *Kalmia* (Fig. 118–5), and *Leucothoe* (Ericaceae). They exert their toxic effects via sodium channels, which they open or close, depending on the toxin.[167] Grayanotoxin I increases membrane permeability to sodium and affected calcium channels in a manner similar to that of veratridine (and batrachotoxin).[78] Grayanotoxins are concentrated in honey made in areas with densely populated grayanotoxin-containing plants, mainly in the Mediterranean. Accounts of poisoning by honey date back to at least 401 B.C., when Xenophon's troops were incapacitated after they consumed honey made from nectar of

Rhododendron luteum.[145] Occasionally, grayanotoxin-containing plants or plant preparations rather than honey cause human poisonings. Bradycardia, hypotension, GI manifestations, mental status changes ("mad honey"), and seizures are described in patients or animals suffering grayanotoxin toxicity.[68]

Antimitotic Alkaloids and Resins: Colchicine, Vincristine, and Podophyllum

Consumption of colchicine from plant sources such as autumn crocus (*Colchicum autumnale*) produces a spectrum of effects, including nausea, vomiting, watery diarrhea, hypotension, bradycardia, electrocardiographic abnormalities, diaphoresis, alopecia, bone marrow depression, acute kidney injury, hepatic necrosis, hemorrhagic acute lung injury, convulsions, and death.[157]

Confusion of the bulbs or leaves of this plant with those of wild onions or garlic occur as a foraging error.[60] Unintentional consumption by children and ingestion for self-harm account for the other cases involving morbidity or mortality. The mechanism of toxicity is disruption of microtubule formation in mitotic cells.[56]

Vincristine and vinblastine are 2 other indole alkaloids that are used as antineoplastics and are both isolated from the Madagascar periwinkle (*Catharanthus roseus*). No reports of poisoning by these alkaloids following ingestion of the plant could be found (Chap. 34).

Podophyllum resin is the dry, alcoholic extract of the rhizomes and roots of mayapple (*Podophyllum peltatum*) (Fig. 118–6). The dry resin consists of up to 20% podophyllotoxin, α- and β-peltatin, desoxypodophyllotoxin, and dehydropodophyllotoxin. These xenobiotics are originally present in the plant as β-D-glucosides. Podophyllum resin containing podophyllin is available by prescription for topical treatment of venereal warts. Its medicinal derivative, etoposide, is used for a range of neoplastic diseases. Podophyllum is used as a popular traditional Chinese medicine. Podophyllotoxins make up 20% of the resin from the roots of mayapple (*P. peltatum*). As a group, they disrupt tubulin formation, producing multisystem organ failure. Poisonings are caused by misidentification and adulteration, possibly because the list of common names by which it is known includes mayapple, as well as mandrake, wild mandrake, American mandrake, and European mandrake.[57] Catharsis is prominent after ingestion, but onset of symptoms may be significantly delayed. Acute, severe sensorimotor neuropathy and bone marrow suppression following transient leukocytosis can occur even after acute exposures and may be directly related to inhibition of microtubule assembly. Lethargy, confusion, encephalopathy, autonomic instability, sensory ataxia, and death are described following large exposures,[114] but poisoning can also occur after "therapeutic" doses of a popular traditional Chinese medicine.[114]

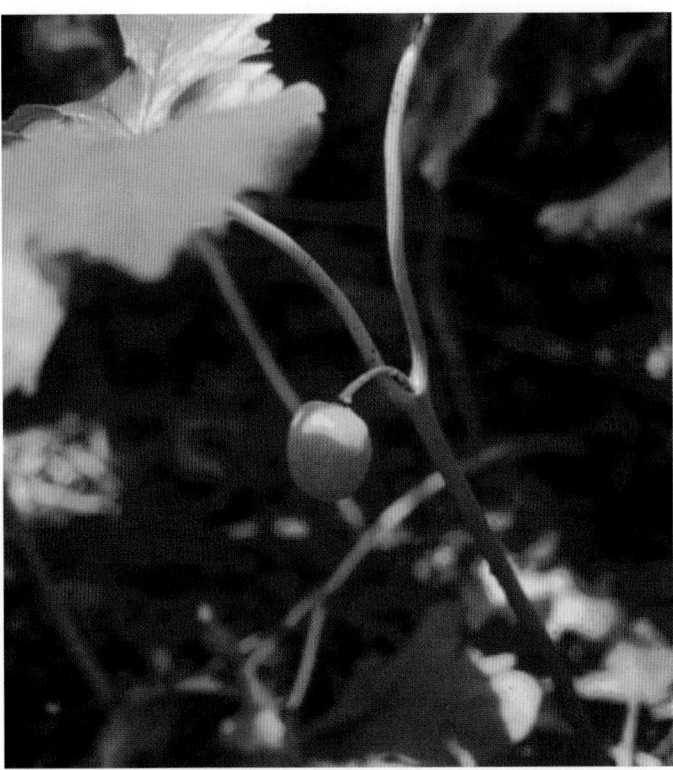

FIGURE 118-6. The mayapple (*Podophyllum peltatum*) develops from an initial nodding flower that grows from the stem of this low-lying ground cover plant. The whole plant contains podophyllotoxin (podophyllin), though the apple is generally considered the least toxic part. *(Used with permission from the Fellowship in Medical Toxicology, New York University School of Medicine, New York City Poison Center.)*

Plant-Induced Dermatitis

A large number of plants result in undesirable dermal, mucous membrane, and ocular effects and they represent the most common adverse effects reported to US poison control centers and occupational health centers. Plant-induced dermal disorders are readily categorized into 4 mechanistic groups, that is, dermatis that results from (1) mechanical injury, (2) irritant molecules that penetrate the skin, (3) allergy, or (4) photosensitivity (direct and hepatogenous) (Chap. 17).[138]

There is much overlap between these categories (some plants can produce all types). Clinicians may have difficulty distinguishing between plant-induced dermatitis and skin disorders[102] or between plant-induced dermatitis and pseudophytodermatitides caused by arthropods, pesticides, or wax (used in fruit and vegetable packaging). Agents that cause adverse skin reactions also cause eye and local gastric mucosal irritation.

Dermatitis from mechanical injury often is combined with primary or allergic contact dermatitis. Stinging nettles (*Urtica dioica* and other species) have a specialized apparatus in the form of an elongated silicious cell (glandular trichome) that acts like a hypodermic syringe to deliver irritant chemicals into the skin. Contact with these stinging hairs shears off the tip of the hair, producing micromechanical injury and releasing irritant contents: acetylcholine, histamine, and 5-hydroxytryptamine.[5] Acute motor polyneuropathy associated with cutaneous exposure to *Urtica ferox* is reported within 48 hours of walking through a patch of the nettles, with recovery occurring over several weeks.[71] The barbed trichomes (spicules) of *Mucuna pruriens* (velvet bean, cowhage) evoke a histamine-independent itch that is mediated by a cysteine protease, mucunain.[87] Workers who handpick pineapples are subject to fissuring and loss of fingerprints after proteolytic enzyme bromelain exposure following dermal abrasion by raphides.

Exposures to commonly available household plants such as dumbcane (*Dieffenbachia* spp), *Philodendron* spp, and *Narcissus* bulbs can lead to mechanical injury and painful microtrauma produced by bundles of tiny

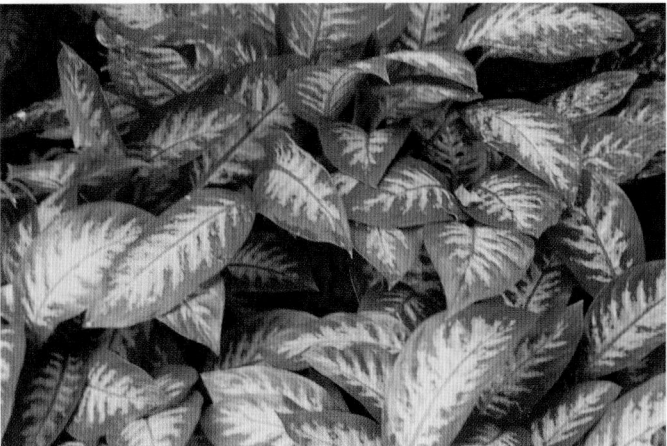

FIGURE 118-7. This dumbcane (*Dieffenbachia* sp) plant is representative of the Arum family, which typically have variegated, waxy leaves. Many contain insoluble crystals of calcium oxalate arranged in idioblasts, which may be ejected following trauma to the leaf. *(Used with permission from the Fellowship in Medical Toxicology, New York University School of Medicine, New York City Poison Center.)*

needlelike calcium oxalate crystals called raphides.[106] Packages of hundreds of raphides called idioblasts contain proteolytic enzymes. *Dieffenbachia* (more than 30 species) (Fig. 118-7) exposures are commonly reported household or malicious plant exposures, although such exposures are rarely serious.[112] When the leaves are chewed, immediate oropharyngeal pain and swelling occur.[4] Severe oral exposures can be excruciating and progress to profuse salivation, dysphagia, and loss of speech. Soothing liquids, ice, parenteral opioids, corticosteroids, and airway protection may be indicated, but antihistamines provide little relief. The edema and pain typically begin to subside after 4 to 8 days. Ocular exposure to the sap may produce chemical conjunctivitis, corneal abrasions, and, rarely, permanent corneal opacifications.

Similar exposures to oxalate raphide–containing household plants in the same family (*Philodendron, Brassaia, Epipremnum aureum, Spathiphyllum,* and *Scheflera* spp) are not as painful as those to dumbcane, presumably because the crystals are packaged differently and do not simultaneously deliver proteolytic enzymes.[106] One exception to their lower severity is a report of death in an 11 month-old following complications arising from esophageal lesions induced by philodendron.[103]

Irritant dermatitis results from low-molecular-weight xenobiotics such as phorbol esters (from Euphorbiaceae) that directly penetrate the skin without antecedent mechanical injury. Similar penetrance is achieved by products of glycoside hydrolysis. For instance, hydrolysis of ranunculin gives rise to anemonin in Ranunculaceae, the buttercup family, and hydrolysis of sinigrin in plants in the mustard family Brassicaceae yields allyl isothiocyanate. Exposures to primary irritants in Brassicaceae and Ranuculaceae usually are mild. Alternatively, airborne contact dermatitis occurs in typically exposed sites such as the upper eyelids; neck; uncovered extremities, including antecubital fossae; and other skin folds (Chap. 17).[108]

Phorbol esters found in spurges (Euphorbiaceae) are contained in milky sap that is capable of producing erythema, desquamation, and bullae. The saps of some species are more irritating than others. For instance, the manchineel tree (*Hippomane mancinella*), found in the Caribbean and Florida, once was planted on graves to deter grave robbers, and juice from the tree has been used to brand animals and to blind people. In addition to dermal and ocular injury,[49] ingestion of some spurges induces severe GI injury. Poinsettia (*Euphorbia pulcherrima*), crown of thorns (*Euphorbia splendens*), candelabra cactus (*Euphorbia lacteal*), and pencil tree (*Euphorbia tirucalli*) are spurges found in the home as holiday or other ornamentation that rarely produce serious injury, despite reputations to the contrary. The poinsettia plant, for instance, gained a reputation of significant toxicity based on a single, inadequately documented case report from Hawaii in 1919, involving the death of a 2-year-old child.[8] In a subsequent case, an 8-month-old child developed oral mucosal burns after chewing poinsettia.[48] Contact dermatitis, irritation of mucous membranes, and GI complaints such as nausea, vomiting, and abdominal pain are rare findings among the many reported exposures to poinsettia.

Allergic contact dermatitis results from type IV hypersensitivity response and, unlike irritant dermatitis, requires prior exposures to the agent before symptoms manifest. The most infamous of these xenobiotics are the urushiol oleoresins derived from catechols that are found in *G. biloba* (Ginkgoaceae) and members of the Proteaceae (eg, *Macadamia integrifolia*) and the Anacardaceae. The latter family is notable for inclusion of poison ivy (*Toxicodendron radicans*), poison oak (*Toxicodendron toxicarium, Toxicodendron diver-silobum*), and poison sumac (*Toxicodendron vernix*),[63] as well as mango (*Mangifera indica*), pistachio (*Pistacia vera*), cashew (*Anacardium occidentale*), and Indian marking nut "Bhilawanol" (*Semecarpus anacardium*). Upon first exposure, urushiol resins penetrate the skin and react with proteins to form antigens to which the body forms antibodies. Upon reexposure to urushiol resins, inflammatory mediators are released, leading to urticaria, itching, swelling, and pain. In extreme cases, these reactions can progress to type I hypersensitivity. Cross-reactivity between allergens is possible, and particular vigilance is required in sensitive individuals.[55] Prevention by removal of exposed objects that act as fomites for the oils and use of protective liniments are appropriate. Therapy includes washing with soap and water, application of topical corticosteroids and, for those at risk for frequent exposure (eg, forestry workers), desensitization (Chap. 17).[63]

Allergic contact dermatitis is the most common plant-induced occupational injury. In the United States, 33% of 462 floral shops surveyed reported that at least one employee had developed contact dermatitis.[136] Reactions are reported following exposure to tulips, Narcissus, Peruvian lily (*Alstroemeria* spp), and primroses (*Primula* spp). Exposure to the glycoside tuliposide A results in "tulip fingers," the dry, painfully fissured hyperkeratosis of fingers observed in horticultural workers who chronically handle tulips.[23] Upon hydrolysis, this compound yields α-methylene-butyrolactone, the true allergen. Cross-reactivity is possible among some of these xenobiotics. *Alstroemeria* spp, a common ornamental called Peruvian lily, contain tuliposide A and thus can cross-react with antigens in those persons already allergic to tulips, producing an allergic contact dermatitis. Primin (2-methoxy-6-*n*-pentyl-*p*-benzoquinone) from members of the Primulaceae family was responsible for the most frequently reported allergic plant dermatitis in northern Europe until workers refused to stock primroses. The "wood cutters dermatitis" of loggers occurs with development of sensitivity to compounds in liverwort (*Frullania* spp), which is cross-reactive to usnic acid in lichens and mosses found on the wood. Cross-reactivity with common weeds such as ragweed (*Ambrosia* spp) or dandelion (*Taraxacum* spp) initiate the risk of hypersensitivity from members of the Compositae family.[82] A myriad of other types of plants are involved in producing occupational dermatitides.[136] Sensitivity to Compositae (daisy family) involves more than 600 sesquiterpene lactones in at least 200 of the 25,000 species in the family and is as ubiquitous as the distribution of species. *Chrysanthemum* allergy is a common occupational hazard in Europe.

Direct photosensitivity dermatitis is produced when compounds such as psoralens or other linear furocoumarins come into direct contact with the skin or are digested and become bloodborne to dermal capillary beds, where they interact with sunlight. These photosensitizing agents are activated by ultraviolet A radiation (320–400 nm), producing singlet oxygen and DNA adducts. In addition to severe sunburnlike symptoms (erythema, epidermal bullae), hyperpigmentation lasting for several months may result from exposure to these compounds. The mechanism by which this reaction is produced is unknown, but depletion of glutathione is postulated to indirectly stimulate melanogenesis by disinhibiting the normally suppressant tyrosinase.[91] More than 200 of these xenobiotics have been identified in at least 15 plant families, including food sources, such as Apiaceae (anise, caraway, carrot, celery, chervil, dill, fennel, parsley, and parsnip), Rutaceae (grapefruit, lemon, lime, bergamot, and orange), Solanaceae (potato), and Moraceae (figs) family.

Hepatogenous photosensitivity is produced when a xenobiotic that normally is harmlessly ingested, absorbed, and hepatically excreted gains access to the peripheral circulation through failure of a liver excretion or detoxification mechanism. An example is the photosensitivity that occurs when phylloerythrin, a product of chlorophyll digestion normally eliminated in the bile, accumulates in the blood as a result of liver dysfunction. The cyanobacterium *Microcystis aeruginosa*, as well as the plants *Lantana camara, Tribulus terrestris*, and *Agave lechuguilla* reportedly cause this type of photosensitization in animals.

SUMMARY

- Plant exposures are among the commonest human exposures but also typically have little morbidity and mortality.
- Plant xenobiotics can be organized by the principles of pharmacognosy (the study of drugs of natural origin).
- Many plants share mechanisms of toxicity with available pharmaceuticals, and many pharmaceuticals are derived from plants.
- Understanding the mechanism of the potential plant toxin exposure will assist in guiding management.
- Confusion among lookalike plants, soundalike common names, and shared clinical findings among different plant species complicates management.
- Some reassurance can be achieved by excluding exposure to the most life-threatening plants.

Acknowledgments

Mary Emery Palmer, MD, and Joseph M. Betz, PhD, contributed to this chapter in previous editions.

REFERENCES

1. Akintonwa A, Tunwashe OL. Fatal cyanide poisoning from cassava-based meal. *Hum Exp Toxicol.* 1992;11:47-49.
2. Alexander RF, et al. A fatal case of solanine poisoning. *Br Med J.* 1948;2:518.
3. Alexandre J, et al. Digitalis intoxication induced by an acute accidental poisoning by lily of the valley. *Circulation.* 2012;125:1053-1055.
4. Altin G, et al. Severe destruction of the upper respiratory structures after brief exposure to a dieffenbachia plant. *J Craniofac Surg.* 2013;24:e245-e247.
5. Anderson BE, et al. Stinging nettle dermatitis. *Am J Contact Dermat.* 2003;14:44-46.
6. Aplin PJ, Eliseo T. Ingestion of castor oil plant seeds. *Med J Aust.* 1997;167:260-261.
7. Arcury TA, et al. Green tobacco sickness and skin integrity among migrant Latino farmworkers. *Am J Ind Med.* 2008;51:195-203.
8. Arnold HL. *Poisonous Plants of Hawaii.* Honolulu: Tongg Publishing Company; 1944.
9. Ascherio A, et al. Outbreak of buckthorn paralysis in Nicaragua. *J Trop Pediatr.* 1992; 38:87-89.
10. Audi J, et al. Ricin poisoning: a comprehensive review. *JAMA.* 2005;294:2342-2351.
11. Babu CK, et al. Alterations in redox potential of glutathione/glutathione disulfide and cysteine/cysteine disulfide couples in plasma of dropsy patients with argemone oil poisoning. *Food Chem Toxicol.* 2008;46:2409-2414.
12. Bandara V, et al. A review of the natural history, toxinology, diagnosis and clinical management of *Nerium oleander* (common oleander) and *Thevetia peruviana* (yellow oleander) poisoning. *Toxicon.* 2010;56:273-281.
13. Barceloux DG. Akee fruit and Jamaican vomiting sickness (*Blighia sapida* Köenig). *Dis Mon.* 2009;55:318-326.
14. Barceloux DG. Cyanogenic foods (cassava, fruit kernels, and cycad seeds). *Dis Mon.* 2009;55:336-352.
15. Barceloux DG. Grass pea and neurolathyrism (*Lathyrus sativus* L.). *Dis Mon.* 2009; 55:365-372.
16. Barker BE, et al. Peripheral blood plasmacytosis following systemic exposure to *Phytolacca americana* (pokeweed). *Pediatrics.* 1966;38:490-493.
17. Bartholomay P, et al. Epidemiologic investigation of an occupational illness of tobacco harvesters in southern Brazil, a worldwide leader in tobacco production. *Occup Environ Med.* 2012;69:514-518.
18. Bick AS, et al. Using advanced imaging methods to study neurolathyrism. *Isr Med Assoc J.* 2016;18:341-345.
19. Blythe WB. Hemlock poisoning, acute renal failure, and the Bible. *Ren Fail.* 1993;15:653.
20. Borsutzky M, et al. Hawaiian baby woodrose: (Psycho-) Pharmacological effects of the seeds of *Argyreia nervosa*. A case-orientated demonstration [in German]. *Nervenarzt.* 2002;73:892-896.
21. Boumba VA, et al. Fatal poisoning from ingestion of *Datura stramonium* seeds. *Vet Hum Toxicol.* 2004;46:81-82.
22. Bradley WG, Mash DC. Beyond Guam: the cyanobacteria/BMAA hypothesis of the cause of ALS and other neurodegenerative diseases. *Amyotroph Lateral Scler.* 2009; 10(suppl 2):7-20.
23. Bruynzeel DP. Bulb dermatitis. Dermatological problems in the flower bulb industries. *Contact Dermatitis.* 1997;37:70-77.

24. Carolino ROG, et al. Convulsant activity and neurochemical alterations induced by a fraction obtained from fruit *Averrhoa carambola* (Oxalidaceae: Geraniales). *Neurochem Int.* 2005;46:523-531.

25. Centers for Disease Control and Prevention (CDC). Anticholinergic poisoning associated with an herbal tea—New York City, 1994. *MMWR Morb Mortal Wkly Rep.* 1995;44:193-195.

26. Chan CK, et al. Star fruit intoxication successfully treated by charcoal haemoperfusion and intensive haemofiltration. *Hong Kong Med J.* 2009;15:149-152.

27. Chan TYK. Aconite poisoning. *Clin Toxicol.* 2009;47:279-285.

28. Chang S-S, et al. Acute Cycas seed poisoning in Taiwan. *J Toxicol Clin Toxicol.* 2004; 42:49-54.

29. Chase GW, et al. Hypoglycin A content in the aril, seeds, and husks of ackee fruit at various stages of ripeness. *J Assoc Off Anal Chem.* 1990;73:318-319.

30. Chiu AS, et al. Does α-amino-β-methylaminopropionic acid (BMAA) play a role in neurodegeneration? *Int J Environ Res Public Health.* 2011;8:3728-3746.

31. Coulson JM, et al. The management of ventricular dysrhythmia in aconite poisoning. *Clin Toxicol (Phila).* 2017;55:313-321.

32. Cox PA, Sacks OW. Cycad neurotoxins, consumption of flying foxes, and ALS-PDC disease in Guam. *Neurology.* 2002;58:956-959.

33. Crone C, et al. Reduced reciprocal inhibition is seen only in spastic limbs in patients with neurolathyrism. *Exp Brain Res.* 2007;181:193-197.

34. Daniele C, et al. Atractylis gummifera L. poisoning: an ethnopharmacological review. *J Ethnopharmacol.* 2005;97:175-181.

35. Dasgupta A. Therapeutic drug monitoring of digoxin: impact of endogenous and exogenous digoxin-like immunoreactive substances. *Toxicol Rev.* 2006;25:273-281.

36. de Jonge H, Vanrenterghem Y. Aristolochic acid: the common culprit of Chinese herbs nephropathy and Balkan endemic nephropathy. *Nephrol Dial Transplant.* 2008; 23:39-41.

37. de Lima Toccafondo Vieira M, Huang S-M. Botanical-drug interactions: a scientific perspective. *Planta Med.* 2012;78:1400-1415.

38. de Silva HA, et al. Multiple-dose activated charcoal for treatment of yellow oleander poisoning: a single-blind, randomised, placebo-controlled trial. *Lancet.* 2003;361: 1935-1938.

39. Debelle FD, et al. Aristolochic acid nephropathy: a worldwide problem. *Kidney Int.* 2008;74:158-169.

40. Deng JF, et al. Acute toxicities of betel nut: rare but probably overlooked events. *J Toxicol Clin Toxicol.* 2001;39:355-360.

41. Dickers KJ, et al. Abrin poisoning. *Toxicol Rev.* 2003;22:137-142.

42. Dittmann E, Wiegand C. Cyanobacterial toxins—occurrence, biosynthesis and impact on human affairs. *Mol Nutr Food Res.* 2006;50:7-17.

43. Doneray H, et al. Clinical outcomes in children with hyoscyamus niger intoxication not receiving physostigmine therapy. *Eur J Emerg Med.* 2007;14:348-350.

44. Eddleston M, et al. Acute yellow oleander (*Thevetia peruviana*) poisoning: cardiac arrhythmias, electrolyte disturbances, and serum cardiac glycoside concentrations on presentation to hospital. *Heart.* 2000;83:301-306.

45. Eddleston M, Haggalla S. Fatal injury in Eastern Sri Lanka, with special reference to cardenolide self-poisoning with *Cerbera manghas* fruits. *Clin Toxicol.* 2008;46:745-748.

46. Eddleston M, et al. Deaths due to absence of an affordable antitoxin for plant poisoning. *Lancet.* 2003;362:1041-1044.

47. Edgar JA, et al. Pyrrolizidine alkaloids in food: a spectrum of potential health consequences. *Food Addit Contam Part A.* 2011;28:308-324.

48. Edwards N. Local toxicity from a poinsettia plant: a case report. *J Pediatr.* 1983;102:404-405.

49. Eke T, et al. The spectrum of ocular inflammation caused by euphorbia plant sap. *Arch Ophthalmol.* 2000;118:13-16.

50. Evans WC, et al. Induction of thiamine deficiency in sheep, with lesions similar to those of cerebrocortical necrosis. *J Comp Pathol.* 1975;85:253-267.

51. Evans WC. *Trease and Evans' Pharmacognosy.* 16th ed. London: Saunders Limited; 2009.

52. Fang H-C, et al. The role of oxalate in star fruit neurotoxicity of five-sixths nephrectomized rats. *Food Chem Toxicol.* 2007;45:1764-1769.

53. Farese RV, et al. Licorice-induced hypermineralocorticoidism. *N Engl J Med.* 1991; 325:1223-1227.

54. Feldman R, et al. 4 cases of poisoning with the extract of yew (*Taxus baccata*) needles [in Polish]. *Pol Arch Med Wewn.* 1988;79:26-29.

55. Fernandez C, et al. Allergy to pistachio: crossreactivity between pistachio nut and other Anacardiaceae. *Clin Exp Allergy.* 1995;25:1254-1259.

56. Finkelstein Y, et al. Colchicine poisoning: the dark side of an ancient drug. *Clin Toxicol.* 2010;48:407-414.

57. Frasca T, et al. Mandrake toxicity. A case of mistaken identity. *Arch Intern Med.* 1997;157:2007-2009.

58. Fu M, et al. Toxicological mechanisms of Aconitum alkaloids. *Pharmazie.* 2006; 61:735-741.

59. Fu PP, et al. Pyrrolizidine alkaloids—genotoxicity, metabolism enzymes, metabolic activation, and mechanisms. *Drug Metab Rev.* 2004;36:1-55.

60. Galland-Decker C, et al. Progressive organ failure after ingestion of wild garlic juice. *J Emerg Med.* 2016;50:55-60.

61. Getahun H, et al. Neurolathyrism risk depends on type of grass pea preparation and on mixing with cereals and antioxidants. *Trop Med Int Health.* 2005;10:169-178.

62. Gilroy DJ, et al. Assessing potential health risks from microcystin toxins in blue-green algae dietary supplements. *Environ Health Perspect.* 2000;108:435-439.

63. Gladman AC. Toxicodendron dermatitis: poison ivy, oak, and sumac. *Wilderness Environ Med.* 2006;17:120-128.

64. Gordon DW, et al. Chaparral ingestion. The broadening spectrum of liver injury caused by herbal medications. *JAMA.* 1995;273:489-490.

65. Grob PJ, et al. Drug-induced pseudolupus. *Lancet.* 1975;2:144-148.

66. Grobosch T, et al. Eight cases of fatal and non-fatal poisoning with *Taxus baccata*. *Forensic Sci Int.* 2013;227:118-126.

67. Grollman AP, et al. Aristolochic acid and the etiology of endemic (Balkan) nephropathy. *Proc Natl Acad Sci U S A.* 2007;104:12129-12134.

68. Gunduz A, et al. Clinical review of grayanotoxin/mad honey poisoning past and present. *Clin Toxicol.* 2008;46:437-442.

69. Hamilton RJ, Goldfrank LR. Poison center data and the Pollyanna phenomenon. *J Toxicol Clin Toxicol.* 1997;35:21-23.

70. Hamilton RJ, et al. Mobitz type I heart block after pokeweed ingestion. *Vet Hum Toxicol.* 1995;37:66-67.

71. Hammond-Tooke GD, et al. Urtica ferox neuropathy. *Muscle Nerve.* 2007;35:804-807.

72. Hanley MJ, et al. The effect of grapefruit juice on drug disposition. *Expert Opin Drug Metab Toxicol.* 2011;7:267-286.

73. Harkrader RJ, et al. The history, chemistry and pharmacokinetics of Sanguinaria extract. *J Can Dent Assoc.* 1990;56(suppl):7-12.

74. Hogan RP. Hemorrhagic diathesis caused by drinking an herbal tea. *JAMA.* 1983; 249:2679-2680.

75. Hsiue TR, et al. Dose-response relationship and irreversible obstructive ventilatory defect in patients with consumption of *Sauropus androgynus. Chest.* 1998;113:71-76.

76. Hui A, et al. A rare ingestion of the Black Locust tree. *J Toxicol Clin Toxicol.* 2004;42:93-95.

77. Ize-Ludlow D. Neurotoxicities in infants seen with the consumption of star anise tea. *Pediatrics.* 2004;114:e653-e656.

78. Jansen SA, et al. Grayanotoxin poisoning: "mad honey disease" and beyond. *Cardiovasc Toxicol.* 2012;12:208-215.

79. Jochimsen EM, et al. Liver failure and death after exposure to microcystins at a hemodialysis center in Brazil. *N Engl J Med.* 1998;338:873-878.

80. Joskow R, et al. Ackee fruit poisoning: an outbreak investigation in Haiti 2000-2001, and review of the literature. *Clin Toxicol.* 2006;44:267-273.

81. Kajiyama Y, et al. Ginkgo seed poisoning. *Pediatrics.* 2002;109:325-327.

82. Kanerva L, et al. Occupational allergic contact dermatitis from Compositae in agricultural work. *Contact Dermatitis.* 2000;42:238-239.

83. Kobusiak-Prokopowicz M, et al. A suicide attempt by intoxication with *Taxus baccata* leaves and ultra-fast liquid chromatography-electrospray ionization-tandem mass spectrometry, analysis of patient serum and different plant samples: case report. *BMC Pharmacol Toxicol.* 2016;17:41.

84. Krakauer J. *Into the Wild.* New York, NY: Anchor Books; 1996.

85. Krenzelok EP, Mrvos R. Friends and foes in the plant world: a profile of plant ingestions and fatalities. *Clin Toxicol (Phila).* 2011;49:142-149.

86. Lachenmeier DW, et al. Thujone—cause of absinthism? *Forensic Sci Int.* 2006;158:1-8.

87. LaMotte RH, et al. Pruritic and nociceptive sensations and dysesthesias from a spicule of cowhage. *J Neurophysiol.* 2009;101:1430-1443.

88. Larson J, et al. Cholestatic jaundice due to ackee fruit poisoning. *Am J Gastroenterol.* 1994;89:1577-1578.

89. Lau CW, et al. Cardiovascular actions of berberine. *Cardiovasc Drug Rev.* 2001;19:234-244.

90. Lee ST, et al. Tremetone and structurally related compounds in white snakeroot (*Ageratina altissima*): a plant associated with trembles and milk sickness. *J Agric Food Chem.* 2010;58:8560-8565.

91. Levin Y, et al. Rare *Jatropha multifida* intoxication in two children. *J Emerg Med.* 2000;19:173-175.

92. Lewis WH, Elvin-Lewis MPF. *Medical Botany: Plants Affecting Human Health.* Hoboken, NJ: John Wiley; 2003.

93. Liebman M, Al-Wahsh IA. Probiotics and other key determinants of dietary oxalate absorption. *Adv Nutr.* 2011;2:254-260.

94. Lieu YK, et al. Carnitine effects on coenzyme A profiles in rat liver with hypoglycin inhibition of multiple dehydrogenases. *Am J Physiol.* 1997;272(3, pt 1):359-366.

95. Lin C-C, et al. Clinical features and management of herb-induced aconitine poisoning. *Ann Emerg Med.* 2004;43:574-579.

96. Lin T-J, et al. Acute poisonings with *Breynia officinalis*—an outbreak of hepatotoxicity. *J Toxicol Clin Toxicol.* 2003;41:591-594.

97. Luh SP, et al. Lung transplantation for patients with end-stage *Sauropus androgynus*-induced bronchiolitis obliterans (SABO) syndrome. *Clin Transplant.* 1999;13:496-503.

98. Lundahl JU, et al. The interaction effect of grapefruit juice is maximal after the first glass. *Eur J Clin Pharmacol.* 1998;54:75-81.

99. Madabushi R, et al. Hyperforin in St. John's wort drug interactions. *Eur J Clin Pharmacol.* 2006;62:225-233.

100. Martinez HR, et al. Clinical diagnosis in *Karwinskia humboldtiana* polyneuropathy. *J Neurol Sci.* 1998;154:49-54.

101. McGee D, et al. Four-year review of cigarette ingestions in children. *Pediatr Emerg Care.* 1995;11:13-16.

102. McGovern TW, et al. Is it, or isn't it? Poison ivy look-a-likes. *Am J Contact Dermat.* 2000;11:104-110.

103. McIntire MS, et al. Philodendron—an infant death. *J Toxicol Clin Toxicol.* 1990;28: 177-183.

104. McTague JA, Forney R. Jamaican vomiting sickness in Toledo, Ohio. *Ann Emerg Med.* 1994;23:1116-1118.

105. Meschler JP, Howlett AC. Thujone exhibits low affinity for cannabinoid receptors but fails to evoke cannabimimetic responses. *Pharmacol Biochem Behav.* 1999;62:473-480.

106. Mezzasalma V, et al. Poisonous or non-poisonous plants? DNA-based tools and applications for accurate identification. *Int J Legal Med.* 2016;131:1-19.

107. Milazzo S, et al. Laetrile treatment for cancer. *Cochrane Database Syst Rev.* 2011; CD005476.

108. Modi GM, et al. Irritant contact dermatitis from plants. *Dermatitis.* 2009;20:63-78.

109. Moertel CG, et al. A clinical trial of amygdalin (Laetrile) in the treatment of human cancer. *N Engl J Med.* 1982;306:201-206.

110. Moritz F, et al. Severe acute poisoning with homemade *Aconitum napellus* capsules: toxicokinetic and clinical data. *Clin Toxicol.* 2005;43:873-876.

111. Morkovsky O, Kucera J. Mass poisoning of children in a nursery school by the seeds of *Laburnum anagyroides* [in Czech]. *Cesk Pediatr.* 1980;35:284-285.

112. Mrvos R, et al. Philodendron/dieffenbachia ingestions: are they a problem? *J Toxicol Clin Toxicol.* 1991;29:485-491.

113. Murphy NG, et al. Anabasine toxicity from a topical folk remedy. *Clin Pediatr (Phila).* 2006;45:669-671.

114. Ng TH, et al. Encephalopathy and neuropathy following ingestion of a Chinese herbal broth containing podophyllin. *J Neurol Sci.* 1991;101:107-113.

115. Ocampo-Roosens LV, et al. Intoxication with buckthorn (*Karwinskia humboldtiana*): report of three siblings. *Pediatr Dev Pathol.* 2007;10:66-68.

116. Oonakahara K, et al. Outbreak of bronchiolitis obliterans associated with consumption of *Sauropus androgynus* in Japan—alert of food-associated pulmonary disorders from Japan. *Respiration.* 2005;72:221-221.

117. Padosch SA, et al. Absinthism: a fictitious 19th century syndrome with present impact. *Subst Abuse Treat Prev Policy.* 2006;1:14.

118. Paine MF, et al. Further characterization of a furanocoumarin-free grapefruit juice on drug disposition: studies with cyclosporine. *Am J Clin Nutr.* 2008;87:863-871.

119. Philippe G, et al. About the toxicity of some *Strychnos* species and their alkaloids. *Toxicon.* 2004;44:405-416.

120. Phillips BJ, et al. A study of the toxic hazard that might be associated with the consumption of green potato tops. *Food Chem Toxicol.* 1996;34:439-448.

121. Pincus SH, et al. Passive and active vaccination strategies to prevent ricin poisoning. *Toxins (Basel).* 2011;3:1163-1184.

122. Rahimi R, Abdollahi M. An update on the ability of St. John's wort to affect the metabolism of other drugs. *Expert Opin Drug Metab Toxicol.* 2012;8:691-708.

123. Ramlakhan SL, Fletcher AK. It could have happened to Van Gogh: a case of fatal purple foxglove poisoning and review of the literature. *Eur J Emerg Med.* 2007;14:356-359.

124. Rao RB, Hoffman RS. Nicotinic toxicity from tincture of blue cohosh (*Caulophyllum thalictroides*) used as an abortifacient. *Vet Hum Toxicol.* 2002;44:221-222.

125. Reynolds T. Hemlock alkaloids from Socrates to poison aloes. *Phytochemistry.* 2005;66:1399-1406.

126. Rich SA, et al. Treatment of foxglove extract poisoning with digoxin-specific Fab fragments. *Ann Emerg Med.* 1993;22:1904-1907.

127. Rizzi D, et al. Clinical spectrum of accidental hemlock poisoning: neurotoxic manifestations, rhabdomyolysis and acute tubular necrosis. *Nephrol Dial Transplant.* 1991; 6:939-943.

128. Robbers JE, et al. *Pharmacognosy and Pharmacobiotechnology.* Baltimore, MD: Lippincott Williams & Wilkins; 1996.

129. Roberge R, et al. The root of evil—pokeweed intoxication. *Ann Emerg Med.* 1986; 15:470-473.

130. Rodrigues TD, et al. Holly berry ingestion: case report. *Vet Hum Toxicol.* 1984;26:157-158.

131. Rosenblatt M, Mindel J. Spontaneous hyphema associated with ingestion of *Ginkgo biloba* extract. *N Engl J Med.* 1997;336:1108.

132. Ruha A-M, et al. Hypertonic sodium bicarbonate for Taxus media-induced cardiac toxicity in swine. *Acad Emerg Med.* 2002;9:179-185.

133. Ruprich J, et al. Probabilistic modelling of exposure doses and implications for health risk characterization: glycoalkaloids from potatoes. *Food Chem Toxicol.* 2009;47:2899-2905.

134. Safadi R, et al. Beneficial effect of digoxin-specific Fab antibody fragments in oleander intoxication. *Arch Intern Med.* 1995;155:2121-2125.

135. Salen P, et al. Effect of physostigmine and gastric lavage in a *Datura stramonium*—induced anticholinergic poisoning epidemic. *Am J Emerg Med.* 2003;21:316-317.

136. Santucci B, Picardo M. Occupational contact dermatitis to plants. *Clin Dermatol.* 1992;10:157-165.

137. Sarris J, et al. Kava: a comprehensive review of efficacy, safety, and psychopharmacology. *Aust N Z J Psychiatry.* 2011;45:27-35.

138. Sasseville D. Clinical patterns of phytodermatitis. *Dermatol Clin.* 2009;27:299-308, vi.

139. Scatizzi A, et al. Acute renal failure due to tubular necrosis caused by wildfowl-mediated hemlock poisoning. *Ren Fail.* 1993;15:93-96.

140. Schellander R, Donnerer J. Antidepressants: clinically relevant drug interactions to be considered. *Pharmacology.* 2010;86:203-215.

141. Schep LJ, et al. Veratrum poisoning. *Toxicol Rev.* 2006;25:73-78.

142. Schep LJ, et al. Poisoning due to water hemlock. *Clin Toxicol.* 2009;47:270-278.

143. Schuurman M, et al. Severe hemolysis and methemoglobinemia following fava beans ingestion in glucose-6-phosphatase dehydrogenase deficiency: case report and literature review. *Eur J Pediatr.* 2009;168:779-782.

144. Shrivastava A, et al. Association of acute toxic encephalopathy with litchi consumption in an outbreak in Muzaffarpur, India, 2014: a case-control study. *Lancet Glob Health.* 2017;5:e458-e466.

145. Silici S, Atayoglu AT. Mad honey intoxication: a systematic review on the 1199 cases. *Food Chem Toxicol.* 2015;86:282-290.

146. Singh R, et al. Epidemic dropsy in the eastern region of Nepal. *J Trop Pediatr.* 1999; 45:8-13.

147. Slifman NR, et al. Contamination of botanical dietary supplements by *Digitalis lanata. N Engl J Med.* 1998;339:806-811.

148. Smith SW, et al. Solanaceous steroidal glycoalkaloids and poisoning by *Solanum torvum*, the normally edible susumber berry. *Toxicon.* 2008;52:667-676.

149. Smith SW, et al. Bidirectional ventricular tachycardia resulting from herbal aconite poisoning. *Ann Emerg Med.* 2005;45:100-101.

150. Snyman T, et al. A fatal case of pepper poisoning. *Forensic Sci Int.* 2001;124:43-46.

151. Spencer PS. Food toxins, AMPA receptors, and motor neuron diseases. *Drug Metab Rev.* 1999;31:561-587.

152. Spiller HA, et al. Retrospective study of mistletoe ingestion. *J Toxicol Clin Toxicol.* 1996;34:405-408.

153. Spina SP, Taddei A. Teenagers with Jimson weed (*Datura stramonium*) poisoning. *CJEM.* 2007;9:467-468.

154. Spoerke DG, Spoerke SE. Three cases of Zigadenus (death camus) poisoning. *Vet Hum Toxicol.* 1979;21:346-347.

155. Staumont G, et al. Changes in colonic motility induced by sennosides in dogs: evidence of a prostaglandin mediation. *Gut.* 1988;29:1180-1187.

156. Suchard JR, et al. Acute cyanide toxicity caused by apricot kernel ingestion. *Ann Emerg Med.* 1998;32:742-744.

157. Sundov Z, et al. Fatal colchicine poisoning by accidental ingestion of meadow saffron-case report. *Forensic Sci Int.* 2005;149:253-256.

158. Teschke R, et al. Herb induced liver injury presumably caused by black cohosh: a survey of initially purported cases and herbal quality specifications. *Ann Hepatol.* 2011;10:249-259.

159. Teschke R, Wolff A. Regulatory causality evaluation methods applied in kava hepatotoxicity: are they appropriate? *Regul Toxicol Pharmacol.* 2011;59:1-7.

160. Tsai M-H, et al. Status epilepticus induced by star fruit intoxication in patients with chronic renal disease. *Seizure.* 2005;14:521-525.

161. Tuncok Y, et al. *Urginea maritima* (squill) toxicity. *J Toxicol Clin Toxicol.* 1995;33: 83-86.

162. Turgut M, et al. Carboxyatractyloside poisoning in humans. *Ann Trop Paediatr.* 2005;25: 125-134.

163. Vargas CP, et al. Getting to the root (*Acorus calamus*) of the problem. *J Toxicol Clin Toxicol.* 1998;36:259-260.

164. Vetter J. Plant cyanogenic glycosides. *Toxicon.* 2000;38:11-36.

165. Vriens J, et al. Herbal compounds and toxins modulating TRP channels. *Curr Neuropharmacol.* 2008;6:79-96.

166. Wang C-F, et al. Early plasma exchange for treating ricin toxicity in children after castor bean ingestion. *J Clin Apher.* 2015;30:141-146.

167. Wang S-Y, Wang GK. Voltage-gated sodium channels as primary targets of diverse lipid-soluble neurotoxins. *Cell Signal.* 2003;15:151-159.

168. Wasfi IA, et al. A fatal case of oleandrin poisoning. *Forensic Sci Int.* 2008;179:e31-e36.

169. Wehner F, Gawatz O. Suicidal yew poisoning—from Caesar to today—or suicide instructions on the internet [in German]. *Arch Kriminol.* 2003;211:19-26.

170. Weisbord SD, et al. Poison on line—acute renal failure caused by oil of wormwood purchased through the Internet. *N Engl J Med.* 1997;337:825-827.

171. West P, Horowitz BZ. Zigadenus poisoning treated with atropine and dopamine. *J Med Toxicol.* 2009;5:214-217.

172. Willaert W, et al. Intoxication with *Taxus baccata*: cardiac arrhythmias following yew leaves ingestion. *Pacing Clin Electrophysiol.* 2002;25(4, pt 1):511-512.

173. Wilson CR, et al. Taxines: a review of the mechanism and toxicity of yew (Taxus spp.) alkaloids. *Toxicon.* 2001;39:175-185.

174. Woldeamanuel YW, et al. Neurolathyrism: two Ethiopian case reports and review of the literature. *J Neurol.* 2012;259:1263-1268.

175. Yamada K, et al. Ptaquiloside, the major toxin of bracken, and related terpene glycosides: chemistry, biology and ecology. *Nat Prod Rep.* 2007;24:798-813.

176. Ye L, et al. Inhibitors of testosterone biosynthetic and metabolic activation enzymes. *Molecules.* 2011;16:9983-10001.

177. Yoshida S, Takayama Y. Licorice-induced hypokalemia as a treatable cause of dropped head syndrome. *Clin Neurol Neurosurg.* 2003;105:286-287.

119 NATIVE (US) VENOMOUS SNAKES AND LIZARDS

Anne-Michelle Ruha and Anthony F. Pizon

EPIDEMIOLOGY

Snakes

More than 3,000 species of snakes are identified worldwide, with nearly 800 species considered venomous. All venomous species are classified taxonomically into one of 4 general groups. These include the families Viperidae, Elapidae, and Colubridae, as well as the Atractaspidinae, a subfamily of the Lamprophiidae family. The United States is home to nearly 30 species and subspecies of venomous snakes (Table 119–1), with many more found throughout Mexico. All belong to either the Crotalinae subfamily of Viperidae or the Elapidae family.

Venomous snakes possess glands that are associated with specialized teeth, or fangs, which allow delivery of venom for the purpose of prey immobilization or defense. Fangs are located in the front of the mouth in most venomous species. In addition to fangs, venomous snakes have rows of small teeth that may cause additional injury during a bite.

The majority of snake species in North America are rear-fanged, nonvenomous members of the Colubridae family. Bites by these species, which include corn snakes, gopher snakes, and garter snakes, are usually harmless. Colubrids do not possess venom glands, but some produce secretions from Duvernoy's glands that contain toxins similar to those found in the venom of venomous species. Although the vast majority of bites by nonvenomous colubrids do not produce symptoms, rare cases of envenomation are documented following a bite by a nonvenomous species.[62]

Venomous snakes are found throughout most of the United States. They are much more common in the southern and western states than in the northern states. Though venomous species are not endemic to Maine, Alaska, or Hawaii, bites are reported in every state except for Hawaii. The true number of bites that occur each year is not accurately known, but an average of 5,000 native venomous snakebites are reported to US poison control centers annually.[49] Mortality is rare in the United States, with fewer than 10 deaths per year reported. Epidemiologic data on snakebites in Mexico is poor, but the number of bites and deaths is thought to be higher. Internationally, snakebites are an important and common cause of morbidity and mortality (Special Considerations: SC10).

The majority of snakebites in the United States occur between April and September, with the peak number reported in July. Men comprise 75% of snakebite victims and children represent about 10% to 15% of reported cases.[49] Most victims are bitten on an extremity, although bites to the torso, face, and tongue also occur. Bites often occur when an individual is purposely handling a known venomous snake. Herpetologists, those who capture and keep wild snakes, and religious snake handlers are at highest risk. Occasionally people are envenomed after killing and decapitating a rattlesnake. This is likely due to persistent reflexes in the venom apparatus.

Snake handlers and collectors are at risk for multiple bites during their lifetime. There is no convincing evidence that immunity develops as a result of repeated envenomation. Victims of repeat bites actually have a greater risk for anaphylaxis because of prior sensitization and the development of IgE antibodies to venom.[45]

Snake enthusiasts often keep nonnative (exotic) species as pets. Approximately 30 to 50 bites from a large variety of exotic venomous snakes are reported to poison control centers each year.[51]

Pit Vipers

The majority of native venomous snakes are members of the Crotalinae subfamily of Viperidae. These crotaline species are variably referred to as crotalids, New World vipers, or pit vipers. The term "pit viper" describes the presence of a pitlike depression behind the nostril that contains a heat-sensing organ used to locate prey. Native pit vipers include the rattlesnakes (genera *Crotalus* and *Sistrurus*) and the cottonmouths and copperheads (genus *Agkistrodon*). These pit vipers can be distinguished from native nonvenomous species by a triangular-shaped head, vertically elliptical pupils, and easily identifiable fangs (Fig. 119–1). Crotalinae have front, mobile fangs that are paired, needlelike structures that can retract on a hingelike mechanism into the roof of the mouth. Rattlesnakes have the longest fangs, reaching 3 to 4 cm. Pit vipers are also identifiable by their scale patterns. Their undersurface has a single row of plates or scales, as opposed to the double row found on nonvenomous species. Rattlesnakes may or may not have rattles, depending on maturity. A rattling sound is often, but not always, heard before a strike. Copperheads and cottonmouths do not have rattles, but shake their tales similarly to rattlesnakes. Cottonmouths, which are also commonly known as water moccasins, are semiaquatic and have a distinct white mouth. Copperheads are known for their reddish-brown (copper) heads and dark hourglass-shaped bands contrasting with a lighter background on their bodies (Fig. 119–2).

Of crotalid bites for which the type of snake is reported, about half are rattlesnake species, and the remainder copperheads and cottonmouths. Rattlesnakes are found throughout most of the United States, but encounters are most common in western and southern states. Rattlesnakes account for the greatest morbidity among the various types of pit vipers. Deaths

Genus	Species	Common Name
TABLE 119–1	**Medically Important Snakes of the United States**	
Crotalinae		
Crotalus	adamanteus	Eastern diamondback rattlesnake
	atrox	Western diamondback rattlesnake
	cerastes	Sidewinder[a]
	cerberus	Arizona black rattlesnake
	horridus	Timber rattlesnake
	lepidus	Rock rattlesnake[a]
	mitchellii	Speckled rattlesnake[a]
	molossus	Black-tailed rattlesnake[a]
	oreganus	Western rattlesnake[a]
	pricei	Twin-spotted rattlesnake[a]
	ruber	Red diamond rattlesnake[a]
	scutulatus	Mojave rattlesnake[a]
	stephensi	Panamint rattlesnake
	tigris	Tiger rattlesnake
	viridis	Prairie rattlesnake[a]
	willardi	Ridgenose rattlesnake[a]
Sistrurus	catenatus	Massasauga[a]
	miliarius	Pygmy rattlesnake[a]
Agkistrodon	contortrix	Copperhead[a]
	piscivorus	Cottonmouth[a]
Elapidae		
Micrurus	fulvius	Eastern coral snake
Micrurus	tener	Texas coral snake[a]

[a]Subspecies identified for this species.

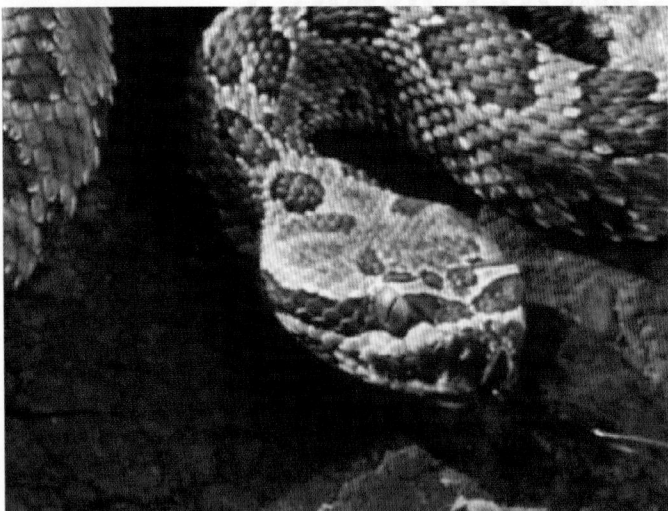

FIGURE 119–1. Pit vipers have a triangular-shaped head, vertically elliptical pupils, and heat-sensing pits behind the nostril.

following snakebite are almost always due to rattlesnakes, although rare deaths are reported from copperhead bites.[41] Copperhead bites are most often reported in the eastern and southeastern United States, although they also occur in the northeast. Cottonmouths are found mainly in the southeastern United States.

Coral Snakes

Coral snakes (genera *Micrurus* and *Micruroides*) represent the Elapidae family in North America. These brightly colored snakes typically have easily identifiable red, yellow, and black bands along the length of their bodies. In the United States, coral snakes and the similarly colored nonvenomous scarlet king snake are often confused. Coral and king snakes can be distinguished by their color patterns. Whereas coral snakes have black snouts, king snakes have red snouts. Both species have red, yellow, and black rings, but in different sequences: the red and yellow rings touch in the coral snake but are separated by black rings in king snakes ("Red on yellow kills a fellow; red on black, venom lack") (Fig. 119–3). This general rule for identifying coral snakes does not apply to Mexican species, some of which have different color patterns.

Elapids possess front-fixed fangs. The fangs of coral snakes are small, and discrete fang marks may not be obvious after envenomation. Coral snakes often latch on to a victim or "chew" for a few seconds in an attempt to deliver venom. A history of this activity may help identify a coral snakebite when the offending reptile cannot be located.

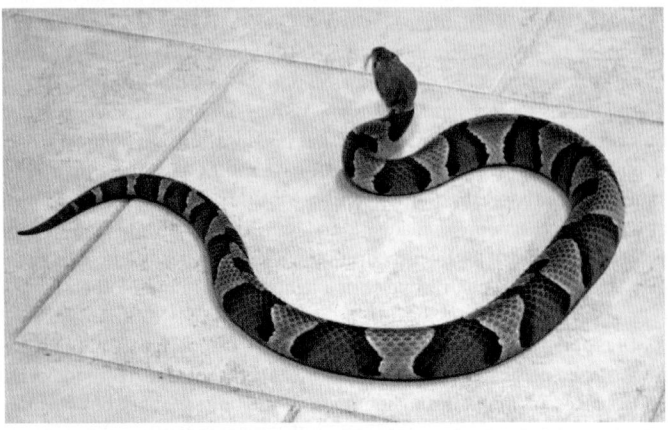

FIGURE 119–2. Copperhead (*Agkistrodon contortrix*). (Used with the permission from Michelle Ruha, MD.)

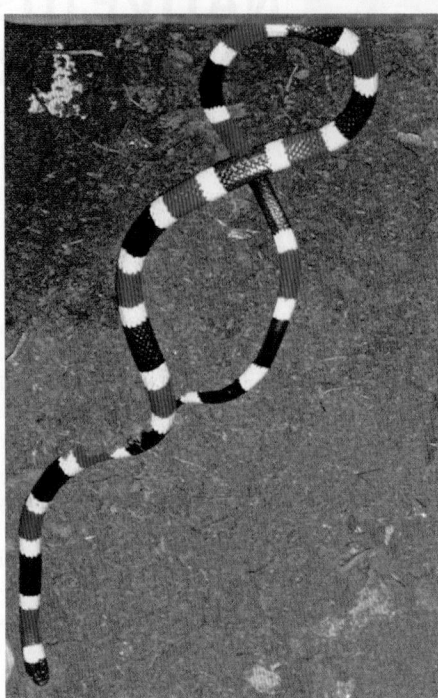

FIGURE 119–3. Coral snake with characteristic black snout and red bands bordered by yellow bands. *(Used with permission from Banner Good Samaritan Medical Center Department of Medical Toxicology.)*

Coral snakes are responsible for approximately 2% of bites reported to US poison control centers.[49] *Micrurus* species are found in 11 southeastern states, where up to 100 bites are reported per year. *Micrurus fulvius* (the Eastern coral snake) is responsible for the greatest morbidity and mortality, whereas *M. tener* (the Texas coral snake) seems to be less dangerous. The Sonoran coral snake (*Micruroides euryxanthus*) does not produce envenomation necessitating medical intervention.[61]

Lizards

There are 2 species of lizard that are known to produce envenomation in humans. These are the Gila monster (*Heloderma suspectum*) (Fig. 119–4), which is native to the desert southwestern United States, and the beaded lizard (*H. horridum*), which is found in Mexico. Both species are members of the Helodermatidae family. Bites by the Gila monster and beaded lizard are extremely uncommon, even in areas where the lizards are endemic. These lizards are slow moving, nocturnal, and thick bodied. Adults reach a maximum length of 60 cm and are generally shy, so bites are relatively rare and usually occur as a result of handling. Bites almost always occur from captive animals, whether found in the wild or kept in a zoo or personal collection. Gila monsters are known for their forceful bites. They can hang on and "chew" for as long as 15 minutes, and they may be difficult to disengage. The great majority of reported cases have involved adult men.

The helodermatid lizards have a less effective venom delivery system than venomous snake species. The lizards possess paired venom glands that are located on either side of the anterior lower mandible. Venom ducts carry the venom from the glands to the base of grooved teeth. When a tooth produces a puncture wound, the venom travels by capillary action into the grooves and then into the wound.[47]

PHARMACOLOGY

Snakes

Snake venom is a complex mixture of proteins, peptides, lipids, carbohydrates, and metal ions. Venom contains a variety of enzymes including phospholipases A_2 (PLA_2s), metalloproteinases (SVMPs), serine proteases, acetylcholinesterases, L–amino acid oxidases, and hyaluronidases. Nonenzymatic proteins include 3-finger toxins (3FTXs), sarafotoxins, disintegrins, and C-type lectins among others. The content and potency of venom in any

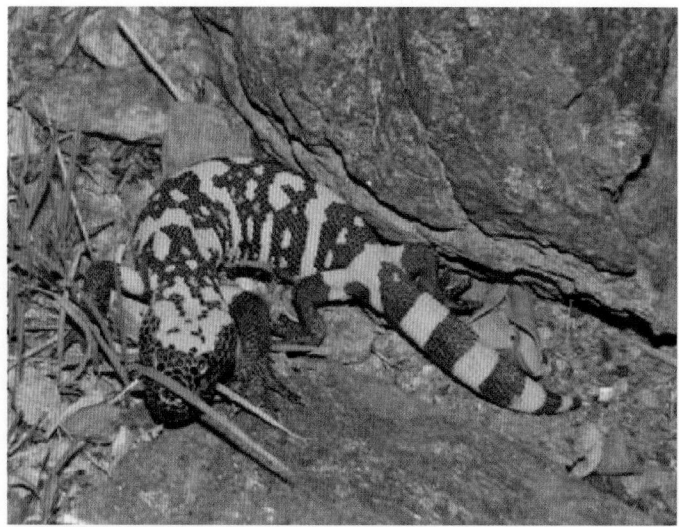

A

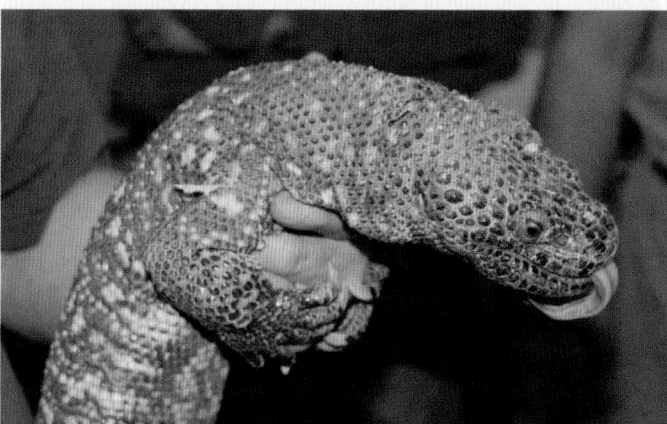

B

FIGURE 119–4. (**A**) Young Gila monster (*Heloderma suspectum*). *(Used with the permission from Steven Curry, MD.)* (**B**) Beaded lizard (*Heloderma horridum*). *(Used with the permission from Michelle Ruha, MD.)*

given snake varies depending on age, diet, and geography. Thus, an adult snake may have significantly different venom composition than a young snake of the same species.[59]

Snakes typically produce about 100 to 200 mg dry venom in a single milking, although some produce several hundred mg to over 1 g.[59] Many venom components are pharmacologically active and target receptors, ion channels, enzymes, or other proteins in mammals. The actions of only a fraction of snake venom components are fully understood. Identification of individual snake venom toxins, understanding of pharmacologic mechanisms, and potential medicinal uses for venom are areas of ongoing research.

Lizards

Helodermatid venom contains a complex mixture of components similar to those of snake venoms, including numerous enzymes such as hyaluronidase, phospholipase A_2, and serotonin.[47,57] Nonenzymatic components include helospectins and helodermin, which are vasoactive peptides that activate adenylate cyclase, and exendin-3 and exendin-4, which stimulate glucose-dependent insulin secretion. Discovery of exendins in *Heloderma* venom lead to development of exenatide (Byetta), a glucagonlike peptide-1 (GLP-1) receptor agonist used in the management of diabetes.[25,57] Another important component of *Heloderma* venom is gilatoxin. Gilatoxin is a serine protease with kallikreinlike activity, thought to be responsible for the hypotension and angioedema that occur in some human envenomations.[57]

PHARMACOKINETICS AND TOXICOKINETICS

Snakes

Very few pharmacokinetic studies of snake venom exist, and much remains unknown regarding absorption, distribution, and elimination of venom following a bite. When a snake bites, venom is usually deposited subcutaneously. In some cases fangs reach muscle or even directly access vasculature. Systemic absorption of venom usually occurs via the lymphatic system. Available human and animal data suggest that venom antigens are absorbed into blood within minutes of envenomation, with peak concentrations detected within 4 hours.[10,31,50] Venom antigen concentrations measured in the first 4 hours following a bite correlate roughly with grade of envenomation.[3,9,31] Venom antigens are also detected in urine as early as 30 minutes after envenomation.[31] After administration of adequate doses of antivenom, venom antigens are no longer detected in blood; however, antigenemia may recur, and such recurrence is associated with reemergence of clinical effects.[31,50]

The elimination half-life of snake venom appears to be long. Following subcutaneous injection of *C. atrox* venom in a rabbit model, mean half-life was 20 hours, and venom was still detectable in blood at 96 hours.[10]

Lizards

Pharmacokinetic studies of helodermatid venom are not available. Clinical reports suggest that venom is absorbed systemically within minutes of a bite.

PATHOPHYSIOLOGY

Snakes

Pit Vipers

Crotaline venom has the potential to simultaneously damage tissue, affect blood vessels and blood, and alter transmission at the neuromuscular junction. It is difficult to attribute specific pathology or pathophysiology to any particular component of snake venom. In fact, clinical effects often occur as the result of several venom components (Table 119–2). For instance, local tissue damage results from venom metalloproteinases and hyaluronidase, which both contribute to swelling through disruption of the extracellular matrix and basement membrane surrounding microvascular endothelial cells.[29] As a result of reduced blood flow through damaged capillaries, they also contribute to myonecrosis, which results primarily from the action of phospholipase A_2 enzymes (PLA_2) on muscle.[29] Additionally, venom metalloproteinases contribute to dermatonecrosis, both directly and through activation of endogenous inflammatory mediators.[29,55]

Venom effects on the hematologic system are especially complex. Numerous components act as anticoagulants, and many others act as procoagulants. Similarly, platelets are inhibited, activated, agglutinated, aggregated,

TABLE 119–2	Major Venom Components of Crotalinae Snakes
General Clinical Effect	**Responsible Venom Components**
Local tissue damage	Metalloproteinases
	Phospholipases A_2
	Hyaluronidase
Coagulation effects[a]	C-type lectinlike proteins
	Metalloproteinases[b]
	Serine proteases[b]
	Phospholipases A_2
Platelet effects[c]	Disintegrins
	C-type lectinlike proteins
	Metalloproteinases
	Phospholipases A_2
Neurotoxic effects	Phospholipases A_2

[a]Venom contains both pro- and anticoagulants, with anticoagulant effects predominating in North American crotaline envenomation. [b]Include thrombinlike enzymes as well as fibrinogenolytic enzymes. [c]Venom may contain factors that inhibit, activate, or affect aggregation of platelets.

or inhibited from aggregating by various venom components. Venom components can be grouped according to certain characteristics, such as structure and enzymatic activity, but as noted above with local tissue damage, components within several groups may contribute to similar effects. For instance, anticoagulants in snake venoms are found among the C-type lectinlike proteins (CLPs), PLA_2 enzymes, serine proteases, and metalloproteinases. Conversely, components within a single group may have many different actions. Various CLPs in venom act as anticoagulants, procoagulants, or platelet modulators. PLA_2 enzymes are especially diverse, acting as anticoagulants and platelet modulators in addition to producing myotoxic and neurotoxic effects. Platelet effects result mainly from the action of disintegrins, although CLPs, PLA_2 enzymes, and other proteinases also have platelet-modulating effects.[40,65]

Specific hematologic effects are species dependent, with no single venom containing all of the identified hemostatically active components. Of particular importance to North American rattlesnake envenomation are the thrombinlike enzymes and fibrinogenolytic enzymes. Thrombinlike enzymes are metalloproteinases and serine proteases that preferentially cleave fibrinopeptide A or fibrinopeptide B from fibrinogen. Unlike thrombin, they do not activate factor XIII. The end result is production of a poorly cross-linked fibrin clot that easily degrades. Multiple other venom components exist, some of which affect the vascular system and contribute to the hypotension that sometimes occurs clinically. Examples include bradykinin-potentiating peptides and vascular endothelial growth factors (Chaps. 20 and 58).[53,65]

Snake neurotoxins act at the neuromuscular junction and do not cross the blood–brain barrier. They are classified as α-neurotoxins, which act postsynaptically, and β-neurotoxins, which act presynaptically. Certain populations of the Mojave rattlesnake, *C. scutulatus*, possess a neurotoxin, Mojave toxin, which is a PLA_2 that acts at the presynaptic terminal of the neuromuscular junction to inhibit acetylcholine release. The presence of Mojave toxin in venom appears to be geographically distributed, with Mojave rattlesnake populations in California and southeast Arizona possessing functional Mojave toxin, and central Arizona populations lacking the neurotoxin.[28,64] Mojave toxin is also identified in the venom of some Southern Pacific rattlesnakes (*C. oreganus helleri*) found in southern California, and envenomations by this species are reported to produce neurologic symptoms in some victims.[14,24]

Coral Snakes

Coral snake venom contains neurotoxins that produce systemic neurotoxicity. Unlike crotaline venom, coral snake venom does not cause local tissue injury. Similar to neurotoxins present in other elapid species, α-neurotoxins bind and competitively block postsynaptic acetylcholine receptors at the neuromuscular junction, leading to weakness and paralysis. Phospholipase A_2 can also cause myotoxicity, although this appears to be of less clinical importance. The LD_{50} of *M. fulvius* venom (0.279 mg/kg) is lower than that of *M. tener* venom (0.779 mg/kg), which corresponds to the more severe effects noted in humans following Eastern coral snake envenomations.[48]

Lizards

The pathophysiology of helodermatid venom is poorly understood. It is suggested that hyaluronidase contributes to spreading of venom throughout tissue.[52] Gilatoxin is believed to produce hypotension and other findings such as angioedema by increasing bradykinin levels.[57]

CLINICAL MANIFESTATIONS

Snakes

The clinical presentation of North American snake envenomation is highly variable and depends upon many factors, including the species of snake, the amount and potency of venom deposited, the location of the bite, and patient factors, such as comorbidities. It is important for the clinician to be familiar with endemic venomous snake species in order to anticipate clinical effects when presented with an envenomed patient. For bites by nonnative species, it is important to identify the species so that specific antivenom can be sought.

Pit Vipers

Envenomation by North American pit vipers is characterized by local swelling and cytotoxic effects. Hematologic effects are common, and there is the potential for development of systemic illness and neurotoxicity. Most patients exhibit only a subset of possible effects of envenomation. In addition, some of the signs and symptoms in a given individual, such as nausea or tachycardia, may be related to fear rather than to envenomation.

The clinical presentation following a pit viper bite can range from benign to life threatening (Table 119–3). One finding common to nearly all victims

TABLE 119–3	Evaluation and Treatment of Crotaline Envenomation			
Extent of Envenomation	*Clinical Observations*	*Antivenom Recommended*[a]	*Other Treatment*	*Disposition*
None ("dry bite")	Fang marks are present, but no local or systemic effects after 8–12 hours	No	Local wound care Tetanus prophylaxis	Discharge after 8–12 hours of observation
Minimal	Minor, nonprogressing, local swelling and discomfort without systemic effects or hematologic abnormalities	No	Local wound care Tetanus prophylaxis	Admit to monitored unit for 24-hour observation
Moderate	Progression of swelling beyond area of bite with or without local tissue destruction, hematologic abnormalities, or non–life-threatening systemic effects	Yes	Intravenous fluids Cardiac monitoring Analgesics Follow laboratory parameters Tetanus prophylaxis	Admit to intensive care unit
Severe	Marked progressive swelling, pain with or without local tissue destruction Systemic effects such as diarrhea, weakness, shock, or angioedema, and/or pronounced thrombocytopenia or coagulopathy	Yes	Intravenous fluids Cardiac monitoring Analgesics Follow laboratory parameters Oxygen Vasopressors Tetanus prophylaxis	Admit to intensive care unit

[a]See Antidotes in Depth: A39 for dosing recommendations.

is the presence of an identifiable disruption of skin integrity. Most commonly, one or 2 distinct punctures are present, though occasionally, patients exhibit multiple punctures, small lacerations, or scratches.

Because pit viper bites result in injection of venom only about 75% of the time, approximately 25% of bites do not result in envenomation and are considered "dry bites." Unfortunately, it is impossible to diagnose a dry bite without an extended period of observation, because some patients have delayed onset of findings for as much as 8 to 10 hours following the bite and some subsequently develop serious illness. Even patients who do present with symptoms require a number of hours for the full extent of clinical illness to become evident. As a general rule, however, it is assumed that envenomation from a pit viper has not occurred if no findings develop within 8 to 10 hours from the time of the bite.

Of the North American pit vipers, rattlesnakes are responsible for the most severe clinical presentations. *Agkistrodon* (cottonmouth and copperhead) bites generally tend to produce less severe local and systemic pathology than rattlesnake bites. Copperhead bites in particular rarely cause systemic effects, and pathology is usually limited to soft tissue swelling without necrosis.[60] However, serious copperhead envenomations occasionally occur, and at least one death is associated with a bite from this species.[49]

Local reactions. Generally, within minutes after pit viper envenomation, the area around the puncture site becomes swollen and painful, and oozing of blood from the wound may occur. Edema stabilizes quickly in mild envenomations, but more commonly, edema will gradually worsen over hours. In severe cases, edema progresses to involve an entire extremity within just a few hours. Swelling can worsen for days when untreated, extending proximally to involve the torso following bites to a distal extremity. Rarely, onset of appreciable swelling is delayed for as long as 10 hours. This is most often noted in lower extremity envenomations.

Ecchymosis may develop early at the wound site. Bites to the feet often exhibit a characteristic bluish tinge over the entire dorsal surface of the foot. Toes remain pink and well perfused, allowing distinction of this ecchymosis from cyanosis (Fig. 119–5). In the days to weeks following the envenomation, ecchymosis will often extend or new ecchymosis develops proximally, even in the absence of significant venom-induced hemotoxicity.

Erythema often develops at the envenomation site and sometimes spreads proximally from the wound along lymphatic pathways. Lymphangitic streaks are rare but may occur early after the envenomation in the absence of infection.

Hemorrhagic blisters (blebs or bullae) often form at the site of a rattlesnake bite. This most commonly occurs after bites to digits but in rare instances occurs at other bite locations or dependent areas distant from the bite (Fig. 119–6). Blebs usually do not appear for several hours after the envenomation but when they do develop they often progress for several days. The tissue underlying blebs is often healthy, but extensive bleb development may signify underlying tissue necrosis (Fig. 119–7).

Myonecrosis is not a feature of most native pit viper envenomations but does sometimes occur. In rare cases, fangs directly penetrate muscle leading to localized necrosis. With subfascial envenomation, there is a risk for compartment syndrome, which could lead to deep tissue necrosis. Compartment

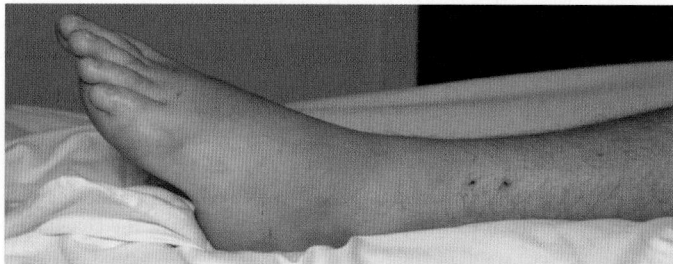

FIGURE 119–5. Rattlesnake bite to the lower leg, with characteristic edema and bluish discoloration of the foot due to ecchymosis. *(Used with the permission from Michelle Ruha, MD.)*

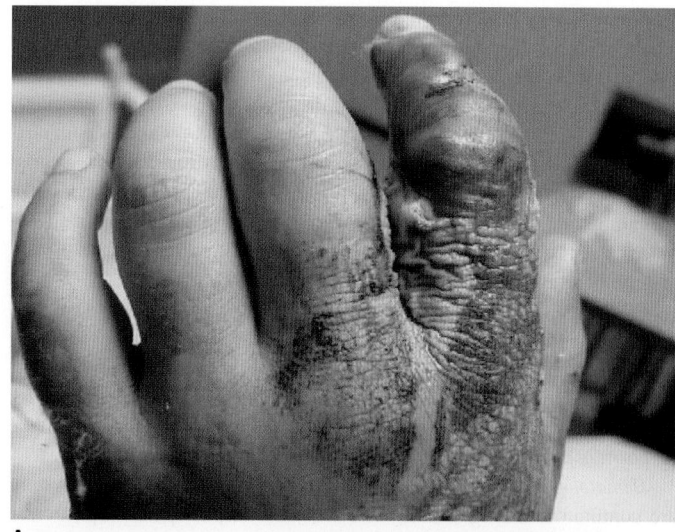

A

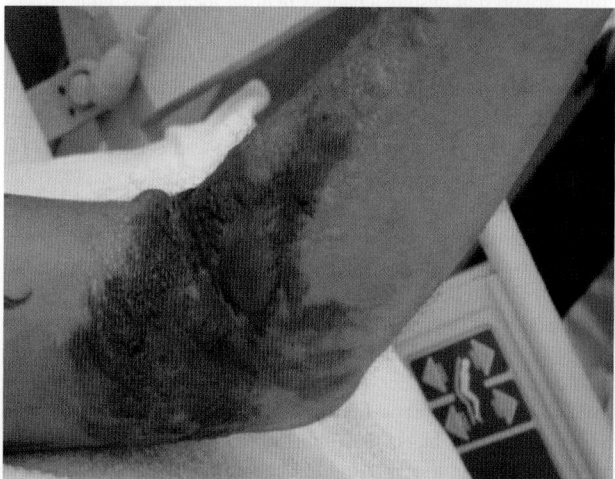

B

FIGURE 119–6. (A) Hemorrhagic bullae involving the entire digit after rattlesnake bite to the second digit. *(Used with the permission from Michelle Ruha, MD.)* **(B)** Hemorrhagic bullae involving the antecubital fossa after rattlesnake bite to the hand. *(Used with the permission from Michelle Ruha, MD.)*

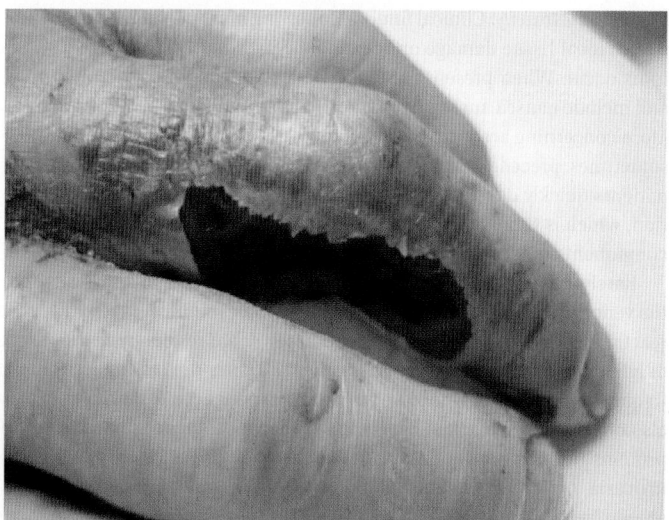

FIGURE 119–7. Debridement of hemorrhagic bullae revealed the underlying tissue to be dark and necrotic in this patient. *(Used with the permission from Michelle Ruha, MD.)*

syndrome is very rare following North American snakebite and cannot be reliably diagnosed in envenomed extremities without directly measuring compartment pressures. More often than not, envenomation simply mimics a compartment syndrome by producing distal paresthesias, tense superficial soft tissue swelling, pain on passive stretch of muscles within a compartment, and muscular weakness. One study using noninvasive vascular arterial studies and skin temperature determinations in patients with rattlesnake envenomation, demonstrated that pulsatile arterial blood flow to an envenomed extremity actually increased after envenomation, even distal to the site of envenomation.[19]

In addition to local myonecrosis, generalized severe rhabdomyolysis occurs in the absence of impressive muscular swelling following some pit viper envenomations. This finding is considered characteristic after envenomation by the Canebrake rattlesnake (*Crotalus horridus atricaudatus*), which was previously classified as a subspecies of the Timber rattlesnake (*C. horridus*). Current prevailing opinion is that they are the same species.[16,56]

Hematologic toxicity. Venom-induced effects on the hematologic system are common following bites by North American pit vipers, in particular rattlesnakes. In rare cases, coagulopathy, thrombocytopenia, or a combination of the 2, are present despite a paucity of other local or systemic effects. The onset, progression, and severity of thrombocytopenia and coagulopathy in patients who exhibit this effect is quite variable. Drops in platelets and fibrinogen are sometimes mild initially, yet continue to worsen for several days following the envenomation. Alternatively, severe decreases in platelet counts (in the 5,000–50,000/mm³ range) and fibrinogen concentrations (to near zero) with immeasurably high prothrombin times (PTs) can occur within minutes to hours of crotaline envenomation. A rise in PT generally follows a drop in fibrinogen, as concentrations of clotting factors remain normal in victims of North American crotaline envenomation with coagulopathy.[15] The likelihood of thrombocytopenia or coagulopathy occurring after a given snakebite depends on the particular species and venom populations present in the geographic area. In the desert southwest, coagulopathy occurs in approximately half and thrombocytopenia in one-third of patients presenting with envenomation.[46] Thrombocytopenia appears to be especially common and often severe after the bite of the Timber rattlesnake (*Crotalus horridus*).[4] The protein crotalocytin that is found in Timber rattlesnake venom causes platelet aggregation and is thought to be at least partially responsible for the thrombocytopenia.

Despite the high rate of hematologic effects following rattlesnake envenomations, the vast majority of patients have no clinical bleeding, even when severe laboratory abnormalities are present. Bleeding appears to be more common when platelets are very low or when both coagulopathy and thrombocytopenia are present and severe.

Systemic toxicity. Clinical findings following most pit viper bites are limited to local tissue damage or hematologic pathology, but systemic symptoms occur. When present, systemic signs and symptoms are often mild and include nausea, metallic taste, restlessness, and nonspecific weakness. More concerning are tachycardia, vomiting, diarrhea, or confusion, which sometimes precede severe systemic toxicity. In the most severe cases, patients quickly develop circulatory shock or airway edema with obstruction, which is thought to be caused by anaphylactoid responses to venom components.

Rarely, patients bitten by crotalids experience classic anaphylaxis from the venom itself, which complicates evaluation or mimics a severe systemic reaction to venom. Previous sensitization to venom results in development of IgE antibodies to venom in these patients. This is thought to occur more frequently in patients who have previously experienced a snakebite, but is also observed in snake handlers who are thought to be sensitized to snake proteins through inhalation or skin contact. The presence of pruritus and urticaria or wheezing, uncommon with envenomation, should suggest anaphylaxis.

There are rare reports of true disseminated intravascular coagulation (DIC) with spontaneous bleeding along with significant hypotension and multiorgan system failure following rattlesnake bite. In such cases of true DIC, the patient has evidence of organ infarction and hemolysis. This is reported after intravascular envenomation.[20]

Neurotoxicity. Although local tissue destruction dominates the picture of Crotalinae envenomations, neurotoxic effects sometimes occur. The Mojave rattlesnake (*C. scutulatus*) is best known for its neurotoxic venom. Some populations of the Mojave rattlesnake possess a neurotoxin, Mojave toxin, which can result in weakness, cranial nerve dysfunction, and respiratory paralysis in victims.[33] The Timber rattlesnake (*C. horridus*) is noted to commonly cause rippling fasciculations of the skin (myokymia), particularly of the facial muscles.[6] Fasciculations are reported following envenomation by several other species of rattlesnake, including the Western diamondback (*C. atrox*), Mojave (*C. scutulatus*), and the Southern Pacific (*C. o. helleri*).[17] Fasciculations involving the shoulders, chest wall, and torso are associated with development of respiratory failure.[58]

Coral Snakes

Coral snake fangs are small and nonmobile, and as a result, bites are less likely than pit viper bites to lead to envenomation. An estimated 40% of patients bitten by a coral snake are subsequently determined to be envenomed, with rates for the Eastern coral snake species possibly higher.[35] The venom of the Eastern coral snake (*Micrurus fulvius*) and Texas coral snake (*M. tener*) are more potent than that of the Sonoran coral snake (*Micruroides euryxanthus*). In fact, there are no reported cases of serious toxicity after the bite of the Sonoran coral snake, which is found primarily in Arizona and western New Mexico.

Coral snake fangs do not always produce easily identifiable puncture wounds. In addition to the absence of a discernable wound in some victims, coral snake envenomations are characterized by potentially serious neurotoxicity without impressive local symptoms. The effects of envenomation are characteristically delayed for a number of hours. One report described a patient who had an asymptomatic period of 13 hours followed by rapid development of paralysis severe enough to require ventilatory support.[35] Neurologic abnormalities reported with coral snake envenomation include paresthesias, slurred speech, ptosis, diplopia, dysphagia, stridor, muscle weakness, fasciculations, and paralysis. The major cause of death is respiratory failure secondary to neuromuscular weakness. Muscle weakness takes weeks to months to resolve completely. With respiratory support, however, paralysis is completely reversible. Pulmonary aspiration is a common sequela in the subacute phase.

Lizards

The rate of envenomation following Gila monster bites is not known, but one case series reported 40% dry bites.[47] *Heloderma* species are known for hanging on to their victims when they bite. Multiple reports are documented where Gila monsters were attached to the victim for up to 15 minutes, and in some cases teeth have broken off in the wound.

Pain is immediate following a bite, and local soft tissue edema often develops within minutes. Swelling extends from the puncture site, though not as commonly or dramatically as occurs following pit viper envenomation. Helodermatid venom does not produce local tissue necrosis, but erythema at the wound site and extension of erythema to an entire extremity is well described. Lymphangitic streaking is also reported.[23,32,52]

Nausea, vomiting, and diaphoresis are reported following helodermatid envenomation. Patients are often tachycardic and hypotension is common. There are numerous reports of upper airway angioedema developing after bites by both Gila monsters and beaded lizards. There is a single report of a young man developing a myocardial infarction after a Gila monster envenomation.[44] This patient also exhibited a coagulopathy although Gila monster venom does not typically produce abnormalities in platelet counts or clotting factors. It is suggested that the coagulopathy occurred as a result of endothelial damage rather than direct effect of venom on the hematologic system.[52] Leukocytosis is common following Gila monster envenomation, with reported white blood cell counts as high as 48,000/mm³.[44]

DIAGNOSTIC TESTING

Snakes

Diagnosis of North American snake envenomation is based on a history of a snakebite and presence of clinical signs of envenomation. There are no available laboratory assays for detection of venom in a wound. Although it is possible to measure blood and urine venom antigen concentrations using enzyme-linked immunosorbent assay (ELISA), this is only available in research settings and is not useful for early diagnosis or clinical management of envenomation.

Platelet counts, fibrinogen concentrations, and PTs are useful in the diagnosis of pit viper envenomation if they are abnormal. However, normal results do not exclude envenomation because thrombocytopenia and coagulopathy do not develop in all patients with pit viper envenomation.

A validated severity score for the objective assessment of crotaline envenomation has been developed and can be useful in a research setting.[21] Its purpose is to assess the clinical condition of patients with snakebite, but it is not intended as a diagnostic tool. Caution should be used when applying this scale because envenomation is a dynamic process and severity can worsen or improve with time, limiting the utility of the score obtained at any given point in time.

Lizards

The diagnosis of helodermatid envenomation is based on the history of a bite and presence of physical examination findings consistent with envenomation. There are no laboratory studies that are available to confirm or exclude the diagnosis, but a complete blood count may reveal leukocytosis.

MANAGEMENT

Snakes

When a patient with a snake bite presents for care, the initial objectives are to determine the presence or absence of envenomation, provide basic supportive therapy, treat the local and systemic effects of envenomation, and limit tissue loss or functional disability (Table 119–3). A combination of medical therapy (mainly supportive care and, often, antivenom) and in some cases conservative surgical treatment (mainly debridement of devitalized tissue), individualized for each patient, will provide the best results. In general, the more rapidly treatment is instituted, the shorter the period of disability.

Pit Vipers

Prehospital care. No first aid measure or specific field treatment has been proven to positively affect outcome following a crotaline envenomation. Prehospital care should generally be limited to immobilization of the affected limb, placement of an intravenous catheter, treatment of life-threatening clinical findings, and rapid transport to a medical facility. If transport time is long and pain is severe, administration of analgesics is recommended. Patients who are volume depleted, vomiting, or experiencing systemic effects such as diarrhea should be given an intravenous fluid bolus. Hypotension that does not quickly respond to a fluid bolus should be treated with epinephrine, since early hypotension is most likely due to anaphylaxis, anaphylactoid reaction to venom, or venom-induced vasodilation. Epinephrine counteracts these effects through stimulation of α-adrenergic receptors on vasculature as well as through inhibition of release of inflammatory mediators.

In the past, various methods were advocated to prevent systemic absorption of venom after snakebites. All of these methods are either ineffective, delay time to definitive care, or are potentially harmful. Such useless and potentially dangerous therapies include tourniquets, incision and suction, venom extractors, electrotherapy, and cryotherapy.[1,12]

Pressure immobilization bandages (PIBs), which are lymphatic-restricting bandages that are applied to the bitten extremity prior to immobilization with a splint, should not be used in patients with North American Crotalinae bites. A randomized, controlled study of pressure immobilization versus observation in a porcine model with intramuscular injection of *Crotalus atrox* venom showed markedly increased compartment pressures in the pressure immobilization group. All animals died in this study, but the pressure immobilization group showed a prolonged time to death as compared to the control group. With local tissue necrosis being the major morbidity associated with pit viper envenomations in humans, not death, the authors concluded that PIB application cannot be recommended as a routine field procedure.[11] The American College of Medical Toxicology, along with 5 other international organizations, released a position statement recommending against use of PIB for North American Crotalinae bites.[2]

Hospital care. When a patient presents to the hospital with history of crotaline snakebite, it is important to first determine whether an envenomation has occurred. Although most patients do show early evidence of envenomation, absence of symptoms at presentation is not uncommon, and not all asymptomatic patients ultimately have "dry" bites. Patients who present with puncture wounds but without swelling or other evidence of envenomation must be observed for delayed onset of symptoms. An observation period of 8 hours for *Agkistrodon* bites and 12 hours for rattlesnake bites is recommended.[38] If no swelling develops, and laboratory study samples drawn at least 8 hours from the time of the bite remain normal and unchanged, the bite is likely "dry" and the patient is safe for discharge from medical care with instructions to return if new pain or swelling develops.

Supportive. The initial in-hospital assessment of North American crotaline envenomation should focus on airway, breathing, and circulation. Patients with evidence of angioedema or with bites to the face or tongue need to be observed closely for signs of airway compromise and intubated early, before swelling progresses to the point of airway obstruction. All patients, regardless of presenting symptoms, should have an intravenous catheter placed in an unaffected extremity and an IV fluid bolus is recommended. Patients presenting with cardiovascular collapse should receive large volumes of fluid. An epinephrine continuous infusion, starting at 0.1 mcg/kg/min and titrating as needed, is the authors' vasopressor of choice for signs of shock following envenomation.

Immobilization of the affected extremity in a padded splint in near-full extension and elevation above the level of the heart to avoid dependent edema is recommended. Although there are no studies to determine the effect of limb elevation on outcome the authors find this helpful because it appears to decrease dependent edema, which contributes to increased pain and physical examination findings concerning for compartment syndrome. The authors maximally elevate affected upper extremities by applying stocking net around the limb and attaching the distal end to a raised IV pole.

Marking the leading edge of swelling with a pen or sequentially measuring extremity circumference will help to identify progression of edema. A baseline complete blood count, PT, and fibrinogen concentration should be obtained initially and repeated in 4 to 6 hours. Patients who are systemically ill should also have electrolytes, creatinine phosphokinase, creatinine, glucose, and urinalysis checked.

A comprehensive physical examination should be done, with emphasis on vital signs, cardiorespiratory and neurologic status, neurovascular status of the affected extremity, and evaluation for evidence of bleeding. Pain should be treated with opioid analgesics as needed, and tetanus prophylaxis should be addressed. The patient should be reassessed frequently with repeat physical examinations, specifically noting any progression of swelling. This is best accomplished by taking serial circumferential measurements of the involved extremity at multiple points proximal to the wound.

Prophylactic antibiotics should not be given, as studies show extremely low (0%–3%) rates of wound infections.[39] There is no indication for corticosteroids or antihistamines in the routine treatment of patients with snakebites, except for treatment of anaphylaxis.

Antivenom. Patients with dry bites or mild envenomations, such as those who present with only localized swelling that fails to progress, do not meet criteria for antivenom[38] (Table 119–3). Patients who present with progressive swelling, thrombocytopenia, coagulopathy, neurotoxicity, or significant systemic toxicity are candidates for antivenom therapy. Antivenom given in a timely manner can reverse coagulopathy and thrombocytopenia and halt progression of local swelling. Antivenom has also been shown to reduces compartment pressure and limits venom-induced decreases in perfusion pressure, potentially preventing the need for fasciotomy.[26,54] There is no evidence, however, that antivenom can prevent or reverse the development of tissue necrosis, so patients should be informed of the risk of tissue loss. This is most commonly noted with rattlesnake bites to the fingers, which occasionally lead to amputation of the digit despite appropriate treatment with antivenom.

Until fall of 2018, the only available FDA-approved antivenom for North American pit viper envenomation is Crotalidae polyvalent immune Fab (Cro-Fab, BTG). Crotalidae polyvalent immune Fab is an ovine-derived Fab fragment antivenom developed from commonly encountered North American pit vipers (*C. atrox, C. adamanteus, C. scutulatus, A. piscivorus*). Crotalidae polyvalent immune Fab is administered IV in an initial dose of 4 to 6 vials reconstituted in 0.9% sodium chloride solution. The recommended starting dose for patients who present with cardiovascular collapse or serious active bleeding is 8 to 12 vials.[38] The infusion is initiated at a slow rate for several minutes, and if no signs of an anaphylactoid reaction develop, increased to complete the infusion over one hour. The patient should be reassessed after completion of the infusion for evidence of continued swelling or worsening thrombocytopenia, and, if present, an additional 4- to 6-vial dose is infused. This process is repeated until control of symptoms is achieved. Fibrinogen and PT are sometimes slower to recover in response to antivenom. If these are the only findings that continue to be abnormal after antivenom, it is reasonable to repeat these studies in 4 hours to determine if redosing of antivenom is necessary. Control is generally considered cessation of progression of swelling and systemic symptoms in addition to improvement in coagulopathy and thrombocytopenia. After control is achieved, maintenance doses of antivenom are given as 2 vials every 6 hours for 3 doses (6 total additional vials after control). Although recommended in the package insert for Crotalidae polyvalent immune Fab, maintenance therapy is not routinely administered by all practitioners.[7] The authors recommend use of maintenance doses unless the patient can be observed closely in the hospital for 18 hours after control of the envenomation is achieved. During this observation period, additional antivenom is given as needed for local or hematologic recurrence.

An alternative antivenom for the treatment of North American rattlesnake envenomation was approved by the FDA in 2015 but is not expected to be available until the fall of 2018. This antivenom, Crotalidae equine immune F(ab')$_2$ (Anavip), is made using venoms of *Bothrops asper* and *Crotalus simus*. A randomized controlled trial comparing Crotalidae polyvalent immune Fab to Crotalidae equine immune F(ab')$_2$ found less late hematologic toxicity in patients who received Crotalidae equine immune F(ab')$_2$.[13] This is likely due to the longer half-life of Fab$_2$ fragments as compared to Fab fragments. The initial dose of Crotalidae equine immune F(ab')$_2$ is 10 vials. After infusion, the patient should be reassessed for further progression of swelling, worsening hematologic toxicity, or continuation of other systemic venom effects, such as neurotoxicity. Additional 10 vial doses are administered until control of the envenomation is achieved. Following control, the patient should be observed for another 18 hours for signs of recurrent venom toxicity. If these occur, additional 4 vial doses of Anavip are given (Antidotes in Depth: A39).[22]

Antivenom administration in children follows the same guidelines as adults, with doses based on clinical presentation and laboratory findings rather than weight. Attention should be paid to total amount of fluid received, and if necessary, antivenom can be reconstituted in a smaller total volume of fluid. Generally, patients with severe snake envenomation have large fluid requirements, and pulmonary edema as a result of antivenom administration has not been reported.

Pregnant patients who meet criteria for treatment should also receive antivenom. Crotalidae polyvalent immune Fab (ovine) and Crotalidae equine immune F(ab')$_2$ are currently listed as pregnancy category C, but the former has been used safely during pregnancy.[36] Given the relative safety of these antivenoms and the potential for fetal demise after envenomation, a low threshold for treatment should be considered. Fetal and maternal monitoring should be carried out throughout the patient's care.[37]

Surgery. Surgery is not routinely indicated following snakebites. An extensive review of the literature failed to identify any evidence to support the use of fasciotomy in the treatment of snakebites.[18] There are reported cases of elevated compartment pressure after pit viper envenomation successfully managed without fasciotomy. When compartment syndrome is suspected, intracompartmental pressures should be measured. It is reasonable to attempt to treat moderately elevated compartment pressures with antivenom initially, but clinical examination and compartment pressures should be followed closely. If compartment pressures are rising despite administration of antivenom or if the patient develops evidence of limb ischemia, fasciotomy is recommended.

Patients with bites to the digit sometimes present with evidence of ischemia. The compromised finger appears cyanotic or pale, tense, and lacks sensation. The small diameter of the digit and limited ability of the skin to expand essentially creates a small compartment. In such cases it is recommended to perform a digital dermotomy, where a longitudinal incision is made through the skin on the medial or lateral aspect of the digit in order to decompress the neurovascular structures. Dermotomy should not be performed prophylactically in cases of digital envenomation, as most patients have good outcome without any surgical intervention.[30]

Debridement of hemorrhagic blebs and blisters is often performed to evaluate underlying tissue and relieve discomfort. Some patients require surgical debridement of necrotic tissue or even amputation of a digit 1 to 2 weeks after the bite. Referral to a hand surgeon is appropriate for patients with evidence of extensive tissue necrosis.

Blood Products. Immeasurably low fibrinogen concentrations, PTs greater than 100 seconds, and platelet counts lower than 20,000/mm^3 are routinely encountered after rattlesnake envenomation. Such abnormal laboratory results alone should not prompt the clinician to treat with blood products in the absence of clinically significant bleeding. The circulating crotaline venom responsible for the thrombocytopenia and coagulopathy is still present and will likely inactivate any transfused components. For this reason, the mainstay of treatment for crotaline envenomation–induced hematopathology is antivenom, not blood products. Correction of coagulopathy, thrombocytopenia, and bleeding is usually achieved with antivenom alone. Rarely, a patient will have clinically significant bleeding, and antivenom alone will not correct the platelets and fibrinogen. In such cases, fresh-frozen plasma, cryoprecipitate, packed red blood cells, or platelet transfusions are recommended to replace losses.

In some cases, thrombocytopenia is difficult, or impossible, to correct with even large amounts of antivenom. The Timber rattlesnake, for example, is known for producing thrombocytopenia resistant to antivenom. The initial correction of platelet counts after treatment is typically transient (lasting only 12–24 hours), with thrombocytopenia sometimes persisting for days to weeks after normalization of other coagulation parameters. In the absence of bleeding, thrombocytopenia is a benign, self-limiting disorder, resolving within 2 to 3 weeks of envenomation. It is best to closely follow patients with resistant thrombocytopenia who are not bleeding, rather than attempt further platelet transfusions or antivenom administration.[42]

Follow-up care. Hospital stays for patients with uncomplicated pit viper envenomations are typically short, lasting approximately 1 to 2 days.[46] Upon discharge from the hospital, patients often have residual swelling and functional disability. Some will have continued progression of hemorrhagic bullae with underlying necrosis. Patients should have an out-patient follow-up evaluation to ensure wounds are healing appropriately and extremity function is returning. If joint mobility does not return to baseline as swelling resolves, the patient should be referred for physical and occupational therapy.

In a significant proportion of rattlesnake bite patients treated with Crotalidae polyvalent immune Fab antivenom, a return of swelling, coagulopathy, or thrombocytopenia is noted days to weeks after initial resolution with effective antivenom treatment. This is termed "recurrence" of venom effect and is attributed to the interrelated kinetics and dynamics of venom and antivenom.[5,46] Simply stated, Fab antivenom has a clinical half-life shorter than that of venom. Administration of maintenance doses of antivenom is used in an attempt to prevent development of recurrent effects. Maintenance doses appear to be effective in preventing recurrence of local swelling in most cases, but many patients develop hematologic recurrence within 3 to 7 days of antivenom treatment despite administration of maintenance doses. Additionally, some patients who never manifested thrombocytopenia or coagulopathy during their hospital presentation later develop the effect, presumably because of initial "masking" of the effect by early antivenom administration. These recurrent or late hematologic effects have been associated with life-threatening bleeding.[34] No risk factors have been identified to predict which patients will develop late thrombocytopenia or coagulopathy.

The most reasonable way to address possible late hematologic effects of crotaline envenomation is careful outpatient follow-up after hospital discharge. Provide careful discharge instructions and consider all patients who have been treated with Crotalidae polyvalent immune Fab antivenom to be at risk for late hematologic toxicity. Patients who use antiplatelet or anticoagulant medications should be continued on these medications only after a careful risk–benefit analysis. Whenever possible the medications should be discontinued until the risk of recurrent or late hematologic toxicity passes. Patients must be warned not to undergo dental or surgical procedures for up to 3 weeks unless platelet and coagulation studies are documented to be normal immediately prior to the procedure. High-risk activities, such as contact sports, should be avoided. All patients with rattlesnake bites should have platelets and coagulation studies measured 2 to 3 days, and again 5 to 7 days, after the last antivenom treatment. If values are abnormal or trending in the wrong direction, the studies should be repeated every few days until normal and stable. Because copperhead envenomation is much less likely to produce severe hemotoxicity, one set of follow-up laboratory studies to screen for late thrombocytopenia or coagulopathy is reasonable in this population. Patients should be advised to avoid surgical procedures and activities that place them at risk for injury. Opinions on when to retreat patients exhibiting late hematologic toxicity with antivenom vary. The general approach of the authors is to retreat any patient with evidence of bleeding, as well as patients with severe isolated thrombocytopenia (platelets <25,000/mm³) or moderate thrombocytopenia (platelets 25,000–50,000/mm³) in combination with severe coagulopathy (fibrinogen <80 mg/dL).[46] Many clinicians choose to observe patients with isolated coagulopathy cautiously as outpatients rather than to retreat them with antivenom. However, if patients with isolated severe coagulopathy have other risk factors for bleeding, such as use of antiplatelet medications, high risk of injury, recent venom-induced shock, or pregnancy, retreatment with antivenom is recommended.

When the decision is made to retreat a patient with late hemotoxicity with antivenom, an initial starting dose of 2 vials is recommended. Late thrombocytopenia appears to be more resistant to antivenom than early venom-induced thrombocytopenia, and it is unclear whether a different mechanism is responsible for the late effect. It is unknown how much antivenom is needed to reverse late thrombocytopenia or at what dose a patient is considered "resistant" to antivenom. Based on anecdotal experience, if platelet counts do not increase after 2 to 3 doses of antivenom, additional antivenom is unlikely to be effective. Response to platelet transfusions is also often poor. Some clinicians give steroids to patients who have not responded to antivenom and platelet transfusions, but there is no evidence to support this treatment, which has not been studied.

Coral Snakes

As with North American pit viper bites, patients who are bitten by North American coral snakes should be taken to a hospital for definitive medical care as soon as possible. There are no field treatments that have been shown to affect outcome in these patients, although use of PIBs is reasonable if transport to a hospital will be prolonged or delayed. Unlike with crotalid bites, worsening of local tissue injury as a result of PIBs is not a concern with coral snakebite. Pressure immobilization bandages delay the systemic absorption of venom from Australian elapid snakes, and a swine model of coral snake envenomation supports a similar effect.[27] Patients who present for care after a PIB has been placed should have the dressing left in place

until resuscitative equipment and personnel are present and, ideally, antivenom is available. The PIB should be checked to ensure it is not functioning as a tourniquet.

Patients with a history concerning for possible Eastern or Texas coral snakebite should be observed for 24 hours in a monitored unit where resuscitative measures, including endotracheal intubation, can be performed. Because neuromuscular weakness and respiratory paralysis can develop quickly, endotracheal intubation is reasonable at the first sign of bulbar paralysis. In the past, treatment with Wyeth Antivenin (*Micrurus fulvius*) (equine origin) North American Coral Snake Antivenin was recommended for all patients in whom there is strong suspicion of coral snakebite, even in the absence of signs of envenomation. This is mainly because paralysis can develop quickly and symptoms may not reverse following antivenom treatment. However, a study comparing patients who received empiric treatment with antivenom to patients who were treated when symptoms developed suggests that a conservative approach (waiting for symptoms to develop before administering antivenom) does not result in worse outcomes for patients.[63] North American Coral Snake Antivenom (Equine) is now available from Pfizer, and administration to asymptomatic patients is listed as a contraindication in the package insert.[43]

If a patient is symptomatic following a coral snake envenomation, antivenom, if available, is indicated. If antivenom is unavailable, supportive care including mechanical ventilation may be necessary for many weeks. Acetylcholinesterase inhibitors have been inconsistently successful in treating patients with South American coral snakebites.[8] If availability of coral snake antivenom is delayed, a trial of neostigmine to reverse the neurotoxic effects of venom is reasonable.

Sonoran coral snakes, indigenous to Arizona and California, have never been reported to cause significant toxicity, and bite victims do not require observation in the hospital or antivenom administration.

Lizards

Management of helodermatid envenomation consists of supportive care. There is no antivenom available against lizard venom. Routine wound care should be performed, and the clinician should look for the presence of teeth in the wound. There is no evidence to guide clinicians when deciding whether to administer antibiotics to patients with erythema surrounding and extending from the bite site. Most case reports describing patients with erythema also report empiric use of antibiotics. There are no reports of confirmed infections following these bites.

Patients who are symptomatic following a bite should be attached to a cardiac monitor and have an intravenous catheter placed. Although serious morbidity from lizard bites is unusual, life-threatening manifestations of envenomation are reported. Angioedema, other evidence of respiratory compromise, or airway obstruction should prompt endotracheal intubation. Hypotension should be treated with intravenous fluid boluses as well as vasopressors such as epinephrine. Epinephrine, corticosteroids, and antihistamines are recommended for the treatment of anaphylactoid reactions.

SUMMARY

- Most native snake envenomations result from bites by Crotalinae species of snakes, also known as pit vipers, and commonly produce local tissue swelling and hematologic toxicity.
- A small percentage of envenomations are due to bites by coral snakes, which are known for producing neurotoxicity without local tissue effects.
- Management of patients with pit viper and coral snake envenomation should focus on aggressive supportive care and specific antivenom when indicated.
- Envenomations by Helodermatid lizards are often associated with local pain, erythema, hypotension, and angioedema.
- Clinicians are encouraged to contact a regional poison control center when a patient presents after a snake or lizard envenomation.

REFERENCES

1. Alberts MB, et al. Suction for venomous snakebite: a study of "mock venom" extraction in a human model. *Ann Emerg Med.* 2004;43:181-186.
2. American College of Medical T, et al. Pressure immobilization after North American Crotalinae snake envenomation. *J Med Toxicol.* 2011;7:322-323.
3. Audebert F, et al. Viper bites in France: clinical and biological evaluation; kinetics of envenomations. *Hum Exp Toxicol.* 1994;13:683-688.
4. Bond RG, Burkhart KK. Thrombocytopenia following timber rattlesnake envenomation. *Ann Emerg Med.* 1997;30:40-44.
5. Boyer LV, et al. Recurrence phenomena after immunoglobulin therapy for snake envenomations: part 2. Guidelines for clinical management with crotaline Fab antivenom. *Ann Emerg Med.* 2001;37:196-201.
6. Brick JF, et al. Timber rattlesnake venom-induced myokymia: evidence for peripheral nerve origin. *Neurology.* 1987;37:1545-1546.
7. BTG. CroFab package insert. http://www.crofab.com/viewpdf.do?documentId=1. Accessed December 20, 2012.
8. Bucaretchi F, et al. Bites by coral snakes (*Micrurus* spp.) in Campinas, State of Sao Paulo, Southeastern Brazil. *Rev Inst Med Trop Sao Paulo. Rev Inst Med Trop Sao Paulo.* 2006;48:141-145.
9. Bucher B, et al. Clinical indicators of envenoming and serum levels of venom antigens in patients bitten by *Bothrops lanceolatus* in Martinique. Research Group on Snake Bites in Martinique. *Trans R Soc Trop Med Hyg.* 1997;91:186-190.
10. Burgess JL, et al. Effects of constriction bands on rattlesnake venom absorption: a pharmacokinetic study. *Ann Emerg Med.* 1992;21:1086-1093.
11. Bush SP, et al. Pressure immobilization delays mortality and increases intracompartmental pressure after artificial intramuscular rattlesnake envenomation in a porcine model. *Ann Emerg Med.* 2004;44:599-604.
12. Bush SP, et al. Effects of a negative pressure venom extraction device (Extractor) on local tissue injury after artificial rattlesnake envenomation in a porcine model. *Wilderness Environ Med.* 2000;11:180-188.
13. Bush SP, et al. Comparison of F(ab')2 versus Fab antivenom for pit viper envenomation: a prospective, blinded, multicenter, randomized clinical trial. *Clin Toxicol (Phila).* 2015;53:37-45.
14. Bush SP, Siedenburg E. Neurotoxicity associated with suspected southern Pacific rattlesnake (*Crotalus viridis helleri*) envenomation. *Wilderness Environ Med.* 1999;10:247-249.
15. Camilleri C, et al. Conservative management of delayed, multicomponent coagulopathy following rattlesnake envenomation. *Clin Toxicol (Phila).* 2005;43:201-206.
16. Carroll RR, et al. Canebrake rattlesnake envenomation. *Ann Emerg Med.* 1997;30:45-48.
17. Clark RF, et al. Successful treatment of crotalid-induced neurotoxicity with a new polyspecific crotalid Fab antivenom. *Ann Emerg Med.* 1997;30:54-57.
18. Cumpston KL. Is there a role for fasciotomy in Crotalinae envenomations in North America? *Clin Toxicol (Phila).* 2011;49:351-365.
19. Curry SC, et al. Noninvasive vascular studies in management of rattlesnake envenomations to extremities. *Ann Emerg Med.* 1985;14:1081-1084.
20. Curry SC, Kunkel DB. Toxicology rounds. Death from a rattlesnake bite. *Am J Emerg Med.* 1985;3:227-235.
21. Dart RC, et al. Validation of a severity score for the assessment of crotalid snakebite. *Ann Emerg Med.* 1996;27:321-326.
22. FDA.gov. Anavip. 2015; Anavip highlights of prescribing information. Accessed September 8, 2015.
23. French RN, et al. Gila monster bite. *Clin Toxicol (Phila).* 2012;50:151-152.
24. French WJ, et al. Mojave toxin in venom of *Crotalus helleri* (Southern Pacific Rattlesnake): molecular and geographic characterization. *Toxicon.* 2004;44:781-791.
25. Furman BL. The development of Byetta (exenatide) from the venom of the Gila monster as an anti-diabetic agent. *Toxicon.* 2012;59:464-471.
26. Garfin SR, et al. The effect of antivenin on intramuscular pressure elevations induced by rattlesnake venom. *Toxicon.* 1985;23:677-680.
27. German BT, et al. Pressure-immobilization bandages delay toxicity in a porcine model of eastern coral snake (*Micrurus fulvius*) envenomation. *Ann Emerg Med.* 2005;45:603-608.
28. Glenn JL, et al. Geographical variation in *Crotalus scutulatus* (Mojave rattlesnake) venom properties. *Toxicon.* 1983;21:119-130.
29. Gutierrez JM, et al. Trends in snakebite envenomation therapy: scientific, technological and public health considerations. *Curr Pharm Des.* 2007;13:2935-2950.
30. Hall EL. Role of surgical intervention in the management of crotaline snake envenomation. *Ann Emerg Med.* 2001;37:175-180.
31. Ho M, et al. Clinical significance of venom antigen levels in patients envenomed by the Malayan pit viper (*Calloselasma rhodostoma*). *Am J Trop Med Hyg.* 1986;35:579-587.
32. Hooker KR, et al. Gila monster envenomation. *Ann Emerg Med.* 1994;24:731-735.
33. Jansen PW, et al. Mojave rattlesnake envenomation: prolonged neurotoxicity and rhabdomyolysis. *Ann Emerg Med.* 1992;21:322-325.
34. Kitchens C, Eskin T. Fatality in a case of envenomation by *Crotalus adamanteus* initially successfully treated with polyvalent ovine antivenom followed by recurrence of defibrinogenation syndrome. *J Med Toxicol.* 2008;4:180-183.
35. Kitchens CS, Van Mierop LH. Envenomation by the Eastern coral snake (*Micrurus fulvius*). A study of 39 victims. *JAMA.* 1987;258:1615-1618.
36. LaMonica GE, et al. Rattlesnake bites in pregnant women. *J Reprod Med.* 2010;55:520-522.
37. Langley RL. Snakebite during pregnancy: a literature review. *Wilderness Environ Med.* 2010;21:54-60.
38. Lavonas EJ, et al. Unified treatment algorithm for the management of crotaline snakebite in the United States: results of an evidence-informed consensus workshop. *BMC Emerg Med.* 2011;11:2.
39. LoVecchio F, et al. Antibiotics after rattlesnake envenomation. *J Emerg Med.* 2002;23:327-328.
40. Lu Q, et al. Snake venoms and hemostasis. *J Thromb Haemost.* 2005;3:1791-1799.
41. Mowry JB, et al. 2015 Annual Report of the American Association of Poison Control Centers' National Poison Data System (NPDS): 33rd Annual Report. *Clin Toxicol (Phila).* 2016;54:924-1109.
42. Odeleye AA, et al. Report of two cases: Rattlesnake venom-induced thrombocytopenia. *Ann Clin Lab Sci.* 2004;34:467-470.
43. Pfizer. North American Coral Snake Antivenin. 2016. http://labeling.pfizer.com/showlabeling.aspx?id=441. Accessed November 2016.
44. Preston CA. Hypotension, myocardial infarction, and coagulopathy following gila monster bite. *J Emerg Med.* 1989;7:37-40.
45. Reimers AR, et al. Are anaphylactic reactions to snake bites immunoglobulin E-mediated? *Clin Exp Allergy.* 2000;30:276-282.
46. Ruha AM, et al. Late hematologic toxicity following treatment of rattlesnake envenomation with crotalidae polyvalent immune Fab antivenom. *Toxicon.* 2011;57:53-59.
47. Russell FE, Bogert CM. Gila monster: its biology, venom and bite—a review. *Toxicon.* 1981;19:341-359.
48. Sanchez EE, et al. Neutralization of two North American coral snake venoms with United States and Mexican antivenoms. *Toxicon.* 2008;51:297-303.
49. Seifert SA, et al. AAPCC database characterization of native U.S. venomous snake exposures, 2001-2005. *Clin Toxicol (Phila).* 2009;47:327-335.
50. Seifert SA, et al. Relationship of venom effects to venom antigen and antivenom serum concentrations in a patient with *Crotalus atrox* envenomation treated with a Fab antivenom. *Ann Emerg Med.* 1997;30:49-53.
51. Seifert SA, et al. Toxic Exposure Surveillance System (TESS)-based characterization of U.S. non-native venomous snake exposures, 1995-2004. *Clin Toxicol (Phila).* 2007;45:571-578.
52. Strimple PD, et al. Report on envenomation by a Gila monster (*Heloderma suspectum*) with a discussion of venom apparatus, clinical findings, and treatment. *Wilderness Environ Med.* 1997;8:111-116.
53. Swenson S, Markland FS Jr. Snake venom fibrin(ogen)olytic enzymes. *Toxicon.* 2005;45:1021-1039.
54. Tanen DA, et al. Crotalidae polyvalent immune Fab antivenom limits the decrease in perfusion pressure of the anterior leg compartment in a porcine crotaline envenomation model. *Ann Emerg Med.* 2003;41:384-390.
55. Teixeira Cde F, et al. Inflammatory effects of snake venom metalloproteinases. *Mem Inst Oswaldo Cruz.* 2005;100(suppl 1):181-184.
56. Uetz P, Hallermann J. *Crotalus horridus* LINNAEUS, 1758. http://reptile-database.reptarium.cz/species?genus=Crotalus&species=horridus&search_param=%28%28taxon%3D%27Crotalinae%27%29%29. Accessed December 20, 2012.
57. Utaisincharoen P, et al. Complete primary structure and biochemical properties of gilatoxin, a serine protease with kallikrein-like and angiotensin-degrading activities. *J Biol Chem.* 1993;268:21975-21983.
58. Vohra R, et al. Fasciculations after rattlesnake envenomations: a retrospective statewide poison control system study. *Clin Toxicol (Phila).* 2008;46:117-121.
59. Vonk FJ, et al. Snake venom: From fieldwork to the clinic: Recent insights into snake biology, together with new technology allowing high-throughput screening of venom, bring new hope for drug discovery. *Bioessays.* 2011;33:269-279.
60. Walker JP, Morrison RL. Current management of copperhead snakebite. *J Am Coll Surg.* 2011;212:470-474; discussion 474-475.
61. Walter FG, et al. Temporal analyses of coral snakebite severity published in the American Association of Poison Control Centers' Annual Reports from 1983 through 2007. *Clin Toxicol (Phila).* 2010;48:72-78.
62. Weinstein SA, Keyler DE. Local envenoming by the Western hognose snake (*Heterodon nasicus*): a case report and review of medically significant Heterodon bites. *Toxicon.* 2009;54:354-360.
63. Wood A, et al. Review of Eastern coral snake (*Micrurus fulvius*) exposures in Florida: 1998-2010. *Clin Toxicol (Phila).* 2012;50:646.
64. Wooldridge BJ, et al. Mojave rattlesnakes (*Crotalus scutulatus*) lacking the acidic subunit DNA sequence lack Mojave toxin in their venom. *Comparative biochemistry and physiology Part B, J Biochem Mol Biol.* 2001;130:169-179.
65. Yamazaki Y, Morita T. Snake venom components affecting blood coagulation and the vascular system: structural similarities and marked diversity. *Curr Pharm Des.* 2007;13:2872-2886.

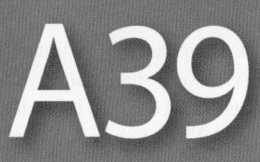

Antidotes in Depth

A39 ANTIVENOM FOR NORTH AMERICAN VENOMOUS SNAKES (CROTALINE AND ELAPID)

Anthony F. Pizon and Anne-Michelle Ruha

INTRODUCTION

In addition to supportive care, antivenom provides definitive management of North American venomous snakebites. In the past, numerous treatments were advocated to prevent systemic absorption or to neutralize venom. These therapies included tourniquets, incision and suction, venom extractors, electrotherapy, and cryotherapy. All of these treatment modalities are either ineffective, delay time to definitive care, or harmful. The focus of treatment for the snakebite victim is a careful assessment, supportive care, evaluating for signs of envenomation, and ultimately, determining the need for antivenom.

HISTORY

Crotalidae Polyvalent Immune Fab (Ovine)

Historically, Wyeth (Marietta, PA) manufactured Antivenin Crotalidae Polyvalent (ACP) for treatment of crotaline snakebites in the United States. It was a poorly purified whole IgG product derived from horse serum with significant risk for acute and delayed allergic reactions.[18] Wyeth stopped production of ACP, and any extant lots expired. Many physicians still recall the use of this product, but new antivenoms have replaced ACP, improving the approach to snakebite treatment. In October 2000, the US Food and Drug Administration (FDA) approved Crotalidae polyvalent immune Fab (Fab antivenom), manufactured by BTG International, marketed as CroFab. This antivenom is derived from sheep serum and formulated as an effective treatment for US Crotalinae species. In addition, because of papain digestion and the affinity purification, which removes extraneous proteins as well as the Fc portion of the antibody, Fab antivenom is a less allergenic alternative to the previously manufactured horse serum product from Wyeth (Table A39–1).[18,37]

Crotalidae Immune F(ab')$_2$ (Equine)

Equine-derived Crotalidae immune F(ab')$_2$ (Anavip; F(ab')$_2$ antivenom) manufactured by Instituto Bioclon, was recently approved by the FDA as an alternative treatment for North American Crotalidae, but its widespread availability is not expected until the fall of 2018. The historical experience with Fab antivenom has revealed the unexpected problem of recurrent

venom effects that occur hours to days after completing treatment. Unlike the Fab antivenom, this F(ab')$_2$ product uses pepsin digestion, which keeps the Fab fragments joined to form a larger antibody complex and, as such, is expected to prolong the duration of action. Therefore, the benefits to this new F(ab')$_2$ antivenom appear to suggest a longer half-life and less recurrent venom effects than the Fab antivenom (Fig. A39–1).[6]

North American Coral Snake Antivenin (Equine)

For decades, Wyeth Laboratories manufactured Antivenin (*Micrurus fulvius*) (Equine), which is more commonly known as North American Coral Snake Antivenin (NACSA), for treatment of envenomations by the eastern coral snake (*Micrurus fulvius*) and Texas coral snake (*Micrurus tener*). Although Wyeth temporarily discontinued production of this antivenom, Pfizer has since acquired Wyeth and began manufacturing this antivenom again. At the time of this writing, Pfizer will only provide the antivenom on an "as needed basis."

PHARMACOLOGY

Mechanism of Action

In general, the mechanism of action of antivenoms remains the same regardless of the preparation (Fab, F(ab)$_2$, or whole IgG). The antibody fragments bind and neutralize venom components. The smaller antibody fragments penetrate tissues and help redistribute the venom from its target tissue.

Crotalidae Polyvalent Immune Fab (Ovine)

Chemistry/Preparation

Crotalidae polyvalent immune Fab (Fab antivenom) is produced by inoculating sheep with the venom of one of the following crotaline snake species: the Eastern diamondback rattlesnake (*Crotalus adamanteus*), Western diamondback rattlesnake (*Crotalus atrox*), cottonmouth (*Agkistrodon piscivorus*), and Mojave rattlesnake (*Crotalus scutulatus*). The species-specific antivenom is then prepared by isolating the antibodies from the sheep serum and digesting the IgG antibodies with papain. The venom-specific Fab antibody fragments are then isolated by affinity purification. This refining process eliminates most of the Fc portion of the immunoglobulin and

TABLE A39–1	Comparison of Crotalid and Elapid Antivenoms				
Antivenom	**Snake Species Used in Production**	**Digestion**	**Origin**	**Recommended Dosing**[a]
Crotalidae Polyvalent Immune Fab (CroFab)	*Crotalus atrox* *C. adamenteus* *C. scutulatus* *Agkistrodon piscivorus*	Papain	Ovine	4–6 vials repeated as needed to achieve control; then 2 vials every 6 h × 3 doses
Crotalidae Immune F(ab')$_2$ (Anavip)	*Bothrops asper* *Crotalus durissus*	Pepsin	Equine	10 vials repeated as needed to achieve control
North American Coral Snake Antivenin	*Micrurus fulvius*	None	Equine	3–5 vials repeated as needed for clinical improvement

[a]As recommended by respective package inserts.

1627

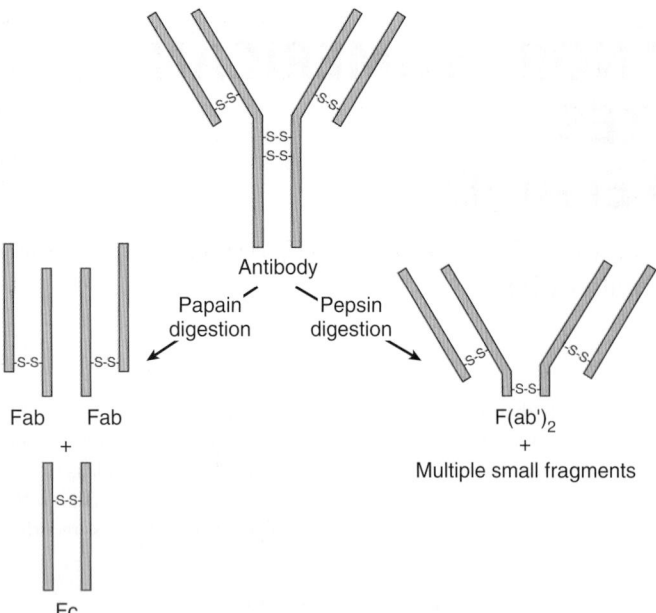

FIGURE A39–1. Antibody fragments produced from various digestion treatments during the production of antivenoms.

other potentially immunogenic sheep proteins. Manufacturing specifications require less than or equal to 1% w/w for Fc fragments and less than or equal to 0.3% w/w for albumin.[16] All 4 species-specific antivenoms are then combined to form the final polyvalent product. The resultant Fab antivenom is less immunogenic and more potent compared to whole IgG antivenoms used previously.[9,14]

Pharmacokinetics

The pharmacokinetics of Fab antivenom is poorly studied. Elimination half-life calculations were performed using only 3 patients' samples. From these data, the half-life was estimated between 12 and 23 hours.[10] Although a similarly prepared and sized ovine Fab product yielded a volume of distribution of 0.3 L/kg, a clearance of 32 mL/min, and an elimination half-life of approximately 15 hours, these parameters are not necessarily applicable to Fab antivenom.[40]

Crotalidae Immune F(ab')₂ (Equine)

Chemistry/Preparation

Crotalidae immune F(ab')₂ (F(ab')₂ antivenom) is manufactured by immunizing horses with the venom of the fer-de-lance (*Bothrops asper*) and the Central American rattlesnake (*Crotalus durissus*). The horse serum is then prepared by pepsin digestion to remove the Fc portion of the antibody creating an F(ab')₂ product. As opposed to the papain digestion to make individual Fab fragments for Fab antivenom, pepsin digestion cleaves the antibody so that Fab fragments remain attached in a V configuration, hence the designation F(ab')₂. The venom-specific antibody fragments are then isolated by nanofiltration and ammonium sulfate precipitation. Each vial contains approximately 120 mg of protein and will neutralize 780 times the LD_{50} of *B. asper* venom and 790 times the LD_{50} of *C. durissus* venom in a mouse assay.[1]

Pharmacokinetics

The pharmacokinetics of F(ab')₂ antivenom provides much longer duration of action than its Fab counterpart. Elimination half-life calculations performed on 13 healthy volunteers provided a mean half-life of 133 hours.[1] Moreover, the F(ab')₂ antivenoms have a similar volume of distribution of 0.2 L/kg, but a much slower clearance of 1.6 mL/min than Fab antivenom. These kinetics suggest that the duration of action of the antivenom is more comparable to the clinical effects of the venom.[6]

North American Coral Snake Antivenin IgG (Equine)

Chemistry/Preparation

North American Coral Snake Antivenin (NACSA) is manufactured by immunizing healthy horses with venom from the Eastern coral snake (*Micrurus fulvius*). The horse serum is then purified and concentrated before it is lyophilized for storage. Unlike Fab and F(ab')₂ antivenoms, NACSA is a whole IgG product.

Pharmacokinetics

The pharmacokinetics of NACSA are unknown and unstudied.

CLINICAL USE

Crotalidae Polyvalent Immune Fab (Ovine)

Although crotalidae polyvalent immune Fab (Fab antivenom) is designed using the venoms of 4 North American crotalids, murine lethality studies demonstrate activity against the venom of 6 other crotaline snake species (*Crotalus viridis helleri*, *C. molossus molossus*, *C. horridus horridus*, *C. horridus atricaudatus*, *Agkistrodon contortrix contortrix*, and *Sistrurus miliarus barbouri*).[9] In addition, numerous case reports document benefit after envenomation by many other North American crotalids.

Some case reports and anecdotal experience report venom effects resistant to Fab antivenom. For instance, thrombocytopenia may not respond to Fab antivenom after envenomations by the red diamond (*C. ruber ruber*) and the timber (*C. horridus horridus*) rattlesnakes.[31] In these cases, the thrombocytopenia often responds to initial doses of Fab antivenom, but a subsequent decline in the platelet count is unaffected by repeat dosing of antivenom. Sometimes severe, platelet counts remain extremely low or undetectable until they rebound approximately a week after the envenomation. In rare cases, despite Fab antivenom therapy, late spontaneous bleeding and laboratory abnormalities occurs beyond 2 weeks.[29] Furthermore, some patients envenomated by the Southern Pacific rattlesnake (*C. viridis helleri*) may have refractory neurotoxicity unresponsive to Fab antivenom.[35] In general, Fab antivenom is used to treat envenomations for all North American pit vipers with expected overall benefit despite the occasional refractory envenomation effects noted in select species.[26]

Following an envenomation, the major indications for Fab antivenom administration are (1) progression of swelling, (2) significant coagulopathy or thrombocytopenia, (3) neuromuscular toxicity, or (4) hemodynamic compromise. These indications permit the clinician to interpret the need for antivenom under varying circumstances. If the prothrombin time is elevated, or the fibrinogen or platelet counts are decreased, we recommend antivenom. Furthermore, antivenom is also recommended when patients demonstrate muscle fasciculations, weakness, or shock.

We recommend against giving antivenom prophylactically to individuals without evidence of envenomation or for localized tissue swelling when other signs of envenomation are absent. This is interpreted as swelling localized to only the bite site or swelling that does not cross a major joint, such as a wrist, elbow, ankle, or knee (Chap. 119).[26] Antivenom is avoided in these circumstances because the risk of antivenom administration outweighs any perceived benefits. Nonetheless, the bedside physician should use their best judgment based on the severity of local swelling before providing antivenom when no other signs are present.

When indications are met, antivenom should be administered as soon as possible. Because antivenom will halt but not reverse swelling, it is anticipated that early administration would reduce pain and loss of function associated with a grossly swollen extremity, as compared to delayed administration. Animal studies demonstrate decreased mortality when antivenom is given immediately after envenomation.[9] Similarly, antivenom benefits diminish with delayed treatment of even a few hours in animal models.[14] Antivenom will not reverse swelling and tissue necrosis that has already occurred, and tissue necrosis often continues to develop despite antivenom administration. Antivenom, at least temporarily, reverses systemic effects, coagulopathy, and platelet defects.[5,11,12,25,37] Although no studies exist comparing outcomes of envenomated patients treated with and without antivenom, it is generally agreed that treatment reduces morbidity in patients with significant crotaline envenomation and in some situations may be a lifesaving therapy.[12] The window of therapeutic efficacy in cases of delayed antivenom administration is unknown.

Crotalidae Immune F(ab′)₂ (Equine)

Although Crotalidae Immune F(ab′)₂ (F(ab′)₂ antivenom) is derived from the venoms of 2 snake species less commonly encountered in North America, F(ab′)₂ antivenom effectively neutralizes the venom from 15 different North American snakes. However, as compared to the Fab counterpart, the dose required for neutralization was higher in nearly every case.[39]

At the time of this writing, F(ab′)₂ antivenom has been used only for research purposes in the treatment of North American rattlesnake bites. Yet, clinical indications for use remain the same as for Fab antivenom. However, this antivenom shows promise as a treatment with less concern for recurrent venom effects in both adult and pediatric patients.[6,23]

North American Coral Snake Antivenin IgG (Equine)

North American Coral Snake Antivenin (NACSA) is the recommended treatment for envenomation by the eastern coral snake (*Micrurus fulvius*) and Texas coral snake (*Micrurus tener*). This antivenom does not treat envenomations from coral snakes found in Mexico, Central America, or South America. Furthermore, bites by the less virulent Arizona coral snake (Sonoran, *Micruroides euryoxanthus*) do not produce significant envenomation requiring treatment with antivenom.[38]

Indications for NACSA administration include the development of any signs or symptoms consistent with coral snake envenomation from the Micrurus genus.[30] Patients with coral snake envenomations typically lack significant local tissue injury. Antivenom administration is recommended following the development of any neurologic abnormalities including, but not limited to, paresthesias, slurred speech, ptosis, diplopia, dysphagia, stridor, muscle weakness, fasciculations, and paralysis. Because anxiety is often associated with a snakebite, true signs of envenomation must be differentiated from the anxiety related to a snake encounter. We recommend against treating patients with NACSA empirically prior to symptom development.[1] At least one study demonstrates that treatment of patients after symptom development was not inferior to an empirical approach.[42]

In the absence of antivenom, the mainstay of treatment consists of aggressive supportive care. In particular, if respiratory failure results from muscle weakness prolonged mechanical intubation is often necessary until neurologic recovery. Paralysis is completely reversible; however, it typically takes weeks to months to resolve completely.[20]

ADVERSE EFFECTS AND SAFETY ISSUES
Crotalidae Polyvalent Immune Fab (Ovine)

Acute hypersensitivity reactions are the most significant safety concerns when administering antivenom to patients. Crotalidae polyvalent immune Fab (Fab antivenom) was specifically designed to have reduced immunogenicity; however, both acute and delayed hypersensitivity reactions are still reported.[7,8] Urticaria, rash, bronchospasm, pruritus, angioedema, anaphylaxis, and delayed serum sickness are all associated with use of this product.[11,40] An early study reported acute reactions in 14.3% of patients receiving this antivenom, but more current studies suggests an incidence of 5% to 6%.[7,12,25]

When antivenom is administered too rapidly, nonimmunogenically mediated anaphylactoid reactions also occur. Most patients appear to tolerate 4 to 6 vials per hour without developing significant anaphylactoid reactions. If the patient requires rapid administration of antivenom because of the severity of the envenomation, H₁ and H₂ histamine receptor antagonists and an epinephrine infusion should be readily available in case symptoms develop. Clinically differentiating between anaphylactoid and anaphylactic reactions may be difficult, especially when antivenom is administered rapidly. Regardless, the treatment remains the same.

For acute anaphylactic reactions (which often occur shortly following initiation of even low doses of antivenom), the antivenom is stopped, and aggressive supportive and pharmacologic therapy begun. Intravenous epinephrine at 2 to 4 mcg/min (0.03–0.06 mcg/kg/min for children) should be initiated and then titrated to effect, as well as corticosteroids and H₁ and H₂ histamine receptor antagonists. After the symptoms of hypersensitivity resolve, the antivenom is restarted only in patients at high risk for significant morbidity or mortality from envenomation. In such cases, the antivenom infusion is restarted at 1 to 2 mL/h, while the epinephrine infusion is continued. The antivenom infusion rate is slowly increased as tolerated. If anaphylaxis recurs, the antivenom is stopped and the epinephrine infusion increased until symptoms resolve. Antivenom can then be restarted while epinephrine is continued at the higher rate. With constant physician monitoring at the bedside and careful titration of epinephrine and antivenom infusions, patients with life-threatening envenomation should tolerate the full antivenom dose. Patients have safely received subsequent doses of antivenom after an acute life-threatening reaction.[27]

In addition to acute allergic reactions, delayed hypersensitivity syndromes in the form of serum sickness are reported. Although most episodes of serum sickness are mild, this syndrome has not been well studied.[18] Typical cases of serum sickness include urticaria, pruritus, and malaise. Arthralgias, lymphadenopathy, and fever also develop. In rare severe cases, glomerulonephritis, vasculitis, myocarditis, and neuritis occur. Delayed hypersensitivity reactions are poorly studied following treatment with Fab antivenom, but are reported to occur in 16% (6/38) of patients in 2 clinical trials.[2,11] This number may be falsely high because all but one of the cases came from a single lot of antivenom that was later found to have a high concentration of Fc antibody fragment contamination.[14] We recommend that patients with serum sickness symptoms receive treatment with 2 mg/kg (a maximum dose of 60 mg per day for adults) of oral prednisone divided into 2 daily doses and tapered over 2 to 3 weeks. Oral H₁ receptor antagonists are reasonable to add for symptomatic treatment as well. The vast majority of patients are managed as outpatients, and most respond favorably to this regimen.

According to the package insert, a known allergy to papaya or papain is a contraindication to the administration of Fab antivenom unless the risks of allergy outweigh the benefits of the administration.[10] Patients with known allergy to papaya or papain appear rare. However, patients who are also allergic to latex or a variety of fruits (banana, avocado, kiwi, apricot, chestnut, grape, passion fruit, and pineapple) may have cross-reactivity with papain.[34] Therefore, we recommend administration of Fab antivenom with caution to any patients with atopy, asthma, or known food allergies.

Crotalidae Immune F(ab′)₂ (Equine)

Although its use in the United States is limited, adverse effects and safety issues remain the same for F(ab′)₂ as for Fab antivenoms. The package insert suggests itching (43%) and nausea (23%) are among the most common adverse effects.[1] In addition, rashes (12%), arthralgias (11%), peripheral edema (8%), myalgias (7%), vomiting (6%), and headache (6%), were observed in clinical trials.[1] Acute and delayed allergies are reported as well.[6] Monitoring for and treatment of these adverse reactions is the same as described for Fab antivenom.

North American Coral Snake Antivenin IgG (Equine)

Acute and delayed hypersensitivity reactions are the most significant safety concerns when providing antivenom products to patients. However, little is published concerning NACSA adverse reactions. The risk of acute hypersensitivity reactions with NACSA is approximately 20%.[42] Wyeth's other equine-derived antivenom product, Antivenin Crotalidae Polyvalent (ACP), caused acute allergies in 20% to 50% of cases and the incidence of delayed hypersensitivity reactions increased with increased doses.[19,41] The exact incidence of hypersensitivity with NACSA is unknown, but approaches 100% when more than 40 vials of ACP were administered.[28] Despite these concerns, severe allergic reactions to NACSA are uncommonly reported, but this may reflect infrequent use and reporting bias.[30,42]

Patients with a known horse serum allergy or who have been treated with equine-derived antivenoms previously should only receive treatment with NACSA if there is a significant risk of severe morbidity or mortality and appropriate management for anaphylactic reactions is readily available.[30] Patients with known horse serum allergies have tolerated equine antivenoms, but they often require more dilute doses of antivenom and pretreatment.[17,27] For these patients we recommend using intravenous H_1 and H_2 receptor antagonists, corticosteroids, and an epinephrine infusion (2–4 mcg/min for adults) prior to antivenom administration. The antivenom is then started at a very low rate of infusion, and if tolerated, the rate is increased. If an acute allergic reaction develops, the antivenom is immediately stopped and the epinephrine drip titrated for symptoms. Only after symptoms abate should the antivenom be restarted by carefully titrating both the antivenom and epinephrine drips. With severe allergic reactions, reserving antivenom for only life-threatening envenomations is recommended. In most cases with severe allergic symptoms, discontinuing antivenom and providing supportive care alone are the preferred recommendations.

PREGNANCY AND LACTATION

Crotalidae Polyvalent Immune Fab (Ovine)

Pregnant patients who meet criteria for treatment should also receive antivenom, which is currently listed as category C, and has been used safely during pregnancy.[21] In the pre-Fab antivenom era, one review of 30 pit viper bites from North American and other international snake species during pregnancy reported 43% fetal demise and 10% maternal mortality.[15] Therefore, given the relative safety of this antivenom and the potential for significant fetal compromise after envenomation, the pregnant patient is approached no differently than the nonpregnant patient. Continuous fetal and maternal monitoring is important as well.[22]

It is unknown if Fab antivenom is excreted in breast milk.

Crotalidae Immune F(ab')₂ (Equine)

Pregnant patients who meet criteria for treatment should also receive antivenom, which is currently listed as category C. No evidence exists concerning use during pregnancy. As mentioned for whole IgG and Fab antivenoms, given the relative safety of this antivenom and the potential for significant fetal compromise after envenomation, the pregnant patient is approached no differently than the nonpregnant patient. Continuous fetal and maternal monitoring is important as well.[22]

It is unknown if F(ab)₂ antivenom is excreted in breast milk.

North American Coral Snake Antivenin (Equine)

Currently NACSA does not have a pregnancy listing. There are no reports of administration of this antivenom in pregnancy. Knowledge of NACSA's safety in pregnancy is unknown. However, other antivenoms have been used safely in pregnancy, and maternal health is often considered of greater concern and risk due to envenomation than the unknown fetal risk associated with antivenom.[4] Considering this, and the severe morbidity associated with coral snake envenomation, we recommend that pregnant patients who meet criteria for treatment receive antivenom. Continuous fetal and maternal monitoring is important as well.

It is unknown if NACSA is excreted in breast milk.

DOSING AND ADMINISTRATION

Crotalidae Polyvalent Immune Fab (Ovine)

A thorough medication history including previous treatment with antivenoms should be obtained. A history of asthma, atopy, or food allergies should be carefully considered when weighing the risks and benefits of antivenom for a particular patient. According to the manufacturer, the only contraindication is an allergy to papaya or papain. These conditions should not exclude the use of antivenom if the patient is suffering from a moderate-to-severe envenomation. Crotalidae polyvalent immune Fab (Fab antivenom) is ovine-derived; therefore, previous reactions to equine-derived antivenoms do not preclude use of this product. In cases of mild envenomation, the risk of allergic reaction to antivenom might outweigh any benefit. Antivenom should be administered in a monitored setting in which resuscitation can be performed

and airway supplies are readily available. Epinephrine, corticosteroids, and antihistamines should be immediately available in the event of a hypersensitivity reaction. If the patient tolerates initial doses without ill effect, subsequent doses may be administered on a medical floor or step-down unit.[26]

Antivenom is packaged in vials as a lyophilized powder, which must be reconstituted. Completely filling each vial with 25 mL of sterile water, rather than the 10 mL advised in the package insert, and then gently hand rolling the vials will result in dissolution times as rapid as one minute. Adding the greater volume also reduces foaming of the product.[10,33] The reconstituted antivenom is further diluted into a 250 mL of 0.9% saline and administered as discussed below.

The initial recommended dose is 4 to 6 vials, which is mixed in 250 mL 0.9% sodium chloride solution and administered over one hour. For patients who present with cardiovascular collapse or life-threatening toxicity we recommend a starting dose of 8 to 12 vials of Fab antivenom.[26] The exact concentration of antivenom is not critical. For children, the total volume of fluid in which the antivenom is diluted can be decreased when necessary.[32] No dosing adjustment is required for children or small adults because the amount of venom requiring neutralization is not dependent on the patient's weight. There is no evidence to support partial doses or infusions of one or 2 vials in minor cases.

In order to avoid serious adverse reactions, the first dose of antivenom is administered cautiously at an escalating rate. We recommend against skin testing. The first dose of antivenom (4–6 vials diluted in 250 mL 0.9% saline) is infused at an initial rate of 10 mL/h while the patient is observed carefully for evidence of hypersensitivity. If after 5 minutes no adverse reactions are witnessed, then the rate is doubled every few minutes, as tolerated by the patient, with the goal of infusing the first dose over one hour. If the patient tolerates the initial dose without adverse effects, subsequent doses can be given at a rate of 250 mL/h without a need for rate titration.

The total dose of antivenom required to control an envenomation varies widely. With the introduction of Fab antivenom, *control* was defined as arrest of local tissue manifestations and return of coagulation parameters, platelet counts, and systemic signs to normal. However, clinical experience demonstrated that some patients have venom-induced coagulopathy and thrombocytopenia resistant to antivenom treatment.[37] Some authors advocate *control* to mean clear improvement in hematologic parameters rather than complete normalization.[37] We find that this definition is more realistic for the subset of patients with difficult-to-treat coagulopathy and thrombocytopenia. After each dose of 4 to 6 vials, prothrombin time, fibrinogen, and platelet counts are measured, and the patient's local injury is reexamined. Multiple doses are often required to achieve control. A retrospective study reported 83% of rattlesnake bites and 98% of copperhead bites obtained control with 12 or fewer vials of Fab antivenom.[43] This study emphasizes the need for multiple antivenom doses in rattlesnake envenomations and typically only one initial dose in copperhead bites in order to gain control. If repeat dosing is necessary to control swelling, but fibrinogen, prothrombin time, and platelets remain normal, these laboratory studies do not need repeating.

After achieving control, maintenance doses of 2 vials every 6 hours are recommended, for a total of 3 doses. The 2 vials are added to 250 mL 0.9% sodium chloride solution and administered over one hour. Because the duration of action of Fab antivenom is less than that of venom, the maintenance doses are provided to preclude recurrence of local manifestations, thrombocytopenia, and coagulopathy. An algorithm for Fab antivenom administration for moderate to severe crotaline envenomation is shown in Fig. A39–2. Although recommended in the CroFab package insert, maintenance therapy is not routinely administered by all practitioners.[10] For example, copperhead envenomations may not require maintenance doses.[26] Because of regional variations in the potency of copperhead venom, we recommend consultation with regional poison control centers in order to provide local practices and receive specific recommendations.

Some patients will demonstrate recurrence of swelling during their maintenance infusions. For this reason, close monitoring of extremity swelling is

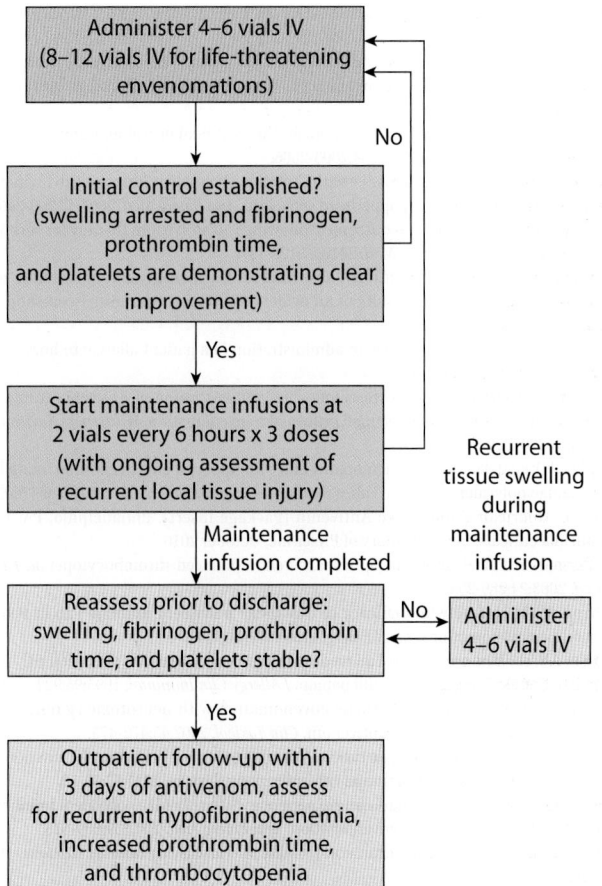

FIGURE A39–2. Algorithm for Crotalidae Polyvalent Immune Fab administration for treatment of moderate-to-severe Crotaline envenomation.

recommended for 18 to 24 hours after apparent control has been achieved. If recurrent swelling occurs, additional doses of 4 to 6 vials are recommended until the swelling again becomes controlled, and then maintenance infusions are resumed.

Despite successful completion of maintenance antivenom doses, some patients also develop a recurrence of coagulopathy and/or thrombocytopenia. Therefore, we recommend repeat prothrombin time, fibrinogen and platelet counts performed 2 to 3 days and again 5 to 7 days in all patients after hospital discharge to ensure late recurrent hematologic effects have not developed. One large retrospective study demonstrated new or recurrent hematologic findings in 32% of patients with rattlesnake envenomations.[36] Another study suggests recurrence is as high as 50%.[3] Close follow-up seems less necessary in copperhead envenomations because hematologic findings are observed less frequently.[24]

Crotalidae Immune F(ab′)$_2$ (Equine)

Prior to administration, the same preparation should occur for F(ab′)$_2$ administration as for Fab antivenoms. However, there are no contraindications listed on the F(ab′)$_2$ package insert.[1] Antivenom should be administered in a monitored setting where resuscitation can be performed and airway supplies are quickly accessed. Epinephrine, corticosteroids, and antihistamines should be immediately available in the event a hypersensitivity reaction occurs.

Antivenom is packaged in vials as a lyophilized powder, which must be reconstituted. Completely filling each vial with 25 mL of sterile water, rather than the 10 mL advised in the package insert, and then gently hand rolling (not shaking) the vials will result in dissolution times as rapid as one minute. Adding the greater volume also reduces foaming of the product.[10,33]

The initial recommended dose of F(ab′)$_2$ is 10 vials, which is mixed in 250 mL 0.9% sodium chloride solution and administered over one hour. For the first 10 minutes, the infusion rate is 25 to 50 mL/h, which is then increased to the full 250-mL/h rate until completion if no allergic reactions develop. Repeat doses of 10 vials are recommended until control is achieved. Clinical trials suggest maintenance dosing is not needed.[6] However, the package insert recommends 4 vials as needed for recurrent venom effects and 18 hours of monitoring after obtaining control. The caveats for Fab antivenom administration (infusion rate and treatment of allergic reactions) apply to F(ab′)$_2$ antivenom.

Recurrent venom effects still occur in 5% to 10% of case.[6] After hospital discharge, outpatient monitoring is still recommended as experience with this antivenom is limited.

North American Coral Snake Antivenin IgG (Equine)

Prior to administration, the same preparation should occur for North American Coral Snake Antivenin (NACSA) administration as for the other antivenoms.

Antivenom is packaged in vials as a lyophilized powder, which must be reconstituted. Completely filling each vial with 25 mL of sterile water, rather than the 10 mL advised in the package insert, and then gently hand rolling (not shaking) the vials will result in dissolution times as rapid as one minute. Adding the greater volume also reduces foaming of the product.[10,33]

The initial recommended dose of NACSA is 3 to 5 vials, which is mixed in 250 mL 0.9% sodium chloride solution and administered over one hour.[30] Additional antivenom doses are indicated for the evolution of any neurologic abnormalities including, but not limited to, paresthesias, slurred speech, ptosis, diplopia, dysphagia, stridor, muscle weakness, fasciculations, and paralysis. The caveats for crotaline antivenom administration (infusion rate and treatment of allergic reactions) apply to coral snake antivenom, except less antivenom is usually required for coral snakes. Up to 10 vials can be administered, although dosing recommendations are vague.

FORMULATION AND ACQUISITION

Crotalidae Polyvalent Immune Fab (Ovine)

Hospitals with native crotaline species within their region should maintain Fab antivenom at all times.[13] Because the timely administration is the cornerstone of treatment, attempting to obtain antivenom at the time of an emergency will likely introduce a significant delay to treatment and exacerbate morbidity.

Crotalidae Immune F(ab′)$_2$ (Equine)

Although this is FDA-approved, the availability of F(ab′)$_2$ is not expected until the fall of 2018.

North American Coral Snake Antivenin IgG (Equine)

In order to obtain NASCA, contact the local poison control center or Pfizer, which currently holds the rights to this antivenom. Poison control centers have access to the online Antivenom Index, which is useful when attempting to locate coral snake antivenom. Otherwise, Pfizer will provide the antivenom on an as needed basis.

SUMMARY

- Antivenom is a significant benefit for some patients envenomated by North American snakes.
- If crotalid snakes are endemic to a catchment area of a hospital, Crotalidae Fab or F(ab′)$_2$ antivenoms should remain stocked and easily accessible at all times.[13]
- In areas endemic with the eastern or Texas coral snake, North American coral snake antivenin (NACSA) should be stocked and immediately accessible at all times.
- Poison control centers have access to the online Antivenom Index, which is useful when attempting to locate antivenom for a coral snake

or a nonnative snake envenomation. Local zoos may also be useful resources when attempting to locate exotic antivenom. Recommendations for these diverse antivenom are difficult to make, but available package instructions should be followed, and preparations should be made to treat hypersensitivity reactions.

REFERENCES

1. Anavip [Package Insert]. Mexico D.F., Mexico: Instituto Bioclon S.A. de C.V.; May 2015.
2. Bogdan GM, et al. Clinical efficacy of two dosing regimens of affinity purified, mixed monospecific crotalid antivenom ovine FAB (CroTAb) [Abstract]. *Acad Emerg Med.* 1997;4:518.
3. Boyer LV, et al. Recurrence phenomena after immunoglobulin therapy for snake envenomations: part 2. Guidelines for clinical management with Crotaline Fab antivenom. *Ann Emerg Med.* 2001;37:196-210.
4. Brown SA, et al. Management of envenomations during pregnancy. *Clin Toxicol.* 2013;51:3-15.
5. Buntain WL. Successful venomous snakebite neutralization with massive antivenom infusion in a child. *J Trauma.* 1983;23:1012-1014.
6. Bush SP, et al. Comparison of F(ab')₂ versus Fab antivenom for pit viper envenomation: a prospective, blinded, multicenter, randomized clinical trial. *Clin Toxicol (Phila).* 2015;53:37-45.
7. Cannon R, et al. Acute hypersensitivity reactions associated with administration of Crotalidae polyvalent immune Fab antivenom. *Ann Emerg Med.* 2008;51:407-411.
8. Clark RF, et al. Immediate and delayed allergic reactions to Crotalidae polyvalent immune Fab (ovine) antivenom. *Ann Emerg Med.* 2002;39:671-676.
9. Consroe P, et al. Comparison of a new ovine antigen binding fragment (Fab) antivenin for United States Crotalidae with the commercial antivenin for protection against venom-induced lethality in mice. *Am J Trop Med Hyg.* 1995;53:507-510.
10. CroFab® [Package Insert]. West Conshohocken, PA: BTG International Inc; March 2012.
11. Dart RC, et al. A randomized multicenter trial of Crotalinae polyvalent immune Fab (ovine) antivenom for the treatment for Crotaline snakebite in the United States. *Arch Intern Med.* 2001;161:2030-2036.
12. Dart RC, McNally J. Efficacy, safety, and use of snake antivenom in the United States. *Ann Emerg Med.* 2001;37:181-188.
13. Dart RC, et al. Insufficient stocking of poisoning antidotes in hospital pharmacies. *JAMA.* 1996;276:1508-1510.
14. Dart RC, et al. Efficacy of post envenomation administration of antivenin. *Toxicon.* 1988;26:1218-1221.
15. Dunnihoo DR, et al. Snake bite poisoning in pregnancy. A review of the literature. *J Reprod Med.* 1992;37:653-658.
16. Gerring D, BTG International Inc, personal communication, January 28, 2013, West Conshohocken, PA.
17. Habib AG. Effect of pre-medication on early adverse reactions following antivenom use in snakebite: a systematic review and meta-analysis. *Drug Saf.* 2011;34:869-880.
18. Howland MA, Smilkstein MJ. Primer on immunology with applications to toxicology. *Contemp Manage Crit Care.* 1991;1:109-145.
19. Jurkovich GJ, et al. Complications of Crotalidae antivenin therapy. *J Trauma.* 1988;28:1032-1037.
20. Kitchen CS, Mierop LHS. Envenomation by the Eastern coral snake (*Micrurus fulvius*). *JAMA.* 1987;258:1615-1618.
21. LaMonica GE, et al. Rattlesnake bites in pregnant women. *J Reprod Med.* 2010;55:520-522.
22. Langley RL. Snakebite during pregnancy: a literature review. *Wilderness Environ Med.* 2010;21:54-60.
23. Lasoff DR, et al. A new F(ab')₂ antivenom for the treatment of crotaline envenomation in children. *Am J Emerg Med.* 2016;34:2003-2006.
24. Lavonas EJ, et al. Initial experience with Crotalidae Polyvalent Immune Fab (ovine) antivenom in the treatment of copperhead snakebite. *Ann Emerg Med.* 2004;43:200-206.
25. Lavonas EJ, et al. Short-term outcomes following Fab antivenom therapy for severe crotaline snakebite. *Ann Emerg Med.* 2010;57:128-137.
26. Lavonas EJ, et al. Unified treatment algorithm for the management of crotaline snakebite in the United States: results of an evidence-informed consensus workshop. *BMC Emerg Med.* 2011;11:2.
27. Loprinzi CL, et al. Snake antivenin administration in a patient allergic to horse serum. *South Med J.* 1983;76:501-502.
28. LoVecchio F, et al. Serum sickness following administration of Antivenin (Crotalidae) Polyvalent in 181 cases of presumed rattlesnake envenomation. *Wilderness Environ Med.* 2003;14:220-221.
29. Miller AD, et al. Recurrent coagulopathy and thrombocytopenia in children treated with crotalidae polyvalent immune Fab: a case series. *Pediatr Emerg Care.* 2010;26:576-582.
30. North American Coral Snake Antivenin [Package Insert]. Philadelphia, PA: Wyeth Pharmaceuticals, Inc, Subsidiary of Pfizer Inc; October 2016.
31. Offerman SR, et al. Biphasic rattlesnake venom-induced thrombocytopenia. *J Emerg Med.* 2003;24:289-293.
32. Pizon AF, et al. Safety and efficacy of Crotalidae polyvalent immune Fab in Pediatric crotaline envenomations. *Acad Emerg Med.* 2007;14:373-376.
33. Quan AN, et al. Improving CroFab reconstitution times. *J Med Tox.* 2008;4:60-61.
34. Quarre J, et al. Allergy to latex and papain. *J Allergy Clin Immunol.* 1995;95:922.
35. Richardson WH, et al. Rattlesnake envenomation with neurotoxicity refractory to treatment with crotaline Fab antivenom. *Clin Toxicol.* 2007;45:472-475.
36. Ruha AM, et al. Late hematologic toxicity following treatment of rattlesnake envenomation with crotalidae polyvalent immune Fab antivenom. *Toxicon.* 2011;57:53-59.
37. Ruha AM, et al. Initial postmarketing experience with crotalidae polyvalent immune Fab for treatment of rattlesnake envenomation. *Ann Emerg Med.* 2002;39:609-615.
38. Russell FE. Bites by the Sonoran coral snake, *Micruroidseuryxanthus. Toxicon.* 1967;5:39-42.
39. Sanchez EE, et al. The efficacy of two antivenoms against the venom of North American snakes. *Toxicon.* 2003;41:357-365.
40. Ward SB, et al. Comparison of the pharmacokinetics and in vivo bioaffinity of DigiTab versus Digibind. *Ther Drug Monit.* 2000;22:599-607.
41. White RR, Weber RA. Poisonous snakebite in central Texas. *Ann Surg.* 1991;213:466-471.
42. Wood A, et al. Review of Eastern coral snake (*Micrurus fulvius*) exposures managed by the Florida Poison Information Center Network: 1998-2010. *Clin Toxicol.* 2013;51:783-788.
43. Yin S, et al. Factors associated with difficulty achieving initial control with Crotalidae Polyvalent Immune Fab antivenom in snakebite patients. *Acad Emerg Med.* 2010;18:46-52.

Keith J. Boesen, Kelly A. Green Boesen,
Nicholas B. Hurst, and Farshad Mazda Shirazi

HISTORY AND EPIDEMIOLOGY

The incidence of snakebites worldwide is difficult to ascertain, as there is no systematic reporting mechanism. This fact, when combined with the variable degree of confirmation of snakebites, makes the estimation of an accurate number extremely difficult. Attempts have been made utilizing available data from case reports in the literature, hospital records, surveys, and existing reporting systems. Current estimates place the worldwide annual incidence of snakebites as high as 5.5 million,[13,44] of which roughly 50% are thought to be from venomous snakes.[8] Estimated annual complications include 400,000 amputations[44] and approximately 100,000 deaths.[13,44]

Snakes, although feared by many, are popular around the world as pets. The desire to keep venomous snakes as pets, which is typically illegal in the United States, and the financial, clinical and ethical implications throughout the world make the trade of exotic creatures third only in sales to drugs and weapons on the international black market. In fact, the estimated annual worth of this trade in the United States alone is at least $15 million.[18]

This Special Consideration will discuss the evaluation and management of patients evenomated in the United States by nonnative snakes (also known as exotic snakes). A review from 2005 through 2011 of the National Poison Data System (NPDS), maintained by the American Association of Poison Control Centers (AAPCC), confirmed 258 exotic snakebites reports, of which 218 were identified by genus and species, from a total of 71 different varieties.[42] The most common envenomations involved male owners bitten in a private residence during feeding or handling the snakes, cleaning the cages, or while milking the snakes for venom.[24,41,42] Of all bites, 82.9% were the result of an Elapidae or Viperidae snakes.[42]

The previous AAPCC study from 1995 to 2004 documented 399 nonnative exposures, of which 350 snakes (87%) were identified by genus and species, comprising at least 77 different varieties. One US expert reported 54 consultations regarding bites from nonnative venomous snakes.[24]

In the most recent AAPCC data, the most common family responsible for envenomations was the Viperidae, making up 43% of these bites. Of the Viperidae, 42 different species were identified, with the top 4 species involved being: gaboon viper (*Bitis gabonica*), bush master (*Lachesis mutus*), the sharpnosed viper (*Deinagkistrodon acutus*), and the hognosed viper (*Bothrops ophroyomegas*). The second most common family responsible for envenomations was the Elapidaes, resulting in 39% of US exotic snakebites. Forty-two percent were from 3 different species: monocellate cobra (*Naja naja kaouthia*), black necked spitting cobra (*Naja nigricollis*), and the Black mamba (*Dendroaspis polylepis*). The monocellate cobra was the most common snake identified during this study (17 envenomations). Of note, 79% of patients were male, the average age was 33 years (7% were 12 years of age or younger), 70% occurred in a private residence, 11% occurred at work, and 10% occurred in a public area.[42]

TAXONOMY

The naming of snakes has evolved and the renaming currently continues at a rapid pace as a result of advances in DNA testing and ongoing research.[29,30,43] There are approximately 2,700 snake species in the world,[29] of which 20% are known to be venomous to humans.[21] Venomous snakes are divided into 4 major families as shown in Table SC10–1.[14,22,29,30,35,43]

The Elapidae family has a wide distribution in primarily tropical or arid desert settings in such continents as Asia, Australia, Africa, North America, and South America, with the sea snakes and sea kraits found in the Pacific and Indian Oceans.[14] Possibly the most well known of this family are the cobras, capable of unique characteristics such as hooding or spitting.[14] In the United States, there are 3 Elapidae snakes; the Eastern coral snake (*Micrurus fulvius fulvius*), the Texas coral snake (*Micrurus fulvius tener*), and the Sonoran coral snake (*Micruuoides euryxanthus*).

The Viperidae family, consisting of the 3 subfamilies Azemiopinae, Viperinae, and Crotalinae, exists throughout the world, with a few exceptions. The majority of the snakes in this family are divided into 2 main categories: Old World vipers (also known as true vipers) and pit vipers.[35]

ANTIVENOM INDEX

The Antivenom Index (AI) was created more than 25 years ago as a joint effort of the Association of Zoos and Aquariums (AZA) and the AAPCC for the purpose of creating a database that would contain the location of all nonnative snake antivenoms stored throughout the zoos in the United States. For many years, this was kept in paper format at the Arizona Poison and Drug Information Center in Tucson, Arizona, and in 2006 it was converted to an electronic database.

The AI can be searched by the common name or the scientific name of the venomous snake. This search will result in a list of possible snakes that match the description of the searched term. From there, a list of antivenoms active against that genus and species will be displayed, including which zoos stock them and how many vials are available. With this information, and help from experts or the closest regional poison control center, it can

TABLE SC10–1 Taxonomy of Snakes

Family	Subfamily	Representative Species
Elapidae	Elipinae	Cobras (*Naja* spp) King cobras (*Ophiophagus hannah*) Mambas (*Dendroaspis* spp) Kraits (*Bungarus* spp) Coral snakes (*Micrurus* spp and *Micruroides* spp)
	Hydrophiinae	Various sea snakes
	Laticaudinae	Sea kraits
Viperidae	Azemiopinae	Fea's viper (*Azemiops feae*)
	Viperinae (Old World vipers)	Russell's viper (*Vipera russelii*) Gaboon viper (*Bitis gabonica*) Saw-scaled viper (*Echis carinatus*) Death adders (*Acanthophis* spp)
	Crotalinae (pit vipers)	Rattlesnakes (*Crotalus* and *Sistrurus* spp) Copperheads (*Agkistrodon* spp)
Atractaspididae		Stiletto snakes (*Atractaspis* spp)
Colubridae		African boomslang (*Dispholidus typus*) Twig snake (*Thelotornis* spp)

be determined where an adequate supply of antivenom exists and what arrangements are necessary to transport the antivenom to the health care facility where the patient in question is receiving care.

Additional information available in the AI includes package inserts for the antivenoms, many of which are translated into English, the expiration dates of the antivenoms, and additional information such as links to various recommendations on the housing, stocking, or administration of antivenoms.

Access to the AI is limited to the AZA and the AAPCC (all poison control centers have access). Association of Zoos and Aquariums members have the ability to input updated stocking information, whereas the AAPCC members can view antivenom supplies. To access the AI, contact the local poison control center at 1-800-222-1222. Southern Florida is unique in the storage and distribution of exotic antivenoms. The Miami-Dade Fire Rescue Venom Response Program maintains one of the largest repositories of exotic antivenoms for public use in the United States. They work with the local Poison Control Center in Miami for the clinical expertise to facilitate treatment of the envenomated patient.

VENOM TOXICITY

Common venom components from the Elapidae and Viperidae families are classified as neurotoxic, hemotoxic, and or myotoxic.[6,20,41] The venom from the Elapidae is associated with neurotoxic effects. Signs and symptoms consistent with neurotoxicity include blurred vision, paresthesias, ptosis, paralysis of facial muscles, difficulty swallowing, respiratory paralysis, and generalized flaccid paralysis.[40] The venom from the Viperidae is more commonly associated with hemotoxicity and myotoxicity, although some species also have neurotoxic effects. The hematologic signs and symptoms associated include petechiae, purpura, ecchymosis, bleeding, and changes in blood coagulation parameters, including platelets and fibrinogen, as well as prothrombin and partial thromboplastin time abnormalities. The activity of Viperidae venom on the clotting cascade occurs at multiple steps throughout the cascade, resulting in varying degrees of severity (Fig. 58–1). The signs and symptoms of myotoxins are consistent with local tissue injury and destruction, including swelling, necrosis, and skin blebs, and are accompanied by elevations of creatine kinase and aminotransferases with possible impairment of kidney function. Although there are some classic differences in the presentation between snakes from the Elapidae and Viperidae families, it is important to note that there are also similarities based on tremendous venom variability found from species to species and in snakes within the same species.[20]

CLINICAL PRESENTATION AND INITIAL MANAGEMENT

It is useful to consult with an expert to help identify the snake and determine specific signs, symptoms, and treatment options. Experts are found within the AAPCC by calling 1-800-222-1222, or a local zoological society or serpentarium.

The clinical presentation of patients with exotic snake envenomation is extremely variable (mentioned in the above section) as the sequelae depend largely on the type of species involved and the same factors that influence the outcome of patients envenomated by better understood local snakes: premorbid condition of the individual, location of the bite, dose of venom delivered, and delay to health care. Local poison control centers or regional experts are likely familiar with species kept in area zoos as part of an emergency response system for treatment of zoo workers. People who maintain these animals as pets and subsequently are envenomated while handling become more difficult to treat. Several basic steps are recommended for the initial management of these patients as outlined in Table SC10–2.[20,41]

Zoological and Exotic Antivenoms

Hospitals in the United States are not permitted to stock antivenoms for exotic snakes that have not been produced for the US market and submitted to the Food and Drug Administration (FDA) process for drug sale and administration. Zoos are permitted to stock antivenoms for the species of snakes locally housed for the purpose of treating an unintentional exposure. When

TABLE SC10–2 General Approach to a Patient With an Exotic Snake Envenomation

Immobilize the bitten limb in a dependent position and rapidly transport the patient to a medical facility. Initiate irrigation with water if the eyes are exposed.

Determine the time and location of bite, and mark the borders. Follow and mark the progression over time.

Determine the species responsible for the bite. If the bite occurred at a zoo, the zoo may have a written plan for management of the specific species ready to accompany the patient (often a zoo employee) that includes the name of species, appropriate first aid, other management guidelines, and any antivenom that is available. Patients who own exotic snakes may know the identity but often use misleading or inaccurate common names. In which case, it is necessary to contact a local herpetologist, who often can be found through the PCC or zoo, to identify the snake.

Standard resuscitation techniques are indicated for cardiovascular or respiratory failure. Initiate volume repletion if there is massive hemorrhage or hypotension.

Physical examination should include evaluation of signs of local envenomation (pain, swelling, bleeding, and bruising), painful and tender enlargement of lymph nodes, hypotension, spontaneous bleeding, ptosis, muscle tone, cranial nerve function, myalgias and a complete neurotoxic assessment. Laboratory assessment should include a complete blood count, coagulation profile, electrolytes and kidney function, creatine kinase, aminotransferase, urinalysis for blood and myoglobin, and an electrocardiogram.

Begin the process of locating, obtaining, and receiving permission to administer antivenom, even if it is unclear that foreign antivenom will be available or required.

Prepare for the treatment of anaphylaxis if foreign antivenom is to be administered.

Because of uncertainties in prediction of clinical evolution and severity of symptom presentation, close monitoring in an intensive care unit is preferred for all patients with exotic envenomations. This will allow for appropriate clinical and laboratory monitoring specific to the needs of the patient. A minimum of 24 hours of hospital observation is recommended to assess delayed evolution of signs or symptoms. Follow up for serum sickness is reasonable.

zoological staff import antivenom from other countries, they must collaborate with the US FDA and the Centers for Biologics Evaluation and Research (CBER). The zoo facility imports the antivenoms with a permit from the US Department of Agriculture. Each state may require additional permits to import/stock non–US FDA-approved antivenoms. To administer the antivenoms to a human, the antivenom must have an Investigational New Drug (IND) Application filed with the US FDA. This can either be done ahead of time or with emergency approval by the US FDA. Investigational New Drug requirements include assignment of one or more local physicians who may administer the antivenom, a record of the name of each product and associated lot numbers, retention of copies of the package insert for each product, and completion of a statement that the antivenom is being imported solely for emergency use and will not be resold.[37] In addition, a Statement of Investigator must be prepared if any changes to the list of approved personnel for administration of the antivenom occur. When the antivenom is administered, a complete case report must be submitted to the director of CBER.

Although zoos are permitted to have antivenom stocked at the facility, a 2008 study demonstrated that of the 106 zoos and 19 aquaria whose representatives responded, only 33 facilities stocked antivenom.[39] In the 10 years prior to the study, zoos and aquaria in the United States reported a total of 39 separate incidents associated with venomous animals. It is unclear why so few facilities with potential for employee exposure do not carry the antivenom required for their local exotic species, as it is possible that a commercially available product could prove essential. Most facilities reported some internal process to respond to an envenomated patient, including coordinating with the PCC, the local emergency medical services, and a local hospital, or have individualized protocols.

The American College of Medical Toxicology (ACMT) recommends that a zoo or facility that houses exotic snakes have a written plan for management of an envenomation.[1] A recent study reviewed and tested the effectiveness of an emergency operation procedure established in Atlanta.[27] Zoo Atlanta, the

Georgia Poison Control Center, and the Grady Health System established a procedure to manage an envenomation resulting from any of the 13 species of snakes housed at the zoo. All 3 organizations participated in the simulated drill and were evaluated on the functional aspects of coordinating patient care from the time of envenomation through stabilization. In this scenario, all personnel involved were previously alerted to the drill and had additional training as to staff expectations. Even in this "best case" scenario that included preparation for a patient with an exotic envenomation, barriers to care were still encountered. For instance, the protocol given to the hospital personnel lacked details about specific signs and symptoms expected, clear instructions for antivenom indication, and specific dosing and reconstitution instructions for the antivenom. There were also some general problems with personnel coordination. This study highlights the importance of having an established plan that includes the zoo facility, a PCC, and the treating institution.

Hospital Use of Exotic Antivenoms

Because exotic antivenoms are not readily available, it is often difficult to obtain the species-specific correct antivenom in the appropriate amount. The PCCs become critical resources during this time. Often they can locate the closest supply and coordinate delivery. In the case of an envenomation at a zoo, the appropriate antivenom may arrive with the patient. In the case of the exotic snake owner, the poison control center may help facilitate acquisition of antivenom from local sources, such as zoos, known to stock the antivenom for emergency use. If there are no local sources, the poison control center staff can easily access the AI to locate the closest available stock of antivenom. In one case report, it took a regional poison control center 5 hours to locate and organize airborne delivery of the appropriate antivenom to the treating facility.[18] A similar report described a 3-hour delay to administration even when the antivenom was present in the local zoo.[10] During that delay, the patient required intubation.

Arranging for transport of the antivenom can be difficult, often requiring fixed wing transportation across state lines. The antivenom must be transported from the zoo, to the airport, and then boarded on a plane. Often, a medical transport team or a commercial airline can assist with the transport. Utilizaiton of commercial airlines often requires extensive justifications, explanations, and authorizations.

Once brought to the facility, a series of steps must occur prior to the patient administration of the non–US FDA-approved antivenom. The treating physician should contact the US FDA to obtain approval to administer the antivenom as an IND under emergency use.[36] Contact numbers are found at http://www.fda.gov/RegulatoryInformation/Guidances/ucm126491.htm.

In addition, the treating physician will need to obtain informed consent from the patient prior to administration. Because the antivenom is considered an investigational product, both the Institutional Review Board (IRB) and Drug and Formulary Committee must be notified and provide approval. Many IRBs have emergency processes to expedite such a request. If such approval cannot be obtained in a clinically relevant time, the IRB must be notified of the emergency treatment within 5 working days of the administration.[1,27] The physician must also complete the appropriate IND paperwork (Form FDA 1571) and submit a comprehensive case report.[37]

In addition to the legalities involved in using an investigational product, there are significant operational and logistical issues necessary to ensure appropriate preparation of the product. The pharmacy department should be notified as soon as possible to allow the staff time to begin investigating preparation and administration instructions. Clinical pharmacists provide additional support for both the treating physician and drug preparation aspects in many emergency departments.[27] The utilization of such individuals can greatly facilitate the medication preparation.

The package insert for the specific antivenom will be most helpful for the pharmacist in the preparation process. Specific instructions on diluents, storage, light or heat sensitivities, compatibility, and rate of administration are usually found in the package insert. If the specific antivenom product is known in advance, the pharmacist can begin to research these issues. Many package inserts are found in the AI and can be obtained with the help of the PCC. However, not all package inserts are in English, and some must be translated or a translated copy must be located.[21] If reconstitution of the antivenom is required, it can take minutes to hours to completely dissolve all the lyophilized particles. In addition to preparation, there is often a significant amount of documentation required when dispensing an IND drug. Having knowledge of the required procedure will expedite the administration of the antivenom.

Other Therapies

In principle, snake venoms should have some commonality, as they share the purposes of immobilizing or killing prey and beginning the digestive process, and have some common genetic linkage. In practicality, many venoms from snakes found from diverse areas of the globe share constituents or antigenic characteristics.[5,7,33,35] It is therefore possible to use antivenoms derived against specific snakes in the treatment of envenomation from other snakes with related venoms. US FDA-approved coral snake antivenom was used in an experimental model of nonnative elapid envenomation.[32] Similarly, US FDA-approved crotalid antivenom demonstrated efficacy against mice treated with venom from *Crotalus durissus terrificus*, *Bothrops atrox*, and *Bitis gabonica*.[23,31] In fact, a single case report demonstrates utilization of this principle of cross reactivity when a patient envenomated by *C. durissus terrificus* was successfully treated with US FDA–approved Crotalidae Polyvalent Immune Fab (CroFab).[19] Such cross-reactivity should never be assumed based on common or taxonomic identification. The manufacturer of Crotalidae Polyvalent Immune Fab has listed experimental cross-reactivity with a number of species in the AI (Table SC10–3). The clinical decision to use Crotalidae Polyvalent Immune Fab for a patient envenomated by a non-US species of snake with known experimental cross-reactivity should be based on the severity of envenomation, the availability of species-specific antivenom, and the risks associated with administration of species-specific antivenom versus the risks of Crotalidae Polyvalent Immune Fab administration (Antidotes in Depth: A39).

The venom of many neurotoxic snakes interferes with neuromuscular transmission similar to neuromuscular blockers used in clinical medicine (Chap. 66). Neostigmine and other cholinesterase inhibitors increase the LD_{50} of animals treated with *Naja haje haje* venom.[11] Additionally, case reports and case series suggest an improvement in neurologic deficits and respiratory failure after neostigmine with or without atropine in humans suffering neurotoxic snake envenomation.[3,9,26,38] In these reports, patients typically received 0.5 to 1 mg of neostigmine IV immediately following pretreatment with 0.5 to 0.6 mg of atropine IV. In some cases, this is repeated every 10 to 30 minutes based on response. Benefits vary and are likely dependent on a number of factors, including differences in the mechanism of neuromuscular blockade between snake species.[2] However, because the complications of atropine and neostigmine at these doses are small and there is a suggestion that they sometimes reverse neuromuscular blockade, administration is reasonable if antivenom is unavailable or delayed. Early trials with mice and intranasal neostigmine use show promise for an alternate route of administration. Animals were injected with an intraperitoneal dose of venom from *Naja naja* at 2.5, 5, and 10 times the LD_{50} with subsequent treatment with neostigmine by nasal administration. Treated mice showed an increase in survival time in all groups, with 10 of 15 mice in the 2.5× LD_{50} group surviving with normal behavior 6 hours after injection of venom.[16] There is one published case report using intranasal neostigmine in a human after being given mivacurium to mimic the mechanism from a neurotoxic envenomation. Using 2 independent, blinded clinicians, the patient demonstrated improvements in visual acuity, ease of swallowing, and neck flexion shortly after administration of intranasal neostigmine (Chap. 66 and Table 66–5).[15]

Tissue and hematologic toxicity are time-dependent effects that would benefit from early intervention. Worldwide, many envenomed individuals have increased morbidity and mortality secondary to delayed time to treatment.[25] Similarly, the lack of readily available antivenoms for nonnative species in the United States also poses a dilemma. Because of delays in acquiring antivenom, as previously discussed, other supportive measures are needed. There has been research attempting to find xenobiotics capable of

TABLE SC10–3	Experimental Cross-Reactivity Between CroFab and Nonnative Snakes is Suggested for these Species[a]		
Genus	*Species and Sub Species*	*Common Name*	*Natural Habitat*
Agkistrodon	*bilineatus bilineatus*	Cantil, common cantil, Mexican moccasin, tropical moccasin, Mexican cantil	Mexico and Central America
	bilineatus howardgloydi	Castellana	Honduras, Nicaragua, and Costa Rica
	bilineatus lemosespinali	Cantil, Mexican moccasin	Mexico and Central America
	bilineatus russeolus	Cantil, common cantil, Mexican moccasin	Mexico and Central America
	bilineatus taylori	Taylor's cantil, ornate cantil	Mexico
Bothriechis	*aurifer*	Yellow-blotched palm pit viper, Guatemalan palm viper	Mexico and Guatemala
	bicolor	Guatemalan palm pit viper, Guatemalan tree viper	Mexico, Guatemala, and Honduras
	rowleyi	Mexican palm pit viper	Mexico
	schlegelii	Eyelash viper	Central and South America
Bothrops	*asper*	Fer-de-lance	Mexico and South America
	moojeni	Brazilian lancehead	Brazil
Crotalus	*basiliscus*	Mexican west coast rattlesnake, Mexican green rattler	Mexico
	cerastes cerastes	Sidewinder, horned rattlesnake, sidewinder rattlesnake	US and Northwestern Mexico
	cerastes cercobombus	Sonoran Desert sidewinder, Sonoran sidewinder	US and Northwestern Mexico
	durissus durissus	South American rattlesnake, tropical rattlesnake	South America
	durissus totonacus	Totonacan rattlesnake	Northern Mexico
	durissus tzabcan	Middle American rattlesnake, Central American rattlesnake, tzabcan	Mexico and Central America
	enyo enyo	Baja California rattlesnake, Lower California rattlesnake	US and Northwestern Mexico
	exsul (Ruber)	Red diamond rattlesnake, red rattlesnake, red diamond snake	Baja California, Mexico
	exsul exsul (Ruber)	Red diamond rattlesnake, red rattlesnake, red diamond snake	Baja California, Mexico
	intermedius gloydi	Oaxacan small-headed rattlesnake	Mexico
	lannomi	Autlán rattlesnake	Mexico
	lepidus castaneus	Rock rattlesnake	US and Mexico
	lepidus klauberi	Banded rock rattlesnake, green rattlesnake, green rock rattlesnake	US and Mexico
	lepidus lepidus	Rock rattlesnake, green rattlesnake, blue rattlesnake	US and Mexico
	lepidus maculosus	Durango rock rattlesnake	Mexico
	lepidus morulus	Rock rattlesnake	Mexico
	mitchelli angelensis	Angel de la Guarda Island speckled rattlesnake	Angel de la Guarda Island, Mexico
	mitchelli mitchelli	Speckled rattlesnake, Mitchell's rattlesnake, white rattlesnake	US and Mexico
	mitchelli muertensis	El Muerto Island speckled rattlesnake	El Muerto Island, Mexico
	mitchelli pyrrhus	Southwestern speckled rattlesnake, Mitchell's rattlesnake	US and Mexico
	molossus estabanensis	San Esteban Island rattlesnake	San Esteban Island, Mexico
	molossus molossus	Northern black-tailed rattlesnake, green rattler	US and Mexico
	molossus nigrescens	Mexican black-tailed rattlesnake	US and Mexico
	molossus oaxacus	Oaxacan black-tailed rattlesnake	Mexico
	polystictus	Mexican lance-headed rattlesnake, lance-headed rattlesnake	Mexico
	pricei miquihuanus	Eastern twin-spotted rattlesnake	Mexico
	pricei pricei	Western twin-spotted rattlesnake	Mexico
	pusillus	Tancitaran dusky rattlesnake	Mexico
	ruber lorenzoensis	San Lorenzo Island rattlesnake	San Lorenzo Island, Mexico
	ruber lucasensis	San Lucan diamond rattlesnake	Mexico
	ruber ruber	Red diamond rattlesnake	US and Mexico
	scutulatus salvini	Huamantlan rattlesnake	Mexico
	scutulatus scutulatus	Mojave rattlesnake	US and Mexico
	stejnegeri	Long-tailed rattlesnake	Mexico
	tigris	Tiger rattlesnake, tiger rattler	US and Mexico
	tortugensis	Tortuga Island diamond rattlesnake, Tortuga Island rattlesnake	Tortuga Island, Mexico

(Continued)

TABLE SC10–3	Experimental Cross-Reactivity Between CroFab and Nonnative Snakes is Suggested for these Species[a] *(Continued)*		
Genus	**Species and Sub Species**	**Common Name**	**Natural Habitat**
	transversus	Cross-banded mountain rattlesnake	Mexico
	triseriatus aquilus	Querétaro dusky rattlesnake, Queretaran dusky rattlesnake	Mexico
	triseriatus armstrongi	Western dusky rattlesnake	Mexico
	triseriatus triseriatus	Dusky rattlesnake	Mexico
	viridis caliginus	Coronado Island rattlesnake	Coronado Island, Mexico
	willardi amabilis	Del Nido ridge-nosed rattlesnake	Mexico
	willardi meridionalis	Southern ridge-nosed rattlesnake	Mexico
	willardi obscurus	Animas ridge-nosed rattlesnake	US and Mexico
	willardi silus	Chihuahuan ridge-nosed rattlesnake	Mexico
	willardi willardi	Arizona ridge-nosed rattlesnake	US and Mexico
Ophryacus	*undulatus*	Mexican horned pit viper, undulated pit viper	Mexico
Porthidium	*dunni*	Dunn's hognosed pit viper	Mexico
	godmani	Godman's montane pit viper, Godman's pit viper	Mexico and Central America
	hespere	Colima hognosed pit viper	Mexico
	nasutum	Rainforest hognosed pit viper, horned hog-nosed viper	Mexico, Central America, and South America
	yucatanicum	Yucatán hognosed pit viper	Mexico
Sistrurus	*ravus*	Mexican pigmy rattlesnake, Mexican pygmy rattlesnake	Mexico

[a]"Cross-reactivity" defined here as experimental evidence supplied by the manufacturer to the Antivenom Index. Although clinical evidence of benefit is lacking, use of Crotalidae Polyvalent Immune Fab is reasonabe in these envenomations based on a risk-to-benefit analysis when species specific antivenom is lacking, delayed, or contraindicated (due to allergy), and the envenomation is a risk to life or limb.

minimizing damage in envenomed patients while awaiting definitive care. Snake venom metalloproteinase (SVMP) and phospholipase A_2 (PLA$_2$) are 2 venom components responsible for some of the hemorrhagic, cytotoxic, and myotoxic effects contributing to morbidity. Research into inhibitors of those agents are ongoing both in vitro and in animal models and shows promise for delaying damaging effects.[4,17,28]

It is important to remember that there is a wide variation in the standards for preparation of antivenoms around the world. Although many products are highly purified antibody fragments, some continue to use whole immunoglobulins that maintain the risk for anaphylaxis. Prior to antivenom administration, preparations must be made to treat anaphylaxis. The appropriate level of nursing care and monitoring should be available, IV access should be secured, and typical drugs (epinephrine, corticosteroids, antihistamines) and airway management equipment should be immediately available.

SUMMARY

- Many venomous snakes are found in homes and zoos far from their native habitats.

- It is essential to develop sophisticated systems of care in collaboration with poison control centers and zoos assuring preparedness for worker or hobbyist injury.

- The use of internationally prepared antivenoms may be both life-saving and hazardous. The risks can be limited and benefits maximized through an understanding of available internationally prepared antivenoms.

- The Antivenom Index, available to poison control centers and the Association of Zoos and Aquariums, provides invaluable information about matching an antivenom to a particular snake, location of antivenoms, package inserts, and available English translations of foreign package inserts.

- The use of antivenoms not US FDA approved must follow the rules for an investigational new drug (IND).

- US Food and Drug Administration approved antivenoms may have cross-reactivity against some nonnative snakes.

- The use of prehospital or preantivenom pressure immobilization in the United States is likely of little benefit. Access to a health care facility capable of critical care interventions is of greater value while awaiting antivenom.

REFERENCES

1. American College of Medical Toxicology. Position Statement: Institutions Housing Venomous Animals. http://www.acmt.net/cgi/page.cgi/zine_service.html?aid=4005&zine=show. Accessed July 15, 2013.
2. Anil A, et al. Role of neostigmine and polyvalent antivenom in Indian common krait (*Bungarus caeruleus*) bite. *J Infect Public Health*. 2010;3:83-87.
3. Banerjee RN, et al. Neostigmine in the treatment of Elapidae bites. *J Assoc Physicians India*. 1972;20:503-509.
4. Baraldi PT, et al. A novel synthetic quinolinone inhibitor presents proteolytic and hemorrhagic inhibitory activities against snake venom metalloproteases. *Biochimie*. 2016;121:179-188.
5. Calvete JJ, et al. Snake venomics and antivenomics of *Bothrops colombiensis*, a medically important pitviper of the *Bothrops* atrox-asper complex endemic to Venezuela: contributing to its taxonomy and snakebite management. *J Proteomics*. 2009;72:227-240.
6. Calvete JJ, et al. Venoms, venomics, antivenomics. *FEBS Lett*. 2009;583:1736-1743.
7. Chiou SH, et al. Characterization and immunological comparison of isoenzymes of phospholipases A2 from snake venoms of different genera and families. *Biochem Int*. 1991;25:1003-1011.
8. Chippaux JP. Snake-bites: appraisal of the global situation. *Bull World Health Organ*. 1998;76:515-524.
9. Gold BS. Neostigmine for the treatment of neurotoxicity following envenomation by the Asiatic cobra. *Ann Emerg Med*. 1996;28:87-89.
10. Gold BS, Pyle P. Successful treatment of neurotoxic king cobra envenomation in Myrtle Beach, South Carolina. *Ann Emerg Med*. 1998;32:736-738.
11. Guieu R, et al. Anticholinesterases and experimental envenomation by Naja. *Comp Biochem Physiol C Pharmacol Toxicol Endocrinol*. 1994;109:265-268.
12. Hantsch C. *Bothrops moojeni* envenomation: a rare situation further complicated by an uncommon horse allergy. *Clin Toxicol*. 2016;54:33.
13. Kasturiratne A, et al. The global burden of snakebite: a literature analysis and modelling based on regional estimates of envenoming and deaths. *PLoS Med*. 2008;5:e218.
14. Kunkel DB, et al. Reptile envenomations. *J Toxicol Clin Toxicol*. 1983;21:503-526.
15. Lewin MR, et al. Reversal of experimental paralysis in human by intranasal neostigmine aerosol suggests a novel approach to the early treatment of neurotoxic envenomation. *Clin Case Rep*. 2013;1:7-15.
16. Lewin MR, et al. Early treatment with intranasal neostigmine reduces mortality in a mouse model of *Naja naja* (Indian Cobra) Envenomation. *J Trop Med*. 2014;2014:1-6.
17. Lewin M, et al. Varespladib (LY315920) appears to be a potent, broad-spectrum, inhibitor of snake venom phospholipase A2 and a possible pre-referral treatment for envenomation. *Toxins (Basel)*. 2016;8. pii: E248.
18. Lubich C, Krenzelok EP. Exotic snakes are not always found in exotic places: how poison centres can assist emergency departments. *Emerg Med J*. 2007;24:796-797.
19. Lynch MJ, et al. Successful treatment of South American rattlesnake (*Crotalus durissus terrificus*) envenomation with Crotalidae polyvalent immune Fab (CroFab). *J Med Toxicol*. 2011;7:44-46.

20. Massey DJ, et al. Venom variability and envenoming severity outcomes of the *Crotalus scutulatus scutulatus* (Mojave rattlesnake) from Southern Arizona. *J Proteomics.* 2012; 75:2576-2587.

21. McNally J, et al. Toxicologic information resources for reptile envenomations. *Vet Clin North Am Exot Anim Pract.* 2008;11:389-401.

22. Mebs D. *Venomous and Poisonous Animals: A Handbook for Biologists, and Toxicologists and Toxinologists, Physicians and Pharmacists.* Boca Raton, FL: CRC Press; 2002.

23. Meggs WJ, et al. Efficacy of North American crotalid antivenom against the African viper *Bitis gabonica* (Gaboon viper). *J Med Toxicol.* 2010;6:12-14.

24. Minton SA. Bites by non-native venomous snakes in the United States. *Wilderness Environ Med.* 1996;7:297-303.

25. Mohapatra B, et al. Snakebite mortality in India: a nationally representative mortality survey. *PLoS Negl Trop Dis.* 2011;5:e1018.

26. Naphade RW, Shetti RN. Use of neostigmine after snake bite. *Br J Anaesth.* 1977; 49:1065-1068.

27. Othong R, et al. Exotic venomous snakebite drill. *Clin Toxicol (Phila).* 2012;50:490-496.

28. Pereañez JA, et al. Glycolic acid inhibits enzymatic, hemorrhagic and edema-inducing activities of BaP1, a P-I metalloproteinase from *Bothrops asper* snake venom: insights from docking and molecular modeling. *Toxicon.* 2013;71:41-48.

29. Pyron RA, et al. The phylogeny of advanced snakes (Colubroidea), with discovery of a new subfamily and comparison of support methods for likelihood trees. *Mol Phylogenet Evol.* 2011;58:329-342.

30. Pyron RA, et al. A phylogeny and revised classification of Squamata, including 4161 species of lizards and snakes. *BMC Evol Biol.* 2013;13:93-146.

31. Richardson WH 3rd, et al. Crotalidae polyvalent immune Fab (ovine) antivenom is effective in the neutralization of South American viperidae venoms in a murine model. *Ann Emerg Med.* 2005;45:595-602.

32. Richardson WH 3rd, et al. North American coral snake antivenin for the neutralization of non-native elapid venoms in a murine model. *Acad Emerg Med.* 2006;13:121-126.

33. Sanz L, et al. Snake venomics of the South and Central American Bushmasters. Comparison of the toxin composition of *Lachesis muta* gathered from proteomic versus transcriptomic analysis. *J Proteomics.* 2008;71:46-60.

34. Seifert S, et al. Toxic Exposure Surveillance System (TESS)-based characterization of U.S. non-native venomous snake exposures, 1995-2004. *Clin Toxicol.* 2007;45:571-578.

35. Uetz P. The reptile database. www.reptile-database.org. Accessed July 15, 2013.

36. US Food and Drug Administration. Emergency use IND requests. https://www.fda.gov/drugs/developmentapprovalprocess/default.htm. Accessed June 27, 2018.

37. US Food and Drug Administration. Information on the use of antivenoms. https://www.fda.gov/biologicsbloodvaccines/developmentapprovalprocess/investigationalnewdrugindordeviceexemptionideprocess/ucm094321.htm. Accessed June 27, 2018.

38. Vital Brazil O, Vieira RJ. Neostigmine in the treatment of snake accidents caused by *Micrurus frontalis*: report of two cases (1). *Rev Inst Med Trop Sao Paulo.* 1996;38:61-67.

39. Vohra R, et al. A pilot study of occupational envenomations in North American zoos and aquaria. *Clin Toxicol (Phila).* 2008;46:790-793.

40. Warrell DA. Venomous bites and stings in the tropical world. *Med J Aust.* 1993;159:773-779.

41. Warrell DA. Commissioned article: management of exotic snakebites. *Q J Med.* 2009; 102:593-601.

42. Warrick BJ, et al. Non-native (exotic) snake envenomations in the U.S., 2005-2011. *Toxins (Basel).* 2014;6:2899-2911.

43. Wiens JJ, et al. Resolving the phylogeny of lizards and snakes (Squamata) with extensive sampling of genes and species. *Biol Lett.* 2012;8:1043-1046.

44. Williams D, et al. The Global Snake Bite Initiative: an antidote for snake bite. *Lancet.* 2010;375:89-91.

45. Yamazaki Y, et al. Wide distribution of cysteine-rich secretory proteins in snake venoms: isolation and cloning of novel snake venom cysteine-rich secretory proteins. *Arch Biochem Biophys.* 2003;412:133-141.

CASE STUDY 12

History A 55-year-old man was working at a textile manufacturing site and developed shortness of breath and a "dusky" skin color. The man had a history of a Barrett's esophagus and obstructive sleep apnea and underwent periodic upper gastrointestinal endoscopy as a screening procedure for esophageal cancer. The foreman who called the rapid response reported that the patient had no complaints before this episode but had been splashed with liquid while connecting a hose coupling to a holding tank containing clothing dye. The identification of the dye was not immediately available, but the employee immediately self-decontaminated with water from an emergency shower before the ambulance arrival. The clothes were removed and disposed of at the work site. No other individuals at the site were potentially exposed.

Physical Examination Upon arrival, the patient had blood pressure, 166/112 mm Hg; pulse, 142 beats/min; respiratory rate, 40 breaths/min; and oxygen saturation, 87% on 4 L/min of oxygen via nasal cannula. Physical examination was notable for an ill-appearing man who could only speak in short sentences. His skin and nailbeds were cyanotic; his chest was clear; and his heart was regular and tachycardic without murmurs, gallops, or rubs.

Initial Management The patient received oxygen via a 100% nonrebreather mask, and bilevel positive airway pressure was started while preparations were made for endotracheal intubation. Although his respiratory rate and pulse improved somewhat, his oxygen saturation remained between 86% and 88%. An electrocardiogram (ECG) was obtained and showed sinus tachycardia without ST-segment or T-wave changes suggestive of ischemia or infarction. His clothes were removed and bagged.

A chest radiograph showed no cardiac or pulmonary disease, and an arterial blood gas (ABG) analysis was obtained. The resident commented that although she was certain that the blood was obtained from an artery, it looked dark as if it were venous blood. The results demonstrated the following: pH, 7.32; PCO_2, 33 mm Hg; PO_2, 426 mm Hg, and oxygen saturation, 100%. The results were interpreted as a primary metabolic acidosis with respiratory compensation (respiratory alkalosis). This corresponded to a serum bicarbonate concentration of approximately 16 mEq/L (Chap. 12) and reinforced the clinical impression that the patient was significantly ill.

What Is the Differential Diagnosis?

This patient presented with hypertension, tachycardia, tachypnea, cyanosis, and decreased oxygen saturation. The most common causes of these findings in a nonindustrial environment are cardiac and pulmonary disease. Hypoxia and cyanosis in a normal environment (breathing a normal FiO_2) can result from a shunt, ventilation–perfusion mismatch, diffusion abnormalities, or pump failure (Chaps. 16 and 28). The absence of underlying heart disease, an unremarkable ECG, pulse and blood pressure that are adequate for tissue perfusion, and clear chest examination essentially excludes these disorders, although laboratory ultrasonographic and radiologic confirmation should be obtained.

The combination of cyanosis with a low oxygen saturation by pulse oximetry, failure to respond to supplemental oxygen, dark-colored blood, and a normal or high PO_2 on the ABG analysis are essentially diagnostic of methemoglobinemia or sulfhemoglobinemia (Chap. 124). When methemoglobinemia is suspected, the color of the blood is related to the methemoglobin level (Fig. CS12–1). Although confirmation can and should be obtained via cooximetry analysis of either venous or arterial blood, the clinical information in this case was sufficient to initiate treatment if cooximetry was either unavailable or delayed.

Treatment Venous blood sent for cooximetry revealed a 43% methemoglobin level. The patient was administered 100 mg of methylene blue by slow intravenous administration (Antidotes in Depth: A43). Within about 5 minutes of starting the infusion, his oxygen saturation by pulse oximetry dropped to 64% without a change in his vital signs. Over the next 15 minutes, his oxygen saturation gradually increased to 99%, and his respiratory rate, heart rate, and blood pressure normalized. His shortness of breath resolved. A repeat methemoglobin level taken 30 minutes after the end of the methylene blue administration was 3%. The patient remained well, and subsequent information from the worksite confirmed that the dye material from the tank was aniline.

After the exposure to aniline was determined, the treating staff and first responders expressed concerns over their potential exposure. Additional concerns were expressed about the possible contamination of the ambulance. Because first responders and providers were not wearing protective equipment and the onset of methemoglobinemia may be delayed, they were all screened for elevated methemoglobin levels. In addition, the ambulance was taken out of service and decontaminated.

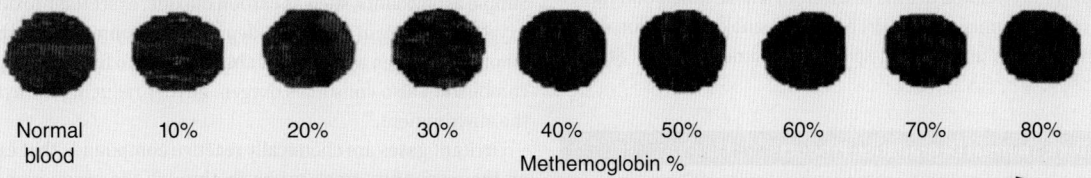

Normal blood   10%   20%   30%   40%   50%   60%   70%   80%

Methemoglobin %

FIGURE CS12–1. The relationship between methemoglobin level and blood color. This figure demonstrates the relationship between methemoglobin level and the color of blood. If anticoagulated blood is placed on a white background, the methemoglobin level can be estimated accurately by comparison with the scale. It is important to note that although normal anticoagulated venous blood oxygenates spontaneously (ie, become redder over time), if exposed to room air, methemoglobin is incapable of extracting oxygen from air and will remain dark over time. *(Reproduced with permission from Shihana F, Dissanayake DM, Buckley NA, et al. A simple quantitative bedside test to determine methemoglobin. Ann Emerg Med. 2010 Feb;55(2):184-189.)*

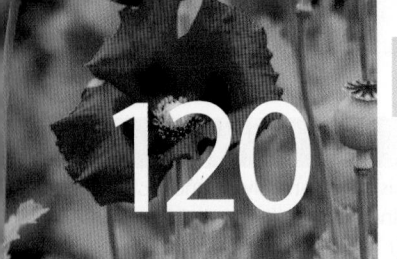
HISTORY AND EPIDEMIOLOGY

Smoke is generated as the result of thermal degradation of a material; it is a complex mixture of heated air containing suspended solid and liquid particles (aerosols), gases, and vapors. Particulates and aerosols typically make these thermal degradation products visible to the naked eye, resulting in the black, acrid substance so often thought of as "smoke"; however, thermal decomposition of common materials also results in the generation of gaseous substances that are invisible to the naked eye. The complex and ever-growing variety of materials used in our environment contributes to the broad spectrum of products present in typical smoke.[32,159] The chemical composition of the parent materials, oxygen availability, and temperature at the time of decomposition all help determine the combustion products found in smoke (Table 120–1).[118,127] As a result of these variabilities, specific thermal degradation products resulting from a fire are difficult to predict; in fact, even the composition of smoke is quite variable within the same fire environment.[127]

Smoke inhalation is a complex medical syndrome involving diverse toxicologic injuries, making care of smoke-injured patients very challenging. These injuries occur both locally within the respiratory tract and systemically. It is, in fact, smoke inhalation—not thermal burns—that is the leading cause of death from fires. Cutaneous burns, however, found concurrently with smoke inhalation complicate airway management and fluid resuscitation and increase the risk of infection. Consequently, burn victims with smoke inhalation injury have higher morbidity and mortality rates than those with burns alone.[47,157,159]

Compared with other industrialized countries, the United States has one of the highest rates of fire-related deaths in the world.[159,168] Throughout the United States, a fire department responds to a fire every 23 seconds.[71] In 2015, the National Fire Protection Agency reported 1,345,500 fire incidents in the United States, and approximately 501,500 of these events were structural fires. There were 3,280 fire-related deaths and 15,700 fire-related injuries reported in 2015.[71] On average, a civilian fire death occurs every 160 minutes, and a civilian injury from a structural fire occurs every 34 minutes.[71] Seventy-eight percent of civilian fire deaths occur in home structural fires.[71] An estimated 50% to 80% of fire-related deaths result from smoke inhalation rather than dermal burns or trauma, and deaths related to smoke inhalation occur much more prevalently in an enclosed-space environment.[23,70,118,180] Studies

indicate that from 10% to more than 40% of patients hospitalized in burn units develop complications of concomitant pulmonary injury.[11,50,74,81] The presence of inhalational injury in burn patients correlates with an increased risk of mortality and decreases the total body surface area (TBSA) of a burn that is needed to lead to death, more than doubling the risk of death per TBSA burn in some studies.[11,50,81]

Disastrous enclosed-space fires are a frequent reminder of the role of inhalation injury in fire deaths. Before 1942, toxic inhalation was not considered in the etiology of morbidity and mortality of structural fire victims. However, in that year, a fire at the Cocoanut Grove Night Club in Boston resulted in a number of fatalities in which victims had no cutaneous burns. This led to the observation that high concentrations of toxic gases are generated in typical enclosed-space structural fires and may result in significant morbidity and mortality.[126] From 1955 to 1972, death from smoke inhalation injury increased threefold and was attributed to abundant use of newer synthetic materials for building and furnishings.[23] From 2006 to 2015 in the United States, an average of 24 catastrophic fires occurred per year, claiming an average of 132 lives each year.[71] Despite improved firefighting resources, mass casualties from smoke inhalation continue. On November 24, 2012, a fire swept through the lower floors of a Bangladesh garment factory, killing 112 and trapping many others on the top floors until rescuers arrived. Hundreds of those trapped above the blaze sustained inhalation injuries.[7] In 2013, 235 people died in a nightclub fire in Brazil when a fire ignited above the concert stage. Smoke inhalation resulted in many of the deaths and forced many others to seek medical treatment.[139] More recently, on December 3, 2016, 36 people were killed when a fire destroyed an Oakland, California, warehouse that was being used to stage a music event.[147] Interestingly, in 2011, explosions caused an unusually high number of catastrophic fires in the United States, highlighting the complex pathologies of fire victims with the potential for victims to have any combination of inhalation injury, burns, and trauma.[6]

PATHOPHYSIOLOGY

Toxic thermal degradation products are classified into three categories: simple asphyxiants, irritant gases, and chemical asphyxiants (Table 120–2). Simple asphyxiants, such as carbon dioxide, exert their toxicity by displacing oxygen, resulting in an oxygen-deprived environment, thereby decreasing the amount of oxygen available for absorption.[59] To further complicate this issue, combustion also consumes oxygen, further reducing the available oxygen in the environment.[59]

Irritant gases are chemically reactive compounds that exert a local effect on the respiratory tract, primarily through the production of acids, alkalis, or reactive oxygen species (ROS) (Chap. 121). Irritant gases affect all levels of the airway, and in general, their damage leads to swelling and obstruction of the airway, ultimately impairing oxygenation. For irritant gases, the degree of water solubility is the most important chemical characteristic in determining the timing and anatomic location of respiratory tract injury. Highly water-soluble xenobiotics, such as ammonia and hydrogen chloride, primarily injure the upper airway by rapidly combining with mucosal water, leaving little of the parent compound to travel farther down the airway. These xenobiotics quickly damage mucosal cells, which subsequently release mediators of inflammation or ROS.[30,96,113,137] This rapid reaction produces early irritation, potentially providing a warning to the victims that the environment is unsafe and prompting escape. After more than a trivial exposure, the intense inflammatory response increases microvascular permeability

TABLE 120–1	Toxic Thermal Degradation Products
Asphyxiants	**Irritants**
Simple	**High Water Solubility (Upper Airway Injury)**
Carbon dioxide	Ammonia
Chemical	Hydrogen chloride
Carbon monoxide	Sulfur dioxide
Hydrogen cyanide	**Intermediate Water Solubility (Upper and Lower Respiratory Tract Injury)**
Hydrogen sulfide	
Oxides of nitrogen	Chlorine
	Isocyanates
	Low Water Solubility (Pulmonary Parenchymal Injury)
	Oxides of nitrogen
	Phosgene

TABLE 120–2	Common Materials and Their Thermal Degradation Products
Materials	*Thermal Degradation Products*
Wool	Ammonia, carbon monoxide, chlorine, cyanide, hydrogen chloride, phosgene
Silk	Ammonia, cyanide, hydrogen sulfide, sulfur dioxide
Nylon	Ammonia, cyanide
Wood, cotton, paper	Acetaldehyde, acetic acid, acrolein, carbon monoxide, formic acid, formaldehyde, methane
Petroleum materials	Acetic acid, acrolein, carbon monoxide, formic acid
Polystyrene	Styrene
Acrylic	Acrolein, carbon monoxide, hydrogen chloride
Plastics	Aldehydes, ammonia, chlorine, cyanide, hydrogen chloride, nitrogen oxides, phosgene,
Polyvinyl chloride	Carbon monoxide, chlorine, hydrogen chloride, phosgene
Polyurethane	Cyanide, isocyanates
Melamine resins	Ammonia, cyanide
Rubber	Hydrogen sulfide, sulfur dioxide
Sulfur-containing materials	Sulfur dioxide
Nitrogen-containing materials	Cyanide, isocyanates, oxides of nitrogen
Fluorinated resins	Hydrogen fluoride
Fire retardant materials	Hydrogen bromide, hydrogen chloride

and allows movement of fluid from the intravascular space into the tissues of the upper airway.[17] This inflammation is potentiated by thermal injury, which, because of the efficient cooling mechanisms of the respiratory tract, primarily occurs in the supraglottic airway. The loosely attached underlying tissue of the supraglottic larynx becomes markedly edematous, causing upper airway obstruction within minutes to hours.[79] The obstruction often progresses to the point of complete upper airway occlusion.[144] Xenobiotics with low water solubility, such as phosgene and oxides of nitrogen, react with the upper respiratory mucosa more slowly and do not elicit the irritation and aversion stimulus that prompts an escape response. These xenobiotics more typically reach the distal lung parenchyma, where they react slowly to create delayed toxic effects. Xenobiotics with intermediate water solubility, such as chlorine and isocyanates, are more likely to result in damage to both the upper and lower respiratory tracts. In addition to water solubility, other factors, such as concentration of the inhaled xenobiotic, duration of exposure, particle size, respiratory rate, absence of protective reflexes, and preexisting disease, influence the region of respiratory tract injury. For example, as the concentration of a highly water-soluble irritant gas increases, more chemical is presented to the lower airway, possibly leading to damage of the lower respiratory tract. In addition, patients with loss of consciousness increase their exposure secondary to their loss of protective reflexes.[8,68] Damage to the tracheobronchial tree is mediated by many of the same mechanisms as those of the pharynx and hypopharynx: inhaled particulates and toxic gases result in deposition of corrosives and oxidants. Direct thermal injury is less likely to occur as a result of the efficient cooling ability of the upper airways.[113] Direct injury to the tracheobronchial tree and an intense inflammatory response, evoked in part by airway nociceptive sensory neurons, leads to an increase in airway resistance from mucosal edema, bronchoconstriction, and accumulation of intraluminal debris and airway secretions.[17,83,102,163] Increased tracheobronchial vascular permeability contributes to interstitial edema of the airways and increased airway resistance. Bronchoconstriction and subsequent wheezing are caused by a reflex response to toxic mucosal injury

and a response to mediators of inflammation.[68,164] Damaged cells release chemotactic factors that stimulate production of an exudate rich in protein, including fibrin and inflammatory cells.[54,169] This injury ultimately results in sloughing of the mucosa, which combines with inflammatory cells and exudate to create casts in the airways.[54] Casts can block both the small and large airways, increasing airway resistance and mechanically preventing passage of oxygen to the alveoli.[43]

Irritant xenobiotics that reach the alveoli injure the lung parenchyma.[119] Corrosives, proteolytic enzymes, reactive free radicals, and mediators of inflammation all contribute to acute respiratory distress syndrome (ARDS).[89,132,164,178] Pathophysiologic changes of ARDS decrease lung compliance and bacterial defenses and lead to ventilation–perfusion mismatch with intrapulmonary shunting, increased extravascular lung water, and microvascular permeability.[40,164,169,173] Lung compliance is further decreased by atelectasis when xenobiotics inactivate pulmonary surfactant.[119,129] In animal studies, patchy atelectasis rapidly occurs after smoke inhalation.[119] In addition, ventilation–perfusion mismatch occurs when pulmonary blood flow is diverted both by hypoxia and vasoactive mediators of inflammation.[98,122] Xenobiotics cause additional injury by impairing clearance by the mucociliary apparatus, altering alveolar macrophage function, and impairing phagocytosis of bacteria, all of which predispose to pulmonary infections and sepsis.[18,55,73,143] The combination of the delayed toxic effects of some inhaled xenobiotics and the slowly developing inflammatory response helps explain the progression of parenchymal injury during the first 24 hours after smoke exposure.

Thermal degradation of organic material produces finely divided carbonaceous particulate matter (soot) suspended in hot gases. These carbonaceous particles adsorb other combustion products from the environment, including metals, aldehydes, organic acids, and other reactive chemicals.[88,137] Soot adheres to the mucosa of the airways, allowing adsorbed irritant xenobiotics to desorb and react with the mucosal surface moisture. The deposition of these particles in the respiratory tract depends on their size, with particles of 1 to 3 μm reaching the alveoli.[111] Irritant gases can also adsorb on aerosol droplets and alter the site of gas deposition.[72] This pattern of chemical deposition and desorption from soot or aerosols appears to worsen inhalational injury by enhancing and prolonging exposure to irritants in a fire environment. Accordingly, experimental animals demonstrate markedly decreased lung injury when exposed to toxic gases from smoke that was filtered to remove particulates.[88]

Nitric oxide plays a significant role in the pathogenesis of smoke inhalation–induced lung injury.[51,108,171] Combined smoke inhalation and burn injury results in an upregulation of inducible nitric oxide synthase (iNOS) mRNA synthesis in animal models and subsequently results in increased activity of iNOS.[51,53,108,152] Increased concentrations of nitric oxide results in myocardial contractile dysfunction with subsequent hypotension.[152] Nitric oxide also increases vascular permeability with resultant edema.[108] One possible mechanism is the formation of the highly reactive peroxynitrite (ONOO⁻) radical from the combination of nitric oxide and ROS, which leads to alveolar capillary membrane damage and subsequent ARDS.[51,108] Inhibition of iNOS reduced lung injury in combined smoke inhalation and burn injury in an ovine model.[52]

Chemical asphyxiants considered are primarily carbon monoxide (CO) and cyanide. These chemical asphyxiants impair extrapulmonary oxygen delivery, or utilization, the route of exposure being commonly smoke inhalation, without much, if any direct pulmonary toxicity, *per se*. Incomplete combustion of organic materials generates CO, which is considered the most common serious acute hazard to victims of smoke inhalation injury (Chap. 122).[1,166] Carbon monoxide binds heme and prevents oxygen from binding to the heme of the hemoglobin tetramer; it also hinders the release of oxygen from any remaining oxygenated hemes, shifting the oxyhemoglobin dissociation curve to the left. Overall, this process creates a functional anemia. Carbon monoxide also works at the tissue level, binding myoglobin in cardiac and skeletal muscle and cytochrome oxidase in all tissues.[38,80,160] The combination of these features impairs aerobic respiration systemically. It also impairs oxygen utilization by the myocardium, contributing to myocardial dysfunction and potentially hypotension, which further hinders oxygen delivery to tissues. Other mechanisms of toxicity induced by CO include induction of oxidative stress and lipid peroxidation of the central nervous system.[160]

Cyanide is produced from combustion of organic nitrogen-containing products that are present in common building materials, such as insulations and laminates.[127] High concentrations of cyanide are measured in air samples from fires, and elevated blood cyanide concentrations occur in both survivors as well as those who die in enclosed space fires.[59,156] Like CO, cyanide impairs aerobic respiration and has at least an additive, if not synergistic, effect with CO in smoke inhalation toxicity (Chaps. 122 and 123).[110,123,136] Combustion of nitrogen-containing materials also generates oxides of nitrogen, which are irritants and rarely induces the formation of methemoglobin (Chap. 124).

Depending on the fuel, other combustion products are aerosolized and act by local irritation or systemic toxicity. Metal oxides, hydrocarbons, hydrogen fluoride, and hydrogen bromide are formed in some fire environments, contributing to toxicity. In addition, antimony, cadmium, chromium, cobalt, gold, iron, lead, and zinc are often recovered from air samples taken during fires and from soot removed from the surface of the trachea and bronchi of fire victims.[19,45] Fires at industrial sites, clandestine drug laboratories, transportation incidents, and natural disasters, (eg, erupting volcanoes) produce additional unique toxic inhalants.

CLINICAL MANIFESTATIONS

The primary clinical problem in smoke inhalation victims is respiratory compromise; therefore, clinical evaluation should specifically address this issue. Additionally, toxicity from inhaled chemicals, such as CO and cyanide, can lead to cardiovascular dysfunction and hypotension and can directly and indirectly impair mental status. Clinical symptoms suggestive of significant smoke exposure include ocular, mouth, and throat irritation. Cough, chest tightness, and complaints of dyspnea are common.

On examination, soot on the body, face, or airway is suggestive of inhalational injury.[66,68] Burns to the face or singed hairs of the head, face, or nasal passages are associated with an increased risk of inhalational injury but are not present in all patients with significant inhalational injury.[66,68,144] Changes in voice and difficulty managing airway secretions are important signs of progressive airway edema. Visualization of the vocal cords by laryngoscopy is sometimes difficult secondary to soot accumulation, secretions, or edema. Ophthalmic examination should occur in all patients who either complain of ocular symptoms or whose symptoms are unable to be obtained because of unresponsiveness. Thermal and chemical injury results in conjunctival injection, corneal ulcerations and blepharospasm. Rhonchi, crackles, and wheezing on chest auscultation are suggestive of inhalational injury, but these finding are often delayed by 24 to 36 hours and are a poor prognostic indicator if present on initial patient presentation.[66,144] Breath sounds, including wheezing, become virtually inaudible in patients with severe bronchospasm because of gravely diminished air movement.

Tachycardia and tachypnea occur secondary to hypoxemia and systemic xenobiotic toxicity. Hypotension occurs secondary to hypoxemia and systemic toxicity and presents with faint or absent peripheral pulses.[152] Altered mental status, including agitation, confusion, or coma, is most often attributable to hypoxia from either pulmonary compromise or cellular hypoxia, but altered consciousness also results from direct effects of systemic xenobiotics, such as CO, or from concomitant trauma or drug or alcohol intoxication.[8]

DIAGNOSTIC TESTING

Diagnostic studies should focus on assessing for airway and pulmonary injury as well as the ability of the patient to oxygenate and ventilate. An arterial blood gas (ABG) analysis with cooximetry and chest radiography (CXR) should be obtained initially in all patients with smoke inhalation. Health care professionals should obtain a rapid lactate concentration in all seriously ill patients with smoke inhalation to aid in evaluation of possible cyanide toxicity.

An ABG analysis assesses both pulmonary function (gas exchange) and blood pH. The presence of metabolic acidosis is an early clue to tissue hypoxia

or cyanide poisoning. Serial measurements of arterial oxygenation and ventilation are helpful in identifying progressive hypoxemia or ventilatory failure. The accuracy of oxygen saturation measurement depends on the method used. Measurement of oxygen saturation by transcutaneous pulse oximetry is unreliable in patients with smoke inhalation because it overestimates oxygen saturation in the presence of carboxyhemoglobin.[9,29,167] Similarly, oxygen saturation calculated from standard ABG analysis is unreliable in the setting of an elevated blood CO concentration. An ABG analysis without cooximetry calculates the saturation of hemoglobin from the PaO_2 and does not account for the dysfunctional carboxyhemoglobin. In the setting of smoke inhalation, oxygen saturation is most accurately determined by cooximetry, which directly measures oxygenated and deoxygenated hemoglobin. Acute respiratory distress syndrome is a common complication of smoke inhalation and is defined as acute onset diffuse alveolar filling with hypoxemia not otherwise explained by congestive heart failure or fluid overload.[4] Acute respiratory distress syndrome is classified as mild, moderate, or severe based on the degree of impairment as determined by the ratio of partial pressure of dissolved oxygen (PO_2) to ratio (Fraction of inspired oxygen {FiO_2}) (Chap. 28).[4]

Cooximetry measures both carboxyhemoglobin and methemoglobin levels and is recommended in those with significant exposure or signs or symptoms of smoke inhalation.[39,179] When using blood sampling, either arterial or venous samples will accurately measure carboxyhemoglobin levels.[99] Noninvasive bedside pulse cooximetry is a rapid screening tool for the detection of CO; its use is becoming more prevalent in clinical practice, although device enhancement will be essential (Chap. 28).[146,150] Unfortunately, the carboxyhemoglobin level alone is a poor predictor of the severity of smoke inhalation because a low or nondetectable level does not exclude the possibility of developing inhalation injury.[105,153] Methemoglobin levels are rarely significantly elevated in fire victims. Because methemoglobin can further reduce oxygen-carrying capacity and contribute to morbidity, methemoglobin levels should also be included in the initial laboratory evaluation.[75,149]

Currently, blood cyanide analysis is of little clinical utility because results of analysis are not typically available for hours or days, and therapy should never await laboratory confirmation of the presence of cyanide. Accurate measurement depends on acquiring the sample soon after exposure because cyanide is rapidly eliminated from the blood.[12,85] Blood pH and lactate are more useful tools in acutely assessing for cyanide exposure. A blood lactate concentration of 10 mmol/L or greater suggests cyanide poisoning, as defined by a blood cyanide concentration of 40 micromol/L (1 mg/L), and supports the administration of empiric antidotal treatment to critically ill fire-exposed patients.[12]

Chest radiography is recommended early in the assessment of patients with smoke inhalation but is an insensitive indicator of pulmonary injury.[134,173] In one series of patients admitted to the intensive care unit (ICU) with smoke inhalation, no significant differences in the duration of either mechanical ventilation or duration in the ICU stay were observed between those who exhibited abnormal findings on the first CXR examination and those without abnormalities.[66] The most frequent abnormal findings on initial CXR are diffuse alveolar and interstitial changes, found in up to 34% of patients.[66] Serial CXR after a baseline study are generally more helpful in detecting evolving pulmonary injury after smoke inhalation (Fig. 120–1).[68] Subtle findings within 24 hours of exposure include perivascular haziness, peribronchial cuffing, bronchial wall thickening, and subglottic edema.[92,158] Widespread airway disease usually occurs more than 24 hours after inhalation injury and typically suggests ARDS, aspiration, infection, or volume overload.[158]

Computed tomography (CT) of the lungs is a more sensitive modality than plain radiography for detecting early pulmonary injury after smoke inhalation.[86,131,141] Computed tomography scanning allows for evaluation of the lung parenchyma and emerging data suggests CT scanning has some value as a "virtual bronchoscopy" for diagnosis and prediction of complications. However, no data are currently available to support improved patient outcomes when using this radiographic modality. Therefore, at this time we recommend against the routine use of CT scanning in patients with smoke inhalation.

In intubated patients, diagnostic fiberoptic bronchoscopy remains the standard in assessing smoke inhalational injury.[154] Bronchoscopy allows for

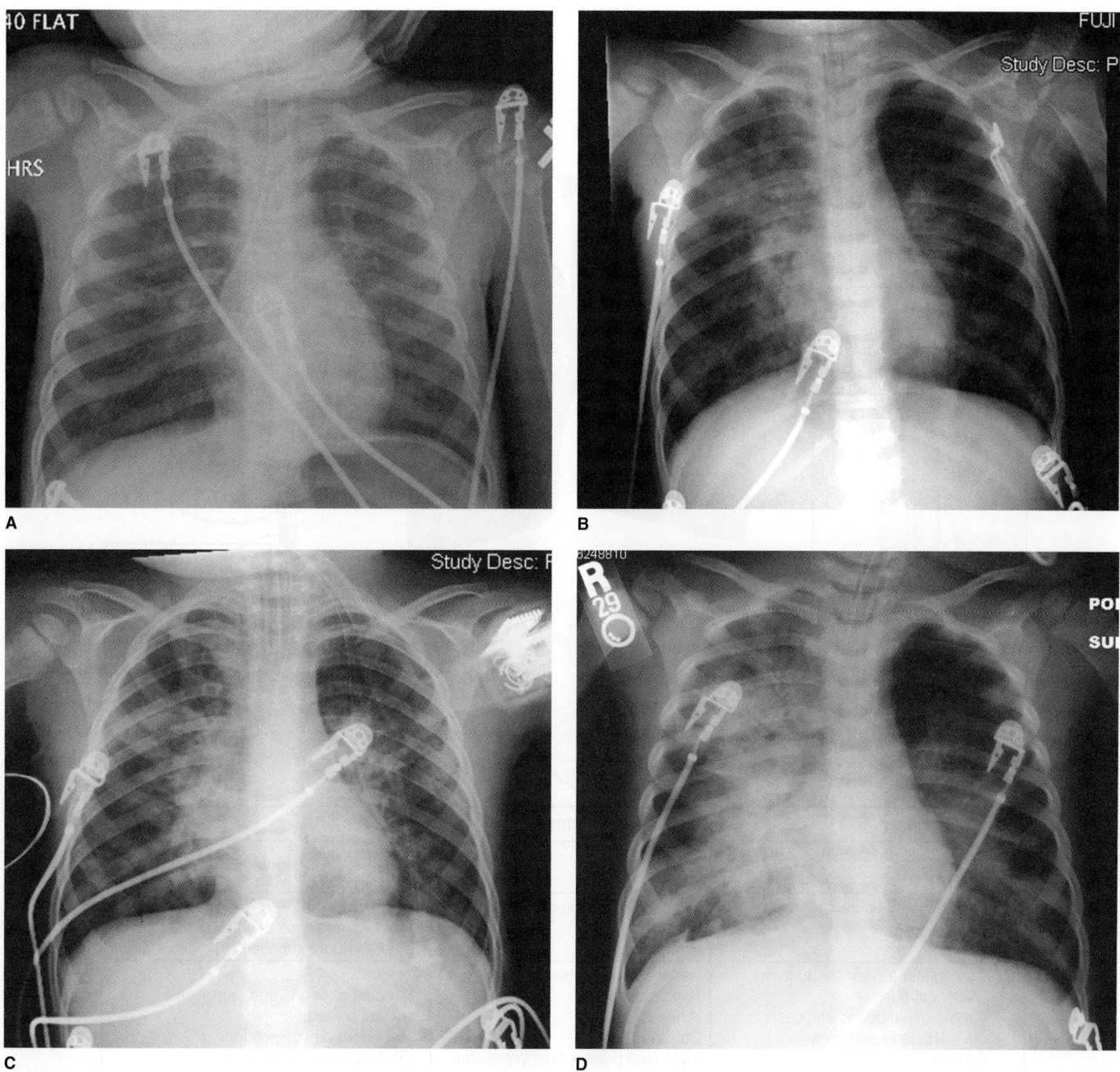

FIGURE 120–1. (**A**) Initial chest radiograph of a 3-year-old boy involved in a structural fire (approximately 60 minutes after the event). (**B**) Chest radiograph approximately 3 hours after exposure demonstrating the appearance of right upper lobe and perihilar infiltrates. (**C**) Evolution of chest radiograph findings approximately 17 hours after initial exposure demonstrating evolution of the right upper and perihilar infiltrates. (**D**) Approximately 60 hours after exposure demonstrating diffuse alveolar and interstitial infiltrates representative of inhalation-induced acute respiratory distress syndrome. *(Used with permission from The University of Virginia Medical Toxicology Fellowship Program.)*

direct visualization of the upper airways, allows for grading of the injury, and helps to determine those at risk for developing inhalational injury.[2,114,154] Bronchoscopy does not visualize the distal airways or lung parenchyma, which helps account for the discrepancies between studies correlating grading of bronchoscopy injury severity and outcome.[154] Early diagnostic bronchoscopy has yet to show an improvement in patient outcome, but because it aids in diagnosis and helps assess the severity of injury, it is reasonable to perform in intubated patients with suspicion of inhalation injury.[2,114,125]

MANAGEMENT

From oxygen acquisition to cellular utilization, the final common pathophysiologic effect from smoke injury is hypoxia. Basic critical care strategies that optimize oxygen delivery and utilization are of primary importance in

treatment. After the patient is removed from the source of exposure and oxygen is administered, the primary problems that the clinician must treat are the effects of thermal injury and irritant gases on the airway and systemic effects of cellular asphyxiants. High-flow humidified oxygen should accompany initial resuscitation in symptomatic patients. In critically ill patients insert two large-bore intravenous (IV) lines and provide appropriate fluid resuscitation as clinically warranted to optimize perfusion and aid in oxygen delivery. The clinical effects of smoke exposure and their appropriate treatment are described in Fig. 120–2.

Critical airway compromise is often present upon initial hospital presentation or develops in the ensuing hours.[67,144] A major pitfall in the management of smoke inhalation is failing to appreciate the possibility of rapid deterioration. History and physical findings help to determine significant

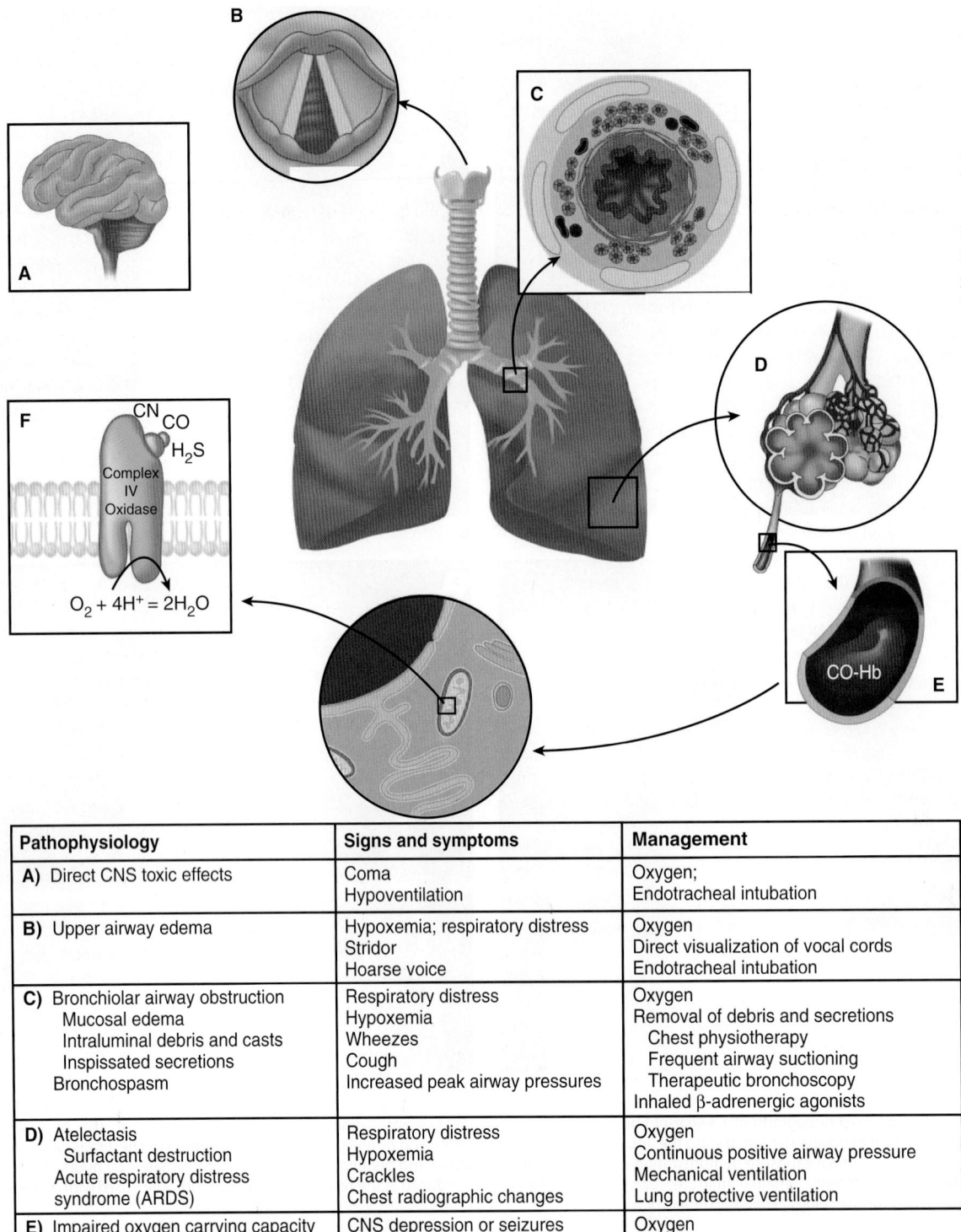

Pathophysiology	Signs and symptoms	Management
A) Direct CNS toxic effects	Coma Hypoventilation	Oxygen; Endotracheal intubation
B) Upper airway edema	Hypoxemia; respiratory distress Stridor Hoarse voice	Oxygen Direct visualization of vocal cords Endotracheal intubation

C) Bronchiolar airway obstruction
   Mucosal edema
   Intraluminal debris and casts
   Inspissated secretions
   Bronchospasm
	Respiratory distress
	Hypoxemia
	Wheezes
	Cough
	Increased peak airway pressures
		Oxygen
		Removal of debris and secretions
		   Chest physiotherapy
		   Frequent airway suctioning
		   Therapeutic bronchoscopy
		Inhaled β-adrenergic agonists

D) Atelectasis Surfactant destruction Acute respiratory distress syndrome (ARDS)	Respiratory distress Hypoxemia Crackles Chest radiographic changes	Oxygen Continuous positive airway pressure Mechanical ventilation Lung protective ventilation
E) Impaired oxygen carrying capacity and delivery (carbon monoxide or methemoglobinemia)	CNS depression or seizures Myocardial ischemia Dysrhythmias Metabolic acidosis	Oxygen Hyperbaric oxygen as clinically indicated Methylene blue as clinically indicated
F) Impaired oxygen use at tissues (cyanide, hydrogen sulfide and/or carbon monoxide)	CNS depression or seizures Myocardial ischemia Dysrhythmias Metabolic acidosis	Oxygen Ensure adequate tissue perfusion Treat suspected cyanide toxicity with cyanide antidote Hyperbaric oxygen as clinically indicated

FIGURE 120–2. The final common pathway from all pathophysiologic changes that occur in smoke inhalation is hypoxia. All treatments should be focused on improving oxygen delivery and oxygen utilization.

thermal injury or smoke exposure and the potential for clinical deterioration. Early airway intervention is recommended as a seemingly patent airway develops progressive obstruction that can make subsequent intubation difficult or impossible. For signs of current or impending airway compromise, upper airway patency must be rapidly established. When obvious oropharyngeal burns are observed, upper airway injury almost certainly is present. Singed hairs of the head, face, or nasal passages and soot or carbonaceous sputum in the oropharynx or nares signify potential for airway edema.

Direct evaluation of the upper airway, preferably with fiberoptic endoscopy, is essential for assessing patients at high risk for inhalation airway injury.[67,68,79] When evidence of upper airway injury exists, early endotracheal intubation should be performed under controlled circumstances, with preparations for advanced or surgical airway interventions in the event that orotracheal intubation cannot be easily established. Other indications for early intubation include coma, stridor, and full-thickness circumferential neck burns.[10,67,68,144] Edema of injured tissue, including that of the airway, is worsened with substantial fluid resuscitation in burned patients; therefore, we recommend early intubation for patients with any amount of inhalation injury and concomitant dermal burns undergoing fluid resuscitation.[67,68,117,144]

Even if overt injuries are not visualized, distal injury is often present and underestimated.[67] Pathophysiologic changes in the lung results in progressive hypoxia over hours to days. Basic treatment of progressive respiratory failure includes continuous positive airway pressure, mechanical ventilation using lung protective strategies, positive end-expiratory pressure (PEEP), and vigorous clearing of pulmonary secretions.[120] Decreased lung compliance is common secondary to cast formation, tissue damage, and atelectasis.[109,120] Recommendations for limiting barotrauma in mechanically ventilated patients include using a low tidal volume (6–8 mL/kg) and PEEP and allowing permissive hypercapnia as necessary.[97,109,159] The fraction of inspired oxygen should be weaned to below 0.4 as rapidly as tolerated to limit oxygen toxicity.[109] Frequent airway suctioning, chest physiotherapy, and therapeutic bronchoscopy clear inspissated secretions, plugs, and casts.[43,109,116] Because xenobiotics and soot can coat the airway in smoke inhalation victims, early bronchoscopy with bronchoalveolar lavage would intuitively be logical in an attempt to decontaminate the airway, similar to irrigation for dermal exposure. However, because only one study suggests that early and scheduled therapeutic bronchoscopy improves overall morbidity in patients with smoke inhalation, we recommend the use of bronchoscopy and bronchoalveolar lavage for therapeutic purposes on a case-by-case basis as needed for clearing airway obstruction.[34]

High-frequency percussive ventilation (HFPV), a method of ventilation that combines a high-frequency low tidal volume with pressure control ventilation, has been studied as an alternative to conventional forms of ventilation in patients with inhalational injury. Studies suggest that HFPV improves lung function by aiding the clearance of intraluminal airway debris and recruiting alveoli.[148] Several studies have investigated the use of HFPV in ventilated patients with inhalational injury. Limited evidence suggests that HFPV decreases peak pulmonary pressures, limits barotrauma, decreases the incidence of pneumonia, and improves the mortality rate in patients with smoke inhalation injury.[37,42,62,109,140] Therefore, HFPV is reasonable to use in patients in whom conventional low tidal volume lung protective strategies fail to provide adequate oxygenation. The role of extracorporeal membrane oxygenation (ECMO) in victims of smoke inhalation is unclear. Although multiple case reports document its use in patients with inhalational injury, there is limited evidence and no high-quality studies to support its use in smoke inhalation injury.[5,128] However, as expertise in the use of ECMO has greatly progressed in recent years, it seems reasonable to use this modality as a rescue therapy in patients failing more conventional ventilation strategies.

Inhaled β_2-adrenergic agonists are the first-line therapy for acute reversible bronchoconstriction resulting from asthma or chronic obstructive pulmonary disease and are recommended to improve oxygenation and ventilation in victims of smoke inhalation. Pathophysiologic changes induced by irritant gases in smoke are similar to those found in asthma, suggesting that β_2-adrenergic agonists would also improve airflow obstruction in smoke

inhalation.[84,104] β_2-Adrenergic agonists also possess antiinflammatory properties, partially through interaction with β-adrenergic receptors on immune cells.[103,172] β_2-Adrenergic agonists also enhance resolution of alveolar edema by modulating the flow of sodium and potassium across cell membranes.[103,172] Limited data in an ovine model suggest that nebulized albuterol improves pulmonary function after smoke inhalation and burn injury.[130] Nebulized epinephrine improved oxygenation and decreased pulmonary vascular permeability in animal models but differs from albuterol in that it provides both α- and β-adrenergic agonist activity.[90,100] Although human data on the efficacy of β_2-adrenergic agonists in smoke inhalation injury are lacking, their role is well established in conditions with reversible bronchoconstriction, animal studies lend support for their use, and the potential benefits greatly outweigh the risks.[130,172] Accordingly, we recommend the use of nebulized albuterol in victims of smoke inhalation injury with evidence of bronchospasm.

Corticosteroids have been used for smoke inhalation in an attempt to limit inflammation and improve outcome. One argument for their use is for the treatment of lung injury induced by oxides of nitrogen. Pulmonary sequelae, including bronchiolitis obliterans, are known to occur after significant exposure to oxides of nitrogen, which are sometimes a prominent component of smoke.[77,93] The mixed xenobiotic exposure from smoke inhalation appears to further complicate the outcome. One early rat study showed a trend toward reduced mortality rates in animals given supraphysiologic doses (25–100 mg/kg) of methylprednisolone; however, other tested corticosteroids (hydrocortisone, dexamethasone, cortisone) failed to demonstrate similar improvement. Consequently, this study failed to effectively prove that corticosteroids reduce mortality rates after rat exposure to smoke.[49] Human studies have also failed to show an improvement in clinical outcome and trend toward worsening outcome.[35,94,121,145] Thus, we do not recommend the routine use of corticosteroids for treatment of patients with smoke inhalation.

A significant amount of pulmonary injury after smoke inhalation is attributable to free radical damage. Smoke inhalation decreases systemic concentrations of the antioxidant vitamin E in sheep models, and treatment with nebulized vitamin E (α- and γ-tocopherol) attenuates smoke inhalation induced pulmonary injury in animal models.[64,112,165,176] Similarly, both nebulized heparin and N-acetylcysteine (NAC) are used by some centers to limit pulmonary damage.[106] Heparin is a glycosaminoglycan with anticoagulant and antiinflammatory properties occasionally used both topically and intravenously in burn treatment. In an ovine model of combined cutaneous burn and smoke inhalation, nebulized heparin combined with recombinant human antithrombin reduced airway obstruction and improved gas exchange.[54] The mechanism is likely attributable to decreased airway inflammation and decreased fibrin deposition and, consequently, decreased cast formation in the airway.[54] Although literature regarding the use of inhaled anticoagulants show variable results, a systematic review of both animal and human clinical data found an association between inhaled anticoagulants and improved mortality from smoke inhalation-associated ARDS.[48,76,106,107] The five human studies included were retrospective analyses of smoke-injured patients treated with nebulized heparin and NAC.[107] At the doses used (typically either 5,000 U or 10,000 U of heparin nebulized every 4 hours), patients did not experience changes in systemic coagulation parameters. However, an additional recent retrospective study demonstrated no difference in mortality or length of ICU stay among patients treated with heparin and NAC and a no treatment control group. In this study, the treatment group had a higher rate of pneumonia compared to the control group.[82] Further data are needed to provide evidence regarding inhalational treatment with heparin, NAC, or both. Although human data are currently limited, with only animal studies and human retrospective data available, it would be reasonable to use nebulize heparin and NAC for the treatment of intubated patients with bronchoscopy confirmed smoke inhalation and associated ARDS.[107] Care should be taken to monitor for pneumonia, which, in one study, had a higher incidence in treated patients.

The initial treatment strategy for patients with CO poisoning should focus on optimizing oxygen delivery to the tissues. Oxygen can be administered by a high-flow tight-fitting mask, endotracheal tube, or hyperbaric oxygen therapy (HBO). Oxygen shortens the half-life of carboxyhemoglobin, the rate of which inversely correlates with the PO_2 of the patient.[135,170] Hyperbaric oxygen can achieve very high arterial oxygen concentrations, enhancing oxygen delivery to tissues and accelerating elimination of CO from blood and tissues.[69,135] Hyperbaric oxygen therapy is recommended as a modality for treatment in certain situations involving CO exposure; however, smoke inhalation injury is much more complex than poisoning solely with CO, such as that caused by a furnace leak.[65] In victims of smoke inhalation, other clinical requirements, such as maintaining a secure airway and the need for additional resuscitative measures to treat ARDS, cardiovascular instability, and metabolic derangements go beyond providing supplemental oxygen to treat CO poisoning. Optimal timing of HBO administration is often during the same period when intensive resuscitative efforts and focused ventilator management are required and could limit attention to these important therapies. Irritant-induced bronchospasm along with exudates and airway casts increase the risk of air trapping, potentially leading to HBO-induced barotrauma.[31,115] In addition, it is known that pulmonary toxicity results from elevated partial pressures of oxygen.[151] Very little information is available to predict the effect of hyperoxygenation on pulmonary toxicity after smoke inhalation.[161,175] The decision to treat a smoke inhalation patient with HBO should take into account risks and other clinical requirements when determining the appropriate therapy because the therapeutic priority is meticulous supportive care and high-flow oxygen therapy. A judicious approach to the treatment of CO poisoning in smoke inhalation is administering 100% oxygen by a tightly fitting mask (or an endotracheal tube if intubated) as long as clinically appropriate (Chap. 122 and Antidotes in Depth: A40).[28,174]

Cyanide is a common product of combustion, with toxic concentrations often measured in fire victims. Because rapid determination of blood cyanide concentrations is not readily available in the prehospital setting or in the emergency department, surrogate markers must be used to help establish the diagnosis. Cyanide poisoning should be suspected in patients involved in enclosed-space fires with evidence of smoke inhalation, particularly in the presence of altered mental status, hemodynamic instability or metabolic acidosis with an elevated lactate concentration.[56,142] Serum lactate concentrations correlate closely with blood cyanide concentrations. In a study of smoke inhalation victims, a blood lactate concentrations of 10 mmol/L was reported to be a sensitive indicator of cyanide toxicity as defined by a blood cyanide concentration above 40 micromol/L (1 mg/L).[12] However, in this study, 26% of fatalities occurred in patients with a blood cyanide concentration less than 40 micromol/L (1 mg/L), possibly because of the compounding effects of cyanide and other toxic products of combustion such as CO. Carboxyhemoglobin levels of more than 10% also correlated with elevated cyanide concentrations.[12] Studies also indicate that smoke inhalation victims with cardiac arrest, those who must be rescued from the environment, and those with soot on the face, oral cavity, neck or carbonaceous sputum are more likely to have elevated blood cyanide concentrations.[12,58] For patients with suspected cyanide poisoning, specific treatment of cyanide toxicity should be implemented while other life support measures are instituted. Systematic reviews of various cyanide antidotes conclude that it is possible to survive even cardiorespiratory arrest caused by cyanide poisoning if the patient is provided optimal supportive care and an appropriate antidote.[124]

Cyanide antidotes function as an adjunct to basic critical care strategies that optimize oxygen delivery and utilization. The components of the classic cyanide antidote kit, amyl nitrite and sodium nitrite, hinder this strategy and therefore should not be routinely used in victims of smoke inhalation. Amyl nitrite and sodium nitrite produce methemoglobinemia, (Chap. 124 and Antidotes in Depth: A43). Unfortunately, methemoglobin is a dysfunctional type of hemoglobin that poorly utilizes oxygen, impairing delivery to the tissues.[44] Impairing oxygen-carrying capacity and oxygen delivery to tissues with nitrite-induced methemoglobinemia is a valid concern in the presence of tissue hypoxia from carboxyhemoglobinemia, lung injury, or other factors. Furthermore, rapid infusion of sodium nitrite causes hypotension secondary to vasodilation.[61]

Hydroxocobalamin is a vitamin B_{12} (cyanocobalamin) precursor that works by chelating cyanide from the cytochrome system and acting as a nitric oxide scavenger. It comes as a red crystalline powder that must be reconstituted and then administered intravenously over 15 minutes.[162] Animal studies focus on poisoning by cyanide salts over cyanide poisoning from smoke inhalation but demonstrate improvement in blood pressure parameters when hydroxocobalamin was compared with the combination of sodium thiosulfate and sodium nitrite, and improved mortality compared with either placebo or sodium thiosulfate alone.[14,15,20] There are no human studies providing head-to-head data on cyanide antidotes in smoke inhalation. Human studies are limited to retrospective or prospective case series that are poorly controlled. Authors of these articles typically report improved survival and few adverse events, but use either historic controls or typically lethal blood concentrations of cyanide as comparison groups, limiting the strength of the evidence.[21,22,57] Side effects of hydroxocobalamin administration include red or pink discoloration of the skin, red discoloration of the urine, and alteration in some laboratory parameters, including carboxyhemoglobin concentrations.[33,91] In addition, certain hemodialysis machines can be adversely affected by red discoloration or the plasma leading to a blood leak error warning.[155] Although the evidence for the use of hydroxocobalamin for patients with cyanide poisoning from smoke inhalation is limited, this antidote appears to be superior to sodium thiosulfate or supportive care alone.[14,15] Because nitrites have a more detrimental side effect profile and are likely detrimental to patients with concomitant CO poisoning, hydroxocobalamin is recommended as first-line therapy when cyanide poisoning is suspected in victims of smoke inhalation.

In the prehospital setting or if unable to obtain a rapid lactate concentration, for patients involved in an enclosed-space fire with signs of inhalation injury and the presence or altered mental status or hemodynamic instability (systolic blood pressure of 90 mm Hg or less), it is reasonable to administer hydroxocobalamin. If a rapid lactate concentration is available, hydroxocobalamin is recommended for to such patients with a lactate concentration greater than or equal to 10 mmol/L. Few data are available to guide clinicians for patients who have evidence of smoke inhalation and the lactate concentration is elevated but less than 10 mmol/L. For patients with an elevated lactate concentration less than 10 mmol/L with altered mental status or hemodynamic instability, it is reasonable to administer hydroxocobalamin. For patients who are hemodynamically stable and without significantly altered mental status and who have an elevated lactate less than 10 mmol/L, it is reasonable to monitor these patients closely while performing resuscitation and considering other causes of the elevated lactate concentration.[3,57,63,101] The initial dose of hydroxocobalamin is 70 mg/kg (5 g in an adult) intravenously, with the option of subsequent dosing of 70 mg/kg (5 g in an adult) intravenously for signs of continued cyanide toxicity or if in cardiac arrest (Chap. 123 and Antidotes in Depth: A41 and A42).[78] It is reasonable to use sodium thiosulfate as adjunctive therapy, but it should not be given concomitantly through the same IV line.[138]

Victims of fires have respiratory compromise and other pathology not directly related to smoke inhalation, such as trauma or other underlying medical problems. Trauma from falls or explosions must be suspected and treatment started simultaneously with treatment of burns and inhalation injury. Comatose patients should be evaluated for other causes of their status and should receive naloxone, thiamine, and hypertonic dextrose as indicated. Inhaled xenobiotics, such as CO directly, cause altered mental status, but drug and ethanol intoxication also contribute significantly to fire fatalities and injuries. Blood ethanol concentrations in fire victims correlate with elevated levels of CO and concentrations of cyanide, suggesting that intoxication impairs escape and prolongs toxic smoke exposure.[8,19,118] Intracranial pathology should be considered and noncontrast head CT scans obtained as clinically indicated.

Xenobiotics often injure the skin or mucous membranes in addition to the respiratory mucosa.[41] The duration of contact of a xenobiotic with tissue is an important factor in determining the extent of chemical injury to the skin and eyes. Rapid removal of soot from the skin or eyes helps to prevent continued injury. The eyes should be evaluated for corneal burns caused by thermal or irritant chemical injury. Patients with signs of ophthalmic irritation should have their eyes irrigated, and dermal decontamination performed as necessary to prevent burns from toxin-laden soot adherent to the skin (Special Considerations: SC2).

SUMMARY

- Smoke inhalation contributes significantly to the morbidity and mortality of fire victims.
- Smoke inhalation is a complex syndrome involving diverse toxicologic injuries. A spectrum of damage occurs, ranging from rapid upper airway occlusion to delayed ARDS.
- The end result of respiratory tract toxicity is tissue hypoxia.
- Goals of treatment should focus on maximizing oxygen delivery while avoiding unnecessary therapies that may hinder oxygenation.
- Early airway management should be implemented for patients with airway compromise. High-flow oxygen will help reverse tissue hypoxia, and fluid resuscitation should be instituted to improve cardiovascular status if indicated.
- Definitive antidotes and procedures for cyanide and carbon monoxide are available in select cases and should be used when appropriate to help stabilize the patient.

REFERENCES

1. Alarie Y. Toxicity of fire smoke. *Crit Rev Toxicol*. 2002;32:259-289.
2. Albright JM, et al. The acute pulmonary inflammatory response to the graded severity of smoke inhalation injury. *Crit Care Med*. 2012;40:1113-1121.
3. Anseeuw K, et al. Cyanide poisoning by fire smoke inhalation: a European expert consensus. *Eur J Emerg Med*. 2013;20:2-9.
4. ARDS Definition Task Force, et al. Acute respiratory distress syndrome: The Berlin definition. *JAMA*. 2012;307:2526-2533.
5. Asmussen S, et al. Extracorporeal membrane oxygenation in burn and smoke inhalation injury. *Burns*. 2013;39:429-435.
6. Badger SG. *Catastrophic Multiple-Death Fires in 2011*. National Fire Protection Association; 2012. NFPA Journal. The magazine of the National Fire Protection Association. https://www.nfpa.org/News-and-Research/Publications/NFPA-Journal/2012/September-October-2012/Features/Catastrophic-Multiple-Death-Fires-in-2011. Last accessed July 10, 2018.
7. Bajaj V. Fatal fire in Bangladesh highlights the dangers facing garment workers. *The New York Times*. http://www.nytimes.com/2012/11/26/world/asia/bangladesh-fire-kills-more-than-100-and-injures-many.html.
8. Barillo DJ, et al. Is ethanol the unknown toxin in smoke inhalation injury? *Am Surg*. 1986;52:641-645.
9. Barker SJ, Tremper KK. The effect of carbon monoxide inhalation on pulse oximetry and transcutaneous PO2. *Anesthesiology*. 1987;66:677-679.
10. Barlett RH, et al. Acute management of the upper airway in facial burns and smoke inhalation. *Arch Surg*. 1976;111:744-749.
11. Barrow RE, et al. Influence of demographics and inhalation injury on burn mortality in children. *Burns*. 2004;30:72-77.
12. Baud FJ, et al. Elevated blood cyanide concentrations in victims of smoke inhalation. *N Engl J Med*. 1991;325:1761-1766.
13. Baud FJ, et al. Value of lactic acidosis in the assessment of the severity of acute cyanide poisoning. *Crit Care Med*. 2002;30:2044-2050.
14. Bebarta VS, et al. Hydroxocobalamin and sodium thiosulfate versus sodium nitrite and sodium thiosulfate in the treatment of acute cyanide toxicity in a swine (sus scrofa) model. *Ann Emerg Med*. 2010;55:345-351.
15. Bebarta VS, et al. Hydroxocobalamin versus sodium thiosulfate for the treatment of acute cyanide toxicity in a swine (sus scrofa) model. *Ann Emerg Med*. 2012;59:532-539.
16. Bebarta VS, et al. Intravenous cobinamide versus hydroxocobalamin for acute treatment of severe cyanide poisoning in a swine (sus scrofa) model. *Ann Emerg Med*. 2014;64:612-619.
17. Bessac BF, Jordt SE. Sensory detection and responses to toxic gases: mechanisms, health effects, and countermeasures. *Proc Am Thorac Soc*. 2010;7:269-277.
18. Bidani A, et al. Early effects of smoke inhalation on alveolar macrophage functions. *Burns*. 1996;22:101-106.
19. Birky MM, Clarke FB. Inhalation of toxic products from fires. *Bull N Y Acad Med*. 1981;57:997-1013.
20. Borron SW, et al. Efficacy of hydroxocobalamin for the treatment of acute cyanide poisoning in adult beagle dogs. *Clin Toxicol*. 2006;44:5-15.
21. Borron SW, et al. Prospective study of hydroxocobalamin for acute cyanide poisoning in smoke inhalation. *Ann Emerg Med*. 2007;49:794-801, 801.e1-2.
22. Borron SW, et al. Hydroxocobalamin for severe acute cyanide poisoning by ingestion or inhalation. *Am J Emerg Med*. 2007;25:551-558.
23. Bowes PC. Casualties attributed to toxic gas and smoke at fires: a survey of statistics. *Med Sci Law*. 1976;16:104-110.
24. Brandt-Rauf PW, et al. Health hazards of fire fighters: exposure assessment. *Br J Ind Med*. 1988;45:606-612.
25. Brenner M, et al. Intramuscular cobinamide sulfite in a rabbit model of sublethal cyanide toxicity. *Ann Emerg Med*. 2010;55:352-363.
26. Brown JE, Birky MM. Phosgene in the thermal decomposition products of poly(vinyl chloride): generation, detection and measurement. *J Anal Toxicol*. 1980;4:166-174.
27. Brown RF, et al. Pathophysiological responses following phosgene exposure in the anaesthetized pig. *J Appl Toxicol*. 2002;22:263-269.
28. Buckley NA, et al. Hyperbaric oxygen for carbon monoxide poisoning. *Cochrane Database Syst Rev*. 2011;CD002041.
29. Buckley RG, et al. The pulse oximetry gap in carbon monoxide intoxication. *Ann Emerg Med*. 1994;24:252-255.
30. Cahalane M, Demling RH. Early respiratory abnormalities from smoke inhalation. *JAMA*. 1984;251:771-773.
31. Cakmak T, et al. A case of tension pneumothorax during hyperbaric oxygen therapy in an earthquake survivor with crush injury complicated by ARDS (adult respiratory distress syndrome). *Undersea Hyperb Med*. 2015;42:9-13.
32. Cark FB. Toxicity of combustion products: current knowledge. *Fire J*. 1983;77:84-101.
33. Carlsson CJ, et al. An evaluation of the interference of hydroxycobalamin with chemistry and co-oximetry tests on nine commonly used instruments. *Scand J Clin Lab Invest*. 2011;71:378-386.
34. Carr JA, Crowley N. Prophylactic sequential bronchoscopy after inhalation injury: results from a three-year prospective randomized trial. *Eur J Trauma Emerg Surg*. 2013;39:177-183.
35. Cha SI, et al. Isolated smoke inhalation injuries: acute respiratory dysfunction, clinical outcomes, and short-term evolution of pulmonary functions with the effects of steroids. *Burns*. 2007;33:200-208.
36. Charan NB, et al. Pulmonary injuries associated with acute sulfur dioxide inhalation. *Am Rev Respir Dis*. 1979;119:555-560.
37. Chung KK, et al. High-frequency percussive ventilation and low tidal volume ventilation in burns: a randomized controlled trial. *Crit Care Med*. 2010;38:1970-1977.
38. Chung Y, et al. Implication of CO inactivation on myoglobin function. *Am J Physiol Cell Physiol*. 2006;290:1616-1624.
39. Clark WR, et al. Smoke inhalation and airway management at a regional burn unit: 1974-1983. Part I: diagnosis and consequences of smoke inhalation. *J Burn Care Rehabil*. 1989;10:52-62.
40. Clark WR Jr, Nieman GF. Smoke inhalation. *Burns Incl Therm Inj*. 1988;14:473-494.
41. Close LG, et al. Acute and chronic effects of ammonia burns on the respiratory tract. *Arch Otolaryngol*. 1980;106:151-158.
42. Cortiella J, et al. High frequency percussive ventilation in pediatric patients with inhalation injury. *J Burn Care Rehabil*. 1999;20:232-235.
43. Cox RA, et al. Airway obstruction in sheep with burn and smoke inhalation injuries. *Am J Respir Cell Mol Biol*. 2003;29:295-302.
44. Curry S. Methemoglobinemia. *Ann Emerg Med*. 1982;11:214-221.
45. Davies JW. Toxic chemicals versus lung tissue—an aspect of inhalation injury revisited. The Everett Idris Evans Memorial Lecture—1986. *J Burn Care Rehabil*. 1986;7:213-222.
46. Decker WJ, Koch HF. Chlorine poisoning at the swimming pool: an overlooked hazard. *Clin Toxicol*. 1978;13:377-381.
47. Demling RH, et al. Oxygen consumption early postburn becomes oxygen delivery dependent with the addition of smoke inhalation injury. *J Trauma*. 1992;32:593-598.
48. Desai MH, et al. Reduction in mortality in pediatric patients with inhalation injury with aerosolized heparin/N-acetylcystine [correction of acetylcystine] therapy. *J Burn Care Rehabil*. 1998;19:210-212.
49. Dressler DP, et al. Corticosteroid treatment of experimental smoke inhalation. *Ann Surg*. 1976;183:46-52.
50. El-Helbawy RH, Ghareeb FM. Inhalation injury as a prognostic factor for mortality in burn patients. *Ann Burns Fire Disasters*. 2011;24:82-88.
51. Enkhbaatar P, et al. Inducible nitric oxide synthase dimerization inhibitor prevents cardiovascular and renal morbidity in sheep with combined burn and smoke inhalation injury. *Am J Physiol Heart Circ Physiol*. 2003;285:2430-2436.
52. Enkhbaatar P, et al. The inducible nitric oxide synthase inhibitor BBS-2 prevents acute lung injury in sheep after burn and smoke inhalation injury. *Am J Respir Crit Care Med*. 2003;167:1021-1026.
53. Enkhbaatar P, Traber DL. Pathophysiology of acute lung injury in combined burn and smoke inhalation injury. *Clin Sci (Lond)*. 2004;107:137-143.
54. Enkhbaatar P, et al. Aerosolized anticoagulants ameliorate acute lung injury in sheep after exposure to burn and smoke inhalation. *Crit Care Med*. 2007;35:2805-2810.
55. Fein A, et al. Pathophysiology and management of the complications resulting from fire and the inhaled products of combustion: review of the literature. *Crit Care Med*. 1980;8:94-98.
56. Fortin JL, et al. Hydroxocobalamin: treatment for smoke inhalation-associated cyanide poisoning. Meeting the needs of fire victims. *JEMS*. 2004;29(8 suppl):18-21.

57. Fortin JL, et al. Prehospital administration of hydroxocobalamin for smoke inhalation-associated cyanide poisoning: 8 years of experience in the Paris fire brigade. *Clin Toxicol (Phila)*. 2006;44(suppl 1):37-44.

58. Geldner G, et al. Report on a study of fires with smoke gas development: determination of blood cyanide levels, clinical signs and laboratory values in victims. *Anaesthesist*. 2013;62:609-616.

59. Grabowska T, et al. Prevalence of hydrogen cyanide and carboxyhaemoglobin in victims of smoke inhalation during enclosed-space fires: a combined toxicological risk. *Clin Toxicol (Phila)*. 2012;50:759-763.

60. Hales CA, et al. Synthetic smoke with acrolein but not HCl produces pulmonary edema. *J Appl Physiol (1985)*. 1988;64:1121-1133.

61. Hall AH, et al. Suspected cyanide poisoning in smoke inhalation: complications of sodium nitrite therapy. *J Toxicol Clin Exp*. 1989;9:3-9.

62. Hall JJ, et al. Use of high-frequency percussive ventilation in inhalation injuries. *J Burn Care Res*. 2007;28:396-400.

63. Hamad E, et al. Case files of the University of Massachusetts Toxicology Fellowship: does this smoke inhalation victim require treatment with cyanide antidote? *J Med Toxicol*. 2016;12:192-198.

64. Hamahata A, et al. Gamma-tocopherol nebulization by a lipid aerosolization device improves pulmonary function in sheep with burn and smoke inhalation injury. *Free Radic Biol Med*. 2008;45:425-433.

65. Hampson NB, Hauff NM. Risk factors for short-term mortality from carbon monoxide poisoning treated with hyperbaric oxygen. *Crit Care Med*. 2008;36:2523-2527.

66. Hantson P, et al. Early complications and value of initial clinical and paraclinical observations in victims of smoke inhalation without burns. *Chest*. 1997;111:671-675.

67. Haponik EF, et al. Acute upper airway injury in burn patients. Serial changes of flow-volume curves and nasopharyngoscopy. *Am Rev Respir Dis*. 1987;135:360-366.

68. Haponik EF, Summer WR. Respiratory complications in burned patients: diagnosis and management of inhalation injury. *J Crit Care*. 1987;2:121-143.

69. Hardy KR, Thom SR. Pathophysiology and treatment of carbon monoxide poisoning. *J Toxicol Clin Toxicol*. 1994;32:613-629.

70. Harwood B, Hall JR. What kills in fires: smoke inhalation or burns? *Fire J*. 1989;84:29-34.

71. Haynes H. NFPA https://www.nfpa.org/News-and-Research/Publications/NFPA-Journal/2016/September-October-2016/Features/2015-US-Fire-Loss-Report. Last accessed July 10, 2018.

72. Henderson RF, Schlesinger RB. Symposium on the importance of combined exposures in inhalation toxicology. *Fund Appl Toxicol*. 1989;12:1-11.

73. Herlihy JP, et al. Impaired alveolar macrophage function in smoke inhalation injury. *J Cell Physiol*. 1995;163:1-8.

74. Herndon DN, et al. Inhalation injury in burned patients: effects and treatment. *Burns Incl Therm Inj*. 1988;14:349-356.

75. Hoffman RS, Sauter D. Methemoglobinemia resulting from smoke inhalation. *Vet Hum Toxicol*. 1989;31:168-170.

76. Holt J, et al. Use of inhaled heparin/*N*-acetylcystine in inhalation injury: does it help? *J Burn Care Res*. 2008;29:192-195.

77. Horvath EP, et al. Nitrogen dioxide-induced pulmonary disease: five new cases and a review of the literature. *J Occup Med*. 1978;20:103-110.

78. Houeto P, et al. Relation of blood cyanide to plasma cyanocobalamin concentration after a fixed dose of hydroxocobalamin in cyanide poisoning. *Lancet*. 1995;346:605-608.

79. Hunt JL, et al. Fiberoptic bronchoscopy in acute inhalation injury. *J Trauma*. 1975;15:641-649.

80. Iheagwara KN, et al. Myocardial cytochrome oxidase activity is decreased following carbon monoxide exposure. *Biochim Biophys Acta*. 2007;1772:1112-1116.

81. Iyun AO, et al. Comparative review of burns with inhalation injury in a tertiary hospital in a developing country. *Wounds*. 2016;28:1-6.

82. Kashefi NS, et al. Does a nebulized heparin/*N*-acetylcysteine protocol improve outcomes in adult smoke inhalation? *Plast Reconstr Surg Glob Open*. 2014;2:e165.

83. Kasten KR. Update on the critical care management of severe burns. *J Intensive Care Med*. 2011;26:223-236.

84. Kinsella J, et al. Increased airways reactivity after smoke inhalation. *Lancet*. 1991;337:595-597.

85. Kirk MA, et al. Cyanide and methemoglobin kinetics in smoke inhalation victims treated with the cyanide antidote kit. *Ann Emerg Med*. 1993;22:1413-1418.

86. Koljonen V, et al. Multi-detector computed tomography demonstrates smoke inhalation injury at early stage. *Emerg Radiol*. 2007;14:113-116.

87. Kwon HP, et al. Comparison of virtual bronchoscopy to fiber-optic bronchoscopy for assessment of inhalation injury severity. *Burns*. 2014;40:1308-1315.

88. Lalonde C, et al. Smoke inhalation injury in sheep is caused by the particle phase, not the gas phase. *J Appl Physiol (1985)*. 1994;77:15-22.

89. LaLonde C, et al. Plasma catalase and glutathione levels are decreased in response to inhalation injury. *J Burn Care Rehabil*. 1997;18:515-519.

90. Lange M, et al. Preclinical evaluation of epinephrine nebulization to reduce airway hyperemia and improve oxygenation after smoke inhalation injury. *Crit Care Med*. 2011;39:718-724.

91. Lee J, et al. Potential interference by hydroxocobalamin on cooximetry hemoglobin measurements during cyanide and smoke inhalation treatments. *Ann Emerg Med*. 2007;49:802-805.

92. Lee MJ, O'Connell DJ. The plain chest radiograph after acute smoke inhalation. *Clin Radiol*. 1988;39:33-37.

93. Lehnert BE, et al. Lung injury following exposure of rats to relatively high mass concentrations of nitrogen dioxide. *Toxicology*. 1994;89:239-277.

94. Levine BA, et al. Prospective trials of dexamethasone and aerosolized gentamicin in the treatment of inhalation injury in the burned patient. *J Trauma*. 1978;18:188-193.

95. Levy DM, et al. Ammonia burns of the face and respiratory tract. *JAMA*. 1964;190:873-876.

96. Lin YS, Kou YR. Acute neurogenic airway plasma exudation and edema induced by inhaled wood smoke in guinea pigs: role of tachykinins and hydroxyl radical. *Eur J Pharmacol*. 2000;394:139-148.

97. Lipes J, et al. Low tidal volume ventilation in patients without acute respiratory distress syndrome: a paradigm shift in mechanical ventilation. *Crit Care Res Pract*. 2012;2012:416862.

98. Loick HM, et al. Smoke inhalation causes a delayed increase in airway blood flow to primarily uninjured lung areas. *Intensive Care Med*. 1995;21:326-333.

99. Lopez DM, et al. Relationship between arterial, mixed venous, and internal jugular carboxyhemoglobin concentrations at low, medium, and high concentrations in a piglet model of carbon monoxide toxicity. *Crit Care Med*. 2000;28:1998-2001.

100. Lopez E, et al. Nebulized epinephrine limits pulmonary vascular hyperpermeability to water and protein in ovine with burn and smoke inhalation injury. *Crit Care Med*. 2016;44:e89-96.

101. MacLennan L, Moiemen N. Management of cyanide toxicity in patients with burns. *Burns*. 2015;41:18-24.

102. Mallory TB, Brickley WJ. Management of the cocoanut grove burns at Massachusetts General Hospital Pathology: with special reference to the pulmonary lesions. *Ann Surg*. 1943;117:865-884.

103. Matthay MA, Abraham E. Beta-adrenergic agonist therapy as a potential treatment for acute lung injury. *Am J Respir Crit Care Med*. 2006;173:254-255.

104. Mellins RB. Respiratory complications of smoke inhalation in victims of fires. *J Pediatr*. 1975;87:1-7.

105. Meyer GW, et al. Hyperbaric oxygen therapy for acute smoke inhalation injuries. *Postgrad Med*. 1991;89:221-223.

106. Miller AC, et al. Influence of nebulized unfractionated heparin and *N*-acetylcysteine in acute lung injury after smoke inhalation injury. *J Burn Care Res*. 2009;30:249-256.

107. Miller AC, et al. Inhaled anticoagulation regimens for the treatment of smoke inhalation-associated acute lung injury: a systematic review. *Crit Care Med*. 2014;42:413-419.

108. Mizutani A, et al. Pulmonary changes in a mouse model of combined burn and smoke inhalation-induced injury. *J Appl Physiol (1985)*. 2008;105:678-684.

109. Mlcak RP, et al. Respiratory management of inhalation injury. *Burns*. 2007;33:2-13.

110. Moore SJ, et al. Severe hypoxia produced by concomitant intoxication with sublethal doses of carbon monoxide and cyanide. *Toxicol Appl Pharmacol*. 1991;109:412-420.

111. Morgan WK. The respiratory effects of particles, vapours, and fumes. *Am Ind Hyg Assoc J*. 1986;47:670-673.

112. Morita N, et al. Aerosolized alpha-tocopherol ameliorates acute lung injury following combined burn and smoke inhalation injury in sheep. *Shock*. 2006;25:277-282.

113. Moritz AR, et al. The effects of inhaled heat on the air passages and lungs: an experimental investigation. *Am J Pathol*. 1945;21:311-331.

114. Mosier MJ, et al. Predictive value of bronchoscopy in assessing the severity of inhalation injury. *J Burn Care Res*. 2012;33:65-73.

115. Murphy DG, et al. Tension pneumothorax associated with hyperbaric oxygen therapy. *Am J Emerg Med*. 1991;9:176-179.

116. Nakae H, et al. Failure to clear casts and secretions following inhalation injury can be dangerous: report of a case. *Burns*. 2001;27:189-191.

117. Navar PD, et al. Effect of inhalation injury on fluid resuscitation requirements after thermal injury. *Am J Surg*. 1985;150:716-720.

118. Nelson GL. Regulatory aspects of fire toxicology. *Toxicology*. 1987;47:181-199.

119. Nieman GF, et al. The effect of smoke inhalation on pulmonary surfactant. *Ann Surg*. 1980;191:171-181.

120. Nieman GF, et al. Positive end expiratory pressure (PEEP) efficacy following wood smoke inhalation [abstract]. *Am Rev Resp Dis*. 1986;133:A347.

121. Nieman GF, et al. Methylprednisolone does not protect the lung from inhalation injury. *Burns*. 1991;17:384-390.

122. Nieman GF, et al. Unilateral smoke inhalation increases pulmonary blood flow to the injured lung. *J Trauma*. 1994;36:617-623.

123. Norris JC, et al. Synergistic lethality induced by the combination of carbon monoxide and cyanide. *Toxicology*. 1986;40:121-129.

124. O'Brien DJ, et al. Empiric management of cyanide toxicity associated with smoke inhalation. *Prehosp Disaster Med*. 2011;26:374-382.

125. Oh JS, et al. Admission chest CT complements fiberoptic bronchoscopy in prediction of adverse outcomes in thermally injured patients. *J Burn Care Res*. 2012;33:532-538.

126. Oliver O. Management of the cocoanut grove burns at the Massachusetts General Hospital. *Ann Surg*. 1943;117:801-802.

127. Orzel RA. Toxicological aspects of firesmoke: polymer pyrolysis and combustion. *Occup Med*. 1993;8:414-429.

128. O'Toole G, et al. Extracorporeal membrane oxygenation in the treatment of inhalation injuries. *Burns*. 1998;24:562-565.

129. Oulton MR, et al. Effects of smoke inhalation on alveolar surfactant subtypes in mice. *Am J Pathol*. 1994;145:941-950.

130. Palmieri TL, et al. Continuous nebulized albuterol attenuates acute lung injury in an ovine model of combined burn and smoke inhalation. *Crit Care Med.* 2006;34:1719-1724.

131. Park MS, et al. Assessment of severity of ovine smoke inhalation injury by analysis of computed tomographic scans. *J Trauma.* 2003;55:417-427.

132. Park MS, et al. Assessment of oxidative stress in lungs from sheep after inhalation of wood smoke. *Toxicology.* 2004;195:97-112.

133. Pauluhn J. Pulmonary irritant potency of polyisocyanate aerosols in rats: comparative assessment of irritant threshold concentrations by bronchoalveolar lavage. *J Appl Toxicol.* 2004;24:231-247.

134. Peitzman AB, et al. Smoke inhalation injury: evaluation of radiographic manifestations and pulmonary dysfunction. *J Trauma.* 1989;29:1232-1238.

135. Peterson JE, Stewart RD. Absorption and elimination of carbon monoxide by inactive young men. *Arch Environ Health.* 1970;21:165-171.

136. Pitt BR, et al. Interaction of carbon monoxide and cyanide on cerebral circulation and metabolism. *Arch Environ Health.* 1979;34:345-349.

137. Prien T, Traber DL. Toxic smoke compounds and inhalation injury—a review. *Burns Incl Therm Inj.* 1988;14:451-460.

138. Reade MC, et al. Review article: management of cyanide poisoning. *Emerg Med Australas.* 2012;24:225-238.

139. Rech TH, et al. Inhalation injury after exposure to indoor fire and smoke: the Brazilian disaster experience. *Burns.* 2016;42:884-890.

140. Reper P, et al. High frequency percussive ventilation and conventional ventilation after smoke inhalation: a randomised study. *Burns.* 2002;28:503-508.

141. Reske A, et al. Computed tomography—a possible aid in the diagnosis of smoke inhalation injury? *Acta Anaesthesiol Scand.* 2005;49:257-260.

142. Riddle K. Hydrogen cyanide: fire smoke's silent killer. *JEMS.* 2004;29(8 suppl 5).

143. Riyami BM, et al. Alveolar macrophage chemotaxis in fire victims with smoke inhalation and burns injury. *Eur J Clin Invest.* 1991;21:485-489.

144. Robinson L, Miller RH. Smoke inhalation injuries. *Am J Otolaryngol.* 1986;7:375-380.

145. Robinson NB, et al. Steroid therapy following isolated smoke inhalation injury. *J Trauma.* 1982;22:876-879.

146. Roth D, et al. Accuracy of noninvasive multiwave pulse oximetry compared with carboxyhemoglobin from blood gas analysis in unselected emergency department patients. *Ann Emerg Med.* 2011;58:74-79.

147. Saincome M. Oakland fire warehouse attendees describe confusing, horrific scene. *Rolling Stone*; 2016. http://www.rollingstone.com/music/news/oakland-fire-warehouse-attendees-describe-horrific-scene-w453695.

148. Salim A, Martin M. High-frequency percussive ventilation. *Crit Care Med.* 2005;33(3 suppl):S241-S245.

149. Schwerd W, Schulz E. Carboxyhaemoglobin and methaemoglobin findings in burnt bodies. *Forensic Sci Int.* 1978;12:233-235.

150. Sebbane M, et al. Emergency department management of suspected carbon monoxide poisoning: role of pulse CO-oximetry. *Respir Care.* 2013;58:1614-1620.

151. Smerz RW. Incidence of oxygen toxicity during the treatment of dysbarism. *Undersea Hyperb Med.* 2004;31:199-202.

152. Soejima K, et al. Role of nitric oxide in myocardial dysfunction after combined burn and smoke inhalation injury. *Burns.* 2001;27:809-815.

153. Sokal JA, Kralkowska E. The relationship between exposure duration, carboxyhemoglobin, blood glucose, pyruvate and lactate and the severity of intoxication in 39 cases of acute carbon monoxide poisoning in man. *Arch Toxicol.* 1985;57:196-199.

154. Spano S, et al. Does bronchoscopic evaluation of inhalation injury severity predict outcome? *J Burn Care Res.* 2016;37:1-11.

155. Stellpflug SJ, et al. Hydroxocobalamin hinders hemodialysis. *Am J Kidney Dis.* 2013;62:395.

156. Stoll S, et al. Concentrations of cyanide in blood samples of corpses after smoke inhalation of varying origin. *Int J Legal Med.* 2017;131:123-129.

157. Tasaki O, et al. of burns on inhalation injury. *J Trauma.* 1997;43:603-607.

158. Teixidor HS, et al. Smoke inhalation: radiologic manifestations. *Radiology.* 1983;149:383-387.

159. The Acute Respiratory Distress Syndrome Network. Ventilation with lower tidal volumes as compared with traditional tidal volumes for acute lung injury and the acute respiratory distress syndrome. the acute respiratory distress syndrome network. *N Engl J Med.* 2000;342:1301-1308.

160. Thom SR. Carbon monoxide-mediated brain lipid peroxidation in the rat. *J Appl Physiol (1985).* 1990;68:997-1003.

161. Thom SR, et al. Smoke inhalation-induced alveolar lung injury is inhibited by hyperbaric oxygen. *Undersea Hyperb Med.* 2001;28:175-179.

162. Thompson JP, Marrs TC. Hydroxocobalamin in cyanide poisoning. *Clin Toxicol (Phila).* 2012;50:875-885.

163. Thorning DR, et al. Pulmonary responses to smoke inhalation: morphologic changes in rabbits exposed to pine wood smoke. *Hum Pathol.* 1982;13:355-364.

164. Traber DL, et al. The pathophysiology of inhalation injury—a review. *Burns Incl Therm Inj.* 1988;14:357-364.

165. Traber MG, et al. Burn and smoke inhalation injury in sheep depletes vitamin E: kinetic studies using deuterated tocopherols. *Free Radic Biol Med.* 2007;42:1421-1429.

166. Treitman RD, et al. Air contaminants encountered by firefighters. *Am Ind Hyg Assoc J.* 1980;41:796-802.

167. Tremper KK, Barker SJ. Using pulse oximetry when dyshemoglobin level are high. *J Crit Illness.* 1988;3:103-107.

168. US Fire Administration National Fire Data Center. Fire death rate trends: an international perspective. *FEMA.* 2011;12:8.

169. Wang CZ, et al. The pathophysiology of carbon monoxide poisoning and acute respiratory failure in a sheep model with smoke inhalation injury. *Chest.* 1990;97:736-742.

170. Weaver LK, et al. Carboxyhemoglobin half-life in carbon monoxide-poisoned patients treated with 100% oxygen at atmospheric pressure. *Chest.* 2000;117:801-808.

171. Westphal M, et al. Neuronal nitric oxide synthase inhibition attenuates cardiopulmonary dysfunctions after combined burn and smoke inhalation injury in sheep. *Crit Care Med.* 2008;36:1196-1204.

172. Wiener-Kronish JP, Matthay MA. Beta-2-agonist treatment as a potential therapy for acute inhalational lung injury. *Crit Care Med.* 2006;34:1841-1842.

173. Wittram C, Kenny JB. The admission chest radiograph after acute inhalation injury and burns. *Br J Radiol.* 1994;67:751-754.

174. Wolf SJ, et al. American College of Emergency Physicians Clinical Policies Subcommittee (Writing Committee) on Carbon Monoxide Poisoning. Clinical policy: critical issues in the evaluation and management of adult patients presenting to the emergency department with acute carbon monoxide poisoning. *Ann Emerg Med.* 2017;69:98-107.e6.

175. Yamaguchi KT, et al. Measurement of free radicals from smoke inhalation and oxygen exposure by spin trapping and ESR spectroscopy. *Free Radic Res Commun.* 1992;16:167-174.

176. Yamamoto Y, et al. Nebulization with gamma-tocopherol ameliorates acute lung injury after burn and smoke inhalation in the ovine model. *Shock.* 2012;37:408-414.

177. Yamamura H, et al. Computed tomographic assessment of airflow obstruction in smoke inhalation injury: relationship with the development of pneumonia and injury severity. *Burns.* 2015;41:1428-1434.

178. Youn YK, et al. Oxidants and the pathophysiology of burn and smoke inhalation injury. *Free Radic Biol Med.* 1992;12:409-415.

179. Zawacki BE, et al. Smoke, burns, and the natural history of inhalation injury in fire victims: a correlation of experimental and clinical data. *Ann Surg.* 1977;185:100-110.

180. Zikria BA, et al. The chemical factors contributing to pulmonary damage in "smoke poisoning." *Surgery.* 1972;71:704-709

History A 29-year-old bank teller presented to the emergency department in cardiopulmonary arrest. While working an evening shift, she entered the bank vault, and the door closed behind her. She called for help but was unable to get assistance, so she pulled the fire alarm to alert security to her presence. When the fire department arrived, she was found unresponsive and pulseless on the floor.

Physical Examination The patient was pulseless on the stretcher with chest compressions in progress. No obvious signs of trauma or other injury were visible.

Initial Management The patient was immediately intubated, chest compressions were continued, and intravenous epinephrine 1 mg of 0.1 mg/mL solution was administered. The patient was still pulseless, and the monitor demonstrated asystole, so defibrillation was not performed.

What is the Differential Diagnosis? This patient presented in cardiopulmonary arrest with no known history of ingestion or overdose after being in a bank vault. This should make a toxic inhalant high on the differential diagnosis list (Chaps. 121 to 123). Simple asphyxiants lead to toxicity purely through the displacement of oxygen from the air. Simple asphyxiants should have no independent pharmacologic activity. The severity of symptoms depends on the degree of hypoxia. A few examples of simple asphyxiants are helium, argon, and methane gases. Carbon dioxide is typically also described as a simple asphyxiant; however, a property of carbon dioxide that differentiates it from other simple asphyxiants is that carbon dioxide acts on the body's chemoreceptors, leading to an increased respiratory rate and therefore a more rapid displacement of oxygen from the body.

Inhalants such as carbon monoxide, cyanide and hydrogen sulfide, on the other hand, work through impairing the ability of the body to use oxygen. Hydrogen sulfide, which is found in sewers, is commonly referred to as a "knockdown gas" (Chap. 123). Hydrogen sulfide is a mitochondrial toxin, and the classic description of exposure to hydrogen sulfide includes several people who serially enter an enclosed space and have cardiac arrest. Another example to consider in a patient who has a rapid cardiac arrest, especially in a young, otherwise healthy individual, is cyanide (Chap. 123).

What Chemical and Laboratory Analyses Help Identify the Cause of This Patient's Presentation? Unfortunately, in someone who is in active cardiopulmonary arrest, laboratory values will unlikely return in a rapid enough time to assist in diagnosis. An elevated lactate concentration is typically associated with chemical asphyxiants; however, in the setting of a patient in active cardiopulmonary arrest, the elevation is not specific. The single most important information to acquire is the background as to how the patient collapsed and to use that history to guide management.

Further Diagnosis and Treatment The treatment for all toxic inhalants is to remove the patient from the exposure and to administer supplemental oxygen as needed. In patients who were otherwise well and present with sudden cardiac arrest, a high suspicion is necessary for cyanide toxicity, and hydroxocobalamin administration is appropriate (Antidotes in Depth: A41). In this case, the history of the cardiac arrest after pulling the fire alarm makes cyanide less likely.

The patient had pulled a fire alarm, while she was enclosed inside a bank vault. Because bank vaults contain currency and monetary instruments, using water is undesirable, and most fire extinguishers are carbon dioxide based. The patient was unable to be resuscitated and was pronounced dead. The medical examiner listed the cause of death as carbon dioxide intoxication.

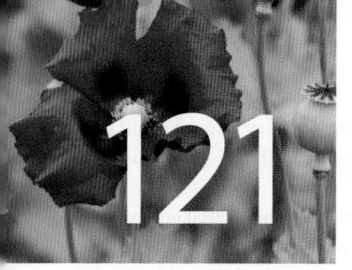

121 SIMPLE ASPHYXIANTS AND PULMONARY IRRITANTS

Lewis S. Nelson and Oladapo A. Odujebe

The respiratory system is responsible for gas exchange, elimination of certain xenobiotics, insensible water loss, temperature regulation, and minor metabolic processes. The principal function of the respiratory system is gas exchange, which occurs in the more than 300 million alveoli that make up approximately 90% of the human lung volume. The average resting adult inhales about 8 L/min of air (a tidal volume of about 500 mL) and averages 16 breaths/min, and this volume can be increased exponentially by increasing the respiratory rate and tidal volume as occurs during exertion. In a 24-hour period, an average adult human at rest will be exposed to 11,500 L of air. There are a number of protective mechanisms within the respiratory system to prevent exposure to xenobiotics, but these mechanisms can be overwhelmed. The principles of respiratory system function are covered extensively in Chap. 28.

The respiratory tract performs several important physiologic functions. Its most important role involves the transfer of oxygen to hemoglobin across the pulmonary endothelium. This transfer facilitates oxygen distribution throughout the body to permit effective cellular respiration. Diverse xenobiotics act at unique points in this distribution pathway to limit or impair tissue oxygenation. For example, whereas opioids and neuromuscular blockers induce hypoventilation, carbon monoxide and methemoglobin inducers prevent loading and unloading of oxygen onto and off hemoglobin. Certain xenobiotics prevent adequate oxygenation of hemoglobin at the level of pulmonary gas exchange. Two mechanistically distinct groups of xenobiotics are capable of interfering with gas exchange: simple asphyxiants and pulmonary irritants. Impairment of transpulmonary oxygen diffusion, regardless of the etiology, reduces the oxygen content of the blood and results in tissue hypoxia.

HISTORY AND EPIDEMIOLOGY

Unlike most xenobiotic exposures, simple asphyxiant and pulmonary irritant poisonings frequently occur on a mass scale due to the magnitude of these exposures. For example, the large-scale emission of carbon dioxide (CO_2) from Lake Nyos, a carbonated volcanic crater lake in Cameroon, West Africa, resulted in nearly 2,000 human deaths and many more livestock deaths (Chap. 2).[8] In this disaster, simple asphyxiation was likely because medical evaluation of both survivors and fatalities demonstrated neither signs of cutaneous or pulmonary irritation nor toxicologic abnormalities.[128] Exposure to compressed liquefied gases, which expand several hundredfold on depressurization or warming, accounts for a substantial number of workplace injuries.[114]

Irritant gases similarly result in mass casualties. For this reason, chlorine and phosgene were used in battle during World War I, resulting in thousands of Allied deaths (Chap. 126). Atmospheric sulfur dioxide and oxides of nitrogen are the primary components of photochemical smog. During the London Fog incident in 1952, 4,000 deaths occurred, primarily from respiratory causes.[102] Similar smog incidents continue to occur around the globe. Relatedly, the diverse irritants found in fire smoke are a major cause of death after smoke inhalation.[113]

Unexpected release of other irritant inhalants leads to large-scale poisoning. In 1984, an inadvertent release of methyl isocyanate (MIC) in Bhopal, India, resulted in immediate and persistent respiratory symptoms in approximately 200,000 local inhabitants, with approximately 2,500 deaths.[82]

Isolated exposures to individuals occur as well, often in workplaces, and more frequently in contained spaces (eg, indoors). Simple asphyxiation as a painless and relatively undetectable method for committing suicide and, paradoxically, for euphoric and erotic experiences, are found in books, on the Internet, and in the medical literature.[39,45,108]

SIMPLE ASPHYXIANTS

Simple asphyxiants work primarily by displacing oxygen from ambient air, unlike chemical asphyxiants, which cause cellular hypoxia and are discussed in Chaps. 122 to 124. Virtually every gas, excluding oxygen, is capable of acting as a simple asphyxiant.

Pathophysiology

Simple asphyxiants displace oxygen from ambient air, thereby reducing the fraction of inspired oxygen (FiO_2) in air to below 21%, and result in a decrease in the partial pressure of oxygen. The partial pressure is a measure of the contribution of oxygen to the total inspired air and is based on both FiO_2 and barometric pressure. For example, because the ambient pressure at sea level (less water vapor, 47 mm Hg) is 713 mm Hg and the percentage of oxygen is 21% (nitrogen 78%), the partial pressure of oxygen in the lungs is 150 mm Hg. However, this relationship is not applicable at other barometric pressures. For example, at the summit of a mountain, the reduced barometric pressure results in a decrease in the partial pressure of oxygen despite a near-normal FiO_2. The barometric pressure decreases in a linear fashion with altitude (above sea level) and increases with descent below sea level. This reduced partial pressure is insufficient to allow adequate oxygen saturation in certain individuals, and supplemental oxygen becomes necessary. As barometric pressure decreases, exposure to simple asphyxiant gases further reduces the oxygen partial pressure to life-threatening levels. Conversely, underwater divers reduce their FiO_2 to below 21% by adding an inert gas, such as helium, to their breathing mixture to avoid oxygen toxicity, yet they maintain adequate oxygenation. This occurs because the elevated barometric pressure increases the partial pressure of oxygen to normal amounts despite the addition of an asphyxiant. However, systemically poisonous gases that enter the breathing mixture would have a magnified effect, given their increased partial pressure at depth.

Conceptually, simple asphyxiants have no pharmacologic activity. For this reason, exceedingly high ambient concentrations of these gases are necessary to produce asphyxia. Asphyxiation typically occurs in confined spaces or with rapid release of large volumes of simple asphyxiants.

Clinical Manifestations

A patient exposed to any simple asphyxiant gas will develop characteristic clinical findings of hypoxia, or lack of oxygen at the cellular level (Table 121–1). These clinical findings are directly related to the reduction in the partial

TABLE 121–1	Clinical Findings Associated with Reduction of Inspired Oxygen
FiO_2[a]	Signs and Symptoms
21	None
16–12	Tachypnea, hyperpnea, (resultant hypocapnia), tachycardia, reduced attention and alertness, euphoria, headache, mild incoordination
14–10	Altered judgment, incoordination, muscular fatigue, cyanosis
10–6	Nausea, vomiting, lethargy, air hunger, severe incoordination, coma
<6	Gasping respiration, seizure, coma, death

[a]At sea level, barometric pressure; appropriate adjustments must be made for altitude and depth exposures.

FiO_2 = fraction of inspired oxygen.

pressure of oxygen in ambient air, which leads to hypoxemia, or low oxygen content of the blood.[128] Cardiovascular and central nervous system (CNS) complications of simple asphyxiants predominate because these organs have the greatest oxygen requirements. As hypoxemia becomes severe, multisystem organ failure and death from tissue hypoxia occur.[28] Postmortem findings are generally minimal, hampering the cause of death determination without historical evidence or advanced laboratory testing.

Exposure to simple asphyxiants does not impair CO_2 exchange, and hypercapnia does not occur. Because dyspnea develops more rapidly from hypercapnia than hypoxemia, the breathlessness associated with physical or simple chemical asphyxiation does not develop until severe hypoxemia intervenes.[75] In these circumstances, victims frequently succumb to hypoxemia without ever developing the expected warning symptoms. In the case of CO_2 inhalation, hypercapnia occurs very rapidly, which itself produces acute cognitive impairment.

Specific Xenobiotics
Noble Gases: Helium, Neon, Argon, and Xenon
Noble gases, which are stored almost exclusively in the compressed form, have numerous industrial and medical roles. Argon is predominantly used as a shielding gas during welding operations, and it is also used in processing titanium and growing crystals. Neon is used in the manufacture of decorative lighting. Xenon, in its radioactive gaseous form, has diagnostic medical applications in ventilation–perfusion scans. Xenon is also used in lighting, solar simulators, digital projectors, and plasma display cells (along with neon). Helium has the lowest molecular weight and is the smallest member of the noble gas family of elements. Because of its lower lipid solubility, helium is often the inert gas used by divers to replace nitrogen to prevent nitrogen narcosis at depth (see Nitrogen). Even using gas mixtures of 50% helium, divers have no adverse effects as long as a normal partial pressure of oxygen is maintained by the mixture at depth. At depth, the quantity (molar quantity, not volume) of air inspired per breath is several-fold greater than at sea level. The lower density of helium than nitrogen results in a lower viscosity of the inhaled air, with a marked decrease in flow resistance. This property of helium is the basis for its use in patients with increased airway resistance (Heliox mixture), such as those with asthma.

Helium is also used in magnetic resonance imaging scanners to keep the coils super cooled. During emergency shutdown of a superconducting electromagnet, an operation known as "quenching," the liquid helium is rapidly boiled from the device and vented into the scanner room.[54] This displaces oxygen from the environment and causes asphyxia. Helium is also used in lung imaging studies and pulmonary function testing. Similarly, the low viscosity of helium has led to its use as an inflation gas for intraaortic balloons, for which rapid inflation and deflation are critical.

All noble gases, when compressed, form cryogenic liquids, which expand rapidly to their gas phase on decompression. Liberation of these gases in closed spaces results in either asphyxiation or freezing injuries, or both.[54] Xenon, unlike the other noble gases, has unique anesthetic properties because of its high lipid solubility and inhibition of N-methyl-D-aspartic acid (NMDA) receptors.[54] The other noble gases have no known direct toxicity.

Short-Chain Aliphatic Hydrocarbon Gases: Methane, Ethane, Propane, and Butane
The short-chain aliphatic hydrocarbon gases are primarily used in the compressed form as fuel.

Methane (CH_4) has no known direct toxicity. Animals can breathe a mixture of 80% methane and 20% oxygen without manifesting hypoxic effects because the FiO_2, and thus their oxygen content, essentially is normal. Methane, also known as "natural gas" and "swamp gas," is present in high ambient concentrations in bogs of decaying organic matter. In addition, compressed natural gas is used as an alternative automotive fuel and poses an asphyxiation hazard if leaked internally. Methane exposure is an occupational hazard for miners who historically carried canaries into their workplace as an "early warning" sign for the presence of toxic gases or

oxygen deficiency. The higher metabolic and respiratory rates of small animals (and children) make them more rapidly susceptible to gas exposures. Methane is also an explosive risk.

Methane is odorless and undetectable without sophisticated equipment. For this reason, natural gas is intentionally adulterated with a small concentration of ethyl mercaptan, a stenching agent, which is responsible for the well-recognized sulfur odor of natural gas. Cooking with natural gas uncommonly causes respiratory symptoms and pulmonary dysfunction.[62] However, methane itself is not the cause because its combustion is generally complete and ambient concentrations are negligible. It is likely that exposure to nitrogen dioxide (NO_2), one of the products of combustion of methane in air the explanation for these symptoms (see Oxides of Nitrogen).

Ethane (C_2H_6) is an odorless component of natural gas and is used as a refrigerant. It has characteristics similar to methane and is occasionally implicated as a simple asphyxiant. Propane (C_3H_8) is widely used in its compressed, liquefied form both as an industrial and domestic fuel and as an industrial solvent. Butane (C_4H_{10}) is a common fuel and solvent. Deliberate butane inhalation from cigarette lighters or air fresheners for recreational purposes, predominantly in adolescents, is associated with cardiovascular dysfunction and cerebral damage (Chap. 81).[110]

Fire-eater's lung (FEL) is a unique form of hydrocarbon pneumonitis caused by aspiration of flammable petrochemical products. Fire-eater's lung occurs after inhalational exposure to the chemicals used to "breathe fire" or "eat fire" during performances. The hydrocarbons are typically low viscosity and disperse throughout bronchioles fairly easily leading to severe lipoid pneumonitis and pneumonia in addition to a systemic inflammatory response. Pulmonary infiltrates occur in as many as 83% of patients studied.[37]

Carbon Dioxide
Although not a simple asphyxiant gas by definition because it produces physiologic effects, CO_2 closely resembles simple asphyxiants from a toxicologic viewpoint. It is used in laboratories as a painless form of animal euthanasia and as a means of large-scale euthanasia of diseased livestock.[94] Carbon dioxide gas has many practical industrial uses, such as production of carbonation in soft drinks. Because it is nonflammable, CO_2 is used as a shielding gas during welding and in commercial fire suppression systems because it safely displace oxygen from the local environment.[44] Dry ice, the frozen form of CO_2, is extremely cold ($-141.3°F$ {$-78.5°C$}) and undergoes conversion from solid to gas without liquefaction, a process known as sublimation. Poisoning occurs when dry ice is allowed to sublimate in a closed space,[19] such as the cabin of a car or in a cold storage room at $39.2°F$ ($4°C$).[32,44] Furthermore, inadvertent connection of respirable gas hoses to CO_2 and other nonrespirable sources is reported in both industrial and medical settings,[63,115] with resultant worker and patient fatalities. This occurrence is uncommon because of mandated engineering controls to prevent the incorrect connection of hose and source terminals.

Pharmacology and pathophysiology. Carbon dioxide, an end product of normal human metabolism, dissolves in the plasma and is in equilibrium with carbonic acid (H_2CO_3). The pH at the central chemoreceptors, reflective of the dissolved carbon dioxide (PCO_2), is responsible for our respiratory drive, and PCO_2 is tightly controlled by the CNS through regulation of breathing.[75] For this reason, exogenous CO_2, combined with oxygen, was at one time used medically as a respiratory stimulant in neonates. Under normal conditions, ambient air contains approximately 0.03% CO_2. When ambient concentrations increase, uptake of CO_2 occurs, which further stimulates respiration thereby further increasing the uptake of ambient CO_2.[27] Accordingly, closed anesthesia systems use scrubbers containing sodium hydroxide (NaOH) to chemically eliminate exhaled CO_2. Failure of the scrubber system results in increasing depth of anesthesia from hypercapnia-induced hyperventilation.

Clinical manifestations. Carbon dioxide produces both acute and subacute poisoning syndromes. The latter occurs during hypoventilation when a patient fails to eliminate endogenous CO_2, develops hypercapnia, and typically presents with gradual somnolence. This is linked to respiratory failure, as in the case of emphysema or opioid poisoning, or at times is iatrogenic, occurring during permissive hypercapnia.[27] Even in experimental models in which a normal FiO_2 is maintained, massive CO_2 inhalation produces CNS and respiratory system manifestations within seconds.[53,61] This occurs because CO_2 is not solely a simple asphyxiant but also possesses protean physiological effects.

Nitrogen Gas

Although nitrogen, like CO_2, produces clinical effects independently of hypoxemia, most poisonings are characterized by the manifestations of a simple asphyxiant. Nitrogen gas is used as a carrier gas for chromatography, as a fertilizer, as a cryogenic gas for surgery, and extensively in manufacturing. Poisoning by nitrogen gas is uncommon but occurs after rapid evaporation of the supercooled liquid.[66,67]

Pharmacology and pathophysiology. Nitrogen is a colorless, odorless, and tasteless gas that makes up 78% by volume of air. Under standard conditions, it is an inert diatomic gas that has no direct physiologic toxicity.

Clinical manifestations. Inadvertent connection of air-line respirator hoses to nitrogen and other inert gas sources results in acute asphyxiation, with unconsciousness occurring in approximately 12 seconds[55,80] and death shortly thereafter. More indolent inhalational poisoning by nitrogen is characterized by impairment of intellectual function and judgment, giddiness, and euphoria, which is qualitatively similar to ethanol intoxication.[83] More severely poisoned patients manifest the spectrum of depressed mental status.[70] Systemic absorption is not rapid, however, and prolonged, high-concentration exposure is required for poisoning. Nitrogen poisoning, also known as *nitrogen narcosis*, occurs in underwater divers while they are breathing air that contains 70% nitrogen. It is sometimes called *rapture of the deep* (*l'ivresse des grandes profondeurs*) and causes many deaths in the subaquatic environment. The underlying mechanism of nitrogen narcosis is unknown, but the simple structure and relatively high lipophilicity of nitrogen suggest a mechanism similar to that of the anesthetic gases.[112] To avoid nitrogen narcosis, a less lipid-soluble inert gas such as helium is generally substituted for nitrogen. Substitution with oxygen, although intuitively logical, is inappropriate because of the risk of oxygen toxicity (see Oxygen).

Dermal exposure to liquid nitrogen produces frostbite because liquid nitrogen is extremely cold and ingestion of liquid nitrogen similarly produces a freezing injury of the gastrointestinal (GI) tract.[130]

Treatment

Treatment of all individuals poisoned by simple asphyxiants begins with immediate removal of the persons from exposure and provision of ventilatory assistance. Provision of supplemental oxygen is preferable, but room air usually suffices. Restoration of oxygenation through spontaneous or mechanical ventilation occurs after only several breaths. Support of vital functions is the mainstay of therapy but is generally unnecessary after a brief exposure. Hyperbaric oxygen therapy offers no benefit.

PULMONARY IRRITANTS

The irritant gases are a heterogeneous group of chemicals that produce toxic effects via a final common pathway: destruction of the integrity of the mucosal barrier of the respiratory tract (Table 121–2).

Pathophysiology

In the lung, irritant chemicals damage both the more prevalent type I pneumocytes and the surfactant-producing type II pneumocytes. Neutrophil influx, recruited in response to macrophage-derived inflammatory cytokines such as tumor necrosis factor (TNF)-α, releases toxic mediators that disrupt the integrity of the capillary endothelial cells.[79] This host defense response results in accumulation of cellular debris and plasma exudate in the alveolar sacs, producing the characteristic clinical findings of the acute respiratory distress syndrome (ARDS). The specific mechanisms by which the irritant gases damage the pulmonary endothelial and epithelial cells vary. Many irritant gases require dissolution in lung water to liberate their

ultimate toxicant, which often is an acid, as occurs when hydrogen chloride gas produces hydrochloric acid. The exact mechanism by which acids damage cells and induce an inflammatory response remains uncertain. Oxidation of intracellular proteins results in rapid cytoskeletal shortening, creating spaces between endothelial cells and allowing fluid movement into the alveolar spaces.[119] Other gases, such as oxygen and ozone, induce pulmonary damage primarily through free radical-mediated oxidative stress on the cellular membranes.[13] Nitrogen dioxide (NO_2) and chlorine are characteristic of a group of gases that produce both acid and free radical oxidants. Furthermore, other respirable xenobiotics, such as metals, injure the respiratory tract through oxidant stress and other mechanisms. Because the precise toxicologic and pathophysiologic effects vary widely depending on the physicochemical properties of the xenobiotic, these mechanisms are covered more completely in the following specific discussions.

By virtue of its use as a chemical weapon, phosgene has received more investigation than the other irritant gases. Although the specific mechanisms of toxicity of the other irritants remain poorly defined, they likely cause injury through a similar process. The acids liberated upon dissolution in the mucosal water react with functional groups on epithelial and endothelial cell membranes and, via cellular messengers, result in a complex inflammatory response.[88,99] Phosgene stimulates the synthesis of lipoxygenase-derived leukotrienes and other cytokines such as TNF-α.[99] Leukotrienes are important chemotactic factors for neutrophils, which accumulate, liberate oxidants, and produce ARDS. Experimentally, ARDS is prevented in rabbits by tomelukast, a leukotriene receptor antagonist, and by methylprednisolone, which blocks leukotriene synthesis, both of which are beneficial postexposure.[51] Ibuprofen, an inhibitor of the arachidonic acid cascade, and xenobiotics capable of reducing neutrophil influx, such as colchicine and cyclophosphamide, reduce lung injury and mortality rates in mice when administered shortly after phosgene exposure.[100] When administered 45 minutes after exposure to phosgene-poisoned rabbits, intratracheal *N*-acetylcysteine (NAC) decreases the formation of leukotrienes by an undefined means and limits the development of ARDS.[101] However, nebulized NAC has not proven successful in the majority of published case material despite some success in basic science research and is not recommended at this time.[46] Intravenous (IV) administration of NAC to patients with mild to moderate ARDS, none of whom had irritant-induced pulmonary damage, improved systemic oxygenation and reduced their need for ventilatory support.[116] However, progression to respiratory failure was not altered. There are no human studies evaluating exposure to chemical irritants and the management of ARDS in patients after a chemical irritant exposure is extrapolated from the ARDS literature. Advanced interventions for reducing the morbidity and mortality associated with non–toxin-induced ARDS such as lung protective strategies, high-frequency ventilation, and prone positioning, widely used in patients with trauma- or sepsis-induced ARDS, have not undergone evaluation in patient with toxin-induced ARDS.[17] Given the pathophysiological and clinical similarities[107] and despite the lack of evidence, it seems reasonable to apply these strategies to patients with inhalational injuries.

Free radicals are highly reactive molecular derivatives, typically from oxygen or nitrogen that bind to and destroy tissue near their site of generation. Through initiation of a lipid peroxidative cascade, free radicals destroy lipid membranes and inhibit energy production through the electron transport chain (Chap. 10). Products of lipid peroxidation and cellular damage initiate neutrophilic influx, presumably in an immunologic response to a pathogen. Ironically, free radicals generated by the invading inflammatory cells contribute to pulmonary damage. Fortunately, the lung has both enzymatic (eg, superoxide dismutase, glutathione peroxidase, catalase) and nonenzymatic (eg, glutathione, ascorbate) antioxidant systems, which detoxify virtually all free radicals present in the lung.[136] However, the oxidant burden imposed by oxidant gases can preempt these detoxifying systems and produce cellular damage. For example, nebulization of manganese superoxide dismutase into the airway 1 hour after smoke inhalation, a form of oxidant lung injury, did not improve lung edema or pulmonary gas exchange.[77]

TABLE 121–2 Characteristics of Common Respiratory Irritants

Gas	Source or Exposure	Solubility (g%)[a]	Detection Threshold (ppm)	Regulatory Standard (ppm)[b]	IDLH[c] (ppm)	STEL (ppm)
Ammonia	Fertilizer, refrigeration, synthetic fiber synthesis	H	5	50	300	35
Cadmium oxide fumes	Welding	I	Odorless	0.005 mg/m³	9 mg/m³ (as Cd)	NA
Carbon dioxide	Exhaust, dry ice sublimation	P	Odorless	5000	40,000	30,000
Chloramine	Bleach plus ammonia	H	NA	NR	NR	NR
Chlorine	Water disinfection, pulp, and paper industry	P	0.3	0.5	10	1
Copper oxide fumes	Welding	I	NA	0.1 mg/m³	100 mg/m³ (as Cu)	NA
Ethylene oxide	Sterilant	H	500	1	800	5
Formaldehyde	Chemical disinfection	H	0.8	0.016	20	2
Hydrogen chloride	Chemical	H	1–5	5	50	5
Hydrogen fluoride	Glass etching, semiconductor industry	H	0.042	3 (as F)	30 (as F)	6
Hydrogen sulfide	Petroleum industry, sewer, manure pits	P	0.025		100	50
Mercury vapor	Electrical equipment, thermometers, catalyst, dental fillings, metal extraction, heating or vacuuming elemental mercury	I	Odorless	0.1 mg/m³	10 mg/m³	0.05
Methane	Natural heating gas, swamp gas	M	Odorless	NR	NR	NR
Methyl bromide	Fumigant	M	20	20	250	NA
Nickel carbonyl	Nickel purification, nickel coating, catalyst	P	1–3	0.001	2 (as Ni)	0.1
Nitrogen		P	Odorless	NR	NR	NR
Nitrogen dioxide	Chemical synthesis, combustion emission	P	0.12	3	20	5
Nitrous oxide	Anesthetic gas, whipping cream dispensers (abuse), racing fuel additive	P	2	25	100	NA
Ozone	Disinfectant, produced by high-voltage electrical equipment	P	0.05	0.1	5	0.1
Phosgene	Chemical synthesis, combustion of chlorinated compounds	P	0.5	0.1	2	0.1
Phosphine	Fumigant, semiconductor industry	P	2	0.3	50	1
Propane	Liquified propane gas	P	Odorless	1000	2100	NR
Sulfur dioxide	Environmental exhaust	H	1	2	100	5
Zinc chloride fumes	Artificial smoke (no longer in use)	H	NA	1 mg/m³	50 mg/m³	2 mg/m³
Zinc oxide	Welding	P	Odorless	5 mg/m³	500 mg/m³	10 mg/m³

[a]g% = grams of gas per 100 mL water; if applicable. Solubility: I = insoluble; P = poor; M = medium; H = high. [b]Standards are either Threshold Limit value-time weighted average (TLV-TWA) set by the American Conference of Governmental Industrial Hygienists (ACGIH) or permissible exposure limits (PELs) set by the Occupational Safety and Health Administration (OSHA). [c]Immediately dangerous to life and health (IDLH): National Institute for Occupational Safety and Health (NIOSH), revised 1995. (Documentation for each IDLH is available at http://www.cdc.gov/niosh/idlh/idlhintr.html.)

F = fluorine; NA = not available; NR = no regulatory standard; STEL = short-term exposure limit (15-minute average not to be exceeded).

Clinical Manifestations

Regardless of the mechanism by which the mucosa is damaged, the clinical presentations of patients exposed to irritant gases are similar.[107] Those exposed to gases that result in irritation within seconds generally develop mucosal injury limited to the upper respiratory tract. The rapid onset of symptoms is usually a sufficient signal to the patient to escape the exposure. Patients present with nasal or oropharyngeal pain in addition to drooling, mucosal edema, cough, or stridor. Conjunctival irritation or chemosis, as well as skin irritation, are often noted because concomitant ocular and cutaneous exposure to the gases usually is unavoidable. Gases that are less rapidly irritating do not typically provide an adequate signal of their presence and therefore do not prompt expeditious escape by the exposed individual. In this case, prolonged breathing allows entry of the toxic gas farther into the bronchopulmonary system, where delayed toxic effects are subsequently noted. Tracheobronchitis, bronchiolitis, bronchospasm, and ARDS are typical inflammatory responses of the airway and represent the spectrum of acute lower respiratory tract injury.

Experimental models assessing the water solubility of a gas to predict the location of its associated lesions generally agree with the clinical data.[15] However, exceptions to this relationship of a gas and its predicted toxicity are common. For example, in situations in which escape from ongoing exposure is prevented, patients develop lower respiratory tract injury after prolonged exposure to acutely irritating gases. Alternatively, rapid onset of upper respiratory irritation occurs in patients after exposure to concentrated gases that are generally associated with delayed signs and symptoms. Exposure to exceedingly high concentrations of any irritant gas produces hypoxemia analogous to that resulting from exposure to a simple asphyxiant.

TABLE 121–3 The Berlin Definition of Acute Respiratory Distress Syndrome[4]

Characteristic	Definition
Timing	Within 1 week of a known clinical insult or new or worsening respiratory symptoms
Chest imaging	Bilateral opacities not fully explained by effusions, lobar or lung collapse, or nodules
Origin of edema	Respiratory failure not fully explained by cardiac failure or fluid overload
	Need objective assessment (eg, echocardiography) to exclude hydrostatic edema if no risk factor is present
Hypoxemia	
Mild	$200 < PaO_2/FiO_2 \leq 300$ with PEEP or CPAP ≥ 5 cm H_2O
Moderate	$100 < PaO_2/FiO_2 \leq 200$ with PEEP ≥ 5 cm H_2O
Severe	$PaO_2/FiO_2 \leq 100$ with PEEP ≥ 5 cm H_2O

CPAP = continuous positive airway pressure; FiO_2 = fraction of inspired oxygen; PEEP = positive end-expiratory pressure; PaO_2 = partial pressure of oxygen.

The most characteristic and serious clinical manifestation of irritant gas exposure is ARDS.[96] Acute respiratory distress syndrome consists of the clinical, radiographic, and physiologic abnormalities caused by pulmonary inflammation and alveolar filling that must be both acute in onset and not attributable solely to pulmonary capillary hypertension as occurs in patients with congestive heart failure.[122] Acute respiratory distress syndrome is a non-specific syndrome resulting from diverse physiologic insults such as sepsis or trauma. Patients with ARDS present with dyspnea, chest tightness, chest pain, cough, frothy sputum, wheezing or crackles, and arterial hypoxemia. Typical radiographic abnormalities include bilateral pulmonary infiltrates with an alveolar filling pattern and a normal cardiac silhouette that differentiate this syndrome from congestive heart failure.

In 2012, the diagnostic criteria for ARDS was updated as a consensus guideline known as the Berlin Definition.[4] The definition created three mutually exclusive strata of ARDS based on the degree of hypoxemia (Table 121–3). Some essential changes of the new definition include acute was defined as 1 week or less, the term *acute lung injury* (ALI) was discontinued, measuring the PaO_2/FiO_2 ratio now requires a specific amount of positive end-expiratory pressure (PEEP), chest radiographic criteria were clarified to improve interrater reliability, the pulmonary capillary wedge pressure (PCWP) criterion was removed, and additional clarity was added to improve the ability to exclude cardiac causes of bilateral infiltrates.

Specific Xenobiotics

Acid- or Base-Forming Gases Highly Water-Soluble Xenobiotics

Ammonia (NH₃). Ammonia is a common industrial and household chemical used in the synthesis of plastics and explosives and as a fertilizer, a refrigerant, and a cleanser. The odor and irritancy are characteristic and serve as an effective warning signals of exposure. Dissolution of NH_3 in water to form the base ammonium hydroxide (NH_4OH) rapidly produces severe upper airway irritation. Patients with exposures to highly concentrated NH_3 or exposures for prolonged periods develop tracheobronchial or pulmonary inflammation. Experimental inhalation of nebulized high-dose ammonia causes ARDS within 2 minutes of exposure.[58] Ultrastructural study of the lungs from two individuals dying acutely of ammonia inhalation revealed marked swelling and edema of type I pneumocytes consistent with ARDS.[16] Chronic inhalation of low concentrations of NH_3 or repetitive exposure to high concentrations of ammonia causes pulmonary fibrosis.[12]

Chloramines. This series of chlorinated nitrogenous compounds (Fig. 121–1) includes monochloramine (NH_2Cl), dichloramine ($NHCl_2$), and trichloramine

A. $3\,NaOCl + 2\,NH_3 \rightarrow NH_2Cl + NHCl_2 + 3\,NaOH$

B. $NH_2Cl + H_2O \rightarrow HOCl + NH_3$
$$HOCl \rightarrow HCl + \{O\}$$

FIGURE 121–1. Chloramine chemistry. (**A**) Sodium hypochlorite (bleach) plus ammonia form monochloramine and dichloramine. (**B**) Chloramine dissolves in water to liberate hypochlorous acid, hydrochloric acid, ammonia, and nascent oxygen {O}, an oxidant.

(NCl_3). The chloramines are most commonly generated by the admixture of ammonia with sodium hypochlorite (NaOCl) bleach, often in an effort to potentiate their individual cleansing powers.[81] Interestingly, the addition of bleach to septic systems results in liberation of the chloramines after the reaction of bleach with urinary nitrogenous compounds.[81] On dissolution of the chloramines in the epithelial lining fluid, hypochlorous acid (HOCl), ammonia, and oxygen radicals are generated, all of which act as irritants. Although less water soluble than ammonia, the chloramines typically promptly result in symptoms. Because these initial symptoms are often mild, however, they often do not prompt immediate escape, resulting in prolonged or recurrent exposure with pulmonary and ocular symptoms predominating.[20] Exposure to trichloramine occurs at indoor swimming pools and is responsible for inducing permeability changes in the pulmonary epithelium, the consequences of which are not yet understood.[25]

Hydrogen chloride (HCl). The largest and most important use of HCl gas is in the production of hydrochloric acid. Dissolution of HCl gas in lung water after inhalation similarly produces hydrochloric acid.[92] Pyrolysis of polyvinyl chloride (PVC), a plastic commonly used in pipe fabrication, generates HCl and is an occupational hazard for firefighters.[113] By adsorbing to respirable carbonaceous particles generated in the fire, HCl is deposited in the alveoli and produces pulmonary toxicity.

Hydrogen fluoride (HF). Hydrogen fluoride and its aqueous form, hydrofluoric acid, are used in the gasoline, glassware, building renovation, and semiconductor industries. Gaseous HF is also liberated, paradoxically by extreme heat, during the release of hydrofluorocarbons from fire suppression systems.[135] Hydrogen fluoride gas dissolves in epithelial lining fluid to form the weak acid hydrofluoric acid. The intact HF molecule is the predominant form in solution, and few free hydronium ions (H_3O^+) are liberated. Low-dose inhalational exposures result in irritant symptoms,[41,132] and large exposures cause bronchial and pulmonary parenchymal destruction.[132] Inhalation results in ARDS, but death usually is related to systemic fluoride poisoning independent of the route of exposure caused by hypocalcemia and hyperkalemia (Chap. 104).[30,135]

Sulfur dioxide and sulfuric acid (SO₂ and H₂SO₄). Sulfur dioxide has multiple industrial applications and is a byproduct found in the smelting and oil refinery industries. It is also generated by the inadvertent mixing of certain chemicals, such as an acid with sodium bisulfite ($NaHSO_3$). Sulfur dioxide is highly water soluble and has a characteristic pungent odor that provides warning of its presence at concentrations well below those that are irritating. In the presence of catalytic metals (Fe, Mn), environmental sulfur dioxide is readily converted to sulfurous acid (H_2SO_3) within water droplets. Sulfurous acid is a major environmental concern and the cause of "acid rain." Exposure to atmospheric sulfur dioxide results in a roughly dose-related bronchospasm, which is most pronounced and difficult to treat in patients with asthma. Inhalation of sulfurous acid or dissolution of sulfur dioxide in epithelial lining fluid produces typical pathologic and clinical findings associated with ARDS.[95] In addition to the effect of acid generation upon dissolution, sulfur dioxide causes oxidative damage to the lungs.[104] Large acute exposure to either xenobiotic produces the expected acute irritant response of both the upper and lower respiratory tracts,[21] and pulmonary dysfunction (see Asthma and Reactive Airways Dysfunction Syndrome) in some persists for several years.[104]

A. $HCl + HOCl \rightarrow Cl_2 + H_2O$

B. $Cl_2 + H_2O \rightarrow 2\, HCl + \{O\}$
$Cl_2 + H_2O \rightarrow HCl + HOCl$

FIGURE 121–2. Chlorine chemistry. **(A)** Formation of chlorine gas from the acidification of hypochlorous acid. **(B)** Dissolution of chlorine in mucosal water to generate both hydrochloric and hypochlorous acids (hydrogen chloride {HCl} and hypochlorous acid {HOCl}) and oxidants {O}.

Intermediate Water-Soluble Xenobiotics

Chlorine (Cl_2). Chlorine gas is a valuable oxidizer with various industrial uses, and occupational exposure is common. Chlorine gas was used as a chemical weapon by both the French and the Germans in World War I (Chap. 126). Although chlorine gas is not generally available for use in the home, domestic exposure to chlorine gas is common. The admixture of an acid to bleach liberates chlorine gas (Fig. 121–2).[85] Because the anionic component of the acid is not involved in the reaction, combining hypochlorite with virtually any acid, such as phosphoric, hydrochloric, or sulfuric acid, results in the release of chlorine gas. As such, inappropriate mixing of cleaning products is the cause of most nonoccupational exposures.[85] Rarely, patients intentionally generate chlorine gas in this manner for purportedly "pleasurable" purposes.[93] Chlorine gas is generated when aging swimming pool chlorination tablets, such as calcium hypochlorite [$Ca(OCl)_2$] or trichloro-s-triazinetrione (TST), decompose[134] or are inadvertently introduced to a swimming pool while swimmers are present.[6,126] Inadvertent mixture of $Ca(OCl)_2$ and TST results in excessive chlorine gas generation, which is also explosive. Acute chlorine toxicity occurs when there is a failure of the system of compressed chlorine gas which is used for direct chlorination of public swimming pools[6] or for drinking water systems. Occasional mass poisoning has occurred during scientific, industrial, or transportation incidents.[56]

The odor threshold for chlorine is low, but distinguishing toxic from permissible air concentrations is difficult until toxicity manifests. The intermediate solubility characteristics of chlorine result in only mild initial symptoms after moderate exposure and allow a substantial time delay, typically several hours, before clinical symptoms develop. Chlorine dissolution in lung water generates HCl and hypochlorous (HOCl) acids. Hypochlorous acid rapidly decomposes into HCl and nascent oxygen (O). The unpaired nascent oxygen atom produces additional pulmonary damage by initiating a free radical oxidative cascade. Although the majority of life-threatening chlorine poisonings occur after acute large exposures, patients with chronic, low-concentration or recurrent and patients with exposure to moderate concentrations often manifest increased bronchial responsiveness[1,42] (see Reactive Airways Dysfunction Syndrome).

Hydrogen sulfide (H_2S). Hydrogen sulfide exposures occur most frequently in the waste management, petroleum, and natural gas industries,[38] although poisoning occurs in asphalt, synthetic rubber, and nylon industry workers as well. Hydrogen sulfide exposure also rarely occurs in hospital workers using acid cleaners to unclog drains clogged with plaster of Paris sludge. The generation of H_2S by mixing household chemicals in a closed automobile, a trend referred to as "detergent suicide," produces a potential threat to the responders.[2] Hydrogen sulfide is a decay product of organic material found in sewers or manure pits. Hydrogen sulfide, hydrogen fluoride, and phosphine are differentiated from the other irritant gases by their ability to produce significant systemic toxicity. Hydrogen sulfide inhibits mitochondrial respiration in a fashion similar to that of cyanide[127] (Chap. 123).

Hydrogen sulfide has the distinctive odor of "rotten eggs," which, although helpful in diagnosis, is not specific. Despite a sensitive odor threshold of several parts per billion,[1] rapid olfactory fatigue ensues, providing a misperception that the exposure and its attendant risk have diminished. At low and moderate concentrations ($\leq$500 ppm), upper respiratory tract mucosal irritation occurs and is the principal toxicity.[118] The rapidity of death in patients exposed to high H_2S concentrations makes it difficult to conclude whether simple asphyxiation or cytochrome oxidase inhibition is causal in most cases. Neither the postmortem H_2S nor thiosulfate concentrations are reliable for determining cause of death.[7]

Phosgene (carbonyl chloride {$COCl_2$}). During World War I, phosgene was an important chemical weapon that produced countless deaths (Chap. 126).[36] Currently, phosgene is used in the synthesis of various organic compounds, such as isocyanates, and it occasionally produces poisoning. It is a byproduct of heating or combustion of various chlorinated organic compounds.

Exposure to phosgene initially produces limited manifestations, but results in acute mucosal irritation after intense exposure. In fact, the pleasant odor of fresh hay, rather than prompting escape, disturbingly promotes prolonged breathing of the toxic gas. The most consequential clinical effect related to phosgene exposure is delayed ARDS.[10] The accumulation of a significant alveolar burden of phosgene due to the lack of a noxious warning property of the gas, explains why the clinical effects generally are severe. Because the onset is typically delayed up to 24 hours, prolonged observation of patients thought to be phosgene-poisoned is warranted. The mechanism of phosgene toxicity occurs by the dissolution of the gas into the fluid of the epithelial lining with resultant liberation of hydrochloric acid and reactive oxygen species (ROS).[10]

Oxidant Gases

Rather than acidic or alkaline metabolites, free radicals mediate the pulmonary toxicity of certain irritant gases. Many of the chemicals discussed participate in both acid–base and oxidant types of injury. However, the clinical distinction between acid- or alkali-forming irritants and oxidants is difficult but is therapeutically relevant.

Oxygen (O_2). Oxygen toxicity is uncommon in the workplace but, ironically, is common in hospitalized patients. Although prolonged, high concentration exposures to O_2 produce CNS and retinal toxicity, pulmonary damage is more common.[111] Several clinical studies indicate that humans can tolerate 100% O_2 at sea level for up to 48 hours without significant acute pulmonary damage.[18,29] Under hyperbaric conditions (2.0 atmospheres absolute), such as during compressed-air diving or while inside a pressurized hyperbaric chamber, oxygen toxicity develops within 3 to 6 hours.[23] Acute respiratory distress syndrome occurs in approximately 5% of patients administered hyperbaric oxygen for therapeutic purposes.[111] Delayed pulmonary fibrosis, presumably from healing of subclinical injury, develops in patients breathing lower concentrations of O_2 at sea level for shorter periods.

Although it appears paradoxical that O_2, an essential molecule, is deleterious at elevated concentrations, it is not. In mitochondria, O_2 plays a critical role as the ultimate acceptor for electrons completing the electron transport chain. This same potent oxidizing activity allows O_2 to remove electrons from other compounds generating the reactive oxygen intermediate.[97]

Generation of ROS, including superoxide (O_2^-), hydroxyl radical (OH·), hydrogen peroxide (HOOH), singlet oxygen (O·), and nitric oxide (NO), produces cellular necrosis, increases pulmonary capillary permeability, and induces apoptosis.[97] Nitric oxide, produced by inducible NO synthase (iNOS) in the setting of oxidative stress, is directly cytotoxic or it can combine with superoxide anions to form the more reactive oxidant peroxynitrite ($ONOO^-$).[57] Experimental prevention of these effects by administration of either parenteral NAC,[129] a chemical antioxidant, or superoxide dismutase, an enzymatic antioxidant,[68] suggests that the mechanism of toxicity relates to the oxidant, or electrophilic, effects of these ROS (Chap. 10). Although several other therapies have shown promise in preventing oxygen-mediated toxicity, none has yet proven to be valuable for patients who already manifest pulmonary toxicity. Current techniques for preventing pulmonary oxygen toxicity emphasize reduction of the inspired oxygen concentration by use of PEEP ventilation. The potential role of liquid ventilation of the lung with perfluorocarbons to prevent or treat pulmonary oxygen toxicity remains under investigation but not highly promising.[40]

Oxides of nitrogen (NO$_x$). Oxides of nitrogen are a series of variably oxidized nitrogenous compounds. The most important substances included in this series are the stable free radicals nitrogen dioxide (NO$_2$) and NO, as well as nitrogen tetroxide (dinitrogen tetroxide {N$_2$O$_4$}), nitrogen trioxide (N$_2$O$_3$), and nitrous oxide (N$_2$O). The oxides of nitrogen are of limited concern in industrial operations, although they are generated during welding and brazing.[24] Nitrogen oxide, in addition to hydrogen cyanide, is produced in the pyrolysis of nitrocellulose, which is a substantial component of radiographic film. For example, a fire in the radiology department of the Cleveland Clinic in 1929 resulted in 125 casualties, with virtually all deaths resulting from cyanide or NO$_2$ gas poisoning.[48] Nitrogen oxide toxicity also occurs when propane-driven ice-cleaning machines are used in indoor ice skating rinks with poor ventilation, thereby allowing accumulation of the generated NO$_2$,[72] or after exposure to high NO$_2$ concentrations in closed space fires, such as in submarines.[78] Nitrogen oxide also causes silo filler's disease, in which the toxic gas generated during decomposition of silage accumulates within the silo shortly after grain storage, eliminating rodents that feast on the grains.[31] In the absence of ventilation, high concentrations of NO$_2$ accumulate in the silo such that an individual entering the silo is rapidly asphyxiated from the depletion of oxygen.[49] Additionally, substantial quantities of NO$_2$ remaining after incomplete ventilation are associated with delayed-onset pulmonary toxicity characteristic of silo filler's disease. Chronic indoor exposure to NO$_2$, generated during cooking or outdoor exposure to photochemical smog, of which the oxides of nitrogen are a component, predisposes individuals to the development or exacerbation of chronic lung diseases.[62]

The various oxides of nitrogen directly oxidize respiratory tract cellular membranes but more typically generate reactive nitrogen intermediates, or radicals, such as ONOO$^-$, which subsequently damage the pulmonary epithelial cells.[90] In addition to generating oxidant cascades, dissolution in respiratory tract water generates nitric acid (HNO$_3$) and NO, which produce injury consistent with other inhaled acids.[52] Antioxidants afford significant protection to environmental oxidant exposure including NO$_2$, indicating an important role of free radicals in the toxicology of these xenobiotics.[69]

Nitric oxide, an endogenous compound important as a neurotransmitter and vasorelaxant, is used clinically exogenously for inhalational therapy to treat pulmonary hypertension and ARDS.[43] In patients with ARDS not resulting from sepsis (although not specifically from inhalational injury), low concentrations of inhaled NO (5 ppm) did not improve the clinical outcome, although its use in premature infants with respiratory distress syndrome is well accepted.[43] Nitric oxide is less soluble in the fluid lining the epithelial surfaces than are the other oxides of nitrogen and produces irritant effects after large exposures.[124] Its pulmonary oxidative toxicity, the manifestations of which are typical of the oxidant gases, is substantially enhanced by conversion to reactive nitrogen intermediates such as ONOO$^-$. This radical selectively interacts with tyrosine to produce nitrotyrosine, which subsequently serves as a marker for oxidant damage. Nitric oxide is absorbed from the lung and is rapidly bound by hemoglobin to form nitrosylhemoglobin, and methemoglobin may also be produced.

Ozone (O$_3$). Ozone is abundant in the stratospheric region found between 5 and 31 miles above the planet. Ozone is formed by the action of ultraviolet light on oxygen molecules, thus reducing the amount of solar ultraviolet irradiation reaching earth. The ozone concentration in passenger aircrafts is at times above regulatory limit, although a specific relationship with the development of clinical effects in airline crew members is elusive.[133] Ozone is an important component of photochemical smog and, as such, contributes to chronic lung disease. It is produced in significant quantities by welding and high-voltage electrical equipment and in more moderate doses by photocopying machines and laser printers. Because of its high electronegativity (only fluorine is higher), ozone is one of the most potent oxidizers available. For this reason, it is used as a bleach, particularly as an alternative to chlorine in water purification and sewage treatment.

The pulmonary toxicity associated with ozone primarily results from its high reactivity toward unsaturated fatty acids and amino acids with

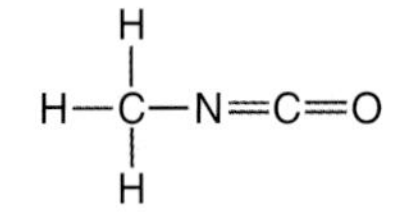

FIGURE 121–3. Methylisocyanate.

sulfhydryl functional groups.[13] Ozonation and free radical damage to the lipid component of the membrane initiate an inflammatory cascade. Reactive nitrogen species are also implicated because NO synthase knockout mice are relatively protected from ozone-induced inflammation and tissue injury.[34] Increased permeability of the pulmonary epithelium results in alveolar filling from the transudation of proteins and fluids characteristic of ARDS.

Miscellaneous Pulmonary Irritants

Methylisocyanate. Methylisocyanate (MIC) (Fig. 121–3) is one of a series of compounds sharing a similar isocyanate (N=C=O) moiety. Toluene diisocyanate (TDI) and diphenyl-methane diisocyanate (MDI) are important chemicals in the polymer industry. In those exposed to MIC in Bhopal, ARDS was evident both clinically and radiographically.[82] Methylisocyanate is a significantly more potent respiratory irritant than the other regularly used isocyanate derivatives such as TDI.

Riot control agents: capsaicin, chlorobenzylidene malononitrile, and chloroacetophenone. Historically, riot control agents (Fig. 126–5), commonly called Mace, consisted primarily of chloroacetophenone (CN) or chlorobenzylidene malononitrile (CS).[9] Both are white solids that are dispersed as aerosols. The dispersion is generally accomplished through mixture with a pyrotechnic agent such as a grenade or with a volatile organic solvent in a personal protection canister. Because the delivery systems of these agents are of limited sophistication and are subject to prevailing environmental conditions, dosing is unpredictable, and unintended self-poisoning is common.[9] After low-concentration exposure, ocular discomfort and lacrimation alone are expected, accounting for the common appellation *tear gas*. The effects are transient, and complete recovery within 30 minutes is typical, although long lasting pulmonary effects are described (see Asthma and Reactive Airways Dysfunction Syndrome). Closed-space or close-range exposure, as well as physical exertion during exposure, is associated with significant ocular toxicity, dermal burns, laryngospasm, ARDS, or death.[120] Because of their high potential for severe toxicity, CN and CS were replaced for civilian use by oleoresin capsicum (OC), also known as *pepper spray* or *pepper mace*. Although capsaicin, its active component, is considerably less toxic, it is occasionally responsible for pneumonitis and death.

Capsaicin interacts with the vanilloid receptor-1 (VR1), which was recently renamed the transient receptor potential vanilloid-1 (TRPV1).[117] Stimulation of this receptor invokes the release of substance P, a neuropeptide involved with transmission of pain impulses. Substance P also induces neurogenic inflammation, which, in the lung, results in ARDS and bronchoconstriction (see Asthma and Reactive Airways Dysfunction Syndrome).

Metal pneumonitis. Acute inhalational exposures to certain metal compounds produce clinical effects identical to those of the chemical irritants. For example, zinc chloride (ZnCl$_2$) fume is used as artificial smoke because of the dense white character of the fume, and an aqueous solution is still used as a soldering flux. Exposure to zinc chloride fumes for just a few minutes is associated with ARDS and death (Chap. 100).[59] Cadmium oxide (CdO) is generated during the burning of cadmium metal in an oxygen-containing environment, as occurs during smelting or welding (Chap. 88). The refining of nickel using carbon monoxide (Mond process) produces nickel carbonyl [Ni(CO)$_4$], a volatile pulmonary oxidant (Chap. 96).[103] Inhalation of volatilized elemental mercury occurs during the vacuuming of mercury spills or home extracting of precious metals (Chap. 95).[87] Although at high concentrations many of these metal exposures produce warning symptoms, severe toxicity may occur even in the absence of warning symptoms. The mechanism of toxicity typically relates to overwhelming oxidant stress with a pronounced inflammatory response as measured by serum cytokine (eg, TNF-α) concentrations, consistent with the role of metals in redox reactions (Chap. 10). Patients with metal-induced pneumonitis present with chest tightness, cough, fever, and signs consistent with ARDS. Metal pneumonitis is distinguishable from other causes of ARDS only by history or, retrospectively, by elevated serum or urine metal concentrations.[3] In particular, metal pneumonitis should be differentiated from the more common and substantially less consequential metal fume fever, discussed later in this chapter. In addition to standard supportive measures, patients with acute metal-induced pneumonitis should be hospitalized, and it is reasonable to administer corticosteroids.[60] Chelation therapy has no documented benefit for treatment of patients with ARDS but is indicated based on conventional indications.

MANAGEMENT

Standard and Supportive Measures

Management of patients with acute respiratory tract injury begins with meticulous support of airway patency by limiting bronchial and pulmonary secretions and maintaining oxygenation. Although various new treatment modalities are available,[17] supportive care remains a cornerstone of therapy. Supplemental oxygen, bronchodilators, and airway suctioning should be used for standard indications. Nitrovasodilators and diuretics have no role in the management of patients with ARDS, although light sedation is recommended as an anxiolytic.[105] Corticosteroid therapy, designed to reduce the inflammatory host defense response, frequently improves surrogate markers of pulmonary damage,[122] such as oxygenation status, but generally offers little outcome enhancement in patients with ARDS.[91] Clinical data on the efficacy of corticosteroids used in human beings exposed to pulmonary irritants are limited and inconclusive.[26] Importantly, most studies of ARDS involve predominantly septic or traumatized patients, with few patients having inhalational poisoning. Because the inflammatory response initiated by bacterial endotoxin differs from that caused by irritant gases, the applicability of these studies to the treatment of poisoned individuals is limited. There is an interesting report of simultaneous, presumably equivalent chlorine exposure in two sisters, with improved outcome in the sister who received steroid treatment.[22] Most available research evaluates parenterally administered corticosteroids, although animal models demonstrate a beneficial effect of nebulized beclomethasone or budesonide after acute chlorine poisoning.[26,50,131] Nebulized budesonide compared to IV betamethasone had similar effects.[26] However, a human pretreatment model of inhaled budesonide fails to document a substantive alteration of the effects of ozone inhalation.[86] Furthermore, most of the aforementioned studies assess acute outcome and not long-term effects in survivors. Because corticosteroids experimentally reduce the late fibroproliferative phase during lung recovery, with additional study, they are thought by some to be beneficial. Overall, there is little reason to suspect any specific benefit of corticosteroids in most poisoned patients. However, because many studies demonstrate little identifiable risk and some potential benefit, corticosteroid use is reasonable whether inhaled or intravenous, and based largely on institutional practices for the management of patients with ARDS.

The clinical similarities among patients with irritant gas exposure and other etiologies of ARDS suggest that similar management principles are reasonable to apply. Although not specifically evaluated in any of these studies, there are sound theoretical reasons to believe that all of these modalities should improve oxygenation in poisoned patients as well. Prone positioning during ventilation; PEEP; early neuromuscular blockade; and low-volume, low-pressure, lung protective strategies are successful in enhancing the oxygenation of patients with ARDS of various causes but are not necessarily successful in improving outcome.[17] Lower tidal volume mechanical ventilation using 6 mL/kg and plateau pressures of 30 cm H_2O attenuated the inflammatory response and resulted in a lower mortality rate and less need for mechanical ventilation than traditional volume ventilation with 12 mL/kg.[84] It is reasonable to reduce the inspired concentration of oxygen to below 50% as rapidly as possible because patients poisoned by irritant gases have enhanced susceptibility to oxygen toxicity as a result of depletion of endogenous antioxidant barriers.[109]

Neutralization Therapy

A therapy unique to several of the acid- or base-forming irritant gases is chemical neutralization. Although contraindicated in acid or alkali ingestion because of concern of an exothermic reaction in the process of neutralization, the large surface area of the lung and the relatively small amount of xenobiotic present allow dissipation of the heat and gas generated during neutralization. Case studies suggest that nebulized 2% sodium bicarbonate is beneficial in patients poisoned by acid-forming irritant gases.[123] The vast majority of these cases involve chlorine gas exposure, and most patients received other symptomatic therapies as well.[5,74] Although there appears to be no specific benefit for patients exposed to chloramine, nebulized bicarbonate therapy appears to be safe and is reasonable to administer. A prospective evaluation of patients poisoned with chloramine and chlorine gas did not show any clinically significant difference between the group getting nebulized sodium bicarbonate and the control group, although there was a small but statistical improvement in forced expiratory volume in 1 second (FEV_1) at 120 and 240 minutes in the group that received nebulized sodium bicarbonate.[5] The sodium bicarbonate solution should be used in a sufficiently dilute form to prevent irritation. Typically, 1 mL of 7.5% or 8.4% sodium bicarbonate solution is added to 3 mL sterile water (resulting in an ~2% solution for nebulization).

Whether nebulized sodium bicarbonate therapy alters the natural course of irritant-induced pulmonary damage remains uncertain. The fact that many irritant gases produce concomitant oxidant injury suggests otherwise. Therefore, patients receiving nebulized bicarbonate therapy require observation beyond the time of symptom resolution. Because administration of neutralizing acids for alkaline irritants, such as ammonia, has not been attempted, we recommend against their use at this time (Antidotes in Depth: A5).

Antioxidants

Antioxidants include reducing agents such as ascorbic acid,[35] N-acetylcysteine, free radical scavengers such as vitamin E, and enzymes such as superoxide dismutase. Studies in humans identify both increased[98] and decreased[11] endogenous antioxidant concentrations in bronchoalveolar lavage fluid in patients with ARDS. Although the concept of treating pulmonary oxidant stress with antioxidants or free radical scavengers is intriguing, most currently available evidence suggests that these xenobiotics offer negligible benefit in humans. The rapid onset of the self-perpetuating destructive effects initiated by redox reactions hinders the success of postexposure therapy. This interpretation is supported by pretreatment models in which antioxidants are effective at preventing or at least limiting the pathologic effects. Use of these and other newer therapies targeted against inflammatory mediators or the oxidative cascade are in the earliest investigative stages and not yet ready to be recommended.

Xenobiotic-Directed Therapy

Patients with inhalational exposure to hydrogen fluoride should undergo frequent electrocardiographic evaluations and correction of serum electrolytes. Administration of nebulized 2.5% calcium gluconate, prepared as 1.5 mL 10% calcium gluconate plus 4.5 mL 0.9% sodium chloride solution or sterile water, is suggested to limit systemic fluoride absorption, and is reasonable to administer. By binding fluoride ion locally, nebulized calcium prevents fluoride-induced cellular and systemic toxicity. Systemic calcium salts should be administered as needed to correct hypocalcemia (Chap. 104 and Antidotes in Depth: A32).

Current therapy for inhalation of capsaicin or of any tear gas, is primarily supportive. Extracorporeal membrane oxygenation was used in children to maintain oxygenation in the presence of severe pulmonary toxicity resulting from capsaicin exposure. There are no antidotes currently available.

Advanced Pharmacologic Therapy
Perfluorocarbon Partial Liquid Ventilation

Partial liquid ventilation involves the intrapulmonary administration of perfluorocarbons, which are inert liquids with low surface tension and excellent oxygen-carrying capacity. Patients with nonchemically induced ARDS have exfoliated tissue, and presumably persistent xenobiotic, effectively lavaged from the bronchopulmonary tree with this method. Perfluorocarbons improve oxygenation and have an antiinflammatory effect, as demonstrated by reduced oxidant lung injury after liquid ventilation in animals. Although perfluorocarbons have interesting potential to be a highly useful therapy in the future, the limited availability, high cost, and lack of demonstrated efficacy of this therapy make it reasonable only if readily available.[40,64]

OTHER INHALED PULMONARY XENOBIOTICS

A particulate, or dust, is a solid dispersed in a gas. Dust is a substantial source of occupational particulate exposure and is an important cause of acute pulmonary toxic syndromes. A respirable particulate must have an appropriately small size (generally <10 microns) and aerodynamic properties to enter the terminal respiratory tree. Nonrespirable particulates, also called *nuisance dusts*, are trapped by the upper airways and are not generally thought to cause pulmonary damage. In distinction from the irritant gases, there is no unifying toxic mechanism among the respirable particulates. Many of the particulate diseases, such as asbestos exposure and its sequelae, are chronic in nature; only the acute and subacute syndromes are discussed here.

Inorganic Dust Exposure

Silicosis, which is pulmonary diseases associated with inhalation of crystalline silica (SiO_2), or quartz, is representative of a range of lung diseases associated with inorganic silica dust inhalation.[71,89] The aftermath of the World Trade Center attack and building collapse resulted in substantial acute silica exposure to residents and rescuers. Exposure-related effects include several acute and delayed-onset pulmonary consequences, such as cough, asthma, chronic obstructive pulmonary disease, and sarcoidlike lung changes.[73,89] More typically, silica exposure occurs in workers involved in occupations in which rock or granite is pulverized, including mining, quarry work, and sandblasting. Although typically a chronic disease, intense subacute silica dust exposure produces acute silicosis in a few weeks and even death within 2 years. The mechanism of toxicity relates to the relentless inflammatory response generated by the pulmonary macrophages.[65] These cells engulf the indigestible particles and are destroyed, releasing their lytic enzymes and oxidative products locally within the pulmonary parenchyma. Patients present with dyspnea, cor pulmonale, restrictive lung findings, and classic radiographic findings. Treatment is limited and includes steroids and supportive care.

Silica combined with other minerals is referred to as *silicates*, the most important of which include asbestos and talc. Talc, or magnesium silicate $[(Mg_3Si_4)O_{10}(OH)_2]$, is widely used in industry, but its use in the home was curtailed over the past two decades because of cases of severe pulmonary injury. Much of the toxicity of talc is related to free silica or asbestos contamination. Improvement after acute massive exposure is sometimes accompanied by progressive pulmonary fibrosis.

Organic Dusts

Inhalation of dusts from cotton or similar natural fibers, usually during the refinement of cotton fibers (byssinosis), produces chest tightness, dyspnea, and fever that typically begin within 3 to 4 hours of exposure. Similar reactions occur after inhalation of hay, silage, grain, hemp, or compost dust. Symptoms often resolve during the workweek but return after a weekend hiatus. Byssinosis is caused by an endotoxin present on the cotton and is not immunologic in nature.[210] "Grain fever" is caused by a respirable compound associated with grain dust, as occurs during harvesting, milling, and transporting.

Hypersensitivity Pneumonitis

Hypersensitivity pneumonitis, also known as extrinsic allergic alveolitis, is the final common pathway for many different organic dust exposures.[125] The name attached to the individual syndrome typically identifies the associated occupation or substrate. For example, *bagassosis* is the term associated with sugar cane (bagasse), and *farmer's lung* is the term associated with moldy hay, although both conditions are caused by thermophilic *Actinomycetes* spp. When associated with puffball mushroom spores (*Lycoperdon* spp), the syndrome is called *lycoperdonosis*; when caused by bird droppings, it is called *bird fancier's lung*. The implicated allergen is capable of depositing in the pulmonary parenchyma and eliciting a cell-mediated (type IV) immunologic response. Clinical findings include fever, chills, and dyspnea beginning 4 to 8 hours after exposure. The chest radiograph is typically normal but also reveals diffuse or discrete infiltrates. Progressive disease is associated with a honeycombing pattern on the radiograph and a restrictive lung disease pattern on formal pulmonary function testing. It is reasonable to administer corticosteroids and recommended to avoid the antigen.

Metal Fume Fever and Polymer Fume Fever

Metal fume fever is a recurrent influenzalike syndrome that develops several hours after exposure to metal oxide fumes generated during welding, galvanizing, or smelting.[47] Although most symptoms of metal fume fever are similar to those expected with irritant gas exposures (dyspnea, cough, chest pain), the presence of fever, typically 100.4°F to 102.2°F (38°C–39°C), distinguishes the syndromes. In addition, patients experience headache, a metallic taste, myalgias, and chills. Direct pulmonary toxicity does not occur, and patients with metal fume fever generally have normal chest radiographs. Interestingly, acute tolerance develops, so repeat daily exposures produce progressively milder symptoms. However, the tolerance disappears rapidly, and after a short work hiatus such as a weekend, the original intensity resumes, thus accounting for the designation "Monday morning fever." Many metal oxides are capable of eliciting this syndrome, but it is noted most frequently in patients who weld galvanized steel, which contains zinc. Metal fume fever also occurs commonly after the high-temperature welding of copper-containing compounds, thus accounting for the historical appellation "brass foundry workers ague." There is a strong association between welding-related metal fume fever and welding-related respiratory symptoms suggestive of occupational asthma.[33] Serum and urine metal concentrations typically are not elevated after the acute event, although they are also found to be chronically elevated following daily occupational exposure. The etiology of metal fume fever is debated, but the syndrome has features suggestive of both an immunologic and a toxic etiology.[47] Antigen release with immunologic response appears to be responsible for the induction of symptoms. On subsequent exposure, proinflammatory cytokines, such as TNF-α, and various interleukins are detected in bronchoalveolar lavage fluid.[70] However, because symptoms often occur with the first exposure to fumes, a direct toxic effect on the respiratory mucosa presumably exists.[122] Exposure to certain metal fumes, such as cadmium oxide or other zinc compounds, produce direct toxic effects on the pulmonary parenchyma.

The management of patients with metal fume fever is supportive and includes analgesics and antipyretics. There is no specific antidote, and chelation therapy we recommend against unless otherwise indicated. For example, patients with ARDS after metal fume inhalation most likely have metal toxicity (eg, cadmium pneumonitis). The natural course of metal fume fever involves spontaneous resolution within 48 hours. Persistent symptoms are rare and should prompt investigation for metal toxicity.

A remarkably similar syndrome occurs subsequent to inhaling pyrolysis products of fluorinated polymers (eg, Teflon), which is aptly termed *polymer fume fever*.[47] Patients develop self-limited influenzalike symptoms several hours after exposure to the fumes. As with metal fumes, very large exposures to polymer fumes result in direct pulmonary toxicity. Supportive care is the therapy of choice.

Asthma and Reactive Airways Dysfunction Syndrome

Asthma, or *reversible airways disease*, is a clinical syndrome that includes intermittent episodes of dyspnea, cough, chest pain or tightness, wheezes on auscultation, and measurable variations in expiratory airflow. Episodes typically are triggered by a xenobiotic or physical stimulus and resolve over several hours with appropriate therapy. The underlying process is immunologic in most cases, with allergen-triggered release of inflammatory mediators

TABLE 121–4 Common Xenobiotic Sensitizers Producing Occupational Asthma

Molecular Weight	Example	Primary Risk Occupations
High		
Proteins	Crab shell protein	Seafood processors
Low		
Acrylate	Plastics	Adhesives, plastics
Glutaraldehyde	Sterilant	Health care workers
Isocyanates	Toluene diisocyanate	Polyurethane foam, automobile painters
Metals	Nickel sulfate	Nickel platers
Trimellitic anhydride	Curing agent for epoxy and paint	Chemical workers
Wood dust	Western red cedar (Thuja plicata)	Foresters, carpenters

causing bronchiolar smooth muscle contraction and subsequent inflammation. Because asthma affects 5% to 10% of the world's population and the triggers often are nonspecific, it is not surprising that work-aggravated asthma is extremely common. The patients are previously sensitized, and the initial irritant exposure causes bronchospasm or similar symptoms. Thus, work-aggravated asthma is discovered early in the worker's employment, and a more appropriate workplace or occupation can be pursued.

Occupational asthma, or asthma occasioned by a workplace exposure to a sensitizing xenobiotic, accounts for perhaps up to 25% of all newly diagnosed asthma in adults.[121] Casual exposure to one of the 250 or more known sensitizers (Table 121–4) is usually associated with a latency period of weeks or months of exposure before symptom onset.[76] After symptoms begin, however, they recur consistently after reexposure to the inciting trigger agent. Occupational asthma with latency is either IgE dependent, in which case it is identical to allergic asthma, or IgE independent.[121] The IgE-dependent form is most commonly associated with high-molecular-weight compounds (>5,000 Da) or with certain haptenic low-molecular-weight agents (eg, acetic anhydride). The low-molecular-weight compounds (eg, nickel, isocyanates) more typically cause IgE-independent disease, which manifests as the delayed reaction pattern of cell-mediated, or type IV, hypersensitivity. Because contact with a trigger is difficult to avoid in either case, reassignment or an outright occupational change is occasionally required. Treatment for exacerbations is comparable to standard asthma therapy and should include bronchodilators and corticosteroids as appropriate.

Acute exposure to irritant gas results in the development of a persistent asthmalike syndrome also termed *reactive airways dysfunction syndrome* (RADS), *irritant-induced asthma*, or *occupational asthma without latency*. Virtually every irritative xenobiotic is reported to cause this syndrome, and those not yet described probably are likely unrecognized. Although asthma typically is associated with massive inhalational exposure, as occurred with irritant dust exposure after the World Trade Center collapse,[73] occasional patients are susceptible to low-level exposure. Reactive airways dysfunction syndrome is often compared to occupational asthma because both disorders are chemically induced and most frequently occur after chemical exposure in the workplace. However, in comparison with those who develop occupational asthma, patients who develop RADS have a lower incidence of atopy and are exposed to agents not typically considered to be immunologically sensitizing.[106] In addition, the airflow improvement with β₂-adrenergic agonist therapy is significantly better in patients with occupational asthma. Bronchial biopsy performed in patients with RADS generally reveals a chronic inflammatory response.[14] Reactive airways dysfunction syndrome also has a neurogenic etiology, as opposed to an immunologic origin as in patients with occupational asthma, which differentiates these clinically similar diseases

on a mechanistic basis. Neurogenic inflammation results from increased vascular permeability, presumably secondary to release of substance P from unmyelinated sensory neurons (C fibers). The role of corticosteroids is undefined, but animal models suggest an antiinflammatory benefit, and they are recommended as for any other patient with acute bronchospasm. Recovery often takes months, with the delay related to either ongoing low level exposures to endopeptidase inhibitors or persistent irritation of impaired tissue by environmental irritants such as pollution.

SUMMARY

- Although the spectrum of xenobiotics capable of causing pulmonary toxicity is large, the pathologic changes are rather limited.
- Gases that have little or no irritant potential or systemic toxicity cause simple asphyxiation, a situation in which the ambient atmosphere has a diminished oxygen concentration.
- Parenchymal irritation occurs after exposure to acid-forming or free radical–generating gases and severe toxicity manifesting such as ARDS occur.
- Reactive airways dysfunction syndrome and occupational asthma are clinically similar diseases that are described in patients after inhalational exposure. Whereas asthma is typically immunologic in origin, RADS is irritant in origin.
- Treatment of all such exposures centers on symptomatic and supportive care, which includes both interventional and pharmacologic interventions. There is little support for corticosteroids, but if used for a short course of therapy, there is limited risk of harm.

REFERENCES

1. Agabiti N, et al. Short term respiratory effects of acute exposure to chlorine due to a swimming pool accident. *Occup Environ Med.* 2001;58:399-404.
2. Anderson AR. Characterization of chemical suicides in the United States and its adverse impact on responders and bystanders. *West J Emerg Med.* 2016;17:680-683.
3. Ando Y, et al. Elevated urinary cadmium concentrations in a patient with acute cadmium pneumonitis. *Scand J Work Environ Health.* 1996;22:150-153.
4. ARDS Definition Task Force, et al. Acute respiratory distress syndrome: the Berlin definition. *JAMA.* 2012;307:2526-2533.
5. Aslan S, et al. The effect of nebulized NaHCO₃ treatment on "RADS" due to chlorine gas inhalation. *Inhal Toxicol.* 2006;18:895-900.
6. Babu RV, et al. Acute respiratory distress syndrome from chlorine inhalation during a swimming pool accident: a case report and review of the literature. *J Intensive Care Med.* 2008;23:275-280.
7. Barbera N, et al. Evaluation of the role of toxicological data in discriminating between H₂S femoral blood concentration secondary to lethal poisoning and endogenous H₂S putrefactive production. *J Forensic Sci.* 2017;62:392-394.
8. Baxter PJ, et al. Lake Nyos disaster, Cameroon, 1986: the medical effects of large scale emission of carbon dioxide? *BMJ.* 1989;298:1437-1441.
9. Blain PG. Tear gases and irritant incapacitants. 1-chloroacetophenone, 2-chlorobenzylidene malononitrile and dibenz[b,f]-1,4-oxazepine. *Toxicol Rev.* 2003;22:103-110.
10. Borak J, Diller WF. Phosgene exposure: mechanisms of injury and treatment strategies. *J Occup Environ Med.* 2001;43:110-119.
11. Bowler RP, et al. Pulmonary edema fluid antioxidants are depressed in acute lung injury. *Crit Care Med.* 2003;31:2309-2315.
12. Brautbar N, et al. Chronic ammonia inhalation and interstitial pulmonary fibrosis: a case report and review of the literature. *Arch Environ Health.* 2003;58:592-596.
13. Bromberg PA. Mechanisms of the acute effects of inhaled ozone in humans. *Biochim Biophys Acta.* 2016;1860:2771-2781.
14. Brooks SM. Reactive airways dysfunction syndrome and considerations of irritant-induced Asthma. *J Occup Environ Med.* 2013;55:1118-1120.
15. Brüning T, et al. Sensory irritation as a basis for setting occupational exposure limits. *Arch Toxicol.* 2014;88:1855-1879.
16. Burns TR, et al. Ultrastructure of acute ammonia toxicity in the human lung. *Am J Forensic Med Pathol.* 1985;6:204-210.
17. Cannon JW, et al. Optimal strategies for severe acute respiratory distress syndrome. *Crit Care Clin.* 2017;33:259-275.
18. Capellier G, et al. Oxygen toxicity and tolerance. *Minerva Anestesiol.* 1999;65:388-392.
19. Centers for Disease Control and Prevention (CDC). Acute illness from dry ice exposure during hurricane Ivan—Alabama, 2004. *MMWR Morb Mortal Wkly Rep.* 2004;53:1182-1183.
20. Centers for Disease Control and Prevention (CDC). Ocular and respiratory illness associated with an indoor swimming pool—Nebraska, 2006. *MMWR Morb Mortal Wkly Rep.* 2007;56:929-932.

21. Charan NB, et al. Pulmonary injuries associated with acute sulfur dioxide inhalation. *Am Rev Respir Dis.* 1979;119:555-560.

22. Chester EH, et al. Pulmonary injury following exposure to chlorine gas: possible beneficial effects of steroid treatment. *Chest.* 1977;72:247-250.

23. Clark JM, Lambertsen CJ. Rate of development of pulmonary O_2 toxicity in man during O_2 breathing at 2.0 ATA. *J Appl Physiol.* 1971;30:739-752.

24. Cosgrove MP. Pulmonary fibrosis and exposure to steel welding fume. *Occup Med (Lond).* 2015;65:706-712.

25. Dang B, et al. Ocular and respiratory symptoms among lifeguards at a hotel indoor waterpark resort. *J Occup Environ Med.* 2010;52:207-213.

26. de Lange DW, Meulenbelt J. Do corticosteroids have a role in preventing or reducing acute toxic lung injury caused by inhalation of chemical agents? *Clin Toxicol (Phila).* 2011;49:61-71.

27. Dean JB, et al. Neuronal sensitivity to hyperoxia, hypercapnia, and inert gases at hyperbaric pressures. *J Appl Physiol.* 2003;95:883-909.

28. DeBehnke DJ, et al. The hemodynamic and arterial blood gas response to asphyxiation: a canine model of pulseless electrical activity. *Resuscitation.* 1995;30:169-175.

29. Deneke SM, Fanburg BL. Normobaric oxygen toxicity of the lung. *N Engl J Med.* 1980;303:76-86.

30. Dote T, et al. Lethal inhalation exposure during maintenance operation of a hydrogen fluoride liquefying tank. *Toxicol Ind Health.* 2003;19:51-54.

31. Douglas WW, et al. Silo-filler's disease. *JMCP.* 1989;64:291-304.

32. Dunford JV, et al. Asphyxiation due to dry ice in a walk-in freezer. *J Emerg Med.* 2009;36:353-356.

33. El-Zein M, et al. Prevalence and association of welding related systemic and respiratory symptoms in welders. *Occup Environ Med.* 2003;60:655-661.

34. Fakhrzadeh L, et al. Deficiency in inducible nitric oxide synthase protects mice from ozone-induced lung inflammation and tissue injury. *Am J Respir Cell Mol Biol.* 2002;26:413-419.

35. Fanucchi MV, et al. Post-exposure antioxidant treatment in rats decreases airway hyperplasia and hyperreactivity due to chlorine inhalation. *Am J Respir Cell Mol Biol.* 2012;46:599-606.

36. Fitzgerald GJ. Chemical warfare and medical response during World War I. *Am J Public Health.* 2008;98:611-625.

37. Franzen D, et al. Fire eater's lung: retrospective analysis of 123 cases reported to a National Poison Center. *Respiration.* 2014;87:98-104.

38. Fuller DC, Suruda AJ. Occupationally related hydrogen sulfide deaths in the United States from 1984 to 1994. *J Occup Environ Med.* 2000;42:939-942.

39. Gallagher KE, et al. Suicidal asphyxiation by using pure helium gas: case report, review, and discussion of the influence of the internet. *Am J Forensic Med Pathol.* 2003;24:361-363.

40. Galvin IM, et al. Partial liquid ventilation for preventing death and morbidity in adults with acute lung injury and acute respiratory distress syndrome. *Cochrane Database Syst Rev.* 2013;CD003707.

41. Gamelli RL. Hydrofluoric acid inhalation injury. *J Burn Care Res.* 2008;29:852-855.

42. Gautrin D, et al. Longitudinal assessment of airway caliber and responsiveness in workers exposed to chlorine. *Am J Respir Crit Care Med.* 1999;160:1232-1237.

43. Gebistorf F, et al. Inhaled nitric oxide for acute respiratory distress syndrome (ARDS) in children and adults. *Cochrane Database Syst Rev.* 2016;CD002787.

44. Gill JR, et al. Environmental gas displacement: three accidental deaths in the workplace. *Am J Forensic Med Pathol.* 2002;23:26-30.

45. Gilson T, et al. Suicide with inert gases: addendum to Final Exit. *Am J Forensic Med Pathol.* 2003;24:306-308.

46. Grainge C, Rice P. Management of phosgene-induced acute lung injury. *Clin Toxicol (Phila).* 2010;48:497-508.

47. Greenberg MI, Vearrier D. Metal fume fever and polymer fume fever. *Clin Toxicol (Phila).* 2015;53:195-203.

48. Gregory KL, et al. Cleveland Clinic Fire Survivorship Study, 1929-1965. *Arch Environ Health.* 1969;18:508-515.

49. Groves JA, Ellwood PA. Gases in forage tower silos. *Ann Occup Hyg.* 1989;33:519-535.

50. Gunnarsson M, et al. Effects of inhalation of corticosteroids immediately after experimental chlorine gas lung injury. *J Trauma.* 2000;48:101-107.

51. Guo YL, et al. Mechanism of phosgene-induced lung toxicity: role of arachidonate mediators. *J Appl Physiol.* 1990;69:1615-1622.

52. Hajela R, et al. Fatal pulmonary edema due to nitric acid fume inhalation in three pulp-mill workers. *Chest.* 1990;97:487-489.

53. Halpern P, et al. Exposure to extremely high concentrations of carbon dioxide. *Ann Emerg Med.* 2004;43:196-199.

54. Harris PD, Barnes R. The uses of helium and xenon in current clinical practice. *Anaesthesia.* 2008;63:284-293.

55. Harrison RJ, et al. Sudden deaths among oil and gas extraction workers resulting from oxygen deficiency and inhalation of hydrocarbon gases and vapors—United States, January 2010-March 2015. *MMWR Morb Mortal Wkly Rep.* 2016;65:6-9.

56. Henry C, et al. Public health consequences from hazardous substances acutely released during rail transit—South Carolina, 2005; selected states, 1999-2004. *MMWR Morb Mortal Wkly Rep.* 2005;293:1968.

57. Hesse A-K, et al. Proinflammatory role of inducible nitric oxide synthase in acute hyperoxic lung injury. *Respir Res.* 2004;5:11.

58. Hojer J, Stauffer K. A placebo-controlled experimental study of steroid inhalation therapy in ammonia-induced lung injury. *J Toxicol Clin Toxicol.* 1999;37:59-67.

59. Hsu H-H, et al. Zinc chloride (smoke bomb) inhalation lung injury: clinical presentations, high-resolution CT findings, and pulmonary function test results. *Chest.* 2005;127:2064-2071.

60. Huang K-L. Systemic Inflammation caused by white smoke inhalation in a combat exercise. *Chest.* 2008;133:722.

61. Ikeda N, et al. The course of respiration and circulation in death by carbon dioxide poisoning. *Forensic Sci Int.* 1989;41:93-99.

62. Jarvis D, et al. Association of respiratory symptoms and lung function in young adults with use of domestic gas appliances. *Lancet.* 1996;347:426-431.

63. Jawan B, Lee JH. Cardiac arrest caused by an incorrectly filled oxygen cylinder: a case report. *Br J Anaesth.* 1990;64:749-751.

64. Kacmarek RM, et al. Partial liquid ventilation in adult patients with acute respiratory distress syndrome. *Am J Respir Crit Care Med.* 2006;173:882-889.

65. Kawasaki H. A mechanistic review of silica-induced inhalation toxicity. *Inhal Toxicol.* 2015;27:363-377.

66. Kernbach-Wighton G, et al. Clinical and morphological aspects of death due to liquid nitrogen. *Int J Legal Med.* 1998;111:191-195.

67. Kim DH, Lee HJ. Evaporated liquid nitrogen-induced asphyxia: a case report. *J Korean Med Sci.* 2008;23:163-165.

68. Kinnula VL, Crapo JD. Superoxide dismutases in the lung and human lung diseases. *Am J Respir Crit Care Med.* 2003;167:1600-1619.

69. Kovacic P, Somanathan R. Pulmonary toxicity and environmental contamination: radicals, electron transfer, and protection by antioxidants. *Rev Environ Contam Toxicol.* 2009;201:41-69.

70. Kuschner WG, et al. Early pulmonary cytokine responses to zinc oxide fume inhalation. *Environ Res.* 1997;75:7-11.

71. Leung CC, et al. Silicosis. *Lancet.* 2012;379:2008-2018.

72. Levy JI, et al. Determinants of nitrogen dioxide concentrations in indoor ice skating rinks. *Am J Public Health.* 1998;88:1781-1786.

73. Lippmann M, et al. Health effects of World Trade Center (WTC) dust: an unprecedented disaster's inadequate risk management. *Crit Rev Toxicol.* 2015;45:492-530.

74. Mackie E, et al. Management of chlorine gas-related injuries from the Graniteville, South Carolina, train derailment. *Disaster Med Public Health Prep.* 2014;8:411-416.

75. Manning HL, Schwartzstein RM. Pathophysiology of dyspnea. *N Engl J Med.* 1995.

76. Mapp CE, et al. Occupational asthma. *Am J Respir Crit Care Med.* 2012;172:280-305.

77. Maybauer MO, et al. Effects of manganese superoxide dismutase nebulization on pulmonary function in an ovine model of acute lung injury. *Shock.* 2005;23:138-143.

78. Mayorga MA. Overview of nitrogen dioxide effects on the lung with emphasis on military relevance. *Toxicology.* 1994;89:175-192.

79. McDonald DM, et al. Endothelial gaps as sites for plasma leakage in inflammation. *Microcirculation.* 1999;6:7-22.

80. Miller TM, Mazur PO. Oxygen deficiency hazards associated with liquefied gas systems: derivation of a program of controls. *Am Ind Hyg Assoc J.* 1984;45:293-298.

81. Minami M, et al. Dangerous mixture of household detergents in an old-style toilet: a case report with simulation experiments of the working environment and warning of potential hazard relevant to the general environment. *Hum Exp Toxicol.* 1992;11:27-34.

82. Mishra PK, et al. Bhopal gas tragedy: review of clinical and experimental findings after 25 years. *Int J Occup Med Environ Health.* 2009;22:193-202.

83. Monteiro MG, et al. Comparison between subjective feelings to alcohol and nitrogen narcosis: a pilot study. *Alcohol.* 1996;13:75-78.

84. Moran JL, et al. Meta-analysis of controlled trials of ventilator therapy in acute lung injury and acute respiratory distress syndrome: an alternative perspective. *Intensive Care Med.* 2005;31:227-235.

85. Mrvos R, et al. Home exposures to chlorine/chloramine gas: review of 216 cases. *South Med J.* 1993;86:654-657.

86. Nightingale JA, et al. No effect of inhaled budesonide on the response to inhaled ozone in normal subjects. *Am J Respir Crit Care Med.* 2000;161(2 Pt 1):479-486.

87. Noble MJ, et al. Inhalational mercury toxicity from artisanal gold extraction reported to the Oregon poison center, 2002-2015. *Clin Toxicol (Phila).* 2016;54:847-851.

88. Pauluhn J, et al. Workshop summary: phosgene-induced pulmonary toxicity revisited: appraisal of early and late markers of pulmonary injury from animal models with emphasis on human significance. *Inhal Toxicol.* 2007;19:789-810.

89. Pavilonis BT, Mirer FE. Respirable dust and silica exposure among World Trade Center cleanup workers. *J Occup Environ Health.* 2017;14:187-194.

90. Persinger RL, et al. Molecular mechanisms of nitrogen dioxide induced epithelial injury in the lung. *Mol Cell Biochem.* 2002;234-235:71-80.

91. Peter JV, et al. Corticosteroids in the prevention and treatment of acute respiratory distress syndrome (ARDS) in adults: meta-analysis. *BMJ.* 2008;336:1006-1009.

92. Promisloff RA, et al. Reactive airway dysfunction syndrome in three police officers following a roadside chemical spill. *Chest.* 1990;98:928-929.

93. Rafferty P. Voluntary chlorine inhalation: a new form of self-abuse? *Br Med J.* 1980;281:1178-1179.

94. Raj M. Humane killing of nonhuman animals for disease control purposes. *J Appl Anim Welf Sci.* 2008;11:112-124.

95. Riechelmann H, et al. Respiratory epithelium exposed to sulfur dioxide—functional and ultrastructural alterations. *Laryngoscope.* 1995;105(3 Pt 1):295-299.

96. Rubenfeld GD, et al. Incidence and outcomes of acute lung injury. *N Engl J Med.* 2005;353:1685-1693.

97. Sanders KA, Sturrock AB. Regulation of oxidant production in acute lung injury. *Chest.* 1999;116(1 suppl):56S-61S.

98. Schmidt R, et al. Alveolar antioxidant status in patients with acute respiratory distress syndrome. *Eur Respir J.* 2004;24:994-999.

99. Sciuto AM, et al. The temporal profile of cytokines in the bronchoalveolar lavage fluid in mice exposed to the industrial gas phosgene. *Inhal Toxicol.* 2003;15:687-700.

100. Sciuto AM, Hurt HH. Therapeutic treatments of phosgene-induced lung injury. *Inhal Toxicol.* 2004;16:565-580.

101. Sciuto AM, et al. Protective effects of *N*-acetylcysteine treatment after phosgene exposure in rabbits. *Am J Respir Crit Care Med.* 1995;151(3 Pt 1):768-772.

102. Scott JA. Fog and deaths in London, December 1952. *Public Health Rep.* 1953;68:474-479.

103. Seet RCS, et al. Inhalational nickel carbonyl poisoning in waste processing workers. *Chest.* 2005;128:424-429.

104. Shadab M, et al. Occupational health hazards among sewage workers: oxidative stress and deranged lung functions. *J Clin Diagn Res.* 2014;8:BC11-BC12.

105. Shah FA, et al. Limiting sedation for patients with acute respiratory distress syndrome—time to wake up. *Curr Opin Crit Care.* 2017;23:45-51.

106. Shakeri MS, et al. Which agents cause reactive airways dysfunction syndrome (RADS)? A systematic review. *Occup Med (Lond).* 2008;58:205-211.

107. Shaver CM, Bastarache JA. Clinical and biological heterogeneity in acute respiratory distress syndrome: direct versus indirect lung injury. *Clin Chest Med.* 2014;35:639-653.

108. Shields LBE, et al. Atypical autoerotic death: part II. *Am J Forensic Med Pathol.* 2005;26:53-62.

109. Sinclair SE, et al. Augmented lung injury due to interaction between hyperoxia and mechanical ventilation. *Crit Care Med.* 2004;32:2496-2501.

110. Sironi L, et al. Recreational inhalation of butane and propane in adolescents: two forensic cases of accidental death. *Forensic Sci Int.* 2016;266:e52-e58.

111. Smerz RW. Incidence of oxygen toxicity during the treatment of dysbarism. *Undersea Hyperb Med.* 2004;31:199-202.

112. Smith CR, Spiess BD. The two faces of Eve: gaseous anaesthesia and inert gas narcosis. *Diving Hyperb Med.* 2010;40:68-77.

113. Stefanidou M, et al. Health impacts of fire smoke inhalation. *Inhal Toxicol.* 2008;20:761-766.

114. Suruda A, Agnew J. Deaths from asphyxiation and poisoning at work in the United States 1984-6. *Br J Industr Med.* 1989;46:541-546.

115. Suruda A, et al. Fatal injuries in the United States involving respirators, 1984-1995. *Appl Occup Environ Hyg.* 2003;18:289-292.

116. Suter PM, et al. *N*-acetylcysteine enhances recovery from acute lung injury in man. A randomized, double-blind, placebo-controlled clinical study. *Chest.* 1994;105:190-194.

117. Szolcsányi J. Forty years in capsaicin research for sensory pharmacology and physiology. *Neuropeptides.* 2004;38:377-384.

118. Tanaka S, et al. Bronchial injury and pulmonary edema caused by hydrogen sulfide poisoning. *Am J Emerg Med.* 1999;17:427-429.

119. Tatsumi T, Fliss H. Hypochlorous acid and chloramines increase endothelial permeability: possible involvement of cellular zinc. *Am J Physiol.* 1994;267(4 Pt 2):H1597-H1607.

120. Thomas RJ, et al. Acute pulmonary effects from o-chlorobenzylidenemalonitrile "tear gas": a unique exposure outcome unmasked by strenuous exercise after a military training event. *Mil Med.* 2002;167:136-139.

121. Trivedi V, et al. Occupational asthma: diagnostic challenges and management dilemmas. *Curr Opin Pulm Med.* 2017;23:177-183.

122. Umbrello M, et al. Current concepts of ARDS: a narrative review. *Int J Mol Sci.* 2017;18:64-20.

123. Vajner JE, Lung D. Acute chlorine gas inhalation and the utility of nebulized sodium bicarbonate. *J Med Toxicol.* 2013;9:259-265.

124. Van Meurs KP, et al. Inhaled NO and markers of oxidant injury in infants with respiratory failure. *J Perinatol.* 2005;25:463-469.

125. Vasakova M, et al. Hypersensitivity pneumonitis: perspectives in diagnosis and management. *Am J Respir Crit Care Med.* 2017;196:680-689.

126. Vohra R, et al. Chlorine-related inhalation injury from a swimming pool disinfectant in a 9-year-old girl. *Pediatr Emerg Care.* 2006;2009:579-580.

127. Volpato GP, et al. Inhaled hydrogen sulfide: a rapidly reversible inhibitor of cardiac and metabolic function in the mouse. *Anesthesiology.* 2008;108:659-668.

128. Wagner GN, et al. Medical evaluation of the victims of the 1986 Lake Nyos disaster. *J Forensic Sci.* 1988;33:12512J.

129. Wagner PD, et al. Protection against pulmonary O_2 toxicity by *N*-acetylcysteine. *Eur Respir J.* 1989;2:116-126.

130. Walsh MJ, et al. Liquid nitrogen ingestion leading to massive pneumoperitoneum without identifiable gastrointestinal perforation. *J Emerg Med.* 2010;38:607-609.

131. Wang J, et al. Inhaled budesonide in experimental chlorine gas lung injury: influence of time interval between injury and treatment. *Intensive Care Med.* 2002;28:352-357.

132. Wing JS, et al. Acute health effects in a community after a release of hydrofluoric acid. *Arch Environ Health.* 1991;46:155-160.

133. Wolkoff P, et al. Pollutant exposures and health symptoms in aircrew and office workers: is there a link? *Environ Int.* 2016;87:74-84.

134. Wood BR. Chlorine inhalation toxicity from vapors generated by swimming pool chlorinator tablets. *Pediatrics.* 1987;79:427-430.

135. Zierold D, Chauviere M. Hydrogen fluoride inhalation injury because of a fire suppression system. *Mil Med.* 2012;177:108-112.

136. Zuo L, et al. Biological and physiological role of reactive oxygen species—the good, the bad and the ugly. *Acta Physiol (Oxf).* 2015;214:329-348.

122 CARBON MONOXIDE

Christian Tomaszewski

Carbon Monoxide (CO)

MW	=	28.01 Da
Gas density	=	0.968 (air = 1.0)
Blood carboxyhemoglobin level		
Nonsmokers	=	1%–2%
Smokers	=	5%–10%
Action level	>	10%
TLV–TWA	=	50 ppm

HISTORY AND EPIDEMIOLOGY

Carbon monoxide (CO) is formed during the incomplete combustion of virtually any carbon-containing compound. Because it is an odorless, colorless, and tasteless gas, it is remarkably difficult to detect in the environment even when present at high ambient concentrations and is a leading cause of poisoning morbidity and mortality in the United States. Based on US national death certificate data, there were 439 annual deaths from unintentional non-fire exposure to CO from 1999 to 2004.[27] The groups with the highest risk were male gender and elderly age, possibly because of occupational exposure and inability to discern CO symptoms, respectively. The CO-related mortality rate has remained essentially unchanged over the years despite increased CO detector use.[22,26,28] More than half of these cases (64%) occurred in homes with faulty furnaces, usually in the fall or winter months. Many clusters were associated with power failures during catastrophic weather, such as ice storms, blizzards, and hurricanes.[24,25] Analysis of the Centers for Disease Control and Prevention wide-ranging online data for epidemiologic research (WONDER) database showed total non–fire-related CO poisoning deaths decreased from 1,967 in 1999 to 1,319 in 2014.[88] Of these non–fire-related deaths, unintentional cases continue at a rate of approximately 450 annually from 1999 to 2015.[29,187]

Just as important as mortality rates are the greater number of survivors from CO poisoning. Despite increased awareness for CO poisoning, there were still an average of 20,636 nonfatal, unintentional, non–fire-related CO exposures treated annually in the United States.[28] More than 40% of cases occurred in the winter, with almost 75% occurring in residences. However, exclusion of intentional and fire-related cases severely underestimates the extent of the problem. Based on firsthand hospital data, a minimum of 50,000 patients with CO poisoning present to US emergency departments (EDs) each year, up to half resulting in hospitalization.[96,111] More recent data using probable and suspected cases suggest that there were more than 230,000 ED visits in 2007 alone that were unintentional and related to non-fire CO poisoning.[112]

The bigger problem with CO poisoning is the associated morbidity that survivors risk even after acute treatment. The most serious complication is persistent or delayed neurologic sequelae (DNS) or delayed neurocognitive sequelae, which occurs in up to 50% of patients with symptomatic acute poisonings.[81,174,226] At 1 year after exposure, of the 1,643 patients not treated with HBO 42% had cognitive sequellae at 6 weeks, 30% at 6 months and 18% at 12 months. Of the 75 treated with HBO 24% had cognitive sequellae at 6 weeks, 17% at 6 months and 14% at 12 months.[228] There is still no highly reliable method of predicting who will have a poor outcome, requiring the threshold for HBO therapy for CO poisoning and follow-up be particularly low.

Potential sources of CO abound in our society, often resulting in unintentional poisoning[28] (Table 122–1). Although CO is found naturally in the body as a byproduct of hemoglobin degradation by heme oxygenase found in the liver and spleen,[47] it is readily available for inhalation from the incomplete combustion of virtually any carbonaceous fuel. Alternatively, absorption (dermal, ingestion, or inhalation) of methylene chloride results in CO toxicity after hepatic metabolism (Chap. 105).[156] Despite catalytic converters and other emission controls, more than 50% of unintentional CO deaths are still caused by motor vehicle exhaust.[45,151] The introduction of catalytic converters with emissions controls is associated with a decrease in suicide attempts and deaths using automobile exhaust.[91] Occupants of motor vehicles are not the only victims of exhaust gases; CO poisoning is also reported in occupants of the beds of pickup trucks and on boats.[22,95,130] Workers are at risk from use of propane-powered equipment indoors such as ice skating rink resurfacers[21,52] and forklifts.[66,104] For optimal performance, propane-powered forklifts are typically adjusted to produce less than 10,000 ppm of CO in exhaust but in fact average more than 30,000 ppm, which could lead to unsafe concentrations in an enclosed warehouse within 1 hour.[67]

In the past 10 years, nonvehicular sources of CO have increasingly accounted for the majority of unintentional poisonings.[151] More than one-third of the deaths from unintentional CO poisoning occur in winter months (December, January, and February) in the US.[29] Predominantly, these involve the burning of charcoal, wood, or natural gas for heating and cooking.[92] Furnaces that burn natural gas (methane or propane) for heating are often implicated, especially when the flue is blocked.[100,101] Gas kitchen stoves are also an important source of CO in indigent populations with marginal heating systems.[101] In fact, the use of gas stoves for supplemental heat is predictive of CO poisoning in patients who present to the ED with headache and dizziness.[100]

Absence of fuel-burning devices is not necessarily protective for CO poisoning. In multifamily homes, CO can diffuse through drywall, which is actually quite porous.[89] During ice storms, blizzards, hurricanes, and other natural disasters with power loss, the indoor use of gasoline-powered generators[115,218] and charcoal-burning grills, the latter particularly in immigrant populations, leads to epidemic CO poisoning outbreaks.[23,25,234]

Fires are another important source of CO exposure, contributing substantially to the approximate 5,613 smoke inhalation deaths each year.[45] Carbon monoxide is considered to be the most common hazard to smoke inhalation victims.[72,186] These cases are further compounded by the high incidence of hydrogen cyanide poisoning (Chap. 123).[84]

TABLE 122–1	Sources of Carbon Monoxide Implicated in Poisonings
Anesthetic absorbents	
Banked blood	
Camp stoves and lanterns	
Charcoal grills	
Coffee roasting	
Fires	
Formic acid decomposition mixed in sulfuric acid	
Gasoline-powered equipment (eg, generators, power washers)	
Ice-resurfacing machines (propane powered)	
Internal combustion engine (boat, car, truck)	
Methylene bromide	
Methylene chloride	
Natural gas combustion furnaces (water heaters, ranges, and ovens)	
Propane powered forklifts	
Underground mine explosions	
Wood pellet storage	

TOXICOKINETICS

Carbon monoxide is readily absorbed after inhalation. The Coburn-Forster-Kane (CFK) model allows approximate prediction of carboxyhemoglobin (COHb) levels based on exposure history.[46,48] A simplification of the model allows for estimation of the equilibrium based on the ambient concentration of CO in ppm: COHb (%) = 100/{1 + (643/ppm CO)}.[214] This assumes that the individual weighs 70 kg and is not anemic. With exponential uptake, it takes more than 4 hours for equilibrium to be attained. Therefore, within minutes of high CO exposures, the arterial COHb level actually overshoots predicted estimates before equilibrium.[9,15] Endogenous production of CO is not factored in because its contribution to COHb is only 2%.

After its absorption, CO is carried in the blood, primarily bound to hemoglobin. The Haldane ratio states that hemoglobin has approximately a 200 to 250 times greater affinity for CO than for oxygen. Therefore, CO is primarily confined to the blood compartment, but eventually up to 15% of total CO body content is taken up by tissue, primarily bound to myoglobin.[46] Therefore, the dissolved CO concentration in the plasma better reflects the ultimate potential for poisoning because it is available for diffusion into all tissue compartments, including the muscle and brain.[135]

Elimination of CO, like absorption, from the blood is modeled mathematically using the CFK model. The equation predicts a half-life of 252 minutes. In actual volunteer studies, means of 249 and 320 minutes breathing room air are reported.[171] With 100% oxygen, these half-lives can be reduced significantly to means ranging 47 to 80 minutes in studies of volunteers who attain COHb levels of 10% to 12%.[171,195] Patients poisoned with CO showed actual mean half-lives ranging from 74 to 131 minutes when treated with 100% oxygen.[226,227]

Methylene chloride, a paint stripper, is another source of CO. It is readily absorbed through the skin or by ingestion or inhalation and is metabolized in the liver to CO.[191] Carboxyhemoglobin levels peak 8 hours or later and range from 10% to 50%.[134,177] Because of ongoing production of CO, the apparent COHb half-life is prolonged to 13 hours in these patients.[176] Carboxyhemoglobin levels after methylene chloride exposure are proportional to the concentration and duration of exposure.[176]

PATHOPHYSIOLOGY

The most obvious deleterious effect of CO is binding to hemoglobin, rendering it incapable of delivering oxygen to the cells. Therefore, despite adequate partial pressures of oxygen in blood (PO_2), there is decreased arterial oxygen content. Further insult occurs because CO causes a leftward shift of the oxyhemoglobin dissociation curve, thus decreasing the offloading of oxygen from hemoglobin to tissue (Fig. 28–2).[180] This results in part from a decrease in erythrocyte 2,3-bisphosphoglycerate (2,3-BPG) concentration. The net effect of all these processes is the decreased ability of oxygen to be delivered to tissue.

Carbon monoxide toxicity cannot be attributed solely to COHb-mediated hypoxia. Neither clinical effects nor the phenomena of delayed neurologic deficits is completely predicted by the extent of binding between hemoglobin and CO.[90,209] Furthermore, such a model fails to explain why even minimal levels of COHb (4%–5%) occasionally result in cognitive impairment. An early study showed that dogs breathing 13% CO died within 1 hour and had COHb levels of 54% to 90%. However, exchange transfusion of this same blood into healthy dogs to reach similar COHb levels caused no untoward effects.[73] Hemorrhaging the dogs to comparable degrees of anemia also produced no adverse effects. The appropriate conclusion was that inherent to CO toxicity is its delivery to target organs such as the brain and heart and that although COHb is easily measured, it rarely has a significant contribution to clinical toxicity. For CO to reach tissue, it has to be dissolved in the plasma rather than bound to hemoglobin.[79,80]

Carbon monoxide interferes with cellular respiration by binding to mitochondrial cytochrome oxidase. Initial studies show that this binding is especially exaggerated under conditions of hypoxia and hypotension. In vitro rat models demonstrate that this oxidative stress causes mitochondrial damage with protein oxidation and lipid peroxidation, particularly in the hippocampus and corpus striatum.[196] In vivo models reveal that CO poisoning causes cell loss in the frontal cortex, which is associated with decrements in learning

and memory.[172] Although no comparable brain studies exist in humans, the peripheral lymphocytes and monocytes of CO-poisoned patients show cytochrome oxidase inhibition accompanied by increased lipid peroxidation.[71,146] In a small clinical series of CO-poisoned patients, normalization of this cytochrome activity lagged behind and seemed to agree better with symptom severity than COHb levels.[147]

Inactivation of cytochrome oxidase is only an initial part of the cascade of inflammatory events that results in ischemic reperfusion injury to the brain after CO poisoning (Fig. A40–1). During recovery from the initial poisoning, white blood cells are attracted to and adhere to the damaged brain microvasculature.[201-203] This attraction is partly attributable to endothelial changes from initial cytochrome oxidase dysfunction, mediated primarily through the free radical nitric oxide (NO).[201,207] Carbon monoxide displaces NO from platelets that in turn form peroxynitrites, which are even stronger inactivators of cytochrome oxidase.[207] Multiple animal studies demonstrate that NO is ultimately responsible for much of the endothelial damage from CO and that NO synthase inhibitors can prevent toxicity.[205,207] The NO formation promotes platelet–neutrophil aggregates that in turn lead to neutrophil adhesion to the brain microvasculature.[202] Myelin peroxidase activation in the area further promotes neutrophil adhesion with degranulation and release of proteases that convert xanthine dehydrogenase to xanthine oxidase, an enzyme that promotes formation of oxygen free radicals.[200] Also, mouse studies suggest that circulating microparticles play a proinflammatory role in activation of neutrophils.[237] The end result of this process is delayed lipid peroxidation of the neurons, and the extent of destruction correlates with decrements in learning in rodents.[200] Rats depleted of xanthine oxidase through a tungsten modified diet show no changes in myelin basic protein and cognitive function after CO poisoning.[98]

Simultaneously, with all this perivascular oxidative stress in the brain, there is activation of excitatory amino acids, which ultimately is responsible for the subsequent neuronal cell loss.[207] In fact, in rat brains, glutamate concentrations increase after CO poisoning. Glutamate is an excitatory amino acid that binds at N-methyl-D-aspartate (NMDA) receptors and causes intracellular calcium release, resulting in delayed neuronal cell death (Chap. 13). Blockade of NMDA receptors prevents the neuronal death and learning deficits that accompany serious CO poisoning in mice.[113] Increases in the glutamate concentrations in rat brain in the first hour after severe CO poisoning are followed by a later increase in hydroxyl radicals.[172] Ultimately, at 1 to 3 weeks, the animals show histologic evidence of both neuronal necrosis and apoptosis in the frontal cortex, globus pallidus, and cerebellum that are accompanied by deficits in learning and memory.

Carbon monoxide neuronal cell death is partly attributable to apoptosis. In bovine pulmonary artery cells, CO exposure is accompanied by activation of caspase-1, a protease implicated in delayed cell death.[206] Confirmatory evidence was provided in the same study because both caspase-1 and NO synthase inhibitors blocked apoptosis. The end result of all these cellular processes is brain injury, particularly in the basal ganglia and hippocampus.[221] In some studies, this is accompanied by learning impairment.[202] Thus, animal models correlate well with what ultimately occurs in victims of serious CO poisoning, namely, persistent or delayed deficits in learning and memory associated with structural changes in the brain.

Myoglobin, another heme protein, binds CO with an affinity about 60 times greater than it binds oxygen.[49] About 10% to 15% of the total body store of CO is extravascular, primarily binding to myoglobin.[15,46] A dog model demonstrates that this binding is enhanced under hypoxic conditions.[49] This binding partially explains the myocardial impairment that occurs in both animal studies and low concentration exposures in patients with ischemic heart disease. The combination of COHb formation, which decreases oxygen-carrying capacity, and reduced myoglobin in the heart, which decreases oxygen extraction, contributes to the preterminal dysrhythmias that occurs in poisoned animals.

Several studies suggest that CO effects on the cardiovascular system are necessary for ischemic reperfusion injury of the brain. Hypotension is an essential component and results from a combination of myocardial depression and vasodilation. Carbon monoxide, perhaps because of its similarity to NO, activates guanylate cyclase, which in turn relaxes vascular smooth muscle. Also, CO further displaces NO from platelets, resulting in additional vasodilation.[205] These factors contribute to the hypotension that occurs in animal experiments with exposure to high concentrations of CO.[73] Such an episode of hypotension leads to syncope, portending a worse clinical outcome.[40] In rhesus monkeys, cerebral white matter lesions correlate better with decreases in blood pressure than with COHb level.[78] Lipid peroxidation of the brain in rats develops 1 hour after a CO exposure that has produced syncope and hypotension.[199] This delay is comparable to the time that is necessary to produce mitochondrial destruction from oxidative stress in rats exposed to CO. In a feline model, central nervous system (CNS) damage from CO is reproduced only when hypoxia is accompanied by an interval of ischemia, confirming the ischemia reperfusion model.[159]

Endogenous CO behaves like NO, binding to guanylate cyclase and thereby increasing cyclic guanosine monophosphate (cGMP) concentrations.[114] Although low endogenous concentrations are physiologic, excessive concentrations of CO from exogenous sources are problematic because CO persists much longer than NO. Carbon monoxide appears to be a neuronal messenger by virtue of the fact that as a gas, it can diffuse and signal adjacent cells.[141]

CLINICAL MANIFESTATIONS

Acute Exposure

The earliest symptoms associated with CO poisoning are often nonspecific and readily confused with other illnesses, typically a viral syndrome[223] (Table 122–2). The initial symptom reported by volunteers within 4 hours of exposure to 200 ppm CO (producing COHb levels of 15%–20%) is headache; shorter exposures at 500 ppm also produce nausea.[192] The incidence of CO poisoning in symptomatic patients presenting to EDs in the winter with an influenzalike illness ranges from 3% to 24% in some series.[61,101] The typical presenting complaints include headache, dizziness, and nausea, and the most frequent exposures occur during the winter, explaining why influenza is the most common misdiagnosis.[61] The most common symptom, headache, is usually described as dull, frontal, and continuous. Carbon monoxide poisoning is also frequently misdiagnosed as food poisoning, gastroenteritis, and even colic in infants. Similar to adults, children tend to develop nonspecific symptoms, complicating diagnosis.

Continued exposure to CO leads to symptoms attributable to oxygen deficiency in the heart. Low-concentration exposures, leading to COHb levels of 2% to 4%, in volunteers with stable angina result in decreased exercise tolerance as well as signs and symptoms of myocardial ischemia.[2] At higher levels (COHb of 6%), there is a greater frequency of premature ventricular contractions during exercise. Myocardial infarction and dysrhythmias are described in victims of CO poisoning, and acute mortality from CO is usually a result of ventricular dysrhythmias.[2,3] Prolonged exposure to CO or high COHb levels are associated with temporary myocardial stunning, manifested as global hypokinesia or Takotsubo cardiomyopathy lasting usually less than 24.[116,118] In some cases stunning, with decreased left ventricular ejection fraction, can last several days and is associated with increased concentrations of β-type natriuretic peptide, lactate, and troponin.[132] Troponin elevations often occur even in the absence of any coronary artery disease or even electrocardiographic (ECG) or echocardiographic changes.[31,55]

These patients have an increased propensity for cardiac mortality, with almost one-third dying within 8 years after serious CO poisoning.[102] A nationwide population based cohort study in Taiwan found an increased incidence of dysrhythmias, mostly paroxysmal tachycardia and ventricular fibrillation, in decade after CO poisoning of 8,381 subjects.[131] Although serious CO exposures are associated with increased long-term mortality beyond 90 days, there was no association with increased cardiac death.[87]

The CNS is the organ system that is most sensitive to CO poisoning. Acutely, otherwise healthy patients may manifest headache, dizziness, and ataxia at COHb levels as low as 15% to 20%, with higher levels or longer exposures causing syncope, seizures, or coma.[223] Focal neurologic findings suggest a cerebrovascular accident. Some cases have diffuse frontal slow-wave activity on electroencephalogram. Within 1 day of exposures that result in coma, many patients show decreased density in the central white matter and globus pallidus on computed tomography (CT) (Fig. 122–1) or magnetic resonance imaging (MRI).[137] Autopsies show involvement of other areas, including the cerebral cortex, hippocampus, cerebellum, and substantia nigra.[129]

Metabolic changes reflect the toxic effects of CO better than any particular COHb level. Patients with mild CO poisoning develop respiratory alkalosis in an attempt to compensate for the reduction in oxygen-carrying capacity and delivery. More substantial exposures result in metabolic acidosis with lactate production that accompanies tissue hypoxia.[189] Even in the absence of hypotension, lactate was an independent predictor of worse mental status and inpatient complications.[30,60,150] The importance of metabolic acidosis was highlighted in a retrospective series of 48 CO-poisoned patients, in whom hydrogen ion concentration was a better predictor of poor recovery during initial hospitalization than was COHb level.[216]

Although the brain and heart are the most sensitive, other organs also manifest the effects of CO poisoning. One-fifth to one-third of patients with severe CO poisoning, particularly those requiring endotracheal intubation, develop pulmonary edema.[82] This is caused by cardiac depression directly from CO or ARDS from associated smoke inhalation.[118,186] This does not appear to be a direct effect of CO on lung tissue because sheep with prolonged exposure to CO, resulting in COHb levels greater than 50%, showed no anatomic or physiologic changes in lung function.[185] Although myonecrosis and even compartment syndromes occur, patients rarely develop acute kidney injury (AKI). Retinal hemorrhages occur with exposures longer than 12 hours.[120] Cherry-red skin coloration occurs only after excessive exposure (2%–3% of cases referred to one hyperbaric center) and represents a combination of CO-induced vasodilation, concomitant tissue ischemia, and failure

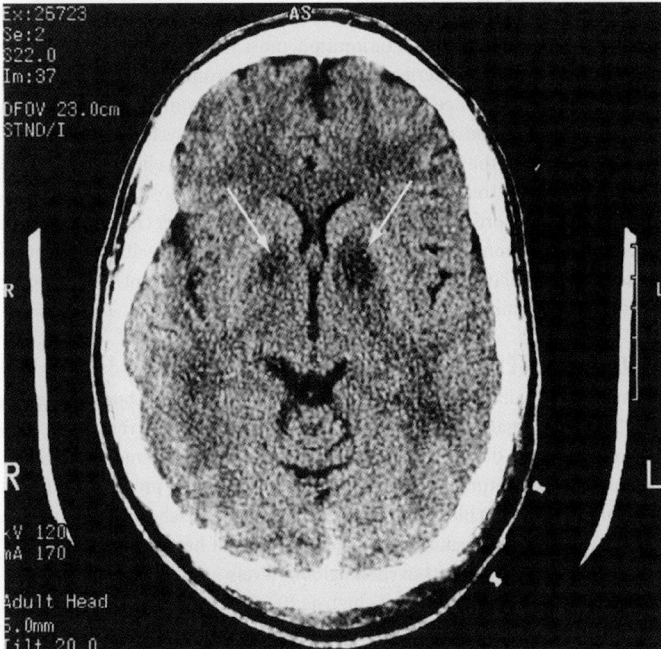

FIGURE 122–1. Computed tomography scan of the brain showing bilateral lesions of the globus pallidus (arrows) in a patient with poor recovery from severe carbon monoxide poisoning. *(Used with permission from the Fellowship in Medical Toxicology, New York University School of Medicine, New York City Poison Center.)*

TABLE 122–2	Clinical Manifestations of Carbon Monoxide Poisoning
Ataxia	Myocardial ischemia
Cardiac dysrhythmias	Nausea
Chest pain	Syncope
Confusion	Tachypnea
Dizziness	Visual blurring
Dyspnea	Vomiting
Headache	Weakness

to extract oxygen from arterial blood.[178] Another classic but uncommon phenomenon is the development of cutaneous bullae after severe exposures. These bullae are thought to be caused by a combination of pressure necrosis and possibly direct CO effects in the epidermis.

NEUROCOGNITIVE SEQUELAE

The persistent or delayed effects of CO poisoning are varied and include dementia, amnestic syndromes, psychosis, parkinsonism, paralysis, chorea, cortical blindness, apraxia and agnosia, peripheral neuropathy, and incontinence.[133,233] If not diagnosed at initial poisoning, neurologic deterioration is delayed and preceded by a lucid period of 2 to 40 days after the initial poisoning.[40] In patients admitted to an intensive care unit (ICU) for severe CO poisoning and treated with 100% oxygen, 14% of survivors had permanent neurologic impairment.[123] In a Korean series of 2,360 CO-poisoned patients, 3% continued to show memory failure or parkinsonian features 1 year after exposure.[40] Another series of 63 seriously poisoned patients showed memory impairment in 43% and deterioration of personality in 33% at 3-year follow-up.[189] Children also develop behavioral and educational difficulties after severe poisoning.[128] However, patients older than 30 years of age are more susceptible to the development of delayed sequelae.[41,228] Most cases of delayed neurocognitive sequelae are associated with loss of consciousness (LOC) in the acute phase of toxicity.[51]

Neurocognitive sequelae probably involve lesions of the cerebral white matter.[75] Weeks after exposure, autopsies show necrosis of the white matter, globus pallidus, cerebellum, and hippocampus. Magnetic resonance imaging studies confirm the damage to the white matter and hippocampus.[70,137,223] Animal studies show that having a markedly elevated COHb level alone cannot cause similar white matter lesions but that there must also be an episode of hypotension.[78,159] The fact that the areas permanently damaged in serious CO poisoning cases are the areas with the poorest vascular supply in the brain is consistent with these findings.

CHRONIC EXPOSURE

Often, patients complain of persistent headaches and cognitive problems after long-term exposure to low concentrations of CO. Unfortunately, to date, there have been no controlled studies demonstrating that in the absence of a severe acute poisoning episode, this type of exposure results in any long-term sequelae. Warehouse workers who are chronically exposed to CO from propane combustion have intermittent problems with headache, nausea, and lightheadedness.[66] Fortunately, unless the individual had an episode of severe poisoning with acute deterioration, most workers achieve resolution of their symptoms.[67] One series of patients with chronic CO poisoning demonstrates a high incidence of headache and memory complaints in addition to motor slowing and memory problems on neuropsychologic testing.[153] Although many of the objective deficits improved with elimination of the exposure and HBO treatment, many continued to have posttraumatic stress and conversion disorders. Although it is uncertain whether chronic exposure to low concentrations of CO causes permanent damage, health care providers should be vigilant for symptomatic individuals to prevent continued or catastrophic outcomes.

DIAGNOSTIC TESTING

The most useful diagnostic test obtainable in a suspected CO poisoning is a COHb level. Normal levels of COHb range from 0% to 5%. Levels at the high end of this range occur in neonates and patients with hemolytic anemia because CO is a natural byproduct of the breakdown of protoporphyrin to bilirubin.[33] Of note, in blood samples from neonates, falsely high COHb levels up to 8% can occur because of interference of fetal hemoglobin with spectroscopy (Chap. 28).[220] Carboxyhemoglobin levels average 6% in one-pack-per-day smokers but may range as high as 10%.[190] Although high COHb levels confirm exposure to CO, particular levels are not necessarily predictive of symptoms or outcome.[90,170]

The usual method for measuring COHb is with a cooximeter, a device that spectrophotometrically reads the percentage of total hemoglobin saturated

with CO. Traditionally, arterial blood was used for this determination; however, venous blood levels are accurate because there is little CO extraction from hemoglobin across the capillary bed.[214] Refrigerated heparinized samples yield accurate COHb levels for months and at room temperature for 28 days, making retrospective clinical and postmortem evaluations reliable.[86,125] The prior administration of hydroxocobalamin, commonly given for cyanide poisoning after smoke inhalation, negatively interferes with COHb levels on selected cooximeters, which could lead to false reassurance.[136,164]

Bedside tests using ammonia or sodium hydroxide are unable to differentiate reliably various levels of COHb versus control participants.[161] Because of the similarities in extinction coefficients, COHb is misinterpreted as oxyhemoglobin on most types of pulse oximetry (Chap. 28).[8] Thus, the pulse oximetry reading is usually normal in the setting of even severe CO poisoning.[85] Some newer pulse oximeters, called pulse cooximeters, have the ability to measure COHb noninvasively.[6] A study in 10 healthy volunteers who inhaled CO at 500 ppm until they reached a peak COHb level of 15% found good agreement between pulse cooximetry and cooximetry.[7] Early models of a commercial bedside pulse cooximeter showed very poor agreement, mischaracterizing half the patients with levels over 15% as lower.[214] Subsequently, two other cohorts of ED patients, using a later model of the same device, found that it measured COHb well, with a bias of 0.6% to 3% and precision of 3.3%.[179,183] Because it tends to overestimate COHb, the authors recommend a normal upper limit of 6.6% as triggering intervention. Because the pulse cooximeter is noninvasive, it can be used for initial screening of ED patients for occult CO poisoning who present with nonspecific symptoms.[37] Likewise, the device is useful for field screening, especially with mass casualties. But because of potential errors with its use, we agree with the American College of Emergency Physicians (ACEP) recent clinical guideline on CO poisoning that recommended it not be used independently to diagnose CO toxicity and therefore cannot substitute for a standard blood COHb measurement.[232]

Breath-sampling methods are used for screening patients.[50,53,64] Cutoffs of 53 ppm in patients breathing air and 43 ppm in those breathing oxygen have a reliability of approximately 80% in predicting COHb levels above 10%.[69] Limited data from French prehospital screening show no correlation between severity of CO poisoning and exhaled CO concentrrations.[109] Therefore, because of its poor reliability, we do not recommend breath sampling for screening of hospitalized CO-poisoned patients.

Some clinical laboratories measure CO directly in blood samples rather than COHb. This technique involves assaying CO directly with infrared spectrophotometry after it is extracted from the blood sample with a manometer. Based on calculations rather than true experimental data, the assumption is made that for a patient with a normal hemoglobin, a CO level of 1 mmol/L corresponds to an 11% COHb concentration. A simpler method to measure serum CO content is to add a known solution of hemoglobin followed by sodium dithionite to form COHb. The resulting COHb is measured spectrophotometrically with the assumption that 1 mole of hemoglobin binds 4 moles of CO. Interestingly, in one study, serum CO ranged from 0.14 to 0.6 mg/L but was the same in smokers (average, 4.6% COHb) and nonsmokers (average, 1% COHb).[230] At this time, further research is required to determine the clinical importance of serum CO content.

Additional laboratory tests are useful in severe poisoning cases. Metabolic acidosis with elevated lactate concentration is a more reliable index of severity than a measurement of the COHb concentration.[189] Unfortunately, even arterial pH does not correlate well with either initial neurologic examination or the COHb level, making it a poor criterion for deciding the need for HBO treatment.[152] Specificity of lactate is low in smoke inhalation victims, in whom it is used to indicate concomitant cyanide poisoning (Chap. 123).

Continuous cardiac monitoring and a 12-lead ECG are essential to identify ischemia or dysrhythmias in symptomatic patients with preexisting coronary artery disease or severe exposure. Mild elevations of creatine phosphokinase are common (ranging 20–1,315 IU/L in one series of 65 cases), usually because of rhabdomyolysis rather than cardiac sources.[184] However, because CO causes myocardial infarction in the presence of normal coronaries,[118] nonspecific increases in troponin concentrations may reflect diffuse cardiac myonecrosis rather than focal coronary artery disease.[34] Congestive heart failure or hypotension can be evaluated with a β-type natriuretic peptide or echocardiography (or both), looking for evidence of myocardial stunning.[33,118] Because of the potential for increased cardiovascular mortality,[102] patients with ECG changes or elevated cardiac markers benefit from further cardiac testing, a stress test, or angiography.

The problem with using COHb levels to base treatment is that there is a wide variation in clinical manifestations across patients with identical COHb levels. Furthermore, particular COHb levels are not predictive of symptoms or final outcome.[142,157,189] In a large prospective study of CO poisoning, COHb levels did not correlate with LOC and were not predictive of delayed neurologic sequelae.[174] Admission COHb levels are inaccurate predictors of peak levels, and the use of nomograms to extrapolate to earlier levels is not validated. Their credibility is also suspect because of the great variability in COHb half-lives and differences in treatment with oxygen. To avert this problem, France equips prehospital personnel with cooximeters (model not stated), which, although imprecise do help them distinguish the severity of poisoining.[109]

Because of the inherent unreliability of COHb levels in predicting outcome, researchers are searching for other surrogate markers. Rats have early increases in glutathione released from erythrocytes, a potential marker for CO oxidative stress that could ultimately lead to brain injury.[208] Another promising marker is serum S100B, a structural protein in astroglia that is released from the brain after hypoxic stress. A series of 38 consecutive patients poisoned with CO showed that those who presented with normal neurologic findings and no LOC had normal S100B concentrations.[17] Patients who presented with LOC and neurologic deficits all had elevated concentrations. Carbon monoxide poisoned rats treated with HBO did not develop elevated S100B concentrations unlike those treated with ambient oxygen therapy.[16] Levels at the target organ, the brain, show that S100B in the cerebrospinal fluid (CSF) predicted extreme neurologic sequelae, that is, persistent vegetative state only.[110] Enolase, a byproduct of neuronal destruction, has a longer half-life than S100B and independently predicts delayed neurologic sequelae.[32] Although markers used for cerebral injury, specifically S100B and neuron-specific enolase, rise after CO poisoning, they have not be shown to be reliable enough to predict final outcome or need for treatment.[1,19,175] A recent pilot study concluded that almost 100 different plasma proteins—cytokines, chemokines, and other biomarkers—increase after CO poisoning in patients; their significance awaits more definitive studies.[204]

NEUROPSYCHOLOGIC TESTING

The extent of neurologic insult from CO can be assessed with a variety of tests. The most basic is documentation of the normal neurologic examination, including a quick mini mental status examination. A more sensitive indicator of the acute effects of CO on cortical function is a detailed neuropsychologic test battery developed specifically for CO patients.[145] The advantages of such testing, which usually takes about 30 minutes, are that it can reliably distinguish 79% of the time between CO-poisoned patients and control participants, and it shows improvement with appropriate HBO treatment.[145] Unfortunately, such testing shows a sensitivity of only 77% and a specificity of 80% for CO poisoning. The patient can show practice effects as well with repeated testing. Another study suggested that the degree of impairment CO patients had on a test of short-term rote and context-aided verbal memory correlated well with the number of HBO treatments needed.[144] The biggest problem with such neuropsychiatric testing is that it is uncertain whether the determined deficits found during the acute CO poisoning phase are at all predictive of the development of neurologic sequelae and therefore the necessity of HBO treatment.

NEUROIMAGING

Acute changes on CT scans of the brain occur within 12 hours of CO exposure that resulted in LOC.[137,148] Symmetric low-density areas in the region of the globus pallidus, putamen, and caudate nuclei are frequently noted.[105] Changes in the globus pallidus and subcortical white matter early within the

first day after poisoning are associated with poor outcomes[167] (Fig. 122–1). Alternatively, in one series of 18 patients, a negative CT within 1 week of admission was associated with favorable outcome.[213] The use of contrast enhances the early isodense changes not visible on initial CT scan[240] but is not routinely performed.

Magnetic resonance imaging is superior to CT in detecting cerebral white matter basal ganglia lesions after CO poisoning.[137] One study found a much higher incidence of periventricular white matter changes on MRIs done within the first day after exposure. However, such changes had no correlation with COHb level or cognitive sequelae.[167] These periventricular changes are more common and probably more sensitive than globus pallidus lesions. Globus pallidus lesions were present on MRI in only one patient (1.4%) in a prospective study of CO-poisoned patients, half of whom had LOC.[105] Diffusion-weighted, or even diffusion tensor imaging MRI, has more promise in detecting changes in subcortical white matter within hours of serious CO poisoning.[10,197] Regardless, neuroimaging usually does not influence patient management and can be reserved for patients who show poor response or have an equivocal diagnosis.

The most promising area of neuroimaging after CO poisoning is the assessment of regional cerebral perfusion.[43,163] Single-photon emission CT (SPECT) gauges regional blood flow noninvasively using an iodine or technetium tracer. In one series of 13 patients with delayed neurologic sequelae (DNS), all cases showed patchy hypoperfusion throughout the cerebral cortex within 11 days of poisoning.[41] These changes in perfusion occur as early as 1 day after poisoning and primarily involve watershed regions such as the temporoparietooccipital area.[58] Perfusion defects on SPECT scanning are associated with neuropsychological impairment months after serious CO poisoning.[70] In a recent series of CO-poisoned patients who required HBO, patients with DNS, rather than persistent neurologic sequelae, were more likely to show frontal hypoperfusion on SPECT scanning.[107,215] Unfortunately, because of the scant availability of the procedure and the lack of comprehensive studies, SPECT scanning is not the definitive tool at this time for determining prognosis or need for HBO. In addition, when imaging patients 1 to 2 years after poisoning, T2-weighted imaging on MRI is more sensitive than SPECT scanning.[38]

Positron emission tomography (PET) can also be used to evaluate regional blood flow as well as oxygen metabolism in the brain after CO exposure. In one series of severely CO-poisoned patients, PET examination after HBO treatment showed increased oxygen extraction and decreased blood flow in the frontal and temporal cortices.[56] Of note, patients with permanent deficits persisted in showing these abnormalities on PET scanning. One delayed PET study demonstrated that increases in dopamine D_2 receptor binding in the caudate and putamen after CO poisoning were improved with bromocriptine, at which time neuropsychiatric symptoms resolved.[239] Although PET scanning cannot be used to predict outcome, abnormalities that persist on the scan are associated with permanent neurologic sequelae. The same is true for proton magnetic resonance spectroscopy in which abnormalities within 1 week of exposure can predict DNS.[126]

Electroencephalograms (EEGs) complement perfusion studies in the evaluation of CO-poisoned patients. Although initial studies demonstrate that many patients have regional EEG abnormalities after poisoning, it is unknown if these are predictive of persistent or delayed neurologic problems. Electroencephalograms mapping may be discrepant relative to SPECT scanning because EEG preferentially demonstrates subcortical lesions.

MANAGEMENT

The mainstay of treatment is initial attention to the airway. One hundred percent oxygen should be provided as soon as possible by either nonrebreather face mask or endotracheal tube. Although concerns have been raised regarding toxicity from excess oxygen, patients poisoned with CO can still have cellular hypoxia despite normal oxygen saturation.[14,85] It is important to remember that a nonrebreathing mask only delivers 70% to 90% oxygen; a positive-pressure mask or an endotracheal tube is necessary to achieve higher oxygen concentrations. The immediate effect of oxygen is to enhance the dissociation of COHb.[180] In volunteers, the half-life of COHb is reduced from a mean of 5 hours (range, 2–7 hours) when breathing room air (21% oxygen) to approximately 1 hour (range, 36–137 minutes) when breathing 100% oxygen at normal atmospheric pressure.[171] Actual poisoned patients show a range in half-lives of 36 to 137 minutes (mean, 85 minutes) when breathing 100% oxygen; the longer elimination half-lives appear to be most often associated with long, low-level exposures.[155,227] With oxygenation and intensive care treatment, hospital mortality rates for serious exposures range from 1% to 30%. The duration of treatment is unclear, with a valid end point being the resolution of symptoms, usually accompanied by a COHb below 5%.

Continuous cardiac monitoring and intravenous (IV) access are necessary in any patient with systemic toxicity from CO poisoning. Hypotension should initially be treated with IV fluids, with the addition of inotropes for persistent myocardial depression. An evaluation for cardiac ischemia, including ECG and cardiac markers, is recommended in symptomatic patients at risk: prolonged exposure (>2 hours), altered mental status, or male gender.[31] Echocardiography is reasonable in such cases; almost three-quarters of CO-poisoned patients with elevated troponins showed cardiomyopathy with global dysfunction or Takotsubo like changes.[33] Standard advanced cardiac life support protocols should be followed for the treatment of patients with life-threatening dysrhythmias. Patients with a depressed mental status should have a rapid blood glucose checked. Animal studies of CO poisoning suggest that hypoglycemia can be deleterious.[168] We recommend not giving sodium bicarbonate for correction of any acidemia unless profound because it will cause left shift of the oxyhemoglobin dissociation curve, further impairing tissue oxygenation.[62]

Hyperbaric Oxygen

Hyperbaric oxygen (HBO) therapy is still the treatment of choice for patients with significant CO exposures.[210] But its most obvious effect is not the most important. One hundred percent oxygen at ambient pressure reduces the half-life of COHb from about 320 minutes to 85 minutes; at 2.5 atmospheres absolute (ATA), it is reduced to 20 minutes.[171,227] Actual CO-poisoned victims treated with HBO have COHb half-lives ranging from 4 to 86 minutes.[155] Hyperbaric oxygen also increases the amount of dissolved oxygen by about 10 times, which is sufficient alone to supply metabolic needs in the absence of hemoglobin (Chap. 28).[12] This is rarely an important clinical issue because most patients are already stabilized and have appreciably decreased COHb with ambient oxygen before preparation for an HBO treatment.

Therefore, HBO is more than just a modality to clear COHb more quickly than ambient oxygen (Antidotes in Depth: A40). More importantly, in rats after LOC from CO exposure, hyperbaric, but not normobaric, oxygen

therapy prevents brain lipid peroxidation.[166] Hyperbaric oxygen therapy prevents ischemic reperfusion injury by a variety of mechanisms. First, in animal models, HBO accelerates regeneration of inactivated cytochrome oxidase, which is the initiating site for CO neuronal damage.[12] Unlike 100% oxygen at room pressure, in clinical trials, HBO was much more effective than room pressure oxygen at restoring mitochondrial function within peripheral white blood cells in CO-poisoned patients.[59] Hyperbaric oxygen also prevents β-integrin–mediated neutrophil adhesion to brain microvascular endothelium, a process essential for amplification of CNS damage from CO.[178] In vitro studies of rat astrocytes show protective effects of HBO versus 100% oxygen in preventing impairment of neurotrophic activity after CO poisoning.[117] All these animal studies explain why HBO, but not 100% oxygen at atmospheric pressure, prevents delayed deficits in a learning and memory maze model.[202]

Clinical studies of the effectiveness of HBO in preventing neurologic damage from CO are not as convincing as basic science studies would suggest. In uncontrolled human clinical series, the incidence of persistent neuropsychiatric symptoms, including memory impairment, ranged from 12% to 43% in patients treated with 100% oxygen and was as low as 0% to 4% in patients treated with HBO.[82,143,154,157]

Additionally, several controlled clinical trials have evaluated the efficacy of HBO in CO poisoning (Table 122–3). The first randomized study of CO poisoning included more than 300 patients and failed to show a benefit from HBO in patients who had no initial LOC.[174] Unfortunately, seriously ill patients were not randomized to surface pressure oxygen; they received either one or three treatments of HBO. Flaws in the study included significant delays to treatment and the use of suboptimal pressure, 2.0 ATA, well below the greater than 2.5 ATA typically used in positive animal and human studies. A smaller (n = 60) controlled study avoided some of these flaws and showed that HBO, at a maximum pressure of 2.8 ATA, decreased delayed neurologic sequelae at 3 to 4 weeks from 23% to 0% in CO-poisoned patients who presented without LOC.[211] However, patients with syncope, a marker of serious poisoning, were excluded. A very small study (n = 26) of patients presenting with Glasgow Coma Scale (GCS) scores above 12 after CO poisoning included almost half with LOC.[63] Randomization to HBO versus 100% normobaric oxygen resulted in decreased EEG abnormalities and less reduction in blood flow reactivity to acetazolamide at 3 weeks. Unfortunately, all of these studies failed to definitively study all CO-poisoned patients, including those with syncope or coma.

The first randomized trial to directly address the issue of HBO efficacy in seriously CO-poisoned patients evaluated 191 CO-poisoned patients referred for HBO treatment.[182] Patients were randomized to a minimum of three daily treatments of HBO (2.8 ATA for 60 minutes) or 100% oxygen at 1.0 ATA for 3 days. Although the HBO group had a higher incidence of persistent

TABLE 122–3	Unfavorable Cognitive Outcome at 4 to 6 Weeks After Exposure to Carbon Monoxide in Randomized Clinical Trials of Hyperbaric Oxygen								
Study	Design	Max HBO Pressure	Time to Treatment	Syncope (%)	Suicide (%)	Treatment	Control	Odds Ratio (95% CI)
Mathieu, et al[143]	HBO for 90 min vs 12-h NBO	2.5 ATA	<12 h	N/A	N/A	69/299	73/276	0.83(0.57–1.22)
Raphael, et al[174]	HBO for 2 h vs 6-h NBO	2.0 ATA	Mean, 7.1 h	0	N/A	51/159	50/148	0.93(0.57–1.49)
Thom, et al[211]	HBO for 2 h vs 100% NBO until asymptomatic	2.8 ATA	Mean, 2.0 h	0	N/A	0/30	7/30	0.05(0.00–0.95)
Scheinkestel, et al[182]	HBO for 1 h vs NBO for 100 min	2.8 ATA	Mean, 7.1 h	53%	69%	30/48	25/40	1.00(0.42–2.38)
Weaver, et al[226]	HBO for 2 h (x3) vs NBO for 2 h (x1)	3.0 ATA	Mean, 5.6 h	53%	31%	19/76	35/76	0.39(0.20–0.78)
Annane, et al[5]	HBO for 2 h vs NBO for 6 h	2.0 ATA	<6 h	97%	0%	33/93	29/86	1.08 (0.58–2.00)

ATA = atmospheres absolute; CI = confidence interval; HBO = hyperbaric oxygen; N/A = not applicable; NBO = normobaric oxygen.

Data from Buckley NA, Juurlink DN, Isbister G, et al. Hyperbaric oxygen for carbon monoxide poisoning. *Cochrane Database Syst Rev.* 2011 Apr 13;(4):CD002041 and Penney DG. Carbon Monoxide Poisoning. New York, NY: CRC Press; 2008.

neurologic sequelae at 1 month, there was no significant difference between the two groups; more than two-thirds of each group had persistent problems. This study, although the largest controlled, randomized study to date, suffered from several flaws. Fewer than half of the patients had follow-up at 1 month. Disproportionate numbers of suicide cases (about two-thirds) and drug toxicity (44%), with accompanying neuropsychologic defects, likely confounded finding any beneficial effect from HBO. Finally, HBO treatment was delayed for 6 hours, making it much less likely to be effective.[82,174]

The landmark randomized, double-blind, placebo-controlled study of 152 CO-poisoned patients identified a beneficial effect of HBO.[226] Most of these patients were ill, with a mean initial COHb level of 25% and a 50% incidence of LOC. Patients were all treated within 24 hours of exposure, but the success of the study might be partially attributable to the rapid mean time to treatment of less than 2 hours. Patients received HBO three times at intervals of 6 to 12 hours, each at 2.0 ATA, except for the first hour of the first treatment, which was at 3.0 ATA. Control patients received sham treatments in the HBO chamber with 100% oxygen at 1.0 ATA. At 6 weeks, the HBO group had a 24% incidence of cognitive sequelae versus 46% in the control group. Based on these data, the number of patients needed to treat to prevent one case of cognitive impairment is only five. Critics of this study point out that the neuropsychiatric tests were not significantly different between the groups except for digit spam and trail making, and there was no difference in activities of daily living. However, untreated patients had increased self-reported memory problems at 6 weeks (51% vs 28%), and the beneficial effect on cognitive sequelae persisted until 12 months.

A more recent study of 179 patients with transient LOC after CO poisoning showed no benefit from a single HBO treatment.[5] Neurologic recovery at 1 month was approximately 60% regardless of HBO or normobaric oxygen. However, the study was done only at 2.0 ATA, and more than 20% of patients were lost to follow-up. The main effect of HBO is to prevent β2 integrins mediated adherence of neutrophils in the brain; this does not occur in animal studies until at least a pressure of 2.8 ATA is attained.[210]

Based on the strong animal and basic science experience, the positive human studies mentioned earlier, and few adverse effects, it is not surprising that the Underwater and Hyperbaric Medical Society (UHMS) recommends HBO for all CO patients with signs of serious toxicity.[224] With the low risk of this procedure,[181,188] almost 1,500 patients are treated with HBO for CO poisoning in the United States each year.[93] Therefore, we believe that HBO is safe and indicated for serious CO poisoning, even though there is still substantial disagreement in the interpretation of the existing evidence regarding its usefulness.[100,138,232]

Indications for Hyperbaric Oxygen Therapy

Although the specific recommendations for HBO after acute CO poisoning are listed (Table 122–4), they are not prospectively evaluated. The patients most likely to benefit are those most at risk for persistent or delayed neurologic sequelae, such as those presenting in coma or with a history of syncope.[121] These are likely clinical markers for the episode of hypotension that are necessary for causing neuronal damage from CO-induced ischemic reperfusion injury in animal models.[78,160] However, syncope is neither

TABLE 122–4	Recommended Indications for Hyperbaric Oxygen[a]

Syncope (transient loss of consciousness)
Coma
Seizure
Altered mental status (Glasgow Coma Scale score <15) or confusion
Carboxyhemoglobin >25%; independent of signs or symptoms
Abnormal cerebellar function
Pregnancy carboxyhemoglobin ≥ 15%
Fetal distress in pregnancy
Equivocal cases with age > 35 years and prolonged exposure (≥24 h).

[a]Patients with these risk factors for cognitive sequelae have the highest potential to benefit from hyperbaric oxygen treatment.

a particularly sensitive nor a specific marker for cognitive sequelae. Patients with long exposures, or "soaking" periods, typically longer than 6 hours, are also at greater risk for neurologic sequelae.[13] The presence of a significant metabolic acidosis is a surrogate marker for CO poisoning.[189,216] Patients who present with decreased level of consciousness, a GCS score of less than 9 in one series, had an odds ratio of 7.0 for the development of neurologic sequelae.[170] Although some authors advocate ongoing myocardial ischemia as an indication for HBO, in our experience, these patients usually already meet neurologic criteria for treatment, such as LOC or ongoing mental status changes. Isolated cardiac ischemia, more importantly, deserves immediate proven myocardial salvaging therapy rather than delayed treatment with HBO.

Some authors advocate treating all patients with COHb levels of 40% or greater with HBO. It is reasonable to use a more conservative level of 25% as an indication for HBO.[94] More important than actual level are patient history and examination. Further analysis of data from the most recent controlled trial demonstrates that in patients not treated with HBO, there were no reliable factors (COHb level, LOC, or base excess) for predicting who progressed to cognitive sequelae.[229] A multivariate analysis showed that of all factors (LOC, age, exposure time, and COHb levels), only age of 36 years or older and CO exposure duration of 24 hours or longer were associated with cognitive dysfunction at 6-week follow-up. More problematic is the incidence of cognitive sequelae in patients without those risk factors: 32% in those younger than age 36 years and 36% in those with less than 24 hours of exposure. In conclusion, it appears that there are no completely reliable predictors for screening out patients who will do well without HBO treatment.

Multiple studies attempted to evaluate serum markers after acute CO poisoning that would predict neurologic sequelae. Although COHb confirms exposure, it does not correlate with future outcome, let alone acute symptoms.[90,228] Multiple serum markers, including cytokines, increase after CO poisoning, but their predictive accuracy is unclear.[204] Although impaired mitochondrial cytochrome function and elevated lipid peroxidation are seen in peripheral lymphocytes and monocytes after clinical CO poisoning, they only confirm CO exposure and are too nonspecific to use as predictors of neurologic sequelae.[71]

Therefore, at this time, it is prudent to refer for HBO treatment those patients with the most serious neurologic symptoms, regardless of their COHb level. Such symptoms include coma, seizures, focal neurologic deficits, altered mental status (GCS score <15), and although controversial, LOC. Patients who have had cardiac arrest from CO poisoning and had the return of spontaneous circulation are poor candidates for HBO therapy because virtually all these cases are fatal.[97] In fact, such deaths from CO poisoning are not contraindication to organ donation (Special Considerations: SC12).

Excluding patients from HBO with milder symptoms after CO poisoning is problematic because even they are susceptible to neurocognitive sequelae. One series of 55 patients with mild poisoning as defined by the absence of LOC and maximum measured COHb level less than 15% found that even one-third of these individuals had neurocognitive sequelae up to 12 months after exposure.[35] This was no different than that occurring in the severely poisoned group, although the milder group had a much longer duration of exposure as well as a greater delay to the evaluation of the COHb level. Brain imaging studies confirm that mild exposures, marked by no LOC and COHb levels lower than 15%, result in visible changes.[70,173] Taken to its logical but impractical conclusion, because even apparently mild cases of CO poisoning have poor neurocognitive outcomes, HBO treatment of every CO-exposed patient, regardless of severity, could be justified.

It is still unclear if mild neurologic effects, such as confusion, headache, dizziness, visual blurring, or abnormal mental status testing on initial presentation after CO poisoning, are prognostic for cognitive sequelae, which would necessitate HBO treatment. These effects simply represent CO poisoning, which at COHb levels approaching 10% in volunteers causes temporary impairment of learning and memory.[4] In one prospective clinical trial of CO poisoning, the incidence of cerebellar dysfunction portended a higher incidence of cognitive sequelae (odds ratio, 5.7; 95% confidence interval {CI},

1.7–19.3).[226] Therefore, difficulties with finger-to-nose, heel-to-shin, rapid alternating hand movements, or even ataxia are recommended indications for HBO. Patients with other mild neurologic findings, such as headache, warrant at least several hours of oxygen by nonrebreather facemask until symptoms resolve. If symptoms do not resolve, HBO is recommended; however, any delay to HBO therapy decreases its efficacy.

A more promising method to discern patients who may respond to HBO is based on the genotype, apolipoprotein E, specifically the isoform ε4.[106] This particular polymorphism allele is present in up to one-quarter of the population, and it is associated with worse neurologic outcome from trauma and stroke. In the presence of CO poisoning, it is associated with lack of response to HBO for preventing neurocognitive sequelae. Further studies support not treating patients with this particular allele, focusing on those with the potential for response to HBO therapy.

Several professional societies have attempted to develop evidence-based guidelines. The American College of Emergency Physicians stated that no clinical variable predicts patients at risk of cognitive sequelae of likelihood to benefit from HBO.[231] The American College of Emergency Physicians guideline recently stated that it remains unclear if HBO provides any added benefit over normobaric oxygen therapy in preventing long-term neurocognitive sequelae.[232] Similarly, the Cochrane Collaboration review on the use of HBO in CO poisoning concluded that because of so much conflicting data, there is insufficient evidence to support HBO for CO poisoning at this time.[18] The collective odds ratio for protective effect at 4 to 6 weeks with HBO versus normobaric oxygen was 0.78 (95% CI 0.54–1.12) based on a collective experience of 1,361 patients in six studies. The most recent guideline from the UHMS states that CO-poisoned patients should be referred for HBO if they have serious poisoning, such as unconsciousness, whether it is transient or persistent; age 36 years or older; or CO exposure duration of 24 hours or longer, even if intermittent.[224] These guidelines are consistent with the prior studies discussed earlier. The UHMS guidelines also state that many physicians treat when neuropsychologic testing results are abnormal or COHb levels are greater than 25% to 30%.

Some authors recommend selective use of HBO because of cost and difficulties in transport if the primary facility lacks a chamber. However, complications that make such transfers and treatment unsafe are rare.[188] At the present time, we routinely recommend HBO for selected patients poisoned by CO based on the indications in Table 122–4. Fortunately, even without HBO, anywhere from one-third to three-quarters of cases with persistent cognitive sequelae resolve over the subsequent year.[40,226]

Delayed Administration of Hyperbaric Oxygen

The optimal timing and number of HBO treatments for CO poisoning is unclear. Patients treated later than 6 hours after exposure tend to have worse outcomes in terms of delayed sequelae (30% versus 19%) and mortality (30% versus 14%).[82] This helps explain the failure of one of the first randomized trials on HBO for CO poisoning, which had a mean time to treatment of over 6 hours after poisoning.[182] Meanwhile, HBO treatments delivered within 6 hours after poisoning in patients with LOC after CO seem to almost completely prevent neurologic sequelae.[241] However, patients benefit even if treated later. In the most recent randomized clinical trial showing beneficial effects of HBO, although all patients were treated within 24 hours of exposure, 38% of patients were treated later than 6 hours after exposure. Therefore, it is reasonable to perform HBO, contingent on transport limitations, within 24 hours of presentation for symptomatic acute poisoning.

One case series suggests beneficial effects for HBO used up to 21 days after exposure, even after patients have developed neuropsychologic sequelae.[154] The problem with studies showing HBO benefits days after an acute poisoning or after chronic poisoning is that these cases are all anecdotal and lack control participants. In fact, delayed neurocognitive sequelae frequently resolve within 2 months in patients with mild CO poisoning,[211] and in those with serious CO poisoning who survive to HBO treatment, one-third resolve within 1 year.[226] It is possible that these delayed or chronic cases simply represent the placebo effect of HBO.

Repeat Treatment with Hyperbaric Oxygen

A randomized clinical trial demonstrated that three HBO treatments within the first 24 hours improved cognitive outcome.[226] Unfortunately, there was no group treated with only one or two HBO sessions in that study. Regardless, it is reasonable to give repeated treatments for patients with persistent symptoms, particularly coma, who do not resolve after their first HBO session. In a pilot study, one HBO treatment was enough to promote almost total mitochondrial cytochrome activity, as measured in peripheral lymphocytes, after CO poisoning.[71] In a nonrandomized retrospective study, CO-poisoned patients who received a second HBO treatment had a reduction in delayed neurologic sequelae from 55% to 18% compared with control participants who had only one treatment.[81]

It is not clear that more HBO treatments are better. A large recent study showed that in seriously poisoned CO patients, two hyperbaric treatments resulted in a worse outcome than one treatment, with complete recovery in 47% versus 68%, respectively.[5] There were serious flaws in that study, including lack of formal neuropsychological testing and the use of only 2.0 ATA of pressure, well below the 3.0 ATA used initially in favorable studies. A recent retrospective nationwide study in Taiwan showed that patients treated for CO poisoning with more than one treatment had lower mortality rates (adjusted hazard ratio of 0.79; 95% CI 0.64–0.95) over the subsequent 4 years, than those receiving only one treatment.[108] With the lack of prospective studies comparing single versus multiple courses of HBO therapy, multiple treatments are not recommended as a routine at this time. The most recent clinical guidelines from the UHMS state that the optimal number of HBO treatments for CO poisoning is unknown and that one should consider reserving multiple treatments for patients who fail to fully recover after one treatment.[224]

Treatment of Pregnant Patients

The management of CO exposure in the pregnant patient is difficult because of the potential adverse effects of both CO and HBO. A literature review of all CO exposures during pregnancy revealed a high incidence of fetal CNS damage and stillbirth after severe maternal poisonings.[217] A series of three severely symptomatic patients who did not receive HBO had adverse fetal outcomes: two stillbirths and one case of cerebral palsy.[122] There are cases of limb malformations, cranial deformities, and a variety of mental disabilities in children poisoned in utero.[20,139,140] A recent epidemiologic study in Guatemala showed that CO exposure from wood smoke during the third trimester was inversely associated with neuropsychological performance at ages 6 to 7 years when corrected for socioeconomic confounders.[59]

Traditionally, it was thought that fetal hemoglobin had a high affinity for CO. Pregnant ewe studies show a delayed but substantive increase in COHb levels in fetuses, exceeding the level and duration of those in the mothers.[140] Thus, it appeared that fetuses were a sink for CO and could be poisoned at concentrations lower than mothers. However, such data do not apply to humans because in vitro work shows that as opposed to sheep, human fetal hemoglobin actually has less affinity for CO than maternal hemoglobin, at a ratio of 0.8. Under conditions of low oxygenation and high 2,3-BPG, as in serious CO poisoning, the affinity of human fetal hemoglobin starts to approach that of maternal.[229] The more important issue with maternal CO exposure is the precipitous decrease in fetal arterial oxygen content that occurs within minutes at CO concentrations of 3,000 ppm.[77] Therefore, the ensuing hypoxia of the fetus, rather than increase in fetal COHb, is of more concern.

Maternal COHb levels do not accurately reflect fetal hemoglobin or tissue concentrations.[51] In primate studies, a single CO exposure insufficient to cause clinical disease in the mother led to intrauterine hypoxia, fetal brain injury, and an increased rate of fetal death.[76,78] In humans, there are a few cases of fetal demise with maternal levels of COHb less than 10%.[20] However, in that series, some mothers were treated with oxygen before their COHb levels were obtained. Another issue with some of these data is that often the mother was chronically "soaked" with CO, making levels difficult to interpret. Rodent studies show that chronic low-level CO exposure in pregnant mothers may result in permanent cognitive deficits in the subsequent progeny.[57]

Because maternal COHb does not necessarily predict fetal demise, clinicians must direct their attention to maternal manifestations of CO toxicity. Multiple case series demonstrate that pregnant women who present with a normal mental status and no LOC after CO poisoning have excellent outcomes in terms of normal deliveries.[20,122] These infants have no subsequent delay in attaining their developmental milestones. Therefore, it appears that mothers who appear well after acute CO poisoning will have good outcomes with respect to their pregnancies.

The bigger dilemma for clinicians is the approach to treatment of seriously symptomatic CO-poisoned pregnant patients. All patients should receive 100% oxygen by face mask, at least until the mother is asymptomatic. However, CO absorption and elimination are slower in the fetal circulation than in the maternal circulation.[140] A mathematical model predicts that elimination of CO from fetuses takes 3.5 times longer than maternal CO elimination.[103] However, because some of these data are based on sheep fetal hemoglobin kinetics, the optimum time for treatment of the mother cannot be recommended at this time.

Unfortunately, pregnant patients were excluded from all prospective trials documenting the efficacy of HBO. However, treatment of pregnant patients with HBO is not without theoretical risk. Animal studies show conflicting results on the effects of HBO on fetal development. Some studies demonstrate that HBO causes developmental abnormalities in the central nervous, cardiovascular, and pulmonary systems of rodent fetuses. This is in marked contrast to the extensive Russian experience, in which hundreds of pregnant women were treated with HBO, apparently without significant perinatal complications and with improvement in fetal and maternal status for their underlying conditions of toxemia, anemia, and diabetes.[149] There are multiple cases where apparently normal infants are born after their pregnant mothers received HBO for mild CO poisoning. However, less than optimal outcomes have occurred in cases of sicker patients in which the mother has had LOC or presented comatose.[65] A 25-year longitudinal study of 406 pregnant women who received HBO for CO poisoning, with many children followed for up to 6 years of age, showed no psychomotor or growth differences between exposed and unexposed control participants.[222] Thus, it appears that HBO should be safe and have the same efficacy for pregnant patients as in nonpregnant patients. There currently is no scientific validation for an absolute level at which to provide HBO therapy for a pregnant patient with CO exposure. Somewhat arbitrarily, we recommend a threshold for HBO in pregnant patients is a COHb level regardless of symptoms of greater then or equal to 15%. Pregnant patients should not be treated any differently if they meet criteria for HBO described above (Table 122–4). Additional criteria include any signs of fetal distress, such as abnormal fetal heart rate.

Treatment of Children

It is suggested that children are more sensitive to the effects of CO because of their increased respiratory and metabolic rate.[39] Epidemiologic studies suggest that children become symptomatic at COHb levels less that 10%, which is lower than commonly expected in adults.[121] The other problem is that these younger patients have unusual presentations. Although most children manifest nausea, headache, or lethargy, an isolated seizure or vomiting is sometimes the only manifestation of CO toxicity in an infant or child.[39]

When interpreting COHb levels in infants, clinicians must be aware of two confounding factors. First, many older cooximeters give falsely elevated COHb levels in proportion to the amount of fetal hemoglobin present.[219] Second, CO is produced during breakdown of protoporphyrin to bilirubin. Therefore, infants normally have higher levels of COHb, which are even higher in the presence of kernicterus. Some neonates not exposed to CO have COHb levels approaching 8%.[220] Thus, before it is assumed that an elevated COHb level implies CO poisoning in an infant, the contribution of jaundice and fetal hemoglobin must be evaluated.

There are alternative clinical markers better than COHb for gauging toxicity in children. An elevated lactate concentration was found in 90.1% of

674 pediatric patients admitted for CO poisoing.[54] Many children with elevated troponin concentrations after CO poisoning had normal ECGs or just subtle transitory T-wave changes from repolarization abnormalities.[162] The echocardiogram is abnormal approximately 50% of patients found to have an elevated troponin concentration, usually showing a temporary decrease in left ventricular function and ejection fraction.[162,198]

Although children are more susceptible to acute toxicity with CO, their long-term outcomes appear to be more favorable than for adults. In one series of 2,360 serious CO cases, all cases of delayed neurologic sequelae occurred in adults older than age 30 years.[40] Another series of CO poisoning demonstrated an incidence of delayed neurologic sequelae of 10% to 20% in children after severe CO poisoning.[39] Increased COHb levels (>25%) in adolescents associated with more severe acute symptoms.[127] One retrospective multivariate analysis showed that prolonged LOC requiring ICU care was the only independent risk factor for delayed neurologic sequelae.[36]

This low incidence of DNS in patients treated only with 100% oxygen at normal pressures is used as an argument to avoid HBO. However, their risk of such sequelae exists, and HBO is used successfully to prevent it.[238] In a recent series of 27 hospitalized children for CO poisoning treated with HBO, only 1 child had minor neurologic sequelae (ie, headache and tinnitus).[119] Deaths in children are often directly related to concomitant smoke inhalation.[42] The CoHb half life with surface pressure oxygen is approximately 44 minutes, faster elimination than occurs in adults.[121] Often, children exposed to CO under similar circumstances with a parent, although appearing well, are treated simultaneously with the sick parent, especially if a multiplace chamber is available.

Novel Neuroprotective Treatments

A variety of neuroprotective therapeutics were tested in animal models. They are targeted primarily at preventing the delayed neurologic sequelae associated with serious CO poisoning. One of the simplest treatments tested is insulin. Hyperglycemia exacerbates neuronal injury from stroke as well as in arrest situations. In CO poisoning of rodents, it is associated with worse neurologic outcome.[138] However, insulin, independent of its glucose-lowering effect, is protective after ischemic insults. In rodent studies, improved neurologic outcome, as measured by locomotor activity, occurs in those with CO poisoning treated with insulin. In light of these findings, it is reasonable to treat documented hyperglycemia with insulin in patients with serious CO poisoning.

Many neuroprotective therapeutics involve blockage of excitatory amino acids that are implicated in neuronal cell death after CO poisoning. Pretreatment of mice with dizocilpine (MK-801), which blocks the action of glutamate at N-methyl-D-aspartate receptors, ameliorates learning, memory, and hippocampal deficits with CO poisoning.[113] Ketamine, another glutamate antagonist, decreases the mortality rate of rats poisoned with CO after carotid ligation.[169] Treatment of mice with various glutamate antagonists prevents learning and memory deficits in a model of CO poisoning.[74] Blockage earlier in the immunologic cascade, with a neuronal NO synthase inhibitor also prevented NMDA receptor activation, thus protecting mice from learning deficits after CO poisoning.[207] Further clinical research is needed before recommending any of these antagonists routinely.

One exciting approach is the use of antioxidants, such as dimethyl sulfoxide and disulfiram, that prevent learning and memory deficits when given after CO poisoning in mice.[74] Use of these or related therapeutics, although promising, awaits further animal testing because of potential adverse effects. Likewise, 3-N-butylphthalide, a celery seed extract, which has a variety of neuroprotective effects, including improved blood flow, antioxidant, and antiapoptosis effects, was adopted from stroke research. A randomized trial of 185 seriously CO-poisoned patients treated with HBO showed that by adding 3-N-butylphthalide 200 mg three times a day orally, neurologic remission improved.[236] Regardless of treatment, both treated and untreated groups showed improvement.

Much of what happens after CO poisoning involves an inflammatory cascade that leads eventually to neurologic sequelae. A recent trial of patients receiving HBO for CO poisoning were randomized to treatment with 5 and 10 mg/day of dexamethasone versus HBO alone.[235] Both dexamethasone groups showed improved scores on mini mental state examination as well as the National Institute of Health Stroke Scale at 4 weeks after poisoning. This was accompanied by a decrease in myelin basic protein in CSF, confirming the antiinflammatory effect of the drug. Erythropoietin is another potential treatment modality for CO poisoning that also decreases the neuronal inflammatory response.[166] A human trial showed that the addition of recombinant erythropoietin daily for 1 week to HBO decreased the incidence of delayed neurologic sequelae from 30% in the HBO alone to 12%.[165]

Other modalities tested in preventing neuronal damage from CO are not successful. Although hypothermia was associated with good outcomes in uncontrolled human trials,[68,158] controlled animal trials actually show an increased mortality rate.[194] Allopurinol, which prevents the formation of free radicals through xanthine oxidase, inhibits lipid peroxidation in CO poisoning when given before exposure.[202] This strategy is not promising because of the necessity for pretreatment.

PREVENTION

Early diagnosis prevents much of the morbidity and mortality associated with CO poisoning, especially in unintentional exposures. The increased quality of home CO-detecting devices allows personal intervention in the prevention of exposure.[124] If a patient presents complaining that his or her CO alarm sounded, it is important to realize that the threshold limit for the alarm is set roughly to approximate a COHb level of 10% at worst. Therefore, manufacturers must have their alarms activate within 189 minutes at 70 ppm CO, 50 minutes at 150 ppm, and 15 minutes at 400 ppm (Underwriters Laboratories, UL2034). Alarms are not designed to activate for prolonged exposures below 30 ppm to prevent epidemic alarming during winter thermal inversions in large cities.[11] Government ordinances for obligatory CO alarms could potentially prevent many poisonings, particularly during winter storms.[23,83] Although most serious CO poisonings are associated with the absence of CO alarms, a small proportion of such patients had alarms, suggesting the need for assessing proper functionality after installation.[44]

Routine laboratory screening of ED patients during the winter is not very efficacious in diagnosing unsuspected CO poisoning; the yield is less than 1% for patients tested in whom the diagnosis of CO exposure was already excluded by history. Instead, selecting patients with CO-related complaints, such as headache, dizziness, or nausea, increases the yield to 5% to 11%.[64,193] During the winter, risk factors such as gas heating or symptomatic cohabitants in patients with influenzalike symptoms such as headache, dizziness, or nausea, particularly in the absence of fever, is the most useful method for deciding when to obtain COHb levels for potential patients.

The issue of symptomatic cohabitants is especially important from a preventive standpoint. Alerting other cohabitants to this danger and effecting evacuation prevents needless morbidity and mortality. This is especially critical for multifamily domiciles, such as hotels, that have resulted in dramatic collective exposures and even deaths.[225] Most communities have multiple resources for onsite evaluation. Usually the local fire department or utility company can either check home appliances or measure ambient CO concentrations with portable monitoring equipment. The current workplace standard for ambient CO exposures is 35 ppm averaged over 8 hours with a ceiling limit of 200 ppm (measured over a 15-minute period).[99] Just a 4-hour exposure to 100 ppm of CO may result in COHb level greater than 10% with symptoms.

SUMMARY

- Unintentional exposures to CO are easily missed or misdiagnosed. Patients with a suspected influenzalike illness should be screened for potential home sources of CO, and symptomatic cohabitants should be alerted.
- Carbon monoxide exposure should be evaluated in patients with unexplained coma, metabolic acidosis, or signs of cardiac ischemia, especially if attempted suicide is suspected.
- Fire victims, in addition to airway complications and potential cyanide and other toxic inhalants may succumb to CO toxicity.

- The mainstay of treatment in CO poisoning is good supportive care with early oxygenation to increase the elimination of COHb.
- Because of the overwhelming clinical successes with HBO and its limited risks, early use of this treatment modality in severe exposures is recommended.
- Discussion with a regional poison control center or hyperbaric facility will help in identifying patients who are most likely to benefit from such treatment.

REFERENCES

1. Akdemir HU, et al. The role of S100B protein, neuron-specific enolase, and glial fibrillary acidic protein in the evaluation of hypoxic brain injury in acute carbon monoxide poisoning. *Hum Exp Toxicol*. 2014;33:1113-1120.
2. Allred EN, et al. Short-term effects of carbon monoxide exposure on the exercise performance of subjects with coronary artery disease. *N Engl J Med*. 1989;321:1426-1432.
3. Allred EN, et al. Effects of carbon monoxide on myocardial ischemia. *Environ Health Perspect*. 1991;91:89-132.
4. Amitai Y, et al. Neuropsychological impairment from acute low-level exposure to carbon monoxide. *Arch Neurol*. 1998;55:845-848.
5. Annane D, et al. Hyperbaric oxygen therapy for acute domestic carbon monoxide poisoning: two randomized controlled trials. *Intensive Care Med*. 2011;37:486-492.
6. Barker SJ, Badal JJ. The measurement of dyshemoglobins and total hemoglobin by pulse oximetry. *Curr Opin Anaesthesiol*. 2008;21:805-810.
7. Barker SJ, et al. Measurement of carboxyhemoglobin and methemoglobin by pulse oximetry: a human volunteer study. *Anesthesiology*. 2006;105:892-897.
8. Barker SJ, Tremper KK. The effect of carbon monoxide inhalation on pulse oximetry and transcutaneous PO2. *Anesthesiology*. 1987;66:677-679.
9. Benignus VA, et al. Prediction of carboxyhemoglobin formation due to transient exposure to carbon monoxide. *J Appl Physiol (1985)*. 1994;76:1739-1745.
10. Beppu T. The role of MR imaging in assessment of brain damage from carbon monoxide poisoning: a review of the literature. *AJNR Am J Neuroradiol*. 2014;35:625-631.
11. Bizovi KE, et al. Night of the sirens: analysis of carbon monoxide-detector experience in suburban Chicago. *Ann Emerg Med*. 1998;31:737-740.
12. Boerema I, et al. [Life without blood]. *Ned Tijdschr Geneeskd*. 1960;104:949-954.
13. Bogusz M, et al. A comparison of two types of acute carbon monoxide poisoning. *Arch Toxicol*. 1975;33:141-149.
14. Brown SD, Piantadosi CA. Recovery of energy metabolism in rat brain after carbon monoxide hypoxia. *J Clin Invest*. 1992;89:666-672.
15. Bruce EN, Bruce MC. A multicompartment model of carboxyhemoglobin and carboxymyoglobin responses to inhalation of carbon monoxide. *J Appl Physiol (1985)*. 2003;95:1235-1247.
16. Brvar M, et al. S100B protein in conscious carbon monoxide-poisoned rats treated with normobaric or hyperbaric oxygen. *Crit Care Med*. 2006;34:2228-2230.
17. Brvar M, et al. S100B protein in carbon monoxide poisoning: a pilot study. *Resuscitation*. 2004;61:357-360.
18. Buckley NA, et al. Hyperbaric oxygen for carbon monoxide poisoning. *Cochrane Database Syst Rev*. 2011:CD002041.
19. Cakir Z, et al. S-100beta and neuron-specific enolase levels in carbon monoxide-related brain injury. *Am J Emerg Med*. 2010;28:61-67.
20. Caravati EM, et al. Fetal toxicity associated with maternal carbon monoxide poisoning. *Ann Emerg Med*. 1988;17:714-717.
21. Centers for Disease Control and Prevention. Carbon monoxide poisoning at an indoor ice arena and bingo hall—Seattle, 1996. *MMWR Morb Mortal Wkly Rep*. 1996;45:265-267.
22. Centers for Disease Control and Prevention. Carbon-monoxide poisoning resulting from exposure to ski-boat exhaust—Georgia, June 2002. *MMWR Morb Mortal Wkly Rep*. 2002;51:829-830.
23. Centers for Disease Control and Prevention. Epidemic carbon monoxide poisoning despite a CO alarm law. Mecklenburg County, NC, December 2002. *MMWR Morb Mortal Wkly Rep*. 2004;2004.
24. Centers for Disease Control and Prevention. Use of carbon monoxide alarms to prevent poisonings during a power outage—North Carolina, December 2002. *MMWR Morb Mortal Wkly Rep*. 2004;53:189-192.
25. Centers for Disease Control and Prevention. Carbon monoxide poisoning from hurricane-associated use of portable generators—Florida, 2004. *MMWR Morb Mortal Wkly Rep*. 2005;54:697-700.
26. Centers for Disease Control and Prevention. Unintentional non-fire-related carbon monoxide exposures—United States, 2001-2003. *MMWR Morb Mortal Wkly Rep*. 2005;54:36-39.
27. Centers for Disease Control and Prevention. Carbon monoxide–related deaths—United States, 1999-2004. *MMWR Morb Mortal Wkly Rep*. 2007;56:1309-1312.
28. Centers for Disease Control and Prevention. Nonfatal, unintentional, non–fire-related carbon monoxide exposures—United States, 2004-2006. *MMWR Morb Mortal Wkly Rep*. 2008;57:896-899.
29. Centers for Disease Control and Prevention. QuickStats: number of deaths resulting from unintentional carbon monoxide poisoning, by month and year—National Vital Statistics System, United States, 2010-2015. *MMWR Morb Mortal Wkly Rep*. 2017;66:234.

30. Cervellin G, et al. Initial blood lactate correlates with carboxyhemoglobin and clinical severity in carbon monoxide poisoned patients. *Clin Biochem.* 2014;47:298-301.

31. Cha YS, et al. Features and predictors of myocardial injury in carbon monoxide poisoned patients. *Emerg Med J.* 2014;31:210-215.

32. Cha YS, et al. Serum neuron-specific enolase as an early predictor of delayed neuropsychiatric sequelae in patients with acute carbon monoxide poisoning. *Hum Exp Toxicol.* 2017;960327117698544.

33. Cha YS, et al. Incidence and patterns of cardiomyopathy in carbon monoxide-poisoned patients with myocardial injury. *Clin Toxicol (Phila).* 2016;54:481-487.

34. Chamberland DL, et al. Transient cardiac dysfunction in acute carbon monoxide poisoning. *Am J Med.* 2004;117:623-625.

35. Chambers CA, et al. Cognitive and affective outcomes of more severe compared to less severe carbon monoxide poisoning. *Brain Inj.* 2008;22:387-395.

36. Chang YC, et al. Risk factors and outcome analysis in children with carbon monoxide poisoning. *Pediatr Neonatol.* 2017;58:171-177.

37. Chee KJ, et al. Finding needles in a haystack: a case series of carbon monoxide poisoning detected using new technology in the emergency department. *Clin Toxicol (Phila).* 2008;46:461-469.

38. Chen NC, et al. Detection of gray matter damage using brain MRI and SPECT in carbon monoxide intoxication: a comparison study with neuropsychological correlation. *Clin Nucl Med.* 2013;38:e53-59.

39. Cho CH, et al. Carbon monoxide poisoning in children. *Pediatr Neonatol.* 2008;49:121-125.

40. Choi IS. Delayed neurologic sequelae in carbon monoxide intoxication. *Arch Neurol.* 1983;40:433-435.

41. Choi IS, et al. Evaluation of outcome of delayed neurologic sequelae after carbon monoxide poisoning by technetium-99m hexamethylpropylene amine oxime brain single photon emission computed tomography. *Euro Neurol.* 1995;35:137-142.

42. Chou KJ, et al. Characteristics and outcome of children with carbon monoxide poisoning with and without smoke exposure referred for hyperbaric oxygen therapy. *Pediatr Emerg Care.* 2000;16:151-155.

43. Chu K, et al. Diffusion-weighted MRI and 99mTc-HMPAO SPECT in delayed relapsing type of carbon monoxide poisoning: evidence of delayed cytotoxic edema. *Eur Neurol.* 2004;51:98-103.

44. Clower JH, et al. Recipients of hyperbaric oxygen treatment for carbon monoxide poisoning and exposure circumstances. *Am J Emerg Med.* 2012;30:846-851.

45. Cobb N, Etzel RA. Unintentional carbon monoxide-related deaths in the United States, 1979 through 1988. *JAMA.* 1991;266:659-663.

46. Coburn RF. The carbon monoxide body stores. *Ann N Y Acad Sci.* 1970;174:11-22.

47. Coburn RF. Endogenous carbon monoxide production. *N Engl J Med.* 1970;282:207-209.

48. Coburn RF. Carbon monoxide uptake and excretion: testing assumptions made in deriving the Coburn-Forster-Kane equation. *Respir Physiol Neurobiol.* 2013;187: 224-233.

49. Coburn RF, Mayers LB. Myoglobin O2 tension determined from measurement of carboxymyoglobin in skeletal muscle. *Am J Physiol.* 1971;220:66-74.

50. Cone DC, et al. Noninvasive fireground assessment of carboxyhemoglobin levels in firefighters. *Prehosp Emerg Care.* 2005;9:8-13.

51. Copel JA, et al. Carbon monoxide intoxication in early pregnancy. *Obstet Gynecol.* 1982;59(6 suppl):26S-28S.

52. Creswell PD, et al. Exposure to elevated carbon monoxide levels at an indoor ice arena—Wisconsin, 2014. *MMWR Morb Mortal Wkly Rep.* 2015;64:1267-1270.

53. Cunnington AJ, Hormbrey P. Breath analysis to detect recent exposure to carbon monoxide. *Postgrad Med J.* 2002;78:233-237.

54. Damlapinar R, et al. Lactate level is more significant than carboxihemoglobin level in determining prognosis of carbon monoxide intoxication of childhood. *Pediatr Emerg Care.* 2016;32:377-383.

55. Davutoglu V, et al. Serum levels of NT-ProBNP as an early cardiac marker of carbon monoxide poisoning. *Inhal Toxicol.* 2006;18:155-158.

56. De Reuck J, et al. A positron emission tomography study of patients with acute carbon monoxide poisoning treated by hyperbaric oxygen. *J Neurol.* 1993;240:430-434.

57. De Salvia MA, et al. Irreversible impairment of active avoidance behavior in rats prenatally exposed to mild concentrations of carbon monoxide. *Psychopharmacology (Berl).* 1995;122:66-71.

58. Denays R, et al. Electroencephalographic mapping and 99mTc HMPAO single-photon emission computed tomography in carbon monoxide poisoning. *Ann Emerg Med.* 1994;24:947-952.

59. Dix-Cooper L, et al. Neurodevelopmental performance among school age children in rural Guatemala is associated with prenatal and postnatal exposure to carbon monoxide, a marker for exposure to woodsmoke. *Neurotoxicology.* 2012;33:246-254.

60. Dogan NO, et al. Can initial lactate levels predict the severity of unintentional carbon monoxide poisoning? *Hum Exp Toxicol.* 2015;34:324-329.

61. Dolan MC, et al. Carboxyhemoglobin levels in patients with flu-like symptoms. *Ann Emerg Med.* 1987;16:782-786.

62. Douglas ME, et al. Alteration of oxygen tension and oxyhemoglobin saturation. A hazard of sodium bicarbonate administration. *Arch Surg.* 1979;114:326-329.

63. Ducasse JL, et al. Non-comatose patients with acute carbon monoxide poisoning: hyperbaric or normobaric oxygenation? *Undersea Hyperb Med.* 1995;22:9-15.

64. Eberhardt M, et al. Noninvasive measurement of carbon monoxide levels in ED patients with headache. *J Med Toxicol.* 2006;2:89-92.

65. Elkharrat D, et al. Acute carbon monoxide intoxication and hyperbaric oxygen in pregnancy. *Intensive Care Med.* 1991;17:289-292.

66. Ely EW, et al. Warehouse workers' headache: emergency evaluation and management of 30 patients with carbon monoxide poisoning. *Am J Med.* 1995;98:145-155.

67. Fawcett TA, et al. Warehouse workers' headache. Carbon monoxide poisoning from propane-fueled forklifts. *J Occup Med.* 1992;34:12-15.

68. Feldman J, et al. Treatment of carbon monoxide poisoning with hyperbaric oxygen and therapeutic hypothermia. *Undersea Hyperb Med.* 2013;40:71-79.

69. Fife CEO, et al. A noninvasive method for rapid diagnosis of carbon monoxide poisoning. *Intern J Emerg Intensive Care Med.* 2001;5:1-8.

70. Gale SD, et al. MRI, quantitative MRI, SPECT, and neuropsychological findings following carbon monoxide poisoning. *Brain Inj.* 1999;13:229-243.

71. Garrabou G, et al. Mitochondrial injury in human acute carbon monoxide poisoning: the effect of oxygen treatment. *J Environ Sci Health C Environ Carcinog Ecotoxicol Rev.* 2011;29:32-51.

72. Gill JR, et al. The happy land homicides: 87 deaths due to smoke inhalation. *J Forensic Sci.* 2003;48:161-163.

73. Gilmer B, et al. Hyperbaric oxygen does not prevent neurologic sequelae after carbon monoxide poisoning. *Acad Emerg Med.* 2002;9:1-8.

74. Gilmer BT, et al. The protective effects of experimental neurodepressors on learning and memory following carbon monoxide poisoning. *J Toxicol Clin Toxicol.* 1999;37:606.

75. Ginsberg MD. Carbon monoxide intoxication: clinical features, neuropathology and mechanisms of injury. *J Toxicol Clin Toxicol.* 1985;23:281-288.

76. Ginsberg MD, Myers RE. Fetal brain damage following maternal carbon monoxide intoxication: an experimental study. *Acta Obstet Gynecol Scand.* 1974;53:309-317.

77. Ginsberg MD, Myers RE. Fetal brain injury after maternal carbon monoxide intoxication. Clinical and neuropathologic aspects. *Neurology.* 1976;26:15-23.

78. Ginsberg MD, et al. Experimental carbon monoxide encephalopathy in the primate. II. Clinical aspects, neuropathology, and physiologic correlation. *Arch Neurol.* 1974; 30:209-216.

79. Goldbaum LR, et al. Mechanism of the toxic action of carbon monoxide. *Ann Clin Lab Sci.* 1976;6:372-376.

80. Goldbaum LR, et al. What is the mechanism of carbon monoxide toxicity? *Aviat Space Environ Med.* 1975;46:1289-1291.

81. Gorman DF, et al. A longitudinal study of 100 consecutive admissions for carbon monoxide poisoning to the Royal Adelaide Hospital. *Anaesth Intensive Care.* 1992; 20:311-316.

82. Goulon M, et al. [Carbon monoxide poisoning and acute anoxia due to inhalation of coal gas and hydrocarbons: 302 cases, 273 treated by hyperbaric oxygen at 2 ata]. *Ann Med Interne (Paris).* 1969;120:335-349.

83. Graber JM, et al. Carbon monoxide: the case for environmental public health surveillance. *Public Health Rep.* 2007;122:138-144.

84. Grabowska T, et al. Prevalence of hydrogen cyanide and carboxyhaemoglobin in victims of smoke inhalation during enclosed-space fires: a combined toxicological risk. *Clin Toxicol (Phila).* 2012;50:759-763.

85. Hampson NB. Pulse oximetry in severe carbon monoxide poisoning. *Chest.* 1998; 114:1036-1041.

86. Hampson NB. Stability of carboxyhemoglobin in stored and mailed blood samples. *Am J Emerg Med.* 2008;26:191-195.

87. Hampson NB. Myth busting in carbon monoxide poisoning. *Am J Emerg Med.* 2016; 34:295-297.

88. Hampson NB. U.S. mortality due to carbon monoxide poisoning, 1999-2014. Accidental and intentional deaths. *Ann Am Thorac Soc.* 2016;13:1768-1774.

89. Hampson NB, et al. Diffusion of carbon monoxide through gypsum wallboard. *JAMA.* 2013;310:745-746.

90. Hampson NB, et al. Symptoms of carbon monoxide poisoning do not correlate with the initial carboxyhemoglobin level. *Undersea Hyperb Med.* 2012;39:657-665.

91. Hampson NB, Holm JR. Suicidal carbon monoxide poisoning has decreased with controls on automobile emissions. *Undersea Hyperb Med.* 2015;42:159-164.

92. Hampson NB, et al. Carbon monoxide poisoning from indoor burning of charcoal briquets. *JAMA.* 1994;271:52-53.

93. Hampson NB, Little CE. Hyperbaric treatment of patients with carbon monoxide poisoning in the United States. *Undersea Hyperb Med.* 2005;32:21-26.

94. Hampson NB, et al. Carbon monoxide poisoning: interpretation of randomized clinical trials and unresolved treatment issues. *Undersea Hyperb Med.* 2001;28:157-164.

95. Hampson NB, Norkool DM. Carbon monoxide poisoning in children riding in the back of pickup trucks. *JAMA.* 1992;267:538-540.

96. Hampson NB, Weaver LK. Carbon monoxide poisoning: a new incidence for an old disease. *Undersea Hyperb Med.* 2007;34:163-168.

97. Hampson NB, Zmaeff JL. Outcome of patients experiencing cardiac arrest with carbon monoxide poisoning treated with hyperbaric oxygen. *Ann Emerg Med.* 2001;38:36-41.

98. Han ST, et al. Xanthine oxidoreductase and neurological sequelae of carbon monoxide poisoning. *Toxicol Lett.* 2007;170:111-115.

99. Health. National Institute for Occupational Safety and Health . *NIOSH Pocket Guide to Chemical Hazards.* In: Department of Health and Human Services Centers for Disease Control and Prevention, National Institute for Occupational Safety and Health, ed. Vol DHHS Publication No. 2005-149. Washington, DC: U.S. Government Printing Offices; 2007.

100. Heckerling PS, et al. Occult carbon monoxide poisoning: validation of a prediction model. *Am J Med.* 1988;84:251-256.
101. Heckerling PS, et al. Predictors of occult carbon monoxide poisoning in patients with headache and dizziness. *Ann Intern Med.* 1987;107:174-176.
102. Henry CR, et al. Myocardial injury and long-term mortality following moderate to severe carbon monoxide poisoning. *JAMA.* 2006;295:398-402.
103. Hill EP, et al. Carbon monoxide exchanges between the human fetus and mother: a mathematical model. *Am J Physiol.* 1977;232:H311-323.
104. Hirsch AE, et al. Carbon monoxide poisonings from forklift use during produce packing operations. *J Agromed.* 2016;21:132-135.
105. Hopkins RO, et al. Basal ganglia lesions following carbon monoxide poisoning. *Brain Inj.* 2006;20:273-281.
106. Hopkins RO, et al. Apolipoprotein E genotype and response of carbon monoxide poisoning to hyperbaric oxygen treatment. *Am J Respir Crit Care Med.* 2007;176:1001-1006.
107. Hou X, et al. Diffusion tensor imaging for predicting the clinical outcome of delayed encephalopathy of acute carbon monoxide poisoning. *Eur Neurol.* 2013;69:275-280.
108. Huang CC, et al. Hyperbaric oxygen therapy is associated with lower short- and long-term mortality in patients with carbon monoxide poisoning. *Chest.* 2017;152:943-953.
109. Hullin T, et al. Correlation between clinical severity and different non-invasive measurements of carbon monoxide concentration: a population study. *PloS One.* 2017;12:e0174672.
110. Ide T, et al. Elevated S100B level in cerebrospinal fluid could predict poor outcome of carbon monoxide poisoning. *Am J Emerg Med.* 2012;30:222-225.
111. Iqbal S, et al. Carbon monoxide-related hospitalizations in the U.S.: evaluation of a web-based query system for public health surveillance. *Public Health Rep.* 2010;125:423-432.
112. Iqbal S, et al. Hospital burden of unintentional carbon monoxide poisoning in the United States, 2007. *Am J Emerg Med.* 2012;30:657-664.
113. Ishimaru H, et al. Effects of N-methyl-D-aspartate receptor antagonists on carbon monoxide-induced brain damage in mice. *J Pharmacol Exp Ther.* 1992;261:349-352.
114. Jackson EB Jr, et al. Pharmacologic modulators of soluble guanylate cyclase/cyclic guanosine monophosphate in the vascular system—from bench top to bedside. *Curr Vasc Pharmacol.* 2007;5:1-14.
115. Johnson-Arbor KK, et al. A comparison of carbon monoxide exposures after snowstorms and power outages. *Am J Prev Med.* 2014;46:481-486.
116. Jung YS, et al. Carbon monoxide-induced cardiomyopathy. *Circ J.* 2014;78:1437-1444.
117. Juric DM, et al. Hyperbaric oxygen preserves neurotrophic activity of carbon monoxide-exposed astrocytes. *Toxicol Lett.* 2016;253:1-6.
118. Kalay N, et al. Cardiovascular effects of carbon monoxide poisoning. *Am J Cardiol.* 2007;99:322-324.
119. Karaman D, et al. Neuropsychological evaluation of children and adolescents with acute carbon monoxide poisoning. *Pediatr Emerg Care.* 2016;32:303-306.
120. Kelley JS, Sophocleus GJ. Retinal hemorrhages in subacute carbon monoxide poisoning. Exposures in homes with blocked furnace flues. *JAMA.* 1978;239:1515-1517.
121. Klasner AE, et al. Carbon monoxide mass exposure in a pediatric population. *Acad Emerg Med.* 1998;5:992-996.
122. Koren G, et al. A multicenter, prospective study of fetal outcome following accidental carbon monoxide poisoning in pregnancy. *Reprod Toxicol.* 1991;5:397-403.
123. Krantz T, et al. Acute carbon monoxide poisoning. *Acta Anaesthesiol Scand.* 1988;32:278-282.
124. Krenzelok EP, et al. Carbon monoxide . . . the silent killer with an audible solution. *Am J Emerg Med.* 1996;14:484-486.
125. Kunsman GW, et al. Carbon monoxide stability in stored postmortem blood samples. *J Anal Toxicol.* 2000;24:572-578.
126. Kuroda H, et al. Altered white matter metabolism in delayed neurologic sequelae after carbon monoxide poisoning: a proton magnetic resonance spectroscopic study. *J Neurol Sci.* 2016;360:161-169.
127. Kurt F, et al. Does age affect presenting symptoms in children with carbon monoxide poisoning? *Pediatr Emerg Care.* 2013;29:916-921.
128. Lacey DJ. Neurologic sequelae of acute carbon monoxide intoxication. *Am J Dis Child.* 1981;135:145-147.
129. Lapresle J, Fardeau M. The central nervous system and carbon monoxide poisoning. II. Anatomical study of brain lesions following intoxication with carbon monoxide (22 cases). *Prog Brain Res.* 1967;24:31-74.
130. LaSala G, et al. The epidemiology and characteristics of carbon monoxide poisoning among recreational boaters. *Clin Toxicol (Phila).* 2015;53:127-130.
131. Lee FY, et al. Carbon monoxide poisoning and subsequent cardiovascular disease risk: a nationwide population-based cohort study. *Medicine.* 2015;94:e624.
132. Lee JH, et al. Incidence and clinical course of left ventricular systolic dysfunction in patients with carbon monoxide poisoning. *Korean Circ J.* 2016;46:665-671.
133. Lee MS, Marsden CD. Neurological sequelae following carbon monoxide poisoning clinical course and outcome according to the clinical types and brain computed tomography scan findings. *Mov Disord.* 1994;9:550-558.
134. Leikin JB, et al. Methylene chloride: report of five exposures and two deaths. *Am J Emerg Med.* 1990;8:534-537.
135. Levasseur L, et al. Effects of mode of inhalation of carbon monoxide and of normobaric oxygen administration on carbon monoxide elimination from the blood. *Hum Exp Toxicol.* 1996;15:898-903.
136. Livshits Z, et al. Falsely low carboxyhemoglobin level after hydroxocobalamin therapy. *N Engl J Med.* 2012;367:1270-1271.
137. Lo CP, et al. Brain injury after acute carbon monoxide poisoning: early and late complications. *AJR Am J Roentgenol.* 2007;189:W205-211.
138. Logue CJ. An inconvenient truth? *Ann Emerg Med.* 2008;51:339-340; author reply 340-332.
139. Longo LD. Carbon monoxide in the pregnant mother and fetus and its exchange across the placenta. *Ann N Y Acad Sci.* 1970;174:312-341.
140. Longo LD, Hill EP. Carbon monoxide uptake and elimination in fetal and maternal sheep. *Am J Physiol.* 1977;232:H324-330.
141. Mannaioni PF, et al. Carbon monoxide: the bad and the good side of the coin, from neuronal death to anti-inflammatory activity. *Inflamm Res.* 2006;55:261-273.
142. Mathieu D, et al. Acute carbon monoxide poisoning. Risk of late sequelae and treatment by hyperbaric oxygen. *J Toxicol Clin Toxicol.* 1985;23:315-324.
143. Mathieu D, et al. Randomized prospective study comparing the effect of HBO versus 12 hours of NBO in non comatose CO poisoned patients: results of the interim analysis. *Undersea Hyperb Med.* 1996;23(suppl):7-8.
144. McNulty JA, et al. Relationship of short-term verbal memory to the need for hyperbaric oxygen treatment after carbon monoxide poisoning. *Neuropsychiatry Neuropsychol Behav Neurol.* 1997;10:174-179.
145. Messier LD, Myers RA. A neuropsychological screening battery for emergency assessment of carbon-monoxide-poisoned patients. *J Clin Psychol.* 1991;47:675-684.
146. Miro O, et al. Oxidative damage on lymphocyte membranes is increased in patients suffering from acute carbon monoxide poisoning. *Toxicol Lett.* 1999;110:219-223.
147. Miro O, et al. Mitochondrial cytochrome c oxidase inhibition during acute carbon monoxide poisoning. *Pharmacol Toxicol.* 1998;82:199-202.
148. Miura T, et al. CT of the brain in acute carbon monoxide intoxication: characteristic features and prognosis. *AJNR Am J Neuroradiol.* 1985;6:739-742.
149. Molzhaninov EVC, et al. Experience and prospects of using hyperbaric oxygenation in obstetrics. Paper presented at Proceedings of the 7th International Congress on Hyperbaric Medicine, Moscow; 1981.
150. Moon JM, et al. The value of initial lactate in patients with carbon monoxide intoxication: in the emergency department. *Hum Exp Toxicol.* 2011;30:836-843.
151. Mott JA, et al. National vehicle emissions policies and practices and declining US carbon monoxide-related mortality. *JAMA.* 2002;288:988-995.
152. Myers RA, Britten JS. Are arterial blood gases of value in treatment decisions for carbon monoxide poisoning? *Crit Care Med.* 1989;17:139-142.
153. Myers RA, et al. Chronic carbon monoxide exposure: a clinical syndrome detected by neuropsychological tests. *J Clin Psychol.* 1998;54:555-567.
154. Myers RA, et al. Subacute sequelae of carbon monoxide poisoning. *Ann Emerg Med.* 1985;14:1163-1167.
155. Myers RAJ, et al. Carbon monoxide half-life study. Paper presented at: *Proceedings of the 9th International Congress on Hyperbaric Medicine*, Flagstaff, AZ; 1987.
156. Nager EC, O'Connor RE. Carbon monoxide poisoning from spray paint inhalation. *Acad Emerg Med.* 1998;5:84-86.
157. Norkool DM, Kirkpatrick JN. Treatment of acute carbon monoxide poisoning with hyperbaric oxygen: a review of 115 cases. *Ann Emerg Med.* 1985;14:1168-1171.
158. Oh BJ, et al. Treatment of acute carbon monoxide poisoning with induced hypothermia. *Clin Exp Emerg Med.* 2016;3:100-104.
159. Okeda R, et al. Comparative study on pathogenesis of selective cerebral lesions in carbon monoxide poisoning and nitrogen hypoxia in cats. *Acta Neuropathol.* 1982;56:265-272.
160. Okeda R, et al. The pathogenesis of carbon monoxide encephalopathy in the acute phase—physiological and morphological correlation. *Acta Neuropathol.* 1981;54:1-10.
161. Otten EJ, et al. An evaluation of carboxyhemoglobin spot tests. *Ann Emerg Med.* 1985;14:850-852.
162. Ozyurt A, et al. Effects of acute carbon monoxide poisoning on ECG and echocardiographic parameters in children. *Cardiovasc Toxicol.* 2017;17:326-334.
163. Ozyurt G, et al. Comparison of SPECT findings and neuropsychological sequelae in carbon monoxide and organophosphate poisoning. *Clin Toxicol (Phila).* 2008;46:218-221.
164. Pace R, et al. Effects of hydroxocobalamin on carboxyhemoglobin measured under physiologic and pathologic conditions. *Clin Toxicol (Phila).* 2014;52:647-650.
165. Pang L, et al. Neuroprotective effects of erythropoietin in patients with carbon monoxide poisoning. *J Biochem Mol Toxicol.* 2013;27:266-271.
166. Pang L, et al. Erythropoietin protects rat brain injury from carbon monoxide poisoning by inhibiting Toll-like receptor 4/NF-kappa B-dependent inflammatory responses. *Inflammation.* 2016;39:561-568.
167. Parkinson RB, et al. White matter hyperintensities and neuropsychological outcome following carbon monoxide poisoning. *Neurology.* 2002;58:1525-1532.
168. Penney DG. Acute carbon monoxide poisoning in an animal model: the effects of altered glucose on morbidity and mortality. *Toxicology.* 1993;80:85-101.
169. Penney DG, Chen K. NMDA receptor-blocker ketamine protects during acute carbon monoxide poisoning, while calcium channel-blocker verapamil does not. *J Appl Toxicol.* 1996;16:297-304.
170. Pepe G, et al. Delayed neuropsychological sequelae after carbon monoxide poisoning: predictive risk factors in the Emergency Department. A retrospective study. *Scand J Trauma Resusc Emerg Med.* 2011;19:16.
171. Peterson JE, Stewart RD. Absorption and elimination of carbon monoxide by inactive young men. *Arch Environ Health.* 1970;21:165-171.

172. Piantadosi CA, et al. Apoptosis and delayed neuronal damage after carbon monoxide poisoning in the rat. *Exp Neurol.* 1997;147:103-114.

173. Porter SS, et al. Corpus callosum atrophy and neuropsychological outcome following carbon monoxide poisoning. *Arch Clin Neuropsychol.* 2002;17:195-204.

174. Raphael JC, et al. Trial of normobaric and hyperbaric oxygen for acute carbon monoxide intoxication. *Lancet.* 1989;2:414-419.

175. Rasmussen LS, et al. Biochemical markers for brain damage after carbon monoxide poisoning. *Acta Anaesthesiol Scand.* 2004;48:469-473.

176. Ratney RS, et al. In vivo conversion of methylene chloride to carbon monoxide. *Arch Environ Health.* 1974;28:223-226.

177. Rioux JP, Myers RA. Hyperbaric oxygen for methylene chloride poisoning: report on two cases. *Ann Emerg Med.* 1989;18:691-695.

178. Risser D, et al. Should coroners be able to recognize unintentional carbon monoxide-related deaths immediately at the death scene? *J Forensic Sci.* 1995;40:596-598.

179. Roth D, et al. Accuracy of noninvasive multiwave pulse oximetry compared with carboxyhemoglobin from blood gas analysis in unselected emergency department patients. *Ann Emerg Med.* 2011;58:74-79.

180. Roughton FJWD. The effect of carbon monoxide on the oxyhemoglobin dissociation curve. *Am J Physiol.* 1944;141:17-31.

181. Sanders RW, et al. Seizure during hyperbaric oxygen therapy for carbon monoxide toxicity: a case series and five-year experience. *J Emerg Med.* 2012;42:e69-72.

182. Scheinkestel CD, et al. Hyperbaric or normobaric oxygen for acute carbon monoxide poisoning: a randomised controlled clinical trial. *Med J Aust.* 1999;170:203-210.

183. Sebbane M, et al. Emergency department management of suspected carbon monoxide poisoning: role of pulse CO-oximetry. *Respir Care.* 2013;58:1614-1620.

184. Shapiro AB, et al. Carbon monoxide and myonecrosis: a prospective study. *Vet Hum Toxicol.* 1989;31:136-137.

185. Shimazu T, et al. Smoke inhalation injury and the effect of carbon monoxide in the sheep model. *J Trauma.* 1990;30:170-175.

186. Shusterman D, et al. Predictors of carbon monoxide and hydrogen cyanide exposure in smoke inhalation patients. *J Toxicol Clin Toxicol.* 1996;34:61-71.

187. Sircar K, et al. Carbon monoxide poisoning deaths in the United States, 1999 to 2012. *Am J Emerg Med.* 2015;33:1140-1145.

188. Sloan EP, et al. Complications and protocol considerations in carbon monoxide-poisoned patients who require hyperbaric oxygen therapy: report from a ten-year experience. *Ann Emerg Med.* 1989;18:629-634.

189. Sokal JA, Kralkowska E. The relationship between exposure duration, carboxyhemoglobin, blood glucose, pyruvate and lactate and the severity of intoxication in 39 cases of acute carbon monoxide poisoning in man. *Arch Toxicol.* 1985;57:196-199.

190. Stewart RD, et al. Carboxyhemoglobin levels in American blood donors. *JAMA.* 1974;229:1187-1195.

191. Stewart RD, Hake CL. Paint-remover hazard. *JAMA.* 1976;235:398-401.

192. Stewart RD, et al. Experimental human exposure to high concentrations of carbon monoxide. *Arch Environ Health.* 1973;26:1-7.

193. Suner S, et al. Non-invasive pulse CO-oximetry screening in the emergency department identifies occult carbon monoxide toxicity. *J Emerg Med.* 2008;34:441-450.

194. Sutariya BB, et al. Hypothermia following acute carbon-monoxide poisoning increases mortality. *Toxicol Lett.* 1990;52:201-208.

195. Takeuchi A, et al. A simple "new" method to accelerate clearance of carbon monoxide. *Am J Respir Crit Care Med.* 2000;161:1816-1819.

196. Taskiran D, et al. Mitochondrial oxidative stress in female and male rat brain after ex vivo carbon monoxide treatment. *Hum Exp Toxicol.* 2007;26:645-651.

197. Teksam M, et al. Diffusion-weighted MR imaging findings in carbon monoxide poisoning. *Neuroradiology.* 2002;44:109-113.

198. Teksam O, et al. Acute cardiac effects of carbon monoxide poisoning in children. *Eur J Emerg Med.* 2010;17:192-196.

199. Thom SR. Carbon monoxide-mediated brain lipid peroxidation in the rat. *J Appl Physiol (1985).* 1990;68:997-1003.

200. Thom SR. Dehydrogenase conversion to oxidase and lipid peroxidation in brain after carbon monoxide poisoning. *J Appl Physiol (1985).* 1992;73:1584-1589.

201. Thom SR. Leukocytes in carbon monoxide-mediated brain oxidative injury. *Toxicol Appl Pharmacol.* 1993;123:234-247.

202. Thom SR, et al. Delayed neuropathology after carbon monoxide poisoning is immune-mediated. *Proc Natl Acad Sci U S A.* 2004;101:13660-13665.

203. Thom SR, et al. Intravascular neutrophil activation due to carbon monoxide poisoning. *Am J Respir Crit Care Med.* 2006;174:1239-1248.

204. Thom SR, et al. Plasma biomarkers in carbon monoxide poisoning. *Clin Toxicol (Phila).* 2010;48:47-56.

205. Thom SR, et al. Role of nitric oxide-derived oxidants in vascular injury from carbon monoxide in the rat. *Am J Physiol.* 1999;276(3 Pt 2):H984-992.

206. Thom SR, et al. Adaptive responses and apoptosis in endothelial cells exposed to carbon monoxide. *Proc Natl Acad Sci U S A.* 2000;97:1305-1310.

207. Thom SR, et al. Neuronal nitric oxide synthase and N-methyl-D-aspartate neurons in experimental carbon monoxide poisoning. *Toxicol Appl Pharmacol.* 2004;194:280-295.

208. Thom SR, et al. Release of glutathione from erythrocytes and other markers of oxidative stress in carbon monoxide poisoning. *J Appl Physiol (1985).* 1997;82:1424-1432.

209. Thom SR, Keim LW. Carbon monoxide poisoning: a review epidemiology, pathophysiology, clinical findings, and treatment options including hyperbaric oxygen therapy. *J Toxicol Clin Toxicol.* 1989;27:141-156.

210. Thom SR, et al. Inhibition of human neutrophil beta2-integrin-dependent adherence by hyperbaric O2. *Am J Physiol.* 1997;272(3 Pt 1):C770-777.

211. Thom SR, et al. Delayed neuropsychologic sequelae after carbon monoxide poisoning: prevention by treatment with hyperbaric oxygen. *Ann Emerg Med.* 1995;25:474-480.

212. Tikuisis P. Modeling the uptake and elimination of carbon monoxide. In: Penney DG, ed. *Carbon Monoxide.* Boca Raton, FL: CRC Press; 1996:45-67.

213. Tom T, et al. Neuroimaging characteristics in carbon monoxide toxicity. *J Neuroimaging.* 1996;6:161-166.

214. Touger M, et al. Performance of the RAD-57 pulse CO-oximeter compared with standard laboratory carboxyhemoglobin measurement. *Ann Emerg Med.* 2010;56:382-388.

215. Tsai CF, et al. The impacts of acute carbon monoxide poisoning on the brain: longitudinal clinical and 99mTc ethyl cysteinate brain SPECT characterization of patients with persistent and delayed neurological sequelae. *Clin Neurol Neurosurg.* 2014;119:21-27.

216. Turner M, et al. Carbon monoxide poisoning treated with hyperbaric oxygen: metabolic acidosis as a predictor of treatment requirements. *J Accid Emerg Med.* 1999;16:96-98.

217. Van Hoesen KB, et al. Should hyperbaric oxygen be used to treat the pregnant patient for acute carbon monoxide poisoning? A case report and literature review. *JAMA.* 1989;261:1039-1043.

218. Van Sickle D, et al. Carbon monoxide poisoning in Florida during the 2004 hurricane season. *Am J Prev Med.* 2007;32:340-346.

219. Vreman HJ, et al. Carbon monoxide and carboxyhemoglobin. *Adv Pediatr.* 1995;42:303-334.

220. Vreman HJ, et al. Interference of fetal hemoglobin with the spectrophotometric measurement of carboxyhemoglobin. *Clin Chem.* 1988;34:975-977.

221. Watanabe S, et al. Transient degradation of myelin basic protein in the rat hippocampus following acute carbon monoxide poisoning. *Neurosci Res.* 2010;68:232-240.

222. Wattel F, et al. [A 25-year study (1983-2008) of children's health outcomes after hyperbaric oxygen therapy for carbon monoxide poisoning in utero]. *Bull Acad Natl Med.* 2013;197:677-694; discussion 695-677.

223. Weaver LK. Clinical practice. Carbon monoxide poisoning. *N Engl J Med.* 2009;360:1217-1225.

224. Weaver LK. Carbon monoxide poisoning. In: Weaver LK, ed. *Hyperbaric Oxygen Therapy Indications.* North Palm Beach, FL: Best Publishing Company; 2014:47-66.

225. Weaver LK, Deru K. Carbon monoxide poisoning at motels, hotels, and resorts. *Am J Prev Med.* 2007;33:23-27.

226. Weaver LK, et al. Hyperbaric oxygen for acute carbon monoxide poisoning. *N Engl J Med.* 2002;347:1057-1067.

227. Weaver LK, et al. Carboxyhemoglobin half-life in carbon monoxide-poisoned patients treated with 100% oxygen at atmospheric pressure. *Chest.* 2000;117:801-808.

228. Weaver LK, et al. Carbon monoxide poisoning: risk factors for cognitive sequelae and the role of hyperbaric oxygen. *Am J Respir Crit Care Med.* 2007;176:491-497.

229. Westphal M, et al. Affinity of carbon monoxide to hemoglobin increases at low oxygen fractions. *Biochem Biophys Res Commun.* 2002;295:975-977.

230. Widdop B. Analysis of carbon monoxide. *Ann Clin Biochem.* 2002;39(Pt 4):378-391.

231. Wolf SJ, et al. Clinical policy: critical issues in the management of adult patients presenting to the emergency department with acute carbon monoxide poisoning. *J Emerg Nurs.* 2008;34:e19-32.

232. Wolf SJ, et al. Clinical policy: critical issues in the evaluation and management of adult patients presenting to the emergency department with acute carbon monoxide poisoning. *Ann Emerg Med.* 2017;69:98-107.e106.

233. Wong CS, et al. Increased Long-term risk of dementia in patients with carbon monoxide poisoning: a population-based study. *Medicine.* 2016;95:e2549.

234. Wrenn K, Conners GP. Carbon monoxide poisoning during ice storms: a tale of two cities. *J Emerg Med.* 1997;15:465-467.

235. Xiang W, et al. Combined application of dexamethasone and hyperbaric oxygen therapy yields better efficacy for patients with delayed encephalopathy after acute carbon monoxide poisoning. *Drug Design Devel Ther.* 2017;11:513-519.

236. Xiang W, et al. Efficacy of N-butylphthalide and hyperbaric oxygen therapy on cognitive dysfunction in patients with delayed encephalopathy after acute carbon monoxide poisoning. *Med Sci Monit.* 2017;23:1501-1506.

237. Xu J, et al. Carbon monoxide inhalation increases microparticles causing vascular and CNS dysfunction. *Toxicol Appl Pharmacol.* 2013;273:410-417.

238. Yarar C, et al. Analysis of the features of acute carbon monoxide poisoning and hyperbaric oxygen therapy in children. *Turk J Pediatr.* 2008;50:235-241.

239. Yoshii F, et al. Magnetic resonance imaging and 11C-N-methylspiperone/positron emission tomography studies in a patient with the interval form of carbon monoxide poisoning. *J Neurol Sci.* 1998;160:87-91.

240. Zeiss J, Brinker R. Role of contrast enhancement in cerebral CT of carbon monoxide poisoning. *J Comput Assist Tomogr.* 1988;12:341-343.

241. Ziser A, et al. Delayed hyperbaric oxygen treatment for acute carbon monoxide poisoning. *Br Med J (Clin Res Ed).* 1984;289:960.

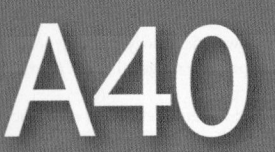

HYPERBARIC OXYGEN

Stephen R. Thom

INTRODUCTION

Hyperbaric oxygen (HBO) is used therapeutically in poisoning by carbon monoxide (CO) (alone or if complicated by cyanide {CN} poisoning), methylene chloride, hydrogen sulfide (H_2S), and carbon tetrachloride (CCl_4). It is also a recognized therapy for air or gas embolism, such as may arise from ingestion of hydrogen peroxide (H_2O_2), and for anemia, a functional form of which arises from oxidants that induce methemoglobinemia.

HISTORY

Hyperbaric medicine became established as a clinical discipline in the latter half of the 20th century with a focus on treatment of decompression sickness. Utilization of hyperbaric chambers has expanded in the past 60 years with improved understanding of basic mechanisms of action. The first case reports of HBO for documented CO poisoning appeared in 1960,[203] and the consistent application of HBO in CO poisoning began in many centers at that time.[200] The first report presenting statistical evidence of the superiority of HBO compared with normobaric oxygen in CO poisoning, as well as a description of the "late syndrome," was published in 1969.[76]

PHARMACOLOGY

Chemistry and Preparation

Pressures applied while patients are in the hyperbaric chamber usually are 2 to 3 atmospheres absolute (ATA); sea level air pressure equals 1 ATA. Treatments generally last for 1.5 to 8 hours, depending on the indication, and are performed one to three times daily. Monoplace (single-person) chambers usually are compressed with pure oxygen. Multiplace (2–14 patients treated simultaneously) chambers are pressurized with air, and patients breathe pure oxygen through a tight-fitting face mask, a head tent, or an endotracheal tube as clinically indicated.

Mechanisms of Action

During treatment, the arterial oxygen tension typically exceeds, 1,500 mm Hg and achieves tissue oxygen tensions of 200 to 400 mm Hg—more than fivefold higher than when breathing air.[214] While one is breathing air under normal environmental conditions, hemoglobin is saturated with oxygen on passage through the pulmonary microvasculature, and the primary effect of HBO is to increase the dissolved oxygen content of plasma. In addition, HBO affects neutrophil adhesion to blood vessels and restores mitochondrial, neutrophil, and immunologic disturbances caused by CO poisoning.

Pharmacokinetics

Oxygen inhaled at hyperbaric pressure is rapidly absorbed. Application of each additional atmosphere of pressure while breathing 100% oxygen increases the dissolved oxygen concentration in the plasma by 2.2 mL O_2/dL (vol%) (Chap. 28). Animal models of focal ischemia suggest that HBO rapidly distributes to target organs to improve penumbral oxygenation.[210] Hyperbaric oxygen increases tissue oxygen concentration and wound oxygen delivery in humans.[182] Regarding pharmaceutical interactions, hyperbaric hyperoxia does not appear to produce appreciable alterations in the pharmacokinetics of pentobarbital, salicylate, or theophylline in canine models[117-119] or gentamicin in healthy human volunteers.[151]

Pharmacodynamics

There are transient benefits from HBO for reducing bubble volume in disorders such as air embolism and oxygenating tissues in conditions in which hemoglobin-based O_2 delivery is impaired. These rather straightforward mechanisms form the basis for using HBO for patients with massive ingestions of H_2O_2 associated with intravascular gas embolism and for life-threatening poisonings from CN, H_2S, and exposure to oxidizers causing methemoglobin. Hyperbaric oxygen is also used for CCl_4 poisoning, in which acute application of oxygen and pressure inhibit the cytochrome P450 oxidase system responsible for producing hepatotoxic free radicals.[30,145] Hyperbaric oxygen also has well-described vasoconstriction effects[340,208,228] compared with dynamic CO-associated effects on cerebral vasodilation.[130]

Recent years have shown that benefits persisting beyond the short period when a patient is in a hyperbaric chamber are related to production of reactive oxygen species (ROS) and reactive nitrogen species.[217,218] Reactive species can have positive and negative effects that depend on the concentration of reactant generated and its intracellular localization. Hence, with regard to HBO, as with any xenobiotic, the precise dose defines the risks and benefits of therapy. Because exposure to hyperoxia in typical clinical HBO protocols is rather brief, most studies show that antioxidant defenses are adequate to avoid tissue injuries.[54,55,183,232]

There are at least four separate therapeutic mechanisms supporting the use of O_2 when treating CO poisoning. Administration of supplemental O_2 is a historical cornerstone for treatment based on reducing body burden of carboxyhemoglobin (COHb). Elevated COHb results in tissue hypoxia, and exogenous O_2 both hastens dissociation of CO from hemoglobin and provides enhanced tissue oxygenation directly through the increased PaO_2. Hyperbaric oxygen causes COHb dissociation to occur at a rate greater than that achievable by breathing 100% O_2 at sea level pressure.[168] Additionally, HBO accelerates restoration of mitochondrial oxidative processes.[28] Among the earliest events observed in both an animal model and in humans with CO poisoning is platelet–neutrophil interactions that mediate intravascular neutrophil activation. These changes precipitate neutrophil adherence to blood vessel walls that initiate vascular changes, leading to a cascade of localized changes in brain that cause neurological dysfunction (Fig. A40–1).[100,219,225] Animal studies indicate that CO-mediated neurologic dysfunction is related to an immune responses to modified myelin basic protein (MBP), impaired neurogenesis associated with diminished production of nerve growth factor, brain-derived neurotrophic factor and neurotrophin-3, and circulating proinflammatory microparticles.[33,35,106,167,210] The presence of MBP in cerebrospinal fluid of CO-poisoned patients appears to serve as a predictive marker for the onset and persistence of CO-mediated encephalopathy.[221]

Timely intervention with HBO in animal models causes rapid improvement in cardiovascular status,[60] leads to lower mortality rates,[171] abrogates changes in MBP, and preserves synthesis of nerve growth factors.[35,106,167,210,239] As a late intervention, approximately 1 month after CO poisoning and the onset of delayed neurologic deterioration, mesenchymal stem cell infusion has been explored to restore neuronal integrity when late use of HBO had no benefit.[201] Benefits of HBO are likely based on improved oxygenation and maintenance of mitochondrial function as well as inhibition of neutrophil adhesion. Exposure to 2.8 to 3.0 ATA O_2 for 45 minutes temporarily inhibits neutrophil adherence to endothelium mediated by the activation-dependent β_2-integrins on the neutrophil membrane in both rodents and humans.[43,107,121,215,226] The ability of HBO to inhibit function of neutrophil β_2-integrin adhesion molecules in animal models forms the basis for amelioration of encephalopathy resulting from CO poisoning, decompression

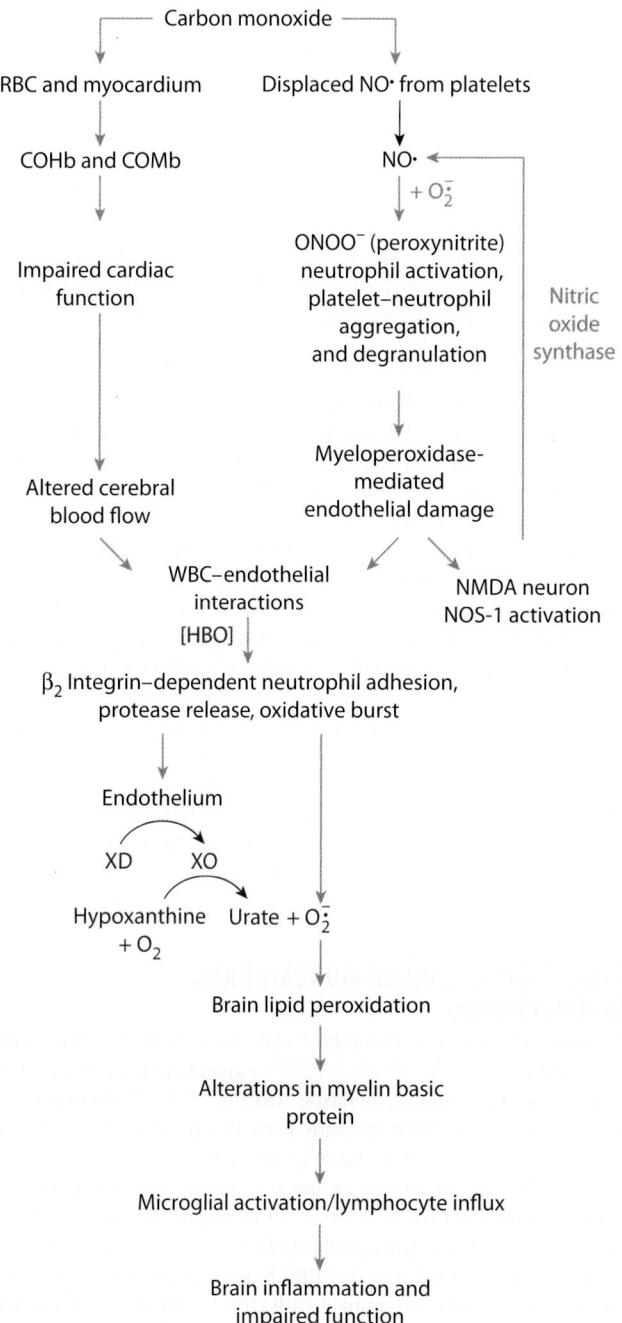

Carbon monoxide

RBC and myocardium   Displaced NO• from platelets

COHb and COMb   NO•

$+ O_2^{\bar{\cdot}}$

ONOO⁻ (peroxynitrite) neutrophil activation, platelet–neutrophil aggregation, and degranulation

Nitric oxide synthase

Impaired cardiac function

Myeloperoxidase-mediated endothelial damage

Altered cerebral blood flow

WBC–endothelial interactions

NMDA neuron NOS-1 activation

[HBO]

β_2 Integrin–dependent neutrophil adhesion, protease release, oxidative burst

Endothelium

XD   XO

Hypoxanthine   Urate $+ O_2^{\bar{\cdot}}$
$+ O_2$

Brain lipid peroxidation

Alterations in myelin basic protein

Microglial activation/lymphocyte influx

Brain inflammation and impaired function

FIGURE A40–1. The pathway demonstrating concurrent events leading to vascular injury with carbon monoxide poisoning and the sequence of events leading to neurologic injuries. COHb = carboxyhemoglobin; COMb = carboxymyoglobin; NMDA = *N*-methyl-D-aspartate neurons; NO• = nitric oxide; NO_2 = nitrite (major oxidation product of NO•); NOS-1 = neuronal nitric oxide synthase; $O_2^{\bar{\cdot}}$ = superoxide radical; ONOO⁻ = peroxynitrite; RBC = erythrocyte; WBC = leukocyte; XD = xanthine dehydrogenase; XO = xanthine oxidase.

sickness, and smoke-induced lung injury, as well as reperfusion injuries of brain, heart, lung, liver, and skeletal muscle.[8,111,144,211,212,215,229,233,238,254,256,257] Hyperbaric oxygen inhibits neutrophil β_2 integrin expression, but not its expression on other circulating leukocytes that proceeds from reactive nitrogen species generation by type 2 nitric oxide synthase and myeloperoxidase present in neutrophil-specific α-granules. That is, the presence of both enzymes within the same granules is required to generate the requisite reactive agents that inhibit neutrophil adherence. The reaction leads to excessive *S*-nitrosylation of cytoskeletal β actin, which in turn impedes the function of β_2 integrins.[221] This leads to modifications in cytoskeletal regulation of a number of proteins[223,224] without reducing neutrophil viability and functions

such as degranulation and oxidative burst in response to chemoattractants remain intact.[215,223,226] It is important to comment that use of HBO at less than 2.8 ATA, as used in several clinical HBO studies, does not inhibit neutrophil adherence functions.[7,91,127]

ROLE IN CARBON MONOXIDE POISONING

Survivors of CO poisoning are faced with potential impairments to cardiac and neurologic functions. Carbon monoxide poisoning causes acute cardiac compromise, including potentially reversible left ventricular dysfunction.[86,129] Survivors appear to exhibit an increased risk for cardiovascular related death in the subsequent 10 years,[88,175] although a study suggests that an excess mortality rate is more closely associated with neurologic and psychological factors.[136] Some patients exhibit acute abnormalities wherein they have impaired consciousness or focal neurologic findings from the time of initial presentation and never recover.[3,49,52,71] Other patients seemingly recover from acute poisoning, but then manifest neurologic or neuropsychiatric abnormalities from 2 days to about 5 weeks after poisoning.[44,57,75,96,140,148,152,161,176,193,196,227,248] Events occurring after a clear or "lucid" interval are termed "subacute" or "delayed" neurologic sequelae. These terms have gained popularity and have some clinical utility, but animal studies suggest neuropathology is more of a continuum. That is, various pathways of injury occur in close proximity, and in some cases, they occur concomitantly.[70,101,149,162,219,220,225]

Since 1960, HBO has been used with increasing frequency for severe CO poisoning because clinical recovery appeared to improve beyond that expected with ambient pressure oxygen therapy. Support for HBO use comes from this experience.[75,76,97,122,147,161,164,181] The clinical efficacy of HBO for acute CO poisoning has been assessed in six prospective, randomized trials published in peer-reviewed journals. Only one clinical trial satisfies all items deemed to be necessary for the highest quality of randomized controlled trials.[248] This double-blinded, placebo-controlled clinical trial involved 152 patients who received treatment with either three sessions of HBO therapy or normobaric O_2 with sham pressurization to maintain blinding. The group treated with HBO had a lower incidence of cognitive sequelae than the group treated with NBO after adjustment for pretreatment cerebellar dysfunction and stratification (odds ratio, 0.45; 95% confidence interval 0.22–0.92; $P = 0.03$).

The only other blinded, prospective, randomized trial was published in 1999, and it involved 191 patients of different severity treated with either daily HBO (2.8 ATA for 60 minutes) with intervening high-flow oxygen for 3 or 6 days versus high flow normobaric oxygen for 3 or 6 days.[188] Additional HBO treatments (up to six daily) were performed in patients without adequate neurologic recovery. The primary outcome measure for this trial was testing performed at completion of treatment (3–6 days) and not from long term follow-up. This study had a high rate of adverse neurologic outcomes in all patients, regardless of treatment assignment. Neurologic sequelae were reported in 74% of HBO-treated patients and in 68% of control participants. No other clinical trial has described this magnitude of neurologic dysfunction. The high incidence may be related to the assessment tool, which could not discern true neurologic impairments from poor test taking related to depression.[189] Suicide attempts with CO represented 69% of cases in this trial. Moreover, 54% of participants were lost to follow-up. Outcomes at 1 month were not reported but were stated to show no difference. Multiple statistical comparisons were reported without apparent planning or the requisite statistical correction. Both treatment arms received continuous supplemental mask O_2 for 3 days between their hyperbaric treatments (both true HBO and "sham"), resulting in greater overall O_2 doses than conventional therapy. Multiple flaws in the design and execution of this study are discussed in the literature, so it is impossible to draw meaningful conclusions from the data.[82,157] Despite these issues, conclusions from this trial were accepted in systematic reviews.[29,252]

Other randomized trials of HBO for CO poisoning were not blinded. The first prospective clinical trial involving HBO therapy did not demonstrate therapeutic benefits.[176] This study was criticized because the authors used a low (insufficient) oxygen partial pressure (2 ATA) versus the more usual protocols with 2.5 to 3 ATA, an unvalidated questionnaire to assess neurologic function, and because nearly half of the patients received hyperbaric treatments more than 6 hours after they were identified.[27] This 1989 study protocol was repeated again in a more recent trial with no modifications despite the criticisms identified more than a decade earlier. Not surprisingly, the outcome was virtually the same. If study results are expressed on an intention-to-treat basis, patients with transient loss of consciousness had an incidence of neurologic sequelae based on the self-assessment questionnaire of 48%, and those treated with HBO had an incidence of 51%. Patients with initial coma who were treated once with HBO had an incidence of sequelae of 47%; patients who were treated with two HBO treatments had an incidence of sequelae of 60% (not significantly different from any of the other groups).[6]

Hyperbaric oxygen was effective in several other prospective investigations. In a trial involving mildly to moderately poisoned patients, 23% of patients (7 of 30) treated with ambient pressure oxygen developed neurologic sequelae, but no patients (0/30; $P < 0.05$) who were treated with HBO (2.8 ATA) developed sequelae.[227] In another prospective, randomized trial, 26 patients were hospitalized within 2 hours of discovery and were equally divided between two treatment groups: ambient pressure oxygen or 2.5 ATA O_2.[57] Three weeks later, patients treated with HBO had significantly fewer abnormalities on electroencephalogram, and single-photon emission computed tomography scans showed that cerebral vessels had nearly normal reactivity to carbon dioxide, in contrast to diminished reactivity in patients treated with ambient pressure oxygen.

In conclusion, the efficacy of HBO for acute CO poisoning is supported in animal trials, and studies provide a mechanistic basis for treatment. In this era of evidence-based medicine, a great deal of emphasis has been placed on systematic reviews, which have stressed the need for new studies because of the range in quality of published clinical trials.[29,252] A practice-based recommendation is that HBO should be administered in all cases of serious acute CO poisoning and normobaric 100% oxygen continued until the time of HBO administration is based on existing studies with the best design that most closely address the actual practical handling of patients.[85] We support this opinion, but readers should note that this perspective is not shared by the American College of Emergency Physicians Clinical Policies Subcommittee.[251] In their policy statement, they conclude that published studies are generally inconclusive.

Carbon monoxide–poisoned patients who receive three HBO treatments within 24 hours after presentation manifest approximately half the rate of cognitive sequelae at 6 weeks, 6 months, and 12 months after treatment as those treated with only normobaric oxygen. Risk factors for long-term cognitive impairment in patients not treated with HBO include age older than 36 years, exposure longer than 24 hours, loss of consciousness, and COHb greater than 25%. Recommendations for children can pose special challenges, but in clinical series, there appear to be no marked differences in clinical manifestations compared with those reported in adults.[64,84,114,172] Pregnancy poses another special situation in that CO readily crosses the placenta and may cause fetal distress and fetal death. Hyperbaric oxygen has been administered safely to pregnant women, but there are no prospective studies of efficacy, in CO poisoned women so standard adult guidelines for treatment are reasonable.

One study demonstrates that HBO was only beneficial in reducing neurologic sequelae among patients who do not possess the apolipoprotein ε4 allele.[93] Because genotype is typically unknown, this report does not alter existing treatment guidelines, but it may become important for future research. Although the basic mechanisms are unknown, it is well established that the apolipoprotein genotype can have profound effects on risk for a variety of neuropathological events.[1,66,150,186] Whether apolipoprotein ε4 modifies the primary pathophysiological insults of CO or the mechanisms of HBO is currently unknown. As of yet, no objective method is available for staging the severity of CO poisoning, although preliminary reports suggest plasma markers may be used in the future.[220] Psychometric screening tests have not proved reliable because abnormalities during the initial screening do not correlate with development of delayed sequelae.[227]

ROLE IN METHYLENE CHLORIDE POISONING

Methylene chloride (CH_2Cl_2) is an organic solvent used commercially in aerosol sprays, as a solvent in plastics manufacturing, in photographic film production, in food processing as a degreaser, and as a paint stripper (eg, for bathtub refinishing).[41] It is readily absorbed through the skin or by inhalation. Immediate effects of methylene chloride are attributable to the direct depressant actions of this solvent on the central nervous system (CNS) and resulting hypoxia. There are two metabolic pathways involved in its metabolism: an oxidative one mediated by cytochrome P450 enzymes, mainly CYP2E1, that appears to involve a metabolic-switch or two-active site process, and another pathway mediated by glutathione (GSH) that involves mainly glutathione S-transferases (GST).[61,206] The P450 pathways generate formyl chloride and CO, with a secondary conjugation of formyl chloride to GSH. The separate GSH–GST pathway involves conjugation of methylene chloride, primarily by metabolism through GST-θ, to generate CO_2 as well as DNA adducts. These GSH–GST conjugation pathway DNA adducts play a role in late-onset carcinogenesis.[241,242] Acute methylene chloride toxicity has many of the same clinical manifestations as CO poisoning.[202] Production of CO is slow, and peak COHb levels of 10% to 50% are reportedly delayed for 8 hours or more.[39,42,62,109,123,140,141,195,206] Effects that are present after 1 hour or more, particularly if the COHb level is elevated, may be partially caused by CO toxicity. Anecdotal reports of HBO treatment for methylene chloride poisoning report both success and failure, which likely reflect additional confounding because of solvent toxicity.[37,115,180,184,255] Hyperbaric oxygen treatment recommendations, using a standard three treatment protocol, follow those in patients meeting the aforementioned considerations in CO poisoning. Additional treatments in the setting of ongoing CO production and persistent or recurring symptoms will likely necessitate additional treatments as the methylene chloride is mobilized from peripheral stores and undergoes metabolism.[124] Prolonged normobaric 100% oxygen therapy is reasonable in patients with HBO contraindicatons.[94,177]

ROLE IN COMBINED CARBON MONOXIDE AND CYANIDE POISONING

Carbon monoxide and CN poisonings can occur concomitantly from smoke inhalation.[4,5,12-15,21,46,51,137,139,155,194,198,244,249] Experimental evidence suggests that they can produce synergistic toxicity.[10,158,165,168,173] Animal studies demonstrate that ambient pressure 100% O_2 can protect against CN toxicity[191] and can enhance CN metabolism to thiocyanate when thiosulfate is used concomitantly.[23] Hyperbaric oxygen also appears to have either direct effects on reducing CN toxicity[50,102,103,127,199,213] or augmenting the effects of other antidotes, including hydroxycobalamin.[34,120,128,191,246] However, animal studies have not uniformly found that HBO improves outcome,[245] and clinical experience regarding CN treatment with HBO is sparse.[3,74,190] In a series of symptomatic smoke inhalation victims with elevated concentrations of both CO and CN who received HBO and treatment for CN involving sodium nitrite and sodium thiosulfate, four of five patients survived without apparent neurologic damage.[89] Clinical case reports in which HBO was used along with standard antidote treatment (sodium nitrite plus sodium thiosulfate) for isolated CN poisonings are equivocal regarding benefit.[74,134,190,230] One case showed dramatic improvement,[230] but another showed none.[134] As one might expect, HBO does not appear to modify blood CN concentrations.[221] Methemoglobin formation with the standard antidote treatment involving nitrite is not thought to generate high enough methemoglobin concentrations to be of concern, but in the setting of concomitant COHb, the additional reduction of oxygen-carrying capacity poses a potential risk.[80,113] Hence, there is a special advantage for hydroxycobalamin use in combined poisonings. Further research in this area is necessary. Because CN is among the most lethal poisons and toxicity is rapid, standard antidotal therapy for isolated CN poisoning is of primary importance. Hyperbaric oxygen is reasonable in any case of dual (CO and CN) poisoning and in CN poisoning when vital signs and mental status do not improve with antidote treatment. Possible use of HBO therapy may change as data on alternative antidotes such as hydroxycobalamin are investigated. When both interventions are administered immediately after CN poisoning, benefits appear to be additive.[120] Some evidence suggests each offers supportive effects on brain metabolism.[127,128]

ROLE IN HYDROGEN SULFIDE POISONING

Hydrogen sulfide binds to cytochrome a-a$_3$. This is similar to CN, although it is more readily dissociated by O$_2$.[207] Clinical manifestations of toxicity are also similar to those of CO and CN.[207] Management of patients with serious H$_2$S poisoning principally involves oxygenation and cardiovascular support, as well as consideration of antidotal therapy with sodium nitrite to induce methemoglobinemia.[68,78,81,163] Hyperbaric oxygen is more effective than sodium nitrite in preventing death in animals.[22] Several clinical reports indicate that HBO, sometimes in conjunction with supplemental oxygen and blood pressure support, appears to be beneficial.[7,16,32,79,131,202,250] Relatively late treatment with HBO (eg, over 9 to 10 hours after poisoning) is reported to be beneficial in some[237] but not all cases.[2,204] No definitive data regarding use of HBO for H$_2$S poisoning are available, but HBO is reasonable when altered mental status or unstable vital signs persist after standard resuscitation measures.

ROLE IN OXIDANT-INDUCED METHEMOGLOBINEMIA

Oxidation of ferrous (2$^+$) heme to the ferric (3$^+$) form renders hemoglobin nonfunctional, and the presence of oxidized hemoglobin varieties causes a left shift of the oxyhemoglobin dissociation curve.[209] Hence, the manifestations of toxicity from acquired methemoglobinemia are usually more severe than those produced by a corresponding degree of anemia. In healthy people, when the fraction of methemoglobin is 10% (approximately 1.5 g/dL), patients generally appear cyanotic but otherwise asymptomatic. With approximately 30% methemoglobin, vague, nonspecific symptoms such as headache, fatigue, dyspnea, tachycardia, and dizziness occur. Unconsciousness is common at levels above 50% and death at 70%. There are numerous anecdotal accounts of clinical improvement with HBO in patients with life-threatening methemoglobinemia.[56,72,73,77,104,126,132,187,243] Ongoing exposure to any oxidants and the potential need for methylene blue to treat methemoglobinemia (Antidotes in Depth: A43) should also be addressed.

ROLE IN CARBON TETRACHLORIDE POISONING

Experimentally induced CCl$_4$ hepatotoxicity is diminished by HBO. Mortality rates were decreased in a number of animal studies,[20,31,156,178] and there are also several case reports of patients surviving potentially lethal ingestions with HBO therapy.[125,205,231,258] Because there are no proven antidotes for CCl$_4$ poisoning, we recommend HBO for patients with confirmed CCl$_4$ exposures. However, there appears to be a delicate balance between oxidative processes that are therapeutic and those that mediate hepatotoxicity.[24] Therefore, when HBO is being performed, it should ideally be instituted before the onset of liver function abnormalities. More recently, N-acetylcysteine (NAC) is effective in limiting liver damage in animals and appears of clinical benefit in humans with massive ingestions.[142,146,234,253] Additive benefit from concomitant use of NAC and HBO was shown in an animal model demonstrating a diminution of toxicity in L-arginine–induced pancreatitis, but there is no experience with CCl$_4$ poisoning.[166]

ROLE IN HYDROGEN PEROXIDE INGESTION

Ingestion of concentrated H$_2$O$_2$ solutions (eg, 35%) can result in venous and arterial gas embolism because of liberation of large volumes of O$_2$. Exposure to household concentrations of H$_2$O$_2$ (3%) has resulted in symptomatic portal venous air embolism on rare occasion.[143] At standard temperature and pressure, ingestion of 1 mL of household 3% H$_2$O$_2$ liberates approximately 10 mL of oxygen gas; by comparison, each milliliter of 35% H$_2$O$_2$ yields 115 mL of oxygen gas.[159] Symptoms vary with the affected organ. Seizures, alterations in mental status, and strokelike manifestations occur with CNS involvement from arterial emboli. Nausea, vomiting, hematemesis, and abdominal pain occur with gastrointestinal and hepatic venous involvement, and acute obstruction of the portal vein, portal venous hypertension, and bowel edema are described.[45,95,135,170,192] Hyperbaric oxygen is a successful

intervention for portal venous gas and in some cases of impaired consciousness and or focal neurologic findings.[9,65,87,105,143,159,170,179,236] Hyperbaric oxygen reduces the volume of offending gas and improves solubility of gas into tissues and plasma.[170] A history of inadvertent ingestion of concentrated H$_2$O$_2$, significant signs or symptoms, or radiologic evidence of gas embolism should prompt patient placement in a Trendelenburg, left lateral decubitus position, administration of 100% oxygen and sufficient fluids to sustain perfusion, and consideration for immediate transportation to the nearest hyperbaric facility. Hyperbaric oxygen to treat gas embolism has demonstrated benefit even if delayed beyond 20 hours.[58]

ADVERSE EFFECTS AND SAFETY ISSUES

Many HBO facilities have equipment and treatment protocols and abilities analogous to those found in an intensive care unit.[110,240,247] The possible capabilities vary, and interventions with HBO should never be undertaken if standard patient support cannot also be achieved. The inherent toxicity of O$_2$ and potential for injury resulting from elevations of ambient pressure must be addressed whenever HBO is used therapeutically. Preexisting conditions that require evaluation for possible management before initiation of HBO include claustrophobia, sinus congestion, and patients with scarred or noncompliant structures in the middle ear, such as otosclerosis.[112] Middle ear barotrauma is the most common adverse effect of HBO treatment,[39] and it occurs in 1.2% to 7% of patients.[48,174,232] When autoinsufflation fails, puncturing the ear drum or tympanostomy tube placement will resolve the problem. Pneumothorax is a rarely reported complication.[25] Toxicity resulting from O$_2$ is manifested by injuries to the CNS, lungs, and eyes. Central nervous system O$_2$ toxicity manifests as a generalized seizure and occurs at an incidence of approximately 1 to 4 per 10,000 patient treatments.[53,88,174] Pulmonary oxygen toxicity typically does not arise when standard treatment protocols are followed.[47,63,90,175] Progressive myopia occurs in some patients undergoing prolonged daily therapy but typically reverses within 6 weeks after treatments are terminated.[138] Nuclear cataracts can form with excessive treatments, exceeding a total of 150 to 200 hours, and they rarely develop with standard treatment protocols.[69,169] Absent onsite hyperbaric capability, the risks of interfacility transportation (eg, clinical decompensation, vehicle crashes) should also factor into decision making.

PREGNANCY AND LACTATION

Hyperbaric oxygen in pregnant patients presents the additional risks of fetal CNS, ocular, pulmonary, and cardiac toxicity.[11] In CO poisoning, these must be weighed against the potentially devastating fetal outcomes such as spontaneous abortion, intrauterine fetal demise, anatomic malformations, CNS injury, respiratory distress, and neonatal jaundice, which occur even in only mildly symptomatic CO-poisoned mothers.[38,116] For these reasons, COHb thresholds (eg, 15%–20%) for HBO therapy are often set lower for the pregnant patients than for other adults in HBO treatment algorithms. The authors of this text recommend treating a pregnant woman with HBO when COHb levels are greater than or equal to 15%. Normal fetal outcomes have followed HBO, even in the setting of severe maternal toxicity, and significant adverse fetal outcomes have followed normobaric oxygen therapy.[116] A summary of more than 700 Russian patients treated with HBO for various hypoxemic states did not find any detrimental HBO effects.[235] Hyperbaric oxygen was used safely in a prospective study of 44 pregnant women poisoned by CO.[59] Multiple other case reports document successful maternal and fetal outcomes in CO-poisoned pregnant patients.[26,67,197] Hyperbaric oxygen was also used successfully in patients with obstetrical procedures complicated by gas embolism.[160] Treatment decisions will ultimately be made on an individual case basis after weighing potential risks and benefits. There are no data regarding the effects of HBO on lactation.

DOSING AND ADMINISTRATION

Hyperbaric oxygen efficacy is a time- and pressure-dependent phenomenon. Rodent and human studies demonstrate that exposure to 2.8 to 3.0 ATA O$_2$ for 45 minutes is required to temporarily inhibit neutrophil adherence to endothelium mediated by the activation-dependent β_2-integrins on the neutrophil membrane and to ameliorate metabolic insults leading to loss of neuronal growth factors.[43,107,121,215,226] Clinical trials using HBO at only 2 ATAs have been unable to demonstrate a benefit of HBO, likely because it is an inadequate dose to achieve biochemical effects on cellular responses as discussed earlier.[6,176] Multiple trials using HBO (2.5 ATA or above) have demonstrated efficacy.[57,148,227,248] One trial using HBO (2.8 ATA) was unable to demonstrate benefit, subject to the previously discussed limitations.[188] If undertaken, HBO therapy (2.5–3.0 ATA, weighted toward the latter) should be provided as early as possible because a mortality benefit is demonstrated if HBO is administered within 6 hours.[76] Clinical trials have initiated therapy within 24 hours of the end of CO exposure.[248] The use of more than one treatment is supported by retrospective and prospective analysis,[75,248] although clinical practice is highly variable in this regard.[35,83]

FORMULATION AND ACQUISITION

Hyperbaric oxygen therapy is provided in monoplace or multiplace chambers, which are considered class II medical devices. For sites not possessing HBO capacity, various online organizational and professional directories may assist in locating hyperbaric facilities in the absence of preexisting HBO transfer protocols.

SUMMARY

- Mechanisms of action and efficacy of HBO are complex and remain an area of active investigation. Research findings are provocative because they highlight the fact that traditional assessments of mechanisms for toxicity of some xenobiotics are incomplete.

- Although the efficacy of HBO for acute CO poisoning is supported in animal trials, questions persist on many issues, including patient selection, optimal dose, and session frequency.

- Hyperbaric oxygen is recommended in serious acute CO poisoning, particularly in cases with end-organ manifestations, recognizing highly varied clinical practice scenarios and preferences.

- Further investigation is required to discern cases where clear benefit arises with HBO treatment and to define the constraints that limit its efficacious use.

- Anecdotal evidence supports HBO therapy in H_2S and CCL_4 poisoning, in oxidant-induced methemoglobinemia, and in H_2O_2 ingestion.

REFERENCES

1. Aamar S, et al. Lesion-induced changes in the production of newly synthesized and secreted apo-E and other molecules are independent of the concomitant recruitment of blood-borne macrophages into injured peripheral nerves. *J Neurochem.* 1992;59:1287-1292.
2. Al-Mahasneh QM, et al. Lack of response to oxygen in a fatal case of hydrogen sulfide poisoning [abstract]. *Vet Hum Toxicol.* 1989;31:353.
3. Anderson E, et al. Effects of low-level carbon monoxide exposure on onset and duration of angina pectoris. *Ann Intern Med.* 1973;79:46-50.
4. Anderson RA, Harland WA. Fire deaths in the Glasgow area. III. The role of hydrogen cyanide. *Med Sci Law.* 1982;22:35-40.
5. Anderson RA, et al. The importance of cyanide and organic nitriles in fire fatalities. *Fire Materials.* 1979;3:91-99.
6. Annane D, et al. Hyperbaric oxygen therapy for acute domestic carbon monoxide poisoning: two randomized controlled trials. *Intensive Care Med.* 2011;37:486-492.
7. Asif MJ, Exline MC. Utilization of hyperbaric oxygen therapy and induced hypothermia after hydrogen sulfide exposure. *Respir Care.* 2012;57:307-310.
8. Atochin D, et al. Neutrophil sequestration and the effect of hyperbaric oxygen in a rat model of temporary middle cerebral artery occlusion. *Undersea Hyperbaric Med.* 2000;27:185-190.
9. Baharnoori M, Lazarou J. A case of acute cerebral gas embolism due to ingestion of hydrogen peroxide. *J Neurol.* 2012;259:381-383.
10. Ballantyne B. Hydrogen cyanide as a product of combustion and a factor in morbidity and mortality from fires. In: Ballantyne B, Marrs T, eds. *Clinical and Experimental Toxicology of Cyanides.* Bristol, UK: John Wright; 1987:248-291.
11. Bar R, et al. Pre-Labor exposure to carbon monoxide: should the neonate be treated with hyperbaric oxygenation? *Clin Toxicol.* 2007;45:579-581.
12. Barillo DJ, et al. Cyanide poisoning in victims of fire: analysis of 364 cases and review of the literature. *J Burn Care Rehabil.* 1994;15:46-57.
13. Barillo DJ, et al. Lack of correlation between carboxyhemoglobin and cyanide in smoke inhalation injury. *Curr Surg.* 1986;43:421-423.
14. Baud F, et al. Cyanide: an unreported cause of neurological complications following smoke inhalation. *BMJ Case Rep.* 2011;pii: bcr0920114881.
15. Baud FJ, et al. Elevated blood cyanide concentrations in victims of smoke inhalation. *N Engl J Med.* 1991;325:1761-1766.
16. Belley R, et al. Hyperbaric oxygen therapy in the management of two cases of hydrogen sulfide toxicity from liquid manure. *Can J Emerg Med.* 2005;7:257-261.
17. Beppu T, et al. Fractional anisotropy in the centrum semiovale as a quantitative indicator of cerebral white matter damage in the subacute phase in patients with carbon monoxide poisoning: correlation with the concentration of myelin basic protein in cerebrospinal fluid. *J Neurol.* 2012;259:1698-1705.
18. Beppu T, et al. 1H-magnetic resonance spectroscopy indicates damage to cerebral white matter in the subacute phase after CO poisoning. *J Neurol Neurosurg Psychiatry.* 2011;82:869-875.
19. Beppu T, et al. Assessment of damage to cerebral white matter fiber in the subacute phase after carbon monoxide poisoning using fractional anisotropy in diffusion tensor imaging. *Neuroradiology.* 2010;52:735-743.
20. Bernacchi A, et al. Protection of hepatocytes with hyperoxia against carbon tetrachloride induced injury. *Toxicol Pathol.* 1984;12:315-323.
21. Birky MM, et al. Correlation of autopsy data and materials in the Tennessee jail fire. *Fire Safety J.* 1979;2:17-22.
22. Bitterman N, et al. The effect of hyperbaric oxygen on acute experimental sulfide poisoning in the rat. *Toxicol Appl Pharmacol.* 1986;84:325-328.
23. Breen PH, et al. Effect of oxygen and sodium thiosulfate during combined carbon monoxide and cyanide poisoning. *Toxicol Appl Pharmacol.* 1995;134:229-234.
24. Brent JA, Rumack BH. Role of free radicals in toxic hepatic injury: I. Free radical biochemistry. *J Toxicol Clin Toxicol.* 1993;31:173-196.
25. Broome JR, Smith DJ. Pneumothorax as a complication of recompression therapy for cerebral arterial gas embolism. *Undersea Biomed Res.* 1992;19:447-455.
26. Brown DB, et al. Hyperbaric oxygen treatment for carbon monoxide poisoning in pregnancy: a case report. *Aviat Space Environ Med.* 1992;63:1011-1014.
27. Brown SD, Piantadosi CA. Hyperbaric oxygen for carbon monoxide poisoning. *Lancet.* 1989:1032-1033.
28. Brown SD, Piantadosi CA. Recovery of energy metabolism in rat brain after carbon monoxide hypoxia. *J Clin Invest.* 1991;89:666-672.
29. Buckley NA, et al. Hyperbaric oxygen for carbon monoxide poisoning. *Cochrane Database Syst Rev.* 2011;13:CD002041.
30. Burk RF, et al. Relationship of oxygen and glutathione in protection against carbon tetrachloride-induced hepatic microsomal lipid peroxidation and covalent binding in the rat. *J Clin Invest.* 1984;74:1996-2001.
31. Burk RF, et al. Hyperbaric oxygen protection against carbon tetrachloride hepatotoxicity in the rat. Association with altered metabolism. *Gastroenterology.* 1986;90:812-818.
32. Burnett WW, et al. Hydrogen sulfide poisoning: review of 5 years' experience. *Can Med Assoc J.* 1977;117:1277-1280.
33. Burns RA, Schmidt SM. Portal venous gas emboli after accidental ingestion of concentrated hydrogen peroxide. *J Emerg Med.* 45, 345-347 (2013).
34. Burrows GE, Way JL. Cyanide intoxication in sheep: therapeutic value of oxygen or cobalt. *Am J Vet Res.* 1977;38:223-227.
35. Byrne BT, et al. Variability in hyperbaric oxygen treatment for acute carbon monoxide poisoning. *Undersea Hyperb Med.* 2012;39:627-638.
36. Byrne B, et al. Hyperbaric oxygen therapy for systemic gas embolism after hydrogen peroxide ingestion. *J Emerg Med.* 2014;46:171-175.
37. Cabrera VJ, et al. Methylene chloride intoxication treated with hyperbaric oxygen therapy. *Am J Med.* 2011;124:e3-4.
38. Caravati EM, et al. Fetal toxicity associated with maternal carbon monoxide poisoning. *Ann Emerg Med.* 1988;17:714-717.
39. Carlson S, et al. Prevention of hyperbaric-associated middle ear barotrauma. *Ann Emerg Med.* 1992;21:1468-1471.
40. Casey DP, et al. Hyperbaric hyperoxia reduces exercising forearm blood flow in humans. *Am J Physiol Heart Circ Physiol.* 2011;300:H1892-H1897.
41. Centers for Disease Control and Prevention (CDC). Fatal exposure to methylene chloride among bathtub refinishers—United States, 2000-2011. *MMWR Morb Mortal Wkly Rep.* 2012;61:119-122.
42. Chang YL, et al. Diverse manifestations of oral methylene chloride poisoning: report of 6 cases. *J Toxicol Clin Toxicol.* 1999;37:497-504.
43. Chen Q, et al. Functional inhibition of rat polymorphonuclear leukocyte B2 integrins by hyperbaric oxygen is associated with impaired cGMP synthesis. *J Pharmacol Exp Ther.* 1996;276:929-933.
44. Choi S. Delayed neurologic sequelae in carbon monoxide intoxication. *Arch Neurol.* 1983;40:433-435.
45. Ciechanowicz R, et al. Acute intoxication with hydrogen peroxide with air emboli in central nervous system—a case report. *Przegl Lek.* 2007;64:339-340.
46. Clark CJ, et al. Blood carboxyhaemoglobin and cyanide levels in fire survivors. *Lancet.* 1981;1:1332-1335.
47. Clark JM, Lambertsen CJ. Rate of development of pulmonary O2 toxicity in man during O2 breathing at 2.0 atm absolute. *J Appl Physiol.* 1971;30:739-768.

48. Clements KS, et al. Complications of tympanostomy tubes inserted for facilitation of hyperbaric oxygen therapy. *Arch Otolaryngol Head Neck Surg.* 1998;124:278-280.

49. Coburn RF, Forman HJ. Carbon monoxide toxicity. In: Fishman AP, et al, eds. *Handbook of Physiology.* Baltimore, MD: Williams & Wilkins; 1987:439-456.

50. Cope C. The importance of oxygen in the treatment of cyanide poisoning. *JAMA.* 1961;175:1061-1064.

51. Copeland AR. Accidental fire deaths: the 5-year metropolitan Dade County experience from 1979 to 1983. *Z Rechtsmed.* 1985;94:71-79.

52. Cramlet SH, et al. Ventricular function following acute carbon monoxide exposure. *J Appl Physiol.* 1975;39:482-486.

53. Davis JC, et al. Hyperbaric medicine: patient selection, treatment procedures, and side-effects. In: Davis JC, Hunt TK, eds. *Problem Wounds.* New York, NY: Elsevier; 1988:225-235.

54. Dennog C, et al. Analysis of oxidative DNA damage and HPRT mutations in humans after hyperbaric oxygen treatment. *Mutation Res.* 1999;431:351-359.

55. Dennog C, et al. Detection of DNA damage after hyperbaric oxygen (HBO) therapy. *Mutagenesis.* 1996;11:605-609.

56. Desusclade S, et al. Methemoglobinemia induced by sodium chlorate: value of hyperbaric oxygen therapy. *Presse Med.* 1994;23:859.

57. Ducasse JL, et al. Non-comatose patients with acute carbon monoxide poisoning: hyperbaric or normobaric oxygenation? *Undersea Hyperbaric Med.* 1995;22:9-15.

58. Dunbar EM, et al. Successful late treatment of venous air embolism with hyperbaric oxygen. *Postgrad Med J.* 1990;66:469-470.

59. Elkharrat D, et al. Acute carbon monoxide intoxication and hyperbaric oxygen in pregnancy. *Intensive Care Med.* 1991;17:289-292.

60. End E, Long CW. Oxygen under pressure in carbon monoxide poisoning. *J Ind Hyg Toxicol.* 1942;24:302-306.

61. Evans MV, Caldwell JC. Evaluation of two different metabolic hypotheses for dichloromethane toxicity using physiologically based pharmacokinetic modeling of in vivo gas uptake data exposure in female B6C3F1 mice. *Toxicol Appl Pharmacol.* 2010;244:280-290.

62. Fagin J, et al. Carbon monoxide poisoning secondary to inhaling methylene chloride. *Br Med J.* 1980;281:1461.

63. Fisher AB, et al. Mechanisms of pulmonary oxygen toxicity. *Lung.* 1984;162:255-259.

64. Foster M, et al. Recurrent acute life-threatening events and lactic acidosis caused by chronic carbon monoxide poisoning in an infant. *Pediatrics.* 1999;104:34-39.

65. French LK, et al. Hydrogen peroxide ingestion associated with portal venous gas and treatment with hyperbaric oxygen: a case series and review of the literature. *Clin Toxicol.* 2010;48:533-538.

66. Friedman G, et al. Apolipoprotein E-epsilon 4 genotype predicts a poor outcome in survivors of traumatic brain injury. *Neurology.* 1999;52:244-248.

67. Gabrielli A, Layon AJ. Carbon monoxide intoxication during pregnancy: a case presentation and pathophysiologic discussion, with emphasis on molecular mechanisms. *J Clin Anesth.* 1995;7:82-87.

68. Gerasimon G, et al. Acute hydrogen sulfide poisoning in a dairy farmer. *Clin Toxicol.* 2007;45:420-423.

69. Gesell L, Trott A. De novo cataract development following a standard course of hyperbaric oxygen therapy. *Undersea Hyperbaric Med.* 2007;34:389-392.

70. Gilmer B, et al. Hyperbaric oxygen does not prevent neurologic sequelae after carbon monoxide poisoning. *Acad Emerg Med.* 2002;9:1-8.

71. Ginsberg MD, Myers RE. Experimental carbon monoxide encephalopathy in the primate. I. Physiologic and metabolic aspects. *Arch Neurol.* 1974;30:202-208.

72. Goldstein GM, Doull J. Treatment of nitrite-induced methemoglobinemia with hyperbaric oxygen. *Proc Soc Exp Biol Med.* 1971;138:137-139.

73. Goldstein GM, Doull J. The use of hyperbaric oxygen in the treatment of p-aminopropiophenone-induced methemoglobinemia. *Toxicol Appl Pharmacol.* 1973;26:247-252.

74. Goodhart GL. Patient treated with antidote kit and hyperbaric oxygen survives cyanide poisoning. *South Med J.* 1994;87:814-816.

75. Gorman DF, et al. A longitudinal study of 100 consecutive admissions for carbon monoxide poisoning to the Royal Adelaide Hospital. *Anaesth Intens Care.* 1992;20:311-316.

76. Goulon M, et al. Carbon monoxide poisoning and acute anoxia due to breathing coal gas and hydrocarbons. *Ann Med Interne (Paris).* 1969;120:335-349. Translated in *J Hyperbaric Med.* 1986;1:23-41.

77. Goulon M, et al. On a case of acquired methemoglobinemia with coma, treated with hyperbaric oxygen and methylene blue. *Rev Neurol (Paris).* 1966;114:376-378.

78. Guidotti TL. Hydrogen sulphide. *Occup Med (London).* 1996;46:367-371.

79. Gunn B, Wong R. Noxious gas exposure in the outback: two cases of hydrogen sulfide toxicity. *Emerg Med (Fremantle).* 2001;13:240-246.

80. Hall AH, et al. Suspected cyanide poisoning in smoke inhalation: complications of sodium nitrite therapy. *J Toxicol Clin Exp.* 1989;9:3-9.

81. Hall AH, Rumack BH. Hydrogen sulfide poisoning: an antidotal role for sodium nitrite? *Vet Hum Toxicol.* 1997;39:152-154.

82. Hampson N. Hyperbaric oxygen for carbon monoxide poisoning. *Med J Aust.* 2000; 172:141-142.

83. Hampson NB, Little CE. Hyperbaric treatment of patients with carbon monoxide poisoning in the United States. *Undersea Hyperb Med.* 2005;32:21-26.

84. Hampson NB, Norkool DM. Carbon monoxide poisoning in children riding in the back of pickup trucks. *JAMA.* 1992;267:538-540.

85. Hampson NB, et al. Practice recommendations in the diagnosis, management and prevention of carbon monoxide poisoning. *Am J Respir Crit Care Med.* 2012;186:1095-1101.

86. Hampso, NB, et al. Increased long-term mortality among survivors of acute carbon monoxide poisoning. *Crit Care Med.* 2009;37:1941-1947.

87. Han ST, et al. Xanthine oxidoreductase and neurological sequelae of carbon monoxide poisoning. *Toxicol Lett.* 2007;170:111-115.

88. Hart GB, Strauss MB. Central nervous system oxygen toxicity in a clinical setting. In: Bove AA, et al, eds. *Undersea and Hyperbaric Physiology IX.* Bethesda, MD: Undersea and Hyperbaric Med Society; 1987:695-699.

89. Hart GB, et al. Treatment of smoke inhalation by hyperbaric oxygen. *J Emerg Med.* 1985;3:211-215.

90. Hart GB, et al. Vital capacity of quadriplegic patients treated with hyperbaric oxygen. *J Am Paraplegia Soc.* 1984;7:113-114.

91. Hendrickson SM, et al. Hyperbaric oxygen therapy for the prevention of arterial gas embolism in food grade hydrogen peroxide ingestion. *Am J Emerg Med.* 2017; 809.e5-809.e8.

92. Henry CR, et al. Myocardial injury and long-term mortality following moderate to severe carbon monoxide poisoning. *JAMA.* 2006;295:398-402.

93. Hopkins R, et al. Apolipoprotein E genotype and response of carbon monoxide poisoning to hyperbaric oxygen treatment. *Am J Respir Crit Care Med.* 2008;176:1001-1006.

94. Horowitz BZ. Carboxyhemoglobinemia caused by inhalation of methylene chloride. *Am J Emerg Med.* 1986;4:48-51.

95. Horowitz BZ. Massive hepatic gas embolism from a health food additive. *J Emerg Med.* 2004;26:229-230.

96. Hsiao CL, et al. Delayed encephalopathy after carbon monoxide intoxication-long term prognosis and correlation of clinical manifestations and neuroimages. *Acta Neurol Taiwan.* 2004;13:64-70.

97. Hsu LH, Wang JH. Treatment of carbon monoxide poisoning with hyperbaric oxygen. *Chinese Med J.* 1996;58:407-413.

98. Ide T, Kamijo Y. Myelin basic protein in cerebrospinal fluid: a predictive marker of delayed encephalopathy from carbon monoxide poisoning. *Am J Emerg Med.* 2008; 26:908-912.

99. Ide T, Kamijo Y. The early elevation of interleukin 6 concentration in cerebrospinal fluid and delayed encephalopathy of carbon monoxide poisoning. *Am J Emerg Med.* 2009;27:992-996.

100. Ischiropoulos H, et al. Nitric oxide production and perivascular tyrosine nitration in brain after carbon monoxide poisoning in the rat. *J Clin Invest.* 1996;97:2260-2267.

101. Ishimaru H, et al. Effects of N-methyl-D-aspartate receptor antagonists on carbon monoxide-induced brain damage in mice. *J Pharmacol Exp Ther.* 1992;261:349-352.

102. Isom GE, Way JL. Effect of oxygen on cyanide intoxication. VI. Reactivation of cyanide inhibited glucose metabolism. *J Pharmacol Exp Ther.* 1974;189:235-243.

103. Ivanov KP. The effect of elevated oxygen pressure on animals poisoned with potassium cyanide. *Pharmacol Toxicol.* 1959;22:476-479.

104. Jansen T, et al. Isobutyl-nitrite-induced methemoglobinemia; treatment with an exchange blood transfusion during hyperbaric oxygenation. *Acta Anaesthesiol Scand.* 2003;47:1300-1301.

105. Juric DM, et al. The effectiveness of oxygen therapy in carbon monoxide poisoning is pressure- and time-dependent: a study on cultured astrocytes. *Toxicol Lett.* 2015;233:16-23.

106. Juric DM, et al. Hyperbaric oxygen preserves neurotrophic activity of carbon monoxide-exposed astrocytes. *Toxicol Lett.* 2016;253:1-6.

107. Kalns J, et al. Hyperbaric oxygen exposure temporarily reduces Mac-1 mediated functions of human neutrophils. *Immunol Lett.* 2002;83:125-131.

108. Kamijo Y, et al. Recurrent myelin basic protein elevation in cerebrospinal fluid as a predictive marker of delayed encephalopathy after carbon monoxide poisoning. *Am J Emerg Med.* 2007;25:483-485.

109. Kaufman D, et al. Methylene chloride report of 5 exposures and 2 deaths. *Vet Hum Toxicol.* 1989:352.

110. Keenan H, et al. Delivery of hyperbaric oxygen therapy to critically ill, mechanically ventilated children. *J Crit Care.* 1998;13:7-12.

111. Kihara K, et al. Effects of hyperbaric oxygen exposure on experimental hepatic ischemia reperfusion injury: relationship between its timing and neutrophil sequestration. *Liver Transpl.* 2005;11:1574-1580.

112. Kindwall EP. *Hyperbaric Medicine Practice.* Flagstaff, AZ: Best Publishing; 1994.

113. Kirk MA, et al. Cyanide and methemoglobin kinetics in smoke inhalation victims treated with the cyanide antidote kit. *Ann Emerg Med.* 1993;22:1413-1418.

114. Klasner AE, et al. Carbon monoxide mass exposure in a pediatric population. *Acad Emerg Med.* 1998;5:992-996.

115. Kobayashi A, et al. Severe optic neuropathy caused by dichloromethane inhalation. *J Ocul Pharmacol Ther.* 2008;24:607-612.

116. Koren G, et al. A multicenter, prospective study of fetal outcome following accidental carbon monoxide poisoning in pregnancy. *Reprod Toxicol.* 1991;5:397-403.

117. Kramer WG, et al. Theophylline pharmacokinetics during hyperbaria and hyperbaric hyperoxia in the dog. *Res Commun Chem Pathol Pharmacol.* 1981;34:381-388.

118. Kramer WG, et al. Salicylate pharmacokinetics in the dog at 6 ATA in air and at 2.8 ATA in 100% oxygen. *Aviat Space Environ Med.* 1983;54:682-684.

119. Kramer WG, et al. Pharmacokinetics of pentobarbital under hyperbaric and hyperbaric hyperoxic conditions in the dog. *Aviat Space Environ Med.* 1983;54:1005-1008.

120. Kuroda H, et al. Novel clinical grading of delayed neurologic sequelae after carbon monoxide poisoning and factors associated with outcome. *Neurotoxicol.* 2015;48:35-43.

121. Labrouche S, et al. Influence of hyperbaric oxygen on leukocyte functions and haemostasis in normal volunteer divers. *Thromb Res.* 1999;96:309-315.

122. Lamy M, Hauguet M. Fifty patients with carbon monoxide intoxication treated with hyperbaric oxygen therapy. *Acta Ahes Belgica.* 1969;1:49-53.

123. Langehennig PL, et al. Paint removers and carboxyhemoglobin. *N Engl J Med.* 1981; 295:1137.

124. Lapoint J, et al. Methylene chloride poisoning with delayed carboxyhemoglobinemia treated with hyperbaric oxygen therapy [abstract]. *Clin Toxicol.* 2012;50:314.

125. Larcan A, Lambert H. Current epidemiological, clinical, biological, and therapeutic aspects of acute carbon monoxide intoxication. *Bull Acad Natl Med (Paris).* 1981; 165:471.

126. Lareng L, et al. Acute, toxic methemoglobinemia from accidental ingestion of nitrobenzene. *Eur J Toxicol Environ Hyg.* 1974;7:12-16.

127. Lawson-Smith P, et al. Effect of acute and delayed hyperbaric oxygen therapy on cyanide whole blood levels during acute cyanide intoxication. *Undersea Hyperbaric Med.* 2011;38:17-26.

128. Lawson-Smith P, et al. Hyperbaric oxygen therapy or hydroxycobalamin attenuates surges in brain interstitial lactate and glucose; and hyperbaric oxygen improves respiratory status in cyanide-intoxicated rats. *Undersea Hyperbaric Med.* 2011;38:223-237.

129. Lee JH, et al. Incidence and clinical course of left ventricular systolic dysfunction in patients with carbon monoxide poisoning. *Korean Circulation J.* 2016;46:665-671.

130. Leffler CW, et al. Carbon monoxide as an endogenous vascular modulator. *Am J Physiol Heart Circ Physiol.* 2011;301:H1-H11.

131. Lindenmann J, et al. Hyperbaric oxygen in the treatment of hydrogen sulphide intoxication. *Acta Anaesthesiol Scand.* 2010;54:784-785.

132. Lindenmann J, et al. Hyperbaric oxygenation in the treatment of life-threatening isobutyl nitrite-induced methemoglobinemia—a case report. *Inhal Toxicol.* 2006;18: 1047-1049.

133. Liner MH, et al. Alveolar gas exchange during simulated breath-hold diving to 20 m. *Undersea Hyperb Med.* 1993;20:27-38.

134. Litovitz TL, et al. Cyanide poisoning treated with hyperbaric oxygen. *Am J Emerg Med.* 1983;1:94-101.

135. Liu TM, et al. Acute paraplegia caused by an accidental ingestion of hydrogen peroxide. *Am J Emerg Med.* 2007;25:90-92.

136. Liu WC, et al. Hyperbaric oxygen therapy alleviates carbon monoxide poisoning-induced delayed memory impairment by preserving brain-derived neurotrophic factor-dependent hippocampal neurogenesis. *Crit Care Med.* 2016;44:e25-e39.

137. Lundquist P, et al. The role of hydrogen cyanide and carbon monoxide in fire casualties: a prospective study. *Forensic Sci Int.* 1989;43:9-14.

138. Lyne AJ. Ocular effects of hyperbaric oxygen. *Trans Ophthalmol Soc UK.* 1978;98:66-68.

139. Madden MR, et al. Respiratory care of the burn patient. *Clin Plast Surg.* 1986;13:29-38.

140. Maeda Y, et al. Effect of therapy with oxygen under high pressure on regional cerebral blood flow in the interval form of carbon monoxide poisoning: observation from subtraction of technetium-99m HMPAOSPECT brain imaging. *Eur Neurol.* 1991;31: 380-383.

141. Mahmud M, Kales S. Methylene chloride poisoning in a cabinet worker. *Environ Health Perspect.* 1999;107:769-772.

142. Maksimchik YZ, et al. Protective effects of N-acetyl-L-cysteine against acute carbon tetrachloride hepatotoxicity in rats. *Cell Biochem Funct.* 2008;26:11-18.

143. Manini A, Harris CR. What is the pertinent finding and an explanation for the cause? *J Med Toxicol.* 2009;5:143-149.

144. Martin JD, Thom SR. Vascular leukocyte sequestration in decompression sickness and prophylactic hyperbaric oxygen therapy in rats. *Aviat Space Environ Med.* 2002; 73:565-569.

145. Marzella L, et al. Effect of hyperoxia on liver necrosis induced by hepatotoxins. *Virchows Arch B Cell Pathol Incl Mol Pathol.* 1986;51:497-507.

146. Mathieson PW, et al. Survival after massive ingestion of carbon tetrachloride treated by intravenous infusion of acetylcysteine. *Hum Toxicol.* 1985;4:627-631.

147. Mathieu D, et al. Acute carbon monoxide poisoning risk of late sequelae and treatment by hyperbaric oxygen. *Clin Toxicol.* 1985;23:315-324.

148. Mathieu D, et al. Randomized prospective study comparing the effect of HBO versus 12 hours NBO in non-comatose CO poisoned patients [abstract]. *Undersea Hyperbaric Med.* 1996;23(suppl):7.

149. Maurice T, et al. Cholecystokinin-related peptides, after systemic or central administration, prevent carbon monoxide-induced amnesia in mice. *J Pharmacol Exp Ther.* 1994;269:665-673.

150. McCarron M, et al. Prospective study of apolipoprotein E genotype and functional outcome following ischemic stroke. *Arch Neurol.* 2000;57:1480-1484.

151. Merritt GJ, Slade JB. Influence of hyperbaric oxygen on the pharmacokinetics of single-dose gentamicin in healthy volunteers. *Pharmacotherapy.* 1993;13:382-385.

152. Meyer BC. Experimentelle erfahrungen uber die kohlenoxydverguftung des zentralnervens systems. *Z Ges Neurol Psychiatr.* 1928;112:187-212.

153. Mileski WJ, et al. Inhibition of leukocyte adherence and susceptibility to infection. *J Surg Res.* 1993;54:349-354.

154. Mileski WJ, et al. Inhibition of CD18-dependent neutrophil adherence reduces organ injury after hemorrhagic shock in primates. *Surgery.* 1990;108:206-212.

155. Mohler SR. Air crash survival: injuries and evacuation toxic hazards. *Aviat Space Environ Med.* 1975;46:86-88.

156. Montani S, Perret C. Oxygenation hyperbare dans l'intoxication experimentale au tetrachlorure de carbon. *Rev Fr Etud Clin Biol.* 1967;12:274-278.

157. Moon R, DeLong E. Hyperbaric oxygen for carbon monoxide poisoning. *Med J Aust.* 1999;170:197-198.

158. Moore SJ, et al. Antidotal use of methemoglobin forming cyanide antagonists in concurrent carbon monoxide/cyanide intoxication. *J Pharmacol Exp Ther.* 1987;242: 70-73.

159. Mullins ME, Beltran JT. Acute cerebral gas embolism from hydrogen peroxide ingestion successfully treated with hyperbaric oxygen. *J Toxicol Clin Toxicol.* 1998;36:253-256.

160. Mushkat Y, et al. Gas embolism complicating obstetric or gynecologic procedures. Case reports and review of the literature. *Eur J Obstet Gynecol Reprod Biol.* 1995;63:97-103.

161. Myers R, et al. Subacute sequelae of carbon monoxide poisoning. *Ann Emerg Med.* 1985;14:1163-1167.

162. Nabeshima T, et al. Carbon monoxide-induced delayed amnesia, delayed neuronal death and change in acetylcholine concentration in mice. *J Pharm Exp Therap.* 1991;256:378-384.

163. Nikkanen H, Burns M. Severe hydrogen sulfide exposure in a working adolescent. *Pediatrics.* 2004;113:927-929.

164. Norkool DM, Kirkpatrick JN. Treatment of acute carbon monoxide poisoning with hyperbaric oxygen: a review of 115 cases. *Ann Emerg Med.* 1985;14:1168-1171.

165. Norris JC, et al. Synergistic lethality induced by the combination of carbon monoxide and cyanide. *Toxicology.* 1986;40:121-129.

166. Onur E, et al. Hyperbaric oxygen and N-acetylcysteine treatment in L-arginine-induced acute pancreatitis in rats. *J Invest Surg.* 2012;25:20-28.

167. Ozyurt A, et al. Effects of acute carbon monoxide poisoning on ECG and echocardiographic parameters in children. *Cardiovasc Toxicol.* 2017;17:326-334.

168. Pace N, et al. Acceleration of carbon monoxide elimination in man by high pressure oxygen. *Science.* 1950;111:652-654.

169. Palmquist BM, et al. Nuclear cataract and myopia during hyperbaric oxygen therapy. *Br J Ophthalmol.* 1984;68:113-117.

170. Papafragkou S, et al. Treatment of portal venous gas embolism with hyperbaric oxygen after accidental ingestion of hydrogen peroxide: a case report and review of the literature. *J Emerg Med.* 2012;43:e21-23.

171. Peirce EC 2nd, et al. Carbon monoxide poisoning: experimental hypothermic and hyperbaric studies. *Surgery.* 1972;72:229-237.

172. Piatt JP, et al. Occult carbon monoxide poisoning in an infant. *Pediatric Emerg Care.* 1990;6:21-23.

173. Pitt BR, et al. Interaction of carbon monoxide and cyanide on cerebral circulation and metabolism. *Arch Environ Health.* 1979;34:354-359.

174. Plafki C, et al. Complications and side effects of hyperbaric oxygen therapy. *Aviat Space Environ Med.* 2000;71:119-124.

175. Pott F, et al. Hyperbaric oxygen treatment and pulmonary function. *Undersea Hyperbaric Med.* 1999;26:225-228.

176. Raphael JC, et al. Trial of normobaric and hyperbaric oxygen for acute carbon monoxide intoxication. *Lancet.* 1989;414-419.

177. Raphael M, et al. Acute methylene chloride intoxication—a case report on domestic poisoning. *Eur J Emerg Med.* 2002;9:57-59.

178. Rapin M, et al. Effect de l'oxygene hyperbare sur la toxicite tetrachlorure de carbone chez le rat. *Rev Fr Etud Clin Biol.* 1967;12:594-599.

179. Rider SP, et al. Cerebral air gas embolism from concentrated hydrogen peroxide ingestion. *Clin Toxicol.* 2008;46:815-818.

180. Rioux JP, Myers RA. Hyperbaric oxygen for methylene chloride poisoning: report on two cases. *Ann Emerg Med.* 1989;18:691-695.

181. Roche L, et al. Comparison de deux groupes de vingt intoxications oxycarbonees traitees par oxygene normobare et hyperbare. *Lyon Med.* 1968;49:1483-1499.

182. Rollins MD, et al. Wound oxygen levels during hyperbaric oxygen treatment in healing wounds. *Undersea Hyperb Med.* 2006;33:17-25.

183. Rothfuss A, et al. Involvement of heme oxygenase-1 (HO-1) in the adaptive protection of human lymphocytes after hyperbaric oxygen (HBO) treatment. *Carcinogenesis.* 2001;22:1979-1985.

184. Rudge FW. Treatment of methylene chloride induced carbon monoxide poisoning with hyperbaric oxygenation. *Mil Med.* 1990;155:570-572.

185. Satran D, et al. Cardiovascular manifestations of moderate to severe carbon monoxide poisoning. *J Am Coll Cardiol.* 2005;45:1513-1516.

186. Saunders A, et al. Association of apolipoprotein E allele epsilon 4 with late-onset familial and sporadic Alzheimer's disease. *Neurology.* 1993;43:1467-1472.

187. Savateev NV, et al. Treatment of sodium nitrite poisoning with oxygen under pressure and Chromosmon. *Voen Med Zh.* 1969;10:42-43.

188. Scheinkestel CD, et al. Hyperbaric or normobaric oxygen for acute carbon monoxide poisoning: a randomised controlled clinical trial. *Med J Aust.* 1999;170:203-210.

189. Schiltz KL. Failure to assess motivation, need to consider psychiatric variables, and absence of comprehensive examination: a skeptical review of neuropsychologic assessment in carbon monoxide research. *Undersea Hyperb Med.* 2000;27:48-50.

190. Scolnick B, et al. Successful treatment of life-threatening propionitrile exposure with sodium nitrite/sodium thiosulfate followed by hyperbaric oxygen. *J Occup Med.* 1993;35:577-580.

191. Sheehy M, Way JL. Effect of oxygen on cyanide intoxication: III Mithridate. *J Pharmacol Exp Ther*. 1968;161:163-168.

192. Sherman SJ, et al. Cerebral infarction immediately after ingestion of hydrogen peroxide solution. *Stroke*. 1994;25:1065-1067.

193. Shimosegawa E, et al. Cerebral blood flow and glucose metabolism measurements in a patient surviving one year after carbon monoxide intoxication. *J Nucl Med*. 1992;33:1696-1698.

194. Shusterman D, et al. Predictors of carbon monoxide and hydrogen cyanide exposure in smoke inhalation patients. *J Toxicol Clin Toxicol*. 1996;34:61-71.

195. Shusterman D, et al. Methylene chloride intoxication in a furniture refinisher. *J Occup Med*. 1990:451-454.

196. Silverman CS, et al. Hemorrhagic necrosis and vascular injury in carbon monoxide poisoning: MR demonstration. *AJNR Am J Neuroradiol*. 1993;14:168-170.

197. Silverman RK, Montano J. Hyperbaric oxygen treatment during pregnancy in acute carbon monoxide poisoning. A case report. *J Reprod Med*. 1997;42:309-311.

198. Silverman SH, et al. Cyanide toxicity in burned patients. *J Trauma*. 1988;28:171-176.

199. Skene WG, et al. Effect of hyperbaric oxygen in cyanide poisoning. In: Brown IW, Cox B, eds. *Proceedings of the Third International Congress on Hyperbaric Medicine*. Washington, DC: National Academy of Sciences, National Research Council; 1966:705-710.

200. Sluijter ME. The treatment of carbon monoxide poisoning by the administration of oxygen at high atmospheric pressure. *Proc R Soc Med*. 1963;56:1002-1008.

201. Smedley BL, et al. Cerebral arterial gas embolism after pre-flight ingestion of hydrogen peroxide. *Diving Hyperb Med*. 2016;46:117-119.

202. Smilkstein MJ, et al. Hyperbaric oxygen therapy for severe hydrogen sulfide poisoning. *J Emerg Med*. 1985:27-30.

203. Smith G, Sharp G. Treatment of carbon-monoxide poisoning with oxygen under pressure. *Lancet*. 1960;276:905-906.

204. Snyder J, et al. Occupational fatality and persistent neurological sequelae after mass exposure to hydrogen sulfide. *Am J Emerg Med*. 1995;13:199-203.

205. Stewart RD, et al. Acute carbon tetrachloride intoxication. *JAMA*. 1963;183:994-997.

206. Stewart RD, Hake CL. Paint remover hazard. *JAMA*. 1976;235:398-401.

207. Stine RJ, et al. Hydrogen sulfide intoxication. *Ann Intern Med*. 1976;85:756-758.

208. Stirban A, et al. Functional changes in microcirculation during hyperbaric and normobaric oxygen therapy. *Undersea Hyperb Med*. 2009;36:381-390.

209. Stolze K, et al. Hydroxylamine and phenol-induced formation of methemoglobin and free radical intermediates in erythrocytes. *Biochem Pharmacol*. 1996;57:1821-1829.

210. Sun L, et al. Hyperbaric oxygen reduces tissue hypoxia and hypoxia-inducible factor-1 alpha expression in focal cerebral ischemia. *Stroke*. 2008;39:1000-1006.

211. Tahepold P, et al. Hyperoxia elicits myocardial protection through a nuclear factor kB-dependent mechanism in the rat heart. *J Thorac Cardiovasc Surg*. 2003;125:650-660.

212. Tahepold P, et al. Pretreating rats with hyperoxia attenuates ischemia-reperfusion injury of the heart. *Life Sci*. 2001;68:1629-1640.

213. Takano T, et al. Effect of hyperbaric oxygen on cyanide intoxication: in situ changes in intracellular oxidation reduction. *Undersea Biomed Res*. 1980;7:191-197.

214. Thom SR. Hyperbaric oxygen therapy. *J Intensive Care Med*. 1989;4:58-74.

215. Thom SR. Functional inhibition of leukocyte B2 integrins by hyperbaric oxygen in carbon monoxide-mediated brain injury in rats. *Toxicol Appl Pharmacol*. 1993;123:248-256.

216. Thom SR. Learning dysfunction and metabolic defects in globus pallidus and hippocampus after CO poisoning in a rat model. *Undersea Hyperbaric Med*. 1997;23:20.

217. Thom SR. Oxidative stress is fundamental to hyperbaric oxygen therapy. *J Appl Physiol*. 2009;106:988-995.

218. Thom SR. Hyperbaric oxygen—its mechanisms and efficacy. *Plast Reconstr Surg*. 2011;127:S131-S141.

219. Thom SR, et al. Delayed neuropathology after carbon monoxide poisoning is immune-mediated. *Proc Natl Acad Sci U S A*. 2004;101:13660-13665.

220. Thom SR, et al. Intravascular neutrophil activation due to carbon monoxide poisoning. *Am J Respir Crit Care Med*. 2006;174:1239-1248.

221. Thom SR, et al. Actin S-nitrosylation inhibits neutrophil beta2 integrin function. *J Biol Chem*. 2008;283:10822-10834.

222. Thom R., et al. Neutrophil beta-2 integrin inhibition by hyperoxia is due to actin S-nitrosylation and delocalized thioredoxin reductase. *Undersea and Hyperbaric Med*. 2010;37:300-301.

223. Thom SR, et al. Thioredoxin reductase linked to cytoskeleton by focal adhesion kinase reverses actin S-nitrosylation and restores neutrophil β(2) integrin function. *J Biol Chem*. 2012;287:30346-30357.

224. Thom SR, et al. Neutrophil beta2 integrin inhibition by enhanced interactions of vasodilator stimulated phosphoprotein with S-nitrosylated actin. *J Biol Chem*. 2011;286:32854-32865.

225. Thom SR, et al. Neuronal nitric oxide synthase and N-methyl-D-aspartate neurons in experimental carbon monoxide poisoning. *Toxicol Appl Pharmacol*. 2004;194:280-295.

226. Thom SR, et al. Inhibition of human neutrophil beta2-integrin-dependent adherence by hyperbaric O2. *Am J Physiol*. 1997;272:C770-C777.

227. Thom SR, et al. Delayed neuropsychologic sequelae after carbon monoxide poisoning: prevention by treatment with hyperbaric oxygen. *Ann Emerg Med*. 1995;25:474-480.

228. Thomas PS, et al. The synergistic effect of sympathectomy and hyperbaric oxygen exposure on transcutaneous PO2 in healthy volunteers. *Anesth Analg*. 1999;88:67-71.

229. Tjarnstrom J, et al. Effects of hyperbaric oxygen treatment on neutrophil activation and pulmonary sequestration in intestinal ischemia-reperfusion in rats. *Eur Surg Res*. 1999;31:147-154.

230. Trapp WG, Lepawsky M. 100% survival in five life-threatening acute cyanide poisoning victims treated by a therapeutic spectrum including hyperbaric oxygen. Paper presented at the First European Conference on Hyperbaric Medicine, Amsterdam, 1983.

231. Truss CD, Killenberg PG. Treatment of carbon tetrachloride poisoning with hyperbaric oxygen. *Gastroenterology*. 1982;82:767-769.

232. Trytko B, Bennett M. Hyperbaric oxygen therapy: complication rates are much lower than authors suggest. *BMJ*. 1999;318:1077-1078.

233. Ueno S, et al. Early post-operative hyperbaric oxygen therapy modifies neutrophile activation. *Hepato Gastroenterology*. 1999;46:1798-1799.

234. Valles EG, et al. N-acetyl cysteine is an early but also a late preventive agent against carbon tetrachloride-induced liver necrosis. *Toxicol Lett*. 1994;71:87-95.

235. Van Hoesen KB, et al. Should hyperbaric oxygen be used to treat the pregnant patient for acute carbon monoxide poisoning? A case report and literature review. *JAMA*. 1989;261:1039-1043.

236. Vander Heide SJ, Seamon JP. Resolution of delayed altered mental status associated with hydrogen peroxide ingestion following hyperbaric oxygen therapy. *Acad Emerg Med*. 2003;10:998-1000.

237. Vicas I, et al. Hydrogen sulfide exposure treated with hyperbaric oxygen (abstract). *Vet Hum Toxicol*. 1989;31:353.

238. Wada K, et al. Repeated hyperbaric oxygen induces ischemic tolerance in gerbil hippocampus. *Brain Res*. 1996;740:15-20.

239. Wang H, et al. Combination of butylphthalide with umbilical mesenchymal stem cells for the treatment of delayed encephalopathy after carbon monoxide poisoning. *Medicine*. 2016;95:49(e5412).

240. Waisman D, et al. Hyperbaric oxygen therapy in the pediatric patient: the experience of the Israel Naval Medical Institute. *Pediatrics*. 1998;102:1-9.

241. Watanabe K, Guengerich FP. Limited reactivity of formyl chloride with glutathione and relevance to metabolism and toxicity of dichloromethane. *Chem Res Toxicol*. 2006;19:1091-1096.

242. Watanabe K, et al. Analysis of SNA adducts formed in vivo in rats and mice from 1,2-dichloromethane, 1,2-dichloroethane, dibromoethane, and dichloromethane using HPLC/accelerator mass spectroscopy and relevance to risk estimates. *Chem Res Toxicol*. 2007;20:1594-1600.

243. Wattel F, et al. Hyperbaric oxygen therapy in the Gernez-Rieux respiratory intensive care unit. Results of the 1,000 first treatments. Outlooks. *Lille Med*. 1974;19(Spec No):333-341.

244. Way JL. Cyanide intoxication and its mechanism of antagonism. *Annu Rev Pharmacol Toxicol*. 1984;24:451-481.

245. Way JL, et al. Effect of oxygen on cyanide intoxication. *Toxicol Appl Pharmacol*. 1972;22:415-421.

246. Way JL, et al. Effect of oxygen on cyanide intoxication. I. Prophylactic protection. *J Pharmacol Exp Ther*. 1966;13:381-382.

247. Weaver LK. Operational use and patient care in the monoplace hyperbaric chamber. *Resp Care Clinics of North America*. 1999;5:51-92.

248. Weaver LK, et al. Hyperbaric oxygen for acute carbon monoxide poisoning. *N Engl J Med*. 2002;347:1057-1067.

249. Wetherill HR. The occurrence of cyanide in the blood of fire victims. *J Forensic Sci*. 1966;11:167-173.

250. Whitcraft DD, et al. Hydrogen sulfide poisoning treated with hyperbaric oxygen. *J Emerg Med*. 1985;3:23-25.

251. Wolf SJ, Maloney, et al. Clinical policy: critical issues in the evaluation and management of adult patients presenting to the emergency department with acute carbon monoxide poisoning. *Ann Emerg Med*. 2017;69:98-107.

252. Wolf FJ, et al. Clinical policy: critical issues in the management of adult patients presenting to the emergency department with acute carbon monoxide poisoning. *Ann Emerg Med*. 2008;51:138-152.

253. Wong CK, et al. Protective effects of N-acetylcysteine against carbon tetrachloride- and trichloroethylene-induced poisoning in rats. *Environ Toxicol Pharmacol*. 2003;14:109-116.

254. Wong HP, et al. Effect of hyperbaric oxygen on skeletal muscle necrosis following primary and secondary ischemia in a rat model. *Surgical Forum*. 1996:705-707.

255. Xu J, et al. Carbon monoxide increases microparticles causing vascular and CNS dysfunction. *Toxicol Appl Pharmacol*. 2013;273:410-417.

256. Yang ZJ, et al. Hyperbaric O2 reduces intestinal ischemia-reperfusion-induced TNF-alpha production and lung neutrophil sequestration. *Eur J Appl Physiol*. 2001;85:96-103.

257. Zamboni WA, et al. Morphologic analysis of the microcirculation during reperfusion of ischemic skeletal muscle and the effect of hyperbaric oxygen. *Plast Reconstr Surg*. 1993;91:1110-1123.

258. Zearbaugh C, et al. Carbon tetrachloride/chloroform poisoning: case studies of hyperbaric oxygen in the treatment of lethal dose ingestion. *Undersea Biomed Res*. 1988;15:44.

123

CYANIDE AND HYDROGEN SULFIDE

Christopher P. Holstege and Mark A. Kirk

Cyanide

MW	=	26.02 Da
Whole blood	<	1 mcg/mL
	<	38.43 µmol/L
Concentrations		
Airborne		
Immediately fatal	=	270 ppm
Life threatening	=	110 ppm >30 minutes
Hydrogen Sulfide		
MW	=	34.08 Da
Airborne		
Odor threshold	=	0.01–0.3 ppm
Olfactory paralysis	=	100–150 ppm
Immediately fatal	=	1,000 ppm

CYANIDE POISONING

History and Epidemiology

Cyanide (CN) exposure is associated with smoke inhalation, laboratory mishaps, industrial incidents, suicide attempts, and criminal activity.[36,106] Cyanide is a chemical group that consists of one atom of carbon bound to one atom of nitrogen by three molecular bonds (C≡N). Inorganic CNs (also known as CN salts) contain CN in the anion form (CN⁻) and are used in industries, such as metallurgy, photographic developing, plastic manufacturing, fumigation, and mining. Common CN salts include sodium CN (NaCN) and potassium cyanide (KCN). Sodium salts react readily with water to form hydrogen cyanide (HCN) gas. Organic compounds that have a cyano group bonded to an alkyl residue are called nitriles. For example, methyl CN is also known as acetonitrile (CH_3CN). Hydrogen cyanide is a colorless gas at standard temperature and pressure with a reported bitter almond odor. Cyanogen gas, a dimer of CN, reacts with water and breaks down into the CN anion. Cyanogen chloride (CNCl) is a colorless gas that is easily condensed; it is a listed agent by the Chemical Weapons Convention.

Many plants, such as the *Manihot* spp, *Linum* spp, *Lotus* spp, *Prunus* spp, *Sorghum* spp, and *Phaseolus* spp, contain cyanogenic glycosides.[111] The *Prunus* species consisting of apricots, bitter almond, cherry, and peaches have pitted fruits containing the glucoside amygdalin. When ingested, amygdalin is biotransformed by intestinal β-D-glucosidase to glucose, benzaldehyde, and CN (Fig. 123–1). Laetrile, which contains amygdalin, was inappropriately suggested to have antineoplastic properties despite a lack of evidence to support such claims.[85] When laetrile was administered by intravenous (IV) infusion, amygdalin bypassed the necessary enzymes in the gastrointestinal (GI) tract to liberate CN and did not cause toxicity. However, ingested laetrile causes CN poisoning. Despite data demonstrating its lack of utility in the treatment of cancer, it still is available via the Internet.

Cassava (*Manihot esculenta*) root is a major source of food for millions of people in the tropics. It is a hardy plant that remains in the ground for up to 2 years and needs relatively little water to survive. Because the shelf life of a cassava root is short after it is removed from the stem, cassava root must be processed and sent to market as soon as it is harvested. However, proper processing must occur to assure the food's safety. Processed cassava is called *Gari*. Linamarin (2-hydroxyisobutyrnitrile-β-D-glucose) is the major cyanogenic glycoside in cassava roots. It is hydrolyzed to hydrogen CN and acetone in two steps during the processing of cassava roots.[114] Whereas soaking

peeled cassava in water for a single day releases approximately 45% of the cyanogens, soaking for 5 days causes 90% loss. If processing is inefficient, linamarin and cyanohydrin, the immediate product of hydrolysis of linamarin, remain in the food.[92] Consumed linamarin is hydrolyzed to cyanohydrin by β-glucosidases of the microorganisms in the intestines. Cyanohydrin present in the food and formed from linamarin then dissociates spontaneously to CN in the alkaline pH of the small intestines.

Iatrogenic CN poisoning occurs during prolonged or high-dose nitroprusside therapy for the management of hypertension. Each nitroprusside molecule contains five CN molecules, which are slowly released in vivo. If endogenous sulfate stores are depleted, as in the malnourished or postoperative patient, CN accumulates even with therapeutic nitroprusside infusion rates.

In 1782, the Swedish chemist Carl Wilhelm Scheele first isolated hydrogen CN. He reportedly died from the adverse health effects of CN poisoning in 1786. Napoleon III was the first to use HCN in chemical warfare, and it was subsequently used on World War I battlefields. During World War II, hydrocyanic acid pellets (brand name Zyklon B) caused more than one million deaths in Nazi gas chambers at Auschwitz, Buchenwald, and Majdanek.

FIGURE 123–1. Biotransformation of cyanogens acetonitrile (**A**) and amygdalin (**B**) to cyanide.

In 1978, KCN was used in a mass suicide led by Jim Jones of the People's Temple in Guyana, resulting in 913 deaths. Other notorious suicide cases include Wallace Carothers, Herman Goring, Heinrich Himmler, and Ramon Sampedro. In 1982, seven deaths resulted from consumption of CN-tainted acetaminophen in Chicago that subsequently led to the requirement of tamper-resistant pharmaceutical packaging. Numerous copycat murders subsequently occurred using CN-tainted capsules, with the last high-profile case occurring in 2010 involving an Ohio emergency medicine physician who murdered his wife with a CN-laden calcium capsule.[16] Cyanide is used for illicit euthanasia.[21] Internet websites provide detailed instructions on how to use various available chemicals to produce HCN.[2] The sale of CN is controlled in various countries, but the expansion of the "deep" or "dark" web enables users to purchase CN more easily with use of virtual money such as the "bitcoin."[79]

The American Association of Poison Control Centers' National Poison Data System reported 1,258 CN exposures from 2011 through 2015 (Chap. 130). One study of poison control center data found that 8.3% of patients with intentional overdoses died, and another 9% developed cardiac arrest but survived; 74% did not receive an antidote, most likely because of the failure of the initial treatment team to recognize the poisoning.[15] The potential for CN poisoning exists after smoke inhalation (ie, recent Kiss nightclub fire in Southern Brazil with more than 200 deaths attributed in part to CN), especially after the combustion of materials such as wool, silk, synthetic rubber, and polyurethane.[45] Ingestion of cyanogenic chemicals (ie, acetonitrile, acrylonitrile, and proprionitrile) is another source of CN poisoning.[108] Acetonitrile (C_2H_3N) and acrylonitrile (C_3H_3N) are themselves nontoxic, but biotransformation via CYP 2E1 liberates CN (Fig. 123–1).[116]

Pharmacology

The dose of CN required to produce toxicity depends on the form of CN, the duration of exposure, and the route of exposure. However, CN is an extremely potent toxin with even small exposures leading to life-threatening symptoms. For example, an adult oral lethal dose of KCN is approximately 200 mg. An airborne concentration of 270 ppm (mcg/mL) of HCN is immediately fatal, and exposures greater than 110 ppm for more than 30 minutes are generally considered life threatening. The current Occupational Safety and Health Administration (OSHA) permissible exposure limit (PEL) for both HCN and cyanogen is 10 ppm as an 8-hour time-weighted average concentration. The immediately dangerous to life or health value for HCN is 50 ppm.

Acute toxicity occurs through a variety of routes, including inhalation, ingestion, dermal, and parenteral. Hydrogen cyanide readily crosses membranes because it has a low molecular weight (27 Da) and is nonionized. After absorption and dissolution in blood, there exists an equilibrium between the CN anion (CN^-) and undissociated HCN. Hydrogen cyanide is a weak acid with a pK_a of 9.21. Therefore, at a physiologic pH of 7.4, it exists primarily as HCN. Rapid diffusion across alveolar membranes followed by direct distribution to target organs accounts for the rapid lethality associated with HCN inhalation.

Toxicokinetics

Cyanide is eliminated from the body by multiple pathways. The major route for detoxification of CN is the enzymatic conversion to thiocyanate. Two sulfurtransferase enzymes, rhodanese (thiosulfate–CN sulfurtransferase) and β-mercaptopyruvate–CN sulfurtransferase, catalyze this reaction. The primary pathway for metabolism is rhodanese, which is widely distributed throughout the body and has the highest concentration in the liver. This enzyme catalyzes the transfer of a sulfane sulfur from a sulfur donor, such as thiosulfate to CN to form thiocyanate. In acute poisoning, the limiting factor in CN detoxification by rhodanese is the availability of adequate quantities of sulfur donors. The endogenous stores of sulfur are rapidly depleted, and CN metabolism slows. Hence, the efficacy of sodium thiosulfate as an antidote stems from its normalization of the metabolic inactivation of CN. The sulfation of CN is essentially irreversible, and the sulfation product thiocyanate has relatively little inherent toxicity. Thiocyanate is eliminated in urine. A number of minor pathways of metabolism (<15% of total) account for CN

elimination, including conversion to 2-aminothiazoline-4-carboxylic acid, incorporation into the 1-carbon metabolic pool, or in combination with hydroxycobalamin to form cyanocobalamin.

Limited human data regarding the CN elimination half-life are available. Elimination follows first-order kinetics, although it varies widely in reports (range, 1.2–66 hours).[10,49,74] Disparity in values results from the number of samples used to perform calculations and the effects of antidotal treatment. The volume of distribution of the CN anion varies according to species and investigator, with 0.075 L/kg reported in humans.[32]

Pathophysiology

Cyanide is an inhibitor of multiple enzymes, including succinic acid dehydrogenase, superoxide dismutase, carbonic anhydrase, and cytochrome oxidase.[82,88] Cytochrome oxidase is an iron-containing metalloenzyme essential for oxidative phosphorylation and hence aerobic energy production. It functions in the electron transport chain within mitochondria, converting catabolic products of glucose into adenosine triphosphate (ATP). Cyanide induces cellular hypoxia by inhibiting cytochrome oxidase at the cytochrome a_3 portion of the electron transport chain (Fig. 123–2). Hydrogen ions that normally would have combined with oxygen at the terminal end of the chain are no longer incorporated. Thus, despite sufficient oxygen supply, oxygen cannot be used, and ATP molecules are no longer formed. Unincorporated hydrogen ions accumulate, contributing to acidemia.

The lactate concentration increases rapidly following CN poisoning because of failure of aerobic energy metabolism. During aerobic conditions, when the electron transport chain is functional, lactate is converted to pyruvate by mitochondrial lactate dehydrogenase. In this process, lactate donates hydrogen moieties that reduce nicotinamide adenine dinucleotide (NAD⁺) to nicotinamide adenine dinucleotide (NADH). Pyruvate then enters the citric acid cycle, with resulting ATP formation. When cytochrome a_3 within the electron transport chain is inhibited by CN, there is a relative paucity of NAD⁺ and predominance of NADH, favoring the reverse reaction, in which pyruvate is converted to lactate.

Cyanide is also a potent neurotoxin. Cyanide exhibits a particular affinity for regions of the brain with high metabolic activity. Central nervous system (CNS) injury occurs via several mechanisms, including impaired oxygen utilization, oxidant stress, and enhanced release of excitatory neurotransmitters. Cranial imaging of survivors of CN poisoning reveals that injury occurs in the most oxygen-sensitive areas of the brains, such as the basal ganglia, cerebellum, and sensorimotor cortex.

Cyanide enhances N-methyl-D-aspartate (NMDA) receptor activity and directly activates the NMDA receptor, which increases release of glutamate and inhibits voltage-dependent magnesium blockade of the NMDA receptor. This NMDA receptor stimulation results in Ca^{2+} entry into the cytosol of neurons. Cyanide also activates voltage-sensitive calcium channels and mobilizes Ca^{2+} from intracellular stores.[61,83,96] As a result, cytosolic Ca^{2+} rises and activates a series of biochemical reactions that lead to the generation of reactive oxygen species (ROS) and nitrous oxide.[71,103] These ROS initiate

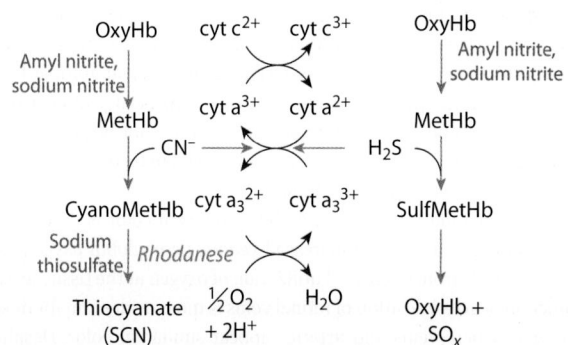

FIGURE 123–2. Pathway of cyanide and hydrogen sulfide toxicity and detoxification. MetHb = methemoglobin; OxyHb = oxyhemoglobin; SulfMetHb = sulfmethemoglobin.

peroxidation of cellular lipids, which, together with CN-induced inhibition of the respiratory chain, adversely affect mitochondrial function, initiating cytochrome c release and execution of apoptosis, necrosis, and subsequent neurodegeneration.[7,95] Experimental studies demonstrate that NMDA inhibitors such as dextrorphan and dizocilpine, antioxidants, and cyclooxygenase inhibitors all protect neurons against CN-induced damage.[58,80,115]

Sulfurtransferase metabolism via rhodanese is crucial for detoxification. However, the aforementioned CN-induced metabolic derangement decreases enzyme detoxification. Decreased ATP and ROS and increased cytosolic Ca^{2+} stimulate protein kinase C activity, which in turn inactivates rhodanese.[4]

Clinical Manifestations
Acute Exposure to Cyanide
The amount, duration of exposure, route of exposure, and premorbid condition of the individual all influence the time to onset and severity of illness. A critical combination of these factors overwhelms endogenous detoxification pathways, allowing CN to diffusely affect cellular function within the body. No reliable pathognomonic symptom or toxic syndrome is associated with acute CN poisoning.[44,60] The initial clinical effects of acute CN poisoning are nonspecific, generalized, and nondiagnostic, thereby making the correct diagnosis difficult to obtain. Clinical manifestations reflect rapid dysfunction of oxygen sensitive organs, with CNS and cardiovascular findings predominating. The time to onset of symptoms typically is seconds with inhalation of gaseous HCN or IV injection of a water-soluble CN salt and several minutes after ingestion of inorganic CN. The clinical effects of cyanogenic chemicals often are delayed, and the time course varies among individuals (range, 3–24 hours), depending on their rate of biotransformation.[108] Clinically apparent CN toxicity occurs within hours to days of initiating nitroprusside infusion, although concurrent administration of thiosulfate or hydroxocobalamin prevents toxicity (Chap. 61).[102]

Central nervous system signs and symptoms are typical of progressive hypoxia and include headache, anxiety, agitation, confusion, lethargy, nonreactive dilated pupils, seizures, and coma. A centrally mediated tachypnea occurs initially followed by bradypnea and apnea.

Cardiovascular responses to CN are complex. Studies of isolated heart preparations and intact animal models show that the principal cardiac insult is slowing of heart rate and loss of contractile force.[9] Several reflex mechanisms, including catecholamine release and central vasomotor activity, modulate myocardial performance and vascular response in patients with CN poisoning.[72] In laboratory investigations, a brief period of increased inotropy caused by reflex compensatory mechanisms occurs before myocardial depression. Clinically, an initial period of tachycardia and hypertension usually occurs followed by hypotension with reflex tachycardia, but the terminal event is consistently bradycardia and hypotension. Ventricular dysrhythmias are rarely reported.

Pulmonary edema is reported at autopsy.[44] Inhalation of HCN is also associated with mild corrosive injury to the respiratory tract mucosa.

Gastrointestinal toxicity occurs after ingestion of inorganic CN and cyanogens and includes abdominal pain, nausea, and vomiting. These symptoms are caused by hemorrhagic gastritis, which is frequently identified on autopsy, and are thought to be secondary to the corrosive nature of CN salts. However, if death occurs rapidly, this gastritis is not seen at autopsy because development of inflammation occurs over time.[44] After ingestion, a smell of bitter almonds is noted in a few reports but should not be relied on to be emitted from the GI system as health care providers in nearly all case reports published do not mention this finding.[30]

Cutaneous manifestations vary. A cherry red skin color is described as a potential finding as a result of increased venous hemoglobin oxygen saturation, which results from decreased utilization of oxygen at the tissue level. The phenomenon of arterialization of retinal veins is more evident on funduscopic examination, where veins and arteries appear similar in color. Despite the inference in the name, CN itself does not directly cause cyanosis. The occurrence of cyanosis is most commonly reported in published case reports and is likely caused by cardiovascular collapse and subsequent poor perfusion.[30]

Delayed Clinical Manifestations of Acute Exposure
Survivors of serious, acute poisoning develop delayed neurologic sequelae. Parkinsonian symptoms, including dystonia, dysarthria, rigidity, and bradykinesia, are most common. Symptoms typically develop over weeks to months, but subtle findings are reported to be present within a few days. Head computed tomography (CT) and magnetic resonance imaging (MRI) consistently reveal basal ganglia damage (globus pallidus, putamen, and hippocampus) with radiologic changes appearing several weeks after onset of symptoms. Whether delayed manifestations result from direct cellular injury or secondary hypoxia is unclear. Extrapyramidal manifestations either progress or resolve. Response to pharmacotherapy with antiparkinsonian drugs is generally disappointing.

Chronic Exposure to Cyanide
Chronic exposure to CN results in insidious syndromes, including tobacco amblyopia, Konzo, and Leber hereditary optic neuropathy. Tobacco amblyopia is a progressive loss of visual function that occurs almost exclusively in men who smoke cigarettes. Affected smokers have lower serum cyanocobalamin and thiocyanate concentrations than unaffected smoking counterparts, suggesting a reduced ability to detoxify CN. Cessation of smoking and administration of hydroxocobalamin often reverse symptoms. Konzo is associated with the consumption of insufficiently processed "bitter" (cyanogenic) cassava. Neurologic manifestations include spastic paraparesis that is often sudden and symmetrical affecting the legs more than the arms. Malnutrition places individuals at greater risk in part caused by low vitamin B_{12} intake.[69] Removal of dietary cassava and institution of vitamin B_{12} therapy is the mainstay of prevention and therapy. Leber hereditary neuropathy, a condition of subacute visual failure affecting men, is thought to be caused by mitochondrial DNA mutations exacerbated by exposure to cyanogenic glycosides.[39]

Chronic exposure to CN is associated with thyroid disorders.[1] Thiocyanate is a competitive inhibitor of iodide entry into the thyroid, thereby causing the formation of goiters and the development of hypothyroidism (Chap. 53). Chronic exposure to CN in animals is associated with hydropic degeneration in hepatocytes and epithelial cells of the renal proximal tubules; however, these morphologic lesions are not linked to functional alternations.[105]

Diagnostic Testing
Because of nonspecific symptoms and delay in laboratory CN confirmation, the clinician must rely on historical circumstances and some initial findings to raise suspicion of CN poisoning and institute therapy (Table 123–1).

Laboratory findings suggestive of CN poisoning reflect the known metabolic abnormalities, which include an increased anion gap metabolic acidosis and elevated lactate concentration. Elevated venous oxygen saturation results from reduced tissue extraction.[63] A venous oxygen saturation above 90% from superior vena cava or pulmonary artery blood indicates decreased oxygen utilization. This finding is not specific for CN and could represent cellular poisoning from other xenobiotics such as carbon monoxide (CO), clenbuterol, hydrogen sulfide (H_2S), and sodium azide or medical conditions such as sepsis, high-output cardiac syndromes, and left-to-right intracardiac shunts.

Hyperlactatemia is found in numerous critical illnesses and typically is a nonspecific finding. However, a significant association exists between blood CN and serum lactate concentrations.[11,12] Arterial blood gas pH correlates inversely with CN concentration.[12] The finding of a small arterial–venous oxygen difference is also suggestive of CN toxicity.

Cyanide results in nonspecific electrocardiographic findings.[37] Rhythm disturbances such as sinus tachycardia, bradydysrhythmias, atrial fibrillation, ventricular tachycardia, and ventricular fibrillation are all reported, as are elevation or depression of the ST segment, shortened ST segments, and fusion of the T wave into the QRS complex.

A determination of the blood CN concentration will confirm toxicity, but this determination is not available in a sufficiently rapid manner to affect initial treatment. It is clinically not possible to obtain the blood CN concentration at the exact time of the exposure when concentrations would be expected to be at peak. Subsequent later testing would be expected to

TABLE 123–1	Cyanide Poisoning: Emergency Management Guidelines

When to Suspect Cyanide

Sudden collapse of laboratory or industrial worker

Fire victim with coma or acidemia

Suicide with unexplained rapid coma or acidemia

Ingestion of artificial nail remover

Ingestion of seeds or pits from *Prunus* spp

Patient with altered mental status, acidemia, and tachyphylaxis to nitroprusside

Supportive Care

Control airway, ventilate, and give 100% oxygen

Crystalloids and vasopressors for hypotension

Administer sodium bicarbonate; titrate according to ABG and serum [HCO_3^-]

Antidotes

1) Hydroxocobalamin (preferred)

Initial adult dose: 5 g IV over 15 min; pediatric dose 70 mg/kg up to 5 g; to be repeated if necessary

or

2) Cyanide Antidote Kit

Amyl nitrite pearls are included in the kit for prehospital use. For hospital management, sodium nitrite is the preferred methemoglobin inducer and is given in lieu of the pearls.

Give sodium nitrite ($NaNO_2$) as a 3% solution over 2–4 min IV: Adult dose: 10 mL (300 mg) (Table 123–2 for pediatric dosing)

Caution: Monitor blood pressure frequently and treat hypotension by slowing infusion rate and giving crystalloids and vasopressors. Obtain methemoglobin level 30 min after dose; excess methemoglobin formation will cause deterioration during therapy. Withhold nitrites if COHb is suspected to be present.

Give sodium thiosulfate (NaS_2O_3) as a 25% solution IV:

Adult dose: 50 mL (12.5 g)

Pediatric dose: 1.65 mL/kg up to 50 mL

Decontamination

Protect health care provider from contamination

Cutaneous: Carefully remove all clothing and flush the skin

Ingestion: Oro- or nasogastric lavage and instill 1 g/kg activated charcoal

Laboratory

ABG

Electrolytes and glucose

Blood lactate

Whole-blood cyanide concentration (for later confirmation only)

ABG = arterial blood gas; COHb = carboxyhemoglobin; IV = intravenous.

---

demonstrate lower concentrations depending on the source of exposure. Whole blood or serum can be analyzed, with most reports using whole blood for CN determination. In mammals, including primates, whole-blood concentrations are twice serum concentrations as a result of CN sequestration in red blood cells. Background whole-blood CN concentrations in smokers are higher than in nonsmokers. Coma and respiratory depression are associated with whole-blood concentrations greater than 2.5 mcg/mL, and death is associated with concentrations greater than 3 mcg/mL depending on the timing of the collection relative to the exposure. Serum thiocyanate concentrations are of limited value in assessing patients with acute poisoning because of a lack of correlation with symptoms but are useful in confirming exposure. Depending on the timing of collection, urinary thiocyanate is used as a marker of CN exposure. More recently, a CN metabolite named 2-aminothiazoline-4-carboxylic acid (ACTA) that is not significantly influenced by putrefaction was found to be a reliable biomarker of CN poisoning because of its long-term stability in biological material.[43]

A semiquantitative assay that uses colorimetric paper test strips immediately detect CN. Cyantesmo test strips currently are used by water treatment facilities to detect CN. An investigation of the utility of these strips in

clinical practice found that the test strips incrementally increased to a deep blue color over a progressively longer portion of the test strip with increasing concentrations of CN in the blood.[100] These strips accurately and rapidly detected, in a semiquantifiable manner, CN concentrations greater than 1 mcg/mL.

Management

Because CN poisoning is rare, it is easy to overlook the diagnosis unless there is an obvious history of exposure. Thus, the most critical steps in treatment are considering the diagnosis in high-risk situations (Table 123–1) and initiating empiric therapy with 100% oxygen and either hydroxycobalamin or the sodium nitrite and sodium thiosulfate combination. The initial care (Table 123–1) of a CN-poisoned patient begins by directing attention to airway patency, ventilatory support, and oxygenation.

Intravenous access should be rapidly obtained and blood samples sent for kidney function, glucose, and electrolyte determinations. A whole-blood CN concentration should be obtained for later confirmation of exposure. Arterial blood gas analysis and serum lactate concentration will help assess acid–base status. Clinicians should initiate crystalloids and vasopressors for hypotension.

First responders should exercise extreme caution when entering potentially hazardous areas such as chemical plants and laboratories where a previously healthy person is "found down." Exposure to CN occurs by multiple routes, including ingestion, inhalation, dermal, and parenteral. For patients with inhalation exposure, removal from the area of exposure is critical. Further decontamination is generally unnecessary. Decontamination of a CN-poisoned patient occurs concurrently with initial resuscitation. The health care provider should always be protected from potential dermal contamination by using personal protective devices such as water-impervious gowns, gloves, and eyewear. For patients with cutaneous exposure, remove their clothing, brush any powder off the skin, and flush the skin with water. Particular attention should be given to open wounds because CN is readily absorbed through abraded skin.

Instillation of activated charcoal often is considered by other authors to be ineffective because of low binding of CN (1 g of activated charcoal only adsorbs 35 mg of CN). However, a potentially lethal oral dose of CN (ie, a few hundred milligrams) is within the adsorptive capacity of a typical 1-g/kg dose of activated charcoal. Preexposure activated charcoal administration improved survival in animals given an LD_{100} dose of KCN.[75] Based on the potential benefits and minimal risks, we recommend activated charcoal in the patient with an intact protected airway.

Although either hydroxocobalamin or sodium nitrite and sodium thiosulfate combination should be administered as soon as CN poisoning is suspected, hydroxocobalamin is preferred. Hydroxocobalamin is a metalloprotein with a central cobalt atom that complexes CN, forming cyanocobalamin (vitamin B_{12}). Cyanocobalamin is eliminated in the urine or releases the CN moiety at a rate sufficient to allow detoxification by rhodanese. One molecule of hydroxocobalamin binds one molecule of CN, yielding a molecular weight binding ratio of 50:1. The US FDA-approved adult starting dose is 5 g administered by IV infusion over 15 minutes. Depending on the severity of the poisoning and the clinical response, a second dose of 5 g is recommended by IV infusion for a total dose of 10 g. Hydroxocobalamin has few adverse effects, which includes rashes and a transient reddish discoloration of the skin, mucous membranes, and urine. No hemodynamic adverse effects other than a potential mild transient rise of blood pressure are observed.

Although no longer available, the CN antidote kit contained amyl nitrite, sodium nitrite, and sodium thiosulfate. Both thiosulfate and nitrite individually have antidotal efficacy when given alone in animal models of CN poisoning, but they have even greater benefit when they are given in combination.[82] Thiosulfate donates the sulfur atoms necessary for rhodanese-mediated CN biotransformation to thiocyanate. The mechanism of nitrite is less clear. Traditional rationale relies on the ability of nitrite to generate methemoglobin. Because CN has a higher affinity for methemoglobin than for cytochrome a_3, cytochrome oxidase function is restored. However, improved hepatic blood flow and nitric oxide (NO) formation are alternative explanations.

TABLE 123–2	Cyanide Pediatric (<25 kg) Sodium Nitrite Guidelines*	
Hemoglobin (g/dL)	**$NaNO_2$ (mg/kg)**	**3% $NaNO_2$ solution (mL/kg)****
7.0	5.8	0.19
8.0	6.6	0.22
9.0	7.5	0.25
10.0	8.3	0.27
11.0	9.1	0.30
12.0	10.0	0.33
13.0	10.8	0.36
14.0	11.6	0.39

^aPediatric thiosulfate dose: 1.65 mL/kg of 25% solution up to 50 mL.

**$NaNO_2$ dosing should not exceed 10 mL.

Adapted with permission from Berlin CM. The treatment of cyanide poisoning in children. *Pediatrics.* 1970 Nov;46(5):793-796.

Amyl nitrite was packaged within glass pearls that are crushed and intermittently inhaled or intermittently introduced into the ventilator system to initiate methemoglobin formation. The amyl nitrite pearls were reserved for cases in which IV access was delayed or not possible. Intravenous sodium nitrite is preferred and is supplied as a 10-mL volume of 3% solution (300 mg). Adverse effects of nitrites include excessive methemoglobin formation and, because of potent vasodilation, hypotension and tachycardia. Avoiding rapid infusion, monitoring blood pressure, and adhering to dosing guidelines limit adverse effects. Because of the potential for excessive methemoglobinemia during nitrite treatment, pediatric dosing guidelines are available (Table 123–2). Sodium thiosulfate was the second component of the CN antidote kit. It is supplied as 50 mL of 25% solution (12.5 g). It is a substrate for the reaction catalyzed by rhodanese that is essentially irreversible, converting a highly toxic entity to a relatively harmless compound. However, thiocyanate has its own toxicity in the presence of kidney failure, including abdominal pain, vomiting, rash, CNS dysfunction and hypothyroidism with chronically elevated concentrations. Thiosulfate itself is not associated with significant adverse reactions. The pediatric dose of thiosulfate is adjusted for weight. The currently available antidote Nithiodote contains both sodium nitrite and sodium thiosulfate in the same concentrations as were available in the CN antidote kit but no longer provides amyl nitrite.

After acetonitrile exposure, administration of disulfiram is proposed by some authorities as an inhibitor of CYP2E1 to prevent the conversion of acetonitrile to cyanohydrin, thereby preventing significant CN formation but there is not enough data to recommend this therapy currently.[31]

The antidote 4-dimethylaminophenol (4-DMAP), rather than sodium nitrite, is also used as a methemoglobin inducer.[50] It generates methemoglobin more rapidly than sodium nitrite, with peak methemoglobin concentrations at 5 minutes after 4-DMAP rather than 30 minutes after sodium nitrite. The dose of 4-DMAP is 3 mg/kg and is coadministered with thiosulfate. As with sodium nitrite, its major adverse effect is excessive methemoglobin formation and potential for hypotension. Cobalt in the form of dicobalt edetate is used as a CN chelator, and it is associated with significant adverse effects such as hypertension, tachycardia, and angioedema.[81] The cobalamin precursor cobinamide is used both prophylactically and therapeutically to treat experimental CN toxicity, and when given at high enough doses, it has rescued animals from CN induced apnea and coma.[23] Cobinamide is an investigational treatment that has a much greater affinity for CN ion than cobalamin.[27] Dimethyl trisulfide (DMTS) acts as a sulfur donor for rhodanese and has efficacy against CN poisoning in animal models and is being explored for prehospital use in humans. Hyperbaric oxygen (HBO) was considered in the past, but recent evidence suggests no benefit in CN poisoning.[78]

In animal models, the antioxidant vitamins A, C, and E diminish the extent of tissue damage caused by subacute CN intoxication.[90] This is especially important in the tropics, where the majority of dietary staples are cyanophoric crops such as cassava. These therapies have no proven utility in acute poisoning and therefore are not recommended.

Patients who do not survive CN poisoning are suitable organ donors. Heart, liver, kidney, pancreas, cornea, skin, and bone have been successfully transplanted after CN poisoning[38] (Special Considerations: SC12).

HYDROGEN SULFIDE POISONING
History and Epidemiology

Hydrogen sulfide exposures are often dramatic and fatal. The American Association of Poison Control Centers' National Poison Data System reported 4,442 exposures from 2011 through 2015 (Chap 130). Only 1,670 of these exposures required evaluation at a health care facility, 573 reported moderate or major effects, and 35 deaths occurred. Most often, serious consequences of H_2S exposures occur through workplace exposures, but they also occur in environmental disasters and suicides.

Bacterial decomposition of proteins generates H_2S, and the gas is produced in many industrial activities. Decay of the sulfur-containing products such as fish, sewage, and manure produce H_2S. Industrial sources include pulp paper mills, heavy-water production, the leather industry, roofing asphalt tanks, vulcanizing of rubber, viscose rayon production, and coke manufacturing from coal.[28] It is a major industrial hazard in oil and gas production, particularly in sour gas fields (natural gas containing sulfur).

Between 1990 and 1999, H_2S poisoning was associated with the deaths of 18% of US construction workers killed by toxic inhalation.[33] Many died while working in confined spaces such as sewers or sewer manholes. Agricultural workers operating near livestock manure storage tanks are at greatest risk of harm from an inhalation exposure.[14,51] Poisoned workers are "knocked down," prompting coworkers to attempt a rescue. Numerous case reports describe multiple victims because the would-be rescuers often themselves become victims when they attempt a rescue in an environment having high concentrations of H_2S.[8,14,33] Studies report that up to 25% of fatalities involve rescuers.[33,40,56] For example, a leaking food waste pipeline in the propeller room of a cruise ship released H_2S, killing 3 workers attempting to repair the pipe. The emergency response resulted in injury to 18 crew members, including a physician and a nurse rushing into the dangerous environment without personal protective equipment.[3]

Occupational Safety and Health Administration and a variety of occupational organizations such as the American Industrial Hygiene Association, the National Institute of Occupational Safety and Health, the American Shipbuilding Association, and the US Chemical Safety Board recognize the serious dangers of H_2S exposures in the workplace and continue to promote safety alerts and educational programs.

Natural sources of H_2S are volcanoes, caves, sulfur springs, and underground deposits of natural gas.[28,99] Hydrogen sulfide is also implicated in several environmental disasters. In 1950, 22 people died, and 320 were hospitalized in Poza Rica, Mexico, when a local natural gas facility inadvertently released H_2S into the air.[84] Hydrogen sulfide claimed nine lives when a sour gas well failed, releasing a cloud of the poisonous gas into the Denver City, Texas community in 1975.[86] In 2003, a gas drilling incident in southwest China released natural gas and a cloud of H_2S into a populated area, killing more than 200 people, injuring 9,000, and necessitating the evacuation of more than 40,000.[118]

More recently, a large number of suicides called "chemical suicides" or "detergent suicides" were attributed to mixing common household chemicals such as pesticides or fungicides and toilet bowl cleaners to create H_2S gas.[70,98] This practice is of concern because the instructions are easily found on Internet sites, precursor chemicals are readily accessible from the cleaning section of many local stores, first responders are at risk of harmful toxic effects from exposure, and the toxic gas can inadvertently expose groups of people in nearby buildings. In Japan, a "chain reaction of suicides" occurred, meaning it escalated nationwide with more than 200 people dead in the first half of 2008.[70] Information resources on the Internet are implicated for the widespread practice and prompted police to request purging these suicide instructions from Internet sites.[54] In the United States, chemical suicides from H_2S are likely underreported but rose from 2 in 2008 to 19 in 2010.[98] In as many as 80% of incidents, first responders report exposures after attempted rescue of victims.[98] Suicide victims using this method to harm themselves inadvertently cause injuries and evacuations because of the toxic gas permeating buildings. One incident in Japan caused 90 people to become ill from the toxic gas as it permeated an apartment building, and another resulted in 350 people evacuating a building.[110]

Pharmacology and Toxicokinetics

Hydrogen sulfide is a colorless gas, more dense than air, with an irritating odor of "rotten eggs." It is highly lipid soluble, a property that allows easy penetration of biologic membranes. Systemic absorption usually occurs through inhalation, and it is rapidly distributed to tissues.[99]

The tissues most sensitive to H_2S are those with high oxygen demand. The systemic toxicity of H_2S results from its potent inhibition of cytochrome oxidase, thereby interrupting oxidative phosphorylation.[28] Hydrogen sulfide binds to the ferric (Fe^{3+}) moiety of cytochrome a_3 oxidase complex with a higher affinity than does CN. The resulting inhibition of oxidative phosphorylation produces cellular hypoxia and anaerobic metabolism.[28]

Cytochrome oxidase inhibition is not the sole mechanism of toxicity. Other enzymes are inhibited by H_2S and contribute to its toxic effects.[99] Besides producing cellular hypoxia, H_2S alters brain neurotransmitter release and neuronal transmission through potassium channel–mediated hyperpolarization of neurons, NMDA receptor potentiation, and has other neuronal inhibitory mechanisms.[91,99] A proposed mechanism of death is poisoning of the brainstem respiratory center through selective uptake by lipophilic white matter in this region.[117] The olfactory nerve is a specific target of great interest. Not only does the toxic gas cause olfactory nerve paralysis, but it also provides a portal of entry into the CNS because of its direct contact with the brain.[119] It is also cytotoxic through formation of reactive sulfur and oxygen species. It also reacts with iron to fuel the Fenton reaction (Chap. 10), causing free radical injury.[109]

In addition to systemic effects, H_2S reacts with the moisture on the surface of mucous membranes to produce intense irritation and corrosive injury. The eyes and nasal and respiratory mucous membranes are the tissues most susceptible to direct injury.[76,119] Despite skin irritation, it has little dermal absorption.

Along with NO and CO, researchers recently recognized H_2S as a signaling molecule of the cardiovascular, renal, inflammatory, and nervous systems, and therefore, they proposed to add H_2S as the "third endogenous gaseous transmitter." Mice inhaling a low dose of H_2S demonstrated a decrease in their metabolic demands, causing them to enter a "suspended animationlike state."[20] This report propelled researchers into studies probing the biosynthesis, metabolism, and physiologic responses of H_2S in hopes of developing future beneficial therapies to combat the adverse consequences of ischemia-reperfusion injury.[26,34,91] Currently, researchers are pursuing the therapeutic potential for H_2S donors for diseases such as ischemia-reperfusion injury in acute stroke and ischemic kidney injury, cisplatin nephrotoxicity, atherosclerosis, heart failure, acute and chronic inflammatory diseases, and Parkinson and Alzheimer diseases.[18,26,34] Researchers' enthusiastic pursuit of a better understanding of H_2S with an intent to create innovative therapies will likely also benefit our understanding of its mechanisms of toxicity and potentially lead to new treatments for toxic exposures.

Inhaled H_2S enters the systemic circulation where, at physiologic pH, it dissociates into hydrosulfide ions (HS^-).[18] After dissociation, hydrosulfide ions interact with metalloproteins, disulfide-containing enzymes, and thio dimethyl S transferase. Hydrogen sulfide and dissociation products are then metabolized by multiple enzymes, including mitochondrial sulfide:quinone oxireductase, sulfur dioxygenase to form sulfate (SO_2^{-4}), and thiosulfate:CN sulfurtransferase (rhodanese) to form thiosulfate (SSO_3^{-2}).[18] The most specific marker of H_2S metabolism is thiosulfate.[18,68] Sulfhemoglobin is not found in significant concentrations in the blood of animals or fatally poisoned humans.[91,94]

TABLE 123–3	Hydrogen Sulfide Poisoning

When to Suspect Hydrogen Sulfide Poisoning

Rapid loss of consciousness ("knocked down") and abrupt awakening
Rapid loss of consciousness ("knocked down") and apnea
Rotten egg odor
Rescue from enclosed space, such as sewer or manure pit
Multiple victims with sudden death
Collapse of a previously healthy worker at work site

Clinical Manifestations

System	Signs and Symptoms
Cardiovascular	Chest pain, bradycardia, sudden cardiac arrest
Central nervous	Headache, weakness, syncope, convulsions, rapid onset of coma ("knockdown")
Gastrointestinal	Nausea, vomiting
Ophthalmic	Conjunctivitis
Pulmonary	Dyspnea, cyanosis, crackles, apnea
Metabolic	Metabolic acidosis, elevated serum lactate

Clinical Manifestations

Acute Manifestations

Hydrogen sulfide poisoning should be suspected whenever a person is found unconscious in an enclosed space, especially if the odor of rotten eggs is noted. The primary target organs of hydrogen sulfide poisoning are those of the CNS, cardiac system, and respiratory system. The clinical findings reported in two large series are listed in Table 123–3.[5,24]

Hydrogen sulfide poisoning has a distinct dose response, and the intensity of exposure likely accounts for the diverse clinical findings in the reports. The odor threshold is between 0.01 and 0.3 ppm, and a strong intense odor is noted at 20 to 30 ppm. Mucous membrane and eye irritation occurs at 20 to 100 ppm. Olfactory nerve paralysis occurs at 100 to 150 ppm rapidly extinguishing the ability to perceive the gas odor at higher concentrations. Prolonged exposure occurs when the extinction of odor recognition is misinterpreted as dissipation of the gas. Strong irritation of the upper respiratory tract and eyes and acute respiratory distress syndrome (ARDS) occur at 150 to 300 ppm. At greater than 500 ppm, H_2S produces systemic effects, including rapid unconsciousness ("knockdown") and cardiopulmonary arrest. At 1,000 ppm, breathing ceases after one to two breaths.[13,47,99]

Hydrogen sulfide reacts with the moisture on the surface of mucous membranes to produce intense irritation and corrosive injury. Mucous membrane irritation of the eye produces keratoconjunctivitis. If exposure persists, damage to the epithelial cells produces reversible corneal ulcerations ("gas eye") and, rarely, irreversible corneal scarring.[76,113] The irritant effects on the respiratory tract include rhinitis, bronchitis, and ARDS.[5,24,119]

Neurologic manifestations are common and often are severe. The rapid and deadly onset of clinical effects of H_2S are termed the "slaughterhouse sledgehammer" effect. In one case series, 75% of 221 patients with acute H_2S exposure lost consciousness at the time of exposure.[24] If a victim is rapidly removed from the exposure, recovery is often prompt and complete. Because unresponsiveness is rapid, trauma from falls should not be overlooked.[5,41] In a report, 7% of patients experiencing a "knockdown" had associated traumatic injuries.[5]

Hypoxia from respiratory compromise contributes secondarily to neurologic effects.[13,28,47,119] Neurologic outcome is quite variable, ranging from no neurologic impairment to permanent sequelae. Delayed neuropsychiatric sequelae are reported after acute exposures.[87] Most evidence suggests that the early rapid CNS effects are direct neurotoxic effects of H_2S, but the permanent neurologic sequelae result from hypoxia secondary to respiratory insufficiency.[13,119] Reported neuropsychiatric changes include memory failure (amnestic syndrome), lack of insight, disorientation, delirium, and dementia.[119] Neurosensory abnormalities include transient hearing impairment, vision loss, and anosmia. Motor symptoms are likely caused by injury to the basal ganglia and result in ataxia, position or intention tremor, and muscle rigidity.[111] Common neuropathologic findings observed on neuroimaging and at autopsy are subcortical white matter demyelination and globus pallidus degeneration.[87]

Animal studies report depressed cardiac contractility producing cardiogenic shock after H_2S exposures.[52,104] Myocardial hypoxia or direct toxic effects of H_2S on cardiac tissue causes cardiac dysrhythmias, myocardial ischemia, or myocardial infarction.[46]

Chronic Manifestations

Most data about chronic low-level exposures to H_2S come from oil and gas industry workers and sewer workers. Mucous membrane irritation seems to be the most prominent problem in patients with low concentration exposures. Workers report nasal, pharyngeal, and eye irritation; fatigue; headache; dizziness; and poor memory with low-concentration, chronic exposures. The chronic irritating effects of H_2S is proposed to be the cause of reduced lung volumes observed in sewer workers.[101] Volunteer studies have not demonstrated significant cardiovascular effects after long-term exposure to concentrations less than 10 ppm.[19] The liver, kidneys, and endocrine system are unaffected. No studies demonstrate increased incidences of cancer with low-level exposures.[28]

Rapid loss of consciousness from H_2S exposure was a well-known and, amazingly, accepted part of the workplace in the gas and oil industry for many years.[57] Some workers experienced repeated "knockdowns," and these workers reported an increased incidence of respiratory diseases and cognitive deficits. Single or repeated high-concentration exposures resulting in unconsciousness cause serious cognitive dysfunction. As noted above, the acute effects of rapid loss of consciousness are most likely caused by H_2S neurotoxicity. Although a clear association exists between knockdown and chronic neurologic sequelae, many of the case reports are complicated by associated apnea or hypoxemia from respiratory failure, asphyxia or exposure to other xenobiotics in a confined space, head injury from a fall, or near drowning in liquid manure or sludge.[119] The association of neurotoxic sequelae are less clear with prolonged low-concentration exposures. Case series suggest that low-concentration exposures cause subtle changes that are only measured by the most sensitive neuropsychiatric tests.[73]

Most effects reported to be associated with long-term exposures are nonspecific, and many of the cases have a poorly documented exposure assessment. Epidemiologic data regarding the effects of low-concentration environmental exposures to H_2S are clouded in populations exposed to complex mixtures of pollutants. Other malodorous sulfur compounds (eg, methyl mercaptan and methyl sulfide) are generated as byproducts of pulp mills. Currently, the association of protracted and low-concentration H_2S exposure with chronic neurologic sequelae remains controversial and needs further study.[47,48,119]

The strong odor of low concentrations of H_2S can magnify irritant effects by triggering a strong psychological response.[119] The odor of H_2S at low concentrations has been the alleged source of mass psychogenic illness cases[42] (Chap. 133). Clinical, epidemiologic, and toxicologic analyses suggested that 943 cases of illness in Jerusalem were caused by the odor of low concentrations of H_2S gas. Symptoms frequently associated with psychogenic illness include headaches; faintness; dizziness; nausea; chest tightness; dyspnea and tachypnea; eye, nose, and throat irritation; weakness; and extremity numbness.[64] Low concentration exposure to H_2S produces nonspecific signs and symptoms that could closely mimic psychogenic illness. Attempting to identify true toxicity from a powerful emotional reaction is extremely difficult.[42] Therefore, symptomatic patients must be assessed for toxicity even when mass psychogenic illness is suspected.

Diagnostic Testing

Only a few inhalation risks are similar to H_2S in their ability to rapidly "knock down" victims. Some examples include low-oxygen environments

in an enclosed space, HCN, volatile nerve agents, and CO. In H_2S poisoning, diagnostic testing is of limited value for clinical decision making after acute exposures, confirmation of acute exposures, occupational monitoring, and forensic analysis after fatal accidents. The etiology is often unclear early in the patient's emergency care and require clinicians to make treatment decisions without confirmatory evidence of poisoning.

Clinicians must base management decisions on history, clinical presentation, and diagnostic tests that infer the presence of H_2S because no method is available to rapidly and directly measure the gas or its metabolites. Circumstances surrounding the patient's illness often provide the best evidence for H_2S poisoning (Table 123–3). At the bedside, the smell of rotten eggs on clothing or emanating from the blood, exhaled air, or gastric secretions suggests H_2S exposure. In addition, darkening of silver jewelry is a clue to exposure. Paper impregnated with lead acetate changes color when exposed to H_2S and is used to detect its presence in the patient's exhaled breath but is not rapidly available.[28]

Specific tests for confirming H_2S exposure are not readily available in clinical laboratories. Therefore, directly measuring the gas in atmospheric air samples by monitoring devices provides stronger evidence of H_2S as the causative substance. Epidemiologic data show H_2S, along with CO and nitrogen (a simple asphyxiant) and oxygen-deficient environments, as some of the most common causes of death and injury from toxic inhalation in confined spaces, especially manholes and sewers.[33] Recognizing confined spaces as extremely hazardous environments, OSHA published the Confined Space Entry Standard to protect workers. It mandates training, rescue procedures, and atmospheric testing before entry, including measuring for the presence of H_2S. Because of OSHA's regulations, most emergency response teams are equipped to investigate toxic environments from hazardous materials incidents using a "four-gas detection unit" that measures H_2S by electrochemical sensors along with measurements for atmospheric oxygen concentration and the presence of explosive gases and CO.[112] In general, the clinician must interpret environmental detection results with caution. Negative results are misleading if toxic gases dissipate before atmospheric air sample collection. False-positive readings occur on field detection devices from interfering gases.[55] Therefore, a positive reading on these devices does not equate to confirmation of that specific gas. Clinical decision making should consider correlation with other circumstantial and clinical data and not rely solely on detection results.

In acute poisoning, readily available diagnostic tests that are biomarkers of H_2S poisoning are useful but are nonspecific. Arterial blood gas analysis demonstrating acidemia with an associated elevated serum lactate concentration is expected, and oxygen saturation should be normal unless ARDS is present. Hydrogen sulfide H_2S, like CN, decreases oxygen consumption and is reflected as an elevated mixed venous oxygen measurement. Because sulfhemoglobin (Chap. 124) typically is not generated in patients with H_2S poisoning, an oxygen saturation gap is not expected.[91,94]

Diagnostic testing for neurologic structure and function show abnormalities for weeks or months in many patients after serious injury from H_2S. Brain MRI and head CT studies demonstrate structural changes, such as globus pallidus degeneration and subcortical white matter demyelination. Neuropsychological testing demonstrates specific abnormalities in cortical functions, such as concentration, attention, verbal abstraction, and short-term retention. Single-photon emission computed tomography (SPECT)/PET brain scans define neurotoxin-induced lesions that correlate well with clinical neuropsychological testing.[25]

No clinically available biological markers or direct measurements of H_2S and its metabolites exist; therefore, confirming poisoning is challenging for clinicians, researchers, and forensic specialists.[91] Whole-blood sulfide concentrations greater than 0.05 mg/L are considered abnormal. Reliable measurements are ensured only if the concentration is obtained within 2 hours after the exposure and analyzed immediately.[99]

In acute exposures, blood and urine thiosulfate concentrations reflect exposure.[68] Urinary thiosulfate excretion is used to monitor chronic low-concentration exposure in the workplace. However, one study could not demonstrate a correlation between the degree of exposure and change in urine thiosulfate from baseline measurements.[35] Another study analyzed the value of blood and urine thiosulfate from data collected in a case series of fatal and nonfatal H_2S victims.[65,67] Because thiosulfate was detected in the urine but sulfide and thiosulfate were not detected in the blood of nonfatal exposures, this report concluded that thiosulfate in urine is the only indicator to prove H_2S poisoning in nonfatal cases.

Sulfide concentrations obtained in postmortem investigations are useful but require rapid sample collection because sulfide concentrations rise with tissue decomposition.[99] In the forensic literature, the detection of elevated thiosulfate concentrations is considered a reliable indicator of H_2S poisoning.[68,77] If death is rapid, urinary thiosulfate concentrations are often not detectable despite blood sulfide and thiosulfate concentrations 10-fold or greater than normal concentrations.[66] At autopsy, a greenish discoloration of the gray matter, viscera, and bronchial secretions is reported.[66,89]

Management

Clinicians faced with victims of "knockdown" syndrome should search for clues, such as victims' activities (eg, working at a manure pit), reports of chemicals detected at the scene by first responders, or suggestive clinical signs. The critical decision is whether to administer specific antidotes empirically. The basic aims are to gather as many facts and suggestive clues as possible, weigh the risk benefits for treatment or not, and treat early in the course, all this while meticulous attention to optimal supportive care is required.

The initial treatment (Table 123–4) is immediate removal of the victim from the contaminated area into a fresh air environment. High-flow oxygen should be administered as soon as possible. Optimal supportive care has the greatest influence on the patient's outcome. Because death from inhalation of H_2S is rapid a limited number of patients reaching the hospital for treatment are reported in the literature. Most patients experience significant delays before receiving treatment. Therefore, specific treatments and antidotal therapies do not show definitive improvement in patient outcome.

The proposed toxic mechanisms, animal studies, and human case reports suggest that oxygen therapy is beneficial for H_2S poisoning.[28,97,119]

TABLE 123–4 Hydrogen Sulfide Poisoning: Emergency Management

Supportive care
Prehospital
   Attempt rescue only if using appropriate respiratory protection
   Move victim to fresh air
   Administer 100% oxygen
   During extrication, evaluate for traumatic injuries from falls
   Apply ACLS protocols as indicated
Emergency department
   Maximize ventilation and oxygenation
   Utilize PEEP or BiPAP for ARDS
   Administer sodium bicarbonate; titrate according to ABG and serum [HCO_3^-]
   Administer crystalloid and vasopressors for hypotension

Antidote
1) It is reasonable to administer sodium nitrite (3% $NaNO_2$) IV over 2–4 min
   Adult dose: 10 mL (300 mg)
   Pediatric dose: Table 123–2; if hemoglobin unknown, presume 7 g/dL for dosing
   Caution:
      Monitor blood pressure frequently
      Obtain methemoglobin level 30 min after dose
OR
2) It is reasonable to administer hydroxocobalamin
   Initial adult dose: 5 g IV over 15 min; pediatric dose 70 mg/kg up to 5 g

ACLS = advanced cardiac life support; ABG = arterial blood gas; ARDS = acute respiratory distress syndrome; Hb = hemoglobin; IV = intravenous; PEEP = positive end-expiratory pressure.

Proposed mechanisms for the beneficial effects of oxygen are competitive reactivation of oxidative phosphorylation by inhibiting H_2S–cytochrome binding, enhanced detoxification by catalyzing oxidation of sulfides and sulfur, and improved oxygenation in the presence of ARDS. Studies demonstrate the binding of H_2S to cytochrome oxidase is readily reversible in the presence of oxygen, and an inverse relationship exists between tissue concentrations of H_2S and oxygen.[29,91] Increased oxygen concentrations enhance the consumption of H_2S through metabolic pathways, while oxygen deprivation results in the accumulation of H_2S in tissue. All patients suspected of H_2S poisoning should receive supplemental oxygen. In case reports, poisoned patients receiving HBO had favorable clinical outcomes.[6] However, no clinical data are available to suggest HBO is superior to normobaric oxygen for acute poisoning or preventing delayed neurologic sequelae. Unless immediately available, the therapeutic priority is meticulous supportive care with high-flow oxygen therapy over transport to a HBO capable facility.

Recognizing similar toxic mechanisms between H_2S and CN, the majority of research focuses on antidotes with high binding affinity to metallocompounds, including methemoglobin inducers (ferric iron) and cobalt-containing compounds. Nitrite-induced methemoglobin protects animals from toxicity of H_2S poisoning in both pre- and postexposure treatment models. Nitrite-generated methemoglobin acts as a scavenger of sulfide. The affinity of H_2S for methemoglobin is greater than that for cytochrome oxidase. When H_2S binds to methemoglobin, it forms sulfmethemoglobin.[17] Because H_2S poisoning is rare, no studies have evaluated the clinical outcomes of patients treated with sodium nitrite. Animal studies suggest that nitrite must be given within minutes of exposure to ensure effectiveness. However, several human case reports showed rapid return of normal sensorium when nitrites were administered soon after exposure.[59,93,107] Sodium nitrite treatment is reasonable to administer to patients with suspected H_2S poisoning who have altered mental status, coma, hypotension, or dysrhythmias but should be given cautiously because of the potential for nitrite-induced hypotension during the infusion. Sodium thiosulfate is of no benefit in the treatment of H_2S. Cobalt compounds, actively pursued as effective CN antidotes, have in vitro and in vivo benefits. Improved outcomes, including restoring depressed cardiac contractility, preventing pulseless electrical activity, and increasing survival, are demonstrated in animals administered hydroxocobalamin.[52,109] Cobinamide, a vitamin B_{12} analog, is actively being investigated for CN poisoning and showing promise as a novel therapy for H_2S.[22,62] Studies in rats and sheep suggest beneficial effects of methylene blue administered soon after H_2S poisoning.[53] Methylene blue administration rapidly restored impaired cardiac contractility and improved neurologic outcomes. The proposed mechanisms for the observed increase in survival of the treated groups included reducing properties, modulating calcium channels, antioxidant effects reducing ROS, and anti-NO effects. Only animal data and case reports are available to guide the use of any of these proposed antidotes.

Treatment of patients with H_2S poisoning requires optimal supportive care. Beyond supportive care, no definitive evidence of significant clinical benefit exists in humans, and additional research is needed to determine efficacy of specific treatments for H_2S poisoning. Because H_2S toxicity is severe and research studies suggest potential benefits of nitrite or hydroxocobalamin therapy, it is reasonable to administer either sodium nitrite or hydroxocobalamin for seriously ill patients exposed to H_2S. If administered, the best available evidence suggests these therapies should be initiated rapidly to be of any appreciable benefit and only after ensuring optimum supportive care.

SUMMARY

- Both CN and H_2S exposures are high-risk xenobiotics.
- There are particular metabolic risks and concerns with regard to exposure to both xenobiotics because they bind specifically to the ferric moiety of the cytochrome a_3 oxidase complex.
- Odor recognition is unreliable and is not a definitive approach to diagnosis.

- The laboratory evaluation usually is not timely for diagnostic purposes.
- Decontamination, removal from the site of exposure, and oxygen are essential with essential personal protection for responders.
- Hydroxocobalamin is the preferred antidote although sodium nitrite is reasonable in the absence of COHb elevation.

REFERENCES

1. Adewusi SR, Akindahunsi AA. Cassava processing, consumption, and cyanide toxicity. *J Toxicol Environ Health*. 1994;43:13-23.
2. Anderson AR. Characterization of chemical suicides in the United States and its adverse impact on responders and bystanders. *West J Emerg Med*. 2016;17:680-683.
3. Anonymous. Deaths and illness from hydrogen sulfide among ship workers. http://publichealth.lacounty.gov/acd/Report.htm.
4. Ardelt BK, et al. Cyanide-induced lipid peroxidation in different organs: subcellular distribution and hydroperoxide generation in neuronal cells. *Toxicology*. 1994;89:127-137.
5. Arnold IM, et al. Health implication of occupational exposures to hydrogen sulfide. *J Occup Med*. 1985;27:373-376.
6. Asif MJ, Exline MC. Utilization of hyperbaric oxygen therapy and induced hypothermia after hydrogen sulfide exposure. *Respir Care*. 2012;57:307-310.
7. Atlante A, et al. Cytochrome c, released from cerebellar granule cells undergoing apoptosis or excytotoxic death, can generate protonmotive force and drive ATP synthesis in isolated mitochondria. *J Neurochem*. 2003;86:591-604.
8. Barbera N, et al. Domino effect: an unusual case of six fatal hydrogen sulfide poisonings in quick succession. *Forensic Sci Int*. 2016;260:e7-10.
9. Barros RC, et al. Cardiovascular responses to chemoreflex activation with potassium cyanide or hypoxic hypoxia in awake rats. *Auton Neurosci*. 2002;97:110-115.
10. Baud FJ, et al. Elevated blood cyanide concentrations in victims of smoke inhalation. *N Engl J Med*. 1991;325:1761-1766.
11. Baud FJ, et al. Relation between plasma lactate and blood cyanide concentrations in acute cyanide poisoning. *BMJ*. 1996;312:26-27.
12. Baud FJ, et al. Value of lactic acidosis in the assessment of the severity of acute cyanide poisoning. *Crit Care Med*. 2002;30:2044-2050.
13. Beauchamp RO Jr, et al. A critical review of the literature on hydrogen sulfide toxicity. *Crit Rev Toxicol*. 1984;13:25-97.
14. Beaver RL, Field WE. Summary of documented fatalities in livestock manure storage and handling facilities—1975-2004. *J Agromedicine*. 2007;12:3-23.
15. Bebarta VS, et al. Seven years of cyanide ingestions in the USA: critically ill patients are common, but antidote use is not. *Emerg Med J*. 2011;28:155-158.
16. Bechtel L, Holstege CP. Forensic analysis of potassium cyanide stored in gelatin capsules. *Clin Toxicol*. 2010;48:614.
17. Beck JF, et al. Nitrite as antidote for acute hydrogen sulfide intoxication? *Am Ind Hyg Assoc J*. 1981;42:805-809.
18. Beltowski J. Hydrogen sulfide in pharmacology and medicine—an update. *Pharmacol Rep*. 2015;67:647-658.
19. Bhambhani Y, et al. Effects of 10-ppm hydrogen sulfide inhalation on pulmonary function in healthy men and women. *J Occup Environ Med*. 1996;38:1012-1017.
20. Blackstone E, et al. H_2S induces a suspended animation-like state in mice. *Science*. 2005;308:518.
21. Blanco PJ, Rivero AG. First case of illegal euthanasia in Spain: fatal oral potassium cyanide poisoning. *Soud Lek*. 2004;49:30-33.
22. Brenner M, et al. The vitamin B12 analog cobinamide is an effective hydrogen sulfide antidote in a lethal rabbit model. *Clin Toxicol (Phila)*. 2014;52:490-497.
23. Broderick KE, et al. Cyanide detoxification by the cobalamin precursor cobinamide. *Exp Biol Med (Maywood)*. 2006;231:641-649.
24. Burnett WW, et al. Hydrogen sulfide poisoning: review of 5 years' experience. *Can Med Assoc J*. 1977;117:1277-1280.
25. Callender TJ, et al. Three-dimensional brain metabolic imaging in patients with toxic encephalopathy. *Environ Res*. 1993;60:295-319.
26. Cao X, Bian JS. The role of hydrogen sulfide in renal System. *Front Pharmacol*. 2016;7:385.
27. Chan A, et al. Cobinamide is superior to other treatments in a mouse model of cyanide poisoning. *Clin Toxicol (Phila)*. 2010;48:709-717.
28. Chou S, et al. *Toxicological Profile for Hydrogen Sulfide*. US Department of Health and Human Services ATSDR; 2006.
29. Collman JP, et al. Using a functional enzyme model to understand the chemistry behind hydrogen sulfide induced hibernation. *Proc Natl Acad Sci U S A*. 2009;106:22090-22095.
30. Cote JL, et al. A systematic review of clinical presentations of cyanide poisoning. *Clin Toxicol*. 2016;54:471.
31. De Paepe P, et al. Disulfiram inhibition of cyanide formation after acetonitrile poisoning. *Clin Toxicol (Phila)*. 2016;54:56-60.
32. Djerad A, et al. Effects of respiratory acidosis and alkalosis on the distribution of cyanide into the rat brain. *Toxicol Sci*. 2001;61:273-282.
33. Dorevitch S, et al. Toxic inhalation fatalities of US construction workers, 1990 to 1999. *J Occup Environ Med*. 2002;44:657-662.
34. Dou Y, et al. The role of hydrogen sulfide in stroke. *Med Gas Res*. 2016;6:79-84.
35. Durand M, Weinstein P. Thiosulfate in human urine following minor exposure to hydrogen sulfide: implications for forensic analysis of poisoning. *Forensic Toxicol*. 2007;25:92-95.
36. Finnberg A, et al. Homicide by poisoning. *Am J Forensic Med Pathol*. 2013;34:38-42.
37. Fortin JL, et al. Cyanide poisoning and cardiac disorders: 161 cases. *J Emerg Med*. 2010;38:467-476.
38. Fortin JL, et al. Successful organ transplantation after treatment of fatal cyanide poisoning with hydroxocobalamin. *Clin Toxicol (Phila)*. 2007;45:468-471.
39. Freeman AG. Optic neuropathy and chronic cyanide toxicity. *Lancet*. 1986;1:441-442.
40. Fuller DC, Suruda AJ. Occupationally related hydrogen sulfide deaths in the United States from 1984 to 1994. *J Occup Environ Med*. 2000;42:939-942.
41. Gabbay DS, et al. Twenty-foot fall averts fatality from massive hydrogen sulfide exposure. *J Emerg Med*. 2001;20:141-144.
42. Gallay A, et al. Belgian coca-cola-related outbreak: intoxication, mass sociogenic illness, or both? *Am J Epidemiol*. 2002;155:140-147.
43. Giebultowicz J, et al. LC-MS/MS method development and validation for quantitative analyses of 2-aminothiazoline-4-carboxylic acid—a new cyanide exposure marker in post mortem blood. *Talanta*. 2016;150:586-592.
44. Gill JR, et al. Suicide by cyanide: 17 deaths. *J Forensic Sci*. 2004;49:826-828.
45. Gragnani A, et al. Response and legislative changes after the Kiss nightclub tragedy in Santa Maria/RS/Brazil: learning from a large-scale burn disaster. *Burns*. 2017;43:343-349.
46. Gregorakos L, et al. Hydrogen sulfide poisoning: management and complications. *Angiology*. 1995;46:1123-1131.
47. Guidotti TL. Hydrogen sulphide. *Occup Med (Oxf)*. 1996;46:367-371.
48. Guidotti TL. Hydrogen sulfide: advances in understanding human toxicity. *Int J Toxicol*. 2010;29:569-581.
49. Hall AH, et al. Nitrite/thiosulfate treated acute cyanide poisoning: estimated kinetics after antidote. *J Toxicol Clin Toxicol*. 1987;25:121-133.
50. Hall AH, et al. Which cyanide antidote? *Crit Rev Toxicol*. 2009;39:541-552.
51. Hallam DM, et al. Manure pit injuries: rare, deadly, and preventable. *J Emerg Trauma Shock*. 2012;5:253-256.
52. Haouzi P, et al. High-dose hydroxocobalamin administered after H2S exposure counteracts sulfide-poisoning-induced cardiac depression in sheep. *Clin Toxicol (Phila)*. 2015;53:28-36.
53. Haouzi P, et al. Developing effective countermeasures against acute hydrogen sulfide intoxication: challenges and limitations. *Ann N Y Acad Sci*. 2016;1374:29-40.
54. Harden B. Japan's latest suicide recipe purged from internet at police request. http://www.irishtimes.com/newspaper/world/2008/0530/1212095650051.html.
55. Hawley C. *Hazardous Materials Air Monitoring and Detection Devices*. 2nd ed. Clifton Park, New York, NY: Delmar Cengage Learning; 2006.
56. Hendrickson RG, et al. Co-worker fatalities from hydrogen sulfide. *Am J Ind Med*. 2004;45:346-350.
57. Hessel PA, et al. Lung health in relation to hydrogen sulfide exposure in oil and gas workers in Alberta, Canada. *Am J Ind Med*. 1997;31:554-557.
58. Himori N, et al. Dextrorphan attenuates the behavioral consequences of ischemia and the biochemical consequences of anoxia: possible role of N-methyl-d-aspartate receptor antagonism and ATP replenishing action in its cerebroprotecting profile. *Psychopharmacology (Berl)*. 1993;111:153-162.
59. Hoidal CR, et al. Hydrogen sulfide poisoning from toxic inhalations of roofing asphalt fumes. *Ann Emerg Med*. 1986;15:826-830.
60. Holstege CP, et al. A case of cyanide poisoning and the use of arterial blood gas analysis to direct therapy. *Hosp Pract (1995)*. 2010;38:69-74.
61. Jensen MS, et al. Preconditioning-induced protection against cyanide-induced neurotoxicity is mediated by preserving mitochondrial function. *Neurochem Int*. 2002;40:285-293.
62. Jiang J, et al. Hydrogen sulfide—mechanisms of toxicity and development of an antidote. *Sci Rep*. 2016;6:20831.
63. Johnson RP, Mellors JW. Arteriolization of venous blood gases: a clue to the diagnosis of cyanide poisoning. *J Emerg Med*. 1988;6:401-404.
64. Jones TF. Mass psychogenic illness: role of the individual physician. *Am Fam Physician*. 2000;62:2649-2653, 2655-2646.
65. Kage S, et al. Fatal hydrogen sulfide poisoning at a dye works. *Leg Med (Tokyo)*. 2004;6:182-186.
66. Kage S, et al. A fatal case of hydrogen sulfide poisoning in a geothermal power plant. *J Forensic Sci*. 1998;43:908-910.
67. Kage S, et al. Fatal and nonfatal poisoning by hydrogen sulfide at an industrial waste site. *J Forensic Sci*. 2002;47:652-655.
68. Kage S, et al. The usefulness of thiosulfate as an indicator of hydrogen sulfide poisoning: three cases. *Int J Legal Med*. 1997;110:220-222.
69. Kambale KJ, et al. Lower sulfurtransferase detoxification rates of cyanide in konzo-A tropical spastic paralysis linked to cassava cyanogenic poisoning. *Neurotoxicology*. 2017;59:256-262.
70. Kamijo Y, et al. A multicenter retrospective survey on a suicide trend using hydrogen sulfide in Japan. *Clin Toxicol (Phila)*. 2013;51:425-428.
71. Kanthasamy AG, et al. Reactive oxygen species generated by cyanide mediate toxicity in rat pheochromocytoma cells. *Toxicol Lett*. 1997;93:47-54.
72. Kawada T, et al. Cyanide intoxication induced exocytotic epinephrine release in rabbit myocardium. *J Auton Nerv Syst*. 2000;80:137-141.

73. Kilburn KH, Warshaw RH. Hydrogen sulfide and reduced-sulfur gases adversely affect neurophysiological functions. *Toxicol Ind Health*. 1995;11:185-197.

74. Kirk MA, et al. Cyanide and methemoglobin kinetics in smoke inhalation victims treated with the cyanide antidote kit. *Ann Emerg Med*. 1993;22:1413-1418.

75. Lambert RJ, et al. The efficacy of superactivated charcoal in treating rats exposed to a lethal oral dose of potassium cyanide. *Ann Emerg Med*. 1988;17:595-598.

76. Lambert TW, et al. Hydrogen sulfide (H2S) and sour gas effects on the eye. A historical perspective. *Sci Total Environ*. 2006;367:1-22.

77. Lancia M, et al. A fatal work-related poisoning by hydrogen sulfide: report on a case. *Am J Forensic Med Pathol*. 2013;34:315-317.

78. Lawson-Smith P, et al. Effect of hyperbaric oxygen therapy on whole blood cyanide concentrations in carbon monoxide intoxicated patients from fire accidents. *Scand J Trauma Resusc Emerg Med*. 2010;18:32.

79. Le Garff E, et al. Cyanide suicide after deep web shopping: a case report. *Am J Forensic Med Pathol*. 2016;37:194-197.

80. Li L, et al. Oxidative stress and cyclooxygenase-2 induction mediate cyanide-induced apoptosis of cortical cells. *Toxicol Appl Pharmacol*. 2002;185:55-63.

81. Marrs TC, Thompson JP. The efficacy and adverse effects of dicobalt edetate in cyanide poisoning. *Clin Toxicol (Phila)*. 2016;54:609-614.

82. Marziaz ML, et al. Comparison of brain mitochondrial cytochrome c oxidase activity with cyanide LD(50) yields insight into the efficacy of prophylactics. *J Appl Toxicol*. 2013;33:50-55.

83. Mathangi DC, Namasivayam A. Calcium ions: its role in cyanide neurotoxicity. *Food Chem Toxicol*. 2004;42:359-361.

84. McCabe L, Clayton GD. Air pollution by hydrogen sulfide in Poza Rica, Mexico; an evaluation of the incident of Nov. 24, 1950. *Arch Ind Hyg Occup Med*. 1952;6:199-213.

85. Milazzo S, Horneber M. Laetrile treatment for cancer. *Cochrane Database Syst Rev*. 2015:CD005476.

86. Morris J. The brimstone battles: death came from a cloud: a silent killer took 9 lives in 1975. Could it happen again? *Houston Chronicle (Special Report, 1997)*. 2000.

87. Nam B, et al. Neurologic sequela of hydrogen sulfide poisoning. *Ind Health*. 2004;42:83-87.

88. Nuskova H, et al. Cyanide inhibition and pyruvate-induced recovery of cytochrome c oxidase. *J Bioenerg Biomembr*. 2010;42:395-403.

89. Oesterhelweg L, Puschel K. "Death may come on like a stroke of lightening": phenomenological and morphological aspects of fatalities caused by manure gas. *Int J Legal Med*. 2008;122:101-107.

90. Okolie NP, Iroanya CU. Some histologic and biochemical evidence for mitigation of cyanide-induced tissue lesions by antioxidant vitamin administration in rabbits. *Food Chem Toxicol*. 2003;41:463-469.

91. Olson KR. A practical look at the chemistry and biology of hydrogen sulfide. *Antioxid Redox Signal*. 2012;17:32-44.

92. Onabolu AO, et al. Ecological variation of intake of cassava food and dietary cyanide load in Nigerian communities. *Public Health Nutr*. 2001;4:871-876.

93. Peters JW. Hydrogen sulfide poisoning in a hospital setting. *JAMA*. 1981;246:1588-1589.

94. Policastro MA, Otten EJ. Case files of the University of Cincinnati fellowship in medical toxicology: two patients with acute lethal occupational exposure to hydrogen sulfide. *J Med Toxicol*. 2007;3:73-81.

95. Prabhakaran K, et al. Caspase inhibition switches the mode of cell death induced by cyanide by enhancing reactive oxygen species generation and PARP-1 activation. *Toxicol Appl Pharmacol*. 2004;195:194-202.

96. Rajdev S, Reynolds IJ. Glutamate-induced intracellular calcium changes and neurotoxicity in cortical neurons in vitro: effect of chemical ischemia. *Neuroscience*. 1994;62:667-679.

97. Ravizza AG, et al. The treatment of hydrogen sulfide intoxication: oxygen versus nitrites. *Vet Hum Toxicol*. 1982;24:241-242.

98. Reedy SJ, et al. Suicide fads: frequency and characteristics of hydrogen sulfide suicides in the United States. *West J Emerg Med*. 2011;12:300-304.

99. Reiffenstein RJ, et al. Toxicology of hydrogen sulfide. *Annu Rev Pharmacol Toxicol*. 1992;32:109-134.

100. Rella J, et al. Rapid cyanide detection using the Cyantesmo kit. *J Toxicol Clin Toxicol*. 2004;42:897-900.

101. Richardson DB. Respiratory effects of chronic hydrogen sulfide exposure. *Am J Ind Med*. 1995;28:99-108.

102. Rindone JP, Sloane EP. Cyanide toxicity from sodium nitroprusside: risks and management. *Ann Pharmacother*. 1992;26:515-519.

103. Shou Y, et al. Cyanide-induced apoptosis involves oxidative-stress-activated NF-kappaB in cortical neurons. *Toxicol Appl Pharmacol*. 2000;164:196-205.

104. Sonobe T, Haouzi P. Sulfide intoxication-induced circulatory failure is mediated by a depression in cardiac contractility. *Cardiovasc Toxicol*. 2016;16:67-78.

105. Sousa AB, et al. Does prolonged oral exposure to cyanide promote hepatotoxicity and nephrotoxicity? *Toxicology*. 2002;174:87-95.

106. Stamyr K, et al. Swedish forensic data 1992-2009 suggest hydrogen cyanide as an important cause of death in fire victims. *Inhal Toxicol*. 2012;24:194-199.

107. Stine RJ, et al. Hydrogen sulfide intoxication. A case report and discussion of treatment. *Ann Intern Med*. 1976;85:756-758.

108. Thier R, et al. Possible impact of human CYP2E1 polymorphisms on the metabolism of acrylonitrile. *Toxicol Lett*. 2002;128(1-3):249-255.

109. Truong DH, et al. Molecular mechanisms of hydrogen sulfide toxicity. *Drug Metab Rev*. 2006;38:733-744.

110. Truscott A. Suicide fad threatens neighbours, rescuers. *CMAJ*. 2008;179:312-313.

111. Tvedt B, et al. Delayed neuropsychiatric sequelae after acute hydrogen sulfide poisoning: affection of motor function, memory, vision and hearing. *Acta Neurol Scand*. 1991;84:348-351.

112. Ursulan S. Confined space entry and compliance. *Occup Health Saf*. 2009;78:32, 34-35.

113. Vanhoorne M, et al. Epidemiological study of eye irritation by hydrogen sulphide and/or carbon disulphide exposure in viscose rayon workers. *Ann Occup Hyg*. 1995;39:307-315.

114. Vetter J. Plant cyanogenic glycosides. *Toxicon*. 2000;38:11-36.

115. Vornov JJ, et al. Delayed protection by MK-801 and tetrodotoxin in a rat organotypic hippocampal culture model of ischemia. *Stroke*. 1994;25:457-464; discussion 464-455.

116. Wang H, et al. Cytochrome P450 2E1 (CYP2E1) is essential for acrylonitrile metabolism to cyanide: comparative studies using CYP2E1-null and wild-type mice. *Drug Metab Dispos*. 2002;30:911-917.

117. Warenycia MW, et al. Acute hydrogen sulfide poisoning. Demonstration of selective uptake of sulfide by the brainstem by measurement of brain sulfide levels. *Biochem Pharmacol*. 1989;38:973-981.

118. Weaver L, Jiang S. China seals gas well after leak. *CNN International*. 2003. http://edition.cnn.com/2003/WORLD/asiapcf/east/12/26/china.gas/index.html.

119. Woodall GM, et al. Proceedings of the Hydrogen Sulfide Health Research and Risk Assessment Symposium October 31–November 2, 2000. *Inhal Toxicol*. 2005;17:593-639.

HYDROXOCOBALAMIN

Mary Ann Howland

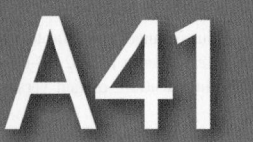

INTRODUCTION

Cyanocobalamin, vitamin B_{12}, is formed when hydroxocobalamin combines with cyanide (CN), quickly dropping CN concentrations and improving hemodynamics. Nitrites and sodium thiosulfate were traditionally used to treat patients with CN toxicity. Nitrites have the disadvantage of purposefully inducing methemoglobin, which is dangerous in a patient with coexistent elevated carboxyhemoglobin (COHb) concentrations, such as in fire victims suspected of having CN toxicity. Based on the mechanism of action of sodium thiosulfate, particularly when used alone, sodium thiosulfate is less effective and works less rapidly than hydroxocobalamin. A study in swine did not show a benefit to sodium thiosulfate as sole therapy or show an added benefit to hydroxocobalamin in a model of intravenous (IV) CN toxicity.[7] Separately, hydroxocobalamin is under investigation for the treatment of hemorrhagic shock.[8,9,12]

HISTORY

The antidotal actions of cobalt as a chelator of CN were recognized as early as 1894.[22,61] Hydroxocobalamin was used as a CN antidote in France for many years, first as a sole agent and then in combination with sodium thiosulfate.[33] Hydroxocobalamin was approved for use in the United States by the Food and Drug Administration (FDA) in December 2006 and is available under the trade name Cyanokit.[21,23]

PHARMACOLOGY

Chemistry

The hydroxocobalamin molecule shares structural similarity with porphyrin, with a cobalt ion at its core. The difference between cyanocobalamin (vitamin B_{12}) and hydroxocobalamin (vitamin B_{12a}) is the replacement of the CN group with an OH group at the active site in the latter.[40,48]

MECHANISM OF ACTION

In experimental models, hydroxocobalamin is successful in protecting against several minimum lethal doses of CN when an equimolar ratio of hydroxocobalamin to CN was used.[1,16,46,56] The cobalt ion in hydroxocobalamin combines with CN in an equimolar fashion to form nontoxic cyanocobalamin—one mole of hydroxocobalamin binds one mole of CN.[45,46] Thus, given the molecular weights of each, 52 g of hydroxocobalamin is needed to bind 1 g of CN.[33] So, a standard 5 g of hydroxocobalamin would be expected to bind 96 mg of CN. Doing a theoretical calculation and assuming a CN simian volume of distribution of 0.25 L/kg, this would mean, in an 80-kg man, 4.8 mg/L or 4.8 mcg/mL.

An ex vivo study using human skin fibroblasts demonstrated that hydroxocobalamin penetrates intracellularly to form cyanocobalamin.[2] In the setting of CN poisoning, hydroxocobalamin removes CN from the mitochondrial electron transport chain, allowing oxidative metabolism to proceed. Hydroxocobalamin also binds structurally similar nitric oxide (NO), a vasodilator, causing vasoconstriction both in the presence and in the absence of CN. This property contributes to its beneficial effects by increasing systolic and diastolic blood pressure and improving the hemodynamic status of CN-poisoned patients.[12,16,29] Other cobalt chelators, such as dicobalt ethylenediaminetetraacetic acid (EDTA), are used both experimentally and clinically in other countries, but their therapeutic index is narrow, especially in the absence of CN. Additionally, idiosyncratic adverse effects make these compounds less advantageous.[45,61]

PHARMACOKINETICS AND PHARMACODYNAMICS

Under an FDA Investigational New Drug permit, the first pharmacokinetic study of IV hydroxocobalamin was performed in the United States and published in 1993.[23,24]

Pharmacokinetic studies must be interpreted in light of the fact that elimination of B_{12a} from the serum compartment reflects the combination of distribution and elimination, as well as chemical conversion to B_{12} in the presence of CN.

Adult volunteers who were heavy smokers were given 5 g of hydroxocobalamin (5%) intravenously. The first four patients received the dose undiluted over 20 minutes.[24] They then received 12.5 g (50 mL of 25% solution) of sodium thiosulfate intravenously infused over 20 minutes. The next 11 patients received the same dose of hydroxocobalamin but diluted with 100 mL water for injection (USP) and infused over 30 minutes. The serum and urine sampling of hydroxocobalamin differed in the two patient groups, yielding somewhat different half-lives (4 versus 1.27 hours). The α distribution half-life was 0.52 hours in patients administered hydroxocobalamin alone. Peak hydroxocobalamin concentrations averaged 813 mcg/mL (604 μmol/L), and volume of distribution (V_d) averaged 0.38 L/kg. A mean of 62% of the hydroxocobalamin dose was recovered in the urine in 24 hours. Whole-blood CN concentrations significantly decreased in all participants after receiving hydroxocobalamin. This study was limited by the short collection time for serum hydroxocobalamin concentrations of only 6 hours, making the pharmacokinetic analysis imprecise.[36,37] A pharmacokinetic study in France[33] was conducted in adult victims of smoke inhalation given hydroxocobalamin, 5 g (5%) by IV infusion over 30 minutes, starting within 30 minutes of patient removal from the fire.[36,37] The α distribution half-life of hydroxocobalamin was 1.86 hours, the elimination half-life of hydroxocobalamin was 26.2 hours based on sampling up to 6 days, and the V_d was 0.45 L/kg. The peak serum cyanocobalamin concentration was 287 mcg/mL (212 μmol/L). In the one patient who was subsequently determined not exposed to CN, the hydroxocobalamin elimination half-life was 13.6 hours, and the V_d was 0.23 L/kg. Renal clearance of hydroxocobalamin was 37% in the CN-exposed patients compared with 62% in the unexposed patient.

In another study in France in which 12 fire victims were suspected of having CN poisoning, the patients received IV hydroxocobalamin 5 g in 100 mL sterile water over 30 minutes.[39] Pretreatment and posttreatment CN concentrations and cyanocobalamin concentrations were analyzed. In patients with CN concentrations less than 1.04 mcg/mL (<40 μmol/L), a linear relationship existed between the blood CN concentration and the formation of cyanocobalamin. In the three patients with blood CN concentration greater than 1.04 mcg/mL (>40 μmol/L), the formation of cyanocobalamin reached a plateau, implying that all the hydroxocobalamin was consumed. When the patient with a blood CN concentration greater than 1.04 mcg/mL (>40 μmol/L) received a second 5-g dose of hydroxocobalamin, the cyanocobalamin concentration subsequently rose.[3,39]

The protein binding and tissue distribution of CN, hydroxocobalamin, and cyanocobalamin likely are different.[38] In addition, hydroxocobalamin probably causes redistribution of CN from the intracellular to the intravascular space.[38]

Cobinamide is a precursor of cobalamin. Compared with hydroxocobalamin, it is capable of binding two CN molecules versus one, is about five times more water soluble, and has a higher affinity for CN, making the effective dose of cobinamide less than hydroxocobalamin. Intravenous cobinamide was effective in rescuing swine brought to apnea with IV CN and at a dose that was one fifth that of hydroxocobalamin.[12a] In a model of oral CN poisoning in rabbits, oral sodium bicarbonate to raise gastric pH along with either oral aquohydroxocobinamide (water and hydroxyl molecules bound to the cobalt moiety) or oral dinitrocobinamide (two nitrite groups bound to the cobalt moiety) both significantly increased survival time.[18,41] Dinitrocobinamide is also being investigated by the intramuscular route and shows promising results in mice and rabbits.

ROLE IN CYANIDE TOXICITY
Animals
The ability of hydroxocobalamin to bind CN and produce beneficial effects on mortality and hemodynamics is demonstrated in many animal species, including rabbits, swine, dogs, and baboons.[34] A study in swine evaluated the effect of hydroxocobalamin plus sodium thiosulfate versus sodium nitrite and sodium thiosulfate in a model using a continuous infusion of CN. There was no difference between the groups with regard to metabolic acidosis with an elevated lactate concentration at times 20 and 40 minutes, cardiac output and pulse rate at 40 minutes, or mortality rate. The mean arterial pressure was higher in the hydroxocobalamin plus sodium thiosulfate group, beginning at 5 minutes and lasting for the entire 40-minute monitoring period.[13] A second CN study in swine done by the same group could not show a benefit to sodium thiosulfate as sole therapy or show an added benefit of sodium thiosulfate to hydroxocobalamin.[11]

Humans
Many case reports and studies in France document the efficacy of hydroxocobalamin combined with sodium thiosulfate for treatment of CN toxicity.[7,17,28,32] An observational case series reviewed 69 adult smoke inhalation victims suspected of CN poisoning who were treated either at the scene of the fire or in the intensive care unit (ICU).[16] They received a median dose of 5 g of hydroxocobalamin, up to a maximum of 15 g, infused as a 5% solution in sterile water for injection over 15 to 30 minutes. Cardiopulmonary arrest occurred in 15 patients, with a mean blood CN concentration of 123 μmol/L (100 μmol/L = 2.7 mcg/mL, a fatal concentration if untreated) and a mean COHb of 30%. Two of these patients survived with normal neurologic function. Of 42 patients with confirmed CN concentrations greater than 39 μmol/L (1 mcg/mL, a potentially fatal concentration), 28 (67%) survived.

The mortality rate contribution from concomitant COHb toxicity is difficult to determine in this study. Of the 69 patients in this study, 57 also received hyperbaric oxygen, complicating the interpretation of the outcome.[16]

An 8-year retrospective analysis of the use of hydroxocobalamin in the prehospital setting concluded that the risk-to-benefit ratio favors its use in smoke inhalation victims suspected of CN poisoning.[26] Of 72 patients in whom survival status could be determined, 30 (42%) survived. Cyanide blood concentrations were not measured in these patients. Although 21 of the 38 patients found in cardiac arrest had hemodynamic improvement, survival was dismal with only 2 patients ultimately surviving. The neurologic function of those two patients was not described.

Hydroxocobalamin also prevented the rise in CN concentration after nitroprusside infusion compared with patients who only received nitroprusside.[19] Nitroprusside contains 5 CN molecules, which produces CN toxicity if given in too high a dose or for too long a duration. When nitroprusside is administered, the use of concomitant hydroxocobalamin prevents CN accumulation and toxicity in both animal models and in humans.[17,19,62] Sodium thiosulfate also prevents nitroprusside-induced CN toxicity (Antidotes in Depth: A42).

There are currently no studies comparing the nitrite plus sodium thiosulfate regimen with hydroxocobalamin in patients with CN poisoning.[53] There are no studies comparing hydroxocobalamin with or without sodium thiosulfate to sodium thiosulfate alone in smoke inhalation victims presumed to be CN toxic.

The kidneys, heart, and liver of a patient who was declared brain dead after third-degree burns and smoke inhalation after a fire were successfully transplanted into four patients.[27] The victim received 10 g of hydroxocobalamin. Whole-blood CN concentrations were later confirmed to be significantly elevated after administration of hydroxocobalamin.

ADVERSE EFFECTS AND SAFETY ISSUES
Hydroxocobalamin has a wide therapeutic index.[16,26,60] Large doses were administered to animals with no adverse effects.[45,51,54] The LD_{50} (median lethal dose in 50% of test subjects) in mice is 2 g/kg.

Red discoloration of mucous membranes, serum, and urine is expected and lasts from 12 hours to many days after therapy.[16,21,26] Patients should be warned to avoid direct sun exposure while their skin remains red for fear of a photosensitivity reaction.[21] Allergic reactions, including anaphylaxis and angioedema, are reported, but serious allergic reactions are rare.[6,7,17,48] Prior chronic exposure to hydroxocobalamin or cyanocobalamin for treatment of vitamin B_{12} deficiency is associated rarely with development of anaphylaxis.[33] A study in 102 healthy volunteers demonstrated that chromaturia is universal, and as the dose increases from 2.5 to 10 g, the incidences of erythema, rash (predominantly acneiform), headache, injection site reaction, nausea, pruritus, chest discomfort, and dysphagia increase.[60] The dermatologic manifestations are quite variable; both immediate in onset or delayed onset with protracted courses occur. Of 102 volunteers randomized to receive hydroxocobalamin, 24 experienced a clinically significant rise in diastolic blood pressures, up to 124 mm Hg. However, only three of them also had clinically significant elevations in systolic blood pressure. These elevations in blood pressure resolved within 4 hours of the end of the infusion. Urinary oxalate crystals were reported in patients receiving hydroxocobalamin whether or not the patient was exposed to CN.[21]

Colorimetric assays are adversely affected because both hydroxocobalamin and cyanocobalamin have an intensely red color. Many clinical chemistry laboratory tests are artificially increased, decreased, or unpredictable.[14,21,52] Hematology tests including hemoglobin, mean corpuscular hemoglobin (MCH), mean corpuscular hemoglobin concentration (MCHC), and basophils are artificially increased.[21] Coagulation tests are unpredictable. Urinalysis tests are usually artificially increased, but pH can also be artificially low with low doses of hydroxocobalamin.[21] An in vitro study found statistically significant alterations in serum concentrations of aspartate aminotransferase (AST), total bilirubin, creatinine, magnesium, and iron after hydroxocobalamin administration.[20] Although an in vitro study demonstrated a considerable false increase in COHb concentrations after hydroxocobalamin administration when measured by cooximetry, other authors suggest that the interference is minimal and results in slight overestimates depending on the instrument and the concentration of hydroxocobalamin.[5,30,42] Inconsequential increases of 1% to 5.7% in the COHb level were reported in another study.[30] However, more worrisome is the report of two instances where the COHb levels were falsely low by a factor of 4 to 14 times.[44] An in vitro experiment using human blood confirmed a substantial false decrease in the COHb concentration depending on the specific cooximeter.[50]

Because of the inaccuracies in laboratory determinations, blood should be drawn before hydroxocobalamin administration whenever possible. This is particularly important in fire victims when COHb concentrations are necessary for management decisions.

Because of the deep red color of hydroxocobalamin, hemodialysis machines often sound a false "blood leak" alarm depending on the wavelength of light that the optical emitter detects. Nephrologists should be aware of this possibility.[4,21,59]

PREGNANCY AND LACTATION

Hydroxocobalamin is FDA Pregnancy Category C. Animal studies are insufficient, and there are no controlled trials in pregnant women. Hydroxocobalamin should be used in pregnant women whose CN toxicity is presumed significant. Under these circumstances, the potential benefit to the mother and fetus outweighs the potential undefined risk to the fetus.[55] A pregnant woman in her fourth week of gestation was inadvertently administered 5 g of hydroxocobalamin during a volunteer study. She went on to deliver a normal healthy baby at term.[21]

DOSING AND ADMINISTRATION

Cyanide Toxicity

The initial dose of hydroxocobalamin in adults is 5 g. Each vial is reconstituted with 200 mL of 0.9% sodium chloride and administered intravenously over 15 minutes. If 0.9% sodium chloride is unavailable, lactated Ringers solution or dextrose 5% in water may be used. Each vial should be inverted or rocked (not shaken) for 60 seconds before administration. The reconstituted solution should be dark red and free of particulate matter and should be used within 6 hours of reconstitution.[21] A second dose of 5 g should be repeated as clinically necessary and infused over 15 minutes to 2 hours depending on patient status.[21] Although not studied in humans, animal studies and human experiences suggest that a faster rate of administration is free of apparent adverse effects.[10,13,35] Based on isolated case reports and animal studies, intraosseous administration is anticipated to be of comparable efficacy to IV administration.[15,25] In children, a dose of 70 mg/kg of hydroxocobalamin up to the adult dose is recommended.[21]

Sodium thiosulfate is often administered in addition to hydroxocobalamin, but the administration of hydroxocobalamin should always take precedence. The sodium thiosulfate is considered to be additive and was used extensively in conjunction with hydroxocobalamin, but a swine model was unable to show added benefit.[11,31,32,43] Hydroxocobalamin and sodium thiosulfate should not be administered simultaneously through the same IV line because the sodium thiosulfate will inactivate the hydroxocobalamin.[38] The adult dose of sodium thiosulfate is 12.5 g (50 mL of 25% solution) and should be administered intravenously as either a bolus injection or infused over 10 to 30 minutes, depending on the severity of the situation. The dose of sodium thiosulfate in children is 1 mL/kg using a 25% solution (250 mg/kg or approximately 30-40 mL/m^2 of body surface area) not to exceed 50 mL (12.5 g) total dose. The dose should be repeated at half the initial dose if manifestations of CN toxicity persist or reappear.[49,58]

Nitroprusside-Induced Cyanide Toxicity

Nitroprusside-induced CN toxicity should be treated like CN toxicity from any other cause: stop the nitroprusside dosage and administer hydroxocobalamin according to the doses and precautions listed. The dose of hydroxocobalamin to prevent CN toxicity from the IV infusion of nitroprusside is not precisely known, but a dose of hydroxocobalamin of 25 mg/h concurrent with nitroprusside administration was sufficient in one study to decrease the red blood cell and serum CN concentrations and to prevent the development of a metabolic acidosis.[62] We recommend continuing the hydroxocobalamin for 10 hours after the discontinuation of the nitroprusside because of a red blood cell CN half-life of 10 hours.[19,62] Hydroxocobalamin should also be used as rescue therapy in the typical dosage. Sodium thiosulfate is used to prevent CN toxicity when mixed with nitroprusside (Antidotes in Depth: A40).

FORMULATION AND ACQUISITION

Cyanokit contains one 250 mL glass vial containing 5 g of lyophilized dark red hydroxocobalamin crystalline powder for injection.[21] The kit also contains one sterile transfer spike, one sterile IV infusion set, one quick reference guide, and one package insert but no diluent.

SUMMARY

- Hydroxocobalamin is effective for CN toxicity generated from all routes of exposure. Intravenous hydroxocobalamin is safe in the setting of a fire when COHb is also expected to be present.
- Hydroxocobalamin affects all laboratory tests that are colorimetric, producing falsely elevated or lowered results. Of particular importance is the significantly falsely diminished assay for COHb.
- Hydroxocobalamin causes a red discoloration of the skin and mucous membranes that lasts hours to days.
- Hydroxocobalamin's deep red color causes many hemodialysis machines to sound a false "blood leak" alarm.

REFERENCES

1. Anonymous. Editorial comment: hydroxocobalamin analysis. *J Toxicol Clin Toxicol.* 1997;35:417.
2. Astier A, Baud FJ. Complexation of intracellular cyanide by hydroxocobalamin using a human cellular model. *Hum Exp Toxicol.* 1996;15:19-25.
3. Astier A, Baud FJ. Simultaneous determination of hydroxocobalamin and its cyanide complex cyanocobalamin in human plasma by high-performance liquid chromatography. Application to pharmacokinetic studies after high-dose hydroxocobalamin as an antidote for severe cyanide poisoning. *J Chromatogr B Biomed Appl.* 1995;667:129-135.
4. Avila J, et al. Pseudo-blood leak? A hemodialysis mystery. *Clin Nephrol.* 2013;79:323-325.
5. Baud F. Clarifications regarding interference of hydroxocobalamin with carboxyhemoglobin measurements in victims of smoke inhalation. *Ann Emerg Med.* 2007;50:625-626.
6. Baud FJ, et al. Elevated blood cyanide concentrations in victims of smoke inhalation. *N Engl J Med.* 1991;325:1761-1766.
7. Beasley DM, Glass WI. Cyanide poisoning: pathophysiology and treatment recommendations. *Occup Med (Lond).* 1998;48:427-431.
8. Bebarta VS, et al. Intraosseous hydroxocobalamin versus intravenous hydroxocobalamin compared to intraosseous whole blood or no treatment for hemorrhagic shock in a swine model. *Am J Disaster Med.* 2015;10:205-215.
9. Bebarta VS, et al. A prospective, randomized trial of intravenous hydroxocobalamin versus whole blood transfusion compared to no treatment for Class III hemorrhagic shock resuscitation in a prehospital swine model. *Acad Emerg Med.* 2015;22:321-330.
10. Bebarta VS, et al. Intraosseous versus intravenous infusion of hydroxocobalamin for the treatment of acute severe cyanide toxicity in a swine model. *Acad Emerg Med.* 2014;21:1203-1211.
11. Bebarta VS, et al. Hydroxocobalamin versus sodium thiosulfate for the treatment of acute cyanide toxicity in a swine model. *Ann Emerg Med.* 2012;59:532-539.
12. Bebarta VS, et al. Hydroxocobalamin and epinephrine both improve survival in a swine model of cyanide-induced cardiac arrest. *Ann Emerg Med.* 2012;60:415-422.
12a. Bebarta VS, et al. Intravenous Cobinamide Versus Hydroxocobalamin for Acute Treatment of Severe Cyanide Poisoning in a Swine (Sus scrofa) Model. *Ann Emerg Med.* 2014;64:612-619.
13. Bebarta VS, et al. Hydroxocobalamin and sodium thiosulfate versus sodium nitrite and sodium thiosulfate in the treatment of acute cyanide toxicity in a swine model. *Ann Emerg Med.* 2010;55:345-351.
14. Beckerman N, et al. Laboratory interference with the newer cyanide antidote: hydroxocobalamin. *Semin Diagn Pathol.* 2009;26:49-52.
15. Borron SW, et al. Hemodynamics after intraosseous administration of hydroxocobalamin or normal saline in a goat model. *Am J Emerg Med.* 2009;27:1065-1071.
16. Borron SW, et al. Prospective study of hydroxocobalamin for acute cyanide poisoning in smoke inhalation. *Ann Emerg Med.* 2007;49:794-801.
17. Braitberg G, Vanderpyl M. Treatment of cyanide poisoning in Australasia. *Emerg Med.* 2000;12:232-240.

18. Chan A, et al. Nitrocobinamide, a new cyanide antidote that can be administered by intramuscular injection. *J Med Chem.* 2015;58:1750-1759.

19. Cottrell JE, et al. Prevention of nitroprusside-induced cyanide toxicity with hydroxocobalamin. *N Engl J Med.* 1978;298:809-811.

20. Curry SC, et al. Effect of the cyanide antidote hydroxocobalamin on commonly ordered serum chemistry studies. *Ann Emerg Med.* 1994;24:65-67.

21. Cyanokit [package insert]. Manufactured by Merck Sante, s.a.s., Semoy, France and distributed by Meridian Medical Technologies, Inc, Columbia, MD; March 2017.

22. Evans CL. Cobalt compounds as antidotes for hydrocyanic acid. *Br J Pharmacol.* 1964;23:455-475.

23. Food and Drug Administration. Listing of orphan drugs. http://www.fda.gov/orphan/designat/alldes.rtf.

24. Forsyth JC, et al. Hydroxocobalamin as a cyanide antidote: safety, efficacy and pharmacokinetics in heavily smoking normal volunteers. *J Toxicol Clin Toxicol.* 1993;31:277-294.

25. Fortin JL, et al. Intraosseous administration of hydroxocobalamin in the acute treatment of cyanide poisoning. *Burns.* 2009;35(suppl):S15-S16.

26. Fortin JL, et al. Prehospital administration of hydroxocobalamin for smoke inhalation-associated cyanide poisoning: 8 years of experience in the Paris Fire Brigade. *Clin Toxicol.* 2006;44:37-44.

27. Fortin JL, et al. Successful organ transplantation after treatment of fatal cyanide poisoning with hydroxocobalamin. *Clin Toxicol.* 2007;45:468-471.

28. Fortin JL, et al. Hydroxocobalamin for poisoning caused by ingestion of potassium cyanide: a case study. *J Emerg Med.* 2010;39:320-324.

29. Gerth K, et al. Nitric oxide scavenging by hydroxocobalamin may account for its hemodynamic profile. *Clin Toxicol.* 2006;44:29-36.

30. Gourlain H, et al. Mesure du CO et de la COHb dans le sang: interferences de l'hydroxocobalamine et du bleu de methylene en CO-oxymetre. *Revue Francaise des Laboratoires.* 1996;282:144-148.

31. Hall AH, et al. Sodium thiosulfate or hydroxocobalamin for the empiric treatment of cyanide poisoning? *Ann Emerg Med.* 2007;49:806-813.

32. Hall AH, Rumack BH. Hydroxycobalamin/sodium thiosulfate as a cyanide antidote. *J Emerg Med.* 1987;5:115-121.

33. Hall AH, et al. Clinical toxicology of cyanide: North American experiences. In: Ballantyne B, Marrs TC, eds. *Clinical and Experimental Toxicology of Cyanides.* Bristol, UK: Wright; 1987:313-333.

34. Hall AH, et al. Which cyanide antidote? *Crit Rev Toxicol.* 2009;39:541-552.

35. Hamad E, et al. Case files of the university of Massachusetts toxicology fellowship: does this smoke inhalation victim require treatment with cyanide antidote. *J Med Toxicol.* 2016;12:192-198.

36. Houeto P, et al. Hydroxocobalamin analysis and pharmacokinetics. Authors' response. *J Toxicol Clin Toxicol.* 1997;35:413-415.

37. Houeto P, et al. Pharmacokinetics of hydroxocobalamin in smoke inhalation victims. *J Toxicol Clin Toxicol.* 1996;34:397-404.

38. Houeto P, et al. Authors' reply to: monitoring of cyanocobalamin and hydroxocobalamin during treatment of cyanide intoxication. *Lancet.* 1995;346:1706-1707.

39. Houeto P, et al. Relation of blood cyanide to plasma cyanocobalamin concentration after a fixed dose of hydroxocobalamin in cyanide poisoning. *Lancet.* 1995;346:605-608.

40. Kaczka EA, et al. Vitamin B$_{12}$: reactions of cyano-cobalamin and related compounds. *Science.* 1950;112:354-355.

41. Lee J, et al. The vitamin B12 analog cobinamide is an effective antidote for oral cyanide poisoning. *J Med Toxicol.* 2016;12:370-379.

42. Lee J, et al. Potential interference by hydroxocobalamin in cooximetry hemoglobin measurements during cyanide and smoke inhalation treatments. *Ann Emerg Med.* 2007;49:802-805.

43. Leybell I, et al. Toxicity, cyanide. http://emedicine.medscape.com/article/814287-overview.

44. Livshits Z, et al. Falsely low carboxyhemoglobin level after hydroxocobalamin therapy. *N Engl J Med.* 2012;367:1270-1271.

45. Marrs TC. Antidotal treatment of acute cyanide poisoning. *Adverse Drug React Acute Poisoning Rev.* 1988;7:179-206.

46. Marrs TC. The choice of cyanide antidotes. In: Ballantyne B, Marrs TC, eds. *Clinical and Experimental Toxicology of Cyanides.* Bristol, UK: Wright; 1987:383-401.

47. Mengel K, et al. Thiosulphate and hydroxocobalamin prophylaxis in progressive cyanide poisoning in guinea-pigs. *Toxicology.* 1989;54:335-342.

48. Meredith TJ, et al, eds. *Antidotes for Poisoning by Cyanide.* New York, NY: Cambridge Press; 1993.

49. Nithiodote [package insert]. Manufactured by Cangene BioPharm, Inc., Baltimore, MD, for Hope Pharmaceuticals, Scottsdale, AZ; 2011.

50. Pace R, et al. Effects of hydroxocobalamin on carboxyhemoglobin measured under physiologic and pathologic conditions. *Clin Toxicol (Phila).* 2014;52:647-650.

51. Posner MA, et al. Hydroxocobalamin therapy of cyanide intoxication in guinea pigs. *Anesthesiology.* 1976;44:157-160.

52. Ranjitkar P, Greene DN. Therapeutic concentrations of hydroxocobalamin interferes with several spectrophotometric assays on the Beckman Coulter DxC and AU680 chemistry analyzers. *Clin Chim Acta.* 2015;450:110-114.

53. Reade MC, et al. Review article: management of cyanide poisoning. *Emerg Med Australas.* 2012;24:225-238.

54. Riou B, et al. Comparison of the hemodynamic effects of hydroxocobalamin and cobalt edetate at equipotent cyanide antidotal doses in conscious dogs. *Intensive Care Med.* 1993;19:26-32.

55. Roderique EJ, et al. Smoke inhalation injury in a pregnant patient: a literature review of the evidence and current best practices in the setting of a classic case. *J Burn Care Res.* 2012;33:624-633.

56. Rose CL, et al. Hydroxo-cobalamin and acute cyanide poisoning in dogs. *Life Sci.* 1965;4:1785-1789.

57. Shepherd G, Velez LI. Role of hydroxocobalamin in acute cyanide poisoning. *Ann Pharmacother.* 2008;42:661-669.

58. Sodium thiosulfate [package insert]. Manufactured by Cangene BioPharma, Inc., Baltimore, MD, for Hope Pharmaceuticals, Scottsdale, AZ; 2012.

59. Sutter M, et al. Hemodialysis complications of hydroxocobalamin: a case report. *J Med Toxicol.* 2010;6:165-167.

60. Uhl W, et al. Safety of hydroxocobalamin in healthy volunteers in a randomized, placebo controlled study. *Clin Toxicol.* 2006;44:17-28.

61. Way JL. Cyanide intoxication and its mechanism of antagonism. *Annu Rev Pharmacol Toxicol.* 1984;24:451-481.

62. Zerbe NF, Wagner BK. Use of vitamin B$_{12}$ in the treatment and prevention of nitroprusside-induced cyanide toxicity. *Crit Care Med.* 1993;21:465-467.

NITRITES (AMYL AND SODIUM) AND SODIUM THIOSULFATE

Mary Ann Howland

INTRODUCTION

Sodium nitrite is an effective cyanide (CN) antidote that acts best when administered in a timely fashion and is followed by sodium thiosulfate. The utility of amyl nitrite, a volatile drug available in ampules that can be broken and administered by inhalation while sodium nitrite is being prepared to administer intravenously, is questioned.[39] This combination of sodium nitrite followed by sodium thiosulfate was the only antidote combination available to treat CN toxicity before the US Food and Drug Administration (FDA) approval of hydroxocobalamin in December 2006. Although there has never been a head-to-head study in humans comparing hydroxocobalamin with the combination for the treatment of CN toxicity, the advantages of hydroxocobalamin are that it works quickly and directly to inactivate CN to form cyanocobalamin. In addition, hydroxocobalamin can be administered to patients with impaired oxygen-carrying capacity from elevated concentrations of carboxyhemoglobin (COHb), methemoglobin, or sulfhemoglobin, making it the preferred CN antidote under most circumstances.

HISTORY

In 1895, Lang reported the efficacy of sodium thiosulfate in detoxifying hydrocyanic acid.[36] The treatment of patients with CN poisoning with methylene blue led to the understanding of the role of methemoglobin in detoxifying CN and the search for better methemoglobin inducers.[22] Experiments in CN-poisoned canines demonstrated the limited role of methylene blue and the efficacy of amyl nitrite, sodium nitrite, and sodium thiosulfate.[12-14] Amyl nitrite administered by inhalation protected canines from up to four minimum lethal doses of sodium CN (a total of 24 mg/kg subcutaneously).[13] In the regimen used, therapy was started within 5 to 7 minutes of exposure and was continued for several hours. The frequency of inhalation was based on clinical response. These experimental results led to the use of inhaled amyl nitrite for patients poisoned by CN. The same authors discovered that intravenous (IV) use of sodium thiosulfate alone protected against three minimum lethal doses of CN in dogs and that the combination of sodium thiosulfate with either inhaled amyl nitrite or IV sodium nitrite protected against 10 to 18 minimum lethal doses, respectively.[12,14]

PHARMACOLOGY OF THE NITRITES
Chemistry

The chemical formula for sodium nitrite is $NaNO_2$ and for amyl nitrite is $C_5H_{11}NO_2$. Sodium nitrite has a molecular weight of 69 Da, and amyl nitrite has a molecular weight of 117 Da. Amyl nitrite is volatile even at low temperatures and is highly flammable.

Mechanism of Action

Cyanide quickly and reversibly binds to the ferric iron in cytochrome oxidase, inhibiting effective energy production throughout the body. The ferric iron in methemoglobin preferentially combines with CN, producing cyanomethemoglobin. This drives the reaction toward cyanomethemoglobin and liberates CN from cytochrome oxidase. Stroma-free methemoglobin is effective against four minimum lethal doses of CN in rats.[65] Nitrites oxidize the iron in hemoglobin to produce methemoglobin. Because nitrites were accepted antidotes for CN poisoning, for many years, methemoglobin formation was assumed to be their sole mechanism of antidotal action.[43,68] Other, faster methemoglobin inducers, such as 4-dimethylaminophenol and hydroxylamine,

also are effective as CN antidotes.[43,66] The production of methemoglobin by nitrite is slow, but when methylene blue is administered to prevent methemoglobin formation, nitrite remains an effective antidote.[43,51,68] This discovery led to the hypothesis that nitrite-induced vasodilation might be part of the mechanism of action and investigators considered the antidotal actions of other vasodilators. The α-adrenergic antagonists and ganglionic blockers demonstrated antidotal activity only when administered with sodium thiosulfate.[68] Experimental evidence in hypoxia- or hypotension-induced organ damage suggests that the benefits of nitrites are related to their conversion to nitric oxide (NO), a potent vasodilator. The conversion to NO occurs only in tissues or blood with the lowest oxygen concentrations.[3,17,48,57] Thus, the major mechanism of action of the nitrites is in their ability to produce large exogenous concentrations of NO, which is proposed to displace CN and compete with CN for binding to cytochrome c oxidase.[10,40,55] Pretreatment with a NO scavenger negated the effects of the nitrite.[41,56] Adding support to this theory is a CN poisoned rabbit model in which IV isosorbide dinitrate was comparable to IV sodium nitrite in short-term survival,[38] clinical scores, blood lactate concentrations, and vital signs without changing methemoglobin concentrations (peak methemoglobin of 7.9% with sodium nitrite).[37] When the cytochrome c oxidase is free of CN, the CN can be detoxified by binding to methemoglobin or to thiosulfate.[11]

PHARMACOLOGY OF SODIUM THIOSULFATE
Chemistry

The chemical formula of sodium thiosulfate is $Na_2S_2O_3$, and the molecular weight is 248 Da. It forms a pentahydrate that is highly water soluble.

Mechanism of Action

The sulfur atom provided by sodium thiosulfate binds to CN with the help of rhodanese (CN sulfurtransferase) and mercaptopyruvate sulfurtransferase.[14,68,70] Sulfane sulfur (a divalent sulfur bound to one other sulfur) is the only sulfur compound that reacts with CN to produce thiocyanate, which is minimally toxic and renally eliminated. The cationic site on rhodanese is essential to cleaving the sulfur–sulfur bond of thiosulfate and forming a sulfur–rhodanese complex that readily reacts with CN.[69] In animal models in multiple species, sodium thiosulfate protects against several minimum lethal doses of CN.[32,43] The addition of rhodanese increases the efficacy of sodium thiosulfate, but the use of rhodanese is impractical in the clinical setting.[43,70] Rhodanese is probably not solely responsible for sulfur–sulfur bond cleavage because rhodanese is largely a mitochondrial enzyme found in the liver and skeletal muscle. Sodium thiosulfate is a divalent ion that poorly crosses membranes.[19,43,46,68,69] It is also suggested that both mercaptopyruvate sulfurtransferase and rhodanese are involved in the formation of sulfane sulfur in the liver from sodium thiosulfate and that serum albumin then carries the sulfane sulfur from the liver to other organs. When CN is present, albumin delivers this sulfur to CN, forming thiocyanate.[33,68,70]

Thiocyanate is much less toxic than CN and is renally eliminated. Although the production of methemoglobin is therapeutic in CN poisoning, it is also potentially life threatening if nitrites are administered to a patient with impaired oxygen-carrying capacity from elevated concentrations of COHb, methemoglobin, or sulfhemoglobin. Because sodium thiosulfate does not compromise hemoglobin oxygen saturation, it should be used without nitrites in circumstances when the formation of methemoglobin would be detrimental, as in patients who have elevated levels of COHb or preexistent methemoglobinemia from smoke inhalation, drug exposure, or congenital dyshemoglobinemias, and when hydroxocobalamin is unavailable. Based on the mechanism of action of sodium thiosulfate, particularly when used alone, it is unlikely to be as effective or work as rapidly as hydroxocobalamin.

Sodium thiosulfate is used prophylactically with nitroprusside (which contains 5 CN ions) to prevent CN toxicity. Sodium thiosulfate is also used to treat calcific uremic arteriolopathy (calciphylaxis), theoretically by increasing the solubility of calcium deposits, inducing vasodilation, and acting as a free radical scavenger.[9,45,53,61]

PHARMACOKINETICS AND PHARMACODYNAMICS OF NITRITES

The pharmacokinetics of sodium nitrite are not established. Most studies were directed at measuring methemoglobin levels rather than nitrite concentrations.[66] In one study, 300 mg of IV sodium nitrite produced peak methemoglobin levels of 10% to 18% in healthy adults and values of 7% when 4 mg/kg was administered.[12,51] Inhalation of crushed amyl nitrite ampules in human volunteers produced insignificant amounts of methemoglobin and caused headache, fatigue, dizziness, and hypotension.[35]

Sodium nitrite administered intramuscularly to dogs was not effective as a CN antidote unless atropine was given as pretreatment.[67] Most likely the rapid reversal of CN-induced bradycardia by atropine facilitated absorption of sodium nitrite, which then was effective.[66,67]

The package insert states that approximately 40% of sodium nitrite is renally eliminated unchanged, and the remainder is metabolized to ammonia and other related molecules.[51]

PHARMACOKINETICS AND PHARMACODYNAMICS OF SODIUM THIOSULFATE

Animal Studies

Sodium thiosulfate is a large divalent anion. Canine studies suggest that sodium thiosulfate rapidly distributes into the extracellular space and then slowly into the cell, perhaps with a carrier facilitating entry into the mitochondria.[30,46] When administered before CN, thiosulfate converted more than 50% of the CN to thiocyanate within 3 minutes and increased the endogenous conversion rate more than 30 times.[64] A canine model using continuous IV infusion of CN to induce a respiratory arrest, demonstrated that the IV administration of 500 mg/kg of sodium thiosulfate decreased the serum CN concentration and restored respirations within 3 minutes.[16] Thiosulfate is filtered and secreted in the kidneys. At low serum concentrations, thiosulfate is subsequently reabsorbed, but at high serum concentrations, filtration and secretion predominate.[21,46]

Human Studies

A volunteer study examined the pharmacokinetics of sodium thiosulfate.[32,46] After injection of 150 mg/kg, the volume of distribution (V_d) was 0.15 L/kg, the distribution half-life was 23 minutes, and the elimination half-life was 3 hours. The peak serum thiosulfate concentration rose 100-fold. Approximately 50% of the drug was eliminated in 18 hours, most of that within the first 3 hours, unchanged in the urine. Baseline thiosulfate concentrations were higher in starved patients and children, presumably because of their higher protein metabolism to thiosulfate.[32]

A study of thiosulfate as a cisplatin neutralizer demonstrated a half-life of 80 minutes and that renal clearance accounted for about 30% of the total clearance.[28,60] Oral sodium thiosulfate is poorly absorbed and acts as a laxative.[46]

A pharmacokinetic study was performed in healthy volunteers as well as hemodialysis (HD) patients both on and off HD.[20] Eight grams of sodium thiosulfate was diluted in 50 mL of 0.9% NaCl and infused over 8 minutes. The use of a population pharmacokinetic model revealed a small V_d (0.226 L/kg), a nonrenal clearance similar to the renal clearance accounting for about 50% of the elimination in both healthy volunteers and HD patients. Total body clearance in the HD patients undergoing HD was double that of the same patients not receiving HD. A one-compartment distribution model was assumed because of the absence of rebound concentrations after HD ended. Oral bioavailability was only about 8% and was calculated after 5 g of the IV solution was diluted in 100 mL of water and ingested rapidly.

ROLE OF NITRITES AND SODIUM THIOSULFATE IN CYANIDE TOXICITY

Maximal benefits of sodium nitrite are realized experimentally when sodium nitrite is given prophylactically, but benefits are still evident even when sodium nitrite is administered after CN poisoning. Sodium nitrite is clearly effective soon after administration, even when methemoglobin levels are low. Thus, a target methemoglobin concentration should not be used to determine the correct dose of sodium nitrite, although care must be taken to avoid excessive methemoglobinemia.[34] Administration of sodium nitrite should always be followed by sodium thiosulfate. Sodium thiosulfate donates a sulfur atom, which, with the help of rhodanese (CN sulfurtransferase) and mercaptopyruvate sulfurtransferase, carries sulfane sulfur to bind to CN, producing thiocyanate. Thiocyanate is a much less toxic substance than CN and is renally eliminated.[13]

As early as 1952, the literature reported 16 CN-poisoned patients who survived after administration of nitrites and sodium thiosulfate.[12] Even patients who were unconscious or apneic survived when given timely cardiopulmonary resuscitation and antidotal therapy.[12] Case reports attest to the ability of amyl nitrite, sodium nitrite, and sodium thiosulfate to reverse the effects of CN if they are administered in a timely fashion.[15,24,71] A 34-year-old man who ingested 1 g of potassium CN became comatose within 45 minutes. One hour after ingestion, he arrived in the emergency department, became apneic, and was intubated. His blood pressure was 134/84 mm Hg and pulse was 84 beats/min, and he had fixed and dilated pupils. At 1 hour, 15 minutes, he was given 300 mg of sodium nitrite intravenously over 20 minutes followed by 12.5 g of sodium thiosulfate. Seizure activity that began just before sodium nitrite infusion resolved rapidly, and by the time the sodium thiosulfate was infused, his pupils were reactive, and spontaneous respirations returned.[24]

In another case, a 4-year-old boy ingested 12 50-mg tablets of laetrile (amygdalin) became unresponsive and developed seizures within 90 minutes.[26] Upon arrival at a second hospital, the patient required intubation, had no measurable blood pressure, and had dilated minimally responsive pupils. Arterial blood gas analysis revealed pH, 6.85; PCO_2, 15 mm Hg; and PO_2, 169 mm Hg on 100% oxygen with an anion gap of 26 mEq/L. His vital signs improved with intermittent inhalation of amyl nitrite pearls. Six hours after ingestion (and 1 hour, 45 minutes after amyl nitrite administration), sodium nitrite and sodium thiosulfate obtained from another hospital were administered. Within 30 minutes of completion of 5 mL (0.33 mL/kg) 3% sodium nitrite solution by IV infusion, spontaneous respirations returned, and his blood pressure and pulse normalized. Over the next 3 hours, his mental status and acid–base status improved. Fifteen hours after ingestion, he was alert, oriented, and extubated. Elevated whole-blood CN concentrations verified the ingestion.

In the few reported cases of CN ingestion treated solely with sodium thiosulfate,[46] the patients had favorable outcomes. However, before sodium thiosulfate administration, we recommend the use of sodium nitrite or preferably hydroxocobalamin.

A study in swine evaluated the effect of hydroxocobalamin plus sodium thiosulfate versus sodium nitrite and sodium thiosulfate in a model using a continuous infusion of CN. There was no difference between the groups with regard to metabolic acidosis with elevated lactate concentrations at times 20 and 40 minutes, in cardiac output and pulse rate at 40 minutes, or in mortality rate. The mean arterial pressure was higher in the hydroxocobalamin plus sodium thiosulfate group, beginning at 5 minutes and lasting for the entire 40-minute monitoring period.[5] A second study in swine was unable to show a benefit to sodium thiosulfate as the sole therapy or to show an added benefit when combined with hydroxocobalamin after IV CN exposure.[4] All 12 swine in the sodium thiosulfate group died compared with only 1 of 12 in the hydroxocobalamin group.

A study using mice, rabbits, and swine demonstrated that intramuscular injection of sodium nitrite and sodium thiosulfate in doses smaller than those used previously were effective in rescuing the animals.[3] The authors comment that the previous dog experiments were likely ineffective because the IM doses were too big in volume, and the model of IV bolus CN with treatment begun at 2 to 3 minutes later prevented the ability to show an effect.

ROLE OF SODIUM THIOSULFATE IN NITROPRUSSIDE-INDUCED CYANIDE TOXICITY

Canine experiments reveal that when a nitroprusside (which contains five CN ions) infusion rate is greater than 0.5 mg/kg/h, CN concentrations in the blood rises. Coadministration of sodium thiosulfate with sodium nitroprusside in a 5:1 molar ratio prevents the rise in CN concentration.[29,46] A 70-kg person administered 3 mcg/kg/min would receive 12.6 mg/h (0.042 mmol/h) of nitroprusside. This would require 52.4 mg (0.211 mmol) of sodium thiosulfate per hour to detoxify the CN liberated from nitroprusside. Prolonged infusion or doses in excess of the detoxifying capability of the body leads to thiocyanate or CN toxicity. Adding 0.5 g of sodium thiosulfate to each 50 mg of nitroprusside is effective in most cases.[8,23,27,31,32] An in vitro study confirms that the admixture of IV nitroprusside with sodium thiosulfate in a 1:10 ratio is chemically and physically stable at room temperature for up to 48 hours.[58] Although this dose of sodium thiosulfate usually is sufficient to prevent CN toxicity from nitroprusside, thiocyanate can accumulate, especially in critically ill patients and in those with kidney insufficiency.[50] Although thiocyanate is relatively nontoxic compared with CN, it produces dose-dependent tinnitus, miosis, hyperreflexia, and hypothyroidism, especially at serum concentrations greater than 60 mcg/mL.[44] Thiocyanate is hemodialyzable. Nitroprusside-induced CN toxicity should be treated by stopping the nitroprusside and administering standard doses of hydroxocobalamin with or without sodium thiosulfate.

ROLE OF SODIUM THIOSULFATE IN CALCIFIC UREMIC ARTERIOLOPATHY (CALCIPHYLAXIS)

Calciphylaxis is a rare vascular disease associated with chronic kidney failure that is defined as calcification of the medial layer of arteries, leading to subcutaneous nodules that typically progress to necrotic skin ulcers.[1,2,9,45,53,61] Sodium thiosulfate in a typical dose of 5 to 25 g IV in adults during or after HD (although some patients reported in a recent case series received daily doses) is used to treat this disease.[45,52] Thiosulfate likely increases the water solubility of calcium, leading to enhanced excretion of calcium thiosulfate, which induces vasodilation and acts as a free radical scavenger.[52,53,61] In a uremic rat model, sodium thiosulfate was able to prevent vascular calcifications but also induced a metabolic acidosis and reduced bone strength.[7,54] A patient being treated for calcific uremic arteriolopathy developed a severe anion gap metabolic acidosis after each repeated dose of sodium thiosulfate.[59] This was also the case in a patient with chronic kidney disease (not on HD) and calciphylaxis receiving IV 25 g daily of sodium thiosulfate. By day 6, the patient had an anion gap metabolic acidosis that went unnoticed and likely caused two episodes of life-threatening acidemia requiring cardiopulmonary resuscitation on days 8 and 11 until the sodium thiosulfate was recognized as the likely cause.[42]

ADVERSE EFFECTS AND SAFETY ISSUES: SODIUM THIOSULFATE

The toxicity of sodium thiosulfate is low. The LD_{50} (median lethal dose in 50% of test subjects) for animals is approximately 3 to 4 g/kg, with death attributed to metabolic acidosis, elevated serum sodium concentration, and decreased blood pressure and oxygenation.[43] Sodium thiosulfate is hyperosmolar, delivering a significant sodium load, resulting in an osmotic diuretic effect.[46] Administering the infusion over 10 to 30 minutes limits some of these adverse effects.[46] Adverse effects associated with therapeutic doses include hypotension, nausea, vomiting, and prolonged bleeding time (1 to 3 days after a single 12.5-g dose) without changes in other hematologic parameters.[46,51,63]

ADVERSE EFFECTS AND SAFETY ISSUES: NITRITES

Amyl nitrite and sodium nitrite work in part by inducing methemoglobinemia, but excessive methemoglobinemia is potentially lethal. Therefore, nitrite dosages must be carefully calculated to avoid excessive methemoglobinemia, especially in cases in which other coexisting conditions, such as COHb, sulfhemoglobin, and anemia, might compromise hemoglobin oxygen saturation.[25,49] Children are particularly at risk for medication errors because of dosage miscalculations. A reported death from methemoglobinemia was caused by the administration of an adult dose of sodium nitrite to a 17-month-old child suspected of ingesting a toxic amount of CN.[6]

Nitrites are potent vasodilators, resulting in transient hypotension. Other common adverse effects include headache, tachycardia, palpitations, dysrhythmias, blurred vision, nausea, and vomiting.[12,51,62]

PREGNANCY AND LACTATION: NITRITES

The nitrites are FDA Pregnancy Category C. There are no adequate studies in pregnant women, and nitrites should only be used in pregnant women when the potential benefit exceeds the potential risk.[51] Hydroxocobalamin would be preferable if available because sodium nitrite has caused fetal death in humans and animals.[51] Fetuses are particularly sensitive to methemoglobinemia with the potential for prenatal hypoxia. High concentrations of nitrites in maternal drinking water have led to teratogenicity.[51]

Hydroxocobalamin is also FDA Pregnancy Category C; however, even with the limited data available, it is the author's impression that it has a lesser risk than nitrite use for a pregnant woman.[18]

It is not known whether nitrites are excreted in breast milk, but the risk is likely to exceed the benefit and is not recommended.

PREGNANCY AND LACTATION: SODIUM THIOSULFATE

Sodium thiosulfate is FDA Pregnancy Category C. No reports of congenital anomalies in infants born to women exposed to sodium thiosulfate during pregnancy are described.[51] Teratogenic effects were not observed in hamster offspring treated with doses of sodium thiosulfate comparable to those that would be used for CN toxicity. Sodium thiosulfate is recommended in pregnant women when the potential benefit outweighs any potential risk. It is not known whether sodium thiosulfate is excreted in breast milk.

DOSING AND ADMINISTRATION OF NITRITES AND SODIUM THIOSULFATE
Adults

Sodium nitrite 300 mg (10 mL of 3% solution) should be administered intravenously at a rate of 2.5 to 5 mL/min. We recommend repeating sodium nitrite at half the initial dose if manifestations of CN toxicity persist or reappear.[51,62]

The cyanide antidote kit is no longer available. It previously contained amyl nitrite, sodium nitrite, and sodium thiosulfate. Since Nithiodote (sodium nitrite and sodium thiosulfate) took its place and no longer contains amyl nitrite, amyl nitrite is no longer recommended. In situations in which only amyl nitrite is available, one amyl nitrite ampule is broken and held in front of the patient's mouth for 15 seconds on and 15 seconds off. Inhalation of amyl nitrite should be discontinued before sodium nitrite administration. The health care provider should be extremely careful not to inhale the amyl nitrite to prevent lightheadedness and syncope.

Immediately after the completion of the sodium nitrite infusion, 50 mL of 25% solution (12.5 g) sodium thiosulfate should be infused intravenously. The same needle and vein are used, and the dose of the thiosulfate should be repeated at half the initial dose if manifestations of CN toxicity persist or reappear.[62]

In situations in which additional methemoglobin formation would be harmful, as in patients with carbon monoxide poisoning, it is recommended to withhold the nitrite and only administer the IV hydroxocobalamin with or without sodium thiosulfate. Hydroxocobalamin has the advantage of rapidly reversing CN toxicity and is usually considered preferable to the combination of sodium nitrite and sodium thiosulfate. The initial dose of hydroxocobalamin in adults is 5 g IV over 15 minutes with a second dose administered if warranted.[51] Care must be taken not to administer the hydroxocobalamin and sodium thiosulfate through the same IV line because a physical incompatibility occurs, inactivating the hydroxocobalamin.

Children

Intravenously infuse 0.2 mL/kg (6 to 8 mL/m² body surface area {BSA}) or 6 mg/kg of 3% sodium nitrite solution at a rate of 2.5 to 5 mL/min, not to exceed 10 mL or 300 mg.[17,18] Based on an in vitro calculation, this dose should be safe for a child with a hemoglobin of 7 g/dL in the absence of other factors that could compromise hemoglobin oxygen saturation, such as COHb or sulfhemoglobin.[2] We recommend repeating sodium nitrite at half the initial dose if manifestations of CN toxicity persist or reappear (Table 123–2).[51,62]

The dose of sodium thiosulfate in children is 1 mL/kg using a 25% solution (250 mg/kg or ~30–40 mL/m² of BSA) not to exceed 50 mL (12.5 g) total dose immediately after administration of sodium nitrite.[51,63] We recommend repeating sodium thiosulfate at half the initial dose if manifestations of CN toxicity persist or reappear. The same needle and vein should be used.

Amyl nitrite inhalation is administered in children at the same dose and with the same precautions as mentioned for adults.

In situations in which additional formation of methemoglobin would be harmful, as in patients with smoke inhalation from a fire in which unknown toxic gases exist, we recommend witholding the nitrite and administering hydroxocobalamin with or without sodium thiosulfate. In children, a dose of 70 mg/kg of hydroxocobalamin up to the adult dose is recommended.[18]

Care must be taken not to administer the hydroxocobalamin and sodium thiosulfate through the same IV line because physical incompatibility occurs, inactivating the hydroxocobalamin.

FORMULATION AND ACQUISITION

Sodium nitrite is available in vials containing 300 mg in 10 mL (3% concentration) of water for injection (USP).[62] Sodium thiosulfate is available in 50-mL vials containing 12.5 g in water for injection (USP).[63] Neither vial contains additives or preservatives. In 2011, the FDA approved Nithiodote, a copackaged vial of sodium nitrite (300 mg in 10 mL water for injection) with one vial of sodium thiosulfate (12.5 g in 50 mL of water) for injection.[51]

SUMMARY

- Intravenous sodium nitrite followed immediately by IV sodium thiosulfate act as CN antidotes.
- Hydroxocobalamin has the advantage of working quickly to reverse CN toxicity and to reduce blood CN concentrations regardless of how they were generated (inhalation, ingestion, or via smoke inhalation from a fire) and is usually preferred over sodium nitrite and thiosulfate.
- The production of methemoglobin by sodium nitrite is both therapeutic in CN poisoning and potentially life threatening if nitrites are administered to a patient with impaired oxygen-carrying capacity from elevated levels of COHb, sulfhemoglobin, or methemoglobin.
- In situations in which additional methemoglobin formation would be harmful, as in patients with carbon monoxide poisoning, the nitrite should be withheld, and IV hydroxocobalamin should be administered.
- Sodium thiosulfate detoxifies CN by forming thiocyanate, which is significantly less toxic than CN and is renally eliminated.
- The action of sodium thiosulfate is slower in onset than hydroxocobalamin or the nitrites.
- Prophylactic administration of sodium thiosulfate in addition to sodium nitroprusside reduces CN toxicity by converting liberated CN to thiocyanate.

REFERENCES

1. Ackermann F, et al. Sodium thiosulfate as first line therapy for calciphylaxis. *Arch Derm.* 143:1336-1337.
2. Baker BL, et al. Calciphylaxis responding to sodium thiosulfate therapy. *Arch Derm.* 2007;143:269-270.
3. Bebarta VS, et al. Sodium nitrite and sodium thiosulfate are effective against acute cyanide poisoning when administered by intramuscular injection. *Ann Emerg Med.* 2017;69:718-725.
4. Bebarta VS, et al. Hydroxocobalamin versus sodium thiosulfate for the treatment of acute cyanide toxicity in a swine model. *Ann Emerg Med.* 2012;59:532-539.
5. Bebarta VS, et al. Hydroxocobalamin and sodium thiosulfate versus sodium nitrite and sodium thiosulfate in the treatment of acute cyanide toxicity in a swine (Sus scrofa) model. *Ann Emerg Med.* 2010;55:345-351.
6. Berlin CM Jr. The treatment of cyanide poisoning in children. *Pediatrics.* 1970;46:793-796.
7. Bourgeois P, De Haes P. Sodium thiosulfate as a treatment for calciphylaxis: a case series. *J Dermatolog Treat.* 2016;27:520-524.
8. Braverman B, et al. Combined use of thiosulfate with nitroprusside during scoliosis surgery [abstract]. *Anesth Analg.* 1983;62: 252-253.
9. Brucculeri M, et al. Long-term intravenous sodium thiosulfate in the treatment of a patient with calciphylaxis. *Semin Dial.* 2005;18:431-434.
10. Cambal LK, et al. Acute, sublethal cyanide poisoning in mice is ameliorated by nitrite alone: complications arising from concomitant administration of nitrite and thiosulfate as an antidotal combination. *Chem Res Toxicol.* 2011;24:1104-1112.
11. Cambal LK, et al. Comparison of the relative propensities of isoamyl nitrite and sodium nitrite to ameliorate acute cyanide poisoning in mice and a novel antidotal effect arising from anesthetics. *Chem Res Toxicol.* 2013;26:828-836.
12. Chen KK, Rose CL. Nitrite and thiosulfate therapy in cyanide poisoning. *JAMA.* 1952: 149:113-119.
13. Chen KK, et al. Amyl nitrite and cyanide poisoning. *JAMA.* 1933;100:1920-1922.
14. Chen KK, et al. Methylene blue, nitrites, and sodium thiosulphate against cyanide poisoning. *Proc Soc Exp Biol Med.* 1933;31:250-252.
15. Chin RG, Calderon Y. Acute cyanide poisoning: a case report. *J Emerg Med.* 2000; 18:441-445.
16. Christel D, et al. Pharmacokinetics of cyanide in poisoning of dogs and the effect of 4-dimethylaminophenol or thiosulfate. *Arch Toxicol.* 1977;38:177-189.
17. Cosby K, et al. Nitrite reduction to nitric oxide by deoxyhemoglobin vasodilates the human circulation. *Nat Med.* 2003;9:1498-1505.
18. Cyanokit [package insert]. Manufactured by Merck Sante, s.a.s., Semoy, France and distributed by Meridian Medical Technologies, Inc, Columbia, MD; March 2017.
19. Devlin DJ, et al. Histochemical localization of rhodanese activity in rat liver and skeletal muscle. *Toxicol Appl Pharmacol.* 1989;97:247-255.
20. Farese S, et al. Sodium thiosulfate pharmacokinetics in hemodialysis patients and healthy volunteers. *Clin J Am Soc Nephrol.* 2011;6:1447-1455.
21. Foulks J, et al. Renal secretion of thiosulfate in the dog. *Am J Physiol.* 1952;168:77-85.
22. Geiger, JC. Cyanide poisoning in San Francisco. *JAMA.* 1932;99:1944-1945.
23. Geiger JC. Methylene blue solutions in potassium cyanide poisoning: report on cases 2 and 3. *JAMA.* 1933;101:269.
24. Hall AH. Nitrite/thiosulfate treated acute cyanide poisoning: estimated kinetics after antidote. *J Toxicol Clin Toxicol.* 1987;25:121-133.
25. Hall AH, et al. Suspected cyanide poisoning in smoke inhalation: complications of sodium nitrite therapy. *J Toxicol Clin Exp.* 1989;9:3-9.
26. Hall AH, et al. Cyanide poisoning from laetrile ingestion: role of nitrite therapy. *Pediatrics.* 1986;78:269-272.
27. Hall VA, Guest JM. Sodium nitroprusside-induced cyanide intoxication and prevention with sodium thiosulfate prophylaxis. *Am J Crit Care.* 1992;1:19-25; quiz 26-27.
28. Hayata S, et al. [Pharmacokinetics of cisplatin and the effect of sodium thiosulfate]. *Gan To Kagaku Ryoho.* 1984;11:2356-2361.
29. Ivankovich AD, Braverman B. Sodium thiosulphate decreases blood cyanide concentration following sodium nitroprusside. *Br J Anaesth.* 1988;60:744-746.
30. Ivankovich AD, et al. Cyanide antidotes and methods of their administration in dogs: a comparative study. *Anesthesiology.* 1980;52:210-216.
31. Ivankovich AD, et al. Prevention of nitroprusside toxicity with thiosulfate in dogs. *Anesth Analg.* 1982;61:120-126.
32. Ivankovich AD, et al. Sodium thiosulfate disposition in humans: relation to sodium nitroprusside toxicity. *Anesthesiology.* 1983;58:11-17.
33. Jarabak R, et al. A chaperone-mimetic effect of serum albumin on rhodanese. *J Biochem Toxicol.* 1993;8:41-48.
34. Johnson WS, et al. Cyanide poisoning successfully treated without therapeutic methemoglobin levels. *Am J Emerg Med.* 1989;7:437-440.
35. Klimmek R, et al. Ferrihaemoglobin formation by amyl nitrite and sodium nitrite in different species in vivo and in vitro. *Arch Toxicol.* 1988;62:152-160.
36. Lang, S. Uber Entgiftung der Blausaure, Arch. f. exper. *Path u Pharmakol.* 1895;36:75-99.
37. Lavon O. Early administration of isosorbide dinitrate improves survival of cyanide poisoned rabbits. *Clin Toxicol (Phila).* 2015;53:22-27.
38. Lavon O, et al. Effectiveness of isosorbide dinitrate in cyanide poisoning as a function of the administration timing. *BMC Pharmacol Toxicol.* 2017;18:13.
39. Lavon O, Bentur Y. Does amyl nitrite have a role in the management of prehospital mass casualty cyanide poisoning? *Clin Toxicol (Phila).* 2010;48:477-484.
40. Leavesley HB, et al. Nitrite mediated antagonism of cyanide inhibition of cytochrome c oxidase in dopamine neurons. *Toxicol Sci.* 2010;115:569-576.
41. Leavesley HB, et al. Interaction of cyanide and nitric oxide with cytochrome c oxidase: implications for acute cyanide toxicity. *Toxicol Sci.* 2008;101:101-111.
42. Mao M, et al. Severe anion gap metabolic acidosis associated with intravenous sodium thiosulfate administration. *J Med Toxicol.* 2013;9:274-277.
43. Marrs TC. The choice of cyanide antidotes. In: Ballantyne B, Marrs TC, eds. *Clinical and Experimental Toxicology of Cyanides.* Bristol, UK: Wright; 1987:383-401.

44. McEvoy GE, ed. *AHFS Drug Information 2005. Nitroprusside*. Bethesda, MD: American Society of Health-System Pharmacists; 2005.

45. Meissner M, et al. Sodium thiosulfate: a new way of treatment for caliphylaxis? *Dermatology*. 2007;214:278-282.

46. Meredith TJ, et al, eds. *Antidotes for Poisoning by Cyanide*. New York, NY: Cambridge Press; 1993.

47. Michenfelder JD, Tinker JH. Cyanide toxicity and thiosulfate protection during chronic administration of sodium nitroprusside in the dog. Correlation with a human case. *Anesthesiology*. 1977; 47: 441-448.

48. Modin A, et al. Nitrite-derived nitric oxide: a possible mediator of "acidic-metabolic" vasodilation. *Acta Physiol Scand*. 2001;171:9-16.

49. Moore SJ, et al. Antidotal use of methemoglobin forming cyanide antagonists in concurrent carbon monoxide/cyanide intoxication. *J Pharmacol Exp Ther*. 1987;242:70-73.

50. Morris AA, et al. Thiocyanate accumulation in critically ill patients receiving nitroprusside infusions. *J Intensive Care Med*. 2016;1-7.

51. Nithiodote [package insert]. Manufactured by Cangene BioPharm, Inc., Baltimore, MD, for Hope Pharmaceuticals, Scottsdale, AZ; 2011.

52. O'Neil B, Southwick AW. Three cases of penile calciphylaxis: diagnosis, treatment strategies, and the role of sodium thiosulfate. *Urology*. 2012;80:5-8.

53. O'Neill WC. Treatment of vascular calcification. *Kidney Int*. 2008;74:1376-1388.

54. Pasch A, et al. Sodium thiosulfate prevents vascular calcifications in uremic rats. *Kidney Int*. 2008;74:1444-1453.

55. Pearce LL, et al. Reversal of cyanide inhibition of cytochrome c oxidase by the auxiliary substrate nitric oxide. *J Biol Chem*. 2003;52:52139-52145.

56. Pearce LL, et al. The antagonism of nitric oxide toward cytochrome oxidase C by CO and Cyanide. *Chem Res Toxicol*. 2008; 21: 2073-2081.

57. Petrikovics I, et al. Past, present and future of cyanide antagonism research: from the early remedies to the current therapies. *World J Methodol*. 2015;5:88-100.

58. Schulz LT, et al. Stability of sodium nitroprusside and sodium thiosulfate 1:10 intravenous admixture. *Hosp Pharm*. 2010;45:779-784.

59. Selk N, Rodby RA. Unexpectedly severe metabolic acidosis associated with sodium thiosulfate therapy in a patient with calcific uremic arteriolopathy. *Semin Dial*. 2011; 24:85-88.

60. Shea M, et al. Kinetics of sodium thiosulfate, a cisplatin neutralizer. *Clin Pharmacol Ther*. 1984;35:419-425.

61. Singh RP, et al. Simulation-based sodium thiosulfate dosing strategies for the treatment of calciphylaxis. *Clin J Am Soc Nephrol*. 2011;6:1155-1159.

62. Sodium Nitrite [package insert]. Manufactured by Cangene BioPharma, Inc, Baltimore, MD, for Hope Pharmaceuticals, Scottsdale, AZ; 2011.

63. Sodium thiosulfate [package insert] Manufactured by Cangene BioPharma, Inc, Baltimore, MD, for Hope Pharmaceuticals, Scottsdale, AZ; 2012.

64. Sylvester DM, et al. Effects of thiosulfate on cyanide pharmacokinetics in dogs. *Toxicol Appl Pharmacol*. 1983;69:265-271.

65. Ten Eyck RP, et al. Stroma-free methemoglobin solution: an effective antidote for acute cyanide poisoning. *Am J Emerg Med*. 1985;3:519-523.

66. Vick JA, Froehlich H. Treatment of cyanide poisoning. *Mil Med*. 1991;156:330-339.

67. Vick JA, Von Bredow JD. Effectiveness of intramuscularly administered cyanide antidotes on methemoglobin formation and survival. *J Appl Toxicol*. 1996;16:509-516.

68. Way JL. Cyanide intoxication and its mechanism of antagonism. *Annu Rev Pharmacol Toxicol*. 1984;24:451-481.

69. Westley J, et al. The sulfurtransferases. *Fundam Appl Toxicol*. 1983;3:377-382.

70. Westley J. Mammalian cyanide detoxification with sulphane sulphur. *Ciba Found Symp*. 1988;140:201-218.

71. Wurzburg H. Treatment of cyanide poisoning in an industrial setting. *Vet Hum Toxicol*. 1996;38:44-47.

124

METHEMOGLOBIN INDUCERS

Dennis P. Price

HISTORY AND EPIDEMIOLOGY

Methemoglobinemia is a disorder of the red blood cells (RBCs). Exposure to various xenobiotics can adversely affect the RBC membrane and intracellular metabolism and, interfere with hemoglobin function. Methemoglobin occurs when the iron atom in hemoglobin loses one electron to an oxidant, and the ferrous (Fe^{2+}) or reduced state of iron is transformed into the ferric (Fe^{3+}) or oxidized state. Although methemoglobin is always present at low concentrations in the body, methemoglobinemia is defined herein as an abnormal elevation of the methemoglobin level above 1%. The ubiquity of oxidants, both in the environment and xenobiotics prescribed in the hospital, has increased the number of cases of reported methemoglobinemia.

Methemoglobin was first described by Felix Hoppe-Seyler in 1864.[42] Subsequently, in 1891, a case of transient drug-induced methemoglobinemia was reported.[85] In the late 1930s, methemoglobinemia was recognized as a predictable adverse effect of sulfanilamide use, and methylene blue was recommended for treatment of the ensuing cyanosis.[56,125] Some authors even recommended concurrent use of methylene blue when sulfanilamides were used.[125] Methylene blue was used prophylactically during general surgery to treat an individual with congenital methemoglobinemia.[7,26] In 1948, an enzyme identified as coenzyme 1 was reported in six patients in two families who had idiopathic methemoglobinemia. The defect in coenzyme 1 (nicotinamide adenine dinucleotide {NADH} methemoglobin reductase) caused cyanosis in the absence of cardiopulmonary disease and responded to ascorbic acid.[44]

Methemoglobinemia is either hereditary or acquired. The hereditary types are rare and grouped into four types depending on their clinical manifestations. To date there are only several hundred reported cases.[57,115] Although the frequency with which xenobiotic-induced methemoglobinemia occurs is unknown, the American Association of Poison Control Centers' annual data over the past 5 years reports approximately 100 yearly uses of methylene blue as an antidote. These data substantially underestimate the incidence of this poisoning because poison control centers are not notified in most cases (Chap. 130).

Methemoglobinemia is relatively common and generally produces no clinical findings. Cooximetry data collected at two teaching hospitals noted a significant number of elevated methemoglobin levels.[4] Of a total of 5,248 cooximetry tests over 28 months on 1,267 patients, 660 tests revealed methemoglobin levels above 1.5% in 414 patients (some patients had more than one test). Thus, 12.5% of all tests and 19.1% of all patients who had cooximetry performed had an abnormal methemoglobin level. A total of 138 patients with peak methemoglobin levels greater than 2% were identified. The mean peak methemoglobin level was 8.4% (range, 2.1%–60.1%), and the patients ranged from 4 days to 86 years of age.[4]

Benzocaine spray accounted for the most seriously poisoned patients ($n = 5$), with a mean peak methemoglobin level of 43.8% (range, 19.1%–60.1%).[4] Dapsone accounted for the largest number of cases ($n = 58$), with a mean peak of 7.6% (range, 2.1%–34.1%). Of the patients who had elevated methemoglobin levels, 8% had symptomatic methemoglobinemia, and approximately one-third received methylene blue. One fatality and three near fatalities were directly attributed to methemoglobinemia. These data likely represent an underestimation of the true number of cases of methemoglobinemia at these institutions because cooximetry was performed only on physician orders for suspected dyshemoglobinemia, and 25% of cases with levels above 2% were found incidentally when cooximetry was performed in the catheterization laboratory to provide data on oxyhemoglobin and deoxyhemoglobin. In addition, not all patients taking dapsone were tested.[4] Extrapolating these

data throughout the country would suggest under reporting and substantial under recognition of this entity with its potential danger. In a 10-year review of topical anesthetic–induced methemoglobinemia, 33 cases of methemoglobinemia were identified. In approximately 95,000 cases in which anesthetics were used topically to facilitate procedures, the rate of methemoglobinemia was low at 0.035%. However, extrapolated to the number of procedures done nationally, this rate would suggest 3,000 cases per year could be expected.[23] These studies suggest underreporting and substantial underrecognition of this entity with its potential danger. Worth noting was that the location of the procedure was a powerful predictor of outcome. Inpatients who likely were sicker had significantly more methemoglobinemia than their outpatient counterparts.

Another study screened a sample of infants younger than 3 months of age who presented to the emergency department with dehydration caused by diarrhea. A small number of patients had elevated levels of methemoglobin.[37] In a large study of children ($n = 2,089$) between the ages of 2 and 5 years old admitted to the hospital for fever, elevated methemoglobin levels were detected in 43% of patients. Levels were assessed using at pulse oximeter calibrated to measure methemoglobin. Vomiting, poor capillary refill, metabolic acidosis with an elevated lactate concentration, severe anemia, and malaria were reported in this population. Higher levels occurred in children who died.[25] Furthermore, the incidence of induced methemoglobinemia in the workplace is poorly documented. A number of reports document several hundred such cases of methemoglobinemia and several more workplace exposures.[15,74,100] Underreporting and underrecognition occur because of the limited symptoms associated with low levels of methemoglobin in most cases. Acute pesticide poisoning leading to methemoglobinemia is common in many parts of the world. In Sri Lanka, a large, multicenter study followed 431 patients with intentional propanil (a herbicide) ingestions and found a 10.7% mortality rate in those with methemoglobinemia.[104] Copper sulfate is another commonly found substance used industrially and as a pesticide that causes both methemoglobinemia and hemolysis.[41,88,113]

Methemoglobin and nitric oxide (NO) are chemically coupled in the RBC. Nitric oxide interacts with oxyhemoglobin and methemoglobin in a complicated and not completely understood fashion. During periods of lowered oxygen delivery to the vascular beds as with acute anemia, NO concentrations fluctuate, and methemoglobin levels rise. Some authors have postulated that this could be an early biomarker of oxidant stress and a predictor of clinical outcome; others suggest that methemoglobin is a mediator of vascular tone.[53,54,119,120]

HEMOGLOBIN PHYSIOLOGY

Hemoglobin consists of four polypeptide chains noncovalently attracted to each other. Each of these subunits carries one heme molecule deeply within the structure. The polypeptide chain protects the iron moiety of the heme molecule from inappropriate oxidation (Fig. 124–1).

The iron is held in position by six coordination bonds. Four of these bonds are between iron and the nitrogen atoms of the protoporphyrin ring with the fifth and sixth bond sites lying above and below the protoporphyrin plane. The fifth site is occupied by histidine of the polypeptide chain. A variety of hemoglobin mutations are attributable to changes in the amino acid sequence of the polypeptide chain, as with hemoglobin M diseases. This influences this protective "pocket," allowing easier iron oxidation (Fig. 124–2), or hemoglobin autooxidation. The sixth coordination site is where most of the activity within hemoglobin occurs. Oxygen transport occurs here, and this site is involved with the formation of methemoglobin or carboxyhemoglobin (Fig. 124–3). It

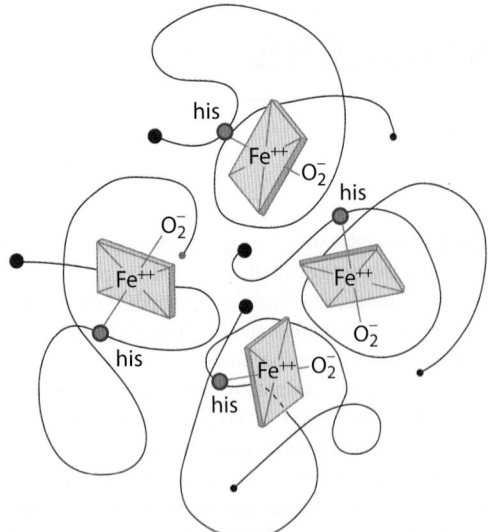

FIGURE 124–1. Hemoglobin molecule symbolically represented with its heme center surrounded by the globin portion of the molecule. his = histidine.

is at this site that an electron is lost to oxidant xenobiotics, transforming iron from its ferrous (Fe^{2+}) to its ferric (Fe^{3+}) state.

Hemoglobin transports an oxygen molecule only when its iron atom is in the reduced ferrous state (Fe^{2+}). During oxygen transport, the iron atom actually transfers an electron to oxygen, thus transporting oxygen as the superoxide charged $Fe^{3+}O_2^-$. When oxygen is released, the ferrous state is restored, and hemoglobin is ready to accept yet another oxygen molecule. Interestingly, a small percentage of oxygen is released from hemoglobin with its shared electron (forming superoxide.O_2^-), leaving iron oxidized (Fe^{3+}). This sixth coordination site becomes occupied by a water molecule. This abnormal unloading of oxygen contributes to the steady-state level of approximately 1% methemoglobin found in normal individuals.

METHEMOGLOBIN PHYSIOLOGY AND KINETICS

Because of the spontaneous and xenobiotic-induced oxidation of iron, the erythrocyte has multiple mechanisms to maintain its normal low concentration of methemoglobin.[13] All these systems donate an electron to the oxidized iron atom. Because of these effective reducing mechanisms, the half-life of methemoglobin acutely formed as a result of exposure to oxidants is between 1 and 3 hours.[62,84] With continuous exposure to the oxidant, the apparent half-life of methemoglobin is prolonged.

Quantitatively the most important reductive system requires NADH, which is generated in the Embden-Meyerhof glycolytic pathway (Fig. 124–4). Nicotinamide adenine dinucleotide serves as an electron donor, and along with the enzyme NADH methemoglobin reductase, reduces Fe^{3+} to Fe^{2+}. There are numerous cases of hereditary deficiencies of the enzyme NADH methemoglobin reductase.[57] Individuals who are homozygotes for this enzyme

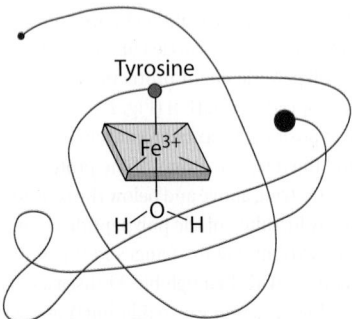

FIGURE 124–2. Hemoglobin M occurs when histidine is replaced by tyrosine in the amino acid sequence of the polypeptide chain. Hemoglobin M is more easily autooxidized (as shown) to methemoglobin.

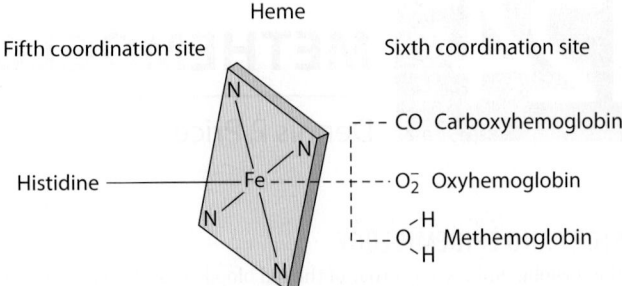

FIGURE 124–3. Heme molecule depicted with its bonding sites. Oxyhemoglobin, carboxyhemoglobin, and methemoglobin all involve the sixth coordination bonding site of iron.

deficiency usually have methemoglobin levels of 10% to 50% under normal conditions without any clinical or xenobiotic stressors. Individuals who are heterozygotes do not ordinarily demonstrate methemoglobinemia except when they are subject to oxidant stress. Additionally, because this enzyme system lacks full activity until approximately 4 months of age, even genetically normal infants are more susceptible than adults to oxidant stress.[3,78,90,127]

Oxidized iron is reduced nonenzymatically using either ascorbic acid or reduced glutathione as electron donors, but this method is slow and quantitatively less important under normal circumstances.

Within the RBC is another enzyme system for reducing oxidized iron that is dependent on the nicotinamide adenine dinucleotide phosphate (NADPH) generated in the hexose monophosphate shunt pathway (Fig. 124–4). Although it is generally accepted that this NADPH-dependent system reduces only a small percentage of methemoglobin under normal circumstances, it plays a more prominent role in maintaining oxidant balance in the cell and is involved in the mechanism of modulating vascular tone during low oxygen delivery to the capillary beds.[54,73,120] Patients with an isolated deficiency of NADPH methemoglobin reductase do not exhibit methemoglobinemia under normal circumstances,[108] perhaps because of the prominence of other cellular protective mechanisms.

However, when the NADPH methemoglobin reductase system is provided with an exogenous electron carrier, such as methylene blue, this system is accelerated and greatly assists in the reduction of oxidized hemoglobin (Antidotes in Depth: A43).

XENOBIOTIC-INDUCED METHEMOGLOBINEMIA

Nitrates and nitrites are powerful oxidizers that are two of the most common methemoglobin-forming compounds. Sources of nitrates and nitrites include well water, food, industrial compounds, and pharmaceuticals. Nitrogen-based fertilizers and nitrogenous waste from animal and human sources may contaminate shallow rural wells. Community-based water serves the majority of Americans; however, there are 37 million private wells in the United States. These wells are not tested regularly and some are shallower than appropriate to prevent contamination from fertilizers.[5,21] The contamination of drinking water occurs mainly with nitrates because nitrites are easily oxidized to the highly soluble nitrates in the environment. Furthermore, foods such as cauliflower, carrots, spinach, and broccoli have high nitrate content, as do preservatives in meat products such as hot dogs and sausage.[6]

The reactions of nitrates that occur both in vivo and in vitro are complex and poorly understood. Ingested nitrates are reduced to nitrites by bacteria in the gastrointestinal (GI) tract (especially in infants) and then can be absorbed, ultimately leading to methemoglobin production. However, this conversion is not essential because nitrates themselves can oxidize hemoglobin.[38,55,114] Some question whether well water consumption alone can cause serious methemoglobinemia in the absence of comorbid disease.[34]

In the past, nitrate-contaminated well water was associated with infant fatalities because of methemoglobinemia.[75,83] A number of reports from the midwestern United States demonstrated the problems of poorly constructed shallow wells that permit contamination by surface waters containing chemicals, pesticides, fertilizers, and microorganisms.[86] In several

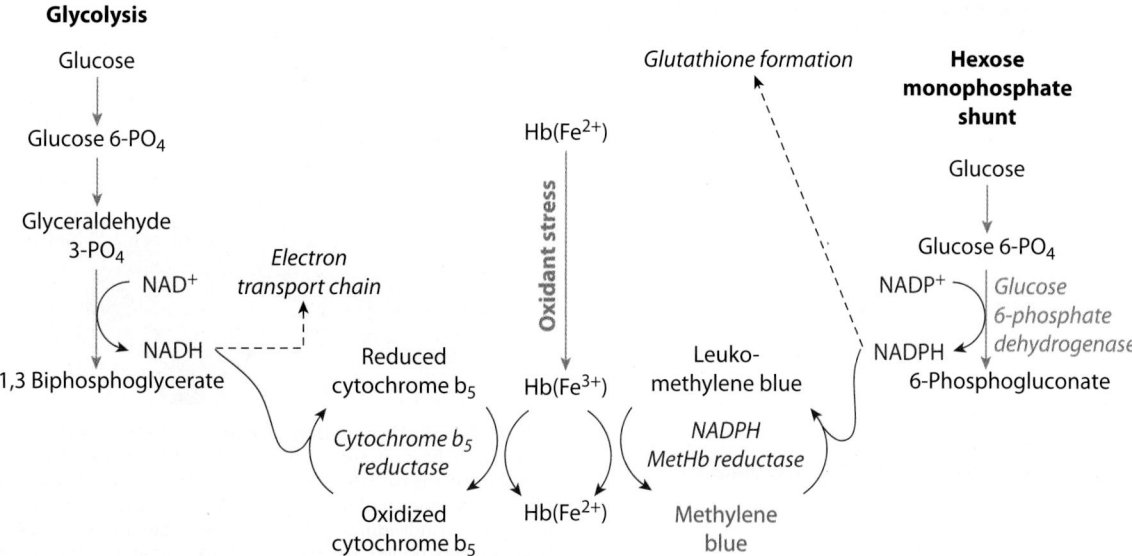

FIGURE 124–4. Role of glycolysis in the Embden-Meyerhof pathway and the role of methylene blue in the reduction of methemoglobin using nicotinamide adenine dinucleotide phosphate (NADPH) generated by the hexose monophosphate shunt. Hb (Fe^{3+}) is methemoglobin.

South Dakota studies, 20% to 50% of wells contained both coliform bacteria and water that exceeded the Environmental Protection Agency standards for permissible quantities of nitrogen as nitrates (10 ppm or 10 mg/L).[65] In New York, 419 wells from rural farms demonstrated elevated concentrations of nitrogen compounds, and 15.7% had well water nitrate concentrations higher than 10 mg/L.[43] In Texas, wells that were studied longitudinally showed increasing nitrate contamination.[21] Governmental programs, such as the Private Well Initiative, are aiming to improve drinking water quality throughout the country.[5]

Nitroglycerin (glyceryl trinitrate) and organic nitrates are more effectively absorbed through mucous membranes and intact skin than from the GI tract. Their onset of action is more rapid, and the total effect is much greater, when mucous membrane or cutaneous absorption occurs.[27,62,97] Aromatic amino and nitro compounds indirectly produce methemoglobin.[68] These xenobiotics do not form methemoglobin in vitro; therefore, they are assumed to do so by in vivo metabolic chemical conversion to some active intermediates.[15,70]

Elevated methemoglobin and carboxyhemoglobin levels are found in victims of fires and automobile exhaust fume poisoning.[12,61,67,79] Heat-induced hemoglobin denaturation in burn patients and the inhalation of oxides of nitrogen from combustion are suggested to be causative factors for methemoglobin formation.

Topical anesthetics are widely used to facilitate multiple procedures and are implicated in the most serious of toxic methemoglobin cases.[1,51] These xenobiotics continue to be a problem despite numerous case studies and recommendations by authors and manufacturers about safe use standards.[28,48,64] Cetacaine spray (14% benzocaine, 2% tetracaine, 2% butylaminobenzoate) and 20% benzocaine sprays commonly produce methemoglobinemia. The dosing recommendations are difficult to comprehend (eg, 0.5-second spray repeat once) and are often ignored. One study showed that the dose is dependent on the residual volume in the canister and the physical orientation of the canister as the spray is being applied.[71]

A review of 52 months of data from the US Food and Drug Administration (FDA) Adverse Event Reporting System demonstrated 132 cases of benzocaine-induced methemoglobinemia. Benzocaine spray was implicated in 107 severe adverse events and two deaths. In 123 cases, the product was a spray. In 69 cases in which the dose was specified, 37 patients received a single spray.[87]

This FDA effort is exclusively based on self-reporting and probably greatly underestimates the extent of the problem.[49] The FDA itself has estimated that approximately 10% of serious events are reported and that some studies show 1% or less serious event reporting.[87]

In one institution, the incidence of benzocaine-induced methemoglobinemia occurring during transesophageal echocardiograms was determined in 28,478 patients over a 90-month period. The incidence was low at 0.067% (1 case per 1,499 patients), with sepsis, anemia, and hospitalization suggested as predisposing factors.[66] During a 32-month period at another institution, an incidence of 0.115% (5 of 4,336) of benzocaine-induced methemoglobinemia was observed.[93] There were no cases of methemoglobinemia in a study of 154 patients receiving lidocaine for bronchoscopy at doses as high as 15 mg/kg. Lidocaine is a much weaker oxidant than benzocaine and is a reasonable substitute in susceptible individuals and is recommended by some authors.[64] In addition to mucosal applications, anesthetics applied topically to skin surfaces produce methemoglobinemia,[22,117] and anesthetics given during delivery to mothers receiving pudendal anesthesia have produced methemoglobinemia in newborns.[121]

Nitric oxide (NO) delivered by inhalation is used to treat persistent pulmonary hypertension of newborns and other cardiopulmonary diseases associated with pulmonary hypertension because it is a potent vasodilator.[105] Despite being a potent oxidant, if NO is used in doses of less than 40 ppm, most patients will maintain methemoglobin levels below 4%.[58,124] Some cases of serious toxicity occurred because of intentional and unintentional overdoses.

Dapsone is implicated as a cause of methemoglobinemia and is used in patients with leprosy and AIDS.[96] Cases of prolonged methemoglobinemia from dapsone ingestion are related to the long half-life of dapsone and the slow conversion to its methemoglobin-forming hydroxylamine metabolites.[30,72] Topical dapsone also produces significant methemoglobinemia.[45,116] Patients receiving dapsone should be carefully monitored for methemoglobinemia.[127] The bladder analgesic phenazopyridine is a commonly reported cause of methemoglobinemia.[24,36,43,89] For this reason, its use should be limited to short periods of time of no more than 3 days and at the lowest dose to improve symptoms. This approach is particularly pertinent in the presence of kidney failure. Predispositions for methemoglobinemia are listed in Tables 124–1 and 124–2.

TABLE 124–1	Some Physiologic and Epidemiologic Factors That Predispose Individuals to Methemoglobinemia	
Acidosis[96,108]		Diarrhea[44,89]
Advanced age[84]		Hospitalization[57,84]
Age <36 mo[24,81,107]		Kidney failure[40]
Anemia[57]		Malnutrition
Concomitant oxidant use[3,69,85]		Sepsis[57,68,84,86]
		Xenobiotics

TABLE 124–2	Common Causes of Methemoglobinemia

Hereditary

Hemoglobin M

NADH methemoglobin reductase deficiency (homozygote and heterozygote)

Acquired

Medications

    Amyl nitrite

    Local anesthetics (benzocaine, lidocaine, prilocaine)

    Dapsone

    Nitric oxide

    Nitroglycerin

    Nitroprusside

    Phenazopyridine

    Quinones (chloroquine, primaquine)

    Sulfonamides (sulfanilamide, sulfathiazide, sulfapyridine, sulfamethoxazole)

Other Xenobiotics

    Aniline dye derivatives (shoe dyes, marking inks)

    Chlorobenzene

    Copper sulfate

    Fires (heat-induced denaturation)

    Organic nitrites (eg, isobutyl nitrite, butyl nitrite)

    Naphthalene

    Nitrates (eg, well water)

    Nitrites (eg, foods)

    Nitrophenol

    Nitrogen oxide gases (occupational exposure in arc welders)

    Propanil[129]

    Silver nitrate

    Trinitrotoluene

    Zopiclone

Pediatric

Reduced NADH methemoglobin reductase activity in infants (<4 mo)

Associated with low birth weight, prematurity, dehydration, acidosis, diarrhea, and hyperchloremia

NADH = nicotinamide adenine dinucleotide.

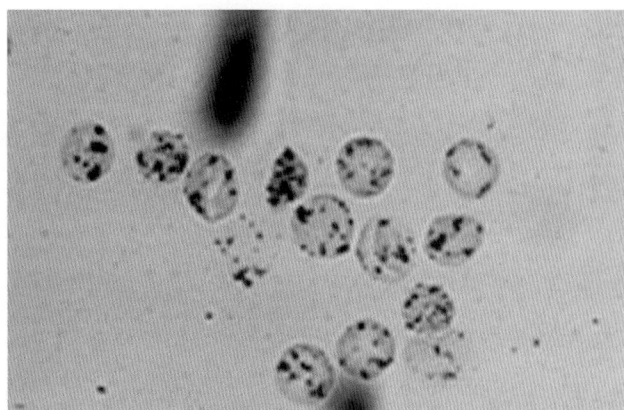

FIGURE 124–5. Heinz bodies are particles of denatured hemoglobin, usually attached to the inner surface of the red blood cell membrane. Xenobiotics that result in the oxidative denaturation of hemoglobin in normal (eg, phenylhydrazine) or glucose-6-phosphate dehydrogenase (G6PD) deficient (primaquine) individuals and unstable hemoglobin mutants are prone to develop these bodies. The Heinz bodies are identified when blood is mixed with a supravital stain, notably crystal violet. The Heinz bodies appear as purple inclusions. *(Reproduced with permission from Lichtman MA. Lichtman's Atlas of Hematology, 1st ed. New York, NY: McGraw-Hill, Inc; 2007.)*

Underlying illness,[37,66,77,93,95] the treatment with xenobiotics for these illnesses,[3,18,70,78,86,94] and the diagnostics and therapeutic modalities[58,85] in patient care all predispose patients to methemoglobinemia. For many individuals, methemoglobin is not caused by one oxidant stressor but rather by a series of stressors that makes methemoglobinemia clinically apparent and potentially predictable.

METHEMOGLOBINEMIA AND HEMOLYSIS

The enzyme defect responsible for most instances of oxidant-induced hemolysis is glucose-6-phosphate dehydrogenase (G6PD) deficiency. Reviews of hemolysis addressed the confusion regarding the relationship between hemolysis and methemoglobinemia.[10,11,40]

Both hemolysis and methemoglobinemia are caused by oxidant stress, and hemolysis sometimes occurs after episodes of methemoglobinemia.[11,96] Certain protective mechanisms involving NADPH and reduced glutathione nonspecifically reduce the oxidant burden and prevent the development of both disorders. Another source of confusion concerning hemolysis and methemoglobinemia is that reduced glutathione is required to protect against both toxic manifestations. Erythrocytes can withstand hemolytic oxidant damage as long as they can maintain adequate concentrations of reduced glutathione, the principal cellular antioxidant. Glutathione is maintained in its reduced form by using NADPH as its reducing agent. Cells with reduced capacity to produce NADPH (ie, erythrocytes of patients with G6PD deficiency

or cells with depleted reduced glutathione or NADPH) are thus susceptible to hemolysis. In the presence of methemoglobinemia, reduced glutathione plays a minor role as a reducing agent, but NADPH is necessary for successful antidotal therapy with methylene blue. This codependence on the reducing power of NADPH links these two disorders. Competition for NADPH by oxidized glutathione and exogenously administered methylene blue is postulated to be the cause of methylene blue–induced hemolysis (ie, competitive inhibition of glutathione reduction). Methylene blue itself is an oxidant, but in an assessment of the hemolytic potency of varied drugs, methylene blue in doses of 390 to 780 mg proved to be only a moderate hemolytic agent.[69] The clinical importance of this phenomenon is uncertain. Although it is easier to consider hemolysis and methemoglobin formation as subclasses of disorders of oxidant stress, they are separate clinical entities sharing limited characteristics.

Oxidative damage to erythrocytes occurs at different locations in the two disorders. Hemolysis occurs when oxidants damage the hemoglobin chain acting directly as electron acceptors or through the formation of hydrogen peroxide or other oxidizing free radicals. This results in oxidants forming irreversible bonds with sulfhydryl group of hemoglobin cause denaturation and precipitation of the globin protein to form Heinz bodies within the erythrocyte (Fig. 124–5). Cells with large numbers of Heinz bodies are removed by the reticuloendothelial system, producing hemolysis. Alternatively, a limited number of oxidants can destroy the erythrocyte membrane directly, causing non–Heinz body hemolysis. Methemoglobinemia does not necessarily progress to hemolysis even if untreated.

Numerous cases describe the occurrence of hemolysis after methemoglobinemia. The combined occurrence is reported with dapsone,[30,64] phenazopyridine,[24,36,46,89] amyl nitrite,[17] copper sulfate,[41] and aniline.[65,68] These instances of combined syndromes may represent the incidental toxicity of an oxidizing agent at both locations or may represent the depletion of all cellular defenses against oxidants. Currently, it is not possible to predict when hemolysis will occur after methemoglobinemia with any degree of certainty, and markers of hemolysis should be followed.

CLINICAL MANIFESTATIONS

The clinical manifestations of methemoglobinemia are related to impaired oxygen-carrying capacity and delivery to the tissue. The clinical manifestations of acquired methemoglobinemia are usually more severe than those produced by a corresponding degree of anemia. This discordance occurs because methemoglobin not only decreases the available oxygen-carrying capacity but also increases the affinity of the unaltered hemoglobin for oxygen. This shifts the oxygen hemoglobin dissociation curve to the left,

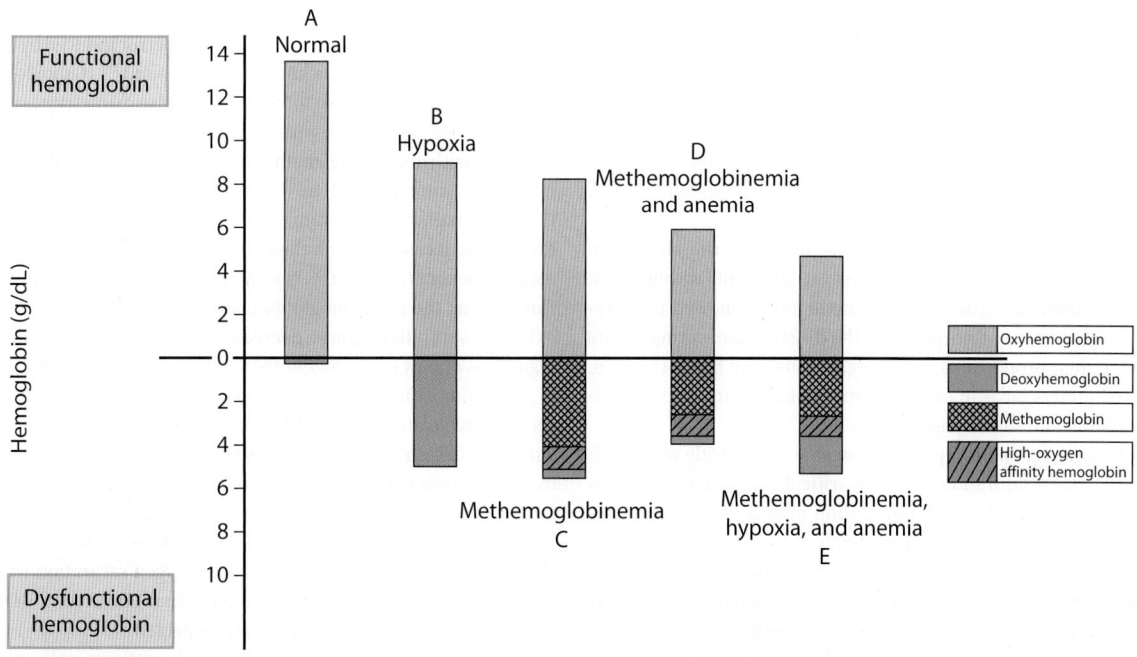

FIGURE 124–6. Clinical manifestations of methemoglobinemia depend on the level of methemoglobin and on host factors such as preexisting disease, anemia, and hypoxemia. Five examples of arterial blood gases and cooximeter analyses are presented. (**A**) Blood gas from a normal individual with 14 g/dL of hemoglobin. Almost all hemoglobin is saturated with oxygen. (**B**) Blood gas from a patient with cardiopulmonary disease producing cyanosis in which only 9 g/dL of hemoglobin is capable of oxygen transport. (**C**) Methemoglobin level of 28% in an otherwise normal individual will reduce hemoglobin available for oxygen transport to less than 9 g/dL (~4 g/dL of methemoglobin and 1.3 g/dL of high oxygen affinity hemoglobin because of the left shift of the oxyhemoglobin dissociation curve). (**D**) Same degree of methemoglobin as in **C** but in a patient with a hemoglobin of 10 g/dL. Only 6 g/dL of hemoglobin would be capable of oxygen transport. (**E**) Methemoglobinemia and anemia to the same degree as **D** but in a patient with hypoxia.

which further impairs oxygen delivery[29] (Chap. 28). This effect is attributed to the formation of heme compounds intermediate between normal reduced hemoglobin (all four iron atoms are ferrous) and methemoglobin, in which one or more of the iron moieties are in the ferric state.[29] The degree to which this high oxygen affinity hemoglobin reduces oxygen delivery to the tissue from arterial blood is unclear but is clinically significant.[19]

Because the symptoms associated with methemoglobinemia are related to impaired oxygen delivery to the tissues, concurrent diseases such as anemia, congestive heart failure, chronic obstructive pulmonary disease, and pneumonia increase the clinical effects of methemoglobinemia (Fig. 124–6).[31] Predictions of symptoms and recommendations for therapy are based on methemoglobin level in previously healthy individuals with normal total hemoglobin concentrations.

Cyanosis is a consistent physical finding in patients with substantial methemoglobinemia and is caused by the deeply pigmented color of methemoglobin. Cyanosis typically occurs when just 1.5 g/dL of methemoglobin is present. This represents only 10% conversion of hemoglobin to methemoglobin if the baseline hemoglobin is 15 g/dL. By contrast, 5 g/dL of deoxyhemoglobin (which represents 33% of the total hemoglobin concentration) is needed to produce the same degree of cyanosis from hypoxia (Table 124–3). The cyanosis associated with methemoglobinemia is both peripheral and central. Patients often appear in less distress or less ill than patients with the same degree of cyanosis secondary to cardiopulmonary causes.

The symptoms of methemoglobinemia are determined not only by the absolute level of methemoglobin but also by its rates of formation and elimination. A level of methemoglobin that is clinically benign when caused by hereditary defects or maintained chronically likely will produce more severe signs when acutely acquired. Healthy subjects lack the compensatory mechanisms that develop over a lifetime in individuals with hereditary compromise, such as erythrocytosis and increased 2,3-bisphosphoglycerate.

DIAGNOSTIC TESTING

For an individual in whom methemoglobinemia is suspected, a source for the oxidant stress should be sought. Arterial blood gas sampling usually reveals blood with a characteristic chocolate brown color. However, in patients who

are clinically stable and not in need of an arterial puncture, a venous blood gas will be accurate in demonstrating the methemoglobin level. The arterial PO_2 should be normal, reflecting the adequacy of pulmonary function to

TABLE 124–3	Signs and Symptoms Typically Associated with Methemoglobin Levels in Healthy Patients with Normal Hemoglobin Concentrations[a]
Methemoglobin Level (%)	**Signs and Symptoms**
1–3 (normal)	None
3–15	Possibly none
	Pulse oximeter reads low SaO_2
	Slate gray cutaneous coloration
15–20	Chocolate brown blood
	Cyanosis
20–50	Dizziness, syncope
	Dyspnea
	Exercise intolerance
	Fatigue
	Headache
	Weakness
50–70	Central nervous system depression
	Coma
	Dysrhythmias
	Metabolic acidosis
	Seizures
	Tachypnea
> 70	Death
	Grave hypoxic symptoms

[a]Associated illness and comorbid diseases produce more severe symptoms at lower levels of methemoglobin.

deliver dissolved oxygen to the blood. However, arterial PO_2 does not directly measure the hemoglobin oxygen saturation (SaO_2) or oxygen content of the blood. When the partial pressure of oxygen is known and oxyhemoglobin and deoxyhemoglobin are the only species of hemoglobin, oxygen saturation can be calculated accurately from the arterial blood gas. If, however, other dyshemoglobins are present, such as methemoglobin, sulfhemoglobin, or carboxyhemoglobin, then the fractional saturation of the different hemoglobin species must be determined by cooximetry in the laboratory.

The cooximeter is a spectrophotometer that identifies the absorptive characteristics of several hemoglobin species at different wavelengths. Because oxyhemoglobin, deoxyhemoglobin, methemoglobin, and carboxyhemoglobin all have different absorptions at the different measuring points of the cooximeter, their proportions and concentrations can be determined. Some newer cooximeters have an expanded spectrum and are able to measure fetal hemoglobin and sulfhemoglobin.[131]

The pulse oximeter applied to a patient's finger at the bedside was developed to estimate oxygen saturation trends in critically ill patients. Its uses have expanded to measuring hemoglobin, carbon monoxide, methemoglobin, pulsus paradoxus, pulse, and wave form analysis to follow volume loading response in shock states.[59,110] The device takes advantage of the unique absorptive characteristics of oxyhemoglobin and deoxyhemoglobin and the different concentrations of these two hemoglobin species during different phases of the pulse. Each manufacturer has calibrated its oximeter using volunteers breathing progressively increasing hypoxic gas mixtures in the absence of a dyshemoglobinemia.[100,112,123] In other words, the oxygen saturation values displayed on the pulse oximeter are derived independently by each manufacturer, who develops a formula using their own software, hardware and sensor. The manufacturer then compares this value with a set of validation data derived from its own experimental population.

Most pulse oximeters in use today use two different wavelengths to determine O_2, saturation and the manufactures do not provide validation data for situations in which any dyshemoglobin is present. All manufactures disclaim accuracy under such circumstances. Similar to cooximetry, the dual-wavelength pulse oximeter reads absorbance of light at wavelengths of 660 and 940 nm, which are selected to efficiently separate oxyhemoglobin and deoxyhemoglobin. However, methemoglobin absorption at these wavelengths is greater than that of either oxyhemoglobin or deoxyhemoglobin.[8,83] Therefore, when methemoglobin is present, the readings become inaccurate. The degree of inaccuracy is unique for each brand of instrument and will be influenced by signal quality, skin temperature, refractive error induced by blood cells, and other factors (eg, finger thickness and perfusion).[102] Hemoglobin variants, of which thousands exist, also interfere with pulse oximetry accuracy as well.[122]

In the dog model, the pulse oximeter oxygen saturation (SpO_2) values decrease with increasing methemoglobin levels. This decrease in SpO_2 is not exactly proportional to the percentage of methemoglobin. However, the pulse oximeter overestimates the level of actual oxygen saturation. For example, in a case in which the methemoglobin level measured in the blood using a cooximeter was 20%, the pulse oximeter indicated an SpO_2 of 90%.[9,118] However, as the methemoglobin concentration approached 30%, the pulse oximeter saturation values decreased to about 85% and then leveled off, regardless of how much higher the methemoglobin level became.[9,118]

From our experience and that of others,[50,101] in humans, much lower levels of oxygen saturation (SpO_2) than 85% can be displayed by pulse oximetry when methemoglobin levels increase above 30%.[63] These differences result from variations in the way different model pulse oximeters deal with methemoglobin interference and perhaps differences between canine and human hemoglobin.[100,101] Therefore, health care professionals must understand how the particular pulse oximeter measures oxygen saturation when methemoglobin levels are elevated and recognize that cooximetry determination is needed when methemoglobinemia is suspected.

Although the pulse oximeter reading in patients with methemoglobinemia is not as accurate as desired, it remains helpful when it is compared with that of the arterial blood gas: if there is a difference between the *measured* oxyhemoglobin saturation of the pulse oximeter (SaO_2) and the *calculated* oxyhemoglobin saturation of the arterial blood gas (SpO_2), then a "saturation gap" exists. The calculated SaO_2 of the blood gas will be greater than the measured SpO_2 if methemoglobin is present (Table 124–4).

Several manufacturers developed pulse oximeters that read multiple wavelengths to identify other hemoglobin species such as methemoglobin, carboxyhemoglobin, and total hemoglobin concentration.[32,33,110,130] Validation studies using human volunteers with these new pulse oximeters suggest that the accuracy for detecting methemoglobin is acceptable.[32,33] Volunteers breathing room air given sodium nitrite at 75% of the recommended cyanide treatment dose developed methemoglobinemia that was detected by the multiwavelength device. There was a spuriously low SpO_2 recorded.[32,33] However, this is not an issue if it alerts the clinician to a potential problem. Certainly,

TABLE 124–4   Hemoglobin Oxygenation Analysis

Measuring Device	Source	What Is Measured	How Data Are Expressed	Benefits	Pitfalls	Insight
Blood gas analyzer	Blood	Partial pressure of dissolved oxygen in whole blood.	PO_2	Also gives information about pH and PCO_2	Calculates SaO_2 from the partial pressure of oxygen in blood; inaccurate if forms of Hb other than OxyHb and DeoxyHb are present	An abnormal Hb form may exist if gap exists between ABG and pulse oximeter
Cooximeter	Blood	Directly measures absorptive characteristics of oxyhemoglobin, deoxyhemoglobin, methemoglobin, and carboxyhemoglobin and in some cases other hemoglobins (fetal hemoglobin, sulfhemoglobin) at different wavelength bands in whole blood.	SaO_2, %MethHb, %CoHb, %OxyHb, %DeoxyHb	Directly measures hemoglobin species	Provides data on hemoglobin only; most instruments will not measure sulfhemoglobin, HbM, and some other forms of Hb	Most accurate method of determining the oxygen content of blood
Pulse oximeter	Monitor sensor on patient	Absorptive characteristics of oxyhemoglobin in pulsatile blood assuming the presence of only OxyHb and DeoxyHb in vivo. Newer pulse oximeters measure methemoglobin.	SpO_2	Moment-to-moment bedside data	Inaccurate data if interfering substances are present (methemoglobin, sulfhemoglobin, carboxyhemoglobin, methylene blue)	Maximum depression, 75%–85% regardless of how much methemoglobin is present

ABG = arterial blood gas; CoHB, carboxyhemoglobin; DeoxyHb = deoxygenated hemoglobin; Hb = hemoglobin; HbM = hemoglobin M; OxyHb = oxygenated hemoglobin; SaO_2 = hemoglobin oxygen saturation; SpO_2 = pulse oximeter oxygen saturation.

in a situation in which xenobiotics known to produce methemoglobinemia are being used such as in the endoscopy or bronchoscopy suite, these devices are useful to determine changes from baseline in methemoglobin.

Methemoglobin produces a color change that can be observed when a drop of blood is placed on absorbant white paper. In one study when various levels of methemoglobin from 10% to 100% were produced in vitro and a drop of each concentration placed on a white background, a color chart was developed that could reliably be used to predict methemoglobin levels.[111] In situations in which laboratory evaluation is limited, such a bedside test is useful because a determination of the exact methemoglobin level is rarely needed.

MANAGEMENT

For most patients with mild methemoglobinemia of approximately 10%, no therapy is necessary other than withdrawal of the offending xenobiotic because reduction of the methemoglobin will occur by normal reconversion mechanisms (NADH methemoglobin reductase). However, in some patients, even small elevations of methemoglobin are problematic because they suggest the individual is at a point at which further oxidant stress will cause methemoglobin levels to increase.[31,53] An individual receiving dapsone with a small elevation of methemoglobin level will likely be more susceptible to clinically significant methemoglobinemia if challenged with a benzocaine-containing anesthetic or an increase in dapsone dose. In the clinical setting, continued absorption, prolonged half-life, and toxic intermediate metabolites will likely prolong methemoglobinemia. Patients should be examined carefully for signs of physiologic stress related to decreased oxygen delivery to the tissue (Fig. 124–7). Obviously, changes in mental status or ischemic chest pain necessitate immediate treatment, but subtle changes in behavior or inattentiveness are also signs of global hypoxia and should be treated. Patients with abnormal vital signs tachycardia and tachypnea or an elevated lactate concentration thought to be caused by tissue hypoxia or the functional anemia of

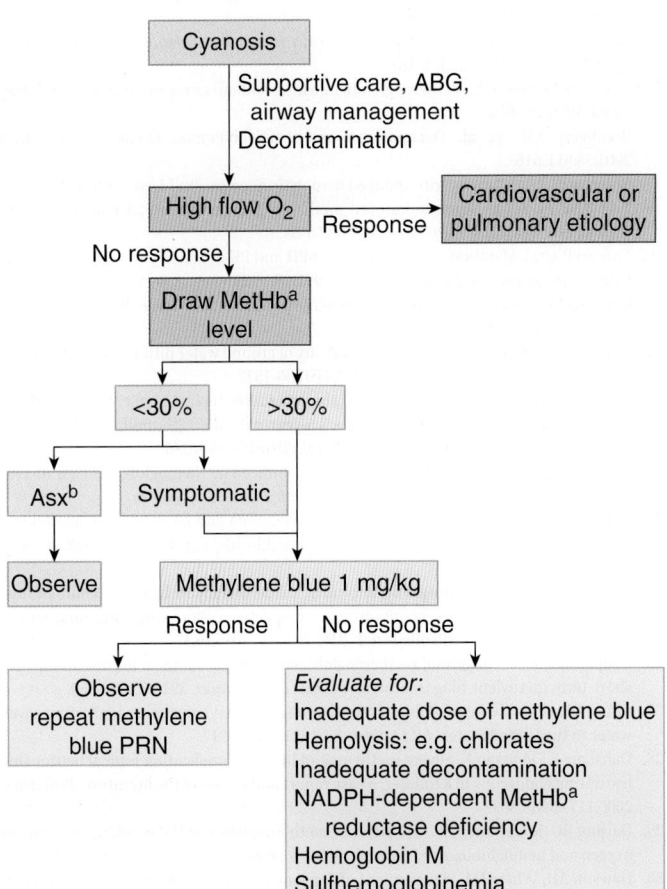

FIGURE 124–7. Toxicologic assessment of a cyanotic patient.
a = MetHb = methemoglobin; b = Asx = asymptomatic.

methemoglobinemia should be treated more aggressively. A mildly elevated methemoglobin level alone generally is not an adequate indication of need for therapy but when levels exceed 30% treatment is invariably indicated.

The most widely accepted treatment of methemoglobinemia is administration of 1 to 2 mg/kg body weight of methylene blue infused intravenously over 5 minutes. This is usually given as 0.1 to 0.2 mL/kg of 1% solution. The use of a slow 5-minute infusion helps prevent painful local responses from rapid infusion. The painful reaction can also be minimized by flushing the intravenous line rapidly with a bolus of at least 15 to 30 mL of fluid after the infusion. Clinical improvement should be noted within minutes of methylene blue administration. If cyanosis has not disappeared within 30-60 minutes of the infusion, then a second dose is recommended (Fig. 124–7). Methylene blue causes a transient decrease in the pulse oximetry reading because its blue color has excellent absorbance at 660 mm.[74,80]

The use of methylene blue in patients with G6PD deficiency is controversial. Deficiency of this enzyme is an estimated 200 million people worldwide. Its incidence in the United States is highest among African Americans (11%),[10] among whom the disease has different degrees of severity. For this reason, G6PD-deficient patients were once excluded from most treatment protocols because methylene blue is a mild oxidant and case reports suggested the toxicity of methylene blue. However, because of the lack of immediate availability of G6PD testing, most patients who need treatment receive methylene blue therapy before their G6PD status is known. Although many patients with G6PD deficiency undoubtedly have been treated unknowingly, few case reports of toxicity are described.

Even the authors of the article most frequently cited as a rationale for withholding methylene blue treatment were unsure whether the methylene blue given to their G6PD-deficient patient produced hemolysis;[106] the dose of methylene blue given to the patient was small, and the patient had taken aniline, which is capable of producing hemolysis. Patients with G6PD deficiency have variable activity of the enzyme and manifest different degrees of disease in response to oxidant stress. For all of these reasons, the judicious use of methylene blue is recommended in most patients with G6PD deficiency and symptomatic methemoglobinemia.

If methylene blue treatment fails to significantly reverse methemoglobinemia, other possibilities should be evaluated. The cause of the oxidant stress may not have been identified and adequately removed, allowing for continuing oxidation. In such situations, decontamination of the gut and skin cleansing must be ensured. Additional doses of methylene blue are also indicated. Patients who have sulfhemoglobinemia or who are deficient in NADPH methemoglobin reductase usually will not improve after methylene blue therapy (Antidotes in Depth: A43).

Theoretically, exchange transfusion or hyperbaric oxygen (HBO) would be expected to be beneficial when methylene blue is ineffective. Both interventions are time consuming and costly, but HBO allows the dissolved oxygen time to protect the patient while endogenous methemoglobin reduction occurs. Ascorbic acid is not recommended in the management of acquired methemoglobinemia if methylene blue is available because the rate at which ascorbic acid reduces methemoglobin is considerably slower than the rate of normal intrinsic mechanisms.[14] Methylene blue has no therapeutic benefit in the presence of sulfhemoglobinemia.[98]

Treatment with dapsone deserves special consideration because of its tendency to produce prolonged methemoglobinemia.[20,72] N-Hydroxylation of dapsone to its hydroxylamine metabolite by a CYP2C9 and CYP3A4 reaction is mainly responsible for methemoglobin formation in both therapeutic and overdose situations. Both the parent compound and its metabolites are oxidants with long half-lives. Cimetidine is a competitive inhibitor in the cytochrome P450 metabolic pathway and reduces methemoglobin concentrations during therapeutic dosing because less dapsone will be metabolized by the route.[103] In situations of overdose, cimetidine in therapeutic doses will likely exert some protective effects and is reasonable to use with methylene blue. When dapsone is therapeutically indicated but low levels of methemoglobin are found, cimetidine is a reasonable method for reducing oxidant stress.

Additionally, cimetidine dosing may need to be adjusted because of the effects it will have on other medications the patient may be taking.

SULFHEMOGLOBIN

Sulfhemoglobin is a variant of hemoglobin in which a sulfur atom is incorporated into the heme molecule but is not attached to iron. The exact location of the sulfur atom in the porphyrin ring is unclear. Sulfhemoglobin is a darker pigment than methemoglobin, producing cyanosis when only 0.5 g/dL of blood is affected. The cyanosis produced is similar to that produced by methemoglobinemia. Sulfhemoglobin also reduces the oxygen saturation determined by the pulse oximeter[2,92] and is characterized in the laboratory by its spectrophotometric appearance and its lack of reaction when cyanide is added to the mixture. Cyanide does not react with sulfhemoglobin but does react with methemoglobin, forming cyanomethemoglobin, which has no adsorption at the spectrums tested. By contrast, the methemoglobin absorption peak will no longer be present after the addition of cyanide, unmasking the sulfhemoglobin as the cause of the abnormal adsorption peak. This technique is not routinely done in clinical laboratories, and the diagnosis often is made based on the patient's failure to improve with methylene blue.[2,76,82,92] In laboratories, isoelectric focusing techniques further define sulfhemoglobin.

Sulfhemoglobin is an extremely stable compound that is eliminated only when RBCs are removed naturally from circulation. Although the oxygen-carrying capacity of hemoglobin is reduced by sulfhemoglobinemia, unlike in methemoglobinemia, there is a decreased affinity for oxygen in the remaining "unaltered" hemoglobin. Therefore, the oxyhemoglobin dissociation curve is shifted to the right. This makes oxygen more available to the tissues. This phenomenon reduces the clinical effect of sulfhemoglobin in the tissues.

Sulfhemoglobin is produced experimentally in vitro by the action of hydrogen sulfide on hemoglobin and was produced in dogs fed elemental sulfur.[98] A number of xenobiotics induce sulfhemoglobin in humans, including acetanilid, phenacetin, nitrates, trinitrotoluene, and sulfur compounds. Most of the xenobiotics that produce methemoglobinemia are reported in various degrees to produce sulfhemoglobinemia. Sulfhemoglobinemia is also recognized in individuals with chronic constipation and in those who abuse laxatives.[98]

Sulfhemoglobinemia usually requires no therapy other than withdrawal of the offending xenobiotic. It appears that patients come to the attention of clinicians earlier because sulfhemoglobinemia produces more cyanosis than does methemoglobinemia. There is no antidote for sulfhemoglobinemia because it results from an irreversible chemical bond that occurs within the hemoglobin molecule. Exchange transfusion would lower the sulfhemoglobin concentration, but this approach usually is unnecessary.

SUMMARY

- Methemoglobinemia is defined as an abnormal level of methemoglobin above 1%.
- Methemoglobinemia is sometimes caused by an acute, oxidant event that overwhelms the protective mechanisms of the host or more commonly and, importantly, as a final clinical manifestation of multiple oxidant stressors.
- Methemoglobinemia is clinically identified by cyanosis without cardiovascular causes, a normal PO_2 on blood gas analysis, chocolate-colored blood, and elevated methemoglobin level on cooximetry.
- Symptoms are usually milder than the appearance of the cyanosis would suggest and can be as minimal as mild fatigue and exertional dyspnea to seizures and central nervous system (CNS) depression depending on degree and coexisting disease.
- Methylene blue therapy is recommended for symptoms of cardiovascular or respiratory distress, any CNS symptoms or findings, metabolic acidosis and patients with methemoglobin levels above 30%.

- Patients with low methemoglobin levels are under oxidant stress and at risk for more serious methemoglobinemia if oxidant stressors persist or increase in their environment.
- Multiwavelength pulse oximeters are becoming more accurate and should be used routinely to monitor patients undergoing procedures in which oxidants, such as benzocaine and lidocaine, are being used.
- Early detection of oxidant stress using methemoglobin as a marker may help in management of critically ill patients.

REFERENCES

1. Aepfelbacher FC, et al. Methemoglobinemia and topical pharyngeal anesthesia. *N Engl J Med*. 2003;348:85-86.
2. Aravindhan N, Chisholm DG: Sulfhemoglobinemia presenting as pulse oximetry desaturation. *Anesthesiology*. 2000;93:883-884.
3. Arrivabene Caruy CA, et al. Perioperative methemoglobinemia. *Minerva Anestesiol*. 2007;73:377-379.
4. Ash-Bernal R, et al. Acquired methemoglobinemia: a retrospective series of 138 cases at two teaching hospitals. *Medicine*. 2004;83:265-273.
5. Backer LC, Tosta N. Unregulated drinking water initiative for environmental surveillance and public health. *J Environ Health*. 2011;73:31-32.
6. Bacon R. Nitrate preserved sausage meat causes an unusual food poisoning incident. *Commun Dis Rep CDR Rev*. 1997;7:R45-R47.
7. Baraka A, et al. Prophylactic methylene blue in a patient with congenital methemoglobinemia. *Can J Anesth*. 2005;52:258-261.
8. Barker SJ, et al. Measurement of carboxyhemoglobin and methemoglobin by pulse oximetry: a human volunteer study. *Anesthesiology*. 2006;105:892-897.
9. Barker SJ, et al. Effects of methemoglobinemia on pulse oximetry and mixed venous oximetry. *Anesthesiology*. 1989;70:112-117.
10. Beutler E. Glucose-6-phosphate dehydrogenase deficiency. *N Engl J Med*. 1991;324: 169-174.
11. Beutler E. The hemolytic effect of primaquine and related compounds: a review. *J Hematol*. 1959;14:103-139.
12. Birky M, et al. Study of biological samples obtained from victims of MGM Grand Hotel fire. *J Anal Toxicol*. 1983;7:265-271.
13. Bodansky O. Methemoglobinemia and methemoglobin producing compounds. *Pharmacol Rev*. 1951;3:144-196.
14. Bolyai JZ, et al. Ascorbic acid and chemically induced methemoglobinemias. *Toxicol Appl Pharmacol*. 1972;21:176-185.
15. Bower PJ, Peterson JN. Methemoglobinemia after sodium nitroprusside therapy. *N Engl J Med*. 1975;293:865.
16. Bradberry SM, et al. Occupational methemoglobinemia. *Occup Environ Med*. 2001;58:611-616.
17. Brandes JC, et al. Amyl nitrite-induced hemolytic anemia. *Am J Med*. 1989;86:252-254.
18. Brar R, et al. Acute Dapsone-induced methemo-globinemia in a 24-year-old woman with ulcerative colitis. *Hosp Phys*. 2007;43:54-58.
19. Caprari P, et al. Membrane alterations in G6PD and PK-deficient erythrocytes exposed to oxidizing agents. *Biol Med Metab Biol*. 1991;45:16-27.
20. Cha YS, et al. Incidence and patterns of hemolytic anemia in acute dapsone overdose. *Am J Emerg Med*. 2016;34:366-369.
21. Chaudhuri S, et al. Spatio-temporal variability of ground water nitrate concentration in Texas: 1960 to 2010. *J Environ Qual*. 2012;41:1806-1817.
22. Cho YS, et al. Seizures and methemoglobinemia after topical application of eutectic mixture of lidocaine and prilocaine on a 3.5-year-old child with molluscum contagiosum and atopic dermatitis. *Pediatr Dermatol*. 2016;33:e284-e285.
23. Chowdhary S, et al. Risk of topical anesthetic-induced methemoglobinemia: a 10-year retrospective case-control study. *JAMA Intern Med*. 2013;173:771-776.
24. Cohen BL, Bovasso GJ. Acquired methemoglobinemia and hemolytic anemia following excessive Pyridium (phenazopyridine hydrochloride) ingestion. *Clin Pediatr*. 1971; 10:537-540.
25. Conroy AL, et al. Methemoglobin and nitric oxide therapy in Ugandan children hospitalized for febrile illness: results from a prospective cohort study and randomized double-blind placebo-controlled trial. *BMC Pediatr*. 2016;16:177.
26. Cooper MS, et al. Congenital methemoglobinemia type II—clinical improvement with short-term methylene blue treatment. *Pediatr Blood Cancer*. 2016;63:558-560.
27. Craun GF, et al. Methemoglobin levels in young children consuming high nitrate well water in the United States. *Int J Epidemiol*. 1981;10:309-317.
28. Dahshan A, Donovan K. Severe methemoglobinemia complicating topical benzocaine use during endoscopy in a toddler: a case report and review of the literature. *Pediatrics*. 2006;117:e806-e809.
29. Darling RC, Roughton FJW. The effect of methemoglobin on the equilibrium between oxygen and hemoglobin. *Am J Physiol*. 1942;137:56-66.
30. Dawson AH, Whyte IM. Management of dapsone poisoning complicated by methemoglobinemia. *Med Toxicol Adverse Drug Exp*. 1989;4:387-392.
31. El-Husseini A, Azarov N. Is threshold for treatment of methemoglobinemia the same for all? A case report and literature review. *Am J Emerg Med*. 2010;28:748.e5-748.e10.

32. Feiner JR, Bickler PE. Improved accuracy of methemoglobin detection by pulse CO-oximetry during hypoxia. *Anesth Analg.* 2010;111:1160-1167.

33. Feiner JR, et al. Accuracy of methemoglobin detection by pulse CO-oximetry during hypoxia. *Anesth Analg.* 2010;111:143-148.

34. Fewtrell L. Drinking water nitrate, methemoglobinemia, and burden of disease: a discussion. *Environ Health Perspect.* 2004;112:1371-1374.

35. Fibuch EE, et al. Methemoglobinemia associated with organic nitrate therapy. *Anesth Analg.* 1979;58:521-523.

36. Fincher ME, Campbell HT. Methemoglobinemia and hemolytic anemia after phenazopyridine hydrochloride (Pyridium) administration in end-stage renal disease. *South Med J.* 1989;82:372-374.

37. Freishtat RJ, et al. A cross-sectional ED survey of infantile subclinical methemoglobinea. *Am J Emerg Med.* 2005;23:574-576.

38. Fung H. Pharmacokinetic determinants of nitrate action. *Am J Med.* 1984;76:22-27.

39. Fung HT, et al. Two cases of methemoglobinemia following zopiclone ingestion. *Clin Toxicol (Phila).* 2008 Feb;46:167-170.

40. Gaetani GD, et al. Intracellular restraint: a new basis for the limitation in response to oxidative stress in human erythrocytes containing low-activity variants of glucose-6-phosphate dehydrogenase. *Proc Natl Acad Sci U S A.* 1974;9:3584-3587.

41. Gamakaranage CS, et al. Complications and management of acute copper sulphate poisoning; a case discussion. *J Occup Med Toxicol.* 2011;6:34.

42. Garrison FH. *An Introduction to the History of Medicine.* 4th ed. Philadelphia, PA: WB Saunders; 1929:566-567.

43. Gelberg KH, et al. Nitrate levels in drinking water in rural New York State. *Environ Res.* 1999;80:34-40.

44. Gibson QH. The reduction of methaemoglobin in red blood cells and studies on the causes of idiopathic methemoglobin. *Biochem J.* 1948;42:13.

45. Graff DM, et al. Case report of methemoglobinemia in a toddler secondary to topical dapsone exposure. *Pediatrics.* 2016;138.

46. Greenberg MS, Wong H. Methemoglobinemia and Heinz body hemolytic anemia due to phenazopyridine hydrochloride. *N Engl J Med.* 1964;271:431-435.

47. Guay J. Methemoglobinemia related to local anesthetics: a summary of 232 episodes. *Anesthesiology.* 2007;107:A640.

48. Gunaratnam NT, et al. Methemoglobinemia related to topical benzocaine use: is it time to reconsider the empiric use of topical anesthesia before sedated EGD? *Gastrointest Endosc.* 2000;52:692-693.

49. Gunter JB. Benefits and risks of local anesthetics in infants and children. *Paediatr Drugs.* 2002;4:649-672.

50. Gupta PM, et al. Benzocaine-induced methemoglobinemia. *South Med J.* 2000;93:83-86.

51. Hahn IH, et al. EMLA-induced methemoglobinemia and systemic topical anesthetic toxicity. *J Emerg Med.* 2004;26:85-88.

52. Hanukoglo A, Danon PN. Endogenous methemoglobinemia associated with diarrheal disease in infancy. *J Pediatr Gastroenterol Nutr.* 1996;23:1-7.

53. Hare GM, et al. Plasma methemoglobin as a potential biomarker of anemic stress in humans. *Can J Anaesth.* 2012;59:348-356.

54. Hare GM, et al. Is methemoglobin an inert bystander, biomarker or a mediator of oxidative stress—the example of anemia? *Redox Biol.* 2013;1:65-69.

55. Harris JC, et al. Methemoglobinemia resulting from absorption of nitrates. *JAMA.* 1979;242:2869-2871.

56. Hartman AF, et al. A study of some of the physiological effects of sulfanilamide. II. Methemoglobin formation and its control. *J Clin Invest.* 1938;17:699-710.

57. Hegesh E, et al. Congenital methemoglobinemia with a deficiency of cytochrome b5. *N Engl J Med.* 1985;314:757-761.

58. Hermon MM, et al. Methemoglobin formation in children with congenital heart disease treated with inhaled nitric oxide after cardiac surgery. *Intensive Care Med.* 2003;29:447-452.

59. Hess DR. Pulse oximetry: beyond SpO2. *Respir Care.* 2016;61:1671-1680.

60. Hjelt K, et al. Methemoglobinemia among neonates in a neonatal intensive care unit. *Acta Paediatr.* 1995;84:365-370.

61. Hoffman RS, Sauter D. Methemoglobinemia resulting from smoke inhalation. *Vet Hum Toxicol.* 1989;31:40-42.

62. Horne MK, et al. Methemoglobinemia from sniffing butyl nitrite. *Ann Intern Med.* 1979;91:417-418.

63. Huang A, et al. Methemoglobinemia following unintentional ingestion of sodium nitrite—New York, 2002. *MMWR Morbid Mortal Wkly Rep.* 2002;51:639-642.

64. Jacka MJ, et al. Methemoglobinemia after transesophageal echocardiography: a life-threatening complication. *J Clin Anesth.* 2006;18:52-54.

65. Johnson CJ, et al. Fatal outcome of methemoglobinemia in an infant. *JAMA.* 1987;257:2796-2797.

66. Kane G, et al. Benzocaine-induced methemoglobinemia based on the Mayo Clinic experience from 28 478 transesophageal echocardiograms: incidence, outcomes, and predisposing factors. *Arch Intern Med.* 2007;167:1977-1982.

67. Katsumata Y, et al. Simultaneous determination of carboxyhemoglobin and methemoglobin in victims of carbon monoxide poisoning. *J Forensic Sci.* 1980;25:546-549.

68. Kearney TE, et al. Chemically induced methemoglobinemia from aniline poisoning. *West J Med.* 1984;140:282-286.

69. Kellermeyer RW, et al. Hemolytic effect of therapeutic drugs: clinical considerations of the primaquine-type hemolysis. *JAMA.* 1962;180:128-134.

70. Kelly KJ, et al. Methemoglobinemia in an infant treated with the folk remedy glycerited asafoetida. *Pediatrics.* 1984;73:717-719.

71. Khorasani A, et al. Canister tip orientation and residual volume have significant impact on the dose of benzocaine delivered by Hurricane Spray. *Anesth Analg.* 2001;92:379-383.

72. Kim YJ, et al. Difference of the clinical course and outcome between dapsone-induced methemoglobinemia and other toxic-agent-induced methemoglobinemia. *Clin Toxicol (Phila).* 2016 Aug;54:581-584.

73. Kinoshita A, et al. Simulation study of methemoglobin reduction in erythrocytes. *FEBS J.* 2007;274:1449-1458.

74. Kirlangitis JJ, et al. False indication of arterial oxygen desaturation and methemoglobinemia following injection of methylene blue in urological surgery. *Mil Med.* 1990;155:260-262.

75. Knobeloch L, et al. Blue babies and nitrate-contaminated well water. *Environ Health Perspect.* 2001;109:12-14.

76. Kouides PA, et al. Flutamide-induced cyanosis refractory to methylene blue therapy. *Br J Haematol.* 1996;94:73-75.

77. Kraft-Jacobss B, et al. Circulating methemoglobin and nitrite/nitrite concentrations as indicators of nitric oxide overproduction in critically ill children with septic shock. *Crit Care Med.* 1997;25:1588-1593.

78. Kreeftenberg H, et al. Methemoglobinemia after low-dose prilocaine in an adult patient receiving barbiturate comedication. *Anesth Analg.* 2007;104:459-460.

79. Laney RF, Hoffman RS. Methemoglobinemia secondary to automobile exhaust fumes. *Am J Emerg Med.* 1992;10:426-428.

80. Larsen VH, et al. The influence of patent blue V on pulse oximetry and haemoximetry. *Acta Anesthesiol Scand Suppl.* 1995;107:53-55.

81. Linz A, et al. Methemoglobinemia: an industrial outbreak among rubber molding workers. *J Occup Environ Med.* 2006;48:523-528.

82. Lu HC, et al. Pseudomethemoglobinemia: a case report and review of sulfhemoglobinemia. *Arch Pediatr Adolesc Med.* 1998;152:803-805.

83. Lukens JN. The legacy of well water methemoglobinemia. *JAMA.* 1987;257:2793-2795.

84. Machabert R, et al. Methaemoglobinemia due to amyl nitrite inhalation: a case report. *Hum Exp Toxicol.* 1994;13:313-314.

85. Mansouri A, Lurie AA. Concise review: methemoglobinemia. *Am J Hematol.* 1993;42:7-12.

86. Methemoglobinemia in an infant—Wisconsin. *MMWR Morbid Mortal Wkly Rep.* 1993;42:217-219.

87. Moore TJ, et al. Reported adverse event cases of methemoglobinemia associated with benzocaine products. *Arch Intern Med.* 2004;164:1192-1196.

88. Naha K, et al. Blue vitriol poisoning: a 10-year experience in a tertiary care hospital. *Clin Toxicol (Phila).* 2012;50:197-201.

89. Nathan DM, et al. Acute methemoglobinemia and hemolytic anemia with phenazopyridine. *Arch Intern Med.* 1977;137:1636-1638.

90. Nathan GD, Oski FA. *Hematology of Infancy and Childhood.* 4th ed. Philadelphia. PA: WB Saunders; 1993:698-731.

91. Nijland R, et al. Notes on the apparent discordance of pulse oximetry and multiwavelength hemoglobin photometry. *Acta Anaesthesiol Scand.* 1995;107:49-52.

92. Noor M, Beutler E. Acquired sulfhemoglobinemia an underreported diagnosis? *West J Med.* 1998;169:386-389.

93. Novaro G, et al. Benzocaine-induced methemoglobinemia. Experience from a high-volume transesophageal echocardiography laboratory. *J Am Soc Echocardiogr.* 2003;16:170-175.

94. Noyes C, et al. Subtle desaturation and preoperative methemoglobinemia. The need for continued vigilance. *Can J Anesth.* 2005;52:771-772.

95. Ohashi k, et al. Elevated methemoglobin in patient with sepsis. *Acta Anaesthesiol Scand.* 1998;48:713-716.

96. Pallais JC, et al. Case records of the Massachusetts General Hospital: case 7-2011: a 52-year-old man with upper respiratory symptoms and low oxygen saturation levels. *N Engl J Med.* 2011;364:957-966.

97. Paris PM, et al. Methemoglobin levels following sublingual nitroglycerin in human volunteers. *Ann Emerg Med.* 1986;15:171-173.

98. Park CM, Nagel RL. Sulfhemoglobinemia: clinical and molecular aspects. *N Engl J Med.* 1984;310:1579-1584.

99. Pollack ES, Pollack CV. Incidence of subclinical methemoglobinemia in infants with diarrhea. *Ann Emerg Med.* 1994;24:652-656.

100. Ralston AC, et al. Potential errors in pulse oximetry. *Anaesthesia.* 1991;46:291-295.

101. Rausch-Madison S, Mohsenifar Z. Methodologic problems encountered with cooximetry in methemoglobinemia. *Am J Med Sci.* 1997;314:203-206.

102. Reynolds KJ, et al. The effects of dyshemoglobins on pulse oximetry: part 1, theoretical approach and part II, experimental results using an in vitro test system. *J Clin Monit.* 1993;9:81-90.

103. Rhodes LE, et al. Cimetidine improves the therapeutic/toxic ratio of dapsone in patients on chronic dapsone therapy. *Br J Dermatol.* 1995;132:257-262.

104. Roberts DM, et al. Clinical outcomes and kinetics of propanil following acute self-poisoning: a prospective case series. *BMC Clin Pharmacol.* 2009;9:3-13.

105. Roberts JD, et al. Inhaled nitric oxide and persistent pulmonary hypertension of the newborn. *N Engl J Med.* 1997;336:605-610.

106. Rosen PJ, et al. Failure of methylene blue treatment in toxic methemoglobinemia. *Ann Intern Med.* 1971;76:83-86.

107. Sager S, et al. Methemoglobinemia associated with acidosis of probable renal origin. *J Pediatr*. 1995;126:59-61.

108. Sass MD, et al. TPNH-methemoglobin reductase deficiency: a new red-cell enzyme defect. *J Lab Clin Med*. 1967;5:760-767.

109. Sekimpi DK, Jones RD. Notifications of industrial chemical cyanosis poisoning in the United Kingdom 1961-80. *Br J Ind Med*. 1986;43:272-279.

110. Shamir MY, et al. The current status of continuous noninvasive measurement of total, carboxy, and methemoglobin concentration. *Anesth Analg*. 2012;114:972-978.

111. Shihana F, et al. A simple quantitative bedside test to determine methemoglobin. *Ann Emerg Med*. 2010;55:184-189.

112. Sinex JE. Pulse oximetry: principles and limitations. *Am J Emerg Med*. 1999;17:59-66.

113. Singh D, et al. Spectrum of unnatural fatalities in the Chandigarh zone of north-west India—a 25 year autopsy study from a tertiary care hospital. *J Clin Forensic Med*. 2003;10:145-152.

114. Smith ER, et al. Mechanism of action of nitrates. *Am J Med*. 1984;76:14-22.

115. Sugahara K, et al. NADH-diaphorase deficiency identified in a patient with congenital methaemoglobinaemia detected by pulse oximetry. *Intensive Care Med*. 1998; 24:706-708.

116. Swartzentruber GS, et al. Methemoglobinemia as a complication of topical dapsone. *N Engl J Med*. 2015;372:491-492.

117. Tran AN, Koo JY. Risk of systemic toxicity with topical lido-caine/prilocaine: a review. *J Drugs Dermatol*. 2014;13:1118-1122.

118. Tremper KK, Barker SJ. Using pulse oximetry when dyshemoglobin levels are high. *J Crit Illness*. 1988;11:103-107.

119. Tsui AK, et al. Reassessing the risk of hemodilutional anemia: some new pieces to an old puzzle. *Can J Anaesth*. 2010;57:779-791.

120. Umbreit J. Methemoglobin—it's not just blue: a concise review. *Am J Hematol*. 2007; 82:134-144.

121. Uslu S, Comert S. Transient neonatal methemoglobinemia caused by maternal pudendal anesthesia in delivery with prilocaine: report of two cases. *Minerva Pediatr*. 2013;65:213-217.

122. Verhovsek M, et al. Unexpectedly low pulse oximetry measurements associated with variant hemoglobins: a systematic review [published correction appears in *Am J Hematol*. 2011;86:722-725]. *Am J Hematol*. 2010;85:882-885.

123. Watcha MF, et al. Pulse oximetry in methemoglobinemia. *Am J Dis Child*. 1989; 143:845-847.

124. Weinberger B, et al. The toxicology of inhaled nitric oxide. *Toxicol Sci*. 2001;59:5-16.

125. Wendel WB. The control of methemoglobinemia with methylene blue. *J Clin Invest*. 1939; 18:179-185.

126. Williams S, et al. Methemoglobinemia in children with acute lymphoblastic leukemia (ALL) receiving dapsone for *Pneumocystis carinii* pneumonia (PCP) prophylaxis: a correlation with cytochrome b5 reductase (Cb5R) enzyme levels. *Pediatr Blood Cancer*. 2005;44:55-62.

127. Wintrobe MM, Lee GR. Unstable hemoglobin disease. In: Lee GR, ed. *Wintrobe's Clinical Hematology*. 10th ed. Baltimore, MD: Williams & Wilkins; 1999:1046-1055.

128. Yano SS, et al. Transient methemoglobinemia with acidosis in infants. *J Pediatr*. 1982;100:415-418.

129. Zamani N, Hassanian-Moghaddam H. RE. Methemoglobin measurements are underestimated by the Radical 7 CO-oximeter: experience from a series of moderate to severe propanil poisonings. *Clin Toxicol (Phila)*. 2017;55:157.

130. Zaouter C, Zavorsky GS. The measurement of carboxyhemoglobin and methemoglobin using a non-invasive pulse CO-oximeter. *Respir Physiol Neurobiol*. 2012;182:88-92.

131. Zijlstra WG, et al. Performance of an automated six-wavelength photometer (Radiometer OSM3) for routine measurement of hemoglobin derivatives. *Clin Chem*. 1988;34:149-152.

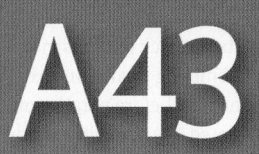

A43

METHYLENE BLUE

Mary Ann Howland

INTRODUCTION

Methylene blue is an extremely effective antidote for acquired methemoglobinemia. Methylene blue has other actions, including the inhibition of nitric oxide synthase and guanylyl cyclase and the inhibition of the generation of oxygen free radicals. These actions likely explain the beneficial effects of methylene blue in the treatment of refractory hypotension, hepatopulmonary syndrome, priapism, sepsis, and malaria; the modulation of streptozocin-induced insulin deficiency; the prevention and treatment of ifosfamide-induced encephalopathy; and the reduction of the development of postsurgical peritoneal adhesions.[15,16,21,24,34,44,53,64]

HISTORY

Methylene blue was initially recommended as an intestinal and urinary antiseptic and subsequently recognized as a weak antimalarial.[20] In 1933, Williams and Challis successfully used methylene blue for the treatment of aniline-induced methemoglobinemia.[69]

PHARMACOLOGY

Chemistry

Methylene blue is tetramethylthionine chloride,[20] a basic thiazine dye with a molecular weight of 319 Da. It is deep blue in the oxidized state and colorless when reduced to leukomethylene blue.

Mechanisms of Action

Methylene blue is an oxidizing agent, which, in the presence of nicotinamide adenine dinucleotide phosphate (NADPH) and NADPH methemoglobin reductase, is reduced to leukomethylene blue (Fig. 124–4). Leukomethylene blue effectively reduces methemoglobin to hemoglobin.[9,20,65] Reduction of methemoglobin via this NADPH pathway is limited under normal circumstances. However, in the presence of methylene blue, the role of the NADPH pathway is dramatically increased and becomes the most efficient means of methemoglobin reduction.

More recent attention has focused on the ability of methylene blue to reverse refractory hypotension from many causes, including drug overdose, vasoplegia, and sepsis.[59,63] Methylene blue inhibits nitric oxide synthase and guanylyl cyclase in vascular smooth muscle. This reduces the amount and effect of nitric oxide. Systemic vascular resistance and cardiac output increase, and the sensitivity of adrenergic receptors to sympathomimetics is enhanced.[12,14,27,36,38,68]

Pharmacokinetics

The pharmacokinetics of methylene blue were studied in animals and human volunteers after intravenous (IV) and oral administration of 100 mg.[9-11,45] Methylene blue exhibits complex pharmacokinetics, consistent with extensive distribution into deep compartments, followed by a slower terminal elimination, with a half-life of 5.25 hours. Peak concentrations after oral administration in healthy volunteers were reached in 1 to 2 hours, but were only approximately 80 to 90 nmol/L, as opposed to 8,000 to 9,000 nmol/L after IV administration.[45] Experiments in rats indicated that the substantial differences in whole-blood concentrations achieved by these routes of administration results from extensive first-pass organ distribution into the intestinal wall and liver after oral administration.[45] Total urinary excretion at 24 hours accounts for 28.6% of the drug after IV administration compared

to 18.5% after oral administration. In both instances, one-third was in the leukomethylene blue form. A phase 1 bioavailability study in healthy volunteers compared plasma and whole-blood concentrations of total methylene blue after 50 mg IV (dissolved in 10 mL of 0.9% sodium chloride over 9.5 min and followed with 10 mL of 0.9% sodium chloride over 30 seconds) and 500 mg orally as an aqueous liquid.[62] The mean plasma and whole-blood concentrations for 50 mg IV were 748 ng/mL and 1,418 ng/mL compared with the mean plasma and whole-blood concentrations for 500 mg oral of 3,905 ng/mL and 3,957 ng/mL; the times to maximum plasma concentrations were 0.5 hours for IV and 2.2 hours for oral; the time to maximum whole blood concentrations for IV were 0.22 hours and 2.2 hours for oral; the half-lives for plasma were similar for IV and oral at 18.3 hours and 18.5 hours, respectively; and the half-lives for whole blood for IV and oral were 13.6 hours and 14.7 hours, respectively. Interindividual variability was significant. The oral bioavailability of methylene blue ranged from 72% to 84% based on plasma and whole-blood analyses respectively. The mean whole blood to plasma concentration ratio was about 1. The most likely explanation for the discrepancies between this study and earlier studies is the improved sensitivity of the analytical technique.

Pharmacodynamics

The onset of action of methylene blue for the reversal of methemoglobin is often within minutes. Maximum effects usually occur by 30 minutes.[22]

ROLE IN XENOBIOTIC-INDUCED METHEMOGLOBINEMIA

Methylene blue is indicated in patients with symptomatic methemoglobinemia. This usually occurs at methemoglobin levels greater than 20%, but symptoms often occur at lower levels in anemic patients or those with cardiovascular, pulmonary, or central nervous system compromise.

Historically, sulfanilamide-induced methemoglobinemia was reversed by methylene blue in IV doses of 1 to 2 mg/kg or oral doses of 65 to 130 mg, given every 4 hours.[22,66] With these regimens, a very rapid fall in methemoglobin was accompanied by disappearance of cyanosis. Subsequent investigations confirmed the effectiveness and safety of IV doses of 1 to 2 mg/kg in reversing the methemoglobinemia produced by sulfanilamide,[66] aniline dye,[13] silver nitrate, benzocaine, nitrites, phenazopyridine, and other xenobiotics.[57,61]

The risk-to-benefit ratio of using methylene blue in a patient for methemoglobinemia must always be weighed as with any other xenobiotic. In this case, the benefit of using methylene blue for a patient with significant methemoglobinemia will almost always outweigh the risk of possibly precipitating serotonin toxicity in a patient taking a selective serotonin reuptake inhibitor (SSRI) (refer to Adverse Events).

Methylene blue is ineffective in the treatment of sulfhemoglobinemia (Chap. 124).

ROLE IN HYPOTENSION

Hypotension refractory to vasopressors occurs in the setting of sepsis, vasoplegia, and drug ingestion. Methylene blue has successfully reversed the low systemic vascular resistance in a few case studies and case reports.[12,14,27,28,32,35,36,38,47,68] A recent review suggests that although blood pressure responds to methylene blue in distributive shock, a prospective study is needed to establish whether better oxygen delivery and improved survival occur.[26]

ADVERSE EFFECTS AND SAFETY ISSUES

The most common diverse effects reported in healthy volunteers when administered 2 mg/kg methylene blue were extremity pain, chromaturia, dysgeusia, dizziness, feeling hot, dizziness, diaphoresis, nausea, skin discoloration, headache, and back pain.[49]

Reports of the paradoxical induction of methemoglobinemia by methylene blue suggest an equilibrium between the direct oxidization of hemoglobin to methemoglobin by methylene blue and its ability (through the NADPH and NADPH methemoglobin reductase pathway and leukomethylene blue production) to reduce methemoglobin to hemoglobin.[4,5] Methylene blue does not produce methemoglobin at doses of 1 to 2 mg/kg. The equilibrium seems to favor the reducing properties of methylene blue unless excessively large doses of methylene blue are administered[3,19,67] or the NADPH methemoglobin reductase system is abnormal. This equilibrium constant varies substantially, as 20 mg/kg IV in dogs and 65 mg/kg intraperitoneally in rats failed to produce methemoglobinemia.[56] In early studies, 50 to 100 mL of a 1% concentration (500-1,000 mg) of methylene blue was used intravenously in volunteers[39] as well as in the treatment of patients with aniline dye-induced methemoglobinemia.[69] In these studies, methemoglobin concentrations, measured when symptoms were most pronounced, were approximately 1.0 g/dL (0.4%-8.3% of total hemoglobin) and unlikely to be solely responsible for the adverse effects demonstrated. Other consequential adverse effects included shortness of breath, tachypnea, chest discomfort, a burning sensation of the mouth and stomach, initial bluish tinged skin and mucous membranes, paresthesias, restlessness, apprehension, tremors, nausea and vomiting, dysuria, and excitation. Urine and vomitus often appears blue in color. These limited studies led to the recommendation to avoid doses higher than 7 mg/kg.

In high doses, methylene blue induces acute hemolytic anemia independent of the presence of methemoglobinemia.[19,33] In dose-response studies in glucose-6-phosphate dehydrogenase (G6PD) deficient homozygous African-American men, daily oral doses of 390 to 780 mg (5.5-11 mg/kg) of methylene blue produced hemolysis,[31] which was comparable with the results after exposure to 15 mg of primaquine base.[31] Because of the sensitivity of neonates due to the presence of hemoglobin F and diminished NADH reductase increases the risk of hemolysis and therefore the smallest effective dose of methylene blue should be used.[24,30] Because any oxidizing agent can independently induce a Heinz body hemolytic anemia, the specific contribution of methylene blue often is difficult to elucidate.[30]

Because methylene blue is a dye, it will transiently alter pulse oximeter readings.[7] Large doses often interfere with the ability to detect a clinical decrease in cyanosis; therefore, repeat cooximeter measurements and arterial or venous blood gas analysis should be used in conjunction with clinical findings to evaluate improvement. Also because of the dye effects, the bispectral index used to assess depth of anesthesia might also be compromised.[49]

Intraamniotic injection of methylene blue results in a number of adverse effects, including infants born with blue skin (with resultant inaccurate pulse oximetry readings),[43] methemoglobinemia, hemolysis, phototoxic skin reactions,[46] or intestinal obstruction.[7,8,29,33,37,42,50,60] One infant exposed in utero at 5.5 weeks was normal at birth.[29] An excessive dose of enterally administered methylene blue that subsequently leaked into the peritoneum of a premature neonate most likely was responsible for a hemolytic anemia appearing 3 days later.[1]

Methylene blue leads to a bluish-green discoloration of the urine and often causes dysuria.[48] Intravenous methylene blue is irritating and exceedingly painful. It may cause local tissue damage even in the absence of extravasation.[50] Subcutaneous and intrathecal administrations are contraindicated.[50]

Recent reviews reveal an association between an encephalopathy and the use of methylene blue for the staining and localization of parathyroid tumors in women receiving serotonin reuptake inhibitors.[41,55,58] Doses of 3 to 7.5 mg/kg were commonly used for this indication.[55] Five of 132 patients in one review developed one or more of the following: confusion, expressive aphasia, lethargy, and vertigo, which lasted from 2 to 3 days. A second review detailed seven patients with signs and symptoms consistent with serotonin toxicity. Finally, a review of 31 published case reports in which patients maintained on SSRIs developed an encephalopathy resembling serotonin toxicity associated with the administration of methylene blue before parathyroid gland surgery concluded that caution was warranted.[55] An in vitro study documented the ability of methylene blue to competitively bind to monoamine oxidase A, raising the possibility that methylene blue might interact with serotonergic xenobiotics by acting as a monamine oxidase inhibitor.[51] Two reviews also conclude that methylene blue has the potential to interact with xenobiotics that elevate serotonin to cause serotonin excess and toxicity in situations not involving parathyroid surgery.[18,40] The US Food and Drug Administration recently added a black box warning of the potential serious or fatal serotonin toxicity when methylene blue is given to patients receiving SSRIs, serotonin-norepinephrine reuptake inhibitors, or monoamine oxidase inhibitors.[49]

High doses of methylene blue (7 mg/kg) have the potential to decrease splanchnic blood flow in the setting of septic shock.[28]

One author suggests that methylene blue directly inactivates lactic acid, giving a potentially false impression of improved perfusion.[14] However, this finding needs confirmation.

Use in Patients with Glucose-6-Phosphate Dehydrogenase Deficiency

Methylene blue is frequently hypothesized to be ineffective in reversing methemoglobinemia in patients with G6PD deficiency[41] because G6PD is essential for generation of NADPH (Chap. 20). Without NADPH, methylene blue cannot reduce methemoglobin. However, G6PD deficiency is an X-linked hereditary deficiency with more than 400 variants. The red blood cells containing the more common G6PD A⁻ variant that are found in 11% of African Americans retain 10% residual activity, mostly in young erythrocytes and reticulocytes. By contrast, the enzyme is barely detectable in those of Mediterranean descent who have inherited the defect. Therefore, it is impossible to predict before the use of methylene blue to which persons will or will not respond and to what extent. Currently, it appears that most individuals have adequate G6PD and express deficiency states in relative terms. This variable expression of their deficiency allows an effective response to most oxidant stresses. In addition, in theory, normal cells might convert methylene blue to leukomethylene blue, which might diffuse into G6PD deficient cells and effectively reduce methemoglobin to hemoglobin.[2]

Before assuming that G6PD deficiency is responsible for a continued elevation of methemoglobin levels despite administration of methylene blue, ongoing xenobiotic absorption and continued methemoglobin production must be excluded. On the other hand, when therapeutic doses of methylene blue fail to have an impact on the methemoglobin levels, the possibility of G6PD deficiency should be evaluated, and further doses of methylene blue should not be administered because of the risk of methylene blue-induced hemolysis. In these cases, exchange transfusion and hyperbaric oxygen are potential alternatives for treating methemoglobinemia (Chap. 124).

PREGNANCY AND LACTATION

Methylene blue was previously listed as a Category X drug in pregnancy. Intraamniotic injection has led to fetal abnormalities, including atresia of the ileum and jejunum, ileal occlusions, hemolytic anemia, hyperbilirubinemia, and methemoglobinemia, and should be avoided. Human data suggest a weak association with developmental toxicity when used orally in the 1970s for treating urinary tract infections in the second and third trimesters.[6]

Intravenous methylene blue should only be used to treat pregnant women with methemoglobinemia when the benefit outweighs the potential risk to the fetus.[49]

There are no data available with regard to use during lactation. However, it is currently recommended to discontinue breastfeeding when methylene blue has been used and not to resume breastfeeding for 8 days after use.[49]

DOSING AND ADMINISTRATION

The dose of methylene blue is 1 mg/kg given IV over 5 minutes followed immediately by a fluid flush of 15 to 30 mL to minimize local pain. This dose can be repeated in 30 to 60 minutes if necessary based on clinical signs and symptoms and a consequential methemoglobin level. If there is no effect after two sequential doses of 1 mg/kg, then subsequent dosing should be halted and the diagnosis reexamined or the possibility of severe G6PD deficiency considered. Methylene blue can be diluted in 50 mL of 5% dextrose in water to decrease the risk of local pain. Sodium chloride should not be used for dilution because the chloride may decrease the solubility of the methylene blue.[49] The appropriate dose of methylene blue in obese patients has not been studied. It is reasonable to theorize that because the effects on methemoglobinemia occur in the blood compartment, each dose of methylene blue should be limited to a maximum dose of 100 mg regardless of the weight of a patient. This dose can be repeated if necessary. In neonates, 0.3- to 1-mg/kg doses often are effective.[17,25] The onset of action is rapid, and maximal effects usually occur within 30 minutes.

Subsequent dosing of methylene blue is often required in conjunction with efforts to decontaminate the gastrointestinal tract when there is continued absorption or slow elimination of the xenobiotic producing the methemoglobinemia, such as with dapsone.

Intraosseous administration of 0.3 mL of 1% solution (1 mg/kg) of methylene blue over 3 to 5 minutes into the anterior tibia of a 6-week-old infant was well tolerated.[24,43] The dose of methylene blue for refractory hypotension is not established. Doses of 1 to 3 mg/kg increase systemic vascular resistance and mean arterial pressure and improve tissue oxygenation.[27] Although doses of 7 mg/kg may produce further increases in mean arterial pressure, this result is associated with a decrease in splanchnic blood flow.[28]

Methylene blue should *not* be administered subcutaneously or intrathecally.

FORMULATION AND ACQUISITION

Methylene blue is available in 10-mL vials of a 1% solution for injection, containing 10 mg/mL (100 mg total in 10 mL) and in a 0.5% solution containing 5 mg/mL (50 mg total in 10 mL).

SUMMARY

- Methylene blue is an effective reducing agent for patients with acquired methemoglobinemia.
- The onset of action for methylene blue in reversing methemoglobinemia is rapid and its adverse reactions are limited.
- After initial control of methemoglobinemia, subsequent doses of methylene blue often are required when methemoglobin-producing xenobiotics with a long duration of effect, such as dapsone, are ingested.
- Methylene blue is being investigated for use in drug-induced vasoplegic shock.

REFERENCES

1. Albert M, et al. Methylene blue: dangerous dye for neonates. *J Pediatr Surg.* 2003; 38:1244-1245.
2. Beutler E, Baluda M. Methemoglobin reduction: studies of the interaction between cell populations and of the role of methylene blue. *Blood.* 1963;22:323-333.
3. Blass N, Fung D. Dyed but not dead—methylene blue overdose. *Anesthesiology.* 1976; 45:458-459.
4. Bodansky O. Mechanism of action of methylene blue in treatment of methemoglobinemia. *JAMA.* 1950;142:923.
5. Bodansky O. Methemoglobinemia and methemoglobin-producing compounds. *Pharmacol Rev.* 1951;3:144-196.
6. Briggs G, et al. *Methylene Blue. Drugs in Pregnancy and Lactation: A Reference Guide to Fetal and Neonatal Risk, Facts & Comparisons.* St. Louis, MO: Wolters Kluwer Health; 2011.
7. Coleman MD, Coleman NA. Drug-induced methaemoglobinemia. *Drug Saf.* 1996;14: 394-405.
8. Crooks J. Haemolytic jaundice in a neonate after intra-amniotic injection of methylene blue. *Arch Dis Child.* 1982;57:872-886.
9. DiSanto AR, Wagner JG. Pharmacokinetics of highly ionized drugs. I: methylene blue—whole blood, urine, and tissue assays. *J Pharm Sci.* 1972;61:598-602.
10. DiSanto AR, Wagner JG. Pharmacokinetics of highly ionized drugs. II: methylene blue—absorption, metabolism and excretion in man and dog after oral absorption. *J Pharm Sci.* 1972;61:1086-1090.
11. DiSanto AR, Wagner JG. Pharmacokinetics of highly ionized drugs. III: methylene blue—blood levels in the dog and tissue levels in the rat following intravenous administration. *J Pharm Sci.* 1972;61:1090-1094.
12. Dumbarton T, et al. Prolonged methylene blue infusion in refractory septic shock: a case report. *Can J Anesth.* 2011;58:401-405.
13. Etteldorf JN. Methylene blue in the treatment of methemoglobinemia in premature infants caused by marking ink. *J Pediatr.* 1951;38:24-27.
14. Evora PR, et al. Methylene blue for vasoplegic syndrome treatment in heart surgery: fifteen years of questions, answers, doubts and certainties. *Rev Bras Cir Cardiovasc.* 2009;24:279-288.
15. Fallon MB. Methylene blue and cirrhosis: pathophysiologic insights, therapeutic dilemmas. *Ann Intern Med.* 2000;133:738-740.
16. Galili Y, et al. Reduction of surgery-induced peritoneal adhesions by methylene blue. *Am J Surg.* 1998;175:30-32.
17. Geiger JC. Cyanide poisoning in San Francisco. *JAMA.* 1932;99:1944-1945.
18. Gillman PK. CNS toxicity involving methylene blue: the exemplar for understanding and predicting drug interactions that precipitate serotonin syndrome. *J Psychopharmacol.* 2010;25:429-436.
19. Goluboff N, Wheaton R. Methylene blue-induced cyanosis and acute hemolytic anemia complicating the treatment of methemoglobinemia. *J Pediatr.* 1961;58:86-89.
20. Goodman LS, Gilman A. *The Pharmacological Basis of Therapeutics.* New York, NY: Macmillan; 1941:869.
21. Haluzik M, et al. Treatment with the NO-synthase inhibitor, methylene blue, moderates the decrease in serum leptin concentration in streptozotocin-induced diabetes. *Endocr Res.* 1999;25:163-171.
22. Hartmann AF, et al. A study of some of the physiological effects of sulfanilamide. II: methemoglobin formation and its control. *J Clin Invest.* 1938;17:699-710.
23. Herman M, et al. Methylene blue by intraosseous infusion for methemoglobinemia. *Ann Emerg Med.* 1999;33:111-113.
24. Hubler J, et al. Methylene blue as a means of treatment for priapism caused by intracavernous injection to combat erectile dysfunction. *Int Urol Nephrol.* 2003;35:519-521.
25. Hjelt K, et al. Methemoglobinemia among neonates in a neonatal intensive care unit. *Acta Pediatr.* 1995;84:365-370.
26. Hosseinian L, et al. Methylene blue: magic bullet for vasoplegia? *Anesth Analg.* 2016; 122:194-201.
27. Jang DH, et al. Methylene blue in the treatment of refractory shock from amlodipine overdose. *Ann Emerg Med.* 2011;58:565-567.
28. Juffermans NP, et al. A dose finding study of methylene blue to inhibit notric oxide actions in the hemodynamics of human septic shock. *Nitric Oxide.* 2010;22:275-280.
29. Katz Z, Lancet M. Inadvertent intrauterine injection of methylene blue in early pregnancy. *N Engl J Med.* 1981;304:1427.
30. Kearney T, et al. Chemically induced methemoglobinemia from aniline poisoning. *West J Med.* 1984;140:282-286.
31. Kellermeyer RW, et al. Hemolytic effect of therapeutic drugs. *JAMA.* 1962;180:128-134.
32. Kirov MY, et al. Infusion of methylene blue in human septic shock: a pilot, randomized, controlled study. *Crit Care Med.* 2001;29:1860-1867.
33. Kirsch I, Cohen M. Heinz body hemolytic anemia from the use of methylene blue in neonates. *J Pediatr.* 1980;96:276-278.
34. Kwok E, Howes D. Use of methylene blue in sepsis: a systematic review. *J Intensive Care Med.* 2006;21:359-363.
35. Levin R, et al. Methylene blue reduces mortality and morbidity in vasoplegic patients after cardiac surgery. *Ann Thorac Surg.* 2004;77:496-499.
36. Lutjen D, Arndt K. Methylene blue to treat vasoplegia due to a severe protamine reaction: a case report. *AANA J.* 2012;80:170-173.
37. McEnerney JK, McEnerney LN. Unfavorable neonatal outcome after intra-amniotic injection of methylene blue. *Obstet Gynecol.* 1983;61:35S-37S.
38. Moncada S, Higgs EA. The discovery of nitric oxide and its role in vascular biology. *Br J Pharmacol.* 2006;147:S193-S201.
39. Nadler JE, et al. Intravenous injection of methylene blue in man with reference to its toxic symptoms and effect on the electrocardiogram. *Am J Med Sci.* 1934;188:15-21.
40. Ng B, Cameron A. The role of methylene blue in serotonin syndrome: a systematic review. *Pschosomatics.* 2010;51:194-200.
41. Ng B, et al. Serotonin syndrome following methylene blue during parathyroidectomy: a case report and literature review. *Can J Anesth.* 2008;55:36-41.
42. Nicolini U, Monni G. Intestinal obstruction in babies exposed in utero to methylene blue. *Lancet.* 1990;336:1258-1259.
43. Orlowski JP, et al. Comparison study of intraosseous, central intravenous, and peripheral intravenous infusions of emergency drugs. *Am J Dis Child.* 1990;144:112-117.
44. Pelgrims J, et al. Methylene blue in the treatment and prevention of ifosfamide-induced encephalopathy: report of 12 cases and a review of the literature. *Br J Cancer.* 2000;82:291-294.
45. Peter C, et al. Pharmacokinetics and organ distribution of intravenous and oral methylene blue. *Eur J Clin Pharmacol.* 2000;56:247-250.
46. Porat R, et al. Methylene blue-induced phototoxicity: an unrecognized complication. *Pediatrics.* 1996;97:717-721.
47. Preiser JC, et al. Methylene blue administration in septic shock: a clinical trial. *Crit Care Med.* 1995:23:259-264.37.
48. Prischl F, et al. Fever, shivering … and blue urine. *Nephrol Dial Transplant.* 1999; 14:2245-2246.
49. ProvayBlue Methylene Blue package insert. Shirley, NY. American Regent; April 2016.
50. Raimer S, et al. Dye rashes. *Cutis.* 1999;63:103-106.

51. Ramsay B, et al. Methylene blue and serotonin toxicity: inhibition of monoamine oxidase A (MAO A) confirms a theoretical prediction. *Br J Pharmacol.* 2007;152: 946-951.

52. Rosen PJ, et al. Failure of methylene blue treatment in toxic methemoglobinemia. *Ann Intern Med.* 1971;76:83-86.

53. Schenk P, et al. Methylene blue improves hepatopulmonary syndrome. *Ann Intern Med.* 2000;133:701-706.

54. Serota FT, et al. The methylene-blue baby. *Lancet.* 1979;2:1142-1143.

55. Shopes E, et al. Methylene blue encephalopathy: a case report and review of the published cases. *AANA J.* 2013;81:215-221.

56. Stossel TP, Jennings RB. Failure of methylene blue to produce methemoglobinemia in vivo. *Am J Clin Pathol.* 1966;45:600-604.

57. Strauch B, et al. Successful treatment of methemoglobinemia secondary to silver nitrate therapy. *N Engl J Med.* 1969;281:257-258.

58. Sweet G, Standiford S. Methylene blue associated encephalopathy. *J Am Coll Surg.* 2007;204:454-458.

59. Tataru AP, et al. A systematic analysis of methylene blue for drug-induced shock in humans. *Clin Toxicol (Phila).* 2017;55:228.

60. Troche BI. Methylene blue baby. *N Engl J Med.* 1989;320:1756-1757.

61. Umbreit J. Methemoglobin—it's not just blue: a concise review. *Am J Hematol.* 2007; 134-144.

62. Walter-Sack I, et al. High absolute bioavailability of methylene blue given in an aqueous oral formulation. *Eur J Clin Pharmacol.* 2009;65:179-189.

63. Warrick BJ, Tataru AP, Smolinske S. A systematic analysis of methylene blue for drug-induced shock. *Clin Toxicol (Phila).* 2016;54:547-555.

64. Weinbroum AA. Methylene blue attenuates lung injury after mesenteric artery clamping/unclamping. *Eur J Clin Invest.* 2004;34:436-442.

65. Wendel WB. The control of methemoglobinemia with methylene blue. *J Clin Invest.* 1939;18:179-185.

66. Wendel WB. Use of methylene blue in methemoglobinemia from sulfanilamide poisoning. *JAMA.* 1937;109:1216.

67. Whitwam JG, et al. Potential hazard of methylene blue. *Anesthesiology.* 1979;34:181-182.

68. Wiklund L, et al. Neuro- and cardioprotective effects of blockade of nitric oxide action by administration of methylene blue. *Ann N Y Acad Sci.* 2007;1122:231-244.

69. Williams JR, Challis FE. Methylene blue as an antidote for aniline dye poisoning. *J Lab Clin Med.* 1933;19:166-171.

125 NANOTOXICOLOGY

Silas W. Smith

HISTORY

Nanotechnology has been serendipitously used by humanity for hundreds of years. Artistically, gold-ruby glass (cranberry glass), present in the Roman Lycurgus cup and later in many church stained glass windows, owes its striking red color and optical properties to gold nanoparticles created when a gold precursor is added to molten silicate glass.[141] Cosmetically, to blacken hair, the Greco-Roman practice of mixing of lead oxide and slaked lime with water created lead sulfite nanocrystals (5 nm), which accumulated in the hair cuticle and cortex.[417] Martially, 17th century Damascus steel sword blades owed their high-quality mechanical properties to carbon nanotubes (CNTs) and cementite (Fe_3C) nanowires found within their structure.[326] Medicinally, specially prepared, "Swarna bhasma," nanosized colloidal gold, has been used as an antirheumatic, antiasthmatic, and antidiabetic in Indian Ayurvedic practice for centuries.[39] Application of the nanosilver colloidal formation "Collargol" as an antiseptic was reported in 1897.[110]

In 1909, Richard Zsigmondy's investigations in colloidal chemistry were translated, and his "ultramicroscope" provided resolution to less than 1 micron, to include ultrafine cigarette smoke particles.[460] Langmuir's detailed experimental work establishing the existence of monatomic films garnered him the Nobel Prize in 1932.[195] In 1959, the physicist Richard Feynman proposed the theoretical framework for "manipulating and controlling things" all the way down to the atomic level.[107] Norio Taniguchi is generally credited with coining the term "nano-technology"—"the processing of separation, consolidation and deformation of materials by one atom or one molecule"—in 1974.[381] The invention of the scanning tunneling microscope in 1981 enabled the visualization of individual atoms and allowed the direct physical manipulation of atomic surfaces.[173] In 1985, Kroto and colleagues reported on a novel, minute crystalline allotropic form of carbon, which had been conceptualized some 15 years previously.[66,188,288] These soccer ball–shaped carbon-60 structures were named "buckminsterfullerenes" after Buckminster Fuller. The discovery of CNTs followed in 1991.[155]

The health and safety of nanotoxicology came to fore during the first consumer recall of a purported nano-based invention.[431] In 2006, the bathroom cleaning product "Magic-Nano" was released in Germany. Within days, more than 110 cases of illness were reported, and several patients were hospitalized with severe respiratory complaints, including acute lung injury. No further episodes of illness occurred after product recall only 3 days after introduction.[168] Although it was ultimately determined that "Magic-Nano" contained no nanoparticles, the incident raised many questions about nanotechnology development, regulation, and health risks.[22,23] More than 1,600 consumer products now incorporate nanotechnology.[388]

PHYSIOCHEMICAL PRINCIPLES

Nanotechnology is defined as the "control and restructuring of matter at the nanoscale, in the size range of approximately 1–100 nanometers, in order to create materials, devices, and systems with fundamentally new properties and functions due to their small structure."[318] The American Society for Testing and Materials (ASTM) International defines an *ultrafine particle* as a particle ranging in size from approximately 0.001 µm (1 nm; 10 Å) to 0.1 µm (100 nm; 1,000 Å) and a *nanoparticle* as an ultrafine particle with lengths in two or three dimensions greater than 0.001 µm (1 nm; 1,000 Å) and smaller than about 0.1 µm (100 nm; 1,000 Å).[8] Alternatively, *nanoparticles* are described as having three nano-scaled dimensions; *nanofibers* have two nano-scaled dimensions; and *nanoplates* have one nano-scaled dimension.

For spherical nanoparticles, as particle diameter decreases, the percentage of molecules on the surface of the nanoparticle increases relative to the total number of molecules. This percentage increases quite steeply below 100 nm.[184]

This provides a large area (high surface to volume ratio) for chemical reactions to occur and for interaction with biologic systems. Furthermore, as particles reach sizes below 100 nm, quantum mechanical principles become manifest, and thus acoustic, diffusion, electrical, magnetic, mechanical, optical, and solubility properties may emerge, which differ from those seen at larger as well as smaller (atomic) scales. Nanoparticles may exist as aggregations (individual particles held together by strong forces) and agglomerations (held together by weak forces such as van der Waals forces and electrostatic and surface tension). The extent of aggregations and agglomerations, particle dispersal, and electrical charge varies, depending on the primary particle constituents and on solvents or media.[35] This imparts additional properties to identical substances even at the nanoparticle level. Whereas C_{60} fullerenes are intensely hydrophobic and essentially insoluble in water, colloidal C_{60} clusters remain mono-dispersed in water as long as electrostatic repulsions are not disrupted by salts.[35] Single elemental materials can also be engineered with complex architecture (eg, gold and platinum nanostars) to alter catalytic activity.[225]

Nanoparticles may be derived "naturally," such as those originating from volcanic explosions, fires, ocean spray, sand storms, and soil and sediment weathering and biomineralization processes.[407] "Incidental" nanosized particles are generated as byproducts of processes such as combustion, cooking, munitions discharge, or welding, or even simply rubbing of bulk solids of C_{60} between fingertips or glass slides.[72] "Engineered" nanomaterials are intentionally created for research purposes or for manufacture for end-use applications. Nanomaterials and nanoparticles include a vast array of structures, such as coatings, composite nanodevices, dendrimers, fullerenes, graphenes, liposomes, nanocrystals, nanogels, nanofibers (nanorods and hollow nanotubes), nanoshells, nanospheres, conducting nanowires, polymeric micelles, quantum dots (QDs) and quantum rods, and supermagnetic particles (Fig. 125–1). They are composed of materials as diverse as their applications, including carbon, lipids, metals and metal oxides (eg, cadmium, cerium, copper, geranium, gold, iron, silver, selenium, titanium, zinc, and zirconium), nucleic acids, polymers, proteins, and combinations thereof.

CURRENT AND PROJECTED APPLICATIONS

Nanotechnologies are currently or anticipated to be incorporated into an ever-widening range of disciplines and industries. These include agriculture; automobile components; chemical and materials science (alloys, catalysts, ceramics, coatings, and thin films); defense; electronics; energy capture and storage; environmental sensing and remediation; human and animal food processing; fuel additives; house-cleaning products; paints, flame-retardants, varnishes, and sealants; pharmaceuticals; textiles; and water purification.[318] Specific human and biomedical applications include biomaterials, cosmetic and external products, diagnostics, drug and gene delivery systems, imaging, immune and transplantation sciences, and oncology therapy.[343] Biomaterial products include creation of scaffolds for in vivo or ex vivo growth to support tissue healing, engineering, and regenerative medicine; coatings to minimize immunogenicity, inhibit specific tissues or cell types, and allow macromolecular repair; and implant engineering in prosthetics to control fibrous tissue formation and biointegration, and implant performance.[112,376,385,386] Nanotechnology is radically advancing imaging capability for specific organs, tumors, sentinel lymph nodes, and vasculature. Molecular imaging now permits differentiation of cellular subcompartments, uptake mechanisms, cell architecture, intracellular trafficking, and single proteins and receptors.[15,127,189] Sunscreens, cosmetics, and conditioners have embraced a range of nanotechnologies. Nanoformulations of TiO_2 and ZnO, which the US Food and Drug Administration (FDA) has

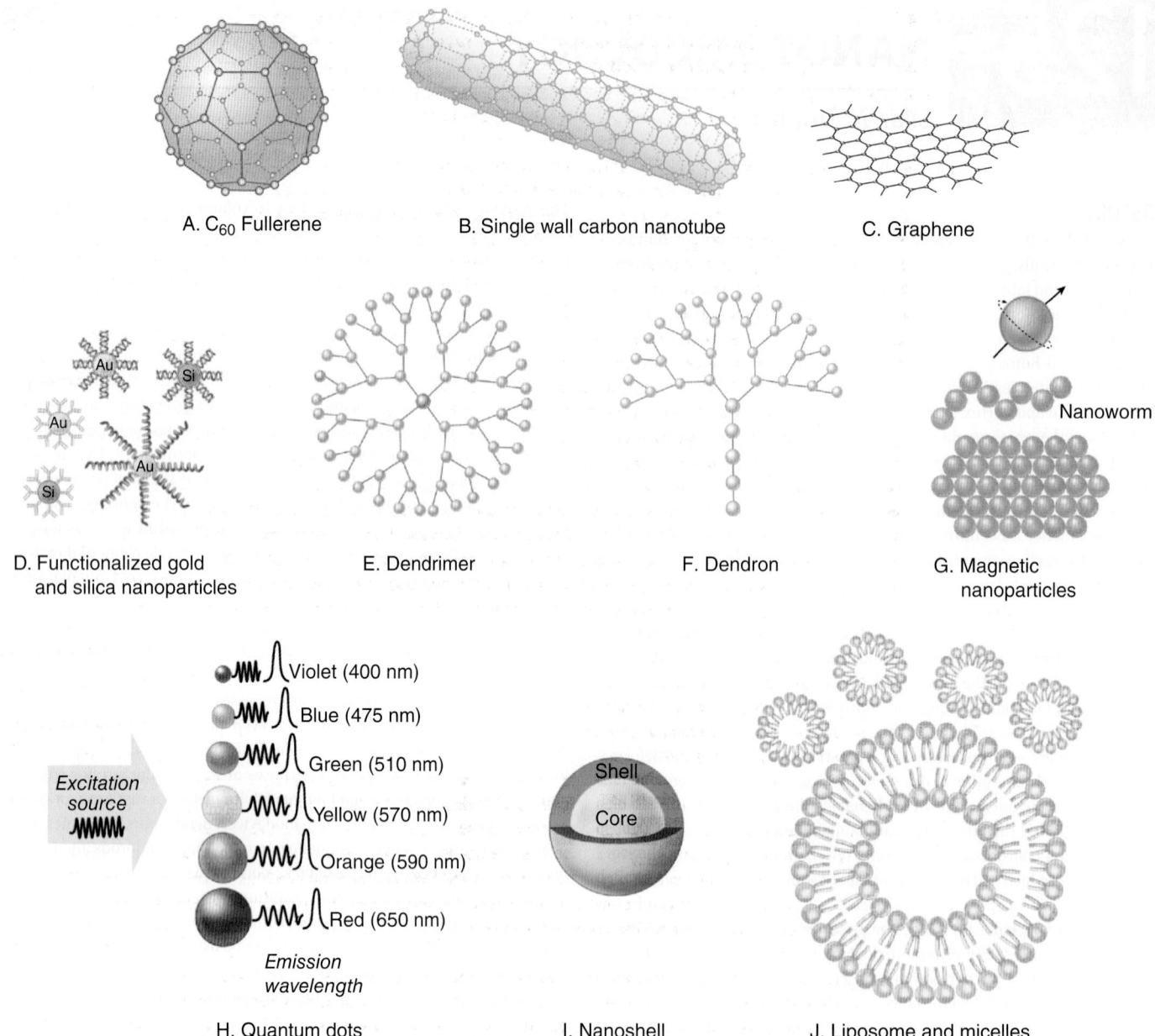

A. C$_{60}$ Fullerene

B. Single wall carbon nanotube

C. Graphene

D. Functionalized gold and silica nanoparticles

E. Dendrimer

F. Dendron

G. Magnetic nanoparticles

Nanoworm

H. Quantum dots

Excitation source

Violet (400 nm)
Blue (475 nm)
Green (510 nm)
Yellow (570 nm)
Orange (590 nm)
Red (650 nm)

Emission wavelength

I. Nanoshell

Shell

Core

J. Liposome and micelles

FIGURE 125–1. Nanoparticles (not to scale). (**A**) C$_{60}$ is a prototypical *fullerene*, or carbon cage, which may enclose additional atoms, ions, or molecular clusters. *Fullerols (fullerenols)* use polyhydroxylation at their surface to improve water solubility. (**B**) *Carbon nanotubes* (*CNTs*) are single-walled (*SWCNTs*) or multiple-walled (*MWCNTs*) cylinders, which are capped at each end and can bundle together into longer and wider agglomerates. (**C**) *Graphene* consists of a single layer of carbon atoms (ie, a sheet) in a hexagonal lattice. (**D**) *Gold nanoparticles* and other nanosized noble metals (eg, silver, copper, platinum) have unusual catalytic, optical, electronic, and (photo)thermal properties and can be conjugated to dyes, antibodies, peptides, and oligonucleotides. (**E**) *Dendrimers* are branched polymers consisting of a central core, an internal branching region, and surface terminal groups; drugs, genes, and imaging agents can be loaded into the inner protected cavities. (**F**) *Dendrons* are wedge-shaped sections of dendrimers with an accessible reactive group. (**G**) Magnetic nanoparticles include *superparamagnetic iron oxide* (*SPIO*) nanoparticles (Fe$_2$O$_3$, Fe$_3$O$_4$), pure metals (Fe and Co), and alloys (CoPt$_3$ and FePt). They are usually surrounded by a shell to minimize agglomeration and chemical reactivity. *Magnetism-engineered iron oxide* (*MEIO*) nanoparticles can be doped with cobalt, manganese, and nickel to create unique magnetism properties. (**H**) *Quantum dots* (*QDs*) and *QRods* (rod-shaped QDs) are semiconductor nanocrystals capable of size-dependent fluorescence with a "tunable" emission spectrum in the 400-nm to 2-μm range. Analogous but chemically inert *Cornell dots* (*CU or C dots*) contain covalently bound fluorescent dyes in a sol—gel-derived silica matrix. (**I**) *Nanoshells* contain a dielectric silica core surrounded by thin metal gold shell. (**J**) *Liposomes* and *micelles* are globular vesicles with hydrophobic and hydrophilic zones composed of phospholipids, sphingolipids, and ceramides or other esters or polymers ranging in size from 25 nm to the micron range. Nanoparticles can be further derivatized, chemically modified, or bioengineered with a variety of detection, imaging, or targeting molecules.

permitted in sunscreens since 1999, provide both aesthetic appeal (sunscreen with transparency, lower viscosity, and improved skin blending) and clinical benefit (more efficient ultraviolet {UV} filtration).[273,431] Wound care is incorporating dressings containing nanocrystalline silver and other delivery systems to improve wound healing through inflammation suppression, upregulation of micronutrients, and antibacterial actions.[260,391,422] Nanotechnology is advancing medical diagnostic capability, detection thresholds, and pathogen sensing, with tagged nanoparticles currently used in commercial genotyping tests and

other assays.[373] Nanoengineering holds the promise of improved pharmacokinetics, solubility, delivery, and targeting of pharmaceuticals, proteins, and genes in a cell-, tissue-, tumor-, or organ-specific manner. New formulations, magnetic drug targeting, thermal ablation, and delivery to incredibly diverse difficult-to-access spaces (eg, intracellular pathogens, tumors, and the central nervous system {CNS}) are being investigated or brought to market.[24,175,351,358,423] Table 125–1 presents selected commercial nanotechnology-based diagnostics, imaging compounds, and therapeutics.

TABLE 125–1   Selected Commercial Nanotechnology-Based Diagnostics and Therapeutics[a]

Xenobiotic	Proprietary Name	Route	Class or Indication	Nanotechnology Platform
Aminosilane–iron oxide	NanoTherm (EU)	IV	Magnetic tumor thermotherapy	SPIO nanoparticle (aminosilane–coated)
Amphotericin	Abelcet, Amphotec, AmBisome	IV	Antifungal	Liposomal
Aprepitant	Emend	PO	Antiemetic	Nanocrystal
Carmustine	Gliadel	Implant	Chemotherapeutic	Degradable solid copolymer
Certolizumab pegol (TNF antagonist)	Cimzia	SC	Immunosuppressant	Polymer protein conjugate
Cytarabine	Depocyt	IV	Chemotherapeutic	Liposomal
Daunorubicin	DaunoXome	IV	Chemotherapeutic	Liposomal
Denileukin diftitox	Ontak	IV	Chemotherapeutic	Diphtheria toxin-antibody-functionalized nanoparticle
Dominant-negative construct of human cyclin-G1 gene	Rexin-G[b] (Philippines)	IV	Chemotherapeutic	Targeted (collagen binding domain) nanoparticle
Doxorubicin	Doxil, Caelyx, Myocet	IV	Chemotherapeutic	Liposomal
Estradiol	Estrasorb	TD	Menopausal symptoms	Micellar nanoparticle
Estradiol	Elestrin	TD	Menopausal symptoms	Calcium phosphate nanoparticles
Fenofibrate	Tricor, Triglide	PO	Antilipidemic	Nanocrystal
Ferucarbotran	Cliavist, Resovist	IV	MRI contrast agent	SPIO nanoparticle (carboxydextran coated)
Ferumoxide	Feridex, Endorem	IV	MRI contrast agent	SPIO nanoparticle (dextran coated)
Ferumoxsil	GastroMARK, Lumirem	IV	MRI contrast agent	SPIO nanoparticle (siloxane coated)
Ferumoxtran-10	Combidex, Sinerem	IV	MRI contrast agent	SPIO nanoparticle (dextran coated)
Ferumoxytol	Feraheme	IV	Iron deficiency anemia of chronic kidney disease	SPIO nanoparticle (polyglucose sorbitol carboxymethyl ether coated)
Glatiramer acetate (L-glutamic acid polymer with L-alanine, L-lysine and L-tyrosine)	Copaxone	SC	Autoimmune disease mitigation (multiple sclerosis)	Polymeric substances
Gold	Verigene	NA	Molecular diagnostics	Oligonucleotide- or antibody-functionalized nanoparticle
Human GM-CSF gene	Reximmune-C	IV	Chemotherapeutic	Targeted nanoparticle
Inactivated hepatitis A (strain RG-SB) virus particles	Epaxal	IM	Vaccine	Virosome
Inactivated influenza (strains A and B) virus particles	Inflexal V	IM	Vaccine	Virosome
Indomethacin	Indaflex (Mexico)	Topical	Antiinflammatory	Nanoparticle emulsion
Insulin (human rDNA origin)	Exubera (discontinued)	Inhalation	Hypoglycemia	Calcium phosphate nanoparticles
Lanthanum carbonate	Fosrenol	PO	Phosphate reduction	Inorganic nanoparticles
Megesterol acetate	Megace ES	PO	Anorexia, cachexia, AIDS-associated weight loss	Nanocrystal
Morphine sulfate	DepoDur	Epidural	Analgesic	Liposomal
Paclitaxel	Genexol-PM[c]	IV	Chemotherapeutic	Polymeric micelle
Paclitaxel (albumin-bound)	Abraxane	IV	Chemotherapeutic	Protein conjugate
Paliperidone palmitate	Invega Sustenna	IM	Antipsychotic	Nanocrystal
Pegademase bovine (PEG-adenosine deaminase)	Adagen	IM	SCID	Polymer protein conjugate

(Continued)

TABLE 125–1	Selected Commercial Nanotechnology-Based Diagnostics and Therapeutics[a] (Continued)			
Xenobiotic	Proprietary Name	Route	Class or Indication	Nanotechnology Platform
Pegaptanib (PEG-anti-VEGF-oligonucleotide)	Macugen	IVit	Aged-related macular degeneration	Polymer protein conjugate
PEG-coated SiO$_2$	NA[d]	IV	Oncology diagnostics	Cornell Dots (C dots)
Pegaspargase	Oncaspar	IM, IV	Chemotherapeutic	Polymer protein conjugate
Pegfilgrastim (PEG-G-CSF)	Neulasta	SC	Chemotherapy-induced neutropenia	Polymer protein conjugate
Peginesatide (erythropoietin receptor agonist)	Omontys[e]	IV, SC	Polycythemic	Polymer protein conjugate
Peginterferon alfa-2b	PegIntron	SC	Antiviral (hepatitis C)	Polymer protein conjugate
Peginterferon alfa-2b	Pegasys	SC	Antiviral (hepatitis B/C)	Polymer protein conjugate
Pegloticase	Krystexxa	IV	Antiuricemic	Polymer protein conjugate
Pegvisomant (PEG-human growth hormone analog)	Somavert	SC	Acromegaly	Polymer protein conjugate
Propofol	Diprivan	IV	Anesthetic	Liposome
Sevelamer HCl (crosslinked with epichlorohydrin)	Renagel	PO	Phosphate reduction	Polymeric crosslinked resin
Silver	Acticoat	Topical	Wound healing	Nanoparticle
Sirolimus	Rapamune	PO	Immunosuppressant	Nanocrystal
Titanium dioxide	Numerous	Topical	Ultraviolet-protectant	Nanoparticle
Thymectacin	Theralux	IV	Chemotherapeutic	Nanocrystal
Vincristine	Marqibo	IV	Chemotherapeutic	Liposomal
Verteporfin	Visudyne	IV	Aged-related macular degeneration	Liposomal

[a]No endorsement is implied. [b]US FDA Orphan Drug Approval but not Marketing Approval. [c]South Korean marketing approval. [d]US Food and Drug Administration investigational new drug approval. [e]Voluntary marketing withdrawal.

EU = European Union; G-CSF = granulocyte-colony stimulating factor; GM-CSF = granulocyte-macrophage colony stimulating factor; IND = investigational new drug; IM = intramuscular; IV = intravenous; IVit = intravitreous; MRI = magnetic resonance imaging; NA = not applicable; PEG = polyethylene glycol; PO = oral; SC = subcutaneous; SCID = severe combined immunodeficiency disease; SPIO = superparamagnetic iron oxide; TD = transdermal; TNF = tumor necrosis factor; VEGF = vascular endothelial growth factor; NA = not available.

EXPOSURE AND DISTRIBUTION

Nanoparticle exposure is anticipated through a variety of mechanisms (Fig. 125–2). Exposure might occur through environmental discharge into air, water, or soil during the primary manufacturing process; disposition of industrial or research waste; mixing, weighing, or dumping powders; active cleaning processes or component replacement between production; or engine combustion. Sanding, machining, wearing and weathering, or disposing of nanomaterial-containing products could also liberate nanoparticles. Exposure might also occur during biologic elimination from a primary target or caused by implant or device wear. Nanoparticles can be consumed and then subsequently transformed, sequestered, re-released to the environment, or potentially accumulate in the food web.[32]

Dermal Exposure

Podoconiosis (endemic nonfilarial, geochemical elephantiasis) is presumed to occur from absorption of various colloid-sized elemental particles in irritant clays (aluminum, silicon, magnesium, iron), which undergo macrophage phagocytosis, induce collagenization of afferent lymphatics, and obliterate them.[70] Thus, transdermal exposure to and disease from certain nanoparticles is assumed established. Nanocompositions in paints and coatings, clothing, transdermal drug delivery devices, topical UV protection products, or proprietary cosmetics are of concern. Nanoparticles can be taken up by human epidermal keratinocytes or cause DNA damage; at issue is whether epidermal penetration to effect such damage actually occurs.[273,337,342] Reviews summarizing studies of TiO$_2$ and ZnO nanoparticles concluded that

dermal penetration for those substances was unlikely beyond the stratum corneum.[273,274] A study of CeO$_2$, silver, and TiO$_2$ nanoparticles applied to a human skin equivalent model did not demonstrate significant dermal irritability and seemed to confirm the protective effect of the stratum corneum.[245] However, TiO$_2$ and ZnO nanoparticles (in currently available sunscreens) can reside in the stratum corneum and follicular sink.[405] Solvents or diseased (eg, psoriatic), injured, or mechanically stressed skin might increase dermal penetration.[405] In experiments simulating heavy industrial solvent exposure, toluene, cyclohexane, or chloroform could transport C$_{60}$ fullerenes across the stratum corneum into viable epidermis.[437] Epidermal and dermal penetration of a phenylalanine-based fullerene amino acid–derivatized peptide occurred via passive diffusion and was enhanced with skin flexion.[333] Oil-water emulsion base products containing diclofenac sodium released nanoparticles capable of reaching human epidermis.[345] Neutral, anionic, or cationic coated commercially available QDs applied to porcine skin at workday exposure doses could attain the epidermis and dermis.[336] Solid lipid nanoparticles were capable of deep penetration in a perfused human skin flap model compared with conventional liposomes and deformable liposomes.[387] Silver nanoparticles cause focal, microscopic inflammation and edema and localize on the surface and in the upper stratum corneum layers when applied topically for 14 days in pigs.[342] Near-infrared QDs intradermally injected in pigs could be followed to sentinel lymph nodes 1 cm below the skin.[178] Intradermally injected CdSe core-CdS capped-PEG nanoparticles remained in the skin and drained via lymphatic ducts to regional lymph nodes and then accumulated in the liver, kidney, spleen, and hepatic lymph nodes.[131]

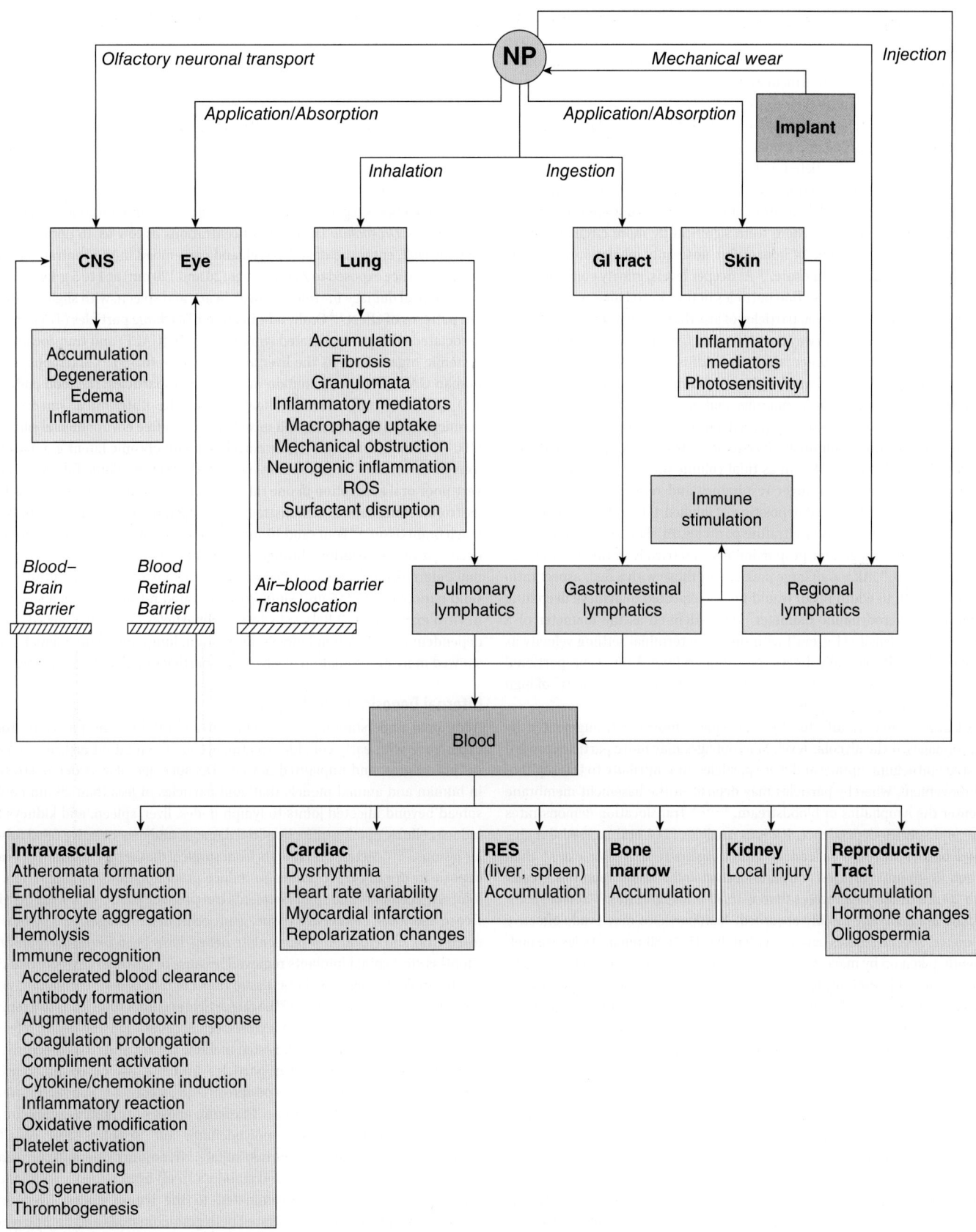

FIGURE 125-2. Potential mechanisms of nanoparticle exposure, distribution, and systemic toxicity. Accumulation may not be limited to the organ systems depicted. CNS, central nervous system; GI, gastrointestinal; NP, nanoparticle; RES, reticuloendothelial system. ROS, reactive oxygen species.

Inhalational Exposure

Nanoparticle aerosols may be generated in manufacturing or research environments. Anthropomorphic ultrafine products are encountered in welding, soldering, cooking fumes, and pollution. As the iron-to-carbon (soot) ratio increases in diesel combustion, the number and size of self-nucleated metallic nanoparticles and larger agglomeration of metallic and carbon particles increase.[197] Carbon fullerenes can be detected in flaming soot after combustion of various hydrocarbon fuels.[361] Combustion-derived nanoparticles carry soluble organic compounds, polycyclic aromatic hydrocarbons, and oxidized transition metals on their surfaces.[242] Secondary nanoparticles can form in the atmosphere via gas-to-particle conversions after nucleation and coagulation or condensation.[29] Intermediate particles (>80 nm and <200 nm) may remain suspended in air for days to weeks.[401]

Deposition of inhaled particles is determined by various factors, including diffusion and inertial impaction. In rat nasal passages, computational fluid dynamics models predicted that 3-nm particles deposited mostly in the anterior nose, and larger 30-nm particles distributed throughout the nasal passages.[116] However, nasal deposition of nanoparticles does not necessarily prevent systemic exposure. There were significantly more circulating iridium nanoparticles in blood 24 hours after nose-only inhalation compared with direct intratracheal exposure.[186] At deeper levels, gravity contributes to greater particle deposition of fine particles in the central airways instead of the lung periphery.[69] However, particles of less than 2,500 nm reach the alveoli, transported from the airway duct by convective bulk flow combined with particle motion from sedimentation and diffusion.[147] Alveolar deposition models indicate a saddle-shaped, volume- and rate-sensitive curve, a minimum particle deposition at 50 microns, and peak deposition at 30 nm and 4,000 nm.[59] Consistent with theory, total deposition fraction of ultrafine aerosols in healthy human volunteers *increased* by as median particle diameter *decreased* from 100 nm to 40 nm as tidal volume increased, and as respiratory flow rate decreased (longer respiratory and retention time).[160] Deep breathing similarly increased deposition of inhaled 100-cm^3 aerosol boluses of ^{99m}Tc–radiolabeled carbon ultrafine particles. In shallow breathing, particles deposit with a greater proportion asymmetrically in the left lung, for unclear reasons.[247] Although large particles or those with a high aspect ratio (ie, high length to width ratio) would not be expected to achieve deep lung penetration, "aerodynamic diameter" (D_{ae})—defined as the diameter of a sphere of unit density (1 g/cm^3) with the same terminal settling velocity as the particle itself—actually determines respirability.[86] As D_{ae} is proportional to the fiber diameter and not to its length, "paradoxical respirability" of high aspect ratio nanoparticles can occur.[86]

Clearance may be affected by mucociliary movement, augmented by macrophages at the alveolar level. Macrophages may move particles toward ciliated epithelium, uptake and store particles, or contribute to transepithelial movement, whereby particles may deposit in the basement membrane or enter the lymphatics or bloodstream.[184,224,278] Translocation demonstrates size- and species-dependence. Iridium particles (2–4 nm) crossed the air–blood barrier to reach secondary target organs to a greater extent than carbon (5–10 nm) particles, and translocation and accumulation was greater with 20-nm iridium aggregates than with 80-nm aggregates.[185] Soluble compounds are generally rapidly absorbed. Nanoparticles may evade effective clearance. Several studies have indicated that 15- to 80-nm particles are inefficiently taken up by macrophages (~20%) but are retained in epithelial cells or interstitium.[278] Prolonged particle pulmonary persistence was seen in one human ultrafine particle inhalation study, accounting for translocation and urinary elimination.[252] In an animal study, at 60 days, 81% of multiwalled carbon nanotubes (MWCNTs) and 36% of ground CNTs administered intratracheally (0.5 mg/rat) could be recovered.[254] In contrast to small particles that transit the visceral pleura, reach the pleural space, and drain into the lymphatic system through chest wall pores (3–8 μm), long nanotubes may travel and embed in the subpleural wall and within subpleural macrophages.[85,335]

Oral Exposure

Multiple nanoparticulate systems are under evaluation for their ability to enhance solubility, permeability, bioadhesion, bioavailability, and efficacy of poorly absorbed drugs, proteins, and vaccines.[75,304,442] Aerosol deposition in the upper aerodigestive tract could provide matter for subsequent swallowing. Indeed, after pulmonary exposure of rats to CeO$_2$, fecal recovery was the highest (71%–90%).[310] Nanoparticles can enter bacteria and living cells, providing a mechanism for food-chain bioaccumulation.[26] Mucus appears to be effective in trapping larger nanoparticles.[310] Nanoparticles can cross either paracellularly (between cells) or transcellularly. Transcellular uptake is thought

primarily to occur at associated lymphoid tissue but may also occur at villi. In general, nanoparticle uptake is enhanced by smaller size and absence of charge.[55,146] Hydrophobicity studies show mixed results (depending on altered permeation through various layers).[176] Similar to skin, inflamed or infected intestinal mucosa can increase permeability and alter experimental results.[193] Nanoparticles can also change intestinal permeability as a result of damage to the integrity of the intestinal barrier.[310] Experimental models have demonstrated that nanoparticles can target (potentially selectively) the gut microbiota and the microbiome, for both beneficial (anti-pathogenic) as well as adverse effects (eg, colitis).[311] Single-walled carbon nanotubes (SWCNTs) ingested by *Drosophila* larvae at concentrations as low as 16 ppm traverse the gut wall, enter the dorsal vessel, and can embed in the central nervous system.[202] Mice exposed to ZnO powder (20 and 120 nm) at 1 to 5 g/kg showed pathological damage in stomach, liver, heart, and spleen, with slightly different patterns of effect.[418] Orally administered TiO$_2$ large particles (475 nm) are associated with gut-associated lymphoid tissue (GALT) and translocated to systemic organs such as the liver and the spleen (6.5%).[159] Macrophages in human GALT frequently contain multiple microparticles: the food additive TiO$_2$ (100–200 nm), aluminosilicates (kaolinite illite, mica, smectite or vermiculite) (<100–400 nm), and mixed aluminum-free environmental silicates (100–700 nm in length).[316] These correlated with chronic latent granulomatous inflammation in susceptible individuals. Water-soluble fullerenes had very poor oral absorption in one rat study. Trace amounts that did cross the gastrointestinal barrier demonstrated prolonged retention and the ability to reach brain tissue.[439] Four- and 10-nm diameter colloidal gold particle uptake occurred by persorption through single enterocytes at villi in the proximal ileum, distal ileum, and Peyer's patch regions of the small intestine.[146] Gold nanoparticles (15 nm) similarly penetrated rat intestine in a separate in vitro experiment.[368] Rats fed silver nanoparticles (~60 nm) showed dose-dependent accumulation kidneys, liver, brain, lungs, and blood; female rats showed more accumulation of silver nanoparticles in all kidney regions.[179]

Internal Deposition and Degradation

Additional understanding of human–particle interactions proceeds from experience with early colloidal treatments for rheumatoid arthritis, surgical procedures, and implanted devices. Decades ago, it was demonstrated in human and animal models that gold particles of less than 20 nm could spread beyond injected joints to lymph nodes, liver, spleen, and kidneys to induce cellular uptake, mitochondrial damage, and degenerative renal tubular lesions.[372,446] Metallic fragments from surgical diathermy instruments can deposit in urinary tract tissues to induce granulomatous inflammation.[144] Joint replacements and spinal implants can produce particulate wear debris. Dense and loose connective tissue, giant cells, macrophages, and phagocytosed iron and chromium particulate debris have been found surrounding stainless steel spinal implants removed because of late operative site pain.[352] In hip implants, periprosthetic tissue may contain cobalt, chromium, and bone cement wear particles.[42,130] Local particle accumulation leads to a repetitive cycle of macrophage phagocytosis, cell degeneration and death; release of intracellular enzymes and ingested metallic debris; and tissue necrosis.[341] Polyethylene micro-sized wear particles promote osteoclast differentiation, which could contribute to periprosthetic osteolysis.[41] Submicron wear particles (including polyethylene; titanium, alloys of titanium–aluminum–vanadium, cobalt–chromium–molybdenum, and stainless-steel cobalt–chromium–nickel–tungsten; barium sulfate; zirconium oxide; and corrosion products of cobalt-chromium and stainless steel) from patients with failed orthopedic replacements disseminated to the lymph nodes, liver, and spleen.[411] Lymph nodes demonstrated both granulomatous and fibrotic reactions and particle-laden macrophages; elevated serum metal concentrations and granulomatous lesions in the liver and spleen were occasionally found. Rare, severe deterioration can produce massive metallosis and systemic metal toxicity.[283] Metal-on-metal hip resurfacing arthroplasty, large head total hip replacement, and non–metal-on-metal dual modular neck total hip replacement create distinct wear and macrophage, lymphocyte, and eosinophil recruitment patterns, with higher blood levels of Co and Cr ions in the metal-on-metal groups caused by generation of a higher total metallic particles burden.[438]

Circulation, Retention, and Elimination

As indicated in the previous sections, circulatory access may occur through intravenous (IV) administration of nanoparticle pharmaceuticals, upper respiratory and pulmonary translocation, intestinal absorption, dermal penetration, or draining lymphatics (Fig. 125–2). In human volunteers, inhaled ^{99m}Tc-labeled ultrafine carbon particles (<100 nm) reached the blood within 1 minute, peaked between 10 and 20 minutes, and persisted for up to 60 minutes.[270] Both hepatic accumulation and urinary excretion occurred. Gold nanomers (30 nm) can be recovered rapidly in blood platelets of the alveolar capillaries after rat intratracheal injection.[20] Aerosolized gold nanoparticles accumulated in more than 20 rat organs and tissues, particularly the lungs, esophagus, kidneys, aorta, spleen, and heart.[451]

Tight junctions (<2 nm) between endothelial cells preclude most nanoparticle exit from systemic circulation. However, organ-specific endothelial characteristics (hepatic fenestrations and splenic discontinuity), transcytosis, or leak-inducing disease conditions (inflammation and cancer) may allow exit of large particles. Reticuloendothelial system (RES) and renal clearance are particle and coating specific.[182,203] Shielding nanoparticles with neutral compounds or those providing steric repulsion or hindrance is thought to impair opsonization with subsequent RES clearance.[289] Neutral charge may also improve renal elimination of certain dendrimers.[2] Size differences of as little as 2 micrometers may shift elimination from renal to hepatic.[180] Prolonged circulation or tumor-retention times are often the goals of nano-based pharmaceuticals, and a large variety of modifications and delivery systems have been described.

DETECTION AND DOSE QUANTIFICATION

Previous sampling of generated aerosols generally focused on the average chemical composition and the mass of all deposited particles, with the exception of asbestos, for which the number of fibers with a specific shape and composition is important.[237] Production of engineered nanoparticles frequently results in a distribution of sizes. Dose assessment is complicated by the multiple differences among nanoparticles and ongoing investigation as to the most appropriate metric to measure: bulk amount (total particulate mass), particle burden (number of particles of a certain size), size distribution, total surface area, surface functional groups, delivered or deposited dose (per cell or other biological unit), internalized dose, or an alternative metric. Measurement approaches include various devices to assess particle mass directly (filter collection with analysis, size-selective static sampling, tapered element oscillating microbalance) or indirectly (via various impactor technologies), direct number assessments (via electron microscopy, optical or condensation particle counters, differential mobility analyzing systems, and scanning mobility particle sizers), and surface area.[101,120,217,237,264,265] The chosen method is critical because mass concentration measurements can demonstrate significant variation compared with particle number counts in industrial settings.[101,309]

TOXICITY

Overview

Certain organisms intentionally synthesize nanoparticles (eg, selenium-respiring bacteria, magnetotactic bacteria, gold nanoparticles in alfalfa).[117,198,285] The diverse nature of the substances, compositions, structures, and physical properties involved in nanotechnology limits generalization regarding possible human effects. Multiple reviews have attempted to address the diverse issues surrounding nanoparticle toxicity, and various schemes have been proposed to categorize nanoparticles.[10,94,137,217,224,277,295,363] One older review reported 428 studies documenting adverse effects of 965 unique nanoparticles.[137] Reviews of a single "class" of nanoparticles have documented both adverse and neutral effects. Inference of systemic biological effects in humans is hindered by the in vitro nature of many experiments. Differences in experimental methodology, cell line, substance concentration, particle size and

geometry, exposure parameters (route, duration, and frequency), duration of observation, and endpoints or surrogate markers have hindered comparisons. Long-term effects data are lacking. Cell-line specific, organ-specific, and species-specific toxicities remain to be fully characterized.

To address these deficiencies, methodologies are being developed to assess nanotechnology risk in a systematic fashion. Classifying nanoparticles based on the results of multidose-range biological assay profiles (adenosine triphosphate content, reducing equivalents, caspase-mediated apoptosis, and mitochondrial membrane potential) in multiple cell lines has been advocated.[360] Other techniques to evaluate toxicity and biological reactivity of nanoparticles have been reviewed and include cellular proliferation, necrosis, and apoptosis assays; reactive oxygen species (ROS) generation and oxidative stress; activation of proinflammatory signaling or other messenger molecules; genotoxicity and gene expression analysis; and in vivo exposure route, short- and long-term effect, tissue localization, biodistribution, and clearance studies.[233,366,374] Studies and models of quantitative structure-activity relationships may take on more importance to profile toxicity as the number of compounds proliferates.[323,428]

Despite the many unknowns, antecedent work within the discipline of particle toxicology has provided extensive epidemiologic and experimental evidence associating airborne pollution particulate matter (PM) with human mortality; cardiovascular, pulmonary, neurologic, and reproductive injury; altered neurocardiac function (decrease heart rate variability and repolarization); and malignancy.[38,77,83,174,300,307,334,412,452] The strength of the association depends on the particle size, type, and the outcome of interest. Similarly, ultrafine particles in home-generated cooking fumes have received attention for their possible role in pulmonary disease, inflammation, and genotoxicity.[244,366,367,415,433] Furthermore, the route of exposure may be disassociated from the primary organ of toxicity. For example, in rats exposed to airborne silver nanoparticles, the most sensitive target organ was the liver.[424]

Genetic or unique susceptibilities to nanoparticles are not well categorized. Preexisting acute or chronic disease (pulmonary disease, cardiac disease, malignancy, infection) or individual genetic variations (resistance to oxidative stress, immune composition, surface or serum proteins) may modify nanoparticle toxicity. For example, after identical ultrafine particle aerosol exposure, patients with chronic obstructive pulmonary disease (COPD) received an increased "dose" (deposition factor, rate, or both) compared with normal participants.[40] Retention of ultrafine particles was similarly higher in patients with COPD than healthy nonsmokers.[252] Patients with preexisting cardiovascular disease or older age show increased susceptibility to concentrated ambient air pollution particles.[77]

Although the following sections generally report "positive" studies to highlight nanotoxicity principles, it is important to acknowledge that many other studies have also produced negative results, and some have challenged the concept of "nano-specific" toxicity.[86] Toxicities identified experimentally must be coupled with an understanding of physicochemical properties (which impact organism and environmental transport) and exposure assessments to appropriately characterize risks.

Specific Factors Affecting Toxicity

Dose

Depending on the nanosubstance, "dose" (particle number or bulk amount) may or may not play a role. Appropriate dose–response curves (linear, supralinear, biphasic, or threshold) for different toxic effects have not yet been described for most particles.[278] For example, anti-*HER2* antibody-tagged silica-gold nanoshells showed no inherent in vitro toxicity to breast adenocarcinoma cells over a range of concentrations and exposure durations.[214] CdSe/ZnS QDs encapsulated in phospholipid block–copolymer micelles injected into *Xenopus* blastospheres were "nontoxic" until doses of 5×10^9 nanocrystals per cell produced "abnormalities."[88] CdSe/ZnS QDs at higher doses (20 nM/L) increased apoptotic cell death and cytokine release.[257] The principal toxicity mechanism changed from intracellular oxidative stress to cadmium ion release as QD concentration increased in another study.[205] Dose-dependent cytotoxicity was seen in human keratinocytes as

SWCNT concentration increased from 0.11 to 10 mcg/mL.[230] Dose- and time-dependent effects were apparent in human peripheral blood lymphocytes exposed to oxidized or pristine MWCNTs.[31] Nano-SiO$_2$ caused cytotoxicity and induced the apoptotic pathway in dose- and time-dependent manners.[447] In zebrafish embryos, silver nanoparticles induced dose-dependent embryotoxicity and multiple developmental abnormalities.[201] Silver nanowires show dose-dependent cytotoxicity from 1.9 mcg/mL to 1,900 mcg/mL in human laryngeal epithelial and cervical carcinoma cells.[1] Carbon black and fullerene (C$_{60}$) manufactured nanoparticles were genotoxic in vitro and in vivo in a dose-dependent manner.[395]

Size and Surface Area

Despite a comparable exposure on a mass-for-mass basis, nanoparticle toxicity may diverge significantly from bulk material. This may occur caused by several factors, including increased surface area, chemical reactivity, or ionization; altered absorption profiles; altered cellular interactions; or access to "protected" intracellular spaces. Cobalt-ferrite particles (6 nm) were more cytotoxic and genotoxic than 10-µm or 120-µm particles.[63] Cytotoxicity of amorphous silica particles increased 33-fold as particle size decreased from 104 nm to 14 nm.[263] Elemental carbon particles (5–10 nm) induced significantly more inflammatory mediators than larger carbon black particles (14 or 51 nm).[17] CoCr nanoparticles generate more superoxide and hydroxyl free radicals and more DNA damage than CoCr microparticles, possibly because of faster dissolving or corrosion within the cell.[293] TiO$_2$ nanotubes (diameter, 15–30 nm) permitted the best cellular adhesion, migration, viability, and differentiation compared with larger 50-nm nanotubes.[298] CdTe QDs of approximately 2 nm, 4 nm, and 6 nm had over a sixfold difference in inhibition of human hepatoma cell growth.[455] CdTe QDs (2.1 nm) can rapidly enter the nucleus of human macrophages, and gold nanoparticles (1 nm) can penetrate cell and nuclear membranes.[259,398] CdTe QDs (2.2 nm) were more cytotoxic than equally charged, larger QDs (5.2 nm).[218] Nano-tungsten carbide-metallic cobalt particles (~80 nm) generated more hydroxyl radicals induced greater oxidative stress and caused faster cell growth/proliferation than fine (4-µm) particles.[79] The toxicity of silver nanoparticles increased as size decreased from 100 nm to 10 nm via multiple mechanisms—cytoplasmic uptake, apoptotic markers, proautophagic proteins, and inflammasome activation all increased.[243] Gold nanoparticles of 1.5 nm were particularly cytotoxic and eliminated stem cell differentiation compared with those that were 4 nm and 14 nm.[353]

Composition

Toxicity may be primarily related to that of the bulk material. Elemental carbon particles (90 nm) were found to be significantly more toxic than diesel exhaust particles of comparable size (120 nm).[360] Redox-active transition metals may pose a particular hazard.[86] Gold, chrysotile asbestos, Al$_2$O$_3$, Fe$_2$O$_3$, ZrO$_2$, and TiO$_2$ nanoparticles differed in cytotoxicity in murine lung macrophage cells.[370] Quantum dot core materials (cadmium, lead, selenium) can be toxic at relatively low concentrations to the plasma membrane, mitochondrion, and nucleus.[58,139,219] Degradation of coated nanoparticles in the acidic and oxidative conditions of endosomes and lysosomes may result in exposure to inherently toxic core materials or ions. Derivitization or degradation may mitigate or exacerbate toxicity. Functionalization with quaternary amines prevented silica mesoporous nanomaterial-induced cellular injury.[383] Conversely, compared with "pristine" SWCNTs, acid-functionalized SWCNTs blocked cell cycling of murine lung epithelium cells and produced a more pronounce inflammatory response in mouse lungs in vivo.[346] Similarly, oxidized MWCNT were significantly more toxic to human T cells than their "pristine" counterparts or carbon black.[31] Decay of certain water-soluble fullerenes produces daughter compounds with increased toxicity in vivo.[21]

Contaminants

Contaminants may introduce or mitigate toxicity. "Doping" intentionally introduces impurities to modify the behavior of materials (eg, electrical properties of semiconductors). Similarly, doping can change the electronic, optical, and magnetic properties of nanocrystals.[275] Nitrogen doping of

MWNTs improved biocompatibility and reduced lethality in mice exposed via multiple routes routes.[47] Nitrogen-doped MWCNTs also proved more biocompatible in *Entamoeba histolytica*.[93]

The manufacturing process may unintentionally instill contamination—atomic or molecular impurities in the nanomaterial structure itself, residual reagents or catalysts, or manufacturing byproducts. Even "purified" SWNT retain significant percentages of cobalt, mobolybdenum, iron, nickel, yttrium, and zinc.[192,229] Consequentially, nonpurified, iron-rich SWCNTs (26 wt.% of iron) generated hydroxyl radicals and lipid hydroperoxides and depleted glutathione more than "purified" SWCNTs (0.23 wt.% of iron).[165] Purified fullerenes generate significantly less biological oxidative damage and adverse mitochondrial effects than unrefined fullerenes.[18,322] Residual contaminants and impurities of substances used in surface modification of QDs are cytotoxic and genotoxic in vitro.[150] Washing off unbound cetyltrimethylammonium bromide eliminated near total lethality of gold nanoparticles modified with this compound.[65] Single-walled carbon nanohorns, prepared from pure graphite without a metal catalyst, showed no skin irritation, eye irritation, or perioral toxicity.[246] Endotoxin contamination during manufacturing and handling is particularly problematic. Endotoxin contamination may lead to misattribution or mischaracterization of particular nanoparticle's toxicologic or immunologic profile.[82] Conversely, nanoparticles may exacerbate endotoxin-mediated toxicities.[82]

Coating and Surfactant Materials

Coating materials may shield toxicity of core compounds or alternatively possess inherent toxicity. They can mediate biocompatibility, duration of circulation, and organ- or cell-specific uptake. For example, various densities of electrostatic poly(glutamic acid)-based peptide coatings altered delivery of cationic polymer-plasmid DNA nanoparticles to the liver, spleen, and bone marrow.[140] Quantum dots coated with carboxylic acids, amines, or polyethylene glycol (PEG) increased uptake by human epidermal keratinocytes in that order, with carboxylic acid coated with QDs demonstrating cytotoxicity 24 hours earlier.[337] Nanoparticle cores of 2-diethylamino ethyl methacrylate polymerized with poly(ethylene glycol) dimethacrylate were significantly more toxic to dendritic cells than cores surrounded by a 2-aminoethyl methacrylate shell.[153] Upon inhalation, SiO$_2$-coated rutile TiO$_2$ nanoparticles but not uncoated rutile or anatase or nanosized SiO$_2$ induced pulmonary neutrophilia and inflammatory markers.[332]

Conversely, covalent materials may reduce toxicity. Dextran coatings decrease iron oxide nanoparticle toxicity (while also mediating superparamagnetic behavior).[359] Carboxylic acid grafting of cobalt-ferrite nanoparticles reduced toxicity by reducing leaching of Co^{2+} into solution.[63] Gelatin coating reduced (but did not eliminate) cytotoxicity of CdTe QDs in human acute monocytic leukemia cells.[43] Polyethylene glycol substituted CdSe core/CdS shell QDs were less cytotoxic extracellularly than "bare" QDs.[50] However, some benign coatings can be rendered cytotoxic by air exposure or photodecomposition.[74]

Nanoparticles tend to aggregate due to attractive forces (Van der Waals), and become progressively difficult to re-disperse as size decreases.[317] Single-walled carbon nanotubes agglomerations induced significantly more adverse effects than identical, well-dispersed SWCNTs.[426] Because CNTs are intensely hydrophobic, solvents or surfactant materials are used to disperse them and avoid clumping, although these materials themselves may be cytotoxic.[426] Exposure to protein-rich biological fluids may change the tendency to agglomerate and therefore produce size-dependent effects. Using surfactants to disperse nanoparticles (eg, SWCNTs) can decrease protein adherence and therefore alter biological effect or fate.[90,122]

Geometry and Architecture

Nanoparticle geometry may modulate toxicity and biological interactions. Previous observations suggested that toxicity might vary with the type of crystalline structure of a given material. For example, asbestos particle shape affects genotoxicity, and inflammatory and mutagenic properties vary by silica type (crystalline or amorphous).[348] Identical concentrations various aluminosilicate zeolite crystals (erionite, mordenite, and synthetic zeolite Y) of 0.1 to 10 micron size produced variant cytotoxicity and hydroxyl radical generation in rat lung macrophages.[102] Material surface defects are important for ROS generation: amorphous TiO_2 crystals were found to generate significantly more ROS than anatase, mixed anatase and rutile, or rutile crystals.[161] In a separate analysis, nano-TiO_2 (anatase) generates more biological oxidative damage than nano-TiO_2 (rutile),[18] and generally anatase nano-TiO_2 is more photocatalytic than the rutile form.[405]

The findings of more significant toxicity from anatase nano-TiO_2 were reproduced in human mesothelial cells. Compared with rutile forms, anatase forms were actively absorbed into cells and generated ROS and oxidative DNA damage.[142]

A high aspect ratio is thought to contribute to nanoparticle pulmonary toxicity, including penetration of the alveolar wall and visceral pleural.[86,241] Single-walled carbon nanotubes produced pulmonary granulomata and inflammation, but nanoparticle carbon black did not.[18,229,365] "Long" (825 nm) CNTs, which were less easily enveloped by macrophages than their 220-nm counterparts, increased the degree of inflammatory response in rats.[344] Asbestos-like pathology was also seen for "long" MWCNT (nanometer diameter, 15+ μm length) in mice.[312] In mice, single-wall nanohorns showed significantly less toxicity than SWCNTs.[222] Nanofibers and graphene nanoplates with high aspect ratios but low aerodynamic diameter can persist to frustrate macrophage engulfment and contribute to toxicity.[349] However, gold nanorods had significantly less cellular uptake than comparable spherical structures.[56] This geometry dependence was reversed upon PEGylation.[228] Long silver nanowires did not show extensive biopersistence, in part because of their transformation to silver salts, although silver was found in subpleural connective tissue and in adjacent subpleural alveolar spaces and septa.[62]

Attachment by HepG2 cells to micelles with PEG copolymer films varied depending on whether PEG polymer was in a "brush" (anchored at one end) or "mushroom" (anchored at both ends) conformation.[153] Compared with control wafers of the same composition, Fe-Co-Ni nanowires hindered macrophage growth and development.[3] Dendritic clusters consisting of aggregated 60-nm nickel nanoparticles produced higher embryonic toxicity than spherical 30-, 60-, and 100-nm particles of the same material.[157]

Additionally, nanoparticles may adsorb varying layers of surrounding biological proteins or lipids, altering their effective size, shape, and density. Curvature and size of the nanoparticle may affect the extent of this "corona" and influence dynamic interactions with bound proteins such as albumin, apolipoprotein, fibrinogen, and complement, which may effect cell entry or receptor interactions.[221,347] Bioassociation may also change nanomaterial properties. Zinc oxide nanoparticles changed particle size, distribution, and charge in the cell culture media.[421] Single-walled carbon nanotubes adsorbed with serum proteins (primarily albumin) had an antiinflammatory effect, which was lost when surfactant-treated SWCNTs precluded adsorption.[90] The same authors found, in contrast, prevention of protein adsorption to amorphous silica particles reduced toxicity. Compared with traditional cell growth media, copper oxide and titanium dioxide nanoparticles in artificial interstitial fluid displayed increased agglomeration, particle deposition, and ROS, and cytotoxicity in human keratinocytes.[48] Conversely, human plasma protein coronas can reduce formation of reactive oxygen and nitrogen species,[61] and pulmonary surfactant mitigates toxicity of silver nanoparticles by reducing silver dissolution into cytotoxic silver ions.[378] Ingested nanoparticles may take on a biocorona derived from food products (eg, β-lactoglobulin–coated gold nanoparticles coingested with milk).[310]

Charge

Surface charge (zeta potential, ζP) may significantly alter the physical characteristics of nanoparticles, biological interactions, or effects. Neutral SWCNT aggregate in aqueous solution; introducing a strong negative charge induces dispersal.[346] Negatively charged nanoparticles permeated model pig skin, which excluded positively charged and neutral particles.[181] Increasing surface charge density alters protein absorption; a positive charge promotes electrostatic association with negatively charged serum proteins.[121,140] Charged nanoparticles are recognized as important inducers of complement

activation.[80] Strongly charged particles can also mediate direct membrane damage (hole formation) in the lipid bilayer.[148,149] Positively charged polystyrene nanospheres induced oxidative stress; those with neutral charge did not.[436] Toxic effects of strongly negatively charged acid-functionalized SWCNTs were abrogated by pretreatment with neutrality-inducing L-lysine.[346] Positive charge mediates actin-dependent amorphous silica nanoparticle movement along filopodia and microvilli like structures.[287] Mouse peritoneal macrophages and human hematopoietic monocytic cells show charge-dependent endocytosis—the higher the negative or positive surface charge of albumin particles, the greater the uptake.[331] An overlap of the conduction band energy (E_c) level of metal oxide nanoparticles with the cellular redox potential (-4.12 to -4.84 eV)—which signifies the permissibility of electron transfers in biological environments—correlated with induction of oxygen radicals, oxidative stress, and inflammation.[453] Also, within lysosomes, positively charged nanoparticles are capable of acting as "proton sponges," enhancing cytoplasmic delivery and inducing cell death signaling.[356] Metal nanoparticles in mixtures can also change each other's charge and therefore the associated corona content and composition and cellular uptake.[76]

pH

pH can affect toxicity by altering charge, solubility, protective or functional groups, bioavailability, and other mechanisms. As pH was dropped from above 6 to 2, the ζP of citrate-stabilized silver nanoparticles dropped from -50 to neutral and resulted in aggregate formation.[97] pH alters the ζP of both microemulsion (3–5 nm) and hydrothermal (8–10 nm) cerium oxide nanoparticles, which in turn alters protein adsorption and cellular uptake.[299] The significant toxicological difference in mice between 23.5-nm and 17-μm copper particles was judged secondary to stomach retention, with persistent depletion of H^+ ions leading to systemic metabolic alkalosis and generation of ionic copper.[240] CdSe core QDs exposed to low-pH simulated gastric fluid decreased cell viability in vitro, possibly caused by degradation of the ZnS shell and increased solubility of cadmium from shell-free particles.[419] Acidic intracellular organelle localization raises degradation and damage concerns; the inflammatory potential of 15 metal/metal oxide nanoparticle correlated with acidic conditions, hypothesized to be related to elimination of the corona in lysosomes to expose a charged surface.[57] Targeted drug delivery employs intentional engineering of pH-responsive nanoparticles. In the acidic environment of the endosome or lysosome (~pH, 4.5), core-shell particles can swell by almost three times, disrupting these structures and allowing cytosolic entry.[153] Alternatively, at altered pH, certain functional groups can be cleaved, resulting in altered charge and improved QD delivery.[249]

Cellular Toxicity

At the cellular level, nanoparticle toxicity has been attributed to multiple mechanisms (Fig. 125–3). Oxidative stress, membrane and cytoskeleton structural alterations, cytoplasmic and nuclear protein interactions, energy failure, photoxicity, autophagy, and genotoxicity have all been described. Nanoparticles may stress cell types differently. This may be due to engineered properties (associated targeting molecules), properties of nanomaterials themselves (size-dependent reticuloendothelial system deposition), or biological processes of target cells (phagocytosis ability, resistance to oxidative stress, cytoskeletal architecture, cell division propensity). Tests in immortalized cell lines may not reflect in vivo findings because of inherent differences in genomic stability or specifically selected traits.

Uptake

Unintended cellular uptake may contribute to toxicity. Depending on the particle architecture, several mechanisms have been described, including phagocytosis or endocytosis (clathrin-mediated, scavenger receptor-mediated, mannose receptor-mediated, Fcγ receptor-mediated, complement receptor-mediated), potocytosis (caveolin dependent), (macro)pinocytosis, and direct cytoplasmic entry.[81,118,268,296,362,390,408] Various types of ammonium-, acetamido-, fluorescein isocyanate-, and methotrexate/fluorescein isocyanate-functionalized SWCNTs and MWCNTs were internalized by a wide

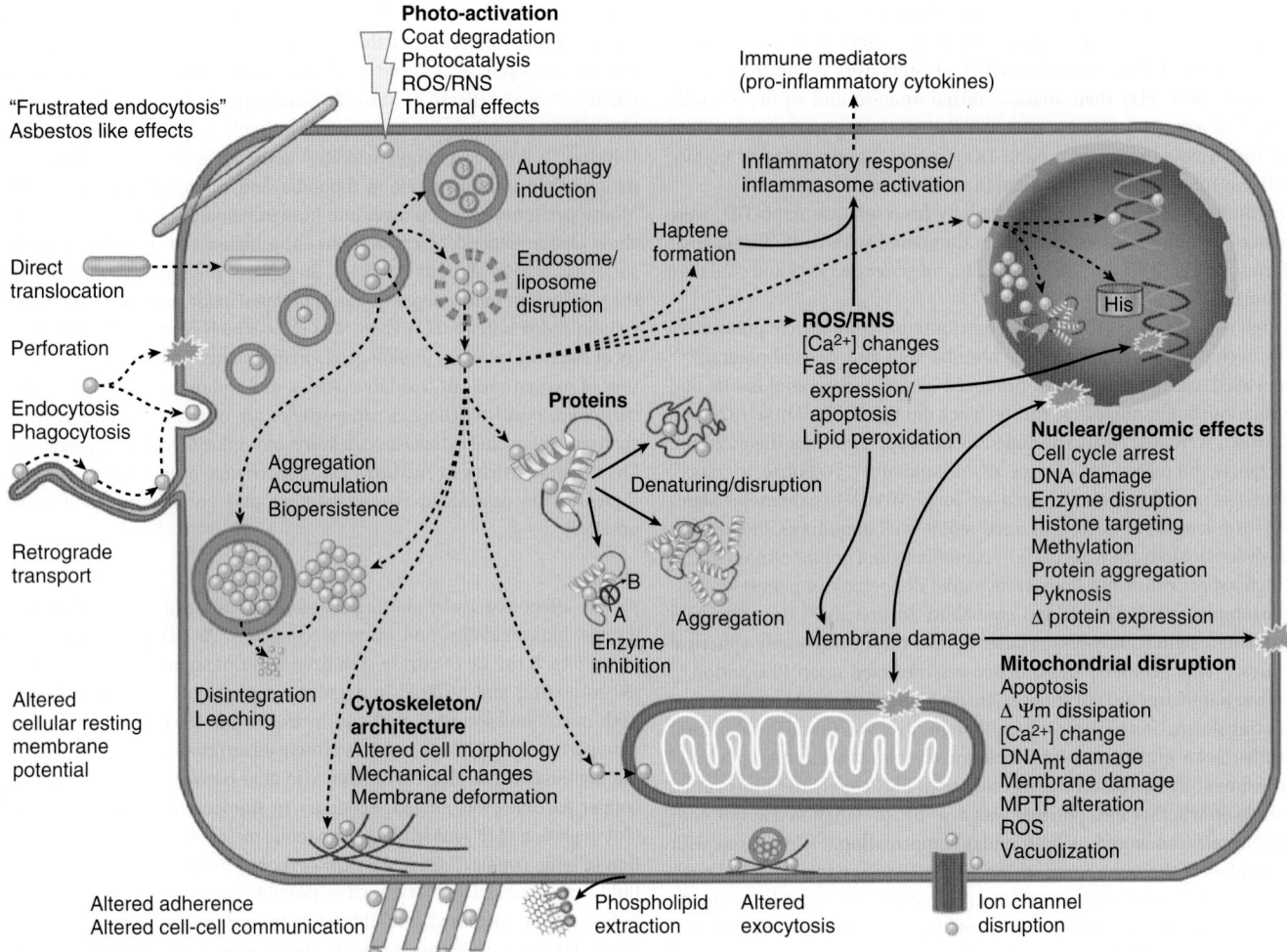

FIGURE 125–3. Potential mechanisms of nanoparticle cellular toxicity. ΔΨm, mitochondrial membrane potential, DNA$_{mt}$, mitochondrial DNA; His, histone; MPTP, mitochondrial permeability transition pore; RNS, reactive nitrogen species; ROS, reactive oxygen species. Additional mechanisms of toxicity may be induced by nanoparticle contaminants.

range of cell lineages (mammalian, fungal, yeast, and bacterial), some of which lack phagocytic and endocytic capacity, and under conditions that block energy dependent pathways.[183] Dextran-coated superparamagnetic iron oxide (SPIO) nanoparticles are taken up by human monocyte-macrophages and concentrated into lysosomes in a nonsaturable manner.[256] Nonendocytic uptake (eg, 78-nm fluorescent polystyrene microspheres and 25-nm gold particles) provides nonmembrane-bound nanoparticles direct access to intracellular proteins, organelles, and DNA.[119]

Engineered nanoparticles, which are capable of endocytosis, would be expected to translocate to distant sites within the body.[94]

Oxidative Stress
Oxidative stress with subsequent lipid peroxidation, DNA damage, and apoptotic or necrotic pathway induction is a significant concern. Biological oxidative damage as assessed by the ferric reducing ability of human serum revealed a diverse capacity for oxidative potential among nanoparticles.[18] Nanoparticles may donate electrons directly to molecular oxygen to produce superoxide, participate in redox cycling and Fenton chemistry, and interact with light to alter electron pairs.[32] Metal oxide nanocompounds (eg, Co_3O_4, Cr_2O_3, Ni_2O_3, Mn_2O_3, and CoO) capable of electron transfers are effectively produce oxygen radicals and oxidative stress.[453] Research findings are complicated by differences in generation of ROS under abiotic conditions versus intracellularly.[436] Biological media may also alter ROS generation.[111] In neuroblastoma cells, CdTe QDs induced lipid peroxidation and Fas cell death receptor upregulation, which could be mitigated by capping QDs with *N*-acetylcysteine (NAC).[58] Adult zebrafish raised in solutions containing

silver nanoparticles demonstrated oxidative injury, apoptosis, and cellular stress response (eg, GSH and p53 induction).[60] Fullerenes have shown more conflicting results. Depending on experimental conditions and purity, they may either induce $O_2^{\cdot-}$ and $\cdot OH$ or possess antioxidant (and anti-eroxidation) activity.[123,440] Single-walled carbon nanotubes and tungsten carbide-cobalt nanoparticles generate ROS and activate pathways leading involved in cytotoxicity and neoplastic transformation.[79,230]

Organelle and Substructure Damage
Nanoparticles may compromise diverse subcellular components. Mitochondrial reduction capacity (eg, MTT assay) is one of the standard in vitro methods to assess nanoparticle toxicity. Nanoparticles' mitochondrial toxicity includes alterations in mitochondrial calcium levels, dissipation of the mitochondrial membrane potential, lipid membrane destruction, and localization within the mitochondria.[58,219,291,436] Small gold nanoparticles (3 nm) can access the voltage-dependent anion channel (porin) to cross the mitochondrial membrane.[338] Induction of the mitochondrial base excision repair pathway enzymes suggests that MWCNTs can induce mitochondrial DNA damage.[457] PAMAM dendrimers (45 nm) can downregulate mitochondrial DNA-encoded genes involved in the maintenance of mitochondrial membrane potential and caused the release of cytochrome C, triggering apoptosis.[200]

Quantum dots (2.1 nm) have been visualized to localize rapidly (<30 min) and preferentially in the nucleus of human macrophages, mediated by endosomal transport along microtubular tracks.[259] Co_3O_4 nanoparticles (45 nm) readily enter cells and their nucleus in vitro.[294] Single-walled carbon nanotubes can accumulate in the cell nucleus by crossing the lipid bilayer.[314] Genotoxic consequences of this migration are described later.

Nanoparticles may cause disruption and compromise integrity of biological membranes by such means as hole formation in the lipid bilayer.[148,149] Alteration in cellular adherence, migration, and actin cytoskeleton or microtubule function and structure have been described after exposure to SWCNTs, gold/citrate, TiO_2, SPIO nanoparticles, and others.[114,125,132,166,305] Calcium-mediated cytoskeletal function (as evidenced by cell stiffening) was altered by ultrafine carbon particles (12 nm, 90 nm) but not by diesel exhaust or urban dust particles.[251] Functional processes may be impaired in the absence of the loss of viability. SiO_2, TiO_2, Ag, and Au, alone or functionalized with either positive or negative side chains, altered exocitosis and decreased secretion of chemical messenger molecules.[216,235] Other protein functions may also be altered by nanoparticles. Copper nanoparticle clusters selectively induced unfolding and precipitation of hemoglobin A0 and E, but almost none occurred with hemoglobin A2.[25] Nanoparticulate anatase TiO_2 (5 nm) can directly bind lactate dehydrogenase and induce protein unfolding.[87] C_{60} fullerene noncompetitively inhibits glutathione peroxidase in a substrate-specific manner.[158] Although relatively high concentrations were required (250 μM), the C_{60} fullerene derivative dendrofullerene selectively inhibited P450 metabolism of progesterone.[109] Graphene nanosheets induce toxicity via numerous mechanisms, including deformation and breaking of peptide α-helix structures and DNA base pairs, direct cutting of cell membranes, and destructive lipid extraction onto the material surface.[456] Modification of protein structures by reactive nanoparticles might also serve as a mechanism for haptene formation and immunoreactivity.

Separately, cadium QDs and other nanoparticles have been found to induce cell death by autophagy (formation and accumulation of QD-containing autophagosomes, followed by lysosome fusion, and degradation of autophagosomes by lysosomes), as opposed to apoptosis.[104] Similarly, carbon nanotubes upregulate autophagy-related genes and autophagosome vacuoles.[399]

Gene Expression and Genotoxicity

Overwhelming nanoparticle toxicity can induce a cascade of expression of genes involved in apoptotic, autophagocytic, or necrotic pathways. Nanoparticles can also upregulate stress- and inflammation-related genes as well as alter expression of genes involved in the cytoskeleton, trafficking, protein degradation, metabolism, growth and division, and detoxification. As a consequence of direct nuclear entry, nanoparticles can aggregate within the nucleus, bind directly to DNA or chaperone proteins, or induce nuclear membrane damage. Gold clusters (1.4 nm) present in growth media can access and directly associate with the major grooves of DNA to induce complete cell death in multiple carcinoma cell lines at concentrations at which cisplatin is only 10% effective[291,398,429] Gold nanoparticles can also alter DNA methylation and hydroxymethylation, leading to cell death and failure of stem cell differentiation.[353] As described earlier, graphene nanosheets can deformation and break DNA base pairs.[456] Nanosilver materials similarly bind with *Escherichia coli* genomic DNA.[445] Some QDs can target histones.[259] Other nanoparticles (eg, SiO_2) can cause clustering of critical enzymes such as topoisomerase I and sequestration of nuclear proteins (histones, splicing factor SC35, nucleolar protein fibrillarin, promyelocytic leukemia body protein and p80 coilin), altering subnuclear architecture.[53] DNA damage also occurs through induction of ROS (compiled by Moller and colleagues[250]). These ROS can affect nuclear DNA mitochondrial DNA differently and can trigger the mitochondria-mediated intrinsic apoptotic pathway.[290,]

Nanoparticle damage may be addressed by base repair and other restorative mechanisms or may be so severe that DNA strand breaks, genome duplication or deletion, chromosomal instability, aneuploidy, malignant transformation, and proliferation occur in vitro and in vivo.[154,397,457] Poorly tumorigenic or benign cells can acquired aggressive metastatic capacity when exposed to TiO_2 nanoparticles.[284] Alternatively, premature senescence was recently described using a C_{60} carboxylated adduct. Such an ability could be protective as a tumor suppression mechanism or compromise organ systems function.[115]

Photothermal Toxicity

Nanoparticles containing photoreactive dyes or intrinsic photothermal properties are useful for imaging and attractive for targeted (chemo)therapy. The approved liposomal verteporfin (benzoporphyrin derivative monoacid ring A) generates $^1O_2$ after activation by low-intensity nonthermal laser light (689 nm). This is believed to induce cell death and prevent the loss of visual acuity in patients with subfoveal choroidal neovascularisation.[172] Similarly, dextran-iron oxide nanoparticles linked to a photosensitizer that generates singlet oxygen caused complete cell death when exposed to specific light wavelengths.[239] Nonmetal graphene QDs irradiated with blue light (470 nm) generated ROS, including singlet oxygen, and killed human glioma cells by causing oxidative stress mechanism.[232] $C_{60}(OH)_{22-26}$, a water-soluble C_{60} derivative under investigation as an antitumor, antibiotic, and drug delivery compound, was only mildly cytotoxic in the dark but was significantly phototoxic to human lens epithelial cells via both type I (free radical) and type II (singlet oxygen) mechanisms under visible light.[427] The concern is that ambient electromagnetic radiation could excite nontherapeutic nanoparticles to generate either ROS or thermal injury. Photolytic conditions have rendered coatings unstable, exposing toxic core metal components.[139] Irradiation of TiO_2, which can act as a photocatalyst, yields both oxidation and reduction reactions.[113] Gold/citrate nanoparticles (13 nm) were capable of easily crossing human dermal fibroblast membranes and absorbing UV radiation.[305] C_{60} fullerenes can generate ROS in the presence of visible light under physiological conditions.[441] The ROS extent depended on C_{60} aggregation and associated stabilizing molecules in the aqueous phase.[199] Phototherapy can be harnessed with other modalities for benefit. Laser phototherapy of gold nanostars coated with polyethylene glycol killed primary tumors (photothermal ablation) in mice, but also successfully led to the death of nontargeted distant tumors when anti-programmed death-ligand 1 immunotherapy was administered.[209]

Miscellaneous Effects

A host of miscellaneous cellular effects are still being characterized. Alterations in cellular resting membrane potential and ion channel functioning by metallic and carbon-based nanoparticles are a particular concern in neuronal tissue.[19,210] Silver nanoparticles caused conformational changes of neuronal voltage-activated sodium currents and produced a hyperpolarizing shift and delayed recovery from inactivation.[211] Quantum dots can provoke intracellular lipid droplet formation caused by accumulation of newly synthesized lipids and downregulation of the β-oxidation of fatty acids.[321] Superparamagnetic iron oxides can generate intracellular gas vesicles.[226] Several nanoparticles have demonstrated ability to stress the endoplasmic reticulum, leading to cell death.[46]

Organ Systems Toxicity

Central Nervous System

A significant concern is nanoparticles' ability to access "protected" spaces: the brain, the eye, and the reproductive tract. Targeted CNS g delivery and imaging using engineered nanoparticles via IV or noninvasive, intranasal ("nose-to-brain") administration shows diagnostic and therapeutic promise (eg, for dementia, Parkinson disease, and stroke).[106,171] However, unintended CNS access is worrisome, particularly because inhaled nanoparticles must first transit the upper respiratory tract. Translocation of insoluble iridium nanoparticles to brain was eightfold higher with nose only inhalation compared with intratracheal inhalation.[186]

Seventy-five years ago, the intranasal inoculation of small viral (nano) particles (the poliomyelitis virus, 25–30 nm) was shown to produce extensive polio invasion of the olfactory bulbs and lesions extending in a continuous series to the brain stem and beyond.[27,28,151,396] Other small viruses (vesicular stomatitis, herpes simplex, and rabies virus) also access retrograde transport from the olfactory bulb to reach deeper brain structures.[327] Anthropomorphic and engineered nanoparticles also may use this mechanism, with variable efficacy. Nanogold particles injected into rabbit olfactory areas demonstrated a direct connection between the olfactory bulb and the cerebrospinal fluid.[67]

Intranasal instillation of SiO2-nanoparticles in rats led to wide distribution, striatal deposition, and a reduction in dopamine activity.[432] In inhalation-exposed rats, ultrafine elemental ^{13}C particles translocated into axons of the olfactory nerve.[279] Rats exposed to aerosolized gold nanoparticles (20 nm) experienced particle distribution to the olfactory bulb and entorhinal cortex.[451] Rats exposed to poorly soluble manganese oxide ultrafine particles (30 nm) showed olfactory bulb uptake and CNS delivery to the striatum, frontal cortex, and cerebellum.[91] Other animal models demonstrated that cadmium, cobalt, manganese, mercury, nickel, and zinc reach the olfactory bulb when applied intranasally, and neuronal connections carry cobalt, manganese, and zinc into deeper brain structures.[37,143,306,394] Children and dogs exposed to pollution show prefrontal white matter hyperintense lesions, which are associated with significant cognitive deficits in children. Ultrafine PM deposition, vascular pathology, and neuroinflammation were evident in the dogs.[44] Chronic respiratory tract inflammation might further diminish nasal respiratory and olfactory barriers and contribute to brain inflammation.[308]

Circulating nanoparticles may reach the brain. The blood–brain barrier (BBB) might be infiltrated via low-density lipoprotein receptor–mediated transcytosis of nanoparticles with nonspecific apolipoprotein adherence, endocytic processes, paracellular aqueous diffusion, or transcellular lipophilic diffusion.[106,355] Intravenously administered water-soluble fullerene and intraabdominally injected nano-TiO$_2$ (5 nm, anatase) migrate to brain in experimental models.[106,439] Nanoparticle entry can produce CNS inflammatory changes, inflammatory gene expression, demyelination, oxidative stress, lipid peroxidation, and NO generation; change neurotransmitter concentrations; and alter mitochondrial energy production.[45,91,213,223,357,454] Cyclooxygenase-2, interleukin (IL)-1β, and CD14 upregulation in the olfactory bulb, frontal cortex, substantia nigrae, and vagus nerves and disruption of the BBB associated with PM deposition were reported in patients exposed to high chronic pollution levels.[45] Similarly, IV and intraperitoneal administration in rats of engineered silver, copper, and aluminum nanoparticles disrupted the ventral brain and proximal frontal cortex BBB to produce brain edema.[357]

Nanoparticles can contribute to secondary excitatory neurotoxicity. Intranasal delivery of carbon black (14 nm) increased olfactory bulb excitatory glutamate levels.[393] Similarly, nano-Ag increased spontaneous excitatory postsynaptic currents and network activity.[212] Given the number of CNS and systemic human amyloidoses, a concerning finding was that polymer nanoparticles, QDs, carbon nanotubes, and cerium nanoparticles all greatly enhanced the rate of β$_2$-microglobulin amyloid fibrillation by decreasing lag time for nucleation.[208] Chronic dietary exposure to TiO$_2$ nanoparticles in juvenile rainbow trout led to brain accumulation and 50% inhibition of Na$^+$,K$^+$-ATPase activity, which did not recover after removal from exposure.[325]

Pulmonary System

The lungs are expected to be the major portal of entry for anthropomorphic nanoparticles and engineered nanoparticles in manufacturing or research settings. Concerns include nanoparticle accumulation and persistent, acute, and chronic inflammation and surfactant disruption. In the bronchial airways, 24-hour retention depends on size fraction, which is negligible for particles greater than 6 μm but increases to 80% at 30 nm.[187] In vitro studies show a variety of effects depending on the particle and experimental model. Canine and human alveolar macrophages uptake of elemental carbon particles (5–10 nm) induced lipid mediators AA, PGE2, LTB4, and 8-isoprostane in a dose-dependent fashion.[17] Single-walled carbon nanotubes activated alveolar macrophages; SWCNTs and C$_{60}$ fullerenes disrupted plasma membranes; and SWCNT and MWCNTs effected antigen processing, presentation, and activation of T lymphocytes.[135] In rat alveolar type II and epithelial cells as well as in human bronchial epithelial cells, nanoparticulate carbon black particles (14 nm) induced dose-dependent proliferation via epidermal growth factor receptor (EGF-R) and β1-integrin membrane receptors, phosphoinositide 3-kinases, and the protein kinase B (Akt) signaling cascade.[409] Cerium oxide nanoparticles can be taken up by human fibroblasts.[207] However, 3-hour exposures to aerosols of this fuel additive, although increasing catalase activity and minimally decreasing glutathione,

did not alter cell viability, ATP content, tumor necrosis factor α (TNF-α) production, glutathione peroxidase activity, or superoxide dismutase activity in rat lung slices.[103] Combustion-derived nanoparticles of organic compounds (1–3 nm) were mutagenic in Ames tests.[354] Positive evidence for carcinogenicity of inhaled nanoparticles has been summarized.[330]

All types of carbon nanotubes and nanofibers are considered a respiratory hazard by the National Institute for Occupational Safety and Health (NIOSH).[266] Carbon nanotubes can produce a variety of adverse effects in animal models, including upper airway mechanical blockage, occlusive airway granulomatas, macrophage uptake and intermacrophage carbon bridges, abnormal macrophage mitoses, type I pulmonary epithelial cell damage, lymphocytic proliferation, multifocal granulomatas, aggregation in alveolar spaces and interstitium, increased inflammatory and oxidative stress biomarkers, fibrinogenic reactions, alveolar wall thickening, bronchiolar epithelial cell hypertrophy, and peribronchial inflammation.[164,192,229,254,266,364,420] At high doses, mice exposed to MWNTs orally, intraperitoneally, or via nasal installation showed essentially no tissue response, but intratracheal administration showed dose-dependent pulmonary tissue invasion, inflammation and granulomata formation, and death.[47] Mice aspirating 40 mcg of SWCNT and acid-functionalized SWCNTs had significantly higher bronchoalveolar lavage cell counts, polymorphonuclear leukocytes, and cytokines (IL-6, TNF-α, and MIP2).[346] Also of concern are MWCNT retention, persistent inflammation, and asbestos like effects suggested by in vitro and in vivo experiments.[312,335,370] A systematic review of 54 animal studies indicated that carbon nanotubes and nanofibers caused adverse pulmonary effects, including inflammation (44 of 54 studies), granulomas (27 of 54), and pulmonary fibrosis (25 of 54), which were similar to other fibrogenic materials such as silica, asbestos, and ultrafine carbon black.[266] Mice receiving both a known initiator chemical plus inhalation exposure to MWCNT were significantly more likely to develop tumors (90% incidence) and have more tumors than mice receiving the initiator chemical alone, suggesting that MWCNT can increase the risk of cancer in mice exposed to a known carcinogen.[266] Fibrosis and bronchioloalveolar hyperplasia (alveolar bronchiolization) can similarly be induced by inhaled CeO$_2$.[350]

Although rats exposed to C$_{60}$ fullerenes nanoparticles (55 nm) for 10 days did not have visible of microscopic pathological lesions, particle burden and BAL protein concentrations were elevated.[11] Intratracheally delivered single wall nanohorns generated no inflammatory response, although nanohorns accumulated and persisted.[246] Intratracheal instillation of ultrafine (<200 nm) particles from combusted coal induced a higher degree of neutrophil inflammation and cytokine levels than did the fine or coarse particles.[128] Rats intratracheally instilled with ultrafine carbon black or TiO$_2$ demonstrated neutrophil recruitment, type II epithelial cell damage, cytotoxicity, impaired macrophage phagocytic ability, and enhanced macrophage sensitivity to chemotactaxins.[328] A summary of nanosized TiO$_2$ particle effects concluded that the crystalline form of has the greatest impact on pulmonary responses, and particle surface area, alumina or amorphous silica coating, and shape have lesser influences on toxicity.[224] Nasal instillation resulted in neutrophil recruitment. Alveolar macrophages took up inhaled elemental silver nanoparticles, and deposition in the alveolar wall was noted.[380] Although particles were rapidly cleared from lungs, there was evidence of circulatory spread. Longer term studies showed significant silver lung persistence, chronic macrophage accumulation and alveolar inflammation, and systemic distribution.[377] The severe toxicity of air-generated polytetrafluoroethylene (PTFE fumes) can be reduced by aging, filtering and preexposure, suggesting nanoparticle upregulation of pulmonary inflammatory cytokines and antioxidants.[163]

Pulmonary surfactant provides low surface tension and can identify and bind targets for phagocytosis. Independent of cellular effects, in vitro lung models suggest that nanoparticle deposition may cause pulmonary surfactant dysfunction during the breathing cycle.[169] The collectins (phagocytosis enhancers), human surfactant protein-A and -D, bind double wall carbon nanotubes in a calcium-dependent manner.[340] Diesel exhaust PM can be solubilized and dispersed in the major component of pulmonary surfactant (dipalmitoyl phosphatidyl choline) and induce genotoxicity in multiple different assays in bacteria and mammals.[340,416]

Humans exposed to nanoparticle-containing welding fumes in a controlled manner immediately increased their IL-6 concentrations in exhaled breath, decreased leukotriene B4 concentrations in nasal lavage samples, and decreased neutrophils and serum IL-8 concentrations the following morning.[78] An early report of uncontrolled workplace exposure to polyacrylic ester nanoparticles and other materials causing retained intracellular nanoparticles, pulmonary inflammation, pulmonary fibrosis, and pleural foreign-body granulomata was criticized for lack of causality and differential diagnosis.[34,369] However, an experimental rat model of polyacrylate/nanosilica nanoparticle exposure reproduced the pulmonary fibrosis and granuloma and pleural and pericardial effusion seen in patients.[458] Also, increased inflammatory and fibrotic biomarkers (IL-1β, IL-6, TNF-α, inflammatory cytokines, and KL-6) were found in nasal lavage–induced sputum and blood serum specimens of workers exposed to MWCNTs.[105] A report of submesothelial deposition of carbon nanoparticles after toner exposure has been criticized for lack of plausibility and causality.[389,425] Nevertheless, officer workers increased nine of 11 biomarkers of lipid oxidation after daily visits to a manufacturing plant's nano-TiO$_2$ production area.[302] Furthermore, nano-TiO$_2$ production rkers demonstrated elevations in all 11 biomarkers of lipid oxidation— malondialdehyde, 4-hydroxy-trans-hexenal, 4-hydroxy-trans-nonenal, 8-isoProstaglandin F2α, and aldehydes C6-C12.[303] These finding complement evidence of DNA and protein oxidative damage in workers exposed to nano-sized iron oxide.[301] Compared with control participants, workers exposed to carbon nanotubes, nanoparticles of titanium dioxide, silicon dioxide, nanosilver, nanogold, nanoclay, nanoalumina and metal oxides demonstrated increased markers of pulmonary injury at the cellular (Clara cell protein 16) and organ system (lung function test) levels, as well as antioxidant and cardiovascular markers (superoxide dismutase, glutathione peroxidase, vascular cell adhesion molecule, and paraoxonase).[206]

Cardiovascular and Hematologic Systems

Ultrafine particles can alter human cardiac function (decreasing heart rate variability and repolarization).[77,138,392,413,452] Heart rate variability provides a measure of cardiac autonomic control; a decrease predicts death in patients with prior myocardial infarction.[392] Significant pulmonary inflammation is not a prerequisite, although autonomic reflexes from pulmonary nerve endings may mediate these effects.[124] Jugular vein or femoral artery administration of silver, copper, and aluminum nanoparticles immediately but transiently slows heart rate.[357] Engineered nanoparticles made of flame soot (Printex 90), spark discharge-generated soot, anatase TiO$_2$, and SiO$_2$ induced catecholamine-mediated dose dependent increases in heart rate and dysarrhythmia in Langendorff heart model systems.[371] Human wood smoke exposure increases levels of serum amyloid A (a cardiovascular risk factor) and factor VIII in plasma.[16] Inhaled TiO$_2$ nanoparticles impair rat coronary arteriole endothelium-dependent vasoreactivity and relaxation, likely caused by microvascular ROS.[196]

Intravascularly, nanoparticle characteristics and concentration determine leukocyte and immune stimulation (detailed in a later section), erythrocyte effects, thrombogenesis, endothelial dysfunction, and atherogenesis. Zinc oxide nanoparticles induced proinflammatory mediators, dyslipidemia, biomarkers of atherosclerogenesis, and aortic pathological damage in human coronary artery endothelial cell systems and in rats.[444]

Dendrimers can adversely alter human erythrocyte morphology, induce clustering, and provoke significant hemolysis.[84,89] Dendrimer generation, concentration, charge, exposure duration, and material type determine the extent to which this occurs. Intravenously provided diesel exhaust particles aggregate within erythrocytes, decreasing counts.[272] Polycationic (but not neutral or anionic) water-soluble fullerene C$_{60}$ derivatives, surfactant stabilized poly(lactic-co-glycolic acid) (PLGA) nanoparticles, and polystyrene nanoparticles all induce significant hemolysis.[30,176,236] The surface silanol groups of silica nanoparticles can induce significant erythrocyte deformation and hemolysis, as can titanium dioxide and silver.[12]

Chitosan–pDNA and uncoated polymer nanoparticles both induce significant hemoagglutination.[140,215]

Engineered and combustion-derived carbon nanoparticles (MWCNTs, SWCNTs, and mixed carbon nanoparticles) stimulated human platelet aggregation, activation of glycoprotein IIb/IIIa, and accelerated the rate of vascular thrombosis in rat carotid arteries.[324] The effect on platelet aggregation was aspirin-resistant but was reduced by low affinity (P2Y12) ADP receptor antagonism. Multiple metal nanoparticles (iron, copper, gold, cadmium sulfide) also induced dose-dependent platelet aggregation through the P2Y12 ADP receptor, an effect was blocked by clopidogrel.[71] Epidemiologic studies support an association between exposure to PM of less than 10 microns and increased risk of deep venous thrombosis.[9] Diesel exhaust particles (20–50 nm) and positively charged polystyrene nanoparticles cause rapid activation of circulating blood platelets and microcirculatory thrombi.[269,271] Healthy volunteers exposed to concentrated ambient air particles increase fibrinogen levels.[126]

Compared with larger particles, ultrafine particles produce larger atherosclerotic lesions, decrease the antiinflammatory effect of high-density lipoprotein, and induce oxidative stress in susceptible animal models.[6] At doses that produced no significant pulmonary inflammatory changes, rats exposed to nano-TiO$_2$ aerosols display systemic impaired endothelium-dependent arteriolar dilation, outright constriction, and decreases in NO bioavailability by increasing local reactive oxidative and nitrosative species.[276]

Immune System

Nanoparticle interaction with the immune system is complex: depending on biophysiochemical properties, nanoparticles can stimulate, silence, or elude immune responses.[459] Most concerning is induction of chronic inflammation. Work in murine macrophage cells lines demonstrated that MWCNTs produced a cytotoxic response nearly identical to asbestos.[370] Commercially and academically available MWCNTs induced asbestos like, length-dependent pathology in mice.[312,406] Multiwalled carbon nanotubes can reach the subpleura in mice after a single inhalation exposure to produce mononuclear cell aggregates and subpleural fibrosis.[335] On the other hand, immune suppression may also occur. Fullerene suppression of mast cell–mediated hypersensitivity reactions appears to proceed from endocytosis, endoplasmic reticulum accumulation, intracellular persistence, and inhibition of calcium and ROS generation.[73] Other nanoparticles, such as polyethylenimines, can induce chronic stress through inflammasome activation, which can promote tumor metastasis.[152]

Particle-specific interactions may yield cellular accumulation, antigen-mediated immune stimulation, inflammatory mediator release, or fibrous or granulomata formation. Mouse granulocyte-macrophage colony formation is now a standard testing methodology for assessing nanoparticle toxicity.[7] Macrophages exposed to Fe-Co-Ni nanowires in vitro increased production of interferon-γ, IL-1α, IL-4, and IL-10.[3] Ultrafine carbon caused macrophages to release[253] lipid mediators arachidonic acid, PGE2, LTB4, and 8-isoprostane.[17] Subcutaneously implanted "hat-stacked" carbon nanofibers in rats generated fibrous connective tissue formation and macrophage recruitment and ingestion without inflammatory response (necrosis, degeneration, or neutrophil infiltration).[449] Intratracheal exposure to nano-sized nickel and cobalt particles induced rat blood neutrophils to release ROS and reactive nitrogen species.[248]

Human volunteer exposures to concentrated ambient particles (<200 nm) increased inflammatory blood mediators.[129] Intravenous administration of ultrafine diesel exhaust particles promoted monocyte and granulocyte proliferation.[272] Other cell lines can also be induced to release inflammatory mediators. Single-walled carbon nanotubes induced human epidermal cells exposed to release IL-8. Multiwalled carbon nanotube introduced in human neonatal epidermal keratinocytes increased IL-8 and IL-1β release.[429]

Direct immune stimulation can also occur. Fullerenes can induce an IgG response capable of cross-reaction with other fullerenes.[33,51] The degree of induced opsonization by various IgG and complement molecules is thought to explain part of the differences seen in blood clearance and tissue distribution of nanoparticles.[289] Upon readministration, PEGylated liposomes have accelerated blood clearance caused by IgM binding; this is inhibited by chemotherapeutics that inhibit B-cell proliferation.[156] In the absence of direct immune stimulation, carbon nanotubes can boost immune response as adjuvants.[292] Indeed, pharmaceutical nanoparticles show promises for eliciting polyclonal and monoclonal antibodies to nonimmunogenic haptens as diverse as herbicides, antibiotics, and vitamins.[231] The flip side to this is that nanoparticles contaminated with hydrophobic metal, glass, and polystyrene particulates can stimulate protein aggregation and immunogenicity, as well as exacerbate production of proinflammatory cytokines induced by endotoxin, a separate common contaminant.[82]

Liposome- and polymer-based therapeutic nanomedicines have been compromised by non–IgE mediated hypersensitivity reactions because of complement system activation, which releases C3a and C5a anaphylatoxins.[5] The drug solubilizer Cremophor EL (polyethoxylated castor oil) forms micelles (8–25 nm) at concentrations above 60 mcg/mL and causes its occasionally severe immune reactions presumable caused by complement activation. Carbon nanotubes can activate human complement via both classical and alternative pathways; C1q binds directly to carbon nanotubes.[339] Surface density of coating materials can also alter complement consumption.[4] Certain dendrimers may also strongly activate the complement system.[226] MnFe$_2$O$_4$ magnetic nanoparticles (10-nm diameter) induce severe inflammatory reactions in mice.[191] The importance of characterizing immune cell subset responses is now recognized. Inhaled carbon nanotubes can induce myeloid-derived suppressor cell accumulation in mice, contributing to tumorogenesis.[82] Microcrystalline silica particles induced a strong Th1 response, and carbon black particles and polystyrene particles induced a mixed Th1:Th2 response.[414] PLGA-based nanoparticles did not induce complement consumption, indicating that this action is nanoparticle specific.[49]

Ocular System

The ocular system is of particular interest because of its immunologic privilege and physiologic characteristics. Therapeutically, nanosuspensions and other constructs show promise for extended release and decreased drug clearance from anterior and posterior ocular structures and diminished systemic drug exposure.[133,320] In vitro studies have shown adverse effects. Silver nanoparticle block the proliferation and migration and inhibit cell survival of bovine retinal endothelial cells.[167] Water-soluble fullerene derivatives are phototoxic to human lens epithelial cells under visible light.[427] Conversely, graphene oxide nanosheets, even when intravitreally injected in rabbits, did not demonstrate significant effects.[443] Conversely, in zebrafish, graphene oxide damaged mitochondria and primarily translocated to the eye, resulting in ocular malformations during embryogenesis.[54] Cerium oxide nanoparticles are reported to offer a protective effect, scavenging reactive oxygen intermediates in rat retina cell culture.[52] In vivo confocal neuroimaging conclusively demonstrated negatively charged nanoparticle-rhodamine formulations injected into rat jugular vein crossed the blood–retinal barrier within 40 minutes.[319] Intravenously administered gold nanoparticles (20 nm) can bypass the blood–retinal barrier to distribute in all retinal layers within 24 hours.[177]

Reproduction and Development

The reproductive effects of nanoparticles are incompletely characterized. One review concluded that nanoparticles can breach the blood–testis barrier and locate in the testes.[238] Subsequent studies using inhaled fluorescent magnetic nanoparticles (50 nm) and injected gold nanoparticles confirmed testicular distribution and persistence.[13,190] Chronic intratracheal administration of carbon black (14 and 56 nm) showed similar partial vacuolation of the seminiferous tubules and decreased daily sperm production.[450] Silver nanoparticles caused dose-dependent mitochondrial impairment and cytotoxicity in spermatogonia in vitro; aluminum nanoparticles caused apoptosis.[36] Gold nanoparticles can penetrate human sperm cells, resulting in fragmentation and dysmotility.[430] Environmental exposure to relevant concentrations of ZnO, TiO$_2$, SiO$_2$ nanoparticles produced reproductive toxicity

in nematodes, which was correlated with ROS production and attenuated with antioxidants (ascorbate and NAC).[434]

Female reproductive effects are less well described. Oral ZnO nanoparticles achieved lactation and placenta transport and resulted in increased postimplantation loss rate, decreased live births, and zinc accumulation in offspring liver and kidney.[162] In perfused human placenta models, PEGylated gold nanoparticles (10–30 nm) were retained mainly in the trophoblastic cell layer and internalized by trophoblastic cells and did not cross in detectable amounts into the fetal circulation over 6 hours of evaluation.[258] Other nanoparticles—particularly MWCNTs and SWCNTs and TiO$_2$-nanoparticles—can cross the placenta to create fetal oxidative stress and inflammation, alter neurodevelopment, alter behavior, and impair learning and memory in offspring in mice and rats.[95] Carbon-based nanomaterials are embryolethal to mice, chickens, and zebrafish, and certain structures such as nanodiamonds impair angiogenesis.[96] Zebrafish embryos exposed to nickel-silica nanomaterials either died or were left with severe malformations or compromised motor function.[227] *Daphnia magna* were unable to reproduce again after exposure during pregnancy to sublethal concentrations of water-stable fullerenes. Less than 10% of daughter daphnids matured after maternal exposure.[382] After exposure to of silver nanoparticles (0.1 or 0.5 mg/L for 3 days), nematode offspring decreased by 70%; oxidative stress was the presumed toxicologic mechanism.[329] In the animal model of organogenesis, medaka (rice fish) eggs easily took up 39.4-nm fluorescent particles and concentrated them in the yolk area and gallbladder during embryonic development.[170] Adults demonstrated diffuse uptake into reproductive organs as well as the brain, liver, intestine, gills, and kidney. Medaka fertilized eggs exposed to silver nanoparticles produced a variety of malformations, including systemic edema, hemostasis, and vertebral, finfold, optic, and cardiac abnormalities over the range of concentrations tested (100–1,000 mcg/L).[435] Altered hormone levels and offspring sex ratios seen in some experimental models of nanoparticle exposure suggest endocrine disruption.[220,261]

Bioaccumulation and Persistence

Nanoparticles can accumulate in certain cells, tissues, or organs to achieve threshold toxicities or leach at a time after the initial exposure. At the cellular level, nanocrystals can be passed to daughter cells upon mammalian cell division.[136,234] Retained fluorescing QDs have been used experimentally to trace *Xenopus* cells from embryo to tadpole stage.[88] Among different fine particles (fiberglass, rock wool, slag wool, asbestos), their biopersistent potential seems to underlie toxic effects.[145] This knowledge drives the concern regarding preliminary studies demonstrating MWCNT persistence, inflammatory induction, and asbestos like pathology.[253,312,335,379] Similarly, the pulmonary biopersistence of aluminum-based nanorods increased with high aspect ratios.[297] Compared with sodium selenite, nano-selenium particles displayed hepatic hyperaccumulation and persistence in fish models, with associated oxidative stress and toxicity.[204] Similarly, uptake, bioconcentration, and alimentary toxicity of TiO$_2$ nanoparticles were demonstrated in crustaceans.[68] Their transmission and bioaccumulation (by a factor of more than 100%% in certain species) up the food chain was also apparent.[448] Nano-crystalline C$_{60}$ had a greater propensity to accumulate in *Daphnia magna* fetuses because of their higher lipid fraction (including the egg sac yolk) and correlated with higher mortality.[382] Even short-term oral exposure may lead to reticuloendothelial accumulation in some animal models.[384]

Although desirable for chemotherapeutic applications, prolonged periods of persistence could allow leaching and toxicity of initially protected materials.[423] Bone marrow deposition of nanoparticles[315] could allow for ongoing systemic exposure. Persistence in other compartments could also permit more extensive distribution (eg, translocation from lung tissue). Dextran-coated ultrasmall SPIO particles currently used in clinical trials are retained by human monocyte-macrophages for days.[255,256] Quantum dots persisted at least 4 months in mice, and those conjugated to bovine serum albumin or coated with mercaptoundecanoic acid underwent negligible elimination in rats.[14,108] Because of intrinsic resistance to lysosomal degradation, inorganic or metal nanoparticles can have extremely low rates of excretion, resulting in long-term accumulation.[423]

ADMINISTRATIVE, REGULATORY, AND RESEARCH ISSUES

The 21st Century Nanotechnology Research and Development Act guides US nanotechnology policy.[410] Elements include federal interagency coordination, establishment of national strategic plans for nanotechnology, and triennial review by the National Research Council; establishment of a public database for funded EHS (environmental, health, and safety), educational and societal dimensions, and nanomanufacturing projects; fiscal support for a Nanotechnology Coordination Office; mandates for research in EHS; development of nomenclature and engineered nanoscale standard reference materials standards; development of standards for detection, measurement, monitoring, sampling, and testing of engineered nanoscale materials for EHS impacts; and nanotechnology education. The National Nanotechnology Initiative (NNI) includes 20 federal departments and agencies with administrative, funding, liaison, regulatory, and research and development roles, including the Department of Defense, National Science Foundation, Department of Education, National Institutes of Health, NIOSH, FDA, National Institute of Standards and Technology (NIST), Occupational Safety and Health Administration, Environmental Protection Agency (EPA), United States Department of Agriculture, and others.[64] In its congressionally mandated role to review federal nanotechnology research and development, the National Nanotechnology Advisory Panel provides ongoing recommendations for development of infrastructure, standards and metrics, and EHS risk analysis concurrent with applications research.[318] International regulatory frameworks continue to evolve.[281]

The detailed NNI strategy for EHS research recommends incorporation of many factors in conducting a nanotechnology risk assessment, including nanomaterials synthesis and use; nanomaterial lifecycle stages (from raw materials through disposal or recycling); transport, transformation, secondary contaminants, and abiotic effects; environmental concentrations; exposure of environmental and biologic systems; internal dose; biologic response; and systemic environmental effects.[64,375,405,406,407] Priority needs included the development of nanomaterial detection methods, certified reference materials, standardized physiochemical assessments, and measurement tools; understanding generalizable toxicologic characteristics of nanomaterials in biologic systems; predictive toxicological profiling; identification of environmental, occupational, and other population exposures and health surveillance; and evaluation of risk management approaches to nanomaterials.[64,375] The National Nanotechnology Coordinated Infrastructure (NNCI), which includes 16 sites, is the latest iteration of NSF supported network of US facilities, universities, and partner organizations for nanofabrication and characterization, education and outreach, and exploration of societal and ethical implications of nanotechnology.[282]

Standards

The NIST is the coordinating agency for instrumentation, metrology, and analytical methods in the United States. Given the broad cross-disciplinary impact of nanomaterials, international standards continue to evolve for nomenclature and terminology, measurements and metrics, reference nanoparticles, toxicity testing and risk assessment tools, and occupational guidelines. The European Centre for Ecotoxicology and Toxicology of Chemicals has proposed a *Decision-Making Framework for the Grouping and Testing of Nanomaterials* (DF4nanoGrouping), which includes three tiers (intrinsic material properties, system-dependent properties and in vitro effects, and in vivo screening) to assign nanomaterials to four main nanoparticles: soluble, biopersistent high aspect ratio, passive, and active nanomaterials.[194] Where available, selected national and international standards relating to these areas are provided in Table 125–2.

Food, Drug, and Device Safety

The FDA regulates food and color additives, drugs, biologics, devices, blood products, and cosmetics to ensure that they are "safe" and unadulterated. The FDA does not regulate "nanotechnology" *per se* and has forgone even adopting regulatory definitions of "nanotechnology," "nanomaterial," "nanoscale," and related terms.[134,403] Rather, marketing authorization occurs

on a product-by-product basis, with further variation for different product-classes. Although the FDA can require manufacturers to provide necessary information (eg, chemistry, manufacturing, active ingredients, pharmacologic and toxicologic results, and particle size) to support decisions regarding pre-market approval, in evaluating the sponsor "claims," the FDA may be unaware that nanotechnology is being used, particularly if no nano-related claims are supplied. In general, the FDA has treated nanomaterial ingredients no differently than bulk material ingredients or products. Guidance has been provided for nanotechnology and nanomaterials issues in industry, cosmetics, food substances, animal feed, and dietary supplements.[402-404] Several countries have excluded engineered nanoparticles from food labeled organic.[401]

Occupational Health and Safety

National Institute for Occupational Safety and Health leads federal agencies in conducting research and providing guidance on the occupational safety and health implications and applications of nanotechnology.[266] National Institute for Occupational Safety and Health has released multiple reports to guide commercial and research entities, including "Approaches to Safe Nanotechnology,"[264] "Building a Safety Program to Protect the Nanotechnology Workforce: A Guide for Small to Medium-Sized Enterprises,"[267] "Filling the Knowledge Gaps for Safe Nanotechnology in the Workplace,"[266] and "General Safe Practices for Working with Engineered Nanomaterials in Research Laboratories."[265] These publications and others identify potential health concerns (nanoparticle dose, deposition, reactivity, toxicity, translocation, and tumorgenicity) and safety issues (fire, explosion, oxidation, and catalytic potential). Recommendations included epidemiology, surveillance, and background nanoaerosol measurements and particle analysis; personnel exposure sampling and medical surveillance; engineering controls with verification and sufficient ventilation; spill response and emergency preparedness; implementation of risk management programs; and use of filters, respirators, and other proper personal protective equipment.[264,267] To address specific risks associated with carbon nanotubes and nanofibers, OSHA recommends that worker exposure not exceed 1.0 mcg/m³ elemental carbon as an 8-hour time-weighted average (TWA), based on the NIOSH-proposed occupational recommended exposure limit (REL).[280] OSHA recommends that worker exposure to TiO_2 nanoscale particles not exceed the NIOSH REL of 0.3 mg/m³, an order of magnitude less than the NIOSH REL of 2.4 mg/m³ for fine TiO_2 particles (>100 nm).[280] The REL for soluble silver compounds and silver metal dust is 0.01 mg/m³, an order of magnitude less than the threshold limit value for metallic silver (0.1 mg/m³) recommended by the American Conference of Governmental Industrial Hygienists (ACGIH). Values for metal fumes may be similarly lower than that for corresponding dusts (eg, a TWA for copper fumes of 0.1 mg/m³ versus 1 mg/m³ for copper dusts). The general federal statute limiting "particulates not otherwise regulated" (also known as "inert or nuisance dusts") to a respirable fraction of 15 millions of particles per cubic foot of air (5 mg/m³) would also apply include nanoparticles, although this is suggested to provide inadequate protection.[92,365] National Institute for Occupational Safety and Health anticipates that properly fit, NIOSH-certified respirators in conjunction with respiratory control programs will protect workers from most inhaled nanoparticles.[264,266] Other occupational professional guidance can be found in national and international guidelines and reviews.[262,286]

Environmental Protection

The EPA is the coordinating federal agency for human nanomaterials environmental research. Nanomaterial applications for environmental remediation and water purification are particularly attractive but require weighing against unintended consequences (eg, nanopollution).[401] Regulation of nanomaterials and the effects of nanotechnology may also come under the EPA's broad authorities under the Clean Air Act (CAA), Pollution Prevention Act (PPA), Clean Water Act (CWA), Safe Drinking Water Act (SDWA), Federal Insecticides and Rodenticides Act (FIFRA), Comprehensive Environmental Response Compensation and Liability Act (CERCLA), National Environmental Policy Act (NEPA), Resource Conservation and Recovery Act (RCRA),

TABLE 125–2	**Selected Nanotechnology Standards[a]**
Nomenclature and Terminology	
ASTM E2456-06(2012)	Standard Terminology Relating to Nanotechnology
ISO/TS 27687:2008	Nanotechnologies – Terminology and Definitions for Nano-Objects – Nanoparticle, Nanofibre and Nanoplate
ISO/TR 11360:2010	Nanotechnologies. Methodology for the classification and categorization of nanomaterials
ISO/TS 80004-1:2010	Nanotechnologies – Vocabulary – Part 1: Core Terms
ISO/TS 80004-2:2015	Nanotechnologies – Vocabulary – Part 2: Nano-objects
ISO/TS 80004-3:2010	Nanotechnologies – Vocabulary – Part 3: Carbon Nano-objects
ISO/TS 80004-4:2011	Nanotechnologies – Vocabulary – Part 4: Nanostructured materials
ISO/TS 80004-5:2011	Nanotechnologies – Vocabulary – Part 5: Nano/Bio Interface
ISO/TS 80004-7:2011	Nanotechnologies – Vocabulary – Part 7: Diagnostics and Therapeutics for Health Care
ISO/TS 80004-11:2017	Nanotechnologies – Vocabulary – Part 11: Nanolayer, Nanocoating, Nanofilm, and Related Terms
ISO/TS 80004-12:2016	Nanotechnologies – Vocabulary – Part 12: Quantum Phenomena in Nanotechnology
ISO/TS 18110:2015	Nanotechnologies – Vocabularies for Science, Technology and Innovation Indicators
Measurements and Metrics	
ASTM E2578-07(2012)	Standard Practice for Calculation of Mean Sizes/Diameters and Standard Deviations of Particle Size Distributions
ASTM E2490-09(2015)	Standard Guide for Measurement of Particle Size Distribution of Nanomaterials in Suspension by Photon Correlation Spectroscopy (PCS)
ASTM E2834-12	Standard Guide for Measurement of Particle Size Distribution of Nanomaterials in Suspension by Nanoparticle Tracking Analysis (NTA)
ASTM E2859-11(2017)	Standard Guide for Size Measurement of Nanoparticles Using Atomic Force Microscopy
ASTM E2859-11(2017)	Standard Guide for Size Measurement of Nanoparticles Using Atomic Force Microscopy
ASTM E2864-13	Standard Test Method for Measurement of Airborne Metal and Metal Oxide Nanoparticle Surface Area Concentration in Inhalation Exposure Chambers using Krypton Gas Adsorption
ASTM E2865-12	Standard Guide for Measurement of Electrophoretic Mobility and Zeta Potential of Nanosized Biological Materials
ISO/TR 18196:2016	Nanotechnologies – Measurement Technique Matrix for the Characterization of Nano-objects
Toxicity Testing and Risk Assessment	
ASTM E2524-08(2013)	Standard Test Method for Analysis of Hemolytic Properties of Nanoparticles
ASTM E2525-08(2013)	Standard Test Method for Evaluation of the Effect of Nanoparticulate Materials on the Formation of Mouse Granulocyte-Macrophage Colonies
ASTM E2526-08(2013)	Standard Test Method for Evaluation of Cytotoxicity of Nanoparticulate Materials in Porcine Kidney Cells and Human Hepatocarcinoma Cells
ASTM E2864-13	Standard Test Method for Measurement of Airborne Metal and Metal Oxide Nanoparticle Surface Area Concentration in Inhalation Exposure Chambers using Krypton Gas Adsorption
ASTM E3025-16	Standard Guide for Tiered Approach to Detection and Characterization of Silver Nanomaterials in Textiles
ISO 10808:2010	Nanotechnologies – Characterization of Nanoparticles in Inhalation Exposure Chambers for Inhalation Toxicity Testing
ISO 29701:2010	Nanotechnologies – Endotoxin Test on Nanomaterial Samples for in Vitro Systems – Limulus Amebocyte Lysate (LAL) test
ISO/TR 13014:2012	Nanotechnologies – Guidance on Physico-Chemical Characterization of Engineered Nanoscale Materials for Toxicologic Assessment
ISO/TR 13121:2011	Nanotechnologies – Nanomaterial Risk Evaluation
ISO/TR 16197:2014	Nanotechnologies – Compilation and description of Toxicological Screening Methods for Manufactured Nanomaterials
ISO/TS 19337:2016	Nanotechnologies – Characteristics of Working Suspensions of Nano-Objects for in Vitro Assays to Evaluate Inherent Nano-Object Toxicity
OECD Test No. 318	Dispersion Stability of Nanomaterials in Simulated Environmental Media
OECD Test No. 412	Subacute Inhalation Toxicity: 28-Day Study
OECD Test No. 413	Subacute Inhalation Toxicity: 90-Day Study
Occupational Health and Safety	
ASTM E2535-07(2013)	Standard Guide for Handling Unbound Engineered Nanoscale Particles in Occupational Settings
ISO/TR 12885:2008	Nanotechnologies – Health and Safety Practices in Occupational Settings Relevant to Nanotechnologies
ISO/TS 12901-1:2012	Nanotechnologies – Occupational Risk Management Applied to Engineered Nanomaterials – Part 1: Principles and Approaches
ISO/TS 12901-2:2014	Nanotechnologies – Occupational Risk Management Applied to Engineered Nanomaterials – Part 2: Use of the Control Banding Approach
ISO/TR 13329:2012	Nanomaterials – Preparation of Material Safety Data Sheet (MSDS)
ISO/TR 18637:2016	Nanotechnologies – Overview of Available Frameworks for the Development of Occupational Exposure Limits and Bands for Nano-objects and their Aggregates and Agglomerates (NOAAs)
ISO/TR 27628:2007	Workplace atmospheres – Ultrafine, nanoparticle and nano-structured aerosols – Inhalation exposure characterization and assessment

[a]No endorsement is implied.

ASTM = ASTM International; ISO = International Organization for Standardization; OECD = Organisation for Economic Co-operation and Development; TR = Technical Report; TS = Technical Specification.

and Toxic Substances Control Act (TSCA).[401] Under TSCA, new nanomaterials are regarded as "chemical substances" subject to review, and the EPA has required reporting by current or planned manufactures, processors, and importers of the specific chemical identity, production volume, methods of manufacture and processing, exposure and release information, and available information concerning environmental and health effects of nanoscale substances.[99,100] The EPA has variously limited use, required personal protective equipment and engineering controls, limited environmental release, and required testing to produce health and environmental effects data. The EPA determined that (nano) silver ion-generating washing machines marketed with bactericidal claims were subject to registration requirements under FIFRA and extended the requirement to copper- and zinc-emitting devices

TABLE 125–3	Selected Nanotechnology Organizational Resources[a]
Organization	**Website**
European Commission, Research in Nanosciences & Technologies	http://ec.europa.eu/research/industrial_technologies/nanoscience-and-technologies_en.html
German Federal Institute for Occupational Safety and Health (BAuA), Innovative Materials	https://www.baua.de/EN/Topics/Safe-use-of-chemicals-and-products/Innovative-materials/Innovative-materials_node.html
International Association of Nanotechnology (IANT)	http://www.ianano.org
National Cancer Institute (NCI), Office for Cancer Nanotechnology Research	https://www.cancer.gov/sites/ocnr
National Center for Earth and Environmental Nanotechnology Infrastructure (NanoEarth)	http://www.nanoearth.ictas.vt.edu
National Institutes of Health (NIH), Nanotechnology at NIH	https://www.nih.gov/research-training/nanotechnology-nih
National Nanotechnology Coordinated Infrastructure (NNCI)[b]	http://www.nnci.net
Organization for Economic Co-operation and Development (OECD), Science and Technology Policy: Nanotechnology	http://www.oecd.org/sti/nano
Project on Emerging Nanotechnologies, Woodrow Wilson International Center for Scholars	http://www.nanotechproject.org
Safenano (UK Institute of Occupational Medicine)	http://www.safenano.org
US Department of Agriculture, National Institute of Food and Agriculture, Nanotoxicology Program	https://nifa.usda.gov/program/nanotechnology-program
US Environmental Protection Agency (EPA), Research on Nanomaterials	https://www.epa.gov/chemical-research/research-nanomaterials
US EPA, Control of Nanoscale Materials under the Toxic Substances Control Act (TSCA)	https://www.epa.gov/reviewing-new-chemicals-under-toxic-substances-control-act-tsca/control-nanoscale-materials-under
US Food and Drug Administration (FDA), Nanotechnology Programs at FDA	https://www.fda.gov/ScienceResearch/SpecialTopics/Nanotechnology/default.htm
US National Institute for Occupational Safety and Health (NIOSH), Workplace Safety & Health Topics, Nanotechnology	https://www.cdc.gov/niosh/topics/nanotech
US National Institute of Standards and Technology (NIST), Nanotechnology	https://www.nist.gov/topics/nanotechnology
US National Nanotechnology Initiative (NNI)	http://www.nano.gov
US National Science Foundation (NSF) National Nanotechnology Initiative	http://www.nsf.gov/crssprgm/nano
US National Toxicology Program (NTP), NTP Nanotechnology Safety Initiative	https://ntp.niehs.nih.gov/results/nano/index.html

[a]Many of these websites are searchable for nano-related developments, policy, research, and toxicology. Websites retrieved October 2, 2017. No endorsement is implied. [b]The NNCI sites are provided at http://www.nnci.net/sites/view-all.

and ion generators in swimming pools.[98] Under FIFRA, it has fined corporations for making unsubstantiated antimicrobial claims with nano-coating technology.[400]

The ongoing rapid evolution of the discipline will mandate constant updating and assessment of available knowledge. A selected list of organizational resources is provided in Table 125–3.

SUMMARY

- Nanotechnology and nanotoxicology represent ever-expanding disciplines.
- Toxicity has been demonstrated at the species level, including in humans.
- The special physiochemical properties of nanoparticles can yield nonintuitive biologic effects, which complicate toxicological assessments.
- Documented cellular and organ systems nanotoxicological mechanisms continue to expand.
- Nanoparticle profiles are incomplete. Although surrogate markers of toxicity are suggestive, human risk remains incompletely characterized across lifecycle stages.
- Appropriate research methodologies, in vitro and in vivo models, risk assessment, and workplace and environmental standards await further exploration and consensus.

REFERENCES

1. Adili A, et al. Differential cytotoxicity exhibited by silica nanowires and nanoparticles. *Nanotoxicology.* 2008;2:1-8.
2. Agashe HB, et al. Investigations on biodistribution of technetium-99m-labeled carbohydrate-coated poly(propylene imine) dendrimers. *Nanomedicine.* 2007;3:120-127.
3. Ainslie KM, et al. Macrophage cell adhesion and inflammation cytokines on magnetostrictive nanowires. *Nanotoxicology.* 2007;1:279.
4. Al-Hanbali O, et al. Concentration dependent structural ordering of poloxamine 908 on polystyrene nanoparticles and their modulatory role on complement consumption. *J Nanosci Nanotechnol.* 2006;6:3126-3133.
5. Andersen A, et al. Complement: alive and kicking nanomedicines. *J Biomed Nanotechnol.* 2009;5:364.
6. Araujo JA, et al. Ambient particulate pollutants in the ultrafine range promote early atherosclerosis and systemic oxidative stress. *Circ Res.* 2008;102:589-596.
7. ASTM International. *ASTM E2525-08 Standard Test Method for Evaluation of the Effect of Nanoparticulate Materials on the Formation of Mouse Granulocyte-Macrophage Colonies.* West Conshohocken, PA: ASTM International; 2008.
8. ASTM International. *ASTM Standard E2456-06(2012). Terminology for Nanotechnology.* West Conshohocken, PA: ASTM International; 2012.
9. Baccarelli A, et al. Exposure to particulate air pollution and risk of deep vein thrombosis. *Arch Intern Med.* 2008;168:920-927.
10. Bakand S, et al. Nanoparticles: a review of particle toxicology following inhalation exposure. *Inhal Toxicol.* 2012;24:125-135.
11. Baker GL, et al. Inhalation toxicity and lung toxicokinetics of C60 fullerene nanoparticles and microparticles. *Toxicol Sci.* 2008;101:122-131.

12. Bakshi MS, Nanotoxicity in systemic circulation and wound healing. *Chem Res Toxicol.* 2017;30:1253-1274.

13. Balasubramanian S, et al. Biodistribution of gold nanoparticles and gene expression changes in the liver and spleen after intravenous administration in rats. *Biomaterials.* 2010;31:2034.

14. Ballou B, et al. Noninvasive imaging of quantum dots in mice. *Bioconj Chem.* 2004;15:79-86.

15. Bao G, et al. Multifunctional nanoparticles for drug delivery and molecular imaging. *Annu Rev Biomed Eng.* 2013;15:253-282.

16. Barregard L, et al. Experimental exposure to wood-smoke particles in healthy humans: effects on markers of inflammation, coagulation, and lipid peroxidation. *Inhal Toxicol.* 2006;18:845-853.

17. Beck-Speier I, et al. Oxidative stress and lipid mediators induced in alveolar macrophages by ultrafine particles. *Free Radic Biol Med.* 2005;38:1080-1092.

18. Bello D, et al. Nanomaterials properties vs. biological oxidative damage: implications for toxicity screening and exposure assessment. *Nanotoxicology.* 2009;3:249-261.

19. Belyanskaya L, et al. Effects of carbon nanotubes on primary neurons and glial cells. *Neurotoxicology.* 2009;30:702.

20. Berry JP, et al. A microanalytic study of particles transport across the alveoli: role of blood platelets. *Biomedicine.* 1977;27:354-357.

21. Beuerle F, et al. Cytoprotective activities of water-soluble fullerenes in zebrafish models. *J Exp Nanosci.* 2007;2:147.

22. Federal Institute of Risk Assessment. Cause of intoxications with nano spray not yet full elucidated [press release]. Berlin, Germany: Federal Institute of Risk Assessment; 2006.

23. Federal Institute of Risk Assessment. Nano particles were not the cause of health problems triggered by sealing sprays! [press release]. Berlin, Germany: Federal Institute of Risk Assessment; 2006.

24. Bhaskar S, et al. Multifunctional nanocarriers for diagnostics, drug delivery and targeted treatment across blood-brain barrier: perspectives on tracking and neuroimaging. *Part Fibre Toxicol.* 2010;7:3.

25. Bhattacharya J, et al. Interaction of hemoglobin and copper nanoparticles: implications in hemoglobinopathy. *Nanomedicine.* 2006;2:191-199.

26. Biswas P, Wu CY. Nanoparticles and the environment. *J Air Waste Manag Assoc.* 2005;55:708-746.

27. Bodian D, Howe HA. An experimental study of the role of neurones in the dissemination of poliomyelitis virus in the nervous system. *Brain.* 1940;63:135-162.

28. Bodian D, Howe HA. The rate of progression of poliomyelitis virus in nerves. *Bull Johns Hopkins Hosp.* 1941;69:79-85.

29. Borm PJ, et al. The potential risks of nanomaterials: a review carried out for ECETOC. *Part Fibre Toxicol.* 2006;3:11.

30. Bosi S, et al. Hemolytic effects of water-soluble fullerene derivatives. *J Med Chem.* 2004;47:6711-6715.

31. Bottini M, et al. Multi-walled carbon nanotubes induce T lymphocyte apoptosis. *Toxicol Lett.* 2006;160:121-126.

32. Boyes WK, et al. A comprehensive framework for evaluating the environmental health and safety implications of engineered nanomaterials. *Crit Rev Toxicol.* 2017;47:767-810.

33. Braden BC, et al. X-ray crystal structure of an anti-Buckminsterfullerene antibody fab fragment: biomolecular recognition of C(60). *Proc Natl Acad Sci U S A.* 2000; 97:12193-12197.

34. Brain JD, et al. To the editors: express concern about the recent paper by Song et al. *Eur Respir J.* 2010;35:226-227.

35. Brant J, et al. Aggregation and deposition characteristics of fullerene nanoparticles in aqueous systems. *J Nanopart Res.* 2005;7:545-553.

36. Braydich-Stolle L, et al. In vitro cytotoxicity of nanoparticles in mammalian germline stem cells. *Toxicol Sci.* 2005;88:412-419.

37. Brenneman KA, et al. Direct olfactory transport of inhaled manganese ((54)MnCl(2)) to the rat brain: toxicokinetic investigations in a unilateral nasal occlusion model. *Toxicol Appl Pharmacol.* 2000;169:238-248.

38. Brook RD, et al. Air pollution and cardiovascular disease: a statement for healthcare professionals from the Expert Panel on Population and Prevention Science of the American Heart Association. *Circulation.* 2004;109:2655-2671.

39. Brown CL, et al. Nanogold pharmaceutics. *Gold Bull.* 2007;40:245-250.

40. Brown JS, et al. Ultrafine particle deposition and clearance in the healthy and obstructed lung. *Am J Respir Crit Care Med.* 2002;166:1240-1247.

41. Brulefert K, et al. Pro-osteoclastic in vitro effect of polyethylene-like nanoparticles: involvement in the pathogenesis of implant aseptic loosening. *J Biomed Mater Res A.* 2016;104:2649-2657.

42. Busse B, et al. Allocation of nonbirefringent wear debris: darkfield illumination associated with PIXE microanalysis reveals cobalt deposition in mineralized bone matrix adjacent to CoCr implants. *J Biomed Mater Res A.* 2008;87:536.

43. Byrne SJ, et al. "Jelly dots": synthesis and cytotoxicity studies of CdTe quantum dot-gelatin nanocomposites. *Small.* 2007;3:1152-1156.

44. Calderon-Garciaduenas L, et al. Air pollution, cognitive deficits and brain abnormalities: a pilot study with children and dogs. *Brain Cogn.* 2008;68:117-127.

45. Calderon-Garciaduenas L, et al. Long-term air pollution exposure is associated with neuroinflammation, an altered innate immune response, disruption of the blood-brain barrier, ultrafine particulate deposition, and accumulation of amyloid beta-42 and alpha-synuclein in children and young adults. *Toxicol Pathol.* 2008;36:289-310.

46. Cao Y, et al. A review of endoplasmic reticulum (ER) stress and nanoparticle (NP) exposure. *Life Sci.* 2017;186:33-42.

47. Carrero-Sanchez JC, et al. Biocompatibility and toxicological studies of carbon nanotubes doped with nitrogen. *Nano Lett.* 2006;6:1609-1616.

48. Cathe DS, et al. Exposure to metal oxide nanoparticles in physiological fluid induced synergistic biological effects in a keratinocyte model. *Toxicol Lett.* 2017;268:1-7.

49. Cenni E, et al. Biocompatibility of poly(D,L-lactide-co-glycolide) nanoparticles conjugated with alendronate. *Biomaterials.* 2008;29:1400-1411.

50. Chang E, et al. Evaluation of quantum dot cytotoxicity based on intracellular uptake. *Small.* 2006;2:1412-1417.

51. Chen BX, et al. Antigenicity of fullerenes: antibodies specific for fullerenes and their characteristics. *Proc Natl Acad Sci U S A.* 1998;95:10809-10813.

52. Chen J, et al. Rare earth nanoparticles prevent retinal degeneration induced by intracellular peroxides. *Nat Nanotechnol.* 2006;1:142.

53. Chen M, von Mikecz A. Formation of nucleoplasmic protein aggregates impairs nuclear function in response to SiO2 nanoparticles. *Exp Cell Res.* 2005;305:51-62.

54. Chen Y, et al. Specific nanotoxicity of graphene oxide during zebrafish embryogenesis. *Nanotoxicology.* 2016;10:42-52.

55. Chen Z, et al. Acute toxicological effects of copper nanoparticles in vivo. *Toxicol Lett.* 2006;163:109-120.

56. Chithrani BD, et al. Determining the size and shape dependence of gold nanoparticle uptake into mammalian cells. *Nano Lett.* 2006;6:662-668.

57. Cho WS, et al. Zeta potential and solubility to toxic ions as mechanisms of lung inflammation caused by metal/metal oxide nanoparticles. *Toxicol Sci.* 2012;126:469-477.

58. Choi AO, et al. Quantum dot-induced cell death involves Fas upregulation and lipid peroxidation in human neuroblastoma cells. *J Nanobiotechnology.* 2007;5:1.

59. Choi J, Kim CS. Mathematical analysis of particle deposition in human lungs: an improved single path transport model. *Inhal Toxicol.* 2007;19:925.

60. Choi J, et al. Induction of oxidative stress and apoptosis by silver nanoparticles in the liver of adult zebrafish. *Aquat Toxicol.* 2010;100:151-159.

61. Choi K, et al. Protein corona modulation of hepatocyte uptake and molecular mechanisms of gold nanoparticle toxicity. *Nanotoxicology.* 2017;11:64-75.

62. Chung KF, et al. Inactivation, clearance, and functional effects of lung-instilled short and long silver nanowires in rats. *ACS Nano.* 2017;11:2652-2664.

63. Colognato R, et al. Analysis of cobalt ferrite nanoparticles induced genotoxicity on human peripheral lymphocytes: comparison of size and organic grafting-dependent effects. *Nanotoxicology.* 2007;1:301.

64. Committee on Technology SoNS, Engineering, and Technology (NSET). *National Nanotechnology Initiative Strategic Plan.* Washington, DC: National Science and Technology Council; 2016.

65. Connor EE, et al. Gold nanoparticles are taken up by human cells but do not cause acute cytotoxicity. *Small.* 2005;1:325-327.

66. Curl RF, et al. How the news that we were not the first to conceive of soccer ball C60 got to us. *J Mol Graph Model.* 2001;19:185-186.

67. Czerniawska A. Experimental investigations on the penetration of 198Au from nasal mucous membrane into cerebrospinal fluid. *Acta Oto-Laryngologica.* 1970;70:58.

68. Dalai S, et al. Acute toxicity of TiO2 nanoparticles to Ceriodaphnia dubia under visible light and dark conditions in a freshwater system. *PloS One.* 2013;8:e62970.

69. Darquenne C, Prisk G. Deposition of inhaled particles in the human lung is more peripheral in lunar than in normal gravity. *Eur J Appl Physiol.*

70. Davey G, et al. Podoconiosis: non-infectious geochemical elephantiasis. *Trans R Soc Trop Med Hyg.* 2007;101:1175-1180.

71. Deb S, et al. Role of purinergic receptors in platelet-nanoparticle interactions. *Nanotoxicology.* 2007;1:93.

72. Deguchi S, et al. Non-engineered nanoparticles of c60. *Sci Rep.* 2013;3:2094.

73. Dellinger A, et al. Uptake and distribution of fullerenes in human mast cells. *Nanomedicine.* 2010;6:575-582.

74. Derfus AM, et al. Probing the cytotoxicity of semiconductor quantum dots. *Nano Lett.* 2004;4:11-18.

75. des Rieux A, et al. Nanoparticles as potential oral delivery systems of proteins and vaccines: a mechanistic approach. *J Control Release.* 2006;116:1-27.

76. Deville S, et al. Interaction of gold nanoparticles and nickel(II) sulfate affects dendritic cell maturation. *Nanotoxicology.* 2016;10:1395-1403.

77. Devlin RB, et al. Elderly humans exposed to concentrated air pollution particles have decreased heart rate variability. *Eur Respir J Suppl.* 2003;40:76S-80S.

78. Dierschke K, et al. Acute respiratory effects and biomarkers of inflammation due to welding-derived nanoparticle aggregates. *Int Arch Occup Environ Health.* 2017;90:451-463.

79. Ding M, et al. Size-dependent effects of tungsten carbide-cobalt particles on oxygen radical production and activation of cell signaling pathways in murine epidermal cells. *Toxicol Appl Pharmacol.* 2009;241:260.

80. Dobrovolskaia MA, et al. Preclinical studies to understand nanoparticle interaction with the immune system and its potential effects on nanoparticle biodistribution. *Mol Pharm.* 2008;5:487-495.

81. Dobrovolskaia MA, McNeil SE. Immunological properties of engineered nanomaterials. *Nat Nanotechnol.* 2007;2:469-478.

82. Dobrovolskaia MA, et al. Current understanding of interactions between nanoparticles and the immune system. *Toxicol Appl Pharmacol.* 2016;299:78-89.

83. Dockery DW, et al. Association of air pollution with increased incidence of ventricular tachyarrhythmias recorded by implanted cardioverter defibrillators. *Environ Health Perspect.* 2005;113:670-674.

84. Domanski DM, et al. Influence of PAMAM dendrimers on human red blood cells. *Bioelectrochemistry.* 2004;63:189-191.

85. Donaldson K, Poland CA. Nanotoxicology: new insights into nanotubes. *Nat Nanotechnol.* 2009;4:708-710.

86. Donaldson K, Poland CA. Nanotoxicity: challenging the myth of nano-specific toxicity. *Curr Opin Biotechnol.* 2013;24:724-734.

87. Duan Y, et al. Interaction between nanoparticulate anatase TiO(2) and LACTATE dehydrogenase. *Biol Trace Elem Res.* 2010;136:302-313.

88. Dubertret B, et al. In vivo imaging of quantum dots encapsulated in phospholipid micelles. *Science.* 2002;298:1759-1762.

89. Duncan R, Izzo L. Dendrimer biocompatibility and toxicity. *Adv Drug Deliv Rev.* 2005;57:2215-2237.

90. Dutta D, et al. Adsorbed proteins influence the biological activity and molecular targeting of nanomaterials. *Toxicol Sci.* 2007;100:303-315.

91. Elder A, et al. Translocation of inhaled ultrafine manganese oxide particles to the central nervous system. *Environ Health Perspect.* 2006;114:1172-1178.

92. Electronic Code of Federal Regulations. *Title 29 (Labor). Subtitle B (Regulations Relating to Labor). Chapter XVII).* Section 1910.1000. Table Z–1—Limits for Air Contaminants. 2008. Washington, DC: Occupational Safety and Health Administration, Department of Labor.

93. Elias AL, et al. Viability studies of pure carbon- and nitrogen-doped nanotubes with *Entamoeba histolytica:* from amoebicidal to biocompatible structures. *Small.* 2007;3:1723-1729.

94. Elsaesser A, Howard CV. Toxicology of nanoparticles. *Adv Drug Deliv Rev.* 2012;64:129-137.

95. Ema M, et al. Developmental toxicity of engineered nanomaterials in rodents. *Toxicol Appl Pharmacol.* 2016;299:47-52.

96. Ema M, et al. Reproductive and developmental toxicity of carbon-based nanomaterials: a literature review. *Nanotoxicology.* 2016;10:391-412.

97. Environment Directorate, Organisation for Economic Co-operation and Development (OECD). *Silver Nanoparticles: Summary of the Dossier. Series on the Safety of Manufactured Nanomaterials.* No. 83. ENV/JM/MONO(2017)31. Paris, France: Organisation for Economic Co-operation and Development (OECD).

98. Environmental Protection Agency. Pesticide Registration; Clarification for Ion-Generating Equipment. *Fed Reg.* 2007;72:54039-54041.

99. Environmental Protection Agency. Toxic Substances Control Act Inventory Status of Carbon Nanotubes. *Fed Reg.* 2008;73:64946-64947.

100. Environmental Protection Agency. Chemical Substances When Manufactured or Processed as Nanoscale Materials; TSCA Reporting and Recordkeeping Requirements. *Fed Reg.* 2017;82:22088-22089.

101. Evans DE, et al. Ultrafine and respirable particles in an automotive grey iron foundry. *Ann Occup Hyg.* 2008;52:9-21.

102. Fach E, et al. Analysis of the biological and chemical reactivity of zeolite-based aluminosilicate fibers and particulates. *Environ Health Perspect.* 2002;110:1087-1096.

103. Fall M, et al. Evaluation of cerium oxide and cerium oxide based fuel additive safety on organotypic cultures of lung slices. *Nanotoxicology.* 2007;1:227.

104. Fan J, et al. Inhibition of autophagy overcomes the nanotoxicity elicited by cadmium-based quantum dots. *Biomaterials.* 2016;78:102-114.

105. Fatkhutdinova LM, et al. Fibrosis biomarkers in workers exposed to MWCNTs. *Toxicol Appl Pharmacol.* 2016;299:125-131.

106. Fernandes C, et al. Nano-interventions for neurodegenerative disorders. *Pharmacol Res.* 2010;62:166-178.

107. Feynman RP. There's plenty of room at the bottom. An invitation to enter a new field of physics. *Eng Sci.* 1960;23:22-36.

108. Fischer HC, et al. Pharmacokinetics of nanoscale quantum dots: in vivo distribution, sequestration, and clearance in the rat. *Adv Functional Mater.* 2006;16:1299-1305.

109. Foley S, et al. Interaction of a water soluble fullerene derivative with reactive oxygen species and model enzymatic systems. *Fullerenes Nanotubes Carbon Nanostruct.* 2002;10:49-67.

110. Fortescue-Brickdale JM. Collargol: a review of some of its clinical applications, with experiments on its antiseptic action. *Bristol Med Chir J (1883).* 1903;21:337-344.

111. Foucaud L, et al. Measurement of reactive species production by nanoparticles prepared in biologically relevant media. *Toxicol Lett.* 2007;174:1-9.

112. Fox K, et al. Recent advances in research applications of nanophase hydroxyapatite. *Chemphyschem.* 2012;13:2495-2506.

113. Fujishima A, et al. Titanium dioxide photocatalysis. *J Photochem Photobiol C Photochem Rev.* 2000;1:1-21.

114. Fujita K, et al. Effects of ultrafine TiO2 particles on gene expression profile in human keratinocytes without illumination: involvement of extracellular matrix and cell adhesion. *Toxicol Lett.* 2009;191:109.

115. Gao J, et al. Fullerene derivatives induce premature senescence: a new toxicity paradigm or novel biomedical applications. *Toxicol Appl Pharmacol.* 2010;244:130-143.

116. Garcia GJM, Kimbell J. Deposition of inhaled nanoparticles in the rat nasal passages: dose to the olfactory region. *Inhal Toxicol.* 2009;21:1165.

117. Gardea-Torresdey JL, et al. Formation and growth of Au nanoparticles inside live alfalfa plants. *Nano Lett.* 2002;2:397-401.

118. Garnett MC, Kallinteri P. Nanomedicines and nanotoxicology: some physiological principles. *Occup Med (Lond).* 2006;56:307-311.

119. Geiser M, et al. Ultrafine particles cross cellular membranes by nonphagocytic mechanisms in lungs and in cultured cells. *Environ Health Perspect.* 2005;113:1555-1560.

120. German Federal Institute for Occupational Safety and Health; German Chemical Industry Association. *Guidance for Handling and Use of Nanomaterials at the Workplace.* Berlin, Germany: Federal Institute for Occupational Safety and Health (Bundesanstalt für Arbeitsschutz und Arbeitsmedizin/BAuA) and the German Chemical Industry Association (Verband der Chemischen Industrie/VCI) 2007.

121. Gessner A, et al. Influence of surface charge density on protein adsorption on polymeric nanoparticles: analysis by two-dimensional electrophoresis. *Eur J Pharm Biopharm.* 2002;54:165-170.

122. Gessner A, et al. Nanoparticles with decreasing surface hydrophobicities: influence on plasma protein adsorption. *Int J Pharm.* 2000;196:245-249.

123. Gharbi N, et al. [60]Fullerene is a powerful antioxidant in vivo with no acute or sub-acute toxicity. *Nano Lett.* 2005;5:2578-2585.

124. Ghelfi E, et al. Cardiac oxidative stress and electrophysiological changes in rats exposed to concentrated ambient particles are mediated by TRP-dependent pulmonary reflexes. *Toxicol Sci.* 2008;102:328-336.

125. Gheshlaghi Z, et al. Toxicity and interaction of titanium dioxide nanoparticles with microtubule protein. *Acta Biochim Biophys Sin (Shanghai).* 2008;40:777.

126. Ghio AJ, et al. Exposure to concentrated ambient air particles alters hematologic indices in humans. *Inhal Toxicol.* 2003;15:1465-1478.

127. Giepmans BN, et al. Correlated light and electron microscopic imaging of multiple endogenous proteins using Quantum dots. *Nat Methods.* 2005;2:743-749.

128. Gilmour MI, et al. Differential pulmonary inflammation and in vitro cytotoxicity of size-fractionated fly ash particles from pulverized coal combustion. *J Air Waste Manag Assoc.* 2004;54:286-295.

129. Gong H Jr, et al. Controlled exposures of healthy and asthmatic volunteers to concentrated ambient particles in metropolitan Los Angeles. *Res Rep Health Eff Inst.* 2003;1-36; discussion 37-47.

130. Goode AE, et al. Chemical speciation of nanoparticles surrounding metal-on-metal hips. *Chem Commun (Camb).* 2012;48:8335-8337.

131. Gopee NV, et al. Migration of intradermally injected quantum dots to sentinel organs in mice. *Toxicol Sci.* 2007;98:249-257.

132. Gupta AK, Gupta M. Cytotoxicity suppression and cellular uptake enhancement of surface modified magnetic nanoparticles. *Biomaterials.* 2005;26:1565-1573.

133. Gupta H, et al. Sparfloxacin-loaded PLGA nanoparticles for sustained ocular drug delivery. *Nanomedicine.* 2010;6:324-333.

134. Hamburg MA. Science and regulation. FDA's approach to regulation of products of nanotechnology. *Science.* 2012;336:299-300.

135. Hamilton RF, et al. Engineered carbon nanoparticles alter macrophage immune function and initiate airway hyper-responsiveness in the BALB/c mouse model. *Nanotoxicology.* 2007;1:104-117.

136. Hanaki K, et al. Semiconductor quantum dot/albumin complex is a long-life and highly photostable endosome marker. *Biochem Biophys Res Commun.* 2003;302:496-501.

137. Hansen SF, et al. Categorization framework to aid hazard identification of nanomaterials. *Nanotoxicology.* 2007;1:243-250.

138. Harder V, et al. Cardiovascular responses in unrestrained WKY rats to inhaled ultrafine carbon particles. *Inhal Toxicol.* 2005;17:29-42.

139. Hardman R. A toxicologic review of quantum dots: toxicity depends on physicochemical and environmental factors. *Environ Health Perspect.* 2006;114:165-172.

140. Harris T, et al. Tissue-specific gene delivery via nanoparticle coating. *Biomaterials.* 2010;31:998.

141. Haslbeck S, et al. Formation of gold nanoparticles in gold ruby glass: the influence of tin. *Hyperfine Interactions.* 2005;165:89-94.

142. Hattori K, et al. Exposure to nano-size titanium dioxide causes oxidative damages in human mesothelial cells: the crystal form rather than size of particle contributes to cytotoxicity. *Biochem Biophys Res Commun.* 2017;492:218-223.

143. Henriksson J, Tjalve H. Manganese taken up into the CNS via the olfactory pathway in rats affects astrocytes. *Toxicol Sci.* 2000;55:392-398.

144. Henry L, et al. Metal deposition in post-surgical granulomas of the urinary tract. *Histopathology.* 1993;22:457.

145. Hesterberg TW, et al. Biopersistence of man-made vitreous fibers and crocidolite asbestos in the rat lung following inhalation. *Fundam Appl Toxicol.* 1996;29:269-279.

146. Hillyer JF, Albrecht RM. Gastrointestinal persorption and tissue distribution of differently sized colloidal gold nanoparticles. *J Pharm Sci.* 2001;90:1927-1936.

147. Hoet PH, et al. Nanoparticles—known and unknown health risks. *J Nanobiotechnology.* 2004;2:12.

148. Hong S, et al. Interaction of poly(amidoamine) dendrimers with supported lipid bilayers and cells: hole formation and the relation to transport. *Bioconjug Chem.* 2004;15:774-782.

149. Hong S, Leroueil PR, Janus EK, et al. Interaction of polycationic polymers with supported lipid bilayers and cells: nanoscale hole formation and enhanced membrane permeability. *Bioconjug Chem.* 2006;17:728-734.

150. Hoshino A, et al. Physicochemical properties and cellular toxicity of nanocrystal quantum dots depend on their surface modification. *Nano Lett.* 2004;4:2163-2169.

151. Howe HA, Bodian D. Poliomyelitis in the chimpanzee: a clinical-pathological study. *Bull Johns Hopkins Hosp.* 1941;69:149-181.

152. Hu Q, et al. Polymeric nanoparticles induce NLRP3 inflammasome activation and promote breast cancer metastasis. *Macromol Biosci.* 2017;17.

153. Hu Y, et al. Cytosolic delivery of membrane-impermeable molecules in dendritic cells using pH-responsive core-shell nanoparticles. *Nano Lett.* 2007;7:3056-3064.

154. Huang S, et al. Disturbed mitotic progression and genome segregation are involved in cell transformation mediated by nano-TiO2 long-term exposure. *Toxicol Appl Pharmacol.* 2009;241:182.

155. Iijima S. Helical microtubules of graphitic carbon. *Nature.* 1991;354:56-58.

156. Ishida T, et al. Accelerated blood clearance of PEGylated liposomes upon repeated injections: effect of doxorubicin-encapsulation and high-dose first injection. *J Control Release.* 2006;115:251-258.

157. Ispas C, et al. Toxicity and developmental defects of different sizes and shape nickel nanoparticles in zebrafish. *Environ Sci Technol.* 2009;43:6349.

158. Iwata N, et al. Effects of C60, a fullerene, on the activities of glutathione s-transferase and glutathione-related enzymes in rodent and human livers. *Fullerenes Nanotubes Carbon Nanostruct.* 1998;6:213.

159. Jani PU, et al. Titanium dioxide (rutile) particle uptake from the rat GI tract and translocation to systemic organs after oral administration. *Int J Pharm.* 1994;105:157-168.

160. Jaques PA, Kim CS. Measurement of total lung deposition of inhaled ultrafine particles in healthy men and women. *Inhal Toxicol.* 2000;12:715-731.

161. Jiang J, et al. Does nanoparticle activity depend upon size and crystal phase? *Nanotoxicology.* 2008;2:33.

162. Jo E, et al. Exposure to zinc oxide nanoparticles affects reproductive development and biodistribution in offspring rats. *J Toxicol Sci.* 2013;38:525-530.

163. Johnston CJ, et al. Pulmonary effects induced by ultrafine PTFE particles. *Toxicol Appl Pharmacol.* 2000;168:208-215.

164. Kagan VE, et al. Nanomedicine and nanotoxicology: two sides of the same coin. *Nanomedicine.* 2005;1:313-316.

165. Kagan VE, et al. Direct and indirect effects of single walled carbon nanotubes on RAW 264.7 macrophages: role of iron. *Toxicol Lett.* 2006;165:88-100.

166. Kaiser JP, et al. Single walled carbon nanotubes (SWCNT) affect cell physiology and cell architecture. *J Mater Sci Mater Med.* 2008;19:1523-1527.

167. Kalishwaralal K, et al. Silver nanoparticles inhibit VEGF induced cell proliferation and migration in bovine retinal endothelial cells. *Colloids Surf B Biointerfaces.* 2009;73:51.

168. Kanarek MS. Nanomaterial health effects part 3: conclusion—hazardous issues and the precautionary principle. *WMJ.* 2007;106:16-19.

169. Kanno S, et al. Effects of eicosane, a component of nanoparticles in diesel exhaust, on surface activity of pulmonary surfactant monolayers. *Arch Toxicol.* 2008;82:841-850.

170. Kashiwada S. Distribution of nanoparticles in the see-through medaka (Oryzias latipes). *Environ Health Perspect.* 2006;114:1697-1702.

171. Kateb B, et al. Nanoplatforms for constructing new approaches to cancer treatment, imaging, and drug delivery: what should be the policy? *NeuroImage.* 2011;54(suppl 1):S106-S124.

172. Keam SJ, et al. Verteporfin: a review of its use in the management of subfoveal choroidal neovascularisation. *Drugs.* 2003;63:2521-2554.

173. Kearnes M, Macnaghten P. Introduction: (re)imagining nanotechnology. *Sci Culture.* 2006;15:279-290.

174. Kettunen J, et al. Associations of fine and ultrafine particulate air pollution with stroke mortality in an area of low air pollution levels. *Stroke.* 2007;38:918-922.

175. Kim BY, et al. Nanomedicine. *N Engl J Med.* 2010;363:2434-2443.

176. Kim D, et al. Interaction of PLGA nanoparticles with human blood constituents. *Colloids Surf B Biointerfaces.* 2005;40:83-91.

177. Kim J, et al. Intravenously administered gold nanoparticles pass through the blood-retinal barrier depending on the particle size, and induce no retinal toxicity. *Nanotechnology.* 2009;20:505101.

178. Kim S, et al. Near-infrared fluorescent type II quantum dots for sentinel lymph node mapping. *Nat Biotechnol.* 2004;22:93-97.

179. Kim W-Y, et al. Histological study of gender differences in accumulation of silver nanoparticles in kidneys of Fischer 344 rats. *J Toxicol Environ Health A.* 2009;72:1279.

180. Kobayashi H, Brechbiel MW. Dendrimer-based macromolecular MRI contrast agents: characteristics and application. *Mol Imaging.* 2003;2:1-10.

181. Kohli AK, Alpar HO. Potential use of nanoparticles for transcutaneous vaccine delivery: effect of particle size and charge. *Int J Pharm.* 2004;275:13-17.

182. Koo OM, et al. Role of nanotechnology in targeted drug delivery and imaging: a concise review. *Nanomedicine.* 2005;1:193-212.

183. Kostarelos K, et al. Cellular uptake of functionalized carbon nanotubes is independent of functional group and cell type. *Nat Nanotechnol.* 2007;2:108-113.

184. Kreyling W, et al. Health implications of nanoparticles. *J Nanopart Res.* 2006;8:543-562.

185. Kreyling W, et al. Size dependence of the translocation of inhaled iridium and carbon nanoparticle aggregates from the lung of rats to the blood and secondary target organs. *Inhal Toxicol.* 2009;21(suppl 1):55.

186. Kreyling WG. Discovery of unique and ENM-specific pathophysiologic pathways: comparison of the translocation of inhaled iridium nanoparticles from nasal epithelium versus alveolar epithelium towards the brain of rats. *Toxicol Appl Pharmacol.* 2016;299:41-46.

187. Kreyling WG, et al. Ultrafine particle-lung interactions: does size matter? *J Aerosol Med.* 2006;19:74-83.

188. Kroto HW, et al. C60: buckminsterfullerene. *Nature.* 1985;318:162-163.

189. Kumar S, et al. Plasmonic nanosensors for imaging intracellular biomarkers in live cells. *Nano Lett.* 2007;7:1338-1343.

190. Kwon J-T, et al. Body distribution of inhaled fluorescent magnetic nanoparticles in the mice. *J Occup Health.* 2008;50:1.

191. Lacava ZGM, et al. Biological effects of magnetic fluids: toxicity studies. *J Magn Magn Mater.* 1999;201:431-434.

192. Lam CW, et al. Pulmonary toxicity of single-wall carbon nanotubes in mice 7 and 90 days after intratracheal instillation. *Toxicol Sci.* 2004;77:126-134.

193. Lamprecht A, et al. Size-dependent bioadhesion of micro- and nanoparticulate carriers to the inflamed colonic mucosa. *Pharm Res.* 2001;18:788-793.

194. Landsiedel R, et al. Safety assessment of nanomaterials using an advanced decision-making framework, the DF4nanoGrouping. *J Nanopart Res.* 2017;19:171.

195. Langmuir I. *Surface Chemistry. Nobel Lectures, Chemistry 1922-1941.* Amsterdam: Elsevier; 1966:287-325.

196. Leblanc AJ, et al. Nanoparticle inhalation impairs coronary microvascular reactivity via a local reactive oxygen species-dependent mechanism. *Cardiovasc Toxicol.* 2010;10:27.

197. Lee D, et al. Characterization of metal-bearing diesel nanoparticles using single-particle mass spectrometry. *J Aerosol Sci.* 2006;37:88-110.

198. Lee H, et al. Controlled assembly of magnetic nanoparticles from magnetotactic bacteria using microelectromagnets arrays. *Nano Lett.* 2004;4:995-998.

199. Lee J, et al. photochemical production of reactive oxygen species by C60 in the aqueous phase during UV irradiation. *Environ Sci Technol.* 2007;41:2529-2535.

200. Lee J-H, et al. Nanosized polyamidoamine (PAMAM) dendrimer-induced apoptosis mediated by mitochondrial dysfunction. *Toxicol Lett.* 2009;190:202.

201. Lee KJ, et al. In Vivo Imaging of transport and biocompatibility of single silver nanoparticles in early development of zebrafish embryos. *ACS Nano.* 2007;1:133-143.

202. Leeuw TK, et al. Single-walled carbon nanotubes in the intact organism: near-IR imaging and biocompatibility studies in Drosophila. *Nano Lett.* 2007;7:2650-2654.

203. Leu D, et al. Distribution and elimination of coated polymethyl [2-14C]methacrylate nanoparticles after intravenous injection in rats. *J Pharm Sci.* 1984;73:1433-1437.

204. Li H, et al. Elemental selenium particles at nano-size (Nano-Se) are more toxic to Medaka (Oryzias latipes) as a consequence of hyper-accumulation of selenium: a comparison with sodium selenite. *Aquat Toxicol.* 2008;89:251.

205. Li KG, et al. Intracellular oxidative stress and cadmium ions release induce cytotoxicity of unmodified cadmium sulfide quantum dots. *Toxicol In Vitro.* 2009;23:1007.

206. Liao HY, et al. Six-month follow-up study of health markers of nanomaterials among workers handling engineered nanomaterials. *Nanotoxicology.* 2014;8(suppl 1):100-110.

207. Limbach LK, et al. Oxide Nanoparticle uptake in human lung fibroblasts: effects of particle size, agglomeration, and diffusion at low concentrations. *Environ Sci Technol.* 2005;39:9370-9376.

208. Linse S, et al. Nucleation of protein fibrillation by nanoparticles. *Proc Natl Acad Sci U S A.* 2007;104:8691.

209. Liu Y, et al. Synergistic Immuno Photothermal Nanotherapy (SYMPHONY) for the treatment of unresectable and metastatic cancers. *Sci Rep.* 2017;7:8606.

210. Liu Z, et al. Action potential changes associated with the inhibitory effects on voltage-gated sodium current of hippocampal CA1 neurons by silver nanoparticles. *Toxicology.* 2009;264:179.

211. Liu Z, et al. Action potential changes associated with the inhibitory effects on voltage-gated sodium current of hippocampal CA1 neurons by silver nanoparticles. *Toxicology.* 2009;264:179-184.

212. Liu Z, et al. Nano-Ag inhibiting action potential independent glutamatergic synaptic transmission but increasing excitability in rat CA1 pyramidal neurons. *Nanotoxicology.* 2012;6:414-423.

213. Long TC, et al. Titanium dioxide (P25) produces reactive oxygen species in immortalized brain microglia (BV2): implications for nanoparticle neurotoxicity. *Environ Sci Technol.* 2006;40:4346-4352.

214. Loo C, et al. Immunotargeted nanoshells for integrated cancer imaging and therapy. *Nano Lett.* 2005;5:709-711.

215. Loretz B, et al. In vitro cytotoxicity testing of non-thiolated and thiolated chitosan nanoparticles for oral gene delivery. *Nanotoxicology.* 2007;1:139.

216. Love SA, Haynes CL. Assessment of functional changes in nanoparticle-exposed neuroendocrine cells with amperometry: exploring the generalizability of nanoparticle-vesicle matrix interactions. *Anal Bioanal Chem.* 2010;398:677-688.

217. Love SA, et al. Assessing nanoparticle toxicity. *Annu Rev Anal Chem (Palo Alto Calif).* 2012;5:181-205.

218. Lovric J, et al. Differences in subcellular distribution and toxicity of green and red emitting CdTe quantum dots. *J Mol Med (Berl).* 2005;83:377-385.

219. Lovric J, et al. Unmodified cadmium telluride quantum dots induce reactive oxygen species formation leading to multiple organelle damage and cell death. *Chem Biol.* 2005;12:1227-1234.

220. Lu X, et al. Nanotoxicity: a growing need for study in the endocrine system. *Small.* 2013;9:1654-1671.

221. Lynch I, Dawson KA. Protein-nanoparticle interactions. *Nano Today.* 2008;3:40-47.

222. Lynch RM, et al. Assessing the pulmonary toxicity of single-walled carbon nanohorns. *Nanotoxicology.* 2007;1:157.

223. Ma L, et al. Oxidative stress in the brain of mice caused by translocated nanoparticulate TiO2 delivered to the abdominal cavity. *Biomaterials.* 2010;31:99.

224. Madl A, Pinkerton K. Health effects of inhaled engineered and incidental nanoparticles. *Crit Rev Toxicol.* 2009;39:629.

225. Mahmoud MA, et al. A new catalytically active colloidal platinum nanocatalyst: the multiarmed nanostar single crystal. *J Am Chem Soc.* 2008;130:4590-4591.

226. Mahmoudi M, et al. A new approach for the in vitro identification of the cytotoxicity of superparamagnetic iron oxide nanoparticles. *Colloids Surf B Biointerfaces.* 2010;75:300.

227. Mahoney S, et al. The developmental toxicity of complex silica-embedded nickel nanoparticles is determined by their physicochemical properties. *PloS One.* 2016;11:e0152010.

228. Malugin A, Ghandehari H. Cellular uptake and toxicity of gold nanoparticles in prostate cancer cells: a comparative study of rods and spheres. *J Appl Toxicol.* 2010;30:212-217.

229. Mangum JB, et al. Single-walled carbon nanotube (SWCNT)-induced interstitial fibrosis in the lungs of rats is associated with increased levels of PDGF mRNA and the formation of unique intercellular carbon structures that bridge alveolar macrophages in situ. *Part Fibre Toxicol.* 2006;3:15.

230. Manna SK, et al. Single-walled carbon nanotube induces oxidative stress and activates nuclear transcription factor-kappaB in human keratinocytes. *Nano Lett.* 2005;5:1676-1684.

231. Maquieira A, et al. Aluminum oxide nanoparticles as carriers and adjuvants for eliciting antibodies from non-immunogenic haptens. *Anal Chem.* 2012;84:9340-9348.

232. Markovic ZM, et al. Graphene quantum dots as autophagy-inducing photodynamic agents. *Biomaterials.* 2012;33:7084-7092.

233. Marquis BJ, et al. Analytical methods to assess nanoparticle toxicity. *Analyst.* 2009;134:425-439.

234. Mattheakis LC, et al. Optical coding of mammalian cells using semiconductor quantum dots. *Anal Biochem.* 2004;327:200-208.

235. Maurer-Jones MA, et al. Functional assessment of metal oxide nanoparticle toxicity in immune cells. *ACS Nano.* 2010;4:3363-3373.

236. Mayer A, et al. The role of nanoparticle size in hemocompatibility. *Toxicology.* 2009;258:139.

237. Maynard AD, Aitken RJ. Assessing exposure to airborne nanomaterials: current abilities and future requirements. *Nanotoxicology.* 2007;1:26-41.

238. McAuliffe ME, Perry MJ. Are nanoparticles potential male reproductive toxicants? A literature review. *Nanotoxicology.* 2007;1:204-210.

239. McCarthy JR, et al. A macrophage-targeted theranostic nanoparticle for biomedical applications. *Small.* 2006;2:983-987.

240. Meng H, et al. Ultrahigh reactivity provokes nanotoxicity: explanation of oral toxicity of nano-copper particles. *Toxicol Lett.* 2007;175:102-110.

241. Mercer RR, et al. Distribution and persistence of pleural penetrations by multi-walled carbon nanotubes. *Part Fibre Toxicol.* 2010;7:28.

242. Mills N, et al. Adverse cardiovascular effects of air pollution. *Nat Clin Pract Cardiovasc Med.* 2009;6:36.

243. Mishra AR, et al. Silver nanoparticle-induced autophagic-lysosomal disruption and NLRP3-inflammasome activation in HepG2 cells is size-dependent. *Toxicol Sci.* 2016;150:473-487.

244. Mitsakou C, et al. Lung deposition of fine and ultrafine particles outdoors and indoors during a cooking event and a no activity period. *Indoor Air.* 2007;17:143-152.

245. Miyani VA, Hughes MF. Assessment of the in vitro dermal irritation potential of cerium, silver, and titanium nanoparticles in a human skin equivalent model. *Cutan Ocul Toxicol.* 2017;36:145-151.

246. Miyawaki J, et al. Toxicity of single-walled carbon nanohorns. *ACS Nano.* 2008;2:213-226.

247. Möller W, et al. Left-to-right asymmetry of aerosol deposition after shallow bolus inhalation depends on lung ventilation. *J Aerosol Med Pulm Drug Deliv.* 2009;22:333.

248. Mö Y, et al. Cytokine and NO release from peripheral blood neutrophils after exposure to metal nanoparticles: in vitro and ex vivo studies. *Nanotoxicology.* 2008;2:79-87.

249. Mök H, et al. Enhanced intracellular delivery of quantum dot and adenovirus nanoparticles triggered by acidic pH via surface charge reversal. *Bioconjug Chem.* 2008;19:797-801.

250. Möller P, et al. Role of oxidative damage in toxicity of particulates. *Free Radic Res.* 2010;44:1.

251. Möller W, et al. Ultrafine particles cause cytoskeletal dysfunctions in macrophages: role of intracellular calcium. *Part Fibre Toxicol.* 2005;2:7.

252. Möller W, et al. Deposition, retention, and translocation of ultrafine particles from the central airways and lung periphery. *Am J Respir Crit Care Med.* 2008;177:426-432.

253. Monteiro-Riviere NA, et al. Surfactant effects on carbon nanotube interactions with human keratinocytes. *Nanomedicine.* 2005;1:293-299.

254. Muller J, Huaux F, et al. Respiratory toxicity of multi-wall carbon nanotubes. *Toxicol Appl Pharmacol.* 2005;207:221-231.

255. Muller K, et al. Effect of ultrasmall superparamagnetic iron oxide nanoparticles (Ferumoxtran-10) on human monocyte-macrophages in vitro. *Biomaterials.* 2007;28:1629-1642.

256. Muller K, et al. Atorvastatin and uptake of ultrasmall superparamagnetic iron oxide nanoparticles (Ferumoxtran-10) in human monocyte-macrophages: implications for magnetic resonance imaging. *Biomaterials.* 2008;29:2656-2662.

257. Muller-Borer BJ, et al. Quantum dot labeling of mesenchymal stem cells. *J Nanobiotechnology.* 2007;5:9.

258. Myllynen P, et al. Kinetics of gold nanoparticles in the human placenta. *Reprod Toxicol.* 2008;26:130.

259. Nabiev I, et al. Nonfunctionalized nanocrystals can exploit a cell's active transport machinery delivering them to specific nuclear and cytoplasmic compartments. *Nano Lett.* 2007;7:3452-3461.

260. Nair LS, Laurencin CT. Nanofibers and nanoparticles for orthopaedic surgery applications. *J Bone Joint Surg Am.* 2008;90(suppl 1):128-131.

261. Nair PM, et al. Differential expression of ribosomal protein gene, gonadotrophin releasing hormone gene and Balbiani ring protein gene in silver nanoparticles exposed Chironomus riparius. *Aquat Toxicol.* 2011;101:31-37.

262. Nanoparticle Task Force ACOEM. Nanotechnology and health. *J Occup Environ Med.* 2011;53:687-689.

263. Napierska D, et al. Size-dependent cytotoxicity of monodisperse silica nanoparticles in human endothelial cells. *Small.* 2009;5:846.

264. National Institute for Occupational Safety and Health (NIOSH). *Approaches to Safe Nanotechnology Managing the Health and Safety Concerns Associated with Engineered Nanomaterials.* Publication No. 2009–125. Cincinnati, OH: US Department of Health and Human Services, Centers for Disease Control and Prevention, National Institute for Occupational Safety and Health; 2009.

265. National Institute for Occupational Safety and Health (NIOSH). *General Safe Practices for Working with Engineered Nanomaterials in Research Laboratories.* Publication No. 2012–147. Cincinnati, OH: US Department of Health and Human Services, Centers for Disease Control and Prevention, National Institute for Occupational Safety and Health; 2012.

266. National Institute for Occupational Safety and Health (NIOSH). *Occupational Exposure to Carbon Nanotubes and Nanofibers.* Current Intelligence Bulletin 65. Cincinnati, OH: US Department of Health and Human Services, Centers for Disease Control and Prevention, National Institute for Occupational Safety and Health; 2013.

267. National Institute for Occupational Safety and Health (NIOSH). *Building a Safety Program to Protect the Nanotechnology Workforce: A Guide for Small to Medium-Sized Enterprises.* DHHS (NIOSH) Publication No. 2016-102. Cincinnati, OH: US Department of Health and Human Services, Centers for Disease Control and Prevention, National Institute for Occupational Safety and Health; 2016.

268. Nel A, et al. Toxic potential of materials at the nanolevel. *Science.* 2006;311:622-627.

269. Nemmar A, et al. Diesel exhaust particles in lung acutely enhance experimental peripheral thrombosis. *Circulation.* 2003;107:1202-1208.

270. Nemmar A, et al. Passage of inhaled particles into the blood circulation in humans. *Circulation.* 2002;105:411-414.

271. Nemmar A, et al. Size effect of intratracheally instilled particles on pulmonary inflammation and vascular thrombosis. *Toxicol Appl Pharmacol.* 2003;186:38-45.

272. Nemmar A, Inuwa IM. Diesel exhaust particles in blood trigger systemic and pulmonary morphological alterations. *Toxicol Lett.* 2008;176:20-30.

273. Newman M, et al. The safety of nanosized particles in titanium dioxide- and zinc oxide-based sunscreens. *J Am Acad Dermatol.* 2009;61:685.

274. Nohynek GJ, et al. Grey goo on the skin? Nanotechnology, cosmetic and sunscreen safety. *Crit Rev Toxicol.* 2007;37:251.

275. Norris DJ, et al. Doped nanocrystals. *Science.* 2008;319:1776-1779.

276. Nurkiewicz T, et al. Pulmonary nanoparticle exposure disrupts systemic microvascular nitric oxide signaling. *Toxicol Sci.* 2009;110:191.

277. Oberdorster G. Safety assessment for nanotechnology and nanomedicine: concepts of Nanotoxicology. *J Intern Med.* 2010;267:89-105.

278. Oberdorster G, et al. Nanotoxicology: an emerging discipline evolving from studies of ultrafine particles. *Environ Health Perspect.* 2005;113:823-839.

279. Oberdorster G, et al. Translocation of inhaled ultrafine particles to the brain. *Inhal Toxicol.* 2004;16:437-445.

280. Occupational Safety and Health Administration (OSHA). *OSHA Fact Sheet. Working Safely with Nanomaterials.* FS-3634. https://www.osha.gov/Publications/OSHA_FS-3634.pdf.

281. OECD. *Regulatory Frameworks for Nanotechnology in Foods and Medical Products: Summary Results of a Survey Activity.* OECD Science, Technology and Industry Policy Papers, No. 4. OECD Publishing. 2013. http://dx.doi.org/10.1787/5k47w4vsb4s4-en.

282. NNCI Coordinating Office. National Nanotechnology Coordinated Infrastructure (NNCI). *Annual Report 2017 (Year 1). NSF Award 1626153.* Atlanta, GA: NNCI Coordinating Office, Georgia Institute of Technology; 2017.

283. Oldenburg M, et al. Severe cobalt intoxication due to prosthesis wear in repeated total hip arthroplasty. *J Arthroplasty.* 2009;24:825.e15.

284. Onuma K, et al. Nano-scaled particles of titanium dioxide convert benign mouse fibrosarcoma cells into aggressive tumor cells. *Am J Pathol.* 2009;175:2171.

285. Oremland RS, et al. Structural and spectral features of selenium nanospheres produced by se-respiring bacteria. *Appl Environ Microbiol.* 2004;70:52-60.

286. Organisation for Economic Co-operation and Development (OECD). *Current Developments on the Safety of Manufactured Nanomaterials—Tour de Table at the 10th Meeting of the Working Party on Manufactured Nanomaterials.* Paris, France: OECD Environment, Health and Safety Publications; 2013.

287. Orr G, et al. Submicrometer and nanoscale inorganic particles exploit the actin machinery to be propelled along microvilli-like structures into alveolar cells. *ACS Nano.* 2007;1:463-475.

288. Osawa E. Superaromaticity. *Kagaku (Kyoto).* 1970;25:854-863.

289. Owens DE 3rd, Peppas NA. Opsonization, biodistribution, and pharmacokinetics of polymeric nanoparticles. *Int J Pharm.* 2006;307:93-102.

290. Paesano L, et al. Markers for toxicity to HepG2 exposed to cadmium sulphide quantum dots; damage to mitochondria. *Toxicology.* 2016;374:18-28.

291. Pan Y, et al. Gold nanoparticles of diameter 1.4 nm trigger necrosis by oxidative stress and mitochondrial damage. *Small.* 2009;5:2067.

292. Pantarotto D, et al. Immunization with peptide-functionalized carbon nanotubes enhances virus-specific neutralizing antibody responses. *Chem Biol.* 2003;10:961-966.

293. Papageorgiou I, et al. The effect of nano- and micron-sized particles of cobalt-chromium alloy on human fibroblasts in vitro. *Biomaterials.* 2007;28:2946-2958.

294. Papis E, et al. Engineered cobalt oxide nanoparticles readily enter cells. *Toxicol Lett.* 2009;189:253-259.

295. Papp T, et al. Human health implications of nanomaterial exposure. *Nanotoxicology.* 2008;2:9-27.

296. Parak WJ, et al. Cell motility and metastatic potential studies based on quantum dot imaging of phagokinetic tracks. *Adv Mater.* 2002;14:882-885.

297. Park EJ, et al. Comparison of subchronic immunotoxicity of four different types of aluminum-based nanoparticles. *J Appl Toxicol.* 2018;38:575-584.

298. Park J, et al. Nanosize and vitality: TiO2 nanotube diameter directs cell fate. *Nano Lett.* 2007;7:1686-1691.

299. Patil S, et al. Protein adsorption and cellular uptake of cerium oxide nanoparticles as a function of zeta potential. *Biomaterials.* 2007;28:4600-4607.

300. Pekkanen J, et al. Particulate air pollution and risk of ST-segment depression during repeated submaximal exercise tests among subjects with coronary heart disease: the Exposure and Risk Assessment for Fine and Ultrafine Particles in Ambient Air (ULTRA) study. *Circulation.* 2002;106:933-938.

301. Pelclova D, et al. Oxidative stress markers are elevated in exhaled breath condensate of workers exposed to nanoparticles during iron oxide pigment production. *J Breath Res.* 2016;10:016004.

302. Pelclova D, et al. Markers of lipid oxidative damage among office workers exposed intermittently to air pollutants including nanoTiO2 particles. *Rev Environ Health.* 2017;32:193-200.

303. Pelclova D, et al. Markers of lipid oxidative damage in the exhaled breath condensate of nano TiO2 production workers. *Nanotoxicology.* 2017;11:52-63.

304. Peng Q, et al. Mechanisms of phospholipid complex loaded nanoparticles enhancing the oral bioavailability. *Mol Pharm.* 2010;7:565-575.

305. Pernodet N, et al. Adverse effects of citrate/gold nanoparticles on human dermal fibroblasts. *Small.* 2006;2:766-773.

306. Persson E, et al. Transport and subcellular distribution of intranasally administered zinc in the olfactory system of rats and pikes. *Toxicology.* 2003;191:97-108.

307. Peters A, Pope CA 3rd. Cardiopulmonary mortality and air pollution. *Lancet.* 2002;360:1184-1185.

308. Peters A, et al. Translocation and potential neurological effects of fine and ultrafine particles a critical update. *Part Fibre Toxicol.* 2006;3:13.

309. Peters TM, et al. The mapping of fine and ultrafine particle concentrations in an engine machining and assembly facility. *Ann Occup Hyg.* 2006;50:249-257.

310. Pietroiusti A, et al. The unrecognized occupational relevance of the interaction between engineered nanomaterials and the gastro-intestinal tract: a consensus paper from a multidisciplinary working group. *Part Fibre Toxicol.* 2017;14:47.

311. Pietroiusti A, et al. New frontiers in nanotoxicology: gut microbiota/microbiome-mediated effects of engineered nanomaterials. *Toxicol Appl Pharmacol.* 2016;299: 90-95.

312. Poland CA, et al. Carbon nanotubes introduced into the abdominal cavity of mice show asbestos-like pathogenicity in a pilot study. *Nat Nanotechnol.* 2008;3:423-428.

314. Porter AE, et al. Direct imaging of single-walled carbon nanotubes in cells. *Nat Nanotechnol.* 2007;2:713-717.

315. Porter CJH, et al. The poloxyethylene/polyoxypropylene block co-polymer Poloxamer-407 selectively redirects intravenously injected microspheres to sinusoidal endothelial cells of rabbit bone marrow. *FEBS Lett.* 1992;305:62-66.

316. Powell JJ, et al. Characterisation of inorganic microparticles in pigment cells of human gut associated lymphoid tissue. *Gut.* 1996;38:390-395.

317. Powers KW, et al. Research strategies for safety evaluation of nanomaterials. Part VI. Characterization of nanoscale particles for toxicological evaluation. *Toxicol Sci.* 2006; 90:296-303.

318. President's Council of Advisors on Science and Technology. *Report to the President and Congress on the Fourth Assessment of the National Nanotechnology Initiative.* Washington, DC: Executive Office of the President; 2012.

319. Prilloff S, et al. In vivo confocal neuroimaging (ICON): non-invasive, functional imaging of the mammalian CNS with cellular resolution. *Eur J Neurosci.* 2010;31:521-528.

320. Prow T. Toxicity of nanomaterials to the eye. *Wiley Interdiscip Rev Nanomed Nanobiotechnol.* 2010;2:317-333.

321. Przybytkowski E, et al. Nanoparticles can induce changes in the intracellular metabolism of lipids without compromising cellular viability. *FEBS J.* 2009;276:6204.

322. Pulskamp K, et al. Carbon nanotubes show no sign of acute toxicity but induce intracellular reactive oxygen species in dependence on contaminants. *Toxicol Lett.* 2007;168:58-74.

323. Puzyn T, et al. Toward the development of "nano-QSARs": advances and challenges. *Small.* 2009;5:2494.

324. Radomski A, et al. Nanoparticle-induced platelet aggregation and vascular thrombosis. *Br J Pharmacol.* 2005;146:882-893.

325. Ramsden C, et al. Dietary exposure to titanium dioxide nanoparticles in rainbow trout, (Oncorhynchus mykiss): no effect on growth, but subtle biochemical disturbances in the brain. *Ecotoxicology.* 2009;18:939.

326. Reibold M, et al. Materials: carbon nanotubes in an ancient Damascus sabre. *Nature.* 2006;444:286-286.

327. Reiss CS, et al. Viral replication in olfactory receptor neurons and entry into the olfactory bulb and brain. *Ann N Y Acad Sci.* 1998;855:751.

328. Renwick LC, et al. Increased inflammation and altered macrophage chemotactic responses caused by two ultrafine particle types. *Occup Environ Med.* 2004;61: 442-447.

329. Roh J-Y, et al. Ecotoxicity of silver nanoparticles on the soil nematode Caenorhabditis elegans using functional ecotoxicogenomics. *Environ Sci Technol.* 2009;43:3933.

330. Roller M. Carcinogenicity of inhaled nanoparticles. *Inhal Toxicol.* 2009;21(suppl 1):144.

331. Roser M. Surface-modified biodegradable albumin nano- and microspheres. II: effect of surface charges on in vitro phagocytosis and biodistribution in rats. *Eur J Pharm Biopharm.* 1998;46:255-263.

332. Rossi E, et al. Airway exposure to silica-coated TiO2 nanoparticles induces pulmonary neutrophilia in mice. *Toxicol Sci.* 2010;113:422.

333. Rouse JG, et al. Effects of mechanical flexion on the penetration of fullerene amino acid-derivatized peptide nanoparticles through skin. *Nano Lett.* 2007;7:155-160.

334. Ruckerl R, et al. Health effects of particulate air pollution: a review of epidemiological evidence. *Inhal Toxicol.* 2011;23:555-592.

335. Ryman-Rasmussen J, et al. Inhaled carbon nanotubes reach the subpleural tissue in mice. *Nat Nanotechnol.* 2009;4:747.

336. Ryman-Rasmussen JP, et al. Penetration of intact skin by quantum dots with diverse physicochemical properties. *Toxicol Sci.* 2006;91:159-165.

337. Ryman-Rasmussen JP, et al. Variables influencing interactions of untargeted quantum dot nanoparticles with skin cells and identification of biochemical modulators. *Nano Lett.* 2007;7:1344-1348.

338. Salnikov V, et al. Probing the outer mitochondrial membrane in cardiac mitochondria with nanoparticles. *Biophys J.* 2007;92:1058-1071.

339. Salvador-Morales C, et al. Complement activation and protein adsorption by carbon nanotubes. *Mol Immunol.* 2006;45:193-201.

340. Salvador-Morales C, et al. Binding of pulmonary surfactant proteins to carbon nanotubes; potential for damage to lung immune defense mechanisms. *Carbon.* 2007;45:607-617.

341. Salvati EA, et al. Particulate metallic debris in cemented total hip arthroplasty. *Clin Orthop Relat Res.* 1993;160.

342. Samberg M, et al. Evaluation of silver nanoparticle toxicity in vivo skin and in vitro keratinocytes. *Environ Health Perspect.* 2010;118:407-413.

343. Sanvicens N, Marco MP. Multifunctional nanoparticles—properties and prospects for their use in human medicine. *Trends Biotechnol.* 2008;26:425-433.

344. Sato Y, et al. Influence of length on cytotoxicity of multi-walled carbon nanotubes against human acute monocytic leukemia cell line THP-1 in vitro and subcutaneous tissue of rats in vivo. *Mol Biosyst.* 2005;1:176-182.

345. Saunders J, et al. A novel skin penetration enhancer: evaluation by membrane diffusion and confocal microscopy. *J Pharm Pharm Sci.* 1999;2:99-107.

346. Saxena RK, et al. Enhanced in vitro and in vivo toxicity of poly-dispersed acid-functionalized single-wall carbon nanotubes. *Nanotoxicology.* 2007;1:291-300.

347. Schaffler M, et al. Serum protein identification and quantification of the corona of 5, 15 and 80 nm gold nanoparticles. *Nanotechnology.* 2013;24:265103.

348. Schins RP. Mechanisms of genotoxicity of particles and fibers. *Inhal Toxicol.* 2002;14:57-78.

349. Schinwald A, et al. Graphene-based nanoplatelets: a new risk to the respiratory system as a consequence of their unusual aerodynamic properties. *ACS Nano.* 2012;6:736-746.

350. Schwotzer D, Ernst et al. Effects from a 90-day inhalation toxicity study with cerium oxide and barium sulfate nanoparticles in rats. *Part Fibre Toxicol.* 2017;14:23.

351. Seleem M, et al. Targeting Brucella melitensis with polymeric nanoparticles containing streptomycin and doxycycline. *FEMS Microbiol Lett.* 2009;294:24.

352. Senaran H, et al. Ultrastructural analysis of metallic debris and tissue reaction around spinal implants in patients with late operative site pain. *Spine.* 2004;29:1618.

353. Senut MC, et al. Size-dependent toxicity of gold nanoparticles on human embryonic stem cells and their neural derivatives. *Small.* 2016;12:631-646.

354. Sgro LA, et al. Toxicological properties of nanoparticles of organic compounds (NOC) from flames and vehicle exhausts. *Environ Sci Technol.* 2009;43:2608.

355. Shah L, et al. Nanotechnology for CNS delivery of bio-therapeutic agents. *Drug Deliv Transl Res.* 2013;3:336-351.

356. Sharifi S, et al. Toxicity of nanomaterials. *Chem Soc Rev.* 2012;41:2323-2343.

357. Sharma H, et al. Influence of nanoparticles on blood-brain barrier permeability and brain edema formation in rats. *Acta Neurochir Suppl.* 2010;106:359.

358. Sharma R, et al. Inhalable microparticles containing drug combinations to target alveolar macrophages for treatment of pulmonary tuberculosis. *Pharm Res.* 2001;18:1405-1410.

359. Shaterabadi Z, et al. High impact of in situ dextran coating on biocompatibility, stability and magnetic properties of iron oxide nanoparticles. *Mater Sci Eng C Mater Biol Appl.* 2017;75:947-956.

360. Shaw SY, et al. Perturbational profiling of nanomaterial biologic activity. *Proc Natl Acad Sci U S A.* 2008;105:7387-7392.

361. Shibuya M, et al. Detection of buckminsterfullerene in usual soots and commercial charcoals. Fullerenes, nanotubes and carbon nanostructures. *Fuller Nanotub Car N.* 1999;7:181-193.

362. Shukla R, et al. Biocompatibility of gold nanoparticles and their endocytotic fate inside the cellular compartment: a microscopic overview. *Langmuir.* 2005;21:10644-10654.

363. Shvedova AA, Kagan VE. The role of nanotoxicology in realizing the 'helping without harm' paradigm of nanomedicine: lessons from studies of pulmonary effects of single-walled carbon nanotubes. *J Intern Med.* 2010;267:106-118.

364. Shvedova AA, et al. Inhalation vs. aspiration of single-walled carbon nanotubes in C57BL/6 mice: inflammation, fibrosis, oxidative stress, and mutagenesis. *Am J Physiol Lung Cell Mol Physiol.* 2008;295:L552.

365. Shvedova AA, et al. Unusual inflammatory and fibrogenic pulmonary responses to single-walled carbon nanotubes in mice. *Am J Physiol Lung Cell Mol Physiol.* 2005;289:L698-L708.

366. Sjaastad AK, et al. Exposure to polycyclic aromatic hydrocarbons (PAHs), mutagenic aldehydes and particulate matter during pan frying of beefsteak. *Occup Environ Med.* 2010;67:228-232.

367. Sjaastad AK, et al. Sub-micrometer particles: their level and how they spread after pan frying of beefsteak. *Indoor Built Environ.* 2008;17:230-236.

368. Sonavane G, et al. In vitro permeation of gold nanoparticles through rat skin and rat intestine: effect of particle size. *Colloids Surf B Biointerfaces.* 2008;65:1-10.

369. Song Y, et al. Exposure to nanoparticles is related to pleural effusion, pulmonary fibrosis and granuloma. *Eur Respir J.* 2009;34:559-567.

370. Soto KF, et al. Comparative in vitro cytotoxicity assessment of some manufactured-nanoparticulate materials characterized by transmission electron microscopy. *J Nanopart Res.* 2005;7:145-169.

371. Stampfl A, et al. Langendorff heart: a model system to study cardiovascular effects of engineered nanoparticles. *ACS Nano.* 2011;5:5345-5353.

372. Stein H, et al. Spread of gold injected into the joints of healthy rabbits. *J Bone Joint Surg Br.* 1976;58-B:496.

373. Stoeva SI, Lee et al. Multiplexed detection of protein cancer markers with biobarcoded nanoparticle probes. *J Am Chem Soc.* 2006;128:8378-8379.

374. Stone V, et al. Development of in vitro systems for nanotoxicology: methodological considerations. *Crit Rev Toxicol.* 2009;39:613.

375. Subcommittee on Nanoscale Science ETNNSaTCCoTC. *National Nanotechnology Initiative. Environmental, Health, and Safety Research Strategy.* Washington, DC: National Science and Technology Council; 2011.

376. Sun L, et al. The nano-effect: improving the long-term prognosis for musculoskeletal implants. *J Long Term Eff Med Implants.* 2012;22:195-209.

377. Sung J, et al. Subchronic inhalation toxicity of silver nanoparticles. *Toxicol Sci.* 2009;108:452.

378. Sweeney S, et al. Pulmonary surfactant mitigates silver nanoparticle toxicity in human alveolar type-I-like epithelial cells. *Colloids Surf B Biointerfaces.* 2016;145:167-175.

379. Takagi A, et al. Induction of mesothelioma in p53+/− mouse by intraperitoneal application of multi-wall carbon nanotube. *J Toxicol Sci.* 2008;33:105-116.

380. Takenaka S, et al. Pulmonary and systemic distribution of inhaled ultrafine silver particles in rats. *Environ Health Perspect.* 2001;109(suppl 4):547-551.

381. Taniguchi N. *On the Basic Concept of "NanoTechnology."* Proceedings of the International Conference on Production Engineering. Tokyo. Part II. Japan Society of Precision Engineering, 1974:18-23.

382. Tao X, et al. Effects of aqueous stable fullerene nanocrystals (nC60) on Daphnia magna: evaluation of sub-lethal reproductive responses and accumulation. *Chemosphere.* 2009;77:1482.

383. Tao Z, et al. Mesoporosity and functional group dependent endocytosis and cytotoxicity of silica nanomaterials. *Chem Res Toxicol.* 2009;22:1869.

384. Tassinari R, et al. Oral, short-term exposure to titanium dioxide nanoparticles in Sprague-Dawley rat: focus on reproductive and endocrine systems and spleen. *Nanotoxicology.* 2014;8:654-662.

385. Tay CY, et al. Micro-/nano-engineered cellular responses for soft tissue engineering and biomedical applications. *Small.* 2011;7:1361-1378.

386. Teixeira LS, et al. Enzyme-catalyzed crosslinkable hydrogels: emerging strategies for tissue engineering. *Biomaterials.* 2012;33:1281-1290.

387. Ternullo S, et al. Going skin deep: a direct comparison of penetration potential of lipid-based nanovesicles on the isolated perfused human skin flap model. *Eur J Pharm Biopharm.* 2017;121:14-23.

388. The Project on Emerging Nanotechnologies, Woodrow Wilson International Center for Scholars. *Consumer Products Inventory. An inventory of nanotechnology-based consumer products introduced on the market.* Washington, DC: Woodrow Wilson International Center for Scholars; 2017. http://www.nanotechproject.org/inventories/consumer.

389. Theegarten D, et al. Submesothelial deposition of carbon nanoparticles after toner exposition: case report. *Diagn Pathol.* 2010;5:77.

390. Thurn KT, et al. Nanoparticles for applications in cellular imaging. *Nanoscale Res Lett.* 2007;2:430-441.

391. Tian J, et al. Topical delivery of silver nanoparticles promotes wound healing. *ChemMedChem.* 2007;2:129-136.

392. Timonen KL, et al. Effects of ultrafine and fine particulate and gaseous air pollution on cardiac autonomic control in subjects with coronary artery disease: the ULTRA study. *J Expo Sci Environ Epidemiol.* 2006;16:332-341.

393. Tin Tin Win S, et al. Changes in neurotransmitter levels and proinflammatory cytokine mRNA expressions in the mice olfactory bulb following nanoparticle exposure. *Toxicol Appl Pharmacol.* 2008;226:192-198.

394. Tjalve H, Henriksson J. Uptake of metals in the brain via olfactory pathways. *Neurotoxicology.* 1999;20:181-195.

395. Totsuka Y, et al. Genotoxicity of nano/microparticles in in vitro micronuclei, in vivo comet and mutation assay systems. *Part Fibre Toxicol.* 2009;6:23.

396. Trask JD, Paul JR. Experimental poliomyelitis in Cercopithecus aethiops sabaeus (the green African monkey) by oral and other routes. *J Exp Med.* 1941;73:453-459.

397. Trouiller B, et al. Titanium dioxide nanoparticles induce DNA damage and genetic instability in vivo in mice. *Cancer Res.* 2009;69:8784.

398. Tsoli M, et al. Cellular uptake and toxicity of Au55 clusters. *Small.* 2005;1:841-844.

399. Tsukahara T, et al. The role of autophagy as a mechanism of toxicity induced by multi-walled carbon nanotubes in human lung cells. *Int J Mol Sci.* 2014;16:40-48.

400. US Environmental Protection Agency Region 9. *US EPA fines Southern California technology company $208,000 for "nano coating" pesticide claims on computer peripherals.* San Francisco, CA: US Environmental Protection Agency, Region 9; 2008.

401. US Environmental Protection Agency Science Policy Council. *Nanotechnology White Paper.* EPA 100/B-07/001. Washington, DC: US Environmental Protection Agency; 2007.

402. US Food and Drug Administration. Guidance for industry: considering whether a Food and Drug Administration-regulated product involves the application of nanotechnology. *Fed Reg.* 2014;79:36534-365535.

403. US Food and Drug Administration. Guidance for industry: safety of nanomaterials in cosmetic products. *Fed Reg.* 2014;79:36532-36533.

404. US Food and Drug Administration. Use of Nanomaterials in Food for Animals; Guidance for Industry; Availability. *Fed Reg.* 2015;80:46587-46588.

405. US Environmental Protection Agency. *Nanomaterial Case Studies: Nanoscale Titanium Dioxide in Water Treatment and in Topical Sunscreen (Final).* EPA/600/R-09/057F. Washington, DC: US Environmental Protection Agency; 2010.

406. US Environmental Protection Agency. *Nanomaterial Case Study: A Comparison of Multiwalled Carbon Nanotube and Decabromodiphenyl Ether Flame-Retardant Coatings Applied to Upholstery Textiles (External Review Draft).* EPA/600/R-12/043A. Washington, DC: US Environmental Protection Agency; 2012.

407. US Environmental Protection Agency. *Nanomaterial Case Study: Nanoscale Silver in Disinfectant Spray (Final Report).* EPA/600/R-10/081F. Washington, DC: US Environmental Protection Agency; 2012.

408. Unfried K, et al. Cellular responses to nanoparticles: target structures and mechanisms. *Nanotoxicology.* 2007;1:52.

409. Unfried K, et al. Carbon nanoparticle-induced lung epithelial cell proliferation is mediated by receptor-dependent Akt activation. *Am J Physiol Lung Cell Mol Physiol.* 2008;294:L358-L367.

410. United States Code. Title 15 C, § 7501: National Nanotechnology Program; December 3, 2003.

411. Urban RM, et al. Dissemination of wear particles to the liver, spleen, and abdominal lymph nodes of patients with hip or knee replacement. *J Bone Joint Surg Am.* 2000;82:457.

412. Valavanidis A, et al. Airborne particulate matter and human health: toxicological assessment and importance of size and composition of particles for oxidative damage and carcinogenic mechanisms. *J Environ Sci Health C Environ Carcinog Ecotoxicol Rev.* 2008;26:339-362.

413. Vallejo M, et al. Ambient fine particles modify heart rate variability in young healthy adults. *J Expos Sci Environ Epidemiol.* 2005;16:125-130.

414. van Zijverden M, Granum B. Adjuvant activity of particulate pollutants in different mouse models. *Toxicology.* 2000;152:69-77.

415. Wallace LA, et al. Source strengths of ultrafine and fine particles due to cooking with a gas stove. *Environ Sci Technol.* 2004;38:2304-2311.

416. Wallace W, et al. Phospholipid lung surfactant and nanoparticle surface toxicity: lessons from diesel soots and silicate dusts. *J Nanopart Res.* 2007;9:23-38.

417. Walter P, et al. Early use of PbS nanotechnology for an ancient hair dyeing formula. *Nano Lett.* 2006;6:2215-2219.

418. Wang B, et al. Acute toxicological impact of nano- and submicro-scaled zinc oxide powder on healthy adult mice. *J Nanopart Res.* 2008;10:263-276.

419. Wang L, et al. Toxicity of CdSe nanoparticles in caco-2 cell cultures. *J Nanobiotechnology.* 2008;6:11.

420. Warheit DB, et al. Comparative pulmonary toxicity assessment of single-wall carbon nanotubes in rats. *Toxicol Sci.* 2004;77:117-125.

421. Warheit DB, et al. Nanoscale and fine zinc oxide particles: can in vitro assays accurately forecast lung hazards following inhalation exposures? *Environ Sci Technol.* 2009;43:7939.

422. Warriner R, Burrell R. Infection and the chronic wound: a focus on silver. *Adv Skin Wound Care.* 2005;18(suppl 1):2-12.

423. Wei A, et al. Challenges and opportunities in the advancement of nanomedicines. *J Control Release.* 2012;164:236-246.

424. Weldon BA, et al. Occupational exposure limit for silver nanoparticles: considerations on the derivation of a general health-based value. *Nanotoxicology.* 2016;10:945-956.

425. Wensing M, et al. A comment on "Theegarten et al. Submesothelial deposition of carbon nanoparticles after toner exposure: case report. Diagnostic Pathology 2010, 5:77." *Diagn Pathol.* 2011;6:20.

426. Wick P, et al. The degree and kind of agglomeration affect carbon nanotube cytotoxicity. *Toxicol Lett.* 2007;168:121-131.

427. Wielgus A, et al. Phototoxicity and cytotoxicity of fullerol in human retinal pigment epithelial cells. *Toxicol Appl Pharmacol.* 2010;242:79.

428. Winkler DA, et al. Applying quantitative structure-activity relationship approaches to nanotoxicology: current status and future potential. *Toxicology.* 2013;313:15-23.

429. Witzmann FA, Monteiro-Riviere NA. Multi-walled carbon nanotube exposure alters protein expression in human keratinocytes. *Nanomedicine.* 2006;2:158-168.

430. Wiwanitkit V, et al. Effect of gold nanoparticles on spermatozoa: the first world report. *Fertil Steril.* 2009;91:e7-8.

431. Wolinsky H. Nanoregulation: a recent scare involving nanotech products reveals that the technology is not yet properly regulated. *EMBO Rep.* 2006;7:858-961.

432. Wu J, et al. Neurotoxicity of silica nanoparticles: brain localization and dopaminergic neurons damage pathways. *ACS Nano.* 2011;5:4476-4489.

433. Wu M, et al. Enhanced sensitivity to DNA damage induced by cooking oil fumes in human OGG1 deficient cells. *Environ Mol Mutagen.* 2008;49:265-275.

434. Wu Q, et al. Comparison of toxicities from three metal oxide nanoparticles at environmental relevant concentrations in nematode Caenorhabditis elegans. *Chemosphere.* 2013;90:1123-1131.

435. Wu Y, et al. Effects of silver nanoparticles on the development and histopathology biomarkers of Japanese medaka (Oryzias latipes) using the partial-life test. *Aquat Toxicol.* 2010;100:160-167.

436. Xia T, et al. Comparison of the abilities of ambient and manufactured nanoparticles to induce cellular toxicity according to an oxidative stress paradigm. *Nano Lett.* 2006;6:1794-1807.

437. Xia X, et al. Skin penetration and kinetics of pristine fullerenes (C60) topically exposed in industrial organic solvents. *Toxicol Appl Pharmacol.* 2010;242:29.

438. Xia Z, et al. Nano-analyses of wear particles from metal-on-metal and non-metal-on-metal dual modular neck hip arthroplasty. *Nanomedicine.* 2017;13:1205-1217.

439. Yamago S, et al. In vivo biological behavior of a water-miscible fullerene: 14C labeling, absorption, distribution, excretion and acute toxicity. *Chem Biol.* 1995;2:385-389.

440. Yamakoshi Y, et al. •OH and O2•- Generation in aqueous C60 and C70 solutions by photoirradiation: an EPR study. *J Am Chem Soc.* 1998;120:12363-12364.

441. Yamakoshi Y, et al. Active oxygen species generated from photoexcited fullerene (C60) as potential medicines: O2-• versus 1O2. *J Am Chem Soc.* 2003;125:12803-12809.

442. Yamanaka Y, Leong K. Engineering strategies to enhance nanoparticle-mediated oral delivery. *J Biomater Sci Polym Ed.* 2008;19:1549.

443. Yan L, et al. Can graphene oxide cause damage to eyesight? *Chem Res Toxicol.* 2012;25:1265-1270.

444. Yan Z, et al. Zinc oxide nanoparticle-induced atherosclerotic alterations in vitro and in vivo. *Int J Nanomedicine.* 2017;12:4433-4442.

445. Yang W, et al. Food storage material silver nanoparticles interfere with DNA replication fidelity and bind with DNA. *Nanotechnology.* 2009;20:85102.

446. Yarom R, et al. Nephrotoxic effect of parenteral and intraarticular gold. Ultrastructure and electron microprobe examination of clinical and experimental material. *Arch Path.* 1975;99:36.

447. Ye Y, et al. Nano-SiO(2) induces apoptosis via activation of p53 and Bax mediated by oxidative stress in human hepatic cell line. *Toxicol In Vitro.* 2010;24:751-758.

448. Yeo MK, Nam DH. Influence of different types of nanomaterials on their bioaccumulation in a paddy microcosm: a comparison of TiO2 nanoparticles and nanotubes. *Environ Pollut.* 2013;178:166-172.

449. Yokoyama A, et al. Biological behavior of hat-stacked carbon nanofibers in the subcutaneous tissue in rats. *Nano Lett.* 2005;5:157-161.

450. Yoshida S, et al. Effect of nanoparticles on the male reproductive system of mice. *Int J Androl.* 2009;32:337.

451. Yu LE, et al. Translocation and effects of gold nanoparticles after inhalation exposure in rats. *Nanotoxicology.* 2007;1:235.

452. Yue W, et al. Ambient source-specific particles are associated with prolonged repolarization and increased levels of inflammation in male coronary artery disease patients. *Mutat Res.* 2007;621:50-60.

453. Zhang H, et al. Use of metal oxide nanoparticle band gap to develop a predictive paradigm for oxidative stress and acute pulmonary inflammation. *ACS Nano.* 2012;6:4349-4368.

454. Zhang L, et al. The dose-dependent toxicological effects and potential perturbation on the neurotransmitter secretion in brain following intranasal instillation of copper nanoparticles. *Nanotoxicology.* 2012;6:562-575.

455. Zhang Y, et al. In vitro and in vivo toxicity of CdTe nanoparticles. *J Nanosci Nanotechnol.* 2007;7:497-503.

456. Zhou R, Gao H. Cytotoxicity of graphene: recent advances and future perspective. *Wiley Interdiscip Rev Nanomed Nanobiotechnol.* 2014;6:452-474.

457. Zhu L, et al. DNA damage induced by multiwalled carbon nanotubes in mouse embryonic stem cells. *Nano Lett.* 2007;7:3592-3597.

458. Zhu X, et al. Polyacrylate/nanosilica causes pleural and pericardial effusion, and pulmonary fibrosis and granuloma in rats similar to those observed in exposed workers. *Int J Nanomedicine.* 2016;11:1593-1605.

459. Zolnik B, et al. Nanoparticles and the immune system. *Endocrinology.* 2010;151:458.

460. Zsigmondy R. *Colloids and the Ultramicroscope. A Manual of Colloid Chemistry and Ultramicroscopy* [translated by J. Alexander]. New York, NY: John Wiley & Sons; 1909.

CHEMICAL WEAPONS

Jeffrey R. Suchard

HISTORY AND EPIDEMIOLOGY

The first well-documented intentional use of chemicals as weapons occurred in 423 B.C. when Spartans besieging Athenian cities burned pitch-soaked wood and brimstone to produce sulfurous clouds.[88] Large-scale chemical warfare began in World War I when the Germans released chlorine near Ypres, Belgium, killing hundreds of people and forcing 15,000 troops to retreat.[19,48] Both sides rapidly escalated the use of toxic gases released from cylinders or by artillery shells, including various pulmonary irritants, lacrimators, arsenicals, and cyanides.

The Germans first used sulfur mustard in 1917, again near Ypres, and caused more than 20,000 deaths or injuries.[48] The Allies soon responded in kind. Sulfur mustard was unequaled in its ability to incapacitate opponents, often resulting in temporary blindness.[9] Injuries far outweighed fatalities, diverting manpower and resources to care for the wounded. By the end of the war, chemical weapons caused more than 1.3 million casualties and approximately 90,000 deaths.[19]

Germany began producing nerve agents just before World War II. Tabun was developed in 1936 by Gerhard Schräder when conducting insecticide research for IG Farbenindustrie.[30,78] Sarin was synthesized in 1938.[30] Between 10,000 and 30,000 tons of tabun and 5 to 10 tons of sarin were produced during World War II. Soman was synthesized in 1944, but no large-scale production facilities were developed. When the Allies discovered these chemical weapons at the end of the war, code names were designated based on the order of their development. Tabun was called GA (the letter G standing for German), sarin was GB, and soman was GD.[30]

In 1952, the British synthesized an even more potent nerve agent while searching for a dichlorodiphenyltrichloroethane (DDT) replacement. This substance was given to the United States for military development and was named VX. The Russians developed a similar nerve agent, variably referred to as VR or "Russian VX."[38] The United States used defoliants and riot control agents in Vietnam and Laos. Iraq used sulfur mustard, tabun, and soman during its war with Iran in the 1980s and may have also used cyanide against the Kurds.[48] More recently, chlorine and sarin were used by government forces in the Syrian civil war, and the Islamic State used sulfur mustard in Syria and Iraq.[87]

Terrorist groups have also used chemical weapons. Sarin was released twice by the Aum Shinrikyo cult in Japan. The first release occurred in Matsumoto in 1994, killing seven and injuring more than 600.[51] A more highly publicized sarin release occurred in the Tokyo subway system in 1995, killing 12 and resulting in more than 5,000 persons seeking medical attention.[75] Cult members have also used VX in assassinations.[50] Chemical weapons are particularly appealing to terrorist groups because the technology and financial outlay required to produce them is much less than for nuclear weapons, and the potential morbidity, mortality, and societal impact remain high (Table 126–1).

Chemical weapons clearly fall within the purview of medical toxicology. Indeed, unlike the diverse xenobiotics widely studied by toxicologists that unintentionally cause poisonings, chemical weapons are specifically designed to kill, injure, or incapacitate. Some compounds generally considered nonlethal, such as tear gas and pepper spray, are therefore also considered chemical weapons. Biological weapons share some characteristics with chemical weapons (Table 126–2) and are covered in Chap. 127, although the issues common to both chemical and biologic weapons are discussed in this chapter.

This chapter focuses on the acute and long-term clinical effects of exposure to chemical weapons, their mechanisms of toxicity, and the medical treatment of individual casualties based on published human case experience. Many other potential subtopics related to chemical (and biologic)

weapons are not specifically reviewed here, including disaster incident command (Chap. 132), chemical and biological weapon (CBW) agent detection, provision of medical care in a chemically contaminated environment, and evidence accumulated from in vitro and ex vivo models of chemical weapons poisoning.

GENERAL CONSIDERATIONS

Physical Properties

The term *war gas* is generally a misnomer. Sulfur mustard and nerve agents are liquids at normal temperatures and pressures, and many riot-control agents are solids. These weapons are most efficiently dispersed as aerosols, which probably leads to the confusion with gases. Some chemical weapons such as chlorine, phosgene, and hydrogen cyanide are true gases, and although they are generally considered obsolete for battlefield use, they might still be used as improvisational chemical weapons, especially in terrorist attacks.

Liquid chemical weapons have a certain degree of volatility and evaporate into poisonous vapors. Volatility is inversely related to persistence, the tendency to remain in the environment. Persistent chemical weapons, such as mustard or VX, contaminate areas for prolonged periods, denying the opponent free movement and use of contaminated material. The toxic hazard from semipersistent weapons such as sarin and nonpersistent agents such as hydrogen cyanide dissipates more rapidly.

Aerosols, gases, and vapors are highly subject to local atmospheric conditions. Less dispersion occurs with atmospheric inversion layers and in the absence of wind, as typically occurs at night or in the early morning. Enclosed spaces also prevent wind dispersion and simple dilution. Except for hydrogen cyanide, chemical weapon (CW) gases and vapors are all more dense than air and collect in low-lying areas.

As a practical example, in the 1995 sarin release in the Tokyo subway system, photos from the attack show severely affected or deceased victims in very close proximity to mildly affected, ambulatory individuals. The number

TABLE 126–1	Unconventional Weapons: Definitions and Acronyms
Chemical warfare	Intentional use of weapons designed to kill, injure, or incapacitate on the basis of toxic or noxious chemical properties.
Biologic warfare	Intentional use of weapons designed to kill, injure, or incapacitate on the basis of microorganisms or xenobiotics derived from living organisms
Terrorism	The unlawful use of force against persons or property to intimidate or coerce a government, the civilian population, or any segment thereof, in furtherance of political or social objectives.
CW	Chemical warfare, or chemical weapon.
BW	Biological warfare, or biological weapon.
CBW	Chemical and/or biological warfare or weapons.
NBC	Nuclear, biological, and/or chemical; usually in reference to weapons.
CBRNE	Chemical, biological, radiologic, nuclear, and explosive; usually in reference to weapons.
WMD	Weapon of mass destruction; nuclear, radiologic, chemical, or biological weapon intended to produce mass casualties.

TABLE 126–2	Chemical versus Biological Weapons: Comparison and Contrast[27]	
Similarities		
Xenobiotics most effectively dispersed in aerosol or vapor forms		
Delivery systems frequently similar		
Movement of xenobiotics highly subject to wind and weather conditions		
Appropriate personal protective equipment prevents illness		
Differences	**Chemical Weapons (CWs)**	**Biological Weapons (BWs)**
Rate at which attack results in illness	Rapid usually minutes to hours	Delayed usually days to weeks
Identifying release	*Relatively easy:* Rapid clinical effects Possible chemical odor Commercially available chemical detectors	*More difficult:* Delayed clinical effects Lack of color, odor, or taste Limited development of real-time detectors
Xenobiotic persistence	Variable Liquids semipersistent to persistent Gases nonpersistent	Generally nonpersistent; most BW xenobiotics are degraded by sunlight, heat, or desiccation (exception: anthrax spores)
Victim distribution	Near and downwind from release point	Victims may be widely dispersed by the time disease is apparent
First responders	EMTs, hazard materials teams, firefighters, law enforcement officers	Emergency physicians and nurses, primary care practitioners, infectious disease physicians, epidemiologists, public health officials (but will likely be same as CW if release is identified immediately)
Decontamination	Critically important in most cases	Not needed in delayed presentations; less important for acute exposures
Medical treatment	Antidotes, supportive care	Vaccines, antibiotics, supportive care
Patient isolation	Unnecessary after adequate decontamination	Crucial for easily communicable diseases (eg, smallpox, pneumonic plague); however, many BW agents are not easily transmissible

EMT = emergency medical technician.

of fatalities could have been much higher had sarin been effectively aerosolized instead of being simply allowed to evaporate. Presumably, sarin concentrations decreased so rapidly as distance from the source increased that few victims were significantly exposed. After removal from high-concentration areas, the victims' bodies posed less threat to bystanders because of dilution and improved ventilation. Even so, some health care professionals were secondarily exposed because the victims were not disrobed before entering the hospitals. Up to 46% of hospital staff in areas with poor ventilation reported symptoms consistent with mild acute poisoning, although cholinesterase activities were not reported.[56,57,60] About one-third of rescue workers in the 1994 Matsumoto sarin incident also developed mild toxicity. Rescuers arriving at the scene later were less likely to develop symptoms,[52] suggesting that the vapor dissipated over time.

Preparation for Chemical and Biological Weapons (CBW) Incidents

A rational medical response to CBW events differs from the common response to isolated toxicologic incidents. Health care professionals must learn about these unconventional weapons and the expected "toxidromes" that they produce.[1] In addition, health care professionals must protect themselves and their facilities first, or ultimately no one will receive care. New medicolegal and ethical considerations will arise in CBW mass casualty events that otherwise infrequently occur. The greatest good for the greatest number of victims may preclude heroic interventions in a few critical patients. Charges of negligence may later arise regarding delays in treatment or failure to diagnose subtle signs of disease even if such actions were unavoidable at the time. Even if physicians become well versed in the appropriate response to CBW incidents, the question remains as to how many will be willing to continue working in the presence of an actual public health disaster.[31] The responses to chemical and biological weapons will also differ, chiefly because of the more immediate nature of the toxic effects of CWs compared with biological weapons[27] (Table 126–2).

Recommendations for sustained health care facility domestic preparedness include improved training to promptly recognize CBW mass casualty events, efforts to protect health care professionals, and establishment of decontamination and triage protocols.[41] Table 126–3 lists some specific recommendations. Several facets of the response to a CBW event are still being refined, such as the optimal choice of personal protective equipment, determining who needs decontamination and by what means, and what is to be done with wastewater produced by mass decontamination.[37,41] On a

TABLE 126–3	Recommendations for Health Care Facility Response to Chemical and/or Biological Warfare or Weapons Incidents

- Immediate access to personal protective equipment for health care professionals
- Decontamination facilities that can be made operational with minimal delay
- Triage of victims into those able to decontaminate themselves (decreasing the workload for health care providers) and those requiring assistance
- Decontamination facilities permitting simultaneous use by multiple persons and providing some measure of visual privacy
- A brief registration process when patients are assigned numbers and given identically numbered plastic bags to contain and identify their clothing and valuables
- Provision of food, water, and psychological support for staff, who will likely be required to perform for extended periods
- Secondary triage to separate persons requiring immediate medical treatment from those with minor or no apparent injuries who are sent to a holding area for observation
- Providing victims with written information regarding the agent involved, potential short- and long-term effects, recommended treatment, stress reactions, and possible avenues for further assistance
- Careful handling of information released to the media to prevent conflicting or erroneous reports
- Instituting postexposure surveillance

TABLE 126–4	Chemical and/or Biological Warfare or Weapons Phone Numbers/Contacts

Centers for Disease Control and Prevention (CDC)

800-CDC-INFO (800-232-4636); https://www.cdc.gov

CDC Emergency Operations Center: 770-488–7100

CDC Division of Preparedness and Emerging Infections: 404-639–0385

US Army Medical Research Institute of Chemical Defense

410-436-3276 (duty hours), 410-436-3277 (Off Duty Hours)

Federal Bureau of Investigation (FBI)

Find your local FBI field office at http://www.fbi.gov/contact-us/field/field-offices

tactical level, communication can be severely impaired by personal protective gear, which points out the need for loudspeakers or other forms of public address.[41,86]

Individual clinicians and hospitals caring for victims of known or suspected CBW incidents should contact their local department of health, which will likely report the incident to outside agencies such as the US Federal Bureau of Investigation and the Centers for Disease Control and Prevention (Table 126–4).

Decontamination

Decontamination serves two functions: (1) to prevent further absorption and spread of a noxious substance on a given casualty and (2) to prevent spread to other persons. CWs that are exclusively gases at normal temperatures and pressures such as chlorine, phosgene, or hydrogen cyanide only require removing the victim from the area of exposure. Isolated aerosol or vapor exposures, as from volatilized nerve agents or sulfur mustard, are also terminated by leaving the area and may require no skin decontamination of the victims.[48,76] The experience in Japan with sarin suggests that clothing should be removed from victims of nerve agent vapor exposure and placed in airtight receptacles, such as sealed plastic bags. Some of the secondary exposures to sarin were thought to have occurred as nerve agent that had condensed on the victims' clothing revaporized into the ambient air, and this caution probably holds true also for sulfur mustard vapor exposures. Removal and isolation of vapor-exposed clothing is therefore a recommended part of thorough decontamination to prevent secondary exposures.

Chemical weapons dispersed as liquids present the greatest need for decontamination. Because nerve agents are highly potent and have rapid onset of effects, some victims with significant dermal contamination will not survive to reach medical care.[76] Liquid-contaminated clothing must be removed, and, if able, victims should remove their own clothing to prevent cross-contamination.

Decontamination should be done as soon as practicable to prevent progression of disease and should occur outside of health care facilities to prevent contamination of the working environment and secondary casualties. Decontamination near the incident scene would be ideal in terms of timeliness, although logistically this will not be possible in many situations. Field decontamination before transport will also help to avoid loss of vehicles from being contaminated and taken out of service. Evidence supports the likelihood that contaminated victims will present to health care facilities on their own or be transported for care without decontamination.[37] In mass casualty incidents, decontamination efforts will benefit from separating victims into those who can remove their own clothing and shower themselves with minimal direction and assistance, and the more seriously affected who will require full assistance. The degree of protective gear required by the decontamination personnel cannot be predicted in advance and may be difficult to objectively determine at the time of the incident. Level C personal protective equipment may be sufficient for most hospital settings when the source is defined (eg, receiving and decontamination areas); however, if health care professionals begin to develop clinical effects, level B gear with supplied air would become necessary (Chap. 132).[58] When the source of the

contamination is not yet known, level B gear should be used. Chemically contaminated victims presenting to a health care facility should, if possible, be denied entrance until decontaminated. Patients who have already entered a health care facility and are only later determined to be a contamination hazard present a more difficult problem. If the situation allows, such patients should be taken outside for decontamination before returning and the previous care area cordoned off until any remaining safety hazard is assessed and eliminated.

Nerve agents are hydrolyzed and inactivated by solutions that release chlorine, such as household bleach, or solutions that are sufficiently alkaline. To avoid potential dermal and mucous membrane injury, we recommend a 1:10 dilution of household bleach in water (producing a 0.5% sodium hypochlorite solution) not only for nerve agents but also for sulfur mustard and many biologic agents.[41,46,78] Alternatives include regular soap and water or copious water alone. Rapid washing is more important than the choice of cleaning solution because 15 to 20 minutes is necessary for hypochlorite solutions to inactivate chemical agents.[41] Care should be taken to clean the hair, intertriginous areas, axillae, and groin.[78]

Decontamination after sulfur mustard exposure is more problematic than for nerve agents. First, it is more likely that significantly contaminated victims will survive to reach medical care because they often remain asymptomatic for several hours. In addition, the biochemical damage becomes irreversible long before symptoms develop. Decontamination within 1 to 2 minutes is the only effective means of limiting tissue damage from mustard.[80] However, the actual means of mustard decontamination are identical to those for nerve agents. Victims must be disrobed and thoroughly showered. Dilute hypochlorite solutions (eg, 0.5% sodium hypochlorite, a 1:10 dilution of household bleach) are used to inactivate mustard, but copious water irrigation will also suffice.[48] Symptomatic victims of mustard exposure should still be decontaminated, although it is unlikely to benefit that particular individual it can prevent the spread of mustard to others.[80] Lewisite and phosgene oxime must also be decontaminated quickly, although they produce immediate effects, making it more likely that victims will present promptly when decontamination is most effective.

We recommend water irrigation for riot control weapon exposures because hypochlorite solutions may exacerbate skin lesions.[48] With small numbers of victims, ocular decontamination after lacrimator exposure is ideally performed with topical anesthesia and a specially designed lens that facilitates irrigation. Inadequately decontaminated patients exposed to lacrimators can produce secondary cases among health care professionals, so any contaminated clothing should be removed and bagged.

Significant issues remain regarding decontamination measures. The number of people potentially requiring decontamination may easily outstrip capacity. Incidents with hundreds or thousands of victims will necessitate communal showers, selective decontamination, or both. Decontamination wastewater should ideally be contained and treated, but few facilities have the capability or funds to do this. However, wastewater is a minor issue because with large-scale CWs events, the wastewater represents only a small percentage of the total environmental impact.[41]

Risk of Exposure

The actual release of chemical or biologic weapons can be characterized as a low-probability, high-consequence event. Potential sources for civilian exposure include terrorist attacks, inadvertent releases from domestic stockpiles, direct military attacks, and industrial events. Terrorists may sabotage military or industrial stockpiles or directly attack the populace. Experience has shown that physicians are much more likely to encounter hoaxes,[12] isolated cases,[67] or limited incidents with a modest number of casualties.[85] Riot control weapons are exceptions, in that treating riot control weapon and pepper spray victims is a routine occurrence in many urban emergency departments (EDs).

Technical and organizational obstacles decrease the chance of major CBW terrorist events. Obtaining or producing chemical or biologic weapons, although simpler than for nuclear weapons, is only part of the process.

Effective dissemination is difficult if the goal is to maximize casualties. Proper milling of biologics to produce stable, respirable aerosols requires technical sophistication probably only attainable with governmental research support. Low-technology attacks such as food contamination, poisoning of livestock, and enclosed-space weapons dispersal appear more likely to occur than attacks resulting in hundreds, thousands, or millions of casualties. Smaller attacks or merely threatening use of chemical or biologic weapons may be equally consequential from a terrorist's perspective if they exert comparable political influence with significant psychosocial impact.

The chemicals most likely to be used militarily appear to be sulfur mustard and the nerve agents. A "low-tech" terrorist attack could involve the release of toxic industrial chemicals, such as chlorine, phosgene, or ammonia gas, as chemical "agents of opportunity."

Psychological Effects

Either the threat or the actual use of CBW agents presents unique psychological stressors. Even among trained persons, a CBW-contaminated environment will produce high stress through the necessity of wearing protective gear, potential exposure to weapons, high workload intensity, defensive posture, and interactions with dead and dying patients. Disorders of mood, cognition, and behavior will be common among exposed or potentially exposed victims as a result of the uncertainty, fear, and panic that may accompany a CBW incident, even a hoax. The psychological casualties will probably outnumber victims requiring medical treatment. Civilians without training to recognize the clinical effects of exposure to CWs, which includes some health care professionals, are likely to confuse somatic symptoms with true exposure. Medical resources may easily be overwhelmed unless triage can identify those who will benefit most from appropriate counseling, education, and psychological support. Psychiatrists and other disaster mental health personnel should be enlisted in plans to manage CBW incidents for their expertise in treating anxiety, fear, panic, somatization, and grief.[15]

In Israel during the Gulf War, anxiety-related somatic reactions to missile attacks were reported in 18% to 38% of persons surveyed,[10] and more than 500 people sought medical attention in EDs for anxiety.[64] Among 5,510 people seeking medical attention after the Tokyo subway sarin release, only about 25% were hospitalized.[75] Some of the "victims" presented days or even weeks after the incident, apparently feeling unwell and thinking they were exposed.[57,61] Civilian survivors of chemical attacks in the 1980 to 1988 Iran–Iraq War report increased symptoms of depression, anxiety, and post-traumatic stress disorder compared with those exposed to low-intensity conventional warfare.[24] In one longitudinal study of American Persian Gulf War veterans, 4.6% reported their belief that they were exposed to CBWs, despite the lack of any convincing evidence of deliberate exposures, nor of unintended exposure to any significant levels of CWs. Greater combat stress was associated with a higher incidence in belief in such exposures.[81] Another study reported a 64% incidence in belief of CBW exposure among Gulf War veterans.[8] Reported indicators supporting these beliefs included receiving an alert, having physical symptoms, and being told to use protective gear. Belief in exposure to biologics correlated with having received an alert about chemicals, suggesting that CW alerts can spread misinformation and confusion among recipients.

Uncontrolled release of information will compound terror and increase psychological casualties. Imagine the influx of patients resulting from a news report suggesting that anyone with dizziness or nausea be checked for cholinesterase inhibitor toxicity or that fever and cough indicate infection with anthrax.

Israeli Experience during the 1990 to 1991 Gulf War

Israel is probably one of the best prepared countries for CBW disasters. In late 1990, the civilian population was supplied with rubber gas masks, atropine syringes, and Fuller's earth decontamination powder.[64] Major Israeli hospitals conduct chemical practice drills every 3 to 5 years.[86] These drills identified several key lessons, including designating specific hospitals for chemical casualties, blocking hospital access to a single guarded entrance

to prevent internal contamination, and extending nurses' authority to initiate treatment by established protocols. The Israeli plan provides two tiers of triage. The first triage occurs outside of the hospital by protected medical personnel who perform only lifesaving interventions, such as intubation, hemorrhage control, and antidotal therapy. Patients are then decontaminated and enter the hospital. Afterward, patients are triaged again according to severity of illness into separate areas where dedicated health care teams provide the appropriate interventions.[69,86]

Thirty-nine ballistic missiles with conventional warheads were launched against Israel from Iraq in early 1991, with only six missiles causing direct casualties. Many more "injuries" resulted from CBW defensive measures and psychological stress than from physical trauma. Of 1,060 injuries reported from EDs during this time period, 234 persons were directly wounded in explosions (most injuries were minor), and there were only two fatalities from trauma.[33,64] More than 200 people presented for medical evaluation after self-injection of atropine, a few requiring admission to the hospital.[3,33,64] About 540 people sought care for acute anxiety reactions. Some suffocated from improperly used gas masks, fell and injured themselves when rushing to rooms sealed against CBW agents, or were poisoned by carbon monoxide in these airtight rooms.[33,64] Increased rates of myocardial infarction and cerebrovascular accidents were also observed.[64] A survey of hospital staff members found that only 42% would report for duty after a CW attack.[70]

Special Populations

Pregnancy does not appear to be a significant factor in the treatment of women victims of CWs. In the Tokyo subway sarin attack, five victims were identified at one hospital as being pregnant. These women were only mildly affected and were admitted for observation. All had healthy babies, the first one born 3 weeks after the incident.[57,59,61] In Israel, no obstetric complications occurred among women wearing gas masks during labor and delivery.[18,64]

Children differ substantially from adults with regard to CWs effects and decontamination efforts. Children breathe at a lower ground elevation above the ground and at a higher rate than adults. Because nearly all CW gases and vapors are heavier than air, children are exposed to higher concentrations than adults in the same exposure setting and generally exhibit symptoms earlier.[4,66,92] Children are also more susceptible to vesicants and nerve agents than adults with equivalent exposures.[65,92] Children have thinner and more delicate skin, allowing for more systemic absorption and more rapid onset of injury with sulfur mustard. Children have lower activity of endogenous detoxifying enzymes, such as paraoxonase, allowing for greater toxicity with nerve agents. Additionally, children with organic phosphorus compound poisoning less frequently exhibit a muscarinic toxic syndrome than adults and often present with isolated central nervous system (CNS) depression.[65]

Decontamination of children is another feature that requires an age-adjusted approach. Children have a larger surface area-to-mass ratio and are more likely to carry a toxic or fatal dose of a CW on their skin. Most children will need assistance and supervision during decontamination procedures; keeping a mother or other adult guardian with a child should help with both decontamination and thermoregulation.[66]

NERVE AGENTS
Physical Characteristics and Toxicity

Nerve agents are extremely potent organic phosphorus compound cholinesterase inhibitors, and are the most toxic of the known CWs (Fig. 126–1).[48] For example, sarin is 1,000-fold more potent in vitro than the pesticide parathion.[76] Aerosol doses of nerve agents causing 50% human mortality (LD_{50}) range from 400 mg-minute/m³ for tabun down to 10 mg-minute/m³ for VX compared with 2,500 to 5,000 mg-minute/m³ for hydrogen cyanide. Dermal exposure LD_{50}s for these compounds range from 1,700 mg for sarin down to only 6 to 10 mg for VX.[48,76] It is noteworthy that these reported values for toxicity are derived from animal data, limited human exposures, or calculations for previously healthy combatant casualties with offensive use. Data from rats exposed to sarin vapor show that Haber's rule (ie, that the time of exposure to a gas multiplied by the concentration required to cause toxicity is a

Military Designation	Common Name	Chemical Name	Chemical Structure
GA	Tabun	Ethyl-*N*, *N*-dimethylphosphoramidocyanidate	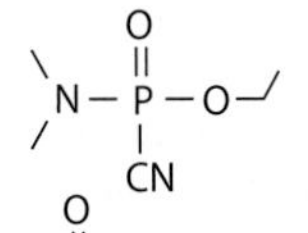
GB	Sarin	Isopropyl-methylphosphonofluoridate	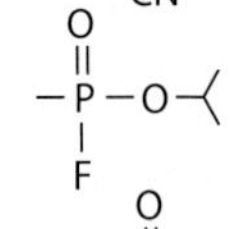
GD	Soman	1, 2, 2-Trimethylpropyl-methyl phosphonofluoridate	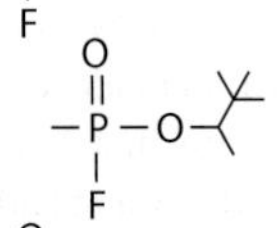
VX	–	*O*-ethyl-*S*-(2-diisopropylaminoethyl)-methylphosphonothiolate	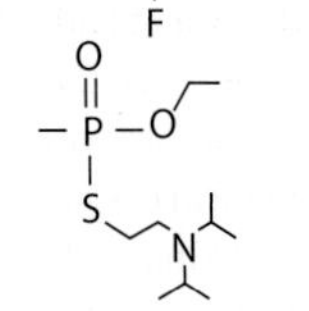

FIGURE 126–1. Nerve agents.

constant) does not hold true across all exposure times, with rats surviving slightly higher concentrations than predicted at the shortest (<10 minutes) and the longest exposure (>200 minutes) times.[49]

Pure nerve agents are clear and colorless. Tabun has a faint fruity odor, and soman is variably described as smelling sweet, musty, fruity, spicy, nutty, or like camphor. Most subjects exposed to sarin and VX were unable to describe the odor.[42,76] The G agents tabun (GA), sarin (GB), and soman (GD) are volatile and present a significant vapor hazard. Sarin is the most volatile, only slightly less so than water. VX is an oily liquid with low volatility and higher environmental persistence.[42,48,76] Other G and V nerve weapons have been developed, including cyclosarin (GF) and Russian VX (VR).

Pathophysiology

The pathophysiology of nerve agents is essentially identical to that from organic phosphorus compound insecticides (Chap. 110), differing only in terms of potency, kinetics, and physical characteristics of the xenobiotics. The resultant toxic syndrome includes muscarinic (salivation, lacrimation, urination, defecation, gastrointestinal {GI} cramping, emesis) and nicotinic (muscle fasciculation, weakness, paralysis) signs, and central effects (loss of consciousness, seizures, respiratory depression).[30,74,78]

Clinical Effects

Nerve agent vapor exposures produce rapid effects, within seconds to minutes, but the effects from liquid exposure are also delayed as the xenobiotic is absorbed through the skin.[76] Vapor or aerosol exposures have historically been more common, whether through experiments or from unintentional releases in the laboratory[74] or in terrorist attacks.[51,61] Aerosol or vapor exposure initially affects the eyes, nose, and respiratory tract. Miosis is common, resulting from direct contact of the xenobiotic with the eye and may persist for several weeks.[74,78] Other ocular effects include conjunctival injection and blurring and dimming of the vision. Dim vision is often ascribed to pupillary constriction, but central neural mechanisms also play a role.[76] Ciliary spasm produces ocular pain, headache, nausea, and vomiting, often exacerbated by near-vision accommodation.[30] Rhinorrhea, airway secretions, bronchoconstriction, and dyspnea occur with increasing exposures. With a large vapor exposure, one or two breaths may produce loss of consciousness within seconds followed by seizures, paralysis, and apnea within minutes.[46]

In the 1995 Tokyo subway sarin incident, ocular effects were most common after sarin vapor exposure, and patients manifested miosis (89%–99% of symptomatic victims), eye pain, dim vision, and decreased visual acuity.[30,61] Other common complaints were cough, throat tightness, nausea, headache, dizziness, chest discomfort, and abdominal cramping.[44,83] Among 111 patients admitted to one hospital, the most common presenting signs and symptoms were miosis (99%), headache (74.8%), dyspnea (63.1%), nausea (60.4%), eye pain (45%), blurred vision (39.6%), dim vision (37.8%), and weakness (36.9%).[57,61] Excessive secretions were less common

because rhinorrhea occurred in approximately one-quarter of patients admitted to one hospital[61] and in none of 58 patients at another.[83] Secondary exposures occurred among emergency medical technicians and hospital personnel in both the Tokyo[44,56,57] and Matsumoto[51,52] terrorist sarin releases, apparently from evaporation of sarin that condensed on the primary victims' clothing.

Liquid nerve agents permeate ordinary clothing, allowing for percutaneous absorption and rendering the clothing of patients' potential hazards to health care personnel before proper decontamination. Mild dermal exposure produces localized sweating and muscle fasciculations after an asymptomatic period lasting up to 18 hours. Moderate skin exposure produces systemic effects with nausea, vomiting, diarrhea, and generalized weakness. Substantial dermal contamination will produce earlier and more severe effects, often with an abrupt onset. Severe toxicity from any route of exposure causes loss of consciousness, seizures, generalized fasciculations, flaccid paralysis, apnea, and/or incontinence.[48,76,78] Cardiovascular effects are less predictable because either bradycardia (muscarinic) or tachycardia (nicotinic) may occur.[46] In the Tokyo sarin event, tachycardia and hypertension were more common than bradycardia.[55,83] Subtle CNS effects can continue for weeks but typically resolve if no anoxic brain injury occurred.

Long-term effects from nerve agent exposure are mostly limited to psychological sequelae.[72] Neither delayed peripheral neuropathy nor the intermediate syndrome are reliably described in humans exposed to these xenobiotics[78,79] Follow-up studies from the Japanese sarin incidents show that neuropathy and ataxia, when initially present, resolved within 3 days to 3 months.[91] The main persistent sequela is posttraumatic stress disorder, found in up to 8% of victims.[29,91]

Treatment of Nerve Agent Exposure
Decontamination

In some critically ill patients, antidotal treatment will be necessary before or during the decontamination process; but generally, decontamination should occur before other treatment is instituted.

Atropine

Atropine (Antidotes in Depth: A35) is the standard anticholinergic antidote for the muscarinic effects of nerve agents.[17] Atropine does not reverse nicotinic effects but does have some central effects and will thus assist in halting seizure activity.[30,42,76]

Atropine is administered parenterally, either by the intravenous (IV) or intramuscular (IM) route, and the dose is determined through titration to effect. The standard adult dose determined by the US military is 2 mg, an amount expected to produce substantial benefit in reversing nerve agent toxicity but one that should be tolerated by a healthy unexposed adult unintentionally receiving the drug.[76] We recommend an initial minimum dose of 2 mg atropine in adults; dosing in children begins at 0.05 mg/kg for mild to moderate symptoms and 0.1 mg/kg for severe symptoms, up to the adult dose.[4] An initial dose of 5 to 6 mg is given for severely poisoned adult patients.[30,76] Repeat doses are given every 2 to 5 minutes until resolution of muscarinic signs of toxicity. Therapeutic endpoints are drying of respiratory secretions and resolution of bronchoconstriction, bradycardia, or seizures (if initially present). Neither reversal of miosis nor development of tachycardia is a reliable marker to guide atropine therapy.[30] The total amount of atropine necessary to treat nerve agent poisoning is often much less than required for organic phosphorus insecticide toxicity of a similar degree. Typically, less than 20 mg is required in the first 24 hours, even in severe cases.[30,76,78] Fewer than 20% of moderately ill patients admitted to one hospital for sarin poisoning in Tokyo required more than 2 mg of atropine.[61] The aforementioned atropine dosing appears to conflict with the experience of an Iranian physician who treated many chemical casualties in the Iran–Iraq War using much higher doses of atropine, starting with 4 mg IV, rapidly titrating by ease of breathing and drying of respiratory secretions, and sometimes giving up to 200 mg. These much higher doses, however, resulted from limited availability of oxime co-antidotal therapy and concern for symptom recurrence during unmonitored victim transport to rearward treatment facilities.[53]

American troops in the 1990 to 1991 Gulf War were issued three MARK I kits for immediate field treatment of nerve agent poisoning. These kits are now also known as NAAKs, for nerve agent antidote kits. Each kit contains two autoinjectors: an AtroPen containing 2 mg of atropine in 0.7-mL diluent and a ComboPen containing 600 mg of pralidoxime chloride (pyridine-2-aldoxime, 2-PAM) in 2 mL of diluent.[76] These autoinjectors permit rapid IM injections of antidote through protective clothing and are given in the lateral thigh.[17] Treatment algorithms guided the number of MARK I kits to administer. In general, conscious casualties not in severe distress self-administer one kit (2 mg of atropine), moderate to severe cases receive three kits (6 mg of atropine) initially, and all receive additional doses as necessary, every 5 to 10 minutes.[17,48,76] A combination atropine (2.1 mg) plus pralidoxime chloride (600 mg) autoinjector is available that gives both drugs with a single injection (Antidotes in Depth: A36).

In a nerve agent mass casualty incident, IV atropine supplies will likely be rapidly depleted from hospital stocks. Alternative sources include atropine from ambulances, ophthalmic and veterinary preparations, or substituting an antimuscarinic such as glycopyrrolate.[30] Facilities expecting large numbers of casualties should store atropine as a bulk powder formulation and rapidly reconstitute it for injection when needed.[20]

Oximes

Oximes are nucleophilic compounds that reactivate organic phosphorus compound–inhibited cholinesterase enzymes by removing the dialkylphosphoryl moiety. The only oxime approved in the United States by the Food and Drug Administration is 2-PAM, a monopyridinium compound. Other pralidoxime salts are used elsewhere, such as the methanesulfonate salt of pralidoxime (P2S) in the United Kingdom and 2-PAM methiodide in Japan. Other oximes include the bispyridinium compounds trimedoxime (TMB4) and obidoxime (toxogonin) used in other European countries.[42,61,76] Oximes should be given in conjunction with atropine because they are not particularly effective in reversing muscarinic effects when given alone. Oximes are the only available nerve agent antidotes that can reverse the neuromuscular nicotinic effects of fasciculations, weakness, and flaccid paralysis (Antidotes in Depth: A36).

Oximes are effective only if administered before irreversible dealkylation, or "aging," of the organic phosphorus compound–cholinesterase complex occurs. Soman has an aging half-life of 2 to 6 minutes in humans.[16] It is unlikely that soman-poisoned victims will reach medical care early enough for oxime therapy to be of great benefit. For comparison, tabun has an aging half-life of about 14 hours, sarin 3 to 5 hours, and VX 48 hours.[16] Pralidoxime is effective against sarin and VX in animal studies. It is ineffectual against tabun because of ineffective nucleophilic attack against that particular agent and not because of aging issues. Obidoxime also is effective against sarin but not against tabun.[42]

The bispyridinium Hagedorn (H-series) oximes, particularly HI-6 and HLö-7, are also studied in the context of nerve agent toxicity.[42] HI-6 appears beneficial against soman poisoning (possibly through direct pharmacologic action or reactivation of aged soman-inhibited ChE) but is not very effective against tabun. HLö-7 has reactivating activity for both soman- and tabun-inhibited ChE and may thus represent a universal oxime antidote for nerve agents. Administration of HI-6 and HLö-7 by autoinjector is difficult because they are not stable in aqueous solution.

For more details about pralidoxime administration, dosing, and adverse events, Antidotes in Depth: A36. The ComboPen autoinjector in MARK I kits contains 600 mg of pralidoxime, which produces a maximal therapeutic serum concentration of 6.5 mcg/mL in average human volunteers.[76] However, when possible, pralidoxime is optimally administered intravenously. Repeat pralidoxime dosing or continuous infusions are less likely to be needed for nerve agents than for organic phosphorus compound insecticides because severe effects are shorter lived in properly decontaminated patients.[30]

Antiepileptics

Severe human nerve agent toxicity rapidly induces convulsions, which persist for a few minutes until the onset of flaccid paralysis. Diazepam is more beneficial than other anticonvulsants and simple γ-aminobutyric acid channel agonists because of its effects on choline transport across the blood–brain barrier and acetylcholine turnover.[42] US military doctrine is to administer 10 mg of diazepam intramuscularly by autoinjector at the onset of severe toxicity whether seizures are present or not. Thus, whenever three MARK I kits are used, a victim is also given diazepam. Additional autoinjectors are given by medical personnel as necessary for seizures.[48] The reason for the IM route of diazepam suggested above is related to timely administration under field conditions. If IV access is feasible, then IV diazepam in 5-mg doses rapidly uptitrated to seizure cessation recommended[42] (Antidotes in Depth: A26). Animal studies suggest that the diazepam dose required to terminate nerve agent seizures may have been underestimated.[45]

Although diazepam is the most well studied benzodiazepine in the treatment of nerve agent toxicity, other medications in the same class such as lorazepam and midazolam have similar or improved beneficial effects in animal studies.[45] Armed service personnel of the United Kingdom are supplied with ComboPens containing atropine sulfate (2 mg); pralidoxime mesylate (P2S; 30 mg); and avizafone (10 mg), a water-soluble prodrug of diazepam.[90]

Pyridostigmine Pretreatment

The first large-scale use of pyridostigmine as a pretreatment for nerve agent toxicity occurred during Operation Desert Storm in 1991.[34] Whereas pyridostigmine is a carbamate acetylcholinesterase inhibitor that is freely and spontaneously reversible, organic phosphorus compound inhibition is permanent after "aging" occurs. Toxicity from rapidly aging weapons such as soman (GD) can probably not be reversed by standard oxime therapy in realistic clinical situations. Almost paradoxically, then, a carbamate can occupy cholinesterase, blocking access of nerve weapons to the active site, and thereby protect the enzyme from permanent inhibition. After nerve agent exposure, pyridostigmine is rapidly hydrolyzed from acetylcholinesterase and can also be easily displaced by oximes, regenerating functional enzyme. Between 20% and 40% cholinesterase inhibition is desired to protect against nerve weapons.[17] Doses of 60 mg of pyridostigmine bromide reduce cholinesterase activity by 28.4% in healthy individuals. Patients with asthma taking 30-mg doses had a mean 24.3% reduction in cholinesterase activity without significant reductions in respiratory function or in response to inhaled atropine.[62] In animal studies, pyridostigmine confers a benefit against soman and tabun but not against sarin or VX.[17] Also, it must be recognized that pyridostigmine is not an antidote but is instead a pretreatment adjunct that greatly enhances the efficacy of atropine and oxime therapy.[78]

US troops in the 1990 to 1991 Gulf War took 30 mg pyridostigmine bromide orally every 8 hours when under threat of nerve agent attack because of concern for potential exposure specifically to soman, which has a short aging half-life. Pyridostigmine pretreatment is not recommended in the civilian sector. Cholinergic side effects, mostly GI, were common but rarely required treatment.[34] Israeli soldiers taking the same dose also reported a range of mostly cholinergic symptoms but also a high incidence (71.4%) of dry mouth, which may be more related to environmental and psychological stressors.[71] Nine Israeli patients were hospitalized during the Gulf War for acute intentional pyridostigmine overdoses.[2] All patients recovered fully, including one patient who self-treated with atropine autoinjectors and presented with anticholinergic toxicity and another who had a cardiac arrest, apparently from coingesting 4,000 mg of propranolol.

VESICANTS

Vesicants are historically designated as "blister agents" because they manifest with blistering of skin and mucous membranes (Fig. 126–2).

Sulfur Mustard

Sulfur mustard is bis(2-chloroethyl) sulfide, a vesicant alkylating compound similar to nitrogen mustards used in chemotherapy. Nineteenth-century scientists described the compound as smelling like mustard, tasting like garlic, and causing blistering of the skin on contact. The Allies of World War I called it Hun Stoffe (also called "German Stuff"), abbreviated as HS and later as just H. Distilled, nearly pure mustard is designated HD. The French called it Yperite, after the site where it was first used, and the Germans called it LOST after the two chemists who suggested its use as a CW, Lommel and Steinkopf. It was also called "yellow cross" after the markings on German artillery shells filled with mustard.[9,14,80] Sulfur mustard caused over 1 million casualties in World War I[21] and was later used by the Italians and Japanese in the 1930s, by Egypt in the 1960s, and by Iraq in the 1980s.[48] About 100,000 Iranians from both military and civilian backgrounds were exposed to vesicant CWs during the latter years of the Iran–Iraq War (1984–1988), many of whom are still suffering long-term effects.[22] Nonbattlefield exposures also occurred among Baltic Sea fishermen while recovering corroding shells dumped after World War II and to persons unearthing or handling old chemical warfare ordinance.[21,54,67,80]

Physical Characteristics

Sulfur mustard is a yellow to brown oily liquid with an odor resembling mustard, garlic, or horseradish. Mustard has relatively low volatility and high environmental persistence. Nonetheless, most historical mustard injuries occurred from vapor exposure, a danger that increases in warmer climates. Mustard vapor is 5.4 times denser than air. Mustard freezes at 57°F (13.9°C), so it is sometimes mixed with other substances, including CW agents such as chloropicrin or Lewisite, to lower the freezing point and permit dispersion as a liquid.[14,48,80]

Pathophysiology

Sulfur mustard toxicity occurs through several mechanisms. First, mustard is an alkylating agent. Mustard spontaneously undergoes intramolecular cyclization to form a highly reactive sulfonium ion that alkylates sulfhydryl (–SH) and amino (–NH₂) groups.[9,14,48,80] This mechanism is the same as occurs with the nitrogen mustards, first developed as cancer chemotherapy agents in the 1940s.[23] The most important acute manifestation is indirect inhibition

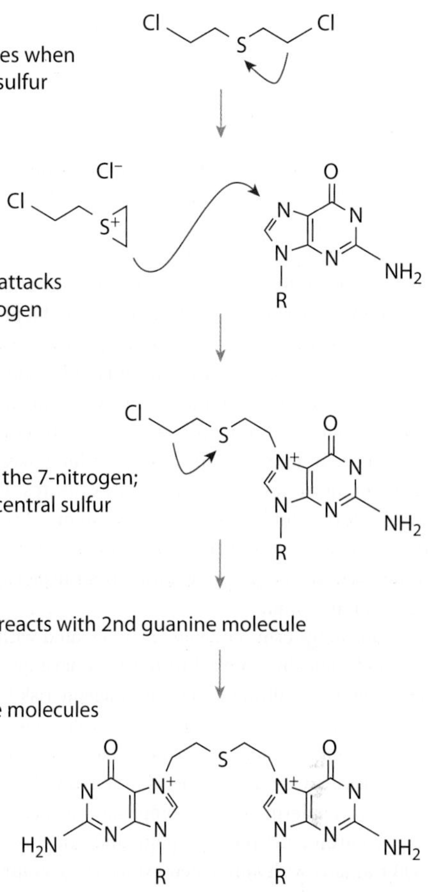

FIGURE 126–3. Mechanism of sulfur mustard toxicity: alkylation and DNA crosslinking.

Sulfur mustard cyclizes when β-carbon attacks sulfur

Cyclic sulfonium ion attacks the guanine 7-nitrogen

Guanine alkylated at the 7-nitrogen; β-carbon attacks central sulfur

Cyclic sulfonium ion reacts with 2nd guanine molecule

Cross-linked guanine molecules

of glycolysis. Sulfur mustard rapidly alkylates and crosslinks purine bases in nucleic acids (Fig. 126–3). DNA repair mechanisms are activated, including the activation of the enzyme poly(ADP-ribose) polymerase,[43] depleting nicotinamide adenine dinucleotide (NAD⁺), which in turn inhibits glycolysis and ultimately leads to cellular necrosis from adenosine triphosphate depletion.[9] Additional mechanisms are likely involved because the inhibition of glycolysis only partially correlates with the depletion of NAD⁺; sulfur mustard may also inhibit glycolysis directly through undetermined mechanisms.[43] Mustard also depletes glutathione, leading to loss of protection against oxidant stress, dysregulation of calcium homeostasis, and further inactivation of sulfhydryl-containing enzymes.[80] Sulfur mustard is also a weak cholinergic agonist.[48,80]

Clinical Effects

The organs most commonly affected by mustard are the eyes, skin, and respiratory tract. During World War I, 80% to 90% of American mustard casualties had cutaneous lesions, 86% had ocular involvement, and 75% had airway injury. Iranian soldiers had more airway (95%) and ocular injuries (92%), and 83% had cutaneous lesions, probably because of the more extensive vaporization occurring in the warmer environment.[9,80] Incapacitation is severe in terms of number of lost man-days, time for lesions to heal, and increased risk of infection. In contrast, the mortality rate is rather low. In World War I, only 2% to 3% of British mustard casualties and fewer than 2% of American casualties died. Fatality rates of 3% to 4% were reported from the Iran–Iraq War.[9] Most deaths occur several days after exposure from respiratory failure, secondary bacterial pneumonia, or bone marrow suppression.

Dermal exposure produces dose-related injury. After a latent period of 4 to 12 hours, victims develop erythema that progresses to vesicles or bullae formation and skin necrosis. Warm, moist, and thin skin is at increased risk of mustard injury, in particular the perineum, scrotum, axillae, antecubital fossae, and neck. The vesicle fluid does not contain mustard because all

Military Designation	Common Name	Chemical Name	Chemical Structure
H, HD	Sulfur mustard	Bis-(2-chloroethyl) sulfide	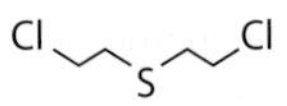
L	Lewisite	2-Chlorovinyldichloroarsine	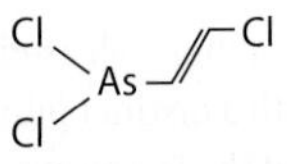
CX	Phosgene oxime	Dichloroformoxime	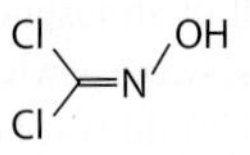

FIGURE 126–2. Vesicants.

chemical reactions are complete within a few minutes. If decontamination is not performed immediately after exposure, injury cannot be prevented. However, later decontamination limits the severity of lesions and further spread of the weapon to develop new lesions. Skin exposure to vapor typically results in first- or second-degree burns, although liquid exposure more commonly results in full-thickness burns.[80] Mustard easily penetrates normal clothing and uniforms, and many soldiers received gluteal, perineal, and scrotal burns from sitting on contaminated objects.

Signs and symptoms of ocular and respiratory tract exposures also occur after a latent period of several hours. Ocular effects include pain, miosis, photophobia, lacrimation, blurred vision, blepharospasm, and corneal damage. Permanent blindness is rare, with recovery generally occurring within a few weeks. Inhalation of mustard results in a chemical tracheobronchitis. Hoarseness, cough, sore throat, and chest pressure are common initial complaints. Bronchospasm and obstruction from sloughed membranes occur in more serious cases, but lung parenchymal damage occurs only in the most severe inhalational exposures. Productive cough associated with fever and leukocytosis is common 12 to 24 hours after exposure and represents a sterile bronchitis or pneumonitis. Nausea and vomiting are common within the first few hours. High-dose exposures also cause bone marrow suppression.[9,48,80]

Various long-term sequelae are associated with sulfur mustard. Factory workers chronically exposed to mustard have increased risk of respiratory tract carcinomas, although the carcinogenic risk from battlefield exposures is more controversial.[21,22,79] Respiratory sequelae include chronic bronchitis, emphysema, tracheobronchomalacia, and bronchiolitis obliterans.[22] Some mustard victims also develop a delayed and often recurrent keratitis.[21,73] Chronic dermatologic complications include scarring, pigmentation changes, chronic neuropathic pain, and pruritus.[21,73] Among approximately 34,000 Iranians with confirmed exposure to sulfur mustard during the war with Iraq, chronic pulmonary sequelae were noted in 42.5%, ocular lesions in 39.3%, and dermatologic lesions in 24.5%.[36]

Treatment

Decontamination is essential in treating the sulfur mustard exposures, even among asymptomatic victims. Further treatment is largely supportive and symptomatic.[9,48,80] Some victims are blinded because of a combination of blepharospasm and corneal edema, which is temporary and completely resolves in most cases. More severe ocular injuries from sulfur mustard are treated with mydriatic and antibiotics drops and applying petroleum jelly to the eyelid edges several times a day.

Several experimental therapies have been proposed for sulfur mustard but are not specifically recommended because of a lack of proven efficacy outside of animal experiments. Antiinflammatory and sulfhydryl-scavenging drugs have shown benefit in animals as prophylactic therapy or if given immediately after exposure.[80] N-Acetylcysteine appears to be a promising therapeutic in cell culture and animal studies, although most of the evidence for its use relates to inhalational aerosol exposures to mustard.[7] Neutropenia from bone marrow suppression, however, should be treated with granulocyte colony–stimulating factor.[47]

Lewisite

Lewisite (2-chlorovinyldichloroarsine) was developed as a less persistent alternative to avoid some shortcomings in the use of sulfur mustard in World War I. Lewisite was never used in combat because the first shipment was en route to Europe when the war ended, and it was intentionally destroyed at sea. British anti-Lewisite (BAL, dimercaprol) was developed as a specific antidote and remains in use for chelation of arsenic and other metals.[42,80]

Pure Lewisite is an oily, colorless liquid. Impure preparations are colored from amber to blue-black to black and have the odor of geraniums. Lewisite is more volatile than mustard and is easily hydrolyzed by water and by alkaline aqueous solutions such as sodium hypochlorite. These properties increase safety for offensive battlefield use, but make maintaining a potent vapor concentration difficult.

Lewisite toxicity is similar to that of sulfur mustard, resulting in dermal and mucous membrane damage, with conjunctivitis, airway injury, and vesiculation. An important clinical distinction is that Lewisite is immediately painful, but initial contact with mustard is not. Other differences are faster onset of inflammatory response and healing of lesions from Lewisite, less secondary infection of Lewisite lesions, and less subsequent pigmentation changes.[80] The mechanisms of Lewisite toxicity are not completely known but appear to involve glutathione depletion and arsenical interaction with enzyme sulfhydryl groups. Nevertheless, Lewisite toxicity is qualitatively and quantitatively different from the arsenic it contains. Treatment consists of decontamination with copious water or dilute hypochlorite solution, supportive care, and BAL. British anti-Lewisite is given parenterally for systemic toxicity and is also used topically for dermal or ophthalmic injuries. Alternative metal chelators that may be used as Lewisite antidotes include dimercaptopropane sulfonate and succimer (2,3-dimercaptosuccinic acid).[42] There is inadequate evidence to recommend one chelating drug over another.

Phosgene Oxime

Although classified as a vesicant, phosgene oxime (dichloroformoxime, or CX) does not cause vesiculation of the skin. CX is more properly an urticant or "nettle" weapon, in that it produces erythema, wheals, and urticaria likened to stinging nettles. Phosgene oxime produces immediate irritation of the skin and mucous membranes. CX has never been used in battle, and little is known about its mechanism or effects on humans.[48,80]

CYANIDES (CHEMICAL ASPHYXIANTS)

Several cyanides have been used as CWs. Historically, the cyanides were classified as "blood agents" because they are first absorbed and then distributed through the body via blood circulation. During World War I, the French used hydrogen cyanide (HCN) and cyanogen chloride (CNCl), designated as agents AC and CK, respectively, without great success; the Austrians introduced cyanogen bromide (CNBr). Cyanide weapons are relatively ineffective because of rapid dispersion and their "all or nothing" biologic activity. An exposed individual either rapidly succumbs to cyanide toxicity or will rapidly recover with minimal sequelae. Mass casualty events from cyanide CW are reported during the Iran–Iraq War and from Iraq's suppression of the Kurds.[5,48]

The clinical effects and treatment of cyanide toxicity are covered elsewhere (Chaps. 123 and 126) and do not differ significantly if used as a weapon. Hydrocyanic acid gas persists for only a few minutes in the atmosphere because it is lighter than air and rapidly disperses. Cyanogen chloride additionally causes ophthalmic and respiratory tract irritation and with sufficiently high exposures is reported to produce delayed acute respiratory distress syndrome (ARDS) in victims who are not rapidly killed.[5,48]

PULMONARY IRRITANTS

Chlorine, phosgene, and diphosgene (DP, trichloromethylchloroformate) were used as war gases in World War I. Chlorine, phosgene, diphosgene, various organohalides, and nitrogen oxides belong to a group of toxic chemicals designated "pulmonary irritants" because they can all induce delayed ARDS from increased alveolar-capillary membrane permeability.[42,48,88] Until chlorine attacks during the Syrian civil war,[87] pulmonary irritants had not been used militarily since 1918. Nevertheless, the risk of chlorine and phosgene exposure remains because of their extensive use in industry and their possible appropriation as terrorist weapons; see Chap. 121 for clinical details because the remainder of this section highlights mass casualty issues regarding these irritant gases.

When released on the battlefield, chlorine forms a yellow-green cloud with a distinct pungent odor detectable at concentrations that are not immediately dangerous. Phosgene is either colorless or seen as a white cloud as a result of atmospheric hydrolysis. Phosgene, which is reported to smell like grass, sweet newly mown hay, corn, or moldy hay, accounted for about 85% of all World War I deaths attributed to CWs.[9,42] Phosgene produces injury by hydrolysis in the lungs to hydrochloric acid and by forming diamides that

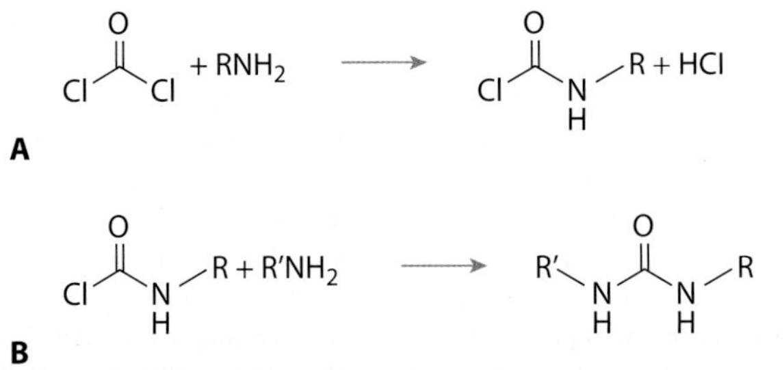

FIGURE 126–4. Proposed mechanism of phosgene toxicity. (**A**) Phosgene reacts with amine group to form an amide, releasing hydrochloric acid. (**B**) A second reaction crosslinks two amine equivalents, forming a diamide.

cross-link cell components (Fig. 126–4). Similar cross-linking reactions occur with hydroxyl and thiol groups. Battlefield exposure triggers cough, chest discomfort, dyspnea, lacrimation, and the peculiar complaint that smoking tobacco produces an objectionable taste. World War I phosgene fatalities were noted to develop a mushroom-shaped efflux of pink foam at their mouths resulting from the acute lung injury. Prolonged observation after phosgene exposure is the rule because some casualties initially appeared well and were discharged, only to return in severe respiratory distress a few hours later.[42,48,88] Exercise appeared to precipitate ARDS in phosgene casualties.[68] For American soldiers in World War I, the average times spent recovering away from the front were 60 days for chlorine and 45.5 days for phosgene.[19]

RIOT CONTROL AGENTS

Riot control agents (Fig. 126–5) are intentionally nonlethal chemicals that temporarily disable exposed individuals through intense irritation of exposed mucous membranes and skin. These weapons are also known as lacrimators, irritants, harassing agents, human repellents, and tear gas. They are solids at normal temperatures and pressures but are typically dispersed as aerosols or as small solid particles in liquid sprays. Common characteristics include rapid onset of effects within seconds to minutes, relatively brief duration after exposure has ceased and the victim is decontaminated, and a high safety ratio (lethal dose versus effective dose).[42,48,77]

Chloroacetophenone (CN) is the active ingredient in the Chemical Mace brand nonlethal weapon.[82] o-Chlorobenzilidene malononitrile (CS) has largely replaced CN because of its higher potency, lower toxicity, and improved chemical stability.[39,77] When used for crowd control, both CN

and CS are disseminated as aerosols or as smoke from incendiary devices. CR (dibenzoxazepine) is a similar weapon with prominent skin irritation. Exposed persons develop burning irritation of the eyes, progressing to conjunctival injection, lacrimation, photophobia, and blepharospasm. Mucous membranes of the upper aerodigestive tracts are frequently also involved. Inhalation causes chest tightness, cough, sneezing, and increased secretions. Dermal exposure causes a burning sensation, erythema, or vesiculation, depending on the dose. Victims generally remove themselves from the offensive environment (which is the primary purpose of their use for "riot control") and recover within 15 to 30 minutes. Deaths are rare and typically occur from respiratory tract complications in closed-space exposures where exiting the area is impossible.[42,48,77]

The biologic mechanism whereby riot control agents exert their effects is less well described than for other CWs. o-Chlorobenzylidene malononitrile (CS) and CN are SN_2 alkylating agents (versus sulfur mustard, an SN_1 alkylator) and react with sulfhydryl-containing compounds and enzymes. For instance, CS reacts rapidly with the disulfhydryl form of lipoic acid, a coenzyme for pyruvate decarboxylase. Pain in the absence of tissue injury is likely to be bradykinin mediated.[48]

Personal protective devices dispensing lacrimator substances also cause chemical injuries in the absence of war or civil unrest. Law enforcement agencies and private citizens have access to products containing CS, CN, or (oleoresin capsicum {OC}, also known as pepper spray). OC is the essential oil derived from pepper plants (*Capsicum anuum*), which contains capsaicin (trans-8-methyl-N-vanillyl-6-noneamide), a naturally occurring lacrimator. Capsaicin activates the TRPV1 receptor, a heat-dependent nociceptor, explaining why exposures are experienced as "hot."[11] Severe skin injuries,[26] respiratory tract injuries, and fatalities are occasionally reported from exposures to these devices, typically only with prolonged or highly concentrated exposures.

Chloropicrin (PS, trichloronitromethane, or nitrochloroform) is another lacrimator that occasionally causes human toxicity through its use as a broad-spectrum fumigant and soil insecticide, as well as a warning agent associated with structural fumigants such as sulfuryl fluoride.[84] 10-Chloro-5,10-dihydrodiphenarsazine (or diphenylaminechlorarsine {DM}) induces vomiting in addition to irritant effects. Because symptoms are delayed, victims remain in the area, and the likelihood of significant absorption is increased. In addition to upper respiratory and ocular irritation, diphenylaminearsine causes more prolonged systemic effects with headache, malaise, nausea, and vomiting.[48,77]

Military Designation	Common Name	Chemical Name	Chemical Formula
CN	Chemical Mace	1-chloroacetophenone	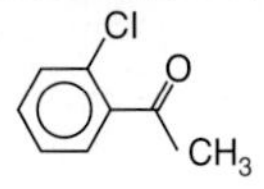
CS	Tear gas	o-chlorobenzylidene malononitrile	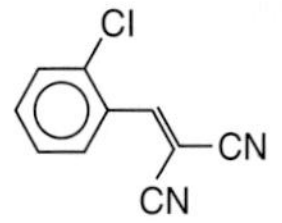
CR	Tear gas DBO	dibenzo[b,f][1,4]oxazepine	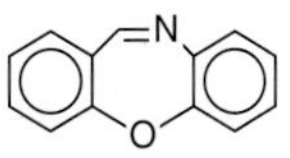
DM	Adamsite	diphenylaminechlorarsine	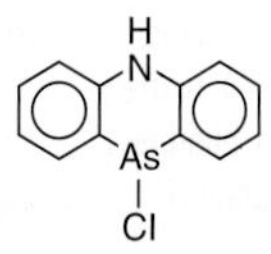
OC	Capsaicin pepper spray	Trans-8-methyl-N-vanillyl-6-noneamide	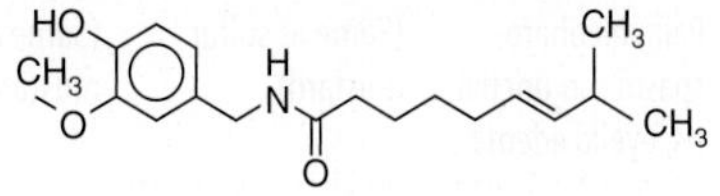

FIGURE 126–5. Riot control agents.

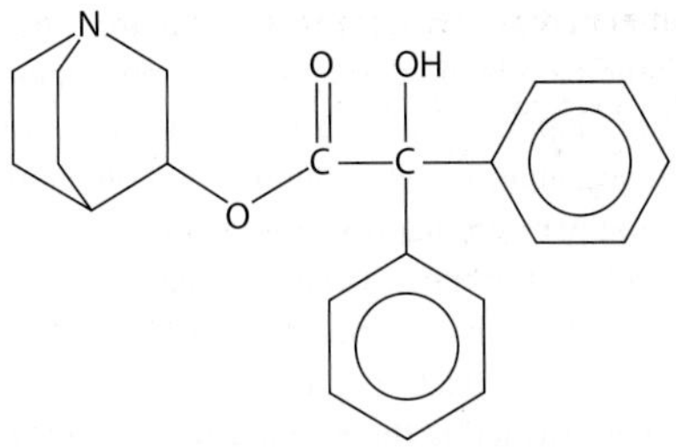

FIGURE 126–6. BZ, 3-quinuclidinyl benzilate (QNB).

The primary treatment for all riot control agents is removal from exposure. Contaminated clothing should be removed and placed in airtight bags to prevent secondary exposures.[39] Skin irrigation with copious cold water should be used for significant dermal exposures.[6,39,40] Symptomatic treatments, such as with topical ophthalmic anesthetics, nebulized bronchodilators, or oral antihistamines and corticosteroids, are indicated for directed therapy in more severely affected victims.[6] Capsaicin-induced dermatitis has been treated variably with immersion in water or oil, vinegar, bleach, lidocaine gel, and topical antacid suspensions.[28,32,82] Cold water produces earlier symptomatic relief, but oil immersion has longer lasting benefits.[32] Given that it is more readily available in most settings, cold water immersion is the treatment of choice.

INCAPACITATING AGENTS

3-Quinuclidinyl benzilate (BZ or QNB; Fig. 126–6) is an antimuscarinic compound that was developed as an incapacitating CW agent. BZ is 25-fold more potent centrally than atropine, with an ID_{50} (dose that incapacitates 50% of

those exposed) of about 0.5 mg. Clinical effects are characteristic for anticholinergics, with drowsiness, poor coordination, and slowing of thought processes progressing to delirium. BZ takes at least 1 hour to produce initial manifestations, peaks at 8 hours, continues to incapacitate for 24 hours, and takes 2 to 3 days to fully resolve.[35] During the Balkan Wars of the 1990s, allegations were made that Bosnian Serbs used BZ against civilians, who reported hallucinations associated with attacks by artillery shells emitting smoke.[25] Agent 15 is a similar incapacitating weapon to BZ, reportedly researched by Iraq prior to the Persian Gulf War but not mass produced or used.[12]

Ultrapotent opioids can be used as incapacitating CWs. In 2002, Russian security forces used a fentanyl derivative (carfentanil or remifentanil) to end a 3-day standoff with terrorists in a Moscow theater in which Chechen rebels held more than 800 hostages.[63,89] A "gas" was introduced into the theater ventilation system, which quickly subdued the occupants. More than 650 of the hostages were hospitalized, and 128 died. Initial news reports suggested the use of BZ, although the clinical findings were more consistent with a CNS depressant. Within a few days, Russian officials stated that a fentanyl derivative was used and was not expected to cause fatalities. The relatively high case fatality rate could be because of multiple factors, including variability in dose, displacement of oxygen by rapid introduction of gas into the building, failure to adequately notify health care teams and supply them with antidotes, and the poor physical condition of the hostages, coupled with their immobility.

Lysergic acid diethylamide (LSD) has also been investigated as an incapacitating weapon.[35] Although effective at very low doses, battlefield use of LSD is impractical because intoxication will not reliably prevent a soldier from participation in combat.

Table 126–5 describes the various toxic syndromes associated with use of CWs.

TABLE 126–5	Chemical Weapons Toxic Syndromes							
			Organ System					
Chemical Weapon	**Onset**	**Eyes**	**Upper Airways and Mucous Membranes**	**Lungs**	**Skin**	**CNS**	**GI Tract**	**Other**
Nerve Agents								
Tabun (GA), Sarin (GB), Soman (GD), VX								
Aerosol/vapor (Mild/moderate exposure)	Rapid (seconds–minutes)	Miosis, eye pain, dim or blurred vision	Rhinorrhea, ↑secretions	Dyspnea, cough, wheezing, bronchorrhea	—	Headache	Nausea, vomiting, abdominal cramps	—
Dermal exposure (mild to moderate exposure)	Delayed (minutes–hours)	—	—	—	Localized sweating	—	—	—
Severe exposure (any route)	As above (by route)	Miosis	↑ Secretions	Apnea	—	Sudden collapse, seizures	Nausea, vomiting, diarrhea, cramping, incontinence	Subjective weakness local muscle fasciculations generalized fasciculations, weakness, flaccid paralysis
Vesicants								
Sulfur mustard (H, HD)	Delayed (hours)	Conjunctivitis, eye pain, blurred vision, blindness (temporary)	Irritation, hoarseness, barky cough, sinus tenderness tracheobronchitis	(More severe exposures) Productive cough, pseudomembrane formation, airway obstruction	Erythema, vesicles, bullae, necrosis	—	Nausea, vomiting	Bone marrow suppression (in severe exposures)
Lewisite (L)	Immediate irritation	Pain, blepharospasm conjunctivitis, eyelid edema	(Same as sulfur mustard)	(Same as sulfur mustard)	Erythema, vesicles	—	—	Shock (in severe exposures)

(Continued)

TABLE 126–5 Chemical Weapons Toxic Syndromes (Continued)

			Organ System					
Chemical Weapon	**Onset**	**Eyes**	**Upper Airways and Mucous Membranes**	**Lungs**	**Skin**	**CNS**	**GI Tract**	**Other**
Phosgene oxime (CX)	Delayed vesication Immediate irritation Delayed urticaria	Pain, corneal damage	Irritation	ARDS	Pain, blanching, erythema, urticaria, necrosis	—	—	—
Toxic Inhalants								
Phosgene (CG) Chlorine (CL)	Immediate Irritation Delayed ARDS	Irritation	Irritation, stridor (Chlorine)	Dyspnea, cough, ARDS	—	—	—	Chlorine effects more rapid than phosgene
Cyanides								
Hydrogen cyanide (AC)	Rapid (seconds–minutes)	—	—	Hyperpnea and then apnea	—	Anxiety, agitation, sudden collapse, seizures	—	—
Cyanogen chloride (CK)	Rapid (seconds–minutes)	Irritation	Irritation	Hyperpnea and then apnea	—	Anxiety, agitation, sudden collapse, seizures	—	—
Riot Control Agents								
Lacrimators (CN, CS) Capsaicin (OC)	Immediate	Pain, lacrimation, blepharospasm, conjunctivitis	Irritation	Cough, chest pain	Burning pain, erythema Vesiculation (severe exposures)	—	Nausea, retching (may occur with CN or CS)	—
Adamsite (DM)	Rapid (minutes)	Irritation	Irritation, sneezing	Cough, chest pain	—	Headache	Nausea, vomiting, abdominal cramps	—
Incapacitating Agents								
3-quinuclidinyl benzilate (BZ)	Delayed (hours)	Mydriasis	Dry mouth	—	—	Anticholinergic delirium	—	—
Ultrapotent opioids	Rapid (seconds–minutes)	Miosis	—	Hypoventilation	—	CNS depression	—	—

— = not an expected major finding; ARDS = acute respiratory distress syndrome; CN = chloroacetophenone; CNS = central nervous system; CS = o-chlorobenzylidene malononitrile; GI = gastrointestinal.

SUMMARY

- Chemical and biological weapons are appealing to terrorist groups because the impact in terms of death, disability, economic losses, panic, and defensive posture remains high.
- The psychological impact of CBW terrorism will likely exceed that for conventional or nuclear weapons.
- Although the probability of incidents resulting in widespread public health disasters appears low, the consequences are high, and substantial preparations must be made in advance.
- Early decontamination is often critical for victims exposed to CWs.
- Nerve agents are potent organic phosphorus compound acetylcholinesterase inhibitors. Toxicity produces cholinergic toxicity, which is treated with antimuscarinics, primarily atropine, and oximes.
- Vesicant CWs induce blistering of the skin and damage to other tissues in contact, such as the eyes or respiratory tract. Sulfur mustard has no specific antidote, but the arsenic containing Lewisite is treated with BAL, a chelator.
- Exposure to chlorine, phosgene, ammonia and some other gases can produce delayed ARDS. Although used on the battlefield in World War I, it is expected that intentional use of these pulmonary irritant gases is now more likely to occur from their use by terrorists as "agents of opportunity."

REFERENCES

1. Alexander GC, et al. Physicians' preparedness for bioterrorism and other public health priorities. *Acad Emerg Med.* 2006;13:1238-1241.
2. Almog S, et al. Acute pyridostigmine overdose: a report of nine cases. *Isr J Med Sci.* 1991;27:659-663.
3. Amitai Y, et al. Atropine poisoning in children during the Persian Gulf crisis: a national survey in Israel. *JAMA.* 1992;268:630-632.
4. Baker MD. Antidotes for nerve agent poisoning: should we differentiate children from adults? *Curr Opin Pediatr.* 2007;19:211-215.
5. Baskin SI, Brewer TG. Cyanide poisoning. In: Sidell FR, et al, eds. *Medical Aspects of Chemical and Biological Warfare.* Washington, DC: Office of the Surgeon General; 1997:271-286.
6. Blaho K, Winbery S. "Safety" of chemical batons. *Lancet.* 1998;352:1633.
7. Bobb AH, et al. N-acetyl-L-cysteine as prophylaxis against sulfur mustard. *Mil Med.* 2005;170:52-56.
8. Brewer NT, et al. Why people believe they were exposed to biological or chemical warfare: a survey of Gulf War veterans. *Risk Analysis.* 2006;2:337-345.
9. Borak J, Sidell FR. Agents of chemical warfare: sulfur mustard. *Ann Emerg Med.* 1992; 21:303-308.
10. Carmell A, et al. Anxiety-related somatic reactions during missile attacks. *Isr J Med Sci.* 1991;27:677-680.
11. Caterina MJ, et al. The capsaicin receptor: a heat-activated ion channel in the pain pathway. *Nature.* 1997;389:816-824.
12. Centers for Disease Control and Prevention. Bioterrorism alleging use of anthrax and interim guidelines for management—United States 1998. *MMWR Morbid Mortal Wkly Rep.* 1999;48:69-74.

13. Central Intelligence Agency. *Intelligence Update: Chemical Warfare Agent Issues During the Persian Gulf War, April 2002.* https://www.cia.gov/library/reports/general-reports-1/gulfwar/cwagents/index.htm#appendixa1.

14. Dacre JC, Goldman M. Toxicology and pharmacology of the chemical warfare agent sulfur mustard. *Pharmacol Rev.* 1996;48:289-326.

15. DiGiovanni C. Domestic terrorism with chemical or biological agents: psychiatric aspects. *Am J Psychiatr.* 1999;156:1500-1505.

16. Dunn MA, et al. Pretreatment for nerve agent exposure. In: Sidell FR, et al, eds. *Medical Aspects of Chemical and Biological Warfare.* Washington, DC: Office of the Surgeon General; 1997:181-196.

17. Dunn MA, Sidell FR. Progress in medical defense against nerve agents. *JAMA.* 1989; 262:649-652.

18. Elchalal U, et al. Delivery with gas mask during missile attack. *Lancet.* 1991;337:242.

19. Fitzgerald GJ. Chemical warfare and medical response during World War I. *Am J Public Health.* 2008;98:611-625.

20. Geller RJ, et al. Atropine availability as an antidote for nerve agent casualties: validated rapid reformulation of high concentration atropine from bulk powder. *Ann Emerg Med.* 2003;41:453-456.

21. Geraci M. Mustard gas: imminent danger or eminent threat? *Ann Pharmacother.* 2008;42:237-246.

22. Ghanei M, Harandi AA. Long term consequences from exposure to sulfur mustard: a review. *Inhal Toxicol.* 2007;19:451-456.

23. Goodman LS, et al. Nitrogen mustard therapy: use of methyl-bis (β-chloroethyl) amine hydrochloride and tris (β-chloroethyl) amine hydrochloride for Hodgkin's disease, lymphosarcoma, leukemia, and certain allied and miscellaneous disorders. *JAMA.* 1946;132:126-32.

24. Hashemian F, et al. Anxiety, depression, and posttraumatic stress in Iranian survivors of chemical warfare. *JAMA.* 2006;296:560-566.

25. Hay A. Surviving the impossible: the long march from Srebrenica. An investigation of the possible use of chemical warfare agents. *Med Confl Surviv.* 1998;14:120-155.

26. Hay A, et al. Skin injuries caused by new riot control agent used against civilians on the West Bank. *Med Confl Surviv.* 2006;22:283-291.

27. Henderson DA. The looming threat of bioterrorism. *Science.* 1999;283:1279-1282.

28. Herman LM, et al. Treatment of mace dermatitis with topical antacid suspension. *Am J Emerg Med.* 1998;16:613-614.

29. Hoffman A. A decade after the Tokyo sarin attack: a review of neurological follow-up of the victims. *Mil Med.* 2007;172:607-610.

30. Holstege CP, et al. Chemical warfare nerve agent poisoning. *Crit Care Clin.* 1997;13: 923-942.

31. Iserson KV, et al. Fight or flight: the ethics of emergency physician disaster response. *Ann Emerg Med.* 2008;51:345-353.

32. Jones LA, et al. Household treatment for "chile burns" of the hands. *J Toxicol Clin Toxicol.* 1987;25:483-491.

33. Karsenty E, et al. Medical aspects of the Iraqi missile attacks on Israel. *Isr J Med Sci.* 1991;27:603-607.

34. Keeler JR, et al. Pyridostigmine used as a nerve agent pretreatment under wartime conditions. *JAMA.* 1991;266:693-695.

35. Ketchum JS, Sidell FR. Incapacitating agents. In: Sidell FR, et al, eds. *Medical Aspects of Chemical and Biological Warfare.* Washington, DC: Office of the Surgeon General; 1997:287-305.

36. Khateri S, et al. Incidence of lung, eye, and skin lesions as late complications in 34,000 Iranians with wartime exposure to mustard agent. *J Occup Environ Med.* 2003; 45:1136-1143.

37. Koenig KL, et al. Health care facility-based decontamination of victims exposed to chemical, biological, and radiological materials. *Am J Emerg Med.* 2008;26:71-80.

38. Kuca K, et al. Inhibition and reactivation of acetylcholinesterase compared with VX agent. *Basic Clin Pharm Tox.* 2006;98:389-394.

39. "Safety" of chemical batons [editorial]. *Lancet.* 1998;352:159.

40. Lee BH, et al. Treatment of exposure to chemical personal protection agents. *Ann Emerg Med.* 1984;13:487-488.

41. Macintyre AG, et al. Weapons of mass destruction events with contaminated casualties: effective planning for health care facilities. *JAMA.* 2000;283:242-249.

42. Marrs TC, et al. Chemical warfare agents. *Toxicology and Treatment.* Chichester, UK: John Wiley & Sons, 1996.

43. Martens ME, Smith WJ. The role of NAD⁺ depletion in the mechanism of sulfur mustard-induced metabolic injury. *Cutan Ocul Toxicol.* 2008;27:41-53.

44. Masuda N, et al. Sarin poisoning in Tokyo subway. *Lancet.* 1995;345:1446.

45. McDonough JH. Midazolam: an improved anticonvulsant treatment for nerve agent-induced seizures. *ADA409494 Proceedings of the 2001 ECBC Scientific Conference on Chemical and Biological Defense Research*, March 6–8, Hunt Valley, MD.

46. Treatment of nerve gas poisoning. *Med Lett Drugs Ther.* 1995;37:43-44.

47. Prevention and treatment of injury from chemical warfare agents. *Med Lett Drugs Ther.* 2002;44:1-4.

48. *Medical Management of Chemical Casualties Handbook.* 4th ed. Proving Ground, MD: US Army Medical Research Institute of Chemical Defense, Chemical Casualty Care Division; 2007. http://www.globalsecurity.org/wmd/library/policy/army/other/mmcc-hbk_4th-ed.pdf.

49. Mioduszewski R, et al. Interaction of exposure concentration and duration in determining acute toxic effects of sarin vapor in rats. *Toxicol Sci.* 2002;66:176-184.

50. Morimoto F, et al. Intoxication of VX in humans. *Am J Emerg Med.* 1999:17:493-494.

51. Morita H, et al. Sarin poisoning in Matsumoto, Japan. *Lancet.* 1995;346:290-293.

52. Nakajima T, et al. Sarin poisoning of a rescue team in the Matsumoto sarin incident in Japan. *Occup Environ Med.* 1997;54:697-701.

53. Newmark J. The birth of nerve agent warfare: lessons from Syed Abbas Foroutan. *Neurology.* 2004;62:1590-1596.

54. Newmark J, et al. Liquid sulfur mustard exposure. *Mil Med.* 2007;172:196-198.

55. Nozaki H, Aikawa N. Sarin poisoning in Tokyo subway. *Lancet.* 1995;345:1446-1447.

56. Nozaki H, et al. Secondary exposure of medical staff to sarin vapor in the emergency room. *Intensive Care Med.* 1995;21:1032-1035.

57. Ohbu S, et al. Sarin poisoning on Tokyo subway. *South Med J.* 1997;90:587-593.

58. Okumura S, et al. Clinical review: Tokyo—protecting the health care worker during a chemical mass casualty event: an important issue of continuing relevance. *Crit Care.* 2005;9:397-400.

59. Okumura T. Organophosphate poisoning in pregnancy. *Ann Emerg Med.* 1997;29:299.

60. Okumura T, et al. The Tokyo subway sarin attack: disaster management, part 2: hospital response. *Acad Emerg Med.* 1998;5:618-624.

61. Okumura T, et al. Report of 640 victims of the Tokyo subway sarin attack. *Ann Emerg Med.* 1996;28:129-135.

62. Ram Z, et al. The effect of pyridostigmine on respiratory function in healthy and asthmatic volunteers. *Isr J Med Sci.* 1991;27:664-668.

63. Riches JR, et al. Analysis of clothing and urine from Moscow theatre siege casualties reveals carfentanil and remifentanil use. *J Anal Tox.* 2012;36:647-656.

64. Rivkind A, et al. Emergency preparedness and response in Israel during the Gulf War. *Ann Emerg Med.* 1998;32:224-233.

65. Rotenberg JS. Diagnosis and management of nerve agent exposure. *Pediatr Ann.* 2003; 32:242-250.

66. Rotenberg JS, et al. Weapons of mass destruction: the decontamination of children. *Pediatr Ann.* 2003;32:260-267.

67. Ruhl CM, et al. A serious skin sulfur mustard burn from an artillery shell. *J Emerg Med.* 1994;12:159-166.

68. Russell D, et al. Clinical management of casualties exposed to lung damaging agents: a critical review. *Emerg Med J.* 2006;23:421-424.

69. Shapira Y, et al. Outline of hospital organization for a chemical warfare attack. *Isr J Med Sci.* 1991;27:616-622.

70. Shapira Y, et al. Willingness of staff to report to their hospital duties following an unconventional missile attack: a state-wide survey. *Isr J Med Sci.* 1991;27:704-711.

71. Sharabi Y, et al. Survey of symptoms following intake of pyridostigmine during the Persian Gulf war. *Isr J Med Sci.* 1991;27:656-658.

72. Sharp D. Long-term effects of sarin. *Lancet.* 2006;367:95-97.

73. Shorati M, et al. Cutaneous and ocular late complications of sulfur mustard in Iranian veterans. *Cutan Ocul Toxicol.* 2007;26:73-81.

74. Sidell FR. Clinical effects of organophosphorus cholinesterase inhibitors. *J Appl Toxicol.* 1994;14:111-113.

75. Sidell FR. Chemical agent terrorism. *Ann Emerg Med.* 1996;28:223-224.

76. Sidell FR. Nerve agents. In: Sidell FR, et al, eds. *Medical Aspects of Chemical and Biological Warfare.* Washington, DC: Office of the Surgeon General; 1997:129-179.

77. Sidell FR. Riot control agents. In: Sidell FR, et al, eds. *Medical Aspects of Chemical and Biological Warfare.* Washington, DC: Office of the Surgeon General; 1997:307-324.

78. Sidell FR, Borak J. Chemical warfare agents: II. Nerve agents. *Ann Emerg Med.* 1992; 21:865-871.

79. Sidell FR, Hurst CG. Long-term health effects of nerve agents and mustard. In: Sidell FR, et al, eds. *Medical Aspects of Chemical and Biological Warfare.* Washington, DC: Office of the Surgeon General; 1997:229-246.

80. Sidell FR, et al. Vesicants. In: Sidell FR, et al, eds. *Medical Aspects of Chemical and Biological Warfare.* Washington, DC: Office of the Surgeon General; 1997:197-228.

81. Stuart JA, et al. Belief in exposure to chemical and biological agents in Persian Gulf War soldiers. *J Nerv Ment Dis.* 2008;196:122-127.

82. Suchard JR. Treatment of capsaicin (Mace?) dermatitis. *Am J Emerg Med.* 1999;17:210-211.

83. Suzuki T, et al. Sarin poisoning in Tokyo subway. *Lancet.* 1995;345:980.

84. TeSlaa G, et al. Chloropicrin toxicity involving animal and human exposure. *Vet Hum Toxicol.* 1986;28:323-324.

85. Török TJ, et al. A large community outbreak of salmonellosis caused by intentional contamination of restaurant salad bars. *JAMA.* 1997;278:389-395.

86. Tur-Kaspa I, et al. Preparing hospitals for toxicological mass casualties events. *Crit Care Med.* 1999;27:1004-1008.

87. UN Security Council. *Third Report of the Organization for the Prohibition of Chemical Weapons–United Nations Joint Investigative Mechanism.* Document S/2016/738. August 24, 2016.

88. Urbanetti JS. Toxic inhalational injury. In: Sidell FR, et al, eds. *Medical Aspects of Chemical and Biological Warfare.* Washington, DC: Office of the Surgeon General; 1997:247-270.

89. Wax PM, et al. Unexpected "gas" casualties in Moscow: a medical toxicology perspective. *Ann Emerg Med.* 2003;41:700-705.

90. Wetherell J, et al. Development of next generation medical countermeasures to nerve agent poisoning. *Toxicology.* 2007;233:120-127.

91. Yanagisawa N, et al. Sarin experiences in Japan: acute toxicity and long-term effects. *J Neurol Sci.* 2006;249:76-85.

92. Yu CE, et al. Vesicant agents and children. *Pediatr Ann.* 2003;32:254-257.

127 BIOLOGICAL WEAPONS

Jeffrey R. Suchard

Expertise in dealing with biological weapons (BWs) requires specific knowledge from the fields of infectious disease, epidemiology, toxicology, and public health. Biological and chemical weapons share many characteristics in common, including intent of use, some dispersion methods, and initial defense based on adequate personal protective equipment and decontamination (Tables 126–2 and 126–3). However, key differences between biological and chemical weapons involve a greater delay in onset of clinical symptoms after exposure to BWs; that is, the incubation period for most BWs is greater than the latent period for most chemical weapons. Decontamination is less crucial for victims exposed to BWs. Additionally, a few BWs can reproduce in the human host and cause secondary casualties, and disease after exposure to certain BWs can be prevented by the timely administration of prophylactic medications.

Biological weapons may be bacteria, fungi, viruses, or toxins derived from microorganisms. Some fungi are listed as potential BWs; however, none are known to have been developed into weapons to date.[72] Because toxin weapons are not living organisms, some authorities classify them as chemical rather than BWs. For the purpose of discussion in this chapter, toxin weapons derived from microorganisms will be considered BWs. Most of these bacterial BWs exert their effects by elaborating protein toxins.

Many diseases caused by BWs are either infrequently encountered in modern clinical medicine, such as anthrax and plague, or no longer occur naturally, such as smallpox. Therefore, health care personnel require specific training in recognizing and managing biological warfare victims. Potential BWs are categorized by their risk of causing mass casualty outbreaks.[14] The high-risk BWs are more easily disseminated or transmitted and may cause high mortality and potential public health disasters; these BWs include smallpox, anthrax, plague, botulism, tularemia, and several hemorrhagic fever viruses. The moderate-risk BWs include Q fever, brucellosis, the equine encephalitis viruses, ricin, and staphylococcal enterotoxin B, all of which are briefly discussed in this chapter.

HISTORY

Biological warfare has ancient roots. Missile weapons poisoned with natural toxins were used as early as 18,000 years ago (Chap. 1). Other uses of biological warfare before the modern era relied mainly on poisoning water supplies with natural toxins or spreading naturally occurring epidemic infections to the enemy by hurling infected corpses over battlements or through the intentional transfer of disease-contaminated goods (eg, smallpox blankets).

During World War I, Germany was the only combatant nation with an active BW program; however, by World War II, many nations had BW research programs, including Japan, the Soviet Union, Germany, France, Britain, Canada, and the United States. The Japanese program included field trials with bubonic plague and conducted BW experiments on prisoners of war and civilians.[35] The American program was founded at Camp Detrick, Maryland, in 1942. Fort Detrick, as it is now known, remains the home of the United States Army Medical Research Institute of Infectious Diseases. Anthrax and botulinum toxins were the foci of American BW development during World War II. The British program was established at Porton Down in 1940, but most of the field testing of anthrax occurred on Gruinard Island off the northern coast of Scotland, resulting in long-term soil contamination with anthrax spores.

In London, in 1978, the Bulgarian exile Georgi Markov was assassinated with a tiny metal pellet fired from a gun designed to appear like an umbrella. He was originally thought to have died from sepsis until the pellet was found at autopsy.[23] After the fall of the Soviet Union, government officials confirmed that the KGB used umbrella guns firing ricin pellets to assassinate Markov and others.

In 1979, an outbreak of human anthrax caused at least 66 fatalities in the Russian city of Sverdlovsk. Autopsies revealed that the deaths were from inhalational anthrax, and epidemiologic investigation demonstrated that almost all the cases occurred downwind from a military facility. These data are consistent only with a release of aerosolized anthrax, which has since been confirmed by Russian authorities.[52]

In the late 1970s and early 1980s, many reports came from Southeast Asia and Afghanistan that Soviet-supported troops were using a BW known as Yellow Rain.[71] Some samples of Yellow Rain were found to contain trichothecene mycotoxins, although controversy remains as to whether this represents intentional biological warfare or was a naturally occurring phenomenon.[63]

During the 1990s, concern arose regarding the use and possible stockpiling of weapons of mass destruction in Iraq.[45] Iraq had an active BW research program, investigating at least five bacteria, one fungus, five viruses, four toxins, and a variety of dispersion methods.[64,74] Thousands of liters of anthrax spores, botulinum toxin, and aflatoxin were produced and weaponized into bombs and as payloads for SCUD missiles.

Biological terrorism and the threat of bioterrorism are now recognized as worldwide, growing public health concerns.[36] In 1984, a large outbreak of salmonellosis was traced to intentional contamination of restaurant salad bars by the Rajneeshee cult in Oregon.[69] The Aum Shinrikyo cult based in Japan investigated the use of cholera and Q fever, unsuccessfully released anthrax spores and botulinum toxin, and even sent members to Africa to obtain the Ebola virus.[56,67] The mere threat of a BW release can terrorize a city, as occurred with several false threats of anthrax spore release in the late 1990s.[13]

In 2001, closely following the September 11, 2001, attack on New York and Washington, DC, a bioterrorist attack occurred in the United States resulting in several cases of inhalational and cutaneous anthrax, with five fatalities. Ricin has also been found in letters and packages and in the possession of would-be terrorists several times, both in the United States and abroad in the post-9/11 era.[62]

GENERAL CONSIDERATIONS

Differences Between Biological Weapons Incidents and Naturally Occurring Outbreaks

Because the clinical effects of BWs are often delayed for several days after exposure, it may be difficult to differentiate an occult BW release from a naturally occurring disease outbreak. Several epidemiologic criteria are proposed to aid in such determinations,[55] many of which should be identifiable in a BW incident (Table 127–1).

To avoid early detection, terrorists might choose to release a BW causing endemic infection or a disease that mimics an endemic infection during its season of peak incidence. In some areas of the United States, for example, a few cases of bubonic plague would not attract notice until, perhaps, dozens or hundreds of cases were identified. An outbreak of inhalational anthrax during the influenza season may similarly be hidden among patients with shared early symptoms until an unusually high mortality rate was evident.[19] By the time the BW outbreak was recognized, the perpetrators could dispose of any physical evidence and flee the area. Alternatively, even a single case of smallpox (anywhere in the world) or Ebola virus disease or Congo-Crimean hemorrhagic fever (in nonendemic areas and unassociated with a known outbreak) should raise suspicion of a BW attack.

TABLE 127–1 Epidemiologic Clues Suggesting Biological Weapon Release

- Large epidemic with unusually high morbidity, mortality, or both
- Epidemic curve (number of cases vs time) showing an "explosion" of cases, reflecting a point source in time rather than insidious onset
- Tight geographic localization of cases, especially downwind of potential release site
- Predominance of respiratory tract symptoms because most BWs are transmitted by aerosol inhalation
- Simultaneous outbreaks of multiple unusual diseases
- Immunosuppressed and elderly persons more susceptible
- Nonendemic infection ("impossible epidemiology")
- Nonseasonal time for endemic infection
- Organisms with unusual antimicrobial resistance patterns, reflecting BW genetic engineering
- Animal casualties concurrent with disease outbreak
- Absence of normal zoonotic disease host
- Low attack rates among persons incidentally working in areas with filtered air supplies or closed ventilation systems, using HEPA masks, or remaining indoors during outdoor exposures
- Delivery vehicle or munitions discovered
- Law enforcement or military intelligence information
- Claim of BW release by a belligerent force

BW = bioweapon; HEPA = high-efficiency particle absorbing.

Preparedness

Many BWs initially produce nonspecific symptoms, and diseases that rarely, if ever, occur in clinical practice. Inhalational anthrax and pneumonic plague, for example, could easily be misdiagnosed as influenza or acute bronchitis. Providers in emergency departments and primary care medicine should be educated to recognize the signs, symptoms, and clinical progression of diseases caused by BW.[60] Clear identification, isolation, and aggressive treatment early after exposure within the first 24 to 48 hours are the best and only means of reducing mortality rates and, in the case of smallpox or plague, preventing secondary or tertiary cases.[27]

Decontamination

Biological weapons are most effective when dispersed by aerosol. Shortly after a known or suspected release of bioaerosols, external decontamination is a relatively minor concern because aerosols sized to reach the lower respiratory tract (<5-μm particles) produce little surface contamination. However, simple removal of clothing will eliminate a high proportion of deposited particles, and subsequent showering with soap and water will probably remove 99.99% of any remaining organisms on the skin.[44] Thus, decontamination after BW aerosol exposure, when needed, is achieved through disrobing and showering with soap and water. This can be done onsite or in the victims' homes and away from health care facilities, thereby reducing strain on disaster response manpower and material in multiple-victim exposures.[27,36,44,60] If there is gross, visible evidence of skin exposure to a BW, victims are decontaminated by thorough irrigation, and, if available, sterilizing the skin with a sporicidal and bactericidal solution (eg, 0.5% sodium hypochlorite) and a final water rinse.[44,60] Contaminated clothing should be removed and placed in airtight bags or containers to prevent resuspension in the air. After an occult BW release, victims are identified late after exposure; decontamination will obviously not be helpful and may only serve to delay care.

BIOLOGICAL WARFARE AGENTS

Starting on September 27, 2001, a 63-year-old Florida man developed malaise, fatigue, fever, chills, anorexia, and diaphoresis. He was admitted to a local hospital on October 2 after presenting with additional complaints of nausea, vomiting, and confusion. Chest radiography showed cardiomegaly, a left perihilar infiltrate, a small left pleural effusion, and a prominent superior mediastinum. Lumbar puncture revealed hemorrhagic meningitis with many gram-positive bacilli. *Bacillus anthracis* was isolated from the

cerebrospinal fluid after only a 7-hour incubation period and from blood cultures within 24 hours. The patient had progressive clinical deterioration and died on hospital day four.[10,42]

On October 4, the US Centers for Disease Control and Prevention (CDC) released a public health message regarding this case, which initially appeared to be an isolated, perhaps naturally occurring sporadic event.[15] Nevertheless, the rarity of inhalational anthrax especially outside of a high-risk occupation, combined with increased suspicion in the wake of the September 11, 2001, attacks led to intense investigation of a potential bioterrorist event. Within days, epidemiologic investigation suggested workplace exposure to anthrax spores, and personnel working in the same building were started on prophylactic ciprofloxacin.[16] On October 12, a case of cutaneous anthrax was reported in New York associated with a suspicious letter opened on September 25.[17] Anthrax cases and environmental contamination were also soon detected in Washington, DC, and in a New Jersey postal facility. The public response to the reports of these serious and fatal cases included misuse and hoarding of antibiotics, purchasing gas masks (often with inappropriate filtering mechanisms for BW), reporting numerous miscellaneous powdery substances, and perpetrating or reporting copycat hoaxes.

By November 7, 2001, a total of 22 cases of anthrax were reported: 10 inhalational and 12 cutaneous.[18] One additional death from inhalational anthrax occurred on November 21, 2001,[4] and a case of cutaneous anthrax also occurred in a laboratory worker analyzing samples obtained during the investigation.[20] In two of the fatal cases, no contact with contaminated letters could be established.[4,54] One infant hospitalized in New York with cutaneous anthrax was initially misdiagnosed as having a brown recluse spider envenomation.[31] The total number of medical victims of anthrax by spring 2002 was 23: 11 cases of inhalational anthrax (with 5 fatalities) and 12 cases of cutaneous anthrax (8 confirmed and 4 suspected).[20]

Bacteria
Anthrax

Anthrax is caused by *Bacillus anthracis*, a gram-positive spore-forming bacillus found in soil worldwide (Figs. 127–1 and 127–2). *B. anthracis* causes disease primarily in herbivorous animals. Human anthrax cases generally occur in farmers, ranchers, and among workers handling contaminated animal carcasses, hides, wool, hair, and bones.[32]

Clinical manifestations. A few clinically distinct forms of anthrax occur, depending on the route of exposure. Cutaneous anthrax results from direct inoculation of spores into the skin via abrasions or other wounds and accounts for about 95% of endemic (naturally occurring) human cases. Patients develop a painless red macule that vesiculates, ulcerates, and forms a 1- to 5-cm brown-black dermatonecrotic eschar surrounded by edema.[49] The eschar color gave rise to the name anthrax, from the Greek word *anthrakos*, meaning "coal." Most skin lesions heal spontaneously, although 10% to 20% of untreated patients progress to septicemia and death. When treated

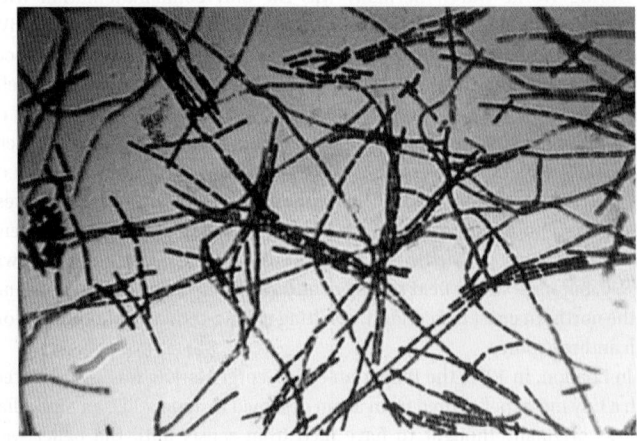

FIGURE 127–1. Anthrax Gram stain.

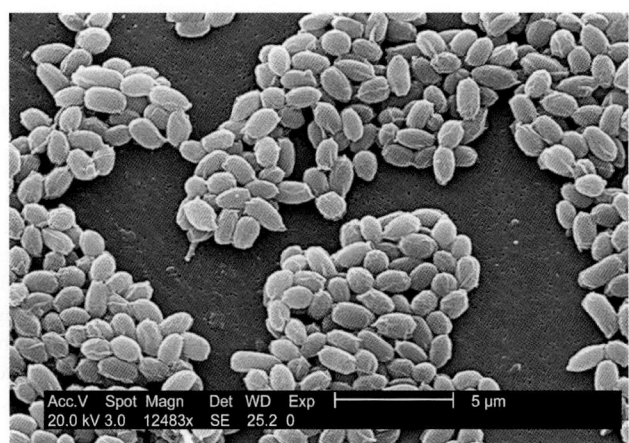

FIGURE 127–2. Anthrax spores.

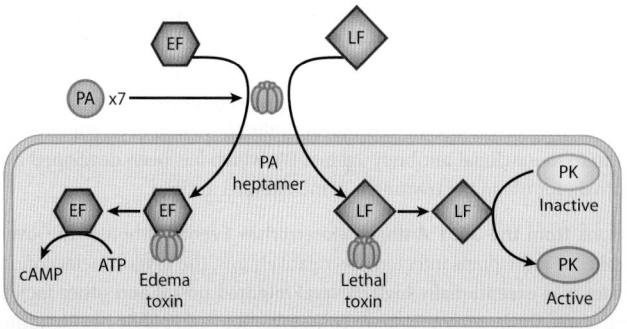

FIGURE 127–3. Model of action of anthrax toxins. Edema factor (EF) and lethal factor (LF) are unable to enter cells until they complex with a protective antigen (PA) heptamer, forming edema toxin and lethal toxin, respectively. When intracellular, release from PA allows EF and LF to exert their intracellular effects. Antibodies against PA confer resistance to the toxic effects of anthrax. ATP = adenosine triphosphate; cAMP = cyclic adenosine monophosphate; PK = protein kinase.

with antibiotics cutaneous anthrax rarely results in fatalities. Anthrax is not transmissible among humans.

Gastrointestinal (GI) anthrax results from ingesting insufficiently cooked meat from infected animals. Patients develop nausea, vomiting, fever, abdominal pain, and mucosal ulcers, which can cause GI hemorrhage, perforation, and sepsis. The mortality rate from GI anthrax is at least 50%, even with antibiotic treatment.[32]

Inhalational anthrax results from exposure to aerosolized *B. anthracis* spores. Although this form of anthrax is very rare, it is so closely associated with occupational exposures that it is called "wool-sorter's disease." Inhalational anthrax is also likely to be the form that occurs in a BW attack because the anthrax spores would be most effectively disseminated by aerosol. After an incubation period of 1 to 6 days, the patient develops fever, malaise, fatigue, nonproductive cough, and mild chest discomfort, which may be easily mistaken for community-acquired pneumonia.[19] The initial symptoms may briefly improve for 2 to 3 days, or the patient may abruptly progress to severe respiratory distress with dyspnea, diaphoresis, stridor, and cyanosis. Bacteremia; shock; metastatic infection such as meningitis, which occurs in about 50% of cases; and death may follow within 24 to 36 hours. Before the 2001 bioterrorist outbreak, the mortality rate from inhalational anthrax was expected to be nearly 100%, even with antibiotics, after symptoms develop.[30,32] With appropriate antibiotic therapy and supportive care, 5 of 11 patients with inhalational anthrax in 2001 died, and although this is still a high mortality rate, it is less than that previously predicted.[40]

Pathophysiology. Inhalational anthrax primarily causes a mediastinitis. Diagnostic imaging typically shows mediastinal widening from enlarged hilar lymph nodes and pleural effusions, although pulmonary parenchymal infiltrates also occur.[40] Inhaled spores are taken up into the lymphatic system, where they germinate and the bacteria reproduce. *B. anthracis* produces three toxins: protective antigen (PA), edema factor, and lethal factor. Protective antigen is so named because antibodies against it protect the individual from the effects of the other two toxins. Protective antigen forms a heptamer that inserts into plasma membranes, facilitating endocytosis of the other two toxins into target cells (Fig. 127–3). Edema factor is a calmodulin-dependent adenylate cyclase. Increased intracellular cyclic adenosine monophosphate (AMP) upsets water homeostasis, leading to massive edema and impaired neutrophil function. Lethal factor is a zinc metalloprotease that stimulates macrophages to release tumor necrosis factor α and interleukin-1β, contributing to death in systemic anthrax infections.[25] The combination of PA plus edema factor is called *edema toxin*, and PA plus lethal factor is *lethal toxin*.[34]

Treatment. The primary antibiotics used to treat anthrax are ciprofloxacin and doxycycline. Although other fluoroquinolones would be expected to have similar activity against anthrax, only the manufacturer of ciprofloxacin applied for and received a US Food and Drug Administration (FDA)–approved

indication for use in this infection. In a mass casualty setting or for postexposure prophylaxis, adults should receive ciprofloxacin 500 mg orally (PO) every 12 hours. Alternate therapies are doxycycline 100 mg PO every 12 hours or amoxicillin 500 mg PO every 8 hours if the anthrax strain is proven susceptible.[40] The recommended duration of therapy is 60 days, stemming from case experience in Sverdlovsk, where some patients developed disease several weeks (6–7 weeks) after the spore release.[52] Children should also be treated with ciprofloxacin (15 mg/kg; maximum, 500 mg/dose) or amoxicillin (80 mg/kg/d divided every 8 hours; maximum, 500 mg/dose). The relative pediatric contraindication to fluoroquinolones is outweighed by the risk of potentially fatal disease. Cutaneous anthrax is treated with the same drugs and doses as for postexposure prophylaxis.

Inhalational anthrax should be treated initially with intravenous antibiotics. Adults receive ciprofloxacin 400 mg intravenously (IV) or doxycycline 100 mg IV every 12 hours, along with one or two additional antibiotics with in vitro activity against anthrax (eg, rifampin, vancomycin, penicillin, ampicillin, chloramphenicol, imipenem, clindamycin, clarithromycin). Children are given ciprofloxacin 10 mg/kg IV (maximum, 400 mg/dose) or doxycycline 2.2 mg/kg IV (maximum, 100 mg/dose) and additional antibiotics, as indicated earlier.[40] However, in a true mass casualty event, when resources are strained and inpatient care is not available for every victim, oral therapy, as described earlier, may be instituted. When clinically appropriate, oral antibiotic therapy can be substituted for IV forms, with a total treatment duration of 60 days. Some patients in the 2001 outbreak were specifically treated with additional antibiotics that inhibit protein synthesis in attempts to reduce bacterial production of toxins.

Raxibacumab is a human monoclonal antibody that blocks binding of the anthrax PA to its host cell receptor. Raxibacumab is approved for treatment of inhalational anthrax in combination with appropriate antibiotics and prophylaxis when alternate therapies are unavailable or not appropriate.[46] Given the high costs of biological therapies, raxibacumab use is likely to be limited to rare individual cases rather than in mass casualty events.

Anthrax vaccine. An effective vaccine against anthrax is available.[33,51,75] In the United States, the Bioport Corporation (formerly Michigan Biologic Products Institute) is licensed by the FDA to produce anthrax vaccine adsorbed (AVA). The vaccine consists of a membrane-sterilized culture filtrate of *B. anthracis* V770-NP1-R, an avirulent, nonencapsulated strain that produces PA, adsorbed to aluminum hydroxide, formulated with benzethonium chloride (preservative) and formaldehyde (stabilizer).[75] In human and animal experiments, the vaccine is highly effective in preventing all forms of anthrax, and the vaccine is recommended for workers in high-risk occupations. As with any vaccine, local reactions to AVA occur in some recipients (up to 20% with mild, local reactions), and self-limited systemic reactions occur more rarely (<1.5%). Women have more frequent injection-site reactions and other adverse events, although this sex difference is also noted with other common vaccines.[34] Serious adverse events are very rare, with only 22 potentially related cases of serious adverse events from more than 1 million doses administered to US Armed Forces.[33] The dosage schedule for AVA is 0.5 mL subcutaneously at 0, 2, and 4 weeks and 6, 12, and 18 months followed by yearly boosters. Preclinical studies have also been conducted on a human monoclonal antibody against PA, which has been developed as an antitoxin for use in the treatment of inhalational anthrax.

Lessons from the 2001 Anthrax Bioterrorism Event. Although the overall number of individuals infected was relatively low, the psychosocioeconomic impact was exceptionally high. Several hundred postal and other facilities were tested for *B. anthracis* spore contamination, and public health authorities recommended antibiotic prophylaxis be initiated for approximately 32,000 persons.[18] Additional indirect costs and effects are more difficult to quantify, including the number of persons self-initiating antibiotic treatment without an evident indication, lost production and wages, environmental and biological sample testing, decontamination efforts, and an international sense of unease.

Published estimates of tens of thousands of deaths from a military-style anthrax attack[43] depend on efficient BW dispersion. The technically easier anthrax letter has clearly proven itself to be a "weapon of mass disruption." As predicted, the psychological impact far exceeded the actual medical consequences, and events with a modest number of medical patients are probably more likely than true mass casualty BW incidents. On the other hand, prior assumptions regarding the clinical aspects of anthrax were not as reliable. The mortality rate, as noted earlier, of inhalational anthrax was 45%, considerably lower than expected. Presentation with fulminant illness, such as sepsis, still appears to be predictive of a fatal outcome, yet the initial phase of illness does not necessarily lead to death if treated with appropriate antibiotics.[6,42,47] Pleural effusions were the most common radiographic abnormality, rather than a widened mediastinum, and pulmonary parenchymal infiltrates were seen in seven patients despite the belief that pneumonia does not commonly occur with inhalation anthrax.[32,42]

Plague

Yersinia pestis is a Gram-negative bacillus (Fig. 127–4) responsible for more than 200 million human deaths and three major pandemics in recorded history.[49,50] Naturally occurring plague is transmitted by flea vectors from rodent hosts or by respiratory droplets from infected animals or humans. Bubonic plague could result from an intentional release of plague-infested fleas. Plague is a particularly frightening BW because it can be released as an aerosol to cause a fulminant communicable form of the disease for which no effective vaccine exists. Antibiotics must be initiated early after exposure because when symptoms develop, mortality rates are reportedly extremely high.

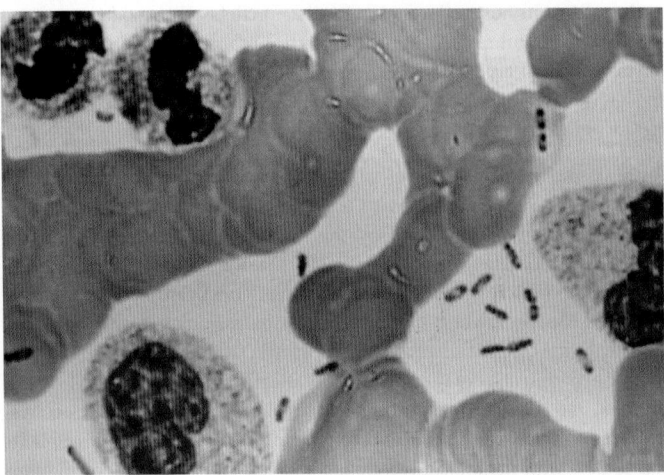

FIGURE 127–4. Dark-stained bipolar ends of *Yersinia pestis* can be seen in this Wright's stain of blood from a patient with plague.

Clinical presentation. Plague occurs in three clinical forms: bubonic, septicemic, and pneumonic. Bubonic plague has an incubation period of 2 to 10 days followed by fever, malaise, and painful, enlarged regional lymph nodes called buboes. The inguinal nodes are most commonly affected, presumably because the legs are more prone to flea bites, although cervical or axillary buboes are more common in children.[59] In the United States, 85% to 90% of human plague patients have the bubonic form, 10% to 15% have a primary septicemic form without lymphadenopathy, and about 1% present with pneumonic plague. Secondary septicemia occurs in 23% of patients presenting with bubonic plague.[50] Various skin lesions at the site of inoculation (pustules, vesicles, eschars, or papules) occur in some patients, although the petechiae and ecchymoses that occur in advanced cases may resemble meningococcemia.[49] Distal gangrene occurs from small artery thromboses, explaining why plague pandemics are sometimes called the Black Death. If left untreated, bubonic plague carries a 60% mortality rate.[49]

Pneumonic plague is an infection of the lungs with *Y. pestis*. Between 5% and 15% of bubonic plague patients develop secondary pneumonic plague through septicemic spread of the organism.[50] Primary pneumonic plague occurs from inhalation of infected respiratory droplets or an intentionally disseminated BW aerosol. The incubation period of pneumonic plague is 2 to 3 days after inhalation. The onset of disease is acute and often fulminant. Patients develop fever, malaise, and cough productive of bloody sputum, rapidly progressing to dyspnea, stridor, cyanosis, and cardiorespiratory collapse. Plague pneumonia is almost always fatal unless treatment is begun with 24 hours of symptom onset.[30]

Diagnosis and treatment. Plague can be diagnosed by various staining techniques, immunologic studies, or culturing the organism from blood, sputum, or lymph node aspirates. *Yersinia pestis* appears as a gram-positive safety pin–shaped bipolar coccobacillus.[30,59] Chest radiographs in patients with pneumonic plague reveal patchy or consolidated bronchopneumonia. Leukocytosis with a left shift is common, as are markers of low-grade disseminated intravascular coagulation and elevations of unconjugated bilirubin and hepatic aminotransferases.[30]

Antibiotic treatment options are similar to those for anthrax. In a mass casualty setting or for postexposure prophylaxis, treatment should be with doxycycline 100 mg or ciprofloxacin 500 mg PO twice daily for adults. Children should be given doxycycline 2.2 mg/kg or ciprofloxacin 20 mg/kg, up to a maximum of the adult doses. Chloramphenicol 25 mg/kg PO four times daily is an alternative. The durations of treatment are 7 days for postexposure prophylaxis and 10 days for mass casualty incidents.[39] Patients with pneumonic plague need to be isolated to prevent secondary cases. Respiratory droplet precautions are necessary in pneumonic plague until the patient has received antibiotics for 3 days.[30] In a contained-casualty setting, patients with pneumonic plague should be treated with parenteral streptomycin or gentamicin; alternative antibiotics include doxycycline, ciprofloxacin, and chloramphenicol.[39] A killed whole-cell vaccine effective against bubonic plague is available, but it does not reliably protect against pneumonic plague in animal studies.[49,51]

Tularemia

Francisella tularensis is a small, aerobic, gram-negative coccobacillus weaponized by the United States and probably other countries as well. Tularemia occurs naturally as a zoonotic disease spread by blood-sucking arthropods or by direct contact with infected animal material. Tularemia in humans may occur in ulceroglandular or typhoidal forms, depending on the route of exposure. Ulceroglandular tularemia is more common, occurring after skin or mucous membrane exposure to infected animal blood or tissues. Patients develop a local ulcer with associated lymphadenopathy, fever, chills, headache, and malaise. Typhoidal tularemia presents with fever, prostration, and weight loss without adenopathy. Exposure to aerosolized bacteria, as used in BW, will most likely result in typhoidal tularemia with prominent respiratory symptoms such as a nonproductive cough and substernal chest discomfort. Diagnosing tularemia is often difficult because the organism is hard to isolate by culture and the symptoms are nonspecific.

Chest radiography may demonstrate infiltrates, mediastinal lymphadenopathy, or pleural effusions.[24,28,30,51]

Antibiotic treatment options are similar to those for anthrax and plague. In mass casualty settings or for postexposure prophylaxis, treatment should be doxycycline 100 mg twice daily or ciprofloxacin 500 mg PO twice daily for 14 days for adults. Pediatric dosing for doxycycline is 2.2 mg/kg or ciprofloxacin 15 mg/kg (maximum, adult dose) twice daily. When dealing with a limited number of casualties, the preferred antibiotics are streptomycin 1 g intramuscularly (IM) twice daily or gentamicin 5 mg/kg IM or IV once daily. Alternatives include parenteral doxycycline, chloramphenicol, and ciprofloxacin.[24]

Brucellosis

Brucellosis could potentially be used as an incapacitating BW because it causes disease with low mortality but significant morbidity. Brucellae (*Brucella melitensis, abortus, suis,* and *canis*) are small, aerobic, gram-negative coccobacilli that generally cause disease in ruminant livestock. Humans develop brucellosis by ingesting contaminated meat and dairy products or by aerosol transmission from infected animals. The United States weaponized *B. suis,* and other countries are also believed to have developed *Brucella* BWs. Brucellosis commonly presents with nonspecific symptoms such as fever, chills, and malaise, with either an acute or insidious onset. Because brucellae are facultative intracellular organisms that localize in the lung, spleen, liver, central nervous system, bone marrow, and synovium, organ-specific signs and symptoms may occur. The diagnosis is made by serologic methods or culture. Because single-drug treatment often results in relapse, combined therapy is indicated. Patients should be given doxycycline 200 mg/day PO, plus rifampin 600 to 900 mg/day PO for 6 weeks, or doxycycline 200 mg/day PO for 6 weeks, with either streptomycin 15 mg/kg twice daily IM or gentamicin 1.5 mg/kg IM every 8 hours for the first 10 days.[30,38,51]

Rickettsiae

Features of rickettsiae favoring their use as BW include environmental stability, aerosol transmission, persistence in infected hosts, low infectious dose, and high associated morbidity and mortality. Rickettsiae that have been weaponized include *Coxiella burnetii,* the causative organism of Q fever, and *Rickettsia prowazekii,* the causative organism of louseborne typhus. Release of *R. prowazekii* into a crowded louse-infested population might induce a typhus outbreak with rapid transmission and a high mortality rate.[3]

Q Fever

Q fever was first described in 1937 and was given its name—Q for "query"—because the causative organism was not then known. Q fever occurs naturally as a self-limited febrile, zoonotic disease contracted from domestic livestock. Q fever is now known to be caused by *Coxiella burnetii,* a unique rickettsi-alike organism that can persist on inanimate objects for weeks to months and can cause clinical disease with the inhalation of only a single organism. These features are of obvious benefit for use as a potential BW. After a 10- to 40-day incubation period, Q fever manifests as an undifferentiated febrile illness, with headache, fatigue, and myalgias. Patchy pulmonary infiltrates on chest radiography that resemble viral or atypical bacterial pneumonia occur in 50% of cases, although only half of patients have cough, and even fewer have pleuritic chest pain. Uncommon complications include hepatitis, endocarditis, meningitis, encephalitis, and osteomyelitis. Patients are generally not critically ill, and the disease can last as long as 2 weeks. Treatment with antibiotics will shorten the course of acute Q fever and can prevent clinically evident disease when given during the incubation period. Tetracyclines are the mainstay of therapy, and either tetracycline 500 mg PO every 6 hours or doxycycline 100 mg PO every 12 hours should be given for 5 to 7 days.[11,30]

Viruses
Smallpox

Smallpox is caused by the variola virus, a large DNA orthopoxvirus (Fig. 127–5) with a host range limited to humans. Before global World Health Organization (WHO) efforts to eradicate naturally occurring smallpox by immunization, recurrent epidemics were common, and the disease

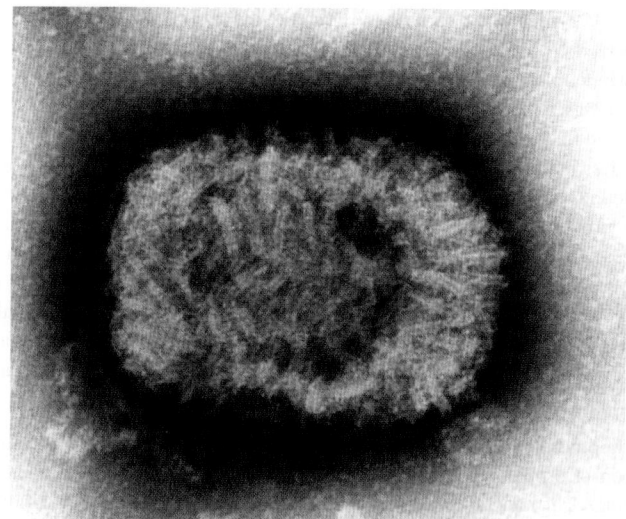

FIGURE 127–5. Variola virus.

carried roughly a 30% fatality rate in unvaccinated populations.[37,48] Smallpox is highly contagious (Fig. 127–6). Outbreaks during the 1960s and 1970s in Europe often resulted in 10 to 20 secondary cases per index case. One German smallpox patient with a cough, isolated in a single room, infected persons on three floors of a hospital.[37] However, the overwhelming majority of secondary infections occur among close family contacts, especially those sleeping in the same room or the same bed.[26]

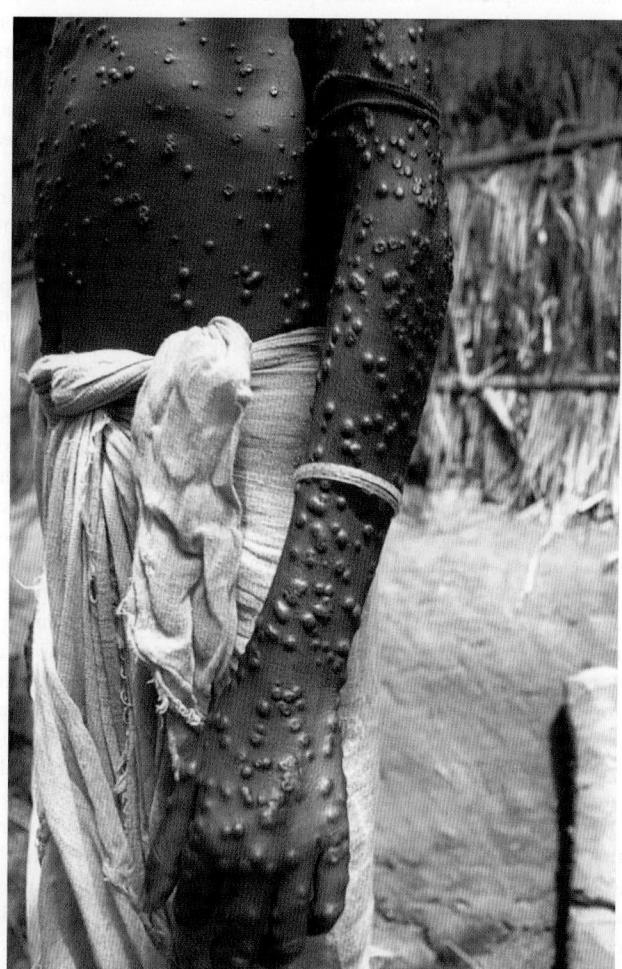

FIGURE 127–6. Smallpox rash demonstrating non-pruritic, synchronous tense vesicles.

In 1980, the United Nations' WHO certified that smallpox was eradicated and recommended ceasing vaccinations and either destroying or transferring remaining stocks of variola virus to one of two designated biosafety level 4 facilities: the CDC in Atlanta or the Russian State Research Center of Virology and Biotechnology.[9] All remaining known variola stocks were scheduled for destruction in 1999; however, before this was done, a WHO resolution called for a delay based on an Institute of Medicine report concluding that live virus should be retained to develop new antivirals or vaccines to protect against any potential future release of smallpox.[65] The Soviet Union is known to have weaponized smallpox, and other countries are believed to maintain stocks of variola virus. In addition to the known stockpiles of smallpox vaccine, several types of new vaccines are being produced.[57,73] Smallpox vaccination for military personnel was reinstated in 2002 and was made available for some civilians in 2003.[21,22]

Pathophysiology. Transmission of smallpox typically occurs through inhalation of droplets or aerosols but may also occur through contaminated fomites. The infectious dose is not known but is probably only a few virions. After a 12- to 14-day incubation period, the patient develops fever, malaise, and prostration with headache and backache. Oropharyngeal lesions appear, shedding virus into the saliva. Two to three days after the onset of fever, a papular rash develops on the face and spreads to the extremities. The fever continues while the rash becomes vesicular and then pustular. Scabs form from the pustules and eventually separate, leaving pitted and hypopigmented scars. Death usually occurs during the second week of the illness. Vaccination before exposure or within 2 to 3 days after exposure provides almost complete protection against smallpox. The disease most likely to be confused with smallpox is chickenpox (varicella). Although the individual lesions of smallpox and varicella are physically indistinguishable, the person infected with smallpox may still be differentiated clinically. The lesions of smallpox should all appear at the same stage of development (synchronous), but chickenpox lesions occur at varying stages (asynchronous). Smallpox lesions tend to be found in a centrifugal distribution (face and distal extremities), but chickenpox lesions are more centripetal, tend to appear first on the trunk and are pruritic.

Two antivirals commercially available in the United States, cidofovir and ribavirin, are effective in vitro against variola.[51] However, current evidence suggests that although cidofovir may prevent smallpox when given within 1 or 2 days of exposure, it is unlikely to be effective after symptoms develop.[37] Even a single case of smallpox should be considered a potential international health emergency and immediately reported to the appropriate public health authorities.

Smallpox vaccination. Rapid postexposure vaccination confers excellent protection against smallpox. The smallpox vaccine uses a live vaccinia virus (derived from cowpox vaccine) rather than the actual variola virus that causes smallpox. Although contracting smallpox from the vaccine is impossible, other adverse reactions may occur. The two most serious reactions are postvaccinal encephalitis and progressive vaccinia. Postvaccinal encephalitis occurs in about three cases per million primary vaccinees. Forty percent of cases are fatal, and some survivors are left with permanent neurologic sequelae. Progressive vaccinia can occur in immunosuppressed individuals and is treated with vaccinia immune globulin (VIG) (Fig. 127–7).[73] Another historically common complication of smallpox vaccination was ocular vaccinia, which typically occurred among health care personnel administering vaccine when it was inadvertently placed in the eye. Ocular vaccinia is also treated with VIG. Because smallpox was eradicated before the emergence of HIV, there is limited clinical experience with smallpox vaccination in patients with AIDS who theoretically are at increased risk of progressive vaccinia.[37,48] However, among 10 individuals with undiagnosed HIV at the time of recent smallpox vaccination, none developed complications.[68] Routine vaccination is contraindicated in immunosuppressed people, persons with a history or evidence of eczema and other chronic dermatitis, close household or sexual contacts of patients with these contraindications, and during pregnancy. Because the vaccine is a live virus, it can be transmitted from the vaccinee to

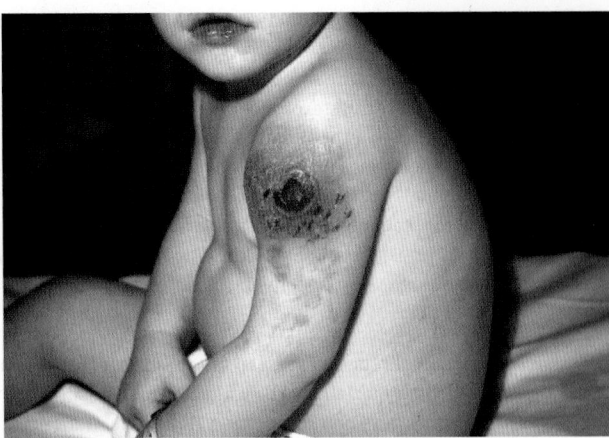

FIGURE 127–7. Progressive vaccinia.

close contacts. Thirty secondary and tertiary cases of vaccinia were reported resulting from recent US military vaccinations.[21] The number of serious adverse events from modern smallpox vaccination is very low;[22] however, rare cardiac complications not reported in previous decades were noted with the recent reinstitution of smallpox vaccination in the early 2000s. More than 1 million military vaccinations given by 2006 resulted in 120 cases of myopericarditis, and 21 cases of myopericarditis occurred among nearly 40,000 civilian vaccine recipients between 2002 and 2003.[57] The number of cardiac ischemic events among vaccinees was not significantly higher than age-matched control participants. After a true exposure to variola, most authorities would agree that the only absolute contraindication to smallpox vaccination is significant impairment of systemic immunity. Concomitant administration of vaccinia immune globulin would be recommended for pregnant women and persons with eczema.[48]

Viral Hemorrhagic Fevers

Several taxonomically diverse RNA viruses produce acute febrile illnesses characterized by malaise, prostration, and increased vascular permeability that can result in bleeding manifestations in the more severely affected patients. Viral hemorrhagic fevers (VHFs) are all highly infectious by the aerosol route, making them candidates for use as BW. These include the viruses causing Lassa fever, dengue, yellow fever, Crimean-Congo hemorrhagic fever, and the Marburg, Ebola virus, and Hanta viruses. Hanta virus is endemic to North America; occasional natural epidemics of human infection occur, which may initially be difficult to differentiate from a BW release. Clinical features, such as the extent of renal, hepatic, and hematologic involvement, vary according to the specific virus, but they all carry the risk of secondary infection through droplet aerosols. Ribavirin is reasonable for some VHFs, but supportive care is the mainstay of therapy.[7,30,41]

Viral Encephalitides

Three antigenically related α viruses of the Togaviridae family pose risks as BWs: western equine encephalitis (WEE), eastern equine encephalitis (EEE), and Venezuelan equine encephalitis (VEE). Birds are the natural reservoir of these viruses, and natural outbreaks occur among equines and humans by mosquito transmission. Eastern equine encephalitis infections are the most severe in humans, with a 50% to 70% fatality rate and high incidence of neurologic sequelae among survivors. Western equine encephalitis is less neurologically invasive, and severe encephalitis from VEE is rare, except in children. Adults infected with VEE usually develop an acute, febrile, incapacitating disease with prolonged recovery. The equine encephalitides have many properties helpful for weaponization, in that they can be produced in large quantities, they are relatively stable and highly infectious to humans as aerosols, and a choice is available between lethal or incapacitating infections.[66]

Venezuelan equine encephalitis is considered the most likely BW threat among the viral encephalitides. After a 1- to 5-day incubation period, victims experience the sudden onset of malaise, myalgias, prostration, spiking fevers, rigors, severe headache, and photophobia. Nausea, vomiting, cough, sore throat, and diarrhea may follow. This acute phase lasts 24 to 72 hours. Between 0.5% and 4% of patients develop encephalitis, with meningismus, seizures, coma, and paralysis, which carries up to a 20% fatality rate. The diagnosis is usually established clinically, although the virus can sometimes be isolated from serum or from throat swabs, and serologic tests are available. The white blood cell count often shows a striking leukopenia and lymphopenia. Treatment is supportive. Person-to-person transmission can theoretically occur from droplet nuclei. Recovery takes 1 to 2 weeks.[30,66]

Toxins

Several toxins derived from bacteria, plants, fungi, and algae could theoretically be used as BWs if produced in sufficient quantities. Because of their high potency, only small amounts would be needed to kill or incapacitate exposed victims. Fortunately, obstacles in manufacturing weaponizable amounts limit the number of toxins that are practical for use as BWs. Discussion here is limited to those toxins known or highly suspected to have been weaponized. Toxins themselves are not living organisms and therefore cannot reproduce; for this reason, they are arguably equivalent to chemical weapons. But because toxin weapons are derived from living organisms, they are categorized here as BWs.

Botulinum Toxin

The United States and some other countries developed botulinum toxin as a potential BW.[1,56,64,74] The two most likely means of using botulinum toxin are by food contamination or by aerosol. Either method would result in the clinical syndrome of botulism (Chap. 38), characterized by multiple bulbar nerve palsies and a symmetric descending paralysis, ending in death from respiratory failure. Inhalational botulism from laboratory incidents has occurred rarely in humans.[53]

Ricin

Ricin is derived from the castor bean plant (*Ricinus communis*) (Chap. 118) and is the only biological toxin to exist naturally in more than microscopic quantities, comprising 1% to 5% of the beans by weight.[8] Its easy accessibility, relative ease of preparation, and low cost may make ricin an attractive BW for terrorists or poor countries. Although ricin has never been used in battle, it has attracted the attention of domestic extremists and terrorists and was used in some politically motivated assassinations.[2,23,29] Ricin is a glycoprotein lectin (or toxalbumin) composed of two protein chains linked by a disulfide bond. The B chain facilitates cell binding and entry of the A chain into cells. The A chain inhibits protein synthesis, inactivating eukaryotic ribosomes by removing an adenine residue from ribosomal RNA.[2]

Clinical toxicity from ricin will vary depending on the dose and route of exposure. Inhalation of aerosolized ricin results in increased alveolar–capillary permeability and airway necrosis after a latent phase of 4 to 8 hours. Ingestion causes GI hemorrhage with necrosis of the liver, spleen, and kidney. Intramuscular administration produces severe local necrosis with extension into the lymphatics. In the absence of specific immunologic testing, differentiating ricin poisoning from sepsis may be difficult because of the presence of leukocytosis and fever. Vaccination of laboratory animals with an investigational toxoid (a modified toxin that does not cause disease but still induces an antibody response) is protective but is not approved for human use.[29]

Staphylococcal Enterotoxin B

Staphylococcal enterotoxin B (SEB) is one of several enterotoxins produced by *Staphylococcus aureus*. Staphylococcal enterotoxin B is recognized as a "superantigen" because of its profound activation of the immune system on exposure to even minute quantities. As a BW, SEB could be ingested through contaminated food or water, resulting in acute gastroenteritis identical to classic staphylococcal food poisoning. If inhaled as an aerosol, SEB produces fever, myalgias, and a pneumonitis after a 3- to 12-hour latent period. Staphylococcal enterotoxin B inhalation can be fatal but more often would simply be incapacitating for several days to weeks. Treatment is supportive.[70]

Exposure to SEB among BWs laboratory personnel has occurred, and even trace amounts unintentionally transferred to the face and eyes may cause conjunctivitis and GI symptoms.[61]

Fungi and Other Fungal Toxins

Fungi may at first appear to be ideal BW, given their relative ease of handling, dissemination, and resistance of spores to physical stressors.[12] The only fungi to be included on lists of microbes with potential use as BWs are *Coccidioides* spp, probably based on the high incidence of symptomatic infection in endemic areas. Nevertheless, the risk of serious disease is low, limiting the utility of *Coccidioides* as an effective weapon.[12,58]

Fungal toxins considered to have potential use as BWs include trichothecene mycotoxins, aflatoxins, and amanita toxins. Although α-amanitin is extremely potent, water soluble, and heat stabile, its use as a weapon would be limited by difficulties in mass production.[58] Aflatoxin would be ineffective on the battlefield because its acute toxicity is uncertain, and the carcinogenetic potential is a delayed phenomenon.[5] However, both of these toxins may still be effective as terror agents.

Trichothecene Mycotoxins

The trichothecene mycotoxins are low-molecular-weight (250–500 Da), nonvolatile compounds produced by filamentous fungi (molds) of various genera, including *Fusarium*, *Myrothecium*, *Phomopsis*, *Trichoderma*, *Tricothecium*, and *Stachybotrys*.[5,71] Tricothecene mycotoxins are unusual among potential BW in that toxicity can occur with exposure to intact skin. Naturally occurring trichothecene toxicity results from ingesting contaminated grains or by inhaling toxin aerosolized from contaminated hay or cotton. Outbreaks of ingested trichothecene toxins result in a clinical syndrome called alimentary toxic aleukia, characterized by gastroenteritis, fevers, chills, bone marrow suppression with granulocytopenia, and secondary sepsis—a syndrome clinically similar to acute radiation poisoning. Survival beyond this stage is characterized by the development of GI and upper airway ulceration and intradermal and mucosal hemorrhage. Trichothecene toxins are potent inhibitors of protein synthesis in eukaryotic cells, producing widespread cytotoxicity, particularly in rapidly proliferating tissues; different trichothecene toxins interfere with initiation, elongation, and termination stages of protein synthesis.[5] Exposure to any mucosal surface results in severe irritation. Dermal exposure can produce inflammatory lesions lasting for 1 to 2 weeks, vesiculation, and, in higher doses, death.[71]

Several reports from the 1970s and 1980s suggested that Soviet-supported forces were using trichothecene mycotoxins, particularly the toxin T-2 (Fig. 127–8), as BW. Aerosol and droplet clouds called Yellow Rain were associated with mass casualty incidents in Southeast Asia.[71] Such incidents would involve multiple routes of exposure, with skin deposition likely being the major site. Early symptoms included nausea, vomiting, weakness, dizziness, and ataxia. Diarrhea would then ensue, at first watery and then becoming bloody. Within 3 to 12 hours, victims would develop dyspnea, cough, chest pain, sore mouths, bleeding gums, epistaxis, and hematemesis. Exposed skin areas would become intensely inflamed, with the appearance of vesicles, bullae, petechiae, ecchymoses, and necrosis.[71]

Nonetheless, evidence that trichothecene mycotoxins were used as BWs was mostly circumstantial. Although T-2 toxin was found in victims'

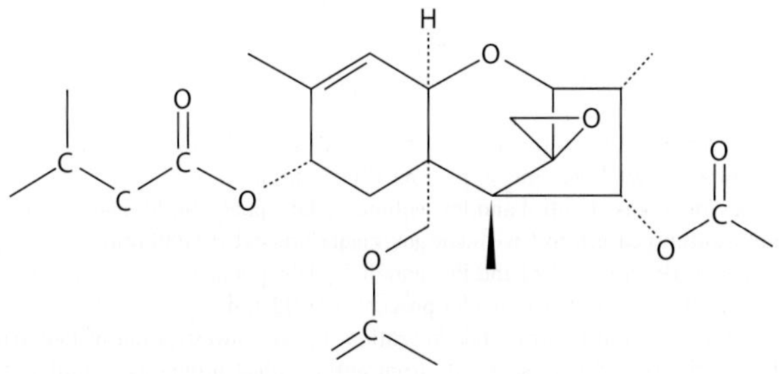

FIGURE 127–8. T-2, a trichothecene mycotoxin.

blood and urine, it was also found in samples from unexposed individuals, probably from baseline ingestion of contaminated foods. Environmental samples containing Yellow Rain droplets were inconsistently found to contain mycotoxins. Eyewitness accounts of Yellow Rain attacks varied widely (including various descriptions of substance's color), and despite the large number of such attacks, no contaminated ordinance or dispersal device was ever recovered.[63] It was also discovered that Yellow Rain droplets were composed mostly of pollen grains. Supporters of the Yellow Rain as BW theory retorted that pollen grains would be an ideal carrier for biotoxins, given that their size is ideal for aerosolization. However, the pollen in Yellow Rain samples did not contain protein, similar to pollen that has been digested by bees. Furthermore, the distribution of pollen species found in Yellow Rain was indistinguishable from the contents of feces of the Asian honeybee, and mass bee defecation resulting in showers of yellow droplets has been observed.[63] The Yellow Rain "bee feces theory" assumes that any mass casualty incidents were from endemic disease outbreaks, other chemical or biological agents not yet identified, or a combination of both.

SUMMARY

- Many biological weapons (BW) are pathogenic bacteria, viruses, or toxins produced by microorganisms.

- Biological weapons share many features with chemical weapons, including that the most effective method of dispersal to cause mass casualties will be via aerosolization. Disease after exposure to many BWs includes respiratory signs and symptoms.

- Victims of BWs exposure may present in a delayed fashion because of the incubation period of the disease. However, with proper identification of the agent, postexposure prophylaxis with antibiotics or vaccination (or both) is possible.

- With typical universal precautions, ill victims from BWs exposure generally do not pose an infection risk to health care providers and others. Notable exceptions include pneumonic plague, smallpox, and the viral hemorrhagic fevers.

REFERENCES

1. Arnon SS, et al. Botulinum toxin as a biological weapon: medical and public health management. *JAMA.* 2001;285:1059-1070.
2. Audi J, et al. Ricin poisoning: a comprehensive review. *JAMA.* 2005;294:2342-2351.
3. Azad AF. Pathogenic rickettsiae as bioterrorism agents. *Clin Infect Dis.* 2007;45:S52-S55.
4. Barakat LA, et al. Fatal inhalational anthrax in a 94-year-old Connecticut woman. *JAMA.* 2002;287:863-8.
5. Bennett JW, Klich M. Mycotoxins. *Clin Microbiol Rev.* 2003;16:497-516.
6. Borio L, et al. Death due to bioterrorism-related inhalational anthrax: report of 2 patients. *JAMA.* 2001;286:2554-2559.
7. Borio L, et al. Hemorrhagic fever viruses as biological weapons: medical and public health management. *JAMA.* 2002;287:2391-2405.
8. Bradberry SM, et al. Ricin poisoning. *Toxicol Rev.* 2003;22:65-70.
9. Bremen JG, Henderson DA. Poxvirus dilemmas—monkeypox, smallpox, and biologic terrorism. *N Engl J Med.* 1998;339:556-559.
10. Bush LM, et al. Index case of fatal inhalational anthrax due to bioterrorism in the United States. *N Engl J Med.* 2001;345:1607-1610.
11. Byrne WR. Fever Q. In: Sidell FR, et al, eds. *Medical Aspects of Chemical and Biological Warfare.* Washington, DC: Office of the Surgeon General; 1997:523-537.
12. Casadevall A, Pirofski LA. The weapon potential of human pathogenic fungi. *Med Mycol.* 2006;44:689-696.
13. Centers for Disease Control and Prevention. Bioterrorism alleging use of anthrax and interim guidelines for management—United States 1998. *MMWR Morbid Mortal Wkly Rep.* 1999;48:69-74.
14. Centers for Disease Control and Prevention. Biological and chemical terrorism: strategic plan for preparedness and response. *MMWR Morbid Mortal Wkly Rep.* 2000; 49(RR04):1-14.
15. Centers for Disease Control and Prevention. Public health message regarding anthrax case. http://www.cdc.gov/media/pressrel/r011004.htm.
16. Centers for Disease Control and Prevention. Update: public health message regarding Florida anthrax case. http://www.cdc.gov/media/pressrel/r011007.htm.
17. Centers for Disease Control and Prevention. Update: public health message regarding anthrax. http://www.cdc.gov/media/pressrel/r011012.htm.
18. Centers for Disease Control and Prevention. Update: investigation of bioterrorism-related anthrax and adverse events from antimicrobial prophylaxis. *MMWR Morbid Mortal Wkly Rep.* 2001;50:973-976.
19. Centers for Disease Control and Prevention. Notice to readers: considerations for distinguishing influenza-like illness from inhalational anthrax. *MMWR Morbid Mortal Wkly Rep.* 2001;50:984-986.
20. Centers for Disease Control and Prevention. Update: cutaneous anthrax in a laboratory worker—Texas 2002. *MMWR Morbid Mortal Wkly Rep.* 2002;51:482.
21. Centers for Disease Control and Prevention. Secondary and tertiary transfer of vaccinia virus among US military personnel—United States and worldwide 2002-2004. *MMWR Morbid Mortal Wkly Rep.* 2004;53:103-105.
22. Centers for Disease Control and Prevention. Update: adverse events following civilian smallpox vaccination—United States 2004. *MMWR Morbid Mortal Wkly Rep.* 2004; 53:106-107.
23. Crompton R, Gall D. Georgi Markov—death in a pellet. *Med Leg J.* 1980;48:51-62.
24. Dennis DT, et al. Tularemia as a biological weapon: medical and public health management. *JAMA.* 2001;285:2763-2773.
25. Dixon TC, et al. Anthrax. *N Engl J Med.* 1999;314:815-826.
26. Eichner M. Case isolation and contact tracing can prevent the spread of smallpox. *Am J Epidemiol.* 2003;158:118-128.
27. Eitzen EM. Education is the key to defense against bioterrorism. *Ann Emerg Med.* 1999;34:221-223.
28. Evans ME, et al, eds. *Medical Aspects of Chemical and Biological Warfare.* Washington, DC: Office of the Surgeon General; 1997:503-512.
29. Franz DR, et al, eds. *Medical Aspects of Chemical and Biological Warfare.* Washington, DC: Office of the Surgeon General; 1997:631-642.
30. Franz DR, et al. Clinical recognition and management of patients exposed to biological warfare agents. *JAMA.* 1997;278:399-411.
31. Freedman A, et al. Cutaneous anthrax associated with microangiopathic hemolytic anemia and coagulopathy in a 7-month-old infant. *JAMA.* 2002;287:869-874.
32. Friedlander AM. Anthrax. In: Sidell FR, et al, eds. *Medical Aspects of Chemical and Biological Warfare.* Washington, DC: Office of the Surgeon General; 1997:467-478.
33. Friedlander AM, et al. Anthrax vaccine: evidence for safety and efficacy against inhalational anthrax. *JAMA.* 1999;282:2104-2106.
34. Grabenstein JD. Countering anthrax: vaccines and immunoglobulins. *Clin Infect Dis.* 2008;46:129-136.
35. Harris S. Japanese biological warfare research on humans: a case study of microbiology and ethics. *Ann N Y Acad Sci.* 1992;666:21-52.
36. Henderson DA. The looming threat of bioterrorism. *Science.* 1999;283:1279-1282.
37. Henderson DA, et al. Smallpox as a biological weapon: medical and public health management. *JAMA.* 1999;281:2127-2137.
38. Hoover DL, Friedlander AM. Brucellosis. In: Sidell FR, et al, eds. *Medical Aspects of Chemical and Biological Warfare.* Washington, DC: Office of the Surgeon General; 1997:513-521.
39. Inglesby TV, et al. Plague as a biological weapon: medical and public health management. *JAMA.* 2000;283:2281-2290.
40. Inglesby TV, et al. Anthrax as a biological weapon 2002: updated recommendations for management. *JAMA.* 2002;287:2236-2252.
41. Jahrling PB. Viral hemorrhagic fevers. In: Sidell FR, et al, eds. *Medical Aspects of Chemical and Biological Warfare.* Washington, DC: Office of the Surgeon General; 1997:591-602.
42. Jernigan JA, et al. Bioterrorism-related inhalational anthrax: the first 10 cases reported in the United States. *Emerg Infect Dis.* 2001;7:933-944.
43. Kaufmann AF, et al. The economic impact of a bioterrorist attack: are prevention and postattack intervention programs justifiable? *Emerg Infect Dis.* 1997;3:83-94.
44. Keim M, Kaufmann AF. Principles for emergency response to bioterrorism. *Ann Emerg Med.* 1999;34:177-182.
45. Knudson GB. Operation Desert Shield: medical aspects of weapons of mass destruction. *Mil Med.* 1991;156:267-271.
46. Kummerfeldt CE. Raxibacumab: potential role in the treatment of inhalational anthrax. *Infect Drug Resist* 2014;7:101-109.
47. Mayer TA, et al. Clinical presentation of inhalational anthrax following bioterrorism exposure: report of 2 surviving patients. *JAMA.* 2001;286:2549-2553.
48. McClain DJ. Smallpox. In: Sidell FR, et al, eds. *Medical Aspects of Chemical and Biological Warfare.* Washington, DC: Office of the Surgeon General; 1997:539-559.
49. McGovern TW, et al. Cutaneous manifestations of biological warfare and related threat agents. *Arch Dermatol.* 1999;135:311-322.
50. McGovern TW, et al, eds. *Medical Aspects of Chemical and Biological Warfare.* Washington, DC: Office of the Surgeon General; 1997:479-502.
51. Abramowicz M. Drugs and vaccines against biological weapons. *Med Lett Drugs Ther.* 1999;41:15-16.
52. Meselson M, et al. The Sverdlovsk anthrax outbreak of 1979. *Science.* 1994;266:1202-1208.
53. Middlebrook JL, Franz DR. Botulinum toxins. In: Sidell FR, et al, eds. *Medical Aspects of Chemical and Biological Warfare.* Washington, DC: Office of the Surgeon General; 1997:643-654.
54. Mina B, et al. Fatal inhalational anthrax with unknown source of exposure in a 61-year-old woman in New York City. *JAMA.* 2001;287:858-862.
55. Noah DL, et al. Biological warfare training: infectious disease outbreak differentiation criteria. *Mil Med.* 1998;163:198-201.
56. Olson KB. Aum Shinrikyo: once and future threat? *Emerg Infect Dis.* 1999;5:513-516.
57. Parrino J, Graham BS. Smallpox vaccines: past, present, and future. *J Allergy Clin Immunol.* 200;118:1320-1326.

58. Paterson RR. Fungi and fungal toxins as weapons. *Mycol Res.* 2006;110:1003-1010.
59. Prentice MB, Rahalison L. Plague. *Lancet.* 2007;369:1196-1207.
60. Richards CF, et al. Emergency physicians and biological terrorism. *Ann Emerg Med.* 1999;34:183-190.
61. Rusnak JM, et al. Laboratory exposures to Staphylococcal enterotoxin B. *Emerg Infect Dis.* 2004;10:1544-1549.
62. Schier JG, et al. Public Health investigation after the discovery of ricin in a South Carolina postal facility. *Am J Public Health.* 2007;97:S152-157.
63. Seeley TD, et al. Yellow rain. *Sci Am.* 1985;253:128-137.
64. Seelos C. Lessons from Iraq on bioweapons. *Nature.* 1999;398:187-188.
65. Shalala DE. Smallpox: setting the research agenda. *Science.* 1999;285:1011.
66. Smith JF, et al. Viral encephalitides. In: Sidell FR, et al, eds. *Medical Aspects of Chemical and Biological Warfare.* Washington, DC: Office of the Surgeon General; 1997: 561-589.
67. Takahashi H, et al. Bacillus anthracis incident, Kameido, Tokyo 1993. *Emerg Infect Dis.* 2004;10:117-120.
68. Tasker SA, et al. Unintended smallpox vaccination of HIV-1-infected individuals in the United States military. *Clin Infect Dis.* 2004;38:1320-1322.
69. Török TJ, et al. A large community outbreak of salmonellosis caused by intentional contamination of restaurant salad bars. *JAMA.* 1997;278:389-395.
70. Ulrich RG, et al. Staphylococcal enterotoxin B and related pyrogenic toxins. In: Sidell FR, et al, eds. *Medical Aspects of Chemical and Biological Warfare.* Washington, DC: Office of the Surgeon General; 1997:621-630.
71. Wannemacher RW, Wiener SL. Trichothecene mycotoxins. In: Sidell FR, et al, eds. *Medical Aspects of Chemical and Biological Warfare.* Washington, DC: Office of the Surgeon General; 1997:655-676.
72. Weinstein RS, Alibek K. *Biological and Chemical Terrorism.* New York, NY: Thieme; 2003.
73. Wittek R. Vaccinia immune globulin: current policies, preparedness, and product safety and efficacy. *Int J Infect Dis.* 2006;10:193-201.
74. Zilinskas RA. Iraq's biological weapons: the past as future? *JAMA.* 1997;278:418-424.
75. Zoon KC. Vaccines, pharmaceutical products, and bioterrorism: challenges for the US Food and Drug Administration. *Emerg Infect Dis.* 1999;5:534-536.

128

RADIATION

Joseph G. Rella

Although the theory of *atomism* originated with the Greeks in the fifth century B.C., it has been only a little more than a century that scientists could describe and measure atoms and the other particles of radiation. Today we use radiation and radionuclides for a vast array of purposes, ranging from mundane household uses such as detecting smoke to powering satellites, treating cancer, and examining the physical properties of individual molecules. Unfortunately, as our knowledge of how to use radiation has expanded, so too has our awareness of radiation as a toxin. Indeed, for three of the last four editions of this text, there has been a significant radiation event that captured the world's attention and demonstrated clearly just how much more we need to know. The particles of radiation, their sources, and the mechanisms by which they pose a health risk are the subjects of the following discussion.

HISTORICAL EXPOSURES

Soon after x-rays were discovered in 1895, a deepening understanding of radiation and radionuclides led to their wider use and their resulting injuries. In the early days of radiation, exposures were small and of low energy, which nevertheless created injuries for a relatively small number of individuals. Clarence Dally was the first known radiation-induced death in 1904 after repeated exposures to Thomas Edison's early fluoroscopes. By 1927, nearly 100 women employed to create illuminated instrument dials became ill or died after exposure to radium-containing paint. Efforts to protect workers such as those by the British Roentgen Society were hampered by limitations on measurement of radiation despite the development in 1908 of the Geiger counter that could detect but not quantify radiation. Much later in 1984 and again in 1987, lack of proper remediation of closed radiation treatment centers led to scavengers releasing sources of ^{60}Co and ^{137}Cs, respectively. In the cobalt incident beginning in Juarez, Mexico, thousands of tiny metal pellets were spilled in a scrapyard and melted with other metals into table legs later shipped throughout Mexico and the United States. In the cesium incident in Goiânia, Brazil, scavengers were fascinated by the bluish glow of the material. Ultimately, 250 individuals were contaminated, 46 patients were treated with a chelator, and 4 died the month after the initial exposure with another dying several years afterward from radiation-induced injuries.

With the advent of the nuclear age, said to have begun with the first detonation of an atomic bomb in New Mexico in July 1945, suddenly the risks of radiation exposure grew to many thousands at once. After the use of the two atomic bombs in Japan at the end of World War II, estimates of dead and injured for both cities were well over 200,000. Most of the deaths were from the bomb blast, but many thousands died from acute radiation syndrome (ARS) and others subsequently from radiation-induced cancers. In addition to the people of those cities who were victims of the bombs, many thousands of military personnel assigned to cleanup tasks or to attend nuclear weapons testing over the following 20 years were also exposed to radiation resulting from nuclear explosions. One relatively well-studied group, the British Nuclear Tests Veterans Association (BNTVA), found that two-thirds of its study group died from neoplasms at ages 50 to 65 years, irrespective of the individual's age at the time of the witnessed explosion.

More recently in the post–nuclear testing era, large radiation incidents occurred at the sites of nuclear reactors. In 1986, the Chernobyl nuclear reactor, built without a hard containment vessel, experienced a series of explosions, releasing an enormous cloud of radioactive material. Thirty-one people died of ARS in the first few weeks after that event, and an unknown number of millions potentially suffered other long-term sequelae in the surrounding geographic area.

On March 11, 2011, a powerful earthquake off the east coast of Japan triggered a destructive tsunami that struck the Fukushima Daiichi nuclear power plant complex, knocking out its own electrical power and disabling the ability to cool its nuclear material. Over the following week, a series of explosions released an amount of radioactive material second only to the Chernobyl incident. Over the intervening time, no conclusive data yet exist describing a change in cancer prevalence, but controversy regarding study methods continues.[14,33,35]

Perhaps one of the most notorious deaths from radiation was that of Alexander Litvinenko, a former Soviet KGB operative who was living in London. On November 1, 2006, shortly after meeting with several men in a public restaurant, Litvinenko experienced nausea and vomiting, prompting a visit to the emergency department (ED). He was treated and released only to return 3 days later for continued vomiting and worsening abdominal pain. Physicians were puzzled by his rapid deterioration, including weight loss, alopecia, hypotension, kidney failure, and leukopenia. He was initially thought to have been poisoned by thallium and later by radioactive thallium. Litvinenko died 22 days later, and it was only after his death that ^{210}Po was discovered to be the cause, heralding what some consider to be a new era of nuclear terrorism.

In the realm of health care, radiologists of the early 20th century used a thorium-containing contrast called Thorotrast in the initial development of angiography. Unfortunately, this xenobiotic accumulated in hepatic tissue, resulting in malignancies and its eventual discontinuance in 1952 (Fig. 8–25). More recently, the steadily increasing use of computed tomography (CT) has led to increased concerns over their safety and potential for stochastic effects. One retrospective study suggests there is a small but measurably increased risk for certain neoplasms in children after the accumulated radiation dose of several CT scans.[31] This topic is discussed in more detail later.

PRINCIPLES OF RADIOACTIVITY

Dating from the 15th century, *radiation* remains defined as energy sent out in the form of waves or particles. Although considered by physicists as incomplete, the particle-wave theory remains a useful model by which to understand the toxic aspects of radiation. Despite the *strong nuclear force* that holds the basic building blocks of atoms together, many isotopes are unstable. Various influences such as quantum fluctuations and the *weak nuclear force* can tip the balance toward instability to transform an isotope. This process can be intentional, as with the criticality events in a nuclear reactor or nuclear bomb, but mainly occurs spontaneously in nature as the process called radioactive decay.

Radioactive Decay

In 1900, Marie Curie discovered that unstable nuclei decay or transform into more stable nuclei (daughters) via the emission of various particles or energy. Radioactive decay occurs mainly through five nuclear mechanisms: emission of gamma rays, alpha particles, beta particles, or positrons or by capture of an electron. The emission of these various particles makes radioactive decay dangerous because these particles *are* ionizing radiation. Each radioisotope has a specific decay energy signature. That is, the emitted particles from a given radioisotope have known energies, which make identification of radiation sources possible.

The half-life ($t_{1/2}$) is the period of time it takes for a radioisotope to lose half of its radioactivity. Every radioisotope has a characteristic half-life, some lasting millionths of a second and others lasting billions of years. In every

TABLE 128–1	Physical Properties of Radioisotopes		
Isotope	*Half-Life*	*Mode of Decay*	*Decay Energy (MeV)*
Radioisotopes of Medicine and Research			
^{2}H	Stable		
^{131}I	8 days	β$^-$	0.97
^{201}Tl	73 hours	EC	0.41
^{99m}Tc	6 hours	IT	0.14
^{133}Xe	5.27 days	β$^-$	0.43
^{67}Ga	78 hours	EC	1.00
^{137}Cs	30.17 years	β$^-$	1.17
^{18}F	109 months	β$^-$, EC	1.65
Military Radioisotopes			
^{3}H	12.26 years	β$^-$	0.02
^{90}Sr	28.79 years	β$^-$	0.55
^{235}U	7.1×10^8 years	α, SF	4.68
^{238}U	4.51×10^9 years	α, SF	4.27
^{210}Po	138 days	α	5.307
^{239}Pu	24,400 years	α, SF	5.24
^{241}Am	470 years	α, γ	5.14/0.02

EC = electron capture; IT = isomeric transition from upper to lower isomeric state; MeV = megaelectron volts; SF = spontaneous fission.

case, the activities of radioactive isotopes diminish exponentially with time (Table 128–1).

Photons are elementary particles that mediate electromagnetic radiation. Depending on their energy, the radiation has different names ranging from extremely long radio waves to high-energy gamma rays.

X-rays and gamma rays are high-energy photons and are only distinguishable by their source. Gamma radiation is emitted by unstable atomic nuclei via radioactive decay and has a fixed wavelength depending on the energy that formed it. X-rays come from atomic processes outside the nucleus. For example, an x-ray machine generates x-rays by accelerating electrons through a large voltage and colliding them into a metal target. The rapid deceleration of electrons in the target generates x-rays, and in general, the higher the voltage, the greater the energy of the x-rays. Because of their nature, high-energy gamma and x-rays can penetrate several feet of insulating concrete.

Beta particles are electrons. They are emitted during beta decay from an unstable radionuclide. Positrons are positively charged electrons and are also emitted during some decay processes. Electrons have less penetrating ability than gamma radiation but can still pass several centimeters into human skin. Beta particles also cause health problems chiefly through incorporation, or internalization into living organisms.

Alpha particles are helium nuclei (two protons and two neutrons) stripped of their electrons and are emitted during alpha decay. These particles are the most easily shielded of the emitted particles mentioned and can be stopped by a piece of paper, skin, or clothing. Unlike beta particles, alpha particles principally cause health effects only when they are incorporated.

Neutrons are primarily released from nuclear processes, although high-energy photon beams used in radiotherapy can also produce them. The natural decay of radionuclides does not include emission of neutrons, which is mainly a health hazard for workers in a nuclear power facility or victims of a nuclear explosion. Unique among the particles of radioactivity, when neutrons are stopped or captured, they can cause a previously stable atom to become radioactive in a process known as neutron activation.

Cosmic rays complete the group of various kinds of radiation. Cosmic rays are streams of electrons, protons, and alpha particles thought to emanate from stars and supernovas. They rain down on the Earth from all directions only to give up their energy as they strike the nuclei of oxygen and nitrogen in the upper atmosphere of the Earth. By the time they reach the Earth, the energy of cosmic radiation is reduced by several orders of magnitude.

Traveling or living at altitude where the atmosphere naturally shields relatively less cosmic radiation naturally means greater exposure to cosmic rays but in general is not considered a significant threat to humans.

Isotopes and nuclides are very closely related terms, and most experts in the field use them interchangeably. Isotopes are two or more species or variants of a particular chemical element (same number of protons) that have different amounts of neutrons (eg, ^{123}I, ^{125}I, ^{127}I, ^{131}I). *Nuclide* is a more general term that may or may not be isotopes of a given element, such as *fissile nuclides* or *primordial nuclides*. Radioisotopes are isotopes that are radioactive, that is, they spontaneously decay and emit energy. Of the iodine nuclides listed previously, ^{123}I, ^{125}I, and ^{131}I are radionuclides. The nuclide ^{127}I is stable (nonradioactive). Finally, radionuclides are simply nuclides that are radioactive.

Ionizing Radiation versus Nonionizing Radiation

Ionizing radiation refers to any radiation with sufficient energy to disrupt an atom or molecule with which it impacts. In this interaction, an electron is removed, or some other decay process occurs, leaving behind a changed atom. Depending on the specifics of the interaction, the chemical bonds become altered, producing ions or highly reactive free radicals. Hydroxyl free radicals, formed by ionizing water, are responsible for biochemical lesions that are the foundation of radiation toxicity.

The space between collisions of ionizing radiation and their target molecules varies with the particle type and its energy. A charged particle, such as an alpha particle, loses kinetic energy through a series of small energy transfers to other atomic electrons in the target medium, such as tissues. Most of the energy deposition occurs in the *infratrack*, a narrow region around the particle track extending about 10 atomic distances. The energy loss per unit length of particle track is called the linear energy transfer (LET), which is expressed in kiloelectron volts per micrometer (keV/μm). Heavy charged particles, such as alpha particles, are referred to as high-LET radiation, and x-rays, gamma rays, and fast electrons are low-LET radiation.

Because of its large size, collisions along the path of an alpha particle are clustered together, impeding its ability to penetrate tissue. By comparison, collisions along the path of gamma rays are spread out, increasing their ability to penetrate tissue. This ability to penetrate tissue and transfer energy accounts for the relative dangers of the forms of radiation and tissue susceptibility.

For a source of radiation to pose a threat to tissue, the ionizing particle must be placed in close proximity to vital components of tissue to inflict damage. High-energy photons penetrate deeply, so they pose a similar risk whether they come from an external source or from an incorporated source. Because alpha particles have much more limited tissue penetration, alpha emitters, radionuclides that radiate these particles, must first be incorporated to pose a threat to tissue. Beta particles similarly have limited tissue penetration and usually are incorporated before damage can occur, although a large external exposure to beta emitters can cause serious cutaneous injury that could be life threatening, as discussed next.

Nonionizing radiation spans a wide spectrum of electromagnetic radiation frequencies. Generally, nonionizing radiation consists of relatively low-energy photons and is used safely in cell phone and television signal transmission, radar, microwaves, and magnetic fields that emanate from high-voltage electricity and metal detectors. Although these are all considered radiation because they each represent energy released from a source, these photons lack the necessary energy required to cause ionization and cellular damage.

Radiation Units of Measure

The amount of radiation to which an object is exposed, that is, the amount emitted from a source that falls on an object, is given in units called roentgens (R), a term that is now considered obsolete. A roentgen is a unit for measuring the quantity of gamma- or x-radiation by measuring the amount of ionization produced in air. As an example, an individual standing at a given distance from the x-ray–generating tube of a particular x-ray machine is exposed, on the skin, to a particular number of roentgens of x-rays (Fig. 128–1).

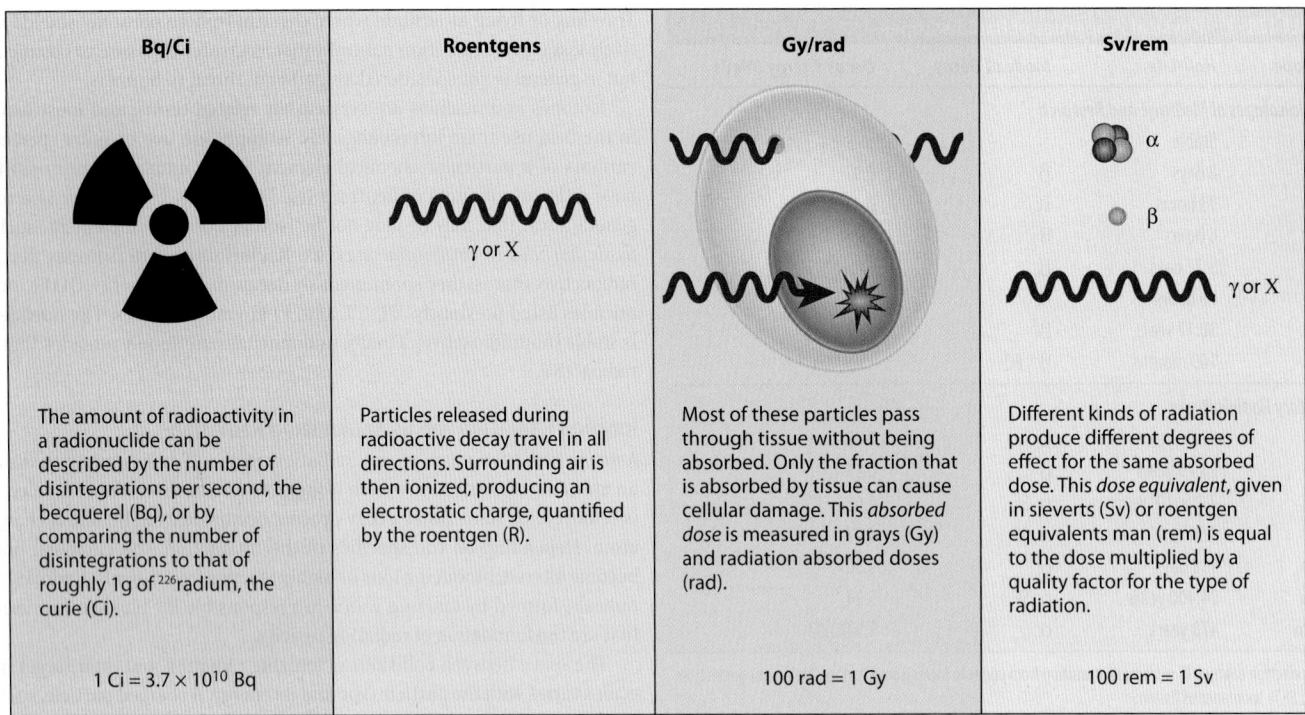

Bq/Ci	Roentgens	Gy/rad	Sv/rem
The amount of radioactivity in a radionuclide can be described by the number of disintegrations per second, the becquerel (Bq), or by comparing the number of disintegrations to that of roughly 1g of ^{226}radium, the curie (Ci).	Particles released during radioactive decay travel in all directions. Surrounding air is then ionized, producing an electrostatic charge, quantified by the roentgen (R).	Most of these particles pass through tissue without being absorbed. Only the fraction that is absorbed by tissue can cause cellular damage. This *absorbed dose* is measured in grays (Gy) and radiation absorbed doses (rad).	Different kinds of radiation produce different degrees of effect for the same absorbed dose. This *dose equivalent*, given in sieverts (Sv) or roentgen equivalents man (rem) is equal to the dose multiplied by a quality factor for the type of radiation.
1 Ci = 3.7 × 10^{10} Bq		100 rad = 1 Gy	100 rem = 1 Sv

FIGURE 128–1. The definitions associated with radiation. Both curies and becquerels describe a quantity of radionuclide in terms of the number of disintegrations rather than mass. Roentgens describes the amount of charge per volume of air ionized by either γ- or x-rays, which indirectly quantifies the amount of radiation in the air around a source. Rads and grays (Gy) describe the fraction of radiation that actually interacts with cellular material and potentially causes injury. Roentgen equivalents man (rem) and sieverts (Sv) calculate the effective dose, taking into account the different particles. For example, a 100-keV alpha particle causes more damage to cellular material than a 100-keV beta particle.

Not all radiation to which an individual is exposed poses a risk for cellular damage. Much of the radiation passes through the body and causes no harm. Only the fraction that is absorbed by the tissue has a chance of causing cellular damage. The International System (SI) unit that describes absorbed radiation is the *gray* (Gy), which has replaced the *rad* (radiation-absorbed dose). One Gy equals 100 rad.

To measure the risk of biologic damage regardless of the type of radiation, the effective dose is given in *sievert* (Sv), which has replaced the *rem* (roentgen equivalent man). One Sv equals 100 rem. This calculation, known as *dosimetry*, takes into account the type of exposure (external or internal, partial or total), the particle or particles involved (eg, alpha, beta, gamma), and the radiosensitivity of the organ or organs exposed. The effective dose is calculated according to the following equation:

$$E = D \times W_R \times W_T$$

where E is the dose in sieverts; D is the absorbed dose in gray; W_R is the radiation weighting factor, also called Q; and W_T is the tissue weighting factor indicating the radiosensitivity of each organ.

In 1910, the *curie* (Ci) became the unit describing the amount of radioactivity in a source. One curie equals 3.7×10^{10} disintegrations per second based on the decay of 1 g of radium. The curie was replaced by the SI unit the *becquerel* (Bq) in which 1 Bq is equivalent to 1 disintegration per second. Thus, 1 Ci is equivalent to 3.7×10^{10} Bq. For example, after the Chernobyl incident, 1.2×10^{19} disintegrations per second of radioactive material was released into the atmosphere. By comparison, the radioactive source of ^{137}Cs in Goiânia contained 50.9×10^{12} Bq (13.7×10^5 mCi) of cesium. A thallium stress test uses 111×10^6 Bq (3 mCi) of ^{201}Tl, and the average indoor concentration of ^{222}Rn in the United States is 55 Bq/m^3 (14.8×10^{-6} mCi).

Protection from Radiation

Shielding refers to the process by which one limits the amount of unwanted ionizing radiation in a given setting. Placing a specific material between a radiation source and a target will limit the amount of ionizing radiation that

will interact with the target. When a particle of ionizing radiation is incident on a material, there exists some probability that it will interact with the material and be attenuated. What happens as a result of this interaction depends on several factors, including the type of particle, its energy, and the atomic number of the target material. The photoelectric effect for photons, Bremsstrahlung for beta particles, and elastic scattering for neutrons are several examples of specific interactions. The shielding equation below allows calculation of the efficacy of shielding

$$I = I_0 e^{-\mu x}$$

where I is the radiation intensity after shielding, I_0 is the radiation intensity before shielding, μ is the linear attenuation coefficient, and x is the thickness material in centimeters. The linear attenuation coefficient is defined as the fraction of photons removed from the radiation field per centimeter of absorber through which it passes. Examples of shielding materials are acrylic, lead, and concrete.

Distance is an important safety factor in limiting radiation exposure. Because of their mass and electric charge, alpha and beta particles have a high probability of interacting with matter, such as the atmosphere. The result is that these particles do not travel more than a few centimeters through air and, in general, moving a few feet from the source of this kind of radiation is enough protection by distance. However, x-rays and gamma rays are uncharged and have no rest mass, greatly reducing their probability of interacting with matter, resulting in an unlimited range in space. Photon radiation that is emitted from a point source diverges from that source to cover an increasingly wider area. The intensity of this radiation follows the inverse square law:

$$\frac{I_1}{I_2} = \frac{(r_2)^2}{(r_1)^2},$$

where I_1 is the initial intensity, I_2 is the final intensity, r_1 is the initial distance from the source, and r_2 is the final distance from the source. For example, if the intensity of radiation 1 m from a source is 1 Gy, its intensity would be 0.11 Gy at 3 m from the source.

Time of exposure is another important safety factor in limiting radiation exposure. Obviously, the longer a person is exposed to radiation, the greater the exposure. The US federal and state regulations based on National Council on Radiation Protection and Measurement (NCRP) and US Food and Drug Administration (FDA) recommendations specify the limits of occupational exposure as well as exposure to patients designed to limit the potentially damaging effects of radiation.

Irradiation, Contamination, and Incorporation

An object is *irradiated* when it is exposed to ionizing radiation. One can be irradiated when handling radioactive isotopes, when undergoing medical diagnostic imaging such as radiography or CT, and during rare exposures to criticality events. These sources of ionizing radiation generate particles that can penetrate tissue well and possibly cause tissue damage. Whole-body irradiation is one in which the entire body is exposed at once. More commonly, shielding devices such as lead aprons and collimation techniques used in radiotherapy limit the amount of exposed tissue to the intended target. The risk of tissue damage depends on the total amount of radiation and the tissue type because different tissue types have their own intrinsic resistance to radiation damage. An irradiated object does not become radioactive itself unless exposed to neutrons, and therefore irradiated individuals pose no risk to others.

The FDA approved irradiation of wheat and flour in 1963. The FDA concluded from 40 years of study that irradiation is a safe and effective process for many foods to control bacteria such as *Escherichia coli*, *Salmonella* spp, and *Campylobacter* spp. Irradiation does not make food radioactive, compromise nutritional quality, or noticeably change the taste, texture, or appearance of food as long as it is applied properly to a suitable product. Organizations that support irradiation of food include the American Medical Association, the Centers for Disease Control and Prevention, and the World Health Organization.

Contamination occurs when a radioactive substance covers an object completely or in part. Several examples include a laboratory or industrial worker who unintentionally spills a radionuclide on clothing or skin or a victim of a radiologic dispersing device, a "dirty bomb," in which a radionuclide is packaged with a conventional explosive and the resultant explosion disperses the radionuclide. In these similar cases, the source of radiation is the nuclide undergoing its normal decay process, and the individual is exposed to particles such as those mentioned in Table 128–1. The risk of tissue damage from the radiation particles is usually quite low, assuming that the contamination is detected and appropriate measures for decontamination are instituted.

Incorporation occurs when a radionuclide is taken up by tissue via some route that permits the radionuclide to enter the body. This principle is used in many diagnostic and therapeutic procedures such as a thallium stress test, gallium scan, or thyroid ablation therapy. Depending on the dose and type of radionuclide, incorporation may lead to tissue damage, as was the situation for several people after the event at Goiânia.

EPIDEMIOLOGY

Everyone is exposed to radiation in one form or another each day (Table 128–2). In the United States, the estimated annual dose equivalent of radiation is now considered to be 6.2 mSv, a number revised sharply upward by the NCRP in 2009.[24] In addition to the naturally occurring sources of radiation in the Earth's crust that make a significant contribution to our overall radiation exposure, the contribution from human-made sources of radiation, specifically medical exposures, has increased greatly over the past few decades.

Exposures to human-made sources of radiation are not required to be reported to poison control centers in most municipalities. Historically, those that have been reported have not resulted in significant morbidity. The American Association of Poison Control Centers National Poison Data System reports an average of about 300 exposures to radiation over the past 20 years. Of the 231 exposures reported in 2015, 77% were unintentional,

TABLE 128–2	Annual Estimated Average Effective Dose Equivalent in the United States		
Source	**Dose^a**		
	mSv/year	*mrem/year*	*% of Total dose*
Natural			
Cosmic	0.27	27	5
Internal	0.31	31	5
Radon^b	2.29	233	37
Terrestrial	0.19	19	3
Subtotal	3.10	310	50
Human-Made			
Consumer products	0.12	12.4	2
Nuclear medicine	0.74	74.4	12
Occupational	<0.01	0.62	0.1
Medical procedures	2.23	223.2	36
Subtotal	3.10	310	50
Total	6.20	620	100

^aAll doses are averages and contain some variability within the measurement.
^bAverage effective dose to bronchial epithelium.
mSv = millisieverts; mrem = millirem.
Data from Mettler FA, Bhargavan M, Faulkner K, et al. Radiologic and nuclear medicine studies in the United States and worldwide: frequency, radiation dose, and comparison with other radiation sources—1950-2007. *Radiology*. 2009 Nov;253(2):520-531.

and 8% involved children younger than 6 years of age. There were no deaths reported to poison control centers from exposure to radioisotopes, and only 5 patients experienced a moderate effect, meaning not life threatening (Chap. 130).[28]

Natural Sources of Radiation

A wide variety of natural sources expose humans on a daily basis to ionizing radiation. Terrestrial sources of radiation originate from radionuclides in the Earth's crust that move into the air and water. These primordial radionuclides, so named because their physical half-lives are comparable with the age of the Earth, include uranium, actinium, and thorium. Geographic areas vary regarding the content of these radionuclides.

Radon, a radioactive noble gas, accounts for most of the human exposure to radiation from natural sources. This gas, a natural decay product of uranium and thorium, enters homes and other buildings from the building materials themselves or through microscopic cracks in the building's structures. With a relatively short half-life of 3.82 days, ^{222}Rn poses a health risk if decay occurs while in the respiratory space and one of its solid daughter isotopes deposits on respiratory tissue. These radon daughters emit alpha particles as they decay and are the principal causes in the associated increased incidence of lung cancer in those exposed to radon. The risk of lung cancer is further increased in heavy smokers who additionally expose their lungs to as much as 200 mSv from ^{210}Po, a radon daughter that is naturally found in tobacco smoke. The US Environmental Protection Agency (EPA) has recommended household-level intervention when ambient radon concentrations exceed 147 Bq/m^3 (4 pCi/L). Individuals can test their own homes for radon with either short-term (<90 days) or long-term (>90 days) commercially available measurement devices.

The second largest natural source of radiation originates from ingested radionuclides, of which ^{40}K, a naturally occurring isotope is the most abundant. Potassium is the seventh most abundant element in the earth's crust, and ^{40}K represents about 0.012% of this naturally occurring element. With a half-life of 1.3 billion years, ^{40}K decays via beta emission and electron capture. Because it is part of the environment, the average amount of ^{40}K in the body is about 3,700 Bq (0.1 μCi), delivering about 0.18 and 0.14 mSv to soft tissue and bone, respectively. The lifetime cancer mortality risk calculated for ^{40}K is

4 in 100,000 from external exposure compared with one in five from the group predicted to die of cancer from all other causes per the US average.

Human-Made Sources

The NCRP report no. 160 sharply increased the estimated annual dose of radiation exposure from human-made sources of radiation largely from the steeply rising use of CT (Table 128–3).[29] Evolving contemporaneously with the computer, CT technology has become extremely efficient and available contributing to the estimate that more than 70 million CT scans were performed in the United States during 2005 and 2006 compared with about 3 million scans in 1980, accounting for more than half of the human-made collective dose.[24] Concern over potential cancer risks stemming from this new volume of exposure centers on children in whom doses are higher despite increasing practice to tailor scans to the size of the patient and because their relatively longer lives make children more likely to manifest slowly developing cancers. One retrospective study conducted over 7 years in Great Britain through the National Health Service examined data for more than 175,000 young patients each in two groups with certain leukemias and brain tumors.[2,31] Based on typical machine settings and estimated absorbed doses, this study found an increased relative risk of these cancers resulting from accumulated doses of just a few CT scans. Importantly, this was one of very few studies on this topic that did not rely on extrapolated data from atomic bomb survivors. Perhaps influenced by data like these accompanied by increased availability of other alternative imaging modalities, such as magnetic resonance imaging, several studies report trends of decreasing use of CT for children.[23,30]

Overall use of other non-CT radiologic studies has increased greatly over the past decades as well. Estimates show 377 million radiologic procedures in the United States in 2006, not including more than 500 million dental radiologic examinations, although these examinations are not thought to

contribute significantly to the overall accumulated dose. Nuclear medicine scans, particularly in the field of cardiology diagnostics, increased sharply as well and account for 4% of all radiologic procedures and 26% of the total collective dose.[24]

Nuclear Occupational Exposure

Estimates of the annual number of workers occupationally exposed to radiation worldwide are several million.[37] On average, the occupations with the highest exposures (about 4 mSv/year) are uranium miners and millers. Overall, as of 1994, the average annual effective dose to monitored workers in the nuclear fuel industry dropped from 4.1 to 1.8 mSv, mainly because of a large decline in underground mining. Despite the many factors that play a role in occupational exposure at more than 1,200 nuclear reactors worldwide, the estimated annual effective dose to measurably exposed workers fell to 2.7 mSv.

Medical occupational exposure principally includes physicians, nurses, radiology technologists, and laboratory workers who receive an additional annual effective dose of about 0.5 mSv, which is decreased from about 1 mSv 25 years ago, possibly because of efforts to improved protection practices. Exposures to health care workers were studied in a wide variety of subspecialties, including cardiology, orthopedics, radiology, urology, and others.[17,39,40] Although each of these fields uses different modalities of radiation that pose different risks to the operator, studies continue to find low overall doses per procedure, suggesting more than 800 procedures would be necessary to approach yearly dose limits.[40] Emergency medicine staff and trauma teams were exposed to higher radiation doses in the past, primarily from holding the cervical spine stable during x-ray studies, but this has largely been replaced by CT. Doses sustained by these staff are well below the upper limits of exposure set by the Nuclear Regulatory Commission (NRC).[11,13] Thus, although the number of CT scans performed continues to rise, the radiation exposure to staff remains low because of collimation and low scatter, as well as proper shielding in properly designed facilities.

Fluoroscopy constitutes less than 10% of all examinations in the United States but remains the largest source of occupational exposure in medicine. Studies of physician exposure to radiation by fluoroscopy used in various procedures, including exploration of the biliary tract, extremity nailing, interventional cardiology, nephrolithotomy, vertebroplasty, and others report, effective doses ranging from 1 to 100 µSv (0.1–10 mrem). Depending on the procedure, doses to the hands, brain, lens of the eye, and thyroid could be much higher placing physicians at greater risk of stochastic effects (see Stochastic versus Deterministic Effects of Radiation) than is suggested by the effective dose.[17,40] Estimated whole-body exposures to these procedures were considered not to exceed the limits established by the Occupational Safety and Health Administration (OSHA) of 50 mSv per year. Although the likelihood of exceeding established radiation limits is low regardless of the procedure and even assuming a reasonable increase in the number of procedures performed, appropriate shielding and safety training are emphasized to minimize the risk of exposure.

Worldwide, nearly 500,000 workers are monitored for exposures during dental radiography, but the annual effective dose averaged over 5 years has declined to 0.05 mSv. Close to 40 million nuclear medicine procedures are performed annually worldwide, but the radiation exposures from this type of procedure are quite small.[24]

Depleted uranium (DU) is used by the US military and by several other governments. Uranium ore mined from the earth is about 99% ^{238}U and 1% ^{235}U. Enrichment involves separating the isotopes—for example, via high-speed gas centrifuge—so that ^{235}U can be used as nuclear fuel and the leftover ^{238}U can be used in munitions. Consequently, although DU is radioactive, it is 40% less so than naturally occurring uranium. External exposure to solid ^{238}U is considered to be negligible, although currently many studies are investigating the potential link between DU and the incidence of leukemias, other cancers, and birth defects.[1] The Depleted Uranium Follow-Up Program that has surveyed exposed veterans since 1994 has not discovered any consistent, clinically significant differences in uranium-health parameters, which includes hematopoiesis, neuroendocrine, and kidney function.[22]

Test	Radionuclide	Amount MBq	Amount mCi	Effective Dose mSv	Effective Dose mrem
Thyroid scan	^{123}I	25	0.68	1.9	191
Cardiac stress-rest test	^{201}Tl	185	5	40.7	4,070
Lung perfusion	^{99m}Tc	185	5	2.0	200
Lung ventilation	^{133}Xe	740	20	0.5	50
Bone scan	^{99m}Tc	1,110	30	6.3	630
Gallium scan	^{67}Ga	150	4.05	15	1,500
Tumor (PET)	^{18}F	740	20	14.1	1,410
Radiographs					
Posteroanterior and lateral study of the chest				0.1	10
Abdomen				0.7	70
Pelvis				0.6	60
Lumbar spine				1.5	150
ERCP				4.0	400
Computed Tomography					
Head				2	200
Cervical spine				3	300
Chest				7	700
Chest for pulmonary embolism				15	1500
Abdomen				8	800
Pelvis				6	600
Coronary angiography				16	1,600

TABLE 128–3 Diagnostic Imaging Procedures: Type and Amount of Radionuclide or Radiation[25]

ERCP = endoscopic retrograde cholangiopancreatography; MBq = megabequerel; mCi = millicuries; mSv = millisievert; mrem = millirem.

EXPOSURE LIMITS

The NRC established the "Standards for Protection against Radiation," which regulates radiation exposures using a twofold system of dose limitation: doses to individuals shall not exceed limits established by the NRC, and all exposures shall be kept *as low as reasonably achievable* (ALARA). The total effective dose equivalent may not exceed 50 mSv/year to reduce the risk of stochastic effects (see Stochastic versus Deterministic Effects of Radiation). The dose to the fetus of a pregnant radiation worker may not exceed 5 mSv over 9 months and should not substantially exceed 0.5 mSv in any 1 month.

REGULATION AND REPORTING

The use of ionizing radiation, radiation sources, and the byproducts of nuclear energy are among the most heavily regulated processes worldwide. Regulations for medical use of radiation derive from multiple international and national organizations. Among the international groups are the United Nations Scientific Committee on the Effects of Atomic Radiation (UNSCEAR), the International Commission on Radiological Protection (ICRP), the Biological Effects of Ionizing Radiation (BEIR) Committee, the International Commission on Radiological Units and Measurements (ICRU), the Radiation Effects Research Foundation (RERF), and the International Radiation Protection Association (IRPA). Because international organizations do not have the authority to enforce their recommendations worldwide, most countries have their own regulatory groups that cooperate internationally. In the United States, the NCRP reviews recommendations from the ICRP and makes recommendations. The NCRP issues BEIR reports that have direct standards for ionizing radiation use. For medical imaging standards, recommendations from the NCRP are considered to be guidelines with which all radiology departments must comply. The goal is to foster a radiation protection program that prevents deterministic effects. Additionally, the Conference of Radiation Control Program Directors (CRCPD) suggests state regulations for control of radiation.

National regulatory agencies include the NRC, EPA, OSHA, and FDA. The NRC also runs an Agreement State Program under which the NRC relinquishes to the States portions of its regulatory authority to license and regulate nuclear materials. The US Department of Transportation (DOT) regulates transport of hazardous materials, including radioactive material.

The NRC, the EPA, and many state governments share the responsibility of licensing and regulating radionuclides in the United States. The Oak Ridge Institute for Science and Education's (ORISE) supports the NRC by maintaining the NRC's website for Radiation Exposure Information and Reporting System (REIRS) and the database of radiation exposure from NRC licensees (http://www.reirs.com). Individual states regulate radioactive substances that occur naturally or are produced by machines, such as linear accelerators or cyclotrons. The EPA oversees the general area of environmental monitoring of radiation. The FDA regulates the design and manufacture of electronic products, inspects diagnostic x-ray equipment, and establishes specific operational standards for x-ray equipment. The NRC regulates medical, academic, and industrial uses of nuclear materials generated by or from a nuclear reactor. The OSHA regulates occupational exposure to radiation and oversees regulations for training programs and "right to know" regulations.

The Oak Ridge Institute for Science and Education's Radiation Emergency Assistance Center/Training Site (REAC/TS) and the International Atomic Energy Agency (IAEA) both maintain radiation incident registries that track US and foreign radiation incidents. Information for the REAC/TS registries is gathered from many sources, including the WHO Radiation Emergency Medical Preparedness and Assistance (REMPAN), IAEA, state health departments, and medical and health physics literature.

PATHOPHYSIOLOGY

Ionizing radiation causes damage to tissue by several mechanisms called direct or indirect effects. *Direct effects* are when particles physically damage the DNA in a cell, which can occur at the sugar phosphate backbone, hydrogen bonds, or base molecules. Although any type of radiation can cause this damage, high-LET radiation is more likely to cause direct effects

owing to its greater probability of interacting with DNA. When this kind of damage occurs, a mutation can arise, which may then result in alteration of a germ line, development of a neoplasm, or cell death. The risk of these consequences overall, however, is low because of the relative paucity of DNA within a cell, the even smaller percentage of active DNA within a given cell, and the ability of DNA to repair itself.

Although DNA represents a low-probability target for radiation, the rest of the cell media represents a higher probability target. *Indirect effects* are when radiation impacts a molecule and creates a reactive species, which then chemically reacts with organic molecules in cells altering their structure or function. These radiation-induced ions are unstable, however, and usually convert to free radicals. Water, which is in great abundance within cells, can transform into a hydroxyl radical (OH·) after interaction with incident radiation. The hydroxyl radical diffuses only a short distance through the cell because of its highly reactive nature and itself causes molecular damage. Indirect effects are predominantly caused by low-LET radiation (x-rays, gamma-rays, and fast electrons).

The bystander effect refers to cellular damage in unirradiated cells that neighbor irradiated cells. As early as the 1940s, there were reports of inactivation of cells by ionization of the surrounding medium. Recently, the use of a single-particle microbeam (a device that can fire a predefined exact number of alpha particles through a particular cell nucleus) demonstrated that cultured cells that were not hit by radiation showed increased chromosome damage, rearrangement, and rate of death. In one experiment, when 10% of cells on a dish were exposed to two or more alpha particles, the resulting frequency of induced oncogenic transformation was indistinguishable from that when all the cells on the dish were exposed to the same number of alpha particles.[27] Studies demonstrate the bystander effect for proton beams, x-rays, and low-LET radiation.[32,34]

Genomic instability is a single mutation followed by a cascade of further mutations altering the fidelity of genomic replication. This modification can be found in cell progeny many generations after irradiation and can have unpredictable outcomes in succeeding generations. Although many hypotheses have been suggested, it appears most likely that the instability is due to irreversible regulatory change in the network of cellular gene products.[12,15,21]

Although any molecule can be damaged in a variety of ways that may lead to cell injury of varying severity, double-stranded breaks in DNA are the type of damage most likely to cause chromosomal aberrations or cell death. The radiosensitivity of the cell is directly related to its rate of proliferation and inversely related to its degree of differentiation.

Thousands of these types of lesions occur daily in the human body. There are several mechanisms by which the body effects its own repair, which forms the basis of fractionated radiation therapy, taking advantage of less efficient repair mechanisms of tumor cells. However, there is evidence that DNA damage induced by radiation is chemically different and more complex from DNA damage that occurs spontaneously, which contributes to a higher rate of mutation than that resulting from spontaneous damage. Dose–response relationships for mutation are approximately linear down to about 25 mGy, the statistical limit of these studies. Although repair mechanisms reduce substantially the radiation risk of mutation, there is no evidence yet that these mechanisms eliminate those risks at low doses, although some question this conclusion.[18]

STOCHASTIC VERSUS DETERMINISTIC EFFECTS OF RADIATION

The radiation damage just described has two consequential results: it kills cells or it alters cells and causes cancer. Injuries that do not require a threshold limit to be exceeded include mutagenic and carcinogenic changes to individual cells in which DNA is the critical and ultimate target. This is the *stochastic effect* of radiation. Theoretically, there is no dose of radiation too small to have the potential of causing cancer in an exposed individual.

Whereas the stochastic effects of radiation can follow less severe exposures, the *deterministic effects* of radiation usually follow a large whole-body exposure, such as a Chernobyl-type event. In terms of cell death, a relatively large number of cells of an organ system must be killed before an effect becomes clinically evident. This number of killed cells constitutes a threshold limit that must be exceeded, and this is what is known as the deterministic or nonstochastic effects of radiation.

To illustrate the differences between stochastic and nonstochastic effects, consider a single alpha particle, emitted from [210]Po, which was incorporated after exposure in a radon-contaminated household. Theoretically, if this particle impacts on an active segment of DNA in a patient's respiratory tract, it could give rise to a cancer—the stochastic effect. In contrast, after exposure to the criticality event in Tokaimura, Japan, the most severely injured worker received 17 Sv of neutron and gamma radiation and experienced so much cell death across so many systems in his body that he died well before any injured yet surviving cells could develop into a cancer—the deterministic effect.

ACUTE RADIATION SYNDROME

The US Army Medical Corps first described ARS in 1946 when victims of the detonations at Hiroshima and Nagasaki were admitted for treatment at Osaka University Hospital.[16] Understanding the features of ARS is essential for managing a patient who is exposed to massive whole-body irradiation, generally considered to be 1 Gy (160 times the average annual exposure) or more. In many cases, a reliable estimate of the radiation dose is difficult, making it more practical to focus on the clinical features of radiation injury and their prognostic utility.

Acute radiation syndrome involves a sequence of events that varies with the severity of the exposure.[41] Generally, more extensive exposures lead to more rapid onset of symptoms and more severe clinical features. Four classic clinical stages are described, which begin with the early prodromal stage of nausea and vomiting. These symptoms begin anywhere from hours to days postexposure. Although the time to onset postexposure is inversely proportional to the dose received, the duration of the prodromal phase is directly proportional to the dose. That is, the greater the dose received, the more rapid the onset of symptoms, and the longer their duration, except in cases in which death follows rapidly. The latent period follows next as an apparent improvement of symptoms, during which time the patient appears to have recovered and has no clinically apparent difficulties. The duration of this stage is inversely related to dose and can last from several days to several weeks. The third stage usually begins in the third to fifth week after exposure and consists of manifest illness described in subsequent paragraphs. If the patient survives this stage, recovery, the fourth stage, is likely but can take weeks to months before it is completed. Those exposed to supralethal amounts of radiation can experience all the phases in a few hours before a rapid death.

These four stages describe the clinical manifestations that can be observed as a result of massive exposure, but the various systems of the body manifest their own injuries, which constitute several subsyndromes. These subsyndromes are not mutually exclusive of one another and often overlap as cell death or damage progresses. Once these subsyndromes are manifest, they often are irreversible.

The cerebrovascular syndrome describes the manifestations of injury to the central nervous system after massive irradiation. This syndrome, after exposure to doses of about 15 to 20 Gy or greater, is characterized by rapid or immediate onset of hyperthermia, ataxia, loss of motor control, apathy, lethargy, cardiovascular shock, and seizures. The mechanism of this injury may be a combination of radiation-induced vascular lesions and free radical–induced neuronal death and cerebral edema.

Despite autopsy evidence of some radiation-induced inflammatory changes to the heart, animal experiments demonstrate that the heart is relatively resistant to high doses of radiation. Cardiovascular shock is more likely because of systemic vascular damage, which can later compound shock resulting from other subsyndromes should the patient survive to that point. A "vascular radiation subsyndrome" might be considered to help explain the hemodynamic changes a patient experiences after a massive dose of radiation.

The pulmonary system is not spared injury from irradiation. Pneumonitis can occur within 1 to 3 months after a dose of 6 to 10 Gy. This can lead to respiratory failure, pulmonary fibrosis, or cor pulmonale months to years later.

The gastrointestinal (GI) syndrome begins after an exposure to about 6 Gy or more when GI mucosal cell injury and death occur. Findings and effects include anorexia, nausea, vomiting, and diarrhea. As the mucosal lining is sloughed, there is persistent bloody diarrhea, hypersecretion of cellular fluids into the lumen, and a loss of peristalsis, which can progress to abdominal distension and dehydration. Destruction of the mucosal lining allows for colonization by enteric organisms with ensuing sepsis.

The hematologic changes that occur after an exposure to about 1 Gy or greater are called the hematopoietic syndrome. Hematopoietic stem cells are highly radiosensitive, in contrast to the more mature erythrocytes and platelets. Lymphocytes are also radiosensitive and can die quickly from cell lysis after an exposure. This contrasts with granulocytes, which endure radiation better. In addition to stem cell death and white blood cell depletion with immunodeficiency, platelets are consumed in gingival and GI microhemorrhages. The main effect of radiation-induced hematopoietic syndrome is pancytopenia, leading to death from sepsis complicated by hemorrhage. The lymphocyte nadir typically occurs 8 to 30 days postexposure, with higher doses achieving earlier nadir.

The cutaneous syndrome, a local radiation injury, can develop early after exposure or can take years to manifest fully. Target cells include all layers, including the epidermis, hair follicle canals, and subcutaneous tissue. Signs and symptoms include bullae, blisters, hair loss, pruritus, ulceration, and onycholysis. Skin injury ranges from epilation beginning at doses of 3 Gy to moist desquamation at about 15 Gy, to necrosis at greater than 50 Gy.

DOSE ESTIMATION

As with other medical management in which determining a specific diagnosis is critical to providing appropriate care, determining an accurate dose of radiation exposure is critical to providing the best care for the irradiated patient because increasing radiation exposure will affect different organ systems, call for different therapies, require different levels of monitoring, and assign different prognoses. Indeed, some consider a dose of 1.5 to 2 Gy to be a critical threshold, beyond which some patients could die from their exposure despite treatment, making the determination of whether a patient has received more than this dose an essential feature of the initial assessment.[9,36] Dose estimation is difficult, however, for a number of reasons, such as the absence of a radiation-monitoring device, exposure to radiation of mixed form (eg, gamma and neutron radiation), and partial shielding of various body parts.

Biodosimetry is the use of physiological, chemical, or biological markers to reconstruct radiation doses to individuals or populations and assess the probability of developing ARS. Key elements of dose estimation include time to onset of vomiting, lymphocyte depletion kinetics, and chromosomal assays. Today there are numerous tools available on the Internet to assist with dosimetry, including the Biological Assessment Tool available at the Armed Forces Radio-biology Research Institute's website (https://www.usuhs.edu/afrri/biodosimetrytools), guidelines from the International Atomic Energy Agency, and the Radiation Emergency Medical Management website (https://www.remm.nlm.gov).

One early response biodosimetry method was developed by REAC/TS that combines post-incident emesis (which could be a sign of psychological stress) with lymphocyte depletion over the first 24 hours.

$$T = N/L + E,$$

where T is the triage score, N/E is the neutrophil/lymphocyte ratio, and E is whether emesis has occurred. E equals 0 if no emesis and E equals 2 if emesis. Based on cases from the REAC/TS registry, for times longer than 4 hours postevent, if T is greater than 3.7, then the patient is deemed at risk of high dose exposure, that is, greater than 2 Gy, and should receive a more extensive hematological evaluation.

The broad ranges of radiation doses that correlate with lymphocyte count are described in the classic Andrews nomogram of 1965. Again, using historic data from exposed patients, a lymphocyte depletion constant was calculated using the equation

$$L(t) = L_0 e^{-K(D)t}$$

where $L(t)$ is the lymphocyte count at time t, L_0 is the lymphocyte count before the exposure (the population mean taken as 2.45×10^9 cells/L), K is the rate constant for a given dose of radiation, and D is the dose of radiation. Solving for $K(D)$ will allow for an accurate estimate of a rapidly delivered, whole-body exposure.

Although there are still other methods of biodosimetry, such as interphase aberrations assessment and electron spin resonance of dental enamel, measurement of chromosomal aberrations has become the gold standard. Introduced in 1966, this technique analyzes the number of dicentric chromosomes that occur after a whole-body exposure to radiation. An exposure to radiation can cause breakage of the DNA molecule in two nonhomologous chromosomes and produce "sticky ends" that recombine end to end. In metaphase, these appear as a single chromosome with two centromeres and are called dicentric. The number of dicentrics in lymphocytes correlates reliably with a given dose of radiation. This assay conforms to International Organization for Standardization (ISO) but suffers from several drawbacks, including reduction of cells for assay in the setting of proliferative cell death, a low mitotic index for irradiated cells, a long time needed for cell cultures to reach metaphase in which dicentrics are measured, and migration of lymphocytes into tissue and the lymphatic system. These complications limit the time available to perform an accurate test as well as make the testing itself a relatively long affair, complicating its potential application to a mass casualty event. The translocation assay uses fluorescence in situ hybridization chromosome-painting technique and is used primarily for estimating doses of historical exposures. Unlike dicentrics, complete translocations persist in cell division and enable dose estimation over years after exposure. In fact, when this technique was used to evaluate the radiation dose experienced by clean-up workers at Chernobyl, the authors concluded that it was likely that recorded doses for these cleanup workers overestimate their average bone marrow doses, perhaps substantially.[19] Another method includes the cytokinesis-block micronucleus (CBMN) assay in which other unstable cell nuclear aberrations form but then disappear over time. This method generates data comparable to dicentric analysis, and when used in a semiautomated fashion, it can greatly improve testing speed.[8] The premature chromosome condensation assay in which chromosomes are stimulated to condense in interphase cells, has been combined experimentally with telomere and centromere staining to reduce greatly the amount of time needed to perform biodosimetry, although this technique is still in an early phase of development.[26] Many of these techniques are not widely available, require incubation times of 48 to 72 hours, and cannot assess for doses greater than 5 Gy.

CARCINOGENESIS

Radiation was recognized as a carcinogen soon after it was initially discovered in 1895. After decades of research, including animal models, epidemiologic studies, and the lifespan studies of Japanese nuclear bomb survivors, radiation was shown to be a "universal carcinogen" able to induce tumor in nearly every tissue type in nearly every species at all ages. In fact, radiation's ability to induce cancer is so well established that the past three decades of research have used radiation-induced tumors to focus on DNA damage and repair mechanisms.

Double-stranded breaks are the biologically important lesion for inducing tumors. Although radiation induces point mutations, it also induces deletions, sometimes of an entire gene. Research on transcription-coupled repair, in which the transcribed strands of expressed genes are more rapidly repaired than the rest of the genome, were shown to be repaired most often by an illegitimate recombination process that is error prone, frequently resulting in the loss of heterozygosity, a "double-hit" mutation. This loss of heterozygosity suggests that radiation-induced carcinogenesis would more likely result from inactivation of a tumor suppressor gene than activation of a proto-oncogene.[20]

COMMONLY ENCOUNTERED RADIONUCLIDES

Most patients who come to medical attention are not exposed to large, whole-body irradiation but rather to small spills in a laboratory or inadvertent exposures from one of many products that are commercially available. With the notable exception of a well-known case of massive americium contamination in

Oak Ridge, Tennessee, and the cesium exposure in Goiânia, Brazil, the vast majority of these types of cases are not reported in the medical literature.

Americium (symbol Am, atomic number 95, and atomic weight 243) was discovered in 1944 in Chicago during the Manhattan Project. Its most stable nuclide, ^{243}Am, has a half-life of more than 7,500 years, although ^{241}Am, with a half-life of 470 years, was the first americium isotope to be isolated. It decays by alpha and gamma emission and will accumulate in bone if incorporated. It is used to test machinery integrity, glass thickness, and in smoke detectors (about 0.26 mcg per detector), in which it ionizes the air between two electrodes and generates an electric current that soot impedes, triggering an alarm. Alpha particles from these detectors are easily absorbed within a few centimeters of the surrounding air and pose little risk. One gram of americium dioxide provides enough americium for more than 5,000 smoke detectors. In 1976, a worker at the Hanford Plutonium Finishing Plant suffered a large ^{241}Am contamination in an explosion at the site. The patient was contaminated with 100 g or 70 MBq (500,000 smoke detectors' worth) in the explosion. He was treated with long-term pentetic acid (DTPA), and despite some leukopenia from the radiation, he survived for 11 years before dying from unrelated cardiac disease.

Cesium (symbol Cs, atomic number 55, and atomic weight 132) was discovered by Bunsen in 1860. It decays by beta and gamma emissions and tends to follow the potassium cycle in nature. It is used as a radiation source in radiation therapy and as a radionuclide source for atomic clocks. Cesium, the radionuclide of the Goiânia incident, comes in the form of a powder, which would make dispersal relatively easy if used in a dirty bomb. Insoluble Prussian blue is the FDA-approved chelator for patients contaminated with cesium (Antidotes in Depth: A31).

Iodine (symbol I, atomic number 53, and atomic weight 126.9) was discovered by Courtois in 1811. Of the 23 isotopes of iodine, ^{127}I is the only one that is stable. ^{129}I and ^{131}I are fission products that are released into the environment during an event. These isotopes will accumulate in thyroid tissue if incorporated and can cause local damage to thyroid tissue. It is this potential for incorporation that prophylaxis with potassium iodide (KI) is indicated in the event of a large exposure.

Polonium (symbol Po, atomic number 84, and atomic weights range from 192 to 218) was discovered by Marie Curie while she was searching for the cause of radioactivity of pitchblende (uranium ore) and was named after her native country of Poland. Polonium has 27 isotopes, the most isotopes of all the elements and all are radioactive. Polonium is a very rarely occurring natural element, and only 100 mcg is found in a ton of uranium ore. Polonium is chiefly manufactured by bombarding ^{210}Bi with neutrons in nuclear reactors, and it exhibits several properties that make it extremely dangerous. The short half-life of ^{210}Po, 138 days, and high specific activity of 4,490 Ci/g means it emits a great deal of high-energy alpha particles (5.3 MeV) that produce 140 W/g. For example, a capsule containing 500 mg of ^{210}Po reaches a temperature of 932°F (500°C). It also demonstrates a high volatility in which 50% vaporizes in 45 hours at 131°F (55°C) and can contaminate a relatively large area even when left alone. Although only a small fraction of absorbed ^{210}Po accumulates in tissue, cumulative doses of radiation can lead to organ systems failure and death. Animal data estimate an LD_{50} (median lethal dose in 50% of test subjects) of 1.3 MBq/kg and that various mammalian species die within 20 days after an ingestion of 1 to 3 GBq. Because of the extreme specific activity of ^{210}Po, this corresponds to a dose of about 0.01 mcg/kg. Currently, there are no specific chelating agents for ^{210}Po. Although there are limited data regarding the effects of ^{210}Po on humans, Alexander Litvinenko's death within 22 days of his poisoning with polonium is similar to animal survival data.

Radon (symbol Rn, atomic number 86, and atomic weights range from 204 to 224) was discovered in 1900 by Dorn and is the heaviest noble gas. ^{222}Radon decays by alpha and gamma emissions. Exposure of radon gas to the pulmonary epithelium is associated with an increased incidence of lung cancer in both uranium miners and in those who dwell in residences with increased concentrations of radon. Damage to bronchial epithelium results from the alpha emissions of radon and radiation from radon daughters that precipitate as solids and remain in the lungs. Good enclosed space ventilation, abstinence from cigarette smoking, and monitoring of radon concentrations help to minimize this risk.

Technetium (symbol Tc, atomic number 43, and atomic weight 98.9) was discovered in 1937 and was the first element to be produced artificially. Unusual among the lighter elements, Tc has no stable isotopes and is therefore found on earth as a product of spontaneous uranium fission. The majority of technetium is extracted from nuclear fuel rods and is used in nuclear medicine for imaging. ^{99m}Technetium (the *m* is for metastable referring to an intermediate energy state) emits gamma rays that are similar to diagnostic x-rays and easy to detect. ^{99m}Technetium decays to ^{99}Tc with a half-life of 6 hours, and the half-life of ^{99}Tc is 2.1×10^5 years, allowing it to be easily eliminated before it decays in turn. Most human contact with Tc is in medical scans in which Tc has a biological half-life of about 1 day. There are no reports of adverse effects resulting from overdose with Tc, and no specific therapy is recommended in that event.

Thallium (symbol Tl, atomic number 81, and atomic weight 204) was discovered by Crookes in 1861. ^{201}Thallium is used for cardiac imaging, has a half-life of 73 hours, and decays by electron capture and gamma emission. Pharmaceutical ^{201}Tl is created in a cyclotron by bombarding thallium with protons creating ^{201}Pb and is shipped in this form, which decays into ^{201}Tl. Because the radioactive decay process is continual, it is recommended to administer the ^{201}Tl close to its *calibration time* to minimize the presence and effects of other radionuclide contaminants. Chelation can be accomplished with Prussian blue (Antidotes in Depth: A31).

Tritium is an isotope of hydrogen whose nucleus contains one proton and two neutrons, and its symbol is ^{3}H. Tritium decays by beta activity and is used in basic science research as a radioactive label, for luminous dials, and self-powered exit signs, which can contain as much as 9.3×10^{11} Bq (25Ci). Tritium has a half-life of 12.3 years. Tritium emits very weak radiation in the form of 18.6 KeV beta particles, which are easily stopped by thin layers of material, and is safe for glow-in-the-dark watches. Tritium is not absorbed as a hydrogen gas, although, when in contact with oxygen it forms tritiated water, which can be absorbed via inhalation or transdermally. The estimated LD$_{50}$ is 3.7×10^{11} Bq (10 Ci) given its extreme specific activity of 9,649 Ci/g. When absorbed as tritiated water, tritium tends to follow the water cycle in humans, providing a whole-body dose if incorporated. However, its biologic half-life is 10 to 12 days, which can be decreased by increasing urine output, greatly limiting its potential toxicity.

MANAGEMENT

Initial Assessment and Early Triage

The initial management of patients exposed to radiation will depend on a number of different factors, including the amount of radiation in the exposure and the number of casualties in the event. Small-scale exposures to radiation still require at least a brief evaluation for burns and trauma, depending on the circumstances surrounding the nature of the exposure. Calls to the poison control center from a residence require referral to emergency services for an expert evaluation of the extent of the contamination of the site and appropriate decontamination measures. Exposures in the laboratory or nuclear medicine suites require referral to the radiation safety officer (RSO) in the building for a similar evaluation.

When considering a local incident involving nuclear material, first responders will likely include a hazardous materials team (HAZMAT) and local police and fire departments. Hospitals should involve their RSO, and public officials will involve a state agency such as the State Department of Environmental Protection. As part of its primary mission for the US Department of Energy, REAC/TS offers consultation with anyone on a 24/7 basis on questions regarding radiation exposure. Its emergency phone number is 865-576-1005 (ask for REAC/TS). For large incidents, other federal agencies will be involved led by the Federal Emergency Management Agency. Additional radiation expertise can be provided via the Department of Energy, and if applicable, the Federal Bureau of Investigation will be called to protect against further threats.

In a mass casualty event, established prehospital plans should be followed to provide the best management for the large numbers of variably injured given that an explosion of potentially catastrophic size also accompanies the radiation exposure. First responders must use universal precautions and should assume that all victims are contaminated; most events will only require C- or D-level protection (Chap. 132). Field triage protocols tailored to the kind of event in question will designate patients as minor, delayed, immediate, or deceased and should not be altered because of radiation exposure.

Preliminary decontamination, including removal of clothing and washing the victim, should be performed before transportation to a medical facility taking care not to contaminate prehospital providers or equipment. Uninjured patients who are contaminated should be relocated upwind of the incident site for further care.

Initial Emergency Department Management

It is not considered a medical emergency to have been irradiated or contaminated; even highly irradiated patients take days to die, which is why standard protocols regarding trauma and other medical complaints continue to be followed even in mass casualty events. In the event of a radiation incident, there will likely be little warning of these patients arriving, and information will be incomplete. Ideally, the ED is divided into clean and dirty areas where the floor of the dirty area is covered by plastic or butcher's paper. Staff should don surgical scrubs, gowns, surgical caps, masks, booties, and face shields. Two sets of gloves should be worn with the inner set taped to the gown. Tape should also close the back of the gown and trousers to the booties. Dosimeters should be worn at the neck for easy access by the RSO, and staff should be reminded that medical personnel have never received a medically significant acute radiation dose when caring for an exposed patient.

Because of the complex nature of radiation and contamination, it will be necessary to call on the various consultation services, who will likely be a part of the hospital medical response team, that can lend their expertise. These services include burn specialists, dermatologists, nuclear medicine specialists, radiation oncologists, hematologists, toxicologists, and the RSO.

When patients arrive to the ED, it is essential to follow an algorithm that takes into account issues of irradiation or contamination and includes data collection specific to biodosimetry. One such algorithm is the REAC/TS patient treatment algorithm at https://orise.orau.gov/reacts/infographics/radiation-patient-treatment-algorithm.pdf. Important patient history includes their location during the incident, duration of the exposure, time interval between exposure and clinical evaluation, occupation of the victim, and whether the patient has had a recent nuclear medicine procedure. Physical examination, in addition to airway, breathing, and circulation, should focus on vital signs, skin (erythema, blisters, desquamation), GI symptoms (abdominal pain and cramping), neurologic findings (ataxia, headache, motor or sensory deficits), and hematologic signs (ecchymoses or petechiae). Vomiting very early after exposure is considered a sign of the central nervous system subsyndrome and is a poor prognostic indicator.

Recommended initial laboratory testing includes baseline complete blood count (CBC) with differential (including an extra sample in a heparinized tube for cytogenetics), serum amylase (increased from specific salivary gland inflammation and degeneration), urinalysis, baseline radiologic assessment of urine, and starting a 24-hour urine collection. Other laboratory tests, if possible, can include blood FLT-3 ligand concentration, blood citrulline, interleukin-6, quantitative granulocyte colony-stimulating factor, and C-reactive protein. Nasal swabs, emesis, and stool should be collected for radiologic monitoring. For patients with persistent vomiting erythema or fever, a repeat CBC with differential is recommended every 4 to 6 hours. If a patient requires surgery, we agree with the Armed Forces Radiobiology Research Institute recommendation that surgery proceed immediately because of the delayed and impaired wound healing associated expected decreases in leukocytes and platelets.

Decontamination

When a patient is medically stable, decontamination should proceed. Patients who were not decontaminated in the prehospital setting but who are grossly contaminated should be fairly easily detected as such by a quick evaluation with an appropriate instrument. As a first step, all clothing should be removed gently by cutting and not tearing as is typically done for trauma patients. Rolling supine patients allows contaminated clothes to be carefully gathered and bagged and marked. Bagged clothes and other contaminated articles should be removed from the ED to a site designated by the RSO so as not to present another source of radiation. A portable dosimeter should assist in external decontamination. After clothing removal, remonitor the patient for contamination, paying attention to exposed areas such as hair. Contaminated hair should be washed with soap and water before washing the body to avoid trickle-down contamination. For patients with contaminated wounds, decontamination should prioritize the wound first, then body orifices around the face, and then intact skin. Always wipe gently away from the wound. Irrigate gently to reduce splashing. Care must be taken not to abrade skin by too vigorous scrubbing or shaving of hair. Contaminated nares can be cleared often by having the patient blow his or her nose. Ideally, all irrigating fluids are collected for analysis, but this will be limited by resources and event details. There should be no eating, drinking, or smoking at the scene of decontamination.

For patients with smaller exposures to radionuclides, such as laboratory workers, decontamination is often the only management technique required to limit injury. Portable dosimeters will identify contaminated areas, which should be sealed off to limit spread of exposure, especially if the radionuclide is in gaseous form. As with larger exposures, contaminated clothing must be removed and collected. Contaminated skin must be washed with lukewarm soap and water, repeatedly if needed.

In evaluating an area where a spill of radioactive material has occurred, a judgment must be made regarding the severity of the incident so that appropriate steps are taken. If a major incident has occurred involving large amounts of radioactive material, a large contaminated area, airborne radioactivity, or spread of radiation outside an authorized area, evacuation, notification of the RSO in an institutional setting, and calling local or regional emergency response personnel are recommended. Minor incidents involve small amounts of radioactive material in which the individual knows how to clean the site, has appropriate decontamination material on hand, and can clean the area in a reasonably short time. Several different decontaminating soaps are commercially available from general stores and many scientific suppliers. These soaps come in the form of concentrated detergents, ready-to-use dispensers, or foaming sprays with which a small spill is quickly wiped clean and disposed of in an appropriate container. Most radiation management sources, such as Radiation Emergency Medical Management (REMM) and REAC/TS, recommend a neutral soap or shampoo.

Medical Decision Making

Exposure to radiation can lead to a complex spectrum of organ damage that can be difficult and confusing for physicians when creating a treatment plan. Establishment of guidance in the form of a *response category* (RC) helps clarify a medical plan and disposition (Table 128–4). After exposure to radiation, quantitative and semiquantitative criteria should be used to describe different degrees of injury to affected organ systems. Combining descriptions of the patient's severity among categories of hematopoietic, cutaneous, GI, and neurovascular subsyndromes allows assignment of a *grade* of injury. For example, a patient with a third-degree cutaneous injury but only first- or second-degree injuries to the other systems would be given an RC grade of 3, giving the cutaneous injury the greatest weighting because its severity would then carry the worst prognosis. This RC grade then suggests a certain level of care whether ambulatory versus inpatient versus intensive care unit, as well as use of specific treatments such as blood transfusion versus colony-stimulating factors (CSFs) versus bone marrow transplantation. (For specific suggestions, refer to the interactive version of this assessment tool at the REMM's website at http://www.remm.nlm.gov.) It is essential to remember that after a mass casualty event, response assets from facilities to medications to personnel may be

diminished significantly and that recommendations using this system can and should be modified in accordance with other recommendations concerning crisis standards of care.[5]

Medical Management

Supportive care quality will determine the extent of the morbidity and mortality. The majority of patients with ARS who succumb usually do so from fluid loss, infection, or bleeding. Irradiated patients require treatment for nausea and vomiting, diarrhea, pain, and fluid and electrolyte losses. Vomiting is thought to occur as a result of serotonin release from damaged gut tissue. The 5-HT$_3$ antagonists, such as ondansetron and granisetron, are the most effective medications to control vomiting. Prolonged antiemetic treatment is usually not necessary because emesis often resolves within 72 hours. Loperamide, anticholinergics, or aluminum hydroxide are reasonable to treat diarrhea. Mild pain should be managed with acetaminophen, but we recommend against the use of aspirin and nonsteroidal drugs because they exacerbate gastric bleeding. An opioid is recommended for the management of more severe pain.

Probiotics is the introduction of selective nonpathogenic strains of *Lactobacillus* and *Bifidobacteria* into the GI tract to suppress the number of pathogens. Experimentally, this technique increased survival in canine and rodent models. Probiotics were used to help care for three men exposed at the incident at Chernobyl, whose survival time was prolonged, although it was not statistically significant when compared, respectively, with case controls. Based on the existing data, it would be reasonable to treat patients who develop diarrhea with probiotics.[4,38]

Intravenous access should be established and maintained with care because these patients are prone to infection. If the patient is expected to become neutropenic and experience a long hospitalization, it would be reasonable to establish central venous access or place a peripherally inserted central catheter to minimize the risk of access-associated infection. Fluid replacement begins with crystalloid solution with the goal of replacing GI losses. The infusion rate will be modified by recorded inputs and outputs and assessment of surface area burns.

Prevention of infection includes attention to several aspects of care. Maintain the patient in a clean environment and institute reverse isolation for patients with at least moderate exposure or when neutrophil counts decline below 1,000/microliter. Prophylactic antibiotics and antifungals are recommended to neutropenic patients, as well as acyclovir or a congener for herpes simplex virus positive patients. If neutropenic patients become febrile we recommend following the Infectious Disease Society of America guidelines for antibiotic choices. It is reasonable to administer broad-spectrum prophylactic antibiotic coverage, including anaerobic coverage for patients with burns.[7,10]

Cutaneous injuries are cared for depending on the nature, location, and extent of the wounds. Care ranges from use of lanolin-free water-based moisturizers to topical steroids to debridement to skin grafting. For patients who develop radiation-induced fibrosis, it is reasonable to treat with pentoxifylline. Surgical consultation or referral to a burn center should be offered early in the clinical course.

Cytokine therapy (CSFs) use in radiation-exposed patients is based on demonstrated enhancement of neutrophil recovery in patients with cancer, a perceived benefit in a small number of radiation-incident victims, and several prospective trials using different animal models involving radiation exposure. These last studies demonstrated not only neutrophil recovery but also a survival advantage. The best outcomes were demonstrated when started less than 24 hours postradiation suggesting CSFs should be started as soon as possible for patients exposed to a survivable dose of radiation who are at risk for hematopoietic syndrome, that is, more than 3 Gy. Additionally, it is reasonable to administer cytokines to vulnerable patients at extremes of age, that is, those younger than 12 years and older adults who are exposed to lower threshold doses.[10]

Use of blood products is required for patients with significant blood loss or for those experiencing radiation-induced aplasia. This latter complication

TABLE 128–4 Grading System for Organ System Dysfunction and Response Category for Disposition[6]

Symptom	Degree 1	Degree 2	Degree 3	Degree 4
Neurovascular System				
Anorexia	Able to eat	Decreased	Minimal	Parenteral
Nausea	Mild	Moderate	Severe	Excruciating
Vomiting	1/day	2–5/day	6–10/day	> 10/day
Fatigue	Able to work	Impaired	Assisted ADLs	No ADL
Fever	(<38°C)	(38°–40°C)	(>40°C) <24 hours	(>40°C) >24 hours
Headache	Minimal	Moderate	Severe	Excruciating
Hypotension (BP, mm Hg) (Adult)	>100/70	<100/70	<90/60	<80 systolic
Cognitive deficits	Minor	Moderate	Major	Complete
Neurological deficits	Barely detectable	Easily detectable	Prominent	Life threatening
Hematopoietic System (all counts × 10⁹/L)				
Lymphocytes	1.5–3.5	0.5–1.5	0.25–1	0.1–0.25
Granulocytes	4–9	< 1ª	< 0.5ª	0–0.5
Platelets	150–350	50–100	0–50	Very lowᵇ
Gastrointestinal System				
Diarrhea				
Frequency (/day)	2–3	4–6	7–9	≥10
Consistency	Bulky	Loose	Loose	Watery
Bleeding	Occult	Intermittent	Persistent	Large, persistent
Abdominal cramps/pain	Minimal	Moderate	Severe	Excruciating
Cutaneous System				
Erythema	Minimal	<10% BSA	10%–40% BSA	>40% BSA
Edema	Asymptomatic	Symptomatic	Secondary dysfunction	Total dysfunction
Blistering	Rare, sterile	Rare, bloody	Bullae, sterile	Bullae, bloody
Desquamation	Absent	Patchy, dry	Patchy, moist	Confluent, moist
Ulceration or necrosis	Epidermal	Dermal	Subcutaneous	Muscle or bone
Hair loss	Absent	Partial	Partial	Complete
Response Category	1	2	3	4
Triage and Monitoring	Ambulatory	Ambulatory vs. Hospitalized	Hospitalized ICU	Hospitalized Specialized hospitalsᶜ
		Supportive care Blood products	Blood products CSFs	Blood products CSFs or SCT

ªAn abortive rise in cell counts begins between days 5 and 10, which lasts about 8 to 12 days. Afterward, cell counts decline slowly reaching a nadir around day 20. ᵇCell counts decline faster reaching lower nadir for more severe exposures at about days 22, 16, and 10 for grades 2 to 4. ᶜ"Specialized hospitals" refers to those with experience in all areas of intensive care medicine, particularly allogenic stem cell transplantation (SCT).
ADL = activity of daily living; BP = blood pressure; BSA = body surface area; CSF = colony-stimulating factor; ICU = intensive care unit.

usually begins several weeks after exposure, allowing for time to identify potential donors. Use of leukoreduced and (ironically) irradiated blood products should be the rule to prevent transfusion-associated graft-versus-host disease. This hyperacute complication can be further complicated by its similarity to radiation-induced organ injury, including fever, pancytopenia, rash or desquamation, diarrhea, and hyperbilirubinemia.

Stem cell transplantation (SCT) can be used to treat patients with severe bone marrow injury, but the decision to use this therapy is very complicated. Currently, it is believed that with aggressive supportive care and early use of CSFs, patients only suffering from hematopoietic syndrome may survive a radiation dose of 7 to 8 Gy, but doses greater than 10 Gy are likely to be fatal, providing a narrow window of opportunity even if an appropriate match could be found. Stem cell transplantation use must also account for other factors, including the manner in which the exposed dose was estimated and its accuracy; the presence of other radiation syndromes; and whether other potentially significant concurrent organ injuries, such as burns or acute respiratory distress syndrome, are present because they have historically accounted for 70% of radiation deaths.[7] Over the past 70 years, radiation incidents have generally produced only small numbers of patients requiring intensive care, the only exceptions being Chernobyl and Goiânia, although with the real threat of terrorism, emergency resources could become severely limited in the face of a large mass casualty event. If conditions were favorable and resources were available, it would be reasonable to attempt SCT in patients with a severe radiation exposure who have an otherwise grave prognosis.

Management of Internal Contamination

Internal contamination is assessed differently from external doses in that they are not measured but rather are calculated. These calculations are performed by a health physicist on samples such as nasal swabs, urine, or stool to estimate how much activity entered the body. Doses are termed *committed doses* defined as the doses received that last more than 50 years because of the internal deposit of the radionuclide. That is, the radionuclide dose is protracted and remains until it decays or is eliminated via normal kinetic processes. These doses are compared with the annual limits on intake (ALIs) provided by the EPA as a benchmark for medical decision making.

Interpretation of committed doses from contaminated wounds requires special conversion factors provided by the NCRP.

Management of internal contamination is isotope dependent. There are more than 8,000 isotopes, making identification of the particular isotope critical. Although both radioactive decay and biologic elimination contribute to an even shorter effective half-life, medical treatment is directed at one of several categories, including reduction of GI absorption, blocking uptake (as with potassium iodide), isotopic dilution (water for tritium), chemical manipulation (sodium bicarbonate for uranium), excision of shrapnel, and chelation. Both NCRP reports No. 65 and No. 161 provide comprehensive information regarding decorporation of radionuclides; however, for the few isotopes of particular concern for industry, the military, and academic and medical centers, potassium iodide and pentetic acid (DTPA) are the most commonly applicable chelators (Antidotes in Depth: A44 and A45).

PROGNOSIS

The prognosis of those exposed to radiation varies with the amount of the exposure, the type of medical care received, and the number of casualties in a given exposure scenario. Survival is inversely proportional to the radiation dose absorbed. Even relatively radioresistant cell types can be killed by high amounts of radiation. Historically, the mean lethal dose required to kill 50% of humans at 60 days ($LD_{50/60}$) was about 3.5 Gy without supportive care. The addition of antibiotics and blood products increases that mean to 6 to 7 Gy. This dose is likely to be even higher for those treated early with CSFs in a specialized hospital. Coexisting traumatic injuries or burns will decrease the $LD_{50/60}$. An acute dose of 20 Gy or more is considered supralethal. Historically, those who were exposed to greater than 10 Gy died despite care including 20 of 21 workers who were exposed anywhere from 6- to 16-Gy at Chernobyl and one worker at Tokaimura who was exposed to 17 Gy and died 3 months postexposure after requiring highly resource and labor-intensive care, including 10 L of fluid daily and extensive transfusion support.

During a catastrophic radiation incident, resources will likely become depleted to the extent that not all patients who require certain medical treatments to survive will be able to receive them. A consistent and transparent method to allocate scarce resources implemented by senior clinicians within their existing legal and ethical constructs should act to maximize the number of patients to survive, the number of life-years saved, and the individuals' chances to live through each of life's stages. The REMM Scarce Resources Triage Tool is available online for assistance in evaluating a patient's prognosis, in which a patient's injury extent may indicate an expectant prognosis assisting clinicians to help those who may survive instead.[5,6,41]

CONSIDERATION OF THE DECEASED

Contaminated bodies should be placed in a temporary morgue that is refrigerated. Use of the hospital morgue will lead to contamination there. These bodies *should not* be cremated because this will only redistribute the nuclear material, which is not destroyed by fire. Respect should be paid to the religious beliefs of family members of the deceased for whom cremation is the custom. Reconciling these personal and cultural beliefs necessitates extreme skill emphasizing cultural, religious and scientific understanding.

PREGNANCY AND RADIATION

When exposure to radiation via medical examination is possible, pregnant women and physicians have exhibited great concern over possible injury to fetuses. In general, radiation effects to an embryo or fetus are dependent on its stage of development and the dose received. The medical decision to perform imaging or a diagnostic procedure that exposes any patient to radiation is always based on a risk-to-benefit analysis with a given patient's situation.

In the normal course of events, uncertainty exists regarding the normal viability of the fertilized ovum in which the estimated baseline risks of birth defects and miscarriage at all stages are 3% and 15%, respectively, for women with normal genetic and reproductive histories. Very early in a pregnancy before implantation, the embryo is in an "all-or-none" period of development in which the greatest risk from radiation is miscarriage but not greater than

baseline risk. Older than this, the fetus is next at greatest risk between 8 to 15 weeks of gestation during which major neuronal migration takes place.

The NCRP considers risk to fetuses to be negligible compared with other risks of pregnancy when the dose to a fetus is less than 50 mGy (5 rad), which corresponds to 50 mSv from x-ray examination, compared with about 6 mSv effective dose from a CT examination of the pelvis. The risk of malformation is increased only at doses above 150 mSv. As mentioned earlier, special attention must be paid to pregnant or potentially pregnant patients when deciding if an examination or procedure involving radiation is considered. Effective doses from various examinations and procedures are known to range from 0.1 mSv from posteroanterior and lateral x-ray examination of the chest to 15 mSv from CT angiography of the chest, to 40.7 mSv from cardiac stress test with ^{201}Tl. The vast majority of routine diagnostic imaging procedures imparts less than 5 mSv to a fetus, increasing baseline risk by about 0.17%, and so is considered to be of negligible risk, but shared decision making should always balance the potential maternal benefit of the radiologic procedure and the potential risk to the fetus.

PEDIATRICS AND RADIATION

The use of CT scanning in children has markedly increased over the past 30 years. Estimates include data that, commensurate with the 20-fold increase in use of CT scans in the United States, the use of CT for pediatric patients has increased by about eight times. The reasons for this increase are many, including greater availability, greater use as a primary diagnostic tool, and an increased perception that the risk of being wrong about a diagnosis is high.[3,24] Estimates calculate an increased risk of lifetime mortality rate in the range of 0.04% for a head CT for a young female patient (1 in 2,500) compared with a normal lifetime cancer mortality risk of 20% (1 in 5). This excess relative risk was supported by a large retrospective study of a pediatric population that found increased incidence of certain leukemias and certain brain tumors attributed to CT scans over a 23-year period.[2,31]

Although radiation is considered to be a weak carcinogen and radiographic studies should continue to be ordered in the best interest of the patient, it is likely that the number of scans performed could safely be diminished without compromising care. Reports on this topic commonly include problems with ordering unnecessary multiple CTs, follow-up CT scans, and CT scans that occur simply because of a lack of communication among the patient, health care professional, and technician. These problems, compounded by inappropriate CT protocol for pediatric patients, suggest that the medical community could be more proactive in reducing the health risk of those in our charge.

SUMMARY

- Ionizing radiation injures humans through the disruption of cellular structure and function that can lead to cell death and or mutagenesis.
- Fortunately, large exposures of radiation to the general population are rare outside of the setting of an armed conflict, and most contaminations that occur are small and easily controlled.
- Recognition of the exposure and thorough decontamination are the critical steps to minimizing the potential toxicity of an exposure.
- Prognosis is based on dose which can be estimated on a number of clinical and laboratory grounds.
- Although consequential, neither contamination nor incorporation should take precedence over the highest priorities of emergency care and urgent surgery.

REFERENCES

1. Al-Hadithi TS, et al. Birth defects in Iraq and plausibility of environmental exposure: a review. *Confl Health.* 2012;6:3.
2. Berrington de González A, et al. Relationship between pediatric CT scans and subsequent risk of leukemia and brain tumors: assessment of the impact of underlying conditions. *Br J Cancer.* 2016;114:388-394.
3. Brenner DJ, Hall EJ. Computed tomography—an increasing source of radiation exposure. *N Engl J Med.* 2007;357:2277-2284.

4. Ciorba MA, et al. Lactobacillus probiotic protects intestinal epithelium from radiation injury in a TLR-2/cyclo-oxygenase-2-dependent manner. *Gut.* 2012;61:829-838.

5. Dainiak N. Hematologic consequences of exposure to ionizing radiation. *Exp Hematol.* 2002;30:513-528.

6. Dainiak N, et al. Literature review and global consensus on management of acute radiation syndrome affecting nonhematopoietic organ systems. *Disaster Med Public Health Prep.* 2011;5:183-201.

7. Dainiak N, et al. The hematologist and radiation casualties. *Hematology.* 2003;2003:473-496.

8. De Sanctis S, et al. Cytokinesis-block micronucleus assay by manual and automated scoring: calibration curves and dose prediction. *Health Phys.* 2014;106:745-749.

9. General medical effects of nuclear weapons: diagnosis, treatment, and prognosis. In: *NATO Handbook on the Medical Aspects of NBC Defensive Operations.* Departments of the Army, the Navy, and the Air Force. https://fas.org/nuke/guide/usa/doctrine/dod/fm8-9/1ch6.htm.

10. Goans RE, Waselenko JK. Medical management of radiological casualties. *Health Phys.* 2005;89:505-512.

11. Gottesman BE, et al. Radiation exposure in emergency physicians working in an urban ED: a prospective cohort study. *Am J Emerg Med.* 2010;28:1037-1040.

12. Hall EJ, Hei TK. Genomic instability and bystander effect induced by high-LET radiation. *Oncogene.* 2003;22:7032-7042.

13. Hassan M, et al. Do we glow? Evaluation of trauma team work habits and radiation exposure. *J Trauma Acute Care Surg.* 2012;73:605-611.

14. Hiranuma Y. Misrepresented risk of thyroid cancer in Fukushima. *Lancet Diabetes Endocrinol.* 2016;4:970-971.

15. Karotki AV, Baverstock K. What mechanisms/processes underlie radiation-induced genomic instability? *Cell Mol Life Sci.* 2012;69:3351-3360.

16. Keller PD. A clinical syndrome following exposure to atomic bomb explosions. *JAMA.* 1946;131:504-506.

17. Kim KP, et al. Occupational radiation doses to operators performing fluoroscopically-guided procedures. *Health Phys.* 2012;103:80-99.

18. Leonard BE, et al. Human lung cancer risks from radon—part III: evidence of influence of combined bystander and adaptive response effects on radon case-control studies—a microdose analysis. *Dose Response.* 2012;10:415-461.

19. Lindholm C, et al. Biodosimetry after accidental radiation exposure by conventional chromosome analysis and FISH. *Int J Radiat Biol.* 1996;70:647-656.

20. Little JB. Radiation carcinogenesis. *Carcinogenesis.* 2000;21:397-404.

21. Lorimore SA, et al. Radiation-induced instability and bystander effects: inter-related nontargeted effects of exposure to ionizing radiation. *Oncogene.* 2003;22:7058-7069.

22. McDiarmid MA, et al. The US Department of Veterans' Affairs depleted uranium exposed cohort at 25 years: longitudinal surveillance results. *Environ Res.* 2017;152:175-184.

23. Menoch M, et al. Trends in computed tomography utilization in the pediatric emergency department. *Pediatrics.* 2012;129:e690-e7.

24. Mettler FA, et al. Radiologic and nuclear medicine studies in the United States and worldwide: frequency, radiation dose, and comparison with other radiation sources—1950-2007. *Radiology.* 2009;253:520-531.

25. Mettler FA, et al. Effective doses in radiology and diagnostic nuclear medicine: a catalog. *Radiology.* 2008;248:254-263.

26. M'kacher R, et al. Detection and automated scoring of dicentric chromosomes in non-stimulated lymphocyte prematurely condensed chromosomes after telomere and centromere staining. *Int J Radiat Biol Phys.* 2015;91:640-649.

27. Morgan WF. Non-targeted and delayed effects of exposure to ionizing radiation: I. Radiation-induced genomic instability and bystander effects in vitro. *Radiat Res.* 2012;178:AV223-AV236.

28. Mowry J, et al. 2015 Annual report of the American Association of Poison Control Centers' National Poison Data System (NPDS): 33rd annual report. *Clin Toxicol.* 2016;54:924-1109.

29. National Council on Radiation Protection and Measurements. *Ionizing Radiation Exposure of the Population of the United States.* Report no. 160. Bethesda, MD: National Council on Radiation Protection and Measurements; 2009.

30. Parker M, et al. Computed tomography and shifts to alternate imaging modalities in hospitalized children. *Pediatrics.* 2015;136:e473-e81.

31. Pearce MS, et al. Radiation exposure from CT scans in childhood and subsequent risk of leukaemia and brain tumours: a retrospective cohort study. *Lancet.* 2012;380:499-505.

32. Persaud R, et al. Demonstration of a radiation-induced bystander effect for low dose low LET beta-particles. *Radiat Environ Biophys.* 2007;46:395-400.

33. Saenko V, et al. Meeting report: the 5th international expert symposium in Fukushima on radiation and health. *Environ Health.* 2017;16:1-5.

34. Sawant SG, et al. The bystander effect in radiation oncogenesis: I. Transformation in C3H 10T1/2 cells in vitro can be initiated in the unirradiated neighbors of irradiated cells. *Radiat Res.* 2001;155:397-401.

35. Takamura N, et al. Radiation and risk of thyroid cancer: Fukushima and Chernobyl. *Lancet Diabetes Endocrinol.* 2016;4:647.

36. Time/dose effects in acute radiation syndrome-acute clinical effects of single-dose exposure of whole-body irradiation. Radiation Emergency Medical Management website. https://www.remm.nlm.gov/nato-doserate0-0_75.htm.

37. UNSCEAR 2008 Report to the General Assembly with Scientific Annexes. *Sources and Effects of Ionizing Radiation. Volume I, Annex B: Exposures of the Public and Workers from Various Sources of Radiation.* United Nations Scientific Committee on the Effects of Atomic Radiation. New York, NY: United Nations; 2010.

38. Urbancsek H, et al. Results of a double-blind, randomized study to evaluate the efficacy and safety of *Antibiophilus* in patients with radiation-induced diarrhoea. *Eur J Gastroenterol Hepatol.* 2001;13:391-396.

39. Vaño E, et al. Radiation exposure to medical staff in interventional and cardiac radiology. *Br J Radiol.* 1998;71:954-960.

40. Vaño E, et al. Estimation of staff lens doses during interventional procedures. Comparing cardiology, neuroradiology, and interventional radiology. *Radiat Prot Dosimetry.* 2015;165:279-283.

41. Waselenko JK, et al. Medical management of the acute radiation syndrome: recommendations of the Strategic National Stockpile Radiation Working Group. *Ann Intern Med.* 2004;140:1037-1051.

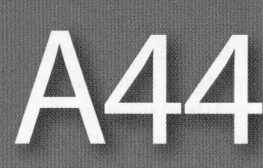
A44

POTASSIUM IODIDE

Joseph G. Rella

INTRODUCTION

Potassium iodide (KI) is the antidote to radioactive iodine that is released into the atmosphere after a nuclear incident. It is approved as a specific competitive inhibitor of thyroid uptake of radioiodine to reduce the risk of thyroid cancer in susceptible populations. The indications for its use are complex, and initiation and maintenance of therapy require great attention to the details of the circumstances of the exposure to limit harm that would result from either under treatment or overtreatment.

HISTORY

Following the study of thyroid cancers in Pacific Islanders who were subjected to fallout from nuclear testing, scientists concluded in 1957 that KI could effectively protect the thyroid from radioactive iodine. The National Council on Radiation Protection and Measurements reported in 1977 that the sudden release of radionuclides, including radioiodine, could affect large numbers of people after a nuclear incident (Fig. A44–1). The following year, the US Food and Drug Administration (FDA) requested the production and storage of KI for the purpose of blocking the effects of radioiodine on the thyroid gland when needed. Although the common terms radioiodine and radioactive iodine are used throughout this text, it is important to note that these are almost exclusively iodide salts containing a radioactive iodine atom rather than molecular iodine that is radioactive. These imprecise terms are retained here for consistency with the medical and lay literature.

PHARMACOLOGY

Chemistry

Iodine is a chemical element, symbol "I," atomic number 53. Its name derives from the Greek *iodes* meaning violet, owing to the violet color of elemental iodine vapor. Similar to other halogens, iodine occurs mainly as a diatomic molecule I_2. Although it is considered a relatively rare element, it is the heaviest essential element used widely in biologic functions. Of 37 iodine isotopes, only ^{127}I is stable. The term *iodide* refers to the ion I^-, which forms inorganic compounds with iodine that is in the oxidation state -1, such as KI.

Mechanism of Action

Neonates, children, and adolescents are particularly susceptible to the toxic effects of radioactive iodine. During the rapid developmental periods for these individuals, there is increasing growth of the thyroid gland, as well as an increase in thyroglobulin and iodothyronine stores. Thyroid tissue also accumulates a larger percentage of exogenously ingested iodide and more efficiently reuses iodine from degraded hormone. This increased activity during human development explains the greater risk for developing thyroid cancer in children compared with adults after exposure to radioactive iodine. During pregnancy, the maternal thyroid gland is stimulated and takes up more iodine compared with in other adults, thus increasing susceptibility in pregnant women to the toxic effects of radioiodine.

Exposure to radioactive iodine occurs via inhalation or via ingestion of contaminated food, as occurred following the Chernobyl incident.

Radioiodine is rapidly absorbed from either the digestive or respiratory tracts. After being incorporated into the thyroid gland, radioiodine exposes thyroid tissue to β and γ emissions, potentially leading to genetic alterations and cancer.[3] This is the stochastic effect of radiation (Chap. 128).

Because the chemical properties of radioactive iodine are unchanged from stable iodine, prophylaxis with KI is effective through the means of isotopic dilution. That is, KI competes with radioactive iodine for the active iodide transport system to reduce the concentration of radioiodine in the serum, making the uptake of radioiodine much less likely, essentially blocking it.

Evacuation and Food Interdiction

Potassium iodide is not a panacea for radiation exposure. Even if appropriately used during a release of ^{131}I, KI will not protect against direct radiation exposure or against other radioactive elements that are included in fallout (ie, cesium and strontium). Depending on radiation levels, communities will be evacuated from areas surrounding a nuclear power plant experiencing a release of radioactive material. Evacuation is most effective if implemented before the passage of a radioactive plume, but this should be guided by dose estimates provided by public health authorities.

The FDA and World Health Organization (WHO) both recommend food interdiction and food control as the principal means to limit public exposure to contamination. Contaminated food that is subsequently canned will ultimately pose no risk to the population if it is stored for sufficient time to allow the radioactive iodine to decay completely. The WHO considers food control to be preferable to iodine prophylaxis and the removal of milk from the diet of some populations to be unfortunate but acceptable.[5,20]

Pharmacokinetics

Dietary iodide is well absorbed from the small intestine under normal conditions. It distributes selectively into the thyroid gland but also to a lesser extent into salivary glands, choroid plexus, and gastric mucosa. Iodine has a volume of distribution of 0.3 L/kg. During pregnancy and lactation, iodide distribution to the mammary glands and ovaries increases.

Iodide that is not concentrated in the thyroid is excreted 80% in urine and 20% in feces, although additional losses via sweat occur and become an important route of loss in warmer climates. Urine iodide concentrations reflect plasma concentrations and have been used for years as a means to assess dietary iodide intake.

Pharmacodynamics

Iodine usually in its ionic form iodide (I^-), is an essential nutrient present in humans in minute total body amounts of 15 to 25 mg. Iodine is required for the synthesis of the thyroid hormones L-thyroxine (T_4) and L-triiodothyronine (T_3), which in turn regulate metabolic processes and determine early growth of most organs, especially the brain. Iodide is actively transported with sodium into thyroid follicular cells, in which it is concentrated 20- to 40-fold compared with its serum concentration. It is then transported into

$$^{235}U + {}^1n \longrightarrow {}^{131}In \xrightarrow{0.28\ s} {}^{131}Sn \xrightarrow{56\ s} {}^{131}Sb \xrightarrow{23\ m} {}^{131}Te \xrightarrow{25\ m} \boxed{^{131}I} \xrightarrow{8.02\ d} {}^{131}Xe$$

FIGURE A44–1. The decay pathway that describes how ^{131}I is derived from nuclear fuel (whether in a bomb or a reactor) and ultimately decays to stable xenon. s = seconds; m = months; d = days. U = uranium; In = indium; Sn = tin; Sb = antimony; Te = tellurium; Xe = xenon; N = neutron.

the follicular lumen, where it iodinates thyroglobulin to form T_4 and T_3 (Chap. 53). Thyroid hormones are metabolized in hepatic and other peripheral tissues (meaning extrathyroid) by sequential deiodination.

ROLE IN RADIOACTIVE IODINE EXPOSURE

Studies over the past 50 years demonstrate that radioactive iodine uptake is effectively blocked by KI supplementation.[2,9,18] In nuclear radiology, administration of iodide-containing contrast media can deliver up to 45 times the recommended daily intake of free iodide and delay the uptake of therapeutic iodine-131 (^{131}I) for several weeks.[10,11] Chernobyl remains the largest experience of KI distribution after a release of radioactive material from a nuclear incident from which data and recommendations are derived. After the incident at Chernobyl, the Polish government distributed nearly 18 million doses of KI to the people in its most affected provinces (in addition to food interdiction), but none was distributed to affected areas of Ukraine and Belarus. Studies of these differently treated populations that were exposed to the radioactive plume clearly demonstrated not only a dose–response relationship between radiation dose and the relative risk of thyroid cancer, but also a threefold reduction of this risk through use of KI supplementation.[3,13] Although some controversy exists regarding increased numbers of detected thyroid cancers possibly because of improved screening, other studies demonstrated the actual increased incidence of these tumors and distinguished radiation-induced cancers from sporadic papillary cancers using genetic analysis.[1,6,7,14]

After the Fukushima incident, the Japanese government gave orders to distribute KI at evacuation sites, but this postexposure prophylaxis did not occur.[15] Data on the aftermath of this event continue to be gathered, but as of 2014, there were no confirmed deleterious effects on the thyroid function of children and adolescents from the emitted radioactivity.[19]

ADVERSE EFFECTS AND SAFETY ISSUES
Thyroidal Effects

Extensive experience with treating goiter and the use of nutritional supplements in the form of iodized salt demonstrates that both hyper- and hypothyroidism result from supplementation with KI.[12] Specifically, treatment with KI is linked to occasional hyperthyroidism, and iodized salt programs are associated with subsequent hypothyroidism and thyroid autoimmunity. Both the prevalence of goiter and subclinical hypothyroidism increase when iodine intake is chronically high. The Wolff-Chaikoff effect, in which high concentrations of iodine inhibit the synthesis of thyroid hormones, is a grave insult to fetal neurologic development in pregnant women treated with KI, which is why we agree with both the FDA and WHO advice against repeat dosing of KI for pregnant women, if possible.[5,20]

A large study in Poland after the Chernobyl incident investigated the risks and benefits of KI prophylaxis. Of the thousands of men, women, and children who were studied, the vast majority of whom received a single dose of KI, no statistical differences were found between treated and untreated groups when thyroid-stimulating hormone (TSH) concentrations were measured among all populations. Additionally, among adults with thyroid disease, no cases of thyrotoxicosis or exacerbation of preexisting thyroid conditions were found. Although pregnant women were not mentioned *per se*, children born in 1986 and examined in the second and third years of life showed no difference in thyroid status compared with those born after radioiodine had disappeared from the environment. In newborns, 12 of 3,214 treated on the second day of life showed transient decreases in serum free T_4 but had no clinical sequelae.[12] Another systematic review of studies reporting adverse effects of iodine used for thyroid blocking, which also did not mention pregnant women, concluded that KI supplementation seemed not to induce severe adverse effects but that scientifically sound studies of this subject are scarce and provide only weak evidence.[17]

Extrathyroidal Effects

Many extrathyroidal effects of KI are described. Sialadenitis, or "iodide mumps," is an inflammation of the salivary glands and appears to be unpredictable. Iododerma is a rare and reversible acneiform eruption related to iodine

ingestion that may result from nonspecific immune stimulation which is similar to bromoderma (Chap. 17).[16] Other reactions reported in association with KI use include gastrointestinal disturbances, fever, and shortness of breath.

Although some reports use imprecise definitions when attributing adverse effects to iodine or iodide-containing medications, "allergy" refers to a specific immune response to target proteins via an immunoglobulin E (IgE) triggered release of cell mediators, such as histamine. There are no studies that demonstrate IgE antibodies to small molecules such as iodine or iodide.

"Allergy" to radiocontrast media is actually an anaphylactoid response to the high osmolarity of these xenobiotics. Anaphylactoid responses manifest by release of similar mediators to anaphylactic response but via non–IgE-mediated pathways. An anaphylactoid response to iodine-containing medications or iodinated contrast materials is predictable in patients with asthma, allergic rhinitis, and food allergies to chocolate, eggs, and milk. Although seafood contains iodide, allergy to fish or shellfish is caused by specific marine proteins and not sensitivity to iodide. Patients manifesting allergic contact dermatitis resulting from iodine-containing cleaning preparations such as povidone–iodine do not react to patch testing with KI. Therefore, when physicians consider the safety of KI dosing in the event of radioactive iodine exposure, reactions to radiocontrast media, seafood, and povidone–iodine should not be interpreted as an allergy to KI. Physicians must also consider that there are inactive ingredients or diluents of the KI formulation as they interpret potential adverse reactions their patients may manifest in response to KI administration.

PREGNANCY AND LACTATION

Potassium iodide is listed in Pregnancy Category D and readily crosses the placenta and distributes into milk. Both the FDA and WHO support the use of KI for pregnant women when the risk is declared substantial by public health authorities.[5,20]

DOSING AND ADMINISTRATION

Based on data from Chernobyl regarding estimated doses and cancer risks in exposed children, the WHO in 1999 and the FDA in 2001 provided recommendations for KI supplementation for various populations, depending on their relative risks (Table A44–1).[5,20] These recommendations remain current and are supported in the text.

Adults older than 40 years of age face a near-zero risk of developing thyroid cancer from exposure to radioactive iodine. For this group, the complications from iodide supplementation, such as goiter or Graves' disease, would likely outweigh any benefit in the setting of relatively mild exposure. However, if public health experts determine that exposure dose is 5 Gy (500 rad) or greater, which is only likely to occur for those living within a 10-mile radius of a nuclear power plant release, KI is recommended.

Adults 18 to 40 years of age are at risk of developing thyroid cancer that is approximately equal to the risks of side effects of a single dose of iodide supplementation, although it should be understood that both risks are very small. The decision to treat should be based on the threshold criteria used as well as the risks of iodide supplementation, such as iodide reactions, or a history of past thyroid disease.

Lactating mothers should take KI when instructed to do so by public health authorities. Potassium iodide is secreted in breast milk and will offer some protection to a neonate, but the risks of treatment are much higher in these patients, requiring greater attention to monitoring, as discussed later.

Pregnant women have increased thyroid uptake of iodide, especially in the first trimester, compared with other adults. Developing fetuses have increased iodide uptake during the second and third trimesters. Because iodide crosses the placenta, fetuses will be exposed to radioactive iodine; thus, supplementation with KI is only recommended at appropriate exposure thresholds.

Children 1 month to 18 years of age are at high risk of thyroid cancer from exposure to radioactive iodine and are at low risk of side effects from supplementation with KI. Therefore, supplementation for children in this age group should begin promptly after official notification of a potential radioactive iodine release.

TABLE A44–1	Threshold Radiation Exposure Doses and Recommended KI Doses for Different Risk Groups				
	Predicted Thyroid Exposure (Gy, rad)				Milliliters of Oral Solution, 65 mg/mL
	Gy	rad	KI Dose (mg)	No of 130-mg Tablets	
Adults >40 yr	≥5	≥500	130	1	2
Adults 18–40 yr	≥0.1	≥10	130	1	2
Pregnant or lactating women	≥0.05	≥5	130	1	2
Children and adolescents 3–18 yr	≥0.05	≥5	65	1/2[a]	1
Children 1 mo to 3 yr	≥0.05	≥5	32	Use KI oral solution[b]	0.5
Birth to 1 mo	≥0.05	≥5	16	Use KI oral solution[b]	0.25

[a]Adolescents approaching adult size (70 kg) should receive a full dose of 130 mg. [b]For smaller, more precise dosing, a potassium iodide (KI) oral solution is available with a dropper marked for 1-mL, 0.5-mL, and 0.25-mL dosing.

Modified with permission from Food and Drug Administration. Guidance. Potassium Iodide as a Thyroid Blocking Agent in Radiation Emergencies. http://www.fda.gov/downloads/Drugs/Guidance ComplianceRegulatoryInformation/Guidances/ucm080542.pdf.

Neonates are at significantly increased risk from exposure to radioactive iodine because of a marked increase in uptake of iodide resulting from neonatal body cooling in the immediate postdelivery period. At the same time, neonates are susceptible to functional blocking by overloading with stable iodide. Therefore, when supplementation is indicated, KI should promptly be given to neonates with critical attention to dosing. The WHO recommends the KI solution be available for maternity wards in the precise dosing for newborns. Because the most critical time period for thyroid blockage is within the first postpartum week, dosing neonates who are older than 1 week should be performed at home by dividing, crushing, or suspending tablets in milk, formula, or water.

Timing of Administration

For full blocking effect, KI should be administered shortly before exposure or as soon as possible afterward. Some models describe the blockade of only 50% of iodide uptake when there is a delay of several hours after an exposure. Depending on the duration and type of risk, administration of KI months after an exposure may also partially reduce thyroid cancer risk.[8,20]

Daily versus Single Dosing

The protective effect of KI lasts for about 24 hours, so it should be dosed daily depending on the dosing estimates for exposure in children aged 1 month to 18 years in whom an ongoing risk is perceived. Groups in whom a single dose is recommended include pregnant women and neonates, in whom there is a significant risk of causing harm to the fetus related to impaired cognitive development. For lactating women, stable iodide will be delivered to the nursing newborn and may cause functional blocking of iodide uptake by an overload of iodine. Therefore, the FDA recommends that lactating mothers not receive repeated doses except during continuing, severe contamination, which would generally be defined by health officials.

As mentioned previously, Chernobyl is the most significant massive release of radioiodine in history and nearly all human experience and recommendations for this type of exposure derive from this one event. Although distribution of radioiodine was uneven in Poland, the air concentration of radioiodine had decreased fourfold 1 week after the first explosion. Therefore, KI prophylaxis was not repeated. It is perhaps based on this experience that it is generally thought that no more than one or two doses of KI would be needed after release of a single radioactive plume, during which other protective measures such as food interdiction or sheltering measures are implemented. Although the possibility exists that many repeated releases of radioactive gas might require prolonged prophylaxis, repeat dosing for days to weeks will usually be unnecessary.

Monitoring

Normal thyroid function is critical for proper brain development in a fetus. Just as a fetus and newborn is susceptible to radioiodine uptake, they are also at risk for development of hypothyroidism from repeat dosing of KI. All neonates who are treated with KI in the first weeks of life should be monitored for changes in TSH, and total T_3 free T_4. Likewise, when a lactating mother requires repeat doses of KI, the nursing infant should also be monitored for the development of hypothyroidism.

FORMULATION AND ACQUISITION

Several manufacturers formulate KI and market them as nonprescription, FDA-approved products with a shelf life of 7 years. Longevity studies over many years demonstrate that the active ingredients of KI are very stable. Recognizing that many state and local governments maintain stockpiles of KI for use in the event of a radiation emergency (KI is also a critical part of the US Strategic National Stockpile), the FDA developed guidelines that manufacturers may use to extend the shelf lives of their products in increments of 2 years.[4] Tablets are available in both 130-mg and 65-mg doses, as well as an oral solution in a concentration of 65 mg/mL. Iodide-containing products *not* considered useful as radioiodine protective treatments include iodized salt, seaweed, and tincture of iodine.

SUMMARY

- Potassium iodide is a safe and effective means of blocking the uptake of ^{131}I after a nuclear catastrophe.
- Firm reliance on the evaluation of health officials of the risk of exposure is vital because the overall likelihood of exposure to the critical radiation threshold is very low, except for those living within 10 miles of a nuclear reactor.
- Exposed persons should strictly adhere to dosing guidelines to minimize the potential risks of KI dosing, especially in pregnant women and newborn children.
- "Iodine allergy" is not a contraindication to KI administration in the setting of a confirmed release of radioactive iodine.
- Food interdiction and environmental evacuation or avoidance of the radioactive plume are preferable to KI prophylaxis in the event of a potential exposure and may obviate the need for KI completely.

REFERENCES

1. Astakhova LN, et al. Chernobyl-related thyroid cancer in children of Belarus: a case-control study. *Radiat Res*. 1998;150:349-356.
2. Blum M, Eisenbud M. Reduction of thyroid irradiation from ^{131}I by potassium iodide. *JAMA*. 1967;200:1036-1040.
3. Cardis E, et al. Risk of thyroid cancer after exposure to ^{131}I in childhood. *J Natl Cancer Inst*. 2005;97:724-732.
4. Food and Drug Administration. *Guidance for Federal Agencies and State and Local Governments. Potassium Iodide Tablets Shelf Life Extension*. Food and Drug Administration, Center for Drug Evaluation and Research (CDER); http://www.fda.gov/downloads/ Drugs/.../Guidances/ucm080549.pdf.

5. Food and Drug Administration. *Guidance. Potassium Iodide as a Thyroid Blocking Agent in Radiation Emergencies.* http://www.fda.gov/downloads/Drugs/GuidanceComplianceRegulatoryInformation/Guidances/ucm080542.pdf.

6. Fridman M, et al. Characteristics of young adults of Belarus with post-Chernobyl papillary thyroid carcinoma: a long-term follow-up of patients with early exposure to radiation at the 30th anniversary of the accident. *Clin Endocrinol.* 2016, 85:971-978.

7. Handkiewicz-Junak D, et al. Gene signature of the post-Chernobyl papillary thyroid cancer. *Eur J Nucl Med Mol Imaging.* 2016,43:1267-1277.

8. Holm L. Thyroid cancer after exposure to radioactive [131]I. *Acta Oncol.* 2006;45:1037-1040.

9. Kunii Y, et al. Inhibitory effect of low-dose inorganic iodine on thyroidal radioactive iodine uptake in healthy Japanese adults. *Endocr J.* 2016;63:21-27.9.

10. Laurie A, et al. Contrast material iodides: potential effects on radioactive iodine thyroid uptake. *J Nucl Med.* 1992;33:237-238.

11. Marraccini P, et al. Prevalence of thyroid dysfunction and effect of contrast medium on thyroid metabolism in cardiac patients undergoing coronary angiography. *Acta Radiologica.* 2013, 54:42-47.11.

12. Nauman J, Wolff J. Iodide prophylaxis in Poland after the Chernobyl reactor accident: benefits and risks. *Am J Med.* 1993;94:524-532.

13. Niedziela M, et al. A prospective study of thyroid nodular disease in children and adolescents in western Poland from 1996 to 2000 and the incidence of thyroid carcinoma relative to iodine deficiency and the Chernobyl disaster. *Pediatr Blood Cancer.* 2004;42:84-92.

14. Port M, et al. A radiation-induced gene signature distinguishes post-Chernobyl from sporadic papillary thyroid cancers. *Radiat Res.* 2007;168:639-649.

15. Schneider AB, Smith JM. Potassium iodide prophylaxis: what have we learned and questions raised by the accident at the Fukushima Daiichi nuclear power plant. *Thyroid.* 2012;22:344-346.

16. Sicherer SH. Risk of severe allergic reactions from the use of potassium iodide for radiation emergencies. *J Allergy Clin Immunol.* 2004;114:1395-1397.

17. Spallek L, et al. Adverse effects of iodine thyroid blocking: a systematic review. *Radiat Prot Dosimetry.* 2012;150:267-277.

18. Sternthal E, et al. Suppression of thyroid radioiodine uptake by various doses of stable iodide. *N Engl J Med.* 1980;303:1083-1088.

19. Watanobe H, et al. The thyroid status of children and adolescents in Fukushima Prefecture examined during 20-30 months after the Fukushima nuclear power plant disaster: a cross-sectional, observational study. *PloS One.* 2014;8:e113804.

20. World Health Organization. Guidelines for iodine prophylaxis following nuclear accidents—update 1999. http://www.who.int/ionizing_radiation/pub_meet/Iodine_Prophylaxis_guide.pdf.

21. Zanzonico PB, Becker DV. Effects of time of administration and dietary iodine levels on potassium iodide (KI) blockade of thyroid irradiation by ^{131}I from radioactive fallout. *Health Phys.* 2000;78:660-667.

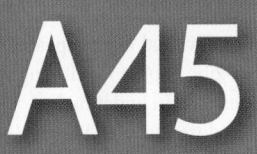

Antidotes in Depth

A45

PENTETIC ACID OR PENTETATE (ZINC OR CALCIUM) TRISODIUM (DTPA)

Joseph G. Rella

INTRODUCTION

Pentetate zinc trisodium and pentetate calcium trisodium (zinc or calcium diethylenetriaminepentaacetate; Zn-DTPA and Ca-DTPA, respectively) are chelators for certain heavy metals and radionuclides. They are recommended for the treatment of internal contamination with plutonium (Pu), americium (Am), and curium (Cm) that occurs after unintentional exposure to these metals or after exposure resulting from a radiation dispersal device or "dirty bomb."

HISTORY

First synthesized in 1954, these chelators were used as investigational therapies to enhance elimination of transuranic elements.[3] Diethylenetriaminepentaacetate is also used for the extraction of metals from soil and as a treatment for iron overload and lead toxicity.[2,9,23] Diethylenetriaminepentaacetate and its derivatives are additionally used to aid with imaging and diagnostics and more recently in chemotherapeutics. Over the past decades, hundreds of human exposures to radionuclides as well as numerous animal studies helped to define the best practices for the use of these chelators, culminating in their approval by the US Food and Drug Administration (FDA) in 2004.

PHARMACOLOGY

Chemistry

Pentetic acid is a synthetic polyaminopolycarboxylic acid with a molecular weight of 393 Da. The calcium trisodium salt weighs 497 Da, and the zinc trisodium salt weighs 522 Da. Pentetic acid is water soluble and bonds stoichiometrically with a central metal ion through the formal donation of one or more of its electrons.

Related Xenobiotics

Several xenobiotics are used in clinical practice to chelate metals. Among these are deferoxamine, dimercaprol (British anti-Lewisite), dimercaptopropane sulfonate, edetate calcium disodium (ethylenediaminetetraacetic acid), penicillamine, Prussian blue, succimer (dimercaptosuccinic acid), and trientine hydrochloride. However, none of these are effective chelators for transuranic metals (elements with atomic numbers greater than 92).

Diethylenetriaminepentaacetate is used to transport gadolinium contrast in magnetic resonance imaging and technetium in nuclear medicine imaging. Other xenobiotics modify the DTPA molecule in conjunction with a monoclonal antibody directed toward specific antigens found on neoplasms, allowing an attached isotope, such as ^{111}In, to deliver site-directed radiation treatment. These related xenobiotics include tiuxetan, pendetide, and pentetreotide.[18]

Mechanism of Action

The conjugate base of pentetic acid has a high affinity for metal cations. Pentetic acid wraps itself around the metal forming up to eight bonds, exchanging its calcium or zinc ions for a metal with greater binding capacity (Fig. A45–1). Remaining water soluble, the chelated complex is then excreted by glomerular filtration into the urine. Diethylenetriaminepentaacetate has specific stability constants for the various elements that it chelates, which presumably explains the different binding efficacies of the calcium and zinc salts.

Pharmacokinetics

Diethylenetriaminepentaacetate is rapidly absorbed via intramuscular, intraperitoneal, and intravenous (IV) routes, but animal studies indicate that DTPA is poorly (< 5%) absorbed by the gastrointestinal (GI) tract. Absorption via the lungs approximates 20% to 30%. Its volume of distribution is small (0.14 L/kg in humans), and it is distributed mainly throughout the extracellular space, although recent data describe a small intracellular activity, particularly in hepatocytes, that explains continued efficacy of delayed protracted treatment. Although some plutonium and americium that is internalized into osteoclasts, bone marrow macrophages, or is still associated with the bone surface is available for chelation by DTPA, that which has been incorporated into the bony mineral matrix is not available for chelation.[7] The plasma half-life is 20 to 60 minutes, although a small fraction is bound to plasma proteins with a half-life of more than 20 hours. Diethylenetriaminepentaacetate undergoes minimal, if any, metabolism. Only a minimal release of acetate is demonstrable, and splitting of ethylene groups has not been detected. Elimination is via glomerular filtration, with more than 95% excreted within 12 hours, and 99% by 24 hours. Although there are no specific data regarding dosing or clearance changes when chelating patients with kidney disease, individuals with kidney disease who receive ^{99m}Tc-DTPA or Gd-DTPA for imaging purposes demonstrate an increased elimination rate of these chelates with hemodialysis. This suggests that hemodialysis might augment transuranic chelate elimination in contaminated patients with kidney disease, and it would be reasonable to use hemodialysis for these patients.[13,24] Fecal excretion is less than 3%.

Pharmacodynamics

Diethylenetriaminepentaacetate increases the urinary elimination rate of certain chelated metals. Animal data show that when treatment is begun within 1 hour of internal contamination, Ca-DTPA resulted in 10-fold greater rate of urinary elimination of plutonium compared with Zn-DTPA. The greatest chelating capacity occurred immediately and for the first 24 hours after contamination while the metal was still circulating and available for chelation. After the initial dose of Ca-DTPA, similar rates of elimination of radionuclide resulted from subsequent treatment with either Ca-DTPA or Zn-DTPA, although continued treatment with Ca-DTPA was associated with

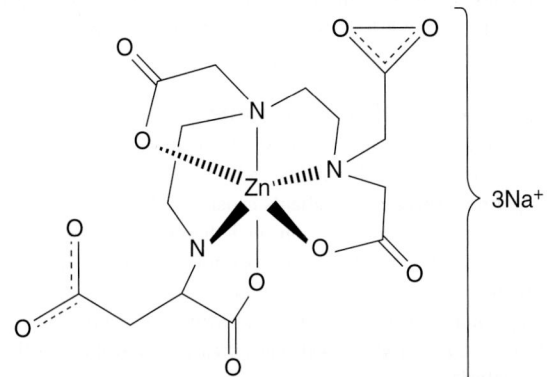

FIGURE A45–1. Trisodium zinc diethylenetriaminepentaacetate, in which a transuranic element (Am, Pu, Cm) is substituted for Zn forming a stable chelate.

much greater toxicity, as described in the later discussion of adverse effects. Animal studies showed that inhalational Ca-DTPA followed by a month-long regimen of Zn-DTPA reduced lung deposits of aerosolized plutonium to 2% of that compared with untreated animals.[19]

ROLE IN RADIONUCLIDE CONTAMINATION

Diethylenetriaminepentaacetate is recommended and FDA approved for suspected contamination via inhalation, dermal, or wound exposure from plutonium, americium, and curium, with the goal of mitigating radionuclide incorporation and local tissue irradiation. For inhaled metals, such as might be experienced after an explosion, treatment with nebulized DTPA is recommended. Depending on the chemistry of the metal (eg, uranium concentrates in renal tissue), this irradiation could possibly lead to development of a malignancy later in life. Chelation is reasonable to increase elimination of the radionuclide and decrease cancer risk, although this risk reduction has only been demonstrated in animals. Increased urinary excretion of transuranic elements is a clinically meaningful endpoint for efficacy of DTPA. We recommend against chelation after ingestion of americium, curium, or plutonium, because increased GI absorption will result.

A report published by the Radiation Emergency Assistance Center/Training Site (REAC/TS) reviewed data from 685 transuranic element exposures, most of which were plutonium, curium, and americium. Most of these exposures (63.5%) were by inhalation, typically a breach of a confined area where workers access the radioactive material via arm-length gloves reaching into a protective box. Ages of the exposed ranged from 10 to 64 years of age. From the 18 patients with the most complete urine bioassay data, the average increase in urine elimination of radionuclide was 39 times the baseline rate after the first dose of DTPA.[19] Although older studies using bone ash showed DTPA ineffective at chelating Pu and Am deposited in bone, in vivo rat studies show reduced retention of actinides possibly by chelating Pu/Am bound to tissue surfaces, but that this is a very small fraction.[7,8] Historical data concerning contaminated workers at nuclear materials production facilities, which included those who received both prolonged and delayed treatments, demonstrated greatly increased urinary excretion of radioactive material.[1,10-12,20,22]

Although data are limited, we agree with REAC/TS recommendation of DTPA for chelating berkelium, californium, cobalt, einsteinium, europium, indium, iridium, manganese, niobium, promethium, ruthenium, scandium, thorium, and yttrium. Pentetic acid salts are not effective in removing antimony, beryllium, bismuth, gallium, lead, mercury, neptunium, platinum, or uranium. Several reports of workers with wounds contaminated by Pu or Am support the practice of surgical decontamination via debridement to decrease absorption of radioactive material. For patients with a discrete wound in which a radioactive fragment is suspected, surgical removal is recommended in addition to chelation therapy.[1,21]

Diethylenetriaminepentaacetate is neither recommended nor approved for treating patients contaminated with uranium or neptunium for several reasons. Diethylenetriaminepentaacetate mobilizes uranium from tissue stores but does not increase urinary elimination.[5,15] Chelating incorporated neptunium is problematic because it forms extremely stable complexes with transferrin, making it very difficult to decorporate.[6,14]

ADVERSE EFFECTS AND SAFETY ISSUES

A review of the clinical data by REAC/TS reported the deaths of three patients with severe hemochromatosis who were treated with up to 4 g of Ca-DTPA per day. Three other patients experienced severe symptoms with similar dosing, including obtundation and lethargy, oral mucosal ulceration, stomatitis, dermatitis, and loss of lower extremity sensation. These reactions resolved upon cessation of Ca-DTPA administration. Injury was attributed to zinc depletion–induced impaired DNA synthesis in organs with rapid cell turnover.[19] Caution is advised when treating individuals with severe hemochromatosis.

No serious toxicity is reported among humans after more than 4,500 Ca-DTPA administrations at recommended doses.[3] Reported adverse reactions include nausea, vomiting, diarrhea, chills, fever, pruritus, and muscle cramps. Transient anosmia was observed in one individual after repeated treatments with Ca-DTPA, also possibly related to zinc depletion, although the specific mechanisms for these adverse reactions remain undefined.

Mice administered 60 times the recommended dose of Ca-DTPA developed severe injuries to kidneys, liver, and the intestines, and deaths occurred.[5] Toxicity was correlated to the total dose and dosing schedule. Fractionated doses increased the mortality rate compared with similar doses given as a single injection. The injuries were believed to result from significant depletion of zinc (Zn) and manganese (Mn) because the same toxicity did not occur when Zn-DTPA was given at the same dose and schedule. These mice data were interpreted to suggest that Zn-DTPA is approximately 30-fold less toxic than Ca-DTPA. Acutely lethal doses of Zn-DTPA were estimated to be 10 g/kg in adult male mice.

Safety

Because of the renal excretion of the radioactive chelate, the kidneys are exposed to potentially higher doses of radiation than other organs, which theoretically increases the risk of malignancy. Additionally, because urine is radioactive during chelation, there are recommendations to use toilets instead of urinals and to flush several times. Any spilled urine or feces should be cleaned promptly and completely, accompanied by thorough hand washing. Patients being chelated should take special care to dispose of any expectorant or breast milk carefully. After nebulization treatments, patients should be cautioned not to swallow any expectorant.

Radiologically contaminated patients do not generally pose a danger to health care personnel. Universal precautions, including a gown, a mask, gloves, a head cover, and booties, effectively protect workers from contaminated material. Urine, feces, blood, expectorant, and breast milk should be collected and disposed of in a safe manner as arranged by health care providers so as not to become a secondary source of contamination. Ambulances, operating rooms, and dialysis machines may become contaminated after providing care to contaminated patients and should be evaluated for decontamination before providing care for the next patient.

DOSING AND ADMINISTRATION

If the contamination route is mixed or unknown, then intravenous Ca-DTPA is recommended. The IV dose of Ca-DTPA is 1 g in adults and 14 mg/kg up to the adult dose as a maximum in children younger than 12 years, administered either undiluted over 3 to 4 minutes, or diluted in 100 to 250 mL D_5W, Ringers lactate, or 0.9% sodium chloride administered over 30 minutes. On the basis of animal studies, it should not be given more slowly.[4] Maintaining normal volume status and frequent voiding should be encouraged to dilute the radioactive chelate and minimize exposure to the bladder. If contamination was solely by inhalation, then we recommend diluting Zn-DTPA 1:1 with sterile water or 0.9% sodium chloride and administering via nebulization.[17]

Although Ca-DTPA is recommended as the initial chelator, Zn-DTPA should be used after the first 24 hours. Animal studies show a 10-fold increased rate of elimination of Pu with Ca-DTPA compared with Zn-DTPA and trace metals, such as zinc, will be severely depleted by continued treatment with Ca-DTPA. After the first 24 hours, Zn-DTPA given daily at the same dose is recommended for continuing therapy because of its sparing effects on the depletion of trace metals and the absence of subsequent liver, kidney, and intestinal injury.

Timing of Administration and Duration of Therapy

Administration of DTPA should be initiated as soon as possible, preferably within the first hour after contamination and is most effective within the first 24 hours, but remains effective as long as radiocontaminants persist and prior to this sequestration in bone and liver.[16] Historically, about 55% of all patients treated with DTPA received only one dose. The decision to continue therapy should be based on radioassay data. This assessment should include collection of 24-hour urine samples, whole-body or chest counting, and close consultation with the hospital radiation safety officer. Assistance is also available from REAC/TS at 865-576–1005; ask for REAC/TS. Current recommendations are to continue chelation until the deposition of contaminant is less than 5% of the maximum permissible body burden for each specific contaminant.[3]

If continued therapy is indicated, a regimen of Zn-DTPA is recommended on the subsequent day. Dosing regimens include Zn-DTPA 1 g intravenously daily up to 5 days per week for the first week. If subsequent chelation therapy is indicated, a twice-a-week regimen is recommended until the excretion rate of the contaminant does not increase with Zn-DTPA administration.[16,17] Continued treatment must be coordinated with a radiation safety officer. For all patients, data regarding vital signs, adverse effects, and bioassay studies should be reported to the drug manufacturer and to REAC/TS.

Monitoring

A complete blood count with differential, blood urea nitrogen, serum electrolytes, and urinalysis, as well as blood and urine radioassays should be obtained before initiating treatment. Daily zinc, manganese, and magnesium monitoring should occur as well as supplementation with zinc. During treatment, repeated blood, urine, and fecal radioassays should be used to monitor elimination.

Patients with Chronic Kidney Disease

Although dose adjustment is currently recommended for patients with chronic kidney disease, kidney disease will impair chelator–ion complex elimination from the body. Hemodialysis is reasonable to increase the rate of chelator elimination in these patients. Because dialyzed radionuclides will contaminate dialysis fluid, care must be exercised during the procedure as well as while discarding fluid and preparing the machine for subsequent patient use. Consultation with the radiation safety officer (RSO) is recommended to assist with discarding waste material, as well as with the overall chelation treatment of the contaminated patient.

PREGNANCY AND LACTATION

Calcium-DTPA is listed as FDA Pregnancy Category C based on animal data. Mouse studies involving doses up to 10 times the recommended dose for Ca-DTPA did not produce harmful effects, but doses of greater than 20 times the recommended dose produced teratogenicity and fetal death. Zinc-DTPA is listed as FDA Pregnancy Category B, also based on mouse data. Doses up to 31 times the recommended dose did not impair fertility or harm to fetuses. There are no human pregnancy outcome data from which to draw conclusions regarding the risk of DTPA. Contaminated pregnant women should begin any treatment with Zn-DTPA as opposed to Ca-DTPA because of perceived risks of the latter chelator for adverse reproductive outcome. However, pregnant women with severe internal contamination in which the risk to the mother and fetus is considered to be high, that is, greater than an expected dose of 200 mSv, it would be reasonable to give Ca-DTPA for a first dose in conjunction with mineral supplements that contain zinc. These chelators do not cross the placental barrier.

There are no studies regarding DTPA excretion in breast milk. However, radiocontaminants are excreted in breast milk. Thus, women with known or suspected contamination should not breastfeed until contamination risk is reduced. Likewise, there are no data regarding safety in lactating women, and data regarding the use in children are extrapolated.

FORMULATION AND ACQUISITION

Diethylenetriaminepentaacetate is available as Ca-DTPA or Zn-DTPA as a sterile solution in 5-mL ampules containing 200 mg/mL (1 g per ampule) for IV use. It should be stored in a cool, dry place with an ambient temperature of between 59°F (15°C) and 86°F (30°C) away from sunlight. Several manufacturers formulate DTPA for IV administration. Five-mL ampules are available singly and in 10 packs. Both chelators are maintained in the US Strategic National Stockpile.

SUMMARY

- Diethylenetriaminepentaacetate is a safe and effective means of chelating americium, curium, and plutonium in a contaminated patient.
- Rapid consultation with a radiation safety officer is recommended to determine the type and degree of contamination, as well as the need for and duration of any treatment.
- In most cases, Ca-DTPA should be started as soon as possible after a contamination, followed by the use of Zn-DTPA if continued treatment is needed.
- Regular monitoring and supplementation of zinc, magnesium, and manganese during therapy is recommended, although the risk of clinically significant depletion is low at therapeutic doses.
- Hemodialysis can increase renal elimination when chelating contaminated patients with kidney disease, although specific data for this use are limited.

REFERENCES

1. Bailey B, et al. An analysis of a puncture wound case with medical intervention. *Radiat Prot Dosimetry.* 2003;105:509-512.
2. Barry M, et al. Quantitative measurement of iron stores with diethylenetriamene pentaacetic acid. *Gut.* 1970;11:891-898.
3. Breitenstein B, et al. DTPA therapy: the US experience 1958-1987. In: Ricks RC, Fry S, eds. *The Medical Basis for Radiation Accident Preparedness II: Clinical Experience and Follow-Up Since 1979.* New York, NY: Elsevier; 1990:397-414.
4. Calder S, et al. Zn-DTPA safety in the mouse fetus. *Health Phys.* 1979;36:524-526.
5. Domingo J, et al. Comparative effects of the chelators sodium 4,5-dihydroxybenzene-1,3-disulfonate (Tiron) and diethylenetriaminepentaacetic acid (DTPA) on acute uranium nephrotoxicity in rats. *Toxicol Appl Pharmacol.* 1997;118:49-59.
6. Fritsch P, et al. Experimental approaches to improve the available chelator treatments for Np decorporation. *J Alloys Compd.* 1998;271:89-92.
7. Grémy O, et al. Decorporation of Pu/Am actinides by chelation therapy: New arguments in favor of an intracellular component of DTPA action. *Radiat Res.* 2016;185:568-579.
8. Guilmette R, et al. Interaction of Pu and Am with bone mineral in vitro. *Radiat Prot Dosimetry.* 1998;79:453-458.
9. Jackson M, Brenton D. DTPA therapy in the management of iron overload in thalassaemia. *J Inher Metab Dis.* 1983;6:97-98.
10. Khokhryakov V, et al. Successful DTPA therapy in the case of [239]Pu penetration via injured skin exposed to nitric acid. *Radiat Prot Dosimetry.* 2003;105:499-502.
11. Lagerquist C, et al. Effectiveness of early DTPA treatments in two types of plutonium exposures in humans. *Health Phys.* 1965;11:1177-1180.
12. Ohlenschlager L, et al. Efficacy of Zn-DTPA and Ca-DTPA in removing plutonium from the human body. *Health Phys.* 1978;35:694-698.
13. Okada S, et al. Safety of gadolinium contrast agent in hemodialysis patients. *Acta Radiol.* 2001;42:339-341.
14. Paquet F, et al. Evaluation of the efficiency of DTPA and other new chelating agents for removing neptunium from target organs. *Int J Radiat Biol.* 1997;71:613-621.
15. Pavlakis N, et al. Deliberate overdose of uranium: toxicity and treatment. *Nephron.* 1996;72:313-317.
16. Pentetate calcium trisodium injection [package insert]. Akorn Pharmaceuticals. http://www.accessdata.fda.gov/drugsatfda_docs/label/2013/021751s008lbl.pdf.
17. Pentetate zinc trisodium injection [package insert]. Akorn Pharmaceuticals. http://www.accessdata.fda.gov/drugsatfda_docs/label/2013/021751s008lbl.pdf.
18. Porziella V, et al. The radioguided ^{111}In-petetreotide surgery in the management of ACTH-secreting bronchial carcinoid. *Eur Rev Med Pharmacol Sci.* 2011;15:587-591.
19. Review of Radiation Emergency Assistance Center/Training Site (REAC/TS) clinical data on the use of calcium DTPA and Zinc DTPA for the treatment of internal radiation contamination. US Food and Drug Administration. http://www.accessdata.fda.gov/drugsatfda_docs/nda/2004/21-749_Pentetate%20Calcium%20and%20Zinc_medr_P2.pdf.
20. Rosen J, et al. Long-term removal of 241Am using Ca-DTPA. *Health Phys.* 1980;39:601-609.
21. Schadilov AE, et al. A case of wound uptake of plutonium isotopes and [241]Am in a human: Application and improvement of the NRCP model. *Health Phys* 2010;99:560-567.
22. Schofield G, et al. Assessment and management of a plutonium contaminated wound case. *Health Phys.* 1974;26:541-554.
23. Soltanpour P, Schwab A. A new soil test for simultaneous extraction of macro- and micro-nutrients in alkaline soils. *Commun Soil Sci Plant Anal.* 1977;8:195-207.
24. Wainer E, et al. Clearance of Tc-99m DTPA in hemodialysis and peritoneal dialysis: concise communication. *J Nucl Med.* 1981;22:768-771.

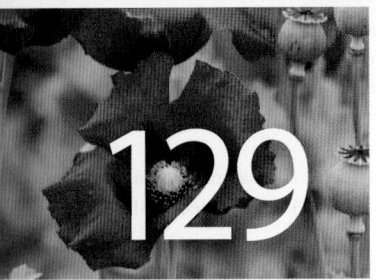

129 POISON PREVENTION AND EDUCATION

Lauren Schwartz

Unintentional poisonings are a global health concern. Pesticides, kerosene, household chemicals, and carbon monoxide are common sources of fatal poisonings.[90] According to the World Health Organization (WHO) International Programme on Chemical Safety: Poison Prevention and Management, in 2012, approximately 193,460 people died worldwide from unintentional poisoning, 84% occurring in low- and middle-income countries. Nearly 1 million people die each year as a result of suicide. Approximately 370,000 deaths result from the deliberate ingestion of pesticides. In addition, an estimated 5 million snakebites occur annually, resulting in at least 100,000 deaths. As of June 2016, only 45% of WHO member states had a poison control center (PCC).

Systematic reviews and meta-analysis conducted of poison prevention studies report that poison prevention interventions improve practices. Interventions that distribute home safety equipment along with education are recommended. However, there is a lack of program outcomes demonstrating a reduction of childhood poisoning rates.[1,37,91] This chapter focuses on programs in the United States that aim to prevent unintentional poisonings and improve access to PCC services.

Healthy People 2020 is a US federal program that outlines the health goals for the nation. These overarching goals are to attain high-quality, longer lives; achieve health equity and eliminate disparities; and create social and physical environments that promote good health and quality of life, healthy development, and healthy behavior across all life stages. Two objectives in the Injury and Violence Prevention section relate to poison prevention. Objective IVP-9 is to reduce poisoning deaths, and Objective IVP-10 is to reduce nonfatal poisonings.[28] Community-based public education programs at PCCs are designed to help meet these public health objectives.

LEGISLATION AND POISON PREVENTION

Since the first PCC was established in 1953, a number of legislative efforts have improved poison prevention and awareness and reduced the number of unintentional poisonings in children. Public education programs at PCCs have been influenced by these federal measures.[80]

National Poison Prevention Week

In 1961, President Kennedy signed Public Law 87–319, designating the third full week of March as National Poison Prevention Week (PPW) to raise awareness of the dangers of unintentional poisonings. Each year, during PPW, PCCs and other organizations across the country create events and activities to promote poison prevention.

Child-Resistant Packaging Act

In 1970, the Poison Prevention Packaging Act was passed. This law requires that the Consumer Product Safety Commission mandate the use of child-resistant containers for toxic household xenobiotics. In 1974, oral prescription medications were included in this requirement. A review of mortality data in children younger than 5 years of age showed a significant decrease in deaths after enactment of the child-resistant packaging legislation.[69,80,86]

Taste-Aversive Xenobiotics and Poison Prevention

Nontoxic taste-aversive xenobiotics are frequently added to products such as shampoos, cosmetics, cleaning products, automotive products, and rubbing alcohol to discourage ingestion.[27] This approach is used primarily to prevent poisoning in children, although in the case of rubbing alcohol, adults are also targeted. The most common taste-aversive xenobiotics are the denatonium salts, particularly denatonium benzoate (Bitrex, benzyldiethyl [(2,6-xylylcarbamoyl) methyl] ammonium benzoate), one of the most bitter-tasting xenobiotics known. The bitter taste of denatonium benzoate can be detected at 50 parts per billion (ppb). This aversive xenobiotic is used in concentrations of 6 to 50 parts per million (ppm), typically 6 ppm in cosmetic products and ethanol-containing household products and 30 to 50 ppm in methanol and ethylene glycol.[9,62] Only limited data are available on the usefulness of taste-aversive xenobiotics for prevention of poisoning. Studies using denatonium benzoate added to liquid detergent and orange juice demonstrate that it can decrease the amount ingested by children.[7,76] However, the degree of taste aversion is not universal. In one study, some children were noted to take more than one sip of denatonium benzoate-containing orange juice.[76] Taste aversion is partially a learned response. Frequently, young children do not find a bitter taste as offensive as do adults.[8] It seems unlikely that taste-aversive xenobiotics will eliminate unintentional ingestions in children because ingestion is required for aversive effects to occur. Taste-aversive xenobiotics are theoretically most beneficial in the prevention of poisoning by toxic and nonaversive xenobiotics, such as ethylene glycol, methanol, paraquat, certain pesticides, acetonitrile, and bromate-containing cosmetics, with which more than one or two sips of the product if ingested can cause significant toxicity. In 1995, in its 1995 Toxic Household Products statute, Oregon became the first state to mandate the addition of an aversive xenobiotic to ethylene glycol- and methanol-containing car products. Unfortunately, analysis of ethylene glycol and methanol exposures before and after the mandate could not demonstrate any difference in children younger than 6 years of age with regard to incidence or severity.[58] Taste-aversive xenobiotics should therefore not be substitutes for other poison prevention modalities.

Toll-Free Access to Poison Control Centers

In 2000, the Poison Control Center Enhancement and Awareness Act (PL 106-174) legislated the goal of nationwide access to PCCs. A toll-free number (800-222-1222) was established in 2001 for all US PCCs.[88] Callers are connected to a regional PCC based on the area code and telephone number exchange. Figure 129–1 displays the national logo incorporated into educational efforts.

ROLE OF PUBLIC EDUCATORS IN POISON CONTROL CENTERS

Public educators in PCCs encompass a range of educational backgrounds, including nurses, physicians, pharmacists, health educators, and teachers. The role of PCC public educators is based on social marketing concepts and encompasses two objectives: health promotion to change behavior and marketing of the PCC.[78] Poison control center public education programs teach poison prevention techniques (primary prevention) and raise awareness about available services in case a poisoning occurs (secondary prevention). Education programs use primary or secondary prevention messages or a combination of both. Primary prevention strategies focus on ways to reduce the risk of exposure. Secondary prevention aims to reduce the effect of an exposure through advice of the PCC.[6,30,39,47] Poison control center public

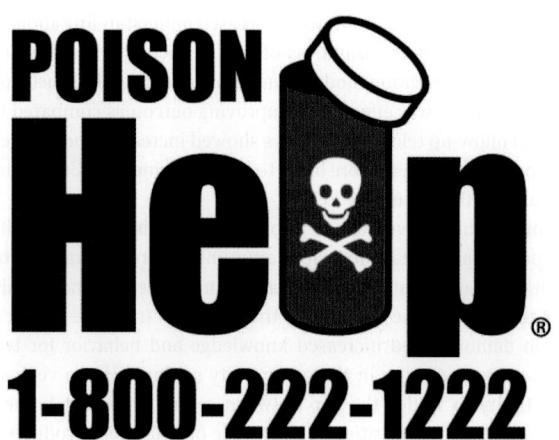

FIGURE 129–1. National toll-free number logo.

educators also provide a range of community-based programs ranging from workshops and health fairs to the production of print materials, videos or DVDs, and awareness campaigns through public service advertising using radio, television, print, and mass transit venues. Social media in health promotion offers an opportunity to further expand the dissemination of health information to diverse audiences through enhanced communication.[56] Poison control center public educators also participate in community health coalitions, working in conjunction with other injury prevention groups such as National Safe Kids, and collaborate with a wide range of community health agencies, substance abuse providers, and others. Caregivers of children younger than age 6 years are often the most important group to reach with education programs. To reach this group, PCC public educators typically work with national programs for families, including Women, Infant and Children (WIC); Head Start; and the Red Cross.

By contrast, individuals older than 65 years of age have not been a priority population for PCC education resources. However, this group is associated with a large number of fatalities reported nationally to PCCs, primarily caused by medication errors.[30] Programs for older adults offer an educational opportunity to reach this high-risk population. Information about medication safety, medication management, and using the PCC as a resource for questions are key messages for PCC public education programs targeting older adults. Collaborative programs with the American Association of Retired Persons (AARP), senior centers, and Departments for the Aging offer an opportunity to provide collaborations focusing on poison prevention and medicine safety programs through educational interventions conducted in senior centers, community agencies, and other groups that serve independently living older adults.

The membership of the American Association of Poison Control Center's Public Education Committee (PEC) includes the PCC public educators from PCCs across the United States and Canada. The mission of the PEC is to provide poison prevention awareness programs in an effort to reduce morbidity and mortality associated with poisoning. Each year, the PEC provides educational sessions at the North American Congress of Clinical Toxicology. Public Education Committee workshops focus on program development, evaluation, grant writing, strategic planning, and other topics of interest to PCC educators.[30]

NEEDS ASSESSMENTS

To develop successful poison education programs, PCC public educators must first analyze demographic data, call volume rates, cultural and language issues, and barriers to calling a PCC. Geographic information systems (GIS) software offers a way for PCCs to map demographic data. The use of this type of software is increasing in public health and can be applied to PCC efforts. The coordination of data retrieval from various data entry programs and the use of GIS software by PCC staff provides access to call rates by zip codes, counties, census tracts, or congressional districts to be used for

planning programs. Health and social services for the targeted community are also well visualized using GIS maps. Using GIS for population-based programs is recommended for developing social marketing campaigns, health education programs, outreach efforts, and coalition building.[68] The study of geographic areas with low call rates enhances the potential for targeted and focused PCC educational programs.

Focus groups, surveys, and interviews provide useful qualitative methods for PCC public educators to identify the perceptions of parents and caregivers about calling the PCC. Barriers regarding PCC utilization include not knowing the PCC number, preference for calling 9-1-1 rather than the PCC, fear of being reported to child welfare agencies, concerns with regard to confidentiality, language difficulties, lack of in-person contact with health care providers, low self-efficacy, and concerns regarding the cost of the call.[2,5,10,31,35,73,84] Each of these barriers must be considered and creatively addressed when planning new programs for reaching caregivers of young children. In one study, 51% of caregivers interviewed in a low-income urban pediatric clinic said that they would immediately take their children to the emergency department (ED) after a possible poisoning exposure.[71] In a separate study, focus group participants stated they would not call the PCC in the case of a poison emergency. Their responses ranking was (1) call the pediatrician, (2) go to the ED, (3) read the label, and (4) call a friend after a poisoning exposure.[31] A focus group with parents provided information to refine a telephone survey concentrating on hazardous household materials and health risks. Feedback from caregivers resulted in a more concise instrument with more targeted questions. In addition, perceptions of the PCC and suggestions for future educational interventions were also gathered from participants.[31] Involving the target audience in the development and testing of information is demonstrated to have improved outcomes when disseminating information.[82]

Follow-up surveys provide a way to analyze factors related to PCC access. English- and Spanish-speaking caregivers in Texas were contacted after an ED visit related to a poisoning exposure in a child. Findings showed that more than half had spoken to PCC staff before the hospital visit. Of those who did not call the PCC, 68% claimed prior knowledge of the PCC yet failed to use it. Significant demographic predictors associated with a failure to call the PCC were being schooled in Mexico and of African American race.[36] Findings from an ethnographic study of 50 Mexican-American mothers with children younger than 5 years of age demonstrated that none had the PCC number in their home.[55]

In person interviews were conducted with parents in the pediatric clinic about poison prevention strategies and awareness of the PCC.[18,22] A pilot study to determine predictors of storage included acculturation, age, gender, and education among Spanish-speaking parents found that less time living in the United States and those with a high school education or less were more likely to store medicines and cleaning products unsafely in the home.[18] Another study conducted with 216 parents and caregivers reported that 80% were aware of the PCC services. However, none knew the 800 number specifically, although many stated they had the number in their home. Of the 42 participants (20% of the sample) unaware of the PCC services, 57% were non-English speakers.[22]

For PCC public educators to plan effective programs with older adults, a needs assessment of the perceived barriers and benefits for this target group related to accessing the PCC is required. Focus groups conducted with older adults show that most do not perceive the PCC as an appropriate service for their concerns but rather as a service for children and parents. Additionally, the participants expressed a very narrow view of what was considered a poison such as bleach and household products. Similar to caregivers of children, older adults repeatedly state that they would call 9-1-1 in an emergency.[11]

POISON EDUCATION PROGRAMS

More than half of the 2 million annual calls to PCCs nationally involve children younger than 6 years of age (Chap. 130). As a result, programs to teach caregivers about primary and secondary prevention techniques have been the major aim of education efforts. Typically, these programs focus on

TABLE 129–1   Poison Prevention Tips

- Identify poisons inside and outside the home.
- Keep poisons out of reach of children in a locked cabinet.
- Keep products in their original containers.
- Never keep food and nonfood items together.
- Install carbon monoxide detectors throughout the home.
- Keep plants out of reach of children and pets.
- Use child-resistant containers.
- Post the poison control center number on all telephones and in all cell phones.

teaching poison prevention (Table 129–1) and raising awareness of PCC services. Poison education programs designed to address barriers to accessing the PCC through community interventions are reported in the literature. In one study, parents at two WIC centers reported an increased comfort level with calling the PCC after a video-based intervention.[35] Interventions have demonstrated an increase in knowledge about PCC messages and poison prevention in the study groups.[34,35,37,46]

Interventions Targeting Health Behavior

Unintentional poisonings can happen even when children are left unattended for a brief period of time (<5 minutes) and a toxic product in use or recently purchased is left within reach of the unattended child.[60] A qualitative study conducted of 65 parents, some whose children had experienced an unintentional poisoning, showed that poison prevention strategies were not consistently implemented in the home. Recommendations included ongoing parent education to reemphasize that "child resistant" is not "childproof" and reinforce safe storage of potentially toxic products, particularly those that are often used.[24] When knowledge and behavior were measured through telephone surveys conducted 3 months after a poison prevention packet was mailed to families of young children who had experienced a poisoning, caregivers were more likely to have the PCC number posted in the home.[35,89]

The ED visit represents an opportunity for poison education programs to work with families to prevent further poisoning exposures.[19] An injury prevention program provided to caregivers of young children after a home injury was effective, particularly regarding retention of poison prevention information and the use of safety devices.[65] A randomized, controlled study measured personalized safety information for parents delivered via computer kiosks in an ED. The intervention group showed significantly higher knowledge of poison storage during follow-up surveys.[25]

The effectiveness of poison prevention education for families who called the PCC after a potential exposure in a young child was also studied. Poison prevention instructions, telephone stickers, and a cabinet lock were sent to the family 1 week after the initial call. Follow-up telephone interviews showed that intervention group recipients reported a higher use of the cabinet lock (59%) and were significantly more likely to post the telephone number for the PCC (78%) than those in the control group who did not receive any poison prevention materials within 2 weeks of the incident.[89]

Poison education programs developed to address caregiver barriers have also been evaluated. An educational video targeting low-income, Spanish-speaking mothers was developed and evaluated. Results showed increased knowledge about the services, staff, and appropriate use of the PCC compared with a control group that attended the regularly scheduled WIC class.[35] Instructor training programs have been designed by a number of PCCs to reach leaders or health educators at community-based organizations to incorporate poison education into their programs for the general population. An evaluation of the "Be Poison Smart" program showed an increase in knowledge and behavior change among service providers after a standardized training session. These reported changes included having the PCC number visibly posted and keeping hazardous products out of reach.[64] Working with community-based services such as WIC presents an opportunity to reach a high-risk population. Pretests and posttests administered to WIC

staff and public health nurses showed increased understanding about poison prevention and increased awareness of PCC services.[66] A randomized trial showed a poison prevention module taught by parenting class instructors in English and Spanish was effective in improving outcomes compared to control group. Follow-up telephone surveys showed increased knowledge about the PCC, participants were more likely to report having the PCC number and behavioral intention to use the PCC.[34]

Community health workers or "promotoras" are involved in health promotion, particularly in hard-to-reach communities. Promotoras are community health educators trained to advocate, promote health, and be culturally aware of the needs of the community they serve.[18] A train-the-trainer model evaluation demonstrated increased knowledge and behavior for teaching healthy homes promotion in the community setting.[48] Home visitors offer an opportunity to bridge the gap between self-report about home safety behavior and direct observation. Safe storage of household products, medicines, and vitamins and posting the PCC number can be addressed through education in the home environment.[45] Focus group participants identified pediatricians as a trusted source of health information for parents.[31,73] The American Academy of Pediatrics (AAP) includes a poison prevention counseling recommendation as part of The Injury Prevention Program (TIPP). The Injury Prevention Program is a safety education program for parents of children newborn through 12 years of age. The TIPP age-related safety sheets include poison prevention advice for parents of children aged 6 to 12 month, 1 to 2 years, and 2 to 4 years.[3] Each safety sheet encourages parents to call the toll-free number for PCCs if the child ingests a potentially poisonous product. It is important that the AAP continues its support for efforts by PCCs to prevent childhood poisonings.[47] In another study, family practitioners and pediatricians were surveyed with respect to poison prevention counseling for parents. Although more than 80% of both groups reported that this was an important topic, family practitioners were less likely than pediatricians to provide poison information during a visit.[23]

Education programs are designed for school-age curricula. The effectiveness of MORE HEALTH, a program to teach kindergarten and third-grade students about poison prevention, was studied.[46] Posttests administered 1 to 2 weeks after the intervention showed increased knowledge in the intervention group of children. Parents of children in the intervention group also self-reported that their homes were more likely to be "poison proofed."

The current opioid epidemic presents a challenging issue for PCC public educators to address with prevention messages. The increased amount of opioids in homes puts both children and teens at risk for exposures. A survey conducted with adults prescribed opioids in the previous year showed that 32% of respondents with children younger than 6 years old reported safe storage in the home. Only 12% of those with children between 7 and 17 years old in the home reported storing these medicines in a locked place.[50] Key messages for parents and caregivers of young children include using a medicine lock box, never storing liquid methadone in a beverage container, storing opioids in original containers, and calling the PCC regarding safe disposal and in case of any exposure.[74] Key messages for those with older children include education about safe storage and the risks for nonmedical use by their children or other teens visiting the home.[50]

Recommendations have been made to develop programs targeting older adults, particularly about potential problems with medication use and storage.[30,43,77] In one study, interviews were conducted with older adults in the ED to assess knowledge of prescription medications. Patients were taking an average of six prescription medications. As the number of medications per patient increases, the likelihood of not knowing one or more medication also rises. Results show that medication management education programs are needed.[15] There has been a shift in the priority of PCC public educators to develop medicine safety programs for older adults.

Community-Wide Interventions

A review of pediatric literature focusing on community-based poisoning prevention programs showed that few studies could be found using poisoning rates as the outcome measure. Additional research to measure community-based poison prevention efforts will be essential to determine the effectiveness of these efforts.[59]

In general, mass mailing of poison information is generally not an effective means to increase call volume for poison exposure or information requests nor is it cost effective.[21,41] Similarly, a distribution of textbook covers with the national logo and PCC information to elementary and secondary schools in low PCC utilization counties was not an effective method for increasing PCC calls.[93] A hospital mailing that combined primary (poison prevention tips) and secondary (telephone stickers) messages was included in an established family health promotion magazine distributed widely in the PCC regional area. This effort resulted in an increased call volume in areas where at least 5% of the residents received the information.[39] In addition, another study result is that overall call volume increased by 11.2% after more than 1 million pieces of literature containing the toll-free number were distributed at sites including EDs, doctor offices, schools, and pharmacies.[40]

An increased number of information calls to the PCC was attributed to a campaign developed to raise community awareness.[79] Media provide a venue for conducting educational activities. Direct mail, radio, television, newspapers, and magazines were incorporated into a media campaign developed to raise awareness in a particular Latino community. A telephone survey conducted before and after the media campaign showed an increase in awareness about the PCC.[2] Although developing this type of program is often costly compared with other educational efforts, the potential audiences are vast. Mass media campaigns are powerful tools used in health promotion and disease prevention efforts.[67] Research shows that a multilevel approach of media campaigns combined with community-based interventions and health education materials influence health behaviors and raise awareness. Additional factors that contribute to successful mass media campaigns include influencing the information environment to maximize exposure, using social marketing strategies, and creating a supportive environment for the target audience to make health changes. Incorporating health education theory and ongoing analyses allow changes midcampaign and assesses outcomes and subsequent media strategies.[67] Radio and television news stations often provide a way to broadcast poison prevention messages during PPW and during periods associated with perceived increased risks to a community.

Social media has become an important venue for expanding health messages and reaching beyond the traditional methods of communication. Although the cost of establishing a social media presence is low, a commitment of staff time and resources are needed to derive the most benefit from these methods of communication.[26,85] There is a need to increase measures of effectiveness of these types of interventions.[38]

The Internet has become a common place for individuals to obtain health information. A survey conducted with parents found that nearly all (98%) used the Internet to search for health information regarding their children. Many used public search engines for obtaining information, raising concerns about reliability and accuracy. Providing education about how to access valid health information is needed.[63] A survey conducted with 21 parents concerning Internet search habits gathered responses to two potential poisoning scenarios; the first one involving a 2-year-old child's exposure to bleach and the other a prescription medicine. Results showed in both scenarios that the parents were most likely to call 9-1-1 in response to the situations. A small number reported that they would be very likely to rely on the Internet. A review of these websites showed that the information presented was often incomplete for poisoning exposures.[32]

Multicultural Populations

Language and culture must be addressed when planning community-based programs. There is a paucity in the published work of PCC public education work in the United States exploring languages other than English and Spanish. Quantitative and qualitative research examining Latino communities and calls to the PCC have been conducted. The findings from interviews with 206 Latino parents at a WIC site showed that 62% had not heard of the local PCC and 77% did not know that the PCC services were free and offered in Spanish.[84] Two other studies examined the call rates in communities

with significant Latino populations. These areas had lower call rates than comparable areas based on demographic and socioeconomic factors.[16,83] Furthermore, a number of studies demonstrate that Spanish-speaking caregivers are less likely to call the PCC because of concerns including confidentiality and language barriers.[2,5,16,33,55] Poison control center public educators need to provide ongoing information about the PCC services to raise awareness and address the barriers to accessing care. In a study conducted with 100 Mexican-American mothers of children younger than 5 years of age, 32% reported that a doctor or nurse would be the initial contact for health advice. Other sources include friends and family (29%), mother, grandmother, mother-in-law (21%), and spouses (17%). Most of the mothers (81%) acknowledged the use of home remedies to treat their children's illnesses.[52] New immigrant families from Mexico and Latin America are at high risk for poisoning exposures. Poison control center education programs should target populations in communities where the impact has the potential to be consequential.[75] Structured interviews conducted with new immigrant Mexican mothers showed that it was common practice for poisonous products to be stored in alternative containers such as water bottles and other beverage containers. This reflects a common practice in Mexico and other developing countries[17] PCC public educators should understand the cultural beliefs of the community and ways to discuss poison prevention with new immigrants.

Qualitative research can help to identify cultural issues when planning targeted education efforts. Monolingual Spanish speaking mothers were more likely to report poor storage of household products, plants, and cleaning supplies. They were also less aware of the PCC and more likely to call 9-1-1.[2] Mexican-born mothers of children younger than 5 years of age were interviewed in their homes about poison prevention techniques. Safe storage was clearly a problem in these homes with 64% of homes having bleach stored within reach of children. The presence of multiple families living in the same home further impedes safe storage practices. In this study, families stored all personal products, including medications and household cleansing agents, with them in their bedrooms rather than in common areas such as the bathroom.[55]

Both language and cultural awareness are important within health communication. Health information needs to address both the beliefs and barriers presented with behavior change. The benefits of a culturally aware and bilingual PCC public educator include their ability to provide programs directly to an audience, building trust by recognizing the distinct needs of the community A lack of bilingual providers was the most significant barrier identified for Spanish-speaking women interviewed about injury prevention techniques.[29] Health education programs including mass media campaigns, designed to accurately reflect the cultural identity—language, beliefs, roles—of the targeted population are more likely to be accepted. Storytelling is also a recommended strategy for health education among many cultures.[53] When asked to provide suggestions for poison prevention education, responses included Spanish radio and video programs as well as brochures that incorporate culturally appropriate values. Incorporating messages into widely recognized media such as telenovelas should also be considered when developing information dissemination channels. Most parents reported interest in learning from PCC staff, doctors, or teachers.[18]

Field testing concepts and materials are important for the development and distribution of appropriate information for multicultural populations. Further work is needed to examine cultural beliefs related to poison prevention and the utilization of the PCC. It is important to address cultural beliefs related to the use of herbal and other complementary medicines.[35] New PCC public education programs are needed to reach multilingual and multicultural communities across the country while also taking into account economic and social needs. Programs are likely to be more successful if individuals trust and view a source as credible, particularly when cultural attitudes and beliefs closely resemble their own.[18,42,53] In addition, "promotoras" or community health workers, should be considered to deliver primary prevention information in the Hispanic community for building relationships with parents and overcoming cultural barriers.[18,48]

Health Literacy and Numeracy

Health literacy is defined as "the degree to which individuals have the capacity to obtain, process, and understand basic health information and services needed to make appropriate health decisions."[82] Health literacy encompasses the ability to read, understand, and discuss medical information. Research from the US Department of Education shows that only 12% of US English-speaking adults have proficient health literacy skills.[82] Older adults, Hispanic adults, immigrants, those with less than a high school degree or GED, and lower socioeconomic groups are at highest risk for low health literacy.[44] People with low functional health literacy abilities are less likely to understand written and verbal health information, medicine labels, and appointment information.[44] This type of health information is often written at reading least 10th grade or higher reading levels.[20] However, 6th grade is the recommended reading level for written medical information. In addition to reading level, use of graphics, font style, color, type size, and layout are important components when developing print material.[20,82] Recommendations for nonprint methods for communicating health information include visuals (posters, fotonovelas, pictographs), action-oriented activities (role-play, theater, storytelling), audiovisuals (videos, DVDs), and improving patient–provider communication.[18,20,61,82]

Warning and medication labels are often difficult to understand. The inability to read these warning labels in English presents a barrier for safe storage and safe use of medication and products.[55] Identification of products often includes brand recognition.[54] Instructions for proper use and warnings may not be understood from the label independent of language. A study evaluating 259 first aid and emergency instructions contained on nonpharmaceutical product labels found many provided inaccurate, inconsistent, or no instructions at all regarding potential exposures. More than half (52%) did not include information regarding product ingestion. In addition, only 39% of products recommended contacting the PCC after an exposure. Standardized emergency information with consistent label placement is recommended.[13] To address medication safety issues, particularly with regard to medication labels, a number of studies have evaluated ways to simplify the information provided. New recommendations for standardized prescription medicine labels incorporate four specific time periods (morning, noon, evening, and bedtime) on the container. Patient provider communication is still needed to reinforce understanding of medication regimens.[87] Similarly, recommendations for improving nonprescription medicine labels have been developed, including larger font size, layout, and use of space.[81,92] Consumer testing of nonprescription medicine labels is recommended to ensure patient understanding of the information provided.[81]

The effects of health numeracy as a distinct component of health literacy are presented in the literature.[57,72] Numeracy is an element of health literacy and involves the ability to use numeric information to make effective health decisions in daily life.[4] Numeracy also includes concepts of risk, probability, and the communication of scientific evidence.[57,70,72] Health-related tasks, including measuring medications, scheduling appointments, and refilling prescriptions, rely on applied numeracy skills.[70,72] Managing multiple prescription and nonprescription regimens frequently leads to medication errors.[87] Poison control center public educators should develop interventions that communicate numerical constructs in simplified and understandable ways. Recommendations for techniques to improve understanding of numeric information include simplifying concepts, using plain language design strategies (larger fonts, use of white space, and appropriate visuals), and using "teach-back" patient understanding strategies.[4,82]

Applying Health Education Principles to Poison Education Programs

Health education involves planning, implementing, and evaluating programs based on theories and models. These models help improve public education interventions for both traditional and social media health promotional approaches.[38,51] There is a need to increase the number of poison educational programs incorporating health education principles. This includes educational efforts designed to reach individuals through community-based programs, mass media, and social media campaigns.

Both the health belief model (HBM) and social cognitive theory (SCT) incorporate the concept of "self-efficacy" and are applicable when designing poison prevention interventions and mass media campaigns. Self-efficacy is the individual's belief that he or she will be able to accomplish the task requested.[14,20,49,67] Many health educators believe that self-efficacy is necessary to enable behavior change. The SCT suggests that individuals, the environment, and behavior are intimately and inextricably interrelated.[49] The HBM suggests that individuals are more likely to make health behavior changes based on perceived risk susceptibility, severity, potential barriers, and self-efficacy. These decisions are made when actions are seen as potentially more beneficial to the individual than the perceived risks associated with surmounting the current barriers.[14,50]

In one study, the HBM approach was used as a framework for poison prevention and for the assessment of barriers to PCC use. Questions for focus group participants were developed based on the principles of HBM—that is, perceived susceptibility, severity, benefits, barriers, and self-efficacy related to the health action requested. Most of the mothers viewed poisoning as an emergency and believed it was a health concern for their children. Cues to action are also a component of the model and involve discussions about poison prevention or related information. Participants recommended using community-based venues and culturally appropriate information to expand awareness about poison prevention and the PCC.[10]

The HBM and SCT approaches were used to develop the questions for focus groups in both English and Spanish. These questions addressed issues related to poison prevention (severity and susceptibility), the services of the PCC (including barriers), and suggestions for education. Focus group participants suggested the use of modeling to reinforce real-life scenarios in which a mother handles the poisoning emergency with the staff at the PCC with a positive outcome.[33] As a result, a video was developed addressing these ideas. Two poisoning situations in which a mother calls the center are depicted. One involves home management (ingestion of bleach), and the second involves taking the child to the ED (swallowing grandmother's antihypertensive pill). The video and correlated teaching guides are available in English and Spanish.[35]

It is important to develop questionnaires that will be accepted and understood by the target population. A Spanish language instrument that addresses home safety beliefs using the HBM framework was developed and tested. Low-income, monolingual, Spanish-speaking mothers of children younger than 4 years of age were interviewed about perceived susceptibility, severity, barriers, and self-efficacy factors affecting unintentional home injuries, including poison prevention measures. Barriers identified include literacy skills and access to bilingual health information.[29]

The HBM supports the idea that a "teachable moment" may be the ideal opportunity to present poison prevention interventions.[25,65] People may be more open to health information after a traumatic experience.[12] Events such as an unintentional poisoning exposure may motivate individuals to behavioral change. Applying HBM principles suggests that individuals will make changes in terms of poison prevention when or if they view the severity and susceptibility of a poisoning to be high in the home. Our goal as PCC public educators is to provide efforts using models that have been tested and evaluated for addressing focused community efforts in each population served by the PCC.

SUMMARY

- Poison control center public educators' efforts must encompass needs assessments, program development, implementation, and evaluation.
- Focus groups with caregivers of young children conducted across the country have consistently identified barriers to calling PCCs. These include calling 9-1-1, fear of being reported to child welfare agencies, and lack of confidence in handling poisoning emergencies.
- Using health education theories and models, programs should be developed that address these barriers and encourage caregivers to use the services of the PCC appropriately.
- Education programs focusing on the needs of older adults and promoting the use of the PCC as a resource for medicine safety should be designed and evaluated.

- A multilevel approach for health communication is needed for poison public education programs.
- Culture, health literacy, health numeracy, and language needs of target populations are important considerations when planning poison education programs.

REFERENCES

1. Achana FA, et al. The effectiveness of different interventions to promote poison prevention behaviours in households with children: a network meta-analysis. *PLoS One.* 2015;10:e0121122.
2. Albertson TE, et al. Regional variations in the use and awareness of the California Poison Control System. *J Toxicol Clin Toxicol.* 2004;42:625-633.
3. American Academy of Pediatrics. The Injury Prevention Program (TIPP). https://patiented.solutions.aap.org/handout-collection.aspx?categoryid=32033.
4. Apter AJ, et al. Numeracy and communication with patients: they are counting on us. *J Gen Intern Med.* 2008;23:2117-2124.
5. Belson M, et al. Childhood pesticide exposures on the Texas-Mexico border: clinical manifestations and poison control center use. *Am J Public Health.* 2003;93:1310-1315.
6. Berlin R. Poison prevention—where can we make a difference? *Acad Emerg Med.* 1997; 4:163-164.
7. Berning CK, et al. Research on the effectiveness of denatonium benzoate as a deterrent to liquid detergent ingestion by children. *Fundam Appl Toxicol.* 1982;2:44-48.
8. Bernstein IL, Webster MM. Learned taste aversions in humans. *Physiol Behav.* 1980;25:363-366.
9. Bitrex P. Bitrex product information. Edinburgh, United Kingdom: Macfarlan Smith; 1989.
10. Brannan JE. Accidental poisoning of children: barriers to resource use in a black, low-income community. *Public Health Nurs.* 1992;9:81-86.
11. C & R R. Seniors' perceptions of the Illinois poison control center. Chicago, IL: Illinois Poison Control Center; May 2002.
12. Caliva M, et al. Frequency of post-poisoning exposure information provided to patients requiring emergency care. *Vet Hum Toxicol.* 1998;40:305-306.
13. Cantrell FL, et al. Inconsistencies in emergency instructions on common household product labels. *J Community Health.* 2013;38:823-828.
14. Champion VL, Skinner CS. The health belief model. In: Glanz K, Rimer BK, Viswanath K, eds. *Health Behavior and Health Education Theory, Research, and Practice.* 4th ed. San Francisco, CA: Jossey-Bass; 2008:45-62.
15. Chung MK, Bartfield JM. Knowledge of prescription medications among elderly emergency department patients. *Ann Emerg Med.* 2002;39:605-608.
16. Clark RF, et al. Evaluating the utilization of a regional poison control center by Latino communities. *J Toxicol Clin Toxicol.* 2002;40:855-860.
17. Crosslin K, Tsai R. Unintentional ingestion of cleaners and other substances in an immigrant Mexican population: a qualitative study. *Inj Prev.* 2016;22:140-143.
18. Crosslin KL, et al. Acculturation in Hispanics and childhood poisoning: are medicines and household cleaners stored properly? *Accid Anal Prev.* 2011;43:1010-1014.
19. Demorest RA, et al. Poisoning prevention education during emergency department visits for childhood poisoning. *Pediatr Emerg Care.* 2004;20:281-284.
20. Doak CC, et al. *Teaching Patients with Low Literacy Skills. 2nd ed.* Philadelphia, PA: JB Lippincott; 1996.
21. Everson G, et al. Ineffectiveness of a mass mailing campaign to improve poison control center awareness in a rural population. *Vet Hum Toxicol.* 1993;35:165-167.
22. George M, Delgaudio A. Poison control center awareness among the parents of pediatric patients in a primary care setting. *J Med Toxicol.* 2011;7:177-178.
23. Gerard JM, et al. Poison prevention counseling: a comparison between family practitioners and pediatricians. *Arch Pediatr Adolesc Med.* 2000;154:65-70.
24. Gibbs L, et al. Understanding parental motivators and barriers to uptake of child poison safety strategies: a qualitative study. *Inj Prev.* 2005;11:373-377.
25. Gielen AC, et al. Using a computer kiosk to promote child safety: results of a randomized, controlled trial in an urban pediatric emergency department. *Pediatrics.* 2007;120:330-339.
26. Gussow L. "My child ate poop!"–how one poison control center established its social media presence. *Clin Toxicol (Phila).* 2015;53:419-420.
27. Hansen SR, et al. Denatonium benzoate as a deterrent to ingestion of toxic substances: toxicity and efficacy. *Vet Hum Toxicol.* 1993;35:234-236.
28. Healthy People 2020. http://www.healthypeople.gov/2020/default.aspx.
29. Hendrickson SG. Beyond translation . . . cultural fit. *West J Nurs Res.* 2003;25:593-608.
30. Institute of Medicine. *Forging a Poison Prevention and Control System.* Washington, DC: National Academies Press; 2004.
31. Kaufman MM, et al. Assessing poisoning risks related to storage of household hazardous materials: using a focus group to improve a survey questionnaire. *Environ Health.* 2005; 4:16.
32. Kearney TE, et al. Investigating the reliability of substance toxicity information found on the Internet in pediatric poisonings. *Pediatr Emerg Care.* 2013;29:1249-1254.
33. Kelly NR, Groff JY. Exploring barriers to utilization of poison control centers: a qualitative study of mothers attending an urban Women, Infants, and Children (WIC) Clinic. *Pediatrics.* 2000;106:199-204.
34. Kelly NR, et al. A randomized controlled trial of a video module to increase U.S. poison control center use by low-income parents. *Clin Toxicol (Phila).* 2014;52:54-62.
35. Kelly NR, et al. Effects of a videotape to increase use of poison control centers by low-income and Spanish-speaking families: a randomized, controlled trial. *Pediatrics.* 2003; 111:21-26.
36. Kelly NR, et al. Assessing parental utilization of the poison control center: an emergency center-based survey. *Clin Pediatr (Phila).* 1997;36:467-473.
37. Kendrick D, et al. Effect of education and safety equipment on poisoning-prevention practices and poisoning: systematic review, meta-analysis and meta-regression. *Arch Dis Child.* 2008;93:599-608.
38. Korda H, Itani Z. Harnessing social media for health promotion and behavior change. *Health Promot Pract.* 2013;14:15-23.
39. Krenzelok EP, et al. Combining primary and secondary poison prevention in one initiative. *Clin Toxicol.* 2008;46:101-104.
40. Krenzelok EP, Mrvos R. Initial impact of toll-free access on poison control center call volume. *Vet Hum Toxicol.* 2003;45:325-327.
41. Krenzelok EP, Mrvos R. Is mass-mailing an effective form of passive poison control center awareness enhancement? *Vet Hum Toxicol.* 2004;46:155-156.
42. Kreuter MW, McClure SM. The role of culture in health communication. *Annu Rev Public Health.* 2004;25:439-455.
43. Kroner BA, et al. Poisoning in the elderly: characterization of exposures reported to a poison control center. *J Am Geriatr Soc.* 1993;41:842-846.
44. Kutner M GE, et al. *The Health Literacy of America's Adults: Results from the 2003 National Assessment of Adult Literacy.* NCES 2006-483. Washington, DC: US Department of Education, National Center for Education Statistics; 2006.
45. Lee LK, et al. Home safety practices in an urban low-income population: level of agreement between parental self-report and observed behaviors. *Clin Pediatr (Phila).* 2012;51:1119-1124.
46. Liller KD, et al. Evaluation of a poison prevention lesson for kindergarten and third grade students. *Inj Prev.* 1998;4:218-221.
47. Lovejoy FH, et al. Poison control centers, poison prevention, and the pediatrician. *Pediatrics.* 1994;94:220-224.
48. Lucio RL, et al. Incorporating what promotoras learn: becoming role models to effect positive change. *J Community Health.* 2012;37:1026-1031.
49. McAlister AL Perry CL, Parcel GS. How individuals, environments, and health behaviors interact Social Cognitive Theory. In: Glanz K, Rimer BK, Viswanath K, eds. *Health Behavior and Health Education Theory, Research, and Practice.* 4th ed. San Francisco, CA: Jossey-Bass; 2008:169-188.
50. McDonald EM, et al. Safe Storage of opioid pain relievers among adults living in households with children. *Pediatrics.* 2017;139.
51. McKenzie JF, Neiger BL, Thackeray R. *Planning, Implementing & Evaluating Health Promotion Programs.* 6th ed. San Francisco, CA: Pearson Education, Benjamin Cummings; 2013.
52. Mikhail BI. Hispanic mothers' beliefs and practices regarding selected children's health problems. *West J Nurs Res.* 1994;16:623-638.
53. Montague E, Perchonok J. Health and wellness technology use by historically underserved health consumers: systematic review. *J Med Internet Res.* 2012;14:e78.
54. Mrvos R, et al. Illiteracy: a contributing factor to poisoning. *Vet Hum Toxicol.* 1993;35:466-468.
55. Mull DS, et al. Household poisoning exposure among children of Mexican-born mothers: an ethnographic study. *West J Med.* 1999;171:16-19.
56. Neiger BL, et al. Use of social media in health promotion: purposes, key performance indicators, and evaluation metrics. *Health Promot Pract.* 2012;13:159-164.
57. Nelson W, et al. Clinical implications of numeracy: theory and practice. *Ann Behav Med.* 2008;35:261-274.
58. Neumann CM, et al. Oregon's Toxic Household Products Law. *J Public Health Policy.* 2000;21:342-359.
59. Nixon J, et al. Community based programs to prevent poisoning in children 0-15 years. *Inj Prev.* 2004;10:43-46.
60. Ozanne-Smith J, et al. Childhood poisoning: access and prevention. *J Paediatr Child Health.* 2001;37:262-265.
61. Parker RM, et al. Health literacy: a policy challenge for advancing high-quality health care. *Health Aff (Millwood).* 2003;22:147-153.
62. Payne HAS, et al. Denatonium benzoate as a bitter aversive additive in ethylene glycol and methanol-based automotive products. Paper presented at: 23rd International Conference on Environmental Systems, Colorado Springs, CO, July 1993.
63. Pehora C, et al. Are parents getting it right? A survey of parents' internet use for children's health care information. *Interact J Med Res.* 2015;4:e12.
64. Polivka BJ, et al. Evaluation of the Be Poison Smart! poison prevention intervention. *Clin Toxicol (Phila).* 2006;44:109-114.
65. Posner JC, et al. A randomized, clinical trial of a home safety intervention based in an emergency department setting. *Pediatrics.* 2004;113:1603-1608.
66. Purello PL, et al. An outreach program to low-income, high risk populations through WIC. *Vet Hum Toxicol.* 1990;32:130-132.
67. Randolph W, Viswanath K. Lessons learned from public health mass media campaigns: marketing health in a crowded media world. *Annu Rev Public Health.* 2004;25:419-437.
68. Riner ME, et al. Public health education and practice using geographic information system technology. *Public Health Nurs.* 2004;21:57-65.

69. Rodgers GB. The safety effects of child-resistant packaging for oral prescription drugs. Two decades of experience. *JAMA.* 1996;275:1661-1665.

70. Rothman RL, et al. Perspective: the role of numeracy in health care. *J Health Commun.* 2008;13:583-595.

71. Santer LJ, Stocking CB. Safety practices and living conditions of low-income urban families. *Pediatrics.* 1991;88:1112-1118.

72. Schapira MM, et al. A framework for health numeracy: how patients use quantitative skills in health care. *J Health Commun.* 2008;13:501-517.

73. Schwartz L, et al. The use of focus groups to plan poison prevention education programs for low-income populations. *Health Promot Pract.* 2003;4:340-346.

74. Schwartz L, et al. Unintentional methadone and buprenorphine exposures in children: developing prevention messages. *J Am Pharm Assoc (2003).* 2017;57:S83-S86.

75. Shepherd G, et al. Language preferences among callers to a regional Poison Control Center. *Vet Hum Toxicol.* 2004;46:100-101.

76. Sibert JR, Frude N. Bittering agents in the prevention of accidental poisoning: children's reactions to denatonium benzoate (Bitrex). *Arch Emerg Med.* 1991;8:1-7.

77. Skarupski KA, et al. A profile of calls to a poison information center regarding older adults. *J Aging Health.* 2004;16:228-247.

78. Spiller HA, Mowry JB. Evaluation of the effect of a public educator on calls and poisonings related to a regional poison control center. *Vet Human Toxicol.* 2004;46:206-208.

79. Sumner D, et al. A project to reduce accidental pediatric poisonings in North Carolina. *Vet Hum Toxicol.* 2003;45:266-269.

80. Swartz MK. Poison prevention. *J Pediatr Health Care.* 1993;7:143-144.

81. Tong V, et al. Design and comprehensibility of over-the-counter product labels and leaflets: a narrative review. *Int J Clin Pharm.* 2014;36:865-872.

82. United States DoHaHS. *National Action Plan to Improve Health Literacy.* OoDPaH, ed. Washington, DC; 2010.

83. Vassilev ZP, et al. Rapid communication: sociodemographic differences between counties with high and low utilization of a regional poison control center. *J Toxicol Environ Health A.* 2003;66:1905-1908.

84. Vassilev ZP, et al. Assessment of barriers to utilization of poison control centers by Hispanic/Latino populations. *J Toxicol Environ Health A.* 2006;69:1711-1718.

85. Vo K, Smollin C. Online social networking and US poison control centers: Facebook as a means of information distribution. *Clin Toxicol (Phila).* 2015;53:466-469.

86. Walton WW. An evaluation of the poison prevention packaging act. *Pediatrics.* 1982;69:1711-1718.

87. Wolf MS, et al. Helping patients simplify and safely use complex prescription regimens. *Arch Intern Med.* 2011;171:300-305.

88. Woolf AD, et al. Preserving the United States's poison control system. *Clin Toxicol (Phila).* 2011;49:284-286.

89. Woolf AD, et al. Poisoning prevention knowledge and practices of parents after a childhood poisoning incident. *Pediatrics.* 1992;90:867-870.

90. World Health Organization. Poisoning prevention and management. http://www.who.int/ipcs/poisons/en.

91. Wynn PM, et al. Prevention of childhood poisoning in the home: overview of systematic reviews and a systematic review of primary studies. *Int J Inj Contr Saf Promot.* 2016;23:3-28.

92. Yin HS, et al. Health literacy assessment of labeling of pediatric nonprescription medications: examination of characteristics that may impair parent understanding. *Acad Pediatr.* 2012;12:288-296.

93. Yudizky M, et al. Can textbook covers be used to increase poison control center utilization? *Vet Hum Toxicol.* 2004;46:285-286.

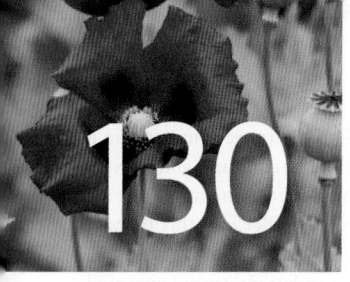

130 POISON CONTROL CENTERS AND POISON EPIDEMIOLOGY

Mark K. Su and Robert S. Hoffman

HISTORY

In 1950, the American Academy of Pediatrics (AAP) created a Committee on Accident Prevention to explore methods to reduce injuries in young children. A subsequent survey by that committee demonstrated that injuries resulting from unintentional poisoning were a significant cause of childhood morbidity. At the same time, there was a realization that a source of reliable information on the active ingredients of common household xenobiotics was lacking and that there were few accepted methods for treating poisoned patients. In response to this void, the first poison control center (PCC) was created in Chicago in 1953.[114] Although initially designed to provide information to health care providers, both the popularity and the success of this center stimulated a PCC movement, which rapidly spread across the country. The myriad of new PCCs not only offered product content information to health care providers but also began to offer first aid and prevention information to members of the community.

In the past 60 years, countless achievements have been realized by a relatively small group of remarkably altruistic individuals. Throughout this time, poison services have remained free to the public, highlighting their essential role in the American public health system. Many of the legislative and educational accomplishments that are chronicled in Chap. 1 have directly reduced the incidence and severity of poisoning in children.[34,109,128] Concurrently, the number, configuration, and specific role of PCCs has shifted in response to public and professional needs.[54,86]

Modern regional PCCs are staffed by highly trained and certified health professionals who are assisted by extensive information systems. Support is provided by 24-hour access to board-certified medical toxicologists and consultants from diverse medical disciplines, the natural sciences, and industry. The American PCC is charged with seven major objectives:

- Maintaining and interpreting a database of xenobiotics
- Providing information and advice to the public and to health professionals
- Collecting epidemiologic data on the incidence and severity of poisoning
- Integrating epidemiologic data as part of the public health surveillance system
- Preventing unnecessary hospitalizations after exposure and thereby cutting health care costs
- Educating health care professionals on the diagnosis and treatment of poisoning
- Contributing to the science of toxicology

In the past, PCCs were evaluated based on the number of incoming calls and measures of community awareness. Current emphasis should be placed on evaluating health outcomes such as intensive care unit (ICU) admissions, length of stay in hospitals, and total health care expenditures. One crucial test of the utility of modern PCCs will be their ability to help reverse the US current trend of increased adult deaths from pharmaceutical poisoning largely driven by prescription opioids.[50,72] This chapter explores some of the critical roles of US poison control centers and attempts to offer a vision of the future. An overview of the composition of PCCs worldwide can be found elsewhere.[107] Unique issues facing PCCs in other countries are discussed in Chap. 136.

MAINTAINING AND INTERPRETING A DATABASE OF XENOBIOTICS

The first toxicology database created in the United States was a set of cumbersome 5″ × 8″ index cards produced in the 1950s by the US National Clearinghouse of Poison Control Centers.[114] When it grew to include more than 16,000 cards, the sheer volume of space required to store this information, and the extensive time necessary to manually search these cards created the necessity of a central repository, such as a PCC. As available information grew, a rapid expansion of information technology occurred, and the unwieldy index card database was privatized and transformed into microfiche. Although this resource was physically smaller, specialized equipment was required, and a search was still time consuming. Numerous encyclopedic and clinical textbooks were written to supplement the database and provide resources for the office or the bedside. With the growth of the computer age and the Internet, the computer product known as POISINDEX was established to replace the microfiche format as the major source of data on the contents of innumerable household and industrial products, drugs, and plant and animal xenobiotics. POISINDEX also provides uniform management strategies for many potentially toxic exposures. Over the years, several proprietary competitors to POISINDEX, such as TOXINZ and TOXBASE, have gained recognition as valuable tools. Additionally, open source programs such as WIKITOX provide free information to both clinicians and members of the public.

With this evolution of information technology, PCCs are no longer perceived as the sole guardians of toxicology information. Although these services are still essential for the public at large and for professionals who are away from their computers or smartphones, a predictable decline in PCC use has paralleled this growth in availability of information. A 1991 study in Utah demonstrated that 82.6% of emergency physicians who had POISINDEX available in their institutions no longer routinely consulted the PCC.[29] A similar 1994 New York State study suggested that 76% of physicians who had POISINDEX in their emergency departments (EDs) perceived that its availability decreased their own use of their PCC.[130]

An initial analysis might suggest that this is an acceptable trend for health care professionals in that it both allows physicians to respond more rapidly to patient needs and for PCCs to be more available to those individuals, especially non–health care professionals, who do not have access to this information system. In fact, one model demonstrated that an integrated voice response system effectively reduced human interactions for medication identification by more than half at one PCC.[80] By extension, it might be suggested that both the public and health care providers can easily access the same information as certified specialists in poison information, making the human interaction nearly obsolete. However, this practice of "not calling" not only undermines the efforts of PCCs to gather epidemiologic data (see later) but also creates a knowledge gap. In other words, the interpretation of the data is as essential (or more essential) than the data itself. For example, some commonly used sources of toxicology information such as the *Physicians' Desk Reference* and material safety data sheets occasionally provide information that is inaccurate, potentially misleading, or severely limited.[21,60,97] Likewise, reviews of drug interaction programs designed for mobile devices demonstrate significant variability between individual programs and inferiority compared with larger online resources.[5,41,105,108] Although the POISINDEX routinely provides more accurate information regarding overdose, it is only updated quarterly and cannot be expected to adapt to ongoing epidemiologic trends such as regional variations in substance use.

The best source for essential new information is skilled professionals who specialize in poisoning. Also, because most databases are designed to provide information about known entities, they perform poorly when dealing with unknown and unclear scenarios, especially long and complex differential diagnoses. For example, consider the case of a clinician caring for a lethargic child whose only medication is Zantac syrup. After other causes of altered mental status are excluded, the clinician considers drug toxicity. Consultation with standard references suggests that altered consciousness would not be expected with use of this medication. However, a certified specialist in poison information at a regional PCC recognizes the potential for drug error, has the physician review the syrup bottle in question, and then calls the pharmacy where the drug was provided. The certified specialist in poison information learns that although the prescription was written for Zantac (ranitidine), the bottle actually contains Zyrtec syrup (cetirizine), which could account for the child's symptoms.

Thus, although originally designed as providers of information, PCCs are valued consultants. They provide content information and interpretation of clinical material, leading to the implementation of appropriate management strategies. This goal can only be achieved through rigorous training and certification and recertification criteria designed to provide valued up-to-date interactions with health care professionals. Access to computer programs may be deceptively inaccurate or superficial compared with a thoughtful human analysis. Computers do not recognize anxiety, inappropriate questions, and other subtle issues that can only be appreciated with human interactions.

Another illustrative example of the value of PCCs can be drawn from the use of flumazenil for benzodiazepine overdose (Chap. 72 and Antidotes in Depth: A25). Although it is easily determined that flumazenil is the antidote for benzodiazepine overdoses, many subtle characteristics of the patient or the overdose often contraindicate its use. A prospective study determined that when flumazenil was used before consultation with the PCC, contraindications to its administration were present in 10 of 14 (71%) cases, resulting in one serious adverse event.[24] In the study mentioned earlier, although physicians with access to the POISINDEX were less likely to call the PCC, 86.7% still thought that using the PCC to gain access to a medical toxicologist was a valued resource.[29] Many PCCs are linked with centers for poison treatment, which are health care facilities that can provide both bedside consultation and unique diagnostic and therapeutic interventions for a subset of patients with severe or complex poisoning.[1] The benefits of consultation are discussed later under Health Care Savings.

PROVIDING INFORMATION AND ADVICE TO THE PUBLIC AND TO HEALTH PROFESSIONALS

Poison Control Centers in the United States interact with the public and health professionals over 2.5 million times annually.[94] Although the financial value of these interactions will be discussed in the next section, two major limitations to the success of PCCs are highlighted in the literature. The first, which should be intuitively obvious, stems from the fact that PCCs are remote from the patient and can therefore only make decisions based on the information provided to them. Although certified specialists in poison information are highly skilled and use a variety of communication styles to obtain the most accurate information,[110] the quality of the information impacts on the utility of their recommendations. The greatest concern here is over estimation of dose. In a 3.5-year study of all children referred by a PCC to a health care facility for determination of either a methanol or an ethylene glycol concentration because of a history of exposure, only 21 of 102 had measurable concentrations.[64] Although this has serious limitations on the interpretation of PCC data,[68] the implications for clinical care are even greater. Likewise, a human volunteer study demonstrated that adults are totally incapable of determining residual volumes in containers or describing the actual volume of semiquantitative descriptors such as "a small mouthful" or "a gulp."[67] Because critical decisions are made based on the history of ingestion or amount ingested, a clear challenge for PCCs is to develop methods to improve the accuracy of this information. Sharing digital imagery is one useful method of assisting caregivers with determination of residual container volumes.

The second challenge involves the gap that exists between recommendations that are made by PCCs and those that are accepted. Two papers highlight this concern. In a 7-year analysis of PCC recommendations for the administration of high-dose insulin and dextrose therapy, the recommended treatment was actually administered only 50% of the time.[53] Similarly, in a 5.5-year study of calcium channel blocker and β-adrenergic antagonist overdoses at a different PCC, high-dose insulin and dextrose therapy was only started in 42% of cases when it was recommended.[45] Because this therapy is considered effective and potentially lifesaving (Antidotes in Depth: A21), PCCs need to evaluate the reasons these recommendations are not accepted and explore methods to improve communication with providers. Similarly, patient compliance with PCCs' recommendations is unknown. Patients may call PCCs directly to request assistance after an exposure occurs. However, because of inaccurate data collection (ie, patient names, telephone numbers), patient outcomes are often unknown because of insufficient follow-up.

COLLECTING POISON EPIDEMIOLOGY DATA

In 2007, the Centers for Disease Control and Prevention (CDC) reported that poisoning fatality surpassed both motor vehicle crashes and firearms to become the leading cause of injury-related fatalities.[7] This trend has continued and is largely influenced by an epidemic of prescription opioid abuse.[72] Understanding the evolving trends in poisoning is essential to the development of enhanced surveillance, prevention, and education programs designed to reduce unintentional poisoning. Although data can be analyzed from numerous sources such as death certificates, hospital discharge coding records, and PCCs, it is essential to recognize the biases that are inherent in each of these reports. Because not all significant poisonings result in either hospitalization or fatality, data from PCCs appear to offer a unique perspective.

Unfortunately, the term "poisoning" is often defined differently and therefore is a confusing term. In this text, "poisoning" is used to denote any exposure to any xenobiotic (drug, toxin, chemical, or naturally occurring substance) that results in injury. Yet the data collected and disseminated by PCCs are defined by the term "exposures."[15-20,93-96] Potential xenobiotic exposures are inevitable given their ubiquity. However, many exposures are of no toxicologic consequence because of the properties of the xenobiotic involved, the magnitude or duration of the exposure, or the uncertainties regarding whether an actual exposure has occurred; therefore, data collected by PCCs represent a limited and ill-defined measure of poisoning.

The situation is further confounded by multiple biases that are introduced by the actual reporting process, which, first and foremost, is voluntary and passive. Because the majority of calls concern self-reported data that originate from the home setting and are never subsequently confirmed, a significant percentage of the data generated to date likely actually represents only potential or possible exposures, which then introduce large statistical errors into the database. This is highlighted by the 21 of 102 children who tested positive for a toxic alcohol discussed earlier.[64] Even though only those 21 children were definitively exposed and potentially poisoned, all 102 were entered into the database as exposures. If these figures are representative of the rest of the data set, they suggest that an actual ingestion does not occur in the vast majority of reported unintentional exposures in children. Also, current events, hoaxes, and media awareness campaigns all influence self-reporting rates.[87] Furthermore, to report a possible exposure, a caller must have a telephone, probably speak English, and have some degree of health literacy and numeracy.[85,127] Although telecommunications devices for hearing impaired individuals and translation services exist, they are rarely used in communications with PCCs. Enhancement of technology to facilitate the accurate exchange of information between certified specialists in poison information and either hearing impaired callers or those who do not speak English is essential to enhance outreach to special populations and those with limited English proficiency and ultimately the success of PCCs. Although text messaging is an interesting option, preliminary data suggest that encounters are too slow and complicated to be productive.[111] Another potential source of PCC notification would be to entertain more active reporting systems automatically triggered directly by hospital laboratory values. Theoretically, with the advent of sophisticated electronic medical record (EMR) systems, PCCs could be sent automatic notifications of patients exposed to xenobiotics. The implementation of this type of system is not currently widespread due to heterogeneity of the EMRs and potential issues with maintaining patient privacy and Health Insurance Portability and Accountability Act (HIPAA) compliance.

Under the present passive system, when hospitals report exposures to the PCC, a comparison of the hospital chart with the PCC record shows good agreement, demonstrating an accurate exchange of information.[70] Unfortunately, a reporting bias similar to that described earlier is well recognized regarding professional use of PCCs and is called the *Pollyanna phenomenon*.[61] For example, when examining New York City Poison Control Center Data from 2011 to 2014, reports of novel psychoactive substances were noted to increase, largely driven by the recent surge in synthetic cannabinoid receptor agonists.[103] Over time, reporting significantly dropped, possibly because of either effective public health interventions or decreased drug supply. In a similar case, during the spring of 1995, PCCs in the northeast United States began to receive numerous reports of severe psychomotor agitation and other manifestations of anticholinergic syndrome in heroin users. In the initial phase of the epidemic, most of the callers requested assistance in establishing a diagnosis and determining possible etiologies and raised questions regarding treatment with physostigmine.[62] Although the epidemic continued for many months, after the media announced that the heroin supply was tainted with scopolamine and clinicians became familiar with the indications and administration of physostigmine, call volume decreased. Stated simply, health care professionals are less likely to call the PCCs regarding issues with which they are familiar, are of little clinical consequence, or are not recognized as being related to a poison. Thus, a bias is introduced that results in a relative overreporting of new and serious events and a relative underreporting of the familiar or very common, unrecognized poisoning and exposures or poisonings that are apparently inconsequential. Numerous comparisons support this contention. Investigators who rely on published data from PCCs as a sole source of epidemiologic information demonstrate a failure to understand the complexity of poisoning data and the aforementioned consequential limitations of PCC-derived data.

Fatal Poisoning

A 4-year study compared deaths from poisoning reported to the Rhode Island medical examiner with those reported to the area PCC.[83] Not surprisingly, the medical examiner reported many more deaths: 369 compared with 45 reported by the PCC. Although the majority of the cases not reported to the PCC were victims who died at home or were pronounced dead on arrival to the hospital or those in whom poisoning was not suspected until the postmortem analysis, 79 patients who subsequently became unreported fatalities were actually admitted to the hospital with a suspected poisoning. In 10 of these cases, the authors concluded that a toxicology consultation might have altered the outcome. Examples of interventions that, if recommended and performed, might have resulted in a more favorable outcome included the proper use of antidotes such as naloxone, *N*-acetylcysteine for acetaminophen poisoning, the cyanide antidote kit, sodium bicarbonate for a cyclic antidepressant overdose, hyperbaric oxygen for carbon monoxide poisoning, hemoperfusion for a theophylline overdose, and hemodialysis for a lithium overdose.

Likewise, when medical examiner data were analyzed in Massachusetts, more than 47% of poison fatalities were not reported to the PCC.[118] A California study evaluating 358 poisoning fatalities reported to the medical examiner showed that only 10 PCC fatalities were reported over a similar time period, demonstrating an even more consequential reporting gap.[9] Again in this study, whereas the majority of underreporting occurred in prehospital deaths (68%), only 5 of 113 hospitalized patients who ultimately died were reported to the PCC. Additionally, a cross-sectional comparison of national mortality data with PCC data for agricultural chemical poisoning demonstrated a similar trend of underreporting to PCCs of seriously poisoned admitted patients who became fatalities.[77] Furthermore, when data for an entire year from the National Center for Health Statistics (NCHS) were compared with the same year of data from the American Association of Poison Control Centers (AAPCC), it was apparent that the AAPCC data captured only about 5% of annual poison fatalities.[69]

More recent analyses highlight a remarkable trend. When 11 states evaluated trends in poison-related mortality rates from 1990 to 2001, an average increase of 145% was noted.[66] A more comprehensive investigation of the National Vital Statistics System (NVSS) accessed via the CDC's Web-based Injury Statistics Query and Reporting System (WISQARS) database demonstrated a 5.5% increase in injury related mortality from 1999 to 2004. The mortality rate from poisoning accounted for 62% of the increase in unintentional injury, 28% of the increase in suicide, 81% of the increase in death from undetermined intent, and more than 50% of the total increase in injury-related mortality.[104] Since 1999, the age-adjusted drug poisoning death rate has increased from 6.1 per 100,000 to 16.3 per 100,000 in 2015.[31] Although the vast majority of poisoning fatalities occur in adults, a review of the entire 2010 AAPCC database only found 74 reported fatalities in children.[25] Focusing on PCC data alone would produce the erroneous assumption that poisoning-related fatalities were not a significant public health concern. In actuality, poisoning is a significant concern considering that other programs designed to reduce deaths from motor vehicle crashes and firearms have been largely successful; however, decades have gone by without a major intervention targeting poison-related fatality.

It is logical to assume that similar disparities exist regarding the reporting of nonfatal poisonings. The resultant gap in public health data needs to be addressed through improved definitions, epidemiology, reporting, and analysis of poison-related data systems. This inequity has developed through a long-standing tradition of PCCs to focus attention and concentrate on the largely benign exposures in children. The emphasis needs to be redirected toward seriously ill poisoning, ICU utilization, and other markers of actual poisoning rather than health care utilization for benign events.

Nonfatal Poisoning

An outreach study in Massachusetts determined that hospitals geographically close to a PCC reported their cases almost twice as often as hospitals remotely located (46% versus 27% of total cases).[32] Additionally, the authors noted that private physicians were less likely to report cases than residents in training. A 1-year retrospective review demonstrated that only 26% (123 of 470) of poisoned patients who were treated in a particular ED were reported to the PCC.[63] Interestingly, only 3% of inhalational exposures were reported compared with 95% of cyclic antidepressant ingestions. The authors also noted, as suggested earlier, that reporting decreased when comparable exposures occurred over a short period of time. Finally, in the physician survey study cited earlier, physicians reported that they would "almost never" contact the PCC for asymptomatic exposures (62.9%), chronic toxicity (50.4%), or simply to assist in establishing a reliable database (90.2%).[29] This statement is most likely accurate even in jurisdictions where reporting of all or select exposures is incorporated into public health laws.

Occupational Exposures

Xenobiotic exposure occurs commonly in the workplace. As a result of the long-recognized association between occupational exposure and illness, a number of federal and state government-funded agencies, such as the National Institute for Occupational Safety and Health (NIOSH), Occupational Safety and Health Act (OSHA), and the Agency for Toxic Substances and Disease Registry (ATSDR), exist to prevent occupational illness, educate the public, and collect data on exposures to occupational xenobiotics. Legislation provides for mandatory reporting in some instances and offers workers job protection for voluntary reporting. Poison control centers also provide information on occupational exposures and collect data. Again, there are discrepancies between the poison information data and the data collected by governmental agencies. A 6-month survey in California noted that only 15.9% of the occupational cases reported to the PCC were captured by a state occupational reporting system.[11] The most common occupational toxicologic illness—dermatitis—was even further underrepresented in these cases. A follow-up study by the same authors demonstrated that more than one-third of calls came directly from the individual worker, 70% of whom were unaware of the link between their occupation and their symptoms.[10]

Although these data suggest that PCCs can provide substantial assistance after occupational exposures, one author expressed concern, noting in a follow-up study that the PCC failed to provide an adequate epidemiologic assessment because an average of 12 other people per workplace who were also potentially exposed in addition to the index case were not identified.[13] A 1999 survey of PCCs concluded that "responses to work-related calls are inadequate" and suggested that written protocols might be helpful.[14]

Adverse Drug Events and Xenobiotic Errors

Although the actual numbers of adverse drug events (ADEs) are a source of controversy, data suggest that a striking number occur each year in the United States, with many resulting in death.[22,35,81] The ease of 24-hour telephone access, combined with the ability to consult with a health professional, make PCCs ideal resources for reporting of ADEs.[38] Yet more than 76% of physicians surveyed stated that they would "almost never" contact the PCC regarding ADEs.[29] Moreover, 30 of 56 (53.6%) PCCs surveyed stated that they had not submitted any of their ADE data to the FDA Med-Watch program.[35] Many of the other centers reported only partial compliance with the MedWatch system.[35]

Prescription drug errors are another source of potential poisoning. Retrospective review of PCC data suggests that many of these errors are reported. In one report, the PCC provided valuable feedback to pharmacists and physicians about these errors. Ideally, reporting to the state board of pharmacy would ensure that proper surveillance and counseling continue. The PCC is ideally suited to perform this function.[116] Unfortunately, although pharmacists are ideally positioned to identify prescribing errors, data suggest that pharmacist utilization of PCCs is poor.[2]

Drugs of Abuse

Poison control centers also collect data on exposures to drugs of abuse and misuse. These data consist largely of calls for information from the concerned public and reports of overdose requiring health care intervention. Although ethanol, tobacco, and caffeine are the most common xenobiotics used in society, these cases are rarely reflected in PCC data, with the exception of unintentional exposures in children. In fact, because most substance abuse does not result in immediate interactions with the health care system, other databases such as the National Institute of Drug Abuse (NIDA) Household Survey (now referred to as the Monitoring the Future Study) might better reflect substance abuse trends. Yet even this database has significant limitations.[8,58] Because PCCs are more focused on immediate health care effects of exposures, it could be argued that only cases in which health care interaction is required are of value in the database. Because PCCs collect data in real time, they are ideally positioned to track emerging trends and report sentinel events. Examples include PCC experiences with trends in opioid abuse among teenagers,[55,123] bath salts,[98] synthetic cannabinoid receptor agonists,[98,102] and tainted cocaine.[124]

Grossly Underreported Xenobiotics

As discussed earlier, there is little doubt that ethanol and tobacco are the most common xenobiotics intentionally used and misused in our society. Although their toxicologic manifestations are acute and severe at times, chronic subclinical poisoning often goes unnoticed for many years. Similarly, based on the 2007 to 2010 National Health and Nutritional Exam Survey, approximately 500,000 American children have lead concentrations above 5 mcg/dL.[30] We must remain cognizant of these large-scale exposures when we read that plants, cleaning products, and cosmetics comprise the most common exposures to xenobiotics;[132] rather, these are the most commonly "reported" exposures.

INTEGRATING EPIDEMIOLOGIC DATA AS PART OF THE PUBLIC HEALTH SURVEILLANCE SYSTEM

With the current limitations of the PCC data, it should be clear that neither the numerator nor the denominator of the actual number of poisonings is easily appreciated. However, analysis of these data for trends has some utility because the inherent biases involved in PCC reporting are probably consistent over many years. Increasingly, PCC data are being used as part of

surveillance and prediction models,[51,132] often that extend beyond poisoning to other public health concerns.[117] Rapid reporting in collaboration with the CDC highlights an essential partnership.[42,59,98] Efforts should be directed to encourage reporting to PCCs by such enhanced access methods as web-based forms for passive reporting, a direct interface between laboratory and hospital databases that actively transmits data to PCCs and linkages to other agencies that collect reports of poisoning such as state and local health departments and medical examiners. Additional resources should be directed at improved case definitions (distinguishing asymptomatic exposure from poisoning) and integration with other essential databases such as MedWatch, NVSS, and NCHS.

Despite its limitations, PCC data have significant utility. It is often an exposure rather than an actual poisoning that provides the impetus for contact with health care. For exposures that are unlikely to be consequential, the PCC can intervene to prevent potentially harmful attempts at home and costly unnecessary visits to health care providers. Interaction with parents at a time of perceived crisis also provides a "teachable moment" (Chap. 129) that may help prevent a more consequential exposure in the future. For exposures that result in poisoning, the period of time immediately after exposure is an ideal moment to initiate first aid measures designed to prevent or lessen the severity of poisoning. For these reasons, the cost, benefits, and efficacy of PCCs, especially regarding home calls, must be measured in terms of exposures and not poisonings.

HEALTH CARE SAVINGS

When visits to pediatric EDs for acute poisoning were analyzed, one study demonstrated that 95% of parents had not contacted the PCC before coming to the hospital, and 64% of these children required no hospital services.[33] In contrast, when parents called the PCC first, fewer than 1% sought emergency services afterward. When 589 callers to one PCC were surveyed, 464 (79%) respondents stated that they would have used the emergency care system if the PCC were unavailable.[74] In a similar study, 36% of callers would have selected a more costly alternative if the PCC were unavailable.[12] Likewise, when primary care providers were surveyed, more than 80% said that they would activate 9-1-1 if there were no PCC.[3] Poison control center data confirm that approximately 75% of reported exposures that originate outside of health care facilities can be safely managed onsite with limited telephone follow-up. Suggesting simple techniques or reassurance can successfully reduce hospital visits for patients who typically call PCCs for what only represents a potential exposure. The use of established protocols, especially for unintentional exposures in children, reduces ED referral rates and unnecessary hospital charges.[65,122] Unfortunately, this approach is not demonstrated to be beneficial for adults.

Limited data suggest that direct bedside consultation and care help reduce length of hospital stay and health care costs.[40] Yet although PCCs operate remotely, in one assessment, consultation with a PCC reduced length of stay by nearly 3 days.[126] Similarly, when the PCC was consulted for patients already in the hospital, length of stay and costs were reduced by 1.9 days and nearly $5,000, respectively.[23] This experience has been replicated outside the United States, where PCC consultation resulted in a decreased length of stay of more than 3 days.[56]

The national average cost to the PCC for a single human exposure call is on the order of $35.[134] A federally funded study concluded that in one year, PCCs reduced the number of patients who were treated but not hospitalized by 350,000 and reduced hospitalizations by an additional 40,000 patients, for a cost savings over more than $3 million.[92] Each call to a PCC prevented at least $175 in subsequent medical costs, providing strong theoretical evidence to support the cost efficacy of PCCs. In fact, two natural experiments support these calculations: In 1988, Louisiana closed its state-sponsored PCC. During the year that followed, the cost of emergency medical services (EMS) for poisoning in Louisiana increased by more than $1.4 million. This additional expenditure represented a greater than threefold increase above the operating cost of that center.[76] Similarly, because of financial disputes in California, direct access to the San Francisco PCC was electronically restricted for one major county, with a recording referring callers instead to the 9-1-1 system for assistance.[106] The result of each blocked call resulted in increased health care costs by approximately $33. Moreover, these calculations cannot account for the unmeasured benefits to society from PCC interventions that reduce waiting times for ambulance availability and hospital treatments because of lower volumes, money saved by the prevention or reduction of injury from early intervention or lives saved by enhancing access to or use of the health care system for seriously poisoned patients. In El Paso, Texas, cooperation between EMS and the PCC was able to reduce ambulance dispatches by 1750 over 5 years.[4] Overall estimates place the rate of return for PCC funding between 11 and 36:1.[71,119] A similar study done in Southern California showed that when the PCC was notified before EMS dispatch, $486,595 and $183,279 were saved in charges and payments, respectively.[82]

However, many barriers prevent a person from calling a PCC, including lack of familiarity with its available services, intellectual and cultural factors, language difficulties, and confidentiality concerns[39,75,85,127] (Chap. 129). Epidemiologic studies demonstrate that areas of increased population density with high percentages of minority inhabitants have lower utilization of PCC services.[125] Additional barriers include the absence of caregiver comfort with the extensive personal contact provided by the health care system and a concern regarding implications of child abuse or neglect when reporting to agencies such as PCC, many of which have governmental ties.[115] Data demonstrate that public educators can help overcome some of these barriers.[120] One good example of an effort to overcome reporting barriers was the institution of a single national toll-free number for poisoning (800-222-1222). Although it is clear that this intervention improved access and increased total calls to the PCC,[79] it has yet to be determined if this has altered the patterns of use (Fig. 129-1).

In terms of alternative ways for PCCs to obtain data on poisoning exposures and assist the public, the use of the internet and mobile devices are being explored. The online platform webPOISONCONTROL was studied as an alternative for the public to obtain emergency advice regarding potential toxic exposures.[84] After using this online platform, user comments suggested advantages, such as not having to call the PCC and overall convenience. Disadvantages included relatively limited guidance and no human interaction for opportunities to ask questions. Thus, although automated online platforms show potential, this study points toward a need for both human interaction and the need to expand communication channels with the public for increased convenience. Another method of PCC contact for the public that is being investigated is the use of texting or chatting. These are alternative methods of communication that have become extremely popular, especially among millennials. Although only a few PCCs currently use texting or chatting, this option is worthy of further investigation as the number of calls to PCCs continues to decrease and other techniques of public engagement become necessary.[121]

PROVIDING EDUCATION FOR THE PUBLIC AND HEALTH PROFESSIONALS

Poison control center staff work closely with physicians, community health educators, community support groups, and parent–teacher associations to develop poison prevention activities.[88] Table 130-1 lists common strategies advocated to prevent poisoning. Poison control centers are also actively involved in enhancing training programs for paramedics,[52] medical students,[73] pharmacy students,[44] and resident physicians[44,100,131] and are an integral part of postgraduate training programs in medical toxicology.

As stated previously, there is an inherent risk in both enhanced public and professional education programs. Currently, the decreased telephone use of a PCC could be both the result of a decrease in the incidence of exposure or poisoning or an enhanced understanding of the prevention, diagnosis, and treatment of poisoning. Although education should never be viewed as detrimental, programs must include an emphasis on the continued use of PCCs to ensure access to current information in a rapidly changing discipline. In actuality, as a result of the ongoing analysis of incoming

TABLE 130–1 Common Strategies Advocated to Help Prevent Poisoning

All xenobiotics should be kept in their original containers. Food and drink containers should never be used for transfer of a xenobiotic.

Never store xenobiotics in unlocked cabinets under the sink. Apply locks to medicine cabinets that are within the reach of a child.

In the absence of a lock, the more toxic xenobiotics should be stored on the highest shelves.

Xenobiotics should never be left in the unlocked glove compartment of the family car.

Parents should buy or accept medication only if it is in a child-resistant container.

Medication should be considered as medicine, not a plaything and certainly not candy.

Adults should not take their medications in front of children:

  This will limit exposure to drug-taking role models that may become objects of imitative behavior.

Unused portions of prescription medications should be discarded, or returned to a pharmacy.

Activated charcoal should be readily available in the home for use if directed by a certified specialist in poison information or clinician. (Particularly for those living in remote areas.)

Children who have ingested a poison will do so again within a year, these children should receive an enhanced level of supervision.

Turn on the light in the room and wear glasses (if appropriate) when taking medications.

calls, the knowledge base has the potential to change as rapidly as the calls are reported. This is far more rapid than can occur in any published literature or electronic database. Thus, additional emphasis should be applied to routine use of the PCC as a public health tool to improve the accuracy of epidemiologic data. Reporting of rare or suspected events can serve as sentinel efforts that help identify consequential adverse drug opportunities long before normal postmarketing surveillance tools identify areas of concern.

On the other hand, outreach programs that advise the public to access free services for inconsequential events would easily overwhelm an already stressed system of responding to incoming calls by demanding an immediate response to the less serious calls in an appropriate time frame. Public education and public health must both be considered to ensure that PCCs are staffed with the appropriate number of skilled individuals to respond not only to daily events but also to address surges in calls that would result from actual epidemics or responses to media announcements. Increasing calls to demonstrate increased use offers no public health advantage if the use is inappropriate or if seriously ill or potentially ill callers lose access to timely responses.

DEVELOPMENT OF FUTURE PUBLIC HEALTH INITIATIVES

The initial public health efforts of PCCs focused on attempts to alter product concentration and to enhance product labeling and packaging. These beneficial endeavors should continue and must evolve. However, current events have also increased PCC activities in preparedness for mass gatherings and disasters resulting from radiologic, biological, and chemical terrorism.[57,78] Additional links with governmental agencies such as the CDC have expanded the role of the PCC in community health. As an example, national PCC data from the National Poison Data System (NPDS) shows that PCC data of exposures related to influenza like illness (ILI) is highly correlated with CDC ILI data.[6] Furthermore, the need for 24-hour rapid access to centralized information, existing data entry and retrieval systems, and links to experts in medical toxicology and emergency medicine helps to place PCCs in critical roles in both local and national initiatives. Important contributions have included development of triage and treatment protocols,[26-28,36,37,43,48,65,89-91,99,101,112,113,129,133] assessments of antidote supplies,[47-49] and disaster preparedness.[46] Table 130-2 summarizes initiatives that require creation or enhancement to improve poisoning epidemiology data. Many of these are discussed extensively in a report from the Institute of Medicine. Lastly, increased awareness of the essential public health role of PCCs by the lay public and policy makers must be accomplished in order to maintain the political and financial support necessary to ensure PCC quality, innovativeness, responsiveness to societal needs and viability.

TABLE 130–2	Goals for Improving Poisoning Epidemiology Data

Identify and remove barriers to reporting.

Create multiple methods of reporting:

Telephone, fax, web based, or e-mail

Simplify communications devices for hearing impaired individuals.

Allow rapid access to translation services.

Enhance awareness of the public health role of poison control centers.

Enhance education of caregivers and health care professionals.

Establish public health legislation requiring professional reporting of exposures.

Distinguish possible exposures from actual exposures to improve the integrity of the database.

Create a category for unconfirmed exposures in the database and encourage its use.

Divide confirmed exposures by certainty:

Confirmed by history

Confirmed by physical examination

Confirmed by quantitative and qualitative laboratory analysis

Integrate the AAPCC database with other databases (eg, the ICD and "E" code systems) and use a standardized data collection instrument.

Automatically interact with hospital and commercial laboratories.

Uplink pharmacy ADE reports, hospital discharges, public health department reports (similarly available with lead screening programs), fire departments and hazardous materials responders, industry workplace exposures, death certificates, and drug abuse monitoring systems.

Provide real-time analysis of incoming data.

Enhance the speed of data collection and reporting.

Analyze data as it is reported to identify emerging trends.

Mandate the use of accepted epidemiologic and statistical analyses of data.

Provide rapid and regular feedback to primary reporters.

Issue timely analyses and reports.

ADE = adverse drug event; AAPCC = American Association of Poison Control Centers; ICD = International Statistical Classification of Diseases and Related Health Problems.

SUMMARY

- Public education efforts help reduce the likelihood of exposure.
- Provision of basic management advice helps to diminish the consequences of a poisoning after an exposure has occurred.
- Reassurance and proper basic management help to curtail unnecessary concern, travel, and use of expensive health care.
- Interactions with health care professionals streamline the care of poisoned patients saving hospital days and health care expenditures.
- Collaboration with public health authorities identify, inform, and help mitigate the consequences of ongoing toxicologic events.
- Data on exposures have been effectively used to create legislation to further limit poisoning by altering contents or improving packaging or labeling.

Acknowledgement

Richard S. Weisman, PharmD, contributed to this chapter in a previous edition.

REFERENCES

1. American Academy of Clinical Toxicology. Facility assessment guidelines for regional toxicology treatment centers. American Academy of Clinical Toxicology. *J Toxicol Clin Toxicol.* 1993;31:211-217.
2. Armahizer MJ, et al. Evaluation of pharmacist utilization of a poison center as a resource for patient care. *J Pharm Pract.* 2013;26:220-227.
3. Austin T, et al. A survey of primary care offices: triage of poisoning calls without a poison control center. *Int J Family Med.* 2012;2012:417823.
4. Baeza SH, et al. Patient outcomes in a poison center/EMS collaborative project. *Clin Toxicol.* 2007;45:622-623.
5. Barrons R. Evaluation of personal digital assistant software for drug interactions. *Am J Health Syst Pharm.* 2004;61:380-385.
6. Beauchamp GA, et al. Relating calls to US poison centers for potential exposures to medications to Centers for Disease Control and Prevention reporting of influenza-like illness. *Clin Toxicol (Phila).* 2016;54:235-240.
7. Bernard SJ, et al. Fatal injuries among children by race and ethnicity—United States, 1999-2002. *MMWR Surveill Summ.* 2007;56:1-16.
8. Biemer PP, Witt M. Repeated measures estimation of measurement bias for self-reported drug use with applications to the National Household Survey on Drug Abuse. *NIDA Res Monogr.* 1997;167:439-476.
9. Blanc PD, et al. Underreporting of fatal cases to a regional poison control center. *West J Med.* 1995;162:505-509.
10. Blanc PD, et al. Occupational illness and poison control centers. Referral patterns and service needs. *West J Med.* 1990;152:181-184.
11. Blanc PD, Olson KR. Occupationally related illness reported to a regional poison control center. *Am J Public Health.* 1986;76:1303-1307.
12. Blizzard JC, et al. Cost-benefit analysis of a regional poison center. *Clin Toxicol (Phila).* 2008;46:450-456.
13. Bresnitz EA. Poison Control Center follow-up of occupational disease. *Am J Public Health.* 1990;80:711-712.
14. Bresnitz EA, et al. A national survey of regional poison control centers' management of occupational exposure calls. *J Occup Environ Med.* 1999;41:93-99.
15. Bronstein AC, et al. 2006 Annual Report of the American Association of Poison Control Centers' National Poison Data System (NPDS). *Clin Toxicol (Phila).* 2007;45:815-917.
16. Bronstein AC, et al. 2010 Annual Report of the American Association of Poison Control Centers' National Poison Data System (NPDS): 28th Annual Report. *Clin Toxicol (Phila).* 2011;49:910-941.
17. Bronstein AC, et al. 2008 Annual Report of the American Association of Poison Control Centers' National Poison Data System (NPDS): 26th Annual Report. *Clin Toxicol (Phila).* 2009;47:911-1084.
18. Bronstein AC, et al. 2009 Annual Report of the American Association of Poison Control Centers' National Poison Data System (NPDS): 27th Annual Report. *Clin Toxicol (Phila).* 2010;48:979-1178.
19. Bronstein AC, et al. 2007 Annual Report of the American Association of Poison Control Centers' National Poison Data System (NPDS): 25th Annual Report. *Clin Toxicol (Phila).* 2008;46:927-1057.
20. Bronstein AC, et al. 2011 Annual report of the American Association of Poison Control Centers' National Poison Data System (NPDS): 29th Annual Report. *Clin Toxicol (Phila).* 2012;50:911-1164.
21. Brubacher JR, et al. Salty broth for salicylate poisoning? Adequacy of overdose management advice in the 2001 Compendium of Pharmaceuticals and Specialties. *CMAJ.* 2002;167:992-996.
22. Budnitz DS, et al. Emergency hospitalizations for adverse drug events in older Americans. *N Engl J Med.* 2011;365:2002-2012.
23. Bunn TL, et al. The effect of poison control center consultation on accidental poisoning inpatient hospitalizations with preexisting medical conditions. *J Toxicol Environ Health A.* 2008;71:283-288.
24. Burda T, et al. Emergency department use of flumazenil prior to poison center consultation. *Vet Hum Toxicol.* 1997;39:245-247.
25. Calello DP, et al. 2010 pediatric fatality review of the National Poison Center database: results and recommendations. *Clin Toxicol (Phila).* 2012;50:25-26.
26. Caravati EM, et al. Ethylene glycol exposure: an evidence-based consensus guideline for out-of-hospital management. *Clin Toxicol (Phila).* 2005;43:327-345.
27. Caravati EM, et al. Elemental mercury exposure: an evidence-based consensus guideline for out-of-hospital management. *Clin Toxicol (Phila).* 2008;46:1-21.
28. Caravati EM, et al. Long-acting anticoagulant rodenticide poisoning: an evidence-based consensus guideline for out-of-hospital management. *Clin Toxicol (Phila).* 2007; 45:1-22.
29. Caravati EM, McElwee NE. Use of clinical toxicology resources by emergency physicians and its impact on poison control centers. *Ann Emerg Med.* 1991;20: 147-150.
30. Centers for Disease Control and Prevention. Blood lead levels in children aged 1-5 years—United States, 1999-2010. *MMWR Morb Mortal Wkly Rep.* 2013;62:245-248.
31. Centers for Disease Control and Prevention. NCHS data on drug-poisoning deaths; 2017. https://www.cdc.gov/nchs/data/factsheets/factsheet_drug_poisoning.htm.
32. Chafee-Bahamon C, et al. Patterns in hospitals' use of a regional poison information center. *Am J Public Health.* 1983;73:396-400.
33. Chafee-Bahamon C, Lovejoy FH Jr. Effectiveness of a regional poison center in reducing excess emergency room visits for children's poisonings. *Pediatrics.* 1983;72:164-169.
34. Chen CN, et al. Pharmacokinetic model for salicylate in cerebrospinal fluid, blood, organs, and tissues. *J Pharm Sci.* 1978;67:38-45.
35. Chyka PA. How many deaths occur annually from adverse drug reactions in the United States? *Am J Med.* 2000;109:122-130.
36. Chyka PA, et al. Salicylate poisoning: an evidence-based consensus guideline for out-of-hospital management. *Clin Toxicol (Phila).* 2007;45:95-131.
37. Chyka PA, et al. Dextromethorphan poisoning: an evidence-based consensus guideline for out-of-hospital management. *Clin Toxicol (Phila).* 2007;45:662-677.
38. Chyka PA, McCommon SW. Reporting of adverse drug reactions by poison control centres in the US. *Drug Saf.* 2000;23:87-93.
39. Clark RF, et al. Evaluating the utilization of a regional poison center by Latino communities. *J Toxicol Clin Toxicol.* 2002;40:855-860.
40. Clark RF, et al. Resource-use analysis of a medical toxicology consultation service. *Ann Emerg Med.* 1998;31:705-709.

41. Clauson KA, et al. Clinical decision support tools: performance of personal digital assistant versus online drug information databases. *Pharmacotherapy.* 2007;27:1651-1658.

42. Clower J. Notes from the field: carbon monoxide exposures reported to poison centers and related to hurricane Sandy—Northeastern United States, 2012. *MMWR Morb Mortal Wkly Rep.* 2012;61:905.

43. Cobaugh DJ, et al. Atypical antipsychotic medication poisoning: an evidence-based consensus guideline for out-of-hospital management. *Clin Toxicol (Phila).* 2007;45:918-942.

44. Cobaugh DJ, et al. Assessment of learning by emergency medicine residents and pharmacy students participating in a poison center clerkship. *Vet Hum Toxicol.* 1997;39:173-175.

45. Darracq MA, Cantrell FL. Hemodialysis and extracorporeal removal after pediatric and adolescent poisoning reported to a state poison center. *J Emerg Med.* 2013;44:1101-1107.

46. Darracq MA, et al. Disaster preparedness of poison control centers in the USA: a 15-year follow-up study. *J Med Toxicol.* 2014;10:19-25.

47. Dart RC, et al. Expert consensus guidelines for stocking of antidotes in hospitals that provide emergency care. *Ann Emerg Med.* 2009;54:386-394 e381.

48. Dart RC, et al. Acetaminophen poisoning: an evidence-based consensus guideline for out-of-hospital management. *Clin Toxicol (Phila).* 2006;44:1-18.

49. Dart RC, et al. Combined evidence-based literature analysis and consensus guidelines for stocking of emergency antidotes in the United States. *Ann Emerg Med.* 2000;36:126-132.

50. Dart RC, et al. Trends in opioid analgesic abuse and mortality in the United States. *N Engl J Med.* 2015;372:241-248.

51. Dasgupta N, et al. Using poison center exposure calls to predict methadone poisoning deaths. *PLoS One.* 2012;7:e41181.

52. Davis CO, et al. Toxicology training of paramedic students in the United States. *Am J Emerg Med.* 1999;17:138-140.

53. Espinoza TR, et al. Hyperinsulin therapy for calcium channel antagonist poisoning: a seven-year retrospective study. *Am J Ther.* 2013;20:29-31.

54. Felberg L, et al. State of the national's poison centers: 1995 American Association of Poison Control Centers Survey of US Poison Centers. *Vet Hum Toxicol.* 1996;38:445-453.

55. Friedman LS. Real-time surveillance of illicit drug overdoses using poison center data. *Clin Toxicol (Phila).* 2009;47:573-579.

56. Galvao TF, et al. Impact of a poison control center on the length of hospital stay of poisoned patients: retrospective cohort. *Sao Paulo Med J.* 2011;129:23-29.

57. Geller RJ, Lopez GP. Poison center planning for mass gatherings: the Georgia Poison Center experience with the 1996 Centennial Olympic Games. *J Toxicol Clin Toxicol.* 1999;37:315-319.

58. Gfroerer J, et al. Studies of nonresponse and measurement error in the national household survey on drug abuse. *NIDA Res Monogr.* 1997;167:273-295.

59. Graber N. Ciguatera fish poisoning—New York City, 2010-2011. *MMWR Morb Mortal Wkly Rep.* 2013;62:61-65.

60. Greenberg MI, et al. Material safety data sheet: a useful resource for the emergency physician. *Ann Emerg Med.* 1996;27:347-352.

61. Hamilton RJ, Goldfrank LR. Poison center data and the Pollyanna phenomenon. *J Toxicol Clin Toxicol.* 1997;35:21-23.

62. Hamilton RJ, et al. A descriptive study of an epidemic of poisoning caused by heroin adulterated with scopolamine. *J Toxicol Clin Toxicol.* 2000;38:597-608.

63. Harchelroad F, et al. Treated vs reported toxic exposures: discrepancies between a poison control center and a member hospital. *Vet Hum Toxicol.* 1990;32:156-159.

64. Harcke HT, et al. Autopsy radiography: digital radiographs (DR) vs multidetector computed tomography (MDCT) in high-velocity gunshot-wound victims. *Am J Forensic Med Pathol.* 2007;28:13-19.

65. Hickey CN, et al. Can a poison center overdose guideline safely reduce pediatric emergency department visits for unintentional beta-blocker ingestions? *Am J Ther.* 2012;19:346-350.

66. Centers for Disease Control and Prevention (CDC). Unintentional and Undetermined Poisoning Deaths-11 States, 1990-2001. MMWR Morb Mortal Wkly Rep. 2004;53;233-238.

67. Hitchings AW, et al. Determining the volume of toxic liquid ingestions in adults: accuracy of estimates by healthcare professionals and members of the public. *Clin Toxicol (Phila).* 2013;51:77-82.

68. Hoffman RS. Understanding the limitations of retrospective analyses of poison center data. *Clin Toxicol (Phila).* 2007;45:943-945.

69. Hoppe-Roberts JM, et al. Poisoning mortality in the United States: comparison of national mortality statistics and poison control center reports. *Ann Emerg Med.* 2000;35:440-448.

70. Hoyt BT, et al. Poison center data accuracy: a comparison of rural hospital chart data with the TESS database. Toxic Exposure Surveillance System. *Acad Emerg Med.* 1999;6:851-855.

71. Jackson BF, et al. Emergency department poisoning visits in children younger than 6 years: comparing referrals by a regional poison control center to referrals by other sources. *Pediatr Emerg Care.* 2012;28:1343-1347.

72. Jones CM, et al. Pharmaceutical overdose deaths, United States, 2010. *JAMA.* 2013;309:657-659.

73. Jordan JK, et al. Poison center rotation for health science students. *Vet Hum Toxicol.* 1987;29:174-175.

74. Kearney TE, et al. Health care cost effects of public use of a regional poison control center. *West J Med.* 1995;162:499-504.

75. Kelly NR, et al. Effects of a videotape to increase use of poison control centers by low-income and Spanish-speaking families: a randomized, controlled trial. *Pediatrics.* 2003;111:21-26.

76. King WD, Palmisano PA. Poison control centers: can their value be measured? *South Med J.* 1991;84:722-726.

77. Klein-Schwartz W, Smith GS. Agricultural and horticultural chemical poisonings: mortality and morbidity in the United States. *Ann Emerg Med.* 1997;29:232-238.

78. Krenzelok EP. Poison centers at the millennium and beyond. *J Toxicol Clin Toxicol.* 2000;38:693-696.

79. Krenzelok EP, Mrvos R. Initial impact of toll-free access on poison center call volume. *Vet Hum Toxicol.* 2003;45:325-327.

80. Krenzelok EP, Mrvos R. A regional poison information center IVR medication identification system: does it accomplish its goal? *Clin Toxicol (Phila).* 2011;49:858-861.

81. Lazarou J, et al. Incidence of adverse drug reactions in hospitalized patients: a meta-analysis of prospective studies. *JAMA.* 1998;279:1200-1205.

82. Levine M, et al. Impact of the use of regional poison control centers in an urban ems dispatch system. *J Med Toxicol.* 2017;13:47-51.

83. Linakis JG, Frederick KA. Poisoning deaths not reported to the regional poison control center. *Ann Emerg Med.* 1993;22:1822-1828.

84. Litovitz T, et al. webPOISONCONTROL: can poison control be automated? *Am J Emerg Med.* 2016;34:1614-1619.

85. Litovitz T, et al. Determinants of U.S. poison center utilization. *Clin Toxicol (Phila).* 2010;48:449-457.

86. Litovitz TL, et al. 1999 annual report of the American Association of Poison Control Centers Toxic Exposure Surveillance System. *Am J Emerg Med.* 2000;18:517-574.

87. LoVecchio F, et al. Media influence on Poison Center call volume after 11 September 2001. *Prehosp Disaster Med.* 2004;19:185.

88. Lovejoy FH Jr, et al. Poison centers, poison prevention, and the pediatrician. *Pediatrics.* 1994;94(2 Pt 1):220-224.

89. Manoguerra AS, et al. Iron ingestion: an evidence-based consensus guideline for out-of-hospital management. *Clin Toxicol (Phila).* 2005;43:553-570.

90. Manoguerra AS, et al. Camphor poisoning: an evidence-based practice guideline for out-of-hospital management. *Clin Toxicol (Phila).* 2006;44:357-370.

91. Manoguerra AS, et al. Valproic acid poisoning: an evidence-based consensus guideline for out-of-hospital management. *Clin Toxicol (Phila).* 2008;46:661-676.

92. Miller TR, Lestina DC. Costs of poisoni.ng in the United States and savings from poison control centers: a benefit-cost analysis. *Ann Emerg Med.* 1997;29:239-245.

93. Mowry JB, et al. 2014 Annual Report of the American Association of Poison Control Centers' National Poison Data System (NPDS): 32nd Annual Report. *Clin Toxicol (Phila).* 2015;53:962-1147.

94. Mowry JB, et al. 2015 Annual Report of the American Association of Poison Control Centers' National Poison Data System (NPDS): 33rd Annual Report. *Clin Toxicol (Phila).* 2016;54:924-1109.

95. Mowry JB, et al. 2012 Annual Report of the American Association of Poison Control Centers' National Poison Data System (NPDS): 30th Annual Report. *Clin Toxicol (Phila).* 2013;51:949-1229.

96. Mowry JB, et al. 2013 Annual Report of the American Association of Poison Control Centers' National Poison Data System (NPDS): 31st Annual Report. *Clin Toxicol (Phila).* 2014;52:1032-1283.

97. Mullen WH, et al. Incorrect overdose management advice in the Physicians' Desk Reference. *Ann Emerg Med.* 1997;29:255-261.

98. Murphy CM, et al. "Bath salts" and "plant food" products: the experience of one regional US poison center. *J Med Toxicol.* 2013;9:42-48.

99. Nelson LS, et al. Selective serotonin reuptake inhibitor poisoning: an evidence-based consensus guideline for out-of-hospital management. *Clin Toxicol (Phila).* 2007;45:315-332.

100. Nelson LS, et al. The benefit of houseofficer education on proper medication dose calculation and ordering. *Acad Emerg Med.* 2000;7:1311-1316.

101. Olson KR, et al. Calcium channel blocker ingestion: an evidence-based consensus guideline for out-of-hospital management. *Clin Toxicol (Phila).* 2005;43:797-822.

102. Palamar JJ, et al. Self-reported use of novel psychoactive substances in a US nationally representative survey: prevalence, correlates, and a call for new survey methods to prevent underreporting. *Drug Alcohol Depend.* 2015;156:112-119.

103. Palamar JJ, et al. Characteristics of novel psychoactive substance exposures reported to New York City Poison Center, 2011-2014. *Am J Drug Alcohol Abuse.* 2016;42:39-47.

104. Paulozzi LJ. Increases in age-group-specific injury mortality—United States, 1999-2004. *MMWR Morb Mortal Wkly Rep.* 2007;56:1281-1284.

105. Perkins NA, et al. Performance of drug-drug interaction software for personal digital assistants. *Ann Pharmacother.* 2006;40:850-855.

106. Phillips KA, et al. The costs and outcomes of restricting public access to poison control centers. Results from a natural experiment. *Med Care.* 1998;36:271-280.

107. Pourmand A, et al. A survey of poison control centers worldwide. *Daru.* 2012;20:13.

108. Robinson RL, Burk MS. Identification of drug-drug interactions with personal digital assistant-based software. *Am J Med.* 2004;116:357-358.

109. Rodgers GB. The safety effects of child-resistant packaging for oral prescription drugs. Two decades of experience. *JAMA.* 1996;275:1661-1665.

110. Rothwell E, et al. Exploring challenges to telehealth communication by specialists in poison information. *Qual Health Res.* 2012;22:67-75.

111. Ryan ML, et al. My Baby Drank Bleach LOL:) NF:(WCUTM?? *Clin Toxicol.* 2010;48.

112. Scharman EJ, et al. Methylphenidate poisoning: an evidence-based consensus guideline for out-of-hospital management. *Clin Toxicol (Phila).* 2007;45:737-752.

113. Scharman EJ, et al. Diphenhydramine and dimenhydrinate poisoning: an evidence-based consensus guideline for out-of-hospital management. *Clin Toxicol (Phila).* 2006;44:205-223.

114. Scherz RG, Robertson WO. The history of poison control centers in the United States. *Clin Toxicol.* 1978;12:291-296.

115. Schwartz L, et al. The use of focus groups to plan poison prevention education programs for low-income populations. *Health Promot Pract.* 2003;4:340-346.

116. Seifert SA, Jacobitz K. Pharmacy prescription dispensing errors reported to a regional poison control center. *J Toxicol Clin Toxicol.* 2002;40:919-923.

117. Simone KE, Spiller HA. Poison center surveillance data: the good, the bad and . . . the flu. *Clin Toxicol (Phila).* 2010;48:415-417.

118. Soslow AR, Woolf AD. Reliability of data sources for poisoning deaths in Massachusetts. *Am J Emerg Med.* 1992;10:124-127.

119. Spiller HA, Griffith JR. The value and evolving role of the U.S. Poison Control Center System. *Public Health Rep.* 2009;124:359-363.

120. Spiller HA, Mowry JB. Evaluation of the effect of a public educator on calls and poisonings reported to a regional poison center. *Vet Hum Toxicol.* 2004;46:206-208.

121. Su MK, et al. North American Congress of Clinical Toxicology (NACCT) Abstracts 2017. *Clin Toxicol.* 2017;55:689-868.

122. Tak CR, et al. The value of a poison control center in preventing unnecessary ED visits and hospital charges: a multi-year analysis. *Am J Emerg Med.* 2017;35:438-443.

123. Tormoehlen LM, et al. Increased adolescent opioid use and complications reported to a poison control center following the 2000 JCAHO pain initiative. *Clin Toxicol (Phila).* 2011;49:492-498.

124. Vagi SJ, et al. Passive multistate surveillance for neutropenia after use of cocaine or heroin possibly contaminated with levamisole. *Ann Emerg Med.* 2013;61:468-474.

125. Vassilev ZP, et al. Rapid communication: sociodemographic differences between counties with high and low utilization of a regional poison control center. *J Toxicol Environ Health A.* 2003;66:1905-1908.

126. Vassilev ZP, Marcus SM. The impact of a poison control center on the length of hospital stay for patients with poisoning. *J Toxicol Environ Health A.* 2007;70:107-110.

127. Vassilev ZP, et al. Assessment of barriers to utilization of poison centers by Hispanic/Latino populations. *J Toxicol Environ Health A.* 2006;69:1711-1718.

128. Walton WW. An evaluation of the Poison Prevention Packaging Act. *Pediatrics.* 1982;69:363-370.

129. Wax PM, et al. beta-blocker ingestion: an evidence-based consensus guideline for out-of-hospital management. *Clin Toxicol (Phila).* 2005;43:131-146.

130. Wax PM, et al. The arrival of the ED-based POISINDEX: perceived impact on poison control center use. *Am J Emerg Med.* 1994;12:537-540.

131. Wolf LR, Hamilton GC. Objectives to direct the training of emergency medicine residents of off-service rotations: toxicology. *J Emerg Med.* 1994;12:391-405.

132. Wolkin AF, et al. Using poison center data for national public health surveillance for chemical and poison exposure and associated illness. *Ann Emerg Med.* 2012;59:56-61.

133. Woolf AD, et al. Tricyclic antidepressant poisoning: an evidence-based consensus guideline for out-of-hospital management. *Clin Toxicol (Phila).* 2007;45:203-233.

134. Youniss J, et al. Characterization of US poison centers: a 1998 survey conducted by the American Association of Poison Control Centers. *Vet Hum Toxicol.* 2000;42:43-53.

131 PRINCIPLES OF OCCUPATIONAL TOXICOLOGY: DIAGNOSIS AND CONTROL

Peter H. Wald

Three workers engaged in the production of mercuric acetate (Chap. 95) were admitted to the hospital within 22 calendar days of each other, 30, 48, and 5 days, respectively, after their last working day. The workers served the same reactor in which elemental mercury was oxidized by peroxide to mercuric oxide and mercuric acetate was formed by the reaction of mercuric oxide with acetic acid. They all presented with neurologic findings, including ataxia, dysarthria, tremor, deteriorating vision, and cerebellar signs. The first 2 workers had rapidly progressive downhill courses to coma that ended in death. The diagnosis of mercury vapor intoxication of the first 2 patients was established 21 and 16 days after their admission, when the third worker was admitted and hospitals were informed about their exposure. Blood mercury concentrations in all 3 patients were approximately 2,000 mcg/L with low urine mercury concentrations. All patients were chelated with penicillamine without any noticeable effect. Organic mercury probably was formed as an unintended byproduct of this reaction. In this reaction, methyl mercury acetate, which is 5.4 times more volatile than mercury vapor, could have been formed. The incorrect diagnosis of mercury vapor exposure in these cases was established even though (1) the observed signs of a rapid irreversible clinical course, ataxia, dysarthria, and constriction of visual fields are rarely present in mercury vapor poisoning and are characteristic of organic mercury poisoning; (2) the degree of deterioration after removal from exposure further implicated organic mercury, not mercury vapor; (3) blood mercury concentrations were in the range associated with severe poisoning in the Iraq methyl mercury epidemic; (4) patients had little response to treatment with penicillamine, the opposite of what is expected with mercury vapor; and (5) the blood-to-urinary mercury concentration ratios were high, but this ratio usually is less than 0.5 in mercury vapor toxicity or in workers exposed to mercury vapor. The other important facet of these cases is the public health implications of this sentinel health event. Three employees in this workplace were affected by this exposure. Further investigation of the workplace revealed that no other workers were affected but also that there were no changing facilities so employees wore their work clothes home. Investigation of their homes revealed elevated environmental mercury concentrations and elevated blood mercury concentrations in family members. Here, an occupational exposure became an environmental exposure for the community.

Many important problems are associated with the diagnosis and treatment of occupational and environmentally caused diseases, including (1) the ability to correctly establish the diagnosis as originating from an exposure, (2) the ability to correctly treat the condition, and (3) the ability to correctly act on any public health issues related to the exposure. The following discussion instructs clinicians on how to assemble adequate information to achieve the appropriate diagnosis and treatment.

TAKING AN OCCUPATIONAL HISTORY

Because time spent at work is a large percentage of many people's day, the occupational health history should be a routine part of the medical history. This is especially true of patients who present to health care with potential xenobiotic exposures. The history should include several brief survey questions. Positive responses then lead to a more detailed occupational and environmental history, which is composed of 3 elements: present work, past work, and nonoccupational exposures.

The Brief Occupational Survey

The following 3 questions should be incorporated into the occupational survey:

■ Exactly what kind of work do you do?

■ Are you exposed to any physical (radiation, noise, extremes of temperature or pressure), chemical (liquids, fumes, vapors, dusts, or mists), or biologic hazards at work (Table 131–1)?

■ Are your symptoms related in any way to starting or being away from work? For example, do the symptoms start when you arrive at work at the beginning of the day or week or when you work at a specific location or during a specific process at work?

Present Work

Collected data on a person's present job reveal what his or her present exposures may be, which can help formulate the differential diagnosis for the

TABLE 131–1	Hazard Classes, Hazard Types, and Several Common Examples Found in the Workplace	
Hazard Class	**Hazard Type**	**Examples**
Physical hazards	Human–machine interfaces	Repetitive motion
		Lifting
		Vibration
		Mechanical trauma, electric shock
	Physical environment	Temperature
		Pressure
		Long or rotating shifts
	Energy	Ionizing radiation: x-ray, ultraviolet
		Nonionizing radiation: infrared, microwave, magnetic fields
		Lasers
		Noise
Chemical hazards	Solvents	Aliphatics, alicyclics, aromatics, alcohols, ketones, ethers, aldehydes, acetates, peroxides, halogenated and nitrogen containing compounds
	Metals	Lead, mercury, cadmium
	Gases	Combustion products, irritants, simple and chemical asphyxiants, oxygen-deficient environments
	Dusts	Organic (wood) and inorganic (asbestos or silica), nano-materials
	Pesticides	Organic chlorine, organic phosphorus, carbamate
	Epoxy resins and polymer systems	Toluene diisocyanate, phthalates
Biologic hazards	Bacteria	*Bacillus anthracis, Legionella pneumophila, Borrelia burgdorferi*
	Viruses	Hepatitis, HIV, Hantavirus
	Mycobacteria	*Mycobacterium tuberculosis*
	Rickettsia and Chlamydia	*Chlamydia psittaci, Coxiella burnetii*
	Fungi	*Histoplasma capsulatum, Coccidioides immitis*
	Parasites	*Echinococcus* spp, *Plasmodium* spp, *Toxoplasma gondii*
	Envenomations	Arthropod, marine, snake
	Allergens	Enzymes, animals, dusts, insects, latex, plant pollen dusts

TABLE 131–2	Components of an Occupational Health History

Current work history
- Specifics of the job
  - Employer's name
  - Type of industry
  - Duration of employment
  - Employment location, hours, and shift changes
  - Description of work process
  - Unusual activities of the job that are occasional (eg, maintenance)
  - Adjacent work processes
  - Employee health, safety, or union contact if available; otherwise manager or supervisor
- Hazardous exposures (Table 132–1)
- Possible health effects
  - Suspicious health problems
  - Temporality of symptoms
  - Specific distribution of symptoms (rash, paresthesias)
  - Affected coworkers
  - Presence or absence of known risk factors (smoking, alcohol)
- Workplace sampling and monitoring
  - Individual or area air monitoring
  - Surface sampling
  - Biologic monitoring
  - Medical surveillance records
- Exposure controls
  - Administrative controls
  - Process engineering controls
    - Enclosure
    - Shielding
    - Ventilation
    - Electrical and mechanically controlled interlocks
  - Personal protective equipment
    - Respirators
    - Protective clothing
    - Earplugs, glasses, gloves, face shields, head and foot protection

Work history (prior)
- Review current work history for all past employment

Nonoccupational exposures
- Secondary employment
- Hobbies
- Outdoor activities
- Residential exposures
- Community contamination
- Habits: tobacco, alcohol, other xenobiotics

employee's complaints. These data should be systematically collected by focusing on 4 areas: specifics of the job, hazardous exposures, health effects, and monitoring and control measures (Table 131–2).

Specifics of the Job

It is not sufficient simply to inquire what the patient does for a living. Similar to health care professionals, workers in other industries have their own jargon. When asked for a job title, a patient may respond with a title that has meaning only in his or her trade. Even if the job title is recognizable, it may not provide any useful information and, in fact, may be misleading. A secretary working in a small plastics manufacturing plant has potential occupational exposures that are quite different from a secretary who works for a law firm.

The important specific information requested should include the name of the employer, type of industry, duration and location of employment,

hours and shift changes, process description (including unusual occasional activities), and adjacent processes. The employer should be able to provide information about materials used at the plant. However, clinicians should always obtain the patient's permission before calling the employer. A patient may be fired or otherwise discriminated against (despite legal protections) for suggesting that health problems are work related.

For patients in whom exposures are expected, it is important to question more closely to learn precisely what happens in the patient's immediate work environment because nearby work processes may contribute other exposures. If possible, the patient should be asked for a diagram of the work area. The patient also should be questioned about job process changes. A previously safe job may have been changed to a potentially dangerous job without a change in the patient's job title.

The patient should describe exactly what he or she does on any given day and for how long. Unusual and nonroutine tasks, such as those performed during overtime, maintenance, or in an emergency, should also be described. The primary job may not involve xenobiotics, but the patient may nevertheless perform tasks that entail unprotected exposure to a toxic xenobiotic.

Hazardous Exposures

The names or types of all xenobiotics to which the patient may be exposed are important in determining potential adverse effects and any relationship to the patient's complaints. It is important to elicit any recent changes in suppliers of these products because even a slight change in the formulation of a xenobiotic may cause adverse effects in an individual who previously had no problems working with that xenobiotic. This information should be obtained from the material safety data sheet (MSDS), an important but not universally reliable source of information. In addition to adverse health effects, the MSDS contains information on chemical reactivity, safety precautions, and other data. As an initial step, the MSDS should be requested and reviewed; however, information provided on health effects should be confirmed using other resources. Four major concerns result from relying solely on the MSDS: (1) some MSDS forms are excellent, but others are incomplete and inadequate; (2) components of a product that are regarded as "trade secrets" do not have to be revealed; (3) components that have important health effects (eg, solvent or solid carriers of the "active ingredients") are often grouped together under "inert ingredients" without being specifically named; and (4) process intermediates or unintended byproducts of a manufacturing process are often not identified. However, if a xenobiotic is believed to be related to a health effect, manufacturers are required to release to a physician all information, including trade secrets and inert components.

Exposures to physical and biologic xenobiotics can be elicited during the review of job processes. Most patients know what they are, or have been, exposed to, even if they do not know the exact name of the xenobiotics or its medical effects.

Health Effects

Significant occupational exposures usually cause medical effects, although some do so only after a substantial latency period. Key areas of inquiry include suspicious health problems, temporality of symptoms, and affected coworkers. These data, combined with workplace monitoring and sampling data, may help in determining whether the patient is experiencing a work-related illness (Table 131–3). Patients may suspect that their illness or complaint is work related, especially when symptoms occur at the workplace and improve or disappear over the weekend or during a vacation. Specific distribution of findings, such as a rash in a bilateral glove pattern, is supportive of an occupational cause. Coworkers with similar complaints (not necessarily of the same severity) should raise suspicion that a workplace exposure is responsible for a particular symptom complex. Diseases such as lung cancer or hepatitis, which occur in the absence of known risk factors such as smoking and alcohol, must be epidemiologically investigated.

TABLE 131–3	Evidence Supporting Work-Relatedness of Occupational Disease

Known or documented exposure to a causative xenobiotic
Symptoms consistent with suspected workplace exposure
Suggestive or diagnostic physical signs
Similar problems in coworkers or workers in related occupations
Temporal relationship of complaints related to work
Confirmatory environmental or biologic monitoring data
Scientific biologic plausibility
Absence of a nonoccupational etiology
Resistance to maximum medical treatment because employee continues to be exposed at work

Workplace Sampling, Monitoring, and Control

Control of workplace hazards begins with an industrial hygiene monitoring program. Employers are required to give results of both area and individual sampling to employees, and these results are potentially valuable to associate presenting symptoms to a workplace exposure. A medical surveillance program that includes periodic spirometry and respiratory questionnaires usually indicates that the patient works with a potential respiratory toxin. A medical surveillance program that includes biologic monitoring for a specific xenobiotic may also provide an immediate clue to the cause of the patient's complaints. Finally, if the patient knows exactly what he or she is working with, the physician can usually quickly determine whether any of the xenobiotics are compatible with the patient's complaints. Many companies do not perform routine industrial hygiene monitoring or medical surveillance. Individuals who become sick or ill at work are often sent to local emergency departments (EDs). In such situations, emergency physicians will need to perform the type of time-consuming, detailed occupational history outlined here or be able to consult or refer immediately to appropriate physicians or clinics.

Portions of Table 131–2 and the following section on Evaluation and Control of Workplace Hazards detail the types of controls typically used in workplaces. It is important to determine whether the workplace uses any of the listed control measures. The existence of control measures usually indicates that the employer recognizes and has attempted to deal with a hazardous exposure.

PAST WORK

It is important not to limit the occupational history to the patient's current workplace and job. Many occupational diseases (asbestosis is the classic example) have long latency periods between xenobiotic exposure and initial development of clinical symptoms. In addition, patients may have been exposed to xenobiotics at work that make them more sensitive to other environmental xenobiotics. For example, someone who developed asthma secondary to a previous workplace exposure may have asthma attacks on exposure to simple irritants in the current workplace. When taking an in-depth occupational history, issues that may be relevant to the current work history as well as for each previous job should be explored.

Nonoccupational Exposures

Workers may be exposed to toxic xenobiotics in the course of pursuing secondary employment, hobbies such as using lead solder for stained glass or electronics or outdoor activities in contaminated or industrial areas. Residential exposures, such as those from gas and wood stoves, chemically treated furniture and fabrics, and pest control, are also relevant. It is important to ask patients about these potential exposures before focusing entirely on exposures in their primary place of employment. This obviously includes relevant issues from the social history, such as tobacco, alcohol, and both licit and illicit drug use.

EVALUATION AND CONTROL OF WORKPLACE HAZARDS
Initial Workplace Evaluation

The Occupational Safety and Health Administration (OSHA) places legal responsibility for providing a safe and healthy workplace on the employer.

The rationale for this placement of responsibility is that the employer is in the best position to make any modifications necessary to prevent additional work-related illness and injury. The physician will likely need to initiate a dialogue with a patient's employer to promote preventive action but should do so only with the patient's informed consent. The initial treating physician should also refer the patient to an occupational medicine specialist who is specifically trained to manage work-related exposures and diseases and initiate prevention programs.

It is important for the health care provider to identify an individual with an appropriate administrative role, such as someone in the company's medical department, the patient's supervisor, the plant's safety officer, or the shop manager. If management is willing, a plant walk-through inspection can provide unique insight and information usually unavailable in an office setting. A walk-through by an occupational medicine specialist makes it easier to understand the work environment, identify safety and health hazards, assess control measures, and recognize opportunities for prevention. It also facilitates a good working relationship with key personnel in management and labor. The physician, who cares for a number of patients who work in the plant or who provides health services to the workers through the company or labor union, should be invited to participate in the walk-through. Assistance with plant inspections can be obtained from occupational health specialists, such as occupational physicians or industrial hygienists.

Industrial Hygiene Sampling and Monitoring

Equipment is available to measure airborne concentrations of toxic xenobiotics, noise levels, radiation levels, temperature, and humidity. Employees can be fitted with pumps and other devices to measure individual exposure concentrations at the breathing zone, where, depending on what controls are used, concentrations may vary from those in the general work area. These results then can be compared with OSHA standards and other available standards to help determine the extent of the hazard and to formulate a control plan. The Occupational and Safety Health Act requires that employers monitor the concentrations of only a few specific hazards, including arsenic, asbestos, benzene, cadmium, chromium, cotton dust, ethylene oxide, formaldehyde, lead, noise, and vinyl chloride. A complete listing of all xenobiotics is available in the OSHA standard *29 CFR 1910 Part Z—Toxic and Hazardous Substances* (http://www.osha.gov/pls/oshaweb/owastand.display_standard_group?p_toc_level=1&p_part_number=1910). In addition, monitoring is required for certain tasks such as hazardous waste operations or entering a confined space that may have an oxygen-deficient atmosphere. Ongoing sampling of the remaining estimated 60,000 xenobiotics used in the workplace is not required. Where industrial hygiene sampling is performed, OSHA's medical access standard gives any exposed worker or his or her representative the right to review and copy all sampling data.

Control of Workplace Exposures

Control of exposures in the workplace has traditionally relied on a hierarchy of methods to protect workers. The preferred solution is complete elimination of the exposure by substitution. When substitution is not possible, the next preferred method consists of shielding for workers to reduce their exposure. The least favored method is personal protective equipment (PPE), which requires a positive action from the worker.

Engineering Controls

Health and safety professionals prefer—and OSHA regulations require when feasible—the use of engineering controls to reduce worker exposure to hazardous xenobiotics. These controls intercept hazards at their source or in the workplace atmosphere before they reach the worker. Engineering controls include redesign or modification of process or equipment to reduce hazardous emissions; isolation of a process through enclosure or shielding; and automation of an operation; and installation of exhaust systems that remove hazardous dusts, fumes, and vapors. Local exhaust systems, such as hoods, are preferable to general dilution ventilation because the former removes contaminants closer to their source and at relatively high rates.

Engineering controls have several advantages over control measures focused on the worker. Properly installed and maintained engineering controls are reliable and consistent, and their effectiveness does not depend on human supervision or interaction. They can simultaneously limit exposure through several routes, such as inhalation and skin absorption. In addition, engineering controls do not place a burden on the worker or interfere with worker comfort or safety.

Work Practices

Work practices are procedures that the worker can follow to limit exposure to hazardous xenobiotics. Examples are the use of high-powered vacuum cleaners instead of compressed air cleaning and pouring techniques that direct hazardous xenobiotics away from the worker. Although not as effective as engineering controls, work practice can be a useful component of an overall hazard control program.

Administrative Controls

Administrative controls reduce the duration of exposure for any individual worker or reduce the total number of workers exposed to a hazardous xenobiotic. Examples are rotating workers into and out of hazardous areas so that no single worker is exposed full time and specific scheduling of procedures likely to generate high concentrations of xenobiotics, such as cleaning or maintenance activities, occurs during nights or weekends. Administrative controls sometimes have the side effect of exposing more workers, albeit at lower doses that limit exposures below action levels.

Personal Protective Equipment

Personal protective equipment, such as respirators, earplugs, gloves, and hard hats, is the least effective but most commonly used control method. Personal protective equipment is the only viable protection strategy when other controls are not practical but can also be used as an additional layer of protection in the presence of engineering controls. Some employers favor PPE over the institution of more costly engineering and administrative controls. Programs that use PPE should have additional Industrial Safety and Hygiene staff or resources to ensure the programs are properly designed and administered.

Respirators and other forms of PPE often are hot, uncomfortable, and awkward to wear and make it difficult for workers to breathe, speak, or hear, depending on the equipment involved. Consequently, workers often remove or only intermittently use the protection. Respirators place extra stress on the heart and the lungs. Both respirators and earplugs limit conversation and therefore present a safety hazard in themselves.

Because PPE does not stop a hazard from entering the environment, the worker is entirely vulnerable to exposure if the equipment fails. In addition, generally only one route of exposure is protected. For example, the commonly used half-mask respirator still leaves the skin and eyes exposed.

Choosing the right piece of PPE is difficult and depends on the nature and extent of the hazard. For example, each type of respirator is rated for the amount of protection it provides; as expected, the cost of a respirator increases with its protection factor. Use of the wrong type of respirator will leave the worker insufficiently protected.

Half-mask respirator cartridges are available in various colors that are coded to the xenobiotic filtered out of the breathing environment. If the wrong cartridge is used, the worker is unprotected from the hazardous contaminant. To be effective, a respirator must be meticulously "fit" to the individual worker. Failure to achieve a proper seal negates the usefulness of respirators. High cheekbones, dentures, scars, perspiration, talking, head movements, and facial hair can prevent a proper seal. These factors often are ignored or overlooked by an employer who adopts a "one-size-fits-all" policy.

Even if each employee is provided the proper respirator, the respiratory protection program may not be effective. The Occupational Safety and Health Act requires that employers institute a program of proper fit testing, cleaning, maintenance, and storage of respirators, which can be at least as costly as the institution of engineering controls.

In some instances, use of PPE may be unavoidable. An employer may need to control a hazardous exposure through a combination of measures, such as engineering controls and PPE. Ideally, the employer is using PPE as a control of last resort and in strict compliance with OSHA standards.

Worker Education and Training

Regardless of the control measures used, workers and supervisors must be educated in the recognition and control of workplace hazards and the prevention of work-related illness and injury. The OSHA Hazard Communication Standard (Table 131–4) requires that employers train workers in ways to detect the presence or release of hazardous xenobiotics, their physical and health hazards, methods of protection against the hazards, and proper emergency procedures, as well as how to read the labeling system and how to read and use an MSDS.

With the passage of federal, state, and local right-to-know laws, many consulting companies now offer hazard communication training. These programs are of uneven quality. Those that tend to focus on acute hazards, ignore chronic effects, and emphasize PPE over other control measures are less effective in both training workers to recognize hazards and ultimately controlling hazardous workplace exposures.

Medical Monitoring

Together with industrial hygiene monitoring, exposure control, and worker education, a medical monitoring program forms the foundation of an effective occupational disease prevention regimen. However, medical monitoring is fraught with technical and ethical pitfalls (Table 131–5). Medical monitoring encompasses both medical screening and medical surveillance.

Medical screening refers to the cross-sectional testing of a population of workers for evidence of excessive exposure or early stages of disease, regardless of relationship to work, that potentially influences the ability to tolerate or perform work.

Preemployment and preplacement physical examinations are another type of medical screening that are often favored by employers. The Americans with Disabilities Act (ADA) and the newer ADA Amendments Act of 2008 (ADAAA) (Table 131–4) regulate the timing, scope, content, and use of these examinations and the information gathered. Comprehensive resources for information on the ADA are available at http://www.adata.org. The ADA prohibits "preemployment" medical examinations and inquiries. After a job offer is made, "preplacement" examinations and inquiries can be conducted to determine whether an applicant can perform a job safely and effectively. The physician evaluates the individual's medical history, current symptoms, and physical laboratory findings to determine whether he or she currently has the physical or mental capacity necessary to perform the essential functions of the job and whether the individual can do so without posing a "direct threat" to the health or safety of him- or herself or others. This threat must be more than theoretical and cannot be based on some future time; the threat must be concrete and relatively immediate.

Few tests and few conditions are good predictors of either the capacity to perform a task or increased susceptibility to a particular exposure. Many workers and their advocates view preplacement examinations as a way for employers to choose the "fittest" worker and to avoid their legally mandated obligation to provide a safe and healthy workplace for all workers. This is not true for most employers. Physicians asked by an employer to perform preplacement examinations should be sure that each component of the examination relates to the actual job the individual is being hired to perform and the actual risks he or she will encounter on the job. Both the law and sound occupational medical practice dictate that the employer's attention and efforts be directed toward redesign of the job and its hazards so that it is safe and healthy for all workers to perform.

Medical surveillance refers to the ongoing evaluation, by means of periodic examinations, of high-risk individuals or potentially exposed workers to detect early pathophysiologic changes indicative of significant exposure. The Occupational Safety and Health Act requires little in the way of medical surveillance, although several OSHA standards require employers to institute

TABLE 131–4	Government Agencies and Their Important Regulatory Authority of the Workplace—A Timeline	
Regulation	**Agency**	**Authority**
Occupational Safety and Health Act (1970)	Department of Labor	Congress passed the Occupational Safety and Health Act and created the Occupational Safety and Health Administration (OSHA) to ensure worker and workplace safety. The goal was to make sure employers provide their workers a place of employment free from recognized hazards to safety and health, such as exposure to toxic xenobiotics, excessive noise levels, mechanical dangers, heat or cold stress, and unsanitary conditions.
		To establish standards for workplace health and safety, the Act also created the National Institute for Occupational Safety and Health (NIOSH) as the research institution for the Occupational Safety and Health Administration. Part 1910.1200 of OSHA established the Hazard Communication Standard (HazCom). The purpose of this section is to ensure that the hazards of all xenobiotics produced or imported are evaluated and that information concerning their hazards is transmitted to employers and employees. This transmittal of information is to be accomplished by means of comprehensive hazard communication programs, which are to include container labeling and other forms of warning, material safety data sheets, and employee training.
Resource Conservation and Recovery Act (RCRA, 1976)	Environmental Protection Agency (EPA)	RCRA (commonly pronounced "rick-rah") gave the EPA the authority to control hazardous waste from "cradle to grave." This includes the generation, transportation, treatment, storage, and disposal of hazardous waste. RCRA also set forth a framework for the management of nonhazardous wastes. The 1986 amendments to RCRA enabled the EPA to address environmental problems that could result from underground tanks storing petroleum and other hazardous xenobiotics. RCRA focuses only on active and future facilities and does not address abandoned or historic sites (see CERCLA).
Hazardous and Solid Waste Amendments (HSWA, 1984)		HSWA (commonly pronounced "hiss-wa"), the Federal Hazardous and Solid Waste Amendments, are the 1984 amendments to RCRA that required the phasing out of land disposal of hazardous waste. Some of the other mandates of this strict law include increased enforcement authority for the EPA, more stringent hazardous waste management standards, and a comprehensive underground storage tank program.
Toxic Substances Control Act (TSCA, 1976)	EPA	TSCA was enacted by Congress to give the EPA the ability to track the 75,000 industrial xenobiotics currently produced or imported into the United States. The EPA repeatedly screens these xenobiotics and can require reporting or testing of those that may pose an environmental or human health hazard. The EPA can ban the manufacture and import of xenobiotics that pose an unreasonable risk.
		Reporting requirements include (1) premanufacturing notification for new xenobiotics, (2) allegation of significant adverse reactions, (3) reporting of health and safety studies, and (4) notification of suspicion of substantial risk to health.
Comprehensive Environmental Response, Compensation, and Liability Act (CERCLA, 1980)	EPA	CERCLA, commonly known as the Superfund Act, was enacted by Congress on December 11, 1980. This law created a tax on the chemical and petroleum industries and provided broad federal authority to respond directly to releases or threatened releases of hazardous xenobiotics that may endanger public health or the environment. Over 5 years, $1.6 billion was collected, and the tax went to a trust fund for cleaning up abandoned or uncontrolled hazardous waste sites. CERCLA (1) established prohibitions and requirements concerning closed and abandoned hazardous waste sites, (2) provided for liability of persons responsible for releases of hazardous waste at these sites, and (3) established a trust fund to provide for cleanup when no responsible party could be identified.
		The law authorizes 2 types of response actions: (1) short-term removals, in which actions may be taken to address releases or threatened releases requiring prompt response, and (2) long-term remedial response actions that permanently and significantly reduce the dangers associated with releases or threats of releases of hazardous xenobiotics that are serious but not immediately life threatening. These actions can be conducted only at sites listed on the EPA's National Priorities List (NPL).
Superfund Amendments and Reauthorization Act (SARA, 1986)	EPA	SARA reflected the EPA's experience in administering the complex Superfund program during its first 6 years and made several important changes and additions to the program. SARA (1) stressed the importance of permanent remedies and innovative treatment technologies in cleaning up hazardous waste sites, (2) required Superfund actions to consider the standards and requirements found in other state and federal environmental laws and regulations, (3) provided new enforcement authorities and settlement tools, (4) increased state involvement in every phase of the Superfund, (5) increased the focus on human health problems posed by hazardous waste sites, (6) encouraged greater citizen participation in making decisions on how sites should be cleaned up, and (7) increased the size of the trust fund to $8.5 billion. SARA also required the EPA to revise the Hazard Ranking System (HRS) to ensure that it accurately assessed the relative degree of risk to human health and the environment posed by uncontrolled hazardous waste sites that may be placed on the NPL. Emergency Planning and Community Right-to-Know Act (EPCRA), also known as Title III of SARA, was enacted by Congress as the national legislation on community safety. This law was designated to help local communities protect public health, safety, and the environment from xenobiotic hazards. The law requires manufacturers to report the amount of toxic xenobiotics released each year (Toxic Release Inventory {TRI}).
		To implement EPCRA, Congress required each state to appoint a State Emergency Response Commission (SERC). The SERCs were required to divide their states into Emergency Planning Districts and to name a Local Emergency Planning Committee (LEPC) for each district.
Americans with Disabilities Act (ADA, 1990) and the ADA Amendments Act of 2008 (ADAAA)	Department of Labor	The ADA was enacted by Congress to establish clear and comprehensive prohibition of discrimination on the basis of disability. The act specifically covers discrimination in the areas of (1) employment, (2) public services, (3) public accommodations and services operated by private entities, and (4) telecommunications. The ADAAA reaffirms Congress' initial intent of the 1990 law to (1) broadly define "disability," (2) use the definition of "handicapped individual" under the Rehabilitation Act of 1973 and (3) state that mitigating measures (eg, insulin for diabetes) shall not be a factor when determining whether an impairment substantially limits a major life activity. The final regulations for the Act were publish in the Federal Register in March 2011. http://www.eeoc.gov/laws/regulations/adaaa_fact_sheet.cfm.

TABLE 131–5   Ethical Code of Conduct
Occupational and environmental health professionals have an obligation to:
Promote a safe and healthy workplace environment.
Uphold ethical standards.
Avoid discrimination.
Maintain professional competence.
Protect patient confidentiality.
Advise and report significant individual and population health while respecting confidentially.
Directly address and disclose conflict of interest issues.

Data from American College of Occupational and Environmental Medicine. Code of Ethics: 2010. http://www.acoem.org/codeofconduct.aspx.

medical surveillance programs, for example, for workers exposed to asbestos, arsenic, cadmium, chromium, vinyl chloride, lead, and ethylene oxide. Depending on the potential exposure, medical surveillance may include a history and physical examination, chest radiography, pulmonary function tests, blood and urine tests, and other laboratory evaluations.

A medical surveillance program may also include biologic monitoring, the purpose of which is not to identify the occurrence of disease but to measure the uptake or presence of a particular xenobiotic or its metabolites in body fluids or organs. Ideally, this occurs before any pathophysiologic damage occurs. Consequently, biologic monitoring is potentially a primary preventive measure. For example, several volatile organic compounds, such as benzene and toluene, if inhaled or absorbed through the skin, produce metabolites that can be measured in urine.

Biologic monitoring has some advantages over air monitoring because biologic monitoring measures the *actual* absorption of a xenobiotic by the body as opposed to ambient concentrations in the workplace. The amount of a chemical absorbed may not be closely correlated to ambient xenobiotics for several reasons, including differences in individual work habits, use and effectiveness of PPE, dermal absorption of xenobiotics unrelated to their concentration in the air, and nonoccupational exposures.

Biologic monitoring, however, has several significant limitations. For most xenobiotics, there are no standards of "normal" or "safe" concentrations against which results can be compared. The timing of specimen collection is critical because different xenobiotics have different biologic half-lives. The storage and handling of specimens and interpretation of results are vulnerable to error. Nevertheless, if carefully designed and implemented, biologic monitoring can be a useful complement to a comprehensive industrial hygiene program.

With the exception of biologic monitoring, medical monitoring programs identify disease processes already underway and therefore are, at best, a form of secondary prevention. If workers are identified as having higher than acceptable exposures, they should be removed from exposure with continuing pay while their internal concentrations decline and while the employer investigates any potential breakdown in the workplace controls. To be an effective preventive measure, these programs must be coordinated with environmental monitoring programs that identify the nature, source, and extent of workplace hazards; implementation of engineering controls and other measures that control hazards as close as possible to the source; and worker education programs that, at a minimum, inform workers of exposures, their effects, and proper control measures.

ETHICAL ISSUES

Physicians delivering occupational medicine services are required to fulfil many often-conflicting roles, including caring for individual employees, protection of groups of employees, ensuring a safe workplace, carrying out mandated regulatory examinations, and confirming the effectiveness of workplace hazard controls. The physician's first role is to do good for the patient or population he or she charged with protecting. Table 131–5 outlines the 7 critical behaviors required for ethical practice

as adopted by the American College of Occupational and Environmental Medicine Medical monitoring programs[1] and preplacement examinations discussed earlier raise issues of doctor–patient confidentiality. Other potential conflicts include access to employee medical records, which should be available only to the corporate medical or first aid department and not to the personnel office and general management. Unless required by statute, employers should never be told the results of history, physical, or diagnostic examinations unless the patient gives his or her written consent. The examining physician need only inform the employer that an individual is or is not capable of performing a particular job with or without specified restrictions. The physician should not disclose diagnostic information about medical conditions. The complex roles of occupational medicine physicians and medical toxicology consultants also require the fulfillment of several additional obligations, which are detailed next.

Obligations of the Health Care Provider to the Individual Patient, Coworkers, Employer, Government, and Community

Occupational diseases and injuries are, in principle, preventable. Physicians who diagnose a work-related disease or injury have an opportunity and an ethical obligation to participate in the identification and control of workplace hazards and the prevention of further occupational illness and injury. Physicians can choose from a range of possible follow-up measures, the goals of which are to prevent recurrence or worsening of the disease or injury in the patient and to prevent the development of disease or injury in other potentially exposed workers. Some of these activities may necessitate contact with occupational medicine physicians, medical toxicologists, industrial hygienists, lawyers, journalists, government officials, management personnel, and union officials.

Obligations to the Patient

Inform the Patient That the Illness May Be Work Related

When the workplace is determined to be a factor in the etiology or aggravation of the patient's illness, this fact and its implications should be discussed with the patient. It should never be assumed that the patient is fully aware of the health risks associated with any workplace exposure. The worker should be provided information regarding the nature of workplace hazards, their health risks, preventive measures, and recommendations regarding continued exposure.

Suggest How the Patient Can Reduce the Exposure

In some cases, the patient should take steps to reduce exposure. Helpful adjustments in work habits include using a respirator or other PPE provided by the employer; using workplace shower and dressing or change rooms to avoid carrying xenobiotics from the workplace to the home; and avoiding ingestion of workplace xenobiotics by careful hand washing before eating or smoking and by taking lunch, coffee, and smoking breaks away from the work station. Obviously, these recommendations assume that the employer provides the appropriate equipment and facilities, which is not always the case. The most effective hazard control measures require significant commitment by, and cooperation from, the employer.

Suggest That the Patient Remove Him- or Herself From the Exposure

The employer may be willing to transfer the patient to a location away from the offending hazard. This may result in a reduction in pay, seniority, or other benefits, which may be compensable under workers' compensation. The employment provisions of the ADA require employers to make "reasonable accommodations" for both work- and non–work-related disabilities. Nevertheless, the employer may not be able to accommodate the patient. The patient should be counseled carefully, and other options should be explored.

Advise the Patient to Notify the Employer

Patients who are experiencing a work-related illness may be entitled to workers' compensation benefits, Social Security disability, or other government-sponsored benefit programs. In addition, they may have a valid claim against the manufacturer of a xenobiotic, a defective product, or another third party. The degree of disability necessary to bring a successful claim varies.

After a patient is informed that he or she has a work-related illness, strict time limits are set in motion, and failure to meet them can preclude the patient from successfully filing a claim or receiving needed benefits. The patient should be advised to provide written notice immediately to his or her employer of a work-related illness (supported by a physician's letter) and to seek advice about statutes of limitations and other requirements. This information is generally available from the State Workers' Compensation Board and is usually required to be provided to the employee by the employer. If a union is available at the workplace, it may be able to advise and assist the patient.

Obligations to Coworkers

A patient with a work-related illness should be advised to inform his or her coworkers about the condition. If the patient belongs to a union, he or she should inform the union representative. If there is no union, the patient may contact OSHA or discuss the situation with the employer.

If the patient is a union member and agrees, the physician can contact the union, which may assist in hazard investigation, identify and warn other workers potentially affected by the hazard, and engage with the employer to take corrective action. The union can help the patient obtain any available benefits.

State based Committees on Occupational Safety and Health (COSH) are coalitions of labor, health, legal professionals, and community and environmental activists working to prevent job-related illnesses and injuries. These groups provide education and technical assistance nationwide on a range of topics, including the health effects of specific hazards, control measures, how to use government agencies, and the legal rights of disabled workers.

Obligations to Notify the Government

Some states have laws that require direct physician reporting of occupational disease. In addition to the federal agencies specifically empowered to protect worker health and safety, physicians may contact the state or local health department, which may initiate action or refer the problem to one of the federal agencies. Many states also require physicians to report any occupational injury or illness to the workers' compensation carrier.

Obligation to Notify the Employer

When treating a patient with an occupational injury or illness, health care providers often are required to report to government agencies, health departments, or insurance carriers. As part of that reporting process, the employer should also be notified. When there is imminent danger to coworkers or the public health, the employer should be contacted to correct the exposure situation.

Obligation to Inform Colleagues and the Public

On occasion, an individual primary care physician or specialist is the first person to suspect a link between a workplace exposure and a serious health problem. This discovery is often referred to as a "sentinel health event." Armed with an increased index of suspicion and the occupational history, the physician will be able to alert workers and companies and prevent the occurrence of a major health problem. Even if the physician chooses not to be involved in subsequent investigation or research, it is important that information about suspected problems and hazards be made available to researchers, workers and employers in similar industrial settings, government agencies, health care professionals.

INFORMATION RESOURCES

Health care professionals require information on industrial toxins in a number of situations, ranging from caring for an acutely ill patient in an ED, when information must be obtained quickly, to caring for a patient with chronic symptoms that may reflect an occupational disease. However, the use of information resources depends on the proper identification of the xenobiotic in question. If the xenobiotic, its generic name, and ingredients are not known, diagnostic and treatment become more difficult.

The practitioner should take a logical approach to seeking information about industrial xenobiotics. First, the xenobiotic must be identified by its generic name. This can be done by reviewing the MSDS or by contacting poison control centers (PCCs), the employer, manufacturer, unions, or government agencies. Material Safety Datasheets also are available by searching online. A good starting point to find MSDSs on the Internet is http://www.ilpi.com/MSDS/index.html, but typing "MSDS" into any online search engine yields a number of sites offering data sheets.

Poison Control Centers

Regional PCCs are able to provide assistance even when the exact chemical name is unknown because information on xenobiotics and their management are cross-referenced by trade name and manufacturer. Moreover, specialists in poison information can usually suggest additional resources. Most PCCs have computerized listings of poisons that are updated regularly. The best-known system is POISINDEX (Truven Health Analytics, Ann Arbor, MI). Subscribers to this system receive quarterly updates of an alphabetically organized listing of approximately 500,000 industrial and nonindustrial xenobiotics. The system includes trade names, the components, and the concentrations, when available, of each xenobiotic listed. These elements are then cross-referenced to management protocols. The name of the manufacturer is also listed and often includes emergency contact numbers if additional information is required.

Employers and Manufacturers

Many state and federal laws require manufacturers to generate, retain, and disclose information that may help physicians care for persons with work-related health problems. Scientific information, exposure data, information on health effects, and collected medical data are included in the types of information that must be retained.

The Chemical Transportation Emergency Center (CHEMTREC; 800-424-9300; http://www.chemtrec.com), sponsored by the Chemical Manufacturers Association, has as its primary responsibility providing information to health care practitioners responding to hazardous spills. However, it also provides information on commercial products found in patients' workplaces. Employers are required to furnish this information to employees in the form of MSDSs.

Workers' Compensation Insurance Carriers

Smaller companies often lack internal health and safety staffs. Workers' compensation or company risk insurance carriers may have valuable information about exposures and controls in the workplace. As a service to their clients, carriers often do walk-throughs and hazards evaluations for clients that lack these resources and suggest appropriate engineering controls. Health care professionals can contact the carrier directly to see what additional information is available.

Regulatory Agencies

The Occupational Safety and Health Act requires chemical manufacturers to create an MSDS for each chemical they produce, and employers who use chemicals must retain the MSDSs in the workplace. Required information includes xenobiotic and common names; physical, safety, and health hazard data; exposure limits; precautions for safe handling and use; generally applicable control measures; and emergency and first aid procedures. The OSHA Hazard Communication Standard requires individual employers to provide employees with information on the xenobiotics used in their workplaces. A call to the plant manager, foreperson, or safety officer may be all that is necessary to determine the name of the xenobiotic in question. Employers may be able to provide information on exposure concentrations in the patient's work environment. In addition, company medical departments (where they exist) may have results of medical testing performed on the patient.

There is an important point to reiterate about MSDSs: health care providers should not rely on these sheets as the sole source of information. The MSDSs are created by the chemical manufacturers as they generate scientific and health data during the course of seeking approval from the Environmental Protection Agency (EPA) to manufacture xenobiotics, and they are not a complete product evaluation. In addition, Section 8(c) of the Toxic Substances Control Act (TSCA) requires chemical manufacturers to report records of significant adverse reactions to human health or the environment. When contacting chemical manufacturers, physicians should ask to speak with a toxicologist, chemist, or someone in the products information department.

Unions

When available, labor unions can be excellent sources of information on xenobiotic exposures. At the local level, union officers, health and safety committee members, and shop stewards may be able to provide MSDSs, exposure data, medical and epidemiologic information, and reports of incidents or cases of interest in a particular plant. The health and safety department of the American Federation of Labor and Congress of Industrial Organizations (http://www.aflcio.org/Issues/Job-Safety) in Washington, DC, can provide information on occupational health and safety activities and advice on which member unions may be of specific help. At the international level, unions often have well-trained health and safety professionals who may provide or suggest sources of helpful information (http://www.ilo.org/global/topics/safety-and-health-at-work/lang--en/index.htm). In addition, some cities and states (http://www.nycosh.org) have a coalition of occupational safety and health groups that may provide information about other known exposed or affected workers.

Government Agencies

A myriad of agencies have some regulatory authority over manufacturing and services industries. These agencies and their important regulatory authority are listed in Table 131–4.

The Occupational Safety and Health Act of the U.S. Department of Labor (http://www.osha.gov) is responsible for setting and enforcing workplace health and safety standards. It is empowered to investigate occupational health and safety complaints and can inspect work sites and levy fines for violations of its standards. In approximately half of the 50 states, the OSHA program is implemented by a state agency. Individual workers, their representatives (unions), or their physicians can file a complaint with the state or federal OSHA program and request an inspection. The clinician may file a complaint with OSHA concerning a hazardous working condition at any time through the OSHA web site at https://www.osha.gov/workers/file_complaint.html. Last accessed July 10, 2018. In an emergency, such as reporting an imminent life threatening situation, contact OSHA immediately using the toll free number 800-321-OSHA (6742) or TTY 877-889-5627. The Occupational Safety and Health Act regulations protect workers from discrimination and punishment by their employer, who may be angered by their filing a complaint.

Some state OSHA agencies have separate enforcement and consultation arms. Thus, companies can request assistance from the occupational health specialists in the consultation branch without fear of reprisal from the enforcement branch. Health care workers should be familiar with the functions of their state agency and workers' rights under the law.

The National Institute for Occupational Safety and Health (NIOSH) of the U.S. Department of Health and Human Services is part of the Centers for Disease Control and Prevention (http://www.cdc.gov/niosh). The National Institute for Occupational Safety and Health is not a regulatory agency and is responsible for researching the causes of occupational disease and injury and methods for their prevention and control, evaluating workplace conditions, recommending exposure limits to OSHA for standard setting, and training occupational health and safety professionals. It is empowered to conduct onsite evaluations of health hazards in response to requests from employee representatives or employers. After conducting these evaluations, NIOSH investigators immediately contact OSHA, the employees, and the employer if they find that the workers are in imminent danger.

As part of the process of recommending exposure standards to OSHA, NIOSH develops comprehensive documents that critically evaluate all available scientific data on particular xenobiotics. These "criteria documents" review the chemical's properties, production methods, uses, and workers at risk as well as studies of exposure effects in humans and animals. Methods of screening, surveillance, and control are presented. The agency periodically issues technical reports and special occupational hazard reviews of specific occupations. In conjunction with OSHA, NIOSH develops and disseminates health hazard alerts to inform employers, employees, and health care professionals of serious health effects of particular xenobiotics.

The EPA (http://www.epa.gov) is charged with protecting the land, air, and water of the nation. The agency administers a number of laws designed to preserve the public health and environment, one of which is the TSCA. This act authorizes the EPA to collect information on xenobiotic risks from manufacturers and processors and to review information on new xenobiotics and new uses of xenobiotics before they are manufactured. Unless designated a trade secret, this information is subject to disclosure and therefore is available. The TSCA assistance office may be most useful when resource materials and government documents contain no information about the xenobiotics or processes in question.

The National Toxicology Program (http://ntp.niehs.nih.gov) is a federal program established in 1978 to develop scientific information on exposure to xenobiotics. The Agency for Toxic Substances and Disease Registry (ATSDR; http://www.atsdr.cdc.gov) was created by Congress in the Comprehensive Environmental Response, Compensation and Liability Act of 1980 (also known as Superfund Act) to implement the health-related sections of laws that protect the public from hazardous wastes and environmental spills of hazardous substances. In 1986, the Superfund Amendments and Reauthorization Act made amendments to the initial enabling legislation of 1980 and broadened the responsibilities of the ATSDR in the areas of health assessment, toxicologic databases, information dissemination, and medical education. One of its offices, the Division of Health Assessment and Consultation, provides emergency response for toxic and environmental disasters, consults in public health emergencies, assesses hazardous waste sites, provides technical assistance to agencies and organizations, and estimates health risks to humans from exposure to hazardous xenobiotics. The program areas in which ATSDR operates include health assessments, toxicologic profiles, emergency response, and exposure and disease registries.

Online Databases

Printed material often is adequate for determining the adverse health effects of xenobiotic exposures, but some resources may be unavailable to physicians, and textbook publications usually lag 2 years or more behind new information. As a result, current findings and reports may be missed if the practitioner relies solely on printed material. The National Library of Medicine (http://www.nlm.nih.gov) sponsors Internet searching of both Medline (PubMed: http://www.ncbi.nlm.nih.gov/pubmed) and a number of databases in the Toxicology Data Network (TOXNET: http://www.toxnet.nlm.nih.gov) that are very useful for finding information about industrial xenobiotics. Additional databases are available for searching on the OSHA, NIOSH, EPA, and ATSDR web sites.

SUMMARY

- Industrial, workplace, and environmental exposures represent a different kind of challenge to primary care and emergency physicians.
- Patients often present with diagnostic dilemmas or with common symptoms that do not respond to the usual medical treatment. The challenge for nonoccupational health professionals is to correctly establish and treat the condition.
- The basic approach to all patients emphasizes additional questions integrated into the medical history and access to printed and electronic information resources that are not part of the usual patient evaluation.
- Exposures to occupational and environmental xenobiotics have public health implications.
- Physicians who make the diagnosis of an occupationally or environmentally related disease have an obligation to prevent further injury, protect the Public Health and follow ethical standards.

REFERENCES

Primary Readings

1. American College of Occupational and Environmental Medicine. Code of Ethics: 2010. http://www.acoem.org/codeofconduct.aspx.
2. Agency for Toxic Substances and Disease Registry. Medical Management Guidelines for Aniline Exposure. https://www.atsdr.cdc.gov/mmg/mmg.asp?id=448&tid=79.
3. Hathaway GJ, et al. *Proctor and Hughes' Chemical Hazards in the Workplace*. 5th ed. New York, NY: John Wiley & Sons; 2014.
4. Stave G, Wald P. *Physical and Biological Hazards in the Workplace*. 3rd ed. New York, NY: John Wiley & Sons; 2016.
5. Stellman JM, ed. *Encyclopedia of Occupational Health and Safety*. 4th ed. Geneva, Switzerland: International Labor Organization; 1998. http://www.iloencyclopaedia.org.
6. Wallace RB, ed. *Maxcy-Rosenau-Last Public Health and Preventive Medicine*. 15th ed. Stamford, CT: Appleton & Lange; 2007.

Additional Readings

1. Burgess WA. *Recognition of Health Hazards in Industry: A Review of Materials and Processes*. 2nd ed. New York, NY: Wiley; 1995.
2. Gosselin RE, et al. *Clinical Toxicology of Commercial Products*. 5th ed. Baltimore, MD: Williams & Wilkins; 1984.
3. Key MM. *Occupational Diseases: A Guide to Their Recognition*. Washington, DC: US Department of Health, Education, and Welfare; 1977. https://www.cdc.gov/niosh/docs/77-181/.
4. Ladou J, Harrison R, Current *Occupational and Environmental Medicine*. 5th ed. New York, NY: McGraw-Hill Education; 2014.
5. Lewis RJ. *Hazardous Chemicals Desk Reference*. 6th ed. New York, NY: Wiley Interscience; 2008.
6. Rose VE, Cohrssen B, eds. *Patty's Industrial Hygiene and Toxicology*. 6th ed. New York, NY: Wiley Interscience; 2010.
7. Sullivan JB, Krieger GR. *Clinical Environmental Health and Toxic Exposures*. 2nd ed. Baltimore, MD: Williams & Wilkins; 2001.

132 HAZARDOUS MATERIALS INCIDENT RESPONSE

Brandy Ferguson and Bradley J. Kaufman

A disaster is typically classified in 2 categories: hazards and threats. Hazards are naturally occurring events, such as blizzards, tornadoes, and flooding. A threat is a human-made event, such a bombing attack or release of a biohazardous agent. Response to an incident must be tailored to the hazard or threat. Whether faced with an earthquake or a hazardous material, incident response must be rapid, effective, and orderly. This chapter focuses on the identification, management, and response to hazardous materials incidents.

According to the US Department of Transportation, a hazardous material is any item or agent that has the potential to cause harm to humans, animals, or the environment, either by itself or through interaction with other agents.[46] These agents can be chemical, radiologic, or biological; moreover, the chemical agents are xenobiotics that can exist in the solid, liquid, or gaseous form.

A hazmat incident can be the result of an unplanned or uncontrolled release of or exposure to a hazardous material. Although there are no specific requirements for an event to be considered a hazardous materials incident, typically, there must be the potential for many people or a large area to be affected. This factor differentiates such an event from the majority of xenobiotic exposures that affect only one person.

In addition, a single event could provide exposure to multiple xenobiotics. Each incident, and the response, is unique, and the response required for chemical, biologic, or radiologic agents might differ substantially. For instance, an event in which a biologic agent is released in a densely populated space, such a concert or sporting event, will likely result in a different response compared with the identical xenobiotic being released in an area with low population density, such as a small town. Emergency managers and health care professionals must consider all possibilities and adjust the incident response based on the specific xenobiotics involved, the route of the exposure, and other variables (eg, time, location, and weather conditions). This chapter discusses the basic principles used for a confined and quickly identifiable hazardous materials incident.

In general, a hazardous materials incident response focuses on the care of patients exposed to xenobiotics in the prehospital setting, prepares for multiple casualties, and emphasizes patient decontamination while at the same time trying to prevent exposure and contamination of first responders and health care professionals.

Every emergency response has the potential to involve hazardous materials, and first responders must always consider this as they approach an incident. For example, an apparently simple motor vehicle crash can release gasoline into the environment, or a train derailment may result in the release of an unknown xenobiotic from a transport container. In the prehospital setting, early identification of a hazardous material event can be difficult, but it is vital to collect as much information as possible to achieve an adequate and efficient response.

DISASTER MANAGEMENT AND RESPONSE

Local resources and agencies provide initial disaster management preparedness and response. Police, fire, and emergency medical services (EMS) provide initial response for an event. If necessary, local agencies can escalate response to the county, state, or federal level. The US Federal Emergency Management Agency (FEMA) within the US Department of Homeland Security is the lead federal agency for emergency management in the United States.

According to FEMA, disaster management contains 4 phases: (1) mitigation, (2) preparedness, (3) response, and (4) recovery. Mitigation measures are plans and efforts that attempt to prevent and reduce or eliminate the effects of a potential hazard from becoming a disaster. A hazard-vulnerability analysis (HVA) determines the hazards or threats most likely to have an impact on a facility. Vulnerability measures weaknesses within a system, and risk determines how much is at stake for a facility. Risk can be calculated using the following equation:

$$Risk = (Likelihood\ of\ occurrence) \times (Impact\ of\ occurrence)$$

An emergency manager at a facility can use these calculations from an HVA to stratify susceptibilities in preparation for disaster mitigation.

Preparedness involves creating action plants to be initiated when a disaster occurs, as well as testing plans with mock exercises and run-throughs. Preplanning is critical to limit damage from an event, and well-developed and tested action plans are necessary for a successful incident response.

The response phase includes the mobilization of appropriate resources and the coordinated management of the incident. A hazardous materials incident response must include the containment of the xenobiotic followed by neutralization, removal, or both. Typically, a response includes multiple trained professionals from various agencies, often including EMS, fire departments, police departments, the Environmental Protection Agency (EPA), the local office of emergency management, and other first responder emergency services personnel. Major hazardous materials events, especially those considered purposeful or the result of a terrorist act, may have responders from multiple federal, state, and local agencies, each with equipment and vehicles, and hundreds of personnel at the scene. These events can be chaotic until control and coordination are achieved. The recovery phase occurs after the immediate needs and threats to human life are addressed in the response phase and entail the restoration of property, infrastructure, and the environment.

Limiting the loss of life is dependent on all responding agencies and personnel working efficiently and effectively together. The coordination of federal, state, and local governments is mandated by the National Incident Management System (NIMS).[10,35] The National Incident Management System uses a systematic approach designed to allow agencies to work together and manage incident response. The National Incident Management System provides for an incident command system (ICS) to be used during a disaster response. Interoperability and compatibility among on-scene assets are dictated by the ICS, which consists of an organizational hierarchy and defines the necessary management components of the overall incident, including mechanisms necessary for controlling personnel, operations, and communications.

The ICS is a standardized, on-scene, all-hazards approach to incident management. The goal of the ICS is to enable a coordinated response among agencies and jurisdictions. It provides a common organizational structure and integrates equipment personnel, facilities, procedures, and communication. During a response, an incident commander (IC) is responsible for managing the incident, establishing objectives, and implementing tactics. Four subsections report to the IC: operations, planning, logistics, and finance and administration. The operations section controls the organizational efforts to reach incident management objectives and directs resources. The planning section supports the incident action planning process, collects and analyzes information, and tracks resources. The logistics section arranges for resources and services, and the finance and administration section monitors costs related to the incident. Each section has an integral role in providing efficient and effective incident response.

Medical professionals are a necessary part of all hazardous materials incident responses because patient assessment and treatment are typically the highest priority. However, as with all mass casualty events, medical professionals, even those with advanced training, must not spontaneously respond to the location of the event.[30] Unsolicited medical personnel at the scene of a hazardous materials incident, although well intentioned, may actually harm the coordinated response and interfere with operational efforts.

The plan for mobilization, management, and use of volunteer medical personnel at the scene of a disaster should be created in advance, especially for events that might reasonably be expected to require resources. Unsolicited medical professionals lack the training and equipment needed to work within a multiagency coordinated operation. Furthermore, they often function outside the organized ICS and most likely lack or are unaware of the necessary personal protective equipment (PPE). By definition, these environments are hazardous; moreover, freelance medical personnel have the potential to become patients themselves, thereby adding to the burden of on-scene rescuers. For instance, although a patient affected by a specific hazardous material may have the same physical findings and treatment indications at the scene or at the hospital, the differences in location often require variation in the medical decision making and patient care. Disaster plans incorporate the use of local medical assets such as hospitals and clinics. Therefore, communities are best served if medical providers respond to their respective institutions during an incident.

RESPONSE COMPONENTS

After the identification of a release of a hazardous material, there must be a notification to emergency response personnel. Typically, someone witnesses the incident, such as a motor vehicle crash in which a tanker trailer is breached, or some resultant effects of the release, such as a fire. The individual activates the emergency response system by calling 9-1-1. Alternatively, an automated detector may activate an emergency response to a hazardous materials incident even before there are easily observable results of the release.

Initially, first responders are often not aware that an incident involves hazardous materials. For instance, a responder to an unconscious patient may be unaware that the cause of the medical emergency was a chemical exposure. First responders must consider that every incident may have a hazardous materials etiology. Awaiting confirmation or exclusion of the presence of a hazardous material can be challenging for responders because they must weigh the possibility of contamination with the urge to treat a critically ill patient. It is important that emergency responders remain vigilant for such situations in care of the patients and themselves.

Extensive knowledge, training, and judgment are requirements for all emergency personnel, especially those responding to a hazardous material incident. They must follow basic response paradigms. Personnel should approach the scene from uphill and upwind if possible. Personnel should not immediately rush to the scene because the rescuer may become an additional victim. Establishment of a perimeter is essential to scene security to prevent uncontaminated individuals from becoming exposed. First responders and prehospital personnel must also consider other aspects of incident response, including the need for escalation to other emergency response agencies, weather and wind conditions, terrain, confinement of the release, intentionality, and the need for rapid rescue and evacuation of casualties. The identification of material, establishment of containment or safety zones, wearing of PPE, decontamination, and medical management of patients are discussed later.

Identification of Hazardous Materials

If the identity of the xenobiotic(s) is known before arrival at the scene, research can begin with review of the physical, chemical, and toxicologic properties of the xenobiotic. If the xenobiotic is not known before arrival at the scene, efforts to obtain this information should begin as soon as safely possible.

Identification of the specific xenobiotic(s) involved is of the highest priority because many of the response components depend on the properties and potential health effects of the xenobiotic itself. Whether the incident involves a mode of transportation (eg, a railcar) or is at a fixed location (eg, a factory

or medical facility), all available information must be used toward material identification. This information can be gleaned from placards, container labels, shipping documents, material safety data sheets (MSDSs), detector devices, personnel at the scene, patients' signs and symptoms, and odors at the scene (eg, the rotten egg smell of hydrogen sulfide).

Because many hazardous materials are transported via railcar or road-trailer, emergency response personnel must always maintain a high index of suspicion when responding to a transportation incident. In the United States, first responders are required to be familiar with the use of the *Emergency Response Guidebook*, which is an aid for quickly identifying the hazards of the material(s) involved in a transportation incident.[46]

Hazardous materials may be categorized in various ways and are often grouped by their harm-causing property. For instance, hazardous materials may be classified as radioactive, flammable, explosive, asphyxiating, pathogenic, and biohazardous. Xenobiotics most commonly encountered at hazardous materials incidents vary from one locale to another and are predominately determined by the major local industries.[49,50] For example, pesticides are the most commonly encountered class of hazardous materials in Fresno County, California, where the major industry is agribusiness. Although most hazardous materials incidents involve only one hazardous material, more than one xenobiotic may be encountered at an incident. One study described 107 hazardous materials incidents involving a total of 156 materials.[50]

For consequential hazardous materials, the vast majority are caused by gases, vapors, or aerosols. In one study, 4 of the 5 most commonly encountered individual chemicals were ammonia, phosphine, sulfur oxides, and hydrogen sulfide.[9] Because they do not adhere to skin, gases do not contaminate people secondarily. Therefore, patients exposed to gases generally do not require decontamination. Inhalation is the most common route of exposure at hazardous materials incidents and was the route of exposure at 73%, accounting for 76% of the exposed patients described in one study.[8,9]

Because the number of hazardous materials is large, it is efficient to group hazardous materials according to their toxicologic characteristics. The International Hazard Classification System (IHCS) is the most commonly used system (Table 132–1).[46,49] Individual hazardous materials studies commonly use their own classification systems, which emphasize the toxicodynamic effects of hazardous materials (eg, systemic asphyxiants), highlighting individual chemicals (eg, ammonia or chlorine) or general classes of chemicals (eg, acids, bases, or volatile organic compounds).[8,9]

Chemical Names and Numbers

Chemical compounds may be known by several names, including the chemical, common, generic, or brand (proprietary) name.[5,6] In a hazardous material response, a chemical may be the sole substance or one of several compounds in a mixture. The Chemical Abstracts Service (CAS) of the American Chemical Society numbers chemicals in order to overcome the confusion regarding multiple names for a single chemical. The CAS assigns a unique CAS registry number (CAS#) to atoms, molecules, and mixtures. For example, the CAS# of methanol is 67–56–1.[35,36] These numbers provide a unique identification system for chemicals and a means for crosschecking chemical names. Identifying a chemical by name and CAS# is critical because one must be as specific as possible about the hazardous material in question. Trade or brand names can be misleading and should not be used in isolation. The SDS describing a product usually lists the chemical name, the CAS#, and the brand name.[29]

Vehicular Placarding: United Nations Numbers, North American Numbers, and Product Identification Numbers

Xenobiotics in each hazard class of the IHCS (Table 132–1) are assigned 4-digit identification numbers, which are known as United Nations, North American, or Product Identification Numbers, and are displayed on characteristic vehicular placards. This system is used by the US Department of Transportation in the *Emergency Response Guidebook*.[46] The IHCS assigns a xenobiotic to a hazard class based on its most dangerous physical characteristic, such as explosiveness or flammability. Other potential hazards

TABLE 132–1   International Hazard Classification System

Class 1: Explosives
Division 1.1: Mass explosion hazard
Division 1.2: Projection hazard
Division 1.3: Predominantly a fire hazard
Division 1.4: No significant blast hazard
Division 1.5: Very insensitive explosives
Division 1.6: Extremely insensitive detonating articles

Class 2: Gases
Division 2.1: Flammable gases
Division 2.2: Nonflammable compressed gases
Division 2.3: Poisonous gases
Division 2.4: Corrosive gases (Canada)

Class 3: Flammable or Combustible Liquids

Class 4: Flammable Solids
Division 4.1: Flammable solid
Division 4.2: Spontaneously combustible materials
Division 4.3: Dangerous when wet materials

Class 5: Oxidizers and Organic Peroxides
Division 5.1: Oxidizers
Division 5.2: Organic peroxides

Class 6: Poisonous Materials and Infectious Substances
Division 6.1: Poison materials
Division 6.2: Infectious substances

Class 7: Radioactive Substances

Class 8: Corrosive Materials

Class 9: Miscellaneous Hazardous Materials

of a xenobiotic, such as its ability to cause cancer or birth defects, are not considered. This system provides very little guidance in treating poisonings caused by hazardous materials.

National Fire Protection Association 704 System for Fixed Facility Placarding

Fixed facilities, such as hospitals and laboratories, use a placarding system that is different from the vehicular placarding system. The National Fire Protection Association (NFPA) 704 system is used at most fixed facilities.[31] The NFPA system uses a diamond-shaped sign that is divided into 4 color-coded quadrants: red, yellow, white, and blue. This system gives incident responders information about the flammability, reactivity, and health effects, as well as other information, such as the water reactivity, oxidizing activity, or radioactivity.

The red quadrant on top indicates flammability; the blue quadrant on the left indicates health hazard; the yellow quadrant on the right indicates reactivity; and the white quadrant on the bottom is for other information, such as OXY for an oxidizing product, W for a xenobiotic that has unusual reactivity with water, and the standard radioactive symbol for radioactive substances. Numbers in the red, blue, and yellow quadrants indicate the degree of hazard: numbers range from 0, which is minimal, to 4, which is severe, and indicate specific levels of hazard. For instance, NFPA 704 defines divinyl benzene with the following values: blue 1 (can cause significant irritation), red 2 (must be moderately heated or exposed to relatively high temperatures before ignition can occur), and yellow 2 (readily undergoes violent chemical changes at elevated temperatures and pressures).

Similar to all placarding systems, this one also has limitations. It does not name the specific hazardous substances in the facility and gives no information about the quantities or locations of the materials.

United Nations

Recognizing that the transport of chemicals often occurs across international boundaries and labels and MSDSs often have different information in different countries, the United Nations developed a chemical classification system in an attempt to harmonize an approach to classification and labeling. The Globally Harmonized System of Classification and Labelling of Chemicals classifies substances and mixtures by their health, environmental, and physical hazards.

CHEMTREC is a service of the Chemical Manufacturers Association providing continuous essential chemical information with regard to shippers, products, and manufacturers. CHEMTREC is available at 800-424-9300 or at http://www.chemtrec.org. Details of an incident are relayed to the shipping or manufacturing 24-hour emergency contact, and they are linked to hazardous materials incident responders. Technical data are available on handling the substance(s) involved, including the physical characteristics, transportation, and disposal.

A regional poison control center is a valuable source of medically relevant information. Other information sources include local and state health departments, the American Conference of Governmental and Industrial Hygienists, the Occupational Safety and Health Administration (OSHA), National Institutes of Occupational Safety and Health (NIOSH), the Agency for Toxic Substances and Disease Registry, and the Centers for Disease Control and Prevention.[1-3,36-38]

Exact identification may not always possible. Hazardous materials responders may be able to classify the hazardous material into one of several major toxicologic classes by identifying a hazardous material toxidrome, allowing providers to reasonably treat patients while protecting themselves and others. For example, it is helpful to recognize irritation of the mucous membranes and upper airway caused by a highly water-soluble irritant gas (Chap. 121) or signs of cholinergic excess caused by organic phosphorus compounds or carbamate poisoning (Chaps. 3 and 110).

Although the exact identity of the hazardous material is usually not known, the physical state of the material (eg, solid, liquid, or gas) may be. Airborne xenobiotics can potentially harm many more victims because of their rapid distribution and ambient nature. Airborne xenobiotics include not only gases and vapors but also the liquid suspensions (eg, fog, aerosols, and mists) and solid suspensions (eg, smoke, fumes, dusts) (Chaps. 28 and 121).

Exposure and Contamination

It is important to note that emergency personnel and equipment can become contaminated at hazardous materials incidents. For example, in one study, a crashed exterminator truck leaked organic phosphorus pesticide onto the street. An ambulance that was responding to the initial call for a motor vehicle crash was contaminated after driving through a puddle of the pesticide.

Primary contamination is contamination of people or equipment caused by direct contact with the initial release of a hazardous material by direct contact at its source of release. Primary contamination occurs whether the hazardous material is a solid, a liquid, or a gas. *Secondary contamination* is contamination of health care personnel or equipment caused by direct contact with a patient or equipment covered with adherent solids or liquids removed from the source of the hazardous material spill. For instance, if a hazardous material remains on a victim (external) or within a victim (internal) or on the body surface or clothing, the person will continue to be exposed and to potentially expose others to the substance until decontamination occurs. If such a patient arrives at a health care facility and is not decontaminated, the hospital and health care providers are at risk for secondary contamination.

Health care professionals should work with hazardous materials personnel to determine whether the hazardous material presents a significant risk of secondary contamination and whether decontamination of the skin and mucous membranes is necessary. Secondary contamination generally occurs only with solids or liquids, but as noted later, some "gaseous" xenobiotics are actually suspended liquids or solids. In general, patients or equipment covered with adherent solid or liquid hazardous materials, including chemical, biological, or radiologic agents, should be decontaminated before transportation to prevent downstream contamination of health care professionals and equipment.[12,20-22,49,50,53]

In terms of cutaneous decontamination, exceptions can exist such as a diaphoretic patient exposed to a highly water-soluble irritant gas (eg, ammonia), which dissolves in sweat. In this case, the primary purpose of decontamination is to prevent or treat the patient's chemical burns caused by caustic action of aqueous ammonium hydroxide on perspiring skin while assuring prevention of secondary contamination of rescuers.

Aerosols are airborne xenobiotics, not gases. Aerosols are suspensions of solids or liquids in air, such as solid dusts or liquid mists, that can cover victims with these adherent solids or liquids, which cause secondary contamination. These patients require decontamination to prevent secondary contamination.

Hazardous Materials Site Operations

Limiting dispersion of the hazardous material is critical to prevent further consequences. The physical state of a material determines how it will spread through the environment and gives clues to the potential route(s) of exposure. Unless moved by physical means such as wind, ventilation systems, or people, solids usually stay in one area. Solids can cause exposures by inhalation of dusts, by ingestion, or rarely by absorption through skin and mucous membranes. Solids that undergo sublimation, changing directly from a solid into a gas without passing through the liquid state, can give off vapors that may cause airborne exposure. Only 2 commonly encountered solids sublime, dry ice (CO_2) and naphthalene. A vapor is defined as a gaseous dispersion of the molecules of a substance that is normally a liquid or a solid at standard temperature and pressure (STP), that is, 32°F (0°C = 273°K) and 1 atm (760 torr = 760 mm Hg = 14.7 psi). Uncontained liquids will spread over surfaces and flow downhill. Liquids that evaporate create a vapor hazard.

The vapor pressure (VP) is useful to estimate whether enough of a solid or liquid will be released in the gaseous state to pose an inhalation risk. Vapor pressure is defined essentially as the quantity of the gaseous state overlying an evaporating liquid or a subliming solid. The lower the VP, the less likely the xenobiotics will volatilize and generate a respirable gas. Conversely, the higher the VP of a chemical, the more likely it will volatilize or generate a respirable gas. Water has a VP of approximately 20 mm Hg at 70°F (21°C), and acetone has a VP of 250 mm Hg at the same temperature. Therefore, acetone evaporates more rapidly than water and poses more of an inhalation risk. Standard reference texts (eg, *NIOSH Pocket Guide to Chemical Hazards and the Merck Index*) list VPs for commonly encountered chemicals.[36,37,46]

Hazardous Materials Scene Control Zones

Scene management is a fundamental feature of hazardous materials incident response. It is almost always necessary to isolate the scene, deny access to the public and the media, and limit access to emergency response personnel to prevent unnecessary contamination. Three control zones are established around a scene and are described by "temperature," "color," or "explanatory terminology" (Table 132–2 and Fig. 132–1). NIOSH, the US EPA, and most US prehospital and hospital health care professionals use the temperature terminology system.[37]

The *hot zone* is the area immediately surrounding a hazardous materials incident. It extends far enough to prevent the primary contamination of people and materials outside this zone. In general, evacuation, but no decontamination or patient care, is carried out in this zone. This is because rescuers are generally hazardous materials technicians who wear level A or

B suits that severely limit their visibility and dexterity. In specific situations, antidotes, such as nerve agents, are administered via autoinjectors.

The *warm zone* is the area surrounding the hot zone and contains the decontamination or access corridor, where victims and the hazardous materials entry team members and their equipment are decontaminated. It includes 2 control points for the access corridor. Many consider initiating therapy at this stage, particularly for chemical weapons, events when multiple casualties are involved as stated earlier. However, with these rare exceptions, medical care should be initiated only after the patient exits into the cold zone.

The *cold zone* is the area beyond the warm zone. Contaminated victims and hazardous materials responders should be decontaminated before entering this area from the warm zone. This is the area where resources are assembled to support the hazardous materials emergency response. The incident command center is usually located in the cold zone, and there is greater ability to provide patient care there. Care provided in this zone includes the primary survey and resuscitation with management of airway (with cervical spine control), breathing, circulation, disability, and exposure with evaluation for toxicity and trauma (ABCDE). Definitive care also includes antidotal treatment for specific poisonings.

Personal Protective Equipment

A critical goal of hazardous materials emergency responders is protecting themselves and the public. Safeguarding hazardous materials responders includes wearing appropriate PPE to prevent exposure to the hazard and prevent injury to the wearer from incorrect use of or malfunction of the PPE equipment.

Donning PPE poses significant health hazards for the provider, including loss of cooling by evaporation, heat stress, physical stress, psychological stress, impaired vision, impaired mobility, and impaired communication. Because of these risks, individuals involved in hazardous materials emergency response must be properly trained regarding the appropriate use, decontamination, maintenance, and storage of PPE. This training includes instruction regarding the risk of permeation, penetration, and degradation of PPE. Personal protective equipment with a self-contained breathing apparatus (SCBA) with a fixed supply of air significantly limits the amount of time the wearer can operate in the hot zone, usually about 20 minutes.

Levels of Protection

The EPA defines 4 levels of protection for PPE: levels A (greatest protection) through D (least protection). The different levels of PPE are designed to provide a choice of PPE, depending on the hazards at a specific hazardous materials incident (Table 132–3).[26,38]

Level A provides the highest level of both respiratory and skin (clothing) protection and provides vapor protection to the respiratory tract, mucous membranes, and skin. This level of PPE is airtight and fully encapsulating, and the breathing apparatus must be worn under the suit.

Level B provides the highest level of respiratory protection and skin splash protection by using chemical-resistant clothing. It does not provide skin vapor protection but does provide respiratory tract vapor protection. Some hospitals have specially trained health care professionals who wear level B PPE when decontaminating patients presenting to the hospital. However, the majority of hospitals are training their frontline emergency department (ED) health care professionals to wear level C PPE when decontaminating contaminated patients who present to the hospital.

Level C protection should be used when the type of airborne xenobiotic is known, its concentration can be measured, the criteria for using air-purifying respirators (APRs) are met, and skin and eye exposures are unlikely. Level C provides skin splash protection, the same as level B; however, level C has a lower level of respiratory protection than levels A and B.

Level D is basically a regular work uniform. It should not be worn when significant chemical respiratory or skin hazards exist. It provides no respiratory protection and minimal skin protection. Level D was specifically developed to show *what not to wear* for chemical protection.

TABLE 132–2	Nomenclatures of the Hazardous Materials Control Zones	
Temperature Terminology System[a]	Color Terminology System	Explanatory Terminology System
Hot zone	Red zone	Exclusion or restricted zone
Warm zone	Yellow zone	Decontamination or contamination reduction zone
Cold zone	Green zone	Support zone

[a]Data from the National Institutes of Occupational Safety and Health and the Environmental Protection Agency.

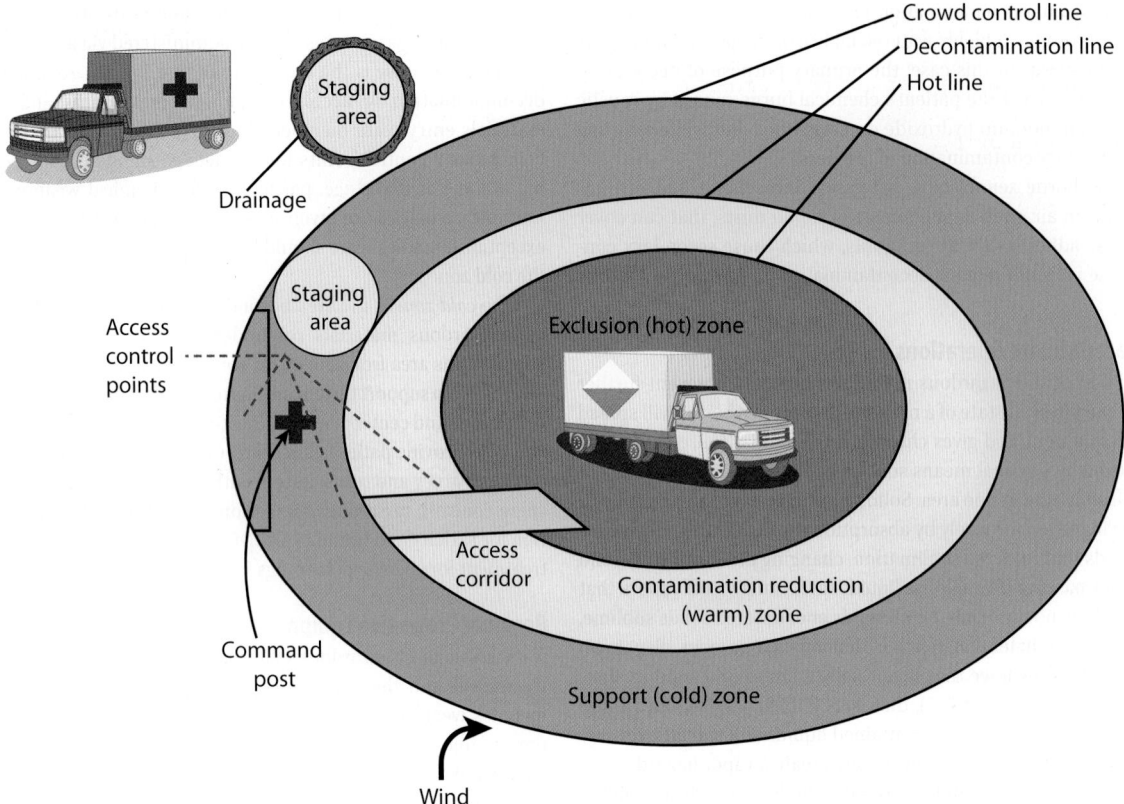

FIGURE 132-1. National Institutes of Occupational Safety and Health/Occupational Safety and Health Administration recommended hazardous materials control zones.

Personal Protective Equipment Respiratory Protection

Personnel must be fit tested before using any respirator. A tiny space between the edge of the respirator and the face of the hazardous materials responder could permit exposure to an airborne hazard. Contact lenses cannot be worn with any respiratory protective equipment. Corrective eyeglass lenses must be mounted inside the facemask of the PPE. The only exception to these general rules is the use of hooded level C powered air purifying respirators (PAPRs) that do not require fit testing and allow individuals to wear their own eyeglasses within the hooded PAPR. This is the reason that most US hospitals prefer hooded PAPRs for their ED personnel who must decontaminate patients.

Level A PPE (Fig. 132–2) mandates the use of a SCBA. A SCBA is composed of a face piece connected by a hose to a compressed air source.

An open-circuit, positive-pressure SCBA is used most often in emergency response and provides clean air from a cylinder to the face piece of the wearer, who exhales into the atmosphere. Thus, a higher air pressure is maintained inside the face piece than outside. This affords the SCBA wearer the highest level of protection against airborne hazards because any leakage will force air out of the face piece and not allow airborne hazards to enter against the higher pressure within the face piece. Disadvantages of the SCBA include its bulkiness and heaviness and a limited time period of respiratory protection because of the limited amount of air in the tank.

A supplied-air respirator (SAR) may be used in level B PPE and differs from SCBA in that air is supplied through a line that is connected to a source

	Protects Skin and Eyes From			Protects Respiratory System From	
Level[a]	Select Vapors and Aerosols	Gases, Vapors, and Aerosols	Oxygen-Deficient Atmospheres	Liquids and Solids	Gases and Vapors
D					
C	+			+	
B	+		+	+	+
A	+	+	+	+	+

TABLE 132–3   Personal Protective Equipment

[a]Level A is a self-contained breathing apparatus (SCBA) worn under a vapor-protective, fully encapsulated, airtight, chemical-resistant suit. Level B is a positive-pressure supplied-air respirator with an escape SCBA worn under a hooded, splash-protective, chemical-resistant suit. Level C is an air-purifying respirator worn with a hooded, splash-protective, chemical-resistant suit. Level D is regular work clothing (offers no protection).

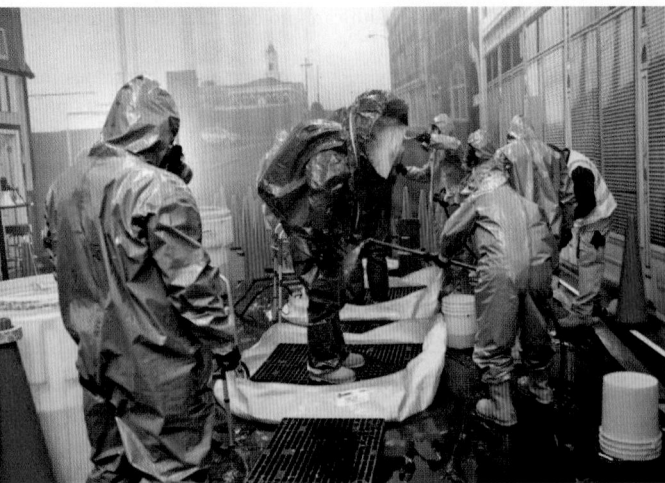

FIGURE 132-2. Individuals wearing level B PPE. (*Reproduced with permission from the Occupational Safety and Health Administration.*)

located away from the contaminated area. Only positive-pressure SARs are recommended for hazardous materials use. One major advantage of SARs over SCBA is that they allow an individual to work for a longer period. However, a hazardous materials worker must stay connected to the SAR and cannot leave the contaminated area by a different exit.

An APR may be used in level C PPE and allows breathing of ambient air after inhalation through a specific purifying canister or filter. There are 3 basic types of APRs: chemical cartridge, disposable, and powered air (PAPR). Although APRs afford the wearer increased mobility, their use is only acceptable when there is sufficient oxygen in the ambient air. The chemical cartridges or canisters purify the air by filtration, adsorption, or absorption. Filters may also be used in combination with cartridges to provide increased protection from particulates such as asbestos. Powered devices reduce the work of breathing, which can significantly limit an individual's performance while wearing PPE.

Decontamination

One of the most important and essential aspects of hazardous materials response is decontamination of patients. Not only does decontamination reduce the health consequences for the patient (by reducing absorption or exposure time), but it also prevents secondary contamination. Decontamination of equipment, the environment, and the entire area (ie, hot zone) is necessary but is secondary in priority to the decontamination of victims.

An estimated 75% to 90% of contaminants can be removed simply by removing clothing and garments. Subsequent decontamination is most commonly accomplished by using water to copiously irrigate the skin of a patient, thereby physically washing off, diluting, or hydrolyzing the xenobiotic. However, the water solubility of a xenobiotic must be considered to determine whether water alone is sufficient for skin decontamination or whether a detergent is needed. The general rule regarding solubility is that "like dissolves like." In other words, a polar solvent, such as water, will dissolve polar substances such as salts. For example, the herbicide paraquat is actually a salt, paraquat dichloride, that is miscible in water. Therefore, if skin is contaminated with paraquat, copious water irrigation is sufficient for skin decontamination. A mild liquid detergent is acceptable but is not necessary. On the other hand, a nonpolar solvent, such as toluene, is not water soluble and is immiscible. Therefore, if skin is contaminated with toluene, water irrigation alone will be insufficient for decontamination, and mild liquid detergent is necessary. Furthermore, copious water is often not available at the site, thereby requiring rescuers to ration the supply and minimize irrigation using the least amount of water necessary. Some solid chemical contaminants react with water and cause an increased hazard. Providers should use care with chemical contaminants because some solid contaminants react with water and create an increased hazard. Some xenobiotics are better removed mechanically by physically wiping it from the skin while avoiding smearing the xenobiotic or abrading the skin. Some contaminants may be chemically "inactivated" by applying another chemical, such as a 0.5% hypochlorite solution (see extensive discussion in Special Considerations: SC2).

All exposed skin, including the skin folds, axillae, genital area, and feet, should be decontaminated. Lukewarm water should be used with gentle water pressure to reduce the risk of hypothermia. Water should be applied systematically from head to toe while the airway is protected.

Exposed, symptomatic eyes should be continuously irrigated with water throughout the patient contact, including transport, if possible. Remember to check for and remove contact lenses.

Removal of internal contamination is often much more problematic. In some cases, specific antidotes are administered to enhance elimination or inactivate the hazardous material. For instance, Prussian blue can trap radioactive cesium in the intestine so that it can be eliminated from the body in the stool rather than be reabsorbed.

Scene Triage

Victim decontamination and movement from a scene requires an organized methodology for categorization of medical severity. The most common

triage method used is the Simple Triage and Rapid Treatment (START) system, although many others exist. This system follows a simple algorithm that allows for a color categorization based upon respiration, perfusion, and mental status: immediate (red), delayed (yellow), walking wounded or minor (green), and deceased or expectant (black). Victims may be initially triaged in the contaminated zone and then retriaged after decontamination. Prehospital providers receive training in START triage and transport patients to a hospital facility according to triage destination. Scene security is an important aspect of scene triage. The decontamination areas must be properly secured by responders (eg, police, EMS) to ensure secure and efficient decontamination of patients. The IC, along with other sections of the ICS, can develop tactics and plans to ensure scene safety.

HAZARDOUS MATERIALS INCIDENT RESPONSE RULES AND STANDARDS

Occupational Safety and Health Administration and the NFPA have developed rules and guidelines, respectively, regarding hazardous materials incident response. Occupational Safety and Health Administration rules are mandated as law and must be followed. Meeting NFPA guidelines will ensure OSHA compliance.[24,31-34,38,41,45,46]

The Superfund Amendments and Reauthorization Act of 1986 (SARA) required OSHA to develop and implement standards to protect employees responding to hazardous materials emergencies. This resulted in the *Hazardous Waste Operations and Emergency Response* standard, 29 CFR 1910.120, or HAZWOPER.[47]

NFPA 471, *Recommended Practice for Responding to Hazardous Materials Incidents*, outlines the following tactical objectives: incident response planning, communication procedures, response levels, site safety, control zones, PPE, incident mitigation, decontamination, and medical monitoring.[32]

NFPA 472, *Standard on Professional Competence of Responders to Hazardous Materials Incidents*, helps define the minimum skills, knowledge, and standards for training outlined in HAZWOPER for 3 types of responders.[33]

Prehospital Hazardous Materials Emergency Response Team Composition, Organization, and Responsibilities
First Responder at the Awareness Level

First responders at the awareness level could be first on the scene at an emergency incident involving hazardous material. They are expected to recognize the presence of hazardous materials, protect themselves, secure the area, and call for better-trained personnel. They must take a safe position and keep other people from entering the area. They must recognize that the level of mitigation exceeds their training and call for a hazardous materials response team. Most basic curricula of emergency medical technicians include this level of first responder training.

First Responder at the Operational Level

These individuals are trained in all competencies of the awareness level and are additionally trained to protect nearby persons, the environment, and exposed property from the effects of hazardous materials releases. Operational level certified individuals are expected to assume a defensive posture, control the release from a safe distance, and keep the hazardous material from spreading. Operational level individuals are trained on the following aspects of material containment: absorption of liquids, containment of the spill, vapor suppression, and vapor dispersion. They do not operate within the hot zone.

Hazardous Materials Technician

Hazardous materials technicians respond to hazardous materials releases, or potential releases, for the purpose of controlling the release. They are trained in the use of chemical-resistant suits, air-monitoring equipment, mitigation techniques, and the interpretation of physical properties of hazardous materials. Technicians are capable of containing an incident, making safe entry into a hazardous environment, determining the appropriate course of action, victim rescue, and cleaning up or neutralizing the incident to return property to a safe and usable status, if possible. These individuals are trained to operate within the hot zone to mitigate the incident. This certification level includes knowledge of hazardous material chemistry, air-monitoring equipment, tools used within the hot zone, and more.

Each of these providers must work in conjunction to ensure effective and efficient incident response, treatment of individuals, scene control, and patient transport to nearby health care facilities.

Advanced Hazardous Materials Components
Advanced Hazardous Materials Providers
Paramedics are trained in the recognition of signs and symptoms caused by exposure to hazardous materials and the delivery of antidotal therapy to victims of hazardous materials poisonings.[24]

The inclusion of such training into a hazardous materials response team is beneficial, not only for the needs of the public but also to protect hazardous materials technicians who make entry into hazardous atmospheres. Ideally, entry into hazardous atmospheres should not be performed until appropriately trained paramedics are on the scene with resuscitative equipment in place, including a drug box containing essential antidotes for specific hazardous materials.[24]

Patient Care Responsibilities of the Prehospital Decontamination Team and the Hazardous Materials Entry Team
Hazardous material incident responders should identify the entry and exit areas by controlling points for the access corridor (decontamination corridor) from the hot zone, through the warm zone, to the cold zone (Fig. 132–1). This corridor should be upwind, uphill, and upstream from the hot zone, if possible. Hazardous materials technician entry team members should remove victims from the contaminated hot zone and deliver patients to the inner control point of the access (decontamination) corridor. Hazardous materials decontamination team members decontaminate patients in the decontamination (access) corridor of the contamination reduction (warm zone).[11,14,18,19,24,27,28,43]

The primary responsibility of the prehospital hazardous materials sector is the protection of the hazardous materials entry team personnel. This is accomplished by researching and recording clinically pertinent information about the hazardous material, remaining available on scene for medical treatment, and assessing individuals before entry into and on exit from a hazardous environment.[24] Documentation of each assessment should be recorded on a prepared form and compared with the exclusion criteria defined by NFPA 471.[24,32]

In some systems, the hazardous materials entry team may include specialized providers who have the ability to provide lifesaving patient care within the hot zone. The ability to perform triage or cardiopulmonary resuscitation or to provide any medical care is greatly limited by the PPE being worn. Therefore, only immediately lifesaving procedures should be considered, such as intubation or antidote administration. In one study, health care professionals were observed performing tasks (laryngotracheal mask placement versus endotracheal intubation, and intravenous cannula insertion versus interosseous needle insertion) with and without CBRN (chemical–biological–radiologic–nuclear) PPE. This study observed 64 clinicians and found that procedure times were slower for endotracheal intubation and intravenous cannula placement, skills requiring more dexterity.

Patient Care Responsibilities of Emergency Medical Services Providers at Hazardous Materials Incidents
Emergency medical services providers who are not part of the hazardous materials team should report to the incident staging area and await direction from the IC. They should approach the site from upwind, uphill, and upstream, if possible.

Emergency medical services providers should remain in the cold zone until properly protected hazardous materials incident responders arrive, decontaminate, and deliver patients to them for further triage and treatment. Emergency medical services providers should evaluate each patient,

triage as appropriate, and move the patient to the appropriate casualty collection point or rapidly transport to the hospital. Exposed victims who are initially asymptomatic should continue to be observed and reassessed for the delayed development of symptoms, and the EMS provider should be prepared to upgrade or downgrade the triage category for the patient. All EMS systems should have protocols in place that direct operations at hazardous materials scenes. Ideally, EMS response for an event with involve direct communication with the EMS medical director or medical control; this physician with assist with coordination of appropriate care with the hospital, regional poison control centers, and toxicologists.

Transportation of patients from the hazardous materials incident is ultimately under the control of the IC but is usually delegated to the prehospital hazardous materials medical sector and EMS providers. Patients with skin contamination should be transported from the hazardous materials site without being properly decontaminated. Before transportation, EMS should notify the receiving hospital of the number of victims being transported and their toxicologic history, patient assessments, and treatment rendered.

Hospital Responsibilities for Hazardous Materials Victims
Ideally, local or regional ED physicians and personnel will receive advanced notification about a hazardous materials incident before any victims arrive at the hospital. This notification to the hospital should occur as early in the event as possible to allow for maximum preparation time. The notification should include, if known, information regarding the event, hazardous materials involved, number and condition of casualties to be transported to the hospital, and estimated time of arrival, as well as information regarding the decontamination completed. Assistance of a poison control center and a medical toxicologist is generally recommended.

Victims may leave an incident scene and subsequently present to a hospital. The hospital must have a preestablished protocol (eg, mass casualty with decontamination response plan) by which hospital response teams will decontaminate patients who arrive at the hospital if not previously decontaminated or if field decontamination is believed to be insufficient.[7,15–17,23,25,40,42,44,48,51,52] Patients who require skin decontamination should be denied entry to the ED until they are decontaminated by an appropriately trained and equipped hazardous materials response team. Again, patient treatment should not be initiated until the patient is in the cold zone. The emergency physician will determine when the patient is safe to enter the ED after carefully assessing the risks and benefits to the decontaminated patient, the other patients in the ED, and the ED health care personnel.

SUMMARY

- Hazardous materials incident response is an integrated, interdisciplinary approach involving prehospital, hospital, poison control center, and public health professionals.
- Most exposures are inhalational, which can be a gas, solid, small suspended particles, or liquid aerosols.
- Prehospital and hospital health care professionals must use appropriate PPE when caring for contaminated patients.
- Decontamination is critical to alter xenobiotic absorption for patients and to prevent secondary contamination of downstream health care professionals and equipment.
- The general principles of toxicology apply regardless of whether a patient is at a hazardous materials incident in a prehospital or hospital setting. Although patient care resources vary among these treatment settings, the fundamental principles of patient care remain the same. All patients should receive a primary survey and resuscitation, emphasizing airway, breathing, and circulation.

REFERENCES
1. Agency for Toxic Substances and Disease Registry. http://www.atsdr.cdc.gov.
2. American Conference of Governmental Industrial Hygienists. http://www.acgih.org.
3. American Conference of Governmental Industrial Hygienists. *2005, TLVs and BEIs.* Cincinnati, OH: ACGIH; 2005.

4. Benson M, et al. Disaster triage: START, then SAVE—a new method of dynamic triage for victims of a catastrophic earthquake. *Prehosp Disaster Med.* 1996;11:117-124.

5. Borak J, et al. *Hazardous Materials Exposure.* Englewood Cliffs, NJ: Brady Publications; 1991.

6. Bronstein AC, Currance PL. *Emergency Care for Hazardous Materials Exposure.* 2nd ed. St. Louis, MO: Mosby-Year Book; 1994.

7. Burgess JL, et al. Hospital preparedness for hazardous materials incidents and treatment of contaminated patients. *West J Med.* 1997;167:387-391.

8. Burgess JL, et al. Hazardous materials exposure information service: development, analysis, and medical implications. *Ann Emerg Med.* 1997;29:248-254.

9. Burgess JL, et al. Hazardous materials incidents: the Washington Poison Center experience and approach to exposure assessment. *J Occup Environ Med.* 1997;39:760-766.

10. Bush GW. *Homeland Security Presidential Directive/HSPD-5.* Washington, DC: The White House; 2003.

11. Cancio LC. Chemical casualty decontamination by medical platoons in the 82d Airborne Division. *Mil Med.* 1993;158:1-5.

12. Centers for Disease Control and Prevention. Public health consequences among first responders to emergency events associated with illicit methamphetamine laboratories, selected states 1996–1999. *MMWR Mortal Morbid Wkly Rep.* 2000;49:1021-1024.

13. CHEMTREC. http://www.chemtrec.org.

14. Domestic Preparedness Program, Defense Against Weapons of Mass Destruction: *Technician-Hospital Provider Course Manual.* Aberdeen, MD: US Army CBDCOM, Domestic Preparedness Office; 1997.

15. Gough AR, Markus K. Hazardous materials protections in practice ED, laws and logistics. *J Emerg Nurs.* 1989;15:477-480.

16. Hall SK. Management of chemical disaster victims. *J Toxicol Clin Toxicol.* 1995;33:609-616.

17. Huff JS. Lessons learned from hazardous materials incidents. *Emerg Care Q.* 1991;7:17-22.

18. Hurst C. *Decontamination.* In: Zatchuk R, ed. Textbook of Military Medicine Washington, DC: US Dept. of Army, Surgeon General, and the Borden Institute 1997:351-359.

19. Kales SN, Christiani DC. Acute chemical emergencies. *N Engl J Med.* 2004;350:800-808.

20. Kales SN, et al. Spirometric surveillance in hazardous materials firefighters: does hazardous materials duty affect lung function? *J Occup Environ Med.* 2001;43:1114-1120.

21. Kales SN, et al. Medical surveillance of hazardous materials response fire fighters: a two-year prospective study. *J Occup Environ Med.* 1997;39:238-247.

22. Kelly KJ, et al. Assessment of health effect in New York City firefighters after exposure to polychlorinated biphenyls (PCBs) and polychlorinated dibenzofurans (PCDFs). The Staten Island transformer fire health surveillance project. *Arch Environ Health.* 2002;57:282-293.

23. Kirk MA, et al. Emergency department response to hazardous materials incidents. *Emerg Med Clin North Am.* 1994;12:461-481.

24. Klein R, Criss EA. Establishing and organizing a hazmat response team. In: Walter FG, et al., eds. *Advanced Hazmat Life Support Provider Manual.* 3rd ed. Tucson, AZ: Arizona Board of Regents; 2003:125-177.

25. Lavoie FW, et al. Emergency department external decontamination for hazardous chemical exposure. *Vet Hum Toxicol.* 1992;34:61-64.

26. Lehmann J. Considerations for selecting personal protective equipment for hazardous materials response. *Disaster Manag Response.* 2002;1:21-25.

27. Leonard RB. Hazardous materials accidents: initial scene assessment and patient care. *Aviat Space Environ Med.* 1993;64:546-551.

28. Levitin HW, Siegelson HJ. Hazardous materials. Disaster medical planning and response. *Emerg Med Clin North Am.* 1996;14:327-348.

29. MSDS SEARCH. http://www.msdssearch.com.

30. National Association of EMS Physicians (NAEMSP) and the American College of Emergency Physicians (ACEP) Joint Position Statement. *Unsolicited Medical Personnel Volunteering at Disaster Scenes;* 2002. *Ann Emerg Med.* 2018;71:e41.

31. National Fire Protection Association. http://www.nfpa.org.

32. Technical Committee on Hazardous Materials Response Personnel. *NFPA 471 Recommended Practice for Responding to Hazardous Materials Incidents.* Quincy, MA: National Fire Protection Association; 1997.

33. National Fire Protection Association Technical Committee on Hazardous Materials Response Personnel. *NFPA 472 Standard on Professional Competence of Responders to Hazardous Materials Incidents.* Quincy, MA: National Fire Protection Association; 2002.

34. National Fire Protection Association Technical Committee on Hazardous Materials Response Personnel. *NFPA 473 Standard for Competencies for EMS Personnel Responding to Hazardous Materials Incidents.* Quincy, MA: National Fire Protection Association; 1997.

35. National Incident Management System. https://www.fema.gov/national-incident-management-system.

36. National Institute for Occupational Safety and Health (NIOSH). *NIOSH Pocket Guide to Chemical Hazards.* Washington, DC: US Government Printing Office for the US Department of Health and Human Services (DHHS) and the National Institute of Occupational Safety and Health (NIOSH); 2004.

37. National Institute of Occupational Safety and Health. http://www.cdc.gov/niosh.

38. Noll G, et al. Personal protective clothing and equipment. In: Daly P, ed. *Hazardous Materials.* Stillwater, OK: Fire Protection Publications; 1995:285-322.

39. Occupational Safety and Health Administration. http://www.osha.gov.

40. Pons P, Dart RC. Chemical incidents in the emergency department: if and when. *Ann Emerg Med.* 1999;34:223-225.

41. Rubin JN. Roles and responsibilities of medical personnel at hazardous materials incidents. *Semicond Saf Assoc J.* 1998;12:25-30.

42. Shapira Y, et al. Outline of hospital organization for a chemical warfare attack. *Isr J Med Sci.* 1991;27:616-622.

43. Sullivan F, et al. Principles and protocols for prevention, evaluation, and management of exposure to hazardous materials. *Emerg Med Rep.* 1998;19:21-32.

44. Tur-Kaspa I, et al. Preparing hospitals for toxicological mass casual- ties events. *Crit Care Med.* 1999;27:1004-1008.

45. US Department of Labor Occupational Safety and Health Administration. https://www.osha.gov/dts/osta/bestpractices/html/hospital_firstreceivers.html.

46. US Department of Transportation (DOT), Transport Canada (TC), Secretariat of Communications and Transportation of Mexico (SCT): *2008 Emergency Response Guidebook.* Washington, DC: DOT, TC, SCT; 2008. http://www.phmsa.dot.gov/static-files/PHMSA/DownloadableFiles/Files/erg2008_eng.pdf.

47. US Government. Title 29, Code of Federal Regulations 1986, Parts 1910.120.

48. Waldron RL II, et al. Radiation decontamination unit for the community hospital. *Am J Roentgenol.* 1981;136:977-981.

49. Walter FG, et al. Hazardous materials incidents in a mid-sized metropolitan area. *Prehosp Emerg Care.* 2003;7:214-218.

50. Walter FG, et al. Hazardous materials incidents: a one-year retrospective review in central California. *Prehospital Disaster Med.* 1992;7:151-156.

51. Young CF, Persell DJ. Biological, chemical, and nuclear terrorism readiness: major concerns and preparedness for future nurses. *Disaster Manag Response.* 2004;2:109-114.

52. Zavotsky KE, et al. Developing an emergency department based special operations team: Robert Wood Johnson University Hospital's experience. *Disaster Manag Response.* 2004;2:35-39.

53. Zeitz P, et al. Frequency and type of injuries in responders of hazardous substances events, 1996 to 1998. *J Occup Environ Med.* 2000;42:1115-1120.

133 RISK ASSESSMENT AND RISK COMMUNICATION

Charles A. McKay

All health care professionals confront questions involving risk on a daily basis. In the area of toxicology, these questions take many forms. An anxious parent with questions about a child's potentially toxic exposure, an urgent consultation for a critically ill patient in the emergency department or intensive care unit, a request to interpret a laboratory test, media requests for information about environmental public health issues, a response to a hazardous materials incident, and biopreparedness education all involve directed communication of information and recommendations. Toxicologists and Certified Specialists in Poison Information (CSPIs) must establish rapport and provide information, instructions, and when appropriate, reassurance, typically by telephone or in short face-to-face interactions. For CSPIs, attribution of a patient's symptoms to one or more potential exposures is further complicated by the absence of visual clues usually available during a clinical evaluation. In addition, the true reason or concern for a call is often difficult to discern, given limited time and incomplete information transfer. Cultural issues also impact perception and communication. All of these situations require a knowledgeable, compassionate, and well-reasoned response to toxicologic concerns.

This chapter focuses on 2 particular components of this response: risk assessment and risk communication. The underlying principles apply equally to individual calls to poison control centers (PCCs), educational outreach to the public and medical professionals, occupational and environmental exposure evaluations, and supportive roles with other public health agencies in terrorism preparedness, environmental public health tracking programs, and research.

RISK ASSESSMENT

In the context of this text, risk assessment is the process of determining the likelihood of toxicity for an individual or group after a perceived exposure to some substance, generally referred to as a xenobiotic. It involves determining the nature and extent of the exposure (ie, xenobiotic, dose, duration, route) and its specific clinical effects, defining an exposure pathway, and assessing the likelihood of effects from a given situation. When available, a published body of knowledge should be applied to some components of risk characterization or assessment. An overview and a number of tools are available through the websites of the US Environmental Protection Agency (EPA) and the Agency for Toxic Substances and Disease Registry (ATSDR) of the Centers for Disease Control and Prevention (CDC).[1,12] However, any given risk assessment is hampered by incomplete information. The exact xenobiotic or mixture, whether there was an actual exposure or just proximity to the xenobiotic (completion of an exposure pathway), the exact dose, and unpredictable features such as host factors (underlying medical conditions or genetic polymorphisms) that could modify the response to a potential exposure, are all potential contributors of uncertainty. Unfortunately, those conducting a risk assessment are affected by their own biases and assumptions in the interpretation of their results, as are the people to whom a risk assessment is communicated. The emotional response to being "poisoned" makes evaluation and attribution even more difficult.

A good example of the practical difficulties involved in a risk assessment is evident from a published description of mass psychogenic illness.[22] In this incident, many individuals at a school complained of odor-triggered nonspecific symptoms such as dizziness, nausea, and palpitations. Symptoms spread, even occurring in some individuals after removal from the building, in a so-called line of sight transmission with no evident dose–response pattern. Extensive testing identified the possibility of potential odor sources, such as dry floor drain traps. However, there was no actual release documented,

and a plausible scenario that would account for significant symptoms could not be identified. When people returned to the school days later, symptoms recurred, again in the absence of documented exposure to any inciting chemical. The extent of investigation of these events is often profound, highlighting the difficulty in appropriate use of potentially unlimited laboratory technology. Yet a complete risk assessment is frequently elusive: our ability to assess a "no-risk" situation is limited. As noted in the letters to the editor of the journal in which the case was published, one can always criticize the methods or conclusions in this and "subsequent and comparable" outbreaks in businesses, hospitals, and mass gatherings.[4,19,30,34]

The fear-arousal cycle that triggers a multitude of "medically unexplained symptoms" precipitates the "maladaptive thoughts, feelings, and behaviors" that characterize "somatic symptom disorder" as described in the *Diagnostic and Statistical Manual of Mental Disorders* (DSM 5) should, in theory, respond to a properly communicated risk assessment. However, any uncertainty will hinder this response. However, any uncertainty will hinder this response. It is stated that "the absence of evidence of harm" is not the same as "the evidence of absence of harm." Both of these positions potentially converge in the face of continued research, data, and debate toward the dichotomous choices of "evidence of harm" or "evidence of safety." Unfortunately, this goal of a refined and improved risk assessment based on accumulating knowledge is polarized in debate and policy as 2 opposing principles: the *Kehoe principle* and the *precautionary principle*. The Kehoe principle is best summarized as "prove something is harmful before excluding a product with known benefits because of concern about potential, unproven future adverse effects." A common example of the use of this principle is the continued marketing of a xenobiotic after another member of the class was removed because of safety issues. More intense scrutiny is indicated, but a class-wide medication recall without evidence of some level of harm by an individual therapeutic drug is very rare. This principle was misused in the past to minimize known risks attributable to environmental lead pollution to delay removal of lead additives from gasoline.[33] Critics of the Kehoe principle suggest that waiting for evidence of harm from a substance results in costly or irreparable damage.

The alternative precautionary principle is often summarized as "where there are threats of serious or irreversible damage, lack of full scientific certainty shall not be used as a reason to postpone cost effective measures to prevent environmental degradation."[27,40] Critics of the precautionary principle often cite the uncertainty of the "threat" and the lack of attention to the "cost" component of the principle, complaining that devotees stifle economic growth and prosperity with unfounded fears rather than reasoned consideration of known data. This principle is commonly extended to potentially harmful situations other than the environment. A common criticism of the precautionary principle is the degree to which alternative actions are evaluated for safety. As an example, concern about thimerosal safety (as a vaccine preservative and source of ethylmercury exposure) in young children led many parents to forego childhood vaccinations. Vaccine manufacturers removed the thimerosal preservative from most routine childhood vaccines. Although this process was accelerated by the theoretical—and, ultimately, unfounded—concerns regarding this source of mercury exposure in young children, the cost of delayed or omitted vaccination was a number of real and preventable serious infectious diseases that occurred, including hepatitis B and measles.[6-8,14]

Although the Kehoe and precautionary principles originated as policy approaches to public health issues, they underlie the automatic or subconscious biases that each individual brings to his or her own personal risk assessment or tolerance. A framework of belief systems and assumptions about life,

TABLE 133–1	Components of Risk Assessment

Hazard Identification

Name and amount of suspected xenobiotic (or general use category if the xenobiotic is unknown)

Exposure Pathway

Proposed route of exposure

Consistency with the nature of the xenobiotic (eg, water-soluble liquid)

Modifying Factors

Environmental factors that would influence systemic availability of the xenobiotic

Patient characteristics (susceptibility or resistance factors), such as:

  Chronic medical conditions

  Possible xenobiotic–drug or other interactions

  Genetically determined receptor physiology (eg, potassium channel or *HERG* mutations predisposing to long QT syndrome)

  Genetic polymorphisms in hepatic or other metabolic pathways

Toxicity Assessment

Compare and contrast organ or systemic effects expected from the particular xenobiotic with existing symptoms

Evaluate both deterministic effects (dose dependent: usually acute or chronic organ injury) and stochastic effects (multifactorial, probabilistic: predominantly carcinogenesis and developmental or transgenerational impact)

justice, and eternity determine the response to uncertain situations.[3,13,17] These underlying worldviews should be considered when discussing risk with an individual and explicitly recognized and addressed in a formal risk assessment. The essential components of a risk assessment for a chemical exposure are listed in Table 133–1.

DIFFERENTIATING PUBLIC HEALTH FROM INDIVIDUAL RISK ASSESSMENT

It is difficult to translate public health risk assessment done for populations by the EPA or other regulatory or advisory organizations to the individual level. Simplistically, the iterative process of adjusting known noncancer adverse exposure outcome limits in an animal model (eg, lowest observed adverse effect level {LOAEL} or no observed effect level {NOEL}) to a safe level of exposure for all humans (including so-called sensitive subpopulations) is arbitrarily set at repetitive multiplicative factors of 10 for each of these extrapolations unless experimental data support a lower multiplier. These are called "uncertainty factors" and are used in the absence of specific information about human exposure to identify a conservative human "safe dose." Thus, a "safe dose" is determined as 0.001 times the animal model LOAEL, reflecting a 10-fold reduction in dose for extrapolation from LOAEL to NOEL, another 10-fold reduction for extrapolation from animal to human, and another 10-fold reduction for potentially "sensitive" human populations. These "uncertainty factors" are actually safety factors for the adverse effect of interest. When individuals exceed these limits, they remain protected by very robust safety factors, and are not—as it is often portrayed—exposing themselves to a defined harm. The dietary guidelines for fish consumption (also known as "fish health advisories") are a good example. Based on concern about exposure to methylmercury and polychlorinated biphenyls, these dietary recommendations rely on epidemiologic studies that suggest subtle neuropsychiatric abnormalities in maternal–fetal pairs (in at least some populations) from levels of fish consumption 10 to 100 times that of the "usual" American diet. Clinical mercury toxicity requires still higher levels of consumption. Although it seems reasonable (precautionary) for pregnant women to limit their intake of certain fish species containing high organic mercury levels, it is inappropriate to avoid fish and the nutrients contained therein because of a misplaced fear of mercury exposure. Furthermore, these risk assessments do not apply to nonpregnant women, children, or men, although they are often generalized to all humans.[2]

The public health modeling concept for cancer health effects risk assessment is even more complex and often misunderstood. In this setting, modeling assumes a linear, no-threshold carcinogenic effect from exposure to a given xenobiotic. Cancer risks from exceedingly small exposures are extrapolated from data in cancer-prone animal models with exposures so large that they are only likely in the experimental setting. This experimental construct ignores the moderating impact of incremental dosing of small amounts over a protracted period of time and potential metabolic and self-repair mechanisms in humans. This aspect of injury surveillance and repair is based on the presence of "cellular chaperones" exemplified by heat-shock protein research.[25] This hormesis effect is modeled as a "U-shaped" dose–response curve whereby low dose exposures are protective against toxicity. Although demonstrated for a number of hazards and exposure settings, hormesis remains controversial as a general concept applicable to risk assessment.[5,21] Even more controversial is the modeling characteristic for "endocrine-disrupters." These xenobiotics have estrogen receptor and other endocrine gland (eg, thyroid) potential interactions during critical pre- and perinatal timeframes, resulting in the potential for adverse effects at low concentrations, although the relevance of reports to actual human exposures is often unclear.[35,40] Modeling of the quantitative or population impact of this "inverted U" dose–response curve is further complicated by confounders, the potential for contradictory effects in different sexes and exposure timeframes; as well as the difficulty of attributing a cancer cause to a single xenobiotic or exposure. It is very difficult to communicate an acceptable cancer risk to a community, even when using the simple linear, no threshold model. The "acceptable risk" in regulatory modeling is a calculation of "one excess cancer in a population of 1 million exposed individuals." Although a limitation of this model is explicit in the footnote that this estimate represents "a plausible upper bound estimate of risk at low dose where true risk is often lower, including zero,"[15] this important caveat is rarely communicated, resulting in the common response by individuals that "an extra cancer is acceptable for you, but not when it is my child."

As this brief review of the principles of regulatory approaches to noncancer and cancer effects demonstrates, risk assessment is often imprecise. Risk characterization for the individual should avoid unfamiliar statistical concepts, aiming instead to communicate the likelihood of significant risk for the exposure actually experienced. The CDC codifies this approach for a community using such escalating terms as "no public health concern," "public health concern," "public health threat," and "immediate risk." Although there is debate about the general use of these terms in isolation (without explicit explanations), a similar approach with an individual would summarize the risk assessment using the phrases "safe," "no adverse effects are expected," "may be of concern—we will need to do some follow-up testing," and "this might be (or is) a problem—let's do the following studies or treatments."

RISK COMMUNICATION

Risk communication consists of an exchange of facts and opinions that allow an individual or a group to make an informed decision regarding a course of action or treatment. Practically, risk communication is a way of translating incomplete knowledge so that individuals can achieve informed decision-making. During a one-on-one interaction with a poisoned individual and his or her family or a caller to the PCC, there is a need to gain the fullest attention or cooperation of the individual. After this occurs, the discussion is usually focused on the risks and benefits of various treatment options (eg, gastrointestinal decontamination) or possible diagnostic modalities (eg, observation versus neuroimaging versus antidote administration). The group dynamics of environmental exposure risk communication at a public meeting are very different. Federal agencies that interact with communities in "Superfund" sites (eg, the EPA and the ATSDR) promulgate principles and practical recommendations for risk communication in this setting. Table 133–2 summarizes general principles of risk communication.

Although some of these recommendations are more applicable to longer term deliberations and interactions, much of the individual communication done by the PCC and medical toxicologists succeeds or fails based on

TABLE 133–2	Principles of Risk Communication[9] and Applicability to the Poison Control Center
Principle	**Applications**
Accept and involve the individual as a partner.	The caller must be involved to obtain the best information possible.
Plan carefully and evaluate your efforts.	There is a very short time to establish rapport with the caller; do not increase the caller's anxiety by asking irrelevant questions or arguing. Monitor your tone; ask for repetition of key information or recommendations.
Listen to the individual's specific concerns.	Why did the person call? Was it for information, treatment recommendations, or reassurance? Make sure the underlying reason for the call is addressed.
Be honest, frank, and open.	If there is uncertainty or there are unknowns, indicate that uncertainty while providing a workable plan.
Work with other credible sources.	Involve medical toxicology backup and other consultants, particularly for questions regarding chronic exposure or effects.
Meet the needs of the media.	If calls involve media notification or contact, make sure the critical information is stated frequently, provide a human context, and avoid sensationalism.
Speak clearly and compassionately.	Remember that the caller was concerned enough to initiate the contact; make sure the call is completed with a clear plan; provide follow-up appropriate to the situation.

these same principles (Table 133–2). Lacking the opportunity for repeated interactions over time to identify and discuss assumptions and biases, toxicologists need to establish credibility, listen to concerns and empathetically respond, admit areas of insufficient knowledge, and commit to follow-up interactions to convey effectively a risk characterization for an individual based on the available knowledge and experience. The scientific terms, rationale, and any extrapolation from modeling (eg, animal data or case series) should be conveyed in an understandable manner to show that appropriate safety factors are incorporated into areas of uncertainty as a risk-diminishing step. The toxicologist should also emphasize that a precautionary action or even taking no action, results in consequences; these need to be evaluated in the total decision-making process. The patient or audience should leave the interaction with a clear understanding of the difference between a short-term risk of symptoms that will resolve or result in serious illness and the degree of certainty about the potential for a long-term consequence.

Multiple examples of the difficulties inherent in risk communication exist. The need to balance rapid, lifesaving response in a disaster with the need for respiratory and skin protection for the responders is a component of every chemical emergency or mass casualty incident. Poor risk communication commonly occurs when the experience and expectations of a community are at odds with the message delivered by an "expert." This dissonance was demonstrated in the messaging surrounding 2 recent public health incidents, both problematic based on sensory clues: public water quality in Flint Michigan and the Elk River West Virginia spill of 4-methylcyclohexane methanol. Initial statements that underplayed the water quality issues in Flint flew in the face of grossly discolored and heavily sedimented water. Although the lead leached from the old water pipes was not the cause of the discoloration, this was not reassuring to disenfranchised residents.[11,23] In West Virginia, residents were told that the water was safe to drink and that concentrations of the contaminant were below detectable concentrations; however, because the odor threshold was below the analytical threshold limit of detection, the water had a noticeable smell.[29]

These examples demonstrate the mistrust and difficulties often present in public health emergencies. Even though no significant acute health effects are attributable to either event, simmering concerns about legacy issues (eg, "chemical alley" in West Virginia) and expressed concern about the long-term consequences of low-level lead exposure in Flint and similarly affected communities (in the absence of measurements early in the crisis) highlight issues of environmental justice and public trust, best characterized as "outrage" (see later).

Effective risk communication must therefore address several questions. The appropriate process is to first obtain the best information available regarding the identification of the xenobiotic and the nature of the exposure and then convey the following:

- Likely **magnitude** of the risk: This includes information on the process by which the person would be exposed (ie, the exposure pathway), such as airborne inhalation or drinking water delivery via a contaminated ground water plume and dose–response, such as: "Does the reported exposure to a particular xenobiotic (amount and duration) approach the exposure amounts reported to cause symptoms?"
- The **urgency** of the risk must also be conveyed along with practical recommendations for simple actions consistent with the level of urgency.
- The **applicability** of a risk characterization also needs to be addressed. Are the animal data applicable to humans? Is the exposure something of concern for an individual?
- **Uncertainties** of the risk assessment: This should include a "worst-case scenario" approach to unknown exposures or uncertainties in the quantity of an absorbed dose. The need for continued observation or follow-up for clinical changes would be expressed here. Individual risk tolerance varies greatly. The same information will be interpreted differently by risk-averse versus risk-tolerant people. A variety of comparisons or communication techniques are used to provide an adequate characterization of risk. It is important to remember that the public and even medical professionals have limited ability to understand and incorporate data that rely on numbers and statistics. This health numeracy limitation is even more prevalent than is limited health literacy (Chap. 129).[36]
- **Management options:** In addition to follow-up and repeated evaluations by a medical toxicologist, the range of choices, associated with their relative benefits or risks, should be presented to the individual or group of individuals. A summary recommendation or opinion from the presenter should emphasize specific steps people can take to decrease exposure or potential toxicity if indicated by the level of risk. This last step is important because uncertainty significantly impacts the ability of an individual to take appropriate action. People should not leave the meeting or interaction with the impression that "no one knows what is going on or what we should do."

APPLICATION OF RISK ASSESSMENT AND COMMUNICATION PRINCIPLES TO TOXICOLOGY

Many home-initiated PCC calls concern nontoxic or minimally toxic xenobiotics potentially ingested by children;[31] however, the common problem of incomplete documentation of the ingestion (unwitnessed ingestions, lack of diagnostic testing) raises the possibility of undertriage of any given call based on misplaced confidence that relies on prior experience. It is generally assumed that the sheer volume of calls provides some reassurance regarding the accuracy of our risk assessment of these xenobiotics, but we should remain cautious in our interpretation of PCC data (Chap. 130).[6,20,35] Given these uncertainties, even calls about nontoxic xenobiotics require communication between the caller and CSPI beyond simple substance identification. The importance of risk assessment and communication principles is demonstrated in the joint position statement[28] on the prehospital management of "minimally toxic substances" crafted by the American Association of Poison Control Centers (AAPCC), the American Academy of Clinical Toxicology

(AACT), and the American College of Medical Toxicology (ACMT). According to the position statement, a CSPI can make a risk assessment that an exposure is benign or minimally toxic only if the following characteristics are true:[28]

- "The information specialist has confidence in the accuracy of the history obtained and the ability to communicate effectively with the caller."
- "The information specialist has confidence in the identity of the product(s) or substance(s) and a reasonable estimation of the maximum amount involved in the exposure."
- "The risks of adverse reactions or expected effects are acceptable to both the information specialist and the caller based on available medical literature and clinical experience."
- "The exposure does not require a health care referral because the worst potential effects are benign and self-limited."

The position statement further notes that patient disposition decisions can be altered by many additional factors, including intent, environment, presence of symptoms (possibly unrelated to the xenobiotic in question), and ongoing review of current recommendations in the face of more data.[28] These points emphasize both the dependence of the CSPI on information derived from the caller and his or her confidence in the level of comprehension of the caller. The caller should understand that his or her exposed child is safe; the expert toxicology communication with the caller should alleviate concern—the extent and detail of the assessment process is guided by the caller's risk tolerance. Toxicologists have developed a number of Web-based consumer tools, attempting to provide simple information outside of direct patient-to-expert consultation. Their utility will depend on the success of implementing these principles.

In the case of a symptomatic patient or a hospital- or physician-initiated contact to a PCC or medical toxicologist, the caller should expect more than just xenobiotic-related information; he or she also expects knowledge and expertise that will provide reassurance or direction for improving the patient's health status. However, merely relaying information regarding the diagnosis, course, and predicted outcome is insufficient. There is often another underlying reason for the call, such as anxiety, uncertainty, or misinformation established through previous experiences or knowledge base. A sense of guilt frequently underlies a parent's call for an inadvertent exposure occurring when a child was unsupervised. A health care professional may have had significant difficulties in the management of a previously poisoned patient. If these issues are not addressed, then the caller will continue seeking reassurance by repeated calls to the PCC or by seeking additional input from other sources, such as family, friends, primary physicians, other health care providers. Any variance in the information obtained from these sources will likely be construed as inconsistencies among supposed experts rather than differences in emphasis with regard to the same information, leading to further uncertainty for the caller. Of further concern, the Internet has become a common source of second opinion for health care. Although many sites are useful, there is no quality control or filter to sort good information from bad or even harmful advice.[16] Table 133–3 lists some barriers to effective risk assessment and communication.

INTERPRETING PUBLIC HEALTH CONCERNS FOR THE INDIVIDUAL

Medical toxicologists and CSPIs frequently encounter callers or individuals at community events or interact with the media regarding public health–related issues, such as heavy metal exposures involving mercury, lead, or arsenic or concerns about "toxic mold," plasticizers, and other environmental xenobiotics. Often these people are concerned that their symptoms or future personal or family health will be adversely impacted by such exposures. Such supposed exposures are usually poorly documented, sometimes also driven by popular media descriptions or litigation, and the risk is virtually impossible to ascertain during a short telephone or personal interaction. In these situations, the individual is best served by referral to a primary care physician with toxicology consultation or directly to a medical toxicology clinic. The data and perceptions can be completely reviewed and a more appropriate risk assessment communicated in those settings. These interactions are very difficult because they are often emotionally and politically charged.[32]

In general, the communication of and response to information depend on a preexisting worldview and prevailing circumstances. The same possible outcome will be perceived as more or less severe depending on factors other than the nature of the outcome itself. Several authors characterized the perceived tolerance to different risks, stratified by features such as familiarity and personal control[13,41] (Table 133–4). The emotional response of individuals confronted with these risks is sometimes characterized as "outrage." One communications specialist posited that "risk = hazard + outrage."[38] He characterizes situations in which there is a significant hazard but little outrage as requiring "precaution advocacy," essentially informing the relevant parties of the need for more action or involvement to reduce risk. On the other end of the spectrum is a situation with little hazard but significant outrage, which requires "outrage management" to address fear or anger that is dissociated from the actual hazard posed by the situation. The greater the degree of familiarity with the particular exposure situation and the greater the voluntary nature of the exposure, the less fear or outrage will be expressed for a given adverse outcome, whether this is an appropriate response or not. Although not necessarily applicable to the initial "fight-or-flight" response to an emergency, these concepts are certainly applicable to the aftermath of these events. Of note, although risk communicators use analogies to place exposures into a context familiar to their audience, one must be careful to avoid equating voluntary and involuntary risk assumption or equating those exposures or risks assumed by one segment of the population unequally. An example of this is the use of a smoking risk analogy when talking to a nonsmoker.

Risk communication is very important in the setting of preparedness for terrorism. Although a great deal of attention and money is directed to improvement of public health infrastructure, reporting and surveillance mechanisms, and response to perceived and actual terrorist acts, less attention has been directed to the process of communicating risk to the individual.[10,26] Although some countries practice public health emergency

TABLE 133–3	Factors That Affect Appropriate Risk Assessment and Effective Risk Communication[13]
Nature of previous encounters with poison control center or health care field	
Lack of prior patient–health care professional relationship	
Incomplete or inadequate response to a prior question	
The provision of information contrary to "popular understanding," cultural background, or media representation	
Loss of credibility	
Lack of appreciation of individual or cultural differences in the perception of risk or the applicability of data	
Incomplete or limited comprehension of scientific or statistical principles	

TABLE 133–4	Factors That Alter the Acceptability of Perceived Risk[13]
More Acceptable	**Less Acceptable**
Natural	Human made
Associated with a trusted source	Not associated with a trusted source
Familiar	Unfamiliar
Voluntary	Involuntary
Potentially beneficial	Limited or absent potential benefit
Statistical (low harm likelihood)	Catastrophic (high harm likelihood)
Fairly distributed or shared by all	Unfairly distributed ("injustice")
Affects adults	Affects children

drills regularly, the United States has concentrated on development of organizational structures and lines of authority, with attention to the importance of outcome-based exercises only recently emphasized.

Maintaining readiness for catastrophic terrorist events (or natural occurrences such as pandemic influenza or storm-related flooding) should use the same risk assessment and communication techniques appropriate for other urgent public health matters. Unfortunately, many factors affect the characterization of risk other than the facts. The importance of presentation style, perception, or the role of the communicator's own biases is exemplified by these 2 composite articles describing the same events:

Event Description 1: Unknown assailants have infiltrated the mail delivery system, resulting in severe illness and deaths of children, healthy adults, and elderly people throughout the country. The initial symptoms can be nonspecific but rapidly progress to death if treatment is not begun early. The medical community routinely fails to diagnose the conditions early, and the government has no system in place to detect this threat after it occurs. The long-ignored public health system is not prepared to deal with the huge burden of preventing illness in those who may have been or will be exposed. Anyone who receives regular mail may be at risk. Tens of thousands of our citizens are taking prophylactic antibiotics "just in case." If you receive any unusual packages or see collections of powder that do not have an obvious explanation, call the police. If you develop a fever, cough, chest pain, or unusual rash, which may not be painful, seek medical attention at once. Tune in to your local news station for more information on this burgeoning threat to our nation's security.

Event Description 2: A small number of individuals in isolated exposure settings have developed illnesses after bioterrorism events. Most people have survived these exposures, particularly with early and proper medical care. The government has developed a case definition, and medical experts have disseminated information to assist the medical community and public in the early recognition of symptoms and signs that are consistent with this exposure. Prophylactic treatment within days of exposure of those in high-risk professions, such as mail handlers at major postal sorting facilities, prevents illness. Unfortunately, there have been a large number of hoaxes and false alarms about possible terrorist events and a lot of understandable fear in the community about nonspecific symptoms. For more information, contact your local health department or obtain information from frequently updated reliable web sites, such as the CDC's Web site.

Both of these paragraphs describe the 2001 anthrax bioterrorism events within the United States, during which a total of 22 people become ill, of whom 5 died from anthrax exposure. The first communication suggests that everyone is at risk and the situation is dire; the communication in the second paragraph is that the risk is isolated (a single individual died who was not in what was recognized as an at-risk setting from the 7 identified mailings), and there is a plan and process being developed to respond to the threat. Whereas the first is sensationalistic, imparting a helpless victim role to the reader, the second provides a framework in which to assess personal risk and access sources of reliable information. Both types of reports were prevalent after the 2001 anthrax attacks. Which report seems more complete, accurate, or useful is determined by the assumptions and perspectives of the reader in addition to the message the author wishes to deliver or response desired. Some would say that communicating a high degree of risk is important to gain the attention of the reader and to ensure that no one ignores a warning. However, the lack of a risk perspective prevents the reader from placing this information in context with the myriad other risk communication messages conveyed on a daily basis. In general, risk communication messages that do not provide a context or comparison to generally familiar activities or risks are more prone to misinterpretation or misapplication. "White powder" events continue throughout the country on a regular basis, but the development of systematic evaluation steps and education by organizations such as the United States Postal Inspection

Service in conjunction with automated environmental sampling at mail handling facilities have decreased the fear of a toxic exposure in this setting. As biopreparedness moves from public health infrastructure development and surveillance improvement to planning and response drills, appropriate message development and risk communication to the public needs continued emphasis.

Informing the public of scientific issues related to complex toxicology principles and risk-to-benefit analysis is also a nonemergency component of risk communication. Clinicians do this every day when interpreting laboratory findings for their patients, as discussed elsewhere in the text (Chaps. 7, 86, and 93). The "press release" examples provided below highlight 2 opposing positions on the recent controversy regarding the herbicide glyphosate (Chap. 109).[18] Read these paragraphs from the perspective of a concerned, but scientifically uninformed parent or school administrator:

Hypothetical Press Release 1: The pesticide in most prevalent use today is a carcinogen. In 2015, the highly respected International Agency for Research on Cancer (IARC) designated glyphosate as a probable human carcinogen, one step away from being labeled a known human carcinogen. Based on evaluation of studies involving cell-based models and experimental animals, as well as human data, the designation puts an end to the longstanding industry claims of low toxicity. Steps should be taken to remove this toxic chemical from the environment and to eliminate exposure, particularly to children on school grounds.

Hypothetical Press Release 2: Glyphosate and its commercial formulations (consisting of the active herbicide and solvents and surfactants added to help it gain and maintain access to plants) have a long history of use throughout the world. They have an excellent safety profile when used as directed. This safety profile is attributable to the dissimilarity between targeted plant and human cell structure. Suicidal ingestions of large amounts of glyphosate formulations can result in fatality, but this is caused by a severe pulmonary reaction to aspirated detergents in the product. A number of organizations in various countries have evaluated decades of data and concluded that glyphosate is unlikely to be a carcinogen. In 2015, a 17-member working group of the international Agency for Research on Cancer (IARC) decided that the weight of evidence supported a probable human carcinogen designation. This anomalous result relied on statistical reevaluation of existing animal experimental data, focusing on lymphomas and rare hemangiosarcomas and human epidemiologic studies. The IARC designation is controversial, considering the likelihood of publication and recall bias in animal and human retrospective studies, respectively. In particular, questions persist regarding the human applicability of cancer-prone animal models at cytotoxic daily doses orders of magnitude in excess of human exposure. These issues speak to the differences between internal and external validity and impact the confidence scientists have in statistical analysis of existing data.

The first statement is direct and identifies a specific action as a desired endpoint. Unfortunately, it mixes "toxicity" and "cancer-causing" without distinguishing the vast difference between these 2 concepts in both dose amount, duration, and mechanism. It makes categorical statements and implies a level of certainty (eg, "human data") without mentioning all the limitations that are involved (eg, bias, extrapolating from experimental models and retrospective epidemiologic assessments). In addition, it implies a progression or proximity in the cancer categories by the false "one step away" analogy. Although short, it is misleading to the point of being false.

The second statement is longer and provides more background and context for the process of decision making or designation, but it concludes without an action step or relevant answer to the implicit question: "Am I at risk?" In addition, for a lay public audience, the statement is much too complex, does not use plain language, and assumes knowledge that is unlikely to be present (eg, regarding specific cancer types, the nature and definitions of bias and editorial process, and the meaning of such concepts as "cytotoxicity"). A shorter statement that removes both the parenthetical partial explanation about mechanism of action and the disconnected statement about suicidal ingestions could be summarized as:

Hypothetical Press Release 2a: *Glyphosate is a weed killer with a long history of safe use throughout the world in the ongoing effort to minimize crop stress and maximize food production. A number of organizations in various countries have evaluated decades of data and concluded that glyphosate is unlikely to be a carcinogen. In 2015, a 17-member working group of the international Agency for Research on Cancer (IARC) reviewed the same published studies and decided that the weight of evidence supported a "probable human carcinogen" designation. The IARC decision is controversial. Many cell-based or experimental animal studies use exposure conditions much more extreme than any usual human exposure, and it is always difficult to sort out the real cause in studies that ask people to recall the nature of daily exposures when evaluating the cause of an illness (this is called "recall bias"). These issues impact scientists' confidence in the application of studies and statistical analysis. An ongoing prospective study has not identified any increased risk of cancer in people who use glyphosate very regularly, which should be even more reassuring to the vast majority of the population who have infrequent or no use of glyphosate.*

Although still lengthy, the last statement provides cautionary remarks that frame the decision-making process. Critics would argue that it is too simplified and omits mention of "low-level exposure" for "susceptible populations" or "susceptible periods of human development." However, the obvious difference in scientific rationale for the first and last example of hypothetical press releases should at least allow a thoughtful conversation in the latter case. It is left to the reader to determine how best to work with media representatives to further this type of risk communication.

SUMMARY

- High-quality risk assessment and effective risk communication are the hallmarks of a successful interaction between the public and PCCs and between a toxicologist and an individual patient, the media, or the public health community.

- A toxicologist's job is to obtain the best information possible regarding potential exposures and then convey that information in an understandable fashion with a detailed risk characterization of the hazard, likelihood of a completed exposure pathway (thus, the likelihood of an actual exposure), possible health effects, and treatment options.

- It is important to clarify the difference between public health standards and individual health risks, with an understanding of the many psychosocial issues that influence perception.

- Information should be provided in a context that allows the individual to prioritize his or her response based on a factual and balanced presentation with respect to his or her health literacy and health numeracy.

REFERENCES

1. Agency for Toxic Substance and Disease Registry. *Public Health Assessment Guidance Manual (2005 update)* 2005. https://www.atsdr.cdc.gov/hac/PHAManual/toc.html.
2. Agency for Toxic Substance and Disease Registry. *Toxicological Profile for Mercury.* http://www.atsdr.cdc.gov/toxprofiles/tp.asp?id=115&tid=24.
3. Ames BN, et al. Nature's chemicals and synthetic chemicals: comparative toxicology. *Proc Natl Acad Sci.* 1990;87:7782-7786.
4. Black D, Murray V. Mass psychogenic illness attributed to toxic exposure at a high school. *N Engl J Med.* 2000;342:1674.
5. Calabrese EJ, Baldwin LA. The frequency of U-shaped dose response in the toxicological literature. *Tox Sci.* 2001;62:330-338.
6. Centers for Disease Control and Prevention. A comprehensive immunization strategy to eliminate transmission of hepatitis B virus transmission in the United States. *MMWR Morbid Mortal Wkly Rep.* 2006;55:1-253.
7. Centers for Disease Control and Prevention. Impact of the 1999 AAP/USPHS joint statement on thimerosal in vaccines on infant hepatitis B vaccination practices. *MMWR Morbid Mortal Wkly Rep.* 2001;50:94-97.
8. Centers for Disease Control and Prevention. Measles cases and outbreaks. https://www.cdc.gov/measles/cases-outbreaks.html.
9. Covello V, Allen F. *Seven Cardinal Rules of Risk Communication.* Washington, DC: US Environmental Protection Agency, Office of Policy Analysis; 1988.
10. Durodié B. Facing the possibility of bioterrorism. *Curr Op Biotech.* 2004;15:264-268.
11. Drake JL. Toxic communication: how the water crisis in Flint corroded the governor's credibility. Public Relations Society of America: The Public Relations Strategist Spring; 2016: http://apps.prsa.org/Intelligence/TheStrategist/Articles/view/11476/1125/Toxic_Communication_How_the_Water_Crisis_in_Flint#.WO7R4ogrKUk.
12. Environmental Protection Agency. *Risk Assessment Website Portal.* http://www.epa.gov/risk.
13. Fischhoff B, et al. *Acceptable Risk.* Cambridge, MA: Cambridge University Press; 1981.
14. Flaherty DK. The vaccine-autism connection: a public health crisis caused by unethical medical practices and fraudulent science. *Ann Pharmacother.* 2011;45:1302-1304.
15. Fowle JR III, Dearfield KL. *Risk Characterization Handbook.* Washington, DC: United States Environmental Protection Agency, Office of Science Policy, Office of Research and Development. EPA 100-B-00-002; 2000. https://www.epa.gov/sites/production/files/2015-10/documents/osp_risk_characterization_handbook_2000.pdf.
16. Fox S. *The Engaged E-Patient Population.* Washington, DC: Pew Internet & American Life Project; 2008. http://www.pewinternet.org/2008/08/26/the-engaged-e-patient-population.
17. Glassner B. *The Culture of Fear: Why Americans Are Afraid of the Wrong Things.* 2nd ed. New York, NY: Basic Books; 2004.
18. Glyphosate. International Agency for Research on Cancer. https://monographs.iarc.fr/ENG/Monographs/vol112/mono112-10.pdf.
19. Goode MD. Mass psychogenic illness attributed to toxic exposure at a high school. *N Engl J Med.* 2000;342:1673-1674.
20. Hamilton RJ, Goldfrank LR. Poison center data and the Pollyanna phenomenon. *J Toxicol Clin Toxicol.* 1997;35:21-23.
21. Hoffman GR. A perspective on the scientific, philosophical, and policy dimensions of hormesis. *Dose Response* 2009;7:1-51.
22. Jones TF, et al. Mass psychogenic illness attributed to toxic exposure at a high school. *N Engl J Med.* 2000;342:96-100.
23. Leber R. The EPA's silent guilty role in the Flint water crisis. *Newsweek* January 25, 2016: http://www.newsweek.com/epa-silent-guilty-role-flint-water-crisis-418957.
24. Longo LD. Environmental pollution and pregnancy: risks and uncertainties for the fetus and infant. *Am J Ob Gynecol.* 1980;137:162-173.
25. Javid B, et al. Structure and function: heat shock proteins and adaptive immunity. *J Immunology* 2007;179:2035-2040.
26. Manning FJ, Goldfrank L, eds. *Preparing for Terrorism: Tools for Evaluating the Metropolitan Medical Response System Program.* Washington, DC: Committee on Evaluation of the Metropolitan Medical Response System Program, Board on Health Sciences Policy, Institute of Medicine; 2002.
27. Martuzzi M, Tickner JA, eds. *The Precautionary Principle: Protecting Public Health, the Environment and the Future of Our Children.* Budapest: Fourth Ministerial Conference on Environment and Health, World Health Organization; 2004. http://www.euro.who.int/__data/assets/pdf_file/0003/91173/E83079.pdf.
28. McGuigan MA. Guideline Consensus Panel. Guideline for the out-of-hospital management of human exposures to minimally toxic substances. *J Toxicol Clin Toxicol.* 2003; 41:907-917.
29. McKay CA, Scharman EJ. Intentional and inadvertent contamination of water, food, and medication. *Emerg Med Clin N Am.* 2015;33:153-177.
30. Miller CS, Ashford NA. Mass psychogenic illness attributed to toxic exposure at a high school. *N Engl J Med.* 2000;342:1673.
31. Mofenson HC, Greensher J. The nontoxic ingestion. *Pediatr Clin North Am.* 1970;17: 583-590.
32. Nanagas K, Kirk M. Perceived poisons. *Med Clin North Am.* 2005;89:1359-1378.
33. Nriagu JO. Clair Patterson and Robert Kehoe's paradigm of "show me the data" on environmental lead poisoning. *Environ Res.* 1998;78:71-78.
34. Page LA, et al. Frequency and predictors of mass psychogenic illness. *Epidemiology.* 2010;21:744-747.
35. Rochester JR, Bolden AL. Bisphenol S and F: a systematic review and comparison of the hormonal activity of Bisphenol A substitutes. *Environ Health Perspect.* 2015;123:643-650.
36. Robertson WO. Poison center data and the Pollyanna phenomenon disputed. *J Toxicol Clin Toxicol.* 1998;36:139-141.
37. Rothman RL, et al. Perspective: the role of numeracy in health care. *J Health Commun.* 2008;13:583-595.
38. Sandman P. The Peter Sandman Risk Communication Website. http://www.psandman.com/index.htm.
39. Slovic P. Perception of risk. *Science.* 1987;236:280-285.
40. Teeguarden JG, Hanson-Drury S. A systematic review of bisphenol A "low dose" studies in the context of human exposure: a case for establishing standards for reporting "low-dose" effects of chemicals. *Food Chem Toxicol.* 2013;62:935-948.
41. Tickner JA, et al. A compass for health: rethinking precaution and its role in science and public health. *Int J Epidemiol.* 2003;32:489-492.

CASE STUDY 14

History A 27-year-old man with a past medical history of opioid dependence who is currently on methadone maintenance therapy was brought into the hospital for a routine medical clearance before arraignment. The patient complained of chest pain and had an electrocardiogram (ECG) that showed ST-segment elevation; however, compared with a prior ECG, it was unchanged (Fig. CS14–1). The patient was admitted for observation.

While he was in the emergency department (ED), the patient developed nausea, vomiting, diarrhea, and abdominal discomfort; he was given 4 mg of intravenous ondansetron. The patient then complained of persistent abdominal discomfort and stated that he was in opioid withdrawal. He was then given 10 mg of methadone intramuscularly. Shortly thereafter, the patient was found unresponsive, he was attached to a cardiac monitor, and the following rhythm (Fig. CS14–2) was obtained:

Physical Examination The patient was pulseless and unresponsive on the stretcher. Active cardiopulmonary resuscitation was in progress.

Initial Management The patient was immediately defibrillated. The patient had return of spontaneous circulation, and then 2 g of magnesium sulfate was administered intravenously. The patient was started on an isoproterenol infusion and is admitted to the critical care unit. An ECG performed after return of spontaneous circulation is shown in Fig. CS14–3.

What Is the Differential Diagnosis?
The patient developed a pulseless rhythm. During this episode, the rhythm strip demonstrated torsade de pointes. Upon evaluation of the postdefibrillation ECG, the patient's QT interval was prolonged. The differential diagnosis for a prolonged QT interval is extensive (Chap. 15). Electrolyte abnormalities, specifically hypokalemia, hypocalcemia, and hypomagnesemia, are common causes of a prolonged QT interval that are easily treatable (Chap. 12).

Although there are hereditary causes of a prolonged QT interval, these are quite rare. The most common cause of a prolonged QT interval is usually medication related and results from potassium channel blockade. The list of medications that prolong the QT interval is quite extensive and includes many common classes; for example, they can be chemotherapeutics, such as arsenic trioxide, antibiotics such as clarithromycin, antidepressants such as citalopram, or antipsychotics such as droperidol and haloperidol. Reviewing the potential for drugs to prolong the QT interval on a website, such as Crediblemeds.org, and also checking for drug interactions should be part of the routine care of patients.

Methadone predictably leads to QT interval prolongation (Chap. 36). The risk of developing a prolonged QT interval is related to the dose of the methadone; the higher the dose taken, the higher the risk. The risk of developing torsade de pointes is additive; as other medication are added,

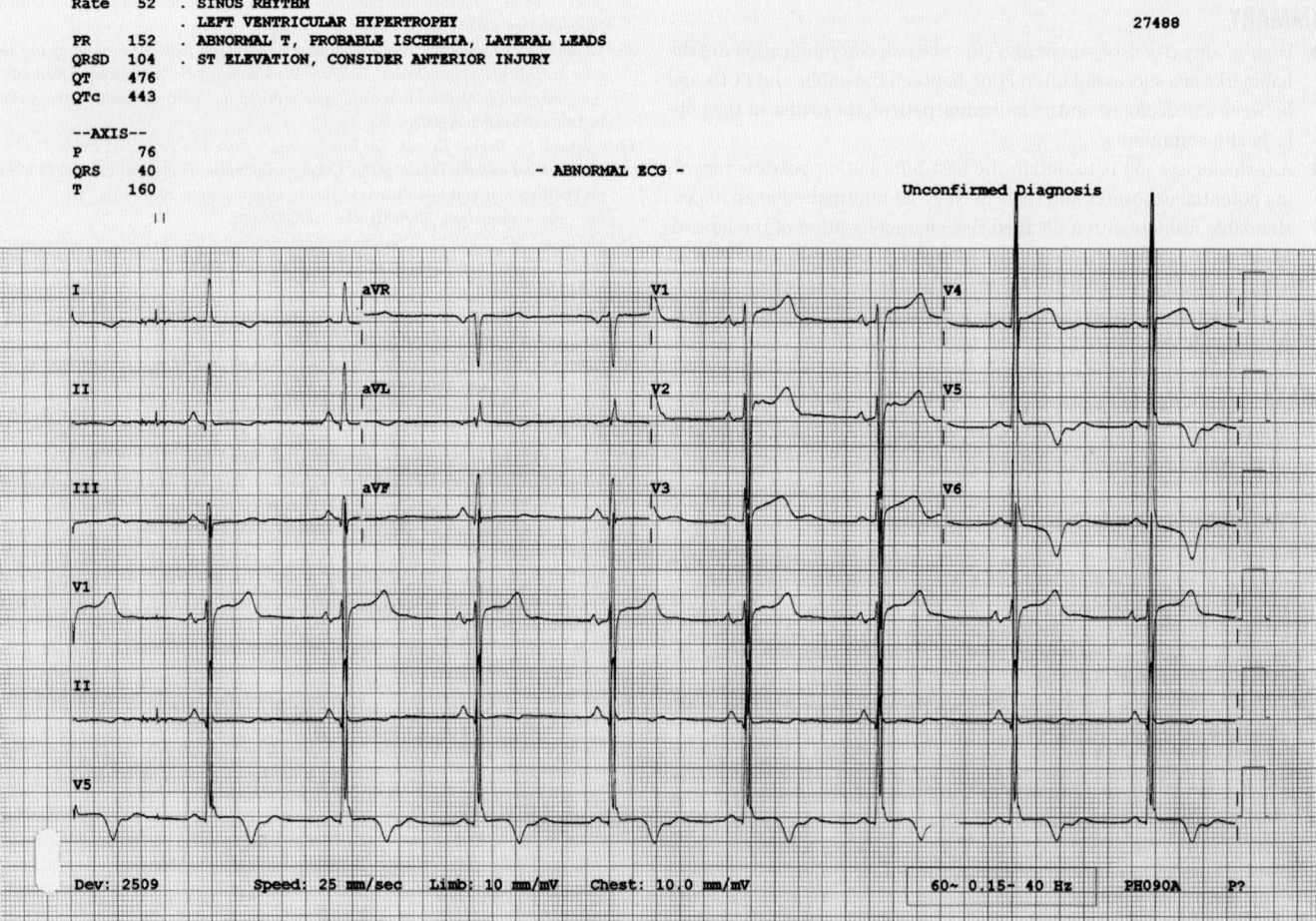

```
Rate    52    . SINUS RHYTHM
              . LEFT VENTRICULAR HYPERTROPHY                              27488
PR     152    . ABNORMAL T, PROBABLE ISCHEMIA, LATERAL LEADS
QRSD   104    . ST ELEVATION, CONSIDER ANTERIOR INJURY
QT     476
QTc    443

--AXIS--
P       76
QRS     40                        - ABNORMAL ECG -
T      160
                                                        Unconfirmed Diagnosis
  | |
```

Dev: 2509   Speed: 25 mm/sec   Limb: 10 mm/mV   Chest: 10.0 mm/mV   60~ 0.15- 40 Hz   PH090A   P?

FIGURE CS14–1. This 27-year-old man was on chronic methadone therapy. His initial electrocardiogram shows a sinus bradycardia.

CASE STUDY 14 (CONTINUED)

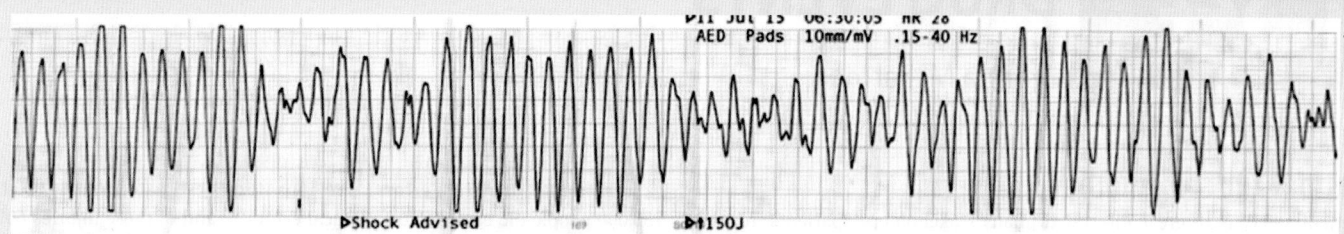

FIGURE CS14–2. A 27-year-old man who chronically received methadone was given 10 mg of methadone intramuscularly for opioid withdrawal and 4 mg of ondansetron for nausea and vomiting. Shortly thereafter he developed torsade de pointes.

the QT interval prolongs, increasing the risk of developing torsade de pointes. Methadone is a particular concern; in addition to the prolonged QT interval, it also leads to a bradycardia, which further increases the risk of torsade de pointes.

Ondansetron, a 5HT$_3$ antagonist that is used commonly in EDs, also prolongs the QT interval. This demonstrates that even a medication that is used several times a day should be checked for an interaction with any other xenobiotic the patient is taking (Chap. 134).

What Clinical and Laboratory Analyses Further Assist in Identifying Causes of the Patient's Presentation? The most important tests in evaluating

patients who have loss of consciousness are vital signs, pulse oximetry, and an EGG. Measuring the QRS complex and QT interval is incredibly important in evaluating the poisoned patient in these circumstances. Serum electrolytes should be checked, specifically, the sodium, potassium, magnesium, and calcium, to evaluate for easily reversible causes of a prolonged QT interval. Often, however, the cause of a prolonged QT interval is best uncovered by performing a thorough history and medication reconciliation.

Further Diagnosis and Treatment The ECG after defibrillation was found to have a markedly prolonged QT interval of 640 ms (Fig. CS14–3). In addition to the prolonged

QT interval, the patient had hypokalemia from his persistent vomiting. The co-administration of ondansetron and methadone, drugs known to cause prolongation of the QT interval, in the setting of hypokalemia was synergistic, leading to torsade de pointes. The most important treatment of torsade de pointes is prevention for which magnesium sulfate was administered. He was administered isoproterenol intravenously to increase the heart rate in the intensive care unit, and he had no further episodes of torsade de pointes. The patient's QT interval narrowed after discontinuation of methadone and ondansetron, and he was transitioned to buprenorphine for his opioid dependence.

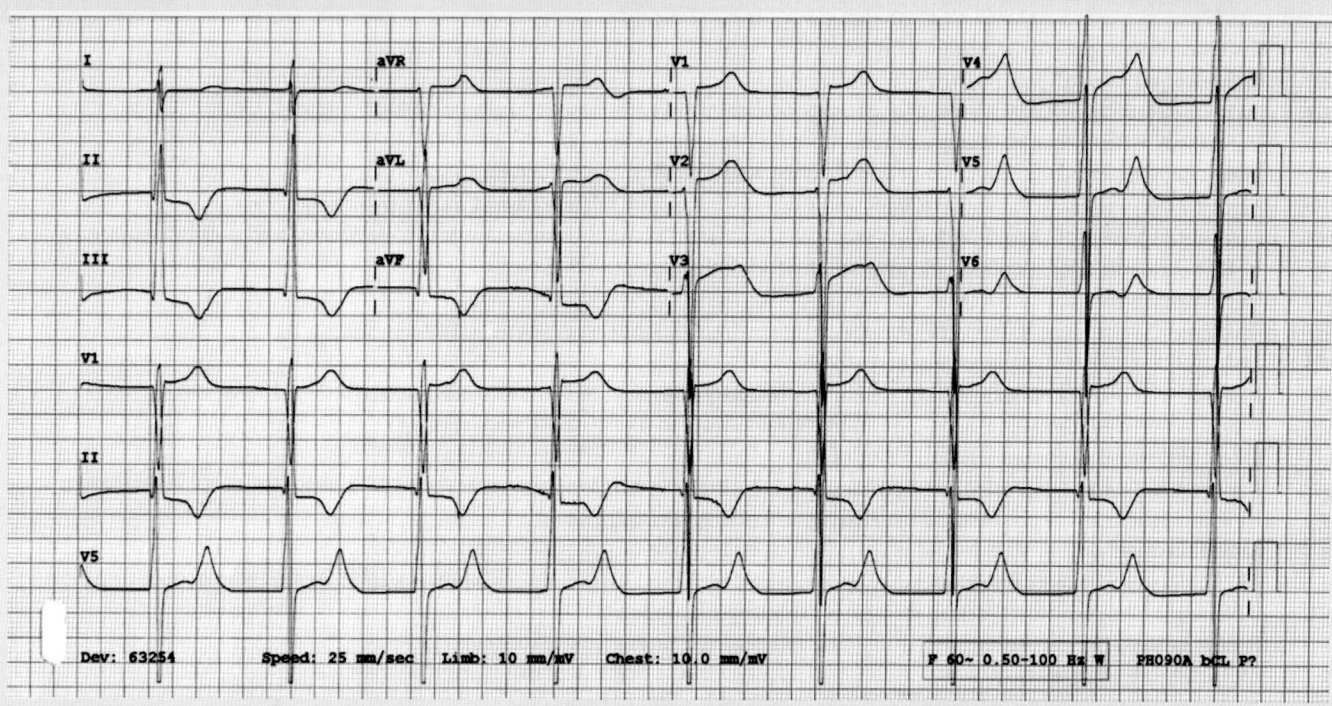

FIGURE CS14–3. A postdefibrillation electrocardiogram of the same 27-year-old man demonstrates a sinus bradycardia and a prolonged QT interval. This was likely caused by a combination of the methadone therapy treatment with, ondansetron, and the hypokalemia that resulted from vomiting.

134 MEDICATION SAFETY AND ADVERSE DRUG EVENTS

Brenna M. Farmer

HISTORY AND EPIDEMIOLOGY

Patient safety is of great interest to many stakeholders—patients, regulatory and accreditation bodies, hospital and health system administrators, and health care professionals. Interest has expanded since the publication of the Institute of Medicine's 1999 report on medical errors and measures necessary to ensure a safer health care system. Its subsequent report in 2001 focus on quality with one aim, to avoid injury to patients and redesign health care, so that safety is a property of the system.[49,53] A 2006 report focused specifically on reducing medication errors and adverse drug effects.[51] These reports and others reveal that medications errors represent up to 25% of all medical errors.[55] Many health care institutions address medication safety through their pharmacy and therapeutics (also commonly called drug and formulary), medication safety, patient safety, and quality improvement committees. Table 134–1 shows a timeline of some important developments in medication safety.

Studies of medical errors, including those involving medications, are of a highly variable quality and usefulness. This occurs in large part because of diverse populations, variable definitions, and multiple study acquisition and analysis methodologies. Despite these differences, studies consistently establish that medical errors cause thousands of deaths each year. Medical errors are a leading cause of death in the United States, with estimates of 251,000 deaths per year. This number is likely an underestimate given how "cause of death" uses ICD 10 codes, on death certificates and does not capture human or system errors.[78] Previous studies estimated that 44,000 to 180,000 people die each year of medical errors[53,71] and of these injuries 60% are probably preventable.[16] With preventable health care harm as a leading cause of death in the United States, the National Patient Safety Foundation has labeled medical error as a public health crisis.[90]

Approximately 9.5 million patients experienced an adverse drug event (ADE) from 2008 to 2011 according to a large retrospective analysis of the Healthcare Cost and Utilization Project's National Inpatient data set. Previous reports estimated that more than 1.5 million preventable ADEs occur each year.[51] An ADE is an untoward event or outcome associated with the therapeutic use of a drug. The definition of ADEs includes medication errors as well as adverse drug reactions and drug interactions. A medication error is "any preventable event that may cause or lead to inappropriate medication use or patient harm while the medication is in the control of the health care professional, patient, or consumer."[89] An adverse drug reaction is a sign or symptom related to use of a medication that results in unpleasant effects when an error has not occurred.

The cost of a single ADE is estimated to be $1,800 to $5,000 at academic and community hospitals.[11,22,23,47] Similarly, length of stay increased from 1.8 to 3 days when an ADE occurred.[47,100] Other studies estimated that the annual cost of ADE morbidity and mortality was greater than $77 to $177 billion in the ambulatory care setting,[33,56] $2 billion in hospitals,[11,23] and $4 billion in nursing homes.[15] These costs exclude legal or other costs that accrue to the patient or their families.

TABLE 134–1	Critical Events in the Evolution of Medication Safety
1820	United States Pharmacopeia (USP) is established in Washington, DC
1906	The Pure Food and Drugs Act is passed by Congress
1927	The Bureau of Chemistry is re-formed into Food, Drug, and Insecticide Administration and the Bureau of Chemistry and Soils
1930	The Food, Drug, and Insecticide Administration was renamed the Food and Drug Administration (FDA)
1962	Kefauver-Harris Drug Amendments passed to ensure drug efficacy and greater drug safety
	President Kennedy proclaims the Consumer Bill of Rights, which includes the right to safety, right to be informed, and right to choose
1963	Representatives from FDA, USP, American Medical Association (AMA), and American Pharmacists Association form the US Adopted Names Council to establish drug nomenclature
1968	The FDA is placed in the Public Health Service after reorganization of the federal government health programs
1970	The FDA requires the first patient package insert
1975	The Institute of Safe Medication Practices's (ISMP) work officially begins with a continuing column in *Hospital Pharmacy*
1987	The first ISMP list of dangerous drug abbreviations is printed in *Nursing '87*
1989	Agency for Health Care Policy and Research (AHCPR) is established as an agency in the Public Health Service in the Department of Health and Human Services
1991	Institute for Healthcare Improvement is founded as a not-for-profit organization to aid in improvement of health care quality
	USP and ISMP create Medication Error Reporting Program (MERP)
1993	A consolidation of several adverse reaction reporting systems is launched as MedWatch, the FDA voluntary reporting system for problems associated with medical products
1996	The National Coordinating Council for Medication Error Reporting and Prevention (NCC MERP) is formed
1997	National Patient Safety Foundation is established with patient safety as its sole purpose
	ISMP founds a subsidiary, Medical Error Recognition and Revision Strategies (Med. E.R.R.S.), to work with drug companies to predict problems with names, labels, and packaging
1998	USP launches MEDMARX, an Internet-accessible medication errors reporting system for hospitals
	Founding members of The Leapfrog Group meet to discuss ways to purchase health care to influence its quality and affordability
	ISMP publishes a list of high alert medications
1999	The Institute of Medicine (IOM) Report *To Err Is Human: Building a Safer Health System*[82] is published
	The Leapfrog Group founding members establish the reduction of preventable medical errors as their initial focus
	The National Quality Forum is created as the President's Advisory Commission on Consumer Protection and Quality in the Health Care Industry
	Agency for Health Care Policy and Research is renamed Agency for Healthcare Research and Quality
2006	IOM Report *Preventing Medication Errors*[83] is published
2007	USP and Quantros, a company that collects data on health care quality, patient safety and accreditation, partner to run MEDMARX

Morbidity and Mortality From Medication Errors and ADEs

Although medication errors are the most common cause of iatrogenic patient injury, less than 2% result in injuries. Poison Control Centers take calls every day for unintentional therapeutic errors related to medications. In 2015, 12.7% of all human exposure calls to poison control were for therapeutic errors.[88] Adverse drug events and medication errors with serious effects lead to 3.1% to 6.2% of all hospital admissions.[69] Nevertheless, the incidence of ADEs in hospitalized patients is estimated to range from 2% to 20%,[22] resulting in 7,000 deaths annually in the United States.[53] A retrospective review of hospital death certificates by ICD 9 and ICD 10 codes from 1983 to 2004 revealed an increase of 361% in fatal medication errors and a 33% increase in deaths from ADEs occurring in a patient's home.[98] The hospital death certificate review also revealed an increase in fatal medication errors 32 times higher when prescription medications were combined with ethanol and or illicit xenobiotics.[98] According to voluntary MedWatch reports to the US Food and Drug Administration (FDA), 17% of reported ADEs were associated with death, 7% were associated with permanent disability, and many others had serious complications. Women and elderly patients were at the highest risk.[85]

Adverse drug events lead to many emergency department (ED) visits and hospitalizations. In one study, 2.5% of all ED visits, for unintentional injuries, are for ADEs and these ADEs make up 6.7% of unintentional injury hospitalizations from the ED.[20] In this study, individuals greater than 65 years of age were at higher risk of unintentional injury and hospitalization.[20] In another study, 59% of ED patients had a medication error occur and 37% of those patients had the error reach them. Factors increasing these errors were boarding patient status, number of medication orders, and number of medications administered.[95] The most recent study of ED visits showed that 27% of ED visits for ADEs lead to hospitalization and reiterated that elderly patients were most at risk.[111]

National Coordinating Council for Medication Error Reporting and Prevention Taxonomy

A useful medication error taxonomy, developed by the National Coordinating Council for Medication Error Reporting and Prevention (NCC MERP), classifies medication errors according to severity of outcome (Fig. 134–1).[89] Importantly, the categories of least severity (A and B) describe circumstances

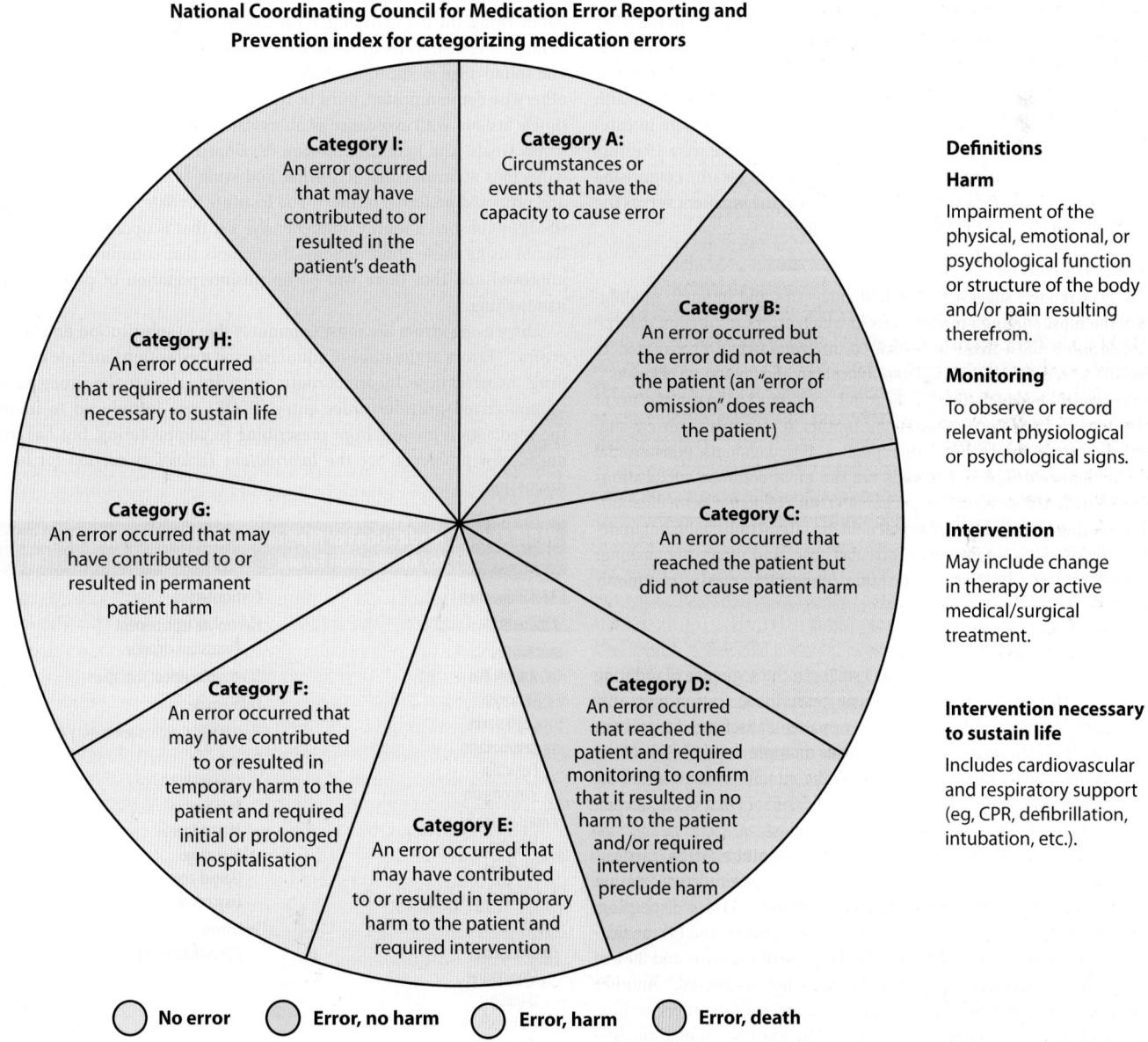

National Coordinating Council for Medication Error Reporting and Prevention index for categorizing medication errors

Category I: An error occurred that may have contributed to or resulted in the patient's death

Category A: Circumstances or events that have the capacity to cause error

Category B: An error occurred but the error did not reach the patient (an "error of omission" does reach the patient)

Category H: An error occurred that required intervention necessary to sustain life

Category G: An error occurred that may have contributed to or resulted in permanent patient harm

Category C: An error occurred that reached the patient but did not cause patient harm

Category F: An error occurred that may have contributed to or resulted in temporary harm to the patient and required initial or prolonged hospitalisation

Category E: An error occurred that may have contributed to or resulted in temporary harm to the patient and required intervention

Category D: An error occurred that reached the patient and required monitoring to confirm that it resulted in no harm to the patient and/or required intervention to preclude harm

Definitions

Harm

Impairment of the physical, emotional, or psychological function or structure of the body and/or pain resulting therefrom.

Monitoring

To observe or record relevant physiological or psychological signs.

Intervention

May include change in therapy or active medical/surgical treatment.

Intervention necessary to sustain life

Includes cardiovascular and respiratory support (eg, CPR, defibrillation, intubation, etc.).

◯ No error   ◯ Error, no harm   ◯ Error, harm   ◯ Error, death

FIGURE 134–1. Diagram showing National Coordinating Council for Medication Error Reporting and Prevention categories of medication errors, ranging from fatal to errors with no impact on patient care. (*© 2001 National Coordinating Council for Medication Error Reporting and Prevention. All rights reserved.*)

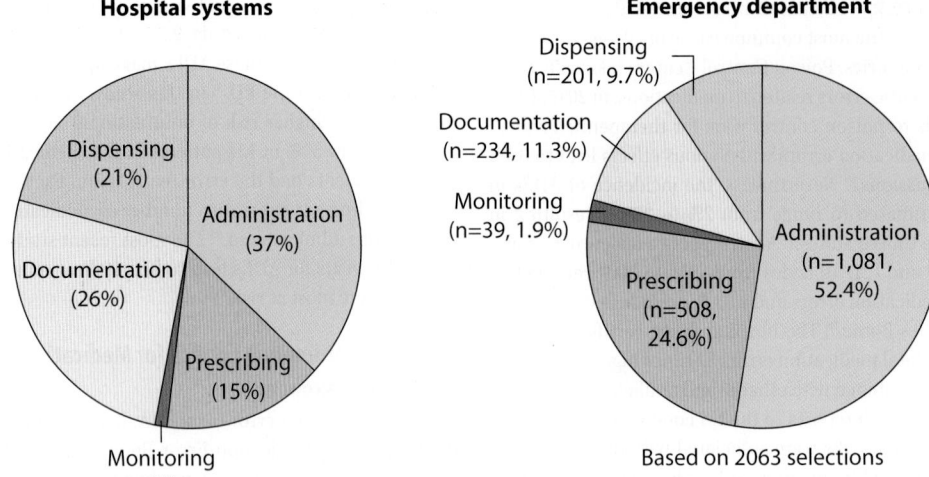

FIGURE 134–2. Diagram showing MEDMARX data for (**A**) hospital systems and (**B**) specifically for the Emergency Department. *(Adapted with permission from United States Pharmacopeial Convention, www.usp.org.)*

or events in which the potential to cause error exists, or the error occurs but does not affect the patient. These "near misses" are so frequent that they serve as a critical source of information related to systems problems and education about medication error, but are typically underreported and underappreciated. In one study of 154,816 errors reported by hospitals and health systems to MEDMARX from 1999 to 2001, most of the errors were in category C (47%) and resulted in no patient injury, whereas there were 19 errors in category I, contributing to or resulting in patient death, comprising 0.01%.[105] See Fig. 134–2 for a comparison of errors in the inpatient versus the ED setting based on the NCC MERP classification.

Medications Involved

The US FDA reports suggest that opioid analgesics and immune modulators are the most common medications in which errors resulted in death.[85] The medications most frequently involved in errors and ADEs reported to MEDMARX were insulin, anticoagulants, morphine, and potassium chloride.[105] These are considered high-alert medications according to the sentinel event alert system of The Joint Commission. Another retrospective review suggests that corticosteroids, chemotherapeutics, anticoagulants, nonsteroidal antiinflammatory drugs, and opioids are the most common medications associated with ADEs.[100] Identifying characteristics of high-risk medications include low therapeutic index, pharmacokinetic interactions, inherent undesirable effects, newly approved or "off-label" use, and direct-to-consumer promotion.[12] Table 134–2 lists medications/medication classes commonly reported.

The Medication Process

The Medication Process comprises the 5 stages in the sequence of ordering a medication to its delivery to the patient: prescribing, transcribing, dispensing, administering, and monitoring.[7] For patients discharged from care, follow-up adds a sixth stage.[28] Each stage yields multiple steps. The potential for error is high, increasing exponentially as the number of steps and their complexity increase. Table 134–3 describes typical errors that occur at each stage in the process, along with prevention strategies.

The greatest number of errors resulting in preventable ADEs (medication errors) occurs at the prescribing stage.[8] In a study of serious medication errors, 39% occurred at prescribing, 12% at transcribing, 11% at dispensing, and 38% at administering.[72] In one study of 17,808 inpatient and ED medication orders, 6.2% of orders written involved a prescribing error and 30% of these were likely to harm the patient if they were not discovered.[14] Another prospective study suggested that up to 43.8% of medication orders on hospital wards had a prescribing error discovered by ward-based pharmacists, independent of the level of prescriber experience.[108] In the ED, most errors occurred in either the prescribing or administering phase.[95]

Transcribing errors usually involve poor communication due to illegible handwriting, the use of trailing zeroes, or inappropriate abbreviations. Poor handwriting also leads to confusion, particularly with regard to look-alike and sound-alike medications.[96] All information, whether printed, spoken, or otherwise communicated, must be transmitted in a clear, unambiguous, and timely fashion with avoidance of abbreviations. In its 2004 National Patient Safety Goals, The Joint Commission developed a minimum list of 5 sets of dangerous abbreviations, acronyms, and symbols that should not be used, and proposed preferred terms.[115] The Institute for Safe Medication Practices (ISMP) published a more comprehensive list that is updated periodically.[54] By not using these abbreviations, the hope is that communication will be improved and that there will be no misinterpretation of poor physician handwriting.

Dispensing errors are most commonly due to substitution and labeling errors.[109] Errors at the stage of administering medications include incorrect drug, incorrect dose, incorrect route, and a drug given to the wrong patient. Computerized provider order entry (CPOE) was introduced to improve the medication process from prescribing to administering, but has introduced new problems. See the *Information Technology* section for further discussion.

TABLE 134–2	Medications or Medication Classes Commonly Responsible for Medication Errors	
Acetaminophen		Corticosteroids
Albuterol		Electrolyte replacement
Antibiotics		Potassium chloride
Amoxicillin		Fluid replacement therapies
Cefazolin		
Cephalexin		Furosemide
Levofloxacin		Nonsteroidal antiinflammatory drugs
Penicillin		Opioids
Vancomycin		Fentanyl
Anticoagulants		Meperidine
Heparin		Methadone
Warfarin		Morphine
Antidiabetics and Hypoglycemics		Opioid-acetaminophen combinations
Aspirin		Oxycodone
Cardiovascular		Sedatives
Clopidogrel		Benzodiazepines
Digoxin		
Inotropes		
Vasopressors		
Chemotherapeutics		

TABLE 134–3 Errors Based on Medication Process Stage and Error-Reducing Strategies

Medication Process Stage	Error-Producing Conditions	Error-Reducing Strategies	Specific IT Error-Reducing Strategies	Introduced Errors	Error-Reducing Strategies
Prescribing	Incomplete knowledge of medication or patient	Increased pharmacist availability Through medication/medical/allergy history Practice conservative prescribing Pediatrics ⠀⠀Accurate weight in kg ⠀⠀Be alert for calculation/ ⠀⠀decimal point errors ⠀⠀Caution with "off-label" use Geriatrics ⠀⠀Consider comorbidities and drug ⠀⠀interactions ⠀⠀Consider possibility of falls with ⠀⠀new medications ⠀⠀Consider renal, hepatic, and ⠀⠀thyroid function Pregnancy ⠀⠀Rule out pregnancy ⠀⠀Careful risk-benefit analysis	Computer Prescriber Order Entry Decision Support Tools ⠀⠀Electronic pharmacopeia ⠀⠀Drug Interactions ⠀⠀Renal Dosing ⠀⠀Age-Related Concerns ⠀⠀Allergy Checks	Incorrect medication selection Wrong patient selection Incorrect data entry Alert Fatigue With "Blow-By" References are often outdated Toxicology information is often lacking Use of free-text order/data entry prevents use of decision support tools Use of multiple systems in one institution—data not updated in all systems (ie, allergy is often only documented in outpatient record and does not cross over to inpatient record)	Pharmacist able to consult and review of prescriber orders TallMan Lettering Active alerts requiring data entry prior to order entry Use of order sets Use a uniform system to prevent loss of important information from one setting to another
Transcribing	Verbal orders Poor penmanship Abbreviations and Symbols	Avoid verbal orders Write legibility, print if necessary Avoid acronyms or prohibited abbreviations Indicate decimal point clearly No trailing zeros Avoid apothecary terms Involve prescriber contact information on order	Electronic order entry		
Dispensing	Dispensing by nurses Dispensing by physicians Patient ID	Nurse dispenses to another nurse and not themselves No dispensing by physicians Check with prescriber if ambiguity in order Check decimal point placement Check weight in kilograms Check allergies Patient ID doubly confirmed Check arithmetic	Bar-code dispensing Automated dispensing cabinets (ADCs)	Inability to scan barcode No barcode devices at bedside Substitutions due to drug shortages Drug override Look-alike errors from small screens unable to show full medication name Stocking errors Dispensing of unit doses instead of patients specific doses	Pharmacist review prior to availability of nurse to obtain from ADC TallMan lettering Use of barcode technology for stocking
Administering	Multiplicity of medications Potency of medications Multiple patients Parenteral administration Medication incompatibilities Physician administration	Challenge orders if necessary Clarify ambiguity or doubt concerning order Consultation with reference materials Consultation with pharmacist Call back verbal orders Avoid physician administration Implement systemic safety checks Engineer intrathecal/intravenous incompatibility	Bar-code medication administration Intelligent infusion pumps	Inability of scanner to read barcode Mismatch of barcodes Drug shortages leading to substitution that do not match order entry exactly Outdated infusion pump libraries Multiple infusion pump devices	Use of drug library based on institution's formulary and guidelines TallMan Lettering
Monitoring	Potent medications Parenteral administration Emergent procedures Complex procedures	Ensure adequate personnel Clearly defined protocols and guidelines: ⠀⠀Procedural sedation ⠀⠀Rapid sequence ventilation ⠀⠀Adequate monitoring time following drug administration	Decision support tools ⠀⠀Drug concentration ⠀⠀monitoring ⠀⠀Other laboratory monitoring ⠀⠀Other vital sign monitoring		
Follow-up	Patients leaving the hospital or health care facility, and especially medicated patients	Medication reconciliation Paper discharge instructions Written information regarding new medications Advise of required follow-up Consider medication effects if a patient is driving Pill counting devices Medications organizing systems			

Monitoring and discharging with follow-up are associated with fewer errors. These phases involve attention to liver and kidney function, checking medication concentrations, and attention to and evaluation of drug interactions and pharmacokinetic interactions.[28] Monitoring must be an ongoing process that begins when the patient receives the medication, regardless of where the patient is in the health care system, and continues as long as the individual continues to have the medication prescribed. In the acute stages of treatment, such as in the hospital or ED, the process is especially important and requires optimal 3-way linkage between the pharmacy, laboratory, and physician.[106] This process must be maintained throughout the individual's continued relationship with the health care system. In the outpatient setting, providers must be aware of signs and symptoms related to adverse drug effects while they are monitoring and following up patients. In a study of 661 patients in 4 primary care practices, patient reports of medication side effects to their physicians led to changed therapies in 76% of cases. A failure to identify medication-related symptoms and change therapy resulted in 21% ameliorable and 2% preventable ADEs. Ameliorable ADEs were defined as those in which "the severity or duration could have been reduced substantially had different actions been taken."[122]

SPECIAL AT-RISK POPULATIONS

Important medication safety issues exist for children and older adults, a problem that is exacerbated by their underrepresentation or exclusion from clinical trials. It is estimated, for example, that only a third of the medications used to treat children are adequately tested in this population.[25] Similar concerns apply to medications used in older adults and those individuals with specific underlying medical conditions that would have excluded them from trials.[48]

Pediatric Considerations

Adverse events involving medications in children occur from the prenatal period through maturation. Errors occur in all settings: the home, ambulatory care, prehospital setting with emergency medical services (EMS), ED, hospital floor, pediatric intensive care unit (PICU), and neonatal intensive care unit (NICU), and by all caregivers. Approximately 1 in 6.4 pediatric orders results in an error that reaches the child.[80] Because of the greater need for dose calculations to allow for weight-based dosing, dose-related errors are more likely to occur in children.[58] Errors also occur in the home environment with nonprescription medications, but the true incidence is unknown. In one survey, the errors associated with home antipyretic use were estimated at almost 50%.[81] These errors were typically associated with underdosing, which is generally of little immediate harm.[104] In the ambulatory care setting, the incidence is unknown but one study identified "numerous" errors in prescription writing in a pediatric clinic.[120] An EMS study determined that 43% of paramedics knew cases in which a dosing error occurred.[44] In the ED, the error rate was estimated at 10% of all pediatric charts.[63] There is an increased risk of errors in children cared for in nonacademic or rural EDs compared with academic or pediatric EDs.[61] A retrospective chart review of 177 pediatric charts in 4 rural EDs identified 84 different medication errors in 69 of the 135 patients who received medications. The outcomes of these errors were in NCC MERP categories A to D (Fig. 134–1).[79] A study of 18 pediatric EDs' voluntary event/incident reporting data showed that 19% of all incidents were related to medication events. A total of 94% were medication errors and 6% were ADRs. Errors included using incorrect weights, duplicate dosing, and miscalculations. Human factors contributed to 84% of the medication errors in this study.[110] See the Factors Affecting Human Performance section for further discussion.

Hospitalized children experience up to 3 times the rate of medication errors and potential ADEs as do adults.[59] The incidence of medication errors of hospitalized children is estimated at about 6% for all orders written; the majority (74%) of these occur at the prescribing stage and approximately 20% are classified as potentially harmful based on a 4-point Likert-type scale developed by the investigators.[37] Pharmacists based on pediatric hospital wards discovered that 5.9% of orders contained a prescribing error and were able to intervene through the order entry system.[30] Generally, children in the intensive care unit are at higher risk for errors compared to adults and hospitalized children not in the ICU, presumably reflecting the increased complexity of disease and the medications used.[61] Incorrect dosing, especially with the intravenous route, is the most commonly reported error. Dosing of antimicrobials and intravenous fluids are the most common medications involved.[29,35,59] Errors and discrepancies found in hospital discharge instructions, with lack of complete medication reconciliation, also lead to patient harm (Chap. 31).[57]

Geriatric Considerations

Medication errors in older adults also occur throughout the health care continuum: in the home, ambulatory care, nursing homes, assisted-living setting, and in the hospital (Chap. 32). Adults older than 65 years of age have a relative risk of 2.37 for drug complications and 4.12 for medication errors compared to adult patients younger than 65 years of age.[16] The incidence of medication error at home with nonprescription medications is unknown but, for reasons outlined below, would be expected to exceed that of the younger adult population. Using a variety of methodologies, ADEs were evaluated for a 12-month period in a multispecialty ambulatory care practice in a cohort of 27,617 Medicare enrollees, equivalent to more than 30,000 person-years of observation. Extrapolating their findings, to the estimated 38 million Medicare enrollees (those ≥65 years), would predict nearly 2 million ADEs annually, of which more than 25% would be considered preventable and about 180,000 fatal or life threatening.[43] One study estimates that there are about 265,802 ED visits in patients older than 65 years of age for ADEs, and 99,628 of these patients require admission to the hospital. In the same study, patients older than 80 years constituted half of those admitted to the hospital. Medications or classes of medications involved in two-thirds of the hospitalizations were diabetic and antithrombotic medications.[18] A more recent study estimates that 34.5% of all ED visits for ADEs were in patients older than 65 years and were more likely to be hospitalized than other age groups. The medications involved were anticoagulants, antidiabetics, hypoglycemics, and opioids.[111]

There are more than 1.5 million nursing home residents in the United States. The average such resident uses 6 different medications, and 20% use 10 or more.[13] Extrapolating the findings of a study of 18 community-based nursing homes in Massachusetts over a 1 year period predicts 350,000 ADEs annually, more than one-half of which would be preventable.[42] Fatal or life-threatening ADEs would represent 20,000 of these predicted events of which 80% would be preventable. Approximately one million other seniors live in assisted-living facilities, and are vulnerable to medication errors for a variety of reasons, including inadequate physician support, inadequately trained staff, and staffing shortages. Adverse drug events cause 10.5% of hospital admissions for geriatric patients and are the most common type of adverse event occurring in hospitalized elderly patients.[72,124] These medications result in nearly 50% of ADE-related visits to the ED but are only prescribed during 9.4% of outpatient visits.[19]

Addressing these issues is becoming ever more important as the US Census Bureau predicts a rise of 62 million in the number of Americans 65 years of age or older by the year 2025 and a 68% increase in the 85 years of age or older population that are at an even higher risk.[6] Advancing age brings with it several important considerations from the point of view of medication safety. Medical comorbidity increases with age, and therefore an increasing likelihood of receiving multiple medications. With more medications, the number of potential errors and interactions increases. Frailty and cognitive decline in older adults result in errors following self-administration. Alterations in medication absorption, metabolism, distribution, and elimination may all affect the efficacy of the medication (Chaps. 9 and 32).

Beers and STOPP/START criteria are methods to determine appropriate medication prescribing for geriatric patients.[3,92] These criteria identify inappropriate prescribing due to increased risk of adverse events with some focus on renal clearance and drug interactions.[3,92] Both criteria have limitations as geriatric patients are underrepresented in clinical drug trials, the recommendations are not individualized and medications on the lists are appropriate for certain conditions such as intravenous diphenhydramine for allergic reactions. The updated Beers list includes conditions when a medication is appropriate for use in the elderly to address this limitation.[3] Additional limitations include that the lists do not include every medication that should be avoided and these lists have not been shown to change morbidity, mortality, or cost.[99] The prevalence of inappropriate medication use in older adults is estimated to be in the 12% to 40% range.[113] One in 5 prescriptions given to elderly individuals are considered inappropriate based on Beers criteria, with diphenhydramine and amitriptyline being the most common medications prescribed inappropriately.[93] Older adult patients medicated with benzodiazepines, for example, have a 4-fold increase in falls (Chap. 32).

RESPONSE TO MEDICATION ERROR

One of the leading causes of medication errors is human performance deficit. See the Factors Affecting Human Performance section later. Almost invariably a human action will precede the ADE, and this temporal contiguity of action and consequence typically generates a tendency to blame someone. In most cases, the blame will fall on the last person to have contact with the patient. In recent years, however, a consensus emerged that blaming people for errors is counterproductive. The number of ADEs that result from egregious behavior is very small, and more often than not an explanation for the fault will be found within the system that allowed the error to occur. Attempts to understand the nature of these faults, and to correct them, while being sensitive to the potential for unintended consequences, is the most appropriate response. Several processes can be used to respond to errors or system-problems. These include root cause analysis, clinical incident analysis, failure mode and effect analysis, and Lean Six Sigma (LSS).

Root cause analysis (RCA), a term originally used to investigate major industrial events, is a technique that provides a structured, process-oriented analysis of sentinel events. The Joint Commission in accredited hospitals mandated its use in 1997. It is a time-consuming process requiring multidisciplinary teams with specialized training, and is subject to bias and methodologic limitations.[118] Nevertheless, a judiciously conducted RCA provides insight into systemic failures underlying the ADE, and identify areas that require change. An alternative approach, a clinical incident analysis protocol, was developed that more appropriately shifts the emphasis from the individual to the system.[117] The clinical incident analysis protocol utilizes 7 factors as the basis for an investigation. Some organizations developed a hybrid combining these 2 approaches. Both RCA and clinical incident analysis are conducted retrospectively, and therefore subject to retrospective bias.

An alternative approach is failure mode and effect analysis (FMEA), which proactively attempts to identify potential errors and to initiate preventive measures. A multidisciplinary group is utilized in the FMEA approach to identify a process or subprocess that needs analysis, to identify the steps of the process and determine the risk/likelihood/severity of failure of each step. Once this phase is accomplished, the team prioritizes a high-risk step and conducts an RCA to make recommendations on redesigning the step. The establishment modifications are analyzed in their performance to determine change and decrease in risk. This process is designed as a quality control and assurance to protect the proceedings from legal investigation.[4]

Other processes are being introduced into the health care industry to improve quality of care and safety and reduce costs. Two such approaches are Lean and Six Sigma, sometimes used together as LSS. Both were initially described in the Toyota Production System and adapted to health care. Define, measure, analyze, improve, and control are all steps related to LSS. It involves defining the process that needs evaluation, determining how to measure the process, analyzing the data collected based on the determined measures, forming an improvement plan based on the

analysis, and putting a new process in place with the goals of developing a lasting culture regarding the newly improved process with elimination of waste.[1,126] Each of these steps has principles to guide the use of LSS. The Agency for Healthcare Research and Quality has specific forms to aid health care facilities when adopting these approaches to safety and improvement.[70]

REDUCING ERRORS

To reduce medication errors, each health care system should simplify, standardize, and stratify processes and communication. The medication process should be carefully automated with computer order entry and bar coding as extensively as the system will permit. Although these information technology solutions will aid the medication process, nothing is perfect and each change introduces new potential problems. See the Information Technology section later. Limitations of attention and vigilance should be understood and the reporting of errors in a nonpunitive environment should be encouraged.[72] Improving information access, error proofing, reducing reliance on memory, enhanced training, and the use of buffers or redundancy in an attempt to prevent errors should also be encouraged.[71] Each time a medication is given, the focus should be "right drug, right dose, right route, right patient, at the right time."

In 2003, the American Academy of Pediatrics Committees on Drugs and on Hospital Care developed a position statement regarding the reduction of medication errors in children. The recommendations can be adapted to all hospital settings and to patients of all ages. These recommendations include appropriate staffing, utilization of the resources in the pharmacy, standardization of hospital equipment and protocols, and the development of a nonpunitive, barrier-free system to report and easily track errors.[114] Other more recent groups also encourage reduction of medication errors and participation in medication safety. The American College of Medical Toxicology encourages medical toxicologists to use their expertise and training to aid health care systems in reduction of errors and other pharmacy and therapeutics issues.[2]

For older adults, prescribers should review medication indications and avoid age bias. Polypharmacy should be limited, with medications prescribed only as necessary. Dosing should be adjusted as needed based on renal and hepatic function as well as drug interactions. Medication review by pharmacists aid in decreasing the use of potentially inappropriate medications and in decreasing the number of medications prescribed (polypharmacy).[83] In the hospital, outside of the ED and emergent situations, pharmacists ought to review all medication orders, when available, and verify the medication as appropriate prior to it being dispensed. Pharmacists can also aid in medication reconciliation at transitions of care and upon hospital discharge to prevent complications of polypharmacy.[40,65]

FACTORS AFFECTING HUMAN PERFORMANCE

Human factors lead to many medication errors. In fact, it is not surprising that human performance deficits are the primary causes of medication errors in such an extremely complex medical environment. A performance deficit means that the individual making the error had the prerequisite knowledge to avoid the error but failed to do so. Performance deficits originate from cognitive failings because of interruptions, distractions, inexperience, or simple overloading. These cognitive errors are discussed below. Other variables contribute to performance deficit, including many ergonomic issues such as workload, resource limitations, and staff shortages. This environment is both burdened and enriched by many inherited properties. Human factors and ergonomics theory draws on a variety of disciplines, including industrial engineering, industrial psychology, cognitive psychology, and information technology. Much should be done to optimize the interface between humans and the work environment and to ensure that systems operate more efficiently. As a general principle, it is preferable if the dominant purpose in designing medical devices and processes is they fit human users, and not forcing the converse. Table 134–4 lists some of the more common human performance deficits. Such errors often manifest as simple slips of action, or

TABLE 134–4	Common Factors That Adversely Affect Human Performance[27,105]
Attentional capture	
Diminished motivation/morale	
Distractions	
Fatigue	
Fragmentation, transitions of care	
Inadequate resource availability (Resource Availability Continuous Quality Improvement Trade-Off)	
Increased work acuity/cognitive load	
Inexperience	
Interruptions	
Poor workplace ergonomics	
Sleep deprivation/debt	

execution failures, arising from distraction by something other than the task at hand.[101] Vigilance is better maintained in individuals who are well rested and working without interruption or distraction in a well-designed environment. Fewer medication errors occur in optimally designed environments.[72]

Human performance deficits such as diminished memory, sleep deprivation, depression, and distractions contribute to errors. Resident physician mood and lack of sleep are also factors in performance deficits. Depressed residents made 6.2 times as many medication errors as nondepressed residents.[34] Sleep deprivation and improper supervision were highlighted initially after the Libby Zion case, in which a patient on phenelzine developed fatal serotonin toxicity following the administration of meperidine by a sleep-deprived and inadequately supervised intern. Interns working a traditional schedule of call every third night with extended work shifts (36 hours) made 35.9% more serious medical errors than those with the current reduced work schedule.[66] In particular, there were 20.8% more serious medication errors during the older work schedules compared with the current reduced hour schedule.[66] In 2008, an Institute of Medicine study addressed resident work hours and patient safety. This report recommended residents be provided with designated sleep time during each day and rest periods each week in order to decrease the risk of fatigue-related medical errors.[52] However, work schedules may not have as much effect on medical errors as once thought. A new study reviewed 2 different work schedules for surgery residents. It found that there was no difference in types of medical errors with a restrictive (standard work schedule based on regulatory guidelines) versus less-restrictive work schedule.[5]

A particularly important goal for human performance deficit is the reduction of cognitive load and distractions. Many medication errors originate from cognitive performance deficits. In the ED, increased cognitive load such as related to increased number of boarding patients, increased number of medication orders, and increased number of medications to be administered all lead to increased medication errors.[95] Further efforts must be directed at strategies to reduce cognitive failure. The adoption of some very simple strategies based on human factors engineering principles will reduce error, such as simplification of the number of steps involved, reducing reliance on memory, applying cognitive forcing strategies,[27] and using cognitive aids. Research into reducing distractions during medication administration focused on adapting principles from the airline industry, "the sterile cockpit principle."[36] This principle limits interruptions and distractions that could interfere with proper performance of a critical task or tasks. In the airline industry, the use of this principle occurs during takeoff, taxi, and landing. In medication administration, this principle involves the use of "do not disturb" signs or vests worn by the nurse administering medications, no conversations to disrupt the medication nurse during this important task, and the other nurses on the unit answering phone calls or patient/family questions. This approach reduces medication administration errors by improving human performance.[36,102] One particularly useful aid to reduce cognitive

load is the color-coded Broselow-Luten system, for pediatric medication dosing.[76] This approach has the potential for further development to improve the safety of nonprescription medications and other potentially dangerous products used in the home.

Another factor that contributes to errors is the assignment of a new role to a provider such as asking physicians to dispense or administer medications. Pharmacists are the only professional group formally trained and experienced in dispensing medication, and not surprisingly, their presence is associated with a lower medication-dispensing error rate.[64,74] Nurses administer medications because they receive such training and the administration should be restricted to them except during specific circumstances such as procedural sedation.[28]

KNOWLEDGE DEFICITS

The 2 most common factors contributing to prescribing errors are related to knowledge deficits. These deficits include lack of knowledge about the medication and about the patient.[72,75] Knowledge deficits are likely due to the number of new medications, dosage formulations, and indications. With the large number of medications prescribed and the continuing and frequent release of new medications, it is difficult to know all of the relevant clinical pharmacology of each medication, including interactions, side effects, and contraindications. Decision support, most commonly in electronic format, should be contemporaneously available to health care professionals to assist in decreasing prescribing errors.[96] However, electronic pharmacopeias, as a form of decision support, have errors and omit warnings, such as discussed with extended-release or long-acting opioids.[67] These tools also need updating by manufacturers for new prescribing information and warnings before prescribers can download and use the update.

Knowledge deficits also affect dosing calculations and drug ordering. This is related in part to the lack of formal medical school education regarding the medication process. Only 10% of medical students answered dose calculation questions correctly in one study.[123] However, students in their final year of training performed much better than students.[123] It is unclear where, when, and how the students obtained the knowledge in the higher years. Specific training is needed in both of these areas of calculation and order writing. Improvements are demonstrated following a short educational intervention,[91] but it is unclear how long this knowledge is retained. Generally, there appears to be a tacit assumption that these skills will be acquired during clinical training, but this study suggested that this knowledge is not acquired independently and that specific training is indicated.

The prevailing emphasis in physician training is on knowledge acquisition. Less time is spent inculcating critical thinking skills and/or teaching reasoning, the assumption being made that these are passively acquired during the process of training. Although this is partially true, it does not exclude opportunities to improve these cognitive faculties by direct intervention.[26]

COMMUNICATION

Improved team communication should result in fewer medication errors. Orders should be written clearly, or CPOE (discussed in detail in the Information Technology section) should be used. Orders should optimally include the indications for the medication. Both generic and trade names should be included in orders so that confusion with look-alike/sound-alike medications is avoided. Abbreviations should have limited use and trailing zeros should be eliminated. Verbal orders should be used sparingly due to the high risk of sound-alike medications and confusion with dosing.[96] If a verbal order is necessary, then it should be restated immediately to the ordering clinician to ensure that it is correct and restated from the physician to the nurse in a "closed loop" communication process.

Communication theory should receive more emphasis in health care training. Good communication skills both within and among disciplines and especially between practitioners and their patients will limit errors. As patients are admitted, transferred within, and discharged from health care facilities, it is essential that precise communication as to what medications, their strengths, doses, and purpose the patient is receiving occur. Any changes that have occurred must be accurately recorded. The medication reconciliation process was adopted by The Joint Commission in 2005 and continues to be an important National Patient Safety Goal. As with other aspects of patient safety, these issues should be formally introduced into the education curriculum. Studies show that pharmacists are an integral part of optimal medication reconciliation.[40,65] Although medication reconciliation may decrease errors in medication histories, it has not been studied for ADEs and few studies link it to decreased health care usage. Efforts to improve documentation of medication reconciliation rather than improved safety efforts are likely the result of the regulatory mandate from the Joint Commission.[96]

INFORMATION TECHNOLOGY

Information technology (IT) in health care has been ponderously slow to develop compared with its use in other organizations, but it is now gathering momentum and has obvious potential to improve patient safety.[9,50] One study estimates that adoption of health IT led to a 22% reduction of adverse drug events with the use of CPOE, decision support, electronic medication administration records, and use of barcode medication reconciliation from 2010 to 2013.[38] However, as considerable gains are made, new technology also introduces new types of errors.[21,125] The US Pharmacopeia announced in 2004 that nearly 20% of 235,159 medication errors reported to MEDMARX involved computerization or automation.[105] One study evaluating CPOE in a tertiary care hospital found that the system actually facilitated a wide variety of medication error risks.[44] Another study conducted by the Pennsylvania Patient Safety Authority found that CPOE facilitated 50% of the medications errors found during a 6-month study period.[68] Common errors associated with order entry include wrong medication selection and input of incorrect data (patient weight, creatinine clearance).[116] Another study identified 24 different types of failures associated with CPOE but suggested that many could be easily corrected, in particular by concentrating on organizational factors.[62] However, more detailed insights offer why process-supporting IT systems fail.[121] Much of the data involved in the medication process are relatively straightforward, amenable to rapid and efficient processing, including crosschecking with patient medication history and evaluating for medication interactions (an example of decision support). A study reviewing 28 trials of point-of-care decision support report showed a 4.2% improvement in patient care with a trend toward better improvement in care when a response was required from prescriber.[112]

Past studies demonstrate that computerized order entry with decision support reduces the incidence of serious medication errors by 50% to 55% once the transitional instability has passed.[10,77] This approach mainly reduces errors at the prescribing stage of the medication process and, while likely to prevent 80% of prescribing errors that led to no patient harm, the errors most likely to cause patient harm is not as amenable to reduction as these errors are related to dispensing, administering, or monitoring.[14]

In high-risk populations, CPOE reduces medication errors. In children, CPOE with substantive decision support reduced ADEs (including medication errors) and potential ADEs in an inpatient pediatrics ward.[45] It also decreased the rate of nonintercepted medication errors by 7% although there was no change in the rate of patient harm.[59,119] In the NICU, CPOE eliminated all calculation errors as decision support included an automatic dosage calculator.[24] However, these decision support systems cannot improve human errors as a result of entering incorrect weights, incorrect units of weight (kilograms versus pounds), or medications entered on the wrong patient.[116] In geriatric medication errors, CPOE resulted in less potentially inappropriate medication prescribing through decision alerts, which led to a pharmacist call to the prescriber that offered alternative choices of medications if possible.[84] Decision support in CPOE also leads to too many alerts when orders are placed, causing alert fatigue and resulting in providers entering an answer to proceed past (or "blow-by") the alert without reading or comprehending the alert. A study reviewing an alert about critical drug–drug interactions with warfarin found that only 19% of providers and 9.7% of pharmacists responding appropriately to the alert and changed the medication order.[82] There is a commercially available software screening system to identify outlier prescribing errors not identified with other clinical decision support tools in CPOE. The outlier alerts would identify high dose, contraindications, and medications never prescribed to specific populations.[107]

Unit dose dispensing systems, usually in association with CPOE and barcoding of medications, reduced monthly errors from 5 to none in an inpatient setting.[39] The package sent from pharmacy is prepared to administer to a specific patient at the appropriate dose, eliminating the need for the nurse to draw up medications resulting in fewer errors. Other dispensing systems, like automated dispensing cabinets (ADCs), are also linked to CPOE, barcoding, and allow for a pharmacist to verify correct drug, correct dose, patient allergies, and use of the medication prior to a drug being dispensed from the cabinet. Theses ADCs can decrease dispensing errors. However, errors occur when using ADCs. One such problem, "drug override," occurs, particularly in an emergency situation or as a work-around. This allows a drug to be dispensed prior to pharmacist verification. Another error, look-alike medication errors, occurs because of the small screens on the ADCs. Errors also occur when the ADCs are stocked such that an incorrect drug is placed in an incorrect bin of the ADC.[41]

Use of barcoding for dispensing and administration of medication ensures that the correct drug is given to the intended patient at the dose intended. Barcoding significantly decreased the relative risk of targeted, preventable ADEs by 47% to 50% in an NICU.[87] The risk of opioid-related ADEs were also reduced when barcode medication administration was implemented.[86] This technique decreases the amount of time nurses spend administering medications in the ICU, allowing them to reallocate that time to other direct patient care activities.[31] As with all technology, new problems arise with the implementation of barcoding and can lead to errors. Such problems range from inability of the scanner to read the barcode on the medication or on the patient identification band, downtime processes, mismatch of barcodes due to new manufacturer barcode, or new or aging scanners, and many more.[32] For a summary of Information Technology, see Table 134-3.

SERVICE-BASED CLINICAL PHARMACISTS

Clinical pharmacists are now employed in high-risk areas such as the ICUs, the pediatrics services, and EDs to identify and prevent medication errors. In one ICU study, the input of a clinical pharmacist during rounds saved an estimated $270,000 annually in costs of rehospitalization due to ADEs.[74] The involvement of a clinical pharmacist in work rounds of an adult ICU reduced preventable ADEs by 66%.[74] The introduction of clinical pharmacists in pediatric services is credited with a 94% reduction of potential ADEs and medication errors.[59] In particular, the addition of pharmacists in the PICUs reduced the serious medication error rate by 80%.[60] Another study showed that pharmacists in 3 EDs identified 2,200 interventions with an estimated savings of $488,000. This savings came from lower-cost medications, reduced length of stay, and fewer readmissions.[103] Similarly a pharmacist reduced the error rate by 67% from 16 errors per 100 medication orders in the control group (without a pharmacist) to 5 errors per 100 medication orders in the intervention group (pharmacist present in the ED).[17] A recent study suggests that the availability of ED pharmacists has even more impact on reducing errors by their assistance for questions, discussion, and consultation rather than in the review of medication orders.[94] And, as previously discussed, hospital pharmacists are able to improve medication reconciliation across the continuum of care for patients.[65]

However, fiscal restrictions will inevitably mitigate against the expansion of service pharmacists as cost–benefit arguments will be applied. An unintended consequence of having a clinical pharmacist present is that nurses, residents, and attending physicians can defer to them and consequently spend less time developing and maintaining their own skills for off-hour periods when such help may not be available.

ROLE OF THE TOXICOLOGIST

Clinical and medical toxicologists are in a unique position to investigate causes and help decrease the incidence of both medication errors and ADEs in the institutions where they work. With their specialized knowledge and training in pharmacology, poisoning, and clinical medicine, both physicians and pharmacists with advanced training in toxicology also aid in the prediction, identification, and management of ADEs. Medical toxicologists should optimally be involved in Pharmacy and Therapeutics and Medication Safety committees (or related efforts) at their institutions. They should educate and collaborate with the providers at their hospitals with regard to means to reduce errors and encourage diligent reporting of medication errors to the hospital and the national databases such as MedWatch at the FDA. They should also encourage drug manufacturers to be diligent in alerting physicians with regard to identified problems.[2]

SUMMARY

- Medications are the principal commerce of modern medicine, and medication safety is of paramount importance to health care systems. The delivery of medications safely to patients is a complex process and is particularly important in pediatrics and geriatrics.
- Health care professionals should be aware of the reasons errors occur and how they are prevented in order to improve patient and medication safety.
- Information technology holds promise for significant improvement in medication safety. Focus should be on CPOE, barcoding, unit dose dispensing, avoidance of look-alike/sound-alike medications, and education.
- Use of clinical pharmacists and updated electronic-based literature should be encouraged.
- Communication and nonpunitive local and national reporting must be encouraged in order to learn from errors.
- Patient safety requires a collaborative effort particularly with the medication manufacturer, but also with federal regulation authorities, independent research organizations, error theorists, hospital administrators and managers, information technologists, nurses, cognitive psychologists, human factors ergonomists, and chronobiologists and all of the health care professionals involved in patient care.
- Clinical and medical toxicologists have a significant role in medication safety.

Acknowledgment

Patrick Crosskerry, MD, PhD, contributed to this chapter in previous editions.

REFERENCES

1. Agency for Healthcare Research and Quality. Lean Hospitals: Six Sigma and Lean Healthcare Forms. innovations.ahrq.gov/content.aspx?id=2148. Published 2008. Accessed May 1, 2014.
2. American College of Medical Toxicology. Medical Toxicologist Participation in Medication Management and Safety Systems. http://acmt.net/cgi/page.cgi/zine_service.html/aid=4129&zine=show. Published 2013. Accessed May 1, 2014.
3. American Geriatric Society 2015 Beers Criteria Update Expert Panel. American Geriatrics Society 2015 updated Beers Criteria for potentially inappropriate medication use in older adults. *J Am Geriatr Soc.* 2015;63:2227-2246.
4. American Society for Healthcare Risk Management. *Strategies and Tips of Maximizing Failure Mode Effects Analysis in Your Organization.* Chicago, IL: American Society for Healthcare Risk Management; 2002.
5. Anderson JE, et al. Restrictions on surgical resident shift length does not impact type of medical errors. *J Surg Res.* 2017;212:8-14.
6. Arnett RH 3rd, et al. National health expenditures 1988: Office of National Cost Estimates. *Health Care Finance Rev.* 1990;11:1-41.
7. Bates DW. Using information technology to reduce rates of medication errors in hospitals. *BMJ.* 2000;320:788-791.
8. Bates DW, et al. Relationship between medication errors and adverse drug events. *J Gen Intern Med.* 1995;10:199-205.
9. Bates DW, Gawande AA. Improving safety with information technology. *N Engl J Med.* 2003;348:2526-2534.
10. Bates DW, et al. Effect of computerized physician order entry and a team intervention on prevention of serious medication errors. *JAMA.* 1998;280:1311-1316.
11. Bates DW, et al. The costs of adverse drug events in hospitalized patients. Adverse Drug Events Prevention Study Group. *JAMA.* 1997;277:307-311.
12. Benjamin DM. Reducing medication errors and increasing patient safety: case studies in clinical pharmacology. *J Clin Pharmacol.* 2003;43:768-783.
13. Bernabei R, et al. Characteristics of the SAGE database: a new resource for research on outcomes in long-term care. SAGE (Systematic Assessment of Geriatric drug use via Epidemiology) Study Group. *J Gerontol A Biol Sci Med Sci.* 1999;54:M25-M33.
14. Bobb A, et al. The epidemiology of prescribing errors: the potential impact of computerized prescriber order entry. *Arch Intern Med.* 2004;164:785-792.
15. Bootman JL, et al. The health care cost of drug-related morbidity and mortality in nursing facilities. *Arch Intern Med.* 1997;157:2089-2096.
16. Brennan TA, et al. Incidence of adverse events and negligence in hospitalized patients. Results of the Harvard Medical Practice Study I. *N Engl J Med.* 1991;324:370-376.
17. Brown JN, et al. Effect of pharmacists on medication errors in an emergency department. *Am J Health Syst Pharm.* 2008;65:330-333.
18. Budnitz DS, et al. Emergency hospitalizations for adverse drug events in older Americans. *N Engl J Med.* 2011;365:2002-2012.
19. Budnitz DS, et al. Medication use leading to emergency department visits for adverse drug events in older adults. *Ann Intern Med.* 2007;147.755-765.
20. Budnitz DS, et al. National surveillance of emergency department visits for outpatient adverse drug events. *JAMA.* 2006;296:1858-1866.
21. Cimino JJ. Improving the electronic health record—are clinicians getting what they wished for? *JAMA.* 2013;309:991-992.
22. Classen D. Medication safety: moving from illusion to reality. *JAMA.* 2003;289:1154-1156.
23. Classen DC, et al. Adverse drug events in hospitalized patients. Excess length of stay, extra costs, and attributable mortality. *JAMA.* 1997;277:301-306.
24. Cordero L, et al. Impact of computerized physician order entry on clinical practice in a newborn intensive care unit. *J Perinatol.* 2004;24:88-93.
25. Cote CJ, et al. Is the "therapeutic orphan" about to be adopted? *Pediatrics.* 1996;98:118-123.
26. Croskerry P. The cognitive imperative: thinking about how we think. *Acad Emerg Med.* 2000;7:1223-1231.
27. Croskerry P. The importance of cognitive errors in diagnosis and strategies to minimize them. *Acad Med.* 2003;78:775-780.
28. Croskerry P, et al. Profiles in patient safety: medication errors in the emergency department. *Acad Emerg Med.* 2004;11:289-299.
29. Crowley E, et al. Medication errors in children: a descriptive summary of medication error reports submitted to the United States Pharmacopeia. *Curr Ther Res Clin Exp.* 2001;26:627-640.
30. Cunningham KJ. Analysis of clinical interventions and the impact of pediatric pharmacists on medication error prevention in a teaching hospital. *J Pediatr Pharmacol Ther.* 2012;17:365-373.
31. Dwibedi N, et al. Effect of bar-code-assisted medication administration on nurses' activities in an intensive care unit: a time-motion study. *Am J Health Syst Pharm.* 2011;68:1026-1031.
32. Early C, et al. Scanning for safety: an integrated approach to improved bar-code medication administration. *Comput Inform Nurs.* 2011;29:TC45-TC52.
33. Ernst FR, Grizzle AJ. Drug-related morbidity and mortality: updating the cost-of-illness model. *J Am Pharm Assoc (Wash).* 2001;41:192-199.
34. Fahrenkopf AM, et al. Rates of medication errors among depressed and burnt out residents: prospective cohort study. *BMJ.* 2008;336:488-491.
35. Folli HL, et al. Medication error prevention by clinical pharmacists in two children's hospitals. *Pediatrics.* 1987;79:718-722.
36. Fore AM, et al. Improving patient safety using the sterile cockpit principle during medication administration: a collaborative, unit-based project. *J Nurs Manag.* 2013;21:106-111.
37. Fortescue EB, et al. Prioritizing strategies for preventing medication errors and adverse drug events in pediatric inpatients. *Pediatrics.* 2003;111:722-729.
38. Furukawa MF, et al. Meaningful use of health information technology and declines in in-hospital adverse drug events. *J Am Med Inform Assoc.* 2017;24:729-736.
39. Gard JW, et al. Reducing antimicrobial dosing errors in a neonatal intensive care unit. *Am J Health Syst Pharm.* 1995;52:1508, 1512-1513.
40. Gleason KM, et al. Results of the Medications at Transitions and Clinical Handoffs (MATCH) study: an analysis of medication reconciliation errors and risk factors at hospital admission. *J Gen Intern Med.* 2010;25:441-447.
41. Grissinger M. Safeguards for using and designing automated dispensing cabinets. *P T.* 2012;37:490-530.
42. Gurwitz JH, et al. Incidence and preventability of adverse drug events in nursing homes. *Am J Med.* 2000;109:87-94.
43. Gurwitz JH, et al. Incidence and preventability of adverse drug events among older persons in the ambulatory setting. *JAMA.* 2003;289:1107-1116.
44. Hersh W. Health care information technology: progress and barriers. *JAMA.* 2004;292:2273-2274.
45. Holdsworth MT, et al. Impact of computerized prescriber order entry on the incidence of adverse drug events in pediatric inpatients. *Pediatrics.* 2007;120:1058-1066.
46. Hoyle JD Jr, et al. Pediatric prehospital medication dosing errors: a national survey of paramedics. *Prehosp Emerg Care.* 2017;21:185-191.

47. Hug BL, et al. The costs of adverse drug events in community hospitals. *Jt Comm J Qual Patient Saf.* 2012;38:120-126.

48. Hutchins LF, et al. Underrepresentation of patients 65 years of age or older in cancer-treatment trials. *N Engl J Med.* 1999;341:2061-2067.

49. Institute of Medicine. *Crossing the Quality Chasm: A New Health System for the 21st Century.* Washington, DC: National Academies Press; 2001.

50. Institute of Medicine. *Health IT and Patient Safety: Building Safer Systems for Better Care.* Washington, DC: National Academies Press; 2012.

51. Institute of Medicine. *Preventing Medication Errors: Quality Chasm Series.* Washington, DC: National Academies Press; 2007.

52. Institute of Medicine. *Resident Duty Hours: Enhancing Sleep, Supervision, and Safety.* Washington, DC: National Academies Press; 2009.

53. Institute of Medicine. *To Err Is Human: Building a Safer Health System.* Washington, DC: National Academies Press; 2000.

54. Institute of Safe Medication Practices. List of error-prone abbreviations, symbols, and dose designations. https://www.ismp.org/Tools/errorproneabbreviations.pdf. Published 2015. Accessed April 28, 2017.

55. Institute of Safe Medication Practices. ISMP Medication Safety Alert! *ISMP Medication Safety Alert!* April 19, 2000: 8.

56. Johnson JA, Bootman JL. Drug-related morbidity and mortality. A cost-of-illness model. *Arch Intern Med.* 1995;155:1949-1956.

57. Johnson KB, et al. Discharging patients with prescriptions instead of medications: sequelae in a teaching hospital. *Pediatrics.* 1996;97:481-485.

58. Kaushal R, et al. How can information technology improve patient safety and reduce medication errors in children's health care? *Arch Pediatr Adolesc Med.* 2001; 155:1002-1007.

59. Kaushal R, et al. Medication errors and adverse drug events in pediatric inpatients. *JAMA.* 2001;285:2114-2120.

60. Kaushal R, et al. Ward-based clinical pharmacists and serious medication errors in pediatric inpatients. Paper presented at Proceedings of the Annual Meeting of the National Academy of Health; June 28, 2003; Nashville, TN.

61. Kaushal R, et al. Pediatric medication errors: what do we know? What gaps remain? *Ambul Pediatr.* 2004;4:73-81.

62. Koppel R, et al. Role of computerized physician order entry systems in facilitating medication errors. *JAMA.* 2005;293:1197-1203.

63. Kozer E, et al. Variables associated with medication errors in pediatric emergency medicine. *Pediatrics.* 2002;110:737-742.

64. Kripalani S, et al. Effect of a pharmacist intervention on clinically important medication errors after hospital discharge: a randomized trial. *Ann Intern Med.* 2012;157:1-10.

65. Kwan JL. Medication reconciliation during transitions of care as a patient safety strategy: a systematic review. *Ann Intern Med.* 2013;158:397-403.

66. Landrigan CP, et al. Effect of reducing interns' work hours on serious medical errors in intensive care units. *N Engl J Med.* 2004;351:1838-1848.

67. Lapoint J, et al. Electronic pharmacopoeia: a missed opportunity for safe opioid use using electronic pharmacopeia. *J Med Toxicol.* 2014;10:15-18.

68. Lawes S, Grissinger M. Medication Errors Attributed to health information technology. *PA-PSRS Patient Saf Advis.* 2017;14:1-8.

69. Lazarou J, et al. Incidence of adverse drug reactions in hospitalized patients: a meta-analysis of prospective studies. *JAMA.* 1998;279:1200-1205.

70. Lean Hospitals. Bringing lean to healthcare. www.leanhospitals.org/downloads.php. Accessed May 1, 2014.

71. Leape LL. Error in medicine. *JAMA.* 1994;272:1851-1857.

72. Leape LL, et al. Systems analysis of adverse drug events. ADE Prevention Study Group. *JAMA.* 1995;274:35-43.

73. Leape LL, et al. The nature of adverse events in hospitalized patients. Results of the Harvard Medical Practice Study II. *N Engl J Med.* 1991;324:377-384.

74. Leape LL, et al. Pharmacist participation on physician rounds and adverse drug events in the intensive care unit. *JAMA.* 1999;282:267-270.

75. Lesar TS, et al. Factors related to errors in medication prescribing. *JAMA.* 1997;277:312-317.

76. Luten R, et al. Managing the unique size-related issues of pediatric resuscitation: reducing cognitive load with resuscitation aids. *Acad Emerg Med.* 2002;9:840-847.

77. Lykowski G, Mahoney D. Computerized provider order entry improves workflow and outcomes. *Nurs Manage.* 2004;35:40G–H.

78. Makary MA, Daniel M. Medical error—the third leading cause of death. *BMJ.* 2016;351:i2139.

79. Marcin JP, et al. Medication errors among acutely ill and injured children treated in rural emergency departments. *Ann Emerg Med.* 2007;50:361-367, 367.e1–367.e2.

80. Marino BL, et al. Prevalence of errors in a pediatric hospital medication system: implications for error proofing. *Outcomes Manag Nurs Pract.* 2000;4:129-135.

81. McErlean MA, et al. Home antipyretic use in children brought to the emergency department. *Pediatr Emerg Care.* 2001;17:249-251.

82. Miller AM, et al. Provider and pharmacist responses to warfarin drug-drug interaction alerts: a study of healthcare downstream of CPOE alerts. *J Am Med Inform Assoc.* 2011;18(suppl 1):i45-i50.

83. Milos V, et al. Improving the quality of pharmacotherapy in elderly primary care patients through medication reviews: a randomised controlled study. *Drugs Aging.* 2013;30:235-246.

84. Monane M, et al. Improving prescribing patterns for the elderly through an online drug utilization review intervention: a system linking the physician, pharmacist, and computer. *JAMA.* 1998;280:1249-1252.

85. Moore TJ, et al. Serious adverse drug events reported to the Food and Drug Administration, 1998-2005. *Arch Intern Med.* 2007;167:1752-1759.

86. Morriss FH Jr, et al. Risk of adverse drug events in neonates treated with opioids and the effect of a bar-code-assisted medication administration system. *Am J Health Syst Pharm.* 2011;68:57-62.

87. Morriss FH Jr, et al. Effectiveness of a barcode medication administration system in reducing preventable adverse drug events in a neonatal intensive care unit: a prospective cohort study. *J Pediatr.* 2009;154:363-368, 368.e1.

88. Mowry JB, et al. 2015 Annual Report of the American Association of Poison Control Centers' National Poison Data System (NPDS): 33rd Annual Report. *Clin Toxicol.* 2016;54:924-1109.

89. National Coordinating Council for Medication Error Reporting and Prevention. About medication errors: medication error category index. http://www.nccmerp.org/medError CatIndex.html. Accessed May 1, 2014.

90. National Patient Safety Foundation. Call to action: preventable healthcare harm is a public health crisis and patient safety requires a coordinated public health response. http://www.npsf.org/page/public_health_crisis. Accessed July 20, 2017.

91. Nelson LS, et al. The benefit of houseofficer education on proper medication dose calculation and ordering. *Acad Emerg Med.* 2000;7:1311-1316.

92. O'Mahony D, et al. STOPP/START criteria for potentially inappropriate prescribing in older adults. Version 2. *Age Ageing.* 2015;44:213-218.

93. Opondo D, et al. Inappropriateness of medication prescriptions to elderly patients in the primary care setting: a systematic review. *PLoS One.* 2012;7:e43617.

94. Patanwala AE, et al. Severity and probability of harm of medication errors intercepted by an emergency department pharmacist. *Int J Pharm Pract.* 2011;19:358-362.

95. Patanwala AE, et al. A prospective observational study of medication errors in a tertiary care emergency department. *Ann Emerg Med.* 2010;55:522-526.

96. Peth HA Jr. Medication errors in the emergency department: a systems approach to minimizing risk. *Emerg Med Clin North Am.* 2003;21:141-158.

97. Pevnick JM, et al. The problem with medication reconciliation. *BMJ Qual Saf.* 2016;25:726-730.

98. Phillips DP, et al. A steep increase in domestic fatal medication errors with use of alcohol and/or street drugs. *Arch Intern Med.* 2008;168:1561-1566.

99. Pharmacist's Letter Detail-Document, STARTing and STOPPing Medications in the Elderly. Pharmacist's Letter/Prescriber's Letter. September 2011.

100. Poudel DR, et al. Burden of hospitalizations related to adverse drug events in the USA: a retrospective analysis from large inpatient database. *Pharmacoepidemiol Drug Saf.* 2017;26:635-641.

101. Reason J. *Human Error.* New York, NY: Cambridge University Press; 1990.

102. Relihan E, et al. The impact of a set of interventions to reduce interruptions and distractions to nurses during medication administration. *Qual Saf Health Care.* 2010;19:e52.

103. Runy LA. Emergency department. Pharmacists in the ED help reduce errors. *Hosp Health Netw.* 2008;82:12, 14.

104. Russell FM, et al. Evidence on the use of paracetamol in febrile children. *Bull World Health Organ.* 2003;81:367-372.

105. Santell JP, et al. Medication errors: experience of the United States Pharmacopeia (USP) MEDMARX reporting system. *J Clin Pharmacol.* 2003;43:760-767.

106. Schiff GD, et al. Linking laboratory and pharmacy: opportunities for reducing errors and improving care. *Arch Intern Med.* 2003;163:893-900.

107. Schiff GD, et al. Screening for medication errors using an outlier detection system. *J Am Med Inform Assoc.* 2017;24:281-287.

108. Seden K, et al. Cross-sectional study of prescribing errors in patients admitted to nine hospitals across North West England. *BMJ Open.* 2013;3.

109. Seifert SA, Jacobitz K. Pharmacy prescription dispensing errors reported to a regional poison control center. *J Toxicol Clin Toxicol.* 2002;40:919-923.

110. Shaw KN, et al. Reported medication events in a paediatric emergency research network: sharing to improve patient safety. *Emerg Med J.* 2013;30:815-819.

111. Shehab N, et al. US emergency department visits for outpatient adverse drug events 2013-14. *JAMA.* 2016;316:2115-2125.

112. Shojania KG, et al. Effect of point-of-care computer reminders on physician behaviour: a systematic review. *CMAJ.* 2010;182:E216-E225.

113. Simon SR, et al. Potentially inappropriate medication use by elderly persons in U.S. Health Maintenance Organizations, 2000-2001. *J Am Geriatr Soc.* 2005;53:227-232.

114. Stucky ER. Prevention of medication errors in the pediatric inpatient setting. *Pediatrics.* 2003;112:431-436.

115. The Joint Commission. *National Patient Safety Goal #2: Communication Prohibited Abbreviations. Joint Commission on Accreditation of Healthcare Organizations,* 2004.

116. Villamañán E, et al. Potential medication errors associated with computer prescriber order entry. *Int J Clin Pharm.* 2013;35:577-583.

117. Vincent C, et al. How to investigate and analyse clinical incidents: clinical risk unit and association of litigation and risk management protocol. *BMJ.* 2000;320:777-781.

118. Wald H, Shojania K. Root cause analysis. In: Shojania KG, et al., eds. *Making Healthcare Safer: A Critical Analysis of Patient Safety Practices. Evidence Report/Technology Assessment No. 43.* University of California at San Francisco–Stanford Evidence-Based Practice Center; 2001:51-56.

119. Walsh KE, et al. Effect of computer order entry on prevention of serious medication errors in hospitalized children. *Pediatrics.* 2008;121:e421-e427.

120. Walson PD, et al. Prescription writing in a pediatric clinic. *Pediatr Pharmacol (New York).* 1981;1:239-244.

121. Wears RL, Berg M. Computer technology and clinical work: still waiting for Godot. *JAMA.* 2005;293:1261-1263.

122. Weingart SN, et al. Patient-reported medication symptoms in primary care. *Arch Intern Med.* 2005;165:234-240.

123. Wheeler DW, et al. Calculation of doses of drugs in solution: are medical students confused by different means of expressing drug concentrations? *Drug Saf.* 2004;27: 729-734.

124. Williamson J, Chopin JM. Adverse reactions to prescribed drugs in the elderly: a multi-centre investigation. *Age Ageing.* 1980;9:73-80.

125. Yasnoff WA, et al. Putting health IT on the path to success. *JAMA.* 2013;309:989-990.

126. Zidel TG. A lean toolbox—using lean principles and techniques in healthcare. *J Healthc Qual.* 2006;28:w1-7-w1-15.

135

DRUG DEVELOPMENT, ADVERSE DRUG EVENTS, AND POSTMARKETING SURVEILLANCE

Louis R. Cantilena*

This chapter will focus on drug-induced diseases that occur as expected or unexpected adverse drug events (ADEs), as a drug–drug interaction or an ADE causing an untoward drug–disease interaction. Also included in this chapter is a brief overview of the drug development process in the United States and specific aspects of the process that relate to the development of antidotes. In addition, a discussion of an approach to the diagnosis of drug-induced disease, monitoring of drug safety postapproval, and the suggested role for the clinical and medical toxicologists in the discovery, reporting, and prevention of ADEs.

Adverse drug events are defined as untoward effects or outcomes associated with use of any dose of a drug whereas an adverse drug reaction refers to harm from a therapeutic dose. In this chapter, the word "drug" will be used for a pharmaceutical product and includes prescription and nonprescription medications, and dietary supplements.

In the United States, all new prescription and nonprescription medications must be shown to be both safe and effective in order to achieve approval by the US Food and Drug Administration (FDA), a prerequisite for marketing and sale. Dietary supplements fall outside of this legal requirement (Chap. 43) and are regulated under the Dietary Supplement Health and Education Act of 1994 (DSHEA).

HISTORY OF THE US DRUG APPROVAL PROCESS

The evolution of drug product regulation in the United States has for the most part, been reactionary; that is, most drug regulations were created in response to medicine-related disasters at various times in our history. Prior to 1900, there was no requirement for a drug or medical device manufacturer to demonstrate that the product actually worked (efficacy), was safe when used as directed, or was made to be within precise manufacturing specifications. In addition, no laws existed that required labeled claims on marketed drug products to be proven valid. Any product could be sold as a company desired and it was left to the consumer or health care professional to determine if the products actually worked and were safe. Initiation of medicinal product regulation and the overall evolution of the US drug law and regulations are closely linked to specific medical product disasters that occurred during the 20th century in the United States. Relatively recent changes in US drug approval law further changed drug review timelines and FDA prioritization of drug application reviews. Most recently, specific incentives to encourage the development of new antimicrobials and novel therapeutics that impart a significant improvement in the effectiveness or safety of drug treatment compared to existing or the current standard of care for the condition have been included in provisions of the FDA authorization legislation.[28] These incentives include extended patent protection or a shortened FDA review timetable that comes with priority review designation.

Examples of the pre-1900—or preregulation—marketed products include aspirin containing heroin sold as cough syrup and wine with cocaine to enhance sales of the alcoholic beverage. There was no legal requirement for systematic testing of products to determine content or the presence of possible adulterants in product formulations. **The Pure Food and Drug Act of 1906** required pharmaceutical manufacturers to meet a standard for the concentration and purity of the drugs they marketed. However, the burden of proof was on the FDA to show that the drug was incorrectly labeled or that the advertising or label was false or misleading. To a large extent this is the current regulatory state for dietary supplements.

The Food, Drug, and Cosmetic Act of 1938 resulted from a tragedy in which more than 100 patients (mostly children) died from poisoning by an excipient used in an oral solution of sulfanilamide, an antibiotic. The Massengil pharmaceutical company added the solvent diethylene glycol to the formulation in an attempt to improve the palatability of a pediatric formulation of a sulfanilamide. Diethylene glycol is a sweet-tasting, but nephrotoxic and neurotoxic hydrocarbon (Special Considerations: SC9). Only after almost a full year of marketing were cases of kidney failure and death reported in sufficient numbers to alert authorities to the extremely toxic nature of the product. The Food, Drug, and Cosmetic Act of 1938 was the result of this medical product disaster and accomplished the following:

- Required companies to list the ingredients on each product label
- Required companies to provide the known risks concerning use of the product to physicians or pharmacists
- Made illegal the misbranding of food or medical products
- For the first time, required companies to test their products for safety before being sold.
- Drugs already marketed before 1938 were exempt from the requirement (Chap. 1).

The Kefauver-Harris Amendments to the Food and Drug Act of 1962 resulted from a drug approval disaster that occurred in Europe and not in the United States. An application in the early 1960s for the approval of thalidomide, a sedative-hypnotic already marketed in Europe at the time, was submitted to the FDA for review and approval. The sedative-hypnotic had a rapid onset and short duration of action, did not affect ventilation, did not cause a morning-after effect, and was inexpensive. Dr Frances Kelsey, a medical officer at the FDA, delayed approval by asking the sponsor to clarify several issues in the reportedly poorly organized new drug application (NDA). In the interim, an unusual teratogenic effect, phocomelia, or limb misdevelopment, was linked to the use of thalidomide in Europe. Congressional hearings on the "almost" approval for marketing in the United States resulted in the **Kefauver-Harris Act of 1962**, which required a drug manufacturer or sponsor to do the following:

- File an investigational new drug (IND) application prior to initiating a clinical study with a drug in humans
- Demonstrate that the drug was effective for the condition that it was being marketed to treat
- Provide adequate directions for safe usage of the drug

The act was not retroactive and drugs that were already on the market were exempt from these new requirements. However, the Waxman-Hatch Act of 1983, among other things, incentivized companies to establish evidence in support of actual indications for an exempt drug. The effects of this incentivization were demonstrated when a small pharmaceutical company studied the use of colchicine in gout, which the company applied for, and subsequently received exclusivity, leading to a 50-fold increase in the price of this ancient drug.[17]

Subsequent US food and drug laws that have primarily affected FDA review and approval of products include the following:

- **The Orphan Drug Act of 1983:** The act provides financial incentives to drug manufacturers to develop drugs for the treatment of rare diseases and conditions.[19] A rare disease is defined as one in which there are

---

*Dr. Cantilena completed work on the chapter shortly before his tragic death.

fewer than 200,000 affected persons in the United States, or one affecting more people, but in which the cost of drug development is likely to exceed any potential sales of the drug. Overall, the Orphan Drug Act has been very successful. As of early 2016, there were 596 approved orphan drugs in the United States, treating approximately 200 rare diseases. In 2016 alone, 9 orphan drugs were approved, which represents 41% of all drugs approved by the FDA in that year. Drug approval via orphan drug designation is incorporated for the approval of antidotes for poisoning. For example, 2 chelators, insoluble Prussian blue and pentetate calcium trisodium, were approved under orphan drug regulations in 2003 and 2004, respectively, for the treatment of exposure to radioactive heavy metals (Antidotes in Depth: A31 and A45). The level of evidence required for efficacy for orphan approval is similar to that required for non-orphan agents but often the type of evidence incorporated in approval decisions is diverse because of the rarity of the respective conditions and/or the ethical barriers to conducting a prospective study. Particularly applicable to the practice of medical toxicology, especially involving making the diagnosis of drug-induced disease, is the fact that the safety database for orphan pathway–approved drugs at the time of product approval is significantly less than that for standard NDAs. The relevance of that is that fewer human exposures, or exposure of the drug candidate to only healthy volunteers, prior to approval could result in the inability to detect less commonly occurring ADEs before marketing. When this occurs, the FDA can require specific postmarketing studies and/or registries of patients who are given the drug therapeutically.

- **The Prescription Drug User Fee Act (PDUFA) of 1992:** The Act requires that manufacturers pay user fees to the FDA for NDAs and regulatory supplements to enable the FDA to hire additional reviewers and accelerate the review process. This Act, which has undergone several revisions (the latest in 2017, covering the FDA until 2022), was originally considered by some to be controversial because of the new working relationships created between industry and regulators, and the concern that it may lead to compromises that are not in the best interest of public health.

- Based on the number of safety-related drug withdrawals from the US market, there does not appear to be evidence of a negative effect of public health safety since the enactment of the PDUFA legislations. An early comparison of review times over the first 4 PDUFA authorizations did not find a substantial improvement in FDA review times.[12] Compared with European Medicines Agency (EMA) and Health Canada—the analogous agencies to FDA in those regions—the FDA already had, and has maintained, significantly shorter review times over the past decade.[12] A more recent review shows that FDA has maintained its advantage for regular reviews submitted through 2010, over the European Medicines Agency (EMA) and the Swissmedic agency.[11] Additionally, although some believe that the shorter review times for FDA approval appear to be associated with an increased likelihood of drug withdrawal and black box label modification of the drug label postapproval,[4,6] others do not concur.[11] The debate on this issue intensified during the controversy involving the cyclooxygenase-2 (COX-2) inhibitor antiinflammatory drugs. This widely publicized withdrawal and press coverage of the related litigation resulted in congressional hearings on the review practices and monitoring of drug safety by the FDA. The legislation evolved to attempt to provide FDA with regulatory authority, adequate funding, and to encourage scientific exchange between the FDA and sponsors of drug products during the drug development process with the goal of improved quality and efficiency of the development process. The sixth reauthorization of the FDA covering the period of 2018 (PDUFA VI, also known as the 21st Century Cures Act, to 2022) was signed into law in late 2016 and is further discussed later in this section.

- **The Dietary Supplement Health and Education Act (DSHEA amendment) of 1994:** The Act removed from FDA the authority to require proof of safety or efficacy prior to marketing of products considered dietary supplements (including herbal remedies). Only when the manufacturer of a product makes a specific health claim, such as "treats congestive heart failure," does the FDA have premarketing approval authority. That is, the use of structure or function claims, such as "supports heart function," obviates the need for FDA approval. Furthermore, rather than placing the burden of proof on the manufacturers for safety and efficacy of a product, the FDA is required to determine that a product is unsafe to prevent sale and distribution in the United States. Few dietary supplements have reached the benchmark of premarketing rigorous proof of efficacy and safety of their product.

- **The FDA Modernization Act of 1997:** In addition to reauthorizing the FDA, this bill put in place mechanisms to improved communication and collaboration between FDA and pharmaceutical sponsors, enhancing label information for practitioners and consumers, as well as allowing FDA to utilize an accelerated drug approval process for the treatment of life-threatening illnesses such as AIDS and cancer if the drug has the potential to address medical needs unmet by currently available drugs. Many of the accelerated drug approvals rely on efficacy results derived from surrogate markers linked to the ultimate indication for the drug. For example, the protease inhibitors were approved on the accelerated track for the treatment of AIDS based on their demonstrated ability to reduce HIV viral load in preapproval clinical studies. Although practical and ultimately useful, subsequent legislation such as the Food and Drug Administration Safety and Innovation Act (FDASIA) refined this process to ensure that confirmatory clinical studies were, in fact, completed in a timely manner by a sponsor of a product approved under the accelerated process.

- **The Animal Efficacy Rule (Animal Rule) in 2002:** The FDA enacted a regulation that allows sponsors to reach approval of some products based on safety testing in humans and efficacy testing in animals.[18] This rule is intended to allow FDA to approve products for serious or life-threatening conditions caused by exposure to lethal or permanently disabling toxic biologic, chemical, radiologic, or nuclear substances. For the indications of treatment of chemical, biologic, or radiologic mass poisonings, such as could be expected in a terrorist attack, testing for efficacy would not be possible for obvious ethical or, in the event of an infectious outbreak, for logistical reasons. The Animal Rule allows the sponsor to establish product efficacy in a validated animal model and then provide human safety data, preapproval in healthy human volunteers. The human safety data would obviously involve administration of therapeutic dosages of the chemical/biologic/radiologic drug in the absence of the poisoning. The sponsor would also be expected to perform a field study post approval, in the event that the indicated exposure occurs naturally for an infectious disease or during an attack.

- **The Pediatric Research Equity Act of 2003:** The Act requires manufacturers to study drugs being submitted for approval for a claimed indication in children. The FDA provides incentives such as patent extension and marketing exclusivity for performing these evaluations. As a result, more data from children are being provided to guide therapeutic use of medications in this patient group, at the expense of allowances for marketing exclusivity to those manufacturers who provide such data.[19]

- **The Food and Drug Administration Amendments Act (FDAAA) of 2007:** This act increased FDA responsibilities and authorizations primarily aimed at improving product safety.[2] Specified deadlines for drug application reviews were added as well as the creation of a priority for FDA review based on indication and potential benefit of the candidate drug for a disease population. Four of the provisions of FDAAA reauthorize past legislation: PDUFA, the Medical Device User Fee Amendments of 2007 (MDUFA), the Pediatric Research Equity Act of 2007 (PREA), and the Best Pharmaceuticals for Children Act of 2007 (BPCA). The Food and Drug Administration Amendments Act gives authorization to FDA to require postmarketing studies, primarily of drug safety, including surveillance and clinical trials, as well as the requirement that sponsors incorporate Risk Evaluation and Mitigation Strategies (REMS) in their proposed marketing activities as a prerequisite for product approval. Risk Evaluation and Mitigation Strategies are a mechanism to allow FDA to require proactive risk surveillance for newly approved products or those in which significant safety signals are detected. The elements of REMS vary considerably among products, and may be applied to both safety concerns and the potential for misuse, as in the case of prescription opioids.[26,49]

Within this FDA reauthorization was a mandate to take the initial steps to set up an active surveillance system utilizing health care claims databases to detect post-approval signals of ADEs. This was called the Mini-Sentinel Pilot Program, which aimed to establish contractual and organizational relationships that could lead to an effective active drug safety surveillance system. The Sentinel program is further discussed below.

The Food and Drug Administration Amendments Act also included a requirement for FDA to ensure that clinical trial information is provided to the National Institute of Health's www.ClinicalTrials.gov web site. Initially there was poor overall compliance with reporting and a significant time lag before most trials were reported into the system.[38] A more recent analysis of ClinicalTrials.gov data, examining the trials completed from 2008 through August, 2012 continues to show poor overall reporting compliance. Industry-funded clinical trials, with FDA oversight demonstrated higher reporting compliance and a shorter time lag compared to NIH-funded, academic studies.[1]

Drug shortages, which have been present for decades, reached crisis levels in 2010. The reasons are multifactorial, but coincide with a time when an empowered FDA began enforcing high manufacturing standards at production sites around the nation and the world.[25] Although some of the concerns leading to plant closure were not associated with patient harm, the proactive stance primarily affected generic drug manufacturers,[7] initially mainly those producing oncology drugs that were unable or unwilling to respond to standard regulations. The shortage of important drugs had significant medical and ethical consequences including delays in care and medication errors. Furthermore, economic consequences of the use of more expensive (and potentially less effective) alternative drugs and development of a "gray" market led to higher costs.[44] Some health systems turned to compounding pharmacies, which were largely unregulated. As this practice grew, new concerns such as interstate transport of compounded medications and safety risks from lax oversight became prominent.[13] This came to light with the highly publicized fungal meningitis outbreak at a compounding facility in Massachusetts ultimately resulting in 64 deaths and significant injury to more than 700 patients given intrathecal corticosteroids that were prepared in this facility.[5]

- **The FDASIA again reauthorized PDUFA (then PDUFA V) in 2012:**[42] This law included 2 noteworthy new FDA responsibilities and authorizations: the establishment of a user fee requirement for generic drugs and for biosimilar (generic-like) biologic products similar to what is called the innovator product for drugs, and a new category of drug application designation called the "breakthrough therapy" designation. The breakthrough designation allows FDA to collaboratively assist drug developers in an expedited review and approval process of a product application when there is preliminary clinical evidence that shows the drug may be a substantial improvement over existing therapies for treatment of patients with serious or life-threatening diseases.[44] Other new initiatives include an active effort to include patient groups representative of the affected populations in the overall FDA review processes and some yet to be determined measures to enhance the safety of the drug supply chain. This act allowed FDA to better regulate foreign drug manufacturing facilities to help alleviate shortages, and to require pharmaceutical companies to make the FDA aware of impending drug shortages. In addition, the provisions of the BCPA and PREA were made permanent.
- **PDUFA VI, also known as the 21st Century Cures Act:** The sixth reauthorization of the FDA covering the period of 2018 to 2022 was signed into law in 2016. Some areas that will likely be emphasized with the

implementation of PDUFA VI include early and further communication between FDA review staff and drug sponsors on priority reviews as well as further development and emphasis on postmarketing drug safety systems and reporting requirements for sponsors. In addition, expanding and making the FDA Sentinel system (see below) for medical product safety surveillance fully operational will likely be brought forward during PDUFA VI, beginning in 2018.

A complete listing of FDA regulatory milestones and drug law history of the FDA is found on the FDA website.[17]

THE DRUG DEVELOPMENT PROCESS

Figure 135–1 is a schematic overview of the process for drug development of a new molecular entity (NME). The process begins with the preclinical evaluation of the candidate drug. During this evaluation, preclinical toxicologic testing is performed in more than one animal species, and other testing includes product stability, assurance that good manufacturing methods are being followed, drug purity, and potential carcinogenicity. Exposure–response relationships for efficacy and nonclinical safety in animal models as well as in vitro receptor binding or surrogate marker effects are often determined at this phase of the evaluation. Generally, for small-molecule (ie, nonbiologic) drugs, the metabolism of the drug in animal and in vitro human systems is determined. Following this preclinical testing, the sponsor submits an IND application to the FDA for approval to initiate human testing. This application contains all relevant data concerning animal and in vitro toxicology testing, product manufacturing and purity, and the clinical protocol for using the drug in the initial human investigation. Within 30 days, the FDA must review the IND application and either allow the proposed human study to proceed or inform the sponsor that additional data or preclinical (eg, animal) study is required before clinical testing of the candidate drug can begin.

The clinical study of new candidate drugs is divided into 4 basic phases.

Phase 1 clinical testing involves a relatively small number of participants with the primary aim of determining the safety and toxicity of the drug. In addition, phase 1 studies will also determine the human pharmacokinetics and metabolism of the drug. Phase 1 studies are normally conducted in 20 to 100 healthy volunteer participants, with the notable exception of phase 1 studies for cancer chemotherapeutics, which enroll only patients with cancer.

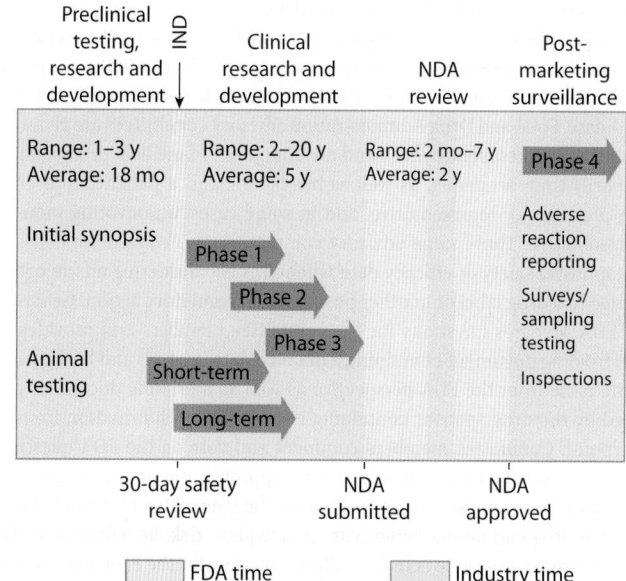

New drug development timeline

| Preclinical testing, research and development | IND | Clinical research and development | NDA review | Post-marketing surveillance |

Range: 1–3 y / Average: 18 mo | Range: 2–20 y / Average: 5 y | Range: 2 mo–7 y / Average: 2 y | Phase 4

Initial synopsis — Phase 1 — Phase 2 — Phase 3

Animal testing — Short-term — Long-term

Adverse reaction reporting / Surveys/sampling testing / Inspections

30-day safety review | NDA submitted | NDA approved

FDA time   Industry time

FIGURE 135–1. Schematic representation of new drug development. FDA = US Food and Drug Administration; IND = Investigational New Drug; NDA = New Drug Application. *(Reproduced with permission from U.S. Food and Drug Administration. U.S. Department of Health and Human Services. www.fda.gov.)*

Phase 2 clinical testing is designed to determine the potential efficacy of the drug candidate in humans, usually at varying levels of exposure to the drug candidate. In this phase, approximately 100 to 300 participants are usually studied. In phase 2 clinical trials, participants generally have the diseases for which the drug is intended or are capable of demonstrating the appropriate, validated, biologic surrogate marker to indicate a meaningful response to the drug. An example of this would be when a drug intended for early treatment of acute coronary syndrome is tested to show that it can inhibit in vivo platelet function after oral dosing in human study participants. In addition to confirming that the drug has the desired effect on the disease state or target disease marker, this phase explores the exposure–response relationships of the candidate drug and metabolites to observed effects in patients. Once the exposure–response relationships are identified, dose selection for phase 3 studies is determined, which is another goal of the phase 2 program. In general, phase 2a studies enroll patients with a mild, or early, form of the disease to limit potential confounding factors that exist in more severe or advance stages of the disease process. Phase 2b studies, in general, focus on patients with a more advanced disease condition, and with the knowledge derived from phase 2a, test doses of the drug candidate that are likely to produce a range of exposures that will further define the target patient exposure of the drug for the phase 3 studies.

Phase 3 clinical drug studies usually involve large-scale clinical trials in the actual, or close-to-the actual patient population for whom the drug is intended. Typically, this phase of drug development will involve testing a treatment cohort versus a control treatment of several hundred to several thousand patients who have the target disease, depending on both the prevalence of the disease and effectiveness of the drug. In some cases, an active comparator is used instead of placebo or in addition to placebo in a 3-arm study depending on the indication. The primary goal of phase 3 studies is to determine the safety and efficacy of the candidate drug in a patient population close to the actual intended patient population in question, under conditions similar to the anticipated medical use. At the completion of phase 3, an NDA or, in the case of a biologic product, a Biologics License Application (BLA) (request for approval to market) is submitted to the FDA. A drug candidate completing phases 1, 2, and 3 can thus be approved for marketing after study in only 2,000 to 4,000 patients. In the setting of a fast-track approval or under the Orphan Drug regulations, substantially fewer patients will receive the drug before its approval for marketing. The relatively small number of human exposures to a new chemical or biologic entity prior to approval for marketing is an important factor that limits the sensitivity of the drug approval process to detect uncommon ADEs.

Toward the end of the review cycle of an NDA, the FDA often seeks the external advice of its constituted advisory committees prior to their approval decision, especially in the setting of an uncertain risk–benefit profile of a drug candidate. Food and Drug Administration advisory committees are generally organized by therapeutic areas and are composed of medical professionals, primarily from academia, as well as biostatisticians, a patient representative, a consumer representative, and in some cases, a nonvoting industry representative. These same advisory committees also convene to consider postapproval safety or efficacy data when FDA is considering an important change to a drug label or another postapproval regulatory action. Generally, the FDA prepares questions for the committee members and provides an FDA briefing document containing a detailed data analysis and background of the issue from the FDA perspective as well as a briefing document prepared by the drug sponsor containing corresponding information from its viewpoint. Committee members comment and vote on the FDA questions during the proceedings. For a new drug approval, one question generally includes a yes or no answer as to whether the committee member believes that the drug can be marketed with an adequate risk–benefit profile. The advisory committee vote is technically nonbinding for the FDA, but the FDA generally follows the advice of the committee. An issue of concern is the fact that some members of FDA advisory committees with perceived conflicts of interest (COI) are granted waivers by FDA to participate in the proceedings.[32] The appearance of conflict of interest on an advisory committee can have

a significant impact on the drug approval process, and the FDA has begun to decrease the number of committee member waivers granted. To limit potential conflicts of interest, the FDA implements a rigorous financial COI screening procedure to limit negative perception of the process. The potential unintended consequence of the elimination or minimization of waivers for committee members to participate in a meeting is that, for some highly specialized medical indications, there are few experts in the country with in-depth knowledge of the condition who may have worked on a study that is being used in the NDA, thus limiting the essential experience and expertise of the committee.

After the NDA or BLA review process and, at times, following an advisory committee meeting about the application, the FDA may issue an approval for marketing the new drug or biological agent. There are certain NDA or BLA applications to FDA that qualify for expedited regulatory pathways such as accelerated approval where conditional approval is granted with the expectation that confirmatory evidence (eg, postapproval clinical trial) will be forthcoming within a specific time. In this case, should the confirmatory trial be unsuccessful, FDA approval is withdrawn. Normal approval for marketing of a drug or biologic agent, granted by the FDA, however, marks the transition point between phase 3 and phase 4 of drug development as discussed separately below.

Phase 4 of the Drug Development Is the Postmarketing Surveillance

Every drug or biologic agent or medical device carries with it some potential risk. If society required that only "completely" safe drugs could be marketed, the drug approval process would likely take decades and few if any new drugs would be made available. The individual and societal cost of adverse drug events, in terms of patient morbidity and mortality is well appreciated. Therefore, the FDA and the pharmaceutical industry must significantly rely on postmarketing surveillance to detect meaningful safety signals associated with the use of a medical product after approval.

The postmarketing surveillance system of the FDA began in the late 1950s after the discovery of cases of aplastic anemia due to chloramphenicol.[14] The process expanded and in 1962 when it became more formalized the drug industry was required for the first time to report ADEs to the FDA. In 1993, the FDA introduced the **MedWatch** system for adverse event reporting. This widely publicized rollout aimed to encourage reporting of ADEs and to simplify the process overall. This system relies on spontaneous reports by health care professionals or patients regarding the occurrence of deleterious effects associated with the use of a medical product. By its nature, this system is passive surveillance. MedWatch reporting to the FDA can be accomplished online, by fax or by telephone. The next important step by the FDA in postapproval monitoring of drug safety came with the passage of the 2007 FDA reauthorization (FDAAA) that included several safety-focused components. The ADE reporting requirements for sponsors became more rigorous, an enabling mechanism for making safety-related changes to the drug label was provided, risk evaluation and mitigation strategies (REMS) surrounding drug approvals were introduced, and the initiation of an active postmarketing risk identification system known as the FDA Sentinel Initiative occurred, which is discussed briefly below.

The FDA postmarketing surveillance system is in place to monitor postapproval drug safety and is intended to detect signals of unanticipated or previously unrecognized adverse events or to identify an at-risk population in whom the safety profile differs from that which was expected based on data collected prior to marketing. Individual pharmaceutical manufacturers are responsible for monitoring the safety of their marketed products and to regularly report any detected ADEs to the FDA. All ADEs reported to the FDA become part of the **FDA Adverse Event Reporting System (FAERS).**[16] The FAERS ADEs database is fully computerized and searchable and contains adverse event reports from human drug and biologic products and medical devices. The data set is made up of sponsor-reported ADEs and MedWatch ADE reports from patients, consumers, physicians, and other health care providers. Approximately 95% of reports in FAERS come from the mandatory reporting from pharmaceutical manufacturers. Since 1969, more than

10 million reports have been filed into FAERS, although since 2013, the FDA has received more than 1 million cases per calendar year into this database (personal communication, Dr Robert Ball, FDA, March 22, 2017).

Because the MedWatch system is passive in nature, the overall rate for spontaneous adverse event reporting is estimated at only 1% to 10%. Despite this, the number of serious adverse events reported to MedWatch continues to increase,[35] although the quality and rigor of the reports are limited.[22] Improved attitudes toward reporting, perhaps due to an appreciation of the risk of error and adverse drug effects, leads to better MedWatch reporting.[21]

The primary goals of the MedWatch system are the following:

- To increase awareness of drug- and device-induced disease.
- To clarify what should (and should not) be reported.
- To facilitate reporting of adverse effects by creating a single system for health professionals to use in reporting ADEs and drug, biologic, and device product problems.
- To provide regular feedback to the health care community about safety issues involving these products.[16]

Establishing causality is not required before submission of a MedWatch report. The FDA is primarily interested in the reporting of serious adverse events, or an ADE previously not associated with the medical product being administered or utilized, whether or not a causal relationship is established. Although any potential ADE should be reported, the FDA strongly encourages reporting of "serious" ADEs, which are events associated with a patient outcome that is one or more of the following:

- Death: If the death is suspected to be a direct result of the adverse event
- Life threatening: If the patient was at substantial risk of dying at the time of the adverse event or the use or continued use of the medical product would result in the patient's death (eg, gastrointestinal hemorrhage, bone marrow suppression, pacemaker failure, and infusion pump failure that permits uncontrolled free flow and results in excessive drug dosing)
- Hospitalization (initial or prolonged): If admission to the hospital or prolongation of a hospital stay resulted from the adverse event (eg, anaphylaxis, pseudomembranous colitis, bleeding that causes or prolongs hospitalization)
- Disability: If the adverse event resulted in a significant, persistent, or permanent change, impairment, damage, or disruption in the patient's body function/structure, physical activities, or quality of life (eg, cerebrovascular accidents caused by drug-induced coagulopathy, toxicity, peripheral neuropathy)
- Congenital anomaly: If there is a suspicion that exposure to a medical product before conception or during pregnancy resulted in an adverse effect on the child (eg, vaginal cancer in female offspring from maternal exposure to diethylstilbestrol during pregnancy or limb malformations in the offspring from thalidomide use during pregnancy)
- Requires intervention to prevent permanent impairment or damage if use of a medical product is suspected to result in a condition requiring medical or surgical intervention to preclude permanent impairment or damage to a patient (eg, acetaminophen overdose–induced hepatotoxicity requiring treatment with *N*-acetylcysteine to prevent permanent liver damage, burns from radiation equipment requiring drug therapy).

Health care professionals are given priority for review by the FDA in the MedWatch system. A well-documented case of a serious adverse event is a significant and useful contribution to the MedWatch system.

Reports of serious ADEs to the FDA or to the manufacturer can become an epidemiologically detectable signal that can trigger a more detailed investigation, several examples of which are provided later in this chapter. On occasion, serious ADEs detected in the AERS database have led to the withdrawal of products from the US market without conducting additional studies.

Currently, the MedWatch program is supported by more than 140 organizations, representing health care professionals and industry collaborating

as MedWatch Partners to help achieve these goals. These organizations include medical societies and organizations such as the American Medical Association (AMA), the American Academy of Clinical Toxicology (AACT), the American Society of Clinical Pharmacology and Therapeutics (ASCPT), the American College of Emergency Physicians (ACEP), the American College of Medical Toxicology (ACMT), and the American Academy of Pediatrics (AAP) that have encouraged their members to report to the MedWatch system. As a requirement for hospital accreditation, the Joint Commission mandates that hospitals collect, analyze, and report significant and unexpected ADEs to the FDA.

The primary limitation of the MedWatch system is the exclusive reliance on spontaneous reporting of ADEs. This passive surveillance system has several important limitations. Significant underreporting is known to occur in such systems. The uncertainty about the significance of a signal in the AERS database is exacerbated by the low estimated rate for adverse event reporting and the fact that the true incidence of the reported ADE is almost never precisely known because the denominator, which is the number of actual exposures to the drug, is rarely accurately known. Despite these limitations, the MedWatch system has detected significant ADEs during the postmarketing period, especially those that have very low background rates.

Drug regulators must rely on passive surveillance systems like the FAERS database to detect potential uncommon or rare but serious ADEs postapproval. Passive surveillance for drug safety signals is useful for serious and rare ADEs. This is primarily because a relatively small number of patients or participants are exposed to the drug during phases 1 to 3 prior to approval for marketing. For example, to detect an uncommon ADE occurring in approximately 1 of 5,000 individuals exposed to a drug with 95% probability that the ADE resulted from exposure to that drug, approximately 15,000 patients would have to be exposed to the drug. In a balanced (equal numbers of drug and placebo recipients) placebo-controlled clinical trial, 30,000 participants would need to be enrolled. Premarketing clinical studies (phases 1, 2, and 3) are usually inadequate to detect rare ADEs, ADEs that are incorrectly diagnosed, or ADEs that result from a drug interaction that were tested in the development program.

An example of a rare ADE not detected until postmarketing involves the drug felbamate, which was approved by the FDA in September 1993 and subsequently found to be associated with aplastic anemia during postmarketing surveillance. Felbamate-induced aplastic anemia was not detected during the drug development program. By July 1994, a total of 9 cases were reported from an estimated 100,000 patients exposed to felbamate in the United States.[37] Most of the aplastic anemia cases occurred in patients who had taken the drug for less than 1 year. The 9 cases represented an approximate 50-fold increase in aplastic anemia over the expected rate in the population with the very low background rate of 2 to 5 cases per million per year, allowing the FDA to attribute this rare condition to exposure to felbamate.

The primary role of the MedWatch system is to generate a hypothesis for potential association of an ADE with a specific drug. These hypotheses are sometimes further tested in subsequent phase 4 investigations. An example of this "hypothesis generation" function of MedWatch was the question of whether phenylpropanolamine (PPA) caused hemorrhagic stroke in patients using nonprescription diet suppressants or cough and cold preparations containing PPA. In the early 1990s, the Spontaneous Reporting System (SRS; now FAERS) detected a potential association of hemorrhagic stroke and nonprescription use of PPA. An industry-sponsored prospective, case–control study was designed to determine if such an association existed. The multicenter study demonstrated that an association did exist, especially for women aged 18 to 49 years. The Nonprescription Drug Advisory Committee (NDAC) of FDA reviewed this study and the associated MedWatch data in 2000 and decided that the evidence supported such an association. The committee advised the FDA to remove PPA from the market, which occurred a short time later. Although the entire process of signal identification from MedWatch to presentation of results from the prospective epidemiologic study required nearly a decade for PPA, the process demonstrates the value of the hypothesis-generating ability of the MedWatch system.

Potential outcomes of the detection of a safety signal for a marketed drug include a drug product label change for a dose reduction in all or certain high-risk patient populations, restriction of the sale of the specific drug to a more medically supervised environment or the development of a patient registry to more closely monitor use, and removal of the drug from the market. These options are further discussed later in this chapter.

Other types of phase 4 safety investigations include clinical studies, comparative studies with the new drug versus a competitor, or a special population study or drug interaction study when suspicion is raised that there may exist a different risk–benefit relationship in certain clinical settings. The enhancement of safety information is the primary goal of most phase 4 studies. Other than the specific prospective, randomized clinical study in patient subpopulations, the methods by which phase 4 safety studies are usually conducted are primarily observational and epidemiologic. The fields of pharmacovigilance and pharmacoepidemiology are often employed in the conduct of phase 4 studies. Attributing a serious ADE to a drug solely from MedWatch reports does occur, but it is much more common for the FAERS database to identify a safety signal, suggesting a possible drug-related safety problem.

Because of the significant limitations of passive surveillance systems for safety reporting, the FDA has initiated an active surveillance system for the detection of drug safety signals in the postapproval time frame. The system, known as Sentinel, was introduced on a small scale in 2008 to establish contracts and organizational relationships to create an active surveillance system within patient claims databases to be able to detect ADEs in marketed medical products. Currently the system consists of an accessible patient claims database that includes more than 100 million US individuals, with access to medical records and laboratory and pharmacy data.[39] The system is configured to ensure privacy and security, with the 18 data partners retaining control of the data (https://www.sentinelinitiative.org/). The FDA was mandated to create an Active Risk Identification and Analysis (ARIA) system in the FDAAA in 2007 and subsequent reauthorization bills for FDA since. Sentinel is an example of the use of real-world evidence for safety collected in an active surveillance setting.[40] Active Risk Identification and Analysis is a subcomponent of Sentinel and uses blinded patient data and a set of analytical tools to probe for safety signals associated with the use of medical products. As this data mining system is further developed, the hope is that FDA's ability to detect and assess meaningful postapproval drug safety problems will be significantly enhanced. The regulatory use of ARIA will help the FDA decide if the sponsor of a newly approved medical product will need to perform a postmarketing required (PMR) study or not. If the ARIA system is likely to detect the safety problem of concern to the FDA, a PMR will not be necessary.

ESTABLISHING THE DIAGNOSIS OF DRUG-INDUCED DISEASE

The recognition and diagnosis of a drug-induced disease, or an ADE, is an essential skill for all practitioners, and especially for clinical and medical toxicologists. The diagnosis of an ADE is typically established as the result of a systematic medical evaluation. One approach to establishing the diagnosis of drug-induced disease involves consideration of 6 related questions concerning the patient's clinical presentation and available medical data, as shown in Table 135–1.

The first question concerns the timing of the onset of the adverse event in relationship to the reported exposure to the drug. Perhaps because of publicity or word of mouth, ADEs are sometimes reported to the FDA MedWatch

TABLE 135–1	Questions to Answer to Help Establish the Diagnosis of an ADE

1. Was the timing of the event appropriate relative to the exposure to the drug?
2. Has the effect noted, which is the suspected ADE, been previously reported?
3. Is there evidence of excessive exposure to the drug?
4. Are there other more likely etiologies responsible for the condition suspected as being an ADE?
5. What is the patient's response to cessation of a suspect drug (dechallenge)?
6. What is the patient's response to rechallenge?

ADE = adverse drug event.

system even when the onset of the adverse event occurs before the first exposure to the suspect drug. A careful reconstruction of the timeline of exposure to the suspected drug and onset of adverse effects is extremely important in assessing causality. The time course differs considerably for different adverse clinical events. An anaphylactic reaction to a drug usually occurs within minutes of exposure, whereas acute kidney injury caused by a drug is not likely to be clinically detectable for up to several days after the exposure. A drug that causes cancer (a carcinogen) may not produce a clinically detectable effect for decades. Establishing a time course that is biologically plausible with the type of ADE event under consideration is an essential first step in the process of making the diagnosis of drug-induced disease.

The second question is whether this adverse effect was reported previously for the suspect drug. An adverse drug effect that occurs commonly is likely to be known before the approval of the drug and therefore is typically found on the initial drug label or other reliable sources of drug information. For example, respiratory depression and mental status changes were well known before the approval of fentanyl, an opioid agonist. Less common ADEs for drugs that have been on the market for a period of time are sometimes found in case reports in the literature and in various medical databases. Many of these will eventually appear in a revised drug label. Previous reports linking the observed adverse effect to drug exposure are very helpful to the clinician trying to establish a sufficient level of probability for causality in the setting of an ADE.

However, in the setting of a newly approved drug or a previously unreported possible ADE, neither previous reports/medical literature nor the drug label will help establish causality. In this setting, the clinician must rely more on what is known of the pharmacology, the pharmacokinetics, and the anticipated pharmacodynamics of the suspect drug and the timing of the appearance and observed time course of the adverse event. The known pharmacology of the drug should include "target" effects as well as "off target" effects. The "target" effects are the intended, therapeutic pharmacology of the drug. Often, in the setting of the evaluation of the poisoned patient, the toxicologist is faced with significant "off-target" pharmacologic effects that become detectable when higher than therapeutic systemic exposure of the suspected drug is present. It is important to put "drug-induced disease" in the differential diagnosis for most patients presenting for medical care. Someone must be the first to report what is ultimately recognized as an ADE. Appropriate vigilance for the possibility of a new ADE significantly increases the probability that a finding can be made early after introduction of a new drug to prevent more widespread drug-induced morbidity or mortality.

The next question to consider is, "Is there evidence of excessive exposure to the drug?" Most ADEs that occur are predictable based on the known pharmacology, targeted and off-target, of the specific drug. Such ADEs are referred to as *type A* ADEs.[5] For example, antihistamines such as diphenhydramine are known to cause significant anticholinergic effects. When a patient presents with mental status changes and other clinical findings consistent with the anticholinergic toxidrome after significant exposure to an antihistamine-containing product, the observed effects are consistent with an ADE attributable to the antihistamine. Occasionally, proof of excess can come from measurement of the drug in serum. In the case of the patient with a history of manic-depression illness, who exhibits nausea, vomiting, tremor, hyperreflexia, and bradycardic dysrhythmias, the measurement of an elevated serum lithium concentration supports the diagnosis of lithium toxicity or an ADE attributable to lithium perhaps as an inadvertent or intentional overdose, drug interaction, or change in patient kidney function resulting in excessive circulating lithium concentration. The latter is an example of a drug–disease interaction when, acute kidney injury, can lead to reduced drug clearance and result in clinical toxicity due to excessive exposure. In any case, knowing the pharmacology of the drug, including the off-target effects, is important for establishing the diagnosis of an ADE.

When an ADE is caused by an allergic mechanism or another mechanism unrelated to the extent of the exposure to the drug, that is, a *type B* ADE, evidence of drug excess usually does not contribute to the diagnosis. In this setting, other factors such as allergy history or pharmacogenetic background are weighed more heavily to support the diagnosis of an ADE. Patients are usually not aware of their genetically determined ability to metabolize or react to medications but most patients will recall a previously experienced allergic reaction.

The next issue to address in considering possible causality is whether there are other more likely etiologies that could be responsible for the observed effects. Although it is important to be appropriately vigilant for possible ADEs, it is equally important not to miss an alternative cause for the patient's condition by automatically attributing the patient's presentation to ADE. Based on the relative probabilities of other potential diagnoses on the differential diagnosis list, the probability of ADE can be estimated. There are certain clinical settings in which establishing an ADE becomes a diagnosis of exclusion. For example, in the case of persistent fever, the assignment of the diagnosis "drug fever" should not be made until a complete search for infectious or other, non–drug-induced causes has excluded this etiology.

A very important factor to consider in contemplating a diagnosis of ADE is "What is the patient's response to cessation of a suspect drug (*dechallenge*)?" In this case, the pharmacokinetics of the drug and the biologic timing of resolution of the specific condition must be carefully considered. In some instances, the resolution of a type A ADE closely follows the pharmacokinetics of the suspect drug. For example, in the case of β-adrenergic antagonist poisoning, cardiac effects resolve in association with decreasing serum concentrations of the drug in question. However, in other instances, onset and resolution of the ADE may not correlate with drug concentrations in the body, for example, in the case of a penicillin rash, which may develop within 1 or 2 days or longer after starting the medication but may take several days to weeks to completely resolve. In this later example of a type B ADE, the resolution of the condition (rash) occurs over a much longer time than would be predicted by the pharmacokinetics of the drug. In this case, the ADE resolution phase, or the toxicodynamic resolution, often significantly lags the toxico- or pharmacokinetic correlation. When a suspected ADE resolves after discontinuation of exposure to the offending drug, along a predictable time course, the result of this dechallenge would support the diagnosis of ADE.

Lastly, the clinician may have the opportunity or medical need to *rechallenge* the patient with the suspect drug. If the rechallenge results in the identical response or effect to that occurred in the initial presentation, this would be considered strong evidence to support a causal relationship for the suspect drug and the adverse event. In the setting of a serious or life-threatening adverse ADE, it is too dangerous to perform a rechallenge with the suspect drug, in which case the response to rechallenge will not be known. In this setting, the weight of evidence previously discussed will then be the only factors available to assess the probability of causality.

FDA REGULATORY ACTIONS REGARDING DRUG SAFETY

When new information about a safety issue for an already marketed drug raises concern at FDA, several regulatory options are available to either attempt to improve the safety margin of the drug or remove the drug from the US market. The most common regulatory action taken by the FDA is modification of the drug label. These modifications can include restrictions as to whom should receive the drug, what doses should be given for which indications or to which patient populations, what type of monitoring should be performed during therapy, and how long treatment should be administered. A survey of safety-related FDA regulatory actions on drug labels over the 20-year period (from 1980 to 1999) revealed that the most common step taken by FDA was dosage reduction of the initially approved therapeutic dosage.[9] When potentially life-threatening safety information is discovered, and the FDA believes that the risk–benefit relationship remains in favor of continued availability of the drug, the FDA can require that a boxed warning (sometimes called a "black box" warning) be carried in the label. A black box warning is the most serious warning placed in the label of a drug. If a black box warning is established, then health care professional advertisements regarding product availability, known as reminder ads, are no longer permitted. Additionally, when the boxed warning is added to the label, the

manufacturer is required in most cases to send a "Dear Doctor" letter to potential prescribers informing them of the new black box warning. Dear Doctor letters may also be required when the FDA requires that prescribers be notified about a significant change in the drug label warning. An example of current medications with recently added black box warnings is antidepressant medication that now must warn about the increased risk of suicidality if children and adolescents are prescribed antidepressants. The antipsychotic clozapine currently has 4 distinct warnings contained in the boxed warning in its drug label for the following attributed ADEs: agranulocytosis, myocarditis, seizures, and "other cardiovascular and respiratory effects."

Another option employed by the FDA is the implementation of restricted availability measures to permit continued availability of the drug but only with specified restrictions. For example, use of the drug isotretinoin (Accutane) requires compliance with a multiple component REMS program called iPLEDGE that includes informed consent, prescriber and dispensing pharmacy registration, serial pregnancy testing if applicable, documentation of patient education, and completion of risk management programs by patients who will receive the medication.[45] This option is more commonly used today when there is concern about "off-label" use. The FDA authority to require companies to submit, prior to drug approval, and execute postapproval, an effective risk management plan is intended to improve both the monitoring and prevention of postapproval adverse drug events and their consequences.

When the FDA believes that a drug can no longer be safely used despite modification of the drug label or any of the aforementioned restrictions, the regulatory threshold is reached to initiate removal of the drug from the market. This occurs when an acceptable risk–benefit relationship for continued availability of a drug product is no longer possible. Table 17–2 in the seventh edition of this text, contains a listing of drug products that were withdrawn or removed from the market. In some cases, such as the withdrawn drug rofecoxib (formally marketed as Vioxx), withdraw occurred because of the recognition of elevated cardiovascular risk.[20] In the case of the COX-2 inhibitor withdrawals, the precipitating factor for withdrawal was the findings of a strong safety signal for excess cardiovascular mortality and morbidity during the conduct of efficacy studies for other potential therapeutic indications for these drugs. The postmarketing surveillance system did not serve as the initial, precipitating data set for regulatory action in this instance.[29,36] The manufacturers voluntarily withdrew most of these COX-2 inhibitors from the US market after they were deemed unsafe by FDA. In most cases, the manufacturer ceases marketing the specific drug after notification by the FDA that regulatory action is being initiated to remove a specific drug from the market. Only very rarely has the FDA itself actually removed a drug from the market. The FDA did implement the removal of phenformin following due process. In the case of ephedra-containing dietary supplements, the FDA removed these products from the market based on their analysis of safety data obtained from the medical literature and from analysis of cases reported to the MedWatch system. In some cases, the pharmaceutical manufacturers file suit against the FDA to fight or delay the planned regulatory action against the product. The manufacturer's legal actions typically prolong the time the product remains on the market because the drug usually continues to be sold, while the legal proceedings and appeals proceed through the courts.

Some legislators and legal experts feel that approval of a drug by FDA should preempt legal action for safety issues identified in the drug labeling. However, the FDA decision-making process regarding drug approval is largely reliant on efficacy and safety data provided by the manufacturer or in the publicly available medical literature. Plaintiff actions, taken against drug and device manufacturers, are sometimes a source of significant publicity and confidential disclosures regarding questionable behaviors practiced by companies that market medicinal products. The patient's right to tort action against a product's manufacturer provides an important mechanism to ensure drug safety following approval and marketing.[10] Recent US Supreme Court appeals have challenged this position seeking to reinforce the legal position of federal preemption. In the case of *Wyeth v. Levine*, the manufacturer appealed to the US Supreme Court to uphold the federal preemption status for FDA-approved

TABLE 135–2 US Drug Product Withdrawals or Removal From the Market for Safety or Lack of Efficacy Concerns

Adenosine	Etretinate	Potassium arsenite
Adrenal cortex	Fenfluramine	Potassium chloride[i]
Alatrofloxacin	Flosequinan	Povidone
Aminopyrine	Gatifloxacin	Propoxyphene
Astemizole	Gelatin[f]	Rapacuronium
Azaribine	Glycerol	Reserpine[j]
Benoxaprofen	Gonadotropin, chorionic[g]	Rofecoxib
Bithionol	Grepafloxacin	Sibutramine
Bromfenac[a]	Mepazine	Sparteine sulfate
Butamben	Metabromsalan	Sulfadimethoxine
Camphorated oil	Methamphetamine	Sulfathiazole[k]
Carbetapentane[b]	Methapyrilene	Suprofen[l]
Casein	Methopholine	Sweet spirits of nitre
Cerivastatin	Methoxyflurane	Tegaserod
Chloramphenicol	Mibefradil	Temafloxacin
Chlorhexidine[c]	Nitrofurazone[h]	Terfenadine
Chlormadinone	Nomifensine	3,3′,4′,5-tetrachlorosalicylanilide
Chloroform	Novobiocin	Tetracycline[m]
Cisapride	Oxyphenisatin	Ticrynafen
Cobalt[d]	Oxyphenisatin	Tribromsalan
Dexfenfluramine	Pemoline	Trichloroethane[n]
Diamthazole	Pergolide	Troglitazone
Dibromsalan	Phenacetin	Trovafloxacin
Diethylstilbestrol	Phenformin	Urethane
Dihydrostreptomycin	Phenylpropanolamine	Valdecoxib
Dipyrone	Pipamazine	Vinyl chloride[o]
Encainide	Polyethylene glycol 3350	Zirconium[p]
Esmolol[e]		Zomepirac

[a]Except ophthalmic solution. [b]Oral gel drug products containing carbetapentane citrate. [c]Tinctures of chlorhexidine gluconate formulated for use as a patient preoperative skin preparation. [d]Except radioactive forms of cobalt and its salts and cobalamin and its derivatives. [e]Products that supply 250 mg/mL of concentrated esmolol per 10-mL ampule. [f]Intravenous drug products containing gelatin. [g]Containing chorionic gonadotropins of animal origin. [h]Except topical drug products formulated for dermatologic application. [i]Solid oral dosage containing potassium chloride that supply 100 mg or more. [j]Products containing more than 1 mg of reserpine. [k]Except for those formulated for vaginal use. [l]Except ophthalmic solutions. [m]Liquid oral drug products formulated for pediatric use containing tetracycline in a concentration greater than 25 mg/mL. [n]Aerosol drug products intended for inhalation containing trichloroethane. [o]Aerosol drug products containing vinyl chloride. [p]Aerosol drug products containing zirconium.

Data from Food and Drug Administration, HHS: Additions and Modifications to the List of Drug Products That Have Been Withdrawn or Removed From the Market for Reasons of Safety or Effectiveness. *Final rule, Fed Regist* 2016 Oct 7;81(195):69668-69677.

drugs.[27] On March 4, 2009, the US Supreme Court ruled that federal law does not preempt this particular plaintiff from seeking and obtaining a judgment from the product manufacturer because the product was approved by the FDA. The case provided the opportunity to debate the extent of protection afforded by the FDA approval status and the issue of product liability litigation as a part of postmarketing surveillance of drug products in the United States.

Over the years, there have been highly publicized drug withdrawals for risk of cardiovascular ADEs such as terfenadine (QT prolongation) or the COX-2 inhibitors (increased risk of major cardiac events such as myocardial ischemia). Until recently, the most common reasons for FDA-initiated drug withdrawals in the United States have been prolongation of the QTc interval followed by drug-induced hepatotoxicity. Advances in nonclinical testing and early-phase human testing have significantly reduced the rate of drug withdrawals for these reasons. These ADEs, as well as the propensity to cause significant drug–drug interactions, occur much less often but are still important examples of drug safety–related regulatory action in the United States.

Prolongation of the QT Interval

Three significant drug withdrawals in the mid- to late 1990s exemplified a serious drug safety issue regarding drug-related prolongation of the QT interval when administered alone or as the result of increasing plasma concentrations due to inhibition of its metabolism by other. The 3 examples in this category are terfenadine (Seldane), astemizole (Hismanal), and cisapride (Propulsid). Several deaths were reported to the MedWatch system for patients taking these medications. In the case of terfenadine, the initial publication of a case report for polymorphic ventricular tachycardia in the setting of routine use of this nonsedating antihistamine with the self-administration of ketoconazole, a known inhibitor of drug metabolism, led to FDA-funded, small prospective clinical studies to confirm a previously unrecognized ability of terfenadine to dramatically alter cardiac repolarization, which led to torsade de pointes. The drug was marketed in 1985, cardiac toxicity was detected in clinical use in 1990,[34] the FDA-funded clinical cardiac safety research was performed in 1991,[24] and, ultimately, the drug was withdrawn from the market in 1998. The medicolegal course of the other 2 drugs is similar except that prospective controlled studies to document the extent of QT interval prolongation were not performed before regulatory action was taken. These early experiences led to new rigorous regulatory requirements and significant preclinical screening and intensive, prospective controlled clinical study of QT interval effects by manufacturers of all drugs worldwide.

These 3 drug withdrawals demonstrated that the preapproval assessment of cardiac repolarization effects at that time was incapable of detecting even the most potent dysrhythmogenic drugs during their respective development and FDA review. Based on this dramatic systematic failure, the FDA (as well as the European and Japanese drug regulatory agencies) now requires a thorough QT study (TQT) for all new molecular entities.[33] These studies are designed to detect as little as a 5-millisecond increase in the corrected QT interval in healthy volunteer participants and must include a positive control to demonstrate the sensitivity of the study to detect this low-level change reliably. Since this new requirement was introduced, no newly approved drugs have subsequently been removed from the US market for QT interval safety reasons, although concern remains about the possibility of effective drugs being discarded early in development by sponsors perceiving excess cardiac QT interval prolongation risk.[3]

Significant Drug–Drug Interactions

Removal of mibefradil (Posicor) is an example of a drug withdrawn from the US market because of postmarketing discovery of a plethora of drug–drug interactions. Mibefradil, a pharmacologically unique calcium channel blocker, was approved by the FDA for the treatment of patients with hypertension and chronic stable angina. The FDA approved mibefradil for marketing in 1997 with the knowledge that the compound possessed the ability to inhibit certain hepatic CYP enzymes; these facts were included on the drug label. The initial labeling for mibefradil specifically listed 3 drug–drug interactions: astemizole, cisapride, and terfenadine (CYP3A pathway interactions). During the one year that mibefradil was marketed, information accumulated regarding drug–drug interactions with many other drugs and CYP pathways. As the in vitro and in vivo drug interaction data continued to accumulate for mibefradil, the FDA made labeling changes and issued a public warning for these potential drug interactions within 5 months of its initial approval. Additionally, the sponsor distributed a letter to health care professionals warning of drug–drug interactions. In the face of a growing and significant list of drug–drug interactions, and a 3-year international study demonstrating no clinical benefit of mibefradil over placebo for congestive heart failure, the FDA initiated regulatory action. In an unprecedented step for a drug with numerous drug interactions, the FDA requested that it be withdrawn from the market approximately one year after it was approved.[41] The FDA felt that the extensive drug–drug interactions could not be addressed by standard drug label instructions and additional public warnings. In the years following, the preclinical study and early human study, of potential human drug–drug interactions has evolved such that discovery of a clinically significant drug–drug interaction postapproval is now relatively uncommon.

Drug-Induced Hepatotoxicity

Another category of ADE of regulatory concern is those drugs that cause hepatotoxicity. In June 1998, the manufacturer of the nonsteroidal antiinflammatory drug (NSAID) bromfenac sodium (Duract) withdrew this drug from the US market.[23] The NDA was submitted for review to the FDA in 1994 and after 28 months of review was approved. The drug was withdrawn approximately 11 months later after postmarketing discovery of significant hepatotoxicity. Although no cases of serious liver injury were reported during premarketing clinical trials, after introduction to the market, a higher incidence of liver enzyme elevation was found in patients who were being treated with the drug. Postapproval exposure of patients to bromfenac generally resulted in longer periods of treatment than that of the participants in the clinical trials. Because of a preapproval concern by the FDA that long-term exposure to bromfenac could cause hepatotoxicity, bromfenac labeling specified that the product was to be used for 10 days or less. This dosing limitation appeared to be inconsistent with the initial approved drug indication for treatment of a chronic condition (eg, osteoarthritis). Information concerning elevated hepatic enzymes was included in the original product labeling. The postmarketing surveillance of this product identified rare cases of hepatitis and liver failure, including some patients who required liver transplantation, among those using the drug for more than the 10 days as specified on the label. In February 1998, approximately 6 months after approval for marketing, the FDA added a black box warning indicating that the drug should not be taken for more than 10 days. Nonetheless, severe injury and death from long-term use of bromfenac sodium continued to be reported, and ultimately, the sponsor agreed to voluntarily withdraw bromfenac sodium from the market. The withdrawal of bromfenac sodium raised several important questions concerning interpretation of "safety laboratory testing," such as liver enzymes during the drug development program, and raised questions to some extent, concerning the effectiveness of drug labeling.

The FDA has issued specific guidance on how to evaluate drug-induced liver injury (DILI) during drug development.[15] As in the case of many other adverse drug effects, severe DILI is uncommon so despite extensive preapproval study, few cases will be found prior to, and even in the postmarketing period. Proper evaluation for evidence of lesser injury such as drug databases may offer insight into the potential for more severe liver injury. One of the common guidelines utilized by FDA is Hy's law, which states that severe liver injury is predicted by laboratory assessment that includes an alanine aminotransferase of more than 3 times the upper limit of normal and a bilirubin of more than twice the upper limit of normal in a patient with no other reason for such an abnormality.[31] Although imperfect, this approach has been demonstrated to be very effective in preventing hepatotoxic new drugs from reaching the US market and has aided our postapproval safety evaluation of already approved drugs that demonstrate a liver toxicity safety signal.

Other Examples of Postmarketing Safety Problems Leading to Drug Withdrawal

One voluntary drug product withdrawal involving 2 separate drugs used in combination is particularly noteworthy as an example of a serious adverse event discovered years after the individual drugs were approved but after a significant increase in the prescription use of these agents as a combination product. The drug fenfluramine was approved in 1973 after an FDA review period of 75 months. A significant increase in prescription use of a combination product of fenfluramine with phentermine, for weight loss (referred to as "fen-phen"), began in the 1990s when clinical data suggested that this drug combination was effective in a weight loss program.[43] However, use of the fen-phen drug combination was never fully approved by the FDA and was therefore considered an "off-label" use of the products. The number of prescriptions for the drug combination soared in the mid-1990s because of the weight loss publications and associated media coverage. In 1997, research from the Mayo Clinic reported 24 cases of an unusual form of cardiac valvular disease causing aortic and mitral regurgitation in patients using the fen-phen combination.[8] The publicity surrounding the potential linkage of this drug combination to an unusual adverse event led to a significant increase in reports of possible adverse events associated with this drug combination. The FDA issued a public health advisory and initiated further epidemiologic studies to ascertain its prevalence. The FDA also encouraged echocardiographic studies of valvular diseases in patients taking fenfluramine or dexfenfluramine either alone or in combination with phentermine. Although at the onset the FDA, the product manufacturers, and the medical community did not expect valvular lesions to be associated with either fenfluramine or dexfenfluramine, the epidemiologic evidence suggested a possible association, leading the FDA to conclude that these drugs should be removed from the US market. The potential association of valvular heart disease with these drugs is an example of the use of a case–control study to explore a possible causal relationship between drug exposure and an ADE. In this case, it is unclear what the strength of the MedWatch signal was for the possible association of cardiac valvular disease with exposure to the fen-phen combination. The association between cardiac valvular lesions and exposure to the drug combination serves as an example of elucidation of a rare, unexpected ADE as the result of a dramatic increase in the number of exposed patients using a product.

ROLE OF THE TOXICOLOGIST IN THE DETECTION AND PREVENTION OF ADVERSE DRUG EVENTS

Toxicologists can play a very important role in ADE diagnosis and prevention, through efforts in patient care, education, and administrative functions. In patient care, it is common for the medical and clinical toxicologists to be the first medical specialists consulted for a patient with a potential ADE. Perhaps more than any other medical specialty, medical and clinical toxicologists are likely to include a thorough medication history that also includes prescription and nonprescription products, as well as dietary supplements. The medical toxicologist's active involvement in the clinical arena, especially in settings in which the initial diagnosis of ADEs can be made, also serves to provide an important role model: the medical toxicologist as an educator to promote the detection, reporting, and prevention of ADEs often in the academic setting of a medical school and affiliated teaching hospitals. Here, the academic toxicologist can champion the inclusion of education in therapeutics in the curriculum for medical and pharmacy students and house officers, and take an active role in the implementation of the instruction. Ensuring that the curriculum in therapeutics includes recognition and prevention of ADEs and medical errors that lead to ADEs could have a significant beneficial impact on the ultimate outcome of the education process toward reduction of preventable ADEs. In addition to making sure that quality information is presented in the curriculum for trainees, the medical toxicologist can often create a special teaching opportunity for this type of education by establishing an elective or, in some cases, a required experience in the curriculum for training in therapeutics that involves recognition and management of ADEs. Participation in a quality learning experience can significantly impact the graduates' knowledge of and attitudes toward therapeutics and risk reduction in patient care. Although the Institute of Medicine report on medical errors[30] did not focus on education initiatives in its main recommendations for reduction of medical errors in the United States, it seems logical that education be considered an important tool to improve medication use and prevent ADEs and medical errors with drugs and devices.

The growth of the discipline of medication safety as part of the increasingly visible overall patient safety initiatives has provided new venues for involvement of both clinical and medical toxicologists. Creation of interdisciplinary teams at many medical centers has allowed a system-oriented approach to the detection, mitigation, and prevention of adverse drug events. These take the form of pharmacy and therapeutics, medication safety, and quality improvement committees and provide important opportunities to impact on the drug-induced disease problem. Proactive interventions include targeted education programs, system modifications to reduce error rates, or a limitation of a specific drug usage to certain units of the organization or by certain specialties.

A well-documented, complete report to MedWatch made by a health care professional is given priority review by the FDA. The medical toxicologist is likely to encounter a significant number of patients with drug-induced disease cases from a diagnostic and management standpoint; therefore, practitioners of the specialty can have a significant impact on ADE reporting. All staff, including medical and clinical toxicologists and their trainees, should always submit an adverse event report locally for appropriate cases they encounter. Hospitals generally do not mandate or request that the reported event be "serious" as a requirement. The FDA MedWatch system requests that the reported events be serious in nature or not previously associated with the medication involved. Other organizations that collect data on medication errors, such as the Institute for Safe Medication Practices, provide valuable insight and support to the drug safety community. They maintain a database, as do poison control centers (PCC), and reporting is voluntary but important. In addition to reporting of the ADE, the toxicologist should promote publication of case reports of all new adverse events or adverse events occurring with newly approved products. Such publication often stimulates appropriate reporting of ADEs from other practitioners and generally raises awareness concerning a new ADE.

Toxicologists already work to facilitate the accurate reporting of PCC data to the National Poison Data System in a timely manner. Poison control center data are invariably considered in the overall safety evaluation of an approved and marketed drug and have obvious value in terms of national security. Accurate case information and causality assignment for ADEs including fatalities by toxicologists working with PCCs can greatly aid regulatory decisions and guide efforts to improve drug safety at the national and international levels. Pharmaceutical sponsors are required to query and report PCC data to the FDA on a periodic basis to add to the safety data set of their respective products. This is especially true for drugs with the potential for abuse and misuse. At the current time, the substance abuse epidemic facing the US, involving increased prevalence of drug abuse, rising national mortality from illicit drug overdose, and expanding availability of potentially deadly "designer" drugs of abuse provides the toxicologist with an opportunity for an even greater role in overall public health.

SUMMARY

- Drug-induced disease is common in both inpatient and outpatient settings.
- Despite significant advances in regulatory science and drug development, ADEs continue to occur in the postmarketing setting and will continue to do so for the foreseeable future in part because of the relatively small number of healthy subjects and patient volunteers who are exposed to a drug or biologic candidate prior to approval.
- Adverse drug events have a significant impact on patient mortality and morbidity in addition to producing a significant burden on the health care system.
- Vigilance for ADEs in routine medical practice will aid in detection and minimization of the negative impact on patients.
- Clinical and medical toxicologists are uniquely qualified and positioned in the health care setting to diagnose and report ADEs.

- Active participation in clinical, teaching, health care, and medical education administrative roles by medical and clinical toxicologists can lead to improved ADE detection and patient clinical outcomes.
- Maintaining a high level of commitment to the ADE recognition, reporting, and education as individuals and as a specialty will ultimately allow toxicologists to make significant contributions to the improvement in patient safety.

REFERENCES

1. Anderson ML, et al. Compliance with results at ClinicalTrials.gov. *N Engl J Med.* 2015;372:1031-1039.
2. Behrman R, et al. New FDA regulation to improve safety reporting in clinical trials. *N Engl J Med.* 2011;365:3-5.
3. Bouvy JC, et al. The cost-effectiveness of drug regulation: the example of thorough QT/QTc studies. *Clin Pharmacol Ther.* 2012;91:281-288.
4. Carpenter D, et al. Drug-review deadlines and safety problems. *N Engl J Med.* 2008;358:1354-1361.
5. CDC. Multistate outbreak of fungal infection associated with injection of methylprednisolone acetate solution from a single compounding pharmacy—United States, 2012. *Morb Mortal Wkly Rep (MMWR).* 2012;61:839-842. https://www.cdc.gov/mmwr/preview/mmwrhtml/mm6141a4.htm?s_cid=mm6141a4_w (accessed March 31, 2017).
6. Chary KV. Expedited drug review process: fast, but flawed. *J Pharmacol Pharmacother.* 2016;7:57-61.
7. Chabner BA. Drug shortages—a critical challenge for the generic-drug market. *N Engl J Med.* 2011;365:2147-2149.
8. Connolly HM, et al. Valvular heart disease associated with fenfluramine-phentermine. *N Engl J Med.* 1997;337:581-588.
9. Cross J, et al. Postmarketing drug dose changes of 499 FDA-approved new molecular entities, 1980-1999. *Pharmacoepidemiol Drug Saf.* 2002;11:439-446.
10. DeAngelis CD, Fontanarosa PB. Prescription drugs, products liability, and preemption of tort litigation. *JAMA.* 2008;300:1939-1941.
11. Dorr P, et al. An analysis of regulatory timing and outcomes for new drug applications submitted to Swissmedic—comparison with the US Food and Drug Administration and the European Medicines Agency. *Therapeutic Innovation & Regulatory Science.* 2016;50:734-742.
12. Downing NS, et al. Regulatory review of novel therapeutics—comparison of three regulatory agencies. *N Engl J Med.* 2012;366:2284-2293.
13. Drazen JM, et al. Compounding errors. *N Engl J Med.* 2012;367:2436-2437.
14. Faich GA. Adverse drug-reaction monitoring. *N Engl J Med.* 1986;314:1589-1592.
15. Food and Drug Administration. Drug-induced liver injury: premarking clinical evaluation. http://www.fda.gov/downloads/Drugs/.../Guidances/UCM174090.pdf. Accessed May 1, 2014.
16. Food and Drug Administration. MedWatch: the FDA safety information and adverse event reporting program. http://www.fda.gov/Safety/MedWatch/default.htm. Accessed May 1, 2014.
17. Food and Drug Administration. Regulatory and milestone information. https://www.fda.gov/AboutFDA/WhatWeDo/History/Milestones/ucm081229.htm. Accessed March 22, 2017.
18. Food and Drug Administration. Animal rule pathway. http://www.raps.org/Regulatory-Focus/News/2015/05/11/22135/FDA-Grants-Approval-to-New-Drug-Under-Rarely-Used-Animal-Rule-Pathway/#sthash.cSoArhZR.dpuf. Accessed March 30, 2017.
19. Food and Drug Administration. http://www.fda.gov/forindustry/developingproductsfor rarediseasesconditions/howtoapplyfororphanproductdesignation/ucm364750.htm.
20. Friedman MA, et al. The safety of newly approved medicines: do recent market removals mean there is a problem? *JAMA.* 1999;281:1728-1734.
21. Gavaza P, et al. Influence of attitudes on pharmacists' intention to report serious adverse drug events to the Food and Drug Administration. *Br J Clin Pharmacol.* 2011;72:143-152.
22. Getz KA, et al. Evaluating the completeness and accuracy of MedWatch Data. *Am J Ther.* 2014;21:442-446.
23. Goldkind L, Laine L. A systematic review of NSAIDs withdrawn from the market due to hepatotoxicity: lessons learned from the bromfenac experience. *Pharmacoepidemiol Drug Saf.* 2006;15:213-220.
24. Honig PK, et al. Terfenadine-ketoconazole interaction. Pharmacokinetic and electrocardiographic consequences. *JAMA.* 1993;269:1513-1518.
25. Issa D; Committee on Oversight and Government Reform. FDA's contribution to the drug shortage crisis. http://oversight.house.gov/report/fdas-contribution-to-the-drug-shortage-crisis/. Published 2012. Accessed May 1, 2014.
26. Jones CM, et al. Addressing prescription opioid overdose data support a comprehensive policy approach. *JAMA.* 2014;312:1733-1734.
27. Kesselheim AS, Studdert DM. The Supreme Court, preemption, and malpractice liability. *N Engl J Med.* 2009;360:559-561.
28. Kesselheim AS. Using market-exclusivity incentives to promote pharmaceutical innovation. *N Engl J Med.* 2010;363:1855-1862.
29. Kim PS, Reicin AS. Rofecoxib, Merck, and the FDA. *N Engl J Med.* 2004;351:2875-2878.

30. Institute of Medicine (US) Committee on Quality of Health Care in America; Kohn LT, et al., eds. *To Err Is Human: Building a Safer Health System.* Washington, DC: National Academies Press; 2000:6.

31. Lewis JH. "Hy's law," the "Rezulin Rule," and other predictors of severe drug-induced hepatotoxicity: putting risk-benefit into perspective. *Pharmacoepidemiol Drug Saf.* 2006;15:221-229.

32. Lurie P, et al. Financial conflict of interest disclosure and voting patterns at Food and Drug Administration Drug Advisory Committee meetings. *JAMA.* 2006;295:1921-1928.

33. Malik M, et al. Thorough QT studies: questions and quandaries. *Drug Saf.* 2010;33:1-14.

34. Monahan BP, et al. Torsades de pointes occurring in association with terfenadine use. *JAMA.* 1990;264:2788-2790.

35. Moore TJ, et al. Serious adverse drug events reported to the Food and Drug Administration, 1998-2005. *Arch Intern Med.* 2007;167:1752-1759.

36. Okie S. Raising the safety bar—the FDA's Coxib Meeting. *N Engl J Med.* 2005;352:1283-1285.

37. Pellock JM. Felbamate in epilepsy therapy: evaluating the risks. *Drug Saf.* 1999;21:225-239.

38. Prayle AP, et al. Compliance with mandatory reporting of clinical trial results on ClinicalTrials.gov: cross sectional study. *BMJ.* 2012;344:d7373.

39. Robb MA, et al. The US Food and Drug Administration's Sentinel Initiative: Expanding the horizons of medical product safety. *Pharmacoepidemiol Drug Saf.* 2012;21:9-11.

40. Sherman RE, et al. Real world evidence—what is it and what can it tell us? *N Engl J Med.* 2016;375:2293-2297.

41. SoRelle R. Withdrawal of Posicor from market. *Circulation.* 1998;98:831-832.

42. Steinbrook R, Sharfstein JM. The FDA Safety and Innovation Act. *JAMA.* 2012;308:1437-1438.

43. Weintraub M, et al. Long-term weight control study. I (weeks 0 to 34). *Clin Pharmacol Ther.* 1992;51:586-594.

44. Woodcock J. Drug development in serious diseases: the new "breakthrough therapy" designation. *Clin Pharmacol Ther.* 2014;95:483-485.

45. Wolverton SE, Harper JC. Important controversies associated with isotretinoin therapy for acne. *Am J Clin Dermatol.* 2013;14:71-76.

136

INTERNATIONAL PERSPECTIVES ON MEDICAL TOXICOLOGY

Sari Soghoian

Poisoning is a worldwide problem, but the major effects are felt in the developing world. At least 150,000 people die every year from acute pesticide poisoning (Chap. 110), and an estimated 20,000 to 94,000 from snake bites,[89] the vast majority of whom live in rural farming areas of lower- and middle-income countries. Hundreds of thousands of people are affected by groundwater arsenic contamination in Bangladesh and India,[155] and outbreaks of poisoning from contaminated food[63] and environmental pollution from poorly regulated industrial activity[40,135] affect whole communities throughout the developing world.

The resources for dealing with these problems are limited in many countries. Public health education about poisons and infrastructure limiting access and exposure to the most highly toxic chemicals are practically absent in much of the developing world. Access to medical care is often limited for financial, cultural, and geographic reasons. Medical toxicology is frequently not a recognized specialty, and patients are usually evaluated by general physicians with little formal training in medical toxicology although often with great experience. Diagnostic facilities are few, effective treatment options even more rare. Where antidotes exist, there is rarely enough knowledge or experience to use them effectively.[22] Intensive care beds for invasive monitoring and long-term ventilatory support are scarce. This chapter outlines some of the major poisoning risks and challenges for medical toxicology in the developing world.

POISONING AND THE GLOBAL BURDEN OF DISEASE

The World Health Organization (WHO) estimates that one in 10 deaths worldwide are due to injury and ranks self-inflicted injury, including poisoning, among the top 15 causes of death.[114,178] Acute and chronic exposure to chemicals caused more than 4.9 million deaths and 86 million disability-adjusted life years (DALYs) worldwide in 2004—more than cancer, sexually transmitted diseases, or diabetes.[135] Children younger than 15 years of age bore more than one-half of this burden.

Tremendous regional disparities in the health impact of poisoning are apparent. The global mortality burden from poisoning is disproportionately shouldered by lower- and middle-income countries. Overall, 75% or more of all poisoning-related deaths occur in the developing world,[76] and an estimated 95% of children who die each year from acute poisoning live in low- and middle-income countries.[130] Children living in Sub-Saharan Africa are at highest risk, with an estimated annual mortality rate of 4 children per 100,000 population.[144] This is double the global average and higher than that in any other region.

These figures are striking, yet most likely underestimate the contribution of poisoning to the global burden of disease and disability. Much of the existing data on poisoning epidemiology from lower-income countries reflects the experience in larger hospital centers. By contrast, most people live in rural areas, and many patients with poisoning never reach such facilities for a variety of financial, cultural, or geographic reasons. For example, logistical difficulty with accessing health care facilities was responsible in part for the high mortality from snakebite noted in one community-based study in Nepal.[151] Social or economic barriers often contribute to "healer shopping" within traditional or spiritual systems, with allopathic medical care delayed or avoided in many African countries.[46,81,125]

Unintentional poisoning risks from occupational, environmental, food, or medication sources are also poorly recognized in communities, or by health care workers.[121] The diagnosis of poisoning is often not suspected if a clear history of exposure is not given, because many symptoms of poisoning mimic infectious or other processes and few medical centers have ready access to laboratory tests for specific poisons. When poisoning is suspect,

many countries lack detailed injury surveillance systems or other standardized reporting mechanisms. The WHO has undertaken several initiatives to improve global poisoning surveillance, including support for poison control center (PCC) development in underrepresented regions worldwide, and the international efforts of the IPCS/INTOX programs to harmonize data collection and reporting terminology represent an important step toward this goal. However, the interpretation of PCC data as evidence of epidemiologic trends must be approached with some caution (Chap. 130).

COMMON XENOBIOTICS AND PATTERNS OF POISONING

Xenobiotics commonly involved in acute poisoning differ substantially among communities, both within and among countries. For example, a comparison of poisoning cases seen at a major public teaching hospital in New York City with 2 large rural hospitals in Sri Lanka found striking differences in the classes of xenobiotics involved. A total of 70% of the patients in New York City were poisoned with pharmaceuticals, and 90% of patients in the Sri Lankan cohort were poisoned with nonpharmaceuticals, primarily pesticides and botanicals, such as yellow oleander, with a 10 times higher case fatality rate.[76] A study comparing poisoning epidemiology in district (rural) and regional (urban) hospitals in Zimbabwe found that poisoning from pesticides was equally common in both settings, but animal envenomation was reported nearly twice as often at the district facilities compared to regional centers, and poisoning with pharmaceuticals was a problem that was uniquely reported at the regional hospital.[160]

Understanding the local patterns and specific risks for poisoning in particular communities is of critical importance because it provides an evidence base for designing and prioritizing strategies to prevent or limit harm. This section reviews some of the more common xenobiotics implicated in poisoning in developing countries worldwide.

Pesticides

Pesticide poisoning is responsible for millions of hospital admissions and at least 150,000 deaths each year (Chap. 110). Most of these deaths occur in Asia, particularly in China and India, and most are related to intentional self-harm.[66] The WHO considers pesticide poisoning to be the single most important means of suicide, accounting for 30% of all suicides worldwide.[177] The total number of deaths worldwide from occupational or unintentional pesticide poisoning is unknown but was estimated nearly 30 years ago at 20,000 per year.[84] Although many classes of pesticides are implicated (Chaps. 109–111), organic phosphorus (OP) pesticides are responsible for the majority of pesticide-related deaths reported in the developing world.[50]

Deliberate self-poisoning with OP pesticides carries a high mortality rate and puts a high intensive care burden on the health care system (Chap. 110). In one study examining the experience in Sri Lanka, OP pesticide poisoning was responsible for 943 of 2,559 (36%) admissions to a secondary hospital for poisoning.[52] The case fatality rate for OP poisoning was 21%, and pesticide poisoned patients occupied 41% of all medical intensive care beds. A systematic review from Iran found that OP compounds were implicated in only 16% of acute poisonings, but with a 13% case fatality rate that accounted for nearly 40% of all poisoning-related mortalities.[148] Similar situations are reported from across the world.[50]

Factors contributing to the high mortality of self-poisoning with pesticides in the developing world include the intrinsic lethality of many pesticides, and health care systems that are poorly prepared to care for such critically ill patients (Table 136–1). Pesticides are often easily available in highly concentrated preparations in rural communities throughout the

TABLE 136-1	Factors Contributing to High Mortality From Self-Poisoning With Pesticides in the Developing World

1. Ease of access to pesticides in rural, agrarian households
2. Poor storage practices
3. Inadequate labeling of lethal pesticide products
4. High potency of pesticides
5. Lack of evidence-based practice guidelines appropriate for resource-poor areas
6. Lack of clear guidelines
7. Distance from and time to health care facilities and resources available at health care facilities

developing world. The ease of drinking liquid pesticides is also a factor facilitating massive intentional ingestions, as are inadequate pesticide storage systems.[93] The extraordinarily high human, economic, and social costs of pesticide-related mortality worldwide reinforce the importance of developing simple, economical, and evidence-based strategies specifically designed to care for acutely poisoned patients in resource limited environments.[21,24]

Envenomation

Envenomation by snakes and other animals represents another significant cause of morbidity and mortality with disproportionate effects in the developing world. Few countries mandate the reporting of animal bites, making it difficult to estimate global incidence, severity, and outcome. Current data estimate that between 421,000 and 1.8 million envenomings and about 20,000 to 94,000 deaths occur globally each year from snakebite, the vast majority of which occur in South Asia, South East Asia, and sub-Saharan Africa.[89] By contrast, less than 100 snakebite deaths per year are estimated to occur in Europe, the United States, Canada, and Australia combined.[32,89] This disparity reflects the combination of increased incidence and decreased access to standards of care for snakebite, such as antivenoms and trained personnel to administer them, among the rural poor in tropical regions.[74]

Snakebites are environmental, household, and important occupational hazards in the rural tropics, particularly within the agricultural sector.[74] Working in large plantations and subsistence farms places rural people in frequent contact with venomous snakes. In Benin, the annual incidence of snake envenomation ranges from 200 in 100,000 in rural villagers to 1,300 in 100,000 in sugarcane plantation workers.[35] With simultaneous changes in global climate and expansion of human settlements, it is likely that the range of venomous snakes will enlarge to include urban areas and regions previously considered too temperate to support them.[77] Snakebites from members of the Elapidae and Viperidae families are responsible for the majority of deaths worldwide, although several other families are also medically important (Colubridae and Atractaspididae species, in particular; Chap. 119 and Special Considerations: SC10).[173]

The global distribution of snakebite is highly correlated with poverty, and the burden of snake envenomation on local economies and health resources can be substantial.[74] In many cases, it is greater than that of other neglected tropical diseases (NTDs) included in the 2009 WHO list.[68,71] The total number of DALYs attributable to snakebites in West Africa is an estimated 319,874 annually, of which more than 90% are associated with early mortality.[71] Throughout the tropics, about 10% of hospital beds are occupied by victims of snakebite, with seasonal and regional variations.[34] During the rainy season in Benin, snakebites account for up to 20% of all hospital admissions, with an estimated case fatality rate of 3% to 6%.[35]

Despite the burden on hospital services, relatively few snakebite victims in the developing world seek allopathic medical care for their injuries.[32,156] For example, a study of rural Philippine rice farmers found that only 8% of cobra (Naja philippinensis) bite victims reached a hospital in the 1980s.[171] A more recent household survey in Bangladesh found that 86% of snakebite victims went to snake charmers for initial management, and only 10% later visited a doctor or hospital.[137] Reliance on traditional healers contributes to morbidity and mortality since many still employ potentially harmful therapeutic techniques such as tourniquet application and making incisions around the

bite site. However, changes in treatment seeking can occur. Studies over the last decade in Sri Lanka show that patients have started going to the hospital rapidly after common krait (Bungarus caeruleus) snakebite, bypassing traditional healers.[97] A study in Ghana found that the incidence of snakebite victims at a district hospital increased significantly after the introduction of a new treatment protocol including early antivenom administration, possibly reflecting increased confidence in the ability of the health care system to manage these cases.[170]

After snakebites, the second most common cause of mortality and morbidity from venomous animals is scorpion stings (Chap. 115 and Antidotes in Depth: A37, A38). Medically important scorpion species are widely distributed throughout the tropics, being particularly common causes of morbidity in North Africa, Mexico, India, and Brazil.[33] The total number of medically significant scorpion stings that occurs annually is unknown; a recent review estimated 1.2 million stings, leading to more than 3,250 deaths (case fatality 0.27%).[33] Other venomous insects, such as Arachnida (spiders) and Hymenoptera (bees, ants, and wasps), are rarely sources of significant mortality on a global scale[83] (Chap. 115).

Herbal and Traditional Medicines

The use of traditional medicine (TM) to treat or prevent health problems is widespread. The WHO estimates that around 80% of the world's population consults traditional healers regularly.[180] Frequently cited reasons for this preference or reliance on TM include financial considerations, sociocultural preferences, beliefs about the relative safety and efficacy of TM compared to allopathic medicines, and mistrust or relative inaccessibility of doctors.[81,125] Traditional practitioners still greatly outnumber medical professionals in many regions. For example, there were an estimated 25 times more traditional healers than physicians practicing in Mali in 2004.[64]

Although TM also encompasses a variety of spiritual, religious, or physical manipulation therapies, it often includes administration of "herbal" remedies orally, topically, or via enema. These are typically prepared using a combination of aqueous plant materials, sometimes mixed with insect or other animal parts, metallic salts, or both. Although traditional medicinal preparations are usually tested by generations of practitioners and the concentrations of active ingredients are generally low, both intentional and unintentional poisonings are common.[29,158,159] In a 2-year retrospective review of acutely poisoned patients from South Africa, TM was the second most common cause of admission (15.8% of cases) and had the highest mortality rate (15.2%), accounting for more than half of all deaths in the series.[87] Traditional medicine was the most common cause of admission (23% of cases) for and death from acute poisoning in a 10-year retrospective review of cases from Zimbabwe.[159]

The specific chemical constituents responsible for TM poisoning vary widely between geographic and cultural areas. Laboratory analysis and ethnopharmacologic surveys in a number of countries have begun to elucidate some of the chemical constituents of commonly prescribed recipes. Interestingly, a review of 41 autopsies in South Africa for which the cause was presumed to be a herbal medicine found that cardiac glycosides were present in 44% of cases.[108] Contamination and erroneous substitution of herbal products is most often the culprit[26] but adulterants are also implicated in poisoning from TM formulations. For example, these are common in traditional Ayurvedic medicines (particularly heavy metals and corticosteroids[67]) and Asian medicines (particularly synthetic pharmaceuticals[58] and heavy metals[28]) (Chap. 43). A Taiwanese study of 2,609 TM samples found that 23% were adulterated with pharmaceutical products such as caffeine, nonsteroidal antiinflammatory drugs, acetaminophen, and diuretics.[80]

Pharmaceuticals

In many lower-income countries, pharmaceuticals are relatively uncommon causes of acute poisoning. However, the incidence appears to be rising in conjunction with larger global demographic shifts toward increased urbanization and industrialization. Access to pharmaceuticals is generally greater among urban dwellers than rural ones, and more people in urban communities have the financial means to buy them. In a retrospective review of poisoning cases admitted to urban versus rural health centers in Zimbabwe, poisoning with pharmaceuticals was uniquely reported at the urban facilities, accounting for more than 15% of poisoning cases at regional hospitals surveyed and none of the cases presenting for care at the district level.[160]

The relative importance of poisoning with pharmaceuticals and the specific xenobiotics involved will likely change as more and more societies develop a "dual burden of disease" pattern including chronic illnesses that require long-term drug therapy.[15,119] Previously the most common xenobiotics implicated in acute poisoning in the developing world were those used to treat tropical infectious diseases. For example, self-poisoning with the antimalarial chloroquine (Chap. 55) is widely reported in Sub-Saharan Africa,[14,136] although this medication is now rarely used so the incidence is expected to decrease. Intentional and unintentional poisoning with the leprosy drug dapsone, as well as the antituberculous drug isoniazid (Chap. 56), are also well reported.[132,162,168]

Criminal poisoning of commuters with benzodiazepines to facilitate robbery is a common problem across South Asia. As many as 300 people are admitted unconscious with this problem to a single university medical unit in Dhaka, Bangladesh, each year.[104] In Pakistan, benzodiazepines are implicated in 60% of drug-facilitated street and public transportation related crimes.[91]

A more general issue of toxicologic concern is the prevalence of poor-quality medicines in use worldwide. Although data estimating the extent of the problem and its impact on health are limited, recent estimates suggest that more than one-third of all medicines on sale in Southeast Asia and Sub-Saharan Africa are substandard or counterfeit.[17,117,118] The major problem with these medications is an absence or subtherapeutic concentration of active ingredient, leading to treatment failures and an increase in drug-resistant pathogens where antimicrobials are involved. However, substandard medications sometimes contain more active ingredients than stated, leading to adverse drug effects,[164] or contain harmful adulterants or contaminants.

Epidemic poisonings from such poor-quality medicines underscore the dangers of inadequate regulation and oversight of pharmaceutical manufacture and sales. Examples include the deaths of more than 120 patients in Karachi, Pakistan, from exposure to a batch of isosorbide mononitrate contaminated with pyrimethamine,[10] the hospitalization of more than 50,000 infants in China with melamine poisoning from adulterated formula,[82] and the numerous epidemics of diethylene glycol poisoning (Special Considerations: SC9) in multiple countries over the past few decades from contaminated glycerine, paracetamol syrups, cough syrups, toothpastes, teething mixtures, and other medications.[16,73,142,154]

Household Products and Chemicals

Poisoning with common household products, such as fuels, cleansing products, rat poisons, insecticides, body care products, and cosmetics, is a global problem. This general category of diverse xenobiotics is consistently implicated as a significant source of unintentional childhood poisoning worldwide. The PC movement that began in the 1950s in North America grew out of an increasing recognition of the child health risks associated with exploratory household poison ingestions. Household chemicals are a similarly well recognized risk for unintentional childhood poisoning internationally.[30,31,56,90,100,120,157] The specific risks are remarkably consistent around the world, including age younger than 6 years (with toddlers younger than 3 years of age most affected), male sex, low socioeconomic status, and unsafe storage practices in the home.

Among specific household products, hydrocarbon poisoning from unintentional ingestion of kerosene (paraffin) is widely reported as the most common cause of pediatric admissions in low-income countries around the world.[20,31,88,95,107] Kerosene is a common fuel used to power stoves and lamps in many relatively poor communities. It is pale in color with an appearance similar to water, and it is often purchased or stored in used beverage containers, making it easy to misidentify (Chap. 105).[57] In Sub-Saharan Africa, household chemicals account for up to 80% of all pediatric admissions for poisoning,[15,31,56,88,123] and kerosene poisoning, specifically, accounts for some 25% to 75% of all poisoning-related hospital visits among children younger than 6 years of age.[56,120,161] Several studies document an increase in poisoning-related admissions during the warmer months of the year,[95] when children are more likely to become thirsty and to drink from any beverage container at hand.

As with other categories of poison, patterns of self-harm using domestic products tend to demonstrate regional particularities. For example, ingestion of caustics is another common scenario implicated in both intentional and unintentional poisoning around the world, and the specific agents most commonly encountered vary by location. In Sierra Leone, children are most likely to ingest alkaline substances such as sodium hydroxide,[39] whereas ingestion of acids is more common in Taiwan[75] and south India.[42] In Hong Kong, there is significant morbidity reported in association with self-poisoning using detergent products such as Dettol (4.8% chloroxylenol, pine oil, and isopropyl alcohol) and Savlon (cetrimide).[27,30] Frequent use of potassium permanganate for self-harm is also reported from Hong Kong.[126,183] Fatal poisoning with hair dye (paraphenylenediamine) is a well-recognized problem in the Middle East, India, and parts of Africa where henna is used cosmetically.[145,146,152]

Plants

Poisonous plants have been used to induce abortion, for recreational intoxication, in homicidal acts, and for self-harm throughout human history (Chap. 118). This section briefly mentions select toxic plants that are most commonly used in self-poisoning, or that have caused epidemic poisoning in the developing world.

Self-poisoning with seeds of plants containing cardioactive steroids are important clinical problems globally. Yellow oleander (*Thevetia peruviana*) kills hundreds of people each year in Sri Lanka and India (Chap. 62).[51,140] Sea mango or suicide tree (*Cerbera* sp) has killed hundreds of people in Kerala, India,[111] and is a focal problem in eastern Sri Lanka.[54] The superb lily (*Gloriosa superba*) contains colchicine alkaloids and is another plant that is used both medicinally and for self-harm in South Asia (Chap. 34).[59,110,133] Numerous plant species contain atropinelike alkaloids, causing an anticholinergic syndrome when ingested. Intentional ingestion of *Datura* species as a recreational drug for their hallucinatory effects[2,61] or as part of traditional medical preparations,[26] and unintentional poisoning from food contamination[131] or plant substitution in meals[48,128] is widely reported from nearly all parts of the globe.[96]

Oduvan (*Cleistanthus collinus*) leaf contains the glycosides cleistanthin A and B, which produce severe hypokalemia and cardiac dysrhythmias.[7] Self-poisoning has killed hundreds of people in South India.[112,149] Poisoning by castor beans (*Ricinus communis*) or other lectin-containing plants such as *Jatropha* spp (African purging nut) is well reported from Africa and South Asia (Chap. 118).[1,44,103]

Ackee tree fruit (*Blighia sapida*), which contains hypoglycin when unripe, is widely consumed as a food source. Epidemics of fatal poisoning with unripe Ackee fruit have occurred throughout the Caribbean and in Africa.[86,105,109] Hypoglycin and its analog methylenecyclopropylglycine (MCPG) were recently implicated in previously unexplained outbreaks of acute toxic encephalopathy linked to litchi fruit consumption in Muzaffarpur, India.[153]

Occupational and Environmental Sources

Poisoning from occupational and environmental sources is a significant global health problem, with disproportionate effects on persons living in lower-income communities around the world. Exposure to "traditional" environmental health hazards, such as indoor air pollution from the combustion of solid fuels, and naturally occurring contaminants in groundwater, soil, and food, is still a major cause of morbidity and mortality in much of the world. Around 50% of the world's people rely on solid fuels such as coal, dung, wood, or crop residues for cooking and heating.[23] Resultant indoor air pollution was estimated to cause 1,965,000 deaths and 41,009,000 DALYs (disability adjusted life years) from lower respiratory tract infections, cancers, and COPD in 2004.[179] Consumption of inorganic arsenic in drinking water and foods affects millions of people worldwide, contributing to the global burden of cancer, cardio- and cerebrovascular disease, diabetes mellitus, and other chronic disease conditions. In Bangladesh, one survey estimated that 9,100 deaths and 125,000 DALYs could be attributed to chronic consumption of arsenic-contaminated groundwater in 2001,[102] and data from another prospective longitudinal study estimated that more than 20% of all deaths in this population are linked to arsenic exposure greater than 10 mcg/L in drinking water.[9] Dental and skeletal fluorosis from excessive fluoride in drinking water is endemic in at least 17 countries worldwide.[60]

Increasingly, modern environmental health hazards (MEHHs) also play a large role in global poisoning risks.[40,122] Modern environmental health hazards include outdoor air pollution from automobiles and factories; soil and water contamination by plastics, heavy metals, pesticides and other industrial chemicals and wastes; radiation hazards; land degradation; and climate change produced by rapid urbanization and industrial development in the absence of strong regulatory controls.[40] These are important sources of both occupational and environmental exposure to a wide range of toxins with acute and chronic health effects. Inadequate safeguards to control the selection, sale, and application of pesticides in parts of Africa and Asia are linked to pesticide poisoning both as an occupational hazard[45,85] and from residues left on food.[6,38,121] Occupational lead poisoning has largely been controlled in developed countries through improved working conditions and occupational health screens, but it remains an enormous problem in developing countries where occupational and environmental health protection measures are often underdeveloped or practically nonexistent.[167,172]

Industrial factories are often placed in urban areas, or the areas around factories are rapidly urbanized, placing large numbers of people at risk not only from pollution but from industrial errors as well. The 1984 Bhopal tragedy in which a Union Carbide pesticide plant malfunctioned, releasing isocyanate gas into the surrounding community and causing an estimated 3,787 deaths and 558,125 injuries, is emblematic of such disasters.[8,150]

Several international agreements on chemical safety provide legal frameworks to mitigate the human and environmental impact of global industrialization; however, the actual implementation of regulatory controls has lagged behind the expansion of toxic exposures. For example, at the governance level a total of 39 Sub-Saharan African countries have ratified the Rotterdam Convention on chemical safety. Yet industrial pollution is now becoming so highly concentrated in growing urban areas that the continent's pollution intensity (pollution generated per unit of production output) is now rated among the world's highest, attesting to significant regional difficulties in enforcing such regulations.[169]

The predominance of informal sector activity in agricultural and industrial work in lower-income countries poses serious regulatory challenges. Fumes and dusts from small-scale domestic businesses involved in smelting, battery recycling or manufacture, welding, pottery, ceramic production, and artisanal mining are common sources of exposure to lead and other heavy metals in developing countries, and put not only workers but whole communities at risk.[167] More recently, unregulated electronic waste (e-waste) recycling, in which salable metals are reclaimed from old electronics by burning, has emerged as a significant human and environmental health hazard in parts of China, West Africa, and India.[4,98,163] Workers are often aware of the health risks, yet economic hardship and lack of alternative employment make them unwilling or unable to change.

Easy access to industrial chemicals from inadequate regulation of packaging and sales also facilitates their use for intentional self-harm. For example, formic and acetic acids are used in the manufacture of rubber, and cases of poisoning are reported from areas surrounding rubber factories in India

and Sri Lanka.[42,139] Copper sulfate is widely used for self-poisoning in parts of South Asia, and carries a high mortality rate because of direct damage to the gastrointestinal tract, hepatorenal failure, and hemolysis (Chap. 92).[115,116] Cyanide self-poisoning has become a commonly used method in Korea over the last 20 years (Chap. 123).[92]

REDUCING THE GLOBAL IMPACT OF POISONING

Regulatory science and the coordinated actions of agencies and programs across multiple sectors play a vital role in preventing or reducing the impact of poisoning in society. An integrated approach is needed, combining the implementation of policies to improve product and environmental safety; development of more robust health information systems to collect reliable data on the burden of poisoning globally; prioritization and funding for research; improving the availability and accessibility of safe and effective treatments; health workforce training in best practices for both acute care and the follow-up of affected patients, including the recognition and management of psychological causes and sequelae; and the design and implementation of community-based education and prevention campaigns.

Timely access to medical care has a major impact on poisoning outcomes. Significant global disparities in the infrastructure to provide acute care and to meet WHO minimum standards for essential emergency supplies exist and must be addressed to improve this.[12,13,78] Lack of human resources for health care is also an enormous problem in many parts of the developing world. There are more than 60 times more physicians per unit population working in North America as compared to Sub-Saharan Africa, and at least 4.3 million more health workers are needed to address critical shortfalls in access to primary medical care globally.[41] Policies and programs encouraging sustainable and equitable health workforce development are urgently needed to address these gaps.

Beyond rectifying the raw numbers deficit, clinical training programs in many low- and middle-income countries must be upgraded to promote broad exposure and specialist development in clinical toxicology and acute care. Input from experts in medical toxicology improves outcomes, reduces hospital stays and health care costs associated with acute poisoning,[25,36,62] but practitioners in many parts of the world have limited or no access to consultation with such specialists. Less than half of all WHO member states have Poison Control Centers, and these are underfunded and understaffed in many countries (Chap. 130).[181] The mission of the International Union of Toxicology is to foster international scientific cooperation, ensure the development of toxicologists, and promote the dissemination of knowledge in toxicology worldwide.[49] Through the efforts of this and other professional societies, an increasing number of local, regional, and international forums now offer educational and professional development opportunities in clinical toxicology around the globe. International collaboration through online forums such as the teleconferencing networks being developed through the Global Educational Toxicology Uniting Project (GETUP) is an important mechanism to bridge the education gaps.[176] Increasing local and international commitment to the growth of emergency medicine in low- and middle-income countries also promises to support the dissemination of scientific knowledge and improve provider competence in advanced resuscitation techniques.[5,11,147]

In addition to global disparities in acute care infrastructure and resources generally, access to antidotes for specific poisons is either lacking or inadequate in much of the world.[3,175] Where antidotes are available, knowledge and experience to know how to use them safely and effectively is often lacking.[24] Poor antidote availability is not unique to the developing world,[43] and many antidotes are considered either adjunctive or unnecessary therapies. However, in certain cases they significantly reduce the need for other medical interventions, and this is particularly important in rural or underdeveloped areas where critical care facilities are not readily available.[134] For example, the most important challenge to improving the treatment of patients with snakebite worldwide is poor antivenom availability, particularly in rural areas where it is most needed to reduce critical delays in administration.[165,166]

Currently, many available antivenoms are prohibitively expensive; ineffective; require refrigeration, which is not practical in rural areas; or have a high rate of adverse reactions. The need for regionally specific formulations makes it difficult to achieve economies of scale that include higher-paying markets.[34,68] Critical evaluation of existing antivenoms and development of new marketing and purchasing strategies that can ensure access to affordable and safe products within the developing world are thus desperately needed (Special Considerations: SC10).[19,22,69,165,166,173,174]

Improving health care access and health system preparedness is only one aspect of the coordinated, multilevel, national, and international public health responses needed to reduce the global impact of poisoning. Prevention and risk reduction efforts must involve locally appropriate community-level education and awareness raising, strong governance to support the design, implementation, and monitoring of regulatory controls, and the involvement of multiple stakeholders and sectors including water, waste management, energy, agriculture, transportation, industry, and civil society. Effective legislative frameworks developed in countries with more advanced public health infrastructure have been successfully disseminated in some cases. For example, between 2000 and 2004 the proportion of people with blood lead concentrations above 10 mcg/dL globally decreased from 20% to 14%, largely because of the widespread phaseout of leaded gasoline.[135] Other strategies, such as pharmaceutical and food safety regulations enacted through the US Food and Drug Administration, have influenced "duplicative legislation" in other countries but continue to pose significant implementation challenges in low- and middle-income countries that lack the necessary financing, human resources, and infrastructure to enforce them well.[129]

Many public health measures with proven efficacy, such as routine lead testing during childhood, the regulation of vehicle emissions, the detection of carbon monoxide, and the incorporation of childproof containers may seem prohibitively resource intensive in many parts of the world. The development of new, low-cost technologies such as solar heating and electrical sources, chemical assays and residue detectors, and electronic devices to identify and track pharmaceuticals hold some promise to reduce global risks for unintentional poisoning. More research is needed to propose and evaluate the effectiveness, acceptability, and sustainability of new and proven poison prevention techniques in resource-limited environments.

Recognizing that self-harm from pesticide ingestion is responsible for a majority of acute poisoning deaths worldwide, public health interventions specifically designed to limit access are an important goal. A minimum pesticide list, based on the WHO essential xenobiotic list initiative, was proposed.[55] Such a list would provide policy makers and farmers with unbiased information about relative risks. However, voluntary initiatives such as international policy statements and industry-sponsored programs often suffer from a lack of resources, a shortage of political will, and nonexistent enforcement mechanisms.[94] A dramatic illustration of an effective national program to reduce pesticide poisoning risks is the ban of all WHO high-risk OP insecticides and the organic chlorine endosulfan in Sri Lanka, which effectively arrested a previously exponential increase in the incidence of pesticide poisoning and halved the national suicide rate between 1995 and 2005 (Chap. 110).[65] This program is estimated to have saved more than 20,000 lives in 10 years.

Ironically, some programs to remove the most environmentally persistent and toxic chemicals from use have inadvertently replaced them with chemicals highly toxic to humans. The replacement of persistent organic chlorine compounds with carbamates in malaria control programs is an example. The opposite effect also occurred, for example, by replacing OP insecticides with pyrethroids to reduce human toxicity.[94] Coordinated pesticide harm reduction strategies should take into account concerns regarding both environmental and human toxicity, and anticipate which xenobiotics will enter into use as replacements as specific chemicals are phased out. A strategy based on industrial hygiene models of a hierarchy of controls has been proposed (Table 136–2).[143]

TABLE 136–2	Hierarchical Strategies to Reduce Pesticide Poisoning Mortality in the Developing World[143]	
E	Most	Eliminate the most highly toxic pesticides
F		Substitute with less toxic, equally effective alternatives
F		Reduce use through improved equipment
I		Isolate people from the hazard
C		Label products and train applicators in safe handling practices
A		Promote use of personal protective equipment
C		
Y	Least	Institute administrative controls

SUMMARY

- Poisoning is common worldwide. Fatal poisoning is disproportionately concentrated in lower- and middle-income countries, where public health systems and acute care resources to detect, manage, prevent, and collect data on poisoning are often less well developed.

- Global poisoning estimates are mostly derived from health care sources in a minority of developing world countries; current data likely underrepresent the true burden and distribution of injuries from poisoning.

- Efforts to develop international poisoning surveillance systems and establish harmonized definitions of poisoning cases will help generate a more complete picture to inform local, national, and international policies and interventions.

- Pesticides are the most important cause of death from acute poisoning worldwide, with a majority of these cases attributable to acts of deliberate self-harm.

- Improving access to health care and health system preparedness to provide acute care is essential to reduce global disparities in poisoning outcomes.

- Randomized controlled trials and cost-effectiveness research are needed to critically evaluate the utility of specific public health and treatment interventions in resource-limited settings.

Acknowledgments

Michael Eddleston, MD, and Aaron Hexdall, MD, contributed to this chapter in previous editions.

REFERENCES

1. Abdu-Aguye I, et al. Acute toxicity studies with *Jatropha curcas* L. *Hum Toxicol.* 1986;5:269-274.
2. Adegoke S, Alo L. *Datura stramonium* poisoning in children. *Niger J Clin Pract.* 2013;16:116.
3. Al-Sohaim SI, et al. Evaluate the impact of hospital types on the availability of antidotes for the management of acute toxic exposures and poisonings in Malaysia. *Hum Exp Toxicol.* 2012;31:274-281.
4. Alabi OA, et al. Comparative evaluation of environmental contamination and DNA damage induced by electronic-waste in Nigeria and China. *Sci Total Environ.* 2012; 423:62-72.
5. Alagappan K, Holliman CJ. History of the development of international emergency medicine. *Emerg Med Clin North Am.* 2005;23:1-10.
6. Amoah P, et al. Pesticide and pathogen contamination of vegetables in Ghana's urban markets. *Arch Environ Contam Toxicol.* 2006;50:1-6.
7. Annapoorani KS, et al. Spectrofluorometric determination of the toxic constituents of *Cleistanthus collinus. J Anal Toxicol.* 1984;8:182-186.
8. [Anonymous]. Calamity at Bhopal. *Lancet.* 1984;2:1378-1379.
9. Argos M, et al. Arsenic exposure from drinking water, and all-cause and chronic-disease mortalities in Bangladesh (HEALS): a prospective cohort study. *Lancet.* 2010; 376:252-258.
10. Arie S. Contaminated drugs are held responsible for 120 deaths in Pakistan. *BMJ.* 2012;34:e951.
11. Arnold JL, Holliman C. Lessons learned from international emergency medicine development. *Emerg Med Clin North Am.* 2005;23:133-147.
12. Awang R, et al. Availability of decontamination, elimination enhancement, and stabilization resources for the management of acute toxic exposures and poisonings in emergency departments in Malaysia. *Intern Emerg Med.* 2011;6:441-448.
13. Baelani I, et al. Availability of critical care resources to treat patients with severe sepsis or septic shock in Africa: a self-reported, continent-wide survey of anesthesia providers. *Crit Care.* 2001;15:1-12.

14. Ball DE, et al. Chloroquine poisoning in Zimbabwe: a toxicoepidemiological study. *J Appl Toxicol.* 2002;22:311-315.
15. Balme K, et al. The changing trends of childhood poisoning at a tertiary children's hospital in South Africa. *S Afr Med J.* 2012;102:142-146.
16. Barr DB, et al. Identification and quantification of diethylene glycol in pharmaceuticals implicated in poisoning epidemics: an historical laboratory perspective. *J Anal Toxicol.* 2007;31:295-303.
17. Bate R, Hess K. Anti-malarial drug quality in Lagos and Accra—a comparison of various quality assessments. *Malar J.* 2010;9:157.
18. Bertolote J, et al. Deaths from pesticide poisoning: are we lacking a global response? *Br J Psychiatry.* 2006;189:201-203.
19. Bhaumik S. Problems with treating snake bite in India. *BMJ.* 2016;103:i103.
20. Bond GR, et al. A clinical decision rule for triage of children under 5 years of age with hydrocarbon (kerosene) aspiration in developing countries. *Clin Toxicol.* 2008;46:222-229.
21. Bond GR, et al. A clinical decision aid for triage of children younger than 5 years and with organophosphate or carbamate insecticide exposure in developing countries. *Ann Emerg Med.* 2008;52:617-622.
22. Brown NI. Consequences of neglect: analysis of the sub-Saharan African snake antivenom market and the global context. *PLoS Negl Trop Dis.* 2012;6:e1670.
23. Bruce N, et al. Air pollution in developing countries: a major environmental and public health challenge. *Bull World Health Organ.* 2000;78:1078-1092.
24. Buckley NA, et al. Where is the evidence for the management of pesticide poisoning—is clinical toxicology fiddling while the developing world burns? *J Toxicol Clin Toxicol.* 2004;42:113-116.
25. Bunn TL, et al. The effect of poison control center consultation on accidental poisoning inpatient hospitalizations with preexisting medical conditions. *J Toxicol Environ Health A.* 2008;71:283-288.
26. Chan TYK. Herbal medicines induced anticholinergic poisoning in Hong Kong. *Toxins (Basel).* 2016;8:80.
27. Chan TY, et al. The risk of aspiration in Dettol poisoning: a retrospective cohort study. *Hum Exp Toxicol.* 1995;14:190-191.
28. Chan TY, Critchley JA. Usage and adverse effects of Chinese herbal medicines. *Hum Exp Toxicol.* 1996;15:5-12.
29. Chan TY, et al. Poisoning due to Chinese proprietary medicines. *Hum Exp Toxicol.* 1995;14:434-436.
30. Chan TYK, et al. Poisoning due to common household products. *Singapore Med J.* 1995;36:285-287.
31. Chibwana C, et al. Childhood poisoning at the Queen Elizabeth Central Hospital, Balatyre, Malawi. *East African Med J.* 2001;78:292-295.
32. Chippaux JP. Snake-bites: appraisal of the global situation. *Bull World Health Organ.* 1998;76:515-524.
33. Chippaux JP, Goyffon M. Epidemiology of scorpionism: a global appraisal. *Acta Trop.* 2008;107:71-79.
34. Chippaux JP, Habib A. Antivenom shortage is not circumstantial but structural. *Trans R Soc Trop Med Hyg.* 2015;109:747-748.
35. Chippaux JP. Snake bite epidemiology in Benin. *Bull Soc Pathol Exot.* 2002;95:172-174.
36. Clark RF, et al. Resource-use analysis of a medical toxicology consultation service. *Ann Emerg Med.* 1998;31:705-709.
37. Clarke EEK, et al. The problems associated with pesticide use by irrigation workers in Ghana. *Occup Med.* 1997;47:301-308.
38. Contini S, et al. Oesophageal corrosive injuries in children: a forgotten social and health challenge in developing countries. *Bull World Health Organ.* 2009;87:950-954.
39. Contini S, et al. Corrosive esophageal injuries in children: a shortlived experience in Sierra Leone. *Int J Pediatr Otorhinolaryngol.* 2007;71:1597-1604.
40. Corvalán C, et al. Health, environment and sustainable development: identifying links and indicators to promote action. *Epidemiology.* 1995;10:656-660.
41. Crisp N. Global health capacity and workforce development: turning the world upside down. *Infect Dis Clin North Am.* 2011;25:359-367.
42. Dalus D, et al. Formic acid poisoning in a tertiary care center in south India: a 2-year retrospective analysis of clinical profile and predictors of mortality. *J Emerg Med.* 2013;44:373-380.
43. Dart RC. Insufficient stocking of poisoning antidotes in hospital pharmacies. *JAMA.* 1996;276:1508-1510.
44. Dayasiri M, et al. Plant poisoning among children in rural Sri Lanka. *Int J Pediatr.* 2017;2017:1-6.
45. de Silva HJ, et al. Toxicity due to organophosphorus compounds: what about chronic exposure? *Trans R Soc Trop Med Hyg.* 2006;100:803-806.
46. de-Graft Aikins A. Healer shopping in Africa: new evidence from rural-urban qualitative study of Ghanaian diabetes experiences. *BMJ.* 2005;331:737.
47. Dewan A, et al. Mass ethion poisoning with high mortality. *Clin Toxicol.* 2008;46:85-88.
48. Disel N, et al. Poisoned after dinner: Dolma with *Datura Stramonium. Turk J Emerg Med.* 2015;15:51-55.
49. Dybing E, et al. Past challenges faced: an overview of current educational activities of IUTOX. *Tox Appl Pharmacol.* 2005;207:S712-S715.
50. Eddleston M. Patterns and problems of deliberate self-poisoning in the developing world. *Q J Med.* 2000;93:715-731.
51. Eddleston M, et al. Epidemic of self-poisoning with seeds of the yellow oleander tree (*Thevetia peruviana*) in northern Sri Lanka. *Trop Med Int Health.* 1999;4:266-273.
52. Eddleston M, et al. Deliberate self-harm in Sri Lanka: an overlooked tragedy in the developing world. *BMJ.* 1998;317:133-135.
53. Eddleston M, et al. Effects of a provincial ban of two toxic organophosphorus insecticides on pesticide poisoning hospital admissions. *Clin Toxicol.* 2012;50:202-209.
54. Eddleston M, Haggalla S. Fatal injury in eastern Sri Lanka, with special reference to cardenolide self-poisoning with *Cerbera manghas* fruits. *Clin Toxicol.* 2008;46:745-748.
55. Eddleston M, et al. Pesticide poisoning in the developing world—a minimum pesticides list. *Lancet.* 2002;360:1163-1167.
56. Edelu BO, et al. Accidental childhood poisoning in Enugu, South-East, Nigeria. *Ann Med Health Sci Res.* 2016;6:168-171.
57. Ellis JB, et al. Paraffin ingestion—the problem. *S Afr Med J.* 1994;84:727-730.
58. Ernst E. Adulteration of Chinese herbal medicines with synthetic drugs: a systematic review. *J Int Med.* 2002;252:107-113.
59. Fernando R, Fernando D. Poisoning with plants and mushrooms in Sri Lanka: a retrospective hospital based study. *Vet Hum Toxicol.* 1990;32:579-581.
60. Fewtrell L, et al. An attempt to estimate the global burden of disease due to fluoride in drinking water. *J Water Health.* 2006;4:533-542.
61. Francis PD, Clarke CF. Angel trumpet lily poisoning in five adolescents: clinical findings and management. *J Paediatr Child Health.* 1999;35:93-95.
62. Galvão TF, et al. Impact of a poison control center on the length of hospital stay of poisoned patients: retrospective cohort. *Sao Paulo Med J.* 2011;129:23-29.
63. Gibb H, et al. World Health Organization estimates of the global and regional disease burden of four foodborne chemical toxins, 2010: a data synthesis. *F1000Res.* 2015;4:1393.
64. Grønhaug TE, et al. Ethnopharmacological survey of six medicinal plants from Mali, West-Africa. *J Ethnobiol Ethnomed.* 2008;4:26.
65. Gunnell D, et al. The impact of pesticide regulations on suicide in Sri Lanka. *Int J Epidemiol.* 2007;36:1235-1242.
66. Gunnell D, et al. The global distribution of fatal pesticide self-poisoning: systematic review. *BMC Public Health.* 2007;7:357.
67. Gupta SK, et al. Misuse of corticosteroids in some of the drugs dispensed as preparations from alternative systems of medicine in India. *Pharmacoepidemiol Drug Saf.* 2000;9:599-602.
68. Gutierrez J, et al. The need for full integration of snakebite envenoming within a global strategy to combat the neglected tropical diseases: the way forward. *PLoS Negl Trop Dis.* 2013;7:7-9.
69. Gutierrez J, et al. Snakebite envenoming from a global perspective: towards an integrated approach. *Toxicon.* 2010;56:1223-1235.
70. Habib A, et al. Cost-effectiveness of antivenoms for snakebite envenoming in Nigeria. *PLoS Negl Trop Dis.* 2015;9:e3381.
71. Habib A, et al. Snakebite is under appreciated: Appraisal of burden from West Africa. *PLoS Negl Trop Dis.* 2015;9:4-11.
72. Hamza M, et al. Cost-effectiveness of antivenoms for snakebite envenoming in 16 countries in West Africa. *PLoS Negl Trop Dis.* 2016;10:1-16.
73. Hanif M, et al. Fatal renal failure caused by diethylene glycol in paracetamol elixir: the Bangladesh epidemic. *BMJ.* 1995;311:88-91.
74. Harrison R, et al. Snake envenoming: a disease of poverty. *PLoS Negl Trop Dis.* 2009;3:e569.
75. Havanond C, Havanond P. Initial signs and symptoms as prognostic indicators of severe gastrointestinal tract injury due to corrosive ingestion. *J Emerg Med.* 2007;33:349-353.
76. Hexdall A, Eddleston M. International perspectives in medical toxicology. In: *Goldfrank's Toxicologic Emergencies.* 8th ed. New York: McGraw-Hill; 2006:1832-1846.
77. Hon KL, et al. Snakebites in children in the densely populated city of Hong Kong: a 10-year survey. *Acta Paediatr.* 2004;93:270-272.
78. Hsia E, et al. Access to emergency and surgical care in sub-Saharan Africa: the infrastructure gap. *Health Policy Plan.* 2012;27:234-244.
79. Huang L, et al. The health effects of exposure to arsenic-contaminated drinking water: a review by global geographic distribution. *Int J Environ Health Res.* 2014;25:432-452.
80. Huang WF, et al. Adulteration by synthetic therapeutic substances of traditional Chinese medicines in Taiwan. *J Clin Pharmacol.* 1997;37:344-350.
81. Hughes GD, et al. The prevalence of traditional herbal medicine use among hypertensives living in South African communities. *BMC Complement Altern Med.* 2013;13:38.
82. Ingelfinger JR. Melamine and the global implications of food contamination. *N Engl J Med.* 2008;359:2745-2748.
83. Isbister GK, et al. Antivenom treatment in arachnidism. *J Toxicol Clin Toxicol.* 2003;41:291-300.
84. Jeyaratnam J. Acute pesticide poisoning: a major global health problem. *World Health Stat Q.* 1990;43:139-144.
85. Jeyaratnam J, et al. Survey of acute pesticide poisoning among agricultural workers in four Asian countries. *Bull World Health Organ.* 1987;65:521-527.
86. Joskow R, et al. Ackee fruit poisoning: an outbreak investigation in Haiti 2000-2001, and review of the literature. *Clin Toxicol (Phila).* 2006;44:267-273.
87. Joubert P. Poisoning admissions of black South Africans. *J Toxicol Clin Toxicol.* 1990;28:85-94.
88. Kasilo OMJ, Nhachi CFB. A pattern of acute poisoning in children in urban Zimbabwe: ten years experience. *Hum Exp Toxicol.* 1992;11:335-340.

89. Kasturiratne A, et al. The global burden of snakebite: a literature analysis and modelling based on regional estimates of envenoming and deaths. *PLoS Med.* 2008;5:e218.

90. Keka A, et al. Acute poisoning in children; changes over the years, data of pediatric clinic department of toxicology. *J Acute Dis.* 2014;3:56-58.

91. Khan T, et al. Drugs-facilitated street and travel related crimes: a new public health issue. *Gomal J Med Sci.* 2014;12:205-209.

92. Ki Lee S, et al. Cyanide poisoning deaths detected at the National Forensic Service headquarters in Seoul of Korea: a six year survey (2005-2010). *Toxicol Res.* 2012;28:195-199.

93. Konradsen F, et al. Pesticide self-poisoning: thinking outside the box. *Lancet.* 2007; 369:169-170.

94. Konradsen F, et al. Reducing acute poisoning in developing countries—options for restricting the availability of pesticides. *Toxicology.* 2003;192:249-261.

95. Korb FA, Young MH. The epidemiology of accidental poisoning in children. *S Afr Med J.* 1985;68:225-228.

96. Krenzelok E. Aspects of Datura poisoning and treatment. *Clin Toxicol.* 2010;48:104-110.

97. Kularatne SAM. Common krait (*Bungarus caeruleus*) bite in Anuradhapura, Sri Lanka: a prospective clinical study, 1996-98. *Postgrad Med J.* 2002;78:276-280.

98. Kuper J, Hojsik M. Poisoning the poor—electronic waste in Ghana. Amsterdam, The Netherlands: Greenpeace International; 2008. http://www.greenpeace.org/raw/content/international/press/reports/poisoning-the-poor-electonic.pdf. Accessed June 27, 2014.

99. Laustsen AH, et al. Recombinant snakebite antivenoms: a cost-competitive solution to a neglected tropical disease? *PLoS Negl Trop Dis.* 2017;11:e0005361.

100. Lin Y, et al. Poison exposure and outcome of children admitted to a pediatric emergency department. *World J Pediatr.* 2011;7:143-149.

101. Liwa A, et al. Traditional herbal medicine use among hypertensive patients in sub-Saharan Africa: a systematic review. *Curr Hypertens Rep.* 2014;16:437.

102. Lokuge KM, et al. The effect of arsenic mitigation interventions on disease burden in Bangladesh. *Environ Health Perspect.* 2004;112:1172-1177.

103. Lucas G. Plant poisoning: a hospital-based study in Sri Lanka. *Indian J Pediatr.* 1997; 64:495-502.

104. Majumder MM, et al. Criminal poisoning of commuters in Bangladesh: prospective and retrospective study. *Forensic Sci Int.* 2008;180:10-16.

105. Malangu N. Contribution of plants and traditional medicines to the disparities and similarities in acute poisoning incidents in Botswana, South Africa and Uganda. *Afr J Tradit Complement Altern Med.* 2014;11:425-438.

106. Mansori K, et al. A case-control study on risk factors for unintentional childhood poisoning in Tehran. *Med J Islamic Rep Iran.* 2016;30:355.

107. Manzar N, et al. The study of etiological and demographic characteristics of acute household accidental poisoning in children—a consecutive case series study from Pakistan. *BMC Pediatr.* 2010;10:28.

108. McVann A, et al. Cardiac glycoside poisoning involved in deaths from traditional medicines. *S Afr Med J.* 1992;81:139-141.

109. Meda HA, et al. Epidemic of fatal encephalopathy in preschool children in Burkino Faso and consumption of unripe ackee (*Blighia sapida*) fruit. *Lancet.* 1999;353: 536-540.

110. Mendis S. Colchicine cardiotoxicity following ingestion of *Gloriosa superba* tubers. *Postgrad Med J.* 1989;65:752-755.

111. Menon M, et al. Clinical profile and management of poisoning with suicide tree: an observational study. *Heart Views.* 2016;17:136-139.

112. Mohan A, et al. *Cleistanthus collinus* poisoning: experience at a medical intensive care unit in a tertiary care hospital in south India. *Ind J Med Res.* 2016;143:793-797.

113. Mohapatra B, et al. Snakebite mortality in India: a nationally representative mortality survey. *PLoS Negl Trop Dis.* 2011;5:e1018.

114. Murray CJ, Lopez AD. Mortality by cause for eight regions of the world: Global Burden of Disease Study. *Lancet.* 1997;349:1269-1276.

115. Naha K, et al. Blue vitriol poisoning: A 10-year experience in a tertiary care hospital. *Clin Toxicol.* 2012;50:197-201.

116. Nastoulis E, et al. Greenish-blue gastric content: literature review and case report on acute copper sulfate poisoning. *Forensic Sci Rev.* 2017;29:77-91.

117. Nayyar GM, et al. Poor-quality antimalarial drugs in southeast Asia and sub-Saharan Africa. *Lancet.* 2012;12:488-496.

118. Newton PN, et al. Impact of poor-quality medicines in the "developing" world. *Trends Pharmacol Sci.* 2010;31:99-101.

119. Nhachi CFB, et al. Aspects of orthodox medicines (therapeutic drugs) poisoning in urban Zimbabwe. *Hum Exp Toxicol.* 1992;11:329-333.

120. Nhachi CFB, Kasilo OMJ. Household chemical poisoning admissions in Zimbabwe's main urban centres. *Hum Exp Toxicol.* 1994;13:69-72.

121. Ntow WJ. Organochlorine pesticides in water, sediment, crops, and human fluids in a farming community in Ghana. *Arch Environ Contam Toxicol.* 2001;40:557-563.

122. Nweke OC, Sanders WH. Modern environmental health hazards: a public health issue of increasing significance in Africa. *Environ Health Perspect.* 2009;117:863-870.

123. Oguche S, et al. Pattern of hospital admissions of children with poisoning in the Sudano-Sahelian North Eastern Nigeria. *Niger J Clin Pract.* 2007;10:111-115.

124. Okuonghae HO, et al. Diethylene glycol poisoning in Nigerian children. *Ann Trop Paediatr.* 1992;12:235-238.

125. Olisa NS, Oyelola FT. Evaluation of use of herbal medicines among ambulatory hypertensive patients attending a secondary health care facility in Nigeria. *Int J Pharm Pract.* 2009;17:101-105.

126. Ong KL, et al. Potassium permanganate poisoning—a rare cause of fatal self poisoning. *J Accid Emerg Med.* 1997;14:43-45.

127. Pac-Kozuchowska E, et al. Patterns of poisoning in urban and rural children: a single center study. *Adv Clin Exp Med.* 2016;25:335-340.

128. Papoutsis I, et al. Mass intoxication with *Datura innoxia*—case series and confirmation by analytical toxicology. *Clin Toxicol.* 2010;48:143-145.

129. Patel M, Miller MA. Impact of regulatory science on global public health. *Kaohsiung J Med Sci.* 2012;28:S5-S9.

130. Peden M, et al. *World Report on Child Injury Prevention.* Geneva: World Health Organization; 2008.

131. Perharic L, et al. Risk assessment of buckwheat flour contaminated by thorn-apple (*Datura stramonium* L.) alkaloids: a case study from Slovenia. *Food Addit Contam Part A Chem Anal Control Expo Risk Assess.* 2013;30:321-330.

132. Prasad R, et al. Dapsone induced methemoglobinemia: intermittent vs continuous intravenous methylene blue therapy. *Indian J Pediatr.* 2008;75:245-247.

133. Premaratna R, et al. *Gloriosa superba* poisoning mimicking an acute infection—a case report. *BMC Pharmacol Toxicol.* 2015;16:27.

134. Pronczuk de Garbino J, et al. Evaluation of antidotes: activities of the International Programme on Chemical Safety. *J Toxicol Clin Toxicol.* 1997;35:333-343.

135. Prüss-Ustüna, et al. Knowns and unknowns on burden of disease due to chemicals: a systematic review. *Environ Health.* 2011;10:9.

136. Queen HF, et al. The rising incidence of serious chloroquine overdose in Harare, Zimbabwe: emergency department surveillance in the developing world. *Trop Doct.* 1999;29:139-141.

137. Rahman R, et al. Annual incidence of snakebite in rural Bangladesh. *PLoS Negl Trop Dis.* 2010;4:1-6.

138. Rajabi M, et al. Corrosive injury of the upper gastrointestinal tract: review of surgical management and outcome in 14 adult cases. *Iranian J Otorhinolar.* 2015;27:15-21.

139. Rajan N, et al. Formic acid poisoning with suicidal intent: a report of 53 cases. *Postgrad Med J.* 1985;61:35-36.

140. Rajapakse S. Management of yellow oleander poisoning. *Clin Toxicol.* 2009;47:206-212.

141. Rapp M, Pdgorny G. Reflections on becoming a specialty and its impact on global emergency medical care: our challenge for the future. *Emerg Med Clin North Am.* 2005;23:259-269.

142. Rentz ED, et al. Outbreak of acute renal failure in Panama in 2006: a case-control study. *Bull World Health Organ.* 2008;86:749-756.

143. Roberts DM, et al. Influence of pesticide regulation on acute poisoning deaths in Sri Lanka. *Bull World Health Organ.* 2003;81:789-798.

144. Ruiz-Casares M. Unintentional childhood injuries in sub-Saharan Africa: an overview of risk and protective factors. *J Health Care Poor Underserved.* 2009;20:51-67.

145. Sampathkumar K, Yesudas S. Hair dye poisoning and the developing world. *J Emerg Trauma Shock.* 2009;2:129-131.

146. Sanchez L, et al. Hair dye poisoning: retrospective analyses of patients admitted to ICU at a rural hospital in India. *Indian J Med Res.* 2016;144:134-137.

147. Schroeder E, et al. Global emergency medicine: a review of the literature from 2011. *Acad Emerg Med.* 2012;19:1196-1203.

148. Shadboorestan A, et al. A systematic review on human exposure to organophosphorus pesticides in Iran. *J Environ Sci Health.* 2016;34:187-203.

149. Shankar V, et al. Epidemiology of *Cleistanthus collinus* (oduvan) poisoning: clinical features and risk factors for mortality. *Int J Inj Cont Saf Promot.* 2009;16:223-230.

150. Sharma DC. Bhopal: 20 years on. *Lancet.* 2005;365:111-112.

151. Sharma SK, et al. Impact of snake bites and determinants of fatal outcomes in southeastern Nepal. *Am J Trop Med Hyg.* 2004;71:234-238.

152. Shigidi M, et al. Clinical presentation, treatment and outcome of paraphenylenediamine induced kidney injury following hair dye poisoning: a cohort study. *Pan Afr Med J.* 2013;19:163.

153. Shrivastava A, et al. Association of acute toxic encephalopathy with litchi consumption in an outbreak in Muzaffarpur, India, 2014: a case-control study. *Lancet.* 2017;17:1-9.

154. Singh J, et al. Diethylene glycol poisoning in Gurgaon, India, 1998. *Bull World Health Organ.* 2001;79:88-95.

155. Singh N, et al. Arsenic in the environment: effects on human health and possible prevention. *J Environ Biol.* 2007;28:359-365.

156. Snow RW, et al. The prevalence and morbidity of snake bite and treatment-seeking behaviour among a rural Kenyan population. *Ann Trop Med Parasitol.* 1994;88:665-671.

157. Srivastava A, et al. An epidemiological study of poisoning cases reported to the National Poisons Information Centre, All India Institute of Medical Sciences, New Delhi. *Hum Exp Toxicol.* 2005;24:279-285.

158. Stewart MJ, et al. The toxicology of African herbal remedies. *Ther Drug Monit.* 1998;20:510-516.

159. Tagwireyi D, et al. Traditional medicine poisoning in Zimbabwe: clinical presentation and management in adults. *Hum Exp Toxicol.* 2002;21:579-586.

160. Tagwireyi D, et al. Differences and similarities in poisoning admissions between urban and rural health centers in Zimbabwe. *Clin Toxicol.* 2006;44:233-241.

161. Tagwireyi D, et al. Pattern and epidemiology of poisoning in the East African region: a literature review. *J Toxicol.* 2016;2016:1-26.

162. Tai W, et al. Coma caused by isoniazid poisoning in a patient treated with pyridoxine and hemodialysis. *Adv Ther.* 2008;25:1085-1088.

163. Tang X, et al. Heavy metal and persistent organic contamination in soil from Wenling: an emerging e-waste recycling city in Taizhou area, China. *J Hazard Mater.* 2010;173:653-660.

164. Taylor RB, et al. Pharmacopoeial quality of drugs supplied by Nigerian pharmacists. *Lancet.* 2001;357:1933-1936.

165. Theakston RDG, Warrell DA. Crisis in snake antivenom supply for Africa. *Lancet.* 2000;356:2104.

166. Theakston RDG, et al. Report of a WHO workshop on the standardization and control of antivenoms. *Toxicon.* 2003;41:541-557.

167. Tong S, et al. Environmental lead exposure: a public health problem of global dimensions. *Bull World Health Organ.* 2000;78:1068-1077.

168. Tracqui A, et al. A case of dapsone poisoning: toxicological data and review of the literature. *J Anal Toxicol.* 1995;19:229-235.

169. UNIDO. *The Industrial Development Report 2004. Industrialization, Environment and the Millennium Development Goals in Sub-Saharan Africa: The New Frontier in the Fight against Poverty.* Vienna: United Nations Industrial Development Organization; 2004.

170. Visser LE, et al. Protocol and monitoring to improve snake bite outcomes in rural Ghana. *Trans R Soc Trop Med Hyg.* 2004;98:278-283.

171. Watt G, et al. Bites by the Philippine cobra (*Naja naja philippinensis*): an important cause of death among rice farmers. *Am J Trop Med Hyg.* 1987;37:636-639.

172. Watts J. Lead poisoning cases spark riots in China. *Lancet.* 2009;374:868.

173. White J, et al. Clinical toxinology—where are we now? *J Toxicol Clin Toxicol.* 2003; 41:263-276.

174. Williams D, et al. The Global Snakebite Initiative: an antidote for snakebite. *Lancet.* 2010;375:89-91.

175. Wium CA, Hoffman BA. Antidotes and their availability in South Africa. *Clin Toxicol.* 2009;47:77-80.

176. Wong A, et al. The Global Educational Toxicology Uniting Project (GETUP): an analysis of the first year of a novel toxicology education project. *J Med Toxicol.* 2015;11:295-300.

177. World Health Organization. *Suicide.* http://www.who.int/mediacentre/factsheets/fs398/en/. Accessed May 15, 2017.

178. World Health Organization. *The Global Burden of Disease; 2004 Update.* Geneva: World Health Organization; 2008.

179. World Health Organization. *Global Health Risks: Mortality and Burden of Diseases Attributable to Selected Major Risks.* Geneva: World Health Organization; 2009. http://www.who.int/healthinfo/global_burden_disease/GlobalHealthRisks_report_full.pdf. Accessed June 27, 2014.

180. World Health Organization. Traditional medicine. http://www.who.int/mediacentre/factsheets/fs134/en/. Accessed April 15, 2017.

181. World Health Organization. *Improving the Availability of Poisons Centre Services in Eastern Africa.* Geneva: World Health Organization; 2015.

182. Yong Y, et al. Collaborative health and enforcement operations on the quality of antimalarials and antibiotics in Southeast Asia. *Am J Trop Med Hyg.* 2015;92:105-112.

183. Young RJ, et al. Fatal acute hepatorenal failure following potassium permanganate ingestion. *Hum Exp Toxicol.* 1996;15:259-261.

137 PRINCIPLES OF EPIDEMIOLOGY AND RESEARCH DESIGN

Alex F. Manini

Galen, an influential physician from the second century, remarked of his clinical trial, "All who drink of this remedy recover in a short time, except those whom it does not help, who all die. Therefore, it is obvious that it fails only in incurable cases." Unfortunately, error in contemporary clinical investigation of poisoning tends to be more insidious than the error in logic in Galen's conclusion, and skillful scrutiny of published research remains an important endeavor.

Advances in medical toxicology are achieved through the scientific method, but must first rely on observations derived from xenobiotic exposures for hypothesis generation. Subsequent research questions are analyzed with epidemiological investigation, and preliminary studies are examined with methodological scrutiny. Initial analytical techniques are improved, and confirmatory studies are performed. Ultimately, models relating cause to effect are formulated.

To optimize patient care, it is useful to grade the quality of available scientific evidence used to justify treatment recommendations. Decisions about how strongly to recommend a medical action will be based on the careful consideration of the risks of leaving a patient untreated, the potential benefits and harms of treatment, the quality of the guiding evidence, a balanced view of resource utilization, and ultimately the values of the person to be treated. The Grading of Recommendations, Assessment, Development, and Evaluation (GRADE) Working Group has provided a framework for assessing and communicating levels of scientific evidence (Table 137–1).[26] An understanding of basic principles of research design and epidemiology is required to interpret published studies and to lay the groundwork for future investigation in toxicology.

EPIDEMIOLOGIC TECHNIQUES AVAILABLE TO INVESTIGATE CLINICAL PROBLEMS

Table 137–2 lists the different study formats discussed below.

Observational Design: Descriptive

Toxicologists rely on good descriptive data regarding the staggering array of xenobiotics that are able to cause injury. Through 2015, the National Poison Data System (NPDS) of the American Association of Poison Control Centers (AAPCC) has amassed a database of more than 50 million human exposures (Chap. 130). Descriptive case reporting serves a valuable purpose in describing the characteristics of a medical condition or procedure and remains a fundamental tool of epidemiologic investigation. A *case report* is a clinical description of a single patient or procedure in a unique context. Case reports are most useful for hypothesis generation. However, single case reports are not always generalizable, as the reported exposure, patients' circumstances, and treatment may be atypical. Certain aspects of a toxicologic case report should be included to maximize their utility and minimize bias.[41] A number of case reports can be grouped on the basis of similarities into a *case series*. Case series can be used to characterize an illness or syndrome, but without a control group they are severely limited in their ability to imply cause and effect. In 1966, a case series of 2 patients with acute liver necrosis following overdose of acetaminophen (APAP)[14] was accompanied by a case report of liver damage and impaired glucose tolerance after APAP overdose,[47] which led to further study and the eventual creation of the Rumack-Matthew nomogram (Chap. 33). The important role for descriptive data in guiding clinical research, focusing educational efforts, and formulating public policy are often underappreciated.

Cross-sectional studies assess a population for the presence or absence of an exposure and condition simultaneously. Such data often provide estimates of prevalence—the fraction of individuals in a population sharing a characteristic or condition at a point in time. These studies are particularly helpful in public health planning and are extremely useful in monitoring common environmental exposures, such as childhood lead poisoning, or population-wide drug use, such as occurs with tobacco, marijuana, and alcohol. A prime example is the US National Health and Nutrition Examination Survey, which demonstrated that the percentage of children with blood lead concentration greater than 10 mcg/dL decreased from 88.2% to 4.4% between 1976 and 1991, after the introduction of unleaded gasoline and paint to reduce populational lead exposure.[5]

An *analysis of secular trend* is a study type that compares changes in illness over time or geography to changes in environmental risk factors. These analyses often lend circumstantial support to a hypothesis; however, because of the environmental nature of their design, individual data on risk factors are not available to allow exclusion of alternative hypotheses also consistent with the data. A prime example of an analysis of secular trends is the finding that there was not a decline in new autism diagnoses after mercury was removed

TABLE 137–1	GRADE System for Evaluating Clinical Recommendations
Strength of Recommendation	**Quality of Evidence**
Strong	High
Weak	Moderate
	Low or very low
Strength/Quality Aggregate	**Implications**
Strong/high	• Recommendation can apply to most patients in most circumstances • Further research is unlikely to change our confidence in the estimate of effect
Strong/moderate	• Recommendation can apply to most patients in most circumstances • Further research (if performed) is likely to have an important impact on our confidence in the estimate of effect and may change the estimate
Strong/low	• Recommendation may change when higher quality evidence becomes available • Further research (if performed) is likely to have an important impact on our confidence in the estimate of effect and is likely to change the estimate
Weak/high	• The best action may differ depending on circumstances or patients or societal values • Further research is unlikely to change our confidence in the estimate of effect
Weak/moderate	• Other alternatives may be equally reasonable • Further research is very likely to have an important impact on our confidence in the estimate of effect and is likely to change the estimate
Weak/low	• Other alternatives may be equally reasonable • Any estimate of effect, for at least one critical outcome, is very uncertain

TABLE 137–2	Epidemiologic Study Designs: Types, Measurements, and Advantages	
Study Design[a]	*Main Measurement*	*Advantages*
Clinical trial	Efficacy	Gold standard for drug development
Noninferiority trial	Safety	Noninferior drugs may be better tolerated, cheaper, or easier to use
Cohort	Incidence, risk factors	Provides more robust evidence of association
		Reduced bias in exposure data
		Can study many outcomes simultaneously
		Allows direct calculation of incidence
		Allows direct calculation of relative risk
Case control	Association	Smaller sample required when outcome is rare
		Reduced bias in outcome data
		Can study many exposures simultaneously
		Allows estimation of relative risk
		May obviate need for long follow-up period
Analysis of secular trends	Population Trends	Examine trends in disease events over time
		Study across different geographic locations
		Can correlate them with trends in putative exposures
Cross sectional	Prevalence	Uncover relationships for future study
		Highly feasible
Case series	Descriptive	Characterize new syndromes or exposures
Case report	Descriptive	Identify signals for hypothesis generation

[a]Study designs are listed in descending order from the design that offers the best epidemiologic evidence for association to that which offers the least evidence.

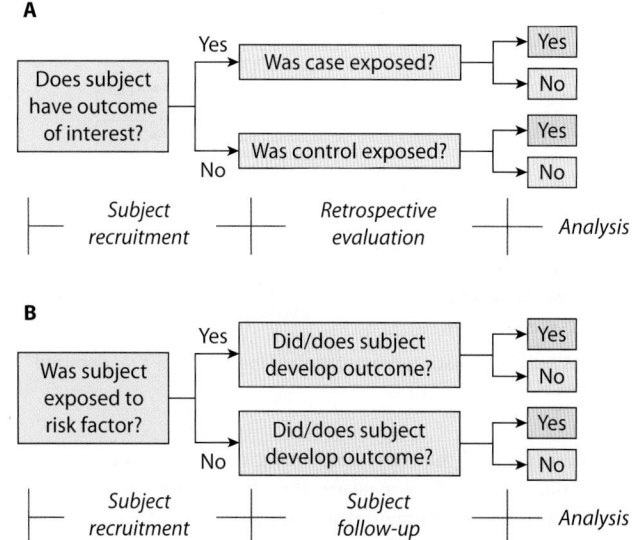

FIGURE 137–1. (**A**) Schematic representation of the case–control study design. Participants with an outcome or condition of interest are selected, along with control participants, and then are evaluated for previous exposure to a risk factor of interest. (**B**) Schematic representation of the cohort study design. Participants are recruited based on the presence or absence of a risk factor or exposure, then followed to see if they develop an outcome.

from vaccines.[44] This investigation found a lack of consistent evidence for an association between autism and thimerosal-containing vaccines.

Observational Design: Analytical

Hypotheses that are generated by theoretical reasoning or anecdotal association require analytical testing. Case–control studies and cohort studies are analytical techniques that use observational data, and each technique has its own advantages and disadvantages (Table 137–2). Case–control studies compare affected, treated, or diseased patients (cases) to nonaffected patients (controls) and evaluate for a difference in prior risk factors or exposures (Fig. 137–1A). Because participants are recruited into the study based on prior presence or absence of a particular outcome, case–control studies are always retrospective in nature. They are especially useful when the outcome being studied is rare, and they enable the investigation of any number of potential etiologies for a single disease.

The connection between CYP2C9 variants and the risk for nonsteroidal antiinflammatory drug (NSAID)–related gastrointestinal hemorrhage served as a prime example of a hypothesis that was well suited to case–control study design. Presence of variants of CYP2C9, the main CYP enzyme involved in the metabolism of NSAIDs, was common; however,

gastrointestinal hemorrhage is generally rare among those taking NSAIDs. Other putative risk factors such as daily NSAID doses were identifiable and could be studied simultaneously. In a case–control analysis of 577 cases who were patients older than 18 years with a diagnosis of upper gastrointestinal (GI) bleeding (UGIB), and 1,343 matched controls, the presence of the CYP2C9*3 variant increased the risk for UGIB associated with NSAID for daily doses greater than 0.5.[16]

Cohort studies compare patients with certain risk factors or exposures to those patients without the exposure, and then follow these cohorts to see which participants develop the outcome of interest (Fig. 137–1B). In this respect, they allow the comparison of *incidence* (the number of new outcomes occurring within a population initially free of disease over a period of time) between populations who share an exposure and populations who do not. They may be retrospective or prospective and enable the study of any number of outcomes from a single exposure. They are particularly well suited to investigations in which the outcome of interest is relatively common. In circumstances when an outcome of interest is very uncommon, such as the case with stroke after phenylpropanolamine use, the large number of study participants required might make a cohort study impractical. A cohort of 981 APAP overdose participants was used retrospectively to investigate whether administration of activated charcoal might be beneficial therapy for APAP poisoning.[9] Participants were separated on the basis of whether or not they were treated with activated charcoal and were subsequently followed to see if they developed concentrations deemed toxic by the Rumack-Matthew nomogram. Perhaps the most famous cohort study was the Framingham Heart Study in which 5,209 residents of Framingham, MA, aged 30 to 62 years, were followed for over 50 years. This study provided a useful tool for studying the incidence of lung cancer, stroke, and cardiovascular disease in those exposed to cigarette smoke and other hazardous xenobiotics.[17]

Experimental Design

Experimental studies are those in which the treatment, risk factor, or exposure of interest can be controlled by the investigator to study differences in outcome between the groups (Fig. 137–2). The prototype is the randomized, blinded, controlled clinical trial. Among epidemiologic study

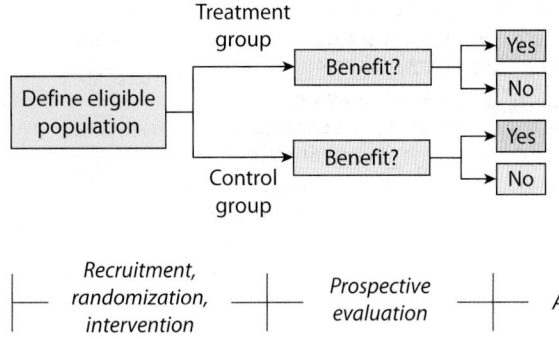

FIGURE 137–2. Schematic representation of the design of a randomized clinical trial.

types, these provide the most convincing demonstration of causality. Clinical trials are used to measure the *efficacy* (the treatment effect within a controlled experimental setting) of treatment regimens and to draw inferences about the *effectiveness* of a treatment applied to the general population. Sometimes a trial can be designed to study drug treatments that are hampered by nonresponders to therapy, expensive drugs, or poorly tolerated regimens. Such trials are termed *noninferiority trials*, and operate on the null hypothesis that the new (study) drug is worse than the control (standard) drug. Thus, finding a difference between groups in a noninferiority trial means that the alternative hypothesis can be accepted that the new drug is not worse than the standard treatment. In this way, noninferiority trials introduce a concept of *equivalence margins* of noninferiority. The term *equivalent* is not used here in the strict sense, but rather to mean that the efficacies of the 2 therapies are close enough so that one cannot be considered superior or inferior to the other. This concept is formalized in the definition of a term called the equivalence margin.

Unfortunately, interventional studies are the most complex to perform, and several questions must be addressed by investigators before performing a clinical trial (Table 137–3). Human clinical trials, despite some recent successes (such as antivenom for scorpion stings),[3] have been traditionally difficult to apply to the practice of toxicology. Table 137–4 lists characteristics of poisoned patients that hamper attempts at performing clinical trials. Volunteer studies, using nontoxic xenobiotics or nontoxic doses of toxic xenobiotics, are often used to circumvent some of the problems in controlling human toxicology studies. However, it is typically difficult to apply results from these studies to the actual clinical context of poisoning. In experimental human studies, activated charcoal reduced absorption of ampicillin by 57%,[46] and had a mortality benefit for yellow oleander poisoning.[15] Taken out of these settings, a trial of single-dose oral activated charcoal was unable to prove benefit to outcome among 1,479 heterogeneous participants presenting to an emergency department

TABLE 137–3	Considerations in Designing a Clinical Trial
What is the question of interest?	
What is the target patient population?	
How will the safety of subjects be assured?	
What is a suitable control group?	
How will outcomes be measured?	
What difference in outcomes between groups is considered important?	
What is the analysis plan?	
How many subjects will be required?	
How will randomization and blinding be achieved and maintained?	
How long a follow-up period will be required?	
How will loss of study subjects be addressed?	
How will treatment compliance be evaluated?	

TABLE 137–4	Difficulties in Utilizing Clinical Trials to Study Human Poisoning
It is unethical to intentionally "poison" subjects.	
Poisoned patients represent a broad spectrum of demographic patterns.	
A wide variety of xenobiotics exist.	
Exposures to any single xenobiotic are usually limited.	
A limited number of poisoned patients are available at any one study site.	
Uncertainty often exists as to type, quantity, and timing of most xenobiotic exposures.	
Poisoning typically results in a relatively short course of illness.	

(ED) for possible poisoning.[33] Unfortunately, none of these studies directly addresses whether activated charcoal reduces morbidity even if administered while the xenobiotic is still in the stomach and amenable to adsorption to activated charcoal.

MEASURES USED TO QUANTIFY THE STRENGTH OF AN EPIDEMIOLOGIC ASSOCIATION

The objective of analytical studies is to define and quantify the degree of statistical dependence between an exposure and an outcome. Such associations are ideally represented by the relative risk of developing an outcome if exposed in comparison to being unexposed. Thus, the *relative risk* can be defined as the incidence of outcome in exposed versus unexposed individuals, and can be calculated directly from cohort and interventional studies. However, in a case–control study, an investigator chooses the numbers of cases and controls to be studied, so true incidence data are not obtained. In case–control studies, an *odds ratio* can be calculated, and the odds ratio will provide an estimate for relative risk in situations in which the outcome is rare, such as when the outcome occurs in fewer than 10% of exposed individuals. Figure 137–3 demonstrates the calculation of relative risk or odds ratio from analytic studies.

A relative risk of 1.0 signifies that an outcome is equally likely to occur whether an individual either is exposed or is not exposed and implies that no association exists between the exposure and the outcome. A relative risk approaching 0 suggests that an exposure is a marker of protection regarding the outcome, and a relative risk approaching infinity suggests the exposure predicts a tendency toward developing the outcome. Among men and women using phenylpropanolamine appetite suppressants, the odds ratio for development of hemorrhagic stroke was 15.9, which indicates a strong association.[26a]

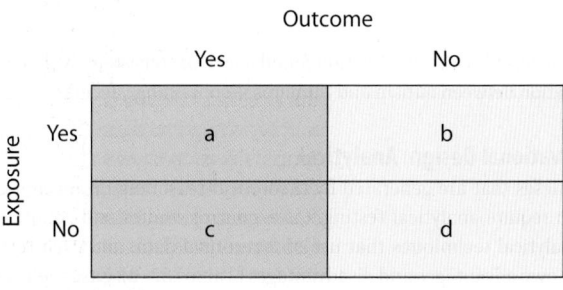

Cohort study

$$\text{Relative risk} = \frac{a}{a+b} \Big/ \frac{c}{c+d}$$

Case-control study

$$\text{Odds ratio} = ad/bc$$

FIGURE 137–3. Use of a 2 × 2 table to calculate or estimate relative risk from analytic studies. In cohort studies, study participants are selected on the basis of exposure. In case–control studies, participants are selected on the basis of outcome. The letters a, b, c, and d represent the number of participants either exposed or unexposed to a "risk factor" or treatment, with or without the outcome of interest. The odds hazard ratios estimate the relative risk if the outcome of interest is rare.

MEASURES USED TO QUANTIFY THE SIGNIFICANCE OF AN EPIDEMIOLOGIC ASSOCIATION

One of the essential features of research in medical toxicology is integration of the available data, whether clinical or experimental, into logical assumptions about how the overall system functions. Systems that are studied in medical toxicology research typically involve either elucidation of how a toxic insult influences normal physiology, or the mechanism and degree to which an antidote mitigates toxicity. Prior to undertaking an interventional study, ethical principles dictate that there must exist clinical *equipoise* regarding whether the intervention will have a benefit; otherwise, it should already be administered to everyone with the condition being studied and not withheld from the placebo group. Thus, a priori hypotheses are tested by performing experiments or by sampling observed data in an organized fashion. If the results are consistent with the predictions, then the hypothesis is retained; if not, then the prior hypothesis is rejected and a new hypothesis is formulated. This process is the basis of the scientific method and is also known as hypothesis testing.

Determination of whether the observed data in a toxicology investigation allow us to retain or refute our a priori hypothesis depends on our ability to gauge the certainty that the data were arrived at by chance. When observing a set of data, investigators can never be 100% certain that what they observed actually happened; it is possible that confounding factors biased what was observed, and it is possible that the observation was made simply by chance. To deal with this problem of interpretation, researchers use statistical methods to evaluate whether their data were arrived at by chance. The presence of an association between 2 factors in any given study has a number of possible explanations (Table 137–5).

To differentiate between differences due to chance and potentially real differences between comparison groups, researchers can use a philosophical approach known as the *null hypothesis*. The null hypothesis involves beginning experiments with the assumption that there is no difference between groups being compared. Thus, any significant deviation from observed and expected results under the null hypothesis allows the investigator to reject the null hypothesis and adopt the alternative hypothesis. The alternative hypothesis to the null is that the groups being compared are significantly different from one another (ie, not the same).

To begin, one must assign a probability percentage or *P* value to the likelihood that their observed results are *really* the case assuming the null hypothesis to be true. With some exceptions, the standard *P* value deemed to represent ability to reject the null hypothesis has historically been set to 5% (or *P* <.05) in epidemiologic science. This value is also termed the alpha (α), the significance level, the *Type 1 error*, and represents the chance of falsely finding a difference between groups when one does not exist. *Type 2 error*, or a beta (β) error, is the possibility that an investigator will be unable to find an association when one is really present. In some cases, investigators must use a *P* value even lower than .05 when testing multiple hypotheses at once, for example, in genetic marker studies examining multiple genes across an entire genome. Such a correction is termed the *Bonferroni correction* and is applied as the *P* value divided by the number of variables being tested at once: *P* = (significance level) / (no. of concurrent variables).[43] The result is a

smaller (ie, more stringent) corrected significance level for studies that test multiple hypotheses at once. For example, if a study protocol uses a genetic "chip" assay to evaluate 50 markers at once for an association with a predetermined disease in a population, the Bonferroni correction would require significance at (0.05)/(50) = 0.001 in order to deem any association to be statistically significant.

Perhaps a more informative description of the significance of an association is provided through the confidence interval (CI). The CI not only provides a test of statistical significance, it also offers information pertaining to the degree (and possible range) of differences observed. In an unbiased study, the 95% CI provides a range between which, if the study could be repeated an infinite number of times, the observed point estimate would fall between the CI 95% of the time. For example, one study reported that no toddlers ingesting one or 2 calcium channel blocker tablets became seriously ill, but a subsequent analysis of the CI around this small set of data demonstrated that the true incidence could be as high as 18%.[36] A CI around a relative risk or odds ratio is not statistically significant if it includes 1.0, and the narrower the CI the more precise the estimate of the magnitude of effect.

The likelihood that a study will find a difference if one truly exists is termed statistical *power* and relates to the likelihood of a false-negative study (Type 2 error). Power of a study is usually preset by an investigator before a study is performed and is typically 80% or 90% to set limits on the number of study participants needed. Table 137–6 lists considerations applicable to the choice of sample size. The sample size of a study is determined by the frequency of the exposure and outcome within the study population, the strength of association deemed clinically relevant, and the amount of error deemed acceptable in the study. Because power is often set relatively low, it is difficult to state that an association does not exist. It is more appropriate to state that a study was unable to reject the null hypothesis to find an association.

Although the clinical significance of an association is ultimately left to the judgment of the individual (or group) interpreting a study, ideally a working definition of clinical significance is developed before a study is performed. The finding of a low *P* value indicates a statistically high level of certainty that a difference between study groups exists, but unfortunately offers no indication that the difference is clinically relevant. This especially becomes problematic to interpret when small actual differences between groups are found to be statistically significant because of large numbers of participants; conversely, impressive associations of cause and effect can seem trivial if few participants are in a study. Therefore, interpretation of statistical versus clinical significance is often required, and may be facilitated either by calculating CIs around the point estimate, or alternatively by estimating the *effect size*.

Calculating the effect size is often used to complement statistical hypothesis testing by providing a quantifiable measure of the strength of a phenomenon. The effect size also plays an important role in power calculations and study sample size requirements. The reporting of effect sizes

TABLE 137–5	Types of Associations Between Exposures and Outcomes That May Be Found With a Clinical Study
No association	The outcome is independent of exposure.
Artifactual association	
Chance	The association demonstrated by the study resulted from random error.
Bias	Systematic error in the study led to the noted association.
Indirect association	The association is real, but not truly cause and effect (confounding).
Causal association	The outcome is dependent on the exposure.

TABLE 137–6	Considerations in Choice of Sample Size	
	Sample Size	
	Large	*Small*
Pros	• Able to detect associations of small magnitude • Less susceptible to some biases • More robust analysis	• Less work • Less cost
Cons	• More work • More cost	• Might not detect associations of small magnitude • More susceptible to biases associated with patient differences

facilitates the interpretation of the substantive, as opposed to the statistical, significance of a research result. Although there are a variety of methods to estimate and calculate effect size, a useful method applicable to many studies in the medical toxicology literature is to calculate the *Cohen's d*. Cohen's *d* is defined as the difference between the means of 2 groups (x_1, x_2) divided by the standard deviation (*s*) of the mean, that is: $d = (x_1 - x_2)/s$. A larger absolute value of *d* represents a stronger effect. Cohen originally defined effect sizes as small, $d \sim 0.2$, medium, $d \sim 0.5$, and large, $d \sim 0.8$.[13] Effect sizes can also be thought of as the average percentile standing of the average treated (or experimental) participant relative to the average untreated (or control) participant; thus, a Cohen's *d* of 0.8 indicates that the mean of the experimental group is at the 80th percentile of the control group. Reporting effect size, by any appropriate method, should generally be considered a good practice when presenting empirical research findings in the field of medical toxicology.

METHODOLOGIC PROBLEMS FOUND WITHIN CLINICAL STUDIES

The calculation of a *P* value or CI to quantify the influence of random error/chance does nothing to assess the adequacy of study design. Clinical research is particularly susceptible to *bias*, defined as systematic error in the collection or interpretation of data. Because such error can lead to inappropriate estimates of the causal relationship between an exposure and an outcome, careful evaluation of potential bias affecting a clinical study is of paramount importance.

Selection bias refers to error introduced into a study by the manner in which participants are selected for inclusion in the study. This type of bias is most problematic for retrospective studies in which exposures and outcomes have both occurred at the time of participant recruitment. Selection bias are introduced into a prospective clinical study if the study fails to enroll potential participants, or if potential participants refuse to participate, on a systematic basis. Selection bias may even influence the results of clinical trials. In a 1995 trial that found no difference in outcome between acutely poisoned patients treated with gastric emptying and patients from whom gastric emptying was withheld, all patients presenting to the ED after acute overdose were enrolled.[39] Because most patients with poisoning exposure are likely to do well with minimal support, selection of patients on this basis might be expected to bias this study to find no effect. Reasoning suggests that the patients most likely to benefit from gastric emptying are those with life-threatening toxic ingestion presenting within the first hour after exposure. Indeed, subgroup analysis of this paper suggests clinical benefit within this group of patients, but without conclusive power.

Information bias refers to error introduced into a study as a result of systematic differences in the quality of data obtained between exposed and unexposed groups, or between those with and without the outcome of interest. Several distinct types of information bias exist. Affected and nonaffected individuals may have differential memories regarding exposures, so recall bias is a concern in retrospective studies. The potential for *recall bias* is often cited as criticism of retrospective case–control studies, such as the seminal study documenting the association between phenylpropanolamine and hemorrhagic stroke, in which patients and families were asked to recollect their phenylpropanolamine use history. Stroke victims and their families might be more vigorous in their recall of exposures than control participants, thus biasing away from the null hypothesis. Similarly, *interviewer bias* occurs if study personnel differ in how they solicit, record, or interpret information as a result of knowledge of participant status regarding exposures or outcomes.

Prospective studies may be limited by loss to follow-up, especially if participants' data are lost from the study for reasons relating to either exposure or outcome (such as when participants withdraw from a study because they are feeling better), or are unable to be contacted because the patients have expired or changed contact information. *Misclassification bias* occurs when investigators incorrectly categorize participants with respect to exposure or

outcome. In a retrospective study of 378 children regarding the predictability of caustic esophageal injury from clinical signs and symptoms, it was found that 11 of 80 asymptomatic children had significant burns.[18] A potential limitation is that "asymptomatic" children were misclassified because of lack of rigorous written documentation of symptoms or signs within the medical charts. In addition, studies that use "cause of death" as an outcome are vulnerable to misclassification as well. For example, in a large study comparing 414 poison control center deaths with 7,050 poisonings in the corresponding vital statistics database, the medical examiner and a medical toxicologist adjudication panel concurred on "cause of death" in only 66%, which the authors interpreted as only fair (ie, less than good) agreement.[29] Thus, when investigators define "cause of death" as their study outcome, their results may be biased depending on which specialists are used to provide the "cause of death" interpretation. Similarly, there are limitations to studies of large administrative databases where the outcome of interest is subject to multiple biases.[31,40]

Bias is best minimized through careful study design. It is important to precisely define the study question and the population at risk and to carefully define rigorous inclusion and exclusion criteria. The outcome should also be defined precisely. During data acquisition the best way to reduce bias is to keep study personnel gathering exposure data blinded to outcome, and vice versa. Often, it is also advisable to keep study participants unaware of their status within a study to the extent that it is ethical (thus, "double-blinded"—neither investigators nor participants are aware of the participants' status within a study). Use of *placebos* or "sham treatments" is a way to facilitate blinding. One of the strongest criticisms of a 1995 trial of hyperbaric oxygen (HBO) for the prevention of delayed neurologic syndromes after CO poisoning[42] has been the failure to blind patients and investigators to the treatment in question,[35] a flaw that was corrected in a follow-up study published in 2002.[40] It is inevitable that some degree of potential bias will be present in any clinical study. Such bias should be reviewed in the analysis, and estimations of its magnitude and direction (bias toward or away from rejection of the null hypothesis) should be considered.

Unlike selection and information biases, which are errors introduced into studies primarily by the investigators or participants, *confounding* is a special type of problem that occurs within a study as a result of interrelationships between the exposure of interest and another exposure. Confounding is a bias wherein an observed association is not a product of cause and effect but instead results from linking of the exposure of interest to another associated exposure. Studies pertaining to adverse effects of drugs of abuse are especially prone to confounding by variables such as concomitant caffeine use, alcohol use, tobacco use, nutritional deficiency, and/or psychiatric illness. Analytic studies often restrict characteristics of enrolled participants or match participant characteristics between comparison groups in an effort to reduce confounding. Accordingly, it has been suggested that future studies on delayed neuropsychiatric manifestations following CO poisoning control for potential confounding from depression and cyanide exposure.[30] During data analysis, confounding can often be controlled through stratification of data into subgroups or through multivariate analysis techniques.

Randomization is of central importance in clinical trials. It prevents selection bias and insures against unintended bias. It is also an important method to ensure that unsuspected confounding factors are equally distributed between treatment groups within interventional studies. The 4 common types of randomization include (1) simple, (2) block, (3) stratified, and (4) unequal randomization. The *simple* method is equivalent to tossing a coin for each participant who enters a trial, such as heads = treatment, tails = placebo. Generally, a random number generator is used for this type of randomization. *Block* randomization is often used to guarantee balance in numbers during a clinical trial. The basic idea of block randomization is to divide potential patients into *m* blocks of size *2n*, randomize each block such that *n* patients are allocated to *A* and *n* to *B*, and then to choose the blocks randomly. Less common is *stratified* randomization to prevent imbalance in prognostic factors that may confound estimating treatment effect. Stratified randomization achieves balance within important subgroups. For example, using block randomization separately for diabetics and nondiabetics in a cardiovascular trial. And finally, *unequal* randomization is used when 2 or more treatments under evaluation have a cost difference such that it is more economically efficient to randomize fewer patients to the expensive treatment and more to the cheaper one.

To improve the reporting of clinical trials, and to improve the recognition and interpretation of biases within them, guidelines referred to as the Consensus Standards of Reporting Trials (CONSORT) have been adopted by many medical journals.[34] The CONSORT guidelines provide a checklist to allow authors to systematically and uniformly report data and limitations. When interpreting published studies, it is also important to consider the potential for *publication bias*. Publication bias refers to the tendency for researchers, editors, and pharmaceutical companies to handle the reporting of studies with positive results differently from those with negative or inconclusive results.[45] Many journals now require that researchers register all planned clinical trials into a registry as a prerequisite for subsequent publication.

EVIDENTIARY CRITERIA USED TO LINK CAUSE AND EFFECT

As is illustrated in Table 137–5, association of an exposure to an illness does not necessarily equate to cause and effect. In assessing causation, it must be determined if bias is present in the selection or measurement of exposure or outcome. If a study is unbiased, then the role of chance in the occurrence of the observed association must be explored. If an association is unbiased, unlikely to result from random error, and is not subject to confounding, then assumptions regarding causation can be derived. Table 137–7 provides a list of evidentiary criteria, first proposed by Bradford Hill in 1965,[22] that are often used to support causation.

In large part due to the inability to perform randomized trials, it is extremely difficult in medical toxicology to prove causal relationships. The goal is to build empiric evidence so that associations can be confirmed or refuted with conviction. However, many toxicologists deem clinical trials unconvincing, such as those investigating benefits from gastric emptying or HBO therapy for CO intoxication, due to the degree of bias present in the relevant published clinical trials. To address this issue, some consensus works (from position papers to formal consensus studies) attempt to provide guidance to clinical toxicologists regarding interventions where equipoise remains despite published clinical trials. For example, the Appraisal of Guidelines for Research and Evaluation (AGREE) Instrument is widely used in consensus guidelines. The instrument in its present form has been updated as "AGREE II" and is composed of 23 items organized into 6 quality domains (scope, stakeholders, rigor, clarity, applicability, independence).[6]

INFERENTIAL STATISTICAL TESTS

As discussed previously, researchers must devise an appropriate statistical test to determine whether or not their data were arrived at by chance, a process known as inferential statistics. Once the significance level has been chosen, the inferential statistical test of choice depends on the type of data that are being collected. It should be noted that using the wrong statistical test for a given set of data will invalidate the reported results of a study; thus, choosing the correct statistical test is of paramount importance for study design, as well as for toxicologists who try to interpret published medical literature.

Once the significance level has been set, then the data must be classified by type. Generally, data are either (1) categoric/nominal (≥2 categories of data with no intrinsic ordering, eg, presence/absence of medical comorbidities), (2) continuous/interval (data along a scale where each value is equidistant from one another, eg, dollar values), or (3) ordinal/ranked (≥2 categories of data with clear intrinsic ordering, eg, grade in high school). The method used to compare groups of data thus depends on whether data are categorical, continuous, or ordinal. Most commonly, categorical data are compared in terms of ratios/percentages (chi-squared test) and continuous data are compared in terms of means (Student t test) or medians (Mann-Whitney U test). As a general rule of thumb, an ideal analysis involves comparing interval/ratio data between groups because these data contain more information than any of the other forms of data. Finally, the number and relatedness of the independent variables for analysis must be determined. Most commonly, 2 unrelated samples are compared to assess for associations. However, there are times when groups are paired or related, such as in clinical trials with before/after data in the same participants. Additionally, it is possible to use more advanced techniques to compare 3 or more independent variables at once (Table 137–8).

Inferential statistical tests are generally classified into parametric versus nonparametric techniques. This distinction is based on the fact that statistical tests make varying assumptions with regard to the population parameters that characterize the distributions for which the test is employed. Parametric tests generally make more stringent assumptions upon the data to produce valid results, while nonparametric tests make few if any assumptions about the data parameters and can thus be thought of as a "backup" test if the parametric assumptions are not met. For example, the t test assumes that the 2 groups being compared are independent of each other and that the dependent variable is continuous and normally distributed along a bell-shaped

TABLE 137–7	Bradford Hill Criteria for Determining Causation
Strength	What degree of relative risk or odds ratio was demonstrated in the analysis?
Consistency	Does the cause and effect hold true in different studies, locations, and populations?
Specificity	Does the effect occur without the cause in question, or vice versa?
Temporality	Does the cause precede the effect?
Biologic gradient	Is there a dose–response effect?
Plausibility	Is the association consistent with the current understanding of the biological system?
Coherence	Is the association compatible with existing theory and knowledge?
Experiment	Was the association demonstrated in a well-designed study?
Analogy	Is there another cause–effect relationship in nature that is similar to the one in question?

TABLE 137–8	Parametric vs Nonparametric Inferential Tests Based on Data Type	
Data Type	**Parametric Test**	**Nonparametric Test**
Continuous/interval		
Related samples	Paired t test	Wilcoxon signed rank
Unrelated samples	Independent samples t test	Mann-Whitney U
≥3 groups	ANOVA	Kruskal Wallis
Correlation	Pearson R	Spearman rho
Nominal/categorical		
Related samples	Chi-squared Fisher exact	McNemar
Unrelated samples	Chi-squared Fisher exact	Mantel Haenszel trend
≥3 groups	Chi-squared	Cochran-Armitage
Correlation	Kappa	Spearman rho
Ordinal/ranked		
Same scales	Not applicable (NA)	Mann Whitney U
Different scales	NA	Wilcoxon signed rank
≥3 groups	NA	Cochran-Armitage
Correlation	Spearman rho	NA

curve (also known as a Gaussian distribution). Similarly, the chi-squared test assumes independent observation from a random selection of a given population with a large enough sample size such that any cell in the resultant 2×2 table is greater than 5. A violation of one or more of these basic assumptions renders the test results invalid and mandates application of the nonparametric versions of these tests. The common parametric and nonparametric tests based on data classifications are summarized in Table 137–8.

EVALUATION OF DIAGNOSTIC TESTS AND CRITERIA

In clinical practice it is often useful to have a test, which may be a laboratory result or clinical paradigm, to help arrive at a diagnosis or predict an outcome. For instance, historical questionnaires, capillary blood lead concentrations, and venous blood lead concentrations might all be used to identify children at risk of neurocognitive injury from plumbism.[10] However, each of these approaches is likely to have certain disadvantages in terms of effort, cost, discomfort, and/or accuracy. Targeting lead evaluation and therapy in children on the basis of exposure history is expected to be easy and inexpensive, but will not identify some children with significant poisoning; thus, the test is susceptible to being falsely negative. Capillary blood testing is more costly and uncomfortable and is susceptible to false-positive test results because of environmental lead dust present on fingertips. The possibility of false-positive or false-negative results must be considered with any diagnostic test (Fig. 137–4).

The utility of diagnostic testing is often described in terms of sensitivity, specificity, predictive value of a positive test (PPV), and predictive value of a negative test (NPV). A cross-sectional design is often used to study diagnostic tests, as we seek to determine the prevalence of positive tests among the diseased (*sensitivity*), and the prevalence of negative tests among the healthy (*specificity*). A perfect test would be highly sensitive and specific, but this is seldom possible. A highly sensitive test is often used in screening programs because they rarely lead to false-negative diagnoses. Specific tests (eg, urine benzoylecgonine for cocaine exposure) are typically used to "rule-in" a

Presence of disease

$$\text{Sensitivity} = \frac{a}{a+c} = \frac{\text{True positives}}{\text{True positives} + \text{False negatives}}$$

$$\text{Specificity} = \frac{d}{b+d} = \frac{\text{True negatives}}{\text{False positives} + \text{True negatives}}$$

$$\text{PPV} = \frac{a}{a+b} = \frac{\text{True positives}}{\text{True positives} + \text{False positives}}$$

$$\text{NPV} = \frac{d}{c+d} = \frac{\text{True negatives}}{\text{False negatives} + \text{True negatives}}$$

PPV = Positive predictive value
NPV = Negative predictive value

FIGURE 137–4. Possible results of diagnostic testing and the statistical characteristics used to describe the utility of diagnostic tests. The letters a, b, c, and d represent the numbers of tested individuals with or without the disease of interest.

TABLE 137–9	Questions to Consider When Evaluating a Study

Research objectives
    What is the study question?
    What is the studied population?
Study design
    What type of study was performed?
    How were participants recruited and enrolled?
    Why were participants excluded?
    What was the nature of the comparison group?
Data accrual
    How were the data collected?
    Are the exposures and outcomes clearly defined?
    Are the observations reliable and reproducible?
    Was randomization and/or blinding used?
    Were participants lost to follow-up?
Analysis
    Are the results statistically significant?
    Are the results clinically significant?
    Are potential confounding variables controlled?
    Was the study powered to detect important differences?
Conclusions
    Are the conclusions justified by data?

diagnosis, as they rarely yield false-positive results. Whereas sensitivity and specificity are inherent properties of a diagnostic test applied to a given population, the probability of disease—based on the results of a test—is highly dependent on the prevalence of disease within the population being tested. The PPV is the probability of having disease in a patient with a positive test; the NPV is the probability of not having disease when the test result is negative. Numerous studies have tried to examine the utility of vomiting, leukocytosis, hyperglycemia, total iron-binding capacity, and radiographic findings in predicting toxicity after acute iron overdose. In a retrospective assessment of 40 adults with oral iron overdose, vomiting was found to predict a serum iron concentration above 300 mcg/dL with a sensitivity rate of 84%, specificity of 50%, NPV of 44%, and PPV of 87%.[37] This suggested that the presence of vomiting should raise concern for iron toxicity but that the lack of vomiting was not particularly useful. Figure 137–4 outlines the calculation of the sensitivity, specificity, PPV, and NPV. It is important to remember that these calculations, too, are subject to bias and are best accompanied by CIs.

SUMMARY

- Medical toxicology has embraced the vision of incorporating evidence-based medicine into practice.
- Randomized clinical trials, although the gold standard study design, have proven difficult to perform within medical toxicology.
- As toxicologists move beyond descriptive data reporting, there remains great potential for scientific advancement in the field of toxicology via hypothesis-testing from observational clinical research.
- Clinical investigators are charged with the imperative to perform studies based on sound epidemiologic principles.
- All studies, by nature of population sampling, are at the mercy of chance, but such random error can be quantified using statistical techniques.
- Systematic error (bias) can be limited, but not entirely excluded, through careful study design.
- Clinicians interpreting published toxicology research need to thoroughly evaluate a study's research objectives, design, data acquisition, analysis, and conclusions before applying the results to patient care (Table 137–9).
- Future epidemiologic investigation should allow more valid conclusions to be drawn regarding the associations between exposures and outcomes, or regarding the value of treatments for poisonings, discussed in the preceding chapters of this text.

REFERENCES

1. AGREE Trust. Development and validation of an international appraisal instrument for assessing the quality of clinical practice guidelines: the AGREE project. *Qual Saf Health Care.* 2003;12:18-23.

2. Albertson TE, et al. Regional variations in the use and awareness of the California Poison Control System. *J Toxicol Clin Toxicol (Phila).* 2004;42:625-633.

3. Anderson KD, et al. A controlled trial of corticosteroids in children with corrosive injury of the esophagus. *N Engl J Med* 1990;323:637-640.

4. Boyer LV, et al. Antivenom for critically ill children with neurotoxicity from scorpion stings. *N Engl J Med* 2009;360:2090-2098.

5. Brody DJ, et al. Blood lead levels in the US population. Phase 1 of the Third National Health and Nutrition Examination Survey (NHANES III, 1988 to 1991). *JAMA.* 1994;272:277-283.

6. Brouwers M, et al; on behalf of the AGREE, Consortium NS. AGREE II: Advancing guideline development, reporting and evaluation in healthcare. In: Can, J MA, eds 2010.

7. Buckler NA, et al. Preformatted admission charts for poisoning admissions facilitate clinical assessment and research. *Ann Emerg Med.* 1999;34(4, pt 1):476-482.

8. Buckley NA, Smith AJ. Evidence-based medicine in toxicology: where is the evidence? *Lancet.* 1996;347:1167-1169.

9. Buckley NA, et al. Activated charcoal reduces the need for *N*-acetylcysteine treatment after acetaminophen (paracetamol) overdose. *J Toxicol Clin Toxicol (Phila).* 1999;37:753-757.

10. Campbell C, Osterhoudt KC. Prevention of childhood lead poisoning. *Curr Opin Pediatr.* 2000;12:428-437.

11. Caravati EM, McElwee NE. Use of clinical toxicology resources by emergency physicians and its impact on poison control centers. *Ann Emerg Med.* 1991;20:147-150.

12. Clark RF, et al. Evaluating the utilization of a regional poison center by Latino communities. *J Toxicol Clin Toxicol (Phila).* 2002;40:855-860.

13. Cohen J. *Statistical Power Analysis for the Behavioral Sciences.* Hillsdale, NJ: Lawrence Erlbaum Associates; 1988.

14. Davidson DG, Eastham WN. Acute liver necrosis following overdose of paracetamol. *Br Med J.* 1966;2:497-499.

15. de Silva HA, et al. Multiple-dose activated charcoal in yellow oleander poisoning. *Lancet.* 2008;371:2171; author reply 2171-2172.

16. Figueiras A, et al. CYP2C9 variants as a risk modifier of NSAID-related gastrointestinal bleeding: a case–control study. *Pharmacogenet Genomics.* 2016;26:66-73.

17. Freund KM, et al. The health risks of smoking. The Framingham Study: 34 years of follow-up. *Ann Epidemiol.* 1993;3:417-424.

18. Gaudreault P, et al. Predictability of esophageal injury from signs and symptoms: a study of caustic ingestion in 378 children. *Pediatrics.* 1983;71:767-770.

19. Hamilton RJ, Goldfrank LR. Poison center data and the Pollyanna phenomenon. *J Toxicol Clin Toxicol (Phila).* 1997;35:21-23.

20. Hansen CK, et al. Analysis and validation of putative substances involved in fatal poisonings. *J Med Toxicol.* 2012;8:94-100.

21. Harchelroad F, et al. Treated vs reported toxic exposures: discrepancies between a poison control center and a member hospital. *Vet Hum Toxicol.* 1990;32:156-159.

22. Hill AB. The environment and disease: association or causation? *Proc R Soc Med.* 1965;58:295-300.

23. Hoppe-Roberts JM, et al. Poisoning mortality in the United States: comparison of national mortality statistics and poison control center reports. *Ann Emerg Med.* May 2000;35:440-448.

24. Hoyt BT, et al. Poison center data accuracy: a comparison of rural hospital chart data with the TESS database. Toxic Exposure Surveillance System. *Acad Emerg Med.* 1999;6:851-855.

25. Institute of Medicine. *Forging a Poison Prevention and Control System.* Washington, DC: National Academies Press; 2004.

26. Kavanagh BP. The GRADE system for rating clinical guidelines. *PLoS Med.* 2009;6:e1000094.

26a. Kernan WN, et al. Phenylpropanolamine and the risk of hemorrhagic stroke. *N Engl J Med.* 2000;343:1826-1832.

27. King J. Hypertension and cerebral haemorrhage after trimolets ingestion. *Med J Aust.* 1979;2:258.

28. Levy A, et al. Unproven ingestion: an unrecognized bias in toxicological case series. *Clin Toxicol (Phila).* 2007;45:946-949.

29. Manini AF, et al. Medical examiner and medical toxicologist agreement on cause of death. *Forensic Sci Int.* 2011;206:71-76.

30. Martin JD, et al. Recognition and management of carbon monoxide poisoning in children. *Clin Pediatr Emerg Med.* 2000;1:244-250.

31. McCaig LF, Burt CW. Understanding and interpreting the National Hospital Ambulatory Medical Care Survey: key questions and answers. *Ann Emerg Med.* 2012;60:716.e1-721.e1.

32. McFee. "The Granny Syndrome" and medication access as significant causes of unintentional pediatric poisoning. *J Toxicol Clin Toxicol (Phila).* 1999;37:593.

33. Merigian KS, Blaho KE. Single-dose oral activated charcoal in the treatment of the self-poisoned patient: a prospective, randomized, controlled trial. *Am J Ther.* 2002;9:301-308.

34. Moher D, et al. The CONSORT statement: revised recommendations for improving the quality of reports of parallel-group randomized trials. *JAMA.* 2001;285:1987-1991.

35. Olson KR, Seger D. Hyperbaric oxygen for carbon monoxide poisoning: does it really work? *Ann Emerg Med.* 1995;25:535-537.

36. Osterhoudt KC, Henretig FM. How much confidence that calcium channel blockers are safe? *Vet Hum Toxicol.* 1998;40:239.

37. Palatnick W, Tenenbein M. Leukocytosis, hyperglycemia, vomiting, and positive X-rays are not indicators of severity of iron overdose in adults. *Am J Emerg Med.* 1996;14:454-455.

38. Polivka BJ, et al. Comparison of poison exposure data: NHIS and TESS data. *J Toxicol Clin Toxicol (Phila).* 2002;40:839-845.

39. Pond SM, et al. Gastric emptying in acute overdose: a prospective randomised controlled trial. *Med J Aust.* 1995;163:345-349.

40. Raven MC, et al. Comparison of presenting complaint vs discharge diagnosis for identifying "nonemergency" emergency department visits. *JAMA.* 2013;309:1145-1153.

41. Ruha AM. The case report: a tool for the toxicologist. *J Med Toxicol.* 2009;5:1-2.

42. Scheinkestel CD, et al. Hyperbaric or normobaric oxygen for acute carbon monoxide poisoning: a randomised controlled clinical trial. *Med J Aust.* 1999;170:203-210.

43. Shaffer JP. Multiple hypothesis testing. *Annu Rev Psychol.* 1995;46:561-584.

44. Stehr-Green P, et al. Autism and thimerosal-containing vaccines: lack of consistent evidence for an association. *Am J Prev Med.* 2003;25:101-106.

45. Sutton AJ, et al. Empirical assessment of effect of publication bias on meta-analyses. *BMJ.* 2000;320:1574.

46. Tenenbein M, et al. Efficacy of ipecac-induced emesis, orogastric lavage, and activated charcoal for acute drug overdose. *Ann Emerg Med.* 1987;16:838-841.

47. Thomson JS, Prescott LF. Liver damage and impaired glucose tolerance after paracetamol overdosage. *Br Med J.* 1966;2:506-507.

48. Vassilev ZP, et al. Rapid communication: sociodemographic differences between counties with high and low utilization of a regional poison control center. *J Toxicol Environ Health A.* 2003;66:1905-1908.

49. Weaver LK, et al. Hyperbaric oxygen for acute carbon monoxide poisoning. *N Engl J Med.* 2002;347:1057-1067.

138 RISK MANAGEMENT AND LEGAL PRINCIPLES

Barbara M. Kirrane

The number and diversity of toxicologic emergencies faced by emergency department (ED) staff have increased steadily since the early 1970s and continue to rise today. This chapter discusses the medicolegal management of patients who are exposed to xenobiotics that alter their ability to think. It also addresses the legal and ethical dilemmas routinely encountered by emergency medicine practitioners.

Patients with toxicologic emergencies require immediate care, and yet are often unable to give consent because their impaired consciousness prevents them from making informed decisions. Treating patients who present with an acute organic impairment manifested by confusion, irrational thought, or even dangerous behavior is very challenging. Emergency practitioners must recognize the medicolegal problems created when the impaired patient refuses treatment and insists on leaving against medical advice. The issue is further complicated by the variations in relevant state laws. Emergency practitioners must become familiar with the legal requirements of informed consent and the essential management necessary to avoid liability for negligence and abandonment within the state in which they practice. Of particular concern are the risk management and liability issues that relate to impaired patients attempting to leave the ED before medical care is complete. The legal requirements of informed consent in emergency settings, the duty to treat, medical malpractice risk, battery, and negligence allegations, are examined here. Guidelines based on generally accepted common law principles are suggested for developing appropriate patient care plans and departmental policies. These issues and principles are best illustrated by case examples.

INFORMED CONSENT

Patient 1

An 18-year-old college student was brought by ambulance to the ED after a friend reported seeing her in the bathroom with slit wrists and an empty bottle of acetaminophen (APAP). In the ED, the patient was alert and oriented to time, place and person. Vital signs were as follows: blood pressure, 120/65 mm Hg; pulse, 95 beats/min; respiratory rate, 16 breaths/min; and temperature, 99.1°F (37.3°C). A rapid bedside glucose concentration was 120 mg/dL. The patient stated that she ingested the APAP approximately 5 hours earlier in an attempt to kill herself. The health care team wished to measure an APAP concentration to determine whether N-acetylcysteine should be administered. The patient refused venipuncture and stated that she would refuse any medications. The physicians informed the patient that she might suffer irreparable damage to her liver and possibly die if not treated immediately. This type of clinical dilemma is the ideal moment to discuss strategies with the local poison control center and medical toxicologist. The poison control center staff will have great experience in addressing complex unorthodox management strategies, suggesting how much time the physician has in the emergency department to achieve a solution without substantially compromising the patient's care and how much of the normal strategy can be altered or eliminated and still render quality care.

Medically treating patients against their will poses a difficult problem. Forcible treatment violates the principle of autonomy and the patient's right to privacy. However, harm to the Satient may ensue if the appropriate evaluation and treatments are not performed. In the case above, the patient gives a history of ingesting a large amount of APAP, which risks causing hepatotoxicity and even death if not treated (Chap. 33). Her refusal to be evaluated raises the important question of whether a physician is ever justified in performing an assessment of someone who is alert and oriented, refuses treatment, yet is poisoned. Do most patients suffering from a mental illness such as depression require treatment against their will? As in this case, if the harm that the patient faces is not immediate, but certain in the near future, does the physician have the duty and authority to treat? General principles of patient autonomy, informed consent and battery will be elucidated here.

A patient's right to choose a course of medical treatment was first recognized in the early twentieth century in a landmark case decided by the New York State (NYS) Court of Appeals in *Schloendorff v. Society of New York Hospital*.[26] Mary Schloendorff was admitted for abdominal pain and was found on physical examination to have a mass. Her physicians offered her a more thorough examination under anesthesia and the option for surgery. Although she consented only to the exploratory surgery, during the procedure the mass was removed. Postoperatively, Schloendorff developed an infection, gangrene, and several fingers had to be amputated. She sued the hospital. In its decision, the Court acknowledged Schloendorff's right to self-determination, and the right to refuse treatment. It stated:

> Every human being of adult years and sound mind has a right to determine what shall be done with his own body and a surgeon who performs an operation without his patient's consent commits an assault, for which he is liable in damages, except in cases of emergency in which the patient is unconscious and it is necessary to operate before consent can be obtained.[26]

This decision formed the foundation for the "Doctrine of Informed Consent." Informed consent serves to protect a patient's autonomy, and creates the concept that each individual has the right to choose a personal course of medical treatment.[45] This includes the right to refuse care, and the right to terminate care already in process. In a nonemergent situation, it is the responsibility of the physician to obtain approval from a patient with decision making capacity or a legally recognized surrogate for those patients lacking such capacity before rendering treatment.

The core elements of the informed consent process consist of (1) an explanation of the treatment or procedure; (2) the disclosure of alternative choices to the proposed intervention; and (3) a discussion of the relevant risks, benefits, and uncertainties associated with each alternative; and (4) the likely outcomes with the various treatment options including the choice of no treatment. This discussion must take place whether the patient is either consenting to a procedure or refusing a recommended procedure. A patient does not automatically assume the risks of rejecting the recommendations of the physician if the patient is not fully apprised of the consequences of his or her decision.[35] Furthermore, it is the duty of the physician to assess how well the patient understands the above information. Before a physician accepts a patient's consent or refusal of care, the patient must demonstrate to the physician an adequate understanding of the nature and consequences of the decision made.

Depending on the state, courts apply one of 2 standards to determine if the information communicated by the physician was sufficient to satisfy common law obligations. The reasonable person standard requires a physician to disclose information that a reasonable person in the same position as the patient would need in order to make an informed decision.[11] The alternative legal approach is the reasonable physician standard, which requires that a physician to reveal information that a reasonable physician in a similar circumstance would disclose to the patient.[11] States vary on which standard they apply, and it is incumbent on physicians to know the legal standard of the state in which they practice.

Courts recognize that the requirement for informed consent has exceptions for situations where physicians do not need to obtain permission before rendering treatment. In *Schloendorff v. Society of New York Hospital*, the Court recognized that consent is not required in emergency situations and is implied. Situations are generally considered emergent if care of the patient would be compromised with a delay in treatment. For example, in New York State, an emergency is defined as a situation that includes both the immediate endangerment of life or health and the need for the immediate alleviation of pain.[32] Physicians need to determine the specific requirements of informed consent in their respective states.

Often well-intended efforts on the part of the physician to fully communicate treatment information to an impaired patient prove ineffectual and then present the practitioner with a medicolegal dilemma. Physicians are frequently unable to discuss in a meaningful way the implications of the proposed treatment with the patient. Nevertheless, there remains a duty to treat the patient who presents with a life-threatening condition or one with the potential for permanent disability. In these situations, consent is considered to be implied, and emergent treatment should be provided. The principle of implied consent is a general tenet of tort law.[22] In our case, although the physicians have explained the risks, they must have a more extensive conversation to determine if the patient is of sound mind. Suicide ideation raises the concern that the patient is not exhibiting rational thought and a thorough investigation needs to take place to determine if the patient has decision-making capacity. Given the fact that timely evaluation and intervention are necessary to prevent hepatotoxicity in overdose, the physician needs to draw blood early even if the patient does not consent, as she is at risk of harm if there is a delay in her care. So in this case, it is essential to begin management by any number of approaches including administering activated charcoal, obtaining blood specimen to assess hepatotoxicity, coagulation profile, basic metabolic and toxicologic evaluation of acetaminophen concentrations and/or initiating *N*-acetylcysteine with or without agreement of the patient. These options are all possible appropriate recommendations for the clinician. Decisions of this complexity should be accomplished with the full support of the local poison control center, a medical toxicologist, and an excellent team in the emergency department.

RISK MANAGEMENT CONSIDERATION AND DOCUMENTATION
Patient 2
A 28-year-old woman was brought to the ED by police who believed she ingested a large quantity of drugs to avoid arrest minutes before their arrival. The triage nurse helped the patient onto a stretcher, brought her to the treatment area, and recorded normal vital signs. The patient became combative and uncooperative as the physician initiated the examination and he verbally ordered that the patient be restrained. The patient was given 40% oxygen via face mask, cardiac monitoring was initiated, and an intravenous line was inserted and 0.9% sodium chloride at a rate of 125 mL/h was administered. A fingerstick glucose was determined to be normal and 100 mg of thiamine were administered intravenously (IV). Three doses of IV diazepam (5 mg) in 5-minute intervals were administered until light sedation was achieved. The physician ordered a basic set of laboratory studies, a urine drug screen and ordered an abdominal radiograph. The laboratory values and the radiographic findings were normal and the urine drug screen was negative. The treatment plan was then to continue monitoring and to reassess the patient at a later time. This was an ideal time for the physician to contact the local poison control center or a medical toxicologist to better understand the management of a body stuffer (Special Considerations: SC5). There are critical decisions to be made immediately: protection of the patient's airway, management of the ingested toxin, and a high level of supervision of the

patient in an intensive care unit (ICU). This case demonstrates inadequate knowledge of the management of an unknown toxin. It demonstrates the risks of management without utilization of available hospital (ICU) and health system resources (Chap. 130).

One hour after arrival the patient's vital signs were blood pressure, 120/70 mm Hg; pulse, 82 beats/min; and respiratory, rate 18 breaths/min. The patient was noted to be stable and was transferred to an observation unit. Oxygen and cardiac monitoring were discontinued. No further orders were written, and the patient remained restrained. Three hours later, the vital signs were blood pressure, 110/60 mm Hg; pulse, 92 beats/min; and respiratory rate, 18 breaths/min. A nursing note stated the patient was resting comfortably.

Forty-five minutes later, at midnight, the initial treating physician completed his shift and informed his replacement that the patient was stable and resting in the observation unit.

At 4:20 AM the patient was found unresponsive, hypotensive, with agonal respirations and with a weakly palpable pulse. The patient felt very hot to the touch and had a rectal temperature of 108°F (42.4°C). Resuscitative efforts were initiated but were unsuccessful. Thirty minutes later, the patient was pronounced dead.

Several important risk management questions frequently arise in emergency medicine malpractice litigation. To prove that a case constitutes medical malpractice, a plaintiff's attorney must show by a preponderance of evidence that a deviation from accepted practice by the physician occurred. The attorney must further demonstrate that this deviation or negligent act or omission by the physician proximately caused the patient's injury. Courts have held that where "there is substantial probability that the [defendant physician's] negligent conduct caused the resulting injury, that sufficient evidence has been developed against [the] physician."[42]

When the attorney for the patient (plaintiff's attorney) introduces evidence to advance the case, the ED record is likely to become the central focus in the medical malpractice trial. The problems associated with an improperly documented ED record are numerous, but they can be minimized if the practitioner is cognizant of risk management principles. Every entry in that record is scrutinized by both parties (plaintiff and defendants). The importance of completing the record with knowledge of risk management implications should be a priority for all health care professionals.

The physician is required to complete a medical record that amply supports the basis for the medical judgments exercised. When a physician opts to complete only a summary statement on the record without noting supporting clinical data or patient history, claims alleging a failure to diagnose will be extremely difficult, if not impossible, to defend. One of the basic tactics of the defense in a medical malpractice case is the argument that the physician's judgment was appropriate given the clinical facts and the patient's history available at that time. Therefore, physicians who do not record supporting clinical data and history undermine their "medical judgment" defense.

Notations in the medical record related to patient monitoring are considered inadequate when those notes do not provide insight into the patient's clinical status. Thus, any note for a restrained patient in the ED for a lengthy period of evaluation, observation, or until an inpatient bed becomes available must include specific clinical data and observations overtime (including relevant laboratory results, radiographic findings, hemodynamic changes, and intravenous medications and solutions). Any deficiencies in this area would undoubtedly be noticed and highlighted at trial by a plaintiff's expert, who usually is a board-certified physician in the same specialty.

Documentation supporting the restraint of an impaired patient against his or her will must include a description of the clinical situation to support such a forcible impediment to the patient's right to liberty and freedom of movement. Such a description should specifically document any manifestation of agitation and/or behavior that might place the patient at risk. The record should incorporate a description of the specific acts of the patient of concern and, most importantly, should comment on the difficulties in providing care to the patient because of those acts. Documentation of patient conduct should be factual, accurate, detailed, and nonjudgmental.

The transition to electronic health records (EHRs) was introduced as a way to improve the health care process by enhancing communication, workflow, decision making, and increasing patient safety while simultaneously decreasing errors. Despite their many actual and potential benefits, EHRs have introduced new concerns not previously encountered in written record keeping. Some of the new errors encountered include poor data display, alert fatigue, wrong order/wrong patient error, and communication failure.[10] An additional concern that could lead to errors and increase physician liability is the potential to overlook pertinent data given the large volume of information that is provided on every aspect of care for each patient regardless of when it took place. For example, every laboratory test that a patient has ever undergone in one hospital system will often be available to the physician as she or he opens the chart to document on a patient's current visit, yet the physician will only want to focus on what is important for the patient's current encounter. The copy and paste function that is often used by providers to save time risks leading to repeating information that is no longer correct.[28] Computerized provider order entry (CPOE) was introduced to improve all aspects of the medication process from prescribing to administration but ultimately introduced new problems. Common errors associated with CPOE include wrong medication selection, incorrect input of patient data, wrong dose or strength selection, and scheduling errors (Chap. 134).[25,43]

To summarize, a well-documented ED record reflecting the practice of accepted risk management principles is the best course to follow for the physician and nursing team managing a difficult overdose situation and one in which legal concerns may appear to present problems in providing proper medical management.

FORCIBLE RESTRAINT OF THE IMPAIRED PATIENT
Patient 3
A 23-year-old woman was found unresponsive on the street and transported to the ED by ambulance. Friends on the scene reported that the patient regularly uses opioids recreationally. In the ED, she was unresponsive and apneic. Oxygen was immediately administered by bag–valve–mask and intravenous access was established. Naloxone was administered, and shortly thereafter the patient regained consciousness. After 20 minutes of care in the ED, the patient became fully alert and oriented, with no evidence of hypoxia or other clinical signs to suggest impaired judgment. The patient stated that she had taken a sustained-release oxycodone and demanded to be discharged immediately.

The ability of a hospital to retain and physically restrain a person who has an altered level of consciousness for evaluation and emergency intervention is generally well supported by state statutes and case law.[11] Reasonably clear guidelines for the management of such impaired patients have evolved from legal precedents governing appropriate medical assessment, from risk management considerations, and from the predictability of patient injury in the event of premature discharge.

A staff decision to allow a treated or partially treated patient with a drug overdose who subsequently becomes alert to return to the community must be based on an assessment of several factors. The initial concern is the capacity of the patient; is the patient able to fully comprehend the current medical situation and associated risks of not receiving treatment? To demonstrate capacity, patients must be able to (1) understand the facts involved in the decision; (2) appreciate the nature and the significance of the decision; (3) weigh the risks and benefits and potential alternatives; and (4) express their choice.[16] The next consideration is that of medical stability. Has the initial process that caused the clinical scenario completed its course? The history of drug use in this patient raises the concern that the underlying toxic metabolic process is not yet resolved, and alteration in mental status, significant respiratory compromise, or other medical symptoms will recur when the naloxone is metabolized, again placing the patient at risk.

Common ED practice and sound legal principles suggest that both the hospital and its staff have a duty to prevent such a person from leaving if the duration of the effect of the involved xenobiotic is longer than that expected for the antidote. Because the duration of effect for naloxone is considerably

shorter than that of sustained-release oxycodone, the physician can predict with reasonable certainty that coma or apnea will recur in the near future. The physician has the duty to inform the individual of the life-threatening nature of the condition, and then to retain, with restraints if necessary, the patient in the hospital until medically stable.

Legal liability in this situation is further reduced if the chart substantiates the medical judgment that was the basis for the decision to retain the patient and, if applicable, the use of restraints. Such documentation should specifically note the likely relapse of the patient into a symptomatic state and that this occurrence could place the patient in a life-threatening situation. When documented in a clear manner, legal challenges to the decision to restrain the patient have a limited chance of success. Sound risk management principles support treatment and detainment. Conversely, prematurely releasing a patient with a significant overdose exposes both the physician and the hospital to a claim of negligence on the grounds of failure to foresee a likely and harmful event. From a practical perspective, the legal risk and liability of the latter scenario is far greater than the former.

In the above case, the patient responded to the opioid antagonist naloxone. Given that there are many different opioids available with variation in half-lives and duration of action, the patient needs to be kept in an acute care setting until the naloxone is metabolized to ensure the patient has not been exposed to a long-acting opioid that will cause recurrent life-threatening toxicity. Once the antidote has worn off the patient must be reassessed to determine possible damage from the initial event (hypoxic brain injury, aspiration, end organ impairment) as well as decision-making capacity and possible underlying psychiatric illness, such as suicidal ideation and the need for a psychiatry consultation. If it is determined that the patient is safe for discharge from the hospital consideration should be made to ensure that available family and social support is arranged and harm reduction including overdose education, naloxone prescriptions for family and friends, and access to counseling and medication-assisted treatment modalities (methadone buprenorphine naltrexone programs) after discharge are performed (Special Considerations: SC6).[12]

BLOOD ALCOHOL CONCENTRATION AND EVIDENCE COLLECTION
Patient 4
A 41-year-old man who was a driver involved in a motor vehicle crash was taken to the ED by ambulance. Two motorists in another vehicle were killed. The patient had no physical complaints, but was transported to the hospital for medical evaluation. On arrival, he was alert and oriented, responded appropriately to all commands, and demonstrated normal motor function and had a normal gait. Police officers suspected that he was driving while intoxicated, but he refused a breath alcohol test at the scene.

The police officers informed the ED staff that he was arrested and might be charged with vehicular homicide. The officers then requested that the emergency physician draw a blood specimen to determine the blood alcohol concentration. The patient stated that he would not allow the ED staff to draw blood for a determination of an alcohol concentration.

In 2015, there were 10,265 people who died in alcohol-related motor vehicle crashes, which comprised 29% of all traffic-related deaths in the United States.[9] In the United States, an alcohol-related motor vehicle crash kills someone every 51 minutes.[9] In 2015, crashes resulting from alcohol-induced impairment were responsible for 16% of fatalities in children younger than 14 years who were killed in motor vehicle crashes.[9] The estimated economic cost of alcohol-impaired motor vehicle crashes in 2015 was $44 billion.[9] The judicial system has historically been one of the most effective tools to combat drunk driving and its effectiveness depends on the ability to identify and punish individuals who violate the law. See Special Considerations: SC11 for more in-depth discussion on "*per se*" limits. It is essential, however, that the collection of evidence does not violate the rights afforded by Constitutional law or specific state law. Does forced phlebotomy for patients suspected of driving while intoxicated violate these protected rights? This has long been debated in the courts, and legal authority specifically brought into question include the Fourth Amendment,[39] the right against unreasonable search and seizure; the Fifth Amendment,[40] the right against self-incrimination, and the Due Process clause of the Fourteenth Amendment.[38] Past court decisions applying Constitutional or statutory law on these issues help guide current clinical practices and also contribute to further evolution of legal standards.

Every state and the District of Columbia have driver "implied consent" laws. When a person obtains a driver's license, he or she consents at the time of acquisition to a chemical alcohol test if suspected of driving while intoxicated. Under implied consent laws, when a person suspected of driving while intoxicated refuses to take an alcohol test, a penalty is imposed. Specific penalties for refusals vary from state to state. At a minimum, the refusal results in suspension or revocation of a driver's license. Some states assign additional fines and penalties for this action. A few states allow the refusal itself to be submitted at trial in support of the prosecution, making it possible to be convicted of an intoxication charge without chemical evidence.[5] Certain states (eg, Texas, Illinois) allow blood tests to be performed on patients as ordered by an officer of the law when there is probable cause that driving while intoxicated resulted in severe injury.[21,33] Other states, such as New York and Wyoming, allow forced blood samples with a warrant issued by a judge.[7,19] State laws in this area vary with respect to amount of force that may be used, requirements of warrants, who may perform the blood draw, and other blood draw restrictions and it is important that the ED staff be familiar with the specific requirements of law in the state in which they practice.[2]

How much force may be used to collect chemical evidence? Does a physician violate human dignity and privacy in obtaining evidence for the State? These issues were addressed by the United States Supreme Court. In *Rochin v. California*,[24] the Court overturned a conviction of drug possession based on violation of the Fourteenth Amendment. In this case, police were informed that Rochin was selling drugs. While entering the home of the defendant, the police witnessed the defendant swallow 2 pills that were lying on the night stand. When the officers failed to recover the pills on the scene, the officers took Rochin to the ED, where they directed the physician to administer an emetic through a nasogastric tube. The capsules were recovered from the vomit, and Mr. Rochin was convicted by the trial court for possessing morphine.[24] The Supreme Court reversed the lower court decision based on Fourteenth Amendment grounds stating that "nor shall any State deprive any person of life, liberty or property, without due process of law."[45] The term *due process* is vague, and is defined on a case-by-case basis; essentially, however, it means that states must use fair legal procedures when depriving an individual of life, liberty, or property. In *Rochin*, the court concluded that forced emesis by a physician was believed to violate "due process," stating:

> This is conduct that shocks the conscience. Illegally breaking into the privacy of the petitioner, the struggle to open his mouth and remove what was there, the forcible extraction of stomach contents—this course of proceeding by agents of government to obtain evidence is bound to offend even hardened sensibilities. They are methods too close to the rack and the screw to permit constitutional differentiation.[24]

The Supreme Court revisited the issues presented in *Rochin* 4 years later in *Breithaupt v. Abram*.[6] Breithaupt was the driver of a truck who killed 3 occupants of another vehicle. In the ED, a police officer requested that a blood alcohol concentration be drawn. The blood, drawn while the patient was unconscious, was above the legal limit for alcohol and the patient was convicted of involuntary manslaughter. Making an analogy to the forced emesis scenario in *Rochin*, Breithaupt argued that the blood draw violated due process because he did not consent to its collection. Justice Clark disagreed, stating "the distinction rests on the fact that there is nothing 'brutal' or 'offensive' when done, as in this case, under the protective eye of a physician" and that the "blood test procedure has become routine in our everyday life."[5,6] Phlebotomy while the patient is unconscious and unable to give consent was determined not to violate the due process clause of the Fourteenth Amendment.

The Supreme Court continued to expand the scope of permissible phlebotomy in *Schmerber v. California*.[27] Schmerber was involved in a motor

vehicle crash in which the police officer suspected he was intoxicated. Unlike the *Breithaupt* case, Schmerber was conscious, and a physician drew a blood sample at the officer's request despite the patient's verbal refusal. The attorney for Schmerber asserted that forced phlebotomy violated several constitutional rights. Specifically, it violated the Fourth, Fifth, and Fourteenth Amendments of the US Constitution. He alleged that forced phlebotomy denied him due process of law, it violated his privilege against self-incrimination, and it violated his right against unreasonable search and seizure.[5,27]

The Supreme Court rejected all of these arguments holding that the phlebotomy did not violate the due process clause because "the extraction was made by a physician in a simple, medically acceptable manner in a hospital environment.... We cannot see that it should make any difference whether one states unequivocally that he objects or resorts to physical violence in protest or is in such condition that he is unable to protest."[27] Furthermore, the court found that the forced blood draw did not violate the Fifth Amendment's Privilege Against Self-Incrimination because the Fifth Amendment only protects evidence of a "testimonial or communicative nature," such as writings or speech. Finally the court found there was no violation of the Fourth and Fourteenth Amendments' protections against unreasonable search and seizure as the delay necessary to obtain a warrant threatened the destruction of evidence.

Considering the "totality of the circumstances" in *Schmerber*, the blood alcohol test fell under the Court's exigent circumstances exception to the general requirement of a warrant.

The percentage of alcohol in the blood begins to diminish shortly after drinking stops as the body eliminates it from the system. Particularly in a case such as this where time elapsed to bring the accused to a hospital and to investigate the scene of the crash, there was no time to seek out a magistrate and secure a warrant.

To ensure compliance with standards set forth in *Schmerber*, the states have tailored laws and regulations governing the seizure of blood for the purpose of blood alcohol testing. Laws generally require the procedure be (1) performed in a reasonable, medically approved manner; (2) incident to a lawful arrest; and (3) based on the belief that the arrestee is intoxicated. It should be remembered that the issues raised by any one case are complex and the application to situations in real time is difficult. Laws and regulations governing blood draws for alcohol testing vary from state to state and are the subject of frequent review and amendment. Medical staff should review with hospital counsel the local laws and regulations that pertain to these issues. The benefits of determining a patient's blood alcohol concentration must be weighed against the risks of the procedure. For example, drawing blood in an agitated patient may place the staff at risk for a needle stick and the patient at risk of vascular injury. It is important to remember that the role of physicians are to be the patient's advocate and they are not serving as representatives of the court. Physicians must order tests they deem to be of clinical benefit and that may assist the court as necessary in obtaining evidence. One way to assist is talking to the agitated patient; if the patient is agitated because of a defense emphasizing that no drinking of alcohol occurred then it would be a good idea to have blood drawn to support that, as refusal of a blood draw is frequently perceived as a presumption of guilt by the court.

It should also be noted that the US Supreme Court in *Missouri v. McNeely* limited the holding of *Schmerber* for warrantless blood alcohol testing.[18] In *McNeely*, the state court in Missouri argued that the metabolism of alcohol over time, by itself, was justification to obtain warrantless blood alcohol testing in the hospital. The US Supreme Court rejected this argument. While the dissipation of alcohol from the bloodstream over time is one of the factors to consider when evaluating the "totality of the circumstances," it does not meet the exigency exception to the warrant requirement by itself. The majority opinion held that "when officers in drunk driving investigations can reasonably obtain a warrant before having a blood sample drawn without significantly undermining the efficacy of the search, the Fourth Amendment mandates that they do so." This does not suggest that a physician should insist on a warrant when an officer requests a blood alcohol test as this is a protection afforded retrospectively by the courts. Familiarity with local regulations is necessary to properly manage requests by law enforcement for blood alcohol testing.

When patients agree to have their blood drawn, it is important that a chain of custody process be carefully followed. The chain of custody process in a legal context refers to the chronological documentation showing the collection, transfer, analysis, and storage of a blood sample from the time it is collected until it is presented at trial. It is used to prevent contamination of evidence. If the proper chain of custody process is not maintained, the evidence collected in general will not be admissible at trial. If the evidence is admissible, and if there are deficits in the chain of custody, the defense attorney will try to cast doubt on the reliability of the information presented.

CONFIDENTIALITY
Patient 5

A 32-year-old woman was fired from her job as a high school mathematics teacher. The school board called for her termination after learning that she had a history of alcohol dependence and had a previous hospitalization for detoxification at the local community hospital. A parent on the school board was also employed as a nurse at the hospital where the teacher had received therapy. The school board member (and nurse) had inadvertently accessed the medical record of the teacher while caring for a patient with the same last name.

The Health Insurance Portability and Accountability Act (HIPAA) was enacted by Congress in 1996 and signed by President Clinton. Initially, the purpose of HIPAA was to increase the portability of health insurance and allow employees to maintain insurance when they changed jobs. The Act called for the establishment of several provisions, among them an electronic database designed to facilitate the exchange of information between health care professionals, insurance companies, and those involved in financial and administrative transactions.[17] However, the idea of developing an electronic database brought to light already growing concerns regarding the maintenance of patient privacy. For the first time, medical records would be accessible to an unlimited number of people working in health care, everyone from bill processors to pharmacists to clinicians. Could the right to privacy be jeopardized by a system designed to increase efficiency?

Prior to HIPAA, individual hospitals or physician offices designed their own methods for maintaining confidential patient information. Records were maintained on computers in some circumstances and on paper in others. Accessibility to that information was largely regulated by state laws and some federal regulations. Ethical codes of conduct also provided guidance. During the 1990s, however, the weaknesses of the existing systems gained attention as multiple high-profile breaches of confidentiality became public. For example, the medical records of a congresswoman were released to the media during her campaign, making her history of depression and a past suicide attempt public knowledge.[30] There were also several cases in which the medical records of hospital employees were read by staff members not involved in the employees' care, health insurance companies released health care information to employers without permission, and physicians released information to pharmaceutical companies that subsequently solicited the patient.[46] These breaches of ethics were each a testament to the fact that the right to privacy needed more stringent regulation. If such breaches occurred in the previous systems for recording personal health information, then it was clearly apparent that further opportunities for transgressions would be created with increased access through an electronic database.

The Privacy Rule of HIPAA has become the most well-publicized aspect of this Act among health care personnel. The Privacy Rule governs the use and disclosure of protected health information in the hands of health care professionals, health plans, and health care clearinghouses.[17] The terminology used in the Privacy Rule is extensively defined. The following is a brief summary of the terms used.

Protected Health Information

Protected health information includes any individually identifiable information concerning the past, present, or future health of an individual including medical information pertaining to assessment and treatment of an individual and payment and billing information. All forms of information, written, oral, or electronic, are protected by this rule. Deidentified data is not considered protected health information.

Covered Entities

The term "covered entities" includes any person or business that provides health-related services or products. All those providing health-related services fall within this provision, including, for example, clinicians, pharmacists, medical equipment providers, and other health care professionals. Companies that provide disability insurance, car insurance, or casualty insurance are not included in the rule.[17,37]

Health Care Clearinghouses

Health care clearinghouses are entities that compile health care information, such as billing companies or data processing centers.

Institutions are required to provide all individuals with written notice of the institutional privacy policy when each individual first seeks medical care. Patients must be informed of how the institution may use and disclose information. The notice must also describe the patients' rights, including the right to access their medical information and their right to file a complaint if they believe their rights were violated. The notice must be written in plain language, and the patient must provide written acknowledgment of receipt of the information in the notice.

The Privacy Rule of HIPAA was not intended to impede health care. There are several exceptions to the nondisclosure rule. A covered entity is permitted to use and disclose protected health information for the purposes of ongoing evaluation and treatment. For example, physicians have the freedom to consult with each other, both within and outside their own institution in order to provide clinical care. Additionally, there are several specific exceptions to the Privacy Rule delineated within the legislation—situations in which protected health information will be and often must be disclosed, even without an individual's permission. For example, activities related to public health, such as reporting communicable diseases; information necessary to report actual or suspected abuse, neglect, or domestic violence; or information pertaining to cadaver organ or tissue donation are all specifically exempt from the Privacy Rule.[13]

Examples of the application of the HIPAA rule occur in everyday emergency medicine. For example, only persons directly involved in a patient's care are allowed to access and view the chart. Occasionally well-recognized politicians, actors and actresses, or even work colleagues seek medical treatment, and previously hospital workers were able to read their medical records. Today, these patients would be protected from the curiosity of medical personnel not directly caring for them. Another example is communication with family, friends, and even law enforcement. Whereas in the past clinical teams periodically discussed questions about a person's health care with anyone who asked, today clinicians may only speak with those individuals to whom the patient specifically has given permission.

The HIPAA Privacy Rule specifically addresses consultations with poison control centers. It states:

> We consider the counseling and follow-up consultations provided by poison control centers with individual providers regarding patient outcomes to be treatment. Therefore, poison control centers and other health care professionals can share protected health information about the treatment of an individual without a business associate contract.[13]

This is important to remember, and individuals seeking assistance from poison control centers to assess risk after exposures to xenobiotics or who need assistance in managing complex cases should never be concerned that they are violating the HIPAA rule by seeking help. The same is true for managing medication safety. The FDA and pharmaceutical industry rely on postmarketing surveillance to obtain further safety information regarding the toxicity of a medication after it has been granted approval for use. The FDA's program MedWatch is a postmarket surveillance tool that relies on reports by health care professionals and/or patients regarding the occurrence of harmful effects associated with the use of a medication or medical device. For a more in-depth discussion of the FDA and MedWatch, see Chaps. 134 and 135. Reports made to MedWatch are in compliance with the HIPAA Privacy Rule, as the rule recognizes the need for public health authorities to have access to protected health information to carry out their mission of ensuring safety and health to the public at large.[36]

Violations of the Privacy Rule are subject to penalties, the severity of which is dependent on the type of infraction. Simple noncompliance will result in financial penalties. Moreover, significant or intentional disclosures of information carries steeper fines in addition to criminal charges and potential imprisonment.[46] In 2009, as part of the economic stimulus plan, the Health Information Technology for Economic and Clinical Health Act (HITECH) under the American Recovery and Reinvestment Act (ARRA) was passed.[23] This Act was primarily created to encourage the use of electronic health records and supporting technology. However, it also widened the scope of privacy and security protections defined by HIPAA. Several notable changes brought forth by this act include an increase in civil penalties for willful neglect, extending up to $250,000 for a single violation, to as much as $1.5 million for repeated or uncorrected violations. Furthermore, HIPAA provisions now apply to business associates. Business associates are defined as persons who, on behalf of a covered entity, perform or assist in performing a function or activity that involves the use or disclosure of individually identifiable health information.

OTHER LEGAL CONSIDERATIONS FOR POISON CONTROL CENTERS AND CERTIFIED SPECIALISTS IN POISON INFORMATION
Patient 6
The poison control center received a call from a concerned mother that her daughter might have ingested one of her grandmother's diabetes medications. The mother stated that the child was acting normally all day at the grandmothers' house, but when the family returned home, the child had become drowsy. When contacted, the grandmother had confirmed that one pill was missing from her purse although she did not know the name of her medication. The poison control center advised that the parents give the child juice and closely observe her over the next 6 hours. Approximately 2 hours later, while sleeping, the child had a seizure. The child continued to seize in the hospital, where medical evaluation revealed hypoglycemia. The patient subsequently suffered permanent neurologic damage. The medication was later identified as glyburide. A negligence action was brought against the poison control center, alleging inappropriate advice and failure to recommend transport to a hospital.

As a general rule, any physician who decides to treat a patient enters into a physician–patient relationship and this creates well-established legal duties. Courts have ruled that the physician–patient encounter need not be a face-to-face interaction to have legal consequences. For example, the absence of physical contact between a physician and patient, as in the practice of radiology and pathology, does not preclude a patient from asserting that a duty of care exists.[6] More particularly and quite relevant to the practice of a poison control center, a New York State court ruled that an initial telephone call from a patient to a physician can be sufficient basis to hold that physician responsible for inappropriate advice or a significant error in judgment.[20] Given these legal precedents, it is clear that contact with a certified specialist of poison information provides sufficient grounds for a subsequent legal action if inappropriate advice was given and that advice was a proximate cause of patient injury.

Standards of Care Applicable in Poison Control Centers
Standards of care applicable to medical toxicologists who supervise or direct a patient's care in a poison control center are examined under the same legal framework as other medical specialists. The basic medical malpractice concepts are universal, with some variations from state to state. Generally, for

patients to prevail in medical malpractice cases, they must demonstrate "by a preponderance of the evidence: (1) that the medical toxicologist's supervision of the care fell below the ordinary standard of care expected of a physician in his [or her] medical specialty, and (2) the existence of a causal relationship between the alleged negligent treatment and the injury sustained."[44] While the standard of care is recognized not to ensure perfection, what constitutes the "ordinary standard of care" has much room for interpretation.

In the 19th century, courts determined what the "ordinary standard of care" was by introducing testimony from physicians practicing in the community where the event occurred. This was known as the strict locality rule.[41] The strict locality rule was intended to prevent the inequities of comparing rural physicians working with limited resources and under exigent conditions from physicians working in large urban hospital settings.[15] In many jurisdictions, however, the strict locality rule was rejected because (1) it was difficult to find an expert witness in a small community to testify against another physician in the community, and (2) the strict locality rule permitted some small medical communities to set unacceptably low standards of care.[41] In response, some states adopted the modified locality rule, which compares the physician in question with physicians practicing "in similar localities."[41] Over time, the basis for the modified locality rule was also called into question. Advances in transportation, communication, and education continued to minimize the disparity between rural and urban medical practice. Most states have abandoned the locality rule altogether, permitting the introduction of evidence of nationwide medical practices. As described by one court:

> [A] physician must exercise that degree of care, skill, and proficiency exercised by reasonably careful, skillful, and prudent practitioners in the same class to which he [or she] belongs, acting under the same or similar circumstances. Rather than focusing on different standards for different communities, this standard uses locality as but one of the factors to be considered in determining whether the doctor acted reasonably.[4]

Although there is movement toward reviewing nationwide medical practices, depending on the jurisdiction where the event occurs, any one of the above rules may apply. In New York, courts allow evidence from the specific locality where the event occurred, from statewide practice, or from nationwide practice.[14]

A discussion of standard of care for certified specialists in poison information should also mention several operational aspects of poison control centers. Certified specialists in poison information are required to have rapid and accurate access to a standard information resource system that contains both basic information and recommendations to deal with most toxic exposures. If a patient were to bring a negligence action against the poison control center, the plaintiff might attempt to demonstrate deviations from the standard recommendations in these resources.

It would be inaccurate to suggest, however, that the care required by a certified specialist in poison information should be measured only by how closely the advice given compares with these standard resources. Frequently, a certified specialist in poison information encounters situations that cannot be managed in accordance with an information system alone, and may seek consultation from a clinical pharmacist or a medical toxicologist working with the poison control center. For example, in this chapter, patient 2 and patient 6 are examples of complicated cases that would involve the expertise of a medical toxicologist. In the above case, the report of only one pill missing and possibly ingested can create a feeling of false reassurance. Life-threatening hypoglycemia can occur after the ingestion of a single pill in children. Additionally, the onset of hypoglycemia may be delayed up to 21 hours after ingestion (Chap. 47).[29] Knowing this, the parents should be advised to bring the patient to a hospital where fingerstick glucoses can be monitored every hour, and dextrose can be administered if necessary. If the certified specialist in poison information were to enlist the help of a medical toxicologist then any subsequent legal proceeding would also carefully review the accuracy of the content of the information provided to the consultant.

State Statutes Limiting Liability of Poison Control Center Consultants

A comprehensive review of state-enacted legislation providing additional liability protection to poison control center consultants is outlined elsewhere.[8] These state statutes provide either immunity from malpractice claims or indemnity for a successful claim against a poison control center consultant. The statutes are state specific and poison control center consultants should review them with local counsel, particularly if the statute has not been challenged in the jurisdiction in question.

Several states have enacted laws granting immunity to poison control center consultants. Immunity is an affirmative defense to medical malpractice liability. In other words, even if a lawsuit were to satisfy all of the elements for a successful malpractice claim, the lawsuit would not lead to compensation for injuries sustained because of this state-conferred protection. Examples of states that have enacted statutes providing immunity include Arkansas, California, Florida, Louisiana, Ohio, Tennessee, and Washington.[1] These statutes are not absolute protections from liability. State statutes granting immunity usually stipulate that the poison control center consultant act in good faith while performing the duties required. In some instances, the poison control center consultant must have been providing information in accordance with protocols established by the poison control center. These laws do not protect against gross negligence, nor do they provide protection against intentional misconduct by the poison control center consultant.

Other states have enacted laws that require the state itself to indemnify poison control center consultants in the case of a successful malpractice claim. In other words, a patient may bring a medical malpractice claim against a poison control center consultant, but if the claim is successful, the state itself compensates the patient rather than the poison control center consultant. States that have enacted indemnity statutes include Illinois and Texas.[48] Statutes providing state indemnification for medical malpractice claims are also limited in that they do not provide protection in the case of gross negligence, nor do they provide indemnity in the case of intentional misconduct.

In addition to state statutes that specifically limit liability for poison control center consultants, it has been argued that some states may hypothetically provide protections under common law or general "public immunity" statutes.[47] Neither poison control centers nor poison control center consultants are specifically delineated under these state laws, but may still be afforded immunity protection. States with general common law or "public immunity" statutes include North Carolina, Missouri, Illinois, Connecticut, and Georgia. Finally, many states have sovereign immunity statutes that afford liability protection to any entity created, funded, and operated by the state. Poison control centers and staff may be considered such an entity and, therefore, granted such protection.

Practices of Regional Poison Control Centers That Can Reduce Potential Liabilities

There are some inherent risks creating potential liability for a poison control center. To minimize these risks and the subsequent risk of civil action against a poison control center, quality assurance and risk management programs should be a regular function. Daily audits or monitoring of the advice given by certified specialists in poison information should be conducted. Such processes enhance care and ensure patient safety for the individual and establish a higher general standard of performance.

The medical toxicologists and clinical pharmacists responsible for supervising the certified specialists in poison information must be able to adequately assess the competence and capabilities of the staff, make recommendations, take corrective actions, and provide suggestions for improvement to involved members. This process is facilitated by such actions as audiotaping calls made to the poison control center, and the subsequent advice given, and reviewing written records maintained by the information specialist on each particular case. Documentation is extremely important because in the event of a lawsuit, the most likely area of dispute will be what was actually said to the patient.

REPORTING IMPAIRED PHYSICIANS

It is well recognized that physicians suffer from substance abuse and misuse disorders just like the general population. Though there are few formalized studies on physician impairment, there are certain factors unique to the medical community, such as knowledge of the medications and ability to prescribe that leads to easier access.[31] Impairment in the medical profession is a serious issue as physicians make daily decisions that affect the health of their patients, and their conduct has the potential to affect the quality and safety of the health care delivered. In 1973, the American Medical Association (AMA) formerly recognized physician impairment in its landmark paper "The Sick Physician: Impairment by Psychiatric Disorders, Including Alcoholism and Drug Dependence."[34] This paper declared that physicians had an ethical obligation to recognize a colleague's impairment due to substance abuse.[3] Subsequently, local, state, and national programs designed to help physicians struggling with impairment were formed. Today there are physician health programs (PHPs) in all 50 states, and they are administered by the state medical boards or medical societies. Physicians may self-refer to these programs or be referred by a colleague or an administrator. These programs seek to provide detection, assessment, and referral to treatment facilities. Physicians entering contracts with PHP can maintain confidentiality and may keep their license after completing treatment and avoids formal disciplinary action.[31] Identifying an impaired colleague may be challenging as physicians can be good at hiding such disorders until it becomes severe. Signs to look for include deteriorating social and interpersonal behaviors, inaccessibility to patients and staff, frequent conflicts with staff members, unexplained absenteeism, and frequent moves to different locations for jobs.[31] Colleagues may be hesitant to report such behaviors because of fear of damaging a career or the fear of confrontation. However, in addition to an ethical obligation as determined by the AMA, many states have laws in place requiring the reporting of impaired colleagues.

SUMMARY

- The risk management and legal issues of an ED with patients exposed to xenobiotics, often with impaired judgment, are complex. The substantial practical challenges in initiating emergent treatment to an individual unable to provide proper informed consent vary depending on individual state laws.
- Medical care is further complicated by the difficulties inherent in documenting these interactions with our patients.
- Both forcible restraint (often desired by the physician) and evidence collection (requested by law enforcement) have significant potential legal ramifications for the care provider.
- Maintaining patient confidentiality outside the ED, despite circumstances often visibly volatile within the department, often seem futile, yet legal obligations to protect patient privacy are stringent.
- A hospital must ensure a close working relationship among the legal department, risk management, and medical personnel. Only in this manner can everyone learn, cooperate, and meet each other's needs in the ever-evolving and challenging clinical scenarios confronted.

Acknowledgments

Walter LeStrange, RN, MPH, MS, Kevin Porter, Esq, and Danius A. Drukteinis contributed to this chapter in previous editions.

REFERENCES

1. A.C.A. §20-13-704 (2004); Cal Health and Saf Code §1799.105 (2005); Fla. Stat. §768.28 (2004); La. R.S.§9:2797.1. (2004); ORC Ann. §3701.20 (2005); Tenn. Code Ann. §68-141-107 (2004); Rev. Code Wash. (ARCW) §18.76.070 (2004).
2. Appel JM. Nonconsensual blood draws and dual loyalty: when bodily integrity conflicts with public health. *Health Care Law Policy.* 2014;17:128-154.
3. Baldisseri MR. Impaired healthcare professional. *Crit Care Med.* 2007;35:s106-s116.
4. *Bates v Meyer,* 565 So.2d 134 (Ala. 1990); *Mann v Cracchiolo,* 38 Cal. 3d 18, 694 P.2d 1134, 210 Cal. Rptr. 762 (Cal. 1985); *Hyles v Cockrill,* 169 Ga.App. 132, 312 S.E.2d 124 (Ga.App. 1983); *Speed v State,* 240 N.W.2d 901 (Iowa 1976); *Blair v Eblen,* 461 S.W.2d 370 (Ky. 1970); *Shilkret v Annapolis Emergency Hosp.,* 276 Md. 187, 349 A.2d 245 (Md. 1975); *Brune v Belinkoff,* 354 Mass. 102, 235 N.E.2d 793 (Mass. 1968); *Hall v Hilburn,* 466 So.2d 856 (Miss. 1985); *Schueler v Strelinger,* 43 N.J. 330, 204 A.2d 577 (N.J. 1964); *Wiggins v Piver,* 276 N.C. 134, 171 S.E.2d 393 (N.C. 1970);

Pharmaseal Lab., Inc., v Goffe, 90 N.M. 753, 568 P.2d 589 (N.M. 1977); *King v Williams*, 276 S.C. 478, 279 S.E.2d 618 (S.C. 1981); *Peterson v Shields*, 652 S.W.2d 929 (Tx. 1983); *Farrow v Health Services Corp.*, 604 P.2d 474 (Utah 1979); *Brown v Koulizakis*, 229 Va. 524, 331 S.E.2d 440 (Va. 1985); *Plaintiff v Parkersburg*, 345 S.E.2d 564 (W.Va. 1986); *Pederson v Dumouchel*, 72 Wash. 2d 73, 431 P.2d 973 (Wash. 1967); *Shier v Freedman*, 58 Wis. 2d 269, 206 N.W.2d 166 (Wis. 1973), modified on other grounds and rehearing denied, 58 Wis. 2d 269, 208 N.W.2d 328.

5. Beauchamp RB. "Shed thou no blood": the forcible removal of blood samples from drunk driving suspects. *South Calif Law Rev.* 1987;60:1115-1141.

6. *Breithaupt v Abram*, 352 US 432 (1957).

7. California Vehicle Code 23612 (West 1996).

8. Curtis JA, Greenberg MI. Legal liability of medical toxicologists serving as poison control center consultants: a review of relevant legal statutes and survey of the experience of medical toxicologists. *J Med Toxicol.* 2009;5:144-148.

9. Department of Transportation (US) NHSA (NHTSA). *Traffic Safety Facts 2015 Data: Alcohol-Impaired Driving.* Washington, DC: NHTSA.

10. Farley HL, et al. Quality and safety implications of emergency department information systems. *Ann Emerg Med.* 2013;62:399-407.

11. Gatter R. Informed consent law and the forgotten duty of physician inquiry. *Loyola Univ Chicago Law J.* 1999;31:557-597.

12. Hawk KF, et al. Reducing fatal opioid overdose: prevention, treatment and harm reduction strategies. *Yale J Biol Med.* 2015;88:235-245.

13. Health Insurance Portability and Accessibility Act of 1996, Pub No L104-191, 110, Stat 1936 (1996). See also 45 CFR 160, 164 (2002).

14. *Hock v United Presbyterian Home*, 236 N.Y.L.J 106 (2006).

15. Johnson JK Jr. An evaluation in the medical standard of care. *Vanderbilt Law Rev.* 1970;729:731-732.

16. Kim SYH. *Evaluation of Capacity to Consent to Treatment and Research.* New York, NY: Oxford University Press; 2010.

17. Kutzko D, et al. HIPAA in real time: practical implications of the federal privacy rule. *Drake Law Rev.* 2003;51:403-450.

18. *Missouri v MCNeely*, 569 U.S. 1 (2013).

19. NY Vehicle and Traffic Law 1194 (McKinney's Consolidated Laws of NY 1996).

20. *O'Neil v Montefiore Hospital*, 11AD 2d 132, 202, NY State 2 D 436 (1960).

21. *People v Ruppel*, 303, 111. App 3d 885, 708, NE2d 824 (4 Dist 1999).

22. Prosser WL. The Law of Torts. Implied Consent. St Paul, MN: West Pub Co; 1984.

23. Public Law 111-5 American Recovery and Reinvestment Act (2009).

24. *Rochin v California*, 342 US 165 (1952).

25. Schiff GD, et al. Computerised physician order entry-related medication errors: analysis of reported errors and vulnerability testing of current systems. *BMJ Qual Saf.* 2015;24:264-271.

26. *Schloendorff v Society of New York Hospital*, 211 NY 125, 105, NE (1914).

27. *Schmerber v California*, 384 US 757 (1966).

28. Sittig DF, Singh H. Legal, ethical, and financial dilemmas in electronic health record adoption and use. *Pediatrics.* 2011;127:e1042-e1047.

29. Spiller HA, et al. Prospective multicenter study of sulfonylurea ingestion in children. *J Pediatr.* 1997;131:141-146.

30. Statement of Janlori Goldman, Deputy Director before Senate Committee on Labor and Human Resources S1360: The Medical Records Confidentiality Act of 1995. http://www .cdt.org/testimony/951114goldman.shtml. Accessed June 27, 2014.

31. Sudan R, Seymour K. The impaired surgeon. *Surg Clin North Am.* 2016;96:89-93.

32. *Sullivan v Montegomery*, 279 NYS: 575 (1935).

33. Texas Transportation Code Ann 724 (Vernon 1991).

34. The sick physician. Impairment by psychaitric disorders, including alcoholism and drug dependence. *JAMA.* 1973;255:684-687.

35. *Truman v Thomas*, 611 P.2d 902 (1980).

36. US Food and Drug Administration. HIPAA compliance for reporters to FDA MedWatch. https://www.fda.gov/safety/medwatch/howtoreport/ucm085589.htm. Accessed July 21, 2017.

37. United States Department of Health and Human Services: Office of Civil Rights. Summary of the HIPAA Privacy Rule. https://www.hhs.gov/ocr/privacysummary.pdf. Accessed April 25, 2005.

38. US Constitution 14th Amendment. http://www.archives.gov/national-archives-experience/ charters/constitution_amendments_11-27.html. Accessed May 1, 2014.

39. US Constitution 4th Amendment. http://www.archives.gov/national-archives-experience/ charters/bill_of_rights_transcript.html. Accessed May 1, 2014.

40. US Constitution 5th Amendment. http://www.archives.gov/national-archives-experience/ charters/bill_of_rights_transcript.html. Accessed May 1, 2014.

41. *Vergara v Doan*, 593 N.E. 185 (Ind. 1992); *Pederson v Dumouchel*, 72 Walsh. 2 d73, 431 P.2d 973, 977 (Wlash. 1967).

42. *Vialva v City of New York*, 118 AD 2d. 701, 499, NY 2d 977 (2nd Dept 1986).

43. Villamañán E, et al. Potential medication errors associated with computer prescriber order entry. *Int J Clin Pharm.* 2013;35:577-583.

44. *Wainwright v Leary*, 623 So.2d 233 (La. 1993).

45. Walter P. The doctrine of informed consent: to inform or not to inform? *St John's Law Rev.* 1997;71:543-589.

46. White RJ Hoffman CA. The privacy standard under the health insurance portability and accountability act: a practcal guide to promote order and avoid potential chaos. *West VA Law Rev.* 2004;106:709-779.

47. Willams CB, et al. State legal statutes for poison center liability. *Clin Toxicol.* 2009;47:736.

48. §5 ILCS 350/1, §5 ILCS 350/2; Tex. Health & Safety Code §777.007 (2004).

139 MEDICOLEGAL INTERPRETIVE TOXICOLOGY

Robert A. Middleberg

One of the potential areas of collaboration for toxicologists is the medicolegal setting. This includes working with forensic toxicologists, medical examiners, law enforcement, lawyers, and regulators. In this arena, interpretive toxicology, whether based on analytical findings or theoretical concepts, is routinely used or required to explain issues in criminal and civil proceedings and as the basis for policy making. Often, the concepts associated with forensic interpretive toxicology are presumed to be associated with deceased individuals. In practice, the preponderance of cases involving toxicologic interpretation involves living people and includes specialty testing such as human performance toxicology. Regardless, interpreting the role, or potential role, of xenobiotics in an adverse outcome is typically not straightforward. For example, the use of generally applied pharmacokinetic equations is usually inappropriate, especially in the postmortem setting, yet it is in widespread practice by individuals unfamiliar with the nuances of case-related issues.[27] Rarely is any given case accurately interpreted solely based on toxicologic assessment. As such, forensic interpretive toxicology generally involves an integrative approach that draws on an understanding of case history in addition to analytical, toxicologic, pathophysiologic, and specimen-related issues. Individuals called on to interpret the role of xenobiotics in any given case must understand the factors that affect such interpretations and associated limitations. Furthermore, although difficult in many situations, they should attempt to have their opinions firmly supported by science. Other chapters in this text (Chaps. 7, 41 and 140, Special Considerations: SC11 and SC12) cover much of the basic science associated with interpretive issues. This section is meant to focus on specific issues as they relate to medicolegal (forensic) interpretive toxicology.

CASE HISTORY

It is reported that case history plays a role in interpreting toxicologic findings in about 70% of cases.[26] A number of specific aspects of a case history will lead a seasoned toxicologist in a direction that narrows the scientific investigative focus and avoids a shotgun approach to defining the role of toxicology in an adverse outcome. Table 139–1 lists some of the more important aspects of the case history that should be evaluated from the outset to begin the interpretive process. Detailed information about the individual should optimally include anthropomorphic information, vocation, hobbies, medical history, timing of events to the extent possible, and other contextual information.[19] As an example of the importance of this information, consider a case in which an individual suspected of drunk driving worked at a company that manufactured chemicals. One of the chemicals known to be handled by the individual was a substance that co-eluted with ethyl alcohol in the gas chromatographic assay used to quantitate the blood alcohol concentration. Without his employment history, the potential for an incorrect interpretation of the data might have occurred.

Unfortunately, toxicology is often not initially considered with respect to field investigation of a case. Therefore, important information is often lost, especially in the case of purposeful poisonings. The longer the time between suspicion of a toxicologic aspect to a case and proper investigation, the greater the chance of lost evidence to achieve an understanding of the situation. The toxicologist can play a key role in mitigating this occurrence. As a significant point of contact with the poisoned individual, the toxicologist has the opportunity to not only ask the individual questions if he or she is conscious, but to also ask police, paramedics, and others questions that could assist in not only treatment of the patient, but also address serious questions that often later arise.

Unlike the confidence in the medical diagnosis of poisoning supported by clinical findings or analytical data, it should be recognized that there is rarely certainty in the use of toxicologic analysis for medicolegal purposes. However, a toxicologist's conclusions and opinions in this setting can only be attained by integrating pieces of information into a coherent analysis of the events.

PREANALYTICAL ISSUES

Ample evidence exists that the major source of error in analytical toxicology is based not on laboratory error, but on preanalytical issues.[20,41] Preanalytical issues are defined as those events that affect an analytical result prior to the specimen(s) arriving at the laboratory. In accordance with ISO (International Organization for Standardization) requirements, mathematical uncertainty should be able to be determined by the analytical testing laboratory.[28] It is an expectation in certain areas of toxicologic testing that such errors be reported for acceptance into legal proceedings.[34] Although laboratory error can usually be relatively easily quantified, the error associated with events surrounding samples before arrival at the laboratory is not so easily measured. The myriad of potential preanalytical factors is summarized in Table 139–2.

Clinical Specimens

With respect to living individuals, where and how specimens are collected from patients, in addition to specimen storage, can adversely affect not only the analytical test but its interpretation as well.[54] For example, although perhaps not protocol, occasionally samples for analysis are collected proximate to the site where medications are administered, such as close to an indwelling antecubital fossa catheter. Contamination of such specimens cannot

TABLE 139–1	Important Aspects of Case History Related to Interpretation of Analytical Findings[19,32]
Aspect	**Information to Be Gathered**
Individual history	Age, gender, weight, nationality, habitus, vocation, hobbies, smoking status, drug abuse history
Medical history	Disease processes, known medications, recent treatments or surgeries, resuscitative efforts, history of snoring (important for cases involving opioids)
Recent activity	Last known activity of the individual; description of behaviors; observations of friends, family, acquaintances, and coworkers
Timing	When did an event occur? How much time between event and specimen collection? When was the patient last seen?
Cohabitants	Vocations, hobbies, medications
Scene	Description (kempt or unkempt) Search results of cabinets, trash cans, pill vials collected, ambient temperature, odors, plants or fungi, recent Internet searches, unusual books or literature, heating pads or hot water bottles
Position and description of body, if found unresponsive	Clothing, covered or uncovered, body temperature, vomitus
Notes or journals	Indications of intent, mindset

TABLE 139–2	Preanalytical Factors That Can Affect Interpretation of Findings[13,64]	
Preanalytical Factor	*Specific Issue*	*Potential Effect*
Specimen source	Site of collection (eg, collection near site of drug administration)	Falsely elevated results
Specimens	Collection tubes or containers to include preservative or anticoagulants used, storage conditions (temperature, humidity), mislabeling	Inability to detect specific analytes Analyte stability Wrong sample tested Addition of analytes not originally present
Contamination issues	Use of inappropriate collection techniques (eg, ethanol-based swabs, lack of metal-free devices and containers)	Introduction of unintended analytes, potential misassignment of poisoning
Postmortem-specific issues	Specimen collection techniques (eg, anatomical source of blood, nonspecified part of a solid organ, collection of only partial amount of gastric contents)	Falsely elevated or depressed analyte concentrations

be excluded and will lead to misinterpretation of findings. Although the treatment of patients is the primary concern during medical emergencies, consideration of potential medicolegal issues should be part of the treating professional's assessment, especially in cases involving children, victims of drug-facilitated sexual assault, motor vehicle operation, workplace incidents, suspected poisoning, and other ill-defined situations. Adequate analysis requires that specimen collection be performed appropriately and consideration given to the types of preservatives used in the collection device. Not all collection devices fit the need for all xenobiotics. For example, although fluoride-containing tubes work well to prevent microorganism-induced ethanol formation, this same preservative will lead to degradation of some organic phosphorus compounds and make the sample totally useless in cases of suspected fluoride poisoning.[1,49] In general, it is good practice to collect both preserved and unpreserved blood samples. Serum samples are generally a good choice from living individuals, but this is analyte specific and certainly not preferred for xenobiotics sequestered in red blood cells. Perhaps the most important precaution in this respect is the collection of specimens for legal blood alcohol determination. Not only are tubes containing fluoride (1%–5% w/v) and oxalate (anticoagulant) necessary, but skin-cleansing swabs containing ethanol should be avoided.[2] Specimen storage conditions can significantly adversely affect analyte stability and specimen integrity. Except for specimens such as hair and nail clippings, specimens for toxicologic analysis should not be maintained at room temperature. Minimally, refrigeration is required, but if it is anticipated that a delay between sample collection and testing will occur, then freezing the samples at –20° or –60°C (the choice of temperature being analyte specific) should be considered, making sure to take precautions to prevent tube cracking.[11] It is recommended that if a specific xenobiotic or class of xenobiotics is suspected, that laboratory personnel should be contacted before specimen collection for guidance on proper collection, preservation, and storage of specimens. Hospitals should have in place a mechanism that ensures retention of specimens beyond the routine time frame for suspect cases. Typically, hospitals maintain specimens from a few days to a few weeks after collection to up to one year or longer in most forensic cases.[46,61] In this regard, all available specimens should be maintained. This is especially important in cases in which death is preceded by a relatively long clinical course. Although it cannot be expected that a hospital maintain specimens under a legal chain of custody, maintaining tubes with original identifier labels often suffices for this purpose.[21]

Postmortem Specimens

In postmortem situations, the potential for sample contamination is substantial, especially in the face of significant trauma. For example, the spread of gastric or intestinal contents containing xenobiotics of interest can contaminate sources of blood collection and visceral organs.[17] Additionally, other postmortem phenomena can mitigate the potential value of laboratory-based testing (Table 139–3) for interpretation purposes (see the Postmortem Redistribution section later). Specimen collection should be done by an experienced pathologist who understands the intricacies of site-specific sample collection. Postmortem blood can be obtained from 2 broadly categorized sources, central (eg, heart) and peripheral sites (eg, femoral and subclavian veins). Not all peripheral sites have the same interpretive value.[56] "Blind stick" samples should not be considered appropriate surrogates for proper dissection and visualization of the specimen source.[42] For example, heart blood should be collected from the right atrium after opening of the pericardial sack, removal of the pericardium, and drying of the heart.[13,65] Although there is no ideal postmortem specimen, femoral vein blood tends to better reflect circulating concentrations of xenobiotics closer to the time of death, but this is not always the case. Even femoral blood is subject to postmortem redistribution (PMR) in a manner similar to other blood sources. Whenever possible, both cardiac and femoral blood should be collected. Because of postmortem changes, heart blood tends to contain higher concentrations of xenobiotics than peripheral blood sites, thus making it a valuable screening specimen but limiting its actual interpretive value. To properly collect femoral vein blood, a dissection and visualization of the femoral vein followed by ligation or clamping of the vessel above the point of collection is recommended to avoid contamination by iliac blood, the latter seemingly representing a cross between peripheral and central blood.[13] Visceral organ specimens are of value in the interpretation of the meaning of blood concentrations in certain situations.[5,43] Although a plethora of data exist regarding toxicologic findings in blood, there tends to be less data regarding tissues. Nevertheless, certain organs are of substantial

TABLE 139–3	Postmortem Phenomena That Can Affect Interpretation of Toxicologic Laboratory Results
Phenomenon	*Potential Effect*
Analyte stability	Can lead to increased or decreased concentrations of analytes (eg, ethanol and cyanide can both form and degrade in specimens); will affect interpretation of results by assuming too much or too little analyte present
Degree and type of decomposition	Can lead to analytical difficulties in recovery of xenobiotics; bacterial metabolism of xenobiotics can alter pre-existing concentrations
Embalming	Can destroy or form xenobiotics or metabolites (eg, cyanide can be destroyed by embalming chemicals; methylation of desmethyl metabolites can occur; can lead to misinterpretation of results)
Entomologic factors	Insect invasion can lead to decreased or altered concentrations of xenobiotics; insects can also be useful to detect xenobiotics in badly decomposed bodies
Plasma vs postmortem blood distribution differences	Blood and plasma concentrations of xenobiotics may differ widely, so reliance on kinetic data in living persons is not comparable to postmortem blood findings; postmortem blood is not the same as whole blood in living individuals
Postmortem redistribution or diffusion	Can lead to increased or decreased concentrations of xenobiotics; misinterpretation of findings
Toxicogenetics	Can lead to unpredictable effects on metabolism; analysis for metabolic status is tenuous as genotype may not equate to phenotype

TABLE 139–4	Potential Value of Postmortem Traditional and Alternative Matrices	
Specimen	**Value**	**Factors Influencing Specimen**
Bile	Accumulates xenobiotics eliminated fecally (eg, opiates); therefore, xenobiotics remain in bile after clearance from blood	Lack of interpretive data; presence of a xenobiotic does not necessarily provide temporal information for exposure
Blood	Largest amount of comparative data; easily obtained	Subject to PMR, diffusion, contamination; blind sticks are suboptimal; xenobiotic concentrations can be a combination of acute and chronic exposure, thus hampering interpretation; back calculation to dose ill-advised
Brain	For certain xenobiotics, some correlation to effects	Very difficult specimen to handle analytically because of fat content
Gastric contents	Assessment of overdose; investigative purposes in tracking pill source; potential high concentrations of xenobiotics	Time dependent; lack of homogeneity of specimen; difficult analytically because of food and other xenobiotics
Hair	Provides exposure history data	Delay between exposure and appearance in hair (~1 week) prevents acute exposure assessment; external contamination; contamination from sweat and sebum
Kidney	High concentrations of xenobiotics cleared renally allows for ease of detection	Lack of interpretive data; xenobiotics accumulate because of specific and nonspecific binding, potentially hampering interpretability
Liver	Contains high concentrations of xenobiotics cleared hepatically; can aid in determination of overdose	Xenobiotics accumulate in liver over time, potentially hampering interpretability; can be affected by both PMR and diffusion; xenobiotics not distributed evenly throughout liver
Urine	Xenobiotics (and metabolites) eliminated renally accumulate in urine; protect xenobiotics from common postmortem degradation factors	Not always present; not always an indicator of acute exposure; analytical issues (deconjugation); no correlation with effects; no back calculation to dose possible
Vitreous humor	Some protection from decompositional changes; ethanol determination; postmortem glucose determination	Delay between appearance of xenobiotic in blood vs vitreous

PMR = postmortem redistribution.

Data from Davis GG; National Association of Medical Examiners and American College of Medical Toxicology Expert Panel on Evaluating and Reporting Opioid Deaths: Complete republication: National Association of Medical Examiners position paper: Recommendations for the investigation, diagnosis, and certification of deaths related to opioid drugs. *J Med Toxicol.* 2014 Mar;10(1):100-106.

value when considering specific xenobiotics (Table 139–4). Specimen collection tubes and storage conditions, although similar to those described with clinical specimens, tend to be more important with postmortem specimens because of continuous postmortem changes in blood pH, autolysis, and cell lysis, which can affect analyte stability, recovery, and interpretation.[61]

Hair collection must be considered in practically all cases of toxicologic concern, especially in those involving children because this specimen can circumvent arguments of incidental exposure and other issues.[47] This specimen, after being collected, requires no special storage conditions and often reflects exposure history for the length of hair growth (~1 cm/mo). Controversy regarding external contamination of hair leading to positive findings, although of some concern, does not impugn the value of this specimen.[27,36]

Lastly, iatrogenic toxicologic injury or death, whether unintentional or purposeful, are often not considered or poorly investigated. The involvement of hospital-based risk management often occurs late and valuable evidence that can either incriminate or exculpate individuals gets destroyed before collection and preservation. Protocols in suspicious cases should exist for the area where the individual was located and considered to be a "crime scene." That is, potential useful evidence, including devices, medications, and other xenobiotics should be gathered and stored.[58]

SPECIAL LABORATORY CONSIDERATIONS

Testing for xenobiotics of interest is varied and inconsistent among laboratories. Hospital-based laboratories tend to be limited in scope compared with toxicology reference laboratories. Even in this latter group, wide variances exist with respect to capability and scope. No interpretation of toxicologic findings should take place without a complete understanding of the testing performed and its limitations in addition to a review of the analytical data by a toxicologist. With the development of robust, widely available analytical tools, inadequate testing with respect to medicolegal interpretive matters should no longer occur.

Ideally, all toxicologic analyses are performed under chain of custody, and all findings are confirmed by a separate and distinct analytical test, with

at least one, such as mass spectrometry, that provides specific molecular identification.[48] This process reduces uncertainty in the utility of a finding for interpretive purposes. For example, the use of gas chromatography to identify ethylene glycol in a hospital-based laboratory led to the wrongful conviction and jailing of a mother for poisoning her infant son. The gas chromatographic peak was actually propionic acid. Remarkably, the reporting of ethylene glycol was duplicated by another laboratory. Post-conviction analysis determined the misidentification of the peak. In this case, the propionic acid resulted from the inborn error of metabolism disease, methylmalonic acidemia. 2,3-Butanediol also co-elutes with ethylene glycol in some gas chromatographic systems.[17,63]

It is uncommon for hospital-based drug testing to be analytically confirmed. However, a positive screen using an immunoassay is rarely sufficient for medicolegal purposes given the general cross-reactivity of these tests. Most hospital laboratory reports include a disclaimer to this effect. Also, most of this testing is performed using urine, so such screening tests are neither quantitative nor interpretable with respect to effects on a given individual.

Today, advanced toxicology laboratories use a combination of tools to help identify xenobiotics of toxicological concern. Many of these tests are performed rapidly and, in some sense, inexpensively compared with the offered breadth of testing. Instruments such as liquid chromatography time of flight mass spectrometry (LC-TOF) have revolutionized broad-based toxicology testing. This technique allows for the rapid screening of a patient sample in minutes covering hundreds of chemically dissimilar compounds with identification using exact mass.[25] Liquid chromatography/tandem mass spectrometry (LC-MS/MS), although somewhat less amenable to broad-based screening, has a similar utility with an easier approach, in general, to quantitative analysis.[44] Both devices will be found in some larger hospital-based laboratories and should help the toxicologist significantly in evaluating potentially poisoned patients.[24] Other instruments, such as inductively coupled plasma mass spectrometry and inductively coupled plasma optical emission spectroscopy used for the analysis of the majority of metals, are typically found in specialty laboratories and most likely will not be cost effective in the hospital laboratory (Chap. 7). In all cases, however, the toxicologist should understand the limitations of these devices that can lead to false-positive and false-negative findings.

CORRELATING FINDINGS OR THEORY TO CASE-RELATED ISSUES

Ultimately, the toxicologist's role in forensic interpretive toxicology is to integrate analytical findings and theory to develop an explanation for an adverse outcome. Although explanations abound, both in concept and practice, plausible explanations are often few. It is rare that findings are simply taken at face value. For example, it is common for identical findings in 2 different cases to have 2 completely distinct interpretations, which should not be surprising or disconcerting. For example, the finding of a high concentration of morphine in the blood of a hospice patient would be expected and often not related to the cause of death, whereas the same concentration in a naïve heroin user would represent a cause of death. Toxicology has been described as both science and art, with the interpretive aspect based in science, knowledge, and experience.[22] Many of the following factors need to be considered in rendering rational opinions.

Problems With Analytical Interpretations

Commonly, individuals render toxicologic opinions without careful review of the analytical data that help form the basis of the opinions. Acceptance of reported results at face value is a fundamental flaw in medicolegal interpretations. It is helpful to review all available information that led to a reported result before interpretation. Table 139–5 lists some of the important facets of analytical data review that lead to incorrectly reported results. Although there is no expectation that the toxicologist be an expert in analytical chemistry, familiarity with the key elements that lead to false-positive, false-negative, or poorly quantified findings should become part of the review process.

TABLE 139–5 | **Important Aspects of Laboratory Data Leading to Reporting of Inaccurate Results**

Factor	Examples	Effects
Inappropriate method validation	Unable to define limit of detection, limit of quantitation, analytical bias and precision, specificity, analyte and analytical stability, potential interferences	No confidence in the ability to produce a defensible result
No or poor analytical method	No written method to follow	Irreproducibility of results; lack of consistent direction to analysts
Lack of proper calibration or control	No controls included in analytical run, reporting results outside of the analytical measurement range, calibrators and controls prepared from the same stock solution	Unreliable results
Analytical characteristics	Poor chromatography, lack of proper internal standard, poor mass spectral characteristics, improper integration of peaks, improper baseline acceptance	Unreliable results
Administrative errors	Wrong demographics, case numbers, dates, etc assigned to the data; improper chain of custody	No confidence that correct patient specimens were tested
Failure to follow standard operating procedures	Specified steps in either administrative or technical standard operating procedures were not followed	Lack of confidence in correct patient specimen tested or in analytical results

Errors ranging from the wrong patient number on the analytical data to poor control and calibration of an analytical run to poorly integrated chromatographic peaks are all examples of errors that invalidate any given finding.

Postmortem Redistribution

There are many factors related to postmortem changes that complicate the interpretation of well-performed toxicologic test results (Chap. 140).[18,19,40,64] However, the importance of PMR, a long-established principle in forensic toxicology, cannot be ignored or underestimated. Although recognized in the early 1980s, Prouty and Anderson authored the first codified report of this phenomenon in 1990.[57] Succinctly, PMR is the term given to changes in site-specific xenobiotic concentrations after death.[53] These xenobiotic movements postmortem generally result in elevated concentrations in common collection sites such as heart blood. The elevation for some xenobiotics are dramatic, giving the appearance of overdose when no such conclusion is supported by other evidence, including analysis of sites of blood collection where PMR may occur to a lesser degree, such as femoral blood. Although instructed to do otherwise, many pathologists still collect heart blood as a sole source of postmortem blood. In attempting to assist in such situations, investigators often publish ratios of heart blood concentrations to femoral blood concentrations over a series of cases from a given laboratory. The common observation is a widespread range of values often encompassing 3- to 5-fold or greater differences in magnitude.[10] The use of such ratios to convert a heart blood concentration to a femoral blood concentration, and by further analogy to a premortem circulating blood concentration, should not be performed. The greatest use of such ratios is to give an idea of the likelihood of PMR for any given xenobiotic based on the mean and range of ratios.[45] Because it cannot be predicted if PMR occurred in any given case and if so to what degree and over what time period, such calculations have no basis for antemortem blood concentration determination. Another confounder to the use of ratios is the possibility that site-specific differences are not due to PMR but merely a reflection of incomplete distribution before death.[19] It is unclear how many of the reported ratios of heart blood to femoral blood actually reflect this process as opposed to true PMR. The proposed mechanisms and influencing factors resulting in PMR are varied and are listed in Table 139–6. It is most likely a combination of factors that lead to PMR in any given case. Interestingly, as noted earlier, PMR is also reported to take place in femoral blood; thus, it should not be taken at face

TABLE 139–6 | **Factors Affecting Postmortem Redistribution[18,53]**

Factor	Issue or Potential Effect
Volume of distribution	Xenobiotics with high volumes of distribution often correlate with a greater degree of PMR; if PMR occurs, it leads to falsely elevated concentrations in fluids and tissues
pH of blood	pH of blood changes postmortem, becoming more acidic; this alters ionization of xenobiotics and promote or hinder PMR
Xenobiotic reservoirs	Organs of high blood content or flow, tissues that specifically or nonspecifically retain analytes (eg, liver, kidney), and holding vessels (eg, GI organs) facilitate movement to blood vessels and neighboring organs
Resuscitative efforts	Some demonstration that xenobiotics move in vivo as a result of resuscitative efforts
Breakdown of barriers	Cellular structural changes cause leaking of xenobiotics from one site to another, including from intracellular sequestration sites
Release of xenobiotics from proteins	Will alter the free to bound ratio, potentially leading to an unreliable reliance on free xenobiotic concentrations
Postmortem metabolism	Leads to decreased or increased concentrations of xenobiotics

GI = gastrointestinal; PMR = postmortem redistribution.

value that any postmortem blood concentration accurately reflects the circulating concentration at and around the time of death.

At one time it was believed that PMR was associated with basic xenobiotics with a large volume of distribution. Seemingly, however, most xenobiotics, including acidic and neutral xenobiotics, undergo PMR. Furthermore, PMR occurs for xenobiotics with wide-ranging volumes of distribution. Still other xenobiotics that would be predicted to undergo PMR have experimental evidence to the contrary.[53] Thus, a priori predictions of PMR for any given xenobiotic without experimental evidence should explicitly state the caveats associated with such a conclusion. It must be stated, however, that PMR does not preclude the interpretation of findings for cause of death determination because the findings represent only one piece of data in a potential myriad of other relevant information.

Another similarly related phenomenon is postmortem diffusion of xenobiotics. In this situation, diffusion of xenobiotics from an area of high concentration to that of a lower concentration occurs. This is most noted when the gastric contents contain a substantial amount of a xenobiotic that migrates across the wall of the stomach into neighboring tissues and blood sources, such as abdominal aorta and iliac vessels. Additionally, perimortem aspiration of gastric contents can lead to significant esophageal, tracheal, and lung concentrations of a xenobiotic, further facilitating diffusion processes.[12,55] One last concern is the administration of drugs via such mechanisms as a central line, whereby it can be reasonably expected that drugs will continue to accumulate in and around the heart postmortem.

Alternative Matrices

Although most discussions regarding interpretive toxicology tend to focus on blood concentrations of xenobiotics, clearly in both the living and the dead, alternative matrices are extremely valuable. It should be recognized that there is no perfect specimen to assess exposure or provide analytical findings in support of impairment. In the living, alternative specimens including hair, oral fluid, and breath are useful. Hair gives a longer window of detection than most other easily obtained specimens.[65] Analytical precautions, such as rinsing procedures, are used to minimize some concerns with hair testing.[59] The utility of hair should not be underestimated, and despite some of its limitations, it can represent the best suited specimen in some cases, such as drug-facilitated sexual assault, especially when more than 24 to 48 hours passed before specimen collection from the time of event, thus often limiting the value of urine or blood testing.[38] In such cases, waiting 1 to 3 months before collecting hair will capture the potential exposure period in growing hair. It is especially useful in children to demonstrate acute versus chronic exposure to xenobiotics.[47] Collection of hair should be from the posterior vertex of the head, which can be easily approximated by drawing an imaginary line over the head connecting the tops of both ears and a line from the bridge of the nose to the nape of the neck.[13,59] The area where the 2 lines meet in the back of the head provides hair that grows most consistently on the head.[37] About a pencil thickness worth of hair should be clipped as closely to scalp as possible.[14] The root ends should be identified either by tying with string or wrapping in foil.[13] Virtually any other sources of hair are suitable for testing, such as pubic and axillary hair, although practical reasons and shorter growth rates tend to make such samples less suitable for testing.

Oral fluid (OF) is gaining ground as a viable specimen type to assess exposure and impairment because obtaining it is noninvasive, and it can be collected at the site of an event, thus eliminating time delays.[5] Such delays will result in clearance of a xenobiotic from other specimen types before collection. Oral fluid is composed of secretions from the parotid, submaxillary, sublingual, and other smaller glands. Numerous specimen collection devices exist today that circumvent the need to expectorate, which is not a desirable means of specimen collection.[51] For the most part, non–protein-bound parent compounds appear in OF, although there are exceptions (eg, benzoylecgonine).[15] Factors that affect how much of a xenobiotic gets into OF include pH of the blood and OF, the pKa of the xenobiotic, and the degree of protein binding. In general, basic xenobiotics get into OF more easily than acidic xenobiotics.[68] Oral fluid has been used for therapeutic

drug–monitoring purposes (eg, theophylline and digoxin).[8] Although some correlations between blood concentrations and a number of xenobiotics have been made, it must be remembered that OF is susceptible to contamination from residual drug in the oral cavity, smoked xenobiotics, and passive exposure.[5,15] Despite its promise, there is variability in OF concentrations of xenobiotics not only within the same individual but also among individuals based on influencing factors that facilitate or inhibit secretion of a xenobiotic into OF.[5] Finally, based on the relatively small specimen volumes after OF collection, specialized testing, including tandem mass spectrometry, is often needed to detect the concentrations of xenobiotics present.

Breath testing for alcohol is a mature subject matter, yet when it comes to impairment, there is a current trend for states to move back to blood alcohol determinations. Legal arguments are the force behind some of this movement.[52] The United States Supreme Court, however, rendered a decision in 2016 whereby blood collection related to driving under the influence can only be obtained after issuance of a search warrant, declaring blood collection to be invasive compared to breath testing. It is unclear how this latter decision will ultimately affect the decision as to what specimen is collected for analysis in driving under the influence cases.[4] In living individuals, particularly in the hospital setting, serum alcohol is typically measured. As such measurements for alcohol are often used in the medicolegal setting, it is imperative that toxicologists understand the differences between blood and serum alcohol concentrations and that such differences are related to attorneys (Special Considerations: SC11 for greater detail).

Breath testing for other xenobiotics is still in its fledgling state. Despite this, the future holds promise for the detection of other xenobiotics in breath with the possibility of roadside breath drug-testing devices.[3] The major advantage of this specimen is not only its lack of invasive nature, but rapid screening capability.

Alternative matrices from decedents are varied and include virtually all fluids and tissues (Table 139–4). Practically speaking, however, other than providing qualitative information, for most matrices, there is little data to support utility of a measured concentration to either allow for independent interpretation or correlation to blood concentrations. Although numerous studies exist that suggest such correlations, rarely is there consistency between studies. Even so, situational use of alternative matrices is sometimes warranted (eg, the use of fat or brain to detect volatiles). A specific exception is vitreous humor (vitreous), a specimen that is often extremely valuable postmortem. Vitreous electrolyte measurements provide data that cannot be gleaned from virtually any other specimen type (Table 139–7).[9] For most xenobiotics, vitreous concentrations lag behind blood concentrations by about 1 or 2 hours. Thereafter, some correlations have been made between vitreous concentrations and those in blood, with the greatest example being ethanol, where there is an approximately 1:1 correlation when equilibrium is reached. Vitreous represents a relatively pristine specimen during

TABLE 139–7	Valuable Normal Vitreous Chemistries	
Analyte	*Factors Affecting Analyte*	*Reported Normal (mmol/L)*
Chloride	Dehydration, water intoxication	105–135
Potassium	Postmortem interval	<15
Sodium	Dehydration, water intoxication	135–150
Urea nitrogen	Dehydration, kidney problems (eg, azotemia)	8–20
Glucose	Hyperglycemia, DKA, hypoglycemia	<200
Ketones	Fasting or starvation, AKA, DKA, isopropanol exposure	None detected

DKA = diabetic ketoacidosis; AKA = alcoholic ketoacidosis.

Data from Collins K. Postmortem Vitreous Analyses. Medscape Reference (updated July 31, 2016) http://emedicine.medscape.com/article/1966150-overview.

decomposition, embalming, exsanguinations, severe peritoneal trauma, and other less ideal situations.[23]

Toxicokinetics, Toxicodynamics, and Drug Interactions

The basics of toxicokinetics (TK) and toxicodynamics (TD) are covered in Chap. 9. The large and unpredictable degree of interindividual variability places practical limits on the use of TK and TD in postmortem interpretation. These same variations affect the pharmacologic response in living patients. Multiple elements related to TK and TD affect the ability to render interpretive opinions of xenobiotics related to an adverse outcome (Table 139–8) and the use of pharmacokinetic and toxicokinetic equations warrants special attention.

Toxicologic emergencies and overdoses alter normal physiologic functions. Liver and kidney dysfunction significantly alter normal TK parameters.[62,66] Coupled with pharmacogenetics, drug–drug or drug–xenobiotic interactions, pathophysiology, and other significant factors, the use of routine TK equations usually leads to grossly under- or overestimates of a specific measured value. Nevertheless, in a living patient, TK equations are useful to estimate certain parameters (eg, dose and, in part, form the basis of such useful tools as nomograms). After death, because of PMR, postmortem diffusion and other issues, the use of TK formulas to predict premortem concentrations or dosing is not generally an acceptable practice. For example, the use of the following formulas will lead to either an absurd dose calculation or an inappropriate estimate of predicted concentration compared with that reported for compounds undergoing significant PMR:[16,29]

$$\text{Dose} = \text{Reported concentration} \times \text{Volume of distribution} \times \text{Body mass}$$

$$\text{Concentration} = \frac{\text{Dose}}{\text{Volume of distribution} \times \text{Body mass}}$$

Nevertheless, such calculations, although ill-advised, are routinely performed and can provide grossly misleading information. "Back extrapolating" from a postmortem concentration to some concentration earlier in time using half-life is fraught with the same perils in that the initial assumption

TABLE 139–8	Factors Affecting the Utility of Toxicokinetic and Toxicodynamic Principles in Interpretive Toxicology[16,18,19,29]
Criterion	**Potential Effect**
Xenobiotic–xenobiotic interactions	Can lead to increased or decreased concentrations of analytes, resulting in serious adverse effects; interactions can take place via increased or decreased metabolism or via competitive interactions at target sites (eg, receptors); can give the appearance of intentional overdose
Idiosyncratic response	There is little or no means of identifying an idiosyncratic response after the fact; can result in serious adverse effects, including fatalities
Pathology or pregnancy	Disease states can alter the toxicokinetic and toxicodynamic profiles for a given xenobiotic and resultant effects; pharmacokinetics and toxicokinetics change in pregnant women (eg, clearance)
Route of administration	Affects body burdens and speed of action of xenobiotics
Tolerance	Can lead to an overestimation of effect of a given xenobiotic concentration; there is no a priori means of determining tolerance
Toxicogenomics	Can lead to unpredictable effects on metabolism; analysis for metabolic status may not be useful because genotype may not equate to phenotype
Toxicokinetic variables	Prevents utility of classic pharmacokinetic or toxicokinetic equations; there is no a priori means of knowing the value for the necessary variables unique to an individual used in equations (eg, clearance)
Trauma or shock	Associated issues, including blood shunting and decreased organ perfusion, can alter toxicokinetic factors

of an unchanged postmortem blood concentration should not be made.[18] Additionally, it is never known how much of any measured blood concentration resulted from single or multiple dosing exposure to a xenobiotic. Despite these and other issues, the toxicologist will be pressured into providing dosing information or predicting a blood concentration during life. The safest avenue in this respect is not to accede to such pressures because the scientific underpinnings are unreliable.

It should be stressed that metabolic drug interaction considerations alone, together, or in conjunction with additional information informs the toxicologist of many varied aspects of exposure and potential effect and outcomes. Often, the metabolic fate of a substance is under genetic control, but it must be understood that genotype does not often relate to phenotype, thus complicating interpretation of toxicologic findings or adversely affecting theoretical interpretive toxicology. Drug interactions occur through varied means, including metabolic inhibition or induction, receptor competition, allosteric modulation, etc. (Chap. 11). All such interactions affect the efficacy and toxicity of a given compound. In some cases, these effects reveal themselves through such factors as ratios of metabolite to parent compound, metabolite to metabolite ratios, etc. One such example is the determination of heroin use from postmortem blood and blood from impaired drivers. In most cases, a ratio of free morphine to free codeine greater than unity is strong evidence that the decedent used heroin. The same appears to hold true in the blood of living people. These latter findings will not hold true when exposure to both heroin and codeine together occurred or when the individual is exposed to both morphine and codeine simultaneously.[7,31]

Assessing Impairment

There exist 2 broad areas of concern with respect to impairment, that from ethanol and that from other xenobiotics. Impairment caused by ethanol has been extensively studied, and general conclusions are usually reached with some confidence. The same cannot be stated for impairment caused by other xenobiotics. Ultimately, conclusions of xenobiotic impairment are based on a number of factors that include physical examination by a trained clinician, dosing information, length of time taking a xenobiotic, co-administered xenobiotics, pathophysiology, observed behaviors, measured concentrations in blood or serum or plasma, and any other useful information.[35] The use of the term "consistent with" is common in assessing impairment in any given individual and might very well be the best opinion that can be offered. Mitigating factors, including tolerance, single versus multiple dosing, reason for the presence of the substance, timing and route of administration, and pathophysiology, all make firm conclusions difficult, especially when blood findings are the first indication of potential impairment (ie, no visible signs of impairment).[30,60] Great care must be exercised in evaluating or predicting impairment from xenobiotics given the implications of such conclusions. There is currently no scientific support for back extrapolation of xenobiotic concentrations based on blood findings. It cannot be stressed enough that urine findings should never be used to assess impairment because the predictive value is limited.[67] Similar to blood ethanol concentration, many states and countries have developed *per se* xenobiotics laws that presume guilt by the presence of certain drugs or metabolites over some prescribed reportable concentration, even in urine, thus mitigating the need for interpretation in most cases. For example, the presence of Δ^9-carboxy-tetrahydrocannabinol, an inactive metabolite of marijuana, is used to convict drivers of impaired driving; for clarity, this is a legal issue, not a scientific, issue.[33,39] Tables and texts that list xenobiotics and determined concentrations in blood and other specimens should only be used as a guide for interpretive purposes because every human toxicologic experience is unique.

REASONABLE MEDICAL CERTAINTY

It is common for experts in the medicolegal setting to be asked to present opinions and conclusions with a reasonable degree of medical or scientific certainty. Although on the surface such a phrase appears to connote some level of confidence in what one opines or concludes, it has been declared a nebulous phrase without true meaning and at its worst, misleading for a trier of fact.[50] The derivation of such a phrase is most likely a legal construct intended to persuade a trier of fact that the particular opinions of the retained expert are somehow weighted to such a degree that no other opinion or conclusion would make sense. However, that 2 toxicologists can give 2 distinctly differing opinions in the same case, both to a reasonable degree of medical certainty, demonstrates the lack of utility of the phrase. It is not common parlance for physicians or scientists to discuss matters with a reasonable degree of medical or scientific certainty and it is unclear why the term should carry into the medicolegal setting. Undoubtedly, there will be a slow retraction from the use of the phrase, but toxicologists can push the measure forward through discussions with attorneys prior to expert report generation or testimony by declaring that use of the phrase cannot be supported in a medical or scientific context.

SUMMARY

- Toxicologists have the opportunity based on both contact with patients and as consultants to be involved with medicolegal cases.

- To properly assess such cases, a holistic approach should be taken that involves the integration of detailed historical information, preanalytical factors and understanding of the analytical work performed (including its limitations), specimen-specific utility, and special aspects that can weaken or strengthen the ability to form medically and scientifically sound conclusions.

- It should be understood that the burden on the toxicologist is not generally "absolute certainty" because this is something that is rarely achievable. However, the toxicologist must develop opinions and conclusions based upon sound medical and scientific principles and, if asked, be able to identify factors that weaken the stated opinions and conclusions.

- The purpose of the proffered opinions and conclusions offered should not be lost, that is, to educate someone or a group of individuals who have to make difficult decisions, some of which infringe on civil liberties and freedoms. In that respect, the burden assumed by toxicologists should be recognized as significant and warrant the same attention to detail with medicolegal opinions as treatment and diagnosis of a poisoned patient.

REFERENCES

1. Amick GD, Habben KH. Inhibition of ethanol production by *Saccharomyces cerevisiae* in human blood by sodium fluoride. *J Forens Sci.* 1997;42:690-692.
2. Anderson WH. Collection and storage of specimens for alcohol analysis: In: Garriott JC, ed. *Garriott's Medicolegal Aspects of Alcohol.* 5th ed. Tucson, AZ: Lawyers & Judges Publishing; 2008:275-283.
3. Beck O et al. Amphetamines detected in exhaled breath from drug addicts: a new possible method for drugs-of-abuse testing. *J Anal Toxicol.* 2010;34:233-237.
4. *Birchfield v North Dakaota*, 579 U.S. (SCOTUS June 23, 2016).
5. Bosker WM, Huestis MA. Oral fluid testing for drugs of abuse. *Clin Chem.* 2009;55:1910-1931.
6. Bynum ND, et al. Postmortem distribution of tramadol, amitriptyline, and their metabolites in a suicidal overdose. *J Anal Toxicol.* 2005;29:401-406.
7. Ceder G, Jones AW. Concentration ratios of morphine to codeine in blood of impaired drivers as evidence of heroin use and not medication with codeine. *Clin Chem.* 2001;47:1980-1984.
8. Choo RE, Huestis MA. Oral fluid as a diagnostic tool. *Clin Chem Lab Med.* 2004;42:1273-1287.
9. Collins K. Postmortem vitreous analyses. Medscape. http://emedicine.medscape.com/article/1966150-overview. Accessed March 12, 2014.
10. Dalpe-Scott M, et al. A comparison of drug concentrations in postmortem cardiac and peripheral blood in 320 cases. *Can J Forens Sci.* 1995;28:113-121.
11. Davis GG. Recommendations for the investigation, diagnosis, and certification of deaths related to opioid drugs. *Acad Forens Pathol.* 2013;3:62-76.
12. DeLetter EA, et al. Post-mortem redistribution of 3,4-methylenedioxymethamphetamine (MDMA, "ecstasy") in the rabbit. Part II: post-mortem infusion in trachea or stomach. *Int J Leg Med.* 2002;116:225-232.
13. Dinis-Oliveira RJ, et al. Collection of biological samples in forensic toxicology. *Toxicol Mech Methods.* 2010;20:363-414.
14. Dolan K, et al. An overview of the use of urine, hair, sweat and saliva to detect drug use. *Drug Alcohol Rev.* 2004;23:213-217.
15. Drummer OH. Drug testing in oral fluid. *Clin Biochem Rev.* 2006;27:147-159.
16. Drummer OH, Karch S. Interpretation of toxicological data. In: Moffat AC, et al., eds. *Clarke's Analysis of Drugs and Poisons.* 4th ed., Vol. 1. London: Pharmaceutical Press; 2011:417-428.
17. Eder AF, et al. Ethylene glycol poisoning: toxicokinetic and analytical factors affecting laboratory diagnosis. *Clin Chem.* 1998;44:168-177.
18. Ferner RE. Post-mortem clinical pharmacology. *Br J Clin Pharmacol.* 2008;66:430-443.
19. Flanagan RJ, Connally G. Interpretation of analytical toxicology results in life and at postmortem. *Toxicol Rev.* 2005;24:51-62.
20. Flanagan RJ, et al. Analytical toxicology: guidelines for sample collection postmortem. *Toxicol Rev.* 2005;24:63-71.
21. Frikke MJ. Evaluation of add-on testing in the clinical chemistry laboratory of a large academic medical center. *Arch Pathol Lab Med.* 2005;129:454; author reply 454.
22. Gallo MA. History and scope of toxicology. In: Klaasen CD, ed. *Casarett and Doull's Toxicology.* 7th ed. New York, NY: McGraw-Hill; 2008:1-10.
23. Garriott JC. Analysis of alcohol in postmortem specimens. In: Garriott JC, ed. *Garriott's Medicolegal Aspects of Alcohol.* 5th ed. Tucson, AZ: Lawyers & Judges Publishing; 2008:217-228.
24. Grebe SK, Singh RJ. LC-MS/MS in the clinical laboratory—where to from here? *Clin Biochem Rev.* 2011;32:5-31.
25. Guale F, et al. Validation of LC-TOF-MS screening for drugs, metabolites, and collateral compounds in forensic toxicology specimens. *J Anal Toxicol.* 2013;37:17-24.
26. Harding-Pink D, Fryc O. Assessing death by poisoning: does the medical history help? *Med Sci Law.* 1991;31:69-75.
27. Huestis MA. Judicial acceptance of hair tests for substances of abuse in the United States courts: scientific, forensic, and ethical aspects. *Ther Drug Monit.* 1996;18:456-459.
28. ISO 15189:2007. *Medical Laboratories—Particular Requirements for Quality and Competence.* 2nd ed. 2007.
29. Jones G. Postmortem toxicology. In: Moffat AC, et al., eds. *Clarke's Analysis of Drugs and Poisons.* 4th ed., Vol. 1. London: Pharmaceutical Press; 2011:176-189.
30. Jones AW, et al. Concentrations of scheduled prescription drugs in blood of impaired drivers: considerations for interpreting the results. *Ther Drug Monit.* 2007;29:248-260.
31. Jones AW, Holmgren A. Concentrations ratios of free-morphine to free-codeine in femoral blood in heroin-related poisoning deaths. *Legal Med.* 2011;13:171-173.
32. Jones AW, Holmgren A. Concentration distributions of the drugs most frequently identified in post-mortem femoral blood representing all causes of death. *Med Sci Law.* 2009;49:257-273.
33. Jones, AW. Driving under the influence of drugs in Sweden with zero concentration limits in blood for controlled substances. *Traf Inj Prev.* 2005;6:317-322.
34. Judge rules against blood alcohol tests. WoodTV. http://www.woodtv.com/dpp/news/michigan/Judge-rules-against-blood-alcohol-tests. Accessed July 15, 2013.
35. Kay GG, Logan BK. *Drugged Driving Expert Panel Report: A Consensus Protocol for Assessing the Potential of Drugs to Impair Driving.* NHTSA. DOT HS 817 438; March 2011.
36. Kintz P. Value of hair analysis in postmortem toxicology. *Forensic Sci Int.* 2004;142:127-134.
37. Kintz P, et al. Hair analysis for drug detection. *Ther Drug Monit.* 2006;28:442-446.
38. Kintz P, et al. Testing for the undetectable in drug-facilitated sexual assault using hair analyzed by tandem mass spectrometry as evidence. *Ther Drug Monit.* 2004;26:211-214.
39. Lacey J, et al. *Drug Per Se Laws: A Review of Their Use in States.* NHTSA. DOT HS 811 317; July 2010.
40. Leikin JB, Watson WA. Post-mortem toxicology: what the dead can and cannot tell us. *J Toxicol Clin Toxicol.* 2003;41:47-56.
41. Linnet K, et al. Dominance of pre-analytical over analytical variation for measurement of methadone and its main metabolite in postmortem femoral blood. *Forensic Sci Int.* 2008;179:78-82.
42. Logan BK, Lindholm G. Gastric contamination of postmortem blood samples during blind-stick sample collection. *Am J Forensic Med Pathol.* 1996;17:109-111.
43. Luckenbill K, et al. Fentanyl postmortem redistribution: preliminary findings regarding the relationship among femoral blood and liver and heart tissue concentrations. *J Anal Toxicol.* 2008;32:639-643.
44. Maurer HH. Multi-analyte procedures for screening for and quantification of drugs in blood, plasma, or serum by liquid chromatography-single stage or tandem mass spectrometry (LC-MS or LC-MS/MS) relevant to clinical and forensic toxicology. *Clin Biochem.* 2005;38:310-318.
45. McIntyre IM, Anderson DT. Postmortem fentanyl concentrations: a review. *J Forensic Res.* 2012;3:1-10.
46. Melanson SF, et al. Evaluation of add-on testing in the clinical chemistry laboratory of a large academic medical center: operational considerations. *Arch Pathol Lab Med.* 2004;128:885-889.
47. Middleberg RA. Poisoning and toxicological issues in infants and children. In: Byard RW, Collins KA, eds. *Handbook of Forensic Pathology of Infancy and Childhood.* Springer; in press.
48. Moffat AC, et al. Introduction to forensic toxicology. In: Jickells S, Negrusz A, eds. *Clarke's Analytical Forensic Toxicology.* London: Pharmaceutical Press; 2008:1-11.
49. Moriya F, et al. Pitfalls when determining tissue distributions of organophosphorus chemicals: sodium fluoride accelerates chemical degradation. *J Anal Toxicol.* 1999;23:210-215.
50. National Commission on Forensic Science. Testimony using the term "Reasonable Scientific Certainty." https://www.justice.gov/ncfs/file/795336/download. Accessed March 15, 2017.
51. O'Neal CL, et al. The effects of collection methods on oral fluid codeine concentrations. *J Anal Toxicol.* 2000;24:536-542.

52. Pennsylvania State Police decide to halt the use of breath testing for DUI. PRWeb. http://www.prweb.com/release/2013/1/prweb10330601.htm. Accessed July 16, 2013.

53. Pélissier-Alicot AL, et al. Mechanisms underlying postmortem redistribution of drugs: a review. *J Anal Toxicol.* 2003;27:533-544.

54. Plebani M, Carraro P. Mistakes in a stat laboratory: types and frequency. *Clin Chem.* 1997;43:1348-1351.

55. Pounder DJ, et al. Postmortem diffusion of drugs from gastric residue: an experimental study. *Am J Forensic Med Pathol.* 1996;17:1-7.

56. Pounder DJ, Jones GR. Post-mortem drug redistribution—a toxicological nightmare. *Forensic Sci Int.* 1990;45:253-263.

57. Prouty RW, Anderson WH. The forensic science implications of site and temporal influences on postmortem blood-drug concentrations. *J Forensic Sci.* 1990;35:243-270.

58. Pyrek KM. Forensic issues in the clinical setting. In: *Forensic Nursing.* Boca Raton, FL: CRC Press; 2006:43-78.

59. Recommendations for hair testing in forensic cases. Society of hair testing. http://www.soht.org/pdf/Consensus_on_Hair_Analysis.pdf. Accessed July 15, 2013.

60. Reisfield GM, et al. The mirage of impairing drug concentration thresholds: a rationale for zero tolerance per se driving under the influence of drugs laws. *J Anal Toxicol.* 2012;36:353-356.

61. *Retention of Laboratory Records and Materials.* College of American Pathologists. http://www.cap.org/apps/cap.portal?_nfpb=true&cntvwrPtlt_actionOverride=%2Fportlets%2FcontentViewer%2Fshow&cntvwrPtlt%7BactionForm.contentReference%7D=policies%2Fpolicy_appPP.html&_pageLabel=cntvwr. Accessed July 15, 2013.

62. Rosenberg J, et al. Pharmacokinetics of drug overdose. *Clin Pharmacokinet.* 1981;6:161-192.

63. Shoemaker JD, et al. Misidentification of propionic acid as ethylene glycol in a patient with methylmalonic acidemia. *J Pediatr.* 1992;120:417-421.

64. Skopp G. Preanalytic aspects in postmortem toxicology. *Forensic Sci Int.* 2004;142:75-100.

65. Stimpfl T, et al. Systematic toxicological analysis: recommendations on sample collection. *TIAFT Bulletin* 2009;XXXIX:10-11.

66. Sue YJ, Shannon M. Pharmacokinetics of drugs in overdose. *Clin Pharmacokinet.* 1992;23:93-105.

67. Toennes SW, et al. Driving under the influence of drugs—evaluation of analytical data of drugs in oral fluid, serum and urine, and correlation with impairment symptoms. *Forensic Sci Int.* 2005;152:149-155.

68. Wille SMR, et al. Relationship between oral fluid and blood concentrations of drugs of abuse in drivers suspected of driving under the influence of drugs. *Ther Drug Monit.* 2009;31:511-519.

SC11

ASSESSMENT OF ETHANOL-INDUCED IMPAIRMENT

Robert B. Palmer

INTRODUCTION

Myriad medical texts describe the medical consequences of acute and chronic ethanol use. The purpose of this discussion is to describe the history and use of assessments of ethanol-induced impairment, primarily in a legal context. Some of the principles described, however, are extrapolated from the legal to the medical setting. Throughout this chapter, the terms *ethanol* and *alcohol* are used interchangeably in order to retain the forensic, legislative, and medical contexts in which the terms are used. Similarly, words such as *drunk* and *punishable* are also occasionally used in this chapter in order to preserve the specific language used in the early studies and legal writings.

HISTORY

Numerous well-designed laboratory studies assessing alcohol-induced impairment are published. However, application of study results to actual cases of possible impaired driving or over service of alcohol in a drinking establishment may be inaccurate without an understanding of the origin of laws governing these activities. Although the intoxicating effects of ethanol have been known for centuries, the advent of mechanized transportation spawned increased public and legal scrutiny. Concern was expressed over the potential adverse safety implications of driving while intoxicated, not just for the impaired driver but also for other persons (passengers, other drivers, pedestrians) and property. Although railroads had regulations against the operation of equipment while intoxicated dating back to at least the 1850s, the first arrest for drunk driving in an automobile was that of a London taxicab driver in 1897.[22] The realization that alcohol intoxicated motor vehicle operators were a public health issue worthy of legal scrutiny soon followed, and legislation was enacted to combat "drunken driving." In 1910, New York was the first US state to enact such a law.[22]

In early laws, "drunken driving" was poorly defined and relied heavily on observable signs of gross intoxication. Attempts at legislative clarification of language resulted in terms that were nearly as nebulous, such as "alcohol-impaired" and "under the influence." Prior to the landmark work by Widmark[67] in Sweden, and by Heise[27] in the United States, evaluations of driver impairment were predominantly based on the "expert" testimony of an evaluating physician and the arresting police officer, as well as behaviors reported by witnesses. These evaluations were observational, rather than scientifically based, and such nonsystematic and nonobjective testimony was often dubious and frequently plagued by exaggeration of behaviors (eg, staggering gait, incoherent speech).

The development of analytical technology capable of measuring the concentration of alcohol in blood gave rise to the idea that diagnosis of intoxication might be assisted by an objective chemical test result. The theory behind this idea being simply, the higher the blood alcohol concentration (BAC), the more drinks the individual must have consumed and, therefore, the greater the degree of impairment. It was, therefore, reasoned that there is a legally punishable limit of alcohol in blood or other biological matrix. Although the assignment of a specific clinical effect to a given BAC is not rigorously applicable to evaluation of an individual case, the general trends when examined across a population formed the foundation of many modern driving while intoxicated (DWI) laws.

Despite centuries' worth of knowledge of the effects of alcohol and decades of efforts to articulate drunk driving standards, a single universal definition of "alcohol intoxicated" does not exist. A typical medical definition focuses on altered mental status, ataxia, or the ability to care for oneself, whereas the focus of a legal definition is on the ability to safely operate a motor vehicle or successfully perform field sobriety tests, or whether the patron of a bar or restaurant should be served additional alcohol. A lay public definition may include parts of both.

Although alcohol intoxication is an important factor in a nearly infinite number of settings, 2 of the most common legal circumstances involving toxicology consultation for alcohol-related issues are (a) alcohol-impaired operation of a motor vehicle and (b) so-called "dram-shop" cases when an already intoxicated individual is served additional alcohol. Discussion of alcohol use in the workplace and alcohol-abstinence monitoring are beyond the scope of this chapter.

PER SE LIMITS

With the advent of analytical measurements capable of quantitatively determining BAC and the increasing public awareness of the dangers associated with drinking and driving, legislation based on BAC began to appear. Although the initial laws did not define the specific BAC that established illegality in the operation of a motor vehicle, they did allow for the use of BAC results as supportive evidence of intoxication. The first states to incorporate BAC into drunk-driving statutes were Indiana and Maine, which did so in 1939.[28] The approach taken by the Indiana legislature resulted in a 3-tiered statute, which stated that a BAC of less than 50 mg/dL was considered presumptive evidence of no intoxication, a BAC between 50 and 100 mg/dL was considered supportive evidence of intoxicated driving, and a BAC of greater than 150 mg/dL was considered *prima facie* (ie, obvious and evident without proof) evidence of guilt. From a legal perspective, *prima facie* evidence shifts the burden of proof from the accuser having to substantiate the charge to the defense to rebut the allegation. It is this legal perspective from which the so-called *per se* standards are derived—that is, an individual whose BAC exceeds a predetermined concentration is deemed guilty of driving while impaired by alcohol, even without any other evidence of intoxication or impairment.

Early drunk-driving standards established in the Uniform Vehicle Code made reference to a BAC at which there was "no doubt of obvious intoxication"; this BAC was defined as 150 mg/dL. However, by 1960, as data regarding alcohol-related motor vehicle crashes became available, most (but not all) states adopted a more rigorous *per se* BAC driving standard of 100 mg/dL.[28] This reduction in the *per se* legal BAC for an alcohol-impaired driving charge was supported by powerful medical and political groups, including the American Medical Association (AMA). Interestingly, the AMA recommendation also noted that some persons were "under the influence" or impaired in their ability to safely operate a motor vehicle at BACs of 50 to 100 mg/dL. Despite newer drinking and driving laws defined on the basis of an objective chemical test, many state laws still contained older vague language such as "intoxicated," "visibly intoxicated," and "obviously intoxicated," which legislators were then forced to define more clearly and objectively.

Different states use different acronyms to apply to alcohol-impaired driving, including DUI (driving under the influence), DUIL (driving under the influence of liquor), DWI (driving while intoxicated), OUI (operating under the influence), OWI (operating while intoxicated), and OMVI (operating a motor vehicle while intoxicated). Regardless of the acronym used, the definitions are effectively the same. Depending on the state, the same terms may also be used in drug-impaired driving, whereas in other states, a separate charge, such as DUID (driving under the influence of drugs) may be applied to nonalcohol drug-related driving impairment.

In 2000, the National Highway Traffic Safety Administration (NHTSA) reported that of 41,471 motor vehicle fatalities, 38.4% were alcohol-related; this corresponded to an average of one alcohol-related traffic fatality every 31 minutes.[69] The 2014 NHTSA data suggest a slight decrease in alcohol-related fatalities, with 31% of fatal motor vehicle crashes involving a driver with a BAC of 80 mg/dL or greater, corresponding to one alcohol-impaired-driving fatality occurring every 53 minutes.[43] However, it must be noted that NHTSA considers any fatal crash in which a driver has a BAC of 80 mg/dL or greater to be an alcohol-impaired driving crash; and, fatalities in these crashes are considered to be due to alcohol-impaired driving.[43] Critics of the NHTSA data claim this method for counting likely overestimates the number of actual fatalities involved in alcohol-related crashes as the mere fact that a driver had consumed alcohol and had a BAC of greater than or equal to 80 mg/dL does not prove crash causality. Nonetheless, there is little argument that alcohol use increases crash risk. Epidemiologic assessments demonstrate that the probability of causing an alcohol-related motor vehicle crash increases slightly at a breath alcohol concentration (BrAC) of 50 mg/dL. The risk of causing a crash is increased by roughly 4-fold at a BrAC of 80 mg/dL, 7-fold at a BrAC of 100 mg/dL, and 25-fold at a BrAC of 150 mg/dL.[5,28] In 1994, a successful campaign, vigorously supported by the AMA and Mothers Against Drunk Driving (MADD), encouraged all states in the US to lower the BAC used to define *per se* intoxicated driving to 80 mg/dL.[22] Although all states technically have the right to set drunk-driving statutes at their discretion, political advocates for more strict alcohol-impaired driving statutes were successful in convincing the US government to require a minimum legal drinking age of 21 years and a mandatory *per se* BAC statute of 80 mg/dL in order to receive federal highway funding.[22] Consequently, as of July 2004, all US states, the District of Columbia, and Puerto Rico conform with federal recommendations defining a BAC of 80 mg/dL as a violation of motor vehicle code. Lower *per se* BACs are applied to interstate commercial drivers (40 mg/dL) and pilots of aircraft (40 mg/dL, with no alcohol consumed within 8 hours prior to acting as pilot in command), as well as minors (10–20 mg/dL, depending on the state, and 20–50 mg/dL in some European countries). Additionally, some US states, such as Colorado, have lower *per se* statutes for the slightly lesser charge of driving while ability impaired (DWAI), which may be invoked when a driver's BAC is between 50 and 80 mg/dL. Some US states also have legal standards defining an "aggravated DUI." Definitions of "aggravated DUI" are variable by state, but some of the actions that may lead to this charge include, committing a DUI while under court order to use an approved ignition interlock device, committing a DUI while the offender's driver's license or driving privileges are suspended, canceled, or revoked because of a prior DUI violation, or committing multiple DUIs in a specified time period (eg, 10 years). States such as Montana have an additional standard that charges an individual with aggravated DUI if the driver's BAC is found to be 160 mg/dL, or more.

Laws addressing *per se* driving under the influence (DUI) limits are based on ethanol concentrations measured in whole blood. BrAC limits (which are arithmetically linked to BAC) are also frequently specified in *per se* statutes. As such, the use of appropriately conducted breath alcohol measurements eliminates the need to collect a blood specimen from a suspect. *Per se* limits, as described above, apply to the ability to safely accomplish specifically defined tasks such as driving an automobile or flying an aircraft. It is, however, imperative to understand that *per se* BACs do *not* define drunkenness or alcohol intoxication in nondriving situations, and their use in circumstances not involving motor vehicle operation is generally inappropriate.

The legal significance of a *per se* limit is that there is no requirement for behavioral evidence of intoxication, as long as the measured BAC exceeds that established by the legislature. Since their enactment, numerous legal arguments have challenged the constitutionality of *per se* drunk-driving laws. Issues including a lack of due process through application of the "void for vagueness" doctrine, reliability of breath testing results, and the distinction between blood alcohol and breath alcohol concentrations have all formed bases for legal challenges to *per se* laws.[22] However, despite such challenges, the courts consistently uphold these laws.

ANALYTICAL CONSIDERATIONS

Accurate measurement of ethanol concentration in various biological matrices can be done using a number of analytical techniques. Historically, Widmark employed wet chemical oxidation, using potassium dichromate and excess sulfuric acid, followed by iodometric titration of the remaining amount of oxidizing agent.[67] Although this method is effective, it is laborious and lacks specificity if other volatiles (eg, methanol, acetone, ether) are present, as these substances are also oxidized, causing a falsely elevated ethanol result. Such wet chemical methods are now obsolete and no longer used in forensic and clinical laboratories.

Enzymatic ethanol assays based on alcohol dehydrogenase (ADH) are commonly used, especially in high-throughput laboratories. The oxidation conditions of enzymatic methods are milder than wet chemical methods. Additionally, acetone, which caused the most troublesome interference with wet chemical methods, is not oxidized by ADH. Interferences by other aliphatic low-molecular-weight alcohols such as methanol and isopropanol occur with ADH isolated from humans and other animals; this interference is reduced by using yeast-derived ADH, which shows greater selectivity for ethanol.[31,64] Specific enzymatic methods used for ethanol analysis in body fluids include enzyme-multiplied immunoassay technique (EMIT), fluorescence polarization immunoassay (FPIA), and radiative energy attenuation (REA), which is related to FPIA (Chap. 7). Comparative study of ethanol determination by REA and gas chromatography shows excellent agreement in precision and accuracy between the 2 techniques.[12] Both high serum lactate and elevated lactate dehydrogenase concentrations interfere with ADH-based methods of ethanol analysis, including providing false-positive results in serum specimens from alcohol-free patients.[3,44]

The greater selectivity for ethanol of gas chromatographic (GC) methods make this technique the mainstay for quantitative analysis in most forensic laboratories. Typically, the GC method involves head space sampling (HS-GC), which capitalizes on the volatility of ethanol, eliminates some potential interferences, and shortens run time. Samples to be run by HS-GC are first diluted (typically 1:5 or 1:10) with an aqueous solution of internal standard. This mixture is then sealed in a crimp-top vial with a rubber septum and gently heated to 122°F to 140°F (50°C–60°C) for 30 to 60 minutes in order to achieve equilibrium of volatiles between the gas and liquid phases. The vapor is then sampled with a syringe by puncturing the rubber septum and the withdrawn vapor injected into the instrument. Heating the sample for too long at a high temperature can result in oxidation from oxyhemoglobin.[56] This problem is solved by the addition of sodium azide or sodium dithionite to block the oxidation or simply reducing the equilibrium temperature to 104°F to 122°F (40°C–50°C).[56] Once chromatographic separation is achieved, various detection methods, including flame ionization (FID), electron capture (EC), and electrochemical sensing are used (Chap. 7). Dual detection (eg, FID and EC) can also be useful in circumstances where a larger number of volatiles may need to be screened.[57]

As ethanol distributes based on total body water, the water content of the matrix will affect the amount of ethanol present in a given volume or mass of biological sample. A common circumstance in which this is observed is in the difference between a whole blood ethanol determination and a plasma or serum ethanol determination. The water content of serum and plasma is 10% to 12% higher than whole blood, meaning that serum or plasma ethanol concentrations will be correspondingly higher than whole blood concentrations. Clinical laboratories most often use serum and plasma for analysis, whereas *per se* DUI statutes are written in terms of whole blood. Therefore, if a comparison is to be made between a serum or plasma analytical result and a legal standard, the result must be converted to an approximated whole blood ethanol concentration. Experimentally determined serum-to-whole blood ethanol ratios range from 1.12 to 1.17, whereas plasma-to-whole blood ethanol ratios range from 1.1 to 1.35.[45] Typically, a ratio of 1.16 is used for this conversion, and no significant difference appears to exist between the serum-to-whole blood and plasma-to-whole blood ratios.[69] Ratios between whole blood and other biological matrices such as urine, saliva, cerebrospinal fluid, vitreous humor, brain, liver, kidney, and bone marrow are published, and a table listing these ratios and the sources from which they are derived is available.[11]

Breath testing is commonly performed to assess BAC because of its relative simplicity and less invasive collection compared to urine or blood. The analytical basis for sampling exhaled breath is that, at equilibrium, alcohol in expired air is present at a predictable ratio with blood. The gas exchange process in the lungs is complex, with significant theoretical variability.[40] In the United States, a blood-to-breath alcohol ratio of 2100:1 is commonly used in the calibration of breath alcohol testing devices, although some experimental evidence suggests that the ratio is actually closer to 2300:1.[17] As such, a systematic underestimation of BAC is expected when breath alcohol results are converted to whole blood alcohol results. Several studies document this underestimation with data from suspected impaired drivers and evidential breath alcohol testing instruments.[20,25] In 1983, Britain adopted a legal limit in breath of 35 mcg/100 mL, which corresponds to a blood alcohol of 80 mg/dL, using a 2300:1 blood-to-breath ratio.[28] Legal statutes that include in their offense definition breath alcohol results expressed in units of grams/210 L of exhaled air eliminate the need to convert breath alcohol to blood alcohol, largely mitigating arguments based on the breath-to-blood ratio.

BREATH-TESTING DEVICES

Three general analytical detection principles have been extensively validated and are currently used in breath alcohol–testing instruments. These are infrared spectroscopy, electrochemical oxidation/fuel cell, and chemical oxidation/photometry.[26] Additionally, combination of multiple technologies is sometimes used, as in infrared/fuel cell dual detectors. Breath-testing instruments are generally divided into 4 broad categories: passive alcohol sensors (PASs), screening devices (preliminary breath testers, {PBTs}), breath alcohol ignition interlock devices (BAIIDs), and evidential breath testers (EBTs).[26]

A PAS device may be concealed in a device such as a modified police flashlight and is used to detect alcohol on or in the immediate vicinity of a subject through passive means (ie, with no requirement for subject cooperation). Breath alcohol ignition interlock devices are used to prevent drinking and driving by requiring the driver to blow into a sensor in order to start the ignition of the vehicle. The devices are typically installed on a court order designed to modify drinking and driving behavior in habitual DUI offenders, with the cost of installation typically borne by the offender. A number of mechanisms are employed to prevent substitution of breath samples, including preset patterns of exhalation or humming while blowing into the sampling tube. Additionally, random rolling retests are required, failure of which result in the vehicle's lights flashing or horn blowing. Neither PAS nor BAIID results are useful for quantitative measurement of breath or blood alcohol for prosecution of a *per se* DUI case.

The PBT and EBT devices are the most common breath alcohol–testing devices encountered in cases of DUI arrest. In this setting, PBT results are used in conjunction with observation and field sobriety tests to establish probable cause for DUI arrest. Although a measured BrAC is often provided as a digital readout on a PBT, in most jurisdictions these results are not admissible as evidence for proceedings other than probable cause hearings. Use of PBT devices is also common in nonlegal settings such as hospital emergency departments, alcohol detoxification units, homeless shelters, and workplaces. As with DUI prosecution, these results are generally used for screening for alcohol presence and not for establishing impairment.

In contrast to PBT results, measurements from an EBT device are admissible in court and administrative proceedings and can be used as the basis for establishment of *per se* DUI cases without the necessity of blood collection and analysis. Although mobile EBT devices are available, most often the EBT is maintained in a fixed location such as a police station. For the results to be considered valid and admissible, the operator of the EBT must be trained and certified, and the operation must be performed using an accepted testing protocol.

Required procedures for the use of EBT devices exist for the subject as well as the instrument. The subject must have a period of alcohol deprivation of at least 15 to 20 minutes during which trained personnel observe him or her to ensure not only that no additional ethanol is consumed but also that no regurgitation, emesis, or eructation occurs, which could result in residual ethanol in the mouth prior to breath alcohol analysis. With respect to the instrument, both blank and control analyses must be performed prior to analysis of the subject sample. A blank analysis, typically done with room air, purges the instrument of contamination from previous samples and demonstrates a lack of environmental contamination. A control analysis is performed on a gaseous ethanol sample of known concentration, usually an ethanol gas canister or wet bath simulator, and demonstrates proper instrument calibration and maintenance. Certification of instrument maintenance of calibration must be documented, demonstrating compliance with applicable rules, regulations, laws, and standards for routine maintenance, troubleshooting, and corrective actions. These documents are then retained for a relevant time period after inspections are complete. Additional documentation for individual cases should include written verification that all steps in the accepted protocol were followed. This documentation also includes automated printouts from the analyzer used, and well as copies of manual checklists.[26]

Beyond the required procedures, additional recommendations include the use of grams/210 L as the reporting units, rather than reporting breath alcohol concentration as a converted blood alcohol concentration of %weight/volume, grams/100 mL, or grams/deciliter. Serial collection and analysis of at least 2 separate sequential breath samples taken 2 to 10 minutes apart should be done in order to demonstrate the absence of residual mouth alcohol, instrument artifacts, frequency interference, and spurious results. Agreement of the serial results must be within prescribed limits (usually, 0.02 g/210 L) to be considered acceptable.[26]

STANDARDIZED FIELD SOBRIETY TESTS

A driver whose BAC exceeds the established legal standard is considered *per se* intoxicated and often convicted without behavioral evidence of intoxication. However, some objective findings of impairment assists in establishing probable cause to demand chemical testing, initiate a DUI arrest, or prosecute a charge of impairment, without invoking *per se* limits. In these settings, results of a specific group of behavioral tests are of value in discriminating and prosecuting or refuting an impaired driving charge, although submitting to these behavioral tests is typically voluntary. Additionally, an objective measurement of alcohol effect is helpful in assessing alcohol-related impairment in nondriving situations, where it is inappropriate to directly apply *per se* standards.

Under a contract with the NHTSA, a group of 15 candidate sobriety tests were evaluated in a laboratory study.[9] From this original group, the investigators developed a series of 3 specific tests that have subsequently been standardized as a test battery, known as standardized "field sobriety tests" (FSTs), for assessing driver impairment in the United States. The 3 tests comprising the standardized FSTs are the one-leg stand (OLS), walk-and-turn (WAT), and horizontal gaze nystagmus (HGN). Descriptions of these tests are provided in Table SC11–1.

A 1981 study of 297 drinking volunteers with BACs ranging from 0 to 180 mg/dL who were evaluated by trained police officers showed adequate interrater reliability (correlations, 0.6–0.8) and test-retest correlations (0.40–0.75).[59] Using all 3 field sobriety tests, the officers were able to distinguish whether BAC was above or below 100 mg/dL in 81% of participants. Test results were observed to generally correlate with BAC. However, the specificity and sensitivity of each individual test was not evaluated. Field sobriety tests are typically associated with physical, rather than mental, ability other than understanding the instructions for each test. Some aspects of variability in cognitive performance correlate moderately and positively with facets of FSTs, especially those tests evaluating reaction time.[16]

TABLE SC11-1	Standardized Field Sobriety Tests	
Test	**Test Description**	**Test Scoring ("clues")**
One-leg stand (OLS)	With the arms at sides, raise one foot at least 6 inches off the ground and stand on the other foot for at least 30 seconds.	4-point scale 1. Putting foot down 2. Hopping 3. Swaying 4. Raising arms Any 2 "clues" is failure.
Walk-and-turn (WAT)	Balance with feet heel-to-toe and listen to test instructions. Walk 9 steps heel-to-toe in a straight line, turn 180 degrees, and walk 9 more steps heel-to-toe, while counting steps, watching feet, and keeping hands at sides.	8-point scale 1. Inability to maintain balance in the starting position 2. Starting too soon (eg, prior to completion of instructions) 3. Stepping off the line 4. Not touching toe to heel 5. Raising arms 6. Improper turn 7. Stopping 8. Wrong number of steps Any 2 "clues" is failure.
Horizontal gaze nystagmus (HGN)	Angle of onset of nystagmus is determined for each eye.	6-point scale (three points for each eye) 1. Lack of smooth pursuit 2. Distinct nystagmus at maximum deviation 3. Onset of nystagmus before 45 degrees Cutoff is 4 "clues."

Adapted with permission from Rubenzer SJ. The standardized field sobriety tests: a review of scientific and legal issues. *Law Hum Behav.* 2008 Aug;32(4):293-313.

In the few studies evaluating the performance of individual FSTs, general correlation between test performance and BAC is observed. Although the correlation magnitudes for the WAT and OLS tests are low, the HGN test showed excellent sensitivity and specificity across a range of BACs.[46] In the control arm (ie, no alcohol ingested and no detectable ethanol in the blood), approximately 50% of the participants were judged to be impaired using the WAT test, whereas in the OLS test, 30% of the participants were rated as impaired. When the BAC was greater than 150 mg/dL, performance on the WAT and OLS tests improved to 78% and 88%, respectively. The rate of false positives (ie, those with a zero BAC who failed the HGN test) was only 3%. As seen with the other FSTs, the sensitivity of the HGN test increased with increasing BAC, being 81% for those with a BAC between 100 and 149 mg/dL and 100% for those with a BAC greater than 150 mg/dL. The presence of horizontal gaze nystagmus, even in alcohol-tolerant drinkers, gives this test an advantage over the WAT and OLS tests in detecting the presence of alcohol.[10] It is noteworthy that balance and coordination can be affected by factors unrelated to alcohol consumption, such as physical disability, age, and nervousness about potential arrest; however, chronic drinkers with substantial alcohol tolerance are reportedly able to complete balance tests with few errors, even with moderate to high BACs.[9]

The 3 tests utilized for field sobriety assessment have some advantages, in that they are standardized and are easily understood by test takers. In addition, personnel administering the tests can be trained in a matter of hours.[39] However, because the test results are only approximately correlated with BAC, their use is limited by the threshold BAC they are able to detect. Predictably, various scientific and legal challenges to the use of the FSTs have also been made. For example, the tests were designed and validated at a time when the *per se* DUI limit in most of the United States was 100 mg/dL; however, that threshold is now 80 mg/dL in every state (and 20–50 mg/dL in many European countries).[39] Because of the variability of psychomotor

effects of alcohol as a result of individual tolerance, FST assessments are generally not allowed as a means of estimating BAC in court proceedings. The effects of fear, fatigue, rehearsal of test performance, the arresting officer's knowledge of estimated BAC prior to administering the standardized FSTs, and various medical conditions have not been fully addressed. It has further been argued that the studies most strongly supporting use of standardized FSTs are those conducted by NHTSA-affiliated investigators and reported in non–peer-reviewed government publications. So contentious has the debate been that some have charged that "the United States Department of Transportation indulged in deliberate fraud in order to mislead the law enforcement and legal communities into believing the test (HGN) was scientifically meritorious and overvaluing its worth in the context of criminal evidence." A comprehensive review detailing this, and other, legal and scientific issues surrounding standardized FSTs was published in 2008.[50] The author concluded that SFTs are not useful in predicting BAC, and that further research is needed to determine whether improvements can be made to the current battery of tests included in FST assessments. Despite arguments of FSTs having limitations, these assessments are still commonly used in arrest and prosecution of alcohol-impaired driving cases.

ESTIMATING THE AMOUNT OF ALCOHOL INGESTED

The kinetic profile of ethanol in the blood has been extensively studied. In general, it is known that when blood ethanol concentration is greater than 20 mg/dL, it follows a zero-order elimination profile and then converts to first-order elimination when the concentration drops below this threshold.[30] In the zero-order portion of the curve, typical elimination rates range from 10 to 20 mg/dL/h in social drinkers. In one study of adult patients in an urban hospital emergency department, nonchronic users of alcohol (n = 9) demonstrated a mean elimination rate of 18.7 mg/dL/h (range, 16.1–21.4), whereas chronic users (n = 15; defined as more than 2 drinks per day, history of delirium tremens, or prior detoxification) had a significantly greater mean elimination rate of 20.3 mg/dL/h (range, 16.1–24.6).[6] Other studies report elimination rates of 30 to 50 mg/dL/h in chronic heavy drinkers due, at least in part, to metabolic enzyme induction.[6,7] Pharmacokinetic calculations in healthy persons often employ a range of elimination rates of 10 to 20 mg/dL/h in order to best bracket individual differences.[7]

The estimation of the number of drinks ingested in order to achieve a given BAC has been extensively studied and is predicated on knowing several case-specific pieces of information. According to the US Department of Agriculture, a standard drink consists of 12 ounces of beer (5% v/v), 5 ounces of wine (12% v/v), or 1.5 ounces of 80-proof spirits (40% v/v); each of these drinks contains approximately 14 g of ethanol.[7,63] The time period over which the ingestion occurred, the time of the last drink, and time of blood alcohol specimen collection must be known. It is helpful to know whether the subject was fasting or had a full stomach at the time of drinking because the presence of food in the stomach slows ethanol absorption.[34,65] Finally, the gender, age, height, and weight of the individual should be known and considered.[7]

Using this information, an estimation of the number of drinks is possible. The original work in which the prediction of ethanol concentrations from known doses was performed by Widmark in 1932 using 20 healthy volunteer moderate drinkers (10 of each gender).[67] This work was translated into English from the original German by Baselt in 1981.[68] The basis of Widmark's work was that the BAC was directly proportional to the administered amount of alcohol ("dose"); the body weight of the subject; and a unitless scaling factor that Widmark referred to as "ρ" (rho), which corrected the subject's body weight for water content. Of note, in present-day pharmacokinetics, Widmark's ρ effectively represents the volume of distribution of ethanol. Because of the differences in body water content between sexes, ρ was determined to be approximately 0.6 in women and 0.7 in men. The original Widmark equation is therefore written as

$$A = C \times \rho \times p$$

where A represents the total amount of ethanol equilibrated in all fluids and tissues at the time of sampling (ie, total dose ingested), C is blood ethanol concentration in grams/kilogram, ρ is the previously described Widmark ρ factor, and p is subject body weight in kilograms. Although the calculation has served well as an estimating tool for more than 80 years, it does have some limitations, principally in the ρ factor. As a result, refinement of Widmark's original ρ was undertaken by others.[7,66] One method for the estimation of total body water (TBW), which takes into account not only gender but also individual age, weight, and height (abbreviated ΣV_d) for men aged 17 to 86 years yields the following equation:

$$\Sigma V_d = 2.44 - (0.09516 \times age) + [0.1074 \times (height \times 2.54)] + [0.3362 \times (weight/2.2045)]$$

For women aged 17 to 84 years, the TBW equation is:

$$\Sigma V_d = -2.097 + [0.1069 \times (height \times 2.54)] + [0.2466 \times (weight/2.2045)]$$

In all persons, the height is measured in inches and the weight is measured in pounds. Note that the equation for men includes a mathematical term derived from age, and the equation for women does not.[66] The significance of this calculation is its ability to be tailored to a specific person, rather than the broad extrapolation of the relatively few subjects in the original study. Inclusion of such individual information improves the accuracy of such calculations.[54]

The need for a more standardized approach to calculations involving alcohol in forensic medicine has been known for decades. One author summarized 20 of the most commonly used alcohol-related calculations.[7] As an example, the following equation is derived to calculate the estimated dose of ethanol necessary to achieve a specific blood alcohol concentration:

$$g\ EtOH = BAC_{target} + [(\beta_{1-n} \times (t_s + t_p)] \times \Sigma V_d / Bl_{H2O}$$

where g EtOH is the ingested dose of ethanol in grams; BAC_{target} is the observed blood alcohol concentration in mg/dL; β_{1-n} is a range of alcohol elimination rates (typically, 10–20 mg/dL/h); t_s is the time from the start of drinking to the last drink; t_p is the range of times from the last drink to the peak BAC (typically, 30–90 minutes); ΣV_d is the Watson TBW, which is the volume of distribution based on age, weight, height and gender; and Bl_{H2O} is the approximate percentage of water in whole blood (80.65%).[7] Noting the inherent variability in terms such as β_{1-n} and absent specific kinetic data from the individual in question, it can be seen that results of such equations are most reasonably presented as a range, rather than a single discrete calculated value.

Some legal arguments have quite incorrectly suggested that ethanol is odorless. Ethanol has a characteristic pleasant smell, with an odor threshold of approximately 50 ppm.[14] The presence or absence of breath alcohol odor is often used by police officers in the decision to proceed further with sobriety testing. In one study, 20 experienced police officers assessed alcohol odor on 14 subjects with BACs ranging from 0 to 130 mg/dL after drinking beer, wine, bourbon, or vodka.[42] Assessments were initiated 30 minutes after cessation of drinking. The strength of breath alcohol odor was determined to be an unreliable indicator of BAC. Correct detection of the presence of alcohol was 85% for BACs at or above 80 mg/dL but declined with decreasing BAC or the presence of food. The authors also noted that there were only small differences in odor intensity as a function of beverage type, meaning fusel oils and other constituents of alcoholic drinks are not the primary determinant of detectable odor after absorption of the beverage.

DRAM SHOP

Liquor liability or "dram shop" laws hold the server of alcoholic beverages liable for damages or injuries caused by an individual who was provided alcohol when such service should have been refused. For example, if a an individual who was already intoxicated, or any minor, is served alcohol and crashes his or her vehicle, the person and/or establishment who served the alcohol may be liable for damages or injuries sustained in the crash.

Interestingly, US dram shop laws were first enacted in the mid-1800s, although they were rarely used. The initial intent of these laws was to provide financial support to the families of persons who had become "habitual

drunkards" through their patronage of a drinking establishment.[52] Repeal of Prohibition in the United States in 1933 shifted laws governing alcohol sales from federal to state control, resulting in state-to-state variability in alcohol availability, criminal and administrative laws, and liquor liability. There was also a move from public focus on habitual drunkenness to the damage caused by impaired drivers, as well as a paradigm shift in the standard for irresponsible service away from serving a "drunkard" to serving an individual who was "visibly intoxicated."[52] The purpose of liquor liability laws has also changed over time. In the 19th century, laws were enacted to punish tavern owners who contributed to the downfall of patrons. By contrast, current application of the laws is typically as a means to compensate innocent victims injured by an intoxicated patron. This action on behalf of the innocent victim is why liquor liability law is sometimes referred to as "third party" liability.

Beginning in the late 1970s and early 1980s, political activists began to take note of dram shop laws as an effective means for prevention of impaired driving (or DWI). Outreach began to bring attention to irresponsible commercial and social service of alcohol. Various drunk-driving prevention strategies emerged, including "server intervention" (ie, the practice of bar or restaurant workers intervening to prevent an intoxicated patron from driving). Interestingly, although the goal of keeping intoxicated patrons from "getting behind the wheel" is certainly praiseworthy, these programs put notably less emphasis on preventing intoxication in the first place. The 1983 Presidential Commission on Drunk Driving recommended dram shop liability and server intervention as drunk-driving prevention strategies, and federal grant funds for state impaired-driving initiatives also listed such programs as qualifying criteria.[1]

Alcoholic Beverage Control agencies in the various states are responsible for reviewing and approving liquor licenses of commercial establishments, collecting taxes, and enforcing criminal and administrative laws prohibiting service to minors and intoxicated persons. Largely as a tool to improve public perception of the industry, the alcoholic beverage producers have largely been responsible for the development of training programs for servers in the retail community. Numerous programs offering Responsible Beverage Service (RBS) training for servers are administered at the state or regional level, or sometimes even sponsored by the server's employer. Calls for greater organization and standardization of RBS programs in the United States have been answered, at least in part, by the Responsible Hospitality Council, whose work has focused on developing minimum standards for legitimate RBS training.[52] Although such standards are often welcomed by regulators, some restaurant associations and owners have expressed concern over cost and compliance standards associated with RBS mandates. Nonetheless, the US legal climate seems to dictate that alcoholic beverages be served in a "responsible" manner and that liability for "overservice" falls on the serving establishment. It is also noteworthy that cases placing liability on individuals serving alcohol socially in their home have been successfully argued.

Direct comparison of the efficacy of dram shop liability laws between states is difficult as liability laws and insurance vary widely. Historically, different states and regions emphasized different areas of alcohol service liability, and it was noted that research played only a minor role in determining server training, with the majority of policy formation arising from political influence.[52] However, even data collected in the 1980s suggested that dram shop laws did result in a statistically significant decline in mortality rates not only for motor vehicle collisions, but also for other alcohol-related causes.[55] A more recent study concluded that dram shop liability and RBS laws were associated with significant reduction in *per capita* beer consumption and fatal crash ratios in drivers under age 21.[53] This begged the question of whether enhanced enforcement of dram shop laws would result in a decrease in excessive alcohol consumption and related consequences. An evaluation of 11 studies concluded that while dram shop laws were effective in reducing alcohol-related harms, the data supporting the efficacy of enhanced enforcement on reduction of alcohol-related harms were mixed and ultimately judged insufficient.[47]

Specific study of alcohol service liability on younger and underage drinkers has also been investigated. Reduction of the legal age for alcohol purchasing from 20 to 18 in New Zealand in December of 1999 resulted in a statistically significant increase in traffic injuries attributable to male drivers aged 15 to 19 years.[33] Review of annual fatal motor vehicle collision data from the United States showed that the most effective interventions for the prevention of underage alcohol-related fatal crashes were those associated with reducing teen drinking, rather than those restricting teen driving.[49] An evaluation of 20 minimum legal drinking age 21 (MLDA-21) laws in order to assess which had an effect on fatal underage drinking and driving traffic crashes.[18] Nine of the laws were associated with a decrease in fatal crash ratios: fake identification support for retailers (−11.9%), use alcohol and lose your driver's license (−7.9%), possession of alcohol (−7.1%), purchase of alcohol (−4.2%), age of the bartender greater than or equal to 21 (−4.1%), responsible beverage service program (−3.8%), zero tolerance 0.02 BAC limits for underage drivers (−2.9%), state dram shop liability (−2.5%), and social host civil liability (−1.7%). Interestingly, 2 laws were associated with a significant increase in fatal underage crash ratios (registration of beer kegs [+9.6%], and prohibition of furnishing alcohol to minors [+7.2%]). The authors concluded that 9 effective MLDA-21 laws were responsible for saving an estimated 1,135 lives annually, though only 5 states have adopted all 9 of these laws.

INTOXICATION AND ESTIMATION OF BLOOD ALCOHOL CONCENTRATION

Neither the characteristic odor of ethanol nor the measurement of various markers of alcohol exposure (eg, ethyl glucuronide, ethyl sulfate, carbohydrate deficient transferrin, and so on) are useful in estimating BAC or degree of intoxication. The ability of an individual to accurately estimate his or her own BAC is poor.[35,51] Drivers who underestimate their own BAC are more impulsive and riskier drivers than those who overestimate their BAC.[36] A lack of accuracy in estimating BAC is also observed in trained medical providers and police officers.[4,13] A large confounding factor in these observations is tolerance. Greater tolerance, as occurs in heavy drinkers and alcoholics, imparts greater difficulty in detecting the clinical effects associated with alcohol intoxication.

Tolerance involves a central adaptation to the intoxicating effects of alcohol. As such, persons with significant tolerance to the effects of ethanol may not manifest signs of intoxication despite having a high BAC. Multiple case reports and case series in the medical literature describe alcoholic individuals with heavy alcohol consumption who have very high BACs but muted or absent clinical effects.[15,24,29,38,48,58] As a result of tolerance in the chronic heavy drinking population, it is often difficult to detect clinical intoxication even though an individual has a high BAC. Critically, this circumstance does not suggest that, even in the clinically sober chronic drinker, driving abilities are unaffected or that the individual is necessarily capable of safely operating a motor vehicle.[4] Furthermore, tolerance has no bearing on the potential prosecution of a DUI case on a *per se* BAC or BrAC basis.

The circumstance is slightly more straightforward in the social drinker. The intensity of the effects of alcohol on the central nervous system (CNS) is generally proportional to the concentration of alcohol in the blood. Dubowski tabulated the stages and effects of acute alcohol intoxication, and these tables are often used in educational programs and some legal proceedings.

However, though useful as a pedagogic tool for explaining the continuum of alcohol intoxication, the table must be used with care as the effects are defined only over a population, thereby making assignment of a specific effect or degree of effect in an individual impossible. The inherent individual variability in the table is apparent in the fact that the BAC ranges for the various stages of alcoholic influence overlap. Furthermore, the population and methods used to compile the table are not described, and the table itself has not been subjected to peer review.

The CNS effects of alcohol intoxication are typically more pronounced on the ascending portion of the blood alcohol kinetic curve than on the descending side due to acute tolerance.[21] In other words, the clinical effect of intoxication is greater during the absorptive arm of the kinetic curve than on the elimination arm, even though the same blood alcohol concentration is measured in both kinetic phases. This principle is known as acute tolerance, or the Mellanby effect.

In a dram shop case, the ultimate question often becomes, what is the typical BAC at which it is more likely than not that the average nontolerant individual will exhibit signs of intoxication (eg, the odor of alcohol on the breath, clumsiness, difficulty walking or maintaining balance, slurred speech, inappropriate behavior) that are apparent to a bystander or untrained casual observer? A 1986 report by the Council on Scientific Affairs of the AMA reviewed 7 studies spanning 50 years that included more than 6,500 participants for identification of BACs at which individuals appeared "drunk" (ie, clinically intoxicated).[2] BACs were stratified by increments of 50 mg/dL, beginning at 0.0 to 50 mg/dL and extending to 401 mg/dL. In the lowest BAC group (0.0–50 mg/dL), observer perceptions of subject drunkenness ranged from 0% to 10%, with an average of 4%. The percentage of individuals determined by observers to be drunk increased steadily from a mean of 32% (range, 14%–68%) at a BAC of 51 to 100 mg/dL to a mean of 62% (range, 47%–93%) at a BAC of 101 to 150 mg/dL. In this latter range, 4 of the 7 studies indicated a perception of drunkenness by less than or equal to 50% of observers. However, in the next BAC increment of 151 to 200 mg/dL, observers judged a mean of 89% (range, 83%–97%) of the drinkers to be drunk. In each of the subsequent higher increments, the mean percentage of persons classified as drunk ranged from 95% to 100% with no individual study value less than 90%. Therefore, it can be reasonably concluded that in a nontolerant individual, a BAC of 151 to 200 mg/dL will more likely than not result in observable signs of drunkenness to a casual observer.

Study of the effects of alcohol on driving performance has been the subject of decades of research. Driving simulators are often used in laboratory studies of impaired driving and have the benefit of easy replication and control of experimental conditions. A number of simulation devices have also been developed including "fatal vision goggles," which provide visual distortion to the wearer in order to simulate the effects of alcohol on visual perception.[41] Additionally, simulators and simulation devices allow study of the effects of impairing substances in populations in which actual drinking is legally or ethically unacceptable (eg, underage prelicensed drivers). However, it is known that driving performance evaluated in a simulator is less sensitive to the effects of alcohol than actual on-the-road driving.[32] Additionally, despite frequent use, many driving simulator tests lack validation and head-to-head comparison with naturalistic driving.[32]

The validity of a police officer detecting intoxication in drivers involved in motor vehicle crashes also increases with increasing BAC. One report examined a total of 1336 subjects over age 15 who were admitted or died at a level 1 trauma center in Seattle during a 5-year period from 1986 to 1993 and in whom both a recorded BAC and a police assessment of sobriety were conducted.[23] The blood alcohol measurement was conducted in the hospital, and it is not expressly stated if the analytical matrix used was whole blood, serum, or plasma. Four categories of sobriety assessment were used by police: (a) had not been drinking, (b) had been drinking–not impaired, (c) had been drinking–sobriety unknown, and (d) had been drinking–impaired. Officers used a battery of specific criteria to judge whether a driver was intoxicated, including odor on the breath, slurred speech, chemosis, poor coordination of motor function, and the ability to simultaneously perform multiple tasks. The greatest number of drivers were in the 2 extreme categories: had not been drinking (n = 746) and had been drinking–impaired (n = 568). A direct correlation between measured BAC and police officer assessment of sobriety was observed. The mean BAC associated with the "had been drinking–impaired" group was 190 mg/dL with a 95% confidence interval (CI) of 180 to 200 mg/dL. Those in the "had been drinking–sobriety unknown" group had a mean BAC of 130 mg/dL (95% CI, 110–150). Among all drivers, police field assessment of sobriety had a positive predictive value of 85% with sensitivity and specificity of 91% and 90%, respectively, demonstrating recognition of drunk driving by police with a high degree of accuracy, especially in the group with the highest BAC.

Another study designed to determine the ability of police officers, who have more training than the average lay person, to make assessments about alcohol intoxication in drinking target subjects without the aid of special testing normally available to them (eg, standardized field sobriety tests or the ability to smell the odor of alcohol on the subject's breath).[8] This study involved 39 police officers who viewed a series of videotaped interviews with 6 volunteer moderate drinkers having targeted BACs in 3 concentration ranges: low (80–90 mg/dL), medium (110–130 mg/dL), and high (150–160 mg/dL). Based on their observations of the taped interviews, the officers answered 3 questions:

1. Has the person been drinking?
2. Was it OK to serve that person one additional drink?
3. Was the person able to drive a car?

Each of the 3 questions could be answered "yes," "no," or "not sure." A fourth question assessed the officers' confidence in their answers as "not sure," "little uncertain," or "positive." Question 2 was to be answered from the perspective of a social host or bartender, not a police officer. None of the police officers had any formal training in the management or service of alcohol to intoxicated people, such as that offered by commercial seller/server training programs like Techniques of Alcohol Management (TAM) or Training for Intervention Procedures (TIPS). With respect to their answers, the police officers were fairly certain that the subjects had been drinking only in the target groups with the highest BAC (150–160 mg/dL). Officers also answered in the affirmative to question 2 (ie, that it was OK to serve the target subject another drink) the majority of the time in the low- and medium-BAC target groups but not in the high BAC target group. The percentage of officers answering affirmatively to this question was 55%, 75%, and 41% for the low, medium, and high target groups, respectively.

Multiple studies have examined the likelihood of on-premise (bars and restaurants) and off-premise (liquor stores, grocery stores, and convenience stores), as well as outdoor events like festivals, to sell alcohol to obviously intoxicated persons (typically, paid professional actors pretending to be drunk).[19,37,60-62] The results are fairly uniform in that the majority of the time the alcohol was sold or served to the individual. Additionally, it was noted that male servers/clerks who appeared younger than age 31 were more likely to make such sales and the sales were more likely to occur in off-premise establishments.[19]

In a typical study, the authors employed 19 actors who were specifically hired based on their ability to feign intoxication. All actors were male and ranged in age from 31 to 59 years, with a mean of 42 years.[61] The actors used a standardized script to attempt to purchase either a single vodka drink after asking what beers were available on tap (on-premise) or a 6-pack of beer (off-premise). Prior to entering the establishment, the actor received specific instructions to demonstrate multiple signs of intoxication, including disheveled hair and clothing, smelling of alcohol, lack of coordination, stumbling, fumbling with money, slurring words, repeating questions, appearing forgetful, and laughing inappropriately. If the actor was asked if he was driving, he responded "no" and if he was asked if he had been drinking, he responded, "I've had a few beers." Attempts at alcohol purchase were made at 223 on-premise and 132 off-premise establishments.

Of the 355 attempts, actors were able to successfully make the alcohol purchase in 280 instances (79%). On-premise establishments served the actors 76% of the time, whereas off-premise establishments allowed the sale 83% of the time. Actors and a nondrinking observer also watched for clues that the server/clerk indicated an awareness or suspicion that the buyer was obviously intoxicated. Verbal indications, including asking the buyer to leave, suggesting a nonalcoholic drink, offering to call a cab, and so on, as well as nonverbal indications, such as staring or rolling of eyes, were recorded. A similar series of observations were made of security staff, other staff/bartenders/cashiers, and other customers. In 51% of the attempted purchases, there was an indication from the server of the recognition of the intoxication of the buyer. Even within the group that recognized signs of apparent intoxication, the alcohol was sold 61% of the time. When the server made no indication of the apparent intoxication, alcohol sales were completed 97% of the time. In 45% of purchase attempts, another staff member or customer made an indication that they believed the buyer was intoxicated. Still, alcohol purchases were completed in 66% of these cases. When no other staff member

or customer indicating an awareness of the buyer's behavior, the actor was served 89% of the time. Details of responsible beverage service (RBS) training for individual servers were not provided, though the authors did comment that such training is an important tool in preventing illegal alcohol sales, especially in younger servers. The authors concluded that sales of alcohol to obviously intoxicated individuals in some US communities is very high and recommended additional study to identify effective training and tools to mitigate such illegal sales.

SUMMARY

- Impaired driving charges may be prosecuted based on BAC and application of a *per se* statute, as well as on observations of impairment such as standardized field sobriety tests (FSTs).
- Analytical techniques capable of accurately measuring alcohol concentration in a variety of biological matrices have been available for decades.
- The ability to accurately predict a BAC after drinking is poor, not only for the drinking individual but also for trained personnel such as police officers and medical professionals.
- Casual observers begin to reliably detect signs of alcohol intoxication in nontolerant persons at a BAC of 150 mg/dL.
- Clinically apparent signs of alcohol intoxication are difficult to detect in individuals with significant tolerance, increasing the probability of driving when BAC exceeds a *per se* value, or "overservice" in a bar or restaurant. Tolerance also seriously limits the applicability of tables correlating BAC with specific clinical effects in an individual case.
- The use of standardized FSTs is the norm for prosecution of impaired driving cases, though this battery of tests has also received significant legal and scientific criticism.
- Of the 3 routinely used FSTs, horizontal gaze nystagmus (HGN) has the best correlation with BAC.

REFERENCES

1. Final Report to the Nation. *Presidential Commission on Drunk Driving.* Washington, DC; 1983.
2. AMA. Alcohol and the driver. Council on Scientific Affairs, Council Report. *JAMA.* 1986;255:522-527.
3. Badcock NR, O'Reilly DA. False positive EMIT-st ethanol screen with post-mortem infant plasma. *Clin Chem.* 1992;38:434.
4. Baker SP, Fisher RS. Alcohol and motorcycle fatalities. *Am J Public Health.* 1977;67:246-249.
5. Borkenstein RF, et al. *The Role of the Drinking Driver in Traffic Accidents: The Grand Rapids Study.* 2nd ed. *Blutalkohol.* vol 11, suppl 1. Hamburg: Steintor-Verlag; 1974: 1-132.
6. Brennan DF, et al. Ethanol elimination rates in an ED population. *Am J Emerg Med.* 1995;13:276-280.
7. Brick J. Standardization of alcohol calculations in research. *Alcohol Clin Exp Res.* 2006;30:1276-1287.
8. Brick J, Carpenter JA. The identification of alcohol intoxication by police. *Alcohol Clin Exp Res.* 2001;25:850-855.
9. Burns M, Anderson EW. A Colorado validation study of the standardized field sobriety test (SFST) battery. Final Report to the Colorado Department of Transportation. NHTSA. 1995.
10. Burns M, Moskowitz H. Psychophysiological tests for DWI arrest: final report. DOT-HS-802-424. 1977.
11. Caplan YH, Goldberger BA. Blood, urine and other fluid and tissue specimens for alcohol analysis. In: Garriott JC, ed. *Garriott's Medicolegal Aspects of Alcohol.* Tucson, AZ: Lawyers and Judges Publishing Company, Inc; 2008:205-215.
12. Caplan YH, Levine B. The analysis of ethanol in serum, blood, and urine: a comparison of the TDx REA ethanol assay with gas chromatography. *J Anal Toxicol.* 1986;10:49-52.
13. Cherpitel C, et al. Clinical assessment compared with breathalyser readings in the emergency room: concordance of ICD-10 Y90 and Y91 codes. *Emerg Med J.* 2005;22:689-695.
14. Cometto-Muniz JE, Cain WS. Relative sensitivity of the ocular trigeminal, nasal trigeminal and olfactory systems to airborne chemicals. *Chem Senses.* 1995;20:191-198.
15. Davis AR, Lipson AH. Central nervous system tolerance to high blood alcohol levels. *Med J Aust.* 1986;144:9-12.
16. Downey LA, et al. The Standardized Field Sobriety Tests (SFST) and measures of cognitive functioning. *Accid Anal Prev.* 2016;86:90-98.
17. Dubowski KM, O'Neill B. The blood/breath ratio of ethanol (Abstract #410). *Clin Chem.* 1979;25:1144.
18. Fell JC, et al. Assessing the impact of twenty underage drinking laws. *J Stud Alcohol Drugs.* 2016;77:249-260.

19. Freisthler B, et al. Evaluating alcohol access and the alcohol environment in neighborhood areas. *Alcohol Clin Exp Res.* 2003;27:477-484.

20. Gainsford AR, et al. A large-scale study of the relationship between blood and breath alcohol concentrations in New Zealand drinking drivers. *J Forensic Sci.* 2006;51:173-178.

21. Garriott JC, Manno JE. Pharmacology and toxicology of ethyl alcohol. In: Garriott JC, ed. *Garriott's Medicolegal Aspects of Alcohol.* 5th ed. Tucson, AZ: Lawyers and Judges Publishing Company, Inc; 2008:25-46.

22. Gore A. Know your limit: how legislatures have gone overboard with per se drunk driving laws and how men pay the price. *Wm & Mary J Women Law.* 2010;16:423-447.

23. Grossman DC, et al. The validity of police assessment of driver intoxication in motor vehicle crashes leading to hospitalization. *Accid Anal Prev.* 1996;28:435-442.

24. Hammond KB, et al. Blood ethanol. A report of unusually high levels in a living patient. *JAMA.* 1973;226:63-64.

25. Harding P, Field PH. Breathalyzer accuracy in actual law enforcement practice: a comparison of blood- and breath-alcohol results in Wisconsin drivers. *J Forensic Sci.* 1987;32:1235-1240.

26. Harding P, Zettl JR. Methods for breath analysis. In: Garriott JC, ed. *Garriott's Medicolegal Aspects of Alcohol.* Tucson, AZ: Lawyers and Judges Publishing Company, Inc; 2008:229-253.

27. Heise HA. Alcohol and automobile accidents. *JAMA.* 1934;103:739-741.

28. Jones AW. Enforcement of drink-driving laws by use of "per se" legal alcohol limits: blood and/or breath concentraiton as evidence of impairment *Alcohol Drugs Driving.* 1988;4:99-112.

29. Jones AW. The drunkest drinking driver in Sweden: blood alcohol concentration 0.545% w/v. *J Stud Alcohol.* 1999;60:400-406.

30. Jones AW. Biochemical and physiological research on the disposition and fate of ethanol in the body. In: Garriott JC, ed. *Garriott's Medicolegal Aspects of Alcohol.* 5th ed. Tucson, AZ: Lawyers and Judges Publishing Company, Inc; 2008:47-155.

31. Jones AW, Pounder DJ. Update on clinical and forensic analysis of alcohol. In: Karch SB, ed. *Forensic Issues in Alcohol Testing.* Boca Raton, FL: CRC Press; 2008:21-64.

32. Jongen S, et al. The sensitivity of laboratory tests assessing driving related skills to dose-related impairment of alcohol: a literature review. *Accid Anal Prev.* 2016;89:31-48.

33. Kypri K, et al. Long-term effects of lowering the alcohol minimum purchasing age on traffic crash injury rates in New Zealand. *Drug Alcohol Rev.* 2017;36:178-185.

34. Lands WE. A review of alcohol clearance in humans. *Alcohol.* 1998;15:147-160.

35. Lansky D, et al. Blood alcohol level discrimination: pre-training monitoring accuracy of alcoholics and nonalcoholics. *Addict Behav.* 1978;3:209-214.

36. Laude JR, Fillmore MT. Drivers who self-estimate lower blood alcohol concentrations are riskier drivers after drinking. *Psychopharmacology (Berl).* 2016;233:1387-1394.

37. Lenk KM, et al. Propensity of alcohol establishments to sell to obviously intoxicated patrons. *Alcohol Clin Exp Res.* 2006;30:1194-1199.

38. Lindblad B, Olsson R. Unusually high levels of blood alcohol? *JAMA.* 1976;236:1600-1602.

39. Martin CS. Measuring acute alcohol impairment. In: Karch SB, ed. *Forensic Issues in Alcohol Testing.* Boca Raton, FL: CRC Press; 2008:1-19.

40. Mason MF, Dubowski KM. Breath-alcohol analysis: uses, methods, and some forensic problems—review and opinion. *J Forensic Sci.* 1976;21:9-41.

41. McCartney D, et al. Using alcohol intoxication goggles (Fatal Vision(R) goggles) to detect alcohol related impairment in simulated driving. *Traffic Inj Prev.* 2017;18:19-27.

42. Moskowitz H, et al. Police officers' detection of breath odors from alcohol ingestion. *Accid Anal Prev.* 1999;31:175-180.

43. NHTSA. Alcohol-impaired driving. *Traffic Safety Facts.* DOT HS-812. Washington, DC: NHTSA; 2015:812, 231:1-7.

44. Nine JS, et al. Serum-ethanol determination: comparison of lactate and lactate dehydrogenase interference in three enzymatic assays. *J Anal Toxicol.* 1995;19:192-196.

45. Payne JP, et al. Observations on the distribution of alcohol in blood, breath and urine. *Br Med J.* 1996;1:196.

46. Perrine MW, et al. Field sobriety tests: Reliability and validity. In: Utzelmann HD et al., eds. *Alcohol, Drugs and Traffic Safety—T92.* Cologne, Germany: TUV Rheinland; 1993.

47. Rammohan V, et al. Effects of dram shop liability and enhanced overservice law enforcement initiatives on excessive alcohol consumption and related harms: two community guide systematic reviews. *Am J Prev Med.* 2011;41:334-343.

48. Roberts JR, Dollard D. Alcohol levels do not accurately predict physical or mental impairment in ethanol-tolerant subjects: relevance to emergency medicine and dram shop laws. *J Med Toxicol.* 2010;6:438-442.

49. Romano E, et al. A comprehensive examination of U.S. laws enacted to reduce alcohol-related crashes among underage drivers. *J Safety Res.* 2015;55:213-221.

50. Rubenzer SJ. The Standardized Field Sobriety Tests: a review of scientific and legal issues. *Law Hum Behav.* 2008;32:293-313.

51. Russ NW, et al. Estimating alcohol impairment in the field: implications for drunken driving. *J Stud Alcohol.* 1986;47:237-240.

52. Saltz RF. The introduction of dram shop legislation in the United States and the advent of server training. *Addiction.* 1993;88(suppl):95S-103S.

53. Scherer M, et al. Effects of dram shop, responsible beverage service training, and state alcohol control laws on underage drinking driver fatal crash ratios. *Traffic Inj Prev.* 2015;16(suppl 2):S59-S65.

54. Seidl S, et al. The calculation of blood ethanol concentrations in males and females. *Int J Legal Med.* 2000;114:71-77.

55. Sloan FA, et al. Effects of prices, civil and criminal sanctions, and law enforcement on alcohol-related mortality. *J Stud Alcohol.* 1994;55:454-465.

56. Smalldon KW, Brown GA. The stability of ethanol in stored blood. II. The mechanism of ethanol oxidation. *Anal Chim Acta.* 1973;66:285-290.

57. Streete PJ, et al. Detection and identification of volatile substances by headspace capillary gas chromatography to aid the diagnosis of acute poisoning. *Analyst.* 1992;117:1111-1127.

58. Sullivan JB Jr, et al. Lack of observable intoxication in humans with high plasma alcohol concentrations. *J Forensic Sci.* 1987;32:1660-1665.

59. Tharp VK, et al. Development and field test of psychophysical tests for DWI arrest: final report. NHTSA, Technical Report DOT-HS-805-864. Washington, DC: NHTSA; 1981.

60. Toomey TL, et al. Illegal alcohol sales and use of alcohol control policies at community festivals. *Public Health Rep.* 2005;120:165-173.

61. Toomey TL, et al. Illegal alcohol sales to obviously intoxicated patrons at licensed establishments. *Alcohol Clin Exp Res.* 2004;28:769-774.

62. Toomey TL, et al. Alcohol sales to pseudo-intoxicated bar patrons. *Public Health Rep.* 1999;114:337-342.

63. USDA. Alcoholic Beverages. In: USDA, ed. *Dietary Guidelines for Americans (Publication #001-000-04719-1).* 6th ed. Washington, DC: US Government Printing Office; 2005.

64. Vasiliades J, et al. Pitfalls of the alcohol dehydrogenase procedure for the emergency assay of alcohol: a case study of isopropanol overdose. *Clin Chem.* 1978;24:383-385.

65. Wagner JG, et al. Estimation of the amount of alcohol ingested from a single blood alcohol concentration. *Alcohol Alcohol.* 1990;25:379-384.

66. Watson PE, et al. Prediction of blood alcohol concentrations in human subjects. Updating the Widmark Equation. *J Stud Alcohol.* 1981;42:547-556.

67. Widmark EMP. *Die theoretischen Grundlagen und die praktische Verwendbarkeit der gerichtlich-medizinischen Alkoholbestimmung.* Berlin: Urban & Schwarzenberg; 1932.

68. Widmark EMP. *Principles and Applications of Medicolegal Alcohol Determination (English translation).* Davis, CA: Biomedical Publications; 1981.

69. Zettl JR. Alcohol determination in point of collection testing. In: Karch SB, ed. *Forensic Issues in Alcohol Testing.* Boca Raton, FL: CRC Press; 2008:119-135.

140 POSTMORTEM TOXICOLOGY

Rama B. Rao and Mark A. Flomenbaum

CASE

A newly hired train conductor sustains irreversible brain injury due to a large subdural hematoma from a train crash. Surgical intervention is deemed futile. After 4 days in the hospital, he is declared dead by neurologic criteria (ie, "brain dead") and removed from life support. An autopsy confirms the brain injury. Postmortem toxicologic samples are obtained from the femoral vein and reveal oxycodone and oxycodone metabolites. As a toxicologist, you are asked to interpret the findings. How do you proceed?

INTRODUCTION

Postmortem toxicology is the study of the identification, distribution, and quantification of xenobiotics after death. This information is used to account for physiologic effects of a xenobiotic at the time of death through its quantification and possible redistribution in the body at the time of autopsy. Several variables cause changes in xenobiotic concentrations during the interval between (1) the time of death and subsequent autopsy and (2) the storage interval between the time of sampling and the time of testing. Toxicologists and forensic experts are frequently asked to interpret postmortem xenobiotic concentrations and decide whether the reported values are meaningful and whether these xenobiotics were incidental or contributory to the cause of death.

The development of the field of forensic toxicology and the improvement of laboratory technology now permit more refined identification and quantification of xenobiotics. The interpretation of postmortem xenobiotic concentrations and their significance, however, continues to evolve.

This chapter reviews factors that affect xenobiotic concentrations identified at autopsy and discusses an approach for interpreting postmortem toxicologic reports as they relate to the cause and manner of death.[39,40,43,45,52-54,61,86,105]

HISTORY AND ROLE OF MEDICAL EXAMINERS

The relationship between antemortem xenobiotic exposures and death has been a subject of investigation for centuries. In 12th-century England, an appointee of the royal court, eventually named the *coroner*, was designated to record and identify causes of death.[78] In suspicious circumstances, coroners investigated poisonings, but scientific methods were primitive, and conclusions regarding such deaths were conjecture at best.

By the mid-19th century, however, techniques for detecting certain xenobiotics in postmortem tissue were developed and focused generally on identifying heavy metals as a cause of death in homicides.[46,78,83,102,108] At that time, coroners were still elected or appointed individuals with little or no medical training. However, with better laboratory techniques and autopsies being performed by trained pathologists, the specialty of forensic medicine continued to develop. In Massachusetts during the late 19th century, these forensically trained pathologists, referred to as *medical examiners*, ultimately replaced the coroner system and were eventually empowered by the state to investigate and determine the cause and manner of death in certain types of unusual or suspicious cases and the medicolegal autopsies became their primary tools.[78] Cause and manner of death are defined below.

Currently, a death may prompt a medicolegal investigation if it serves the interests of the state through either the criminal justice or public health systems.[89] Information from the circumstances of the death are integrated with laboratory data and a medicolegal autopsy when human remains are available. In the United States, the requirements for performing a medicolegal autopsy vary substantially by jurisdiction.[4,50]

Some US jurisdictions use elected or appointed personnel with variable or no medical training to determine the cause and manner of death. These are usually termed coroner systems. The coroner is usually not a physician but may have other qualifications. Other jurisdictions require that physicians or other medically trained personnel determine the cause and manner of death and perform a medicolegal autopsy if they deem it necessary. These providers are medical examiners, and their training requirements also vary by jurisdiction. The strictest and most robust regulations specify that autopsies are performed exclusively by forensic pathologists. These are physicians with board certification in forensic pathology. The specific training and performance standards of forensic pathologists are well described elsewhere.[1,89]

As of 2016 in the United States, death investigations are the responsibility of a coroner in 14 states, a medical examiner in 20 states, or some combination of coroner and medical examiner in the remainder.[4] For the purposes of this chapter, the person performing the medicolegal autopsy will be referred to broadly as the medical examiner.

The purpose of the death investigation is to determine the *cause* and *manner* of death. The *cause of death* is the etiologically specific pathophysiologic aberration that is ultimately responsible for death to occur (Table 140–1). For example, the presence of cyanide in the toxicologic evaluation is sufficient to establish cardiorespiratory arrest from cyanide poisoning. The *manner of death* is an explanation of how the death occurred, or the circumstances surrounding the terminal events. It broadly distinguishes natural from nonnatural (or violent) deaths. Nonnatural deaths, depending on the jurisdiction, can be divided into several categories (Table 140–2). With the identification of cyanide, the manner of death cannot be considered natural because a poisoning is a "chemically traumatic" (violent) event. The medical examiner must make the best determination of the manner of death based on the available evidence.[108,115] An unintentional exposure can be classified as an *accident* (a legal term for some unintentional nonnatural deaths), and intentional self-injury can be classified as a *suicide*. If the circumstances indicate an exposure due to the acts of another person, the manner of death can be classified as a *homicide*.

Determination of the manner of death has important consequences. Homicide necessitates involvement of law enforcement officials for further investigation. Cases deemed suicide not only impact survivors psychologically but also can nullify some life insurance payments. Conversely, a case deemed an "accident" can invoke a double-indemnity insurance clause. Assignment of financial responsibility for workplace deaths can be similarly affected when xenobiotics are identified in the postmortem specimens of involved workers.

Recognition of xenobiotic-related deaths also has significant public health consequences. The findings may identify fatal drug reactions, preventable errors, or rapidly fatal epidemics associated with illicit xenobiotic use or malicious intent activities. In cases of occupational and environmental xenobiotic-related fatalities, interventions can be implemented to prevent subsequent morbidity and mortality. In addition, the gross and microscopic autopsy findings can elucidate mechanisms of xenobiotic toxicity.

TABLE 140–1	Information Used by Forensic Pathologists
Autopsy	
Evidence from the crime scene	
Laboratory investigations	
Medical consultants	
Available history	
Medical records	
Police reports	
Interviews with contacts	

TABLE 140–2	Categories of Manner of Death
Natural	
Nonnatural	
Homicide	
Suicide	
Accident*	
Therapeutic complication[a]	
Undetermined	

[a]Not all jurisdictions recognize therapeutic complication as a manner of death.

*A legal term described in the text.

TABLE 140–3	Postmortem Biochemical Changes Over the First 3 Days[a]		
Increased	**Decreased**	**Stable[b]**	**Variable**
Amino acids	Cl⁻	BUN/Cr (vitreous)	Lipids
Ammonia	Glucose	Cholinesterases	T_3
Ca^{2+}, K^+, Mg^{2+}	Na^+	Cortisol (serum)	
Epinephrine	pH	Proteins (serum)	
Aspartate aminotransferases	T_4	Sulfates	
Insulin (especially right heart blood)			

[a]In refrigerated bodies. [b]Whole blood is typically utilized unless otherwise reported.

BUN = blood urea nitrogen; Cr = creatinine; T_3 = triiodothyronine; T_4 = thyroxine.

Postmortem toxicologic techniques can be used in other types of investigations as well. For example, if carboxyhemoglobin is identified in burned human remains from an airplane crash, a cabin fire before descent is more probable than deaths due to a fire on impact. This type of postmortem analysis is useful in the reconstruction of events leading to the crash.[10,57,66,106]

THE TOXICOLOGIC INVESTIGATION

Ordinarily, toxicologic samples are collected as part of an autopsy. In the hospital, when a death is assumed to be from natural causes, the hospital pathologist can perform an autopsy with the consent of the family. In a medicolegal investigation, however, the medical examiner determines the need for an autopsy and has statutory authority to act on that determination independent of familial consent or wishes. A "complete autopsy" is one that "completely" answers the questions needed to determine cause and manner of death; and usually includes gross external and internal inspection of the body and organs and often includes microscopical analyses as well as tissue and fluid sampling for microbiologic and toxicologic testing. Occasionally, only fluid samples are obtained along with an external inspection of the body if a complete autopsy is either unnecessary or the family has valid legal or religious grounds for objecting to an internal examination.

The precise list of xenobiotics screened in postmortem samples varies greatly by jurisdiction and by individual preference of the medical examiner, and is often case specific. Investigations in large cities routinely screen for hundreds of illicit, therapeutic, and environmental xenobiotics. Occasionally, the suspicions of the medical examiner or death scene investigator warrant specific assays that are performed only upon special request.

The sampling of fluid and tissue can be obtained minutes to years after death. The *postmortem interval*, defined as the time between death and autopsy, is important, but many other factors will influence the extent of bodily decomposition. Some of these factors include environmental conditions such as ambient temperature, humidity, aerobic versus anaerobic surroundings, immersion in water,[67] type of local flora and fauna, and the body habitus and metabolic state immediately prior to death. Samples for testing can be collected from a body during advanced stages of decomposition, after exhumation from graves, or even after embalming.[10,39,40,47,85] Knowing the condition of the body at the time of sampling assists in interpreting the toxicologic findings. These postmortem changes are reviewed below.

DECOMPOSITION AND POSTMORTEM BIOCHEMICAL CHANGES

The first stage of decomposition is autolysis, during which endogenous enzymes are released and normal mechanisms maintaining cellular integrity fail.[60] Chemicals move across compromised and leaky cellular membranes down relative concentration gradients. Glycolysis continues in the red blood cells until intracellular glucose is depleted and lactate is produced. Ultimately, intracellular ions and proteins are released into the blood, and tissue and blood acidemia develops leading to the biochemical changes described in Table 140–3.[108]

The next stage of decomposition in most normal environments is putrefaction. This stage involves digestion of tissue by bacterial organisms, which typically colonize the bowel or respiratory system. Later, additional organisms can be introduced by insects or other external sources. As the putrefactive process advances, the colors of the skin and organs change; epithelial blebs may form and separate from the underlying dermis; and gases accumulate, resulting in foul odors and bloating.[108]

If death occurs in a very warm, dry climate, such as a desert or comparably arid environment, the body can desiccate so rapidly that putrefactive changes do not occur. This results in mummification and produces a lightweight cadaver with a tight, dry skin enveloping a prominent bony skeleton.[108]

If the environment is very cold and devoid of oxygen, such as at great depths under water, putrefaction will be slowed. Anoxic decomposition of fatty tissues occurs, forming a white, cheesy material known as adipocere.

Another phase of decomposition, anthropophagia, occurs in unprotected environments where insects or large animals feed on the remains.[108]

Because most postmortem changes result from chemical reactions that are temperature dependent, increased temperatures will accelerate the process and cooler temperatures will retard it. In general, morgue refrigerators achieve low enough temperatures (40°F {4°C}) to prevent further gross decomposition and many of its associated postmortem changes.

Another means of altering natural decomposition is embalming, a process of chemically preserving tissues that can be performed in a variety of ways.[48,49] Typically, blood is drained through large vessel pumps, and embalming fluid is injected intravascularly to perfuse and preserve the face or other tissues. Intracavitary spaces can be injected with the preserving substances, and solid organs are sometimes removed. Some authorities regulate the contents of the embalming fluid specifically to avoid confounding postmortem analysis. Most embalming fluid in the United States consists of formaldehyde, sodium borate, sodium nitrate, glycerin, water, and colorants.

SAMPLES USED FOR TOXICOLOGIC ANALYSIS

Unless the medical examiner has other suspicions about a death, only standard autopsy samples will be obtained from an otherwise intact body.[26,39,40,55,62,90] These typically include samples of blood, gastric contents, bile, urine, and occasionally solid organs such as the liver or brain. Less commonly, vitreous humor and/or cerebrospinal fluid is obtained for analysis (Table 140–4). Antemortem specimens, if available, can be used for evaluation and comparison. These specimen analyses are reviewed in greater detail below.

TABLE 140–4	Sampling Sites[18,23,27,39,53,100]		
Routine	**Infrequent**	**Uncommon**
Bile	Antemortem blood	Casket fluid
Blood	Cerebrospinal fluid	Extravasated fluid
Brain	Fat	Extravasated blood
Gastric contents	Hair	Insect larvae
Liver	Kidneys	Pupae casings
	Muscle, nails, skin	
	Vitreous humor	

Blood

Postmortem cell lysis limits the concept of plasma concentrations, and "blood" concentrations are reported instead. Most commonly, a single site such as femoral or subclavian blood is sampled unless an unusual xenobiotic with nonuniform distribution is suspected of causing the death. In patients with a prolonged postmortem interval and in cases where intravascular blood is coagulated, right heart blood can serve as an alternative sample.

Other sources of blood are sometimes available. These frequently include antemortem samples often from time of hospital admission and occasionally extravasated blood, which is unlikely to undergo extensive metabolism. Intracranial clots, in particular, serve as useful comparative samples in patients with a prolonged survival period after exposure to a xenobiotic.[68]

In advanced states of decomposition, blood from the abdominal or thoracic cavities is less useful for some testing because it can be contaminated by bacteria or other substances that can affect xenobiotic metabolism, recovery, or analysis.

Vitreous Humor

Because of the relatively avascular and acellular nature of the fluid, the vitreous humor is well protected from the early decompositional changes that typically occur in blood.[18,21-24,27] When bodies are immediately refrigerated, creatinine, blood urea nitrogen, and sodium can be reliably approximated from vitreous humor samples for up to 3 or 4 days. Potassium concentrations are less reliable because cell lysis causes intracellular release. When vitreous glucose is elevated, hyperglycemia at the time of death can be assumed. A low vitreous glucose concentration, however, is a less reliable indicator of the antemortem serum glucose concentration, because a low vitreous glucose concentration can be attributable to either antemortem hypoglycemia or postmortem glycolysis even in the relatively avascular vitreous.

The aqueous content of the vitreous is normally higher than that of blood and can affect the partitioning of certain water-soluble xenobiotics, such as ethanol.

Urine

Urine may be available during the autopsy and can reveal renally eliminated xenobiotics or their metabolites. Because the bladder serves as a reservoir in which metabolism is unlikely to occur, the concentrations of xenobiotics obtained during the autopsy reflect antemortem urine concentrations. An isolated urine sample is of limited quantitative value but can be useful when compared with other sample sites.

Gastric Contents

The contents of the stomach are measured and grossly inspected for color, odor, and the presence or absence of pill fragments, food particles, activated charcoal, and other foreign materials.[105] Typically, gastric concentrations of xenobiotics are reported as milligrams of substance per gram of total gastric contents. Xenobiotic-induced pylorospasm, diminished intestinal motility, or decreased splanchnic blood flow may all decrease gastric emptying and affect the quantitative values obtained from sampling different parts of the gastrointestinal tract. Pills and pill fragments from modified release drugs are sometimes identified on autopsy after oral overdose in some cases after surviving several days postingestion.[75]

Solid Organs and Other Sources

Xenobiotic concentrations in solid organs, such as the liver and brain, are usually reported as milligrams of substance per kilogram of tissue. Other tissue samples, including hair and nails, are used for thiol-avid xenobiotics such as metals. Rarely, tracheal aspirates of gases can be analyzed to confirm inhalational exposures when circumstances warrant testing. Pleural fluid analysis of postmortem xenobiotics typically yields qualitative results in decomposed bodies because redistribution of xenobiotics from the stomach and intestines can occur.[34,97] Cerebrospinal fluid (CSF) is inconsistently collected at autopsy and is not relevant in most cases. The ratios of CSF to heart blood are described for a number of xenobiotics, but data are limited antemortem because of the lack of published information, cause of death, or time of last exposure.

OTHER SAMPLING SOURCES

In an embalmed body, either the organs or tissues that remain relatively unembalmed, such as deep leg muscle,[70] or the embalming fluid itself can be used for analysis. When a body is disinterred, soil samples are usually obtained from above and below the coffin to validate identification of xenobiotics that leeched into, or out from the body.[85]

On rare occasions, cremated remains, often referred to as *cremains*, are the only source of sampling available. Most battery-containing metallic implants, such as pacemakers, are removed before cremation to prevent explosions or environmental hazards.[107] Other metallic implants such as joint prostheses are removed in whole or in part after cremation depending on the particular alloy. Only dental remains, particulate matter, and occasionally calcified blood vessels are available for analysis.[5,114] In most cremations performed in the United States, the incineration process is followed by mechanical grinding to yield a fine particulate matter.[114] The ability to extract xenobiotics from cremains is markedly limited at best, and little published data are available on the subject. A technique to identify heavy metals such as lead from cremains was described, but is not routinely used.[5,114]

ENTOMOTOXICOLOGY

A variety of anthropophagic insect species can demonstrate the presence of xenobiotics.[2,44,64,65] This process of analysis is termed *entomotoxicology*. In putrefied bodies or bodies that have undergone anthropophagy, fluids and even insect parts can be analyzed. Forensic entomologists collect samples of these insects from the remains. After considering the stage of insect life, environmental conditions, and the season, the approximate time of death can be extrapolated. The family of flies Calliphoridae, such as the common blow fly, is attracted to unprotected remains by a very fine scent that develops in the cadaver within hours of death. The adult fly lays eggs on mucosal surfaces or in open wounds. After the eggs hatch, the larvae feed on the decomposing tissue. Larval samples can then be examined for the presence of xenobiotics. To achieve accurate analysis, these samples must be preserved immediately after collection because living larvae can continue to metabolize certain xenobiotics. In the next phase of their life cycle, the larvae undergo pupation, secreting a substance that encloses them into pupal casings until they hatch as adults. These pupal casings are often found in the soil beneath the body or in the body cavities. Some xenobiotics are identified in the pupal casings long after the adult fly has emerged and flown away (Table 140–5).[91]

INTERPRETATION OF POSTMORTEM TOXICOLOGY RESULTS

After fluid and tissue samples are collected and analyzed for the presence of xenobiotics, the process of interpreting these results begins. This complex task attempts to account for the clinical effects of a xenobiotic at the time of death by integrating medical history, autopsy, death-scene findings, and toxicologic reports. Multiple confounding variables can affect the final concentrations of xenobiotics from the time of death to the time of testing after the autopsy. Variables include the nature, metabolism, and distribution of the xenobiotic; the body habitus and state of health of the decedent prior to death; physical and environmental variables during the postmortem

TABLE 140–5 Xenobiotics Reported From Larvae and Pupal Casings
Benzoylecgonine
Cocaine
Heroin
Malathion
Mercury
Methamphetamine
Morphine
Nortriptyline
Oxazepam
Phenobarbital
Triazolam

TABLE 140–6	Considerations in Interpreting Postmortem Xenobiotic Concentrations		
Xenobiotic Dependent	*Decedent Dependent*	*Autopsy Dependent*	*Other*
Pharmacokinetic considerations	Comorbid conditions	Handling and preservation	Laboratory techniques
State of absorption or distribution	Tolerance	Postmortem interval: State of preservation	Evidence at scene
at time of death	Pharmacogenetic variability	or decomposition	Previously published tissue concentrations
Postmortem redistribution		Sample sites	
Postmortem metabolism		Specimens sampled	
Pharmacodynamic considerations			
Expected clinical effects			
Synergistic interactions			
Postmortem xenobiotic stability during			
Putrefaction			
Preservation			

interval; the techniques of sampling and analysis; and other variables of the autopsy (Tables 140–6 and 140–7).

Variables Relating to the Xenobiotic

Postmortem Redistribution

The xenobiotic concentration in blood can be higher during the time of sampling at autopsy than at the actual time death occurred if significant postmortem redistribution occurs.[56,88,113-120] Redistribution typically occurs with xenobiotics that have large volumes of distribution and when postmortem changes result in release of intracellular xenobiotic into the extracellular compartment.[94] For example, amitriptyline can be released from tissue stores into the blood as autolysis progresses, resulting in a significantly higher blood concentration at the autopsy than at the actual time of death.

TABLE 140–7	Xenobiotic Stability and Laboratory Recovery[12,14,25,30,79,87,88,96]

Quantitative recovery affected by preservatives
  As, Ag, Cu, Hg, Pb
  Carbon monoxide
  Cyanide
  Ethchlorvynol
  Nortriptyline (converted to amitriptyline in fixatives)

Chemical stability in formalin	Labile
Stable	Desipramine
Diazepam	
Phenobarbital	
Phenytoin (30 d)	
Succinylcholine	

Chemical stability in putrefying liver	Labile
Stable	*o,p*-Aminophenols
Acetaminophen	Chlordiazepoxide
Amitriptyline	Chlorpromazine
Barbiturates	Clonazepam
Chloroform	Malathion
Clemastine	Metronidazole
Dextropropoxyphene	Nitrofurazone
Diazepam	Nitrazepam
Doxepin	*p*-Nitrophenol
Flurazepam	Obidoxime
Glutethimide	Perphenazine
Hydrochlorothiazide	Trifluoperazine
Imipramine	
Lorazepam	
Methaqualone	
Morphine	
Nicotine	
Paraquat	
Pentachlorophenol	
Plant alkaloids	
Quinine	
Strychnine	

If postmortem redistribution is not considered, xenobiotic concentrations obtained during the autopsy can be misinterpreted as being supratherapeutic or even toxic, and the cause of death can be inappropriately attributed to this xenobiotic.

Postmortem Metabolism

Less commonly, xenobiotic concentration can decrease secondary to postmortem metabolism. For example, cocaine continues to be degraded after death by endogenous enzymes such as cholinesterases in the blood, which continue to function in postmortem tissue and in vitro. Unless blood is collected immediately after death and placed in tubes containing enzyme inhibitors such as sodium fluoride, the concentration of cocaine will decrease, and the analysis will not accurately reflect the concentration of the drug at the time of death.[61,76,106,111] All available information regarding postmortem redistribution or metabolism of a specific xenobiotic must be evaluated for the proper interpretation of the toxicologic results.

State of Absorption and Distribution

Both in the living and deceased, the state of absorption, distribution, and other toxicokinetic principles affect the apparent concentration of a sampled xenobiotic. For a xenobiotic with minimal postmortem metabolism or redistribution, the phase of absorption is suggested by the relative quantity of the xenobiotic in different fluids and solid organs. For example, a high concentration of xenobiotic in the gastric contents, with progressively lower concentrations in the liver, blood, vitreous, and brain, suggests an early phase of absorption at the time of death. When a xenobiotic is orally administered and the tissue concentration is highest in the liver, the relationship suggests a postabsorption phase but a predistribution concentration. A concentration found to be highest in the urine suggests that the xenobiotic was in an elimination phase at the time of death. Although this approach has limitations, it is important for correlating the state of absorption and the expected clinical course of the xenobiotic. Unfortunately, multiple samples are not always available at the time of autopsy or the interpretation of reports, and opportunities for subsequent sampling are often limited.

Xenobiotic Properties

Xenobiotic chemical composition affects partitioning into fat or water compartments and total body burden is poorly captured when sampling the blood compartment. The significance of this and partitioning of blood to serum is uncertain.[74] Xenobiotic stability refers to the ability of a xenobiotic to maintain its molecular integrity despite postmortem changes such as decomposition of the body, adverse storage conditions, or the lack of preservatives.[7,15,17,58,59,64,74,100,109,116-119]

Postmortem xenobiotic stability was assessed in homogenized liver tissue infused with various concentrations of xenobiotics.[109] The samples were allowed to putrefy outdoors, and sequential sampling of xenobiotic concentrations was performed. The xenobiotics that decreased in concentration as putrefaction progressed were considered labile, and samples with a constant concentration were considered stable. The authors proposed that the chemical characteristics of a xenobiotic determine its stability. For example, labile xenobiotics share the molecular configuration of an oxygen–nitrogen bond, thiono groups, or aminophenols. Conversely, chemical structures that enhance stability include single-bonded sulfur groups, carbon–oxygen and carbon–nitrogen bonds, and sulfur–oxygen and hydrogen–nitrogen bonds. Although not explicitly studied in otherwise intact but putrefying bodies, logically, a less stable xenobiotic can be recovered in a lower concentration than the actual concentration at the time of death. This must be considered when information regarding stability is available and the body of a decedent is in an advanced stage of decomposition.

Xenobiotic Chemical Reactions

An artifact can result from a chemical reaction with a xenobiotic added during the postmortem interval, such as embalming fluid.[41] In a study of xenobiotic-spiked blood and formalin in test tubes, amitriptyline was formed by the methylation of nortriptyline.[29,119] Identification of amitriptyline, which was not present at the time of death, could confuse the interpretation of toxicologic analyses.

Expected Clinical Effects of the Xenobiotic

For a fatality to be attributed to a xenobiotic, the expected clinical course from the exposure should be consistent with the autopsy findings. For example, what are the implications of a person found dead minutes after ingesting pills, if a large concentration of acetaminophen (APAP) is identified in both the gastric contents and blood but not in other tissues at autopsy?[99] Although suicidal intent can be supported by this finding, the onset of death within minutes is inconsistent with a fatality due to an APAP overdose. Thus, another cause of death must be sought. Interpretation of postmortem toxicology must also incorporate clinically relevant consequences of xenobiotic interactions. For example, the combined ingestion of phenobarbital and ethanol can cause fatal respiratory depression. Although neither are necessarily fatal alone, their additive effects must be acknowledged during toxicologic interpretation.

Variables Related to the Decedent

Comorbid Conditions

The clinical response to a xenobiotic can be affected by acquired and inherited physiologic conditions that are not always identified or identifiable on autopsy. A thorough medical history is important and can assist in interpreting the clinical effects of a xenobiotic exposure. Similarly, certain clinical conditions can produce substances that interfere with postmortem laboratory assays. For example, an individual with a critical illness can produce digoxinlike immunoreactive substances (DLIS), which may cross-react with the postmortem digoxin assay.[8] Without knowledge of DLIS production, the results can confound toxicologic analysis (Chap. 62).

Tolerance

Tolerance is an acquired condition in which increasingly higher xenobiotic concentrations are required to produce a given clinical effect. It is an important consideration for deaths in the presence of opioids, ethanol, and sedative–hypnotics. For example, respiratory depression and death from methadone is easily diagnosed in an opioid-naive individual with a history of methadone exposure and methadone-positive postmortem samples. However, the same methadone concentrations in a patient on chronic methadone maintenance therapy will not produce the same outcome. Unfortunately, no autopsy markers are available to indicate tolerance, and no biochemical or histologic markers are available during autopsy that can be used to predict clinically dangerous xenobiotic concentrations in a tolerant individual.[30] Complex postmortem assays analyzing opioid receptors are not routinely used.[38] Postmortem assessment of tolerance ultimately depends on knowledge of the patient, pharmacokinetics of the xenobiotic, and the best judgment of the investigator.

Pharmacogenetics

There is genetic variability in the expression of certain metabolic enzymes. For example, pharmacogenetic differences in metabolic enzymes such as CYP2D6 can affect the metabolism of codeine to morphine. Individuals with duplicate alleles for CYP2D6 may be ultra-rapid metabolizers, rendering them susceptible to morphine toxicity despite generally acceptable dosing of the parent compound codeine. Deaths in young children are reported from bioaccumulation of morphine. In such cases, postmortem blood analysis can reveal an elevated concentration of morphine, the codeine metabolite, and raise suspicion for a malicious overdose. Postmortem genotyping can provide an alternate explanation. Such distinctions are not routinely identifiable on autopsy.[19,31,32] Postmortem evaluation of frozen tissue or blood can also identify genetic predisposition of long-QT syndromes that can be consequential in both the diagnosis of sudden death that can be considered along with toxicologic data, but such testing is not routine across jurisdictions.[71]

Variables Relating to the Autopsy

State of Decomposition

In bodies with advanced stages of decomposition, xenobiotics diffuse from depot compartments such as the stomach urinary or gall bladders into adjacent tissues and blood vessels and secondarily affect sample concentrations near sites of origin of diffusion.[25,39,68,81,82,93-95]

During putrefaction, bacteria cause fermentation of endogenous carbohydrates, resulting in ethanol formation. In decedents without gross evidence of putrefaction, especially those in cool, dry environments, endogenous ethanol production is minimal.[24,30,84] With a longer postmortem interval or in an environment that is more conducive to ethanol production, the distinction between endogenous and exogenous sources of ethanol becomes more difficult. Sampling from multiple sites is often useful in making the distinction, but not definitive.[110] The pattern of ethanol detected in the blood and absent from the urine and vitreous samples is more suggestive of postmortem ethanol production. However, postmortem ethanol production may occur in the vitreous in decedents with hyperglycemia at the time of death and significant putrefaction at autopsy. A comprehensive review of interpreting postmortem ethanol concentrations is available elsewhere.[68,84]

Handling of the Body or Samples

Inappropriate handling of the body can result in artifacts.[99,101] In one reported case, methanol was detected in the vitreous humor of a decedent after embalming.[14] The methanol was subsequently traced to a spray cleanser that likely settled on the surface of open eyes during washing of the body.

In addition, inappropriate handling of samples can affect xenobiotic concentrations. In one study, autopsy blood was obtained from a diabetic man who died of bronchopneumonia. The samples were stored at 40°F (4°C) and tested at 2 and 5 days postmortem. The blood ethanol increased from 0.4 to 3.5 g/L due to an inadequate addition of fluoride preservative to the samples. The combination of inadequate preservation, hyperglycemia (vitreous glucose of 996 mg/dL), and bacterial sepsis created an ideal environment for ethanol production by fermentation.[68]

In the United States, heavy metals are currently banned for use in embalming because they can contaminate subsequent evaluation for metal poisoning. Formalin can also affect stability or quantitative identification of some xenobiotics. When necessary, an analysis of the embalming fluid used in the body or soil samples from around disinterred bodies may facilitate the toxicologic investigation.[21,36,116,118,119]

Autopsy Findings

In many xenobiotic-related deaths, the anatomic findings are nonspecific,[116] but in some cases, the autopsy does reveal confirmatory or supportive findings. A large quantity of undigested pills in the stomach is consistent with an intentional overdose, and suicide should be considered as the manner of death. Centrilobular hepatic necrosis can be found in decedents with a history of acetaminophen overdose. The autopsy can also reveal other findings such as coronary artery narrowing, chronic hypertensive changes, renal abnormalities, or a clinically silent myocardial injury. Such information is useful to assess the potential effects of a xenobiotic in a patient with previously undiagnosed conditions. In other cases, the absence of a chronic condition can be strongly suggestive of a xenobiotic-related death. For example, a decedent with an autopsy finding of aortic dissection in the absence of chronic hypertensive findings or other predisposing conditions suggests a xenobiotic-induced hypertensive crisis as can occur from the use of cocaine or other sympathomimetics.

Artifacts Related to Sampling Sites

Site-specific differences in postmortem xenobiotic blood concentrations are common.[37] For example, blood obtained from femoral vessels can have low glucose concentrations because of postmortem glycolysis, but the blood glucose concentration removed from the right heart chambers can be high as a result of perimortem release of liver glycogen stores. Concentrations between heart, femoral, and subclavian samples vary significantly.[80] As noted above, hyperglycemic conditions are more reliably assessed from sampling the vitreous humor because it is an acellular fluid and in an environment that is relatively protected from diffusion artifacts in the early postmortem interval. An elevated vitreous glucose concentration strongly suggests antemortem hyperglycemia. The individual interpreting the toxicologic report must know the exact site from which the sample was taken.[22,62]

Ideally, samples from more than one site would be available for comparison; fortunately, multiple site sampling is now a standard procedure required for accreditation. In decedents with minimal putrefaction or decomposition, comparison of concentrations from different sites can reveal important information regarding the extent of xenobiotic absorption at the time of death and acute versus chronic exposure.[11-13,28,32,52-54,77,87,90,93,96-98,103,110,112]

Other Considerations

Published therapeutic, toxic, and fatal xenobiotic concentrations from autopsy samples as well as postmortem redistribution data are available to aid in the interpretation of these specimens.[6,73] However, the conditions associated with reported concentrations ("average" range) do not necessarily permit comparisons with the concentrations of the particular case under investigation. Thus, these resources although valuable, should not be accepted as absolute values that specifically define either toxic or therapeutic concentrations. Similarly, formulas available for assessing xenobiotic doses or concentrations in the living are not usually applicable when analyzing postmortem samples.

Other Limitations

Although there are generalized standards of practice in forensic investigations, specimen collection and laboratory methodologies may vary.[3,6] Some xenobiotic concentrations may be falsely elevated or depressed depending on the chosen methodology.[33,77] Descriptions of specific toxicology laboratory techniques are beyond the scope of this chapter, but these variables must also be considered in the interpretations of results. Other limitations may include a lack of information relating to the circumstances of death, or the possible compromise in specimen handling to maintain proper chain-of-custody for evidence that is often of paramount importance in medicolegal autopsies.[39,40]

Case Discussion

Interpreting the oxycodone concentrations obtained from postmortem femoral samples requires information about the medical and behavioral health of the decedent before death, medication history, interviews with family, coworkers, scene investigation, and thorough review of all medications administered during the hospital stay. A subsequent evaluation revealed a previously undisclosed history of opioid misuse syndrome and recent discharge from an opioid rehabilitation program. A review of hospital records revealed that no oxycodone was administered in the hospital. The scene investigation and evaluation of the train and rails revealed no clear mechanical failure. The concern is for illicit oxycodone use. Samples of blood from the subdural hematoma revealed high concentrations of oxycodone. Although there may be postmortem drug redistribution, extravasated blood is generally protected from these changes and likely more closely related to antemortem concentrations. Ideally, a sample of blood from admission or recovered from the blood bank should be sent for forensic toxicologic studies. A family member subsequently came forward, having found a bottle of pills with

the markings of oxycodone in the decedent's home. The family member remarked that he seemed unusually drowsy prior to leaving for work and they were suspicious for relapsed opioid misuse. A coworker confirmed that he seemed lethargic and asked if he was "okay." An analysis of the tablets revealed that the pills were oxycodone. The cause of death was deemed traumatic brain injury due to blunt force injury while intoxicated by oxycodone. The manner of death was deemed an accident, the legal term for a nonnatural, unintentional death.

SUMMARY

- Accurate interpretation of postmortem toxicology reports requires an understanding of the potential biochemical changes that affect these samples.
- It is exceptionally difficult to make an absolute correlation between the xenobiotic concentrations of postmortem blood and tissue to the concentrations in comparable samples from the actual time of death.
- Postmortem toxicology is an evolving discipline that permits identification of the most likely cause and manner of xenobiotic-related deaths.
- Progress in this field will depend on the continued collaboration between the treating physicians, medical and forensic toxicologists, and medical examiners.

REFERENCES

1. Accreditation council. American College of Graduate Medical Education. https://www.acgme.org/Portals/0/PFAssets/ProgramRequirements/310_forensic_path_07012017_TCC.pdf. Accessed June 20, 2017.
2. Amendt J, et al. Forensic entomology. *Naturwissenschaften.* 2004;91:51-56.
3. Andollo W. Quality assurance in postmortem toxicology. In: Karch SB, ed. *Drug Abuse Handbook.* Boca Raton, FL: CRC Press; 1998:953-969.
4. Anonymous. Centers for Disease Control and Prevention. *https://www.cdc.gov/phlp/publications/coroner/death.html.* Accessed June 20, 2017.
5. Barry M. Metal residues after cremation. *BMJ.* 1994;308:390.
6. Baselt RC, ed. *Disposition of Toxic Drugs and Chemicals in Man.* 8th ed. Foster City, CA: Biomedical Publications; 2009.
7. Battah AH, Hadidi KA. Stability of trihexyphenidyl in stored blood and urine specimens. *Int J Legal Med.* 1998;111:111-114.
8. Bentur Y, et al. Postmortem digoxin-like immunoreactive substance (DLIS) in patients not treated with digoxin. *Hum Exp Toxicol.* 1999;18:67-70.
9. Berryman HE, et al. Recognition of cemetery remains in the forensic setting. *J Forensic Sci.* 1991;36:230-237.
10. Blackmore DJ. Aircraft accident toxicology: UK experience 1967–1972. *Aerospace Med.* 1974;45:987-994.
11. Bonnichsen R, et al. Toxicological data on phenothiazine drugs in autopsy cases. *J Legal Med.* 1970;67:158-169.
12. Briglia EJ, et al. The distribution of ethanol in postmortem blood specimens. *J Forensic Sci.* 1993;38:1019-1021.
13. Caplan YH, Levine B. Vitreous humor in the evaluation of postmortem blood ethanol concentrations. *J Anal Toxicol.* 1990;14:305-307.
14. Caughlin J. An unusual source for postmortem findings of methyl ethyl ketone and methanol in two homicide victims. *Forensic Sci Int.* 1994;67:27-31.
15. Chace DH, et al. Factors affecting the loss of carbon monoxide from stored blood samples. *J Anal Toxicol.* 1986;10:181-189.
16. Chamberlain RT. Role of the clinical toxicologist in court. *Clin Chem.* 1996;42:1337-1341.
17. Chikasue F, et al. Cyanide distribution in five fatal cyanide poisonings and the effect of storage conditions on cyanide concentration in tissue. *Forensic Sci Int.* 1988;38:173-183.
18. Choo-Kang E, et al. Vitreous humor analytes in assessing the postmortem interval and the antemortem clinical status. *West Med J.* 1983;32:23-26.
19. Ciszkowski C, et al. Codeine, ultrarapid-metabolism genotype, and postoperative death. *N Engl J Med.* 2009;361:827-828.
20. Clark MA, Jones JW. Studies on putrefactive ethanol production. I: lack of spontaneous ethanol production in intact human bodies. *J Anal Toxicol.* 1982;27:366-371.
21. Coe JI. Comparative postmortem chemistries of vitreous humor before and after embalming. *J Forensic Sci.* 1976;21:583-586.
22. Coe JI. Postmortem chemistry of blood, cerebrospinal fluid, and vitreous humor. *Legal Med Ann.* 1977;76:55-92.
23. Coe JI. Use of chemical determinations on vitreous humor in forensic pathology. *J Forensic Sci.* 1972;17:541-546.
24. Coe JI, Sherman RE. Comparative study of postmortem vitreous humor and blood alcohol. *J Forensic Sci.* 1970;15:185-190.
25. Cook DS, et al. Estimating the antemortem drug concentrations from postmortem drug samples: the influence from postmortem redistribution. *J Clin Pathol.* 2000;53:282-285.
26. Craig PH. Standard procedures for sampling—a pathologist's prospective view. *Clin Toxicol.* 1979;15:597-603.

27. Daae LN, et al. Determination of glucose in human vitreous humor. *J Legal Med.* 1978;80:287-290.

28. Davis GL. Postmortem alcohol analyses of general aviation pilot fatalities, Armed Forces Institute of Pathology 1962-1967. *Aerospace Med.* 1973;44:80-83.

29. Dettling RJ, et al. The production of amitriptyline from nortriptyline in formaldehyde-containing solutions. *J Anal Toxicol.* 1990;14:325-326.

30. Devgun MS, Dunbar JA. Post-mortem estimation of gamma-glutamyl transferase in vitreous humor and its association with chronic abuse of alcohol and road-traffic deaths. *Forensic Sci Int.* 1985;28:179-180.

31. Druid H, Holmgren P. A compilation of fatal and control concentrations of drugs in postmortem femoral blood. *J Forensic Sci.* 1997;42:79-87.

32. Druid H, et al. Cytochrome P450 2D6 (CYP2D6) genotyping on postmortem blood as a supplementary tool for interpretation of forensic toxicological results. *Forensic Sci Int.* 1999;99:25-34.

33. Drummer OH. Postmortem toxicology of drugs of abuse. *Forensic Sci Int.* 2004; 142:101-113.

34. Drummer OH, Gerostamoulos J. Postmortem drug analysis: analytical and toxicological aspects. *Ther Drug Monit.* 2002;24:199-209.

35. Ernst MF, et al. Evaluation of medicolegal investigators' suspicions and positive toxicology findings in 100 drug deaths. *J Anal Toxicol.* 1982;27:61-65.

36. Falconer B, Moller M. The determination of carbon monoxide in blood treated with formaldehyde. *J Legal Med.* 1971;68:17-19.

37. Felby S, Olsen J. Comparative studies of postmortem barbiturate and meprobamate in vitreous humor, blood and liver. *J Forensic Sci.* 1969;14:507-514.

38. Ferrer-Alcon M, et al. Decreased immunodensities of μ opioid receptors, receptor kinases, GRK 2/6 and β-arrestin-2 in postmortem brains of opioid addicts. *Mol Brain Res.* 2004;121:114-122.

39. Flanagan RJ, Connally G. Interpretation of analytical toxicology results in life and at postmortem. *Toxicol Rev.* 2005;24:51-62.

40. Flanagan RJ, et al. Analytical toxicology: guidelines for sample collection postmortem. *Toxicol Rev.* 2005;24:63-71.

41. Fomey RB, et al. Extraction, identification and quantitation of succinylcholine in embalmed tissue. *J Anal Toxicol.* 1982:6:115-119.

42. Forrest AR. Obtaining samples at post mortem examination for toxicological and biochemical analyses. *J Clin Pathol.* 1993;46:292-296.

43. Garriott JC. Interpretive toxicology. *Clin Lab Med.* 1983;3:367-384.

44. Goff ML, Lord WD. Entomotoxicology. A new area for forensic investigation. *Am J Forensic Med Pathol.* 1994;15:51-57.

45. Goldman P, Ingelfinger JA. Completeness of toxicological analyses. *JAMA.* 1980; 243:2030-2031.

46. Goulding R. Poisoning as a fine art. *Med Legal J.* 1978;46:6-17.

47. Grellner W, Glenewinkel F. Exhumations: synopsis of morphologic findings in relation to the postmortem interval. Survey on a 20-year the literature. *Forensic Sci Int.* 1997; 90:139-159.

48. Halmai J. Common thyme (*Thymus vulgaris*) as employed for the embalming. *Ther Hungarica.* 1972;20:162-165.

49. Hanzlick R. Embalming, body preparation, burial, and disinterment. *Pathology.* 1994;15:122-131.

50. Hanzlick R. Medical examiner and coroner systems: history and trends. *JAMA.* 1998;279:870-874.

51. Hearn WL, et al. Site dependent postmortem changes in blood cocaine concentrations. *J Forensic Sci.* 1991;36:673-684.

52. Hearn WL, Walls HC. Common methods in postmortem toxicology. In: Karch SB, ed. *Drug Abuse Handbook.* Boca Raton, FL: CRC Press; 1998:890-926.

53. Hearn WL, Walls HC. Introduction to postmortem toxicology. In: Karch SB, ed. *Drug Abuse Handbook.* Boca Raton, FL: CRC Press; 1998:863-873.

54. Hearn WL, Walls HC. Strategies for postmortem toxicological investigation. In: Karch SB, ed. *Drug Abuse Handbook.* Boca Raton, FL: CRC Press; 1998:926-953.

55. Helper BR, Isenschmid DS. Specimen selection, collection, preservation, and security. In: Karch SB, ed. *Drug Abuse Handbook.* Boca Raton, FL: CRC Press; 1998:873-889.

56. Hilberg T, et al. Postmortem drug redistribution—human cases related to results in experimental animals. *J Forensic Sci.* 1999;44:3-9.

57. Hill IR. Toxicological findings in fatal aircraft accidents in the United Kingdom. *Am J Forensic Med Pathol.* 1986;7:322-326.

58. Høiseth G, et al. Disappearance of ethyl glucuronide during heavy putrefaction. *Forensic Sci Int.* 2008;176:147-151.

59. Høiseth G, et al. In vitro formation of ethanol in autopsy samples containing fluoride ions. *Int J Legal Med.* 2008;122:63-66.

60. Iwasa Y, Onaya T. Postmortem changes in the level of calcium pump triphosphatase in rat heart sarcoplasmic reticulum. *Forensic Sci Int.* 1988;39:13-22.

61. Jones GR. Interpretation of postmortem drug levels. In: Karch SB, ed. *Drug Abuse Handbook.* Boca Raton, FL: CRC Press; 1998:970-985.

62. Jones GR, Pounder DJ. Site dependence of drug concentrations in postmortem blood—a case study. *J Anal Toxicol.* 1987;11:186-190.

63. Karch SB. Introduction to the forensic pathology of cocaine. *Am J Forensic Med Pathol.* 1991;12:126-131.

64. Karger B, et al. Analysis of 155 consecutive forensic exhumations with emphasis on undetected homicides. *Int J Legal Med.* 2004;118:90-94.

65. Kintz P, et al. Fly larvae and their relevance in forensic toxicology. *Am J Forensic Med Pathol.* 1990;11:63-65.

66. Klette K, et al. Toxicological findings in military aircraft fatalities from 1986-1990. *Forensic Sci Int.* 1992;53:143-148.

67. Krompecher T. Experimental evaluation of rigor mortis. v. Effect of various temperatures on the evolution of rigor. *Forensic Sci Int.* 1981;17:19-26.

68. Kugelberg FC, Jones AW. Interpreting results of ethanol analysis in postmortem specimens: a review of the literature. *Forensic Sci Int.* 2007;165:10-29.

69. Kunsman GW, et al. Fluvoxamine distribution in postmortem cases. *Am J Forensic Med Pathol.* 1999;20:78-83.

70. Langford AM, et al. Drug concentration in selected skeletal muscles. *J Forensic Sci.* 1998;43:22-27.

71. Lee AF, et al. Postmortem genetic diagnosis of long QT syndrome in a case of sudden unexplained pediatric death of a young child. A case report and overview of regional guidelines for genetic testing. *Br Columbia Med J.* 2014;56:486-491.

72. Levine BS, et al. Postmortem forensic toxicology. *Clin Lab Med.* 1990;10:571-589.

73. Lewin JF, et al. Computer storage of toxicology methods and postmortem drug determinations. *Forensic Sci Int.* 1983;23:225-232.

74. Linnet K. Post-mortem drug concentrations for the non-intoxicated state. A review. *J Forensic Legal Med.* 2012;19;245-249.

75. Livshits Z, et al. Retained drugs in the gastrointestinal tracts of deceased victims of oral drug overdose. *Clin Toxicol (Phila).* 2015;53:113-118.

76. Logan BK, et al. Lack of predictable site-dependent differences and time-dependent changes in postmortem concentrations of cocaine, benzoylecgonine, and cocaethylene in humans. *J Anal Toxicol.* 1997;20:23-31.

77. Long C, et al. Comparison of analytical methods in the determination of two venlafaxine fatalities. *J Anal Toxicol.* 1997;21:166-169.

78. Mellen PF, Bouvieer EC. Nineteenth-century Massachusetts coroner inquests. *Am J Forensic Med Pathol.* 1996;17:207-210.

79. Messite J, Stellman SD. Accuracy of death certificate completion. *JAMA.* 1996; 275:794-796.

80. Molina DK, Hargrove VM. Should postmortem subclavian blood be considered a peripheral or central sample. *Am J Forensic Med Pathol.* 2013;34:155-158

81. Moriya F, Hashimoto Y. Postmortem diffusion of drugs from the bladder into femoral blood. *Forensic Sci Int.* 2001;123;248-253.

82. Moriya F, Hashimoto Y. Redistribution of basic drugs into cardiac blood from surrounding tissues during early stages postmortem. *J Forensic Sci.* 1999;44:10-16.

83. Niyogi SK. Historic development of forensic toxicology in America up to 1978. *Am J Forensic Med Pathol.* 1980;1:249-264.

84. O'Neal CL, Poklis A. Postmortem production of ethanol and factors that influence interpretation: a critical review. *Am J Forensic Med Pathol.* 1996;17:8-20.

85. Oxley DW. Examination of the exhumed body and embalming artifacts. *Med Legal Bull.* 1984;33:1-7.

86. Peat MA. Advances in forensic toxicology. *Clin Lab Med.* 1998;18:263-278.

87. Peclet C, et al. The use of vitreous humor levels of glucose, lactic acid and blood levels of acetone to establish antemortem hyperglycemia in diabetics. *Forensic Sci Int.* 1994; 65:1-6.

88. Pelissier-Alicot AL, et al. Mechanisms underlying postmortem redistribution of drugs: a review. *J Anal Toxicol.* 2003;27:533-544.

89. Peterson GF, Clark SC. Forensic autopsy forensic standards. *Am J Forensic Med Pathol.* 2006;27:200-225.

90. Pla A, et al. A fatal case of oral ingestion of methanol. Distribution in postmortem tissues and fluids including pericardial fluid and vitreous humor. *Forensic Sci Int.* 1991;49:193-196.

91. Polson CJ, et al. *The Essentials of Forensic Medicine.* 4th ed. Oxford, UK: Pergamon; 1985:3-39.

92. Pounder DJ. Forensic entomo-toxicology. *Forensic Sci Soc.* 1991;31:469-472.

93. Pounder DJ, et al. Electrolyte concentration differences between left and right vitreous humor samples. *J Forensic Sci.* 1998;43:604-607.

94. Pounder DJ, Davies JI. Zopiclone poisoning: tissue distribution and potential for postmortem diffusion. *Forensic Sci Int.* 1994;65:177-183.

95. Pounder DJ, et al. Postmortem diffusion of drugs from gastric residue: an experimental study. *Am J Forensic Med Pathol.* 1996;17:1-7.

96. Prouty RW, Anderson WH. A comparison of postmortem heart blood and femoral blood ethyl alcohol concentrations. *J Anal Toxicol.* 1987;11:191-197.

97. Prouty RW, Anderson WH. The forensic science implications of site and temporal influences on postmortem blood-drug concentrations. *J Forensic Sci.* 1990;35:243-270.

98. Ritz S, et al. Measurement of digitalis-glycoside levels in ocular tissues. *Int J Legal Med.* 1992;105:155-159.

99. Rivers RL. Embalming artifacts. *J Forensic Sci.* 1978;23:531-535.

100. Robertson MD, Drummer OR. Stability of nitrobenzodiazepines in postmortem blood. *J Forensic Sci.* 1998;43:5-8.

101. Rohrig TP. Comparison of fentanyl concentrations in unembalmed and embalmed liver samples. *J Anal Toxicol.* 1998;22:253.

102. Rosenfeld L. Alfred Swaine Taylor (1806-1880), pioneer toxicologist—and a slight case of murder. *Clin Chem.* 1985;31:1235-1236.

103. Schonheyder RC, Renriques U. Postmortem blood cultures. Evaluation of separate sampling of blood from the right and left cardiac ventricle. *APMIS.* 1997;105:76-78.

104. Schoning P, Strafuss AC. Analysis of postmortem canine blood, cerebrospinal fluid, and vitreous humor. *Am J Vet Res.* 1981;42:1447-1449.

105. Skopp G. Preanalytic aspects in postmortem toxicology. *Forensic Sci Int.* 2004;142:75-100.

106. Smith PW, et al. Toxicological findings in aircraft accident investigation. *Aerospace Med.* 1970;41:760-762.

107. Smith TO, et al. The potential dangers of medical devices with current cremation practices. *Eur Geriatr Med.* 2012;3:97-102.

108. Spitz WU, ed. *Spitz's and Fischer's Medicolegal Investigation of Death.* Springfield, IL: Charles C. Thomas; 1993.

109. Stevens HM. The stability of some drugs and poisons in putrefying human liver tissues. *J Forensic Sci Soc.* 1984;24:577-589.

110. Stone BE, Rooney PA. A study using body fluids to determine blood alcohol. *J Anal Toxicol.* 1984;8:95-96.

111. Tardiff K, et al. Analysis of cocaine positive fatalities. *J Forensic Sci.* 1989;34:53-63.

112. Vermeulen T. Distribution of paroxetine in three postmortem cases. *J Anal Toxicol.* 1998;22:541-544.

113. Vorpahl TE, Coe JI. Correlation of antemortem and postmortem digoxin levels. *J Forensic Sci.* 1978;23:329-334.

114. Warren MW, et al. Evidence of arteriosclerosis in cremated remains. *Am J Forensic Med Pathol.* 1999;20:277-280.

115. Wetli CV. Investigation of drug-related deaths—an overview. *Am J Forensic Med Pathol.* 1984;5:111-120.

116. Winek CL, et al. The stability of several compounds in formalin fixed tissues and formalin-blood solutions. *Forensic Sci Int.* 1990;44:159-168.

117. Winek CL, Wahba WW. The role of trauma in postmortem blood alcohol determination. *Forensic Sci Int.* 1995;74:213-214.

118. Winek CL, et al. Determination of ethchlorvynol in body tissues and fluids after embalmment. *Forensic Sci Int.* 1988;37:161-166.

119. Winek CL, et al. The study of tricyclic antidepressants in formalin fixed human liver and formalin solutions. *Forensic Sci Int.* 1993;61:175-183.

120. Worm K, et al. Citalopram concentrations in samples from autopsies and living persons. *Int J Legal Med.* 1998;111:188-190.

Special Considerations

ORGAN PROCUREMENT FROM POISONED PATIENTS

Rama B. Rao

Xenobiotics cause brain death as a result of the unique vulnerabilities of the central nervous system. With supportive care, however, many such patients are suitable candidates for organ donation.[11,12,38,47]

Early identification of potential donors is critical because the viability of transplantable tissue diminishes as duration from the time of brain or cardiac death prolongs.[30]

Donor identification by clinicians is one barrier. Among a group of toxicologists given scenarios of brain death from poisoning due to cocaine or carbon monoxide, toxicologists had variable perceptions of donor and organ suitability.[45] Such inconsistency can affect the potential pool of donors in patients with clinical signs of brain death.

Some xenobiotic poisonings can confound clinical assessments of brain stem function and mimic brain death (Table SC12-1). Published brain death protocols require exclusion of poisoning,[12,43,49] but limited guidance is provided.[44] Obtaining and interpreting xenobiotic concentrations is complex and, in many circumstances, not feasible. Few xenobiotics have timely and readily available assays. This is further complicated when the exposure history is unknown. Determining brain death from novel psychoactive substances (NPS) and illicit synthetic opioids is especially challenging. Routine testing for many NPS is often unavailable or uninterpretable, further complicating decisions regarding donor suitability.

Other methods of establishing brain death are utilized such as cerebral blood flow. The effects of xenobiotics on these studies are not well described.[34]

Once brain death is established, organ procurement personnel assist in obtaining familial consent, deciding which organs are most suitable for transplant, and maximizing physiological support and perfusion until organ procurement occurs.[47] The protocols following controlled or uncontrolled donation after cardiac arrest are socially complicated and practiced extensively in Europe.[42]

Successful transplantation of organs is reported from poisoned donors associated with a variety of xenobiotics (Tables SC12-2 and SC12-3).[2,3,6,8,11,12,18,26,29,36,38-41,46] Although some xenobiotics are highly toxic, such as cyanide and carbon monoxide (CO), transfer of clinical poisoning to the organ recipient is not reported. This is likely caused by several factors, including xenobiotic metabolism, tissue redistribution or binding prior to procurement, as well as the means of handling organs during the transplantation process. For example, some xenobiotic clearance occurs in the myocardium during organ rinsing and cardiopulmonary bypass.[35] Furthermore, individual organs do not uniformly manifest toxicity following specific xenobiotic insults. For example, the heart of a CO-poisoned donor was examined after a transplantation failed for technical reasons. The myocardium did not demonstrate histologic signs of CO poisoning.[41] A comprehensive review with organ-specific procurement recommendations post-CO poisoning is presented elsewhere.[4]

Probably more critical to transplantation success is adequate tissue perfusion and well-maintained cellular morphology. For example, patients suffering brain death from acetaminophen poisoning are not suitable liver donors given the hepatoxicity. Alternatively, xenobiotics considered toxic to organ function by impairing enzymes resulted in successful transplantation if the cellular structure is otherwise maintained. For example, a death from cardioactive steroid poisoning did not preclude successful heart transplantation even when the donor had a bradydysrhythmia, an elevated serum digoxin concentration, and required cardiopulmonary resuscitation.[41] Similarly, the liver of a patient poisoned with brodifacoum was transplanted after administration of fresh-frozen plasma and vitamin K_1. The recipient's international normalized ratio (INR) post-transplant was 2 and corrected rapidly with supportive care. Recipient concentrations of brodifacoum were not reported and not clearly causative of the elevated INR.[35] In both examples, the target of toxicity was enzymatic and the tissue morphology was otherwise minimally affected. Organs from a patient who suffered hypoxic brain death after malathion poisoning were procured and successfully transplanted 2 weeks after the exposure, at which time no further evidence

TABLE SC12–1	Xenobiotic Mimics* of Clinical Brain Death
Amitriptyline[48]	
Baclofen[34]	
Barbiturates[44]	
Bupropion[33]	
Lidocaine[37]	
Phorate[34]	
Snake envenomation[24,34] (Old World)**	
Valproic acid[1]	
Vecuronium[44]	

*Based on reported cases

** Case from India, species not identified

TABLE SC12–2	Organs Transplanted After Donor Poisonings
Organ	**Xenobiotics Identified in Donors**
[a]Cornea[a,2,27,29,30,35]	Brodifacoum, cyanide
Heart[9,16,29,32]	Acetaminophen, β-adrenergic antagonists, alkylphosphate, benzodiazepines, brodifacoum, carbamazepine, carbon monoxide, chlormethiazole, cyanide, digitalis, digoxin, ethanol, glibenclamide, insulin, meprobamate, methanol, propoxyphene, thiocyanate
Kidney[a,3,5,7,12,29,30]	Acetaminophen, brodifacoum, carbon monoxide, *Conium maculatum*, cyanide, ethylene glycol, insulin, malathion, methanol, cyclic antidepressants
Liver[5,7,8,12,16]	Brodifacoum, carbon monoxide, *Conium maculatum*, cyanide, ethylene glycol, insulin, malathion, methanol, methaqualone, cyclic antidepressants
Lung[6,8,16,29,31,35]	Brodifacoum, carbon monoxide, methanol
Pancreas[7,8,12,29]	Acetaminophen, brodifacoum, carbon monoxide, *Conium maculatum*, cyanide, ethylene glycol, methanol, cyclic antidepressants
Skin[8,31]	Cyanide, methanol

[a]Can be cadaveric procurement.

TABLE SC12–3	Xenobiotic-Related Deaths With Successful Organ Donation
β-Adrenergic antagonists	Ethanol
Alkylphosphate	Ethylene glycol
Barbiturates	Glibenclamide
Benzodiazepines	Ibuprofen
Brodifacoum	Insulin
Carbamazepine	Malathion
Carbon monoxide	Methaqualone
Cardioactive steroids	Meprobamate
Chlormethiazole	Methanol
Conium maculatum	Nicotine
Cyanide	Opioids
Cyclic antidepressants	Propoxyphene

of acute cholinergic toxicity was present.[6] Most transplant failures from poisoned donors are due to rejection, sepsis, or technical reasons. The one-year survival in recipients from poisoned donors approximates that from nonpoisoned donors. One series reported at 75% survival.[15] In another review, 5-year survival rates were between 33% and 100%, with heart transplant recipients the lowest.[17]

In the United States, the waitlist for organs exceeds 100,000.[10] Since 2003, the percentage of organ donors due to drug overdose increased 350%, largely due to the opioid epidemic.[10] Despite concerns about infectious disease transmission from these donors, the risk of dying while on the waitlist is substantially higher. Finding consensus on the ethics of procuring organs from this vulnerable population is challenging.

Ideally, a comprehensive international registry of transplants from poisoned donors will be established to improve understanding of transplants from such patients. Patients who suffer brain death from poisoning are potentially suitable donors when cellular infrastructure is preserved.[22,24-26,28,38,47] Consideration for organ procurement should not be defined or limited by the xenobiotic.

SUMMARY

- Organ procurement from poisoned donors often reaches success rates similar to nonpoisoned donors when carefully selected.
- Clinically significant xenobiotic concentrations are not reported in organ recipients.
- Adequate tissue perfusion is important for the viability of a transplanted organ, regardless of the primary toxicologic insult.

REFERENCES

1. Auineger K, et al. Case report: valproic acid intoxication imitating brain death. *Am J Emerg Med.* 2009;27:1177.e5-1177.e6.
2. Basu PK. Experimental and clinical studies on corneal grafts from donors dying of drug overdose: a review. *Cornea.* 1984-85;3:262-267.
3. Brown PW, et al. Successful cadaveric transplantation from a donor who died of cyanide poisoning. *Br Med J Clin Res.* 1987;294:1325.
4. Busche MN, et al. Solid organ procurement from donors with carbon monoxide poisoning and/or burn—a systematic review. *Burns.* 2011;37:814-822.
5. de Tourtchaninoff M, et al. Brain-death diagnosis in misleading conditions. *Q J Med.* 1999;92:404-414.
6. Dribben WH, Kirk MA. Organ procurement and successful transplantation after malathion poisoning. *J Toxicol Clin Toxicol.* 2001;39:633-636.
7. Evrard P, et al. Successful double lung transplantation with a graft obtained from a methanol-poisoned donor. *Chest.* 1999;115:1458-1459.
8. Foster PF, et al. Successful transplantation of donor organs from a hemlock poisoning victim. *Transplantation.* 2003;76:874-876.
9. Garcia JH, et al. Successful organ transplantation from donors poisoned with a carbamate insecticide. *Am J Transplant.* 2010;10:1490-1492.
10. Goldberg DS, et al. Improving organ utilization to help overcome the tragedies of the opioid epidemic. *Am J Transplant.* 2016;16:2836-2841.
11. Hantson P. Organ donation after fatal poisoning: an update and recent literature data. *Adv Exp Med Biol.* 2004;550:207-213.
12. Hantson P, et al. Multimodality evoked potentials as a valuable technique for brain death diagnosis in poisoned patients. *Transplant Proc.* 1997;29:3345-3346.
13. Hantson P, et al. Successful liver transplantation with a graft from a methanol-poisoned donor. *Transpl Int.* 1996;9:437.
14. Hantson P, et al. Outcome following organ removal from poisoned donors in brain death status: a report of 12 cases and review of the literature. *J Toxicol Clin Toxicol.* 1995;33:709-712.
15. Hantson P, Mahieu P. Organ donation after fatal poisoning. *Q J Med.* 1999;92: 415-418.
16. Hantson P, et al. Organ transplantation after fatal cyanide poisoning. *Clin Transplant.* 1999;13:72-73.
17. Hantson P, et al. Strategies to increase the lung donors' pool. *Eur Respir J.* 2004;24: 889-890.
18. Hantson P, et al. Fatal methanol poisoning and organ donation: experience with seven cases in a single center. *Transplant Proc.* 2000;32:491-492.
19. Hantson P, et al. Methanol poisoning and organ transplantation. *Transplantation.* 1999;68:165-166.
20. Hantson P, et al. Heart donation after fatal acetaminophen poisoning. *J Toxicol Clin Toxicol.* 1997;35:325-326.
21. Hantson P, et al. Organ transplantation from victims of carbon monoxide poisoning. *Ann Emerg Med.* 1996;27:673-674.
22. Hantson P, et al. Outcome following organ removal from poisoned donors: experience with 12 cases and a review of the literature. *Transpl Int.* 1995;8:185-189.
23. Hantson P, et al. Organ procurement after evidence of brain death in victims of acute poisoning. *Transplant Proc.* 1997;29:3341-3342.
24. John J, et al. Snakebite mimicking brain death. *Cases J.* 2008;1:16.
25. Jones AL, Simpson KJ. Drug abusers and poisoned patients: a potential source of organs for transplantation? *Q J Med.* 1998;91:589-592.
26. Kalliomaki J, et al. A case report of successful kidney donation after brain death following nicotine intoxication. *Transplant Proc.* 2017;49:229-231.
27. Koerner MM, et al. Extended donor criteria: use of cardiac allografts after carbon monoxide poisoning. *Transplantation.* 1997;63:1358-1360.
28. Leikin JB, et al. The toxic patient as a potential organ donor. *Am J Emerg Med.* 1994;12:151-154.
29. Lindquist TD, et al. Cyanide poisoning victims as corneal transplant donors. *Am J Ophthalmol.* 1988;106:354-355.
30. Lopez-Navidad A, Caballero F. Extended criteria for organ acceptance: strategies for achieving organ safety and for increasing organ pool. *Clin Transplant.* 2003;17:308-324.
31. Luckraz H, et al. Improved outcome with organs from carbon monoxide poisoned donors for intrathoracic transplantation. *Ann Thorac Surg.* 2001;72:709-713.
32. Mariage JL, et al. Organ donation following fatal organophosphate poisoning. *Transpl Int.* 2012;25:e71-e72.
33. Mundi JP, et al. Dilated and unreactive pupils and burst suppression on electroencephalography due to bupropion overdose. *J Intensive Care Med.* 2012;27:384-388.
34. Neavyn MJ, et al. ACMT Position Statement: determining brain death in adults after drug overdose. *J Med Toxicol.* 2017;13:271-273.
35. Ornstein DL, et al. Successful donation and transplantation of multiple organs after fatal poisoning with brodifacoum, along-acting anticoagulant rodenticide: case report. *Transplantation.* 1999;67:475-478.
36. Ravishankar DK, et al. Organ transplant from a donor who died of cyanide poisoning. *Clin Transplant.* 1998;12:142-143.
37. Richard IH, et al. Non-barbiturate drug induced reversible loss of brainstem reflexes. *Neurology.* 1998;51:639-640.
38. Shennib H, et al. Successful transplantation of a lung allograft from a carbon monoxide poisoning victim. *J Heart Lung Transplant.* 1992;11:68-71.
39. Smith JA, et al. Successful heart transplantation with cardiac allografts exposed to carbon monoxide poisoning. *J Heart Lung Transplant.* 1992;11:698-700.
40. Swanson-Bieraman B, et al. Successful donation and transplantation of multiple organs from a victim of cyanide poisoning. *J Toxicol Clin Toxicol.* 1993;31:95-99.
41. Tenderich G, et al. Hemodynamic follow-up of cardiac allografts from poisoned donors. *Transplantation.* 1998;66:1163-1167.
42. Wall SP, et al. NYC UDCDD Study Group. Derivation of the uncontrolled donation after circulatory determination of death protocol for New York city. *Am J Transplant.* 2011;11:1417-1426.
43. Wijdicks EF. The diagnosis of brain death. *N Engl J Med.* 2001;3444:1215-1221.
44. Wijdicks EF, et al. American Academy of Neurology. Evidence-based guideline update: determining brain death in adults: report of the Quality Standards Subcommittee of the American Academy of Neurology. *Neurology.* 2010;74:1911-1918.
45. Wood DM, et al. Using drug-intoxicated deaths as potential organ donors: impressions of attendees at the ACMT 2014 Annual Scientific Meeting. *J Med Toxicol.* 2014;10:360-363.
46. Wood DM, et al. Poisoned patients as potential organ donors: postal survey of transplant centres and intensive care units. *Crit Care (London).* 2003;7:147-154.
47. Wood KE, et al. Care of the potential organ donor. *N Engl J Med.* 2004;351:2730-2739.
48. Yang KL, Dantker DR. Reversible brain death—a manifestation of amitriptyline overdose. *Chest.* 1991;99:1037.
49. Youn TA, Greer DM. Brain death and management of a potential organ donor in the intensive care unit. *Crit Care Clin.* 2014;30:813-831.

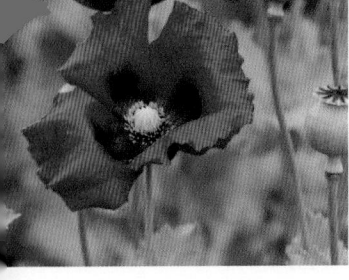

INDEX

Note: Page numbers followed by f and t indicate figures and tables, respectively.

A

AACT (American Academy of Clinical Toxicology), 11, 11t
AAPCC (American Association of Poison Control Centers), 11, 11t. *See also* Antivenom Index
Abacavir (ABC), 144, 831
    diabetes insipidus caused by, 195t
    hypersensitivity reactions to, HLA and, 329
    and methanol metabolism, 1428
ABAT (American Board of Applied Toxicology), 11t, 12
Abbolipid, 684–685
Abbonus, Petrus, 4
ABCB1 gene, and codeine toxicity, 441
ABCDX classification, of pregnancy risk, 431
Abciximab, 323, 899
    adverse effects and safety issues, 900
    dosage and administration, 899
    mechanism of action, 898f
    pharmacokinetics, 899
    and thrombocytopenia, 324
ABCs of initial management, 33, 34f
ABC transporters, 144, 168, 173
    and transplacental transfer, 432
Abdomen
    deep viscera, thermosensitivity, 411
    diagnostic imaging, 127–130, 129t
    examination, 38
    trauma to, 38
Abdominal compartment syndrome, 391
Abdominal pain
    cocaine use and, 1127
    in ketamine users, 1215–1216
    lead-induced, 1296
    in paraquat poisoning, 1475–1476
    in thallium toxicity, 1351
Abdominal radiography, 127
    in arsenic toxicity, 1244
    in bismuth toxicity, 1256
    in body packers, 117, 120f
    of caustic injury, 1391
    in iron ingestion, 671, 672f
    phenothiazines on, 1040
    in toxicologic emergencies, 129t
    for unknown xenobiotic ingestion, 47f
    with xenobiotic exposure, 115t
Abemaciclib, 349f
    cell cycle phase specificity, 761f
Abetalipoproteinemia, vitamin E deficiency in, 661
AB-FUBINACA, structure, 1112f
ABMT (American Board of Medical Toxicology), 11t, 12
AbobotulinumtoxinA (Dysport), 578–579
Abortifacients, 297, 302–304, 303t, 838. *See also specific xenobiotic*
    herbal, 303, 303t
    overdose, 304
AB-PINACA, structure, 1112f
Abrin, 1598t, 1608, 1608f
    as abortifacient, 303t
Abruptio placentae, cocaine use and, 440
Abrus precatorius (jequirity pea, rosary pea), 1598t, 1608f, 1609
    as abortifacient, 303t

Absinthe (*Artemisia absinthium*), 627–628, 1598t, 1608
    history of, 9
    toxicity, 648
        diagnostic tests for, 634
        treatment, 634
Absinthes. *See* Wormwood
Absinthism, 1608
Absorbed dose (radiation), 1764, 1764f
Absorption, 140–144, 167. *See also* Activated charcoal; *specific xenobiotic*
    administration route and, 140–141, 144
    bioavailability and, 140, 140f
    cutaneous, in neonates, 442
    definition, 140
    in elderly, 461
    extent of, 140. *See also* Bioavailability
    factors affecting, 167
    formulation and, 143
    gastric, lipid solubility and, 142, 143f
    gastric bypass and, 148
    gastrointestinal. *See* Gastrointestinal absorption
    gastrointestinal transit time and, 143
    ionization and, 142, 143f
    lipid solubility and, 142, 143f
    in neonates, 442
    in obese patients, 148
    postmortem, 1887
    rate (k_a), 140, 140f
        and peak plasma concentrations, 152
        pharmacokinetic effects, 152, 152t
    transdermal, 271
    transport proteins and, 173
Absorption rate constant (k_a), 140, 140f
    and peak plasma concentrations, 152
    pharmacokinetic effects, 152, 152t
Acacia confusa, 1077
Acadesine, and adenosine, 230t, 231
Acamprosate, 1172
    mechanism of action, 227t
Acanthaster planci (crown-of-thorns sea star), 1573–1574
Acanthophis spp. (death adders), 1633t
Acanthoscurria spp., 1547
Acanthospermum hispidum (bristly starbur), as abortifacient, 303t
Acarbose
    adverse effects and safety issues, 699–700
    history of, 694
    mechanism of action, 695
    pharmacokinetics and toxicokinetics, 697t
    pharmacology, 695
    structure, 695f
Acari, 1540f. *See also* Ticks
Acceptable risk, 1815
Accident, death as, 1884
Accommodation, visual, 357, 365
Acebutolol
    overdose/poisoning
        clinical manifestations, 931–932
        management, 936
    pharmacokinetics, 930
    pharmacology, 927t
    potassium channel blockade, 930, 932

Acenocoumarin, 885
Acetaldehyde, 145t, 159, 168, 168f, 805
    in disulfiram-ethanol reaction, 1173, 1173f, 1174
    ethanol metabolism and, 1144–1145, 1145f
    fomepizole and, 1174
    as thermal degradation product, 1641t
    toxicity, 1146
Acetaldehyde adducts, 1146
Acetaminophen, 472–491
    absorption, 472
        administration route and, 472
        extended-release preparations and, 49, 51f–52f
    and acute liver failure with uncertain diagnosis, 480
    adsorption to activated charcoal, 77
    analgesic activity, 472
    antidote for, 35t, 44t, 58t, 482, 492–497. *See also* *N*-Acetylcysteine (NAC)
    antiinflammatory activity, 472
    antiplatelet effects, 472
    antipyretic activity, 472
    chronic use, ethanol and, 480
    and CNS depression, 474
    concentration, early measurement, 477
    cyanide-tainted, 1685
    diethylene glycol (DEG) in, 681
    effects on liver, 328
    elimination half-life, 473
    elixir, diethylene glycol contamination, 19, 20t
    enhanced elimination, 484–485
    exposure, categories, 475–476
    extended-release
        gastrointestinal absorption and, 49, 51f–52f
        risk assessment after, 477–478
    extracorporeal elimination, 91, 91f, 97t
    gastrointestinal decontamination for, 48–49, 50t–51t, 54t–55t, 58t–59t, 60, 77–78, 85
    glucuronyltransferase deficiency and, 329
    glutathione and, 473
    and hepatocellular necrosis, 331
    hepatotoxicity, 147, 160, 163, 474–475
        biomarkers in, 481
        definition, 475
        ethanol and, 1146
        isoniazid and, 852
        liver transplantation for, 483
        pathophysiology, 474
        in pregnancy, 435, 436t
    hepatotoxicity risk assessment
        with *N*-acetylcysteine antidotal therapy, 482–483
        after acute overdose, Rumack-Matthew nomogram for, 476, 477f
        when nomogram is not applicable, 477–479
    history of, 472
    ingestion
        earliest possible time for, 476–477
        unknown time of, risk determination with, 477–478
    intravenous
        overdose, 478
        toxicokinetics, 473
    laboratory testing for, 101t, 102, 516
        indications for, 37

1895

Acetaminophen (*Cont.*):
mechanism of action, 472
metabolism, 172, 175, 330, 473
N-acetyl-*p*-benzoquinoneimine in, 160, 163, 163f, 172, 174, 473, 473f. *See also* N-Acetyl-*p*-benzoquinoneimine (NAPQI)
nephrotoxicity, 474–475
and "nomogram crossing," 478
oral, toxicokinetics, 473
pancreatitis caused by, 295t
pediatric exposure, risk determination after, 479
pharmacokinetics, 145t, 472–473, 478
pharmacology, 472
physicochemical properties, 472
in pregnancy, 434–435, 436f
risk determination after, 479–480
repeated supratherapeutic ingestions
history and physical examination in, 479
laboratory investigation in, 479
risk determination after, 478
self-poisoning with, 376
serum concentration, interpretation, 153
structure, 472
teratogenicity, 434
time to peak, 472
toxicity (overdose/poisoning), 472, 1852
N-acetylcysteine for, 482, 492–497. *See also* N-Acetylcysteine
activated charcoal for, cohort study, 1853
acute
ethanol and, 480
hepatotoxicity risk assessment after, Rumack-Matthew nomogram for, 476, 477f
risk determination after, 476–477
antidote for, 35t, 44t, 58t
biomarkers in, 481
in children, risk determination after, 479
chronic, risk determination after, 478
clinical and laboratory findings with, 32, 36t, 474–475
CYP inducers and, 480
deaths caused by, 475
diagnostic tests for, 475–481
and risk determination, with antidotal therapy, 482–483
ethanol and, 480
extracorporeal therapies for, 91, 91f, 97t
fetal risk in, 479–480
gastrointestinal decontamination for, 481
initial testing in, 480
150 line for, 476, 477f
liver support devices for, 96
liver transplantation after, 483
management, 58t, 77–78, 91, 481–485, 484t
miRNA-122 in, 481
in neonate, 495
ongoing monitoring and testing in, 480–481
pathophysiology, 473–474
in pregnancy, 39
prognosis for, 483–484
risk determination in, 475–477
after acute overdose, 476–477, 477f
after chronic overdose, 478
in children, 479
with extended-release preparation, 4770478
in pregnancy, 479–480
with unknown time of ingestion, 477–478
when nomogram is not applicable, 477–479
Rumack-Matthew nomogram and, 476, 477f
screening for, principles, 475–477

stages, 474–475
supportive care for, 481–482
survival after, prediction, 483–484, 483t–484t
King's College Criteria and, 483–484, 483t–484t
treatment line for, 476–477, 477f
in unclear risk scenarios, 481
whole-bowel irrigation and, 63
toxic metabolite, 174, 174t
toxicokinetics, 473
volume of distribution, 145t, 472
Acetanilide, 472
sulfhemoglobin from, 1710
Acetazolamide
adverse effects and safety issues, 658
and gustatory dysfunction, 365
for idiopathic intracranial hypertension, 658
and normal anion gap metabolic acidosis, 191t
and thiamine pharmacokinetics, 1158
Acetic acid(s), 168, 512t, 1388t
odor, 364t
self-harm with, 1847
as thermal degradation product, 1641t
Acetoacetate, 1148f, 1150–1151
Acetochlor, 1472
in herbicides, 1467t
Acetohexamide, pharmacokinetics and toxicokinetics, 697t
Acetone, 1423, 1423f
biotransformation, 172
blood:gas partition coefficient, 1195t
and creatinine assays, 1425
elimination, 1195t
inhaled, 1193t. *See also* Inhalant(s)
odor, 37, 364t
pharmacokinetics, 1194
Acetonitrile, 1684. *See also* Cyanide(s)
biotransformation to cyanide, 1684, 1684f, 1685, 1688
taste-aversive xenobiotics in, 1782
N-Acetyl-*p*-aminophenol, 472. *See also* Acetaminophen
N-Acetyl aspartate, in toluene leukoencephalopathy, 1199
Acetylation, in biotransformation, 170
L-Acetylcarnitine, therapeutic uses, 228
Acetylcholine (ACh), 203, 206–208, 805. *See also* Cholinergic neurotransmission
aluminum and, 1224
in central nervous system, 206
chemistry, 162, 163f
definition, 206
functions, 206
and gastric acid secretion, 742, 743f
γ-hydroxybutyrate and, 1189
inactivation, 206, 206f
metabolism, 755–756, 1488f
nicotine and, 1206
and pancreatic function, 292
in peripheral nervous system, 206
release, 206, 206f
adenosine and, 229
inhibitors, 207, 207t
lead and, 1295
modulators, 207, 207t, 208
prevention, 206
thiamine and, 1158
xenobiotics causing, 207, 207t
and sexual function, 300
in skeletal muscle excitation-contraction coupling, 1018, 1019f
structure, and muscarine, 1587

synthesis, 206, 206f
and thermoregulation, 412
Acetylcholine receptors
muscarinic, 206f, 207
subtypes, 207
nicotinic, 206–207, 206f, 239
agonists and antagonists, 206f
distribution, 239
neuromuscular blockers and, 1018–1019, 1019f
neuromuscular junction, 206–207, 206f, 207
neuronal, 206–207, 206f, 207
nicotine and, 239, 1206
structure, 239
subtypes, 239
Acetylcholinesterase (AChE), 206, 206f
activity, 1488f, 1489–1490
carbamates and, 755–756, 1487
inhibition, 207–208, 755–756, 1489–1490
by organic phosphorus compound, 208, 1487, 1489f, 1508–1509
reactions, 162, 163f
reactivation, 1487, 1508
with pralidoxime, 1487, 1510
red blood cell level, interpretation, 1495t
in snake venom, 1618
Acetylcholinesterase inhibitors, 755–756, 1503, 1508. *See also* Organic phosphorus compounds
antidote for, 35t, 1503, 1508
as nerve agents, 1504
for neuromuscular blockade reversal, 1025–1026, 1026t
Acetyl-coenzyme A (acetyl-CoA), 175–177, 954–955, 1148f, 1150, 1157–1158, 1157f
and fatty acid metabolism, 178–179
structural similarity to SMFA and fluoroacetamide, 1533, 1533f
trivalent arsenic and, 1238
Acetylcysteine. *See* N-Acetylcysteine (NAC)
N-Acetylcysteine (NAC), 492–500, 1656
for acetaminophen toxicity, 482, 492–497
dosage and administration, 482, 494
dose adjustment, 483, 497
duration of therapy, 482, 494, 496
hepatotoxicity risk assessment with, 482–483
history of, 492
IV, specific indications for, 494
150 line and, 476, 477f
mechanism of action, 482, 492
oral *vs.* IV, 493–494
in pregnancy, 494
protocols for, 482, 494–496, 496t–497t
Rumack-Matthew nomogram and, 476, 477f, 494
treatment line and, 476–477, 477f, 497
in unclear risk scenarios, 481
for acrylonitrile toxicity, 494
with activated charcoal, 58t, 493
for acute liver failure, 495
adverse effects and safety issues, 495
for amatoxin-induced liver toxicity, 494–495, 1585
amide, 492
as antineoplastic, 494
availability and storage, 44t
for bipolar disorder, 495
for bismuth toxicity, 1257
and boron excretion, 494
and cadmium excretion, 494
for cadmium toxicity, 494
for carbon tetrachloride toxicity, 492, 494, 1679
for cardiac injury, 494
chemistry, 165, 492

for children, 493
for chloroform toxicity, 492, 494
and chromium excretion, 494
for chromium toxicity, 1271
for chronic obstructive pulmonary disease, 494
for cisplatin nephrotoxicity, 494
for clove oil toxicity, 492, 494
and cobalt excretion, 494
for cobalt toxicity, 1278–1279
for contrast-induced nephropathy, 495
in copper poisoning, 1287
for cyclopeptide-containing mushroom toxicity, 492, 494–495
for cyclophosphamide toxicity, 494
for 1,2-dichloropropane toxicity, 494
dosage and administration, 495–497
    intravenous vs. oral, 493–494
    in patients weighing < 40 kg, 497
for doxorubicin toxicity, 494
effervescent formulation, 492–493, 497
    adverse effects and safety issues, 495
    dosage and administration, 497
    sodium in, 495
elimination half-life, 493
    in neonates, 495
for eugenol toxicity, 494
formulations, 492, 497
and gold excretion, 494
for *Helicobacter pylori* infection, 495
hemodialysis and, 95, 497
and hepatic graft procurement, 494
for hepatorenal syndrome, 494–495
for ifosfamide-induced nephrotoxicity, 494
indications for, 32, 35t, 44t, 492, 496
intravenous
    adverse effects and safety issues, 495
    dosage and administration, 497
    for fulminant hepatic failure, 494
    for intolerance of oral preparation, 494
    loading dose, 495
    vs. oral, 493–495
    pharmacokinetics, 493
    precautions with, 497
    in pregnancy, 494
    specific indications for, 494
    three-bag protocol, 493, 494t, 496, 497t
liposomal, 492
loading dose, 494t, 495, 496t
for lung injury, 494
mechanism of action, 227t, 228, 474, 482, 492
and metal excretion, 494
for metal phosphide poisoning, 1459
for methyl bromide poisoning, 1461
and methylmercury excretion, 494
monitoring with, 496–497
for multiorgan failure in trauma and sepsis, 494
for myocardial infarction, 494
nebulized, for smoke inhalation, 1645
for necrotizing enterocolitis, 495
in neonates, 495
for nonacetaminophen toxicity, 494–495
for obese adults, 493, 497
odor, 364t
as oncologic chemopreventive, 494
oral
    absorption, 493
    adverse effects and safety issues, 495
    bioavailability, 493
    vs. intravenous, 493–495
    loading dose, 494t, 495, 496t

maintenance dose, 495, 496t
    pharmacokinetics, 493
overdose/poisoning, 495
for pennyroyal toxicity, 492, 494
pharmacokinetics and pharmacodynamics, 492–493
pharmacology, 492–494
for phosgene exposure, 1653
for phosphorus ingestion, 1531
postcardiac surgery use, 494
in pregnancy and lactation, 39, 435, 436t, 479–480, 495
and prevention of aminoglycoside-induced ototoxicity, 823
for propanil poisoning, 1473
protein binding, 492
for pulegone toxicity, 494
related xenobiotics, 492
rescue, with high-dose acetaminophen therapy, 495
for ricin toxicity, 494
shortage, 43
for sickle cell disease, 495
for spinal injury, 494
stocking, recommended level, 44t
structure, 492
for sulfur mustard exposure, 1748
supplies, 42
therapeutic uses, 228
transplacental transfer, 495
for traumatic brain injury, 494
for valproic acid-related liver failure, 492, 494
volume of distribution, 492
for zidovudine toxicity, 494
for zinc toxicity, 1365
Acetylenes, 1410. *See also* Hydrocarbons
    physicochemical properties, 159
Acetyl fentanyl, 529
N-Acetyl-β-glucosaminidase, in acute kidney injury, 396
N-Acetylglutamate, 180f, 181
N-Acetylglutamate synthetase, 180f, 181
Acetylhydrazine, 851f, 853
Acetylisoniazid, 850
Acetylmorphine, 145t
    urine screening assays for, performance characteristics, 111t
N-Acetyl-*p*-benzoquinoneimine (NAPQI), 145t, 330, 473, 473f, 492
    in acetaminophen overdose, 160, 172, 174, 473–474
    binding to hepatocyte proteins, protein adducts as indicators of, 481
    chemistry, 163, 163f, 165
    reactions with hepatocyte proteins, 163, 163f
N-Acetyl-D,L-penicillamine (NAP), for mercury poisoning, 1330
N-Acetylprocainamide (NAPA), 866t, 868
Acetylsalicylate. *See* Aspirin; Nonsteroidal antiinflammatory drugs (NSAIDs)
Acetylsalicylic acid
    enteric-coated, gastrointestinal evacuation, 84
    history of, 638
    structure, 555
N-Acetyltransferase-2 (NAT2), 850
Achillea millefolium (yarrow), 645t
Achlorhydria, 294
Acid(s). *See also* Caustics; *specific acid*
    adsorption to activated charcoal, 76
    anionic, 141
    Arrhenius definition, 160
    Brønsted-Lowry definition, 160–161

cationic, 141
    definition, 160–161, 1388
    dermal toxicity, 271
    desorption (dissociation) from activated charcoal, 77
    endogenous, 165
    exogenous, 165
    exposure to, pathophysiology, 1389–1390
    gastrointestinal perforation caused by, 127
    ingestion
        clinical manifestations, 1390–1391
        worldwide, 1846
    injury caused by
        clinical presentation, 1390–1391
        endoscopic evaluation, 1390, 1390t, 1391
    ionization, 161
    Lewis, 160–161
    nonionized, 141–142
    ophthalmic decontamination for, 72–73
    ophthalmic exposure to, irrigating solution for, 359t
    ophthalmic toxicity, 356f
    organic, 1410. *See also* Hydrocarbons
    predictors of injury with, 1390–1391
    production, by irritant gases, 1653
    strength, vs. concentration, 161, 161t
    strong, 158, 161
    weak, 158, 161
        dissociation constant for, 141
        enhanced elimination, 93
        ionization, and passive diffusion, 141
        membrane transport, 142
Acid–base abnormality(ies), 37, 189. *See also* Electrolyte abnormality(ies); Fluid abnormalities; Ketoacidosis; Metabolic acidosis; Metabolic alkalosis; Respiratory acidosis; Respiratory alkalosis
    correction, hemodialysis for, 95
    definitions, 189–190
    delta gap ratio (Δ anion gap/Δ [HCO$_3^-$]) in. *See* Delta gap ratio (Δ anion gap/Δ [HCO$_3^-$])
    with hypokalemia, 198
    mixed, 190, 192
        delta gap ratio (Δ anion gap/Δ [HCO$_3^-$]) in, 192
    primary
        compensation, 190
        determination, 190
    secondary, 190
Acid–base chemistry, 160–161
Acidemia
    cardiac effects, 254–255
    caustic ingestion and, 1391
    definition, 190
    in DEG poisoning, 1446–1447
    effects on oxygenation, 403f
    in strychnine poisoning, 1537–1538
α$_1$-Acid glycoprotein
    cyclic antidepressant binding to, 1045
    xenobiotic binding to, 146
Acidifying agents, and normal anion gap metabolic acidosis, 191t
Acid- or base-forming gases, 1655, 1658. *See also* *specific xenobiotic*
Acidosis. *See also* Ketoacidosis; Metabolic acidosis; Renal tubular acidosis (RTA); Respiratory acidosis
    definition, 190
    intracellular, and muscle fatigue, 621
Acid phosphatase
    in Hymenoptera venom, 1551, 1551t
    zinc in, 1362–1363

Acifluorfen, 1468t

Acinus, hepatic, 327, 328f
  functional zones, 327, 328f

Ackee tree (*Blighia sapida*) fruit, 1591, 1609. *See also*
    Hypoglycin
  and gluconeogenesis, 176t, 178
  self-poisoning with, 1846
  toxicity, 1598t

Aclonifen, 1468t

Acne
  with anabolic-androgenic steroids, 618
  gymnasium, 618

Acneiform lesions
  sedative-hypnotic overdose and, 1086t
  xenobiotics causing, 274t

Aconitase, 177
  suicide inhibitor of, 1533–1534

Aconite (*Aconitum*, monkshood), 1611
  cardiotoxicity, magnesium for, 877
  historical perspective on, 1–3, 5t, 6–8

Aconite alkaloids, 640t
  uses and toxicities, 640t, 648

Aconitine, 640t, 1597, 1598t
  bradycardia caused by, 263
  cardiotoxicity, 256, 1611
  mechanism of action, 933f
  and sodium channels, 1611–1612
  and voltage-gated calcium channels, 244f, 245

Aconitum spp., 639, 1598t. *See also* Aconite
    (*Aconitum*, monkshood)

Aconitum carmichaelii, 640t

Aconitum kusnezoffii (Caowu), 640t

Aconitum napellus, 640t
  toxicity, 1598t

Acorus calamus (sweet flag, calamus), 1598t, 1610

Acquired immunodeficiency syndrome (AIDS).
    See HIV-infected (AIDS) patients

Acremonium spp., 824

Acrids, 6

Acrinathrin, 1520t

Acrodermatitis enteropathica, 1362

Acrodynia, 11, 1324, 1326–1327

Acrolein
  in herbicides, 1467t
  as thermal degradation product, 1641t

Acromelic acids, 1583t, 1589t
  structure, 1591

Acroosteolysis, 122, 122t

Acrylamide, overdose/poisoning, clinical and
    laboratory findings with, 36t

Acrylate, and occupational asthma, 1660, 1660t

Acrylic, thermal degradation products, 1641t

Acrylonitrile, 174t. *See also* Cyanide(s)
  biotransformation to cyanide, 1685
  toxicity, *N*-acetylcysteine for, 494

Actaea racemosa (black cohosh), 651, 1611

Actin, myocardial cell, 262, 928, 928f, 946

Actinia equina (beadlet anemone), 1567t

Actinides, 156f

Actinodendron plumosum (Hell's fire anemone), 1567t

Actinomyces, hypersensitivity pneumonitis caused by,
    399t, 1659

Actinoporins, 1570

Actin-tropomyosin helix, 262, 263f

Action potential(s), 206–207. *See also* Compound
    muscle action potential (CMAP); Sensory
    nerve action potential (SNAP)
  cardiac, 254–258, 254f
    ion channels and, 245–246, 245f
    phases, 245–246, 245f

prolonged duration, 254f

compound, polyethylene glycol (PEG) and,
    686–687

propagation, 203–204

Activated charcoal, 7, 33, 56–61. *See also* Multiple-dose
    activated charcoal (MDAC)
  for acetaminophen toxicity, 481
  acquisition, 80
  for β₂-adrenergic agonist toxicity, 990
  adsorption to, 56–57, 57f, 60, 60f, 76, 86
  adverse effects, 61, 79
  for amphetamine toxicity, 1104–1105, 1104t
  for antimony toxicity, 1233–1234
  for antithrombotic overdose/poisoning, 888t
  for apixaban-induced coagulopathy, 895
  for arsenic poisoning, 1244
  and aspiration pneumonitis, 61
  availability and storage, 44t
  for barium ingestion, 1455
  for bismuth toxicity, 1256–1257
  for body packers, 548
  for calcium channel blocker toxicity, 948
  with cathartics, 77, 84
  chemistry, 76
  for chemotherapeutic toxicity, 764
  in children, 60–61, 79, 452
  for chromium toxicity, 1271
  clinical trials, difficulties with, 1854
  contraindications and complications, 57, 61,
    61t, 79
  for cyanide poisoning, 1687
  for cyclic antidepressant toxicity, 1049, 1051
  for decongestant ingestion, 750–751
  for dermal decontamination, 72
  desorption (drug dissociation from), 77
  discovery, 7
  for disulfiram toxicity, 1175
  dosage and administration, 60, 60f, 79
  effect on oral therapeutics, 61
  efficacy, 57, 58t–59t, 76–78, 84–85
  with ethanol, 61, 77
  with evacuants, 77
  flavoring agents for, 61, 79
  formulation, 80
  with gastric emptying, 53, 54t–55t, 77
  gastrointestinal transit time for, 76
  for herbicide poisoning, 1471
  history of, 76
  home use, 60, 79
  hospital use, 79
  for hypoglycemic overdose, 701
  indications for, 35t, 44t, 61t
  in lactation, 79
  with magnesium citrate, 77
  mechanism of action, 56–57, 57f, 76
  for mercury poisoning, 1329
  for methotrexate overdose, 769
  for methylxanthine toxicity, 990
  for mushroom ingestion, 1590–1592
  for nicotine ingestion, 1207
  for organic phosphorus compound and carbamate
    poisoning, 1498
  palatability of, improving, 60–61, 79
  for paraquat poisoning, 1474f, 1476–1477
  pharmacodynamics, 76–77
  pharmacokinetics, 76
  pharmacology, 76
  for phencyclidine toxicity, 1217
  for plant poisoning, 1606
  in polydrug ingestions, 57, 60

with polyethylene glycol, 77
  pore sizes, 76
  in post-bariatric surgery patients, 64
  in pregnancy, 79
  prehospital use, 57–60, 79
  preparation, 76
  related formulations, 77
  for ricin poisoning in children, 1609
  risk:benefit assessment with, 76, 78–79
  for rivaroxaban-induced coagulopathy, 895
  for salicylate toxicity, 561
  for sedative-hypnotic overdose, 1087
  single-dose, 77–78
    pharmacokinetic effects, 152
  for SMFA ingestion, 1534
  with sorbitol, 61, 76–77, 80
  for SSRI overdose, 1057
  stocking, recommended level, 44t
  in strychnine poisoning, 1537
  studies of, 50t–51t, 53, 57, 58t–59t, 77
  supplies, 42
  surface areas, 76
  for thallium poisoning, 1353
    and Prussian blue, in vitro comparison,
      1357–1358
  time frame for use, 49, 57, 77–78
  trends in use, 48, 64–65
  and whole-bowel irrigation, 85
    interactions, 77
  and xenobiotic, ratio of, 60, 60f, 76–77, 79
  xenobiotics bound by, 76
  xenobiotics not bound by, 76

Activated clotting time, 890

Activated partial thromboplastin time (aPTT), 321,
    890, 893

Active Risk Identification and Analysis (ARIA) system,
    1838

Active transport, 141–142, 141f, 142

Acute care, access to, global disparities in, 1847

Acute coronary syndrome
  cocaine-related, 1129
  dabigatran and, 893
  rivaroxaban for, 894

Acute generalized exanthematous pustulosis,
    276, 276t

Acute interstitial nephritis, 391f, 392–394
  antimonials and, 1232
  clinical presentation, 393–394
  metals causing, 397t
  pathology, 393, 394f
  progression to chronic, 395
  xenobiotic-induced, 393–394, 394t

Acute kidney injury (AKI), 391–395
  and acute tubular necrosis, differentiation,
    393, 393t, 397
  amphetamine-induced, 1104
  with anticholinesterase poisoning, 1491–1493
  in arsenic poisoning, 1241
  bismuth-related, 1256
  cannabinoid-induced, 1117
  with colchicine poisoning, 503t
  deferoxamine overdose and, 678
  in DEG poisoning, 1444, 1446
  in ethylene glycol poisoning, 1424
  fluoroquinolones and, 826
  glomerular causes, 391–392
  in heatstroke, 421
  laboratory investigation, 396–397
  lithium-induced, 1068
  in methanol poisoning, 1424

NSAIDs and, 514–515
postrenal, 394–395
quinine-induced, 840
renal, 391–394
salicylates and, 558
sodium stibogluconate and, 1232
staging criteria, 391, 391t
in strychnine poisoning, 1537–1538
tubulointerstitial causes, 391–392
vancomycin-induced, 828
vascular causes, 391
Acute lung injury (ALI), 401
Acute myelogenous leukemia, all-*trans*-retinoic acid
    (ATRA), 656
Acute myeloid leukemia (AML), 320
Acute promyelocytic leukemia (APML)
    arsenic trioxide for, 1237–1238. *See also* Arsenic
        trioxide (white arsenic)
    all-*trans*-retinoic acid for, 656
Acute promyelocytic leukemia differentiation
        syndrome, 656, 658
Acute radiation syndrome (ARS), 13, 1762, 1768
    clinical manifestations, 1768
    subsyndromes, 1768
Acute renal failure. *See* Acute kidney injury (AKI)
Acute respiratory distress syndrome (ARDS), 37, 115t,
        123, 125f, 125t, 165, 401
    activated charcoal and, 79
    antimonials and, 1232
    in arsenic poisoning, 1241
    Berlin definition, 401, 1655, 1655t
    bipyridyl compounds and, 1475
    cadmium-induced, 1260
    calcium channel blockers and, 401, 402t
    carbon monoxide and, 401, 402t
    and cardiogenic pulmonary edema, differentiation,
        402
    catecholamine hypothesis, 401
    chlorhexidine-induced, 1368
    chromium-induced, 1270
    clinical manifestations, 1655
    cocaine-induced, 401, 402t
    with colchicine poisoning, 503, 503t
    cyclic antidepressants and, 402t, 1046–1047
    deferoxamine and, 678
    diagnosis, 401, 406
    diuretics and, 401
    in drug-induced hypersensitivity syndrome,
        277–278
    fatality rate, 401
    fluid management in, 401
    inhalational nickel exposure and, 1335–1336
    inhalational zinc toxicity and, 1363, 1365
    inhalation-induced, 1196, 1643f
    irritant gas exposure and, 402t, 1643f, 1654–1655
    lipid emulsion and, 1007
    management, 1653, 1657–1659
    mechanical ventilation in, 401, 407
    in mercury poisoning, 1326
    metal pneumonitis and, 1658
    methylxanthines and, 988
    morphine and, 401
    naloxone and, 540
    NSAID overdose and, 516
    opioid-related, 402t, 525
    in paraquat poisoning, 1475
    pathogenesis, 401
    pathophysiology, 401, 1641, 1653
    phosphine gas and, 1458
    positive end-expiratory pressure for, 401

salicylate-induced, 401, 402t, 558
sedative-hypnotics and, 401, 402t
severity, classification, 401, 1642
smoke inhalation and, 402t, 1641–1642, 1643f
toxin-induced, management, 1653
treatment, 402, 407–408, 1653
whole-bowel irrigation and, 85
xenobiotic-induced, 401–402, 402t, 1653
Acute tubular necrosis, 390f, 392
    in acetaminophen toxicity, 474
    and acute kidney injury, differentiation, 393, 393t,
        397
    bismuth-related, 1256
    copper poisoning and, 1286
    inhalational nickel exposure and, 1335–1336
    pathology, 392, 392f
    pathophysiology, 392, 392f
    shock, metals causing, 397t
    sodium stibogluconate and, 1232
    toxic, metals causing, 397t
    xenobiotics causing, 390f, 392, 392t
Acute tubulointerstitial nephritis (ATIN), from NSAIDs,
        515
Acyclovir, 829
    nephrotoxicity, 829
    renal effects, 390f
Adalimumab
    and posterior reversible encephalopathy syndrome,
        132
    and rhabdomyolysis, 393t
Adam. *See* 3,4-Methylenedioxymethamphetamine
        (MDMA, Adam, molly, ecstasy, XTC)
Adams, Samuel Hopkins, 9
Adamsite, 1749f
    toxic syndrome caused by, 1751t
ADAMTS13, 324
Adaptive immunity, 319
Adderpike (*Trachinus draco*), 1576
Addiction, 236–237. *See also specific xenobiotic*
    and dependence, differentiation, 236
Addiction medicine, 12
Additives, pharmaceutical. *See* Pharmaceutical
        additives
Adduct(s), 163
Adefovir, diabetes insipidus caused by, 195t
Adelfa. *See* Oleander
Adenoma(s), hepatic, 333
Adenosine, 203, 229–231, 873
    and acetylcholine release, 229
    action of, 229
    adverse effects and safety issues, 867t, 873
    in brain, 229
    and dopamine, 229
    extracellular, 229
    and glutamate release, 229
    methylxanthines and, 986
    pharmacokinetics, 867t
    pharmacology, 867t
    release, 229, 229f, 239
    reuptake, 229, 229f
        inhibitors, 230, 230t
    reverse transport, 229f, 230
    and seizure termination, 230
    synthesis, 229, 229f
    transport, 229–230, 229f
Adenosine agonists
    direct, 230, 230t
    and ethanol, 231
    indirect, 230–231, 230t
Adenosine antagonists, 230t, 231

methylxanthines as, 986
Adenosine deaminase, 229
    inhibitors, 230t, 231
Adenosine diphosphate receptor inhibitors, 899
    antidotes and treatment strategies for, 888t
    laboratory testing for, 888t
    mechanism of action, 898f
Adenosine kinase, 229, 229f
    inhibition, 231
Adenosine receptor(s), 229, 229f, 230
    A_1, 229f, 230, 239
    A_2, 229f, 230, 239
    A_3, 229f, 230
    affinity for adenosine, caffeine and, 239
    benzodiazepines and, 1084
    in spinal cord, 231
    xenobiotics affecting, 230–231, 230t
Adenosine reuptake inhibitors, 899
    antidotes and treatment strategies for, 888t
    laboratory testing for, 888t
    mechanism of action, 898f
Adenosine triphosphatase (ATPase)
    calcium, organic chlorine insecticides and, 1517
    copper (Menkes), 1284
    sodium, potassium, 203
        myocardial, 245, 245f
        organic chlorine insecticides and, 1516f, 1517
        thallium and, 1350
    in thermoregulation, 411
Adenosine triphosphate (ATP)
    hydrolysis, 177, 178f
    and insulin release, 694–695, 696f, 953, 953f
    metabolism
        adenosine and, 229, 229f
        cyanide and, 1685–1686
    in oxidative metabolism, 168
    synthesis, 175, 177, 707–708, 1006, 1157–1158, 1157f
        inhibitors, 176t
Adenosine triphosphate-binding cassette transporters.
        See ABC transporters
Adenylate cyclase, 204, 209, 213, 217, 220, 229f, 230, 238,
        260–261
    activation, by lizard venom, 1619
    inhibitors, 899, 1503
    in opioid receptor signal transduction, 522f
Adequate daily intake, for vitamins, 655t
Adhesives, inhaled, 1193t. *See also* Inhalant(s)
ADH gene family, 1144–1145, 1151
Adipocere, 1885
Adipocytes, beige, 606
Adipose tissue
    brown, 606
    cannabinoids in, 112
    in obese patients, 148
Administration. *See also specific xenobiotic*
    of medication, and errors, 1824–1826, 1825t
Administration route
    and absorption, 140–141, 144
    and interpretive toxicology, 1873t
Adolapin, 1551
Adolescent(s). *See also* Children
    solvent abuse by, 1409
Adonis microcarpa (pheasants eye), 979
ADP-arsenate, 1239, 1239f
ADP ribosyl cyclase, 217
Adrenal hemorrhage, with colchicine poisoning, 503
α-Adrenergic agonist(s)
    $α_1$-
        cardiac effects, 258t, 263t, 264
        decongestants as, 749, 749f

α-Adrenergic agonist(s) (*Cont.*):
  α$_2$-, 208, 211t, 212, 239
    cardiac effects, 256, 258t, 263t, 264, 924, 924t
    decongestants as, 749, 749f
    effects on vital signs, 29t–31t
    and female sexual dysfunction, 302f
    and glutamate release, 228
    mechanism of action, 210, 210f, 238f
    ophthalmic use, systemic toxicity with, 360
  decongestants as, 749, 749f
  effect on thermoregulation, 412–413, 413t
  ergot and ergot alkaloids and, 806, 807t
  and myocardial ischemia and infarction, 249
  and ST segment, 249
β-Adrenergic agonist(s). *See also specific xenobiotic*
  β$_2$-
    cardiac effects, 264
    effects on vital signs, 29t
    inhaled, 985
      for smoke inhalation, 1645
    selective, 985–993. *See also specific xenobiotic*
      adverse effects and safety issues, 986
      cardiovascular effects, 988, 990–991
      gastrointestinal effects, 988
      inhaled, 985
      metabolic effects, 989, 991
      pharmacokinetics, 987
      pharmacology, 986–987
      tachyphylaxis with, 986
      toxicity, 985–992
    toxicity
      activated charcoal for, 990
      gastrointestinal decontamination for, 990
      management, 989–992
      spectrum, 986
  cardiac effects, 264
  effects on vital signs, 30t
  immunologic effects, 929
  metabolic effects, 929
  noncardiac effects, 929
  overdose/poisoning
    dysrhythmias in, 255
    and organ donation, 1893t
  and potassium balance, 199
  for venomous caterpillar exposure, 1554
Adrenergic antagonist(s)
  α-. *See* α-Adrenergic antagonist(s)
  β-. *See* β-Adrenergic antagonist(s)
  for alcohol withdrawal, 1169
α-Adrenergic antagonist(s), 211t, 212
  α$_1$-
    antipsychotics as, 1034t, 1035
    effects on vital signs, 30t
    and male sexual function, 299f
  α$_2$-, 208, 212
    and cholinergic neurotransmission, 206f, 207t
    effects on vital signs, 29t
    and male sexual function, 299f
    physiologic effects, 212
  for α-adrenergic agonist overdose, 751
  diabetes insipidus caused by, 195, 195t
  indications for, 751
  priapism caused by, 301, 301t
β-Adrenergic antagonist(s), 211t, 212, 926–940. *See also specific xenobiotic*
  β$_1$-, cardiac effects, 258t
  β$_2$-
    action, 929–930
    cardiac effects, 258t
  adrenergic blocking activity, 927t, 930

for akathisia, 1036
antidote for, 35t
bioavailability, 927t
and calcium transport, 1405
cardiovascular effects, 247–248, 256, 263–265, 924, 924t
for cocaine-associated chest pain, 1129
and cocaine toxicity, risks of, 1129
combined products, 931–932
contraindications to, 1129
for dysrhythmias, in inhalant abuse, 1199
effect on thermoregulation, 412–413, 413t
effects on vital signs, 29t–30t
elimination half-life, 927t
for glaucoma, 926
history of, 926
hypoglycemia caused by, 698
indications for, 926
for inhalant-related dysrhythmias, 1199
intrinsic sympathomimetic activity, 930, 932
lipid solubility, 930, 932
Log D, 927t
and male sexual dysfunction, 299f
membrane-stabilizing effects, 927t, 930, 932, 936
metabolism, 927t
and neuromuscular blockers, interactions, 1021t
ophthalmic, 926, 927t, 932
  pharmacology, 927t, 931
  systemic toxicity with, 360
partial agonist activity, 927t, 930, 932
pediatric delayed toxicity, 452
pharmacokinetics, 927t, 930–931
pharmacology, 926–930, 927t, 930–931
potassium channel blockade, 930, 932
protein binding, 927t
β$_1$ selectivity, 927t, 930–932
structures, 926f
sustained-release, 932
and thiazide diuretics, combined, 931
for thyrotoxicosis, 817
and tinnitus, 370t
toxicity (overdose/poisoning), 198
  calcium for, 933, 933f, 1405
  cardiac effects, 258, 709, 924, 925f, 953–954
  case study, 924, 925f
  catecholamines for, 934, 942
  clinical manifestations, 931–932
  diagnostic tests for, 932
  epidemiology, 926
  experimental treatments, 935
  extracorporeal treatment, 935
  gastrointestinal decontamination for, 932–933
  glucagon for, 933, 941–942
  high-dose insulin for, 942, 953–958
  insulin and glucose for, 933–934, 933f
  lipid emulsion for, 1007
  management, 44t–45t, 709, 924, 932–936, 933f
  mechanical life support in, 935
  membrane-stabilizing effects and, 936
  mortality rate for, 926
  observation in, 936
  pathophysiology, 931
  peripheral vasodilation and, 936
  phosphodiesterase inhibitors for, 934–935
  sodium bicarbonate for, 568t
  ventricular pacing for, 935
vasodilating effects, 927t, 930–932, 936
volume of distribution, 91, 927t
Adrenergic blockers. *See* Adrenergic antagonist(s)
Adrenergic receptor(s), 208–210, 260–262

α-. *See* α-Adrenergic receptor(s)
β-. *See* β-Adrenergic receptor(s)
cellular physiology, 260–261, 261f
physiological effects, 263t
subclasses, physiologic effects, 261–262
α-Adrenergic receptor(s), 206f, 208–210
  α$_1$-, 209–210, 261–262, 262f, 264
    cyclic antidepressants and, 1044
    subtypes, 209
  α$_2$-, 209–210, 261–262
    activation, 210f, 212
    central and peripheral, 206f, 209–210, 209f, 212, 239
    subtypes, 209, 212
  and bladder function, 304, 305f
  cardiac effects, 264, 265t
  dopamine and, 212
  types, 209
β-Adrenergic receptor(s), 206f, 208–209
  β$_1$-, 208–209, 261–262, 261t
    cardiac, 928
    heart and, 929, 929f
  β$_2$-, 208–209, 261–262, 261t
    cardiac, 928–929
    stimulation of, 929
  β$_3$-, 208–209, 261, 261t, 929
  and bladder function, 304, 305f
  cardiac, 928–929, 929f
  dopamine and, 212
  in heart, 929
  in immune system, 929
  metabolic effects of, 929
  polymorphism, 209
  and smooth muscle relaxation, 929
  types and functions, 208, 261–262, 261t, 928
Adrenocorticotropic hormone (ACTH)
  and sexual function, 304
  and thermoregulation, 412
Adrenopituitary function, lead and, 1296
Adverse drug events (ADEs). *See also* FDA Adverse Event Reporting System (FAERS); Medication errors; *specific xenobiotic*
  ameliorable, 1826
  costs, 1822
  cytochrome P450 and, 170
  data collection on, 1792, 1842
  definition, 1822, 1833
  detection, toxicologist's role in, 1841–1842
  diagnosis, establishing, 1838–1839, 1838t
  drug approval process and, 1833–1835
  in elderly, 460, 463–464, 1823
    age distribution, 460
    comorbidity and, 464
    complicated medication regimens and, 464
    inadequate premarketing research and, 465
    medication/xenobiotic interactions and, 465–466
    polypharmacy and, 464
    prescriber lack of knowledge and, 464
    prescribing medications too soon and, 464–465
    prevalence, 460
    risk factors for, 464–466
  epidemiology, 1822
  geriatric considerations, 1826–1827
  incidence, 1822
  morbidity and mortality caused by, 1822–1823
  pediatric considerations, 1826
  preventable, 1826
  prevention, toxicologist's role in, 1841–1842
  rare, 1837, 1841
  reporting requirements, 1836

serious, characteristics of, 1837
toxicologists' role in, 1830, 1841–1842
type A, 1838
type B, 1838–1839
Adverse drug reaction, definition, 1822
Aedes aegypti, 1522
Aerosols
definition, 1809
secondary contamination with, 1809
in smoke, 1640–1641
Aerozine-50, 863
Aesculin (esculoside, esculin), 1610
Aesculus hippocastanum (horse chestnut), 642t, 1598t, 1610
Affective disorders, and suicide, 378–379
Affinity constant (K_m), 1440
Aflatoxin, 332
in biological warfare, 1759
and fatty acid metabolism, 176t
Aflatoxin B, 174t
African boomslang (*Dispholidus typus*), 1633t
Africanized honeybees, 1551
African rue. *See* Syrian rue (*Peganum harmala*)
Afterdepolarization
delayed, 255, 970
electrophysiology, 253t, 254, 254f
and dysrhythmias, 254–255
early, 251, 254f, 255–256, 1265
electrophysiology, 253t, 254, 254f
Afterdrop, 418
Agathosma betulina (buchu), 640t
uses and toxicities, 640t
Agatoxin, and calcium channels, 945t
Agave, 1598t
Agave lechequilla, 1598t
Agency for Toxic Substances and Disease Registry (ATSDR), 12, 1804, 1808
website, information from, 1814
Agent 15, 1750
Agent Orange, 17, 17t, 1480
Ageratina altissima (white snakeroot), 1611
Ageusia, 365, 365t
Aggrenox, 899
Aggression. *See also* Violence
cocaine and, 1127
Aging. *See* Elderly; Geriatric principles
Agitation, 33–36
amphetamine-induced, 1103–1104
management, 1104–1105, 1104t
antihistamine-related, management, 748
in arylcyclohexylamine toxicity, management, 1217
benzodiazepines for, 1138–1139
cannabinoid-induced, 1117
cocaine and, 1127–1128
cyclic antidepressants and, 1046–1047
hallucinogen-induced, 1184
inhalant-induced, 1200
poisoning/overdose causing, 36t
therapeutics for, 35t
in toxidromes, 29t
treatment, 385–387
Agkistrodon bilineatus bilineatus, 1636t
Agkistrodon bilineatus howardgloydi, 1636t
Agkistrodon bilineatus lemosespinali, 1636t
Agkistrodon bilineatus russeolus, 1636t
Agkistrodon bilineatus taylori, 1636t
Agkistrodon contortrix (copperhead), 1617, 1617t, 1618f, 1633t. *See also* Pit vipers (Crotalinae)
envenomation

clinical manifestations, 1621
deaths caused by, 1618
geographic distribution, 1618
Agkistrodon piscivorus (cottonmouth), 1617, 1617t. *See also* Pit vipers (Crotalinae)
antivenom, 1627–1631, 1627t
envenomation, clinical manifestations, 1621
geographic distribution, 1618
Agkistrodon rhodostoma. *See* Malayan pit viper (*Calloselasma rhodostoma*)
Aglycones, 639, 969, 1597, 1598t, 1603t, 1604, 1606
Agmatine, 212
Agnosia, carbon monoxide poisoning and, 1665
Agomelatine, mechanism of action, 218
Agranulocytosis, 319–320
antipsychotic-induced, 1039
chemotherapeutic-related, management, 764
herbal causing, 647
idiosyncratic xenobiotic-induced, 320, 320t
NSAID-induced, 516
quinine-induced, 840
thioamide-induced, 818
AGREE Instrument, 1857
Agrippina, 2
AH-7921, 529
AH25086, 808
AIDS. *See* HIV-infected (AIDS) patients
Aimovig, 809
Air, free intraperitoneal, 127
Air embolism, hyperbaric oxygen for, 1676, 1679
Air fresheners, inhaled, 1193, 1193t. *See also* Inhalant(s)
Air pollution
indoor, in developing world, 1847
outdoor, 1798
toxic gases in, 16, 16t, 17. *See also specific gas*
Air potato (*Breynia officinalis*), 1611
Air-purifying respirator (APR), 1810–1811, 1810t
Airspace filling, 123
diagnostic imaging, 115t
diffuse, 115t, 123, 125f, 125t
focal, 123–125, 125f, 125t
multifocal, 125, 125t, 126f
Airway
edema, smoke inhalation and, 1641–1642, 1645
management
with caustic exposure, 1392–1393
in poisoned patient, 403
with smoke inhalation, 1643–1645, 1644f
obstruction, 400
irritant gases and, 1641
with smoke inhalation, 1645
patency, 400
Ajoene, 642t
Akathisia, 344
antipsychotic-induced, 1036, 1037t
SSRIs and, 1058
tardive, 1036
treatment, 1036, 1037t
Akt, 1065–1066, 1066f
Alachlor, 1472
in herbicides, 1467t
structure, 1472f
toxicity, clinical manifestations, 1473
Alacramyn, 1549
Alanine, 179–181
and NMDA receptor, 227t
β-Alanine, as glycine agonist, 223
Alanine aminotransferase, 181
in acetaminophen toxicity, 480–481
elevation, methotrexate-related, 768

in heatstroke, 422
in liver injury, 327–328, 334, 335t
ALARA (as low as reasonably achievable), for radiation exposure, 1767
Albendazole, 829
for HIV-related infections, 830t
Albiglutide, 607t, 694. *See also* Dieting xenobiotics and regimens
pharmacokinetics and toxicokinetics, 696, 697t
pharmacology, 696
Albumin
cobalt binding, 1273
in dialysis, for Wilson disease, 1289
and doping analysis, 623
in liver support devices, 96
serum
age-related changes in, 462
and anion gap, 191
in liver injury, 334–335, 335t
xenobiotic binding to, 146
Albumin Cobalt Binding (ACB) test, 1273
Albuterol, 985
pharmacokinetics, 987
pharmacology, 986
quaternary ammonium compounds in, 1374
for smoke inhalation, 1645
and tinnitus, 370t
toxicokinetics, 987
Alcohol(s), 8, 1410. *See also* Ethanol (alcohol); *specific alcohol*
as antiseptics, 1368, 1369t, 1372
breath odor from, 38
chemistry, 165–166
dermatologic effects, 269
disasters due to, 21–22, 21t, 1430
ethyl. *See* Ethanol (alcohol)
as functional groups, 165–166
laboratory testing for, 101t
nomenclature, 165
oxidation, 168
pancreatitis caused by, 295t
pharmacokinetics, 145t
primary, 165–166, 1422
secondary, 165–166, 1422
tertiary, 165
toxic. *See* Toxic alcohol(s)
Alcohol abuse and alcoholism, 1151–1152. *See also* Ethanol (alcohol)
and acetaminophen toxicity, 480
and affective disorders, 1152
and aggression and violence, 384–385
cardiovascular abnormalities in, 126
cerebellar atrophy in, 134
deaths caused by, 1143–1144
definition, 1151
and depression, 1152
diagnosis
Alcohol Use Disorders Identification Test for, 1151–1152, 1152t
CAGE questions for, 1151, 1151t
Michigan Alcoholism Screening Test (MAST) for, 1151, 1151t
diffuse airspace filling in, 125t
in elderly, 466–467
epidemiology, 1143–1144
and erectile dysfunction, 300
gastrointestinal perforation in, 127
genetics, 1151
head trauma in, imaging, 131, 132t, 134f
history and epidemiology, 1165

Alcohol abuse and alcoholism (*Cont.*):
  hospitalization for, indications for, 1150–1151
  lifetime risk for, in men, 1165
  magnesium in, 878
  neuronal atrophy in, 131
  organ system effects, 1146, 1147t
  pathophysiology, 1146, 1165
  screening for, 1151
  and suicidality/suicide, 378, 1152
  therapeutics for, 35t, 1152
  thiamine deficiency in, 878, 1157, 1160
  treatment, 1152
Alcohol dehydrogenase (ADH), 159, 166, 166f,
    1144–1145, 1285t, 1422
  activity, 168, 168f
  age-related changes in, 461
  antihistamines and, 744
  in diethylene glycol metabolism, 1444, 1445f
  ethanol affinity for, 1440
  ethanol assays based on, 1877
  in ethanol metabolism, 1428
  in ethylene glycol metabolism, 1422, 1423f, 1428
  genes for, 1144–1145
  γ-hydroxybutyrate and, 1188–1189, 1189f
  inhibition, 1144
    ethanol and, 1440
    fomepizole and, 1428, 1435, 1440
    for toxic alcohol poisoning, 1428
  in isopropanol metabolism, 1423, 1423f
  in methanol metabolism, 1422, 1423f, 1428
  pyrazole and, 1435
  in spectrochemical testing, 103
  zinc in, 1362
Alcohol dependence, 1166
  gabapentin for, 1170
  lifetime risk for, in men, 1165
Alcohol hangover, 1143. *See also* Ethanol (alcohol)
Alcohol herbicides, 1467t
Alcoholic beverages. *See* Ethanol (alcohol)
Alcoholic hallucinosis, 1166
Alcoholic ketoacidosis (AKA), 37, 192, 709, 1146, 1149
  clinical and laboratory findings in, 36t
  clinical features, 1150–1151
  hyperventilation caused by, 400t
  management, 193, 1151, 1160–1161
  pathophysiology, 179, 1150
  thiamine for, 1160–1161
Alcoholics Anonymous (AA), 381
Alcoholic tremulousness, 1166
Alcohol intoxication. *See* Ethanol (alcohol),
    intoxication
Alcoholism. *See* Alcohol abuse and alcoholism
Alcohol-related birth defects (ARBD), 438
Alcohol-related motor vehicle crash(es)
  costs of, 1862
  deaths caused by, 1143–1144, 1862, 1877
  driver involved in, and permissible phlebotomy,
    1862–1864
  incidence, 1862, 1877
Alcohol-related neurodevelopmental disorder (ARND),
    438
Alcohol test, for drunk driving, 1876–1877
Alcohol use disorder (AUD), 1151–1152, 1151t
  DSM-5 criteria for, 380, 380t
Alcohol Use Disorders Identification Test (AUDIT,
    AUDIT-C), 1151–1152, 1152t
Alcohol withdrawal, 222, 236t, 237, 1165–1171
  and agitation/violence, 385
  benzodiazepine-resistant, 1165, 1168–1169
  benzodiazepines for, 1138

clinical and biochemical predictors, 1167
clinical manifestations, 36t, 1165–1166
diagnostic criteria for, 1165, 1166t
diagnostic tests for, 1167
DSM-V criteria for, 1165, 1166t
early uncomplicated, clinical manifestations, 1166
effects on vital signs, 29t–31t
in elderly, 467
genetics and, 1166–1167
history and epidemiology, 1165
hyperthermia in, 27, 27t
and ICU admission, 1168–1169
and kindling phenomenon, 1165
laboratory findings in, 36t, 1167
magnesium for, 878
management, 1167–1170
  historical perspective on, 1165
outpatient management, 1167
pathophysiology, 1165
in postsurgical and trauma patients, 1165
resistant
  and ICU admission, 1168
  management, 1168–1170
and rhabdomyolysis, 393
risk factors for, 1166–1167
seizures in, 228, 237, 1165–1166
  management of, 1167
  predictive factors, 1167
severity, 1165–1166
  assessment, 1166
  risk factors for, 1166–1167
therapeutics for, 35t
timing, 1165
toxic syndrome caused by, 29t
Alcohol withdrawal syndrome (AWS), 1165
Aldehyde(s), 166, 166f, 1369t, 1410
  oxidation, 168
  as thermal degradation product, 1641t
Aldehyde dehydrogenase (ALDH), 168
  in diethylene glycol metabolism, 1444, 1445f
  disulfiram and, 1173, 1173f
  disulfiram metabolites and, 1173
  in ethanol metabolism, 1144–1145, 1145f
  in ethylene glycol metabolism, 1422, 1423f
  γ-hydroxybutyrate and, 1188, 1189f
  inhibition, by cyclopropanone hydrate and coprine,
    1587
  inhibitors, 1173, 1173f
  in methanol metabolism, 1422, 1423f
Aldehyde herbicides, 1467t
Aldehyde oxidase, 768
Alder buckthorn (*Rhamnus frangula*), 1602t
Alderlin, 926
ALDH gene family, 1144–1145, 1151
Aldicarb, 1450
  food contamination with, 599
  toxicity (poisoning), 1510
    epidemics, 1487
    management, 1498
Aldohexose, 707
Aldrin, 1514
  physicochemical properties, 1515t
  structure, 1516f
Alendronate, skeletal effects, imaging, 119, 123f
Aleurites fordii (tung seed). *See* Tonka bean (*Dipteryx*
    odorata, D. oppositifolia)
Aleurites moluccana (tung seed). *See* Tonka bean
    (*Dipteryx odorata, D. oppositifolia*)
Alexander of Tralles, 501
Alexander VI (Pope), 4

Alexandrian senna. *See* Senna
Alexipharmaca, 1t, 2–3
Alfalfa (*Medicago sativa*), uses and toxicities, 640t
Algae, 1597
  blue-green, 1601t
    Anabaena, 1598t, 1601t
    Aphanizomenon, 1598t
    Microcystis, 1601t
Alimentary toxic aleukia, 1759
Aliphatic hydrocarbons. *See* Hydrocarbons, aliphatic
Aliphatics, adsorption to activated charcoal, 76
Aliskiren, 965, 1070
  as antihypertensive, 959t, 965
  contraindications to, 965
Alkadienes, 1410. *See also* Hydrocarbons
Alkalemia
  definition, 190
  effects on oxygenation, 403f
Alkali(s). *See also* Caustics; *specific xenobiotic*
  definition, 1388
  dermal toxicity, 271
  exposure to, pathophysiology, 1389, 1389f
  gastrointestinal perforation caused by, 127
  ingestion
    clinical manifestations, 1390–1391
    worldwide, 1846
  injury caused by
    clinical presentation, 1390–1391
    endoscopic evaluation, 1390, 1390t, 1391
  ophthalmic decontamination for, 72–73
  ophthalmic exposure to, irrigating solution for, 359t
  ophthalmic toxicity, 356f
  predictors of injury with, 1390–1391
Alkali disease, 1339. *See also* Selenium
Alkali metal(s), 156f, 157
Alkaline earth metals, 156f, 157
Alkaline phosphatase
  in liver injury, 334, 335t
  zinc in, 1362
Alkalinity. *See* pH
Alkalinization. *See also* Sodium bicarbonate (NaHCO₃)
  plasma, rationale for, 560f
  rationale for, 560f
  for salicylate toxicity, 562, 562f, 563
  serum, for salicylate toxicity, 562, 562f
  for toxic alcohol poisoning, 1430
  urine. *See* Urine, alkalinization
Alkaloids. *See also specific alkaloid*
  anticholinergic, 2, 1604. *See also* Belladonna
    alkaloids
  antimitotic, 1612
  cholinergic, 1605
  definition, 1597
  indole, 1612
  isoquinoline, 1605
  mescaline, 1605
  nicotinelike, 1604–1605
  plant, 639, 1597, 1598t–1603t, 1604–1606
  psychotropic, 1605
  pyridine, 1607
  steroidal, 1604
  taxine-derived, 1612
  veratrum, 1603t, 1611
Alkalosis. *See also* Metabolic alkalosis; Respiratory
    alkalosis
  and anion gap, 191t
  definition, 190
Alkanes, 165–166, 165f, 1410. *See also* Hydrocarbons
Alkenes, 165, 1410. *See also* Hydrocarbons
Alkermes, 539

Alkoxyl radical, structure, 160t
Alkylating agents, 349f, 759, 760t, 761f. *See also*
      Antineoplastics; *specific xenobiotic*
   antidotes for, 760t
   mechanism of action, 350f, 759, 761, 761f–762f
   overdose/poisoning, clinical and laboratory findings
      with, 36t
   site of action, 762f
   teratogenicity, 429t
Alkyl lead, 1294
Alkyl mercury compounds
   absorption, 1325
   poisoning, clinical manifestations, 1327
   tissue distribution, 1325
Alkyl nitrites
   as aphrodisiacs, 304t
   inhaled volatile, 1193–1194
      clinical manifestations of, 1199t
      pharmacology, 1195, 1195t
      use/abuse, clinical manifestations, 1198–1199
Alkylphosphate poisoning, and organ donation, 1893t
Alkyl selenides, 1340
Alkyl sulfonates, enhanced elimination, 764
Alkynes, 165, 1410
Alleles, 169
Allenic norleucine, 1582t, 1589t, 1593
   structure, 1590
Allergens
   in contact dermatitis, 279
   inhaled. *See also specific allergen*
      imaging, 115t
   respiratory effects, 399t
Allergic contact dermatitis, 274t. *See also* Contact
      dermatitis
   plant-induced, 1613–1614
      as occupational injury, 1614
Allergic reactions. *See also* Allergy(ies)
   antimonials and, 1233
   therapeutics for, 35t
Allergic rhinitis, urticating hairs of tarantula and, 1547
Allergy(ies)
   to antimicrobials, 821
   to ant stings, 1552
   to caterpillars, 1553
   to Hymenoptera venom, 1552
   jellyfish stings and, 1569
   with local anesthetics, 997
   to mushrooms, 1594
   to penicillins, 823
   to protamine, 919–920
   to sulfonamides, 827
Allethrin, 1519, 1520t
   structure, 1520f
Alliaria officinalis (horseradish root), 1607
Alliin, 642t
Allium porrum (leeks), 1611
Allium sativum (garlic)
   pharmacologic interactions, 646t
   uses and toxicities, 642t
   volatile oils in, 639
Allium tricoccum (ramps), 1606
Allium ursinum (wild garlic), *Colchicum autumnale*
      (autumn crocus) and, confusion, 501
Allocryptopine, 650t
Allopurinol
   acute interstitial nephritis caused by, 394t
   for carbon monoxide poisoning, 1672
   in drug-induced hypersensitivity syndrome, 278
   hepatitis caused by, 330
   renal effects, 390f

Alloxan
   and pancreatic dysfunction, 295t
   site of action, 173f
Alloxydim, in herbicides, 1467t
All-*trans*-retinoic acid (ATRA)
   for acute myelogenous leukemia, 656
   for acute promyelocytic leukemia, 656
   for myelodysplastic syndrome, 656
Allyl alcohol
   effects on liver, 328
   in herbicides, 1467t
N-Allylnorcodeine, 538
N-Allylnormorphine, 538
Almond, 1602t
Almotriptan, 217, 808–809, 808t
Alnico, 1273
Aloe (*Aloe vera, A. barbadensis, Aloe* spp.), 608t, 1598t
   glycosides in, 639
   as laxative, 83
   uses and toxicities, 640t
Alogliptin
   pharmacokinetics and toxicokinetics, 697t
   pharmacology, 696
Aloinosides, 1598t
Alopecia
   in arsenic poisoning, 1241
   chemotherapeutics and, 761
   in colchicine poisoning, 503, 503t
   differential diagnosis, 1353
   poisoning/overdose causing, 36t
   in thallium toxicity, 1351–1352
   in zinc deficiency, 1363
Alosetron, 218
Alpha (α) (type I error), 1855
Alpha particles, 1762–1763
Alprazolam. *See also* Sedative-hypnotics
   duration of action, 1137
   gastrointestinal decontamination for, 54t
   pharmacokinetics and toxicokinetics, 145t, 1085t
   volume of distribution, 145t
   withdrawal, 1088
Alprostadil
   adverse effects and safety issues, 300
   for erectile dysfunction, 300
   mechanism of action, 300
Alquist, Raymond, 926
Alstroemeria spp. (Peruvian lily), 1614
Altamisa. *See* Feverfew (*Tanacetum parthenium*)
Altered mental status (AMS), 194
   cathartics causing, 85
   definition, 33
   in elderly, 460
   hypercalcemia and, 199
   hypoglycemia and, 707–708, 710
   management of patient with, 33–37, 34f, 707, 1149,
      1862
   smoke inhalation and, 1642
   spectrum, 33
   in toxidromes, 28, 29t
   and violence/agitation, 384
Alternative hypothesis, 1855
Alternative medicine. *See specific herb; specific treatment*
Alum, 1223–1224
Alumina, 1223
Aluminosis, 1223–1225
Aluminoxamine, 1225
Aluminum, 1223–1227
   absorption, 1224
   alkyl of, dermal decontamination for, precautions
      with, 72

   in alum, 1223–1224
   in antacids, 1223, 1225
   antidote for, 35t
   in brain, 1224–1225
      normal concentration, 1225
   chemistry, 1223
   contamination of dialysates, 98–99
   dermal absorption, from antiperspirants, 1224
   dietary intake, 1224
   elimination half-life, 1224
   excretion, 1224
   in gems, 1223
   history and epidemiology, 1223
   inhaled, pulmonary absorption, 1224
   isotopes, 1223
   metabolism, 1224
   neurotoxicity, 1224–1225
   as occupational toxin, 1223
   in ores, 1223
   oxidation state, 1223
   physicochemical properties, 1223
   products containing, 1223
   serum, normal concentration, 1223, 1225
   in sucralfate, 1223, 1225
   tissue distribution, 1224
   toxicity, 98
      acute
         clinical manifestations, 1224
         management, 1225
      chelation therapy for, 1225
      chronic
         clinical manifestations, 1224–1225
         management, 1225
      clinical manifestations, 1224–1225
      CNS effects, 1224
      deferoxamine for, 677–678
      diagnostic tests for, 1225
      hematologic effects, 1224
      historical perspective on, 1223
      management, 1225
      multisystem manifestations, 1225
      musculoskeletal effects, 1224
      pathophysiology, 1224
      pulmonary effects, 1224
   toxicokinetics, 1223–1224
   urine
      measurement, 1225
      normal concentration, 1223, 1225
   volume of distribution, 1224
   whole blood, normal concentration, 1223, 1225
Aluminum citrate, for ethylene glycol poisoning, 1430
Aluminum hydroxide, 1225
   in antacids, 1223
   effect on thyroid hormones and function, 814t, 817
   for levothyroxine overdose, 817
Aluminum phosphide, 1450, 1457
   odor, 364t
   physicochemical properties, 1457
   toxic dose, 1458
   toxicity (poisoning)
      clinical manifestations, 1458
      epidemiology, 1457
      magnesium for, 879
      management, 709
      prognosis for, 1459
      treatment, 1459–1460
Aluminum salts, as neurotoxins, 1223
Alveolar–arterial (A–a) oxygen gradients, 400, 408f
Alveolar partial pressure of carbon dioxide ($PACO_2$),
      408f

Alveolar partial pressure of oxygen (PAO$_2$), 399–400, 408f
Alvimopan, 84
  contraindications to, 542
  dosage and administration, 542
  indications for, 542
Alzheimer disease, 756
  aluminum and, 1223–1224
  copper and, 1283
  glutamate and, 224
  pathophysiology, 1295
  treatment, 228
AM2201, 1111, 1112f
  acute toxicity, 1117
  metabolism, 1116f
AM4113, 611
Amabiline, 640t
Amanita spp.
  geographic distribution, 1581
  hepatotoxicity, management, 1586
  poisoning with
    deaths caused by, 1581
    multiple-dose activated charcoal in, 61
  protective tissues, 1584f
  toxin exposure, liver support devices for, 96
Amanita abrupta, 1590
Amanita franchetti, 1582t, 1591
Amanita gemmata, 1582t, 1588
Amanita muscaria (fly agaric), 3, 1178–1179, 1582t, 1587–1588, 1589f
Amanita ocreata, 1586
Amanita pantherina, 1179, 1582t, 1587–1588
Amanita phalloides, 2, 5t, 6, 600, 1581–1583, 1582t, 1583f, 1586, 1594
  poisoning with
    activated charcoal for, 1584–1585
    multiple-dose activated charcoal in, 61, 1586
    treatment, 1584–1586
Amanita proxima, 1582t, 1590
Amanita pseudoporphyria, 1582t, 1590
Amanita smithiana, 600, 1582t, 1590–1591, 1590f, 1593
Amanita tenuifolia, 1582t
Amanita verna, 1581
Amanita virosa, 1581, 1582t, 1583f, 1586, 1594
α-Amanitin, 1583–1585
  as biological weapon, 1759
  mechanism of action, 167, 1583
  structure, 1581
  transporter-mediated uptake, 173, 1583
β-Amanitin, 1583–1584
Amantadine
  cardiac effects, 248, 258t
  and dopamine reuptake, 214
  for drug-induced parkinsonism, 1037
  effects on QRS complex, 567–569
  and levodopa, combined, 228
  mechanism of action, 227t, 228
  and prolonged QT interval, 253t
  syrup, sorbitol in, 688t
  toxicity, sodium bicarbonate for, 568t, 569
Amaranthaceae, 1610
Amaryllidaceae, 1598t, 1601t
Amatoxin(s), 1581–1584, 1593
  clinical and laboratory findings with, 36t, 1589t
  extracorporeal elimination, 97t
  hepatotoxicity
    N-acetylcysteine for, 494–495, 1585
    treatment, 1584–1586
  mushrooms containing, 1582t

Amberlite XAD-2, 96
Amberlite XAD-4, 96
Amblyopia, quinine, 361
Ambrosia spp. (ragweed), 1614
Ambroxol, for paraquat poisoning, 1474f, 1476
American Academy of Clinical Toxicology (AACT), 11, 11t
American Academy of Pediatrics (AAP)
  Committee on Accident Prevention, 1789
  The Injury Prevention Program, 1784
American Association of Poison Control Centers (AAPCC), 11, 11t. *See also* Antivenom Index
American Board of Applied Toxicology (ABAT), 11t, 12
American Board of Medical Toxicology (ABMT), 11t, 12
American cancer pokeweed (*Phytolacca americana*), 1601t
American College of Medical Toxicology (ACMT), 11t, 12
American cone flower. *See* Echinacea (*Echinacea angustifolia, E. purpurea*)
American Conference of Governmental and Industrial Hygienists, 1808
American dog tick (*Dermacentor variabilis*), 1550
American dwarf palm tree. *See* Saw palmetto (*Serenoa repens*)
American holly, 642t
American mistletoe (*Phoradendron* spp.), 1601t, 1609
American nightshade. *See* Pokeweed (*Phytolacca americana, P. decandra*)
American nightshade (*Solanum americanum*), 1602t
American pennyroyal. *See* Pennyroyal (*Mentha pulegium, Hedeoma pulegioides*)
American podophyllum. *See* Podophyllin; Podophyllum (*Podophyllum* spp.)
Americans with Disabilities Act (ADA), 1800, 1801t
Americans with Disabilities Act Amendment Act of 2008 (ADAAA), 1800, 1801t
Americium (Am)
  antidote for, 35t
  chemistry, 1769
  contamination, in Oak Ridge TN, 1769
  DTPA for, 1779–1781, 1779f
  internal contamination by, management, 44t
  radioactive, 1769
Amethopterin, 775. *See also* Methotrexate
Ametryn poisoning, 1483
Amiben. *See* Chloramben
Amide(s), 1410. *See also* Hydrocarbons
  structure, 1472f
Amide herbicides, 1467t
Amifostine, 367
  for cisplatin toxicity, 764
Amikacin, 821–823
  and neuromuscular blockers, interactions, 1021t
  toxicity, clinical manifestations, 822t
Amiloride. *See also* Diuretics, potassium-sparing
  for diabetes insipidus, 196
  for hypertension, 963
  and thiamine pharmacokinetics, 1158
Amines, 1075
  biogenic
    amphetamines and, 1099–1100, 1100f
    reuptake, cocaine and, 1125
  lipophilic, and ATP synthesis, 176t
  secondary, 1044, 1044t
  tertiary, 1044, 1044t
Amino acid(s), 179–181. *See also* Excitatory amino acid (EAA) neurotransmitters
  essential, 179

  in gluconeogenesis, 178
  postmortem changes, 1885t
  synthesis, 175
L-Amino acid decarboxylase (AADC), 215, 216f
L-Amino acid oxidase(s), in snake venom, 1618
Amino alcohols, 836–842
  antimalarial mechanism, 836, 837f, 838t
γ-Aminobutyric acid. *See* GABA
γ-Aminobutyric acid receptors. *See* GABA receptor(s)
Aminocaproic acid, 321f, 884f, 897
  adverse effects and safety issues, 897
  and fibrinolysis, 323
  for fibrinolytic overdose/poisoning, 888t
1-Aminocyclopropanol, 1582t, 1588f
2-Amino-2-deoxyglucose, uses and toxicities, 642t
Aminoglutethimide, 617, 618f
  effect on thyroid hormones and function, 814t
Aminoglycosides, 821–823
  acute interstitial nephritis caused by, 394t
  acute tubular necrosis caused by, 392
  adverse drug reactions with therapeutic use, 821
  adverse effects and safety issues, 821, 822t
  cranial neuropathy caused by, 346t
  dosage and administration, in obese patients, 148
  excipients, adverse effects, 821
  extracorporeal elimination, 97t
  formulations, 821
  hypocalcemia caused by, 199
  hypomagnesemia caused by, 877
  mechanism of action, 822t
  nephrotoxicity, 392, 394t, 821–822
  and neuromuscular blockers, interactions, 1021t
  and NSAIDs, interactions, 514t
  ototoxicity, 366f, 821–823
  renal effects, 390f
  and tinnitus, 370t
  toxicity (overdose/poisoning), 821, 822t
    clinical and laboratory findings with, 36t, 576t, 822t
2*R*-Amino-5-hexynoic acid, 1591
2*R*-Amino-4,5-hydroxy-5-hexynoic acid, 1582t, 1589t, 1591
α-Amino-3-hydroxy-5-methyl-4-isoxazole propionate. *See* AMPA
5-Aminoimidazole-4-carboxamide ribonucleotide (AICAR) transformylase, methotrexate and, 767
Aminoindanes, and serotonin toxicity, 1058t
5-Aminolevulinic acid (ALA), 314, 314f
Aminolevulinic acid dehydratase, 314, 314f
δ-Aminolevulinic acid dehydrogenase, aluminum and, 1224
Aminolevulinic acid synthetase (ALAS), 314, 314f
6-Aminonicotinamide, and tinnitus, 370t
1,2-Amino-4-pentynoic acid, 1590
Aminophylline
  elimination, multiple-dose activated charcoal and, 62, 78
  intrathecal administration
    clinical manifestations, 793
    inadvertent overdose and unintentional exposures due to, 795t
  therapeutic use, 985
  in neonates, 985
β-Aminopropionitrile (BAPN), 1601t, 1609
Aminopterin, 775, 782
  teratogenicity, 429t, 433
4-Aminopyridine, mechanism of action, 933f
Aminopyridines, and acetylcholine release, 207, 207t
Aminopyrine, 647

4-Aminoquinolines, 836, 842–844
  antimalarial mechanism, 836, 837f, 838t, 842
8-Aminoquinolines, 836, 844–845, 847
  antimalarial mechanism, 837f, 838t
para-Aminosalicylic acid
  adverse effects and safety issues, 853t, 857–858
  monitoring with, 853t
  pharmacokinetics, 857
  for tuberculosis, 857–858
Aminosilane-iron oxide, SPIO nanoparticles, 1719t
2-Aminothiazoline-4-carboxylic acid (ACTA), 1687
Aminotransferases. *See also specific enzyme*
  hepatic, in liver injury, 334, 335t
Amiodarone, 871–873
  adverse effects and safety issues, 867t, 872–873
  ARDS caused by, 402t
  benzyl alcohol in, 683t
  cranial neuropathy caused by, 346t
  effect on thyroid hormones and function, 813f, 814t
  and fatty acid metabolism, 176t
  hepatotoxicity, 332
  for hypothermia, 417
  and loratadine, interactions, 746
  ophthalmic toxicity, 356f
  overdose/poisoning
    chest X-ray findings in, 115t, 125t, 126, 126f
    clinical and laboratory findings with, 36t
    multiple-dose activated charcoal in, 61
  pharmacokinetics, 867t
  pharmacology, 867t, 871–872
  skin discoloration caused by, 273
  structure, 872f
  teratogenicity, 429t
  and thyroid hormone synthesis, 813f
  torsade de pointes caused by, magnesium for, 878
Amisulpride, 218. *See also* Antipsychotics
  clinical and toxicologic effects, 1034t
  dosage and administration, 1033t
  mechanism of action, 1035
  overdose/poisoning, 1040
  pharmacokinetics, 1033t
Amitriptyline, 1044, 1044t. *See also* Cyclic
        antidepressants
  adsorption to activated charcoal, 76
  elimination, multiple-dose activated charcoal and, 78
  inappropriate prescribing of, 1827
  inhibition of glucuronidation, 172
  Log D, 1045
  metabolite, 145t, 147
  pharmacokinetics and toxicokinetics, 145t, 1045
  pharmacology, 1044
  pulmonary effects, 1046–1047
  skin discoloration caused by, 273
  toxicity (overdose/poisoning)
    chronic, 1048
    lipid emulsion for, 1006–1007
    magnesium for, 877
    management, 1050
    multiple-dose activated charcoal in, 61
    sodium bicarbonate for, 567–569
  volume of distribution, 145t
Amitrole poisoning, clinical manifestations, 1483
Amlodipine
  excretion, 946
  mechanism of action, 945
  pharmacokinetics, 946t
  pharmacology, 945
  poisoning, lipid emulsion for, 1006
  structure, 945
  volume of distribution, 946, 946t

Ammonia, 333–334, 1388t, 1655
  airway injury by, 1640, 1640t
  detection threshold, 1654t
  exposure to, pathophysiology, 1389
  immediately dangerous to life and health (IDLH),
        1654t
  postmortem changes, 1885t
  regulatory standard for, 1654t
  serum, in liver disease, 335, 335t
  short-term exposure limit (STEL), 1654t
  and sodium hypochlorite (bleach), 1655
  sources, 1654t
  in terrorism, 1744
  as thermal degradation product, 1641t
  and urea cycle, 180f, 181
  water solubility, 1654t
Ammonium, excretion, and urinary anion gap, 193
Ammonium aluminum sulfate. *See* Alum
Ammonium bifluoride, synthesis, 1397
Ammonium chloride, and normal anion gap metabolic
        acidosis, 191t
Ammonium compounds, quaternary. *See* Quaternary
        ammonium compounds
Ammonium ferric ferrocyanide, 1357
Ammonium fluoride, 1397
Ammonium hydroxide, 1388t, 1655
  exposure to, pathophysiology, 1389
Ammonium sulfamate, 1468t
Amnestic shellfish poisoning, 593t, 595–596
Amnestic syndrome
  carbon monoxide poisoning and, 1665
  hydrogen sulfide poisoning and, 1689–1690
Amobarbital. *See also* Sedative-hypnotics
  pharmacokinetics, 1085t
Amodiaquine, 842
  antimalarial mechanism, 838t
  pharmacokinetics, 844
  structure, 844
  toxicity, 844
Amorphophallus konjac (glucomannan). *See also*
        Dieting xenobiotics and regimens
  uses and toxicities, 642t
Amoxapine, 1044. *See also* Cyclic antidepressants
  and dopamine receptors, 215
  and GABA receptors, 222
  pharmacology, 1045
  structure, 1044t
  and tinnitus, 370t
  toxicity, 1048
Amoxicillin, 823–824
Amoxicillin-clavulanic acid, and drug-induced liver
        injury, 823–824
AMPA, 225
AMPA receptor(s), 225, 719
  and excitotoxicity, 225
AMPA receptor antagonists, 227t, 228
AMPA receptor modulators, 227t
Amphetamine(s), 145t, 1099–1110, 1178, 1180. *See also*
        specific xenobiotic
  absorption, 1102
  abuse, 1099
  adverse effects and safety issues, 608t
  ARDS caused by, 402t
  as athletic performance enhancers, 621
  bioavailability, administration route and, 1102
  body packers, 85, 1105
  brain changes caused by, imaging, 132t
  clinical effects, 1102
  contaminants, 1104
  cranial neuropathy caused by, 346t

  as decongestant, 748
  definition, 1099
  distribution, 1102
  and dopamine reuptake, 214
  and dopaminergic activity, 214
  elimination, 1102
  elimination half-life, 1102
  gas chromatography-mass spectrometry, 1104
  gastrointestinal decontamination for, 1104–1105,
        1104t
  halogenation, 1102, 1102t
  history of, 748, 1099
  hyperventilation caused by, 400t
  immunoassays for, 1104
  intravenous injection, necrotizing angiitis caused
        by, 128
  laboratory testing for, 101, 101t
  and male sexual dysfunction, 299f
  mechanism of action, 204, 208, 210, 210t, 218, 608t,
        1099, 1100f
  metabolism, 1102
  monoamine oxidase inhibitor effect, 1100
  movement disorders with, dopamine and, 214
  neurotoxicity, 1102, 1102t, 1103
  and neurotransmission, 343
  ophthalmic toxicity, 361t
  pharmacokinetics and toxicokinetics, 145t, 1102
  pharmacology, 1099–1102
  receptor activity, 1099–1100, 1100f, 1101t
  regulation, 608t, 1099
  renal effects, 390f
  and rhabdomyolysis, 393, 393t
  screening for, 110, 112
  serotonergic, 1100, 1101t, 1102
  and serotonin toxicity, 1058t, 1079
  structure, 610f, 1076f, 1099, 1101t
  strychnine as adulterant in, 1536
  substituted, mechanism of action, 218
  therapeutic uses, 1099
  toxicity (overdose/poisoning)
    acute, 1103–1104, 1103t
    cardiovascular effects, 1103–1104, 1103t
    chronic, 1103, 1103t, 1104
    clinical manifestations, 36, 36t, 1103–1104, 1103t
    CNS effects, 1103–1104, 1103t
    diagnostic tests for, 1104
    management, 1104–1105, 1104t
    pathophysiology, 1102–1103
    vascular effects, 1103, 1103t
  toxicokinetics, 1182
  transport, 210
  urine screening assays for, performance
        characteristics, 111t
  volume of distribution, 145t, 1102
Amphotericin (amphotericin B), 160, 828–829
  acute tubular necrosis caused by, 390f, 392
  adverse effects associated with therapeutic use,
        828–829
  ARDS caused by, 402t
  diabetes insipidus caused by, 195, 195t
  dosage and administration, 828
  formulation, lipid emulsion in, 1004
  formulations, 828
  for HIV-related infections, 830t
  hypomagnesemia caused by, 877
  lipid carrier formulation, 684, 684t
  liposomal, 1719t
  mechanism of action, 822t, 828
  pharmacology, 822t
  renal effects, 392f

Amphotericin (amphotericin B) (*Cont.*):
site of action, 173f
structure, 828
and tinnitus, 370t
toxicity (overdose/poisoning), 822t
in infants and children, 828–829
Amphoteric salts, in emergency rinsing solution, 73
Ampicillin, 823–824
Amprenavir, propylene glycol in, 687
Amrinone
for β-adrenergic antagonist toxicity, 934–935
glucagon with, 942
and gustatory dysfunction, 365
AMT. *See* α-Methyltryptamine (AMT)
Amycolatopsis mediterranei, 854
Amygdalin, 1, 640t, 1602t, 1607, 1684
biotransformation to cyanide, 144, 1684, 1684f
toxicity, 648
toxic metabolite, 144, 1684, 1684f
Amylin, 696
Amylin analogs, 696, 700
overdose, hospitalization for, 702
pharmacokinetics and toxicokinetics, 696, 697t
Amyl nitrite, 1700–1701
adverse effects and safety issues, 1700
as aphrodisiac, 304t
chemistry, 1698
for cyanide poisoning, 1646, 1687–1688, 1687t
and methemoglobinemia, with hemolysis, 1706
odor, 364t
pharmacokinetics and pharmacodynamics, 1699
in poppers, 1193t, 1194. *See also* Inhalant(s)
clinical effects, 1198
Amyotrophic lateral sclerosis (ALS), 340
BMAA and, 227–228
cyanobacteria and, 227–228
glutamate and, 224
treatment, 228
Amyotrophic lateral sclerosis-parkinsonism dementia
complex (ALS-PDC), 1607
Amytal, site of action, 173f
Anabaena spp. (blue-green algae), 1598t, 1601t, 1609
Anabasine, 1604
Anabolic [term], definition, 616
Anabolic-androgenic steroids (AAS), 616–619,
616t–617t. *See also* Steroid(s), anabolic
administration, 617
bridging therapy with, 617
and cancer, 617
cardiovascular effects, 617–618
cycling, 617
dermatologic effects, 618
endocrine effects, 618
endogenous, 617
exogenous, 617
gingival hyperplasia with, 618
hepatic effects, 618
infectious complications, 618
musculoskeletal effects, 618
neuropsychiatric effects, 618
plateauing with, 617
stacking, 617
use, clinical manifestations, 617–618
Anabolic process, definition, 616
Anabolic Steroid Control Act of 2004, 617
Anabolic steroids. *See* Steroid(s), anabolic
Anabolic xenobiotics, as athletic performance
enhancers, 616–619
Anacardiaceae, 1598t, 1603t, 1614
Anacardium occidentale (cashew), 1598t, 1614

Anagen effluvium, 274t, 281
Anagyrine, 1601t
Analatro, 1543–1544, 1559–1560
safety, 1560
Analbis, 1255
Analgesia, opioid-induced, 521
Analgesic abuse nephropathy, 515
Analgesic nephropathy, 395, 395f
Analgesics
combinations, renal effects, 390f
history of, 555
and monoamine oxidase inhibitors, safety
considerations, 1079, 1079t
opioid, 521. *See also* Opioid(s)
pancreatitis caused by, 295t
pharmacokinetics, 145t
Analysis of secular trends, 1852–1853, 1853t
Analytic toxicology, 6
Anandamide, structure, 1112f
Anaphase-promoting complex (APC), 350
Anaphe venata caterpillar, 345, 1553
Anaphylactic reactions/anaphylaxis, 273
chlorhexidine-related, 1368
classification, 823, 823t
crotalid venom and, 1622
drug-induced, 21
fire ant stings and, 1552
with foodborne toxins or toxicity, 600–601, 600t
Hymenoptera stings and, 1551
to iodinated contrast media, 1776
to mushrooms, 1594
Neofibularia exposure and, 1574
neuromuscular blockers and, 1019
with nonsteroidal antiinflammatory drugs,
514t, 515
pathophysiology, 823, 824f
penicillins and, 823, 823t
protamine and, 919–920
to radiocontrast media, 1776
snake antivenom and, 1637
to snakebite, 1617
spider antivenom and, 1560
Anaphylactoid reactions
with 50% dextrose, 709
with foodborne toxins or toxicity, 600–601, 600t
with intravenous *N*-acetylcysteine, 495
with intravenous vitamin K₁, 916
with nonsteroidal antiinflammatory drugs, 514t, 515
with sulfites, 757
Anaphylaxis. *See* Anaphylactic reactions/anaphylaxis
Anaplasmosis, 1550
Anasatin, 1600t
Anascorp, 1549, 1563
adverse effects and safety issues, 1565
dosage and administration, 1565
formulation, 1565
pregnancy category, 1565
Anastrazole, 617, 618f
Anavip, 1624, 1627–1631, 1627t
Ancrod, 883
adverse effects and safety issues, 900
mechanism of action, 900
proposed therapeutic uses, 900
Andexanet alfa, 888t, 908, 911–913
adverse effects and safety issues, 896, 912
availability, 913
dosage and administration, 912
for factor Xa inhibitor–induced coagulopathy, 896
history of, 912
mechanism of action, 912

pharmacokinetics and pharmacodynamics, 912
pharmacology, 912
in pregnancy and lactation, 912
Andexxa, 912–913
Androctonus spp., 1548, 1548t
antivenoms, 1564t, 1565
Androctonus crassicauda, envenomation, treatment,
1563
Androgenic [term], 616
Androgen receptor blockers, 299f
Androgens. *See also specific androgen*
decreased, in men, exacerbated or unmasked by
xenobiotics in elderly, 463, 463t
effect on thyroid hormones and function, 813f, 814t
for female sexual dysfunction, 302
infertility caused by, 297t, 298f
and pancreatic dysfunction, 295t
priapism caused by, 301t
teratogenicity, 429t
Andromachus, 1t, 2–3
Andromedotoxins. *See* Grayanotoxins
Androstenedione, 618f, 619
Anemia
aplastic, 311–312, 311t, 352–353
felbamate-induced, 1837
idiosyncratic, 311
inborn, 311
NSAID-induced, 516
in arsenic poisoning, 1241
hemolytic. *See also* Hemolysis
NSAID-induced, 516
quinine-induced, 840
xenobiotic-induced, 174
hypoplastic, 353
iron deficiency, 669
in lead-exposed children, 1315–1316
treatment, 670
macrocytic, 318–319
megaloblastic, 318–319
thiamine-responsive, 1158
microcytic
aluminum and, 1223–1225
in dialysis patients, 1223
oxygen content of blood in, 402–403, 402f
post-chemotherapy, new-onset, 352–353
and pulse oximetry, 404, 404t
sideroblastic, reversible, coin ingestion and, 1363
sodium stibogluconate and, 1232
sports, 621
vitamin D toxicity and, 661
Anemones, 1567, 1567t, 1568. *See also* Cnidaria
(jellyfish)
sponges colonized with, 1573
Anemonia sulcata (European stinging anemone),
1567t
stings, clinical manifestations, 1569
Anemonin, 1613
Anesthesia [term], 1011
Anesthesia, general, 1011. *See also specific xenobiotic*
Anesthetic(s). *See also* Inhalational anesthetic(s); Local
anesthetic(s)
fluorinated, renal effects, 390f
general, effects on vital signs, 31t
halogenated
abuse, 1016
long-term use in ICUs, 1016
metabolism, 172
history of, 994
intravenous (IV), effects on vital signs, 31t
oral, cranial neuropathy caused by, 346t

topical, and methemoglobin formation, 1703, 1705
volatile, 1011
binding by activated charcoal, 76
Anesthetic gas, waste, chronic exposure to, 1016
Anethum graveolens (dill), as early emetic, 4
Aneurin, 1157
Aneurysm(s)
cerebral, 132f
injection drug use and, 132f
mycotic, rupture, imaging, 132t
Angel de la Guarda Island speckled rattlesnake
(*Crotalus* spp.), 1636t
Angel dust. See Phencyclidine (PCP)
Angelica polymorpha (Dong Quai), uses and toxicities,
641t
Angelica sinensis (Dong Quai), as abortifacient, 303t
Angel's trumpet, 1181–1182
Angioedema
with *N*-acetylcysteine, 495
airway obstruction caused by, 399t, 400
angiotensin-converting enzyme inhibitor–induced,
963–964
in drug-induced hypersensitivity syndrome, 277
food toxins and, 600t
hereditary, 963–964
NSAID-induced, 515
Angiogenesis
copper and, 1283
tumor, 761
Angiosarcoma, hepatic, 333, 334t
Angiosperms, 1597
Angiotensin-converting enzyme inhibitors (ACEI)
angioedema caused by, 963–964
as antihypertensives, 959t, 963–964
and colchicine, interactions, 502
effects on vital signs, 29t
and gustatory dysfunction, 365, 365t
hyperkalemia caused by, 251
overdose/poisoning, 964
pancreatitis caused by, 295t
renal effects, 391
respiratory effects, 399t
structure, 963
teratogenicity, 429t
Angiotensin I, 963
Angiotensin II, 93, 963
mechanism of action, 933f
Angiotensin receptor blockers (ARBs, Angiotensin II
receptor blockers)
as antihypertensives, 959t, 964–965
CYP enzymes and, 170
effects on vital signs, 29t
hyperkalemia caused by, 251
and male sexual function, 299f
mechanism of action, 964
overdose/poisoning, 964
pancreatitis caused by, 295t
pharmacokinetics, 964
renal effects, 391
teratogenicity, 429t
Anhydroecgonine methyl ester (AEME), 1125
Anilide derivative herbicides, 1467t, 1472–1473, 1472f
extracorporeal removal, 1473
pharmacokinetics, 1472
self-poisoning with, 1472
toxicity
clinical manifestations, 1472–1473
diagnostic tests for, 1473
management, 1473
pathophysiology, 1472

toxicokinetics, 1472
Aniline
exposure to
case study, 1639
management, 1639
metabolism, 172
and methemoglobinemia, with hemolysis, 1706
Aniline dyes
neonatal poisoning with, 453
pediatric poisoning with, 453
Anilofos, 1468t
Animal Efficacy Rule (2002), 1834
Animal poisons, 1–2
Animal Rule, 1834
Animas ridge-nosed rattlesnake (*Crotalus* spp.), 1637t
Anion(s)
extracellular, 190
monovalent, effect on thyroid hormones and
function, 814t
normally present, 190
unmeasured, 190–191, 191t, 192
Anion exchange resins, 96
Anion gap. See also Delta gap ratio (Δ anion gap/Δ
[HCO₃⁻]); Metabolic acidosis
calculation, 190–191
clinical applications, 191
high, causes, 191, 191t
hypoalbuminemia and, 191
increased, polyethylene glycol (PEG) and, 687
in liver disease, 335t
low, causes, 191, 191t
normal, 190–191
with metabolic acidosis, 193
and osmol gap, reciprocal relationship, 1426, 1426f
reliability, 191
in toxic alcohol poisoning, 1423, 1426
in risk stratification, 1427
urinary, 193
xenobiotics and, 191, 191t
Anion gap acidosis, 166
Anion gap ratio, 192
Anion inhibitors, and thyroid function, 814t
Aniracetam, 227t, 228
Anisakiasis, 597t, 600
Anisakis simplex, 600
Anisatin, 1608
Anise, Japanese star (*Illicium anisatum*), 1600t
Aniseed, 2
Anisindione, 885
Anisocoria, physiologic, 357
Anisodamine, for organic phosphorus compound
poisoning, 1497
Anistreplase, 884, 896–897
Anisylcyclohexylamines, 1211
ANIT. See α-Naphthyl-isothiocyanate (ANIT)
Anmi, 2
Annelida, 1573–1574
Annulus, of mushrooms, 1584f, 1593
Anopheles mosquito
DDT-resistant, 836
and malaria, 836
Anorectics, 606. See also Dieting xenobiotics and
regimens
Anorexia, lead-induced, 1296
Anorexia-cachexia syndrome, in HIV-infected (AIDS)
patients, cannabinoids for, 1113
Anorexia nervosa, and thiamine deficiency, 1160
Anosmia, 363–364, 364t
congenital, 364
intranasal zinc and, 1363

Antacids
aluminum in, 1223, 1225
gastrointestinal effects, 292f
Antagonism, 755
Anterior chamber of eye, 356
Anthomedusae, 1567
Anthoxanthum odoratum (sweet vernal grass),
1598t
Anthozoa, 1567–1568, 1567t. See also Cnidaria
(jellyfish)
actinoporins, 1570
characteristics, 1567t
venom, toxins in, 1569
Anthracene, 1410
Anthracyanins, 1602t
Anthracyclines, 354. See also specific xenobiotic
antidote for, 764
cardiovascular toxicity, 762–763, 763t
chemistry, 160
as chemotherapeutics, 760t
adverse effects and safety issues, 760t
antidote for, 760t
overdose/poisoning, 760t
extravasation, 802, 803t
antidotes for, 803
mechanism of action, 761
neutropenia caused by, 762
toxicity, 763
and trastuzumab, interactions, 763
Anthraquinone(s), 639, 640t–641t, 644t
as laxatives, 83, 1607
Anthraquinone glycosides, 1597, 1598t–1599t, 1602t,
1607
Anthrax (*Bacillus anthracis*), 1754–1756
bioterrorism event with, risk communication in,
1818
2001 bioterrorist attack with, 1754, 1756
clinical manifestations of, 1754–1755
cutaneous, 268
gram stain for, 1754, 1754f
occupational diseases caused by, 23
pathophysiology, 1755, 1755f
spores, 1754, 1755f
treatment, 1755
vaccine against, 1755–1756
Anthropophagia, 1885
Anti-activated protein C aptamer, 896
Antiandrogens, 617. See also specific xenobiotic
and male sexual dysfunction, 299f
Antiarachnid serum, 1546
Antibacterials, 821–828. See also specific xenobiotic
history of, 821
pharmacology, 822t
toxicity, organ system manifestations, 829t
Antibiotic(s). See also Antimicrobials; specific
antibiotic
acute interstitial nephritis caused by, 393, 394t
adverse effects and safety issues, in elderly, 465
and anion gap, 191t
antibacterial. See Antibacterials
antineoplastic, 759, 760t. See also Antineoplastics;
specific xenobiotic
antitumor, 349f, 761f
for caustic injury, 1390t, 1394
as chemotherapeutics, 759, 760t
adverse effects and safety issues, 760t
antidotes for, 760t
overdose/poisoning, 760t
dialysis and, 95
and erectile dysfunction, 300

Antibiotic(s) (*Cont.*):
  for hydrocarbon pulmonary toxicity, 1416–1417
  for malaria, 836
    antimalarial mechanism, 837f, 838t, 846
  ophthalmic, 359–360
  pancreatitis caused by, 295t
  as photoallergens, 280
  polypeptide, and neuromuscular blockers, interactions, 1021t
  for tuberculosis, 858
Antibody(ies) (Ab), therapeutic use, 147
Antibody fragments, therapeutic use, 147
Anticholinergic alkaloids, in plants, 2, 651, 1604. *See also* Belladonna alkaloids
Anticholinergic effects, antipsychotic-induced, 1034t, 1035
Anticholinergic poisoning syndrome, 1504
Anticholinergics. *See also specific anticholinergic*
  for acute dystonia, 1036, 1037t
  for akathisia, 1036, 1037t
  antidote for, 35t
  and dopamine reuptake, 214
  for drug-induced parkinsonism, 1037, 1037t
  effects on vital signs, 29t–31t
  and erectile dysfunction, 300
  hyperventilation caused by, 400t
  ileus caused by, imaging, 127, 129f, 129t
  and male sexual dysfunction, 299f
  renal effects, 390f
  toxicity (overdose/poisoning), 756
    clinical and laboratory findings with, 36t, 37–38, 576t, 1183
    in heroin users, 21t, 22
    management, 45t
    plants causing, 1181
    treatment, 1184
  toxic syndrome caused by, 28, 29t, 30
Anticholinergic syndrome
  antihistamines associated with, 745–746
  case study, 736–737, 736f–737f
  management, 748
Anticholinergic toxidrome, 207
Anticholinesterase(s), 207–208. *See also* Acetylcholinesterase inhibitors; *specific anticholinesterase*
  carbamate, 208
  centrally acting, and neuromuscular blockers, interactions, 1021t
  deaths caused by, 1486
  inhibition, by carbamates, 1489
  for neuromuscular blockade reversal, 1025–1026, 1026t
  non-carbamate, reversible, 208
  oral, for central anticholinergic syndrome, 748
  peripherally acting, and neuromuscular blockers, interactions, 1021t
  pharmacology, 1025, 1026t
  self-poisoning with, 1487
  toxicity (poisoning)
    epidemiology, 1486–1487
    unintentional, 1487
    WHO classification, 1486, 1486t
Anticholinesterase inhibitors, and neurotransmission, 343
Anticoagulant aptamers, 896
Anticoagulants, 322. *See also* Long-acting anticoagulant rodenticide(s) (LAARs); *specific anticoagulant*
  adverse effects and safety issues, in elderly, 464–465
  cerebral hemorrhage caused by, imaging, 132t

history of, 883
and NSAIDs, interactions, 514t
overdose/poisoning
  clinical and laboratory findings with, 36t
  management, 46t
physiology, 884f
priapism caused by, 301t
renal effects, 391
rodenticide
  antidote for, 35t, 1453t
  clinical and laboratory findings with, 36t, 1453t
  long-acting, 1453t
  short-acting, 1453t
skin necrosis caused by, 279, 279f
vitamin K cycle and, 885–886, 885f
warfarinlike, 885–890
Anticoagulation
  for continuous renal replacement therapy, 97
  with hemodialysis, 95
Anticonvulsant(s). *See* Antiepileptics
Anticonvulsant hypersensitivity syndrome (AHS). *See* Drug-induced hypersensitivity syndrome (DIHS)
Antidepressant Overdose Risk Assessment (ADORA), 1051
Antidepressants. *See also* Cyclic antidepressants; Tricyclic antidepressants; *specific xenobiotic*
  antimuscarinic properties, 756
  atypical, 1054, 1060–1064. *See also specific xenobiotic*
    definition, 1060
    discontinuation syndrome, 1061
    overdose/poisoning
      clinical manifestations, 1056–1057, 1057t
      management, 1057–1058
    receptor activity, 1056, 1056f, 1057t
  cardiac effects, 258t
  discontinuation syndrome, 1061
  and erectile dysfunction, 300
  mechanism of action, 218
    receptor sensitivity hypothesis of, 1044
  noradrenergic, site of action, 1054, 1056f
  obstructive nephropathy caused by, 394
  overdose/poisoning
    clinical and laboratory findings with, 32
    clinical manifestations, 1056–1057, 1057t
    gastrointestinal decontamination for, 58t
  pharmacokinetics and toxicokinetics, 145t
  priapism caused by, 301t
  self-poisoning with, 376, 1044
  and suicide, 379
  and tinnitus, 370t
Antidiabetics, 694–706. *See also specific xenobiotic*
  history of, 694
  hypoglycemia caused by, pathophysiology, 697–698
  and metabolic acidosis with elevated lactate concentration, 703–704
  noninsulin, pharmacokinetics and toxicokinetics, 697t
  pharmacokinetics and toxicokinetics, 696, 697t
  pharmacology, 694–696
  structure, 695f
  xenobiotics reacting with, 698t
Antidiuretic hormone (ADH), 194. *See also* Syndrome of inappropriate antidiuretic hormone secretion (SIADH)
  in diabetes insipidus, 195
  excess, 189
  release, factors affecting, 195
  renal effects, 389
  secretion

and hyponatremia, 196
  increased, exacerbated or unmasked by xenobiotics in elderly, 463, 463t
Antidotes. *See also specific antidotes and xenobiotics*
  access to, global disparities in, 1847
  administration, strategies for, 46t
  alternatives for, 43
  cost, 43
  early, 1t. *See also* Mithridatum; Theriacs
  essential, 43
  indications for, 35t
  labeling, 43
  local availability, 42–43
  national availability, 43
  needs assessment for, 43
  in pregnancy, 39
  in pregnancy and lactation, 434
  shortages, 43
  stocking, 33, 35t, 41–47, 44t–46t
    hazard vulnerability assessment and, 43
    strategies for, 46t
  substitutes for, 43
  universal, early quests for, 2–3
  for xenobiotic-induced respiratory dysfunction, 407
Antidote treatment nerve agent autoinjector (ATNAA), 1506, 1511
Antidysrhythmics, 865–875. *See also specific xenobiotic*
  adverse effects and safety issues, 866t–867t
  cardiac effects, 248f, 258, 258t
  class I, 866–871, 866t–867t
    antidote for, 35t
    bradycardia with, 924, 924t
    mechanism of action, 865f, 866–868
  class IA, 866t, 868–869
    contraindications to, 974
    structure, 868f
    toxicity, management, 869
  class IB, 866t, 868–871
    structure, 869f
    toxicity, management, 870–871
  class IC, 866t–867t, 871
    toxicity, management, 871
  class II, 867t
  class III, 867t, 871–873
    mechanism of action, 871
  class IV, 867t, 873
  classification, 865–866
  contraindications to, 747, 1040, 1050, 1130
  for cyclic antidepressant toxicity, 1049t, 1050
  effects on QRS complex, 567–569
  effects on vital signs, 29t
  history of, 865
  mechanism of action, 865, 865f
  pharmacokinetics, 866t–867t
  pharmacology, 866t–867t
  and prolonged QT interval, 253t, 256
  toxicity (overdose/poisoning)
    ECG changes in, 250, 567–569
    sodium bicarbonate for, 567–569, 568t, 569
  and voltage-gated calcium channels, 244f, 245
Antiemetic(s), 217
  for chemotherapeutic-related vomiting, 764
  mechanism of action, 218
  for methylxanthine-induced vomiting, 990
  with whole-bowel irrigation, 86
Antiepileptics, 719–731. *See also specific xenobiotic*
  acute interstitial nephritis caused by, 394t
  adverse effects and safety issues, 727–728, 727t
  for alcohol withdrawal, 1169

broad *vs.* narrow spectrum, 719
calcium channel blockade by, 719, 720f, 720t
and calcium channels, 244f, 245, 719, 720f, 720t
cross-reactivity, 277
drug-induced hypersensitivity syndrome with, 277, 727–728, 727t
drug interactions with, 723t
excitatory amine blockade by, 719, 720f, 720t
GABA potentiation by, 719, 720f, 720t
hepatitis caused by, 330
history of, 719
hypocalcemia caused by, 199
indications for, 719
mechanism of action, 222, 230, 719, 720t
for nerve agent exposure, 1746
pancreatitis caused by, 295t
pharmacokinetics and toxicokinetics, 721t
pharmacology, 719, 720f, 720t
and pregnancy complications, 719
sodium channel blockade by, 719, 720f, 720t
and suicide risk, 719
synaptic vesicle protein 2A (SV2A) binding by, 719, 720t
teratogenicity, 434
therapeutic uses, 719
and tinnitus, 370t
for xenobiotic-induced seizures, 1138
Antiestrogens, 617. *See also specific xenobiotic*
Anti-factor VIIa aptamer, 896
Anti-factor IX aptamer, 896
Antifolates, 354
for malaria, 836
adverse effects and safety issues, 846
antimalarial mechanism, 837f, 838t, 846
Antifreeze, 1421. *See also* Ethylene glycol; Toxic alcohol(s)
fluorescein in, 1427
Antifungals, 828–829. *See also specific xenobiotic*
azole. *See* Azole antifungals
history of, 821
pharmacology, 822t
and prolonged QT interval, 253t
and tinnitus, 370t
toxicity, organ system manifestations, 829t
Antiglaucoma drugs. *See also specific xenobiotic*
ophthalmic use, systemic toxicity with, 360
Antiglycemics, 694–706
hypoglycemia caused by, pathophysiology, 697–698
and metabolic acidosis with elevated lactate concentration, 703–704
pharmacokinetics and toxicokinetics, 696, 697t
xenobiotics reacting with, 698t
Antihistamines, 738–748. *See also specific xenobiotic*
abuse/misuse, pathophysiology, 744
adverse effects and safety issues, 738–739
antimuscarinic properties, 756
atypical, 743
availability, 738–739
cardiac effects, 258t
and ethanol, interactions, 1144, 1146t
exposure to, trends in, 738
fatal concentrations, assessment, 747
H$_1$, 741–742
absorption, 743
abuse, pathophysiology, 744
adverse effects and safety issues, 739, 744
antimuscarinic effects, 746
classification, 741–742
contraindications to, 746
dermal absorption, 743

distribution, 743
dose modification in liver or kidney disease, 744
drug interactions with, 744
duration of action, 744
effects, 745t
elimination half-life, 744
excretion, 744
first-generation, 741–742
effects, 745t
pharmacokinetics and toxicokinetics, 745t
mechanism of action, 741–742
metabolism, 743–744
pediatric pharmacokinetics, 744
pharmacokinetics and toxicokinetics, 743–744, 745t
pregnancy categories, 746
receptor occupancy, 742
second-generation, 742
effects, 745t
pharmacokinetics and toxicokinetics, 745t
sedating *vs.* nonsedating, 742, 746
sedative effects, 742
structure, 740f, 742
teratogenicity, 746
topical, toxicity, 743
toxicity (overdose/poisoning)
cardiovascular effects, 746
clinical manifestations, 744–746
in elderly, 746
neurologic effects, 745–746
pathophysiology, 744
volume of distribution, 743
H$_2$
absorption, 744
adverse effects and safety issues, 739
drug interactions with, 744
elimination half-life, 744
excretion, 744
and gastric acid secretion, 742, 743f
mechanism of action, 742
metabolism, 744
pharmacokinetics and toxicokinetics, 745t
pharmacology, 742
structure, 742, 742f
toxicity (overdose/poisoning)
clinical manifestations, 746
pathophysiology, 744
H$_3$, 742
H$_4$, 743
histamine receptor physiology and, 739–740. *See also* Histamine receptor(s)
history of, 738–739
mortality rate for, 738–739
pediatric poisoning with, 738–739
pharmacokinetics and toxicokinetics, 743–744, 745t
and prolonged QT interval, 253t
recreational use, 738
for seabather's eruption, 1572
sedation caused by, management, 747
for serotonin toxicity, 1059
and suicide, 739
third-generation, 742
and tinnitus, 370t
toxicity (overdose/poisoning)
diagnostic tests for, 746–747
management, 747–748
use of, 738–739
for venomous caterpillar exposure, 1554
Antihypertensives, 959t. *See also specific xenobiotic*
α$_2$-adrenergic agonists as, 959t

β-adrenergic antagonists as, 926–940, 959t
angiotensin-converting enzyme inhibitors as, 959t, 963–964
angiotensin II receptor blockers as, 959t
calcium channel blockers as, 959t. *See also* Calcium channel blockers
cardiac effects, 256
centrally acting, 959–961
overdose/poisoning
clinical manifestations, 960
diagnostic tests for, 960
management, 960–961
pathophysiology, 960
pharmacokinetics, 959–960
pharmacology, 959
withdrawal, 961
direct renin inhibitors as, 959t
diuretics as, 959t, 963
and erectile dysfunction, 300
ganglionic blockers as, 959t
imidazoline agonists as, 959t
and male sexual dysfunction, 299f
mechanism of action, 212
and NSAIDs, interactions, 514t
peripheral α$_1$-adrenergic antagonists as, 959t
peripheral adrenergic neuron antagonists as, 959t
pharmacologically related xenobiotics, 959t
priapism caused by, 301t
renal effects, 390f
sympatholytics as, 959t
vasodilators as, 959t
Antiinflammatory agents, for sulfur mustard exposure, 1748
Antimalarials, 836–849. *See also specific xenobiotic*
classification, 836
genetic polymorphisms and, 847
history of, 836
hypoglycemia caused by, octreotide for, 715
metabolic interactions, 839t, 847
pharmacokinetics, 839t
resistance to, 836, 849
self-poisoning with, 1846
skin discoloration caused by, 273
volume of distribution, 838
Antimetabolites, 759, 760t, 767. *See also* Antineoplastics; *specific xenobiotic*
adverse effects and safety issues, 760t
antidotes for, 760t
overdose/poisoning, 760t
Antimicrobials. *See also* Antibacterials; Antibiotic(s); Antifungals; Antimalarials; Antiparasitics; Antituberculous medications; Antivirals; *specific xenobiotic*
acute interstitial nephritis caused by, 393, 394t
adverse drug events related to, 821
allergy to, 821
cardiac effects, 258t
and disulfiramlike reactions, 1174t
drug interactions with, 821
excipients, adverse effects, 821
history of, 821
for HIV/AIDS and related infections, 829–832, 830t–831t
hypomagnesemia caused by, 877
iatrogenic complications with, 821
ophthalmic use, systemic toxicity with, 360
pharmacology, 821, 822t
and prolonged QT interval, 253t
renal effects, 390f
resistance to, 821

Antimicrobials (*Cont.*):
  and tinnitus, 370t
  toxicity, organ system manifestations, 829t
  toxicology, 821
Antimigraine medications, 805–811, 805t. *See also specific xenobiotic*
  abortive, 805t
  prophylactic, 805t
Antimitotic(s), 759, 760t. *See also* Colchicine; Podophyllin; Vinblastine; Vincristine
  toxicity (overdose/poisoning), 507t
Antimony, 1228–1236, 1780
  absorption, 1229–1230
  biomethylation, 1230
  carcinogenicity, 1232t, 1233
  chemistry, 1228–1229
  in cigarette smoke, 1228
  in cosmetics, 1228
  decontamination, 1233–1234
  ECG changes caused by, 1232–1233
  elemental, 1228
  excretion, 1230
  exposure to, sources, 1228
  genotoxicity, 1232t, 1233
  historical perspective on, 1–2, 5t, 6, 12
  history and epidemiology, 1228
  for HIV-related infections, 830t
  industrial uses, 1228
  inorganic compounds, 1228–1229
  medicinal use, historical perspective on, 1228
  metabolism, 1230
  metal fume fever caused by, 1232
  nephrotoxicity, 397t
  occupational exposure to, 1228, 1230
  ophthalmic effects, 1230
  oxidation states, 1228, 1230
  permissible exposure limits, 1228, 1229t
  pharmacology, 1229
  physicochemical properties, 1228
  regulations and advisories for, 1229t
  serum, normal concentration, 1228, 1233
  as thermal degradation product, 1642
  tissue distribution, 1230
  toxicity
    cardiovascular effects, 1231t, 1232
    chelation therapy for, 1234
    clinical manifestations, 1230–1233, 1231t–1232t
    dermatologic effects, 1231t, 1233
    diagnostic tests for, 1233
    in firefighters, 1229–1230
    gastrointestinal effects, 1230, 1231t
    hematologic effects, 1231t, 1232–1233
    hepatic effects, 1231t, 1232
    imaging in, 1233
    immunologic effects, 1233
    local irritation in, 1230, 1231t
    metabolic effects, 1233
    musculoskeletal effects, 1232t, 1233
    neurologic effects, 1231t–1232t, 1233
    pathophysiology, 1230
    renal effects, 1231t, 1232
    reproductive effects, 1233
    respiratory effects, 1231t, 1232
    supportive care for, 1234
    treatment, 1233–1234
  toxicokinetics, 1229–1230
  urine
    clinical significance, 1232–1233
    normal concentration, 1228, 1233

Antimony-a,a′-dimercaptopotassium succinate (TWSb), 1309
Antimony oxide, 1228
Antimony oxychloride, 1229
Antimony pentachloride/pentoxide, 1228–1230, 1232
  toxicity, clinical manifestations, 1231t–1232t
Antimony pneumoconiosis, 1232
Antimony potassium tartrate, 4
  toxicity, clinical manifestations, 1231t–1232t
Antimony spots, 1233
Antimony sulfide, 1228
Antimony trioxide, 1228–1230, 1232–1233
  carcinogenicity, 1233
  toxicity, clinical manifestations, 1231t–1232t
Antimony trisulfide, carcinogenicity, 1233
Antimuscarinic(s), 1503. *See also specific xenobiotic*
  cranial neuropathy caused by, 346t
  mechanism of action, 343
  in neuromuscular blockade reversal, 1025, 1026t
  for organic phosphorus compound poisoning, 1496–1497
  pharmacology, 1025, 1026t
  toxicity (overdose/poisoning)
    clinical and laboratory findings with, 36, 756
    cutaneous findings in, 189
    physostigmine for, 755–756
Antimuscarinic syndrome, 1038
  central, treatment, 1041
Antimuscarinic toxidrome, 207
Antimycin A
  and electron transport, 176t
  site of action, 173f
Antineoplastics, 759, 760t. *See also* Chemotherapeutics; *specific xenobiotic*
  antidotes for. *See specific antidote*
  classification, 759, 760t
Antioxidants, 661. *See also* N-Acetylcysteine (NAC); β-Carotene; SOD (superoxide dismutase); Vitamin C; Vitamin E
  for carbon monoxide poisoning, 1671
  in cyanide poisoning, 1688
  indications for, 661
  for metal phosphide poisoning, 1459
  for paraquat poisoning, 1474f, 1476–1477
  for pulmonary irritant exposure, 1658
  and silver exposure management, 1347
Antiparasitics, 829, 1228–1229
  and tinnitus, 370t
Antiperspirants, aluminum absorption from, 1224
Antipharmakon, 2
α₂-Antiplasmin, 322, 896
Antiplatelet agents, 323–324, 883, 897–899, 898f. *See also specific xenobiotic*
  antidotes and treatment strategies for, 888t
  coagulopathy caused by, management, 900
  laboratory assessment, 888t, 900
  reversal, 900
Antiplatelet antibodies, 324
Antipsychotics, 1032–1043. *See also specific xenobiotic*
  adverse effects and safety issues, 1032, 1036–1039, 1036t, 1039. *See also* Extrapyramidal syndromes (EPS)
    during therapeutic use, 1036–1039, 1036t
  for agitated/violent behavior, 386
  for amphetamine toxicity, 1104–1105
  anticholinergic effects, 1034t, 1035
  antimuscarinic properties, 756
  atypical, 1032–1034, 1033t
    cardiac effects, 258t
    for chemotherapeutic-related vomiting, 764

  clinical and toxicologic effects, 1034t
  extrapyramidal effects, 214–215
  mechanism of action, 214
  off-label uses, 1033–1034
  and QT interval, 253t
  self-poisoning with, 376
  for serotonin toxicity, 1059
  and sudden cardiac death, 253
  benzamides, 1033t
  benzepines, 1033t
  benzisothiazole, 1033t
  benzisoxazole, 1033t
  cardiac effects, 258t
  classification, 1032–1034, 1033t
  for cocaine toxicity, 1128
  conventional, 1032–1033
  dibenzo-oxine pyrroles, 1033t
  and dopaminergic transmission, 1032–1035
  ECG changes caused by, 1039
  effects on vital signs, 30t
  enhanced elimination, 1041
  and erectile dysfunction, 300
  for ethanol-induced agitation, 386
  extrapyramidal effects, 214
  and female sexual dysfunction, 302f
  first-generation, 1032–1033
  for hallucinogen-induced agitation, 1184
  high-potency, 1032
  history of, 1032
  idiosyncratic effects, 1032, 1039
  imidazolidinone, 1033t
  indications for, 1149
  indole, 1033t
  for inhalant-induced psychosis, 1200
  low-potency, 1032
  and male sexual dysfunction, 299f
  mechanism of action, 218, 1034–1035
  mechanism of toxicity, 1032
  medical clearance for, 375
  muscarinic effects, 1034t, 1035
  pharmacokinetics and toxicokinetics, 1035–1036
  priapism caused by, 301t
  and prolactin, 299f
  and prolonged QT interval, 256
  quinolinones, 1033t
  and rhabdomyolysis, 393t
  second-generation, 1032
  and serotonergic transmission, 1032–1033, 1035
  and sudden cardiac death, 253
  therapeutic uses, 1033–1034
  third-generation, 1032–1033
  and tinnitus, 370t
  toxicity (overdose/poisoning), 1032
    acute, 1039
    cardiovascular complications, treatment, 1040
    clinical and laboratory findings with, 32, 36t
    diagnostic tests for, 1039–1040
    epidemiology, 1032
    fatalities with, 1032
    gastrointestinal decontamination for, 1040
    magnesium for, 878
    management, 1040–1041
    monitoring in, 1040
  traditional, 1032
  typical, 1032–1034, 1033t
    clinical and toxicologic effects, 1034t
  volume of distribution, 91
Antipyrimidine, 354
Antiretrovirals, 831–832
  hepatotoxicity, 331–332

and methadone, interactions, 172
pancreatitis caused by, 295t
and prolonged QT interval, 253t
Antiseptics, 1368–1372, 1369t. *See also specific xenobiotic*
  definition, 1368
  history of, 1368
  potassium permanganate, 1319
Antistasin, 883, 894
Antistasinlike proteins, 883
Antisyphilis therapy, imaging findings after, 117f, 132f
Antithrombin, 884, 884f, 919
Antithrombin agonists, 890–891. *See also* Heparin
  antidotes and treatment strategies for, 888t
  laboratory testing for, 888t
Antithrombin III, 322
Antithrombotics, 883–907
  adverse events with, 883
  antidotes and treatment strategies for, 888t
  clinical applications, 883
  coagulopathy caused by, treatment, 887–889, 888t
  indications for, 883
  ingestion, management, 885
  laboratory testing for, 888t
  oral, pharmacology, 892, 893t
  physiology, 883–884
  toxicity (overdose/poisoning)
    epidemiology, 883
    management, 885
Antithyroid medications, 814–815, 814t, 818. *See also* Iodide(s); Thioamides; *specific xenobiotic*
  and gustatory dysfunction, 365
  history of, 812
Antituberculous medications, 850–861. *See also specific xenobiotic*
  adverse effects and safety issues, 850
  and hepatocellular necrosis, 331
  history of, 850
Antitumor antibiotics, 349f
Antitussives. *See also specific xenobiotic*
  opioid, 521. *See also* Codeine; Dextromethorphan
Antivenin. *See* Antivenom(s)
Antivenin [term], vs. antivenom, 1559
Antivenom(s)
  administration routes, 1559–1560
  antidotal fraction (IgG, Fab, F(ab')₂), 1559
  availability, global disparities in, 1847–1848
  box jellyfish (*Chironex fleckeri*), 1570, 1575t
  crotalid, 1627–1631, 1627t
  elapid, 1627–1631, 1627t
    for xenobiotic-induced respiratory dysfunction, 407
  equine-derived
    adverse effects and safety issues, 1560–1561, 1565
    pharmacokinetics and pharmacodynamics, 1559
  exotic snake
    hospital use, 1635
    zoological, 1634–1635
  Fc fragment, 1559
  indications for, 35t
  mechanism of action, 1627
  Micrurus fulvius, phenol in, 685t
  production, 1559
  scorpion, 1563–1566, 1564t
    adverse effects and safety issues, 1565
    availability and storage, 44t
    cost-effectiveness, 1565
    dosage and administration, 1565
    formulation, 1565
    indications for, 44t
    pharmacokinetics and pharmacodynamics, 1563

pharmacology, 1563
  in pregnancy, 1565
  stocking, recommended level, 44t
  worldwide availability, 1564t–1565t
  sea snake (CSL), 1575–1576, 1575t
  snake
    international use, 1845
    phenol in, 685t
  spider, 1559–1562. *See also specific spider*
    administration routes, 1559–1560
    adverse effects and safety issues, 1560–1561
    chemistry, 1559
    history of, 1559
    Latrodectus, 44t
    mechanism of action, 1559
    pharmacokinetics and pharmacodynamics, 1559–1561
    pharmacology, 1559
    preparation, 1559
    worldwide availability, 1560t
  stonefish, 1575t, 1578
  supplies, 42
Antivenom [term], vs. antivenin, 1559
Antivenom Index, 1561, 1565–1566, 1633–1635
  access to, 1634
Antivirals, 829. *See also specific antiviral*
  diabetes insipidus caused by, 195t
  history of, 821
Anti-Xa assay, 890–891
Ants, 1540, 1551–1552, 1845
  stings, allergy to, 1552
ANTU. *See* α-Naphthylthiourea (ANTU)
Anuria, sudden, 394
Anxiety
  amphetamine-induced, 1103
  glutamate and, 224–227
  perinatal, 433–434
  SSRIs and, 1058
  and suicidality, 378–379
  in toxidromes, 29t
Anxiolytics. *See also* Sedative-hypnotics; *specific xenobiotic*
  definition, 1084
Aortic dissection, 122
  amphetamine-related, 126
  cocaine-related, 115t, 126, 128f
Aortoesophageal fistula, after caustic injury, 1391
APACHE II score, and liver transplantation for acetaminophen poisoning, 483–484, 484t
Apamin, 1551, 1551t
  and voltage-gated potassium channels, 244f, 245, 1551
APAP. *See* Acetaminophen
Apes, bezoars from, 3
Aphanizomenon (blue-green algae), 1598t
Aphonopelma hentzi, 1547
Aphrodisiacs, 297, 304, 304t. *See also specific aphrodisiac*
  toxicity, 304, 304t
Apiaceae, 1599t, 1614
Apids. *See* Honeybee (*Apis mellifera*)
Apiol, 643t
Apis mellifera (honeybee). *See* Honeybee (*Apis mellifera*)
Apixaban, 321f, 883, 884f, 894–896
  adverse effects and safety issues, 894
    in elderly, 465
  laboratory investigation and, 888t, 895
  overdose/poisoning
    clinical manifestations, 895

gastrointestinal decontamination for, 50t, 78
    treatment strategies for, 888t
  pharmacology, 893t, 895
  reversal agent for, 912–913
Aplastic anemia. *See* Anemia, aplastic
APML syndrome, 1243
Apocrine glands, 270
Apocynaceae, 1599t, 1602t
Apocynum cannabinum (dogbane), 969, 979
Apomorphine
  mechanism of action, 214
  and sexual function, 304
  sublingual
    adverse effects and safety issues, 301
    for erectile dysfunction, 301
    for female sexual dysfunction, 302
    pharmacokinetics, 301
Apoponax, 2
Apoptosis
  in acetaminophen toxicity, 474
  arsenic trioxide and, 1237–1238
  cadmium-related, 1259
  cytokines and, 311
  hepatocellular, 328, 330
  lead-induced, 1294–1295
  neuronal, carbon monoxide poisoning and, 1664
Apparent half-life, 151
Apple (*Malus*), seeds, 1602t
Apple of Peru. *See* Jimsonweed (*Datura stramonium*)
Appraisal of Guidelines for Research and Evaluation (AGREE) Instrument, 1857
Apraclonidine
  benzalkonium chloride in, 682t
  ophthalmic use, systemic toxicity with, 360
Apraxia, carbon monoxide poisoning and, 1665
Aprepitant, nanocrystal, 1719t
Apricot pits (*Prunus armeniaca*)
  cyanogenic glycosides in, 640t, 1602t, 1607, 1684
  uses and toxicities, 640t
Aprotinin, and fibrinolysis, 323
Aptamers, anticoagulant, 896
Aptiganel, 227t
A-200 Pyrinate shampoo, ophthalmic exposure to, 359
Aquadots, 1188
Aquaporins, 194, 389
Aqua toffana, 5t, 6
Aqueous humor, 356
Aquifoliaceae, 1600t
Aquohydroxocobinamide, 1695
Arabinoside, 349f
  cell cycle phase specificity, 761f
Araceae, 1598t, 1600t–1603t, 1610
Arachidonic acid (AA), 897, 941
  acetaminophen and, 472
  metabolism, 511, 513f
N-Arachidonoyl dopamine, structure, 1112f
2-Arachidonoylglycerol (2AG), structure, 1112f
2-Arachidonyl glyceryl ether, structure, 1112f
Arachnida, 1540, 1540f, 1845. *See also* Scorpions; Spiders; Ticks
Arachnidism, 1540
  history and epidemiology, 1540–1541
Arachnids. *See also* Spiders
  and insects, differences between, 1540
Araliaceae, 1598t, 1600t
Araneae, 1540, 1540f. *See also* Spiders
Araneism, 1540
Aranha Armadeira (*Phoneutria nigriventer*), 1540
Arcaine, 227t
Arctic hysteria, 654–655

Arctium lappa (burdock root), 640t
Arctium minus (burdock root), 640t
Area under the curve (AUC), 143, 151, 152f
Areca catechu (betel nut), 1598t, 1605
   uses and toxicities, 640t
Arecaceae, 1598t
Areca nut, uses and toxicities, 640t
Arecoline, 640t, 648–649, 1598t, 1605
Arformoterol, 985
Argasidae, 1550
Argatroban, 321f, 892, 892f
   anticoagulant effect, 884f
      laboratory investigation, 893
   coagulopathy caused by, treatment, 893–894
   indications for, 891
   laboratory testing for, 888t, 893
   overdose/poisoning, treatment strategies for, 888t
Argemone mexicana (Mexican pricklepoppy, prickly
      poppy), 650t, 1598t, 1605
Argemone oil, 1605
Arginase, 180f, 181
Arginine hydrochloride, and normal anion gap
      metabolic acidosis, 191t
Arginine vasopressin, 194. *See also* Antidiuretic
      hormone (ADH)
Arginosuccinate, 180f, 181
Argiotoxin, 227t
Argon
   as simple asphyxiant, 400t, 1650, 1652
   uses, 1652
Argyreia spp., 1598t
Argyreia nervosa (Hawaiian baby wood rose),
      1179, 1179t, 1181t, 1182, 1598t, 1605
Argyria, 273, 1344, 1346–1347, 1346f
   histopathology, 1347
   localized, 1344, 1347
   treatment, 1347
Aripiprazole. *See also* Antipsychotics
   clinical and toxicologic effects, 1034t
   dosage and administration, 1033t
   for inhalant-induced psychosis, 1200
   mechanism of action, 1035
   pharmacokinetics, 1033t
   priapism caused by, 301t
Aristocholic acid, 613
Aristolochia (*Aristolochia fangi, A. clematis, A. fangji,*
      A. reticulata), 1598t, 1610
   as abortifacients, 303, 303t
Aristolochia (*Aristolochia fangchi, A. clematis, A.*
      reticulata), uses and toxicities, 640t
Aristolochiaceae, 1598t
Aristolochia fangji, 613
Aristolochic acid(s), 639, 640t, 1598t, 1610
   as abortifacient, 303t
   toxicity, 648
Aristolochic acid nephropathy, 1610
Aristophanes, 632
Aristotle, 1t, 2
Arizona black rattlesnake (*Crotalus cerberus*), 1617t
Arizona ridge-nosed rattlesnake (*Crotalus* spp.), 1637t
Arkansas tarantula (*Dugesiella hentzi*), 1547
Armed Forces Radio-biology Research Institute,
      website, 1768
Armillariella mellea (honey mushroom), 1594
Armstrong, Robert, 5t
Aromatase inhibitors, 617, 618f
Aromatic acid herbicides, 1467t
Aromatic hydrocarbons. *See* Hydrocarbons, aromatic
Aromatics, adsorption to activated charcoal, 76
Arrestins, 205

Arrhenius, Svante, 160
Arrhythmia, definition, 865
Arrow poisons, 1. *See also specific poison*
Arsenate, 1237
   and ATP production, 176t
   and glycolysis, 175, 176t, 177f
   laboratory measurement, 1243
   metabolism, 1240, 1240f
   pathophysiologic effects, 1239, 1239f
   physicochemical properties, 157–158
   site of action, 173f
Arsenic, 1237–1250
   absorption, 1239–1240
   antidote for, 3, 35t
      unicorn horn as, 3
   in antimony ore, 1230
   antisyphilis therapy, imaging findings after, 117f, 132f
   beer contamination with, 21, 21t
   Borgias' use of, 4
   in breast milk, 1240
   carcinogenicity, 1239, 1242
   cardiac effects, 258t, 1239, 1241, 1243
   chemistry, 157–158, 1237
   in chemotherapeutics, 1237. *See also* Arsenic trioxide
      (white arsenic)
   childhood exposure to, adverse effects, 1242
   in dietary supplements, 647–648
   in drinking water, 1237, 1242–1243. *See also* Health
      Effects of Arsenic Longitudinal Study
      (HEALS)
      and QT prolongation, 1239
   early use of, 1–2, 4, 4t–5t, 6, 6t, 12
   elemental, 1237
   elimination, 1240
      folic acid and, 775
   exposure to, sources, 1237, 1237t
   fetal effects, 1241
   in food, 18t, 19, 1237
   food contamination with, 599–600
   gaseous, 1237
   gastrointestinal effects, 1241–1243
   groundwater contamination with, 18t, 19, 1847
      in India and Bangladesh, 1844
   hair, tests for, 1244
   hematologic effects, 1242–1244
   hepatic effects, 334, 1241–1243
   hepatotoxicity, 1252
   and hERG channels, 253
   history and epidemiology, 1237
   inorganic
      absorption, 1239–1240
      exposure to, sources, 1237, 1237t
      toxicity
         acute, 1241–1242
         chronic, 1242–1243
         clinical manifestations, 1241–1243
   intentional poisoning with, 1237, 1244
   in utero exposure to, adverse effects, 1242
   mass poisoning with, 1237
   metabolism, 1240, 1240f
   methylation, folates and, 777
   nail changes caused by, 282
   nail tests for, 1244
   nephrotoxicity, 390f, 397t
   neurotoxicity, 343, 1241, 1243–1244
   odor, 364t
   organic
      absorption, 1240
      exposure to, sources, 1237, 1237t
   ototoxicity, 1241

pentavalent, 1237
   toxicity, pathophysiology, 1239, 1239f
pentavalent form, 158
pharmacokinetics, 1239–1241
pharmacology, 1237–1238
physicochemical properties, 1237
physiology, 1237–1238
regulations and guidelines for, 1237, 1238t
in rice, 1237
skin discoloration caused by, 273
speciation, 1243
tests for, 4t, 6
therapeutic use, 1237
toxicity (overdose/poisoning)
   abdominal radiographs in, 1244
   chelation therapy for, 1244–1245, 1245f, 1245t,
      1251–1253
   chronic, diagnostic tests for, 1243–1244
   clinical and laboratory findings with, 36t,
      1241–1243, 1241f–1242f
   death caused by, 1241
   diagnostic imaging, 116, 1244
   diagnostic tests for, 1243–1244
   dimercaprol for. *See* Dimercaprol (BAL, British
      anti-Lewisite)
   gastrointestinal decontamination for, 1244
   hemodialysis in, 1245
   management, 44t, 46t, 775, 777, 1244–1245,
      1245f, 1245t
      nutritional supplementation in, 1245
   metallic taste in, 1241
   pathophysiology, 1238–1239
   and QT interval, 253
   subacute, 1242
   whole-bowel irrigation for, 1234, 1244
toxicokinetics, 1239–1241
transplacental transfer, 1240
trivalent, 158
   toxicity, pathophysiology, 1238–1239, 1239f
urine
   in chronic toxicity, 1244
   in contaminated meat consumers, 19
   factors affecting, 1243
   interpretation, 1243–1244
   measurement, 1243
   normal concentration, 19, 1237
   in poisoning, 1243
   specimen collection for, 1243
   in subacute toxicity, 1244
   and vascular disease, 1239
water contamination with, 777
whole blood
   normal concentration, 1237
   in poisoning, 1243
Arsenic acid, dermal absorption, 1240
Arsenic Act (1851), 6
Arsenical dermatitis, 38, 1242, 1242f, 1251
Arsenical herbicides, 1467t
Arsenicals. *See also* Arsenic
   as chemical weapon, 1741
   and selenium toxicity, 1342
Arsenic compounds
   pharmacology, 1237–1238
   regulations and guidelines for, 1237, 1238t
Arsenic trioxide (white arsenic), 158, 1237. *See also* Arsenic
   absorption, 1240
   for acute promyelocytic leukemia, 1237–1238
   adverse effects, 762–763, 763t, 1243
   cardiovascular toxicity, 253t, 762–763, 763t
   elimination half-life, 1240

EPA regulation of, 765
estimated fatal dose, 1452t
historical perspective on, 5t, 6
LD$_{50}$ for, 1240
mechanism and site of action, 762f
pharmacokinetics, 1240–1241, 1240f
physicochemical properties, 1452t
and QT interval, 253t, 762–763, 763t
in rodenticides, 1452t
tissue distribution, 1240
toxicity (overdose/poisoning)
    antidote and/or treatment, 1452t
    clinical manifestations, 1452t
    magnesium for, 878
    onset, 1452t
    whole-bowel irrigation for, 85
toxic mechanism, 1452t
Arsenious acid, food contamination with, 21, 21t
Arsenite, 158, 1237
and citric acid cycle, 176t
laboratory measurement, 1243
metabolism, 1240, 1240f
Arsenobetaine (AsB), 1237, 1241, 1243
Arsenopyrite, 1339. See also Selenium
Arsenosugars, 1237
Arsine, 1233
hemolysis caused by, 317–318
overdose/poisoning, hyperkalemia caused by, 251
Arteether, 845
Artemesia absinthium (wormwood). See Wormwood
Artemether, 845
antimalarial mechanism, 838t
Artemisia absinthium (absinthe), 9, 627–628, 650t,
    1598t, 1608. See also Wormwood
Artemisia annua (sweet wormwood), 638, 845
for malaria, 638, 647
Artemisia dracunculus, 643t
Artemisia lactiflora, 643t
Artemisia (Artemesia) toxicity, 648
Artemisia vulgaris, 643t
Artemisinin, 638, 647, 836, 845
adverse effects and safety issues, 845
antimalarial mechanism, 838t, 845
derivatives, 845
overdose/poisoning, clinical manifestations, 845
pharmacokinetics, 839t, 845
structure, 845
toxicodynamics, 845
Artemisinin-based combination therapy (ACT), 836,
    842, 844, 847
formulations, 845
Artemisone, antimalarial mechanism, 838t
Arterial blood gases
analysis, 36–37, 190
    in cyanide poisoning, 1687, 1687t
    smoke inhalation and, 1642
physiochemistry, in hypothermia, 417
Arterial partial pressure of carbon dioxide (PaCO$_2$), 408f
Arterial partial pressure of oxygen (PaO$_2$), 399–400, 408f
Artesunate, 638, 647, 845
antimalarial mechanism, 838t
toxicity, 648
Arthropoda (phylum), 1540
taxonomy, 1540, 1540f
Arthropods, 1540–1566, 1540t. See also Hymenoptera;
    Spiders; specific arthropod
bites, definition, 1540
biting
    stinging, or nettling, 1540t
        history and epidemiology, 1540–1541

stings, definition, 1540
taxonomy, 1540
Arthroprosthetic cobaltism, 1273, 1275–1276
and cardiac disorders, 1275
and dermatitis, 1277
laboratory investigation, 1278
management, 1279
and neurologic disorders, 1275
and thyroid abnormalities, 1275
treatment, 1278–1279
Artificial tears, benzalkonium chloride in, 682t
Arylcyclohexylamines. See also Ketamine;
    Methoxetamine; Phencyclidine (PCP)
and biogenic amine reuptake complex, 1213
clinical effects, 1214–1216, 1215f
designer, 1211
neuropsychiatric effects, 1214–1215
and NMDA receptors, 1213–1214
pathophysiology, 1213–1214
and sensory processing, 1213
sites of activity, 1213
toxicity, management, 1217–1218
Arylhexamines, 1178
Aryl hydrocarbon receptor (AhR), 170–171
Aryl mercury compounds, 1324t–1325t
absorption, 1325
poisoning, clinical manifestations, 1327
tissue distribution, 1325
Asarin, 1598t, 1609–1610
Asarum arifolium, 1610
Asarum europaeum, 1610
Asbestos, 12, 1659
calcified pleural plaques caused by, 115t, 126, 127f
occupational diseases caused by, 23, 23t
physicochemical properties, 160
respiratory effects, 399t, 401
Asbestosis, 23, 23t, 126
calcified pleural plaques in, imaging, 115t, 126,
    127f
chest radiograph perfusion score in, 1277
diagnostic imaging, 115t, 125t, 126, 127f
pulmonary effects, imaging, 115t, 125t
Ascending tonic-clonic syndrome (ATCS), 794
Asclepiadaceae, 1598t
Asclepias spp. (milkweed), 969, 1598t
Asclepias curassavica (redheaded cotton-bush), 979
Asclepias syriaca (common milkweed), 969
Asclepin, 1598t
Ascorbic acid, 662. See also Vitamin C
hepatoprotective effects, with antimonial therapy,
    1232
for propanil poisoning, 1473
Asenapine. See also Antipsychotics
clinical and toxicologic effects, 1034t
dosage and administration, 1033t
mechanism of action, 1035
pharmacokinetics, 1033t
Aseptic lymphocyte-dominated vasculitis-associated
    lesion (ALVAL), 1276
Asian flush, 273, 744, 1145
Asian medicine
adulterants in, and poisoning, 1845
heavy metals in, 1845
synthetic pharmaceuticals in, 1845
Asians, ADH and ALDH gene variants in, 1144–1145
Asiatic acid, 642t
Asiaticoside, 642t
Asoxime (HI-6), structure, 1508
L-Asparaginase, 759, 760t
and fibrinolysis, 322–323

mechanism and site of action, 762f
neurotoxicity, 763
Aspartate, 179
Aspartate aminotransferase
in acetaminophen toxicity, 480–481
elevation, methotrexate-related, 768
in heatstroke, 422
in liver injury, 327–328, 334, 335t
postmortem changes, 1885t
Aspartic acid, 595, 595f
mechanism of action, 227t
Aspergillosis, in HIV-infected (AIDS) patients,
    830t–831t
Aspergillus, mycotoxins, 174t
Asphalt. See also Hydrocarbons
injuries caused by, 1416
Asphyxiants
chemical, 1640–1642, 1640t, 1748
    effects on oxygenation, 403, 403f
inert (noble) gases as, 158
simple, 400, 400t, 1640, 1640t, 1650–1653
    clinical effects, 1651–1652, 1651t
    from combustion, 1640, 1640t
    management, 1653
    pathophysiology, 1651
Asphyxiation
causes, 1196
nitrous oxide abuse and, 1199
Aspiration pneumonitis, 37, 58t, 401, 540
activated charcoal and, 61, 79
diagnosis, 401
hypercalcemia and, 199
imaging, 115t, 123, 125t
multiple-dose activated charcoal and, 62
with organic phosphorus compound poisoning,
    1490–1491, 1492f
whole-bowel irrigation and, 85
Aspirin. See also Nonsteroidal antiinflammatory drugs
    (NSAIDs); Salicylate(s)
absorption, 555
    prevention, 85
adverse effects and safety issues, 555, 561, 899
antiplatelet effects, 323, 555, 897–899
    mechanism of action, 898f
antithrombotic properties, 883
cardiovascular benefits, 899
cerebral hemorrhage caused by, imaging, 132t
for cocaine-associated chest pain, 1129
contraindications to, 817
and cyclooxygenase, 555
and ethanol, interactions, 1146t
gastrointestinal effects, 558
hematologic effects, 516
high-dose, 899
historical perspective on, 8, 555, 638
low-dose, 899
metabolism, 555
for niacin-induced flushing, 273, 664
ototoxicity, 561
percent nonionized, pH and, 142t
pharmacokinetics, 145t, 555
pharmacology, 555
and Reye syndrome, 557
in stroke prevention, 899
tablets, gastric outlet obstruction caused by, 128
therapeutic uses, 555
toxicity (overdose/poisoning), 559–561
    in elderly, case study, 459
    epidemiology, 555
    pathophysiology, 557–558

Aspirin (*Cont.*):
    toxicokinetics, 555–556, 556f
    volume of distribution, 145t, 555
Aspirin-phenacetin-caffeine (APC), renal effects, 558
Aspirin-sensitive asthmatic, 515
Assessment
    bedside, 28
    emergency, 28
Association of Occupational and Environmental Clinics
        (AOEC), recommendations for lead-exposed
        workers, 1300, 1301t
Association of Zoos and Aquariums. *See also*
        Antivenom Index
    Antivenom Index, 1561, 1565–1566
AST-120, 77
Astemizole, 21, 171
    cardiotoxicity, 746
    pharmacology, 742
    QT interval prolongation by, 1840
Asteraceae, 1598t–1600t, 1602t–1603t
Asthenosoma spp., 1573
Asthenospermia, 298
Asthma, 987, 1659–1660
    aluminum-induced, 1223–1225
    aspirin-intolerant, 230
    aspirin-sensitive, 515
    cobalt-associated, 1276
    cocaine and, 8, 1126
    irritant-induced, 1660
    nickel exposure and, 1336
    occupational (work-related), 403, 1660, 1660t
        treatment, 407
        without latency, 1660
    potroom, 1223, 1225
    quinine and, 840
    work-aggravated, 403
Astoria stokesii (Stokes' sea snake), 1574
Astragalus spp. (locoweed), 1598t
Astragalus (*Astragalus membranaceus*), uses and
        toxicities, 640t
Astragalus lentiginosis (spotted locoweed), 1606
Astringents, 6
Astrocytes, 340–341
Astrogalasides, 640t
Astrovirus, foodborne illness caused by, 592t
Asulam, in herbicides, 1467t
Asystole, 256, 263
    physostigmine and, 756
Ataxia, 345
    carbon monoxide poisoning and, 1665
    in toxidromes, 29t
Atazanavir, 831–832
    crystalluria caused by, 395
    and methadone, interactions, 172
Atelectasis, smoke inhalation and, 1641
Atenolol
    extracorporeal elimination, 97t
    overdose/poisoning
        clinical manifestations, 931–932
        lipid emulsion for, 1006
    pharmacokinetics, 930
    pharmacology, 927t
    structure, 926f
    for thyrotoxicosis, 817
Atenolol-chlorthalidone, 931
Atheroemboli, acute kidney injury caused by, 391
Atherogenesis, cocaine and, 1125, 1127
Atherosclerosis, 661
    cadmium and, 1261
    carbon disulfide and, 1175

Athletes, sudden death in, 623
Athlete's biological passport, 623
Athletic performance enhancers, 616–626. *See also*
        specific xenobiotic
    capillary gas chromatography-mass spectrometry,
        622
    history of, 616
    isotope ratio mass spectrometry, 622
    laboratory detection, 621–623
    neurocognitive enhancement as, 623
    and sudden death, 623
    and testosterone-to-epitestosterone ratio, 622
    World Anti-Doping Agency Code on, 616, 616t
Atom(s)
    definition, 155
    functional groups, 165–166
Atomic bombs, 1762
Atomic mass, definition, 155
Atomic number, 156f
    definition, 155
Atomic weight, 156f
    definition, 155
Atomism, 1762
Atomoxetine, mechanism of action, 211, 227t, 228,
        1056f
Atopic dermatitis, 278
Atorvastatin
    CYP enzymes and, 170
    as P-glycoprotein inhibitor, 173
Atovaquone, 845–846
    adverse effects and safety issues, 846
    antimalarial mechanism, 838t, 845–846
    for HIV-related infections, 830t
    overdose, 846
    pharmacokinetics, 839t
    structure, 845
Atovaquone–proguanil combination, 846
ATP. *See* Adenosine triphosphate (ATP)
ATP-binding cassette transporters, 341
ATP synthase, 177
ATRA. *See* all-*trans* Retinoic acid
Atractaspididae, 1633t, 1845
Atractaspidinae, 1617
Atractaspis spp. (stiletto snakes), 1633t
Atractylis gummifera (thistle), 1598t, 1607
    uses and toxicities, 640t
Atractyloside, 176t, 1597, 1598t, 1607
    site of action, 173f
Atracurium. *See also* Neuromuscular blockers
    benzyl alcohol in, 683t
    and histamine release, 1019
    mechanism of action, 207
    pharmacokinetics, 1019
    pharmacology, 1020t, 1024–1025
ATRA syndrome, 656, 658
Atrax spp. (funnel web spider). *See also* Funnel web
        spider (*Atrax* spp., *Hadronyche* spp.)
    antivenom, worldwide availability, 1560t
Atrax robustus, 1548. *See also* Funnel web spider (*Atrax*
        spp., *Hadronyche* spp.)
Atrazine, 1471, 1482–1483
    dermal absorption, 1483
    metabolism, 1482–1483
    metabolites, 1482
    pharmacokinetics and toxicokinetics, 1482–1483
    pharmacology, 1482
    poisoning
        clinical manifestations, 1483
        management, 1483
    structure, 1482f

Atrial fibrillation
    cardioactive steroid toxicity and, 972t, 974
    ethanol and, 1148
    hypothermia and, 416
    magnesium for, 877
Atrial flutter, cardioactive steroid toxicity and, 972t,
        974
Atrial tachycardia
    cardioactive steroid toxicity and, 972
    magnesium for, 877
Atrioventricular (AV) dissociation, 248, 972
Atrioventricular (AV) junctional block, 972
Atrioventricular (AV) nodal block, 258, 972
Atrioventricular (AV) node, 246, 248, 926, 928f, 945,
        947, 970
    dysfunction, exacerbated or unmasked by
        xenobiotics in elderly, 463, 463t
Atropa belladonna (belladonna). *See also* Atropine;
        Belladonna (*Atropa belladonna*)
    uses and toxicities, 1598t
AtroPen Auto-Injector, 1506, 1746
Atrophic gastritis, exacerbated or unmasked by
        xenobiotics in elderly, 463, 463t
Atrophy, skin, 269t
Atropine, 2, 640t, 642t–643t, 650t, 651, 755, 1181, 1181t,
        1182, 1604
    absorption, 1504
    adverse effects and safety issues, 1504–1505
    as antidote, 1503–1508
    antidote for, 755
    autoinjector, 1506
    availability and storage, 44t, 1746
    for calcium channel blocker toxicity, 948–949
    for carbamate poisoning, 1498
    for carbamate toxicity, 1504
    cardiac effects, 255
    for cardioactive steroid poisoning, 973
    for chemical weapons nerve agents, 1505–1506
    chemistry, 1503
    clinical effects, 1503
    distribution, 1504
    dosage and administration, 1505–1506
        for chemical weapons nerve agents, 1505–1506
        in children, 1505
    duration of action, 1504
    elimination, 1504
    elimination half-life, 1182, 1504
    formulation and acquisition, 1506
    and glycopyrrolate, comparison, 1503f
    history of, 1503
    indications for, 35t, 44t, 751, 1503
    for local anesthetic–induced bradycardia, 1001
    mechanism of action, 1503–1504
    for metal phosphide poisoning, 1460
    for muscarine-containing mushroom poisoning, 1587
    nebulized, 1504
    in nerve agent antidote kit, 1746
    for nerve agents, 1745–1746
    for neurotoxic snake envenomation, 1635
    obstructive nephropathy caused by, 394
    onset of action, 1504
    ophthalmic effects, 1504
    for organic phosphorus compound poisoning,
        1496–1497, 1504
        dosage and administration, 1505
    for organic phosphorus insecticide poisoning, 1504
    for organic phosphorus nerve agent poisoning,
        1504–1506
    pharmacodynamics, 1504
    pharmacokinetics, 1504

pharmacology, 1025, 1026t, 1183, 1503–1504
poisoning, 756
and pralidoxime, synergism, 1509
in pregnancy and lactation, 1505
serum concentration, 1504
shortage, 43
stocking, recommended level, 44t, 1746
in Strategic National Stockpile, 1506
structure, 1503
sublingual, 1504
supplies, 42
volume of distribution, 1504
for xenobiotic-induced respiratory dysfunction, 407
Atropine challenge, 1495
Atropine-diphenoxylate, pediatric delayed toxicity, 452
Attention-deficit/hyperactivity disorder
glutamate and, 224
treatment, 228
Atypical antidepressants. See Antidepressants, atypical;
specific xenobiotic
Aum Shinrikyo cult, 1753
Aura, migraine, 805
Australian estuarine stonefish (Synanceja trachynis),
1576, 1576t, 1577–1578
antivenom, 1575t
Australian marsupial tick (Ixodes holocyclus), 1550
Australian redback spider. See Latrodectus hasselti
Australian stinging sponge (Neofibularia mordens), 1573
Autism
copper and, 1283
glutamate and, 224
thimerosal and, 689, 1327–1328
vaccines and, 689, 1852–1853
Autlán rattlesnake (Crotalus spp.), 1636t
Autoinjectors, in nerve agent antidote kit, 1746
Autologous blood transfusions, as doping, 319
Automated dispensing cabinets (ADCs), 1829
Automaticity, cardiac
and dysrhythmias, 254–255
increased/enhanced, 254–255
triggered, 255
Automobile exhaust fumes, and methemoglobin
formation, 1705
Autonomic failure, hypoglycemia-associated, 698, 708
Autonomic instability, hallucinogen-induced, 1184
Autonomic nervous system, 260
cardioactive steroids and, 970
and hemodynamics, 260–262
hypoglycemia and, 698
Autonomy, principle of, 1860
Autophagy, induction
lithium and, 1067f
nanoparticles and, 1726f, 1727
Autopotentiation, 1078
Autopsy, medicolegal, 1885
Autoreceptors, 205–206, 205f, 207, 215, 216f, 220
somatodendritic, 205, 205f, 215, 216f
terminal, 205–206, 205f
Autumn crocus (Colchicum autumnale), 1599t, 1612.
See also Colchicine
uses and toxicities, 640t
Avanafil
for erectile dysfunction, 301
pharmacokinetics, 301
Avascular necrosis. See also Osteonecrosis
imaging, 115t, 122, 124f
Averrhoa carambola (star fruit, carambola), 1611
Avizafone, in nerve agent antidote, 1746
Axon(s), 340
Axonopathies, 345–346

Ayahuasca, 640t, 647, 1178, 1180
with Banisteriopsis caapi, 647, 649
DMT in, 641t, 647
MAOI activity, 1077
and serotonin toxicity, 1058t
Ayurvedic medicine
adulterants in, poisoning caused by, 1845
conessine in, 742
contaminants and, 647–648
corticosteroids in, 1845
lead exposure in, 1293, 1304
and mercury poisoning, 1327
metals in, 1293, 1845
Swarna bhasma in, 1717
AZA (Association of Zoos and Aquariums). See
Antivenom Index
Azalea spp. (azalea), 1598t, 1612
Azatadine, pharmacology, 742
Azathioprine
acute interstitial nephritis caused by, 394t
pancreatitis caused by, 295t
Azelastine
elimination half-life, 744
pharmacology, 742
Azelastine hydrochloride, benzalkonium chloride in,
682
Azemiopinae, 1633t, 1633t
Azemiops feae (Fea's viper), 1633t
Azides
and electron transport, 176t
site of action, 173f
Azinphos-methyl, 1488t
Azithromycin, 826–827
antimalarial mechanism, 838t
for HIV-related infections, 830t
Azole antifungals, 829. See also Imidazoles; Triazoles;
specific xenobiotic
and vincristine, interactions, 506
Azoospermia, 298
Aztreonam, 825
and GABA receptor, 222
Azure B, 1077

B
Babesiosis, 1550
BabyBIG, 582
Bachelor's button. See Feverfew (Tanacetum
parthenium)
Bacillus anthracis, 1754–1756, 1755f
Bacillus cereus
foodborne infection, 592t, 599
gastroenteritis, 597, 597t
steatosis caused by, 332
Bacitracin toxicity, organ system manifestations, 829t
Baclofen
for alcohol withdrawal, 1170
bradycardia with, 924, 924t
effects on vital signs, 30t
GABAB agonism by, 1084
and GABAB receptors, 238
for γ-hydroxybutyrate (GHB) withdrawal, 1191
hypoventilation caused by, 400t
for inhalant withdrawal, 1200
intrathecal, 794, 798
inadvertent overdose and unintentional
exposures due to, 795t
withdrawal, 222
mechanism of action, 222
overdose/poisoning, 222, 238, 1094
physostigmine and, 756

renal impairment and, 389
withdrawal, 222, 238, 1138
GABAB receptor in, 238
Bacterial infection(s), propofol and, 1090
Bacteriostatic saline for injection, benzyl alcohol in,
683, 683t
Bacteriostatic water for injection, benzyl alcohol in,
683, 683t
Bagassosis, 1659
Bagging, 1193, 1196
Baja California rattlesnake (Crotalus spp.), 1636t
BAL. See Dimercaprol (BAL, British anti-Lewisite)
Bala (Sida cordifolia), 1602t
Balanced salt solution, benzalkonium chloride in,
682
Balfour, John, 755
Balkan endemic nephropathy, 1610
Ballismus, mercury-associated, 1327
Balloon plant (Gomphocarpus physocarpus, G.
fruticosus), 979
Balucanat. See Tung and tung seed (Aleurites
moluccana, A. fordii)
Bancroftian filariasis, 1522
Band 3 anion-exchange protein, 312
Banded rock rattlesnake (Crotalus spp.), 1636t
Baneberry. See Black cohosh (Actaea racemosa);
Black cohosh (Cimicifuga racemosa)
Banisteriopsis caapi (caapi), 650t, 1077, 1180
uses and toxicities, 640t, 647, 649
Bannal (Cytisus scoparius), 640t
Barbaloin, 640t, 1598t
Barberry (Berberis spp.), 1598t, 1605
Barbital, 1087
gastric absorption, lipid solubility and, 143f
Barbiturate blisters, 1086
Barbiturates. See also Sedative-hypnotics; specific
xenobiotic
absorption, 1087
for agitation, in thyrotoxicosis, 817
for alcohol withdrawal, 1168
for amphetamine toxicity, 1104–1105, 1104t
for cocaine toxicity, 1128
cranial neuropathy caused by, 346t
drug interactions with, 1085, 1087
effects on vital signs, 31t
focal brain lesions caused by, 131
and GABA receptor, 221
history of, 1084, 1135
for γ-hydroxybutyrate (GHB) withdrawal, 1191
hypoventilation caused by, 400t
laboratory testing for, 36t, 101t, 1086t
lipid solubility, 1087
for local anesthetic–induced seizures, 1000
and male sexual dysfunction, 299f
ophthalmic effects, 361
overdose/poisoning
clinical and laboratory findings in, 36t, 1086t
deaths caused by, 1087
extracorporeal therapies for, 91, 91f
and organ donation, 1893t
pharmacodynamics and toxicodynamics, 1084
pharmacokinetics and toxicokinetics, 1084–1087
protein binding, 1085
and pyridoxine, combined, for INH-induced seizures,
863
screening for, 113
structure, 1087
urine screening assays for, performance
characteristics, 111t
withdrawal, 237

Barbituric acid, 1087
Barcoding, in medication dispensing and administration, 1829
Bariatric surgery, 613
  effects on gastrointestinal tract, 293
  effects on pharmacokinetics, 148, 293
  patients who have undergone, gastrointestinal decontamination in, 64
  and thiamine deficiency, 1157, 1160
Baricity, and intrathecal administration, 793
Barite, 1454
Baritosis, 1454
Barium acetate, 1454
  common uses, 1454t
  solubility, 1454t
Barium and barium salts
  absorption, 1454
  chemistry, 157, 1454, 1454t
  common uses, 1454, 1454t
  as contrast agent, 127–128, 130f
  decontamination, 1455
  elimination, enhancement, 1455
  estimated fatal dose, 1452t
  fumes, 1454
  history of, 1454
  ingestion, 1454
  inhalation, 1454
  lethal dose, 1454
  nephrotoxicity, 397t
  occupational exposure to, 1454
  physicochemical properties, 1452t, 1454
  in rodenticides, 1452t
  serum
    normal concentration, 1454
    in toxicity, 1454
  solubility, 1454, 1454t
  toxicity
    antidote and/or treatment, 1452t
    clinical manifestations, 1452t, 1455
    diagnostic tests for, 1455
    epidemiology, 1454
    management, 1455
    onset, 1452t
    pathophysiology, 1455
  toxic mechanism, 1452t
  toxicokinetics, 1454–1455
Barium arsenate, 1454
Barium carbonate, 1454
  common uses, 1454t
  solubility, 1454t
Barium chloride, 1454
  common uses, 1454t
  ingestion, 1454
  solubility, 1454t
Barium chromate, 1268t, 1454
Barium dioxide, 1454
Barium fluoride, 1454
  common uses, 1454t
  solubility, 1454t
Barium hydroxide, 1454
Barium nitrate, 1454
  common uses, 1454t
  solubility, 1454t
Barium oxalate, 1454
Barium oxide, 1454
  common uses, 1454t
  solubility, 1454t
Barium permanganate, 1319
Barium styphnate, common uses, 1454t
Barium sulfate, 1454

common uses, 1454t
intravasation, 1454–1455
  management, 1455
intravenous administration, 1455
solubility, 1454t
Barium sulfide/polysulfide, 1454
  common uses, 1454t
  solubility, 1454t
Bark scorpion (Centruroides exilicauda). See Centruroides exilicauda (bark scorpion)
Barnish tree. See Tung and tung seed (Aleurites moluccana, A. fordii)
Barometric pressure, 399, 1651
Baroreceptor dysfunction, exacerbated or unmasked by xenobiotics in elderly, 463, 463t
Barotrauma, 400–401
  inhalant abuse and, 1196
Bartlett, Adelaide, 5t
Basal ganglia
  barium toxicity and, 1455
  focal necrosis, 132t
  hypoxic damage to, 131
  imaging, 115t, 131, 132t
  in methanol poisoning, 1424
  thiamine-biotin-responsive disease, 1158
Base(s)
  adsorption to activated charcoal, 76
  anionic, 141
  Arrhenius definition, 160
  Brønsted-Lowry definition, 160–161
  cationic, 141
  definition, 160–161
  ionization, 161
  Lewis, 160–161
  nonionized, 141
  strength of, vs. concentration, 161, 161t
  weak
    dissociation constant for, 142
    ionization, and passive diffusion, 141
    membrane transport, 142
Base (bulb), of mushrooms, 1584f
Base-forming gases, 1655, 1658. See also specific xenobiotic
Basement membrane zone, 270, 270f
Basitrichous isorhiza, 1568
Basophils, 319
Batfish, 1576
"Bath salts." See Cathinone(s)
Batrachotoxin, 1612
  clinical effects, 576t
  and voltage-gated calcium channels, 244f, 245
Battered child, 454
Batteries, button, 1389
Bauxite, 1223
Bazett formula, for corrected QT, 251
BB-22, 1112f
Beaded lizard (Heloderma horridum), 1618, 1619f
Beadlet anemone (Actinia equina), 1567t
Beaked sea snake (Enhydrina schistosa), 1574–1575
  antivenom, 1575t
Beau lines, 274t, 281f, 282
Bebulin, 910
Beclomethasone dipropionate, nasal spray, benzalkonium chloride in, 682
Becquerel (Bq), 1764, 1764f
Bedaquiline
  adverse effects and safety issues, 858
  dosage and administration, 858
  drug interactions with, 858
  monitoring with, 858

pharmacokinetics, 858
pharmacology, 858
Bee (Apis mellifera), 1540, 1551–1552, 1845. See also Honeybee (Apis mellifera)
  stings, 3
  venom
    and rhabdomyolysis, 393
    uses and toxicities, 640t
Bee bread. See Borage (Borago officinalis)
Beecher, Henry, 1018
Beef liver, vitamin A toxicity from, 655
Bee plant. See Borage (Borago officinalis)
Bee pollen (Apis mellifera), uses and toxicities, 640t
Beer, cobalt sulfate in, 1143, 1273–1275
Beer drinkers' cardiomyopathy, 21, 22t, 1143, 1273–1275
Beer foam stabilizer, 1143. See also Cobalt
Beers criteria, 460, 1826–1827
Beetles, as aphrodisiacs, 304
Beggar's button. See Burdock root (Arctium lappa, A. minus)
Behavioral disturbances, and diagnostic assessment, 375
Belladonna (Atropa belladonna), 1503. See also Atropine
  as aphrodisiac, 304
  early poisoning with, 2, 4, 5t, 6
  uses and toxicity, 1598t
Belladonna alkaloids, 1178, 1179t, 1181, 1598t, 1600t–1602t, 1604
  clinical effects, 1183, 1604
  toxicokinetics, 1182
Bel Zaard, 3
Benazolin, in herbicides, 1467t
Benefin. See Benfluralin
Benfluralin, 1468t
Benfotiamine, 1158
Ben-Gay, wintergreen oil in, 634
Benign prostatic hyperplasia (BPH), 305
Bensulide, 1468t
Benzaldehyde, CNS effects, 1196
Benzalkonium chloride (BAC), 681–682, 682t, 1369t, 1388t
  antimicrobial activity, 681
  chemistry, 681
  nasopharyngeal toxicity, 682
  in ophthalmic medications, 681–682, 682t
  ophthalmic toxicity, 682
  oropharyngeal toxicity, 682
  as sterilant, 1374
  structure, 681
Benzedrine, 1099
Benzedrine Inhaler, 748
Benzene, 12, 174t, 1410. See also Hydrocarbons, aromatic
  aplastic anemia caused by, 22, 23t
  biotransformation, 172
  effects on liver, 328
  in gasoline, 1410
  infertility caused by, 297t
  inhaled, 1193t
  and leukemia, 320
  pharmacology, 1194
  and tinnitus, 370t
  toxicity, 1415
  toxicokinetics, 1411t
  uses, 1409t
  viscosity, 1409t
Benzo[a]pyrene, 7
  CYP and, 171
  toxic metabolite, 174t

Benzocaine. *See also* Local anesthetic(s)
  and methemoglobinemia, 994, 997
  structure, 995f
  topical, poisoning with, 994
Benzocaine spray, methemoglobinemia caused by,
    1703, 1705
Benzodiazepine(s), 1087–1088, 1135–1142. *See also*
    Sedative-hypnotics
  for acute dystonia, 1036, 1037t
  and adenosine reuptake, 230–231
  administration route, 1136–1137
  adverse effects and safety issues, 1088, 1139–1140
  for agitated/violent behavior, 386
  for agitation
    with hallucinogens, 1184
    in thyrotoxicosis, 817
  for akathisia, 1036, 1037t
  for alcohol withdrawal, 1138, 1168
    symptom-triggered administration, 1168
  for alcohol withdrawal seizures, 1167
  for amphetamine toxicity, 1104–1105, 1104t
  for anticholinergic syndrome, 748
  antidote for, 35t
  and antipsychotic, combined, for agitated/violent
    behavior, 386
  binding sites in brain, 1087–1088
  for black widow spider envenomation, 1543
  chemistry, 1135
  for chemotherapeutic-related vomiting, 764
  and chloride channels, 1135, 1136f
  for chloroquine toxicity, 1139
  for cocaine-associated agitation, 386
  for cocaine-associated chest pain, 1139
  for cocaine toxicity, 1128, 1139
  for conscious sedation, flumazenil and,
    1094–1095
  for cyclic antidepressant toxicity, 1049t
  deaths caused by, 1084
  diluents, 1137t
  and drug-facilitated crime, in developing world,
    1846
  drug interactions with, 1085
  duration of action, 1137–1138, 1137t
  elimination, 1137–1138
  for emergence reactions, 1217
  and ethanol, interactions, 1149
  and female sexual dysfunction, 302f
  formulations, 1137t
  and GABA receptors, 221, 1084, 1087–1088, 1094,
    1135
  gastrointestinal decontamination for, 54t, 58t, 77
  for hallucinogen-related adverse effects, 1184
  hepatic metabolism, 1137t, 1138
  history of, 719, 1084, 1087, 1094, 1135
  for γ-hydroxybutyrate (GHB) withdrawal, 1138, 1191
  immunoassays for, 105
  inappropriate prescribing of, 1827
  indications for, 35t, 728, 1149
  for inhalant-induced agitation, 1200
  laboratory testing for, 36t, 101
  for lead encephalopathy, in children, 1302
  for local anesthetic–induced seizures, 1000
  and male sexual dysfunction, 299f
  mechanism of action, 221
  metabolites, 1088, 1137t, 1138
  for nerve agent toxicity, 1746
  neuroadaptation and, 237
  for neuroleptic malignant syndrome, 1038–1039
  for organic phosphorus compound poisoning, 1498
  overdose/poisoning, 1086

clinical and laboratory findings with, 36t
  flumazenil for, 1094–1098, 1095t, 1790. *See also*
    Flumazenil
  management, 44t, 1095, 1790
  and organ donation, 1893t
  pathophysiology, 1095
paradoxical reactions to, 1087, 1139
  flumazenil for, 1095, 1139
for penicillin-induced seizures, 823
pharmacodynamics and toxicodynamics, 1084,
    1136–1138, 1137t
pharmacokinetics and toxicokinetics, 1084–1088,
    1136–1138, 1137t
pharmacology, 1136–1138, 1137t
physostigmine and, 756
for priapism, 301
protein binding, 1085
for psychomotor agitation, 1138–1139
and pyridoxine, combined, for INH-induced seizures,
    863
receptor activity, 1084
for resistant alcohol withdrawal, 1168–1169
reversal, seizures after, 1095
screening for, 110, 112–113
for sedative-hypnotic withdrawal, 1138
self-poisoning with, 376
and serotonergic pathways, 1084
for serotonin toxicity, 1059
shortage, 43
for status epilepticus, 1137t, 1138
structure, 1087, 1135, 1135f
for strychnine poisoning, 1537–1538
for suicidal patient, 379
suicide with, 466
for sympathomimetic poisoning, 751
tolerance, 1088
urine screening assays for, performance
    characteristics, 111t
for venomous caterpillar exposure, 1553
withdrawal, 222, 237, 1088, 1138
  and agitation/violence, 385
for xenobiotic-induced seizures, 1138
Benzodiazepine antagonist, history of, 1094
Benzodiazepine derivatives, history of, 1094
Benzodiazepine receptor(s), 342, 1135–1136
  central, 1135–1136
  flumazenil and, 1094
  peripheral, 1136, 1136f
  type 1 (BZ$_1$), 1135
  type 2 (BZ$_2$), 1135
  type 3 (BZ$_3$), 1135
Benzodiazepine receptor agonists, 1084
Benzoic acid, 683, 683f
Benzonitrile, and ATP synthesis, 176t
Benzophenone-3, as photoallergen, 280
p-Benzoquinone, and citric acid cycle, 176t
Benzothiazole herbicides, 1467t
Benzoylecgonine (BE), 1124, 1125f, 1139. *See also* Cocaine
  assays for, 112
  laboratory testing for, 1127–1128
  trimethylsilyl (TMS) derivative of (TMS-BE), mass
    spectrometry, 107, 108f
Benzoylmethylecgonine, 1124. *See also* Cocaine
Benzphetamine, for weight loss, 608t
Benztropine, 756
  for acute dystonia, 1036
  for akathisia, 1036
  availability and storage, 44t
  and dopamine reuptake, 214
  indications for, 44t

mechanism of action, 211
  stocking, recommended level, 44t
Benzyl alcohol, 683, 683f, 683t
  diagnostic tests for, 1425
  epidural exposure to, 683
  in folic acid preparations, 779
  gasping (baby, neonatal) syndrome from, 20–21, 20t,
    442, 452, 683, 1430
  intrathecal exposure to, 683
  in intravenous solutions, 1430
  metabolism, 683, 683f
  neurotoxicity, 683
  pharmacokinetics, 683
  structure, 683
  toxicity, in neonates, 779
N-Benzyl-oxy-methyl (NBOME), 1179
Berberidaceae, 1599t, 1602t
Berberine, 641t–642t, 1598t–1601t, 1605
Berberis spp. (barberry), 1598t, 1605
Bergamottin, 1599t, 1609–1610
  xenobiotic interactions, 1611
Bergapten, 644t
Bergerine, 650t
Beriberi
  dry, 1157, 1159
  Shoshin, 1159
  wet, 1157, 1159
Berinert, 964
Beriplex, 910
Berkelium, chelator for, 1780
Berlin blue. *See* Prussian blue
Bernard, Claude, 4t, 7, 1018
Bertrand, Grand Marshall, 4t, 7
Berylliosis, 1276
  imaging in, 115t, 125t
Beryllium, 1780. *See also* Berylliosis
  hepatic effects, 334t
  nephrotoxicity, 390f, 397t
Berzelius, Jöns, 1339
Best Pharmaceuticals for Children Act (BPCA) of 2007,
    1834
Betadine. *See* Povidone-iodine
Beta (β) error, 1855
Beta particles, 1762–1763
Betaxolol
  benzalkonium chloride in, 682t
  ophthalmic use, systemic toxicity with, 360
  pharmacokinetics, 930
  pharmacology, 927t
  toxicity (overdose/poisoning)
    clinical manifestations, 931–932
    management, 936
  vasodilating effects, 930–931
Betel nut (*Areca catechu*), 1598t, 1605
  and discoloration of teeth and gums, 293t
  toxicity, 648–649
  uses and toxicities, 640t
Bethanechol, 1495t, 1496
Betrixaban, 894
Betula lenta (sweet birch), 634
Bevacizumab, and posterior reversible encephalopathy
    syndrome, 132
Bezoars, 3–4
  bowel obstruction caused by, 127, 129t
  definition, 143, 294
  diagnosis, 294
  effects from, 294
  imaging, 294
  removal, 294
  xenobiotics forming, 143t

1918   INDEX

Bhang, 3. *See also* Cannabis (*Cannabis*, marijuana, bhang)
Bhilawanol, 1614
Bhopal disaster, 16, 16t, 1486, 1651, 1657, 1847
Bialaphos, 1468t. *See also* Organic phosphorus compounds
Bias, 1856–1857
    information, 1856
    interviewer, 1856
    misclassification, 1856
    publication, 1857
    recall, 1856
    selection, 1856
Bicalutamide, as androgen receptor blocker, 299f
Bicarbonate. *See* Sodium bicarbonate (NaHCO₃)
Bicuculline, and GABA receptor, 222
Bifenox, 1468t
Bifenthrin, 1520t. *See also* Pyrethroids
Bifeprunox, mechanism of action, 1035
Biguanides. *See also specific xenobiotic*
    history of, 694
    and metabolic acidosis with elevated lactate concentration, 703–704
    pharmacokinetics and toxicokinetics, 697t
    pharmacology, 695
    structure, 695f
Bilanafos. *See* Bialaphos
Bile, postmortem collection, 1870t
Bile acids
    enterohepatic recirculation, 327
    transport systems, 327
Bile acid sequestrant(s), 92
    for levothyroxine overdose, 817
Bile alcohol, C27, 640t
Bile canaliculi, 329f
    xenobiotics that target, 330
Bile cancer, 327
Bile duct(s), xenobiotic-induced damage to, 331t
Bile duct epithelia, 327
Bile transport proteins, 330
Bilevel positive airway pressure (BiPAP), 407
Biliary tract, xenobiotics that target, and liver injury, 330
Bilirubin
    elimination, multiple-dose activated charcoal in, 78
    in liver injury, 334, 335t
Biliverdin, 315
Bilobalide, 642t
Bindeez, 1188
Bioallethrin, 1520t. *See also* Pyrethroids
Bioavailability (F), 140, 140f. *See also specific xenobiotic*
    definition, 143
    in elderly, 461
    factors affecting, 143f, 144
    oral, 148
    P-glycoprotein and, 173
Biochanin A, 1603t
Biochemistry, 167–181
    definition, 161
Biodosimetry, 1768–1769
Biogenic amine reuptake complex, arylcyclohexylamines and, 1213
Biogenic amines. *See also specific amine*
    amphetamines and, 1099–1100, 1100f
    reuptake, cocaine and, 1125
Biological Assessment Tool, 1768
Biological Effects of Ionizing Radiation (BEIR) Committee, 1767
Biological weapons (BW), 1741t–1742t, 1753–1761. *See also specific xenobiotic*
    bacterial, 1754–1757

and chemical weapons, comparison, 1742, 1742t, 1753
    decontamination for, 1743, 1754
    epidemiologic clues to, 1754t
    history of, 1753
    low-tech attacks using, 1744
    and naturally occurring outbreaks, differences between, 1753, 1754t
    preparedness for, 1754
    risk of exposure to, 1743–1744
    toxins, 1759–1760
    viral, 1757–1759
Biologic hazards, workplace, 1797, 1797t
Biologics License Application (BLA), 1836
Biologic warfare, 1741t
Biomaterials, nanotechnology in, 1717
Bioresmethrin, 1520t. *See also* Pyrethroids
Biosimilar products, 1835
Bioterrorism. *See also* Biological weapons (BW); *specific xenobiotic*
    food poisoning and, 602
    preparedness for, risk communication in, 1817–1818
Biotin, 654
    carboxylation, trivalent arsenic and, 1238
Biotransformation, 147, 167–168
    phase I reactions in, 147
    phase II reactions in, 147
Bioweapons. *See* Biological weapons (BW)
Bipolar disorder
    N-acetylcysteine for, 495
    and suicide, 378–379
Bipyridyl herbicides, 1467t, 1473–1478
Bird fancier's lung, 1659
Bird's foot (*Trigonella foenumgraecum*), 641t
Birgus latro L. (coconut crab), 979
Birthwort (*Aristolochia*)
    as abortifacient, 303t
    uses and toxicities, 640t
Bishydroxycoumarin, 883, 885
Bismacine, 1255
Bismuth, 1255–1258, 1780
    absorption, 1255
    antisyphilis therapy, 1255
        imaging findings after, 132f
    apparent half-life in urinary excretion, 1255
    apparent plasma half-life, 1255
    blood
        and illness severity, 1256
        normal concentration, 1255
        in toxicity, 1256
    cellular uptake, 1255
    in central nervous system, 1255
    chemistry, 1255
    distribution half-life, 1255
    drug interactions with, 1257
    effects on *Helicobacter pylori*, 1255
    elimination, 1255
    encephalopathy caused by, 1255–1256, 1256t
        differential diagnosis, 1256, 1256t
        imaging in, 1256
    history and epidemiology, 1255
    imaging, 116f
    nephrotoxicity, 390f, 397t, 1255
    neurotoxicity, 1255–1256
    ototoxicity, 1256
    pentavalent, 1255
    pharmacokinetics, 1255
    physicochemical properties, 1255, 1256t
    radiopacity, 1256
    serum, normal concentration, 1255

serum-to-blood ratio, 1255
    sulfhydryl binding, 1255
    therapeutic uses, 1255
    tissue concentration, and illness severity, 1256
    tissue distribution, 1255
    toxicity (overdose/poisoning)
        abdominal radiographs in, 1256
        N-acetylcysteine for, 1257
        chelation therapy for, 1257
        clinical and laboratory findings with, 36t
        diagnosis, 1256
        EEG in, 1256
        pathophysiology, 1255–1256
        treatment, 1256–1257
    toxicology, 1255
    transport in body, 1255
    trivalent, 1255
    urine, normal concentration, 1255
Bismuth bicitropeptide, physicochemical properties, 1256t
Bismuth citrate, 1255
Bismuth lines, 273
Bismuth salts
    physicochemical properties, 1255, 1256t
    therapeutic uses, 1255
Bismuth subcarbonate, physicochemical properties, 1256t
Bismuth subcitrate, colloidal, and PPIs, interactions, 1257
Bismuth subgallate, 1255
    physicochemical properties, 1256t
Bismuth subnitrate
    methemoglobinemia caused by, 1257
    physicochemical properties, 1256t
Bismuth subsalicylate, 557, 1255
    physicochemical properties, 1256t
    and salicylate toxicity, 1257
    toxicity, 1256
Bismuth thioglycollate, 1255
Bismuth triglycollamate, physicochemical properties, 1256t
Bisoprolol
    overdose/poisoning, clinical manifestations, 931–932
    pharmacokinetics, 930
    pharmacology, 927t
Bisoprolol-hydrochlorothiazide, 931
Bisphosphonates
    for hypercalcemia, 199
    ophthalmic toxicity, 356f
    skeletal effects, imaging, 119, 123f
Bispyribac, 1471
    in herbicides, 1467t
Bis(2-chloroethyl) sulfide (sulfur mustard). *See* Sulfur mustard
"Bite cells," 317
Bites. *See also specific predator*
    arthropod, definition, 1540
    snake. *See* Snakebite(s)
    spider, 1540–1547. *See also* Spiders
Bitis gabonica (Gaboon viper), 1633t
Bitolterol, 985
Bitter almond
    cyanogenic glycosides in, 1684
    odor, 364t
Bitter fennel (*Foeniculum vulgare*), 641t
Bitter melon (*Momordica charantia*), as abortifacient, 303t
Bitter orange (*Citrus aurantium*), 606, 607t, 610, 649, 1599t, 1605. *See also* Dieting xenobiotics and regimens
    uses and toxicities, 640t

Bittersweet woody nightshade (*Solanum dulcamara*), 1602t

Bitter yam (*Dioscorea bulbifera*), 1611

Bivalirudin, 321f, 892, 892f

  anticoagulant effect, 884f

    laboratory investigation, 893

    laboratory testing for, 888t, 893

    overdose/poisoning, treatment strategies for, 888t

Black, James, 926

Black box warning, 21, 1839

Black cohosh (*Actaea racemosa*), 1611

  hepatotoxicity, 651

Black cohosh (*Cimicifuga racemosa*)

  as abortifacient, 303t

  resins in, 639

  uses and toxicities, 640t

Black copper oxide, 1284t

Blackfoot disease, 1241–1242

Black hellebore (*Helleborus niger*), 1600t

Blackjack disease, 1270

BlackLeaf 40, 1203

Black locust (*Robinia pseudoacacia*), 1602t, 1609

Black mamba (*Dendroaspis polylepis*), 1633

Black morel (*Morchella angusticeps*), 1594

Black mustard (*Brassica nigra*), 1598t

Black necked spitting cobra (*Naja nigricollis*), 1633

Black nightshade (*Solanum nigrum*), 1602t

Black phosphorus, chemistry, 1528

Black snakeroot. *See* Black cohosh (*Actaea racemosa*)

Black stone (*Bufo bufo gargarizans, Bufo bufo melanosticus*), 649

  as aphrodisiac, 649

  psychoactive properties, 650t

  uses and toxicities, 641t

Black-tailed rattlesnake (*Crotalus molossus*), 1617t

Black tar heroin, 527. *See also* Heroin

Black vomit nut (*Jatropha curcas*), 1601t

Black widow spider (*Latrodectus mactans*), 12, 1540, 1540t, 1541–1544, 1541f

  antivenom, 35t, 44t, 1543, 1559–1561

    adverse effects and safety issues, 1560–1561

    availability and storage, 44t, 1561

    dosage and administration, 1561

    formulation, 1561

    indications for, 44t

    pregnancy category, 1561

    shortage, 43, 1560

    stocking, recommended level, 44t

    use in pregnancy, 1560

  appearance, 1541–1542, 1541f, 1542t

  and brown recluse, comparative characteristics, 1542t

  envenomation. *See also* Latrodectism

    antivenom for, 35t, 44t, 1559–1561

    clinical effects, 1542–1543, 1542t

    diagnostic tests for, 1543

    grading system for, 1543

    pathophysiology, 1542, 1542t

    in pregnancy, 1561

    priapism caused by, 301t, 1543

      treatment, 1560

    prognosis for, 1543

    treatment, 1542t, 1543–1544

  F(ab′)₂ fragment antivenom, 1543–1544, 1559

  venom

    and acetylcholine release, 207, 207t, 1542

    components, 1542, 1542t

    and neurotransmitter release, 1542

    sympathomimetic action, 211

Black Widow Spider Antivenin (BW-AV), 1559–1561

Blackwort (*Symphytum*), 641t

Bladder

  anatomy, 304–307

  dysfunction

    exacerbated or unmasked by xenobiotics in elderly, 463, 463t

    xenobiotic-induced, 394, 394t

  innervation, 304

  physiology, 304

Blandy, Mary, 5t, 6

Bleach (sodium hypochlorite)

  as disinfectant, 1368

  exposure to, pathophysiology, 1389

Bleeding. *See also* Hemorrhage

  dabigatran and, 892

  with factor Xa inhibitors, 895

  fibrinolytics and, 897

  gastrointestinal

    aspirin and, 899

    NSAIDs and, 515

  in heatstroke, 421

  intracerebral, cocaine-related, 1126

  in liver disease, 335

  NSAIDs and, 516

  xenobiotic-induced, in elderly, 465

Bleeding time

  laboratory assessment, 900

  NSAIDs and, 516

Bleomycin

  adverse effects and safety issues, 760t, 762

  ARDS caused by, 402t

  nail changes caused by, 281

  pulmonary/thoracic effects, imaging, 115t, 125t, 126

  respiratory effects, 399t

  scleroderma-like reaction with, 281

  skin discoloration caused by, 273

Blepharitis, in pyridoxine deficiency, 663

Bligh, William, 1609

Blighia sapida (Ackee fruit), 1598t, 1609

  toxicity, 1598t

Blindness

  cortical

    carbon monoxide poisoning and, 1665

    xenobiotic exposures and, 357t

  in methanol poisoning, 1423

  poisoning/overdose causing, 36t

  quinine-induced, 840

  xenobiotics causing, 361

Blind staggers, 1339. *See also* Selenium

Blister agents. *See* Vesicants

Blister beetles, 276, 640t, 1554. *See also* Cantharidin

Blistering diseases, 276

Blistering reactions, 276

Blood, 310. *See also* Coagulation; Hematologic principles

  alteration, before doping analysis, 622

  arterial, pH, 190

  oxygen-carrying capacity, factors affecting, 402–403

  oxygen content, calculation, 402, 402f

  pH, 190

    and cyclic antidepressants, 1045

  postmortem collection and analysis, 1869, 1870t, 1885–1886

  postmortem redistribution, 1869, 1870t, 1871–1872, 1871t

Blood agents (cyanide), 1748

Blood alcohol (ethanol) concentration, 38, 1876–1877

  antihistamines and, 744

  blood sample for, and chain of custody, 1864

  and driver involved in motor vehicle crash, 1862–1864

  in elderly, 461

  estimation, intoxication and, 1881–1882

  evidence collection for, 1862–1864

  measurement, 1877–1878

  and motor vehicle crashes, 1144, 1862–1864, 1877

  per se laws and, 1144, 1873, 1876–1878

  predictive value for alcohol withdrawal, 1167

  warrantless testing, 1863

Blood–brain barrier, 167, 173, 215, 228, 341

  antimuscarinics and, 1503

  factors affecting, 342

  manganese and, 1320

Blood–cerebrospinal fluid (CSF) barrier, 341

Blood doping, 319. *See also* Doping

Blood flow, effects on pharmacokinetics/toxicokinetics, 144

Blood gas analysis, 189, 405. *See also* Arterial blood gases

Blood:gas partition coefficient, 1194

  of inhalants, 1194, 1195t

Blood pressure. *See also* Hypertension; Hypotension

  caffeine and, 988

  control, for monoamine oxidase inhibitor toxicity, 1080

  evaluation, 37

  factors affecting, 264

  in initial assessment, 189

  normal, by age, 28t

  and pulse rate, 30

  support, in MAOI overdose, 212

  xenobiotics affecting, 29, 29t

Blood products, for radiation-exposed patients, 1771–1772

Bloodroot (*Sanguinaria canadensis*), 1543t, 1605

Blood tests, in initial management, 37

Blood transfusions

  autologous, as doping, 319

  indications for, 885, 900

Blood urea nitrogen (BUN), 37, 189

  corticosteroids and, 396

  in differential diagnosis of high anion gap metabolic acidosis, 192

  postmortem changes, 1885t

  in renal disorders, 396

Bloodwort. *See* Yarrow (*Achillea millefolium*)

"Blow," 162. *See also* Cocaine

Blow fly, in entomotoxicology, 1886, 1886t

Blue-blooded animals, 1285

Bluebottle (*Physalia utriculus*), 1567, 1567t, 1570. *See also* Cnidaria (jellyfish)

Blue cohosh (*Caulophyllum thalictroides*), 1599t, 1604

  as abortifacient, 303t

  uses and toxicities, 640t

Blue ginseng. *See* Blue cohosh (*Caulophyllum thalictroides*)

Blue-green algae, 1601t

  Anabaena, 1598t, 1601t

  Aphanizomenon, 1598t

  and ciguatoxin, 593

  microcystins in, 1609

  Microcystis, 1601t

Blue Man, 1346

Blue Mystic. *See* 2C-T-7

Blue rattlesnake (*Crotalus* spp.), 1636t

Blue-ringed octopus (*Hapalochlaena maculosa*), 1572, 1572f

  tetrodotoxin in, 596

Blue skin color. *See also* Cyanosis
  poisoning/overdose causing, 36t
Blue star. *See* Morning glory
Bluestone, 1284t
Blue vitriol, 1284t
Blue vomitus, causes, 1286
B lymphocytes, 319
Body composition, in elderly, 461, 461t
Body mass index (BMI), 148, 148t
  and mortality, 606
Body packers, 117, 295, 545–547, 545t, 546f. *See also*
    specific xenobiotic
  bowel obstruction in, 127, 545
    diagnostic imaging, 115t, 120f, 122f, 129t
  clinical manifestations in, 545
  cocaine toxicity in, 63–64, 85, 545–547, 1128–1129
  composition of packages in, 545, 545t
  definition, 545
  double breasting by, 546
  gastrointestinal evacuation in, 85, 547
  gastrointestinal perforation in, 545, 546f
  imaging, 115t, 117, 122f, 129t, 546–547, 546f
    double condom sign in, 546
  laboratory evaluation, 546
  legal considerations with, 549
  management, 85, 547, 547f
  opioid, management, 534
  packet rupture in, 63–64
  pregnant, 547
  residual packets in, imaging, 117
  surgery for, 63–64, 547, 547f
  whole-bowel irrigation for, 63, 85
Body size, determination, equations for, 148t
Body stuffers, 85, 545t, 547–549. *See also specific*
    xenobiotic
  clinical manifestations in, 548
  cocaine in, 1128–1129
  composition of packages in, 545t, 548
  definition, 117, 545
  imaging, 117, 121f, 548
  laboratory evaluation, 548
  legal considerations with, 549
  management, 548–549, 1861
Body surface area (BSA), 148t
Body temperature. *See* Thermoregulation
Boehmite, 1223
Boerhaave syndrome, 126
Bohr effect, 316
Boletus spp.
  deaths caused by, 1581
  GI toxins in, 1589
Boletus eastwoodiae, 1582t
Boletus luridus, 1583t, 1592
Bologna, theriac production in, 2
Bombus spp. *See* Bumblebees (*Bombus* spp.)
Bond(s), 158–159, 174
  carbon, 161
  covalent, 159, 162
  electrovalent, 158–159
  in hydrocarbons, 165
  hydrogen, 159
  ionic, 158–159
  noncovalent, 159
  polar, 159
  representation, 162
Bone(s)
  aluminum in, 1224
  cadmium and, 1260, 1260t
  calcium in, 1405
  growth, lead and, 1296

lead in, 1294, 1296, 1298
  measurement, 1300
Bone density
  focal loss of, xenobiotic-induced, 122t
    imaging, 119–122, 124f
  increased, xenobiotic-induced, 122t
    imaging, 119, 122f–123f
Bone marrow, 310, 353
Bone marrow suppression
  chemotherapeutics and, 761
  chloramphenicol and, 826
  nitrous oxide and, 1012
  sulfonamides and, 827
  xenobiotic-induced, 402
Bone metabolism, lead and, 1296
Bone mineral density, inhalants and, 1197
Boneset (*Eupatorium perfoliatum*), 640t
  uses and toxicities, 640t
Bonferroni correction, 1855
Bookoo. *See* Buchu (*Agathosma betulina*)
Borage (*Borago officinalis*), 1598t
  uses and toxicities, 640t
Boraginaceae, 1598t, 1603t, 1605
Borax, 1369t, 1375
Bordeaux solution, 1284t, 1287
Borderline personality disorder, and suicidality, 378
Borgia, Cesare, 5t
Boric acid, 1369t, 1375, 1388t
  absorption, 1375
  clinical and laboratory findings with, 36t
  dermal effects, 278
  ingestion, 1375
  sources, 1375
  toxicity, 1375
    clinical effects, 1375
    management, 1375
Boron, 640t
  excretion, *N*-acetylcysteine and, 494
  uses and toxicities, 640t
Bortezomib
  intrathecal administration, inadvertent overdose
      and unintentional exposures due to, 795t
  peripheral neuropathy with, 763
Botanical poisoning, in developing world, 1844
Bothriechis aurifer, 1636t
Bothriechis bicolor, 1636t
Bothriechis rowleyi, 1636t
Bothriechis schlegelii, 1636t
Bothrops asper (fer-de-lance), 1636t
  antivenom, 1627t, 1628–1631
Bothrops moojeni, 1636t
Botkin, Cordelia, 5t
Botox, 578–579
Botulinum antitoxin
  adverse effects and safety issues, 581
  availability and storage, 44t
  dosage and administration, 581
  efficacy, 581
  indications for, 35t, 44t
  mechanism of action, 581
  sources, 581
  stocking, recommended level, 44t
  for xenobiotic-induced respiratory dysfunction, 407
Botulinum toxin/neurotoxin (BoNT), 574
  and acetylcholine release, 207, 207t
  as biological weapon, 574–575, 1759
  cosmetic preparations, 578–579
  cranial neuropathy caused by, 346t
  duration of action, 575

effects on vital signs, 30t
  for hyperhidrosis, 273
  hypoventilation caused by, 400t
  lethal dose, 575
  mechanism of action, 343, 1018
  and neuromuscular blockers, interactions, 1021t
  pharmacokinetics and toxicokinetics, 575
  physicochemical properties, 575, 576f
  pregnancy category, 582
  respiratory effects, 399t, 400
  serotypes, 574–575
    receptor specificity, 575
    subtypes, 575
  and skeletal muscle excitation-contraction coupling,
      1019f
  therapeutic uses, 578–579
  type A, therapeutic, 578–579
Botulism, 574–585, 593t, 1759
  adult intestinal colonization
    clinical manifestations, 578
    epidemiologic assessment in, 580, 580t
    laboratory investigation, 580, 580t
  bacteriology, 574–575
  botulinum antitoxin for, 581
  CDC assistance with, 582
  clinical and laboratory findings in, 36t, 596
  Clostridium argentinense, 575
  Clostridium baratii, 575
  Clostridium botulinum, 574–575
  Clostridium butyricum, 575
  diagnostic testing for, 578–579
  differential diagnosis, 596
    nontoxicologic, 576–577, 576t
    toxicologic, 576–577, 576t
  edrophonium testing and, 578–579
  electrophysiologic testing in, 580, 580f
  epidemiologic assessment in, 580, 580t
  epidemiology, 574–575
  foodborne, 596
    CDC case definition, 578
    clinical manifestations, 576–577
    epidemiologic assessment in, 580, 580t
    epidemiology, 574
    laboratory investigation, 580, 580t
    prognosis, 582
  gastrointestinal decontamination for, 581
  and Guillain-Barré syndrome, differentiation,
      576–577, 577t
  history of, 574
  iatrogenic, clinical manifestations, 578–579
  incubation period, 575, 596
  infant, 442, 575
    clinical manifestations, 577–578
    epidemiologic assessment in, 580, 580t
    epidemiology, 574, 578
    incubation period, 575
    laboratory investigation, 580, 580t
    prevention, 582
    toxin causing, 574
    treatment, 582
  inhalational, 574
    clinical manifestations, 578
  laboratory testing in, 36t, 580, 580t, 596
  long-term sequelae, 582
  management, 35t, 44t, 581–582, 596
    botulinum antitoxin in, 581
  and Miller Fisher variant of Guillain-Barré
      syndrome, differentiation, 576–577, 577t
  pathophysiology, 575
  in pregnancy, 582

prevention, 574, 582
prognosis, 582
reporting, 582
supportive care in, 581
surveillance, 582
wound. *See* Wound botulism
Botulism immune globulin, 582
Bouncing bet. *See Saponaria officinalis* (soapwort)
Bowel distension, 127, 129f
Bowel infarction, 127, 129f
Bowel ischemia, in cocaine toxicity, 1127, 1130
Bowel obstruction, 127
    in body packers, 127
        diagnostic imaging, 115t, 122f, 129t
    in body stuffers, 548
        diagnostic imaging, 115t, 122f, 127, 129t
Bowel sounds, 38
Bowen's disease, from arsenic, 1242
Bowman capsule, 389, 390f
Box jellyfish, 1567t. *See also Chironex fleckeri* (box jellyfish,
        sea wasp); *Chiropsalmus quadrumanus* (box
        jellyfish); Cnidaria (jellyfish)
    antivenom, 1570, 1575t
    stings, epidemiology, 1569
Boyle, Robert, 1421
Brachypelma spp., 1547, 1547f
Brachyponera spp., 1552
Bracken fern (*Pteridium* spp.), 1602t, 1608
Bradycardia (bradydysrhythmias), 28–30, 248, 256–258
    in arsenic poisoning, 1241
    atropine-induced, 1503, 1505
    calcium channel blocker–induced, 948
    cannabinoid-associated, 1117
    cardioactive steroid toxicity and, 972
    central α_2-adrenoceptor activation in, 210, 210f, 212
    and hypotension
        case study, 924, 925f
        differential diagnosis, 924, 924t
    management, 35t, 44t
    with neuromuscular blockade reversal, 1025, 1026t
    NSAID overdose and, 516
    sotalol-induced, 936
    SSRIs and, 1058
    in strychnine poisoning, 1537
    succinylcholine and, 1020
    xenobiotic-induced, in elderly, 463, 463t
    xenobiotics causing, 30t, 263, 263t, 953–954
Bradykinesia, 344
Bradykinin, as vasodilator, 945
Bradypnea, 30, 189, 399
    opioid-induced, 28
    xenobiotics causing, 30t
Brain
    aluminum in, 1224–1225
    anatomic imaging, 133
    atrophy in, imaging, 132t
    computed tomography of, in toxicologic
        emergencies, 132t
    development, lead and, 1295
    focal lesions, computed tomography of, 130, 132t
    functional imaging, 133
    manganese and, 1320
    mass lesions, computed tomography of, 132t
    mercury in, 1326
    methylmercury in, 1326
    specimen, postmortem collection and analysis,
        1870t, 1885
Brain death
    and organ donation, 1892
    xenobiotic mimics of, 1892, 1892t

Brain stem, α_2-adrenoceptor activation in, 210, 210f
Brandt, George, 1273
Brandt, Hennig, 1528
Brass, 1283
Brassaia spp. (*Schefflera* spp., umbrella tree), 1598t,
        1613
Brass chills, 1286
Brass foundry workers' ague, 1362, 1659
Brassicaceae, 1598t, 1613
Brassica nigra (black mustard), 1607
    toxicity, 1598t
Brassica oleracea var. capitata (cabbage), 1598t
Brazilian armed spider, 1540
Brazilian huntsman (*Phoneutria fera*), 1540
Brazilian lancehead (*Bothrops moojeni*), 1636t
Brazilian scorpion (*Tityus serrulatus*), 1549f
Brazilian wandering spider (*Phoneutria nigriventer*),
        envenomation by, priapism caused by, 301t
Brazil nuts, selenium content, 1339
Breakthrough therapy, 1835
Breast cancer
    DDT and, 1518
    parabens and, 685
Breast-feeding
    arsenic exposure and, 1240
    cesium exposure and, 1360
    dimercaprol and, 1252
    ethanol (alcohol) and, 1441
    fomepizole and, 1437
    by lead-exposed mothers, 1252, 1294, 1305, 1305t,
        1312
    succimer and, 1252
    thallium exposure and, 1360
    toxic alcohols and, 1441
    xenobiotic exposure and, 440–441
Breast milk
    magnesium in, 879
    pyridoxine in, 863
    pyrrolizidine alkaloids in, 1605
    thiamine in, 1160–1161
    vitamin E in, 661
    xenobiotics in, 440–441
        concentration of, estimation, 440–441
Breath alcohol concentration (BrAC)
    legal limits and, 1878
    measurement, 1877–1878
    and motor vehicle crashes, 1877
    reporting units, 1878
    testing devices for, 1878
Breath alcohol ignition interlock devices (BAIIDs), 1878
Breath analysis bedside test, for carbon monoxide
        poisoning, 1666
Breathing, assessment, 36
Breath odor, 37–38
Breath sounds
    auscultation, 37
    smoke inhalation and, 1642
Breath testing, 1872. *See also* Breath alcohol
        concentration (BrAC)
Breithaupt v. Abram, 1863
Brentuximab vedotin, mechanism of action, 761
Brevetoxin, 595
    and voltage-gated calcium channels, 244f, 245
Breynia officinalis, 1611
Bridging, of steroids, 617
Bridion, 1025
Brief Michigan Alcoholism Screening Test (MAST),
        1151, 1151t
Brimonidine, ophthalmic use, systemic toxicity with,
        360

Brimonidine/timolol, benzalkonium chloride in, 682t
Brindleberry (*Garcinia cambogia*), uses and toxicities,
        642t
Bristle worms, 1573–1574
Bristly starbur (*Acanthospermum hispidum*), as
        abortifacient, 303t
Britannicus, 2, 5t
British anti-Lewisite. *See* Dimercaprol (BAL, British
        anti-Lewisite)
British Nuclear Tests Veterans Association (BNTVA),
        cancers among, 1762
Brittle stars, 1573–1574
Broccoli, xenobiotic interactions, 1611
Brodifacoum
    pharmacokinetics, 146t
    pharmacology, 886
    physicochemical properties, 1453t
    in rodenticides, 1453t
    toxicity (overdose/poisoning), 887
        antidote and/or treatment for, 1453t
        clinical manifestations, 1453t
        management, 915–917
        onset, 1453t
        and organ donation, 1893t
        treatment, 889
    toxic mechanism, 1453t
    volume of distribution, 146t
Bromadiolone poisoning, lipid emulsion for, 1006
Bromates. *See also specific xenobiotic*
    cosmetics containing, taste-aversive xenobiotics
        in, 1782
    ototoxicity, 366f
    and tinnitus, 370t
Bromethalin
    physicochemical properties, 1453t
    in rodenticides, 1453t. *See also* Rodenticides
    toxicity
        antidote and/or treatment for, 1453t
        clinical manifestations, 1453t
        onset, 1453t
    toxic mechanism, 1453t
Bromfenac sodium, 171
    anaphylaxis caused by, 21
    hepatotoxicity, 1841
Bromides, 1084, 1088. *See also* Sedative-hypnotics
    and chloride assays, 1088
    extracorporeal elimination, 97t
    mass poisoning with, 1088
    pharmacokinetics, 1088
    toxicity (overdose/poisoning), 1088
        clinical findings in, 1086t
        clinical manifestations, 1088
    volume of distribution, 91, 97t
Bromism, and anion gap, 191t
Bromo. *See* 2C-B
Bromobenzene
    and hepatocellular necrosis, 331
    hepatotoxicity, ethanol and, 329
Bromobutide, in herbicides, 1467t
2-Bromo-2-chloro-1,1,1-trifluroethane. *See also*
        Halothane
    chemistry, 162, 162f
Bromocriptine
    duration of action, 807t
    elimination half-life, 807t
    for erectile dysfunction, 304
    indications for, 807t
    labeling, 43
    mechanism of action, 214
    and olfactory dysfunction, 364

Bromocriptine (*Cont.*):
pharmacokinetics, 807t
renal effects, 390f
and serotonin toxicity, 218
withdrawal, and neuroleptic malignant syndrome, 215
Bromoderma, 1088
4-Bromo-2,5-dimethoxy-amphetamine (DOB), 1101t, 1102. *See also* Amphetamine(s)
4-Bromo-2,5-dimethoxyphenethylamine (2CB). *See* 2CB
Bromo-dragonFLY, 1100, 1107
clinical effects, 1183
deaths caused by, 1107
history of, 1107
structure, 1107
toxicity, 1107
4-Bromo-2,5-methoxyphenylethylamine (2CB, MFT), 1099, 1101t. *See also* Amphetamine(s); 2CB
Bromophos, 1488t
Bromoxynil, 1468t
Brompheniramine
pediatric exposure to, 738
pharmacology, 742
Bronchiolitis obliterans
activated charcoal and, 79
Sauropus androgynus and, 1611
Bronchoalveolar lavage (BAL), 73
Bronchodilators. *See also specific xenobiotic*
for xenobiotic-induced respiratory dysfunction, 407
Bronchorrhea, 125t
and fluid balance, 194
Bronchoscopy, fiberoptic, in smoke inhalation, 1642–1643, 1645
Bronchospasm, 399t, 400
with *N*-acetylcysteine, 495
cocaine-induced, 1126
food toxins and, 600t
smoke inhalation and, 1642
treatment, 407
Bronze, 1283
Broom and broom top (*Cytisus scoparius*), 1599t, 1604
psychoactive properties, 650t
uses and toxicities, 640t
Broselow-Luten system, and pediatric medication dosing, 1828
Brown button spider. *See* Brown widow spider (*Latrodectus geometricus*)
Browning, Elizabeth Barrett, 8, 519
Brown recluse spider (*Loxosceles reclusa*), 1540t
antivenom, 1546, 1559–1561
appearance, 1542t, 1544f
and black widow, comparative characteristics, 1542t
envenomation
antiloxoscelic serum for, 1546
antivenom antibodies for, animal studies, 1546, 1560
antivenom for, 1546, 1559–1561
clinical effects, 1542t, 1544, 1544f
diagnostic tests for, 1545
in head and neck, clinical effects, 1545
pathophysiology, 1542t, 1544
in pregnancy, 1561
red, white, and blue reaction with, 1545
treatment, 1542t, 1545–1546, 1545t
venom, hemolytic activity, 1544, 1546
Brown widow spider (*Latrodectus geometricus*), 1541, 1541f, 1543, 1559–1560
Brucella abortus, 1757
Brucella canis, 1757

Brucella melitensis, 1757
Brucella suis, 1757
Brucellosis, 1757
Brucine, 1536, 1603t, 1605
structure, 1536
Brugada ECG pattern, 260, 1048, 1050
in cyclic antidepressant poisoning, 568, 1046
xenobiotics and
Internet resource on, 260
physiology, 260
Brugada syndrome, 260
in cyclic antidepressant poisoning, 1046, 1048
Brugmansia, as hallucinogen, 1179t, 1181–1183
Bruisewort. *See also Saponaria officinalis* (soapwort)
Symphytum, 641t
Bruxism, amphetamine-related, 1104
Bryophyllum tubiflorum (mother of millions), 979
Bubonic plague (*Yersinia pestis*), 1756, 1756f
Bucco. *See* Buchu (*Agathosma betulina*)
Buchu (*Agathosma betulina*), 640t
uses and toxicities, 640t
Bucindolol
pharmacology, 927t, 930–931
toxicity (overdose/poisoning)
clinical manifestations, 932
management, 936
vasodilating effects, 930–931
Buckeye. *See* Horse chestnut (*Aesculus hippocastanum*)
Buckminsterfullerenes, 1717
Buckthorn, 608t, 1610
alder, *Rhamnus frangula*, 1602t
clinical effects, 576t
Karwinskia humboldtiana, 1601t
Rhamnus frangula, uses and toxicities, 640t
Bucku. *See* Buchu (*Agathosma betulina*)
Buddhist's rosary bead (*Abrus precatorius*), 1598t. *See also* Rosary pea (*Abrus precatorius*)
Budesonide
benzalkonium chloride in, 682
inhaled, for acute respiratory distress syndrome, 1658
nasal spray, benzalkonium chloride in, 682
Buenoano, Judias, 5t, 12
Bufadienolide, 973, 1180, 1453t
toxicity, 649
Bufalin, 979
Bufo spp., 979, 1180, 1181t
Bufo alvarius (Sonoran Desert toad, Colorado River toad), 1180
Bufo bufo gargarizans (Ch'an su), 641t, 649, 650t
Bufo bufo melanosticus (Ch'an su), 641t, 649, 650t
psychoactive properties, of 650t
secretions, as aphrodisiacs, 304t, 649, 1180
uses and toxicities, 641t, 649
Bufodienolides, 641t
Bufotenin, 641t, 649, 650t
Bufotenine, 1180
chemical structure, 1180f, 1589
Bufotoxin, as aphrodisiac, 304t
Bugbane. *See* Black cohosh (*Actaea racemosa*); Black cohosh (*Cimicifuga racemosa*)
Buku. *See* Buchu (*Agathosma betulina*)
Bulk flow, 97, 141, 141f
Bulla (pl., bullae), 269t
cutaneous, carbon monoxide poisoning and, 1666
Bullet(s), lead absorption from, 1294, 1299f
imaging, 117, 119f, 1299f
interventions for, 1301
Bullous dermatosis, 276
Bullous eruptions, NSAID-induced, 515

Bullrout (*Notesthes robusta*), 1576, 1576t, 1577
Bumblebees (*Bombus* spp.), 1540t, 1551–1552
Bumetanide, 963. *See also* Diuretics, loop
benzyl alcohol in, 683t
and tinnitus, 370t
Bundle branch block, 248, 258
Bungarotoxin, clinical effects, 576t
Bungarus spp. (kraits), 1633t
Bupivacaine. *See also* Local anesthetic(s)
cardiovascular toxicity, 999–1000
CNS toxicity, 998
fast on–slow off kinetics with, 999
history of, 994
injection, parabens in, 685t
intrathecal administration, inadvertent overdose and unintentional exposures due to, 795t
lipid carrier formulation, 684t
liposomal, 996
minimal IV toxic dose, 998t
neurotoxicity, 995
overdose/poisoning, lipid emulsion for, 1004, 1007
pharmacology, 996t
seizures caused by, management, 1000
structure, 995f
and tinnitus, 370t
Buprenorphine, 530, 539. *See also* Opioid(s)
characteristics, 526t
immunoassays for, 112
mechanism of action, 227t, 228
for medication-assisted treatment of opioid addiction, 530
for neonatal opioid withdrawal, 439
for opioid overdose, 542
for opioid use disorder, 552
pharmacodynamics, 539
pharmacology, 530
reversal, 541–542
screening for, 110
Bupropion, 1055t
adverse effects and safety issues, 1061
cardiac effects, 248f
clinical and laboratory findings with, 36t
and CYPs, 1055t
and dopamine reuptake, 214
ECG changes caused by, 1057t, 1061
and female sexual function, 302
indications for, 1061
and lamotrigine, combined poisoning with, lipid emulsion for, 1006
mechanism of action, 1056f, 1061
metabolite, 112, 145t, 147
pharmacokinetics, 145t
priapism caused by, 301t
receptor activity, 1057t
seizures caused by, 1057t, 1061
and serotonin toxicity, 1058t
and sexual function, 304
structure, 1061
therapeutic uses, 1061
toxicity (overdose/poisoning), 1061
lipid emulsion for, 1006–1007
sodium bicarbonate for, 568t, 569
volume of distribution, 145t
for weight loss, 612
Bupropion/naltrexone, 606, 607t, 612. *See also* Dieting xenobiotics and regimens
adverse effects and safety issues, 612
pharmacology, 612
Burdock root (*Arctium lappa, A. minus*), 640t
uses and toxicities, 640t

Burn(s)
  alkali, 271
  chemical, 72, 271
    decontamination procedures and, 73
  corrosive, decontamination procedures and, 73
  hydrofluoric acid toxicity and, 1397, 1400–1401
  with inhalant use, 1197
  and methemoglobin formation, 1705
  ophthalmic, 72–73, 358–360
    disposition of patient with, 360
  phosphorus-induced, 1528, 1530
  and smoke inhalation, 1640, 1642, 1645
  thermal, 271
Burn patients, hyponatremia in, 196
Burton line, 1298
Bushi, 640t. *See also* Aconite (*Aconitum*, monkshood)
Bushman's poison (*Carissa acokanthera*), 979
Bush master (*Lachesis mutus*), 1633
Bush tea (*Crotalaria spectabilis, Heliotropium
    europaeum*), 642t
Business associates
  definition, 1865
  and health information privacy, 1865
Buspirone
  extrapyramidal effects, 215
  for inhalant dependence, 1200
  mechanism of action, 217
  and serotonin toxicity, 1058t
Busulfan (busulphan)
  adverse effects and safety issues, 760t
  diagnostic tests for, 763
  infertility caused by, 297t
  neutropenia caused by, 762
  ophthalmic toxicity, 356f
  overdose, 760t
  pulmonary/thoracic effects, imaging, 115t, 125t,
    126
  teratogenicity, 429t
Butabarbital. *See also* Sedative-hypnotics
  pharmacokinetics, 1085t
Butachlor, 1472
  in herbicides, 1467t
  structure, 1472f
  toxicity, clinical manifestations, 1473
Butamifos, 1468t
Butane (*n*-butane), 1652
  cardiotoxicity, 1196
  inhaled, 1193t. *See also* Inhalant(s)
    blood:gas partition coefficient, 1195t
    elimination, 1195t
    metabolites, 1195t
  isomers, 165, 165f
1,3-Butanediol, and leukemia, 320
Butanediol and 1,4-butanediol (1,4-BD), 1188, 1189f
  synonyms for, 1190t
  toxicity (overdose/poisoning), 1188
    clinical findings in, 1086t
  on toy beads, 1188
  withdrawal, 1138
Butane hash oil (BHO), 1113
Butanoic acid, 165
Buthus spp., 1548, 1548t
  antivenoms, 1564t, 1565
Buthus occitanus, antivenom, 1565
Buthus quinquestriatus, pancreatitis caused by, 295t
Buthus tamulus, antivenom, 1565
Butoconazole, 829
Butorphanol. *See also* Opioid(s)
  characteristics, 526t
  pruritus caused by, 273

2-Butoxyethanol, fomepizole for, 1436
Butralin, 1468t
Butroxydim, in herbicides, 1467t
Buttercups (*Ranunculus*), 1602t
  as abortifacient, 303t
Butterflies, 1552–1554
  larval. *See* Caterpillars
Butterfly ray, 1576
Button batteries, 1389
Butyl Cellosolve. *See* 2-Butoxyethanol
n-Butyl mercaptan, congenital anosmia for, 364
Butyl nitrite
  as aphrodisiac, 304t
  inhaled, 1193t, 1194
  odor, 364t
  in poppers, clinical effects, 1198
Butylone, and serotonin toxicity, 1058t
3-*N*-Butylphthalide, for carbon monoxide poisoning, 1671
γ-Butyrolactone (GBL), 1188–1189, 1189f
  overdose, clinical findings in, 1086t
  synonyms for, 1190t
  withdrawal, 1138
Butyrophenones, 1032, 1033t
  contraindications to, 1128–1129
  mechanism of action, 214
  and neuroleptic malignant syndrome, 215
  priapism caused by, 301t
Butyrylcholinesterase, 206
  activity, 1490
    as indicator of anticholinesterase toxicity, 1494
    interpretation, 1494, 1495t
  inhibition, 1489–1490
    by organic phosphorus compounds, 1487, 1508–1509
Butyryl fentanyl, 529
BW (biological weapons), 1741t
Byers, Eben, 24
Byssinosis, 1659
Bystander effect, 1767

C
C-4 (explosive), 1482
Caapi (*Banisteriopsis caapi*), uses and toxicities, 640t,
    647, 649, 650t, 1077, 1180
Cabbage (*Brassica oleracea* var. capitata), 1598t
Cabbage head (*Stomolophus meleagris*), 1567t
Cabbage palm. *See* Saw palmetto (*Serenoa repens*)
Cabergoline, 806
  cardiac effects, 806–807
  mechanism of action, 214
CACNA1S protein, and malignant hyperthermia, 1023
Cacodylic acid, 1240. *See also* Dimethylarsinic acid
Cacogeusia, 365
Cacosmia, 364, 364t
Cactus (*Cactus* spp.)
  mescaline in, 1180
  toxicity, 1598t
Cadmium, 1259–1263
  absorption, 1259
  biologic half-life, 1259
  and calcium channels, 945t
  carcinogenicity, 1261
  cardiovascular effects, 1261
  cation, and electron transport, 176t
  in dietary supplements, 647–648
  and discoloration of teeth and gums, 293t
  elemental, 1259
  excretion, *N*-acetylcysteine and, 494
  exposure to
    environmental, 1259
    hobby-related, 1259

  occupational, 1259, 1261, 1261t
  food contamination with, 1259
  fumes, pulmonary toxicity, 1260. *See also* Cadmium
    oxide
  gastrointestinal effects, 1260, 1260t
  hepatotoxicity, 1261
  history and epidemiology, 1259
  ingestion, 1260
    management, 1261
  inhalation. *See also* Cadmium oxide
    management, 1261–1262
  metallothionein and, 1259, 1261–1262
  musculoskeletal effects, 1260, 1260t
  nephrotoxicity, 390f, 397t, 1260–1261, 1261t
  neurotoxicity, 1261
  and olfactory dysfunction, 364
  permissible exposure limit, 1261
  physicochemical properties, 1259
  pulmonary effects, 1260, 1260t
  renal effects, 1259–1260, 1260t, 1261, 1261t
  as thermal degradation product, 1642
  tissue distribution, 1259
  toxicity
    N-acetylcysteine for, 494
    acute, 1260
      management, 1261–1262
    chelation therapy and, 1261–1262
    chronic, 1260–1261
      management, 1262
    clinical manifestations, 1260–1261
    diagnostic testing for, 1261
    management, 1261–1262
    pathophysiology, 1259–1260, 1260t
      cellular, 1259
      organ system, 1259–1260, 1260t
  toxicokinetics, 1259
  urine
    clinical significance, 1261
    normal concentration, 1259
    in workplace exposure risk assessment, 1261, 1261t
  uses, 1259
  volume of distribution, 1259
  water contamination with, 18t, 19
  whole blood
    normal concentration, 1259
    in smokers, 1259
    in workplace exposure risk assessment, 1261,
      1261t
Cadmium chloride, ingestion, 1260
Cadmium iodide, ingestion, 1260
Cadmium oxide, 1259, 1657–1658
  fumes, 1259
    bioavailability, 1259
    immediately dangerous to life and health (IDLH),
      1654t
    inhalation, 1260
    pneumonitis caused by, 1260–1262
    pulmonary toxicity, management, 1261–1262
    regulatory standard for, 1654t
    water solubility, 1654t
Cadmium sulfide, 1259
Caffeine, 606, 643t, 650t. *See also* Methylxanthines
  and adenosine, 239
  as adenosine antagonist, 231
  as athletic performance enhancer, 621
  beverages containing, 985
  and blood pressure, 988
  cardiovascular effects, 988
  chronic use, adverse effects and safety issues, 989
  in cocaine, 1130

Caffeine (*Cont.*):
in common products, 985, 986t
elimination half-life, neonatal, 442
extracorporeal elimination, 97t
metabolism, neonatal, 442
neuropsychiatric effects, 988
pharmacokinetics, 987
pharmacology, 986
physicochemical properties, 985
plant sources, 1599t–1601t
pulmonary effects, 988
structure, 985
as theophylline metabolite, in neonates, 146t
therapeutic use, in neonates, 985
and tinnitus, 369, 370t
tolerance, 239
toxicity, 987–989
chronic, 986
diagnostic tests for, 989
epidemiology, 985
toxicokinetics, 987
for weight loss, 608t
withdrawal, 986, 989
clinical findings in, 239
Caffeine-induced disorders, 986
Caffeine-related disorder, unspecified, 986
Caffeine use disorder, 986
Caffeinism, 986
Cage convulsant, 602
CAGE questions, 1151, 1151t
Cahn-Ingold-Prelog rules, 164
Cajanus cajan (pigeon pea), as abortifacient, 303t
Calabar bean (*Physostigma venenosum*), 755, 1486,
1601t, 1605. *See also* Physostigmine
in insecticides. *See* Insecticides
Caladium spp. (caladium), 1598t
Calamus (*Acorus calamus*), 1598t
Calcific uremic arteriolopathy (calciphylaxis), sodium
thiosulfate in, 1699–1700
Calcineurin, nephrotoxicity, 391
Calcineurin inhibitors. *See also* Cyclosporine;
Tacrolimus
and normal anion gap metabolic acidosis, 191t
renal effects, 391
Calcinosis cutis, 1406
Calcitonin, for vitamin D toxicity, 661
Calcitonin gene-related peptide (CGRP) antagonists,
809
Calcitriol, 659–661
Calcium
abnormalities, 199, 199t
absorption, gastric bypass and, 148
for β-adrenergic antagonist toxicity, 1405
adverse effects and safety issues, 1406
albumin binding, 1403
antidotal, 1403–1408
units for, 1403
balance, renal regulation of, 389
blood
ionized, 1403
normal concentration, 1403
protein-bound, 1403
body stores, 199, 1403
in bone, 1405
in breast milk, 1406
for calcium channel blocker toxicity, 1404, 1404t
in cardiac cycle, 926–928, 928f
cardiomyocyte flow, 928, 928f, 946–947, 946f, 970,
971f
chemistry, 157, 164, 1403

for citrate toxicity, 1406
in coagulation, 883, 884f
concentration gradient, 946–947, 946f, 1403
cytosolic, cyanide and, 1685–1686
dosage and administration, 1404t, 1406
effect on thyroid hormones and function, 814t
excretion, 1403
in extracellular fluid, 1403
glucagon and, 941–942
and glutamate excitotoxicity, 225, 226f
homeostasis, vitamin D in, 659–660
for hydrofluoric acid toxicity, 1399–1401, 1405
hydrofluoric acid toxicity and, 1397, 1398f
for hyperkalemia, 1406
for hypermagnesemia, 200, 1405
for hypocalcemia
from ethylene glycol, 1405
from fluoride-releasing products, 1405
from hydrofluoric acid toxicity, 1405
from phosphate exposures, 1405
and insulin release, 696f, 953, 953f
intraarterial therapy with, for hydrofluoric acid
toxicity, 1399–1400
intracellular, 209, 261–263, 1403
dysrhythmias caused by, 255–256
intradermal therapy with, for hydrofluoric acid
toxicity, 1399
intraosseous administration, 1406
intravenous therapy with, for hydrofluoric acid
toxicity, 1399
mechanism of action, 1404
membrane transport, 203
myocardial, 1403–1404
in myocardial contractility, 245, 1404
in neurotransmission, 205–206, 205f, 207
in pacemaker function, 246
pharmacodynamics, 1404
pharmacokinetics, 1403–1404
physiological actions, 946–947, 946f, 1403–1404
lead and, 1294–1295
physiology, 199
postmortem changes, 1885t
in pregnancy and lactation, 1406
renal reabsorption, 1403
as second messenger, and withdrawal syndrome, 237
serum
ECG changes caused by, 250, 250f
in ethylene glycol poisoning, 1427
supplementation
for lead-exposed breastfeeding mother, 1305
for lead-exposed pregnant patient, 1304–1305
in pregnancy, 1406
total, corrected, 1403
transdermal delivery, for hydrofluoric acid dermal
toxicity, 1399
transport systems, cadmium and, 1259
units for, 1405
Calcium acetate, uses, 1403
Calcium/calmodulin-dependent protein kinase II
(CaMKII), in nicotine withdrawal, 239
Calcium carbimide, and disulfiramlike reactions, 1174t
Calcium carbonate, 1403, 1406
suspension, sorbitol in, 688t
Calcium channel(s), 261–263
antidysrhythmics and, 865, 866t–867t, 869, 871
cardiovascular, 262–263, 262f
cyanide and, 1685–1686
high-voltage, 719
and insulin release, 696f, 713, 953, 953f
ligand-gated, 945

lipid emulsion and, 1005
low-voltage, 719
L-type, 203, 228, 245, 262, 945, 945t, 953, 953f
blockers, 945t
in cardiac cycle, 928, 928f
and malignant hyperthermia, 1023
myocardial, 245, 245f
of myocardial cell membrane, 245
NMDA, PCP binding site, 228
N-type, 203, 228, 719, 945, 945t
in opioid receptor signal transduction, 522f
P/Q-type, 203, 719
P-type, 945, 945t
Q-type, 945, 945t
R-type, 203, 719, 945, 945t
ryanodine receptor, 245, 262
T-type, 245, 719, 945, 945t
voltage-gated, 203, 719, 953, 953f
blockers, 945, 945t
distribution, 945, 945t
ethanol and, 237
functions, 945, 945t
insecticides and, 1521
subtypes, 945, 945t
subunits, 945
Calcium channel blockers, 262, 945–952. *See also
specific xenobiotic*
absorption, 946
and adenosine reuptake, 231
adverse effects and safety issues, 867t
antidote for, 35t
and antimalarial resistance, 836
ARDS caused by, 401, 402t
benzothiazepine, pharmacology, 946t
bradycardia with, 924, 924t
cardiac effects, 247, 256, 258t, 945, 947–948
cardiovascular effects, 203
classification, 945, 946t
combined products, 945
dihydropyridine, 945, 946t
pharmacology, 946t
distribution, 946
drug interactions with, 946
effects on vital signs, 29t–30t
excretion, 946
formulations, 945
and gingival hyperplasia, 293
and gustatory dysfunction, 365
history of, 945
for hyperthyroidism, 817
indications for, 945
and insulin secretion, 292, 953–954, 953f
intestinal ischemia and infarction caused by,
diagnostic imaging, 127, 129t
mechanism of action, 263, 945
metabolic effects, 953–954, 954f
metabolism, 946
myocardial effects, 947–948, 948f, 950
and neuromuscular blockers, interactions, 1021t
nondihydropyridine, 945, 946t
ophthalmic toxicity, 361t
pediatric delayed toxicity, 452
pharmacokinetics, 867t, 946
pharmacology, 867t, 945
phenylalkylamine, pharmacology, 946t
structure, 945
toxicity (overdose/poisoning), 207
adjunctive hemodynamic support for, 950
adjunctive pharmacotherapy for, 950
atropine for, 948–949

calcium for, 949, 1404–1405
cardiac effects, 258, 953–954
clinical and laboratory findings in, 37, 947, 1404
diagnostic tests for, 947
disposition with, 950–951
epidemiology, 945
factors affecting, 947
gastrointestinal decontamination for, 948
glucagon for, 941–942, 949
high-dose insulin for, 949, 953–958
inotropes for, 950
intestinal ischemia in, 127, 129t
lipid emulsion for, 949–950, 1007
management, 44t–45t, 709, 947–950, 1404
pathophysiology, 947
pediatric, 946–947
pharmacotherapy for, 948
vasopressors for, 950
toxicokinetics, 946
vasodilatory effects, 945, 947
volume of distribution, 946, 946t
Calcium chloride
administration route for, 1406
adverse effects and safety issues, 1406
availability and storage, 44t
calcium content, 1403
chemistry, 1403
extravasation, 1406
history of, 1403
indications for, 35t, 44t
intravenous
adult dose, 1404, 1404t
pediatric dose, 1404t
10% solution, 1404t
pharmacokinetics, 1403–1404
stocking, recommended level, 44t
uses, 1403
Calcium chromate, 1268t
Calcium citrate, 1403
Calcium clock, 926, 928f
Calcium complex formation, 199
Calcium cyanide, 1457
Calcium-dependent calcium release, 928
Calcium disodium EDTA. See Edetate calcium
disodium (calcium disodium versenate,
CaNa₂EDTA)
Calcium disodium ethylenediaminetetraacetate
(CaNa₂EDTA). See Edetate calcium disodium
(calcium disodium versenate, CaNa₂EDTA)
Calcium disodium versenate (CaNa₂). See Edetate
calcium disodium (calcium disodium
versenate, CaNa₂EDTA)
Calcium fluoride, 1397
Calcium gel, 1406
for hydrofluoric acid dermal toxicity, 1399, 1405
Calcium glubionate, 1403
Calcium gluconate
adverse effects and safety issues, 1406
availability and storage, 44t
calcium content, 1403
chemistry, 1403
in decontamination of hydrofluoric acid exposure, 73
dosage and administration, 1406
drug interactions with, 1406
extravasation, 1406
eye drops, for hydrofluoric acid exposure, 1400
history of, 1403
for hydrogen fluoride inhalation, 1658
for hyperkalemia, 1406
indications for, 35t, 44t

intraarterial therapy with, for hydrofluoric acid
toxicity, 1399–1400
intravenous
adult dose, 1404, 1404t
Bier block using, for hydrofluoric acid toxicity,
1400, 1405
for hydrofluoric acid systemic toxicity, 1400
pediatric dose, 1404t
10% solution, 1404t
nebulized, for hydrofluoric acid inhalational toxicity,
1400, 1405
pharmacokinetics, 1403–1404
for selenium hexafluoride exposure, 1342
stocking, recommended level, 44t
topical, 1406
for hydrofluoric acid dermal toxicity, 1399, 1405
uses, 1403
for venomous caterpillar exposure, 1553–1554
Calcium glycerophosphate, 1403
Calcium hypochlorite, 1656
Calcium-induced calcium release, 928, 947
Calcium iodide, 818
Calcium lactate, 1403
Calcium oxalate crystals
aluminum citrate and, 1430
in ethylene glycol poisoning, 1424, 1427
plants with, 1613, 1613f
Calcium oxide
dermal decontamination for, 272
fumes, sources, 1654t
Calcium phosphide, 1457
physicochemical properties, 1457
Calcium polycarbophil, 1403
Calcium salts
formulation, 1404t, 1406
for hydrofluoric acid ingestion, 1400, 1405
for hyperkalemia, 199
intravenous, for hydrofluoric acid systemic toxicity,
1400, 1405
mechanism of action, 933f
oral, uses, 1403
for SMFA or fluoroacetamide poisoning, 1534
Calcium sensitizers, mechanism of action, 933f
Calcium-sodium antiporter (NCX), 928, 928f, 970, 971f
Calcium trisodium pentetate
availability and storage, 44t
indications for, 35t, 44t
stocking, recommended level, 44t
California buckeye. See Horse chestnut
(Aesculus hippocastanum)
California hellebore (Veratrum californicum), 1603t
California poppy (Eschscholtzia californica), 650t
California sculpin (Scorpaena guttata), 1576, 1576t
Californidine, 650t
Californium, chelator for, 1780
Callilepsis laureola (impila), 643t, 1607
Calliphoridae, in entomotoxicology, 1886, 1886t
Calloselasma rhodostoma (Malayan pit viper), 900
Calmodulin, calcium binding, 946
Calomel (mercurous chloride), 648
Calotropis spp. (crown flower), 1598t
Calotropis procera (King's crown), 979
Calpain inhibitor, 368
Caltrop (Tribulus terrestris), 1603t
Calvin Klein. See Ketamine, and cocaine, combined
Camellia sinensis (green tea), 642t, 1599t. See also
Methylxanthines
cAMP, in opioid receptor signal transduction, 522f
Camphor, 628–629, 644t, 1380–1381, 1410
from Cinnamomum camphora, 1380

diagnostic testing for, 1381
hepatotoxicity, 1381
history and epidemiology, 1380
hyperventilation caused by, 400t
laboratory identification, 1385, 1385t
in lavender, 630
NIOSH Immediately Dangerous To Life or Health
Concentration, 1381
occupational exposure to, 1380
odor, 364t
permissible exposure limit, 1381
pharmacokinetics, 1380–1381
pharmacology, 1380
products containing, 1380
short-term exposure limit, 1381
structure, 1380
threshold limit value, 1381
toxic dose, 1381
toxicity
case study, 339
clinical manifestations, 36t, 1381
laboratory findings with, 36t, 1381
management, 1381
pathophysiology, 1381
treatment, 634–635
toxicokinetics, 1380–1381
transdermal absorption, 271
transplacental transfer, 1381
uses, 1380
Camphorated oil, 1380
cAMP response element-binding protein (CREB),
238, 238f
Camptotheca acuminata, 761
Camptothecins, 761
adverse effects and safety issues, 760t
mechanism and site of action, 762f
overdose/poisoning, 760t
Campylobacter spp., 597, 597t
Campylobacter jejuni, foodborne infection, 597t, 599
CaNa₂EDTA. See Edetate calcium disodium (calcium
disodium versenate, CaNa₂EDTA)
Canagliflozin
pharmacokinetics and toxicokinetics, 697t
pharmacology, 696
L-Canavanine, 640t
Cancer
anabolic-androgenic steroids and, 617
radiation-induced, 1762, 1769
risk, CT and, 1766
risk assessment, 1815
xenobiotics causing, 12
Cancer jalap. See Pokeweed (Phytolacca americana,
P. decandra)
Candelabra cactus (Euphorbia lacteal), 1613
Candesartan, CYP enzymes and, 170
Candidiasis, in HIV-infected (AIDS) patients, 830t
Candleberry. See Tung and tung seed (Aleurites
moluccana, A. fordii)
Candlenut. See Tung and tung seed (Aleurites
moluccana, A. fordii)
Canebrake rattlesnake (Crotalus horridus atricaudatus),
envenomation, and rhabdomyolysis, 1622
Cangrelor, 323, 899
Cannabidiol (CBD), 1112f, 1113
mechanism of action, 227t
Cannabigerol, 1112f
Cannabinoid(s), 1111–1123, 1178
absorption, 1113–1114
abuse, 1118
for acute pain, 1111–1113

Cannabinoid(s) (*Cont.*):
acute use, adverse effects and safety issues, 1117
in adipose tissue, 112
adverse effects and safety issues, 1117–1118
management, 1120
for anorexia-cachexia syndrome in HIV-infected (AIDS) patients, 1113
cardiovascular effects, 1117
as cellular messengers, 1113, 1114f
for chronic pain, 1111–1113
chronic use, adverse effects and safety issues, 1117–1118
clinical effects, 1115–1117
definition, 1113
dependence, 1118
diagnostic tests for, 1119–1120
distribution, 1114–1115
effects on vital signs, 31t
endocrine effects, 1118
excretion, 1115, 1115f
gas chromatography-mass spectrometry for, 1119–1120
hair testing for, 1120
immunoassays for, 112, 1119–1120
xenobiotics or conditions interfering with, 1119–1120, 1119t
immunologic effects, 1117
medical uses, 1111–1113
metabolism, 1115
metabolites, 1115, 1116f
neurobehavioral effects, 1118
odor, 364t
pharmacokinetics and toxicokinetics, 1113–1115
pharmacology, 1113
physiological effects, 1115–1117
in pregnancy and lactation, 1117–1118
psychological effects, 1115
reproductive effects, 1117–1118
respiratory effects, 1117
saliva testing for, 1120
screening for, 110
serum concentration, and time of exposure, 1120
sweat testing for, 1120
synthetic, 112, 1111–1123
and agitation/violence, 385
aminoalkylindole, 1112f
classical, 1112f
effects on vital signs, 30t
indazole, 1112f
acute toxicity, 1117
indole, 1112f
nonclassical, 1112f
acute toxicity, 1117
metabolites, 1115, 1116f
renal effects, 393, 393t
time of exposure to, 1120
toxicity, acute, 1117
urine screening assays for, performance characteristics, 111t
withdrawal, 1118
Cannabinoid antagonist(s), 1112f
Cannabinoid hyperemesis syndrome, 1118
Cannabinoid receptor(s), 239, 1111, 1113, 1114f, 1116f
Cannabinoid receptor agonists, 1113
dependence, 239
discontinuation syndrome, 239
synthetic, clinical and laboratory findings with, 36t
Cannabinol, 1111, 1113
Cannabinomimetic, 1113
Cannabis (*Cannabis*, marijuana, bhang)

abuse, 1118
adverse effects and safety issues, management, 1120
in antiquity, 3
C. indica, 2, 1113
early use and abuse, 2
C. sativa, 1113, 1599t
definition, 1113
dependence, 1118
and driving, 1118–1119
historical perspective on, 9, 1111
and hyperemesis syndrome, 1118
ingestion, by children, 1117
odor, 364t
in pregnancy and lactation, 1117–1118
priapism caused by, 301t
regulation, 1111
serum concentration, and time of exposure, 1120
smoking, and barotrauma, 401
time of exposure to, 1120
toxicity
acute, 1117
pediatric, 1117
use
by elderly, 467
epidemiology, 1111
withdrawal, 1118
Cannonball jellyfish (*Stomolophus meleagris*), 1567t
Canthacur Plus, 1554
Canthacur PS, 1554
Cantharellus cibarius (chanterelle), 1589
Cantharidin, 276, 640t, 1554
as aphrodisiac, 304t, 1554
mechanism of action, 1554
poisoning
clinical manifestations, 1554
diagnostic tests for, 1554
pathophysiology, 1554
treatment, 1554
priapism caused by, 301t, 1554
uses and toxicities, 640t, 1554
Cantharis vesicatoria, 1554
uses and toxicities, 640t
Cantharone, 1554
Cantils (*Agkistrodon* spp.), 1636t
Caowu, 640t. *See also* Aconite (*Aconitum*, monkshood)
Cap (pileus), of mushrooms, 1584f, 1593
Capacity
assessment, 373–374
sliding scale of, 374
in suicide and self-poisoning, 377–378
Cape. *See* Aloe (*Aloe vera, A. barbadensis, Aloe* spp.)
Capecitabine
adverse effects and safety issues, 760t
antidote for, 35t, 764, 771, 771f, 772
folates and, 777
mechanism and site of action, 762f, 771, 771f
pharmacology, 771
structure, 771
toxicity (overdose/poisoning), 760t
clinical manifestations, 772
diagnostic tests for, 772
management, 46t, 772
pathophysiology, 771–772
uridine triacetate for, 771, 771f, 772, 789–791
ultra-metabolizers, 771
Cape periwinkle. *See* Periwinkle (*Catharanthus roseus*)
Capillary gas chromatography-mass spectrometry, of athletic performance enhancers, 622
Capital punishment, poisons/drugs used in, 13
Capnography, 403–405, 405f

Capreomycin
adverse effects and safety issues, 853t, 858
monitoring with, 853t
for tuberculosis, 853t, 858
Caprifoliaceae, 1602t
Capsaicin, 1599t, 1609–1610, 1657
chemical name and structure, 1749f
inhalation, treatment, 1658
mechanism of action, 1749
ophthalmic exposure to, irrigating solution for, 359t
ophthalmic toxicity, 356f
pruritus caused by, 273
as pulmonary irritant and riot control agent, 1749–1750, 1749f, 1751t
source, 1749
toxic syndrome caused by, 1751t
Capsaicin pepper spray, 1749–1750, 1749f
toxic syndrome caused by, 1751t
Capsicum spp. (capsicum, cayenne pepper), 1599t
Capsicum annuum (capsicum, cayenne pepper), 1610
capsaicin from, 1749
uses and toxicities, 1599t
Capsicum frutescens (capsicum, cayenne pepper), 1599t
Captopril. *See also* Angiotensin-converting enzyme inhibitors (ACEI)
dermal effects, 276
Capulincillo (*Karwinskia humboldtiana*), 1601t, 1610
Caput medusae, 272
Carbachol, 1495t, 1496
Carbamate(s), 1450. *See also* Insecticides
absorption, 1489
anticholinesterase inhibition by, 1489
coformulants, 1490
decontamination for, 1498
delayed neurotoxicity, 1494
effects on vital signs, 30t
and ethanol, interactions, 1146t
history of, 1486
in homicides, 1487
hypoventilation caused by, 400t
pharmacokinetics and toxicokinetics, 1489
pharmacology, 1487
structure, 755f, 1489f
tissue distribution, 1489
toxicity (overdose/poisoning)
acute, clinical manifestations, 1493
atropine for, 1504
case fatality for, 1486
clinical effects, 576t
diagnostic tests for, 1495
epidemiology, 1486–1487
gastrointestinal decontamination for, 54t, 78
management, 45t, 1498–1499
organic chlorines and, 1515
pathophysiology, 1489–1490, 1490f
pralidoxime for, 1510
Carbamate inhibitors. *See* Neostigmine; Physostigmine
Carbamazepine, 719–721
and acetaminophen toxicity, 480
acute interstitial nephritis caused by, 394t
for alcohol withdrawal, 1169
and adenosine reuptake, 231
adverse effects and safety issues, 727–728, 727t
cardiac effects, 248f, 258t
and CYP induction, 171
drug-induced hypersensitivity syndrome with, 277, 727–728, 727t
drug interactions with, 723t, 827, 852
effect on thyroid hormones and function, 814t
elimination, multiple-dose activated charcoal and, 78

and enterohepatic circulation, 172
and female sexual dysfunction, 302f
and GABA receptor, 222
history of, 719
indications for, 719
laboratory testing for, 36t, 101t, 102
mechanism of action, 208, 211, 218, 222, 231, 720f, 720t
metabolism and effects on CYP enzymes, 722t
and neuromuscular blockers, interactions, 1021t
pancreatitis caused by, 295t
pharmacokinetics and toxicokinetics, 719–721, 721t
pharmacology, 203, 719, 720t
and pregnancy complications, 719
protein-binding characteristics, 110, 110t
and suicide risk, 719
syrup, sorbitol in, 688t
teratogenicity, 429t
and tinnitus, 370t
toxicity (overdose/poisoning)
    clinical and laboratory findings in, 36t, 721
    diagnostic tests for, 721
    extracorporeal therapies for, 91f, 95–96, 97t
    gastrointestinal decontamination for, 86
    hemodialysis for, 95
    hemoperfusion for, 96
    lipid emulsion for, 1006
    management, 38, 721
    multiple-dose activated charcoal in, 61
    and organ donation, 1893t
    sodium bicarbonate for, 568t, 569
    whole-bowel irrigation and, 63
Carbamoyl phosphate synthetase-1, 181
    in urea cycle, 180f
Carbanilate herbicides, 1467t
Carbapenems, 825
Carbaryl
    history of, 1486
    poisoning, 1510
        management, 1498
Carbenicillin, and anion gap, 191t
Carbetamide, in herbicides, 1467t
Carbidopa, scleroderma-like reaction with, 281
Carbofuran, 1489
Carbohydrates
    for insulin reactions, 701
    myocardial metabolism and, 953–955
    oral, for hypoglycemia, 710
Carbol-fuchsin solution, toxicity, organ system
        manifestations, 829t
Carbolic acid. See Phenol
β-Carbolines, 212
Carbon
    chemical properties, 161
    oxidation, 168
    reduction, 168
    stereogenic (chiral), 164
Carbon bond(s), 161
Carbon dioxide
    as asphyxiant, 400, 1640, 1650, 1652–1653
        mass casualties from, 1651
    elimination, 399
    immediately dangerous to life and health (IDLH),
        1654t
    intoxication, 1652
        acute, 1652–1653
        case study, 1650
        clinical manifestations, 1652–1653
        subacute, 1652–1653
    mass casualties from, 16, 16t
    partial pressure (PCO$_2$), 399

in hypothermia, 417
partial pressure of (PCO$_2$), 190
pathophysiology, 1652
pharmacology, 1652
in pulmonary gas exchange, 399
regulatory standard for, 1654t
respiratory effects, 399t
short-term exposure limit (STEL), 1654t
as simple asphyxiant, 400t, 1650
sources, 1654t
uses, 1652
water solubility, 1654t
Carbon disulfide, 1172–1173, 1172f
    clinical and laboratory findings with, 36t
    and disulfiramlike reactions, 1174t
    in disulfiram neurotoxicity, 1175
    and dopamine-β-hydroxylase, 1175
    elimination half-life, 1173
    excretion, 1173
    exposure to, clinical manifestations, 1175
    hepatic injury caused by, 1174
    industrial use, 1175
    infertility caused by, 297t, 298f
    as insecticide, 1175
    neurotoxicity, 1175
    odor, 364t
    ototoxicity, 368
    as pesticide, 1175
    physicochemical properties, 1175
Carbonic anhydrase
    inhibition, by cyanide, 1685
    zinc in, 1362
Carbon microspheres, 77
Carbon monoxide, 1650, 1663–1675. See also
        Carboxyhemoglobin
    antidote for, 35t
    ARDS caused by, 401, 402t
    as asphyxiant, 1641–1642
    chemistry, 1663
    clinical manifestations
        with acute exposure, 1665, 1665f
        with chronic exposure, 1666
    in coal fumes, as early poison, 2
    diagnostic testing for, 1666–1667
    early description of, 4
    effects on oxygenation, 403f
    effects on vital signs, 31t
    and electron transport, 176t, 177
    elimination, 1664
    elimination half-life, 1664
    and fetal survival, 1679
    from fires, 16, 16t, 1641
    in genocidal killings, 17, 17t
    heme binding, 1641
    and high anion gap metabolic acidosis, 191t
    historical perspective on, 4t, 1663
    hyperbaric oxygen for
        delayed administration, 1670
        in pregnancy, 1670
        repeat treatment, 1670
    hyperventilation caused by, 400t
    hypothermia caused by, 412
    management
        in children, 1671
        novel neuroprotective treatments for, 1671–1672
        in pregnancy, 1670–1671
    from methylene chloride metabolism, 1195t, 1197,
        1663–1664, 1678
    neurotoxicity, 160, 343, 1664–1666, 1676–1677
    ophthalmic effects, 361

physicochemical properties, 1663
poisoning, 160
    brain computed tomography in, 1665, 1665f
    carboxyhemoglobin level in, 1666–1667
    cardiac monitoring in, 1666–1667
    in children, 1671
    clinical manifestations, 36t, 576t, 1665–1666,
        1665t
    deaths caused by, 1663
    diagnostic imaging in, 115t, 131, 132t, 134, 134f,
        1665, 1665f, 1667
    epidemiology, 1663
    hyperbaric oxygen for, 1668–1670, 1668t–1669t,
        1676–1683
    with inhalational anesthetics, 1015–1016
    laboratory findings with, 36t, 1666–1667, 1686
    management, 1667–1672
    neurocognitive sequelae, 1666, 1677–1678
    neuroimaging findings in, 131, 132t, 134, 134f,
        1665, 1665f, 1667
    neuropsychologic testing in, 1667
    non-fire-related, epidemiology, 1663
    and organ donation, 1893t
    outcomes with, predictive markers for, 1667
    pathophysiology, 1641–1642, 1664–1665, 1676,
        1677f
    in pregnancy, 39, 437, 1679
    prevention, 1672
    sequelae, 1663
    treatment, 1645–1646
    unintentional, 1663
    with waterpipes, 1205
and respiratory rate, 30
and rhabdomyolysis, 393, 393t
site of action, 173f
smoke inhalation and, 1641–1642, 1663
sources, 1663, 1663t
teratogenicity, 429t
tests for, 7
as thermal degradation product, 1641t
and toxic leukoencephalopathy, 133
toxicokinetics, 1664
Carbon nanotubes, 1717
Carbon tetrachloride (CCl$_4$), 174t. See also
        Hydrocarbons, halogenated
    blood:gas partition coefficient, 1195t
    dermal absorption, 1411
    diagnostic imaging, 117–118
    and disulfiramlike reactions, 1174t
    effects on liver, 328
    elimination, 1195t
    hepatic effects, 334t
    and hepatocellular necrosis, 331
    hepatotoxicity, 175, 175f, 1196, 1679
        ethanol and, 329
    metabolism, 172, 175, 175f
        by hepatocytes, 175, 175f
    metabolites, 1195t
    ototoxicity, 368
    toxicity, 1415
        N-acetylcysteine for, 492, 494, 1679
        hyperbaric oxygen for, 1679
    toxicokinetics, 1411t
    uses, 1409t
    viscosity, 1409t
Carbonyl atoms, 163
Carbonyl group, 166, 166f
Carbonyl iron, 669–670, 670t
Carbonyl sulfide, Coca-Cola contamination with, 19
Carbophenothion, 1488t

Carboplatin
   adverse effects and safety issues, 760t
   antidote for, 760t
   overdose/poisoning, 760t
   vomiting with, 762
Carbosulfan, 1489
Carbowax, 686
5-Carboxamidotryptamine (5-CT), 808
γ-Carboxyglutamate, 885
Carboxyhemoglobin, 316–317, 1694, 1699, 1703, 1704f
   blood level
      action level, 1663
      in nonsmokers, 1663
      in smokers, 1663
   in carbon monoxide poisoning, 1664–1667, 1676, 1677f
   detection, 1708
   effects on oxygenation, 403
   elevated, inhalant-induced, management, 1199–1200
   evaluation, 37
   fetal, 437
   hydroxocobalamin and, 1695–1696
   laboratory measurement, 101t, 102–103, 1642, 1666
   levels, prediction, 1664
   measurement, 1666–1667
   methylene chloride and, 1664, 1678
   in pregnancy, 39
   TLV-TWA, 1663
Carboxyhemoglobinemia
   hydrocarbon-induced, 1415
   and pulse oximetry, 404, 404t
Carboxylesterases, inhibition, 1489
Carboxylic acids, 166, 166f, 512t, 1610
   chemistry, 165
   elimination, 167
   as functional groups, 165
   nomenclature, 165
Carboxypeptidase G₁, 782
Carboxypeptidase G₂. *See also* Glucarpidase
      (carboxypeptidase G₂)
   history of, 782
Carboxypeptidase G₃, 782
Carboxyatractyloside, 1607
Carburetor cleaner, inhaled, 1193t, 1197, 1422. *See also* Inhalant(s)
   clinical manifestations of, 1199t
   management, 1437
   in pregnancy, 1437
Carcinogen(s)
   cobalt as, 1276
   nickel as, 1336
   universal, radiation as, 1769
   xenobiotics activated to, 174t
Carcinogenesis, 661
   fetal xenobiotic exposure and, 433
   radiation-induced, 1769
Carcinogenicity
   of anabolic-androgenic steroids, 617
   of antimonials, 1232t, 1233
   of antimony, 1232t, 1233
   of arsenic, 1239, 1242
   of cadmium, 1261
   of chromium, 1268–1270
   of ethylene oxide, 1374
   of formaldehyde, 1373
   of lead, 1294–1295
   of paradichlorobenzene, 1385
   of radiation, 1767
Carcinoid syndrome, 21, 273
Cardenolides, 969, 1598t

Cardiac arrest, ropivacaine and, 1001
Cardiac Arrhythmia Suppression Trials, 865
Cardiac conduction abnormalities. *See also specific abnormality*
   fluoride poisoning and, 1398
   xenobiotics causing, 256, 258, 258t
Cardiac conduction system, 926–928, 928f, 970, 971f, 972t
Cardiac contractility, 970, 971f, 972t
   decreased, 263–264
Cardiac cycle, 926–930, 928f, 970, 971f, 972t
   myocyte calcium flow and contractility in, 928, 928f, 946–947, 946f, 970, 971f
Cardiac excitation, 928, 928f, 970, 971f, 972t
Cardiac glycosides, 645, 1597, 1600t, 1606. *See also* Cardioactive steroids
Cardiac muscle, mushroom toxin affecting, 1589t, 1591
Cardiac output, 402
   xenobiotics affecting, 403
Cardiac pacing, for local anesthetic–induced bradycardia, 1001
Cardioactive steroids, 644t, 645, 969–976
   antidote for, 35t, 44t
   and calcium salts, interactions, 199, 974
   cardiac effects, 248, 256, 258t, 973–975
   chemistry, 969
   drug interactions with, 970
   ECG changes caused by, 250, 258
   effects on autonomic nervous system, 970
   effects on cardiac electrophysiology, 970, 971f, 972t
   effects on vital signs, 30t
   electrophysiologic effects, 970, 971f, 972t
   extracorporeal removal, 975
   in foxglove, 642t
   gastrointestinal absorption, prevention, 64
   laboratory detection, 109
   mechanism of action, 970, 971f
   and neuromuscular blockers, interactions, 1021t
   ophthalmic toxicity, 356f
   pharmacokinetics, 969–970, 969t
   pharmacology, 971f
   physicochemical properties, 969
   from plants, 969, 973
   positive inotropic effect, 970, 971f, 972t
   serum concentration, 972–973
      factors affecting, 973
      interpretation, 973
   structure, 969
   from toads, 969, 973, 1180
   toxicity (overdose/poisoning), 198, 924
      acute, 971–972
         management, 973
      cardiac manifestations, 972, 972t
      cardiac therapeutics for, 973–974
      cardioversion for, 974
      chronic, 971–972
      clinical and laboratory findings with, 37
      diagnostic tests for, 972–973
      digoxin-specific antibody fragments for, 973, 974t, 977–982
      dysrhythmias caused by, 255
      electrolyte abnormalities with, 972, 974–975
      electrolyte therapy for, 974–975
      epidemiology, 969
      external pacemaker for, 974
      gastrointestinal decontamination for, 973
      hyperkalemia caused by, 251, 1406
      management, 973–975, 1404
      manifestations, 970–972
         noncardiac, 971–972

and organ donation, 1893t
   pharmaceutically induced, 969
   sources, 969
   toxicology, 971f
Cardiogenic shock, xenobiotics causing, 953–954
Cardiomyocyte(s)
   calcium flow and, 928, 928f, 946–947, 946f, 970, 971f
   catecholamine-induced damage to, cocaine and, 1127
   contractility, calcium and, 262–263
Cardiomyopathy
   with alcoholism, 1275
   amphetamine-induced, 1103–1104
   anthracyclines and, 763, 763t
   beer drinkers', 21t, 22, 1143, 1273–1275f
   chemotherapeutic-related, 762–763, 763t
   chronic ethanol use and cobalt in, 1274
   cobalt-induced, tests for, 1277
   cocaine-associated, 1127
   dilated
      diagnostic imaging, 115t, 126
      inhalant-induced, 1196
   with malnutrition, 1275
   and sudden death in athletes, 623
   Takotsubo, from cocaine, 1127
   xenobiotics causing, 263–264, 264f
Cardiopulmonary arrest, *case study*, 1650
Cardiopulmonary bypass, for local anesthetic cardiotoxicity, 1000–1001
Cardiopulmonary resuscitation
   for hypothermia with cardiac arrest, 417
   for local anesthetic cardiotoxicity, 1000
Cardiotoxicity. *See also specific xenobiotic*
   of aconitine, 1611
   antihistamines associated with, 746
   of cesium, 1264–1265
   chemotherapeutic-related, 762–763, 763t
   of chloral hydrate, 1088
   of Cnidaria envenomation, 1570–1571
   of colchicine, 502–503, 503t
   factors affecting, 260
   of hydrocarbons, 1412–1413
   of inhalants, 1194, 1196
   of lead, 1295–1296
   of local anesthetics, 998–1000
   of propylene glycol, 687
   sedative-hypnotic overdose and, 1086–1087, 1086t
   of toluene, 1194
Cardiovascular abnormalities
   in arsenic poisoning, 1241
   imaging, 126, 128f
Cardiovascular disease, prevention, aspirin in, 899
Cardiovascular system, physiology, 260
Cardiovascular xenobiotics, poisoning with, epidemiology, 945
Cardioversion
   for cardioactive steroid toxicity, 974
   for cyclic antidepressant toxicity, 1049t
Carfentanil, 529
   deaths from, 21t, 22
   as incapacitating agent, 1750
   Russian military's use of, 17, 17t
   structure, 529, 529f
Carisoprodol, 1088–1089
Carissa acokanthera (bushman's poison), 979
Carissa laxiflora (conkerberry), 979
Carissa spectabilis (wintersweet), 979
Carmustine, 760t
   degradable solid copolymer, 1719t

as local irritant, 802
    mechanism of action, 353
    neutropenia caused by, 762
    overdose/poisoning, chest X-ray findings in, 125t
L-Carnitine, 732–735
    availability and storage, 45t
    chemistry, 732
    concentrations, 733
    deficiency, 732
    dosage and administration, 726, 732–734
    elimination half-life, 732
    exogenous
        adverse effects and safety issues, 733
        pharmacokinetics, 732
    formulation and acquisition, 734
    history of, 732
    homeostasis, 732
    indications for, 35t, 45t, 726, 732
    labeling, 43
    mechanism of action, 732
    metabolism, 732
    overdose, 733
    pharmacology, 732
    in pregnancy and lactation, 733
    serum, normal concentration, 732
    stocking, recommended level, 45t
    structure, 732
    synthesis, 732
    for valproic acid–induced hepatotoxicity, 726,
        732–733
    for valproic acid–induced hyperammonemia, 726,
        732–733
    volume of distribution, 732
Carnitine acylcarnitine translocase, 732
Carnitine palmitoyltransferase, 732
Carnitor, 732
α-Carotene, 272
β-Carotene, 272, 655, 661
    overdose/poisoning, clinical and laboratory findings
        in, 36t
    pharmacokinetics, 656
Carotenoids, 272, 642t
    absorption, 656
    foods with, 655
Carothers, Wallace, 1685
Carotenemia, 272, 272f
Carp bile (Ctenopharyngodon idellus, Cyprinus carpio),
        uses and toxicities, 640t
Carpenter bee (Xylocopa spp.), 1540t
Carpenter's grass. See Yarrow (Achillea millefolium)
Carrier-mediated transport, 141
Carrisyn. See Aloe (Aloe vera, A. barbadensis, Aloe spp.)
Carrots, odor, 364t
Carson, Rachel, 11, 1514
Carteolol
    benzalkonium chloride in, 682t
    ophthalmic use, systemic toxicity with, 360
    pharmacology, 927t, 930
    toxicity (overdose/poisoning)
        clinical manifestations, 932
        management, 936
    vasodilating effects, 930–931
Carukia barnesi (Irukandji jellyfish), 1567, 1567t, 1569,
        1571. See also Cnidaria (jellyfish)
    stings, management, 1569
Carvedilol
    overdose/poisoning
        clinical manifestations, 932
        lipid emulsion for, 1006
        management, 936

pharmacokinetics, 930
    pharmacology, 927t
    vasodilating effects, 930–931
Carybdea alata (Hawaiian box jellyfish), 1567t. See also
        Cnidaria (jellyfish)
Carybdea rastoni stings, management, 1569
Carybdeidae, 1567
Caryophyllum. See also Clove oil (Syzygium
        aromaticum)
    uses and toxicities, 641t
Casanthranol, 83
Cascara (Cascara sagrada), 608t, 612
    uses and toxicities, 641t, 1599t
Cascarosides, 1599t
Case-control studies, 1853, 1853f, 1853t, 1854, 1854f
Case history, and medicolegal interpretive toxicology,
        1868, 1868t
Case reports, 1852, 1853t
Case series, 1852, 1853t
Cashew (Anacardium occidentale)
    allergic contact dermatitis from, 1614
    toxicity, 1598t
Caspase inhibitor, 368
Caspofungin, for HIV-related infections, 830t
Cassava (Manihot esculenta), 1601t, 1607, 1684, 1686,
        1688
    neurotoxicity, 343
Cassia acutifolia (senna). See Senna
Cassia angustifolia (senna). See Senna
Cassia senna (senna). See Senna
Castellana (Agkistrodon spp.), 1636t
Castellani paint, 686
Castor bean (Ricinus communis), 1602t, 1608f
    in biologic warfare, 1759
    self-poisoning with, 1846
Castor oil, 83
Cat. See Methcathinone (cat, Jeff, khat, ephedrone)
Catabolic pathways, 175
Catalase, 175, 1285t
    activity, 168, 168f
    and mercury, 1325
    pyrazole and, 1435
Catalepsy, with arylcyclohexylamine toxicity, 1215
Cataracts, 356, 357t
Cataria (Nepeta cataria), 641t
Catatonia, disulfiram-induced, 1175
Catechins, 642t
Catecholamine hypothesis, of acute respiratory distress
        syndrome (ARDS), 401
Catecholaminelike excess, in thyrotoxicosis,
        management, 817
Catecholamines, 1075. See also specific catecholamine
    for β-adrenergic antagonist toxicity, 934
    amphetamines and, 1099, 1100f
    excess, 263
        cardiac effects, 255
    in heatstroke, 422
    and hypertension, 210
    metabolism, 208
    methylxanthines and, 986
    reuptake, cocaine and, 1125
Catechol-O-methyltransferase (COMT), 208, 209f,
        213, 213f, 1075
    inhibitors, 212, 214
    substrates for, 214
Catechol-O-methyltransferase (COMT) inhibitors,
        212. See also Entacapone; Tolcapone
Catechols, 1410
Caterpillars, 1552–1554
    envenomation

clinical manifestations, 1553
        pathophysiology, 1553
        pruritic reaction to, 1553
        stinging reaction to, 1553
        treatment, 1553–1554
    nettling, 1540t
    stinging, 1553
    urticating hairs, 1552–1553
    venom, composition, 1553
Catfish, 1576
    marine, 1576–1577
Catha edulis (khat), 1106, 1605. See also
        Amphetamine(s)
    uses and toxicities, 643t, 1599t
Catharanthus roseus (periwinkle), 505, 1599t, 1612
    antimitotic alkaloids from. See also Vinblastine;
        Vinca alkaloids; Vincristine
    antimitotic alkaloids from, 505
    psychoactive properties, 650t
    use and toxicities, 643t
Cathartic bowel, exacerbated or unmasked by
        xenobiotics in elderly, 463, 463t
Cathartics, 63, 83. See also specific xenobiotic
    abuse, 612–613
    with activated charcoal, 63, 77, 84, 1353
    adverse effects, 85
    clinical and laboratory findings with, 36t
    and electrolyte abnormalities, 62
    history of, 83
    and hypernatremia, 195, 195t
    magnesium-containing, 199
    pharmacokinetics, 84
    renal effects, 390f, 391
    saline, 83
        mechanism of action, 84
        pharmacodynamics, 84
Cathine (norpseudoephedrine), 643t, 1605. See also
        Amphetamine(s)
Cathinone(s) (benzylketoamphetamine), 643t, 1106–
        1107, 1599t, 1605. See also Amphetamine(s)
    as aphrodisiac, 304t
    and serotonin toxicity, 1058t
    synthetic, 1099, 1102, 1106–1107
    and agitation/violence, 385
Cations
    and electron transport, 176t
    extracellular, 190
    normally present, 190
    unmeasured, 190–191, 191t
Catmint (Nepeta cataria), 641t, 650t
Catnip (Nepeta cataria)
    psychoactive properties, 650t
    uses and toxicities, 641t
    volatile oils in, 639
Cauda equina syndrome, lidocaine and, 997
Caulophyllum thalictroides (blue cohosh), 1604
    as abortifacient, 303t
    uses and toxicities, 1599t
Causation
    assessment, 1855t, 1857
    Bradford Hill criteria for, 1857, 1857t
Caustics, 1388–1396. See also specific caustic
    absorption, systemic, 1391
    acid, 1388
        exposure to, pathophysiology, 1389–1390, 1389f
    alkali, 1388
        exposure to, pathophysiology, 1389, 1389f
    burns caused by, 1388
    child-resistant containers for, 1388
    clinical and laboratory findings with, 36t

Caustics (*Cont.*):
decontamination, 1392
definition, 1388
esophageal effects, 293. *See also* Esophageal injuries
exposure to
in adults, 1388, 1390–1391
age distribution, 1388
in children, 1388, 1390–1391
epidemiology, 1388
pathophysiology, 1388–1390
routes, 1388
gastrointestinal effects, 292f
gastrointestinal perforation caused by, 127
history of, 1388
ingestion
adjunctive therapy for, 1394
clinical manifestations, 1390–1391
contrast esophagram, 127–128
diagnostic imaging, 115t, 1391, 1392f
diagnostic tests for, 1391–1392
dilutional therapy for, 1393
disposition of patients with, 1394
endoscopic evaluation, 1390, 1390t, 1391–1392
gastrointestinal decontamination for, 1393
laboratory investigation, 36t, 1391
management, 1392–1395
predictors of injury, 1390–1391
surgical management, 1393–1394
injury caused by
acute management, 1392–1393
airway management with, 1392–1393
clinical presentation, 1390–1391
endoscopic evaluation, 1390, 1390t
factors affecting, 1388
management, animal studies, 1394
predictors, 1390–1391
steroids for, 1390t, 1394
legislation about, 1388
neutralization, 1393
ocular effects, management, 1395
ophthalmic exposure to, 358, 1389
irrigating solution for, 359t
management, 1395
ophthalmic toxicity, 356f, 361t
predictors of injury with, 1390–1391
products containing, 1388, 1388t
respiratory effects, 399t
self-poisoning with, worldwide, 1846
sources of, 1388, 1388t
toxicity, systemic, 1388, 1391
Caution, on rodenticide label, 1450t, 1453t
Cayenne pepper (*Capsicum frutescens, C. annuum*), 1599t
2C-B, 1179t, 1180–1181, 1181t, 1182, 1184
chemical structure, 1180f
clinical effects, 1183
2CB. *See* 4-Bromo-2,5-methoxyphenylethylamine (2CB, MFT)
2C-B-FLY, clinical effects, 1183
CBRNE (chemical, biological, radiologic, nuclear, and explosive), 1741t
CBW (chemical and biological weapons), 1741t
2C-C, 1181
CCA wood preservative, 1268–1269
2C-D, 1181
2C-E, 1181
CEDIA (cloned enzyme donor immunoassay), 104–105
Cefaclor, 824–825
Cefadroxil, 824–825
Cefamandole, 825f

and vitamin K antagonism, 916
Cefazolin, 824–825
Cefdinir, 824–825
Cefditoren, 824–825
Cefepime, 824–825
Cefixime, 824–825
Cefotaxime, 824–825
Cefotetan, 824–825
Cefotiam, intrathecal administration, inadvertent overdose and unintentional exposures due to, 795t
Cefoxitin, 824–825
Cefpodoxime, 824–825
Cefprozil, 824–825
Ceftaroline, 824–825
Ceftazidime, 824–825
Ceftibuten, 824–825
Ceftolozane, 824–825
Ceftriaxone, 824–825
and calcium salts, adverse interactions, 1406
and EAAT2 activity, 225
intrathecal administration, inadvertent overdose and unintentional exposures due to, 795t
mechanism of action, 227t
Cefuroxime, 824–825
Celastraceae, 1599t
Celebrex, 511
Celecoxib, 514
pharmacology, 512t
Celiprolol
overdose/poisoning
clinical manifestations, 932
management, 936
pharmacokinetics, 930
pharmacology, 927t
vasodilating effects, 930–931
Cell cycle, 349, 349f
gap phases, 349
interphase, 349
Cell senescence, 350
Cell surface antigens, 311
Cellular chaperones, 1815
Cellular chemokine receptor (Ccr5) antagonist, 832
Cellular injury, mechanisms, 173–175
Cellulose acetate (Adsorba), 96
Cementite, 1717
Centella asiatica (gotu kola), 642t
Centers for Biologics Evaluation and Research (CBER), 1634
Centers for Disease Control and Prevention (CDC), 1808
classification of community (public health) risk, 1815
contact information, 1743t
emergency number for, 1360
website, information from, 1814
Centipedes (*Chilopoda*), 1540t
Central American rattlesnake (*Crotalus* spp., *Crotalus durissus*), 1636t
antivenom, 1627t, 1628–1631
Central anticholinergic syndrome
antihistamines associated with, 746
management, 748
Central Asian pine-tree lappet moth, 1553
Central nervous system (CNS), 340
aluminum in, 1224–1225
carbon monoxide poisoning and, 1665
chlorobutanol and, 683–684
copper in, 1286
depression, antihypertensive-related, 960–961

disorders, diagnostic imaging in, 130–135
functional pathways, 340
hydrocarbons and, 1413–1414
infection, 38
differential diagnosis, 1299
empiric treatment, 1299
inhalants and, 1196
muscarinic agonists and, 207
muscarinic blockade and, 207
neurons, 340
nicotinic receptor agonists and antagonists and, 207
thallium and, 1351
toxicity. *See also* Seizures
sulfonamides and, 827
Central nervous system (CNS) depressants
alkaloidal, 1605
and erectile dysfunction, 300
Central nervous system (CNS) stimulants, alkaloidal, 1605
Central pontine myelinolysis. *See* Osmotic demyelination syndrome (ODS)
Central venous pressure, in heatstroke, 420–421
Centruroides spp., 1540t, 1548, 1548t
antivenom, 35t, 44t, 1563–1565, 1564t
availability and storage, 44t
indications for, 44t
stocking, recommended level, 44t
Centruroides elegans, 1563, 1564t
Centruroides exilicauda (bark scorpion), 1548–1549, 1548t–1549t
antivenom, 35t, 44t, 1563–1565, 1564t
envenomation, treatment, 1563
Centruroides gertschi, 1563, 1564t. *See also Centruroides exilicauda* (bark scorpion)
Centruroides limpidus, 1549, 1563, 1564t
Centruroides meisei, 1563, 1564t
Centruroides noxius, 1563, 1564t
Centruroides sculpturatus. See Centruroides exilicauda (bark scorpion)
Centruroides suffusus, 1563, 1564t
Centruroides vittatus, 1548
CEP72 gene, 505
Cephaelis acuminata (ipecac), 1599t
Cephaelis ipecacuanha (ipecac), 1599t, 1605
Cephalexin, 824–825
pharmacokinetics, oral zinc salts and, 1363
Cephaline, 1599t, 1605
Cephalopholis boenak (grouper fish), vitamin A toxicity from, 655
Cephalopoda, 1572
Cephalosporins, 824–825
adverse drug reactions with therapeutic use, 824
cephem nucleus, 824
cross-hypersensitivity, 824
and ethanol, interactions, 1146t
and GABA receptor, 222
mechanism of action, 822t
N-methylthiotetrazole side-chain effects, 824–825, 825f
seizures caused by, 824–825
toxicity (overdose/poisoning), 822t
Cephalothin, 825f
Ceramic glaze, leaded, imaging, 116, 117f
Ceramides, 269, 271
Cerapachys spp., 1552
Cerbera spp., self-poisoning with, 1846
Cerbera manghas (sea mango), 969, 979, 1606
self-poisoning with, 1846
Cerbera odollam (pong-pong "suicide" tree), 979

Cerebellar atrophy, 134
diagnostic imaging, 115t, 131, 132t
Cerebellitis, cyclic antidepressant overdose and, 1047
Cerebral atrophy, diagnostic imaging, 131, 132t
Cerebral blood flow
positron emission tomography of, 134
single-photon emission computed tomography of, 134
Cerebral edema, 93, 131, 161, 195
with N-acetylcysteine, 495
in ethylene glycol poisoning, 1424
in lead encephalopathy, management, 1303
thallium and, 1351
Cerebral hypoxia, focal lesions caused by, 131
Cerebrospinal fluid (CSF)
circulation, 793
pH, 142t
production, 793
specimens, postmortem collection and analysis, 1886
volume, 793
xenobiotic recovery from, 794
xenobiotics intentionally delivered to, 793, 793t
Cerebrovascular accident, with prothrombin complex
concentrate, 909
Cerebrovascular disease, arsenic and, 1242
Cerebrovascular syndrome, radiation-induced, 1768
Cerivastatin, 171
rhabdomyolysis caused by, 21
Certified Specialists in Poison Information (CSPIs), 1814
legal considerations for, 1865–1866
in risk assessment, 1816–1817
Certolizumab pegol, polymer protein conjugate, 1719t
Cereulide, mitochondrial injury from, 331
Ceruloplasmin, 146, 160, 1284, 1285t, 1287
Cesium, 1264–1267
absorption, 1264
adsorption, in vitro studies, 1359
antidote for, 35t
in brachytherapy, 1264
in brain, imaging, 1265
in breast milk, 1360
cardiotoxicity, 1264–1265
chemistry, 1769
contamination by, 1762
dermal decontamination for, precautions with, 72
elemental, 1264
elimination, 1264–1265, 1359
elimination half-life, 1264
history and epidemiology, 1264
industrial uses, 1264
isotopes, 1264, 1359
mass exposure to, 23t, 24, 1264
nonradioactive
poisoning with, in humans, Prussian blue for,
1266, 1359
toxicity, 1359
occupational exposure to, 1264
pharmacokinetics, 1264–1265
pharmacology, 1264
physicochemical properties, 1264
poisoning with, 1357
cardiovascular effects, 1265
clinical manifestations, 1265
death from, 1359
diagnostic tests for, 1265
electrolyte abnormalities in, 1265
gastrointestinal effects, 1265
management, 46t, 92, 1265–1266, 1359–1360
neurologic effects, 1265
pathophysiology, 1265, 1359
Prussian blue for, 1266, 1359–1360

radioactive, 1264, 1769
in breast milk, 1265
dermal absorption, 1265
detection, 1265
poisoning with
in humans, Prussian blue for, 1266, 1359
management, 1265–1266
sources, 1359
therapeutic uses, 1264
transplacental transfer, 1265
tissue distribution, 1264
toxicokinetics, 1264–1265
urine
measurement, 1265
normal concentration, 1264
in toxicity, 1265
whole blood
measurement, 1265
normal concentration, 1264
in toxicity, 1265
Cesium chloride
adverse effects, 1264
in cancer treatment, 1264
cardiovascular toxicity, 1265
gastrointestinal effects, 1265
neurologic effects, 1265
purported therapeutic uses, 1264
toxicity, 1266, 1359
Cesium oxide, 1264
Cetacaine spray, methemoglobinemia from, 1705
Cetirizine
adverse effects and safety issues, 746
dose modification in liver or kidney disease, 744
metabolism, 743
pharmacokinetics and toxicokinetics, 745t
pharmacology, 742
and QT interval prolongation, 746
structure, 740f
toxicity, clinical manifestations, 744
Cetrimonium bromide. See Quaternary ammonium
compounds
Cetylev, 495, 497
Chaat, 643t
Chacocine, 1604
Chaconine, 1602t–1603t
Chacruna (Psychotria viridis), 641t, 647, 649, 650t, 1180
Chain of custody
in blood sample for blood alcohol (ethanol)
concentration, 1864
in drug screening, 111
in forensic interpretive toxicology, 1870
Chalcocite, 1283
Chalcopyrite, 1283, 1284t, 1339
Chalcosis lentis, 1287
Chalepesin, as abortifacient, 303t
Chamaemelum nobile, 641t
Chamois, bezoars from, 3
Chamomile (Chamomilla recutita), volatile oils in,
639
Chamomile (Matricaria recutita, Chamaemelum
nobile), uses and toxicities, 641t
Changcao. See Bitter orange (Citrus aurantium)
Channel receptors, 204, 204t
Ch'an Su (Bufo bufo gargarizans, Bufo bufo
melanosticus), 649
as aphrodisiac, 649
psychoactive properties, 650t
uses and toxicities, 641t
Chanterelle (Cantharellus cibarius), 1589
Chaparral (Larrea tridentata), 1610

hepatotoxicity, 651
uses and toxicities, 641t
CharcoAid G, 79
Charcoal, 4t. See also Activated charcoal
early use of, 7
history of, 76
Charcot-Marie-Tooth disease, 342
Chasing the dragon, 21t, 22, 343, 527–528, 1223. See
also Heroin
and toxic leukoencephalopathy, 133
Chatinine, 650t
Chechen rebels, chemical used against, 17, 17t
Checkerberry oil, 634
Cheilosis, in pyridoxine deficiency, 663
Chelation. See also specific chelator
for aluminum toxicity, 1225
of antimony, 1234
for arsenic toxicity, 1244–1245, 1245f, 1245t
for bismuth toxicity, 1257
for cadmium toxicity, 1261–1262
of chromium, 1271
definition, 1315
for lead poisoning, 1302, 1303t
for manganese toxicity, 1321
for mercury poisoning, 1330
for neonates of lead-exposed mothers, 1305
of nickel, 1337
of radionuclides, renal exposure during, 1780
for selenium toxicity, 1342
contraindications to, 1342
teratogenicity, 1305
for thallium poisoning, 1354–1355
for zinc toxicity, 1365
Chelators, 147, 1779. See also
Diethylenetriaminepentaacetic acid (DTPA);
Pentetate calcium trisodium (Ca-DTPA);
Pentetate zinc trisodium (Zn-DTPA); specific
chelator
effects on bioavailability, 144
mechanism of action, 164–165
pharmacokinetic effects, 152
Chelicerae, of spiders, 1540
Chelirubine, 650t
Chemical, biological, radiologic, nuclear, and explosive
(CBRNE), 1741t
Chemical Abstracts Services (CAS), registry numbers
for chemicals, 1807
Chemical and biological weapons (CBW), 1741t. See
also Biological weapons (BW); Chemical
weapons (CW)
atropine for, 1505–1506
incidents
personal protective gear for, 1742–1743, 1742t
preparation for, 1742–1743, 1742t
triage in, 1742, 1742t
Israeli experience with (1990–1991 Gulf War), 1744
low-tech attacks using, 1744
metal phosphides as, 1457
psychological effects, 1744
Chemical disasters, antidote availability in, 42
Chemical hazards. See also Hazardous materials
incident response
workplace, 1797, 1797t
Chemical Mace, 1749–1750, 1749f
Chemical reactivity, 155–157
Chemical restraint, 386
Chemicals
CAS registry numbers for, 1807
Globally Harmonized System of Classification and
Labelling of Chemicals for, 1808

Chemicals (*Cont.*):
 household, poisoning with, in developing world, 1846
 industrial, self-harm with, 1847
Chemical safety, international agreements on, 1847
Chemical Transportation Emergency Center (CHEMTREC), 1803, 1808
Chemical warfare, 1741t
 in World War I, 17, 17t
Chemical weapons (CW), 1741–1752, 1741t. *See also* Nerve agents; Pulmonary irritants; Riot control agents; Vesicants; *specific xenobiotic*
 aerosols
  gases, and vapors, 1741–1742
   and children, 1744
    decontamination for, 1743
 atropine for, 1505–1506. *See also* Atropine
 and biological weapons, comparison, 1742, 1742t, 1753
 and children, 1744
 decontamination for, 1743
 history of, 1486, 1741
 liquid, 1741
  decontamination for, 1743
 low-tech attacks using, 1744
 persistence, 1741
 physical properties, 1741–1742
 and pregnancy, 1744
 preparation for, 1742–1743, 1742t
 risk of exposure to, 1743–1744
 toxic syndromes caused by, 1750t–1751t
 volatility, 1741
 war gases in, 1741
Chemistry, 155
 acid-base, 160–161
 inorganic, 155–161. *See also* Periodic Table of the Elements
 organic, 161–166
Chemoreceptor trigger zone (CTZ), 214, 217–218, 1034
Chemotherapeutics, 759–766. *See also specific xenobiotic*
 agranulocytosis caused by, management, 764
 alkylating agents, 759, 760t
 antibiotics, 759, 760t
 antimetabolites, 759, 760t, 767
 antimitotics, 759, 760t
 antimony-based, 1228
 arsenic in, 1237. *See also* Arsenic trioxide (white arsenic)
 cardiovascular toxicity, 762–763, 763t
 cell cycle nonspecific, 349, 349f, 350, 354, 761f
 cell cycle specificity, 349, 349f, 350, 759, 761f
 and cell injury, 350
 classification, 759, 760t
 dermatologic effects, 762
 diagnostic tests for, 763
 and DNA damage, 350
 enhanced elimination, 764
 EPA-regulated, 765
 and erectile dysfunction, 300
 exposure to
  epidemiology, 759
  mortality rate for, 759
  in pregnancy, 764
 extravasation, 762, 802, 803t
 and female sexual dysfunction, 302f
 and fibrinolysis, 322–323
 focal brain lesions caused by, 131
 and gustatory dysfunction, 365
 and hair loss, 281

hematopoietic toxicity, 311
hypomagnesemia caused by, 877
indications for, 759
infertility caused by, 297t, 298f
injury to cell lines from selected tissues, 351–354
intrathecal administration, 794
irritant, extravasation, 802
and male sexual dysfunction, 299f
mechanism of action, 761, 762f
metabolism, genetic polymorphisms and, 759
monoclonal antibodies, 759, 760t, 761f
nephrotoxicity, 763
neurotoxicity, 343
and olfactory dysfunction, 364
platinum-based, 759, 760t
and posterior reversible encephalopathy syndrome, 132
protein kinase inhibitors, 759, 760t, 761f
pulmonary/thoracic effects, imaging, 115t, 125t, 126
renal effects, 390f
resistance to, P-glycoprotein and, 144
sites of action, 759, 761, 761f–762f
skin discoloration caused by, 273
and tinnitus, 370t
topoisomerase inhibitors, 759, 760t
toxicity (overdose/poisoning)
 clinical manifestations, 761–763, 763t
 diagnosis, 763
 epidemiology, 759
 genetic polymorphisms and, 759, 771
 iatrogenic, 759
 management, 763–764
 patient-specific factors affecting, 759
and toxic leukoencephalopathy, 133
vesicant, extravasation, 802
in workplace, 764–765
Chemsex, 1188
CHEMTREC (Chemical Transportation Emergency Center), 1803, 1808
Chenopodiaceae, 1603t, 1610
Chernobyl disaster, 23t, 24, 1264, 1359, 1762, 1772, 1775–1776
Cherry, *Prunus*, cyanogenic glycosides in, 1684
Chest pain, 122
 cannabinoid-associated, 1117
 cocaine-related, 126, 128f, 249, 1127–1128
  benzodiazepines for, 1139
 in thallium toxicity, 1351
Chest radiograph perfusion score, 1276–1277
Chest radiography, 125t
 of caustic injury, 1391
 in cocaine toxicity, 125t
 in injection drug use (IDU), 125t, 126f
 in metal phosphide poisoning, 1459
 for poisoned patient, 407
 of pulmonary and other thoracic complications, 115t, 122–126
 in respiratory disorders, 401, 406
 in smoke inhalation, 1642, 1643f
 smoke inhalation and, 1642, 1643f
 in strychnine poisoning, 1537
 in toxicologic emergencies, 125t
 xenobiotics on, 115t
Chest wall, muscle weakness or rigidity, xenobiotic-induced, 400
Chewable vitamins, childhood poisoning with, 669
Chewing tobacco, 1204t, 1205. *See also* Nicotine
Chickling peas (*Lathyrus sativus*), 227
Chihuahuan ridge-nosed rattlesnake (*Crotalus* spp.), 1637t

Chikungunya, 1522
Child abuse, 454–455
 medical, 455, 455t
Childhood cirrhosis, 1287
Childhood poisoning. *See* Pediatric poisoning
Child Protection Act (1966), 10t, 11
Children. *See also* Pediatric poisoning
 N-acetylcysteine use in, 493
 activated charcoal use in, 79, 452
 acute liver failure in, 480
 ADEs and medication errors in, 1826
  prevention, 1829
  reduction/prevention, 1827
 carbon monoxide poisoning in, 1671
 chemical weapons and, 1744
 critically ill, and thiamine deficiency, 1160
 CT use in
  and cancer risk, 1766, 1773
  and radiation exposure, 1766, 1773
 decontamination, 1744
 disulfiram toxicity in, 1175
 enhanced elimination in, 452
 exchange transfusions in, 98, 452
 gastrointestinal decontamination in, 452
 hemodialysis in, 452
 historical mass casualties affecting, 453
 inhalant abuse among, 1193
 medication dosing for, Broselow-Luten system, 1828
 mushroom ingestion by, 1581, 1592
 obesity in, 606
 ophthalmic exposures, systemic toxicity with, 360
 orogastric lavage in, 452
 pesticide poisoning in, *case study*, 1450–1451
 poisoning and, worldwide, 1844
 poisoning with household products and chemicals, global aspects, 1846
 poison prevention aimed at, 1784
  taste-aversive xenobiotics in, 1782
 radiation exposure, 1773
 ricin poisoning in, 1608–1609
 salicylate toxicity in, 563–564
 in sub-Saharan Africa, morbidity and mortality rates, 1844
 unintentional poisoning of, 9
 unusual/idiosyncratic reactions to xenobiotics, 452–453
 vital signs in, 28, 28t
 whole-bowel irrigation in, 63, 86
 xenobiotic exposures, NEISS data on, 448–449
 xenobiotic ingestion
  characteristics, 448
  gastrointestinal decontamination for, 452
  history-taking with, 451
  and time to presentation, 57
 xenobiotics that are toxic in small quantities in, 452, 452t
 xenobiotics with delayed toxicity in, 452
Child-resistant closures/containers, 451, 1782
Child-Resistant Packaging Act, 1782
Chimney sweeps, scrotal cancer in, 7, 23t
China, opium abuse in, 8
China bark. *See Cinchona* spp.; Quinine
Chinese bird spider toxin, and voltage-gated calcium channels, 244f, 245
Chinese blue, 1357
Chinese cucumber (*Trichosanthes kirilowii*), 1609
Chinese cucumber root (*Trichosanthes kirilowii*), 641t
Chinese herb nephropathy, 613, 1610
Chinese herbs, acute interstitial nephritis caused by, 394t

Chinese medicines, traditional. *See also specific*
        medicines
    podophyllum resin in, 1612
Chinese restaurant syndrome, 600
Chinese star anise (*Illicium verum*), 1608
CHIPES (mnemonic), 114
Chiral carbon, 164
Chiral center, 147
Chiral structures, 147, 164, 164f
Chiral switching, 147
Chirodropidae, 1567
    deaths caused by, 1568
Chironex fleckeri (box jellyfish, sea wasp), 1567–1568.
        See also Cnidaria (jellyfish)
    antivenom, 1575t
    cardiotoxin, 1570–1571
    envenomation
        clinical manifestations, 1569
        management, 1569–1571
    venom, toxins in, 1569
Chiropsalmus spp., 1567t. *See also* Cnidaria (jellyfish)
    venom, cardiotoxicity, 1570
Chiropsalmus quadrigatus (box jellyfish), 1567t. *See also*
        Cnidaria (jellyfish)
Chiropsalmus quadrumanus (box jellyfish), 1567t, 1568.
        See also Cnidaria (jellyfish)
    venom, cardiotoxicity, 1570
Chi-squared test, 1857–1858
Chitin, in urticarial hairs of tarantulas, 1547
Chitosamine (glucosamine, 2-amino-2-deoxyglucose),
        uses and toxicities, 642t
Chitosan, 606, 607t. *See also* Dieting xenobiotics and
        regimens
Chittern bark (*Cascara sagrada*), 1599t. *See also*
        Cascara (*Cascara sagrada*)
Chlomethoxyfen, 1468t
Chloracne, 13, 16t, 17–18, 271, 271f, 1414
Chloral hydrate, 1088. *See also* Sedative-hypnotics
    abuse, 8–9
    with alcohol/ethanol (Mickey Finn), 8, 1085, 1085f,
        1146
    cardiotoxicity, 1088
    in children, 1088
    and disulfiramlike reactions, 1174t
    elimination half-life, in children, 1088
    and ethanol, interactions, 1146t
    historical perspective on, 8–9, 1084
    odor, 364t, 1086t
    pharmacokinetics, 145t, 1085, 1085t, 1088
    radiopacity, 114
    structure, 1088
    toxicity (overdose/poisoning), clinical findings in,
        1086–1088, 1086t
    volume of distribution, 145t
Chloramben, in herbicides, 1467t
Chlorambucil, 760t
    EPA regulation of, 765
    infertility caused by, 297t
    neurotoxicity, 763
    teratogenicity, 429t
Chloramine, 1655, 1655f
    sources, 1654t
    toxicity, and dialysis, 98–99
    water solubility, 1654t
Chloramphenicol, 825–826
    adverse effects with therapeutic use, 825–826
    bone marrow suppression with, 826
    and ethanol, interactions, 1146t
    extracorporal elimination, 825
    gray baby syndrome from, 442, 452–453

    mechanism of action, 822t, 825
    overdose, 822t, 825
    pharmacokinetics, 825
    structure, 825
    thimerosal in, 690
    toxicity, 822t
p-Chloraniline, 1368
Chlorates, 1369t, 1375–1376
Chlorobenzilate, physicochemical properties, 1515t
Chlorbutol. *See* Chlorobutanol
Chlordane
    enterohepatic circulation, interruption, 64
    fat-to-serum ratio for, 1515
    metabolism, 1515
    physicochemical properties, 1515t
Chlordecone, 1514
    absorption, 1514
    and ATP synthesis, 176t
    chronic exposure to, clinical manifestations, 1518
    elimination, 1515
    enterohepatic/enteroenteric recirculation, 1516
    hepatic effects, 334t
    infertility caused by, 297t, 298f
    mechanism of toxicity, 1517
    metabolism, 1515
    occupational disease from, 23, 23t
    physicochemical properties, 1515t
    poisoning, management, 1519
    site of action, 173f
    structure, 1516f
Chlordiazepoxide, 1087. *See also* Benzodiazepine(s);
        Sedative-hypnotics
    for alcohol withdrawal, 1138, 1168
    duration of action, 1137
    hepatic metabolism, 1137t, 1138
    history of, 1084, 1135
    metabolites, 1088
    pharmacokinetics, 1085t
Chlordimeform, hemorrhagic cystitis caused by, 306
Chlorfenapyr
    acute ingestion, case-fatality ratio, 1519
    mechanism of action, 1519
    poisoning
        clinical manifestations, 1519
        onset, 1519
    structure, 1519
Chlorfenvinphos, 1488t
Chlorhexidine, 1368, 1369t
    absorption, 1368
    as antiseptic, 1368
    clinical effects, 1368
    and discoloration of teeth and gums, 293t
    exposure to, management, 1368
    and gustatory dysfunction, 365
Chloride
    assays, bromides and, 1088
    and GABA neurotransmission, 221–222
    postmortem changes, 1885t
    vitreous, normal concentration, 1872t
Chloride channel, 204, 205f, 218–219, 220f
    glycinergic, strychnine and, 1536
    organic chlorine insecticides and, 1516–1517, 1517f
    voltage-gated, insecticides and, 1521
Chloride (Cl⁻) ions
    membrane transport, 203
    and metabolic acidosis, 191
    and metabolic alkalosis, 194, 194t
Chloride shift, 316
Chlorine, 1653
    airway injury by, 1640t, 1641

    as antiseptic, 1369t, 1372
    as chemical weapon, 17t, 1741, 1748–1749
    chemistry, 1656, 1656f
    decontamination for, 1743
    detection threshold, 1654t
    diffuse airspace filling from, 123, 125t
    immediately dangerous to life and health (IDLH),
        1654t
    inhalation, sodium bicarbonate for, 568t, 571
    odor, 1656, 1748
    organic, 1450
        and ATP production, 176t
    pulmonary toxicity, 160
        management, 407
    regulatory standard for, 1654t
    short-term exposure limit (STEL), 1654t
    sources, 1654t
    in Syrian civil war, 17, 1741, 1748
    in terrorism, 1744
    as thermal degradation product, 1641t
    toxic syndrome caused by, 1751t
    in warfare, 17, 17t, 1651
    water solubility, 1654t
Chlormethiazole
    as glycine agonist, 223
    poisoning, and organ donation, 1893t
Chloroacetophenone (CN, Mace), 1657, 1749–1750,
        1749f
    ophthalmic exposure to, 359
para-Chloroamphetamine, 1102
Chlorobenzilate
    absorption, 1514
    metabolism, 1515
o-Chlorobenzylidene malononitrile, 1749, 1749f
Chlorobenzylidene malononitrile, (CS), 364t, 1657
    odor, 364t
Chlorobutanol, 683–684, 683t, 863, 1161
    CNS toxicity, 683–684
    lethal dose, 683
    odor, 683
    ophthalmic toxicity, 684
    physicochemical properties, 683
    structure, 683–684
    therapeutic uses, 683
2-Chlorodeoxyadenosine, mechanism and site of
        action, 762f
Chloroform (CHCl₃), 4t–5t, 7, 174t, 1410
    abuse, 8
    diagnostic imaging, 117–118
    hepatotoxicity, 1196
    history of, 1011
    odor, 364t
    tests for, 7
    toxicity, *N*-acetylcysteine for, 492, 494
4-Chloro-2-methylphenoxyacetic acid (MCPA), 1471,
        1480–1482. *See also* Phenoxy herbicides
    mechanism of toxicity, 1481
    pharmacokinetics and toxicokinetics, 1481
    structure, 1481f
    toxicity, mortality rate for, 1482
Chlorophacinone, 885
    physicochemical properties, 1453t
    in rodenticides, 1453t
    toxicity
        antidote and/or treatment for, 1453t
        clinical manifestations, 1453t
        onset, 1453t
        toxic mechanism, 1453t
m-Chlorophenylpiperazine (mCPP), 218
Chlorophors, as antiseptics, 1369t, 1372

Chlorophyllum esculentum, 1582t, 1589
Chlorophyllum molybdites, 1582t, 1589
Chlorophytum comosum (spider plant), 1599t
Chloropicrin, 1462, 1749
Chloroprocaine. *See also* Local anesthetic(s)
  minimal IV toxic dose, 998t
  neurotoxicity, 997
  pharmacology, 966t
Chloroquine, 842–844
  as abortifacient, 838
  antidote for, 35t
  antimalarial mechanism, 838t
  cardiac effects, 258t
  hypoglycemia caused by, 715
  pharmacokinetics, 839t, 843
  and prolonged QT interval, 253t
  self-poisoning with, 1846
  structure, 842, 1139, 1139f
  and tinnitus, 370t
  toxicity
    benzodiazepines for, 1139
    clinical manifestations, 843
    management, 843–844
    pathophysiology, 843
    sodium bicarbonate for, 568t
  toxicodynamics, 843
Chlorothiazide, and thiamine pharmacokinetics,
    1158
Chlorothion, 1488t
Chloroxylenol, 1373–1374
Chlorpheniramine
  abuse/misuse, pathophysiology, 744
  elimination, 744
  elimination half-life, 744
  pediatric exposure to, 738
  pharmacokinetics and toxicokinetics, 745t
  pharmacology, 742
  structure, 740f
Chlorphenoxy herbicides. *See also* Phenoxy herbicides
  toxicity (overdose/poisoning), alkalinization for,
    570
Chlorproguanil, antimalarial mechanism, 838t
Chlorpromazine. *See also* Antipsychotics
  adverse effects and safety issues, 1039
  for alcohol withdrawal, 1168
  cholestasis caused by, 330
  clinical and toxicologic effects, 1034t
  and cyclic antidepressants, structural similarity,
    1032, 1034f
  dosage and administration, 1033t
  history of, 1032
  mechanism of action, 227t, 228
  nicotinic receptor blockade by, 207
  ophthalmic toxicity, 356f
  pharmacokinetics, 1033t
  pharmacology, 1032
  and seizures, 1168
  for serotonin toxicity, 1059
  skin discoloration caused by, 273
  toxicity (overdose/poisoning), 1032
    gastrointestinal decontamination for, 86
Chlorpropamide. *See also* Sulfonylureas
  adverse effects and safety issues, 699
  antidote for, 35t
  and disulfiramlike reactions, 1174t
  enhanced elimination, urine alkalinization for, 93
  and ethanol, interactions, 1146t
  exposure, in children, hypoglycemia caused by, 699
  pharmacokinetics and toxicokinetics, 697t
  structure, 695f

toxicity (overdose/poisoning)
  hypoglycemia caused by, 699
  octreotide for, 715
  sodium bicarbonate for, 568t
Chlorprothixene. *See also* Antipsychotics
  dosage and administration, 1033t
  pharmacokinetics, 1033t
Chlorpyrifos, 1488t, 1509–1510
  absorption, 1487
  cytochrome P450 enzymes and, 1489
  pharmacokinetics and toxicokinetics, 146t
  toxicity, solvent and, 1490
  volume of distribution, 146t
Chlorthal, in herbicides, 1467t
Chlorthalidone, 963. *See also* Diuretics, thiazide
Chlorthiamid, in herbicides, 1467t
Chocolate (*Theobroma cacao*, theobromine), 985.
    See also Methylxanthines; Theobromine
    (chocolate)
Cholecalciferol (vitamin D₃). *See* Vitamin D
    (cholecalciferol and ergocalciferol); Vitamin
    D₃ (cholecalciferol)
Cholecystokinin (CCK), 290t, 292
Cholelithiasis, laboratory investigation, 335t
Cholera, 597, 597t
Cholestasis, 327–328, 330, 334t
  intrahepatic, 330
  laboratory investigation, 335t
  xenobiotic-induced, 330–331, 331t
Cholestyramine, 92
  for chlordecone poisoning, 1519
  for digoxin, digitoxin, and chlordane overdose, 64
  effect on thyroid hormones and function, 814t, 817
  for levothyroxine overdose, 817
Choline acetyltransferase, 206
  aluminum and, 1224
Cholinergic crisis, 1488. *See also* Cholinergic syndrome
  management, 1498
Cholinergic nervous system, 206f
Cholinergic neurotransmission. *See also* Acetylcholine
    (ACh)
  xenobiotics affecting, 206f, 207, 207t
Cholinergic poisoning
  categories, 1495, 1495t
  differential diagnosis, 1495–1496
Cholinergic receptors, subtypes, 1503
Cholinergics. *See also specific xenobiotic*
  cardiac effects, 258t
  cranial neuropathy caused by, 346t
  diagnostic imaging, 115t
  effect on thermoregulation, 412, 413t
  effects on vital signs, 29t
  toxicity (overdose/poisoning)
    clinical and laboratory findings in, 36t
    cutaneous findings in, 189
  toxic syndrome caused by, 29t
Cholinergic syndrome, 1487, 1491, 1492f. *See also*
    Cholinergic crisis
  pathophysiology, 1489–1490, 1490f
  pralidoxime for, 1509
Cholinesterase, 755–756
  activity, interpretation, 1495t
  plasma, inhibition, 755–756
    by organic phosphorus compound, 1508–1509
  postmortem changes, 1885t
Cholinesterase inhibitors, 2, 1495, 1495t, 1503. *See
    also* Insecticides; Organic phosphorus
    compounds; *specific xenobiotic*
  antidote for, 35t
  carbamate. *See also* Carbamate(s)

structure, 755f
  contraindications to, 1041
  ophthalmic effects, 1504
  overdose/poisoning, management, 44t–45t
Cholinesterase sponges, 1498
Choline transporter (ChT), 206, 206f
Cholinolytics, 207t
Cholinomimetics, 207t, 1495t, 1496
Chondrichthyes, 1576
Chondrodendron spp. (tubocurare, curare), 1599t, 1605.
    See also Curare
Chondrodendron tomentosum, 1605
Chondroitin sulfate, heparin contaminated with, 891
Chondrosclerosis, 122t
  lead-induced, 119
Chorea, 344
  carbon monoxide poisoning and, 1665
Choreoathetosis
  amphetamine-induced, 1103–1104
  cocaine and, 1127
  dopamine and, 213–214
  mercury-associated, 1327
Christison, Robert, 4t, 6, 8
Christmas cactus (*Schlumbergera bridgesii*), 1602t
Christmas rose (*Helleborus niger*), 1600t
Chromacine, 1255
Chromated copper arsenate (CCA) wood preservative,
    1268–1269
Chromated cupric arsenate, 1283, 1284t
Chromatography, 102, 103t, 105–106. *See also* Gas
    chromatography (GC); High-performance
    liquid chromatography (HPLC); Thin-layer
    chromatography (TLC)
  detectors for, 106
  interferences in, 109
  liquid-liquid extraction for, 105
  mobile phase for, 105
  modalities for, 105–106
  principles of, 105
  retention time in, 105, 107
  sample preparation for, 105
  solid-phase extraction for, 105
  stationary phase for, 105
  xenobiotic identification in, 106
  xenobiotic quantification in, 106
Chromatopsia, 972
Chrome holes, 1270
Chromic acid, 1268t
  dermal burns, 1270
Chromic chloride, 1268t
Chromic fluoride, 1268t
Chromic oxide, 1268t
Chromite ore, 1268t
Chromium
  absorption, 1269
  carcinogenicity, 1269–1270
  distribution, 1269
  in drinking water, 1268–1269
  elemental, 1268
  elimination, 1269
  excretion, 1269
    N-acetylcysteine and, 494
  exposure to
    environmental, 1268–1269
    medical device, 1269
    occupational, 1269, 1269t, 1270
  extracorporeal elimination, 1271
  in food, 1268
  forms, 1268, 1268t
  in hair and nails, 1270–1271

hexavalent, 1268
  absorption, 1269
  carcinogenicity, 1268
  permissible exposure limit, 1269
  reduction, 1268
  toxicity, pathophysiology, 1270
history and epidemiology, 1268
industrial uses, 1268
inhalation, 1270
nephrotoxicity, 397t
oxidative states, 1268
pharmacokinetics, 1269
pharmacology, 1268
physicochemical properties, 1268
respiratory effects, 1270
serum
  clinical significance, 1270
  normal concentration, 1268
as thermal degradation product, 1642
toxicity, 1268, 1275
  N-acetylcysteine for, 1271
  acute, clinical manifestations, 1270
  chelation therapy for, 1271
  chronic, clinical manifestations, 1270
  clinical manifestations, 1270
  decontamination for, 1271
  diagnostic tests for, 1270–1271
  management, 1271
  pathophysiology, 1269–1270
toxicokinetics, 1269
trivalent, 1268
  absorption, 1269
  toxicity, pathophysiology, 1269–1270
urine
  clinical significance, 1270
  normal concentration, 1268
whole blood
  clinical significance, 1270
  normal concentration, 1268
Chromium picolinate, 607t, 1268t
Chromosome(s)
  dicentric, radiation exposure and, 1769
  premature condensation, radiation exposure and, 1769
  translocation assay, radiation exposure and, 1769
Chronic interstitial nephritis
  metals causing, 397t
  xenobiotic-induced, 395, 395f
Chronic kidney disease (CKD), 395
  and aluminum toxicity, 1223–1225
  causes, 395
  classification, 395, 395t
  and diethylenetriaminepentaacetic acid (DTPA) use, 1781
  in elderly, and adverse events, 464–465
  lithium-induced, 1068
  porous carbon microsphere compounds used in, 77
  stages, 395, 395t
  xenobiotic-induced, 395, 395f
Chronic obstructive pulmonary disease, N-acetylcysteine for, 494
Chronic renal failure. See Chronic kidney disease (CKD)
Chrysanthemum (chrysanthemum), 1599t
  allergy to, 1521, 1614
Chrysanthemum cinerariaefolium, 1519. See also Pyrethrins
Chrysanthemum vulgare. See Tanacetum vulgare (tansy)
Chrysaora quinquecirrha (sea nettle), 1568. See also Cnidaria (jellyfish)

dermal reaction to, pathophysiology, 1569
envenomation, management, 1569, 1571
venom, cardiotoxicity, 1570
Chrysene, 174t
Chrysiasis, 273
Chrysophanol, 641t
Chuanwu, 640t
Chuan wu (Bufo bufo gargarizans, Bufo bufo melanosticus), uses and toxicities, 637t
Chuen-Lin (Coptis chinensis, Coptis japonicum), 641t
Chui Fong Tou Ku Wan, 647
Church-flower. See Periwinkle (Catharanthus roseus)
Chvostek sign, 189
Chymotrypsin, inhibition, 1489
2C-I, 1181
Cicero, 2
Cicuta douglasii (western water hemlock), cicutoxin in, 1610
Cicuta maculata (water hemlock)
  cicutoxin in, 1610
  odor, 364t
  toxicity, 1599t
Cicutoxin, 1599t, 1610–1611
  and GABA, 222
  odor, 364t
Cider, lead contamination, 18t, 19
Cidex, 1369t
Cidex OPA, 1369t
Cidofovir, diabetes insipidus caused by, 195t
Cigar, nicotine content and delivery, 1204, 1204t
Cigarette lighter fluid, 1193t. See also Inhalant(s)
Cigarettes. See also Nicotine
  disease burden from, 1203
  electronic. See e-cigarettes
  ingestion, by children, 1204, 1207
  nicotine content and delivery, 1204, 1204t
  soakage water, and suicide, 1204
Ciguateralike poisoning, 595
Ciguatera poisoning, 592–595, 593t
  clinical and laboratory findings with, 36t, 593–594, 593t
  diagnostic tests for, 594
  prevention, 596
  treatment, 593t, 594–595
Ciguatoxin, 592–595, 593t
  effects on vital signs, 30t
  physicochemical properties, 593, 594f
  and voltage-gated calcium channels, 244f, 245
Cilastatin, 825
Ciliary body, 356
Cilostazol, 899
  mechanism of action, 898f
Cimetidine
  absorption, 744
  acute interstitial nephritis caused by, 394t
  adverse effects and safety issues, 739
  as androgen receptor blocker, 299f
  contraindications to, 990
  and dapsone, 846–847, 1709–1710
  drug interactions with, 744
  elimination, 744
  and ethanol, interactions, 1144–1145, 1146t
  history of, 739
  infertility caused by, 297t, 298f
  and lidocaine, interactions, 996
  metabolism, 744
  and metformin, interactions, 144
  overdose/poisoning, clinical manifestations, 746
  pharmacokinetics and toxicokinetics, 745t
  and procainamide, interactions, 144

for propanil poisoning, 1473
structure, 742, 742f
syrup, sorbitol in, 688t
volume of distribution, 744
Cimicifuga racemosa (black cohosh)
  as abortifacient, 303t
  resins in, 639
  uses and toxicities, 640t
Cinchona spp., 1599t
  as abortifacient, 303t
  bark, 641t, 836, 838. See also Quinine
Cinchona alkaloids. See Quinidine; Quinine
Cinchona calisaya (quinine), 644t
Cinchona ledgeriana (quinine), 641t
Cinchona succirubra (quinine), 641t
Cinchonism, 370, 839–840, 1599t, 1602t
1,8-Cineole, 630
Cinnabar (mercuric sulfide). See Mercury
Cinnabarinic acid, 227t
Cinnamaldehyde, 650t
Cinnamomum camphora, 628, 650t, 1380. See also Camphor
Cinnamon, psychoactive properties, 650t
Cinobufagin, 979
Cinobufotalin, 979
Ciprofloxacin
  adverse effects and safety issues, in elderly, 465
  benzalkonium chloride in, 682t
  and GABA receptor, 222
  hypoglycemia caused by, 715
  and methadone, interactions, 172
  seizures caused by, 826
  structure, 826
  and tizanidine, interactions, 171
Ciproxifan, 742
Ciraparantag, 888t, 894
Circadian rhythm, 217
Cirrhosis, 331t, 333, 334t
  alcoholic, 333
  bleeding risk in, 335
  laboratory investigation, 335t
Cisapride, 21, 171
  and hERG channels, 245
  QT interval prolongation by, 1840
Cisatracurium. See also Neuromuscular blockers (NMBs)
  pharmacology, 1020t, 1024–1025
Cisplatin, 349f, 761f
  acute tubular necrosis caused by, 390f, 392
  adverse effects and safety issues, 760t
  antidote for, 760t, 764
  clinical and laboratory findings with, 36t
  cranial neuropathy caused by, 346t
  diagnostic tests for, 763
  enhanced elimination, 764
  hypomagnesemia caused by, 877
  and kidney failure, 763
  as local irritant, 802
  nephrotoxicity
    N-acetylcysteine for, 494
    magnesium for, 877
  ophthalmic toxicity, 356f, 361t
  ototoxicity, 366f, 370t, 763
  peripheral neuropathy with, 763
  and posterior reversible encephalopathy syndrome, 132
  and tinnitus, 370t
  toxicity (overdose/poisoning), 760t, 763
    management, 764
  vomiting with, 762

Citalopram, 218, 1054
  and CYPs, 1056
  mechanism of action, 1056f
  metabolite, 145t, 147
  pharmacokinetics and toxicokinetics, 145t, 1055t
  and QT interval, 253, 253t
  receptor activity, 1057t
  structure, 1054f
  toxicity (overdose/poisoning)
    clinical manifestations, 1056–1057
    ECG changes in, 235, 253t, 1056–1057, 1057t
    gastrointestinal decontamination for, 51t, 64
    management, 1057
    seizures with, 1056–1057, 1057t
    sodium bicarbonate for, 568t, 569
  volume of distribution, 145t
Citrate
  and aluminum, 1224
  in blood products, 1406
  cation binding to, 1406
  excess, hypocalcemia caused by, 199
  and laboratory tests, 102
  physiologic functions, 1406
  toxicity, 1406
Citric acid cycle, 168, 173, 173f, 175–177, 707–708, 1006,
      1144, 1157–1159, 1157f
  inhibitors, 168, 175, 176t
  salicylates and, 557
  sodium monofluoroacetate and, 1533
  toxins in, 173, 173f
  trivalent arsenic and, 1238
Citronella oil, comparative efficacy and toxicity, 1523t
Citrovorum factor, 775. See also Leucovorin (folinic acid)
Citrulline, 180f, 181
Citrus spp., xenobiotic interactions, 1611
Citrus aurantium (bitter orange), 606, 607t, 610, 649,
      748, 1599t, 1605. See also Dieting xenobiotics
      and regimens
  uses and toxicities, 640t
Citrus paradisi (grapefruit), 1599t, 1607
  xenobiotic interactions, 1599t, 1610–1611
Civil War, US, opioid use and abuse in, 8
CK. See Ketamine, and cocaine, combined
CKD-EPI formula, 393t
CL 303268, 1519
Clarithromycin, 826–827
  adverse effects and safety issues, in elderly, 465
  and colchicine, interactions, 502
  for HIV-related infections, 830t
  metabolite, as CYP inhibitor, 171
  as P-glycoprotein inhibitor, 173
Claudius (Roman Emperor), 2, 5t
Claviceps paspali (ergot), 1599t. See also Ergot and
      ergot alkaloids
Claviceps purpurea (ergot), 18, 18t, 805–806, 1178–1179,
      1599t. See also Ergot and ergot alkaloids
  as abortifacient, 303t
Clavicipitaceae, 1599t
Clay(s), antidotal, 3
Clean Air Act (1963), 10t, 12
  and nanotechnology, 1731
Clean Air Act (England), 17
Clean Water Act (1972), 10t
  and nanotechnology, 1731
Clearance, 151
  compartment model for, 151–152, 152f
  definition, 151
  endogenous, and enhanced elimination techniques,
      92
  hepatic, 147–148

  model independent, 151–152, 152f
  oral, 148
  physiological model for, 151–152, 152f
  of xenobiotics
    calculation, 95
    in hemodialysis, 94–95, 95t
Cleistanthins, 1846
Cleistanthus collinus, and normal anion gap metabolic
      acidosis, 191t
Clenbuterol, 606, 619, 985
  adverse effects and safety issues, 608t
  in bodybuilding, 986
  in food supply, 986
  in heroin, 528
  hyperthermia induced by, 412
  in illicit drugs, 986
  mechanism of action, 608t
  pharmacokinetics, 987
  poisoning, 986
    epidemics, 986
    laboratory findings with, 1686
  regulation, 608t
  toxicokinetics, 987
Cleopatra, 1t, 2
Cleveland Clinic, toxic gas disaster, 16, 16t
Clevidipine, pharmacokinetics, 946t
Climbing knotwood (Polygonum multiflorum), 641t
Clindamycin, 827
  antimalarial mechanism, 838t
  for HIV-related infections, 830t
  and tinnitus, 370t
  toxicity, organ system manifestations, 829t
Clinical Institute Withdrawal Assessment of Alcohol
      Scale, Revised (CIWA-Ar), 1166–1167
Clinical testing, of new candidate drugs, 1835–1836,
      1835f
Clinical trials, 1835–1836, 1835f, 1853–1854, 1853t
  design, 1853–1854, 1854f, 1854t
  randomized, 1853–1854, 1854f, 1856–1857
  reporting on, regulation, 1835
  in toxicology, 1854, 1854t
Clioquinol, 20, 20t, 1287
  cranial neuropathy caused by, 346t
Clitocybe spp., 1503
  antidote for, 35t
Clitocybe acromelalga, 1583t, 1591
Clitocybe amoenolens, 1583t, 1591
Clitocybe claviceps, 1583t, 1592
Clitocybe dealbata, 1587, 1587f
Clitocybe illudens, 1587. See also Omphalotus olearius
Clitocybe nebularis, 1582t
Clobenpropit, 742
Clofarabine, mechanism and site of action, 762f
Clomeprop, in herbicides, 1467t
Clomethiazole, mechanism of action, 222
Clomiphene, athletes' use of, 617
Clomipramine, 1044, 1044t. See also Cyclic
      antidepressants
  overdose/poisoning
    gastrointestinal decontamination for, 54t
    management, 1050
  and serotonin toxicity, 1058t
  and sexual function, 304
Clonazepam, 1087. See also Benzodiazepine(s);
      Sedative-hypnotics
  duration of action, 1137
  pharmacokinetics, 1085t
  and serotonergic pathways, 1084
  toxicity (overdose/poisoning), 1087
    laboratory finding in, 112

Cloned enzyme donor immunoassay (CEDIA), 104–105
Clonidine
  adverse effects and safety issues, in children, 453
  for alcohol withdrawal, 1169
  antidote for, 35t
  as antihypertensive, 959–961
  deaths caused by, in children, 960
  and glutamate release, 228
  hyperthermia induced by, 412
  hypoglycemia caused by, 715
  hypoventilation caused by, 400t
  intrathecal administration, 794
  and male sexual dysfunction, 299f
  mechanism of action, 212, 239
  for neonatal opioid withdrawal, 439
  and opioids, cross-tolerance, 239
  for opioid withdrawal, 239
  overdose/poisoning, 32
    in children, 959
    clinical and laboratory findings in, 36t, 960
    diagnostic tests for, 960
    management, 960–961
    pathophysiology, 960
  pharmacokinetics, 959–960
  pharmacology, 959
  transdermal patch, ingestion, whole-bowel irrigation
      for, 85
  withdrawal
    α_2-adrenergic receptors in, 239
    clinical findings in, 239
Clonus
  in strychnine poisoning, 1536–1537
  in toxidromes, 29t
Clopidogrel, 899
  as antiplatelet agent, 899
  antiplatelet effects, 323
  mechanism of action, 898f
  metabolism, 170
Clopyralid, in herbicides, 1467t
Clorazepate. See also Benzodiazepine(s);
      Sedative-hypnotics
  pharmacokinetics, 1085t
Clorgyline, 1077
  mechanism of action, 218
  and serotonin toxicity, 1058t
Clostridial infections (Clostridium), 574–580. See also
      Botulism
Clostridium argentinense, 575
Clostridium baratii, 575
Clostridium botulinum, 592t, 596
  culture, 580
  detection, 580
  infection, 574–580. See also Botulism
Clostridium butyricum, 575
Clostridium perfringens, 592, 592t
  gastroenteritis, 597, 597t
Clothing, contaminated, removal, 72
Clotrimazole, 829
Clove (Syzygium aromaticum)
  psychoactive properties, 650t
  uses and toxicities, 641t
Clove oil (Syzygium aromaticum), 629–630
  toxicity
    N-acetylcysteine for, 492, 494
    treatment, 635
Clover, sweet (Melilotus spp.), 1601t
Cloxacillin, acute interstitial nephritis caused by,
      394t
Clozapine. See also Antipsychotics
  adverse effects and safety issues, 1039

clinical and laboratory findings with, 36t
clinical and toxicologic effects, 1034t
dosage and administration, 1033t
drug interactions with, 827
extrapyramidal effects, 215
and glycine reuptake, 223
history of, 1032
mechanism of action, 227t, 1035
pharmacokinetics, 1033t
priapism caused by, 301t
self-poisoning with, 376
and sudden cardiac death, 253
warnings related to, 1839
Club drugs, 1178. *See also* Ketamine
Clusiaceae, 1600t
Cluster designation (CD), 311
Cnidae, 1567
Cnidaria (jellyfish), 1567–1572
    Anthozoa, 1567–1568, 1567t
    clinical manifestations, 1568f
    Cubozoa, 1567, 1567t
    dermatitis caused by, 1568–1570
        clinical manifestations, 1569
        diagnosis, 1569
        management, 1569–1570
        pathophysiology, 1569
    envenomation
        cardiotoxicity, 1570–1571
        deaths caused by, 1568
    habitats and geographic distribution, 1567t, 1568
    Hydrozoa, 1567, 1567t
    postenvenomation syndromes, 1569
    Scyphozoa, 1567–1568, 1567t
    sponges colonized with, 1574
    stings
        epidemiology, 1568–1569
        prevention, 1569
    venom, toxins in, 1569
Cnidocil, 1567, 1568f
Cnidocysts, 1567
Coagulation, 320
    abnormal, evaluation, 322t
    in heatstroke, 420–421
    laboratory investigation, 320–322, 322t
    xenobiotic-induced defects in, 322
Coagulation cascade, inhibitors, 885
Coagulation factors, 883. *See also specific factor*
    in liver injury, 335
    salicylates and, 558
Coagulation pathways, 883–884, 884f, 897
Coagulative necrosis, 271
Coagulopathy
    amphetamine-induced, 1104
    development, 884–885
    evaluation, 322t
    in heatstroke, 420–421
    in liver disease, 335
    and liver transplantation for acetaminophen
        poisoning, 483–484
    in methanol poisoning, 1429
    vitamin K antagonist–induced, treatment, 887–889,
        888t
Coal dust, pulmonary effects, 401
    chest X-ray findings in, 125t
Coal fumes (carbon monoxide). *See* Carbon monoxide
Coal gas, 1409. *See also* Hydrocarbons
Coal tar, 7, 1409–1410. *See also* Hydrocarbons
Cobalamin, 654
    oxidation, 1199
Cobalt, 1273–1282

absorption, 1273
acute exposure
    clinical manifestations, 1274–1275
    management, 1278–1279
and arthroprosthetic cobaltism, 1273, 1275–1276
    management, 1279
beer drinkers' cardiomyopathy caused by, 21t, 22,
    1143, 1273–1275
bioavailability, 1273
carcinogenesis with, 1276
cardiovascular effects, 1274–1275
cellular uptake, 1273
chelation therapy for, 1278–1279
chelator for, 1780
chemistry, 1273
chronic exposure
    clinical manifestations, 1275–1277
    prevention, 1279
contamination by, 1762
as cyanide chelator, 1694
decontamination for, 1278
dermatologic effects, 1277
distribution, 1273
elemental, 1273
elimination, 1273–1274, 1277
endocrine effects, 1274–1275
and erythrocytosis, 319
excretion, *N*-acetylcysteine and, 494
gastrointestinal effects, 1275
hematologic effects, 1274–1275
history and epidemiology, 1273
inorganic, 1273, 1277
neurologic effects, 1274–1275
occupational exposure, 1276–1277
    prevention, 1279
occupational exposure to, 1273
organic, 1273, 1277
pathophysiology, 1274
physicochemical properties, 1273
plasma protein binding, 1273
pulmonary effects, 1274, 1276–1277
in radionuclides, 1273
renal effects, 1276
reproductive effects, 1276
retinal effects, 1275
serum
    interpretation, 1277–1278
    normal concentration, 1273, 1278
    testing for, 1277–1278
testing for, 1277–1278
as thermal degradation product, 1642
and thyroid hormone synthesis, 813f
toxicity (overdose/poisoning), 1274
    N-acetylcysteine for, 1278–1279
    acute management, 1278–1279
    cardiac studies in, 1277
    clinical manifestations, 1274–1275
        with acute exposure, 1274–1275
        with chronic exposure, 1275–1277
    diagnostic testing for, 1277–1278
    diffuse airspace filling in, 125t
    pulmonary testing in, 1277
    soft tissue imaging in, 1277
    treatment, 1278–1279
toxicokinetics, 1273–1274
in urine, 1277–1278
    interpretation, 1273–1274, 1277–1278
    normal concentration, 1273, 1278
uses of, 1273
whole blood level, 1278

Cobalt-beer cardiomyopathy, 21t, 22, 1143, 1273–1275
Cobaltite, 1273
Cobaltous chloride, 1273
Cobaltous sulfate, 1273
Cobalt salts, and pancreatic dysfunction, 295t
Cobalt stearate, 1273
Cobalt sulfate, 1273–1275
Cobbler (*Gymnapistes marmoratus*), 1576, 1576t,
    1577–1578
Cobinamide, 1688, 1695
Cobra (*Naja philippinensis*), bites, management, 1845
Cobras (*Naja* spp.), 1633, 1633t
    envenomation, 1t
    snakestones from, 3
Coburn-Forster-Kane (CFK) model, 1664
Coca (*Erythroxylum coca*), 8, 1124, 1600t
    in antiquity, 3, 1124
    local anesthesia with, 994
Coca-Cola
    carbonyl sulfide contamination, 19
    cocaine in, 8
Cocaethylene, 165, 165f, 1125, 1145
Cocaine, 4t, 1124–1134, 1600t. *See also* Local
        anesthetic(s)
    absorption, administration route and, 140–141, 1124
    acute coronary syndrome caused by, 1129
    administration route
        and absorption, 140–141, 1124
        pharmacologic effects, 1124, 1124t
    adsorption to activated charcoal, 76
    adulterants, 1130
    agitation caused by, 386
    antidote for, 35t
    ARDS caused by, 401, 402t
    and asthma, 1126
    and atherogenesis, 1125
    bioavailability, 545
    body packers, 63–64, 85, 545–547, 1128–1129
        whole-bowel irrigation in, 63
    in body stuffers, 548, 1128–1129
    brain changes caused by, imaging, 132t, 134
    bronchospasm caused by, 1126
    cardiac effects, 248f, 249, 255–256, 258t, 1127
    cardiovascular effects, 1145
    cessation of use, 1128
    chest pain associated with, 126, 128f, 249, 1127–1128
        benzodiazepines for, 1139
    contaminants, 1130
    crack
        and aortic dissection, 126, 128f
        and barotrauma, 401
        brain changes caused by, imaging, 132t
        case study, 27
        diffuse alveolar hemorrhage caused by, 123
        esophageal effects, 1126
        gastrointestinal perforation caused by, 127
        levamisole-adulterated, 329
        oropharyngeal effects, 1126
        pharmacology, 1124
        and pneumomediastinum, 126, 128f
    crack rocks, in body stuffers, 548
    cutting agents, 1130
    and dopamine receptor downregulation, 134
    and dopamine reuptake, 214
    duiluents, 1130
    duration of action, administration route and, 1124t
    dysrhythmias associated with, 1126
    effects on cerebral blood flow, imaging, 134
    effects on cerebral glucose metabolism, imaging, 134
    end-organ toxicity, 1126

Cocaine (*Cont.*):
and ethanol, reaction, 165, 165f, 1125, 1145
ethyl, 1125
and female sexual dysfunction, 302f
fetal effects, 1127
focal cortical perfusion defects caused by, imaging, 134
free-base, 1124
hematologic effects, 1126
hepatotoxicity, 1127
and heroin, combined (speedball), 524
history of, 3, 8, 1124
as local anesthetic, 994
hyperventilation caused by, 400t
intestinal ischemia and infarction caused by, 127
intracerebral hemorrhage caused by, 130–131
intravenous injection, necrotizing angiitis caused by, 128
laboratory testing for, 101t
levamisole-adulterated, 279, 279f
and male sexual dysfunction, 299f
mechanism of action, 208, 210, 210t, 211, 218
metabolism, 206, 1022, 1124–1125, 1125f
metabolites, 1124–1125, 1125f
molecular structure, 162, 162f
neuropsychiatric effects, 1127
and neurotransmission, 343
and neurotransmitter reuptake, 204, 1125
obstetric effects, 1127
onset of action, administration route and, 140–141, 1124t
ophthalmic toxicity, 356f, 361, 361t
opioid combined with, 28
oxidative stress caused by, 1125
peak action, administration route and, 1124t
peak concentration, administration route and, 140–141, 1124t
perinatal effects, 440
pharmacokinetics, 145t
pharmacology, 996t, 1124–1125
physicochemical properties, 1124
plasma, disulfiram and, 1173
posttoxicity syndrome, 236–237
in pregnancy, 440, 1127
prenatal exposure to, long-term effects, 440
priapism caused by, 301t
protein binding, 1124
pruritus caused by, 273
pulmonary artery spasm caused by, 401
pulmonary effects, 1126–1127
and QT interval, 253t
respiratory effects, 401
and rhabdomyolysis, 393, 393t
screening for, 110, 112
and serotonin toxicity, 1058t
smoking, respiratory effects, 401
street names for, 162
structure, 994, 995f, 1124
strychnine as adulterant in, 1536
subarachnoid hemorrhage caused by, imaging, 115t, 132t
sympathomimetic effects, 211
teratogenicity, 429t, 440
therapeutic uses, 1124
toxicity, 994
abdominal effects, 1127
benzodiazepines for, 1139
in body packers, 63–64
cardiovascular effects, 1125–1127, 1145
chest radiographic findings in, 125t

clinical manifestations, 36, 36t, 1126–1127
abdominal, 1127
cardiovascular, 1127
central nervous system, 1126
in eyes, nose, and throat, 1127
general, 1126
musculoskeletal, 1127
neuropsychiatric, 1127
obstetric, 1127
pulmonary, 1126–1127
CNS effects, 1125, 1125f, 1126
cutaneous findings in, 189
decontamination for, 1129
diagnostic imaging, 115t, 125t, 132t
diagnostic tests for, 1127–1128
diffuse airspace filling in, 125t
disposition of patients with, 1130
ECG changes in, 250
effects on vital signs, 1126
gastrointestinal decontamination for, 86
lipid emulsion for, 1006
management, 1128–1130
nasal effects, 1126
neurotransmitter effects, 1125, 1125f
ophthalmic effects, 1126
pathophysiology, 1125–1126, 1125f
sodium bicarbonate for, 568t, 569
supportive care for, 1128–1129
urine screening assays for, performance characteristics, 111t
use, epidemiology, 1124
vasospasm caused by, 1125–1127, 1129
volume of distribution, 145t
and washed-out syndrome, 343, 1128
withdrawal, 236–237
Cocaine hydrochloride, 1124
Coccidioides spp., in biological warfare, 1759
Coccidioidomycosis, in HIV-infected (AIDS) patients, 830t
Cochlea, 366–367, 366f
Cochlear duct, 366
Cochlear implantation, 368
Cochlear-vestibular function, 363
Cockcroft-Gault formula, 148, 393t, 397
Cocklebur (*Xanthium strumarium*), 1607
Cocktail purpura, 840
Cocoa (*Theobroma cacao*), 985, 1603t. *See also* Methylxanthines
Cocoanut Grove Nightclub fire, 16, 16t, 1640
Coconut crab (*Birgus latro L.*), 979
Codeine, 519, 526. *See also* Opioid(s)
antitussive effects, 521
and breastfeeding, 441
characteristics, 526t
metabolism, 170, 172, 526, 527f
and opioid assays, 532
pancreatitis caused by, 295t
pruritus caused by, 273
talc retinopathy from, 361
ultrametabolizer, and breastfeeding, 441
urine screening assays for, performance characteristics, 111t
Cod liver oil, 1410
Coenzyme 1, 1703
Cofactors, 910
in redox reactions, 168
Coffee (*Coffea arabica*), 985, 1599t. *See also* Methylxanthines
Cognitive deficits, in thallium toxicity, 1351
Cohen's *d*, 1856

Cohort studies, 1853, 1853f, 1853t, 1854, 1854f
Cohosh
black. *See* Black cohosh
blue. *See* Blue cohosh
Coin ingestion
management, 64
zinc toxicity with, 1363–1364
Cola spp. (cola nut, kola nut), 643t, 1599t. *See also* Methylxanthines
Cola acuminata (kola nut)
psychoactive properties, 650t
use and toxicities, 643t
Cola nitida, 1599t
Colchicine, 501–504, 640t, 1599t–1600t, 1612
absorption, 501
adverse effects and safety issues, 501
antibodies, 504
ARDS caused by, 402t
deaths caused by, 501
diabetes insipidus caused by, 195, 195t
diagnostic testing for, 503
drug interactions with, 502
elimination half-life, 502
and gustatory dysfunction, 365
history of, 501
mechanism of action, 502
metabolism, 502
neurotoxicity, 343
and other antimitotics, in overdose, comparison, 507t
pharmacokinetics and toxicokinetics, 501–502
pharmacology, 501
for phosgene exposure, 1653
plant sources, 501
protein binding, 501
regulation, 501
and rhabdomyolysis, 393t
structure, 501
therapeutic uses, 501
tissue distribution, 502
toxic dose, 502
toxicity (overdose/poisoning)
clinical and laboratory findings in, 36t, 502–503, 503t
epidemiology, 501
multiple-dose activated charcoal in, 61
pathophysiology, 502
timing of onset, 503t
treatment, 503–504, 503t
cytokines in, 311, 504
volume of distribution, 501
Colchicine-binding domain, 502
Colchicum, 501
Colchicum autumnale (autumn crocus), 1612. *See also* Colchicine
Allium ursinum (wild garlic) and, confusion, 501
uses and toxicities, 640t, 1599t
Cold (common). *See* Common cold
Cold (temperature), thermoregulatory response to, 414
Coldargan, 1347
Cold medications. *See also* Antihistamines; Decongestants; Expectorants; *specific xenobiotic*
adverse effects and safety issues, 738
effects on drug abuse screening, 112
exposure to, trends in, 738
fatalities associated with, 748
pediatric poisoning with, 738
use in children, restriction, 738

Cold receptors, 411

Cold zone, in hazardous materials incident response, 1809, 1809t, 1810f

Coleridge, Samuel Taylor, 8, 519

Colistimethate toxicity, organ system manifestations, 829t

Colistin sulfate toxicity, organ system manifestations, 829t

Colestipol
    for digoxin, digitoxin, and chlordane overdose, 64
    effect on thyroid hormones and function, 814t, 817
    for levothyroxine overdose, 817

Colima hognosed pit viper (*Porthidium* spp.), 1637t

Colistin, acute interstitial nephritis caused by, 394t

Colitis, in drug-induced hypersensitivity syndrome, 278

Collargol, 1717

Collecting duct, renal, 389, 390f

Colloidal silver proteins (CSPs), 1344
    ingestion, for health supplementation, 1346–1347

Colloids, and osmotic nephrosis, 392

Colocynth, wild, as abortifacient, 303t

Colony-forming unit-erythroid, 352

Colony-forming unit-fibroblast, 353

Colony-forming unit-granulocyte-macrophage, 352

Colony-forming unit-megakaryocyte, 352

Colony-stimulating factors (CSFs), 311

Colorado tick fever, 1550

Color vision, 356
    abnormalities, 356
    xenobiotic exposures and, 357t

Colostomy, bismuth preparations used with, 1255

Coltsfoot (*Tussilago farfara*), 1603t
    uses and toxicities, 641t

Colubridae, 1617, 1633t, 1845

Columbus, Christopher, 1203

Colyte, 86

Coma, 708
    atypical cyclic antidepressants and, 1048
    case study, 32
    causes, 32, 32t
    with colchicine poisoning, 503
    cyclic antidepressant overdose and, 1047
    diagnostic testing with, 1086
    in hydrazide- or hydrazine-related toxicity,
            pyridoxine for, 863
    hypoglycemic, 33, 37
    management, 33
    sedative-hypnotic overdose and, 1086t
    in thallium toxicity, 1351
    ventilatory management in, 36

Coma bullae, 277

Combat Methamphetamine Act (2006), 748

Combat Methamphetamine Epidemic Act (2005), 10t

Comb-footed spider (*Steatoda* spp.), 1544

Combination chemotherapy, infertility caused by, 297t

ComboPen, 1746

Combustion products
    common materials and, 1641t
    in smoke, 1640, 1640t
    toxic, 1640, 1640t

Comedone, 269t

Comfrey (*Symphytum* spp.), 651, 1603t
    hepatic venoocclusive disease caused by, 332
    uses and toxicities, 641t

Common bile duct, 327, 328f

Common buckthorn (*Cascara sagrada*), 1599t. *See also*
            Cascara (*Cascara sagrada*)

Common cantil (*Agkistrodon* spp.), 1636t

Common carp (*Cyprinus carpio*), 640t

Common cold. *See also* Cold medications
    zinc for, 1362

Common fennel (*Foeniculum vulgare*), 641t

Common kingslayer (*Malo kingi*), 1567

Common milkweed (*Asclepias syriaca*), 969

Common name, 162

Common nightshade (*Solanum nigrum*), 1602t

Common willow (*Salix alba*), 644t

Communication, and medication errors, 1828–1829

Compact fluorescent bulbs
    broken, disposal, 1329
    mercury in, 1324

Compartmental modeling, 149–151, 149f

Compartment syndrome
    abdominal, 391
    carbon monoxide poisoning and, 1665
    dantrolene and, 1030
    diphenhydramine and, 746
    of latrodectism, 1543
    snakebite and, 1621–1622, 1624
    with stonefish stings, 1578
    theophylline overdose and, 989

Complement activation-related pseudoallergy
            (CARPA), 1006

Complementary and alternative medicine (CAM).
            See specific herb; specific therapy

Complement inhibition, for paraquat poisoning, 1474f, 1476

Complete blood count, 37

Compositaceae, 1598t–1599t, 1603t

Compositae, 1600t, 1602t, 1605, 1614

Compound(s)
    definition, 155
    nonpolar, 159
    physicochemical properties, 159
    polar, 159

Compound 1080, 1533–1535. *See also* Sodium
            monofluoroacetate (SMFA, compound 1080)

Compound 1081, 1533–1535. *See also* Sodium
            fluoroacetamide (compound 1081)

Compound A, 1015

Compounding pharmacies, safety considerations, 1835

Compound muscle action potential (CMAP), in arsenic
            poisoning, 1244

Compound Q (*Trichosanthes kirilowii*)
    as abortifacient, 303t
    uses and toxicities, 641t

Comprehensive Addiction and Recovery Act (CARA),
            10t, 552

Comprehensive Drug Abuse and Control Act (1970), 10t

Comprehensive Environmental Response,
            Compensation, and Liability Act (CERCLA,
            Superfund), 10t, 12, 1801t, 1804
    and nanotechnology, 1731

Compulsive behavior, amphetamine-induced, 1104

Computed tomography (CT)
    abdominal, 128
        in body packers, 117, 120f, 546, 546f
    of bezoars, 294
    in carbon monoxide poisoning, 1665, 1665f, 1667
    of caustic injury, 1391
    of cesium-exposed brain, 1265
    chest, in bipyridyl compound poisoning, 1476
    cranial (head), 130
        emergency, 130–131, 132f–134f
        in ethanol-tolerant patient, 1149
        in methanol poisoning, 1424, 1427
        noncontrast, in toxicologic emergencies, 132t
        threshold for, 1149
    in toxicologic emergencies, 132t

and detection of ingested xenobiotics, 53
in liver disease, 336
of lungs, in smoke inhalation, 1642
of mesenteric ischemia, 127, 129f
of neurodegenerative disorders, 131
radiation exposure in, 1762, 1766, 1766t, 1773
ring enhancement on, 131, 134f
of soft tissue changes, 122
for unknown xenobiotic ingestion, 47f
of xenobiotics, 115t

Computerized provider order entry (CPOE), 1824, 1829, 1862

Computer keyboard duster, inhaled, 1193, 1193t. *See
            also* Inhalant(s)
    toxicity, 1197

Conatokins, mechanism of action, 227t

Concanavalin A, mechanism of action, 227t

Concentration(s), 140, 140f
    calculation, 1873
    decreasing (decay), 149
    determination, 149
    free vs. protein-bound drug and, 109–110, 110t
    and management, 109
    nonlinear pharmacokinetics and, 149–150, 150f
    pathology affecting, 109–110
    peak plasma, 152
    plasma, 140
        and clearance, 151
        maximum predicted, 146
    prognostic value, 109
    serum, 140
        interpretation, 152–153
    at steady state (Cpss), 151–152
    therapeutic, 109
    total, 109–110
    toxic, 109

Concentration–effect relationships, 109
    and laboratory test results, 109

Concretion
    and interpretation of serum concentration, 153
    and peak plasma concentrations, 152
    xenobiotics forming, 143t

Conduction (cardiac). *See* Cardiac conduction system

Conduction (for heat transfer), 411

Conduction (nerve). *See* Nerve conduction

Cone snails, 1572–1573
    geographic distribution, 1572

Conessine, 742

Conference of Radiation Control Program Directors
            (CRCPD), 1767

Confidence interval (CI), 1855

Confidentiality, 1864–1865

Confidex, 910

Confined Space Entry Standard (OSHA), 1690

Confounding, 1856

Confusion
    cocaine and, 1127
    in elderly, *case study*, 459
    xenobiotic-induced, in elderly, 463, 463t

Congeners
    in alcoholic beverages, and hangover syndrome,
            1143
    types, 1143

Congestive heart failure (CHF), 189, 263–264
    loop diuretics for, and thiamine replacement, 1160
    thiamine deficiency and, 1157, 1159–1160
    xenobiotic-induced, in elderly, 463, 463t
    from xenobiotics, 125t

γ-Coniceine, 1605

Coniine, 1495t, 1496, 1599t, 1604–1605

(CTR1), 368
Copper triethanolamine complex, 1284t

Coppolino, Carl, 5t, 1018
Coprine, 1582t, 1587–1588, 1589t
    inhibition of aldehyde dehydrogenase,
        1587–1588
    structure, 1588f
Coprinopsis atramentaria, 1582t, 1587, 1588f
Coprinopsis insignis, 1582t
Coprinus spp., 1587–1588, 1588f
    ethanol and, 1146t, 1587–1588
Coprinus atramentarius, 1587, 1594. *See also*
        Coprinopsis atramentaria
Coprinus comatus (shaggy mane), 1587, 1588f
Coptis spp. (goldenthread), 641t, 1599t
Coptis chinensis (Chuen-Lin), 641t
Coptis japonicum (Chuen-Lin), 641t
Coral snakes (*Micrurus* spp., *Micruroides* spp.), 1633t
    antivenom, 1625
        use for nonnative elapid envenomation, 1635
    bites, 1618
        pressure immobilization bandages for, 1625
    color patterns, 1618, 1618f
    envenomation
        clinical manifestations, 1622
        pathophysiology, 1620
        treatment, 1625
    geographic distribution, 1618
    venom, neurotoxin in, 1620
Cordyline spp., 633
Cornea, 356, 356f
    abnormalities, 356
    abrasions, 359
    chemical injury, 1642, 1647
    cocaine effects on, 1126
    damage, methicillin and, 823
    deposits in, xenobiotic exposures and, 357t
    erosions, 359
    inflammation, xenobiotic exposures and, 357t
    smoke and, 1642
    thermal injury, 1642, 1647
    transplantation of, from poisoned patients,
        1892–1893, 1892t
Corneal argyrosis, 1344, 1347
Corn mint oil, 632
Corn snake, 1617
Coronado Island rattlesnake (*Crotalus* spp.), 1637t
Coronary artery bypass grafting, protamine in, 919–921
    dosage and administration, 920
Coroners, 1884
Corrosives, 6, 271
Cortex, renal, 389
Cortical atrophy, diagnostic imaging, 115t
Cortical spreading depression, 805
Corticosteroid(s)
    for acute promyelocytic leukemia differentiation
        syndrome, 658
    for acute respiratory distress syndrome, 1658
    for caustic injury, 1390t, 1394
    clinical and laboratory findings with, 36t
    diagnostic imaging, 115t
    effect on thyroid hormones and function,
        814t, 817
    for hydrocarbon pulmonary toxicity, 1416–1417
    for hyperthyroidism, 817
    for idiopathic intracranial hypertension, 658
    intrathecal injection, polyethylene glycol (PEG) in,
        686–687
    nasal sprays, benzalkonium chloride in, 682
    and olfactory dysfunction, 364
    ophthalmic toxicity, 356f
    pancreatitis caused by, 295t

for paraquat poisoning, 1474f, 1477
for retinal injury in methanol poisoning, 1430
for seabather's eruption, 1571–1572
for smoke inhalation, 1645
for thyroxine overdose, 817
for venomous caterpillar exposure, 1554
Corticotropin-releasing factor (CRF), in nicotine
        withdrawal, 239
Cortinarines, 1589
Cortinarius gentilis, 1582t
Cortinarius orellanus, 1582t, 1590
Cortinarius rubellus, 1582t, 1590, 1590f
Cortisol, serum, postmortem changes, 1885t
Corymbia citriodora, 1524
Cosmic rays, 1763
Costill, O.H., 4t, 6
Cotinine, 1204
    clearance, 1204
    elimination half-life, 1204
    tests for, 1207
    urinary, 1207
Cotransport, 707
Cotton
    byssinosis caused by, 1659
    thermal degradation products, 1641t
Cottonmouth (*Agkistrodon piscivorus*), 1617, 1617t. *See
        also* Snakebite(s)
    antivenom, 1627–1631, 1627t
    envenomation, clinical manifestations, 1621
    geographic distribution, 1618
Cotton plants (*Gossypium* spp.), 1600t
Cottonseed oil (*Gossypium* spp.), 1600t, 1608
Cough medicines. *See also specific xenobiotic*
    adverse effects and safety issues, 738
    exposure to, trends in, 738
    fatalities associated with, 748
    pediatric poisoning with, 738
    unintentional exposures, 748
    use in children, restriction, 738
Cough syrup, diethylene glycol contamination,
        19, 20t, 681
Coughwort (*Tussilago farfara*), 641t
Coumadin. *See* Warfarin
Coumafuryl, 885. *See also* Warfarin
    physicochemical properties, 1453t
    in rodenticides, 1453t
    toxicity
        antidote and/or treatment for, 1453t
        clinical manifestations, 1453t
    toxic mechanism, 1453t
Coumaphos, 1488t
Coumarin(s), 641t, 644t–645t, 1597, 1598t, 1600t, 1603t,
        1609–1610
Council of Ten, 4
Couplons, 262, 928
Covalence, 159
Covalent bond(s), 159, 162
Covered entities, 1864
Cowhage (*Mucuna pruriens*), 1613
Cows, bezoars from, 3
COX. *See* Cyclooxygenase (COX)
Coxibs, 511
Coxiella burnetii, 1757
Coyotillo (*Karwinskia humboldtiana*), 1601t, 1610
CP 47,497, structure, 1112f
CP 55,940, structure, 1112f
2C-P, 1181
C-peptide, serum, 700–701, 701t
CPOE (computerized provider order entry),
        1824, 1829, 1862

Crab's eye (*Abrus precatorius*), 1598t. *See also* Rosary
        pea (*Abrus precatorius*)
Crack cocaine. *See* Cocaine, crack
Crack crash, 236–237
Crack dancing, 1127
Crack eye, 361
Crack lung, 1127
Cranberry glass, 1717
Cranial nerve(s)
    abnormalities
        in ethylene glycol poisoning, 1424–1425
        in thallium toxicity, 1351
    in gustation, 365
    in olfaction, 364
Cranial neuropathies, xenobiotic-induced, 345, 346t
Crassula spp. (jade plant), 1599t
Crataegus spp. (hawthorn), 642t
    xenobiotic interactions, 1611
Crataegus laevigata (hawthorn), 642t
Crataegus monogyna (hawthorn), 642t
Crataegus oxyacantha (hawthorn), 642t
Cream, Thomas Neville, 5t, 6
Creatine, as athletic performance enhancer, 619
Creatinine
    elevation, methotrexate-related, 768
    measurement, Jaffe reaction for, paraquat and
        diquat and, 1475–1476
    in renal disorders, 396–397
    serum
        in bipyridyl compound poisoning, 1475
        in differential diagnosis of high anion gap
            metabolic acidosis, 192
        in ethylene glycol poisoning, 1427
Creatinine clearance, 151, 397
    calculation, 393, 393t
    estimated, 393, 393t
Crediblemeds.org, 1820
Cremains, 1886
Creolin, 686, 1373
Creosol, sources of, 1388t
Creosote
    odor, 364t
    sources, 1388t
Cresol(s), 1373–1374, 1410
Cretinism, 812, 818
Creutzfeldt-Jakob disease (CJD), 908
    variant, 908
Crigler-Najjar syndrome, hyperbilirubinemia in, 334
Crime, drug-facilitated, 736–737
    in developing world, 1846
Crimean-Congo hemorrhagic fever, as biological
        weapon, 1758
Crime scene, 1870
Crippen, Harvey, 5t, 6
Crisis intervention, 379–380
Crisis management team, 385
Critical illness
    blood glucose control in, 710
    hyperglycemia in, 698
    myopathy, 1025, 1025t
    polyneuropathy, 1025, 1025t
Critical items, cleaning, 1368
Crocus, autumn (*Colchicum autumnale*). *See also*
        Colchicine
    uses and toxicities, 640t, 1599t
CroFab, 1624, 1627–1631, 1627t, 1635
Cronstedt, Axel Fredrik, 1333
Cross-banded mountain rattlesnake (*Crotalus* spp.),
        1637t
Cross-sectional studies, 1852, 1853t

Crotalaria spp. (rattlebox), 651, 1599t, 1605
Crotalaria and *C. spectabilis* (heliotrope), 642t
  hepatic venoocclusive disease caused by, 332
Crotalidae (pit viper) bites. *See also* Snakebite(s)
  antivenom for, 35t
    availability and storage, 44t
    indications for, 44t
    stocking, 43
      recommended level, 44t
  management, 44t
Crotalidae immune F(ab')₂ (equine), 1624, 1627, 1627t
  advantages, 1627
  adverse effects and safety issues, 1629
  chemistry, 1628
  clinical use, 1629
    in pregnancy and lactation, 1630
  dosage and administration, 1631
  formulation and acquisition, 1631
  history of, 1627
  pharmacokinetics, 1628
  preparation, 1627–1628, 1628f
Crotalidae polyvalent immune Fab (ovine), 1624, 1627, 1627t
  adverse effects and safety issues, 1629
  chemistry, 1627–1628
  clinical use, 1628–1629
    in pregnancy and lactation, 1630
  cross-reactivity, 1635
  dosage and administration, 1630–1631, 1631f
  formulation and acquisition, 1631
  history of, 1627
  pharmacokinetics, 1628
  preparation, 1627–1628
Crotalids. *See also* Pit vipers (Crotalinae)
  antivenoms, 35t, 1624, 1627, 1627t
Crotalinae, 1617, 1617t, 1633, 1633t. *See also* Pit vipers (Crotalinae)
  antivenom, phenol in, 685t
Crotaline snake envenomation, antivenom for, 35t, 1624, 1627, 1627t
Crotalocytin, 1622
Crotalus spp. (rattlesnakes), 1617t, 1633t. *See also* Snakebite(s)
Crotalus adamanteus (Eastern diamondback rattlesnake), 1617t
  antivenom, 1627–1631, 1627t
Crotalus atrox (Western diamondback rattlesnake), 1617t
  antivenom, 1627–1631, 1627t
  envenomation, neurotoxicity, 1622
  venom, elimination half-life, 1619
Crotalus basilicus, 1636t
Crotalus cerastes (sidewinder), 1617t
Crotalus cerastes cerastes, 1636t
Crotalus cerastes cercobombus, 1636t
Crotalus cerberus (Arizona black rattlesnake), 1617t
Crotalus durissus (Central American rattlesnake), antivenom, 1627t, 1628–1631
Crotalus durissus durissus, 1636t
Crotalus durissus totonacus, 1636t
Crotalus durissus tzabcan, 1636t
Crotalus enyo enyo, 1636t
Crotalus exsul (Ruber), 1636t
Crotalus exsul exsul (Ruber), 1636t
Crotalus horridus (timber rattlesnake), 1617t
  envenomation
    neurotoxicity, 1622
    and rhabdomyolysis, 1622
    thrombocytopenia caused by, 1622, 1624

Crotalus intermedius gloydi, 1636t
Crotalus lannomi, 1636t
Crotalus lepidus (rock rattlesnake), 1617t
Crotalus lepidus castaneus, 1636t
Crotalus lepidus klauberi, 1636t
Crotalus lepidus lepidus, 1636t
Crotalus lepidus maculosus, 1636t
Crotalus lepidus morulus, 1636t
Crotalus mitchelli angelensis, 1636t
Crotalus mitchellii (speckled rattlesnake), 1617t
Crotalus mitchelli mitchelli, 1636t
Crotalus mitchelli muertensis, 1636t
Crotalus mitchelli pyrrhus, 1636t
Crotalus molossus (black-tailed rattlesnake), 1617t
Crotalus molossus estabanensis, 1636t
Crotalus molossus molossus, 1636t
Crotalus molossus nigrescens, 1636t
Crotalus molossus oaxacus, 1636t
Crotalus oreganus (western rattlesnake), 1617t
Crotalus polystictus, 1636t
Crotalus pricei (twin-spotted rattlesnake), 1617t
Crotalus pricei miquihuanas, 1636t
Crotalus pricei pricei, 1636t
Crotalus pusillus, 1636t
Crotalus ruber (red diamond rattlesnake), 1617t
Crotalus ruber lorenzoensis, 1636t
Crotalus ruber lucasensis, 1636t
Crotalus ruber ruber, 1636t
Crotalus scutalatus salvini, 1636t
Crotalus scutulatus (Mojave rattlesnake), 1617t, 1636t. *See also* Snakebite(s)
  antivenom, 1627–1631, 1627t
  neurotoxin from, 1620, 1622
  venom, neurotoxicity, 1622
Crotalus stejnegri, 1636t
Crotalus stephensi (panamint rattlesnake), 1617t
Crotalus tigris (tiger rattlesnake), 1617t, 1636t
Crotalus tortugensis, 1636t
Crotalus transversus, 1637t
Crotalus triseriatus aquilus, 1637t
Crotalus triseriatus armstrongi, 1637t
Crotalus triseriatus triseriatus, 1637t
Crotalus viridis (prairie rattlesnake), 1617t
Crotalus viridis caliginus, 1637t
Crotalus willardi (ridgenose rattlesnake), 1617t
Crotalus willardi amabilis, 1637t
Crotalus willardi meridionalis, 1637t
Crotalus willardi obscurus, 1637t
Crotalus willardi silus, 1637t
Crotalus willardi willardi, 1637t
Croton (*Croton tiglium, Croton* spp.), 1599t
Croton and croton oil (*Croton tiglium, Croton* spp.), 2
Croton oil, 1599t
Crotoxyphos, 1488t
Crown flower (*Calotropis* spp.), 1598t
Crown of thorns (*Euphorbia splendens*), 1613
Crown-of-thorns sea star (*Acanthaster planci*), 1573–1574
Crufomate, 1488t
Cryoprecipitate, for fibrinolytic overdose/poisoning, 888t
Cryptococcosis, in HIV-infected (AIDS) patients, 830t
Cryptosporidiosis, 592t
  in HIV-infected (AIDS) patients, 830t–831t
Cryptostegia grandifolia (rubber vine), 979
Crystalloids, for cyanide poisoning, 1687, 1687t
Crystalluria, xenobiotic-induced, 305, 306t, 394–395, 394t
2C-series (amphetamine), 1107

CS syndrome, pyrethroid-induced, 1519
2C-T-2, 1181
2C-T-4, 1181
2C-T-7, 1179t, 1182, 1184
  chemical structure, 1180f
  clinical effects, 1183
Ctenopharyngodon idellus (carp bile), 640t
Ctesias, 3
Cubozoa, 1567, 1567t. *See also* Cnidaria (jellyfish)
  characteristics, 1567t
  stings
    epidemiology, 1569
    management, 1569
    venom, toxins in, 1569
Cullen, Charles, 13
Cumaru. *See* Tonka bean (*Dipteryx odorata, D. oppositifolia*)
Cumulative blood lead index, 1300
Cup moths (*Doratifera* spp.), 1552
Cupping glasses, 3
Cuprea bark (*Remijia pedunculata*), 1602t
Cupric acetoarsenite, 1284t
Cupric arsenite, 1284t
Cupric chloride, 1284t
  basic, 1284t
Cupric hydroxide, 1284t
Cupricin, 1284t
Cupric oxide, 1284t
Cupric salts, 1283–1284
Cupric sulfate, 1284t
  basic, 1284t
Cuprite, 1283, 1284t
Cuprous cyanide, 1284t
Cuprous oxide, 1284t
Cuprous salts, 1283–1284. *See also* Copper
Curacao. *See* Aloe (*Aloe vera, A. barbadensis, Aloe* spp.)
Curare, 4t, 7, 756, 1605–1606
Curare (*Chondrodendron* spp., *Curarea* spp., *Strychnos* spp.), 1018. *See also* Neuromuscular blockers (NMBs)
  history of, 1018
  toxicity, 1599t
Curarea (tubocurare, curare), 1599t. *See also* Curare (*Chondrodendron* spp., *Curarea* spp., *Strychnos* spp.)
Curcin, 1601t–1602t
Curie (Ci), 1764, 1764f
Curie, Marie, 1762, 1769
Curium
  DTPA for, 35t, 1779–1781, 1779f
  internal contamination by, management, 44t
Curved arrows, in chemical reactions, 162, 163f
Cutaneous exposure, toxic. *See also* Skin; *specific xenobiotic*
  management, 39
Cutaneous syndrome, radiation-induced, 1768
Cutaneous T-cell lymphoma (CTCL), 278
Cutoff values, for drug screening, 110
Cuttlefish, 1572
CW (chemical weapons), 1741t
CX (phosgene oxime). *See* Phosgene oxime (CX)
Cycasin, 1599t, 1607
Cyanea capillata (lion's mane, hair jellyfish), 1567t, 1568
  stings, management, 1569
Cyanide(s), 1684–1688
  activated charcoal binding to, 76
  airborne
    immediately fatal, 1684–1685
    life threatening, 1684–1685

antidote for, 35t, 1646, 1685, 1687t
  supplies, 42
as asphyxiant, 1642, 1748
blood, 1686–1687
  laboratory measurement, 1642, 1687
brain changes caused by, imaging, 131, 132t, 1686
with carbon monoxide
    additive or synergistic effects, 1642, 1678
    hyperbaric oxygen for, 1676, 1678–1679
as chemical weapon, 1741, 1748
decontamination for, 1687, 1687t
detoxification, 167, 1685, 1685f, 1686
effects on vital signs, 29t–30t, 1686
and electron transport, 176t, 177, 1685
elimination, 1685
elimination half-life, 1685
exposure to
  routes, 1685, 1687
  sources, 1684
and high anion gap metabolic acidosis, 191, 191t,
    1686
historical perspective on, 4t–5t, 6, 1684–1685
hyperventilation caused by, 400t
inhalation, 1650
  management, 1687
Internet sources for, 1685
lethal dose, 1685
in mass suicide, 24
mechanism of action, 221
murders using, 1685
neurotoxicity, 343, 1685–1686
and NMDA receptor, 1685
odor, 37, 364t
pharmacokinetics, 146t
pharmacology, 1685
physicochemical properties, 159, 1684
production, from amygdalin, 144, 1684, 1684f
and respiratory rate, 30
as sedative, 8
self-poisoning with, 1847
serum, 1687
site of action, 173f, 1685
from smoke inhalation, 1642, 1685
suicide using, 1685
sulfation, 1685
tests for, 7, 1686–1687, 1687t
as thermal degradation product, 1641t
toxicity (overdose/poisoning), 1684–1688
  acute, 1686, 1687t
    delayed manifestations, 1686
  biomarker for, 1687
  blood lactate in, 1642, 1685–1686, 1687t
  chronic, 1686
  clinical presentation, 16, 36t, 1686, 1687t
  diagnostic tests for, 1642, 1686–1687, 1687t
  ECG changes in, 1686
  epidemiology, 1684–1685
  hydroxocobalamin for, 1646, 1650, 1687, 1687t,
    1694–1696, 1698–1699
  laboratory findings with, 36t, 1642, 1686–1687,
    1687t
  management, 45t–46t, 1646, 1650, 1687t, 1694,
    1699–1700
  nitroprusside and, 1684, 1686, 1695–1696, 1700
  and organ donation, 1688, 1695, 1893t
  pathophysiology, 1685–1686, 1685f
  sodium bicarbonate for, 568t
  from sodium nitroprusside, 962
  sources, 1685
  supportive care for, 1687, 1687t

toxicokinetics, 146t, 1685
toxic syndromes caused by, 1751t
volume of distribution, 146t
in warfare, 1684
whole blood, 1684, 1687
Cyanide antidote kit, 1646, 1687–1688, 1687t, 1700
  cost, 43
  indications for, 35t
  stocking, 43
Cyanide salts, 1684
Cyanoacrylate adhesives, ophthalmic exposure to,
    irrigating solution for, 359, 359t
Cyanobacteria. See also Blue-green algae
  hepatogenous photosensitivity caused by, 1614
Cyanocobalamin, 1273, 1685, 1687, 1694. See also
    Vitamin B$_{12}$
  nitrous oxide abuse and, 1199
Cyanofenphos, 1488t
Cyanogen bromide, as chemical weapon, 1748
Cyanogen chloride (CK), as chemical weapon, 1684, 1748
  toxic syndrome caused by, 1751t
Cyanogen gas, 1684
  permissible exposure limit, 1685
Cyanogenic glycosides, 1–2, 639, 1597, 1601t–1602t,
    1607, 1684
  in apricot pits (Prunus armeniaca), 640t, 1602t
  in cassava (Manihot esculenta), 1684, 1686, 1688
  in cherry (Prunus), 1602t
Cyanohydrin, 1684, 1688
Cyanokit, 1694, 1696
Cyanomethemoglobin, 1698, 1710
Cyanophosphates, 1487, 1488t. See also Organic
    phosphorus compounds
Cyanosis, 38, 1686, 1703
  causes, 272
  clinical significance, 272
  in herbicide poisoning, 1473
  with hydrocarbon toxicity, 1412, 1417
  management, 1709, 1709f
  in methemoglobinemia, 1707
  in sulfhemoglobinemia, 1710
  toxicologic assessment, 1709, 1709f
Cyantesmo test strips, 1687
Cyanuric acid, 601
Cycad toxins, 1607
Cycasin, 1599t, 1607
Cycas circinalis (queen sago, indu, cycad),
    1599t, 1607
Cycas micronesica, 227
Cyclic adenosine monophosphate (cAMP), 209, 213,
    220, 260–261, 261f
  in cardiac physiology, 928–929, 929f
  glucagon and, 941
  methylxanthines and, 986
  in neurotransmission, 204
  in nicotine withdrawal, 239
  in thermoregulation, 411
  and water balance, 194
  and withdrawal syndrome, 237
Cyclic adenosine monophosphate (cAMP) modulators,
    899
Cyclic antidepressants, 1044–1053. See also Tricyclic
    antidepressants
  absorption, 1045
  and adenosine reuptake, 231
  and α$_1$-adrenergic receptors, 1044
  antidote for, 35t
  ARDS caused by, 402t, 1046–1047
  atypical, toxicity, 1048
  cardiovascular effects, 248f, 256, 258t, 1045–1047

  classification, 1044, 1044t
  CNS toxicity, 1047
  definition, 1044
  discontinuation syndrome, 1047
  and dopamine receptors, 215
  effects on vital signs, 29t–30t
  elimination, 1045
  elimination half-life, 1045
  enhanced elimination, 1051
  and erectile dysfunction, 300
  and ethanol, interactions, 1146t
  and female sexual dysfunction, 302f
  and GABA receptors, 222, 1045
  and histamine receptors, 1044
  history of, 1044
  hypoventilation caused by, 400t
  ileus caused by, imaging, 129t
  indications for, 1044
  Log D, 1045
  Log P, 1045
  and male sexual dysfunction, 299f
  mechanism of action, 211, 218, 1044
  metabolism, 1045, 1048
  and muscarinic acetylcholine receptors, 1044
  and norepinephrine reuptake, 1044
  and pancuronium, 1022t
  pharmacokinetics, 1045
  pharmacology, 1044–1045
  phototoxicity, 281f
  physostigmine and, 756
  poor metabolizers, 1045
  and prolonged QT interval, 256, 1046
  and QT interval, 253t, 256, 1048
  self-poisoning with, 376
  and serotonin reuptake, 1044
  serum concentration, factors affecting, 1045
  and sodium channels, 1044–1045, 1045f
  structure, 1044, 1044t
  and sudden death in children, 1048
  suicide with, 466
  and tinnitus, 370t
  toxicity (overdose/poisoning), 161
    acute, 1047
    anticholinergic effects in, 1047
    chronic, 1047–1048
    clinical and laboratory findings with, 36t, 37,
      1047–1049
    deaths caused by, 1047
      laboratory investigation, 1048–1049
    diagnostic tests for, 1048–1049
    ECG changes in, 248–249, 249f, 250, 254,
      1045–1047, 1046f, 1047–1048, 1047f, 1048
    epidemiology, 1044
    gastrointestinal complications, 1047
    gastrointestinal decontamination for, 1049
    hospital admission criteria in, 1051
    inpatient cardiac monitoring with, 1051
    lipid emulsion for, 1007
    magnesium for, 877
    management, 46t, 90, 1049–1051
    and organ donation, 1893t
    pathophysiology, 1045–1047
    pulmonary complications, 1046–1047
    QRS complex in, 248–249, 249f, 567–569,
      1045–1046, 1046f–1047f
    refractory, management, 1049t
    sodium bicarbonate for, 567–569, 568t
    therapeutics for, 37
  toxicokinetics, 1045
  volume of distribution, 91, 1045

Cyclin A, 350
Cyclin-dependent kinases, 350
Cyclin E, 350
Cyclines, antimalarial mechanism, 838t
Cycling, of steroids, 617
Cyclin-G1 gene, dominant-negative construct, 1719t
Cyclizine
    history of, 739
    and pancreatic dysfunction, 295t
Cyclobenzaprine, cardiac effects, 258t
Cyclodienes, 1514–1519
    absorption, 1514
    acute exposure to, clinical manifestations, 1517
    mechanisms of toxicity, 1517–1518
    physicochemical properties, 1515t
    resistance to, 1517
Cycloguanil, 846
    antimalarial mechanism, 838t
Cyclohexamine, 1211, 1211t
    DEA class, 1211
Cyclohexane, 1410
Cyclohexane oxime herbicides, 1467t
Cyclohexanone, 643t
    and hypotension, 1491
    toxicity, 1493
Cyclohexyl nitrite, inhaled, 1193t, 1194
Cycloolefins, 1410. See also Hydrocarbons
Cyclooxygenase (COX)
    acetaminophen and, 472
    COX-1, 511, 513f, 897
        aspirin and, 323
        hyperforin and, 646t, 647
    COX-2, 511, 513f, 897
        acetaminophen and, 472
        aspirin and, 323
    NSAIDs and, 511, 513f
Cyclooxygenase inhibitors, 897–899
    antidotes and treatment strategies for, 888t
    laboratory testing for, 888t
Cyclooxygenase-1 (COX-1) inhibitors, 555. See also
        Nonsteroidal antiinflammatory drugs
        (NSAIDs)
Cyclooxygenase-2 (COX-2) inhibitors, 294, 323, 511,
        513f. See also Nonsteroidal antiinflammatory
        drugs (NSAIDs)
    acute interstitial nephritis caused by, 394t
    as antiplatelet xenobiotics, 323
    cardiovascular risk with, 514, 1839–1840
    gastrointestinal effects, 513
    market withdrawal of, 1839–1840
    pharmacology, 512t, 513f
Cycloparaffins, 1410. See also Hydrocarbons
Cyclopentadiene, 1410
Cyclopentolate, benzalkonium chloride in, 682t
Cyclopeptide(s)
    mushrooms containing, 492, 494–495, 1581–1584,
        1582t
    toxicity
        N-acetylcysteine for, 492, 494–495
        clinical manifestations, 1582t, 1583
        treatment, 1582t, 1583–1585
Cyclophosphamide, 13, 760t
    cardiovascular toxicity, 762–763, 763t
    diagnostic tests for, 763
    EPA regulation of, 765
    and hair loss, 281
    hemorrhagic cystitis caused by, 306
    hepatic venoocclusive disease caused by, 332
    infertility caused by, 297t
    metabolism, 171

    nail changes caused by, 281–282
    neurotoxicity, 763
    for paraquat poisoning, 1474f, 1477
    for phosgene exposure, 1653
    and posterior reversible encephalopathy syndrome,
        132
    pulmonary/thoracic effects, imaging, 125t, 126
    teratogenicity, 429t
    toxicity, N-acetylcysteine for, 494
    toxic metabolite, 174t
    vomiting with, 762
Cycloplegics, 360
Cyclopropanone hydrate, 1588f
    inhibition of aldehyde dehydrogenase, 1587–1588
Cycloprop-2-enecarboxylic acid, 1582t, 1589t, 1591
Cyclosarin, 1745
Cycloserine
    adverse effects and safety issues, 853t, 857
    effects on NMDA channels, 857
    and isoniazid, interactions, 853t
    monitoring with, 853t
    overdose, 857
    pregnancy class, 857
D-Cycloserine, 228
    mechanism of action, 227t
Cyclosporine
    and colchicine, interactions, 502
    drug interactions with, 827
    elimination, multiple-dose activated charcoal and,
        78
    and gingival hyperplasia, 293
    hepatotoxicity, 330
    hypomagnesemia caused by, 877
    ophthalmic toxicity, 356f
    and posterior reversible encephalopathy syndrome,
        135f
    protein-binding characteristics, 110t
    renal effects, 390f, 391
    and vincristine, interactions, 506
Cyclothiazide, mechanism of action, 227t, 228
Cyclotrimethylenetrinitramine. See RDX
        (cyclotrimethylenetrinitramine)
Cycloxydim, in herbicides, 1467t
Cyfluthrin, 1520t. See also Pyrethroids
Cyhalofop, in herbicides, 1467t
Cyhalothrin, 1520t. See also Pyrethroids
Cyhexatin, and ATP production, 176t
Cypermethrin, 1519, 1520t. See also Pyrethroids
    absorption, 1521
Cyprinol, 640t
Cyprinus carpio (common carp), 640t
Cyproheptadine
    availability and storage, 44t
    indications for, 35t, 44t, 742
    labeling, 43
    mechanism of action, 218
    and pancreatic dysfunction, 295t
    pharmacokinetics and toxicokinetics, 745t
    for serotonin syndrome, 1184
    for serotonin toxicity, 1059, 1081
    stocking, recommended level, 44t
    structure, 740f
    supplies, 43
Cyproterone acetate, hepatotoxicity, 618
CYP system. See Cytochrome P450 (CYP) enzymes
Cyromazine, 1482
Cystatin, 1603t
Cystatin C, serum
    in acute kidney injury, 396
    in bipyridyl compound poisoning, 1475

Cysteamine, 492
    structure, 492
Cystitis, ketamine-induced, 1215–1216, 1215f,
        1217–1218
Cytarabine
    adverse effects and safety issues, 760t
    intrathecal administration, inadvertent overdose
        and unintentional exposures due to, 795t
    lipid carrier formulation, 684t
    liposomal, 1719t
    mechanism and site of action, 350, 759, 762f
    and olfactory dysfunction, 364
Cytidine deaminase, 771
Cytisine, 1206, 1601t, 1604
Cytisus laburnum (laburnum, golden chain), 1601t,
        1604
Cytisus scoparius (broom), 1599t, 1604
    psychoactive properties, 650t
    uses and toxicities, 640t
Cytoadhesins, 323
Cytochrome(s), 167
Cytochrome c oxidase, 1285t
    cyanide binding to, 1698
    inhibition, formate and, 1424
Cytochrome oxidase
    inactivation, by carbon monoxide, 1664
    inhibition
        by cyanide, 1685, 1685f, 1698
        by hydrogen sulfide, 1689, 1691
Cytochrome P450 (CYP) enzymes, 144, 147, 328
    and acetaminophen, 473, 480
    activity, 167f, 168
    amphetamines and, 1102
    antidysrhythmics and, 866t–867t, 870–871
    antiepileptics and, 722t
    antihistamines and, 744
    antimalarials and, 839t, 847
    antipsychotics and, 1035–1036
    antituberculous medications and, 850–852,
        855, 858
    atypical antidepressants and, 1054–1056, 1055t
    autoantibodies, and liver injury, 330
    autoinduction, 1087
    azole antifungals and, 829
    barbiturates and, 1087
    caffeine and, 987
    and calcium channel blockers, 946
    characteristics, 169, 169t
    and colchicine, 502
    cyclic antidepressants and, 1045, 1048
    CYP1A1
        characteristics, 171
        in placenta, 432
        toxic activation by, 174, 174t
    CYP1A2
        characteristics, 169, 169t, 170–171
        inducers/induction, 184
        inhibitors, 184
        substrates, 184
        toxic activation by, 174t
    CYP2A6, induction, 171
    CYP3A4, 502
        characteristics, 169, 169t, 171–172
        and drug–drug interactions, 946
        gastric bypass and, 148
        inducers/induction, 171, 187
        inhibitors, 172, 187
        and plant–xenobiotic interactions, 1610–1611
        substrates, 187–188
        toxic activation by, 174, 174t

CYP2B6
  characteristics, 169t, 171
  inducers, 184
  inhibitors, 184
  substrates, 184
  toxic activation by, 174, 174t
CYP2C9
  characteristics, 169, 169t, 170–172
  inducers/induction, 171, 185
  inhibitors, 171, 185
  substrates, 185
  toxic activation by, 174, 174t
CYP2C19
  characteristics, 169, 169t, 171–172
  inducers, 185
  inhibitors, 185
  substrates, 185
  toxic activation by, 174t
CYP2C8, toxic activation by, 174t
CYP2C9 variants, and NSAID-related upper
    gastrointestinal bleeding, 1853
CYP2D6, 147, 1102
  characteristics, 169, 169t, 170, 172
  inducers/induction, 171, 186
  inhibitors, 186
  polymorphism, 1102
  substrates, 186
  toxic activation by, 174, 174t
  and ultrarapid opioid metabolism, 526
CYP2E1, 168f, 169, 330–331
  characteristics, 169, 169t, 172
  disulfiram and, 1173
  ethanol and, 1144–1145, 1145f, 1146, 1440
  fomepizole and, 1435
  and free radical formation, 175
  inducers, 186
  and inhalants, 1195, 1195t, 1197
  inhibitors, 186
  in liver zone 3, 328–329, 328f
  substrates, 186
  toxic activation by, 174, 174t
CYP2F1, toxic activation by, 174t
and dapsone metabolism, 1709
disulfiram and, 1172–1173
and drug–drug interactions, 170
and drug–xenobiotic interactions, 170
and ethanol, 480
ethanol and, 1144–1145, 1145f, 1146, 1440
families, 168–169
  inducible, 170
fetal, 435
fomepizole and, 1435
functions, 168
gene family, 147, 168
genetic polymorphism and, 169t, 170, 172
grapefruit juice and, 170, 172, 1610
induction/inducers, 169–171, 184–188
  and acetaminophen toxicity, 480
and inhalants, 1194–1195, 1195t
inhibition/inhibitors, 169, 171, 184–188
isoniazid and, 850–852
and ketamine, 1212
lidocaine and, 996
and long-acting vitamin K antagonists, 890
macrolides and, 827
menthol and, 632
and methadone, 529–530
and methoxetamine, 1212
monoamine oxidase inhibitors and, 1077, 1079
and nicotine, 1204

nomenclature for, 168–169
and opioid metabolism, 526, 527f
and organic phosphorus compounds, 1489
organ/tissue distribution, 169, 169t
oxidation reaction, 167, 167f
and phencyclidine, 1212
phenobarbital and, 1087
and phosphodiesterase inhibitors, 301
piperonyl butoxide and, 1521
and plant–xenobiotic interactions, 1610–1611
and porphyrias, 314
pulegone and, 632
and pyrrolizidine alkaloids, 651, 1605
quinine and, 838
rifamycins and, 855
St. John's wort and, 646–647, 646t, 647f, 1610–1611
and sedative-hypnotics, 1085–1086
selective serotonin reuptake inhibitors and,
    1054–1056, 1055t
and strychnine metabolism, 1536
subfamilies, 168
  substrate specificity, 169
substrate specificity, 169–170, 184–188
theophylline and, 987
and thujone, 627
toxic activation by, 174, 174t
and warfarin, 886
in xenobiotic metabolism, 292–293
Cytokine(s), 311
  in heatstroke, 420
  therapy with, for radiation-exposed patients, 1771
Cytokine receptor family, 311
Cytokinesis-block micronucleus (CBMN) assay,
    radiation exposure and, 1769
Cytomegalovirus, in HIV-infected (AIDS) patients,
    830t–831t
Cytosine, 349f
  cell cycle phase specificity, 761f
Cytosine arabinoside, ARDS caused by, 402t
Cytosolic enzymes, 167
Cytotoxic xenobiotics. See also specific xenobiotic
  teratogenicity, 432

D
2,4-D (2,4-dichlorophenoxyacetic acid), 17, 1466,
    1480–1482. See also Phenoxy herbicides
  in Agent Orange, 17, 1480
  chloracne caused by, 271
  enhanced elimination, urine alkalinization for, 93
  mechanism of toxicity, 1481
  pharmacology, 1481
  structure, 1481f
Dabigatran, 321f, 884f, 892, 892f
  adverse effects and safety issues, 883, 892–893
  antidote for, 35t, 888t, 908
  coagulopathy caused by, treatment, 893–894
  laboratory testing for, 888t
  overdose/poisoning
    antidotes and treatment strategies for, 888t
    gastrointestinal decontamination for, 54t
    management, 45t
  pharmacology, 893t
  reversal agent, 908. See also Idarucizumab
Dacarbazine, 349f
  adverse effects and safety issues, 760t
  as local irritant, 802
Dacriose, 682
Dactinomycin
  adverse effects and safety issues, 760t
  extravasation, 802

intrathecal administration, inadvertent overdose
    and unintentional exposures due to, 795t
Daidzein, 644t
Dakin solution, 1369t
Dalapon, 1468t
Dalfampridine, for botulism, 581
Dally, Clarence, 1762
Dalteparin, 890
  antidotes and treatment strategies for, 888t, 891
  laboratory testing for, 888t
  reversal, 921
Damiana (Turnera diffusa), psychoactive properties,
    650t
DAMPA (2,4-diamino-N(10)-methylpteroid acid), 768,
    782, 783f, 785–786
  laboratory measurement, 769, 769t
  toxicity, sodium bicarbonate for, 568t
Danaparoid, indications for, 891
Danbury shakes, 1324
DanceSafe, 1184
Dandelion (Taraxacum officinale), 1599t, 1614
  resins in, 639
Danger, rodenticide, labeling as, 1450t, 1452t–1453t
Dangerous Drugs Act (1920), 8
Danshen (Salvia miltiorrhiza), pharmacologic
    interactions, 646t
Dantrium, 1030
Dantrolene (sodium), 1029–1031
  absorption, 1029
  adverse effects and safety issues, 1029–1030
  for antipsychotic malignant syndrome, 1029
  availability and storage, 44t
  dosage and administration of, 1030
  for ecstasy overdose, 1029
  elimination half-life, 1029
  formulation, 1030
  for heat stroke, 1029
  history of, 1029
  for hyperthermic syndromes, 1029
  indications for, 35t, 44t, 1029
  for intrathecal baclofen withdrawal, 1029
  for malignant hyperthermia, 1023, 1024t, 1029–1031
  for MAOI interaction, 1029
  for MAOI overdose, 1029
  mechanism of action, 1029
  metabolism, 1029
  for neuroleptic malignant syndrome, 1039
  and neuromuscular blockers, interactions, 1021t
  pharmacokinetics, 1029
  pharmacology, 1029
  in pregnancy and lactation, 1030
  for serotonin toxicity, 1029, 1081
  and skeletal muscle excitation-contraction coupling,
    1019f
  for skeletal muscle spasticity, 1029–1030
  stocking, recommended level, 44t
  structure, 1029
  supplies, 42
  for thyroid storm, 1029
  and verapamil, interactions, 1030
Dapagliflozin
  pharmacokinetics and toxicokinetics, 697t
  structure, 695f
Daphne genkwa, as abortifacient, 303t
Dapsone
  adverse effects and safety issues, 846, 1546
  antimalarial mechanism, 838t, 846
  as aphrodisiac, 304t
  for brown recluse spider bites, 1545–1546
  cimetidine and, 846–847

Dapsone (*Cont.*):
  elimination, multiple-dose activated charcoal and, 78
  for HIV-related infections, 830t
  metabolism, 1472
  methemoglobinemia caused by, 174, 174t, 846–847, 1703, 1705, 1709
    with hemolysis, 1706
  overdose/poisoning, multiple-dose activated charcoal in, 61, 846
  pharmacokinetics, 839t, 846
  poisoning with, 1846
  and tinnitus, 370t
  toxic metabolites, 174, 174t
Dapsone hydroxylamine, 846
  toxicodynamics, 846
Darbopoetin, 620
Darunavir, 831–832
Da suan. *See Allium sativum* (garlic)
Dasyatidae, 1576
Dasyatis americana, 1576
Data
  categorical/nominal, 1857, 1857t
  continuous/interval, 1857, 1857t
  ordinal/ranked, 1857, 1857t
  types, 1857, 1857t
Database(s)
  online, 1804
  toxicology, 1789–1790
Date-rape drugs, Internet sources, 1210
Datura. *See* Jimsonweed (*Datura stramonium*)
Datura spp., 1181
  as aphrodisiac, 304
  self-poisoning with, 1846
Datura inoxia, as hallucinogen, 1181
Datura stramonium (jimsonweed, stramonium, locoweed), 2, 638, 1179t, 1181, 1181t, 1600t, 1604, 1604f
  alkaloids in, 639, 1604
  as hallucinogen, 1604
  psychoactive properties, 650t
  toxicokinetics, 1182
  use and toxicity, 643t
Daunomycin, EPA regulation of, 765
Daunorubicin, 760t
  extravasation, 802
  liposomal, 1719t
  mechanism and site of action, 762f
Davy, Humphry, 8, 1011, 1403, 1454
Day of week, and violence, 385
DDC. *See* Diethyldithiocarbamate
DDT (dichlorodiphenyltrichloroethane), 1514–1519
  absorption, 1514
  acute exposure to, clinical manifestations, 1517
  in adipose tissue, 1518
  and ATP production, 176t
  and breast cancer, 1518
  elimination, 1515
  hazards associated with, 1514
  history of, 1514
  laboratory testing for, 1518
  and malaria, 836
  mechanisms of toxicity, 1517–1518, 1521
  metabolism, 1515
  physicochemical properties, 1515t
  serum, 1518
  structure, 1516f
  temperature coefficient, 1521
  tissue distribution, 1515
  toxicokinetics, 1514–1516

Dead in bed syndrome, 708
Deadly nightshade (*Atropa belladonna*), 1179t, 1181
Dead man's bells. *See* Foxglove (*Digitalis* spp.)
Deafness, poisoning/overdose causing, 36t
Dealkylation, 168
Death(s). *See also* Brain death; Sudden (cardiac) death; Sudden sniffing death; Suicide
  as accident, 1884
  adverse drug events and, 1822–1823
  cause of, 1884
  fetal, xenobiotics and, 432–433
  manner of, 1884, 1885t
  medical errors and, 1822–1823
  medication errors and, 1822–1823
  natural vs. nonnatural, 1884, 1885t
  and organ donation, 1892–1893, 1892t–1893t
  pediatric poisoning and, 448–450
  from poisoning
    data collection on, 1791
    prevention, 1791
    trends in, 1791
    unreported, 1791
  snakebite-related, global burden of, 1844
  xenobiotic-related, 1884
    with successful organ donation, 1893t
    worldwide, 1844
Death adders (*Acanthophis* spp.), 1633t
Death camas (*Zigadenus* spp.), 1612
Death investigations, 1884
Debrisoquine, 329
  pharmacokinetics, 172
Decamethylene diguanide, and pancreatic dysfunction, 295t
Decay, radioactive. *See* Radioactive decay
Dechallenge, response to, 1838t, 1839
Decibel (dB) scale, 368
Decongestants, 738, 748–751
  α-adrenergic, 749, 749f
  adverse effects and safety issues
    in children, 453
    epidemiology, 748–749
  cardiovascular toxicity, 750
    management, 751
  duration of action, 749t
  effects on drug abuse screening, 112
  fatality rates with, 748
  history of, 748
  imidazoline, 749, 749t
    pharmacokinetics and toxicokinetics, 750
    structure, 749, 750f
    toxicity
      clinical manifestations, 750
      management, 750–751
      pathophysiology, 750
  neurologic toxicity, 750
    management, 751
  pharmacokinetics and toxicokinetics, 749–750
  pharmacology, 749, 749f, 749t
  recreational use, 738
  respiratory toxicity, 750
    management, 751
  sympathomimetic, 749, 749f, 749t
    pharmacokinetics and toxicokinetics, 749–750
    toxicity
      clinical manifestations, 750
      pathophysiology, 750
  therapeutic effects, 749t
  toxicity, 749t
    diagnostic tests for, 750

  epidemiology, 748–749
  management, 750–751
Decontamination, 35t. *See also* Gastrointestinal decontamination
  in arylcyclohexylamine toxicity, 1217
  for biological weapons, 1754
  for chemical weapons, 1743
  of children, 1744
  for cocaine, 1129
  definition, 71
  dermal, 71–72
    for corrosive exposure, 73
    by dilution, 72
    emergency rinsing solution for, 73
    by neutralization, 72
    for phenol exposure, 74
    by physical removal, 72
    precautions with, 72
    for unknown xenobiotics, 74
  environmental, for spilled mercuy compounds, 1329
  gastrointestinal. *See* Gastrointestinal decontamination
  for hazardous materials, 71
  inhalational exposures and, 73
  and off-gassing, 72
  ophthalmic, 71–73
    for unknown xenobiotics, 74
  for organic phosphorus compound and carbamate poisoning, 1498
  pulmonary, 71, 73
  and secondary contamination, 71–72
  for unknown xenobiotics, 74
  wastewater from, 1743
Deep venous thrombosis, treatment/prevention, 890
Deepwater Horizon oil spill, 1409
DEET (*N,N*-diethyl-3-methylbenzamide), 1522–1524
  absorption, 1523
  efficacy, 1522, 1523t
  formulations, 1522–1523
  mechanism of action, 1522
  safety, 1523–1524
  with sunscreen, combined, 1524
  toxicity
    clinical manifestations, 1523–1524
    pathophysiology, 1523
    treatment, 1524
  toxicokinetics, 1523
Deferasirox
  adverse effects and safety issues, 676
  as iron chelator, 673
  physicochemical properties, 676
  and thallium toxicity, 1355
  therapeutic uses, 676
Deferiprone
  adverse effects and safety issues, 676
  as iron chelator, 673
  physicochemical properties, 676
  therapeutic uses, 676
  and zinc chelation, 1365
Deferoxamine (deferoxamine mesylate), 676–680, 1779
  adverse effects and safety issues, 673, 678
  affinity constant
    for aluminum, 676
    for iron, 676
  for aluminum-induced encephalopathy, 1224–1225
  for aluminum toxicity, 676–678, 1225
  availability and storage, 44t
  chemistry, 676
  contraindications to, 1321
  cranial neuropathy caused by, 346t

effects on bioavailability, 144
and ferrophilic organism infection, 671, 678
formulation and acquisition, 679
hemodialysis and, 677
history of, 676
and hypotension, 678
indications for, 35t, 44t
for iron poisoning, 672–673, 672f, 676–677
  animal studies, 677
  dosing recommendations, 677
  duration of dosing, 677
  intramuscular vs. intravenous administration, 677
mechanism of action, 676–677, 676f
ophthalmic toxicity, 356f, 678
overdose, and acute kidney injury, 678
for paraquat poisoning, 1474f, 1477
pharmacokinetics and pharmacodynamics, 677
pharmacology, 676–677
physicochemical properties, 676
in pregnancy and lactation, 39, 434–437, 678
and prevention of aminoglycoside toxicity, 823
related chelators, 676
stocking, 43
  recommended level, 44t
structure, 676
supplies, 42
and thallium toxicity, 1355
and urinary color change, 672, 672f, 678–679
use in pregnancy, 674
and *Yersinia* infection, 671
Degreasing agents, inhaled, 1193t. *See also* Inhalant(s)
Dehalogenation, 168
Dehydroepiandrosterone (DHEA), 618–619, 618f
  for female sexual dysfunction, 302
Dehydrogenation, 168
5′-Deiodinase, 812, 813f
  inhibitors, 814t
Deionization, for water purification, 99
Delamanid, 858
de la Pommerais, Edmond, 5t
Delavirdine, 831
Delayed afterdepolarization (DAD), 255, 970
  electrophysiology, 253t, 254, 254f
Delayed rectifier currents, blockade, by antipsychotics, 1034t, 1035
Delayed-release formulation, and gastrointestinal absorption, 143
Delirium, 33–36
  amphetamine-induced, management, 1104–1105, 1104t
  anticholinergic, management, 748
  with colchicine poisoning, 503
  cyclic antidepressants and, 1046–1047
  in elderly, 460
    case study, 459
  salicylate-induced euglycemic, reversal by dextrose, 698
  in thallium toxicity, 1351
  in toxidromes, 29t
  and violence, 384–385
Delirium tremens (DT), 1165
  clinical characteristics, 1166
  magnesium for, 878
  resistant, management, 1168–1169
  risk factors for, 1167
  and seizures, 1166
Del Nido ridge-nosed rattlesnake (*Crotalus* spp.), 1637t
Delphinium spp. (larkspur), 1600t, 1611
Δ anion gap/Δ [HCO$_3^-$]. *See* Delta gap ratio (Δ anion gap/Δ [HCO$_3^-$])

Delta gap ratio (Δ anion gap/Δ [HCO$_3^-$]), 190, 192
Deltamethrin, 1519, 1520t. *See also* Pyrethroids
  elimination, 1521
  structure, 1520f
Deltorphin, 521
Delysidas, 1178
De Materia Medica. *See* Dioscorides
Demeclocycline, 827
  diabetes insipidus caused by, 195, 195t
  for SIADH, 197
de Medici, Catherine, 4, 5t
Dementia
  carbon monoxide poisoning and, 1665
  dialysis, 1223–1224
  exacerbated or unmasked by xenobiotics in elderly, 463, 463t
  treatment, 1077
  and unintentional poisoning, 466
  and violence, 385
Demeton, 1488t
Demorphin, 521
Demyelinating disease(s), zinc and, 1364
Demyelination, 131
Denatonium benzoate, 451, 1782
Denatonium salts, 1782
Dendrimer, 1718f
Dendrites, 340
Dendroaspis spp. (mambas), 1633t
Dendrolimiasis, 1553
Dendron, 1718f
Dengue fever, 1522
  as biological weapon, 1758
Denileukin diftitox, nanoparticles, 1719t
Dent, Charles, 1178
Dental amalgam, 1324, 1326
  silver, and argyria, 1347
Dental radiography, radiation exposure in, 1766
Deodorants, inhaled, 1193, 1193t. *See also* Inhalant(s)
Deodorizers (room), inhaled, 1193t. *See also* Inhalant(s)
Deoxyhemoglobin, laboratory measurement, 103
Deoxythymidine monophosphate (dTMP), 789
Deoxyuridine monophosphate (dUMP), 789
Department of Labor, regulatory authority in workplace, 1801t, 1804
Department of Veterans Affairs, mandatory reversal agents, 42
Dependence, 236–237
  and addiction, differentiation, 236
  physiologic, 236
Depolarization
  myocardial, 245–254, 245f, 970, 971f
  neuronal, 203, 205, 205f
Depression
  alcoholism and, 1152
  epidemiology, 1054
  glutamate and, 224
  ketamine for, 1211
  monoamine hypothesis of, 1044, 1075
  pathophysiology, 1054, 1056
  perinatal, 433–434
  postpartum, 433–434
  and suicidality, 378–379
  treatment, 215, 228
  xenobiotic-induced, 344, 344t
de Quincey, Thomas, 8, 519
Dermabond, ophthalmic exposure to, irrigating solution for, 359
Dermacentor spp., 1550
Dermal decontamination, 272
  flushing for, 72

Dermal-epidermal junction (DEJ), 269–270, 270f
Dermal exposure, 269
Dermal toxicity, direct, 271
Dermatitis
  antimonials and, 1233
  arsenical, 38, 1242, 1242f, 1251
  capsaicin-induced, treatment, 1750
  Cnidaria, 1568–1570
  cobalt and, 1277
  contact. *See* Contact dermatitis
  copper and, 1283
  differential diagnosis, 1613
  hydrocarbon-induced, 1414
  inhalant abuse and, 1197
  irritant, 1613
  methotrexate-related, 768
  nickel, 1277, 1333–1335, 1335f, 1335t
    disulfiram for, 1176
    testing for, 1336–1337
  occupational, plant-induced, 1614
  phototoxic, 274t, 276
  plant-induced, 1598t–1603t, 1613–1614
    differential diagnosis, 1613
  in pyridoxine deficiency, 663
  in zinc deficiency, 1362–1363
Dermatologic examination, 269
Dermatologic principles, 269–283
Dermatotoxicity, xenobiotic-induced, 273–281, 274t
Dermis, 269, 270f
N-Desalkylquetiapine, 145t
Desert tea (*Ephedra* spp.). *See also* Ephedra (*Ephedra* spp.)
  uses and toxicities, 641t, 649
Desethylamodiaquine, 844
Desferrioxamine, supplies, 42
Desflurane, 1011, 1015
  with carbon dioxide absorbers, 1015–1016
  carbon monoxide poisoning with, 1015–1016
  pharmacology, 1410
  structure, 1011f
Deshayes, Catherine, 5t, 6
Designer drug poisoning, 21t, 22
Desipramine, 145t, 1044, 1044t, 1045. *See also* Cyclic antidepressants
  Log D, 1045
  mechanism of action, 227t, 228
  pharmacokinetics and toxicokinetics, 145t
  pharmacology, 1044
  skin discoloration caused by, 273
  toxicity, sodium bicarbonate for, 567
  volume of distribution, 145t
Desirudin, 884f, 891–892, 892f
Deslafaxine, mechanism of action, 1056f
Deslanoside toxicity, epidemiology, 969
Desloratadine, 746
  dose modification in liver or kidney disease, 744
  elimination half-life, 743
  metabolism, 743
  pharmacokinetics and toxicokinetics, 745t
  pharmacology, 742
  volume of distribution, 743
Desmedipham, in herbicides, 1467t
Desmethylcitalopram, 145t, 147
Desmethyldoxepin, 145t
Desmopressin, 888t
  adverse effects and safety issues, 900
  for diabetes insipidus, 195–196
  and fibrinolysis, 323
  indications for, 900
  mechanism of action, 900

Desmoteplase, 897
Dessicants, 271
Desvenlafaxine, 1060
    ECG changes caused by, 1057t
    pharmacokinetics, 1055t
    receptor activity, 1057t
    seizures caused by, 1057t
    structure, 1060
Detergents
    cationic, 1389
    dermatologic effects, 269
    household, ingestion, 1389
    ophthalmic exposure to, 359
    self-poisoning with, 1846
Deterministic effect, 432
    of radiation, 1767–1768
Detoxification, 167–168, 172–173. *See also*
        Biotransformation
Dettol, self-poisoning with, 1846
Developed countries, trends in poisonings in, 48
Developing world
    drug-facilitated crime in, 1846
    envenomations in, 1845–1846
    household products and chemicals in, 1846
    occupational and environmental exposures in,
        1846–1847
    pesticide poisoning in, prevention strategies, 1848, 1848t
    pharmaceuticals in, 1845–1846
    plant poisoning in, 1846
    poisoning-related deaths in, 1844
    poisoning risks and challenges in, 1844–1851
    substandard medications in, 1846
    traditional medicine in, 1845
    trends in poisonings in, 48
    xenobiotic ingestion in, gastrointestinal
        decontamination for, 59t
Devil's claw, as abortifacient, 303t
Devonshire colic, 18t, 19
Dexamethasone
    for acute promyelocytic leukemia differentiation
        syndrome, 658
    benzalkonium chloride in, 682t
    for carbon monoxide poisoning, 1672
Dexfenfluramine, 611
    adverse effects and safety issues, 21, 608t
    cardiotoxicity, 21
    market withdrawal, 608t
    mechanism of action, 608t
Dexmedetomidine, 961, 1090. *See also*
        Sedative-hypnotics
    and α$_2$-adrenergic receptors, 239
    adverse effects and safety issues, 210, 1090
    for alcohol withdrawal, 1169
    contraindications to, 1090
    indications for, 210, 239, 1090
    mechanism of action, 239
    pharmacodynamics, 1084
    pharmacokinetics, 1085t
    pharmacology, 1090
    for sedation, 1084
    withdrawal, 239
        clinical findings in, 239
        treatment, 239
Dexrazoxane, 760t, 764
    for anthracycline extravasation, 803
    mechanism of action, 803
    shortage, 43
Dextran
    and doping analysis, 623
    and osmotic nephrosis, 392

Dextroamphetamine, 1099
Dextromethorphan, 531–532. *See also* Opioid(s)
    antitussive effects, 521
    characteristics, 526t
    chemical structure, 1210
    clinical and laboratory findings with, 36t
    immunoassays for, 112
    laboratory detection, 113
    mechanism of action, 218, 227t, 228
    and phencyclidine, structural similarity, 532, 532f
    recreational use, 738
    and serotonin toxicity, 1058t, 1079
Dextromethorphan hydrobromine, 1088
Dextropropoxyphene poisoning, multiple-dose
        activated charcoal in, 61
Dextrorotatory entantiomers, 164
Dextrorphan, mechanism of action, 227t, 228
Dextrose, 707–712
    adverse effects and safety issues, 709–710
    for alcoholic ketoacidosis, 709
    availability and storage, 44t
    and blood glucose, 707
    definition, 707
    dosage and administration, 710, 710t
    empiric treatment with, 708–709
    in ethanol disorders, 709
    formulations, 710, 710t
    with high-dose insulin therapy, 709, 956
    history of, 707
    in hyperkalemia, 709
    hypertonic, indications for, 37
    for hypoglycemia, 33, 701–702, 707–710
    indications for, 38, 44t, 403, 1040, 1149
    for insulin overdose, 701–702
    pharmacodynamics, 707–708
    pharmacokinetics, 707
    in pregnancy and lactation, 710
    for quinine overdose, 840
    reversal of salicylate-induced euglycemic delirium,
        698
    for salicylate poisoning, 562, 709
    stocking, recommended level, 44t
    structure, 707
    supplies, 43
    in water, indications for, 35t
Diabetes insipidus (DI), 194–196, 395–396
    causes, 195, 195t
    diagnosis, 195
    lithium-induced, 189, 195, 195t, 1068, 1070
    nephrogenic, 195–196
        lithium-induced, 1068, 1070
    neurogenic, 195–196
    tetracyclines and, 827
    treatment, 195–196
    xenobiotic-induced, 195–196, 195t
Diabetes mellitus (DM)
    antimonials and, 1233
    arsenic and, 1242
    counterregulatory hormone response in, 698–699
    hypoglycemia in, management, 701
    hypoglycemia unawareness in, 699
    insulin receptors in, 708
    malicious, surreptitious, or unintentional insulin
        overdose in, 700–701
    neuropathy in, 342
    type 2, insulin resistance in, 696
Diabetic ketoacidosis, 37, 198, 1149–1150
    antipsychotic-induced, 1039
    clinical and laboratory findings in, 36t
    differential diagnosis, 192

    euglycemic, 192
    management, 193
Diacylglycerol (DAG), 209
Diadema spp., 1573
Diagnostic and Statistical Manual of Mental Disorders
    criteria
        for alcohol use disorder (AUD), 380, 380t
        for alcohol withdrawal, 1165, 1166t
        for withdrawal syndrome, 236–237
    definitions of female sexual dysfunction, 302
    diagnoses of substance use disorders, 380
    terminology for substance use, 236
Diagnostic imaging, 114–139
    abdominal, 127–130, 129t
    in CNS disorders, 130–135
    in fluorosis, 119, 123f
    for known xenobiotics, 114–118
        in containers, 120f–121f
        ultrasonography in, 114
    in lead poisoning, 119, 122f, 122t
    of neurologic problems, 130–135
    of pulmonary and other thoracic complications,
        115t, 122–126
    radiation exposure in, 1766, 1766t
    for radiolucent xenobiotics, 118, 121f
    of skeletal changes, 119–122, 122t
    of soft tissue changes, 122
    for unknown xenobiotics, 47f, 114, 116f
    for xenobiotics in containers, 117, 120f
Diagnostics, nanotechnology in, 1718, 1719t–1720t
Diagnostic test(s)
    evaluation, 1858, 1858f
    negative predictive value (NPV), 1858, 1858f
    positive predictive value (PPV), 1858, 1858f
    sensitivity, 1858, 1858f
    specificity, 1858, 1858f
Diallylacetic acid, 1255
Dialysis. *See* Hemodialysis (HD)
Dialysis dementia, 1223–1224
Dialysis encephalopathy syndrome, 1223–1224
    treatment, 1225
Dialysis fluid, aluminum contamination,
        1223, 1225
Dialyzer, 93–94
3,4-Diaminopyridine, for botulism, 581
Dianethole, 641t
Diaphoresis
    poisoning/overdose causing, 36t
    in toxidromes, 28, 29t
Diarrhea
    activated charcoal and, 79
    in arsenic poisoning, 1241
    causes, 597
    with colchicine poisoning, 502, 503t
    foodborne, 597
    food poisoning with, 596–598, 597t
    and hypernatremia, 195
    infectious, 597
    and normal anion gap metabolic acidosis, 193
    poisoning/overdose causing, 36t
    sorbitol-induced, 689
    in thallium toxicity, 1351
    and thiamine deficiency, 1160
    in toxidromes, 29t
    xenobiotic-induced, 294, 597
    in zinc deficiency, 1363
Diarsenic trisulfide, 1237. *See also* Arsenic
Diarylethylamines, 1211
Diastole, 264
    calcium flow in, 928, 928f, 970

Diatoms, and shellfish poisoning, 595
Diazepam. *See also* Benzodiazepine(s); Sedative-hypnotics
    for acute dystonia, 1036
    administration route, 1136–1137
    adverse effects and safety issues, 1139–1140
    for agitated/violent behavior, 386
    for agitation, 1138–1139
        in thyrotoxicosis, 817
    for alcohol withdrawal, 1168
        symptom-triggered administration, 1168
    for amphetamine toxicity, 1104–1105, 1104t
    benzyl alcohol in, 683, 683t
    cardiovascular effects, 1139
    for chloroquine toxicity, 1139
    for cocaine-associated chest pain, 1139
    for cocaine toxicity, 1128
    for conscious sedation, flumazenil and, 1094–1095
    dosage and administration, 1137t
    duration of action, 1137–1138, 1137t
    for emergence reactions, 1217
    flumazenil and, 1094–1095
    hepatic metabolism, 1137t, 1138
    injection, propylene glycol in, 687t, 688
    laboratory detection, 112
    lipophilicity, 1137
    metabolism, 169
    metabolites, 1088, 1137t, 1138
    for neonatal opioid withdrawal, 439
    for nerve agent toxicity, 1746
    onset of action, 1137, 1137t
    pharmacodynamics, 1137–1138, 1137t–1138t
    pharmacokinetics, 1085t, 1137–1138, 1138t
    pharmacology, 1136–1138, 1137t
    for resistant alcohol withdrawal, 1168–1169
    respiratory effects, 1140
    for sedative-hypnotic withdrawal, 1138
    for status epilepticus, 1137t
    structure, 1094
    for strychnine poisoning, 1537–1538
    suicide with, 466
    teratogenicity, 429t
    volume of distribution, 91
Diazinon, 1488t, 1509–1510
    cytochrome P450 enzymes and, 1489
Diazoxide
    adverse effects and safety issues, 702
    as antihypertensive, 962
    hypoglycemia caused by, octreotide for, 714
    mechanism of action, 227t
    ophthalmic toxicity, 361t
    overdose/poisoning, 962
    and pancreatic dysfunction, 295t
    site of action, 713
Dibenzodiazepine, 1033t
Dibenzothiazepine, 1033t
Dibenzoxazepine, 1033t, 1749, 1749f
Dibromochloropropane (DBCP), 1457
    infertility caused by, 23, 23t, 297t, 298f
Dibucaine, history of, 994
Dicamba, 1466
    in herbicides, 1467t
Dicapthon, 1488t
Dicarboximide. *See* Norbormide (dicarboximide)
Dichapetalum braunii, 1533
Dichapetalum cymosum, 1533
Dichlobenil, 1468t
Dichlofenthion
    pharmacokinetics and toxicokinetics, 1488
    poisoning, clinical manifestations, 1490–1491

Dichloramine, 1655
3,4-Dichloroaniline, 1472, 1472f, 1473
p-Dichlorobenzene, odor, 364t
1,2-Dichloro-1,1-difluoroethane, inhaled
    cardiotoxicity, 1196
    metabolites, 1195t
Dichlorodiphenyl dichloroethylene (DDE)
    and breast cancer, 1518
    metabolism, 1515
Dichlorodiphenyltrichloroethane (DDT). *See* DDT (dichlorodiphenyltrichloroethane)
2,4-Dichlorophenoxyacetic acid (2,4-D). *See* 2,4-D (2,4-dichlorophenoxyacetic acid)
3,4-Dichlorophenylhydroxylamine, 1472, 1472f
1,2-Dichloropropane toxicity, *N*-acetylcysteine for, 494
Dichloropropene, 1461–1462
    clinical effects, 1458t
    exposure to, sources, 1461
    history of, 1461
    industrial uses, 1457t
    physicochemical properties, 1457t
    poisoning
        clinical manifestations, 1461
        diagnostic tests for, 1462
        treatment, 1462
    toxicodynamics, 1461
    toxicokinetics, 1461
    uses, 1461
Dichlorvos, 1488t, 1509–1510
Dicitratobismuthate, physicochemical properties, 1256t
Diclofenac
    adverse effects and safety issues, 515
    and ATP synthesis, 176t
    cardiovascular risk with, 514
    chronic hepatitis caused by, 333
    pharmacology, 511, 512t
Diclosulam, in herbicides, 1467t
Dicloxacillin, 823–824
Dicobalt ethylenediaminetetraacetic acid, 1694
Dicofol
    absorption, 1514
    metabolism, 1515
    physicochemical properties, 1515t
Dicrotophos, 1488t
Dicumarol, 885, 1601t
Didanosine, 831. *See also* Nucleoside analogs
    hepatotoxicity, 332
    pancreatitis caused by, 294, 295t
Dieffenbachia spp. (dumbcane), 1600t, 1613, 1613f
Dieldrin, 1514–1515
    absorption, 1514
    fat-to-serum ratio for, 1515
    metabolism, 1515
    physicochemical properties, 1515t
    tissue distribution, 1515
Dienochlor, 1514
    metabolism, 1515
    physicochemical properties, 1515t
Dietary fibers, 611
Dietary guidelines. *See also specific nutrient*
    for fish, 1815
Dietary Supplement Health and Education Act (DSHEA), 10t, 21, 638–639, 1833–1834
Dietary supplements. *See also specific supplement*
    adulteration, 639, 645
        with pharmaceuticals, 647
    adverse effects and safety issues, 639
    coadministration, 647

    contaminants, 639, 645
        metals and minerals as, 647–648
    health claims for, 639
    hepatotoxins in, 651
    herbs as, 638. *See also* Herbal preparations; *specific herb*
    history of, 638
    hospital policies on, 639
    labeling, 639
    vs. medications, 638
    pharmacokinetics and toxicokinetics, 645
    pharmacologic interactions, 645–647, 646t
    pharmacologic synergy, 647
    pharmacology, 639–647
    plant- and animal-derived, 638–653
    preparation, 645
    recalls/bans, 639
    regulation, 638–639, 1833
    sales, 638
    use, 638, 654
Dieter's teas, 612
    adverse effects and safety issues, 608t
    mechanism of action, 608t
    regulation, 608t
Diethylamine, 1172, 1172f
Diethyldithiocarbamate (DDC), 1172, 1172f
    and copper-dependent enzymes, 1173
    and disulfiram reaction, 1337
    mechanism of action, 212
    metabolism, 1172, 1172f
    as metal chelator, 1173
    for nickel-carbonyl poisoning, 1176
    for nickel poisoning, 1173, 1337
Diethyldithiomethylcarbamate (MeDDC), 1172
Diethylene glycol (DEG), 9, 1422, 1444–1449
    absorption, 1444
    antidote for, 35t
    chemical structure, 1444
    as contaminant, 1846
    cranial neuropathy caused by, 346t
    drug contaminations with, 19, 20t, 453, 681
    elimination, 1445
    exposure to
        management, 1447–1448
        sources, 1444
    extracorporeal elimination, 97t
    fomepizole and, 1436–1437
    history of, 1444
    mass poisonings with, 1444–1447
    in medications, 1444
    metabolism, 1444–1445, 1445f
    metabolites, 1436–1437, 1444–1445, 1445f
    nephrotoxicity, 1436, 1444, 1446–1447
    neurotoxicity, 1436, 1444, 1446–1447
    osmotic diuretic effects, 1445
        management, 1447
    pediatric poisoning with, 453
    physicochemical properties, 1444
    in sulfanilamide, 1833
    tissue distribution, 1444
    toxic dose, 1445–1448
    toxicity
        clinical manifestations, 1446–1447
        diagnostic tests for, 1447
        epidemiology, 1444
        management, 45t
        outcomes, 1447
        pathophysiology, 1446
        treatment, 1447–1448
    uses, 1444
    volume of distribution, 1444

Diethylenetriamine, 227t
Diethylenetriaminepentaacetic acid (DTPA), 35t
  absorption, 1779
  adverse effects and safety issues, 1780
  for americium exposure, 1769
  for cadmium toxicity, 1261
  chemistry, 1779
  chronic kidney disease and, 1781
  dosage and administration, 1780–1781
  formulation and acquisition, 1781
  history of, 1779
  indications for, 35t
  mechanism of action, 1779, 1779f
  nebulized, 1780
  pharmacodynamics, 1779–1780
  pharmacokinetics, 1779
  pharmacology, 1779
  plasma half-life, 1779
  for plutonium, americium, and curium, 1779–1781, 1779f
  in pregnancy and lactation, 1781
  for radionuclide contamination, 1780
  related xenobiotics, 1779
  uses, 1779
  for zinc toxicity, 1365
Diethyl ether, GABA receptors and, 237
N,N-Diethyl-3-methylbenzamide. *See* DEET (*N,N*-diethyl-3-methylbenzamide)
Diethylprimaquine, antimalarial mechanism, 838t
Diethylpropion, 607, 607t. *See also* Dieting xenobiotics and regimens
Diethylstilbestrol (DES)
  abortion caused by, 297t
  infertility caused by, 297t, 428
  in utero exposure to, 20, 20t, 428, 433
  teratogenicity, 20, 20t, 428, 429t
Dieting xenobiotics and regimens, 606–615. *See also specific xenobiotic*
  advances in (future directions for), 613
  expenditures on, 606
  fibers and other supplements as, 607t
  GLP-1 agonist, 607t
  history of, 606
  nonpharmacologic interventions in, 613
  pharmacology, 606
  serotonergic, 607t
  sympathomimetic, 606–610, 607t
Difenacoum, 885
  pharmacology, 886
  physicochemical properties, 1453t
  in rodenticides, 1453t
  toxicity
    antidote and/or treatment for, 1453t
    clinical manifestations, 1453t
    onset, 1453t
  toxic mechanism, 1453t
Differentiation syndrome, 1243
Diffusing capacity abnormalities, 401–402
Diffusion
  facilitative, 707
  Fick's law of, 141, 569
  passive, 141, 141f
  postmortem, of xenobiotics, 1872
  rate, 141
  transplacental, 431
Diffusion coefficient (D), 141
Diffusion theory, 569
Diflunisal
  enhanced elimination, urine alkalinization for, 93
  toxicity, sodium bicarbonate for, 568t

Difluoroethane, inhaled, 1193, 1193t
  clinical findings with, 1199t
  pharmacokinetics, 1194
  toxicity, 1197
1,3-Difluoro-2-propanol (ethylene glycol monobutyl ether), fomepizole for, 1436
Digibind. *See* Digoxin-specific antibody fragments (DSFab)
DigiFab. *See* Digoxin-specific antibody fragments (DSFab)
Digitalin, in foxglove, 642t
Digitalis, 4t–5t, 6–7
Digitalis spp. (foxglove), 1606. *See also* Cardioactive steroids; Digoxin
  lanatosides, 979
  uses and toxicities, 641t–642t
Digitalis effect, on ECG, 250, 250f, 258, 970, 972f
Digitalis lanata (foxglove), 613, 1600t, 1606
  uses and toxicities, 641t
Digitalis lutea (foxglove), uses and toxicities, 641t
Digitalis purpurea (foxglove), 1600t
  uses and toxicities, 641t
Digitoxin, 1600t, 1606
  elimination, multiple-dose activated charcoal and, 78
  enterohepatic circulation, interruption, 64
  in foxglove, 642t
  pharmacokinetics, 970
  pharmacology, 969t
  toxicity (overdose/poisoning)
    digoxin-specific antibody fragments for, 977–982
    epidemiology, 969
    multiple-dose activated charcoal in, 61
Diglycolic acid (DGA), 1444–1446, 1445f
  toxic dose, 1446
Digoxigenin, 969
Digoxin, 6t, 873, 1600t, 1606. *See also Digitalis* spp. (foxglove)
  administration route, 867t
  binding, by cholestyramine, 92
  bioavailability, 173
  for calcium channel blocker toxicity, 950
  cardiac effects, 248
  drug interactions with, 970
  ECG changes caused by, 250, 250f
  elimination, multiple-dose activated charcoal and, 78
  elixir, sorbitol in, 688t
  enterohepatic circulation, interruption, 64
  in foxglove, 642t
  iatrogenic toxicity, 152
  infertility caused by, 298f
  ingestion, DSFab dose calculation with
    in adults, 980, 980t
    in children, 980, 980t
  injection, propylene glycol in, 687t
  intrafetal, as abortifacient, 303t
  laboratory detection, 101t, 102, 109
  mechanism of action, 933f
  membrane transport, 168
  and NSAIDs, interactions, 514t
  pharmacokinetics, 145t, 970
  pharmacology, 969t
  physicochemical properties, 969
  poisoners' use of, 12–13
  presystemic metabolism, 144
  and prolactin, 299f
  protein-binding characteristics, 110, 110t
  renal impairment and, 389
  serum concentration, 972–973

DSFab dose calculation with
  in adults, 980, 981t
  in children, 980, 981t
  free, 973
  interpretation, 153
  measurement after DSFab administration, 981–982
  total, 973
  and thiamine pharmacokinetics, 1158
  toxicity (overdose/poisoning), 970
    cardiac manifestations, 972, 972t
    clinical and laboratory findings in, 37
    diagnostic tests for, 972–973
    digoxin-specific antibody fragments for, 977–982. *See also* Digoxin-specific antibody fragments (DSFab)
    measurement of serum digoxin after, 981–982
    epidemiology, 969
    macrolide-induced, 827
    magnesium for, 877
    management, 1404
    multiple-dose activated charcoal in, 61
    risk factors for, 969
  two-compartment model for, 153f
  volume of distribution, 91, 145t
Digoxin-dicarboxymethoxylamine (DDMA), 977
Digoxin immune Fab
  shortage, 43
  stocking, 43
Digoxin-specific antibody fragments (DSFab), 977–984
  administration, measurement of serum digoxin concentration after, 981–982
  adverse effects and safety issues, 980
  availability and storage, 44t
  for cardioactive steroid poisoning, 973, 974t, 1404, 1406, 1606
  chemistry, 977
  for digoxin toxicity, 978–979
  dosage and administration, 980–981, 981t
  dose calculation, 980, 980t–981t
  formulation and acquisition, 982
  history of, 977
  indications for, 35t, 44t, 973, 974t, 979–980
  mechanism of action, 977
  with other cardioactive steroids, 979
  pharmacodynamics, 978
  pharmacokinetics, 977–978
  pharmacology, 977–978
  in pregnancy and lactation, 980
  preparation, 977
  stocking, 43
    recommended level, 44t
  supplies, 42
Dihydralazine, hepatotoxicity, 330
Dihydroartemisinin, 836, 845
  antimalarial mechanism, 838t
  pharmacokinetics, 839t
Dihydroergotamine
  cardiac effects, 806–807
  duration of action, 807t
  elimination half-life, 807t
  indications for, 807t
  pharmacology and pharmacokinetics, 806, 807t
Dihydrofolate, 767, 775
Dihydrofolate reductase, 775
  inhibitor, 767, 767f
    antidote for, 775
    toxicity, folates for, 777
Dihydrolipoamide, trivalent arsenic and, 1238, 1239f
Dihydrolipoamide acetyltransferase, trivalent arsenic and, 1239f

Dihydrolipoamide dehydrogenase, trivalent arsenic and, 1239f
Dihydropyridine receptor, and malignant hyperthermia, 1023
Dihydropyridines
    mechanism of action, 945, 945t
    vasodilatory effects, 947
Dihydropyrimidine dehydrogenase (DPD), 789, 791
    genetic polymorphisms and, 759, 771
Dihydrotestosterone, 618f, 619
1,2-Dihydroxy-3,4-epoxy-1,2,3,4-tetrahydronaphthalene, 1382, 1382f
Diiodotyrosine, 813f
N,N-Diisopropyl-5-methoxytryptamine (5-MeO-DiPT), 1179t, 1180, 1181t, 1184. *See also* Foxy Methoxy
    toxicokinetics, 1182
Diltiazem
    in cocaine, 1130
    and colchicine, interactions, 502
    drug interactions with, 946
    ECG changes caused by, 258
    for hyperthyroidism, 817
    mechanism of action, 945, 945t
    metabolism, 946
    myocardial effects, 947
    pharmacokinetics and toxicokinetics, 145t, 946t
    pharmacology, 945
    structure, 945
    toxicity (overdose/poisoning)
        calcium for, 1404
        lipid emulsion for, 1006
        pathophysiology, 953
    volume of distribution, 145t, 946, 946t
Diluents
    in cocaine, 1130
    definition, 1130
    toxicity caused by, 1086
Dilute thrombin time (dTT), 893
Dimaval. *See* 2,3-Dimercapto-1-propanesulfonic acid (DMPS)
Dimebon, mechanism of action, 227t
Dimefox, 1488t
Dimenhydrinate
    abuse/misuse, pathophysiology, 744
    antimuscarinic effects, 742
    history of, 738–739
    pharmacology, 741–742
    structure, 740f
    toxicity, sodium bicarbonate for, 568t
Dimercaprol (BAL, British anti-Lewisite), 1309, 1748, 1779
    adverse effects and safety issues with, 1252
    for antimony toxicity, 1234
    for arsenic toxicity, 1244–1245, 1245f, 1245t, 1251–1253
    availability and storage, 44t
    for bismuth toxicity, 1257
    and breast-feeding, 1252
    and CaNa₂EDTA, combined, 1251–1253, 1316–1317
        for zinc toxicity, 1365
    chelator effect, maintenance, sodium bicarbonate with, 568t, 571, 1252
    chemistry, 1251
    for copper poisoning, 1287
    dosage and administration, 1251–1253, 1253t
    excretion, 1251
    history of, 1251, 1330
    indications for, 35t, 44t, 1251
    intravenous infusion, 1252
    and iron, 1252

LD₅₀, 1252
    for lead poisoning, 1251–1253, 1253t, 1292, 1302
        in adults, 1253, 1303t, 1304
        in children, 1252–1253, 1253t, 1302–1303, 1303t
    mechanism of action, 164–165, 1251
    for mercury poisoning, 1251–1253, 1325t, 1330
    for methyl bromide poisoning, 1461
    and peanut allergy, 1252
    pharmacokinetics, 1251
    physicochemical properties, 1251
    pregnancy category, 1252
    for selenium toxicity, contraindications to, 1342
    stocking, recommended level, 44t
    tissue distribution, 1251
    urine alkalinization with, 571, 1252–1253
Dimercaptopropane sulfonate (DMPS), 1287, 1779
    challenge testing, in arsenic poisoning, 1243
    for paraquat poisoning, 1474f, 1476
2,3-Dimercapto-1-propanesulfonic acid (DMPS), 1309–1314
    adverse effects and side effects, 1309
    for antimony toxicity, 1234
    for arsenic poisoning, 1244–1245, 1245f, 1245t, 1311
    for bismuth toxicity, 1257
    for cadmium toxicity, 1261
    chemistry, 1309
    and copper, 1285, 1285f, 1287
    history of, 1309
    indications for, 1309
    LD₅₀, 1252
    for mercury poisoning, 1330
    pharmacology, 1309
    structure, 1309
    for thallium toxicity, 1355
    for zinc toxicity, 1365
Dimethachlor, in herbicides, 1467t
Dimethenamid, in herbicides, 1467t
Dimethicone, 1416
Dimethoate, 1488t, 1509–1510
    pharmacokinetics and toxicokinetics, 1488
    poisoning, clinical features, 1491
Dimethoate EC40, toxicity, solvent and, 1490
2,5-Dimethoxy-4-iodoamphetamine (DOI), 1107
    and serotonin receptors, 1182
2,5-Dimethoxy-4-methylamphetamine (DOM), 1107
2,5-Dimethoxy-4-N-propylthiophenethylamine. *See* 2C-T-7
2,4-Dimethoxy-4-(n)-propylthiophenylethylamine (2C-T7), 1105
Dimethrin, 1520t. *See also* Pyrethroids
4-Dimethylaminophenol (4-DMAP), for cyanide poisoning, 1688, 1698
4-(Dimethylamino)phenol p-benzoquinone, and gluconeogenesis, 176t
1,3-Dimethylamylamine, hepatotoxicity, 651
Dimethylarsinic acid, 1240–1241, 1240f
    absorption, 1240
    in herbicides, 1467t
    laboratory measurement, 1243
    LD₅₀ for, 1240–1241
Dimethylether, chemistry, 164, 164f
Dimethylformamide
    and disulfiramlike reactions, 1174t
    hepatotoxicity, 331, 334, 334t
        ethanol and, 329
    steatosis caused by, 332
Dimethylglyoxime spot test, for nickel, 1337
1,1-Dimethylhydrazine (UDMH)
    seizures caused by, pyridoxine for, 862
    toxicity, pyridoxine for, 863

Dimethylmercury, 157, 1324, 1324t. *See also* Mercury
    cranial neuropathy caused by, 346t
    poisoning, 1324, 1328
        pathophysiology, 1326
Dimethylselenide, 1340
    chemistry, 1339t
Dimethyl sulfoxide (DMSO)
    for anthracycline extravasation, 803
    beneficial properties, 803
    for carbon monoxide poisoning, 1671
    mechanism of action, 803
    odor, 364t
    plus calcium salts, for hydrofluoric acid dermal toxicity, 1399
Dimethyl trisulfide (DMTS), 1688
Dimethyltryptamine, 1077
    chemical structure, 1589
N,N-Dimethyltryptamine (DMT), 641t, 647, 649, 650t, 1179, 1179t, 1180, 1180f, 1181t, 1184
    toxicokinetics, 1181t, 1182
1,3-Dimethyluric acid, 146t
Dinitramine, 1468t
Dinitroaniline herbicides, 1468t
Dinitrocobinamide, 1695
Dinitrophenol (DNP), 1468t
    adverse effects and safety issues, 608t, 611
    and ATP synthesis, 176t, 177–178
    clinical and laboratory findings with, 36t
    effects on vital signs, 30t–31t
    and electron transport, 176t
    hyperventilation caused by, 400t
    mechanism of action, 608t, 611
    regulation, 608t
    site of action, 173f
    structure, 611
    for weight loss, 611
    yellow skin caused by, 272
Dinoflagellates
    and ciguatoxin, 593
    and shellfish poisoning, 595
Dinoterb, 1468t
Diols, 1422
Dioscorea bulbifera (bitter yam), 1611
Dioscorides, 1t, 2, 501, 632, 637–638, 1292
Diosgenin, 1603t
Diosma. *See* Buchu (*Agathosma betulina*)
Diosmin, 640t
Dioxathion, 1488t
Dioxin, 6t, 13
    in Agent Orange, 17, 17t, 1480–1481
    chloracne caused by, 271, 271f
    disaster caused by, 16–17, 16t
    pancreatitis caused by, 294, 295t
    poisoning, management, 1519
    poisoning with, of Viktor Yushchenko, 6t, 13
Dioxygenase(s), 167
Dip. *See* Snuff
Dipeptidylpeptidase-4 (DPP-4) inhibitors
    pharmacokinetics and toxicokinetics, 697t
    pharmacology, 696
    structure, 695f
Diphacinone, 885
    physicochemical properties, 1453t
    in rodenticides, 1453t
    toxicity
        antidote and/or treatment for, 1453t
        clinical manifestations, 1453t
        onset, 1453t
        toxic mechanism, 1453t

Diphenadione, 885

Diphenamid, in herbicides, 1467t

Diphenhydramine, 755
  abuse/misuse, pathophysiology, 744
  for acute dystonia, 1036
  anesthetic properties, 742
  antimuscarinic effects, 742
  availability and storage, 44t
  cardiac effects, 248f
  and dopamine reuptake, 214
  elimination, 744
  exposure to, 739
  history of, 738–739
  inappropriate prescribing of, 1827
  indications for, 35t, 44t
  laboratory detection, 113
  mechanism of action, 211
  metabolism, 743–744
  pharmacokinetics and toxicokinetics, 743, 745t
  pharmacology, 741–742
  and prolonged QT interval, 253t
  rhabdomyolysis with, 746
  sedative effects, 742, 746
  stocking, recommended level, 44t
  structure, 740f
  toxic concentration in children, 747
  toxicity (overdose/poisoning)
    case study, 736–737, 736f–737f
    clinical manifestations, 744, 746
    laboratory findings in, 109
    lipid emulsion for, 1006
    sodium bicarbonate for, 568t, 569
  for venomous caterpillar exposure, 1554

Diphenidine, 1211

Diphenoxylate, 531
  characteristics, 526t

Diphenylaminearsine, 1749, 1749f

Diphenylbutylpiperidines, 1033t

Diphenylether herbicides, 1468t

Diphenylmethane (bisacodyl), 83

Diphenyl-methane diisocyanate, 1657

Diphosgene, as chemical weapon, 1748–1749

Diphosphine, odor, 1457

Diphtheria, clinical features, 576t

Diphyllobothriasis (fish tapeworm disease), 600

Diphyllobothrium (fish tapeworms), 600

Dipivefrin, ophthalmic use, systemic toxicity with, 360

Diplopia, 358
  nonophthalmic xenobiotics causing, 361

Dipraglurant, 227t

Dipteryx odorata (tonka bean). *See* Tonka bean
  (*Dipteryx odorata, D. oppositifolia*)

Dipteryx oppositifolia (tonka bean). *See* Tonka bean
  (*Dipteryx odorata, D. oppositifolia*)

Dipyridamole, 899
  and adenosine receptor, 230
  antiplatelet effects, 323–324, 899
  and aspirin, combined, 899
  mechanism of action, 231, 898f

Diquat, 1466, 1467t, 1473–1478
  elimination, 1474
  pharmacokinetics, 1474
  pharmacology, 1473–1474
  poisoning
    clinical manifestations, 1475
    diagnostic tests for, 1475
    mortality rate for, 1473
    multiple-dose activated charcoal in, 61
  structure, 1473f
  toxicokinetics, 1474

Direct factor Xa inhibitors
  adverse effects and safety issues, in elderly, 465
  antidotes and treatment strategies for, 888t
  laboratory testing for, 888t

Direct oral anticoagulant(s) (DOACs), 892
  coagulopathy caused by
    activated prothrombin complex concentrate for, 910
    prothrombin complex concentrate for, 908–911
  priapism caused by, 301t
  prothrombin complex concentrate for, 910
  reversal, 908. *See also* Prothrombin complex concentrate (PCC)

Direct renin inhibitors, as antihypertensives, 959t, 965

Direct thrombin inhibitors (DTIs), 321f, 883, 884f, 891–894
  anticoagulant effect, laboratory investigation, 893
  antidotes and treatment strategies for, 888t
  bivalent, 892, 892f
  coagulopathy caused by, treatment, 893–894
  laboratory testing for, 888t, 893
  overdose/poisoning, clinical manifestations, 892–893
  pharmacology, 892, 892f
  univalent, 892, 892f

Disability-adjusted life years (DALYs)
  indoor air pollution and, in developing world, 1847
  poisoning and, worldwide, 1844
  snakebites and, in West Africa, 1845

Disaccharides, 707

Disaster(s), types, 1806

Disaster management and response, 1806–1807
  mitigation phase, 1806
  preparedness phase, 1806
  recovery phase, 1806
  response phase, 1806

Disaster preparedness, 1806

Disconjugate gaze, xenobiotic exposures causing, 357t

Disease
  dual burden of, 1846
  global burden of, poisoning and, 1844

Dishwasher detergent, ingestion, 1389

Disinfectants, 1369t, 1372–1374
  definition, 1368
  history of, 1368
  odor, 364t

Disintegration, in gastrointestinal absorption, 143, 143f

Disintegrins, in snake venom, 1618, 1619t, 1620

Disodium EDTA, 1315, 1317

Disopyramide
  adverse effects and safety issues, 866t, 869
  extracorporeal elimination, 97t
  pharmacokinetics, 866t
  pharmacology, 866t
  structure, 868f
  toxicity (overdose/poisoning)
    multiple-dose activated charcoal in, 61
    sodium bicarbonate for, 568t

Disorientation, cocaine and, 1127

Dispensing errors, 1824, 1825t

Dispholidus typus (African boomslang), 1633t

Disseminated intravascular coagulation (DIC), 885, 908
  chromium-induced, 1270
  with colchicine poisoning, 503
  with prothrombin complex concentrate, 909
  quinine-induced, 840
  rattlesnake bites and, 1622

Dissociation constant(s), 141–142

Dissolution, in gastrointestinal absorption, 143, 143f

Distal tubule, 389, 390f

Distance, in radiation protection, 1764–1765

Distribution, xenobiotic, 141, 141f, 144–147, 167
  in elderly, 461–462
  factors affecting, 144, 167
  postmortem, 1887

Disulfiram, 1172–1177
  absorption, 1172
  adverse drug events with, 1174
  for alcoholism, 1152, 1172–1173
  and aldehyde dehydrogenase, 1173, 1173f
  as antidote, 1176
  in cancer treatment, 1172
  for carbon monoxide poisoning, 1671
  clinical and laboratory findings with, 36t
  cytochrome P450 and, 1172–1173
  deaths associated with, 1172
  and dopamine-β-hydroxylase, 1173, 1175
  and dopamine levels, 1173, 1175
  dosage and administration, 1172
  drug interactions with, 1173
  elimination, 1173
  elimination half-life, 1173
  enzyme inhibition by, 1173, 1173f
  excretion, 1173
  fomepizole and, 1436
  hepatotoxicity, 1174–1176
  history and epidemiology, 1172
  interaction with ethanol, 1146t
    effects on vital signs, 30t
  mechanism of action, 212
  metabolism, 1172, 1172f
  metabolites, 1172–1173, 1172f
  neurotoxicity, 1174–1175
  for nickel carbonyl toxicity, 1337
  for nickel dermatitis, 1176
  odor, 364t
  ophthalmic toxicity, 356f
  pharmacokinetics, 1172–1173
  pharmacology, 1172–1173
  and pregnancy, 1175
  seizures caused by, 1175
  serum, 1172
  and serum cholesterol, 1175
  site of action, 1173, 1173f
  teratogenicity, 1175
  toxicity (overdose/poisoning), 1172
    acute, 1174
      diagnostic tests for, 1175
      management, 1175
      in children, 1175
    chronic, 1174–1175
      diagnostic tests for, 1175
      management, 1175–1176
    diagnostic tests for, 1175
    management, 1175–1176

Disulfiram-ethanol reaction, 1146t, 1173–1174
  acetaldehyde in, 1173, 1173f, 1174
  clinical manifestations, 1173–1174
  complications, 1173
  cytochrome P450 system in, 1172–1173
  deaths associated with, 1172–1173
  duration, 1174
  ECG changes in, 1173
  effects on vital signs, 30t
  fomepizole and, 1436
  household products causing, 1173, 1173t
  hypotension with, 1173–1174
  management of, 1174. *See also* Fomepizole
  pharmacokinetics, 1173
  pharmacology, 1173

Disulfiramlike reactions, 1146t, 1174, 1174t
  mushrooms and, 1587–1588, 1594

sulfonylurea-induced, 699
  xenobiotics causing, 1174, 1174t
Disulfoton, 1488t
Diterpenes, 1597
Dithiocarb (sodium diethyldithiocarbamate), and
        thallium chelation, 1354–1355
Dithiocarbamates, and cadmium toxicity, 1262
Dithizone (diphenylthiocarbazone), and thallium
        chelation, 1354–1355
Diuresis
  forced, 38, 92–93
    for cardioactive steroid toxicity, 975
  and glucarpidase therapy, 785
  for hypercalcemia, 199
Diuretics. See also specific xenobiotic
  abuse, and rhabdomyolysis, 393
  acute interstitial nephritis caused by, 394t
  as antihypertensives, 959t, 963
  as athletic performance enhancers, 621
  clinical and laboratory findings with, 36t
  dermal effects, 276t
  diabetes insipidus caused by, 195
  and fluid balance, 194
  and gustatory dysfunction, 365
  hypercalcemia caused by, 250
  for hypertension, 963
  hypomagnesemia caused by, 200, 877, 963
  and hyponatremia, 196, 963
  loop, 963. See also specific xenobiotic
    clinical and laboratory findings with, 36t
    for congestive heart failure, and thiamine
        replacement, 1160
    cranial neuropathy caused by, 346t
    for hypermagnesemia, 200
    for hypertension, 963
  ototoxicity, 366f
  overdose/poisoning, 963
  pancreatitis caused by, 295t
  potassium-sparing, 963. See also specific
        xenobiotic
    hyperkalemia caused by, 251
    for hypertension, 963
  renal effects, 390f, 391
  thiazide, 963. See also specific xenobiotic
    acute interstitial nephritis caused by, 394t
    and β-adrenergic antagonists, combined, 931
    for diabetes insipidus, 196
    for hypertension, 963
    and male sexual dysfunction, 299f
    mechanism of action, 227t
  and tinnitus, 369, 370t
  and urine for doping analysis, 623
  and urine specific gravity, 189
Divalent metal transporter (DMT1), 1294
  and manganese, 1320
Divers
  inert gas used by, 1651–1653
  nitrogen poisoning in, 1653
Divicine, 1607
Diviner's sage. See Salvia (Salvia divinorum, S.
        miltiorrhizae)
Divinyl ether, 1011
Dizocilpine (MK-801)
  for carbon monoxide poisoning, 1671
  mechanism of action, 227t, 228
  and NMDA receptors, 237, 1213–1214
  prevention of thallium-induced CNS effects,
        1351
Dizziness
  carbon monoxide poisoning and, 1665
  inhalant-induced, 1196

DM. See Adamsite
DMPS. See 2,3-Dimercapto-1-propanesulfonic acid
        (DMPS)
DMSA. See Succimer (2,3-dimercaptosuccinic acid,
        DMSA)
DMT. See N,N-Dimethyltryptamine (DMT)
DNA
  chemotherapeutics and, 761, 762f
  damage to
    antimonials and, 1233
    arsenicals and, 1239
    chemotherapeutics and, 350, 350f
    radiation-induced, 1767
  double-strand break, 350–351
  fluoropyrimidines and, 771–772, 771f
  methylation
    lead and, 1294
    and withdrawal syndrome, 237
  radiation exposure and, 1767
  repair mechanisms, 350–351
  replication, 349–350
    checkpoints that regulate, 350–351
  single-strand breaks, 351
  synthesis, 767
DNA ligase, 350
DNA polymerase, 349–351
  zinc in, 1362
DNOC (4,6-dinitro-o-cresol), 1468t
Dobell solution, 1369t
Dobutamine
  for β-adrenergic antagonist toxicity, 935
  for calcium channel blocker toxicity, 950
  enantiomers, 165
Docetaxel, adverse effects and safety issues, 760t
Dock (Rumex spp.), 1602t
Documentation, and risk management, 1861
Dofetilide
  adverse effects and safety issues, 867t, 872
  as antidysrhythmic, 872
  indications for, 872
  magnesium with, 877
  pharmacokinetics, 867t
  pharmacology, 867t
Dogbane (Apocynum cannabinum), 969, 979
Dog cloves. See Saponaria officinalis (soapwort)
Dog daisy. See Yarrow (Achillea millefolium)
Dogfish shark, 1576
Dolasetron, mechanism of action, 218
Dolutegravir, 832
Domoic acid, 227, 343, 595, 595f
  mechanism of action, 221, 227t
  toxicosis, 227
DOM/STP, 1101t. See also Amphetamine(s)
Donepezil, 1495, 1503
  acetylcholinesterase inhibition by, 208, 756
  indications for, 1041
  and neuromuscular blockers, interactions, 1021t
  oral, for central anticholinergic syndrome, 748
Dong Quai (Angelica polymorpha), uses and toxicities,
        641t
Dong Quai (Angelica sinensis), as abortifacient, 303t
Dopa, synthesis, 208, 209f
L-Dopa
  and serotonin, 218
  and thyroid hormone synthesis, 813f
  withdrawal, and neuroleptic malignant syndrome,
        215
DOPA decarboxylase, 208, 214–215
Dopamine, 203, 208, 209f, 212–215, 1180
  adenosine and, 229
  amphetamines and, 1099, 1100f, 1101

in brain, 212–213
  for calcium channel blocker toxicity, 950
  cellular responses to, 213, 213f
  contraindications to, 212, 1081
  disulfiram and, 1173, 1175
  effect on thyroid hormones and function, 814t
  γ-hydroxybutyrate and, 223, 1189
  for hypothermia, 417–418
  intravenous, mechanism of action, 211–212
  and movement disorders, 344
  nicotine and, 1206
  in nicotine withdrawal, 239
  norepinephrine and, 209f, 211–212
  release, 209f, 212–213, 213f
    lead and, 1295
  reuptake, 213, 213f
    cocaine and, 1125
    inhibition, 214, 214t
  reuptake transporters, 204
  and serotonin, 215, 218
  and sexual function, 298, 300, 304
  synthesis, 208, 213
  and thermoregulation, 412
Dopamine agonists, 214, 214t
  clinical and laboratory findings with, 36t
  direct, 214, 214t
  for drug-induced parkinsonism, 1037, 1037t
  and male sexual function, 299f
  receptor affinity, 214
Dopamine antagonists, 214–215, 214t
  indirect, 214t, 215
  receptor affinity, 214
Dopamine D₁-like receptors, 213
Dopamine D₂-like receptors, 213–214
Dopamine β-hydroxylase, 208, 209f, 1285t
  carbon disulfide and, 1175
  disulfiram and, 1173, 1175
  inhibition, 211t, 212, 1173
Dopamine hypothesis, 1034–1035
Dopamine receptor(s), 204–205, 212–214, 213f
  cocaine and, 134
  hallucinogens and, 1182
  increased sensitivity, xenobiotics causing, 214, 214t
  and thermoregulation, 412
  upregulation, by dopamine antagonists, 215
Dopamine reuptake transporter (DAT), 1056f
Dopaminergic neurotransmission
  agonists, 214, 214t
  antagonists, 214–215, 214t
  xenobiotics affecting, 214–215, 214t
Dopamine transporter (DAT), 213, 213f, 214
  amphetamines and, 1103
  inhibition, 215
Doping, 616. See also Athletic performance enhancers
  with autologous blood transfusions, 319
Doripenem, 825
Dorzolamide/timolol, benzalkonium chloride in, 682t
Dose, calculation, 1873
Dose–response concept, 4, 4t
Dose–response curve
  inverted U, 1815
  U-shaped, 1815
Dosimetry, 1764
Dosing body weight, 148
Doss, Nannie, 5t
Dosulepin, toxicity (overdose/poisoning)
  lipid emulsion for, 1006
  multiple-dose activated charcoal in, 61
Double breasting, by body packers, 546
Double condom sign, 546
Double-peak phenomenon, 144

Douglas fir tussock moth (*Orgyria pseudotsugata*), 1553
Dover, Thomas, 7
Dover's powder, 7, 519
Dow 1X-2, 96
Doxapram, for xenobiotic-induced respiratory dysfunction, 407
Doxazosin, 962
Doxepin, 1044, 1044t. *See also* Cyclic antidepressants
    cardiac effects, 248f
        Log D, 1045
    pharmacokinetics and toxicokinetics, 145t
    pharmacology, 203
    poisoning, lipid emulsion for, 1006
    volume of distribution, 145t
Doxorubicin, 760t
    adverse effects and safety issues, 762
    chemistry, 160
    effects on mitochondrial inner membrane, 176t
    enhanced elimination, 764
    extravasation, 802–803
    and free radical formation, 175
    and hair loss, 281
    intrathecal administration, inadvertent overdose and unintentional exposures due to, 795t
    lipid carrier formulation, 684t
    liposomal, 1719t
    mechanism and site of action, 762f
    metabolism, 175
    nail changes caused by, 281–282
    renal effects, 390f, 391
    toxicity (overdose/poisoning)
        N-acetylcysteine for, 494
        diffuse airspace filling in, 125t
    vomiting with, 762
Doxycycline, 827
    antimalarial mechanism, 838t
    and discoloration of teeth and gums, 293t
    and tinnitus, 369
Doxylamine
    clinical and laboratory findings with, 36t
    for nausea and vomiting of pregnancy, 663
    pharmacokinetics and toxicokinetics, 745t
    pharmacology, 741–742
    and pyridoxine, for nausea and vomiting of pregnancy, 663
    rhabdomyolysis with, 393t, 746
    sedative effects, 742
    structure, 740f
    toxicity, clinical manifestations, 744
DP. *See* Diphosgene
DPESA, for zinc poisoning, 1365
Dr. Tucker's Asthma Specific, 8
Dracotoxin, 1577
Drain cleaner(s), and toxic gas poisoning, 1233
Dram shop laws, 1880–1881
Drinking water
    arsenic in, 1237, 1242. *See also* Health Effects of Arsenic Longitudinal Study (HEALS)
        and QT prolongation, 1239
    nitrates in, 1704–1705
Driving, cannabis and, 1118–1119
Driving under the influence (DUI), 1876–1877
Driving under the influence of liquor (DUIL), 1876
Driving while intoxicated (DWI), 1876
Dronabinol, 1113
    structure, 1112f
Dronedarone, 871–872
    adverse effects and safety issues, 867t
    pharmacokinetics of, 867t
    pharmacology, 867t, 871–872

Droperidol. *See also* Antipsychotics
    for agitated/violent behavior, 386
        dosage and administration, 386
    cardiac effects, 258t
    dosage and administration, 1033t
    indications for, 1149
    pharmacokinetics, 1033t
    and QT interval, 253t
Drug(s)
    labeling, 9
    overdose, deaths from, 21t, 22
    plasma protein binding by, 109–110, 110t
    removal or withdrawal from market, for safety and/or efficacy concerns, 1839–1840, 1840t
    shortages, 43
Drug abuse screening tests, 102, 105, 110–112
    and chain of custody, 111
    in chronic pain patients, 111–112
    confirmatory testing in, 110–111
    cutoff concentrations in, 110, 112
    duration of positivity after last use, 112
    metabolites measured in, 112
    performance characteristics, 111t, 112–113
    specimen validity and, 111
    workplace, 110–112
Drug approval process, U.S., 1833–1835
Drug development, 1835–1838, 1835f
Drug discontinuation syndrome
    antidepressants and, 1061
    cyclic antidepressants and, 1047
    monoamine oxidase inhibitors and, 1080
    in neonates, 1061
    SSRIs and, 237, 239, 1061
Drug–drug interactions, 13, 21, 147. *See also specific drugs*
    CYP enzymes in, 1840. *See also* Cytochrome P450 (CYP) enzymes
    cytochrome P450 and, 170–171
    FDA regulatory action due to, 1840–1841
    in interpretive toxicology, 1873, 1873t
    transporters and, 144
Drug Enforcement Administration (DEA), 10t
Drug eruptions
    exanthematous, 274t
        extreme, 276
    maculopapular, 274t
Drug-Free Federal Workplace Program (1986), 10t
Drug-induced disease. *See also* Adverse drug events (ADEs)
    diagnosis, establishing, 1838–1839
Drug-induced hypersensitivity syndrome (DIHS), 277–278, 278f, 727–728, 727t
    with antituberculous medications, 855
    reporting requirements, 728
Drug-induced liver injury (DILI)
    amoxicillin-clavulanic acid and, 823–824
    evaluation, FDA policy on, 1841
    prediction, 329
Drug laws, historical perspective on, 8
Drug reactions, 278
    bullous, 276
    cutaneous, xenobiotic-induced, 273–281, 274t
    urticarial, xenobiotic-induced, 273–274
Drug reaction with eosinophilia and systemic symptoms (DRESS), 277, 727t. *See also* Drug-induced hypersensitivity syndrome (DIHS)
Drug rehabilitation, and thiamine deficiency, 1160
Drug safety, 9
Drug safety signals, postapproval, 1836–1838, 1841
Drug shortages, 1835

Drugs of abuse
    data collection on, 1792
    pharmacokinetics and toxicokinetics, 145t
    street names for, 162
Drug–xenobiotic interactions. *See also* Drug–drug interactions
    cytochrome P450 and, 170
Drunk driving, evidence of, 1876–1877
Drunkenness. *See* Alcohol abuse and alcoholism; Ethanol (alcohol)
Dry cleaning agents, inhaled, 1193t. *See also* Inhalant(s)
Dry ice, 1652
    sublimation, 1809
Dry mouth, antipsychotic-induced, 1039
DTPA (diethylenetriaminepentaacetic acid). *See* Diethylenetriaminepentaacetic acid (DTPA)
Due process, 1863
Dulaglutide, 607t, 694. *See also* Dieting xenobiotics and regimens
    pharmacokinetics and toxicokinetics, 696, 697t
    pharmacology, 696
Duloxetine, 1060
    mechanism of action, 1056f
    overdose/poisoning, multiple-dose activated charcoal in, 61
    pharmacokinetics, 1055t
    receptor activity, 1057t
    seizures caused by, 1057t
DUMBBELS mnemonic, 1491
Dumbcane (*Dieffenbachia*), 1613, 1613f
Dunn's hognosed pit viper (*Porthidium* spp.), 1637t
Duodenum, pH, 142t
DuoDote Autoinjector System, 1511
Dupuytren, Baron Guillaume, 4t, 7
Durango rock rattlesnake (*Crotalus* spp.), 1636t
Durham-Humphrey Amendment (1951), 10t
Dusky rattlesnake (*Crotalus* spp.), 1637t
Dust(s)
    definition, 1659
    in developing world, 1847
    ignition upon contact with air, 72
    inhaled
        inorganic, 1659
        organic, 1659
    nuisance, 1659
    and occupational health and safety, 1731
Dusting, 1193
Dutasteride
    as androgen receptor blocker, 299f
    and doping analysis, 623
Duvernoy's gland, of snakes, 1617
DVD head cleaner, inhaled, 1193t. *See also* Inhalant(s)
Dye
    aniline
        neonatal poisoning with, 453
        pediatric poisoning with, 453
    hair, self-poisoning with, 1846
Dynein, 340
Dynorphin, 520
Dynorphin peptides
    mechanism of action, 227t
    opioid antagonists and, 539
Dyserythropoiesis, arsenic and, 1244
Dysesthesias, poisoning/overdose causing, 36t
Dysgeusia, 365, 365t
Dysiherbaine, mechanism of action, 227t
Dyslipidemia, antipsychotic-induced, 1039
Dysosmia, 364, 364t
Dyspepsia, NSAIDs and, 515

Dysphagia, xenobiotic-induced, 293, 293t
Dysphoria, hallucinogen-induced, 1184
Dyspigmentation, xenobiotic-induced, 273
Dyspnea
  with *N*-acetylcysteine, 495
  cannabinoid-induced, 1117
  dantrolene and, 1030
Dysport, 578–579
Dysrhythmias, cardiac, 37, 254–258. *See also specific*
    dysrhythmia
  anabolic-androgenic steroids and, 617–618
  antihistamine-related, 746
    management, 747
  antimonials and, 1232
  in arsenic poisoning, 1239, 1241–1242
  atypical cyclic antidepressants and, 1048
  bupivacaine-induced, 999
    treatment, 1000
  in carbamate poisoning, 1491
  carbon monoxide poisoning and, 1664–1665
  cardioactive steroid toxicity and, 972, 972t, 974
  cesium-induced, 1265
  chemotherapeutics and, 762–763, 763t
  chloral hydrate-induced, 1087–1088
  cocaine-associated, 1126
    management, 1130
  with colchicine poisoning, 502
  in cyclic antidepressant poisoning, 567–569, 1046,
    1046f, 1047
  definition, 865
  digoxin-related, magnesium for, 877
  ethanol and, 1148
  in ethylene glycol poisoning, 1424
  fluoride poisoning and, 1398, 1400
  with hydrocarbon toxicity, 1412, 1417
  hydrogen sulfide poisoning and, 1690
  hypercalcemia and, 199
  hypermagnesemia and, 200
  hypoglycemia-induced, 699, 708
  hypomagnesemia and, 200, 249, 253t, 256, 258t, 970,
    1820
  in hypothermia, 416, 416f
  inhalants and, 1194, 1196, 1199
  initiation and propagation, 254–255, 255f
  lead-induced, 1298
  with long QT interval. *See* Torsade de pointes
  macrolides and, 826–827
  magnesium for, 877
  MAOI-induced, 1078
    management, 1081
  mechanisms, 254–255, 255f
  methadone and, 1820–1821, 1820f–1821f
  in methylxanthine poisoning, 988
  with naloxone-induced opioid reversal, 540
  NSAID overdose and, 516
  organic chlorine insecticides and, 1517
  in organic phosphorus compound poisoning, 1491
  propofol and, 1089
  with QT dispersion, 253
  quinidine and, 838
  quinine and, 838
  reentry (reentrant), 255, 255f, 256
  risk, corrected QT as predictor of, 251
  with sea snake envenomation, 1575
  sodium monofluoroacetate and, 1533–1534
  with succinylcholine, 1020
  from sympathomimetic decongestants, 750–751
  ventricular, 255–256
  vitamin D toxicity and, 661
  volatile hydrocarbons and, 1196
  wide-complex, in cyclic antidepressant toxicity,
    management, 567–569, 1049–1050, 1049t
  xenobiotic-induced, magnesium for, 877–878
  xenobiotics causing, 263, 263t–264t
  with ziconotide therapy, 1573
Dystonia (dystonic reactions)
  acute
    antipsychotic-induced, 1036, 1037t
    dopamine and, 213
    management, 44t
    treatment, 1036, 1037t
    xenobiotic-induced, 344
  with arylcyclohexylamine toxicity, 1215
  cocaine and, 1127
  SSRIs and, 1058
  therapeutics for, 35t

E
E-506, 5t
Eagle ray, 1576
Ear(s). *See also* Hearing
  anatomy and physiology, 365–367
  blast injury to, 369
  sound conduction in, 365–366, 366f
Early afterdepolarization (EAD), 251, 254f, 255–256
  electrophysiology, 253t, 254, 254f
Early repolarization, 249, 250f
Earthworms, anticoagulants from, 883
Eastern coral snake (*Micrurus fulvius*), 1617t, 1618,
    1633
  antivenom for, 35t, 1627t, 1628–1631
  envenomation
    clinical manifestations, 1622
    treatment, 1625
  venom, LD$_{50}$, 1620
Eastern diamondback rattlesnake (*Crotalus
    adamanteus*), 1617t
  antivenom, 1627–1631, 1627t
Eastern equine encephalitis (EEE), as biological
    weapon, 1758
Eastern teaberry (*Gaultheria procumbens*), 634
Eastern twin-spotted rattlesnake (*Crotalus* spp.), 1636t
Eating disorders, and thiamine deficiency, 1160
Eau Medicinale, 501
Ebastine, pharmacology, 742
Ebers Papyrus, 1, 3, 519, 627, 638, 969
Ebola virus, as biological weapon, 1758
Ecallantide, 964
Ecarin clotting time (ECT), 893
Eccles, John, 1018
Eccrine glands, 270
Ecgonine methyl ester (EME), 1124, 1125f
Echimidine, 641t
Echinacea (*Echinacea angustifolia, E. purpurea*)
  preparations, 639
  uses and toxicities, 641t
Echinacoside, 641t
Echinodermata, 1573
Echinoderms, 1573–1574
  foodborne illness caused by, 596
Echinothrix spp., 1573
Echis carinatus (saw-scaled viper), 1633t
Echocardiography, 402
  indications for, 406
  in metal phosphide poisoning, 1459
  with xenobiotic exposure, 115t
Echogenicity, ultrasound, 114
Echol's Roach Powder, 1350
Echothiophate, ophthalmic use, systemic toxicity with,
    360
Echothiophate iodide, 1488t
e-cigarettes, 1203–1206
  deaths associated with, 1204
  and nicotine poisoning, 1206
Eclampsia, and posterior reversible encephalopathy
    syndrome, 132
Econazole, 829
Ecstasy (amphetamine). *See*
    3,4-Methylenedioxymethamphetamine
    (MDMA, Adam, molly, ecstasy, XTC)
Ectopic beats, 255
Eculizumab, for quinine-induced thrombotic
    microangiopathy, 847
Edema, 38
  xenobiotic-induced, in elderly, 463, 463t
Edema toxin, 1755
Edetate calcium disodium (calcium disodium versenate,
    CaNa$_2$EDTA), 1287, 1315–1318, 1779
  adverse effects and safety issues with, 1316
  as antidote
    availability and storage, 44t
    cost, 43
    indications for, 44t
    stocking, recommended level, 44t
    supplies, 43
  chemistry, 1315
  for cobalt toxicity, 1278–1279
  and dimercaprol, combined, 1251, 1316–1317
    for zinc toxicity, 1365
  with DMPS, 1317
  dosing and administration, 1316–1317, 1317t
  elimination, 1315
  formulation, 1317
  half-life, 1315
  history of, 1315
  indications for, 35t, 1315
  intramuscular administration, 1316–1317
  intravenous administration, 1316–1317
  LD$_{50}$, 1252
  lead chelation by, 1315
  for lead poisoning, 1292, 1302, 1312, 1315
    in adults, 1303t, 1304
    animal studies, 1315
    in breastfeeding mothers, 1316
    in children, 1302–1304, 1303t, 1315
    dosage and administration, 1316–1317, 1317t
    efficacy, 1315–1316
    in pregnancy, 1316
    renal toxicity with, 1316
  and manganese excretion, 1321
  mechanism of action, 1315
  mobilization test with, 1315
  for neonates of blood-exposed mothers, 1305
  pharmacokinetics and pharmacodynamics, 1315
  pharmacology, 1315
  structure, 1315
  with succimer, 1312, 1317
  volume of distribution, 1315
  and zinc depletion, 1316
  for zinc toxicity, 1365
Edoxaban, 321f, 883, 884f, 894–896
  adverse effects and safety issues, 894–895
  efficacy, 894
  laboratory testing for, 888t
  overdose/poisoning, treatment strategies for, 888t
  pharmacology, 893t, 895
Edrophonium
  acetylcholinesterase inhibition by, 208
  contraindications to, 1041
  mechanism of action, 579

Edrophonium (*Cont.*):
  for neuromuscular blockade reversal, 1025, 1026t
  and neuromuscular blockers, interactions, 1021t
Edrophonium testing
  and botulism, 578–579
  and myasthenia gravis, 578
Education
  poison, 1782–1788
    global disparities in, 1847
    health education principles in, 1786
    health literacy in, 1786
    health numeracy in, 1786
    programs for, 1783–1786
    for public and health professionals, 1793, 1793t
    public health initiatives for, 1793, 1794t
  worker, and occupational exposure control, 1800, 1801t
Edward I (King), 17
Edwardsiella lineata, larvae, and seabather's eruption,
    1571
Eels, ciguatoxinlike neurotoxin in, 595
Efavirenz, 831
  and prolonged QT interval, 253t
E-Ferol, 681
Effective dose (radiation), 1764
Effectiveness, assessment, 1854
Effect size, 1855–1856
Efficacy
  assessment, 1854
  definition, 1854
Eggs (rotten), odor, 364t
Ehrlichiosis, 1550
Eicosanoids, 511, 513f
Einsteinium, chelator for, 1780
Einthoven, Willem, 246
Einthoven triangle, 246, 246f–247f
ELA-Max, 996
Elapidae (coral snakes), 1617–1618, 1633, 1633t. *See also*
    Coral snakes (*Micrurus* spp., *Micruroides* spp.)
  antivenom
    availability and storage, 44t
    indications for, 44t
    stocking, recommended level, 44t
    for xenobiotic-induced respiratory dysfunction, 407
  bites, 1617t. *See also* Snakebite(s)
    epidemiology, 1633
  geographic distribution, 1633
  neurotoxins
    α-, nicotinic receptor blockade by, 207
    β-, and acetylcholine release, 207
  venom
    effects on vital signs, 30t
    hypoventilation caused by, 400t
    toxicity, 1634
Elapids, 1574. *See also* Elapidae (coral snakes)
  antivenoms, 1627, 1627t
Elapinae, 1633t
Elderberry (*Sambucus* spp.), 1602t
  uses and toxicities, 641t
Elderly
  absorption in, 461
  ADEs and medication errors in, 1826–1827
    reduction/prevention, 1827
  adverse drug events (ADEs) and, 463–464, 1823
  alcohol abuse and alcoholism in, 466–467
  alcohol withdrawal in, 467
  body composition in, 461, 461t
  cannabis use by, 467
  confusion in, *case study*, 459
  delayed toxicity in, 460
  delirium in, 460
    case study, 459

distribution of xenobiotics in, 461–462
falls in, 460
hepatic metabolism in, 462
illicit drug use in, 466–467
intentional poisoning in, 466
loperamide abuse/misuse in, 466
medication errors and, 1823
mental status changes in, 460
neuroleptic malignant syndrome in, 464
neurotoxins and, 342
opioid abuse/misuse in, 466
outdated and discontinued medications used by, 466
overdose/poisoning in, *case study*, 459
pathology exacerbated or unmasked by xenobiotics
    in, 463, 463t
pharmacodynamics in, 463
pharmacokinetics in, 461–463, 461t
physiologic changes exacerbated or unmasked by
    xenobiotics in, 463, 463t
poison prevention aimed at, 1783–1784
polypharmacy and, 464–465, 1827
and potentially inappropriate medications (PIMs), 460
"renal" dosing in, 462–463, 462t
renal function in, 462–463
    and potential xenobiotic toxicity, 462–463, 462t
salicylate toxicity in, *case study*, 459
substance abuse in, 466–467
substance withdrawal in, 467
suicide in, 466
therapeutic errors and, 463–464
and thiamine deficiency, 1160
toxic exposures in
  clinical presentation, 460
  lethality, 460
  prevalence, 460
  risk factors for, 460
  underrecognition, 460
  xenobiotics associated with, 460, 461t
toxicity in
  admission criteria with, 467–468
  management, 467
  prevention, 467
  timing of discharge with, 467–468
trauma in, substance abuse and, 466–467
unintentional poisoning in, 463–464
Electrocardiography (ECG), 27, 37, 244, 246–254
  with anticholinergic toxicity, 736, 737f
  antihistamine toxicity and, 746
  antimonials and, 1232–1233
  antipsychotic overdose and, 1039
  in arsenic poisoning, 1244
  basic electrophysiology, 245f, 246
  Brugada pattern, 249–250, 250f
    in cyclic antidepressant poisoning, 568, 1046
  in calcium channel blocker poisoning, 947
  in carbon monoxide oisoning, 1666–1667
  of cardiac cycle, 245, 245f
  clinical applications, 189, 246
  in cyanide poisoning, 1686
  in cyclic antidepressant overdose/poisoning, 568, 1048
  digitalis effect on, 250, 250f, 258, 970, 972f
  dysrhythmias in. *See* Dysrhythmias, cardiac; *specific
    dysrhythmia*
  early repolarization abnormality, 249, 250f
  ectopy on, 255
  electrophysiology, 246–254
  fluoride poisoning and, 1398
  history of, 246
  hyperkalemia and, 198–199
  hypermagnesemia and, 200
  hypocalcemia and, 199, 250

hypokalemia and, 198, 251, 252f
in hypothermia, 416, 416f
intervals, 247, 247f
J point, 247f, 249
  elevation, 249, 250f
J wave, 249
leads, 246–247, 246f–247f
in metal phosphide poisoning, 1458–1459
in methanol poisoning, 1427
nickel poisoning and, 1335
normal, 247f
Osborn wave, 249
overdose/poisoning and, 254
pediatric
  abnormal, 258
  normal, 258
phosphorus and, 1529
in poisoned patient, 266
PQ segment, 248
PR interval, 247f, 248, 251, 252f
  abnormal, 248
  electrophysiology, 248
P wave, 247–248, 247f, 251, 252f
  abnormal, 247–248
  electrophysiology, 247
  notched, 247, 247f
QRS complex, 246, 247f, 248–249, 251, 252f
  abnormal, 248–249, 248f–249f
  in cyclic antidepressant poisoning, 248–249, 249f,
    567–569, 1045, 1046f–1047f
  electrophysiology, 248
  in infants < 6 months old, 249
  prolonged
    atypical antidepressants and, 1056, 1057t
    citalopram toxicity and, 1056–1057, 1057t
    escitalopram toxicity and, 1056–1057, 1057t
    tachydysrhythmia associated with, 256, 257f
  terminal portion, 248–249, 249f
  widened, 258, 567–569
    antipsychotic-induced, 1034t
QT dispersion on, 253
QT interval, 247f, 249, 251–253, 252f, 1820–1821,
    1821f
  abnormal, 251–253
  age and, 251
  corrected (QTc), 251
    dispersion, 253
  electrophysiology, 251
  factors affecting, 251
  gender and, 251
  heart rate and, 251
  inhalants and, 1196
  measurement, 251
  nickel poisoning and, 1335
  prolonged, 251–253, 253f, 253t, 254, 254f, 258,
    877–878, 1335, 1820–1821, 1821f
    acebutolol-induced, 930
    antipsychotic-induced, 1034t, 1035
    arsenic and, 1239, 1241
    atypical antidepressants and, 1056, 1057t
    cesium-induced, 1264–1265, 1359
    cetirizine-induced, 746
    citalopram toxicity and, 1056–1057, 1057t
    cyclic antidepressants and, 256, 1046
    escitalopram toxicity and, 1056–1057, 1057t
    fluoroquinolones and, 826
    macrolides and, 826–827
    NSAID overdose and, 516
    quinine and, 838–839
    sotalol-induced, 930
    telithromycin and, 827

QT interval dispersion, inhalants and, 1196
QT Interval Nomogram, 251, 253f
QU interval, 254
    abnormal, 254
Q wave, 248–249
    in infant, 258
R waves, in infant, 258
    screening, 32
    sine wave on, 251, 252f
    ST segment, 247f, 249–251, 252f
        abnormal, 249–250, 249f–250f
        electrophysiology, 249
    S wave, in infant, 258
    in thallium toxicity, 1351
    T wave, 247f, 248, 250–251
        abnormal, 251
        in children, 258
        electrophysiology, 250–251
        notched, 253, 254f
        persistent juvenile pattern, 258
    U wave, 247f, 251, 252f, 253–254, 254f
        abnormal, 254
        electrophysiology, 254
    waves, 247, 247f
Electrochemical detectors, 106
Electroconvulsive therapy, for neuroleptic malignant
        syndrome, 1039
Electroencephalography
    in bismuth encephalopathy, 1256
    in carbon monoxide poisoning, 1667
Electrolyte(s). See also specific electrolyte
    fluoride poisoning and, 1398
    laboratory investigation, 37
    replacement, for SMFA or fluoroacetamide
        poisoning, 1534
    serum, 189
        in differential diagnosis of high anion gap
            metabolic acidosis, 192
Electrolyte abnormalities, 189, 197–200. See also Acid–
        base abnormality(ies); specific electrolyte
    in alcoholic patients, 1167
    cardiac effects, 254–255
    cardioactive steroids and, 972, 974–975
    cathartics causing, 77
    cesium chloride and, 1265
    correction, hemodialysis for, 95
    and enhanced elimination of xenobiotics, 90
    with gastrointestinal decontamination, 62
    hypoventilation caused by, 399, 400t
    multiple-dose activated charcoal and, 79
    phosphorus and, 1529
    and prolonged QT interval, 251–253, 253t, 256,
        1820–1821, 1821f
    in SMFA or fluoroacetamide poisoning, 1534
    xenobiotic-induced, 197–200
Electromyography (EMG)
    in botulism, 580
    in diagnosis of anticholinesterase poisoning, 1495
Electron(s), 1763
    capture, 1762
    in chemical reactions, 155
    unpaired, and free radicals, 174
    valence, 159
Electron deficiency, of electrophiles, 162
    absolute, 162
    relative, 162
Electronegativity, of elements, 158, 158f
Electronegativity difference, 159, 162
Electroneutrality, law of, 190
Electronic health records (EHRs), 1862, 1865
Electron impact (EI) ionization, 107

Electron transport chain, 168, 175, 177–178
    at ATP synthase, 177
        inhibitors, 176t
    at complex I, 177
        inhibitors, 176t
    at complex II, 177
    at complex IV, 177
        inhibitors, 176t
    at complex III, inhibitors, 176t
    cyanide and, 177, 1685
Electrophiles, 162–164
    hard, 164
    soft, 164
Electrophysiology
    basic, of electrocardiogram, 245f, 246. See also
            Electrocardiography (ECG)
    cardiac, 244, 246–258
Electroplating, cobalt in, 1273
Electroretinography, in methanol poisoning, 1423–1424
Electrospray ionization (ESI), 107
Electrovalent bond(s), 158–159
Element(s). See also Periodic Table of the Elements
    definition, 155
    family of, 155
    groups of, 155
    physicochemical properties, 157
    transition, 155
Elemicin, 631, 1179t, 1181t, 1183, 1601t
    structure, 1183f
Elephant tranquilizer. See Phencyclidine (PCP)
Eletriptan, 217, 808–809, 808t
Elimination
    enhanced, 90–100
        case reporting, improving, 92
        in children, 452
        clinical effects, 92
        efficacy, 90
        endogenous clearance rates and, 92
        evidence of, evaluation, 92
        frequency of use, by modality, 90, 90t
        indications for, 90–91
        pharmacokinetics and, 91
        recommendations for, 90
        serum concentration and, 92
        techniques for, 90, 90t, 92–98, 147
        time frame for, 92
        toxicokinetic efficacy, 91–92
        volume of distribution and, 91
    inhibition, techniques for, 147
    rate, pharmacokinetic effects, 152, 152t
    of xenobiotics, 147–148
        factors affecting, 147
        transport proteins and, 173
Elimination rate constant, 140, 150
Eliprodil, 227t, 228
Eliquis. See Apixaban
Elk River, West Virginia, water quality in, risk
        communication and, 1816
Elm (Ulmus rubra, U. fulva), 644t
El Muerto Island speckled rattlesnake (Crotalus spp.),
        1636t
Elvitegravir, 832
Embalming, 1885
Embalming fluid, 1885
    analysis, 1886
Embden-Meyerhof glycolysis, 312, 313f, 1704, 1705f
Emboli, septic, diagnostic imaging, 115t, 125, 125t,
        126f, 131, 132t
Embryopathy, warfarin, 890
Emergence reaction, 1216
    management, 1217

Emergency, definition, 1861
Emergency Medical Treatment and Labor Act (1986),
        42, 375
Emergency Planning and Community Right-to-Know
        Act, 1801t
Emergency Planning Districts, 1801t
Emergency Response Guidebook, 1807
Emergency rinsing solution, 73
Emesis
    early methods, 4
    induction, 3
Emetics. See also specific xenobiotic
    abuse, 612–613
    ancient use of, 3
    renal effects, 391
    tartar, 4
Emetine, 4t, 7, 613, 1599t, 1605
EMIT immunoassay. See Enzyme-multiplied
        immunoassay technique (EMIT)
EMLA (eutectic mixture of local anesthetics), 996
Emodin, 641t, 1599t
Empacho, 648
Empagliflozin, pharmacokinetics and toxicokinetics,
        697t
Emphysema, 401
Emtricitabine, 831
Emulsin, 1602t
Enalaprilat, benzyl alcohol in, 683t
Enantiomer(s), 147, 164, 164f
    agonist vs. antagonist, 165
    dextrorotatory, 164
    levorotatory, 164
    R and S, 164, 164f
Encainide, 865
    and prolonged QT interval, 256
    toxicity (overdose/poisoning)
        ECG changes in, 250
        sodium bicarbonate for, 568t
Encephalitis
    clinical manifestations, 577t
    in drug-induced hypersensitivity syndrome,
            277
    infectious, focal brain lesions caused by, 131
    viral, as biological weapon, 1758–1759
Encephalopathy
    aluminum-induced, 1223–1225
    in arsenic poisoning, 1241
    bismuth-induced, 1255–1256, 1256t
        differential diagnosis, 1256, 1256t
        imaging in, 1256
    in carbon monoxide poisoning, 1676–1677, 1677f
    chemotherapeutic-related, management, 764
    with colchicine poisoning, 503
    differential diagnosis, 1256, 1256t
    disulfiram-induced, 1175
    hepatic, flumazenil for, 1094–1096
    lead
        acute, 1295, 1295f, 1297–1298
        in adults, 1298
            treatment, 1303t, 1304
        in children, 1297
            treatment, 1302–1303, 1303t
        clinical characteristics, 1297
        diagnosis, 1298–1300
        gold mining and, 1293
        laboratory findings in, 1300
        mortality rate for, 1297
        neurologic sequelae, 1297, 1297f
        treatment, 1310–1311, 1316–1317
            in adults, 1303t, 1304
            in children, 1302–1303, 1303t

Encephalopathy (*Cont.*):
    mushroom ingestions causing, 1583t, 1592
    paradichlorbenzene-induced, 1384–1385
    posthypoglycemic, 710
    Wernicke. *See* Wernicke encephalopathy
Endemic ALS-Parkinson disease in Guam, 227–228
Endocannabinoid(s), 1111, 1112f, 1113
Endocannabinoid receptor antagonists, 606, 611–612
Endocannabinoid receptor inverse agonists, 611–612
Endocannabinoid system (ECS), 611–612
Endocrine disorders, lithium-induced, 1068–1069
Endocrine disrupting substances, 685, 1815
    in dietary supplements, 649
Endocrine disruptors, 649, 685, 1815
Endocrine xenobiotics, combined, ophthalmic toxicity,
    361t
Endocytosis, 141, 141f, 142
Endogenous digitalis-like substances (EDLIS), 979
Endogenous digoxinlike immunoreactive substance
    (EDLIS), 973
Endolymph, 366
Endoperoxides, antimalarial mechanism, 837f, 838t,
    845
Endorphins, 519–520
    nicotine and, 1206
    opioid antagonists and, 539
    and thermoregulation, 412
Endoscopy
    in body stuffers, 548
    of caustic injury, 1390–1392, 1390t
    fiberoptic, in smoke inhalation, 1642–1643, 1645
    in gastrointestinal decontamination, 53, 63–64
Endosulfan, 1514
    acute exposure to, clinical manifestations, 1517
    metabolism, 1515
    odor, 1518
    physicochemical properties, 1515t, 1518
Endothall, 1554
Endothelial cells, hepatic, 327, 329f
Endothelin, mechanism of action, 933f
Endotoxin, and hemodialysis, 99
Endotracheal intubation, 36
Endrin, 1514
    metabolism, 1515
    physicochemical properties, 1515t
Energy drinks, 985, 986t
Energy metabolism. *See also* Adenosine triphosphate
    (ATP)
    cellular, 175
Enflurane, 1011
    abuse, 1016
    elimination, 167
    pharmacology, 1410
    structure, 1011f
Enfuvirtide, 832
English hawthorn (*Crataegus oxyacantha*), 642t
English holly, 642t
English yew (*Taxus* spp.), 1603t
Enhanced elimination. *See* Elimination, enhanced
Enhydrina schistosa (beaked sea snake), 1574
    antivenom, 1575t
Enkephalins
    and gastrointestinal tract, 290t
    opioid antagonists and, 539
Enolase, in carbon monoxide poisoning, 1667
Enolic acid(s), pharmacology, 512t
Enoxacin, and GABA receptor, 222
Enoxaparin, 890
    adverse effects and safety issues, in elderly, 465
    antidotes and treatment strategies for, 888t, 891

    laboratory testing for, 888t
    overdose/poisoning, clinical manifestations, 890
    reversal, 921
Enoximone
    for β-adrenergic antagonist toxicity, 934–935
    for calcium channel blocker toxicity, 948
Entacapone
    indications for, 214
    mechanism of action, 212
Entactogen(s), 1105–1106. *See also* Hallucinogens
    definition, 1178
Enteric-coated preparations, radiopacity, 114
Enteric coating, and absorption, 143
Enteritis, xenobiotic-induced, 294, 294t
Enterohepatic circulation, 172, 327
    Prussian blue and, 1357
    of xenobiotics, 144
        interruption, 64
Entero-Vioform, 20
Entheogen. *See also* Hallucinogens
    definition, 1178
Entomotoxicology, 1886, 1886t
Envenomations
    arthropod, 1540–1558. *See also* Arthropods
    in developing world, 1844–1845
    marine, 1567–1580. *See also* Marine envenomations
    scorpion. *See* Scorpions
    snake. *See* Snakebite(s)
    spider, 1540–1547. *See also* Spiders
    suction therapy for, 3–4
Environmental exposures, in developing world,
    1846–1847
Environmental Protection Agency, U.S. (EPA), 10t, 12, 1804
    chemotherapeutics regulated by, 765
    and nanotechnology, 1731–1733
    and radiation regulation, 1767
    regulatory authority, in workplace, 1801t, 1804
    website, information from, 1814
Environmental toxicology, origins, 11–12
Enzymatic assays, for ethanol, 1877
Enzyme(s), 167
    cytochrome, 168–169. *See also* Cytochrome P450
        (CYP) enzymes
    cytosolic, 167
    genetic polymorphism, 170
    hepatic, 167
    inducible, 172
    inhibition
        competitive, 171
        noncompetitive, 171
        reversible vs. irreversible, 171
    microsomal, 167
    in phase I reactions, 147
    in phase II reactions, 147
    and presystemic metabolism of xenobiotics, 144
    in spectrochemical testing, 103
    xenobiotic-metabolizing, and bioavailability, 144
Enzyme-linked immunosorbent assay (ELISA), for
    Loxosceles venom, 1545
Enzyme-multiplied immunoassay technique (EMIT),
    104–105, 104f
    for ethanol, 1877
    interference in, 105
Eosinophilia, 320
Eosinophilia myalgia syndrome, 20t, 21, 217, 320, 346
    from tryptophan, 20t, 21, 281, 320
Eosinophils, 319–320
EPA toxicity classification, of pesticides, 1450, 1450t
Ephedra (*Ephedra* spp.), 607–608, 608t, 639, 748, 1600t,
    1605

    adverse effects and side effects, 21
    E. nevadensis (Mormon tea)
        psychoactive properties, 650t
        uses and toxicities, 641t, 649
    E. sinensis, 1600t
    uses and toxicities, 641t, 649
Ephedra alkaloids, 608
Ephedraceae, 1600t
Ephedra sinica, 608t
Ephedrine, 641t, 649, 650t, 1600t, 1602t, 1605. *See also*
    Amphetamine(s)
    brain changes caused by, imaging, 132t
    cardiac effects, 256
    duration of action, 749t
    history of, 748, 1099
    mechanism of action, 211
    and methamphetamine synthesis, 1105
    monitoring, insports, 748
    pharmacology, 749
    recreational use, 748
    structure, 606, 610f, 749f
    therapeutic effects, 749t
    toxicity, 749t
        clinical manifestations, 750
L-Ephedrine, 112
Ephedrone. *See also* Methcathinone (cat, Jeff, khat,
    ephedrone)
    abuse, 1320
Epicauta vittata, 1554
Epidemic polyarthritis, mosquitoes and, 1522
Epidemiologic association
    artifactual, 1855, 1855t
    causal, 1855, 1855t
    indirect, 1855, 1855t
    significance of, measurement, 1855–1856
    strength of, measurement, 1853t, 1854
    types of, 1855, 1855t
Epidemiologic study(ies)
    advantages, 1853t
    designs, 1853t
    evaluation, 1859, 1859t
    measurements, 1853t
    observational
        analytical, 1853, 1853t
        descriptive, 1852–1853, 1853t
    power of, 1855
    sample size for, 1855, 1855t
    types, 1853t
Epidemiology
    poison, 1789–1794
        adverse drug events and, 1792
        data collection on, 1790–1792
        data on, in public health surveillance system,
            1792
        in developing world, 1844
        drugs of abuse and, 1792
        fatal poisonings and, 1791
        improvement, 1793, 1794t
        nonfatal poisonings and, 1791
        occupational exposures and, 1791–1792
        underreported exposures and, 1792
        xenobiotic errors and, 1792
    techniques in, 1852–1854, 1853t
Epidermal growth factor (EGF), 761f
Epidermal growth factor receptor(s) (EGFR), 761
Epidermal growth factor receptor antagonists,
    hypomagnesemia caused by, 877
Epidermis, 269, 270f
    basal layer, 269–270, 270f
    granular layer, 269, 270f

horny layer, 269, 270f
layers, 269, 270f
spinous layer, 269, 270f
Epidural abscess, spinal, imaging, 122, 124f
Epigallocatechin gallate (EGCG), 642t
Epigenetics, and withdrawal syndrome, 237
Epilepsy
  epidemiology, 719
  generalized, 719
  glutamate and, 224
  history of, 719
  partial, 719
Epinephrine, 203, 206f, 208–212, 260, 926, 985
  absorption, in obese patients, 148
  for calcium channel blocker toxicity, 950
  chemistry, 165
  cost, 43
  effects on vital signs, 30t
  enantiomers, 165
  and fatty acid metabolism, 178–179
  for hypothermia, 417
  injection, chlorobutanol in, 683t
  and local anesthetics, combined, adverse effects and
     safety issues, 996
  and pancreatic dysfunction, 295t
  postmortem changes, 1885t
  for quinine overdose, 840
  release, 206f, 208
  reuptake, cocaine and, 1125
  shortage, 43
  structure, 1099
  for venomous caterpillar exposure, 1554
Epipodophyllotoxin, 760t
  extravasation, 803t
Epipremnum aureum (pothos), 1600t, 1613
Epirubicin, 760t
  extravasation, 802–803
Epistratos, 3
Epothilones, mechanism and site of action, 762f
Epoxide reductase, 885f, 886
Epoxy resins, scleroderma-like reaction with, 281
Epping jaundice, 18, 18t
Eprosartan, CYP enzymes and, 170
Epsom salt, 83, 876
Eptifibatide, 323, 899
  adverse effects and safety issues, 900
  dosage and administration, 899
  mechanism of action, 898f
Equilibrative nucleoside transporters (ENTs), 229, 229f
Equivalence margins, 1854
Equivalent, definition, 158, 1854
Erectile dysfunction
  causes, 300
  definition, 300
  epidemiology, 300
  treatment, 304
    xenobiotics for, 300–301
    xenobiotic-induced, 299f, 300, 300t
Erection (penile). *See also* Erectile dysfunction
  physiology, 298, 299f
  xenobiotics that improve, 299f
Erenumab-aooe, 809
Erethism, 1324, 1327
Ergine, 643t, 650t, 1179, 1179t, 1181t
Ergocalciferol (vitamin D₂). *See* Vitamin D
    (cholecalciferol and ergocalciferol)
Ergonovine, 1179. *See also* Ergot and ergot alkaloids
  duration of action, 807t
  elimination half-life, 807t
  history of, 806

indications for, 807t
pharmacology and pharmacokinetics, 806, 807t
Ergotamine(s), 18, 21, 805–806, 1599t. *See also* Ergot
    and ergot alkaloids
  as abortifacients, 303t
  brain changes caused by, imaging, 132t
  cardiac effects, 806–807
  duration of action, 807t
  elimination half-life, 807t
  indications for, 807t
  intravenous injection, necrotizing angiitis caused
    by, 128
  pharmacology and pharmacokinetics, 806, 807t
  structure, 806f
Ergot and ergot alkaloids, 4t, 7, 805–807, 1178. *See also*
    Claviceps purpurea (ergot); Ergotism; *specific*
    alkaloid
  as α-adrenergic agonists, 806, 807t
  amine, 806, 806f
  amino acid, 806, 806f
  cardiac effects, 249, 256, 806–807
  central effects, 806, 807t
  in *Claviceps purpurea*, 1599t
  clinical and laboratory findings with, 36t
  and dopaminergic receptors, 806, 807t
  drug interactions with, 806
  effects on vital signs, 29t–30t
  epidemics caused by, 18, 18t
  in grains, 805–806
  history of, 805–806
  intestinal ischemia and infarction caused by, 127, 129t
  mechanism of action, 217
  ophthalmic toxicity, 356f, 361t
  pancreatitis caused by, 294
  peripheral effects, 806, 807t
  pharmacokinetics, 806, 807t
  pharmacology, 806, 807t
  renal effects, 390f
  and serotonergic receptors, 806–807, 807t
  vascular effects, 806
  as vasoconstrictors, 806
Ergotism, 806–807, 1178. *See also* Ergot and ergot
    alkaloids
  clinical manifestations, 806–807, 807t
  convulsive, 806
  epidemics, 18, 18t
  gangrenous, 18
  treatment, 807
Ergotoxine, 806
Ericaceae, 1598t, 1602t
Erlotinib
  adverse effects and safety issues, 760t, 762
  overdose/poisoning, 760t
Erosion, cutaneous, 269t
Erowid.org, 1178
Error(s). *See also* Medication errors
  in analytical toxicology, preanalytical issues and,
    1868–1870, 1869t
  with antimicrobials, 821
  in computerized provider order entry (CPOE), 1862
  in electronic health records, 1862
  in laboratory test results, 153
  medical, 13, 1822
    deaths caused by, 1822–1823
  in medicolegal interpretive toxicology, factors
    leading to, 1871, 1871t
  prescribing, data collection on, 1792
  stages of medication process and, 1824–1826, 1825t
Ertapenem, 825
Erucism, 1552–1554

Erythema, with *N*-acetylcysteine, 495
Erythema multiforme, 273–275, 274t, 275f, 276
  Neofibularia exposure and, 1574
Erythema nodosum, jellyfish sting and, 1569
Erythema of the 9th day, 1255
Erythrocyte(s), 312, 352–353
  basophilic stippling in, lead and, 1295, 1295f
  for dabigatran-induced coagulopathy, 894
  lead and, 1295
  mature, 312
  membrane-associated enzymes, 312
  metabolism in, 312–313, 313f
  methylmercury in, 1326
  oxidative stress in, 178, 178f
  and oxygen-carbon dioxide exchange, 315–316
  spondylolysis, copper and, 1285
  structural proteins, 312
  transport proteins, 312
  trivalent arsenicals and, 1239
Erythrocyte protoporphyrin concentration, 1299
Erythrocytosis, 319
Erythroderma, 274t, 278
Erythromelalgia, 1583t, 1591–1592
Erythromycin
  adverse effects associated with xenobiotic
    interactions, 827
  metabolite, as CYP inhibitor, 171
  as promotility agent, 84
  and pyloric stenosis, 442
  structure, 826
  and vincristine, interactions, 506
Erythromycin estolate, cholestasis caused by, 330
Erythron, 312–319
Erythropoiesis, cobalt-related, 1274
Erythropoiesis-stimulating proteins, 620
Erythropoietin (EPO), 312
  for anemia associated with chemotherapy, 764
  as athletic performance enhancer, 319, 620–621
    and sudden death, 623
  for carbon monoxide poisoning, 1672
  competition effect and, 622
  overdose, 620
  testing for, 621
  in urine testing for doping, 622–623
Erythroxylum coca (coca), 8, 1124, 1600t. *See also*
    Cocaine
  local anesthesia with, 994
Escape rhythm, 255
Escherichia coli
  enterohemorrhagic (EHEC), 598–599
  enterotoxigenic, 597, 597t
  hemorrhagic, 597t
  invasive, 597, 597t
  O157:H7, 598–599
  shigatoxin-producing (STEC), 592t
Escholtzine, 650t
Eschscholtzia californica (California poppy), 650t
Escitalopram, 1054
  cardiac effects, 257f
  mechanism of action, 1056f
  overdose/poisoning
    clinical manifestations, 1056–1057
    ECG changes in, 1056–1057, 1057t
    gastrointestinal decontamination for, 64
    magnesium for, 878
    management, 1057
    seizures with, 1056–1057, 1057t
  pharmacokinetics, 1055t
  and QT interval, 253, 253t
  receptor activity, 1057t

Esculin (esculoside, aesculin), 642t, 1610
Esculoside, 1598t, 1609–1610
Esere ordeal, 755
Eserine, 755. *See also* Physostigmine
Esfenvalerate, 1520t. *See also* Pyrethroids
Esketamine, mechanism of action, 227t
Eslicarbazepine (eslicarbazepine acetate)
    adverse effects and safety issues, 727t
    drug-induced hypersensitivity syndrome with, 727t
    drug interactions with, 723t
    mechanism of action, 720f, 720t
    metabolism and effects on CYP enzymes, 722t
    pharmacokinetics and toxicokinetics, 721, 721t
    pharmacology, 719, 720t
Esmolol
    for inhalant-related dysrhythmias, 1199
    and neuromuscular blockers, interactions, 1021t
    overdose/poisoning, clinical manifestations, 931–932
    pharmacokinetics, 930
    pharmacology, 927t
Esophageal carcinoma, after caustic injury, 1391
Esophageal dilation, 1394–1395
Esophageal injuries, caustic, 1389–1390, 1389f. *See also* Esophageal stricture(s)
    clinical manifestations, 1390
    diagnostic imaging, 1391, 1392f
    disposition of patients with, 1394
    endoscopic evaluation, 1390, 1390t, 1391
    evaluation, 1391
    grading, 1390, 1390t
        and disposition of patients, 1394
    management, 1390, 1390t
    predictors, 1391
    stricture formation with, 1390, 1390t, 1391
Esophageal malignancy, 293
Esophageal obstruction, 128
Esophageal perforation, 127–128
    imaging, 115t, 127–128, 129t
Esophageal stent/stenting, for caustic injury, 1390t, 1394
Esophageal stricture(s), 293
    caustic injury and, 1390, 1390t, 1391
    chronic treatment, 1394–1395
    diagnostic imaging, 115t, 127, 130f
Esophageal webs, 293
Esophagitis, xenobiotic-induced, 293, 293t
Esophagram, contrast, 127–128, 130f
Esophagus, 290–291
    ulcers, xenobiotic-induced, 293, 293t
Espand. *See* Syrian rue (*Peganum harmala*)
Essential (ethereal) oils, 627–637, 1380, 1410, 1597. *See also* Volatile oils; *specific oil*
    definition, 637
    history of, 637
    toxicity
        diagnostic tests for, 634
        treatment, 634–635
Esters, 1410. *See also* Hydrocarbons
Estradiol
    calcium phosphate nanoparticles, 1719t
    micellar nanoparticle, 1719t
Estradiol-levonorgestrel, as abortifacient, 303t
Estramustine, mechanism and site of action, 762f
Estrogen(s). *See also* Phytoestrogen(s)
    effect on thyroid hormones and function, 813f, 814t
    for female sexual dysfunction, 302
    and fibrinolysis, 323
    as glutamate scavenger, 229
    and male sexual dysfunction, 299f

pancreatitis caused by, 295t
plant, 641t
and sexual function, 298, 300
Eszopiclone, 1089. *See also* Sedative-hypnotics
    history of, 1084
    pharmacokinetics, 1085t
Etauine, 847
Ethacrynic acid, 963. *See also* Diuretics, loop
    and tinnitus, 369, 370t
Ethalfluralin, 1468t
Ethambutol, 856
    adverse effects and safety issues, 853t
    contraindications to, 853t, 856
    and gustatory dysfunction, 365
    for HIV-related infections, 830t
    mechanism of action, 856
    monitoring with, 853t
    ocular toxicity, 856
    ophthalmic toxicity, 356f
    pharmacokinetics, 856
    pharmacology, 856
    resistance to, 856
    structure, 856
    toxicity (overdose/poisoning)
        clinical manifestations, 36t, 856
        management, 856
Ethane, 1652
    chemistry, 165–166
    as simple asphyxiant, 400t
Ethanol (alcohol), 162, 1143–1156. *See also* Alcohol abuse and alcoholism; Alcoholic ketoacidosis (AKA); Antiseptics; Disulfiram
    absorption, 1144, 1149, 1440
    and acetaminophen, 480, 1146
    with activated charcoal, 77
    and adenosine, 231
    affinity for alcohol dehydrogenase, 1440
    agitation caused by, 385–386
    for alcohol dehydrogenase inhibition, 1428
    for alcohol withdrawal, 1169
    as antidote, 1440–1443
        vs. fomepizole, 1437, 1442
        adverse effects and safety issues, 1441
        dosage and administration, 1440–1441, 1441t–1442t
        ethanol tolerance and, 1440–1441, 1441t–1442t
        formulation and acquisition, 1442
        hemodialysis and, 1441, 1441t–1442t
        history of, 1440
        loading dose, 1440, 1441t–1442t
        mechanism of action, 1440
        monitoring with, 1440–1441
        pharmacokinetics, 1440–1441
        in pregnancy, 1441
    as antiseptic, 1368, 1369t
    Asian flush caused by, 273, 744, 1145
    availability and storage, 44t
    blood concentrations. *See* Blood alcohol (ethanol) concentration
    brain atrophy caused by, 132t
    and breast-feeding, 441, 1441
    breath odor, 1148, 1880
    breath testing for, 1149, 1872, 1877–1878
        devices for, 1878
        temperature and, 414
    chemistry, 164, 164f, 165–166, 1422
    childhood poisoning with, 1143
    with chloral hydrate (Mickey Finn), 8, 1085, 1085f, 1146
    chronic consumption
        and cardiomyopathy, 1274

and clinical assessment, 38
    cobalt and, 1274
    therapeutics for, 35t
clearance, 1145
clinical and laboratory findings with, 36t
as CNS depressant, 413, 1146–1147
and cocaine, reaction, 165, 165f, 1125, 1145
in cologne, 1143
in common products, 1143
content, of beverages, 1143, 1143t, 1879
and CYP enzymes, 1144–1145, 1145f, 1146, 1440
deaths caused by, 1165
for DEG poisoning, 1448
diabetes insipidus caused by, 195, 195t
dialysis and, 95
disease burden caused by, 1165
disulfiram-like reaction with, 1174, 1174t
dysrhythmias caused by, 1148
effect on thermoregulation, 413–414, 413t
effects on vital signs, 29t–31t
elimination, 1143t, 1144–1145, 1441, 1879
    first-order kinetics, 1145
    zero-order kinetics, 1145
enhanced elimination, 1149
and erectile dysfunction, 300
for ethylene glycol poisoning, 1441
    history of, 1440
and fatty acid metabolism, 179
and female sexual dysfunction, 302f
first-pass metabolism, antihistamines and, 744, 1144
and fomepizole, pharmacokinetic interactions, 1435
in food extracts/flavorings, 1143
and GABA receptors, 221, 236f, 237, 1096, 1146
and gluconeogenesis, 178, 179f
as glycine agonist, 223
in hand sanitizers, 1143, 1149
harmful effects, 1144
hepatic effects, 334
and hepatotoxicity of other xenobiotics, 329
history of, 1143–1144
hyperventilation caused by, 400t
hypoglycemia caused by, 698, 1150–1151
    in children, 453, 709
    hospitalization for, 702
hypomagnesemia caused by, 200, 877–878
hypoventilation caused by, 400t
impairment due to. *See* Ethanol-induced impairment
indications for, 35t, 44t
inebriation with, 1423
    acute clinical features, 1146–1148
    differential diagnosis, 1148
    habituation and, 1147–1148
    management, 1149
    signs and symptoms, 1148
infertility caused by, 297t, 298f
infusion, adverse effects, 1428
ingestion, estimation, 1879–1880
intoxication, 236f
    acute clinical features, 1146–1148
    diagnostic tests for, 1149
    disinhibition in, 1147
    and estimation of blood alcohol concentration, 1881–1882
    flumazenil for, 1094, 1096
    history of, 1876
    hospitalization for, indications for, 1150–1151
    management, 1149
    pathophysiology, 1146
intravenous administration, 1440–1441, 1441t

laboratory tests for, 36t, 101t, 102, 1149
and male sexual dysfunction, 299f
in mass suicide, 24
mechanism of action, 1440
metabolism, 38, 159, 168–169, 168f, 172, 175, 178–179, 1144–1146, 1145f, 1148f, 1422
for methanol poisoning, 1441
history of, 1440
millimole/milligram equivalent, 1440
in mouthwash, 1143, 1149
mushrooms and, 1587–1588, 1594
neuroadaptation and, 237
and neurotransmitter function, 1165
nicotinic receptor blockade by, 207
and NMDA receptors, 227t, 228, 236f, 237, 1146, 1165
and NSAIDs, interactions, 514t
odor, 364t, 1880
oral administration, 1440–1441, 1442t
pharmacokinetics, 1440
and osmol gap, 193
oxidative metabolism, 166, 166f, 1146
and oxidative stress, 1146
pancreatitis caused by, 295t
peak effect, in elderly, 461
pesticide coingestion with, 1490
pharmacokinetics, hypothermia and, 413–414
pharmacokinetics and toxicokinetics, 145t, 1144–1145, 1440–1441, 1879
pharmacology, 1440–1441
physicochemical properties, 1143t
plasma-to-whole blood ratios, 1877–1878
poikilothermic effect, 413
and potassium channels, 1194
in pregnancy, 437–438
pregnancy category, 1441
prenatal exposure to, detection, 1149
proof number, 1442
protective effect against ischemic heart disease, 1144
and respiratory depression, 386, 1149
and rhabdomyolysis, 393, 393t
sales, to intoxicated persons, 1882
saliva testing for, 1149
"sensible" or "responsible" drinking, 1144
serum, 1145. See also Blood alcohol (ethanol) concentration
assessment, in toxic alcohol poisoning, 1426
calculation, 1143t
and coma, 1147
dose of ethanol and, 1143t
in habitual drinkers, 1143t, 1145
habituation and, 1143t, 1147–1148
in inebriated patients, 1143t, 1145
interpretation, 1149
in occasional drinkers, 1143t, 1145
in tolerant drinkers, 1143t, 1145
serum-to-whole blood ratios, 1877
shortage, 43
for SMFA ingestion, 1534
10% solution
dosage and administration, 1440–1441, 1441t
formulation and acquisition, 1442
intravenous administration, 1441, 1441t
monitoring with, 1440
20% solution
formulation and acquisition, 1442
oral administration, 1441, 1442t
spectrochemical testing for, 103
standard drink of, 1143t
stocking, 43
recommended level, 44t

structure, 1440
supplies, 43
teratogenicity, 429t, 432, 437–438, 1441
and thiamine absorption, 1158
tolerance, 236f, 237, 1147, 1165, 1881
functional, 1147
metabolic, 1147
NMDA glutamate receptors in, 228, 236f
and thermoregulation, 414
for toxic alcohol poisoning, 1428
comparison with fomepizole, 1437, 1442
toxicity (overdose/poisoning), 166
diagnostic imaging in, 115t
extracorporeal therapies for, 91
and organ donation, 1893t
toxic syndrome caused by, 29t
transdermal absorption, 271
transplacental transfer, 1144
underage drinking and, 1880–1881
in vanilla extract, 1143
and violence, 385
vitreous, correlation with blood concentration, 1872
volume of distribution, 145t, 1143t, 1440
withdrawal. See Alcohol withdrawal
xenobiotic interactions with, 1145–1146, 1146t
Ethanol-induced impairment
assessment, 1876–1883
dram shop laws and, 1880–1881
history of, 1876
per se laws and, 1144, 1873, 1876–1878
standardized field sobriety tests for, 1878–1879, 1879t
Ethchlorvynol
ARDS caused by, 402t
odor, 1086t
overdose, clinical findings in, 1086t
Ether
abuse, 8
history of, 1011
Ethereal oils. See Essential (ethereal) oils
Ethers, 1410. See also Hydrocarbons
glycol, chemistry, 1422
Ethical code of conduct, 1802–1803, 1802t
Ethical considerations, in interventional studies, 1855
Ethionamide, 1488t
adverse effects and safety issues, 853t, 857
and cycloserine, interactions, 853t
monitoring with, 853t
pharmacokinetics, 857
pregnancy class, 857
structure, 857
for tuberculosis, 857
Ethisterone, teratogenicity, 430t
Ethosuximide, protein-binding characteristics, 110t
2-Ethoxyethanol, infertility caused by, 297t
Ethyl acetate, inhaled, 1193t
Ethyl alcohol. See Ethanol (alcohol)
Ethylbenzoylecgonine, 1125, 1145
Ethyl biscoumacetate, 885
Ethyl carbamate, 174t
Ethyl chloride, 1011
inhaled, 1193t
Ethylenediaminetetra-acetic acid (EDTA)
history of, 1315
and laboratory tests, 102
Ethylene dibromide, 174t, 1457
Ethylene glycol, 1444. See also Toxic alcohol(s)
affinity for alcohol dehydrogenase, 1440
antidote for, 35t
bioavailability, 1422
chemistry, 166, 1422

cranial neuropathy caused by, 346t
crystalluria caused by, 395
in DEG metabolism, 1444, 1445f
diagnostic tests for, 1425
effects on vital signs, 30t
elimination, 1422–1423, 1436
fomepizole and, 1436
enhanced elimination, 90
enzymatic assay for, 1425
extracorporeal elimination, 91f, 97t
focal brain lesions caused by, 131
gas chromatography and, 1870
and high anion gap metabolic acidosis, 191t
history of, 1421
hyperventilation caused by, 400t
hypocalcemia caused by, 199
calcium for, 1405
hypoventilation caused by, 400t
ingestion
epidemiology, 1421
sodium bicarbonate for, 568t, 571
inhalation, 1422
laboratory testing for, 101t, 103–104
metabolism, 165, 1422, 1423f, 1440
ethanol and, 1440
nephrotoxicity, 1424
neurotoxicity, 1424
and osmol gap, 193
pharmacokinetics, 146t
physicochemical properties, 1421t
serum, 1425
taste-aversive xenobiotics added to, 1782
toxicity (overdose/poisoning), 166
adjunctive therapy for, 1430
assay for, 1425
clinical manifestations, 36t, 1483
death in, 1425
end-organ manifestations, 1424–1425
extracorporeal therapies for, 91f, 97t
lactate concentration in, 1426–1427
magnesium and thiamine for, 878
management, 38, 44t–46t
metabolic acidosis in, 1423, 1426
and organ donation, 1893t
in pregnant women, 1430, 1441
pyridoxine for, 862–863
thiamine for, 1160–1161
urinalysis in, 192
urinary calcium oxalate crystals in, 1427
toxicokinetics/toxicodynamics, 1422–1423
transdermal exposure to, 1422
volume of distribution, 146t, 1422
Ethylene glycol butyl ether, 1422
Ethylene glycol methyl ether, 1422
Ethylene glycol monobutyl ether, fomepizole for, 1436
Ethylene oxide, 1369t, 1374, 1457
abortion caused by, 297t
carcinogenicity, 1374
detection threshold, 1654t
immediately dangerous to life and health (IDLH), 1654t
infertility caused by, 297t, 298f
and leukemia, 320
mutagenicity, 1374
regulatory standard for, 1654t
short-term exposure limit (STEL), 1654t
sources, 1654t
as sterilant, 1368
toxicity, 1374
water solubility, 1654t

Ethyl glucuronide, 1144, 1149
    urinary, and detection of ethanol use, 1149
Ethyl mercaptan, in natural gas, 1652
Ethylmercury, 689–690, 1324t. *See also* Mercury
    pharmacokinetics, 689
N-Ethylnorketamine (N-EK), 1211, 1211t, 1212
Ethylparabens, 685
Ethyl parathion, 1510
N-Ethyl-1-phenylcyclohexylamine. *See* Cyclohexamine
Ethyl sulfate, 1144, 1149
    urinary, and detection of ethanol use, 1149
Ethyl vinyl ether, 1011
Etidocaine. *See also* Local anesthetic(s)
    CNS toxicity, 998
    history of, 994
    minimal IV toxic dose, 998t
    pharmacology, 996t
    pharmacology of, 966t
Etilefrin hydrochloride, ingestion, endoscopic
        management, 64
Etodolac, pharmacology, 512t
Etomidate, 1018
    adverse effects and safety issues, 1090
    formulations, 1090
    and GABA receptors, 221, 1084
    indications for, 1090
    injection, propylene glycol in, 688
    mechanism of action, 221
    overdose, clinical findings in, 1086t
    pharmacokinetics, 1085t, 1090
    and propylene glycol, 687t, 1090
    structure, 1090
Etoposide, 504, 760t, 1612. *See also* Podophyllin
    benzyl alcohol in, 683t
    extravasation, 802
    injection, polyethylene glycol (PEG) in, 686t
    mechanism and site of action, 762f
    pharmacology, 504
Etravirine, 831
Etretinate, teratogenicity, 428, 430t
Eubacterium lentum, and digoxin metabolism, 970
Eucalyptol, 630, 1600t
Eucalyptus spp. (eucalyptus), 1600t
Eucalyptus citriodora, 1524
Eucalyptus globulus, 630
Eucalyptus globus (eucalyptus), 1600t
Eucalyptus oil, 630
Eugenia aromatica (clove), 629
Eugenol, 629–630, 641t, 650t
    toxicity, *N*-acetylcysteine for, 494
Euglycemia, maintaining, after initial control of
        hypoglycemia, 701–702
Eupatorium perfoliatum (boneset), 640t
Eupatorium rugosum. See White snakeroot (*Ageratina
        altissima*)
Euphorbia spp. (poinsettia), 1600t
Euphorbiaceae, 1598t–1602t, 1609, 1613
Euphorbia lacteal (candelabra cactus), 1613
Euphorbia pulcherrima (poinsettia), 1600t, 1613–1614
Euphorbia splendens (crown of thorns), 1613
Euphorbia tirucalli (pencil tree), 1613
Euphoria
    inhalant-induced, 1196
    opioid-induced, 521
Euphorics, 7
Europe, poison control center movement in, 11, 11t
European Association for Poison Control Centers
        (EAPCC), 11, 11t
European elderberry (*Sambucus nigra*), 1607
European mandrake (*Mandragora officinarum*), 1601t

European mistletoe (*Viscum album*), 1603t, 1609
European mountain ash (*Sorbus aucuparia*), 688
European stinging anemone (*Anemonia sulcata*), 1567t
    stings, clinical manifestations, 1569
European viper, venom, 6
European weeverfish (*Trachinus*), 1576
European widow spider (*Latrodectus tredecimguttatus*),
        1540–1541, 1542t, 1543, 1559
European willow (*Salix alba*), 644t
Europium, chelator for, 1780
Eurycoma longifolia Jack, as aphrodisiac, 304
Eustrongyloides anisakis (roundworms), 600
Evacuants, 83. *See also* Whole-bowel irrigation (WBI)
    with activated charcoal, 77
Evaporation, 411
Eve. *See* 3,4-Methylenedioxyethamphetamine (MDEA,
        Eve)
Evening primrose (*Oenothera biennis*), 641t
Evidence, quality of, grading, 1852, 1852t
Evidence-based medicine, 33
Evidential breath testers (EBTs), 1878
e-waste, 1847
Exanthem, in drug-induced hypersensitivity syndrome,
        277
Exchange resins, cationic, and potassium balance, 199
Exchange transfusion, 38
    in children, 98, 452
        for iron poisoning, 674
    for copper poisoning, 1289
    in herbicide poisoning, 1473
    indications for, 98
    in infants, 98
    for iron poisoning in children, 674
    in neonates, 98
        of blood-exposed mothers, 1305
    plasma protein binding and, 147
    volume of distribution and, 147
    xenobiotics amenable to, 98
Excipients, 681. *See also* Pharmaceutical additives
    FDA and, 681
    functions, 681
    generally recognized as safe (GRAS), 681
    potential systemic toxicity, 681, 681t
Excitants, 7
Excitation-contraction coupling, skeletal muscle, 1018,
        1019f
Excitatory amino acid (EAA) neurotransmitters, 340, 342
Excitatory amino acid transporters (EAATs), 204, 225,
        226f, 228
    EAAT3, opioids and, 238
Excitotoxicity, 341–342
Excretion. *See also specific xenobiotic*
    organs involved in, 147
    renal, 148, 148t
    of xenobiotics, 147–148
Exenatide, 607t, 1619. *See also* Dieting xenobiotics and
        regimens
    history of, 694
    overdose/poisoning, hypoglycemia caused by, 700
    pharmacokinetics and toxicokinetics, 696, 697t
    pharmacology, 696
Exendins, in helodermatid venom, 1619
Exfoliative dermatitis, xenobiotics in, 278
Exothermic reaction, 271
Expectorants, 738
Experimental study(ies). *See also* Clinical trials
    design, 1853–1854
Exposure
    route of, and toxicity, 167
    time of, in radiation protection, 1765

Extended-release formulation, and gastrointestinal
        absorption, 143
Extensive metabolizer, 170
Extracellular fluid (ECF), 93, 389
    and hemofiltration, 97
    volume, 189
        and hyponatremia, 196
    volume overload, 93
Extracellular matrix, 310
Extracorporeal albumin dialysis, for amanitin
        poisoning, 1586
Extracorporeal life support (ECLS)
    for β-adrenergic antagonist toxicity, 935
    for cyclic antidepressant toxicity, 1049t, 1050
    for local anesthetic toxicity, 1000–1001
    for zinc chloride inhalational toxicity, 1365
Extracorporeal membrane oxygenation (ECMO)
    for ARDS, 401
    for calcium channel blocker toxicity, 950
    for cyclic antidepressant toxicity, 1049t, 1050
    for smoke inhalation, 1645
    venoarterial
        for aluminum phosphide poisoning, 1460
        for β-adrenergic antagonist toxicity, 935
        for local anesthetic cardiotoxicity, 1001
Extracorporeal treatment(s) (ECTRs), 90, 90t. *See also*
        Elimination, enhanced; *specific therapy*
    algorithm for, 98f
    annual reported use of, 90, 90t
    for cardioactive steroid toxicity, 975
    case reporting, improving, 92
    of chromium toxicity, 1271
    clinical effects, 92
    for glufosinate poisoning, 1479
    indications for, 90–91
    and laboratory test results, 153
    for lithium toxicity, 1070–1071
    for methotrexate toxicity, 770–771
    for methylxanthine toxicity, 991–992, 992t
    for monoamine oxidase inhibitor toxicity, 1081
    for paraquat poisoning, 1477
    pharmacokinetics and, 91
    recommendations for, 90
    for selenium toxicity, 1342
    for thallium poisoning, 1354
    for thyroid hormone overdose and thyroid storm,
        817–818
    toxicokinetics and, 91
    volume of distribution and, 91, 147
    xenobiotics cleared by, 90, 91f
        characteristics, 91–92, 97t
Extracorporeal Treatments in Poisoning (EXTRIP),
        guidelines for methanol poisoning, 1429,
        1429t
Extraction ratio (ER), 95
Extraocular muscles, examination, 356
Extrapyramidal symptoms, 214, 218
    cyclic antidepressant overdose and, 1047
Extrapyramidal syndromes (EPS), 1032, 1036–1037, 1037t
Extravasation, xenobiotic, 802–804
    antidotal therapy for, 803
    associated factors, 802
    chemotherapeutics and, 762
    in children, 802
    clinical manifestations, 802
    management, 802–803, 803t
    outcomes, factors affecting, 802
    prevention, 802
    of radiocontrast agents
        diagnostic imaging, 119, 121f

prevention, 119
treatment, 119
risk factors for, 802
Extremity(ies), examination, 38
Extrinsic allergic alveolitis, 1659
Extrinsic pathway, 320, 321f, 883, 884f, 897
Eye(s), 356–362. *See also* Pupil(s)
anatomy, 356, 356f
chemical injury, 358
direct toxins, 358–360
examination, 356
illicit drug use and, 361
injury
Ballen classification, 360
caustic
clinical manifestations, 1390
management, 1395
disposition of patient with, 360
in fire victims, 1646–1647
hydrofluoric acid and, 1398
Roper-Hall modification of Ballen classification, 360
irrigation, 39–40, 72–73
aqueous solutions for, 358
for caustic exposure, 1395
duration of, 359, 359t
exposure-specific solutions for, 358–359, 359t
for hydrofluoric acid exposure, 1400
nanoparticles in, 1721f, 1730
in paraquat poisoning, 1475
pH
normal, 1395
testing, 1395
pH check, 39–40, 73, 1395
toxic exposures, 39–40
from nonophthalmic xenobiotics, 360–361, 361t
urticating hairs of tarantula and, 1547–1548
xenobiotic exposure, classic findings in, 357t
Eye drops, systemic toxicity with, 360
Eyelash viper (*Bothriechis* spp.), 1636t
Eye movement, abnormalities, 358
nonophthalmic xenobiotics causing, 361
Ezogabine, 721–722
adverse effects and safety issues, 722, 727t
drug interactions with, 723t
metabolism and effects on CYP enzymes, 722t
pharmacokinetics and toxicokinetics, 721t
pharmacology, 719, 720t

F
Fabaceae, 1598t–1603t, 1605
Fabric softener, 1389
Facial edema
arsenic trioxide and, 1243
in drug-induced hypersensitivity syndrome, 277
Facial grimacing, antipsychotic-induced, 1036
Facial nerve, palsy, unilateral, in arsenic poisoning, 1241
Facial trismus, in strychnine poisoning, 1536–1537
Facies latrodectismica, 1543
Facilitated exchange diffusion, 211
Facilitated transport, 141–142, 141f, 142
Factor II, 884f, 885, 885f
pharmacokinetics, after prothrombin complex concentrate administration, 908, 909t
in prothrombin complex concentrate, 908, 908t
Factor V, 883–884, 884f, 885, 1285t
Factor VII, 320, 884f, 885, 885f
activated, 897
antibodies to, 885

pharmacokinetics, after prothrombin complex concentrate administration, 908, 909t
in prothrombin complex concentrate, 908, 908t
Factor VIII, 883–884, 884f, 885, 900
activated, intrinsic tenase complex with, 320
antibodies to, 885
Factor IX, 320, 883–884, 884f, 885, 885f, 897
pharmacokinetics, after prothrombin complex concentrate administration, 908, 909t
in prothrombin complex concentrate, 908, 908t
Factor X, 320, 883–884, 884f, 885, 885f, 890
activated (Xa), 883–884, 884f. *See also* Factor Xa inhibitors
recombinant human, 908
activation, 883
pharmacokinetics, after prothrombin complex concentrate administration, 908, 909t
in prothrombin complex concentrate, 908, 908t
Factor XI, 885
antibodies to, 885
Factor XII (Hageman factor), 883, 885
Factor XIII, 884f
antibodies to, 885
Factor VIIa, recombinant, 911
Factor eight inhibitor bypassing activity (FEIBA), 887, 894, 910
Factor Xa inhibitors, 321f, 883, 908
antidote for, 895–896
bleeding with, 895
coagulopathy caused by, treatment, 895–896
laboratory investigation and, 895
overdose/poisoning
clinical manifestations, 895
gastrointestinal decontamination for, 78, 895
pharmacokinetics, 895–896
pharmacology, 894–895
reversal agent for, 896, 912–913
Factory and Workshop Act (1895), 23
FADH, 173f
FAERS (FDA Adverse Event Reporting System), 1836–1837
Failure mode and effect analysis (FMEA), 1827
Fairy cap. *See* Foxglove (*Digitalis* spp.)
Fairy finger. *See* Foxglove (*Digitalis* spp.)
Fall crocus (*Colchicum autumnale*), uses and toxicities, 640t
Falls, in elderly, 460
False hellebore, 1603t
Famciclovir, 829
Family Smoking Prevention and Tobacco Control Act (2009), 10t, 1205–1206
Famotidine
absorption, 744
elimination, 744
metabolism, 744
overdose/poisoning, 746
pharmacokinetics and toxicokinetics, 745t
structure, 742, 742f
volume of distribution, 744
Fanconi anemia, 311
Fanconilike syndrome
lead-induced, 1298
salicylates and, 558
Fanconi syndrome, tetracyclines and, 827
Fangchi (*Aristolochia fangji*), uses and toxicities, 640t
Farmer's lung, 125, 125t, 1659
Faroe Islands, methylmercury exposure studies in, 1328
Fasciculations, methylxanthine-induced, 989, 991
Fast on–fast off kinetics, 999
Fast on–slow off kinetics, 999

Fat absorption blockers, 611. *See also* Dieting xenobiotics and regimens
Fatal poisonings. *See also* Death(s); *specific xenobiotic*
data collection on, 1791
Fat emulsion. *See* Lipid emulsion
Fat overload syndrome, 1007
Fatty acid ethyl esters, 1144, 1149
Fatty acid metabolism, 178–179, 1148f, 1150
inhibitors, 176t
Fava beans, 1603t, 1607
and glucose-6-phosphate dehydrogenase deficiency, 318
Favism, 1607
Fazekas, Suzanne, 5t
FDA. *See* Food and Drug Administration (FDA)
FDA Adverse Event Reporting System (FAERS), 728, 1836–1837
FDA Modernization Act (1997), 10t, 1834
FD&C #1 dye, clinical and laboratory findings with, 36t
Fear-arousal cycle, 1814
Fea's viper (*Azemiops feae*), 1633t
Feather, as emetic device, 3
Featherfew. *See* Feverfew (*Tanacetum parthenium*)
Featherfoil. *See* Feverfew (*Tanacetum parthenium*)
Feather hydroid, 1569
Febrifuge plant. *See* Feverfew (*Tanacetum parthenium*)
Fecal impaction, xenobiotic-induced, in elderly, 463, 463t
Federal Anti-Tampering Act (1983), 10t
Federal Bureau of Investigation (FBI), contact information, 1743t
Federal Caustic Poison Act (1927), 9, 10t
Federal Emergency Management Agency (FEMA), 1806
Federal Hazardous Substances Labeling Act (1960), 10t, 11
Federal Insecticide, Fungicide, and Rodenticide Act (FIFRA), 10t, 1450, 1525
and nanotechnology, 1731–1733
Feeding tubes, for caustic injury, 1394
Felbamate
aplastic anemia caused by, 1837
history of, 719
mechanism of action, 222, 227t, 228
Felodipine, pharmacokinetics, 946t
Felon herb (*Artemisia* spp.), 643t
Fenamic acid(s), pharmacology, 512t
Fenchone, 641t
Fenfluramine, 606, 608t, 611, 816
cardiotoxicity, 21
overdose/poisoning, whole-bowel irrigation for, 85
and phentermine, combined, safety problems with, 1841
Fenfluramine-phentermine (Fen-Phen), adverse effects and side effects, 21
Fenitrothion, 1509–1510
Fenobam, 227t
Fenobucarb, 1489
Fenofibrate, nanocrystal, 1719t
Fenoldopam, effect on dopamine receptors, 214
Fenoprofen, pharmacology, 512t
Fenoxaprop-*P*-ethyl, 1471
Fen-phen, safety problems with, 1841
Fenpropathrin, 1519, 1520t
Fentanyl, 519, 528–529, 539. *See also* Opioid(s)
characteristics, 526t
and chest wall rigidity, 400
deaths caused by, 21t, 22, 519
immunoassays for, 112
respiratory effects, 399t

Fentanyl (*Cont.*):
  and serotonin toxicity, 1058t
  structure, 529, 529f
  toxicity, in illicit drug users, 21t, 22
  transdermal patch, ingestion, whole-bowel irrigation
      for, 85
Fentanyl analogs, 528–529
  characteristics, 526t
  deaths from, 21t, 22
  structure, 529, 529f
Fentanyl derivative(s)
  as incapacitating agent, 1750
  opioid antagonists and, 541
Fenthion, 1488t, 1509–1510
  pharmacokinetics and toxicokinetics, 1488
  poisoning
      atropine for, 1505
      clinical manifestations, 1490–1491
Fenthion EC50, toxicity, 1490
Fenton reaction, 157, 157f, 160, 670, 1285, 1285f
  manganese and, 1320
Fenugreek (*Trigonella foenumgraecum*), 641t
Fenvalerate, 1519, 1520t. *See also* Pyrethroids
  elimination, 1521
  structure, 1520f
Fer-de-lance (*Bothrops asper*), 1636t
  antivenom, 1627t, 1628–1631
Fern, bracken (*Pteridium* spp.), 1602t
Ferric carboxymaltose, 670t
Ferric chloride (FeCl₃), 669
Ferric gluconate, 670, 670t
Ferric hydroxide, 670
Ferrihemoglobin, 316
Ferrioxamine, 672, 674, 676, 676f
  pharmacokinetics and pharmacodynamics, 677
Ferritin, 160, 315, 315f
Ferroportin, 315, 315f
Ferrous chloride, 670t
Ferrous fumarate, 669, 670t
Ferrous gluconate, 669, 670t
Ferrous lactate, 670t
Ferrous sulfate, 669, 670t
  effect on thyroid hormones and function, 814t
  infant drops, sorbitol in, 688t
  ingestion, 127
      diagnostic imaging, 114–116, 116f
Ferroxidase, 1284, 1285t
Fertility
  female, 302–304
      xenobiotics affecting, 297t
  male, 297–302
      xenobiotics affecting, 297t, 298f
Ferucarbotran, SPIO nanoparticles, 1719t
Ferumoxide, SPIO nanoparticles, 1719t
Ferumoxsil, SPIO nanoparticles, 1719t
Ferumoxtran-10, SPIO nanoparticles, 1719t
Ferumoxytol, 670t
  SPIO nanoparticles, 1719t
Fetal alcohol spectrum disorders (FASD), 438
Fetal alcohol syndrome (FAS), 432, 438, 1198, 1441
  partial, 438
Fetal death, xenobiotics and, 432–433
Fetal solvent syndrome (FSS), 1198
Fetid nightshade (henbane, *Hyoscyamus niger*)
  Theophrastus on, 2
  use and toxicity, 642t
Fetus
  death, xenobiotics and, 432–433
  xenobiotic exposure, 428
  xenobiotic transfer to, placental regulation, 431–432

Fever, 30, 122. *See also specific xenobiotic*
  in arsenic poisoning, 1241
  tarantula bites and, 1547
Feverfew (*Tanacetum parthenium*), 641t
Fever tree. *See Cinchona* spp.
Feverwort (*Eupatorium perfoliatum*), 640t
Fexofenadine
  dose modification in liver or kidney disease, 744
  history of, 739
  metabolism, 743
  pharmacokinetics and toxicokinetics, 745t
  pharmacology, 742
  structure, 740f
  toxicity, clinical manifestations, 744
Feynman, Richard, 1717
Fiber(s), dietary, 611
Fibrates, and colchicine, interactions, 502
Fibrin, 883
Fibrinogen, 883
Fibrinogen concentration, 320–322
Fibrinolysis, 322
  xenobiotic-induced defects in, 322–323, 322t
  xenobiotics and, 322, 322t
Fibrinolytic pathways, 321f, 884, 884f
Fibrinolytics, 896–897
  adverse effects and safety issues, 897
  antidotes and treatment strategies for, 888t, 897
  contraindications to, 897
  hemorrhagic complications, 897
      treatment, 897
  laboratory testing for, 888t
Fibrosis
  hepatic, 328, 331t, 333, 334t
  retroperitoneal, xenobiotic-induced, 394, 394t
Fick's law of diffusion, 141, 569
Fidaxomicin, 826–827
Fiddleback spider. *See* Brown recluse spider
      (*Loxosceles reclusa*)
Fiddlehead fern. *See* Ostrich fern (*Matteuccia
      struthipteris*)
Field sobriety tests, standardized, 1878–1879, 1879t
Filtration, 142
Final Exit, 24
Finasteride
  as androgen receptor blocker, 299f
  and doping analysis, 623
Fingernails. *See* Nail(s)
FiO₂, 399, 405
  decreased, 399–400
      clinical findings associated with, 1651, 1651t
  in mechanical ventilation, 407
Fire(s)
  carbon monoxide poisoning from, 16, 16t
  deaths related to, epidemiology, 1640
  enclosed-space, 1640
  incidence, in United States, 1640
  injuries caused by, 1640
  victims, management, 1646
Fire ants, 1551–1552
  bites, and rhabdomyolysis, 393
  envenomation (stings)
      clinical manifestations, 1552
      large local reactions to, 1552
      local reactions to, 1552
      pathophysiology, 1552
      systemic reactions to, 1552
  imported, in United States, 1552
  venom, composition, 1551t, 1552
Fire coral (*Millepora alcicornis*), 1567, 1567t
  envenomation, clinical manifestations, 1569

Fire-eater's lung, 1652
Firefighters, antimony toxicity in, 1229–1230
Fire-retardant materials, thermal degradation
      products, 1641t
Fire sponge (*Tedania ignis*), 1573–1574
Fireworks, phosphorus in, 1528
First-order reactions, 149–151, 150f, 151t
First-pass effect, 140, 144
First-pass metabolism, 143f
  CYP enzymes in, 169, 172
  gastric bypass and, 148
First responders
  at awareness level, training and responsibilities,
      1811
  at operational level, training and responsibilities,
      1811
Fish
  mercury in, 18t, 19, 1328, 1815
  odor, 364t
  spiny, 1576, 1576f, 1576t
      toxins from, 1577
      wounds from, management, 1578
  venomous, 1576–1578, 1576f, 1576t
Fish health advisories, 1815
Fish-liver oils, vitamin A in, 654–655
Fish odor syndrome, 365
Fish tapeworms (*Diphyllobothrium*), 600
Fixed drug eruptions, 276–277, 277f, 1086
  bullous, 277
  generalized, 277
Fixed oils, 645
Flag root (*Acorus calamus*), 1598t
Flame ionization detector (FID), 106
Flamprop, in herbicides, 1467t
Flannel moth caterpillar (*Megalopyge crispata*),
      1552
Flatulence, with whole-bowel irrigation, 85
Flavin adenine dinucleotide (FADH₂), 175, 177
Flavin monoxygenase, 168
Flavokwain A and B, 643t
Flavonoids, 643t, 1597
Flecainide, 865, 871
  adverse effects and safety issues, 866t, 871
  pharmacokinetics, 866t
  pharmacology, 866t
  and prolonged QT interval, 256
  toxicity (overdose/poisoning)
      ECG changes in, 250
      lipid emulsion for, 1006
      magnesium for, 878
      sodium bicarbonate for, 568t
Fleckenstein, Albrecht, 945
Flibanserin, 217
  contraindications, 302
  for hypoactive sexual desire disorder, 302
Flint, Michigan, water quality in, risk communication
      and, 1816
Flour, for dermal decontamination, 72
Flow cytometry, 900
Floxacillin, cholestasis caused by, 330
Floxuridine, 771
Fluchloralin, 1468t
Flucloxacillin, hepatic effects, HLA and, 329
Fluconazole, 829
  dosage and administration, renal replacement
      therapy and, 390
  for HIV-related infections, 830t
  and prolonged QT interval, 253t
  structure, 829
  teratogenicity, 429t

Flucythrinate, 1520t. *See also* Pyrethroids

Flucytosine, for HIV-related infections, 830t

Fludarabine
  adverse effects and safety issues, 760t
  mechanism and site of action, 762f

Flufenacet, in herbicides, 1467t

Fluid abnormalities, 194. *See also* Hypovolemia

Fluid balance
  abnormalities, 194. *See also* Hypernatremia;
      Hyponatremia
  factors affecting, 194

Fluid challenge, 37

Fluid loss(es), 189, 194
  chemotherapeutic-related, 764
  and hypernatremia, 195, 195t

Fluindione, and colchicine, interactions, 502

Flumazenil, 1094–1098
  adverse effects and safety issues, 1087, 1096–1097
  availability and storage, 44t
  for benzodiazepine overdose, 1088, 1094–1098,
      1095t, 1790
  in conscious sedation, 1094–1095
  contraindications to, 1051, 1096–1097, 1097t, 1790
  dosage and administration, 1097
  drug interactions with, 222
  for ethanol intoxication, 1094, 1096
  formulation, 1097
  and GABA receptor, 1094
  for hepatic encephalopathy, 334, 1094–1096
  history of, 1094
  indications for, 35t, 44t, 1087, 1094
  injection, parabens in, 685t
  mechanism of action, 222, 231, 1094
  for oral hypnotic toxicity, 1089
  for paradoxical reactions to benzodiazepines,
      1095, 1139
  for paradoxical reactions to midazolam, 1095
  pharmacodynamics, 1094, 1095t
  pharmacokinetics, 1088, 1094, 1095t
  pharmacology, 1094
  physicochemical properties, 1094, 1095t
  precautions with, 1088
  in pregnancy and lactation, 1097
  stocking, recommended level, 44t
  structure, 1094
  supplies, 42

Flumetsulam, in herbicides, 1467t

Flunisolide nasal spray, benzalkonium chloride in,
    682

Flunitrazepam, 466. *See also* Benzodiazepine(s);
    Sedative-hypnotics
  pharmacokinetics, 1085t

Fluopropanate, 1468t

Fluorescein, in antifreeze, 1427

Fluorescence polarization immunoassay (FPIA),
    for ethanol, 1877

Fluoride
  chemistry, 164
  and discoloration of teeth and gums, 293t
  enhanced elimination, urine alkalinization for, 93
  food contamination with, 599–600
  hypocalcemia caused by, 199, 199t, 1398, 1405
  serum, 1398
  toxicity (poisoning), 1397
    hyperkalemia caused by, 251
    management, 44t, 1405
    sodium bicarbonate for, 568t

Fluoride ions
  decontamination, in acidic environment, 73
  volume of distribution, 91

Fluoride-releasing xenobiotics, exposure, magnesium
    for, 879

Fluorides (fluoride salts)
  antidote for, 35t
  extracorporeal elimination, 97t

Fluorinated resins, thermal degradation products,
    1641t

Fluorine, 158
  physicochemical properties, 1397

Fluoroacetamide (compound 1081), 1450
  chemical structure, 1533, 1533f
  and citric acid cycle, 175
  history of, 1533
  poisoning
    clinical manifestations, 1533
    diagnostic tests for, 1534
    pathophysiology, 1533
    treatment, 1534
  toxicokinetics and toxicodynamics, 1533
  uses, 1533

Fluoroacetate, 763
  and citric acid cycle, 176t
  metabolism, 168, 173
  site of action, 173f

Fluoroacetyl CoA (FAcCoA), 175

Fluorocarbons, inhaled, 1193t

Fluorocitrate, 168, 175–177, 1533–1534

Fluorodeoxyuridine monophosphate (5-FdUMP), 789

Fluoroglycofen, 1468t

Fluorometers, 106

Fluorophosphates, 1487, 1488t

Fluoropyrimidine(s), 767. *See also* Capecitabine;
      Floxuridine; 5-Fluorouracil; Tegafur
  indications for, 771
  toxicity, 771
    clinical manifestations, 790
    uridine triacetate for, 789–791

Fluoroquinolones
  acute interstitial nephritis caused by, 394t
  and acute kidney injury, 826
  adverse effects with therapeutic use, 826
  effects on bone and cartilage, 826
  and GABA receptor, 222, 826
  hepatotoxicity, 826
  mechanism of action, 822t, 826
  overdose, 822t, 826
  and pregnancy outcomes, 826
  and prolonged QT interval, 253t
  renal effects, 390f
  and seizures, 826
  structure, 826
  and tendon rupture, 826
  toxicity, 822t

Fluoroscope, 1762

Fluoroscopy, radiation exposure in, 1766

Fluorosis, skeletal, imaging, 115t, 119, 122t, 123f

5-Fluorouracil
  adverse effects and safety issues, 760t, 762
  antidote for, 35t, 764, 772
  cardiovascular toxicity, 762–763, 763t
  diagnostic tests for, 763
  efficacy, (6R)-5,10-methylene-THF and, 776
  as local irritant, 802
  mechanism and site of action, 173, 762f
  nail changes caused by, 282
  neurotoxicity, 763
  pharmacology, 771
  structure, 771
  toxicity (overdose/poisoning), 760t
    clinical manifestations, 772

diagnostic tests for, 772
genetic polymorphisms and, 759, 771
leucovorin and, 775
management, 46t, 772
pathophysiology, 771–772
sex differences in, 759
uridine triacetate for, 789–791
transport in body, 142

Fluorouracil prodrugs, toxicity, uridine triacetate for,
    789–791

Fluorouridine triphosphate (FUTP), 789–790

Fluoxetine, 218, 1054
  CYP enzymes and, 169–170, 1055t, 1056
  and CYP induction, 171
  and MAOI, 1077
  mechanism of action, 204, 228, 1056f
  metabolite, 1055t, 1058
  pharmacokinetics, 1055t
  receptor activity, 1057t
  seizures caused by, 1057t
  structure, 1054f
  toxicity (overdose/poisoning)
    gastrointestinal decontamination for, 86
    sodium bicarbonate for, 568t, 569

Flupentixol. *See also* Antipsychotics
  dosage and administration, 1033t
  pharmacokinetics, 1033t

Fluphenazine. *See also* Antipsychotics
  clinical and toxicologic effects, 1034t
  dosage and administration, 1033t
  pharmacokinetics, 1033t

Flurazepam. *See also* Benzodiazepine(s);
    Sedative-hypnotics
  pharmacokinetics, 1085t
  structure, 1139, 1139f
  suicide with, 466

Flurbiprofen
  hematologic effects, 516
  pharmacology, 512t

Fluroxene, 1011

Flushing
  with *N*-acetylcysteine, 495
  clinical significance, 273
  food toxins and, 600t
  menopausal, 273
  niacin-induced, 664
  nontoxicologic causes, 273
  physiology, 273
  in toxidromes, 29t
  xenobiotics causing, 273

Flutamide, as androgen receptor blocker, 299f

Fluticasone, benzalkonium chloride in, 682

Fluvalinate, 1519, 1520t. *See also* Pyrethroids

Fluvastatin, CYP enzymes and, 170

Fluvoxamine, 1054
  and CYPs, 1055t, 1056
  mechanism of action, 1056f
  pharmacokinetics, 1055t
  receptor activity, 1057t
  seizures caused by, 1057t
  structure, 1054f

Flux coupling, 707

Fly agaric (*Amanita muscaria*), 3

Flying saucers. *See* Morning glory

Foeniculum vulgare (fennel), 641t

Folate(s), 775–781. *See also* Folic acid; Leucovorin
    (folinic acid)
  absorption, gastric bypass and, 148
  for arsenic toxicity, 777
  biochemistry, 775

Folate(s) (*Cont.*):
  deficiency
    and arsenic toxicity, 777
    and megaloblastic anemia, 318–319
  definition, 775
  dietary, 776
  for dihydrofolate reductase inhibitor toxicity, 777
  and formate clearance, 1429
  glucarpidase activity and, 782, 783f
  for methanol poisoning, 775, 1429, 1436
  for methanol toxicity, 776–777
  pharmacology, 775
  supplementation, for arsenic exposure, 777
  in toxic alcohol poisoning, 1429–1430
Folate antagonist(s), 759
Folate inhibitors, for malaria, 836
Folic acid, 654, 775–781
  adverse effects and safety issues with, 777
  and arsenic elimination, 775
  deficiency, teratogenicity, 433
  formulation and acquisition, 779
  history of, 775
  for methanol toxicity, 779
  pharmacology, 775
  in pregnancy and lactation, 777
  structure, 775
  supplementation
    in alcoholic patients, 1167
    for arsenic exposure, 777
    in pregnancy, 433
  supplies, 42
Folinic acid (leucovorin). *See* Leucovorin (folinic acid)
Folk medicine, lead exposure in, 1293, 1304
Follicle-stimulating hormone (FSH), 297–298, 302
Follow-up, of medication, and errors, 1825t, 1826
Fomepizole, 1435–1439
  adverse effects and safety issues, 1437
  for alcohol dehydrogenase inhibition, 1428, 1435, 1440
  for aldehyde dehydrogenase inhibition by coprine-containing mushrooms, 1588
  availability and storage, 45t
  and breast-feeding, 1437
  for butoxyethanol overdose, 1437
  chemistry, 1435
  for DEG poisoning, 1447–1448
  dialysis and, 95
  for diethylene glycol toxicity, 1436–1437
  for disulfiram-ethanol reaction, 1174, 1435–1436
  dosage and administration, 1428, 1437–1438
    kidney function and, 1437–1438
  and ethanol, pharmacokinetic interactions, 1436
  for ethylene glycol monobutyl ether overdose, 1437
  for ethylene glycol poisoning, 1428, 1435–1436
    vs. ethanol, 1437
  formulation, 1438
  hemodialysis clearance, 1436
  history of, 1435
  indications for, 35t, 45t, 193
  inhibition of DEG metabolism, 1444–1446
  LD_{50}, 1437
  mechanism of action, 1174, 1428, 1435
  for methanol poisoning, 1428, 1435–1436
    vs. ethanol, 1437
  pharmacokinetics, 1435–1436
  pharmacology, 1435–1436
  in pregnancy and lactation, 1437
  stocking, 43
    recommended level, 45t
  structure, 1435

supplies, 43
  for toxic alcohol poisoning, 1428
    vs. ethanol, 1437, 1442
Fondaparinux, 321f, 884f
  coagulopathy caused by, management, 896
  dosage and administration, 896
  laboratory testing for, 888t
  overdose/poisoning, treatment strategies for, 888t
  pharmacokinetics, 896
Fontana, Felice, 4t, 6
Food, Drug, and Cosmetic Act (1938), 9, 10t, 19, 453, 1833
Food, irradiation of, 1765
Food additives
  anaphylaxis from, 601
  illegal, 601–602
Food and Drug Administration (FDA), 9, 10t. *See also* FDA Modernization Act (1997)
  Adverse Event Reporting System (FAERS), 728
  advisory committees, 1836
  Animal Rule, 1834
  Dear Doctor letters, 1839
  and dietary supplements, 638–639
  drugs approved by, federal preemption status and, 1839–1840
  and excipients, 681
  Investigational New Drug (IND) application, for exotic snake antivenom, 1634–1635
  and nanotechnology, 1731
  and new drug applications, 1836. *See also* New drug application (NDA)
  nonprescription monograph rule, 738
  pregnancy classification scheme, 431
  review and approval of drugs, 1833–1835
  thorough QT study (TQT) requirement, 1840
Food and Drug Administration Amendments Act (FDAAA) of 2007, 1834–1835
Food and Drug Administration Safety and Innovation Act (2012), 43, 1834
Foodborne illness. *See also* Food poisoning
  causes, 592, 592t
  epidemiology, 597, 598t
  food additives and, 601–602
  incubation period, 597, 597t
  marine, prevention, 596
  and multiorgan system dysfunction, 598–599
  mushroom-induced, 600
  with neurologic symptoms, 592–596, 593t
    differential diagnosis, 592, 593t
  onset, 597, 597t
  plant-related, 602
  prevention, 602
  vegetable-related, 602
  xenobiotic-related, 599–600
Food disasters, 18–19, 18t
Food poisoning, 592–605
  bacteriology, 592, 592t
  and bioterrorism, 602
  clinical manifestations, 577t
  with diarrhea, 596–598, 597t
  epidemiology, 592, 592t
  history of, 592
  parasite-associated, 592, 592t
  steatosis caused by, 332
  viral, 592, 592t
Food Safety Modernization Act (2010), 639
Foreign body(ies)
  in gastrointestinal tract, 295
  ingested. *See also* Body packers; Body stuffers
    diagnostic imaging, 128, 129t
  in stomach, 295

Foreign materials, embolization to eye, 361t
Forensic interpretive toxicology, 1868–1875, 1884
Forensic pathologists, inforation used by, 1884, 1884t
Forensic toxicology, father of, 7
Formaldehyde, 1369t, 1388t, 1457
  as carcinogen, 1373
  chemistry, 168
  detection threshold, 1654t
  as disinfectant, 1368, 1372–1373
  immediately dangerous to life and health (IDLH), 1654t
  off-gassing, in FEMA trailers, 1373
  and olfactory dysfunction, 364
  poisoning, clinical manifestations, 1483
  regulatory standard for, 1654t
  short-term exposure limit (STEL), 1654t
  sources, 1654t
  as thermal degradation product, 1641t
  water solubility, 1654t
Formalin, 1369t, 1372–1373
Formate
  clearance, 1429–1430
    by hemodialysis, 1428–1429
  and cytochrome c oxidase inhibition, 1424
  and electron transport, 176t
  elimination, 1428–1429
  enhanced elimination, urine alkalinization for, 93
  serum, 1425
    methanol metabolism and, 1436
    in methanol poisoning, prognostic significance, 1427
  site of action, 173f
Formic acid, 146t, 165–166, 166f, 775–776, 1388t
  enzymatic assay for, 1425
  self-harm with, 1847
  as thermal degradation product, 1641t
  toxicity, 166
    sodium bicarbonate for, 568t
  undissociated, toxicity, 1430
Formication, in alcohol withdrawal, 1166
Formononetin, 1603t
Formoterol, 985
  pharmacology, 986
Fosamine, 1468t
Fosamprenavir, 831–832
Foscarnet
  diabetes insipidus caused by, 195, 195t
  for HIV-related infections, 830t
  and QT interval, 253t
Fosphenytoin
  advantages, 724
  mechanism of action, 720t
  pharmacokinetics and toxicokinetics, 724
  and phenytoin, conversion factor, 724
  toxicity (overdose/poisoning)
    clinical manifestations, 724
    management, 725
Fo-Ti (*Polygonum multiflorum*), 641t
Foundry workers' ague, 1286
Four-gas detection unit, 1690
Foxglove (*Digitalis* spp.), 969, 1600t. *See also* Cardioactive steroids; Digoxin
  cardiac glycosides in, 645
  uses and toxicities, 642t
Foxy Methoxy, 1179t, 1180, 1181t.
    See also N,N-Diisopropyl-5-methoxytryptamine (5-MeO-DiPT)
Fracking, 1409
  hydraulic fluid in, abuse, 1421

Fractional absorption (F), 143

Fractional sodium excretion, 393, 393t, 397

Fractional urea excretion, 393, 393t

Fractionated plasma separation, albumin adsorption, and hemodialysis. *See also* Prometheus system
  for acetaminophen removal, 485

Fractionated plasma separation and adsorption system (FPSA), for amanitin poisoning, 1586

Fraction of inspired oxygen. *See* FiO_2

Fracture(s)
  bisphosphonate-related, 119, 123f
  SSRIs and, 1058

Fragrances, as photoallergens, 280

Framingham Heart Study, 1853

Framingham linear regression analysis, for corrected QT, 251

Francisella tularensis, 1756–1757

Frangipani (*Plumeria rubra*), 979

Frangula bark (*Rhamnus frangula*), 1602t

Frangulins, 1602t

Franklin, Benjamin, 501, 1292

Free-drug concentration, 109–110, 110t

Free drug monitoring, 109–110, 110t

Free fatty acids (FFA), 178–179

Free radicals, 157, 174–175
  and cobalt toxicity, 1274
  definition, 159–160
  production, by irritant gases, 1653

Free radical scavengers, for pulmonary irritant exposure, 1658

French honeysuckle (*Galega officinalis*), uses and toxicities, 642t

French lilac (*Galega officinalis*), 694
  uses and toxicities, 642t

Freon, 1410
  inhaled, 1193t. *See also* Inhalant(s)

Fresh-frozen plasma (FFP)
  for angioedema, 964
  for anticoagulant reversal, 887, 888t, 910–911
  for antithrombotic overdose/poisoning, 888t
  for dabigatran-induced coagulopathy, 894

Freud, Sigmund, 8
  on cocaine, 1124

Fridericia formula, for corrected QT, 251

Froben, Wilhelm, 1011

Frostbite, 271, 418
  with ingalant abuse, 1197

Frovatriptan, 217, 808–809, 808t

Fructose, 707
  absorption, 707
  dietary, and fructose intolerance, 689

Fructose 1,6-diphosphate, for β-adrenergic antagonist toxicity, 935

Fructose intolerance. *See also* Hereditary fructose intolerance (HFI)
  dietary, 689

Fructus aurantii. See Bitter orange (*Citrus aurantium*)

Fruity smell, sweet, 364t

Frullania spp. (liverwort), 1614

Fry. *See* Phencyclidine (PCP)

Fugu, tetrodotoxin in, 596

Fukushima nuclear plant, radiation disaster, 23t, 24, 1264, 1762, 1776

Fuller, Buckminster, 1717

Fuller Earth
  for dermal decontamination, 72
  for paraquat poisoning, 1474f, 1477

Fullerenes, 1717, 1718f

Fuller's herb. *See Saponaria officinalis* (soapwort)

Fumagillin, for HIV-related infections, 830t

Fumasol, 885

Fumes
  in developing world, 1847
  and occupational health and safety, 1731

Fumigants, 1457–1465. *See also specific fumigant*
  clinical effects, 1458t
  gaseous, 1457, 1457t
  history of, 1457
  industrial uses, 1457t
  inhalation, 1457
  liquid, 1457, 1457t
  methyl bromide. *See* Methyl bromide
  physicochemical properties, 1457, 1457t
  solid, 1457

Functional groups, in organic chemistry, 165–166, 165f–166f, 168

Funduscopy, 356
  abnormalities on, xenobiotic exposures causing, 357t

Fungi and fungal toxins, 2, 1581, 1606. *See also* Mushrooms
  in biological warfare, 1759–1760

Fungicides
  and disulfiramlike reactions, 1174t
  thiocarbamate, 1487

Funiculosin, and electron transport, 176t

Funk, Casimir, 1157

Funnel web spider (*Atrax* spp., *Hadronyche* spp.), 1540, 1548
  antivenom, 1560, 1560t
    dosage and administration, 1561

Furacin, 687

Furanocoumarin, as abortifacient, 303t

Furano neoclerodane diterpenes, 642t

Furanyl fentanyl, 529
  structure, 529, 529f

Furazolidone, 1077

Furocoumarins, 643t–644t

Furosemide, 963. *See also* Diuretics, loop
  acute interstitial nephritis caused by, 394t
  dermal effects, 276t
  effect on thyroid hormones and function, 814t
  and gustatory dysfunction, 365
  for hypermagnesemia, 200
  for idiopathic intracranial hypertension, 658
  intrathecal administration, inadvertent overdose and unintentional exposures due to, 795t
  and neuromuscular blockers, interactions, 1021t
  solution, sorbitol in, 688t
  and thiamine deficiency, 1160
  and thiamine pharmacokinetics, 1158
  and tinnitus, 369, 370t

Fursultiamine, 1158

Fusarium spp., in biological warfare, 1759

Fusion inhibitors, 832

G

GA (military designation). *See* Tabun

GABA (gamma-aminobutyric acid), 203, 218–222, 719, 720f, 720t, 862
  antipsychotics and, 1035
  in brain, 218
  degradation, modulation, 220–221
  in hepatic encephalopathy, 1096
  and γ-hydroxybutyrate, 1188–1189
  hypoglycins and, 1609
  imipenem and, 825
  inhibition, 218
  monoamine oxidase inhibitors and, 1078

in nicotine withdrawal, 239
  organic chlorine insecticides and, 1516–1517
  penicillins and, 823
  physiologic effects, 218
  release, 218
    lead and, 1295
  reuptake, 218
    inhibitors, 221t, 222
  reuptake transporters, 204
  and sexual function, 304
  in spinal cord, 218
  structure, 1588
  synthesis, 218, 219f, 663
    isoniazid and, 220, 851, 852f
    modulation, 220–221
    xenobiotics affecting, 220–222, 221t

GABA agonists, 221–222, 221t, 1517, 1517f
  direct, 221, 221t
  indirect, 221–222, 221t, 1517f

GABA antagonists, 221t, 222, 1517f
  direct, 221t, 222
  indirect, 221t, 222

$GABA_A$ withdrawal, 222

$GABA_B$ withdrawal, 222

GABAergic neurotransmission
  ethanol and, 221, 236f, 237, 1096, 1146, 1165
  in hepatic encephalopathy, 1096

GABA neurotransmission, chloride and, 221–222

Gabapentin
  adverse effects and safety issues, 727t
  for alcohol dependence, 1170
  for alcohol withdrawal, 1169–1170
  drug interactions with, 723t
  history of, 719
  indications for, 722, 728
  mechanism of action, 221, 228, 720f, 720t
  metabolism and effects on CYP enzymes, 722t
  overdose/poisoning
    clinical manifestations, 722
    management, 722
  pharmacokinetics and toxicokinetics, 721t, 722
  pharmacology, 719, 720t
  pregnancy category, 722
  renal failure and, 389
  therapeutic serum concentration, 722
  withdrawal, 722, 1138

GABA receptor(s), 218–220, 219f, 219t
  benzodiazepines and, 221, 1084, 1087–1088, 1094, 1135
  distribution, 237
  ethanol and, 221, 236f, 237, 1096, 1146, 1165
  $GABA_A$, 204, 218–220, 219f, 219t, 220f
    agonists, 221–222, 221t
    antagonists, 221t, 222, 1516–1517
    barbiturates and, 237
    benzodiazepines and, 237, 1135, 1136f, 1517
    binding sites, 237, 1135, 1136f
    ethanol and, 1146, 1165
    isoforms, and benzodiazepine binding, 1135
    kava lactones and, 1607
    loreclezole and, 237
    and neurosteroids, 1135–1136, 1136f
    organic chlorine insecticides and, 1516–1517
    picrotoxin and, 237, 1516, 1517f
    propofol and, 237
    pyrethroids and, 1521
    sedative-hypnotics and, 1084
    structure and subtypes, 219–220, 1084, 1135, 1136f
    subunits, 237, 1084, 1135, 1136f

GABA receptor(s) (*Cont.*):
GABA$_B$, 204, 218–220, 219f, 219t
  agonists, 238
  antagonists, 221t, 222
  baclofen and, 238
  GHB and, 238
  kava lactones and, 1607
  structure, 238
inhalants and, 1194
nicotine and, 1206
in peripheral nervous system, 1084
sedative-hypnotics and, 1084
structure, 219–220, 238, 1084, 1135, 1136f
subtypes, 237
subunits, 237, 1084, 1135, 1136f
GABA receptor-chloride channel
  ethanol and, 236f, 1165
  organic chlorine insecticides and, 1516–1517
  pyrethroids and, 1521
GABA-transaminase (GABA-T), 218, 219f, 220–221,
  719, 862
GABA transporter, GAT-1, 719, 720f
Gaboon viper (*Bitis gabonica*), 1633, 1633t
Gadolinium
  intrathecal administration, inadvertent overdose
    and unintentional exposures due to, 795t
  nephrotoxicity, 397t
  renal impairment and, 389–390
Gadolinium-DTPA, 1779
G agents. *See also* Cyclosarin; Sarin; Soman; Tabun
  physical characteristics, 1745
Galactorrhea, antipsychotic-induced, 1039
Galactose, 707
Galantamine
  acetylcholinesterase inhibition by, 208, 756
  indications for, 1041
  mechanism of action, 207
Galega officinalis (French lilac), 694
Galega officinalis (goat's rue), uses and toxicities, 642t
Galegine, 642t
Galen, 1t, 2–3, 1852
Galene, 2
Galerina spp., hepatotoxicity, management, 1586
Galerina autumnalis, 1581, 1582t
Galerina marginata, 1581, 1582t
Galerina venenata, 1581, 1582t
Galium odoratum (woodruff), 645t
Galium triflorum (sweet-scented bedstraw), 1600t
Gallamine, intrathecal administration, inadvertent
  overdose and unintentional exposures due
  to, 795t
Gallium, 1780
Galvanization, 1364
Gambierdiscus toxicus, and ciguatoxin, 593
Gamblegram, 190
Gamma-benzene hexachloride, 1514
Gamma rays, 1762–1763
Ganciclovir, for HIV-related infections, 830t
Ganglionic blockers, 756, 961
Gap junctions, in cardiac sensitization, 1412–1413
Garcinia (*Garcinia cambogia*), 606, 607t, 651. *See also*
  Dieting xenobiotics and regimens
  uses and toxicities, 641t–642t
Garcinia cambogia (Garcinia), 606, 607t. *See also*
  Dieting xenobiotics and regimens
  hepatotoxicity, 651
  uses and toxicities, 641t–642t
Garden parsley (*Petroselinum crispum*), 643t
Garden sage. *See Salvia officinalis* (sage)
Gari, 1684. *See also* Cassava (*Manihot esculenta*)

Garlic
Allium sativum
  odor, 364t
  pharmacologic interactions, 646t
  uses and toxicities, 642t
  volatile oils in, 639
wild (*Allium ursinum*), *Colchicum autumnale*
  (autumn crocus) and, confusion, 501
Garrod, Alfred, 4t, 7
Garter snake (*Thamnophis* spp.), 1617
Gas(es). *See also* Asphyxiants; *specific gas*
  acid- or base-forming, 1655. *See also specific*
    xenobiotic
    neutralization therapy for, 1658
  compressed liquified, 1652
    exposure to, 1651
  and dermal decontamination, 71–72
  inert (noble), 155, 156f
    as asphyxiants, 158, 1652
    physicochemical properties, 158
    uses, 1652
  intestinal. *See* Intestinal gas
  irritant, 400, 401t, 1640–1641, 1651, 1653–1659. *See*
    also Pulmonary irritants; *specific xenobiotic*
    ARDS caused by, 402t, 1643f, 1654–1655
    clinical effects, 1654–1655
    diagnostic imaging, 115t
    diffuse airspace filling from, 125t
    inhalation, 123
    water solubility, 1640, 1640t, 1654, 1654t, 1655–1656
  ophthalmic decontamination for, 72–73
  oxidant, 1656–1657
  short-chain aliphatic hydrocarbon, 1652
  in smoke, 1640
  toxic, in antiquity, 2
Gas chromatography (GC), 102, 103t, 106
  detectors used in, 106
  electron impact ionization in, 107
  in ethanol measurement, 1149, 1877
  ethylene glycol and, 1870
  head space sampling, in ethanol measurement, 1877
  limitations, 106
  principles of, 106
Gas chromatography/mass spectrometry (GC/MS),
  102, 103t
  in drug abuse screening tests, 110–111
Gas disasters, 16–17
Gas embolism, hyperbaric oxygen for, 1676, 1679
Gasoline. *See also* Hydrocarbons, aliphatic
  chemistry, 165, 1410
  constituents, 1410
  GABA receptors and, 237
  inhaled, 1193, 1193t. *See also* Inhalant(s)
    clinical effects, 1198
    methylcyclopentadienyl manganese tricarbonyl
      (MMT) in, 1319
  toxic exposure, diagnostic imaging, 118, 121f
  uses, 1409t
  viscosity, 1409t
Gasping syndrome (gasping baby syndrome), 20–21,
  20t, 442, 452
  from benzyl alcohol, 20–21, 20t, 683, 1430
Gastric acid, secretion, 742, 743f
Gastric contents
  postmortem collection and analysis, 1870t,
    1885–1886
  residual, after overdose/poisoning, 49, 51t
  tube aspiration of, 56
Gastric emptying, 49, 50t, 291. *See also* Orogastric
  lavage

age-related changes in, 461
delayed
  and absorption, 143
  concretions and bezoars causing, 143, 143t
  pylorospasm and, 143, 143t
  and interpretation of serum concentration, 153
  pharmacokinetic effects, 152
  procedures for, studies, 55t
Gastric fluid, pH, 142t
Gastric hemorrhage, xenobiotic-induced, in elderly,
  463, 463t
Gastric lavage. *See also* Orogastric lavage
  in antimony toxicity, 1233
  for DEG poisoning, 1447
  early use of, 7
Gastric outlet obstruction, 128, 129t
Gastric parietal cell, hydrogen ion secretion in, 742, 743f
Gastric perforation, imaging, 127–128, 129f, 129t
Gastrin, 290t
  and gastric acid secretion, 742, 743f
Gastrin-releasing peptide (GRP), 290t
Gastritis
  atrophic, exacerbated or unmasked by xenobiotics
    in elderly, 463, 463t
  xenobiotic-induced, 293–294, 294t
Gastroenteritis, in arsenic poisoning, 1241
Gastrointestinal absorption, 142–143, 143f. *See also*
  Absorption
  extended-release preparations and, 49, 51f–52f
  factors affecting, 49
  formulations and, 49
  immediate-release preparations and, 49, 52f
  of liquids, 49
  in neonates, 442
  prevention, 84–85. *See also* Gastrointestinal
    decontamination
    activated charcoal and, 57, 76–77
    adjunctive methods for, 64
    techniques for, 48–70
  sites, 56–57, 57f, 77
  of solids, 49
Gastrointestinal contents, residual, after overdose/
  poisoning, 49, 51t
Gastrointestinal decontamination, 33, 38, 45t, 48–70.
  See also Activated charcoal; Multiple-dose
  activated charcoal (MDAC); Orogastric
  lavage; Whole-bowel irrigation (WBI)
  for acetaminophen toxicity, 481
  adequacy, imaging evaluation, 116, 116f
  adjunctive methods for, 64
  for β$_2$-adrenergic agonist toxicity, 990
  for amphetamine toxicity, 1104–1105, 1104t
  in antiquity, 3
  for botulism, 581
  for calcium channel blocker toxicity, 948
  cathartics in, 63
  in children, 63, 452
  clinical endpoints for, 64
  controversy and debates about, 48, 65
  in copper poisoning, 1287
  for cyclic antidepressant toxicity, 1049
  in 18th and 19th centuries, 7
  endoscopy in, 53, 63–64
  gastric emptying and, 49, 50t, 53, 54t–55t, 77
  general guidance for, 64–65
  for iron ingestion, 671–672, 672f
  for lithium toxicity, 1069–1070
  for methylxanthine toxicity, 989–990
  for monoamine oxidase inhibitor toxicity, 1080
  in overdose/poisoning, 84–85

patient management and, 39
in polydrug ingestions, 57, 60
position statements on, 48, 65
in post-bariatric surgery patients, 64
in pregnancy, 63
recommendations for, 48, 65
for salicylate toxicity, 561
for sedative-hypnotic overdose, 1087
studies of, difficulties, 48, 65
surgical, 63–64
time frame for, 49, 50t–51t
trends in, 48, 64–65
for zinc toxicity, 1365
Gastrointestinal dialysis, 78, 84, 92
Prussian blue and, 1357
Gastrointestinal evacuation. *See* Gastrointestinal
decontamination
Gastrointestinal hemorrhage, 127
chromium-induced, 1270
NSAIDs and, 515
sedative-hypnotic overdose and, 1086t
Gastrointestinal motility
activated charcoal and, 76
cathartics and, 84
evacuants and, 84
factors affecting, 49, 50t–51t
Gastrointestinal obstruction, 129t
Gastrointestinal perforation, 127, 129f, 129t
Gastrointestinal principles, 287–296
Gastrointestinal tract
age-related changes in, 461
anatomy, 287, 288f, 289–292
antimicrobial toxicity and, 829t
cadmium and, 1260, 1260t
cardioactive steroid toxicity and, 971
foreign bodies in, 295
immune system and, 287–288
innervation, 287, 289f
microbiology, 287–288
mushroom toxins affecting, 1589, 1589t
pathology, 293–295
physiology, 289–292
postoperative effects on, 293
regulatory substances, 288–289, 290t
structure, 287
in xenobiotic metabolism, 292–293
Gastrointestinal transit time, 143
Gastropoda, 1572–1573
Gastroscopy, 64
Gastrotomy, 64
Gat (*Catha edulis*), uses and toxicities, 643t
Gatifloxacin, 464, 826
hypoglycemia caused by, 715
Gatorade, and PEG, mixture, 86–87
Gaultheria oil, 634
Gaultheria procumbens (Eastern teaberry, wintergreen),
634. *See also* Wintergreen
Gaultier, M., 11
Gaussian distribution, 1857–1858
Gaze, disconjugate, xenobiotic exposures causing, 357t
GB (military designation). *See* Sarin
GD (military designation). *See* Soman
Gefitinib
adverse effects and safety issues, 760t, 762
overdose/poisoning, 760t
Geiger counter, 1762
Gelsinger, Jesse, 13
Gemcitabine, mechanism and site of action, 762f
Gemifloxacin, 826
Gemtuzumab, 760t

Gene doping, 616t
definition, 623
Gene expression, nanoparticles and, 1726f, 1727
General anesthesia, 1011–1012. *See also* Anesthetic(s);
specific xenobiotic
Generally recognized as safe (GRAS), excipients, 681
Gene therapy, 13
Genetic polymorphisms, 169
antimalarials and, 847
and cytochrome P450 enzymes, 169t, 170, 172
for membrane transporters, 173
Genin, 969
Genistein, 644t
Genitourinary principles, 297–309
Genomic instability, radiation and, 1767
Genotoxicity
of antimony, 1232t, 1233
of nanoparticles, 1726f, 1727
Gentamicin, 821–823
benzalkonium chloride in, 682t
and neuromuscular blockers, interactions, 1021t
parabens in, 685
serum concentration, interpretation, 153
structure, 821
toxicity, clinical manifestations, 822t
Gentian (*Gentiana lutea*), 1611
Gentian violet, toxicity, organ system manifestations,
829t
Gentiobiosyloeandrin, 643t
Geometric isomer(s), 164
Geophagia, lead exposure from, in pregnancy, 1304
Gepirone, mechanism of action, 217
Geriatric principles, 460–471. *See also* Elderly
Germander (*Teucrium chamaedrys*), 613
hepatotoxicity, 651
uses and toxicities, 642t
Germanium, nephrotoxicity, 390f, 397t
German Stuff, 1748
GF (military designation). *See* Cyclosarin
Ghrelin, 290t, 606
Giardia lamblia. See Giardiasis
Giardiasis, 592t, 597
Gibbite, 1223
Gifblaar (*Dichapetalum cymosum*), 1533
Gila monster (*Heloderma suspectum*), 1618, 1619f.
See also Lizards
bites, 1622
envenomation, 1622
Gilatoxin, 1619
Gilbert syndrome, 329, 334, 722
hyperbilirubinemia in, 172
Gilles de la Tourette syndrome, 213–214
Gills (lamellae), of mushrooms, 1584f, 1593
Ginger (*Zingiber officinale*), 642t
Ginger Jake paralysis, 21t, 22
Gingival hyperplasia, 293
with anabolic-androgenic steroids, 618
Gingko (*Gingko biloba*), 1607, 1614
pharmacologic interactions, 646t
seizures caused by, 220–221
uses and toxicities, 642t, 1600t
xenobiotic interactions, 1611
Gingkoaceae, 1600t, 1614
Gingkolide(s), 642t, 1600t, 1607
B, as glycine antagonist, 223
Ginseng (*Panax ginseng, P. quinquefolius, P.
pseudoginseng*), 639
as aphrodisiac, 304, 304t
pharmacologic interactions, 646t
preparations, 639

and serotonin toxicity, 1058t
uses and toxicities, 642t
Ginsenin, 642t
Ginsenosides, 642t
Girard, 6
Gitalin toxicity, epidemiology, 969
Gitaloxin, in foxglove, 642t
Gitoxin, in foxglove, 642t
Glade Air Freshener, inhaled, cardiotoxicity, 1196
Glasgow Coma Scale (GCS), 37
Glasgow Modified Alcohol Withdrawal Scale (GMAWS),
1166
Glatiramer acetate, polymeric substances, 1719t
Glauber, Johann, 83
Glaucoma, cannabinoids for, 1113
Glaze, ceramic, leaded, imaging, 116, 117f
Glial cells, 340–341
Glibenclamide, overdose/poisoning
octreotide for, 715
and organ donation, 1893t
Gliclazide
hypoglycemia caused by, octreotide for, 714–715
overdose/poisoning, octreotide for, 715
Glifozins, 707
Glimepiride
overdose/poisoning, octreotide for, 715
pharmacokinetics and toxicokinetics, 696, 697t
Glipizide
exposure, in children, hypoglycemia caused by, 699
hypoglycemia caused by, octreotide for, 714–715
overdose/poisoning, octreotide for, 715
pediatric delayed toxicity, 452
pharmacokinetics and toxicokinetics, 696, 697t
structure, 695f
Gliptins
history of, 694
overdose/poisoning
hospitalization for, 702
hypoglycemia caused by, 700
pharmacokinetics and toxicokinetics, 696
Global Educational Toxicology Uniting Project
(GETUP), 1847
Globally Harmonized System of Classification and
Labelling of Chemicals, 1808
Globin chain, oxidation, 317
Globin synthesis, 313–314
Glomerular filtration, 389
Glomerular filtration rate (GFR), 92–93, 194, 389
age-related changes in, 462–463
in chronic kidney disease, 395, 395t
estimated, 393t, 397
laboratory assessment, 396–397
neonatal, 442
in obese patients, 148
occult reduction, in elderly, 462–463
Glomeruli, renal, 389
Glomerulonephritis
hydrocarbon inhalation and, 1196
membranous, mercurials and, 1326
Gloriosa superba (glory lily, meadow saffron, superb
lily). *See also* Colchicine
Ipomoea batatas (sweet potatoes) and, confusion,
501
primary toxicity, 1600t
self-poisoning with, 1846
Glossitis, in pyridoxine deficiency, 663
GLQ-223 (*Trichosanthes kirilowii*), 641t
Glucagon, 941–944
for β-adrenergic antagonist toxicity, 35t, 924, 933,
941–942

Glucagon (*Cont.*):
adverse effects and safety issues with, 942–943
as antidote, 941–944
availability and storage, 45t
for calcium channel blocker toxicity, 941–942, 949
cardiovascular effects, 941–942
chemistry, 941
dosage and administration, 942
and fatty acid metabolism, 178–179
formulation and acquisition, 942
as glutamate scavenger, 229
history of, 941
for hypoglycemia, 701, 941–942
indications for, 35t, 45t, 924
labeling, 43
mechanism of action, 941
pancreatic, 941
and pancreatic dysfunction, 295t
pharmacokinetics and pharmacodynamics, 941
pharmacology, 941–942
with phosphodiesterase inhibitors and calcium, 942
in pregnancy and lactation, 942
preparation, 941
secretion, 292
and smooth muscle relaxation, 941, 943
stocking, recommended level, 45t, 943
supplies, 42, 943
tachyphylaxis with, 941
volunteer studies, 941–942
and warfarin, interactions, 943
Glucagon-like peptide-1 (GLP-1), 290t, 696, 696f
Glucagon-like peptide-1 (GLP-1) agonists, 606, 607t. *See also* Dieting xenobiotics and regimens
Glucagon-like peptide-1 (GLP-1) analogs
overdose/poisoning
hospitalization for, 702
hypoglycemia caused by, 700
pharmacokinetics and toxicokinetics, 696, 697t
Glucagonoma, 943
Glucagon receptors, 941
physiologic effects, 262
Glucantime. *See* Meglumine antimoniate
Glucarpidase (carboxypeptidase G₂), 764, 782–788
adverse effects and safety issues with, 785
availability and storage, 45t
chemistry, 782
dosage and administration, 786
efficacy trials, 782–784, 784t
formulation and acquisition, 786
history of, 782
immunogenicity, 785
indications for, 35t, 45t, 782
intrathecal, 785–786
for intrathecal methotrexate, 770, 778–779
lactose intolerance and, 785
leucovorin and, 777, 784–785
mechanism of action, 782, 783f
for methotrexate toxicity, 760t, 770, 783–785
monitoring with, 786
pharmacodynamics, 782–783, 784t
pharmacokinetics, 782
pharmacology, 782–783
in pregnancy and lactation, 786
production, 782
stocking, recommended level, 45t
Glucocorticoid(s). *See also specific glucocorticoid*
effect on thyroid hormones and function, 814t
and neuromuscular blockers, interactions, 1021t
and pancreatic dysfunction, 295t
for vitamin D toxicity, 661

Glucomannan (*Amorphophallus konjac*), 607t, 611. *See also* Dieting xenobiotics and regimens
uses and toxicities, 642t
Gluconeogenesis, 175, 178, 179f
inhibitors, 176t
trivalent arsenic and, 1238–1239
Glucosamine (chitosamine), uses and toxicities, 642t
Glucose, 175
absorption, 707
for β-adrenergic antagonist toxicity, 933–934
blood, 32–33, 37, 175, 189
in critical illness, 710
dextrose and, 707
in differential diagnosis of high anion gap metabolic acidosis, 192
normal fasting range, 694
rapid point-of-care testing, 707
testing, 708
in brain, 175
continuous monitoring, 709
definition, 707
discordant serum and CSF concentrations, salicylates and, 557
homeostasis, 707
intolerance, antipsychotic-induced, 1039
metabolism, 175
inhibitors, 176t
salicylates and, 557
physicochemical properties, 694
postmortem changes, 1885t
serum, in toxic alcohol poisoning, 1427
vitreous, normal concentration, 1872t
D-Glucose, 707. *See also* Dextrose
Glucose dehydrogenase pyrroloquinolinequinone (GDH-PQQ), 709
Glucose-dependent insulinotropic polypeptide (GIP), 290t
Glucose-6-phosphate dehydrogenase (G6PD), 178, 178f, 312, 1285
copper poisoning and, 1287
deficiency, 170, 312–313, 318, 318t, 1473
and dimercaprol therapy, 1252
epidemiology, 1709
fava beans and, 1607
and hemolysis, 1706
and malaria, 844–845
management, 1709
methemoglobinemia in, 178
methylene blue use in, 1714
vetch seeds and, 1607
trivalent arsenic and, 1238
Glucose (uptake) transporters, 696f, 707
GLUT-1, 341
calcium-channel blockers and, 953–954, 954f
GLUT3, 707
GLUT4, 707
GLUT5, 707
α-Glucosidase inhibitors. *See also* Antidiabetics
history of, 694
overdose, management, 702
pharmacokinetics and toxicokinetics, 697t
pharmacology, 695f
β-Glucuronidase
activity, 172
pretreatment, in benzodiazepine screening, 113
Glucuronidation, 172
Glucuronides, 144
Glucuronyl transferase, 172, 826
deficiency, 329
Glues, inhaled, 1193, 1193t. *See also* Inhalant(s)
Glue sniffer's rash, 1197, 1414

Glufosinate, 228, 1468t, 1471, 1478–1479
chemical structure, 1478f
diabetes insipidus caused by, 195, 195t
extracorporeal removal, 1479
gastrointestinal decontamination, 1479
nomogram for, 1478, 1478f
pharmacokinetics, 1478
pharmacology, 1478
poisoning
case fatality rate, 1478
clinical manifestations, 1478
diagnostic tests for, 1478–1479
management, 1479
pathophysiology, 1478
toxicokinetics, 1478
Glutamate, 179, 181, 203, 223–229
and adenosine, 224–225
carbon monoxide poisoning and, 1664
and dopamine, 224–225
in GABA synthesis, 218, 219f, 223
in neurologic disorders, 224
nicotine and, 1206
in nicotine withdrawal, 239
physiologic functions, 224
in psychiatric disorders, 224
release, 225, 226f
adenosine and, 229
prevention, 227t, 228
in withdrawal syndromes, 237
reuptake, 225, 226f
xenobiotics increasing, 227t
reuptake transporters, 204
and serotonin, 224–225
synthesis, 225, 226f
uptake, inhibitors, 227t
Glutamate agonists, 227–228, 227t
Glutamate antagonists, 224, 227t, 228–229
for carbon monoxide poisoning, 1671
Glutamate-cystine exchanger (SLC7A11), 225
Glutamate decarboxylase (GAD), 220–221
Glutamate-oxaloacetate transaminase, as glutamate scavenger, 229
Glutamate-pyruvate transaminase, as glutamate scavenger, 229
Glutamate receptor(s), 205, 224–227
AMPA, 225, 226f
ionotropic, 225, 227f
kainate, 205, 225, 226f
metabotropic, 225–227, 226f
negative allosteric modulators for, 225–227, 227t
NMDA. *See* NMDA (*N*-methyl-D-aspartate) glutamate receptor
positive allosteric modulators for, 227
upregulation, withdrawal and, 237
Glutamate receptor antibody(ies), 229
Glutamate-related excitotoxicity, 224
Glutamatergic neurotransmission, 225, 226f
ethanol and, 1165
Glutamate scavengers, 227t, 229
Glutamic acid, 595, 595f, 862
Glutamic acid decarboxylase (GAD), 218, 219f, 862
Glutaminase, 225, 226f
Glutamine, 181, 225, 226f
Glutamine synthase, 225, 226f
γ-Glutamyl cycle, 474, 475f
Glutaraldehyde, 1369t
clinical effects, 1374–1375
exposure to, management, 1375
and occupational asthma, 1660, 1660t
occupational exposure to, 1374

pharmacology, 1374
  as sterilant, 1368, 1374–1375
Glutathione, 160, 1285, 1285f
  in acetaminophen toxicity, 160, 172, 330, 473–474
  in carbon monoxide poisoning, 1667
  conjugates, 172
  and hemolysis, 1706
  oxidized, 1340
  for paraquat poisoning, 1474f, 1477
  precursors, 492
  and prevention of aminoglycoside toxicity, 823
  reduced, trivalent arsenic and, 1238–1239
  reduction, 168, 178, 1285f, 1340
  structure, 492
  synthesis, 492
  thallium and, 1351
Glutathione peroxidase, 1340
  selenium as cofactor for, 1339
Glutathione reductase, 1285, 1285f
  trivalent arsenic and, 1238
Glutathione S-transferase (GST), 172, 1340
Glutathione synthase, trivalent arsenic and, 1238
Glutethimide. See also Sedative-hypnotics
  mechanism of action, 221–222
  overdose, clinical findings in, 1086t
Glyburide
  exposure, in children, hypoglycemia caused by,
    699
  overdose/poisoning, octreotide for, 715
  pharmacokinetics and toxicokinetics, 696, 697t
  structure, 695f
Glycemic control
  in critical illness, 698
  and risk of hypoglycemia, 697–698
Glycemic threshold, 699
  for counterregulatory response, 708
Glycerin, diethylene glycol contamination, 19, 20t
Glycerol, in gluconeogenesis, 178
Glycerol monoacetate (monacetin), for SMFA or
    fluoroacetamide poisoning, 1534
Glycine, 179, 203, 223, 224f
  and hyponatremia, 196
  inhibition, by strychnine, 1536
  release, 223
  reuptake, 223
    inhibitors, 227t
  and spinal cord, 344
Glycine agonists, 223, 224t
Glycine antagonists, 223, 224t, 227t, 228
Glycine Cl⁻ channels, 223
  xenobiotics affecting, 223, 224t
Glycine max (soy isoflavone), 644t
Glycine receptors, 223
  inhalants and, 1194
Glycine (reuptake) transporters, 204, 224f
  GLYT-1, 223
  GLYT-2, 223
Glycitein, 644t
Glycocalyx, of platelets, 323
Glycogen, 707
Glycogen synthase kinase-3 (GSK-3), 1065–1067, 1066f
  lithium and, 1065–1067, 1066f
Glycol(s), 639, 1422
  acute tubular necrosis caused by, 390f
  chemistry, 166
  definition, 166
  renal effects, 390f
Glycolate
  fomepizole and, 1436
  and lactate laboratory evaluation, 192

Glycol ethers
  chemistry, 1422
  infertility caused by, 297t, 298f
Glycolic acid, 146t, 165, 1423f
  acidosis caused by, 1423
  enzymatic assay for, 1425
  laboratory test for, 1425
Glycolysis, 175, 177f, 178, 179f, 707
  anaerobic, 177, 178f
  in erythrocyte, 312, 313f
  inhibitors, 176t
  pentavalent arsenic and, 1239, 1239f
  in postmortem changes, 1885
Glycone, 1597, 1606
Glycoprotein(s). See also P-glycoprotein
  GP Ia, 898f
  GP Ib-V-IX, 323, 898f
  GP IIb/IIIa, 323, 897, 898f
  GP VI, 898f
  platelet, 323, 897, 898f
Glycoprotein hormones, as athletic performance
    enhancers, 619–620
Glycoprotein IIb-IIIa fibrinogen receptor, 323, 897, 898f
Glycoprotein IIb/IIIa inhibitors, 323, 899–900
  adverse effects and safety issues, 899–900
  antidotes and treatment strategies for, 888t
  efficacy, 899–900
  laboratory testing for, 888t
  mechanism of action, 898f
Glycopyrrolate, 1503
  atropine and, comparison, 1503f
  benzyl alcohol in, 683t
  for organic phosphorus compound poisoning,
    1496–1497
  pharmacology, 1025, 1026t
Glycosides, 639, 644t
  anthraquinone, 639, 1597, 1598t–1599t, 1602t, 1607
  cardiac. See Cardiac glycosides
  cyanogenic. See Cyanogenic glycosides
  definition, 1597
  lactone, 639
  in plants, 1606–1607
  saponin, 1597, 1606
  steroidal, 1597
  from yew, 1612
O-Glycosides, 1599t
Glycyrrhiza spp., 1606
Glycyrrhiza glabra (licorice), 1600t, 1606
  glycosides in, 639
  hyponatremia from, 196
  use and toxicities, 643t, 649
Glycyrrhizic acid, and hyponatremia, 196
Glycyrrhizin, 643t, 649, 1600t, 1606, 1608
Glyoxylic acid, 165, 878
Glyphosate, 1466, 1468t, 1471, 1479–1480
  carcinogenicity, risk communication about,
    1818–1819
  exposure, risk communication about, 1818–1819
  pharmacokinetics, 1479
  pharmacology, 1479
  structure, 1479f
  toxicity (overdose/poisoning)
    clinical manifestations, 1479–1480
    diagnostic tests for, 1480
    management, 1480
    pathophysiology, 1479–1480
    risk communication about, 1818–1819
  toxicokinetics, 1479
Gnetaceae, 1600t
Goat's rue (Galega officinalis), uses and toxicities, 642t

Goatweed. See St. John's wort (Hypericum perforatum)
Gobo. See Burdock root (Arctium lappa, A. minus)
Goddard, James, 9
Godfrey's cordial, 519
Godman's montane pit viper (Porthidium spp.), 1637t
Godman's pit viper (Porthidium spp.), 1637t
God's flesh. See Psilocybe spp.
God's sacred mushroom. See Psilocybe spp.
Goiânia, Brazil, cesium exposure in, 1762, 1764–1765,
    1769, 1772
Goiter, 812
  cobalt-induced, 1273, 1275
  iodide-induced, 818
Goji (Lycium barbarum, L. chinense), 642t
Gold
  antidote for, 35t
  excretion, N-acetylcysteine and, 494
  membranous glomerulonephropathy caused by,
    391, 392f
  nanoparticles, 1717, 1718f, 1719t
  nephrotoxicity, 397t
  as thermal degradation product, 1642
Golden chain (Cytisus laburnum, Laburnum
    anagyroides), 1601t, 1604
Goldenseal (Hydrastis canadensis), 1600t, 1605
  alkaloids in, 639
  use and toxicities, 642t
Golden Seal tea, 622
Goldenthread (Coptis spp.), 641t, 1599t
Gold mining, mercury exposure in, 1324
GoLYTELY, 86–87
Gomphocarpus physocarpus, G. fruticosus (balloon
    plant), 979
Gonadotropin-releasing hormone (GnRH), 297–298, 302
Gonadotropin-releasing hormone (GnRH) agonists,
    and female sexual dysfunction, 302f
Goodpasture syndrome, 1414
Gopher snakes, 1617
Gordolobo yerba (Senecio longiloba, S. aureus, S.
    vulgaris, S. spartoides), 642t
Goring, Herman, 1685
Gossypium spp. (cotton, cottonseed oil), 1600t
Gossypol, 1600t, 1608
Gotu kola (Centella asiatica), 642t
Goulding, Roy, 11
Gou qi zi. See Goji (Lycium barbarum, L. chinense)
Gout
  colchicine for, 501
  diuretic-induced, 963
  lead-induced, 2, 1295
  saturnine, 1295, 1298
Government agencies, as information resources, 1801t,
    1804
Governmental poisoner, 5t
GP IIb-IIIa antagonists. See Glycoprotein IIb/IIIa
    inhibitors
G protein(s), 204, 521, 522f
  α chain, 204
  β chain, 204
  γ chain, 204
  families, 204
  G_{I/o}, 204, 207–208, 213, 217, 238
  G_q, 204
  G_s, 204, 208, 213, 217, 238, 261–262
  subunits, 204, 238
G protein complex, 260–261, 262f
G protein–coupled receptor (GCPR), lithium and,
    1065–1066, 1067f
G protein-coupled receptors, 204–205, 204t, 206f,
    218–220, 219t

G protein kinases (GPKs), 205

GRADE (Grading of Recommendations Assessment, Development, and Education), system for evaluating clinical recommendations, 1852, 1852t

Graft-versus-host disease, acute, 276, 276t

Grain fever, 1659

Grains, ergot in, 805–806

Grammostola spp., 1547

Gramoxone Inteon, 1474–1475

Granisetron
mechanism of action, 218
for methylxanthine-induced vomiting, 990
and serotonin toxicity, 1058t

Granulocyte colony-stimulating factor (G-CSF), 818
for agranulocytosis caused by chemotherapeutics, 764
for colchicine toxicity, 504
for sulfur mustard-associated neutropenia, 1748

Granulocyte-macrophage colony-stimulating factor (GM-CSF)
for agranulocytosis caused by chemotherapeutics, 764
gene, targeted nanoparticle, 1719t
for methotrexate overdose, 769–770

Granulocytes, 319. *See also* Agranulocytosis

Granuloma(s), hepatic, 330

Granulomatous hepatitis, 333, 334t
xenobiotic-induced, 331t

Grapefruit (*Citrus paradisi*), 1599t, 1607
xenobiotic interactions, 1599t, 1610–1611

Grapefruit juice, and CYP enzymes, 170, 172, 1610

Graphene, 1718f

Grass carp (*Ctenopharyngodon idellus*), 640t

Grass pea (*Lathyrus sativus*), 343, 1601t, 1609

Graves disease, 812, 815
management, 818

Gray (Gy), 1764, 1764f

Grayanotoxins, 1598t, 1602t, 1612f
and sodium channels, 1611–1612
and voltage-gated calcium channels, 244f, 245

Gray baby syndrome, 442, 452–453, 825–826

Great burdock. *See* Burdock root (*Arctium lappa, A. minus*)

Greater blue-ringed octopus (*Hapalochlaena lunulata*), 1572, 1572f

Greater weeverfish (*Trachinus draco*), 1576–1577

Great keyhole limpet (*Megathura crenulata*), 977

Grecian foxglove (*Digitalis lanata*), 1600t

Greek hay seed (*Trigonella foenumgraecum*), 641t

Greenhead ant, 1552

Green orange. *See* Bitter orange (*Citrus aurantium*)

Green rattler (*Crotalus* spp.), 1636t

Green rattlesnake (*Crotalus* spp.), 1636t

Green rock rattlesnake (*Crotalus* spp.), 1636t

Green tea (*Camellia sinensis*), 642t, 1599t. *See also* Methylxanthines; *specific plant*
extract, hepatotoxicity, 651

Green tobacco sickness, 1203, 1206–1207, 1604

Grew, Nehemiah, 83, 876

Griffith, Harold, 1018

Grijns, Gerrir, 1157

Griseofulvin
and ethanol, interactions, 1146t
toxicity, organ system manifestations, 829t

Groundberry oil, 634

Groundsel (*Crotalaria spectabilis, Heliotropium europaeum*), 642t

Groundsel (*Senecio* spp.), 1602t. *See also Senecio* spp.

Grouper fish, vitamin A toxicity from, 655

Growth factors, 311, 761f
myeloid, for agranulocytosis caused by chemotherapeutics, 764
tumor, 761

Growth hormone (GH)
human
adverse effects and safety issues, 619–620
as athletic performance enhancer, 619–620
testing for, 620
and pancreatic dysfunction, 295t
secretion, lead and, 1296

Gualougen (*Trichosanthes kirilowii*), 641t

Guanabenz, 959–961
pharmacokinetics, 960

Guanethidine
adverse effects and safety issues, 961
mechanism of action, 961
priapism caused by, 301t
structure, 961

Guanfacine, 959–961
and glutamate release, 228
pharmacokinetics, 960

Guanidine
and acetylcholine release, 207, 207t
for botulism, 581

Guanosine diphosphate (GDP), 204

Guanosine triphosphatase (GTPase), 204

Guanosine triphosphate (GTP), 175, 204

Guanylhistamine, history of, 739

Guarana (*Paullinia cupana*), 607t, 985, 1601t. *See also* Caffeine; Dieting xenobiotics and regimens

Guar gum, for weight loss, 608t

Guatemalan palm-pit viper (*Bothriechis* spp.), 1636t

Guatemalan palm viper (*Bothriechis* spp.), 1636t

Guatemalan tree viper (*Bothriechis* spp.), 1636t

Guijui. *See* Podophyllum (*Podophyllum* spp.)

Guillain-Barré syndrome, 1550
botulism and, differentiation, 576–577, 577t
clinical manifestations, 577t
differential diagnosis, 1353, 1414
Miller Fisher variant, botulism and, differentiation, 576–577, 577t
and neuromuscular blockade, 1020

Guizhou (*Artemisia* spp.), 643t

Gula, 1, 1t

Gulf War illness (GWI), 17t

Gum, nicotine, 1204t, 1205

Gum metal, 1283

Gummiferin, 640t, 1598t

Gums (gingiva) discoloration
poisoning/overdose causing, 36t
xenobiotics causing, 293, 293t

Gun bluing solution, 1339, 1339t, 1341

Gustation, 363, 365. *See also* Taste
dysfunction, classification, 365
physiology, 365

Gustin/carbonic anhydrase VI, 1362

"Gut dialysis." *See* Multiple-dose activated charcoal (MDAC)

Gutzeit, Max, 4t, 6

Guvacine, mechanism of action, 222

GX (glycine xylidide), 866t, 870

Gymnapistes marmoratus (cobbler), 1576, 1576t, 1577–1578

Gymnasium acne, 618

Gymnopilus penetrans, poisoning with, multiple-dose activated charcoal in, 61

Gymnopilus spectabilis, 1582t, 1588, 1589f

Gymnosperms, 1597, 1600t

Gymnuridae, 1576

Gynecomastia
lavender oil and, 631, 633–634
tea tree oil and, 633–634
xenobiotic-induced, in elderly, 463, 463t

Gynura segetum (T'u-san-chi), use and toxicities, 644t

Gypsy moth caterpillar (*Lymantria dispar*), 1553

Gyromitra spp., 852
clinical and laboratory findings with, 36t
hyperventilation caused by, 400t
toxicity, management, 46t

Gyromitra ambigua, 1582t, 1586

Gyromitra esculenta (false morel), 1582t, 1586, 1586f
monomethylhydrazine (MMH) in, 862
poisoning with, pyridoxine for, 862–863

Gyromitra infula, 1582t, 1586

Gyromitrin, 852, 862, 1581, 1582t, 1586–1587, 1587f, 1589t

H

Haber's rule, 1744–1745

Haber-Weiss reaction, 157, 157f, 160, 670, 1285, 1285f

Haddon Matrix, 450

Hadronyche spp. (funnel web spider), 1548. *See also* Funnel web spider (*Atrax* spp., *Hadronyche* spp.)
antivenom, worldwide availability, 1560t

Haementeria officinalis (Mexican leech), 883

Haff disease, 596

Hageman factor, 885. *See also* Factor XII

Hai-ge-tan (clamshell powder), contaminants in, 648

Hair
arsenic in, 1244
growth, 271
anagen phase, 271
catagen phase, 271
telogen phase, 271
mercury in, 1329, 1329t
specimen collection and analysis, 1244, 1872
postmortem, 1870, 1870t, 1885

Hair cells, of organ of Corti, 366, 366f, 368
noise-induced toxicity in, 368–369
outer, ototoxins and, 367

Hair dye, self-poisoning with, 1846

Hair follicle, 271

Hair jellyfish (*Cyanea capillata*), 1567t, 1568

Hair loss, 274t, 281

Hair spray, inhaled, 1193t. *See also* Inhalant(s)

Haldane effect, 316

Haldane ratio, 1664

Half-life, 150
apparent, 151
and CYP induction, 171
and enzyme inhibition, 171
of radioactive particles, 1762–1763, 1763t

Halides, 158
acyl, 1410
organic, 1410. *See also* Hydrocarbons

Halitoxin, 1574

Hallucinations
in alcohol withdrawal, 1166
amphetamine-induced, 1103
management, 1104–1105, 1104t
cocaine and, 1127
definition, 1178
and illusions, differentiation, 1178
inhalant-induced, 1196
ketamine-induced, 1214
poisoning/overdose causing, 36t
in toxidromes, 29t

Hallucinogen persisting perception disorder (HPPD), 1178, 1184–1185

Hallucinogens, 1178–1187. *See also* Salvia (*Salvia divinorum, S.*); *specific hallucinogen*
adverse psychiatric effects, 1183–1184
in antiquity, 3
classification, 1178
clinical effects, 1183–1184
cross-tolerance, 1183
cryptomarkets for, 1178
designer, 1178
EEG abnormalities caused by, 1182
historical perspective on, 9, 1178
hyperthermia caused by, 27, 1184
Internet and, 1178
laboratory findings with, 1184
long-term effects, 1184–1185
and out-of-body experiences, 1184
pharmacology, 1181t, 1182–1183
psychological effects, 1183
structural classifications, 1178, 1179t
therapeutic uses, 1178
toxicity, treatment, 1184
toxicokinetics, 1181–1182
and trauma, 1183
unclassified, 1178
use
    epidemiology, 1178–1179
    trends in, 1179
Halofantrine, 838t
adverse effects and safety issues, 842
pharmacokinetics, 839t
structure, 842
toxicity
    clinical manifestations, 842
    management, 842
Halogenated aliphatic herbicides, 1468t
Halogenated anesthetic, as glycine agonist, 223
Halogenated hydrocarbons. *See* Hydrocarbons, halogenated
Halogens, 156f. *See also specific xenobiotic*
physicochemical properties, 158
Haloperidol
for agitated/violent behavior, 386
    dosage and administration, 386
cardiac effects, 258t
clinical and toxicologic effects, 1034t
dosage and administration, 1033t
for hallucinogen-induced agitation, 1184
and hERG channels, 245
for inhalant-induced psychosis, 1200
mechanism of action, 214, 227t
pharmacokinetics, 1033t
pharmacology, 1032
poisoning, lipid emulsion for, 1006
and QT interval, 253t
and sudden cardiac death, 253
and tinnitus, 370t
Halophosphates, 1488t
Halothane, 162, 1011
abuse, 1016
chemistry, 164–165
and hepatocellular necrosis, 331
hepatotoxicity, 174t, 1014–1015
history of, 1011
idiosyncratic liver injury caused by, 330
ingestion, 1016
intravenous injection, 1016
mechanism of toxicity, 1014–1015, 1014f
metabolism, 1014, 1014f
molecular structure, 162, 162f
pharmacology, 1410

R and *S* enantiomers, 164–165, 164f
structure, 1011f
trade name, 162
Halothane hepatitis, 1014–1015
Haloxon, 1488t
Halsted, William, 8
Hamburg blue. *See* Prussian blue
Hamburger thyrotoxicosis, 812
Hamilton, Alice, 4t, 7
Hand-and-foot syndrome, 772
Hand-foot skin reaction, kinase inhibitors and, 762
Hanford Plutonium Finishing Plant, americium contamination, 1769
Hanta virus, as biological weapon, 1758
Hapalochlaena lunulata (greater blue-ringed octopus), 1572
Hapalochlaena maculosa (blue-ringed octopus), 1572, 1572f
    tetrodotoxin in, 596
Hapalopilus rutilans, 1583t, 1592
Happy Land Social Club fire, 16, 16t
Haptoglobin, serum, decreased, 317
Harassing agents, 1749
Hard metal disease, 1273
    cobalt-associated, 1276–1277
    definition, 1276
    diagnosis, 1277
Hareburr. *See* Burdock root (*Arctium lappa, A. minus*)
Harington, Charles R., 812
Harm, absence of evidence of, vs. evidence of absence of, 1814
Harmal. *See* Syrian rue (*Peganum harmala*)
Harmala alkaloids, 643t–644t, 649, 650t, 1077
Harmaline, 640t, 649
    and serotonin toxicity, 1058t
Harmaline alkaloids, 1077
Harmane, 212
Harmine, 640t, 649
Harmine alkaloids, 1178, 1180
    and serotonin toxicity, 1058t
Harrison Narcotics Act (1914), 8, 10t, 1124
Harrison Narcotic Tax Act (1914), 519
HAS-BLED score, 886
Hashish, 1111, 1179t
    body packers, 85
    historical perspective on, 9
    in mummies, 3
Hatter's shakes, 22, 23t, 1324. *See also* Mercury
Haw (*Crataegus* spp.), 642t
Hawaiian baby wood rose (*Argyreia nervosa*), 1179t, 1181t, 1598t, 1605
    lysergamides in, 1179
    toxicokinetics, 1182
Hawthorn (*Crataegus* spp.), 642t
    xenobiotic interactions, 1611
Hay, odor, 364t
Hazard(s), definition, 1806
Hazard classes, 1797, 1797t
Hazardous agents
    NIOSH definition, 764
    NIOSH list, 764
Hazardous and Solid Waste Amendments (HSWA, 1984), 1801t
Hazardous incident response. *See* Hazardous materials incident response
Hazardous materials (hazmat)
    biological, 1806
    CAS registry number (CAS#), 1807
    chemical, 1806
    chemical names, 1807

classification, 1807, 1808t
contamination
    primary, 1808
    secondary, 71–72, 1808
decontamination for, 71, 1808–1809, 1811
definition, 1806
exposure to, 1808
fixed facility placarding for, National Fire Protection Association 704 system, 1808
identification, 1807–1808
information on, sources, 1808
North American numbers, 1807–1808
prehospital management, 71
Product Identification Numbers, 1807–1808
radiologic, 1806
and transportation incidents, 1807
United Nations numbers, 1807–1808
vehicle placarding for, 1807–1808
Hazardous materials emergency. *See* Hazardous materials incident response
Hazardous materials incident response, 1806–1813. *See also* Hazardous materials (hazmat)
    activation, 1807
    advanced hazardous materials providers in, 1812
    agencies involved in, 1806
    components, 1807–1811
    decontamination in, 71, 1808–1809, 1811
        prehospital, 1812
    emergency medical services providers in, patient care responsibilities, 1812
    focus of, 1806
    goals, 1806
    hazardous material entry team in, patient care responsibilities, 1812
    identification of hazardous materials in, 1807
    incident command system (ICS) for, 1806
    medical personnel and, 1806–1807
    paradigms for, 1807
    personal protective equipment in, 1807, 1809–1811, 1810f, 1810t
    personnel involved in, 1806
    prehospital decontamination team in, patient care responsibilities, 1812
    prehospital response team, composition, organization, and responsibilities, 1811–1812
    responders in, 1806
    rules and standards for, 1811–1812
    scene control zones, 1809, 1809t, 1810f
    scene triage in, 1811
    site operations, 1809
    victims, hospital responsibilties for, 1812
Hazardous materials technician, training and responsibilities, 1811–1812
Hazardous Material Transportation Act (1972), 10t
Hazardous Waste Operations and Emergency Response (HAZWOPER), 1811
Hazard Ranking System, 1801t
Hazard types, 1797, 1797t
Hazard-vulnerability analysis (HVA), 1806
Hazmat. *See* Hazardous materials
HAZWOPER (Hazardous Waste Operations and Emergency Response), 1811
Headache. *See also* Migraine headaches
    carbon monoxide poisoning and, 1665
    cocaine-related, 1126
    food toxins and, 600t
    inhalant-induced, 1196
    medication overuse, 515
    poisoning/overdose causing, 36t

Health belief model (HBM), 1786

Health care, access to, global disparities in, 1847

Health care clearinghouses, 1864–1865

Health care providers, as poisoners, 12–13

Health Effects of Arsenic Longitudinal Study (HEALS), 1242–1243, 1245

Health information, protected, 1864

Health Information Technology for Economic and Clinical Health Act (HITECH), 1865

Health Insurance Portability and Accountability Act (HIPAA), 1864

  and history-taking from friend or relative, 38

Health literacy, 454, 1786

Health numeracy, 454, 1786

Healthy People 2020, 1782

Hearing, 365–369. *See also* Ototoxicity

  physiology, 365–367

Hearing loss

  blast injury and, 369

  in elderly, and unintentional poisoning, 466

  irreversible, 367

    xenobiotics causing, 367t

  noise-induced, 368–369

  occupation-related, 368

  opioids and, 524

  reversible, 367, 367t

  sudden, recreational drug use and, 368

Heart. *See also* Cardiac *entries*

  absolute refractory period, 251

  anabolic-androgenic steroids and, 617–618

  electric axis of, factors affecting, 248

  refractory period, 246

  relative refractory period, 246, 251

Heart block, 256, 263

  antihypertensive-related, 960

  complete, 248

  xenobiotics causing, 256, 258t

Heart disease, exacerbated or unmasked by xenobiotics in elderly, 463, 463t

Heart failure, cadmium and, 1261

Heart murmur(s), 37

Heart rate

  abnormalities. *See also* specific abnormality(ies)

    xenobiotics causing, 263, 263t–264t

  assessment, in poisoned patient, 266t

  determinants, 926, 928, 928f

  in initial assessment, 189

  pediatric, 258

  and QT interval, 251

  regulation, 255, 926, 928f

Heart transplantation, from poisoned patients, 1892–1893, 1892t

Heartwort (*Aristolochia fangji*), uses and toxicities, 640t

Heat

  generation, in uncoupled oxidative phosphorylation, 178

  transfer, 411

Heat receptors, 411

Heat-shock proteins, 367, 420, 1815

Heat stress, thermoregulation and, 419

Heatstroke, 30–31. *See also* Hyperthermia

  clinical findings in, 421–422

  coagulopathy in, 420–421

  cooling measures for, 422–423, 423t

  definition, 418

  diagnosis, 418

  ECG changes in, 420–421

  epidemiology, 419

  exertional, 419

  gastrointestinal effects, 420–421

  and heat intolerance subsequently, 422

  inflammatory mediators in, 420

  laboratory findings in, 422

  neuropsychiatric effects, 420–421

  nonexertional, 419

  pathophysiology, 420–421, 421t

  signs and symptoms, 418

  treatment, 422–423, 423t

  types, 419

  xenobiotics and, 422

Heat transfer, 411

Heavenly blue. *See* Morning glory

Heavens Gate mass suicide, 24

Heavy fuel oil. *See also* Hydrocarbons, aliphatic

  uses, 1409t

  viscosity, 1409t

Heavy metals, 157–158. *See also* specific metal

  chemistry, 157

  definition, 157

  diagnostic imaging, 115t, 116–117

  in folk medicine, 1293

  food contamination with, 18t, 19

  radiopacity, 114

  tests for, 7

  and tinnitus, 369

Heberden, William, 3

Hedeoma pulegioides. See Pennyroyal (*Mentha pulegium, Hedeoma pulegioides*)

Hederacoside C, 1600t

Hederagenin, 1600t

Hedera helix (common ivy), 1600t

α-Hederin, 1600t

Hedysarum alpinum (wild potato), 1600t

Heinz bodies, 1285, 1383, 1458, 1706, 1706f, 1714

Helicobacter pylori, 513

  bismuth and, 1255, 1257

Heliotrope

  Crotalaria spectabilis, 642t

  Heliotropium spp. (ragwort), 651, 1600t, 1605

    H. europaeum, 642t

      hepatic venoocclusive disease caused by, 332

Heliox, 1652

Helium, 1650

  in divers' gas mixture, 1652

  inhaled, 1193

  physicochemical properties, 1652

  as simple asphyxiant, 400t

  uses, 1652

Hellebore

  black (*Helleborus niger*), 1600t

  Veratrum album, 1603t

  Veratrum californicum, 1603t

  Veratrum viride, 979, 1603t, 1611

Helleborus niger (black hellebore, Christmas rose), 1600t

Helleborus orientalis, 1

Hellebrin, 1600t

HELLP syndrome, 324

Hell's fire anemone (*Actinodendron plumosum*), 1567t

Heloderma horridum (beaded lizard), 1618, 1619f

Heloderma suspectum (Gila monster), 1618, 1619f, 1622

Helodermatidae, 1618

Helodermin, 1619

Helospectins, 1619

Hematemesis, management, 990

Hematin, as tubulotoxin, 393

Hematologic principles, 310–326. *See also* Hemostasis

Hematopoiesis, 310–311

  aluminum and, 1224

  bone marrow in, 310

  cytokines in, 311

  principles of, 310, 310f

  stem cells in, 310, 310f

Hematopoietic progenitor cells, 310, 310f

Hematopoietic stem cells, 310, 310f

Hematopoietic syndrome, radiation-induced, 1768

Hematotoxicity, of lead, 1295, 1295f

Hematuria, 306, 307t, 397

Heme, 313

Heme oxygenase, 315

Heme synthesis, 314, 314f

Hemichromes, 1458

Hemihemoglobin, 316

Hemiplegia, hypoglycemic, 708

Hemlock

  poison (*Conium maculatum*), 1, 1t, 2, 7–8

    toxicity, 1599t

  water (*Cicuta maculata*)

    odor, 364t

    toxicity, 1599t

Hemlock water dropwort (*Oenanthe crocata*), cicutoxin in, 1610

Hemochromatosis, 669

Hemoconcentration, in heatstroke, 422

Hemocyanin, 1285

Hemodiafiltration, 97

Hemodialysis (HD), 33, 90, 90t, 93–95

  for absorbed toxins, 38

  for acetaminophen elimination, 484

  N-acetylcysteine and, 95, 484, 497

  for β-adrenergic antagonist toxicity, 935

  for aluminum-induced encephalopathy, 1224

  in aluminum toxicity, 1225

  for amanitin exposure, 1586

  anticoagulation with, 95

  in arsenic poisoning, 1245

  for barbiturate poisoning, 1087

  in barium toxicity, 1455

  for cardioactive steroid toxicity, 975

  for chemotherapeutic toxicity, 764

  in children, 452

  and chromium, 1271

  clearance of xenobiotics with, 94–95, 95t

  contraindications to, 91

  for copper clearance, 1289

  in copper poisoning, 1287

  for cyclic antidepressant toxicity, 1051

  for dabigatran removal, 894

  deferoxamine and, 677

  for DEG poisoning, 1447–1448

  dialysate for, 95

    contamination, 98–99

  dialysis membranes for, 94

  effects on therapeutics, 95

  endotoxin and, 99

  for ethanol poisoning, 1149

  for fluoride clearance, 1401

  frequency of use, 90, 90t

  for glufosinate poisoning, 1479

  and hemoperfusion, combined, 96, 96f

    for thallium poisoning, 1354

  high-flux, 94–95, 99

  for hypercalcemia, 199

    in vitamin D toxicity, 661

  for hypermagnesemia, 200

  and hypotension, 95

  indications for, 90, 94

  for lithium toxicity, 1070–1071, 1070t

  for methanol poisoning, 1428–1429, 1429t

  for methotrexate toxicity, 770–771

for methyl bromide poisoning, 1461
for methylxanthine poisoning, 991–992, 992t
for organic phosphorus compound and carbamate poisoning, 1498
for paraquat poisoning, 1474f, 1476–1477
and pharmacokinetics, 390
plasma protein binding and, 147
and potassium balance, 199
principles of, 93
procedure for, 94
for salicylate toxicity, 562–563, 563t
schematic layout, 94f
for selenium toxicity, 1342
for thallium poisoning, 1354
and thiamine deficiency, 1160
and thiamine repletion, 1160
for toxic alcohol poisoning, 1428–1429
   duration, 1429
   and fomepizole, 1437–1438
toxicology, 98–99
for triazine herbicide poisoning, 1483
vascular access for, 94
volume of distribution and, 91, 147
water for, 98–99
for xenobiotic removal, clinical effects, 92
xenobiotics amenable to, characteristics, 95, 95t
xenobiotics cleared by, 90, 91f
Hemodilution, and anion gap, 191t
Hemodynamics, 260–267. See also Blood pressure; Hypertension; Hypotension
adrenergic receptors in, 260–262
autonomic nervous system and, 260–262
Hemodynamic status, assessment, in poisoned patient, 265–266, 266t
Hemofiltration (HF), 90, 90t, 96–97
continuous techniques, 97–98. See also specific technique
principles of, 96–97
xenobiotics amenable to, characteristics, 95t, 97
Hemoglobin, 313–315
abnormal, 316–317, 402–403
   and pulse oximetry, 404
autooxidation, 1703
laboratory measurement, 103
oxygenation, xenobiotics affecting, 1651
oxygenation analysis, 1708, 1708t
oxygen binding, 316
and oxygen-carbon dioxide exchange, 315–316
as oxygen transporter, 402–403, 1704
physiology, 1703–1704
precipitation, 1285
renal effects, 390f
structure, 1703, 1704f
total concentration, detection, 1708
Hemoglobinemia, 317
Hemoglobin M, 1703–1704, 1704f
Hemoglobinuria, 317
copper poisoning and, 1286
renal effects, 393
Hemolysis, 170, 178, 178f, 317–318
with N-acetylcysteine, 495
with anilide compound toxicity, 1472
chlorhexidine-induced, 1368
chromium-induced, 1270
copper and, 1285–1286
hydrocarbon-associated, 1414
immune-mediated, 317t
lead-induced, 1295
in metal phosphide poisoning, 1458
metals causing, 397t

methemoglobinemia and, 1706, 1706f
methylene blue and, 1714
naphthalene-induced, 1382–1384
non-immune-mediated, 317–318, 317t
paradichlorbenzene-induced, 1384–1385
phosphine gas and, 1458
renal effects, 393
sodium chlorate and, 1376
stibine and, 1233
sulfonamides and, 827
xenobiotic-induced, 402
Hemolytic anemia
NSAID-induced, 516
quinine-induced, 840
xenobiotic-induced, 174
Hemolytic uremic syndrome (HUS), 317, 324, 598–599
acute kidney injury caused by, 391
Hemoperfusion (HP), 33, 90, 90t
for absorbed toxins, 38
for amanitin exposure, 1586
for cardioactive steroid toxicity, 975
charcoal, 95
   annual reported use of, 90, 90t
   limitations, 96
   schematic layout, 94f
for chemotherapeutic toxicity, 764
complications, 96
for cyclic antidepressant toxicity, 1051
effects on therapeutics, 96
frequency of use, 90
for glufosinate poisoning, 1479
and hemodialysis, combined, 96, 96f
   for thallium poisoning, 1354
layout for, 94f, 95–96, 96f
limitations, 96
for methotrexate toxicity, 770–771
for methylxanthine poisoning, 991–992, 992t
for organic phosphorus compound and carbamate poisoning, 1498
for paraquat poisoning, 1474f, 1476–1477
plasma protein binding and, 147
procedure for, 96
resin, 96
   annual reported use of, 90, 90t
for salicylate toxicity, 562–563
for thyroxine overdose, 818
volume of distribution and, 147
xenobiotics amenable to, characteristics, 95t, 96
Hemoperitoneum, cocaine and, 1127
Hemopexin, 315
Hemophagocytic syndrome and liver failure, in ethylene glycol poisoning, 1424
Hemophilia, 885
Hemorrhage. See also Bleeding; Subarachnoid hemorrhage
adrenal, with colchicine poisoning, 503
gastric, xenobiotic-induced, in elderly, 463, 463t
gastrointestinal, 127
   chromium-induced, 1270
   NSAIDs and, 515
   sedative-hypnotic overdose and, 1086t
intracerebral
   cocaine-related, 1126
      diagnostic imaging, 115t
      computed tomography of, 130
      imaging, 115t, 130, 132t
intracranial, in ethylene glycol poisoning, 1424
intraparenchymal, computed tomography of, 132t
retinal, carbon monoxide poisoning and, 1665
vitreous, 356

Hemorrhagic cystitis, 306
alum therapy for, 1223–1224
cyclophosphamide-related, 306
Hemorrhagic gastritis, in isopropyl alcohol toxicity, 1425
Hemorrhagic syndrome, for venomous caterpillar exposure, 1552–1554
Hemorrhagic tracheobronchitis, in isopropanol aspiration, 1425
Hemosiderinuria, 317
Hemostasis, 320–322, 321f
Hemotoxicity, of Viperidae venom, 1634
Hemozoin, 836
Hemp products, 112
Henbane (Hyoscyamus niger), 2, 1179t, 1600t
as aphrodisiac, 304
use and toxicity, 642t
Henderson-Hasselbalch equation, 76, 93, 141–142
Henry VIII (King of England), 4
Heparin, 322, 890–891. See also Antithrombin agonists; Low-molecular-weight heparin (LMWH)
antidote for, 35t, 891, 919–923
chemistry, 890
chondroitin sulfate contamination, 891
with hemodialysis, 95
history of, 883
low-molecular-weight. See Low-molecular-weight heparin (LMWH)
mechanism of action, 884f, 890, 919
nebulized, for smoke inhalation, 1645
nonbleeding complications with, 891
overdose/poisoning
   clinical manifestations, 36t, 890
   management, 46t
   protamine dosing for, 921
pharmacology, 890
in pregnancy and lactation, 431
priapism caused by, 301t
rebound, 920
resistance, 891
reversal
   alternatives to protamine for, 920
   protamine for, 919–923
      dosage and administration, 920–921
skin necrosis caused by, 279
therapy with, monitoring, 890–891
unfractionated, 883, 890–891
   antidote for, 891
   antidotes and treatment strategies for, 888t
   for cocaine-associated myocardial infarction, 1129
   laboratory testing for, 888t
Heparinase, 890
Heparin-hydrogel, 96
Heparin-induced thrombocytopenia (HIT), 324, 887, 891, 908
Heparin-induced thrombocytopenia and thrombosis syndrome (HITTS), 887, 891–892, 908
Heparinoids, 322
Hepatic artery, 327, 328f
Hepatic encephalopathy, 333–334, 342–343
GABA in, 1096
in Reye syndrome, 557
stages, 333, 333t
Hepatic extraction ratio, 144, 147t, 148
Hepatic lobule, 327
Hepatic metabolism, 144, 147, 292–293, 327. See also Cytochrome P450 (CYP) enzymes
age-related changes in, 462
Hepatic portal venous gas, 128, 130f

Hepatic principles, 327–338. *See also* Liver
Hepatic tumors, 333
    laboratory findings with, 335t
    xenobiotic-induced, 331t
Hepatic veins, 327
Hepatic venoocclusive disease. *See* Venoocclusive
       disease, hepatic
Hepatitis, 327–328, 330
    in arsenic poisoning, 1241
    autoimmune, 331t
    cholestatic, antipsychotic-induced, 1039
    chronic, 333
       laboratory investigation, 335t
    dantrolene and, 1030
    disulfiram-induced, 1174
    granulomatous, 333, 334t
       xenobiotic-induced, 331t
    halothane, 330, 1014–1015
    immune-mediated toxic, 330
    isoniazid-induced, 852–854
    macrolide-related, 827
    in methanol poisoning, 1427
    xenobiotic-induced, 330–331
Hepatitis A
    foodborne illness caused by, 592t
    virosome, 1719t
Hepatitis B, 334
Hepatitis B immune globulin (HBIG), mercury toxicity
       caused by, 1372
Hepatitis C, 334
Hepatobiliary dysfunction, in ketamine users, 1216
Hepatocellular carcinoma, 333
Hepatocellular necrosis, 328, 330–331
    acute, 331, 331t, 334t
       focal, laboratory findings in, 335t
       massive, laboratory findings in, 335t
    centrilobular (zone 3), 328–329, 329f
       acetaminophen and, 330
Hepatocytes, 327, 329f
    copper in, 1284–1286
    injury, in alcoholic liver disease, 1146
Hepatogenous photosensitivity, 1613–1614
Hepatorenal syndrome, 391
    N-acetylcysteine for, 494–495
Hepatotoxicity, 127, 174, 174t. *See also* Drug-induced
       liver injury; *specific xenobiotic*
    of acetaminophen, 147, 160, 163, 474–475
       biomarkers in, 481
       definition, 475
       ethanol and, 1146
       isoniazid and, 852
       liver transplantation for, 483
       pathophysiology, 474
       in pregnancy, 435, 436t
    of *Actaea racemosa* (black cohosh), 1611
    of amatoxins
       N-acetylcysteine for, 494–495, 1585
       treatment, 1584–1586
    of amiodarone, 332
    of anabolic steroids, 330
    of antimonials, 1232
    of antiretrovirals, 331–332
    of arsenic, 1252
    of black cohosh (*Actaea racemosa*), 651
    of *Breynia officinalis*, 1611
    of bromfenac sodium, 1841
    of bromobenzene, ethanol and, 329
    of cadmium, 1261
    of camphor, 1381
    of carbon tetrachloride, 175, 175f, 1196, 1679
       ethanol and, 329

    of chaparral (*Larrea tridentata*), 651
    of chloroform, 1196
    of cocaine, 1127
    of copper, 1285–1286
    of cyclosporine, 330
    of cyproterone acetate, 618
    development, factors affecting, 329–330
    of didanosine, 332
    of dihydralazine, 330
    of 1,3-dimethylamylamine, 651
    of dimethylformamide, 331, 334, 334t
       ethanol and, 329
    of *Dioscorea bulbifera* (bitter yam), 1611
    of disulfiram, 1174–1176
    drug-induced, 21, 35t
       FDA policy and, 1841
    enzyme function and, 329
    of fluoroquinolones, 826
    of *Galerina* spp., management, 1586
    of *Garcinia cambogia* (Garcinia), 651
    of germander (*Teucrium chamaedrys*), 651
    of green tea extract, 651
    of halothane, 174t, 1014–1015
    of hydrocarbons, 1414
    of hydrochlorofluorocarbons, 331
    of Hydroxycut, 651
    of hypoglycin, 331
    of inhalants, 1196
    of inhaled volatile hydrocarbons, 1196
    of isoniazid, 850–851, 851f, 852–854
       risk factors for, 331
    of kava extracts, 651, 1607
    of *Lepiota* spp., 1586
    of linoleic acid, 651
    of LipoKinetix, 651
    of Ma huang, 651
    management, 44t
    of margosa oil, 331
    of methotrexate, 332, 332f, 768
    of methyltestosterone, 330
    mushrooms and, 1593
    NSAID-induced, 514t, 515, 1841
    of OxyELITE, 651
    of pennyroyal, 651
    of phenytoin, 330
    of phosphorus, 1529
    of pioglitazone, 331
    of pyrrolizidine alkaloids, 1605
    of rifampin, 330
    of rosiglitazone, 331
    of solvents, 331
       ethanol and, 329
    of SSRIs, 1058
    of sulfonamides, 827
    of tetracyclines, 331–332, 827
    of thiazolidinediones, 331
    of thorium dioxide, 127
    of toluene, 1196
    of trichloroethane, 1196
    of trichloroethylene, 1196
    of troglitazone, 21, 331
    of usnic acid, 651
    of valproic acid, 331–332, 332f, 726, 732–733
       N-acetylcysteine for, 492, 494
       L-carnitine for, 726, 732–733
    of vinyl chloride, 1414
    of vitamin A, 656–657, 657f, 658
       diagnosis, 658
    xenobiotic metabolites and, 329
    of zalcitabine, 332
    of zidovudine, 332

Hepatotoxins. *See also specific xenobiotic*
    in dietary supplements, 651
    idiosyncratic, 329
    intrinsic, 329
Hepcidin, 315, 315f
Heptachlor, 1514
    metabolism, 1515
    physicochemical properties, 1515t
Heptachlor epoxide, 1515
Heptest, 895
Herba epimedii, as aphrodisiac, 304
Herbal balls, contaminants in, 648
Herbal ecstasy, 748
Herbalife, hepatotoxicity, 651
Herbal preparations, 638–653. *See also specific herb;*
       specific preparation
    abortifacient, 303, 303t
    adverse effects and safety issues, in elderly, 465
    coadministration, 647
    hepatic injury associated with, 333
    and hepatocellular necrosis, 331
    nephrotoxic, 390f
    psychoactive xenobiotics in, 650t
    in traditional medicine, 1845
    uses and toxicity, 640t–645t, 650t
    for weight loss, 613
Herbal synergy, 647
Herb grass. *See* Rue (*Ruta graveolens*)
Herbicides, 1466–1485. *See also specific herbicide*
    acute exposure to/poisoning with, 1466
       dermal decontamination for, 1471
       diagnosis, 1471
       gastrointestinal decontamination for, 1471
       initial management, 1471
       laboratory investigation, 1471
       occupational and secondary exposures with,
          1471–1472
       pathophysiology, 1471
    alcohol, 1467t
    aldehyde, 1467t
    amide, 1467t, 1472–1473
    anilide derivative, 1467t, 1472–1473, 1472f
    applications, 1467t–1470t
    aromatic acid, 1467t
    arsenical, 1467t
    arsenic-containing, overdose/poisoning,
       whole-bowel irrigation for, 85
    availability, 1466–1471
    benzothiazole, 1467t
    bipyridyl, 1467t, 1473–1478
    carbanilate, 1467t
    chemical classes, 1467t–1470t
    chlorophenoxy
       antidote for, 35t
       effects on vital signs, 31t
       poisoning with, sodium bicarbonate for,
          568t, 570
    chlorphenoxy, toxicity (overdose/poisoning),
       alkalinization for, 570
    chronic exposure to, 1466
    classification, 1466, 1467t–1470t
    clinical effects, 1467t–1470t
    coformulants in, 1466
    combination preparations, 1466
    cyclohexane oxime, 1467t
    deaths caused by, 1466
    definition, 1466
    dinitroaniline, 1468t
    dinitrophenol, 1468t
    diphenylether, 1468t
    exposure to

epidemiology, 1466–1471
    treatments and supportive care for, 1467t–1470t
halogenated aliphatic, 1468t
history of, 1466
imidazolinone, 1468t
inorganic, 1468t
LD$_{50}$, 1466
mechanism of action, 1466, 1467t–1470t
mechanism of human toxicity, 1466
nitrile, 1468t
nosocomial poisoning with, 1471–1472
occupational exposures, 1471–1472
organic phosphorus, 1468t
phenoxy (2,4-D and MCPA), 17, 1469t, 1480–1482
poisoning with, 1466
pyrazole, 1469t
pyridazine, 1469t
pyridazinone, 1469t
pyridine, 1469t
regulatory considerations, 1471
secondary exposures, 1471–1472
selective targeting, 1471
self-poisoning with, 1471
thiadiazol, and ATP synthesis, 176t
thiocarbamate, 1469t, 1487
triazine, 1469t, 1482–1483. See also Atrazine
triazinone, 1469t
triazole, 1469t
triazolone, 1469t
triazolopyrimidine, 1469t
uracil, 1470t
urea, 1470t
usage data, 1467t–1470t
WHO hazard classification, 1466, 1467t–1470t
Herb of grace. See Rue (Ruta graveolens)
Herbs. See Herbal preparations; specific herb
Hereditary fructose intolerance (HFI)
    adverse effects of sucrose, fructose, and sorbitol in, 689
    epidemiology, 689
    pathophysiology, 689
Hereditary hemochromatosis, 315
Hereditary orotic aciduria (HOA), 789
hERG (Human Ether-à-go-go Related Gene), 245, 253, 256, 877
Hermodice carunculata (bristle worm), 1573
Heroin, 5t
    adulterants, 528
    base, 527
    bioavailability, 545
    body packers, 85, 545–547
        management, 64
        whole-bowel irrigation in, 63
    characteristics, 526t
    "chasing the dragon" with, 21t, 22, 343, 527–528, 1223
    chemistry, 527
    clenbuterol in, 528
    and cocaine, combined (speedball), 524
    contaminants, 528
        ophthalmic complications, 361
    effect on thyroid hormones and function, 814t
    focal brain lesions caused by, 131
    heated on aluminum foil, 21t, 22
    historical perspective on, 8
    history of, 519
    inhalation, and toxic leukoencephalopathy, 133
    injection, vascular lesions from, 132f
    intranasal administration, 527
    intravenous use, 527
    medical interventions for, 552
    metabolism, 527, 527f

murder using, 12
opioid antagonists and, 541
pharmacokinetics, 145t
quinine-containing, 361, 528
and rhabdomyolysis, 393t
safe injection sites and, 552
salt, 527
scopolamine tainting, 528
screening for, 112
smoking, 527
street names for, 162
strychnine as adulterant in, 528, 1536
substitutes for, 528
synthesis, 519
talc retinopathy from, 361
toxicity (overdose/poisoning)
    deaths caused by, 22, 527, 551
    epidemiology, 551
    naloxone for, 527
    prevention and management, naloxone education program for, 551
    risk factors for, 527
volume of distribution, 145t
withdrawal, neonatal, 439
Heroin-assisted treatment, 552
He shou-wu (Polygonum multiflorum), 641t
Hesperidin, 640t
Heteroreceptors, 206, 215, 220
Hexachlorobenzene, food contamination with, 18, 18t
Hexachlorocyclohexane, 1514
    physicochemical properties, 1515t
γ-Hexachlorocyclohexane. See Lindane
Hexachlorophene, 1369t
    neurotoxicity, 343
    transdermal absorption, 271
Hexafluorine, 1399
Hexamethonium, 13
Hexane (n-hexane)
    blood:gas partition coefficient, 1195t
    elimination, 1195t
    in gasoline, 1198, 1410
    inhaled, 1193t
        clinical manifestations, 1197–1198, 1199t
    metabolites, 1195t, 1414–1415, 1415f
    neurotoxicity, 1200, 1414–1415, 1415f
    peripheral neuropathy caused by, 1414
    toxicokinetics, 1411t
2,5-Hexanedione, 1195t, 1197, 1414–1415, 1415f
    chemical properties, 162, 162f
Hexose monophosphate shunt, 178, 178f, 312–313, 313f, 1704, 1705f
HI-6, 1746
Hibiclens (chlorhexidine), 1369t
Hickory tussock caterpillar (Lophocampa caryae), 1552
High altitude, acclimitization, and oxygenation, 403f
High-dose insulin (HDI)
    for β-adrenergic antagonist toxicity, 933–934, 933f, 953–958
    adverse effects and safety issues, 955–956
    for bupivacaine cardiotoxicity, 1001
    for calcium channel blocker toxicity, 949, 953–958, 1404
    dosage and administration, 956
    for drug-induced cardiovascular toxicity, 953–958
    indications for, 709
    labeling, 43
    and lipid emulsion, 1007
    mechanism of action, 709, 954–955, 954f
    for metal phosphide poisoning, 1459
    monitoring with, 956
    pharmacokinetics and pharmacodynamics, 955

High-frequency percussive ventilation, for smoke inhalation, 1645
High-mobility group Box-1 (HMGB-1), in acetaminophen hepatotoxicity, 481, 484
High-molecular-weight kininogen (HMWK), in coagulation, 883–884, 884f
High-performance liquid chromatography (HPLC), 103t, 106, 106f
    advantages, 106
    C-18 columns, 106
    detectors used in, 106
    disadvantages, 106
    electrospray ionization in, 107
    internal standard for, 106, 106f
    reverse-phase partitioning for, 106
    xenobiotic detection in, 106
    xenobiotic quantification in, 106
Hilar adenopathy, imaging, 115t, 126
Himmler, Heinrich, 1685
Hippocastanaceae, 1598t
Hippocratic Corpus, 638
Hippomane mancinella (manchineel tree), 1613
Hippurate, excretion, 1196
Hippuric acid, 1195t, 1196
    urinary, 1199
Hippus, 358
Hirasawa, Sadamichi, 5t
Hiroshima atomic bombing, radiation effects from, 23t, 24
Hirudin, 883, 891–894, 892f
Hirudo medicinalis (medicinal leech), anticoagulants from, 883
Histamine, 738, 805
    action on H$_1$ receptor, 741f
    and gastric acid secretion, 742, 743f
    and gastrointestinal tract, 290t
    release, neuromuscular blockers and, 1019
    structure, 740f
Histamine antagonists. See also Antihistamines
    gastrointestinal effects, 292f
Histamine receptor(s)
    H$_1$, 739
    H$_2$, 739–740
    H$_3$, 739–740
    H$_4$, 739–740
    inverse agonists vs. antagonists, 740–741, 741f
    subtypes, 739–740
Histamine receptor blockade, 44t
Histamine receptor blockers. See Antihistamines
Histidine decarboxylase, inhibitors, 743
Histone(s), modification, and withdrawal syndrome, 237
Histone acetyltransferase, and opioid tolerance, 238–239
Histone deacetylase, and opioid tolerance, 238–239
Histone deacetylase inhibitors, mechanism and site of action, 762f
Histoplasmosis, in HIV-infected (AIDS) patients, 830t
History, 1–15. See also specific xenobiotic
    early (antiquity), 1–3, 1t
    in Medieval and Renaissance periods, 3–6, 4t, 5t
    18th and 19th century, 6–9
    20th century, 9–13, 10t, 11t
    21st century, 10t, 11t, 13
History-taking, 38–39. See also Occupational history taking
    in initial assessment, 189
HIV-infected (AIDS) patients
    anorexia-cachexia syndrome in, cannabinoids for, 1113
    antimicrobials for, 829–832, 830t–831t

HIV-infected (AIDS) patients (*Cont.*):
antimonial therapy in, adverse effects, 1230, 1232
management/treatment, 829–830
neuropathy in, 342
ophthalmic complications in, 361
opportunistic infections in, antimicrobial treatment for, 830t–831t
and thiamine deficiency, 1160
tuberculosis in, 855
HLö-7, 1746
HMG Co-A reductase inhibitors
clinical and laboratory findings with, 36t
CYP enzymes and, 170
pancreatitis caused by, 295t
and rhabdomyolysis, 393, 393t
HMIT, 707
Hobo spider (*Eratigena agrestis*), 1540, 1546–1547
venom, differences in European and American spiders, 1546
Hoch, Johann, 5t
Hofmann, Albert, 9, 1178
Hog. *See* Phencyclidine (PCP)
Hognosed viper (*Bothrops ophroyomegas*), 1633
Hoigne syndrome, 824
Holiday heart syndrome, 1148
Holly (*Ilex* spp.), toxicity, 642t, 1600t, 1606–1607
Holmes, Oliver Wendell, 1011
Holocyclotoxin, cranial neuropathy caused by, 346t
Holothurin, 1574
Holy fire, 806
Homatropine, 1503
ophthalmic effects, 1504
Homer, 1, 1t
Homicide, 1884
Homocysteine, serum, in alcoholism, 1167
Homolycorin, 1601t
Homoquinolinic acid, mechanism of action, 227t
Honey
grayanotoxins in, 1612
pyrrolizidine alkaloids in, 1605
Honeybee (*Apis mellifera*), 1540t, 1551–1552. *See also* Bee (*Apis mellifera*)
venom, composition, 1551, 1551t
Honey mushroom (*Armillariella mellea*), 1594
Hookahs, 1205
Hopelessness, and suicidality, 378
Hopewell epidemic, 1518–1519
Hops (*Humulus lupulus*), 650t
Horizontal eye gaze nystagmus (HGN), 1878–1879, 1879t
Hormesis effect, 1815
Hormonal therapy, as abortifacient, 303t
Hormone(s). *See also specific hormone*
androgenic, and hepatic tumors, 333
exogenous, and erectile dysfunction, 300
hypothalamic, and thermoregulation, 412
Hormone antagonists, mechanism and site of action, 762f
Horned hog-nosed viper (*Porthidium* spp.), 1637t
Horned rattlesnake (*Crotalus* spp.), 1636t
Hornets, 1540, 1540t, 1551–1552
venom, composition, 1551, 1551t
Horse chestnut (*Aesculus hippocastanum*), 642t, 1598t, 1610
Horsehoof (*Tussilago farfara*), 641t
Horseradish root (*Alliaria officinalis*), 1607
Horseradish tree (*Moringa oleifera*), as abortifacient, 303t
Hort, 7
Hospitalization, psychiatric, medical clearance for, 375

Hot water immersion (HWI)
for cone snail envenomation, 1573
for crown-of-thorns starfish envenomation, 1574
for jellyfish stings, 1570–1571
for sea urchin envenomation, 1574
for stingray stings, 1578
Hot zone, in hazardous materials incident response, 1809, 1809t, 1810f
Hourglass spider (black widow, *Latrodectus mactans*). *See also* Black widow spider (*Latrodectus mactans*)
antivenom, 35t, 44t
Household products, poisoning with, in developing world, 1846
Housing First, 1152
HU210, structure, 1112f
Huamantlan rattlesnake (*Crotalus* spp.), 1636t
Huang-lien (*Coptis chinensis, C. japonica*), 641t
Huang qi (*Astragalus membranaceus*), 640t
Huffer's eczema, 1197, 1414
Huffing, 1193, 1422
Human chorionic gonadotropin (hCG)
as athletic performance enhancer, 620
for weight loss, 606, 608t
Human epidermal growth factor receptor 2 (HER2), 761
Human Ether-à-go-go Related Gene (hERG), 245, 253, 256, 877
Human factors, in medication errors, 1827–1828, 1828t
Human growth hormone (hGH). *See* Growth hormone (GH)
Human immunodeficiency virus. *See* HIV-infected (AIDS) patients
Human leukocyte antigen(s) (HLA), 311
and drug-induced liver injury, 329
and hypersensitivity, 329
Human performance. *See also* Athletic performance enhancers
deficits, and medication errors, 1827–1828, 1828t
factors affecting, 1827–1828, 1828t
Human repellents, 1749
Humulone, 650t
Humulus lupulus (hops), 650t
Hun Stoffe (HS, H), 1748
Huntington disease, glutamate and, 224
Hyaluronidase, 640t
in brown recluse spider venom, 1544
for calcium gluconate extravasation, 1406
for extravasation injury, 802–803
in Hymenoptera venom, 1551, 1551t
in lizard venom, 1619
in sea snake venom, 1575
in snake venom, 1618–1619, 1619t
Hydoxybenzene. *See* Phenol
2′-Hydroxynicotine, 1204
Hydralazine
as antihypertensive, 962
and gustatory dysfunction, 365
metabolism, 170
overdose/poisoning, 962
diagnostic imaging, 115t
priapism caused by, 301t
SLE induced by, 126
Hydrangea (*Hydrangea* spp.), 642t, 1607
H. arborescens, 642t
H. paniculata, 642t, 650t
Hydrangin, 642t, 650t
Hydrastine, 642t, 1600t, 1605
Hydrastis canadensis (goldenseal), 1600t, 1605
alkaloids in, 639
use and toxicities, 642t

Hydration, 168
initial assessment, 189
Hydrazides, 862
Hydrazine, 850–851, 851f, 852–853
poisoning with, management, pyridoxine in, 862–863
seizures caused by, 220
toxicity, 220
Hydro. *See* Phencyclidine (PCP)
Hydrocarbon pneumonitis, 1196, 1200, 1652
with insecticide poisoning, 1491, 1492f
management, 1416
radiographic evidence, 1412, 1413f
Hydrocarbons, 165
absorption, 1411
alicyclic, 1410
aliphatic, 1193. *See also* Gasoline; Naphtha
absorption, 1411
definition, 1410
inhaled, 1193t
toxicokinetics, 1411, 1411t
unsubstituted, 1410
aromatic, 1193, 1410. *See also* Benzene; Toluene; Xylene
absorption, 1411
elimination, 1194–1195
heterocyclic, 1410
inhaled, 1193t
polycyclic, 1410
polynuclear, 1410
toxicokinetics, 1411, 1411t
aspiration, 123–125, 125f, 165
bioassays for, 1416
bonds in, 165
cardiac effects, 1412–1413
cardiotoxicity, 1412–1413
chemistry, 165–166, 1410
chlorinated. *See* Organic chlorine (organochlorine) insecticides
classification, 1409t
CNS effects, 1413–1414
combustion, health effects, 1409
common products containing, 1409, 1409t
cyclic, definition, 1410
decontamination, 1416
definition, 1193, 1410
dermal toxicity, 271
dermatologic effects, 269, 1414–1415
diagnostic imaging, 115t
distillation, 1409
elimination, 1411, 1411t
elimination half-lives, 1411, 1411t
environmental exposure to, 1409
exposure to
in children, 1409
epidemiology, 1409
flammability, 1416
fluorinated
cardiotoxicity, 1196
toxicity, 1197, 1197f–1198f
focal airspace filling from, 125t
gastrointestinal effects, 1414
halogenated, 1011, 1014–1015. *See also* Carbon tetrachloride; Methylene chloride; Tetrachloroethylene; Trichloroethylene
cardiac effects, 255
clinical and laboratory findings with, 36t
diagnostic imaging, 117–118
elimination, 1194–1195
and hepatocellular necrosis, 331
history of, 1011

pharmacokinetics, 1194
pharmacology, 1410
and potassium currents, 1410
toxicokinetics, 1411, 1411t
hematologic effects, 1414
hepatotoxicity, 1414
history of, 1409
in hydraulic fluids for fracking, 1409
illness caused by
at-risk populations, 1409
epidemiology, 1409
immunologic effects, 1414
ingestion, management, 1417
inhalation, 1411
inhaled volatile, 165, 1193, 1409
and calcium currents, 1410
cardiotoxicity, 1196
clinical effects, 1196–1198
hepatotoxicity, 1196
neurochemical activity, 1410
and neuronal tissue, 1410
pharmacology, 1194, 1195t
teratogenicity, 1198
toxicokinetics, 1411
use/abuse, clinical manifestations, 1196–1198, 1197f–1198f
withdrawal, 1198
metabolites, 1411, 1411t
mixtures, 1409
neurotoxicity, 1414–1415, 1415f
occupational exposure to, 1409
and olfactory dysfunction, 364
oxygenated, 1410
partition coefficients, 1411, 1411t
peripheral neuropathy caused by, 1414
pharmacology, 1410
physical properties, 1410
poisoning, 7, 165. See also Hydrocarbons, toxicity
polyaromatic, and CYP induction, 171
polycyclic, and CYP enzymes, 170
pulmonary toxicity, 1412
management, 1416–1417
radiographic evidence, 1412, 1413f
receptor-ligand interaction, 1410
renal effects of, 1414
respiratory effects, 399t
saturated, 1410
skin exposure to, toxicokinetics, 1411
soft tissue injection, 1414–1415
substituted, 1193
as thermal degradation product, 1642
and tinnitus, 370t
toxicity
diagnostic tests for, 1416
disposition of patients with, 1417
epidemiology, 1409
factors affecting, 1410
management, 1416–1417
pathophysiology, 1412–1415
respiratory effects, 1412
symptom development, time course, 1417
toxicokinetics, 1411, 1411t
unsaturated, 1410
vapors, dermal absorption, 1411
viscosity, 1409t
dynamic (absolute), 1412
kinematic, 1412
volatility, 1412
Hydrochloric acid, 291, 1388t, 1656, 1656f
ingestion, laboratory investigation, 1391

and normal anion gap metabolic acidosis, 191t
production, by antimony reaction with water, 1230
Hydrochlorofluorocarbons, hepatotoxicity, 331
Hydrochlorothiazide, 963. See also Diuretics, thiazide
hypercalcemia caused by, 250
Hydrocodone, 528. See also Opioid(s)
characteristics, 526t
DEA class, 553
and hearing loss, 524
metabolism, 172
regulation, 553
screening for, 110
urine screening assays for, performance characteristics, 111t
Hydrocortisone, for vitamin D toxicity, 661
Hydrocotyle. See Gotu kola (Centella asiatica)
Hydrocyanic acid, 1748
Nazis' use of, 1684
Hydrocyanite, 1284t
Hydrofluoric acid (HF), 1388t, 1397–1402
absorption, 1397–1398
antidote for, 35t
chemistry, 1397
decontamination procedures for, 73, 1399–1400
dermal toxicity, 271
digital exposure to, management, 1399–1400
disaster involving, 16, 16t, 1397
exposure
clinical presentation, 246
dermal effects, 1397, 1398f, 1399–1400
epidemiology, 1397
management, 879, 1399–1401
ophthalmic effects, 1398, 1400
severity, assessment, 1398
fatalities caused by, 1398
history of, 1397
hypocalcemia caused by, 199, 1405
ingestion
clinical effects, 1397–1398
management, 1400
inhalation, 1398, 1400
ophthalmic exposure to, irrigating solution for, 359, 359t
ophthalmic injury caused by, 1398
ophthalmic toxicity, 356f
pathophysiology, 1397
physicochemical properties, 1397
poisoning
diagnostic tests for, 1398–1399
ECG changes in, 1398–1399
epidemiology, 1397
gastrointestinal effects, 1397–1398, 1400
local effects, 1397–1398
management, 44t, 879, 1399–1401
synthesis, 1397
systemic toxicity, 1397
assessment, 1398
management, 1400–1401
uses, 1397
Hydrofluorocarbons, inhaled, 1193t
Hydrogen
production, in ATP hydrolysis, 177
as simple asphyxiant, 400t
Hydrogen bond(s), 159
Hydrogen bromide, as thermal degradation product, 1641t, 1642
Hydrogen chloride, 160, 1653, 1655
airway injury by, 1640, 1640t
detection threshold, 1654t

immediately dangerous to life and health (IDLH), 1654t
pulmonary exposure to, management, 407
regulatory standard for, 1654t
short-term exposure limit (STEL), 1654t
sources, 1654t
as thermal degradation product, 1641t
water solubility, 1654t
Hydrogen cyanide, 1457, 1684. See also Cyanide(s)
as chemical weapon, 1741, 1748
congenital anosmia for, 364
decontamination for, 1743
from fires, 16, 16t
in genocidal killings, 17, 17t
LD$_{50}$, 1744
odor, 1684
permissible exposure limit, 1685
physicochemical properties, 1684–1685
poisoning, clinical manifestations, 1686
toxic syndrome caused by, 1751t
in warfare, 1684
Hydrogen fluoride, 1655
detection threshold, 1654t
immediately dangerous to life and health (IDLH), 1654t
inhalation, treatment, 1658
physicochemical properties, 158
regulatory standard for, 1654t
short-term exposure limit (STEL), 1654t
sources, 1654t
as thermal degradation product, 1641t, 1642
water solubility, 1654t
Hydrogen halides, 158
Hydrogen peroxide, 159–160, 175f, 1368–1370, 1369t, 1656
commercial uses, 1368
dilute, 1368–1370
gas
formation, 1370
as sterilant, 1368
home uses, 1368
as hyperoxygenation therapy, 1370
ingestion, 128, 130f, 1370
hyperbaric oxygen for, 1679
liquid, as disinfectant, 1368
oxygen embolization caused by, 1370
structure, 160t
toxicity, 1370
clinical effects, 1370
diagnosis, 1370
management, 1370
mechanisms, 1370
Hydrogen selenide
chemistry, 1339–1340, 1339t
inhalation, 1340–1341
olfactory fatigue to, 1341
Hydrogen sulfide, 1656, 1688–1691
airborne
immediately fatal, 1684
olfactory paralysis caused by, 1684
antidote for, 35t, 1691, 1691t
brain changes caused by, imaging, 131, 132t
chemical suicide with, 1688
Coca-Cola contamination with, 19
detection threshold, 1654t, 1684
detergent suicide with, 1688
detoxification, 1685f
diffuse airspace filling from, 123
dissociation products, 1689
effects on vital signs, 30t

Hydrogen sulfide (*Cont.*):
and electron transport, 176t, 177
as endogenous gaseous transmitter, 1689
environmental disasters caused by, 1688
exposure to
sources and settings for, 1688, 1690
workplace, 1688, 1690
and high anion gap metabolic acidosis, 191t
history of, 1688–1689
hyperventilation caused by, 400t
immediately dangerous to life and health (IDLH), 1654t
inhalation, 1650, 1688–1689
as knockdown gas, 1650, 1689t, 1690–1691
mass casualties from, 16, 16t, 1688
mechanism of toxicity, 1689
methemoglobin binding, 1691
odor, 37, 364t, 1656, 1689, 1689t, 1690
ophthalmic toxicity, 356f
pharmacology, 1689
physicochemical properties, 1684, 1689
poisoning
clinical manifestations, 1679, 1689–1690, 1689t
deaths caused by, 1688
diagnostic tests for, 1690–1691
emergency management, 1691, 1691t
epidemiology, 1688–1689
hyperbaric oxygen for, 1676, 1679, 1691
laboratory findings with, 1686
pathophysiology, 1685f
vs. psychogenic illness, 1690
rescuers as victims in, 1688
treatment, 1691, 1691t
production, 1688
short-term exposure limit (STEL), 1654t
sources, 1654t, 1688
natural, 1688
suicide with, 1688–1689
Internet instructions for, 1688–1689
therapeutic potential, 1689
as thermal degradation product, 1641t
toxicokinetics, 1689
water solubility, 1654t
Hydrohalidic halides, 158
Hydrolysis, 168
for chemical weapons exposure, 72
Hydromorphone, 528. *See also* Opioid(s)
in capital punishment, 13
characteristics, 526t
urine screening assays for, performance
characteristics, 111t
Hydronephrosis, 397
Hydronium ion, 160, 1655
5-Hydroperoxyeicosatetraenoic acid (5-HPETE),
511, 513f
Hydrophiinae, 1574–1575, 1633t
Hydrophis curtus (spine-bellied sea snake), 1575
Hydrophis cyanocintus, 1575
Hydrosulfide ions, 1689
Hydroxocobalamin, 1273, 1694–1697
adverse effects and safety issues, 1687, 1695–1696
availability and storage, 45t
chemistry, 1694
clinical and laboratory findings with, 36t
for cyanide poisoning, 1646, 1650, 1687, 1687t,
1694–1696, 1698–1699
animal studies, 1695
dosage and administration, 1687
human studies, 1695
dosage and administration, 1696, 1700–1701
in children, 1701

effects on laboratory tests, 1695–1696
elimination half-life, 1694
formulation and acquisition, 1696
for hemorrhagic shock, 1694
history of, 1694
for hydrogen sulfide poisoning, 1691, 1691t
indications for, 35t, 45t
mechanism of action, 1694
for nitroprusside-induced cyanide toxicity, 962–963,
1686, 1695–1696
pharmacokinetics and pharmacodynamics,
1694–1695
in pregnancy, 1696, 1700
red color, 1695–1696
stocking, recommended level, 45t
structure, 1694
4-Hydroxyamphetamine, 145t
p-Hydroxybenzoic acid, 685
Hydroxybupropion, 145t, 147, 1061
β-Hydroxybutyrate, 1150–1151
γ-Hydroxybutyrate (GHB), 203, 1188–1192
adverse effects, 1190
analogs, 238, 1188–1189, 1190t
and chemsex, 1188
clinical effects, 1190
CNS depression caused by, 1190
DEA class, 1188
deaths related to, 1188
degradation, 223, 223f
dependence, 1190
diagnostic tests for, 1190–1191
and dopamine, 223
effects on vital signs, 30t–31t
endogenous, 222, 1188–1189
pharmacology, 1188
exogenous, 1189
pharmacology, 1188
and GABA_B receptors, 223, 238, 1188–1189
history of, 1188
metabolism, 1188–1189, 1189f
as neuromdulator, 1189
overdose, 1190
clinical findings in, 1086t
ECG changes in, 1190
laboratory investigation, 1190–1191
pharmacokinetics, 1189–1190
pharmacology, 1188
physicochemical properties, 1188
physostigmine and, 756
regulation, 606
respiratory depression caused by, 1190
reuptake transporter, 223
serum
clinical significance, 1190
normal concentration, 1190
in succinic semialdehyde dehydrogenase
deficiency, 1190
and sleep, 1189
street name for, 162
structure, 1188
synonyms for, 1190t
synthesis, 223, 223f, 1188–1189, 1189f
therapeutic uses, 1188
tolerance, 223, 1190
toxicity, 222–223, 606, 756
clinical manifestations, 1190
epidemiology, 1188
management, 1191
toxicokinetics, 1189–1190
urine, normal concentration, 1190

use, trends in, 1188
withdrawal, 223, 238, 1138, 1191
γ-Hydroxybutyrate (GHB) receptors, 223, 238,
1188–1189
γ-Hydroxybutyric acid (GHB). *See* γ-Hydroxybutyrate
(GHB)
Hydroxychloroquine, 842–844
antimalarial mechanism, 838t
hypoglycemia caused by, 715
and QT interval, 253t
structure, 843
therapeutic uses, 842
and tinnitus, 370t
toxicity (overdose/poisoning)
clinical manifestations, 843
lipid emulsion for, 1006
management, 843–844
pathophysiology, 843
sodium bicarbonate for, 568t
Hydroxycitric acid, 642t
4-Hydroxycoumarin derivatives, 886
Hydroxycoumarins, 885–890. *See also* Warfarin; *specific
xenobiotic*
in rodenticides, 1453t
Hydroxycut, hepatotoxicity, 651
Hydroxy-DAMPA, 782, 783f
5-Hydroxydantrolene, 1029
elimination half-life, 1029
2-Hydroxyethoxyacetaldehyde, 1444–1445, 1445f
2-Hydroxyethoxyacetic acid (HEAA), 1444–1446,
1445f
Hydroxyethyl starch, and osmotic nephrosis, 392
2-Hydroxyiminomethyl-1-methyl pyridinium chloride
(2-PAM). *See* Pralidoxime
4-Hydroxyisoleucine, 641t
4-Hydroxylalprazolam, 145t
α-Hydroxylalprazolam, 145t
Hydroxylamine, 850, 1508, 1698
Hydroxylation, 168
Hydroxyl radical, 160, 174, 1285f, 1656
formation, 175, 175f
radiation-induced, 1767
structure, 160t
p-Hydroxymethamphetamine, 145t
7-Hydroxy methotrexate, 768
laboratory measurement, 769, 769t
1-Hydroxymethyl pyrrolizidine, 1605
Hydroxymethyl starch, and doping analysis, 623
7-Hydroxymitragynine, 649, 1181, 1181t, 1183
4-Hydroxy-2-nonenal (HNE), 1146
p-Hydroxynorephedrine, 145t
17β-Hydroxysteroid dehydrogenase, 618f, 619
5-Hydroxytryptamine (5-HT). *See* Serotonin (5-HT)
5-Hydroxytryptophan (5-OHT), 215, 216f, 217
Hydroxyurea, 349f
cell cycle phase specificity, 761f
mechanism and site of action, 762f
nail changes caused by, 281
γ-Hydroxyvaleric acid (GHV), 1190t
Hydroxyzine
for alcohol withdrawal, 1168
in cocaine, 1130
elimination half-life, 744
history of, 739
pharmacokinetics and toxicokinetics, 745t
pharmacology, 742
priapism caused by, 301t
structure, 740f
Hydrozoa, 1567, 1567t. *See also* Cnidaria (jellyfish)
actinoporins, 1570

characteristics, 1567t
stings, 1569
Hylenex, 803
Hymenoptera, 1541, 1551–1552, 1845
  envenomation (stings)
    clinical manifestations, 1551
    pathophysiology, 1551
    treatment, 1552
  taxonomy, 1551, 1551f
  venom, composition, 1551, 1551t
Hyoscine, 5t, 6, 642t
Hyoscyamine, 2, 642t–643t, 651, 756, 1181, 1181t, 1503, 1604
  elimination half-life, 1182
  pharmacology, 1183
Hyoscyamus niger (henbane), 2, 1600t
  use and toxicity, 642t
Hyperadrenergic crisis, monoamine oxidase inhibitors and, 1078, 1078t, 1079
Hyperalgesia, opioid-related, 523–524
Hyperammonemia, 342
  L-carnitine for, 35t, 726, 732–733
  valproic acid–induced, 181, 335, 726, 732–733
  xenobiotics causing, 181, 181t
Hyperbaric oxygen, 1676–1683
  adverse effects and safety issues, 1679
  for air or gas embolism, 1676, 1679
  and aluminum phosphide poisoning, 1460
  for carbon monoxide plus cyanide poisoning, 1676, 1678–1679
  for carbon monoxide poisoning, 1646, 1663, 1668–1670, 1668t–1669t, 1676–1683
    in children, 1671
    delayed administration, 1670
    in pregnancy, 437, 1670–1671
    repeat treatment, 1670
  for carbon tetrachloride poisoning, 1676, 1679
  chambers, 1676
  in cyanide poisoning, 1688
  dosage and administration, 1679–1680
  formulation and acquisition, 1680
  hepatic benefits, 329
  history of, 1676
  with hydrocarbon toxicity, 1417
  for hydrogen peroxide ingestion, 1676, 1679
  for hydrogen sulfide poisoning, 1676, 1679, 1691
  indications for, 35t, 407
  mechanism of action, 1676
  for methemoglobinemia, in dapsone toxicity, 846
  for methylene chloride poisoning, 1676, 1678
  middle ear barotrauma caused by, 1679
  for oxidant-induced methemoglobinemia, 1679
  and oxygen content of blood, 402f, 403
  pharmacodynamics, 1676–1677
  pharmacokinetics, 1676
  pharmacology, 1676
  in pregnancy, 39, 1679
  therapy with, for brown recluse spider bites, 1546
Hyperbilirubinemia
  in Gilbert syndrome, 172
  in liver injury, 334
  in metal phosphide poisoning, 1458
  methotrexate-related, 768
  neonatal, multiple-dose activated charcoal in, 78
  unconjugated (indirect), 317
Hypercalcemia, 189, 1403–1404
  adverse effects, 1406
  and anion gap, 191t
  definition, 1406
  ECG changes in, 250, 250f

leucovorin and, 783
phosphorus and, 1529
signs and symptoms, 199
toxin-induced, saline diuresis for, 93
vitamin A toxicity and, 657
vitamin D toxicity and, 660–661
xenobiotic-induced, 199, 199t, 250
Hypercalciuria
  cadmium-induced, 1260
  vitamin D and, 660
Hypercapnia, 1652
  clinical effects, 1652–1653
Hypercarbia, in poisoned patient, 403
Hypercarotenemia, 272, 657
Hyperchloremia, with hypokalemia, 198
Hyperemesis gravidarum, and thiamine deficiency, 1160
Hyperforin, 644t, 647, 1600t, 1610
  in St. John's wort, 1610
  xenobiotic interactions, 1611
Hyperglycemia
  antipsychotic-induced, 1039
  in calcium channel blocker poisoning, 947
  chronic, 708
  in critical illness, 698, 710
  diuretic-induced, 963
  glucagon-induced, 942
  and hyponatremia, 196
  in metal phosphide poisoning, 1458
  in methanol poisoning, 1427
  in theophylline overdose, 989, 991
  therapeutics for, 35t
  xenobiotics causing, 953
Hyperhidrosis, treatment, 273
Hypericin, 644t, 1600t
Hypericum perforatum. *See* St. John's wort (*Hypericum perforatum*)
Hyperinsulinemia, quinine-induced, 838, 840
Hyperkalemia, 189
  and anion gap, 191t
  calcium for, 1406
  cardiac manifestations, 198–199, 256
  cardioactive steroid toxicity and, 972, 974
  causes, 198, 198t
  clinical manifestations, 577t
  dextrose for, 709
  diagnosis, 198
  digoxin overdose and, 972
  diuretic-induced, 963
  ECG changes in, 247, 251, 252f, 1406
  fluoride poisoning and, 1398
  intravenous insulin for, 709
  management, sodium polystyrene sulfonate in, 1069
  phosphate excess causing, management, 1405
  phosphorus and, 1529
  QRS complex in, 249
  in strychnine poisoning, 1537
  succinylcholine-induced, 1022
  therapeutics for, 35t
  treatment, 199
  xenobiotic-induced, 197–199, 198t
    sodium bicarbonate for, 568t
Hyperlactatemia, 191, 1686
  management, 193
  propylene glycol and, 688
Hyperlipidemia
  after lipid meulsion therapy, 1007–1008
  and hyponatremia, 196
Hypermagnesemia, 157, 189, 199–200, 879
  and acetylcholine release, 207, 207t

and anion gap, 191t
calcium for, 1405
cardiac effects, 200, 249, 258t, 1405
cathartics causing, 77, 85
causes, 199, 200t
clinical manifestations, 577t, 876
ECG changes in, 200, 249, 1405
gastrointestinal decontamination and, 85
iatrogenic, 879
in kidney disease, 876
management, 44t
multiple-dose activated charcoal and, 62, 79
QRS complex in, 249
respiratory effects, 400
signs and symptoms, 199–200
therapeutics for, 35t
treatment, 200
Hypernatremia, 189, 194–195
  in diabetes insipidus, 195–196
  diagnosis, 195
  gastrointestinal decontamination and, 85
  multiple-dose activated charcoal and, 62, 79
  orogastric lavage and, 56
  in strychnine poisoning, 1537
  treatment, 195
  with whole-bowel irrigation, 85
  xenobiotics causing, 194–195, 195t
Hyperoside, 642t
Hyperosmolality, polyethylene glycol (PEG) and, 687
Hyperosmolarity, propylene glycol and, 687–688
Hyperostosis deformans, with fluorosis, 119
Hyperoxygenation therapy, 1370. *See also* Hydrogen peroxide
Hyperparathyroidism, and hypercalcemia, lithium-induced, 1068
Hyperphosphatemia
  gastrointestinal decontamination and, 85
  management, 1405
  phosphorus and, 1529
Hyperpigmentation, 273
  tetracyclines and, 827
Hyperpnea, 30, 399
Hyperprolactinemia, antipsychotic-induced, 1039
Hyperreflexia, 189
  in strychnine poisoning, 1536–1537
Hypersensitivity. *See also* Drug-induced hypersensitivity syndrome (DIHS)
  antihistamines and, 746
  antimonials and, 1233
  antipsychotic-induced, 1039
  to arsenic, 1241
  chemotherapeutic-related, 762, 802
  delayed, 279
  and flushing, 273
  human leukocyte antigen (HLA) and, 329
  to Hymenoptera venom, 1552
  to liposomes, 1006
  and liver injury, 330
  with nonsteroidal antiinflammatory drugs, 514t, 515
  plant-induced allergic contact dermatitis and, 1614
  prothrombin complex concentrate and, 909
  quinine-induced, 840
  renal effects, 390f
  rifampin and, 855
  sulfonamides and, 827
  tetracyclines and, 827
Hypersensitivity pneumonitis, 1659
  imaging, 115t, 125–126, 125t
  sulfonamides and, 827

Hypertension, 959
  amphetamine-induced, management, 1104–1105,
    1104t
  barium-induced, 1455
  catecholamines and, 210
  cocaine and, 1129
  decongestant-induced, 750–751
  food toxins and, 600t
  in imidazoline toxicity, 961
  lead-related, 1295–1296, 1298
  malignant
    acute kidney injury caused by, 391
    and posterior reversible encephalopathy
      syndrome, 132
  MAOI-induced, 1078
    management, 1080
  and pulse rate, 30
  in strychnine poisoning, 1537
  in thallium toxicity, 1351
  xenobiotics causing, 29, 29t, 264, 265t
Hypertensive crisis, of MAOI-food interaction, clinical
    and laboratory findings in, 36t
Hyperthermia, 30, 418–423. See also Heatstroke;
    Malignant hyperthermia
  amphetamine-induced, 1104
    management, 1104–1105, 1104t
  antihistamine-related, 746
    management, 747
  approach to patient with, 27
  in arylcyclohexylamine toxicity, management,
    1217
  cocaine and, 1128
  complications, 27, 27t
  cooling measures for, 422–423, 423t
  dantrolene sodium for, 1029
  differential diagnosis, 419–420, 419t, 1038
  dissociative anesthetics and, 1214
  effects on oxygenation, 403f
  etiology, 27, 27t
  hallucinogen-related, 27, 1184
  life-threatening, 30, 37, 412
    case study, 27
  management, 37
  in MAOI toxicity, 1078, 1078t, 1080
  in neuroleptic malignant syndrome, 420
  organic chlorine insecticides causing, 1517
  in serotonin toxicity, 420
  in strychnine poisoning, 1537–1538
  in thyrotoxicosis, 815
    management, 817
  xenobiotic-induced
    ambient temperature and, 412
    in animals, species differences, 412
    in elderly, 463, 463t
  xenobiotics causing, 31t, 412–414, 413t
Hyperthyroidism, 816
  epidemiology, 812
  iodide-induced, 818
  pathophysiology, 814–815
  potassium iodide and, 1776
  xenobiotics and, 814t
Hypertonicity, methylxanthine-induced, 989, 991
Hypertonic saline, for cyclic antidepressant toxicity,
    1049–1050, 1049t
Hyperuricemia, diuretic-induced, 963
Hyperventilation, 30, 189
  for cyclic antidepressant toxicity, 1050
  for local anesthetic–induced seizures, 1000
  methylxanthines and, 988
  xenobiotic-induced, 299, 300t

Hypervitaminosis A
  clinical and laboratory findings in, 36t
  skeletal changes in, 122t
Hypervitaminosis D, skeletal changes in, 122t
Hyphema, 356
Hypnotics, 7
Hypoactive sexual desire disorder, flibanserin for, 302
Hypoalbuminemia, and anion gap, 191, 191t
Hypocalcemia, 189, 1403
  aminoglycoside-induced, 199
  and anion gap, 191t
  antiepileptic-induced, 199
  citrate excess and, 199
  ECG changes in, 199, 250
  in ethylene glycol toxicity, 199, 1424
    calcium for, 1405
  fluoride-induced, 199, 199t, 1398, 1405
    calcium for, 1405
  gastrointestinal decontamination and, 85
  in hydrofluoric acid toxicity, 199, 1405
    calcium for, 1405
  and hypomagnesemia, 200
  magnesium therapy and, 879
  management, 44t
  methylxanthine toxicity and, 991
  oxalic acid and, 1405
  phosphate excess causing, 199
    calcium for, 1405
  phosphorus and, 1529
  and prolonged QT interval, 253, 253t, 256, 1820
  signs and symptoms, 199
  in strychnine poisoning, 1537
  vitamin D deficiency and, 660
  xenobiotic-induced, 164, 199, 199t
Hypocaloric diets, for weight loss, 612
Hypochlorhydria, 294
Hypochlorite, 160
  0.5% solution, for dermal decontamination, 72
Hypochlorous acid, 1655–1656, 1656f
  structure, 160t
Hypocretins, 708, 1090
Hypodermis, 269, 270f
Hypogeusia, 365, 365t
Hypoglycemia, 37. See also Antidiabetics
  β-adrenergic antagonists and, 698
  altered mental status from, 707–708, 710
  antidiabetic-induced, pathophysiology, 697–698
  antiglycemic-induced, 697–698
  antimalarial-induced, octreotide for, 715
  autonomic failure associated with, 698, 708
  cardiovascular effects, 699
  causes, 694, 694t, 697
  chloroquine-induced, 715
  chlorpropamide-induced, 699
    in children, 699
  ciprofloxacin-induced, 715
  clinical, 698
  clinical manifestations, 36t, 697–698, 707–708
  clonidine-induced, 715
  complications, 709
  definition, 708
  delayed or prolonged, in overdose situations,
    699–700, 702
  detection
    blood for, 708–709
    reagent strips for, 700, 708–709
  dextrose for, 33, 701–702, 707–710
  in diabetes mellitus, 708
    management, 701
  diagnostic tests for, 700

  diazoxide-induced, 714
  dysrhythmias in, 699, 708
  ethanol-induced, 698, 1150–1151
    in children, 453, 709
    hospitalization for, 702
  exenatide and, 700
  fasting, laboratory investigation, 700–701, 701t
  focal brain lesions caused by, 131
  gatifloxacin-induced, 715
  gliclazide-induced, octreotide for, 714–715
  glipizide-induced
    in children, 699
    octreotide for, 714–715
  gliptins and, 700
  glucagon for, 701, 941–942
  glucagon-induced, 942
  glucagon-like peptide-1 GLP-1 analogs and, 700
  glyburide exposure and, in children, 699
  hospitalization for, 702–703
  hydroxychloroquine-induced, 715
  hypothermia in, 699
  imidazoline-induced, 715
  initial control of, euglycemia maintenance after,
    701–702
  insulin-induced, 694, 696, 698–699, 955–956
    hospitalization for, 702
  insulin overdose and, 699
    hospitalization for, 702
  insulin-related, 694, 696, 698–699, 955–956
    hospitalization for, 702
  insulin secretagogue-induced, therapeutics for, 35t,
    713–718
  intentionally self-induced, hospitalization for, 702
  in kidney failure, 702
  laboratory findings in, 36t
  levofloxacin-induced, 715
  liraglutide-induced, 700
  in liver failure, 702
  management, 33, 44t, 701–702, 710
    octreotide in, 702, 714–715. See also Octreotide
  meglitinide-induced, 702, 713–718
    octreotide for, 715
  in metal phosphide poisoning, 1458
  metformin-induced, 699
  misdiagnosis, 700
  mortality rate for, 699
  nalidixic acid-induced, 715
  nateglinide-induced, 700
  neuropsychiatric effects, 698–699, 708
  nocturnal, 708
  nonketotic, 697
  numerical, 698–699, 708–709
  octreotide as antidote for, 702, 713–718
    clinical use of, for insulin suppression, 714–715
    dosage and administration, 702
    effect on insulin secretion, 713–715
  oral carbohydrates for, 710
  outcomes with, 699
  pathophysiology, 697–698
  phentolamine-induced, 715
  quinine-induced, 713–718, 840
    management, 840
  quinolone-induced, 713–718
  rebound, 709–710
  recurrent, 701
  repaglinide-induced, 700
  repeated, 708
  risk of, glycemic control and, 697–698
  salicylate-induced, 698, 709
  in salicylate poisoning, 709

in starvation, 702
sulfonylurea-induced, 694, 696, 698–699, 702, 709–710, 713–718
  in children, 699
    hospitalization for, 702
    octreotide for, 714–715
therapeutics for, 35t
trivalent arsenic and, 1238–1239
of unknown etiology, hospitalization for, 702
xenobiotic-related, 178
yohimbine-induced, 715
Hypoglycemia unawareness, 698–699, 708
Hypoglycemics, 694–706
cranial neuropathy caused by, 346t
effects on vital signs, 31t
history of, 694
hypoglycemia caused by, pathophysiology, 697–698, 697t
maintaining euglycemia after initial control with, 701–702
and metabolic acidosis with elevated lactate concentration, 703–704
oral, and ethanol, interactions, 1146t
overdose/poisoning, management, 701
pancreatitis caused by, 295t
pharmacokinetics and toxicokinetics, 696, 697t
pharmacology, 694–696
potentiation by interaction with other xenobiotics, 697, 698t
xenobiotics reacting with, 698t
Hypoglycin, 332, 1591, 1598t, 1846. *See also* Ackee tree (*Blighia sapida*) fruit
and fatty acid metabolism, 176t
hepatotoxicity, 331
Hypoglycin A, 1609
and fatty acid metabolism, 179
and gluconeogenesis, 176t, 178, 179f
Hypoglycin B, 1609
Hypokalemia, 157
β_2-adrenergic agonist toxicity and, 989, 991
and anion gap, 191t
barium-induced, 1455
cardiac effects, 198, 251, 252f, 970
cardioactive steroid toxicity and, 974
cesium chloride and, 1265
chloroquine-induced, 843–844
clinical manifestations, 198, 577t
differential diagnosis, 1455
diuretic-induced, 963
ECG changes in, 198, 251, 252f
fluoride poisoning and, 1398–1399
gastrointestinal decontamination and, 85
glucagon-induced, 942–943
in heatstroke, 422
hyperchloremia with, 198
and hypomagnesemia, 198, 200
  cardiac effects, 254
hypophosphatemia with, 198
and ileus, 198
insulin and, 699, 956
licorice and, 1606
metabolic alkalosis with, 198
in metal phosphide poisoning, 1458
in methylxanthine overdose, 989, 991
and QT interval, 253, 253t, 256, 1820–1821, 1821f
quinine-induced, 840
respiratory effects, 400
rhabdomyolysis and, 198, 393
in strychnine poisoning, 1537
toluene and, 1196–1197

treatment, 198
ventricular tachycardia and, 198
weakness and, 198
  in toluene abusers, 1197
xenobiotic-induced, 197–199, 198t
Hypokalemic periodic paralysis, clinical manifestations, 577t
Hypomagnesemia, 189
β_2-adrenergic agonist toxicity and, 989
and anion gap, 191t
cardiac effects, 200, 249, 253t, 256, 258t, 970, 1820
cardioactive steroid toxicity and, 975
cesium chloride and, 1265
clinical manifestations, 876
diuretic-induced, 200, 877, 963
ethanol-related, 200, 877–878
hypocalcemia and, 200
with hypokalemia, 198, 200
  cardiac effects, 254
magnesium for, 200, 876–877
methylxanthine toxicity and, 989, 991
and prolonged QT interval, 253t, 256, 1820
QRS complex in, 249
signs and symptoms, 200
therapeutics for, 35t
treatment, 200
and Wernicke encephalopathy, 1159
xenobiotic-induced, 200, 200t
  magnesium for, 876–877
Hyponatremia, 189, 196, 724
artifactual, 196
in burn patients, 196
carbamazepine-induced, 721
causes, 196, 196t
diuretic-induced, 196, 963
with ethanol therapy, 1440–1441
glycine and, 196
glycyrrhizic acid and, 196
and hyperglycemia, 196
and hyperlipidemia, 196
lithium and, 196
management, 197
multiple myeloma and, 196
SIADH and, 196–197
silver nitrate and, 196
SSRIs and, 1058
with whole-bowel irrigation, 85
xenobiotic-induced, 196, 196t
  in elderly, 463, 463t
Hypopharynx, 289–290
Hypophosphatemia
β_2-adrenergic agonist toxicity and, 989
barium toxicity and, 1455
in heatstroke, 422
with hypokalemia, 198
methylxanthine toxicity and, 989, 991
and rhabdomyolysis, 393, 393t
Hypopnea, 30, 189, 399
Hypoprothrombinemia
cephalosporin-induced, 824–825
salicylate-induced, 558
Hypopyon, 356
Hyporeflexia, in toxidromes, 29t
Hyposmia, 363–364, 364t
Hypotension, 189
with *N*-acetylcysteine, 495
angiotensin-converting enzyme inhibitor–induced, 964
angiotensin II receptor blocker–induced, 964
antihistamine-related, management, 747
antihypertensive-related, 960–961

antipsychotic-induced, 1034t
  management, 1040
and bradycardia
  case study, 924, 925f
  differential diagnosis, 924, 924t
calcium channel blocker–induced, 948
carbon monoxide poisoning and, 1664–1665
cardiac effects, 254–255
cathartics causing, 77
central α_2-adrenoceptor activation in, 210, 210f, 212
chemotherapeutic-related, management, 764
cyclic antidepressants and, 1046
  management, 1049t, 1050–1051
cyclohexanone and, 1491
deferoxamine and, 678
with disulfiram-ethanol reaction, 1173–1174
food toxins and, 600t
in heatstroke, 420–421
hemodialysis and, 95
with hydrocarbon toxicity, 1417
in hypothermia, 417
management, 37
  in MAOI overdose, 212, 1081
MAOI-induced, 212, 1078
  management, 212, 1081
methylene blue for, 964, 1713, 1715
multiple-dose activated charcoal and, 79
NSAID overdose and, 516
ophthalmic toxicity, 361t
orthostatic
  xenobiotic-induced, in elderly, 463, 463t
  xenobiotics causing, 29
phosphodiesterase inhibitors and nitrates, combined, and, 301
in pregnant patient, 39
protamine-related, 919–920
and pulse rate, 30
smoke inhalation and, 1642
sotalol-induced, 936
in strychnine poisoning, 1537
theophylline-induced, 988, 991
therapeutics for, 35t
tubocurarine-induced, 1019
verapamil-induced, calcium salts and, 1404
xenobiotics causing, 29, 29t, 264–265, 265t, 403
  heart rate and ECG abnormalities associated with, 265, 265t
Hypothalamus
thermoregulatory role, 411
and thyroid function, 812, 813f
Hypothermia, 30–31, 414–418
amiodarone for, 417
antihypertensive-related, 960
arterial blood gas physiochemistry in, 417
carbon monoxide and, 412, 1672
with cardiac arrest, management, 417
clinical manifestations, 415–416, 415t
and DIC, 885
dopamine for, 417–418
dysrhythmias in, 416, 416f
effects on oxygenation, 403f, 416
epidemiology, 414
epinephrine for, 417
ethanol-induced, 413–414, 413t
as glutamate scavenger, 229
in hypoglycemia, 699
hypotension in, 417
management, 37, 416–417
metabolic changes in, 415
organic phosphorus compounds and, 412

Hypothermia (*Cont.*):
　and oxyhemoglobin dissociation curve, 416
　pharmacology in, 415
　physiologic manifestations, 415–416, 415t
　predisposing factors, 414, 414t
　prognosis for, 418
　QRS complex in, 249
　rewarming for, 418
　　underlying illness and, 414–415, 415f
　sedative-hypnotic overdose and, 1086, 1086t
　underlying illness and, 414–415
　vasopressin for, 417
　and ventricular fibrillation, 416
　xenobiotic-induced, in elderly, 463, 463t
　xenobiotics causing, 31t, 412–414, 413t
Hypothyroidism
　amiodarone-induced, 872
　autoimmune, in drug-induced hypersensitivity
　　　syndrome, 278
　cobalt-related, 1274–1275
　in elderly, 812
　epidemiology, 812
　goitrous, 815
　iodide-induced, 818
　neonatal, epidemiology, 812
　pathophysiology, 815
　potassium iodide and, 1776
　treatment, 813
　xenobiotics and, 814t
Hypoventilation, 30, 189
　case study, 32
　chest wall weakness/rigidity and, 400
　metabolic alkalosis and, 194
　neuromuscular blockers and, 1019
　in poisoned patient, approach to, 403
　xenobiotic-induced, 299, 300t
Hypovolemia, with colchicine poisoning, 502–503, 503t
Hypoxemia, 173f, 405
　and pulse oximetry, 404, 404t
　simple asphyxiants and, 1652
Hypoxia
　acute tubular necrosis caused by, 392
　cardiac effects, 254–255
　cerebral, focal lesions caused by, 131
　clinical manifestations, 1651–1652, 1651t
　inhalant-induced, 1196
　ophthalmic toxicity, 356f, 361
　in poisoned patient, 403
　simple asphyxiants and, 1651–1652, 1651t
　in smoke inhalation, 1642–1643
Hypoxic encephalopathy, 541
Hypoxic ventilatory response (HVR), neuromuscular
　　blockers and, 1019
Hy's law, 1841
Hysteresis, 152
Hysteroscopy, and hyponatremia, 196

I
Iatrogenic toxicity, 152
Ibn Wahshiya, 1t, 3
Iboga (*Tabernanthe iboga*), 642t
Ibogaine, 642t, 650t
　cardiac effects, *case study*, 242–243
Ibotenic acid, 221, 228, 1179, 1582t, 1588, 1589t
　effect on NMDA receptors, 1588
　mechanism of action, 227t, 1588
　structure, 1588
Ibuprofen
　adverse effects and safety issues, 515
　binding, by cholestyramine, 92

　cardiovascular risk with, 514
　hematologic effects, 516
　history of, 511
　ingestion, management, 516
　pharmacokinetics and toxicokinetics, 512
　pharmacology, 511, 512t
　for phosgene exposure, 1653
　poisoning, and organ donation, 1893t
Ibutilide, 872–873
　adverse effects and safety issues, 867t
　magnesium with, 877
　pharmacokinetics, 867t
　pharmacology, 867t
Icatibant, 964
Ice (methamphetamine), 1099
Ice packs, for jellyfish stings, 1569–1570
Ice-water bath, 27
Idanediones, 885
Idarubicin, 760t
　extravasation, 802
Idarucizumab, 888t, 892–894, 908, 911–912
　adverse effects and safety issues, 912
　availability and storage, 45t, 912
　chemistry, 911
　for dabigatrin reversal in ischemic stroke, 912
　dosage and administration, 912
　history of, 911
　indications for, 35t, 45t
　mechanism of action, 911
　pharmacokinetics and pharmacodynamics, 911–912
　pharmacology, 911
　in pregnancy and lactation, 912
　stocking, recommended level, 45t
　before thrombolytic therapy in ischemic stroke, 912
Ideal body weight (IBW), equations for, 148t
Idioblasts, 1613, 1613f
Idiopathic copper toxicosis, 1287
Idiopathic intracranial hypertension (IIH), 657
　clinical manifestations, 658
　treatment, 658
Idiosyncratic response, 1873t
Ifenprodil, 227t, 228
　indications for, 228
　mechanism of action, 227t
　and NMDA receptors, 228
Ifosfamide, 760t
　acute tubular necrosis caused by, 392
　antidote for, 35t, 764
　diabetes insipidus caused by, 195t
　diagnostic tests for, 763
　and kidney failure, 763
　metabolism, 171
　nephrotoxicity, *N*-acetylcysteine for, 494
　neurotoxicity, 763
　toxicity, 763
Ignatia (*Strychnos* spp.), 1603t
Ignis sacer, 18
Ileostomy, bismuth preparations used with, 1255
Ileum, pH, 142t
Ileus
　activated charcoal and, 79
　adynamic, 127, 129f
　in body stuffers, 548
　colonic, 129f
　diagnostic imaging, 115t, 127, 129f, 129t
　hyperkalemia and, 198
　hypokalemia and, 198
　postoperative, alvimopan for, 542
Ilex spp. (holly), 642t, 1600t, 1606–1607
Ilex aquifolium, 642t

Ilex opaca, 642t
Ilex paraguariensis (maté, yerba maté, Paraguay tea),
　　1600t
　psychoactive properties, 650t
　use and toxicities, 643t
Ilex vomitoria, 642t
Illiciaceae, 1600t
Illicit drug use
　disasters, 21–22, 21t
　in elderly, 466–467
　ophthalmic complications, 361
Illicium spp., 1608
Illicium anisatum (Japanese star anise), 1600t, 1608
Illicium verum (Chinese star anise), 1608
Illusions
　definition, 1178
　hallucinogen-induced, 1184
Illy, 1212
Iloperidone. *See also* Antipsychotics
　clinical and toxicologic effects, 1034t
　dosage and administration, 1033t
　pharmacokinetics, 1033t
Iloprost, for frostbite, 418
Imaging
　in antimonial toxicity, 1233
　of bezoars, 294
　of body packers, 115t, 117, 120f, 122f, 129t, 546–547,
　　546f
　of gastrointestinal foreign bodies, 295
　in liver disease, 336
　nanotechnology in, 1717
Imazamethabenz, 1468t
Imazapyr, 1466, 1468t
Imazaquin, 1468t
Imazethapyr, 1468t
Imazosulfuron toxicity, clinical manifestations, 1473
Imidazoles, 829
　mechanism of action, 822t
　overdose, 822t
　toxicity, 822t
Imidazoline(s). *See also specific xenobiotic*
　abuse, 748
　adverse effects and safety issues, in children, 453
　cardiac effects, 256
　centrally acting, 959–961
　as decongestants, 748–751, 749t
　history of, 748
　hypoglycemia caused by, 715
　pharmacology, 749, 749t
　structure, 749, 750f
Imidazoline agonists, central, 961
Imidazoline-binding sites, 212
Imidazoline derivatives, mechanism of action, 212
Imidazoline receptor(s), 749
Imidazolinone herbicides, 1468t
Imipenem, 825
　and GABA receptor, 222
　seizures caused by, 823
Imipramine, 1044. *See also* Cyclic antidepressants
　history of, 1044
　Log D, 1045
　pharmacokinetics and toxicokinetics, 145t, 1045
　pharmacology, 1044
　plasma protein binding by, 146
　poisoning, lipid emulsion for, 1006
　and serotonin toxicity, 1058t
　skin discoloration caused by, 273
　structure, 1044t
　torsade de pointes caused by, magnesium for, 878
　volume of distribution, 145t

Imiprothrin, 1520t. *See also* Pyrethroids
Immobilization, and rhabdomyolysis, 393, 393t
Immune checkpoint inhibitors
  as chemotherapeutics, mechanism and site of
    action, 762f
  respiratory effects, 399t
Immune response, zinc and, 1362
Immune system
  β-adrenergic antagonists and, 929
  antimicrobial toxicity and, 829t
  mushroom toxins affecting, 1589t
Immunity
  adaptive, 319
  innate, 319
Immunoassays, 102, 103t, 104–105, 104f–105f
  antihistamines affecting, 746
  competitive, 104
  cross-reactivity, 105
  drug-screening, 110–111
    performance characteristics, 111t, 112–113
  for ethanol, 1149, 1877
  heterogeneous, 104, 104f
  homogenous, 104
  metabolites and, 105
  noncompetitive, 104
  sensitivity, 103t, 105
  specificity, 103t, 105
  urine drug-screening, performance characteristics,
    111t, 112–113
Immunoglobulin G (IgG) replacement therapy,
    thimerosal in, 690
Immunomodulators, for tuberculosis, 858
Immunosuppressants
  hypomagnesemia caused by, 877
  pancreatitis caused by, 295t
  for paraquat poisoning, 1474f, 1477
  and posterior reversible encephalopathy syndrome,
    132
Impaired physician, reporting, 1866
Impairment
  assessment, 1873
  ethanol-induced
    assessment, 1876–1883
    dram shop laws and, 1880–1881
    history of, 1876
    per se laws and, 1144, 1873, 1876–1878
    standardized field sobriety tests for, 1878–1879,
      1879t
IMPase (inositol 1-monophosphatase), lithium and,
    1066
Impila (*Callilepsis laureola*), 643t
Implant(s)
  chromium-containing, 1269
  cobalt-containing
    failure, 1276–1277
    management of, recommendations/guidelines
      for, 1277
    radiologic evaluation, 1277
  metal-on-metal, 1269, 1273, 1275–1276
  metal-on-polyethylene, 1276
Impotence. *See* Erectile dysfunction
Inamrinone, for calcium channel blocker toxicity,
    948
Inborn errors of metabolism, 181
Incapacitating agents, 1750
  toxic syndromes caused by, 1751t
Incarceration, and thiamine deficiency, 1160
Incense blends, cannabinoids in, 1111, 1117
Incidence, 1853t
  definition, 1853

IncobotulinumtoxinA (Xeomin), 578–579
Incontinence, carbon monoxide poisoning and, 1665
Incretins, 694, 696
  synthetic analogs, 694
Indandiones, in rodenticides, 1453t
Inderal, history of, 926
India, ancient, poisons in, 2
Indian bean (*Abrus precatorius*), 1598t. *See also* Rosary
    pea (*Abrus precatorius*)
Indian marking nut (*Semecarpus anacardium*), 1614
Indian pennywort. *See* Gotu kola (*Centella asiatica*)
Indian podophyllum. *See* Podophyllin; Podophyllum
    (*Podophyllum* spp.)
Indian poke, 1603t
Indian snakeroot (*Rauwolfia serpentina*), 1602t
Indian squill, 1603t
Indian stonefish (*Synanceja horrida*), 1576, 1576t, 1577
Indian tobacco (*Lobelia inflata*), 1601t, 1604
  use and toxicities, 643t
Indian valerian (*Valeriana officinalis*), 644t
Indinavir, 831–832
  inhibition of glucuronidation, 172
Indium, chelator for, 1780
Indobufen
  hematologic effects, 516
  pharmacology, 512t
Indole alkaloids, 650t
Indolealkylamines (tryptamines), 1179–1180
  chemical structure, 1180f
  pharmacology, 1182–1183
  structure, 1179, 1180f
Indoleamines, 1075
Indoles, 217
Indomethacin
  and ATP synthesis, 176t
  cardiovascular risk with, 514
  nanoparticle emulsion, 1719t
  pharmacology, 511, 512t
  and tinnitus, 369
  as tocolytic, 514
Indu (*Cycas circinalis*), 1599t
Inductively coupled plasma (ICP), 107
Industrial hygiene sampling and monitoring, 1799
Industrialization, human and environmental impact,
    1847
Inebriants, 7
Infant(s), exchange transfusions in, 98
Infant botulism. *See* Botulism, infant
Infant formula, melamine in, 18t, 19, 453, 601, 1846
Infant soy formula, effect on thyroid hormones and
    function, 814t
Infection(s)
  after sea urchin envenomation, 1574
  anabolic-androgenic steroids and, 618
  intracerebral, 131
  ophthalmic involvement in, 361
  opportunistic, in HIV-infected (AIDS) patients,
    antimicrobial treatment for, 830t–831t
Infectious endocarditis, 37, 125
Inferential statistical tests, 1857–1858, 1857t
  nonparametric, 1857–1858, 1857t
  parametric, 1857–1858, 1857t
Infertility
  antimonials and, 1233
  female, lead and, 1298
  male, lead and, 1296, 1298
  xenobiotic-induced, 297, 297t
Inflammation, irritant gases and, 1640–1641
Inflammatory mediators, in heatstroke, 420
Inflammatory response, 159, 174

urticating hairs of tarantula and, 1547–1548
Influenza, virosome, 1719t
Influenza like illness (ILI), 1793
Information, on xenobiotics, sources, 1814
Information bias, 1856
Information resources
  employers and manufacturers as, 1803
  government agencies as, 1801t, 1804
  for occupational toxicology, 1801t, 1803–1804
  online databases as, 1804
  poison control centers as, 1782–1786, 1803
  regulatory agencies as, 1801t, 1803–1804
  unions as, 1804
  worker's compensation insurance carriers as,
    1803
Information technology, for medication error
    prevention, 1825t, 1829
Informed consent, 1860–1861
  reasonable person standard, 1860–1861
  reasonable physician standard, 1861
Infratrack, 1763
INH. *See* Isoniazid (INH)
Inhalant(s), 1193–1202. *See also specific inhalant*
  blood:gas partition coefficient, 1194, 1195t
  cardiotoxicity, 1194, 1196
  and CYP system, 1194–1195, 1195t
  dependence, 1198
    management, 1200
  and dysrhythmias, 1194, 1196, 1199
  elimination, 1194–1195, 1195t
  and GABA receptors, 1194
  laboratory tests for, 1199
  metabolites, 1194, 1195t
  and motor activity, 1194
  pharmacokinetics, 1194–1195, 1195t
  and potassium channels, 1196
  tolerance, 1198
  toxic, *case study*, 1650
  toxic syndromes caused by, 1751t
  use/abuse
    clinical manifestations of, 1195–1199, 1199t
    CNS depression with, 1196
    common, 1193–1194, 1193t
    constituent chemicals in, 1193t
    diagnostic tests for, 1199
    management, 1199–1200
    pharmacology, 1194, 1195t
  withdrawal, 1198
    management, 1200
Inhalational anesthetic(s), 1011–1017. *See also specific*
    xenobiotic
  abuse, 1016
  with carbon dioxide absorbers, 1015–1016
  carbon monoxide poisoning with, 1015–1016
  history of, 1011
  for lead encephalopathy, in children, 1302
  lipid solubility, 1410
  long-term use in ICUs, 1016
  malignant hyperthermia with, 1023
  and neuromuscular blockers, interactions, 1021t
  pharmacodynamics, 1194
  pharmacokinetics, 1012, 1194
  pharmacology, 1011–1012, 1194, 1410
  and sodium channels, 1410
  structure, 1011f
  waste, chronic exposure to, 1016
Inhalational pulmonary xenobiotic disorders
  pulmonary irritants in. *See* Pulmonary irritants
  simple asphyxiants in, 400, 400t. *See also*
    Asphyxiants, simple

Initial patient assessment, 189
Injection drug use (IDU). *See also* Intravenous drug use (IVDU)
  abdominal complications, 128
  aneurysms caused by, 132f
  chest radiographic findings in, 125t, 126f
  diagnostic imaging for, 115t, 122, 124f, 125t, 126f, 132f
  infectious complications, imaging, 122
  neurologic complications, 131
  pleural disorders in, 126
  skeletal changes in, 122t
    imaging, 122, 124f
  vascular complications, 128–130, 132f
Injury Prevention Program, The (TIPP), 1784
Inkberry. *See* Pokeweed (*Phytolacca americana, P. decandra*)
Inky caps, 1587
Innate immunity, 319
Innovator product, 1835
Inocybe spp., 1503, 1582t, 1587
  antidote for, 35t
Inocybe geophylla, 1587
Inocybe iacera, 1587
Inocybe lanuginosa, 1587
Inorganic acids, 271
Inorganic chemistry. *See* Chemistry, inorganic
Inositol 1,4-bisphosphate 1-phosphatase (IPPase), lithium and, 1066, 1067f
Inositol depletion, lithium and, 1066–1067, 1067f
Inositol 1-monophosphatase (IMPase), lithium and, 1066, 1067f
Inositol triphosphate (IP$_3$), 209, 945, 1066, 1067f
Inotropes
  for β-adrenergic antagonist toxicity, 933, 933f
  for calcium channel blocker toxicity, 950
  and fluid balance, 194
Inotropy
  cardioactive steroids and, 970, 971f, 972t
  decreased, xenobiotics causing, 953–954
  methylxanthines and, 988
Insane root. *See* Henbane (*Hyoscyamus niger*)
Insect(s). *See also specific insect*
  bites, 1541
  biting, stinging, and nettling, 1540, 1540t
Insecta, 1540
Insecticides, 1504, 1514–1527. *See also* DEET; Insect repellents; Pyrethrins; Pyrethroids; *specific insecticide*
  coformulants, 1490
  food contamination with, 599–600, 602
  and GABA receptor, 1521
  hemorrhagic cystitis caused by, 306
  in homicides, 1487
  labeling, legal standards for, 1525
  mass poisoning with, 1487
  neonicotinoids in, 1203
  nicotine in, 1203
  nicotinic, antidote for, 755
  organic phosphorus compounds and carbamates, 1486–1502
  organochlorine, 222. *See also* Organic chlorine insecticides
  poisoning
    case fatality rate for, 1486
    epidemiology, 1486–1487
  resistance to, 1521
  terrorist use of, 1486
Insect repellents, 1522–1525
  comparative efficacy and toxicity, 1523t
  public believes about, 1524

Institute for Safe Medication Practices, best practice re antidotes, 42
Institute of Medicine (IOM)
  report on medical errors, 13
  report on poison control services, 11t
Insulin. *See also* High-dose insulin (HDI)
  actions, 694, 707
  for β-adrenergic antagonist toxicity, 933–934, 933f
  adverse effects and safety issues, 698–699, 955–956
  antibodies, 700–701, 701t
  aspart, characteristics, 698t
  as athletic performance enhancer, 620
  calcium phosphate nanoparticles, 1719t
  for carbon monoxide poisoning, 1671
  characteristics, 698t
  chemistry, 953–954
  designer, 694
  detemir, characteristics, 698t
  and fatty acid metabolism, 178–179
  forms of, characteristics, 698t
  glargine, characteristics, 698t
  glulisine, characteristics, 698t
  as glutamate scavenger, 229
  history of, 694, 953
  hypoglycemia caused by, 694, 696, 698–699, 955–956
    hospitalization for, 702
  hypokalemia caused by, 699, 956
  indications for, 35t
  intermediate-acting, characteristics, 698t
  intravenous, in hyperkalemia, 709
  laboratory detection, 622
  lente, characteristics, 698t
  lispro, characteristics, 698t
  long-acting, characteristics, 698t
  maintaining euglycemia after initial control with, 701–702
  NPH, characteristics, 698t
  overdose/poisoning, 696, 701–702
    death after, 699
    hypoglycemia caused by, 699
      hospitalization for, 702
    malicious, surreptitious, or unintentional, 700–701
      hospitalization for, 702
    management, 701
    and organ donation, 1893t
  pharmacokinetics and toxicokinetics, 696
  pharmacology, 694, 953
  physiology, 953–954, 953f
  postmortem changes, 1885t
  and potassium balance, 199
  in pregnancy and lactation, 956
  presystemic metabolism, 144
  protamine, allergy and, 920
  rapid-acting, 694
    characteristics, 698t
  reactions, carbohydrates for, 701
  regular
    availability and storage, 45t
    characteristics, 698t
    indications for, 45t
    stocking, recommended level, 45t
  release, regulation, 694, 696f
  secretion, 292, 700, 953–954, 953f
    octreotide and, 713–715
    somatostatin and, 713
    stimulation by lizard venom, 1619
  short-acting, characteristics, 698t
  suppression, octreotide for, 713–715. *See also* Octreotide, as antidote for hypoglycemia

  synthesis, 694
  ultralente, characteristics, 698t
Insulin-like growth factor(s)
  IGF-1, as athletic performance enhancer, 620
  secretion, lead and, 1296
Insulinoma, 700, 701t, 708
Insulin resistance
  in type 2 diabetes, 696
  xenobiotics causing, 953
Insulin suppression test, octreotide in, 714
Integral sign, 149
Integrase inhibitor, 832
Intellectual disability, glutamate and, 224
Intensive care unit, admission to, 40
  indications for, 40t
Intercellular signaling, and withdrawal syndrome, 237
Interferon(s) (IFN), IFN-alpha, cranial neuropathy caused by, 346t
Interleukin(s) (IL), effect on thyroid hormones and function, 814t
Intermediate syndrome, 1493, 1498, 1509
Intermezzo, 1084, 1089
Internal concealment of xenobiotics, 545–550, 545t
  in body packers, 545–547, 545t, 546f
  in body stuffers, 547–549
  legal principles and, 549
International Commission on Radiological Protection (ICRP), 1767
International Commission on Radiological Units and Measurement (ICRU), 1767
International Hazard Classification System (IHCS), 1807, 1808t
International normalized ratio (INR), 320–322, 335, 883
  with *N*-acetylcysteine, 495
  elevated
    management, 889, 889t
    vitamin K$_1$ for, 915, 917
    warfarin-related, vitamin K$_1$ for, 915, 917
  and liver transplantation for acetaminophen poisoning, 483–484
  monitoring, in anticoagulant toxicity, 887
International perspectives on toxicology, 1844–1851
International Radiation Protection Association (IRPA), 1767
International Sensitivity Index (ISI), 321
International Union of Pure and Applied Chemistry (IUPAC), nomenclature system, 155, 161–162
International Union of Toxicology, 1847
Internet
  date-rape drugs on, 1210
  ketamine on, 1210
  poison information on, 1785
Interpretive toxicology, forensic (medicolegal), 1868–1875
Interstitial lung disease(s), imaging, 115t, 123, 125, 125t, 126, 126f
Interstitial pneumonitis, diagnostic imaging, 115t
Interviewer bias, 1856
Intestinal epithelial cells, 353–354, 354f
Intestinal gas, intramural, 127–128, 129f, 129t
Intestinal ischemia, 128
Intestinal obstruction
  activated charcoal and, 79
  in body packer, imaging, 115t, 120f
Intestinal pseudo-obstruction, activated charcoal and, 79
Intra-aortic balloon pump
  for calcium channel blocker toxicity, 950
  for circulatory failure, in aluminum phosphide poisoning, 1460

Intracerebral hemorrhage
  cocaine-related, 1126
    diagnostic imaging, 115t
  computed tomography of, 130
  imaging, 115t, 130, 132t
Intracranial hemorrhage, in ethylene glycol poisoning, 1424
Intracranial hypertension (increased ICP)
  in lead encephalopathy, management, 1303
  xenobiotics associated with, 658, 658t
Intralipid, 684, 1004
Intraparenchymal hemorrhage, computed tomography of, 132t
Intrathecal administration, 793–801
  advantages, 793
  complications, 793
  errors in, 793, 798–799
    prevention, 799
  factors affecting, 793
  inadvertent overdose and unintentional exposures due to, 795t–798t
  indications for, 793
  overrinfusion in, 798–799
  pump malfunctions and, 794–799
  toxicity
    causes, 793
    clinical manifestations, 793
  underinfusion in, 793
  xenobiotics intentionally used, 793, 793t
Intravenous drug use (IVDU). *See also* Injection drug use (IDU)
  intracerebral lesions with, imaging, 132t
  multifocal airspace filling in, 125t
  respiratory effects, 399t
Intravenous lipid emulsion (ILE). *See* Lipid emulsion
Intrinsic pathway, 320, 321f, 883, 884f
Intubation
  for poisoned patient, 407
  salicylate toxicity and, 563
Inverted V sign, 1199
Investigational New Drug (IND) application, 1833, 1835, 1835f
  for exotic snake antivenom, 1634–1635
Involutin, 1583t, 1589t, 1592
Iodide(s)
  dietary, pharmacokinetics, 1775
  effect on thyroid hormones and function, 814t, 818
  excretion, 1775
  for hyperthyroidism, 818
  pharmacodynamics, 1775
  potassium. *See* Potassium iodide (KI)
  in pregnancy, 818
  tissue distribution, 1775
    in pregnancy and lactation, 1775
  urinary, 1775
Iodide (SSKI), indications for, 35t
Iodide mumps, 818, 1776
Iodide salts, containing radioactive iodine, 1775
Iodide trapping, 812
Iodinated compounds, clinical and laboratory findings with, 36t
Iodine, 1369t, 1370–1371, 1388t
  absorption, 1370–1371
  "allergy," 1776
  antidote for, 35t
  chemistry, 1769
  clinical effects, 1371
  deficiency, 812, 815
  elemental, 1370
  free, 1370

in Fukushima nuclear plant disaster, 23t, 24
  ingestion, management, 1371
  isotopes, 1769
  molecular, 1370
  nuclides, 1763
  pharmacodynamics, 1775
  radioactive
    antidote for, 35t, 45t
    definition, 1775
    and thyroid function, 814t
  teratogenicity, 429t
  and thyroid function, 813f, 814t
Iodine-123, in SPECT, 133
Iodine-containing products, teratogenicity, 429t
Iodism, 818
  and anion gap, 191t
Iodoacetate, and glycolysis, 176t
Iododerma, 1776
2-(4-Iodo-2,5-dimethoxyphenyl)-*N*-[(2-methoxyphenyl)methyl]ethanamine (2C-I-NBOMe, N-Bomb), 1107
Iodomethane, 1462
Iodophors, 1368, 1369t, 1370–1371
  clinical effects, 1371
  ingestion, management, 1371
Iodothyronine 5-deiodinases, 1340
Iohexol, intrathecal administration, inadvertent overdose and unintentional exposures due to, 795t
Io moth (*Automeris io*), 1552
Ion(s), 158–159
  properties, 158
  solvation of, 159
  spectator, 157
Ion channels, 203, 204t, 209. *See also specific channel*
  activation, 203
  cardiac, 244
    xenobiotics and, 254
  inactivation, 203
  ligand-gated, 203–204, 218–219, 220f, 945
  myocardial, 256
  and myocardial cell action potential, 245–246, 245f
  of myocardial cell membrane, 244–245
  recovery, 203
  resting, 203
  voltage-gated, 203
Ionic bond(s), 158–159
Ionization
  of acids, 161
  of bases, 161
  hard, 107
  for mass spectrometry, 107
  soft, 107
  and xenobiotic absorption, 142, 143f, 167
Ionization constant, 161
Ionizing radiation. *See* Radiation, ionizing
Ionotropic receptors, 204
Ion trapping, 93, 148, 167, 204, 560f, 569
  and breast milk xenobiotic accumulation, 440
  pharmacokinetic effects, 152
  in teratogenesis, 431–432
Iopanidol, intrathecal administration, inadvertent overdose and unintentional exposures due to, 795t
Iopanoic acid, 818
  effect on thyroid hormones and function, 814t, 818
Ioxitalamate contrast, intrathecal administration, inadvertent overdose and unintentional exposures due to, 795t
Ioxynil, 1468t

Ipecac (syrup), 33, 452, 613, 1605
  from *Cephaelis ipecacuanha*, 1599t, 1605
  gastrointestinal perforation caused by, 127
  studies of, 55t
Ipecacuanha, 4
Ipe roxo (*Tabebuia* spp.), 643t
iPLEDGE program, 656, 1839
Ipodate, effect on thyroid hormones and function, 814t
Ipomoea spp., 1601t, 1605–1606
Ipomoea batatas (sweet potatoes), *Gloriosa superba* (glory lily) and, confusion, 501
Ipomoea purga (jalap), 643t
Ipomoea purpurea (morning glory), use and toxicities, 643t
Ipomoea tricolor (morning glory), 1601t
Ipomoea violacea (morning glory), 1179t
  lysergamides in, 1179
  psychoactive properties, 650t
  use and toxicities, 643t
Ipratropium bromide, 1503
  quaternary ammonium compounds in, 1374
Ipsapirone, mechanism of action, 217
IR3535, 1524
  comparative efficacy and toxicity, 1523t
Irbesartan, CYP enzymes and, 170
Iridium, chelator for, 1780
Irinotecan, 329, 349f, 760t
  cell cycle phase specificity, 761f
  toxicity, genetic polymorphisms and, 759
Iris (eye), 356, 356f, 357
Iron, 669–675
  absorption, 315, 669
    gastric bypass and, 148
    vitamin C and, 662
  antidote for, 35t
  carbonyl, 669–670, 670t
  chemistry, 157, 159
  diagnostic imaging, 115t, 116f, 671
  effects on vital signs, 29t–30t
  ferric, 669, 1703–1704, 1704f
  ferrous, 669, 1703–1704, 1704f
  formulations, 670t
  gastrointestinal perforation caused by, 127
  in hemoglobin, 1703, 1704f
  and hemostasis, 670
  and high anion gap metabolic acidosis, 191t
  history of, 669
  homeostasis, 314
  hyperventilation caused by, 400t
  laboratory testing for, 101t, 102, 671
  and manganese, competition for ligands, 1319–1321
  and metabolic acidosis, 670
  metabolism, 314–315, 315f
  myocardial effects, 670
  nephrotoxicity, 390f, 397t
  ophthalmic toxicity, 356f
  overdose/poisoning
    abdominal radiography in, 671, 672f
    adjunctive therapies, 674
    anemia in, 671
    in children, 669
    clinical presentation, 36t, 192, 670–671
    decision analysis in, algorithm for, 673f
    deferoxamine for, 672–673, 673f
    diagnostic tests for, 671
    epidemiology, 669
    experimental therapies for, 673
    fatalities with, 669
    gastrointestinal decontamination for, 671–672, 672f

Iron, overdose/poisoning (*Cont.*):
  laboratory investigation, 671
  latent stage, 670
  local effects in, 670
  management, 44t
  metabolic acidosis in, 671
  pathophysiology, 670
  patient disposition with, 673–674
  in pregnancy, 39, 435–437, 674, 678
  saturation of plasma proteins in, 147
  and shock, 670–671
  shock stage, 670–671
  whole-bowel irrigation for, 63, 85, 436–437
  oxidized, 1704, 1704f
    reduction, 1704
  parenteral, 670, 670t
  pharmacokinetics, 669–670
  pharmacology, 669–670
  physicochemical properties, 669
  polysaccharide, 669–670, 670t
  radiopacity, 114
  replacement, 670
  serum, 671
    normal concentration, 669
  supplementation
    contraindications to, in dimercaprol therapy, 1252
    dimercaprol and, 1312
    for manganism, 1321
    safety considerations in, 669
    succimer and, 1312
    warning labels in, 669
  supplements, 669
  as thermal degradation product, 1642
  toxic dose, 669
  toxicokinetics, 669–670
  transport, 146
Iron-binding capacity, laboratory measurement, 101t, 102, 671
Iron chelators, 673. *See also* Deferoxamine
Iron cycle, 314–315, 315f
Iron deficiency anemia. *See* Anemia
Iron dextran, 670, 670t
Iron salts, 669
Iron sucrose, 670, 670t
  and metal phosphide poisoning, 1460
Iron tablets, ingested, imaging, 114–116, 116f
Irradiation, 1765. *See also* Radiation
Irrigation, whole-bowel. *See* Whole-bowel irrigation (WBI)
Irritable bowel syndrome (IBS)
  constipation-predominant, 217
  diarrhea-predominant, 217–218
Irritant(s), 6
  botanical, clinical and laboratory findings with, 36t
  chemical, respiratory effects, 399t
  ophthalmic toxicity, 356f
  respiratory, 1640–1641, 1640t, 1653–1658
Irritant dermatitis, 280, 1613
Irritant gases. *See* Gas(es), irritant; Pulmonary irritants
Irritant toxins, from combustion, 1640–1641, 1640t
Irukandji jellyfish (*Carukia barnesi*), 1567, 1567t, 1569, 1571. *See also* Cnidaria (jellyfish)
  priapism caused by, 301t
  stings, management, 1569
Irukandji syndrome, 1571
Irwin, Steve, 1576
Isavuconazonium, 829
Iscador, 643t
Ischemia-reperfusion injury, 1689
Ischemic heart disease, carbon disulfide and, 1175

Islet amyloid polypeptide (IAPP), inhibition by silver nanoparticles, 1346
Islets of Langerhans, 292
Isobarbaloin, 640t
Iso-barbaloin, 1598t
Isobenzan, physicochemical properties, 1515t
Isobutane, 165, 165f
Isobutyl nitrite
  as aphrodisiac, 304t
  inhaled, 1193t, 1194
  pharmacology, 1195
  in poppers, clinical effects, 1198
Isocarboxazid, 1076–1077. *See also* Monoamine oxidase inhibitors (MAOIs)
  discontinuation syndrome, 1080
  and GABA receptors, 222
  and serotonin toxicity, 1058t
  structure, 1076f
Isocyanates, 763
  airway injury by, 1640t, 1641
  and occupational asthma, 1660, 1660t
  as thermal degradation product, 1641t
Isoflurane, 1011, 1015
  and adenosine receptor, 230
  with carbon dioxide absorbers, 1015–1016
  carbon monoxide poisoning with, 1015–1016
  for ICU sedation, 1016
  and neuromuscular blockers, interactions, 1021t
  pharmacology, 1410
  recovery time improvement, lipid emulsion for, 1006
  for status epilepticus, 1016
  structure, 1011f
Isolation (seclusion), 387
Isomer(s)
  constitutional, 164
  definition, 164
  geometric, 164
  optical, 164, 164f
Isomerism, 164
  geometric, 164
Isometheptene
  adverse effects and safety issues, 809
  for migraine, 809
  pharmacology, 809
Isomylamine, 805
Isoniazid (INH), 850–854
  absorption, 850
  and acetaminophen toxicity, 480
  activation, 850
  antidote for, 35t, 8564
  diagnostic imaging, 115t
  drug interactions with, 852, 853t
  effects on CYP2E1 in liver, 851–852
  effects on GABA, 220, 851–852, 852f, 854
  elimination, 850
  and ethanol, interactions, 1146t
  food interactions with, 852, 853t
  and hepatocellular necrosis, 331
  hepatotoxicity, 850–851, 851f, 852–854
    risk factors for, 331
  and high anion gap metabolic acidosis, 191t, 852
  history of, 850
  HIV enteropathy and, 853t
  hyperventilation caused by, 400t
  injection, chlorobutanol in, 683t
  mechanism of action, 850
  mechanism of toxicity, 851–852
  metabolism, 170, 850–851, 851f
  monitoring with, 853t, 854

  neurotoxicity, 851f, 852–854
  ophthalmic toxicity, 356f
  optic neuritis with, 853
  pancreatitis caused by, 295t
  pharmacokinetics, 850–851
  pharmacology, 850
  in pregnancy and lactation, 852
  and pyridoxine, 663
  and rhabdomyolysis, 393
  seizures caused by, 852–854, 862
    management, 854, 863
    management of, 663
  SLE induced by, 126, 853
  slow, intermediate, and fast acetylators, 850–851
  toxicity, 1138, 1846
    acute, 853t, 854
    chronic, 853t, 854
    clinical manifestations, 36t, 192, 852–853, 853t
    diagnostic tests for, 853–854
    management, 46t, 854, 862
    pathophysiology, 851–852, 852f
    pyridoxine for, 854, 862–863
    pyridoxine stocking and, 43, 854
  and vincristine, interactions, 506
  volume of distribution, 850
Isonicotinic acid, 850–851
Isonicotinic acid hydrazide. *See* Isoniazid (INH)
Isoprene, polymers, 1410
Isopropanol (isopropyl alcohol), 162, 166, 1369t
  as antiseptic, 1368
  chemistry, 1422
  history of, 1421–1422
  hyperventilation caused by, 400t
  hypoventilation caused by, 400t
  ingestion, 37
    epidemiology, 1422
  metabolism, 1423, 1423f, 1437
  odor, 364t
  oxidative metabolism, 166, 166f
  physicochemical properties, 1421t
  serum, 1425
  toxicity, 166
    end-organ manifestations, 1425
    extracorporeal therapies for, 91f, 97t
    ketosis without acidosis in, 1423
    toxicokinetics/toxicodynamics, 1422–1423
    volume of distribution, 1422
Isopropyl paraoxon, 1488t
Isopropyl parathion, 1488t
Isoproterenol, 985
  for β-adrenergic antagonist toxicity, 934
  for calcium channel blocker toxicity, 950
  cardiac effects, 988
  contraindications to, 974
  and myocardial infarction, 988
Isoproterenol 30%, asthma deaths due to, 20t
Isoquercitrin cyanogenic glycoside, 641t
Isoquinolones, 650t
Isosorbide mononitrate, pyrimethamine contamination, 1846
Isosporiasis, in HIV-infected (AIDS) patients, 831t
Isosthenuria, 189
Isotaxine B, 1612
Isotope(s), 1762–1763
  definition, 155
Isotope ratio mass spectrometry, of athletic performance enhancers, 622
Isotretinoin (Accutane), 656
  FDA risk management program on, 1839
  teratogenicity, 430t, 658

Isovaleric acid, congenital anosmia for, 364
Isoxaben, in herbicides, 1467t
Isradipine, pharmacokinetics, 946t
Israel, experience with chemical and biological weapons (1990–1991 Gulf War), 1744
Istradefylline, 231
Itai-itai, 18t, 19, 1259–1260
Ito cells, 327, 329f
Itraconazole, 829
    as CYP inhibitor, 171
    for HIV-related infections, 830t
    and methadone, interactions, 172
    and prolonged QT interval, 253t
    and vincristine, interactions, 506
Ivermectin, 829
    as glycine agonist, 223
    mechanism of action, 222
Ivy (Hedera helix), 1600t
Ixodes holocyclus (Australian marsupial tick), 1550
Ixodidae, 1550

J

Jaborandi (Pilocarpus jaborandi), 1601t
Jack-o'-lantern (Omphalotus illudens), 1589
Jackson, Chevalier, 9
Jacobine, 645
Jacobs, Rosemary, 1346f
Jade plant (Crassula spp.), 1599t
Jaffe reaction, paraquat and diquat and, 1475–1476
Jake leg, 22
Jake walk, 22
Jalap (Ipomoea purga), 643t
Jaligonic aci, 644t
Jamaican vomiting sickness, 178, 332, 1609
Jamestown weed. See Jimsonweed (Datura stramonium)
Japan, nuclear disaster in, 24
Japanese star anise (Illicium anisatum), 1600t, 1608
Jarisch-Herxheimer reaction, 824
Jatropha spp., 1609
    self-poisoning with, 1846
Jatropha curcas (black vomit nut, physic nut, purging nut), toxicity, 1601t
Jaundice, 272, 330
    causes, differentiation, 1287
JC virus, 216
Jeff. See Methcathinone (cat, Jeff, khat, ephedrone)
Jellyfish, 1567, 1567t. See also Cnidaria (jellyfish)
    pelagic, 1567
    poisons from, 1
    stings, prevention, 1569
    true, 1568. See also Scyphozoa
Jequirity pea (Abrus precatorius), 1598t, 1609. See also Rosary pea (Abrus precatorius)
    as abortifacient, 303t
Jervell and Lange-Nielsen syndrome, 838–839
Jesuit bark. See Cinchona spp.
Jimsonweed (Datura stramonium), 1600t, 1604, 1604f. See also Datura stramonium (jimsonweed, stramonium, locoweed)
    use and toxicity, 643t
JNJ 38518168, 743
JNJ 397588979, 743
Johnson, Enid, 1018
John's wort. See St. John's wort (Hypericum perforatum)
Joint Commission, medication management requirements, 42
Jones, Jim, 5t, 1685
Jones, John, 7
Jones, Stan, 1346
Jonestown, Guyana mass suicide, 24

Joro spider toxins, 227t
Jukes, Edward, 4t, 7
Jukes syringe, 4t, 7
Jumper ant (Myrmecia spp.), 1552
Jumping spider (Phidippus), bites, necrotic wounds with, 1545
Juniper (Juniperus spp.)
    J. macropoda, 650t
    J. sabina, as abortifacient, 303t
Jurema (Mimosa hostilis), 650t
JWH-018, 1111, 1112f
    acute toxicity, 1117
    metabolism, 1116f
JWH-073, 1111, 1112f
JWH200, 1112f
JWH 250, 1112f
JWH-122, acute toxicity, 1117
JWH-210, acute toxicity, 1117

K

"K." See Ketamine
Kainate, 227
Kainate receptor(s), 227, 719
    antagonists, 227t
    modulators, 227t
Kainic acid, 595, 595f
Kallikrein, in coagulation, 883
Kallmann syndrome, 364
Kalmia latifolia (mountain laurel), 1612, 1612f
Kanamycin, 821–823
    toxicity, clinical manifestations, 822t
Kaposi sarcoma, conjunctival, 361
Karenia brevis, and shellfish poisoning, 595
Karwinskia humboldtiana (buckthorn), 1601t, 1610
Karwinskia toxins, 1609–1610
Karyorrhexis, arsenic and, 1244
Kashin-Beck disease, 1339
Kat, 643t
Katz, Bernard, 1018
Kava kava (Piper methysticum), 1178, 1179t, 1602t, 1607
    extract, hepatotoxicity, 651
    pharmacologic interactions, 646t
    psychoactive properties, 650t
    use and toxicity, 643t
Kava lactones, 643t, 650t, 1607
Kaveri (Gingko biloba). See Gingko (Gingko biloba)
Kawain, 1602t
Kayser-Fleischer rings, 1286–1287
Kcentra, 908, 910
    dosage and administration, 909, 909t
Kefauver-Harris Act of 1962, 1833
Kefauver-Harris Drug Amendments (1962), 10t, 1833
Kehoe principle, 1814
Kelsey, Frances, 1833
Kepone. See Chlordecone
Kepone shakes, 1518
Keratin-18, in acetaminophen hepatotoxicity, 481
Keratinocyte, 269
Keratinosomes, 269
Kernicterus, 342
Kerosene, 1409–1410. See also Hydrocarbons, aliphatic
    ingestion, 1409
        by children, worldwide, 1846
    uses, 1409t
    viscosity, 1409t
Keshan disease, 1339
"Ket." See Ketamine
Ketaject, 1210
Ketalar, 1210
Ketamine, 1179t, 1210–1221

abuse, epidemiology, 1210–1211
adverse effects, 1211
for agitated/violent behavior, 386
for alcohol withdrawal, 1170
analogs, 1211, 1211t
antidepressant effect, 1211, 1214
antiepileptic effect, 1213
available forms, 1212
for carbon monoxide poisoning, 1671
chemical structure, 1210
chemistry, 1211
chlorobutanol in, 684
and cocaine, combined, 1212
for cocaine toxicity, 1128
DEA class, 1211
dependence, 1216
diagnostic tests for, 1217
EEG changes caused by, 1217
elimination half-life, 1212
emergence reaction with, 1216–1217
enantiomers, 1211
ethanol tolerance and, 228
and glutamate release, 228
hepatobiliary dysfunction with, 1216
and heroin, combined, 1212
history and epidemiology, 1210–1211
indications for, 386
and k-hole, 1214
laboratory detection, 113
and male sexual dysfunction, 299f
and MDMA, combined, 1212
mechanism of action, 227t, 386
medical uses, 1210–1211
metabolism, 1212
molecular structure, 1211
neurotoxicity, 1182
nicotinic receptor blockade by, 207
and NMDA receptors, 228, 386, 1213–1214
for pain, 1211
pharmacokinetics, 1212
and respiratory depression, 1214
respiratory effects, 1214
sources, 1210
street names, 1212
toxicity
    blood pressure in, 1214
    cardiopulmonary effects, 1214
    cholinergic/anticholinergic effects in, 1215
    clinical and laboratory findings with, 36t, 1214–1217
    diagnostic testing for, 1216–1217
    heart rate in, 1214
    lower urinary tract syndrome in, 1215–1216, 1215f, 1217–1218
    management, 1217–1218
    neuropsychiatric effects, 1214–1215, 1217
    tachycardia in, 1214
    urologic effects, 1215–1216, 1215f, 1217–1218
    vital signs in, 1214
toxicokinetics, 1212
withdrawal, 1216
xenobiotics combined with, 1212
Ketanserin, mechanism of action, 212, 218
Ketavet, 1210
Ketoacidosis. See also Alcoholic ketoacidosis (AKA)
    diabetic. See Diabetic ketoacidosis
    euglycemic, SGLT2 inhibitor therapy and, 700
    and high anion gap metabolic acidosis, 191t, 192
    management, 193
    starvation, clinical and laboratory findings in, 36t

Ketoconazole, 829
    and colchicine, interactions, 502
    infertility caused by, 298f
    and prolonged QT interval, 253t
    and terfenadine, interactions, 172
α-Ketoglutarate, 177, 181, 218, 219f, 862, 1158–1159, 1533
    for SMFA or fluoroacetamide poisoning, 1534
α-Ketoglutarate dehydrogenase, 177
    arsenicals and, 1238–1239
    inhibitors, 1274
    magnesium and, 878
    thiamine and, 1158–1159, 1158f
Ketolide antibiotics, 826–827
    mechanism of action, 822t
    overdose, 822t, 827
    toxicity, 822t
Ketones, 165–166, 166f, 697, 1410. See also
        Hydrocarbons
    nitroprusside test for, 1150–1151
    oxidation, 168
    serum, 189
        elevated, 191, 191t
    urine, 192
        assay for, 1149
    vitreous, normal concentration, 1872t
Ketoprofen, pharmacology, 512t
Ketorolac
    benzalkonium chloride in, 682t
    hematologic effects, 516
    pharmacology, 511, 512t
Ketotifen, pharmacology, 742
Ketum. See Kratom (Mitragyna speciosa)
Kew tree (Gingko biloba). See Gingko (Gingko biloba)
Khat. See Methcathinone (cat, Jeff, khat, ephedrone)
Khat (Catha edulis), 1106, 1605
    uses and toxicities, 643t, 1599t
Kidney(s). See also Nephrotoxicity; Renal entries;
        Renal principles
    anatomy, 389
    antimicrobial toxicity and, 829t
    cadmium and, 1259–1260, 1260t
    excretion via, 148, 148t
    function, 389
        age-related changes in, 462–463
        evaluation, 396–397
        neonatal, 442
        in obese patients, 148
    functional toxic disorders, 395–396
    lead and, 1295
    medullary pyramids, 389
    mushroom toxins affecting, 1589t, 1590–1591
    physiology, 389, 390f
    specimens, postmortem collection, 1870t
    thallium toxicity and, 1351–1352
    toluene abuse and, 1196
    toxic injury, risk/susceptibility, 390
    xenobiotic excretion by, 147–148
    xenobiotics and, 389–396
    zinc toxicity and, 1363
Kidney disease. See also Acute kidney injury (AKI);
        Chronic kidney disease (CKD)
    enhanced elimination techniques in, 90
    and forced diuresis, 93
    hemofiltration in, 97
    pharmacokinetic effects, 389
Kidney Disease: Improving Global Outcomes
        (KDIGO)
    classification of chronic kidney disease, 395, 395t
    staging criteria for acute kidney injury, 391, 391t

Kidney failure. See also Acute kidney injury (AKI);
        Chronic kidney disease (CKD)
    bismuth-related, 1255
    chemotherapeutics and, 763
    copper poisoning and, 1286
    and high anion gap metabolic acidosis, 191t, 192
    hypoglycemia caused by, hospitalization for, 702
    management, 193–194
    and neurotoxicity, 342
    and xenobiotic clearance, 389
Kidney injury, acute. See Acute kidney injury (AKI)
Kidney injury molecule-1, urinary, in acute kidney
        injury, 396
Kidney transplantation, from poisoned patients,
        1892–1893, 1892t
Kijitsu. See Bitter orange (Citrus aurantium)
Kim Jong-nam, 6t, 13
Kinase inhibitors, 761
    adverse effects and safety issues, 762
Kindling hypothesis, 237
Kindling phenomenon, alcohol withdrawal and, 1165
Kinesin, 340
King cobras (Ophiophagus hannah), 1633t
King Mithridates VI, 1t, 2
King's College Criteria, and liver transplantation
        for acetaminophen poisoning, 483–484,
        483t–484t
King's crown (Calotropis procera), 979
King snake, color patterns, 1618
Kinins, in vespid venom, 1551
Kircher, Athanasius, 3
KJ. See Phencyclidine (PCP)
Klamath weed. See St. John's wort (Hypericum
        perforatum)
Klear, 622
K_m (Michaelis-Menten dissociation constant), 167, 169
Knitbone (Symphytum spp.), 641t
Knockdown gas, hydrogen sulfide as, 1650, 1689t,
        1690–1691
Knowledge, deficits, and medication errors, 1828
Kobert, Rudolf, 4t
Kohl, 1228
Kolanin, 643t, 650t
Kola nut (Cola spp.), 1599t
    psychoactive properties, 650t
    use and toxicities, 643t
Koller, Karl, 1124
Kombucha (Manchurian tea), 643t
Konjac (Amorphophallus konjac), 642t
Konjac mannan (Amorphophallus konjac), 642t
Korsakoff, Sergei, 1157
Korsakoff psychosis, 177, 1159
    epidemiology, 1160
Kozo, 1686
Kraits (Bungarus spp.), 1633t
    bites, management, 1845
Kratom (Mitragyna speciosa), 643t, 649, 650t, 1178,
        1179t, 1181
    clinical effects, 1183
    pharmacology, 1181t, 1183
    toxicokinetics, 1182
Krazy Glue, ophthalmic exposure to, irrigating solution
        for, 359
Krebs cycle, 954–955. See also Citric acid cycle
Kuandong hua (Tussilago farfara), 641t
KULT mnemonic, 191
Kupfernickel, 1333
Kupffer cells, 327, 329f, 1146
    and liver injury, 330
Kus es Salahin, 643t

Kynurenic acid
    and glycine antagonism, 228
    and NMDA receptor, 227t
Kyushin (Bufo bufo gargarizans, Bufo bufo
        melanosticus), 649
    as aphrodisiac, 649
    psychoactive properties, 650t
    uses and toxicities, 641t

L
LAARs. See Long-acting anticoagulant rodenticide(s)
        (LAARs)
Labeling, 9, 10t, 11
    of antidotes, 43
    black box warning in, 1839
    of dietary supplements, 639
    FDA regulatory actions on, 1839
    inadequacies, 1786
    and poison education, 1786
    and poison prevention, 1786
    Pregnancy and Lactation Labeling Rule (PLLR) for,
        431
    of pregnancy risk, 431
    signal words in, 40, 1450t
Labeling of Hazardous Art Materials Act (1988), 10t
Labetalol
    indications for, 751
    injection, parabens in, 685t
    intrathecal administration, inadvertent overdose
        and unintentional exposures due to, 795t
    overdose/poisoning, clinical manifestations, 932
    pharmacology, 927t, 930–931
    priapism caused by, 301t
    toxicity, management, 936
    vasodilating effects, 930–931
Laboratory errors, 108, 153
Laboratory principles, 101–113
Laboratory proficiency, 101–102
Laboratory test(s), 189
    analyte range, 103t
    analytical phase, errors in, 108
    cost, 103t
    cross-reactivity in, 109
    diagnostic, 102
    for drug-abuse screening, 110–113
    errors in, 108, 153
    exposure information from, 102
    interferences in, 109
    medicolegal considerations with, 102
    menu, 101
    methods for, 102–107
    in poisoned patient, 266t
    postanalytical phase, errors in, 108
    preanalytical phase, errors in, 108
    qualitative, 109
    quantitative, 103t, 109
    send-out vs. in-house, 102
    sensitivity, 103t
    specificity, 103t
    specimens for, 102
    speed, 103t
    toxicology, routinely available, 101–102, 101t
    turn-around times, 101
    use of, 102
    xenobiotic identification by, 102
Labor unions, as information resource, 1804
Laburnum (Cytisus laburnum, Laburnum anagyroides),
        1601t, 1604
La Cantarella, 4, 5t
Lacosamide

adverse effects and safety issues, 727t
history of, 719
mechanism of action, 720f, 720t
metabolism and effects on CYP enzymes, 722t
overdose/poisoning
clinical manifestations, 722
management, 722
pharmacokinetics and toxicokinetics, 721t, 722
pharmacology, 719, 720t
therapeutic serum concentration, 722
Lacquer, odor, 364t
Lacrimators (tear gas), 1749
as chemical weapon, 1741
decontamination for, 1743
ophthalmic exposure to, 359
toxic syndrome caused by, 1751t
Lactaldehyde, 687
β-Lactam antibiotics, 823–825
adverse effects associated with therapeutic use, 825
cross-hypersensitivity, 825
overdose, 822t, 825
pharmacology, 822t
renal effects, 390, 394t
structure, 825
toxicity, 822t
Lactarius spp., 1582t, 1589
Lactate, 177, 178f
assays for, 103
assessment, in poisoned patient, 266
barium toxicity and, 1455
blood
in cyanide poisoning, 1642, 1685–1686, 1687t
in high anion gap metabolic acidosis, 192
in brain energy metabolism, 707–708
calcium-channel blockers and, 954
concentration, in toxic alcohol poisoning,
1426–1427
and high anion gap metabolic acidosis, 191t
in postmortem changes, 1885
production, in propylene glycol metabolism, 1427
salicylates and, 557
serum, 189
elevated, 191, 191t
and liver transplantation for acetaminophen
poisoning, 483–484
in methanol poisoning, prognostic significance,
1427
smoke inhalation and, 1642
in strychnine poisoning, 1537
in toxic alcohol poisoning, 1426
volume of distribution, 192
Lactate dehydrogenase (LDH), 175
in heatstroke, 422
serum, increased, 317
Lactation
activated charcoal and, 79
cesium exposure and, 1360
thallium exposure and, 1360
whole-bowel irrigation in, 86
Lactic acid, 165
propylene glycol metabolism and, 687
Lactic acidosis
clinical and laboratory findings in, 36t
and high anion gap metabolic acidosis, 192
metformin-associated, 699, 703–704
correction, hemodialysis for, 90, 95
phenformin-induced, 694
propylene glycol metabolism and, 1430
Lactone glycosides, 639
Lactones, 643t

kava, 1602t, 1607
terpene, 1607
Lactose, 707
Lactose intolerance, and glucarpidase therapy, 785
Lactrodectus spp., 1540
Lactuca sativa (wild lettuce), 645t, 650t
Lactuca virosa (wild lettuce), 645t
Lactulose, 83
and hepatic encephalopathy, 334
and hypernatremia, 195, 195t
mechanism of action, 84
pharmacokinetics, 84
Ladostigil, 1077
Lady's thimble. *See* Foxglove (*Digitalis* spp.)
Laetiporus sulfureus, 1594
Laetrile, 1607, 1684
poisoning, management, 1699
Lagenaria breviflora, as abortifacient, 303t
Lagoa crispata, 1553
Lake Mounoun, Cameroon, 400
Lake Nyos, Cameroon, 16, 16t, 400
Lambert-Eaton myasthenic syndrome (LEMS), 207, 579
clinical manifestations, 577t
Lamellae, of mushrooms, 1584f, 1593
Lamellar granules, 269
Lamiaceae, 1600t–1601t
Lamivudine, 831
Lamotrigine
adverse effects and safety issues, 727–728, 727t
cardiac effects, 248f
drug-induced hypersensitivity syndrome with, 278,
727–728, 727t
drug interactions with, 723t
elimination, multiple-dose activated charcoal and,
62
history of, 719
indications for, 722
for inhalant dependence, 1200
mechanism of action, 218, 227t, 228, 720f, 720t
metabolism and effects on CYP enzymes, 722t
pharmacokinetics and toxicokinetics, 721t, 722
pharmacology, 719, 720t
pregnancy category, 722
and pregnancy complications, 719
and suicide risk, 719
therapeutic serum concentration, 722
toxicity (overdose/poisoning)
clinical manifestations, 722
gastrointestinal decontamination for, 58t, 77
lipid emulsion for, 1006
management, 722
multiple-dose activated charcoal in, 61
sodium bicarbonate for, 568t, 569
Lampona (white tail spider). *See* White tail spider
(*Lampona* spp.)
Lamprophiidae, 1617
Lamson, George Henry, 5t, 6
Lanatoside C, toxicity, epidemiology, 969
Lanatosides, 979, 1600t
Lance-headed rattlesnake (*Crotalus* spp.), 1636t
Landru, Henri Girard, 5t
Langerhans cells, 279
Lanoteplase, 897
Lanreotide, 713–714, 716
Lantadene A and B, 1601t
Lantana camara (lantana), 1601t
hepatogenous photosensitivity caused by, 1614
Lanthanides, 156f
Lanthanum carbonate, nanoparticles, 1719t
Lapacho (*Tabebuia*), 643t

Lapachol, 643t
Laparotomy, 63–64
Lapatinib, 763
Lapemis hardwickii, 1575
La poudre de succession, 5t, 6
Lappa. *See* Burdock root (*Arctium lappa, A. minus*)
Laquer(s), inhaled, 1193t. *See also* Inhalant(s)
Large intestine(s), 291–292
Larkspur (*Delphinium* spp.), 1600t
Laropiprant, for niacin-induced flushing, 664
Larrea tridentata (chaparral), 1610
uses and toxicities, 641t
Laryngeal dystonia, antipsychotic-induced, 1036
Laryngospasm, 399t, 400
with arylcyclohexylamine toxicity, 1215
with ketamine, 1215
Lasiocarpine, 641t
Lasiodora spp., 1547
Lasmiditan, 809
Lassa fever, as biological weapon, 1758
Latherwort. *See Saponaria officinalis* (soapwort)
Lathyrins, 1609
Lathyrism, 343, 1607
neurogenic, 227
Lathyrus sativus (grass pea), 343, 1609
toxicity, 1601t
Laticauda laticaudata, 1575
Laticauda semifasciata, 1575
Laticaudinae, 1574–1575, 1633t
Latrodectism, 1542–1543
clinical manifestations, 1542t, 1543
diagnostic tests for, 1543
Latrodectus spp., antivenom, 1543, 1559–1561
worldwide availability, 1560t
Latrodectus bishopi, 1541, 1559
Latrodectus cinctus, 1541
Latrodectus geometricus. See Brown widow spider
(*Latrodectus geometricus*)
Latrodectus hasselti, 1541, 1541f, 1542t
antivenom (RBS-AV), 1544, 1559–1560
Latrodectus hesperus. See Western black widow spider
(*Latrodectus hesperus*)
Latrodectus indistinctus, 1542t
Latrodectus lugubris, 1559
Latrodectus mactans (black widow spider). *See* Black
widow spider (*Latrodectus mactans*)
Latrodectus tredecimguttatus. See European widow
spider (*Latrodectus tredecimguttatus*)
Latrodectus variolus, 1541, 1559
Latrophilin, 1542
Latrotoxin, 345
sympathomimetic action, 211
α-Latrotoxin, 1542, 1542t
Laudanosine, 1018
from neuromuscular blocking drugs, 1025
Laudanum, 7, 519
Laughing gas, 1011. *See also* Nitrous oxide
Laundry detergent pods, ingestion, 1389
Laundry powder ingestion, 1389
Lauraceae. *See* Sassafras (*Sassafras albidum*)
Laurier rose. *See* Oleander
Lavandula angustifolia, 630–631
Lavandula latifolia, 630
Lavandula stoechas, 630
Lavandula x intermedia, 630
Lavender, 630–631
Lavender oil, 630–631, 633–634
La Voisine, 6
Laws. *See also* Legislation; *specific law*
per se, 1144, 1873, 1876–1878

Laxatives, 83
  adverse effects, 85
  classification and mechanism of action, 83
  hypomagnesemia caused by, 877
  misuse/abuse, 612–613
    and rhabdomyolysis, 393
Lead, 1–2, 4, 4t, 7, 1292–1308, 1780. *See also* Heavy
    metals
  abortion caused by, 297t
  absorption, 1294, 1311–1312, 1316
  and aging-related disorders, 1298
  antidote for, 35t
  as aphrodisiac, 304t
  in battery cases, 11
  biologic half-lives, 1294
  blood (concentration)
    in adults, 1293, 1297t, 1298
    chelation therapy and, 1311
    in children, 1293, 1296–1297, 1296t, 1304
      follow-up for, 1300, 1301t
    and encephalopathy, 1297
    and intellectual development, 1296
    as marker of brain lead, 1310
    measurement, 1299
      succimer and, 1311–1312
    in neonates of blood-exposed mothers, 1305
    OSHA standards for, 1300, 1301t
    in pregnancy, screening and follow-up for,
      1304
    screening, 1299
    threshold of concern, 1292, 1296
  body burden, measurement, 1300
  in bone, 1294, 1296
    measurement, 1300
  and breastfeeding, 441
  in breast milk, 1252, 1294, 1305, 1305t, 1312
  calcium-mimetic properties, 1294–1295
  carcinogenicity, 1294–1295
  cardiotoxicity, 1295–1296, 1298
  in central nervous system, 1294
  chemistry, 158, 164, 1293
  children exposed to, but asymptomatic,
    management, 1303t, 1304
  contamination of alcoholic beverages, 1143
  in cosmetics, 1228
  cutaneous absorption, 1294
  diagnostic imaging, 115t, 116, 117f, 119, 119f, 122f,
    122t, 1299f, 1300, 1300f
  in dietary supplements, 647–648
  and discoloration of teeth and gums, 293t
  distribution, 1294
  in drinking water, 1292
  as early poison, 2
  elimination, therapeutic manipulation, 147
  endocrine toxicity, 1296, 1298
  excretion, 1294
  exposure, interventions for, 1300–1302, 1302t,
    1304
  and fertility, 1296
  fetal exposure to, 1294, 1304
  food and water poisoning with, 18t, 19
  food contamination with, 599–600
  in gasoline, 1293
  gastrointestinal absorption, 1294
  gastrointestinal toxicity, 1296, 1298
  hematotoxicity, 1295, 1295f, 1298
  history and epidemiology, 1292–1293
  infertility caused by, 297t, 298f
  ingested
    absorption, 1294, 1302

  imaging, 1299f–1300f
  management, 1302
  inhaled, absorption, 1294
  inorganic, 1294
    physicochemical properties, 1293
    poisoning, clinical manifestations, 1296–1298
  isotopes, 1293
  metallic, 1294
    physicochemical properties, 1293
  mitogenic effects, 1294
  in moonshine, 1298
  mutagenic effects, 1294
  neonatal exposure to, 1294
  nephrotoxicity, 390f, 397t, 1295, 1298
  neurocognitive effects, in children, 1296
  neurotoxicity, 1295, 1295f, 1297–1298, 1297f
  occupational exposure, 23, 23t
    health-based management recommendations for,
      1300, 1301t
    interventions for, 1300–1302, 1302t
    screening for, 1300, 1301t
    surveillance recommendations for, 1300, 1301t
  ophthalmic toxicity, 356f, 361t, 1298
  organic, 1293–1294
    poisoning, clinical manifestations, 1298
  in paint, 115t, 116, 122f, 1292, 1292t
  pathophysiology, 1294–1296
  perinatal exposures, 1292
  pharmacology, 1294
  physicochemical properties, 1292–1293
  poisoning
    acute, 1298
    in adults, 1297–1298, 1297t
      treatment, 1304–1305
    biomolecular mechanisms in, 1294
    chelation therapy for, 1252–1253, 1253t, 1292,
      1300, 1302, 1303t
      in adults, 1253, 1303t, 1304–1305
      in pregnancy, 1305, 1312
      teratogenicity, 1305
    in children, 1292–1293, 1296–1297, 1296t
      risk factors for, 1298
      treatment, 1252–1253, 1253t, 1302–1304
      uncommon presentations, 1297
    clinical diagnosis in symptomatic patients,
      1298–1299
    clinical manifestations, 36t, 1296–1298
    differential diagnosis, 1298
    ECG changes in, 1298
    historical perspective on, 1292
    imaging in, 119, 119f, 122f, 122t, 1296,
      1296f–1297f, 1299f, 1300, 1300f
    laboratory findings with, 36t, 1299–1300
    management, 44t, 46t, 1300–1305
      in neonates of blood-exposed mothers, 1305
    occupational, in developing world, 1798
    in pregnancy, 1304–1305, 1312
    presumptive treatment, 1299
    prevention, 1300, 1852
    screening for, 1300, 1301t
    whole-bowel irrigation for, 63, 85, 1300f, 1302
  provoked challenge urine testing for, 1300
  psychiatric effects, 1298
  pulmonary absorption, 1294
  reproductive toxicity, 1292, 1296, 1298
  skeletal effects, 1296, 1296f
    imaging, 119, 119f, 122f, 122t, 1296, 1296f
  smelting, 1293
  soft tissue absorption/uptake, 1294
  sources, 116

  additional/exotic, 1293, 1293t
  environmental, 1292–1293, 1292t
  occupational and recreational, 1292–1293, 1293t
  subclinical toxicity, in children, 1292, 1296–1297,
    1296t, 1303t, 1304
  susceptibility to, genetic polymorphisms and, 1294
  in teeth, 1294
  teratogenicity, 429t
  as thermal degradation product, 1642
  transplacental transfer, 1294, 1304
  transport in body, 142
  and vital signs, 29t
  whole blood level, 1292
Lead acetate, 1292
Lead arthrogram, 119f
Lead-based Paint Poison Prevention Act (1973), 10t
Lead carbonate, 1292
Lead chromate, 1268t, 1293
Leaded ceramic glaze, ingested, imaging, 116, 117f
Leaded paint chips
  imaging, 115t, 116, 122f, 1300f
  ingestion (pica), 1292, 1300f
Lead encephalopathy
  acute, 1295, 1295f, 1297–1298
  in adults, 1298
    treatment, 1303t, 1304
  in children, 1297
    treatment, 1302–1303, 1303t
  clinical characteristics, 1297
  diagnosis, 1298–1300
  gold mining and, 1293
  laboratory findings in, 1300
  mortality rate for, 1297
  neurologic sequelae, 1297, 1297f
  treatment, 1310–1311, 1316–1317
    in adults, 1303t, 1304
    in children, 1302–1303, 1303t
Lead lines, 273, 1296, 1296f, 1300
  imaging, 119, 122f, 122t
Lead mercury, 5t
Lead oxide, 1293
Lead-pipe rigidity, 1038
Lead salts, 1292
Lead sulfite, nanocrystals, 1717
Lean, 1827
Lean body mass, in obese patients, 148
Lean body weight (LBW), equations for, 148t
Leary, Timothy, 1178
Leaving groups, 755, 755f
  in organic phosphorus compounds, 1487, 1487f,
    1488t
Leber hereditary optic neuropathy, 1686
Lectin(s), 643t, 1597, 1598t, 1601t–1603t, 1608–1609,
    1846
  definition, 1597
  ricinlike, 1608–1609
Lectinlike proteins, C-type, in snake venom, 1618,
    1619t, 1620
Leech, anticoagulants from, 883
Leeks (*Allium porrum*), 1611
Lefarge, Marie, 5t, 6
Left lateral decubitus position, for pregnant patient, 39
Legalon SIL, for amatoxin-induced liver toxicity, 1585
Legislation. *See also* Laws; *specific law*
  on drug review and approval, 1833–1835
  early, 9
  and global public health, 1848
  important, 10t
  for poison prevention, 1782
Legumaceae, 1601t, 1603t

Lehman, Betsy, 13
Lehmann, Christa Ambros, 5t
Leishmaniasis
 in HIV-infected (AIDS) patients, 830t
 treatment, 1229
  antimony in, 1228, 1230, 1232
 visceral, treatment, antimony toxicity in, 1228, 1230, 1232
Leiurus spp., 1548, 1548t
 antivenom, 1563, 1564t
Leiurus quinquestriatus
 antivenom, 1563, 1564t, 1565
 geographic distribution, 1563
Lens, 356, 356f
 abnormalities, 356
 deposits in, xenobiotic exposures and, 357t
Lepidium meyenii, as aphrodisiac, 304
Lepidoptera, 1552–1554
 larval. *See* Caterpillars
Lepidopterism, 1552–1554
Lepiota spp., 1581–1583
 hepatotoxicity, management, 1586
Lepiota brunneoincarnata, 1581, 1586
Lepiota helveola, 1581, 1582t, 1586
Lepiota josserandi, 1581, 1582t
Lepirudin, 891–894
 indications for, 891
Leptin, 271, 606
Leptospermum spp., 633
Lesser weeverfish (*Trachinus vipera*), 1576–1577
Lethal toxin, 1755
Lettuce, wild (*Lactuca sativa, L. virosa*), 645t, 650t
Lettuce opium. *See* Lettuce, wild (*Lactuca sativa, L. virosa*)
Leuconostoc citrovorum, 775
Leucotomy, 1032
Leucovorin (folinic acid), 764, 775–781
 adverse effects and safety issues with, 777
 as antidote, 775–779
  dosage and administration, 777–779, 778t
  for methotrexate, 769–770, 775, 777–778
 for antifolate overdose, 846
 availability and storage, 45t
 dialysis and, 770–771
 for dihydrofolate reductase inhibitor toxicity, 777
 dosage and administration, 777–779
 and 5-fluorouracil toxicity, 775
 and formate clearance, 1429
 formulation and acquisition, 779
 glucarpidase and, 777, 782, 783f, 784–785
 history of, 789
 indications for, 35t, 45t
 intramuscular, pharmacokinetics, 776
 intrathecal
  inadvertent overdose and unintentional exposures due to, 795t
  toxicity, 776–777, 794
 intravenous, pharmacokinetics, 776
 mechanism of action, 767, 767f
 for methanol toxicity, 776–777, 779
 for methotrexate toxicity, 760t
 for nitrous oxide toxicity, 1200
 oral, pharmacokinetics, 776
 for pemetrexed toxicity, 779
 pharmacokinetics, 776
 pharmacology, 775
 in pregnancy and lactation, 777
 with pyrimethamine, 777
 rescue, for methotrexate, 770, 775–776, 783, 789
  dosage and administration, 778, 778t, 779f

shortage, 43
 stocking, recommended level, 45t
 structure, 775
 supplies, 42
 with trimetrexate glucuronate, 777
Leu-enkephalin, 520
Leukemia(s), 320
 acute myelogenous, all-*trans*-retinoic acid for, 656
 acute myeloid (AML), 320
 acute promyelocytic (APML)
  arsenic trioxide for, 1237–1238
  all-*trans*-retinoic acid for, 656
 arsenicals for, 1237–1238
 benzene and, 320
Leukemoid reaction(s)
 arsenic trioxide and, 1243
 in ethylene glycol poisoning, 1424
Leukocytes, 319–320
 polymorphonuclear, 319–320
Leukocytosis
 with colchicine poisoning, 502, 503t
 in methylxanthine overdose, 989
Leukoencephalopathy, 343
 chemotherapeutic-related, 763
 inhalant-induced, 133, 1196, 1199
 methotrexate-induced, 763, 768
 paradichlorbenzene-induced, 1384–1385
 progressive multifocal, 216
 reversible. *See* Reversible posterior leukoencephalopathy
 spongiform. *See* Spongiform leukoencephalopathy
 toluene-induced, 133, 1196, 1199–1200, 1412
 toxic, 133
Leukon, 319–320
Leukonychia, 274t, 281f, 282
Leukopenia
 in arsenic poisoning, 1241
 chemotherapeutic-related, 762
 with colchicine poisoning, 502, 503t
 in metal phosphide poisoning, 1458
 methotrexate-related, 768
Leukotriene(s) (LT), 511, 513f
 in acute respiratory distress syndrome, 1653
Leupeptin, 368
Levalbuterol, 985
Levallorphan, 538
Levamisole
 cocaine adulterated with, 279, 279f, 329, 1130
 respiratory effects, 399t
 toxicity, 1130
  clinical and laboratory findings with, 36t
Level of consciousness
 altered, management of patient with, 1862
 depressed, 33–36, 189
Levetiracetam
 adverse effects and safety issues, 727–728, 727t
 drug-induced hypersensitivity syndrome with, 727–728, 727t
 drug interactions with, 723t
 history of, 719
 indications for, 723
 for lead encephalopathy, in children, 1302
 mechanism of action, 720f, 720t
 metabolism and effects on CYP enzymes, 722t
 pharmacokinetics and toxicokinetics, 721t, 723
 pharmacology, 719, 720t
 pregnancy category, 723
 and suicide risk, 719
 therapeutic serum concentration, 723
 toxicity

clinical manifestations, 723
 management, 723
Levobunolol
 benzalkonium chloride in, 682t
 ophthalmic use, systemic toxicity with, 360
 pharmacology, 927t
Levobupivacaine, 1001
Levocabastine
 elimination half-life, 744
 pharmacology, 742
Levocabnastine hydrochloride, benzalkonium chloride in, 682
Levocarnitine. *See* L-Carnitine
Levocetirizine, 746
 dose modification in liver or kidney disease, 744
 metabolism, 743
 pharmacokinetics and toxicokinetics, 745t
 pharmacology, 742
Levodopa
 COMT inhibitors and, 214
 effect on thyroid hormones and function, 814t
 and manganism, 1321
 and olfactory dysfunction, 364
 and serotonin toxicity, 218
Levofloxacin, 826
 hypoglycemia caused by, 715
Levoleucovorin, 775
 adverse effects and safety issues, 777
 dosage and administration, 777–778
 formulation and acquisition, 779
 intrathecal, toxicity, 776–777
 pharmacokinetics, 776
 pharmacology, 775
Levomilnacipran, 1060
 pharmacokinetics, 1055t
 receptor activity, 1057t
Levonorgestrel, as abortifacient, 303t
Levorotatory entantiomers, 164
Levorphanol, 538. *See also* Opioid(s)
 characteristics, 526t
Levosimendan
 for β-adrenergic antagonist toxicity, 935
 mechanism of action, 933f
Levothyroxine, 813. *See also* Thyroid hormone(s)
 overdose, 815
  diagnostic tests for, 816
Lewin, Louis, 4t
Lewisite, 1251, 1330
 antidote, 1748
 chemical name and structure, 1747f
 odor, 1748
 physical characteristics, 1748
 toxicity, 1748
 toxic syndrome caused by, 1750t
Lewy body dementia, exacerbated or unmasked by xenobiotics in elderly, 463, 463t
Lex Cornelia, 1t
Lhermitte sign, 1199
Libido
 decreased female, 302f
 decreased male, 298–300, 299f
  xenobiotics causing, 300t
Licarbazepine, 723–724
 therapeutic serum concentration, 724
Lichenification, 269t
Licorice (*Glycyrrhiza glabra*), 649, 1600t, 1606
 glycosides in, 639
 and hyponatremia, 196
 pharmacologic interactions, 646t
 use and toxicities, 643t

Lidocaine. *See also* Local anesthetic(s)
  administration routes for, 144
  adverse effects and safety issues, 866t, 870
  as antidysrhythmic, 869–871
  for antipsychotic cardiotoxicity, 1040
  ARDS caused by, 402t
  for bupivacaine cardiotoxicity, 1000
  for cardioactive steroid poisoning, 973–974
  for cesium-induced dysrhythmias, 1265
  for cyclic antidepressant toxicity, 1049t, 1050
  drug interactions with, 996
  epinephrine, fentanyl, intrathecal administration,
        inadvertent overdose and unintentional
        exposures due to, 796t
  fast on–fast off kinetics with, 999
  history of, 994
  liposomal formulation, 996
  metabolism
    patient age and, 996
    and toxicity, 998
  methemoglobinemia caused by, 997
  minimal IV toxic dose, 998t
  and neuromuscular blockers, interactions, 1021t
  neurotoxicity, 997
  pharmacokinetics, 866t
  pharmacology, 866t, 995, 996t
  plasma protein binding by, 146
  protein-binding characteristics, 110t
  serum concentration, and signs and symptoms of
        toxicity, 998, 998f
  for stingray envenomation, 1578
  structure, 869f, 995f
  and tinnitus, 370t
  topical, for jellyfish stings, 1569
  toxicity, diagnostic tests for, 1000
  transient neurologic symptoms with, 997
Lidocaine-prilocaine cream, methemoglobinemia
        associated with, 997
Ligament calcification
  with fluorosis, 115t, 119
  imaging, 115t
Ligand-gated ion channels (LGICs), 203–204, 218–219,
        220f, 945
  structure, 204
  subunits, 204
Ligands, 170
  nuclear receptor binding by, 170–171
Ligatoxin, 1601t
Lighter fluid, inhaled, 1193
Light transmission aggregometry, 900
Lignans, 1597, 1609–1610
Lignins, 1597, 1609–1610
Ligroin, 1410
Lilac, French (*Galega officinalis*), 642t, 694
Lilac daphne, as abortifacient, 303t
Liliaceae, 1598t–1601t, 1603t
Lily
  glory (*Gloriosa superba*). *See Gloriosa superba* (glory
        lily, meadow saffron, superb lily)
  Peruvian (*Alstroemeria* spp.), 1614
  superb (*Gloriosa superba*). *See Gloriosa superba*
        (glory lily, meadow saffron, superb lily)
Lily of the valley (*Convallaria majalis*), 979, 1606, 1606f
  cardiac glycosides in, 969, 979
  toxicity, 1599t
Limb ischemia
  cocaine and, 1127
  in cocaine toxicity, 1127, 1130
Limited reactions, 1036
Limonene, 1410

Linaclotide, 84
Linagliptin
  pharmacokinetics and toxicokinetics, 697t
  pharmacology, 696
Linalool, 630–631
Linalyl acetate, 630–631
Linamarin, 1601t, 1607, 1684
  neurotoxicity, 343
Lincosamides, 827
  mechanism of action, 822t
  overdose, 822t
  toxicity, 822t
Lind, James, 662
Lindane, 1514–1519
  absorption, 1514
  acute exposure to, clinical manifestations, 1517
  contraindications to, 1518
  elimination, 1515–1516
  fat-to-serum ratio for, 1515
  history of, 1514
  mechanisms of toxicity, 1517–1518
  metabolism, 1515
  physicochemical properties, 1515t
  regulation of, 1518
  serum
    clinical significance, 1518
    in toxicity, 1518
  sources, 1514
  structure, 1516f
  toxicity, risk factors for, 1517–1518
  toxicokinetics, 1514–1516
Linear energy transfer (LET), 1763
Linear IgA dermatosis, 276, 276t
Linear processes, 149
Line of sight transmission, 1814
Linezolid, 218, 1077
  MAO inhibition by, 212
  mechanism of action, 822t
  ophthalmic toxicity, 356f
  overdose, 822t
  and serotonin toxicity, 1058t
  toxicity, 822t
Linoleic acid, 641t, 1005
  hepatotoxicity, 651
Linolenic acid, 1005
Linseed oil, 3
Linuche unguiculata (thimble jellyfish), 1567t. *See also*
        Cnidaria (jellyfish)
  larvae, and seabather's eruption, 1568, 1571–1572
Linum spp., cyanogenic glycosides in, 1684
Lionfish (*Pterois*), 1576, 1576t, 1577, 1577f
Lion's mane, 1567t, 1568. *See also* Cnidaria (jellyfish);
        Stomolophus nomurai (lion's mane)
Liothyronine, 813
Lipase, 1007
  serum, in methanol poisoning, 1427
Lipid complex, 684, 684t
Lipid conduit, 1004–1005
Lipid emulsion, 684, 684t, 1004–1010
  for β-adrenergic antagonist toxicity, 934
  adverse effects and safety issues, 1007–1008
  for aluminum phosphide poisoning, 1460
  for antipsychotic cardiotoxicity, 1040
  availability and storage, 45t
  for calcium channel blocker toxicity, 949–950
  chemistry, 1004
  for cyclic antidepressant toxicity, 1049t, 1050–1051
  dosage and administration, 1008
  droplet sizes, 1004, 1006
  effects on analytical test results, 1007–1008

  elimination half-life, 1006
  formulation and acquisition, 1008
  and high-dose insulin, 1007
  history of, 1004
  hyperlipidemia caused by, 1007–1008
  and increased absorption of xenobiotics, 1007
  indications for, 35t, 45t, 747, 1004
  interactions with other antidotes, 1007
  and ion channel activation, 1005
  for local anesthetic toxicity, 1001, 1004, 1006
  mechanism of action, 1004–1006
  modulation of intracellular metabolism, 1004–1005
  for non-local anesthetic toxicity, 1004, 1006–1007
  for organic phosphorus compound poisoning,
        1498
  pancreatitis caused by, 1007
  pharmacodynamics, 1006
  pharmacokinetics, 1006
  pharmacology, 1004
  physicochemical properties, 684–685
  in pregnancy and lactation, 1008
  preparation, 1004
  priapism caused by, 301t
  pulmonary toxicity, 1007
  recommendations for, 1007
  respiratory effects, 399t
  shortage, 43
  stocking, recommended level, 45t
Lipid-lowering resins, for digoxin, digitoxin, and
        chlordane overdose, 64
Lipid peroxidation, 160, 174–175
  carbon monoxide poisoning and, 1664–1665
  irritant gases and, 1653
Lipids, postmortem changes, 1885t
Lipids and lipid carriers, as pharmaceutical additives,
        684–685, 684t
Lipid sink, 1004–1005
Lipid solubility
  and breast milk xenobiotic accumulation, 440
  and xenobiotic absorption, 142, 143f
Lipid sponge, 1004–1005
Lipoamide, trivalent arsenic and, 1238, 1239f
Lipoic acid, 643t
α-Lipoic acid, 643t
Lipoid pneumonia, 1415–1416
LipoKinetix, 608t, 639
  hepatotoxicity, 651
Lipolysis, 179
Lipophilicity
  and intrathecal administration, 793
  and xenobiotic metabolism, 167
Liposomes, 684, 684t, 1718f
  hypersensitivity to, 1006
5-Lipoxygease (5-LOX) inhibitors, 294
Lipoxygenase, in arachidonic acid metabolism, 511,
        513f
Liqui-Char, 79
Liquid(s), exposure to, 1809
Liquid chromatography, 106. *See also* High-performance
        liquid chromatography (HPLC)
Liquid chromatography/tandem mass spectrometry
        (LC/MS/MS), 107, 109f, 1870
Liquid chromatography/tandem mass spectroscopy
        (LC/MS/MS), 103t
Liquid chromatography time of flight mass
        spectrometry (LC-TOF), 1870
Liquid ecstasy, 162
Liraglutide, 606, 607t, 694. *See also* Dieting xenobiotics
        and regimens
  overdose/poisoning, hypoglycemia caused by, 700

pharmacokinetics and toxicokinetics, 697t
pharmacology, 612, 696
Lispro, 694. *See also* Insulin
Lister, Joseph, 1368, 1375
Listeria monocytogenes, 592t
  foodborne infection, 599
Listeriosis, 599
Litchi fruit, 1846
Literacy, and poison education, 1786
Lithium, 109, 1065–1074
  alkyl of, dermal decontamination for, precautions
      with, 72
  chemistry, 157
  clearance, and extracorporeal removal, 92
  cranial neuropathy caused by, 346t
  dermal decontamination for, precautions with, 72
  diabetes insipidus caused by, 189, 195, 195t, 1068,
      1070
  ECG changes caused by, 250–251, 1069
  effect on thyroid hormones and function, 813f, 814t,
      1068–1069
  endocrinopathy caused by, 1068–1069
  enhanced elimination, 90, 92
  extracorporeal elimination, 91f, 92, 97t, 1070–1071,
      1070t
  fetal effects, 1069
  gastrointestinal absorption, prevention, 64
  and gingival hyperplasia, 293
  and glutamate reuptake, 227t
  history of, 1065
  and hyponatremia, 196
  indications for, 1065
  laboratory testing for, 101t, 102
  leukocytosis caused by, 1069
  and male sexual dysfunction, 299f
  nephrotoxicity, 390f, 397t
  and neuromuscular blockers, interactions, 1021t
  neurotoxicity, systemic manifestations, 1068–1069
  and neutrophil count, 1069
  and NSAIDs, interactions, 514t
  pharmacokinetics and toxicokinetics, 145t, 1067
  pharmacology, 1065–1067, 1066f
  physicochemical properties, 1065
  priapism caused by, 301t
  protein-binding characteristics, 110t
  and serotonin toxicity, 1058t
  serum concentration
    interpretation, 153
    therapeutic, for bipolar disorder, 1065
  for SIADH, 197
  therapeutic uses, 1065
  and tinnitus, 370t
  toxicity
    acute, 1068
    acute-on-chronic, 1068
    and anion gap, 191t
    chronic, 1068
    clinical manifestations, 36, 36t, 1067–1068
    diagnostic tests for, 1069
    ECG changes caused by, 250–251
    extracorporeal elimination for, 91f, 92, 97t,
        1070–1071, 1070t
    fluid and electrolytes for, 1070
    gastrointestinal decontamination for, 85,
        1069–1070
    management, 38, 92–93, 1069–1071
    whole-bowel irrigation for, 1069
  volume of distribution, 91, 145t
Lithium carbonate, teratogenicity, 429t
Lithospermate B, 644t

Litvinenko, Alexander, poisoning, 6t, 13, 1762, 1769
Liver. *See also entries under* Hepatic
  antimicrobial toxicity and, 829t. *See also*
      Drug-induced liver injury
  blood flow, and xenobiotic elimination, 148
  blood supply to, 327
  cell types in, 327, 329f
  enzymes in, 167
    in liver injury, 334
  in ethanol metabolism, 1144–1145, 1145f
  fatty, laboratory findings with, 335t
  functions, 327
  metabolic zones of, 327, 328f
  morphology, 327
  mushroom toxins affecting, 1589t, 1590
  neoplasms, xenobiotic-induced, 331t
  raw, smell of, 364t
  specimens, postmortem collection and analysis,
      1870t, 1886
  structural unit, 327
  vitamin A in, 655
  xenobiotic metabolism by, 144, 147, 292–293
Liver dialysis, 96. *See also* Molecular Adsorbent
      Recirculating System (MARS)
  for acetaminophen removal, 484–485
Liver disease
  alcoholic, 1146
  coagulopathy in, 335
  evaluation of patient with, 334–336, 335t
  infiltrative, laboratory findings in, 335t
  prothrombin complex concentrate in, 910
Liver failure
  acute, 333. *See also* Hepatotoxicity
    acetaminophen and, 480
      N-acetylcysteine for, 495
    in children, 480
    with uncertain diagnosis, 480
  amatoxin-induced, 1584–1586
  with colchicine poisoning, 503
  fulminant, intravenous *N*-acetylcysteine and, 494
  hypoglycemia caused by, hospitalization for, 702
  nonacetaminophen-related, *N*-acetylcysteine for, 495
  treatment, 96
Liver function tests, 37
  in methanol poisoning, 1427
Liver injury. *See also* Hepatotoxicity
  anatomic localization, factors affecting, 328–329
  autoimmune, 330
  biochemical patterns in, 334–335, 335t
  immune-mediated, 330
  mechanisms, 330
  mitochondrial injury and, 330
  morphologic manifestations, 330–333
  occupational exposures associated with, 334, 334t
  toxic
    clinical presentation, 333–334
    management, 336
    types, 327–328
Liver support devices, 96
LiverTox, 329
Liver transplantation, 336
  for acetaminophen poisoning, 483
    APACHE II score and, 483–484, 484t
    King's College Criteria and, 483–484, 483t–484t
    MELD score and, 484, 484t
    SOFA score and, 484, 484t
  after amatoxin poisoning, 1586
  in copper poisoning, 1287–1288
  for disulfiram-induced liver failure, 1175
  organ procurement, *N*-acetylcysteine and, 494

  from poisoned patients, 1892–1893, 1892t
  for Wilson disease, 1287
Liverwort, *Frullania* spp., 1614
Lizards, venomous, 1618
  envenomation
    clinical manifestations, 1622
    diagnosis, 1623
    management, 1625
  venom
    components, 1619
    pharmacokinetics, 1619
    pharmacology, 1619
Llamas, bezoars from, 3
LMWH. *See* Low-molecular-weight heparin (LMWH)
Lobelia (*Lobelia inflata*), use and toxicities, 643t, 650t
Lobelia inflata (Indian tobacco), 1601t, 1604
Lobeline, 643t, 650t, 1495t, 1496, 1601t, 1604
Lobenzarit, diabetes insipidus caused by, 195, 195t
Lobster skin, 278
Local anesthetic(s), 994–1003. *See also specific*
      xenobiotic
  absorption, systemic, 995–996
  acute reactions to, 1000t
  adjuvant catecholamines in, reaction to, 1000t
  allergic reactions to, 997, 1000t
  amide, 994
    metabolism, 996, 998
    pharmacology, 996t
    structure, 995f
    toxicity, 998
  antidote for, 35t
  approximate allowable subcutaneous doses, 996t
  cardiac effects, 258t
  cardiovascular toxicity, 998–1000
    treatment, 1000–1001
  clinical applications, 994
  CNS toxicity, 998–999
    treatment, 1000
  and coagulation, 995
  in cocaine, 1130
  cranial neuropathy caused by, 346t
  cytotoxicity in nerve cells, 997
  dermal absorption, 996
  distribution, 995–996
  dosage and administration, 994, 1001
  duration of action, 995–996, 996t
  elimination, 995
  and epinephrine, combined, adverse effects and
      safety issues, 996
  esters, 994
    metabolism, 996
      and toxicity, 998
    pharmacology, 996t
    structure, 995f
  high spinal or epidural block, manifestations, 1000t
  history of, 994
  iatrogenic poisoning, 994
  and immune system, 995
  intermediate chain length, 995, 995f
  intravascular injection, clinical manifestations,
      1000t
  lipid solubility, 995
  local disposition, 995
  long-acting, 996
  maximal dose, 997–998
  mechanism of action, 994, 995f
  metabolism
    patient age and, 996
    and toxicity, 998
  methemoglobinemia caused by, 997

Local anesthetic(s), (*Cont.*):
  minimal IV toxic doses, 998t
  mixtures, 996
  and monoamine oxidase inhibitors, safety
      considerations, 1079, 1079t
  neurotoxicity, 997
  nicotinic receptor blockade by, 207
  onset of action, 995
  pharmacokinetics, 995–997
  pharmacology, 994–995
  pK$_a$, 995, 996t
  potency, 995, 996t
  protein binding, 995, 996t
  regional side effects and tissue toxicity, 997
  and respiratory system, 995
  seizures caused by, 996, 998–999
  serum concentration, factors affecting, 997
  skeletal muscle changes caused by, 997
  and sodium channels, 994, 995f, 999
  structure, 994, 995f
  systemic disposition, 995
  systemic side effects, 997–1000
  and tinnitus, 370t
  topical, 996
  toxicity (overdose/poisoning), 994
    diagnostic tests for, 1000
    lipid emulsion for, 1001, 1004, 1006–1007
    management, 45t
    resuscitation for, 1006
    systemic, 997–1000
      prevention, 1001
      treatment, 1000–1001
  vasodilatory effects, 996
  vasopressor syncope with, 1000t
  and voltage-gated calcium channels, 244f, 245
Local Emergency Planning Committee (LEPC), 1801t
Locoism, 1606
Locoweed, 1600t. *See also Datura stramonium*
    (jimsonweed, stramonium, locoweed)
  Astragalus spp., 1598t
  Astragalus lentiginosis (spotted locoweed), 1606
  Oxytropis spp., 1601t, 1606
  Sida carpinifolia, 1602t, 1606
  Swainsonia spp., 1603t
Locus ceruleus, 208, 212
  α_2-adrenoceptor activation in, 210, 210f, 212
Locusta, 2, 5t
Lodenafil, for erectile dysfunction, 301
Loganiaceae, 1603t
Log D, 141, 927t, 1045
Log P, 141
Lomotil, pediatric delayed toxicity, 452
Lomustine, 760t
  neurotoxicity, 763
London dispersion forces, 159
London fog, 17
London Fog incident (1952), 1651
Lone Star tick (*Amblyomma americanum*), 1550
Long-acting anticoagulant rodenticide(s) (LAARs),
    overdose/poisoning, management,
    915–917
Long QT syndrome. *See also* Electrocardiography (ECG)
  torsade de pointes in, magnesium for, 878
Long-tailed rattlesnake (*Crotalus* spp.), 1636t
Long-term potentiation, 237
Lonomia achelous, 1553–1554
  exposure to, treatment, 1554
Lonomia obliqua, 1552–1554
  exposure to, treatment, 1554
Lonomia saturniid, 1553

Lonomin V, 1553
Loop diuretics. *See* Diuretics, loop
Loop of Henle, 389, 390f
Loperamide, 531. *See also* Opioid(s)
  abuse/misuse, in elderly, 466
  cardiotoxicity, 246, 253, 257f
  characteristics, 526t
  and hERG channels, 253
  overdose/poisoning, ECG changes in, 254f
  P-glycoprotein and, 173
  and QT interval, 253t
Lophophora williamsii (peyote, mescal buttons), 1601t,
    1605
  ancient use of, 3
Loranthaceae, 1601t, 1603t
Loratadine
  and amiodarone, interactions, 746
  dose modification in liver or kidney disease, 744
  pharmacokinetics and toxicokinetics, 745t
  pharmacology, 742
  structure, 740f
  toxicity, clinical manifestations, 744
Lorazepam. *See also* Benzodiazepine(s);
    Sedative-hypnotics
  for acute dystonia, 1036
  administration route, 1136
  for agitated/violent behavior, 386
  for agitation with ketamine, 1217
  for alcohol withdrawal, 1168
    symptom-triggered administration, 1168
  for alcohol withdrawal seizures, 1167
  benzyl alcohol in, 683t
  in cirrhosis, 1139
  for cocaine-associated chest pain, 1139
  dosage and administration, 1137t
  duration of action, 1137–1138, 1137t
  hepatic metabolism, 1137t, 1138
  injection
    polyethylene glycol (PEG) in, 686t
    propylene glycol in, 687t, 688
  laboratory detection, 113
  lipophilicity, 1137
  metabolites, 1138
  for nerve agent toxicity, 1746
  onset of action, 1137, 1137t
  pharmacokinetics and pharmacodynamics, 1085t,
      1137–1138, 1137t–1138t
  pharmacology, 1136–1138, 1137t
  propylene glycol in, 1086
  for status epilepticus, 1137t, 1138
  for strychnine poisoning, 1537–1538
  withdrawal, 1088
  for xenobiotic-induced seizures, 1138
Lorcaserin, 606, 607t. *See also* Dieting xenobiotics and
    regimens
  adverse effects and safety issues, 611
  pharmacology, 611
  for weight loss, 611
Losartan, CYP enzymes and, 170
Loss of heterozygosity (LOH), radiation and, 1769
LOST, 1748
Lotus spp., cyanogenic glycosides in, 1684
Louche effect, 627
Louis XIV (King of France), 2, 6
Louseborne typhus, weaponized, 1757
Lovastatin, CYP enzymes and, 170
Love Canal (New York), 12
Love stone (*Bufo bufo gargarizans, Bufo bufo
    melanosticus*), 649
  as aphrodisiac, 649

psychoactive properties, 650t
  uses and toxicities, 641t
Lower California rattlesnake (*Crotalus* spp.), 1636t
Lower esophageal sphincter (LES), 290–291
Lower urinary tract syndrome (LUTS), ketamine-
    associated, 1215–1216, 1215f, 1217–1218
Lowest observed adverse effect level (LOAEL), 1815
Low-molecular-weight heparin (LMWH), 321f, 322,
    884f, 890–891. *See also* Heparin
  adverse effects and safety issues, in elderly, 464–465
  antidotes and treatment strategies for, 888t, 891
  for cocaine-associated myocardial infarction, 1129
  contraindications to, 891
  history of, 883
  laboratory testing for, 888t
  monitoring, 464–465, 891
  overdose/poisoning, clinical manifestations, 890
  pharmacokinetics, 890
  pharmacology, 890
  in pregnancy and lactation, 890
  priapism caused by, 301t
  reversal, protamine for, 919–923
    dosage and administration, 920–921
  skin necrosis caused by, 279
  toxicology, 890
Loxapine, 1045. *See also* Antipsychotics
  clinical and toxicologic effects, 1034t
  dosage and administration, 1033t
  mechanism of action, 1035
  pharmacokinetics, 1033t
Loxosceles spp., 1540
  antivenom, 1559–1561
    worldwide availability, 1560t
  geographic distribution, 1544
Loxosceles arizonica, 1544, 1560
Loxosceles bergeri, 1542t
Loxosceles boneti, antivenom, 1560
Loxosceles deserta, 1544
Loxosceles devia, 1544
Loxosceles gaucho, 1542t, 1546
  venom, detection, 1545
Loxosceles intermedia, 1544–1546
Loxosceles laeta, 1542t, 1546, 1560
Loxosceles parrami, 1542t
Loxosceles pilosa, 1542t
Loxosceles reclusa. *See* Brown recluse spider (*Loxosceles
    reclusa*)
Loxosceles rufescens, 1542t, 1544
  antivenom, 1560
Loxosceles spiniceps, 1542t
Loxosceles unicolor, 1560
Loxoscelism
  clinical spectrum, 1545
  systemic, 1545
  treatment, 1546, 1560
Lozenges, nicotine, 1204t, 1205
LSD. *See* Lysergic acid diethylamide (lysergide, LSD)
LSS (Lean and Six Sigma), 1827
Lubiprostone, 84
Lucibufagin, 969
Ludlow, Fitz Hugh, 9
Lugol solution, 818, 1369t
Lumbar puncture
  in alcoholic patients, 1167
  contraindications to, 1299, 1303
  indications for, 38
Lumefantrine, 838t
  adverse effects and safety issues, 842
  pharmacokinetics, 839t
  structure, 842

Lung(s). *See also* Pulmonary *entries*
  aluminum in, 1224
  cadmium and, 1260, 1260t
  computed tomography, in smoke inhalation, 1642
  and fluid balance, 194
  functions, 399
  ground-glass opacification, in bipyridyl compound
     poisoning, 1476
  smoke inhalation-induced injury, 1640–1642
Lung cancer
  cadmium-related, 1261
  chromium-related, 1270
Lung disease
  arsenic and, 1242
  cadmium-induced, 1260
Lung injury. *See also* Acute lung injury (ALI)
  N-acetylcysteine for, 494
Lung point, 406
Lung transplantation, from poisoned patients, 1892–
  1893, 1892t
Lupine (*Lupinus* spp.), 1601t
Lupinus latifolius (lupine), 1601t
Lupulone, 650t
Lupus syndrome, xenobiotic-induced, imaging, 115t,
  126
Lurasidone. *See also* Antipsychotics
  clinical and toxicologic effects, 1034t
  dosage and administration, 1033t
  mechanism of action, 1035
  pharmacokinetics, 1033t
Lusitropy, 929
Lutein, 272, 642t
Luteinizing hormone (LH), 297–298, 302
  for erectile dysfunction, 304
Lychee fruit, and gluconeogenesis, 176t, 178
Lycium barbarum (Goji), 642t
Lycium sinense (Goji), 642t
Lycopene, 272
Lycopenemia, 272
Lycoperdon spp., hypersensitivity pneumonitis caused
  by, 1659
Lycoperdon gemmatum, 1583t, 1592
Lycoperdonosis, 1592, 1659
Lycoperdon perlatum, 1583t, 1592, 1592f
Lycoperdon pyriforme, 1583t, 1592, 1592f
Lycopersicon (tomato, green), 1601t
Lycorine, 1601t
Lycosa tarantula, 1540
Lycotonum, 1597
Lye (sodium hydroxide), exposure to, pathophysiology,
  1389
Lyme disease, 1550
  bismacine for, adverse effects, 1255
  case study, 268, 268f
Lymphadenopathy, 126
  imaging, 115t
Lymphocyte(s), 319
  alterations, in heatstroke, 422
  hepatic, 327
Lymphocyte transformation test, for loxoscelism, 1545
Lymphoid cells, 310
Lymphoma(s), HIV-associated, 131, 132t
Lyon hypothesis, 318
Lysergamides, 1178, 1179t
  clinical effects, 1183–1184
  and dopamine receptors, 1182
  naturally occurring, 1179
  pharmacology, 1182–1183
  and serotonin receptors, 1182
  synthetic, 1179

Lysergic acid, 805
Lysergic acid amide, 1178, 1598t, 1605
D-Lysergic acid amide, 643t, 650t
Lysergic acid derivatives, 1598t, 1601t
Lysergic acid diethylamide (lysergide, LSD), 9, 1179t,
  1605
  bad trip with, 1179
  blotter paper for, hallucinogens in, 1179
  chemical structure, 1589
  cross-tolerance with other hallucinogens, 1183
  DEA class, 1179
  flashbacks with, 1184
  historical perspective on, 1178
  as incapacitating agent, 1750
  laboratory detection, 1184
  long-term effects, 1184–1185
  mechanism of action, 217
  and NMDA receptor, 1182
  pharmacology, 1181t
  physicochemical properties, 1179
  and rhabdomyolysis, 393t
  screening for, 110
  and serotonin receptors, 1182
  and serotonin toxicity, 1058t
  structure, 1179f
  synthesis, 9
  tolerance, 1183
  toxicity (overdose/poisoning), clinical
     manifestations, 36t, 1183
  toxicokinetics, 1181, 1181t
  use, epidemiology, 1178–1179
Lysergic acid ethylamide, 1605
Lysergic acid hydroxyethylamide, 1179, 1179t
  structure, 1179f
Lysine hydrochloride, and normal anion gap metabolic
  acidosis, 191t
Lysol disinfectant, as abortifacient, 303t
Lysophospholipases, 1509
Lysosomal storage disease, swainsonine and, 1606
Lysyl oxidase, 1285t

M
M30, 1077
M-291, for dermal decontamination, 72
Maca, as aphrodisiac, 304
Macarpine, 650t
MacArthur Competence Assessment Tool for
  Treatment (MacCAT-T), 374, 374t
Mace, 631
Mace (chloroacetophenone), 1749–1750, 1749f
  chemical name and structure, 1749f
  as pulmonary irritant, 1657
Mace (*Myristica fragrans*), 1601t. *See also Myristica
  fragrans* (mace, nutmeg)
α_2-Macroglobulin, 322
Macrogol, 83, 686
Macrolide antibiotics, 826–827
  adverse effects associated with xenobiotic
    interactions, 827
  as antimalarials, 836
    antimalarial mechanism, 838t
  cardiac effects, 258t, 826–827
  end-organ effects, 827
  mechanism of action, 822t
  ototoxicity, 366f
  and prolonged QT interval, 253t
  toxicity (overdose/poisoning), 822t, 826
    clinical and laboratory findings in, 36t
Macular edema, xenobiotic exposures and, 357t
Macule, 269t

Maculotoxin, 1572
Madagascar periwinkle (*Catharanthus roseus*), 1599t,
  1612
  psychoactive properties, 650t
  use and toxicities, 643t
Madarosis, from crack cocaine, 1126
Madecassic acid, 642t
Mafenide acetate, and normal anion gap metabolic
  acidosis, 191t
Magdalena. *See* Periwinkle (*Catharanthus roseus*)
Magendie, Francois, 4t
Magenta paint, 686
Magic mint. *See* Salvia (*Salvia divinorum, S.
  miltiorrhizae*)
Magic mushrooms. *See* Psilocybin mushrooms
  (*Psilocybe*)
Magic-Nano, 1717
Magnesium, 873, 876–882
  abnormalities, 199–200, 200t
  for alcohol withdrawal, 1169
  alkyl of, dermal decontamination for, precautions
    with, 72
  antidysrhythmic effects, 877
  and calcium channels, 876–877
  cardiac effects, 248, 876
  in cardiac toxin overdose/poisoning, 877–878
  for cardioactive steroid poisoning, 975
  chemistry, 157, 876
  clinical and laboratory findings with, 36t
  as coenzyme, 876, 878
  for cyclic antidepressant overdose, 877
  dermal decontamination for, 272
  dosage and administration, 879–880
  dust, dermal decontamination for, precautions
    with, 72
  for eclampsia/preeclampsia, 877
  effect on early afterdepolarizations, 251
  effects on vital signs, 30t
  elimination, 876
  for ethanol disorders, 878
  fluoride binding to, 1397
  for fluoride-releasing xenobiotic exposure, 879
  formulation and acquisition, 880
  history of, 876
  for hydrofluoric acid poisoning, 879
  for hydrofluoric acid systemic toxicity, 1400–1401
  iatrogenic toxicity, 199
  indications for, 876
  infusion
    adverse effects, 200
    monitoring, 200
  and neuromuscular blockers, interactions, 1021t
  and NMDA receptors, 227t, 876–877
  for organic phosphorus compound poisoning, 1498
  for pesticide poisoning, 878–879
  pharmacokinetics, 876
  physiology, 199, 876
  postmortem changes, 1885t
  in pregnancy and lactation, 879
  serum
    ethanol and, 1148–1149
    normal concentration, 876
  supplementation, 200
  and thiamine, 878
  tissue distribution, 876
  total body, 876
  for xenobiotic-induced hypomagnesemia, 877
Magnesium chloride
  for hydrofluoric acid exposure, 879
  for hypomagnesemia, 200, 876

Magnesium citrate, 83–84, 86
  with activated charcoal, 77
  for hypomagnesemia, 876
  pharmacodynamics, 84
Magnesium hydroxide, 83–84
  in antacids, 1223
  for hypomagnesemia, 876
Magnesium lactate, for hypomagnesemia, 200
Magnesium oxide, 200
  for hypomagnesemia, 876
Magnesium phosphide, 1457
  physicochemical properties, 1457
Magnesium salts
  for hydrofluoric acid toxicity, 1400
  intravenous, for hydrofluoric acid systemic toxicity, 1400
Magnesium sulfate, 83–84, 199
  for aconite poisoning, 877
  adverse effects and safety issues, 879
  for alcoholic patients, 1167
  for amitriptyline poisoning, 877
  for barium ingestion, 1455
  for cardiovascular poisonings, 877
  chemistry, 876
  for cyclic antidepressant toxicity, 1049t, 1050
  for digoxin toxicity, 877
  dosage and administration, 200, 879–880
  formulation and acquisition, 880
  history of, 876
  for hypomagnesemia, 876
  indications for, 35t, 876, 1040
  intrathecal administration, inadvertent overdose
      and unintentional exposures due to, 796t
  for metal phosphide poisoning, 1459
  pharmacodynamics, 84
  pharmacokinetics, 876
  in pregnancy and lactation, 879
  preparation, 876
  and seizure management in organic phosphorus
      compound poisoning, 878–879
  for torsade de pointes, 878
Magnetic microparticle chemiluminescent competitive
    immunoassay, 104f
Magnetic resonance imaging (MRI)
  of body packers, 546–547
  in carbon monoxide poisoning, 1667
  cranial, 130–133, 133f
  in inhalant-induced leukoencephalopathy, 1196, 1199
  in liver disease, 336
  in manganism, 1321
  in methanol poisoning, 1424, 1427
  of neurodegenerative disorders, 131
  in Parkinson disease, 1321
  in posterior reversible encephalopathy syndrome, 131–133
  of spinal cord, 131
    inverted V sign, 1199
  of stroke, 133f
  in toluene leukoencephalopathy, 1196, 1199
  T1-weighted, of basal ganglia, 1321
  of white matter lesions, 131
  of xenobiotics, 115t
  in zinc toxicity and copper deficiency, 1364–1365
Magnolia officinalis, acute interstitial nephritis caused
    by, 394t
Mahonia spp. (Oregon grape), 1601t, 1605
Ma-huang, 607, 608t, 1600t
  hepatotoxicity, 651
  uses and toxicities, 641t, 649

Ma Huang (*Coptis* spp.), 641t, 748
Maidenhair tree (*Gingko biloba*). *See* Gingko
    (*Gingko biloba*)
Maimonides, Moses, 1t, 3
Major depressive disorder
  epidemiology, 1054
  and suicide, 378–379
Major tranquilizers, 1032. *See also* Antipsychotics
MALA. *See* Metabolic acidosis, with elevated lactate
    concentration
Malabsorption
  and thiamine deficiency, 1160
  vitamin E deficiency in, 661
Malachite, 1283
Malaoxon, 146t, 1487, 1508
Malaria, 836, 1522
  control, 1514
  deaths from, 836
  glucose-6-phosphate dehydrogenase (G6PD)
      deficiency and, 844–845
  prophylaxis, 842
  treatment, 638, 647
    and hemolytic anemia, 318
  vaccine, 847
Malaria drugs, 836–849. *See also* Antimalarials
Malathion, 1488t, 1509–1510
  cytochrome P450 enzymes and, 1489
  food contamination with, 599
  pharmacokinetics and toxicokinetics, 146t
  pharmacology, 1487
  poisoning, and organ donation, 1893t
  volume of distribution, 146t
Malayan pit viper (*Calloselasma rhodostoma*), 900
Malignancy. *See also* Tumor lysis syndrome; *specific
    malignancy*
  and thiamine deficiency, 1160
Malignant hyperthermia, 31, 31t, 420, 1020
  clinical manifestations, 1029
  dantrolene for, 1029–1031
  differential diagnosis, 1023
  genetic disorders and, 1023
  management, 44t, 76
  pathophysiology, 1029
  prevention, 76, 1029–1031
  succinylcholine-induced, 1023–1024, 1024t
  therapeutics for, 35t
  treatment, 1023, 1024t
  xenobiotics causing, 1023
Malignant Hyperthermia Association of the
    United States, 1024
  registry, 1030
  website, 1030
Mallory bodies, 332
Mallory-Weiss syndrome, 126
Malo kingi (common kingslayer), 1567
Malonate, site of action, 173f
Malondialdehyde, 160, 1146
Malpractice, medical, 1861, 1865
Maltose, 707
Malvaceae, 1602t
Mambas (*Dendroaspis* spp.), 1633t
Management, of overdose/poisoning. *See also specific
    xenobiotic*
  in acute overdose/poisoning, 33–38
  algorithm for, 33, 34f
  altered mental status and, 33–37, 34f
  antidotes for, 35t
  with cutaneous exposure, 39
  disposition of patient in, 40
  eliminating absorbed xenobiotics in, 38

initial, for suspected exposure, 33
intentional exposures and, 39
nontoxic exposures and, 40
normal mental status and, 38–39
ophthalmic exposures and, 39–40
optimal outcome in, ensuring, 40–41
pitfalls, 38
reassessment in, 38
therapeutics for, 35t
Mana of St. Nicholas of Bari, 5t
Manchineel tree (*Hippomane mancinella*), 1613
Manchurian tea (kombucha), 643t
Mancozeb, 1487
Mandibular necrosis, from white phosphorus,
    22–23, 23t
Mandragora officinarum (mandrake), 2, 638,
    1601t
  as aphrodisiac, 304, 304t
  psychoactive properties, 650t
Mandrake, 1
  Mandragora officinarum (true mandrake, European
      mandrake), 2, 304, 304t, 638, 1601t
    psychoactive properties, 650t
  Podophyllum. See Podophyllin; Podophyllum
      (*Podophyllum* spp.)
Maneb, 1487
Manganese, 1319–1323
  absorption, 1319–1320
  brain changes caused by, 1320
    imaging, 131, 132t, 1320–1321
  in breast milk, 1319
  chelator for, 1780
  chemistry, 157, 1319
  cognitive effects, 1319–1320
  deficiency, 1319
  dietary sources, 1319
  divalent, 1319–1320
  in drinking water, 1319–1320
  elemental, 1319
  elimination, 1320
  elimination half-life, 1320
  as enzyme cofactor, 1319
  excretion, 1320–1321
  fluoride binding to, 1397
  history and epidemiology, 1319
  ionized, 1319
  and iron, competition for ligands, 1319–1321
  in metalloproteins, 1319
  movement disorder caused by, 1320–1321
  neurodevelopmental effects, 1319–1320
  neurotoxicity, 1320
  occupational exposure to, 1319–1320
  oxidation states, 1319–1320
  pharmacology, 1319
  physicochemical properties, 1319
  physiology, 1319–1320
  psychiatric effects, 1319–1320
  serum, 1319–1320
    normal concentration, 1319
  tissue distribution, 1320
  toxicity
    chelation therapy for, 1321
    clinical manifestations, 1320–1321, 1320t
    diagnostic imaging, 115t, 131, 132t, 1321
    diagnostic testing for, 1321
    pathophysiology, 1320
    sources, 1319
    treatment, 1321
  transport, 1319–1320
  trivalent, 1319–1320

urine, 1321
  normal concentration, 1319
use of, 1319
whole blood, 1319–1320
  clinical utility, 1321
  factors affecting, 1321
  normal concentration, 1319
Manganese chloride, 1319
Manganese dioxide, 1319
Manganese exporter protein SLC30A10, mutations, 1320–1321
Manganese-iron alloys, 1319
Manganese madness, 1320
Manganese oxide, 1319
  inhalation
    metal fume fever caused by, 1321
    neuropsychiatric syndrome caused by, 1319
Manganese sulfate, 1319
Manganism. *See also* Manganese, toxicity
  definition, 1319
Mangifera indica, contact dermatitis from, 1614
Mango, contact dermatitis from, 1614
Mania, xenobiotic-induced, 344, 344t
Manihot spp., 1601t, 1684
Manihot esculenta (cassava, manihot, tapioca), 1601t, 1607, 1684, 1686, 1688
Mannitol
  with activated charcoal, 1353
  and osmotic nephrosis, 392
  and thiamine pharmacokinetics, 1158
Mann-Whitney *U* test, 1857
Manzanilla (chamomile), uses and toxicities, 641t
MAOI. *See* Monoamine oxidase inhibitors (MAOIs)
Maprotiline, 1044. *See also* Cyclic antidepressants
  and GABA receptors, 222
  pharmacology, 1045
  structure, 1044t
  toxicity, 1048
Maqianzi, 651, 1536, 1605
Maraviroc, 832
Marburg virus, as biological weapon, 1758
Marcasite, 1339
Marchioness de Brinvilliers, 4–6, 5t
Margosa oil
  hepatotoxicity, 331
  steatosis caused by, 332
Mariani, Angelo, 8
Maria pastora. *See* Salvia (*Salvia divinorum, S. miltiorrhizae*)
Marijuana, 1179t. *See also* Cannabinoid(s); Cannabis (*Cannabis*, marijuana, bhang)
  abuse, 1118
  adverse effects and safety issues, management, 1120
  definition, 1113
  dependence, 1118
  and hyperemesis syndrome, 1118
  medical uses, 1111–1113
  passive inhalation, tests for, 1119
  phencyclidine (PCP) and, combined, 1212
  in pregnancy and lactation, 1117–1118
  regulation, 1111
  street names for, 162
Marijuana Tax Act (1937), 10t
Marine envenomations, 1567–1580
  annelid, 1573–1574
  Cnidaria (jellyfish), 1567–1572, 1567t
  echinoderm, 1573–1574
  fish, 1576–1578, 1576t
  invertebrate, 1567–1574

Mollusca, 1572–1573, 1573t
  sea snake, 1574–1576
  sponge (Porifera), 1573–1574
  vertebrate, 1574–1578
Marinobufagenin, 979
MARK I Nerve Agent Antidote Kit, 1506, 1511, 1746
Markov, Georgi, 5t, 12, 1753
Marsh, James, 4t, 6
Marsh test, 6
Martin's Rat Stop liquid, 1350
Masai hunters, 1
Masking xenobiotics, added to urine before doping analysis, 622–623
Massasauga (*Sistrurus catenatus*), 1617t
Masseter muscle rigidity (MMR), 1024
Massive transfusion protocols (MTP), 885
Mass psychogenic illness, 1814
Mass spectrometer (MS), 106–107
  components, 107
  ion detector for, 107
  ion source for, 107
  mass analyzer for, 107
  quadrupole, 107, 107f
Mass spectrometry, 107. *See also* Tandem mass spectrometry
  ionization modalities for, 107
  scanning mode, 107
  selected ion monitoring (SIM) mode, 107
Mass suicide by poison, 24
Mass-to-charge (m/z) ratio, 107
Mastocytosis, 273
Mastoparans, 1551
Matches, phosphorus in, 1528
Maté (*Ilex paraguariensis*), 1600t
  psychoactive properties, 650t
  use and toxicities, 643t
Material safety data sheets (MSDS)
  information from, 1797, 1803–1804
  limitations, 1789, 1797, 1803–1804
  worker education about, 1800
Materia Medica, 1, 1t. *See also* Dioscorides
Matricaria recutita (chamomile), uses and toxicities, 641t
Matsutake, 1590, 1590f
Matter, definition, 155
Matteuccia struthipteris (ostrich fern), 643t
Matthew, Henry, 11
Mauve stinger (*Pelagia noctiluca*), 1567, 1567t, 1568. *See also* Cnidaria (jellyfish)
Maximum inspiratory pressure (MIP), 406
Mayapple (*Podophyllum peltatum*, mandrake), 504, 1602t, 1612, 1613f. *See also* Podophyllin
  as abortifacient, 303t
Maybrick, Florence, 5t, 6
Maybush (*Crataegus* spp.), 642t
Maypop (*Passiflora incarnata*), 643t, 650t
Mazindol, 607, 607t. *See also* Dieting xenobiotics and regimens
M cells, cardiac, electrophysiology, 253–254
MCPA, and fatty acid metabolism, 179
MDEA. *See* 3,4-Methylenedioxyethamphetamine (MDEA, Eve)
MDMA. *See* 3,4-Methylenedioxymethamphetamine (MDMA, Adam, molly, ecstasy, XTC)
MDRD formula, 393t, 397
MDR1 gene, 144
Mead, Richard, 4t
Meadow saffron
  Colchicum autumnale. See also Colchicine
    uses and toxicities, 640t

Gloriosa superba, primary toxicity, 1600t. *See also* *Gloriosa superba* (glory lily, meadow saffron, superb lily)
Meadow sage. *See Salvia officinalis* (sage)
Mean arterial pressure (MAP), 264
Mebendazole, 829
Mechanical ventilation
  for ARDS, 401
  for hydrocarbon pulmonary toxicity, 1416–1417
  for poisoned patient, 407
  salicylate toxicity and, 563
  smoke inhalation and, 1645
Mechlorethamine, 760t
  extravasation, 802–803, 803t
  mechanism of action, 350f
  teratogenicity, 429t
Meclofenamate, pharmacology, 512t
Mecoprop (MCPP), 1480
  structure, 1481f
Medea, 501
Medicago sativa (alfalfa), 640t
Medical child abuse, 455, 455t
Medical Device User Fee Amendments (MDUFA) of 2007, 1834–1835
Medical errors, 13. *See also* Adverse drug events (ADEs); Medication errors
Medical examiners, 6–7, 1884
Medical toxicology
  historical perspective on, 9, 11t, 12
  nonphysician practitioners, 12
  postgraduate education in, 12
  as specialty, 11t, 12
Medication(s)
  vs. dietary supplements, 638
  substandard, in developing world, 1846
Medication errors, 13. *See also* Adverse drug events (ADEs)
  causes, 1827
  in children, 1826
  communication and, 1828–1829
  data collection on, 1792, 1842
  deaths from, medications involved in, 1824
  definition, 1822
  in elderly, 463–464, 1823, 1826–1827
  examples, 453t
  human factors in, 1827–1828, 1828t
  incidence, 1822
  in inpatient vs. emergency department settings, 1824, 1824f
  knowledge deficits and, 1828
  medications involved in, 1824, 1824t
  morbidity and mortality caused by, 1822–1823
  and pediatric poisoning, 453–454
  prevalence, 1822
  prevention, 454, 1827
    information technology and, 1825t, 1829
  reduction, 1827
  response to, 1827
  stages of medication process and, 1824–1826, 1825t
  taxonomy, of National Coordinating Council for Medication Error Reporting and Prevention, 1823–1824, 1823f–1824f
  toxicologists' role in, 1830
  underreporting, 1824
Medication overuse headache, 515
Medication Process, 1824–1826
  stages, 1824
    errors at, 1824–1826, 1825t
Medication reconciliation, 1829

Medication safety, 1822–1832, 1864–1865. *See also* Adverse drug events (ADEs)
  concerns about, and removal or withdrawal from market, 1839–1840, 1840t
  evolution of, critical events in, 1822t
  FDA regulatory actions on, 1839–1840, 1840t
  history of, 1822, 1822t
  monitoring, by FDA, 1834
  postmarketing problems with, leading to drug withdrawal from market, 1839–1841, 1840t
  toxicologists' role in, 1830, 1841–1842
Medicinal drug disasters, 19–21, 20t
Medicolegal considerations
  in product liability litigation about FDA-approved medications, 1839–1840
  in toxicologic emergencies, 1860
Medicolegal interpretive toxicology, 1868–1875
  alternative matrices in, 1870t, 1872–1873
  case history and, 1868, 1868t
  inaccurate results, factors leading to, 1871, 1871t
  preanalytical issues in, 1868–1870, 1869t
  special laboratory considerations in, 1870–1871
Medicolegal investigation, 1885
Medieval period, toxicology in, 3–6
Mediterranean squill, 1603t
Medline, 1804
Medroxyprogesterone
  as CYP inhibitor, 171
  depot, polyethylene glycol (PEG) in, 686t
Medullary pyramids, 389
MedWatch Partners, 1837
MedWatch system, 1836–1838, 1841–1842, 1865
  hypothesis generation in, 1837
Mees lines, 38, 274t, 282, 1351, 1353
  arsenic and, 1241–1242
  causes, 1241–1242, 1241f
  thallium-induced, 1351–1352
Mefenacet
  in herbicides, 1467t
  toxicity, clinical manifestations, 1473
Mefenamic acid
  effect on thyroid hormones and function, 814t
  pharmacology, 512t
Mefloquine, 838t
  pharmacokinetics, 839t, 841
  structure, 841
  toxicity
    clinical manifestations, 841
    management, 841–842
  toxicodynamics, 841
Mefluidide, in herbicides, 1467t
Mefolinate, 776
Megathura crenulata (great keyhole limpet), 977
Megestrol acetate, nanocrystals, 1719t
Meglitinides
  hypoglycemia caused by, 702, 713–718
    octreotide for, 715
  maintaining euglycemia after initial control with, 701
  mechanism of action, 696f
  overdose
    hospitalization for, 702
    management, 702
  pharmacokinetics and toxicokinetics, 697t
  structure, 695f
Meglumine antimoniate
  adverse effects, 1230–1233
  ECG changes caused by, 1232
  ototoxicity, 1233

  pancreatitis caused by, 1230
  toxicity, clinical manifestations, 1231t–1232t
MEGX (monoethylglycylxylidide), 866t, 870
  chemical structure, 869f
Melaleuca spp., 633
Melaleuca alternifolia (tea tree), 633
Melaleuca oil, 633
Melamine, 1482
  in human food, 19, 601
  in infant formula, 18t, 19, 453, 601, 1846
  in pet food, 19
  thermal degradation products, 1641t
Melanin, xenobiotic binding to, 146
Melanocortin, and sexual function, 298, 300
Melanocyte-stimulating hormone (MSH), and thermoregulation, 412
Melanonychia, 281
Melanosis coli, 613
Melarsoprol, 1237
  adverse effects, 1238
  mechanism of action, 1238
  pharmacology, 1238
  therapeutic uses, 1238
Melatonin, 215, 1084, 1090, 1179
Melatonin receptor agonists, 1084
Meldonium, as athletic performance enhancer, 620
Melhase, Margaret, 1264
Melilotus spp. (sweet clover), 1601t
Melittin, in honeybee venom, 1551, 1551t
Mellanby effect, 1147
Mellitin, 640t
Meloxicam
  cardiovascular risk with, 514
  pharmacology, 512t
Melphalan, 760t
  EPA regulation of, 765
Memantine
  and levodopa, combined, 228
  mechanism of action, 227t, 228
  and NMDA receptors, 228
Membrane(s)
  cell, reactive oxygen species and, 160
  structure, 141
  xenobiotic diffusion through, 141, 141f
Membrane-associated enzymes, in erythrocyte, 312
Membrane potentials, 203
Membrane transport, 141–142, 141f, 167
Membrane transporters, 168, 172–173
Memory, deficits
  carbon monoxide poisoning and, 1665
  in elderly, and unintentional poisoning, 466
  in thallium toxicity, 1351
Menadione (vitamin K_3), effects on mitochondrial inner membrane, 176t
Mendeleev, Dmitri, 155
Meningitis
  aseptic
    in drug-induced hypersensitivity syndrome, 277
    NSAIDs and, 515
    sulfonamides and, 827
  in HIV-infected (AIDS) patients, ophthalmic complications, 361
Menkes ATPase, 1284
Menkes kinky-hair syndrome, 1284
Mental illness. *See also specific disorder*
  and hospitalization, 379
  and involuntary commitment, 379
  perinatal, 433–434
  and suicide, 377–379
  and violence, 385

Mental status, altered. *See* Altered mental status (AMS)
Mentha arvensis, 632
Mentha piperita (peppermint), 632
Mentha pulegium (pennyroyal), 1601t
  as abortifacient, 303t
  use and toxicities, 643t
Menthol, 632–633, 1410
2-MeO-diphenidine, 1211
2-MeO-ketamine (2-MK), 1211, 1211t, 1212
3-MeO-PCE. *See* Methoxieticyclidine
Meperidine (MPPP, methylphenylpropionoxypiperidine), 174, 532. *See also* Opioid(s)
  characteristics, 526t
  immunoassays for, 112
  mechanism of action, 218, 227t, 228
  metabolite, 147
  seizures caused by, 539
  and serotonin toxicity, 1058t, 1079
  talc retinopathy from, 361
Mephedrone, 1106–1107
  and chemsex, 1188
Mephobarbital. *See also* Sedative-hypnotics
  pharmacokinetics, 1085t
Mephyton, 917
Mepivacaine. *See also* Local anesthetic(s)
  history of, 994
  minimal IV toxic dose, 998t
  pharmacology, 996t
  structure, 995f
  and tinnitus, 370t
Meprobamate, 1088–1089. *See also* Sedative-hypnotics
  history of, 1135
  mechanism of action, 222, 227t, 228
  overdose, 1087
    clinical findings in, 1086–1087, 1086t
  pharmacokinetics, 1085
  poisoning, and organ donation, 1893t
  structure, 1088
Mepyramine, pharmacology, 741–742
Merbromin, 1368, 1369t, 1372
Mercaptans, odor, 364t
Mercaptoethane sulfonate, 764
Mercaptopurine (6-mercaptopurine), 349f
  adverse effects and safety issues, 760t
  cell cycle phase specificity, 761f
  mechanism and site of action, 762f
  overdose/poisoning, 760t
β-Mercaptopyruvate-cyanide sulfurtransferase, 1685
Mercaptopyruvate sulfurtransferase, 1698–1699
Mercurialism, in hatters, 22, 23t, 1324
Mercurials, 1369t, 1372. *See also* Mercury
  organic, 157
  organification, 1325–1326
Mercurial salivation, 1324. *See also* Mercury
Mercuric acetate, production, 1797
Mercuric bichloride, 1372
Mercuric chloride, 1324, 1324t, 1368, 1388t. *See also* Mercury
  absorption, 1325
  adsorption to activated charcoal, 76
  exposure to, management, 1393
  ingestion, 1327
    management, 1329
  lethal dose, 1327
  ophthalmic toxicity, 361t
  poisoning, treatment, 1330
Mercuric oxide, 116, 1324. *See also* Mercury
  overdose/poisoning, whole-bowel irrigation for, 85

Mercuric sulfide (cinnabar), 1324
   teratogenicity, 429t
Mercurochrome, 1369t, 1372
Mercurothiolate, 689
Mercurous chloride (calomel), 1324, 1324t. *See also*
      Mercury
   absorption, 1325
Mercury, 1324–1332, 1780. *See also* Heavy metals
   absorption, 1325
   antidote for, 35t
   aspiration, 1326
      management, 1329
   biotransformation, 1325–1326
   in breast milk, 1328
   cation, and electron transport, 176t
   in central nervous system, 1325–1326
   chemistry, 157
   dermal absorption, 1325
   diagnostic imaging, 115t, 116–117, 118f, 128
   in dietary supplements, 647–648
   elemental, 1324–1325, 1324t
      absorption, 1325
      clearance, 1325t
      diagnostic testing for, 1329, 1329t
      elimination, 1326
      elimination half-life, 1326
      exposure to, differential characteristics, 1325,
         1325t
      poisoning
         chelation therapy for, 1330
         clinical manifestations, 1325, 1325t, 1326–1327
         treatment, 1325t, 1329
      subcutaneous or intravenous injection, 1327,
         1327f, 1329
      tissue distribution, 1325, 1325t
   elimination, 1326
      chelation and, 1330
   exposure to
      differential characteristics, 1325, 1325t
      sources, 1324, 1324t
   in fish, 1328, 1815
   fish contaminated with, 18t, 19
   focal brain lesions caused by, 131
   forms, 1324–1325, 1324t–1325t
   in hair, 1329, 1329t
   historical perspective on, 2, 7, 1324
   ingestion, 1325, 1325t, 1327
   inhalation, 157, 1325, 1325t, 1326
      management, 1329
   inorganic, 1324–1325, 1324t
      absorption, 1325
      clearance, 1325t
      diagnostic testing for, 1329, 1329t
      elimination, 1326
      elimination half-life, 1326
      exposure to, differential characteristics, 1325,
         1325t
      nephrotoxicity, 1327
      neurotoxicity, 1327
      poisoning
         chelation therapy for, 1253, 1330
         clinical manifestations, 1325, 1325t, 1327–1328
         treatment, 1325t, 1329
      tissue distribution, 1325, 1325t
   intramuscular, management, 1329
   intrathecal administration, inadvertent overdose
        and unintentional exposures due to, 796t
   mercuric form, 157, 1324t, 1325, 1327
   mercurous form, 157, 1324t, 1325, 1327
   nephrotoxicity, 390f, 392f, 397t

occupational diseases caused by, 23
ophthalmic toxicity, 356f
organic, 1324–1325, 1324t
   absorption, 1325
   clearance, 1325t
   diagnostic testing for, 1329, 1329t
   elimination, 1326
   elimination half-life, 1326
   exposure to
      differential characteristics, 1325, 1325t
      management, 1329
   poisoning
      chelation therapy for, 1330
      clinical manifestations, 1325, 1325t, 1328
      detection, 1329
      treatment, 1325t, 1329
   tissue distribution, 1325–1326, 1325t
in paint, 1324
physicochemical properties, 1324
poisoning
   chelation therapy for, 1252–1253, 1330
   chronic, 1327
   clinical manifestations, 36t, 1325t, 1326–1328
   epidemiology, 1324
   laboratory investigation in, 36t, 1328–1329, 1329t
   management, 44t, 46t, 1329–1330
   pathophysiology, 1326
   subacute, 1327, 1329
   subclinical, 1329
   whole-bowel irrigation in, 63, 1329
   subcutaneous, 1327, 1327f
      management, 1329
tests for, 4t, 36t, 1328–1329, 1329t
tissue distribution, 1325–1326
toxicokinetics, 1324–1325, 1325t
urine
   clinical significance, 1329–1330
   measurement, 1328–1329, 1329t
   normal concentration, 1324
whole blood, 1325
   clinical significance, 1329–1330
   measurement, 1328–1329, 1329t
   normal concentration, 1324
Mercury bichloride, 4, 7
Mercury decontamination kit, 1329
Mercury nitrate, occupational poisoning with, 22, 23t
Mercury vapor, 1657
   exposure to, 1326
      management, 1329
   immediately dangerous to life and health (IDLH),
        1654t
   intoxication, 1797
   permissible exposure limit, 1326
   regulatory standard for, 1654t
   short-term exposure limit (STEL), 1654t
   sources, 1654t
   water solubility, 1654t
Meropenem, 825
Merphos, 1488t
Merthiolate(s), 689, 1327, 1369t, 1372
Meru, 2
Mesalamine, pancreatitis caused by, 295t
Mesalazine, diabetes insipidus caused by, 195, 195t
Mescal buttons (*Lophophora williamsii*), 1601t
Mescaline, 1179t, 1180, 1181t, 1601t, 1605
   chemical structure, 1180f
   cross-tolerance with other hallucinogens, 1183
   mechanism of action, 217
   toxicokinetics, 1182
Mesenteric ischemia, imaging, 127, 129f, 129t

MESNA, 760t
Mesobuthus spp., antivenoms, 1564t, 1565
Mesobuthus tamulus, antivenom, 1565
Meso-2,3-dimercaptosuccinic acid (DMSA). *See*
      Succimer (2,3-dimercaptosuccinic acid,
      DMSA)
Mesoridazine. *See also* Antipsychotics
   clinical and toxicologic effects, 1034t
   dosage and administration, 1033t
   pharmacokinetics, 1033t
   toxicity, 1032
      sodium bicarbonate for, 568t, 569
Mesothelioma, 115t, 126
Messenger RNA (mRNA), and withdrawal syndrome, 237
Metabisulfites, foodborne, 600t
Metabolic abnormalities. *See also specific abnormality*
   antipsychotic-induced, 1039
   carbon monoxide poisoning and, 1665
   cardiac effects, 254–255
   ethanol and, 1146
   and prolonged QT interval, 256
Metabolic acidosis, 161, 191
   in acetaminophen toxicity, 474
   acute, 193
   adverse effects, 193
   in aluminum phosphide poisoning, 1459
   amphetamine-induced, 1104
   anion gap
      NSAIDs and, 515
      toluene and, 1196
      in toxic alcohol poisoning, 1423, 1426
   barium-induced, 1455
   carbon monoxide poisoning and, 1665
   caustic ingestion and, 1391
   chromium-induced, 1270
   chronic, 193
   correction, hemodialysis for, 90, 95
   definition, 190
   in DEG poisoning, 1446
   diagnosis, 191
   with elevated lactate concentration, 703–704
      albuterol and, 989
      clinical manifestations, 703
      management, 703–704
      metformin-associated, 699, 703–704
      phenformin-associated, 703
      theophylline and, 989
   and enhanced elimination of xenobiotics, 90
   fluoride poisoning and, 1398
   high anion gap, 32
      causes, 191, 191t
      caustic ingestion and, 1391
      delta gap ratio (Δ anion gap/Δ [HCO$_3^-$]) in, 192
      differential diagnosis, 192
      poisoning/overdose causing, 36t
   hyperchloremic, 191
   with hyperlactatemia, metformin-associated, 90, 95,
      699, 703–704
   and hyperventilation, 30
   impaired oxidative metabolism and, 177
   iron and, 670
   life-threatening, sodium bicarbonate for, 568t,
      570–571
   management, 46t, 193–194
   in metal phosphide poisoning, 1458
   non-anion gap (hyperchloremic), with ethylene
      glycol poisoning, 1423f
   normal anion gap
      causes, 191, 191t
      differential diagnosis, 193

Metabolic acidosis (*Cont.*):
  with 5-oxoprolinemia and 5-oxoprolinuria, in
      acetaminophen toxicity, 474
  polyethylene glycol (PEG) and, 687
  propylene glycol and, 688
  respiratory compensation in, 190
  salicylates and, 399
  in strychnine poisoning, 1537
  toluene and, 1196
  in toxic alcohol poisoning, 191t, 1423, 1426
Metabolic alkalosis, 189, 194
  adverse effects, 194
  approach to patient with, 194
  causes, 194, 194t
  chloride-resistant, 194, 194t
  chloride-responsive, 194, 194t
  compensation for, 190, 194
  correction, hemodialysis for, 95
  definition, 190
  gastrointestinal decontamination and, 85
  with hypokalemia, 198
Metabolic syndrome, antipsychotic-induced, 1039
Metabolism. *See also specific xenobiotic*
  aerobic, 177
  β-adrenergic antagonists and, 929
  phase I. *See* Phase I reactions
  phase II. *See* Phase II reactions
  postmortem, 1887
Metabolite(s)
  active, 145t–146t, 147
  cellular injury by, 174, 174t
  as CYP inhibitors, 171
  glucuronidated, laboratory detection, 112–113
  hepatic conjugated, 144
  and laboratory test results, 153
  screening for, in drug abuse testing, 110
  toxic, 144, 167, 174, 174t
Metabolizer(s)
  extensive, 170
  intermediate, 170
  phenotypes, 170
  poor, 170
  ultrarapid, 170, 172
Metachlor toxicity, clinical manifestations, 1473
Metal(s), 156f. *See also specific metal*
  alkali, 156f, 157
  alkaline earth, 156f, 157
  alkyl, dermal decontamination for, precautions
      with, 72
  characteristics, 155
  clinical and laboratory findings with, 36t
  contact dermatitis from, 279
  dermal decontamination for, precautions with, 72
  in dietary supplements, 647–648
  excretion, *N*-acetylcysteine and, 494
  and free radical formation, 174–175, 175f
  heavy. *See* Heavy metals; *specific metal*
  nephrotoxicity, 390f, 397, 397t
  and occupational asthma, 1660, 1660t
  overdose/poisoning, 38
  solid alkali, dermal decontamination for,
      precautions with, 72
  transition, 156f, 157
    long-term exposure to, 160
    mutagenic effects, 160
    in redox reactions, 160
  transuranic, 1779–1781
Metal allergy, 1333
Metal fume fever (MFF), 1286, 1362, 1365, 1659
  antimony oxides and, 1232

clinical manifestations, 1659
copper-induced, 1286
manganese oxide and, 1321
zinc and, 1364
Metal ions, ophthalmic toxicity, 356f
Metallic taste, 365, 365t
Metalloestrogen(s), antimonials as, 1233
Metalloids, 156f
  characteristics, 155
  chemistry, 158
Metalloprotease(s), in Cnidaria venom, 1569
Metalloproteinase(s), in snake venom, 1618–1620,
      1619t, 1637
Metallosis, 1275–1276
  definition, 1275
Metallothionein, 160, 340, 1285–1287, 1363
  and cadmium, 1259, 1261–1262, 1363
  and copper, 1284, 1363
  and mercury, 1325, 1363
  and silver, 1363
  xenobiotic binding to, 146
  and zinc, 1363
Metal oxides, as thermal degradation product, 1642
Metal phosphides, 1457–1460
  absorption, 1458
  history of, 1457
  ingestion, 1457–1458
  odor, 1458
  physicochemical properties, 1457
  poisoning
    N-acetylcysteine for, 1459
    clinical manifestations, 1458
    diagnostic tests for, 1458–1459
    ECG changes in, 1458–1459
    epidemiology, 1457
    mortality rate for, 1459
    prognosis for, 1459
    toxicological analyses in, 1459
    treatment, 1459–1460
  toxic dose, 1458
  toxicodynamics, 1458
  toxicokinetics, 1457–1458
Metal pneumonitis, 1657–1658
Metal salts, unintentional ingestion, 600
Metaphyseal bands, 122t. *See also* Lead lines
  causes, 1300
  imaging, 115t
  lead-induced, imaging, 119, 122f, 122t
  xenobiotics causing, 119
Metaproterenol, 985
  and tinnitus, 370t
Metazachlor, in herbicides, 1467t
Met-enkephalin, 520
Metformin
  adverse effects and safety issues, 612
  cimetidine and, interactions, 144
  enhanced elimination, 90
  extracorporeal elimination, 97t, 704
  and high anion gap metabolic acidosis, 191t
  history of, 694
  hyperventilation caused by, 400t
  lactic acidosis from, 90, 95
  mechanism of action, 695, 703, 703f
  and metabolic acidosis with elevated lactate
      concentration, 699, 703–704
  overdose/poisoning
    clinical and laboratory findings in, 36t
    extracorporeal treatment for, 97t, 704
    hospitalization for, 702
    hypoglycemia caused by, 699

outcomes with, 703
    sodium bicarbonate for, 568t, 571
  pharmacokinetics and toxicokinetics, 697t
  pharmacology, 695
  structure, 695f
  and thiamine deficiency, 1160
  volume of distribution, 704
  for weight loss, 606, 612
Metformin-associated metabolic acidosis with
      hyperlactatemia, 90, 95, 699, 703–704
Methabenzthiazuron, in herbicides, 1467t
Methacholine, 1495t, 1496
Methadone, 519, 529–530, 539. *See also* Opioid(s)
  cardiac effects, 246, 253f, 253t, 258t, 924, 1820–1821,
      1820f–1821f
  characteristics, 526t
  effect on thyroid hormones and function, 814t
  and ethanol, interactions, 1146t
  and hearing loss, 524
  ileus caused by, 129f
  immunoassays for, 112
  injection, chlorobutanol in, 683t
  mechanism of action, 227t, 228
  metabolism, 172
  for neonatal opioid withdrawal, 439
  for opioid use disorder, 552
  pharmacokinetics, 145t
  and prolonged QT interval, 1820–1821, 1821f
  and propoxyphene, structural similarity, 532,
      532f
  and QT interval, 253f, 253t, 1820–1821, 1821f
  screening for, 110
  solution, sorbitol in, 688t
  talc retinopathy from, 361
  urine screening assays for, performance
      characteristics, 111t
  volume of distribution, 145t
  withdrawal, neonatal, 439
Methadone maintenance treatment programs
      (MMTPs), 529–530, 552
Methamidophos, 1487
  pharmacokinetics and toxicokinetics, 1488
Methamphetamine(s), 1180. *See also* Amphetamine(s)
  abuse, 1099
  bioavailability, administration route and, 1102
  in body stuffers, 85, 548
  and chemsex, 1188
  clinical effects, 1102
  contaminants, 1105
  deaths caused by, 1099
  elimination, 1102
  history of, 1099, 1105
  illicit synthesis, 738
  oral pathology from, 293
  percent nonionized, pH and, 142t
  pharmacokinetics, 1105
  pharmacokinetics and toxicokinetics, 145t
  pharmacology, 1105
  production, 1105
  pruritus caused by, 273
  street names, 1105
  structure, 1099, 1105
  synthesis, phosphorus in, 1528
  therapeutic uses, 1105
  toxicokinetics, 1182
  urine screening assays for, performance
      characteristics, 111t
  vascular lesions from, 132f
  volume of distribution, 145t, 1102
L-Methamphetamine, 112

Methane
  chemistry, 159, 166
  exposure to, 1652
  physicochemical properties, 1652
  as simple asphyxiant, 400t, 1650
  sources, 1654t
  as thermal degradation product, 1641t
  water solubility, 1654t
Methanol, 4t, 7, 162, 1421–1430. *See also* Toxic
        alcohol(s)
  affinity for alcohol dehydrogenase, 1440
  and anion gap, 193
  antidote for, 35t, 775
  brain changes caused by, imaging, 131, 132t
  breath test for, 1425
  chemistry, 165–166, 168, 1422
  clearance, 1423
  common products containing, 1421
  cranial neuropathy caused by, 346t
  diagnostic tests for, 1425
  effects on vital signs, 30t
  enhanced elimination, 90
  enzymatic assay for, 1425
  epidemic poisoning with, 21t, 22, 1421t, 1430
  and formate toxicity, management, 776–777
  and high anion gap metabolic acidosis, 191t
  history of, 1421
  hyperventilation caused by, 400t
  hypoventilation caused by, 400t
  inhaled/inhalation, 1193t, 1422. *See also* Inhalant(s)
        toxicity, 1197
  laboratory testing for, 36t, 101t, 103–104, 1425
  metabolism, 775, 1422, 1423f, 1436, 1440
        ethanol and, 1440
  neurotoxicity, 1424
  occupational exposure to, 1422
  ophthalmic toxicity, 356, 356f, 358, 361, 361t
  and osmol gap, 193
  oxidative metabolism, 166, 166f
  pancreatitis caused by, 295t
  permissible exposure limit, 1422
  pharmacokinetics, 146t
  physicochemical properties, 1421t
  retinal toxicity, 1423–1424
        corticosteroids for, 1430
  serum, 1425
        and toxicity, 1425
  taste-aversive xenobiotics added to, 1782
  toxic epidemics, 1421
  toxicity (poisoning), 166
        acute kidney injury in, 1424
        adjunctive therapy for, 1429
        anion gap in, in risk stratification, 1427
        clinical presentation, 36t, 192
        CNS lesions in, 1424
        coagulopathy in, 1429
        ECG changes in, 1427
        end-organ manifestations, 1423–1424
        epidemics, 21t, 22, 1421t, 1430
        extracorporeal therapies for, 91f, 97t
        folate and, 776
        hemodialysis for, 1428–1429, 1429t
        laboratory investigation, 36t, 1425
        lactate concentration in, 1426–1427
        management, 38, 44t–45t, 776–777, 779,
              1199–1200, 1428–1429, 1429t
        and metabolic acidosis, 191t, 1426
        and organ donation, 1893t
        osmol gap in, in risk stratification, 1427
        outcomes with, predictors, 1427

  in pregnant women, 1430, 1441
  retinal toxicity, 1423–1424
        sodium bicarbonate for, 568t
  and toxic leukoencephalopathy, 133
  toxicokinetics/toxicodynamics, 1422–1423
  transdermal exposure to, 1422
  uses, 1421
  volume of distribution, 91, 146t, 1422
Methapyrilene, 739
Methaqualone
  and GABA receptor, 221–222
  hemorrhagic cystitis caused by, 306
  mechanism of action, 221–222
  poisoning, and organ donation, 1893t
  screening for, 110
Methcathinone (cat, Jeff, khat, ephedrone),
        1099, 1106–1107. *See also* Amphetamine(s)
  clinical effects, 1101t
  manganese in, 1319, 1321
  structure, 1101t
Methemoglobin, 316, 1646, 1703
  agents producing, effects on vital signs, 30t
  assessment, 37
  blood level, and blood color, 1639, 1639f, 1709
  detection, 1708
  effects on oxygenation, 403, 403f
  half-life, 1704
  in hydrogen sulfide poisoning, 1691
  kinetics, 1704, 1705f
  laboratory testing for, 101t, 102–103, 1642
  normal concentration, 1704
  physiology, 1704
  production, 159, 178
  stroma-free, for cyanide poisoning, 1698
Methemoglobinemia, 472, 1698–1699, 1703. *See also*
        Methemoglobin inducers
  acquired, 1703, 1706t
  alkyl nitrite inhalation and, 1198
  with anilide compound toxicity, 1472
  aniline dyes and, 453
  benzocaine-induced, 994, 1703, 1705
  bismuth subnitrate and, 1257
  case study, 1639
  causes, 1705–1706, 1706t
  in children, 1703
  chlorhexidine-induced, 1368
  clinical manifestations, 1706–1707, 1707f, 1707t
  clinical presentation, 36t, 1198, 1679
  congenital, 1703
  copper and, 1285–1286
  dapsone-induced, 846–847, 1703, 1705–1706, 1709
  definition, 1703
  diagnostic tests for, 1707–1709
  epidemiology, 1703
  in G6PD deficiency, 178
  and hemolysis, 1706, 1706f
  hereditary, 1703, 1706t
  idiopathic, 1703
  inhalant-induced, management, 1199–1200
  laboratory findings in, 36t
  local anesthetics and, 997
  management, 35t, 45t, 1199–1200, 1473, 1639,
        1700–1701, 1709–1710, 1713
        hyperbaric oxygen for, 1679
  in metal phosphide poisoning, 1458
  methylene blue for, 997
  naphthalene-induced, 1382–1384
  nitrite-induced, 1646, 1691, 1698–1701
  NSAID-induced, 516
  oxidant-induced, 1679

  paradichlorbenzene-induced, 1384–1385
  pediatric, causes, 1706t
  phosphine gas and, 1458
  predisposing factors, 1705–1706, 1705t
  and pulse oximetry, 404, 404t
  sodium chlorate and, 1376
  sulfonamides and, 827
  topical anesthetic-induced, 1703, 1705
  workplace exposures and, 1703
  xenobiotic-induced, 174, 174t, 1700–1701,
        1703–1706, 1706t
        methylene blue for, 1713
Methemoglobin inducers, 1698, 1703–1712. *See also*
        Methemoglobinemia
  for cyanide poisoning, 1687–1688, 1698
  hyperventilation caused by, 400t
Methemoglobin reductase, 178
Methicillin
  acute interstitial nephritis caused by, 394t
  corneal damage with, 823
Methimazole, 818
  adverse effects and safety issues, 818
  effect on thyroid hormones and function,
        813f, 814t, 817
  for hyperthyroidism, 817
  pharmacokinetics, 818
  teratogenicity, 429t
Methionine, 492, 1326
  for nitrous oxide toxicity, 1200
  structure, 492
Methionine synthase, 1012, 1013f
Meth mouth, 293
Methohexital. *See also* Sedative-hypnotics
  pharmacokinetics, 1085t
Methomyl poisoning, 1510
  management, 1498
Methosfolan, 1488t
Methotrexate, 349f, 767–771
  as abortifacient, 302, 303t
  absorption, 767
  adverse effects and safety issues, 760t, 762
  antidote for, 35t, 760t, 764, 770, 775. *See also*
        Glucarpidase (carboxypeptidase G$_2$);
        Leucovorin (folinic acid)
  antiinflammatory effect, 767
  benzyl alcohol in, 683t
  bioavailability, 767
  cell cycle phase specificity, 761f
  chemistry, 776
  cirrhosis caused by, 333
  clearance, 767–768
  concentration, rapid calculation, 778, 778t
  cranial neuropathy caused by, 346t
  crystalluria caused by, 395
  CSF concentration, measurement, 769–770
  diagnostic tests for, 763
  dosage and administration, 767
  elimination, 768
  elimination half-life, 767–768, 778
  enhanced elimination, urine alkalinization for, 93
  extracorporeal elimination, 97t, 770–771
  and fibrinolysis, 323
  glucarpidase activity and, 782, 783f
  hepatotoxicity, 332, 332f, 768
  high-dose, 767–768
        adverse effects and safety issues, 783–785
        management, 783–785
  immunoassays, glucarpidase and, 786
  indications for, 767
  infertility caused by, 297t

Methotrexate (*Cont.*):
intracellular, 785
intrathecal, 768–770
inadvertent overdose and unintentional exposures due to, 796t
overdose, management, 778–779, 786, 794
toxicity, 763
and kidney failure, 763
leucovorin rescue for, 767–768, 770, 775–776, 783, 789
dosage and administration, 778, 778t, 779f
leukoencephalopathy caused by, 763, 768
mechanism and site of action, 759, 762f, 767, 767f, 775–776
nail changes caused by, 282
nephrotoxicity, 768
neurotoxicity, 763, 768
and NSAIDs, interactions, 514t
peak plasma concentrations, 767
pharmacokinetics, 777
pharmacology, 767–768
pulmonary/thoracic effects, imaging, 125t, 126
rebound, 785
renal effects, 390f
rescue agent, 770
leucovorin as, 770, 775–776. *See also* Leucovorin (folinic acid)
(6*R*)-5,10-methylene-THF as, 776
structure, 767
teratogenicity, 429t
and tinnitus, 370t
toxicity (overdose/poisoning), 760t, 763
alkalinization for, 568t, 570
clinical manifestations, 768
diagnostic tests for, 768–769, 769t
gastrointestinal decontamination for, 785
leucovorin for, 770, 777–778. *See also* Leucovorin (folinic acid)
management, 45t, 764, 769–770, 778, 785
pathophysiology, 768
risk factors for, 767
sodium bicarbonate for, 568t
toxic threshold, 777
volume of distribution, 768
Methotrimeprazine. *See also* Antipsychotics
dosage and administration, 1033t
pharmacokinetics, 1033t
Methoxetamine, 1211, 1211t
chemical structure, 1210
chemistry, 1211
diagnostic tests for, 1217
and glutamate receptors, 228
mechanism of action, 227t
metabolism, 1212
metabolites, 1212
and m-hole, 1214–1215
and NMDA receptor, 228
pharmacokinetics, 1212
street names for, 1212
toxicity, 1212
Methoxieticyclidine, 1211, 1211t
para-Methoxyamphetamine (PMA), 1099–1100, 1101t, 1106. *See also* Amphetamine(s)
N-2-Methoxybenzylphenylethylamines, 1107
Methoxychlor
absorption, 1514
metabolism, 1515
physicochemical properties, 1515t
5-Methoxydimethyl tryptamine (5-MeO-DMT), 1179–1181, 1181t

2-Methoxyethanol, infertility caused by, 297t
Methoxyethylmercury, 1324t. *See also* Mercury
Methoxyflurane, 1011
diabetes insipidus caused by, 195, 195t
nephrotoxicity, 1015
para-Methoxymethamphetamine (PMMA), 1099, 1106
4-Methoxypyridoxine, 220–221, 1600t, 1607
Methscopolamine, 756
Methyl acetate, 1421
β-Methylamino-L-alanine (BMAA), 227–228, 227t, 340
Methylarsonic acid (MAA, MSMA), in herbicides, 1467t
Methylated hydrazines
poisoning with, pyridoxine for, 862–863
seizures caused by, 862
Methylatropine bromide, 1503
Methyl bromide, 1457, 1460–1461
clinical effects, 36t, 1458t, 1460–1461
detection threshold, 1654t
exposure limits, 1516
history of, 1460
immediately dangerous to life and health (IDLH), 1654t
industrial uses, 1457t
inhalation, 1460–1461
laboratory findings with, 36t
metabolism, 1460
occupational exposure to, 1460
odor, 364t
physicochemical properties, 1457t, 1460
poisoning
N-acetylcysteine for, 1461
clinical manifestations, 1460–1461
diagnostic tests for, 1461
epidemiology, 1460
treatment, 1461
regulatory standard for, 1654t
sources, 1654t
toxicodynamics, 1460
toxicokinetics, 1460
water solubility, 1654t
N-Methyl-1-(3,4-methylenedioxyphenyl)-2-butanamine (MBDB), 1105
Methylbutenol, 650t
Methyl *n*-butyl ketone (MBK)
metabolites, 1414–1415, 1415f
neurotoxicity, 1414–1415, 1415f
peripheral neuropathy caused by, 1414
N-Methylcarbamate, mechanism of action, 208
Methyl-CCNU, renal effects, 390f
Methylcellulose, 83
Methyl chloride, inhaled, 1193t
Methylcobalamin, 157
Methyl cyanide, 1684
Methylcyclopentadienyl manganese tricarbonyl (MMT), 1319
N-Methylcytisine, 640t, 1599t, 1604
Methylcytosine, as abortifacient, 303t
N-Methyl-D-aspartate (NMDA) glutamate receptor. *See* NMDA (*N*-methyl-D-aspartate) glutamate receptor
4-Methyl-2,5-dimethoxyamphetamine (DOM/STP), 1101t. *See also* Amphetamine(s)
Methyldopa, 959–961
cirrhosis caused by, 333
and gustatory dysfunction, 365
injection, parabens in, 685t
and male sexual dysfunction, 299f
pancreatitis caused by, 295t
pharmacokinetics, 960
and prolactin, 299f

SLE induced by, 126
α-Methyldopa, mechanism of action, 212
α-Methyldopamine, 960
Methylecgonide, 1125
Methylene [term], 1421
Methylene blue, 218, 1713–1716
for ACEI-induced hypotension, 964
adverse effects and safety issues, 1714
for angiotensin II receptor blocker–induced hypotension, 964
availability and storage, 45t
for β-adrenergic antagonist toxicity, 935
and breastfeeding, 1714
for calcium channel blocker toxicity, 950
chemistry, 1713
dosage and administration, 1709, 1709f, 1714–1715
fetal effects, 1714
formulation and acquisition, 1715
in glucose-6-phosphate dehydrogenase (G6PD) deficiency, 1714
and hemolysis, 1714
history of, 1703, 1713
for hydrogen sulfide poisoning, 1691
for hypotension, 964, 1713, 1715
for ifosfamide toxicity, 764
indications for, 35t, 45t, 1703
induction of methemoglobinemia, 1714
intrathecal administration, inadvertent overdose and unintentional exposures due to, 796t
MAO inhibition by, 212, 1714
mechanism of action, 1705f, 1706, 1713
for metal phosphide poisoning, 1459
for methemoglobinemia, 997, 1473, 1639, 1703, 1709, 1709f, 1713
in dapsone toxicity, 846
for nitrogen mustard toxicity, 760t
pharmacodynamics, 1713
pharmacokinetics, 1713
pharmacology, 1713
in pregnancy, 1714
for priapism, 302
and serotonin toxicity, 1058t, 1714
shortage, 43
and splanchnic blood flow in septic shock, 1714–1715
stocking, recommended level, 45t
supplies, 42
teratogenicity, 429t, 1714
Methylene chloride, 174t, 1415, 1664. *See also* Hydrocarbons, halogenated
blood:gas partition coefficient, 1195t
carbon monoxide from, 1195t, 1197, 1663–1664, 1678
elimination, 1195t
inhaled, 1193t. *See also* Inhalant(s)
clinical manifestations of, 1199t
metabolites, 1195t, 1197
poisoning
hyperbaric oxygen for, 1676, 1678
pathophysiology, 1678
toxicokinetics, 1411t
uses, 1409t
viscosity, 1409t
Methylenecyclopropylacetic acid, and gluconeogenesis, 176t, 178
Methylenecyclopropylglycine (MCPG), 1846
Methylenedianiline
food contamination with, 18, 18t
hepatic effects, 334t
Methylene dibromide, 1415

3,4-Methylenedioxyamphetamine (MDA), 1099, 1101t, 1105. *See also* Amphetamine(s)
  detection, 112
4,5-Methylenedioxyamphetamine (MMDA), 631
3,4-Methylenedioxyethamphetamine (MDEA, Eve), 1101t, 1105. *See also* Amphetamine(s)
3,4-Methylenedioxymethamphetamine (MDMA, Adam, molly, ecstasy, XTC), 162, 1099, 1101t, 1102, 1179, 1179t, 1180. *See also* Amphetamine(s)
  and ADH secretion, 189
  adverse effects and safety issues, 1106
  content, websites monitoring, 1184
  detection, 112
  elimination, 1102
  elimination half-life, 1102
  formulations, 1106
  history of, 1105
  long-term effects, 1106
  mechanism of action, 218
  metabolism, 1102, 1106
  metabolites, 1106
  regulation, 1106
  screening for, 110
  serotonergic effects, 1100
  and serotonin toxicity, 1058t
  street names for, 1105
  structure, 1099, 1105
  strychnine as adulterant in, 1536
  therapeutic uses, 1178
  toxicokinetics, 1182
Methylenedioxypyrovalerone (MDPV), 1106–1107
Methylene ketone peroxide, 1388t
6-Methylergoline, 806
Methylergonovine, 806
  duration of action, 807t
  elimination half-life, 807t
  indications for, 807t
  overdose/poisoning, 304
  pharmacokinetics, 807t
  structure, 806f
Methylethyl ketone, inhaled, 1193t
3-Methylfentanyl, 21t, 22
Methyl-fluorophosphonylcholines, 1508
N-Methyl-*N*-formylhydrazine, 1587, 1587f
N-Methyl-*N*-formylhydrazones, 1586–1587
N-Methylglycine. *See* Sarcosine
Methylglyoxal, 687
Methyl hippuric acid, 1199
R-α-Methylhistamine, 739
Methylhomatropine, 1503
3-Methylindole, 174t
Methyl iodide, 818
  cranial neuropathy caused by, 346t
  poisoning with, 1462
  toxicity, 818
Methylisocyanate, 1657, 1657f
  in Bhopal disaster, 16, 16t, 1486, 1651, 1657
Methyllycaconitine, 1600t
Methyl malonic acidemia, 455
Methylmercury, 157, 689, 1324, 1324t. *See also* Mercury
  absorption, 1325
  in brain, 1326
  elimination, 1326
  in erythrocytes, 1326
  excretion, *N*-acetylcysteine and, 494
  mass poisoning with, 18t, 19, 1324, 1328
  neurotoxicity, 1325–1326, 1328
  poisoning, 1324
    chelation therapy for, 1330

clinical manifestations, 1328
  diagnostic testing for, 1329
  management, 1252
  pathophysiology, 1326
  prenatal exposure to, 1326, 1328
  teratogenicity, 429t
  tissue distribution, 1326
Methyl mercury acetate, 1797
Methylnaltrexone, 84, 538–539
  characteristics, 526t
  dosage and administration, 542
  formulation and acquisition, 542
  indications for, 540
  for opioid-induced constipation, 295
Methyl nonyl ketone. *See* 2-Undecanone
α-Methylnorepinephrine, 960
Methylone, and serotonin toxicity, 1058t
Methylparabens, 685, 997
  structure, 685
Methylparaoxon, acetylcholinesterase inhibition by, 1489f
Methyl parathion, 1510
Methylphenidate
  and dopamine reuptake, 214
  and dopaminergic activity, 214
  elimination half-life, 1102
  mechanism of action, 211
  priapism caused by, 301t
  talc retinopathy from, 361
  and tinnitus, 370t
  volume of distribution, 1102
Methylphenylpropionoxypiperidine (MPPP), 22, 174
1-Methyl-4-phenylpyridinium (MPP⁺), 215
  effects on mitochondrial inner membrane, 176t
  and electron transport, 176t
  site of action, 173f
Methylphenyltetrahydropiperidine (MPTP), 340, 343
  parkinsonism caused by, 21t, 22, 174
1-Methyl-4-phenyl-1,2,3,6-tetrahydropyridine (MPTP), 215
4-Methylpyrazole. *See* Fomepizole
Methyl salicylate, 556–557
  odor, 37, 364t
  structure, 634
  toxicity, 559–561
  in wintergreen, 634
Methyl salicylic acid, structure, 555
Methyltestosterone
  for female sexual dysfunction, 302
  hepatotoxicity, 330
N-Methylthiotetrazole side-chain, of cephalosporins, 824–825, 825f
α-Methyltryptamine (AMT), 1179, 1179t, 1180, 1182, 1184
Methylxanthines, 985–993
  as adenosine antagonists, 231, 239, 986
  cardiac effects, 255
  cardiovascular effects, 988
    management, 990–991
  and cerebrovascular tone, 988
  chronic use, 989
  clinical and laboratory findings with, 36t
  CNS toxicity, management, 991
  effects on vital signs, 29t–30t
  enhanced elimination, 991–992
  gastrointestinal effects, 988
    management, 990
  history of, 985
  hyperventilation caused by, 400t
  musculoskeletal effects, 988–989, 991

  neuropsychiatric effects, 988
    management, 991
  pharmacology, 986
  as phosphodiesterase inhibitors, 986
  pulmonary effects, 988
  respiratory effects, 399, 399t
  seizures caused by, 231, 988, 991
  teratogenicity, 989
  toxicity, 987–989
    activated charcoal for, 989–990
    acute, 986
    acute on chronic, 986
    chronic, 986, 989
    diagnostic tests for, 989
    epidemiology, 985
    hypocalcemia and, 991
    management, 989–992
    orogastric lavage for, 989–990
    spectrum, 986
    supraventricular tachycardia in, 988, 990–991
    whole-bowel irrigation for, 990
  vasopressor effects, 988
Methysergide
  bioavailability, 807t
  duration of action, 807t
  elimination half-life, 807t
  indications for, 807t
  mechanism of action, 218
  obstructive nephropathy caused by, 394
  pharmacokinetics, 807t
  for serotonin toxicity, 1059
Methysticine yangonin, 1602t
Metipranolol
  ophthalmic use, systemic toxicity with, 360
  pharmacology, 927t
Metoclopramide
  extrapyramidal effects, 214
  mechanism of action, 217–218
  for methylxanthine-induced vomiting, 990
  and neuroleptic malignant syndrome, 215
  and prolactin, 299f
  as promotility agent, 84
  and serotonin toxicity, 1058t
Metolachlor, 1472
  in herbicides, 1467t
  toxicity, clinical manifestations, 1473
Metolachlor-S, 1472
Metoprolol
  overdose/poisoning, clinical manifestations, 931–932
  pharmacokinetics, 930
  pharmacology, 927t
  structure, 926f
  for thyrotoxicosis, 817
Metoprolol-chlorthalidone, 931
Metoprolol-hydrochlorothiazide, 931
Metosulam, in herbicides, 1467t
Metrifonate, acetylcholinesterase inhibition by, 208
Metronidazole
  and ethanol, interactions, 1146t
  pancreatitis caused by, 295t
  and tinnitus, 370t
  toxicity, organ system manifestations, 829t
Mevinphos, 1488t, 1508
Mexican black-tailed rattlesnake (*Crotalus* spp.), 1636t
Mexican cantil (*Agkistrodon* spp.), 1636t
Mexican green rattler (*Crotalus* spp.), 1636t
Mexican horned pit viper (*Ophryacus undulatus*), 1637t
Mexican lance-headed rattlesnake (*Crotalus* spp.), 1636t

Mexican leech (*Haementeria officinalis*), 883
Mexican moccasins (*Agkistrodon* spp.), 1636t
Mexican palm pit viper (*Bothriechis* spp.), 1636t
Mexican pigmy (pygmy) rattlesnake (*Sistrurus ravus*), 1637t
Mexican pricklepoppy (*Argemone mexicana*), 1598t, 1605
Mexican prickly poppy (*Argemone mexicana*), 650t
Mexican redknee tarantula (*Brachypelma smithi*), 1547f
Mexican rue. *See* Syrian rue (*Peganum harmala*)
Mexican west coast rattlesnake (*Crotalus* spp.), 1636t
Mexiletine, 870–871
    adverse effects and safety issues, 866t, 870
    pharmacokinetics, 866t
    pharmacology, 866t
    structure, 869f
Meyer-Overton lipid solubility theory, 1012, 1410
Mibefradil, 21, 171, 945t
    drug interactions with, 946, 1840–1841
    pharmacology, 945
Micelles, 1718f
Michaelis-Menten dissociation constant. *See* K_m (Michaelis-Menten dissociation constant)
Michaelis-Menten equation, 149–150
Michigan Alcoholism Screening Test (MAST), 1151, 1151t
Mickey Finn, 8, 1085, 1085f, 1146
Miconazole, 829
Microciona prolifera (red sponge), 1573
Microcystic aeruginosa, hepatogenous photosensitivity caused by, 1614
Microcystins, 1601t, 1609
Microcystis spp. (blue-green algae), 1601t, 1609
Microfiche technology, in poison information, 11, 11t
Microglia, 340–341
β_2-Microglobulin
    urinary loss
        cadmium-induced, 1260
        chromium and, 1270
    in workplace cadmium exposure risk assessment, 1261, 1261t
Microparticle capture immunoassay, 105, 105t
Micro-RNA (miRNA)
    miRNA-122, in acetaminophen overdose, 481
    and withdrawal syndrome, 237
Microsomal enzymes, 167
Microsomal ethanol oxidizing system (MEOS), 168f
Microsome(s), 167
Microsporidiosis, in HIV-infected (AIDS) patients, 830t
Microtubule-associated proteins (MAP), 502
Microtubules
    physiologic functions, 502
    xenobiotics affecting, 501–502
Micruroides spp. (coral snake), 1633t
Micrurus spp. (coral snakes), 1633t
Micrurus fulvius (Eastern coral snake), 1617t, 1618
    antivenom, 35t, 1627t, 1628–1631
        phenol in, 685t
        shortage, 43
    envenomation
        clinical manifestations, 1622
        treatment, 1625
    venom, LD$_{50}$, 1620
Micrurus tener (Texas coral snake), 1617t, 1618, 1620
    antivenom for, 35t, 1628–1631
    envenomation
        clinical manifestations, 1622
        treatment, 1625
Micturition
    neurophysiology, 304
    physiology, 304, 305f

Midazolam. *See also* Benzodiazepine(s); Sedative-hypnotics
    administration route, 1136
    adverse effects and safety issues, 1139–1140
    for agitation, 386, 1138–1139
        in thyrotoxicosis, 817
    for alcohol withdrawal, 1168
    for amphetamine toxicity, 1104–1105, 1104t
    benzyl alcohol in, 683t
    in capital punishment, 13
    cardiovascular effects, 1139
    for cocaine toxicity, 1128
    for conscious sedation, flumazenil and, 1094–1095
    for cyclic antidepressant toxicity, 1049t, 1051
    dosage and administration, 1137t
    drug interactions with, 1085–1086
    duration of action, 1137, 1137t
    flumazenil and, 1094–1095
    hepatic metabolism, 1137t, 1138
    indications for, 27, 1149
    and itraconazole, interactions, 1086
    lipophilicity, 1137
    metabolites, 1137t
    for nerve agent toxicity, 1746
    onset of action, 1137, 1137t
    paradoxical reactions to, flumazenil for, 1095
    pharmacokinetics and pharmacodynamics, 1085t, 1137–1138, 1137t–1138t
    pharmacology, 1136–1138, 1137t
    respiratory effects, 1140
    for status epilepticus, 1137t, 1138
    structure, 1094
    for strychnine poisoning, 1537–1538
    for violent behavior, 386
    for xenobiotic-induced seizures, 1138
Middle Ages, toxicology in, 3–6
Middle American rattlesnake (*Crotalus* spp.), 1636t
Midrin, 809
Midsummer daisy. *See* Feverfew (*Tanacetum parthenium*)
Miescher, Friedric, 919
Mifepristone, as abortifacient, 302, 303t
Miglitol
    adverse effects and safety issues, 699
    mechanism of action, 695
    pharmacokinetics and toxicokinetics, 697t
    pharmacology, 695
Migraine headaches
    aura with, 805
    chronic, 805
    classic (with aura), 805
    common (without aura), 805
    complications of, 805
    diagnostic criteria for, 805
    episodic syndromes that may be associated with, 805
    genetic component, 805
    5-HT$_1$ receptors and, 216
    medications for, 805–811, 805t. *See also* Antimigraine medications; *specific xenobiotic*
        serotonin toxicity caused by, 809
    pathophysiology, 805
    probable, 805
    treatment, 216
Milacemide
    mechanism of action, 228
    and NMDA receptor, 227t
Milk. *See also* Breast milk
    hypercalcemia caused by, 199
Milk alkali syndrome, 250

Milk of magnesia, 83
Milk sickness, 1611
Milk thistle (*Silybum marianum*), silymarin from, for amatoxin-induced liver toxicity, 1585
Milk-to-plasma (M/P) ratio, 440
Milk vetch root (*Astragalus membranaceus*), 640t
Milkweed (*Asclepias* spp.), 969, 1598t
Millepora alcicornis (fire coral), 1567, 1567t. *See also* Cnidaria (jellyfish)
    envenomation, clinical manifestations, 1569
Millimolar concentration, 1440
Milnacipran, 1060
    pharmacokinetics, 1055t
    receptor activity, 1057t
    and serotonin toxicity, 1058t
Milrinone
    for β-adrenergic antagonist toxicity, 934–935
    for calcium channel blocker toxicity, 948
    glucagon with, 942
Mimosa hostilis (Jurema), 650t
Minamata Bay, mercury contamination, 1324–1326, 1328
Mineral blue. *See* Prussian blue
Mineral oil, 83, 1410
    contraindications to, 85
Mineral poisons, early, 2, 4
Minerals. *See also specific mineral*
    in dietary supplements, 647–648
    supplements, use, 654
Mineral seal oil. *See also* Hydrocarbons, aliphatic
    uses, 1409t
    viscosity, 1409t
Mineral spirits. *See also* Hydrocarbons, aliphatic
    uses, 1409t
    viscosity, 1409t
Miners, pulmonary disease in, 7
Minimum alveolar concentration (MAC), 1012
Minimum legal drinking age 21 (MLDA-21), 1881
Mini-Sentinel Pilot Program, 1835
Minocycline, 827
    adverse effects and safety issues, 827
    and calcium salts, adverse interactions, 1406
    diabetes insipidus caused by, 195t
    mechanism of action, 227t, 228
    skin discoloration caused by, 273
Minoxidil
    as antihypertensive, 962
    overdose/poisoning, 962
Miosis, 356, 358
    cholinesterase inhibitors and, 1503–1504
    opioids and, 524
    poisoning/overdose causing, 36t
    sarin and, 358
    xenobiotic exposures causing, 357t, 358
Miotics, systemic toxicity, 360
Mipafox, 1488t
MiraLAX, 86–87
Mirex, 1514
    absorption, 1514
    enterohepatic/enteroenteric recirculation, 1516
    mechanism of toxicity, 1517
    metabolism, 1515
    physicochemical properties, 1515t
Mirodenafil, for erectile dysfunction, 301
Mirtazapine, 1055t, 1060–1061
    adverse effects and safety issues, 1061
    and CYPs, 1055t, 1056
    ECG changes caused by, 1057t
    mechanism of action, 212, 218, 1056f, 1060
    overdose/poisoning, 1061

receptor activity, 1057t, 1060–1061
and serotonin toxicity, 1058t
structure, 1060
Misclassification bias, 1856
Mismatch repair, 351
Misoprostol
as abortifacient, 302, 303t
overdose/poisoning, 304
teratogenicity, 303, 429t
Missouri v. McNeely, 1863
Mistletoe
American (*Phoradendron leucarpum*), 643t, 1601t
European (*Viscum album*), 643t, 1603t
Mistletoe brown tail moth (*Euproctis edwardsi*), 1552
Mitchell's rattlesnake (*Crotalus* spp.), 1636t
Mithridates, 3
Mithridatum, 1t, 2–4
Mitiglinide, 715
Mitochondria, 177
ADP/ATP antiporter, inhibitors, 176t
damage to, 159
disruption by nanoparticles, 1726, 1726f
dysfunction
in organic phosphorus compound poisoning,
1490
steatosis with, 332
inner membrane, 177
inhibitors, 176t
lead-induced injury, 1294–1295
manganese and, 1320
thallium and, 1350
Mitochondrial injury, 330–331
laboratory findings in, 335t
Mitochondrial membrane potential, 177
Mitomycin (mitomycin C)
adverse effects and safety issues, 760t
EPA regulation of, 765
extravasation, 802, 803t
antidote for, 803
mechanism and site of action, 762f
and vincristine, interactions, 506
Mitotane, effect on thyroid hormones and function,
814t
Mitoxantrone
adverse effects and safety issues, 760t
overdose/poisoning, 760t
Mitragyna speciosa (kratom). *See* Kratom
(*Mitragyna speciosa*)
Mitragynine, 643t, 649, 650t, 1181, 1181t, 1184
pharmacology, 1183
Mixed-function oxidases, 167
Mixture(s)
definition, 155
racemic, 165
Mizolastine, pharmacology, 742
2-MK. *See* 2-MeO-ketamine (2-MK)
Moclobemide, 1075. *See also* Monoamine oxidase
inhibitors (MAOIs)
gastrointestinal decontamination for, 54t
mechanism of action, 218
overdose, 1079
and serotonin toxicity, 1058t
structure, 1076f
Model for Endstage Liver Disease (MELD), and
liver transplantation for acetaminophen
poisoning, 484, 484t
Modern lipid hypothesis, 1410
Modified release
definition, 143
and gastrointestinal absorption, 143

and peak plasma concentrations, 152
and serum concentration interpretation, 153
Modified-release formulations, absorption, gastric
bypass and, 148
Mo-Go, 1350
Mojave rattlesnake (*Crotalus* spp.), 1617t, 1636t. *See
also* Snakebite(s)
antivenom, 1627–1631, 1627t
neurotoxin from, 1620, 1622
venom, neurotoxicity, 1622
Mojave toxin, 1620, 1622
Molar mass, definition, 155
Molds, 1581
Molecular Adsorbent Recirculating System (MARS),
96, 1289
for acetaminophen removal, 484–485
for amanitin poisoning, 1586
for calcium channel blocker toxicity, 950
Molecular imaging, 1717
Moli, 2
Molindone, and tinnitus, 370t
Molineux, Roland, 5t, 6
Molluscum contagiosum, cantharidin therapy for,
1554
Molly. *See* 3,4-Methylenedioxymethamphetamine
(MDMA, Adam, molly, ecstasy, XTC)
Molybdenum salts, for Wilson disease, 1286–1287
Mometasone, benzalkonium chloride in, 682
α-Momorcharin, as abortifacient, 303t
Momordica charantia (bitter melon), as abortifacient,
303t
Mond, Ludwig, 1333
Monday morning fever, 1659
Monitoring, of medication, and errors, 1825t, 1826
Monitoring the Future Study, 1792
Monkshood (*Aconitum, Aconitum napellus*), 2, 1598t.
See also Aconite (*Aconitum*, monkshood)
6-Monoacetylmorphine, 112
Monoamine(s), 1075
Monoamine hypothesis, of depression, 1044, 1075
Monoamine neurotransmitter(s), 1075
Monoamine oxidase (MAO), 208, 209f, 213, 213f, 1285t
and dopamine, 1075t, 1076
and epinephrine, 1075t
first-generation, 1076–1077
history of, 1075
irreversible, 1076–1077
isoenzymes, 208, 208t
inhibitor specificity and, 211–212
isoforms, 1075, 1075t
localization, 1075, 1075t
substrate affinity, 1075, 1075t
metabolic activity, 174
nonselective, 1076–1077
and norepinephrine, 1075–1076, 1075t
and serotonin, 215, 216f, 217–218, 1075, 1075t
and tyramine, 1075t
Monoamine oxidase inhibitors (MAOIs), 211–212, 218,
1054, 1075–1083. *See also specific xenobiotic*
acetylinic, 1076f
adrenergic action, 211
adrenergic crises with, 211
amphetamine, 1076–1077, 1076f
benzamide, 1076f
and blood pressure, 29
chemistry, 1075
clinical and laboratory findings with, 36t
CNS manifestations, management, 1081
discontinuation syndrome, 1080
dopamine and, 214

drug interactions with, 1079, 1079t
dysrhythmias caused by, 1078
management, 1081
effects on vital signs, 29t, 31t
and erectile dysfunction, 300
experimental, 1077
extracorporeal elimination, 1081
and female sexual dysfunction, 302f
first-generation, enzyme systems inhibited by, 1077
food interactions with, clinical and laboratory
findings in, 36t
and GABA receptors, 222
history of, 1075
hydrazide, 1076–1077, 1076f
toxicity, pathophysiology, 1078
and male sexual dysfunction, 299f
MAO-A, 1076–1077
MAO-B, 1076–1077
mechanism of action, 208, 210–212, 210t,
1075–1076, 1076f
methylene blue and, 1714
naturally occurring, 1077
and neurotransmission, 343
nonselective, 1075
nonspecific, 211
and norepinephrine, 1078
pharmacokinetics and toxicokinetics, 1077
pharmacology, 1075–1077
reversible, 1075, 1077
second-generation, 1077
selective, 1075, 1077
and serotonin toxicity, 1058–1059, 1058t
specificity, 211–212
third-generation, 1077
toxicity (overdose/poisoning), 1078
cardiovascular effects, 1078, 1078t
clinical manifestations, 1078, 1078t
dermatologic effects, 1078, 1078t
diagnostic tests for, 1080
epidemiology, 1075
gastrointestinal decontamination for, 1080
gastrointestinal effects, 1078, 1078t
hyperthermia in, 1078, 1078t, 1080
management, 212, 1080–1081
neurologic effects, 1078, 1078t
ophthalmologic effects, 1078, 1078t
pathophysiology, 1078
patient disposition with, 1081
sympathomimetic findings in, 211
and tricyclic antidepressants, combined, 212
and tyramine, 1077
Monobactams, 825
Monocellate cobra (*Naja naja kaouthia*), 1633
Monochloramine, 1655
Monoclonal antibody(ies)
as chemotherapeutics, 759, 760t, 761, 761f
mechanism and site of action, 762f
extravasation, 802
radioactive isotope conjugates, 761
and rhabdomyolysis, 393t
therapeutic, and posterior reversible encephalopathy
syndrome, 132
against tumor growth factor receptors, 761
xenobiotic conjugates, 761
Monocrotophos, 602, 1509
Monocytes, 319
Monofluoroacetate, 1450
Monohydroxycarbazepine, 723
Monoiodotyrosine, 813f
Monomethylarsenous acid, 1240–1241, 1240f

Monomethylarsonic acid (MMA), 1240, 1240f
  laboratory measurement, 1243
  LD$_{50}$ for, 1240–1241
Monomethylarsonic acid reductase, 1240, 1240f
Monomethylhydrazine (MMH), 852, 1582t, 1587, 1587f
  effects on GABA, 220
  seizures caused by, pyridoxine for, 862
  toxicity
    clinical manifestations, 863
    pyridoxine for, 862–863
Monooxygenases, 167
Monosaccharides, 707
Monosodium glutamate (MSG), 600, 600t
  adverse effects and safety issues, 600
  gastrointestinal effects, 600, 600t
  metabolic effects, 600
  neurotoxicity, 600
  pharmacokinetics, 600
  shudder attacks caused by, 600
Monoterpenes, 1597
Monteplase, 897
Mood disorders
  and suicidality, 378
  xenobiotic-induced, 344, 344t
Moonflower, as hallucinogen, 1181
Moonshine, 1143
Moraceae, 1614
Morbakka, stings, management, 1569
Morchella spp. (morel), 1586, 1586f
Morchella angusticeps (black morel), 1594
Morchella esculenta (morel), 1586, 1594
Morel (*Morchella*), 1586, 1586f, 1594
Moricizine, 865, 870–871
  adverse effects and safety issues, 866t, 870
  pharmacokinetics, 866t
  pharmacology, 866t
  structure, 869f
Moringa oleifera (horseradish tree), as abortifacient, 303t
Mormon tea (*Ephedra nevadensis*)
  psychoactive properties, 650t
  uses and toxicities, 641t, 649
Morning glory, 1605. *See also* Ololiuqui
  Argyreia spp., 1598t
  Ipomoea tricolor, 1601t
  Ipomoea violacea, 1179t
    lysergamides in, 1179
    psychoactive properties, 650t
    use and toxicities, 643t
  Rivea corymbosa, lysergamides in, 1179
  seeds, hallucinogens in, toxicokinetics, 1182
  Turbina corymbosa, 1178
Morphine, 526. *See also* Opioid(s)
  characteristics, 526t
  chlorobutanol in, 684
  cutoff concentration, in drug abuse screening, 112
  historical perspective on, 7–8, 638
  history of, 519
  intrathecal administration
    clinical manifestations, 793
    inadvertent overdose and unintentional
      exposures due to, 796t–797t
    overdose, 798
  isolation, 519
  metabolism, 526, 527f
  for neonatal opioid withdrawal, 439
  pharmacokinetics, 145t
  plant source, 1601t
  pruritus caused by, 273
  structure, 519, 538

urine screening assays for, performance
    characteristics, 111t
  volume of distribution, 145t
Morphine glucuronide, urinary concentration, 112
Morphine 3-glucuronide, 145t
Morphine 6-glucuronide, 145t
Morphine-scopolamine combination, 22
Morphine sulfate
  lipid carrier formulation, 684t
  liposomal, 1719t
Morton, William, 1011
Mosquito(es)
  attractants, 1522
  control, 1522
    aerial spraying for, pyrethroids in, 1520
  disease transmission by, 1522
  repellents, 1522
Mosquito plant. *See* Pennyroyal (*Mentha pulegium, Hedeoma pulegioides*)
Moth(s), 1552–1554
  larval. *See* Caterpillars
Mothballs and moth repellents, 1380
  camphor in, 1380
  diagnostic imaging, 118
  laboratory identification, 1385, 1385t
  odor, 364t
  radiographic appearance, 1385, 1385t
Motherisk, 431
Mother of millions (*Bryophyllum tubiflorum*), 979
Moth flakes, 1380
Motilin, 290t
Motion sickness, 739, 742
Motor neuropathy, in thallium toxicity, 1351
Motor vehicle fatalities
  ethanol and, 1143–1144, 1862, 1877
  NHTSA data on, 1877
Mountain laurel (*Kalmia latifolia*), 1612, 1612f
Mountain tea, 634
Movement and tone disorders. *See also specific disorder*
  with arylcyclohexylamine toxicity, 1215
  cocaine and, 1127
  opioid-induced, 524
  SSRIs and, 1058
  xenobiotic-induced, 344
Moxa (*Artemisia* spp.), 643t
Moxalactam, and vitamin K antagonism, 916
Moxifloxacin, 826
Moxonidine, 961
MPTP. *See* Methylphenyltetrahydropiperidine (MPTP)
MT-45, 529
Mucin, 292
Mucositis
  chemotherapeutics and, 761–762
  methotrexate-related, 768
Mucous membranes
  initial assessment, 189
  in toxidromes, 28, 29t
Mucuna pruriens (cowhage, velvet bean), 1613
MUDPILES mnemonic, 191
Mugwort (*Artemisia* spp.), 643t
Mules. *See* Body packers; Heroin; Opioid(s)
Multidrug resistance, 144
Multidrug-resistant (MDR) proteins, 341
Multiple chemical sensitivity (MCS), pyrethroid
    exposure and, 1522
Multiple-dose activated charcoal (MDAC), 33, 61–62, 78
  adverse effects, 79, 85
  for antimony toxicity, 1234
  contraindications and complications, 62, 62t
  for dapsone overdose, 846

definition, 61
dosage and administration, 62, 62t, 80
efficacy, 78
and enterohepatic circulation, 172
frequency of use, 90
for "gastrointestinal dialysis," 61, 78
indications for, 60–61, 62t, 78
mechanism of action, 78
for methotrexate overdose, 769
for methylxanthine toxicity, 990–991
pharmacokinetic effects, 152
for phenobarbital toxicity, 570
position paper on, 90
in post-bariatric surgery patients, 64
for quinine overdose, 841
recommendations for, 62
risk:benefit assessment with, 78–80
with 70% sorbitol, 85
studies of, 59t, 61, 78
for thallium poisoning, 78, 1353
trends in use of, 64–65
Multiple myeloma
  and anion gap, 191t
  and hyponatremia, 196
Multiple sclerosis, 207
  zinc and, 1364
Multivitamins and multiminerals (MVMMs)
  injection, propylene glycol in, 687, 687t
  pediatric, propylene glycol in, 687–688
  use, 654
Mummies
  cocaine in, 3
  hashish in, 3
Mummification, 1885
Munchausen syndrome by proxy. *See* Medical child abuse; Pediatric condition falsification
Munitions, white phosphorus in, 1528
Mupirocin ointment, polyethylene glycol (PEG) in, 686t
Murder
  arsenic use in, 6, 12
  by poisoners
    in Medieval and Renaissance periods, 4–6
    in recent history, 12
Muriatic acid, 1388t
Muscarine, 1582t, 1587, 1589t
  structure, 1587
Muscarinic antagonists
  antipsychotics as, 1034t, 1035
  and gastric acid secretion, 743f
  gastrointestinal effects, 292f
Muscarinic receptors, 206f, 207, 1503
  acetylcholine and, 1587
  agonists, 207
  antagonists, 207, 207t
  and bladder function, 304, 305f
  muscarine and, 1587
  neuromuscular blocking agents and, 1019–1020
  and thermoregulation, 412
Muscarinics
  cardiac effects, 248
  cholinergic, cranial neuropathy caused by, 346t
Muscazone, 1179
Muscimol, 1179, 1582t, 1588, 1589t
  and GABA receptor, 221, 228, 1588
  structure, 1588
Muscle biopsy, for malignant hyperthermia diagnosis, 1023–1024
Muscle contraction(s), in strychnine poisoning, 1536–1537
  management, 1537–1538

Muscle injury, with anticholinesterase poisoning, 1491–1493
Muscle toxicity, xenobiotic-induced, 346, 346t
Muscular dystrophy, and neuromuscular blockade, 1020
Muscular twitching, sedative-hypnotic overdose and, 1086t
Mushrooms, 1581–1596. *See also specific mushroom*
　allergy to, 1594
　base (bulb), 1584f
　cap (pileus), 1584f, 1593
　classification and management, 1581, 1582t–1583t
　and disulfiramlike reactions, 1174t
　encephalopathy caused by, 1583t, 1592
　gastroenterotoxic, 600
　gills (lamellae), 1584f, 1593
　group I, cyclopeptide-containing, 1581–1586, 1582t
　group II, gyromitrin-containing, 1581, 1582t, 1586–1587, 1586f, 1589t
　　antidote for, 35t
　group III, muscarine-containing, 1582t, 1587, 1587f, 1589t
　group IV, coprine-containing, 1582t, 1587–1588, 1588f, 1589t
　group V, ibotenic acid- and muscimol-containing, 1582t, 1588, 1589f, 1589t
　group VI, psilocybin-containing, 1582t, 1588–1589, 1589f, 1589t
　group VII, gastrointestinal toxin-containing, 1582t, 1589, 1589t
　group VIII, orellanine- and orellinine-containing, 1582t, 1589t, 1590, 1590f
　group IX, allenic norleucine-containing, 1582t, 1589t, 1590–1591, 1590f
　group X, cycloprop-2-enecarboxylic acid-containing, 1582t, 1589t, 1591
　group XI, 2R-amino-4,5-hydroxy-5-hexynoic acid and 2R-amino-5-hexynoic acid-containing, 1582t, 1589t, 1591
　group XII, acromelic acid-containing, 1583t, 1589t, 1591–1592
　group XIII, polyporic acid-containing, 1583t, 1589t, 1592
　group XIV, involutin-containing, 1583t, 1589t, 1592
　group XV, lycoperdonosis-inducing, 1583t, 1592
　hallucinogenic, 9, 1178–1179, 1588–1589. *See also specific mushroom*
　　ancient use of, 3
　　deaths caused by, 1581
　identification, 1593
　ingestion by children, 1581, 1592
　muscarinic, 1495t, 1496
　　antidote for, 35t
　mycelium, 1584f
　myths and science, 1594
　and nephrotoxicity, 1589t, 1590–1591, 1593
　partial veil, 1584f
　protective tissues, 1584f
　psychoactive, 1179
　ring (annulus), 1584f, 1593
　scales, 1584f
　spore print from, 1593
　stem (stipe), 1584f, 1593
　toxicity
　　clinical findings in, 1582t–1583t
　　disposition of patients with, 1593
　　epidemiology, 1581
　　factors affecting, 1594
　　mortality rate for, 1581, 1582t–1583t

　overview, 1582t–1583t
　primary site, 1582t–1583t
　time of onset of symptoms, 1582t–1583t, 1589t
　treatment, 1582t–1583t, 1592–1593
　xenobiotics involved in, 1582t–1583t, 1589t
　universal veil, 1584f, 1593–1594
　unknown, 1593
　veil, 1584f, 1593–1594
　volva, 1584f, 1593
Mustard
　black (*Brassica nigra*), 1598t
　liquid vesicant, in warfare, 17, 17t
Mustard agents. *See also* Nitrogen mustards; Sulfur mustard; *specific agents*
　dermal decontamination for, 72
Mustard gas, 1251
　in Iran–Iraq war (1980s), 17, 17t
　in warfare, 17, 17t
Mustard oil, edible, argemone oil in, 1605
Musty smell, 364t
Mutagenicity
　of ethylene oxide, 1374
　of radiation, 1767
Myasthenia gravis, 207, 342
　clinical manifestations, 577t
　edrophonium testing in, 578
　and neuromuscular blockade, 1020
Mycelium, of mushrooms, 1584f
Mycobacterium avium complex, in HIV-infected (AIDS) patients, 830t
Mycobacterium marinum, 1574
Mycobacterium tuberculosis, 850
Mycophenolate mofetil
　binding, by cholestyramine, 92
　protein-binding characteristics, 110t
　teratogenicity, 430t
Mycotoxins, 174t
　and ATP production, 176t
　as biological weapons, 1759–1760, 1759f
Mydriasis, 356–358, 357t
　antihistamines associated with, 746
　cocaine use and, 1126
　poisoning/overdose causing, 36t
　xenobiotic exposures causing, 357–358, 357t
Mydriatics, systemic toxicity, 360
Myelin basic protein, in carbon monoxide poisoning, 1676, 1677f
Myelodysplastic syndrome, 353
Myeloid cells, 310
Myeloneuropathy
　nitrous oxide abuse and, 1199–1200
　progressive, zinc and, 1364
Myelopathy, 131
　infectious, clinical manifestations, 577t
　inflammatory, clinical manifestations, 577t
Myeloperoxidase, 319
Myelosuppression
　antihistamines associated with, 744
　chemotherapeutic-related, 764
　vincristine-related, 506
Myliobatidae, 1576
Myobloc, 578–579
Myocardial cell(s)
　action potential, ion channels and, 245–246, 245f
　depolarization/repolarization, 245–254, 245f, 254–255, 970, 971f, 1045
　membrane, ion channels, 244–245, 244f
　refractory, 246
　relatively refractory, 246
　resting, 245, 245f

Myocardial depression
　antipsychotic-induced, 1034t, 1035
　xenobiotic-induced
　　high-dose insulin for, 953–958
　　pathophysiology, 953–954
Myocardial infarction
　N-acetylcysteine for, 494
　anabolic-androgenic steroids and, 617–618
　carbon monoxide poisoning and, 1665
　in clenbuterol poisoning, 988
　cocaine-associated, 1124, 1127–1128
　　management, 1129
　dabigatran and, 892–893
　ECG changes in, 249, 249f
　hydrogen sulfide poisoning and, 1690
　in methylxanthine poisoning, 988
　with prothrombin complex concentrate, 909
　ST elevation (STEMI), 249, 249f
　vincristine-induced, 506
Myocardial ischemia
　Albumin Cobalt Binding (ACB) test for, 1273
　carbon monoxide poisoning and, 1665
　cocaine-associated, 1127–1128, 1139
　dysrhythmias caused by, 256
　ECG changes after, 251
　ethanol and, 1148
　hydrogen sulfide poisoning and, 1690
　in methylxanthine poisoning, 988
　NSAID overdose and, 516
　propofol and, 1089
　ST segment in, 249
Myocarditis
　antipsychotic-induced, 1039
　inhalant-induced, 1196
Myoclonic syndrome, propofol and, 1089
Myoclonus
　with arylcyclohexylamine toxicity, 1215
　bismuth-induced, 1256
　cyclic antidepressant overdose and, 1047
　methylxanthine-induced, 989, 991
　SSRIs and, 1058
Myoglobin
　carbon monoxide poisoning and, 1664
　excretion, 393
　renal effects, 390f
Myoglobinuria, 93
　PCP toxicity and, 1217
　renal effects, 393
　with sea snake envenomation, 1575
Myoinositol, lithium and, 1066–1067
Myokymia, rattlesnake bites and, 1622
Myonecrosis
　carbon monoxide poisoning and, 1665
　pit viper envenomation and, 1621–1622
Myoneuropathy, with colchicine poisoning, 503, 503t
Myopathy(ies)
　with colchicine poisoning, 503, 503t
　critical illness, 1025, 1025t
　disuse (cachectic), 1025, 1025t
　of latridectism, 1543
　and succinylcholine toxicity, 1022
　xenobiotic-induced, 346, 346t
Myopia, xenobiotic exposures and, 357t
Myosin, 262, 263f
　myocardial cell, 928, 928f
Myostatin, 623
Myotoxicity
　mushrooms causing, 1591
　with sea snake envenomation, 1575
　of Viperidae venom, 1634

Myristica fragrans (mace, nutmeg), 631, 643t, 1178, 1179t, 1181, 1181t, 1601t
ancient use of, 3
as aphrodisiac, 304t
clinical effects, 1183
nutmeg, psychoactive properties, 650t
pharmacology, 1183
psychoactive properties, 650t
toxicokinetics, 1182
Myristicin, 631, 643t, 650t, 1179t, 1181t, 1183–1184, 1601t
structure, 631, 1183f
Myrmecia spp., 1552
Myrothecium spp., in biological warfare, 1759
Myrtle. *See* Periwinkle (*Catharanthus roseus*)
Mysteria (*Colchicum autumnale*), uses and toxicities, 640t
Myxedema, 812

N

Nabilon, structure, 1112f
Nabiximol, 1113
Nabumetone, pharmacology, 512t
NADH dehydrogenase, 173f
NADH methemoglobin reductase, 1703–1704, 1709
NADH:NAD⁺ ratio, 179
cytosolic, 178
Nadolol
elimination, multiple-dose activated charcoal and, 78
overdose/poisoning, multiple-dose activated charcoal in, 61
pharmacology, 927t
Nadolol-bendrofluethiazide, 931
NADPH methemoglobin reductase, 1704, 1705f, 1709
Nadroparin, 890
Nafcillin, 823–824
Nagasaki atomic bombing, radiation effects from, 23t, 24
Naglexol, characteristics, 526t
Nail(s)
arsenic in, 1244
defects, thallium-induced, 1351
growth, 271
hyperpigmentation, 281
specimen, postmortem collection and analysis, 1885
xenobiotic-induced changes, 274t, 281–282
Nail plate, 271, 281
Nail polish remover, inhaled, 1193t. *See also* Inhalant(s)
Nairobi eye, 1554
Naja spp. (cobras), 1633t
envenomation, treatment, 1635
Naked lady (*Colchicum autumnale*). *See* Colchicine
Nalbuphine. *See also* Opioid(s)
characteristics, 526t
effects on kappa receptor, 521
Nalidixic acid, hypoglycemia caused by, 715
Nalmefene. *See also* Opioid antagonist(s)
for alcoholism, 1152
structure, 538
Nalorphine, 538. *See also* Opioid(s)
effects on kappa receptor, 521
Naloxegol, 84, 538. *See also* Opioid antagonist(s)
dosage and administration, 542
formulation and acquisition, 542
indications for, 540
for opioid-induced constipation, 295
pharmacokinetics, 539
Naloxone, 28, 538. *See also* Opioid antagonist(s)
administration, by laypersons, 539, 552
adverse effects and safety issues, 540

availability and storage, 45t
bioavailability, administration route and, 539
for buprenorphine reversal, 542
for bystander administration, 539, 551–552
characteristics, 526t
for clonidine poisoning, 961
community-based approaches using, effectiveness, 551
controversies regarding, 551–552
cost, 43
dosage and administration, 538–539, 541–542
duration of action, 539–540
effect on runner's high, 523
elimination half-life, 539
formulation and acquisition, 542
and harm reduction approaches to overdose prevention and overdose reversal, 551–553
history of, 538
for imidazoline toxicity, 750
indications for, 32–33, 35t, 37–38, 45t, 84, 403, 538, 1040, 1149, 1191
injection, parabens in, 685t
intranasal, 541–542
low dose, 541
metabolism, 539
nebulized, 541
observation period with, 540–541
onset of action, administration route and, 539, 541
for opioid-induced constipation, 295
for opioid-induced seizures, 539
and opioid toxicity, pharmacokinetic mismatch, 540–541
for opioid toxicity, 527, 539, 1862
dosage and administration, 533–534, 534t
pharmacokinetics, 538–539
policies regarding, 552
in pregnancy and lactation, 39, 434, 541
prehospital administration, 541, 551–552
shortage, 43
stocking, 43
recommended level, 45t
structure, 538
take-home, 539
titrated dosing, 538
for xenobiotic-induced respiratory dysfunction, 407
Naltrexone, 1172. *See also* Opioid antagonist(s)
absorption, 539
for alcoholism, 1152
characteristics, 526t
dosage and administration, 541–542
duration of action, 540
elimination half-life, 539
in ethanol abstinence, 540
extended-release injectable suspension, 539, 552
formulation and acquisition, 542
indications for, 84, 538
metabolism, 539
for opioid abstinence, 539–540
for opioid use disorder, 552
pharmacokinetics, 538–539
precautions with, 533–534
in pregnancy and lactation, 541
structure, 538
volume of distribution, 539
Name(s)
product, 162
trade, 162
trivial, 162
Nanofibers, definition, 1717

Nanomaterials
engineered, 1717
structures, 1717, 1718f
types, 1717, 1718f
Nanoparticles, 157
aerodynamic diameter (D_ae), 1722
aerosols, 1721–1722
agglomerations, 1717
aggregations, 1717
and autophagy induction, 1726f, 1727
bioaccumulation, 1730
in bone marrow, 1730
cardiovascular effects, 1721f, 1729
cellular toxicity, 1725–1727, 1726f
miscellaneous mechanisms, 1727
in central nervous system (CNS), 1721f, 1727–1728
circulation, 1721f, 1722–1723
combustion-derived, 1721–1722
definition, 1717
dermal exposure, 1720
detection, 1723
developmental effects, 1730
distribution, 1721f, 1722
dose assessment, 1723
elimination, 1723
exposure to, 1720–1723, 1721f
fetal effects, 1730
functionalized gold, 1717, 1718f, 1719t
functionalized silver, 1717, 1718f
genotoxicity, 1726f, 1727
hematologic effects, 1721f, 1729
in immune system, 1721f, 1729–1730
incidental, 1717
inhalation, 1721–1722, 1721f, 1728–1729
internal deposition and degradation, 1722–1723
magnetic, 1718f
materials, 1717, 1718f
mitochondrial disruption by, 1726, 1726f
naturally derived, 1717
nuclear effects, 1726–1727, 1726f
in ocular system, 1721f, 1730
oral exposure, 1722
organelle and substructure damage by, and cellular toxicity, 1726–1727, 1726f
organ systems toxicity, 1721f, 1727–1730
paracellular uptake, 1722
persistence, 1730
photothermal toxicity, 1726f, 1727
in pulmonary system, 1721f, 1728–1729
reproductive effects, 1721f, 1730
retention, 1723
structures, 1717, 1718f
systemic toxicity, 1721f
toxicity, 1721f, 1723–1730
charge and, 1725
coating and surfactant materials and, 1724
composition and, 1724
contaminants and, 1724
dose and, 1723–1724
factors affecting, 1723–1725
geometry and architecture and, 1724–1725
pH and, 1725
size and, 1724
surface area and, 1724
transcellular uptake, 1722
types of, 1717, 1718f
uptake, and cellular toxicity, 1725–1726, 1726f
Nanoplates, definition, 1717
Nanorods, 1717
Nanoshell, 1718f

Nanotechnology
  administrative issues, 1731–1733
  applications, 1717–1718, 1719t–1720t
  and biomaterials, 1717
  definition, 1717
  and device safety, 1731
  and drug safety, 1731
  and environmental protection, 1731–1733
  and food safety, 1731
  history of, 1717
  and occupational health and safety, 1731
  organizational resources, 1733, 1733t
  physiochemical principles, 1717
  regulatory issues, 1731–1733
  research issues, 1731–1733
  standards, 1731, 1732t
  in therapeutics, 1718, 1719t–1720t
Nanotoxicology, 13, 157, 1717–1740
  history of, 1717
  overview, 1723
  principles, 1723
Nanotubes, 1717
  carbon, 1717, 1718f
    and occupational health and safety, 1731
Nanoworm, 1718f
Naphazoline
  adverse effects and safety issues, in children, 453
  benzalkonium chloride in, 682t
  duration of action, 749t
  history of, 748
  structure, 750f
  therapeutic effects, 749t
  toxicity, 749t
    clinical manifestations, 750
    management, 750–751
Naphtha. See also Hydrocarbons, aliphatic
  uses, 1409t
  viscosity, 1409t
Naphthalene, 1381–1384, 1410. See also Hydrocarbons
  history and epidemiology, 1381
  laboratory identification, 1385, 1385t
  metabolism, 1382, 1382f
  metabolites, 1382, 1382f
  NIOSH Immediately Dangerous To Life or Health
      Concentration, 1382
  odor, 364t
  permissible exposure limit, 1382
  pharmacokinetics, 1382, 1382f
  pharmacology, 1382
  products containing, 1381
  radiographic appearance, 1385, 1385t
  short-term exposure limit, 1382
  structure, 1380
  sublimation, 1809
  threshold limit value, 1382
  toxicity, 1381
    clinical manifestations, 1383
    diagnostic tests for, 1383
    management, 1383–1384
    pathophysiology, 1383
  toxicokinetics, 1382
1,2-Naphthalene oxide, 1382, 1382f
Naphthenes, 1410
1-Naphthol, 1382, 1382f
1,2-Naphthoquinone, 1382, 1382f
1,4-Naphthoquinone, 1382
Naphthoquinone derivative, 643t
Naphthoquinones, 845–846
  antimalarial mechanism, 837f, 838t
  effects on mitochondrial inner membrane, 176t

2-Naphthylamine, 174t
β-Naphthylamine, bladder tumors from, 22, 23t
Naphthylamine mustard, EPA regulation of, 765
α-Naphthyl-isothiocyanate (ANIT)
  cholangitis and polymorphonucleocyte infiltration
      caused by, 330
  cholestasis caused by, 330
α-Naphthylthiourea (ANTU)
  estimated fatal dose, 1453t
  physicochemical properties, 1453t
  in rodenticides, 1453t. See also Rodenticides
  toxicity
    antidote and/or treatment for, 1453t
    clinical manifestations, 1453t
    toxic mechanism, 1453t
Naples, poisoners in, 6
NAPQI. See N-Acetyl-p-benzoquinoneimine (NAPQI)
Napropamide, in herbicides, 1467t
Naproxen
  adverse effects and safety issues, 515
  cardiovascular risk with, 514
  pharmacokinetics and toxicokinetics, 511–512
  pharmacology, 511, 512t
Naratriptan, 217, 808–809, 808t
  as 5HT$_{1F}$ agonist, 809
Narcissus spp., 1601t, 1613
  allergic contact dermatitis from, 1614
Narcolepsy, treatment, 606, 1188, 1190
Narcotic(s), 6. See also specific narcotic
  definition, 519
  regulation, 8
Narcoticoacrids, 6
Narcotics Anonymous (NA), 381
Naringen, 1599t, 1607
Naringenin, 1597, 1599t, 1609–1610
  xenobiotic interactions, 1611
Naringin, 1610
Nasal decongestants. See also Decongestants
  adverse effects and safety issues, in children, 453
Nasal septum, perforation, cocaine-related, 1126
Nasogastric intubation
  for hydrofluoric acid ingestion, 1400
  for organic phosphorus compound and carbamate
      poisoning, 1498
Nasogastric lavage, for DEG poisoning, 1447
Nasopharyngeal carcinoma, formaldehyde and, 1373
Nateglinide, 715
  hypoglycemia caused by, 700
  overdose/poisoning, octreotide for, 715
  pharmacokinetics and toxicokinetics, 697t
  pharmacology, 696
National Academy of Clinical Biochemists (NACB)
      guidelines, for toxicology assays, 101–102
National Center for Environmental Health, 12
National Clearinghouse for Poison Control Centers, 9, 11t
National Coordinating Council for Medication Error
      Reporting and Prevention (NCC MERP),
      medication error taxonomy, 1823–1824,
      1823f–1824f
National Council on Radiation Protection and
      Measurement (NCRP), 1765–1767
National Electronic Injury Surveillance System (NEISS),
      data on xenobiotic exposures in children,
      448–449
National Environmental Policy Act, and
      nanotechnology, 1731
National Fire Protection Association (NFPA)
  rules and guidelines for hazardous materials
      incident response, 1811–1812
  704 system for fixed facility placarding, 1808

National Health and Nutrition Examination Survey
      (NHANES), 1852
National Highway Traffic Safety Administration
      (NHTSA)
  data on motor vehicle fatalities, 1877
  on per se serum ethanol concentrations, 1144
  and standardized field sobriety tests, 1878–1879
National Incident Management System (NIMS), 1806
National Institute for Occupational Safety and Health
      (NIOSH), 1801t, 1804, 1808
  criteria documents, 1804
  list of hazardous drugs, 764
National Institute of Drug Abuse (NIDA), drug
      screening, 110
National Library of Medicine (NLM), 1804
National Nanotechnology Initiative (NNI), 1731
National Poison Database System (NPDS), 11
National Poison Prevention Week, 11, 11t
National Preparedness Guidelines, antidotal
      provisioning and administration in, 42
National Toxicology Program (NTP), 1804
Natural gas, 1410, 1652
  and hydrogen sulfide poisoning, 1688
  sulfur-containing (sour gas), 1688
Natural killer (NK) cells, hepatic, 327, 329f, 330
Naturopaths, 638
Nausea
  with N-acetylcysteine, 495
  cannabinoids for, 1113
  with colchicine poisoning, 502, 503t
  hypercalcemia and, 199
Navy beans, imaging, 116f
NBC (nuclear, biological, and/or chemical), 1741t
N-Bomb, 1107
Near-death experience, with arylcyclohexylamine
      toxicity, 1214–1215
Nebivolol
  and erectile dysfunction, 300
  mechanism of action, 209
  overdose/poisoning, clinical manifestations,
      931–932
  pharmacokinetics, 930
  pharmacology, 927t
  poisoning, lipid emulsion for, 1006
  toxicity, management, 936
  vasodilating effects, 930–931
Necrosis. See also Avascular necrosis; Hepatocellular
      necrosis
  with brown recluse spider bite, 268, 1545
    pathophysiology, 1544
  coagulative, 271
  with fire ant stings, 1552
  spider bites producing, 268, 1545
    differential diagnosis, 1546
Necrotizing angiitis, 128
Necrotizing enterocolitis, N-acetylcysteine for, 495
Necrotizing fasciitis
  after stonefish sting, 1578
  NSAIDs and, 516
Necrotizing vasculitis, amphetamines and, 1103–1104
Nectar of the gods. See Allium sativum (garlic)
Nefazodone, 171, 1060
  adverse effects and safety issues, 1060
  and CYPs, 1055t, 1056
  mechanism of action, 218
  overdose/poisoning, 1060
  pharmacokinetics, 1055t
  receptor activity, 1057t, 1060
  and serotonin toxicity, 1058t
  and sexual function, 304

Negative allosteric modulators (NAMs), for glutamate receptors, 225–227, 227t
Negative inspiratory force (NIF), 404, 406
Negative predictive value (NPV), of diagnostic test, 1858, 1858f
N-EK. *See* *N*-Ethylnorketamine
Nelfinavir, 831–832
　pancreatitis caused by, 295t
Nematocysts, 1567, 1568f
Nemzyl alcohol, in physostigmine preparations, 757
Neocycasin, 1607
Neodysiherbaine A, mechanism of action, 227t
Neofibularia mordens (Australian stinging sponge), 1573
Neofibularia nolitangere (poison-bun sponge, touch-me-not sponge), 1573–1574
Neomycin, 821–823
　contact dermatitis caused by, 280
　mechanism of action, 227t
　and tinnitus, 369
　toxicity, clinical manifestations, 822t
Neon, as simple asphyxiant, 1652
Neonatal abstinence syndrome (NAS), 439
Neonatal (serotonin) abstinence syndrome (NSAS), 1061
Neonatal gasping syndrome, 20–21, 20t, 683, 1430
Neonate(s)
　N-acetylcysteine and, 495
　exchange transfusions in, 98
　hemorrhage in, vitamin K and, 916
　neurotoxins and, 342
　poisoning in, management, 442
　toxicologic problems in, 441–442
　unusual/idiosyncratic reactions to xenobiotics, 452–453
Neonicotinoids, in insecticides, 1203
Neosaxitoxin, clinical effects, 576t
Neostigmine, 755–756, 1487, 1495
　acetylcholinesterase inhibition by, 208
　contraindications to, 1041
　intrathecal administration, inadvertent overdose and unintentional exposures due to, 797t
　for neuromuscular blockade reversal, 1025, 1026t
　and neuromuscular blockers, interactions, 1021t
　for neurotoxic snake envenomation, 1635
　structure, 755f
　for tetrodotoxin poisoning, 596
　for xenobiotic-induced respiratory dysfunction, 407
Neostigmine methylsulfate injection, phenol in, 685t
Nepeta cataria (catnip)
　psychoactive xenobiotics in, 650t
　uses and toxicities, 641t
　volatile oils in, 639
Nepetalactone, 641t, 650t
Nephritis
　acute interstitial. *See* Acute interstitial nephritis
　chronic interstitial. *See* Chronic interstitial nephritis
Nephrocalcinosis, diagnostic imaging, 129t
Nephrogenic diabetes insipidus (NDI). *See* Diabetes insipidus (DI)
Nephrolithiasis
　cadmium exposure and, 1260
　vitamin C and, 662–663
　vitamin D and, 660–661
Nephron, xenobiotics affecting, 390, 390f
Nephropathy
　analgesic abuse, 515
　aristolochic acid, 1610
　Balkan endemic, 1610
　Chinese herb, 1610

phosphate-induced, gastrointestinal decontamination and, 85
　warfarin-related, 890
Nephrotic syndrome, 390f
　clinical features, 391
　metals causing, 397t
　pathophysiology, 391
　xenobiotics causing, 391, 392t
Nephrotoxicity, 368
　of acetaminophen, 474–475
　of acyclovir, 829
　of aminoglycosides, 392, 394t, 821–822
　of amphotericin B, 828–829
　of antimony, 397t
　of arsenic, 390f, 397t
　of barium and barium salts, 397t
　of beryllium, 390f, 397t
　of bismuth, 390f, 397t, 1255
　of cadmium, 390f, 397t, 1260–1261, 1261t
　of calcineurin, 391
　of chemotherapeutics, 763
　of chromium, 397t
　of cisplatin
　　N-acetylcysteine for, 494
　　magnesium for, 877
　of copper, 397t, 1286
　of diethylene glycol, 1436, 1444, 1446–1447
　of ethylene glycol, 1424
　of fluoroquinolones, 826
　of gadolinium, 397t
　of germanium, 390f, 397t
　of gold, 397t
　of hydrocarbons, 1414
　of ifosfamide, *N*-acetylcysteine for, 494
　of iron, 390f, 397t
　of lead, 390f, 397t, 1295, 1298
　of lithium, 390f, 397t
　of mercury, 390f, 392f, 397t, 1327
　of metals, 390f, 397, 397t
　of methotrexate, 768
　of methoxyflurane, 1015
　mushrooms and, 1589t, 1590–1591, 1593
　of platinum, 397t
　of polyethylene glycol (PEG), 686
　of propylene glycol, 688
　of silicon, 397t
　of sodium stibogluconate, 1232
　of streptozocin, 763
　of tetracyclines, 827
　of thallium, 397t
　of uranium, 392, 397t
　of vancomycin, 828
Neptunium, 1780
Neramexane, mechanism of action, 227t
Neriifolin, 979
Neriin, 643t
Nerium oleander (oleander), 979, 1601t
　cardiac glycosides in, 969, 979
　cardioactive steroids in, 64, 973
　poisoning, digoxin-specific antibody fragments for, 979
　use and toxicities, 643t
Nero (Roman Emperor), 2
Nerve agent antidote kits (NAAKs), 1746
Nerve agents, 1504, 1744–1747. *See also specific agent*
　aerosol/vapor, toxic syndrome caused by, 1750t
　aging half-life, 1746
　antidote availability for, 42, 1746
　chemical names, 1745f
　chemical structures, 1745f

and children, 1744
　CNS penetration, 1508
　decontamination for, 1743, 1745
　dermal decontamination for, 72, 1743
　dermal exposure to, toxic syndrome caused by, 1750t
　long-term effects, 1745
　physical characteristics, 1744–1745
　pretreatment for, 1746–1747
　psychological effects, 1745
　severe exposure to, toxic syndrome caused by, 1750t
　toxicity, 1744–1745
　　clinical effects, 1745
　　pathophysiology, 1745
　toxic syndromes caused by, 1750t
　treatment
　　antiepileptics for, 1746
　　atropine for, 1505–1506, 1745–1746
　　pralidoxime for, 1511
　in warfare, 1741
Nerve conduction, 203
　in arsenic poisoning, 1244
　in botulism, 580
Nerve growth protein, serum, ethanol and, 237
Nervous system. *See also* Central nervous system (CNS); Peripheral nervous system (PNS)
　cells, 340–341
　mushroom toxins affecting, 1589t
　neuroprotective mechanisms, 341
Nettles (*Urtica dioica*), 1613
Neural tube defects, 433, 846
Neurasthenia, mercury-induced, 1327
Neuroadaptation, to xenobiotics, mechanisms involved in, 237
Neuroblastoma, 433
Neurocognitive enhancement, for athletic performance enhancements, 623
Neurodegenerative disorders, xenobiotic-mediated, imaging in, 131–133, 132t, 134f–135f
Neuroglycopenia, 698–699
　in diabetes mellitus, 708
　salicylate-induced, 708–709
　signs and symptoms, 708
Neurokinin NK₁ receptor antagonist, for chemotherapeutic-related vomiting, 764
Neurolathyrism, 227, 1607, 1609
Neuroleptic malignant syndrome, 31, 31t, 215, 218, 344, 420, 1037–1039
　diagnostic criteria for, 1038, 1038t
　differential diagnosis, 1038
　in elderly, 464
　incidence, 1037
　manifestations, 1038
　pathophysiology, 1037
　rhabdomyolysis with, 393
　risk factors for, 1038
　and serotonin toxicity, differentiation, 1059–1060, 1059t
　treatment, 1038–1039
Neuroleptics, 1032. *See also* Antipsychotics
Neurologic principles, 340–348
Neuromodulators, 203. *See also specific neuromodulator*
Neuromuscular blockade (NMB)
　for cyclic antidepressant toxicity, 1049t, 1051
　depolarizing, 1018
　hypoventilation caused by, 400t
　mechanism of, 1018
　nondepolarizing, 1018
　　for strychnine poisoning, 1538
　pharmacologic reversal, 1025–1026, 1026t
　selection of agent for, 1026

residual, 1025, 1025t
reversal agent, 46t
for serotonin toxicity, 1059
Neuromuscular blockers (NMBs), 756, 1018–1028. See also specific xenobiotic
and anaphylaxis, 1019
autonomic side effects, 1019–1020
clinical effects, 576t
complications, 1019–1020
and consciousness, 1019
depolarizing (DNMB), 1018, 1020t. See also Succinylcholine
pharmacology, 1020t
effects on vital signs, 30t
and histamine release, 1019
history of, 1018
interactions
with other xenobiotics, 1020, 1021t–1022t
with pathologic conditions, 1020
for local anesthetic–induced seizures, 1000
mechanisms of action, 1018, 1020t
nondepolarizing (NDNMB), 1018, 1020t
diagnostic tests for, 1027
inhibition, xenobiotics causing, 1021t
pharmacology, 1020t, 1024–1025
potentiation, xenobiotics causing, 1021t
prolonged effect, xenobiotics causing, 1021t, 1022
and response to subsequent nondepolarizer administration, 1021t
shortened effect, xenobiotics causing, 1021t
toxicity, 1025
onset of action, 1019, 10120t
pharmacokinetics, 1018–1019
pharmacology, 1020t
phase II block, 1020
and pupillary light reflex, 1019
and respiratory control, 1019
respiratory effects, 400
respiratory-sparing effect, 1019
and skeletal muscle excitation-contraction coupling, 1019f
Neuromuscular junction (NMJ), 342
dysfunction, with insecticide poisoning, 1491, 1492f, 1493
signal transmission at, 1018, 1019f
transmission at, xenobiotic-induced changes in, 345
Neuromuscular transmission, mechanism of, 1018, 1019f
Neuron(s), 340
anatomic structure, 340
apoptosis, carbon monoxide poisoning and, 1664
cyanide and, 1685–1686
depolarization, 203, 205, 205f
dopaminergic, 212–213
MPTP-induced destruction, 215
excitation, 205, 205f
excitatory, 236
first-order, 805
functions, 340
inhibition, 205–206, 205f
inhibitory, 236
manganese uptake and efflux, 1320
noradrenergic, 208, 209f
physiology, 203–206
repolarization, 203, 205f
resting membrane potential, 203
second-order, 805
serotonergic, 215, 1054, 1056f
thermosensitive, 411, 412f
third-order, 805

Neuronopathies, 345–346
Neuron-specific enolase, in carbon monoxide poisoning, 1667
Neuropathic pain
glutamate and, 224
treatment, 231
Neuropathy(ies), 342, 345–346. See also Polyneuropathy
with colchicine poisoning, 503, 503t
differential diagnosis, 1353
disulfiram-induced, 1174–1175
postoperative, after nerve block, 997
pyridoxine-induced, 863
Neuropeptides, inflammatory, 805
Neuropeptide Y, and thermoregulation, 412
Neuroplasticity, 340
Neuro polyvalent antivenom (NPAV), for sea snake envenomation, 1575
Neuroprotective mechanisms, of nervous system, 341
Neuropsychiatric disorders, cardioactive steroid toxicity and, 971
Neurosteroids
and GABA$_A$ function, 1135–1136, 1136f
modulation, and withdrawal syndrome, 237
withdrawal from, 222
Neurotoxicity
administration route and, 341
of aluminum, 1224–1225
of amphetamines, 1102, 1102t, 1103–1104
of antimicrobials, 829t
of antivirals, 829
of arsenic, 1241, 1243–1244
of benzyl alcohol, 683
of bismuth, 1255–1256
of bupivacaine, 995
of cadmium, 1261
of camphor, 1381
of carbon disulfide, 1175
chemical properties of xenobiotics and, 341
of chemotherapeutics, 763
of chloroprocaine, 997
crotalid bites and, 1622
of cyanide, 1685
delayed
carbamates and, 1494
organic phosphorus compounds and, 1493–1494, 1509
determinants, 341
of disulfiram, 1174–1175
of Elapidae venom, 1634
of ethylene glycol, 1424
extraaxial organ dysfunctiona and, 342–343
of hydrocarbons, 1414–1415, 1415f
of isoniazid, 852–854
of ketamine, 1182
of lead, 1295, 1295f, 1297–1298, 1297f
of lithium, 1068
of local anesthetics, 997
of manganese, 1320
mechanisms, 343
of methanol, 1424
of methotrexate, 768
of methylmercury, 1325–1326, 1328
of monosodium glutamate (MSG), 600
neurologic comorbidities and, 342
of nitrous oxide, 1199
of paradichlorobenzene, 1384–1385
patient characteristics and, 342
of phencyclidine, 1182
of phosphorus, 1529–1530
of polyethylene glycol (PEG), 686–687

of propylene glycol, 687
of pyridoxine (vitamin B$_6$), 663
of sodium stibogluconate, 1233
of tetrodotoxin, 596
vinblastine-related, 506
vincristine-related, 505–506
of Viperidae venom, 1634
xenobiotic interactions and, 342
Neurotoxic principles, 341–343
Neurotoxic shellfish poisoning (NSP), 593t, 595
Neurotoxin(s)
α-, in snake venom, 1620
β-, in snake venom, 1620
mechanism of action, 343
in sea snake venom, 1575
of sea urchins, 1574
Neurotransmission, 203–206, 340
calcium in, 205–206, 205f, 207
cholinergic, xenobiotics affecting, 206f, 207, 207t
dopaminergic, 208
agonists, 214, 214t
antagonists, 214–215, 214t
xenobiotics affecting, 214–215, 214t
enhancement, by xenobiotics, 343
GABAergic
ethanol and, 221, 236f, 237, 1096, 1146, 1165
in hepatic encephalopathy, 1096
glutamatergic, 225, 226f
ethanol and, 1165
impairment, by xenobiotics, 343
noradrenergic, 208
potassium in, 205, 205f
serotonergic, 208, 215
xenobiotics affecting, 217–218, 217t
sodium in, 205, 205f, 206–207
tonic inhibitory, 236
Neurotransmitter(s), 203, 340
degradation, 208
in drug-induced hallucinations, 1182
excitatory, 205, 205f
hydrogen sulfide and, 1689
inhibitory, 205f
lead and, 1294–1295
movement into vesicles, 203–204
release, 203
inhibition, 205–206, 205f
prevention, 205, 205f
reuptake, 204
storage, 208
synthesis, 208
and thermoregulation, 412
uptake, 208
vesicle transport, 203–204, 208
Neurotransmitter receptor(s), 203–205, 204t
Neutralization therapy, for pulmonary irritant exposure, 1658
Neutrons, 1763
Neutropenia, 319–320
chemotherapeutic-related, 762
management, 764
methotrexate-related, management, 770
vancomycin-induced, 828
Neutrophil gelatinase-associated lipocalin (NGAL), in acute kidney injury, 396
Neutrophilic eccrine hidradenitis, 270f
Neutrophils, 319–320
Nevirapine, 831
Newborn. See Neonate(s)
New drug application (NDA), 1833–1834, 1835f, 1836

New molecular entity (NME), 1835
New World vipers. *See* Pit vipers (Crotalinae)
New Zealand, methylmercury exposure studies in, 1328
Nexus. *See* 2C-B
n-hexane. *See* Hexane (*n*-hexane)
Niacin. *See* Nicotinic acid (niacin, vitamin B_3)
Nicander of Colophon, 1–2, 1t, 2–3
Nicardipine
    for amphetamine toxicity, 1104–1105, 1104t
    indications for, 751
    pharmacokinetics, 946t
Niccolite, 1333
Nickel, 1333–1338
    absorption, 1334
    in air/atmosphere, 1333
    allergy, 1333–1335
        testing for, 1336–1337
    alloys containing, 1333
    in breast milk, 1334
    as carcinogen, 1336
    chelation therapy for, 1336–1337
    chemistry, 1333
    contact dermatitis from, 279
    cutaneous manifestations with, 1277
    dermal absorption, 1334, 1336
    dermatitis caused by, 1176, 1277, 1333–1335,
        1335f, 1335t
        management, 1337
        primary, 1335
        secondary, 1335
        testing for, 1336–1337
    in dialysis water, 1336
    dietary intake, 1334
    dimethylglyoxime spot test for, 1337
    divalent, 1334
    in drinking water, 1333
    elemental, 1333
    elimination, 1334
    excretion, 1334
    exposure, 1333–1334
        acute, clinical manifestations, 1334–1335
        chronic, 1336
        management, 1337
        sources, 1333
    exposure limits, 1336, 1336t
    forms, 1333
    free, testing metal surfaces for, 1337
    half-lives of, 1334
    in herbal medicine, 1334
    history and epidemiology, 1333
    ingestion, 1334, 1336
    inhalational poisoning, 1334–1336
    in lungs, 1334
    medical devices containing, 1335
    occupational exposures to, 1333, 1335
    ores, 1333
    in orthodontics, 1335
    parenteral administration, 1336
    physicochemical properties, 1333
    poisoning
        diagnostic testing for, 1336–1337
        management, 1337
        pulmonary symtoms, management, 1337
    refining, Mond process, 1657
    serum, 1334
        factors affecting, 1336
        measurement, 1336
        normal concentration, 1333
        in poisoning, 1336

    in soil, 1333
    tissue distribution, 1334
    total body burden, 1334
    toxicokinetics, 1333–1334
    transplacental transport, 1334
    urine, 1334
        factors affecting, 1336
        measurement, 1336
        normal concentration, 1333
    whole blood, factors affecting, 1336
Nickel (coin), 1333
Nickel carbonyl, 1333, 1657–1658
    absorption, 1333
    chemistry, 1333
    deaths caused by, 1335
    decontamination, 1337
    detection threshold, 1654t
    exposure limits, 1336t
    immediately dangerous to life and health (IDLH), 1654t
    inhalational exposure, 1335
    myocarditis caused by, 1335
    neurologic symptoms caused by, 1335
    occupational disasters related to, 1333
    odor, 1333
    pneumonitis caused by, 1335
    regulatory standard for, 1654t
    short-term exposure limit (STEL), 1654t
    sources, 1654t
    toxicity (poisoning), 1333
        chelation therapy for, 1337
        DDC for, 1176
        diagnostic testing in, 1336
        severity classification, 1336
        signs and symptoms, 1334t, 1335
        treatment, 1337
    water solubility, 1654t
Nickel chloride, 1334
Nickeloplasmin, 1334
Nickel oxide, 1333–1334
    as carcinogen, 1336
Nickel subsulfide, 1334
    as carcinogen, 1336
    exposure limit, 1336t
Nickel sulfate, 1333–1334
    as carcinogen, 1336
Nickel sulfide, 1333–1334
Nicotiana and *Nicotiana tabacum* (tobacco), 1203,
        1601t, 1604. *See also* Nicotine; Tobacco
    psychoactive xenobiotics in, 650t
Nicotiana glauca (tree tobacco), 1604
Nicotinamide adenine dinucleotide (NAD), 168, 173f,
        175, 177, 850
    depletors, 173f
    in gluconeogenesis, 178
    in oxidative metabolism, 168
    oxidized (NAD^+), 168, 168f, 175, 178
        in spectrochemical testing, 103
Nicotinamide adenine dinucleotide phosphate
        ($NADPH/NADP^+$), 1704, 1705f
    and hemolysis, 1706
    and methemoglobinemia, 1706
    in oxidation-reduction, 168, 168f
    production, 178, 178f
    in spectrochemical testing, 103
    synthesis, 1158
Nicotine, 642t, 650t, 1203–1209, 1495t, 1496, 1601t,
        1604–1605
    absorption, 1203–1204, 1204t
    blood levels, 1204
        in toxicity, 1207

    and breastfeeding, 441
    in breast milk, 1204
    clearance, 1204
    clinical effects, dose dependency, 1206
    dermal exposure to. *See also* Green tobacco sickness
        management, 1207
    diagnostic testing for, 1207
    effects on vital signs, 29t–30t
    elimination, 1204, 1204t
    elimination half-life, 1204, 1204t
    exposure to
        clinical manifestations, 1206–1207
        management, 1207
        occupational, 1203
    food contamination with, 18t, 19
    gum, 1204t, 1205
    history and epidemiology, 1203
    hypoventilation caused by, 400t
    inhaler, 1205
    in insecticides, 1203
    LD_{50}, 1204
    lethal dose, 1604
    liquid preparations, 1203, 1204t, 1205
        death associated with, 1204
        and poisoning, 1206–1207
    lozenges, 1204t, 1205
    metabolism, 1204, 1204t
    nasal spray, 1204t
    odor, 364t
    patch(es), 1204t, 1205
        absorption from, 1207
        nicotine elimination with, 1204
    pathophysiology, 1206
    pediatric exposure to, sources, 1203
    pharmacology and pharmacokinetics, 1203–1204,
        1204t
    physicochemical properties, 1203
    in plants, 1203
    protein binding by, 1204, 1204t
    renal excretion, 1204
    seizures caused by, 1206
    serum, in smokers, 1207
    and skeletal muscle excitation-contraction coupling,
        1019f
    sources, 1204–1206, 1204t
    spray, 1205
    tolerance, 1204
    toxicity (overdose/poisoning), 207
        acute, 1207, 1207t
            diagnostic testing for, 1207
            management, 1207
        in children, 1204
        clinical manifestations, 1206–1207, 1207t
        diagnostic testing for, 1207
        doses associated with, 1204
        management, 1207
        and organ donation, 1893t
        sources, 1604
    transplacental transfer, 1204
    uses, 1204–1206
    withdrawal, 239
Nicotine alkaloids, 1495t, 1496
Nicotine-derived nitrosamine ketone (NNK), 174t
Nicotine glucuronide, 1204
Nicotine-1-*N*-oxide, 1204
Nicotine receptor partial agonists, 1203, 1206
Nicotine sulfate, 1203
Nicotinic acid (niacin, vitamin B_3), 654, 664
    adverse effects and safety issues, 622, 664
    for alteration of urine test results, 622

in common products, 986t
dietary sources, 664
flushing caused by, 273, 664
formulations, 664
history of, 664
pharmacokinetics, 664
pharmacology, 664
physicochemical properties, 664
recommended dietary allowance or adequate daily
    intake for, 655t
structure, 850
toxicokinetics, 664
and urine testing for illicit drugs, 664
Nicotinic receptors (nAchr), 204, 206–207, 206f, 1503
agonists, 206f, 207, 207t
antagonists, 206f, 207, 207t
neuromuscular blockers at, 1018–1019, 1019f
Nicotinics, in dietary supplements, 648–649
Nicotinism, 1604
Niemann, Albert, 4t, 8, 994, 1124
Nifedipine
as CYP inhibitor, 171
excretion, 946
pharmacokinetics, 145t, 946t
pharmacology, 945
toxicokinetics, 145t
and vincristine, interactions, 506
volume of distribution, 145t, 946, 946t
Night blindness, 656
Nightshade, fetid, stinky (henbane, *Hyoscyamus niger*)
Theophrastus on, 2
use and toxicity, 642t
Nikolsky sign, 274–275
Nimesulide, pharmacology, 512t
Nimodipine
and adenosine reuptake, 231
mechanism of action, 227t
pharmacokinetics, 946t
Niobium, chelator for, 1780
Nisoldipine, pharmacokinetics, 946t
Nitazoxanide, for HIV-related infections, 830t
Nithiodote, 1688, 1700–1701
Nitrates
effects on vital signs, 29t
excess, and anion gap, 191t
and methemoglobin formation, 1704–1705
organic, absorption, 1705
sources, 1704
sulfhemoglobin from, 1710
transdermal absorption, 271
water contaminated with, 1704–1705
Nitrazepam, 466
Nitrazine paper, for ocular pH check, 1395
Nitrefazole, and disulfiramlike reactions, 1174t
Nitric acid, 1657
Nitric oxide (NO), 160, 1656
and electron transport, 176t
and gastrointestinal tract, 290t
and glycolysis, 176t
mechanism of action, 227t
production, nitrites and, 1698
release, amlodipine and, 945
for respiratory dysfunction, 407
and sexual function, 300, 304
in smoke inhalation-induced lung injury, 1641
structure, 160t
toxicity, 1705f
Nitric oxide (NO) donors, 1195
Nitric oxide synthase (NOS), 1656
endothelial, 945, 954, 954f

inducible, in smoke inhalation-induced lung injury,
    1641
inhibitor, for carbon monoxide poisoning,
    1664, 1671
Nitrile herbicides, 1468t
Nitriles, 1684
Nitrites, 1694, 1698–1702. *See also* Amyl nitrite; Sodium
    nitrite
adverse effects and safety issues, 1646, 1687t, 1700
and breast-feeding, 1700
chemistry, 1698
for cyanide poisoning, 1699–1700
dosage and administration, in adults, 1700–1701
effects on vital signs, 29t
mechanism of action, 1698
methemoglobinemia from, 1646, 1687t, 1698–1699.
    See also Methemoglobinemia
and methemoglobin formation, 1704
odor, 364t
pharmacokinetics and pharmacodynamics, 1699
pharmacology, 1698
in pregnancy, 1700
and sodium thiosulfate, for cyanide poisoning,
    1699
sources, 1704
Nitrobenzene, odor, 364t
Nitrocellulose, 1657
Nitrochloroform, 1749
Nitrofurantoin
acute interstitial nephritis caused by, 394t
chronic hepatitis caused by, 333
diagnostic imaging, 115t, 125–126, 125t
and ethanol, interactions, 1146t
infertility caused by, 297t, 298f
mechanism of action, 822t
polyethylene glycol (PEG) in, 687
toxicity (overdose/poisoning), 822t
    chest X-ray findings in, 125–126, 125t
    organ system manifestations, 829t
Nitrogen. *See also* Reactive nitrogen species
chemistry, 168
gas
    physicochemical properties, 1653
    as simple asphyxiant, 400t, 1653
    uses, 1653
liquid, 271
materials containing, thermal degradation products,
    1641t
metabolism, 179–181
poisoning with, 1653
water solubility, 1654t
Nitrogen dioxide, 1652–1653
detection threshold, 1654t
diffuse airspace filling from, 123, 125t
from fire, 16, 16t
immediately dangerous to life and health (IDLH),
    1654t
regulatory standard for, 1654t
respiratory effects, 399t
short-term exposure limit (STEL), 1654t
sources, 1654t
structure, 160t
water solubility, 1654t
Nitrogen mustards, 354, 1748
adverse effects and safety issues, 760t
antidotes for, 760t
enhanced elimination, 764
mechanism of action, 761
neurotoxicity, 763
overdose/poisoning, 760t

teratogenicity, 429t
and tinnitus, 370t
Nitrogen narcosis, 1653
Nitrogen oxides, 1642, 1657
airway injury by, 1640t, 1641
and methemoglobin formation, 1705
in smog, 1651
as thermal degradation product, 1641t
Nitrogen-phosphorus detectors, for gas
    chromatography, 106
Nitroglycerin, 1195
absorption, 1705
administration routes for, 144
for amphetamine toxicity, 1104–1105, 1104t
for cocaine-associated chest pain, 1129, 1139
cranial neuropathy caused by, 346t
for erectile dysfunction, 304
injection, propylene glycol in, 687t, 688
Nitronium cation, structure, 160t
Nitropropionic acid, mechanism of action, 227t
Nitroprusside, 962–963
cyanide poisoning from, 1684, 1686, 1695–1696, 1700
effects on vital signs, 29t
sodium thiosulfate prophylactic use with, 1699–1700
structure, 962
Nitroprusside test, for ketones, 1150–1151
1-Nitropyrene, 174t
N-Nitrosamines
biotransformation, 172
effects on liver, 328
effects on mitochondrial inner membrane, 176t
N-Nitrosodiethylamine, 174t
N-Nitrosodimethylamine, 174t
metabolism, 172
Nitrosoureas, 349f, 354, 761f
adverse effects and safety issues, 760t
and kidney failure, 763
neurotoxicity, 763
overdose/poisoning, 760t
Nitrous oxide, 1011–1014
abuse, 8
    and barotrauma, 401
antinociceptive effects, 1195
blood:gas partition coefficient, 1195t
cardiovascular effects, 1013
clinical and laboratory findings with, 36t
deaths associated with, 1199
detection threshold, 1654t
elimination, 1194, 1195t
hematologic effects, 1012, 1013f
history of, 1011
immediately dangerous to life and health (IDLH),
    1654t
immunologic effects, 1013
inhalation, 1193t, 1194
    clinical manifestations, 36t, 1199, 1199t
and kappa opioid receptor, 1195
mechanism of action, 1195
neurologic effects, 1012–1013, 1013f
neurotoxicity, 343, 1199
pharmacodynamics, 1195
pharmacokinetics, 1195
pharmacology, 1195
regulatory standard for, 1654t
sources, 1654t
spinal cord lesions caused by, 131
structure, 1011f
toxicity, 1012–1014
    treatment, 1014
water solubility, 1654t

Nitzschia pungens, and shellfish poisoning, 595
Niu bang zi. *See* Burdock root (*Arctium lappa, A. minus*)
Nizatidine
    pharmacokinetics and toxicokinetics, 745t
    structure, 742, 742f
NMDA (*N*-methyl-D-aspartate) glutamate receptor, 225,
        226f–227f, 236f, 719
    in alcohol intoxication, tolerance, and withdrawal,
        227t, 228, 236f
    aminoglycosides and, 821–822
    antagonists, 227t, 228
        neurotoxicity, prevention, 1182
    cyanide and, 1685
    ethanol and, 227t, 228, 236f, 237, 1146, 1165
    in excitotoxicity, 225
    and glutamatergic neurotransmission, 225, 227f
    hallucinogens and, 1182
    inhalants and, 1194
    ketamine and, 386
    lead and, 1295
    magnesium and, 876–877
    modulators, 227t
    opioids and, 238, 521
    phencyclidine and, 228, 1213–1214
    phencyclidine and ketamine at, 1213–1214
    sedative-hypnotics and, 1084
    thallium and, 1351
Noble gases. *See* Gas(es), inert (noble); *specific gas*
Nociceptin, 519, 521
Nociceptin receptor, opioid, 520t, 521
Nocitoxin, 1577
Nodal escape rhythm, 247
Nodularia spumigena, 1609
Nodularins, 1609
Nodule (skin), 269t
Noise
    characteristics, 368
    definition, 368
    hearing loss caused by, 368–369
    permissible exposure levels (OSHA), 368, 369t
Nomenclature
    of alcohols, 165
    of carboxylic acids, 165
    chemical, 155
    for cytochrome P450, 168–169
    of organic chemistry, 161–162, 162f
    of thiols, 165
Noncovalent bond(s), 159
Noncritical items, cleaning, 1368
Nondihydroguaiaretic acid, 641t
Nonfatal poisonings, data collection on, 1791
Noninferiority trial, 1853t, 1854
Nonionizing radiation, 1763
Nonlinear processes, 149–150, 150f
Nonmetals, 156f
    characteristics, 155
    physicochemical properties, 158
Nonnucleoside reverse transcriptase inhibitors, 831
Nonpolar compounds, 159
Nonprescription drug(s)
    adverse effects and safety issues, in elderly, 465–466
    use, 738
Nonsteroidal antiinflammatory drugs (NSAIDs),
        511–518. *See also* Salicylate(s); *specific NSAID*
    absorption, 511
    acute interstitial nephritis caused by, 393, 394t
    anaphylactoid and anaphylactic reactions with,
        514t, 515
    antiplatelet effects, 514
    cardiovascular effects, 516

cardiovascular risk with, 514
cerebral hemorrhage caused by, imaging, 132t
CNS effects, 514–515, 514t
and colchicine, interactions, 502
dermatologic effects, 514t, 515
drug interactions with, 514t
and electrolytes, 514t, 515
elimination half-life, 511, 512t
and GABA receptor, 222
gastrointestinal effects, 512–513, 515
gastrointestinal toxicity, 512–513, 514t
and gustatory dysfunction, 365
hematologic effects, 514, 514t, 515–516
hepatotoxicity, 514t, 515, 1841
history of, 511
immunologic effects of, 514t, 515
with ionizable groups, and ATP synthesis, 176t
and medication overuse headache, 515
metabolism, 511
neurologic effects, 514–515, 514t
nonselective, cardiovascular risk with, 514
ototoxicity, 366f
overdose/poisoning
    clinical manifestations, 514–516
    diagnostic tests for, 516
    epidemiology, 511
    management, 516
    pathophysiology, 512–514, 514t
pancreatitis caused by, 295t
pharmacokinetics and toxicokinetics, 511–512, 512t
pharmacology, 511, 512t, 555
as photoallergens, 280
in pregnancy and lactation, 515
pulmonary effects, 514t, 516
renal effects, 390f, 391, 395, 395f, 513–514, 514t, 515
and tinnitus, 370t
as tocolytics, 514
and upper gastrointestinal bleeding, 1853
Nontoxic exposures, identification, 40
Nonylphenol ethoxylate, 1466
No observed effect level (NOEL), 1815
Norbormide (dicarboximide)
    estimated fatal dose, 1453t
    physicochemical properties, 1453t
    in rodenticides, 1453t. *See also* Rodenticides
    toxicity
        antidote and/or treatment for, 1453t
        clinical manifestations, 1453t
        toxic mechanism, 1453t
Norcocaine, 145t, 1124, 1125f
Nordiazepam, 1138
Nordihydroguaiaretic acid (NDGA), 1609–1610
Norephedrine, 145t
Norepinephrine (NE), 203, 206f, 208–212, 260, 1180
    actions, 208
    amphetamines and, 1099–1101, 1100f
    for calcium channel blocker toxicity, 950
    chemistry, 165
    for cyclic antidepressant toxicity, 1050
    cytoplasmic, 210–211
    displacement from nerve ending, 211
    dopamine and, 211–212
    enantiomers, 165
    facilitated exchange diffusion of, 211
    indications for, 35t
    nicotine and, 1206
    release, 206f, 208, 209f, 210
        prevention, 211t, 212
        xenobiotics that prevent, 211t, 212
    reuptake, 208, 209f

cocaine and, 1125
    inhibitors, 210t, 211
        competitive, 210t, 211
        noncompetitive, 210t, 211
    reverse transport out of neuron, 210–211
    and serotonin, 1054, 1056f
    and sexual function, 300, 304
    synthesis, 208, 209f
    and thermoregulation, 412
    in vasoconstriction, 209–210
Norepinephrine/dopamine reuptake inhibitor (NDRI),
        1061. *See also* Bupropion
    metabolites, 1055t
    pharmacokinetics, 1055t
Norepinephrine (reuptake) transporter (NET), 208,
        209f, 211, 213, 1056f
    inhibition
        competitive, 211
        noncompetitive, 211
Norethindrone, teratogenicity, 430t
Norfloxacin, 826
    and GABA receptor, 222
Norfluoxetine, 1055t, 1058
    clearance, 1058, 1077
    and CYPs, 1056
Norketamine, 1212
Normeperidine, 147
Nornicotine, 1204
Norovirus, foodborne illness caused by, 592t
Noroxycodone, 145t
North American coral snake (*Micrurus fulvius*),
        antivenom for, 1625, 1627, 1627t
    shortage, 43
North American Coral Snake Antivenin (Equine), 1625,
        1627, 1627t
    adverse effects and safety issues, 1629–1630
    chemistry, 1628
    clinical use, 1629
        in pregnancy and lactation, 1630
    dosage and administration, 1631
    formulation and acquisition, 1631
    history of, 1627
    preparation, 1628
North American Coral Snake Antivenom, 1625.
        See also North American Coral Snake
        Antivenin (Equine)
Northern black-tailed rattlesnake (*Crotalus* spp.), 1636t
Northwestern brown spider. *See* Hobo spider (*Eratigena
        agrestis*)
Nortriptyline, 145t, 147, 1044–1045. *See also* Cyclic
        antidepressants
    elimination, multiple-dose activated charcoal and, 78
    Log D, 1045
    pharmacology, 1044
    structure, 1044t
Norverapamil, 145t
Nosebleed (plant). *See* Feverfew (*Tanacetum
        parthenium*); Yarrow (*Achillea millefolium*)
Nostoc, 1609
Notechis scutatus (terrestrial tiger snake), antivenom,
        1575, 1575t
Notesthes robusta (bullrout), 1576, 1576t, 1577
n- prefix, 165, 165f
Nuclear, biological, and/or chemical (NBC), 1741t
Nuclear dust, 278
Nuclear excision repair, 351
Nuclear medicine, radiation exposure in, 1766, 1766t
Nuclear receptors
    genetic polymorphisms for, 171
    as transcription factors, 170–172

Nuclear Regulatory Commission (NRC), 1766–1767
Nuclear scintigraphy. *See also* Positron emission tomography (PET); Single-photon emission computed tomography (SPECT)
    of CNS, 130, 133–134
    ligands for, 133
    principles of, 133
Nucleophiles, 162–164
    hard, 164
    site-directed, 162
    soft, 164
Nucleoside analog reverse transcriptase inhibitors, 831
Nucleoside analogs, and fatty acid metabolism, 179
Nucleoside reverse transcriptase inhibitors (NRTIs), hyperventilation caused by, 400t
Nucleotides
    lesions, 351
    pyridine, in oxidation, 168
Nucleus tractus solitarius (NTS), 212
    α_2-adrenoceptor activation in, 210f
Nuclides, 1763
    fissile, 1763
    primordial, 1763
Null hypothesis, 1855
NuLYTELY, 86
Nutmeg, 643t, 1601t. *See also Myristica fragrans* (mace, nutmeg)
Nutmeg liver, 332
Nutmeg oil, 631
Nutritional deficiencies, in alcoholic patients, 1167
Nuttalliellidae, 1550
Nut theriac, 1t
Nux vomica (*Strychnos* spp.), 1603t
Nyctalopia, 656
Nylon, thermal degradation products, 1641t
Nystagmus, 37, 358
    jerk, 358
    nonophthalmic xenobiotics causing, 361
    pendular, 358
    poisoning/overdose causing, 36t
    in strychnine poisoning, 1536–1537
    xenobiotic exposures causing, 357t, 358
Nystatin, toxicity, organ system manifestations, 829t

O

Oak (*Quercus* spp.), 1602t
Oak Ridge Institute for Science and Education (ORISE), 1767
Oaxacan black-tailed rattlesnake (*Crotalus* spp.), 1636t
Oaxacan small-headed rattlesnake (*Crotalus* spp.), 1636t
Obesity. *See also* Bariatric surgery; Dieting xenobiotics and regimens
    adult patient with, *N*-acetylcysteine for, 493, 497
    in children, 606
    definition, 148, 610t
    endocrine and neuroendocrine pathways, 609f
    epidemiology, 606
    health effects, 606
    management, nonpharmacologic interventions in, 613
    and mortality, 606
    and xenobiotic elimination, 148
Obidoxime (Toxogonin, LuH-6), 1487, 1508–1509, 1746
    for organic phosphorus compound poisoning, 1497–1498
    structure, 1508
O'Bryan, Ronald Clark, 5t
Observational study(ies)

analytical, 1853, 1853f, 1853t
    descriptive, 1852–1853, 1853t
Obsessive-compulsive disorder (OCD), glutamate and, 224–227
Obstructive nephropathy, 390f, 394–395, 394t
    laboratory investigation, 397
Occupational exposures. *See also specific xenobiotic*
    associated with liver injury, 334, 334t
    and asthma, 403, 1660, 1660t
    data collection on, 1791–1792
    in developing world, 1846–1847
    diagnosis, 1797
    ethical issues with, 1802–1803
    health effects, 1797, 1798t
    and secondary (environmental) exposure, 1797
    treatment, 1797
Occupational history taking, 1797–1799
    brief occupational survey in, 1797, 1797t
    components, 1798t
    hazardous exposures in, 1797t, 1798, 1798t
    health effects in, 1798, 1798t
    job specifics in, 1798, 1798t
    nonoccupational exposures in, 1798t, 1799
    past work (work history) in, 1798t, 1799
    present work in, 1797–1798
    workplace sampling and monitoring in, 1798t, 1799
Occupational medicine, 4t, 7
    ethical considerations in, 1802–1803, 1802t
Occupational Safety and Health Act, 10t, 12, 1800, 1801t, 1803–1804
Occupational Safety and Health Administration (OSHA), 12, 1799, 1801t, 1808
    Confined Space Entry Standard, 1690
    contact information, 1804
    Hazard Communication Standard, 1800, 1801t, 1803
    monitoring and sampling requirements, 1799
    permissible noise exposure levels, 368, 369t
    radiation exposure limits, 1766
    and radiation regulation, 1767
    rules and guidelines for hazardous materials incident response, 1811–1812
    toxic and hazardous substances list, 1799
Occupational toxicology
    information resources for, 1801t, 1803–1804
    origin of, 7
Occupation-related chemical disasters, 22–23, 23t
OcPlex, 910
Octaplex, 909–910
Octaplex 500, 910
Octaplex 1000, 910
Octopus, 1572
Octreotide, 696f, 713–718. *See also* Somatostatin
    adverse effects and safety issues, 702, 715
    as antidote for hypoglycemia, 702, 713–718
        clinical use of, for insulin suppression, 714–715
        dosage and administration, 702
        effect on insulin secretion, 713–715
    availability and storage, 45t
    chemical structure, 713
    depot formula, 716
    dosage and administration, 702, 715–716
    drug interactions with, 715
    effects on insulin secretion, mechanism of action, 713–714
    elimination, 714
    elimination half-life, 714
    formulation, 716
    history of, 713
    indications for, 35t, 45t, 713

for insulin suppression, 714–715
        labeling, 43
        long-acting release (LAR), 716
            kinetics, 714
        monitoring with, 702, 715
        pharmacokinetics, 714
        pharmacology, 713–714
        for PHHI, 715
        physiologic effects, 713–714
        in pregnancy and lactation, 715
        for quinine overdose, 840
        receptor affinity, 713–714
        shortage, 43
        stocking, recommended level, 45t
        storage, 716
        volume of distribution, 714
N-Octyl bicycloheptene dicarboximide, 1520
Octylphenoxyethoxyethyl ether sulfonate, 1373–1374
Ocular exposures. *See* Eye(s); *specific xenobiotic*
Oculogyric crisis, antipsychotic-induced, 1036
Odadaic acid, 1574
Odds ratio, 1854, 1854f
Odland bodies, 269
Odontobuthus spp., antivenoms, 1564t
Odontomachus spp., 1552
Odoroside A, 643t
Odor recognition, clinical use, 363, 364t
Oduvan (*Clistanthus collinus*), self-poisoning with, 1846
Odyssey, 1–2
Oenanthe crocata (hemlock water dropwort), cicutoxin in, 1610
Oenothera biennis (evening primrose), 641t
Off-gassing, and decontamination, 72
Ofloxacin, 826
    benzalkonium chloride in, 682t
    and GABA receptor, 222
Ohio buckeye. *See* Horse chestnut (*Aesculus hippocastanum*)
Oil. *See specific oil*
    essential. *See* Essential (ethereal) oils
Oil disease, 18, 18t
Oil folliculitis, 1414
Oil of citronella, 1525
Oil of evening primrose, 641t
Oil of lemon eucalyptus (PMD, *p*-menthane-3,8-diol), 1524
    comparative efficacy and toxicity, 1523t
Oil of savin, as abortifacient, 303t
Oil of wintergreen, 37, 556–557, 634
    toxicity, 559–561
        diagnostic tests for, 634
        treatment, 635
Olanzapine, 218. *See also* Antipsychotics
    adverse effects and safety issues, 1039
    for agitated/violent behavior, 386
    cardiac effects, 258t
    clinical and toxicologic effects, 1034t
    contraindications to, 387
    dosage and administration, 1033t
    extrapyramidal effects, 215
    mechanism of action, 1035
    pharmacokinetics, 1033t
    priapism caused by, 301t
    and respiratory depression, 387
    self-poisoning with, 376
    and sudden cardiac death, 253
Older adults, poison prevention aimed at, 1783–1784
Old maid. *See* Periwinkle (*Catharanthus roseus*)
Olea europaea (olive), 645

Oleander, 4, 1606
cardiac glycosides in, 645
Nerium oleander, 643t, 979, 1601t. *See also* Cardioactive steroids
cardiac glycosides in, 969, 979
poisoning, digoxin-specific antibody fragments for, 979
use and toxicities, 643t
yellow (*Thevetia peruviana*), 979, 1603t, 1606, 1606f. *See also* Cardioactive steroids
cardiac glycosides in, 969, 979
overdose/poisoning, 78
gastrointestinal decontamination for, 59t, 61–62, 78
self-poisoning with, 1846
Oleandrigenin, 973, 979
Oleandrin, 643t, 973, 979, 1601t
Olefins, 1410. *See also* Hydrocarbons
Oleic acid, 1004–1005
Oleoresin, 644t
Oleoresin capsicum (OC, pepper spray), 1749–1750, 1749f, 1751t
ophthalmic exposure to, 359
Olestra, for organic chlorine toxicity, 1519
Oleyl anilide, 19
Olfaction, 363–365
disorders
central etiologies, 364
peripheral etiologies, 364
xenobiotics and, 364, 364t
zinc and, 1362
disturbances, cadmium and, 1261
impairment
classification, 363–364
conductive causes, 363–364
etiology, 363–364
evaluation, 364–365
perceptive causes, 363–364
xenobiotics causing, 293t
Olfactory receptors, 363
Oligodendrocytes, 340–341
Oligomycin, site of action, 173f
Olive (*Olea europaea*), oil, 645
Ololiuqui (morning glory seeds), 1178–1179, 1179t. *See also* Lysergamides
Olopatadine, pharmacology, 742
Omegaven, 684
Omeprazole, and CYP induction, 171
Omphalotus illudens (jack-o'-lantern), 1589
Omphalotus olearius, 1582t, 1587, 1587f, 1589
OnabotulinumtoxinA (Botox), 578–579
Oncologic centers, antidote needs assessment for, 43
Oncologic principles, 349–355. *See also* Chemotherapeutics
Ondansetron
adverse effects and safety issues, 990
injection, parabens in, 685t
mechanism of action, 218
metabolism, 172
for methylxanthine-induced vomiting, 990
and QT interval, 253t, 1820–1821, 1821f
and serotonin toxicity, 1058t
One-compartment model, 149–151, 149f–150f
One-leg stand (OLS), 1878–1879, 1879t
Online databases, 1804
Oogenesis, xenobiotics and, 302
Operating a motor vehicle while intoxicated (OMVI), 1876
Operating under the influence (OUI), 1876
Operating while intoxicated (OWI), 1876

Ophiophagus hannah (king cobras), 1633t
Ophryacus undulatus, 1637t
Ophthalmia nodosa, 1547, 1553–1554
clinical spectrum (types), 1553
treatment, 1553
Ophthalmic examination, 356
Ophthalmic exposures, management, 39–40
Ophthalmic medications
benzalkonium chloride in, 681–682, 682t
preservatives for, 682
topical, systemic toxicity with, 360
Ophthalmic principles, 356–362. *See also* Eye(s)
Ophthalmologic assessment and management, after ocular xenobiotic exposure, 73
Ophthalmoplegia, 345, 358
Opiate(s). *See also* Opioid(s)
definition, 519
immunoassays for, cross-reactivity in, 112
laboratory testing for, 101t
urine screening assays for
cross-reactivity in, 112
performance characteristics, 111t, 112
Opioid(s), 4t, 519–537, 1605. *See also specific opioid*
abstinence, opioid antagonists for, 539–540
abuse deterrent formulations, 519
abuse-deterrent immediate-release, 519
abuse/misuse, 12, 521–523
in elderly, 466
historical perspective on, 7–8
addiction, 521–523
management, 529–530
medication-assisted treatment, 529–530. *See also* Buprenorphine; Methadone
adulterants, and opioid assays, 532
adverse effects and safety issues, 521–524
low-dose opioid antagonists and, 539
analgesic effects, 521
antidote for, 35t
administration, 533–534, 534t
antitussive effects, 521
for black widow spider envenomation, 1543
body packers, management, 534
bradycardia with, 924, 924t
cardiac effects, 256
cardiovascular effects, 523t, 525
characteristics, 526t
for children, historical perspective on, 8
chronic use, medication-assisted therapy for, 529–530. *See also* Buprenorphine; Methadone
classification, 526t
congeners, and opioid assays, 532
constipation caused by, 84, 295, 524, 538, 540, 542
cross-reactivity, 532, 532f
deaths caused by, 519
definition, 519
dermatologic effects, 523t
detoxification, rapid and ultrarapid, 239, 534
drug testing for, 532–533
effect on thermoregulation, 412–413, 413t
effects on vital signs, 29t–31t
endocrine effects, 523t, 524
endogenous
opioid antagonists and, 539–540
and sexual function, 304
and ethanol, interactions, 1146t
euphoria caused by, 521
and female sexual dysfunction, 302f
forensic testing for, 532–533
formulations, 519
and GABAergic neurotransmission, 238

gastrointestinal effects, 523t, 524
and hearing loss, 524
history of, 519
and hyperalgesia, 523–524
hypoventilation caused by, 400t
immediate effects, 238, 238f
immunoassays for, 105
infertility caused by, 297t, 298f
intrathecal administration, 794, 798
laboratory tests for, 532–533
cross-reactivity and, 532, 532f
factors affecting, 532
long-term effects, 238, 238f
and male sexual dysfunction, 299f
mechanism of action, 231
metabolism, 526, 527f
and miosis, 524
misuse or diversion, detection, 111–112
and monoamine oxidase inhibitors, safety considerations, 1079, 1079t
movement disorders with, 524
natural, 526t
neurologic effects, 523t
and NMDA receptors, 238, 521
for noncancer pain, regulation, 111
ophthalmic effects, 361, 523t, 524
pharmacology, 520–521
receptor subtypes in, 520–521, 520t
physostigmine and, 756
and pinpoint pupil, 524
potency, 526t
in pregnancy, 438–440
prenatal exposure to, long-term effects, 439–440
prescriber practice reforms and, 553
prescription, laboratory identification, 111–112
pulmonary effects, 523t, 525
rapid detoxification for, 239, 534
regulation, 519, 553
respiratory depression caused by, 524–525
respiratory effects, 399, 525
and rhabdomyolysis, 393
screening for, 110
seizures caused by, 525
self-poisoning with, 376
semisynthetic, 519, 526t
structure, 519
synthetic, 519, 526t. *See also specific opioid*
deaths caused by, 519
immunoassays for, cross-reactivity in, 112
tamper-resistant formulations, 519
teratogenicity, 438–440
therapeutic effects, 521
therapeutic misuse, 522
therapeutic uses, 519
tolerance, 238–239
toxic effects, 524–525
toxicity (overdose/poisoning), 924
ARDS in, 123, 125t, 401, 402t
clinical and laboratory findings in, 36, 36t, 37, 521–525, 523t
deaths from, 21t, 22, 551
diagnosis, 533
diagnostic imaging in, 115t
differential diagnosis, 533
diffuse airspace filling in, 125t
epidemiology, 551
ileus caused by, 127, 129f, 129t
management, 45t, 84, 533–534
harm reduction approaches to, 551–553
naloxone for, 1862

opioid antagonists for, 539
and organ donation, 1893t
in pregnancy, 434
prevention, harm reduction approaches to,
551–553
primary prevention, 551
rates, 551
reversal, harm reduction approaches to, 551–553
risk factors for, 551
secondary prevention, 551
toxic syndrome caused by, 29t
ultrapotent
as incapacitating agents, 1750
toxic syndrome caused by, 1751t
ultrarapid detoxification for, 239, 534
for venomous caterpillar exposure, 1553
withdrawal, 238–239, 533–534, 534t, 539–541
antagonist-precipitated, 534
clinical and laboratory findings with, 7, 36t
effects on vital signs, 29t
iatrogenic, management, 541
intentional iatrogenic, 239
naloxone-precipitated, 239, 540
neonatal, 439, 541
precipitated, 239, 540
in pregnancy and lactation, 541
symptoms, 7
toxic syndrome caused by, 29t
withdrawal syndrome, 238
Opioid agonist antagonist, 526t
Opioid agonists, 526t, 539
deaths caused by, 519
duration of action, 540
partial, 526t
Opioid antagonist(s), 538–544. *See also* Nalmefene;
Naloxone; Naltrexone
adverse effects and safety issues, 540–541
for alcoholism, 1152
for captopril overdose/poisoning, 540
characteristics, 526t
chemistry, 538
for clonidine overdose/poisoning, 540
diabetes insipidus caused by, 195, 195t
dosage and administration, 541–542
in children, 541
in ethanol abstinence, 540
for ethanol toxicity, 540
formulation and acquisition, 542
full, 526t
history of, 538
mechanism of action, 538
observation period with, 540–541
for opioid abstinence, 539–540
for opioid toxicity, 533–534, 539, 541–542
and overshoot phenomenon, 540
peripherally restricted, 538, 540
pharmacodynamics, 539
pharmacokinetics, 538–539
pharmacology, 538–539
and pituitary hormone release, 540
in pregnancy and lactation, 541
receptor activity, 538–539
receptor affinity, 541
for valproic acid overdose/poisoning, 540
Opioid epidemic, in United States, 519, 553
Opioid receptor(s), 238–239, 520–521, 520t
cochlear, 368
delta, 521, 538–539
dynorphin/kappa, ethanol and, 237
kappa, 520–521, 520t, 538–539

nitrous oxide and, 1195
salvinorin A and, 1182
mu, 520, 520t, 538–539
nociceptin/orphanin FQ, 520t, 521
ethanol and, 237
nomenclature for, 520, 520t
opioid antagonist affinity for, 541
signal transduction mechanisms, 521, 522f
subtypes, 520–521, 520t
Opioid toxic syndrome, 524–525, 924
Opioid use disorder, 521–523, 523t
treatment, 551
counseling-only approaches, 552–553
extended-release natrexone for, 552
as overdose prevention, 552–553
Opisthotonus, in strychnine poisoning, 1536–1537
Opium, 519. *See also* Opioid(s)
abuse, 519
in antiquity, 3
early abuse, 5t, 7–8
eating of, 8
gastric lavage for, development, 7
history and early use of, 1, 6–7
odor, 364t
overdose, early description of, 4
as sedative, 8
smoking of, 8
in theriacs, 2–3
Opium poppy (*Papaver somniferum*), 519
Opium Wars, 519
Opportunistic infections, in HIV-infected (AIDS)
patients, antimicrobial treatment for,
830t–831t
Opsoclonus, xenobiotic exposures causing, 357t
Optical coherence tomography, in methanol poisoning,
1424
Optical isomer(s), 164, 164f
Optical tests, 103
Optic cortex, 356
Optic disc, in methanol poisoning, 1423–1424
Optic nerve, 356, 356f
methanol-induced toxicity, 1423–1424
Optic neuritis
with isoniazid, 853
in thallium toxicity, 1351
Optic neuropathy
in thallium toxicity, 1351
xenobiotic exposures and, 357t
Oral contraceptives
adverse effects, 127
and hepatic tumors, 333
infertility caused by, 297t
mesenteric ischemia caused by, diagnostic imaging,
129t
overdose/poisoning, 304
presystemic metabolism, 144
and tinnitus, 370t
Oral fluid, specimen collection, 1872
Oral pain, in paraquat poisoning, 1475–1476
Oral pathology, 293, 293t
Orange root. *See* Goldenseal (*Hydrastis canadensis*)
Orbitals, 155
Orb weaver spider (*Argiope*)
bites, necrotic wounds with, 1545
venom, and EAAT2 activity, 225
Ordeal bean (*Physostigma venenosum*), 1601t
Ordeal bean (*Tanghinia venenifera*), 979
Oregon grape (*Mahonia* spp.), 1601t, 1605
Orellanine, 1582t, 1589t, 1590, 1593
structure, 1589

Orellinine, 1582t, 1589t, 1590
Orexin(s), 708, 1084, 1090
Orexin agonism, 238
Orexin receptor(s), 238
Orexin receptor antagonist, 1084
Orfila, Bonaventure, 4t, 6
Organ donation, after cyanide poisoning, 1688, 1695,
1893t
Organic acids, 271. *See also* Hydrocarbons; *specific acid*
Organic acid transport (OAT) protein, 341
Organic anion transporters (OATs), 144, 148, 148t
Organic anion transporting polypeptides (OATPs), 144
Organic cation transporters (OCTs), 144, 148, 148t, 368
Organic chemistry, 161–166
bonding in, 161–162
definition, 161
functional groups in, 165–166, 165f–166f
nomenclature in, 161–162, 162f
Organic chlorine insecticides, 1514–1519
absorption, 1514
acute oral toxicity, 1515t
body burden, 1515
chronic exposure to, clinical manifestations, 1518
classification, 1514, 1515t
decontamination, 1518–1519
diagnostic information on, 1515t, 1518
drug interactions with, 1517
elimination, 1515–1516
enterohepatic/enteroenteric recirculation, 1516
EPA-registered uses, 1515t, 1518
estrogenic effects, 1518
excretion, 1516
sucrose polyester (olestra) and, 1519
exposure to, clinical manifestations, 1517–1518
fat-to-serum ratios for, 1515
hazards associated with, 1514
history of, 1514
laboratory testing for, 1518
mechanisms of toxicity, 1517–1518
metabolism, 1515
odors, 1515t, 1518
physicochemical properties, 1514, 1515t
radiopacity, 1518
structure, 1516f
tissue distribution, 1515
toxicity, management, 1518–1519
toxicokinetics, 1514–1516, 1515t
Organic molecules, adsorption to activated charcoal,
76
Organic phosphorus compounds, 1450. *See also*
Herbicides; Nerve agents; *specific compound*
acetylcholinesterase inhibition by, 208, 1487, 1489f,
1508–1509
activation, rate, 1487
aging, 1487, 1509–1510
antidote for, 35t, 45t
behavioral toxicity, 1494
bronchorrhea caused by, 123, 125t
butyrylcholinesterase inhibition by, 1487
case fatality for, 1486
chemical structure, 1488t
as chemical weapons, 1487
chemistry, 162, 163f
and children, 1744
chlorinated, 1488t
classification, 1487, 1488t
CNS penetration, 1508
coformulants, 1490
coingestion with ethanol, 1490
decontamination for, 1498

Organic phosphorus compounds (*Cont.*):
delayed neurotoxicity, 1493–1494, 1509
dermal absorption, 1487
dermal decontamination for, 72
dialkoxy, 1488t
diamino, 1488t
diethoxy, 1487, 1488t, 1509–1510
dimethoxy, 1487, 1488t, 1509–1510
direct-acting, 1487
effects on vital signs, 30t
extracorporeal elimination, 1498
gastrointestinal decontamination for, 54t–55t
as herbicides, 1468t
history of, 1486
in homicides, 1487
hypothermia caused by, 412
hypoventilation caused by, 400t
leaving groups, 1487, 1487f, 1488t
lipid solubility, 1487, 1491
lipophilicity, 1488
mechanism of action, 208
mixed substituent, 1488t
with multiple constituents, 1488t
as nerve agents, 1504
and neuromuscular blockers, interactions, 1021t
odor, 37, 364t
oxon, 1487, 1490
pancreatitis caused by, 295t
pharmacokinetics and toxicokinetics, 146t,
        1487–1489
pharmacology, 1487, 1487f
and QT interval, 253t
and recurrent cholinergic crisis, 1488
respiratory effects, 400
self-poisoning with, 1486–1487
    in developing world, 1844
solvents with, 1490
    and pharmacokinetics, 1487–1488
structure, 1487, 1487f, 1510
substituted dialkoxy, 1488t
substituted triphenyl, 1488t
thion, 1488–1490
tissue distribution, 1488
toxicity (poisoning), 123
    acute, 1487
        clinical manifestations, 1490–1493
    antimuscarinic therapy for, 1496–1497
    atropine for, 1504
    benzodiazepines for, 1498
    chronic, 1487, 1494
    clinical manifestations, 37, 576t, 1490–1494
    cutaneous findings in, 189
    in developing world, 1844
    diagnostic tests for, 1494–1495, 1495t
    disposition with, 1498
    epidemiology, 1486–1487
    gastrointestinal decontamination for, 78
    magnesium for, 878–879
    management, 1496–1498
    and neuromuscular junction (NMJ) dysfunction,
        1491, 1492f, 1493
    occupational, 1487
    onset of symptoms, 1490–1491
    organic chlorines and, 1515
    oximes for, 1497–1498
    pathophysiology, 1489–1490
    pralidoxime for, 1510
    prehospital events in, 1486, 1490
    pulmonary complications, 1491, 1492f
    respiratory system toxicity in, 1491, 1492f

transdermal absorption, 271
triphenyl, 1488t
trithioalkyl, 1488t
volume of distribution, 91
Organic solvents, hydrocarbon. *See* Hydrocarbons
Organochlorines, transdermal absorption, 271
Organ of Corti, 366, 366f
ototoxins and, 367
Organogenesis, 432, 432f
teratogens and, 432–433
Organophosphate, 1486
Organotins, and ATP production, 176t
Organ procurement, from poisoned patients,
        1892–1893, 1892t
Orgasmic dysfunction (female), xenobiotics and,
        302, 302f
Orlistat, 606, 607t, 611. *See also* Dieting xenobiotics and
        regimens
Ornate cantil (*Agkistrodon* spp.), 1636t
Ornithine, 180f, 181
Ornithine aminotransferase, deficiency, cranial
        neuropathy caused by, 346t
Ornithine transcarbamylase deficiency, 13, 181
Ornithodorus (louse), 1550
Orogastric lavage, 4t, 33, 51–56
    with activated charcoal, 53, 54t–55t
    adverse effects, 56
    for barium ingestion, 1455
    for calcium channel blocker toxicity, 948
    in children, 452
    complications, 56
    contraindications to, 53, 56t
    for cyclic antidepressant toxicity, 1049
    effects on xenobiotic absorption, 53, 54t–55t
    efficacy, factors affecting, 51–53
    gastrointestinal perforation in, 129f
    indications for, 53, 56t
    for iron poisoning, 671–672
    for methylxanthine toxicity, 989–990
    in post-bariatric surgery patients, 64
    for sedative-hypnotic overdose, 1087
    in strychnine poisoning, 1537
    studies, 53, 54t–55t
    technique for, 53, 56t
    time frame for, 49, 53
    trends in use of, 48, 53, 64–65
    tube size for, 52f, 53, 56t
    volume of fluid used in, 53–56, 56t
Oropharynx, 289–290
Orphan Drug Act of 1983, 1833–1834
Orphanin FQ, 519, 521
Orphenadrine
    and dopamine reuptake, 214
    history of, 738
    mechanism of action, 211, 227t, 228
    pharmacology, 741–742
    toxicity, sodium bicarbonate for, 568t
Orpiment, 1237
Orthostatic hypotension, xenobiotic-induced, 29
    in elderly, 463, 463t
Orthotoluidine, hemorrhagic cystitis caused by,
        306
Oryzalin, 1468t
    in herbicides, 1467t
Osborn wave, 416, 416f
Oscillatoria, 1609
OSHA. *See* Occupational Safety and Health
        Administration (OSHA)
Osler, William, 401
Osmolality

definition, 192
measurement, 193
plasma, 194
serum, 189
    factors affecting, 104
    and hyponatremia, 196
    measured, 103–104
urine, 189
Osmolar gap
propylene glycol and, 688
serum, 101
Osmolarity
calculation, 192–193
definition, 192
serum, calculated, 103–104
Osmol gap, 192–193
    and anion gap, reciprocal relationship, 1426, 1426f
    calculation, 103
    elevated, causes, 193
    ethanol and, 1149
    normal, 193
    serum, and determination of volatiles, 103–104
    toxic alcohol ingestion and, 192–193
    in toxic alcohol poisoning, 1426
        in risk stratification, 1427
Osmometry, 193
Osmotic demyelination syndrome (ODS), 197, 963
    reversible, in ethylene glycol poisoning, 1424
Osmotic nephrosis, 392
Osteolathyrism, 1609
Osteomalacia
    aluminum and, 1223–1225
    cadmium-induced, 1259–1260
    in dialysis patients, 1223
    vitamin D deficiency and, 660
Osteomyelitis, 119–122
    xenobiotic-related, imaging, 115t, 119–122, 124f
Osteonecrosis, 119–122, 124f
Osteopathy, aluminum and, 1224–1225
Osteopenia, cadmium exposure and, 1260
Osteophytosis
    with fluorosis, 115t, 119
    imaging, 115t, 119
Osteoporosis
    cadmium exposure and, 1260
    diagnostic imaging, 115t
    heparin and, 891
    vitamin A toxicity and, 657
Osteosclerosis
    with fluorosis, 115t, 119
    imaging, 115t, 119
Ostrich fern (*Matteuccia struthipteris*), 643t
Otaheite. *See* Tung and tung seed (*Aleurites moluccana,
        A. fordii*)
Otolaryngologic principles, 363–372. *See also*
        Gustation; Hearing; Olfaction
Ototoxicity, 367–368, 367t. *See also specific xenobiotic*
    of acetaminophen, 368
    of acetazolamide, 367t
    of aminoglycosides, 366f, 367–368, 367t, 821–823
    of antimicrobials, 367t
    of arsenic, 367t, 368, 1241
    of bismuth, 1256
    of bleomycin, 367t
    of bromates, 366f, 367t, 368
    of bumetanide, 367, 367t
    of carbon disulfide, 368
    of carbon monoxide, 367t, 368
    of carbon tetrachloride, 368
    of carboplatin, 367

of chemotherapeutics, 367, 367t
of chloroquine, 367t
of cisplatin, 366f, 367, 367t, 763
of cocaine, 367, 367t, 368
of diuretics, 366f, 367, 367t
of erythromycin, 367t, 368
of ethacrynic acid, 367, 367t
of furosemide, 367, 367t
of gentamicin, 367–368
of heroin, 367–368
of hydrocarbons, 367t
of kanamycin, 367
of lead, 367t, 368
of macrolides, 366f
of mannitol, 367t
of meglumine antimoniate, 1233
of mercury, 367t, 368
of methadone, 368
of neomycin, 367
of nitrogen mustard, 367t
of NSAIDs, 366f, 367, 367t
of opioids, 367t, 368
of oxaliplatin, 367
of propylene glycol, 687
quinine-induced, 366f, 367, 367t, 838–840
of salicylates, 366f, 367, 367t, 558
of streptomycin, 367
of styrene, 367t, 368
of toluene, 367t, 368
of trichloroethylene, 368
of vancomycin, 366f, 368
of vinblastine, 367, 367t
of vincristine, 367, 367t
of xylene, 367t, 368
Ouabain, 979
    toxicity, epidemiology, 969
Ouch-ouch disease (itai-itai), 18t, 19, 1259–1260
Out-of-body experience, with arylcyclohexylamine
        toxicity, 1214–1215
Outrage, 1817
Overshoot phenomenon, 540
Overweight. See also Dieting xenobiotics and regimens
    definition, 148, 610t
Ovid, 1
Ovulation, 302
Oxacillin, 823–824
Oxalate(s), 1602t–1603t
    dietary sources, 1610
    overdose/poisoning, management, 44t
    in plants, 1610
    serum, 1425
    urine, 1425
    vitamin C metabolism and, 662–663
Oxalate raphides, 1598t, 1600t–1603t, 1610
Oxalic acid, 146t, 165–166, 1388t, 1602t, 1610
    in ethylene glycol poisoning, 1424
    and hypocalcemia, 1405
    toxicity, 166
Oxaliplatin
    adverse effects and safety issues, 760t
    antidote for, 760t
    cranial neuropathy caused by, 346t
    overdose/poisoning, 760t
Oxaloacetate, as glutamate scavenger, 229
Oxalosis, 395
    cranial neuropathy caused by, 346t
    vitamin C and, 662–663
L-β-N-Oxalyl-α,β-diaminopropionic acid (ODAP)
    and AMPA receptors, 227
    mechanism of action, 227, 227t

Oxaprozin, pharmacology, 512t
Oxatomide, dyskinesia caused by, 742
Oxazepam, 1138. See also Sedative-hypnotics
    in immunoassays, 112
    pharmacokinetics, 1085t
    suicide with, 466
Oxazolidine-2,4-diones, teratogenicity, 430t
Oxcarbazepine (MHD)
    adverse effects and safety issues, 727–728, 727t
    drug-induced hypersensitivity syndrome with,
        727–728, 727t
    drug interactions with, 723t
    elimination, multiple-dose activated charcoal and,
        62
    gastrointestinal decontamination for, 58t, 77
    history of, 719
    mechanism of action, 720f, 720t
    metabolism and effects on CYP enzymes, 722t
    overdose/poisoning
        clinical manifestations, 724
        diagnostic tests for, 724
        management, 724
    pharmacokinetics and toxicokinetics, 721t, 723–724
    pharmacology, 719, 720t
    pregnancy category, 723
    and pregnancy complications, 719
    priapism caused by, 301t
    and suicide risk, 719
    therapeutic serum concentration, 724
Oxicams, pharmacology, 512t
Oxidant stress
    and hemolysis, 1706
    and methemoglobin levels, 1703–1704, 1706
Oxidase(s), NADPH-dependent, 168
Oxidation, 168. See also Reduction/oxidation (redox)
        reactions
    of alcohols, 165
    definition, 159
β-Oxidation, 179, 180f
Oxidation-reduction. See Reduction/oxidation (redox)
        reactions
Oxidation state, 159
Oxidative chlorination, for chemical weapons
        exposure, 72
Oxidative metabolism, 175, 177–178
    xenobiotics that inhibit, sites of action, 173f
Oxidative phosphorylation, 175, 177–178
    arsenicals and, 1238–1239
    inhibition, by hydrogen sulfide, 1689
    uncoupled, 177–178
Oxidative stress, 159, 174, 178, 178f, 1172
    ethanol and, 1146
    and nanoparticle cellular toxicity, 1726, 1726f
    naphthalene-induced, 1382–1383
    in organic phosphorus compound poisoning, 1490
Oxides of nitrogen. See Nitrogen oxides
Oxidizing agents, 159, 174, 271
Oxidizing species, 174
Oximes, 1487, 1508. See also Acetylcholinesterase
        inhibitors; specific oxime
    bispyridium Hagedorn (H-series), 1746
    for carbamate poisoning, 1498
    CNS penetration, 1508
    H series (Hagedorn), 1508
    for nerve agent exposure, 1746
    for organic phosphorus compound poisoning, 1497
Oxprenolol
    overdose/poisoning
        clinical manifestations, 932
        management, 936

    pharmacokinetics, 930
    pharmacology, 927t
Oxybenzone, as photoallergen, 280
2,2-Oxybisacetic acid. See Diglycolic acid (DGA)
Oxychlordane, 1515
Oxycodone. See also Opioid(s)
    characteristics, 526t
    gastrointestinal decontamination for, 58t
    and hearing loss, 524
    immunoassays for, 105
        cross-reactivity in, 112
    pharmacokinetics, 145t
    screening for, 110
    urine screening assays for, performance
        characteristics, 111t
    volume of distribution, 145t
Oxydemeton methyl, pharmacokinetics and
        toxicokinetics, 1488
OxyELITE, hepatotoxicity, 651
Oxyfluorfen, 1468t
Oxygen. See also Reactive oxygen species (ROS)
    biradical nature, 159
    chemistry, 159
    distribution, xenobiotics affecting, 1651
    for hydrogen sulfide poisoning, 1691, 1691t
    hyperbaric. See Hyperbaric oxygen
    indications for, 33, 37, 1040
    inspired. See FiO₂
    molecular, 159, 174–175
    partial pressure, 1651, 1708, 1708t
    partial pressure (PO₂), 399, 405
        decreased, clinical significance, 405
    partial pressure (PCO₂), in hypothermia, 417
    physiologic role, 159
    pulmonary damage caused by, 1653
    in pulmonary gas exchange, 399
    singlet, 1656
        structure, 160t
    for smoke inhalation, 1643, 1644f
    supplemental, for poisoned patient, 406–407
    therapy with
        for cyanide poisoning, 1687, 1687t
        indications for, 1149
    toxicity, 1656
    toxicologic role, 159
    transport, 399
        xenobiotics affecting, 1651
    use, 399
        xenobiotics affecting, 399, 399t
Oxygenated hydrocarbons. See Hydrocarbons
Oxygenation
    assessment, 36–37
    xenobiotics affecting, 1651
Oxygen-carbon dioxide exchange, 315–316
Oxygen content of blood
    calculation, 402, 402f
    factors affecting, 402–403
Oxygen saturation
    laboratory measurement, 101t, 1642, 1708
    pulse oximetry values, 1708, 1708t
    smoke inhalation and, 1642
    venous, elevated, 1686
Oxyhemoglobin, 1703, 1704f
    laboratory measurement, 103
Oxyhemoglobin dissociation curve, 316, 403, 403f, 404
    carbon monoxide and, 1641, 1664
    hypothermia and, 416
    metabolic alkalosis and, 194
    oxidized hemoglobin and, 1679
    sulfhemoglobin and, 1710

β-*N*-Oxylamino-ʟ-alanine (BOAA), 343, 1601t, 1609
  and AMPA receptors, 227, 343, 1609
Oxymetazoline, 959–961
  adverse effects and safety issues, in children, 453
  duration of action, 749t, 750
  nasal spray, benzalkonium chloride in, 682
  structure, 750f
  therapeutic effects, 749t
  toxicity, 749t
    clinical manifestations, 750
Oxymorphone, 145t, 528, 538. *See also* Opioid(s)
  characteristics, 526t
  urine screening assays for, performance
      characteristics, 111t
Oxytocin
  for erectile dysfunction, 304
  and sexual function, 304
Oxytropis spp. (locoweed), 1601t, 1606
Oysters, as aphrodisiacs, 304
Ozone, 1657
  detection threshold, 1654t
  immediately dangerous to life and health (IDLH),
      1654t
  pulmonary damage caused by, 1653
  regulatory standard for, 1654t
  short-term exposure limit (STEL), 1654t
  sources, 1654t
  structure, 160t
  water solubility, 1654t

P
P450. *See* Cytochrome P450 (CYP) enzymes
Pabrinex, 1161
Pacemaker cells
  cardiac, 926, 928f
  depolarization, 254–255
  electrophysiology, 255
  myocardial, 245–246
  refractory, 246
  relatively refractory, 246
  resting, 245, 245f
Pacemaker currents, cardiac, 926, 928f
Pacific urchin (*Tripneustes*), 1574
Pacific yew (*Taxus brevifolia*), 1603t, 1612
Packaging, in preventing pediatric poisoning, 748
Paclitaxel, 349f, 1612
  adverse effects and safety issues, 760t
  albumin-bound, 1719t
  bioavailability, 173
  cell cycle phase specificity, 761f
  peripheral neuropathy with, 763
  polymeric micelle, 1719t
  protein conjugate, 1719t
Pad zahr, 3
Paganini, Niccolò, mercury poisoning in, 1324
Pain
  abdominal. *See* Abdominal pain
  acute, cannabinoids for, 1111–1113
  in arsenic poisoning, 1241
  bismuth-related, 1256
  chest. *See* Chest pain
  chronic, cannabinoids for, 1111–1113
  hydrofluoric acid toxicity and, 1397, 1400
  musculoskeletal, antimonials and, 1233
  neuropathic
    glutamate and, 224
    treatment, 231
  oral, in paraquat poisoning, 1475–1476
  tarantula bites and, 1547
  in thallium toxicity, 1351

Pain fibers, local anesthetics and, 994–995
Paint
  inhaled, 1193t. *See also* Inhalant(s)
  lead in, 115t, 116, 122f, 1292, 1292t. *See also* Lead
  mercury in, 1324. *See also* Mercury
  radium-containing, 1762
  spray, inhaled, 1193, 1193t. *See also* Inhalant(s)
Paint chips, leaded
  imaging, 115t, 116, 122f, 1300f
  ingestion (pica), 1292, 1300f
Painter syndrome, 1412
Paint thinner, inhaled, 1193t, 1197. *See also* Inhalant(s)
Palamnaeus spp., antivenoms, 1564t
Palbociclib, 349f
  cell cycle phase specificity, 761f
Palinopsia, 1185
Paliperidone. *See also* Antipsychotics
  clinical and toxicologic effects, 1034t
  dosage and administration, 1033t
  mechanism of action, 1035
  pharmacokinetics, 1033t
Paliperidone palmitate, nanocrystal, 1719t
Palmer, William, 5t, 6
Palonosetron, 218
Pamidronate, for vitamin D toxicity, 661
Pamiteplase, 897
Panacea, 1t
Panaeolus spp., 1179
Panaeolus cyanescens, 1588
Panamint rattlesnake (*Crotalus stephensi*), 1617t
Panax ginseng (ginseng), 639
  as aphrodisiac, 304t
  uses and toxicities, 642t
Panaxin, 642t
Panax pseudoginseng
  as aphrodisiac, 304t
  uses and toxicities, 642t
Panax quinquefolius (ginseng), 639
  as aphrodisiac, 304t
  uses and toxicities, 642t
Pancreas, 292
  α-cells, xenobiotics affecting, 294, 295t
  β-cells, xenobiotics affecting, 294–295, 295t
  xenobiotics affecting, 294–295, 295t
Pancreas transplantation, from poisoned patients,
      1892–1893, 1892t
Pancreatic cancer, 273
Pancreatic dysfunction, xenobiotics associated with,
      295, 295t
Pancreatitis
  acute, 294
  antimony-related, 1230
  in arsenic poisoning, 1241
  causes, 294
  with colchicine poisoning, 503
  lipid emulsion and, 1007
  in methanol poisoning, 1424, 1427
  mortality rate for, 294
  risk factors for, 294
  severity, 294
  xenobiotic-induced, 294–295, 295t
Pancuronium
  adverse effects and safety issues, 1019–1020
  in capital punishment, 13
  drug interactions with, 1021t–1022t
  murder using, 12
  pharmacology, 1020t
  and response to succinylcholine, 1021t
Pancytopenia
  of aplastic anemia, 311

chemotherapy-related, 311
  with colchicine poisoning, 502, 503t
  methotrexate-related, 768
    management, 770
  NSAID-induced, 516
  radiation-induced, 311
Pane, Ramon, 1203
Panic disorder, new-onset, SSRIs and, 1058
Pantothenic acid, 654
Papaver (poppy), 1605. *See also Papaver somniferum*
      (opium poppy)
Papaveraceae, 1598t, 1602t
Papaverine
  and adenosine receptor, 230
  adverse effects and safety issues, 300
  chlorobutanol in, 684
  for erectile dysfunction, 300
  mechanism of action, 300
  and phentolamine, combined, for erectile
      dysfunction, 300
  priapism caused by, 301t
  Sauropus androgynous and, 1611
Papaver somniferum (opium poppy), 519, 638, 1601t
  historical perspective on, 2–3
Paper, thermal degradation products, 1641t
Paperbark oil, 633
Paperbark trees, 633
Paper wasps, 1540t
Papilledema, xenobiotic exposures causing, 357t
Papule, 269t
Para-aminobenzoic acid (PABA), from local anesthetic
      metabolism, 996–997
Para-aminosalicylate, adsorption to activated charcoal,
      76–77
Parabens
  estrogenic and anti-androgenic effects, 685
  as pharmaceutical additives, 685, 685t
  spermicidal effects, 685
  uses, 685
Parabuthus spp., 1548, 1548t
  antivenoms, 1564t, 1565
Paracelsus, 4, 4t, 7, 519, 812, 1011, 1228
Paracetamol, 472. *See also* Acetaminophen
Paracoccidioidomycosis, in HIV-infected (AIDS)
      patients, 830t
Paradichlorobenzene
  carcinogenicity, 1385
  history and epidemiology, 1384
  laboratory identification, 1385, 1385t
  moth repellents, imaging, 118
  neurotoxicity, 1384–1385
  pharmacokinetics, 1384
  pharmacology, 1384
  radiographic appearance, 1385, 1385t
  structure, 1380
  toxicity
    clinical manifestations, 1384
    diagnostic tests for, 1384
    management, 1385
    pathophysiology, 1384
  toxicokinetics, 1384
  workplace standards for, 1385
Paraffin(s), 1410. *See also* Hydrocarbons
  definition, 1410
  medicinal, 1410
  toxicokinetics, 1411t
Paraffin wax, 1410
Paragalegine, 642t
Paraguay tea (*Ilex paraguariensis*), 643t, 1600t
Parahydroxybenzoic acids. *See* Parabens

Parakeratosis, 269
Paraldehyde
    clinical and laboratory findings with, 36t
    and high anion gap metabolic acidosis, 191t
    history of, 1084
    hyperventilation caused by, 400t
    odor, 364t
Paralysis
    acute ascending flaccid, differential diagnosis, 1550
    ascending, with sea snake envenomation, 1575
    barium-induced, 1455
    carbon monoxide poisoning and, 1665
    flaccid, 345
    Ginger Jake, 21t, 22
    hypokalemic periodic, clinical manifestations, 577t
    skeletal muscle, mechanisms, 1018, 1019f
    tick, 1550
        clinical manifestations, 577t
Paralytics, cranial neuropathy caused by, 346t
Paralytic shellfish poisoning, 593t, 595
    clinical features, 576t
Paramethadione, teratogenicity, 430t
Paraoxon, 144, 1487, 1508. See also Organic phosphorus compounds
    toxicity, magnesium for, 878–879
Paraoxonase, 1489, 1508
    inhibition, 1489
Paraphenylenediamine
    contact dermatitis caused by, 280
    self-poisoning with, 1846
Parapodia, of bristle worms, 1574
Paraquat, 1466–1471, 1467t, 1473–1478
    absorption, 1474
    antidotes for, 1474f, 1477
    and ATP production, 176t
    chemistry, 160
    clearance, and extracorporeal removal, 92
    effects on mitochondrial inner membrane, 176t
    and electron transport, 176t
    elimination, 1474–1475
    enhanced elimination, 90, 92
    extracorporeal removal, 92, 97t, 1477
    formulation with emetic, 1474
    and free radical formation, 175
    gastrointestinal decontamination for, 1477
    laboratory testing for, 101
    mechanisms of toxicity, 1473–1474, 1474f
    pharmacokinetics, 1474
    pharmacology, 1473–1474
    plasma concentration
        nomogram for, 1475, 1476f
        prognostic significance, 1475, 1476f
    poisoning
        ARDS in, 123, 125t, 401
        clinical manifestations, 1475
        diagnostic tests for, 1475
        diffuse airspace filling caused by, 125t
        extracorporeal elimination for, 92, 97t, 1477
        mortality rate for, 1473
        pathophysiology, 1475
        prognosis for, 1475–1477
        treatment, 1474f, 1476–1478
    pulmonary toxicity, 160, 1475–1476
    and redox cycling, 1474, 1474f
    respiratory effects, 399t
    self-poisoning with, 1473
    structure, 1473f
    taste-aversive xenobiotics added to, 1782
    toxicokinetics, 1474

Pararamose, 1553–1554
Parasite(s)
    foodborne, 592t, 597
    intestinal, 600
Parasympathetic nervous system, 260
Parathion, 5t, 144, 1488t, 1504, 1509
    cytochrome P450 enzymes and, 1489
    history of, 1486
    pancreatitis caused by, 294
    pharmacology, 1487
    terrorist use of, 1486
    tissue distribution of, 1488
    toxicity (poisoning), 1486
        case fatality rate for, 1486
        onset of symptoms in, 1490
        prehospital events in, 1486
Parathion ethyl, 1509
Parathion-methyl, 1488t
Parathyroid hormone (PTH), and aluminum deposition in bone, 1224
Pare, Ambroise, 4, 4t
Paregoric, 519, 628, 1380. See also Opioid(s)
    characteristics, 526t
    for neonatal opioid withdrawal, 439
Parenteral nutrition, and thiamine deficiency, 1158, 1160
Paresthesias
    in methylmercury poisoning, 1329
    poisoning/overdose causing, 36t
    in pyrethroid poisoning, 1521–1522
Pargyline. See also Monoamine oxidase inhibitors (MAOIs)
    structure, 1076f
Paris blue. See Prussian blue
Paris green, 1284t
Parkinson disease, 340, 342–343
    copper and, 1283
    early-onset, and dementia, 230
    exacerbated or unmasked by xenobiotics in elderly, 463, 463t
    glutamate and, 224–227
    imaging in, 1320–1321
    and manganism, comparison, 1320–1321
    pesticides and, 1494
    treatment, 212, 214, 228, 231, 1075, 1077
Parkinsonism (Parkinson syndrome)
    with anticholinesterase poisoning, 1491
    antipsychotic-induced, 1037, 1037t
        treatment, 1037, 1037t
    barium toxicity and, 1455
    cadmium and, 1261
    carbon monoxide poisoning and, 1665
    cyanide poisoning and, 1686
    disulfiram-induced, 1175
    dopamine and, 213
    in ethylene glycol poisoning, 1424
    in methanol poisoning, 1424
    MPTP-induced, 21t, 22, 174, 343
    pathophysiology, 1295
    SSRIs and, 1058
    xenobiotic-induced, 342, 344–345, 345t
        in elderly, 463, 463t
Paromomycin, 821–823
    for HIV-related infections, 831t
Parosmia, 364, 364t
Paroxetine, 218, 1054
    CYP enzymes and, 169–170, 1055t, 1056
    mechanism of action, 1056f
    pharmacokinetics, 1055t
    receptor activity, 1057t

    seizures caused by, 1057t
    structure, 1054f
    teratogenicity, 430t
Paroxysmal nocturnal hemoglobinuria, 324
Parsley (Petroselinum crispum), 2, 643t
Parthenolide, 641t
Partial pressure of inspired oxygen (PiO$_2$), 408f
Partial thromboplastin time (PTT), 320–322, 883
    prolonged, 885
Particle size, and toxicity, 157
Particle-wave theory, 1762
Particulates. See also specific xenobiotic
    inhaled. See Pneumoconiosis
    nonrespirable, 1659
    respirable, 1659
    in smoke, 1640
Partition coefficient(s), 1194, 1411
    of inhalants, 1194, 1195t
Partition constant/ratio (K$_{ow}$), 141
partyflock.nl, 1184
Pasireotide, 713–714, 716
Passiflora spp., 1607
Passiflora incarnata, 643t, 650t
Passion flower, 643t, 650t
Passive alcohol sensors (PASs), 1878
Passive diffusion, 141, 141f
Passive hemagglutination inhibition test (PHAI), for loxoscelism, 1545
Patch (skin lesion), 269t
Patent medications, 647
Pathology, and interpretive toxicology, 1873t
Patiromer, and potassium balance, 199
Pauling, Linus, 158
Paullinia cupana (guarana), 607t, 985, 1601t. See also Dieting xenobiotics and regimens
Pausinystalia yohimbe (yohimbe), 645t, 650t, 1601t
Pavor mortis, of latrodectism, 1543
Paxillus involutus, 1582t–1583t, 1592
Pay-loo-ah, lead in, 647
PCE. See Cyclohexamine
PCP. See Phencyclidine (PCP)
PCPy. See Rolicyclidine
PCPy. See Rolicyclidine
Peace lily (Spathiphyllum spp.), 1603t
Peaches and peach pits, 1602t, 1684
Peak plasma concentrations, 152
Peanut allergy, and dimercaprol therapy, 1252
Peanut (Arachis hypogaea) oil, 645
Pears, pits, 1602t
Pediatric condition falsification, anticoagulant poisoning in, 887
Pediatric poisoning. See also Children
    by age group, 448, 449t
    behavioral factors affecting, 450
    deaths caused by, 448–450
    economic cost, 450
    environmental factors affecting, 450
    epidemiology, 448–450, 449t
    Haddon Matrix and, 450
    hospitalization rates for, 448–449
    with illicit substances, 455
    injury phase, 450–451
    intentional, 448, 454–455
        characteristics, 455
    medication errors and, 453–454
    outcomes with, 448–449, 449t
    passive exposure and, 448, 455
    patient (host), xenobiotic (agent), and environment in, 450–451
    peak age of, 448

Pediatric poisoning (*Cont.*):
  physical factors affecting, 450
  postinjury phase, 450
  preinjury phase, 450–451
  prevention, 451
  risk factors for, 450–451
  suicidal, 448
  unintentional, 450–451
    epidemiology, 448
  unsupervised exposures and, 448
  unusual/idiosyncratic reactions to xenobiotics and,
    452–453
  by xenobiotic type, 448, 449t
Pediatric principles, 448–458. *See also specific*
    xenobiotic
Pediatric Research Equity Act of 2003, 1834
Pediatric Research Equity Act of 2007, 1834
Pedicellariae, of sea urchins, 1573–1574
Pediculus humanus, 1550
Peganum harmala (Syrian rue), 644t, 650t, 1077
  and serotonin toxicity, 1058t
Pegaptanib, polymer protein conjugate, 1720t
Pegaspargase, polymer protein conjugate, 1720t
PEG-coated SiO_2, Cornell dots, 1720t
Pegedemase bovine, polymer protein conjugate, 1719t
Pegfilgrastim, polymer protein conjugate, 1720t
Peginesatide, polymer protein conjugate, 1720t
Peginterferon alfa-2a, PEG molecular weight in, 686t
Peginterferon alfa-2b, polymer protein conjugate,
    1720t
Pegloticase, polymer protein conjugate, 1720t
Pegnivacogin, 896
Pegvisomant, polymer protein conjugate, 1720t
Pegylation, 686
Pelagia noctiluca (mauve stinger), 1568. *See also*
    Cnidaria (jellyfish)
Pelagia noctiluca (mauve stinger, purple-striped
    jellyfish), 1567t
Pelamis platurus (yellow-bellied sea snake), 1574–1575
Peliosis hepatis, 331t, 618
Peltzman effect, 527
Pemberton, J.S., 8
Pemetrexed
  hydrolysis, by glucarpidase, 785
  mechanism and site of action, 762f, 775
  toxicity, management, 779
Pemoline
  dopamine release by, 214
  volume of distribution, 1102
Pemphigoid, 276t
  drug-induced, 276
Pemphigus, 276t
  paraneoplastic, 276, 276t
  penicillin and, 823
  xenobiotic-triggered, 276t
Pemphigus foliaceus, 270f
Pemphigus vulgaris, 270f, 276, 277f
Penbutolol
  overdose/poisoning, clinical manifestations, 932
  pharmacology, 927t, 930
Pencil tree (*Euphorbia tirucalli*), 1613
Pendetide, 1779
Pendimethalin, 1468t
Penicillamine, 1779
  dermal effects, 276, 276t
  and gustatory dysfunction, 365
  overdose/poisoning, chest X-ray findings in, 125t
  renal effects, 390f
  teratogenicity, 430t
D-Penicillamine, 1285

adverse effects and side effects, 1287, 1302
  in bismuth toxicity, 1257
  for copper poisoning, 1287
  effects on bioavailability, 144
  indications for, 35t
  for lead poisoning, 1302
  for mercury poisoning, 1330
  and Prussian blue, combined, for thallium toxicity,
    1354, 1358
  teratogenicity, 1289
  and thallium chelation, 1354
  for Wilson disease, 1286–1287
Penicillin(s), 823–824. *See also specific penicillin*
  adverse effects, with therapeutic use, 823
  allergy to, 823
  anaphylactic reactions with, 823, 823t
  antistaphylococcal, 823–824
  cholestasis caused by, 330
  dermal effects, 276
  and GABA receptor, 222
  history of, 821
  Hoigne syndrome caused by, 824
  intrathecal administration, inadvertent overdose
    and unintentional exposures due to, 797t
  Jarisch-Herxheimer reaction with, 824
  mechanism of action, 822t
  nucleus, structure, 823
  overdose, 822t, 823
  renal effects, 390f
  seizures caused by, 222, 823
  toxicity, 822t
Penicillin G, 823–824
  for amatoxin-induced liver toxicity, 1585
Penicillin V, 823–824
Penicilliosis, in HIV-infected (AIDS) patients, 830t
Penile erection. *See also* Erectile dysfunction
  physiology, 298, 299f
Pennies
  ingestion, management, 1365
  zinc in, 1363–1365
Pennyroyal (*Mentha pulegium, Hedeoma pulegioides*),
    632, 639, 1600t–1601t
  as abortifacient, 303t, 632
  hepatotoxicity, 651
  toxicity, *N*-acetylcysteine for, 492, 494
  use and toxicities, 643t
Pennyroyal oil, 631–632
  toxicity
    diagnostic tests for, 634
    treatment, 635
Pentachlorophenol, 178
  and ATP synthesis, 176t
  and electron transport, 176t
  hospital laundry poisoning from, 20t
  hyperventilation caused by, 400t
Pentamidine
  acute tubular necrosis caused by, 392
  cardiac effects, 258t
  for HIV-related infections, 831t
  hypomagnesemia caused by, 877
  mechanism of action, 227t, 228
  and pancreatic dysfunction, 295t
  and prolonged QT interval, 253t
Pentanochlor, in herbicides, 1467t
Pentasaccharide, as anticoagulant, 896
  antidotes and treatment strategies for, 888t
  laboratory testing for, 888t
Pentazocine
  characteristics, 526t
  effects on kappa receptor, 521

injection, parabens in, 685t
scleroderma-like reaction with, 281
and serotonin toxicity, 1058t
talc retinopathy from, 361
Pentetate calcium trisodium (Ca-DTPA), 1779–1781
  adverse effects and safety issues, 1780
  dosage and administration, 1780–1781
  formulation and acquisition, 1781
  orphan drug designation and, 1834
  pharmacodynamics, 1779–1780
  in pregnancy and lactation, 1781
Pentetate zinc trisodium (Zn-DTPA), 1779–1781, 1779f.
    See also Diethylenetriaminepentaacetic acid
    (DTPA)
  adverse effects and safety issues, 1780
  dosage and administration, 1780–1781
  formulation and acquisition, 1781
  pharmacodynamics, 1779–1780
  in pregnancy and lactation, 1781
Pentetic acid (DTPA), 1779–1781, 1779f
  as antidote for radiation poisoning, 1773
Pentetrotide, 1779
Pentobarbital. *See also* Sedative-hypnotics
  in capital punishment, 13
  injection, propylene glycol in, 688
  pharmacokinetics, 1085t
Pentobarbital sodium, injection, propylene glycol in,
    687t
Pentostan. *See* Sodium stibogluconate
Pentostatin, adverse effects and safety issues, 760t
Pepper, odor, 364t
Pepper mace, 1657
Peppermint oil, 632–633
Pepper spray, 1657, 1749–1750, 1749f, 1751t
  ophthalmic exposure to, 359
    irrigating solution for, 359t
Peptic ulcer disease (PUD), xenobiotic-induced,
    293–294, 294t
Peptic ulcer perforation, imaging, 127
Peptide hormones, as athletic performance enhancers,
    619–620
Peptides. *See also specific peptide*
  definition, 1597
  in plants, 1597, 1608–1609
Peracetic acid, as sterilant, 1368
Perampanel, 227t, 229
  adverse effects and safety issues, 727t
  drug interactions with, 723t, 724
  mechanism of action, 720f, 720t, 724
  metabolism and effects on CYP enzymes, 722t
  overdose/poisoning, 724
  pharmacokinetics and toxicokinetics, 721t, 724
  pharmacology, 719, 720t
Perchloroethylene
  pharmacology, 1410
  scleroderma-like reaction with, 281
Perfluorocarbon partial liquid ventilation, 1658–1659
Performance enhancers, athletic, 616–626. *See also*
    Athletic performance enhancers
Pergolide, 806
  cardiac effects, 806–807
Perhexiline
  and fatty acid metabolism, 176t
  liver injury caused by, 329
Pericardial effusions, imaging, 115t, 126
Pericarditis
  antimonials and, 1232
  in arsenic poisoning, 1241
Perilymph, 366
Period(s), in periodic table of elements, 155, 156f

Periodic Table of the Elements, 155, 156f
  nomenclature for, 155
  periodicity, definition, 155
Peripheral α₁-adrenergic antagonists, as
    antihypertensives, 959, 962
Peripheral nervous system (PNS)
  hydrocarbons and, 1414
  muscarinic agonists and, 207
  muscarinic blockade and, 207
  nicotinic receptor agonists and antagonists and, 207
  thallium and, 1351
Peripheral neuropathy(ies)
  after periphetral nerve block, 997
  in arsenic poisoning, 1241
  carbon monoxide poisoning and, 1665
  chemotherapeutic-related, 763
  in DEG poisoning, 1446
  disulfiram-induced, 1175
  in ethylene glycol poisoning, 1424–1425
  lead-induced, 1295, 1297–1298
  sensory, with gastrointestinal complaints,
    differential diagnosis, 1222, 1222t
  sodium stibogluconate and, 1233
  thallium-induced, 1351
  xenobiotic-induced, 345–346
Peripheral polyradiculoneuropathy, in ethylene glycol
    poisoning, 1424
Peritoneal dialysis (PD), 38
  annual reported use of, 90, 90t
  and chromium, 1271
  and copper poisoning, 1289
  efficacy, 93
  indications for, 93
  and pharmacokinetics, 390
  and potassium balance, 199
  technique for, 93
Peritonitis, activated charcoal and, 79
Periwinkle (Catharanthus roseus), 1599t
  psychoactive properties, 650t
  use and toxicities, 643t
Permanganates, 1319
Permeabilizing agents, site of action, 173f
Permethrin, 1519, 1520t
  safety, 1520
  structure, 1520f
  uses, 1520
Peroxidase, 175
  acetaminophen and, 472
Peroxidase-catalase system, in hepatic peroxisomes, in
    ethanol metabolism, 1144–1145, 1145f
Peroxide tone, acetaminophen and, 472
Peroxisome proliferator activator receptor(s) (PPAR),
    PPAR-γ
  agonists, and opioid tolerance and withdrawal, 238
  opioids and, 238
Peroxisomes, hepatic, in ethanol metabolism,
    1144–1145, 1145f
Peroxyl radical, structure, 160t
Peroxynitrite anion, 160, 1656
  structure, 160t
Perphenazine. See also Antipsychotics
  clinical and toxicologic effects, 1034t
  dosage and administration, 1033t
  pharmacokinetics, 1033t
Per se xenobiotic laws, 1144, 1873, 1876–1878
Persistence
  of chemical weapons, 1741
  definition, 1741
Persistent organic chemicals, 1518
Personality disorders, and violence, 385

Personal protective equipment (PPE), 71
  for chemical weapons, 1742, 1742t, 1743
  in hazardous materials incident response, 1807,
    1809–1811, 1810f, 1810t
  in hydrofluoric acid poisoning management, 1400
  levels, 71, 1809, 1810t
  and respiratory protection, 1810–1811
  and workplace exposure control, 1800
  and zinc inhalation, 1365
Peruvian bark. See Cinchona spp.
Peruvian lily (Alstroemeria spp.), allergic contact
    dermatitis from, 1614
Peruvian torch cactus (Trichocereus peruvianus), 1180
Pesticides, 12, 1503. See also Fumigants; Insecticides
  coingestion with ethanol, 1490
  deaths caused by, 1486
    global burden of, 1844
  definition, 1450
  Environmental Protection Agency (EPA) toxicity
    classification, 1450, 1450t
  eye irritation by, 1450t
  LC₅₀, inhalation, 1450t
  LD₅₀, 1466
    dermal, 1450t
    oral, 1450t
  and methemoglobinemia, 1703
  pancreatitis caused by, 295t
  pediatric poisoning with, case study, 1450–1451
  poisoning, in developing world, 1844
    prevention strategies, 1848, 1848t
  rat LD₅₀, 1486, 1486t
  regulation, 1450
  self-poisoning with, 1844–1845, 1845t
  skin irritation by, 1450t
  taste-aversive xenobiotics in, 1782
  toxicity
    gastrointestinal decontamination for, 59t
    WHO classification, 1486, 1486t
  WHO classification, 1450, 1486t
Pet food, melamine in, 19
Petroleum, 1410
  distillates, 1409–1410
  thermal degradation products, 1641t
Petroselinum crispum (parsley), 643t
Petrus Abbonus, 1t
Peyote (Lophophora williamsii), 1178, 1180, 1181t,
    1601t, 1605
  ancient use of, 3
  toxicokinetics, 1182
P-glycoprotein, 144, 168, 173, 341–342
  age-related changes in, 461
  calcium channel blockers and, 946
  and colchicine, 502
  gene for, 144
  inducers, 144
  induction, for paraquat poisoning, 1474f, 1477
  inhibitors, 144, 173
  and plant–xenobiotic interactions, 1610–1611
  rifampin and, 855
  St. John's wort and, 646
  in xenobiotic metabolism, 293
pH, 160. See also Acid–base abnormality(ies)
  of acid/base solutions, 161, 161t
  arterial, 190
  of body fluids, 142t
  manipulation, pharmacokinetic effects, 152
  ocular, checking, 39–40, 73
  postmortem changes, 1885t
  renal regulation of, 389
  and respiratory drive, 399

  urinary, manipulation, 93. See also Urine,
    acidification; Urine, alkalinization
  venous, 190
  and xenobiotic absorption, 142
  and xenobiotic adsorption to activated charcoal, 76
  and xenobiotic desorption (dissociation) from
    activated charcoal, 77
Phalloidin, 1583
Phallotoxins, 1581–1583
  mushrooms containing, 1582t
Phantastics, 7
Phantosmia, 364, 364t
Pharmaceutical additives, 681–693. See also specific
    additive
  functions, 681
  toxicity, history of, 681
Pharmaceuticals, poisoning with, in developing world,
    1845–1846
Pharmacist(s)
  clinical, service-based, 1829
  medication review by, 1827
Pharmacobezoars, 49
  endoscopic removal, 64
  formation, 49, 51f–52f
Pharmacodynamics. See also specific xenobiotic
  definition, 109, 140
  in elderly, 463
  and laboratory test results, 109
Pharmacogenetics, 172
  in postmortem toxicology, 1888
Pharmacognosy, 1597
Pharmacokinetics
  bariatric surgery and, 148, 293
  definition, 109, 140
  in elderly, 461–463, 461t
  factors affecting, 140
  hemodialysis and, 390
  kidney disease and, 389
  and laboratory test results, 109
  neonatal, 442
  peritoneal dialysis and, 390
  in pregnancy, 428
  of xenobiotics with significant morbidity and
    mortality, 145t–146t
Pharmacy Act (1868), 8
Phase II block, 1020
Phase III metabolism, 172
Phaseolus spp., cyanogenic glycosides in, 1684
Phase I reactions, 147, 168
Phase II reactions, 147, 168, 172
Phase III reactions, 168
Pheasants eye (Adonis microcarpa), 979
Phenacetin, 472
  in cocaine, 1130
  sulfhemoglobin from, 1710
Phenazopyridine, methemoglobinemia caused by,
    1705
  with hemolysis, 1706
Phenbenzamine, history of, 738
Phencyclidine (PCP), 1179, 1179t, 1210–1221
  absorption, 1211
  and agitation/violence, 385
  analogs, 1211, 1211t
    and NMDA receptors, 1213–1214
  available forms, 1212
  brain changes caused by, imaging, 132t
  chemical structure, 1210
  chemistry, 1211
  cigarettes dipped in, 1212
  CNS effects, duration, 1212

Phencyclidine (PCP) (*Cont.*):
DEA class, 1210–1211
decontamination for, 1217
dependence, 1216
derivatives, 1210
and dextromethorphan, structural similarity, 532, 532f
diagnostic tests for, 1216–1217
duration of effects, 1211–1212
effects on vital signs, 29t–31t
elimination, 1212
emergence reaction with, 1216–1217
enzyme immunoassay for, 1216
history and epidemiology, 1210–1211
hyperthermia caused by, 27, 27t
laboratory testing for, 101, 101t
leaf mixtures, 1212
in marijuana cigarettes, 1212
mechanism of action, 210, 210t, 211, 227t
metabolism, 1212
neurotoxicity, 343, 1182
nicotinic receptor blockade by, 207
and NMDA receptors, 228, 1213–1214
pharmacokinetics, 1211–1212
and respiratory depression, 1214
and rhabdomyolysis, 393t
screening for, 110, 113
as street drug, 1210
street names for, 1210
tolerance, 1216
toxicity, 211
agitation in, management, 1217
blood pressure in, 1214
cardiopulmonary effects, 1214
clinical manifestations, 36t, 1214–1217
and dysrhythmias, 1214
heart rate in, 1214
hyperthermia in, 1214
and hypoventilation, 1214
management, 1217–1218
neuropsychiatric effects, 1214–1215
vital signs in, 1214
toxicokinetics, 1211–1212
urine screening assays for, performance characteristics, 111t
withdrawal, 1216
Phendimetrazine, for weight loss, 606, 608t
Phenelzine, 1076–1077. *See also* Monoamine oxidase inhibitors (MAOIs)
and neuromuscular blockers, interactions, 1021t
priapism caused by, 301t
and serotonin toxicity, 1058t
structure, 1076f
Phenformin
and high anion gap metabolic acidosis, 191t
history of, 694
hyperventilation caused by, 400t
lactic acidosis caused by, 694
and metabolic acidosis with elevated lactate concentration, 703
pharmacokinetics and toxicokinetics, 697t
structure, 695f
Phenibut, and GABA receptor, 222
Phenindione, 885
Pheniramine, pharmacology, 742
Phenmedipham, in herbicides, 1467t
Phenobarbital. *See also* Sedative-hypnotics
and acetaminophen toxicity, 480
acute interstitial nephritis caused by, 394t
for agitation, in thyrotoxicosis, 817

for alcohol withdrawal, 222
antidote for, 35t
and CYP induction, 171
drug contamination with, 20, 20t
drug-induced hypersensitivity syndrome with, 277, 727–728
effect on thyroid hormones and function, 814t, 817
elimination, multiple-dose activated charcoal and, 78
enhanced elimination, urine alkalinization for, 93
and enterohepatic circulation, 172
and female sexual dysfunction, 302f
and gingival hyperplasia, 293
history of, 719
indications for, 35t
laboratory testing for, 101t, 102
for lead encephalopathy, in children, 1302
in mass suicide, 24
mechanism of action, 221
metabolism and effects on CYP enzymes, 722t
for neonatal opioid withdrawal, 439
pharmacokinetics, 145t, 721t, 1085t, 1087
protein-binding characteristics, 110t
for resistant alcohol withdrawal, 1169
serum assays for, 113
toxicity (overdose/poisoning)
alkalinization for, 570
clinical and laboratory findings with, 32
extracorporeal elimination for, 97t
lipid emulsion for, 1006
management, 38
multiple-dose activated charcoal for, 61, 570, 1087
sodium bicarbonate for, 568t
toxicokinetics, 145t, 721t
volume of distribution, 91, 145t
for xenobiotic-induced seizures, 1138
Phenobarbital sodium, injection, propylene glycol in, 687t
Phenol(s) (carbolic acid), 642t, 1373, 1388t, 1410
antimicrobial activity, 685
cutaneous absorption, 271, 685–686, 1411
decontamination, 74, 272, 1416
dermal absorption, 271, 685–686, 1411
dermal decontamination for, 74, 272
as disinfectants, 1368
history of, 1368
nonsubstituted, 1369t
ophthalmic exposure to, irrigating solution for, 359, 359t
ophthalmic toxicity, 356f
as pharmaceutical additive, 685–686, 685t
pharmacokinetics, 685
physicochemical properties, 685
from plants, 1597, 1598t–1603t, 1609–1610
poisoning, 1373
structure, 685
substituted, 1369t, 1373–1374
and ATP synthesis, 176t
and electron transport, 176t
TAR (titratable acid/alkaline reserve), 1388
transdermal absorption, 271, 685–686, 1411
uses, 73
Phenolic glucuronide, 634
Phenol/resorcinol/fuchsin, toxicity, organ system manifestations, 829t
Phenothiazines, 1032
on abdominal radiography, 1040
aliphatic, 1032, 1033t
and antimalarial resistance, 836
cardiac effects, 248f, 258t

for chemotherapeutic-related vomiting, 764
clinical and laboratory findings with, 36t
contraindications to, 990, 1128–1129, 1217
and cyclic antidepressants, structural similarity, 1032, 1034f
effects on immunoassays for tricyclic antidepressants, 1040
effects on vital signs, 29t
and ethanol, interactions, 1146t
mechanism of action, 214
and neuroleptic malignant syndrome, 215
piperazine, 1032, 1033t
piperidine, 1032, 1033t
priapism caused by, 301t
and QT interval, 253t
radiopacity, 114
and thermoregulation, 413
Phenothrin, 1519, 1520t. *See also* Pyrethroids
Phenoxy acid, 1466
Phenoxybenzamine, 926
Phenoxy herbicides, 17, 1469t, 1480–1482, 1481f. *See also* Herbicides
absorption, 1481
mechanism of toxicity, 1481
pharmacokinetics and toxicokinetics, 1481
rernal clearance, 1481
tissue distribution, 1481
toxicity
clinical manifestations, 1481
diagnostic tests for, 1482
management, 1482
mortality rate for, 1482
pathophysiology, 1481
Phenprocoumon, 885
Phentermine, 606, 607t, 1102. *See also* Dieting xenobiotics and regimens
detection, 112
elimination, 1102
elimination half-life, 1102
and fenfluramine, combined, safety problems with, 1841
volume of distribution, 1102
Phentermine/topiramate, 606–607, 607t. *See also* Dieting xenobiotics and regimens
pharmacology, 610
for weight loss, 610
Phentolamine
for amphetamine toxicity, 1104–1105, 1104t
and disulfiramlike reactions, 1174t
for erectile dysfunction, 300
hypoglycemia caused by, 715
indications for, 35t, 751
mechanism of action, 210, 300
priapism caused by, 301t
Phenylalkalamines, 217
β-Phenyl-γ-amino butyric acid. *See* Phenibut
Phenylarsine oxide, 1239
Phenylbutazone, 647
elimination, multiple-dose activated charcoal and, 78
hematologic effects, 516
inhibition of glucuronidation, 172
overdose/poisoning, multiple-dose activated charcoal in, 61
pharmacology, 512t
Phenylephrine
benzalkonium chloride in, 682t
duration of action, 749t
pharmacokinetics and toxicokinetics, 749
pharmacology, 749

for priapism, 301
therapeutic effects, 749t
toxicity, 749t
Phenylethanolamine-*N*-methyl-transferase, 208
Phenylethylamines (amphetamines), 1099, 1178, 1179t.
See also Amphetamine(s)
clinical effects, 1183–1184
DEA class, 1180–1181
designer, 1180–1181
endogenous, 1180
exogenous, 1180
laboratory findings with, 1184
and NMDA receptor, 1182
pharmacology, 1182–1183
and serotonin receptors, 1182
and serotonin toxicity, 1058t
structure, 1105
structure modification, 1101–1102, 1102t
toxicity, clinical manifestations, 1183
Phenylic acid. *See* Phenol(s) (carbolic acid)
Phenylic alcohol. *See* Phenol(s) (carbolic acid)
β-Phenylisopropylamine, 1099. *See also*
Amphetamine(s)
Phenylmercury, 1324t. *See also* Mercury
Phenylpropanoids
definition, 1597
from plants, 1597, 1598t–1602t, 1609–1610
Phenylpropanolamine (norephedrine), 606–607
adverse effects and safety issues, 608t
brain changes caused by, imaging, 132t
cardiovascular effects, management, 751
and hemorrhagic stroke, 1837, 1854
hemorrhagic stroke associated with, 748
market withdrawal, 608t
mechanism of action, 608t
pharmacology, 749
stroke caused by, 21
structure, 610f, 749f
toxicity, clinical manifestations, 750
Phenyl-2-propanone (P2P), 1105
Phenytoin
and acetaminophen toxicity, 480
acute interstitial nephritis caused by, 394t
adjusted concentration, calculation, 146
adverse effects and safety issues, 724, 727–728,
727t, 866t
albumin binding by, 146
for cardioactive steroid poisoning, 973–974
choreoathetosis with, 214
clearance, and extracorporeal removal, 92
contraindications to, 1051
drug-induced hypersensitivity syndrome with,
277, 278f, 727–728, 727t
drug interactions with, 723t, 852
effect on thyroid hormones and function, 814t
elimination, multiple-dose activated charcoal and,
78
and ethanol, interactions, 1146t
and female sexual dysfunction, 302f
and fosphenytoin, conversion factor, 724
free vs. protein-bound, 146
and gingival hyperplasia, 293
and gustatory dysfunction, 365
hepatotoxicity, 330
history of, 719, 724
iatrogenic toxicity, 152
injection, propylene glycol in, 687, 687t
laboratory testing for, 101t
mechanism of action, 231, 720f, 720t
metabolism and effects on CYP enzymes, 722t, 724

and neuromuscular blockers, interactions, 1021t
pharmacokinetics, 721t, 724, 866t
in elderly, 462
pharmacology, 719, 720t, 866t
plasma protein binding by, 109
pregnancy category, 724
pregnancy outcomes with, 724
protein-binding characteristics, 110, 110t
respiratory effects, 399t
for seizures, in alcoholic patients, 1167
and suicide risk, 719
teratogenicity, 430t
therapeutic serum concentration, 724
toxicity (overdose/poisoning)
clinical manifestations, 36t, 724
diagnostic imaging, 115t, 126
diagnostic tests for, 724
extracorporeal elimination for, 92, 97t
gastrointestinal decontamination for, 86
hilar lymphadenopathy caused by, 126
liver support devices for, 96
management, 724
multiple-dose activated charcoal in, 61
toxic metabolite, 174t
toxicokinetics, 721t, 724
and vincristine, interactions, 506
Pheochromocytoma, 273
glucagon and, 943
Philanthotoxins, 227t
Philodendron spp., 1601t, 1613
Phlebotomy, for blood alcohol testing, and driver
involved in motor vehicle crash, 1862–1864
Phocomelia, thalidomide-induced, 1833
Phomopsis spp., in biological warfare, 1759
Phoneutria nigriventer (Brazilian wandering spider),
envenomation by, priapism caused by,
301t
Phoradendron spp. (mistletoe), 643t, 1601t, 1609
Phorate, 1488t
Phoratoxin, 1601t
Phorbol esters, 1600t
Phosgene (carbonyl chloride), 1656
airway injury by, 1640t, 1641, 1748–1749
ARDS caused by, 401
as chemical weapon, 1741, 1748–1749
decontamination for, 1743
detection threshold, 1654t
diffuse airspace filling caused by, 123, 125t
exposure, *N*-acetylcysteine for, 1653
immediately dangerous to life and health (IDLH),
1654t
mechanism of toxicity, 1653, 1748–1749, 1749f
odor, 364t, 1748
physical characteristics, 1748
as pulmonary irritant, 1748–1749
regulatory standard for, 1654t
respiratory effects, 399t
short-term exposure limit (STEL), 1654t
sources, 1654t
in terrorism, 1744
as thermal degradation product, 1641t
toxicity, clinical effects, 1749
toxic syndrome caused by, 1751t
in warfare, 17, 17t, 1651, 1656, 1748–1749
water solubility, 1654t
Phosgene oxime (CX)
chemical name and structure, 1747f
clinical effects, 1748
toxic syndrome caused by, 1751t
as urticant, 1748

Phosinothricin (glufosinate). *See* Glufosinate
Phosphamidon, 1488t
Phosphate, 1486
balance, renal regulation of, 389
excess, hypocalcemia caused by, 199
calcium for, 1405
inorganic, pentavalent arsenic and, 1239, 1239f
Phosphate binders, aluminum-containing, 1225
Phosphate of soda, 83
Phosphatidylinositol 3-kinase (PI3K), 953–954, 954f
calcium-channel blockers and, 953–954, 954f
Phosphides, poisoning with, magnesium for, 879
Phosphine (phosphine gas), 1457–1460, 1529
absorption, 1458
clinical effects, 1458t
and electron transport, 176t
elimination half-life, 1458
history of, 1457
immediately dangerous to life and health (IDLH), 1654t
industrial uses, 1457t
odor, 1457
physicochemical properties, 1457, 1457t
recommended exposure limit, 1458
regulatory standard for, 1654t
self-poisoning with, 879
short-term exposure limit (STEL), 1458, 1654t
sources, 1654t
tissue distribution, 1458
toxicity
clinical manifestations, 1458
epidemiology, 1457
mechanisms, 1458
prognosis for, 1459
toxicological analyses in, 1459
treatment, 1459–1460
toxicodynamics, 1458
toxicokinetics, 1458
uses, 1457
water solubility, 1654t
Phosphodiesterase inhibitors, 899
for β-adrenergic antagonist toxicity, 934–935
adverse effects and safety issues, 301
antidotes and treatment strategies for, 888t
for calcium channel blocker toxicity, 948
drug interactions with, 301
effects on vital signs, 29t
for erectile dysfunction, 301
glucagon with, 942
laboratory testing for, 888t
and male sexual function, 299f
mechanism of action, 898f, 933f
methylxanthines as, 986
and nitrates, hypotension caused by, 301
ophthalmic toxicity, 356f
pharmacokinetics, 301
priapism caused by, 301t
Phosphofructokinase, antimony and, 1229
Phospholamban, 262
in cardiac physiology, 928–929, 929f
Phospholipase A, phospholipase A_2 (PLA, PLA_2), 897
and archidonic acid metabolism, 511, 513f
in Cnidaria venom, 1569
in Hymenoptera venom, 1551, 1551t
in lizard venom, 1619
in sea snake venom, 1575
in sea star venom, 1574
in snake venom, 1618–1620, 1619t, 1637
Phospholipase C (PLC)
inhibitors, 1503
in neurotransmission, 204

Phospholipidosis, diagnostic imaging, 115t, 125t
Phospholipids, 141
  in lipid emulsion, 1004
Phosphoric acid, 1388t
Phosphorofluoridates, history of, 1486
Phosphorus, 1528–1532. *See also* Organic phosphorus
      compounds
  Borgias' use of, 4
  burns caused by, 1528, 1530
  central nervous system effects, 1529–1530
  chemistry, 168, 1528
  dermal exposure to
    clinical manifestations, 1530
    decontamination for, 1531
    management, 1530–1531
  diagnostic testing for, 1530
  early use of, 5t
  ECG changes caused by, 1529
  elemental
    estimated fatal dose, 1452t
    physicochemical properties, 1452t
    in rodenticides, 1452t
    toxicity
      antidote and/or treatment, 1452t
      clinical manifestations, 1452t
      onset, 1452t
      toxic mechanism, 1452t
  gastrointestinal exposure to, management, 1531
  hepatic effects, 334t
  hepatotoxicity, 1529
  history of, 1528
  ingestion
    N-acetylcysteine for, 1531
    cardiovascular effects, 1529
    gastrointestinal effects, 1529
    management, 1530–1531
  in methamphetamine synthesis, 1528
  neurotoxicity, 1529–1530
  occupational diseases caused by, 23
  odor, 364t
  organic. *See* Organic phosphorus compounds
  pharmacokinetics, 1528
  pharmacology, 1528
  physicochemical properties, 1528
  poisoning
    clinical manifestations, 1452t, 1529–1530
    diagnosis, 1530
    electrolyte disturbances caused by, 1529
    management, 1530–1531
  renal effects, 1529
  serum, normal concentration, 1528
  sources, 1388t
  toxicokinetics, 1528
  white. *See* White phosphorus
Phosphorus pentoxide, 1528
Phosphorus trioxide, 1528
Phosphorylcholines, 1487, 1488t
Phossy jaw, 22–23, 23t, 1528
Photinus spp., 969
Photoallergens, 280
Photoallergic reactions, 280
Photoanethole, 641t
Photons, 1763
Photopatch test, 280
Photopsia, 972
Photosensitivity, 274t
  antipsychotic-induced, 1039
  NSAID-induced, 515
  pathophysiology, 280
  plant-induced, 1600t–1601t, 1603t, 1613–1614

  direct, 1613–1614
  hepatogenous, 1613–1614
  xenobiotics causing, 280, 281f
Phototoxic dermatitis, 274t, 276, 280
Phrenic nerveparalysis, in arsenic poisoning, 1241
ortho-Phthalaldehyde, as disinfectant, 1368, 1369t, 1375
Phylloerythrin, 1601t
  hepatogenous photosensitivity caused by, 1614
Physalia spp.
  stings, epidemiology, 1569
  venom, cardiotoxicity, 1570
Physalia physalis (Portuguese man-of-war), 1567, 1567t,
      1568, 1568f, 1571. *See also* Cnidaria (jellyfish)
  deaths caused by, 1568
  dermal reaction to, pathophysiology, 1569
  stings, management, 1569
Physalia utriculus (bluebottle), 1567, 1567t, 1570.
      See also Cnidaria (jellyfish)
Physical examination
  of conscious patient, 39
  in inital assessment, 189
Physical hazards, workplace, 1797, 1797t
Physician health programs (PHPs), 1866
Physician impairment, reporting, 1866
Physician–patient relationship, legal considerations, 1865
Physicians, as poisoners, 6, 12
Physicians' Desk Reference (PDR), limitations, 1789
Physick, Philip, 4t, 7
Physic nut
  Jatropha curcas, 1601t
  Ricinus communis, 1602t
    in biologic warfare, 1759
Physostigma venenosum (calabar bean, ordeal bean),
      1, 755, 1486, 1601t, 1605.
      See also Physostigmine
Physostigmine (physostigmine salicylate), 1, 755–758,
      1487, 1601t, 1605
  adverse effects and safety issues, 756–757
  for anticholinergic poisoning, 748, 1604
  antidote for, 35t, 755
  for antihistamine overdose, 748
  for antimuscarinic toxicity, 756
  for antipsychotic overdose, 1041
  for atropine overdose/poisoning, 755, 1505
  availability and storage, 45t
  for belladonna alkaloid poisoning, 1184
  cardiac effects, 756
  for central antimuscarinic syndrome, 1041
  chemistry, 165
  contraindications to, 748, 755–756, 1051
  dosage and administration, 748, 757
  drug interactions with, 756–757
  enantiomers, 165
  excess, 28
  formulation, 757
  history of, 755, 1486
  indications for, 35t, 45t, 736
  as ketamine antagonist, 1215
  mechanism of action, 207–208
  monitoring with, 748
  pharmacokinetics and pharmacodynamics, 756
  in pregnancy and lactation, 757
  stocking, recommended level, 45t
  structure, 755f
Phytocannabinoids, 1111, 1112f, 1113
  pharmacokinetics and toxicokinetics, 1113–1115
Phytodermatitis, 280
Phytoestrogen(s), 644t
  as abortifacient, 303t
  in red clover, 1603t

Phytolacca americana (pokeweed), 644t, 1601t, 1608f,
      1609
Phytolaccaceae, 1601t
Phytolacca decandra (pokeweed), 644t
Phytolaccagenic acid, 644t
Phytolaccatoxin, 1601t, 1608f
Phytolaccigenin, 644t
Phytotoxins, 644t
Pibloktoq, 654–655
Pica, lead exposure from, in pregnancy, 1304
Picardin (Bayrepel, KBR3023), 1524
  comparative efficacy and toxicity, 1523t
Picric acid, yellow skin caused by, 272
Picrotin, 222
Picrotoxin
  and GABA receptor, 222
  as glycine antagonist, 223
Picrotoxinin, 222
Piedras della cobra de Capelos, 3
Pigeon breeder's lung, 125, 125t
Pigeon pea (*Cajanus cajan*), as abortifacient, 303t
Pigmentation, skin, xenobiotic-induced alterations, 273
Pigment blue 27. *See* Prussian blue
Pigmenturia, renal effects, 393
pillreports.net, 1184
Pilocarpine, 1495t, 1496, 1503, 1601t, 1605
  benzalkonium chloride in, 682t
  ophthalmic use, systemic toxicity with, 360
Pilocarpus jaborandi (pilocarpus, jaborandi), 1601t,
      1605
Pilocarpus pinnatifolius, 1601t
Piloerection, in response to cold, 414
Pilosebaceous follicle, 270–271
Pilot whales
  mercury in, 1328
  PCBs in, 1328
Pimobendan
  for β-adrenergic antagonist toxicity, 935
  mechanism of action, 933f
Pimozide. *See also* Antipsychotics
  clinical and toxicologic effects, 1034t
  dosage and administration, 1033t
  pharmacokinetics, 1033t
  and QT interval, 253t
Pinang (*Areca catechu*), uses and toxicities, 640t
Pindolol
  overdose/poisoning, clinical manifestations, 932
  pharmacology, 927t, 930
  structure, 926f
Pindone
  physicochemical properties, 1453t
  in rodenticides, 1453t
  toxicity
    antidote and/or treatment for, 1453t
    clinical manifestations, 1453t
    onset, 1453t
    toxic mechanism, 1453t
Pineapples, dermatitis caused by, 1613
Pinellia, 748
Pinene and α-pinene, 1380, 1410. *See also* Camphor
Pine oil, 633, 1410
  toxicity, 1415
Pine processionary caterpillars (*Thaumetopoea
      pityocampa*), 1552–1553
Piney thistle (*Atractylis*), 640t
Pink disease, 1324, 1327
Pinlang (*Areca catechu*), uses and toxicities, 640t
Pinna, 3
Pinpoint pupil, opioids and, 524
Pinus spp., 633

Pioglitazone
    adverse effects and safety issues, 700
    hepatotoxicity, 331
    pharmacokinetics and toxicokinetics, 697t
Piperacillin, 823–824
Piperaquine, 842
    antimalarial mechanism, 838t
    pharmacokinetics, 839t
    structure, 844
    toxicity, 844
Piperine, pharmacologic interactions, 646t
Piper longum Linn. See Piperine
Piper methysticum (kava kava), 650t, 1602t, 1607
    psychoactive properties, 650t
    use and toxicity, 643t
Piper nigrum Linn. See Piperine
Piperonyl butoxide, 1515, 1519–1520
    absorption, 1520
    metabolism, 1521
Piperophos, 1468t
Pipotiazine. *See also* Antipsychotics
    dosage and administration, 1033t
    pharmacokinetics, 1033t
Piracetam, mechanism of action, 227t
Pirbuterol, 985
Pirfenidone, for paraquat poisoning, 1474f, 1476
Piroxicam
    adverse effects and safety issues, 515
    and ATP synthesis, 176t
    overdose/poisoning, multiple-dose activated
        charcoal in, 61
    pharmacology, 511, 512t
Piso, William, 4, 4t
Pistachio (*Pistacia vera*), 1614
Pistacia vera, 1614
Pit cells, hepatic, 327, 329f
Pitolisant, 742
Pituitary, and thyroid function, 812, 813f
Pit vipers (Crotalinae), 1617–1618, 1617t, 1618f, 1633,
        1633t
    antivenom, 35t, 1623–1625
        for children, 1624
        in pregnancy, 1624
    bites
        pressure immobilization bandages for, 1623
        surgery for, 1624
    distingushing features, 1617, 1618f
    dry bites, 1620t, 1621
    envenomation
        antivenom for, 1620t
        blood products for, 1624
        clinical manifestations, 36t, 1620–1622, 1620t,
            1621f
        coagulation effects, 1619–1620, 1619t,
            1624–1625
        diagnosis, 1623
        ecchymosis caused by, 1621, 1621f
        edema caused by, 1621, 1621f
        evaluation, 1620t
        follow-up care for, 1624–1625
        hematologic toxicity, 1622, 1624–1625
        hemorrhagic bullae/blebs caused by, 1621,
            1621f
        hospital care for, 1623
        local reactions to, 1621–1622, 1621f
        local tissue damage in, 1619, 1619t
        management, 1620t, 1623–1625
        myonecrosis caused by, 1621–1622
        neurotoxicity, 1619–1620, 1619t, 1622
        pathophysiology, 1619–1620

platelet effects, 1619–1620, 1619t, 1624–1625
        prehospital care for, 1623
        return/recurrence of symptoms after antivenom
            therapy, 1624–1625
        rhabdomyolysis caused by, 1622
        systemic toxicity, 1622
        treatment, 1623–1625
    neurotoxins, and acetylcholine release, 207, 207t
    venom, components, 1619, 1619t
PK 11195, structure, 1139, 1139f
pK$_a$, 142, 161, 167
pK$_b$, 161
Placebos, 1856
Placenta, xenobiotic transfer across, 431–432
Plague (*Yersinia pestis*), 1756, 1756f
Plancitoxin, 1574
Plantago spp., 1602t
Plant growth regulators, 1466
PLANTOX database, 1597
Plants, 1597–1616. *See also* Herbal preparations;
        specific plant
    with anticholinergic effects, 1598t, 1600t–1603t
    and approach to exposed patient, 1603–1604
    with carcinogenic effects, 1598t–1599t, 1602t
    with cardiac toxicity, 1598t–1603t
    with cardiovascular effects, 1598t–1601t
    with cholinergic effects, 1598t, 1601t
    contact dermatitis caused by, 1598t–1603t,
        1613–1614
    dermatitis caused by, 1598t–1603t, 1613–1614
        allergic, 1599t–1600t, 1603t, 1613
        cytotoxic, 1598t–1603t
        irritant, 1598t–1599t, 1613
        mechanical, 1598t–1603t, 1613
    early poisons from, 1–2
    exposures, epidemiology, 1597
    families, 1597–1603
    and food poisoning, 602
    with gastrointestinal toxicity, 1598t–1603t
    hallucinogenic, 4t
    with hematologic toxicity, 1598t, 1600t–1601t,
        1603t
    with hepatic effects, 1598t–1603t
    hepatic injury associated with, 333
    identification, 1597–1603
    with metabolic effects, 1598t–1603t
    with neurotoxic effects, 1598t–1603t
    nicotine in, 1203
    with nicotinic effects, 1599t, 1601t
    nomenclature, 638
    with oxytocic effects, 1598t–1601t
    photosensitivity caused by, 1600t–1601t, 1603t,
        1613–1614
    with renal effects, 1598t–1603t
    with respiratory effects, 1599t–1601t
    and risk assessment, 1603–1604
    self-poisoning with, in developing world, 1846
    with skeletal effects, 1601t
    with urologic effects, 1602t–1603t
    xenobiotic interactions with, 1611
    xenobiotics from
        alcohol, 1599t, 1610–1611
        alkaloid, 1597, 1598t–1603t, 1604–1606
        amino acid, 1598t, 1601t–1603t
        carbohydrate, 1602t
        carboxylic acid, 1598t, 1600t–1603t, 1610
        cardioactive steroid, 1598t–1601t, 1603t
        classification, 1597, 1598t–1603t
        clinical effects, 1598t–1603t, 1604
        diterpene, 1599t

glucosinolate, 1598t
        glycoalkaloid, 1601t–1602t, 1604
        glycoside group, 1597, 1598t–1599t, 1602t–1603t,
            1606–1607. *See also* Cardiac glycosides
            anthraquinone, 1597, 1598t–1599t, 1602t, 1607
            cyanogenic, 1–2, 1597, 1601t–1602t, 1607
            saponin, 1597, 1598t, 1600t, 1603t, 1606, 1606f
        history of, 1597
        isothiocyanate, 1598t
        lectin, 1597, 1598t, 1601t–1603t, 1608–1609
        lignan, 1603t
        oleoresin, 1599t, 1602t
        peptide, 1597, 1598t, 1601t–1603t, 1608–1609
        phenol, 1597, 1598t–1603t, 1609–1610
        phenylpropanoid, 1597, 1598t–1602t,
            1609–1610
        polypeptide, 1603t
        protein, 1597, 1598t, 1601t–1603t, 1608–1609
        resins, 1597, 1599t, 1602t, 1607–1608
        and sodium channels, 1611–1612
        terpene, 1597
        terpenoid, 1598t–1603t, 1607–1608
        tropane alkaloid, 1599t
        unidentified, 1611
Plant toxicology
    animal studies, 1597
    human data, 1597
Plaque (skin), 269t, 277f
Plasma
    dithionate test for paraquat or diquat, 1475, 1477
    pH, 142t
Plasma cholinesterase (PChE), 206
    in cocaine metabolism, 1124–1125, 1125f
    genetic variants, 1022
    inhibitors, 1020, 1021t, 1022
Plasma exchange
    for acetaminophen removal, 484
    for ricin poisoning in children, 1609
    for vinblastine overdose, 507
Plasma expanders, and doping analysis, 623
Plasmapheresis, 38
    for acetaminophen removal, 484
    for chemotherapeutic toxicity, 764
    for thyroxine overdose, 818
    for vincristine overdose, 507
    xenobiotics amenable to, 98
Plasma protein(s)
    as carriers, 146
    saturation of, 147
    as storage depots, 146
    xenobiotic binding to, 109–110, 110t, 144, 146
        and extracorporeal elimination of xenobiotics, 147
        and laboratory test results, 153
Plasmin, 896–897
Plasminogen, 896–897
Plasminogen activator, 321f, 896–897
Plasminogen activator inhibitor (PAI), 321f, 322
Plasmodium spp., 836
    chloroquine-resistant, 836, 846
    life cycle, 836, 837f
    and antimalarial effects, 837f, 838t
Plasmodium falciparum, 647, 836, 837f, 837t
Plasmodium knowlesi, 836, 837t
Plasmodium malariae, 837f, 837t
Plasmodium ovale, 836, 837t
Plasmodium vivax, 836, 837f, 837t
Plastics
    contact dermatitis from, 280t
    thermal degradation products, 1641t
Plateauing, 617

Platelet(s), 323–324
  activation, 321f, 323, 897
  adhesion, 323, 897
  aggregation, 323, 897, 898f
  in coagulation, 883
  dysfunction, salicylate-induced, 558
  function, 883
    laboratory assessment, 900
    NSAIDs and, 514, 514t, 516
    renal dysfunction and, 900
    SSRIs and, 1058
  structure, 323
Platelet-activating factor, 323
Platelet-derived growth factor receptor (PDGFR), 761
Platelet factor-4, 324
Platelet transfusion, 900
Platinum, 1780
  nephrotoxicity, 397t
Platinum analogs, mechanism and site of action, 762f
Platinum-based complex(es)
  antidotes for, 760t
  as chemotherapeutics, 759, 760t
  neutropenia caused by, 762
Plecanatide, 84
Pleural disorders, imaging, 115t, 126, 127f
Pleural effusions, imaging, 115t, 126
  ultrasound in, 406
Pleuritis, in arsenic poisoning, 1241
Pleurocybella porrigens, 1583t, 1592
Pliny the Elder, 637, 1165
Plotosus lineatus (marine catfish), 1576
Plumbism, 1292. *See also* Lead; Lead, poisoning
Plumeria rubra (frangipani), 979
Plums, pits, 1602t
Plutonium
  DTPA for, 35t, 1779–1781, 1779f
  inhalation, bronchoalveolar lavage for, 73
  internal contamination by, management, 44t
Pneumatic treatment, 1011
Pneumococcal vaccine, phenol in, 685t
Pneumoconiosis
  antimony, 1232
  imaging, 125t, 126
Pneumocystis jiroveci pneumonia, in HIV-infected
    (AIDS) patients, 830t–831t, 846
Pneumocyte(s)
  type I, 399
  type II, 399
Pneumomediastinum, 122, 126, 128f–129f
  cocaine and, 1126–1127
  imaging, 115t, 122, 126, 128f–129f, 406
Pneumonic plague (*Yersinia pestis*), 1756, 1756f
Pneumonitis. *See also* Aspiration pneumonitis
  antimonials and, 1232
  cadmium-induced, 1260
  hydrocarbon, 1196, 1200, 1652
    with insecticide poisoning, 1491, 1492f
    management, 1416
    radiographic evidence, 1412, 1413f
  hypersensitivity, 1659
    imaging, 115t, 125–126, 125t
    sulfonamides and, 827
  inhalant-induced, 1196
  interstitial, diagnostic imaging, 115t
  metal, 1657–1658
  nickel carbonyl and, 1335
Pneumopericardium, cocaine and, 1126–1127
Pneumoperitoneum, imaging, 127, 129t
Pneumothorax, 122, 126, 400–401
  cocaine and, 1126–1127

  imaging, 115t, 122, 126, 406
  ultrasound of, 406
Pneumotoxicity, 174t
PNU (*N3*-pyridylmethyl-*N′-p*-nitrophenylurea, Vacor)
  estimated fatal dose, 1452t
  physicochemical properties, 1452t
  in rodenticides, 1452t
  site of action, 173f
  toxicity
    antidote and/or treatment, 1452t
    clinical manifestations, 1452t
    onset, 1452t
  toxic mechanism, 1452t
Poaceae, 1598t
Podoconiosis, 1720
Podophyllin, 504–505, 1597, 1602t, 1609–1610, 1612,
    1613f. *See also* Podophyllum (*Podophyllum*
    spp.)
  as abortifacient, 303t
  active compounds in, 504
  brain changes caused by, 131, 505
  definition, 504
  derivatives, 504
  history of, 504
  laboratory analysis for, 505
  and other antimitotics, in overdose, comparison,
    507t
  pharmacokinetics and toxicokinetics, 504
  pharmacology, 504
  toxic dose, 504
  toxicity (overdose/poisoning)
    clinical presentation, 504–505
    management, 505
    pathophysiology, 504
  transdermal absorption, 271
Podophyllotoxin, 501, 505, 643t, 1612, 1613f
  structure, 501, 504
Podophyllum (*Podophyllum* spp.), 504
  P. emodi (wild mandrake), 504, 1602t
  P. peltatum (mayapple, mandrake), 504, 638, 1602t,
    1612, 1613f
    as abortifacient, 303t
  P. pleianthum, 504
  toxicity, management, cytokines for, 311
Podophyllum resin, 504, 1612. *See also* Podophyllin
Poikilothermia, 31
  definition, 413
  ethanol-induced, 413
Poinsettia (*Euphorbia pulcherrima*), 1600t, 1613–1614
POISINDEX, 11, 1789, 1803
Poison(s). *See also specific xenobiotic*
  classification of, early, 6
  fast vs. slow, 1
  hematotoxic effects, 3–4
  historical perspective on, 1
  neurotoxic effects, 4
Poison [term], 1
Poison-bun sponge (*Neofibularia nolitangere*),
    1573–1574
Poison Control Center Enhancement and Awareness
    Act, 11, 11t, 1782
Poison control (information) centers(s) (PCC), 9–11,
    11t, 1789–1794
  and collection of epidemiologic data, 1790–1792
  consultants, liability of, state statutes limiting, 1866
  consultation with, 1803
    Privacy Rule and, 1864
    value of, 1789–1790
  in developing world, 1844, 1847
  in disposition of patients, 40

  as education providers, 1793, 1793t
  health care savings from, 1792–1793
  and health professionals, 1790
  history of, 1789
  information from, 1803
  legal considerations for, 1865–1866
  and medicolegal considerations, 1860–1861
  needs assessment by, 1783
  objectives, 1789
  and public, 1790
  public educators in, 1782–1783
  in public health initiatives, 1793
  in public health surveillance system, 1792
  public immunity protection and, 1866
  recommendations by
    vs. acceptance, 1790
    compliance with, 1790
  regional
    practices that reduce potential liabilities, 1866
    standards for, 11, 11t
  in risk assessment, 1816–1817
  and risk communication, 1815–1817, 1816t
  standards of care applicable to, 1865
  toll-free access to, 11, 1782, 1783f
  value/importance, 1789–1790
  worldwide numbers, 1782
Poison education, 1782–1788, 1793, 1793t
  community-based, 1783–1785
  health education principles in, 1786
  health literacy in, 1786
  health numeracy in, 1786
  for multicultural populations, 1785
  programs for, 1783–1786
  in public health initiatives, 1793, 1794t
  for schoolchildren, 1784
  for Spanish speakers, 1784–1785
  targeting health behavior, 1784
Poison epidemiology, 1789–1794
  adverse drug events and, 1792
  data collection on, 1790–1792
  data on, in public health surveillance system, 1792
  fatal poisonings and, 1791
  improvement, 1793, 1794t
  nonfatal poisonings and, 1791
  occupational exposures and, 1791–1792
Poisoners, 5t–6t
  Medieval and Renaissance, 4–6
  in recent history, 12
Poison hemlock (*Conium maculatum*), 1599t, 1605
  hypoventilation caused by, 400t
Poison information centers. *See* Poison control
    (information) centers(s) (PCC)
Poisoning
  diagnosis, 6
  fatal, 1791. *See also* Death(s)
  self-. *See* Self-poisoning
  suicide by. *See* Suicide
Poisoning [term], definition, 1790
Poison ivy (*Toxicodendron* spp.), 1603t, 1614
Poison oak (*Toxicodendron* spp.), 1603t, 1614
Poison prevention, 1782–1788, 1793, 1793t
  community-based, 1783–1785
  education about, 1782–1786
  legislation for, 1782
  for multicultural populations, 1785
  taste-aversive xenobiotics and, 1782
Poison Prevention Packaging Act (1970), 10t, 11,
    451, 1782
Poison sumac (*Toxicodendron* spp.), 1603t, 1614
Poison tobacco. *See* Henbane (*Hyoscyamus niger*)

Poke. *See* Pokeweed (*Phytolacca americana, P. decandra*)

Pokeweed (*Phytolacca americana, P. decandra*), 644t, 1601t, 1608f, 1609

Pokeweed mitogen, 644t, 1609

Polar bear liver, vitamin A toxicity from, 654–655

Polar bond(s), 159

Polar compounds, 159

Polar groups, 165

Poliomyelitis, clinical manifestations, 577t

Pollucite, 1264

Pollution
    air. *See* Air pollution
    industrial, 1847

Pollution intensity, in Africa, 1847

Pollution Prevention Act, and nanotechnology, 1731

Pollyanna phenomenon, 1791

Polonium
    chemistry, 1769
    radioisotopes, 1769

Polonium-210, 6t, 13, 1762, 1769

Polyamine agonist, 227t

Polyamine antagonism, 227t, 228

Polybrominated biphenyls (PBBs), food contamination with, 18, 18t

Polycarbophil, 83

Polychaetae, 1573–1574

Polychlorinated biphenyls (PCBs)
    chloracne caused by, 271
    estrogenic effects, 1518
    infertility caused by, 297t
    in rice oil disease, 18, 18t
    teratogenicity, 430t

Polychlorinated dibenzofurans (PCDFs), in rice oil disease, 18, 18t

Polychromasia, 317

Polycyclic aromatic hydrocarbons, 23t. *See also* Hydrocarbons

Polycythemia, cobalt-related, 1274

Polydipsia, 195
    psychogenic, and hyponatremia, 196

Polyethylene glycol (PEG)
    with activated charcoal, 77
    adverse effects, 85
    for bismuth toxicity, 1256–1257
    chemistry, 83
    dosage and administration, 86
    electrolyte lavage solution, 686
        PEG molecular weight in, 686, 686t
    and fluid,electrolyte, and acidbase disturbances, 687
    and Gatorade, mixture, 86–87
    high-molecular-weight, pharmacokinetics, 686
    history of, 83
    and hypernatremia, 195
    low-molecular-weight
        absorption, 686
        adverse effects and safety issues, 686
        pharmacokinetics, 686
    mechanism of action, 84
    medical applications, 83
    molecular weight, 83
    nephrotoxicity, 686
    neurotoxicity, 686–687
    palatability, improving, 86–87
    as pharmaceutical additive, 686–687, 686t
    pharmacokinetics, 84
    physicochemical properties, 686
    production, 83
    rinsing with, for phenol exposure, 74
    in whole-bowel irrigation formulations, 86–87

Polyethylene glycol (PEG) asparaginase, intrathecal administration, inadvertent overdose and unintentional exposures due to, 797t

Polyethylene glycol electrolyte lavage solutions (PEG-ELS), 83
    adverse effects, 85
    availability and storage, 45t
    for GI tract decontamination, 33
    indications for, 35t, 45t
    mechanism of action, 84
    stocking, recommended level, 45t
    in whole-bowel irrigation, 62–63, 84

Polyethylene glycol-industrial methylated spirits, rinsing with, for phenol exposure, 74

Polygonaceae, 1602t, 1610

Polygonum multiflorum (Fo-Ti), 641t

PolyHEMA, 96

Polymer fume fever, 1659

Polymorphism, 170

Polymorphonuclear leukocytes, 319–320
    hepatic, 330

Polymyositis, clinical manifestations, 577t

Polymyxin, and neuromuscular blockers, interactions, 1021t

Polymyxin B, for amanitin poisoning, 1585–1586

Polymyxin B sulfate, toxicity, organ system manifestations, 829t

Polymyxin B sulfate/trimethoprim, benzalkonium chloride in, 682t

Polyneuropathy, 342. *See also* Neuropathy(ies)
    of critical illness, 1025, 1025t
    gasoline inhalation and, 1198

Polynucleotide phosphorylase, cobalt and, 1274

Polypharmacy, elderly and, 464–465, 1827

Polyphenols, 1600t

Polypodiaceae, 1602t

Polyporic acid, 1583t, 1589t, 1592

Polyquaternium-1, 682

Polyradiculopathy, clinical manifestations, 577t

Polysaccharide iron, 669–670, 670t

Polystyrene, thermal degradation products, 1641t

Polyunsaturated fatty acids (PUFAs)
    neuroprotection by, and mercury-containing seafood consumption, 1328
    oxidative stress and, 174

Polyurethane, thermal degradation products, 1641t, 1685

Polyuria, causes, 195

Polyvinyl chloride
    scleroderma-like reaction with, 281
    thermal degradation products, 1641t

Polyvinylpyrrolidone-isopropyl alcohol, rinsing with, for phenol exposure, 74

Pommerais, 6

Pompeii, Italy, 16, 16t

Pong-pong ("suicide") tree (*Cerbera odollam*), 979

Poplar (*Populus* spp.), 1602t

Poppers, 1193t, 1194. *See also* Inhalant(s)

Poppers retinopathy, 1198–1199

Poppy
    Papaver spp., 1605
    Papaver somniferum, 519, 1601t
    prickly (*Argemone mexicana*), 650t
    seeds, ingestion, and opioid assays, 532

Popstpartum period, acute poisoning in, 433–434

Populus spp. (poplar), 1602t

Porifera, 1573–1574

Porphylleren-MC16, 879

Porphyria, 314
    absinthe and, 627

Porphyria cutanea tarda, 18, 18t

Portal triad, 327

Portal vein, 327, 328f

Porthidium dunni, 1637t

Porthidium godmani, 1637t

Porthidium hespere, 1637t

Porthidium nasutum, 1637t

Porthidium yucatanicum, 1637t

Port Jackson shark, 1576

Portland cement ingestion, management, 64

Portuguese man-of-war (*Physalia physalis*), 1567, 1567t, 1568, 1568f, 1571. *See also* Cnidaria (jellyfish)
    deaths caused by, 1568
    stings, management, 1569

Posaconazole, 829

Positive allosteric modulators (PAMs), for glutamate receptors, 227

Positive end-expiratory pressure (PEEP), 407, 1656
    for ARDS, 401

Positive predictive value (PPV), of diagnostic test, 1858, 1858f

Positron emission tomography (PET)
    in carbon monoxide poisoning, 1667
    of cerebellar atrophy, 134
    of CNS, 130
    indications for, 134
    of inhalant-exposed animals, 1194
    isotopes used in, 133
    in Parkinson disease, 1320
    principles of, 133–134
    with xenobiotic exposure, 115t

Positrons, 1760, 1763

Posterior chamber of eye, 356

Posterior reversible encephalopathy syndrome (PRES), 131–133, 135f

Posthypoglycemic encephalopathy, 710

Postmarketing surveillance, 1836–1838, 1864–1865

Postmortem interval, 1885

Postmortem redistribution, 1869, 1870t, 1871–1872, 1871t, 1873t, 1887

Postmortem toxicology, 1884–1891
    alternative matrices in, 1870t, 1872–1873
    artifacts related to sampling sites in, 1889
    autopsy and, 1888–1889
    case study, 1884, 1889
    clinical effects of xenobiotic and, 1888
    comorbid conditions and, 1888
    decomposition and postmortem biochemical changes in, 1885, 1885t
    decomposition state and, 1888
    entomotoxicology in, 1886, 1886t
    handling of body or samples and, 1888
    limitations, 1889
    pharmacogenetics and, 1888
    postmortem absorption and, 1887
    postmortem distribution and, 1887
    postmortem metabolism and, 1887
    postmortem redistribution and, 1869, 1870t, 1871–1872, 1871t, 1873t, 1887
    results, interpretation, 1886–1889, 1887t
    samples used for toxicologic analysis in, 1885–1886, 1885t
    tolerance and, 1888
    uses, 1884–1885
    xenobiotic chemical reactions and, 1888
    xenobiotic concentrations in, published data on, 1889
    xenobiotic properties and, 1887–1888, 1887t
    xenobiotic stability and laboratory recovery in, 1887, 1887t

Postpartum blues, 433–434
Postpartum psychosis, 433–434
Postsynaptic excitation, 205, 205f
Postsynaptic inhibition, 205, 205f
Posttoxicity syndrome, 236–237
Posttraumatic stress disorder (PTSD)
    glutamate and, 224
    nerve agents and, 1745
Posturing, abnormal, 37
Potamotrygonidae, 1576
Potassium
    absorption, 198
    balance, renal regulation of, 389
    cardiac effects, 258t
    for cardioactive steroid poisoning, 974
    chemistry, 157–158
    dermal decontamination for, precautions with, 72
    excretion, 198
    intracellular:extracellular ratio, 198
    intravenous (IV), infusion rate for, 198
    membrane transport, 203
    in neurotransmission, 205, 205f
    postmortem changes, 1885t
    serum, 197–198
        abnormalities. See also Hyperkalemia;
            Hypokalemia
            xenobiotic-induced, 197–199, 198t, 956
        ECG changes caused by, 251, 252f
    supplementation/replacement, 198
        in barium toxicity, 1455
        hyperkalemia caused by, 251, 956
        for quinine overdose, 840
    for thallium poisoning, 1353–1354
    total body, 197–198
    vitreous, normal concentration, 1872t
Potassium-40, radiation from, 1765–1766
Potassium aluminum sulfate. See Alum
Potassium atractylate, 640t
Potassium atractylatelike compound, 643t
Potassium bromide, as early sedative-hypnotic, 8–9
Potassium channel(s)
    antidysrhythmics and, 865, 866t–867t, 868–869,
        871
    cardiac, arsenic and, 1239
    delayed rectifier, 245
        arsenic and, 1239
        blockade by antipsychotics, 1034t, 1035
        cesium and, 1264
        myocardial, 245
    ethanol and, 1194
    funny (I_{Kf}), 245, 247
    genes for, 245
    hERG-encoded subunit, xenobiotics and, 245, 253,
        256, 877
    hyperpolarization-activated (I_{Kh}), 245, 247
    inhalants and, 1196
    and insulin release, 696f, 713, 715
    inward rectifier, arsenic and, 1239
    myocardial, 245, 245f
        xenobiotics affecting, 258
    of myocardial cell membrane, 245
    in opioid receptor signal transduction, 522f
    opioids and, 238, 238f
    quinine and, 838–839
    rapidly activating (I_{Kr}), 245
    slowly activating (I_{Ks}), 245
    α-subunit, 244, 244f, 245
    toluene and, 1194
    voltage-gated, 244, 244f
        structure, 244f, 245

Potassium channel blockers
    β-adrenergic antagonists as, 932, 9930
    and QT interval, 251–253
Potassium channel complex(es), 245
Potassium chlorate, 1369t
Potassium chloride, 6t, 12, 198
    in capital punishment, 13
    intrathecal administration
        clinical manifestations, 793
        inadvertent overdose and unintentional
            exposures due to, 797t
    overdose/poisoning, whole-bowel irrigation for, 85
    solution, sorbitol in, 688t
    tablets, gastric outlet obstruction caused by, 128
Potassium compounds, clinical and laboratory findings
    with, 36t
Potassium cyanide, 5t, 1684
    lethal dose, 1685
    mass suicide using, 1685
Potassium dichromate, 1268t
Potassium hydroxide, 1388t
Potassium iodide (KI), 817–818
    adverse effects and safety issues, 1776
    as antidote
        for radiation poisoning, 1773, 1775
        for radioactive iodine, 1769, 1775
    availability and storage, 45t
    chemistry, 1775
    dosage and administration, 1776–1777, 1777t
        daily vs. single dosing in, 1777
        monitoring, 1777
        timing of administration in, 1777
    extrathyroidal effects, 1776
    formulation and acquisition, 1777
    indications for, 45t
    mechanism of action, 1775
    pharmacology, 1775
    prophylactic, for radiation exposure, 1775
    stocking, recommended level, 45t
    thyroidal effects, 1776
    and thyroid function, 1775
Potassium permanganate, 1319, 1369t, 1371–1372,
        1388t
    clinical effects, 1371–1372
    ingestion, 1371–1372
        management, 1372
    self-poisoning with, 1846
Potassium phosphate, 198
Potassium salts, overdose/poisoning, 198
Potassium sorbate, 682
Potassium-sparing diuretics. See Diuretics,
        potassium-sparing
Potatoes
    green (Solanum tuberosum), 1603t, 1604
    Solanum americanum, 1603t
    wild (Hedysarum alpinum), 1600t
Potentially inappropriate medications (PIMs), 460
Pothos (Epiprenum aureum), 1600t, 1613
Potroom asthma, 1223, 1225
Potroom palsy, 1223
Pott, Percivall, 4t, 22
Povidone-iodine, 1369t, 1370
    and hypernatremia, 195, 195t
Power, statistical, 1855
PPSB-HT Nichiyaku Profilnine, 910
PPSB S.D., 910
Pradaxa. See Dabigatran
Praescutata viperina, 1575
Prairie rattlesnake (Crotalus viridis), 1617t
Pralidoxime chloride (2-PAM, Protopam), 1508–1513

    acquisition, 1511
    adverse effects and safety issues, 1510
    as antidote, 1508–1513
    and atropine
        combination therapy with, 1510–1511
        synergism, 1509
    autoinjector administration, 1511
        adverse effects and safety issues, 1510
        pharmacokinetics, 1509
    availability and storage, 45t
    for carbamate poisoning, 1498–1499
    for carbamate toxicity, 1510
    chemistry, 162, 163f, 1508
    CNS penetration, 1509
    dosage and administration, 1511
    duration of treatment with, 1511
    excretion, 1509
    formulation, 1511
    indications for, 35t, 45t
    intramuscular administration, 1511
        pharmacokinetics, 1509
    intravenous administration, 1511
        pharmacokinetics, 1509
    loading dose, 1511
    maintenance infusion, 1511
    mechanism of action, 162, 1508–1509
    for metal phosphide poisoning, 1460
    in nerve agent antidote kit, 1746
    for nerve agent exposure, 1746
    oral administration, pharmacokinetics, 1509
    for organic phosphorus poisoning, 1497–1498,
        1504
        cholinesterase reactivation after, 1508
        efficacy, time of administration and, 1510
        human trials, 1510
    pharmacokinetics, two-compartment model, 1509
    pharmacology, 1508
    in pregnancy and lactation, 1510
    related xenobiotics, 1508
    serum, therapeutic concentration, 1509
    stocking, 43
        recommended level, 45t
    in Strategic National Stockpile, 1511
    structure, 1508
    supplies, 42–43
    toxicokinetics, 1509
    volume of distribution, 1509
    for xenobiotic-induced respiratory dysfunction,
        407
Pralidoxime iodide, 1508, 1511
Pralidoxime salts, for nerve agent exposure, 1746
Prallethrin, 1520t. See also Pyrethroids
Pramipexole, mechanism of action, 214
Pramlintide, 694, 700
    pharmacokinetics and toxicokinetics, 696, 697t
    pharmacology, 696
Prasugrel, 899
    antiplatelet effects, 323
    mechanism of action, 898f
Pravastatin, CYP enzymes and, 170
Praxbind, 892. See also Idarucizumab
Prayer beans (Abrus precatorius), 1598t. See also Rosary
        pea (Abrus precatorius)
Praziquantel, 829
Prazosin, 961–962
    with scorpion antivenom, for scorpion
        envenomation, 1565
Prealbumin, serum, in liver injury, 335
Precaution advocacy, 1817
Precautionary principle, 1814

Protamine chloride, 919
Protamine sulfate, 919
Proteaceae, 1614
Protease(s), added to urine before doping analysis, 622
Protease inhibitors, 831–832, 1489. *See also specific xenobiotic*
 bioavailability, 173
 clinical and laboratory findings with, 36t
 crystalluria caused by, 395
 and fatty acid metabolism, 176t, 179
 and male sexual dysfunction, 299f
 and rifampin, 855
Protected health information, 1864
Protective antigen, 1755
Protein(s). *See also* Plasma protein(s); *specific protein*
 definition, 1597
 membrane, 141
 metabolism, 179–181
 and occupational asthma, 1660, 1660t
 from plants, 1597, 1608–1609
 serum, postmortem changes, 1885t
 tissue, xenobiotic affinity for, 146
 transport, 172–173
 xenobiotic binding to, 144
Protein, serum, age-related changes in, 462
Protein adducts, as indicator of organophosphate exposure, 1495
Protein C, 321f, 322, 885f
 in coagulation, 884, 884f
 deficiency, 889–890
 pharmacokinetics, after prothrombin complex concentrate administration, 908, 909t
 in prothrombin complex concentrate, 908, 908t
Protein kinase(s), and withdrawal syndrome, 237
Protein kinase A (PKA), 208, 220, 261
 in cardiac physiology, 928–929, 929f
Protein kinase B (PKB), 953–954, 954f
 calcium-channel blockers and, 953–954, 954f
 insulin and, 955
Protein kinase C (PKC)
 cyanide and, 1686
 lead and, 1294–1295
Protein kinase inhibitors, 761
 adverse effects and safety issues, 760t
 as chemotherapeutics, 759, 760t, 761f
 mechanism and site of action, 762f
 overdose/poisoning, 760t
Protein reserve, age-related changes in, 462
Protein S, 321f, 322
 in coagulation, 884, 884f–885f
 pharmacokinetics, after prothrombin complex concentrate administration, 908, 909t
 in prothrombin complex concentrate, 908, 908t
Proteinuria, cadmium and, 1259–1260
Protein Z, 321f
 in coagulation, 884, 884f–885f
Prothiofos, 1487
ProthoRAAS, 910
Prothrombin, 883, 884f
Prothrombin complex concentrate (PCC), 908–911
 activated, 887, 908, 910–911
 adverse effects and safety issues, 908–909
 for apixaban-induced coagulopathy, 895
 availability, 910
 components, 908, 908t
 contraindications to, 887, 908
 for dabigatran-induced coagulopathy, 894
 for direct oral anticoagulants, 910
 disease transmission in, 908
 dosage and administration, 887, 909, 909t

 for edoxaban-induced coagulopathy, 895
 for factor Xa inhibitor–induced coagulopathy, 895–896
 for fondaparinux-induced coagulopathy, 896
 formulations, 908
 four-factor, 887, 888t, 908, 908t
  availability and storage, 46t
  indications for, 46t
  vs. plasma, 910
  stocking, recommended level, 46t
  vs. three-factor, 909–910
 history of, 908
 in liver disease, 910
 mechanism of action, 908
 nonactivated, 908
 pharmacokinetics and pharmacodynamics, 908, 909t
 pharmacology, 908
 in pregnancy and lactation, 909
 for rivaroxaban-induced coagulopathy, 895
 three-factor, 908, 908t
  availability and storage, 46t
  vs. four-factor, 909–910
  indications for, 46t
  stocking, recommended level, 46t
 in trauma, 910
 for VKA-induced coagulopathy, 887, 888t
Prothrombin Complex Octapharm, 910
Prothrombinex-HT, 910
Prothrombin time (PT), 320–322, 335, 883
 elevated, vitamin K₁ for, 915, 917
 in liver injury, 335, 335t
Prothromblex, 910
Prothromblex NF, 910
Prothromblex Total, 910
Prothromblex Total NF, 910
Prothromplex Immuno Tim 4, 910
Protoanemonin, 644t, 1602t
Protogonyaulax catanella, and shellfish poisoning, 595
Protogonyaulax tamarensis, and shellfish poisoning, 595
Proton(s), 160
 production, in ATP hydrolysis, 177
Proton pump inhibitors (PPIs)
 acute interstitial nephritis caused by, 393, 394t
 and bismuth preparations, interactions, 1257
 for caustic injury, 1394
 and gastric acid secretion, 743f
 gastrointestinal effects, 292f
 hypomagnesemia caused by, 877
Protopine, 650t
Protoplasmic proteins, 271
Protoporphyrin IX, 314, 314f
Protozoa, and ciguatoxin, 593
Protriptyline, 1044, 1044t. *See also* Cyclic antidepressants
Protromplex TIM3, 910
Provando et riprovando, 3
Proximal tubule, 389, 390f
Prucalopride, 84
Prunus spp., 1602t, 1607
 cyanogenic glycosides in, 1684
Prunus armeniaca (apricot), 1602t
 uses and toxicities, 640t
Pruritus
 causes, 273
 cholestatic, opioid antagonists for, 540
 clinical significance, 273
 morphine-induced, opioid antagonists for, 540
 neurally mediated, xenobiotics causing, 273
 NSAID-induced, 515

Pruritus ani, with whole-bowel irrigation, 85
Prussian blue, 92, 1357–1361, 1779
 acquisition, 1360
 adsorption of thallium, in vitro, 1357
 adverse effects, 1360
 availability and storage, 46t
 cesium adsorption, 1266
  in vitro, 1359
 cesium binding, 1266, 1357
 as cesium chelator, 1769
 for cesium poisoning, 1266, 1357, 1359–1360
  animal data on, 1359
  dosage and administration, 1359–1360
  in humans, 1359
 chemistry, 1357, 1357f
 cyanide release from, 1360
 dosage and administration, 1266
 and enterohepatic circulation, 1357
 formulation, 1360
 history of, 1357
 indications for, 35t, 46t
 insoluble, 1357
  chemical structure, 1357f
  elimination, 1357
  formulation, 1360
 orphan drug designation and, 1834
 penicillamine and, combined, for thallium toxicity, 1354, 1358
 pharmacology, 1357
 potassium binding, 1357
 pregnancy category, 1360
 for radiocesium poisoning, 1266
 rubidium binding, 1357
 shelf life, 1360
 soluble (colloidal), 1357
  absorption, 1357
 stocking, recommended level, 46t
 synonyms for, 1357
 thallium binding by, 1357
 for thallium poisoning, 1354, 1357–1358
  and activated charcoal, in vitro comparison, 1357–1358
  animal data on, 1358
  dosage and administration, 1358
  end point for, 1358
  in humans, 1358
Prussic acid (cyanide), 8. *See also* Cyanide(s)
Psathyrella foenisecii, 1582t, 1588
Pseudoaneurysm, 128, 130f
Pseudocholinesterase, 206, 1022
Pseudochromhidrosis, 272, 272f, 273
Pseudoephedrine, 112, 641t
 adverse effects and safety issues, in children, 748
 brain changes caused by, imaging, 132t
 and dopaminergic activity, 214
 duration of action, 749t
 in *Ephedra*, 649
 history of, 748
 in illicit synthesis of methamphetamines, 738
 liquid, sorbitol in, 688t
 monitoring, insports, 748
 pediatric exposure to, 738
 pharmacokinetics and toxicokinetics, 749–750
 pharmacology, 749
 therapeutic effects, 749t
 toxicity, 749t
  clinical manifestations, 750
Pseudo-hypoaldosteronism, licorice and, 1606
Pseudohyponatremia, 196
Pseudolymphoma, imaging, 115t

Pseudonitzschia australis, 595

Pseudoporphyria, 276

Pseudoterranova decipiens, 600

Pseudotumor, metallosis and, 1276

Psilocin, 1179t, 1182, 1582t
  chemical structure, 1180f, 1588–1589
  pharmacology, 1181t

Psilocybe spp., 9, 1179, 1588–1589, 1589f. *See also*
    Psilocybin mushrooms (*Psilocybe*)

Psilocybe caerulipes, 1589f

Psilocybe cubensis, 1582t, 1588

Psilocybe cyanescens, 1582t, 1588, 1589f

Psilocybe mexicana, 9, 1178

Psilocybin, 9, 1179, 1179t, 1182, 1582t, 1588–1589, 1589t
  chemical structure, 1180f, 1588
  cross-tolerance with other hallucinogens, 1183
  effect on 5-HT receptors, 1588
  mechanism of action, 217
  pharmacology, 1181t
  therapeutic uses, 1178

Psilocybin mushrooms (*Psilocybe*), 1179–1180, 1181t,
    1588–1589, 1589f
  history of, 9, 1178
  toxicokinetics, 1182

Psoas abscess, 128

Psoralen, 641t, 643t, 1609–1610

Psoriasis, 278

Psychedelic [term], 1178

Psychedelic drugs, 1178. *See also* Hallucinogens

Psychiatric assessment
  comprehensive, 378
  initial, with self-poisoning, 377

Psychiatric illness. *See also* Mental illness
  and suicide, 378–379

Psychiatric patient, medical evaluation before
    admission, 375

Psychiatric principles, 373–383

Psychological autopsy, 378

Psychosis, 33–36, 1182
  amphetamine-induced, 1103
  antihistamine-related, management, 748
  belladonna alkaloids causing, 1183
  cannabinoid-induced, 1117
  carbon monoxide poisoning and, 1665
  cyclic antidepressants and, 1047
  glutamate and, 227
  hallucinogen-induced, 1184
  inhalant-induced, 1200
  postpartum, 433–434
  and suicide, 378–379
  in thallium toxicity, 1351
  and violence, 385
  xenobiotic-induced, 344, 344t

Psychotria viridis (chacruna), 641t, 647, 649, 650t, 1180

Psychotropics. *See also* specific xenobiotic
  skin discoloration caused by, 273

Psyllium, 83, 1602t

Ptaquilosides, 1602t, 1608

Pteridium spp. (bracken fern), 1602t, 1608

Pteridium aquilinum (bracken fern), 1608

Pterois spp. (lionfish), 1576, 1576t, 1577, 1577f

Pterois lunulata, 1576, 1576t

Pterois volitans, 1576, 1576t, 1577, 1577f, 1578

Publication bias, 1857

Public health
  vs. individual risk assessment, 1815
  interventions, in resource-limited settings, 1848

Public Health Security and Bioterrorism Preparedness
    and Response Act (2002), 10t

Puffball mushrooms, 1592, 1592f

Puffer fish, tetrodotoxin in, 596

Pulegone, 632, 640t, 643t, 1600t–1601t
  as abortifacient, 303t
  structure, 631
  toxicity, *N*-acetylcysteine for, 494

Pulmonary artery catheter, 402

Pulmonary edema, 37, 93
  carbon monoxide poisoning and, 1665
  cardiogenic, 402, 406
    differentiation from ARDS, 402
    treatment, 402
  neurogenic, 401
  noncardiogenic, 401. *See also* Acute lung injury (ALI)
  ultrasound in, 406

Pulmonary embolism
  metallic (mercury), diagnostic imaging, 117, 118f
  with prothrombin complex concentrate, 909
  septic, 125, 125t, 126f
  treatment/prevention, 890

Pulmonary fibrosis
  aluminum and, 1224–1225
  cadmium-induced, 1260
  diagnostic imaging, 115t
  nickel exposure and, 1336

Pulmonary function testing, 406

Pulmonary gas exchange, 399
  xenobiotics affecting, 1651

Pulmonary hypertension, amphetamine-induced, 1103

Pulmonary infarction, cocaine use and, 1127

Pulmonary infiltrates, cannabinoid-induced, 1117

Pulmonary injury, and respiratory rate, 30

Pulmonary irritants, 1640–1641, 1640t, 1653–1658
  acid- or base-forming gases, 1655, 1658. *See also*
      specific xenobiotic
  characteristics, 1653, 1654t
  as chemical weapon, 1741, 1748–1749
  effects on vital signs, 30t
  pathophysiology, 1653
  toxic syndromes caused by, 1751t

Pulmonary xenobiotic disorders, inhalational,
    simple asphyxiants in, 400, 400t. *See also*
    Asphyxiants, simple

Pulsatilla spp., 1602t

Pulse cooximeter, 404

Pulse oximeter, 404, 1708, 1708t
  multiwavelength, 1708–1709

Pulse oximetry, 36, 103, 403–404, 407
  factors affecting, 404, 404t
  in initial assessment, 189
  in methemoglobinemia, 1708
  methylene blue and, 1714
  sulfhemoglobin and, 1710

Pulse pressure, methylxanthines and, 988

Pulse rate. *See also* Bradycardia (bradydysrhythmias);
    Tachycardia
  blood pressure and, 30
  evaluation, 37
  normal, by age, 28t
  temperature and, 30
  xenobiotics affecting, 29–30, 30t

Pulvis Doveri, 519

Puncture vine (*Tribulus terrestris*), 1603t

Puncturevine, as aphrodisiac, 304t

Pupil(s)
  constriction, 357
  dilation, 357–358
  examination, 356
  size, in toxidromes, 28, 29t
  size and reactivity, 37, 357–358
  unequal, 357

Pupura, poisoning/overdose causing, 36t

Pure Food and Drug Act (1906), 9, 10t, 1833

Pure red cell aplasia, 319

Purgatives, 83. *See also* specific xenobiotic

Purging nut
  Jatropha spp., 1601t, 1846
  Ricinus communis, 1602t
    in biologic warfare, 1759

Purine analogs, 173
  as chemotherapeutics, 760t

Purine nucleotides, synthesis, 767

Purple cone flower. *See* Echinacea (*Echinacea
    angustifolia, E. purpurea*)

Purple foxglove (*Digitalis purpurea*), 1600t. *See also*
    Foxglove (*Digitalis*)

Purple glove syndrome, 724

Purple-striped jellyfish (*Pelagia noctiluca*). *See* Mauve
    stinger (*Pelagia noctiluca*)

Purple toe syndrome, 889–890

Purpura, 278–279, 278f
  levamisole-induced, 279, 279f

Pushu Laishi, 910

Puss caterpillar (*Megalopyge opercularis*), 1552–1553

Pustule, 269t

Putrefaction, 1885, 1888

Putrefiants, 6

Putrescine, for paraquat poisoning, 1474f, 1477

P value, 1855

Pygmy rattlesnake (*Sistrurus miliarius*), 1617t

Pylorospasm, 143, 143t

Pyracantha spp., 1607

Pyramiding, 617

Pyrantel pamoate, 829

Pyrazinamide, 856–857
  adverse effects and safety issues, 853t
  dosage and administration, 853t
  and isoniazid, interactions, 853t
  monitoring with, 853t
  pharmacokinetics, 856–857
  pharmacology, 856
  pregnancy category, 857
  structure, 856
  toxicity, management, 857

Pyrazole
  adverse effects, 1435
  and alcohol dehydrogenase inhibition, 1435

Pyrazole herbicides, 1469t

Pyrazolones, pharmacology, 512t

Pyrethrins, 1519–1522
  absorption, 1520
  allergic reactions to, 1521
  exposure to, pathophysiology of, 1521
  history of, 1519
  mechanism of action, 1519
  metabolism, 1521
  structure, 1520f
  synthetic. *See* Pyrethroids
  tissue distribution, 1521
  toxicokinetics, 1520–1521

Pyrethroids, 1519–1522
  absorption, 1521
  aerial spraying, for mosquito control, 1520
  classification, 1519
  dermal exposure to, clinical manifestations, 1522
  elimination, 1521
  exposure to
    chronic, 1522
    pathophysiology of, 1521
  generations, 1519–1520, 1520f, 1520t
  ingestion, clinical manifestations, 1522

metabolism, 1521
metabolites, in urine, 1521
poisoning
    clinical manifestations, 1521–1522
    treatment, 1522
structures, 1519, 1520f
tissue distribution, 1521
toxicokinetics, 1520–1521
type I, 1519
    poisoning, clinical manifestations, 1521–1522
    structure, 1520f
    temperature coefficient, 1521
type II, 1519–1520
    poisoning, clinical manifestations, 1521–1522
    structure, 1520f
    temperature coefficient, 1521
and voltage-gated calcium channels, 244f, 245
Pyrethrum, 1519
  LD$_{50}$, 1521
Pyrexia, 30
Pyridazine herbicides, 1469t
Pyridazinone herbicides, 1469t
Pyridine herbicides, 1469t
Pyridinium compounds, in detergent, 1389
Pyridostigmine, 755, 1487, 1495
  acetylcholinesterase inhibition by, 1745
  contraindications to, 1041
  mechanism of action, 208
  as nerve agent pretreatment, 1746–1747
  for neuromuscular blockade reversal, 1025, 1026t
  overdose/poisoning, 1747
Pyridoxal, 663, 862
Pyridoxal kinase, 221
Pyridoxal phosphate (PLP), 218, 219f, 220, 663
Pyridoxal-5′-phosphate (PLP), 851, 862
  as coenzyme, 862
  inhibitors, seizures caused by, pyridoxine for, 862
Pyridoxamine, 663, 862
Pyridoxine (hydrochloride, vitamin B$_6$), 218, 219f, 220,
    654, 663
  absorption, 862
  adverse effects and safety issues, 863
  availability and storage, 46t
  benzodiazepines and, 1138
  chemistry, 862
  chlorobutanol in, 683t
  as coenzyme, 862
  in common products, 986t
  deficiency, 862
    isoniazid-induced, 851
    pathophysiology, 663
  dietary sources, 663
  dosage and administration, 863
  and doxylamine, combined, for nausea and vomiting
    of pregnancy, 663
  drug interactions with, 863
  in ethylene glycol metabolism, 1422, 1423f, 1429
  for ethylene glycol poisoning, 863
  formulation, 864
  for gyromitrin toxicity, 1587
  history of, 663
  for hydrazide- and hydrazine-induced seizures,
    862–863
  indications for, 35t, 46t, 862, 1138
  and isoniazid, 663
  for isoniazid overdose, 862–863
  mechanism of action, 862
  metabolism, 862
  for nausea and vomiting of pregnancy, 663
  neurotoxicity, 663

pharmacokinetics, 862
pharmacology, 663, 862
physicochemical properties, 663
in pregnancy and lactation, 863
recommended dietary allowance or adequate daily
    intake for, 655t
stocking, 43, 864
  recommended level, 46t
storage, 43
structure, 663, 850, 862
therapeutic uses, 663
in toxic alcohol poisoning, 1429–1430
toxicity (overdose/poisoning)
  clinical manifestations, 663
  pathophysiology, 663
volume of distribution, 862
Pyridoxine kinase, 218, 219f, 220
Pyridoxine phosphokinase, 862
N3-Pyridylmethyl-N′-p-nitrophenylurea. See PNU
    (N3-pyridylmethyl-N′-p-nitrophenylurea,
    Vacor)
Pyrilamine, 1035
  history of, 738
Pyrimethamine
  adverse effects and safety issues, 846
  antimalarial mechanism, 838t, 846
  for HIV-related infections, 831t
  mechanism of action, 759, 775
  overdose, 846
  pharmacokinetics, 839t
  structure, 846
  toxicity, management, 777
Pyrimidine-5′-nucleotidase, 1295
Pyrimidine analogs, 173
  adverse effects and safety issues, 760t
Pyriminobac, in herbicides, 1467t
Pyrinuron (Vacor), overdose, 43
Pyrithiobac, in herbicides, 1467t
Pyritinol, 862
Pyrolusite, 1319
Pyrroles, 1519
1-(1-Phenylcyclohexyl)pyrrolidine. See Rolicyclidine
Pyrrolizidine alkaloids, 639, 640t–642t, 644t, 651,
    1598t–1600t, 1602t–1603t, 1605
  in breast milk, 1605
  clinical and laboratory findings with, 36t
  concentration in plant, factors affecting, 645
  hepatotoxicity, 1605
  in honey, 1605
  teratogenicity, 1605
  toxicity, 645
  variations, 645
Pyruvate, 175, 1157–1158, 1157f
  in gluconeogenesis, 178
  as glutamate scavenger, 229
  metabolism, 177, 178f, 181
    cyanide and, 1685
Pyruvate decarboxylase, 175, 177
Pyruvate dehydrogenase, 177, 878, 954
  trivalent arsenic and, 1238, 1239f
Pyruvate dehydrogenase complex, thiamine and, 1157,
    1157f
Pyruvate kinase, thallium and, 1350

Q

Q fever (Coxiella burnetii), 1757
Qing hao (Artemisia annua, sweet wormwood), for
    malaria, 638, 647
Qinghaosu (artemisinin), 836
Qsymia, 607, 610

QT interval, and thorough QT study (TQT)
    requirement, 1840
QT Interval Nomogram, 251, 253f
QT interval prolongation, 246
  by astemizole, 1840
  case study, 1820–1821, 1821f
  by cisapride, 1840
  drug-related, and drug withdrawal from market,
    1840
  FDA regulatory action due to, 1840
  information sources on, 1820
  by methadone, 1820–1821, 1821f
  by terfenadine, 1840
  workup of patient with, 242
  xenobiotics associated with, 242–243, 243t, 1820
QT liability, 877
Quadriplegic myopathy, acute, of intensive care
    patients, 346
Quantum dots, 1717, 1718f
Quantum rods, 1717
Quantum shells, 155
Quaternary ammonium compounds, 1369t, 1374
  as disinfectants, 1368
  toxicity, 1374
Quaternary ammonium salts, in cationic detergents,
    1389
Queen sago (Cycas circinalis), 1599t
Quercetin, 642t
Quercitrin, 642t
Quercus spp. (oak), 1602t
Queretaran dusky rattlesnake (Crotalus spp.), 1637t
Querétaro dusky rattlesnake (Crotalus spp.), 1637t
Quetiapine, 218. See also Antipsychotics
  cardiac effects, 246, 257t, 258t
  clinical and toxicologic effects, 1034t
  dosage and administration, 1033t
  extrapyramidal effects, 215
  gastrointestinal decontamination for, 51t, 58t
  mechanism of action, 1035
  overdose/poisoning
    gastrointestinal decontamination for, 64, 77
    multiple-dose activated charcoal in, 61
  pharmacobezoar, formation, 49, 52f
  pharmacokinetics, 145t, 1033t
  poisoning, lipid emulsion for, 1006
  priapism caused by, 301t
  and QT interval, 253t
  self-poisoning with, 376
  and sudden cardiac death, 253
  volume of distribution, 145t
Quicksilver, 324t, 1324. See also Mercury
Quid, 1605
Quinaquina. See Cinchona spp.
Quinazoline alkaloids, 644t, 650t
Quinclorac, in herbicides, 1467t
Quinghao, 845
Quinidine, 1602t
  adverse effects and safety issues, 866t, 868–869
  antidote for, 35t
  as antidysrhythmic, 868–869
  cardiac effects, 248f, 567
  cardiotoxicity, 567
  contraindications to, 974
  for fluoride toxicity, 1401
  inhibition of glucuronidation, 172
  pharmacokinetics, 866t
  pharmacology, 838, 866t
  plant source, 1599t
  and prolonged QT interval, 256
  protein-binding characteristics, 110t

Quinidine (*Cont.*):
structure, 868f
and tinnitus, 370t
torsade de pointes caused by, magnesium for, 878
toxicity (overdose/poisoning)
ECG changes in, 247, 247f
pathophysiology, 838–839
sodium bicarbonate for, 568t
volume of distribution, 91, 838
Quinidine gluconate injection, phenol in, 685t
Quinidine syncope, 838, 868
Quinine, 641t, 836, 838–841
as abortifacient, 303t, 838
amblyopia caused by, 361
antimalarial mechanism, 838t
cardiac effects, 258t, 838–840
management, 840
from *Cinchona*, 641t
cranial neuropathy caused by, 346t
dermal effects, 840
and discoloration of teeth and gums, 293t
elimination, multiple-dose activated charcoal and, 78
enhanced elimination, 841
gastrointestinal effects, 839
hyperinsulinemia with, 840
hypoglycemia caused by, 713–718, 840
lethal dose, 839
ophthalmic effects, 839–840
management, 841
ophthalmic toxicity, 356, 356f, 358, 361, 361t
ototoxicity, 366f, 840
pharmacokinetics, 838, 839t
in pregnancy and lactation, 838
retinal toxicity, 839, 841
serum, and clinical effects, 839
structure, 838, 868f
teratogenicity, 430t
therapeutic uses, 838
thrombotic microangiopathy caused by, 840, 847
and tinnitus, 369–370, 370t, 840
toxicity (overdose/poisoning), 304
clinical manifestations, 36t, 839–840
diagnostic tests for, 840
management, 840–841
multiple-dose activated charcoal in, 61, 841
pathophysiology, 838–839
sodium bicarbonate for, 568t, 569
toxicokinetics, 838
toxic-to-therapeutic ratio, 839
and vision, 839–840
Quinmerac, in herbicides, 1467t
Quinolinium compounds, in cationic detergents, 1389
Quinolones
cardiac effects, 258t
clinical and laboratory findings with, 36t
hypoglycemia caused by, 713–718
Quinoxalinediones, mechanism of action, 227t
Quinpirole, and sexual function, 304
3-Quinuclidinyl benzilate (BZ, QNB), 1750, 1750f
toxic syndrome caused by, 1751t
Quisqualate (*Quisqualis indica*), mechanism of action, 227t
Qut (*Catha edulis*), uses and toxicities, 643t

R
Rabbitfish, 1576
Rabbit syndrome, 1373
Rabies vaccine, neurotoxicity, 343
Racemic mixture, 165

Racetams, mechanism of action, 227t
Raclopride. *See also* Antipsychotics
dosage and administration, 1033t
pharmacokinetics, 1033t
Rad, 1764, 1764f
Radiation, 1762–1774
absorbed dose, 1764, 1764f
annual estimated average effective dose equivalent in United States, 1765t
biodosimetry, 1768–1769
in initial emergency department management, 1770
bystander effect with, 1767
and carcinogenesis, 1769
clinical and laboratory findings with, 36t
committed doses, 1772
contamination, 1765
definition, 1762
in diagnostic imaging, 1762
dose, and lymphocyte count, 1768–1769
dose equivalent, 1764f
dose estimation, 1768–1769
effective dose, 1764
exposure
and children, 1773
deceased contaminated bodies, disposition, 1773
decontamination for, 1770–1771
direct effects, 1767
epidemiology, 1765–1766, 1765t
and evacuation, 1775
and food interdiction, 1775
grade of injury with, 1771, 1772t
indirect effects, 1767
initial assessment, 1770
initial emergency department management, 1770
as low as reasonably achievable (ALARA), 1767
management, 1770–1773
potassium iodide in, 1775–1777. *See also* Potassium iodide (KI)
medical decision making with, 1771, 1772t
medical management, 1771–1772
pathophysiology, 1767
prognosis for, 1773
response category for, 1771, 1772t
supportive care for, 1771
threshold dose for potassium iodide administration, 1776–1777, 1777t
time of, 1765
triage, 1770, 1772t
exposure limits, 1767
and genomic instability, 1767
hematopoietic toxicity, 311
high-LET, 1763, 1767
historical exposures to, 1762
internal contamination by, management, 1772–1773
ionizing, 1763
vs. nonionizing, 1763
exposure to, 1765
infertility caused by, 297t, 298f
teratogenicity, 430t
$LD_{50/60}$, 1773
low-LET, 1763, 1767
nonionizing, 280
occupational exposure to, 1766
pregnancy and, 1773
protection from, 1764–1765, 1775
regulation and reporting on, 1767
sources
human-made, 1765, 1765t, 1766, 1766t
natural, 1765–1766, 1765t

stochastic *vs.* deterministic effects, 1767–1768
units of measure, 1763–1764
Radiation (of heat), 411
Radiation disasters, 23–24, 23t
Radiation Effects Research Foundation (RERF), 1767
Radiation Emergency Assistance Center/Training Site (REAC/TS), 1767–1768, 1770, 1780–1781
emergency number for, 1360
Radiation Emergency Medical Management, website, 1768
Radiation Emergency Medical Preparedness and Assistance (REMPAN), 1767
Radiation Exposure Information and Reporting System (REIRS), 1767
Radiative energy attenuation (REA), in ethanol measurement, 1877
Radical(s), 174
Radioactive decay, 1762–1763, 1763t
Radioactive isotopes, antidote for, 35t
Radioactivity, principles, 1762–1765
Radiocontrast agents. *See also specific xenobiotic*
extravasation of, diagnostic imaging, 119, 121f
Radiogardase, 1357. *See also* Prussian blue
acquisition, 1360
formulation, 1360
Radiography, 114
abdominal, 127
in arsenic toxicity, 1244
in bismuth toxicity, 1256
in body packers, 117, 120f
of caustic injury, 1391
in iron ingestion, 671, 672f
phenothiazines on, 1040
in toxicologic emergencies, 129t
for unknown xenobiotic ingestion, 47f
with xenobiotic exposure, 115t
of caustic injury, 1391, 1392f
chest, 125t
of caustic injury, 1391
in cocaine toxicity, 125t
in injection drug use (IDU), 125t, 126f
in metal phosphide poisoning, 1459
for poisoned patient, 407
of pulmonary and other thoracic complications, 115t, 122–126
in respiratory disorders, 401, 406
in smoke inhalation, 1642, 1643f
in strychnine poisoning, 1537
in toxicologic emergencies, 125t
with xenobiotic exposure, 115t
xenobiotics on, 115t
dental, radiation exposure in, 1766
of hydrocarbon pneumonitis, 1412, 1413f
mothballs and moth repellents on, 1385, 1385t
naphthalene on, 1385, 1385t
paradichlorobenzene on, 1385, 1385t
radiation exposure in, 1766, 1766t
of soft tissue abnormalities, 122
stingray spines on, 1578
Radioimmunoassay(s) (RIA), 104
Radioiodine
absorption, 1775
decay pathway, 1775f
definition, 1775
protection against
iodides not useful as, 1777
potassium iodide in, 1775–1777
sources, 1775
Radioisotope(s)
definition, 155, 1763

half-life, 1762–1763, 1763t
in medicine and research, 1763t
military, 1763t
physical properties, 1762–1763, 1763t
Radionuclides
commonly encountered, 1769–1770
contamination by, 1765
definition, 1763
in diagnostic imaging, 1766, 1766t
history of, 1762
incorporation, 1765
Radiopacity
factors affecting, 114
intrinsic, 114
in vitro, 114
of xenobiotics, 114
Radithor, 23–24, 23t
Radium, toxic exposure to, 23, 23t
Radix bupleuri, 647
Radix valerianae (*Valeriana officinalis*), 644t
Radon, 158, 1765, 1765t, 1769–1770
Ragweed, allergic reactions to, 1521, 1614
Ragwort, *Heliotropium* spp., 1600t, 1605
Rainforest hognosed pit viper (*Porthidium* spp.), 1637t
Rajiformes, 1576
Raleigh, Sir Walter, 1018
Raloxifene, 617
Raltegravir, 832
Raltitrexed, hydrolysis, by glucarpidase, 785
Ramaria rufescens, 1582t, 1591
Ramazzini, Bernadino, 4t, 22
Ramelteon, 1090. *See also* Sedative-hypnotics
history of, 1084
pharmacodynamics, 1084
pharmacokinetics, 1085t
Ram-goat rose. *See* Periwinkle (*Catharanthus roseus*)
Ramps (*Allium tricoccum*), 1606
Rand, Benjamin Howard, 4t, 7
Randomization
block, 1856
in clinical trials, 1856–1857
simple, 1856
stratified, 1856–1857
unequal, 1856–1857
Ranitidine
absorption, 744
acute interstitial nephritis caused by, 394t
and alcohol dehydrogenase inhibition, 1428
drug interactions with, 744
elimination, 744
and ethanol, interactions, 744, 1146t
and ethanol metabolism, 1144
history of, 739
metabolism, 744
overdose/poisoning, 746
pharmacokinetics and toxicokinetics, 745t
structure, 742, 742f
volume of distribution, 744
RANKL inhibitors, hypomagnesemia caused by, 877
Ranunculaceae, 1598t–1602t, 1605, 1613
Ranunculin, 1602t, 1613
Ranunculus spp. (buttercups), 1602t
as abortifacients, 303t
Rapastinel (GLYX-13), 228
and NMDA receptor, 227t
Rapeseed oil, contaminated, 18–19, 18t, 281
Raphides, 1613
Rapid acetylators, 170
Rapid opioid detoxification, 239, 534
Rapoport-Luebering shunt, 312, 313f

Rapture of the deep, 1653
Rare disease(s), 1833–1834
Rasagiline, 1077
mechanism of action, 212
Rasa shastra, 648, 1293
Rash
antimonials and, 1233
in arsenic poisoning, 1241
bismuth-related, 1255
Raspberry ketone, 607t, 610. *See also* Dieting xenobiotics and regimens
structure, 610f
Rate constant (k), 150
Ratfish, 1576
Rat root (*Acorus calamus*), 1598t
Rattlebox (*Crotalaria* spp.), 1599t
Rattlebox (*Heliotropum europaeum*), 642t
Rattlesnakes (*Crotalus* spp., *Sistrurus* spp.), 1617, 1633t
bites. *See also* Snakebite(s)
deaths caused by, 1617–1618
killed and decapitated snake and, 1617
envenomation
clinical manifestations, 1621
hematologic toxicity, 1622
venom, neurotoxicity, 1622
Rauwolfia serpentina (snakeroot), 1602t
psychoactive properties, 650t
Rave parties, 1099, 1178
ketamine at, 1210
Raynaud syndrome, 281
Rays, 1576
RBCs. *See* Erythrocyte(s)
RCS-4, 1112f
RDX (cyclotrimethylenetrinitramine), 1482
and GABA, 222
Reabsorption, renal, 389
Reactive airways dysfunction syndrome (RADS), 403, 1660
Reactive nitrogen species, 159–160
structure, 160t
Reactive oxygen species (ROS), 157, 157f, 159–160, 174, 670, 1172, 1656
copper and, 1285, 1285f, 1286
cyanide-induced, 1685–1686
iron-induced, 670
irritant gases and, 1640
manganese and, 1320
in naphthalene metabolism, 1382, 1382f
paraquat and, 1474, 1474f, 1477
production, by irritant gases, 1653
structure, 160t
toluene-induced, 1196
trivalent arsenic and, 1238
Reactive species, 159–160. *See also* Reactive nitrogen species; Reactive oxygen species (ROS)
definition, 159
detoxification, 160
formation, 160
structure, 160t
REAC/TS. *See* Radiation Emergency Assistance Center/ Training Site (REAC/TS)
Reagent strip testing, for blood glucose measurement, 700, 708–709
Realgar, 1237
Reasonable medical certainty, 1873–1874
Recall bias, 1856
Receptor(s). *See also specific receptor*
endocytosis, and withdrawal syndrome, 237
and withdrawal syndrome, 237

Rechallenge, by suspect drug, 1838t, 1839
Recombinant activated factor VII (rFVIIa), for anticoagulant overdose, 887, 891, 894–896
Recombinant tissue plasminogen activator (rt-PA), 884
Recommended dietary allowances (RDAs), for vitamins, 655t
Recovery, of ion channels, 203
Rectal prolapse, cathartic-induced, 85
Rectifying channels, 245
Redback widow spider. *See Latrodectus hasselti*
Red bark. *See Cinchona* spp.
Red blood cell(s). *See* Erythrocyte(s)
Red blood cell acetylcholinesterase, activity
as indicator of anticholinesterase toxicity, 1494–1495, 1495t
interpretation, 1494–1495, 1495t
Red cell aplasia, pure, 319
Red cell distribution width (RDW), 317
Red clover (*Trifolium pratense*), 1603t
Red copper oxide, 1284t
Red diamond rattlesnake (*Crotalus ruber*), 1617t, 1636t
Red elm (*Ulmus rubra*), 644t
Red flower oil, 634
Redheaded cotton-bush (*Asclepias curassavica*), 979
Redi, Francesco, 3
Red man syndrome, 273, 828
Red-moss sponge, 1574
Redotex, 816
Redox cycling, 160, 1274
paraquat and, 1474, 1474f
Redox potential, ethanol metabolism and, 1146
Redox reactions. *See* Reduction/oxidation (redox) reactions
Red periwinkle (*Catharanthus roseus*). *See* Periwinkle (*Catharanthus roseus*)
Red phosphorus, 1528–1532
chemistry, 1528
toxicity, pathophysiology, 1529
Red rattlesnake (*Crotalus* spp.), 1636t
Red River snake root (*Aristolochia* spp.), 1598t
Red rock cod (*Scorpaena cardinalis*), 1576t
Red skin color, poisoning/overdose causing, 36t
Red sponge (*Microciona prolifera*), 1573
Red squill (*Urginea maritima*), 644t, 969, 979, 1603t
physicochemical properties, 1453t
in rodenticides, 1453t. *See also* Rodenticides
toxicity
antidote and/or treatment for, 1453t
clinical manifestations, 1453t
onset, 1453t
toxic mechanism, 1453t
Red tides, 595–596
Reducing agent, 159, 271
5α-Reductase inhibitor(s), 644t
Reduction, 168
definition, 159
Reduction/oxidation (redox) reactions, 159–160, 168
copper-containing enzymes and, 1284–1285, 1285t
iron in, 670
transition metals in, 157, 160
Red valerian (*Valeriana officinalis*), 644t
Reef stonefish (*Synanceja verrucosa*), 1576, 1576t, 1577
Reentry dysrhythmias, 255, 255f, 256
Refeeding syndrome, and thiamine deficiency, 1160
Reflex(es), abnormal, 37
Refractory cells, 246

Regadeoson, and adenosine receptor, 230, 230t
Regulatory agencies, 1801t, 1804
Regulatory initiatives, 9, 10t
Reinsch, Hugo, 4t, 6
Relapsing fever, 1550
  tick-borne, 1550
Relative risk
  definition, 1854
  estimation, 1853t, 1854, 1854f
Rem (roentgen equivalent man), 1764, 1764f
Remacemide, mechanism of action, 227t
Remifentanil
  as incapacitating agent, 1750
  Russian military's use of, 17, 17t
Remijia pedunculata (cuprea bark), 1602t
Remoxipride. *See also* Antipsychotics
  clinical and toxicologic effects, 1034t
  dosage and administration, 1033t
  pharmacokinetics, 1033t
Renaissance, toxicology in, 3–6
Renal artery(ies), 389
  stenosis, 397
Renal calculi, diuretic-induced, 963
Renal carcinoma, 273
Renal cortex, 389, 390f
Renal disorders. *See also specific disorder*
  functional toxic, 395–396
  history-taking in, 396
  laboratory investigation, 396–397
  patient evaluation for, 396–397
  physical examination in, 396
  and urine specific gravity, 189
Renal failure. *See* Kidney failure
Renal fascia, 389
Renal function. *See also* Kidney(s), function
  evaluation, 396–397
Renal injury, acute. *See* Acute kidney injury (AKI)
Renal medulla, 389, 390f
Renal pelvis, 389
Renal principles, 389–398. *See also* Kidney(s);
        Nephrotoxicity
Renal tubular acidosis (RTA), 395–396
  management, 193–194
  and normal anion gap metabolic acidosis, 193
  sodium stibogluconate and, 1232
  toluene and, 1196
Renal tubular dysfunction, metals causing, 397t
Renin, serum, lead poisoning and, 1295–1296
Renin-angiotensin-aldosterone system, 963, 963f, 965
Renin-angiotensin system, activation, gastrointestinal
        decontamination and, 85
Ren shen (ginseng), uses and toxicities, 642t
Repaglinide, 715
  history of, 694
  hypoglycemia caused by, 700
  pharmacokinetics and toxicokinetics, 696, 697t
  pharmacology, 696
  structure, 695f
Replisome (DNA), 349
Repolarization
  early, 249, 250f
  myocardial, 245–254, 245f, 970, 971f
  neuronal, 203, 205f
Reproduction. *See also* Fertility; Teratogen(s);
        Teratogenesis; Teratogenicity
  antimonials and, 1233
Reproductive and perinatal principles, 428–447.
        See also Pregnancy; *specific xenobiotic*
  in females, 428
  in males, 428

Reproductive system
  female, xenobiotics and, 302–304, 302t
  male, xenobiotics and, 297–301
Rescue agent. *See also specific agent*
  definition, 770
Research subjects, protection, 13
Reserpine, 650t, 961, 1602t
  adverse effects and safety issues, 961
  mechanism of action, 208, 211t, 212, 215, 218
Resins, 639, 1597, 1599t, 1602t, 1607–1608
  antimitotic, 1612
  fluorinated, thermal degradation products, 1641t
  in hemoperfusion, 96
  in poisoning management, 90, 90t, 92
  urushiol, 1614
Resmethrin, 1520t. *See also* Pyrethroids
Resource Conservation and Recovery Act (RSRA), 10t,
        1801t
  and nanotechnology, 1731
Respiration, neuromuscular blockers and, 1019
Respiratory acidosis, 189
  compensation for, 190
  definition, 190
  in strychnine poisoning, 1537
Respiratory alkalosis, 189
  carbon monoxide poisoning and, 1665
  compensation for, 190
  definition, 190
  methylxanthines and, 988–989
  renal compensation for, 190
  salicylates and, 399
Respiratory arrest, methylxanthines and, 988
Respiratory center, 399
Respiratory depression
  after naloxone administration, 541
  benzodiazepines and, 386, 1139–1140
  dissociative anesthetics and, 1214
  ethanol and, 386, 1149
  inhalant-induced, 1196
  opioid-induced, 524–525
    management, 541–542
  propofol and, 1089
  sedative-hypnotics and, 1086–1087
Respiratory depth, 399
Respiratory drive, xenobiotics and, 299, 299t
Respiratory dysfunction, in poisoned patient
  antidotal therapy for, 407–408
  approach to, 403–406
  history-taking for, 404
  physical examination in, 404
  treatment, 406–408
Respiratory echange ratio, 408f
Respiratory failure
  in barium toxicity, 1455
  metabolic alkalosis and, 194
  methylxanthines and, 988
  smoke inhalation and, 1645
Respiratory irritants, 1640–1641, 1640t, 1653–1658
  characteristics, 1653, 1654t
  detection threshold, 1654t
  exposure to, clinical manifestations, 1654–1655
  immediately dangerous to life and health (IDLH),
        1654t
  regulatory standards for, 1654t
  short-term exposure limits (STEL), 1654t
  sources, 1654t
  water solubility, 1640, 1640t, 1654, 1654t, 1655–1656
Respiratory muscle weakness, 406. *See also* Chest wall
Respiratory pattern, in initial assessment, 189
Respiratory principles, 399–410

Respiratory rate, 399. *See also* Bradypnea; Tachypnea
  assessment, 36
    in poisoned patient, 266t
  decreased, 399–400
  in initial assessment, 189
  normal, 30, 1651
    by age, 28t
  xenobiotics affecting, 30t
Respiratory-sparing effect, of neuromuscular blockers,
        1019
Respiratory tract
  injury
    caustic, clinical manifestations, 1390
    irritant gases and, 1640–1641, 1640t
    thermal, 1640–1641
  physiology, 1651
Restaurant syndromes, 600
Restraint
  chemical, 386
  forcible, of impaired patient, 1862
    documentation supporting, 1861
  physical, for violent patient, 387
Retention time (t$_R$), 105, 107
Reteplase, 896–897
Reticulocytosis, 317
  cobalt-related, 1274
Retigabine. *See* Ezogabine
Retina, 356, 356f
  injury to, xenobiotic exposures and, 357t
  in methanol poisoning, 1423–1424
    corticosteroids and, 1430
  quinine and, 839, 841
  veins, arterialization, in cyanide poisoning, 1686
Retinal (vitamin A), 655
11-*cis*-Retinal, 656
Retinal hemorrhage, carbon monoxide poisoning and,
        1665
Retinoic acid, 655–656
all-*trans* Retinoic acid, mechanism and site of action,
        762f
Retinoic acid syndrome, 656, 1243
Retinoids, 655–656. *See also* Vitamin A
  excess, pathophysiology, 656–657
  hypercalcemia caused by, 250
  teratogenicity, 430t
Retinoid X receptor (RXR), 170
Retinol, 655. *See also* Vitamin A
  serum, normal concentration, 656
Retinol activity equivalents (RAEs), 655
Retinol-binding protein, 656
  urinary loss, cadmium-induced, 1260
Retinol dehydrogenase, 1437
Retinyl esters, 655–656
Retrobulbar neuropathy, xenobiotic exposures and, 357t
Retroperitoneal fibrosis, xenobiotic-induced, 394, 394t
Reverse osmosis, for water purification, 99
Reverse T$_3$, 812
Reversible inhibitors of monoamine oxidase-A
        (RIMAs), 1077
Reversible leukoencephalopathy. *See* Reversible
        posterior leukoencephalopathy
Reversible osmotic demyelination syndrome, in
        ethylene glycol poisoning, 1424
Reversible posterior leukoencephalopathy
  ophthalmic effects, 361t
  xenobiotic exposures and, 357t
Revonto, 1030
Rewarming
  active external, 418
  active internal, 418

for frostbite, 418
for hypothermia, 418
 underlying illness and, 414–415, 415f
passive external, 418
Reye syndrome, 557
Rhabdomyolysis, 93, 393t, 1020
amphetamine-induced, 1104
antihistamine-related, 746
 management, 747
in arsenic poisoning, 1241
barium toxicity and, 1455
cocaine and, 1127–1128
with colchicine poisoning, 503, 503t
hallucinogen-induced, 1184
hypokalemia and, 198, 393
hypophosphatemia and, 393, 393t
insect venom and, 393, 393t
methylxanthine-induced, 989, 991
mushrooms and, 393t
phencyclidine toxicity and, 1217
pit viper envenomation and, 1622
renal effects, 393
simvastatin and, 171
snake venom and, 393t, 1622
in strychnine poisoning, 1537–1538
xenobiotic-induced, 21, 27, 36t, 393, 393t
 sodium bicarbonate for, 568t
Rhamnaceae, 1599t, 1602t
Rhamnus frangula, 1602t
 uses and toxicities, 640t
Rhamnus purshiana, uses and toxicities, 641t
Rhein, 641t
Rhein anthrones, 1602t
Rheum spp. (rhubarb), 1602t
Rheum officinale (rhubarb), 1602t
Rhinitis medicamentosa, 1347
rho (ρ), Widmark's, 1879–1880
Rhodanase, 167, 1685
Rhodanese, 1686–1687, 1689, 1698–1699
 and cyanide detoxification, 1685, 1685f
 deficiency, 1686
Rhododendron, 1602t, 1612
Rhododendron luteum, 1612
Rhodophyllus spp., GI toxins in, 1589
Rhubarb (*Rheum officinale, Rheum* spp.), 1602t
Rhytidoponera metallica, 1552
Ribociclib, 349f
 cell cycle phase specificity, 761f
Riboflavin, 654
 thallium and, 1351
Ribosome(s), thallium and, 1351
Ribotide, 212
Rice oil disease, 18, 18t
Richmond Agitation Sedation Scale (RASS), 1166–1168
Ricin, 5t, 12, 1597, 1602t, 1608–1609, 1608f, 1753
 as abortifacient, 303t
 as biological weapon, 1608, 1759
 mechanism of action, 167
 toxicity (poisoning)
  N-acetylcysteine for, 494
  in children, 1608–1609
  in US government buildings, 17, 17t
Ricinus communis, 1602t, 1608f
 as abortifacient, 303t
 in biologic warfare, 1759
 self-poisoning with, 1846
Rickets, 659
 vitamin D deficiency and, 660
Rickettsiae, 1757

Rickettsia prowazekii, 1757
Ridgenose rattlesnake (*Crotalus willardi*), 1617t
Rifabutin, 854–855
 effect on thyroid hormones and function, 814t
 for HIV-related infections, 831t
 ophthalmic toxicity, 356f
 pregnancy class, 855
Rifampin, 854–855
 acute interstitial nephritis caused by, 394f, 394t
 adverse effects and safety issues, 853t
 cholestasis caused by, 330
 and CYP induction, 171
 diabetes insipidus caused by, 195, 195t
 drug interactions with, 853t, 855
 effect on thyroid hormones and function, 814t
 elimination half-life, 855
 hepatotoxicity, 330
 HIV medications and, 853t
 monitoring with, 853t
 pharmacokinetics and toxicokinetics, 854–855
 pregnancy class, 855
 and protease inhibitors, 855
 renal effects, 390f
 structure, 854
 toxicity
  acute, 855
  chronic, 855
  clinical manifestations, 855
  diagnostic tests for, 855
  management, 855
Rifamycins, 854–855
 drug interactions with, 855
 and HIV medications, 855
 pharmacology, 854
Rifapentine, 854–855
 pregnancy class, 855
Rifaximin, and hepatic encephalopathy, 334
Right to refuse treatment, 1860
Rig-Veda, 1, 1178
Riker Sedation Anesthesia Scale (SAS), 1166, 1168
Rilmenidine, 961
Rilpivirine, 831
Riluzole, mechanism of action, 227t, 228
RimabotulinumtoxinB (Myobloc), 578–579
Rimonabant, 606, 608t, 611
 structure, 1112f
Ring (annulus), of mushrooms, 1584f, 1593
Riot control agents
 chemical names and structures, 1749f
 as chemical weapons, 1741, 1749–1750
 decontamination for, 1743, 1750
 exposure to, treatment, 1743, 1750
 military designations, 1749f
 as pulmonary irritants, 1657
 toxic syndromes caused by, 1751t
Risk
 acceptable, 1815
 applicability, communication about, 1816
 calculation, 1806
 definition, 1806
 as hazard + outrage, 1817
 magnitude, communication about, 1816
 perceived, acceptability, factors affecting, 1817, 1817t
 urgency, communication about, 1816
Risk assessment
 for cancer, 1815
 components, 1814, 1815t
 definition, 1814
 difficulties, 1814

factors affecting, 1817, 1817t
individual, *vs.* public health, 1815
for noncancer effects, 1815
in toxicology, 1816–1817
uncertainties and, 1814–1815
 communication about, 1816
Risk communication, 1815–1816, 1816t
 factors affecting, 1817, 1817t
 interpreting public health concerns for individual in, 1817–1819, 1817t
 terrorism and, 1817–1818
 in toxicology, 1816–1817
Risk Evaluation and Mitigation Strategies (REMS), 1834–1835, 1839
Risk factors, assessment, 1853t
Risk management, 1861–1862
 options for, communication about, 1816
Risperidone. *See also* Antipsychotics
 cardiac effects, 258t
 clinical and toxicologic effects, 1034t
 dosage and administration, 1033t
 extrapyramidal effects, 215
 and female sexual dysfunction, 302f
 for hallucinogen-induced agitation, 1184
 for inhalant-induced psychosis, 1200
 mechanism of action, 1035
 pharmacokinetics, 1033t
 priapism caused by, 301t
 and sudden cardiac death, 253
Risus sardonicus
 with arylcyclohexylamine toxicity, 1215
 in strychnine poisoning, 1536–1537
Ritanserin, mechanism of action, 218
Ritodrine, 985
 toxicity, 986
Ritonavir, 831–832
 and colchicine, interactions, 502
 and methadone, interactions, 172
 and serotonin toxicity, 1058t
Rituximab
 and posterior reversible encephalopathy syndrome, 132
 and rhabdomyolysis, 393t
Rivaroxaban, 321f, 884f, 894–896
 adverse effects and safety issues, 894
  in elderly, 465
 efficacy, 894
 gastrointestinal decontamination for, 50t
 laboratory testing for, 888t, 895
 overdose/poisoning
  clinical manifestations, 895
  gastrointestinal decontamination for, 78
  treatment strategies for, 888t
 pharmacology, 893t, 894–895
 reversal agent for, 912–913
Rivastigmine, 1495, 1503
 acetylcholinesterase inhibition by, 208, 756
 mechanism of action, 208
 oral, for central anticholinergic syndrome, 748
River ray, 1576
Rizatriptan, 217, 808–809, 808t
RNA, fluoropyrimidines and, 771–772, 771f
RNA polymerase, zinc in, 1362
RNA primase, 349–350
Robin (robinia lectin), 1602t
Robinia pseudoacacia (black locust), 1602t, 1609
Roche, Ellen, 13
Rochin v. California, 1863
Rocket fuel, poisoning with, pyridoxine for, 862–863

Rock hard (*Bufo bufo gargarizans, Bufo bufo melanosticus*), 649
  as aphrodisiac, 649
  psychoactive properties, 650t
  uses and toxicities, 637t
Rock parsley (*Petroselinum crispum*), 643t
Rock rattlesnake, 1617t, 1636t
Rocky Mountain spotted fever, 324, 1550
Rocky Mountain wood tick (*Dermacentor andersoni*), 1550
Rocuronium
  and anaphylaxis, 1019
  pharmacology, 1020t
  and response to subsequent nondepolarizer administration, 1021t
  and response to succinylcholine, 1021t
  reversal, sugammadex for, 1025–1026, 1026f
  reversal agent, 46t
Rodenticides, 1457. *See also* Long-acting anticoagulant rodenticide(s) (LAARs); *specific rodenticide*
  anticoagulant
    antidote for, 35t
    clinical and laboratory findings with, 36t
  and citric acid cycle, 175
  EPA toxicity classification, 1450, 1450t
  food contamination with, 599–600, 602
  high toxicity ("danger"), 1450t, 1452t–1453t
  labeling of
    caution, 1450t, 1453t
    danger, 1450t, 1452t–1453t
    warning, 1450t, 1453t
  low toxicity ("caution"), 1450t, 1453t
  moderate toxicity ("warning"), 1450t, 1453t
  pharmacokinetics, 146t
  phosphorus as, 1528
  poisoning, 886–887
  regulation, 1450
  toxicity, management, 45t
  vitamin K antagonists as, 886
  warfarin poisoning from. *See* Warfarin
Roentgen (R), 1763, 1764f
Rofecoxib (Vioxx), 465, 511, 514, 1839
  adverse effects and side effects, 21
Roid rage, 618
Rokan (*Gingko biloba*). *See* Gingko (*Gingko biloba*)
Rolicyclidine (PCPy), 1211, 1211t
  DEA class, 1211
Rolipram, glucagon with, 942
Roman Empire
  lead poisoning in, 2
  poisoners in, 2
Roman vitriol, 1284t
Rome, poisoners in, 4
Roncovite, 1273
R on T phenomena, 256
Room deodorizers, inhaled, 1193t, 1194. *See also* Inhalant(s)
Root cause analysis (RCA), 1827
Rope (burnt), smell of, 364t
Ropinirole, mechanism of action, 214
Ropivacaine. *See also* Local anesthetic(s)
  cardiac arrest associated with, 1001
  cardiovascular toxicity, 999
  history of, 994
  pharmacology, 996t
Rosaceae, 1602t, 1607
Rosa laurel. *See* Oleander
Rosary pea (*Abrus precatorius*), 1598t, 1608f, 1609
Rosary seeds (*Ricinus communis*), 1602t
  in biologic warfare, 1759

Rose bay. *See* Oleander
Rose eye, 1341
Rose francesca. *See* Oleander
Rosiglitazone
  adverse effects and safety issues, 700
  hepatotoxicity, 331
  pharmacokinetics and toxicokinetics, 697t
Rosiglitazone maleate, structure, 695f
Rotavirus, foodborne illness caused by, 592t
Rotenone
  and electron transport, 176t
  site of action, 173f
Rotterdam Convention, 1847
Rou dou kou. *See Myristica fragrans* (mace, nutmeg)
Round ray, 1576
Roundup. *See* Glyphosate
Roundworms
  intestinal infestations, 600
  larvae, illness caused by, 597
Royal jelly (*Apis mellifera*), 640t
Rubber
  synthetic, thermal degradation products, 1685
  thermal degradation products, 1641t
Rubber vine (*Cryptostegia grandifolia*), 979
Rubbing alcohol, 162, 1369t. *See also* Isopropanol (isopropyl alcohol)
Rubiaceae, 1599t–1602t
Rubidium, dermal decontamination for, precautions with, 72
Rue (*Ruta graveolens*), 644t
Rufinamide
  adverse effects and safety issues, 725, 727–728, 727t
  drug-induced hypersensitivity syndrome with, 727–728, 727t
  drug interactions with, 723t, 725
  mechanism of action, 720f, 720t
  metabolism and effects on CYP enzymes, 722t
  pharmacokinetics and toxicokinetics, 721t
  pharmacology, 719, 720t
  therapeutic serum concentration, 725
Rufinamine, 227t
Rumack-Matthew nomogram, 476, 477f, 494, 1852–1853
Rumex spp. (dock), 1602t
"Runner's high," 523
Russell's viper (*Vipera russelii*), 1633t
Russian cocktail, manganese in, 1319
Russian comfrey (*Symphytum* spp.), uses and toxicities, 641t
Russian VX, 1741, 1745
Russula subnigricans, 1582t, 1591
Rustic treacle. *See Allium sativum* (garlic)
Rutaceae, 1599t, 1601t, 1614
Ruta graveolens (rue), 644t
  as abortifacient, 303t
Ruthenium, chelator for, 1780
Rutin, 642t, 1597
Ryanodex, 1030
Ryanodine receptor(s) (RYR), 262, 262f, 945, 946f, 947
  cardiac (RYR-2), 1029
  in cardiac physiology, 928–929
  dantrolene and, 1029
  and malignant hyperthermia, 1023, 1029
RYR1 gene, and malignant hyperthermia, 1023

S

Sabal. *See* Saw palmetto (*Serenoa repens*)
Sacred bark (*Cascara sagrada*), uses and toxicities, 1599t
Sacred earth, 3

Sac spider (*Cheiracanthium*), bites, necrotic wounds with, 1545
Saddleback caterpillar (*Sibine stimulata*), 1552
Safe Drinking Water Act (1974), 10t
  and nanotechnology, 1731
Safe injection sites, 552
S.A.F.E.S.T. approach, for violent patient, 387, 387t
Safety. *See also specific xenobiotic*
  medication, 1822–1832. *See also specific xenobiotic*
Saffron
  as aphrodisiac, 304
  meadow, *Colchicum autumnale. See also* Colchicine
    uses and toxicities, 640t
Safrole, 641t, 1179t, 1183
  structure, 1183f
Sage (*Salvia officinalis*), 644t
St. Anthony's fire, 18, 806. *See also* Ergot and ergot alkaloids
St. Ignatius bean (*Strychnos* spp.), 1603t
St. John's wort (*Hypericum perforatum*), 4, 144, 644t, 1600t
  and CYP enzymes, 170, 646–647, 646t, 647f, 1610–1611
  hyperforin and hypericin in, 646–647, 1610
  MAOI activity, 646, 646t, 1077
  pharmacologic interactions, 646–647, 646t, 647f
  and serotonin toxicity, 646, 646t, 1058t, 1611
  xenobiotic interactions with, 646–647, 646t, 647f, 1610–1611
Salamanders, poisons from, 1
Salem witchcraft trials, 18, 18t, 1178
Salicaceae, 1602t
Salicin, 555, 638, 644t, 1597, 1602t, 1607
Salicyl acid, 634
Salicylate(s), 555–566, 634, 1410. *See also* Nonsteroidal antiinflammatory drugs (NSAIDs)
  and acid-base balance, 557, 559
  adverse effects and safety issues, 608t
  antidote for, 35t
  antiinflammatory effects, 555
  and ATP synthesis, 176t
  chemistry, 161
  clearance, and extracorporeal removal, 91–92
  effect on thyroid hormones and function, 814t
  effects on vital signs, 30t–31t
  elimination
    multiple-dose activated charcoal and, 78
    therapeutic manipulation, 147
  enhanced elimination, 90
    urine alkalinization for, 93, 562, 562f, 563, 569–570
  extracoporeal removal, 562–563, 563t
  and fatty acid metabolism, 176t
  and fluid balance, 194
  gastric irritant effects, 558
  gastrointestinal effects, 558
  hematologic effects, 558
  and high anion gap metabolic acidosis, 191t
  history of, 555
  hyperventilation caused by, 400t
  hypoglycemia caused by, 698, 709
  laboratory testing for, 101t, 102–103
  mechanism of action, 608t
  metabolic effects, 557
  metabolism, 555
  neuroglycopenia caused by, 708–709
  ototoxicity, 366f, 558, 561
  for paraquat poisoning, 1474f, 1477
  pharmacokinetics, 555
  pharmacology, 555
  plasma protein binding by, 146

pulmonary effects, 558
renal effects, 558
respiratory effects, 399, 399t
and respiratory rate, 30
serum concentration
    analysis, 560
    factors affecting, 560
    interpretation, and correlation with toxicity,
        560–561
    reporting (units for), 560
    therapeutic, 555
    toxic, 555
site of action, 173f
and tinnitus, 369–370, 370t
topical, 556–557
toxicity (overdose/poisoning), 161, 178
    activated charcoal for, 561
    acute, 558–559, 559t
    adrenergic effects, 557
    ARDS in, 123, 125t, 401, 402t
    bismuth subsalicylate and, 1257
    chronic, 559, 559t
    clinical manifestations, 36, 36t, 558–559, 559t,
        560–561
    cranial neuropathy caused by, 346t
    diagnostic imaging in, 115t, 123, 125t
    diffuse airspace filling in, 125t
    in elderly, case study, 459
    epidemiology, 555
    evaluation and diagnostic tests for, 559–561
    extracorporeal therapies for, 91, 91f, 92, 97t
    fluid replacement for, 561–562
    and "forced diuresis," 561
    gastrointestinal decontamination for, 86, 561
    glucose supplementation for, 562
    hemodialysis for, 94, 562–563, 563t
    hepatic effects, 557
    hypoglycemia in, 698, 709
    intubation and, 563
    management, 38, 46t, 148, 167, 561–564
    mechanical ventilation and, 563
    neurologic effects, 557
    oxygen consumption in, 557
    pediatric considerations, 563–564
    in pregnancy, 564
    saturation of plasma proteins in, 147
    sedation and, 563
    serum and urine alkalinization for, 562, 562f, 563,
        569–570
    serum salicylate concentration and pH
        monitoring in, 563
    sodium bicarbonate for, 568t
    toxicokinetics, 555–556, 556f
    urine alkalinization for, 93
    and vitamin K antagonism, 916
    volume of distribution, 91
Salicylic acid, 145t, 556–557
    chemistry, 161
    physicochemical properties, 555
    salicin hydrolysis and, 1607
    serum concentration, therapeutic, 555
    toxicity, organ system manifestations, 829t
Salicylism, 1602t
    diagnosis, 192
    sodium bicarbonate for, 569–570
    and tinnitus, 370, 561
Salicyluric acid, 634
Saline cathartics, 83
Saliva, pH, 142t
Salivation, poisoning/overdose causing, 36t

Salix spp. (willow), 555, 1602t
Salix alba (white willow), 644t
Salmeterol, 985
    pharmacology, 986–987
Sal mirabile, 83
Salmonella spp., 592, 592t, 597–598, 597t
    and bioterrorism, 602
    dairy contaminated with, 602
Salmonella enterica, 592t, 597–598
Salmonella typhimurium, and bioterrorism, 602
Salt(s). See also specific salt
    depletion
        gastrointestinal decontamination and, 85
        multiple-dose activated charcoal and, 79
    and hypernatremia, 194–195
Salt loading, and thiamine pharmacokinetics, 1158
Salvia (Salvia divinorum, S. miltiorrhizae), 644t, 650t,
        1178–1179, 1179t, 1181, 1181t
    clinical effects, 1183
    pharmacologic interactions, 646t
    toxicokinetics, 1182
Salvia officinalis (sage), 644t
Salvinorin A, 1181t
    effects on kappa receptor, 521
    and kappa opioid receptor, 1182
    laboratory detection, 1184
    pharmacology, 1182
    structure, 1183f
Salvinorum A, 644t, 650t
Sambucus spp. (elder, elderberry), 639, 1602t
    uses and toxicities, 641t
Sambucus nigra (European elderberry), 1607
Sambunigirn, 641t
(S)-Sambunigrin, 1607
Sammarco, Thomas, 1018
Sampedro, Ramon, 1685
Sand dollars, 1573–1574
San Esteban Island rattlesnake (Crotalus spp.), 1636t
Sanguinaria canadensis (bloodroot), 1543t, 1605
Sanguinarine, 650t, 1598t, 1602t, 1605
San Lorenzo Island rattlesnake (Crotalus spp.), 1636t
San Lucan diamond rattlesnake (Crotalus spp.), 1636t
San Pedro cactus (Trichocereus pachanoi), 3, 1180
Sapa, 1292
Sapindaceae, 1598t, 1601t
Saponaria officinalis (soapwort), 644t
Saponin glycosides, 639, 1597, 1598t, 1600t, 1603t,
        1606, 1606f
Saponins, 642t, 644t, 650t, 1600t
    steroidal, 1603t
    toxic, of sea stars, 1574
Saquinavir, 831–832
Saquinavir mesylate, ritonavir-boosted, and prolonged
        QT interval, 253t
Sarafotoxins, in snake venom, 1618
Sarcosine, 227t, 228
Sarin, 1488t, 1508
    aging half-life, 1746
    chemical name and structure, 1745f
    clinical effects, 1745
    decontamination for, 1743
    history of, 1486, 1741
    long-term effects, 1745
    ophthalmic effects, 358
    physical characteristics, 1745
    secondary exposure to, 1742, 1745
    in Syrian civil war, 17, 17t, 1741
    terrorists' use of, 17, 17t, 1741
    Tokyo subway incident with, 71, 1741–1742,
        1744–1745

toxicity, 1744
    magnesium for, 878–879
    toxic syndrome caused by, 1750t
SARMs (selective androgen receptor modulators),
        617
Sarsasapogenin, 1598t
Sassafras (Sassafras albidum), 644t
Sassafras oil, 644t
Saturation gap, 1708
Sauropus androgynous, 1611
Savayasa. See Edoxaban
Savin, as abortifacient, 303t
Savlon, self-poisoning with, 1846
Saw palmetto (Serenoa repens), use and toxicities,
        644t, 649
Saw-scaled viper (Echis carinatus), 1633t
Saxagliptin
    pharmacokinetics and toxicokinetics, 697t
    pharmacology, 696
Saxitoxin, 595
    clinical effects, 576t
    and voltage-gated calcium channels, 244f, 245
Saxitoxinlike toxin, 1598t
Saybolt universal seconds (SUS), 1412
S100B, serum, in carbon monoxide poisoning, 1667
Scala tympani, 366, 366f
Scala vestibuli, 366, 366f
Scale (skin lesion), 269t
Scales, of mushrooms, 1584f
Scandium, chelator for, 1780
Scanning tunneling microscope (STM), 1717
Scar, 269t
Scarlet sage. See Salvia officinalis (sage)
Schecoids, 1540t
Scheele, Carl Wilhelm, 1684
Scheele green, 1284t
Schefflera spp. (umbrella tree), 1602t, 1613
Schistosomiasis
    and bladder tumors, 1233
    treatment, antimony in, 1228–1229
Schizoaffective disorder, and suicide, 378–379
Schizophrenia
    glutamate and, 224
    negative symptoms, 1032–1033
    positive symptoms, 1032, 1034
    and suicide, 378–379
    treatment, 215
        history of, 1032
    and violence, 385
Schloendorff v. Society of New York Hospital, 1860–1861
Schmerber v. California, 1863
Schou, Mogens, 1065
Schradan, 1488t
Schräder, Gerhard, 1741
Schwann cells, 340–341
Scientific method, 1855
Scillaren (scillaren A, B), 644t, 969, 1603t
Sclera, 356
Scleroderma, 281
    acute kidney injury caused by, 391
Scleroderma-like reactions, cutaneous, 281
Scoke. See Pokeweed (Phytolacca americana, P.
        decandra)
Scombroid poisoning, 273, 600t, 601
    clinical and laboratory findings with, 36t
Scopolamine, 2, 643t, 650t, 651, 755–756, 1181, 1181t,
        1182, 1503, 1604
    elimination half-life, 1182
    heroin adulterated with, 21t, 22, 1181
    pharmacology, 1183

Scorpaena (scorpionfish), 1576, 1576t
Scorpaena cardinalis (red rock cod, scorpionfish), 1576t
Scorpaena guttata (California sculpin), 1576, 1576t
Scorpaenidae, 1576, 1576t
  envenomation, pathophysiology, 1577
Scorpio maurus, antivenoms, 1564t
Scorpiones, 1540f
Scorpionfish, 1576, 1576t
Scorpions, 1540, 1540t, 1548–1550
  antivenoms, 1563–1566, 1564t
    history of, 1563
    worldwide availability, 1564t–1565t
  deaths caused by, 1845
  envenomation
    grades, 1549, 1549t
    management, 44t
    pathophysiology, 1548–1549
  envenomation by, priapism caused by, 301t
  geographic distribution, 1845
  stings, 3, 1548
    management, 1845
    untreated, 1565
  telson, 1548, 1549f
  of toxicologic importance, 1548, 1548t
  venom
    components, 1548–1549
    pancreatitis caused by, 294
Scorpion toxin(s)
  and voltage-gated calcium channels, 244f
  and voltage-gated potassium channels, 244f, 245
Scotch broom (*Cytisus scoparius*), 1599t–1600t
  uses and toxicities, 640t
Scotch mercury. *See* Foxglove (*Digitalis* spp.)
Screening. *See also* Drug abuse screening tests; *specific xenobiotic*
  for alcohol abuse and alcoholism, 1151, 1151t
  brief intervention, and referral to treatment (SBIRT), 381, 1151
Scurvy
  clinical manifestations, 662
  prevention, vitamin C for, 662
  risk factors for, 662
Scyllatoxin, and voltage-gated potassium channels, 245
Scyphozoa, 1567–1568, 1567t. *See also* Cnidaria (jellyfish)
  characteristics, 1567t
Sea anemone toxin(s)
  and late sodium channel, 251
  and voltage-gated calcium channels, 244f, 245
Sea bather's eruption (SBE), 1568, 1571–1572
Seaborg, Glenn, 1264
Seacat (*Trachinus draco*), 1576
Sea cucumbers, 1573–1574
Seafood, mercury in, 1324, 1328
Sea grape (*Ephedra* spp.). *See also* Ephedra (*Ephedra* spp.)
  uses and toxicities, 641t, 649
Sea hares, poisons from, 1
Sea kraits, 1633t
  geographic distribution, 1633
Seal liver, vitamin A toxicity from, 655
Sea mango (*Cerbera manghas*), 969, 979
  self-poisoning with, 1846
Sea nettle (*Chrysaora quinquecirrha*), 1567, 1567t, 1568. *See also* Cnidaria (jellyfish)
Sea onion, 644t, 979, 1603t. *See also* Squill (*Urginea maritima, U. indica*)
Seasickness, 739

Sea snakes, 1574–1576, 1633t
  antivenom (CSL), 1575–1576, 1575t
  envenomation
    clinical manifestations, 1575
    deaths caused by, 1574
    diagnostic tests for, 1575
    epidemiology, 1574
    management, 1575
    pathophysiology, 1575
  geographic distribution, 1574, 1633
  venom
    composition, 1575
    terrestrial antivenom cross-reactivity with, 1575
Season, and violence, 385
Seasonal ataxia, 1553–1554
Sea stars, 1573–1574
Sea urchins, 1573–1574
  foodborne illness caused by, 596
Sea wasp, 1567. *See also Chironex fleckeri* (box jellyfish, sea wasp)
Sebaceous glands, 270–271
Seborrheic dermatitis, in pyridoxine deficiency, 663
Seclusion, 387
Secobarbital. *See also* Sedative-hypnotics
  gastric absorption, lipid solubility and, 143f
  pharmacokinetics, 1085t
Second messengers
  and opioids, 238
  and withdrawal syndrome, 237
Secretin, 290t, 292
Secundus, Munro, 7
Sedation
  after naloxone administration, 541
  for agitated/violent behavior, 386
  antipsychotic-induced, 1039
  central α$_2$-adrenoceptor activation in, 210, 210f, 212
  for cocaine toxicity, 1128–1129
  and respiratory depression, 386–387
  salicylate toxicity and, 563
  SSRIs and, 1058
Sedative-hypnotics, 1084–1093, 1085t. *See also specific xenobiotic*
  additive and synergistic effects, 1085
  for alcohol withdrawal, 1168
  ARDS caused by, 402t
  barbiturate, 1084, 1085t
  benzodiazepine, 1084, 1085t
  cardiac effects, 256
  cross-tolerance, 1086
  deaths caused by, 1084
  definition, 1084
  dependence, 1086
  drug interactions with, 1085–1086
  effect on thermoregulation, 412–413, 413t
  effects on vital signs, 29t–31t
  elimination, 1085
  and ethanol, interactions, 1146t
  gastrointestinal decontamination for, 54t
  history of, 8–9, 1084, 1135
  hypoventilation caused by, 400t
  lipophilicity, 1084–1086
  mechanism of action, 210
  metabolism, 1085
  metabolites, 1084–1085
  and monoamine oxidase inhibitors, safety considerations, 1079, 1079t
  for neonatal opioid withdrawal, 439
  nonbenzodiazepine, 1084
    structure, 1135

  ophthalmic effects, 361
  pharmacokinetics and toxicokinetics, 145t, 1084–1086
  respiratory effects, 399t
  and rhabdomyolysis, 393
  tolerance, 1086
  toxicity (overdose/poisoning), 1084
    additive effects and, 1085
    clinical manifestations, 36, 1086, 1086t
    death caused by, 1086–1087
    diagnostic tests for, 1086
    gastrointestinal decontamination for, 1087
    head trauma caused by, imaging, 132t
    lipid emulsion for, 1006
    management, 1086–1087
    observation with, 1087
    synergism and, 1085
  toxic syndrome caused by, 29t
  withdrawal, 1086
    benzodiazepines for, 1138
    clinical and laboratory findings in, 36t
    effects on vital signs, 29t–31t
    hyperthermia in, 27, 27t
    therapeutics for, 35t
    toxic syndrome caused by, 29t
Seddon, Federick Henry, 5t, 6
Seducaps, 684
Seizures
  with *N*-acetylcysteine, 495
  adenosine and, 230
  after benzodiazepine reversal, 1095
  alcohol-related, magnesium and, 878
  in alcohol withdrawal, 222, 878, 1166
  aluminum and, 1224–1225
  amphetamine-induced, 1103
    management, 1104–1105, 1104t
  antihistamines associated with, 746
    management, 747
  antipsychotic-induced, 1039
    management, 1041
  in arsenic poisoning, 1241
  with arylcyclohexylamine toxicity, 1215
  atypical antidepressants and, 1048, 1056, 1057t
  baclofen withdrawal, 238
  barium toxicity and, 1455
  bupivacaine–induced, management, 1000
  camphor-induced, 628–629, 1381
  cannabinoid-induced, 1117
  cephalosporin-induced, 824–825
  ciprofloxacin-induced, 826
  citalopram toxicity and, 1056–1057, 1057t
  cocaine-related, 1126
  with colchicine poisoning, 503
  in cyclic antidepressants toxicity, 1046–1047
  in cyclic antidepressant toxicity, management, 1049t, 1051
  disulfiram-induced, 1175
  escitalopram toxicity and, 1056–1057, 1057t
  ethanol-related, 1148
  fluoroquinolones and, 826
  generalized, 719
  in glufosinate poisoning, 1478–1479
  hallucinogen-induced, 1184
  head trauma caused by, imaging, 132t
  hydrazide-induced, pyridoxine for, 862–863
  hydrazine-induced, pyridoxine for, 862–863
  ibuprofen-induced, 515
  imipenem-related, 825
  inhalant-induced, 1196
  isoniazid-induced, 852

management, 663
    pyridoxine for, 862–863
local anesthetic–induced, 998, 1000
in MAOI overdose, 1078
methylxanthine-induced, 231, 988, 991
neonatal, in opioid withdrawal, 439
nerve agent-induced, treatment, 1746
nickel exposure and, 1336
nicotine-induced, 1206
opioid-induced, 525, 539
organic chlorine insecticides causing, 1517, 1519
in organic phosphorus compound poisoning,
        magnesium and, 878–879
partial, 719
penicillin-induced, 823
in pesticide poisoning, 1450–1451
poisoning/overdose causing, 36t
propylene glycol and, 687
pyridoxal-5′-phosphate inhibitors causing,
        pyridoxine for, 862
in pyridoxine deficiency, 663
pyridoxine-responsive, in neonates, 862
and rhabdomyolysis, 393, 393t
in SMFA or fluoroacetamide poisoning, 1533–1534
SSRI toxicity and, 1056, 1057t
and strychnine poisoning, differentiation, 1537
termination, adenosine and, 230
theophylline-induced, 231, 988, 991
therapeutics for, 35t
in toxidromes, 29t
treatment, history of, 719
with venlafaxine overdose, decontamination
        strategy and, 86
vinblastine-related, 506
vincristine-related, 506
xenobiotic-induced, 37, 222, 343–344, 344t, 1450
    benzodiazepines for, 1138
Selection bias, 1856
Selective androgen receptor modulators (SARMs),
        athletes' use of, 617
Selective estrogen receptor modulators (SERMs),
        athletes' use of, 617
Selective progesterone receptor modulator, as
        abortifacient, 303t
Selective serotonin reuptake inhibitors (SSRIs), 218,
        1054–1064. See also xenobiotic
    adverse effects after therapeutic dosages, 1058–1060
    CYP enzymes and, 169–170
    death caused by, laboratory investigation, 1057–1058
    discontinuation syndrome, 237, 239, 1061
    and erectile dysfunction, 300
    extrapyramidal effects, 218
    and female sexual dysfunction, 302f
    gastrointestinal decontamination for, 77
    hepatotoxicity, 1058
    history of, 1054
    and male sexual dysfunction, 299f
    metabolites, 1054–1056, 1055t
    methylene blue and, 1714
    overdose/poisoning, 1044
        clinical manifestations, 1056–1057, 1057t
        management, 1057–1058
    pharmacokinetics, 1054–1056, 1055t
    and QT interval, 253
    receptor activity, 1056, 1056f, 1057t
    and rhabdomyolysis, 393t
    and serotonin toxicity, 1058t, 1079
    site of action, 1054, 1056f
    structure, 1054f
    for suicidal patient, 379

therapeutic uses, 1054
    toxicokinetics, 1054–1056
    with triptans, and serotonin toxicity, 809, 1058t,
        1059
    withdrawal, 237, 239
Selegiline, 1075, 1077. See also Monoamine oxidase
        inhibitors (MAOIs)
    mechanism of action, 212
    overdose, 1078
    structure, 1076f
Selenate, 1340, 1340f
Selenide(s), 1340f
    alkyl, 1340
Selenious acid, 1340, 1388t
    absorption, 1340
    chemistry, 1339t
    dermal exposure to, 1341
    ingestion, 1341
    toxicokinetics, 1340
Selenite, 1340f
    toxicokinetics, 1340
Selenium, 1339–1343
    absorption, 1340
    for argyria, 1347
    in breast milk, 1340
    chemistry, 1339–1340, 1339t
    decontamination, 1342
    deficiency, 1339
        effects, metals that modify, 1340
        modification of chemical toxicity by, 1340
        pathophysiology, 1340
    dietary sources, 1339
    in dietary supplements, 647–648
    elemental, 1339–1340
        absorption, 1340
        allotropes, 1339
        bioavailability, 1340
    elimination, 1340
    embryotoxic effects, 1342
    excess, effects, metals that modify, 1340
    exposure, sources, 1339
    gray, 1339
    hair
        clinical significance, 1342
        normal concentration, 1339
    history and epidemiology, 1339
    inhalational exposure to, 1341
    inorganic, 1339–1340
        absorption, 1340
        ECG changes caused by, 1341
        ingestion, 1341
        toxicity, 1341
    metabolism, 1340, 1340f
    odor, 364t, 1339t, 1340
    oral exposure to, 1341
    organic, 1339
        absorption, 1340
    oxidation states, 1339, 1339t
    for paraquat poisoning, 1474f, 1476
    pharmacokinetics, 1340
    pharmacology, 1340
    physicochemical properties, 1339
    physiologic functions, 1339
    recommended daily allowance for, 1339
    red amorphous powder, 1339
    red crystalline, 1339
    regulations and advisories on, 1340t
    as respiratory irritant, 1341
    serum
        average concentration, 1342

normal concentration, 1339
    in poisoning, 1342
    in selenosis, 1342
and silver tolerance, 1347
in soil, 1339
supplementation, adverse effects, 1339, 1342
supplement containing, toxicity caused by, 1341
teratogenicity, 1342
toxic dose, 1340
toxicity
    acute, 1340–1341
    biochemistry of, 1341
    chelation therapy for, 1342
    chronic, 1339, 1341–1342. See also Selenosis
    clinical manifestations, 36t, 1341–1342
    diagnostic testing for, 1342
    laboratory findings with, 36t, 1342
    management, 1342
    pain management in, 1342
    pathophysiology, 1340–1341
    supportive care for, 1342
toxicokinetics, 1340
transport, 1340
urine
    normal concentration, 1339, 1342
    in poisoning, 1342
    in selenosis, 1342
uses of, 1339, 1339t
whole blood
    normal concentration, 1339
    in selenosis, 1342
Selenium compounds
    absorption, 1340
    burns caused by, pain management for, 1342
    chemistry, 1339t
    uses of, 1339, 1339t
Selenium dioxide
    chemistry, 1339t
    dermal exposure to, 1341
    inhalation, 1340–1341
    ophthalmic exposure to, 1341
    oral exposure to, 1341
Selenium disulfide, in shampoo, 1342
    absorption, 1340
Selenium hexafluoride, 1341–1342
    chemistry, 1339t
Selenium oxide
    inhalational exposure to, 1341
    oral exposure to, 1341
    toxicokinetics, 1340
Selenium oxychloride
    chemistry, 1339t
    dermal exposure to, 1341
Selenium sulfide, 1339
    chemistry, 1339t
    toxicity, organ system manifestations, 829t
Selenocysteine, 1340
Selenomethionine, 1340–1341
Selenoproteins, 1340, 1340f
Selenosis, 1339. See also Selenium, toxicity
    causes, 1341
    clinical manifestations, 1341–1342
    environmental exposures and, 1341–1342
    hair in, 1341
    industrial exposures and, 1342
    nails in, 1341
Self-contained breathing apparatus (SCBA),
        1810–1811, 1810t
Self-determination, right to, 1860
Self-incrimination, 1863

Self-injurious behavior, 375–376
  nonfatal, epidemiology, 376
Selfotel, mechanism of action, 227t
Self-poisoning, 376–377, 377t. *See also* Suicide
  capacity and, 377–378
  epidemiology, 375
  initial psychiatric management of, 377
  with pesticides, 1844–1845, 1845t
  suspected, *case example*, 377, 377t
Semecarpus anacardium (Indian marking nut), 1614
Semicritical items, cleaning, 1368
Semustine, 760t
  and kidney failure, 763
Senco Corn Mix, 1350
Senecio spp., 642t, 645, 651, 1605
  groundsel, 1602t
  hepatic venoocclusive disease caused by, 332
Senecionine, 174t, 645
Seneciphylline, 645
Senkirkine, 641t, 645
Senna, 608t, 612, 1599t
  Cassia acutifolia, C. angustifolia
    glycosides in, 639
    uses and toxicity, 644t
Sennosides, 83, 644t, 1599t, 1607
Sensitive subpopulations, 1815
Sensitivity, of diagnostic test, 1858, 1858f
Sensorineural hearing loss, zinc gluconate and
    corticosteroids for, combined, 1362
Sensory nerve action potential (SNAP), in arsenic
    poisoning, 1244
Sensory neuropathy
  sodium stibogluconate and, 1233
  in thallium toxicity, 1351, 1353
Sentinel system, 1838
Sepsis, chemotherapeutic-related, management,
    764
September 11, 2001, attacks, dust and chemical
    exposure in, 17, 17t
Septic emboli
  CNS involvement, 131, 132t
  diagnostic imaging, 115t, 125, 125t, 126f, 131, 132t
  respiratory effects, 399t, 401
Septics, 6
Septic shock, opioid antagonists for, 540
Sequential Organ Failure Assessment (SOFA), and
    liver transplantation for acetaminophen
    poisoning, 484, 484t
Séquin, Armand, 519
SERCA2a, 928–929
Serenoa repens (saw palmetto), 649
  use and toxicities, 644t, 649
Serine, as glycine agonist, 223
D-Serine, and NMDA receptor, 227t
L-Serine, and NMDA receptor, 227t
Serine protease(s), in snake venom, 1618, 1619t, 1620
SERMs (selective estrogen receptor modulators), 617
Sernyl, 1210. *See also* Phencyclidine (PCP)
Sernylan, 1210. *See also* Phencyclidine (PCP)
Serotonergic agents. *See also* Dieting xenobiotics and
    regimens
  for alcoholism, 1152
  indications for, 610
  for weight loss, 606, 610–611
Serotonergic neurotransmission, 208, 215
  benzodiazepines and, 1084
  xenobiotics affecting, 217–218, 217t
Serotonin (5-HT), 203, 208, 215–218, 1054, 1179
  amphetamines and, 1099–1100, 1103
  cardiovascular effects, 215

in central nervous system, 215
chemical structure, 1588–1589
and dopamine, 215
in enterochromaffin cells, 215
lithium and, 217t
in lizard venom, 1619
lysergamides' chemical similarity to, 1179f
and male sexual dysfunction, 300
metabolism, 215, 216f, 217
  inhibitors, 217t
nicotine and, 1206
and norepinephrine, 1054, 1056f
peripheral, 215
physiologic functions, 215, 1182
in platelets, 215
and psychiatric disorders, 215
release, 215, 216f
  enhancers, 217t
reuptake, 215, 216f
  inhibitors, 217t, 218
reuptake transporters, 204
and sexual function, 304
and suicidality, 378
synthesis, 208, 215, 216f
  enhancers, 217t
and thermoregulation, 412
toxicity, methylene blue and, 1714
tryptamines' chemical similarity to, 1179, 1180f
uptake
  enhancers, 217t
  inhibitors, 217t
Serotonin agonist/partial agonist/reuptake inhibitors.
    See Nefazodone; Trazodone
Serotonin agonists, 217–218, 217t
  5HT$_{1P}$, 809
  triptans as, 808–809, 808f
Serotonin antagonist/partial agonist/reuptake
    inhibitors (SARI), 1055t, 1056f, 1060
Serotonin antagonists, 217t, 218
Serotonin behavioral syndrome. *See* Serotonin toxicity
Serotonin hyperactivity syndrome. *See* Serotonin
    toxicity
Serotonin-norepinephrine reuptake inhibitors (SNRIs),
    1056f, 1060. *See also specific xenobiotic*
  metabolites, 1055t
  methylene blue and, 1714
  pharmacokinetics, 1055t
  and serotonin toxicity, 1079
Serotonin (5-HT) receptor(s), 205, 215–217, 216f,
    610–611, 1054
  amphetamines and, 1103
  hallucinogens and, 1182
  5-HT$_1$, 215–216, 216f
    genes for, 215
    subtypes, 215
  5-HT$_2$, 216
    ethanol and, 237
    hallucinogens and, 1182
    subunits, 216
  5-HT$_3$, 216–217, 216f
  5-HT$_4$, 217
  5-HT$_5$, 217
  5-HT$_6$, 217
  5-HT$_7$, 217
  5HT$_{1P}$ agonists, 809
  promotility agents and, 84
  subtypes, 215, 1182
  triptans and, 808–809, 808f
Serotonin receptor antagonists, for chemotherapeutic-
    related vomiting, 764

Serotonin reuptake inhibitors (SSRIs). *See* Selective
    serotonin reuptake inhibitors (SSRIs)
Serotonin reuptake inhibitors/partial receptor
    agonists (SPARI), 1055t, 1056f, 1060. *See also*
    Vilazodone; Vortioxetine
Serotonin syndrome. *See* Serotonin toxicity
Serotonin toxicity, 29t, 218, 344, 1038, 1054, 1058–1060
  causes, 1058–1059, 1058t, 1079
  clinical and laboratory findings in, 36t, 218, 1079
  cyproheptadine for, 1081
  dantrolene for, 1081
  diagnosis, 1059, 1059t, 1079
  diagnostic criteria for, 1059, 1059t
  effects on vital signs, 29t, 31t
  hallucinogen-induced, 1183–1184
  hyperthermia in, 31, 420
  management, 35t, 44t, 218, 742, 1059
  manifestations, 1059, 1059t
  migraine medications and, 809
  monoamine oxidase inhibitors and, 1078, 1078t,
      1079
  and neuroleptic malignant syndrome,
      differentiation, 1059–1060, 1059t
  pathophysiology, 1058–1059
  St. John's wort and, 1611
  with triptans plus SSRIs, 809
  xenobiotics causing, 218
Serotonin transporter (SERT), 215, 216f, 1054, 1056,
    1056f
  amphetamines and, 1103
Serpents, blood of, 1
Sertindole, 218. *See also* Antipsychotics
  clinical and toxicologic effects, 1034t
  dosage and administration, 1033t
  mechanism of action, 1035
  pharmacokinetics, 1033t
Sertraline, 218, 1054
  CYP enzymes and, 170, 1055t, 1056
  gastrointestinal decontamination for, 50t
  mechanism of action, 1056f
  overdose/poisoning, gastrointestinal
      decontamination for, 77–78
  pharmacokinetics, 1055t
  receptor activity, 1057t
  seizures caused by, 1057t
  structure, 1054f
Serum
  alkalinization, 161
    for cyclic antidepressant toxicity, 1049–1050,
        1049t
  osmolality, 189
  pH, therapeutic manipulation, 147, 161
Serum assay(s)
  quantitative, basic, 101, 101t
  specimens for, 102
Serum glutamic-oxaloacetic transaminase (SGOT), 862
Serum sickness, with spider antivenom, 1560
Sesamin, 1520
Sesquiterpene lactones, 1599t
  contact dermatitis from, 279
Sesquiterpenes, 643t, 1597, 1608
Sethoxydim, in herbicides, 1467t
Set point, hypothalamic, 411
Sevelamer hydrochloride, polymeric crosslinked resin,
    1720t
Seven bark (*Hydrangea paniculata*), 642t
7-Up, lithium in, 1065
Severity Index of Paraquat Poisoning (SIPP), 1475, 1477
Seville orange. *See* Bitter orange (*Citrus aurantium*)
Sevoflurane, 1011, 1015

and adenosine receptor, 230
defluorination, 1015
for ICU sedation, 1016
low-flow, 1015
metabolism, 1015
pharmacology, 1410
structure, 1011f
Sexual dysfunction, 297
female, 302
DSM-5 definitions, 302
treatment, 302
xenobiotics causing, 302, 302f
male, 298–300
xenobiotics causing, 300t
Seychelles, methylmercury exposure studies in, 1328
SF-ADB-PINACA, structure, 1112f
Shamans, 638
Sharks, venomous, 1576
Sharpnosed viper (*Deinagkistrodon acutus*), 1633
Shellfish poisoning, 595–596
paralytic, clinical and laboratory findings in, 36t
prevention, 596
Shennong Bencaojing, 638
Shen Nung, 1t
Sherrington, Charles, 1018
Shielding (radiation), 1764
Shigalike toxin, 598–599
Shigella spp., 592, 592t, 597, 597t. *See also* Shigellosis
Shigellosis
and bioterrorism, 602
immune response in, zinc and, 1362
Shikimic acid, 642t
Shipman, Harold, 5t, 12
Shisha, 1205
Shivering, 414
Shock
cardiogenic, xenobiotics causing, 953–954
and interpretive toxicology, 1873t
therapeutics for, 35t
Shoe polish, odor, 364t
Shohl solution, indications for, 194
Sho-rengyo. *See* St. John's wort (*Hypericum perforatum*)
Sho-saiko-to, 647
Shoshin beriberi, 1159
Shudder attacks, caused by monosodium glutamate, 600
Sialadenitis, iodide-induced, 1776
Sibutramine, 606, 611
adverse effects and safety issues, 608t
market withdrawal, 608t
mechanism of action, 608t
and serotonin toxicity, 1058t
Sick euthyroid, 812–813
Sickle cell disease, *N*-acetylcysteine for, 495
Sida carpinifolia (locoweed), 1602t, 1606
Sida cordifolia (bala), 748, 1602t, 1605
Sidewinder (*Crotalus* spp.), 1617t, 1636t
Sierra mazateca. *See* Salvia (*Salvia divinorum, S. miltiorrhizae*)
Sievert, 1764, 1764f
Signal words, 40, 1450t
Sildenafil
for erectile dysfunction, 301
for female sexual dysfunction, 302
pharmacokinetics, 301
SILENT (syndrome of irreversible lithium-effectuated neurotoxicity), 1068
Silent Spring, 11, 1514
Silexan (lavender), 630
Silibinin

for amatoxin-induced liver toxicity, 1585–1586
mechanism of action, 1585
Silica
crystalline, inhalation, 1659
pulmonary effects, diagnostic imaging, 115t, 125t
respiratory effects, 399t, 401
scleroderma-like reaction with, 281
Silicates, 1659
Silicon, nephrotoxicity, 397t
Silicone polymers, 1416
Silicosis, 126, 1659
chest X-ray findings in, 115t, 125t
Silk, thermal degradation products, 1641t, 1685
Silo filler's disease, 123, 125t
Silver
ancient use of, 1344
antimicrobial effects, 1344–1345, 1345t
bactericidal effects, 1344–1345
in burn treatment, 1345
clinical and laboratory findings with, 36t
in coins, 1344
and discoloration of teeth and gums, 293t
disinfectant characteristics, 1345
elimination, 1345
elimination half-life, 1345
excretion, 1345
exposure to, epidemiology, 1344
fecal
normal concentration, 1347
in workers exposed to silver, 1347
hair, 1347
history of, 1344
ingestion, management, 1347
medicinal uses, 1344–1345, 1345t
nanoparticles, 1718, 1720t
nephrotoxicity, 390f, 397t
occupational exposure to, 1344
pharmacology, 1345
physicochemical properties, 1344
serum, 1347
normal concentration, 1344, 1347
in workers exposed to silver, 1347
tissue distribution, 1345
toxicity. *See also* Argyria
diagnostic tests for, 1347
emergency management, 1347
pathophysiology, 1345
systemic manifestations, 1345, 1346t
transport, 1345
urine, 1347
normal concentration, 1344, 1347
in workers exposed to silver, 1347
uses of, 1344
Silver acetate, and smoking cessation, 1344, 1345t
Silver iodide, in rainmaking, 1344
Silver nanoparticles, 1344
antitumor properties, 1345
cytotoxicity, 1345
dental applications, 1345
inhibition of amyloid-mediated pathology, 1346
Silver nanowire, 1344
Silver nitrate
and hyponatremia, 196
for phosphorus dermal exposure, 1531
Silver selenide, 1347
Silver sulfadiazine, 1345, 1345t, 1347
propylene glycol in, 688
toxicity, organ system manifestations, 829t
Silybum marianum (milk thistle), silymarin from, for amatoxin-induced liver toxicity, 1585

Silymarin, for amatoxin-induced liver toxicity, 1585
Simazine, structure, 1482f
Simple Triage and Rapid Treatment (START), 1811
Simpson, James, 1011
Simvastatin
CYP enzymes and, 170
metabolism, 171
Sinclair, Upton, *The Jungle*, 9
Single-pass albumin dialysis (SPAD), 96, 1289
for acetaminophen removal, 485
Single-photon emission computed tomography (SPECT)
in carbon monoxide poisoning, 1667
of CNS, 130
indications for, 134
isotopes used in, 133
in Parkinson disease, 1320
principles of, 133
with xenobiotic exposure, 115t
Sinigrin, 1598t, 1607, 1613
Sinoatrial (SA) node, 246, 248, 945, 947, 970
dysfunction, exacerbated or unmasked by xenobiotics in elderly, 463, 463t
pacemaker cells in, 926, 928f
Sinus arrest, 247
Sinus bradycardia, 255–256, 263
methadone and, 1820, 1820f
Sinus node, 247, 255
Sinusoids, hepatic, 327
Sinus tachycardia, 255–256, 263
antipsychotic-induced, management, 1040
in cyclic antidepressant poisoning, 1046, 1046f, 1047
xenobiotics causing, 255
Siphonophorae, 1567
Sirolimus
nanocrystals, 1720t
and normal anion gap metabolic acidosis, 191t
Sistrurus spp. (rattlesnakes), 1633t
Sistrurus catenatus (massasauga), 1617t
Sistrurus miliarius (pygmy rattlesnake), 1617t
Sistrurus ravus, 1637t
Sitagliptin
overdose/poisoning, 700
pharmacokinetics and toxicokinetics, 697t
pharmacology, 696
structure, 695f
Six Sigma, 1827
Ska Maria, 1181
Skates, 1576
Skeletal changes, xenobiotic-related, diagnostic imaging, 119–122, 122t
Skeletal fluorosis, 1197, 1197f–1198f
Skeletal muscle
excitation-contraction coupling in, 1018, 1019f
mushroom toxin affecting, 1589t, 1591
paralysis, mechanisms, 1018, 1019f
spasticity, dantrolene for, 1029–1030
Skin. *See also* Cutaneous *entries*
anatomy, 269–271
antimicrobial toxicity and, 829t
antimonials and, 1233
in arsenic poisoning, 1241–1243, 1242f
micronutrients and, 1245
arteriovenous framework, 270, 270f
barrier function, 269
bluish-gray, in argyria, 1346–1347, 1346f
color
carbon monoxide poisoning and, 1665–1666
cyanide poisoning and, 1686
decontamination, by physical removal, 72
examination, 269

Skin (*Cont.*):
and fluid balance, 194
histology, 269–271, 270f
histopathology, 269, 270f
initial assessment, 189
injury, in fire victims, 1646–1647
physiology, 269–271
pigmentation changes
antipsychotic-induced, 1039
arsenic and, 1242–1243
bismuth and, 1256
xenobiotic-induced, 273
reactive units, 269, 270f
rinsing, for decontamination, 72
signs of systemic disease, 272–273
superficial reactive unit, 269, 270f
surface area, 269
surface film, 269
thermosensitivity, 411, 412f
trivalent arsenicals and, 1239
xenobiotic absorption through, factors affecting,
1411
Skin lesion(s), 269, 269t
descriptions/terminology, 269t
Skin necrosis
anticoagulant-induced, 279, 279f
with spider envenomation, 268, 268f, 1544–1545
warfarin-related, 279, 279f, 889–890
Skin odor, 37
Skin-popping scars, 38
Skin transplantation, from poisoned patients,
1892–1893, 1892t
Skip lesions, with acid ingestion, 1389–1390
Slang nut, 1536
Sleep aids, 1089
Sliding scale, of capacity, 374
Slimming pills, 816
Slippery elm (*Ulmus rubra, U. fulva*), 644t
Slippery root (*Symphytum* spp.), 641t
Slit-lamp examination, 356
Slow acetylators, 170
SLUD mnemonic, 1491
"Smack," 162
Small intestine(s), 291–292
pH, 142t
transit time in, 143
Smallpox
as biological weapon, 1757–1758
clinical manifestations, 1757, 1757f
pathophysiology, 1758
secondary infections, 1757
vaccination, 1758, 1758f
SMART program, 656
Smell. *See also* Olfaction
disorders, zinc and, 1362
Smell test(s), 364–365
Smelter shakes, 1362
SMFA. *See* Sodium monofluoroacetate (SMFA,
compound 1080)
Smilagenin, 1598t
Smith, Madeline, 5t
Smog
components, 1651
toxic gases in, 16t, 17
Smoke, toxic components, 1640, 1640t
Smoke inhalation, 1640–1649, 1651, 1663, 1665, 1685
ARDS caused by, 402t, 1641–1642, 1643f
bronchoalveolar lavage for, 73
burns and, 1640–1641, 1645
chest radiography in, 1642, 1643f

clinical manifestations, 1642, 1644f
deaths caused by, 1640
diagnostic testing for, 1642–1643, 1643f
epidemiology, 1640
hypoxia in, 1642–1643
management, 1643–1647, 1644f, 1694–1695
mass casualties from, 1640
pathophysiology, 1640–1642, 1644f
respiratory effects, 399t
toxic thermal degradation products in, 1604t,
1640, 1641t
Smokeless tobacco, 1203, 1205. *See also* Nicotine
Smoking. *See also* Nicotine
drug interactions with, 1204
in pregnancy and lactation, 441
teratogenicity, 430t
and tobacco amblyopia, 1686
yellow skin caused by, 272
Smoking cessation, products for, 1206
nicotine in, 1203
Smoky air, 17
Snake(s), 1617–1632. *See also* Sea snakes; Snakebite(s);
Snake venom(s); *specific snake*
envenomation
clinical manifestations, 1620–1622, 1620t, 1621f
diagnosis, 1623
expert help for, 1634
management, 1623–1625
pathophysiology, 1619–1620
exotic (nonnative), 1617, 1633–1638
antivenoms for
hospital use, 1635
Investigational New Drug (IND) application for,
1634–1635
zoological, 1634–1635
bites, epidemiology, 1633
envenomation
clinical presentation, 1634–1637
general approach for, 1634, 1634t
initial management, 1634–1637
geographic distribution, 1633
identification, expert help for, 1634
medically important, in United States, 1617, 1617t
nonvenomous, envenomation by, 1617
as pets, 1633
taxonomy, 1633, 1633t
venomous
exotic (nonnative), 1617, 1633–1638
fangs, 1617
geographic distribution in United States, 1617
as pets, 1633
taxonomy, 1617
teeth, 1617
Snakebite(s)
annual incidence, 1782
antivenoms for, global disparities in, 1847–1848
complications, worldwide occurrence, 1633
deaths caused by, 1617, 1782
worldwide (global burden), 1633, 1844
in developed countries, 1845
in developing world, 1845
early therapies for, 4
epidemiology, 1617, 1633, 1845
incidence, worldwide, 1633
management
antivenom in, international use of, 1845
in developing world, 1845
pit vipers (Crotalinae), antivenom for, 35t
repeat (multiple), 1617
risk factors for, 1617

seasonal occurrence, 1617
snakestone therapy for, 3
Snake gourd (*Trichosanthes kirilowii*), as abortifacient,
303t
Snakeroot
Echinacea. *See* Echinacea (*Echinacea angustifolia,
E. purpurea*)
Rauwolfia serpentina, psychoactive properties,
650t
Snakestones, 3
Snake venom(s). *See also* Ancrod
as anticoagulants, 900
biologic activity, 900
components, 1618–1619
early history of, 1
elimination half-life, 1619
hemostatic effects, 900
historical perspective on, 1, 4t, 7
pharmacokinetics, 1619
pharmacology, 1618–1619
Snare complex, 203
SNARE proteins, and botulinum toxin, 575, 576f
Sniffing (inhalant), 1193
Sniffing bar, 363
Snow, John, 1011
Snowfield vision, in methanol poisoning, 1423
Snuff, 1204t, 1205
Soap, for dermal decontamination, 72
Social cognitive theory (SCT), 1786
Socotrine. *See* Aloe (*Aloe vera, A. barbadensis, Aloe* spp.)
Socrates, 1t, 2
SOD (superoxide dismutase), 159–160, 175, 1285t,
1656
inhibition, by cyanide, 1685
manganese in, 1319
for paraquat poisoning, 1474f, 1477
zinc in, 1362
Soda lime, and carbon monoxide poisoning with
inhalational anesthetics, 1015–1016
Soda loading, 621
Sodium. *See also* Fractional sodium excretion
chemistry, 157
dermal decontamination for, precautions with, 72
in extracellular space, 194
intake, and hypernatremia, 194–195, 195t
membrane transport, 203
in neurotransmission, 205, 205f, 206–207
postmortem changes, 1885t
reabsorption, 389
serum, 194. *See also* Hypernatremia; Hyponatremia
in SIADH, 197
vitreous, normal concentration, 1872t
Sodium acetate
adverse effects and side effects, 43
and anion gap, 191t
for cyclic antidepressant toxicity, 1050
Sodium arsenite
meat contamination with, 19
toxicity, management, 1252
Sodium azide
hepatic effects, 334t
poisoning, laboratory findings with, 1686
Sodium bicarbonate (NaHCO₃), 567–573
adverse effects and safety issues, 571
as antidote and therapy, 567–571, 568t
indications for, 27
for antipsychotic overdose, 1040
as athletic performance enhancer, 621
availability and storage, 46t
and calcium salts, adverse interactions, 1406

for chlorine gas inhalation, 571
for chlorphenoxy herbicide poisoning, 570
for cocaine toxicity, 1130
contraindications to, 569–570, 1430
for cyclic antidepressant toxicity, 1049–1050, 1049t
dosage and administration, 571–572
excretion, in respiratory alkalosis, 190
formulations, 572
indications for, 32, 35t, 46t, 567, 568t
inhaled, 407
for life-threatening metabolic acidosis, 570–571
for local anesthetic cardiotoxicity, 1001
loss, and normal anion gap metabolic acidosis, 193
mechanism of action, 567–569, 568t, 1040
for metformin toxicity, 571
for methotrexate toxicity, 570
nebulized, for pulmonary irritant exposure, 1658
pharmacology, 567
for phenobarbital toxicity, 570
and potassium balance, 199
in pregnancy and lactation, 571
for quinine overdose, 840
for salicylate toxicity, 569–570
serum, 190. *See also* Delta gap ratio (Δ anion gap/Δ
    [HCO$_3^-$])
site of action, 567–569, 568t
stocking, recommended level, 46t
structure, 567
supplies, 43
therapy with, in metabolic acidosis, 193–194
for toxic alcohol ingestions, 571
in toxic alcohol poisoning, 1430
for urine alkalinization, 38, 93
uses in toxicology, 567–569, 568t
volume of distribution, 192
Sodium borates, 1375, 1388t
Sodium carbonates, 1388t
Sodium channel(s)
    activation, 995
    alpha subunits, 719
    antidysrhythmics and, 865, 865f, 866–868, 866t–867t,
        869, 871
    antipsychotic blockade of, management, 1040
    blockade, ECG changes in, 736, 737f
    classes, 995
    cyclic antidepressants and, 1044, 1045f
    fast, blockade, by antipsychotics, 1034t, 1035
    in hyperkalemia, 1406
    inactivation, 995
    ligand-gated, 204
    lipid emulsion and, 1005
    local anesthetics and, 994, 995f, 999
    and malignant hyperthermia, 1023
    myocardial, 245–246, 245f, 999
        and dysrhythmias, 256
        xenobiotics affecting, 258
    of myocardial cell membrane, 244–245
    opioids and, 238, 238f
    organic chlorine insecticides and, 1516, 1516f
    plant xenobiotics and, 1611–1612
    pyrethrins and pyrethroids and, 1521
    resting, 995
    structure, 244, 244f
    α-subunit, 244–245, 244f
        receptor sites, 244–245, 244f
        xenobiotics binding to, 244–245, 244f
    use-dependent blockade, 838
    voltage-gated, 203, 244, 719
        activation, 1516, 1516f
        insecticides and, 1521

xenobiotic interactions with
    altered, 567–569
    sodium bicarbonate and, 567–569
Sodium channel agonists, mechanism of action, 933f
Sodium channel blockers. *See also specific xenobiotic*
    antidote for, 35t
    cardiac effects, 248–249
    cardiotoxicity, sodium bicarbonate for, 567–569,
        568t
    effects on QRS complex, 567–569
    overdose/poisoning, ECG changes in, 250
    and QT interval, 251–253
    therapeutics for, 37
Sodium chlorate (NaClO$_3$), 1369t, 1375–1376, 1468t
Sodium chloride
    and hypernatremia, 194–195, 195t
    0.9% solution, supplies, 43
Sodium citrate
    and anion gap, 191t
    and hypernatremia, 194–195, 195t
    indications for, 194
Sodium cyanide, 1457, 1684
Sodium-dependent glucose transporter(s), 707
    SGLT2, inhibitors, 707
Sodium dithionate, test for paraquat or diquat,
    1475–1477
Sodium ethylmercurithiosalicylate, 689
Sodium ferric ferrocyanide, 1357
Sodium fluoride, 1397
    poisoning with, 1397
    toxicity, 1398–1399
Sodium fluoroacetamide (compound 1081), in
        rodenticides, 1452t
    estimated fatal dose, 1452t
    physicochemical properties, 1452t
    toxicity
        antidote and/or treatment, 1452t
        clinical manifestations, 1452t
        onset, 1452t
        toxic mechanism, 1452t
Sodium fluoroacetate, and citric acid cycle, 175
Sodium glucose cotransporter 2 (SGLT2) inhibitors,
        694
    adverse effects and safety issues, 700
    overdose, hospitalization for, 702
    pharmacokinetics and toxicokinetics, 696, 697t
    pharmacology, 696
    structure, 695f
Sodium hydroxide (lye), 1388t. *See also* Caustics
    exposure to, pathophysiology, 1389f
    ingestion, worldwide, 1846
Sodium hypochlorite (bleach), 1369t, 1372, 1388t
    and ammonia, 1655
    in decontamination, 1743
    exposure to, pathophysiology, 1389
    and hypernatremia, 194–195, 195t
Sodium iodide, 818
Sodium lactate, 567
    and anion gap, 191t
Sodium metabisulfite, 757
    in physostigmine preparations, 757
Sodium monofluoroacetate (SMFA, compound 1080),
        1533–1535
    chemical structure, 1533, 1533f
    estimated fatal dose, 1452t
    history of, 1533
    hyperventilation caused by, 400t
    lethal dose, 1533
    physicochemical properties, 1452t
    as rodenticide, 1452t, 1533

toxicity (overdose/poisoning)
    antidote and/or treatment, 1452t
    clinical manifestations, 1452t, 1533
    diagnostic tests for, 1534
    onset, 1452t
    pathophysiology, 1533
    treatment, 1534
    toxic mechanism, 1452t
    toxicokinetics and toxicodynamics, 1533
    uses, 1533
Sodium nitrite
    adverse effects and safety issues, 1700
    availability and storage, 46t
    chemistry, 1698
    for cyanide poisoning, 1646, 1687–1688, 1687t,
        1699–1700
    dosage and administration
        in adults, 1700
        pediatric, 1688, 1688t, 1701
    formulation and acquisition, 1701
    for hydrogen sulfide poisoning, 1691, 1691t
    indications for, 46t
    pharmacokinetics and pharmacodynamics,
        1699
    stocking, recommended level, 46t
Sodium nitroprusside, 962–963, 1195
Sodium oleate, 1004
Sodium oxybate, 1188
Sodium penicillin, and anion gap, 191t
Sodium perborate, 682, 1369t
Sodium permanganate, 1319
Sodium phosphates, 83, 1388t
    adverse effects, 85
    pharmacodynamics, 84
    pharmacokinetics, 84
Sodium picosulfate, 83
    adverse effects, 86
    mechanism of action, 84
    pharmacokinetics, 84
Sodium polystyrene sulfonate (SPS), 92
    for hyperkalemia, 1069
    for lithium or thallium overdose/poisoning, 64
    and potassium balance, 199
    thallium binding by, 1354
Sodium salts, and hypernatremia, 194–195, 195t
Sodium selenate, chemistry, 1339, 1339t
Sodium selenite, chemistry, 1339, 1339t
Sodium silicates, 1388t
Sodium stibogluconate, 1228
    adverse effects, 1229–1233
    ECG changes caused by, 1232
    hematologic effects, 1232
    for leishmaniasis, 1229
    nephrotoxicity, 1232
    toxicity, clinical manifestations, 1231t–1232t
    toxicokinetics, 1230
Sodium succinate, for SMFA or fluoroacetamide
        poisoning, 1534
Sodium sulfate
    for barium ingestion, 1455
    as cathartic, 83–84
        pharmacodynamics, 84
Sodium thiopental, in capital punishment, 13
Sodium thiosulfate, 962, 1694, 1698–1702
    adverse effects and safety issues, 1700
    availability and storage, 46t
    and breast-feeding, 1700
    in calcific uremic arteriolopathy (calciphylaxis),
        1699–1700
    chemistry, 1698

Sodium thiosulfate (*Cont.*):
  for cyanide poisoning, 1685, 1687–1688, 1687t, 1699–1700
  dosage and administration, 1687t
    in adults, 1700–1701
    in children, 1701
  formulation and acquisition, 1701
  indications for, 46t
  mechanism of action, 1698–1699
  for mechlorethamine extravasation, 803
  pharmacokinetics and pharmacodynamics, 1699
  pharmacology, 1698–1699
  in pregnancy, 1700
  prophylactic use with nitroprusside, 1699–1700
  stocking, recommended level, 46t
  volume of distribution, 1699
Sof Zia, 682
Soladulcidine, 1602t
Solanaceae, 1597, 1598t–1603t, 1604, 1614
Solanidine, 1604
Solanine, 1602t–1603t, 1604
Solanum americanum (American nightshade), 1602t
Solanum dulcamara (bittersweet woody nightshade), 1602t
Solanum nigrum (black nightshade, common nightshade), 1602t
Solanum tuberosum (potato, green), 1603t, 1604
Solasodine, 1602t
Soldiers' disease, 8
Solenopsins, 1552
Solenopsis invicta, 1552
Solenopsis richteri, 1552
Solid(s)
  exposure to, 1809
  sublimation, 1809
Solubility product constant (K$_{sp}$), 158
Solute carrier class (SLC) transporters, and transplacental transfer, 432
Solvate, 159
Solvents. *See also specific solvent*
  abuse, 1409
  chemistry, 1410
  chronic exposure to, cerebral atrophy caused by, 131
  cranial neuropathy caused by, 346t
  dermal absorption, 1411
  focal brain lesions caused by, 131
  hepatic effects, 334, 334t
  hepatotoxicity, 331
    ethanol and, 329
  inhaled, 1193
    toxicity, 1410
  and nanoparticle epidermal penetration, 1720
  ophthalmic exposure to, 359
  organic, 1410
    scleroderma-like reaction with, 281
  volatile, GABA receptors and, 237
Soma (*Amanita muscaria*), 3, 1178
Soma (of neuron), 340
Soman
  aging half-life, 1746
  chemical name and structure, 1745f
  history of, 1486, 1741
  odor, 1745
  physical characteristics, 1745
  toxic syndrome caused by, 1750t
Somatic symptom disorder, 1814
Somatostatin, 702, 713. *See also* Octreotide
  actions, 713
    effect on thyroid hormones and function, 813f, 814t
    gastrointestinal effects, 290t, 292f

history of, 713
  and insulin secretion, 713–715
  and pancreatic dysfunction, 295t
  secretion, 292
Somatostatin receptor ligands (SRLs), 713–714
Somatostatin receptors, 713
Somnolence, cannabinoid-associated, 1117
Son-before-the-father (*Colchicum autumnale*). *See* Colchicine
Sonoran coral snake (*Micruroides euryxanthus*), 1618, 1622, 1625, 1633
Sonoran Desert sidewinder (*Crotalus* spp.), 1636t
Sonoran sidewinder (*Crotalus* spp.), 1636t
Soot
  nanoparticles in, 1721
  skin decontamination for, 1647
  and smoke inhalation, 1641–1642
Sorafenib, 761
  adverse effects and safety issues, 760t, 762
  overdose/poisoning, 760t
Sorbitol (D-glucitol)
  with activated charcoal, 77
  adverse effects, 79, 85
  cathartic effects, 689
  and fructose intolerance, 689
  gastrointestinal toxicity, 689
  and hypernatremia, 195, 195t
  mechanism of action, 84
  as pharmaceutical additive, 688–689, 688t
  pharmacodynamics, 84
  pharmacokinetics, 84, 688–689
  sources, 688
  structure, 688
Sorbus aucuparia, 688
Sorghum spp., cyanogenic glycosides in, 1684
Soro antiaracnídico, 1565, 1565t
Soro antiscorpiônico, 1565, 1565t
Sotalol
  ECG changes caused by, 258
  pharmacology, 927t, 930
  potassium channel blockade, 930, 932
  toxicity (overdose/poisoning)
    management, 936
    multiple-dose activated charcoal in, 61
Sound pressure levels (SPLs), 368
Sour orange. *See* Bitter orange (*Citrus aurantium*)
South American rattlesnake (*Crotalus* spp.), 1636t
Southern fire ant (*Solenopsis* spp.), 1540t
Southern Pacific rattlesnakes (*Crotalus oreganus helleri*)
  envenomation, neurotoxicity, 1622
  Mojave toxin in, 1620
Southern ridge-nosed rattlesnake (*Crotalus* spp.), 1637t
Southwestern speckled rattlesnake (*Crotalus* spp.), 1636t
Soy isoflavone (*Glycine max*), 644t
Space of Disse, 329f
Space sickness, 739
Spanish fly (*Cantharis vesicatoria*), 640t, 1554. *See also* Cantharidin
  strychnine as adulterant in, 1536
  uses and toxicities, 640t
Spara, Hieronyma, 5t
Sparteine, 1599t, 1604
L-Sparteine, 640t
Spasmodic torticollis, antipsychotic-induced, 1036
Spathiphyllum spp. (peace lily), 1603t, 1613
Specialist in Poison Information (SPI), 11, 11t
"Special K." *See* Ketamine
Specificity, of diagnostic test, 1858, 1858f

Specimens
  clinical
    collection, 1868–1869, 1869t
    preservation, 1869
    storage, 1869
    postmortem, 1869–1870, 1869t–1870t
  for toxicology laboratory, 102
Speckled rattlesnake (*Crotalus* spp.), 1617t, 1636t
Spectator ion, 157
Spectrochemical tests, 103, 103t
  endpoint method, 103
  indirect, 103
  kinetic method, 103
Spectrometry, direct, 103
Spectrophotometer, 106
Spectrophotometric tests, 103
Spectrophotometry, 106
Spectrum. *See* 2C-B
Speed runs, 1104
Spermatogenesis, xenobiotics affecting, 297–298, 297t, 298f
Spermidine, for paraquat poisoning, 1477
Spermine, and NMDA receptor, 227t
Spherocytosis, 317
Sphingomyelinase D, in brown recluse spider venom, 1542t, 1544
Spice blends, cannabinoids in, 1117
Spicewood oil, 634
Spider plant (*Chlorophytum comosum*), 1599t
Spiders, 1540–1547, 1540t. *See also specific spider*
  anatomy, 1540
  antivenoms for, 1559–1561. *See also* Antivenom(s); *specific spider*
  bites, 3
    diagnosis/misdiagnosis, 268, 1541, 1544–1545
  chelicerae, 1540
  envenomation by, priapism caused by, 301t
  history and epidemiology, 1540–1541
  as hunters, 1540
  of medical importance, 1540, 1541t
    North American, 1541t
  mygalomorph. *See* Funnel web spider (*Atrax* spp., *Hadronyche* spp.); Tarantulas
  necrotic envenomation, 268, 268f, 1544–1545
  stings, diagnosis, 1541
  as trappers, 1540
  venom, AMPA receptor antagonists in, 228
  venomous, 1540
Spider toxin(s), and voltage-gated calcium channels, 244f
Spinach (*Spinacia oleracea*), 1603t
Spinacia oleracea (spinach), 1603t
Spinal cord
  focal lesions in, 131
  injury, polyethylene glycol (PEG) and, 686–687
    magnetic resonance imaging, inverted V sign, 1199
  thallium and, 1351
Spinal injury, *N*-acetylcysteine for, 494
Spindle assembly checkpoint (SAC), 350–351
Spine-bellied sea snake (*Hydrophis curtus*), 1575
Spinothalamic tract, in thermoregulation, 411
Spironolactone. *See also* Diuretics, potassium-sparing
  as androgen receptor blocker, 299f, 300
  dermal effects, 276t
  and female sexual dysfunction, 302f
  and gustatory dysfunction, 365
  for hypertension, 963
  infertility caused by, 298f
  and prolactin, 299f
  and thiamine pharmacokinetics, 1158

Splenic abscess, 128
Splenic infarction, 128
Sponge diver's disease, 1574
Sponges, 1573–1574
Spongiform leukoencephalopathy, from heroin use, 21t, 22, 1223
Spore print, 1593
Spores, mushroom, 1583t, 1589t, 1592–1593
Sporocysts, 1568
Sports anemia, 621
Spot removers, inhaled, 1193t. *See also* Inhalant(s)
Spotted locoweed (*Astragalus lentiginosis*), 1606
Spot tests, 103, 103t
Spray paint, inhaled, 1193, 1193t. *See also* Inhalant(s)
Spreading wave of oligemia, 805
Spurges, 1613
Squawmint. *See* Pennyroyal (*Mentha pulegium, Hedeoma pulegioides*)
Squaw root. *See* Black cohosh; Blue cohosh
Squaw tea (*Ephedra* spp.), uses and toxicities, 641t, 649
Squid, 1572
Squill (*Urginea maritima, U. indica*), 644t, 969, 979, 1603t, 1606
SR 144,528, structure, 1112f
SR (sarcoplasmic reticulum) calcium release channels, 928, 928f
Stabilized oxychloride complex, 682
Stachybotrys spp., in biological warfare, 1759
Stacking, of steroids, 617
Staffordshire beer epidemic, 21, 21t, 1237
Stalinon affair, 20, 20t
Standardized field sobriety tests, for ethanol-induced impairment, 1878–1879, 1879t
Standards of care
    and medical malpractice, 1865
    ordinary, 1865
    for poison information specialists, 1865
    strict locality rule and, 1865
Staphylococcal enterotoxin B (SEB), as biological weapon, 1759
Staphylococcal scalded skin syndrome, 275, 276t
Staphylococci (*Staphylococcus* spp.), foodborne infection, 592t, 597, 597t, 599
Staphylococcus aureus
    enterotoxin, 592
    gastroenteritis, 597
    propofol and, 1090
Star anise
    health risks caused by, 1608
    Japanese (*Illicium anasatum*), 1600t
    seizures caused by, 1608
Starch, 707
    in cocaine, 1130
    oral, for iodine poisoning/overdose, 35t
Star fruit (*Averrhoa carambola*), 1611
Stargazers, 1576
Starvation, hypoglycemia caused by, hospitalization for, 702
Starvation ketoacidosis, 192
Starvation ketosis, 1149
State Emergency Response Commission (SERC), 1801t
State-sponsored poisoners, 6t
Statins
    and colchicine, interactions, 502
    and rhabdomyolysis, 393
Station nightclub fire, 16, 16t
Status epilepticus, 237
    benzodiazepines for, 1137t, 1138
    case study, 339

in cyclic antidepressant toxicity, management, 1051
    EEG findings in, 230
    organic chlorine insecticides causing, 1517, 1519
    xenobiotic-induced, 339, 339t, 343–344, 1450
Stavudine, 831
Steady state, 151–152
    concentration achieved at, 151–152
Steatoda spp. *See* Comb-footed spider (*Steatoda* spp.)
Steatohepatitis, 331t, 332, 334t
    antipsychotic-induced, 1039
Steatosis, 179, 180f, 331–332, 331t
    alcoholic, 328
    hepatic, 327–328
    laboratory findings with, 335t
    macrovesicular, 331t, 332, 332f
    microvesicular, 331t, 332, 332f
    with mitochondrial dysfunction, 332
    nonalcoholic, 331
Stellate cells, hepatic, 327, 329f, 330
Stem (stipe), of mushrooms, 1584f, 1593
Stem cells
    fate, 352
    functions, 352
    hematopoietic, 310, 310f, 352–353, 352f
        chemotherapy and, 353
        niche for, 352–353, 352f
        response to stress, 353
    intestinal, 353–354, 354f
        response to stress, 354
    multipotent mesenchymal, 310
    niche for, 352
    properties, 352
    tissue-specific, 310
    transplantation
        for radiation-exposed patients, 1772
        for vision loss in methanol poisoning, 1430
Stephania tetrandra, 613
    acute interstitial nephritis caused by, 394t
Sterculiaceae, 1599t, 1603t
Stereochemistry, toxicologic and pharmacologic importance, 164–165
Stereogenic carbon, 164
Stereoisomerism, 164, 164f
    and CYP substrate affinity, 169
Stereoisomers, 164, 164f
Sterigmatocystin, 174t
Sterilants, 1369t, 1374–1375
    definition, 1368
Steroid(s). *See also* Anabolic-androgenic steroids (AAS); *specific steroid*
    anabolic
        definition, 617
        and female sexual dysfunction, 302f
        and hepatic tumors, 333
        hepatotoxicity, 330
        infertility caused by, 297t, 298f
        and male sexual dysfunction, 299f
        regulation, 617
        use, 616
    androgenic, use, 616
    cardioactive. *See* Cardioactive steroids
    clinical and laboratory findings with, 36t
    nicotinic receptor blockade by, 207
    plant sources, 1600t
    topical, for extravasation injury, 803
Steroidal glycosides, 1597
Stevens-Johnson syndrome, 274–277, 1309
    NSAID-induced, 515
    sulfonamides and, 827
Stibanate, cranial neuropathy caused by, 346t

Stibine
    chemistry, 1233
    hemolysis caused by, 317–318
    toxicity, 1231t–1232t, 1233
        clinical manifestations, 1231t–1232t
        treatment, 1234
Stibnite, 1228
Stiff person syndrome, 228
Stiletto snakes (*Atractaspis* spp.), 1633t
Stimulants. *See also specific stimulant*
    antidote for, 35t
    as athletic performance enhancers, 621
    pharmacokinetics and toxicokinetics, 145t
Stinger nets, 1569
Stingfish (*Trachinus draco*), 1576
Stinging nettles (*Urtica dioica*), 1613
    pruritus caused by, 273
Stingose, 1569
Stingrays, 1576–1578
    envenomation, pathophysiology, 1577
    poisons from, 1
    spines, radiography, 1578
    wounds from, management, 1578
Stings
    arthropod, definition, 1540
    scorpion. *See* Scorpions
Stinking rose. *See Allium sativum* (garlic)
Stinky nightshade. *See* Henbane (*Hyoscyamus niger*)
Stipe, of mushrooms, 1584f, 1593
Stiripentol, mechanism of action, 720f, 720t
Stochastic effect, 432
    of radiation, 1767–1768
Stoddard solvent, 1410
Stokes' sea snake (*Astotia stokesii*), 1574
Stomach, 291
    caustic injuries to, 1389, 1389f
    foreign bodies in, 295
Stomach pump, 7
Stomatitis
    in pyridoxine deficiency, 663
    sulfonamides and, 827
Stomolophus spp., venom, cardiotoxicity, 1570
Stomolophus meleagris (cabbage head, cannonball jellyfish), 1567t
Stomolophus nomurai (lion's mane), 1567t, 1568
Stone (*Bufo bufo gargarizans, Bufo bufo melanosticus*)
    psychoactive properties, 650t
    uses and toxicities, 641t
Stonefish, 1576, 1576f, 1576t
    antivenom, 35t, 1575t, 1578
    envenomation, 35t
    pathophysiology, 1577
Stonustoxin (SNTX), 1577
Stool
    adult, pH, 142t
    black, bismuth-induced, 1256
    of infants/children, pH, 142t
STOPP/START, 460
STOP/START criteria, 1826–1827
Storage depot, of xenobiotic, 146
STP. *See* 2,5-Dimethoxy-4-methylamphetamine (DOM)
Stramonium, 643t. *See also* Jimsonweed (*Datura stramonium*)
Stratum corneum, 269, 270f
Stratum germinativum, 269–270, 270f
Stratum granulosum, 269, 270f
Stratum spinosum, 269, 270f
Street drugs. *See specific drug*
Street names, for drugs, 162

Streptococci (*Streptococcus* spp.), group A, foodborne infection, 592t, 599
Streptokinase, 883–884, 896–897
 ARDS caused by, 402t
Streptomyces spp., tetracyclines from, 827
Streptomyces nodosus, 828
Streptomyces pilosus, 673, 676
Streptomyces venezuelae, 825
Streptomycin, 821–823
 teratogenicity, 430t
 and tinnitus, 369
 toxicity, clinical manifestations, 822t
Streptozocin, 760t
 EPA regulation of, 765
 nephrotoxicity, 763
 pancreatic damage caused by, 295
 and pancreatic dysfunction, 295t
Streptozotocin, diabetes insipidus caused by, 195, 195t
Stress-vulnerability model, 384
Stria vascularis, 366
Stroke
 clinical manifestations, 577t
 cocaine-related, 1126, 1130
 hemorrhagic, drug-induced, 21, 748
 imaging, 130–131, 133f
 ischemic, in cocaine toxicity, 1130
 prevention
  aspirin in, 899
  rivaroxaban for, 894
Strontium
 dermal decontamination for, 272
 dust, dermal decontamination for, precautions with, 72
 overdose/poisoning, whole-bowel irrigation for, 85
Strophanthin, 1599t
Structolipid, 684
Strychnine, 344, 651, 1450, 1536–1539, 1603t, 1605
 absorption, 1536
 and chest wall rigidity, 400
 cranial neuropathy caused by, 346t
 effect on glycinergic chloride channels, 1536
 elimination, 1536
 estimated fatal dose, 1452t
 as glycine antagonist, 223
 historical perspective on, 1, 4t–5t, 6–7, 1536
 hypoventilation caused by, 400t
 lethal dose, 1536
 metabolism, 1536
 pharmacokinetics, 146t
 physicochemical properties, 1452t
 plant sources, 1536
 in rodenticides, 1452t, 1536
 structure, 1536
 tissue distribution, 1536–1537
 toxicity (overdose/poisoning)
  antidote and/or treatment, 1452t
  clinical manifestations, 36t, 1452t, 1536–1537
  diagnostic testing for, 1537
  differential diagnosis, 1537
  epidemiology, 1536
  hypocalcemia in, 1537
  management, 1537–1538
  mortality rate for, 1536
  onset, 1452t
  pathophysiology, 1536
  sources, 1536
 toxic mechanism, 1452t
 toxicokinetics, 1536
 volume of distribution, 146t, 1536–1537

Strychnos spp. (tubocurare, curare), 1599t, 1605
Strychnos ignatii (ignatia, St. Ignatius bean), 1536, 1603t
Strychnos nux-vomica (poison nut, strychnine), 2, 651, 1536, 1603t, 1605
 glycine inhibition by, 1605
Strychnos tiente, 1536
Strychnos toxifera, 1018
Student *t* test, 1857
Study(ies). *See* Clinical trials; Epidemiologic study(ies)
Stupefacients, 6
Stupor, with colchicine poisoning, 503
Styrene, 174t
 infertility caused by, 297t
 as thermal degradation product, 1641t
Styrol, and leukemia, 320
Subacute myelooptic neuropathy (SMON), 20, 20t
Subarachnoid hemorrhage
 cocaine-related, 1126
  diagnostic imaging, 115t, 132t
 computed tomography of, 130, 132f
 imaging, 115t, 130, 132f, 132t
Subcritine, 1574
Subcutis, 269, 270f, 271
Subdural hematoma, diagnostic imaging, 115t, 131, 132t, 134f
Sublimate, corrosive, 4
Sublimation
 of dry ice, 1652
 of solid, 1652
Substance abuse. *See also specific substance*
 data collection on, 1792
 in elderly, 466–467
 screening tests for, 110–113. *See also* Drug abuse screening tests
Substance Abuse and Mental Health Services Administration (SAMHSA), 110–111, 111t
Substance use
 DSM-5 terminology for, 236
 and violence, 384–385
Substance use disorder(s), 380–381
 DSM-5 diagnoses, 380
 glutamate and, 224
 neurobiology, 380–381
 treatment, 381
Substance withdrawal
 in elderly, 467
 glutamate and, 224
Substituents, 162, 164, 164f
Succimer (2,3-dimercaptosuccinic acid, DMSA), 1285, 1309–1314, 1779
 advantages, 1309
 adverse effects, 1311–1312
 for antimony toxicity, 1234
 arsenic chelation by, 1309
 for arsenic toxicity, 1244–1245, 1245f, 1245t, 1309, 1311
 availability and storage, 46t
 and breast-feeding, 1252
 cadmium chelation by, 1309, 1309f
 for cadmium toxicity, 1261
 with CaNa$_2$EDTA, 1312
 chemistry, 1309
 for copper poisoning, 1287
 dosage and administration, 1312, 1313t
  for adults, 1312, 1313t
  for children, 1312, 1313t
 effects, 144
 elimination, 1309
 formulation, 1312
 history of, 1309

 indications for, 35t, 46t, 1309
 LD$_{50}$, 1252
 lead chelation by, 1309, 1309f
 for lead encephalopathy
  in adults, 1311
  in children, 1310–1311
 for lead poisoning, 1302, 1309–1311
  in adults, 1303t, 1304, 1310
  in children, 1303–1304, 1303t, 1309–1310, 1316
  modeling of plasma pharmacokinetics in, 1310
  utility/efficacy, 1310
 mechanism of action, 164–165, 1309
 for mercury poisoning, 1309, 1309f, 1311, 1325t, 1330
 metabolism, 1309–1310
 overdose, 1312
 pharmacokinetics and pharmacodynamics, 1309–1310
 pharmacology, 1309
 related chelators, 1309
 renal clearance, 1310
 stocking, recommended level, 46t
 structure, 1309
 supplies, 43
 for thallium toxicity, 1355
 therapy with
  and elimination of essential elements, 1311
  monitoring, 1311
 urinary excretion, 1309
 use in pregnancy, 1312
Succinate dehydrogenase, thallium and, 1350
Succinic acid dehydrogenase, inhibition, by cyanide, 1685
Succinic semialdehyde (SSA), 218
Succinic semialdehyde dehydrogenase (SSAD), 221
 deficiency, 222, 1190
Succinylcholine, 5t–6t, 12
 adverse effects and safety issues, 1020
 and anaphylaxis, 1019
 cardiac effects, 1020
 and cocaine, 1128
 contraindications to, 1020, 1128
 diagnostic tests for, 1027
 drug interactions with, 1021t–1022t
 dysrhythmias with, 1020
 and histamine release, 1019
 history of, 1018
 hyperkalemia caused by, 1022
 malignant hyperthermia with, 1023
 mechanisms of action, 207, 1018, 1019f
 metabolism, 206
 muscle spasms with, 1024
 and pancuronium, 1022t
 pharmacology, 1020, 1020t
 potentiation, xenobiotics causing, 1021t
 prolonged effect, xenobiotics causing, 1021t
 and skeletal muscle excitation-contraction coupling, 1019f
 toxicity, 1020
 and vecuronium, 1022t
Succinylmonocholine, diagnostic tests for, 1027
Sucralfate
 aluminum in, 1223, 1225
 effect on thyroid hormones and function, 814t, 817
 for levothyroxine overdose, 817
Sucrose. *See* Sugar(s) (sucrose)
Sucrose polyester, for organic chlorine toxicity, 1519
Sudden (cardiac) death
 anabolic-androgenic steroids and, 617–618
 antimonials and, 1232
 antipsychotics and, 1035

in athletes
  athletic performance enhancers and, 623
  cardiac anomalies and, 623
  medical causes, 623
in children, cyclic antidepressants and, 1048
with colchicine poisoning, 502–503, 503t, 504
succinylcholine-induced, 1022–1023
xenobiotics and, 253
Sudden sniffing death, 1193–1194, 1196, 1412–1413
Sugammadex, 1025–1026, 1026f
  availability and storage, 46t
  dosage and administration, 1026
  indications for, 46t
  stocking, recommended level, 46t
Sugar(s) (sucrose), 707
  definition, 707
  dietary, and fructose intolerance, 689
  simple, 707
Suicidal gesture, 375–376
Suicidal ideation, 375
  assessment, 378
  in pregnancy, 433–434
Suicidal patient, initial management, 37
Suicide, 1884
  alcoholism and, 1152
  antiepileptics and, 719
  capacity and, 377–378
  in children, 448
  cigarette soakage water and, 1204
  completed, 377
    epidemiology, 377
  definition, 375
  in elderly, 466
  epidemiology, 375
  factors associated with protective effects against, 376t
  nicotine patches and, 1205
  with pesticides, 1844–1845, 1845t
  in pregnancy, 433–434
  prevention, 379–380
  psychiatric illness and, 378–379
  risk
    antidepressants and, 1054
    assessment, 378
  risk factors for, 375, 376t
  by self-poisoning, 376
Suicide attempt, 376
  assessment, 378
  epidemiology, 377
  initial psychiatric management of, 377
  as predictor of completed suicide, 377
  "serious," 376
  treatment, 379–380
Suicide tree, self-poisoning with, 1846
Sulfacetamide, ophthalmic solution, parabens in, 685t
Sulfa derivatives, and tinnitus, 370t
Sulfadiazine, for HIV-related infections, 831t
Sulfadoxine
  for malaria, 836, 846
    antimalarial mechanism, 838t
    structure, 846
Sulfamethoxazole, structure, 827
Sulfamylon, and normal anion gap metabolic acidosis, 191t
Sulfane sulfur, 1698–1699
Sulfanilamide
  diethylene glycol (DEG) in, 681, 1833
  elixir of, 9
    diethylene glycol in, 19, 20t, 453
Sulfasalazine

dermal effects, 276
infertility caused by, 297t, 298f
mechanism of action, 227t
Sulfates, postmortem changes, 1885t
Sulfathiazole, phenobarbital contamination, 20, 20t
Sulfation, 172
Sulfhemoglobin, 317, 1689, 1710
  chemistry, 1710
  effects on oxygenation, 403, 403f
  and pulse oximetry, 404, 1710
Sulfhemoglobinemia, 1639, 1709–1710
  xenobiotics causing, 1710
Sulfhydryl-scavenging drugs, for sulfur mustard exposure, 1748
Sulfide:quinone oxireductase, 1689
Sulfinpyrazone, acute interstitial nephritis caused by, 394t
Sulfonamides, 827
  acute interstitial nephritis caused by, 394t
  adverse effects associated with therapeutic use, 827
  as antimalarials, 836
    adverse effects and safety issues, 846
    antimalarial mechanism, 838t, 846
  cholestasis caused by, 330
  crystalluria caused by, 395
  drug-induced hypersensitivity syndrome with, 277–278
  hepatotoxicity, 827
  mechanism of action, 822t, 827
  metabolism, 170
  ophthalmic toxicity, 356f
  overdose, 822t, 827
  and pancreatic dysfunction, 295t
  pancreatitis caused by, 295t
  renal effects, 390f
  toxicity, 822t
  urine alkalinization for, 93
p-Sulfonatocalix-[4]arene, for paraquat poisoning, 1474f, 1476
Sulfonyl, history of, 1084
Sulfonylureas
  adverse effects and safety issues, 698–699
  and disulfiramlike reactions, 1174t
  exposure, in children, hypoglycemia caused by, 699
  history of, 694
  hypoglycemia caused by, 694, 696, 698–699, 702, 709–710, 713–718
    hospitalization for, 702
    octreotide for, 714–715
  ingestion
    by children, hospitalization for, 702–703
    diagnosis, 700–701, 701t
  and insulin secretion, 292
  maintaining euglycemia after initial control with, 701
  mechanism of action, 694–695, 696f
  and NSAIDs, interactions, 514t
  pediatric delayed toxicity, 452
  pharmacokinetics and toxicokinetics, 696, 697t
  pharmacology, 694–695
  site of action, 713
  structure, 695f
  toxicity (overdose/poisoning), 700–701, 701t
    management, 45t, 702
    octreotide for, 715
Sulfur
  and argyria, 1347
  chemistry, 164–165, 168
  dermal decontamination for, 272

dust, dermal decontamination for, precautions with, 72
and high anion gap metabolic acidosis, 191t
materials containing, thermal degradation products, 1641t
Sulfur compounds, sulfhemoglobin from, 1710
Sulfur dioxide, 1655
  detection threshold, 1654t
  diffuse airspace filling caused by, 123
  immediately dangerous to life and health (IDLH), 1654t
  regulatory standard for, 1654t
  short-term exposure limit (STEL), 1654t
  in smog, 16t, 17, 1651
  sources, 1654t
  as thermal degradation product, 1641t
  water solubility, 1654t
Sulfur dioxygenase, 1689
Sulfuric acid, 1388t, 1655
  esophageal injury caused by, 1390
Sulfur mustard, 1747–1748
  chemical name and structure, 1747f
  as chemical weapon, 1741, 1748
  and children, 1744
  decontamination for, 1743, 1748
  dermal decontamination for, 72
  exposure, N-acetylcysteine for, 1748
  history of, 1747
  long-term effects, 1748
  mechanism of toxicity, 1747, 1747f
  ophthalmic exposure to, 358
  physical characteristics, 1747
  toxicity
    clinical effects, 1747–1748
    ocular injury in, 1747–1748
    pathophysiology, 1747
    treatment, 1748
  toxic syndrome caused by, 1750t
Sulfurous acid, 1655
Sulfurtransferases, 1685–1686, 1698
Sulfuryl fluoride
  clinical effects, 1458t
  exposure to
    clinical manifestations, 1462
    diagnostic tests for, 1462
    treatment, 1462
  history of, 1462
  industrial uses, 1457t
  physicochemical properties, 1457t
  toxicodynamics, 1462
  toxicokinetics, 1462
Sulindac
  adverse effects and safety issues, 515
  pharmacology, 512t
Sulla, 1t
Sulpiride. See also Antipsychotics
  dosage and administration, 1033t
  pharmacokinetics, 1033t
Sumac, poison (Toxicodendron spp.), 1603t
Sumatriptan, 808–809, 808t
  adverse effects and safety issues, 215, 809
  mechanism of action, 217
  and serotonin toxicity, 1058t
  structure, 808f
Sumatriptan/naproxen, 808
Sunitinib, 761
  adverse effects and safety issues, 762
Sunscreens, 280
  nanotechnology in, 1717–1718
Supercools. See Phencyclidine (PCP)

Superfund Amendments and Reauthorization Act (SARA), 10t, 1801t, 1804, 1811
"Super K." *See* Ketamine
Superoxide, 159–160, 174, 175f, 1274, 1656
  structure, 160t
Superoxide dismutase (SOD), 159–160, 175
  for phosphorus ingestion, 1531
Superwarfarins, 886
  history of, 883
  and vitamin K antagonism, 916
Supplements. *See specific supplement*
Supplied-air respirator (SAR), 1810–1811, 1810t
Supraventricular tachycardia
  in methylxanthine toxicity, 988, 990–991
  treatment, 230
Suramin, 1228
  neurotoxicity, 343
Surface-connected canalicular system (SCCS), 323
Surface tension, 1412
Surfactants
  in herbicides, 1466
  ophthalmic exposure to, 359
Surgery
  for body packers, 63–64
  for gastrointestinal decontamination, 63–64
Surma, 1228
Sustained-release preparations, radiopacity, 114
Suvorexant, 1084, 1090. *See also* Sedative-hypnotics
  pharmacokinetics, 1085t
Swainsonia spp. (locoweed), 1603t
Swainsonia canescens, 1606
Swainsonine, 1598t, 1600t–1603t, 1606
Swamp gas, 1652
Swango, Michael, 12, 1018
Swarna bhasma, 1717
Swayback, 1364
Sweat glands, 411–412
Sweating
  clinical significance, 273
  xenobiotic-induced, 273
Swedish green, 1284t
Sweet birch (*Betula lenta*), 634
Sweet birch oil, 634
Sweet clover (*Melilotus* spp.), 1601t
Sweet elder (*Sambucus* spp.), uses and toxicities, 641t
Sweet fennel (*Foeniculum vulgare*), 641t
Sweet flag (*Acorus calamus*), 1598t, 1610
Sweet fruity smell, 364t
Sweet oil of vitriol, 1011
Sweet potatoes (*Ipomoea batatas*), *Gloriosa superba* (glory lily) and, confusion, 501
Sweet-scented bedstraw (*Galium triflorum*), 1600t
Sweet vernal grass (*Anthoxanthum odoratum*), 1598t
Sweet woodruff (*Galium odoratum*), 645t
Sweet wormwood (*Artemisia annua*), 638, 647–648, 845
Sydenham, Thomas, 7
Sympathetic nerve terminal, 1075–1076, 1076f
Sympathetic nervous system, 260
Sympatholytics, 210, 211t, 212
  for alcohol withdrawal, 1169
  as antihypertensives, 959t, 961–962
  direct antagonists, 211t, 212
Sympathomimetics, 210–212, 210t. *See also* Dieting xenobiotics and regimens
  addiction caused by, 213–214
  adverse effects and safety issues, 608–610
  brain changes caused by, imaging, 130–131, 132t
  cardiac effects, 255
  in cocaine, 1130
  craving caused by, 213–214
  as decongestants, pharmacology, 749, 749f, 749t

direct-acting, 210, 210t
  effects on vital signs, 29t–31t
  herbal, 610
  indirect-acting, 210–211, 210t, 214, 214t, 218
  intestinal ischemia and infarction caused by, 127
    imaging, 129t
  intracerebral hemorrhage caused by, 130–131
  mixed-acting, 210, 210t, 211, 214
  ophthalmic toxicity, 356f
  pharmacology, 608, 610f
  respiratory effects, 399
  reuptake inhibitors, 211
  and tinnitus, 370t
  toxicity (overdose/poisoning)
    clinical and laboratory findings in, 36, 36t, 37
    cutaneous findings in, 189
  for weight loss, 606
Sympathomimetic toxic syndrome, 27, 29t, 30, 750
Symphytine, 641t
Symphytum spp. (comfrey), 651, 1603t
  hepatic venoocclusive disease from, 332
  uses and toxicities, 641t
Synanceja spp., 1576, 1576f, 1576t
Synanceja horrida (Indian stonefish), 1576, 1576t, 1577
Synanceja trachynis (Australian estuarine stonefish), 1576, 1576t, 1577–1578
  antivenom, 1575t
Synanceja verrucosa (reef stonefish), 1576, 1576t, 1577
Synaptic localization, and withdrawal syndrome, 237
Synaptic pruning, lead and, 1295
Synaptosomal-associated protein (SNAP)-25, 575, 576f
Syndrome of inappropriate antidiuretic hormone secretion (SIADH), 194, 197, 395–396
  causes, 196t, 197
  diagnosis, 197
  and hyponatremia, 196–197
  with lead encephalopathy, 1302–1303
  SSRIs and, 1058
  sulfonylurea-induced, 699
  treatment, 197
  vincristine and, 763
  vincristine-related, 506–507
Syndrome of irreversible lithium-effectuated neurotoxicity (SILENT), 1068
Synephrine, 610, 640t, 1599t, 1605
p-Synephrine, 610, 610f
Synesthesia
  hallucinogen-induced, 1183–1184
  lysergamides and, 1179
Synthetic erythropoiesis protein, 620
Synthroid, 813
Syrian rue (*Peganum harmala*), 644t, 649, 650t, 1077
  and serotonin toxicity, 1058t
Syrup of ipecac. *See* Ipecac (syrup)
Syrup of poppies, 7
Systemic lupus erythematosus (SLE), drug-induced, 115t, 126
Systemic sclerosis, antimonials and, 1233
Systemic vascular resistance, 264
System to Manage Accutane-Related Teratogenicity (SMART), 656
Systole, 264
  calcium flow in, 928, 928f, 970
Syzygium aromaticum (clove)
  psychoactive properties, 650t
  uses and toxicities, 641t

T

T_3. *See* Triiodothyronine (T_3)
T_4. *See* Thyroxine (T_4)
Tabebuia spp. (Pau d'Arco), 643t

Tabernanthe iboga, 642t, 650t
Tabex. *See* Cytisine
Tabun, 1487, 1488t, 1741
  aging half-life, 1746
  chemical name and structure, 1745f
  history of, 1486
  LD_{50}, 1744
  odor, 1745
  physical characteristics, 1745
TachoSil, 910
Tachycardia, 28–30, 189
  in anticholinergic toxicity, 30
  cannabinoid-induced, 1117
  catecholamine-induced, 926
  in cyclic antidepressant poisoning, 1046, 1046f, 1047
  in heatstroke, 420–421
  in ketamine toxicity, 1214
  smoke inhalation and, 1642
  in strychnine poisoning, 1537
  in sympathomimetic toxicity, 30
  in thallium toxicity, 1351
  wide-complex, in cyclic antidepressant poisoning, 1046, 1046f, 1047
  xenobiotics causing, 30t, 217, 263, 264t
Tachydysrhythmias, 255–256
  supraventricular, 255–256
    xenobiotics causing, 255t
  ventricular, 255–256
    xenobiotics causing, 255t
Tachypnea, 28, 30, 399
  with methylxanthine overdose, 989
  smoke inhalation and, 1642
  xenobiotics causing, 30t
Tacrine
  acetylcholinesterase inhibition by, 208, 756
  indications for, 1041
  mechanism of action, 207
  oral, for central anticholinergic syndrome, 748
Tacrolimus
  hypomagnesemia caused by, 877
  neurotoxicity, 343
  and normal anion gap metabolic acidosis, 191t
  and posterior reversible encephalopathy syndrome, 132
  protein-binding characteristics, 110t
  and QT interval, 253t
  renal effects, 391
Tadalafil
  adverse effects and safety issues, 301
  for erectile dysfunction, 301
  pharmacokinetics, 301
Tafenoquinone, 847
Taft, William, 8
Taheebo tea (*Tabebuia* spp.), 643t
Takaki, Kanehiro, 1157
Takotsubo cardiomyopathy, 750, 1127
  carbon monoxide poisoning and, 1665
  from cocaine, 1127
Talampanel, 227t, 228–229
Talc, 1659
  intravenous injection, 401
Talcosis, 125t, 126
Talc retinopathy, 361
Talcum powder, neonatal toxicity caused by, 442
Talepetrako. *See* Gotu kola (*Centella asiatica*)
Tamapin, and voltage-gated potassium channels, 245
Tamoxifen, 617
  effect on thyroid hormones and function, 814t
Tanacetum parthenium (feverfew), 641t
Tanacetum vulgare (tansy), 1603t, 1608
Tanakan (*Gingko biloba*). *See* Gingko (*Gingko biloba*)
Tancitaran dusky rattlesnake (*Crotalus* spp.), 1636t

Tandem mass spectrometry, 107, 109f. *See also* Liquid chromatography/tandem mass spectrometry (LC/MS/MS)
Tanghinia venenifera (Ordeal bean), 979
Tango and Cash, 21t, 22
Taniguchi, Norio, 1717
Tannins, 1597, 1609–1610
Tansy (*Tanacetum vulgare*), 1603t, 1608
Tapantadol, characteristics, 526t
Tapentadol, 530–531
Tapioca (*Manihot esculentus*), 1601t
Tar. *See also* Hydrocarbons
  injuries caused by, 1416
TAR (titratable acid/alkaline reserve), 1388
Taranabant, 611
Tarantism, 1540
Tarantulas, 1547–1548, 1547f
  bites, 1547
  envenomation
    clinical manifestations, 1547
    pathophysiology, 1547
  geographic distribution, 1547
  urticating hairs, 273, 1547–1548
Taraxacum officinale (dandelion), 1599t, 1614
  resins in, 639
Tardive dyskinesia, 214
  antipsychotic-induced, 1037, 1037t
  dopamine antagonists and, 215
  treatment, 1037, 1037t
Taricha spp., tetrodotoxin in, 596
Tartar emetic, 1309
  chelation therapy for, 1234
  clearance, 1230
  medicinal use, historical perspective on, 1228
  toxicity, 1229
Tartrazine, foodborne, 600t
Tasimelteon, 1090. *See also* Sedative-hypnotics
  history of, 1084
  pharmacodynamics, 1084
  pharmacokinetics, 1085t
Taste. *See also* Gustation
  aversion, as learned response, 1782
  disorders, zinc and, 1362
Taste-aversive xenobiotics, 1782
Taste buds, 365
Taste receptors, 365
Tasters, 2
Taurine
  in common products, 986t
  as glycine agonist, 223
Tawell, John, 5t, 6
Taxaceae, 1603t
Taxanes, 760t
  extravasation, 802
  mechanism and site of action, 762f
  scleroderma-like reaction with, 281
Taxicatine, 1612
Taxine, 645t, 1603t, 1612f
  and sodium channels, 1611–1612
Taxol (taxol A and B), 1612. *See also* Paclitaxel
Taxus spp. (yew), 645t, 1603t, 1612, 1612f
Taylor's cantil (*Agkistrodon* spp.), 1636t
TCDD. *See also* Dioxin
  in Agent Orange, 17
Tchaad, 643t
TCP. *See* Tenocyclidine
Tea (*Camellia sinensis*), 1599t
Teaberry, 634
Tear gas, 1749, 1749f. *See also* Lacrimators (tear gas)
  inhalation, treatment, 1658
Tear gas DBO, 1749, 1749f

Tears, pH, 142t
Tea tree oil, 633–634
Tebonin (*Gingko biloba*). *See* Gingko (*Gingko biloba*)
Tebutam, in herbicides, 1467t
Tecadenoson, and adenosine receptor, 230, 230t
Technetium
  chemistry, 1770
  sources, 1770
  uses, 1766t, 1770
Technetium-DTPA, 1779
Technetium-99m, in SPECT, 133
Techno parties, 1099
Tedania ignis (fire sponge), 1573–1574
Teeth, discoloration, xenobiotics causing, 293, 293t
Teething formula, diethylene glycol contamination, 19–20, 20t, 681
Tefluthrin, 1520t. *See also* Pyrethroids
Tegafur, 771, 771f
  folates and, 777
  toxicity, uridine triacetate for, 789–791
Tegaserod, 84
  mechanism of action, 217
Tegenaria agrestis. *See* Hobo spider (*Eratigena agrestis*)
Telazol, 1211
Telithromycin, 826–827
  adverse effects and safety issues, 827
Tellurium, 1339
  odor, 364t
Telmisartan, and muscle performance, 623
Telogen effluvium, 274t, 281
Temazepam, 1138. *See also* Sedative-hypnotics
  gastrointestinal decontamination for, 54t
  pharmacokinetics, 1085t
Temephos, 1486, 1488t
Temozolomide
  diabetes insipidus caused by, 195, 195t
  mechanism and site of action, 762f
  overdose/poisoning, 760t
Temperature, 30–31. *See also* Fever; Hyperthermia; Hypothermia
  assessment, 30
    in poisoned patient, 266t
  body, control of. *See* Thermoregulation
  core, 30, 37
  measurement, 37
  normal, 28
  oral, normal, 28
  and pulse rate, 30
  rectal
    accuracy, 30
    normal, 28
  and violence, 385
  xenobiotics affecting, 31t
Tenase, 320
Tendon rupture, fluoroquinolones and, 826
Tenecteplase, 896–897
Teniposide, 504, 760t. *See also* Podophyllin
  mechanism and site of action, 762f
  pharmacology, 504
Tenocyclidine, 1211, 1211t
Tenofovir (TDF)
  diabetes insipidus caused by, 195t
  renal effects, 395
Tenofovir alafenamide (TAF), 395
Tenorite, 1284t
Teonanacatl (psilocybin mushroom), 9, 1178. *See also* Psilocybin
TEPP, 1488t
Teratogen(s). *See also specific xenobiotic*
  dose-response curve for, 432
  human, 428, 429t–430t

Teratogenesis
  as deterministic phenomenon, 432
  ion trapping in, 431–432
  mechanisms, 433
  with single high-dose exposure, 434
Teratogenicity, 428
  chelation and, 1305
  of diethylstilbestrol (DES), 20, 20t
  of disulfiram, 1175
  of ethanol (alcohol), 1441
  of isotretinoin (Accutane), 658
  of methylxanthines, 989
  of penicillamine, 1289
  of pyrrolizidine alkaloids, 1605
  of selenium, 1342
  of thalidomide, 1833
  of thallium, 1353
  of vitamin A, 658
Teratospermia, 298
Terazosin, 962
Terbutaline, 985
  pharmacokinetics, 987
  for priapism, 301–302
  toxicity, 986
Terconazole, 829
Terfenadine, 21, 171
  adverse effects and safety issues, 739
  cardiotoxicity, 746
  cardiovascular risk with, 1840
  and hERG channels, 245
  history of, 739
  pharmacology, 742
  QT interval prolongation by, 1840
Terpenes, 1410, 1597. *See also* Hydrocarbons
  acyclic, 1410
  cyclic, 1410
  toxicity, 1415
Terpenoids, 640t, 1598t–1603t, 1607–1608
Terpinen-4-ol, 630
Terra sigillata, 3
Terrestrial tiger snake (*Notechis scutatus*), antivenom, 1575–1576, 1575t
Terrorism, 1741t
  agents of opportunity in, 1744
  biological, 1753–1761. *See also* Biological weapons (BW)
  chemical, 17, 17t, 1741. *See also* Chemical weapons (CW); *specific xenobiotic*
  preparedness for, risk communication in, 1817–1818
Testicular xenobiotics, 297t, 298
Testosterone, 298, 617, 618f, 619
  clearance, 617
  for female sexual dysfunction, 302
  metabolism, 170
  musculoskeletal effects, 618
  priapism caused by, 301t
  and sexual function, 298–300
Testosterone:epitestosterone (T:E) ratio, 170, 622
Tetanospasmin, 344
  cranial neuropathy caused by, 346t
  effects on vital signs, 30t
  as glycine antagonist, 223, 1536
  mechanism of action, 223
  poisoning, pathophysiology, 1536
Tetanus
  and chest wall rigidity, 400
  clinical manifestations, 577t
  differential diagnosis, 1537
Tetanus toxin
  effect on glycinergic chloride channels, 1536
  hypoventilation caused by, 400t
  poisoning, pathophysiology, 1536

Tetany, 194

Tetra-arsenic tetrasulfide, 1237

Tetrabenazine
  mechanism of action, 215, 218
  for tardive dyskinesia, 1037

Tetracaine. *See also* Local anesthetic(s)
  gel preparation, 996
  history of, 994
  methemoglobinemia caused by, 997
  minimal IV toxic dose, 998t
  pharmacology, 996t
  structure, 995f

2,3,7,8-Tetrachlorodibenzo-*p*-dioxin (TCDD).
        See also Dioxin
  in Agent Orange, 1480–1481
  and CYP induction, 171

Tetrachloroethane, hepatic effects, 334t

Tetrachloroethylene. *See also* Hydrocarbons,
        halogenated
  dermal absorption, 1411
  hepatic effects, 334t
  inhaled, 1193t
  toxicokinetics, 1411t
  uses, 1409t
  viscosity, 1409t

Tetracycline(s), 827
  acute interstitial nephritis caused by, 394t
  adverse effects associated with therapeutic use, 827
  as antimalarials, 836
    antimalarial mechanism, 838t
  and discoloration of teeth and gums, 293, 293t
  and fatty acid metabolism, 176t
  fixed drug eruption with, 277f
  hepatotoxicity, 331–332, 827
  mechanism of action, 822t
  nephrotoxicity, 827
  oral, and thimerosal, interactions, 690
  pancreatitis caused by, 295t
  structure, 827
  teratogenicity, 430t
  and tinnitus, 370t
  toxicity (overdose), 822t, 827

Tetraethyl lead (TEL), 1198, 1293
  absorption, 1294
  pharmacology, 1294
  toxicity
    clinical manifestations, 1298
    treatment, 1304

Tetraethylpyrophosphate (TEPP), 1504
  history of, 1486

Tetrafluoroethane, inhaled, 1193t
  clinical manifestations of, 1199t

Tetrahydrocannabinoic acid (THC-COOH),
        immunoassays for, 112

Tetrahydrocannabinoids, 3, 1179t
  as glycine agonists, 223
  laboratory testing for, 101

Tetrahydrocannabinol (THC), 611, 1111, 1113, 1179t,
        1599t, 18733
  absorption, 1113–1114
  distribution, 1114–1115
  excretion, 1115, 1115f
  metabolism, 1115
  pharmacokinetics and toxicokinetics, 1113–1115
  screening tests for, 1119–1120
    xenobiotics or conditions interfering with,
        1119–1120, 1119t
  serum concentration, and time of exposure, 1120
  structure, 1112f
  and thujone, structural similarity, 1608
  time of exposure to, 1120

Tetrahydrofolate, 767, 767f, 775–776

Tetrahydrofuran (THF), 1190t

Tetrahydrogestrinone (THG), 622

Tetrahydroharmine, 640t

Tetrahydrozoline, 959–961
  adverse effects and safety issues, in children, 453
  benzalkonium chloride in, 682t
  duration of action, 749t
  structure, 750f
  therapeutic effects, 749t
  toxicity, 749t
    clinical manifestations, 750

Tetramethrin, 1519, 1520t. *See also* Pyrethroids

Tetramethylene disulfotetramine, 1452t

Tetramethyl lead, 1293

Tetramine, 1450, 1534
  estimated fatal dose, 1452t
  food contamination with, 18t, 19, 602
  physicochemical properties, 1452t
  in rodenticides, 1452t
  toxicity
    antidote and/or treatment, 1452t
    clinical manifestations, 1452t
    onset, 1452t
  toxic mechanism, 1452t

Tetrathiomolybdate, 1284, 1287

Tetrazoline toxicity, management, 750–751

Tetrodotoxin (TTX), 1180
  in blue-ringed octopus, 596, 1572
  clinical effects, 576t
  effect on skeletal muscle excitation-contraction
        coupling, 1018
  effects on vital signs, 30t
  fish sources of, 596
  hypoventilation caused by, 400t
  and neuromuscular transmission, 596
  neurotoxicity, 596
  in newts and salamanders, 596
  physicochemical properties, 596
  poisoning with, 343, 596
  and skeletal muscle excitation-contraction coupling,
        1019f
  and voltage-gated calcium channels, 244f, 245

Teucrium chamaedrys (germander), 613
  uses and toxicities, 642t

Texan snake root (*Aristolochia* spp.), 1598t

Texas coral snake (*Micrurus fulvius tener*), 1633

Texas coral snake (*Micrurus tener*), 1617t, 1618, 1620
  antivenom for, 35t, 1628–1631
  envenomation
    clinical manifestations, 1622
    treatment, 1625

Textbooks, of clinical toxicology, 11

Thalamic filtering, 1182

Thalgrain, 1350

Thalidomide, teratogenicity, 20, 20t, 430t, 431, 1833

Thallic ions, 1350

Thallium, 5t–6t, 12, 116, 1350–1356, 1450
  absorption, 1350
  antidote for, 35t, 1452t
  bioavailability, 1350
  in breast milk, 1360
  chemistry, 157–158, 1350, 1770
  cranial neuropathy caused by, 346t
  decontamination, 1353
  elimination, 1350
  elimination half-life, 1350
  enhanced elimination, 92
  estimated fatal dose, 1452t
  excretion, 1350
  exposure to, sources, 1350

  gastrointestinal absorption, prevention, 64
  in hair, 1352, 1352f
  and hair loss, 281
  history and epidemiology, 1350
  imaging, 1353
  ingestion, 1350
  inhalation, 1350
  Mees lines caused by, 1351–1353
  nail changes caused by, 282
  nephrotoxicity, 397t
  occupational exposure to, 1350
  odor, 364t
  ophthalmic toxicity, 356f
  physicochemical properties, 1350, 1452t
  radioactive
    exposure to, animal data on, 1358
    Prussian blue and, 1358
  as radioactive contrast agent, 1350, 1358
  ringworm treatment, toxicity, 20, 20t, 1350
  in rodenticides, 1350, 1452t
  teratogenicity, 1353
  tissue distribution, 1350
  toxicity (overdose/poisoning), 1357
    activated charcoal for, and Prussian blue, in vitro
        comparison, 1357–1358
    assessment, 1353
    case study, 1222
    chelation therapy for, 1354–1355
    clinical manifestations, 36t, 576t, 1351–1353,
        1352t, 1452t
    death caused by, 1351
    diagnosis, 1353
    differential diagnosis, 1353
    epidemiology, 1350
    extracorporeal treatment for, 1354
    laboratory findings with, 36t, 1353
    management, 38, 46t, 92, 1353–1355, 1354t,
        1358, 1452t
    multiple-dose activated charcoal for, 78, 1353
    onset, 1452t
    pathophysiology, 1350–1351
    potassium for, 1353–1354
    in pregnancy, 1353
    Prussian blue for, 1354, 1357–1358
    tests for, 1353
  toxic mechanism, 1452t
  toxicokinetics, 1350
  transport in body, 142
  urine
    measurement, 1353
    normal concentration, 1350, 1353
  volume of distribution, 1350
  whole blood, normal concentration, 1350

Thallium-201
  calibration time, 1770
  in cardiac imaging, 1766t, 1770

Thallium cardiac stress test, 158

Thallium salts
  chemistry, 1350
  historical perspective on, 1350
  inorganic, 1350
  organic, 1350

Thallium sulfate, 1350

Thallotoxicosis, 1350. *See also* Thallium

Thallous ions, 1350–1351

Theaceae, 1599t

Thea sinensis, 985. *See also Camellia sinensis*
        (green tea); Methylxanthines

Thelotornis spp. (twig snake), 1633t

Theobroma cacao (cocoa), 985, 1603t. *See also*
        Methylxanthines

Theobromine (chocolate), 643t, 650t, 1603t. *See also*
    Methylxanthines
  in common products, 986t
  in energy and sports drinks, 986
  pharmacokinetics, 987
  physicochemical properties, 985
  structure, 985
  toxicity (poisoning), 987–989
    in bears, 986
    in dogs and small animals, 986
  toxicokinetics, 987
Theophrastus, 1t, 2
Theophylline. *See also* Methylxanthines
  and adenosine, 239
  as adenosine antagonist, 231
  cardiovascular effects, 988
  clearance, and extracorporeal removal, 92, 992
  CNS toxicity, management, 991
  in common products, 986t
  drug interactions with, 827, 852
  elimination, multiple-dose activated charcoal and,
      78
  enhanced elimination, 90, 991–992
  and GABA receptor, 222
  gastrointestinal effects, 988
  and high anion gap metabolic acidosis, 191t
  laboratory testing for, 101t, 102
  and neuromuscular blockers, 1022t
  and pancuronium, 1022t
  pharmacokinetics, 146t, 987
  physicochemical properties, 985
  plant source, 1599t
  protein-binding characteristics, 110t
  pulmonary effects, 988
  and rhabdomyolysis, 393
  seizures caused by, 231, 988, 991
  structure, 985
  therapeutic use, 985
    in neonates, 985
  and tinnitus, 370t
  toxicity (overdose/poisoning), 987–989
    diagnostic tests for, 989
    epidemiology, 985
    extracorporeal therapies for, 91f, 92, 97t, 991–992
    gastrointestinal decontamination for, 86
    hemoperfusion for, 96
    liver support devices for, 96
    management, 38
    multiple-dose activated charcoal in, 61, 990
    whole-bowel irrigation for, 85, 990
  toxicokinetics, 146t, 987
  volume of distribution, 91, 146t
  whole-bowel irrigation and, 63
Therapeutic drug monitoring (TDM), 101, 108–110
  drugs amenable to, characteristics, 109
  free vs. protein-bound drug and, 109–110, 110t
  immunoassays for, 105
  requirements for, 109
Therapeutic range, 152
Therapeutic Use Exemptions (TUE), 616
Theriaca, 2
Theriac of Andromachus, 1t
Theriacs, 2–4
Thermogenesis
  nonshivering, 414
  shivering for, 414
Thermometer(s), mercury-containing, 1324
Thermoregulation
  disease processes and, 414
    exacerbated or unmasked by xenobiotics in
        elderly, 463, 463t

and heat stress, 419
  neurotransmitters and, 412
  physiology, 411, 412f
  in response to cold, 414
  sweat glands in, 411–412
  vasomotor responses in, 411
  xenobiotic effects on, 412–414
Thermoregulatory principles, 411–427
Thermo-transient receptor potential (TRP) channels,
    628–629, 628f–629f, 630, 632
Thevetia peruviana (yellow oleander), 979, 1603t, 1606,
    1606f. *See also* Cardioactive steroids
  cardiac glycosides in, 969, 979
  overdose/poisoning, 78
    gastrointestinal decontamination for, 59t,
        61–62, 78
Thevetin, 1603t, 1606f
Thiabendazole, and tinnitus, 370t
Thiaminase, site of action, 173f
Thiamine (thiamine hydrochloride, vitamin B₁),
    654, 709, 1157–1163
  absorption, 1158
    ethanol and, 1158
    gastric bypass and, 148
  administration route, 1160
    and pharmacokinetics, 1158
  adverse effects and safety issues, 1160
  for alcoholic ketoacidosis, 1160–1161
  availability and storage, 46t
  biochemistry, 1157–1158, 1157f
  and citric acid cycle, 177, 1157–1159, 1157f
  for congestive heart failure treated with loop
      diuretics, 1160–1161
  deficiency, 177, 179, 1157, 1351
    alcoholism and, 878, 1157, 1160
    Anaphe venata caterpillar and, 345, 1553
    clinical manifestations, 1159–1160
    cranial neuropathy caused by, 346t
    effects on vital signs, 30t–31t
    epidemiology, 1160
    in ethanol disorders, 878
    management, 46t
    ophthalmic effects, 358
    pathophysiology, 1158–1159
    risk factors for, 1157–1158, 1160
    treatment, 35t
  dietary requirement, 1158
  dietary sources, 1157
  dosage and administration, 1161, 1279
  drug interactions with, 1158
  elimination, 1158
  in ethylene glycol metabolism, 1422, 1423f, 1429
  for ethylene glycol poisoning, 1160–1161
    magnesium with, 878
  formulation and acquisition, 1161
  history of, 1157
  indications for, 33, 35t, 37, 46t, 403, 1040, 1149,
      1279
  injection, chlorobutanol in, 683t
  pharmacokinetics, 1158
  pharmacology, 1157–1158
  physiologic functions, 1157
  in pregnancy and lactation, 1160–1161
  recommended daily consumption, 1158
  replacement, 1161
  for seasonal ataxia, 1554
  stocking, recommended level, 46t
  structure, 1158
  supplementation, in alcoholic patients, 1167
  in toxic alcohol poisoning, 1429–1430
  for Wernicke encephalopathy, 1159–1161

Thiamine propyl disulfide, 1158
Thiamine pyrophosphate, trivalent arsenic and,
    1239f
Thiamine transporters
  high-affinity (THTR1), 1158
  low-affinity (THTR2), 1158–1159
Thiazide diuretics. *See* Diuretics, thiazide
Thiazolidinedione derivatives, pharmacokinetics and
    toxicokinetics, 697t
Thiazolidinediones
  hepatotoxicity, 331
  mechanism of action, 696
  overdose, management, 702
  pharmacology, 696
  structure, 695f
Thienobenzodiazepine, 1033t
Thienopyridines, as antiplatelet xenobiotics, 323
Thimble jellyfish (*Linuche unguiculata*), 1567t
  larvae, and seabather's eruption, 1568
Thimerosal, 1324, 1368, 1369t, 1372
  antibacterial activity, 689
  as antiseptic, 689
  and autism, 689, 1327–1328
  in common medications, 689t
  intramuscular exposure to, toxicity, 690
  mercury poisoning from, 689–690, 1327
  metabolites, 689
  ophthalmic exposure to, toxicity, 690
  oral exposure to, toxicity, 690
  and oral tetracycline, interactions, 690
  as pharmaceutical additive, 689–690, 689t
  pharmacokinetics, 689
  regulatory guidelines for, 689
  structure, 689
  topical exposure to, toxicity, 690
  uses, 689
  in vaccines, 689, 1327–1328
Thin-layer chromatography (TLC), 103t
Thioamides, 818
  adverse effects and safety issues, 818
  effect on thyroid hormones and function,
      814t, 817
  for hyperthyroidism, 817
  overdose, 818
  in pregnancy, 818
Thiocarbamate herbicides, 1469t
Thioctic acid (lipoic acid), 643t
  for amatoxin-induced liver toxicity, 1585
Thiocyanate, 146t, 167, 962, 1685, 1698–1700. *See also*
    Cyanide(s)
  serum, 1687
  and thyroid disorders, 1686
  and thyroid hormone synthesis, 813f
  urinary, 1687
Thioguanine
  adverse effects and safety issues, 760t
  mechanism and site of action, 762f
Thiolated resin, for mercury poisoning, 1330
Thiol group, and bullous drug reaction, 276, 276t
Thiols
  chemistry, 165
  as functional groups, 165
  nomenclature, 165
Thiopental
  gastric absorption, lipid solubility and, 143f
  for local anesthetic–induced seizures, 1000
  transplacental transfer, 431
Thioperamide, 739, 742
1-(1-(Thiophen-2-yl)cyclohexyl)piperidine. *See*
    Tenocyclidine
Thioredoxin reductase, 1340

Thioridazine. *See also* Antipsychotics
  clinical and toxicologic effects, 1034t
  dosage and administration, 1033t
  extrapyramidal effects, 215
  and male sexual dysfunction, 300
  mechanism of action, 227t
  pharmacokinetics, 1033t
  pharmacology, 1032
  skin discoloration caused by, 273
  and sudden cardiac death, 253
  toxicity, 1032
    sodium bicarbonate for, 568t, 569
Thiosalicylate, 689
Thiosulfate, 1689
  blood, 1690–1691
  for cisplatin toxicity, 764
  urinary, 1690–1691
Thiosulfate:CN sulfurtransferase. *See* Rhodanese
Thiothixene. *See also* Antipsychotics
  dosage and administration, 1033t
  pharmacokinetics, 1033t
Thioxanthenes, 1033t
Thiram analogs
  and disulfiramlike reactions, 1174t
  and ethanol, interactions, 1146t
Third spacing, 189
Thirst, 194
Thistle (*Atractylis gummifera*), 1598t
Thiuram analogs, and disulfiramlike reactions, 1174t
Thiurams, contact dermatitis from, 279
Thorium, 127
  chelator for, 1780
Thorium dioxide, 127, 129f
  diagnostic imaging, 115t
  and hepatic tumors, 333
  hepatotoxicity, 127
Thornapple, 650t. *See also* Jimsonweed
        (*Datura stramonium*)
Thorotrast, 20, 20t, 1762. *See also* Thorium dioxide
Thorough QT study (TQT) requirement, 1840
Thoroughwort (*Eupatorium perfoliatum*), 640t
Threat(s), definition, 1806
3-finger toxins (3FTXs), in snake venom, 1618
Throatwort. *See* Foxglove (*Digitalis* spp.)
Thrombin, 322, 883, 884f
  binding sites, 892, 892f
Thrombin receptor inhibitors, 900
Thrombin time, 320–322
Thrombocytopenia
  in arsenic poisoning, 1241
  caused by pit viper bite, 1622, 1624–1625
  causes, 324
  chemotherapeutic-related, management, 764
  drug-induced, 891. *See also* Heparin-induced
        thrombocytopenia (HIT)
    differential diagnosis, 324
  heparin-induced, 324, 908
  in heparin-induced thrombocytopenia and
        thrombosis syndrome (HITTS), 887,
        891–892, 908
  methotrexate-related, 768
  NSAID-induced, 515–516
  postoperative, 891
  quinine-induced, 840
  and thrombosis, heparin-induced, 908
  vancomycin-induced, 828
  xenobiotic-induced, 324, 324t
Thrombocytopenic purpura, 324
  idiopathic, 324
Thrombocytosis, 317

β-Thromboglobulin, 323
Thrombolytics, 883–884, 896–897. *See also specific*
        xenobiotic
Thrombosis
  desmopressin-induced, 900
  physiology, 884
  with prothrombin complex concentrate, 909
Thrombotic microangiopathy
  quinine-induced, 840
    eculizumab for, 847
  xenobiotics causing, 391, 391t
Thrombotic thrombocytopenic purpura (TTP), 317,
        323–324
  acute kidney injury caused by, 391
Thromboxane A$_2$ (TXA$_2$), 323
  in arachidonic acid metabolism, 511, 513f
  serum, assay, 900
Thromboxane A$_2$ (TXA$_2$) synthase inhibitors, 900
Thrombus, formation, 897, 898f
Thuja plicata (Western red cedar), and occupational
        asthma, 1660t
Thujone, 644t–645t, 650t, 1598t, 1603t, 1608
  α-, 9, 627
    and GABA, 222, 627
  β-, 9, 627
  and GABA receptor, 222, 627
  structure, 627
Thymectacin, nanocrystals, 1720t
Thymidylate synthase, 789
  genetic polymorphisms, 771
  inhibitor, 767, 767f
Thyroglobulin, 813f
Thyroid cancer
  medullary, 273
  risk, by age group and radiation dose, 1776–1777,
        1777t
Thyroid function tests, 816, 816t
Thyroid gland
  abnormalities
    cobalt and, 1275
    cyanide and, 1686
  historical perspective on, 812
  lead and, 1296
  physiology, 812–813
  radioiodine in, protection against, potassium iodide
        for, 1775–1777
Thyroid hormone(s), 812–820. *See also specific hormone*
  cardiac effects, 255, 815
  chronic toxicity, 815–816
  diagnostic tests for, 816, 816t
  effects on vital signs, 30t–31t
  and energy enhancement, 816
  infertility caused by, 297t
  pharmacokinetics and toxicokinetics, 812–814, 813f,
        813t
  preparation, 813
  synthesis, 812, 813f, 1775–1776
    cobalt and, 1274
  toxicity (overdose/poisoning), 815
    clinical manifestations, 36t, 815–816
    management, 816–818
  unintentional ingestion, management, 816–817
  and weight loss, 606, 816
  xenobiotic interactions, 813–814, 814t
Thyroiditis, 814–815
Thyroid medications, 812–820. *See also specific*
        xenobiotic
  pharmacokinetics and toxicokinetics, 813–814
  xenobiotic interactions, 813–814, 814t
Thyroid-releasing hormone (TRH), 812, 813f

Thyroid-stimulating hormone (TSH), 812–813, 813f
  in screening for thyroid function, 816, 816t
Thyroid storm, 814–815
  management, 817–818
Thyrotoxic crisis, 814
Thyrotoxicosis, 814–816
  amiodarone-induced, 872
  cardiovascular symptoms in, management, 817
  catecholaminelike excess in, management, 817
  hamburger, 812
Thyrotoxicosis factitia, 814, 816
Thyrotropin-releasing hormone (TRH), and
        thermoregulation, 412
Thyroxine (T$_4$), 1340
  free, tests for, 816, 816t
  history of, 812
  overdose, 815
  pharmacokinetics, 813t
  pharmacology, 812–813
  physiologic functions, 812–813
  postmortem changes, 1885t
  preparation, 813
  structure, 813f
  synthesis, 812, 1775–1776
  total, by radioimmunoassay, 816, 816t
  unintentional ingestion, management, 816–817
Thyroxine-binding globulin (TBG), 813f
Tiagabine, 725
  adverse effects and safety issues, 727t
  drug interactions with, 723t
  history of, 719
  indications for, 728
  mechanism of action, 222, 720f, 720t, 725
  metabolism and effects on CYP enzymes, 722t
  overdose/poisoning
    clinical manifestations, 725
    management, 725
  pharmacokinetics and toxicokinetics, 721t, 725
  pharmacology, 719, 720t
  pregnancy category, 725
  and suicide risk, 719
  therapeutic serum concentration, 725
Tianeptine, mechanism of action, 218
Tic(s), 344
Ticagrelor, 323, 883, 899
  mechanism of action, 898f
Ticarcillin, 823–824
  and prevention of aminoglycoside toxicity, 823
Tick paralysis, 1550
  clinical manifestations, 577t
Ticks, 1540, 1550
  families, 1550
  hard, 1550
  infective diseases caused by, 1550
  removal, 1550
  soft, 1550
Tick seeds (*Ricinus communis*), 1602t
  in biologic warfare, 1759
Tick toxicosis, 1550
Ticlopidine, 899
  as antiplatelet agent, 899
  antiplatelet effects, 323
  mechanism of action, 898f
Tidal volume, 1651
  decreased, 399–400
Tiger Balm
  camphor in, 628
  wintergreen oil in, 634
Tiger rattlesnake (*Crotalus tigris*), 1617t, 1637t
Tiletamine, 228, 1211

Timber rattlesnake (*Crotalus horridus*), 1617t
  envenomation
    neurotoxicity, 1622
    and rhabdomyolysis, 1622
    thrombocytopenia caused by, 1622, 1624
Times Beach (Missouri), 12
Time to presentation, after overdose, 57–60
Timolol
  adverse effects and safety issues, 360
  benzalkonium chloride in, 682t
  ophthalmic use, systemic toxicity with, 360
  pharmacology, 927t
Tincture of iodine, 1369t, 1370
Tinnitus, 369–370, 561
  etiologies, 369–370, 370t
  poisoning/overdose causing, 36t
  quinine and, 369–370, 370t, 840
  in salicylism, 370, 561
  xenobiotics causing, 369–370, 370t, 561
Tinzaparin, reversal, 891, 921
Tioconazole, 829
Tiotropium, 1503
Tipranavir, 831–832
Tirofiban, 323, 899
  adverse effects and safety issues, 900
  mechanism of action, 898f
Tissue factor, 897, 898f
Tissue plasminogen activator (t-PA), 322, 883, 896–897
Tissue plasminogen activator inhibitors (PAIs), 896–897
Titanium
  dermal decontamination for, 272
  dust, dermal decontamination for, precautions
    with, 72
Titanium dioxide, nanocrystals, 1720t
Titratable acid/alkaline reserve (TAR), 1388
Ti tree, 633
Ti tree oil, 633
Tityus spp., 1548, 1548t, 1549, 1549f
  antivenom, 1563–1565, 1565t
  geographic distribution, 1563
Tityus discrepans, pancreatitis caused by, 295t
Tityus serrulatus, antivenom, 1563–1565, 1565t
Tiuxetan, 1779
Tizanidine
  and ciprofloxacin, interactions, 171
  and glutamate release, 228
  indications for, 228
T lymphocytes, 319
Toadfish, 1576
Toads. *See also Bufo* spp.
  hallucinogens from, 1180
  licking, 649
  poisons from, 1
Tobacco, 1203. *See also* Nicotine
  dermal exposure to, in harvesting, 1203, 1206
  in home remedies, 1206
  Indian (*Lobelia inflata*), 1600t
    use and toxicities, 643t
  infertility caused by, 297t, 298f
  MAO-B activity in, 1077
  Nicotiana spp., 650t, 1203, 1601t. *See also* Nicotine
  Nicotiana tabacum, 1203, 1601t
  nitrosamine in, 174t
  odor, 364t
  oral products, 1205
  poison (*Hyoscyamus niger*). *See* Henbane
    (*Hyoscyamus niger*)
  smokeless, 1205
  smoking, respiratory effects, 401
  in traditional medicine, 1206

Tobacco amblyopia, 1686
Tobramycin, 821–823
  benzalkonium chloride in, 682t
  ophthalmic ointment, chlorobutanol in, 683t
  toxicity, clinical manifestations, 822t
Tocainide
  adverse effects and safety issues, 866t
  pharmacokinetics, 866t
  pharmacology, 866t
  structure, 869f
Tocolytic(s)
  indomethacin as, 514
  NSAIDs as, 514
α-Tocopherol. *See* Vitamin E
all-rac-α-Tocopherol, 661
Tocopherols, 661
Tocotrienols, 661
Toenails. *See* Nail(s)
Toffana, Madame Giulia, 5t, 6
Togaviridae, 1758
Tolazamide, pharmacokinetics and toxicokinetics, 697t
Tolazoline
  and disulfiramlike reactions, 1174t
  history of, 748
Tolbu, overdose/poisoning, octreotide for, 715
Tolbutamide
  and disulfiramlike reactions, 1174t
  pharmacokinetics and toxicokinetics, 697t
Tolcapone
  indications for, 214
  mechanism of action, 212, 214
  withdrawal, and neuroleptic malignant syndrome, 215
Tolerance, 236. *See also specific xenobiotic*
  alcohol, 1881
  definition, 153, 1086
  and interpretive toxicology, 1873t
  in postmortem toxicology, 1888
  sedative-hypnotic, 1086
  to xenobiotics, 152–153
Tolguacha. *See* Jimsonweed (*Datura stramonium*)
Toll-free access to poison centers, 1782, 1783f
Tolmetin
  adverse effects and safety issues, 515
  pharmacology, 511, 512t
Toluene. *See also* Hydrocarbons, aromatic
  blood:gas partition coeffcient, 1195t
  and bone mineral density, 1197
  brain changes caused by, 131, 132t
  cardiotoxicity, 1194, 1196
  CNS effects, 1196
  dependence, 1198
  elimination, 1195t
  GABA receptors and, 237
  hepatotoxicity, 334t, 1196
  and high anion gap metabolic acidosis, 191t, 193
  inhaled, 1193, 1193t. *See also* Inhalant(s)
    pharmacology of, 1194
  kidney toxicity, 1196
  leukoencephalopathy caused by, 133, 1196, 1199–
    1200, 1412
  metabolites, 1195t, 1199
  and normal anion gap metabolic acidosis, 191t, 193
  ophthalmic toxicity, 356f, 1197
  pharmacokinetics, 1194
  pharmacology, 1410
  and potassium channels, 1194
  renal effects, 1414
  toxicity (overdose/poisoning), 1415
    clinical manifestations, 36t, 1199t
  toxicokinetics, 1411t

uses, 1409t
  viscosity, 1409t
Toluene diisocyanate, 1657
Toluene leukoencphalopathy, 1196, 1412
Toluidine blue, for methemoglobinemia, 1473
Tolvaptan
  diabetes insipidus caused by, 195t
  for SIADH, 197
Tomatidine, 1601t
Tomatine, 1601t
Tomato, green, *Lycopersicon* spp., 1601t
Tomelukast, 1653
Tongkat ali, as aphrodisiac, 304
Tongue, protrusion, antipsychotic-induced, 1036
Tonic inhibition, 236
Tonka bean (*Dipteryx odorata, D. oppositifolia*),
  644t, 645, 1600t
Tonquin bean. *See* Tonka bean (*Dipteryx odorata*,
  D. oppositifolia)
Topiramate, 725
  adverse effects and safety issues, 727t
  for alcoholism, 1152
  cardiac effects, 248f
  drug interactions with, 723t
  and gingival hyperplasia, 293
  history of, 719
  for idiopathic intracranial hypertension, 658
  indications for, 725, 728
  mechanism of action, 222, 227t, 720f, 720t, 725
  metabolism and effects on CYP enzymes, 722t
  and normal anion gap metabolic acidosis, 191t
  overdose/poisoning
    clinical manifestations, 725
    diagnostic tests for, 725
    management, 725
  pharmacokinetics and toxicokinetics, 721t, 725
  pharmacology, 719, 720t
  pregnancy category, 725
  pseudochromhidrosis caused by, 272, 272f, 273
  and suicide risk, 719
  therapeutic serum concentration, 725
Topoisomerase inhibitors, 759
  mechanism of action, 761
Topotecan, 349f, 760t
  cell cycle phase specificity, 761f
  mechanism of action, 761
Toreforant, 743
Torqosmia, 364
Torsade de pointes, 242–243, 243f, 246, 251, 253–256,
  257f, 877–878
  antidysrhythmics and, 866t–867t, 868–869, 872–873
  antimonials and, 1232
  antipsychotic-induced, 1034t, 1035
  arsenic and, 1239
  in arsenic poisoning, 1241
  arsenic trioxide and, 762–763, 763t
  case study, 1820–1821, 1821f
  cesium-induced, 1265, 1359
  in cyclic antidepressant toxicity, management, 1049t
  drug interactions causing, 172
  fluoroquinolones and, 826
  inhalant abuse and, 1196
  methadone and, 172
  risk factors for, 1820–1821, 1821f
  sotalol-induced, 930
  therapeutics for, 35t
  xenobiotics associated with, 242, 243t
Tortuga Island rattlesnake (*Crotalus* spp.), 1636t
Total body burden, 146
Total body clearance, 151

Total body water (TBW), estimation, 1880

Total iron-binding capacity (TIBC), 671

Total parenteral nutrition
octreotide and, 715
zinc in, 1362–1363

Totonacan rattlesnake (*Crotalus* spp.), 1636t

Touch-me-not sponge (*Neofibularia nolitangere*), 1573

Touery, Pierre, 4t, 7

Toxalbumins, 1597, 1608–1609, 1608f

Toxaphene, 1514
absorption, 1514
acute exposure to, clinical manifestations, 1517
mechanism of toxicity, 1517
metabolism, 1515
odor, 1518
physicochemical properties, 1515t, 1518

TOXBASE, 1789

Toxic alcohol(s), 1421–1434. *See also* Ethylene glycol;
Isopropanol (isopropyl alcohol); Methanol
absorption, 1422
and breast-feeding, 1441
chemistry, 1422
definition, 1422
dermal absorption, 1422
diagnostic tests for, 101, 103–104, 1425–1427
distribution, 1422
elimination, 1422–1423, 1440
enhanced elimination, 90
hemodialysis for, 95
history and epidemiology, 1421–1422
inebriation with, 1423
ingestion, 1422
in children, 1427
risk assessment for, 1427
sodium bicarbonate for, 568t, 571
inhalation, 1422
laboratory testing for, 101, 103–104, 1425
metabolism, 1422–1423
millimole/milligram equivalents, 1440
and osmol gap, 192–193, 1426
poisoning
acute CNS effects, 1423
adjunctive therapy for, 1429–1430
alcohol dehydrogenase inhibition for, 1428
clinical manifestations, 1423–1424
epidemics, 1430
ethanol concentration in, 1426
hemodialysis for, 1428–1429
laboratory investigation, 1425
lactate concentration in, 1426–1427
management, 193, 1427–1430
metabolic acidosis in, 1423, 1426
osmol gap in, 192–193, 1426
pathophysiology, 1423–1424
in pregnant women, 1430
projected maximum serum concentration, formula
for, 1427
toxicokinetics/toxicodynamics, 1422–1423

Toxic epidermal necrolysis (TEN), 270f, 274t, 275–276,
275f, 277
with colchicine poisoning, 503
NSAID-induced, 515

Toxic Exposure Surveillance System (TESS), 11

Toxic leukoencephalopathy, 133

Toxicodendron spp., 279, 1603t

Toxicodendron diversilobum, 1603t, 1614

Toxicodendron radicans, 1603t, 1614

Toxicodendron toxicarium, 1603t, 1614

Toxicodendron vernix, 1603t, 1614

Toxicodynamics. *See also specific xenobiotic*

definition, 140
in interpretive toxicology, 1873, 1873t

Toxicogenomics, 13
and interpretive toxicology, 1873t

Toxic oil syndrome, 18–19, 18t, 281, 320, 346

Toxicokinetics, 109. *See also* Absorption; *specific
xenobiotic*
classical versus physiological compartment,
149–151
definition, 140
factors affecting, 140
in interpretive toxicology, 1873, 1873t
of xenobiotics with significant morbidity and
mortality, 145t–146t

Toxicologic investigation, postmortem. *See
Postmortem toxicology*

Toxicologists
of antiquity, 1
and medication safety, 1830

Toxicology. *See also* Medical toxicology
analytic, 6
clinical trials in, 1854, 1854t
environmental, 11–12
global disparities in, 1847
medicolegal interpretive. *See* Medicolegal
interpretive toxicology
medieval, 3–6
modern, father of, 6
postmortem. *See* Postmortem toxicology
in Renaissance, 3–6
in 21st century, 13
in 18th and 19th centuries, 4t, 6–9
in 20th century, 9–13

Toxicology [term], 1

Toxicology databases, 1789–1790

Toxicology Data Network, 1804

Toxicology screening (tox screen), 101–102
communication and, 102
xenobiotics detected by, 102
xenobiotics not detected by, 102

Toxicology test(s). *See also* Laboratory test(s); *specific
xenobiotic*
communication and, 102
for drug abuse screening, 110–113, 111t
menu, 102
routinely available, 101–102, 101t
tier-1 (basic), 101, 101t
turn-around times, 102
two-tiered approach to, 101

Toxicology treatment center(s), regional, 12

Toxic Substances Control Act (TSCA), 10t, 1801t,
1804
and nanotechnology, 1732

Toxic syndromes, 29t
clinical presentation, 29, 29t
with combination of xenobiotics, 28–29
reassessment in, 38
signs and symptoms, 28, 29t
unexpected or atypical findings in, 29

Toxidromes (toxic syndromes), 28, 260

Toxiferines, 1018

Toxification, 167

Toxifile, 11

Toxin T-514, 1601t

TOXINZ, 1789

TOXNET, 1804

Toxogonin, 1746

Toxoplasma gondii, in HIV-infected (AIDS) patients,
830t–831t

Toxoplasmosis, 597

brain changes caused by, imaging, 132t
HIV-associated, 131, 132t
pyrimethamine therapy for, leucovorin with, 777

Tox screen. *See* Toxicology screening (tox screen)

TPESA, for zinc toxicity, 1365

Trace of burning, 622

Tracheal fluid, specimen, postmortem collection and
analysis, 1885

Tracheoesophageal fistula (TEF), after caustic injury, 1391

Trachinidae, 1576, 1576t

Trachinine, 1577

Trachinus (European weeverfish), 1576

Trachinus draco (greater weeverfish), 1576–1577

Trachinus vipera (lesser weeverfish), 1576–1577

Trachynilysin (TLY), 1577

Track marks, 38

Tractus solitarius, 212

Trade names, 162

Traditional medicine, 638
herbal remedies in, 1845
poisoning caused by, 1845
preference for, or reliance on, worldwide, 1845

Tralkoxydim, in herbicides, 1467t

Tralomethrin, 1520t. *See also* Pyrethroids

Tramadol, 530–531. *See also* Opioid(s)
characteristics, 526t
immunoassays for, 112
intrathecal administration, inadvertent overdose
and unintentional exposures due to, 797t
mechanism of action, 218, 227t, 228
metabolism, 172
pruritus caused by, 273
seizures caused by, 539
and serotonin toxicity, 1058t, 1079

Tranexamic acid, 321f, 884f, 897
adverse effects and safety issues, 897
and fibrinolysis, 323
for fibrinolytic overdose/poisoning, 888t
intrathecal administration, inadvertent overdose
and unintentional exposures due to, 797t

Tranquilizers. *See also* Antipsychotics
major, 1032
minor, 1084

Transanethole, 641t

Transcribing error(s), 1824, 1825t

Transdermal absorption, 271

Transdermal patches, 271

Transesophageal echocardiography, with xenobiotic
exposure, 115t

Transferrin, 146, 314–315, 315f, 669
and aluminum, 1224
cobalt binding, 1273–1274
laboratory measurement, 101t
and manganese, 1319–1320

Transfusion, exchange. *See* Exchange transfusion

Transient ischemic attacks, cocaine-related, 1126

Transient neurologic symptoms, from local anesthetics,
997

Transient receptor potential cation channel subfamily
V member 1 (TRPV1) receptors, 472, 1118

Transient receptor potential vanilloid subtype 1
(TRPV1) channel, 628–629, 628f–629f

Transketolase, 878
genetic variant, 1159
thiamine and, 1158

Transplantation, of organs from poisoned patients,
1892–1893, 1892t

Transport
active, 141–142, 141f
carrier-mediated, 141

facilitated, 141–142, 141f
membrane, 141–142, 141f, 167
Transporter proteins. *See* Transport proteins (transporters)
Transporters. *See* Transport proteins (transporters)
Transport inducers, 144
Transport inhibitors, 144
Transport proteins (transporters), 172–173
cell membrane, for neurotransmitters, 204
in erythrocyte, 312
neurotransmitter reuptake, 204
SLC1, 204
SLC6, 204
toxicologic significance, 204
vesicular, for neurotransmitters, 203–204
Transurethral resection of prostate (TURP), glycine irrigation in, and hyponatremia, 196
Tranylcypromine, 1076–1077, 1100. *See also* Monoamine oxidase inhibitors (MAOIs)
as CYP inhibitor, 171
discontinuation syndrome, 1080
and GABA receptors, 222
structure, 1076f
and tinnitus, 370t
Trastuzumab, 760t
and anthracyclines, interactions, 763
Trauma
abdominal, 38
cocaine and, 1127
in elderly, substance abuse and, 466–467
hallucinogen-related, 1183
head, 37, 131, 134f
imaging, 131, 132t, 134f
and interpretive toxicology, 1873t
laboratory findings in, 102
and olfactory dysfunction, 364
prothrombin complex concentrate in, 910
Traumatic brain injury
N-acetylcysteine for, 494
and violence, 385
Trazodone, 1060
ECG changes caused by, 1057t
mechanism of action, 218, 1056f
overdose/poisoning, 1060
priapism caused by, 301, 301t
receptor activity, 1057t, 1060
seizures caused by, 1057t
and serotonin toxicity, 1058t
and sexual function, 304
Tree tobacco (*Nicotiana glauca*), 1604
Tremetone, 1611
Tremor(s), 189
lithium-induced, 1068
mercury-associated, 1327
methylxanthine-induced, 989
organic chlorine insecticides causing, 1517
poisoning/overdose causing, 36t
in toxidromes, 29t
xenobiotic-induced, 345
Tres pasitos, 1450
Tretinoin (all-*trans*-retinoic acid), 656
Triacylglycerol, 178
Triage, in hazardous materials incident, 1811
Triamterene. *See also* Diuretics, potassium-sparing
for hypertension, 963
1,3,5-Triazine, 1482, 1482f
Triazine herbicides, 1469t, 1482–1483.
See also Atrazine
poisoning

clinical manifestations, 1483
diagnostic tests for, 1483
management, 1483
Triazinone herbicides, 1469t
Triazolam. *See also* Sedative-hypnotics
pharmacokinetics, 1085t
suicide with, 466
Triazoles, 829
in herbicides, 1469t
mechanism of action, 822t
overdose, 822t
toxicity, 822t
Triazolone herbicides, 1469t
Triazolopyrimidine herbicides, 1469t
Tribulus terrestris, 1603t
as aphrodisiac, 304t
hepatogenous photosensitivity caused by, 1614
Trichinella spp. *See* Trichinosis
Trichinosis, 592t, 597
Trichloramine, 1655
Trichlorfon, 1488t
2,3,6-Trichlorobenzoic acid (2,3,6-TBA), in herbicides, 1467t
Trichloroethane
dependence, 1198
hepatotoxicity, 334t, 1196
inhaled, clinical manifestations of, 1199t
1,1,1-Trichloroethane (TCE)
blood:gas partition coefficient, 1195t
elimination, 1195t
inhaled, 1193t
metabolites, 1195t
odor, 364t
pharmacology, 1194
toxicokinetics, 1411t
Trichloroethanol, 145t, 683–684, 1085, 1088, 1146
elimination half-life, in children, 1088
mechanism of action, 222
receptor activity, 1084
Trichloroethylene, 174t, 1011, 1410. *See also* Hydrocarbons, halogenated
blood:gas partition coefficient, 1195t
cardiotoxicity, 1196
and disulfiramlike reactions, 1174t
elimination, 1195t
hepatotoxicity, 1196
inhaled, 1193t
clinical manifestations of, 1199t
metabolites, 1195t
ototoxicity, 368
peripheral neuropathy caused by, 1414
pharmacology, 1194, 1410
scleroderma-like reaction with, 281
toxicity, 1415
toxicokinetics, 1411t
uses, 1409t
viscosity, 1409t
Trichloromethylchloroformate. *See* Diphosgene
Trichloromethyl radical, 1195t, 1196
Trichloronitromethane, 1749
2,4,5-Trichlorophenoxyacetic acid (2,4,5-T), 1480
in Agent Orange, 17, 1480
structure, 1481f
3,5,6-Trichloro-2 pyridinol, 146t
Trichloro-*S*-triazinetrione, 1656
Trichoderma spp., in biological warfare, 1759
Tricholoma spp.
GI toxins in, 1589
rhabdomyolysis from, 393t
Tricholoma equestre, 1582t, 1591

clinical and laboratory findings with, 36t
Tricholoma flavovirens, 1591
Tricholoma magnivelare, 1590, 1590f
Tricholoma muscarium, 1582t
Trichosanthes spp., 1609
Trichosanthes kirilowii, 1609
as abortifacient, 303t
uses and toxicities, 641t
Trichosanthin, 641t
as abortifacient, 303t
Trichothecene mycotoxins, as biological weapons, 1581, 1759–1760, 1759f
Tricothecium spp., in biological warfare, 1759
Tricyclic antidepressants, 1044
and antimalarial resistance, 836
elimination, therapeutic manipulation, 147
gastrointestinal decontamination for, 54t
history of, 1044
ileus caused by, 127
immunoassays for, 109
indications for, 1044
laboratory testing for, 101, 101t, 105
and monoamine oxidase inhibitors, combined, 212
overdose/poisoning
lipid emulsion for, 1006
physostigmine and, 756
pharmacology, 1044–1045
Trientine
adverse effects and side effects, 1287
for copper poisoning, 1287
for Wilson disease, 1286–1287
Trientine hydrochloride, 1779
Triethylene glycol, fomepizole for, 1436
Triethyl lead, 1294
Triethyltin, 20, 20t
Trifluoperazine. *See also* Antipsychotics
clinical and toxicologic effects, 1034t
dosage and administration, 1033t
pharmacokinetics, 1033t
Trifluralin, 1468t
Trifolium pratense (red clover), 1603t
Trigeminocervical complex, 805
Trigger beats, 255
Triglyceresin vegetable oil, 1410
Triglycerides, 178–179
and immune function, 685
in lipid emulsion, 1004
in parenteral nutrition emulsions, 685
Trigonella foenumgraecum (fenugreek), 641t
Trigonoside, 640t
Trihexyphenidyl
and dopamine reuptake, 214
mechanism of action, 211
Triiodothyronine (T$_3$), 1340
cardiac effects, 815
free, tests for, 816, 816t
history of, 812
pharmacokinetics, 813t
pharmacology, 812–813
physiologic functions, 812–813
postmortem changes, 1885t
preparation, 813
structure, 813f, 872f
synthesis, 812, 1775–1776
total, by radioimmunoassay, 816, 816t
unintentional ingestion, management, 816–817
TriLyte, 86
Trimedoxime (TMB4), 1746
Trimetallic anhydride, and occupational asthma, 1660, 1660t

Trimethadione, teratogenicity, 430t
Trimethaphan, 756, 961
   ganglionic blocking by, 207
   mechanism of action, 207
   nicotinic receptor blockade by, 207
Trimethoprim
   antimalarial mechanism, 838t, 846
   mechanism of action, 759
   teratogenicity, 430t
Trimethoprim-sulfamethoxazole
   adverse effects and safety issues, in elderly, 465
   hepatitis caused by, 330
   for HIV-related infections, 831t
   injection, propylene glycol in, 687t
   mechanism of action, 825
   overdose, 825
   toxicity, 825
2,4,5-Trimethoxyamphetamine, 1101t
3,4,5-Trimethoxyamphetamine (TMA), 631
Trimethylamine, congenital anosmia for, 364
Trimethylaminuria, 365
Trimethylammoniobutanoate, 732
Trimethyllysine, 732
Trimethylselenide, 1340, 1340f
Trimethyltin, contamination with, 20
Trimetrexate, for HIV-related infections, 831t
Trimetrexate glucuronate, 777
Trimipramine, 1044, 1044t
Trinder test, 103
Trinitrotoluene, sulfhemoglobin from, 1710
Triorthocresyl phosphate (TOCP), 1488t. *See also*
       Organic phosphorus compounds
   cooking oil contamination with, 18t, 22
   Jamaican ginger contamination by, 21t, 22
   neurotoxicity, 22
Tripelennamine, pharmacology, 741–742
Tripneustes (Pacific urchin), 1574
Tripotassium dicitratobismuthate (TDC), toxicity,
      1256
Triptans, 217, 808–809, 808t
   adverse effects and safety issues, 808–809
   mechanism of action, 808, 808f
   for migraine abortive therapy, 805
   pharmacology and pharmacokinetics, 808, 808t
   with selective serotonin reuptake inhibitors, and
      serotonin toxicity, 809, 1058t, 1059, 1079
   and serotonergic receptors, 808–809, 808f
   structure, 808f
   vasoconstriction caused by, 808–809
Tritanomaly, in thallium toxicity, 1351
Triterpene glycosides, 640t
Triterpenes, 1597
Triterpenoids, 1600t
Tritium
   chemistry, 1770
   uses, 1770
Tritoqualine, 743
Trivial name, 162
Trogia venenata, 1582t, 1591
Troglitazone
   adverse effects and safety issues, 700
   hepatotoxicity, 21, 331
   history of, 694
Trohexyphenidyl, 756
Troleandomycin, 827
   and CYP induction, 171
Tropane alkaloids, 651, 1178, 1181, 1503
Tropical moccasin (*Agkistrodon* spp.), 1636t
Tropical rattlesnake (*Crotalus* spp.), 1636t
Tropicamide, benzalkonium chloride in, 682t
Troponin, 262, 263f, 947, 988

in cardiac physiology, 928, 929f
   serum, 1427
Trousseau sign, 189
True sage. *See Salvia officinalis* (sage)
Trunnionosis, 1276
Trypanosomiasis, African, treatment, 1237
Trypanothione reductase, 1229
Tryptamines (indolealkylamines), 1178, 1179t
   chemical structure, 1180f
   clinical and laboratory findings with, 36t
   clinical effects, 1183–1184
   endogenous, 1179
   exogenous, naturally occurring, 1179
   pharmacology, 1182–1183
   synthetic, 1180
L-Tryptophan, 215
   absorption, 217
   eosinophilia myalgia syndrome from, 20t, 21, 281, 320
   and serotonin toxicity, 1058t, 1079
Tryptophan hydroxylase, 215, 216f
Tryptophan-rich sensory protein (TSPO), 1136, 1136f,
      1139
   cocaine use and, 1139
T's and blues, 738
T syndrome, pyrethroid-induced, 1519
T-2 toxin, 1759, 1759f
T-tubules, 262
Tuberculosis. *See also* Antituberculous medications
   drug-resistant, treatment, 858
   epidemiology, 850
   extensively drug-resistant (XDR), 850, 857
   history of, 850
   in HIV-infected (AIDS) patients, 850, 855
   multidrug-resistant (MDR), 850, 857–858
   risk factors for, 850
Tuberomammillary nucleus
   α_2-adrenoceptor activation in, 210f
   histaminergic neurons in, 210f
Tubocurare (*Chondrodendron* spp., *Curarea* spp.,
      Strychnos spp.), 1599t
Tubocurarine, 1599t
   hypotension caused by, 1019
   mechanism of action, 207
D-Tubocurarine, 1018
D-Tubocurarine chloride, 1605–1606
Tubulointerstitial nephropathy, lithium-induced, 1068
Tularemia (*Francisella tularensis*), 1550, 1756–1757
Tulip fingers, 1614
Tuliposide (ragweed), contact dermatitis from, 279
Tuliposide A, 1614
Tulips, allergic contact dermatitis from, 1614
Tullidora (*Karwinskia humboldtiana*), 1601t, 1610
Tumor, skin, 269t
Tumor lysis syndrome, 392, 394
Tumor necrosis factor (TNF) inhibitors, neurotoxicity,
      343
Tung and tung seed (*Aleurites moluccana, A. fordii*), 644t
Tungsten carbide, 1273, 1276–1277
Turkish rue. *See* Syrian rue (*Peganum harmala*)
Turmeric root. *See* Goldenseal (*Hydrastis canadensis*)
Turnbull's blue. *See* Prussian blue
Turnera diffusa (damiana), psychoactive properties, 650t
Turpentine, 633. *See also* Hydrocarbons, aliphatic
   odor, 364t
   uses, 1409t
   viscosity, 1409t
T'u-san-chi (*Gynura segetum*), use and toxicities, 644t
Tussilagin, 641t
Tussilago farfara (coltsfoot), 1603t
   uses and toxicities, 641t
21st Century Cures Act, 1835

Twig snake (*Thelotornis* spp.), 1633t
Twilight sleep, 22
Twin-spotted rattlesnake (*Crotalus pricei*), 1617t
Two-compartment model, 149–151, 149f–150f
Tylenol, mixed with cyanide, 5t, 12, 20t
Type 1 error, 1855
Type 2 error, 1855
Typewriter correction fluids, inhaled, 1193, 1193t. *See
     also* Inhalant(s)
Typhoid fever, 597
Typhoid Vi vaccine, phenol in, 685t
Typhus, louseborne, weaponized, 1757
Tyramine, 805
   adrenergic action, 211
   foodborne toxicity caused by, 600t
Tyrosinase, 1285t
Tyrosine, 1180
Tyrosine hydroxylase, 208, 209f
Tyrosine iodase, cobalt and, 1274
Tyrosine kinase(s), 761f
   inhibitors, 761f
      adverse effects and safety issues, 762
Tyrosine kinase family, 311
Tzabcan (*Crotalus* spp.), 1636t

U

U-47700, 529, 551
   structure, 529, 529f
U-50488, 529
Udenafil, for erectile dysfunction, 301
UDP-glucuronsyltransferase
   inducers, 172
   inhibitors, 172
UDP-glucuronsyltransferase 2B17 (UGT2B17), genetic
      polymorphism, 170
Ulcer(s)
   cutaneous, 269t
   esophageal, xenobiotic-induced, 293, 293t
   gastroduodenal, 513
      NSAIDs and, 515
Ulinastatin, for paraquat poisoning, 1476
Ulipristal, as abortifacient, 303t
Ulmus fulva (slippery elm), 644t
Ulmus rubra (slippery elm), 644t
Uloboridae, 1540
Ultrafine particle, 1717
Ultramicroscope, 1717
Ultrarapid opioid detoxification (UROD), 239, 534
Ultrasound (ultrasonography), 114, 115t
   abdominal, in body packers, 117, 120f
   bedside
      indications for, 406
      in respiratory disorders, 406
   and detection of gastric tablets and tablet residues,
      53
   in liver disease, 336
   renal, 397
   of soft tissue changes, 122
   of xenobiotics in containers, 117
Uman Complex, 910
Uman-Complex D.I., 910
Umbelliferae, 1599t
Umbrella tree (*Brassaia* spp.), 1598t
Umbrella tree (*Schefflera* spp.), 1602t
Uncertainties, and risk assessment, 1814–1815
Uncertainty factors, 1815
Uncouplers, 177
   site of action, 173f
2-Undecanone (BioUD, methyl nonyl ketone), 1523t,
      1524–1525
   comparative efficacy and toxicity, 1523t

Undecylenate salt, toxicity, organ system manifestations, 829t
Undecylenic acid, toxicity, organ system manifestations, 829t
Underreported xenobiotics, and epidemiologic data, 1792
Undulated pit viper (*Ophryacus undulatus*), 1637t
Unfractionated heparin (UFH). *See also* Heparin history of, 883
Unicorn horn, 4
Unidentified poisoner, 5t
Unintentional poisoning
    global incidence, 1782
    prevention, 1782–1788
Unions, as information resource, 1804
United Nations Scientific Committee on the Effects of Atomic Radiation (UNSCEAR), 1767
Unknown overdose, 41
Upper GI series, 127–128, 129t
UR144, 1112f
Uracil, 789
Uracil herbicides, 1470t
Uracil mustard, EPA regulation of, 765
Uranium, 1780
    depleted, 1766
        exposure to, renal protection after, sodium bicarbonate for, 571
    dermal decontamination for, 272
    dust, dermal decontamination for, precautions with, 72
    elimination, sodium bicarbonate and, 568t
    nephrotoxicity, 392, 397t
URB 597, structure, 1112f
Urea. *See also* Fractional urea excretion
    elimination, 180f
    formation, 180f
    in renal disorders, 396–397
Urea cycle, 180f, 181
    SMFA or fluoroacetamide and, 1533
Urea formaldehyde resins, contact dermatitis caused by, 279
Urea herbicides, 1470t
Urea nitrogen. *See also* Blood urea nitrogen (BUN)
    vitreous, normal concentration, 1872t
Uremia
    clinical and laboratory findings in, 36t
    and high anion gap metabolic acidosis, 191t
Urethane, history of, 1084
Urginea spp., 1606
Urginea indica, 1603t
Urginea maritima (red squill), 644t, 969, 979, 1603t, 1606. *See also* Squill (*Urginea maritima, U. indica*)
    physicochemical properties, 1453t
    in rodenticides, 1453t
    toxicity
        antidote and/or treatment for, 1453t
        clinical manifestations, 1453t
        onset, 1453t
        toxic mechanism, 1453t
Uridine diphosphate glucuronosyltransferase, genetic polymorphisms and, 759
Uridine monophosphate (UMP), 789
Uridine monophosphate synthetase (UMPS), 789
Uridine phosphorylase, 789–790
Uridine triacetate, 760t, 764, 789–792
    adverse effects and safety issues, 772, 791
    availability and storage, 46t
    chemistry, 789
    dosage and administration, 772, 791
    formulation and acquisition, 791–792

history of, 789
indications for, 35t, 46t, 772, 789
mechanism of action, 789
pharmacokinetics and pharmacodynamics, 789–790
pharmacology, 789
in pregnancy and lactation, 791
stocking, recommended level, 46t
structure, 789
Uridine triphosphate, 789
Urinalysis
    abnormalities in, 305–306
    in acute kidney injury, 397
    in diabetes insipidus, 195
    in differential diagnosis of high anion gap metabolic acidosis, 192
    for prohibited xenobiotics, in athletes, 622–623
    in renal disorders, 396–397
Urinary abnormalities, 304–305, 305f, 306t
Urinary bladder, ketamine and, 1216
Urinary incontinence, 304, 305f, 306t
    SSRIs and, 1058
    xenobiotic-induced, in elderly, 463, 463t
    xenobiotics causing, 217
Urinary retention, 38, 304–305, 306t
    antipsychotic-induced, 1039
    in toxidromes, 28, 29t
    xenobiotic-induced, in elderly, 463, 463t
Urinary system, 304–307
Urinary tract obstruction
    lower, 394
    upper, 394
    xenobiotics in, 390f, 394–395, 394t
Urination
    neurophysiology, 304
    physiology, 304, 305f
Urine
    acidification, 38, 93
        contraindications to, 1212, 1217
    alkalinization, 33, 38, 93, 161, 167
        complications, 93
        in dimercaprol therapy, 571
        with dimercaprol therapy, 1252–1253
        and fluoride excretion, 1400–1401
        frequency of use, 90
        with glucarpidase therapy, 785
        for methotrexate overdose, 769
        and PCP toxicity, 1217
        and phenobarbital elimination, 1087
        for phenoxy herbicide toxicity, 1482
        position paper on, 90
        principles of, 148
        for salicylate toxicity, 93, 562, 562f, 563, 569–570
    alteration, before doping analysis, 622
    color, abnormal, 305–306, 307t
    color change with deferoxamine therapy, 672, 672f, 678–679
    dipstick test, 189
    discolored, sedative-hypnotic overdose and, 1086t
    dithionate test for paraquat or diquat, 1475–1476
    drug concentration in, factors affecting, 110
    electrolytes in, 189
    ferric chloride test, 192
    fluorescent
        in antifreeze poisoning, 1427
        in ethylene glycol poisoning, 192
    formation, 389
    ketones in, 192
    osmolality, 189
    pH, 142t
        and drug concentration, 110

and phencyclidine elimination, 1212
    therapeutic manipulation, 147, 161
    screening, for drugs of abuse, 102, 105, 110, 111t, 112–113
    sediment, microscopic examination, 397
    specific gravity, assessment, 189
    specimens, postmortem collection and analysis, 1870t, 1885–1886
    volume
        in diabetes insipidus, 195
        and drug concentration, 110
Urine assay(s)
    qualitative, basic, 101, 101t
    specimens for, 102
Urine Luck, 622
Urobilinogen, 334
Urochloralic acid, 1088
Urokinase, 883–884, 896–897
Urolophidae, 1576
Urolophus halleri, 1576
Urtica dioica (stinging nettles), 1613
Urtica ferox, 1613
Urticaria, 273
    with *N*-acetylcysteine, 495
    food toxins and, 600t
    NSAID-induced, 515
    warfarin-related, 889–890
    xenobiotic-induced, 273–274
Urticating hairs
    of caterpillars, 1552–1553
    pruritus caused by, 273
    on tarantulas, 273, 1547–1548
Urushiol, contact dermatitis from, 279
Urushiol oleoresins, 1598t–1600t, 1603t, 1614
Use dependence, 868
Use-dependent blockade, 838
Usnic acid, 1614
    hepatotoxicity, 651
US Strategic National Stockpile, 1360
Uveitis, nonophthalmic xenobiotics causing, 360

V

Vaccines
    and autism, 689, 1852–1853
    malaria, 847
    thimerosal in, 689, 1327–1328
Vaccinia immune globulin, 1758
Vacor. *See also* PNU (*N*3-pyridylmethyl-*N*'-*p*-nitrophenylurea, Vacor)
    and pancreatic dysfunction, 295t
Vagina, pH, 142t
Vagus nerve, and cardiac function, 247–248
Valacyclovir, 829
Valbenazine, for tardive dyskinesia, 1037
Valdecoxib, market withdrawal, 514
Valence shells, 155
Valepotriates, 644t
Valeric acid, 644t
Valerian (*Valeriana officinalis*), 644t, 650t
γ-Valerolactone (GHL), 1190t
    overdose, clinical findings in, 1086t
Valganciclovir, for HIV-related infections, 831t
Valinomycin, and ATP synthesis, 176t
Valone
    physicochemical properties, 1453t
    in rodenticides, 1453t
    toxicity
        antidote and/or treatment for, 1453t
        clinical manifestations, 1453t
        onset, 1453t
        toxic mechanism, 1453t

Valproate
  for lead encephalopathy, in children, 1302
  mechanism of action, 221–222
  plasma protein binding by, 109
  protein-binding characteristics, 110, 110t
Valproic acid (VPA)
  adverse effects and safety issues, 727t
  for agitated/violent behavior, 386
  for alcohol withdrawal, 1169
  antidote for, 35t
  clearance, and extracorporeal removal, 92
  diabetes insipidus caused by, 195t
  drug interactions with, 723t, 852
  elimination, multiple-dose activated charcoal and,
      78
  and fatty acid metabolism, 176t
  and gingival hyperplasia, 293
  hepatotoxicity, 331–332, 332f, 726, 732–733
      N-acetylcysteine for, 492, 494
      L-carnitine for, 726, 732–733
  history of, 719
  hyperammonemia caused by, 335
      L-carnitine for, 732–733
  indications for, 725, 728
  laboratory testing for, 101t, 102
  mechanism of action, 720f, 720t
  metabolism and effects on CYP enzymes, 722t
  pancreatitis caused by, 295t
  pharmacokinetics and toxicokinetics, 721t, 725–726,
      726f
  pharmacology, 719, 720t, 1066–1067
  pregnancy category, 725
  and pregnancy complications, 719
  and serotonin toxicity, 1058t
  site of action, 173f
  and suicide risk, 719
  teratogenicity, 430t
  therapeutic serum concentration, 726
  toxicity (overdose/poisoning)
      clinical manifestations, 726
      diagnostic tests for, 726
      extracorporeal therapies for, 91, 91f, 92, 97t
      hemodialysis for, 95
      hyperammonemia in, 181
      liver support devices for, 96
      management, 38, 45t, 733–734
      multiple-dose activated charcoal in, 61
      pathophysiology, 726
  toxic metabolite, 174t
  toxicokinetics, and extracorporeal removal, 91
  transplacental transfer, 431
  volume of distribution, 91
Valsartan, CYP enzymes and, 170
Valvular heart disease
  amphetamine-induced, 1103
  drug-induced, 21
Vancomycin
  acute interstitial nephritis caused by, 394t
  adverse effects and safety issues, 273
      with therapeutic use, 828
  clinical and laboratory findings with, 36
  dermal effects, 276t
  mechanism of action, 822t
  nephrotoxicity, 828
  ototoxicity, 366f
  overdose, 822t, 828
  renal effects, 390f
  renal impairment and, 389
  serum concentration, interpretation, 153
  structure, 828

  and tinnitus, 370t
  toxicity, 822t
Van der Waals forces, 159
Van Gogh, Vincent, 9
Vanilla extract, ethanol in, 1143
Vapor(s)
  definition, 1809
  and dermal decontamination, 71–72
  exposure to, 1809
  in smoke, 1640
Vapor pressure, 1809
Vapreotide, 713–714, 716
Vardenafil
  adverse effects and safety issues, 301
  for erectile dysfunction, 301
  pharmacokinetics, 301
Varencicline, mechanism of action, 239
Varenicline, 1203, 1206
  adverse effects, 1206
  overdose, 1206
Variola virus
  as biological weapon, 1757–1758, 1757f
  remaining stocks, 1758
Varnish(es), inhaled, 1193t. See also Inhalant(s)
Vascular disease, arsenic and, 1242
Vascular endothelial growth factor (VEGF), 761f
Vascular endothelial growth factor receptor (VEGFR),
      761
Vascular lesions, abdominal, imaging, 128–130
Vascular radiation subsyndrome, 1768
Vascular subendothelial collagen, 883, 884f
Vasculitis
  acute kidney injury caused by, 391
  cutaneous, 278–279, 278f
  leukocytoclastic, 278
  renal, 390f
  urticarial, 278
  xenobiotics causing, 274t, 278–279, 278f
Vasoactive intestinal peptide (VIP), 290t
Vasoconstriction
  dopamine-induced, 211–212
  in response to cold, 414
  serotonin-induced, 215
  therapeutics for, 35t
  in thermoregulation, 411
  triptan-induced, 808–809
Vasoconstrictors, ophthalmic toxicity, 356f
Vasodilation
  physiology, 954, 954f
  serotonin-induced, 215
  in thermoregulation, 411
Vasodilators
  for amphetamine toxicity, 1104–1105, 1104t
  as antihypertensives, 959t
  direct, 962–963
  and ethanol, interactions, 1146t
Vasomotor responses, to thermoregulatory input, 411
Vasoplegic syndrome, therapeutics for, 35t
Vasopressin
  for β-adrenergic antagonist toxicity, 935
  for calcium channel blocker toxicity, 950
  for cyclic antidepressant toxicity, 1051
  for diabetes insipidus, 196
  for hypothermia, 417
  injectable, chlorobutanol in, 683t
  precautions with, 1040
  and thermoregulation, 412
Vasopressin receptor antagonists, diabetes insipidus
      caused by, 195t
Vasopressors. See also specific vasopressor

  for calcium channel blocker toxicity, 950
  for cyanide poisoning, 1687, 1687t
Vasospasm, cocaine-induced, 1129
Vaughan-Williams classification, of antidysrhythmics,
      865–866
Vecuronium
  drug interactions with, 1021t–1022t
  pharmacology, 1020t
  and response to subsequent nondepolarizer
      administration, 1021t
  and response to succinylcholine, 1021t
  reversal, sugammadex for, 1025–1026
  reversal agent, 46t
Vegetable antimony (Eupatorium perfoliatum), 640t
Vegetable poisons, early, 2, 4
Vegetables, and food poisoning, 602
Veil, mushroom, 1584f, 1593–1594
Veisalgia, 1143
Velerine alkaloids, 650t
Vellorita (Colchicum autumnale), uses and toxicities, 640t
Velvet bean (Mucuna pruriens), 1613
Venezuelan equine encephalitis (VEE), as biological
      weapon, 1758–1759
Venice, poisoners in, 4
Venice treacle, 2
Venlafaxine, 1060
  and CYP enzymes, 171, 1056
  ECG changes caused by, 1057t
  mechanism of action, 211, 1056f
  pharmacokinetics, 1055t
  and QT interval, 253t
  receptor activity, 1057t, 1060
  seizures caused by, 1057t
  structure, 1060
  and serotonin toxicity, 1058t, 1079
  toxicity (overdose/poisoning), 376, 1060
      gastrointestinal decontamination for, 64, 77, 86
      lipid emulsion for, 1006
      seizures with, decontamination strategy and, 86
      sodium bicarbonate for, 568t
      whole-bowel irrigation in, 63
Venom. See also Envenomations; Snakebite(s); specific
      organism; specific venom
  cranial neuropathy caused by, 346t
  pancreatitis caused by, 295t
Venom proteins, and coagulation, 884f
Venoocclusive disease, hepatic, 330, 331t, 332
  plant alkaloids causing, 332, 1605
Venous insufficiency, exacerbated or unmasked by
      xenobiotics in elderly, 463, 463t
Venous thromboembolism
  anabolic-androgenic steroids and, 617–618
  antipsychotic-induced, 1039
  apixaban for, 894
  prevention, 891–892
  rivaroxaban for, 894
  treatment, 891–892
Ventilation, 36
  assessment, 36–37
  mechanical, 36
Ventilation-perfusion (V/Q) mismatch, 401, 405
Ventricular dysrhythmias
  cardioactive steroid toxicity and, 972, 972t, 974
  hypermagnesemia and, 200
Ventricular ectopy, cardioactive steroid toxicity and,
      972, 972t
Ventricular escape rhythm, 247
Ventricular fibrillation, 251, 877
  in cyclic antidepressant poisoning, 1047
  hydrofluoric acid and, 1398

hypothermia and, 416
inhalant abuse and, 1196, 1199
NSAID overdose and, 516
Ventricular tachycardia, 251, 253, 255–256, 877
bidirectional, 256, 256f
cardioactive steroid toxicity and, 972, 972t
in cyclic antidepressant poisoning, 1047
hypokalemia and, 198
NSAID overdose and, 516
polymorphic, 877–878
Ventrolateral medulla (VLM), 212
α_2-adrenoceptor activation in, 210f
Ventrolateral preoptic nucleus (VLPO)
α_2-adrenoceptor activation in, 210f
GABAergic neurons in, 210f
Verapamil
for Cnidaria cardiotoxicity, 1570–1571
and colchicine, interactions, 502
and dantrolene, interactions, 1030
drug interactions with, 946
ECG changes caused by, 258
excretion, 946
gastrointestinal decontamination for, 54t
history of, 945
hypotension caused by, calcium salts and, 1404
mechanism of action, 945, 945t
metabolism, 946
myocardial effects, 947
overdose/poisoning
calcium for, 1404–1405
gastrointestinal decontamination for, 86
multiple-dose activated charcoal in, 61
pathophysiology, 953
whole-bowel irrigation for, 85
pharmacobezoar, formation, 52f
pharmacokinetics, 145t, 946t
pharmacology, 945
poisoning, lipid emulsion for, 1006
structure, 945
toxicokinetics, 145t
volume of distribution, 145t
whole-bowel irrigation and, 63
Veratridine, 1603t, 1612
and sodium channels, 1611
and voltage-gated calcium channels, 244f, 245
Veratrum album (hellebore), 2, 1603t
Veratrum alkaloids, 1603t, 1611
Veratrum californicum, 1603t
Veratrum viride, 979, 1603t, 1611
Verbal de-escalation, with violent patient, 385
Verpa bohemica, 1594
Verrucotoxin (VTX), 1577
Verteporfin, liposomal, 1720t
Vesicants, 271, 1747–1748
chemical names and structures, 1747f
and children, 1744
military designations, 1747f
toxic syndromes caused by, 1750t–1751t
Vesicle, 269t
Vesicle-associated membrane protein (VAMP), 575, 576f
Vesicular acetylcholine transporter (VAChT), 203–204, 206
Vesicular GABA transporter (VGAT), 203, 218, 219f
Vesicular glutamate transporters (VGluTs), 204
Vesicular monoamine transporter
inhibition, 215
VMAT1, 203, 213
VMAT2, 203, 208, 209f, 210, 213–215, 216f
Vesicular transporters, for neurotransmitters, 203–204, 206

Vesiculobullous lesions, xenobiotics in, 274t, 276, 276t
Vespids, 1511–1552, 1540t, 1551t
Vetch, 1603t, 1607
VIAAT. See Vesicular GABA transporter (VGAT)
Vibrio cholerae, foodborne illness caused by, 597t
Vibrio parahaemolyticus, 592t, 1574
foodborne illness caused by, 597
Vibrio vulnificus, 592t
Vicia fava, 1603t, 1607
and glucose-6-phosphate dehydrogenase deficiency, 318
Vicia sativa, 1603t, 1607
Vicine, 1603t, 1607
Vick's Vapo-Rub, camphor in, 628
Victoria (Queen of England), 1011
Video cassette recorder head cleaner, inhaled, 1193t.
See also Inhalant(s)
Vienna green, 1284t
Vietnam War, opioid abuse in, 8
Vigabatrin
adverse effects and safety issues, 727t
drug interactions with, 723t
history of, 719
mechanism of action, 221, 720f, 720t, 726
metabolism and effects on CYP enzymes, 722t
pharmacokinetics and toxicokinetics, 721t, 726
pharmacology, 719, 720t
pregnancy category, 726
therapeutic serum concentration, 726
toxicity
clinical manifestations, 726
management, 726
Vilazodone, 1060
mechanism of action, 217, 1056f
pharmacokinetics, 1055t
receptor activity, 1057t
seizures caused by, 1057t
structure, 1060
Vinblastine, 349f, 505–507, 644t, 1612. See also
Antineoplastics
adverse effects and safety issues, 760t
cell cycle phase specificity, 761f
dosage and administration, 505
intrathecal, 505
neurotoxicity, 506
and other antimitotics, in overdose, comparison, 507t
structure, 501
therapeutic uses, 505
and tinnitus, 370t
toxic dose, 506
toxicity (overdose/poisoning), 760t
clinical presentation, 506
laboratory investigation, 506
management, 506–507
pathophysiology, 505
Vinblastine binding site, 505
Vinca (Catharanthus roseus). See Catharanthus roseus
(periwinkle)
Vinca alkaloids, 354, 501, 505–507
adverse effects and safety issues, 760t
ARDS caused by, 402t
extravasation, 802–803, 803t
history of, 505
mechanism and site of action, 762f
peripheral neuropathy with, 763
toxicity (overdose/poisoning), 760t, 763
Vinca rosea. See Catharanthus roseus (periwinkle)
Vincristine, 349f, 505–507, 644t, 1612
adverse effects and safety issues, 760t
cell cycle phase specificity, 761f

cranial neuropathy caused by, 346t
diagnostic tests for, 763
dosage and administration, 505
drug interactions with, 506
elimination, 505
and hair loss, 281
intrathecal, 505
inadvertent overdose and unintentional
exposures due to, 797t–798t
management, 794
toxicity, 763, 794
liposomal, 1720t
mechanism of action, 350, 759
nail changes caused by, 282
neurotoxicity, 343, 505–506, 763
and other antimitotics, in overdose, comparison,
507t
peripheral neuropathy with, 763
pharmacokinetics, 505–506
plant source, 1599t
and posterior reversible encephalopathy syndrome,
132
structure, 501
therapeutic uses, 505
toxic dose, 506
toxicity (overdose/poisoning), 760t
clinical presentation, 506
epidemiology, 505
laboratory investigation, 506
management, 506–507
pathophysiology, 505
Vindesine
adverse effects and safety issues, 760t
overdose/poisoning, 760t
Vinegar
for Cnidaria stings, 1569, 1571
odor, 364t
for seabather's eruption, 1571–1572
Vineyard sprayer's lung, 1287
Vin Mariani, 8
Vinorelbine, overdose/poisoning, multiple-dose
activated charcoal in, 61
Vinyl chloride, 12, 174t
acroosteolysis caused by, 122, 122t
hepatic effects, 334, 334t
and hepatic tumors, 333
hepatotoxicity, 1414
and leukemia, 320
metabolism, 172
occupational exposure to, 23, 23t
Vinyl GABA. See Vigabatrin
Violence, 384–388
additional factors in, 385
alternative etiologies, 385
assessment of patient, 384–385
de-escalation for, 385
differential diagnosis, 384
in emergency department, 384
in hospital, types, 384
mental illness and, 385
physical restraint for, 387
prediction, 384
psychopharmacologic interventions for, 385–387
risk assessment for, 384
S.A.F.E.S.T. approach for, 387, 387t
stress-vulnerability model and, 384
substance use and, 384–385
treatment, 384–387
warning signs for, 387, 387t
workplace, 384

Violets, odor, 364t
Violin spider, 1540. *See also* Brown recluse spider
     (*Loxosceles reclusa*)
Viper(s). *See also* Pit vipers (Crotalinae); Viperidae
     antivenom, supplies, 43
     New World. *See* Pit vipers (Crotalinae)
     Old World (true), 1633, 1633t
Vipera russelii (Russell's viper), 1633
Viperidae, 1617, 1633, 1633t. *See also* Pit vipers
     (Crotalinae)
     bites, epidemiology, 1633, 1845
     geographic distribution, 1633
     venom, toxicity, 1634
Viperinae, 1633, 1633t
Viper's bugloss (*Crotalaria spectabilis, Heliotropum
     europaeum*), 642t
Viral encephalitis
     as biological weapon, 1758–1759
     mosquito-borne, 1522
Viral hemorrhagic fevers, 1758
     as biological weapon, 1758
Viral infection, and anosmia/hyposmia, 364
Virol A, and GABA receptor, 222
Virotoxins, 1583
Virus(es)
     foodborne illness caused by, 592t, 597
     transmission, by prothrombin complex concentrate,
          908–909
Viscaceae, 1601t, 1603t
Viscera, thermosensitivity, 411
Viscotoxins, 643t
Viscum album (mistletoe), 643t, 1603t, 1609
Viscumin, 1603t
Vision
     cardioactive steroid toxicity and, 971–972
     phosphodiesterase inhibitors and, 301
Vision loss
     cocaine use and, 1126
     in elderly, and unintentional poisoning, 466
     in methanol poisoning, 1423
          corticosteroids for, 1430
          stem cell transplantation for, 1430
     nonophthalmic xenobiotics causing, 360–361,
          361t
Visual acuity, 356
     decreased, poisoning/overdose causing, 36t
Vital signs, 28–29
     assessment, in poisoned patient, 265–266,
          266t
     in children, 28, 28t
     in initial assessment, 189
     normal, by age, 28, 28t
     normalcy of, factors affecting, 28
     recording, 28
     in toxidromes, 28, 29t
Vitamin(s), 654–668. *See also specific vitamin*
     adequate daily intake for, 655t
     adverse effects and safety issues, 654
     deficiency
          health effects, 654
          neurologic effects, 342
          risk factors for, 654
     definition, 654
     excess intake, 654
     exposure to, epidemiology, 654
     fat-soluble, 654
     recommended dietary allowances for, 654, 655t
     supplementation, 654
     water-soluble, 654
          dialysis and, 95
          repletion, for dialysis patient, 1160

Vitamin A, 654–658
     absorption, vitamin E and, 662
     cirrhosis caused by, 333
     in cyanide poisoning, 1688
     deficiency, 656
     dietary sources, 654–656
     hepatic accumulation, 656, 657f
     hepatotoxicity, 656–657, 657f, 658
          diagnosis, 658
     history of, 654–656
     hypercalcemia caused by, 250
     and idiopathic intracranial hypertension, 657
     injection, chlorobutanol in, 683t
     metabolism, kidney disease and, 657–658
     pharmacokinetics, 656
     pharmacology, 656
     physicochemical properties, 654
     recommended dietary allowance or adequate daily
          intake for, 655t, 656
     structure, 654
     teratogenicity, 430t, 658
     toxicity, 654–655. *See also* Hypervitaminosis A
          acute, 657
          chronic, 657
          clinical manifestations, 333, 657–658
          diagnostic tests for, 658
          management, 658
          musculoskeletal effects, 657
          pathophysiology, 656–657
     toxicokinetics, 656
Vitamin B$_1$. *See* Thiamine (thiamine hydrochloride,
     vitamin B$_1$)
Vitamin B$_3$. *See* Nicotinic acid (niacin, vitamin B$_3$)
Vitamin B$_6$. *See* Pyridoxine (hydrochloride, vitamin B$_6$)
Vitamin B$_9$. *See* Folic acid
Vitamin B$_{12}$, 654. *See also* Cyanocobalamin
     absorption, gastric bypass and, 148
     in common products, 986t
     deficiency
          and megaloblastic anemia, 318–319
          xenobiotics and, 319
     nitrous oxide abuse and, 1199
     for nitrous oxide toxicity, 1200
     oxidation and inactivation, 1012, 1013f
     and urine cobalt concentration, 1277
Vitamin B-17. *See* Laetrile
Vitamin B$_{12a}$. *See* Hydroxocobalamin
Vitamin BT. *See* L-Carnitine
Vitamin C, 654, 662–663
     as antioxidant, 662
     for common cold, 662
     in cyanide poisoning, 1688
     dietary sources, 662
     history of, 662
     overdose, clinical manifestations, 662–663
     for paraquat poisoning, 1477
     pharmacokinetics, 662
     pharmacology, 662
     physicochemical properties, 662
     physiologic functions, 662
     prooxidant effect, 662
     recommended dietary allowance or adequate daily
          intake for, 655t
     as reducing agent, 662
     structure, 662
     therapeutic uses, 662
     toxicokinetics, 662
Vitamin D (cholecalciferol and ergocalciferol),
     654, 659–661
     deficiency, 659–660
          hypocalcemia and, 660

dietary sources, 659
food fortified with, 659
history of, 659
indications for, 659
metabolism, 659
pharmacokinetics, 659–660
pharmacology, 659–660
physicochemical properties, 659, 1453t
physiologic functions, 659–660, 660f
recommended dietary allowance or adequate daily
     intake for, 655t, 659
in rodenticides, 659, 1453t. *See also* Rodenticides
structure, 659
supplementation, 659
synthesis, 659, 660f
teratogenicity, 430t
therapeutic uses, 659
toxic dose, 660
toxicity, 659. *See also* Hypervitaminosis D
     antidote and/or treatment for, 1453t
     clinical manifestations, 660–661, 1453t
     diagnostic tests for, 661
     ECG changes in, 661
     hypercalcemia caused by, 199, 199t
     onset, 1453t
     pathophysiology, 660
     treatment, 661
toxic mechanism, 1453t
toxicokinetics, 659–660
Vitamin D$_2$ (ergocalciferol), 659
     absorption, gastric bypass and, 148
     overdose/poisoning, diabetes insipidus caused by, 195
Vitamin D$_3$ (cholecalciferol), 659
     hypercalcemia caused by, 199, 199t, 250
     in rodenticides, 659, 1453t
Vitamin D-binding protein, 659
Vitamin E, 654, 661–662
     as antioxidant, 662
     as aphrodisiac, 304
     in breast milk, 661
     in cyanide poisoning, 1688
     deficiency, 661
     dietary sources, 661
     dose, and adverse effects, 662
     high doses
          clinical manifestations, 662
          pathophysiology, 662
     history of, 661
     for metal phosphide poisoning, 1459
     nebulized, for smoke inhalation, 1645
     for paraquat poisoning, 1477
     pharmacokinetics, 661–662
     pharmacology, 661–662
     physicochemical properties, 661
     physiologic functions, 662
     and polysorbate emulsifiers, 681
     prooxidant effect, 662
     recommended dietary allowance or adequate daily
          intake for, 655t
     and silver tolerance, 1347
     structure, 661
     therapeutic uses, 661
     topical, for cutaneous paresthesias in topical
          pyrethroid exposure, 1522
     toxicokinetics, 661–662
     as vitamin K antagonist, 662
Vitamin K (phylloquinone), 915
     adverse effects and safety issues, 654
     concentrations, warfarin therapy and, 915
     cycling, inhibition, 915. *See also* Warfarin
     daily requirement for, 915

deficiency, 885, 915–916
  diagnostic tests for, 916
  xenobiotic-induced, 916
dietary, pharmacokinetics, 915
fetal stores, 916
shortage, 43
supplies, 42
synthesis, 915
vitamin E and, 662
"Vitamin K." *See* Ketamine
Vitamin K antagonists (VKAs), 884f, 885–890, 908
  antidotes and treatment strategies for, 888t
  coagulopathy caused by
    activated prothrombin complex concentrate for, 910
    recombinant factor VIIa for, 911
    treatment, 887–889, 888t
  dosage and administration, 886
  ingestions
    clinical manifestations, 886–887
    intentional vs. unintentional, 886–887
  laboratory testing for, 887, 888t
  long-acting, 886
    overdose/poisoning, 886–887
      treatment, 889
  nonbleeding complications with, 889–890
  overanticoagulation with
    management, 889, 889t
    risk factors for, 889
  overdose/poisoning, clinical manifestations, 886–887
  pharmacology, 886
  as rodenticides, 886
  and vitamin K deficiency, 916
Vitamin K_1 (phytonadione), 915–918
  administration route, 889, 915–916
    and pharmacodynamics, 916
    and pharmacokinetics, 915–916
  adverse effects and safety issues, 916
  for anticoagulant overdose, 887–889, 888t, 915–918
  availability and storage, 45t
  dosage and administration, 917
  formulation and acquisition, 917
  indications for, 35t, 45t, 915
  intravenous administration, anaphylactoid reaction with, 916
  mechanism of action, 915
  pharmacodynamics, 916
  pharmacokinetics, 915–916
  pharmacology, 915
  in pregnancy and lactation, 916
  for rodenticide anticoagulant poisoning, 915–917
  stocking, recommended level, 45t
  structure, 915
  synthesis, 915
Vitamin K_2 (menaquinones), 915
Vitamin K cycle, 885–886, 885f
Vitamin K_3 (menadione), 915
Vitamin K_4 (menadiol sodium diphosphate), 915
Vitamin K 2,3-epoxide, 885f, 886
Vitamin K 2,3-epoxide reductase, 885f, 886
Vitamin K epoxide reductase complex 1 (VKORC1), 885f, 886
Vitamin K quinone, 885f, 886
Vitamin K reductase, inhibitors, 916
Vitexin, 642t
Vitreous hemorrhage, 356
Vitreous humor, 356
  normal chemistries, 1872, 1872t
  specimens, postmortem collection and analysis, 1870t, 1872–1873, 1886

Vitronectin, 323
Vivitrol, 539
Vodka, as ethanol source, 1442
Volatile anesthetics, 1011
Volatile hydrocarbons. *See* Hydrocarbons
Volatile oils, 639, 641t–642t. *See also* Essential (ethereal) oils
Volatile substance use, 1193. *See also* Inhalant(s)
Volatility, 1412
Volcanic eruption, toxic gases in, 16, 16t
Volume depletion, with colchicine poisoning, 502, 503t
Volume expansion theory, 1012
Volume of distribution (V_d), 144–146. *See also specific xenobiotic*
  definition, 91
  in elderly, 461–462
  and extracorporeal elimination of xenobiotics, 91, 147
Volume replacement
  for alcoholic patients, 1167–1168
  for cocaine toxicity, 1128–1129
Volume status, assessment, in poisoned patient, 265–266, 266t
Volva, mushroom, 1584f, 1593
Vomit button (*Strychnos* spp.), 1603t
Vomiting
  with *N*-acetylcysteine, 495
  activated charcoal and, 61, 79
  β_2-adrenergic agonist toxicity and, 988
  with arylcyclohexylamine toxicity, 1215
  cannabinoids for, 1113
  chemotherapeutic-related, 762
    management, 764
  with colchicine poisoning, 502, 503t
  in copper poisoning, 1287
  forceful, gastrointestinal perforation in, 127
  hypercalcemia and, 199
  methotrexate-related, 768
  methylxanthine-induced, 988, 990
  with multiple-dose activated charcoal, 62
  in nicotine toxicity, 1206–1207
  in thallium toxicity, 1351
  with whole-bowel irrigation, 85
  withdrawal-associated, 540
von Anrep, Vassili, 1124
von Willebrand factor, 323–324, 514, 897, 898f, 900
Voraxaze, 782, 786. *See also* Glucarpidase (carboxypeptidase G_2)
Voriconazole, 829
  for HIV-related infections, 831t
Vortioxetine, 1060
  and CYPs, 1056
  mechanism of action, 218
  receptor activity, 1057t
  structure, 1060
VR, 1741, 1745
VX, 6t, 13, 1508, 1741
  aging half-life, 1746
  chemical name and structure, 1745f
  LD_{50}, 1744

W
W-18, 551
Walckenaer spider. *See* Hobo spider (*Eratigena agrestis*)
Walk-and-turn (WAT) test, 1878–1879, 1879t
Wall germander (*Teucrium chamaedrys*), uses and toxicities, 642t
Warburg effect, 708
Warfare, 17, 17t
Warfarin, 322, 885–890, 908
  adverse effects and safety issues, in elderly, 465

adverse events with, 883
antidote for, 35t
drug interactions with, 827, 852
duration of action, 886
elevated INR with, vitamin K_1 for, 915
elimination half-life, 886
embryopathy, 890
enantiomers, 886
estimated fatal dose, 1453t
and ethanol, interactions, 1146t
and glucagon, interactions, 943
history of, 883
laboratory assessment, 887, 888t
mechanism of action, 886
metabolism, 171–172
nephropathy caused by, 890
pharmacology, 886, 893t
physicochemical properties, 1453t
plasma protein binding by, 146
priapism caused by, 301t
in rodenticides, 1453t
skin necrosis caused by, 279, 279f, 889–890
stereoisomers, and CYP substrate affinity, 169
teratogenicity, 429t, 431
toxicity (overdose/poisoning)
  antidote and/or treatment for, 1453t
  clinical manifestations, 886–887, 1453t
  management, 45t
  treatment strategies for, 888t
toxic mechanism, 1453t
transplacental transfer, 431
vitamin K and, 654, 916
Warfarinlike anticoagulants, 885–890
War gases, 1741
Warm zone, in hazardous materials incident response, 1809, 1809t, 1810f
Warning, on rodenticide labels, 1450t, 1453t
Warning label(s), 9
Washed out syndrome, 236–237, 1128
Wasps, 1540, 1551–1552, 1845
  stings, 3
  thread-waisted, 1540t
  venom
    AMPA receptor antagonists in, 228
    composition, 1551, 1551t
    and rhabdomyolysis, 393
Water. *See also* Drinking water
  amphoteric nature, 160
  balance, renal regulation of, 389
  depletion
    gastrointestinal decontamination and, 85
    multiple-dose activated charcoal and, 79
  excess intake, and hyponatremia, 196
  for hemodialysis, 98–99
  pH, 160
  purification, 99
  restriction, in SIADH, 197
  rinsing with
    for corrosive exposures, 73
    for dermal decontamination, 72–73
    for hydrofluoric acid exposures, 73
    for ophthalmic decontamination, 72–73
    for phenol exposure, 74
    for unknown xenobiotic exposure, 74
  for skin decontamination, 272
  tritiated, 1770
  xenobiotics that react to, 72
Water balance
  alterations, xenobiotic-induced, 194
  factors affecting, 194
Water deficit, estimation, 195

absorption, 1363
  defect in, 1362
in air, 1364
alkyl of, dermal decontamination for, precautions
    with, 72
blood, 1362
  normal concentration, 1362
  testing for, 1364
cation, and electron transport, 176t
chelation, and gustatory dysfunction, 365
chemistry, 1362
for common cold, 1362
and copper poisoning, 1287
deficiency, 1362–1363
  and cadmium-induced tumors, 1261
  risk factors for, 1362
in denture cream, 1362, 1364
dermal decontamination for, 272, 1365
dietary intake, and kidney stones, 1364
dietary sources, 1362
in dietary supplements, 647–648
in drinking water, 1364
dust, dermal decontamination for, precautions
    with, 72
for erectile dysfunction, 304
and fetal development, 1362
and GABA receptors, 222
and gene expression, 1362
and gustatory function, 1362
history and epidemiology, 1362
and immune response, 1362
industrial uses, 1364
inhalational toxicity, 1363, 1365
  management, 1365
intranasal use, and anosmia, 1363
and metal fume fever, 1364
metallic, ignition when wet, 1365
in metalloenzymes, 1362
metallothionein and, 1363
occupational exposure to, 1364
occupational threshold limit value-time-weighted
    average, 1364
and olfactory function, 1362
oxidation states, 1362
in pennies, 1363–1365
pharmacology, 1362
physicochemical properties, 1362
physiology, 1362–1363
plasma protein binding, 1363
recommended dietary allowances, 1362
salivary, 1362
serum, 1362
  normal concentration, 1362
supplementation, 1362
  in pregnancy, 1362
as thermal degradation product, 1642
tissue distribution, 1363
in total parenteral nutrition, 1362–1363
toxicity
  N-acetylcysteine for, 1365
  acute, clinical manifestations, 1363
  chelation therapy for, 1365
  chronic, clinical manifestations, 1363–1364
  clinical manifestations, 1363–1364
  from coin ingestion, 64
  and copper deficiency, 1365
  diagnostic imaging in, 1364

diagnostic tests for, 1364–1365
  management, 1365
toxicokinetics, 1363
urine
  normal concentration, 1362, 1364
  testing for, 1364
for Wilson disease, 1363–1364
Zinc acetate
  for common cold, 1362
  for Wilson disease, 1285–1287, 1363
Zinc carbonate, 1362
Zinc chloride, 1362, 1388t
  exposure to, management, 1393
  fumes, 1657–1658
    immediately dangerous to life and health (IDLH),
      1654t
    regulatory standard for, 1654t
    respiratory effects, 399t
    short-term exposure limit (STEL), 1654t
    sources, 1654t
    water solubility, 1654t
  inhalational toxicity, 399t, 1363
    management, 1365
    prevention, 1365
  renal effects, 1363
  TAR (titratable acid/alkaline reserve), 1388
  toxicity, 1363
  water solubility, 1363
Zinc fever, 1362
Zinc fingers, 1362
Zinc gluconate
  for common cold, 1362
  and corticosteroids, combined, for sensorineural
    hearing loss, 1362
  intranasal use, and anosmia, 1363
Zinc oxide, 1362–1364
  dermal effects, 1363
  immediately dangerous to life and health (IDLH),
    1654t
  inhalational toxicity, 1363–1364
    management, 1365
    prevention, 1365
  and metal fume fever, 1364
  regulatory standard for, 1654t
  short-term exposure limit (STEL), 1654t
  sources, 1654t
  water solubility, 1363, 1654t
Zinc phosphate, and rhabdomyolysis, 393
Zinc phosphide, 1450, 1457
  estimated fatal dose, 1452t
  odor, 364t
  physicochemical properties, 1452t, 1457
  in rodenticides, 1452t
  toxic dose, 1458
  toxicity (poisoning)
    antidote and/or treatment, 1452t
    clinical manifestations, 1452t, 1458
    onset, 1452t
    toxic mechanism, 1452t
Zinc salts, 1363
  inhalational toxicity, 1363
  and metal fume fever, 1364
  toxicity, acute, 1363
  water solubility, 1363
Zinc sulfate, 1362
  intranasal use, and anosmia, 1363
  for olfactory disorders, 1362

renal effects, 1363
  toxicity (poisoning), 1363
    whole-bowel irrigation for, 85
Zinc sulfide, 1362
Zinc swayback, 1362, 1364
Zingerone, 642t
Zingiber officinale (ginger), 642t
Zion, Libby, 13
Ziprasidone, 218. *See also* Antipsychotics
  clinical and toxicologic effects, 1034t
  dosage and administration, 1033t
  extrapyramidal effects, 215
  and female sexual dysfunction, 302f
  for hallucinogen-induced agitation, 1184
  mechanism of action, 1035
  overdose/poisoning, 1040
  pharmacokinetics, 1033t
  priapism caused by, 301t
  and QT interval, 253t
ZIP transporter protein, and manganese, 1320
Zirconium
  dermal decontamination for, 272
  dust, dermal decontamination for, precautions
    with, 72
Zolazepam, 228, 1211
Zoledronate, acute interstitial nephritis caused by,
    394t
Zoledronic acid, for vitamin D toxicity, 661
Zolmitriptan, 217, 808–809, 808t
Zolpidem, 1086, 1089. *See also* Sedative-hypnotics
  and GABA receptors, 221, 1084
  history of, 1084
  overdose/poisoning, flumazenil for, 1094
  pharmacokinetics, 1085t
  pharmacology, 237
  structure, 1089, 1135
  withdrawal from, 222, 1138
Zonisamide
  adverse effects and safety issues, 612, 727t
  drug interactions with, 723t
  history of, 719
  mechanism of action, 720f, 720t, 726
  metabolism and effects on CYP enzymes, 722t
  pharmacokinetics and toxicokinetics, 721t, 727
  pharmacology, 719, 720t
  pregnancy category, 726
  and suicide risk, 719
  therapeutic serum concentration, 727
  toxicity
    clinical manifestations, 727
    management, 727
  for weight loss, 612
Zoo(s), exotic snake antivenoms in, 1634–1635
Zooids, 1567
Zopiclone, 1089
  and GABA receptors, 221, 1084
  history of, 1084
  structure, 1135
  withdrawal from, 222, 1138
Zotepine, 218
Zsigmondy, Richard, 1717
Zuclopenthixol. *See also* Antipsychotics
  dosage and administration, 1033t
  pharmacokinetics, 1033t
Zwanizer, Anna Maria, 5t
Zygacine, and sodium channels, 1612
Zyklon B gas, 17, 17t, 1684. *See also* Cyanide(s)

Common Toxicology Laboratory Concentrations (serum unless otherwise noted)

	Conventional	SI		Conventional	SI
Acetaminophen*	10–30 mcg/mL	66–199 μmol/L	Lithium*	0.6–1.2 mEq/L	0.6–1.2 mmol/L
Arsenic (blood)	<5 mcg/L	<0.0665 μmol/L	Mercury (blood)	<10 mcg/L	<50 nmol/L
Arsenic (urine)	<50 mcg/L	<0.665 μmol/L	Mercury (urine)	<20 mcg/L	<100 nmol/L
Caffeine	1–10 mcg/mL	5.2–51 μmol/L	Methanol[c]	<25 mg/dL	<7.8 mmol/L
Carbamazepine	4–12 mg/L	17–51 μmol/L	Methemoglobin	<3%	<3%
Carboxyhemoglobin (blood)	<2%	<2%	Phenobarbital*	15–40 mg/L	65–172 μmol/L
Cyanide (blood)	<1 mcg/mL	<38.5 μmol/L	Phenytoin*	10–20 mg/L	40–79 μmol/L
Digoxin[a],*	0.8–2 ng/mL	1.1–2.6 nmol/L	Salicylates[c],*	15–30 mg/dL	1.1–2.2 mmol/L
Ethanol[b]	80 mg/dL	17.4 mmol/L	Thallium (blood)	<2.0 mcg/L	<9.78 nmol/L
Ethlyene glycol[c]	<25 mg/dL	<4 mmol/L	Thallium (urine)	<5.0 mcg/L	<24.5 nmol/L
Iron*	80–180 mcg/dL	14–32 μmol/L	Theophylline*	5–15 mcg/mL	27.8–83 μmol/L
Lead (blood)	<10 mcg/dL	<0.48 μmol/L	Thiocyanate	<30 mcg/mL	<100 μmol/L
Lidocaine*	1.5–5 mcg/mL	6.4–21.4 μmol/L	Valproic acid*	50–120 mg/L	347–832 μmol/L

*Therapeutic, generally accepted normal or nonaction concentrations (no symbol) are listed. Please see the appropriate chapter for details regarding specific situations. Normal ranges vary by laboratory.
[a]The therapeutic concentration of digoxin for heart failure is 0.5 to 0.9 ng/mL, but toxicity is usually present only when the concentration is >2 ng/mL. [b]This value is the "per se" concentration for ethanol above which motor vehicle operators are considered legally impaired in the United States. [c]Concentration must be interpreted with respect to the serum pH and clinical status.
*See acetaminophen nomogram (page 477).

Common Standard Blood/Serum Laboratory Concentrations

	Conventional	SI		Conventional	SI
Ammonia	10–80 mcg/dL	6–47 μmol/L	Glucose	60–99 mg/dL	3.3–6.1 mmol/L
Alanine aminotransferase (ALT, SGPT)	7–41 U/L	0.12–0.70 μkat/L	Lactate	<18 mg/dL	<2 mmol/L
			Magnesium	1.3–2.1 mEq/L	0.65–1.05 mmol/L
Aspartate aminotransferase (AST, SGOT)	12–38 U/L	0.20–0.65 μkat/L	PCO₂ (art)	35–45 mm Hg	4.7–6.0 kPa
			PCO₂ (ven)	45–55 mm Hg	6.0–7.33 kPa
Bicarbonate	18–24 mEq/L	18–24 mmol/L	pH (art)	7.35–7.45	7.35–7.45
Blood urea nitrogen	7–18 mg/dL	2.5–6.4 mmol/L	pH (ven)	7.33–7.40	7.33–7.40
Calcium	8.4–10.2 mg/dL	2.10–2.55 mmol/L	PO₂ (art)	90–100 mm Hg	12–13.3 kPa
Chloride	98–106 mEq/L	98–106 mmol/L	PO₂ (ven)	30–50 mm Hg	4.0–6.67 kPa
Creatinine	0.6–1.2 mg/dL	0.053–0.106 mmol/L	Phosphorus	3–4.5 mg/L	1–1.4 mmol/L
Creatine kinase (total)			Potassium	3.5–5.2 mEq/L	3.5–5 mmol/L
Females	39–238 U/L	0.66–4.0 μkat/L	Sodium	135–145 mEq/L	135–145 mmol/L
Males	51–294 U/L	0.87–5.0 μkat/L			

art = arterial; ven = venous.

PCO_2, PO_2

Clinical and Laboratory Findings in Poisoning and Overdoses

Agitation	Antimuscarinics,[a] ethanol and sedative–hypnotic withdrawal, hypoglycemia, lithium, phencyclidine, sympathomimetics,[b] synthetic cannabinoids
Alopecia	Alkylating agents, radiation, selenium, strontium, thallium
Ataxia	Benzodiazepines, carbamazepine, carbon monoxide, ethanol, hypoglycemia, lithium, mercury, nitrous oxide, phenytoin
Blindness or decreased visual acuity	Caustics (direct), cocaine, cisplatin, mercury, methanol, quinine, thallium
Blue skin	Amiodarone, FD&C #1 dye, methemoglobin, silver, sulfhemoglobin
Constipation	Antimuscarinics,[a] botulism, lead, opioids, thallium (severe)
Deafness, tinnitus	Aminoglycosides, carbon disulfide, cisplatin, loop diuretics, macrolides, metals, opioids, quinine, salicylates
Diaphoresis	Amphetamines, cholinergics,[c] ethanol and sedative–hypnotic withdrawal, hypoglycemia, opioid withdrawal, salicylates, serotonin toxicity, sympathomimetics[b]
Diarrhea	Arsenic and other metals/metalloids, boric acid (blue-green), botanical irritants, cathartics, cholinergics,[c] colchicine, iron, lithium, opioid withdrawal, radiation
Dysesthesias, paresthesias	Acrylamide, arsenic, ciguatera, cocaine, colchicine, n-hexane, thallium
Gum discoloration	Arsenic, bismuth, hypervitaminosis A, lead, mercury

(Continued)